2018
ICD-10-CM
FOR HOSPITALS

INCLUDES NETTER'S ANATOMY ART

Carol J. Buck
MS, CPC, CCS-P

Former Program Director
Medical Secretary Programs
Northwest Technical College
East Grand Forks, Minnesota

ELSEVIER

ELSEVIER

3251 Riverport Lane
St. Louis, Missouri 63043

2018 ICD-10-CM HOSPITAL EDITION

ISBN: 978-0-323-43072-2

International Standard Book Number: 978-0-323-43072-2

Content Strategist: Brandi Graham
Content Development Manager: Luke Held
Associate Content Development Specialist: Anna Miller
Publishing Services Manager: Jeffrey Patterson
Project Manager: Lisa A. P. Bushey
Designer: Maggie Reid

Printed in Canada

 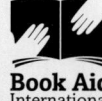
Last digit is the print number: 9 8 7 6 5 4 3 2 1

DEDICATION

To all the brave medical coders who transitioned the nation into a new coding system.
Decades of waiting finally concluded with the implementation of I-10,
and you have been the pioneers leading the way.

With greatest appreciations for your efforts!

Carol J. Buck, MS, CPC, CCS-P

DEVELOPMENT OF THIS EDITION

Query Team

Patricia Cordy Henricksen, MS, CHCA, CPC-I, CPC, CCP-P, ASC-PM
Auditing and Coding Educator
Soterion Medical Services
Lexington, Kentucky

Jackie Grass Koesterman, CPC
Coding and Reimbursement Specialist
Grand Forks, North Dakota

Kathleen Buchda, CPC, CPMA
Revenue Recognition
New Richmond, Wisconsin

Editorial Consultant

Jenna Price, CPC
President
Price Editorial Services, LLC
St. Louis, Missouri

Elsevier/MC Strategies Revenue Cycle, Coding and Compliance Staff

"Experts in providing e-learning on revenue cycle, coding and compliance."

Deborah Neville, RHIA, CCS-P
Director

Lynn-Marie D. Wozniak, MS, RHIT
Content Manager

Sandra L. Macica, MS, RHIA, CCS, ROCC
Content Manager

CONTENTS

GUIDE TO USING THE 2018 ICD-10-CM FOR HOSPITALS

Medical coding has long been a part of the health care profession. Through the years medical coding systems have become more complex and extensive. Today, medical coding is an intricate and immense process that is present in every health care setting. The increased use of electronic submissions for health care services only increases the need for coders who understand the coding process.

2018 ICD-10-CM for Hospitals, Professional Edition was developed to help meet the needs of coding professionals at all levels by offering a comprehensive coding text at a reasonable price.

All material strictly adheres to the latest government versions available at the time of printing. Updates from the *Definitions of Medicare Code Edits* (MCE) will be posted to the companion website (www. codingupdates.com) when available.

Illustrations and Items

The ICD-10-CM Tabular List contains illustrations, pictures, and items to assist you in understanding difficult terminology, diseases/conditions, or coding in a specific category. Items are always printed in ▆▆▆▆▆ ink so that the added material is not mistaken for official notations or instructions. ▆▆▆▆▆ ink is used for other annotations in the text. Your ideas on what other descriptions or illustrations should be in future editions of this text are always appreciated.

Instructional Notations

Includes Notes

Includes

The word 'Includes' appears immediately under certain categories to further define, or give examples of, the content of the category.

Excludes Notes

The ICD-10-CM has two types of excludes notes. Each note has a different definition for use, but they are both similar in that they indicate that codes excluded from each other are independent of each other.

Excludes1

A type 1 Excludes note is a pure excludes. It means "NOT CODED HERE!" An Excludes1 note indicates that the code excluded should never be used at the same time as the code above the Excludes1 note. An Excludes1 is for use when two conditions cannot occur together, such as a congenital form versus an acquired form of the same condition.

Excludes2

A type 2 Excludes note represents "NOT INCLUDED HERE." An Excludes2 note indicates that the condition excluded is not part of the condition it is excluded from but a patient may have both conditions at the same time. When an Excludes2 note appears under a code, it is acceptable to use both the code and the excluded code together.

Code First/Use Additional Code notes (etiology/manifestation paired codes)

Certain conditions have both an underlying etiology and multiple body system manifestations due to the underlying etiology. For such conditions the ICD-10-CM has a coding convention that requires the underlying condition be sequenced first, followed by the manifestation. Wherever such a combination exists, there is a "use additional code" note at the etiology code, and a "code first" note at the manifestation code. These instructional notes indicate the proper sequencing order of the codes, etiology followed by manifestation.

In most cases the manifestation codes will have in the code title, "in diseases classified elsewhere." Codes with this title are a component of the etiology/manifestation convention. The code title indicates that it is a manifestation code. "In diseases classified elsewhere" codes are never permitted to be used as first-listed or principal diagnosis codes. They must be used in conjunction with an underlying condition code, and they must be listed following the underlying condition.

Use additional

The words indicate an instructional note that another code may be needed.

Code first

The words indicate an instructional note that directs the coder to sequence the underlying condition before the manifestation.

Code also

A "code also" note instructs that two codes may be required to fully describe a condition, but the sequencing of the two codes is discretionary, depending on the severity of the conditions and the reason for the encounter.

7th characters and placeholder X

For codes less than 6 characters that require a 7th character a placeholder X should be assigned for all characters less than 6. The 7th character must always be the 7th character of a code.

Annotated

Throughout the manual, revisions, additions, and deleted codes or words are indicated by the following symbols:

⮕ **Revised:** Revisions within the line or code from the previous edition are indicated by the arrow.

▶ **New:** Additions to the previous edition are indicated by the triangle.

~~deleted~~ **Deleted:** Deletions from the previous edition are struck through.

ICD-10-CM Tabular List Symbols

● **Use Additional Character(s):** The red stop sign cautions that the code requires additional character(s) to ensure the greatest specificity.

X For codes less than 6 characters that require a 7th character, a placeholder X should be assigned for all characters less than 6. The 7th character must always be the 7th character of a code.

● **Unacceptable Principal Diagnosis:** These codes have a blue dot before them and give additional information or describe the circumstances affecting the health care encounter but are unacceptable as principal diagnosis in the *Definitions of Medicare Code Edits* (MCE) for inpatient admission.

OGCR The *Official Guidelines for Coding and Reporting* symbol includes the placement of a portion of a guideline as that guideline pertains to the code by which it is located. The complete OGCR are located in Part I.

🐾🐾 Indicates **complications and comorbidities and major complications and comorbidities** according to the *Medicare Severity Diagnosis Related Groups (MS-DRGs), Definitions Manual*.

(Ex:) Indicates exclusions to complications and comorbidities (CC) and major complications and comorbidities (MCC) for both primary and secondary diagnoses, according to the *Medicare Severity Diagnosis Related Groups (MS-DRGs), Definitions Manual*. Each exclusion will indicate the corresponding PDX Collection, and the collections that list all of the excluded codes appear in Appendix A.

PDX as its own CC/MCC Indicates a combination code that when assigned as the Principal Diagnosis, it includes a condition that also qualifies as a CC/MCC according to the *Medicare Severity Diagnosis Related Groups (MS-DRGs), Definitions Manual*.

🩸 HAC is a **Hospital-Acquired Condition** that, when present as a secondary diagnosis in an inpatient setting, is a higher cost, higher volume, or both and results in a higher MS-DRG assignment according to the *Medicare Severity Diagnosis Related Groups (MS-DRGs), Definitions Manual*.

🌓 **Manifestation Code:** Describes the manifestation of an underlying disease, not the disease itself, and therefore should not be assigned as a principal diagnosis, according to the *Definitions of Medicare Code Edits* (MCE).

Age conflict: The *Definitions of Medicare Code Edits* (MCE) detects inconsistencies between a patient's age and diagnosis. For example, a 5-year-old patient with benign prostatic hypertrophy or a 78-year-old pregnant female.

The diagnosis is clinically and virtually impossible in a patient of the stated age. Therefore, either the diagnosis or the age is presumed to be incorrect. There are four age categories for diagnoses in the *Definitions of Medicare Code Edits* (MCE):

N • Newborn. Age of 0 years; a subset of diagnoses intended only for newborns and neonates (e.g., fetal distress, perinatal jaundice).

P • Pediatric. Age range is 0-17 years inclusive (e.g., Reye's syndrome, routine child health exam).

M • Maternity. Age range is 12-55 years inclusive (e.g., diabetes in pregnancy, antepartum pulmonary complication).

A • Adult. Age range is 15-124 years inclusive (e.g., senile delirium, mature cataract).

♀♂ **Sex conflict:** *Definitions of Medicare Code Edits* (MCE) detects inconsistencies between a patient's sex and any diagnosis or procedure on the patient's record. For example, a male patient with cervical cancer (diagnosis) or a female patient with a prostatectomy (procedure). In both instances, the indicated diagnosis or the procedure conflicts with the stated sex of the patient. Therefore, either the patient's diagnosis, procedure, or sex is presumed to be incorrect.

Key words

Highlight identifies key words within similar code descriptions in a particular category.

Coding Clinic Identifies the year, quarter, and page number that presents information about an ICD-10-CM code in the American Hospital Association's *Coding Clinic®* for ICD-10-CM.

Visit codingupdates.com for the full list of 2017 Present on Admission codes.

SYMBOLS AND CONVENTIONS

ICD-10-CM Tabular

Use Additional Character(s): The red stop sign cautions you that the code requires additional character(s) to ensure greatest specificity.

Volume 1, Tabular List

● **K22   Other diseases of esophagus**
   Excludes2   esophageal varices (I85.-)

X ● **V00.01   Pedestrian on foot injured in collision with roller-skater**

A02.20   Localized salmonella infection, unspecified

Placeholder X: The red X reminds you that for codes less than 6 characters that require a 7th character, a placeholder X should be assigned to all characters less than 6.

Unspecified: These codes are for use when the information in the medical record is insufficient to assign a more specific code. For those categories for which an unspecified code is not provided, the "other specified" code may represent both other and unspecified.

Unacceptable Principal Diagnosis: These codes have a blue dot before them and are not permitted as a first-listed or principal diagnosis. They must be assigned in conjunction with an underlying condition code, and they must be listed following the underlying condition.

● **B95.0   Streptococcus, group A, as the cause of diseases classified elsewhere**

A48.3   Toxic shock syndrome
   Use additional code to identify the organism (B95, B96)

Use additional code: Located at the etiology code and directs you to assign a manifestation code.

Code first indicates the etiology code is to be first-listed before the manifestation code.

B39   Histoplasmosis
   Code first associated AIDS (B20)

Notes define terms or give coding instructions.

E34.0   Carcinoid syndrome
   Note: May be used as an additional code to identify functional activity associated with a carcinoid tumor.

Codes or index entries are for purposes of illustration only and may not be current.

OGCR Section I.C.6.B.5.

OGCR: The *Official Guidelines for Coding and Reporting* are placed near the codes to which they refer and are highlighted.

Neoplasm Related Pain Code G89.3 is assigned to pain documented as being related, associated or due to cancer, primary or secondary malignancy, or tumor. This code is assigned regardless of whether the pain is acute or chronic.

I70.2   **Atherosclerosis of native arteries of the extremities**
Mönckeberg's (medial) sclerosis

Use additional code, if applicable, to identify chronic total occlusion of artery of extremity (I70.92)

code, if applicable, directs the coder to other conditions that may be appropriate to report.

I74   **Arterial embolism and thrombosis**
Includes   embolic infarction
embolic occlusion
thrombotic infarction
thrombotic occlusion

The word "and" should be interpreted to mean either "and" or "or" when it appears in a statement.

Bold typeface is used on all codes and titles.

I83.001   **Varicose veins of unspecified lower extremity with ulcer of thigh**

"with" should be interpreted to mean "associated with" or "due to."

K73.2   Chronic active hepatitis, not elsewhere classified

"not elsewhere classified" or **NEC** identifies a code that is assigned only when the information at hand specifies a condition for which no more specific code is available.

"not otherwise specified" or **NOS** is equivalent to unspecified.

W13.9   Fall from, out of or through building, not otherwise specified

Codes or index entries are for purposes of illustration only and may not be current.

Excludes1 means "NOT CODED HERE!" An Excludes1 note indicates that the code excluded should never be assigned at the same time as the code above the Excludes1 note.

M19 Other and unspecified osteoarthritis

Excludes1 polyarthritis (M15.-)

Excludes2 arthrosis of spine (M47.-)
hallux rigidus (M20.2)
osteoarthritis of spine (M47.-)

Excludes2 represents "NOT INCLUDED HERE." An Excludes2 note indicates that the condition excluded is not part of the condition represented by the code, but a patient may have both conditions at the same time and it is acceptable to use both the code and the excluded code together, when appropriate.

Includes: This note appears immediately under a three-character code title to further define, or give examples of, the content.

A06 Amebiasis

Includes   infection due to Entamoeba histolytica

E26.01 Conn's syndrome
Code also adrenal adenoma (D35.0)

Code also instructs that two codes may be required to fully describe a condition, but this note does not provide sequencing direction.

Codes titled "other" or "other specified" are for use when the information in the medical record provides detail for which a specific code does not exist.

E25.8 Other adrenogenital disorders

O00.2 Ovarian pregnancy   M

Maternity DX (Diagnosis) for ages 12-55 according to the *Definitions of Medicare Code Edits* (MCE).

P02.20 Newborn (suspected to be) affected by unspecified morphological and functional abnormalities of placenta   N

Newborn, Age 0, according to the *Definitions of Medicare Code Edits* (MCE).

L21.0 Seborrhea capitis   P
Cradle cap

Pediatric Age, 0-17, according to the *Definitions of Medicare Code Edits* (MCE).

G30.1 Alzheimer's disease with late onset   A

Adult Age, 15-124, according to the *Definitions of Medicare Code Edits* (MCE).

Females Only according to the *Definitions of Medicare Code Edits* (MCE).

B37.3 Candidiasis of vulva and vagina ♀

C60.1 Malignant neoplasm of glans penis ♂

Males Only according to the *Definitions of Medicare Code Edits* (MCE).

Codes or index entries are for purposes of illustration only and may not be current.

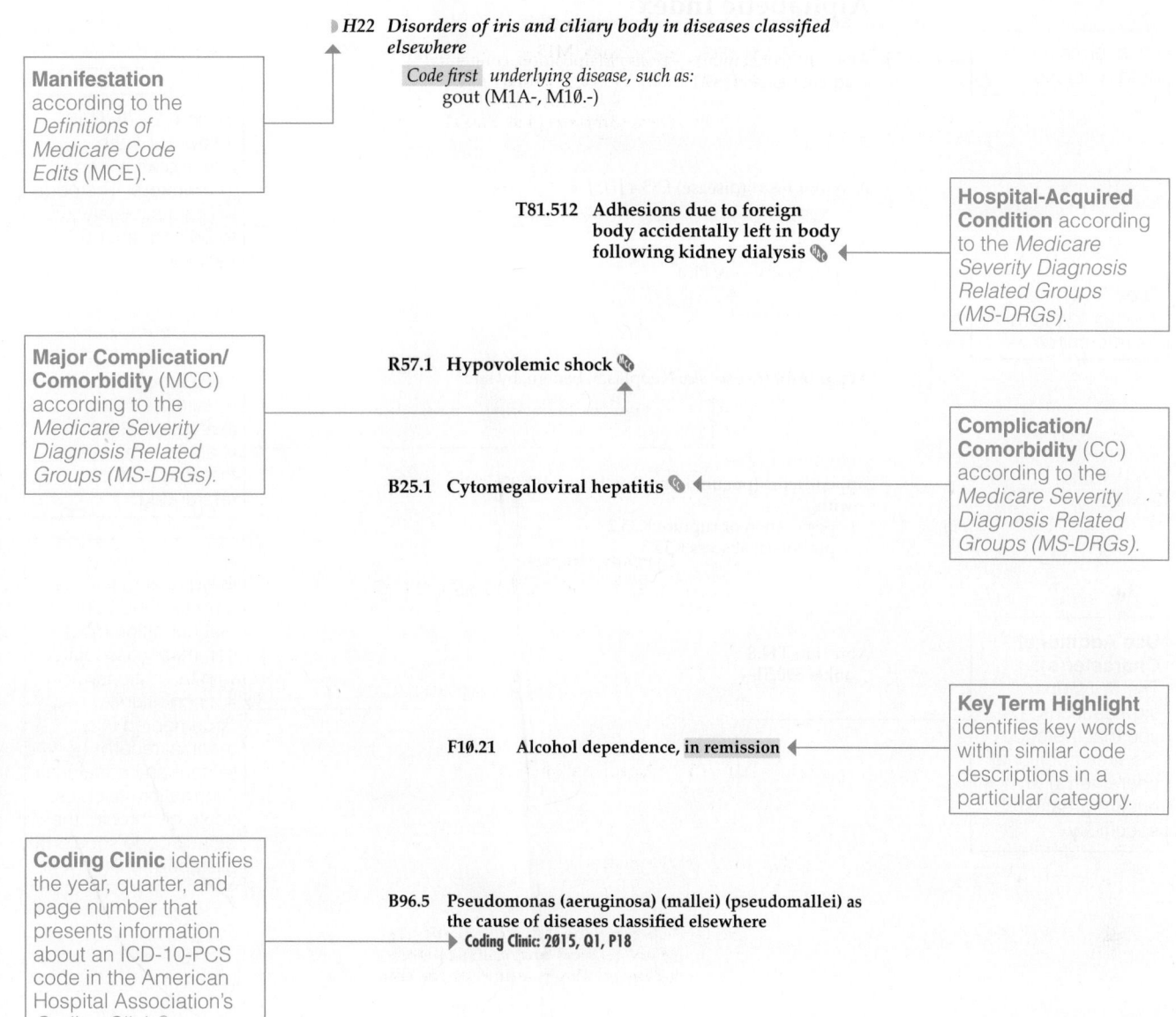

Manifestation according to the *Definitions of Medicare Code Edits* (MCE).

H22 *Disorders of iris and ciliary body in diseases classified elsewhere*
　　Code first *underlying disease, such as:*
　　　gout (M1A-, M1Ø.-)

T81.512 Adhesions due to foreign body accidentally left in body following kidney dialysis

Hospital-Acquired Condition according to the *Medicare Severity Diagnosis Related Groups (MS-DRGs).*

Major Complication/ Comorbidity (MCC) according to the *Medicare Severity Diagnosis Related Groups (MS-DRGs).*

R57.1 Hypovolemic shock

B25.1 Cytomegaloviral hepatitis

Complication/ Comorbidity (CC) according to the *Medicare Severity Diagnosis Related Groups (MS-DRGs).*

F1Ø.21 Alcohol dependence, in remission

Key Term Highlight identifies key words within similar code descriptions in a particular category.

Coding Clinic identifies the year, quarter, and page number that presents information about an ICD-10-PCS code in the American Hospital Association's *Coding Clinic®.*

B96.5 Pseudomonas (aeruginosa) (mallei) (pseudomallei) as the cause of diseases classified elsewhere
　▶ Coding Clinic: 2Ø15, Q1, P18

Codes or index entries are for purposes of illustration only and may not be current.

Alphabetic Index

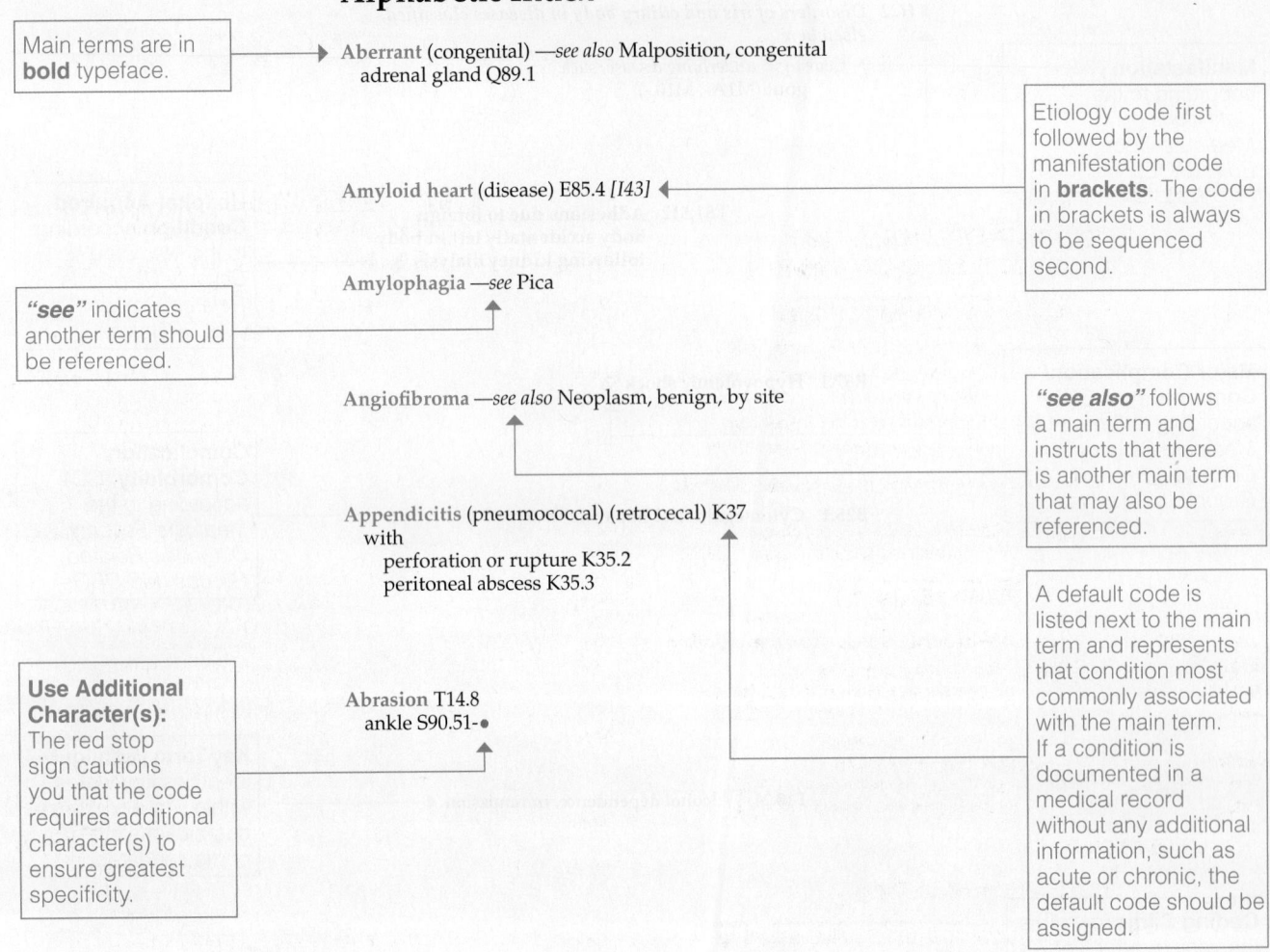

Main terms are in **bold** typeface.

Aberrant (congenital) —*see also* Malposition, congenital
    adrenal gland Q89.1

Etiology code first
followed by the
manifestation code
in **brackets**. The code
in brackets is always
to be sequenced
second.

Amyloid heart (disease) E85.4 *[I43]*

Amylophagia —*see* Pica

"see" indicates
another term should
be referenced.

Angiofibroma —*see also* Neoplasm, benign, by site

"see also" follows
a main term and
instructs that there
is another main term
that may also be
referenced.

Appendicitis (pneumococcal) (retrocecal) K37
    with
        perforation or rupture K35.2
        peritoneal abscess K35.3

A default code is
listed next to the main
term and represents
that condition most
commonly associated
with the main term.
If a condition is
documented in a
medical record
without any additional
information, such as
acute or chronic, the
default code should be
assigned.

**Use Additional
Character(s):**
The red stop
sign cautions
you that the code
requires additional
character(s) to
ensure greatest
specificity.

Abrasion T14.8
    ankle S90.51-•

Codes or index entries are for purposes of illustration only and may not be current.

CHAPTER 1

CERTAIN INFECTIOUS AND PARASITIC DISEASES (A00-B99)

INTESTINAL INFECTIOUS DISEASES (A00-A09)

A04.7   Enterocolitis due to Clostridium difficile

New   A04.71   **Enterocolitis due to Clostridium difficile, recurrent**

New   A04.72   **Enterocolitis due to Clostridium difficile, not specified as recurrent**

A05   Other bacterial foodborne intoxications, not elsewhere classified

Revised   **Excludes1**   Clostridium difficile foodborne intoxication and infection (A04.7-)

HELMINTHIASES (B65-B83)

B81   Other intestinal helminthiases, not elsewhere classified

Revised   **Excludes1**   angiostrongyliasis due to:
New   Angiostrongylus cantonensis (B83.2)
New   Parastrongylus cantonensis (B83.2)

B81.3   **Intestinal angiostrongyliasis**
Revised   Angiostrongyliasis due to:
New   Angiostrongylus costaricensis (B83.2)
New   Parastrongylus costaricensis (B83.2)

CHAPTER 2

NEOPLASMS (C00-D49)

MALIGNANT NEOPLASMS OF ILL-DEFINED, OTHER SECONDARY AND UNSPECIFIED SITES (C76-C80)

C79   Secondary malignant neoplasm of other and unspecified sites

Deleted   **Excludes2**   lymph node metastases (C77.0)

C79.11   **Secondary malignant neoplasm of bladder**
New   **Excludes2**   lymph node metastases (C77.0)

C86.4   **Blastic NK-cell lymphoma**
New   Blastic plasmacytoid dendritic cell neoplasm (BPDCN)

Revised   C96.2   **Malignant mast cell neoplasm**
Deleted   Aggressive systemic mastocytosis
Deleted   Mast cell sarcoma
Revised   **Excludes1**   indolent mastocytosis (D47.02)
New   C96.20   **Malignant mast cell neoplasm, unspecified**
New   C96.21   **Aggressive systemic mastocytosis**
New   C96.22   **Mast cell sarcoma**
New   C96.29   **Other malignant mast cell neoplasm**

NEOPLASMS OF UNCERTAIN BEHAVIOR, POLYCYTHEMIA VERA AND MYELODYSPLASTIC SYNDROMES (D37-D48)

Revised   D47.0   **Mast cell neoplasms of uncertain behavior**
Deleted   Indolent systemic mastocytosis
Deleted   Mast cell tumor NOS
Deleted   Mastocytoma NOS
     Excludes1
Deleted   malignant mast cell tumor (C96.2)
Deleted   mastocytosis (congenital) (cutaneous) (Q82.2)
New   congenital cutaneous mastocytosis (Q82.2-)
New   histiocytic neoplasms of uncertain behavior (D47.Z9)
New   malignant mast cell neoplasm (C96.2-)

New   D47.01   **Cutaneous mastocytosis**
New   Diffuse cutaneous mastocytosis
New   Maculopapular cutaneous mastocytosis
New   Solitary mastocytoma
New   Telangiectasia macularis eruptiva perstans
New   Urticaria pigmentosa
New   **Excludes1**   congenital (diffuse) (maculopapular) cutaneous mastocytosis (Q82.2)
New   congenital urticaria pigmentosa (Q82.2)
New   extracutaneous mastocytoma (D47.09)

New   D47.02   **Systemic mastocytosis**
New   Indolent systemic mastocytosis
New   Isolated bone marrow mastocytosis
New   Smoldering systemic mastocytosis
New   Systemic mastocytosis, with an associated hematological non-mast cell lineage disease (SM-AHNMD)
New   Code also if applicable, any associated hematological non-mast cell lineage disease, such as:
New   acute myeloid leukemia (C92.6-, C92.A-)
New   chronic myelomonocytic leukemia (C93.1-)
New   essential thrombocytosis (D47.3)
New   hypereosinophilic syndrome (D72.1)
New   myelodysplastic syndrome (D46.9)
New   myeloproliferative syndrome (D47.1)
New   non-Hodgkin lymphoma (C82-C85)
New   plasma cell myeloma (C90.0-)
New   polycythemia vera (D45)
New   **Excludes1**   aggressive systemic mastocytosis (C96.21)
New   mast cell leukemia (C94.3-)

New   D47.09   **Other mast cell neoplasms of uncertain behavior**
New   Extracutaneous mastocytoma
New   Mast cell tumor NOS
New   Mastocytoma NOS
New   Mastocytosis NOS

CHAPTER 3

DISEASES OF THE BLOOD AND BLOOD-FORMING ORGANS AND CERTAIN DISORDERS INVOLVING THE IMMUNE MECHANISM (D50-D89)

APLASTIC AND OTHER ANEMIAS AND OTHER BONE MARROW FAILURE SYNDROMES (D60-D64)

	D63.0	Anemia in neoplastic disease
Deleted		**Excludes1** anemia due to antineoplastic chemotherapy (D64.81)
New		**Excludes2** anemia due to antineoplastic chemotherapy (D64.81)

CERTAIN DISORDERS INVOLVING THE IMMUNE MECHANISM (D80-D89)

	D89.4	Mast cell activation syndrome and related disorders
Revised		**Excludes1** aggressive systemic mastocytosis (C96.21)
Revised		congenital cutaneous mastocytosis (Q82.2)
Deleted		indolent systemic mastocytosis (D47.0)
Deleted		malignant mastocytoma (C96.2)
New		(non-congenital) cutaneous mastocytosis (D47.01)
New		(indolent) systemic mastocytosis (D47.02)
New		malignant mast cell neoplasm (C96.2-)
New		malignant mastocytoma (C96.29)
Deleted		mastocytoma (D47.0)
Deleted		systemic mastocytosis associated with a clonal hematologic non-mast cell lineage disease (SM-AHNMD) (D47.0)
New		mast cell sarcoma (C96.22)
New		mastocytoma NOS (D47.09)
New		other mast cell neoplasms of uncertain behavior (D47.09)
New		systemic mastocytosis associated with a clonal hematologic non-mast cell lineage disease (SM-AHNMD) (D47.02)

CHAPTER 4

ENDOCRINE, NUTRITIONAL AND METABOLIC DISEASES (E00-E89)

DIABETES MELLITUS (E08-E13)

New	E11.1	Type 2 diabetes mellitus with ketoacidosis
New	E11.10	Type 2 diabetes mellitus with ketoacidosis without coma
New	E11.11	Type 2 diabetes mellitus with ketoacidosis with coma

	E13	Other specified diabetes mellitus
Deleted		**Excludes1** type 2 diabetes mellitus (E11.-)
	E13.00	Other specified diabetes mellitus with hyperosmolarity without nonketotic hyperglycemic-hyperosmolar coma (NKHHC)
New		**Excludes2** type 2 diabetes mellitus (E11.-)

OTHER DISORDERS OF GLUCOSE REGULATION AND PANCREATIC INTERNAL SECRETION (E15-E16)

	E16.0	Drug-induced hypoglycemia without coma
Revised		**Excludes1** diabetes with hypoglycemia without coma (E09.649)

METABOLIC DISORDERS (E70-E88)

	E78.00	Pure hypercholesterolemia, unspecified
New		(Pure) hypercholesterolemia NOS
	E83.11	Hemochromatosis
New		**Excludes1** GALD (P78.84)
New		Gestational alloimmune liver disease (P78.84)
New		Neonatal hemochromatosis (P78.84)

	E85	Amyloidosis
Deleted		**Excludes1** Alzheimer's disease (G30.0-)
New		**Excludes2** Alzheimer's disease (G30.0-)
	E85.0	Non-neuropathic heredofamilial amyloidosis
New		Code also associated disorders, such as:
New		autoinflammatory syndromes (M04.-)
New		**Excludes2** Transthyretin-related (ATTR) familial amyloid cardiomyopathy (E85.4)
	E85.1	Neuropathic heredofamilial amyloidosis
New		Transthyretin-related (ATTR) familial amyloid polyneuropathy
	E85.4	Organ-limited amyloidosis
New		Transthyretin-related (ATTR) familial amyloid cardiomyopathy
	E85.8	Other amyloidosis
New	E85.81	Light chain (AL) amyloidosis
New	E85.82	Wild-type transthyretin-related (ATTR) amyloidosis
New		Senile systemic amyloidosis (SSA)
New	E85.89	Other amyloidosis

CHAPTER 5

MENTAL, BEHAVIORAL AND NEURODEVELOPMENTAL DISORDERS (F01-F99)

MENTAL DISORDERS DUE TO KNOWN PHYSIOLOGICAL CONDITIONS (F01-F09)

	F06.31	Mood disorder due to known physiological condition with depressive features
New		Depressive disorder due to known physiological condition, with depressive features
	F06.32	Mood disorder due to known physiological condition with major depressive-like episode
New		Depressive disorder due to known physiological condition, with major depressive-like episode
	F06.33	Mood disorder due to known physiological condition with manic features
New		Bipolar and related disorder due to a known physiological condition, with manic features
New		Bipolar and related disorder due to known physiological condition, with manic- or hypomanic-like episodes

F13.959 **Sedative, hypnotic or anxiolytic use, unspecified with sedative, hypnotic or anxiolytic-induced psychotic disorder, unspecified**

Revised   Sedative, hypnotic, or anxiolytic-induced psychotic disorder, without use disorder

F13.97 **Sedative, hypnotic or anxiolytic use, unspecified with sedative, hypnotic or anxiolytic-induced persisting dementia**

Revised   Sedative, hypnotic, or anxiolytic-induced major neurocognitive disorder, without use disorder

F13.980 **Sedative, hypnotic or anxiolytic use, unspecified with sedative, hypnotic or anxiolytic-induced anxiety disorder**

Revised   Sedative, hypnotic, or anxiolytic-induced anxiety disorder, without use disorder

F13.981 **Sedative, hypnotic or anxiolytic use, unspecified with sedative, hypnotic or anxiolytic-induced sexual dysfunction**

Revised   Sedative, hypnotic, or anxiolytic-induced sexual dysfunction disorder, without use disorder

F13.982 **Sedative, hypnotic or anxiolytic use, unspecified with sedative, hypnotic or anxiolytic-induced sleep disorder**

Revised   Sedative, hypnotic, or anxiolytic-induced sleep disorder, without use disorder

F13.988 **Sedative, hypnotic or anxiolytic use, unspecified with other sedative, hypnotic or anxiolytic-induced disorder**

Revised   Sedative, hypnotic, or anxiolytic-induced mild neurocognitive disorder

New   F14.11 **Cocaine abuse, in remission**
New   Cocaine use disorder, mild, in early remission
New   Cocaine use disorder, mild, in sustained remission

New   F14.21 **Cocaine dependence, in remission**
New   Cocaine use disorder, moderate, in early remission
New   Cocaine use disorder, moderate, in sustained remission
New   Cocaine use disorder, severe, in early remission
New   Cocaine use disorder, severe, in sustained remission

New   F15.11 **Other stimulant abuse, in remission**
New   Amphetamine type substance use disorder, mild, in early remission
New   Amphetamine type substance use disorder, mild, in sustained remission
New   Other or unspecified stimulant use disorder, mild, in early remission
New   Other or unspecified stimulant use disorder, mild, in sustained remission

New   F15.21 **Other stimulant dependence, in remission**
New   Amphetamine type substance use disorder, moderate, in early remission
New   Amphetamine type substance use disorder, moderate, in sustained remission
New   Amphetamine type substance use disorder, severe, in early remission
New   Amphetamine type substance use disorder, severe, in sustained remission
New   Other or unspecified stimulant use disorder, moderate, in early remission
New   Other or unspecified stimulant use disorder, moderate, in sustained remission
New   Other or unspecified stimulant use disorder, severe, in early remission
New   Other or unspecified stimulant use disorder, severe, in sustained remission

New   F15.288 **Other stimulant dependence with other stimulant-induced disorder**
Revised   Amphetamine or other stimulant use disorder, moderate, with amphetamine or other stimulant-induced obsessive-compulsive or related disorder
Revised   Amphetamine or other stimulant use disorder, severe, with amphetamine or other stimulant-induced obsessive-compulsive or related disorder

F15.959 **Other stimulant use, unspecified with stimulant-induced psychotic disorder, unspecified**
Revised   Amphetamine or other stimulant-induced psychotic disorder, without use disorder

New   F16.11 **Hallucinogen abuse, in remission**
New   Other hallucinogen use disorder, mild, in early remission
New   Other hallucinogen use disorder, mild, in sustained remission
New   Phencyclidine use disorder, mild, in early remission
New   Phencyclidine use disorder, mild, in sustained remission

F16.21   Hallucinogen dependence, in remission

New   Other hallucinogen use disorder, moderate, in early remission

New   Other hallucinogen use disorder, moderate, in sustained remission

New   Other hallucinogen use disorder, severe, in early remission

New   Other hallucinogen use disorder, severe, in sustained remission

New   Phencyclidine use disorder, moderate, in early remission

New   Phencyclidine use disorder, moderate, in sustained remission

New   Phencyclidine use disorder, severe, in early remission

New   Phencyclidine use disorder, severe, in sustained remission

F17.201   Nicotine dependence, unspecified, in remission

New   Tobacco use disorder, mild, in early remission

New   Tobacco use disorder, mild, in sustained remission

New   Tobacco use disorder, moderate, in early remission

New   Tobacco use disorder, moderate, in sustained remission

New   Tobacco use disorder, severe, in early remission

New   Tobacco use disorder, severe, in sustained remission

F17.211   Nicotine dependence, cigarettes, in remission

New   Tobacco use disorder, cigarettes, mild, in early remission

New   Tobacco use disorder, cigarettes, mild, in sustained remission

New   Tobacco use disorder, cigarettes, moderate, in early remission

New   Tobacco use disorder, cigarettes, moderate, in sustained remission

New   Tobacco use disorder, cigarettes, severe, in early remission

New   Tobacco use disorder, cigarettes, severe, in sustained remission

F17.221   Nicotine dependence, chewing tobacco, in remission

New   Tobacco use disorder, chewing tobacco, mild, in early remission

New   Tobacco use disorder, chewing tobacco, mild, in sustained remission

New   Tobacco use disorder, chewing tobacco, moderate, in early remission

New   Tobacco use disorder, chewing tobacco, moderate, in sustained remission

New   Tobacco use disorder, chewing tobacco, severe, in early remission

New   Tobacco use disorder, chewing tobacco, severe, in sustained remission

F17.291   Nicotine dependence, other tobacco product, in remission

New   Tobacco use disorder, other tobacco product, mild, in early remission

New   Tobacco use disorder, other tobacco product, mild, in sustained remission

New   Tobacco use disorder, other tobacco product, moderate, in early remission

New   Tobacco use disorder, other tobacco product, moderate, in sustained remission

New   Tobacco use disorder, other tobacco product, severe, in early remission

New   Tobacco use disorder, other tobacco product, severe, in sustained remission

New   **F18.11   Inhalant abuse, in remission**

New   Inhalant use disorder, mild, in early remission

New   Inhalant use disorder, mild, in sustained remission

F18.21   Inhalant dependence, in remission

New   Inhalant use disorder, moderate, in early remission

New   Inhalant use disorder, moderate, in sustained remission

New   Inhalant use disorder, severe, in early remission

New   Inhalant use disorder, severe, in sustained remission

New   **F19.11   Other psychoactive substance abuse, in remission**

New   Other (or unknown) substance use disorder, mild, in early remission

New   Other (or unknown) substance use disorder, mild, in sustained remission

F19.21   Other psychoactive substance dependence, in remission

New   Other (or unknown) substance use disorder, moderate, in early remission

New   Other (or unknown) substance use disorder, moderate, in sustained remission

New   Other (or unknown) substance use disorder, severe, in early remission

New   Other (or unknown) substance use, severe, in sustained remission

---

SCHIZOPHRENIA, SCHIZOTYPAL, DELUSIONAL, AND OTHER NON-MOOD PSYCHOTIC DISORDERS (F20-F29)

F25.0   Schizoaffective disorder, bipolar type

Deleted   Schizophreniform psychosis, manic type

F25.1   Schizoaffective disorder, depressive type

Deleted   Schizophreniform psychosis, depressive type

F28   Other psychotic disorder not due to a substance or known physiological condition

New   Other specified schizophrenia spectrum and other psychotic disorder

F29   Unspecified psychosis not due to a substance or known physiological condition

New   Unspecified schizophrenia spectrum and other psychotic disorder

MOOD [AFFECTIVE] DISORDERS (F30-F39)

F31   Bipolar disorder
New   **Includes**   bipolar I disorder
New   bipolar type I disorder
    F31.2   Bipolar disorder, current episode manic severe with psychotic features
New   Bipolar I disorder, current or most recent episode manic with psychotic features
    F31.5   Bipolar disorder, current episode depressed, severe, with psychotic features
New   Bipolar I disorder, current or most recent episode depressed, with psychotic features
    F31.8   Other bipolar disorders
        F31.81   Bipolar II disorder
New   Bipolar disorder, type 2
    F31.9   Bipolar disorder, unspecified
New   Manic depression

    F33.3   Major depressive disorder, recurrent, severe with psychotic symptoms
New   Major depressive disorder, recurrent, with psychotic features

ANXIETY, DISSOCIATIVE, STRESS-RELATED, SOMATOFORM AND OTHER NONPSYCHOTIC MENTAL DISORDERS (F40-F48)

    F40.1   Social phobias
New   Social anxiety disorder

Revised   **F41.0   Panic disorder [episodic paroxysmal anxiety]**

    F44.4   Conversion disorder with motor symptom or deficit
New   Conversion disorder with abnormal movement
New   Conversion disorder with speech symptoms
New   Conversion disorder with swallowing symptoms
New   Conversion disorder with weakness/paralysis
    F44.5   Conversion disorder with seizures or convulsions
New   Conversion disorder with attacks or seizures
    F44.6   Conversion disorder with sensory symptom or deficit
New   Conversion disorder with anesthesia or sensory loss
New   Conversion disorder with special sensory symptoms

BEHAVIORAL SYNDROMES ASSOCIATED WITH PHYSIOLOGICAL DISTURBANCES AND PHYSICAL FACTORS (F50-F59)

F50   Eating disorders
New   **Excludes1**   feeding problems of newborn (P92.-)
    F50.8   Other eating disorders
New   **F50.82   Avoidant/restrictive food intake disorder**
    F50.9   Eating disorder, unspecified
New   Feeding or eating disorder, unspecified
New   Other specified feeding disorder

    F51.3   Sleepwalking [somnambulism]
New   Non-rapid eye movement sleep arousal disorders, sleepwalking type
    F51.4   Sleep terrors [night terrors]
New   Non-rapid eye movement sleep arousal disorders, sleep terror type

    F52.0   Hypoactive sexual desire disorder
New   Male hypoactive sexual desire disorder
        F52.21   Male erectile disorder
New   Erectile disorder
        F52.22   Female sexual arousal disorder
New   Female sexual interest/arousal disorder

DISORDERS OF ADULT PERSONALITY AND BEHAVIOR (F60-F69)

    F63.0   Pathological gambling
New   Gambling disorder

    F64.8   Other gender identity disorders
New   Other specified gender dysphoria
    F64.9   Gender identity disorder, unspecified
New   Gender dysphoria, unspecified

    F65.0   Fetishism
New   Fetishistic disorder
    F65.1   Transvestic fetishism
New   Transvestic disorder
    F65.2   Exhibitionism
New   Exhibitionistic disorder
    F65.3   Voyeurism
New   Voyeuristic disorder
    F65.4   Pedophilia
New   Pedophilic disorder

        F65.51   Sexual masochism
New   Sexual masochism disorder
        F65.52   Sexual sadism
New   Sexual sadism disorder

        F65.81   Frotteurism
New   Frotteuristic disorder
        F65.89   Other paraphilias
New   Other specified paraphilic disorder
    F65.9   Paraphilia, unspecified
New   Paraphilic disorder, unspecified

PERVASIVE AND SPECIFIC DEVELOPMENTAL DISORDERS (F80-F89)

    F81.0   Specific reading disorder
New   Specific learning disorder, with impairment in reading

    F81.2   Mathematics disorder
New   Specific learning disorder, with impairment in mathematics

        F81.81   Disorder of written expression
New   Specific learning disorder, with impairment in written expression

BEHAVIORAL AND EMOTIONAL DISORDERS WITH ONSET USUALLY OCCURRING IN CHILDHOOD AND ADOLESCENCE (F90-F98)

    F90.0   Attention-deficit hyperactivity disorder, predominantly inattentive type
New   Attention-deficit/hyperactivity disorder, predominantly inattentive presentation
    F90.1   Attention-deficit hyperactivity disorder, predominantly hyperactive type
New   Attention-deficit/hyperactivity disorder, predominantly hyperactive impulsive presentation
    F90.2   Attention-deficit hyperactivity disorder, combined type
New   Attention-deficit/hyperactivity disorder, combined presentation

CHAPTER 6

DISEASES OF THE NERVOUS SYSTEM (G00-G99)

INFLAMMATORY DISEASES OF THE CENTRAL NERVOUS SYSTEM (G00-G09)

G00 Bacterial meningitis, not elsewhere classified

Revised   **Excludes1**   bacterial meningoencephalitis (G04.2)
Revised   bacterial meningomyelitis (G04.2)
Deleted   meningomyelitis (G04.2)

SYSTEMIC ATROPHIES PRIMARILY AFFECTING THE CENTRAL NERVOUS SYSTEM (G10-G14)

G10 Huntington's disease

New   Code also dementia in other diseases classified elsewhere without behavioral disturbance (F02.80)

         G12.21 Amyotrophic lateral sclerosis
Deleted   Progressive spinal muscle atrophy
New   **G12.23 Primary lateral sclerosis**
New   **G12.24 Familial motor neuron disease**
New   **G12.25 Progressive spinal muscle atrophy**
         G12.29 Other motor neuron disease
Deleted   Familial motor neuron disease
Deleted   Primary lateral sclerosis

EXTRAPYRAMIDAL AND MOVEMENT DISORDERS (G20-G26)

         G21.19 Other drug induced secondary parkinsonism
New   Other medication-induced parkinsonism

         G25.71 Drug induced akathisia
New   Tardive akathisia

OTHER DEGENERATIVE DISEASES OF THE NERVOUS SYSTEM (G30-G32)

         G31.84 Mild cognitive impairment, so stated
New   Mild neurocognitive disorder

EPISODIC AND PAROXYSMAL DISORDERS (G40-G47)

         G47.24 Circadian rhythm sleep disorder, free running type
New   Circadian rhythm sleep disorder, non-24-hour sleep-wake type

         G47.31 Primary central sleep apnea
New   Idiopathic central sleep apnea

         G47.33 Obstructive sleep apnea (adult) (pediatric)
New   Obstructive sleep apnea hypopnea

         G47.61 Periodic limb movement disorder
Deleted   Periodic limb movement disorder

     G47.8 Other sleep disorders
New   Other specified sleep-wake disorder

     G47.9 Sleep disorder, unspecified
New   Unspecified sleep-wake disorder

OTHER DISORDERS OF THE NERVOUS SYSTEM (G89-G99)

G92 Toxic encephalopathy
New   *Code first* if applicable, drug induced (T36-T50)

G93.7 Reye's syndrome
New   *Code first* (poisoning due to salicylates, if applicable (T39.0-, with sixth character 1-4)
Deleted   (T39.0-), if salicylates-induced
New   Use additional code for adverse effect due to salicylates, if applicable (T39.0-, with sixth character 5)

CHAPTER 7

DISEASES OF THE EYE AND ADNEXA (H00-H59)

DISORDERS OF EYELID, LACRIMAL SYSTEM AND ORBIT (H00-H05)

Revised   **H02.05 Trichiasis without entropion**
Revised   **H02.051 Trichiasis without entropion right upper eyelid**
Revised   **H02.052 Trichiasis without entropion right lower eyelid**
Revised   **H02.053 Trichiasis without entropion right eye, unspecified eyelid**
Revised   **H02.054 Trichiasis without entropion left upper eyelid**
Revised   **H02.055 Trichiasis without entropion left lower eyelid**
Revised   **H02.056 Trichiasis without entropion left eye, unspecified eyelid**
Revised   **H02.059 Trichiasis without entropion unspecified eye, unspecified eyelid**

GLAUCOMA (H40-H42)

H42 Glaucoma in diseases classified elsewhere
      Code first underlying condition, such as:
New   glaucoma (in) diabetes mellitus (E08.39, E09.39, E10.39, E11.39, E13.39)
Deleted   **Excludes2**   glaucoma (in) diabetes mellitus (E08.39, E09.39, E10.39, E11.39, E13.39)

DISORDERS OF VITREOUS BODY AND GLOBE (H43-H44)

New   **H44.2A Degenerative myopia with choroidal neovascularization**
New   Use Additional code for any associated choroid disorders (H31.-)
New   **H44.2A1 Degenerative myopia with choroidal neovascularization, right eye**
New   **H44.2A2 Degenerative myopia with choroidal neovascularization, left eye**
New   **H44.2A3 Degenerative myopia with choroidal neovascularization, bilateral eye**
New   **H44.2A9 Degenerative myopia with choroidal neovascularization, unspecified eye**
New   **H44.2B Degenerative myopia with macular hole**
New   **H44.2B1 Degenerative myopia with macular hole, right eye**
New   **H44.2B2 Degenerative myopia with macular hole, left eye**
New   **H44.2B3 Degenerative myopia with macular hole, bilateral eye**
New   **H44.2B9 Degenerative myopia with macular hole, unspecified eye**
New   **H44.2C Degenerative myopia with retinal detachment**
New   Use Additional code to identify the retinal detachment (H33.-)
New   **H44.2C1 Degenerative myopia with retinal detachment, right eye**
New   **H44.2C2 Degenerative myopia with retinal detachment, left eye**
New   **H44.2C3 Degenerative myopia with retinal detachment, bilateral eye**
New   **H44.2C9 Degenerative myopia with retinal detachment, unspecified eye**

New		H44.2D	Degenerative myopia with foveoschisis
New		H44.2D1	Degenerative myopia with foveoschisis, right eye
New		H44.2D2	Degenerative myopia with foveoschisis, left eye
New		H44.2D3	Degenerative myopia with foveoschisis, bilateral eye
New		H44.2D9	Degenerative myopia with foveoschisis, unspecified eye
New	H44.2E		Degenerative myopia with other maculopathy
New		H44.2E1	Degenerative myopia with other maculopathy, right eye
New		H44.2E2	Degenerative myopia with other maculopathy, left eye
New		H44.2E3	Degenerative myopia with other maculopathy, bilateral eye
New		H44.2E9	Degenerative myopia with other maculopathy, unspecified eye

VISUAL DISTURBANCES AND BLINDNESS (H53-H54)

New	H54.0X		Blindness, both eyes, different category levels
New		H54.0X3	Blindness right eye, category 3
New		H54.0X33	Blindness right eye category 3, blindness left eye category 3
New		H54.0X34	Blindness right eye category 3, blindness left eye category 4
New		H54.0X35	Blindness right eye category 3, blindness left eye category 5
New		H54.0X4	Blindness right eye, category 4
New		H54.0X43	Blindness right eye category 4, blindness left eye category 3
New		H54.0X44	Blindness right eye category 4, blindness left eye category 4
New		H54.0X45	Blindness right eye category 4, blindness left eye category 5
New		H54.0X5	Blindness right eye, category 5
New		H54.0X53	Blindness right eye category 5, blindness left eye category 3
New		H54.0X54	Blindness right eye category 5, blindness left eye category 4
New		H54.0X55	Blindness right eye category 5, blindness left eye category 5

New		H54.113	Blindness right eye category 3, low vision left eye
New		H54.1131	Blindness right eye category 3, low vision left eye category 1
New		H54.1132	Blindness right eye category 3, low vision left eye category 2
New		H54.114	Blindness right eye category 4, low vision left eye
New		H54.1141	Blindness right eye category 4, low vision left eye category 1
New		H54.1142	Blindness right eye category 4, low vision left eye category 2
New		H54.115	Blindness right eye category 5, low vision left eye
New		H54.1151	Blindness right eye category 5, low vision left eye category 1
New		H54.1152	Blindness right eye category 5, low vision left eye category 2
New		H54.121	Low vision right eye category 1, blindness left eye
New		H54.1213	Low vision right eye category 1, blindness left eye category 3
New		H54.1214	Low vision right eye category 1, blindness left eye category 4
New		H54.1215	Low vision right eye category 1, blindness left eye category 5
New		H54.122	Low vision right eye category 2, blindness left eye
New		H54.1223	Low vision right eye category 2, blindness left eye category 3
New		H54.1224	Low vision right eye category 2, blindness left eye category 4
New		H54.1225	Low vision right eye category 2, blindness left eye category 5

New	H54.2X	Low vision, both eyes, different category levels	
New	H54.2X1	Low vision, right eye, category 1	
New		H54.2X11	Low vision right eye category 1, low vision left eye category 1
New		H54.2X12	Low vision right eye category 1, low vision left eye category 2
New	H54.2X2	Low vision, right eye, category 2	
New		H54.2X21	Low vision right eye category 2, low vision left eye category 1
New		H54.2X22	Low vision right eye category 2, low vision left eye category 2
New	H54.413	Blindness, right eye, category 3	
New		H54.413A	Blindness right eye category 3, normal vision left eye
New	H54.414	Blindness, right eye, category 4	
New		H54.414A	Blindness right eye category 4, normal vision left eye
New	H54.415	Blindness, right eye, category 5	
New		H54.415A	Blindness right eye category 5, normal vision left eye
New	H54.42A	Blindness, left eye, category 3-5	
New		H54.42A3	Blindness left eye category 3, normal vision right eye
New		H54.42A4	Blindness left eye category 4, normal vision right eye
New		H54.42A5	Blindness left eye category 5, normal vision right eye
New	H54.511	Low vision, right eye, category 1-2	
New		H54.511A	Low vision right eye category 1, normal vision left eye
New		H54.512A	Low vision right eye category 2, normal vision left eye

New	H54.52A	Low vision, left eye, category 1-2	
New		H54.52A1	Low vision left eye category 1, normal vision right eye
New		H54.52A2	Low vision left eye category 2, normal vision right eye

CHAPTER 9

DISEASES OF THE CIRCULATORY SYSTEM (I00-I99)

HYPERTENSIVE DISEASES (I10-I16)

I11   Hypertensive heart disease
Revised   **Includes**   any condition in I50.-, I51.4-I51.9 due to hypertension

ISCHEMIC HEART DISEASES (I20-I25)

Revised   I21   Acute myocardial infarction
Revised   **Excludes2**   subsequent type 1 myocardial infarction (I22.-)

I21.0   **ST elevation (STEMI) myocardial infarction of anterior wall**
New   Type 1 ST elevation myocardial infarction of anterior wall

I21.1   **ST elevation (STEMI) myocardial infarction of inferior wall**
New   Type 1 ST elevation myocardial infarction of inferior wall

I21.2   **ST elevation (STEMI) myocardial infarction of other sites**
New   Type 1 ST elevation myocardial infarction of other sites

I21.3   **ST elevation (STEMI) myocardial infarction of unspecified site**
Deleted   Myocardial infarction (acute) NOS
New   Type 1 ST elevation myocardial infarction of unspecified site

I21.4   **Non-ST elevation (NSTEMI) myocardial infarction**
New   Type 1 non-ST elevation myocardial infarction

New   I21.9   **Acute myocardial infarction, unspecified**
New   Myocardial infarction (acute) NOS

New   I21.A   **Other type of myocardial infarction**

New   I21.A1   **Myocardial infarction type 2**
New   Myocardial infarction due to demand ischemia
New   Myocardial infarction secondary to ischemic imbalance

New   Code also the underlying cause, if known and applicable, such as:
New   anemia (D50.0-D64.9)
New   chronic obstructive pulmonary disease (J44.-)
New   heart failure (I50.-)
New   paroxysmal tachycardia (I47.0-I47.9)
New   renal failure (N17.0-N19)
New   shock (R57.0-R57.9)

New	**I21.A9**	**Other myocardial infarction type**
New		Myocardial infarction associated with revascularization procedure
New		Myocardial infarction type 3
New		Myocardial infarction type 4a
New		Myocardial infarction type 4b
New		Myocardial infarction type 4c
New		Myocardial infarction type 5
New		*Code first, if applicable, postprocedural myocardial infarction following cardiac surgery (I97.190), or postprocedural myocardial infarction during cardiac surgery (I97.790)*
New		Code also complication, if known and applicable, such as:
New		(acute) stent occlusion (T82.897-)
New		(acute) stent stenosis (T82.857-)
New		(acute) stent thrombosis (T82.867-)
New		cardiac arrest due to underlying cardiac condition (I46.2)
New		complication of percutaneous coronary intervention (PCI) (I97.89)
New		occlusion of coronary artery bypass graft (T82.218-)

	I22	**Subsequent ST elevation (STEMI) and non-ST elevation (NSTEMI) myocardial infarction**
New	**Includes**	subsequent type 1 myocardial infarction
New	**Excludes1**	subsequent myocardial infarction, type 2 (I21.A1)
New		subsequent myocardial infarction of other type (type 3) (type 4) (type 5) (I21.A9)

	I24.8	**Other forms of acute ischemic heart disease**
New	**Excludes1**	myocardial infarction due to demand ischemia (I21.A1)

	I25.7	**Atherosclerosis of coronary artery bypass graft(s) and coronary artery of transplanted heart with angina pectoris**
Deleted	**Excludes1**	embolism or thrombus of coronary artery bypass graft(s) (T82.8-)
	I25.710	**Atherosclerosis of autologous vein coronary artery bypass graft(s) with unstable angina pectoris**
New		**Excludes2** embolism or thrombus of coronary artery by-pass graft(s) (T82.8-)

	I25.82	**Chronic total occlusion of coronary artery**
Revised	**Excludes1**	acute coronary occlusion with myocardial infarction (I21.0-I21.9, I22.-)
Revised		acute coronary occlusion without myocardial infarction (I24.0)

	I27.0	**Primary pulmonary hypertension**
New		Heritable pulmonary arterial hypertension
New		Idiopathic pulmonary arterial hypertension
New		Primary group 1 pulmonary hypertension
New		Primary pulmonary arterial hypertension
		Excludes1
Deleted		pulmonary hypertension NOS (I27.2)
Deleted		secondary pulmonary hypertension (I27.2)
New		persistent pulmonary hypertension of newborn (P29.30)
New		pulmonary hypertension NOS (I27.20)
New		secondary pulmonary arterial hypertension (I27.21)
New		secondary pulmonary hypertension (I27.29)

	I27.2	**Other secondary pulmonary hypertension**
Deleted		Pulmonary hypertension NOS
New		**Excludes1** Eisenmenger's syndrome (I27.83)
New	**I27.20**	**Pulmonary hypertension, unspecified**
New		Pulmonary hypertension NOS
New	**I27.21**	**Secondary pulmonary arterial hypertension**
New		(Associated) (drug-induced) (toxin-induced) pulmonary arterial hypertension NOS
New		(Associated) (drug-induced) (toxin-induced) (secondary) group 1 pulmonary hypertension
New		Code also associated conditions if applicable, or adverse effects of drugs or toxins, such as:
New		adverse effect of appetite depressants (T50.5X5)
New		congenital heart disease (Q20-Q28)
New		human immunodeficiency virus [HIV] disease (B20)
New		polymyositis (M33.2-)
New		portal hypertension (K76.6)
New		rheumatoid arthritis (M05.-)
New		schistosomiasis (B65.-)
New		Sjögren syndrome (M35.0-)
New		systemic sclerosis (M34.-)
New	**I27.22**	**Pulmonary hypertension due to left heart disease**
New		Group 2 pulmonary hypertension
New		Code also associated left heart disease, if known, such as:
New		multiple valve disease (I08.-)
New		rheumatic mitral valve diseases (I05.-)
New		rheumatic aortic valve diseases (I06.-)
New	**I27.23**	**Pulmonary hypertension due to lung diseases and hypoxia**
New		Group 3 pulmonary hypertension
New		Code also associated lung disease, if known, such as:
New		bronchiectasis (J47.-)
New		cystic fibrosis with pulmonary manifestations (E84.0)
New		interstitial lung disease (J84.-)
New		pleural effusion (J90)
New		sleep apnea (G47.3-)

New	I27.24	Chronic thromboembolic pulmonary hypertension
New		Group 4 pulmonary hypertension
New		Code also associated pulmonary embolism, if applicable (I26.-, I27.82)
New	I27.29	Other secondary pulmonary hypertension
New		Group 5 pulmonary hypertension
New		Pulmonary hypertension with unclear multifactorial mechanisms
New		Pulmonary hypertension due to hematologic disorders
New		Pulmonary hypertension due to metabolic disorders
New		Pulmonary hypertension due to other systemic disorders
New		Code also other associated disorders, if known, such as:
New		chronic myeloid leukemia (C92.10-C92.22)
New		essential thrombocythemia (D47.3)
New		Gaucher disease (E75.22)
New		hypertensive chronic kidney disease with end stage renal disease (I12.0, I12.11, I13.2)
New		hyperthyroidism (E05.-)
New		hypothyroidism (E00-E03)
New		polycythemia vera (D45)
New		sarcoidosis (D86.-)
New	I27.83	Eisenmenger's syndrome
New		Eisenmenger's complex
New		(Irreversible) Eisenmenger's disease
New		Pulmonary hypertension with right to left shunt related to congenital heart disease
New		Code also underlying heart defect, if known, such as:
New		atrial septal defect (Q21.1)
New		Eisenmenger's defect (Q21.8)
New		patent ductus arteriosus (Q25.0)
New		ventricular septal defect (Q21.0)
	I27.89	Other specified pulmonary heart diseases
Deleted		Eisenmenger's complex
Deleted		Eisenmenger's syndrome
Deleted		**Excludes1** Eisenmenger's defect (Q21.8)

OTHER FORMS OF HEART DISEASE (I30-I52)

	I30	Acute pericarditis
New		**Excludes1** viral pericarditis due to Coxsakie virus (B33.23)
	I34	Nonrheumatic mitral valve disorders
Revised		**Excludes1** mitral valve disorder specified as congenital (Q23.2, Q23.9)
	I49	Other cardiac arrhythmias
Deleted		**Excludes1** bradycardia NOS (R00.1)
New		**Excludes2** bradycardia NOS (R00.1)
	I49.8	Other specified cardiac arrhythmias
New		Brugada syndrome

	I50		Heart failure
Revised	I50.1		Left ventricular failure, unspecified
	I50.2		Systolic (congestive) heart failure
New			Heart failure with reduced ejection fraction [HFrEF]
New			Systolic left ventricular heart failure
New			Code also end stage heart failure, if applicable (I50.84)
	I50.3		Diastolic (congestive) heart failure
New			Diastolic left ventricular heart failure
New			Heart failure with normal ejection fraction
New			Heart failure with preserved ejection fraction [HFpEF]
New			Code also end stage heart failure, if applicable (I50.84)
	I50.4		Combined systolic (congestive) and diastolic (congestive) heart failure
New			Combined systolic and diastolic left ventricular heart failure
New			Heart failure with reduced ejection fraction and diastolic dysfunction
New			Code also end stage heart failure, if applicable (I50.84)
New	I50.8		Other heart failure
New	I50.81		Right heart failure
New			Right ventricular failure
New		I50.810	Right heart failure, unspecified
New			Right heart failure without mention of left heart failure
New			Right ventricular failure NOS
New		I50.811	Acute right heart failure
New			Acute isolated right heart failure
New			Acute (isolated) right ventricular failure
New		I50.812	Chronic right heart failure
New			Chronic isolated right heart failure
New			Chronic (isolated) right ventricular failure
New		I50.813	Acute on chronic right heart failure
New			Acute on chronic isolated right heart failure
New			Acute on chronic (isolated) right ventricular failure
New			Acute decompensation of chronic (isolated) right ventricular failure
New			Acute exacerbation of chronic (isolated) right ventricular failure
New		I50.814	Right heart failure due to left heart failure
New			Right ventricular failure secondary to left ventricular failure
New			Code also the type of left ventricular failure, if known (I50.2-I50.43)
New			**Excludes1** Right heart failure with but not due to left heart failure (I50.82)

New		I50.82	**Biventricular heart failure**
New			Code also the type of left ventricular failure as systolic, diastolic, or combined, if known **(I50.2-I50.43)**
New		I50.83	**High output heart failure**
New		I50.84	**End stage heart failure**
New			Stage D heart failure
New			Code also the type of heart failure as systolic, diastolic, or combined, if known (I50.2-I50.43)
New		I50.89	**Other heart failure**
		I50.9	**Heart failure, unspecified**
Deleted			Biventricular (heart) failure NOS
Deleted			Right ventricular failure (secondary to left heart failure)

CEREBROVASCULAR DISEASES (I60-I69)

Deleted	**Excludes1**	transient cerebral ischemic attacks and related syndromes (G45.-)

I60   Nontraumatic subarachnoid hemorrhage

Deleted	**Includes**	ruptured cerebral aneurysm

Revised		I63.211	Cerebral infarction due to unspecified occlusion or stenosis of right vertebral artery
Revised		I63.212	Cerebral infarction due to unspecified occlusion or stenosis of left vertebral artery
Revised		I63.22	Cerebral infarction due to unspecified occlusion or stenosis of basilar artery
Revised		I63.323	Cerebral infarction due to thrombosis of bilateral anterior cerebral arteries
Revised		I63.333	Cerebral infarction to thrombosis of bilateral posterior cerebral arteries
Revised		I63.513	Cerebral infarction due to unspecified occlusion or stenosis of bilateral middle cerebral arteries
Revised		I63.523	Cerebral infarction due to unspecified occlusion or stenosis of bilateral anterior cerebral arteries
Revised		I63.533	Cerebral infarction due to unspecified occlusion or stenosis of bilateral posterior cerebral arteries
		I63.9	Cerebral infarction, unspecified
New		**Excludes2**	transient cerebral ischemic attacks and related syndromes (G45.-)

	I67.4	**Hypertensive encephalopathy**
New	**Excludes2**	insufficiency, NOS, of precerebral arteries (G45.2)

I69   Sequelae of cerebrovascular disease

Deleted	**Excludes1**	transient ischemic attack (TIA) (G45.9)	
		I69.322	**Dysarthria following cerebral infarction**
New		**Excludes2**	transient ischemic attack (TIA) (G45.9)
		I69.351	**Hemiplegia and hemiparesis following cerebral infarction affecting right dominant side**
New		**Excludes2**	transient ischemic attack (TIA) (G45.9)

DISEASES OF ARTERIES, ARTERIOLES AND CAPILLARIES (I70-I79)

I72   Other aneurysm

New	**Excludes2**	precerebral artery, congenital (nonruptured) (Q28.1)

DISEASES OF VEINS, LYMPHATIC VESSELS AND LYMPH NODES, NOT ELSEWHERE CLASSIFIED (I80-I89)

Revised		I82.811	Embolism and thrombosis of superficial veins of right lower extremity
Revised		I82.812	Embolism and thrombosis of superficial veins of left lower extremity
Revised		I82.819	Embolism and thrombosis of superficial veins of unspecified lower extremity
Revised		I83.811	Varicose veins of right lower extremity with pain
Revised		I83.812	Varicose veins of left lower extremity with pain
Revised		I83.819	Varicose veins of unspecified lower extremity with pain
Revised		I83.891	Varicose veins of right lower extremity with other complications
Revised		I83.892	Varicose veins of left lower extremity with other complications
Revised		I83.899	Varicose veins of unspecified lower extremity with other complications

OTHER AND UNSPECIFIED DISORDERS OF THE CIRCULATORY SYSTEM (I95-I99)

I96   Gangrene, not elsewhere classified

Deleted	**Excludes1**	gangrene in diabetes mellitus (E08-E13 with .52)
New	**Excludes2**	gangrene in diabetes mellitus (E08-E13 with .52)

		I97.190	**Other postprocedural cardiac functional disturbances following cardiac surgery**
New			Use Additional code, if applicable, for type 4 or type 5 myocardial infarction, to further specify disorder

CHAPTER 10

DISEASES OF THE RESPIRATORY SYSTEM (J00-J99)

INFLUENZA AND PNEUMONIA (J09-J18)

J09 **Influenza due to certain identified influenza viruses**
New   **Excludes1** influenza A/H1N1 (J10.-)

Revised   **J15.6** **Pneumonia due to other Gram-negative bacteria**
New   Pneumonia due to other aerobic Gram-negative bacteria

CHRONIC LOWER RESPIRATORY DISEASES (J40-J47)

J44 **Other chronic obstructive pulmonary disease**
Deleted   **Excludes2** lung diseases due to external agents (J60-J70)

    J44.0 **Chronic obstructive pulmonary disease with acute lower respiratory infection**
Deleted   Use additional code to identify the infection
New   Code also to identify the infection

    J44.1 **Chronic obstructive pulmonary disease with (acute) exacerbation**
New   **Excludes2** lung diseases due to external agents (J60-J70)

    J44.9 **Chronic obstructive pulmonary disease, unspecified**
New   **Excludes2** lung diseases due to external agents (J60-J70)

J45 **Asthma**
Deleted   **Excludes1** lung diseases due to external agents (J60-J70)

    J45.909 **Unspecified asthma, uncomplicated**
New   **Excludes2** lung diseases due to external agents (J60-J70)

OTHER RESPIRATORY DISEASES PRINCIPALLY AFFECTING THE INTERSTITIUM (J80-J84)

J84 **Other interstitial pulmonary diseases**
Deleted   **Excludes1** lung diseases due to external agents (J60-J70)
New   **Excludes2** lung diseases due to external agents (J60-J70)

INTRAOPERATIVE AND POSTPROCEDURAL COMPLICATIONS AND DISORDERS OF RESPIRATORY SYSTEM, NOT ELSEWHERE CLASSIFIED (J95)

    J95.02 **Infection of tracheostomy stoma**
     Use additional code to identify type of infection, such as:
Revised   cellulitis of neck (L03.221)

CHAPTER 11

DISEASES OF THE DIGESTIVE SYSTEM (K00-K95)

DISEASES OF ORAL CAVITY AND SALIVARY GLANDS (K00-K14)

K04.7 **Periapical abscess without sinus**
Deleted   Periapical abscess without sinus

K06.0 **Gingival recession**
Revised   Gingival recession (postinfective) (postprocedural)
New   **K06.01** **Gingival recession, localized**
New   **K06.010** **Localized gingival recession, unspecified**
      Localized gingival recession, NOS
New   **K06.011** **Localized gingival recession, minimal**
New   **K06.012** **Localized gingival recession, moderate**
New   **K06.013** **Localized gingival recession, severe**
New   **K06.02** **Gingival recession, generalized**
New   **K06.020** **Generalized gingival recession, unspecified**
      Generalized gingival recession, NOS
New   **K06.021** **Generalized gingival recession, minimal**
New   **K06.022** **Generalized gingival recession, moderate**
New   **K06.023** **Generalized gingival recession, severe**

OTHER DISEASES OF INTESTINES (K55-K64)

K55.3 **Necrotizing enterocolitis**
Revised   **Excludes2** necrotizing enterocolitis due to Clostridium difficile (A04.7-)

K56 **Paralytic ileus and intestinal obstruction without hernia**
Revised   **Excludes1** postprocedural intestinal obstruction (K91.3-)
Deleted   intestinal obstruction with hernia (K40-K46)

K56.0 **Paralytic ileus**
Revised   **Excludes1** obstructive ileus NOS (K56.69-)
Revised **K56.5** **Intestinal adhesions [bands] with obstruction (postinfection)**
Revised   Peritoneal adhesions [bands] with intestinal obstruction (postinfection)
New   **K56.50** **Intestinal adhesions [bands], unspecified as to partial versus complete obstruction**
New   Intestinal adhesions with obstruction NOS
New   **K56.51** **Intestinal adhesions [bands], with partial obstruction**
New   Intestinal adhesions with incomplete obstruction
New   **K56.52** **Intestinal adhesions [bands] with complete obstruction**

	K56.60	Unspecified intestinal obstruction
Deleted		Intestinal obstruction NOS
New	K56.600	Partial intestinal obstruction, unspecified as to cause
New		Incomplete intestinal obstruction, NOS
New	K56.601	Complete intestinal obstruction, unspecified as to cause
New	K56.609	Unspecified intestinal obstruction, unspecified as to partial versus complete obstruction
New		Intestinal obstruction NOS
New	K56.690	Other partial intestinal obstruction
New		Other incomplete intestinal obstruction
New	K56.691	Other complete intestinal obstruction
New	K56.699	Other intestinal obstruction unspecified as to partial versus complete obstruction
New		Other intestinal obstruction, NEC

K56.7   Ileus, unspecified

Revised	**Excludes1**	obstructive ileus (K56.69-)
New	**Excludes2**	intestinal obstruction with hernia (K40-K46)

K59.3   Megacolon, not elsewhere classified

Revised	**Excludes1**	megacolon (due to) (in) Clostridium difficile (A04.7-)

DISEASES OF PERITONEUM AND RETROPERITONEUM (K65-K68)

K66.0   Peritoneal adhesions (postprocedural) (postinfection)

Revised	**Excludes1**	peritoneal adhesions with intestinal obstruction (K56.5-)

OTHER DISEASES OF THE DIGESTIVE SYSTEM (K90-K95)

K90.0   Celiac disease
Celiac gluten-sensitive enteropathy

Revised		

K90.4   Other malabsorption due to intolerance

Revised	**Excludes2**	celiac gluten-sensitive enteropathy (K90.0)

New	K91.30	Postprocedural intestinal obstruction, unspecified as to partial versus complete
New		Postprocedural intestinal obstruction NOS
New	K91.31	Postprocedural partial intestinal obstruction
New		Postprocedural incomplete intestinal obstruction
New	K91.32	Postprocedural complete intestinal obstruction

CHAPTER 12

DISEASES OF THE SKIN AND SUBCUTANEOUS TISSUE (L00-L99)

RADIATION-RELATED DISORDERS OF THE SKIN AND SUBCUTANEOUS TISSUE (L55-L59)

L57   Skin changes due to chronic exposure to nonionizing radiation

Revised		Use additional code to identify the source of the ultraviolet radiation (W89)

OTHER DISORDERS OF THE SKIN AND SUBCUTANEOUS TISSUE (L80-L99)

	L89.019	Pressure ulcer of right elbow, unspecified stage
Revised		Healing pressure ulcer of right elbow, unspecified stage
	L89.029	Pressure ulcer of left elbow, unspecified stage
Revised		Healing pressure ulcer of left elbow, unspecified stage
	L89.619	Pressure ulcer of right heel, unspecified stage
Revised		Healing pressure ulcer of right heel, unspecified stage

L92.9   Granulomatous disorder of the skin and subcutaneous tissue, unspecified

New	**Excludes2**	umbilical granuloma (P83.81)
New	L97.105	Non-pressure chronic ulcer of unspecified thigh with muscle involvement without evidence of necrosis
New	L97.106	Non-pressure chronic ulcer of unspecified thigh with bone involvement without evidence of necrosis
New	L97.108	Non-pressure chronic ulcer of unspecified thigh with other specified severity
New	L97.115	Non-pressure chronic ulcer of right thigh with muscle involvement without evidence of necrosis
New	L97.116	Non-pressure chronic ulcer of right thigh with bone involvement without evidence of necrosis
New	L97.118	Non-pressure chronic ulcer of right thigh with other specified severity
New	L97.125	Non-pressure chronic ulcer of left thigh with muscle involvement without evidence of necrosis
New	L97.126	Non-pressure chronic ulcer of left thigh with bone involvement without evidence of necrosis
New	L97.128	Non-pressure chronic ulcer of left thigh with other specified severity

New	L97.205	Non-pressure chronic ulcer of unspecified calf with muscle involvement without evidence of necrosis
New	L97.206	Non-pressure chronic ulcer of unspecified calf with bone involvement without evidence of necrosis
New	L97.208	Non-pressure chronic ulcer of unspecified calf with other specified severity
New	L97.215	Non-pressure chronic ulcer of right calf with muscle involvement without evidence of necrosis
New	L97.216	Non-pressure chronic ulcer of right calf with bone involvement without evidence of necrosis
New	L97.218	Non-pressure chronic ulcer of right calf with other specified severity
New	L97.225	Non-pressure chronic ulcer of left calf with muscle involvement without evidence of necrosis
New	L97.226	Non-pressure chronic ulcer of left calf with bone involvement without evidence of necrosis
New	L97.228	Non-pressure chronic ulcer of left calf with other specified severity
New	L97.305	Non-pressure chronic ulcer of unspecified ankle with muscle involvement without evidence of necrosis
New	L97.306	Non-pressure chronic ulcer of unspecified ankle with bone involvement without evidence of necrosis
New	L97.308	Non-pressure chronic ulcer of unspecified ankle with other specified severity
New	L97.315	Non-pressure chronic ulcer of right ankle with muscle involvement without evidence of necrosis
New	L97.316	Non-pressure chronic ulcer of right ankle with bone involvement without evidence of necrosis
New	L97.318	Non-pressure chronic ulcer of right ankle with other specified severity
New	L97.325	Non-pressure chronic ulcer of left ankle with muscle involvement without evidence of necrosis
New	L97.326	Non-pressure chronic ulcer of left ankle with bone involvement without evidence of necrosis
New	L97.328	Non-pressure chronic ulcer of left ankle with other specified severity
New	L97.405	Non-pressure chronic ulcer of unspecified heel and midfoot with muscle involvement without evidence of necrosis
New	L97.406	Non-pressure chronic ulcer of unspecified heel and midfoot with bone involvement without evidence of necrosis
New	L97.408	Non-pressure chronic ulcer of unspecified heel and midfoot with other specified severity
New	L97.415	Non-pressure chronic ulcer of right heel and midfoot with muscle involvement without evidence of necrosis
New	L97.416	Non-pressure chronic ulcer of right heel and midfoot with bone involvement without evidence of necrosis
New	L97.418	Non-pressure chronic ulcer of right heel and midfoot with other specified severity
New	L97.425	Non-pressure chronic ulcer of left heel and midfoot with muscle involvement without evidence of necrosis
New	L97.426	Non-pressure chronic ulcer of left heel and midfoot with bone involvement without evidence of necrosis
New	L97.428	Non-pressure chronic ulcer of left heel and midfoot with other specified severity
New	L97.505	Non-pressure chronic ulcer of other part of unspecified foot with muscle involvement without evidence of necrosis
New	L97.506	Non-pressure chronic ulcer of other part of unspecified foot with bone involvement without evidence of necrosis
New	L97.508	Non-pressure chronic ulcer of other part of unspecified foot with other specified severity
New	L97.515	Non-pressure chronic ulcer of other part of right foot with muscle involvement without evidence of necrosis
New	L97.516	Non-pressure chronic ulcer of other part of right foot with bone involvement without evidence of necrosis
New	L97.518	Non-pressure chronic ulcer of other part of right foot with other specified severity
New	L97.525	Non-pressure chronic ulcer of other part of left foot with muscle involvement without evidence of necrosis
New	L97.526	Non-pressure chronic ulcer of other part of left foot with bone involvement without evidence of necrosis
New	L97.528	Non-pressure chronic ulcer of other part of left foot with other specified severity

New	L97.805	Non-pressure chronic ulcer of other part of unspecified lower leg with muscle involvement without evidence of necrosis
New	L97.806	Non-pressure chronic ulcer of other part of unspecified lower leg with bone involvement without evidence of necrosis
New	L97.808	Non-pressure chronic ulcer of other part of unspecified lower leg with other specified severity
New	L97.815	Non-pressure chronic ulcer of other part of right lower leg with muscle involvement without evidence of necrosis
New	L97.816	Non-pressure chronic ulcer of other part of right lower leg with bone involvement without evidence of necrosis
New	L97.818	Non-pressure chronic ulcer of other part of right lower leg with other specified severity
New	L97.825	Non-pressure chronic ulcer of other part of left lower leg with muscle involvement without evidence of necrosis
New	L97.826	Non-pressure chronic ulcer of other part of left lower leg with bone involvement without evidence of necrosis
New	L97.828	Non-pressure chronic ulcer of other part of left lower leg with other specified severity
New	L97.905	Non-pressure chronic ulcer of unspecified part of unspecified lower leg with muscle involvement without evidence of necrosis
New	L97.906	Non-pressure chronic ulcer of unspecified part of unspecified lower leg with bone involvement without evidence of necrosis
New	L97.908	Non-pressure chronic ulcer of unspecified part of unspecified lower leg with other specified severity
New	L97.915	Non-pressure chronic ulcer of unspecified part of right lower leg with muscle involvement without evidence of necrosis
New	L97.916	Non-pressure chronic ulcer of unspecified part of right lower leg with bone involvement without evidence of necrosis
New	L97.918	Non-pressure chronic ulcer of unspecified part of right lower leg with other specified severity

New	L97.925	Non-pressure chronic ulcer of unspecified part of left lower leg with muscle involvement without evidence of necrosis
New	L97.926	Non-pressure chronic ulcer of unspecified part of left lower leg with bone involvement without evidence of necrosis
New	L97.928	Non-pressure chronic ulcer of unspecified part of left lower leg with other specified severity
New	L98.415	Non-pressure chronic ulcer of buttock with muscle involvement without evidence of necrosis
New	L98.416	Non-pressure chronic ulcer of buttock with bone involvement without evidence of necrosis
New	L98.418	Non-pressure chronic ulcer of buttock with other specified severity
New	L98.425	Non-pressure chronic ulcer of back with muscle involvement without evidence of necrosis
New	L98.426	Non-pressure chronic ulcer of back with bone involvement without evidence of necrosis
New	L98.428	Non-pressure chronic ulcer of back with other specified severity
New	L98.495	Non-pressure chronic ulcer of other sites with muscle involvement without evidence of necrosis
New	L98.496	Non-pressure chronic ulcer of other sites with bone involvement without evidence of necrosis
New	L98.498	Non-pressure chronic ulcer of other sites with other specified severity

CHAPTER 13

DISEASES OF THE MUSCULOSKELETAL SYSTEM AND CONNECTIVE TISSUE (M00-M99)

This chapter contains the following blocks:

Deleted	M04	Autoinflammatory syndromes
Deleted	M97	Periprosthetic fracture around internal prosthetic joint

SYSTEMIC CONNECTIVE TISSUE DISORDERS (M30-M36)

Revised	M33.0	Juvenile dermatomyositis
Revised	M33.00	Juvenile dermatomyositis, organ involvement unspecified
Revised	M33.01	Juvenile dermatomyositis with respiratory involvement
Revised	M33.02	Juvenile dermatomyositis with myopathy
New	M33.03	Juvenile dermatomyositis without myopathy
Revised	M33.09	Juvenile dermatomyositis with other organ involvement

Revised	M33.1	Other dermatomyositis
New		Adult dermatomyositis
Revised	M33.10	Other dermatomyositis, organ involvement unspecified
Revised	M33.11	Other dermatomyositis with respiratory involvement
Revised	M33.12	Other dermatomyositis with myopathy
New	M33.13	Other dermatomyositis without myopathy
New		Dermatomyositis NOS
Revised	M33.19	Other dermatomyositis with other organ involvement
New	M33.93	Dermatopolymyositis, unspecified without myopathy

SPONDYLOPATHIES (M45-M49)

New	M48.061	Spinal stenosis, lumbar region without neurogenic claudication
New		Spinal stenosis, lumbar region NOS
New	M48.062	Spinal stenosis, lumbar region with neurogenic claudication

DISORDERS OF MUSCLES (M60-M63)

	M62.5	Muscle wasting and atrophy, not elsewhere classified
Revised	**Excludes1**	progressive muscular atrophy (G12.21)

CHAPTER 14

DISEASES OF THE GENITOURINARY SYSTEM (N00-N99)

RENAL TUBULO-INTERSTITIAL DISEASES (N10-N16)

	N13	Obstructive and reflux uropathy
Revised	**Excludes2**	hydronephrosis with ureteropelvic junction obstruction (Q62.11)

ACUTE KIDNEY FAILURE AND CHRONIC KIDNEY DISEASE (N17-N19)

	N18.9	Chronic kidney disease, unspecified
Revised		Chronic uremia NOS
New		Diffuse sclerosing glomerulonephritis NOS

OTHER DISORDERS OF KIDNEY AND URETER (N25-N29)

	N25	Disorders resulting from impaired renal tubular function
Deleted	**Excludes1**	metabolic disorders classifiable to E70-E88
	N25.0	Renal osteodystrophy
New	**Excludes2**	metabolic disorders classifiable to E70-E88
	N25.81	Secondary hyperparathyroidism of renal origin
New	**Excludes2**	metabolic disorders classifiable to E70-E88
	N28.1	Cyst of kidney, acquired
Revised		Cyst (multiple) (solitary) of kidney, (acquired)

OTHER DISEASES OF THE URINARY SYSTEM (N30-N39)

Revised	N35.112	Postinfective bulbous urethral stricture, not elsewhere classified, male
Revised	N35.113	Postinfective membranous urethral stricture, not elsewhere classified, male
Revised	N35.114	Postinfective anterior urethral stricture, not elsewhere classified, male

DISORDERS OF BREAST (N60-N65)

New	N63.0	Unspecified lump in unspecified breast
New	N63.1	Unspecified lump in the right breast
New	N63.10	Unspecified lump in the right breast, unspecified quadrant
New	N63.11	Unspecified lump in the right breast, upper outer quadrant
New	N63.12	Unspecified lump in the right breast, upper inner quadrant
New	N63.13	Unspecified lump in the right breast, lower outer quadrant
New	N63.14	Unspecified lump in the right breast, lower inner quadrant
New	N63.2	Unspecified lump in the left breast
New	N63.20	Unspecified lump in the left breast, unspecified quadrant
New	N63.21	Unspecified lump in the left breast, upper outer quadrant
New	N63.22	Unspecified lump in the left breast, upper inner quadrant
New	N63.23	Unspecified lump in the left breast, lower outer quadrant
New	N63.24	Unspecified lump in the left breast, lower inner quadrant
New	N63.3	Unspecified lump in axillary tail
New	N63.31	Unspecified lump in axillary tail of the right breast
New	N63.32	Unspecified lump in axillary tail of the left breast
New	N63.4	Unspecified lump in breast, subareolar
New	N63.41	Unspecified lump in right breast, subareolar
New	N63.42	Unspecified lump in left breast, subareolar

NONINFLAMMATORY DISORDERS OF FEMALE GENITAL TRACT (N80-N98)

	N80.8	Other endometriosis
New		Endometriosis of thorax
	N81.2	Incomplete uterovaginal prolapse
Revised	**Excludes1**	cervical stump prolapse (N81.85)
	N94.3	Premenstrual tension syndrome
Deleted		Premenstrual dysphoric disorder

INTRAOPERATIVE AND POSTPROCEDURAL COMPLICATIONS AND DISORDERS OF GENITOURINARY SYSTEM, NOT ELSEWHERE CLASSIFIED (N99)

Revised	N99.111	Postprocedural bulbous urethral stricture, male
Revised	N99.112	Postprocedural membranous urethral stricture, male
Revised	N99.113	Postprocedural anterior bulbous urethral stricture, male

CHAPTER 15

PREGNANCY, CHILDBIRTH AND THE PUERPERIUM (O00-O9A)

PREGNANCY WITH ABORTIVE OUTCOME (O00-O08)

	O00.10	Tubal pregnancy without intrauterine pregnancy
New	O00.101	Right tubal pregnancy without intrauterine pregnancy
New	O00.102	Left tubal pregnancy without intrauterine pregnancy
New	O00.109	Unspecified tubal pregnancy without intrauterine pregnancy
New	O00.111	Right tubal pregnancy with intrauterine pregnancy
New	O00.112	Left tubal pregnancy with intrauterine pregnancy
New	O00.119	Unspecified tubal pregnancy with intrauterine pregnancy
New	O00.201	Right ovarian pregnancy without intrauterine pregnancy
New	O00.202	Left ovarian pregnancy without intrauterine pregnancy
New	O00.209	Unspecified ovarian pregnancy without intrauterine pregnancy
New	O00.211	Right ovarian pregnancy with intrauterine pregnancy
New	O00.212	Left ovarian pregnancy with intrauterine pregnancy
New	O00.219	Unspecified ovarian pregnancy with intrauterine pregnancy

MATERNAL CARE RELATED TO THE FETUS AND AMNIOTIC CAVITY AND POSSIBLE DELIVERY PROBLEMS (O30-O48)

New	O36.83	Maternal care for abnormalities of the fetal heart rate or rhythm
New	O36.831	Maternal care for abnormalities of the fetal heart rate or rhythm, first trimester
New	O36.832	Maternal care for abnormalities of the fetal heart rate or rhythm, second trimester
New	O36.833	Maternal care for abnormalities of the fetal heart rate or rhythm, third trimester
New	O36.839	Maternal care for abnormalities of the fetal heart rate or rhythm, unspecified trimester

OTHER OBSTETRIC CONDITIONS, NOT ELSEWHERE CLASSIFIED (O94-O9A)

	O99.1	Other diseases of the blood and blood-forming organs and certain disorders involving the immune mechanism complicating pregnancy, childbirth and the puerperium
New		**Excludes1** hemorrhage with coagulation defects (O45.-, O46.0-, O67.0, O72.3)
Deleted		**Excludes2** hemorrhage with coagulation defects (O45.-, O46.0-, O67.0, O72.3)

CHAPTER 16

CERTAIN CONDITIONS ORIGINATING IN THE PERINATAL PERIOD (P00-P96)

NEWBORN AFFECTED BY MATERNAL FACTORS AND BY COMPLICATIONS OF PREGNANCY, LABOR, AND DELIVERY (P00–P04)

	P00.2	Newborn affected by maternal infectious and parasitic diseases
Deleted		**Excludes1** infections specific to the perinatal period (P35-P39)
New		**Excludes2** infections specific to the perinatal period (P35-P39)

RESPIRATORY AND CARDIOVASCULAR DISORDERS SPECIFIC TO THE PERINATAL PERIOD (P19-P29)

	P24.01	Meconium aspiration with respiratory symptoms
Revised		Use additional code to identify any secondary pulmonary hypertension, if applicable (I27.2-)
	P24.11	Neonatal aspiration of (clear) amniotic fluid and mucus with respiratory symptoms
Revised		Use additional code to identify any secondary pulmonary hypertension, if applicable (I27.2-)
	P24.21	Neonatal aspiration of blood with respiratory symptoms
Revised		Use additional code to identify any secondary pulmonary hypertension, if applicable (I27.2-)
	P24.31	Neonatal aspiration of milk and regurgitated food with respiratory symptoms
Revised		Use additional code to identify any secondary pulmonary hypertension, if applicable (I27.2-)
	P24.81	Other neonatal aspiration with respiratory symptoms
Revised		Use additional code to identify any secondary pulmonary hypertension, if applicable (I27.2-)
P27		Chronic respiratory disease originating in the perinatal period
Deleted		**Excludes1** respiratory distress of newborn (P22.0-P22.9)
New		**Excludes2** respiratory distress of newborn (P22.0-P22.9)

	P29.3	Persistent fetal circulation
Deleted		Delayed closure of ductus arteriosus
Deleted		(Persistent) pulmonary hypertension of newborn
New	P29.30	Pulmonary hypertension of newborn
New		Persistent pulmonary hypertension of newborn
New	P29.38	Other persistent fetal circulation
New		Delayed closure of ductus arteriosus

DIGESTIVE SYSTEM DISORDERS OF NEWBORN (P76-P78)

New	P78.84	Gestational alloimmune liver disease
New		GALD
New		Neonatal hemochromatosis
New		**Excludes1** hemochromatosis (E83.11-)

CONDITIONS INVOLVING THE INTEGUMENT AND TEMPERATURE REGULATION OF NEWBORN (P80-P83)

	P83.8	Other specified conditions of integument specific to newborn
Deleted		Bronze baby syndrome
Deleted		Neonatal scleroderma
Deleted		Urticaria neonatorum
New	P83.81	Umbilical granuloma
New		**Excludes2** Granulomatous disorder of the skin and subcutaneous tissue, unspecified (L92.9)
New	P83.88	Other specified conditions of integument specific to newborn
New		Bronze baby syndrome
New		Neonatal scleroderma
New		Urticaria neonatorum

OTHER DISORDERS ORIGINATING IN THE PERINATAL PERIOD (P90-P96)

	P91.6	Hypoxic ischemic encephalopathy [HIE]
New		**Excludes1** Neonatal cerebral depression (P91.4)
New		Neonatal cerebral irritability (P91.3)
New		Neonatal coma (P91.5)
New	P91.81	Neonatal encephalopathy
New	P91.811	Neonatal encephalopathy in diseases classified elsewhere
New		*Code first underlying condition, if known, such as:*
New		congenital cirrhosis (of liver) (P78.71)
New		intracranial nontraumatic hemorrhage of newborn (P52.-)
New		kernicterus (P57.-)
New	P91.819	Neonatal encephalopathy, unspecified
New	P91.88	Other specified disturbances of cerebral status of newborn
	P92	Feeding problems of newborn
New		**Excludes1** eating disorders (F50.-)

CHAPTER 17

CONGENITAL MALFORMATIONS, DEFORMATIONS AND CHROMOSOMAL ABNORMALITIES (Q00-Q99)

CONGENITAL MALFORMATIONS OF THE CIRCULATORY SYSTEM (Q20-Q28)

	Q21.8	Other congenital malformations of cardiac septa
Deleted		**Excludes1** Eisenmenger's complex (I27.8)
Deleted		Eisenmenger's syndrome (I27.8)
New		Code also if applicable:
New		Eisenmenger's complex (I27.83)
New		Eisenmenger's syndrome (I27.83)
	Q25.49	Other congenital malformations of aorta
New		Aortic arch
New		Bovine arch

CONGENITAL MALFORMATIONS OF GENITAL ORGANS (Q50-Q56)

New	Q53.111	Unilateral intraabdominal testis
New	Q53.112	Unilateral inguinal testis
New	Q53.13	Unilateral high scrotal testis
New	Q53.211	Bilateral intraabdominal testes
New	Q53.212	Bilateral inguinal testes
New	Q53.23	Bilateral high scrotal testes

CONGENITAL MALFORMATIONS OF THE URINARY SYSTEM (Q60-Q64)

Revised	Q64.12	Cloacal exstrophy of urinary bladder

OTHER CONGENITAL MALFORMATIONS (Q80-Q89)

	Q82.2	Congenital cutaneous mastocytosis
Revised		
Deleted		Urticaria pigmentosa
New		Congenital diffuse cutaneous mastocytosis
New		Congenital maculopapular cutaneous mastocytosis
New		Congenital urticaria pigmentosa
		Excludes1
Deleted		malignant mastocytosis (C96.2)
New		cutaneous mastocytosis NOS (D47.01)
New		diffuse cutaneous mastocytosis (with onset after newborn period) (D47.01)
New		malignant mastocytosis (C96.2-)
New		systemic mastocytosis (D47.02)
New		urticaria pigmentosa (non-congenital) (with onset after newborn period) (D47.01)

CHAPTER 18

SYMPTOMS, SIGNS AND ABNORMAL CLINICAL AND LABORATORY FINDINGS, NOT ELSEWHERE CLASSIFIED (R00-R99)

SYMPTOMS AND SIGNS INVOLVING THE CIRCULATORY AND RESPIRATORY SYSTEMS (R00-R09)

	R06.03	Acute respiratory distress
New		
	R09.0	Asphyxia and hypoxemia
Deleted		**Excludes1** hypercapnia (R06.4)
New		**Excludes2** hypercapnia (R06.89)

SYMPTOMS AND SIGNS INVOLVING THE GENITOURINARY SYSTEM (R30-R39)

New   R39.83   Unilateral non-palpable testicle

New   R39.84   Bilateral non-palpable testicles

SYMPTOMS AND SIGNS INVOLVING COGNITION, PERCEPTION, EMOTIONAL STATE AND BEHAVIOR (R40-R46)

R40.222   **Coma scale, best verbal response, incomprehensible words**

New   Incomprehensible sounds (2-5 years of age)

New   Moans/grunts to pain; restless (<2 years old)

R40.223   **Coma scale, best verbal response, inappropriate words**

New   Inappropriate crying or screaming (< 2 years of age)

New   Screaming (2-5 years of age)

R40.224   **Coma scale, best verbal response, confused conversation**

New   Inappropriate words (2-5 years of age)

New   Irritable cries (< 2 years of age)

R40.225   **Coma scale, best verbal response, oriented**

New   Cooing or babbling or crying appropriately (< 2 years of age)

New   Uses appropriate words (2- 5 years of age)

R40.232   **Coma scale, best motor response, extension**

New   Abnormal extensor posturing to pain or noxious stimuli (< 2 years of age)

New   Extensor posturing to pain or noxious stimuli (2-5 years of age)

R40.233   **Coma scale, best motor response, abnormal**

New   Abnormal flexure posturing to pain or noxious stimuli (0-5 years of age)

New   Flexion/decorticate posturing (< 2 years of age)

R40.234   **Coma scale, best motor response, flexion withdrawal**

New   Withdraws from pain or noxious stimuli (0-5 years of age)

R40.235   **Coma scale, best motor response, localizes pain**

New   Localizes pain (2-5 years of age)

New   Withdraws to touch (< 2 years of age)

R40.236   **Coma scale, best motor response, obeys commands**

New   Normal or spontaneous movement (< 2 years of age)

New   Obeys commands (2-5 years of age)

R41.9   **Unspecified symptoms and signs involving cognitive functions and awareness**

New   Unspecified neurocognitive disorder

GENERAL SYMPTOMS AND SIGNS (R50-R69)

R53.8   **Other malaise and fatigue**

Deleted   **Excludes1**   exhaustion and fatigue due to depressive episode (F32.-)

R53.83   **Other fatigue**

New   **Excludes2**   exhaustion and fatigue due to depressive episode (F32.-)

R57   **Shock, not elsewhere classified**

Deleted   **Excludes1**   septic shock (R65.21)

R57.0   **Cardiogenic shock**

New   **Excludes2**   septic shock (R65.21)

R60   **Edema, not elsewhere classified**

Deleted   **Excludes1**   nutritional edema (E40-E46)

R60.1   **Generalized edema**

New   **Excludes2**   nutritional edema (E40-E46)

R63.3   **Feeding difficulties**

New   Picky eater

New   **Excludes1**   eating disorders (F50.-)

R68.13   **Apparent life threatening event in infant (ALTE)**

New   Brief resolved unexplained event (BRUE)

ABNORMAL FINDINGS ON EXAMINATION OF BLOOD, WITHOUT DIAGNOSIS (R70-R79)

R79   **Other abnormal findings of blood chemistry**

Deleted   **Excludes1**   abnormality of fluid, electrolyte or acid-base balance (E86-E87)

R79.1   **Abnormal coagulation profile**

New   **Excludes2**   abnormality of fluid, electrolyte or acid-base balance (E86-E87)

CHAPTER 19

INJURY, POISONING AND CERTAIN OTHER CONSEQUENCES OF EXTERNAL CAUSES (S00-T88)

This chapter contains the following blocks:

Deleted
T20-T32	Burns and corrosions

INJURIES TO THE HEAD (S00-S09)

S00.531   **Contusion of lip**

Revised   Hematoma of lip

S00.532   **Contusion of oral cavity**

Revised   Bruise of oral cavity

S01.85   **Open bite of other part of head**

Revised   **Excludes1**   superficial bite of other part of head (S00.87)

		S04.0	Injury of optic nerve and pathways
Revised			Use additional code to identify any visual field defect or blindness (H53.4-, H54.-)
Revised		S04.031	Injury of optic tract and pathways, right side
Revised		S04.032	Injury of optic tract and pathways, left side
Revised		S04.039	Injury of optic tract and pathways, unspecified side
Revised		S04.041	Injury of visual cortex, right side
Revised		S04.042	Injury of visual cortex, left side
Revised		S04.049	Injury of visual cortex, unspecified side

S06 Intracranial injury

New — Note: 7th characters D and S do not apply to codes in category S06 with 6th character 7 - death due to brain injury prior to regaining consciousness, or 8 - death due to other cause prior to regaining consciousness.

INJURIES TO THE WRIST, HAND AND FINGERS (S60-S69)

Revised	S62.311	Displaced fracture of base of second metacarpal bone, left hand
Revised	S62.317	Displaced fracture of base of fifth metacarpal bone, left hand
Revised	S62.341	Nondisplaced fracture of base of second metacarpal bone, left hand
Revised	S62.347	Nondisplaced fracture of base of fifth metacarpal bone, left hand
Revised	S62.62	Displaced fracture of middle phalanx of finger
Revised	S62.620	Displaced fracture of middle phalanx of right index finger
Revised	S62.621	Displaced fracture of middle phalanx of left index finger
Revised	S62.622	Displaced fracture of middle phalanx of right middle finger
Revised	S62.623	Displaced fracture of middle phalanx of left middle finger
Revised	S62.624	Displaced fracture of middle phalanx of right ring finger
Revised	S62.625	Displaced fracture of middle phalanx of left ring finger
Revised	S62.65	Nondisplaced fracture of middle phalanx of finger
Revised	S62.650	Nondisplaced fracture of middle phalanx of right index finger
Revised	S62.651	Nondisplaced fracture of middle phalanx of left index finger
Revised	S62.652	Nondisplaced fracture of middle phalanx of right middle finger
Revised	S62.653	Nondisplaced fracture of middle phalanx of left middle finger

Revised	S63.12	Subluxation and dislocation of interphalangeal joint of thumb
Revised	S63.121	Subluxation of interphalangeal joint of right thumb
Revised	S63.122	Subluxation of interphalangeal joint of left thumb
Revised	S63.123	Subluxation of interphalangeal joint of unspecified thumb
Revised	S63.124	Dislocation of interphalangeal joint of right thumb
Revised	S63.125	Dislocation of interphalangeal joint of left thumb
Revised	S63.126	Dislocation of interphalangeal joint of unspecified thumb
Deleted	S63.13	Subluxation and dislocation of proximal interphalangeal joint of thumb
Deleted	S63.131	Subluxation of proximal interphalangeal joint of right thumb
Deleted	S63.132	Subluxation of proximal interphalangeal joint of left thumb
Deleted	S63.133	Subluxation of proximal interphalangeal joint of unspecified thumb
Deleted	S63.134	Dislocation of proximal interphalangeal joint of right thumb
Deleted	S63.135	Dislocation of proximal interphalangeal joint of left thumb
Deleted	S63.136	Dislocation of proximal interphalangeal joint of unspecified thumb
Deleted	S63.14	Subluxation and dislocation of distal interphalangeal joint of thumb
Deleted	S63.141	Subluxation of distal interphalangeal joint of right thumb
Deleted	S63.142	Subluxation of distal interphalangeal joint of left thumb
Deleted	S63.143	Subluxation of distal interphalangeal joint of unspecified thumb
Deleted	S63.144	Dislocation of distal interphalangeal joint of right thumb
Deleted	S63.145	Dislocation of distal interphalangeal joint of left thumb
Deleted	S63.146	Dislocation of distal interphalangeal joint of unspecified thumb
	S63.259	Unspecified dislocation of unspecified finger
Revised		Unspecified dislocation of unspecified finger with unspecified laterality
	S63.279	Dislocation of unspecified interphalangeal joint of unspecified finger
Revised		Dislocation of unspecified interphalangeal joint of unspecified finger without specified laterality

INJURIES TO THE HIP AND THIGH (S70-S79)

	S72	Fracture of femur
Revised		**Excludes2** periprosthetic fracture of prosthetic implant of hip (M97.0-)
Revised	S73.03	Other anterior subluxation and dislocation of hip
Revised	S73.04	Central subluxation and dislocation of hip

INJURIES TO THE KNEE AND LOWER LEG (S80-S89)

	S82	Fracture of lower leg, including ankle
Revised		**Excludes2** periprosthetic fracture of prosthetic implant of knee (M97.0-)

INJURIES TO THE ANKLE AND FOOT (S90-S99)

Revised	S92.52	Fracture of middle phalanx of lesser toe(s)
Revised	S92.521	Displaced fracture of middle phalanx of right lesser toe(s)
Revised	S92.522	Displaced fracture of middle phalanx of left lesser toe(s)
Revised	S92.523	Displaced fracture of middle phalanx of unspecified lesser toe(s)
Revised	S92.524	Nondisplaced fracture of middle phalanx of right lesser toe(s)
Revised	S92.525	Nondisplaced fracture of middle phalanx of left lesser toe(s)
Revised	S92.526	Nondisplaced fracture of middle phalanx of unspecified lesser toe(s)

INJURIES INVOLVING MULTIPLE BODY REGIONS (T07)

	T07	Unspecified multiple injuries
New		The appropriate 7th character is to be added to code T07
New		A initial encounter
New		D subsequent encounter
New		S sequela
Revised		**Excludes1** injury NOS (T14.90)

INJURY OF UNSPECIFIED BODY REGION (T14)

	T14	Injury of unspecified body region
New		The appropriate 7th character is to be added to each code from category T14
New		A initial encounter
New		D subsequent encounter
New		S sequela
	T14.8	Other injury of unspecified body region
New		Wound NOS

BURNS AND CORROSIONS CONFINED TO EYE AND INTERNAL ORGANS (T26-T28)

	T27.3	Burn of respiratory tract, part unspecified
Deleted		*Code first (T51-T65) to identify chemical and intent for codes T27.4-T27.7*
	T27.4	Corrosion of larynx and trachea
New		*Code first (T51-T65) to identify chemical and intent*
	T27.6	Corrosion of other parts of respiratory tract
New		*Code first (T51-T65) to identify chemical and intent*
	T27.7	Corrosion of respiratory tract, part unspecified
New		*Code first (T51-T65) to identify chemical and intent*
	T28.4	Burns of other and unspecified internal organs
New		*Code first (T51-T65) to identify chemical and intent*
	T28.49	Burn of other internal organ
Deleted		*Code first (T51-T65) to identify chemical and intent for T28.5-T28.9-*
	T28.5	Corrosion of mouth and pharynx
New		*Code first (T51-T65) to identify chemical and intent*
	T28.6	Corrosion of esophagus
New		*Code first (T51-T65) to identify chemical and intent*
	T28.7	Corrosion of other parts of alimentary tract
New		*Code first (T51-T65) to identify chemical and intent*
	T28.8	Corrosion of internal genitourinary organs
New		*Code first (T51-T65) to identify chemical and intent*
	T28.9	Corrosions of other and unspecified internal organs
New		*Code first (T51-T65) to identify chemical and intent*

POISONING BY, ADVERSE EFFECTS OF AND UNDERDOSING OF DRUGS, MEDICAMENTS AND BIOLOGICAL SUBSTANCES (T36-T50)

	T43.205	Adverse effect of unspecified antidepressants
New		Antidepressant discontinuation syndrome

OTHER AND UNSPECIFIED EFFECTS OF EXTERNAL CAUSES (T66-T78)

	T76.2	Sexual abuse, suspected
Deleted		Sexual abuse, suspected

COMPLICATIONS OF SURGICAL AND MEDICAL CARE NOT ELSEWHERE CLASSIFIED (T80-T88)

	T80.69	Other serum reaction due to other serum
New		Code also, if applicable, arthropathy in hypersensitivity reactions classified elsewhere (M36.4)
	T84.01	Broken internal joint prosthesis
Revised		**Excludes1** periprosthetic joint implant fracture (M97-)
	T85.623	Displacement of artificial skin graft and decellularized allodermis
Deleted		Displacement of artificial skin graft and decellularized allodermis

CHAPTER 20

EXTERNAL CAUSES OF MORBIDITY (V00-Y99)

This chapter contains the following blocks:

Deleted	X50	Overexertion and strenuous or repetitive movements

OTHER LAND TRANSPORT ACCIDENTS (V80-V89)

New   V86.05   Driver of 3- or 4-wheeled all-terrain vehicle (ATV) injured in traffic accident

New   V86.06   Driver of dirt bike or motor/cross bike injured in traffic accident

New   V86.15   Passenger of 3- or 4-wheeled all-terrain vehicle (ATV) injured in traffic accident

New   V86.16   Passenger of dirt bike or motor/cross bike injured in traffic accident

New   V86.25   Person on outside of 3- or 4-wheeled all-terrain vehicle (ATV) injured in traffic accident

New   V86.26   Person on outside of dirt bike or motor/cross bike injured in traffic accident

New   V86.35   Unspecified occupant of 3- or 4-wheeled all-terrain vehicle (ATV) injured in traffic accident

New   V86.36   Unspecified occupant of dirt bike or motor/cross bike injured in traffic accident

New   V86.45   Person injured while boarding or alighting from a 3- or 4-wheeled all-terrain vehicle (ATV)

New   V86.46   Person injured while boarding or alighting from a dirt bike or motor/cross bike

New   V86.55   Driver of 3- or 4-wheeled all-terrain vehicle (ATV) injured in nontraffic accident

New   V86.56   Driver of dirt bike or motor/cross bike injured in nontraffic accident

New   V86.65   Passenger of 3- or 4-wheeled all-terrain vehicle (ATV) injured in nontraffic accident

New   V86.66   Passenger of dirt bike or motor/cross bike injured in nontraffic accident

New   V86.75   Person on outside of 3- or 4-wheeled all-terrain vehicle (ATV) injured in nontraffic accident

New   V86.76   Person on outside of dirt bike or motor/cross bike injured in nontraffic accident

New   V86.95   Unspecified occupant of 3- or 4-wheeled all-terrain vehicle (ATV) injured in nontraffic accident

New   V86.96   Unspecified occupant of dirt bike or motor/cross bike injured in nontraffic accident

New   V86.99   Unspecified occupant of other special all-terrain or other off-road motor vehicle injured in nontraffic accident

Deleted   All-terrain motor-vehicle accident NOS

Deleted   Unspecified occupant of dirt bike injured in nontraffic accident

SLIPPING, TRIPPING, STUMBLING AND FALLS (W00-W19)

Revised   **Excludes2**   fall into fire (X00-X04, X08)

EXPOSURE TO INANIMATE MECHANICAL FORCES (W20-W49)

Revised   W29.8   Contact with other powered hand tools and household machinery

CONTACT WITH HEAT AND HOT SUBSTANCES (X10-X19)

Revised   **Excludes1**   exposure to fire and flames (X00-X08)

   X19   Contact with other heat and hot substances

Revised   **Excludes1**   objects that are not normally hot, e.g., an object made hot by a house fire (X00-X08)

EXPOSURE TO FORCES OF NATURE (X30-X39)

   X32   Exposure to sunlight

New   **Excludes2**   radiation-related disorders of the skin and subcutaneous tissue (L55-L59)

CHAPTER 21

FACTORS INFLUENCING HEALTH STATUS AND CONTACT WITH HEALTH SERVICES (Z00-Z99)

This chapter contains the following blocks:

Deleted	Z19	Hormone sensitivity malignancy status

PERSONS ENCOUNTERING HEALTH SERVICES FOR EXAMINATIONS (Z00-Z13)

   Z03   Encounter for medical observation for suspected diseases and conditions ruled out

New   **Excludes1**   encounter for observation and evaluation of newborn for suspected diseases and conditions ruled out (Z05.0-)

Deleted   newborn observation for suspected condition, ruled out (P00-P04)

   Z05   Encounter for observation and evaluation of newborn for suspected diseases and conditions ruled out

Revised   This category is to be used for newborns, within the neonatal period (the first 28 days of life), who are suspected of having an abnormal condition, but without signs or symptoms, and which, after examination and observation, is ruled out.

Deleted   **Excludes2**   newborn observation for suspected condition, related to exposure from the mother or birth process (P00-P04)

RESISTANCE TO ANTIMICROBIAL DRUGS (Z16)

Z16   Resistance to antimicrobial drugs

Deleted   **Excludes1**   Methicillin resistant Staphylococcus aureus infection in diseases classified elsewhere (B95.62)

Z16.12   Extended spectrum beta lactamase (ESBL) resistance

New   **Excludes2**   Methicillin resistant Staphylococcus aureus infection in diseases classified elsewhere (B95.62)

PERSONS ENCOUNTERING HEALTH SERVICES IN CIRCUMSTANCES RELATED TO REPRODUCTION (Z30-Z39)

Revised   Z31.5   Encounter for procreative genetic counseling

Z36   Encounter for antenatal screening of mother

New   **Includes**   Encounter for placental sample (taken vaginally)

New   Screening is the testing for disease or disease precursors in asymptomatic individuals so that early detection and treatment can be provided for those who test positive for the disease.

Deleted   **Excludes1**   abnormal findings on antenatal screening of mother (O28.-)

New   **Excludes2**   abnormal findings on antenatal screening of mother (O28.-)

New   Z36.0   Encounter for antenatal screening for chromosomal anomalies

New   Z36.1   Encounter for antenatal screening for raised alphafetoprotein level

New   Encounter for antenatal screening for elevated maternal serum alphafetoprotein level

New   Z36.2   Encounter for other antenatal screening follow-up

New   Non-visualized anatomy on a previous scan

New   Z36.3   Encounter for antenatal screening for malformations

New   Screening for a suspected anomaly

New   Z36.4   Encounter for antenatal screening for fetal growth retardation

New   Intrauterine growth restriction (IUGR) / small-for-dates

New   Z36.5   Encounter for antenatal screening for isoimmunization

New   Z36.8   Encounter for other antenatal screening

New   Z36.81   Encounter for antenatal screening for hydrops fetalis

New   Z36.82   Encounter for antenatal screening for nuchal translucency

New   Z36.83   Encounter for fetal screening for congenital cardiac abnormalities

New   Z36.84   Encounter for antenatal screening for fetal lung maturity

New   Z36.85   Encounter for antenatal screening for Streptococcus B

New   Z36.86   Encounter for antenatal screening for cervical length

New   Screening for risk of pre-term labor

New   Z36.87   Encounter for antenatal screening for uncertain dates

New   Z36.88   Encounter for antenatal screening for fetal macrosomia

New   Screening for large-for-dates

New   Z36.89   Encounter for other specified antenatal screening

New   Z36.8A   Encounter for antenatal screening for other genetic defects

New   Z36.9   Encounter for antenatal screening, unspecified

Z3A   Weeks of gestation

Revised   *Code first complications of pregnancy, childbirth and the puerperium (O09-O9A)*

ENCOUNTERS FOR OTHER SPECIFIC HEALTH CARE (Z40-Z53)

Revised   Z40.02   Encounter for prophylactic removal of ovary(s)

New   Encounter for prophylactic removal of ovary(s) and fallopian tube(s)

New   Z40.03   Encounter for prophylactic removal of fallopian tube(s)

Z43   Encounter for attention to artificial openings

Deleted   **Excludes1**   artificial opening status only, without need for care (Z93.-)

Z43.1   Encounter for attention to gastrostomy

New   **Excludes2**   artificial opening status only, without need for care (Z93.-)

Z45   Encounter for adjustment and management of implanted device

Deleted   **Excludes1**   presence of prosthetic and other devices (Z95-Z97)

Z45.018   Encounter for adjustment and management of other part of cardiac pacemaker

New   **Excludes2**   presence of prosthetic and other devices (Z95-Z97)

Z48   Encounter for other postprocedural aftercare

New   **Excludes1**   encounter for aftercare following injury - code to Injury, by site, with appropriate 7th character for subsequent encounter

PERSONS WITH POTENTIAL HEALTH HAZARDS RELATED TO SOCIOECONOMIC AND PSYCHOSOCIAL CIRCUMSTANCES (Z55-Z65)

Z63.0   Problems in relationship with spouse or partner

New   Relationship distress with spouse or intimate partner

Z65.8   Other specified problems related to psychosocial circumstances

New   Religious or spiritual problem

BODY MASS INDEX [BMI] (Z68)

Revised   Z68.1   Body mass index (BMI) 19.9 or less, adult

PERSONS ENCOUNTERING HEALTH SERVICES IN OTHER CIRCUMSTANCES (Z69-Z76)

Z69.010 **Encounter for mental health services for victim of parental child abuse**

New Encounter for mental health services for victim of child abuse by parent

New Encounter for mental health services for victim of child neglect by parent

New Encounter for mental health services for victim of child psychological abuse by parent

New Encounter for mental health services for victim of child sexual abuse by parent

Z69.011 **Encounter for mental health services for perpetrator of parental child abuse**

New Encounter for mental health services for perpetrator of parental child neglect

New Encounter for mental health services for perpetrator of parental child psychological abuse

New Encounter for mental health services for perpetrator of parental child sexual abuse

Z69.020 **Encounter for mental health services for victim of non-parental child abuse**

New Encounter for mental health services for victim of non-parental child neglect

New Encounter for mental health services for victim of non-parental child psychological abuse

New Encounter for mental health services for victim of non-parental child sexual abuse

Z69.021 **Encounter for mental health services for perpetrator of non-parental child abuse**

New Encounter for mental health services for perpetrator of non-parental child neglect

New Encounter for mental health services for perpetrator of non-parental child psychological abuse

New Encounter for mental health services for perpetrator of non-parental child sexual abuse

Z69.11 **Encounter for mental health services for victim of spousal or partner abuse**

New Encounter for mental health services for victim of spouse or partner neglect

New Encounter for mental health services for victim of spouse or partner psychological abuse

New Encounter for mental health services for victim of spouse or partner violence, physical

Z69.12 **Encounter for mental health services for perpetrator of spousal or partner abuse**

New Encounter for mental health services for perpetrator of spouse or partner neglect

New Encounter for mental health services for perpetrator of spouse or partner psychological abuse

New Encounter for mental health services for perpetrator of spouse or partner violence, physical

New Encounter for mental health services for perpetrator of spouse or partner violence, sexual

Z69.81 **Encounter for mental health services for victim of other abuse**

New Encounter for mental health services for perpetrator of non-spousal adult abuse

New Encounter for mental health services for victim of non-spousal adult abuse

New Encounter for mental health services for victim of spouse or partner violence, sexual

Z71.8 **Other specified counseling**

Deleted **Excludes2** counseling for genetics (Z31.5)
Deleted counseling for procreative management (Z31.6-)

New **Z71.82** **Exercise counseling**

New **Z71.83** **Encounter for nonprocreative genetic counseling**

New **Excludes1** counseling for procreative genetics (Z31.5)
New counseling for procreative management (Z31.6)

PERSONS WITH POTENTIAL HEALTH HAZARDS RELATED TO FAMILY AND PERSONAL HISTORY AND CERTAIN CONDITIONS INFLUENCING HEALTH STATUS (Z77-Z99)

Z79.81 **Long term (current) use of agents affecting estrogen receptors and estrogen levels**

Revised **Excludes1** hormone replacement therapy (Z79.890)

Revised **Z79.890** **Hormone replacement therapy**

Z83.71 **Family history of colonic polyps**

Deleted **Excludes1** family history of malignant neoplasm of digestive organs (Z80.0)

New **Excludes2** family history of malignant neoplasm of digestive organs (Z80.0)

| | Z87.41 | **Personal history of dysplasia of the female genital tract** |
| *Revised* | **Excludes1** | personal history of intraepithelial neoplasia III of female genital tract (Z86.001, Z86.008) |

	Z91	**Personal risk factors, not elsewhere classified**
New	**Excludes2**	female genital mutilation status (N90.81-)
	Z91.19	**Patient's noncompliance with other medical treatment and regimen**
New		Nonadherence to medical treatment

New	Z91.84	**Oral health risk factors**
New	Z91.841	**Risk for dental caries, low**
New	Z91.842	**Risk for dental caries, moderate**
New	Z91.843	**Risk for dental caries, high**
New	Z91.849	**Unspecified risk for dental caries**

	Z95	**Presence of cardiac and vascular implants and grafts**
Deleted	**Excludes1**	complications of cardiac and vascular devices, implants and grafts (T82.-)
New	**Excludes2**	complications of cardiac and vascular devices, implants and grafts (T82.-)

PART I

Introduction

ICD-10-CM Official Guidelines for Coding and Reporting 2018
Narrative changes appear in bold text
Items <u>underlined</u> have been moved within the guidelines since the 2017 version
***Italics* are used to indicate revisions to heading changes**

The Centers for Medicare and Medicaid Services (CMS) and the National Center for Health Statistics (NCHS), two departments within the U.S. Federal Government's Department of Health and Human Services (DHHS) provide the following guidelines for coding and reporting using the International Classification of Diseases, 10th Revision, Clinical Modification (ICD-10-CM). These guidelines should be used as a companion document to the official version of the ICD-10-CM as published on the NCHS website. The ICD-10-CM is a morbidity classification published by the United States for classifying diagnoses and reason for visits in all health care settings. The ICD-10-CM is based on the ICD-10, the statistical classification of disease published by the World Health Organization (WHO).

These guidelines have been approved by the four organizations that make up the Cooperating Parties for the ICD-10-CM: the American Hospital Association (AHA), the American Health Information Management Association (AHIMA), CMS, and NCHS.

These guidelines are a set of rules that have been developed to accompany and complement the official conventions and instructions provided within the ICD-10-CM itself. The instructions and conventions of the classification take precedence over guidelines. These guidelines are based on the coding and sequencing instructions in the Tabular List and Alphabetic Index of ICD-10-CM, but provide additional instruction. Adherence to these guidelines when assigning ICD-10-CM diagnosis codes is required under the Health Insurance Portability and Accountability Act (HIPAA). The diagnosis codes (Tabular List and Alphabetic Index)

have been adopted under HIPAA for all healthcare settings. A joint effort between the healthcare provider and the coder is essential to achieve complete and accurate documentation, code assignment, and reporting of diagnoses and procedures. These guidelines have been developed to assist both the healthcare provider and the coder in identifying those diagnoses that are to be reported. The importance of consistent, complete documentation in the medical record cannot be overemphasized. Without such documentation accurate coding cannot be achieved. The entire record should be reviewed to determine the specific reason for the encounter and the conditions treated.

The term encounter is used for all settings, including hospital admissions. In the context of these guidelines, the term provider is used throughout the guidelines to mean physician or any qualified health care practitioner who is legally accountable for establishing the patient's diagnosis. Only this set of guidelines, approved by the Cooperating Parties, is official.

The guidelines are organized into sections. Section I includes the structure and conventions of the classification and general guidelines that apply to the entire classification, and chapter-specific guidelines that correspond to the chapters as they are arranged in the classification. Section II includes guidelines for selection of principal diagnosis for non-outpatient settings. Section III includes guidelines for reporting additional diagnoses in non-outpatient settings. Section IV is for outpatient coding and reporting. It is necessary to review all sections of the guidelines to fully understand all of the rules and instructions needed to code properly.

ICD-10-CM Official Guidelines for Coding and Reporting

Section I. Conventions, general coding guidelines and chapter specific guidelines

A. Conventions for the ICD-10-CM
  1. The Alphabetic Index and Tabular List
  2. Format and Structure:
  3. Use of codes for reporting purposes
  4. Placeholder character
  5. 7th Characters
  6. Abbreviations
    a. Alphabetic Index abbreviations
    b. Tabular List abbreviations
  7. Punctuation
  8. Use of "and"
  9. Other and Unspecified codes
    a. "Other" codes
    b. "Unspecified" codes
  10. Includes Notes
  11. Inclusion terms
  12. Excludes Notes
    a. Excludes1
    b. Excludes2
  13. Etiology/manifestation convention ("code first", "use additional code" and "in diseases classified elsewhere" notes)
  14. "And"
  15. "With"
  16. "See" and "See Also"
  17. "Code also note"
  18. Default codes
  19. Code assignment and Clinical Criteria
B. General Coding Guidelines
  1. Locating a code in the ICD-10-CM
  2. Level of Detail in Coding
  3. Code or codes from A00.0 through T88.9, Z00-Z99.8
  4. Signs and symptoms
  5. Conditions that are an integral part of a disease process
  6. Conditions that are not an integral part of a disease process
  7. Multiple coding for a single condition
  8. Acute and Chronic Conditions
  9. Combination Code
  10. Sequela (Late Effects)
  11. Impending or Threatened Condition
  12. Reporting Same Diagnosis Code More than Once
  13. Laterality
  14. Documentation for BMI, Depth of Non-pressure ulcers, Pressure Ulcer Stages, Coma Scale, and NIH Stroke Scale
  15. Syndromes
  16. Documentation of Complications of Care
  17. Borderline Diagnosis
  18. Use of Sign/Symptom/Unspecified Codes
C. Chapter-Specific Coding Guidelines
  1. Chapter 1: Certain Infectious and Parasitic Diseases (A00-B99)
    a. Human Immunodeficiency Virus (HIV) Infections
    b. Infectious agents as the cause of diseases classified to other chapters
    c. Infections resistant to antibiotics
    d. Sepsis, Severe Sepsis, and Septic Shock
    e. Methicillin Resistant *Staphylococcus aureus* (MRSA) Conditions
    f. Zika virus infection
  2. Chapter 2: Neoplasms (C00-D49)
    a. Treatment directed at the malignancy
    b. Treatment of secondary site
    c. Coding and sequencing of complications
    d. Primary malignancy previously excised
    e. Admissions/Encounters involving chemotherapy, immunotherapy and radiation therapy
    f. Admission/encounter to determine extent of malignancy
    g. Symptoms, signs, and abnormal findings listed in Chapter 18 associated with neoplasms
    h. Admission/encounter for pain control/management
    i. Malignancy in two or more noncontiguous sites
    j. Disseminated malignant neoplasm, unspecified
    k. Malignant neoplasm without specification of site
    l. Sequencing of neoplasm codes
    m. Current malignancy versus personal history of malignancy
    n. Leukemia, Multiple Myeloma, and Malignant Plasma Cell Neoplasms in remission versus personal history
    o. Aftercare following surgery for neoplasm
    p. Follow-up care for completed treatment of a malignancy
    q. Prophylactic organ removal for prevention of malignancy
    r. Malignant neoplasm associated with transplanted organ
  3. Chapter 3: Disease of the blood and blood-forming organs and certain disorders involving the immune mechanism (D50-D89)
  4. Chapter 4: Endocrine, Nutritional, and Metabolic Diseases (E00-E89)
    a. Diabetes mellitus
  5. Chapter 5: Mental, Behavioral and Neurodevelopmental disorders (F01 – F99)
    a. Pain disorders related to psychological factors
    b. Mental and behavioral disorders due to psychoactive substance use
  6. Chapter 6: Diseases of the Nervous System (G00-G99)
    a. Dominant/nondominant side
    b. Pain - Category G89
  7. Chapter 7: Diseases of the Eye and Adnexa (H00-H59)
    a. Glaucoma
    b. Blindness
  8. Chapter 8: Diseases of the Ear and Mastoid Process (H60-H95)
  9. Chapter 9: Diseases of the Circulatory System (I00-I99)
    a. Hypertension
    b. Atherosclerotic Coronary Artery Disease and Angina
    c. Intraoperative and Postprocedural Cerebrovascular Accident
    d. Sequelae of Cerebrovascular Disease
    e. Acute myocardial infarction (AMI)

10. Chapter 10: Diseases of the Respiratory System (J00-J99)
    a. Chronic Obstructive Pulmonary Disease [COPD] and Asthma
    b. Acute Respiratory Failure
    c. Influenza due to certain identified influenza viruses
    d. Ventilator associated Pneumonia
11. Chapter 11: Diseases of the Digestive System (K00-K95)
12. Chapter 12: Diseases of the Skin and Subcutaneous Tissue (L00-L99)
    a. Pressure ulcer stage codes
    b. Non-Pressure Chronic Ulcers
13. Chapter 13: Diseases of the Musculoskeletal System and Connective Tissue (M00-M99)
    a. Site and laterality
    b. Acute traumatic versus chronic or recurrent musculoskeletal conditions
    c. Coding of Pathologic Fractures
    d. Osteoporosis
14. Chapter 14: Diseases of Genitourinary System (N00-N99)
    a. Chronic kidney disease
15. Chapter 15: Pregnancy, Childbirth, and the Puerperium (O00-O9A)
    a. General Rules for Obstetric Cases
    b. Selection of OB Principal or First-listed Diagnosis
    c. Pre-existing conditions versus conditions due to the pregnancy
    d. Pre-existing hypertension in pregnancy
    e. Fetal Conditions Affecting the Management of the Mother
    f. HIV Infection in Pregnancy, Childbirth and the Puerperium
    g. Diabetes mellitus in pregnancy
    h. Long term use of insulin and oral hypoglycemics
    i. Gestational (pregnancy induced) diabetes
    j. Sepsis and septic shock complicating abortion, pregnancy, childbirth and the puerperium
    k. Puerperal sepsis
    l. Alcohol and tobacco use during pregnancy, childbirth and the puerperium
    m. Poisoning, toxic effects, adverse effects and underdosing in a pregnant patient
    n. Normal Delivery, Code O80
    o. The Peripartum and Postpartum Periods
    p. Code O94, Sequelae of complication of pregnancy, childbirth, and the puerperium
    q. Termination of Pregnancy and Spontaneous abortions
    r. Abuse in a pregnant patient
16. Chapter 16: Certain Conditions Originating in the Perinatal Period (P00-P96)
    a. General Perinatal Rules
    b. Observation and Evaluation of Newborns for Suspected Conditions not Found
    c. Coding Additional Perinatal Diagnoses
    d. Prematurity and Fetal Growth Retardation
    e. Low birth weight and immaturity status
    f. Bacterial Sepsis of Newborn
    g. Stillbirth

17. Chapter 17: Congenital malformations, deformations, and chromosomal abnormalities (Q00-Q99)
18. Chapter 18: Symptoms, signs, and abnormal clinical and laboratory findings, not elsewhere classified (R00-R99)
    a. Use of symptom codes
    b. Use of a symptom code with a definitive diagnosis code
    c. Combination codes that include symptoms
    d. Repeated falls
    e. Coma scale
    f. Functional quadriplegia
    g. SIRS due to Non-Infectious Process
    h. Death NOS
    i. NIHSS Stroke Scale
19. Chapter 19: Injury, poisoning, and certain other consequences of external causes (S00-T88)
    a. Application of 7th Characters in Chapter 19
    b. Coding of Injuries
    c. Coding of Traumatic Fractures
    d. Coding of Burns and Corrosions
    e. Adverse Effects, Poisoning, Underdosing and Toxic Effects
    f. Adult and child abuse, neglect and other maltreatment
    g. Complications of care
20. Chapter 20: External Causes of Morbidity (V00-Y99)
    a. General External Cause Coding Guidelines
    b. Place of Occurrence Guideline
    c. Activity Code
    d. Place of Occurrence, Activity, and Status Codes Used with other External Cause Code
    e. If the Reporting Format Limits the Number of External Cause Codes
    f. Multiple External Cause Coding Guidelines
    g. Child and Adult Abuse Guideline
    h. Unknown or Undetermined Intent Guideline
    i. Sequelae (Late Effects) of External Cause Guidelines
    j. Terrorism Guidelines
    k. External cause status
21. Chapter 21: Factors influencing health status and contact with health services (Z00-Z99)
    a. Use of Z codes in any healthcare setting
    b. Z Codes indicate a reason for an encounter
    c. Categories of Z Codes

Section II. Selection of Principal Diagnosis

A. Codes for symptoms, signs, and ill-defined conditions
B. Two or more interrelated conditions, each potentially meeting the definition for principal diagnosis
C. Two or more diagnoses that equally meet the definition for principal diagnosis
D. Two or more comparative or contrasting conditions
E. A symptom(s) followed by contrasting/comparative diagnoses
F. Original treatment plan not carried out
G. Complications of surgery and other medical care
H. Uncertain Diagnosis

GUIDELINES (ICD-10-CM)

I. Admission from Observation Unit
    1. Admission Following Medical Observation
    2. Admission Following Post-Operative Observation
J. Admission from Outpatient Surgery
K. Admissions/Encounters for Rehabilitation

Section III. Reporting Additional Diagnoses

A. Previous conditions
B. Abnormal findings
C. Uncertain Diagnosis

Section IV. Diagnostic Coding and Reporting Guidelines for Outpatient Services

A. Selection of first-listed condition
    1. Outpatient Surgery
    2. Observation Stay
B. Codes from A00.0 through T88.9, Z00-Z99
C. Accurate reporting of ICD-10-CM diagnosis codes
D. Codes that describe symptoms and signs
E. Encounters for circumstances other than a disease or injury
F. Level of Detail in Coding
    1. ICD-10-CM codes with 3, 4, 5, 6, or 7 characters
    2. Use of full number of characters required for a code
G. ICD-10-CM code for the diagnosis, condition, problem, or other reason for encounter/visit
H. Uncertain diagnosis
I. Chronic diseases
J. Code all documented conditions that coexist
K. Patients receiving diagnostic services only
L. Patients receiving therapeutic services only
M. Patients receiving preoperative evaluations only
N. Ambulatory surgery
O. Routine outpatient prenatal visits
P. Encounters for general medical examinations with abnormal findings
Q. Encounters for routine health screenings

Appendix I: Present on Admission Reporting Guidelines

Section I. Conventions, general coding guidelines and chapter specific guidelines

The conventions, general guidelines and chapter-specific guidelines are applicable to all health care settings unless otherwise indicated. The conventions and instructions of the classification take precedence over guidelines.

A. **Conventions for the ICD-10-CM**
The conventions for the ICD-10-CM are the general rules for use of the classification independent of the guidelines. These conventions are incorporated within the Alphabetic Index and Tabular List of the ICD-10-CM as instructional notes.

  1. **The Alphabetic Index and Tabular List**
The ICD-10-CM is divided into the Alphabetic Index, an alphabetical list of terms and their corresponding code, and the Tabular List, a structured list of codes divided into chapters based on body system or condition. The Alphabetic Index consists of the following parts: the Index of Diseases and Injury, the Index of External Causes of Injury, the Table of Neoplasms and the Table of Drugs and Chemicals.
    See Section I.C2. General guidelines
    See Section I.C.19. Adverse effects, poisoning, underdosing and toxic effects

  2. **Format and Structure:**
The ICD-10-CM Tabular List contains categories, subcategories and codes. Characters for categories, subcategories and codes may be either a letter or a number. All categories are 3 characters. A three-character category that has no further subdivision is equivalent to a code. Subcategories are either 4 or 5 characters. Codes may be 3, 4, 5, 6 or 7 characters. That is, each level of subdivision after a category is a subcategory. The final level of subdivision is a code. Codes that have applicable 7th characters are still referred to as codes, not subcategories. A code that has an applicable 7th character is considered invalid without the 7th character.
The ICD-10-CM uses an indented format for ease in reference

  3. **Use of codes for reporting purposes**
For reporting purposes only codes are permissible, not categories or subcategories, and any applicable 7th character is required.

  4. **Placeholder character**
The ICD-10-CM utilizes a placeholder character "X". The "X" is used as a placeholder at certain codes to allow for future expansion. An example of this is at the poisoning, adverse effect and underdosing codes, categories T36-T50. Where a placeholder exists, the X must be used in order for the code to be considered a valid code.

  5. **7th Characters**
Certain ICD-10-CM categories have applicable 7th characters. The applicable 7th character is required for all codes within the category, or as the notes in the Tabular List instruct. The 7th character must always be the 7th character in the data field. If a code that requires a 7th character is not 6 characters, a placeholder X must be used to fill in the empty characters.

  6. **Abbreviations**
    a. **Alphabetic Index abbreviations**
    NEC "Not elsewhere classifiable"
      This abbreviation in the Alphabetic Index represents "other specified". When a specific code is not available for a condition the Alphabetic Index directs the coder to the "other specified" code in the Tabular List.
    NOS "Not otherwise specified"
      This abbreviation is the equivalent of unspecified.

b. **Tabular List abbreviations**

NEC "Not elsewhere classifiable"
This abbreviation in the Tabular List represents "other specified". When a specific code is not available for a condition, the Tabular List includes an NEC entry under a code to identify the code as the "other specified" code.

NOS "Not otherwise specified"
This abbreviation is the equivalent of unspecified.

7. **Punctuation**

[ ] Brackets are used in the Tabular List to enclose synonyms, alternative wording or explanatory phrases. Brackets are used in the Alphabetic Index to identify manifestation codes.

( ) Parentheses are used in both the Alphabetic Index and Tabular List to enclose supplementary words that may be present or absent in the statement of a disease or procedure without affecting the code number to which it is assigned. The terms within the parentheses are referred to as nonessential modifiers. The nonessential modifiers in the Alphabetic Index to Diseases apply to subterms following a main term except when a nonessential modifier and a subentry are mutually exclusive, the subentry takes precedence. For example, in the ICD-10-CM Alphabetic Index under the main term Enteritis, "acute" is a nonessential modifier and "chronic" is a subentry. In this case, the nonessential modifier "acute" does not apply to the subentry "chronic".

: Colons are used in the Tabular List after an incomplete term which needs one or more of the modifiers following the colon to make it assignable to a given category.

8. **Use of "and".**
See Section I.A.14. Use of the term "And"

9. **Other and Unspecified codes**

a. **"Other" codes**
Codes titled "other" or "other specified" are for use when the information in the medical record provides detail for which a specific code does not exist. Alphabetic Index entries with NEC in the line designate "other" codes in the Tabular List. These Alphabetic Index entries represent specific disease entities for which no specific code exists so the term is included within an "other" code.

b. **"Unspecified" codes**
Codes titled "unspecified" are for use when the information in the medical record is insufficient to assign a more specific code. For those categories for which an unspecified code is not provided, the "other specified" code may represent both other and unspecified.
See Section I.B.18 Use of Signs/Symptom/Unspecified Codes

10. **Includes Notes**
This note appears immediately under a three-character code title to further define, or give examples of, the content of the category.

11. **Inclusion terms**
List of terms is included under some codes. These terms are the conditions for which that code is to be used. The terms may be synonyms of the code title, or, in the case of "other specified" codes, the terms are a list of the various conditions assigned to that code. The inclusion terms are not necessarily exhaustive. Additional terms found only in the Alphabetic Index may also be assigned to a code.

12. **Excludes Notes**
The ICD-10-CM has two types of excludes notes. Each type of note has a different definition for use but they are all similar in that they indicate that codes excluded from each other are independent of each other.

a. **Excludes1**
A type 1 Excludes note is a pure excludes note. It means "NOT CODED HERE!" An Excludes1 note indicates that the code excluded should never be used at the same time as the code above the Excludes1 note. An Excludes1 is used when two conditions cannot occur together, such as a congenital form versus an acquired form of the same condition.

An exception to the Excludes1 definition is the circumstance when the two conditions are unrelated to each other. If it is not clear whether the two conditions involving an Excludes1 note are related or not, query the provider. For example, code F45.8, Other somatoform disorders, has an Excludes1 note for "sleep related teeth grinding (G47.63)," because "teeth grinding" is an inclusion term under F45.8. Only one of these two codes should be assigned for teeth grinding. However psychogenic dysmenorrhea is also an inclusion term under F45.8, and a patient could have both this condition and sleep related teeth grinding. In this case, the two conditions are clearly unrelated to each other, and so it would be appropriate to report F45.8 and G47.63 together.

b. **Excludes2**
A Type 2 Excludes note represents "Not included here." An excludes2 note indicates that the condition excluded is not part of the condition represented by the code, but a patient may have both conditions at the same time. When an Excludes2 note appears under a code, it is acceptable to use both the code and the excluded code together, when appropriate.

13. **Etiology/manifestation convention ("code first", "use additional code" and "in diseases classified elsewhere" notes)**
Certain conditions have both an underlying etiology and multiple body system manifestations

due to the underlying etiology. For such conditions, the ICD-10-CM has a coding convention that requires the underlying condition be sequenced first, if applicable, followed by the manifestation. Wherever such a combination exists, there is a "use additional code" note at the etiology code, and a "code first" note at the manifestation code. These instructional notes indicate the proper sequencing order of the codes, etiology followed by manifestation.

In most cases the manifestation codes will have in the code title, "in diseases classified elsewhere." Codes with this title are a component of the etiology/ manifestation convention. The code title indicates that it is a manifestation code. "In diseases classified elsewhere" codes are never permitted to be used as first-listed or principal diagnosis codes. They must be used in conjunction with an underlying condition code and they must be listed following the underlying condition. See category F02, Dementia in other diseases classified elsewhere, for an example of this convention.

There are manifestation codes that do not have "in diseases classified elsewhere" in the title. For such codes, there is a "use additional code" note at the etiology code and a "code first" note at the manifestation code and the rules for sequencing apply.

In addition to the notes in the Tabular List, these conditions also have a specific Alphabetic Index entry structure. In the Alphabetic Index both conditions are listed together with the etiology code first followed by the manifestation codes in brackets. The code in brackets is always to be sequenced second.

An example of the etiology/manifestation convention is dementia in Parkinson's disease. In the Alphabetic Index, code G20 is listed first, followed by code F02.80 or F02.81 in brackets. Code G20 represents the underlying etiology, Parkinson's disease, and must be sequenced first, whereas code F02.80 and F02.81 represent the manifestation of dementia in diseases classified elsewhere, with or without behavioral disturbance.

"Code first" and "Use additional code" notes are also used as sequencing rules in the classification for certain codes that are not part of an etiology/manifestation combination.

See Section I.B.7. Multiple coding for a single condition.

14. "And"
The word "and" should be interpreted to mean either "and" or "or" when it appears in a title.

For example, cases of "tuberculosis of bones", "tuberculosis of joints" and "tuberculosis of bones and joints" are classified to subcategory A18.0, Tuberculosis of bones and joints.

15. "With"
The word "with" **or "in"** should be interpreted to mean "associated with" or "due to" when it appears in a code title, the Alphabetic Index, or an instructional note in the Tabular List. The classification presumes a causal relationship

between the two conditions linked by these terms in the Alphabetic Index or Tabular List. These conditions should be coded as related even in the absence of provider documentation explicitly linking them, unless the documentation clearly states the conditions are unrelated **or when another guideline exists that specifically requires a documented linkage between two conditions (e.g., sepsis guideline for "acute organ dysfunction that is not clearly associated with the sepsis").**

For conditions not specifically linked by these relational terms in the classification **or when a guideline requires that a linkage between two conditions be explicitly documented** provider documentation must link the conditions in order to code them as related.

The word "with" in the Alphabetic Index is sequenced immediately following the main term, not in alphabetical order.

16. "See" and "See Also"
The "see" instruction following a main term in the Alphabetic Index indicates that another term should be referenced. It is necessary to go to the main term referenced with the "see" note to locate the correct code.

A "see also" instruction following a main term in the Alphabetic Index instructs that there is another main term that may also be referenced that may provide additional Alphabetic Index entries that may be useful. It is not necessary to follow the "see also" note when the original main term provides the necessary code.

17. "Code also" note
A "code also" note instructs that two codes may be required to fully describe a condition, but this note does not provide sequencing direction. **The sequencing depends on the circumstances of the encounter.**

18. Default codes
A code listed next to a main term in the ICD-10-CM Alphabetic Index is referred to as a default code. The default code represents that condition that is most commonly associated with the main term, or is the unspecified code for the condition. If a condition is documented in a medical record (for example, appendicitis) without any additional information, such as acute or chronic, the default code should be assigned.

19. Code assignment and Clinical Criteria
The assignment of a diagnosis code is based on the provider's diagnostic statement that the condition exists. The provider's statement that the patient has a particular condition is sufficient. Code assignment is not based on clinical criteria used by the provider to establish the diagnosis.

B. General Coding Guidelines

1. Locating a code in the ICD-10-CM
To select a code in the classification that corresponds to a diagnosis or reason for visit documented in a medical record, first locate the

term in the Alphabetic Index, and then verify the code in the Tabular List. Read and be guided by instructional notations that appear in both the Alphabetic Index and the Tabular List.

It is essential to use both the Alphabetic Index and Tabular List when locating and assigning a code. The Alphabetic Index does not always provide the full code. Selection of the full code, including laterality and any applicable 7th character can only be done in the Tabular List. A dash (-) at the end of an Alphabetic Index entry indicates that additional characters are required. Even if a dash is not included at the Alphabetic Index entry, it is necessary to refer to the Tabular List to verify that no 7th character is required.

2. **Level of Detail in Coding**
   Diagnosis codes are to be used and reported at their highest number of characters available.

   ICD-10-CM diagnosis codes are composed of codes with 3, 4, 5, 6 or 7 characters. Codes with three characters are included in ICD-10-CM as the heading of a category of codes that may be further subdivided by the use of fourth and/or fifth characters and/or sixth characters, which provide greater detail.

   A three-character code is to be used only if it is not further subdivided. A code is invalid if it has not been coded to the full number of characters required for that code, including the 7th character, if applicable.

3. **Code or codes from A00.0 through T88.9, Z00-Z99.8**
   The appropriate code or codes from A00.0 through T88.9, Z00-Z99.8 must be used to identify diagnoses, symptoms, conditions, problems, complaints or other reason(s) for the encounter/visit.

4. **Signs and symptoms**
   Codes that describe symptoms and signs, as opposed to diagnoses, are acceptable for reporting purposes when a related definitive diagnosis has not been established (confirmed) by the provider. Chapter 18 of ICD-10-CM, Symptoms, Signs, and Abnormal Clinical and Laboratory Findings, Not Elsewhere Classified (codes R00.0 - R99) contains many, but not all codes for symptoms.
   See Section I.B.18 Use of Signs/Symptom/ Unspecified Codes

5. **Conditions that are an integral part of a disease process**
   Signs and symptoms that are associated routinely with a disease process should not be assigned as additional codes, unless otherwise instructed by the classification.

6. **Conditions that are not an integral part of a disease process**
   Additional signs and symptoms that may not be associated routinely with a disease process should be coded when present.

7. **Multiple coding for a single condition**
   In addition to the etiology/manifestation convention that requires two codes to fully describe a single condition that affects multiple body systems, there are other single conditions that also require more than one code. "Use additional code" notes are found in the Tabular List at codes that are not part of an etiology/manifestation pair where a secondary code is useful to fully describe a condition. The sequencing rule is the same as the etiology/manifestation pair, "use additional code" indicates that a secondary code should be added, **if known.**

   For example, for bacterial infections that are not included in chapter 1, a secondary code from category B95, Streptococcus, Staphylococcus, and Enterococcus, as the cause of diseases classified elsewhere, or B96, Other bacterial agents as the cause of diseases classified elsewhere, may be required to identify the bacterial organism causing the infection. A "use additional code" note will normally be found at the infectious disease code, indicating a need for the organism code to be added as a secondary code.

   "Code first" notes are also under certain codes that are not specifically manifestation codes but may be due to an underlying cause. When there is a "code first" note and an underlying condition is present, the underlying condition should be sequenced first, **if known.**

   "Code, if applicable, any causal condition first," notes indicate that this code may be assigned as a principal diagnosis when the causal condition is unknown or not applicable. If a causal condition is known, then the code for that condition should be sequenced as the principal or first-listed diagnosis.

   Multiple codes may be needed for sequela, complication codes and obstetric codes to more fully describe a condition. See the specific guidelines for these conditions for further instruction.

8. **Acute and Chronic Conditions**
   If the same condition is described as both acute (subacute) and chronic, and separate subentries exist in the Alphabetic Index at the same indentation level, code both and sequence the acute (subacute) code first.

9. **Combination Code**
   A combination code is a single code used to classify:
   Two diagnoses, or
   A diagnosis with an associated secondary process (manifestation)
   A diagnosis with an associated complication
   Combination codes are identified by referring to subterm entries in the Alphabetic Index and by reading the inclusion and exclusion notes in the Tabular List.

   Assign only the combination code when that code fully identifies the diagnostic conditions involved or when the Alphabetic Index so directs. Multiple coding should not be used when the classification provides a combination code that clearly identifies all of the elements documented in the diagnosis. When the combination code lacks necessary specificity in describing the manifestation or complication, an additional code should be used as a secondary code.

10. Sequela (Late Effects)

A sequela is the residual effect (condition produced) after the acute phase of an illness or injury has terminated. There is no time limit on when a sequela code can be used. The residual may be apparent early, such as in cerebral infarction, or it may occur months or years later, such as that due to a previous injury. Examples of sequela include: scar formation resulting from a burn, deviated septum due to a nasal fracture, and infertility due to tubal occlusion from old tuberculosis. Coding of sequela generally requires two codes sequenced in the following order: the condition or nature of the sequela is sequenced first. The sequela code is sequenced second.

An exception to the above guidelines are those instances where the code for the sequela is followed by a manifestation code identified in the Tabular List and title, or the sequela code has been expanded (at the fourth, fifth or sixth character levels) to include the manifestation(s). The code for the acute phase of an illness or injury that led to the sequela is never used with a code for the late effect.

See Section I.C.9. Sequelae of cerebrovascular disease
See Section I.C.15. Sequelae of complication of pregnancy, childbirth and the puerperium
See Section I.C.19. Application of 7th characters for Chapter 19

11. Impending or Threatened Condition

Code any condition described at the time of discharge as "impending" or "threatened" as follows:

If it did occur, code as confirmed diagnosis.

If it did not occur, reference the Alphabetic Index to determine if the condition has a subentry term for "impending" or "threatened" and also reference main term entries for "Impending" and for "Threatened."

If the subterms are listed, assign the given code.

If the subterms are not listed, code the existing underlying condition(s) and not the condition described as impending or threatened.

12. Reporting Same Diagnosis Code More than Once

Each unique ICD-10-CM diagnosis code may be reported only once for an encounter. This applies to bilateral conditions when there are no distinct codes identifying laterality or two different conditions classified to the same ICD-10-CM diagnosis code.

13. Laterality

Some ICD-10-CM codes indicate laterality, specifying whether the condition occurs on the left, right or is bilateral. If no bilateral code is provided and the condition is bilateral, assign separate codes for both the left and right side. If the side is not identified in the medical record, assign the code for the unspecified side.

When a patient has a bilateral condition and each side is treated during separate encounters, assign the "bilateral" code (as the condition still exists on both sides), including for the encounter to treat the first side. For the second encounter for treatment after one side has previously been treated and the condition no longer exists on that side, assign the appropriate unilateral code for the side where the condition still exists (e.g., cataract surgery performed on each eye in separate encounters). The bilateral code would not be assigned for the subsequent encounter, as the patient no longer has the condition in the previously-treated site. If the treatment on the first side did not completely resolve the condition, then the bilateral code would still be appropriate.

14. Documentation for BMI, Depth of Non-pressure ulcers, Pressure Ulcer Stages, Coma Scale, and NIH Stroke Scale

For the Body Mass Index (BMI), depth of non-pressure chronic ulcers, pressure ulcer stage, coma scale, and NIH stroke scale (NIHSS) codes, code assignment may be based on medical record documentation from clinicians who are not the patient's provider (i.e., physician or other qualified healthcare practitioner legally accountable for establishing the patient's diagnosis), since this information is typically documented by other clinicians involved in the care of the patient (e.g., a dietitian often documents the BMI, a nurse often documents the pressure ulcer stages, and an emergency medical technician often documents the coma scale). However, the associated diagnosis (such as overweight, obesity, acute stroke, or pressure ulcer) must be documented by the patient's provider. If there is conflicting medical record documentation, either from the same clinician or different clinicians, the patient's attending provider should be queried for clarification.

The BMI, coma scale, and NIHSS codes should only be reported as secondary diagnoses.

15. Syndromes

Follow the Alphabetic Index guidance when coding syndromes. In the absence of Alphabetic Index guidance, assign codes for the documented manifestations of the syndrome. Additional codes for manifestations that are not an integral part of the disease process may also be assigned when the condition does not have a unique code.

16. Documentation of Complications of Care

Code assignment is based on the provider's documentation of the relationship between the condition and the care or procedure, unless otherwise instructed by the classification. The guideline extends to any complications of care, regardless of the chapter the code is located in. It is important to note that not all conditions that occur during or following medical care or surgery are classified as complications. There must be a cause-and-effect relationship between the care provided and the condition, and an indication in the documentation that it is a complication. Query the provider for clarification, if the complication is not clearly documented.

17. Borderline Diagnosis

If the provider documents a "borderline" diagnosis at the time of discharge, the diagnosis is coded as confirmed, unless the classification provides a specific entry (e.g., borderline diabetes). If a borderline condition has a specific index entry in ICD-10-CM, it should be coded as such. Since borderline conditions are not uncertain diagnoses, no distinction is made between the care setting (inpatient versus outpatient). Whenever the documentation is unclear regarding a borderline condition, coders are encouraged to query for clarification.

18. **Use of Sign/Symptom/Unspecified Codes**
Sign/symptom and "unspecified" codes have acceptable, even necessary, uses. While specific diagnosis codes should be reported when they are supported by the available medical record documentation and clinical knowledge of the patient's health condition, there are instances when signs/symptoms or unspecified codes are the best choices for accurately reflecting the healthcare encounter. Each healthcare encounter should be coded to the level of certainty known for that encounter.

If a definitive diagnosis has not been established by the end of the encounter, it is appropriate to report codes for sign(s) and/or symptom(s) in lieu of a definitive diagnosis. When sufficient clinical information isn't known or available about a particular health condition to assign a more specific code, it is acceptable to report the appropriate "unspecified" code (e.g., a diagnosis of pneumonia has been determined, but not the specific type). Unspecified codes should be reported when they are the codes that most accurately reflect what is known about the patient's condition at the time of that particular encounter. It would be inappropriate to select a specific code that is not supported by the medical record documentation or conduct medically unnecessary diagnostic testing in order to determine a more specific code.

C. **Chapter-Specific Coding Guidelines**
In addition to general coding guidelines, there are guidelines for specific diagnoses and/or conditions in the classification. Unless otherwise indicated, these guidelines apply to all health care settings. Please refer to Section II for guidelines on the selection of principal diagnosis.

1. **Chapter 1: Certain Infectious and Parasitic Diseases (A00-B99)**

   a. **Human Immunodeficiency Virus (HIV) Infections**

   1) **Code only confirmed cases**
   Code only confirmed cases of HIV infection/illness. This is an exception to the hospital inpatient guideline Section II, H.

   In this context, "confirmation" does not require documentation of positive serology or culture for HIV; the provider's diagnostic statement that the patient is HIV positive, or has an HIV-related illness is sufficient.

2) **Selection and sequencing of HIV codes**

   (a) **Patient admitted for HIV-related condition**
   If a patient is admitted for an HIV-related condition, the principal diagnosis should be B20, Human immunodeficiency virus [HIV] disease followed by additional diagnosis codes for all reported HIV-related conditions.

   (b) **Patient with HIV disease admitted for unrelated condition**
   If a patient with HIV disease is admitted for an unrelated condition (such as a traumatic injury), the code for the unrelated condition (e.g., the nature of injury code) should be the principal diagnosis. Other diagnoses would be B20 followed by additional diagnosis codes for all reported HIV-related conditions.

   (c) **Whether the patient is newly diagnosed**
   Whether the patient is newly diagnosed or has had previous admissions/encounters for HIV conditions is irrelevant to the sequencing decision.

   (d) **Asymptomatic human immunodeficiency virus**
   Z21, Asymptomatic human immunodeficiency virus [HIV] infection status, is to be applied when the patient without any documentation of symptoms is listed as being "HIV positive," "known HIV," "HIV test positive," or similar terminology. Do not use this code if the term "AIDS" is used or if the patient is treated for any HIV-related illness or is described as having any condition(s) resulting from his/her HIV positive status; use B20 in these cases.

   (e) **Patients with inconclusive HIV serology**
   Patients with inconclusive HIV serology, but no definitive diagnosis or manifestations of the illness, may be assigned code R75, Inconclusive laboratory evidence of human immunodeficiency virus [HIV].

   (f) **Previously diagnosed HIV-related illness**
   Patients with any known prior diagnosis of an HIV-related illness should be coded to B20. Once a patient has developed an HIV-related illness, the patient should always be assigned code B20 on every subsequent admission/encounter. Patients previously diagnosed with any HIV illness (B20) should never be assigned to R75 or Z21, Asymptomatic human immunodeficiency virus [HIV] infection status.

   (g) **HIV Infection in Pregnancy, Childbirth and the Puerperium**
   During pregnancy, childbirth or the puerperium, a patient admitted (or presenting for a health care encounter) because of an HIV-related illness should receive a principal diagnosis code of O98.7-, Human immunodeficiency [HIV] disease complicating pregnancy, childbirth and the puerperium, followed by B20 and the code(s) for the HIV-related illness(es). Codes from Chapter 15 always take sequencing priority.

Patients with asymptomatic HIV infection status admitted (or presenting for a health care encounter) during pregnancy, childbirth, or the puerperium should receive codes of O98.7- and Z21.

(h) Encounters for testing for HIV

If a patient is being seen to determine his/her HIV status, use code Z11.4, Encounter for screening for human immunodeficiency virus [HIV]. Use additional codes for any associated high risk behavior.

If a patient with signs or symptoms is being seen for HIV testing, code the signs and symptoms. An additional counseling code Z71.7, Human immunodeficiency virus [HIV] counseling, may be used if counseling is provided during the encounter for the test.

When a patient returns to be informed of his/her HIV test results and the test result is negative, use code Z71.7, Human immunodeficiency virus [HIV] counseling.

If the results are positive, see previous guidelines and assign codes as appropriate.

b. Infectious agents as the cause of diseases classified to other chapters

Certain infections are classified in chapters other than Chapter 1 and no organism is identified as part of the infection code. In these instances, it is necessary to use an additional code from Chapter 1 to identify the organism. A code from category B95, Streptococcus, Staphylococcus, and Enterococcus as the cause of diseases classified to other chapters, B96, Other bacterial agents as the cause of diseases classified to other chapters, or B97, Viral agents as the cause of diseases classified to other chapters, is to be used as an additional code to identify the organism. An instructional note will be found at the infection code advising that an additional organism code is required.

c. Infections resistant to antibiotics

Many bacterial infections are resistant to current antibiotics. It is necessary to identify all infections documented as antibiotic resistant. Assign a code from category Z16, Resistance to antimicrobial drugs, following the infection code only if the infection code does not identify drug resistance.

d. Sepsis, Severe Sepsis, and Septic Shock

1) Coding of Sepsis and Severe Sepsis

(a) Sepsis

For a diagnosis of sepsis, assign the appropriate code for the underlying systemic infection. If the type of infection or causal organism is not further specified, assign code A41.9, Sepsis, unspecified organism.

A code from subcategory R65.2, Severe sepsis, should not be assigned unless severe sepsis or an associated acute organ dysfunction is documented.

(i) Negative or inconclusive blood cultures and sepsis
Negative or inconclusive blood cultures do not preclude a diagnosis of sepsis in patients with clinical evidence of the condition, however, the provider should be queried.

(ii) Urosepsis
The term urosepsis is a nonspecific term. It is not to be considered synonymous with sepsis. It has no default code in the Alphabetic Index. Should a provider use this term, he/she must be queried for clarification.

(iii) Sepsis with organ dysfunction
If a patient has sepsis and associated acute organ dysfunction or multiple organ dysfunction (MOD), follow the instructions for coding severe sepsis.

(iv) Acute organ dysfunction that is not clearly associated with the sepsis
If a patient has sepsis and an acute organ dysfunction, but the medical record documentation indicates that the acute organ dysfunction is related to a medical condition other than the sepsis, do not assign a code from subcategory R65.2, Severe sepsis. An acute organ dysfunction must be associated with the sepsis in order to assign the severe sepsis code. If the documentation is not clear as to whether an acute organ dysfunction is related to the sepsis or another medical condition, query the provider.

(b) Severe sepsis

The coding of severe sepsis requires a minimum of 2 codes: first a code for the underlying systemic infection, followed by a code from subcategory R65.2, Severe sepsis. If the causal organism is not documented, assign code A41.9, Sepsis, unspecified organism, for the infection. Additional code(s) for the associated acute organ dysfunction are also required.

Due to the complex nature of severe sepsis, some cases may require querying the provider prior to assignment of the codes.

2) Septic shock

(a) Septic shock generally refers to circulatory failure associated with severe sepsis, and therefore, it represents a type of acute organ dysfunction.

For all cases of septic shock, the code for the systemic infection should be sequenced first, followed by code R65.21, Severe sepsis with septic shock or code T81.12, Postprocedural septic shock. Any additional codes for the other acute organ dysfunctions should also be assigned. As noted in the sequencing instructions in the Tabular List, the code for septic shock cannot be assigned as a principal diagnosis.

3) Sequencing of severe sepsis

If severe sepsis is present on admission, and meets the definition of principal diagnosis, the underlying systemic infection should be assigned as principal diagnosis followed by the appropriate code from subcategory R65.2 as required by the sequencing rules in the Tabular List. A code from subcategory R65.2 can never be assigned as a principal diagnosis.

When severe sepsis develops during an encounter (it was not present on admission) the underlying systemic infection and the appropriate code from subcategory R65.2 should be assigned as secondary diagnoses.

Severe sepsis may be present on admission but the diagnosis may not be confirmed until sometime after admission. If the documentation is not clear whether severe sepsis was present on admission, the provider should be queried.

4) Sepsis and severe sepsis with a localized infection

If the reason for admission is both sepsis or severe sepsis and a localized infection, such as pneumonia or cellulitis, a code(s) for the underlying systemic infection should be assigned first and the code for the localized infection should be assigned as a secondary diagnosis. If the patient has severe sepsis, a code from subcategory R65.2 should also be assigned as a secondary diagnosis. If the patient is admitted with a localized infection, such as pneumonia, and sepsis/severe sepsis doesn't develop until after admission, the localized infection should be assigned first, followed by the appropriate sepsis/severe sepsis codes.

5) Sepsis due to a postprocedural infection

(a) Documentation of causal relationship

As with all postprocedural complications, code assignment is based on the provider's documentation of the relationship between the infection and the procedure.

(b) Sepsis due to a postprocedural infection

For such cases, the postprocedural infection code, such as, T80.2, Infections following infusion, transfusion, and therapeutic injection, T81.4, Infection following a procedure, T88.0, Infection following immunization, or O86.0, Infection of obstetric surgical wound, should be coded first, followed by the code for the specific infection. If the patient has severe sepsis the appropriate code from subcategory R65.2 should also be assigned with the additional code(s) for any acute organ dysfunction.

(c) Postprocedural infection and postprocedural septic shock

In cases where a postprocedural infection has occurred and has resulted in severe sepsis the code for the precipitating complication such as code T81.4, Infection following a procedure, or O86.0, Infection of obstetrical surgical wound should be coded first followed by code R65.20, Severe sepsis

without septic shock. A Code for the systemic infection should also be assigned.

If a postprocedural infection has resulted in postprocedural septic shock, the code for the precipitating complication such as code T81.4, Infection following a procedure, or O86.0, Infection of obstetrical surgical wound should be coded first followed by code T81.12-, Postprocedural septic shock. A code for the systemic infection should also be assigned.

6) Sepsis and severe sepsis associated with a noninfectious process (condition)

In some cases a noninfectious process (condition), such as trauma, may lead to an infection which can result in sepsis or severe sepsis. If sepsis or severe sepsis is documented as associated with a noninfectious condition, such as a burn or serious injury, and this condition meets the definition for principal diagnosis, the code for the noninfectious condition should be sequenced first, followed by the code for the resulting infection. If severe sepsis is present, a code from subcategory R65.2 should also be assigned with any associated organ dysfunction(s) codes. It is not necessary to assign a code from subcategory R65.1, Systemic inflammatory response syndrome (SIRS) of non-infectious origin, for these cases.

If the infection meets the definition of principal diagnosis it should be sequenced before the non-infectious condition. When both the associated non-infectious condition and the infection meet the definition of principal diagnosis either may be assigned as principal diagnosis.

Only one code from category R65, Symptoms and signs specifically associated with systemic inflammation and infection, should be assigned. Therefore, when a non-infectious condition leads to an infection resulting in severe sepsis, assign the appropriate code from subcategory R65.2, Severe sepsis. Do not additionally assign a code from subcategory R65.1, Systemic inflammatory response syndrome (SIRS) of non-infectious origin.

See Section I.C.18. SIRS due to non-infectious process

7) Sepsis and septic shock complicating abortion, pregnancy, childbirth, and the puerperium

See Section I.C.15. Sepsis and septic shock complicating abortion, pregnancy, childbirth and the puerperium

8) Newborn sepsis

See Section I.C.16. f. Bacterial sepsis of Newborn

e. Methicillin Resistant Staphylococcus aureus (MRSA) Conditions

1) Selection and sequencing of MRSA codes

(a) Combination codes for MRSA infection

When a patient is diagnosed with an infection that is due to methicillin resistant *Staphylococcus aureus* (MRSA), and that infection has a combination code that includes the causal organism (e.g., sepsis, pneumonia) assign the appropriate combination code for the condition (e.g., code A41.02, Sepsis due to Methicillin resistant Staphylococcus aureus or code J15.212, Pneumonia due to Methicillin resistant Staphylococcus aureus). Do not assign code B95.62, Methicillin resistant Staphylococcus aureus infection as the cause of diseases classified elsewhere, as an additional code because the combination code includes the type of infection and the MRSA organism. Do not assign a code from subcategory Z16.11, Resistance to penicillins, as an additional diagnosis.

See Section C.1. for instructions on coding and sequencing of sepsis and severe sepsis.

(b) Other codes for MRSA infection

When there is documentation of a current infection (e.g., wound infection, stitch abscess, urinary tract infection) due to MRSA, and that infection does not have a combination code that includes the causal organism, assign the appropriate code to identify the condition along with code B95.62, Methicillin resistant Staphylococcus aureus infection as the cause of diseases classified elsewhere for the MRSA infection. Do not assign a code from subcategory Z16.11, Resistance to penicillins.

(c) Methicillin susceptible Staphylococcus aureus (MSSA) and MRSA colonization

The condition or state of being colonized or carrying MSSA or MRSA is called colonization or carriage, while an individual person is described as being colonized or being a carrier. Colonization means that MSSA or MSRA is present on or in the body without necessarily causing illness. A positive MRSA colonization test might be documented by the provider as "MRSA screen positive" or "MRSA nasal swab positive".

Assign code Z22.322, Carrier or suspected carrier of Methicillin resistant Staphylococcus aureus, for patients documented as having MRSA colonization. Assign code Z22.321, Carrier or suspected carrier of Methicillin susceptible Staphylococcus aureus, for patient documented as having MSSA colonization. Colonization is not necessarily indicative of a disease process or as the cause of a specific condition the patient may have unless documented as such by the provider.

(d) MRSA colonization and infection

If a patient is documented as having both MRSA colonization and infection during a hospital admission, code Z22.322, Carrier or suspected carrier of Methicillin resistant Staphylococcus aureus, and a code for the MRSA infection may both be assigned.

f. Zika virus infections

1) Code only confirmed cases

Code only a confirmed diagnosis of Zika virus (A92.5, Zika virus disease) as documented by the provider. This is an exception to the hospital inpatient guideline Section II, H.

In this context, "confirmation" does not require documentation of the type of test performed; the physician's diagnostic statement that the condition is confirmed is sufficient. This code should be assigned regardless of the stated mode of transmission.

If the provider documents "suspected", "possible" or "probable" Zika, do not assign code A92.5. Assign a code(s) explaining the reason for encounter (such as fever, rash, or joint pain) or Z20.828, Contact with and (suspected) exposure to other viral communicable diseases.

2. Chapter 2: Neoplasms (C00-D49)
General guidelines

Chapter 2 of the ICD-10-CM contains the codes for most benign and all malignant neoplasms. Certain benign neoplasms, such as prostatic adenomas, may be found in the specific body system chapters. To properly code a neoplasm it is necessary to determine from the record if the neoplasm is benign, in-situ, malignant, or of uncertain histologic behavior. If malignant, any secondary (metastatic) sites should also be determined.

Primary malignant neoplasms overlapping site boundaries

A primary malignant neoplasm that overlaps two or more contiguous (next to each other) sites should be classified to the subcategory/ code .8 ('overlapping lesion'), unless the combination is specifically indexed elsewhere. For multiple neoplasms of the same site that are not contiguous such as tumors in different quadrants of the same breast, codes for each site should be assigned.

Malignant neoplasm of ectopic tissue

Malignant neoplasms of ectopic tissue are to be coded to the site of origin mentioned, e.g., ectopic pancreatic malignant neoplasms involving the stomach are coded to **malignant neoplasm of** pancreas, unspecified (C25.9).

The neoplasm table in the Alphabetic Index should be referenced first. However, if the histological term is documented, that term should be referenced first, rather than going immediately to the Neoplasm Table, in order to determine which column in the Neoplasm Table is appropriate. For example, if the documentation indicates "adenoma," refer to the term in the Alphabetic Index to review the entries under this term and the instructional note to "see also neoplasm, by site, benign." The table provides the proper code based on the type of neoplasm and the site. It is important to select the proper column in the table that corresponds to the type of neoplasm. The Tabular List should then be referenced to verify that the correct code has been selected from the table and that a more specific site code does not exist.

See Section I.C.21. Factors influencing health status and contact with health services, Status, for information regarding Z15.0, codes for genetic susceptibility to cancer.

a. Treatment directed at the malignancy

If the treatment is directed at the malignancy, designate the malignancy as the principal diagnosis.

The only exception to this guideline is if a patient admission/encounter is solely for the administration of chemotherapy, immunotherapy or **external beam** radiation therapy, assign the appropriate Z51.— code as the first-listed or principal diagnosis, and the diagnosis or problem for which the service is being performed as a secondary diagnosis.

b. Treatment of secondary site

When a patient is admitted because of a primary neoplasm with metastasis and treatment is directed toward the secondary site only, the secondary neoplasm is designated as the principal diagnosis even though the primary malignancy is still present.

c. Coding and sequencing of complications

Coding and sequencing of complications associated with the malignancies or with the therapy thereof are subject to the following guidelines:

1) Anemia associated with malignancy

When admission/encounter is for management of an anemia associated with the malignancy, and the treatment is only for anemia, the appropriate code for the malignancy is sequenced as the principal or first-listed diagnosis followed by the appropriate code for the anemia (such as code D63.∅, Anemia in neoplastic disease).

2) Anemia associated with chemotherapy, immunotherapy and radiation therapy

When the admission/encounter is for management of an anemia associated with an adverse effect of the administration of chemotherapy or immunotherapy and the only treatment is for the anemia, the anemia code is sequenced first followed by the appropriate codes for the neoplasm and the adverse effect (T45.1X5, Adverse effect of antineoplastic and immunosuppressive drugs).

When the admission/encounter is for management of an anemia associated with an adverse effect of radiotherapy, the anemia code should be sequenced first, followed by the appropriate neoplasm code and code Y84.2, Radiological procedure and radiotherapy as the cause of abnormal reaction of the patient, or of later complication, without mention of misadventure at the time of the procedure.

3) Management of dehydration due to the malignancy

When the admission/encounter is for management of dehydration due to the malignancy and only the dehydration is being treated (intravenous rehydration), the dehydration is sequenced first, followed by the code(s) for the malignancy.

4) Treatment of a complication resulting from a surgical procedure

When the admission/encounter is for treatment of a complication resulting from a surgical procedure, designate the complication as the principal or first-listed diagnosis if treatment is directed at resolving the complication.

d. Primary malignancy previously excised

When a primary malignancy has been previously excised or eradicated from its site and there is no further treatment directed to that site and there is no evidence of any existing primary malignancy, a code from category Z85, Personal history of malignant neoplasm, should be used to indicate the former site of the malignancy. Any mention of extension, invasion, or metastasis to another site is coded as a secondary malignant neoplasm to that site. The secondary site may be the principal or first-listed with the Z85 code used as a secondary code.

e. Admissions/Encounters involving chemotherapy, immunotherapy and radiation therapy

1) Episode of care involves surgical removal of neoplasm

When an episode of care involves the surgical removal of a neoplasm, primary or secondary site, followed by adjunct chemotherapy or radiation treatment during the same episode of care, the code for the neoplasm should be assigned as principal or first-listed diagnosis.

2) Patient admission/encounter solely for administration of chemotherapy, immunotherapy and radiation therapy

If a patient admission/encounter is solely for the administration of chemotherapy, immunotherapy or **external beam** radiation therapy assign code Z51.∅, Encounter for antineoplastic radiation therapy, or Z51.11, Encounter for antineoplastic chemotherapy, or Z51.12, Encounter for antineoplastic immunotherapy as the first-listed or principal diagnosis. If a patient receives more than one of these therapies during the same admission more than one of these codes may be assigned, in any sequence.

The malignancy for which the therapy is being administered should be assigned as a secondary diagnosis.

If a patient admission/encounter is for the insertion or implantation of radioactive elements (e.g., brachytherapy) the appropriate code for the malignancy is sequenced as the principal or first-listed diagnosis. Code Z51.∅ should not be assigned.

3) Patient admitted for radiation therapy, chemotherapy or immunotherapy and develops complications

When a patient is admitted for the purpose of **external beam** radiotherapy, immunotherapy or chemotherapy and develops complications such as uncontrolled nausea and vomiting or dehydration, the principal or first-listed diagnosis is Z51.∅, Encounter for antineoplastic radiation therapy, or Z51.11, Encounter for antineoplastic chemotherapy, or Z51.12, Encounter for antineoplastic immunotherapy followed by any codes for the complications.

When a patient is admitted for the purpose of insertion or implantation of radioactive elements (e.g., brachytherapy) and develops complications such as uncontrolled nausea and vomiting or dehydration, the principal or first-listed diagnosis is the appropriate code for the malignancy followed by any codes for the complications.

13

f. Admission/encounter to determine extent of malignancy

When the reason for admission/encounter is to determine the extent of the malignancy, or for a procedure such as paracentesis or thoracentesis, the primary malignancy or appropriate metastatic site is designated as the principal or first-listed diagnosis, even though chemotherapy or radiotherapy is administered.

g. Symptoms, signs, and abnormal findings listed in Chapter 18 associated with neoplasms

Symptoms, signs, and ill-defined conditions listed in Chapter 18 characteristic of, or associated with, an existing primary or secondary site malignancy cannot be used to replace the malignancy as principal or first-listed diagnosis, regardless of the number of admissions or encounters for treatment and care of the neoplasm.

See section I.C.21. Factors influencing health status and contact with health services, Encounter for prophylactic organ removal.

h. Admission/encounter for pain control/ management

See Section I.C.6. for information on coding admission/ encounter for pain control/management.

i. Malignancy in two or more noncontiguous sites

A patient may have more than one malignant tumor in the same organ. These tumors may represent different primaries or metastatic disease, depending on the site. Should the documentation be unclear, the provider should be queried as to the status of each tumor so that the correct codes can be assigned.

j. Disseminated malignant neoplasm, unspecified

Code C80.0, Disseminated malignant neoplasm, unspecified, is for use only in those cases where the patient has advanced metastatic disease and no known primary or secondary sites are specified. It should not be used in place of assigning codes for the primary site and all known secondary sites.

k. Malignant neoplasm without specification of site

Code C80.1, Malignant (primary) neoplasm, unspecified, equates to Cancer, unspecified. This code should only be used when no determination can be made as to the primary site of a malignancy. This code should rarely be used in the inpatient setting.

l. Sequencing of neoplasm codes

1) Encounter for treatment of primary malignancy

If the reason for the encounter is for treatment of a primary malignancy, assign the malignancy as the principal/first-listed diagnosis. The primary site is to be sequenced first, followed by any metastatic sites.

2) Encounter for treatment of secondary malignancy

When an encounter is for a primary malignancy with metastasis and treatment is directed toward the metastatic (secondary) site(s) only, the metastatic site(s) is designated as the principal/

first-listed diagnosis. The primary malignancy is coded as an additional code.

3) Malignant neoplasm in a pregnant patient

When a pregnant woman has a malignant neoplasm, a code from subcategory O9A.1-, Malignant neoplasm complicating pregnancy, childbirth, and the puerperium, should be sequenced first, followed by the appropriate code from Chapter 2 to indicate the type of neoplasm.

4) Encounter for complication associated with a neoplasm

When an encounter is for management of a complication associated with a neoplasm, such as dehydration, and the treatment is only for the complication, the complication is coded first, followed by the appropriate code(s) for the neoplasm.

The exception to this guideline is anemia. When the admission/encounter is for management of an anemia associated with the malignancy, and the treatment is only for anemia, the appropriate code for the malignancy is sequenced as the principal or first-listed diagnosis followed by code D63.0, Anemia in neoplastic disease.

5) Complication from surgical procedure for treatment of a neoplasm

When an encounter is for treatment of a complication resulting from a surgical procedure performed for the treatment of the neoplasm, designate the complication as the principal/ first-listed diagnosis. See guideline regarding the coding of a current malignancy versus personal history to determine if the code for the neoplasm should also be assigned.

6) Pathologic fracture due to a neoplasm

When an encounter is for a pathological fracture due to a neoplasm, and the focus of treatment is the fracture, a code from subcategory M84.5, Pathological fracture in neoplastic disease, should be sequenced first, followed by the code for the neoplasm.

If the focus of treatment is the neoplasm with an associated pathological fracture, the neoplasm code should be sequenced first, followed by a code from M84.5 for the pathological fracture.

m. Current malignancy versus personal history of malignancy

When a primary malignancy has been excised but further treatment, such as an additional surgery for the malignancy, radiation therapy or chemotherapy is directed to that site, the primary malignancy code should be used until treatment is completed.

When a primary malignancy has been previously excised or eradicated from its site, there is no further treatment (of the malignancy) directed to that site, and there is no evidence of any existing primary malignancy, a code from category Z85, Personal history of malignant neoplasm, should be used to indicate the former site of the malignancy.

See Section I.C.21. Factors influencing health status and contact with health services, History (of)

n. Leukemia, Multiple Myeloma, and Malignant Plasma Cell Neoplasms in remission versus personal history

The categories for leukemia, and category C90, Multiple myeloma and malignant plasma cell neoplasms, have codes indicating whether or not the leukemia has achieved remission. There are also codes Z85.6, Personal history of leukemia, and Z85.79, Personal history of other malignant neoplasms of lymphoid, hematopoietic and related tissues. If the documentation is unclear, as to whether the leukemia has achieved remission, the provider should be queried.

See Section I.C.21. Factors influencing health status and contact with health services, History (of)

o. Aftercare following surgery for neoplasm

See Section I.C.21. Factors influencing health status and contact with health services, Aftercare

p. Follow-up care for completed treatment of a malignancy

See Section I.C.21. Factors influencing health status and contact with health services, Follow-up

q. Prophylactic organ removal for prevention of malignancy

See Section I.C. 21, Factors influencing health status and contact with health services, Prophylactic organ removal

r. Malignant neoplasm associated with transplanted organ

A malignant neoplasm of a transplanted organ should be coded as a transplant complication. Assign first the appropriate code from category T86.-, Complications of transplanted organs and tissue, followed by code C80.2, Malignant neoplasm associated with transplanted organ. Use an additional code for the specific malignancy.

3. Chapter 3: Disease of the blood and blood-forming organs and certain disorders involving the immune mechanism (D50-D89)

Reserved for future guideline expansion

4. Chapter 4: Endocrine, Nutritional, and Metabolic Diseases (E00-E89)

a. Diabetes mellitus

The diabetes mellitus codes are combination codes that include the type of diabetes mellitus, the body system affected, and the complications affecting that body system. As many codes within a particular category as are necessary to describe all of the complications of the disease may be used. They should be sequenced based on the reason for a particular encounter. Assign as many codes from categories E08 – E13 as needed to identify all of the associated conditions that the patient has.

1) Type of diabetes

The age of a patient is not the sole determining factor, though most type 1 diabetics develop the condition before reaching puberty. For this reason type 1 diabetes mellitus is also referred to as juvenile diabetes.

2) Type of diabetes mellitus not documented

If the type of diabetes mellitus is not documented in the medical record the default is E11.-, Type 2 diabetes mellitus.

3) Diabetes mellitus and the use of insulin oral hypoglycemics

If the documentation in a medical record does not indicate the type of diabetes but does indicate that the patient uses insulin, code E11, Type 2 diabetes mellitus, should be assigned. **An additional code should be assigned from category Z79 to identify the long-term (current) use of insulin or oral hypoglycemic drugs. If the patient is treated with both oral medications and insulin, only the code for long-term (current) use of insulin should be assigned. Code Z79.4 should not be assigned if insulin is given temporarily to bring a type 2 patient's blood sugar under control during an encounter.**

4) Diabetes mellitus in pregnancy and gestational diabetes

See Section I.C.15. Diabetes mellitus in pregnancy.
See Section I.C.15. Gestational (pregnancy induced) diabetes

5) Complications due to insulin pump malfunction

(a) Underdose of insulin due to insulin pump failure

An underdose of insulin due to an insulin pump failure should be assigned to a code from subcategory T85.6, Mechanical complication of other specified internal and external prosthetic devices, implants and grafts, that specifies the type of pump malfunction, as the principal or first-listed code, followed by code T38.3X6-, Underdosing of insulin and oral hypoglycemic [antidiabetic] drugs. Additional codes for the type of diabetes mellitus and any associated complications due to the underdosing should also be assigned.

(b) Overdose of insulin due to insulin pump failure

The principal or first-listed code for an encounter due to an insulin pump malfunction resulting in an overdose of insulin, should also be T85.6-, Mechanical complication of other specified internal and external prosthetic devices, implants and grafts, followed by code T38.3X1-, Poisoning by insulin and oral hypoglycemic [antidiabetic] drugs, accidental (unintentional).

6) Secondary diabetes mellitus

Codes under categories E08, Diabetes mellitus due to underlying condition, E09, Drug or chemical induced diabetes mellitus and E13, Other specified diabetes mellitus, identify complications/manifestations associated with secondary diabetes mellitus. Secondary diabetes is always caused by another condition or event (e.g., cystic fibrosis, malignant neoplasm of pancreas, pancreatectomy, adverse effect of drug, or poisoning).

(a) Secondary diabetes mellitus and the use of insulin or hypoglycemic drugs
For patients with secondary diabetes mellitus who routinely use insulin or oral hypoglycemic drugs, an additional code from category Z79 should be assigned to identify the long-term (current) use of insulin or oral hypoglycemic drugs. If the patient is treated with both oral medications and insulin, only the code for long-term (current) use of insulin should be assigned. Code Z79.4 should not be assigned if insulin is given temporarily to bring a type 2 patient's blood sugar under control during an encounter.

(b) Assigning and sequencing secondary diabetes codes and its causes
The sequencing of the secondary diabetes codes in relationship to codes for the cause of the diabetes is based on the Tabular List instructions for categories E08, E09 and E13.

(i) Secondary diabetes mellitus due to pancreatectomy For postpancreatectomy diabetes mellitus (lack of insulin due to the surgical removal of all or part of the pancreas), assign code E89.1, Postprocedural hypoinsulinemia. Assign a code from category E13 and a code from subcategory Z90.41-, Acquired absence of pancreas, as additional codes.

(ii) Secondary diabetes due to drugs Secondary diabetes may be caused by an adverse effect of correctly administered medications, poisoning or sequela of poisoning.
See section I.C.19.e for coding of adverse effects and poisoning, and section I.C.20 for external cause code reporting.

5. **Chapter 5: Mental, Behavioral and Neurodevelopmental disorders (F01 – F99)**

a. Pain disorders related to psychological factors
Assign code F45.41, for pain that is exclusively related to psychological disorders. As indicated by the Excludes 1 note under category G89, a code from category G89 should not be assigned with code F45.41

Code F45.42, Pain disorders with related psychological factors, should be used with a code from category G89, Pain, not elsewhere classified, if there is documentation of a psychological component for a patient with acute or chronic pain.
See Section I.C.6. Pain

c. Mental and behavioral disorders due to psychoactive substance use

1) In Remission
Selection of codes for "in remission" for categories F10-F19, Mental and behavioral disorders due to psychoactive substance use (categories F10-F19 with -11, -.21) requires the provider's clinical judgment. The appropriate codes for "in remission" are assigned only on the basis of

provider documentation (as defined in the Official Guidelines for Coding and Reporting), **unless otherwise instructed by the classification.**

Mild substance use disorders in early or sustained remission are classified to the appropriate codes for substance abuse in remission, and moderate or severe substance use disorders in early or sustained remission are classified to the appropriate codes for substance dependence in remission.

2) Psychoactive Substance Use, Abuse and Dependence
When the provider documentation refers to use, abuse and dependence of the same substance (e.g. alcohol, opioid, cannabis, etc.), only one code should be assigned to identify the pattern of use based on the following hierarchy:
- If both use and abuse are documented, assign only the code for abuse
- If both abuse and dependence are documented, assign only the code for dependence
- If use, abuse and dependence are all documented, assign only the code for dependence
- If both use and dependence are documented, assign only the code for dependence.

3) Psychoactive Substance Use *Disorders*
As with all other diagnoses, the codes for psychoactive substance use **disorders** (F10.9-, F11.9-, F12.9-, F13.9-, F14.9-, F15.9-, F16.9-) should only be assigned based on provider documentation and when they meet the definition of a reportable diagnosis (see Section III, Reporting Additional Diagnoses). The codes are to be used only when the psychoactive substance use is associated with a **physical,** mental or behavioral disorder, and such a relationship is documented by the provider.

6. **Chapter 6: Diseases of the Nervous System (G00-G99)**

a. Dominant/nondominant side
Codes from category G81, Hemiplegia and hemiparesis, and subcategories, G83.1, Monoplegia of lower limb, G83.2, Monoplegia of upper limb, and G83.3, Monoplegia, unspecified, identify whether the dominant or nondominant side is affected. Should the affected side be documented, but not specified as dominant or nondominant, and the classification system does not indicate a default, code selection is as follows:
- For ambidextrous patients, the default should be dominant.
- If the left side is affected, the default is non-dominant.
- If the right side is affected, the default is dominant.

b. Pain - Category G89

1) General coding information
Codes in category G89, Pain, not elsewhere classified, may be used in conjunction with codes from other categories and chapters to provide more detail about acute or chronic pain and neoplasm-related pain, unless otherwise indicated below.

If the pain is not specified as acute or chronic, post-thoracotomy, postprocedural, or neoplasm-related, do not assign codes from category G89.

A code from category G89 should not be assigned if the underlying (definitive) diagnosis is known, unless the reason for the encounter is pain control/management and not management of the underlying condition.

When an admission or encounter is for a procedure aimed at treating the underlying condition (e.g., spinal fusion, kyphoplasty), a code for the underlying condition (e.g., vertebral fracture, spinal stenosis) should be assigned as the principal diagnosis. No code from category G89 should be assigned.

(a) Category G89 Codes as Principal or First-Listed Diagnosis

Category G89 codes are acceptable as principal diagnosis or the first-listed code:

- When pain control or pain management is the reason for the admission/encounter (e.g., a patient with displaced intervertebral disc, nerve impingement and severe back pain presents for injection of steroid into the spinal canal). The underlying cause of the pain should be reported as an additional diagnosis, if known.
- When a patient is admitted for the insertion of a neurostimulator for pain control, assign the appropriate pain code as the principal or first-listed diagnosis. When an admission or encounter is for a procedure aimed at treating the underlying condition and a neurostimulator is inserted for pain control during the same admission/encounter, a code for the underlying condition should be assigned as the principal diagnosis and the appropriate pain code should be assigned as a secondary diagnosis.

(b) Use of Category G89 Codes in Conjunction with Site Specific Pain Codes

(i) Assigning Category G89 and Site-Specific Pain Codes

Codes from category G89 may be used in conjunction with codes that identify the site of pain (including codes from chapter 18) if the category G89 code provides additional information. For example, if the code describes the site of the pain, but does not fully describe whether the pain is acute or chronic, then both codes should be assigned.

(ii) Sequencing of Category G89 Codes with Site-Specific Pain Codes

The sequencing of category G89 codes with site-specific pain codes (including chapter 18 codes), is dependent on the circumstances of the encounter/admission as follows:

- If the encounter is for pain control or pain management, assign the code from category G89 followed by the code identifying the specific site of pain (e.g., encounter for pain management for acute neck pain from trauma is assigned code G89.11, Acute pain due to trauma, followed by code M54.2, Cervicalgia, to identify the site of pain).
- If the encounter is for any other reason except pain control or pain management, and a related definitive diagnosis has not been established (confirmed) by the provider, assign the code for the specific site of pain first, followed by the appropriate code from category G89.

2) Pain due to devices, implants and grafts
See Section I.C.19. Pain due to medical devices

3) Postoperative Pain

The provider's documentation should be used to guide the coding of postoperative pain, as well as *Section III. Reporting Additional Diagnoses* and *Section IV. Diagnostic Coding and Reporting in the Outpatient Setting.*

The default for post-thoracotomy and other postoperative pain not specified as acute or chronic is the code for the acute form.

Routine or expected postoperative pain immediately after surgery should not be coded.

(a) Postoperative pain not associated with specific postoperative complication

Postoperative pain not associated with a specific postoperative complication is assigned to the appropriate postoperative pain code in category G89.

(b) Postoperative pain associated with specific postoperative complication

Postoperative pain associated with a specific postoperative complication (such as painful wire sutures) is assigned to the appropriate code(s) found in Chapter 19, Injury, poisoning, and certain other consequences of external causes. If appropriate, use additional code(s) from category G89 to identify acute or chronic pain (G89.18 or G89.28).

4) Chronic pain

Chronic pain is classified to subcategory G89.2. There is no time frame defining when pain becomes chronic pain. The provider's documentation should be used to guide use of these codes.

5) Neoplasm Related Pain

Code G89.3 is assigned to pain documented as being related, associated or due to cancer, primary or secondary malignancy, or tumor. This code is assigned regardless of whether the pain is acute or chronic.

This code may be assigned as the principal or first-listed code when the stated reason for the admission/encounter is documented as pain control/pain management. The underlying neoplasm should be reported as an additional diagnosis.

When the reason for the admission/encounter is management of the neoplasm and the pain associated with the neoplasm is also documented, code G89.3 may be assigned as an additional diagnosis. It is not necessary to assign an additional code for the site of the pain.

See Section I.C.2 for instructions on the sequencing of neoplasms for all other stated reasons for the admission/ encounter (except for pain control/pain management).

6) Chronic pain syndrome

Central pain syndrome (G89.Ø) and chronic pain syndrome (G89.4) are different than the term "chronic pain," and therefore codes should only be used when the provider has specifically documented this condition.

See Section I.C.5. Pain disorders related to psychological factors

7. Chapter 7: Diseases of the Eye and Adnexa (HØØ-H59)

a. Glaucoma

1) Assigning Glaucoma Codes

Assign as many codes from category H4Ø, Glaucoma, as needed to identify the type of glaucoma, the affected eye, and the glaucoma stage.

2) Bilateral glaucoma with same type and stage

When a patient has bilateral glaucoma and both eyes are documented as being the same type and stage, and there is a code for bilateral glaucoma, report only the code for the type of glaucoma, bilateral, with the seventh character for the stage.

When a patient has bilateral glaucoma and both eyes are documented as being the same type and stage, and the classification does not provide a code for bilateral glaucoma (i.e. subcategories H4Ø.1Ø, H4Ø.11 and H4Ø.2Ø) report only one code for the type of glaucoma with the appropriate seventh character for the stage.

3) Bilateral glaucoma stage with different types or stages

When a patient has bilateral glaucoma and each eye is documented as having a different type or stage, and the classification distinguishes laterality, assign the appropriate code for each eye rather than the code for bilateral glaucoma.

When a patient has bilateral glaucoma and each eye is documented as having a different type, and the classification does not distinguish laterality (i.e. subcategories H4Ø.1Ø, H4Ø.11 and H4Ø.2Ø), assign one code for each type of glaucoma with the appropriate seventh character for the stage.

When a patient has bilateral glaucoma and each eye is documented as having the same type, but different stage, and the classification does not distinguish laterality (i.e. subcategories H4Ø.1Ø, H4Ø.11 and H4Ø.2Ø), assign a code for the type of glaucoma for each eye with the seventh character for the specific glaucoma stage documented for each eye.

4) Patient admitted with glaucoma and stage evolves during the admission

If a patient is admitted with glaucoma and the stage progresses during the admission, assign the code for highest stage documented.

5) Indeterminate stage glaucoma

Assignment of the seventh character "4" for "indeterminate stage" should be based on the clinical documentation. The seventh character "4" is used for glaucomas whose stage cannot be clinically determined. This seventh character should not be confused with the seventh character "Ø", unspecified, which should be assigned when there is no documentation regarding the stage of the glaucoma.

b. Blindness

If "blindness" or "low vision" of both eyes is documented but the visual impairment category is not documented, assign code H54.3, Unqualified visual loss, both eyes. If "blindness" or "low vision" in one eye is documented but the visual impairment category is not documented, assign a code from H54.6-, Unqualified visual loss, one eye. If "blindness" or "visual loss" is documented without any information about whether one or both eyes are affected, assign code H54.7, Unspecified visual loss.

8. Chapter 8: Diseases of the Ear and Mastoid Process (H6Ø-H95)

Reserved for future guideline expansion

9. Chapter 9: Diseases of the Circulatory System (IØØ-I99)

a. Hypertension

The classification presumes a causal relationship between hypertension and heart involvement and between hypertension and kidney involvement, as the two conditions are linked by the term "with" in the Alphabetic Index. These conditions should be coded as related even in the absence of provider documentation explicitly linking them, unless the documentation clearly states the conditions are unrelated.

For hypertension and conditions not specifically linked by relational terms such as "with," "associated with" or "due to" in the classification, provider documentation must link the conditions in order to code them as related.

1) Hypertension with Heart Disease

Hypertension with heart conditions classified to I5Ø.- or I51.4-I51.9, are assigned to, a code from category I11, Hypertensive heart disease. Use additional code(s) from category I5Ø, Heart failure, to identify the type(s) of heart failure in those patients with heart failure.

The same heart conditions (I5Ø.-, I51.4-I51.9) with hypertension are coded separately if the provider has specifically documented a different cause. Sequence according to the circumstances of the admission/encounter.

2) Hypertensive Chronic Kidney Disease

Assign codes from category I12, Hypertensive chronic kidney disease, when both hypertension and a condition classifiable to category N18, Chronic kidney disease (CKD), are present. CKD should not be coded as hypertensive if the physician has specifically documented a different cause.

The appropriate code from category N18 should be used as a secondary code with a code from category I12 to identify the stage of chronic kidney disease.

See Section I.C.14. Chronic kidney disease.

If a patient has hypertensive chronic kidney disease and acute renal failure, an additional code for the acute renal failure is required.

3) Hypertensive Heart and Chronic Kidney Disease

Assign codes from combination category I13, Hypertensive heart and chronic kidney disease, when there is hypertension with both heart and kidney involvement. If heart failure is present, assign an additional code from category I50 to identify the type of heart failure.

The appropriate code from category N18, Chronic kidney disease, should be used as a secondary code with a code from category I13 to identify the stage of chronic kidney disease.

See Section I.C.14. Chronic kidney disease.

The codes in category I13, Hypertensive heart and chronic kidney disease, are combination codes that include hypertension, heart disease and chronic kidney disease. The Includes note at I13 specifies that the conditions included at I11 and I12 are included together in I13. If a patient has hypertension, heart disease and chronic kidney disease then a code from I13 should be used, not individual codes for hypertension, heart disease and chronic kidney disease, or codes from I11 or I12.

For patients with both acute renal failure and chronic kidney disease an additional code for acute renal failure is required.

4) Hypertensive Cerebrovascular Disease

For hypertensive cerebrovascular disease, first assign the appropriate code from categories I60-I69, followed by the appropriate hypertension code.

5) Hypertensive Retinopathy

Subcategory H35.0, Background retinopathy and retinal vascular changes, should be used with a code from category I10 – I15, Hypertensive disease to include the systemic hypertension. The sequencing is based on the reason for the encounter.

6) Hypertension, Secondary

Secondary hypertension is due to an underlying condition. Two codes are required: one to identify the underlying etiology and one from category I15 to identify the hypertension. Sequencing of codes is determined by the reason for admission/encounter.

7) Hypertension, Transient

Assign code R03.0, Elevated blood pressure reading without diagnosis of hypertension, unless patient has an established diagnosis of hypertension. Assign code O13.-, Gestational [pregnancy-induced] hypertension without

significant proteinuria, or O14.-, Pre-eclampsia, for transient hypertension of pregnancy.

8) Hypertension, Controlled

This diagnostic statement usually refers to an existing state of hypertension under control by therapy. Assign the appropriate code from categories I10-I15, Hypertensive diseases.

9) Hypertension, Uncontrolled

Uncontrolled hypertension may refer to untreated hypertension or hypertension not responding to current therapeutic regimen. In either case, assign the appropriate code from categories I10-I15, Hypertensive diseases.

10) Hypertensive Crisis

Assign a code from category I16, Hypertensive crisis, for documented hypertensive urgency, hypertensive emergency or unspecified hypertensive crisis. Code also any identified hypertensive disease (I10-I15). The sequencing is based on the reason for the encounter.

10) Pulmonary Hypertension

Pulmonary hypertension is classified to category I27, Other pulmonary heart diseases. For secondary pulmonary hypertension (I27.1, I27.2-), code also any associated conditions or adverse effects of drugs or toxins. The sequencing is based on the reason for the encounter.

b. Atherosclerotic Coronary Artery Disease and Angina

ICD-10-CM has combination codes for atherosclerotic heart disease with angina pectoris. The subcategories for these codes are I25.11, Atherosclerotic heart disease of native coronary artery with angina pectoris and I25.7, Atherosclerosis of coronary artery bypass graft(s) and coronary artery of transplanted heart with angina pectoris.

When using one of these combination codes it is not necessary to use an additional code for angina pectoris. A causal relationship can be assumed in a patient with both atherosclerosis and angina pectoris, unless the documentation indicates the angina is due to something other than the atherosclerosis.

If a patient with coronary artery disease is admitted due to an acute myocardial infarction (AMI), the AMI should be sequenced before the coronary artery disease.

See Section I.C.9. Acute myocardial infarction (AMI)

c. Intraoperative and Postprocedural Cerebrovascular Accident

Medical record documentation should clearly specify the cause-and-effect relationship between the medical intervention and the cerebrovascular accident in order to assign a code for intraoperative or postprocedural cerebrovascular accident.

Proper code assignment depends on whether it was an infarction or hemorrhage and whether it occurred intraoperatively or postoperatively. If it was a cerebral hemorrhage, code assignment depends on the type of procedure performed.

d. Sequelae of Cerebrovascular Disease

1) Category I69, Sequelae of Cerebrovascular disease

Category I69 is used to indicate conditions classifiable to categories I60-I67 as the causes of sequela (neurologic deficits), themselves classified elsewhere. These "late effects" include neurologic deficits that persist after initial onset of conditions classifiable to categories I60-I67. The neurologic deficits caused by cerebrovascular disease may be present from the onset or may arise at any time after the onset of the condition classifiable to categories I60-I67.

Codes from category I69, Sequelae of cerebrovascular disease, that specify hemiplegia, hemiparesis and monoplegia identify whether the dominant or nondominant side is affected. Should the affected side be documented, but not specified as dominant or nondominant, and the classification system does not indicate a default, code selection is as follows:

- For ambidextrous patients, the default should be dominant.
- If the left side is affected, the default is non-dominant.
- If the right side is affected, the default is dominant.

2) Codes from category I69 with codes from I60-I67

Codes from category I69 may be assigned on a health care record with codes from I60-I67, if the patient has a current cerebrovascular disease and deficits from an old cerebrovascular disease.

3) Codes from category I69 and Personal history of transient ischemic attack (TIA) and cerebral infarction (Z86.73)

Codes from category I69 should not be assigned if the patient does not have neurologic deficits.

See Section I.C.21. 4. History (of) for use of personal history codes

e. Acute myocardial infarction (AMI)

1) Type 1 ST elevation myocardial infarction (STEMI) and non ST elevation myocardial infarction (NSTEMI)

The ICD-10-CM codes for **type 1** acute myocardial infarction (AMI) identify the site, such as anterolateral wall or true posterior wall. Subcategories I21.0-I21.2 and code I21.3 are used for **type 1** ST elevation myocardial infarction (STEMI). Code I21.4, Non-ST elevation (NSTEMI) myocardial infarction, is used for **type 1** non ST elevation myocardial infarction (NSTEMI) and nontransmural MIs.

If **a type 1** NSTEMI evolves to STEMI, assign the STEMI code. If **a type 1** STEMI converts to NSTEMI due to thrombolytic therapy, it is still coded as STEMI.

For encounters occurring while the myocardial infarction is equal to, or less than, four weeks old, including transfers to another acute setting or a postacute setting, and the myocardial infarction meets the definition for "other diagnoses" (see

Section III, Reporting Additional Diagnoses), codes from category I21 may continue to be reported. For encounters after the 4 week time frame and the patient is still receiving care related to the myocardial infarction, the appropriate aftercare code should be assigned, rather than a code from category I21. For old or healed myocardial infarctions not requiring further care, code I25.2, Old myocardial infarction, may be assigned.

2) Acute myocardial infarction, unspecified

Code **I21.9, Acute myocardial infarction, unspecified,** is the default for unspecified acute myocardial infarction **or unspecified type**. If only **type 1** STEMI or transmural MI without the site is documented, assign code I21.3, **ST elevation (STEMI) myocardial infarction of unspecified site**.

3) AMI documented as nontransmural or subendocardial but site provided

If an AMI is documented as nontransmural or subendocardial, but the site is provided, it is still coded as a subendocardial AMI.

See Section I.C.21.3 for information on coding status post administration of tPA in a different facility within the last 24 hours.

4) Subsequent acute myocardial infarction

A code from category I22, Subsequent ST elevation (STEMI) and non ST elevation (NSTEMI) myocardial infarction, is to be used when a patient who has suffered **a type 1 or unspecified** AMI has a new AMI within the 4 week time frame of the initial AMI. A code from category I22 must be used in conjunction with a code from category I21. The sequencing of the I22 and I21 codes depends on the circumstances of the encounter.

Do not assign code I22 for subsequent myocardial infarctions other than type 1 or unspecified. For subsequent type 2 AMI assign only code I21.A1. For subsequent type 4 or type 5 AMI, assign only code I21.A9.

5) Other Types of Myocardial Infarction

The ICD-10-CM provides codes for different types of myocardial infarction. Type 1 myocardial infarctions are assigned to codes I21.0-I21.4.

Type 2 myocardial infarction, and myocardial infarction due to demand ischemia or secondary to ischemic balance, is assigned to code I21.A1, Myocardial infarction type 2 with a code for the underlying cause. Do not assign code I24.8, Other forms of acute ischemic heart disease for the demand ischemia. Sequencing of type 2 AMI or the underlying cause is dependent on the circumstances of admission. When a type 2 AMI code is described as NSTEMI or STEMI, only assign code I21.A1. Codes I21.01-I21.4 should only be assigned for type 1 AMIs.

Acute myocardial infarctions type 3, 4a, 4b, 4c and 5 are assigned to code I21.A9, Other myocardial infarction type.

The "Code also" and "Code first" notes should be followed related to complications, and for coding of postprocedural myocardial infarctions during or following cardiac surgery.

10. **Chapter 10: Diseases of the Respiratory System (J00-J99)**

    a. **Chronic Obstructive Pulmonary Disease [COPD] and Asthma**

       1) **Acute exacerbation of chronic obstructive bronchitis and asthma**

    The codes in categories J44 and J45 distinguish between uncomplicated cases and those in acute exacerbation. An acute exacerbation is a worsening or a decompensation of a chronic condition. An acute exacerbation is not equivalent to an infection superimposed on a chronic condition, though an exacerbation may be triggered by an infection.

    b. **Acute Respiratory Failure**

       1) **Acute respiratory failure as principal diagnosis**

    A code from subcategory J96.0, Acute respiratory failure, or subcategory J96.2, Acute and chronic respiratory failure, may be assigned as a principal diagnosis when it is the condition established after study to be chiefly responsible for occasioning the admission to the hospital, and the selection is supported by the Alphabetic Index and Tabular List. However, chapter-specific coding guidelines (such as obstetrics, poisoning, HIV, newborn) that provide sequencing direction take precedence.

       2) **Acute respiratory failure as secondary diagnosis**

    Respiratory failure may be listed as a secondary diagnosis if it occurs after admission, or if it is present on admission, but does not meet the definition of principal diagnosis.

       3) **Sequencing of acute respiratory failure and another acute condition**

    When a patient is admitted with respiratory failure and another acute condition, (e.g., myocardial infarction, cerebrovascular accident, aspiration pneumonia), the principal diagnosis will not be the same in every situation. This applies whether the other acute condition is a respiratory or nonrespiratory condition. Selection of the principal diagnosis will be dependent on the circumstances of admission. If both the respiratory failure and the other acute condition are equally responsible for occasioning the admission to the hospital, and there are no chapter-specific sequencing rules, the guideline regarding two or more diagnoses that equally meet the definition for principal diagnosis (*Section II, C.*) may be applied in these situations.

    If the documentation is not clear as to whether acute respiratory failure and another condition are equally responsible for occasioning the admission, query the provider for clarification.

    c. **Influenza due to certain identified influenza viruses**

    Code only confirmed cases of influenza due to certain identified influenza viruses (category J09), and due to other identified influenza virus (category J10). This is an exception to the hospital inpatient guideline Section II, H. (Uncertain Diagnosis).

    In this context, "confirmation" does not require documentation of positive laboratory testing specific for avian or other novel influenza A or other identified influenza virus. However, coding should be based on the provider's diagnostic statement that the patient has avian influenza, or other novel influenza A, for category J09, or has another particular identified strain of influenza, such as H1N1 or H3N2, but not identified as novel or variant, for category J10.

    If the provider records "suspected" or "possible" or "probable" avian influenza, or novel influenza, or other identified influenza, then the appropriate influenza code from category J11, Influenza due to unidentified influenza virus, should be assigned. A code from category J09, Influenza due to certain identified influenza viruses, should not be assigned nor should a code from category J10, Influenza due to other identified influenza virus.

    d. **Ventilator associated Pneumonia**

       1) **Documentation of Ventilator associated Pneumonia**

    As with all procedural or postprocedural complications, code assignment is based on the provider's documentation of the relationship between the condition and the procedure.

    Code J95.851, Ventilator associated pneumonia, should be assigned only when the provider has documented ventilator associated pneumonia (VAP). An additional code to identify the organism (e.g., Pseudomonas aeruginosa, code B96.5) should also be assigned. Do not assign an additional code from categories J12-J18 to identify the type of pneumonia.

    Code J95.851 should not be assigned for cases where the patient has pneumonia and is on a mechanical ventilator and the provider has not specifically stated that the pneumonia is ventilator-associated pneumonia. If the documentation is unclear as to whether the patient has a pneumonia that is a complication attributable to the mechanical ventilator, query the provider.

       2) **Ventilator associated Pneumonia Develops after Admission**

    A patient may be admitted with one type of pneumonia (e.g., code J13, Pneumonia due to Streptococcus pneumonia) and subsequently develop VAP. In this instance, the principal diagnosis would be the appropriate code from categories J12-J18 for the pneumonia diagnosed at the time of admission. Code J95.851, Ventilator associated pneumonia, would be assigned as an additional diagnosis when the provider has also documented the presence of ventilator associated pneumonia.

11. **Chapter 11: Diseases of the Digestive System (K00-K95)**

    Reserved for future guideline expansion

12. **Chapter 12: Diseases of the Skin and Subcutaneous Tissue (L00-L99)**

   a. **Pressure ulcer stage codes**

   1) **Pressure ulcer stages**

   Codes from category L89, Pressure ulcer, identify the site of the pressure ulcer as well as the stage of the ulcer.

   The ICD-10-CM classifies pressure ulcer stages based on severity, which is designated by stages 1-4, unspecified stage and unstageable.

   Assign as many codes from category L89 as needed to identify all the pressure ulcers the patient has, if applicable.

   2) **Unstageable pressure ulcers**

   Assignment of the code for unstageable pressure ulcer (L89.--0) should be based on the clinical documentation. These codes are used for pressure ulcers whose stage cannot be clinically determined (e.g., the ulcer is covered by eschar or has been treated with a skin or muscle graft) and pressure ulcers that are documented as deep tissue injury but not documented as due to trauma. This code should not be confused with the codes for unspecified stage (L89.--9). When there is no documentation regarding the stage of the pressure ulcer, assign the appropriate code for unspecified stage (L89.--9).

   3) **Documented pressure ulcer stage**

   Assignment of the pressure ulcer stage code should be guided by clinical documentation of the stage or documentation of the terms found in the Alphabetic Index. For clinical terms describing the stage that are not found in the Alphabetic Index, and there is no documentation of the stage, the provider should be queried.

   4) **Patients admitted with pressure ulcers documented as healed**

   No code is assigned if the documentation states that the pressure ulcer is completely healed.

   5) **Patients admitted with pressure ulcers documented as healing**

   Pressure ulcers described as healing should be assigned the appropriate pressure ulcer stage code based on the documentation in the medical record. If the documentation does not provide information about the stage of the healing pressure ulcer, assign the appropriate code for unspecified stage.

   If the documentation is unclear as to whether the patient has a current (new) pressure ulcer or if the patient is being treated for a healing pressure ulcer, query the provider.

   For ulcers that were present on admission but healed at the time of discharge, assign the code for the site and stage of the pressure ulcer at the time of admission.

   6) **Patient admitted with pressure ulcer evolving into another stage during the admission**

   If a patient is admitted **to an inpatient hospital** with a pressure ulcer at one stage and it progresses to a higher stage, two separate codes should be assigned: one code for the site and stage of the ulcer on admission and a second code for the same ulcer site and the highest stage reported during the stay.

   b. **Non-Pressure Chronic Ulcers**

   1) **Patients admitted with non-pressure ulcers documented as healed**

   No code is assigned if the documentation states that the non-pressure ulcer is completely healed.

   2) **Patients admitted with non-pressure ulcers documented as healing**

   Non-pressure ulcers described as healing should be assigned the appropriate non-pressure ulcer code based on the documentation in the medical record. If the documentation does not provide information about the severity of the healing non-pressure ulcer, assign the appropriate code for unspecified severity.

   If the documentation is unclear as to whether the patient has a current (new) non-pressure ulcer or if the patient is being treated for a healing non-pressure ulcer, query the provider.

   For ulcers that were present on admission but healed at the time of discharge, assign the code for the site and severity of the non-pressure ulcer at the time of admission.

   3) **Patient admitted with non-pressure ulcer that progresses to another severity level during the admission**

   If a patient is admitted to an inpatient hospital with a non-pressure ulcer at one severity level and it progresses to a higher severity level, two separate codes should be assigned: one code for the site and severity level of the ulcer on admission and a second code for the same ulcer site and the highest severity level reported during the stay.

13. **Chapter 13: Diseases of the Musculoskeletal System and Connective Tissue (M00-M99)**

   a. **Site and laterality**

   Most of the codes within Chapter 13 have site and laterality designations. The site represents the bone, joint or the muscle involved. For some conditions where more than one bone, joint or muscle is usually involved, such as osteoarthritis, there is a "multiple sites" code available. For categories where no multiple site code is provided and more than one bone, joint or muscle is involved, multiple codes should be used to indicate the different sites involved.

   1) **Bone versus joint**

   For certain conditions, the bone may be affected at the upper or lower end, (e.g., avascular necrosis of bone, M87, Osteoporosis, M80, M81). Though the portion of the bone affected may be at the joint, the site designation will be the bone, not the joint.

   b. **Acute traumatic versus chronic or recurrent musculoskeletal conditions**

   Many musculoskeletal conditions are a result of previous injury or trauma to a site, or are recurrent conditions. Bone, joint or muscle conditions that are the result of a healed injury are usually found in chapter 13. Recurrent bone, joint or muscle conditions are also usually found in chapter 13. Any current, acute injury should be coded to the appropriate injury code from chapter 19. Chronic or recurrent conditions should generally be coded with a code from chapter 13. If it is difficult to determine from the documentation in the record which code is best to describe a condition, query the provider.

c. Coding of Pathologic Fractures

7th character A is for use as long as the patient is receiving active treatment for the fracture. While the patient may be seen by a new or different provider over the course of treatment for a pathological fracture, assignment of the 7th character is based on whether the patient is undergoing active treatment and not whether the provider is seeing the patient for the first time.

7th character, D is to be used for encounters after the patient has completed active treatment **for the fracture and is receiving routine care for the fracture during the healing or recovery phase**. The other 7th characters, listed under each subcategory in the Tabular List, are to be used for subsequent encounters for treatment of problems associated with the healing, such as malunions, nonunions, and sequelae.

Care for complications of surgical treatment for fracture repairs during the healing or recovery phase should be coded with the appropriate complication codes.

See Section I.C.19. Coding of traumatic fractures.

d. Osteoporosis

Osteoporosis is a systemic condition, meaning that all bones of the musculoskeletal system are affected. Therefore, site is not a component of the codes under category M81, Osteoporosis without current pathological fracture. The site codes under category M80, Osteoporosis with current pathological fracture, identify the site of the fracture, not the osteoporosis.

1) Osteoporosis without pathological fracture

Category M81, Osteoporosis without current pathological fracture, is for use for patients with osteoporosis who do not currently have a pathologic fracture due to the osteoporosis, even if they have had a fracture in the past. For patients with a history of osteoporosis fractures, status code Z87.310, Personal history of (healed) osteoporosis fracture, should follow the code from M81.

2) Osteoporosis with current pathological fracture

Category M80, Osteoporosis with current pathological fracture, is for patients who have a current pathologic fracture at the time of an encounter. The codes under M80 identify the site of the fracture. A code from category M80, not a traumatic fracture code, should be used for any patient with known osteoporosis who suffers a fracture, even if the patient had a minor fall or trauma, if that fall or trauma would not usually break a normal, healthy bone.

14. Chapter 14: Diseases of Genitourinary System (N00-N99)

a. Chronic kidney disease

1) Stages of chronic kidney disease (CKD)

The ICD-10-CM classifies CKD based on severity. The severity of CKD is designated by stages 1-5. Stage 2, code N18.2, equates to mild CKD; stage 3, code N18.3, equates to moderate CKD; and stage 4, code N18.4, equates to severe CKD. Code N18.6, End stage renal disease (ESRD), is assigned when the provider has documented end-stage-renal disease (ESRD).

If both a stage of CKD and ESRD are documented, assign code N18.6 only.

2) Chronic kidney disease and kidney transplant status

Patients who have undergone kidney transplant may still have some form of chronic kidney disease CKD because the kidney transplant may not fully restore kidney function. Therefore, the presence of CKD alone does not constitute a transplant complication. Assign the appropriate N18 code for the patient's stage of CKD and code Z94.0, Kidney transplant status. If a transplant complication such as failure or rejection or other transplant complication is documented, see section I.C.19.g for information on coding complications of a kidney transplant. If the documentation is unclear as to whether the patient has a complication of the transplant, query the provider.

3) Chronic kidney disease with other conditions

Patients with CKD may also suffer from other serious conditions, most commonly diabetes mellitus and hypertension. The sequencing of the CKD code in relationship to codes for other contributing conditions is based on the conventions in the Tabular List.

See I.C.9. Hypertensive chronic kidney disease.
See I.C.19. Chronic kidney disease and kidney transplant complications.

15. Chapter 15: Pregnancy, Childbirth, and the Puerperium (O00-O9A)

a. General Rules for Obstetric Cases

1) Codes from chapter 15 and sequencing priority

Obstetric cases require codes from chapter 15, codes in the range O00-O9A, Pregnancy, Childbirth, and the Puerperium. Chapter 15 codes have sequencing priority over codes from other chapters. Additional codes from other chapters may be used in conjunction with chapter 15 codes to further specify conditions. Should the provider document that the pregnancy is incidental to the encounter, then code Z33.1, Pregnant state, incidental, should be used in place of any chapter 15 codes. It is the provider's responsibility to state that the condition being treated is not affecting the pregnancy.

2) Chapter 15 codes used only on the maternal record

Chapter 15 codes are to be used only on the maternal record, never on the record of the newborn.

3) Final character for trimester

The majority of codes in Chapter 15 have a final character indicating the trimester of pregnancy. The timeframes for the trimesters are indicated at the beginning of the chapter. If trimester is not a component of a code it is because the condition always occurs in a specific trimester, or the concept of trimester of pregnancy is not applicable. Certain codes have characters for only certain trimesters because the condition does not occur in all trimesters, but it may occur in more than just one.

Assignment of the final character for trimester should be based on the provider's documentation of the trimester (or number of weeks) for the current admission/encounter. This applies to the assignment of trimester for pre-existing conditions as well as those that develop during or are due to the pregnancy. The provider's documentation of the number of weeks may be used to assign the appropriate code identifying the trimester.

Whenever delivery occurs during the current admission, and there is an "in childbirth" option for the obstetric complication being coded, the "in childbirth" code should be assigned.

4) Selection of trimester for inpatient admissions that encompass more than one trimester

In instances when a patient is admitted to a hospital for complications of pregnancy during one trimester and remains in the hospital into a subsequent trimester, the trimester character for the antepartum complication code should be assigned on the basis of the trimester when the complication developed, not the trimester of the discharge. If the condition developed prior to the current admission/encounter or represents a pre-existing condition, the trimester character for the trimester at the time of the admission/encounter should be assigned.

5) Unspecified trimester

Each category that includes codes for trimester has a code for "unspecified trimester." The "unspecified trimester" code should rarely be used, such as when the documentation in the record is insufficient to determine the trimester and it is not possible to obtain clarification.

6) 7th character for Fetus Identification

Where applicable, a 7th character is to be assigned for certain categories (O31, O32, O33.3 - O33.6, O35, O36, O40, O41, O60.1, O60.2, O64, and O69) to identify the fetus for which the complication code applies.

Assign 7th character "0":
- For single gestations
- When the documentation in the record is insufficient to determine the fetus affected and it is not possible to obtain clarification.
- When it is not possible to clinically determine which fetus is affected.

b. Selection of OB Principal or First-listed Diagnosis

1) Routine outpatient prenatal visits

For routine outpatient prenatal visits when no complications are present, a code from category Z34, Encounter for supervision of normal pregnancy, should be used as the first-listed diagnosis. These codes should not be used in conjunction with chapter 15 codes.

2) Supervision of High-Risk Pregnancy

Codes from category O09, Supervision of high-risk pregnancy, are intended for use only during the prenatal period. For complications during the labor or delivery episode as a result of a high-risk pregnancy, assign the applicable complication codes from Chapter 15. If there are no complications during the labor or delivery episode, assign code O80, Encounter for full-term uncomplicated delivery.

For routine prenatal outpatient visits for patients with high-risk pregnancies, a code from category O09, Supervision of high-risk pregnancy, should be used as the first-listed diagnosis. Secondary chapter 15 codes may be used in conjunction with these codes if appropriate.

3) Episodes when no delivery occurs

In episodes when no delivery occurs, the principal diagnosis should correspond to the principal complication of the pregnancy which necessitated the encounter. Should more than one complication exist, all of which are treated or monitored, any of the complications codes may be sequenced first.

4) When a delivery occurs

When an obstetric patient is admitted and delivers during that admission, the condition that prompted the admission should be sequenced as the principal diagnosis. If multiple conditions prompted the admission, sequence the one most related to the delivery as the principal diagnosis. A code for any complication of the delivery should be assigned as an additional diagnosis. In cases of cesarean delivery, if the patient was admitted with a condition that resulted in the performance of a cesarean procedure, that condition should be selected as the principal diagnosis. If the reason for the admission was unrelated to the condition resulting in the cesarean delivery, the condition related to the reason for the admission should be selected as the principal diagnosis.

5) Outcome of delivery

A code from category Z37, Outcome of delivery, should be included on every maternal record when a delivery has occurred. These codes are not to be used on subsequent records or on the newborn record.

c. Pre-existing conditions versus conditions due to the pregnancy

Certain categories in Chapter 15 distinguish between conditions of the mother that existed prior to pregnancy (pre-existing) and those that are a direct result of pregnancy. When assigning codes from Chapter 15, it is important to assess if a condition was pre-existing prior to pregnancy or developed during or due to the pregnancy in order to assign the correct code.

Categories that do not distinguish between pre-existing and pregnancy-related conditions may be used for either. It is acceptable to use codes specifically for the puerperium with codes complicating pregnancy and childbirth if a condition arises postpartum during the delivery encounter.

d. Pre-existing hypertension in pregnancy

Category O10, Pre-existing hypertension complicating pregnancy, childbirth and the puerperium, includes codes for hypertensive heart and hypertensive chronic kidney disease. When assigning one of the O10 codes that includes hypertensive heart disease or hypertensive chronic kidney disease, it is necessary to add a secondary code from the appropriate hypertension category to specify the type of heart failure or chronic kidney disease.

See Section I.C.9. Hypertension.

e. Fetal Conditions Affecting the Management of the Mother

1) Codes from categories O35 and O36

Codes from categories O35, Maternal care for known or suspected fetal abnormality and damage, and O36, Maternal care for other fetal problems, are assigned only when the fetal condition is actually responsible for modifying the management of the mother, i.e., by requiring diagnostic studies, additional observation, special care, or termination of pregnancy. The fact that the fetal condition exists does not justify assigning a code from this series to the mother's record.

2) In utero surgery

In cases when surgery is performed on the fetus, a diagnosis code from category O35, Maternal care for known or suspected fetal abnormality and damage, should be assigned identifying the fetal condition. Assign the appropriate procedure code for the procedure performed.

No code from Chapter 16, the perinatal codes, should be used on the mother's record to identify fetal conditions. Surgery performed in utero on a fetus is still to be coded as an obstetric encounter.

f. HIV Infection in Pregnancy, Childbirth and the Puerperium

During pregnancy, childbirth or the puerperium, a patient admitted because of an HIV-related illness should receive a principal diagnosis from subcategory O98.7-, Human immunodeficiency [HIV] disease complicating pregnancy, childbirth and the puerperium, followed by the code(s) for the HIV-related illness(es).

Patients with asymptomatic HIV infection status admitted during pregnancy, childbirth, or the puerperium should receive codes of O98.7- and Z21, Asymptomatic human immunodeficiency virus [HIV] infection status.

g. Diabetes mellitus in pregnancy

Diabetes mellitus is a significant complicating factor in pregnancy. Pregnant women who are diabetic should be assigned a code from category O24, Diabetes mellitus in pregnancy, childbirth, and the puerperium, first, followed by the appropriate diabetes code(s) (E08-E13) from Chapter 4.

h. Long term use of insulin and oral hypoglycemics

See section I.C.4.a.3 for information on the long term use of insulin and oral hypoglycemic.

i. Gestational (pregnancy induced) diabetes

Gestational (pregnancy induced) diabetes can occur during the second and third trimester of pregnancy in women who were not diabetic prior to pregnancy. Gestational diabetes can cause complications in the pregnancy similar to those of pre-existing diabetes mellitus. It also puts the woman at greater risk of developing diabetes after the pregnancy. Codes for gestational diabetes are in subcategory O24.4, Gestational diabetes mellitus. No other code from category O24, Diabetes mellitus in pregnancy, childbirth, and the puerperium, should be used with a code from O24.4.

The codes under subcategory O24.4 include diet controlled, insulin controlled, and controlled by oral hypoglycemic drugs. If a patient with gestational diabetes is treated with both diet and insulin, only the code for insulin-controlled is required. If a patient with gestational diabetes is treated with both diet and oral hypoglycemic medications, only the code for "controlled by oral hypoglycemic drugs" is required. Code Z79.4, Long-term (current) use of insulin or code Z79.84, Long-term (current) use of oral hypoglycemic drugs, should not be assigned with codes from subcategory O24.4.

An abnormal glucose tolerance in pregnancy is assigned a code from subcategory O99.81, Abnormal glucose complicating pregnancy, childbirth, and the puerperium.

j. Sepsis and septic shock complicating abortion, pregnancy, childbirth and the puerperium

When assigning a chapter 15 code for sepsis complicating abortion, pregnancy, childbirth, and the puerperium, a code for the specific type of infection should be assigned as an additional diagnosis. If severe sepsis is present, a code from subcategory R65.2, Severe sepsis, and code(s) for associated organ dysfunction(s) should also be assigned as additional diagnoses.

k. Puerperal sepsis

Code O85, Puerperal sepsis, should be assigned with a secondary code to identify the causal organism (e.g., for a bacterial infection, assign a code from category B95-B96, Bacterial infections in conditions classified elsewhere). A code from category A40, Streptococcal sepsis, or A41, Other sepsis, should not be used for puerperal sepsis. If applicable, use additional codes to identify severe sepsis (R65.2-) and any associated acute organ dysfunction.

l. Alcohol and tobacco use during pregnancy, childbirth and the puerperium

1) Alcohol use during pregnancy, childbirth and the puerperium

Codes under subcategory O99.31, Alcohol use complicating pregnancy, childbirth, and the puerperium, should be assigned for any pregnancy case when a mother uses alcohol during the pregnancy or postpartum. A secondary code from category F10, Alcohol related disorders, should also be assigned to identify manifestations of the alcohol use.

2) Tobacco use during pregnancy, childbirth and the puerperium

Codes under subcategory O99.33, Smoking (tobacco) complicating pregnancy, childbirth, and the puerperium, should be assigned for any pregnancy case when a mother uses any type of tobacco product during the pregnancy or postpartum. A secondary code from category F17, Nicotine dependence, should also be assigned to identify the type of nicotine dependence.

m. Poisoning, toxic effects, adverse effects and underdosing in a pregnant patient

A code from subcategory O9A.2, Injury, poisoning and certain other consequences of external causes complicating pregnancy, childbirth, and the puerperium, should be sequenced first, followed by the appropriate injury, poisoning, toxic effect, adverse effect or underdosing code, and then the additional code(s) that specifies the condition caused by the poisoning, toxic effect, adverse effect or underdosing.

See Section I.C.19. Adverse effects, poisoning, underdosing and toxic effects.

n. Normal Delivery, Code O80

1) Encounter for full term uncomplicated delivery

Code O80 should be assigned when a woman is admitted for a full-term normal delivery and delivers a single, healthy infant without any complications antepartum, during the delivery, or postpartum during the delivery episode. Code O80 is always a principal diagnosis. It is not to be used if any other code from chapter 15 is needed to describe a current complication of the antenatal, delivery, or perinatal period. Additional codes from other chapters may be used with code O80 if they are not related to or are in any way complicating the pregnancy.

2) Uncomplicated delivery with resolved antepartum complication

Code O80 may be used if the patient had a complication at some point during the pregnancy, but the complication is not present at the time of the admission for delivery.

3) Outcome of delivery for O80

Z37.0, Single live birth, is the only outcome of delivery code appropriate for use with O80.

o. The Peripartum and Postpartum Periods

1) Peripartum and Postpartum periods

The postpartum period begins immediately after delivery and continues for six weeks following delivery. The peripartum period is defined as the last month of pregnancy to five months postpartum.

2) Peripartum and postpartum complication

A postpartum complication is any complication occurring within the six-week period.

3) Pregnancy-related complications after 6 week period

Chapter 15 codes may also be used to describe pregnancy-related complications after the peripartum or postpartum period if the provider documents that a condition is pregnancy related.

4) Admission for routine postpartum care following delivery outside hospital

When the mother delivers outside the hospital prior to admission and is admitted for routine postpartum care and no complications are noted, code Z39.0, Encounter for care and examination of mother immediately after delivery, should be assigned as the principal diagnosis.

5) Pregnancy associated cardiomyopathy

Pregnancy associated cardiomyopathy, code O90.3, is unique in that it may be diagnosed in the third trimester of pregnancy but may continue to progress months after delivery. For this reason, it is referred to as peripartum cardiomyopathy. Code O90.3 is only for use when the cardiomyopathy develops as a result of pregnancy in a woman who did not have pre-existing heart disease.

p. Code O94, Sequelae of complication of pregnancy, childbirth, and the puerperium

1) Code O94

Code O94, Sequelae of complication of pregnancy, childbirth, and the puerperium, is for use in those cases when an initial complication of a pregnancy develops a sequelae requiring care or treatment at a future date.

2) After the initial postpartum period

This code may be used at any time after the initial postpartum period.

3) Sequencing of Code O94

This code, like all sequela codes, is to be sequenced following the code describing the sequelae of the complication.

q. Termination of Pregnancy and Spontaneous abortions

1) Abortion with Liveborn Fetus

When an attempted termination of pregnancy results in a liveborn fetus assign code Z33.2, Encounter for elective termination of pregnancy and a code from category Z37, Outcome of Delivery.

2) Retained Products of Conception following an abortion

Subsequent encounters for retained products of conception following a spontaneous abortion or elective termination of pregnancy, **without** complications are assigned O03.**4, Incomplete spontaneous,** abortion **without complication** or codes O07.4, Failed attempted termination of pregnancy without complication. This advice is appropriate even when the patient was discharged previously with a discharge diagnosis of complete abortion. **If the patient has a specific complication associated with the spontaneous abortion or elective termination of pregnancy in addition to retained products of conception, assign the appropriate complication in category O03 or O07 instead of code O03.4 or O07.4**

3) Complications leading to abortion
Codes from Chapter 15 may be used as additional codes to identify any documented complications of the pregnancy in conjunction with codes in categories in **O04**, O07 and O08.

r. Abuse in a pregnant patient
For suspected or confirmed cases of abuse of a pregnant patient, a code(s) from subcategories O9A.3, Physical abuse complicating pregnancy, childbirth, and the puerperium, O9A.4, Sexual abuse complicating pregnancy, childbirth, and the puerperium, and O9A.5, Psychological abuse complicating pregnancy, childbirth, and the puerperium, should be sequenced first, followed by the appropriate codes (if applicable) to identify any associated current injury due to physical abuse, sexual abuse, and the perpetrator of abuse.
See Section I.C.19. Adult and child abuse, neglect and other maltreatment.

16. **Chapter 16: Certain Conditions Originating in the Perinatal Period (P00-P96)**
For coding and reporting purposes the perinatal period is defined as before birth through the 28th day following birth. The following guidelines are provided for reporting purposes

a. General Perinatal Rules

1) Use of Chapter 16 Codes
Codes in this chapter are never for use on the maternal record. Codes from Chapter 15, the obstetric chapter, are never permitted on the newborn record. Chapter 16 codes may be used throughout the life of the patient if the condition is still present.

2) Principal Diagnosis for Birth Record
When coding the birth episode in a newborn record, assign a code from category Z38, Liveborn infants according to place of birth and type of delivery, as the principal diagnosis. A code from category Z38 is assigned only once, to a newborn at the time of birth. If a newborn is transferred to another institution, a code from category Z38 should not be used at the receiving hospital.

A code from category Z38 is used only on the newborn record, not on the mother's record.

3) Use of Codes from other Chapters with Codes from Chapter 16
Codes from other chapters may be used with codes from chapter 16 if the codes from the other chapters provide more specific detail. Codes for signs and symptoms may be assigned when a definitive diagnosis has not been established. If the reason for the encounter is a perinatal condition, the code from chapter 16 should be sequenced first.

4) Use of Chapter 16 Codes after the Perinatal Period
Should a condition originate in the perinatal period, and continue throughout the life of the patient, the perinatal code should continue to be used regardless of the patient's age.

5) Birth process or community acquired conditions
If a newborn has a condition that may be either due to the birth process or community acquired and the documentation does not indicate which it is, the default is due to the birth process and the code from Chapter 16 should be used. If the condition is community-acquired, a code from Chapter 16 should not be assigned.

6) Code all clinically significant conditions
All clinically significant conditions noted on routine newborn examination should be coded. A condition is clinically significant if it requires:
- clinical evaluation; or
- therapeutic treatment; or
- diagnostic procedures; or
- extended length of hospital stay; or
- increased nursing care and/or monitoring; or
- has implications for future health care needs

Note: The perinatal guidelines listed above are the same as the general coding guidelines for "additional diagnoses", except for the final point regarding implications for future health care needs. Codes should be assigned for conditions that have been specified by the provider as having implications for future health care needs.

b. Observation and Evaluation of Newborns for Suspected Conditions not Found

1) Use of Z05 codes
Assign a code from category Z05, Observation and evaluation of newborns and infants for suspected conditions ruled out, to identify those instances when a healthy newborn is evaluated for a suspected condition that is determined after study not to be present. Do not use a code from category Z05 when the patient has identified signs or symptoms of a suspected problem; in such cases code the sign or symptom.

2) Z05 on Other than the Birth Record
A code from category Z05 may also be assigned as a principal or first-listed code for readmissions or encounters when the code from category Z38 code no longer applies. Codes from category Z05 are for use only for healthy newborns and infants for which no condition after study is found to be present.

3) Z05 on a birth record
A code from category Z05 is to be used as a secondary code after the code from category Z38, Liveborn infants according to place of birth and type of delivery.

GUIDELINES (ICD-10-CM)

c. Coding Additional Perinatal Diagnoses

1) Assigning codes for conditions that require treatment

Assign codes for conditions that require treatment or further investigation, prolong the length of stay, or require resource utilization.

2) Codes for conditions specified as having implications for future health care needs

Assign codes for conditions that have been specified by the provider as having implications for future health care needs.

Note: This guideline should not be used for adult patients.

d. Prematurity and Fetal Growth Retardation

Providers utilize different criteria in determining prematurity. A code for prematurity should not be assigned unless it is documented. Assignment of codes in categories P05, Disorders of newborn related to slow fetal growth and fetal malnutrition, and P07, Disorders of newborn related to short gestation and low birth weight, not elsewhere classified, should be based on the recorded birth weight and estimated gestational age.

When both birth weight and gestational age are available, two codes from category P07 should be assigned, with the code for birth weight sequenced before the code for gestational age.

e. Low birth weight and immaturity status

Codes from category P07, Disorders of newborn related to short gestation and low birth weight, not elsewhere classified, are for use for a child or adult who was premature or had a low birth weight as a newborn and this is affecting the patient's current health status.

See Section I.C.21. Factors influencing health status and contact with health services, Status.

f. Bacterial Sepsis of Newborn

Category P36, Bacterial sepsis of newborn, includes congenital sepsis. If a perinate is documented as having sepsis without documentation of congenital or community acquired, the default is congenital and a code from category P36 should be assigned. If the P36 code includes the causal organism, an additional code from category B95, Streptococcus, Staphylococcus, and Enterococcus as the cause of diseases classified elsewhere, or B96, Other bacterial agents as the cause of diseases classified elsewhere, should not be assigned. If the P36 code does not include the causal organism, assign an additional code from category B96. If applicable, use additional codes to identify severe sepsis (R65.2-) and any associated acute organ dysfunction.

g. Stillbirth

Code P95, Stillbirth, is only for use in institutions that maintain separate records for stillbirths. No other code should be used with P95. Code P95 should not be used on the mother's record.

17. Chapter 17: Congenital malformations, deformations, and chromosomal abnormalities (Q00-Q99)

Assign an appropriate code(s) from categories Q00-Q99, Congenital malformations, deformations, and chromosomal abnormalities when a malformation/deformation or chromosomal abnormality is documented. A malformation/deformation/or chromosomal abnormality may be the principal/first-listed diagnosis on a record or a secondary diagnosis.

When a malformation/deformation/or chromosomal abnormality does not have a unique code assignment, assign additional code(s) for any manifestations that may be present.

When the code assignment specifically identifies the malformation/deformation/or chromosomal abnormality, manifestations that are an inherent component of the anomaly should not be coded separately. Additional codes should be assigned for manifestations that are not an inherent component.

Codes from Chapter 17 may be used throughout the life of the patient. If a congenital malformation or deformity has been corrected, a personal history code should be used to identify the history of the malformation or deformity. Although present at birth, malformation/deformation/or chromosomal abnormality may not be identified until later in life. Whenever the condition is diagnosed by the physician, it is appropriate to assign a code from codes Q00-Q99.

For the birth admission, the appropriate code from category Z38, Liveborn infants, according to place of birth and type of delivery, should be sequenced as the principal diagnosis, followed by any congenital anomaly codes, Q00-Q99.

18. Chapter 18: Symptoms, signs, and abnormal clinical and laboratory findings, not elsewhere classified (R00-R99)

Chapter 18 includes symptoms, signs, abnormal results of clinical or other investigative procedures, and ill-defined conditions regarding which no diagnosis classifiable elsewhere is recorded. Signs and symptoms that point to a specific diagnosis have been assigned to a category in other chapters of the classification.

a. Use of symptom codes

Codes that describe symptoms and signs are acceptable for reporting purposes when a related definitive diagnosis has not been established (confirmed) by the provider.

b. Use of a symptom code with a definitive diagnosis code

Codes for signs and symptoms may be reported in addition to a related definitive diagnosis when the sign or symptom is not routinely associated with that diagnosis, such as the various signs and symptoms associated with complex syndromes. The definitive diagnosis code should be sequenced before the symptom code.

Signs or symptoms that are associated routinely with a disease process should not be assigned as additional codes, unless otherwise instructed by the classification.

c. Combination codes that include symptoms

ICD-10-CM contains a number of combination codes that identify both the definitive diagnosis and common symptoms of that diagnosis. When using one of these combination codes, an additional code should not be assigned for the symptom.

d. Repeated falls

Code R29.6, Repeated falls, is for use for encounters when a patient has recently fallen and the reason for the fall is being investigated.

Code Z91.81, History of falling, is for use when a patient has fallen in the past and is at risk for future falls. When appropriate, both codes R29.6 and Z91.81 may be assigned together.

e. Coma scale

The coma scale codes (R40.2-) can be used in conjunction with traumatic brain injury codes, acute cerebrovascular disease or sequelae of cerebrovascular disease codes. These codes are primarily for use by trauma registries, but they may be used in any setting where this information is collected. The coma scale may also be used to assess the status of the central nervous system for other non-trauma conditions, such as monitoring patients in the intensive care unit regardless of medical condition. The coma scale codes should be sequenced after the diagnosis code(s).

These codes, one from each subcategory, are needed to complete the scale. The 7th character indicates when the scale was recorded. The 7th character should match for all three codes.

At a minimum, report the initial score documented on presentation at your facility. This may be a score from the emergency medicine technician (EMT) or in the emergency department. If desired, a facility may choose to capture multiple coma scale scores.

Assign code R40.24, Glasgow coma scale, total score, when only the total score is documented in the medical record and not the individual score(s).

f. Functional quadriplegia
GUIDELINE HAS BEEN DELETED EFFECTIVE OCTOBER 1, 2017

g. SIRS due to Non-Infectious Process

The systemic inflammatory response syndrome (SIRS) can develop as a result of certain non-infectious disease processes, such as trauma, malignant neoplasm, or pancreatitis. When SIRS is documented with a noninfectious condition, and no subsequent infection is documented, the code for the underlying condition, such as an injury, should be assigned, followed by code R65.10, Systemic inflammatory response syndrome (SIRS) of non-infectious origin without acute organ dysfunction, or code R65.11, Systemic inflammatory response syndrome (SIRS) of non-infectious origin with acute organ dysfunction. If an associated acute organ dysfunction is documented, the appropriate code(s) for the specific type of organ dysfunction(s) should be assigned in addition to code R65.11. If acute organ dysfunction is documented, but it cannot be determined if the acute organ dysfunction is associated with SIRS or due to another condition (e.g., directly due to the trauma), the provider should be queried.

h. Death NOS
Code R99, Ill-defined and unknown cause of mortality, is only for use in the very limited circumstance when a patient who has already died is brought into an emergency department or other healthcare facility and is pronounced dead upon arrival. It does not represent the discharge disposition of death.

i. NIHSS Stroke Scale
The NIH stroke scale (NIHSS) codes (R29.7- -) can be used in conjunction with acute stroke codes (I63) to identify the patient's neurological status and the severity of the stroke. The stroke scale codes should be sequenced after the acute stroke diagnosis code(s).

At a minimum, report the initial score documented. If desired, a facility may choose to capture multiple stroke scale scores.

See Section I.B.14. for information concerning the medical record documentation that may be used for assignment of the NIHSS codes.

19. **Chapter 19: Injury, poisoning, and certain other consequences of external causes (S00-T88)**

    ### a. Application of 7th Characters in Chapter 19
    Most categories in chapter 19 have a 7th character requirement for each applicable code. Most categories in this chapter have three 7th character values (with the exception of fractures): A, initial encounter, D, subsequent encounter and S, sequela. Categories for traumatic fractures have additional 7th character values. While the patient may be seen by a new or different provider over the course of treatment for an injury, assignment of the 7th character is based on whether the patient is undergoing active treatment and not whether the provider is seeing the patient for the first time.

    For complication codes, active treatment refers to treatment for the condition described by the code, even though it may be related to an earlier precipitating problem. For example, code T84.50XA, Infection and inflammatory reaction due to unspecified internal joint prosthesis, initial encounter, is used when active treatment is provided for the infection, even though the condition relates to the prosthetic device, implant or graft that was placed at a previous encounter.

    7th character "A", initial encounter is used for each encounter where the patient is receiving active treatment for the condition.

    7th character "D" subsequent encounter is used for encounters after the patient has completed active treatment of the condition and is receiving routine care for the condition during the healing or recovery phase.

    The aftercare Z codes should not be used for aftercare for conditions such as injuries or poisonings, where 7th characters are provided to identify subsequent care. For example, for aftercare of an injury, assign the acute injury code with the 7th character "D" (subsequent encounter).

    7th character "S", sequela, is for use for complications or conditions that arise as a direct result of a condition, such as scar formation after a burn. The scars are sequelae of the burn. When using 7th character "S", it is necessary to use both

GUIDELINES (ICD-10-CM)

the injury code that precipitated the sequela and the code for the sequela itself. The "S" is added only to the injury code, not the sequela code. The 7th character "S" identifies the injury responsible for the sequela. The specific type of sequela (e.g. scar) is sequenced first, followed by the injury code.

See Section I.B.10. Sequelae, (Late Effects)

b. Coding of Injuries

When coding injuries, assign separate codes for each injury unless a combination code is provided, in which case the combination code is assigned. **Codes from category** T07, Unspecified multiple injuries should not be assigned in the inpatient setting unless information for a more specific code is not available. Traumatic injury codes (S00-T14.9) are not to be used for normal, healing surgical wounds or to identify complications of surgical wounds.

The code for the most serious injury, as determined by the provider and the focus of treatment, is sequenced first.

1) Superficial injuries

Superficial injuries such as abrasions or contusions are not coded when associated with more severe injuries of the same site.

2) Primary injury with damage to nerves/blood vessels

When a primary injury results in minor damage to peripheral nerves or blood vessels, the primary injury is sequenced first with additional code(s) for injuries to nerves and spinal cord (such as category S04), and/or injury to blood vessels (such as category S15). When the primary injury is to the blood vessels or nerves, that injury should be sequenced first.

c. Coding of Traumatic Fractures

The principles of multiple coding of injuries should be followed in coding fractures. Fractures of specified sites are coded individually by site in accordance with both the provisions within categories S02, S12, S22, S32, S42, S49, S52, S59, S62, S72, S79, S82, S89, S92 and the level of detail furnished by medical record content.

A fracture not indicated as open or closed should be coded to closed. A fracture not indicated whether displaced or not displaced should be coded to displaced.

More specific guidelines are as follows:

1) Initial vs. Subsequent Encounter for Fractures

Traumatic fractures are coded using the appropriate 7th character for initial encounter (A, B, C) for each encounter where the patient is receiving active treatment for the fracture. The appropriate 7th character for initial encounter should also be assigned for a patient who delayed seeking treatment for the fracture or nonunion.

Fractures are coded using the appropriate 7th character for subsequent care for encounters after the patient has completed active treatment of the fracture and is receiving routine care for the fracture during the healing or recovery phase.

Care for complications of surgical treatment for fracture repairs during the healing or recovery phase should be coded with the appropriate complication codes.

Care of complications of fractures, such as malunion and nonunion, should be reported with the appropriate 7th character for subsequent care with nonunion (K, M, N,) or subsequent care with malunion (P, Q, R).

Malunion/nonunion: The appropriate 7th character for initial encounter should also be assigned for a patient who delayed seeking treatment for the fracture or nonunion.

The open fracture designations in the assignment of the 7th character for fractures of the forearm, femur and lower leg, including ankle are based on the Gustilo open fracture classification. When the Gustilo classification type is not specified for an open fracture, the 7th character for open fracture type I or II should be assigned (B, E, H, M, Q).

A code from category M80, not a traumatic fracture code, should be used for any patient with known osteoporosis who suffers a fracture, even if the patient had a minor fall or trauma, if that fall or trauma would not usually break a normal, healthy bone.

See Section I.C.13. Osteoporosis.

The aftercare Z codes should not be used for aftercare for traumatic fractures. For aftercare of a traumatic fracture, assign the acute fracture code with the appropriate 7th character.

2) Multiple fractures sequencing

Multiple fractures are sequenced in accordance with the severity of the fracture.

d. Coding of Burns and Corrosions

The ICD-10-CM makes a distinction between burns and corrosions. The burn codes are for thermal burns, except sunburns, that come from a heat source, such as a fire or hot appliance. The burn codes are also for burns resulting from electricity and radiation. Corrosions are burns due to chemicals. The guidelines are the same for burns and corrosions.

Current burns (T20-T25) are classified by depth, extent and by agent (X code). Burns are classified by depth as first degree (erythema), second degree (blistering), and third degree (full-thickness involvement). Burns of the eye and internal organs (T26-T28) are classified by site, but not by degree.

1) Sequencing of burn and related condition codes

Sequence first the code that reflects the highest degree of burn when more than one burn is present.

a. When the reason for the admission or encounter is for treatment of external multiple burns, sequence first the code that reflects the burn of the highest degree.

b. When a patient has both internal and external burns, the circumstances of admission govern the selection of the principal diagnosis or first-listed diagnosis.

c. When a patient is admitted for burn injuries and other related conditions such as smoke inhalation and/or respiratory failure, the circumstances of admission govern the selection of the principal or first-listed diagnosis.

2) Burns of the same local site
Classify burns of the same local site (three-character category level, T20-T28) but of different degrees to the subcategory identifying the highest degree recorded in the diagnosis.

3) Non-healing burns
Non-healing burns are coded as acute burns.
Necrosis of burned skin should be coded as a non-healed burn.

4) Infected Burn
For any documented infected burn site, use an additional code for the infection.

5) Assign separate codes for each burn site
When coding burns, assign separate codes for each burn site. Category T30, Burn and corrosion, body region unspecified is extremely vague and should rarely be used.

6) Burns and Corrosions Classified According to Extent of Body Surface Involved
Assign codes from category T31, Burns classified according to extent of body surface involved, or T32, Corrosions classified according to extent of body surface involved, when the site of the burn is not specified or when there is a need for additional data. It is advisable to use category T31 as additional coding when needed to provide data for evaluating burn mortality, such as that needed by burn units. It is also advisable to use category T31 as an additional code for reporting purposes when there is mention of a third-degree burn involving 20 percent or more of the body surface.

Categories T31 and T32 are based on the classic "rule of nines" in estimating body surface involved: head and neck are assigned nine percent, each arm nine percent, each leg 18 percent, the anterior trunk 18 percent, posterior trunk 18 percent, and genitalia one percent. Providers may change these percentage assignments where necessary to accommodate infants and children who have proportionally larger heads than adults, and patients who have large buttocks, thighs, or abdomen that involve burns.

7) Encounters for treatment of sequela of burns
Encounters for the treatment of the late effects of burns or corrosions (i.e., scars or joint contractures) should be coded with a burn or corrosion code with the 7th character "S" for sequela.

8) Sequelae with a late effect code and current burn
When appropriate, both a code for a current burn or corrosion with 7th character "A" or "D" and a burn or corrosion code with 7th character "S" may be assigned on the same record (when both a current burn and sequelae of an old burn exist).

Burns and corrosions do not heal at the same rate and a current healing wound may still exist with sequela of a healed burn or corrosion.
See Section I.B.10. Sequela, (Late Effects)

9) Use of an external cause code with burns and corrosions
An external cause code should be used with burns and corrosions to identify the source and intent of the burn, as well as the place where it occurred.

e. Adverse Effects, Poisoning, Underdosing and Toxic Effects
Codes in categories T36-T65 are combination codes that include the substance that was taken as well as the intent. No additional external cause code is required for poisonings, toxic effects, adverse effects and underdosing codes.

1) Do not code directly from the Table of Drugs
Do not code directly from the Table of Drugs and Chemicals. Always refer back to the Tabular List.

2) Use as many codes as necessary to describe
Use as many codes as necessary to describe completely all drugs, medicinal or biological substances.

3) If the same code would describe the causative agent
If the same code would describe the causative agent for more than one adverse reaction, poisoning, toxic effect or underdosing, assign the code only once.

4) If two or more drugs, medicinal or biological substances
If two or more drugs, medicinal or biological substances are reported, code each individually unless a combination code is listed in the Table of Drugs and Chemicals.

5) The occurrence of drug toxicity is classified in ICD-10-CM as follows:
(a) Adverse Effect
When coding an adverse effect of a drug that has been correctly prescribed and properly administered, assign the appropriate code for the nature of the adverse effect followed by the appropriate code for the adverse effect of the drug (T36-T50). The code for the drug should have a 5th or 6th character "5" (for example T36.0X5-) Examples of the nature of an adverse effect are tachycardia, delirium, gastrointestinal hemorrhaging, vomiting, hypokalemia, hepatitis, renal failure, or respiratory failure.

(b) Poisoning
When coding a poisoning or reaction to the improper use of a medication (e.g., overdose, wrong substance given or taken in error, wrong route of administration), first assign the appropriate code from categories T36-T50. The poisoning codes have an associated intent as their 5th or 6th character (accidental, intentional self-harm, assault and undetermined). If the intent of the poisoning is unknown or unspecified, code the intent as accidental intent. The undetermined

intent is only for use if the documentation in the record specifies that the intent cannot be determined. Use additional code(s) for all manifestations of poisonings.

If there is also a diagnosis of abuse or dependence of the substance, the abuse or dependence is assigned as an additional code.

Examples of poisoning include:

(i) Error was made in drug prescription Errors made in drug prescription or in the administration of the drug by provider, nurse, patient, or other person.

(ii) Overdose of a drug intentionally taken If an overdose of a drug was intentionally taken or administered and resulted in drug toxicity, it would be coded as a poisoning.

(iii) Nonprescribed drug taken with correctly prescribed and properly administered drug.
If a nonprescribed drug or medicinal agent was taken in combination with a correctly prescribed and properly administered drug, any drug toxicity or other reaction resulting from the interaction of the two drugs would be classified as a poisoning.

(iv) Interaction of drug(s) and alcohol. When a reaction results from the interaction of a drug(s) and alcohol, this would be classified as poisoning.

See Section I.C.4. if poisoning is the result of insulin pump malfunctions.

(c) Underdosing

Underdosing refers to taking less of a medication than is prescribed by a provider or a manufacturer's instruction. For underdosing, assign the code from categories T36-T50 (fifth or sixth character "6").

Codes for underdosing should never be assigned as principal or first-listed codes. If a patient has a relapse or exacerbation of the medical condition for which the drug is prescribed because of the reduction in dose, then the medical condition itself should be coded.

Noncompliance (Z91.12-, Z91.13-) or complication of care (Y63.6-Y63.9) codes are to be used with an underdosing code to indicate intent, if known.

(d) Toxic Effects

When a harmful substance is ingested or comes in contact with a person, this is classified as a toxic effect. The toxic effect codes are in categories T51-T65.

Toxic effect codes have an associated intent: accidental, intentional self-harm, assault and undetermined.

f. Adult and child abuse, neglect and other maltreatment

Sequence first the appropriate code from categories T74 (Adult and child abuse, neglect and other maltreatment, confirmed) or T76 (Adult and child abuse, neglect and other maltreatment, suspected) for abuse, neglect and other maltreatment, followed by any accompanying mental health or injury code(s).

If the documentation in the medical record states abuse or neglect it is coded as confirmed (T74.-). It is coded as suspected if it is documented as suspected (T76.-).

For cases of confirmed abuse or neglect an external cause code from the assault section (X92-Y09) should be added to identify the cause of any physical injuries. A perpetrator code (Y07) should be added when the perpetrator of the abuse is known. For suspected cases of abuse or neglect, do not report external cause or perpetrator code.

If a suspected case of abuse, neglect or mistreatment is ruled out during an encounter code Z04.71, Encounter for examination and observation following alleged physical adult abuse, ruled out, or code Z04.72, Encounter for examination and observation following alleged child physical abuse, ruled out, should be used, not a code from T76.

If a suspected case of alleged rape or sexual abuse is ruled out during an encounter code Z04.41, Encounter for examination and observation following alleged adult rape or code Z04.42, Encounter for examination and observation following alleged child rape, should be used, not a code from T76.

See Section I.C.15. Abuse in a pregnant patient.

g. Complications of care

1) General guidelines for complications of care

(a) Documentation of complications of care
See Section I.B.16. for information on documentation of complications of care.

2) Pain due to medical devices
Pain associated with devices, implants or grafts left in a surgical site (for example painful hip prosthesis) is assigned to the appropriate code(s) found in Chapter 19, Injury, poisoning, and certain other consequences of external causes. Specific codes for pain due to medical devices are found in the T code section of the ICD-10-CM. Use additional code(s) from category G89 to identify acute or chronic pain due to presence of the device, implant or graft (G89.18 or G89.28).

3) Transplant complications

(a) Transplant complications other than kidney
Codes under category T86, Complications of transplanted organs and tissues, are for use for both complications and rejection of transplanted organs. A transplant complication code is only assigned if the complication affects the function

of the transplanted organ. Two codes are required to fully describe a transplant complication: the appropriate code from category T86 and a secondary code that identifies the complication.

Pre-existing conditions or conditions that develop after the transplant are not coded as complications unless they affect the function of the transplanted organs.

See I.C.21. for transplant organ removal status
See I.C.2. for malignant neoplasm associated with transplanted organ.

(b) Kidney transplant complications
Patients who have undergone kidney transplant may still have some form of chronic kidney disease (CKD) because the kidney transplant may not fully restore kidney function. Code T86.1- should be assigned for documented complications of a kidney transplant, such as transplant failure or rejection or other transplant complication. Code T86.1- should not be assigned for post kidney transplant patients who have chronic kidney (CKD) unless a transplant complication such as transplant failure or rejection is documented. If the documentation is unclear as to whether the patient has a complication of the transplant, query the provider.

Conditions that affect the function of the transplanted kidney, other than CKD, should be assigned a code from subcategory T86.1, Complications of transplanted organ, Kidney, and a secondary code that identifies the complication.

For patients with CKD following a kidney transplant, but who do not have a complication such as failure or rejection, *see section I.C.14. Chronic kidney disease and kidney transplant status*.

4) Complication codes that include the external cause
As with certain other T codes, some of the complications of care codes have the external cause included in the code. The code includes the nature of the complication as well as the type of procedure that caused the complication. No external cause code indicating the type of procedure is necessary for these codes.

5) Complications of care codes within the body system chapters
Intraoperative and postprocedural complication codes are found within the body system chapters with codes specific to the organs and structures of that body system. These codes should be sequenced first, followed by a code(s) for the specific complication, if applicable.

20. Chapter 20: External Causes of Morbidity (V00-Y99)
The external causes of morbidity codes should never be sequenced as the first-listed or principal diagnosis.

External cause codes are intended to provide data for injury research and evaluation of injury prevention strategies. These codes capture how the injury or health condition happened (cause), the intent (unintentional or accidental; or intentional, such as suicide or assault), the place where the event occurred the activity of the patient at the time of the event, and the person's status (e.g., civilian, military).

There is no national requirement for mandatory ICD-10-CM external cause code reporting. Unless a provider is subject to a state-based external cause code reporting mandate or these codes are required by a particular payer, reporting of ICD-10-CM codes in Chapter 20, External Causes of Morbidity, is not required. In the absence of a mandatory reporting requirement, providers are encouraged to voluntarily report external cause codes, as they provide valuable data for injury research and evaluation of injury prevention strategies.

a. General External Cause Coding Guidelines

1) Used with any code in the range of A00.0-T88.9, Z00-Z99
An external cause code may be used with any code in the range of A00.0-T88.9, Z00-Z99, classification that **represents** a health condition due to an external cause. Though they are most applicable to injuries, they are also valid for use with such things as infections or diseases due to an external source, and other health conditions, such as a heart attack that occurs during strenuous physical activity.

2) External cause code used for length of treatment
Assign the external cause code, with the appropriate 7th character (initial encounter, subsequent encounter or sequela) for each encounter for which the injury or condition is being treated.

Most categories in chapter 20 have a 7th character requirement for each applicable code. Most categories in this chapter have three 7th character values: A, initial encounter, D, subsequent encounter and S, sequela. While the patient may be seen by a new or different provider over the course of treatment for an injury or condition, assignment of the 7th character for external cause should match the 7th character of the code assigned for the associated injury or condition for the encounter.

3) Use the full range of external cause codes
Use the full range of external cause codes to completely describe the cause, the intent, the place of occurrence and if applicable, the activity of the patient at the time of the event, and the patient's status, for all injuries, and other health conditions due to an external cause.

4) Assign as many external cause codes as necessary
Assign as many external cause codes as necessary to fully explain each cause. If only one external code can be recorded, assign the code most related to the principal diagnosis.

5) The selection of the appropriate external cause code
The selection of the appropriate external cause code is guided by the Alphabetic Index of External Causes and by Inclusion and Exclusion notes in the Tabular List.

6) External cause code can never be a principal diagnosis

An external cause code can never be a principal (first-listed) diagnosis.

7) Combination external cause codes

Certain of the external cause codes are combination codes that identify sequential events that result in an injury, such as a fall which results in striking against an object. The injury may be due to either event or both. The combination external cause code used should correspond to the sequence of events regardless of which caused the most serious injury.

8) No external cause code needed in certain circumstances

No external cause code from Chapter 20 is needed if the external cause and intent are included in a code from another chapter (e.g. T36.0X1- Poisoning by penicillins, accidental (unintentional)).

b. Place of Occurrence Guideline

Codes from category Y92, Place of occurrence of the external cause, are secondary codes for use after other external cause codes to identify the location of the patient at the time of injury or other condition.

Generally, a place of occurrence code is assigned only once, at the initial encounter for treatment. However, in the rare instance that a new injury occurs during hospitalization, an additional place of occurrence code may be assigned. No 7th characters are used for Y92. Only one code from Y92 should be recorded on a medical record.

Do not use place of occurrence code Y92.9 if the place is not stated or is not applicable.

c. Activity Code

Assign a code from category Y93, Activity code, to describe the activity of the patient at the time the injury or other health condition occurred.

An activity code is used only once, at the initial encounter for treatment. Only one code from Y93 should be recorded on a medical record.

The activity codes are not applicable to poisonings, adverse effects, misadventures or sequela.

Do not assign Y93.9, Unspecified activity, if the activity is not stated.

A code from category Y93 is appropriate for use with external cause and intent codes if identifying the activity provides additional information about the event.

d. Place of Occurrence, Activity, and Status Codes Used with other External Cause Code

When applicable, place of occurrence, activity, and external cause status codes are sequenced after the main external cause code(s). Regardless of the number of external cause codes assigned, there should be only one place of occurrence code, one activity code, and one external cause status code assigned to an encounter.

e. If the Reporting Format Limits the Number of External Cause Codes

If the reporting format limits the number of external cause codes that can be used in reporting clinical data, report the code for the cause/intent most related to the principal diagnosis. If the format permits capture of additional external cause codes, the cause/intent, including medical misadventures, of the additional events should be reported rather than the codes for place, activity, or external status.

f. Multiple External Cause Coding Guidelines

More than one external cause code is required to fully describe the external cause of an illness or injury. The assignment of external cause codes should be sequenced in the following priority:

If two or more events cause separate injuries, an external cause code should be assigned for each cause. The first-listed external cause code will be selected in the following order:

External codes for child and adult abuse take priority over all other external cause codes.

See Section I.C.19., Child and Adult abuse guidelines.

External codes for terrorism events take priority over all other external cause codes except child and adult abuse.

External cause codes for cataclysmic events take priority over all other external cause codes except child and adult abuse and terrorism.

External cause codes for transport accidents take priority over all other external cause codes except cataclysmic events, child and adult abuse and terrorism.

Activity and external cause status codes are assigned following all causal (intent) external cause codes.

The first-listed external cause code should correspond to the cause of the most serious diagnosis due to an assault, accident, or self-harm, following the order of hierarchy listed above.

g. Child and Adult Abuse Guideline

Adult and child abuse, neglect and maltreatment are classified as assault. Any of the assault codes may be used to indicate the external cause of any injury resulting from the confirmed abuse.

For confirmed cases of abuse, neglect and maltreatment, when the perpetrator is known, a code from Y07, Perpetrator of maltreatment and neglect, should accompany any other assault codes.

See Section I.C.19. Adult and child abuse, neglect and other maltreatment

h. Unknown or Undetermined Intent Guideline

If the intent (accident, self-harm, assault) of the cause of an injury or other condition is unknown or unspecified, code the intent as accidental intent. All transport accident categories assume accidental intent.

1) Use of undetermined intent

External cause codes for events of undetermined intent are only for use if the documentation in the record specifies that the intent cannot be determined.

i. Sequelae (Late Effects) of External Cause Guidelines

1) Sequelae external cause codes

Sequela are reported using the external cause code with the 7th character "S" for sequela. These codes

should be used with any report of a late effect or sequela resulting from a previous injury.
See Section I.B.10. Sequela, (Late Effects)

2) Sequela external cause code with a related current injury

A sequela external cause code should never be used with a related current nature of injury code.

3) Use of sequela external cause codes for subsequent visits

Use a late effect external cause code for subsequent visits when a late effect of the initial injury is being treated. Do not use a late effect external cause code for subsequent visits for follow-up care (e.g., to assess healing, to receive rehabilitative therapy) of the injury when no late effect of the injury has been documented.

j. Terrorism Guidelines

1) Cause of injury identified by the Federal Government (FBI) as terrorism

When the cause of an injury is identified by the Federal Government (FBI) as terrorism, the first-listed external cause code should be a code from category Y38, Terrorism. The definition of terrorism employed by the FBI is found at the inclusion note at the beginning of category Y38. Use additional code for place of occurrence (Y92.-). More than one Y38 code may be assigned if the injury is the result of more than one mechanism of terrorism.

2) Cause of an injury is suspected to be the result of terrorism

When the cause of an injury is suspected to be the result of terrorism a code from category Y38 should not be assigned. Suspected cases should be classified as assault.

3) Code Y38.9, Terrorism, secondary effects

Assign code Y38.9, Terrorism, secondary effects, for conditions occurring subsequent to the terrorist event. This code should not be assigned for conditions that are due to the initial terrorist act.

It is acceptable to assign code Y38.9 with another code from Y38 if there is an injury due to the initial terrorist event and an injury that is a subsequent result of the terrorist event.

k. External cause status

A code from category Y99, External cause status, should be assigned whenever any other external cause code is assigned for an encounter, including an Activity code, except for the events noted below. Assign a code from category Y99, External cause status, to indicate the work status of the person at the time the event occurred. The status code indicates whether the event occurred during military activity, whether a non-military person was at work, whether an individual including a student or volunteer was involved in a non-work activity at the time of the causal event.

A code from Y99, External cause status, should be assigned, when applicable, with other external cause codes, such as transport accidents and falls. The external cause status codes are not applicable to poisonings, adverse effects, misadventures or late effects.

Do not assign a code from category Y99 if no other external cause codes (cause, activity) are applicable for the encounter.

An external cause status code is used only once, at the initial encounter for treatment. Only one code from Y99 should be recorded on a medical record.

Do not assign code Y99.9, Unspecified external cause status, if the status is not stated.

21. Chapter 21: Factors influencing health status and contact with health services (Z00-Z99)

Note: The chapter specific guidelines provide additional information about the use of Z codes for specified encounters.

a. Use of Z codes in any healthcare setting

Z codes are for use in any healthcare setting. Z codes may be used as either a first-listed (principal diagnosis code in the inpatient setting) or secondary code, depending on the circumstances of the encounter. Certain Z codes may only be used as first-listed or principal diagnosis.

b. Z Codes indicate a reason for an encounter

Z codes are not procedure codes. A corresponding procedure code must accompany a Z code to describe any procedure performed.

c. Categories of Z Codes

1) Contact/Exposure

Category Z20 indicates contact with, and suspected exposure to, communicable diseases. These codes are for patients who do not show any sign or symptom of a disease but are suspected to have been exposed to it by close personal contact with an infected individual or are in an area where a disease is epidemic.

Category Z77, Other contact with and (suspected) exposures hazardous to health, indicates contact with and suspected exposures hazardous to health.

Contact/exposure codes may be used as a first-listed code to explain an encounter for testing, or, more commonly, as a secondary code to identify a potential risk.

2) Inoculations and vaccinations

Code Z23 is for encounters for inoculations and vaccinations. It indicates that a patient is being seen to receive a prophylactic inoculation against a disease. Procedure codes are required to identify the actual administration of the injection and the type(s) of immunizations given. Code Z23 may be used as a secondary code if the inoculation is given as a routine part of preventive health care, such as a well-baby visit.

3) Status

Status codes indicate that a patient is either a carrier of a disease or has the sequelae or residual of a past disease or condition. This includes such things as the presence of prosthetic or mechanical devices resulting from past treatment. A status code is informative, because the status may affect the course of treatment and its outcome. A status code is distinct from a history code. The history code indicates that the patient no longer has the condition.

A status code should not be used with a diagnosis code from one of the body system chapters, if the diagnosis code includes the information provided by the status code. For example, code Z94.1, Heart transplant status, should not be used with a code from subcategory T86.2, Complications of heart transplant. The status code does not provide additional information. The complication code indicates that the patient is a heart transplant patient.

For encounters for weaning from a mechanical ventilator, assign a code from subcategory J96.1, Chronic respiratory failure, followed by code Z99.11, Dependence on respirator [ventilator] status.

The status Z codes/categories are:

Z14   Genetic carrier
Genetic carrier status indicates that a person carries a gene, associated with a particular disease, which may be passed to offspring who may develop that disease. The person does not have the disease and is not at risk of developing the disease.

Z15   Genetic susceptibility to disease Genetic susceptibility indicates that a person has a gene that increases the risk of that person developing the disease.

Codes from category Z15 should not be used as principal or first-listed codes. If the patient has the condition to which he/she is susceptible, and that condition is the reason for the encounter, the code for the current condition should be sequenced first. If the patient is being seen for follow-up after completed treatment for this condition, and the condition no longer exists, a follow-up code should be sequenced first, followed by the appropriate personal history and genetic susceptibility codes. If the purpose of the encounter is genetic counseling associated with procreative management, code Z31.5, Encounter for genetic counseling, should be assigned as the first-listed code, followed by a code from category Z15. Additional codes should be assigned for any applicable family or personal history.

Z16   Resistance to antimicrobial drugs
This code indicates that a patient has a condition that is resistant to antimicrobial drug treatment. Sequence the infection code first.

Z17   Estrogen receptor status

Z18   Retained foreign body fragments

Z19   Hormone sensitivity malignancy status

Z21   Asymptomatic HIV infection status This code indicates that a patient has tested positive for HIV but has manifested no signs or symptoms of the disease.

Z22   Carrier of infectious disease Carrier status indicates that a person harbors the specific organisms of a disease without manifest symptoms and is capable of transmitting the infection.

Z28.3   Underimmunization status

Z33.1   Pregnant state, incidental This code is a secondary code only for use when the pregnancy is in no way complicating the reason for visit. Otherwise, a code from the obstetric chapter is required.

Z66   Do not resuscitate
This code may be used when it is documented by the provider that a patient is on do not resuscitate status at any time during the stay.

Z67   Blood type

Z68   Body mass index (BMI)
As with all other secondary diagnosis codes, the BMI codes should only be assigned when they meet the definition of a reportable diagnosis (see Section III, Reporting Additional Diagnoses).

Z74.01   Bed confinement status

Z76.82   Awaiting organ transplant status

Z78   Other specified health status
Code Z78.1, Physical restraint status, may be used when it is documented by the provider that a patient has been put in restraints during the current encounter. Please note that this code should not be reported when it is documented by the provider that a patient is temporarily restrained during a procedure.

Z79   Long-term (current) drug therapy
Codes from this category indicate a patient's continuous use of a prescribed drug (including such things as aspirin therapy) for the long-term treatment of a condition or for prophylactic use. It is not for use for patients who have addictions to drugs. This subcategory is not for use of medications for detoxification or maintenance programs to prevent withdrawal symptoms in patients with drug dependence (e.g., methadone maintenance for opiate dependence). Assign the appropriate code for the drug dependence instead.

Assign a code from Z79 if the patient is receiving a medication for an extended period as a prophylactic measure (such as for the prevention of deep vein thrombosis) or as treatment of a chronic condition (such as arthritis) or a disease requiring a lengthy course of treatment (such as cancer). Do not assign a code from category Z79 for medication being administered for a brief period of time to treat an acute illness or injury (such as a course of antibiotics to treat acute bronchitis).

Z88   Allergy status to drugs, medicaments and biological substances Except: Z88.9, Allergy status to unspecified drugs, medicaments and biological substances status

Z89   Acquired absence of limb

Z90   Acquired absence of organs, not elsewhere classified

Z91.0-   Allergy status, other than to drugs and biological substances

Z92.82   Status post administration of tPA (rtPA) in a different facility within the last 24 hours prior to admission to a current facility Assign code Z92.82, Status post administration of tPA (rtPA) in a different facility within the last 24 hours prior to admission to current facility, as a secondary diagnosis when a patient is received by transfer into a facility and documentation indicates they were administered tissue plasminogen activator (tPA) within the last 24 hours prior to admission to the current facility. This guideline applies even if the patient is still receiving the tPA at the time they are received into the current facility. The appropriate code for the condition for which the tPA was administered (such as cerebrovascular disease or myocardial infarction) should be assigned first. Code Z92.82 is only applicable to the receiving facility record and not to the transferring facility record.

Z93	Artificial opening status
Z94	Transplanted organ and tissue status
Z95	Presence of cardiac and vascular implants and grafts
Z96	Presence of other functional implants
Z97	Presence of other devices
Z98	Other postprocedural states

Assign code Z98.85, Transplanted organ removal status, to indicate that a transplanted organ has been previously removed. This code should not be assigned for the encounter in which the transplanted organ is removed. The complication necessitating removal of the transplant organ should be assigned for that encounter.

See section I.C.19. for information on the coding of organ transplant complications.

Z99	Dependence on enabling machines and devices, not elsewhere classified

Note: Categories Z89-Z90 and Z93-Z99 are for use only if there are no complications or malfunctions of the organ or tissue replaced, the amputation site or the equipment on which the patient is dependent.

4) History (of)

There are two types of history Z codes, personal and family. Personal history codes explain a patient's past medical condition that no longer exists and is not receiving any treatment, but that has the potential for recurrence, and therefore may require continued monitoring.

Family history codes are for use when a patient has a family member(s) who has had a particular disease that causes the patient to be at higher risk of also contracting the disease.

Personal history codes may be used in conjunction with follow-up codes and family history codes may be used in conjunction with screening codes to explain the need for a test or procedure. History codes are also acceptable on any medical record regardless of the reason for visit. A history of an illness, even if no longer present, is important information that may alter the type of treatment ordered.

The history Z code categories are:

Z80	Family history of primary malignant neoplasm
Z81	Family history of mental and behavioral disorders
Z82	Family history of certain disabilities and chronic diseases (leading to disablement)
Z83	Family history of other specific disorders
Z84	Family history of other conditions
Z85	Personal history of malignant neoplasm
Z86	Personal history of certain other diseases
Z87	Personal history of other diseases and conditions
Z91.4-	Personal history of psychological trauma, not elsewhere classified
Z91.5	Personal history of self-harm
Z91.81	**History of falling**
Z91.82	**Personal history of military deployment**
Z92	Personal history of medical treatment Except: Z92.0, Personal history of contraception Except: Z92.82, Status post administration of tPA (rtPA) in a different facility within the last 24 hours prior to admission to a current facility

5) Screening

Screening is the testing for disease or disease precursors in seemingly well individuals so that early detection and treatment can be provided for those who test positive for the disease (e.g., screening mammogram).

The testing of a person to rule out or confirm a suspected diagnosis because the patient has some sign or symptom is a diagnostic examination, not a screening. In these cases, the sign or symptom is used to explain the reason for the test.

A screening code may be a first-listed code if the reason for the visit is specifically the screening exam. It may also be used as an additional code if the screening is done during an office visit for other health problems. A screening code is not necessary if the screening is inherent to a routine examination, such as a pap smear done during a routine pelvic examination.

Should a condition be discovered during the screening then the code for the condition may be assigned as an additional diagnosis.

The Z code indicates that a screening exam is planned. A procedure code is required to confirm that the screening was performed.

The screening Z codes/categories:

Z11	Encounter for screening for infectious and parasitic diseases
Z12	Encounter for screening for malignant neoplasms
Z13	Encounter for screening for other diseases and disorders Except: Z13.9, Encounter for screening, unspecified
Z36	Encounter for antenatal screening for mother

6) Observation

There are three observation Z code categories. They are for use in very limited circumstances when a person is being observed for a suspected condition that is ruled out. The observation codes are not for use if an injury or illness or any signs or symptoms related to the suspected condition are present. In such cases the diagnosis/symptom code is used with the corresponding external cause code.

The observation codes are to be used as principal diagnosis only. The only exception to this is when the principal diagnosis is required to be a code from category Z38, Liveborn infants according to place of birth and type of delivery. Then a code from category Z05, Encounter for observation and evaluation of newborn for suspected diseases and conditions ruled out, is sequenced after the Z38 code. Additional codes may be used in addition to the observation code, but only if they are unrelated to the suspected condition being observed.

Codes from subcategory Z03.7 Encounter for suspected maternal and fetal conditions ruled out, may either be used as a first-listed or as an additional code assignment depending on the case. They are for use in very limited circumstances on a maternal record when an encounter is for a suspected maternal or fetal condition that is ruled out during that encounter (for example, a maternal or fetal condition may be suspected due to an abnormal test result). These codes should not be used when the condition is confirmed. In those cases, the confirmed condition should be coded. In addition, these codes are not for use if an illness or any signs or symptoms related to the suspected condition or problem are present. In such cases the diagnosis/symptom code is used.

Additional codes may be used in addition to the code from subcategory Z03.7, but only if they are unrelated to the suspected condition being evaluated.

Codes from subcategory Z03.7 may not be used for encounters for antenatal screening of mother. *See Section I.C.21. Screening.*

For encounters for suspected fetal condition that are inconclusive following testing and evaluation, assign the appropriate code from category O35, O36, O40 or O41.

The observation Z code categories:

Z03 Encounter for medical observation for suspected diseases and conditions ruled out

Z04 Encounter for examination and observation for other reasons Except: Z04.9, Encounter for examination and observation for unspecified reason

Z05 Encounter for observation and evaluation of newborn for suspected diseases and conditions ruled out

7) Aftercare

Aftercare visit codes cover situations when the initial treatment of a disease has been performed and the patient requires continued care during the healing or recovery phase, or for the long-term consequences of the disease. The aftercare Z code should not be used if treatment is directed at a current, acute disease. The diagnosis code is to be used in these cases.

Exceptions to this rule are codes Z51.0, Encounter for antineoplastic radiation therapy, and codes from subcategory Z51.1, Encounter for antineoplastic chemotherapy and immunotherapy. These codes are to be first-listed, followed by the diagnosis code when a patient's encounter is solely to receive radiation therapy, chemotherapy, or immunotherapy for the treatment of a neoplasm. If the reason for the encounter is more than one type of antineoplastic therapy, code Z51.0 and a code from subcategory Z51.1 may be assigned together, in which case one of these codes would be reported as a secondary diagnosis.

The aftercare Z codes should also not be used for aftercare for injuries. For aftercare of an injury, assign the acute injury code with the appropriate 7th character (for subsequent encounter).

The aftercare codes are generally first-listed to explain the specific reason for the encounter. An aftercare code may be used as an additional code when some type of aftercare is provided in addition to the reason for admission and no diagnosis code is applicable. An example of this would be the closure of a colostomy during an encounter for treatment of another condition.

Aftercare codes should be used in conjunction with other aftercare codes or diagnosis codes to provide better detail on the specifics of an aftercare encounter visit, unless otherwise directed by the classification. Should a patient receive multiple types of antineoplastic therapy during the same encounter, code Z51.0, Encounter for antineoplastic radiation therapy, and codes from subcategory Z51.1, Encounter for antineoplastic chemotherapy and immunotherapy, may be used together on a record. The sequencing of multiple aftercare codes depends on the circumstances of the encounter.

Certain aftercare Z code categories need a secondary diagnosis code to describe the resolving condition or sequelae. For others, the condition is included in the code title.

Additional Z code aftercare category terms include fitting and adjustment, and attention to artificial openings.

Status Z codes may be used with aftercare Z codes to indicate the nature of the aftercare. For example code Z95.1, Presence of aortocoronary bypass graft, may be used with code Z48.812, Encounter for surgical aftercare following surgery on the circulatory system, to indicate the surgery for which the aftercare is being performed. A status code should not be used when the aftercare code indicates the type of status, such as using Z43.0, Encounter for attention to tracheostomy, with Z93.0, Tracheostomy status.

The aftercare Z category/codes:

Z42   Encounter for plastic and reconstructive surgery following medical procedure or healed injury

Z43   Encounter for attention to artificial openings

Z44   Encounter for fitting and adjustment of external prosthetic device

Z45   Encounter for adjustment and management of implanted device

Z46   Encounter for fitting and adjustment of other devices

Z47   Orthopedic aftercare

Z48   Encounter for other postprocedural aftercare

Z49   Encounter for care involving renal dialysis

Z51   Encounter for other aftercare and medical care

8) Follow-up

The follow-up codes are used to explain continuing surveillance following completed treatment of a disease, condition, or injury. They imply that the condition has been fully treated and no longer exists. They should not be confused with aftercare codes, or injury codes with a 7th character for subsequent encounter, that explain ongoing care of a healing condition or its sequelae. Follow-up codes may be used in conjunction with history codes to provide the full picture of the healed condition and its treatment. The follow-up code is sequenced first, followed by the history code.

A follow-up code may be used to explain multiple visits. Should a condition be found to have recurred on the follow-up visit, then the diagnosis code for the condition should be assigned in place of the follow-up code.

The follow-up Z code categories:

Z08   Encounter for follow-up examination after completed treatment for malignant neoplasm

Z09   Encounter for follow-up examination after completed treatment for conditions other than malignant neoplasm

Z39   Encounter for maternal postpartum care and examination

9) Donor

Codes in category Z52, Donors of organs and tissues, are used for living individuals who are donating blood or other body tissue. These codes are only for individuals donating for others, not for self-donations. They are not used to identify cadaveric donations.

10) Counseling

Counseling Z codes are used when a patient or family member receives assistance in the aftermath of an illness or injury, or when support is required in coping with family or social problems.

The counseling Z codes/categories:

Z30.0-   Encounter for general counseling and advice on contraception

Z31.5   Encounter for **procreative** genetic counseling

Z31.6-   Encounter for general counseling and advice on procreation

Z32.2   Encounter for childbirth instruction

Z32.3   Encounter for childcare instruction

Z69   Encounter for mental health services for victim and perpetrator of abuse

Z70   Counseling related to sexual attitude, behavior and orientation

Z71   Persons encountering health services for other counseling and medical advice, not elsewhere classified

Z76.81   Expectant mother prebirth pediatrician visit

11) Encounters for Obstetrical and Reproductive Services

See Section I.C.15. Pregnancy, Childbirth, and the Puerperium, for further instruction on the use of these codes.

Z codes for pregnancy are for use in those circumstances when none of the problems or complications included in the codes from the Obstetrics chapter exist (a routine prenatal visit or postpartum care). Codes in category Z34, Encounter for supervision of normal pregnancy, are always first listed and are not to be used with any other code from the OB chapter.

Codes in category Z3A, Weeks of gestation, may be assigned to provide additional information about the pregnancy. Category Z3A codes should not be assigned for pregnancies with abortive outcomes (categories O00-O08), elective termination of pregnancy (code **Z33.2**), nor for postpartum conditions, as category Z3A is not applicable to these conditions. The date of the admission should be used to determine weeks of gestation for inpatient admissions that encompass more than one gestational week.

The outcome of delivery, category Z37, should be included on all maternal delivery records. It is always a secondary code. Codes in category Z37 should not be used on the newborn record.

Z codes for family planning (contraceptive) or procreative management and counseling should be included on an obstetric record either during the pregnancy or the postpartum stage, if applicable.

Z codes/categories for obstetrical and reproductive services:

Z30   Encounter for contraceptive management

Z31   Encounter for procreative management

Z32.2   Encounter for childbirth instruction

Z32.3   Encounter for childcare instruction

Z33   Pregnant state

Z34   Encounter for supervision of normal pregnancy

Z36   Encounter for antenatal screening of mother

Z3A   Weeks of gestation

Z37   Outcome of delivery

Z39   Encounter for maternal postpartum care and examination

Z76.81   Expectant mother prebirth pediatrician visit

GUIDELINES (ICD-10-CM)

12) Newborns and Infants

See Section I.C.16. Newborn (Perinatal) Guidelines, for further instruction on the use of these codes.

Newborn Z codes/categories:

Z76.1 Encounter for health supervision and care of foundling

Z00.1- Encounter for routine child health examination

Z38 Liveborn infants according to place of birth and type of delivery

13) Routine and administrative examinations

The Z codes allow for the description of encounters for routine examinations, such as, a general check-up, or, examinations for administrative purposes, such as, a pre-employment physical. The codes are not to be used if the examination is for diagnosis of a suspected condition or for treatment purposes. In such cases the diagnosis code is used. During a routine exam, should a diagnosis or condition be discovered, it should be coded as an additional code. Pre-existing and chronic conditions and history codes may also be included as additional codes as long as the examination is for administrative purposes and not focused on any particular condition.

Some of the codes for routine health examinations distinguish between "with" and "without" abnormal findings. Code assignment depends on the information that is known at the time the encounter is being coded. For example, if no abnormal findings were found during the examination, but the encounter is being coded before test results are back, it is acceptable to assign the code for "without abnormal findings." When assigning a code for "with abnormal findings," additional code(s) should be assigned to identify the specific abnormal finding(s).

Pre-operative examination and pre-procedural laboratory examination Z codes are for use only in those situations when a patient is being cleared for a procedure or surgery and no treatment is given.

The Z codes/categories for routine and administrative examinations:

Z00 Encounter for general examination without complaint, suspected or reported diagnosis

Z01 Encounter for other special examination without complaint, suspected or reported diagnosis

Z02 Encounter for administrative examination
Except: Z02.9, Encounter for administrative examinations, unspecified

Z32.0- Encounter for pregnancy test

14) Miscellaneous Z codes

The miscellaneous Z codes capture a number of other health care encounters that do not fall into one of the other categories. Certain of these codes identify the reason for the encounter; others are for use as additional codes that provide useful information on circumstances that may affect a patient's care and treatment.

Prophylactic Organ Removal

For encounters specifically for prophylactic removal of an organ (such as prophylactic removal of breasts due to a genetic susceptibility to cancer or a family history of cancer), the principal or first-listed code should be a code from category Z40, Encounter for prophylactic surgery, followed by the appropriate codes to identify the associated risk factor (such as genetic susceptibility or family history).

If the patient has a malignancy of one site and is having prophylactic removal at another site to prevent either a new primary malignancy or metastatic disease, a code for the malignancy should also be assigned in addition to a code from subcategory Z40.0, Encounter for prophylactic surgery for risk factors related to malignant neoplasms. A Z40.0 code should not be assigned if the patient is having organ removal for treatment of a malignancy, such as the removal of the testes for the treatment of prostate cancer.

Miscellaneous Z codes/categories:

Z28 Immunization not carried out
Except: Z28.3, Underimmunization status

Z29 Encounter for other prophylactic measures

Z40 Encounter for prophylactic surgery

Z41 Encounter for procedures for purposes other than remedying health state
Except: Z41.9, Encounter for procedure for purposes other than remedying health state, unspecified

Z53 Persons encountering health services for specific procedures and treatment, not carried out

Z55 Problems related to education and literacy

Z56 Problems related to employment and unemployment

Z57 Occupational exposure to risk factors

Z58 Problems related to physical environment

Z59 Problems related to housing and economic circumstances

Z60 Problems related to social environment

Z62 Problems related to upbringing

Z63 Other problems related to primary support group, including family circumstances

Z64 Problems related to certain psychosocial circumstances

Z65 Problems related to other psychosocial circumstances

Z72 Problems related to lifestyle
Note: These codes should be assigned only when the documentation specifies that the patient has an associated problem

Z73 Problems related to life management difficulty

Z74 Problems related to care provider dependency Except: Z74.01, Bed confinement status

Z75   Problems related to medical facilities and other health care

Z76.0   Encounter for issue of repeat prescription

Z76.3   Healthy person accompanying sick person

Z76.4   Other boarder to healthcare facility

Z76.5   Malingerer [conscious simulation]

Z91.1-   Patient's noncompliance with medical treatment and regimen

Z91.83   Wandering in diseases classified elsewhere

Z91.84-   **Oral health risk factors**

Z91.89   Other specified personal risk factors, not elsewhere classified

15) Nonspecific Z codes

Certain Z codes are so non-specific, or potentially redundant with other codes in the classification, that there can be little justification for their use in the inpatient setting. Their use in the outpatient setting should be limited to those instances when there is no further documentation to permit more precise coding. Otherwise, any sign or symptom or any other reason for visit that is captured in another code should be used.

Nonspecific Z codes/categories:

Z02.9   Encounter for administrative examinations, unspecified

Z04.9   Encounter for examination and observation for unspecified reason

Z13.9   Encounter for screening, unspecified

Z41.9   Encounter for procedure for purposes other than remedying health state, unspecified

Z52.9   Donor of unspecified organ or tissue

Z86.59   Personal history of other mental and behavioral disorders

Z88.9   Allergy status to unspecified drugs, medicaments and biological substances status

Z92.0   Personal history of contraception

16) Z Codes That May Only be Principal/First-Listed Diagnosis

The following Z codes/categories may only be reported as the principal/first-listed diagnosis, except when there are multiple encounters on the same day and the medical records for the encounters are combined:

Z00   Encounter for general examination without complaint, suspected or reported diagnosis
Except: Z00.6

Z01   Encounter for other special examination without complaint, suspected or reported diagnosis

Z02   Encounter for administrative examination

Z03   Encounter for medical observation for suspected diseases and conditions ruled out

Z04   Encounter for examination and observation for other reasons

Z33.2   Encounter for elective termination of pregnancy

Z31.81   Encounter for male factor infertility in female patient

Z31.83   Encounter for assisted reproductive fertility procedure cycle

Z31.84   Encounter for fertility preservation procedure

Z34   Encounter for supervision of normal pregnancy

Z39   Encounter for maternal postpartum care and examination

Z38   Liveborn infants according to place of birth and type of delivery

Z40   **Encounter for prophylactic surgery**

Z42   Encounter for plastic and reconstructive surgery following medical procedure or healed injury

Z51.0   Encounter for antineoplastic radiation therapy

Z51.1-   Encounter for antineoplastic chemotherapy and immunotherapy

Z52   Donors of organs and tissues Except: Z52.9, Donor of unspecified organ or tissue

Z76.1   Encounter for health supervision and care of foundling

Z76.2   Encounter for health supervision and care of other healthy infant and child

Z99.12   Encounter for respirator [ventilator] dependence during power failure

Section II. Selection of Principal Diagnosis

The circumstances of inpatient admission always govern the selection of principal diagnosis. The principal diagnosis is defined in the Uniform Hospital Discharge Data Set (UHDDS) as "that condition established after study to be chiefly responsible for occasioning the admission of the patient to the hospital for care."

The UHDDS definitions are used by hospitals to report inpatient data elements in a standardized manner. These data elements and their definitions can be found in the July 31, 1985, Federal Register (Vol. 50, No, 147), pp. 31038-40.

Since that time the application of the UHDDS definitions has been expanded to include all nonoutpatient settings (acute care, short term, long term care and psychiatric hospitals; home health agencies; rehab facilities; nursing homes, etc). The UHDDS definitions also apply to hospice services (all levels of care).

In determining principal diagnosis, coding conventions in the ICD-10-CM, the Tabular List and Alphabetic Index take precedence over these official coding guidelines.
(See Section I.A., Conventions for the ICD-10-CM)

The importance of consistent, complete documentation in the medical record cannot be overemphasized. Without such documentation the application of all coding guidelines is a difficult, if not impossible, task.

A. Codes for symptoms, signs, and ill-defined conditions

Codes for symptoms, signs, and ill-defined conditions from Chapter 18 are not to be used as principal diagnosis when a related definitive diagnosis has been established.

B. Two or more interrelated conditions, each potentially meeting the definition for principal diagnosis.

When there are two or more interrelated conditions (such as diseases in the same ICD-10-CM chapter or manifestations characteristically associated with a certain disease) potentially meeting the definition of principal diagnosis, either condition may be sequenced first, unless the circumstances of the admission, the therapy provided, the Tabular List, or the Alphabetic Index indicate otherwise.

C. Two or more diagnoses that equally meet the definition for principal diagnosis

In the unusual instance when two or more diagnoses equally meet the criteria for principal diagnosis as determined by the circumstances of admission, diagnostic workup and/or therapy provided, and the Alphabetic Index, Tabular List, or another coding guidelines does not provide sequencing direction, any one of the diagnoses may be sequenced first.

D. Two or more comparative or contrasting conditions.

In those rare instances when two or more contrasting or comparative diagnoses are documented as "either/or" (or similar terminology), they are coded as if the diagnoses were confirmed and the diagnoses are sequenced according to the circumstances of the admission. If no further determination can be made as to which diagnosis should be principal, either diagnosis may be sequenced first.

E. A symptom(s) followed by contrasting/comparative diagnoses

GUIDELINE HAS BEEN DELETED EFFECTIVE OCTOBER 1, 2014

F. Original treatment plan not carried out

Sequence as the principal diagnosis the condition, which after study occasioned the admission to the hospital, even though treatment may not have been carried out due to unforeseen circumstances.

G. Complications of surgery and other medical care

When the admission is for treatment of a complication resulting from surgery or other medical care, the complication code is sequenced as the principal diagnosis. If the complication is classified to the T80-T88 series and the code lacks the necessary specificity in describing the complication, an additional code for the specific complication should be assigned.

H. Uncertain Diagnosis

If the diagnosis documented at the time of discharge is qualified as "probable", "suspected", "likely", "questionable", "possible", or "still to be ruled out", or other similar terms indicating uncertainty, code the condition as if it existed or was established. The bases for these guidelines are the diagnostic workup, arrangements for further workup or observation, and initial therapeutic approach that correspond most closely with the established diagnosis.

Note: This guideline is applicable only to inpatient admissions to short-term, acute, long-term care and psychiatric hospitals.

I. Admission from Observation Unit

1. Admission Following Medical Observation

When a patient is admitted to an observation unit for a medical condition, which either worsens or does not improve, and is subsequently admitted as an inpatient of the same hospital for this same medical condition, the principal diagnosis would be the medical condition which led to the hospital admission.

2. Admission Following Post-Operative Observation

When a patient is admitted to an observation unit to monitor a condition (or complication) that develops following outpatient surgery, and then is subsequently admitted as an inpatient of the same hospital, hospitals should apply the Uniform Hospital Discharge Data Set (UHDDS) definition of principal diagnosis as "that condition established after study to be chiefly responsible for occasioning the admission of the patient to the hospital for care."

J. Admission from Outpatient Surgery

When a patient receives surgery in the hospital's outpatient surgery department and is subsequently admitted for continuing inpatient care at the same hospital, the following guidelines should be followed in selecting the principal diagnosis for the inpatient admission:

- If the reason for the inpatient admission is a complication, assign the complication as the principal diagnosis.
- If no complication, or other condition, is documented as the reason for the inpatient admission, assign the reason for the outpatient surgery as the principal diagnosis.
- If the reason for the inpatient admission is another condition unrelated to the surgery, assign the unrelated condition as the principal diagnosis.

K. Admissions/Encounters for Rehabilitation

When the purpose for the admission/encounter is rehabilitation, sequence first the code for the condition for which the service is being performed. For example, for an admission/encounter for rehabilitation for right-sided dominant hemiplegia following a cerebrovascular infarction, report code I69.351, Hemiplegia and hemiparesis following cerebral infarction affecting right dominant side, as the first-listed or principal diagnosis.

If the condition for which the rehabilitation service is no longer present, report the appropriate aftercare code **as the first-listed or principal diagnosis, unless the rehabilitation service is being provided following an injury. For rehabilitation services following active treatment of an injury, assign the injury code with the appropriate seventh character for subsequent encounter** as the first-listed or principal diagnosis.

For example, if a patient with severe degenerative osteoarthritis of the hip, underwent hip replacement and the current encounter/admission is for rehabilitation, report code Z47.1, Aftercare following joint replacement surgery, as the first-listed or principal diagnosis. **If the patient requires rehabilitation post hip replacement for right intertrochanteric femur fracture, report code S72.141D, Displaced intertrochanteric fracture of right femur, subsequent encounter for closed fracture with routine healing, as the first-listed or principal diagnosis.**

See Section I.C.21.c.7, Factors influencing health states and contact with health services, Aftercare.

See Section I.C.19.a for additional information about the use of 7th characters for injury codes.

Section III. Reporting Additional Diagnoses

GENERAL RULES FOR OTHER (ADDITIONAL) DIAGNOSES

For reporting purposes the definition for "other diagnoses" is interpreted as additional conditions that affect patient care in terms of requiring:

clinical evaluation; or

therapeutic treatment; or

diagnostic procedures; or

extended length of hospital stay; or

increased nursing care and/or monitoring.

The UHDDS item #11-b defines Other Diagnoses as "all conditions that coexist at the time of admission, that develop subsequently, or that affect the treatment received and/or the length of stay. Diagnoses that relate to an earlier episode which have no bearing on the current hospital stay are to be excluded." UHDDS definitions apply to inpatients in acute care, short-term, long term care and psychiatric hospital setting. The UHDDS definitions are used by acute care short-term hospitals to report inpatient data elements in a standardized manner. These data elements and their definitions can be found in the July 31, 1985, Federal Register (Vol. 50, No, 147), pp. 31038-40.

Since that time the application of the UHDDS definitions has been expanded to include all nonoutpatient settings (acute care, short term, long term care and psychiatric hospitals; home health agencies; rehab facilities; nursing homes, etc). The UHDDS definitions also apply to hospice services (all levels of care).

The following guidelines are to be applied in designating "other diagnoses" when neither the Alphabetic Index nor the Tabular List in ICD-10-CM provide direction. The listing of the diagnoses in the patient record is the responsibility of the attending provider.

A. Previous conditions

If the provider has included a diagnosis in the final diagnostic statement, such as the discharge summary or the face sheet, it should ordinarily be coded. Some providers include in the diagnostic statement resolved conditions or diagnoses and status-post procedures from previous admission that have no bearing on the current stay. Such conditions are not to be reported and are coded only if required by hospital policy.

However, history codes (categories Z80-Z87) may be used as secondary codes if the historical condition or family history has an impact on current care or influences treatment.

B. Abnormal findings

Abnormal findings (laboratory, x-ray, pathologic, and other diagnostic results) are not coded and reported unless the provider indicates their clinical significance. If the findings are outside the normal range and the attending provider has ordered other tests to evaluate the condition or prescribed treatment, it is appropriate to ask the provider whether the abnormal finding should be added.

Please note: This differs from the coding practices in the outpatient setting for coding encounters for diagnostic tests that have been interpreted by a provider.

C. Uncertain Diagnosis

If the diagnosis documented at the time of discharge is qualified as "probable", "suspected", "likely", "questionable", "possible", or "still to be ruled out" or other similar terms indicating uncertainty, code the condition as if it existed or was established. The bases for these guidelines are the diagnostic workup, arrangements for further workup or observation, and initial therapeutic approach that correspond most closely with the established diagnosis.

Note: This guideline is applicable only to inpatient admissions to short-term, acute, long-term care and psychiatric hospitals.

Section IV. Diagnostic Coding and Reporting Guidelines for Outpatient Services

These coding guidelines for outpatient diagnoses have been approved for use by hospitals/ providers in coding and reporting hospital-based outpatient services and provider-based office visits. Guidelines in Section I, Conventions, general coding guidelines and chapter-specific guidelines, should also be applied for outpatient services and office visits.

Information about the use of certain abbreviations, punctuation, symbols, and other conventions used in the ICD-10-CM Tabular List (code numbers and titles), can be found in Section IA of these guidelines, under "Conventions Used in the Tabular List." Section I.B. contains general guidelines that apply to the entire classification. Section I.C. contains chapter-specific guidelines that correspond to the chapters as they are arranged in the classification. Information about the correct sequence to use in finding a code is also described in Section I.

The terms encounter and visit are often used interchangeably in describing outpatient service contacts and, therefore, appear together in these guidelines without distinguishing one from the other.

Though the conventions and general guidelines apply to all settings, coding guidelines for outpatient and provider reporting of diagnoses will vary in a number of instances from those for inpatient diagnoses, recognizing that:

The Uniform Hospital Discharge Data Set (UHDDS) definition of principal diagnosis does not apply to hospital-based outpatient services and provider-based office visits.

Coding guidelines for inconclusive diagnoses (probable, suspected, rule out, etc.) were developed for inpatient reporting and do not apply to outpatients.

A. Selection of first-listed condition
In the outpatient setting, the term first-listed diagnosis is used in lieu of principal diagnosis.

In determining the first-listed diagnosis the coding conventions of ICD-10-CM, as well as the general and disease specific guidelines take precedence over the outpatient guidelines.

Diagnoses often are not established at the time of the initial encounter/visit. It may take two or more visits before the diagnosis is confirmed.

The most critical rule involves beginning the search for the correct code assignment through the Alphabetic Index. Never begin searching initially in the Tabular List as this will lead to coding errors.

1. Outpatient Surgery
When a patient presents for outpatient surgery (same day surgery), code the reason for the surgery as the first-listed diagnosis (reason for the encounter), even if the surgery is not performed due to a contraindication.

2. Observation Stay
When a patient is admitted for observation for a medical condition, assign a code for the medical condition as the first-listed diagnosis.

When a patient presents for outpatient surgery and develops complications requiring admission to observation, code the reason for the surgery as the first reported diagnosis (reason for the encounter), followed by codes for the complications as secondary diagnoses.

B. Codes from A00.0 through T88.9, Z00-Z99
The appropriate code(s) from A00.0 through T88.9, Z00-Z99 must be used to identify diagnoses, symptoms, conditions, problems, complaints, or other reason(s) for the encounter/visit.

C. Accurate reporting of ICD-10-CM diagnosis codes
For accurate reporting of ICD-10-CM diagnosis codes, the documentation should describe the patient's condition, using terminology which includes specific diagnoses as well as symptoms, problems, or reasons for the encounter. There are ICD-10-CM codes to describe all of these.

D. Codes that describe symptoms and signs
Codes that describe symptoms and signs, as opposed to diagnoses, are acceptable for reporting purposes when a diagnosis has not been established (confirmed) by the provider. Chapter 18 of ICD-10-CM, Symptoms, Signs, and Abnormal Clinical and Laboratory Findings Not Elsewhere Classified (codes R00-R99) contain many, but not all codes for symptoms.

E. Encounters for circumstances other than a disease or injury
ICD-10-CM provides codes to deal with encounters for circumstances other than a disease or injury. The Factors Influencing Health Status and Contact with Health Services codes (Z00-Z99) are provided to deal with occasions when circumstances other than a disease or injury are recorded as diagnosis or problems.

See Section I.C.21. Factors influencing health status and contact with health services.

F. Level of Detail in Coding
1. ICD-10-CM codes with 3, 4, 5, 6 or 7 characters
ICD-10-CM is composed of codes with 3, 4, 5, 6 or 7 characters. Codes with three characters are included in ICD-10-CM as the heading of a category of codes that may be further subdivided by the use of fourth, fifth, sixth or seventh characters to provide greater specificity.

2. Use of full number of characters required for a code
A three-character code is to be used only if it is not further subdivided. A code is invalid if it has not been coded to the full number of characters required for that code, including the 7th character, if applicable.

G. ICD-10-CM code for the diagnosis, condition, problem, or other reason for encounter/visit
List first the ICD-10-CM code for the diagnosis, condition, problem, or other reason for encounter/visit shown in the medical record to be chiefly responsible for the services provided. List additional codes that describe any coexisting conditions. In some cases the first-listed diagnosis may be a symptom when a diagnosis has not been established (confirmed) by the physician.

H. Uncertain diagnosis
Do not code diagnoses documented as "probable", "suspected," "questionable," "rule out," or "working diagnosis" or other similar terms indicating uncertainty. Rather, code the condition(s) to the highest degree of certainty for that encounter/visit, such as symptoms, signs, abnormal test results, or other reason for the visit.

Please note: This differs from the coding practices used by short-term, acute care, long-term care and psychiatric hospitals.

I. Chronic diseases
Chronic diseases treated on an ongoing basis may be coded and reported as many times as the patient receives treatment and care for the condition(s)

J. Code all documented conditions that coexist
Code all documented conditions that coexist at the time of the encounter/visit, and require or affect patient care treatment or management. Do not code conditions that were previously treated and no longer exist. However, history codes (categories Z80-Z87) may be used as secondary codes if the historical condition or family history has an impact on current care or influences treatment.

K. Patients receiving diagnostic services only

For patients receiving diagnostic services only during an encounter/visit, sequence first the diagnosis, condition, problem, or other reason for encounter/visit shown in the medical record to be chiefly responsible for the outpatient services provided during the encounter/visit. Codes for other diagnoses (e.g., chronic conditions) may be sequenced as additional diagnoses.

For encounters for routine laboratory/radiology testing in the absence of any signs, symptoms, or associated diagnosis, assign Z01.89, Encounter for other specified special examinations. If routine testing is performed during the same encounter as a test to evaluate a sign, symptom, or diagnosis, it is appropriate to assign both the Z code and the code describing the reason for the non-routine test.

For outpatient encounters for diagnostic tests that have been interpreted by a physician, and the final report is available at the time of coding, code any confirmed or definitive diagnosis(es) documented in the interpretation. Do not code related signs and symptoms as additional diagnoses.

Please note: This differs from the coding practice in the hospital inpatient setting regarding abnormal findings on test results.

L. Patients receiving therapeutic services only

For patients receiving therapeutic services only during an encounter/visit, sequence first the diagnosis, condition, problem, or other reason for encounter/visit shown in the medical record to be chiefly responsible for the outpatient services provided during the encounter/visit. Codes for other diagnoses (e.g., chronic conditions) may be sequenced as additional diagnoses.

The only exception to this rule is that when the primary reason for the admission/encounter is chemotherapy or radiation therapy, the appropriate Z code for the service is listed first, and the diagnosis or problem for which the service is being performed listed second.

M. Patients receiving preoperative evaluations only

For patients receiving preoperative evaluations only, sequence first a code from subcategory Z01.81, Encounter for pre-procedural examinations, to describe the pre-op consultations. Assign a code for the condition to describe the reason for the surgery as an additional diagnosis. Code also any findings related to the pre-op evaluation.

N. Ambulatory surgery

For ambulatory surgery, code the diagnosis for which the surgery was performed. If the postoperative diagnosis is known to be different from the preoperative diagnosis at the time the diagnosis is confirmed, select the postoperative diagnosis for coding, since it is the most definitive.

O. Routine outpatient prenatal visits

See Section I.C.15. Routine outpatient prenatal visits.

P. Encounters for general medical examinations with abnormal findings

The subcategories for encounters for general medical examinations, Z00.0- **and encounter for routine child health examination, Z00.12-,** provide codes for with and without abnormal findings. Should a general medical examination result in an abnormal finding, the code for general medical examination with abnormal finding should be assigned as the first-listed diagnosis. An examination with abnormal findings refers to a condition/diagnosis that is newly identified or a change in severity of a chronic condition (such as uncontrolled hypertension, or an acute exacerbation of chronic obstructive pulmonary disease) during a routine physical examination. A secondary code for the abnormal finding should also be coded.

Q. Encounters for routine health screenings

See Section I.C.21. Factors influencing health status and contact with health services, Screening

Appendix I
Present on Admission Reporting Guidelines

Introduction

These guidelines are to be used as a supplement to the *ICD-10-CM Official Guidelines for Coding and Reporting* to facilitate the assignment of the Present on Admission (POA) indicator for each diagnosis and external cause of injury code reported on claim forms (UB-04 and 837 Institutional).

These guidelines are not intended to replace any guidelines in the main body of the *ICD-10-CM Official Guidelines for Coding and Reporting*. The POA guidelines are not intended to provide guidance on when a condition should be coded, but rather, how to apply the POA indicator to the final set of diagnosis codes that have been assigned in accordance with Sections I, II, and III of the official coding guidelines. Subsequent to the assignment of the ICD-10-CM codes, the POA indicator should then be assigned to those conditions that have been coded.

As stated in the Introduction to the ICD-10-CM Official Guidelines for Coding and Reporting, a joint effort between the healthcare provider and the coder is essential to achieve complete and accurate documentation, code assignment, and reporting of diagnoses and procedures. The importance of consistent, complete documentation in the medical record cannot be overemphasized. Medical record documentation from any provider involved in the care and treatment of the patient may be used to support the determination of whether a condition was present on admission or not. In the context of the official coding guidelines, the term "provider" means a physician or any qualified healthcare practitioner who is legally accountable for establishing the patient's diagnosis.

These guidelines are not a substitute for the provider's clinical judgment as to the determination of whether a condition was/was not present on admission. The provider should be queried regarding issues related to the linking of signs/symptoms, timing of test results, and the timing of findings.

Please see the CDC website for the detailed list of ICD-10-CM codes that do not require the use of a POA indicator **(https://www.cdc.gov/nchs/icd/icd10cm.htm)** **(https://www.cms.gov/Medicare/Coding/ICD10/2018-ICD-10-CM-and-GEMs.html)**. The **codes and categories** on this exempt list **are** for circumstances regarding the healthcare encounter or factors influencing health status that do not represent a current disease or injury or **that describe conditions that** are always present on admission.

General Reporting Requirements

All claims involving inpatient admissions to general acute care hospitals or other facilities that are subject to a law or regulation mandating collection of present on admission information.

Present on admission is defined as present at the time the order for inpatient admission occurs—conditions that develop during an outpatient encounter, including emergency department, observation, or outpatient surgery, are considered as present on admission.

POA indicator is assigned to principal and secondary diagnoses (as defined in Section II of the Official Guidelines for Coding and Reporting) and the external cause of injury codes.

Issues related to inconsistent, missing, conflicting or unclear documentation must still be resolved by the provider.

If a condition would not be coded and reported based on UHDDS definitions and current official coding guidelines, then the POA indicator would not be reported.

Reporting Options

Y - Yes

N - No

U - Unknown

W - Clinically undetermined

Unreported/Not used - (Exempt from POA reporting)

Reporting Definitions

Y = present at the time of inpatient admission

N = not present at the time of inpatient admission

U = documentation is insufficient to determine if condition is present on admission

W = provider is unable to clinically determine whether condition was present on admission or not

Timeframe for POA Identification and Documentation

There is no required timeframe as to when a provider (per the definition of "provider" used in these guidelines) must identify or document a condition to be present on admission. In some clinical situations, it may not be possible for a provider to make a definitive diagnosis (or a condition may not be recognized or reported by the patient) for a period of time after admission. In some cases it may be several days before the provider arrives at a definitive diagnosis. This does not mean that the condition was not present on admission. Determination of whether the condition was present on admission or not will be based on the applicable POA guideline as identified in this document, or on the provider's best clinical judgment.

If at the time of code assignment the documentation is unclear as to whether a condition was present on admission or not, it is appropriate to query the provider for clarification.

Assigning the POA Indicator

Condition is on the "Exempt from Reporting" list

Leave the "present on admission" field blank if the condition is on the list of ICD-10-CM codes for which this field is not applicable. This is the only circumstance in which the field may be left blank.

POA Explicitly Documented

Assign Y for any condition the provider explicitly documents as being present on admission.

Assign N for any condition the provider explicitly documents as not present at the time of admission.

Conditions diagnosed prior to inpatient admission

Assign "Y" for conditions that were diagnosed prior to admission (example: hypertension, diabetes mellitus, asthma)

Conditions diagnosed during the admission but clearly present before admission

Assign "Y" for conditions diagnosed during the admission that were clearly present but not diagnosed until after admission occurred.

Diagnoses subsequently confirmed after admission are considered present on admission if at the time of admission they are documented as suspected, possible, rule out, differential diagnosis, or constitute an underlying cause of a symptom that is present at the time of admission.

Condition develops during outpatient encounter prior to inpatient admission

Assign Y for any condition that develops during an outpatient encounter prior to a written order for inpatient admission.

Documentation does not indicate whether condition was present on admission

Assign "U" when the medical record documentation is unclear as to whether the condition was present on admission. "U" should not be routinely assigned and used only in very limited circumstances. Coders are encouraged to query the providers when the documentation is unclear.

Documentation states that it cannot be determined whether the condition was or was not present on admission

Assign "W" when the medical record documentation indicates that it cannot be clinically determined whether or not the condition was present on admission.

Chronic condition with acute exacerbation during the admission

If a single code identifies both the chronic condition and the acute exacerbation, see POA guidelines pertaining to codes that contain multiple clinical concepts.

If a single code only identifies the chronic condition and not the acute exacerbation (e.g., acute exacerbation of chronic leukemia), assign "Y."

Conditions documented as possible, probable, suspected, or rule out at the time of discharge

If the final diagnosis contains a possible, probable, suspected, or rule out diagnosis, and this diagnosis was based on signs, symptoms or clinical findings suspected at the time of inpatient admission, assign "Y."

If the final diagnosis contains a possible, probable, suspected, or rule out diagnosis, and this diagnosis was based on signs, symptoms or clinical findings that were not present on admission, assign "N".

Conditions documented as impending or threatened at the time of discharge

If the final diagnosis contains an impending or threatened diagnosis, and this diagnosis is based on symptoms or clinical findings that were present on admission, assign "Y".

If the final diagnosis contains an impending or threatened diagnosis, and this diagnosis is based on symptoms or clinical findings that were not present on admission, assign "N".

Acute and Chronic Conditions

Assign "Y" for acute conditions that are present at time of admission and N for acute conditions that are not present at time of admission.

Assign "Y" for chronic conditions, even though the condition may not be diagnosed until after admission.

If a single code identifies both an acute and chronic condition, see the POA guidelines for codes that contain multiple clinical concepts.

Codes That Contain Multiple Clinical Concepts

Assign "N" if at least one of the clinical concepts included in the code was not present on admission (e.g., COPD with acute exacerbation and the exacerbation was not present on admission; gastric ulcer that does not start bleeding until after admission; asthma patient develops status asthmaticus after admission).

Assign "Y" if all of the clinical concepts included in the code were present on admission (e.g., duodenal ulcer that perforates prior to admission).

For infection codes that include the causal organism, assign "Y" if the infection (or signs of the infection) were present on admission, even though the culture results may not be known until after admission (e.g., patient is admitted with pneumonia and the provider documents Pseudomonas as the causal organism a few days later).

Same Diagnosis Code for Two or More Conditions

When the same ICD-10-CM diagnosis code applies to two or more conditions during the same encounter (e.g. two separate conditions classified to the same ICD-10-CM diagnosis code):

Assign "Y" if all conditions represented by the single ICD-10-CM code were present on admission (e.g. bilateral unspecified age-related cataracts).

Assign "N" if any of the conditions represented by the single ICD-10-CM code was not present on admission (e.g. traumatic secondary and recurrent hemorrhage and seroma is assigned to a single code T79.2, but only one of the conditions was present on admission).

Obstetrical conditions

Whether or not the patient delivers during the current hospitalization does not affect assignment of the POA indicator. The determining factor for POA assignment is whether the pregnancy complication or obstetrical condition described by the code was present at the time of admission or not.

If the pregnancy complication or obstetrical condition was present on admission (e.g., patient admitted in preterm labor), assign "Y".

If the pregnancy complication or obstetrical condition was not present on admission (e.g., 2nd degree laceration during delivery, postpartum hemorrhage that occurred during current hospitalization, fetal distress develops after admission), assign "N".

If the obstetrical code includes more than one diagnosis and any of the diagnoses identified by the code were not present on admission assign "N".

(e.g., Category O11, Pre-existing hypertension with pre-eclampsia)

Perinatal conditions

Newborns are not considered to be admitted until after birth. Therefore, any condition present at birth or that developed in utero is considered present at admission and should be assigned "Y". This includes conditions that occur during delivery (e.g., injury during delivery, meconium aspiration, exposure to streptococcus B in the vaginal canal).

Congenital conditions and anomalies

Assign "Y" for congenital conditions and anomalies except for categories Q00-Q99, Congenital anomalies, which are on the exempt list. Congenital conditions are always considered present on admission.

External cause of injury codes

Assign "Y" for any external cause code representing an external cause of morbidity that occurred prior to inpatient admission (e.g., patient fell out of bed at home, patient fell out of bed in emergency room prior to admission).

Assign "N" for any external cause code representing an external cause of morbidity that occurred during inpatient hospitalization (e.g., patient fell out of hospital bed during hospital stay, patient experienced an adverse reaction to a medication administered after inpatient admission).

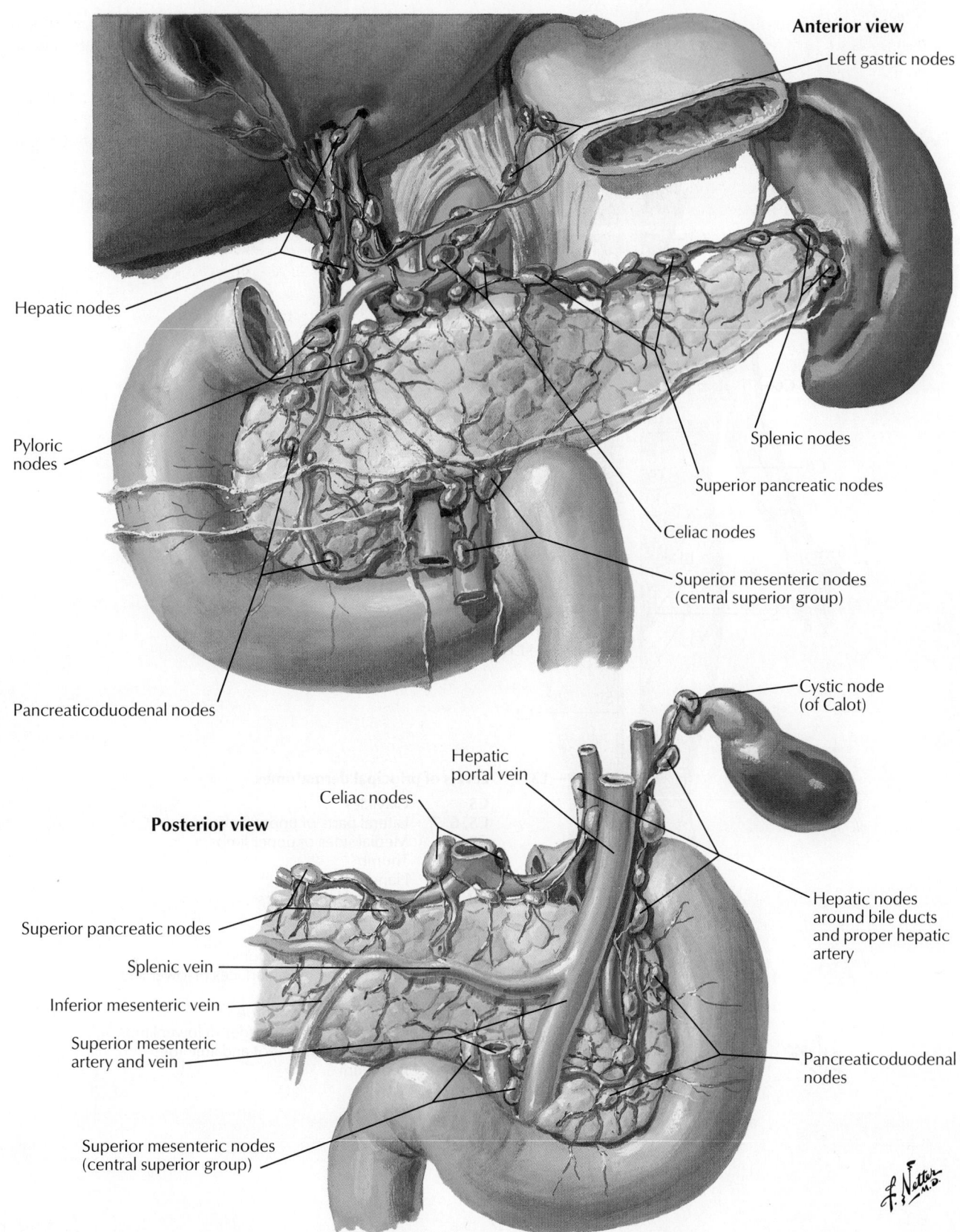

Anterior view

Left gastric nodes

Hepatic nodes

Pyloric nodes

Pancreaticoduodenal nodes

Splenic nodes

Superior pancreatic nodes

Celiac nodes

Superior mesenteric nodes (central superior group)

Cystic node (of Calot)

Posterior view

Hepatic portal vein

Celiac nodes

Superior pancreatic nodes

Splenic vein

Inferior mesenteric vein

Superior mesenteric artery and vein

Superior mesenteric nodes (central superior group)

Hepatic nodes around bile ducts and proper hepatic artery

Pancreaticoduodenal nodes

Plate 315 Lymph Vessels and Nodes of Pancreas. (Netter: Atlas of Human Anatomy, 4 ed, 2006, Saunders.)

Dermatome pattern

Levels of principal dermatomes

C5	Clavicles
C5, 6, 7	Lateral parts of upper limbs
C8; T1	Medial sides of upper limbs
C6	Thumb
C6, 7, 8	Hand
C8	Ring and little fingers
T4	Level of nipples
T10	Level of umbilicus
T12	Inguinal or groin regions
L1, 2, 3, 4	Anterior and inner surfaces of lower limbs
L4, 5; S1	Foot
L4	Medial side of great toe
L5; S1, 2	Outer and posterior sides of lower limbs
S1	Lateral margin of foot and little toe
S2, 3, 4	Perineum

Plate 164 Dermatomes. (Netter: Atlas of Human Anatomy, 4 ed, 2006, Saunders.)

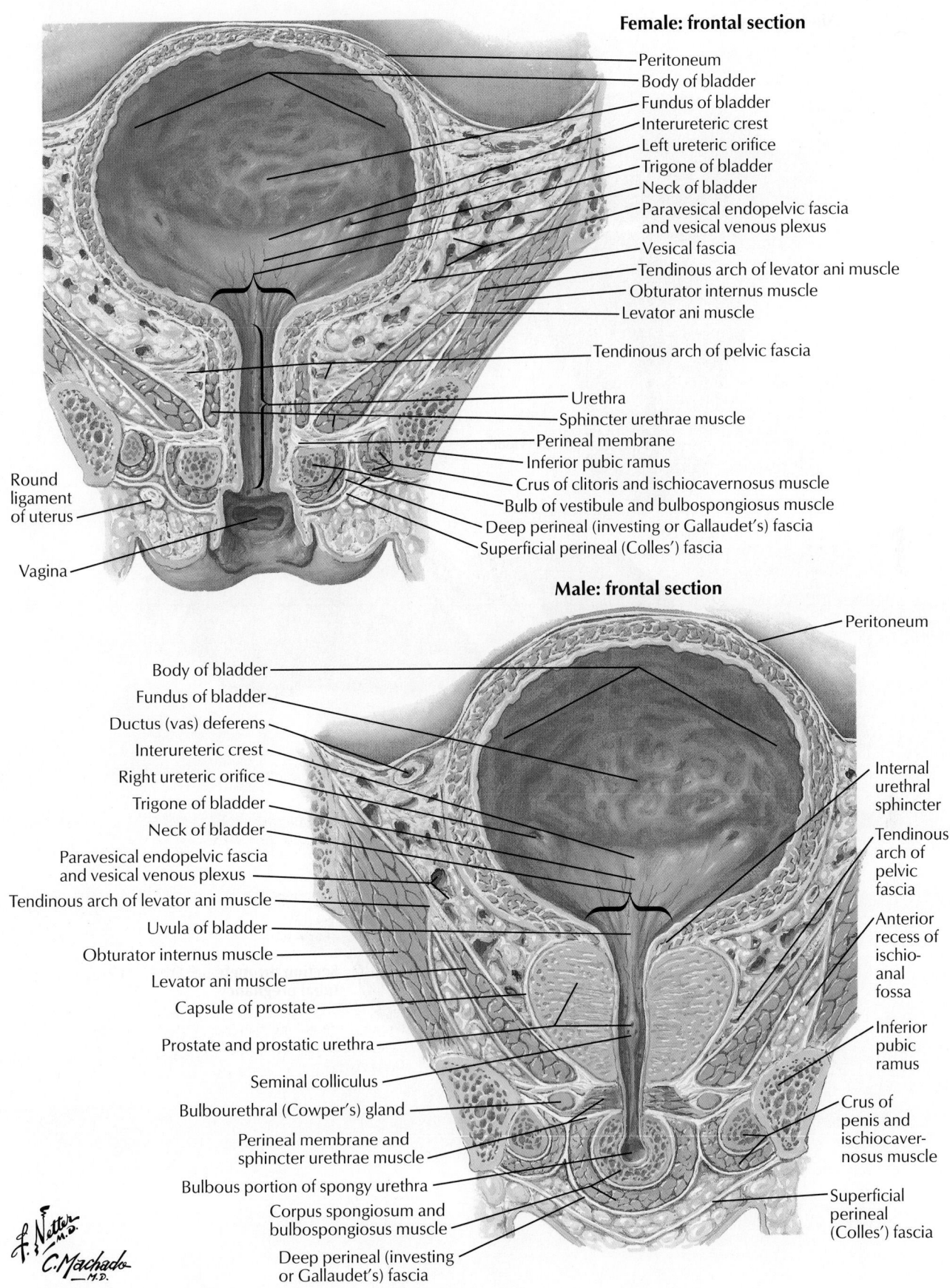

Female: frontal section

- Peritoneum
- Body of bladder
- Fundus of bladder
- Interureteric crest
- Left ureteric orifice
- Trigone of bladder
- Neck of bladder
- Paravesical endopelvic fascia and vesical venous plexus
- Vesical fascia
- Tendinous arch of levator ani muscle
- Obturator internus muscle
- Levator ani muscle
- Tendinous arch of pelvic fascia
- Urethra
- Sphincter urethrae muscle
- Perineal membrane
- Inferior pubic ramus
- Crus of clitoris and ischiocavernosus muscle
- Bulb of vestibule and bulbospongiosus muscle
- Deep perineal (investing or Gallaudet's) fascia
- Superficial perineal (Colles') fascia

Round ligament of uterus

Vagina

Male: frontal section

- Body of bladder
- Fundus of bladder
- Ductus (vas) deferens
- Interureteric crest
- Right ureteric orifice
- Trigone of bladder
- Neck of bladder
- Paravesical endopelvic fascia and vesical venous plexus
- Tendinous arch of levator ani muscle
- Uvula of bladder
- Obturator internus muscle
- Levator ani muscle
- Capsule of prostate
- Prostate and prostatic urethra
- Seminal colliculus
- Bulbourethral (Cowper's) gland
- Perineal membrane and sphincter urethrae muscle
- Bulbous portion of spongy urethra
- Corpus spongiosum and bulbospongiosus muscle
- Deep perineal (investing or Gallaudet's) fascia

- Peritoneum
- Internal urethral sphincter
- Tendinous arch of pelvic fascia
- Anterior recess of ischio-anal fossa
- Inferior pubic ramus
- Crus of penis and ischiocavernosus muscle
- Superficial perineal (Colles') fascia

Plate 366 Urinary Bladder: Female and Male. (Netter: Atlas of Human Anatomy, 4 ed, 2006, Saunders.)

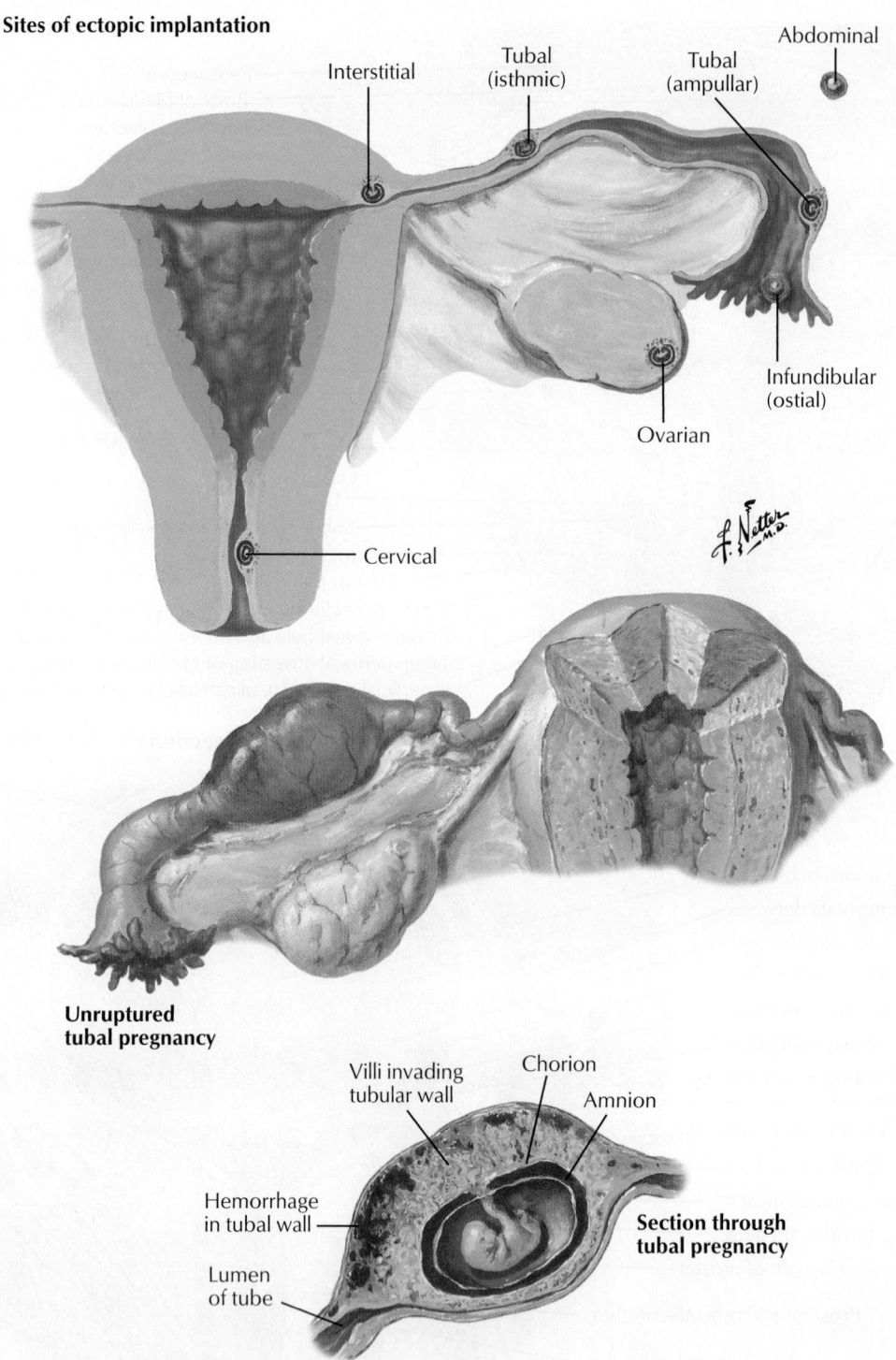

Sites of ectopic implantation

Interstitial

Tubal (isthmic)

Tubal (ampullar)

Abdominal

Infundibular (ostial)

Ovarian

Cervical

Unruptured tubal pregnancy

Villi invading tubular wall

Chorion

Amnion

Hemorrhage in tubal wall

Lumen of tube

Section through tubal pregnancy

Plate 375   Ectopic Pregnancy. (Netter: Atlas of Human Anatomy, 4 ed, 2006, Saunders.)

Skin of penis

Superficial fascia of penis (Colles' fascia)

Deep (Buck's) fascia of penis

Testicular artery

Ductus deferens

Artery to ductus deferens

Genital branch of genitofemoral nerve

Pampiniform (venous) plexus

Epididymis

Appendix of epididymis

Appendix of testis

Testis (covered by visceral layer of tunica vaginalis)

Parietal layer of tunica vaginalis

Superficial inguinal ring

External spermatic fascia

Cremaster muscle and fascia

Septum of scrotum (formed by dartos fascia)

Superficial (dartos) fascia of scrotum

Skin of scrotum

Superficial (dartos) fascia of scrotum

External spermatic fascia

Cremaster muscle and fascia

Internal spermatic fascia

Parietal layer of tunica vaginalis

Epididymis

Testis (covered by visceral layer of tunica vaginalis)

Skin of scrotum

Plate 387 Scrotum and Contents. (Netter: Atlas of Human Anatomy, 4 ed, 2006, Saunders.)

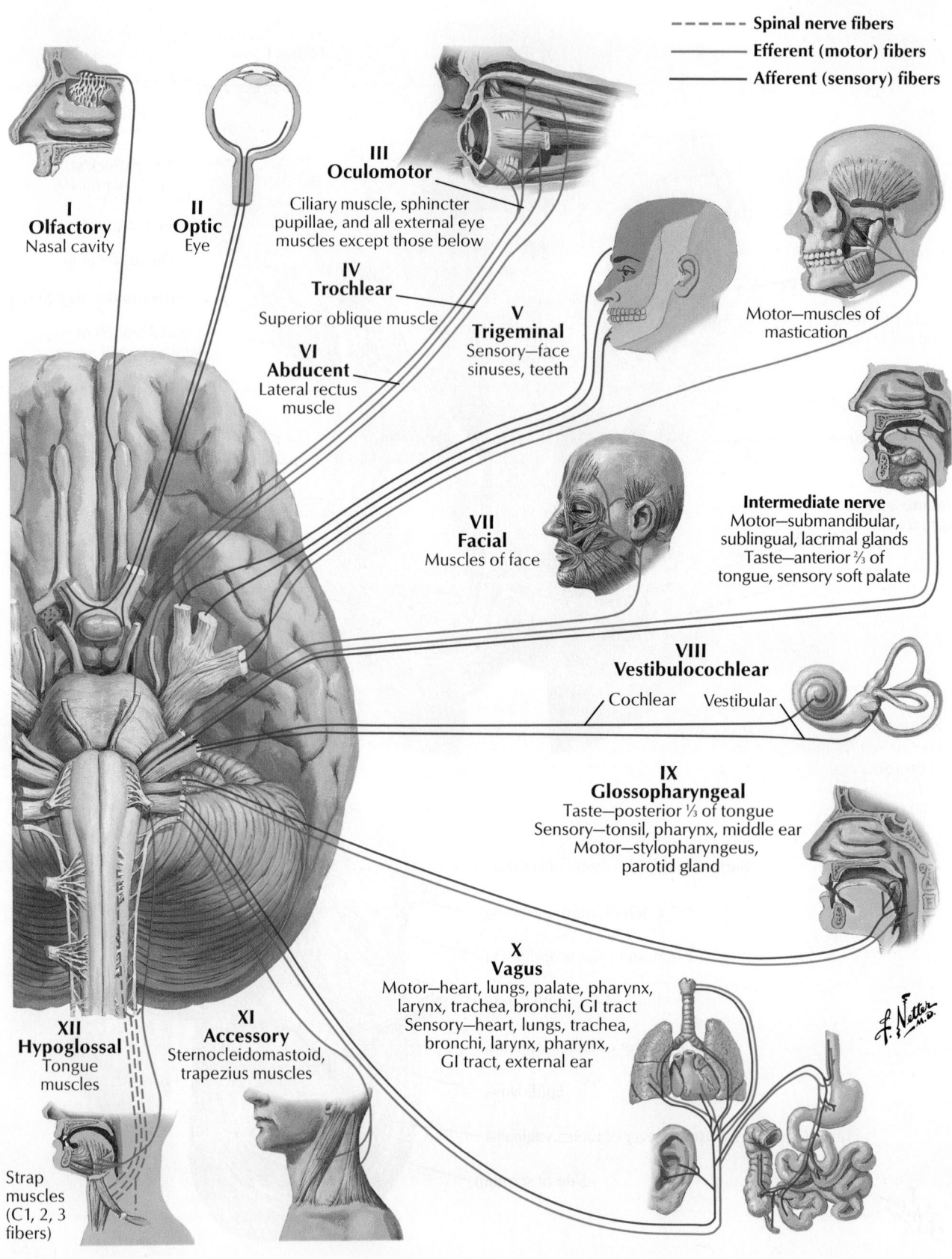

---- Spinal nerve fibers
—— Efferent (motor) fibers
—— Afferent (sensory) fibers

I
Olfactory
Nasal cavity

II
Optic
Eye

III
Oculomotor
Ciliary muscle, sphincter pupillae, and all external eye muscles except those below

IV
Trochlear
Superior oblique muscle

V
Trigeminal
Sensory—face sinuses, teeth

VI
Abducent
Lateral rectus muscle

Motor—muscles of mastication

VII
Facial
Muscles of face

Intermediate nerve
Motor—submandibular, sublingual, lacrimal glands
Taste—anterior ⅔ of tongue, sensory soft palate

VIII
Vestibulocochlear
Cochlear   Vestibular

IX
Glossopharyngeal
Taste—posterior ⅓ of tongue
Sensory—tonsil, pharynx, middle ear
Motor—stylopharyngeus, parotid gland

X
Vagus
Motor—heart, lungs, palate, pharynx, larynx, trachea, bronchi, GI tract
Sensory—heart, lungs, trachea, bronchi, larynx, pharynx, GI tract, external ear

XII
Hypoglossal
Tongue muscles

XI
Accessory
Sternocleidomastoid, trapezius muscles

Strap muscles (C1, 2, 3 fibers)

f. Netter M.D.

Plate 118 Cranial Nerves (Motor and Sensory Distribution): Schema. (Netter: Atlas of Human Anatomy, 4 ed, 2006, Saunders.)

Superior view

Supratrochlear nerve

Medial rectus muscle

Superior oblique muscle

Infratrochlear nerve

Nasociliary nerve

Trochlear nerve (IV)

Common tendinous ring

Ophthalmic nerve (V₁)

Optic nerve (II)

Internal carotid artery and nerve plexus

Oculomotor nerve (III)

Trochlear nerve (IV)

Abducent nerve (VI)

Tentorium cerebelli

Medial branch } Supraorbital nerve
Lateral branch

Levator palpebrae superioris muscle

Superior rectus muscle

Lacrimal gland

Lacrimal nerve

Lateral rectus muscle

Frontal nerve

Maxillary nerve (V₂)

Meningeal branch of maxillary nerve

Mandibular nerve (V₃)

Lesser petrosal nerve

Meningeal branch of mandibular nerve

Greater petrosal nerve

Trigeminal (semilunar) ganglion

Tentorial (meningeal) branch of ophthalmic nerve

Superior view:
levator palpebrae superioris, superior rectus, and superior oblique muscles partially cut away

Supratrochlear nerve *(cut)*

Supraorbital nerve branches *(cut)*

Infratrochlear nerve

Anterior ethmoidal nerve

Optic nerve (II)

Posterior ethmoidal nerve

Superior branch of oculomotor nerve (III) *(cut)*

Nasociliary nerve

Internal carotid plexus

Trochlear nerve (IV) *(cut)*

Oculomotor nerve (III)

Abducent nerve (VI)

Long ciliary nerves

Short ciliary nerves

Lacrimal nerve

Ciliary ganglion

Parasympathetic root of ciliary ganglion (from inferior branch of oculomotor nerve)

Sympathetic root of ciliary ganglion (from internal carotid plexus)

Sensory root of ciliary ganglion (from nasociliary nerve)

Branches to inferior and medial rectus muscles

Abducent nerve (VI)

Inferior branch of oculomotor nerve (III)

Lacrimal nerve

Frontal nerve *(cut)*

Ophthalmic nerve (V₁)

Plate 86 Nerves of Orbit. (Netter: Atlas of Human Anatomy, 4 ed, 2006, Saunders.)

Anterior (palmar) view

Musculocutaneous nerve { Lateral antebrachial cutaneous nerve }

Medial antebrachial cutaneous nerve

Radial nerve { Superficial branch }

Palmar branch

Ulnar nerve

Palmar digital branches

Median nerve { Palmar branch / Palmar digital branches }

Posterior (dorsal) view

Lateral antebrachial cutaneous nerve } **Musculocutaneous nerve**

Medial antebrachial cutaneous nerve

Posterior antebrachial cutaneous nerve

Division between ulnar and radial nerve innervation on dorsum of hand is variable.

Radial nerve

Dorsal branch and dorsal digital branches

Superficial branch and dorsal digital branches

Ulnar nerve

Proper palmar digital branches

Proper palmar digital branches } **Median nerve**

Plate 472 Cutaneous Innervation of Wrist and Hand. (Netter: Atlas of Human Anatomy, 4 ed, 2006, Saunders.)

Anterior view

Deltoid muscle

Coracobrachialis muscle

Biceps brachii muscle { Short head (*cut*)
Long head (*cut*)

Musculocutaneous nerve

Brachialis muscle

Biceps brachii muscle (*cut*) and tendon

Lateral antebrachial cutaneous nerve (from musculocutaneous nerve)

Radial nerve { Deep branch
Superficial branch

Supinator muscle

Brachioradialis muscle

Radial artery

Pronator teres muscle (*partially cut*)

Median nerve

Flexor pollicis longus muscle

Flexor carpi radialis tendon (*cut*)

Flexor retinaculum (transverse carpal ligament)

Superficial branch of radial nerve

Recurrent (motor) branch of median nerve to thenar muscles

Common palmar digital branches of median nerve

Proper palmar digital branches of median nerve

Intercostobrachial nerve

Medial brachial cutaneous nerve

Radial nerve

Ulnar nerve

Medial antebrachial cutaneous nerve

Median nerve

Brachial artery

Bicipital aponeurosis

Humeral head (*cut*) } Pronator teres muscle
Ulnar head

Flexor carpi radialis muscle (*cut*)

Humeroulnar head } Flexor digitorum superficialis muscle (*cut*)
Radial head

Flexor digitorum profundus muscle

Flexor carpi ulnaris muscle

Ulnar artery and nerve

Dorsal branch of ulnar nerve

Flexor digitorum superficialis tendons (*cut*)

Deep palmar branch of ulnar artery and deep branch of ulnar nerve

Superficial branch of ulnar nerve

Superficial palmar arch (*cut*)

Common palmar digital branch of ulnar nerve

Communicating branch of median nerve with ulnar nerve

Proper palmar digital branches of ulnar nerve

Plate 473 Arteries and Nerves of Upper Limb. (Netter: Atlas of Human Anatomy, 4 ed, 2006, Saunders.)

Lateral cutaneous branch of subcostal nerve

Inguinal ligament (Poupart's)

Superficial circumflex iliac vein

Femoral branches of genitofemoral nerve

Lateral femoral cutaneous nerve

Saphenous opening (fossa ovalis)

Fascia lata

Anterior cutaneous branches of femoral nerve

Patellar nerve plexus

Branches of lateral sural cutaneous nerve (from common fibular [peroneal] nerve)

Deep fascia of leg (crural fascia)

Superficial fibular (peroneal) nerve
Medial dorsal cutaneous branch

Intermediate dorsal cutaneous branch

Small saphenous vein and lateral dorsal cutaneous nerve (from sural nerve)

Lateral dorsal digital nerve and vein of 5th toe

Dorsal metatarsal veins

Dorsal digital nerves and veins

Superficial epigastric vein

Ilioinguinal nerve (scrotal branch) (usually passes through superficial inguinal ring)

Genital branch of genitofemoral nerve

Femoral vein

Superficial external pudendal vein

Accessory saphenous vein

Great saphenous vein

Cutaneous branches of obturator nerve

Infrapatellar branch of saphenous nerve

Saphenous nerve (terminal branch of femoral nerve)

Great saphenous vein

Dorsal digital nerves

Dorsal venous arch

Dorsal digital nerve and vein of medial side of great toe

Dorsal digital branch of deep fibular (peroneal) nerve

Plate 544 Superficial Nerves and Veins of Lower Limb: Anterior View. (Netter: Atlas of Human Anatomy, 4 ed, 2006, Saunders.)

Lateral cutaneous branch of iliohypogastric nerve

Iliac crest

Medial clunial nerves (from dorsal rami of S1, 2, 3)

Superior clunial nerves (from dorsal rami of L1, 2, 3)

Inferior clunial nerves (from posterior femoral cutaneous nerve)

Perforating cutaneous nerve (from dorsal rami of S1, 2, 3)

Branches of posterior femoral cutaneous nerve

Branches of lateral femoral cutaneous nerve

Accessory saphenous vein

Branch of femoral cutaneous nerve

Branch of cutaneous branch of femoral nerve

Terminal branches of posterior femoral cutaneous nerve

Great saphenous vein

Lateral sural cutaneous nerve (from common fibular [peroneal] nerve)

Small saphenous vein

Sural communicating nerve

Branches of saphenous nerve

Medial sural cutaneous nerve (from tibial nerve)

Sural nerve

Lateral calcaneal branches of sural nerve

Medial calcaneal branches of tibial nerve

Lateral dorsal cutaneous nerve (continuation of sural nerve)

Plantar cutaneous branches of medial plantar nerve

Plantar cutaneous branches of lateral plantar nerve

Plate 545 Superficial Nerves and Veins of Lower Limb: Posterior View. (Netter: Atlas of Human Anatomy, 4 ed, 2006, Saunders.)

NETTER'S ANATOMY ILLUSTRATIONS

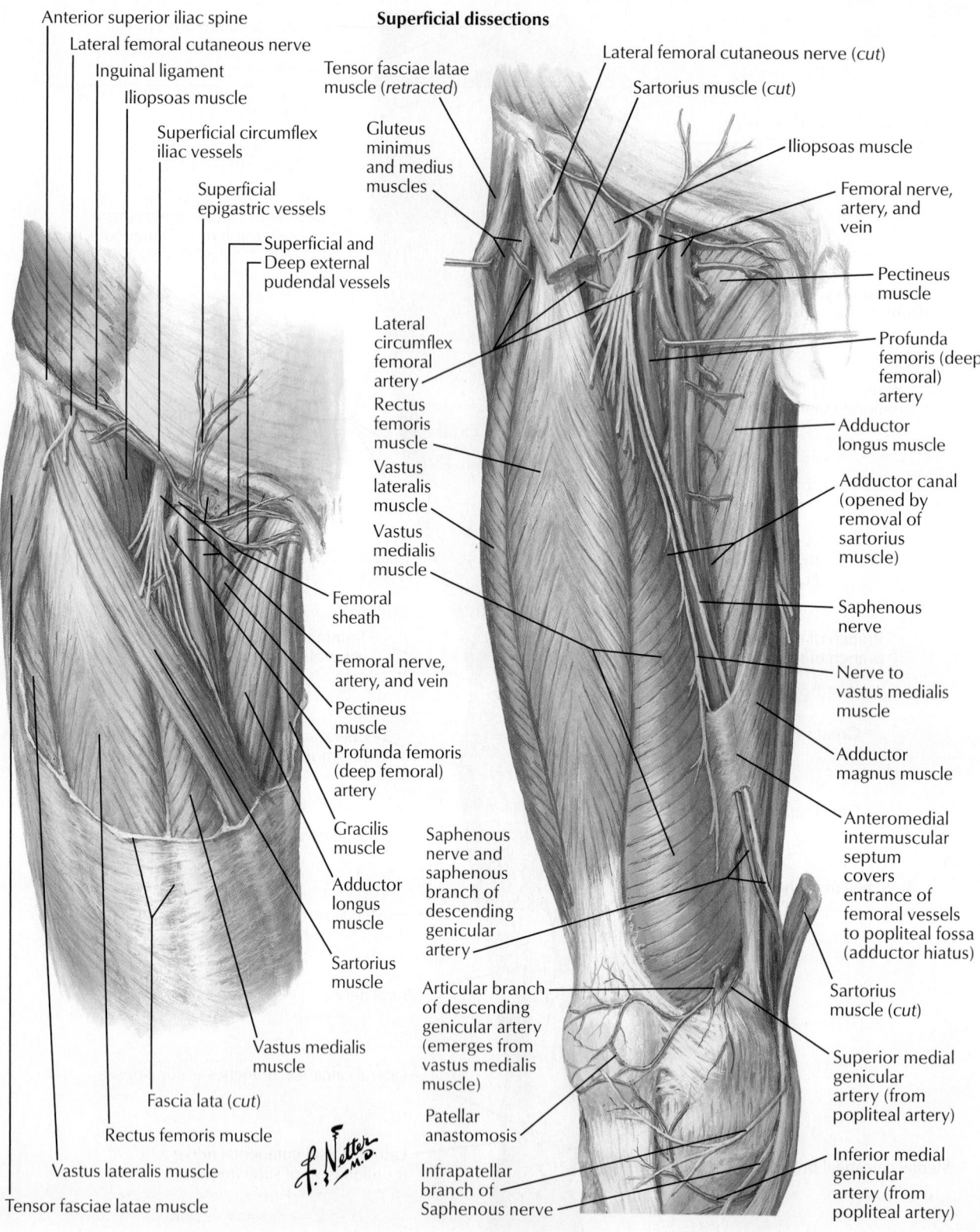

Anterior superior iliac spine
Lateral femoral cutaneous nerve
Inguinal ligament
Iliopsoas muscle
Superficial circumflex iliac vessels
Superficial epigastric vessels
Superficial and Deep external pudendal vessels

Superficial dissections

Tensor fasciae latae muscle (*retracted*)
Gluteus minimus and medius muscles
Lateral circumflex femoral artery
Rectus femoris muscle
Vastus lateralis muscle
Vastus medialis muscle
Femoral sheath
Femoral nerve, artery, and vein
Pectineus muscle
Profunda femoris (deep femoral) artery
Gracilis muscle
Adductor longus muscle
Sartorius muscle
Vastus medialis muscle
Fascia lata (*cut*)
Rectus femoris muscle
Vastus lateralis muscle
Tensor fasciae latae muscle

Saphenous nerve and saphenous branch of descending genicular artery
Articular branch of descending genicular artery (emerges from vastus medialis muscle)
Patellar anastomosis
Infrapatellar branch of Saphenous nerve

Lateral femoral cutaneous nerve (*cut*)
Sartorius muscle (*cut*)
Iliopsoas muscle
Femoral nerve, artery, and vein
Pectineus muscle
Profunda femoris (deep femoral) artery
Adductor longus muscle
Adductor canal (opened by removal of sartorius muscle)
Saphenous nerve
Nerve to vastus medialis muscle
Adductor magnus muscle
Anteromedial intermuscular septum covers entrance of femoral vessels to popliteal fossa (adductor hiatus)
Sartorius muscle (*cut*)
Superior medial genicular artery (from popliteal artery)
Inferior medial genicular artery (from popliteal artery)

Plate 500 Arteries and Nerves of Thigh: Anterior Views. (Netter: Atlas of Human Anatomy, 4 ed, 2006, Saunders.)

Deep dissection

Deep circumflex iliac artery

Lateral femoral cutaneous nerve

Sartorius muscle (*cut*)

Iliopsoas muscle

Tensor fasciae latae muscle (*retracted*)

Gluteus medius and minimus muscles

Femoral nerve

Rectus femoris muscle (*cut*)

Ascending, transverse and descending branches of Lateral circumflex femoral artery

Medial circumflex femoral artery

Pectineus muscle (*cut*)

Profunda femoris (deep femoral) artery

Perforating branches

Adductor longus muscle (*cut*)

Vastus lateralis muscle

Vastus intermedius muscle

Rectus femoris muscle (*cut*)

Saphenous nerve

Anteromedial intermuscular septum (*opened*)

Vastus medialis muscle

Quadriceps femoris tendon

Patella and patellar anastomosis

Medial patellar retinaculum

Patellar ligament

External iliac artery and vein

Inguinal ligament (Poupart's)

Femoral artery and vein (*cut*)

Pectineus muscle (*cut*)

Obturator canal

Obturator externus muscle

Adductor longus muscle (*cut*)

Anterior branch and Posterior branch of obturator nerve

Quadratus femoris muscle

Adductor brevis muscle

Branches of posterior branch of obturator nerve

Adductor magnus muscle

Gracilis muscle

Cutaneous branch of obturator nerve

Femoral artery and vein (*cut*)

Descending genicular artery
Articular branch
Saphenous branch

Adductor hiatus

Sartorius muscle (*cut*)

Adductor magnus tendon

Adductor tubercle on medial epicondyle of femur

Superior medial genicular artery (from popliteal artery)

Infrapatellar branch of Saphenous nerve

Inferior medial genicular artery (from popliteal artery)

Plate 501 Arteries and Nerves of Thigh: Posterior View. (Netter: Atlas of Human Anatomy, 4 ed, 2006, Saunders.)

61

Deep dissection

Superior clunial nerves

Gluteus maximus muscle (*cut*)

Medial clunial nerves

Inferior gluteal artery and nerve

Pudendal nerve

Nerve to obturator internus
(and superior gemellus)

Posterior femoral
cutaneous nerve

Sacrotuberous ligament

Ischial tuberosity

Inferior clunial nerves (*cut*)

Adductor magnus muscle

Gracilis muscle

Sciatic nerve

Muscular branches of sciatic nerve

Semitendinosus muscle (*retracted*)

Semimembranosus muscle

Sciatic nerve

Articular branch

Adductor hiatus

Popliteal vein and artery

Superior medial genicular artery

Medial epicondyle of femur

Tibial nerve

Gastrocnemius muscle (medial head)

Medial sural cutaneous nerve

Small saphenous vein

Iliac crest

Gluteal aponeurosis and
gluteus medius muscle (*cut*)

Superior gluteal artery and nerve

Gluteus minimus muscle

Tensor fasciae latae muscle

Piriformis muscle

Gluteus medius muscle (*cut*)

Superior gemellus muscle

Greater trochanter of femur

Obturator internus muscle

Inferior gemellus muscle

Gluteus maximus muscle (*cut*)

Quadratus femoris muscle

Medial circumflex femoral
artery

Vastus lateralis muscle
and iliotibial tract

Adductor minimus part of
adductor magnus muscle

1st perforating artery (from
profunda femoris artery)

Adductor magnus muscle

2nd and 3rd perforating arteries
(from profunda femoris artery)

4th perforating artery (from
profunda femoris artery)

Long head (*retracted*) ⎫
Short head   ⎬ Biceps femoris
                  ⎭ muscle

Superior lateral genicular artery

Common fibular (peroneal) nerve

Plantaris muscle

Gastrocnemius muscle (lateral head)

Lateral sural cutaneous nerve

Plate 502   Arteries and Nerves of Thigh: Posterior View. (Netter: Atlas of Human Anatomy, 4 ed, 2006, Saunders.)

62

Horizontal section

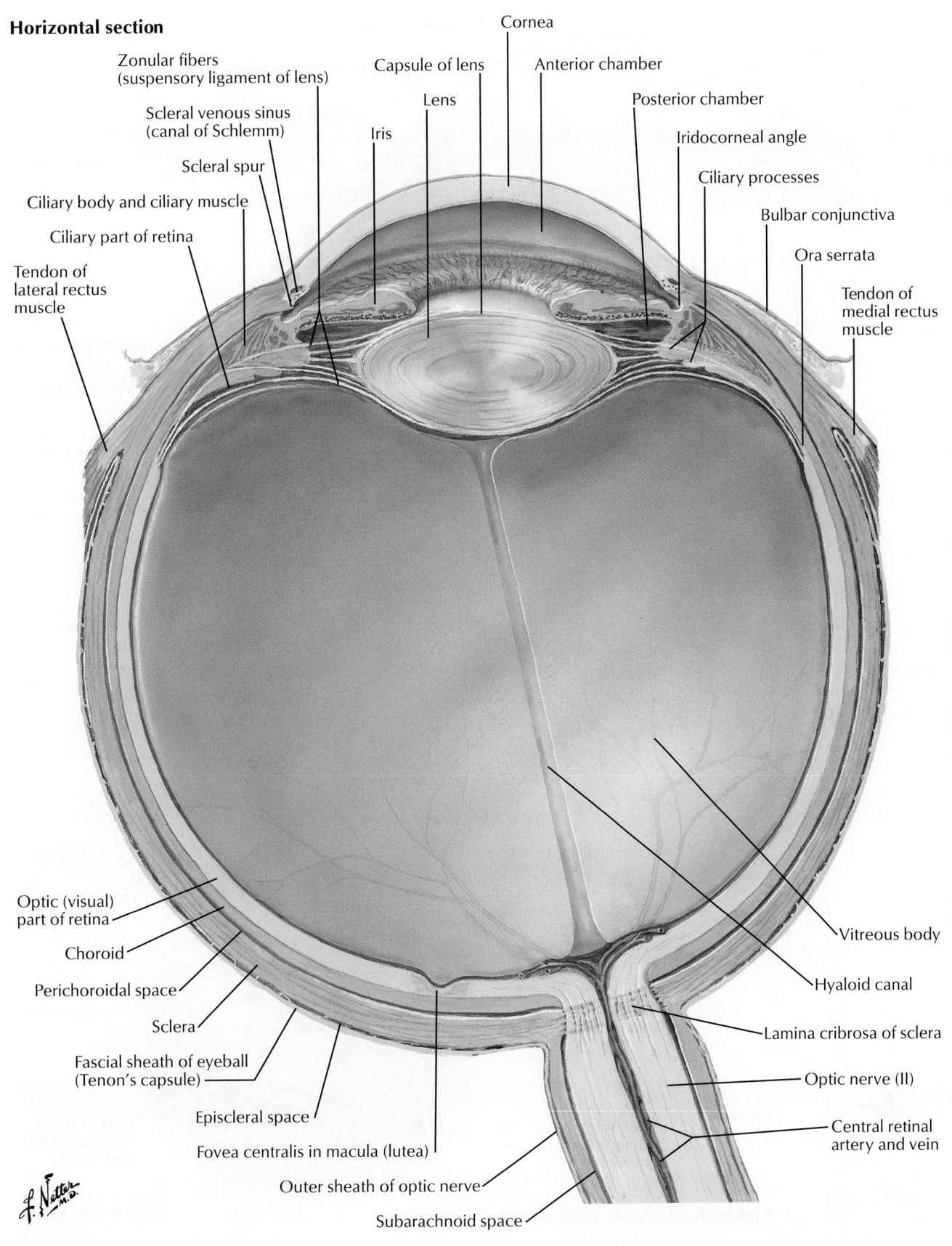

Zonular fibers (suspensory ligament of lens)

Scleral venous sinus (canal of Schlemm)

Scleral spur

Ciliary body and ciliary muscle

Ciliary part of retina

Tendon of lateral rectus muscle

Capsule of lens

Iris

Lens

Cornea

Anterior chamber

Posterior chamber

Iridocorneal angle

Ciliary processes

Bulbar conjunctiva

Ora serrata

Tendon of medial rectus muscle

Optic (visual) part of retina

Choroid

Perichoroidal space

Sclera

Fascial sheath of eyeball (Tenon's capsule)

Episcleral space

Fovea centralis in macula (lutea)

Outer sheath of optic nerve

Subarachnoid space

Vitreous body

Hyaloid canal

Lamina cribrosa of sclera

Optic nerve (II)

Central retinal artery and vein

NETTER'S ANATOMY ILLUSTRATIONS

Plate 87 Eyeball. (Netter: Atlas of Human Anatomy, 4 ed, 2006, Saunders.)

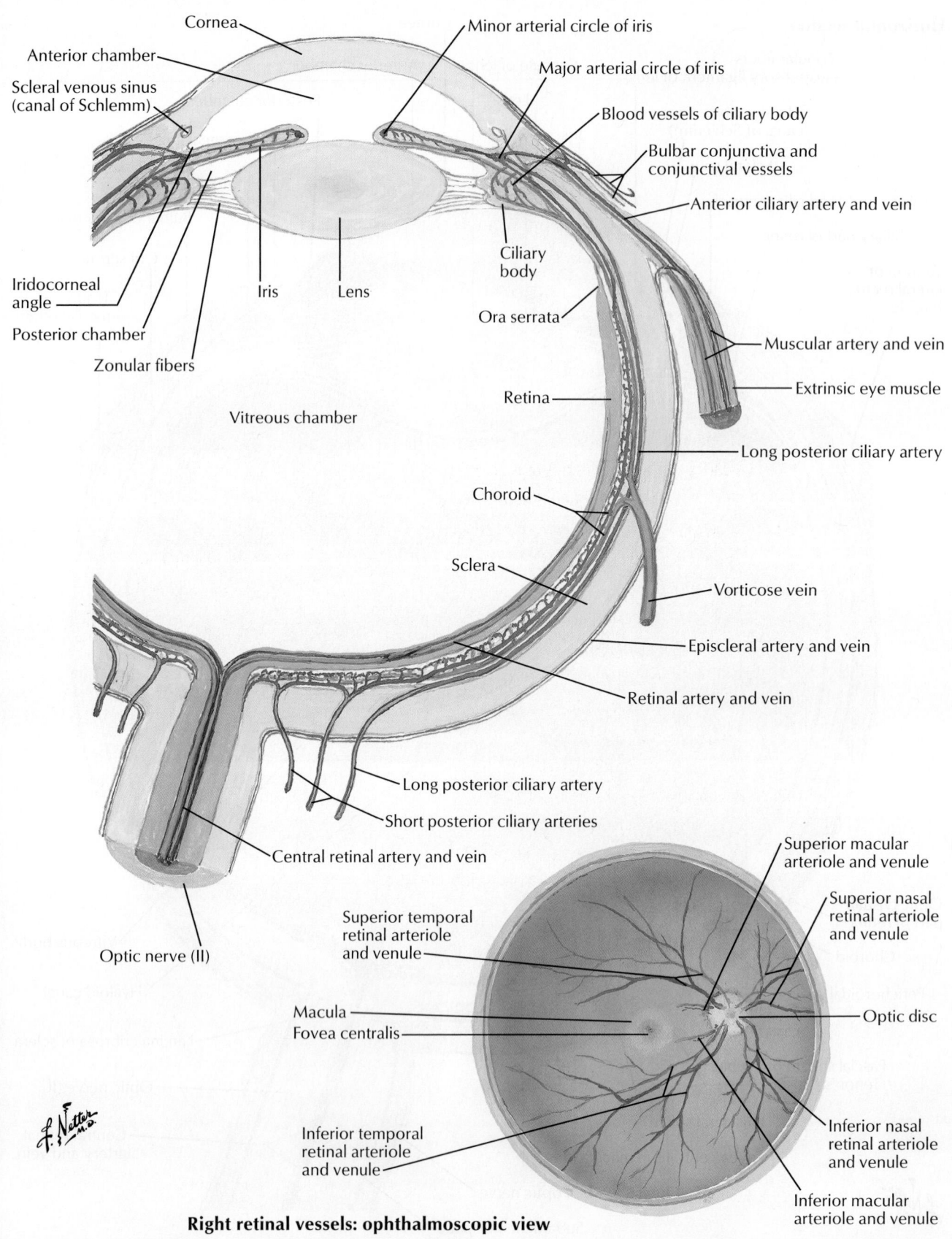

Cornea

Anterior chamber

Scleral venous sinus
(canal of Schlemm)

Minor arterial circle of iris

Major arterial circle of iris

Blood vessels of ciliary body

Bulbar conjunctiva and
conjunctival vessels

Anterior ciliary artery and vein

Iridocorneal
angle

Posterior chamber

Zonular fibers

Iris

Lens

Ciliary
body

Ora serrata

Retina

Choroid

Sclera

Vitreous chamber

Muscular artery and vein

Extrinsic eye muscle

Long posterior ciliary artery

Vorticose vein

Episcleral artery and vein

Retinal artery and vein

Long posterior ciliary artery

Short posterior ciliary arteries

Central retinal artery and vein

Optic nerve (II)

Superior temporal
retinal arteriole
and venule

Macula

Fovea centralis

Inferior temporal
retinal arteriole
and venule

Superior macular
arteriole and venule

Superior nasal
retinal arteriole
and venule

Optic disc

Inferior nasal
retinal arteriole
and venule

Inferior macular
arteriole and venule

Right retinal vessels: ophthalmoscopic view

Plate 90   Intrinsic Arteries and Veins of Eye. (Netter: Atlas of Human Anatomy, 4 ed, 2006, Saunders.)

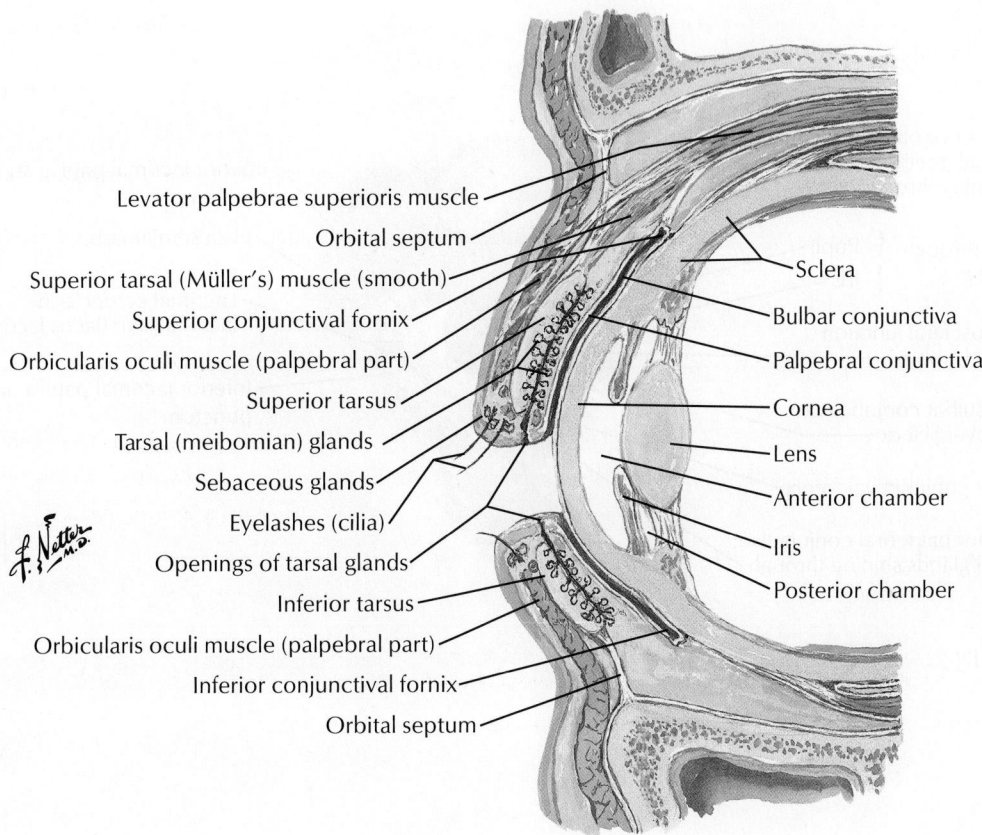

Levator palpebrae superioris muscle

Orbital septum

Superior tarsal (Müller's) muscle (smooth)

Superior conjunctival fornix

Orbicularis oculi muscle (palpebral part)

Superior tarsus

Tarsal (meibomian) glands

Sebaceous glands

Eyelashes (cilia)

Openings of tarsal glands

Inferior tarsus

Orbicularis oculi muscle (palpebral part)

Inferior conjunctival fornix

Orbital septum

Sclera

Bulbar conjunctiva

Palpebral conjunctiva

Cornea

Lens

Anterior chamber

Iris

Posterior chamber

Plate 81, Middle Eyelids. (Netter: Atlas of Human Anatomy, 4 ed, 2006, Saunders.)

Superior palpebral conjunctiva:
tarsal (meibomian) glands
shining through

Seen through { Pupil
cornea { Iris

Corneoscleral junction
(corneal limbus)

Bulbar conjunctiva
over sclera

Inferior conjunctival fornix

Inferior palpebral conjunctiva:
tarsal glands shining through

Superior lacrimal papilla and
punctum

Plica semilunaris

Lacrimal caruncle in
lacrimal lake (lacus lacrimalis)

Inferior lacrimal papilla and
punctum

Plate 81, Upper Eyelid. (Netter: Atlas of Human Anatomy, 4 ed, 2006, Saunders.)

Superior lacrimal papilla and punctum

Orbital part of lacrimal gland

Palpebral part of lacrimal gland

Excretory ducts of lacrimal gland

Plica semilunaris

Lacrimal caruncle

Inferior lacrimal papilla and punctum

Lacrimal canaliculi

Lacrimal sac

Nasolacrimal duct

Opening of nasolacrimal duct

Superior lacrimal papilla and punctum

Frontal bone (*cut away*)

Orbital part of lacrimal gland

Palpebral part of lacrimal gland

Excretory ducts of lacrimal gland

Plica semilunaris and lacrimal lake

Lacrimal caruncle

Inferior lacrimal papilla and punctum

Opening of nasolacrimal duct

Lacrimal canaliculi

Lacrimal sac

Nasolacrimal duct

Middle nasal concha

Nasal cavity

Inferior nasal concha (*cut*)

Inferior nasal meatus

Plate 82   Lacrimal Apparatus. (Netter: Atlas of Human Anatomy, 4 ed, 2006, Saunders.)

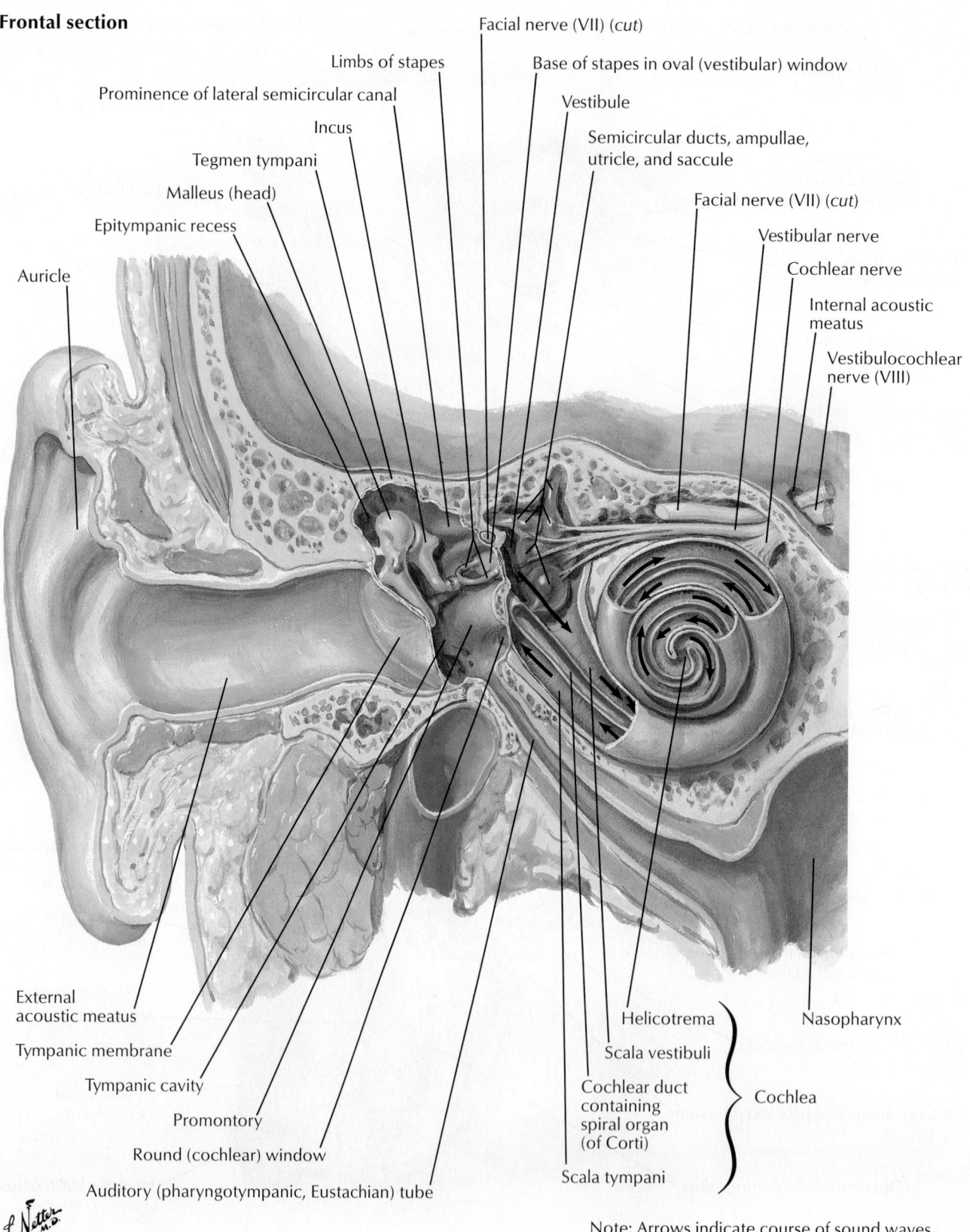

Facial nerve (VII) (*cut*)

Limbs of stapes

Base of stapes in oval (vestibular) window

Prominence of lateral semicircular canal

Vestibule

Incus

Semicircular ducts, ampullae, utricle, and saccule

Tegmen tympani

Malleus (head)

Facial nerve (VII) (*cut*)

Epitympanic recess

Vestibular nerve

Auricle

Cochlear nerve

Internal acoustic meatus

Vestibulocochlear nerve (VIII)

External acoustic meatus

Tympanic membrane

Tympanic cavity

Promontory

Round (cochlear) window

Auditory (pharyngotympanic, Eustachian) tube

Helicotrema

Scala vestibuli

Cochlear duct containing spiral organ (of Corti)

Scala tympani

Cochlea

Nasopharynx

Note: Arrows indicate course of sound waves.

Plate 92   Pathway of Sound Reception. (Netter: Atlas of Human Anatomy, 4 ed, 2006, Saunders.)

68

Medial wall of tympanic cavity: lateral view

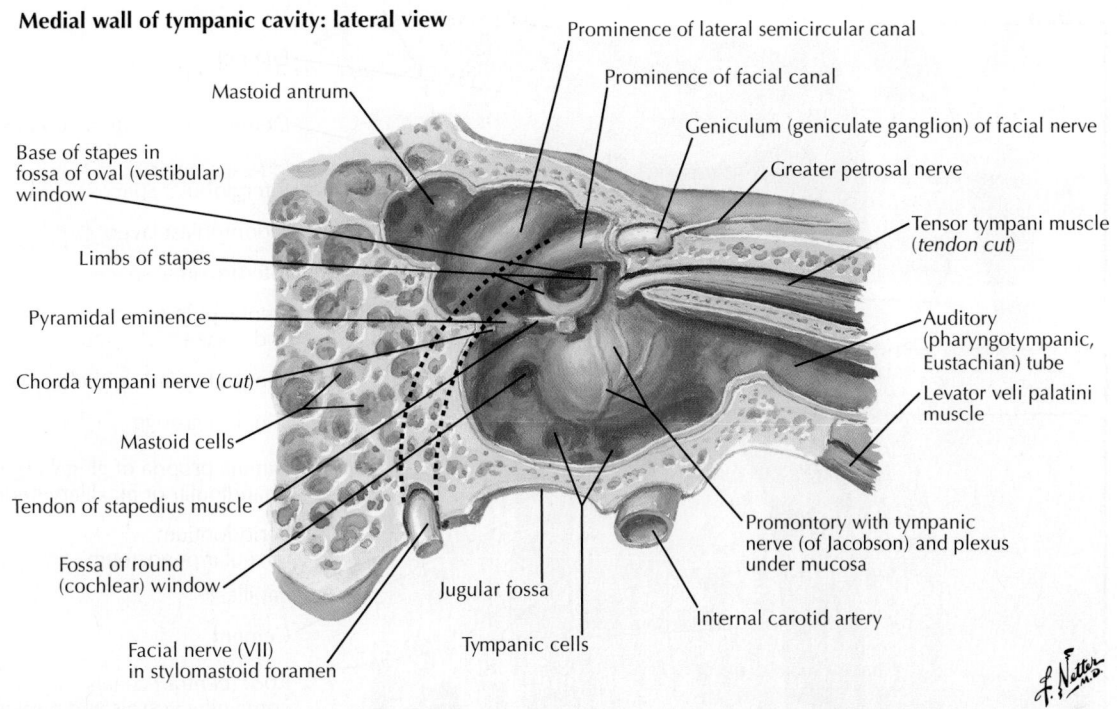

Prominence of lateral semicircular canal

Prominence of facial canal

Mastoid antrum

Geniculum (geniculate ganglion) of facial nerve

Greater petrosal nerve

Base of stapes in fossa of oval (vestibular) window

Tensor tympani muscle (*tendon cut*)

Limbs of stapes

Auditory (pharyngotympanic, Eustachian) tube

Pyramidal eminence

Levator veli palatini muscle

Chorda tympani nerve (*cut*)

Mastoid cells

Tendon of stapedius muscle

Promontory with tympanic nerve (of Jacobson) and plexus under mucosa

Fossa of round (cochlear) window

Internal carotid artery

Jugular fossa

Tympanic cells

Facial nerve (VII) in stylomastoid foramen

Plate 94   Tympanic Cavity. (Netter: Atlas of Human Anatomy, 4 ed, 2006, Saunders.)

Otoscopic view of right tympanic membrane

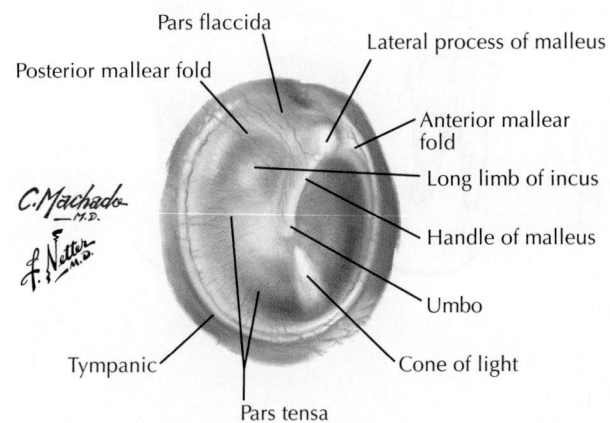

Pars flaccida

Posterior mallear fold

Lateral process of malleus

Anterior mallear fold

Long limb of incus

Handle of malleus

Umbo

Tympanic

Cone of light

Pars tensa

Plate 93   Tympanic Cavity. (Netter: Atlas of Human Anatomy, 4 ed, 2006, Saunders.)

Dissected right bony labyrinth (otic capsule): membranous labyrinth removed

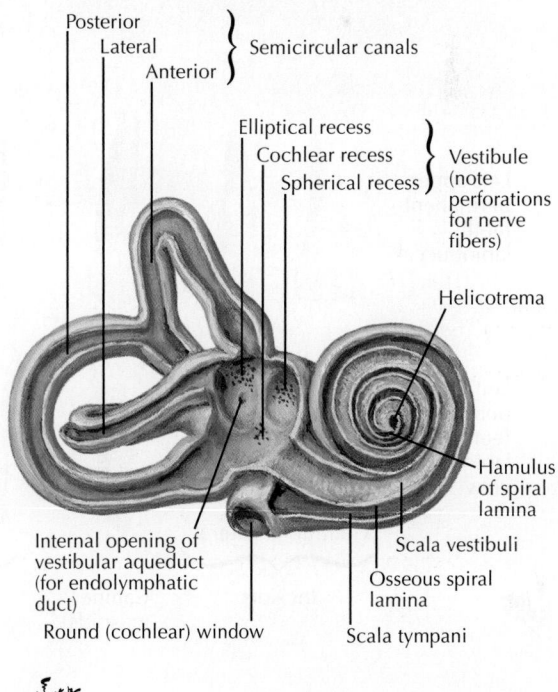

Posterior

Lateral

Anterior

Semicircular canals

Elliptical recess

Cochlear recess

Spherical recess

Vestibule (note perforations for nerve fibers)

Helicotrema

Hamulus of spiral lamina

Scala vestibuli

Osseous spiral lamina

Scala tympani

Internal opening of vestibular aqueduct (for endolymphatic duct)

Round (cochlear) window

Plate 95   Bony Membranous Labyrinth. (Netter: Atlas of Human Anatomy, 4 ed, 2006, Saunders.)

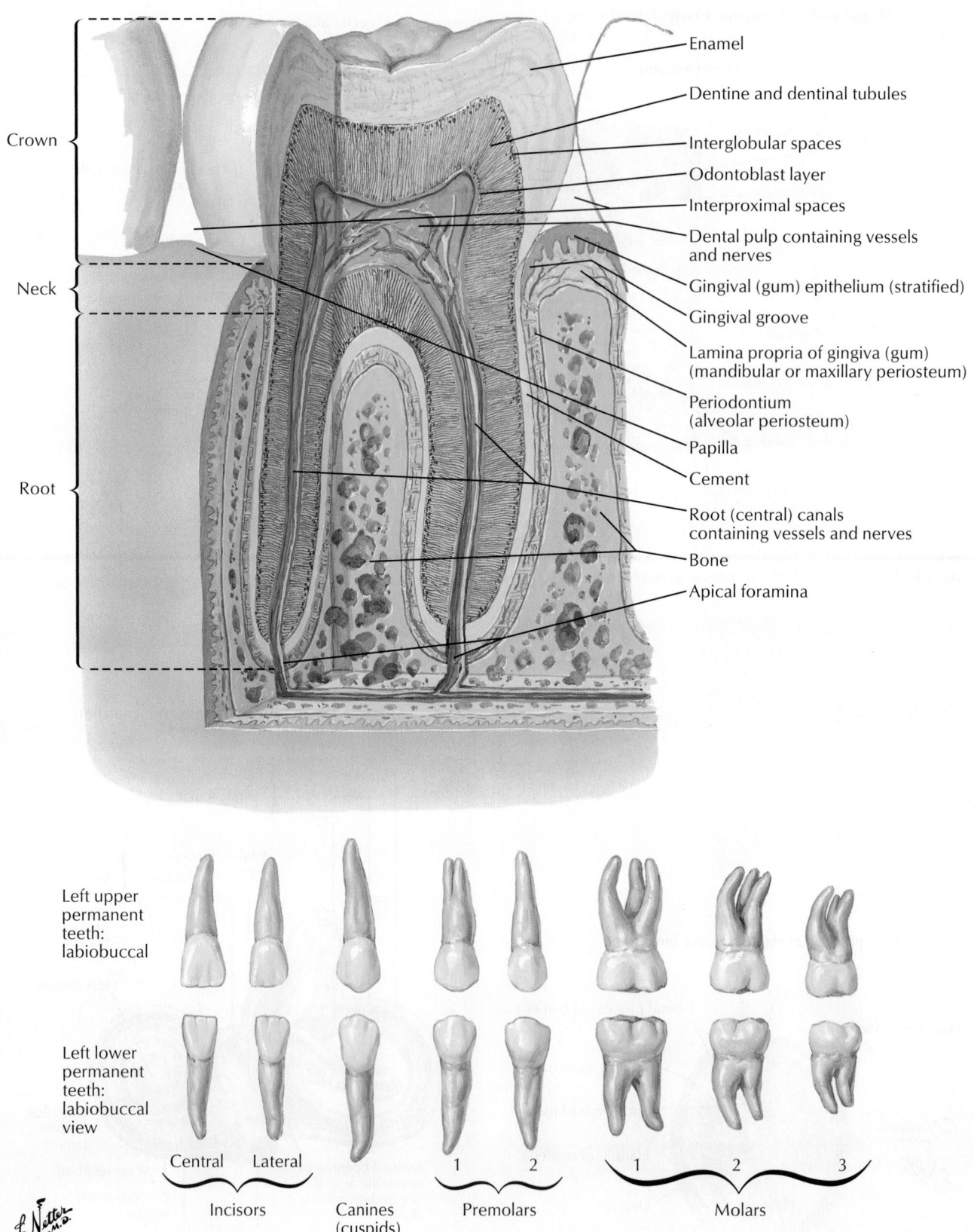

Crown

Neck

Root

Enamel

Dentine and dentinal tubules

Interglobular spaces

Odontoblast layer

Interproximal spaces

Dental pulp containing vessels and nerves

Gingival (gum) epithelium (stratified)

Gingival groove

Lamina propria of gingiva (gum) (mandibular or maxillary periosteum)

Periodontium (alveolar periosteum)

Papilla

Cement

Root (central) canals containing vessels and nerves

Bone

Apical foramina

Left upper permanent teeth: labiobuccal

Left lower permanent teeth: labiobuccal view

Central   Lateral

Incisors

Canines (cuspids)

1   2

Premolars

1   2   3

Molars

Plate 57   Teeth. (Netter: Atlas of Human Anatomy, 4 ed, 2006, Saunders.)

Tongue

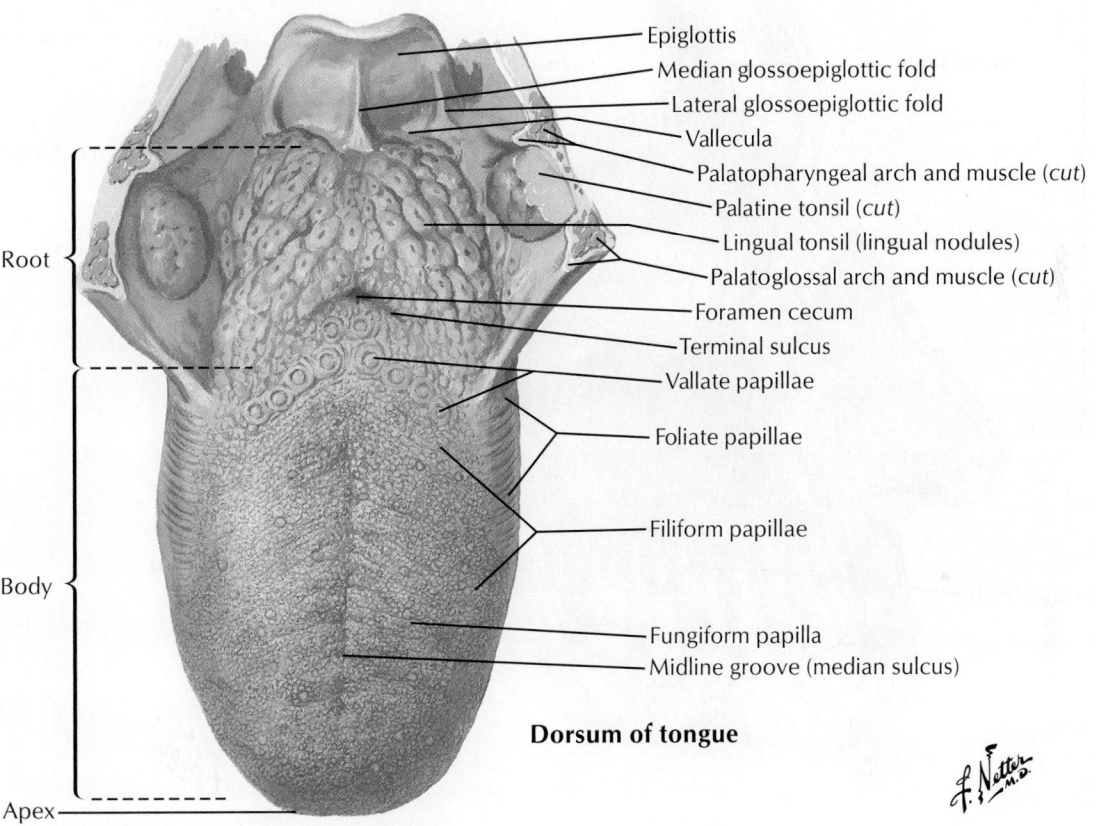

Epiglottis

Median glossoepiglottic fold

Lateral glossoepiglottic fold

Vallecula

Palatopharyngeal arch and muscle (*cut*)

Palatine tonsil (*cut*)

Lingual tonsil (lingual nodules)

Palatoglossal arch and muscle (*cut*)

Foramen cecum

Terminal sulcus

Vallate papillae

Foliate papillae

Filiform papillae

Fungiform papilla

Midline groove (median sulcus)

Root

Body

Apex

Dorsum of tongue

Plate 58 Tongue. (Netter: Atlas of Human Anatomy, 4 ed, 2006, Saunders.)

71

Frontal sinus

Opening into middle nasal meatus

Orbit

Pterygopalatine fossa

Maxillary sinus

Roots of teeth

Lateral dissection

Plate 49   Paranasal Sinuses. (Netter: Atlas of Human Anatomy, 4 ed, 2006, Saunders.)

72

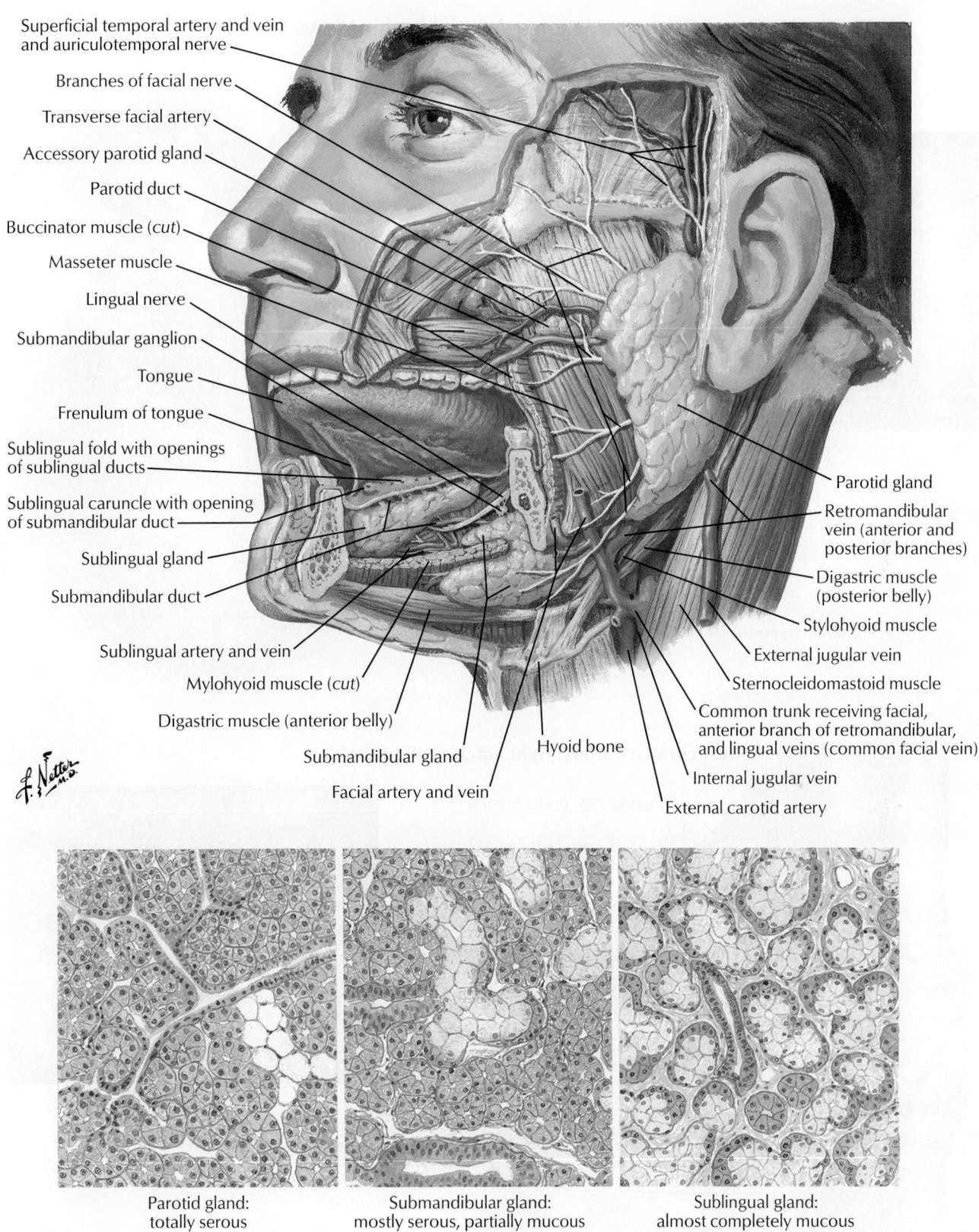

Superficial temporal artery and vein
and auriculotemporal nerve

Branches of facial nerve

Transverse facial artery

Accessory parotid gland

Parotid duct

Buccinator muscle (*cut*)

Masseter muscle

Lingual nerve

Submandibular ganglion

Tongue

Frenulum of tongue

Sublingual fold with openings
of sublingual ducts

Sublingual caruncle with opening
of submandibular duct

Sublingual gland

Submandibular duct

Sublingual artery and vein

Mylohyoid muscle (*cut*)

Digastric muscle (anterior belly)

Submandibular gland

Facial artery and vein

Hyoid bone

Parotid gland

Retromandibular
vein (anterior and
posterior branches)

Digastric muscle
(posterior belly)

Stylohyoid muscle

External jugular vein

Sternocleidomastoid muscle

Common trunk receiving facial,
anterior branch of retromandibular,
and lingual veins (common facial vein)

Internal jugular vein

External carotid artery

Parotid gland:
totally serous

Submandibular gland:
mostly serous, partially mucous

Sublingual gland:
almost completely mucous

Plate 61 Salivary Glands. (Netter: Atlas of Human Anatomy, 4 ed, 2006, Saunders.)

Coronary Arteries: Arteriographic Views

Right coronary artery: left anterior oblique view

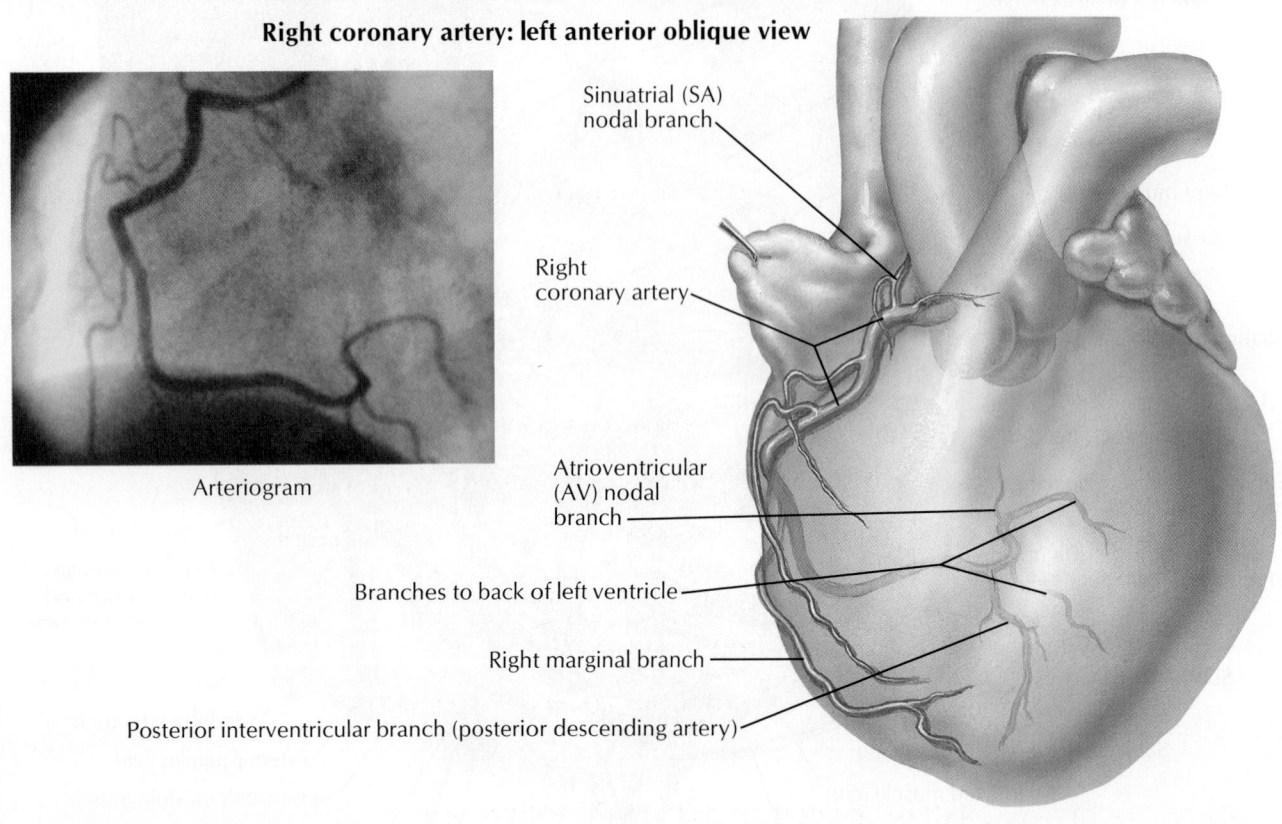

Arteriogram

Sinuatrial (SA) nodal branch

Right coronary artery

Atrioventricular (AV) nodal branch

Branches to back of left ventricle

Right marginal branch

Posterior interventricular branch (posterior descending artery)

Right coronary artery: right anterior oblique view

Sinuatrial (SA) nodal branch

Conus (arteriosus) branch

Right coronary artery

Right marginal branch

Arteriogram

Atrioventricular (AV) nodal branch

Right posterolateral branches (to back of left ventricle)

Posterior interventricular branch (posterior descending artery)

Plate 218 Coronary Arteries: Arteriographic Views. (Netter: Atlas of Human Anatomy, 4 ed, 2006, Saunders.)

Left coronary artery: left anterior oblique view

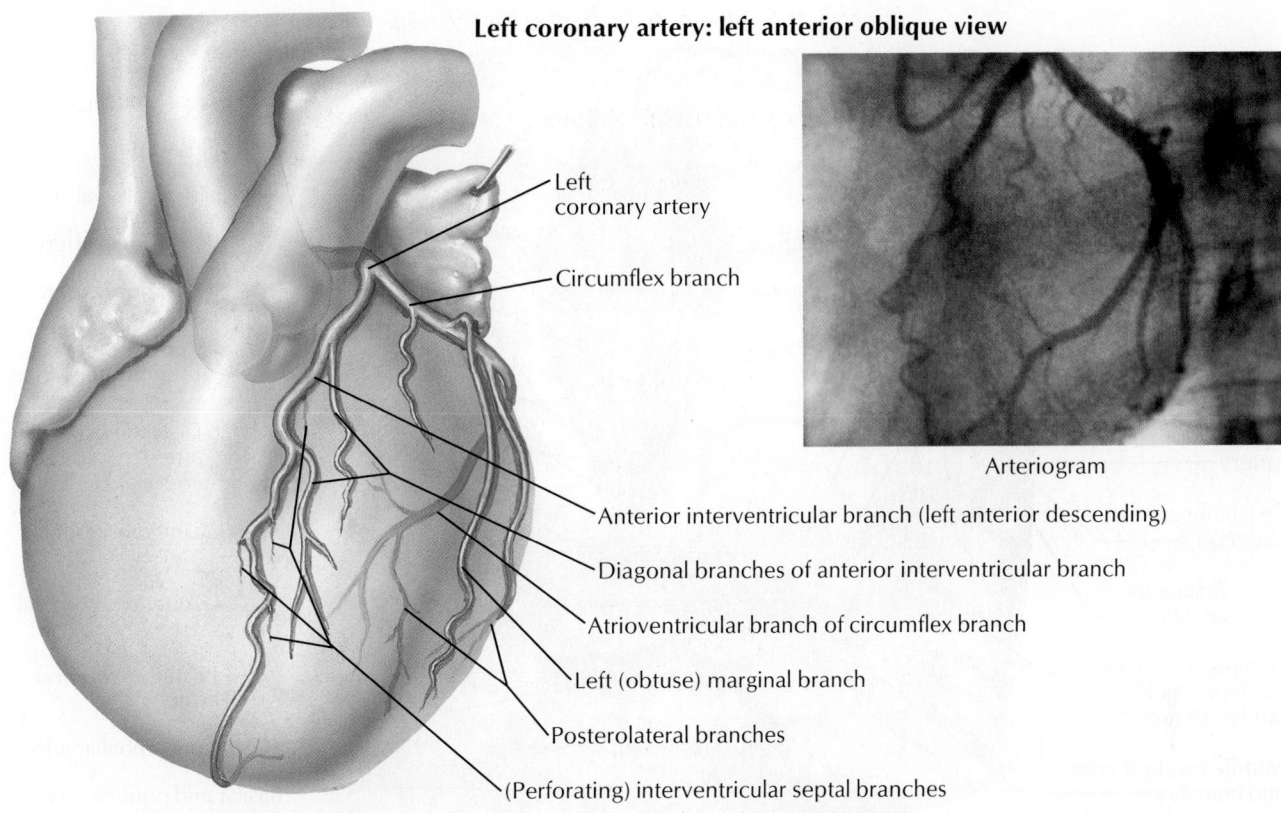

Left coronary artery

Circumflex branch

Arteriogram

Anterior interventricular branch (left anterior descending)

Diagonal branches of anterior interventricular branch

Atrioventricular branch of circumflex branch

Left (obtuse) marginal branch

Posterolateral branches

(Perforating) interventricular septal branches

Left coronary artery: right anterior oblique view

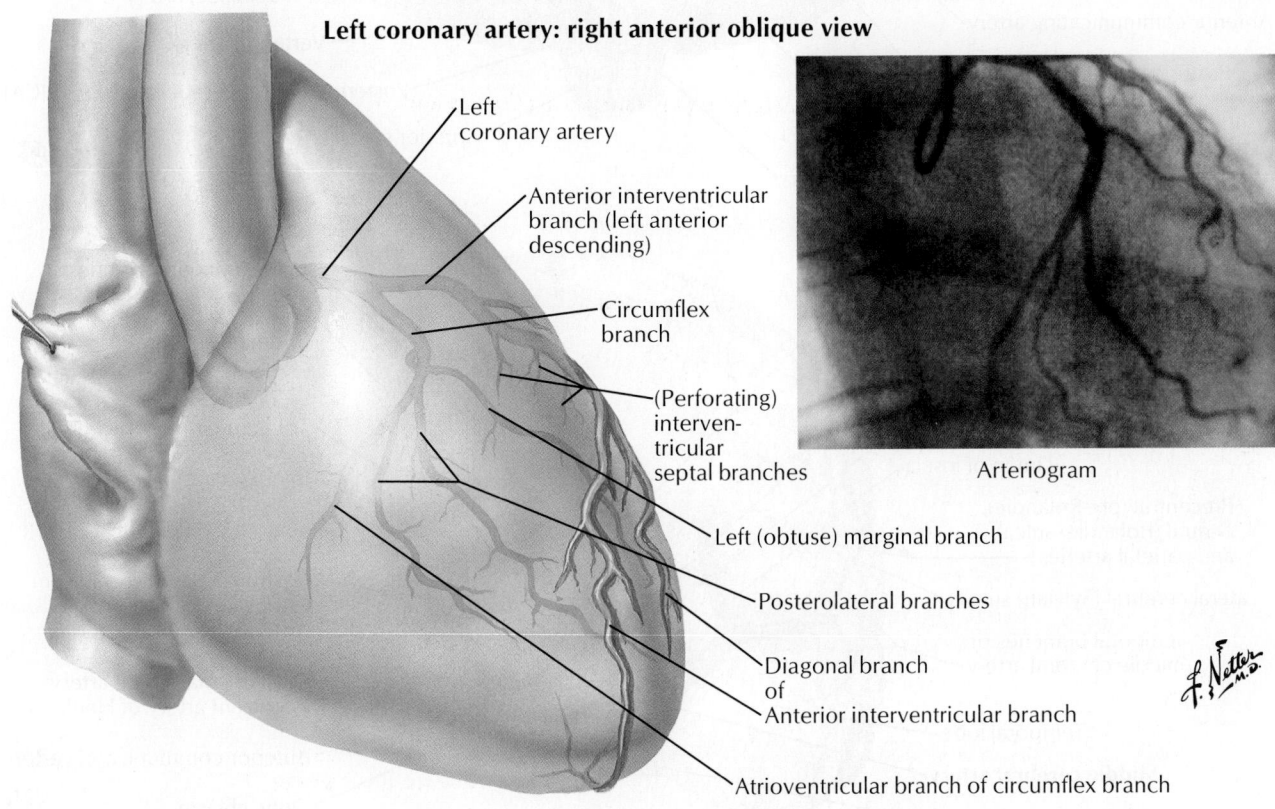

Left coronary artery

Anterior interventricular branch (left anterior descending)

Circumflex branch

(Perforating) interventricular septal branches

Arteriogram

Left (obtuse) marginal branch

Posterolateral branches

Diagonal branch of Anterior interventricular branch

Atrioventricular branch of circumflex branch

NETTER'S ANATOMY ILLUSTRATIONS

Corpus callosum

Anterolateral central
(lenticulostriate) arteries

Lateral frontobasal
(orbitofrontal) artery

Prefrontal artery

Precentral (pre-Rolandic)
and central (Rolandic)
sulcal arteries

Anterior parietal
(postcentral sulcal)
artery

Posterior parietal
artery

Branch to
angular gyrus

Temporal branches
(anterior, middle,
and posterior)

Middle cerebral artery
and branches
(deep in lateral cerebral
[Sylvian] sulcus)

Anterior communicating artery

Posterior communicating artery

Anterior inferior cerebellar artery (AICA)

Posterior spinal artery

Paracentral artery

Medial frontal branches

Pericallosal artery

Callosomarginal artery

Polar frontal artery

**Anterior cerebral
arteries**

Medial frontobasal
(orbitofrontal) artery

Distal medial striate
artery (recurrent
artery of Heubner)

Internal carotid
artery

Anterior choroidal
artery

**Posterior cerebral
artery**

Superior cerebellar artery

Basilar and pontine arteries

Labyrinthine (internal
acoustic) artery

Vertebral artery

Posterior inferior cerebellar artery (PICA)

Anterior spinal artery

Corpus striatum
(caudate and lentiform nuclei)

Anterolateral central
(lenticulostriate) arteries

Insula (island of Reil)

Limen of insula

Precentral (pre-Rolandic),
central (Rolandic) sulcal,
and parietal arteries

Lateral cerebral (Sylvian) sulcus

Temporal branches of
middle cerebral artery

Temporal lobe

Middle cerebral artery

Internal carotid artery

Falx cerebri

Callosomarginal arteries
and
Pericallosal arteries
(branches of anterior
cerebral arteries)

Trunk of corpus callosum

Internal capsule

Septum pellucidum

Rostrum of corpus callosum

Anterior cerebral arteries

Distal medial striate artery
(recurrent artery of Heubner)

Anterior communicating artery

Optic chiasm

Plate 141 Arteries of Brain: Frontal View and Section. (Netter: Atlas of Human Anatomy, 4 ed, 2006, Saunders.)

76

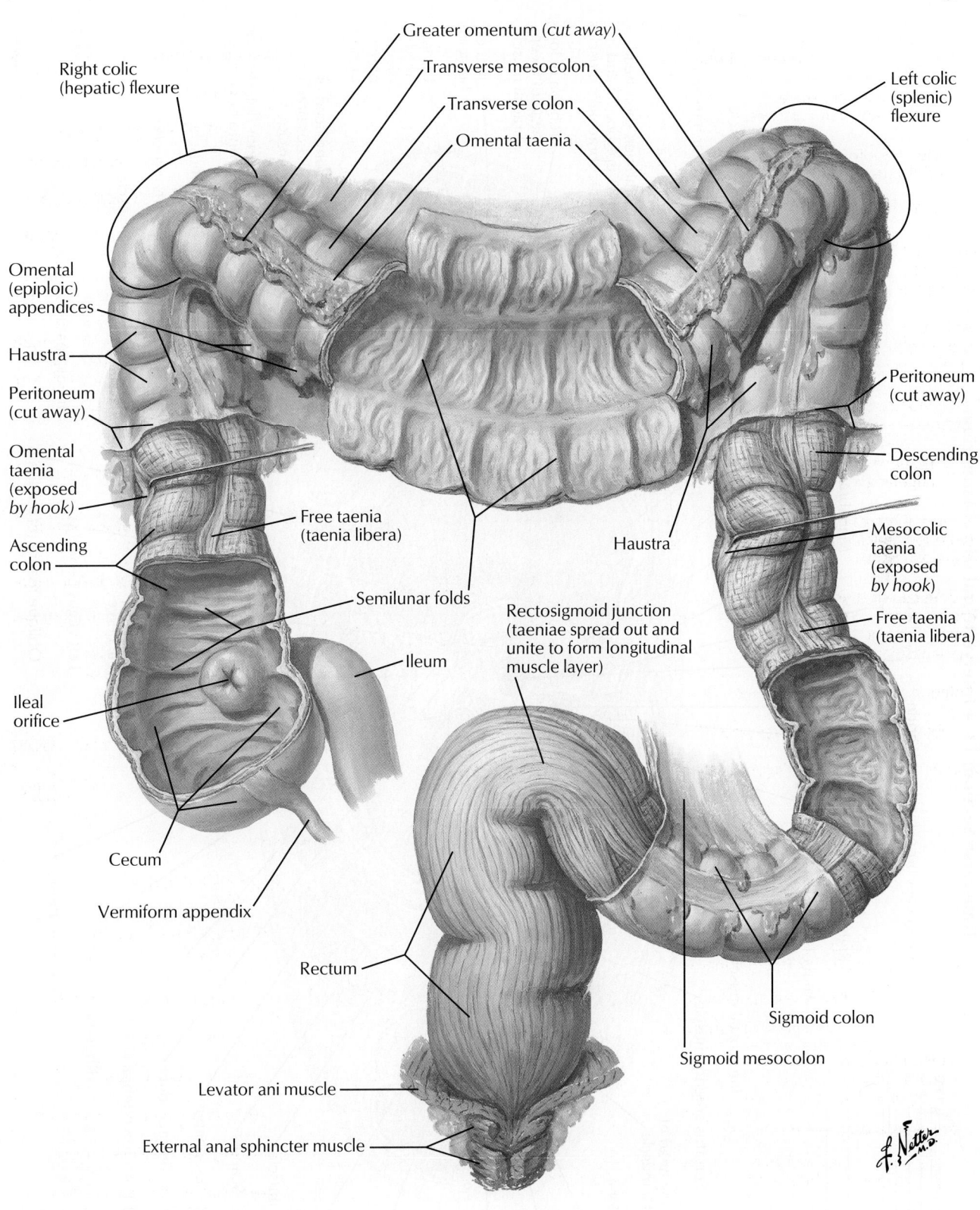

Right colic
(hepatic) flexure

Greater omentum (*cut away*)

Transverse mesocolon

Transverse colon

Omental taenia

Left colic
(splenic)
flexure

Omental
(epiploic)
appendices

Haustra

Peritoneum
(cut away)

Omental
taenia
(exposed
by hook)

Ascending
colon

Ileal
orifice

Cecum

Vermiform appendix

Free taenia
(taenia libera)

Semilunar folds

Ileum

Peritoneum
(cut away)

Descending
colon

Haustra

Mesocolic
taenia
(exposed
by hook)

Free taenia
(taenia libera)

Rectosigmoid junction
(taeniae spread out and
unite to form longitudinal
muscle layer)

Rectum

Sigmoid colon

Sigmoid mesocolon

Levator ani muscle

External anal sphincter muscle

Plate 284   Mucosa and Musculature of Large Intestine. (Netter: Atlas of Human Anatomy, 4 ed, 2006, Saunders.)

Transverse Section: T3–4 Intervertebral Disc, Manubrium

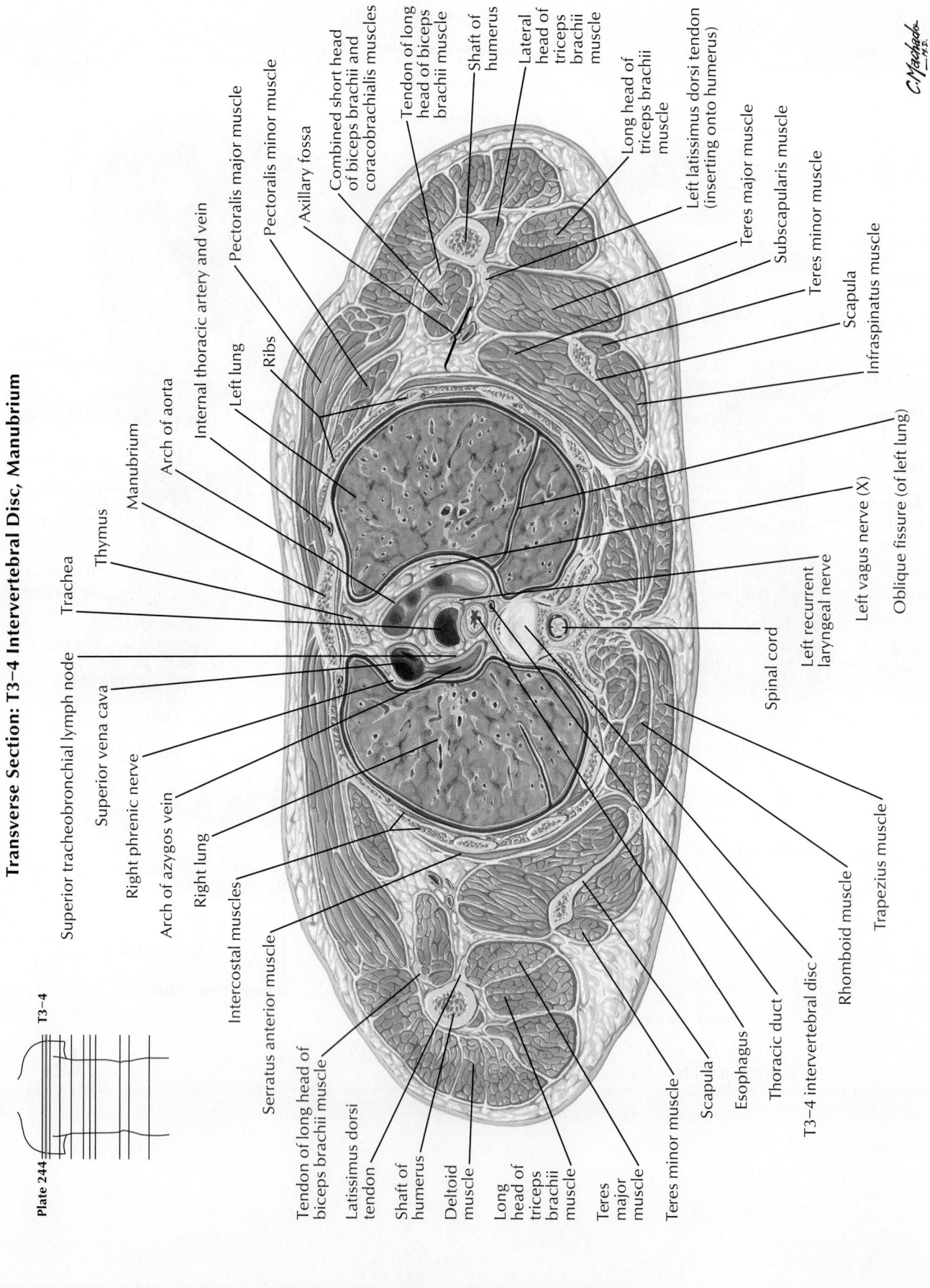

Plate 244 Cross Section of Thorax at T3-4 Disc Level. (Netter: Atlas of Human Anatomy, 4 ed, 2006, Saunders.)

Right knee in extension: posterior view

Adductor tubercle on medial epicondyle of femur

Medial condyle of femur (articular surface)

Medial meniscus

Tibial collateral ligament

Medial condyle of tibia

Posterior cruciate ligament

Anterior cruciate ligament

Posterior meniscofemoral ligament

Lateral condyle of femur (articular surface)

Popliteus tendon

Fibular collateral ligament

Lateral meniscus

Head of fibula

Plate 509   Knee: Cruciate and Collateral Ligaments. (Netter: Atlas of Human Anatomy, 4 ed, 2006, Saunders.)

Paramedian (sagittal) dissection

Ureter

Uterine (fallopian) tube

Ovary

Ligament of ovary

Round ligament of uterus

Broad ligament (*cut*)

Superior pubic ramus (*cut*)

Inferior pubic ramus (*cut*)

Ischiocavernosus muscle

Body of clitoris

Labia minora

Labium majus

Rectouterine pouch (of Douglas)

Peritoneum (*cut edge*)

Vesicouterine pouch

Rectum

Ureter

Urinary bladder

Vagina

Pelvic diaphragm (levator ani muscle)

Deep transverse perineal muscle (*cut*)

External anal sphincter muscle

Median (sagittal) section

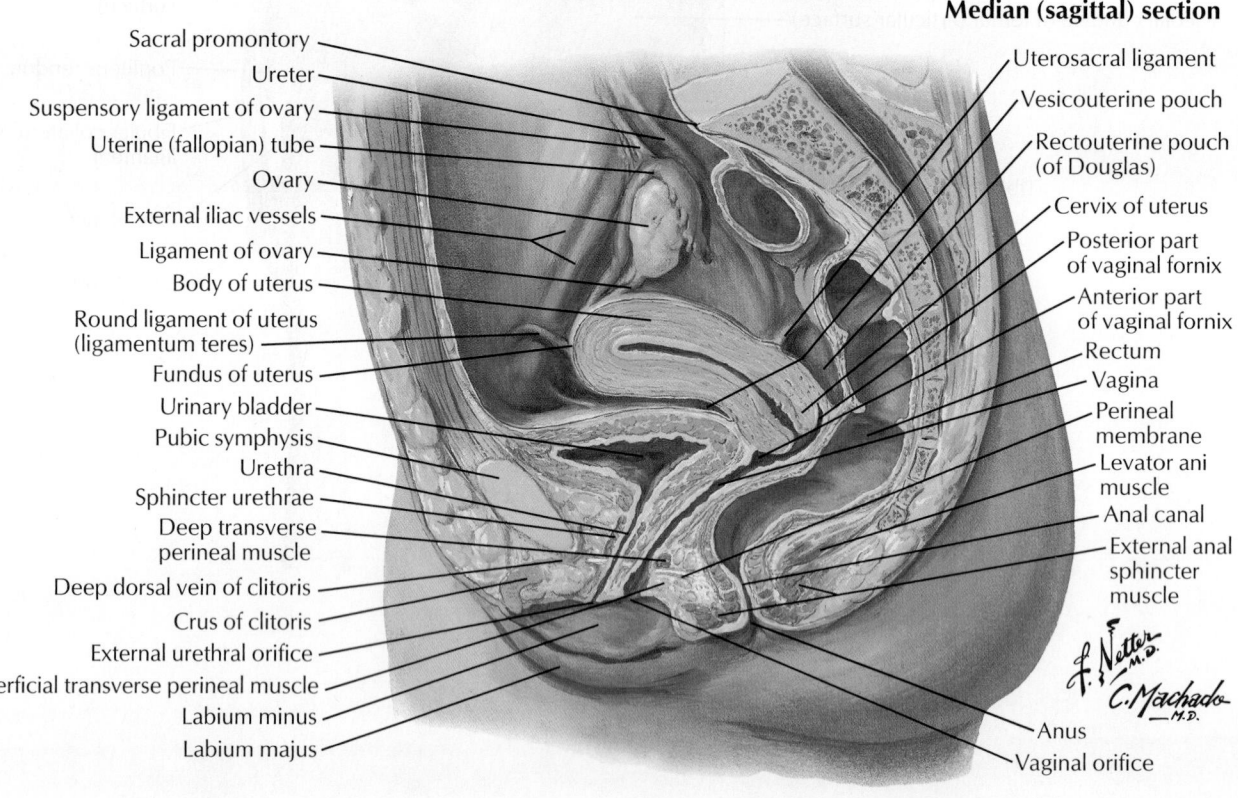

Sacral promontory

Ureter

Suspensory ligament of ovary

Uterine (fallopian) tube

Ovary

External iliac vessels

Ligament of ovary

Body of uterus

Round ligament of uterus (ligamentum teres)

Fundus of uterus

Urinary bladder

Pubic symphysis

Urethra

Sphincter urethrae

Deep transverse perineal muscle

Deep dorsal vein of clitoris

Crus of clitoris

External urethral orifice

Superficial transverse perineal muscle

Labium minus

Labium majus

Uterosacral ligament

Vesicouterine pouch

Rectouterine pouch (of Douglas)

Cervix of uterus

Posterior part of vaginal fornix

Anterior part of vaginal fornix

Rectum

Vagina

Perineal membrane

Levator ani muscle

Anal canal

External anal sphincter muscle

Anus

Vaginal orifice

Plate 360   Pelvic Viscera and Perineum: Female. (Netter: Atlas of Human Anatomy, 4 ed, 2006, Saunders.)

PART II

Alphabetic Index

A

Aarskog's syndrome Q87.1
Abandonment —*see* Maltreatment
Abasia (-astasia) (hysterical) F44.4
Abderhalden-Kaufmann-Lignac syndrome
(cystinosis) E72.04
Abdomen, abdominal —*see also* condition
acute R10.0
angina K55.1
muscle deficiency syndrome Q79.4
Abdominalgia —*see* Pain, abdominal
Abduction contracture, hip or other joint —*see*
Contraction, joint
Aberrant (congenital) —*see also* Malposition,
congenital
adrenal gland Q89.1
artery (peripheral) Q27.8
basilar NEC Q28.1
cerebral Q28.3
coronary Q24.5
digestive system Q27.8
eye Q15.8
lower limb Q27.8
precerebral Q28.1
pulmonary Q25.79
renal Q27.2
retina Q14.1
specified site NEC Q27.8
subclavian Q27.8
upper limb Q27.8
vertebral Q28.1
breast Q83.8
endocrine gland NEC Q89.2
hepatic duct Q44.5
pancreas Q45.3
parathyroid gland Q89.2
pituitary gland Q89.2
sebaceous glands, mucous membrane,
mouth, congenital Q38.6
spleen Q89.09
subclavian artery Q27.8
thymus (gland) Q89.2
thyroid gland Q89.2
vein (peripheral) NEC Q27.8
cerebral Q28.3
digestive system Q27.8
lower limb Q27.8
precerebral Q28.1
specified site NEC Q27.8
upper limb Q27.8
Aberration
distantial —*see* Disturbance, visual
mental F99
Abetalipoproteinemia E78.6
Abiotrophy R68.89
Ablatio, ablation
retinae —*see* Detachment, retina
Ablepharia, ablepharon Q10.3
Abnormal, abnormality, abnormalities —*see
also* Anomaly
acid-base balance (mixed) E87.4
albumin R77.0
alphafetoprotein R77.2
alveolar ridge K08.9
anatomical relationship Q89.9
apertures, congenital, diaphragm
Q79.1
auditory perception H93.29-●
diplacusis —*see* Diplacusis
hyperacusis —*see* Hyperacusis
recruitment —*see* Recruitment, auditory
threshold shift —*see* Shift, auditory
threshold
autosomes Q99.9
fragile site Q95.5
basal metabolic rate R94.8
biosynthesis, testicular androgen
E29.1
bleeding time R79.1

Abnormal, abnormality, abnormalities —
(Continued)
blood level (of)
cobalt R79.0
copper R79.0
iron R79.0
lithium R78.89
magnesium R79.0
mineral NEC R79.0
zinc R79.0
blood pressure
elevated R03.0
low reading (nonspecific) R03.1
blood sugar R73.09
blood-gas level R79.81
bowel sounds R19.15
absent R19.11
hyperactive R19.12
brain scan R94.02
breathing R06.9
caloric test R94.138
cerebrospinal fluid R83.9
cytology R83.6
drug level R83.2
enzyme level R83.0
hormones R83.1
immunology R83.4
microbiology R83.5
nonmedicinal level R83.3
specified type NEC R83.8
chemistry, blood R79.9
C-reactive protein R79.82
drugs —*see* Findings, abnormal, in blood
gas level R79.81
minerals R79.0
pancytopenia D61.818
PTT R79.1
specified NEC R79.89
toxins —*see* Findings, abnormal, in
blood
chest sounds (friction) (rales) R09.89
chromosome, chromosomal Q99.9
with more than three X chromosomes,
female Q97.1
analysis result R89.8
bronchial washings R84.8
cerebrospinal fluid R83.8
cervix uteri NEC R87.89
nasal secretions R84.8
nipple discharge R89.8
peritoneal fluid R85.89
pleural fluid R84.8
prostatic secretions R86.8
saliva R85.89
seminal fluid R86.8
sputum R84.8
synovial fluid R89.8
throat scrapings R84.8
vagina R87.89
vulva R87.89
wound secretions R89.8
dicentric replacement Q93.2
ring replacement Q93.2
sex Q99.8
female phenotype Q97.9
specified NEC Q97.8
male phenotype Q98.9
specified NEC Q98.8
structural male Q98.6
specified NEC Q99.8
clinical findings NEC R68.89
coagulation D68.9
newborn, transient P61.6
profile R79.1
time R79.1
communication —*see* Fistula
conjunctiva, vascular H11.41-●
coronary artery Q24.5
cortisol-binding globulin E27.8
course, eustachian tube Q17.8

Abnormal, abnormality, abnormalities —
(Continued)
creatinine clearance R94.4
cytology
anus R85.619
atypical squamous cells cannot
exclude high grade squamous
intraepithelial lesion (ASC-H)
R85.611
atypical squamous cells of undetermined
significance (ASC-US) R85.610
cytologic evidence of malignancy
R85.614
high grade squamous intraepithelial
lesion (HGSIL) R85.613
human papillomavirus (HPV) DNA test
high risk positive R85.81
low risk postive R85.82
inadequate smear R85.615
low grade squamous intraepithelial
lesion (LGSIL) R85.612
satisfactory anal smear but lacking
transformation zone R85.616
specified NEC R85.618
unsatisfactory smear R85.615
female genital organs —*see* Abnormal,
Papanicolaou (smear)
dark adaptation curve H53.61
dentofacial NEC —*see* Anomaly, dentofacial
development, developmental Q89.9
central nervous system Q07.9
diagnostic imaging
abdomen, abdominal region NEC R93.5
biliary tract R93.2
bladder R93.41
breast R92.8
central nervous system NEC R90.89
cerebrovascular NEC R90.89
coronary circulation R93.1
digestive tract NEC R93.3
gastrointestinal (tract) R93.3
genitourinary organs R93.8
head R93.0
heart R93.1
intrathoracic organ NEC R93.8
kidney R93.42-●
limbs R93.6
liver R93.2
lung (field) R91.8
musculoskeletal system NEC R93.7
renal pelvis R93.41
retroperitoneum R93.5
site specified NEC R93.8
skin and subcutaneous tissue R93.8
skull R93.0
urinary organs specified NEC R93.49
ureter R93.41
direction, teeth, fully erupted M26.30
ear ossicles, acquired NEC H74.39-●
ankylosis —*see* Ankylosis, ear ossicles
discontinuity —*see* Discontinuity, ossicles,
ear
partial loss —*see* Loss, ossicles, ear (partial)
Ebstein Q22.5
echocardiogram R93.1
echoencephalogram R90.81
echogram —*see* Abnormal, diagnostic
imaging
electrocardiogram [ECG] [EKG] R94.31
electroencephalogram [EEG] R94.01
electrolyte —*see* Imbalance, electrolyte
electromyogram [EMG] R94.131
electro-oculogram [EOG] R94.110
electrophysiological intracardiac studies
R94.39
electroretinogram [ERG] R94.111
erythrocytes
congenital, with perinatal jaundice
D58.9
feces (color) (contents) (mucus) R19.5

Abnormal, abnormality, abnormalities —
(Continued)
finding —see Findings, abnormal, without
diagnosis
fluid
amniotic —see Abnormal, specimen,
specified
cerebrospinal —see Abnormal,
cerebrospinal fluid
peritoneal —see Abnormal, specimen,
digestive organs
pleural —see Abnormal, specimen,
respiratory organs
synovial —see Abnormal, specimen,
specified
thorax (bronchial washings) (pleural
fluid) —see Abnormal, specimen,
respiratory organs
vaginal —see Abnormal, specimen, female
genital organs
form
teeth K00.2
uterus —see Anomaly, uterus
function studies
auditory R94.120
bladder R94.8
brain R94.09
cardiovascular R94.30
ear R94.128
endocrine NEC R94.7
eye NEC R94.118
kidney R94.4
liver R94.5
nervous system
central NEC R94.09
peripheral NEC R94.138
pancreas R94.8
placenta R94.8
pulmonary R94.2
special senses NEC R94.128
spleen R94.8
thyroid R94.6
vestibular R94.121
gait —see Gait
hysterical F44.4
gastrin secretion E16.4
globulin R77.1
cortisol-binding E27.8
thyroid-binding E07.89
glomerular, minor —see also N00-N07 with
fourth character .0 N05.0
glucagon secretion E16.3
glucose tolerance (test) (non-fasting)
R73.09
gravitational (G) forces or states (effect of)
T75.81
hair (color) (shaft) L67.9
specified NEC L67.8
hard tissue formation in pulp (dental)
K04.3
head movement R25.0
heart
rate R00.9
specified NEC R00.8
shadow R93.1
sounds NEC R01.2
hemoglobin (disease) —see also Disease,
hemoglobin D58.2
trait —see Trait, hemoglobin, abnormal
histology NEC R89.7
immunological findings R89.4
in serum R76.9
specified NEC R76.8
increase in appetite R63.2
involuntary movement —see Abnormal,
movement, involuntary
jaw closure M26.51
karyotype R89.8
kidney function test R94.4
knee jerk R29.2
leukocyte (cell) (differential) NEC D72.9

Abnormal, abnormality, abnormalities —
(Continued)
liver
▶liver function test R94.5
loss of
height R29.890
weight R63.4
mammogram NEC R92.8
calcification (calculus) R92.1
microcalcification R92.0
Mantoux test R76.11
movement (disorder) —see also Disorder,
movement
head R25.0
involuntary R25.9
fasciculation R25.3
of head R25.0
spasm R25.2
specified type NEC R25.8
tremor R25.1
myoglobin (Aberdeen) (Annapolis) R89.7
neonatal screening P09
oculomotor study R94.113
palmar creases Q82.8
Papanicolaou (smear)
anus R85.619
atypical squamous cells cannot
exclude high grade squamous
intraepithelial lesion (ASC-H)
R85.611
atypical squamous cells of undetermined
significance (ASC-US) R85.610
cytologic evidence of malignancy
R85.614
high grade squamous intraepithelial
lesion (HGSIL) R85.613
human papillomavirus (HPV)
DNA test
high risk positive R85.81
low risk postive R85.82
inadequate smear R85.615
low grade squamous intraepithelial
lesion (LGSIL) R85.612
satisfactory anal smear but lacking
transformation zone R85.616
specified NEC R85.618
unsatisfactory smear R85.615
bronchial washings R84.6
cerebrospinal fluid R83.6
cervix R87.619
atypical squamous cells cannot
exclude high grade squamous
intraepithelial lesion (ASC-H)
R87.611
atypical squamous cells of undetermined
significance (ASC-US) R87.610
cytologic evidence of malignancy
R87.614
high grade squamous intraepithelial
lesion (HGSIL) R87.613
inadequate smear R87.615
low grade squamous intraepithelial
lesion (LGSIL) R87.612
non-atypical endometrial cells R87.618
satisfactory cervical smear but
lacking transformation zone
R87.616
specified NEC R87.618
thin preparaton R87.619
unsatisfactory smear R87.615
nasal secretions R84.6
nipple discharge R89.6
peritoneal fluid R85.69
pleural fluid R84.6
prostatic secretions R86.6
saliva R85.69
seminal fluid R86.6
sites NEC R89.6
sputum R84.6
synovial fluid R89.6
throat scrapings R84.6

Abnormal, abnormality, abnormalities —
(Continued)
Papanicolaou (smear) (Continued)
vagina R87.629
atypical squamous cells cannot
exclude high grade squamous
intraepithelial lesion (ASC-H)
R87.621
atypical squamous cells of
undetermined significance
(ASC-US) R87.620
cytologic evidence of malignancy
R87.624
high grade squamous intraepithelial
lesion (HGSIL) R87.623
inadequate smear R87.625
low grade squamous intraepithelial
lesion (LGSIL) R87.622
specified NEC R87.628
thin preparation R87.629
unsatisfactory smear R87.625
vulva R87.69
wound secretions R89.6
partial thromboplastin time (PTT) R79.1
pelvis (bony) —see Deformity, pelvis
percussion, chest (tympany) R09.89
periods (grossly) —see Menstruation
phonocardiogram R94.39
plantar reflex R29.2
plasma
protein R77.9
specified NEC R77.8
viscosity R70.1
pleural (folds) Q34.0
posture R29.3
product of conception O02.9
specified type NEC O02.89
prothrombin time (PT) R79.1
pulmonary
artery, congenital Q25.79
function, newborn P28.89
test results R94.2
pulsations in neck R00.2
pupillary H21.56-●
function (reaction) (reflex) —see Anomaly,
pupil, function
radiological examination —see Abnormal,
diagnostic imaging
red blood cell(s) (morphology) (volume)
R71.8
reflex —see Reflex
renal function test R94.4
response to nerve stimulation R94.130
retinal correspondence H53.31
retinal function study R94.111
rhythm, heart —see also Arrhythmia
saliva —see Abnormal, specimen, digestive
organs
scan
kidney R94.4
liver R93.2
thyroid R94.6
secretion
gastrin E16.4
glucagon E16.3
semen, seminal fluid —see Abnormal,
specimen, male genital organs
serum level (of)
acid phosphatase R74.8
alkaline phosphatase R74.8
amylase R74.8
enzymes R74.9
specified NEC R74.8
lipase R74.8
triacylglycerol lipase R74.8
shape
gravid uterus —see Anomaly, uterus
sinus venosus Q21.1
size, tooth, teeth K00.2
spacing, tooth, teeth, fully erupted
M26.30

A

Abnormal, abnormality, abnormalities —
    (Continued)
specimen
    digestive organs (peritoneal fluid) (saliva)
        R85.9
        cytology R85.69
        drug level R85.2
        enzyme level R85.0
        histology R85.7
        hormones R85.1
        immunology R85.4
        microbiology R85.5
        nonmedicinal level R85.3
        specified type NEC R85.89
    female genital organs (secretions) (smears)
        R87.9
        cytology R87.69
            cervix R87.619
                human papillomavirus (HPV) DNA
                    test
                    high risk positive R87.810
                    low risk positive R87.820
                    inadequate (unsatisfactory) smear
                        R87.615
                    non-atypical endometrial cells
                        R87.618
                    specified NEC R87.618
            vagina R87.629
                human papillomavirus (HPV) DNA
                    test
                    high risk positive R87.811
                    low risk positive R87.821
                    inadequate (unsatisfactory) smear
                        R87.625
            vulva R87.69
        drug level R87.2
        enzyme level R87.0
        histological R87.7
        hormones R87.1
        immunology R87.4
        microbiology R87.5
        nonmedicinal level R87.3
        specified type NEC R87.89
    male genital organs (prostatic secretions)
        (semen) R86.9
        cytology R86.6
        drug level R86.2
        enzyme level R86.0
        histological R86.7
        hormones R86.1
        immunology R86.4
        microbiology R86.5
        nonmedicinal level R86.3
        specified type NEC R86.8
    nipple discharge —see Abnormal,
        specimen, specified
    respiratory organs (bronchial washings)
        (nasal secretions) (pleural fluid)
        (sputum) R84.9
        cytology R84.6
        drug level R84.2
        enzyme level R84.0
        histology R84.7
        hormones R84.1
        immunology R84.4
        microbiology R84.5
        nonmedicinal level R84.3
        specified type NEC R84.8
    specified organ, system and tissue NOS
        R89.9
        cytology R89.6
        drug level R89.2
        enzyme level R89.0
        histology R89.7
        hormones R89.1
        immunology R89.4
        microbiology R89.5
        nonmedicinal level R89.3
        specified type NEC R89.8
    synovial fluid —see Abnormal, specimen,
        specified

Abnormal, abnormality, abnormalities —
    (Continued)
specimen (Continued)
    thorax (bronchial washings) (pleural
        fluids) —see Abnormal, specimen,
        respiratory organs
    vagina (secretion) (smear) R87.629
    vulva (secretion) (smear) R87.69
    wound secretion —see Abnormal,
        specimen, specified
spermatozoa —see Abnormal, specimen, male
    genital organs
sputum (amount) (color) (odor) R09.3
stool (color) (contents) (mucus) R19.5
    bloody K92.1
    guaiac positive R19.5
synchondrosis Q78.8
thermography —see also Abnormal,
    diagnostic imaging R93.8
thyroid-binding globulin E07.89
tooth, teeth (form) (size) K00.2
toxicology (findings) R78.9
transport protein E88.09
tumor marker NEC R97.8
ultrasound results —see Abnormal, diagnostic
    imaging
umbilical cord complicating delivery O69.9
urination NEC R39.198
urine (constituents) R82.90
    bile R82.2
    cytological examination R82.8
    drugs R82.5
    fat R82.0
    glucose R81
    heavy metals R82.6
    hemoglobin R82.3
    histological examination R82.8
    ketones R82.4
    microbiological examination (culture)
        R82.79
    myoglobin R82.1
    positive culture R82.79
    protein —see Proteinuria
    specified substance NEC R82.99
        chromoabnormality NEC R82.91
    substances nonmedical R82.6
uterine hemorrhage —see Hemorrhage,
    uterus
vectorcardiogram R94.39
visually evoked potential (VEP) R94.112
white blood cells D72.9
    specified NEC D72.89
X-ray examination —see Abnormal,
    diagnostic imaging
Abnormity (any organ or part) —see Anomaly
Abocclusion M26.29
    hemolytic disease (newborn) P55.1
    incompatibility reaction ABO —see
        Complication(s), transfusion,
        incompatibility reaction, ABO
Abolition, language R48.8
Aborter, habitual or recurrent —see Loss (of),
    pregnancy, recurrent
Abortion (complete) (spontaneous) O03.9
    with
        retained products of conception —see
            Abortion, incomplete
    attempted (elective) (failed) O07.4
        complicated by O07.30
            afibrinogenemia O07.1
            cardiac arrest O07.36
            chemical damage of pelvic organ(s)
                O07.34
            circulatory collapse O07.31
            cystitis O07.38
            defibrination syndrome O07.1
            electrolyte imbalance O07.33
            embolism (air) (amniotic fluid) (blood
                clot) (fat) (pulmonary) (septic)
                (soap) O07.2
            endometritis O07.0

Abortion (Continued)
    attempted (Continued)
        complicated by (Continued)
            genital tract and pelvic infection O07.0
            hemolysis O07.1
            hemorrhage (delayed) (excessive) O07.1
            infection
                genital tract or pelvic O07.0
                urinary tract tract O07.38
            intravascular coagulation O07.1
            laceration of pelvic organ(s) O07.34
            metabolic disorder O07.33
            oliguria O07.32
            oophoritis O07.0
            parametritis O07.0
            pelvic peritonitis O07.0
            perforation of pelvic organ(s) O07.34
            renal failure or shutdown O07.32
            salpingitis or salpingo-oophoritis O07.0
            sepsis O07.37
            shock O07.31
            specified condition NEC O07.39
            tubular necrosis (renal) O07.32
            uremia O07.32
            urinary tract infection O07.38
            venous complication NEC O07.35
                embolism (air) (amniotic fluid) (blood
                    clot) (fat) (pulmonary) (septic)
                    (soap) O07.2
    complicated (by) (following) O03.80
        afibrinogenemia O03.6
        cardiac arrest O03.86
        chemical damage of pelvic organ(s) O03.84
        circulatory collapse O03.81
        cystitis O03.88
        defibrination syndrome O03.6
        electrolyte imbalance O03.83
        embolism (air) (amniotic fluid) (blood clot)
            (fat) (pulmonary) (septic) (soap) O03.7
        endometritis O03.5
        genital tract and pelvic infection O03.5
        hemolysis O03.6
        hemorrhage (delayed) (excessive) O03.6
        infection
            genital tract or pelvic O03.5
            urinary tract O03.88
        intravascular coagulation O03.6
        laceration of pelvic organ(s) O03.84
        metabolic disorder O03.83
        oliguria O03.82
        oophoritis O03.5
        parametritis O03.5
        pelvic peritonitis O03.5
        perforation of pelvic organ(s) O03.84
        renal failure or shutdown O03.82
        salpingitis or salpingo-oophoritis
            O03.5
        sepsis O03.87
        shock O03.81
        specified condition NEC O03.89
        tubular necrosis (renal) O03.82
        uremia O03.82
        urinary tract infection O03.88
        venous complication NEC O03.85
            embolism (air) (amniotic fluid) (blood
                clot) (fat) (pulmonary) (septic)
                (soap) O03.7
    failed —see Abortion, attempted
    habitual or recurrent N96
    ➡with current abortion —see categories
        O03-O04
        without current pregnancy N96
        care in current pregnancy O26.2-●
    incomplete (spontaneous) O03.4
        complicated (by) (following) O03.30
            afibrinogenemia O03.1
            cardiac arrest O03.36
            chemical damage of pelvic organ(s)
                O03.34
            circulatory collapse O03.31
            cystitis O03.38

▶ New   ⇒ Revised   ~~deleted~~ Deleted   ● Use Additional Character(s)

Abortion *(Continued)*
  incomplete *(Continued)*
    complicated *(Continued)*
      defibrination syndrome O03.1
      electrolyte imbalance O03.33
      embolism (air) (amniotic fluid) (blood
          clot) (fat) (pulmonary) (septic)
          (soap) O03.2
      endometritis O03.0
      genital tract and pelvic infection O03.0
      hemolysis O03.1
      hemorrhage (delayed) (excessive)
          O03.1
      infection
        genital tract or pelvic O03.0
        urinary tract O03.38
      intravascular coagulation O03.1
      laceration of pelvic organ(s) O03.34
      metabolic disorder O03.33
      oliguria O03.32
      oophoritis O03.0
      parametritis O03.0
      pelvic peritonitis O03.0
      perforation of pelvic organ(s) O03.34
      renal failure or shutdown O03.32
      salpingitis or salpingo-oophoritis O03.0
      sepsis O03.37
      shock O03.31
      specified condition NEC O03.39
      tubular necrosis (renal) O03.32
      uremia O03.32
      urinary infection O03.38
      venous complication NEC O03.35
        embolism (air) (amniotic fluid) (blood
            clot) (fat) (pulmonary) (septic)
            (soap) O03.2
  induced (encounter for) Z33.2
    complicated by O04.80
      afibrinogenemia O04.6
      cardiac arrest O04.86
      chemical damage of pelvic organ(s)
          O04.84
      circulatory collapse O04.81
      cystitis O04.88
      defibrination syndrome O04.6
      electrolyte imbalance O04.83
      embolism (air) (amniotic fluid) (blood
          clot) (fat) (pulmonary) (septic)
          (soap) O04.7
      endometritis O04.5
      genital tract and pelvic infection O04.5
      hemolysis O04.6
      hemorrhage (delayed) (excessive) O04.6
      infection
        genital tract or pelvic O04.5
        urinary tract O04.88
      intravascular coagulation O04.6
      laceration of pelvic organ(s) O04.84
      metabolic disorder O04.83
      oliguria O04.82
      oophoritis O04.5
      parametritis O04.5
      pelvic peritonitis O04.5
      perforation of pelvic organ(s) O04.84
      renal failure or shutdown O04.82
      salpingitis or salpingo-oophoritis O04.5
      sepsis O04.87
      shock O04.81
      specified condition NEC O04.89
      tubular necrosis (renal) O04.82
      uremia O04.82
      urinary tract infection O04.88
      venous complication NEC O04.85
        embolism (air) (amniotic fluid) (blood
            clot) (fat) (pulmonary) (septic)
            (soap) O04.7
  missed O02.1
  spontaneous —*see* Abortion (complete)
      (spontaneous)
    threatened O20.0
  threatened (spontaneous) O20.0

Abortion *(Continued)*
  tubal O00.10-
    with intrauterine pregnancy O00.11-
Abortus fever A23.1
Aboulomania F60.7
Abrami's disease D59.8
Abramov-Fiedler myocarditis (acute isolated
    myocarditis) I40.1
Abrasion T14.8
  abdomen, abdominal (wall) S30.811
  alveolar process S00.512
  ankle S90.51-●
  antecubital space —*see* Abrasion, elbow
  anus S30.817
  arm (upper) S40.81-●
  auditory canal —*see* Abrasion, ear
  auricle —*see* Abrasion, ear
  axilla —*see* Abrasion, arm
  back, lower S30.810
  breast S20.11-●
  brow S00.81
  buttock S30.810
  calf —*see* Abrasion, leg
  canthus —*see* Abrasion, eyelid
  cheek S00.81
    internal S00.512
  chest wall —*see* Abrasion, thorax
  chin S00.81
  clitoris S30.814
  cornea S05.0-●
  costal region —*see* Abrasion, thorax
  dental K03.1
  digit(s)
    foot —*see* Abrasion, toe
    hand —*see* Abrasion, finger
  ear S00.41-●
  elbow S50.31-●
  epididymis S30.813
  epigastric region S30.811
  epiglottis S10.11
  esophagus (thoracic) S27.818
    cervical S10.11
  eyebrow —*see* Abrasion, eyelid
  eyelid S00.21-●
  face S00.81
  finger(s) S60.41-●
    index S60.41-●
    little S60.41-●
    middle S60.41-●
    ring S60.41-●
  flank S30.811
  foot (except toe(s) alone) S90.81-●
    toe —*see* Abrasion, toe
  forearm S50.81-●
    elbow only —*see* Abrasion, elbow
  forehead S00.81
  genital organs, external
    female S30.816
    male S30.815
  groin S30.811
  gum S00.512
  hand S60.51-●
  head S00.91
    ear —*see* Abrasion, ear
    eyelid —*see* Abrasion, eyelid
    lip S00.511
    nose S00.31
    oral cavity S00.512
    scalp S00.01
    specified site NEC S00.81
  heel —*see* Abrasion, foot
  hip S70.21-●
  inguinal region S30.811
  interscapular region S20.419
  jaw S00.81
  knee S80.21-●
  labium (majus) (minus) S30.814
  larynx S10.11
  leg (lower) S80.81-●
    knee —*see* Abrasion, knee
    upper —*see* Abrasion, thigh

Abrasion *(Continued)*
  lip S00.511
  lower back S30.810
  lumbar region S30.810
  malar region S00.81
  mammary —*see* Abrasion, breast
  mastoid region S00.81
  mouth S00.512
  nail
    finger —*see* Abrasion, finger
    toe —*see* Abrasion, toe
  nape S10.81
  nasal S00.31
  neck S10.91
    specified site NEC S10.81
    throat S10.11
  nose S00.31
  occipital region S00.01
  oral cavity S00.512
  orbital region —*see* Abrasion, eyelid
  palate S00.512
  palm —*see* Abrasion, hand
  parietal region S00.01
  pelvis S30.810
  penis S30.812
  perineum
    female S30.814
    male S30.810
  periocular area —*see* Abrasion, eyelid
  phalanges
    finger —*see* Abrasion, finger
    toe —*see* Abrasion, toe
  pharynx S10.11
  pinna —*see* Abrasion, ear
  popliteal space —*see* Abrasion, knee
  prepuce S30.812
  pubic region S30.810
  pudendum
    female S30.816
    male S30.815
  sacral region S30.810
  scalp S00.01
  scapular region —*see* Abrasion, shoulder
  scrotum S30.813
  shin —*see* Abrasion, leg
  shoulder S40.21-●
  skin NEC T14.8
  sternal region S20.319
  submaxillary region S00.81
  submental region S00.81
  subungual
    finger(s) —*see* Abrasion, finger
    toe(s) —*see* Abrasion, toe
  supraclavicular fossa S10.81
  supraorbital S00.81
  temple S00.81
  temporal region S00.81
  testis S30.813
  thigh S70.31-●
  thorax, thoracic (wall) S20.91
    back S20.41-●
    front S20.31-●
  throat S10.11
  thumb S60.31-●
  toe(s) (lesser) S90.416
    great S90.41-●
  tongue S00.512
  tooth, teeth (dentifrice) (habitual) (hard
      tissues) (occupational) (ritual)
      (traditional) K03.1
  trachea S10.11
  tunica vaginalis S30.813
  tympanum, tympanic membrane —*see*
      Abrasion, ear
  uvula S00.512
  vagina S30.814
  vocal cords S10.11
  vulva S30.814
  wrist S60.81-●
Abrism —*see* Poisoning, food, noxious,
    plant

Abruptio placentae O45.9-●
  with
    afibrinogenemia O45.01-●
    coagulation defect O45.00-●
      specified NEC O45.09-●
    disseminated intravascular coagulation
      O45.02-●
    hypofibrinogenemia O45.01-●
  specified NEC O45.8-●
Abruption, placenta —see Abruptio placentae
Abscess (connective tissue) (embolic) (fistulous)
    (infective) (metastatic) (multiple)
    (pernicious) (pyogenic) (septic) L02.91
  with
    diverticular disease (intestine) K57.80
      with bleeding K57.81
      large intestine K57.20
        with
          bleeding K57.21
          small intestine K57.40
            with bleeding K57.41
      small intestine K57.00
        with
          bleeding K57.01
          large intestine K57.40
            with bleeding K57.41
    lymphangitis - code by site under
      Abscess
  abdomen, abdominal
    cavity K65.1
    wall L02.211
  abdominopelvic K65.1
  accessory sinus —see Sinusitis
  adrenal (capsule) (gland) E27.8
  alveolar K04.7
    with sinus K04.6
  amebic A06.4
    brain (and liver or lung abscess) A06.6
    genitourinary tract A06.82
    liver (without mention of brain or lung
      abscess) A06.4
    lung (and liver) (without mention of brain
      abscess) A06.5
    specified site NEC A06.89
    spleen A06.89
  anerobic A48.0
  ankle —see Abscess, lower limb
  anorectal K61.2
  antecubital space —see Abscess, upper limb
  antrum (chronic) (Highmore) —see Sinusitis,
      maxillary
  anus K61.0
  apical (tooth) K04.7
    with sinus (alveolar) K04.6
  appendix K35.3
  areola (acute) (chronic) (nonpuerperal)
      N61.1
    puerperal, postpartum or gestational —see
      Infection, nipple
  arm (any part) —see Abscess, upper limb
  artery (wall) I77.89
  atheromatous I77.2
  auricle, ear —see Abscess, ear, external
  axilla (region) L02.41-●
    lymph gland or node L04.2
  back (any part, except buttock) L02.212
  Bartholin's gland N75.1
    with
      abortion —see Abortion, by type
        complicated by, sepsis
      ectopic or molar pregnancy O08.0
    following ectopic or molar pregnancy O08.0
  Bezold's —see Mastoiditis, acute
  bilharziasis B65.1
  bladder (wall) —see Cystitis, specified type
      NEC
  bone (subperiosteal) —see also Osteomyelitis,
      specified type NEC
    accessory sinus (chronic) —see Sinusitis
    chronic or old —see Osteomyelitis, chronic
    jaw (lower) (upper) M27.2

Abscess (Continued)
  bone (Continued)
    mastoid —see Mastoiditis, acute,
      subperiosteal
    petrous —see Petrositis
    spinal (tuberculous) A18.01
      nontuberculous —see Osteomyelitis,
        vertebra
  bowel K63.0
  brain (any part) (cystic) (otogenic) G06.0
    amebic (with abscess of any other site) A06.6
    gonococcal A54.82
    pheomycotic (chromomycotic) B43.1
    tuberculous A17.81
  breast (acute) (chronic) (nonpuerperal)
      N61.1
    newborn P39.0
    puerperal, postpartum, gestational —see
      Mastitis, obstetric, purulent
  broad ligament N73.2
    acute N73.0
    chronic N73.1
  Brodie's (localized) (chronic) M86.8X-●
  bronchi J98.09
  buccal cavity K12.2
  bulbourethral gland N34.0
  bursa M71.00
    ankle M71.07-●
    elbow M71.02-●
    foot M71.07-●
    hand M71.04-●
    hip M71.05-●
    knee M71.06-●
    multiple sites M71.09
    pharyngeal J39.1
    shoulder M71.01-●
    specified site NEC M71.08
    wrist M71.03-●
  buttock L02.31
  canthus —see Blepharoconjunctivitis
  cartilage —see Disorder, cartilage, specified
      type NEC
  cecum K35.3
  cerebellum, cerebellar G06.0
    sequelae G09
  cerebral (embolic) G06.0
    sequelae G09
  cervical (meaning neck) L02.11
    lymph gland or node L04.0
  cervix (stump) (uteri) —see Cervicitis
  cheek (external) L02.01
    inner K12.2
  chest J86.9
    with fistula J86.0
    wall L02.213
  chin L02.01
  choroid —see Inflammation, chorioretinal
  circumtonsillar J36
  cold (lung) (tuberculous) —see also
      Tuberculosis, abscess, lung
    articular —see Tuberculosis, joint
  colon (wall) K63.0
  colostomy K94.02
  conjunctiva —see Conjunctivitis, acute
  cornea H16.31-●
  corpus
    cavernosum N48.21
    luteum —see Oophoritis
  Cowper's gland N34.0
  cranium G06.0
  cul-de-sac (Douglas') (posterior) —see
      Peritonitis, pelvic, female
  cutaneous —see Abscess, by site
  dental K04.7
    with sinus (alveolar) K04.6
  dentoalveolar K04.7
    with sinus K04.6
  diaphragm, diaphragmatic K65.1
  Douglas' cul-de-sac or pouch —see
      Peritonitis, pelvic, female
  Dubois A50.59

Abscess (Continued)
  ear (middle) —see also Otitis, media,
      suppurative
    acute —see Otitis, media, suppurative,
      acute
    external H60.0-●
  entamebic —see Abscess, amebic
  enterostomy K94.12
  epididymis N45.4
  epidural G06.2
    brain G06.0
    spinal cord G06.1
  epiglottis J38.7
  epiploon, epiploic K65.1
  erysipelatous —see Erysipelas
  esophagus K20.8
  ethmoid (bone) (chronic) (sinus) J32.2
  external auditory canal —see Abscess, ear,
      external
  extradural G06.2
    brain G06.0
      sequelae G09
    spinal cord G06.1
  extraperitoneal K68.19
  eye —see Endophthalmitis, purulent
  eyelid H00.03-●
  face (any part, except ear, eye and nose)
      L02.01
  fallopian tube —see Salpingitis
  fascia M72.8
  fauces J39.1
  fecal K63.0
  femoral (region) —see Abscess, lower limb
  filaria, filarial —see Infestation, filarial
  finger (any) —see also Abscess, hand
    nail —see Cellulitis, finger
  foot L02.61-●
  forehead L02.01
  frontal sinus (chronic) J32.1
  gallbladder K81.0
  genital organ or tract
    female (external) N76.4
    male N49.9
      multiple sites N49.8
      specified NEC N49.8
  gestational mammary O91.11-●
  gestational subareolar O91.11-●
  gingival —see Peridontitis, aggressive,
      localized
  gland, glandular (lymph) (acute) —see
      Lymphadenitis, acute
  gluteal (region) L02.31
  gonorrheal —see Gonococcus
  groin L02.214
  gum —see Peridontitis, aggressive, localized
  hand L02.51-●
  head NEC L02.811
    face (any part, except ear, eye and nose)
      L02.01
  heart —see Carditis
  heel —see Abscess, foot
  helminthic —see Infestation, helminth
  hepatic (cholangitic) (hematogenic)
      (lymphogenic) (pylephlebitic) K75.0
    amebic A06.4
  hip (region) —see Abscess, lower limb
  ileocecal K35.3
  ileostomy (bud) K94.12
  iliac (region) L02.214
    fossa K35.3
  infraclavicular (fossa) —see Abscess, upper
      limb
  inguinal (region) L02.214
    lymph gland or node L04.1
  intestine, intestinal NEC K63.0
    rectal K61.1
  intra-abdominal —see also Abscess,
      peritoneum K65.1
➣ postprocedural T81.4
      retroperitoneal K68.11
    intra-muscular, postprocedural T81.42

Abscess *(Continued)*
  intracranial G06.0
  intramammary —*see* Abscess, breast
  intraorbital —*see* Abscess, orbit
  intraperitoneal K65.1
  intrasphincteric (anus) K61.4
  intraspinal G06.1
  intratonsillar J36
  ischiorectal (fossa) K61.3
  jaw (bone) (lower) (upper) M27.2
  joint —*see* Arthritis, pyogenic or pyemic
    spine (tuberculous) A18.01
      nontuberculous —*see* Spondylopathy,
        infective
  kidney N15.1
    with calculus N20.0
      with hydronephrosis N13.6
    puerperal (postpartum) O86.21
  knee —*see also* Abscess, lower limb
    joint M00.9
  labium (majus) (minus) N76.4
  lacrimal
    caruncle —*see* Inflammation, lacrimal,
      passages, acute
    gland —*see* Dacryoadenitis
    passages (duct) (sac) —*see* Inflammation,
      lacrimal, passages, acute
  lacunar N34.0
  larynx J38.7
  lateral (alveolar) K04.7
    with sinus K04.6
  leg (any part) —*see* Abscess, lower limb
  lens H27.8
  lingual K14.0
    tonsil J36
  lip K13.0
  Littre's gland N34.0
  liver (cholangitic) (hematogenic)
    (lymphogenic) (pylephlebitic) (pyogenic)
    K75.0
    amebic (due to Entamoeba histolytica)
      (dysenteric) (tropical) A06.4
      with
        brain abscess (and liver or lung
          abscess) A06.6
        lung abscess A06.5
  loin (region) L02.211
  lower limb L02.41-●
  lumbar (tuberculous) A18.01
    nontuberculous L02.212
  lung (miliary) (putrid) J85.2
    with pneumonia J85.1
      due to specified organism (*see*
        Pneumonia, in (due to))
    amebic (with liver abscess) A06.5
      with
        brain abscess A06.6
        pneumonia A06.5
  lymph, lymphatic, gland or node (acute) —*see*
    also Lymphadenitis, acute
    mesentery I88.0
  malar M27.2
  mammary gland —*see* Abscess, breast
  marginal, anus K61.0
  mastoid —*see* Mastoiditis, acute
  maxilla, maxillary M27.2
    molar (tooth) K04.7
      with sinus K04.6
    premolar K04.7
    sinus (chronic) J32.0
  mediastinum J85.3
  meibomian gland —*see* Hordeolum
  meninges G06.2
  mesentery, mesenteric K65.1
  mesosalpinx —*see* Salpingitis
  mons pubis L02.215
  mouth (floor) K12.2
  muscle —*see* Myositis, infective
  myocardium I40.0
  nabothian (follicle) —*see* Cervicitis
  nasal J32.9
  nasopharyngeal J39.1

Abscess *(Continued)*
  navel L02.216
    newborn P38.9
      with mild hemorrhage P38.1
      without hemorrhage P38.9
  neck (region) L02.11
    lymph gland or node L04.0
  nephritic —*see* Abscess, kidney
  nipple N61.1
    associated with
      lactation —*see* Pregnancy, complicated by
      pregnancy —*see* Pregnancy, complicated
        by
  nose (external) (fossa) (septum) J34.0
    sinus (chronic) —*see* Sinusitis
  omentum K65.1
  operative wound T81.4
  orbit, orbital —*see* Cellulitis, orbit
  otogenic G06.0
  ovary, ovarian (corpus luteum) —*see*
    Oophoritis
  oviduct —*see* Oophoritis
  palate (soft) K12.2
    hard M27.2
  palmar (space) —*see* Abscess, hand
  pancreas (duct) —*see* Pancreatitis, acute
  parafrenal N48.21
  parametric, parametrium N73.2
    acute N73.0
    chronic N73.1
  paranephric N15.1
  parapancreatic —*see* Pancreatitis, acute
  parapharyngeal J39.0
  pararectal K61.1
  parasinus —*see* Sinusitis
  parauterine (*see also* Disease, pelvis,
    inflammatory) N73.2
  paravaginal —*see* Vaginitis
  parietal region (scalp) L02.811
  parodontal —*see* Peridontitis, aggressive,
    localized
  parotid (duct) (gland) K11.3
    region K12.2
  pectoral (region) L02.213
  pelvis, pelvic
    female —*see* Disease, pelvis, inflammatory
    male, peritoneal K65.1
  penis N48.21
    gonococcal (accessory gland) (periurethral)
      A54.1
  perianal K61.0
  periapical K04.7
    with sinus (alveolar) K04.6
  periappendicular K35.3
  pericardial I30.1
  pericecal K35.3
  pericemental —*see* Peridontitis, aggressive,
    localized
  pericholecystic —*see* Cholecystitis, acute
  pericoronal —*see* Peridontitis, aggressive,
    localized
  peridental —*see* Peridontitis, aggressive,
    localized
  perimetric —*see also* Disease, pelvis,
    inflammatory N73.2
  perinephric, perinephritic —*see* Abscess,
    kidney
  perineum, perineal (superficial) L02.215
    urethra N34.0
  periodontal (parietal) —*see* Peridontitis,
    aggressive, localized
    apical K04.7
  periosteum, periosteal —*see also*
    Osteomyelitis, specified type NEC
    with osteomyelitis —*see also* Osteomyelitis,
      specified type NEC
      acute —*see* Osteomyelitis, acute
      chronic —*see* Osteomyelitis, chronic
  peripharyngeal J39.0
  peripleuritic J86.9
    with fistula J86.0

Abscess *(Continued)*
  periprostatic N41.2
  perirectal K61.1
  perirenal (tissue) —*see* Abscess, kidney
  perisinuous (nose) —*see* Sinusitis
  peritoneum, peritoneal (perforated)
    (ruptured) K65.1
    with appendicitis K35.3
    pelvic
      female —*see* Peritonitis, pelvic, female
      male K65.1
    postoperative T81.4
    puerperal, postpartum, childbirth O85
    tuberculous A18.31
  peritonsillar J36
  perityphlic K35.3
  periureteral N28.89
  periurethral N34.0
    gonococcal (accessory gland) (periurethral)
      A54.1
  periuterine —*see also* Disease, pelvis,
    inflammatory N73.2
  perivesical —*see* Cystitis, specified type NEC
  petrous bone —*see* Petrositis
  phagedenic NOS L02.91
    chancroid A57
  pharynx, pharyngeal (lateral) J39.1
  pilonidal L05.01
  pituitary (gland) E23.6
  pleura J86.9
    with fistula J86.0
  popliteal —*see* Abscess, lower limb
  postcecal K35.3
  postlaryngeal J38.7
  postnasal J34.0
  postoperative (any site) T81.4
    retroperitoneal K68.11
  postpharyngeal J39.0
  posttonsillar J36
  post-typhoid A01.09
  pouch of Douglas —*see* Peritonitis, pelvic,
    female
  premammary —*see* Abscess, breast
  prepatellar —*see* Abscess, lower limb
  prostate N41.2
    gonococcal (acute) (chronic) A54.22
  psoas muscle K68.12
  puerperal - code by site under Puerperal,
    abscess
  pulmonary —*see* Abscess, lung
  pulp, pulpal (dental) K04.01
    irreversible K04.02
    reversible K04.01
  rectovaginal septum K63.0
  rectovesical —*see* Cystitis, specified type NEC
  rectum K61.1
  renal —*see* Abscess, kidney
  retina —*see* Inflammation, chorioretinal
  retrobulbar —*see* Abscess, orbit
  retrocecal K65.1
  retrolaryngeal J38.7
  retromammary —*see* Abscess, breast
  retroperitoneal NEC K68.19
    postprocedural K68.11
  retropharyngeal J39.0
  retrouterine —*see* Peritonitis, pelvic, female
  retrovesical —*see* Cystitis, specified type NEC
  root, tooth K04.7
    with sinus (alveolar) K04.6
  round ligament —*see also* Disease, pelvis,
    inflammatory N73.2
  rupture (spontaneous) NOS L02.91
  sacrum (tuberculous) A18.01
    nontuberculous M46.28
  salivary (duct) (gland) K11.3
  scalp (any part) L02.811
  scapular —*see* Osteomyelitis, specified type
    NEC
  sclera —*see* Scleritis
  scrofulous (tuberculous) A18.2
  scrotum N49.2

Abscess *(Continued)*
  seminal vesicle N49.0
  septal, dental K04.7
    with sinus (alveolar) K04.6
  serous —*see* Periostitis
  shoulder (region) —*see* Abscess, upper limb
  sigmoid K63.0
  sinus (accessory) (chronic) (nasal) —*see also*
      Sinusitis
    intracranial venous (any) G06.0
  Skene's duct or gland N34.0
  skin —*see* Abscess, by site
  specified site NEC L02.818
  spermatic cord N49.1
  sphenoidal (sinus) (chronic) J32.3
  spinal cord (any part) (staphylococcal) G06.1
    tuberculous A17.81
  spine (column) (tuberculous) A18.01
    epidural G06.1
    nontuberculous —*see* Osteomyelitis,
        vertebra
  spleen D73.3
    amebic A06.89
⇒ stitch T81.4
  subarachnoid G06.2
    brain G06.0
    spinal cord G06.1
  subareolar —*see* Abscess, breast
  subcecal K35.3
  subcutaneous —*see also* Abscess, by site
    pheomycotic (chromomycotic) B43.2
    postprocedural T81.41
  subdiaphragmatic K65.1
  subdural G06.2
    brain G06.0
      sequelae G09
    spinal cord G06.1
  subgaleal L02.811
  subhepatic K65.1
  sublingual K12.2
    gland K11.3
  submammary —*see* Abscess, breast
  submandibular (region) (space) (triangle) K12.2
    gland K11.3
  submaxillary (region) L02.01
    gland K11.3
  submental L02.01
    gland K11.3
  subperiosteal —*see* Osteomyelitis, specified
      type NEC
  subphrenic K65.1
⇒ postoperative T81.4
  suburethral N34.0
  sudoriparous L75.8
  supraclavicular (fossa) —*see* Abscess, upper
      limb
  suprapelvic, acute N73.0
  suprarenal (capsule) (gland) E27.8
  sweat gland L74.8
  tear duct —*see* Inflammation, lacrimal,
      passages, acute
  temple L02.01
  temporal region L02.01
  temporosphenoidal G06.0
  tendon (sheath) M65.00
    ankle M65.07-•
    foot M65.07-•
    forearm M65.03-•
    hand M65.04-•
    lower leg M65.06-•
    pelvic region M65.05-•
    shoulder region M65.01-•
    specified site NEC M65.08
    thigh M65.05-•
    upper arm M65.02-•
  testis N45.4
  thigh —*see* Abscess, lower limb
  thorax J86.9
    with fistula J86.0
  throat J39.1
  thumb —*see also* Abscess, hand
    nail —*see* Cellulitis, finger

Abscess *(Continued)*
  thymus (gland) E32.1
  thyroid (gland) E06.0
  toe (any) —*see also* Abscess, foot
    nail —*see* Cellulitis, toe
  tongue (staphylococcal) K14.0
  tonsil(s) (lingual) J36
  tonsillopharyngeal J36
  tooth, teeth (root) K04.7
    with sinus (alveolar) K04.6
    supporting structures NEC —*see*
        Peridontitis, aggressive, localized
  trachea J39.8
  trunk L02.219
    abdominal wall L02.211
    back L02.212
    chest wall L02.213
    groin L02.214
    perineum L02.215
    umbilicus L02.216
  tubal —*see* Salpingitis
  tuberculous —*see* Tuberculosis, abscess
  tubo-ovarian —*see* Salpingo-oophoritis
  tunica vaginalis N49.1
  umbilicus L02.216
  upper
    limb L02.41-•
    respiratory J39.8
  urethral (gland) N34.0
  urinary N34.0
  uterus, uterine (wall) —*see also* Endometritis
    ligament —*see also* Disease, pelvis,
        inflammatory N73.2
    neck —*see* Cervicitis
  uvula K12.2
  vagina (wall) —*see* Vaginitis
  vaginorectal —*see* Vaginitis
  vas deferens N49.1
  vermiform appendix K35.3
  vertebra (column) (tuberculous) A18.01
    nontuberculous —*see* Osteomyelitis,
        vertebra
  vesical —*see* Cystitis, specified type NEC
  vesico-uterine pouch —*see* Peritonitis, pelvic,
      female
  vitreous (humor) —*see* Endophthalmitis,
      purulent
  vocal cord J38.3
  von Bezold's —*see* Mastoiditis, acute
  vulva N76.4
  vulvovaginal gland N75.1
  web space —*see* Abscess, hand
⇒ wound T81.4
  wrist —*see* Abscess, upper limb
Absence (of) (organ or part) (complete or
    partial)
  adrenal (gland) (congenital) Q89.1
    acquired E89.6
  albumin in blood E88.09
  alimentary tract (congenital) Q45.8
    upper Q40.8
  alveolar process (acquired) —*see* Anomaly,
      alveolar
  ankle (acquired) Z89.44-•
  anus (congenital) Q42.3
    with fistula Q42.2
  aorta (congenital) Q25.41
  appendix, congenital Q42.8
  arm (acquired) Z89.20-•
    above elbow Z89.22-•
      congenital (with hand present) —*see*
          Agenesis, arm, with hand present
          and hand —*see* Agenesis, forearm,
              and hand
      below elbow Z89.21-•
      congenital (with hand present) —*see*
          Agenesis, arm, with hand present
          and hand —*see* Agenesis, forearm,
              and hand
      congenital —*see* Defect, reduction, upper
          limb

Absence *(Continued)*
  arm *(Continued)*
    shoulder (following explantation of
        shoulder joint prosthesis) (joint) (with
        or without presence of antibiotic-
        impregnated cement spacer) Z89.23-•
    congenital (with hand present) —*see*
        Agenesis, arm, with hand present
  artery (congenital) (peripheral) Q27.8
    brain Q28.3
    coronary Q24.5
    pulmonary Q25.79
    specified NEC Q27.8
    umbilical Q27.0
  atrial septum (congenital) Q21.1
  auditory canal (congenital) (external) Q16.1
  auricle (ear), congenital Q16.0
  bile, biliary duct, congenital Q44.5
  bladder (acquired) Z90.6
    congenital Q64.5
  bowel sounds R19.11
  brain Q00.0
    part of Q04.3
  breast(s) (and nipple(s)) (acquired) Z90.1-•
    congenital Q83.8
  broad ligament Q50.6
  bronchus (congenital) Q32.4
  canaliculus lacrimalis, congenital Q10.4
  cerebellum (vermis) Q04.3
  cervix (acquired) (with uterus) Z90.710
    with remaining uterus Z90.712
    congenital Q51.5
  chin, congenital Q18.8
  cilia (congenital) Q10.3
    acquired —*see* Madarosis
  clitoris (congenital) Q52.6
  coccyx, congenital Q76.49
  cold sense R20.8
  congenital
    lumen —*see* Atresia
    organ or site NEC —*see* Agenesis
    septum —*see* Imperfect, closure
  corpus callosum Q04.0
  cricoid cartilage, congenital Q31.8
  diaphragm (with hernia), congenital Q79.1
  digestive organ(s) or tract, congenital Q45.8
    acquired NEC Z90.49
    upper Q40.8
  ductus arteriosus Q28.8
  duodenum (acquired) Z90.49
    congenital Q41.0
  ear, congenital Q16.9
    acquired H93.8-•
    auricle Q16.0
    external Q16.0
    inner Q16.5
    lobe, lobule Q17.8
    middle, except ossicles Q16.4
      ossicles Q16.3
    ossicles Q16.3
  ejaculatory duct (congenital) Q55.4
  endocrine gland (congenital) NEC Q89.2
    acquired E89.89
  epididymis (congenital) Q55.4
    acquired Z90.79
  epiglottis, congenital Q31.8
  esophagus (congenital) Q39.8
    acquired (partial) Z90.49
  eustachian tube (congenital) Q16.2
  extremity (acquired) Z89.9
    congenital Q73.0
    knee (following explantation of knee joint
        prosthesis) (joint) (with or without
        presence of antibiotic-impregnated
        cement spacer) Z89.52-•
    lower (above knee) Z89.619
      below knee Z89.51-•
    upper —*see* Absence, arm
  eye (acquired) Z90.01
    congenital Q11.1
    muscle (congenital) Q10.3

▶ New   ⇒ Revised   ~~deleted~~ Deleted   • Use Additional Character(s)

Absence *(Continued)*
  eyeball (acquired) Z90.01
  eyelid (fold) (congenital) Q10.3
    acquired Z90.01
  face, specified part NEC Q18.8
  fallopian tube(s) (acquired) Z90.79
    congenital Q50.6
  family member (causing problem in home)
    NEC —*see also* Disruption, family Z63.32
  femur, congenital —*see* Defect, reduction,
    lower limb, longitudinal, femur
  fibrinogen (congenital) D68.2
    acquired D65
  finger(s) (acquired) Z89.02-•
    congenital —*see* Agenesis, hand
  foot (acquired) Z89.43-•
    congenital —*see* Agenesis, foot
  forearm (acquired) —*see* Absence, arm, below
    elbow
  gallbladder (acquired) Z90.49
    congenital Q44.0
  gamma globulin in blood D80.1
    hereditary D80.0
  genital organs
    acquired (female) (male) Z90.79
    female, congenital Q52.8
      external Q52.71
      internal NEC Q52.8
    male, congenital Q55.8
  genitourinary organs, congenital NEC
    female Q52.8
    male Q55.8
  globe (acquired) Z90.01
    congenital Q11.1
  glottis, congenital Q31.8
  hand and wrist (acquired) Z89.11-•
    congenital —*see* Agenesis, hand
  head, part (acquired) NEC Z90.09
  heat sense R20.8
  hip (following explantation of hip joint
    prosthesis) (joint) (with or without
    presence of antibiotic-impregnated
    cement spacer) Z89.62-•
  hymen (congenital) Q52.4
  ileum (acquired) Z90.49
    congenital Q41.2
  immunoglobulin, isolated NEC D80.3
    IgA D80.2
    IgG D80.3
    IgM D80.4
  incus (acquired) —*see* Loss, ossicles, ear
    congenital Q16.3
  inner ear, congenital Q16.5
  intestine (acquired) (small) Z90.49
    congenital Q41.9
      specified NEC Q41.8
    large Z90.49
      congenital Q42.9
        specified NEC Q42.8
  iris, congenital Q13.1
  jejunum (acquired) Z90.49
    congenital Q41.1
  joint
    acquired
      hip (following explantation of hip joint
        prosthesis) (with or without
        presence of antibiotic-impregnated
        cement spacer) Z89.62-•
      knee (following explantation of knee
        joint prosthesis) (with or without
        presence of antibiotic-impregnated
        cement spacer) Z89.52-•
      shoulder (following explantation of
        shoulder joint prosthesis) (with or
        without presence of antibiotic-
        impregnated cement spacer)
        Z89.23-•
    congenital NEC Q74.8
  kidney(s) (acquired) Z90.5
    congenital Q60.2
      bilateral Q60.1
      unilateral Q60.0

Absence *(Continued)*
  knee (following explantation of knee joint
    prosthesis) (joint) (with or without
    presence of antibiotic-impregnated
    cement spacer) Z89.52-•
  labyrinth, membranous Q16.5
  larynx (congenital) Q31.8
    acquired Z90.02
  leg (acquired) (above knee) Z89.61-•
    below knee (acquired) Z89.51-•
    congenital —*see* Defect, reduction, lower
      limb
  lens (acquired) —*see also* Aphakia
    congenital Q12.3
    post cataract extraction Z98.4-•
  limb (acquired) —*see* Absence, extremity
  lip Q38.6
  liver (congenital) Q44.7
  lung (fissure) (lobe) (bilateral) (unilateral)
    (congenital) Q33.3
    acquired (any part) Z90.2
  menstruation —*see* Amenorrhea
  muscle (congenital) (pectoral) Q79.8
    ocular Q10.3
  neck, part Q18.8
  neutrophil —*see* Agranulocytosis
  nipple(s) (with breast(s)) (acquired) Z90.1-•
    congenital Q83.2
  nose (congenital) Q30.1
    acquired Z90.09
  organ
    of Corti, congenital Q16.5
    or site, congenital NEC Q89.8
      acquired NEC Z90.89
  osseous meatus (ear) Q16.4
  ovary (acquired)
    bilateral Z90.722
    congenital
      bilateral Q50.02
      unilateral Q50.01
    unilateral Z90.721
  oviduct (acquired)
    bilateral Z90.722
    congenital Q50.6
    unilateral Z90.721
  pancreas (congenital) Q45.0
    acquired Z90.410
      complete Z90.410
      partial Z90.411
      total Z90.410
  parathyroid gland (acquired) E89.2
    congenital Q89.2
  patella, congenital Q74.1
  penis (congenital) Q55.5
    acquired Z90.79
  pericardium (congenital) Q24.8
  pituitary gland (congenital) Q89.2
    acquired E89.3
  prostate (acquired) Z90.79
    congenital Q55.4
  pulmonary valve Q22.0
  punctum lacrimale (congenital) Q10.4
  radius, congenital —*see* Defect, reduction,
    upper limb, longitudinal, radius
  rectum (congenital) Q42.1
    with fistula Q42.0
    acquired Z90.49
  respiratory organ NOS Q34.9
  rib (acquired) Z90.89
    congenital Q76.6
  sacrum, congenital Q76.49
  salivary gland(s), congenital Q38.4
  scrotum, congenital Q55.29
  seminal vesicles (congenital) Q55.4
    acquired Z90.79
  septum
    atrial (congenital) Q21.1
    between aorta and pulmonary artery Q21.4
    ventricular (congenital) Q20.4
  sex chromosome
    female phenotype Q97.8
    male phenotype Q98.8

Absence *(Continued)*
  skull bone (congenital) Q75.8
    with
      anencephaly Q00.0
      encephalocele —*see* Encephalocele
      hydrocephalus Q03.9
        with spina bifida —*see* Spina
          bifida, by site, with
          hydrocephalus
      microcephaly Q02
  spermatic cord, congenital Q55.4
  spine, congenital Q76.49
  spleen (congenital) Q89.01
    acquired Z90.81
  sternum, congenital Q76.7
  stomach (acquired) (partial) Z90.3
    congenital Q40.2
  superior vena cava, congenital
    Q26.8
  teeth, tooth (congenital) K00.0
    acquired (complete) K08.109
      class I K08.101
      class II K08.102
      class III K08.103
      class IV K08.104
      due to
        caries K08.139
          class I K08.131
          class II K08.132
          class III K08.133
          class IV K08.134
        periodontal disease K08.129
          class I K08.121
          class II K08.122
          class III K08.123
          class IV K08.124
        specified NEC K08.199
          class I K08.191
          class II K08.192
          class III K08.193
          class IV K08.194
        trauma K08.119
          class I K08.111
          class II K08.112
          class III K08.113
          class IV K08.114
    partial K08.409
      class I K08.401
      class II K08.402
      class III K08.403
      class IV K08.404
      due to
        caries K08.439
          class I K08.431
          class II K08.432
          class III K08.433
          class IV K08.434
        periodontal disease K08.429
          class I K08.421
          class II K08.422
          class III K08.423
          class IV K08.424
        specified NEC K08.499
          class I K08.491
          class II K08.492
          class III K08.493
          class IV K08.494
        trauma K08.419
          class I K08.411
          class II K08.412
          class III K08.413
          class IV K08.414
  tendon (congenital) Q79.8
  testis (congenital) Q55.0
    acquired Z90.79
  thumb (acquired) Z89.01-•
    congenital —*see* Agenesis, hand
  thymus gland Q89.2
  thyroid (gland) (acquired) E89.0
    cartilage, congenital Q31.8
    congenital E03.1

Absence *(Continued)*
  toe(s) (acquired) Z89.42-●
    with foot —*see* Absence, foot and
        ankle
    congenital —*see* Agenesis, foot
    great Z89.41-●
  tongue, congenital Q38.3
  trachea (cartilage), congenital Q32.1
  transverse aortic arch, congenital
      Q25.49
  tricuspid valve Q22.4
  umbilical artery, congenital Q27.0
  upper arm and forearm with hand present,
      congenital —*see* Agenesis, arm, with
      hand present
  ureter (congenital) Q62.4
    acquired Z90.6
  urethra, congenital Q64.5
  uterus (acquired) Z90.710
    with cervix Z90.710
    with remaining cervical stump
        Z90.711
    congenital Q51.0
  uvula, congenital Q38.5
  vagina, congenital Q52.0
  vas deferens (congenital) Q55.4
    acquired Z90.79
  vein (peripheral) congenital NEC
      Q27.8
    cerebral Q28.3
    digestive system Q27.8
    great Q26.8
    lower limb Q27.8
    portal Q26.5
    precerebral Q28.1
    specified site NEC Q27.8
    upper limb Q27.8
  vena cava (inferior) (superior), congenital
      Q26.8
  ventricular septum Q20.4
  vertebra, congenital Q76.49
  vulva, congenital Q52.71
  wrist (acquired) Z89.12-●
Absorbent system disease I87.8
Absorption
  carbohydrate, disturbance K90.49
  chemical —*see* Table of Drugs and
      Chemicals
    through placenta (newborn) P04.9
      environmental substance P04.6
      nutritional substance P04.5
      obstetric anesthetic or analgesic drug
          P04.0
  drug NEC —*see* Table of Drugs and
      Chemicals
    addictive
      through placenta (newborn) P04.49
        cocaine P04.41
    medicinal
      through placenta (newborn) P04.1
    through placenta (newborn) P04.1
      obstetric anesthetic or analgesic drug
          P04.0
  fat, disturbance K90.49
    pancreatic K90.3
  noxious substance —*see* Table of Drugs and
      Chemicals
  protein, disturbance K90.49
  starch, disturbance K90.49
  toxic substance —*see* Table of Drugs and
      Chemicals
  uremic —*see* Uremia
Abstinence symptoms, syndrome
  alcohol F10.239
    with delirium F10.231
  cocaine F14.23
  neonatal P96.1
  nicotine —*see* Dependence, drug, nicotine,
      with, withdrawal
  opioid F11.93
    with dependence F11.23

Abstinence symptoms, syndrome *(Continued)*
  psychoactive NEC F19.939
    with
      delirium F19.931
      dependence F19.239
        with
          delirium F19.231
          perceptual disturbance F19.232
        uncomplicated F19.230
      perceptual disturbance F19.932
    uncomplicated F19.930
  sedative F13.939
    with
      delirium F13.931
      dependence F13.239
        with
          delirium F13.231
          perceptual disturbance F13.232
        uncomplicated F13.230
      perceptual disturbance F13.932
    uncomplicated F13.930
  stimulant NEC F15.93
    with dependence F15.23
Abulia R68.89
Abulomania F60.7
Abuse
  adult —*see* Maltreatment, adult
    as reason for
      couple seeking advice (including
          offender) Z63.0
  alcohol (non-dependent) F10.10
    with
      anxiety disorder F10.180
      intoxication F10.129
        with delirium F10.121
        uncomplicated F10.120
      mood disorder F10.14
      other specified disorder F10.188
      psychosis F10.159
        delusions F10.150
        hallucinations F10.151
      sexual dysfunction F10.181
      sleep disorder F10.182
      unspecified disorder F10.19
    counseling and surveillance Z71.41
    ▶in remission (early) (sustained) F10.11
  amphetamine (or related substance) —*see*
      Abuse, drug, stimulant NEC
  analgesics (non-prescribed) (over the counter)
      F55.8
  antacids F55.0
  antidepressants —*see* Abuse, drug,
      psychoactive NEC
  anxiolytic —*see* Abuse, drug, sedative
  barbiturates —*see* Abuse, drug, sedative
  caffeine —*see* Abuse, drug, stimulant NEC
  cannabis, cannabinoids —*see* Abuse, drug,
      cannabis
  child —*see* Maltreatment, child
  cocaine —*see* Abuse, drug, cocaine
  drug NEC (non-dependent) F19.10
    with sleep disorder F19.182
    amphetamine type —*see* Abuse, drug,
        stimulant NEC
    analgesics (non-prescribed) (over the
        counter) F55.8
    antacids F55.0
    antidepressants —*see* Abuse, drug,
        psychoactive NEC
    anxiolytics —*see* Abuse, drug, sedative
    barbiturates —*see* Abuse, drug, sedative
    caffeine —*see* Abuse, drug, stimulant NEC
    cannabis F12.10
      with
        anxiety disorder F12.180
        intoxication F12.129
          with
            delirium F12.121
            perceptual disturbance F12.122
          uncomplicated F12.120
        other specified disorder F12.188

Abuse *(Continued)*
  drug NEC *(Continued)*
    cannabis *(Continued)*
      with *(Continued)*
        psychosis F12.159
          delusions F12.150
          hallucinations F12.151
        unspecified disorder F12.19
      ▶in remission (early) (sustained) F12.11
    cocaine F14.10
      with
        anxiety disorder F14.180
        intoxication F14.129
          with
            delirium F14.121
            perceptual disturbance F14.122
          uncomplicated F14.120
        mood disorder F14.14
        other specified disorder F14.188
        psychosis F14.159
          delusions F14.150
          hallucinations F14.151
        sexual dysfunction F14.181
        sleep disorder F14.182
        unspecified disorder F14.19
      ▶in remission (early) (sustained) F14.11
    counseling and surveillance Z71.51
    hallucinogen F16.10
      with
        anxiety disorder F16.180
        flashbacks F16.183
        intoxication F16.129
          with
            delirium F16.121
            perceptual disturbance F16.122
          uncomplicated F16.120
        mood disorder F16.14
        other specified disorder F16.188
        perception disorder, persisting
            F16.183
        psychosis F16.159
          delusions F16.150
          hallucinations F16.151
        unspecified disorder F16.19
      ▶in remission (early) (sustained) F16.11
    hashish —*see* Abuse, drug, cannabis
    herbal or folk remedies F55.1
    hormones F55.3
    hypnotics —*see* Abuse, drug, sedative
    inhalant F18.10
      with
        anxiety disorder F18.180
        dementia, persisting F18.17
        intoxication F18.129
          with delirium F18.121
          uncomplicated F18.120
        mood disorder F18.14
        other specified disorder F18.188
        psychosis F18.159
          delusions F18.150
          hallucinations F18.151
        unspecified disorder F18.19
      ▶in remission (early) (sustained) F18.11
    ▶in remission (early) (sustained) F19.11
    laxatives F55.2
    LSD —*see* Abuse, drug, hallucinogen
    marihuana —*see* Abuse, drug, cannabis
    morphine type (opioids) —*see* Abuse, drug,
        opioid
    opioid F11.10
      with
        intoxication F11.129
          with
            delirium F11.121
            perceptual disturbance F11.122
          uncomplicated F11.120
        mood disorder F11.14
        other specified disorder F11.188
        psychosis F11.159
          delusions F11.150
          hallucinations F11.151

▶ New ⇒ Revised ~~deleted~~ Deleted ● Use Additional Character(s)

Abuse *(Continued)*
  drug NEC *(Continued)*
    opioid *(Continued)*
      with *(Continued)*
        sexual dysfunction F11.181
        sleep disorder F11.182
        unspecified disorder F11.19
      ▶in remission (early) (sustained) F11.11
    PCP (phencyclidine) (or related substance) —
        see Abuse, drug, hallucinogen
    psychoactive NEC F19.10
      with
        amnestic disorder F19.16
        anxiety disorder F19.180
        dementia F19.17
        intoxication F19.129
          with
            delirium F19.121
            perceptual disturbance F19.122
          uncomplicated F19.120
        mood disorder F19.14
        other specified disorder F19.188
        psychosis F19.159
          delusions F19.150
          hallucinations F19.151
        sexual dysfunction F19.181
        sleep disorder F19.182
        unspecified disorder F19.19
    sedative, hypnotic or anxiolytic F13.10
      with
        anxiety disorder F13.180
        intoxication F13.129
          with delirium F13.121
          uncomplicated F13.120
        mood disorder F13.14
        other specified disorder F13.188
        psychosis F13.159
          delusions F13.150
          hallucinations F13.151
        sexual dysfunction F13.181
        sleep disorder F13.182
        unspecified disorder F13.19
      ▶in remission (early) (sustained) F13.11
    solvent —*see* Abuse, drug, inhalant
    steroids F55.3
    stimulant NEC F15.10
      with
        anxiety disorder F15.180
        intoxication F15.129
          with
            delirium F15.121
            perceptual disturbance F15.122
          uncomplicated F15.120
        mood disorder F15.14
        other specified disorder F15.188
        psychosis F15.159
          delusions F15.150
          hallucinations F15.151
        sexual dysfunction F15.181
        sleep disorder F15.182
        unspecified disorder F15.19
      ▶in remission (early) (sustained) F15.11
    tranquilizers —*see* Abuse, drug, sedative
    vitamins F55.4
  hallucinogens —*see* Abuse, drug, hallucinogen
  hashish —*see* Abuse, drug, cannabis
  herbal or folk remedies F55.1
  hormones F55.3
  hypnotic —*see* Abuse, drug, sedative
  inhalant —*see* Abuse, drug, inhalant
  laxatives F55.2
  LSD —*see* Abuse, drug, hallucinogen
  marihuana —*see* Abuse, drug, cannabis
  morphine type (opioids) —*see* Abuse, drug,
      opioid
  non-psychoactive substance NEC F55.8
    antacids F55.0
    folk remedies F55.1
    herbal remedies F55.1
    hormones F55.3
    laxatives F55.2

Abuse *(Continued)*
  non-psychoactive substance NEC *(Continued)*
    steroids F55.3
    vitamins F55.4
  opioids —*see* Abuse, drug, opioid
  PCP (phencyclidine) (or related substance) —
      see Abuse, drug, hallucinogen
  physical (adult) (child) —*see* Maltreatment
  psychoactive substance —*see* Abuse, drug,
      psychoactive NEC
  psychological (adult) (child) —*see* Maltreatment
  sedative —*see* Abuse, drug, sedative
  sexual —*see* Maltreatment
  solvent —*see* Abuse, drug, inhalant
  steroids F55.3
  vitamins F55.4
Acalculia R48.8
  developmental F81.2
Acanthamebiasis (with) B60.10
  conjunctiva B60.12
  keratoconjunctivitis B60.13
  meningoencephalitis B60.11
  other specified B60.19
Acanthocephaliasis B83.8
Acanthocheilonemiasis B74.4
Acanthocytosis E78.6
Acantholysis L11.9
Acanthosis (acquired) (nigricans) L83
  benign Q82.8
  congenital Q82.8
  seborrheic L82.1
    inflamed L82.0
  tongue K14.3
Acapnia E87.3
Acarbia E87.2
Acardia, acardius Q89.8
Acardiacus amorphus Q89.8
Acardiotrophia I51.4
Acariasis B88.0
  scabies B86
Acarodermatitis (urticarioides) B88.0
Acarophobia F40.218
Acatalasemia, acatalasia E80.3
Acathisia (drug induced) G25.71
Accelerated atrioventricular conduction I45.6
Accentuation of personality traits (type A) Z73.1
Accessory (congenital)
  adrenal gland Q89.1
  anus Q43.4
  appendix Q43.4
  atrioventricular conduction I45.6
  auditory ossicles Q16.3
  auricle (ear) Q17.0
  biliary duct or passage Q44.5
  bladder Q64.79
  blood vessels NEC Q27.9
    coronary Q24.5
  bone NEC Q79.8
  breast tissue, axilla Q83.1
  carpal bones Q74.0
  cecum Q43.4
  chromosome(s) NEC (nonsex) Q92.9
    with complex rearrangements NEC Q92.5
      seen only at prometaphase Q92.8
    13 —*see* Trisomy, 13
    18 —*see* Trisomy, 18
    21 —*see* Trisomy, 21
    partial Q92.9
    sex
      female phenotype Q97.8
  coronary artery Q24.5
  cusp(s), heart valve NEC Q24.8
    pulmonary Q22.3
  cystic duct Q44.5
  digit(s) Q69.9
  ear (auricle) (lobe) Q17.0
  endocrine gland NEC Q89.2
  eye muscle Q10.3
  eyelid Q10.3
  face bone(s) Q75.8
  fallopian tube (fimbria) (ostium) Q50.6

Accessory *(Continued)*
  finger(s) Q69.0
  foreskin N47.8
  frontonasal process Q75.8
  gallbladder Q44.1
  genital organ(s)
    female Q52.8
      external Q52.79
      internal NEC Q52.8
    male Q55.8
  genitourinary organs NEC Q89.8
    female Q52.8
    male Q55.8
  hallux Q69.2
  heart Q24.8
    valve NEC Q24.8
      pulmonary Q22.3
  hepatic ducts Q44.5
  hymen Q52.4
  intestine (large) (small) Q43.4
  kidney Q63.0
  lacrimal canal Q10.6
  leaflet, heart valve NEC Q24.8
  ligament, broad Q50.6
  liver Q44.7
    duct Q44.5
  lobule (ear) Q17.0
  lung (lobe) Q33.1
  muscle Q79.8
  navicular of carpus Q74.0
  nervous system, part NEC Q07.8
  nipple Q83.3
  nose Q30.8
  organ or site not listed —*see* Anomaly, by site
  ovary Q50.31
  oviduct Q50.6
  pancreas Q45.3
  parathyroid gland Q89.2
  parotid gland (and duct) Q38.4
  pituitary gland Q89.2
  preauricular appendage Q17.0
  prepuce N47.8
  renal arteries (multiple) Q27.2
  rib Q76.6
    cervical Q76.5
  roots (teeth) K00.2
  salivary gland Q38.4
  sesamoid bones Q74.8
    foot Q74.2
    hand Q74.0
  skin tags Q82.8
  spleen Q89.09
  sternum Q76.7
  submaxillary gland Q38.4
  tarsal bones Q74.2
  teeth, tooth K00.1
  tendon Q79.8
  thumb Q69.1
  thymus gland Q89.2
  thyroid gland Q89.2
  toes Q69.2
  tongue Q38.3
  tooth, teeth K00.1
  tragus Q17.0
  ureter Q62.5
  urethra Q64.79
  urinary organ or tract NEC Q64.8
  uterus Q51.2
  vagina Q52.10
  valve, heart NEC Q24.8
    pulmonary Q22.3
  vertebra Q76.49
  vocal cords Q31.8
  vulva Q52.79
Accident
  birth —*see* Birth, injury
  cardiac —*see* Infarct, myocardium
  cerebral I63.9
  cerebrovascular (embolic) (ischemic)
      (thrombotic) I63.9
    aborted I63.9

Accident *(Continued)*
  cerebrovascular *(Continued)*
    hemorrhagic —*see* Hemorrhage,
      intracranial, intracerebral
    old (without sequelae) Z86.73
      with sequelae (of) —*see* Sequelae,
        infarction, cerebral
    coronary —*see* Infarct, myocardium
    craniovascular I63.9
    vascular, brain I63.9
Accidental —*see* condition
Accommodation (disorder) —*see also* condition
  hysterical paralysis of F44.89
  insufficiency of H52.4
  paresis —*see* Paresis, of accommodation
  spasm —*see* Spasm, of accommodation
Accouchement —*see* Delivery
Accreta placenta O43.21-●
Accretio cordis (nonrheumatic) I31.0
Accretions, tooth, teeth K03.6
Acculturation difficulty Z60.3
Accumulation secretion, prostate N42.89
Acephalia, acephalism, acephalus, acephaly
  Q00.0
Acephalobrachia monster Q89.8
Acephalochirus monster Q89.8
Acephalogaster Q89.8
Acephalostomus monster Q89.8
Acephalothorax Q89.8
Acerophobia F40.298
Acetonemia R79.89
  in Type 1 diabetes E10.10
    with coma E10.11
Acetonuria R82.4
Achalasia (cardia) (esophagus) K22.0
  congenital Q39.5
  pylorus Q40.0
  sphincteral NEC K59.8
Ache(s) —*see* Pain
Acheilia Q38.6
Achillobursitis —*see* Tendinitis, Achilles
Achillodynia —*see* Tendinitis, Achilles
Achlorhydria, achlorhydric (neurogenic) K31.83
  anemia D50.8
  diarrhea K31.83
  psychogenic F45.8
  secondary to vagotomy K91.1
Achluophobia F40.228
Acholia K82.8
Acholuric jaundice (familial)
    (splenomegalic) —*see also* Spherocytosis
  acquired D59.8
Achondrogenesis Q77.0
Achondroplasia (osteosclerosis congenita) Q77.4
Achroma, cutis L80
Achromat (ism), achromatopsia (acquired)
    (congenital) H53.51
Achromia, congenital —*see* Albinism
Achromia parasitica B36.0
Achylia gastrica K31.89
  psychogenic F45.8
Acid
  burn —*see* Corrosion
  deficiency
    amide nicotinic E52
    ascorbic E54
    folic E53.8
    nicotinic E52
    pantothenic E53.8
  intoxication E87.2
  peptic disease K30
  phosphatase deficiency E83.39
  stomach K30
    psychogenic F45.8
Acidemia E87.2
  argininosuccinic E72.22
  isovaleric E71.110
  metabolic (newborn) P19.9
    first noted before onset of labor P19.0
    first noted during labor P19.1
    noted at birth P19.2

Acidemia *(Continued)*
  methylmalonic E71.120
  pipecolic E72.3
  propionic E71.121
Acidity, gastric (high) K30
  psychogenic F45.8
Acidocytopenia —*see* Agranulocytosis
Acidocytosis D72.1
Acidopenia —*see* Agranulocytosis
Acidosis (lactic) (respiratory) E87.2
  in Type 1 diabetes E10.10
    with coma E10.11
  kidney, tubular N25.89
  lactic E87.2
  metabolic NEC E87.2
    with respiratory acidosis E87.4
    late, of newborn P74.0
  mixed metabolic and respiratory,
    newborn P84
  newborn P84
  renal (hyperchloremic) (tubular)
    N25.89
  respiratory E87.2
    complicated by
      metabolic
        acidosis E87.4
        alkalosis E87.4
Aciduria
  argininosuccinic E72.22
  glutaric (type I) E72.3
    type II E71.313
    type III E71.5-●
  orotic (congenital) (hereditary) (pyrimidine
    deficiency) E79.8
    anemia D53.0
Acladiosis (skin) B36.0
Aclasis, diaphyseal Q78.6
Acleistocardia Q21.1
Aclusion —*see* Anomaly, dentofacial,
  malocclusion
Acne L70.9
  artificialis L70.8
  atrophica L70.2
  cachecticorum (Hebra) L70.8
  conglobata L70.1
  cystic L70.0
  decalvans L66.2
  excoriée (des jeunes filles) L70.5
  frontalis L70.2
  indurata L70.0
  infantile L70.4
  keloid L73.0
  lupoid L70.2
  necrotic, necrotica (miliaris) L70.2
  neonatal L70.4
  nodular L70.0
  occupational L70.8
  picker's L70.5
  pustular L70.0
  rodens L70.2
  rosacea L71.9
  specified NEC L70.8
  tropica L70.3
  varioliformis L70.2
  vulgaris L70.0
Acnitis (primary) A18.4
Acosta's disease T70.29
Acoustic —*see* condition
Acousticophobia F40.298
Acquired —*see also* condition
  immunodeficiency syndrome (AIDS)
    B20
Acrania Q00.0
Acroangiodermatitis I78.9
Acroasphyxia, chronic I73.89
Acrobystitis N47.7
Acrocephalopolysyndactyly Q87.0
Acrocephalosyndactyly Q87.0
Acrocephaly Q75.0
Acrochondrohyperplasia —*see* Syndrome,
  Marfan's

Acrocyanosis I73.8
  newborn P28.2
    meaning transient blue hands and feet -
      omit code
Acrodermatitis L30.8
  atrophicans (chronica) L90.4
  continua (Hallopeau) L40.2
  enteropathica (hereditary) E83.2
  Hallopeau's L40.2
  infantile papular L44.4
  perstans L40.2
  pustulosa continua L40.2
  recalcitrant pustular L40.2
Acrodynia —*see* Poisoning, mercury
Acromegaly, acromegalia E22.0
Acromelalgia I73.81
Acromicria, acromikria Q79.8
Acronyx L60.0
Acropachy, thyroid —*see* Thyrotoxicosis
Acroparesthesia (simple) (vasomotor) I73.89
Acropathy, thyroid —*see* Thyrotoxicosis
Acrophobia F40.241
Acroposthitis N47.7
Acroscleriasis, acroscleroderma,
    acrosclerosis —*see* Sclerosis, systemic
Acrosphacelus I96
Acrospiroma, eccrine —*see* Neoplasm, skin,
  benign
Acrostealgia —*see* Osteochondropathy
Acrotrophodynia —*see* Immersion
ACTH ectopic syndrome E24.3
Actinic —*see* condition
Actinobacillosis, actinobacillus A28.8
  mallei A24.0
  muris A25.1
Actinomyces israelii (infection) —*see*
  Actinomycosis
Actinomycetoma (foot) B47.1
Actinomycosis, actinomycotic A42.9
  with pneumonia A42.0
  abdominal A42.1
  cervicofacial A42.2
  cutaneous A42.89
  gastrointestinal A42.1
  pulmonary A42.0
  sepsis A42.7
  specified site NEC A42.89
Actinoneuritis G62.82
Action, heart
  disorder I49.9
  irregular I49.9
    psychogenic F45.8
Activated protein C resistance D68.51
Activation
  mast cell (disorder) (syndrome) D89.40
    idiopathic D89.42
    monoclonal D89.41
    secondary D89.43
    specified type NEC D89.49
Active —*see* condition
Acute —*see also* condition
  abdomen R10.0
  gallbladder —*see* Cholecystitis, acute
Acyanotic heart disease (congenital) Q24.9
Acystia Q64.5
Adair-Dighton syndrome (brittle bones and
    blue sclera, deafness) Q78.0
Adamantinoblastoma —*see* Ameloblastoma
Adamantinoma —*see also* Cyst, calcifying
    odontogenic
  long bones C40.90
    lower limb C40.2-●
    upper limb C40.0-●
  malignant C41.1
    jaw (bone) (lower) C41.1
      upper C41.0
  tibial C40.2-●
Adamantoblastoma —*see* Ameloblastoma
Adams-Stokes (-Morgagni) disease or
  syndrome I45.9
Adaption reaction —*see* Disorder, adjustment

▶ New ➡ Revised ~~deleted~~ Deleted ● Use Additional Character(s)

Addiction —*see also* Dependence F19.2Ø
  alcohol, alcoholic (ethyl) (methyl) (wood)
    (without remission) F1Ø.2Ø
    with remission F1Ø.21
  drug —*see* Dependence, drug
  ethyl alcohol (without remission) F1Ø.2Ø
    with remission F1Ø.21
  heroin —*see* Dependence, drug, opioid
  methyl alcohol (without remission) F1Ø.2Ø
    with remission F1Ø.21
  methylated spirit (without remission) F1Ø.2Ø
    with remission F1Ø.21
  morphine(-like substances) —*see*
    Dependence, drug, opioid
  nicotine —*see* Dependence, drug, nicotine
  opium and opioids —*see* Dependence, drug,
    opioid
  tobacco —*see* Dependence, drug, nicotine
Addisonian crisis E27.2
Addison's
  anemia (pernicious) D51.Ø
  disease (bronze) or syndrome E27.1
    tuberculous A18.7
  keloid L94.Ø
Addison-Biermer anemia (pernicious) D51.Ø
Addison-Schilder complex E71.528
Additional —*see also* Accessory
  chromosome(s) Q99.8
    21 —*see* Trisomy, 21
  sex —*see* Abnormal, chromosome, sex
Adduction contracture, hip or other joint —*see*
    Contraction, joint
Adenitis —*see also* Lymphadenitis
  acute, unspecified site LØ4.9
  axillary I88.9
    acute LØ4.2
    chronic or subacute I88.1
  Bartholin's gland N75.8
  bulbourethral gland —*see* Urethritis
  cervical I88.9
    acute LØ4.Ø
    chronic or subacute I88.1
  chancroid (Hemophilus ducreyi) A57
  chronic, unspecified site I88.1
  Cowper's gland —*see* Urethritis
⇒ due to Pasteurella multocida (P. septica)
    A28.Ø
  epidemic, acute B27.Ø9
  gangrenous LØ4.9
  gonorrheal NEC A54.89
  groin I88.9
    acute LØ4.1
    chronic or subacute I88.1
  infectious (acute) (epidemic) B27.Ø9
  inguinal I88.9
    acute LØ4.1
    chronic or subacute I88.1
  lymph gland or node, except mesenteric I88.9
    acute —*see* Lymphadenitis, acute
    chronic or subacute I88.1
  mesenteric (acute) (chronic) (nonspecific)
    (subacute) I88.Ø
  parotid gland (suppurative) —*see* Sialoadenitis
  salivary gland (any) (suppurative) —*see*
    Sialoadenitis
  scrofulous (tuberculous) A18.2
  Skene's duct or gland —*see* Urethritis
  strumous, tuberculous A18.2
  subacute, unspecified site I88.1
  sublingual gland (suppurative) —*see*
    Sialoadenitis
  submandibular gland (suppurative) —*see*
    Sialoadenitis
  submaxillary gland (suppurative) —*see*
    Sialoadenitis
  tuberculous —*see* Tuberculosis, lymph gland
  urethral gland —*see* Urethritis
  Wharton's duct (suppurative) —*see*
    Sialoadenitis
Adenoacanthoma —*see* Neoplasm, malignant,
  by site

Adenoameloblastoma —*see* Cyst, calcifying
  odontogenic
Adenocarcinoid (tumor) —*see* Neoplasm,
  malignant, by site
Adenocarcinoma —*see also* Neoplasm,
  malignant, by site
  acidophil
    specified site —*see* Neoplasm, malignant,
      by site
    unspecified site C75.1
  adrenal cortical C74.Ø-●
  alveolar —*see* Neoplasm, lung, malignant
  apocrine
    breast —*see* Neoplasm, breast, malignant
    in situ
      breast DØ5.8-●
      specified site NEC —*see* Neoplasm, skin,
        in situ
      unspecified site DØ4.9
    specified site NEC —*see* Neoplasm, skin,
      malignant
    unspecified site C44.99
  basal cell
    specified site —*see* Neoplasm, skin,
      malignant
    unspecified site CØ8.9
  basophil
    specified site —*see* Neoplasm, malignant,
      by site
    unspecified site C75.1
  bile duct type C22.1
    liver C22.1
    specified site NEC —*see* Neoplasm,
      malignant, by site
    unspecified site C22.1
  bronchiolar —*see* Neoplasm, lung, malignant
  bronchioloalveolar —*see* Neoplasm, lung,
    malignant
  ceruminous C44.29-●
  cervix, in situ (*see also* Carcinoma, cervix
    uteri, in situ) DØ6.9
  chromophobe
    specified site —*see* Neoplasm, malignant,
      by site
    unspecified site C75.1
  diffuse type
    specified site —*see* Neoplasm, malignant,
      by site
    unspecified site C16.9
  duct
    infiltrating
      with Paget's disease —*see* Neoplasm,
        breast, malignant
      specified site —*see* Neoplasm,
        malignant, by site
      unspecified site (female) C5Ø.91-●
        male C5Ø.92-●
    specified site —*see* Neoplasm, malignant,
      by site
    unspecified site
      female C56.9
      male C61
  eosinophil
    specified site —*see* Neoplasm, malignant,
      by site
    unspecified site C75.1
  follicular
    with papillary C73
    moderately differentiated C73
    specified site —*see* Neoplasm, malignant,
      by site
    trabecular C73
    unspecified site C73
    well differentiated C73
  Hurthle cell C73
  in
    adenomatous
      polyposis coli C18.9
  infiltrating duct
    with Paget's disease —*see* Neoplasm,
      breast, malignant

Adenocarcinoma (*Continued*)
  infiltrating duct (*Continued*)
    specified site —*see* Neoplasm, malignant,
      by site
    unspecified site (female) C5Ø.91-●
      male C5Ø.92-●
  inflammatory
    specified site —*see* Neoplasm, malignant,
      by site
    unspecified site (female) C5Ø.91-●
      male C5Ø.92-●
  intestinal type
    specified site —*see* Neoplasm, malignant,
      by site
    unspecified site C16.9
  intracystic papillary
  intraductal
    breast DØ5.1-●
    noninfiltrating
      breast DØ5.1-●
      papillary
        with invasion
          specified site —*see* Neoplasm,
            malignant, by site
          unspecified site (female) C5Ø.91-●
            male C5Ø.92-●
        breast DØ5.1-●
        specified site NEC —*see* Neoplasm, in
          situ, by site
        unspecified site DØ5.1-●
      specified site NEC —*see* Neoplasm, in
        situ, by site
      unspecified site DØ5.1-●
    papillary
      with invasion
        specified site —*see* Neoplasm,
          malignant, by site
        unspecified site (female) C5Ø.91-●
          male C5Ø.92-●
      breast DØ5.1-●
      specified site —*see* Neoplasm, in situ,
        by site
      unspecified site DØ5.1-●
    specified site NEC —*see* Neoplasm, in situ,
      by site
    unspecified site DØ5.1-●
  islet cell
    with exocrine, mixed
      specified site —*see* Neoplasm,
        malignant, by site
      unspecified site C25.9
    pancreas C25.4
    specified site NEC —*see* Neoplasm,
      malignant, by site
    unspecified site C25.4
  lobular
    in situ
      breast DØ5.Ø-●
      specified site NEC —*see* Neoplasm, in
        situ, by site
      unspecified site DØ5.Ø-●
    specified site —*see* Neoplasm, malignant,
      by site
    unspecified site (female) C5Ø.91-●
      male C5Ø.92-●
  mucoid —*see also* Neoplasm, malignant, by site
    cell
      specified site —*see* Neoplasm,
        malignant, by site
      unspecified site C75.1
  nonencapsulated sclerosing C73
  papillary
    with follicular C73
    follicular variant C73
    intraductal (noninfiltrating)
      with invasion
        specified site —*see* Neoplasm,
          malignant, by site
        unspecified site (female) C5Ø.91-●
          male C5Ø.92-●
      breast DØ5.1-●

Adenocarcinoma *(Continued)*
  papillary *(Continued)*
    intraductal *(Continued)*
      specified site NEC —*see* Neoplasm, in situ, by site
      unspecified site D05.1-●
    serous
      specified site —*see* Neoplasm, malignant, by site
      unspecified site C56.9
  papillocystic
    specified site —*see* Neoplasm, malignant, by site
    unspecified site C56.9
  pseudomucinous
    specified site —*see* Neoplasm, malignant, by site
    unspecified site C56.9
  renal cell C64-●
  sebaceous —*see* Neoplasm, skin, malignant, by site
  serous —*see also* Neoplasm, malignant, by site
    papillary
      specified site —*see* Neoplasm, malignant, by site
      unspecified site C56.9
  sweat gland —*see* Neoplasm, skin, malignant
  water-clear cell C75.0
Adenocarcinoma-in-situ —*see also* Neoplasm, in situ, by site
  breast D05.9-●
Adenofibroma
  clear cell —*see* Neoplasm, benign, by site
  endometrioid D27.9
    borderline malignancy D39.10
    malignant C56-●
  mucinous
    specified site —*see* Neoplasm, benign, by site
    unspecified site D27.9
  papillary
    specified site —*see* Neoplasm, benign, by site
    unspecified site D27.9
  prostate —*see* Enlargement, enlarged, prostate
  serous
    specified site —*see* Neoplasm, benign, by site
    unspecified site D27.9
  specified site —*see* Neoplasm, benign, by site
  unspecified site D27.9
Adenofibrosis
  breast —*see* Fibroadenosis, breast
  endometrioid N80.0
Adenoiditis (chronic) J35.02
  with tonsillitis J35.03
  acute J03.90
    recurrent J03.91
    specified organism NEC J03.80
      recurrent J03.81
    staphylococcal J03.80
      recurrent J03.81
    streptococcal J03.00
      recurrent J03.01
Adenoids —*see* condition
Adenolipoma —*see* Neoplasm, benign, by site
Adenolipomatosis, Launois-Bensaude E88.89
Adenolymphoma
  specified site —*see* Neoplasm, benign, by site
  unspecified site D11.9
Adenoma —*see also* Neoplasm, benign, by site
  acidophil
    specified site —*see* Neoplasm, benign, by site
    unspecified site D35.2
  acidophil-basophil, mixed
    specified site —*see* Neoplasm, benign, by site
    unspecified site D35.2

Adenoma *(Continued)*
  adrenal (cortical) D35.00
    clear cell D35.00
    compact cell D35.00
    glomerulosa cell D35.00
    heavily pigmented variant D35.00
    mixed cell D35.00
  alpha-cell
    pancreas D13.7
    specified site NEC —*see* Neoplasm, benign, by site
    unspecified site D13.7
  alveolar D14.30
  apocrine
    breast D24-●
    specified site NEC —*see* Neoplasm, skin, benign, by site
    unspecified site D23.9
  basal cell D11.9
  basophil
    specified site —*see* Neoplasm, benign, by site
    unspecified site D35.2
  basophil-acidophil, mixed
    specified site —*see* Neoplasm, benign, by site
    unspecified site D35.2
  beta-cell
    pancreas D13.7
    specified site NEC —*see* Neoplasm, benign, by site
    unspecified site D13.7
  bile duct D13.4
    common D13.5
    extrahepatic D13.5
    intrahepatic D13.4
    specified site NEC —*see* Neoplasm, benign, by site
    unspecified site D13.4
  black D35.00
  bronchial D38.1
    cylindroid type —*see* Neoplasm, lung, malignant
  ceruminous D23.2-●
  chief cell D35.1
  chromophobe
    specified site —*see* Neoplasm, benign, by site
    unspecified site D35.2
  colloid
    specified site —*see* Neoplasm, benign, by site
    unspecified site D34
  duct
  eccrine, papillary —*see* Neoplasm, skin, benign
  endocrine, multiple
    single specified site —*see* Neoplasm, uncertain behavior, by site
    two or more specified sites D44-●
    unspecified site D44.9
  endometrioid —*see also* Neoplasm, benign
    borderline malignancy —*see* Neoplasm, uncertain behavior, by site
  eosinophil
    specified site —*see* Neoplasm, malignant, by site
    unspecified site D35.2
  fetal
    specified site —*see* Neoplasm, benign, by site
    unspecified site D34
  follicular
    specified site —*see* Neoplasm, benign, by site
    unspecified site D34
  hepatocellular D13.4
  Hurthle cell D34
  islet cell
    pancreas D13.7
    specified site NEC —*see* Neoplasm, benign, by site
    unspecified site D13.7

Adenoma *(Continued)*
  liver cell D13.4
  macrofollicular
    specified site —*see* Neoplasm, benign, by site
    unspecified site D34
  malignant, malignum —*see* Neoplasm, malignant, by site
  microcystic
    pancreas D13.6
    specified site NEC —*see* Neoplasm, benign, by site
    unspecified site D13.6
  microfollicular
    specified site —*see* Neoplasm, benign, by site
    unspecified site D34
  mucoid cell
    specified site —*see* Neoplasm, benign, by site
    unspecified site D35.2
  multiple endocrine
    single specified site —*see* Neoplasm, uncertain behavior, by site
    two or more specified sites D44-●
    unspecified site D44.9
  nipple D24-●
  papillary —*see also* Neoplasm, benign, by site
    eccrine —*see* Neoplasm, skin, benign, by site
  Pick's tubular
    specified site —*see* Neoplasm, benign, by site
    unspecified site
      female D27.9
      male D29.20
  pleomorphic
    carcinoma in —*see* Neoplasm, salivary gland, malignant
    specified site —*see* Neoplasm, malignant, by site
    unspecified site C08.9
  polypoid —*see also* Neoplasm, benign
    adenocarcinoma in —*see* Neoplasm, malignant, by site
    adenocarcinoma in situ —*see* Neoplasm, in situ, by site
  prostate —*see* Neoplasm, benign, prostate
  rete cell D29.20
  sebaceous —*see* Neoplasm, skin, benign
  Sertoli cell
    specified site —*see* Neoplasm, benign, by site
    unspecified site
      female D27.9
      male D29.20
  skin appendage —*see* Neoplasm, skin, benign
  sudoriferous gland —*see* Neoplasm, skin, benign
  sweat gland —*see* Neoplasm, skin, benign
  testicular
    specified site —*see* Neoplasm, benign, by site
    unspecified site
      female D27.9
      male D29.20
  tubular —*see also* Neoplasm, benign, by site
    adenocarcinoma in —*see* Neoplasm, malignant, by site
    adenocarcinoma in situ —*see* Neoplasm, in situ, by site
    Pick's
      specified site —*see* Neoplasm, benign
      unspecified site
        female D27.9
        male D29.20
  tubulovillous —*see also* Neoplasm, benign, by site
    adenocarcinoma in —*see* Neoplasm, malignant, by site
    adenocarcinoma in situ —*see* Neoplasm, in situ, by site

▶ New   ⟹ Revised   ~~deleted~~ Deleted   ● Use Additional Character(s)

Adenoma *(Continued)*
  villous —*see* Neoplasm, uncertain behavior,
      by site
    adenocarcinoma in —*see* Neoplasm,
        malignant, by site
    adenocarcinoma in situ —*see* Neoplasm, in
        situ, by site
  water-clear cell D35.1
Adenomatosis
  endocrine (multiple) E31.20
    single specified site —*see* Neoplasm,
        uncertain behavior, by site
  erosive of nipple D24-●
  pluriendocrine —*see* Adenomatosis,
      endocrine
  pulmonary D38.1
    malignant —*see* Neoplasm, lung,
        malignant
  specified site —*see* Neoplasm, benign, by site
  unspecified site D12.6
Adenomatous
  goiter (nontoxic) E04.9
    with hyperthyroidism —*see* Hyper-
        thyroidism, with, goiter, nodular
    toxic —*see* Hyperthyroidism, with, goiter,
        nodular
Adenomyoma —*see also* Neoplasm, benign, by
    site
  prostate —*see* Enlarged, prostate
Adenomyometritis N80.0
Adenomyosis N80.0
Adenopathy (lymph gland) R59.9
  generalized R59.1
  inguinal R59.0
  localized R59.0
  mediastinal R59.0
  mesentery R59.0
  syphilitic (secondary) A51.49
  tracheobronchial R59.0
    tuberculous A15.4
      primary (progressive) A15.7
  tuberculous —*see also* Tuberculosis, lymph
      gland
    tracheobronchial A15.4
      primary (progressive) A15.7
Adenosalpingitis —*see* Salpingitis
Adenosarcoma —*see* Neoplasm, malignant, by
    site
Adenosclerosis I88.8
Adenosis (sclerosing) breast —*see*
    Fibroadenosis, breast
**Adenovirus, as cause of disease classified
    elsewhere** B97.0
Adentia (complete) (partial) —*see* Absence,
    teeth
Adherent —*see also* Adhesions
  labia (minora) N90.89
  pericardium (nonrheumatic) I31.0
    rheumatic I09.2
  placenta (with hemorrhage) O72.0
    without hemorrhage O73.0
  prepuce, newborn N47.0
  scar (skin) L90.5
  tendon in scar L90.5
Adhesions, adhesive (postinfective) K66.0
  ⟹with intestinal obstruction K56.50
    ▶complete K56.52
    ▶incomplete K56.51
    ▶partial K56.51
  abdominal (wall) —*see* Adhesions, peritoneum
  appendix K38.8
  bile duct (common) (hepatic) K83.8
  bladder (sphincter) N32.89
  bowel —*see* Adhesions, peritoneum
  cardiac I31.0
    rheumatic I09.2
  cecum —*see* Adhesions, peritoneum
  cervicovaginal N88.1
    congenital Q52.8
    postpartal O90.89
      old N88.1

Adhesions, adhesive *(Continued)*
  cervix N88.1
  ciliary body NEC —*see* Adhesions, iris
  clitoris N90.89
  colon —*see* Adhesions, peritoneum
  common duct K83.8
  congenital —*see also* Anomaly, by site
    fingers —*see* Syndactylism, complex, fingers
    omental, anomalous Q43.3
    peritoneal Q43.3
    tongue (to gum or roof of mouth) Q38.3
  conjunctiva (acquired) H11.21-●
    congenital Q15.8
  cystic duct K82.8
  diaphragm —*see* Adhesions, peritoneum
  due to foreign body —*see* Foreign body
  duodenum —*see* Adhesions, peritoneum
  ear
    middle H74.1-●
  epididymis N50.89
  epidural —*see* Adhesions, meninges
  epiglottis J38.7
  eyelid H02.59
  female pelvis N73.6
  gallbladder K82.8
  globe H44.89
  heart I31.0
    rheumatic I09.2
  ileocecal (coil) —*see* Adhesions, peritoneum
  ileum —*see* Adhesions, peritoneum
  intestine —*see also* Adhesions, peritoneum
  ⟹with obstruction K56.50
    ▶complete K56.52
    ▶incomplete K56.51
    ▶partial K56.51
  intra-abdominal —*see* Adhesions, peritoneum
  iris H21.50-●
    anterior H21.51-●
    goniosynechiae H21.52-●
    posterior H21.54-●
    to corneal graft T85.898
  joint —*see* Ankylosis
    knee M23.8X
    temporomandibular M26.61-●
  labium (majus) (minus), congenital Q52.5
  liver —*see* Adhesions, peritoneum
  lung J98.4
  mediastinum J98.59
  meninges (cerebral) (spinal) G96.12
    congenital Q07.8
    tuberculous (cerebral) (spinal) A17.0
  mesenteric —*see* Adhesions, peritoneum
  nasal (septum) (to turbinates) J34.89
  ocular muscle —*see* Strabismus, mechanical
  omentum —*see* Adhesions, peritoneum
  ovary N73.6
    congenital (to cecum, kidney or omentum)
        Q50.39
  paraovarian N73.6
  pelvic (peritoneal)
    female N73.6
      postprocedural N99.4
    male —*see* Adhesions, peritoneum
    postpartal (old) N73.6
    tuberculous A18.17
  penis to scrotum (congenital) Q55.8
  periappendiceal —*see also* Adhesions,
      peritoneum
  pericardium (nonrheumatic) I31.0
    focal I31.8
    rheumatic I09.2
    tuberculous A18.84
  pericholecystic K82.8
  perigastric —*see* Adhesions, peritoneum
  periovarian N73.6
  periprostatic N42.89
  perirectal —*see* Adhesions, peritoneum
  perirenal N28.89
  ⟹peritoneum, peritoneal (postinfective)
    ⟹with obstruction (intestinal) K56.50
      ▶complete K56.52

Adhesions, adhesive *(Continued)*
  peritoneum, peritoneal *(Continued)*
    with obstruction *(Continued)*
      ▶incomplete K56.51
      ▶partial K56.51
    congenital Q43.3
    pelvic, female N73.6
      postprocedural N99.4
    postpartal, pelvic N73.6
    ▶postprocedural K66.0
    to uterus N73.6
  peritubal N73.6
  periureteral N28.89
  periuterine N73.6
  perivesical N32.89
  perivesicular (seminal vesicle) N50.89
  pleura, pleuritic J94.8
    tuberculous NEC A15.6
  pleuropericardial J94.8
  postoperative (gastrointestinal tract) K66.0
    ⟹with obstruction —*see also* Obstruction,
        intestine, postoperative K91.30
      due to foreign body accidentally left
          in wound —*see* Foreign body,
          accidentally left during a procedure
    pelvic peritoneal N99.4
    urethra —*see* Stricture, urethra,
        postprocedural
    vagina N99.2
  postpartal, old (vulva or perineum) N90.89
  preputial, prepuce N47.5
  pulmonary J98.4
  pylorus —*see* Adhesions, peritoneum
  sciatic nerve —*see* Lesion, nerve, sciatic
  seminal vesicle N50.89
  shoulder (joint) —*see* Capsulitis, adhesive
  sigmoid flexure —*see* Adhesions, peritoneum
  spermatic cord (acquired) N50.89
    congenital Q55.4
  spinal canal G96.12
  stomach —*see* Adhesions, peritoneum
  subscapular —*see* Capsulitis, adhesive
  temporomandibular M26.61-●
  tendinitis —*see also* Tenosynovitis, specified
      type NEC
    shoulder —*see* Capsulitis, adhesive
  testis N44.8
  tongue, congenital (to gum or roof of mouth)
      Q38.3
    acquired K14.8
  trachea J39.8
  tubo-ovarian N73.6
  tunica vaginalis N44.8
  uterus N73.6
    internal N85.6
    to abdominal wall N73.6
  vagina (chronic) N89.5
    postoperative N99.2
  vitreomacular H43.82-●
  vitreous H43.89
  vulva N90.89
Adiaspiromycosis B48.8
Adie (-Holmes) pupil or syndrome —*see*
    Anomaly, pupil, function, tonic pupil
⟹**Adiponecrosis neonatorum** P83.88
Adiposis —*see also* Obesity
  cerebralis E23.6
  dolorosa E88.2
Adiposity —*see also* Obesity
  heart —*see* Degeneration, myocardial
  localized E65
Adiposogenital dystrophy E23.6
Adjustment
  disorder —*see* Disorder, adjustment
  implanted device —*see* Encounter (for),
      adjustment (of)
  prosthesis, external —*see* Fitting
  reaction —*see* Disorder, adjustment
Administration of tPA (rtPA) in a different
    facility within the last 24 hours prior to
    admission to current facility Z92.82

Admission (for) —*see also* Encounter (for)
  adjustment (of)
    artificial
      arm Z44.00-●
        complete Z44.01-●
        partial Z44.02-●
      eye Z44.2
      leg Z44.10-●
        complete Z44.11-●
        partial Z44.12-●
    brain neuropacemaker Z46.2
      implanted Z45.42
    breast
      implant Z45.81
      prosthesis (external) Z44.3
    colostomy belt Z46.89
    contact lenses Z46.0
    cystostomy device Z46.6
    dental prosthesis Z46.3
    device NEC
      abdominal Z46.89
      implanted Z45.89
        cardiac Z45.09
          defibrillator (with synchronous
            cardiace pacemaker) Z45.02
          pacemaker (cardiac
            resynchronization therapy
            (CRT-P)) Z45.018
          pulse generator Z45.010
          resynchronization therapy
            defibrillator (CRT-D) Z45.02
        hearing device Z45.328
          bone conduction Z45.320
          cochlear Z45.321
        infusion pump Z45.1
        nervous system Z45.49
          CSF drainage Z45.41
          hearing device —*see* Admission,
            adjustment, device, implanted,
            hearing device
          neuropacemaker Z45.42
          visual substitution Z45.31
        specified NEC Z45.89
        vascular access Z45.2
        visual substitution Z45.31
      nervous system Z46.2
        implanted —*see* Admission,
          adjustment, device, implanted,
          nervous system
      orthodontic Z46.4
      prosthetic Z44.9
        arm —*see* Admission, adjustment,
          artificial, arm
        breast Z44.3
        dental Z46.3
        eye Z44.2
        leg —*see* Admission, adjustment,
          artificial, leg
        specified type NEC Z44.8
      substitution
        auditory Z46.2
          implanted —*see* Admission,
            adjustment, device, implanted,
            hearing device
          nervous system Z46.2
            implanted —*see* Admission,
              adjustment, device, implanted,
              nervous system
          visual Z46.2
            implanted Z45.31
      urinary Z46.6
    hearing aid Z46.1
      implanted —*see* Admission, adjustment,
        device, implanted, hearing device
    ileostomy device Z46.89
    intestinal appliance or device NEC Z46.89
    neuropacemaker (brain) (peripheral nerve)
      (spinal cord) Z46.2
      implanted Z45.42
    orthodontic device Z46.4
    orthopedic (brace) (cast) (device) (shoes)
      Z46.89

Admission (*Continued*)
  adjustment (*Continued*)
    pacemaker (cardiac resynchronization
      therapy (CRT-P))
      cardiac Z45.018
        pulse generator Z45.010
      nervous system Z46.2
        implanted Z45.42
    portacath (port-a-cath) Z45.2
    prosthesis Z44.9
      arm —*see* Admission, adjustment,
        artificial, arm
      breast Z44.3
      dental Z46.3
      eye Z44.2
      leg —*see* Admission, adjustment,
        artificial, leg
      specified NEC Z44.8
    spectacles Z46.0
  aftercare (*see also* Aftercare) Z51.89
    postpartum
      immediately after delivery Z39.0
      routine follow-up Z39.2
    radiation therapy (antineoplastic) Z51.0
  attention to artificial opening (of) Z43.9
    artificial vagina Z43.7
    colostomy Z43.3
    cystostomy Z43.5
    enterostomy Z43.4
    gastrostomy Z43.1
    ileostomy Z43.2
    jejunostomy Z43.4
    nephrostomy Z43.6
    specified site NEC Z43.8
      intestinal tract Z43.4
      urinary tract Z43.6
    tracheostomy Z43.0
    ureterostomy Z43.6
    urethrostomy Z43.6
  breast augmentation or reduction Z41.1
  breast reconstruction following mastectomy
    Z42.1
  change of
    dressing (nonsurgical) Z48.00
    neuropacemaker device (brain) (peripheral
      nerve) (spinal cord) Z46.2
      implanted Z45.42
    surgical dressing Z48.01
  circumcision, ritual or routine (in absence of
    diagnosis) Z41.2
  clinical research investigation (control)
    (normal comparison) (participant) Z00.6
  contraceptive management Z30.9
  cosmetic surgery NEC Z41.1
  counseling (*see also* Counseling)
    dietary Z71.3
    gestational carrier Z31.7
    HIV Z71.7
    human immunodeficiency virus Z71.7
    nonattending third party Z71.0
    procreative management NEC Z31.69
  delivery, full-term, uncomplicated O80
    cesarean, without indication O82
  desensitization to allergens Z51.6
  dietary surveillance and counseling Z71.3
  ear piercing Z41.3
  examination at health care facility (adult) —
    see also Examination Z00.00
    with abnormal findings Z00.01
    clinical research investigation (control)
      (normal comparison) (participant)
      Z00.6
    dental Z01.20
      with abnormal findings Z01.21
    donor (potential) Z00.5
    ear Z01.10
      with abnormal findings NEC Z01.118
    eye Z01.00
      with abnormal findings Z01.01
    general, specified reason NEC Z00.8
    hearing Z01.10
      with abnormal findings NEC Z01.118

Admission (*Continued*)
  examination at health care facility (*Continued*)
    postpartum checkup Z39.2
    psychiatric (general) Z00.8
      requested by authority Z04.6
    vision Z01.00
      with abnormal findings Z01.01
  fitting (of)
    artificial
      arm —*see* Admission, adjustment,
        artificial, arm
      eye Z44.2
      leg —*see* Admission, adjustment,
        artificial, leg
    brain neuropacemaker Z46.2
      implanted Z45.42
    breast prosthesis (external) Z44.3
    colostomy belt Z46.89
    contact lenses Z46.0
    cystostomy device Z46.6
    dental prosthesis Z46.3
    dentures Z46.3
    device NEC
      abdominal Z46.89
      nervous system Z46.2
        implanted —*see* Admission,
          adjustment, device, implanted,
          nervous system
      orthodontic Z46.4
      prosthetic Z44.9
        breast Z44.3
        dental Z46.3
        eye Z44.2
      substitution
        auditory Z46.2
          implanted —*see* Admission,
            adjustment, device, implanted,
            hearing device
        nervous system Z46.2
          implanted —*see* Admission,
            adjustment, device, implanted,
            nervous system
        visual Z46.2
          implanted Z45.31
    hearing aid Z46.1
    ileostomy device Z46.89
    intestinal appliance or device NEC Z46.89
    neuropacemaker (brain) (peripheral nerve)
      (spinal cord) Z46.2
      implanted Z45.42
    orthodontic device Z46.4
    orthopedic device (brace) (cast) (shoes)
      Z46.89
    prosthesis Z44.9
      arm —*see* Admission, adjustment,
        artificial, arm
      breast Z44.3
      dental Z46.3
      eye Z44.2
      leg —*see* Admission, adjustment,
        artificial, leg
      specified type NEC Z44.8
    spectacles Z46.0
  follow-up examination Z09
  intrauterine device management Z30.431
    initial prescription Z30.014
  mental health evaluation Z00.8
    requested by authority Z04.6
  observation —*see* Observation
  Papanicolaou smear, cervix Z12.4
    for suspected malignant neoplasm Z12.4
  plastic and reconstructive surgery following
    medical procedure or healed injury NEC
    Z42.8
  plastic surgery, cosmetic NEC Z41.1
  postpartum observation
    immediately after delivery Z39.0
    routine follow-up Z39.2
  poststerilization (for restoration) Z31.0
    aftercare Z31.42
  procreative management Z31.9
  prophylactic (measure) —*see also* Encounter,
    prophylactic measures

▶ New   ⇒ Revised   ~~deleted~~ Deleted   ● Use Additional Character(s)

Admission *(Continued)*
  prophylactic *(Continued)*
    organ removal Z40.00
      breast Z40.01
      ▶fallopian tube(s) Z40.03
        ▶with ovary(s) Z40.02
      ⟹ovary(s) Z40.02
      specified organ NEC Z40.09
      testes Z40.09
    vaccination Z23
  psychiatric examination (general) Z00.8
    requested by authority Z04.6
  radiation therapy (antineoplastic) Z51.0
  reconstructive surgery following medical
    procedure or healed injury NEC Z42.8
  removal of
    cystostomy catheter Z43.5
    drains Z48.03
    dressing (nonsurgical) Z48.00
    implantable subdermal contraceptive Z30.46
    intrauterine contraceptive device Z30.432
    neuropacemaker (brain) (peripheral nerve)
      (spinal cord) Z46.2
      implanted Z45.42
    staples Z48.02
    surgical dressing Z48.01
    sutures Z48.02
    ureteral stent Z46.6
  respirator [ventilator] use during power
    failure Z99.12
  restoration of organ continuity
    (poststerilization) Z31.0
    aftercare Z31.42
  sensitivity test —*see also* Test, skin
    allergy NEC Z01.82
    Mantoux Z11.1
  tuboplasty following previous sterilization
    Z31.0
    aftercare Z31.42
  vasoplasty following previous sterilization
    Z31.0
    aftercare Z31.42
  vision examination Z01.00
    with abnormal findings Z01.01
  waiting period for admission to other facility
    Z75.1
Adnexitis (suppurative) —*see* Salpingo-oophoritis
Adolescent X-linked adrenoleukodystrophy
  E71.521
Adrenal (gland) —*see* condition
Adrenalism, tuberculous A18.7
Adrenalitis, adrenitis E27.8
  autoimmune E27.1
  meningococcal, hemorrhagic A39.1
Adrenarche, premature E27.0
Adrenocortical syndrome —*see* Cushing's,
  syndrome
Adrenogenital syndrome E25.9
  acquired E25.8
  congenital E25.0
  salt loss E25.0
Adrenogenitalism, congenital E25.0
Adrenoleukodystrophy E71.529
  neonatal E71.511
  X-linked E71.529
    Addison only phenotype E71.528
    Addison-Schilder E71.528
    adolescent E71.521
    adrenomyeloneuropathy E71.522
    childhood cerebral E71.520
    other specified E71.528
Adrenomyeloneuropathy E71.522
Adventitious bursa —*see* Bursopathy, specified
  type NEC
Adverse effect —*see* Table of Drugs and
  Chemicals, categories T36-T50, with 6th
  character 5
Advice —*see* Counseling
Adynamia (episodica) (hereditary) (periodic)
  G72.3
Aeration lung imperfect, newborn —*see*
  Atelectasis

Aerobullosis T70.3
Aerocele —*see* Embolism, air
Aerodermectasia
  subcutaneous (traumatic) T79.7
Aerodontalgia T70.29
Aeroembolism T70.3
Aerogenes capsulatus infection A48.0
Aero-otitis media T70.0
Aerophagy, aerophagia (psychogenic) F45.8
Aerophobia F40.228
Aerosinusitis T70.1
Aerotitis T70.0
Affection —*see* Disease
Afibrinogenemia —*see also* Defect, coagulation
  D68.8
  acquired D65
  congenital D68.2
  following ectopic or molar pregnancy
    O08.1
  in abortion —*see* Abortion, by type,
    complicated by, afibrinogenemia
  puerperal O72.3
African
  sleeping sickness B56.9
  tick fever A68.1
  trypanosomiasis B56.9
    gambian B56.0
    rhodesian B56.1
Aftercare —*see also* Care Z51.89
  following surgery (for) (on)
    amputation Z47.81
    attention to
      drains Z48.03
      dressings (nonsurgical) Z48.00
        surgical Z48.01
      sutures Z48.02
    circulatory system Z48.812
    delayed (planned) wound closure Z48.1
    digestive system Z48.815
    explantation of joint prosthesis (staged
      procedure)
      hip Z47.32
      knee Z47.33
      shoulder Z47.31
    genitourinary system Z48.816
    joint replacement Z47.1
    neoplasm Z48.3
    nervous system Z48.811
    oral cavity Z48.814
    organ transplant
      bone marrow Z48.290
      heart Z48.21
      heart-lung Z48.280
      kidney Z48.22
      liver Z48.23
      lung Z48.24
      multiple organs NEC Z48.288
      specified NEC Z48.298
    orthopedic NEC Z47.89
    planned wound closure Z48.1
    removal of internal fixation device
      Z47.2
    respiratory system Z48.813
    scoliosis Z47.82
    sense organs Z48.810
    skin and subcutaneous tissue Z48.817
    specified body system
      circulatory Z48.812
      digestive Z48.815
      genitourinary Z48.816
      nervous Z48.811
      oral cavity Z48.814
      respiratory Z48.813
      sense organs Z48.810
      skin and subcutaneous tissue Z48.817
      teeth Z48.814
    specified NEC Z48.89
    ⟹spinal Z47.89
    teeth Z48.814
  fracture — code to fracture with seventh
    character D

Aftercare *(Continued)*
  involving
    removal of
      drains Z48.03
      dressings (nonsurgical) Z48.00
      staples Z48.02
      surgical dressings Z48.01
      sutures Z48.02
    neuropacemaker (brain) (peripheral nerve)
      (spinal cord) Z46.2
      implanted Z45.42
  orthopedic NEC Z47.89
  postprocedural —*see* Aftercare, following
    surgery
After-cataract —*see* Cataract, secondary
Agalactia (primary) O92.3
  elective, secondary or therapeutic O92.5
Agammaglobulinemia (acquired (secondary))
  (nonfamilial) D80.1
  with
    immunoglobulin-bearing B-lymphocytes
      D80.1
    lymphopenia D81.9
  autosomal recessive (Swiss type) D80.0
  Bruton's X-linked D80.0
  common variable (CVAgamma) D80.1
  congenital sex-linked D80.0
  hereditary D80.0
  lymphopenic D81.9
  Swiss type (autosomal recessive) D80.0
  X-linked (with growth hormone deficiency)
    (Bruton) D80.0
Aganglionosis (bowel) (colon) Q43.1
Age (old) —*see* Senility
Agenesis
  adrenal (gland) Q89.1
  alimentary tract (complete) (partial) NEC
    Q45.8
    upper Q40.8
  anus, anal (canal) Q42.3
    with fistula Q42.2
  aorta Q25.41
  appendix Q42.8
  arm (complete) Q71.0-●
    with hand present Q71.1-●
  artery (peripheral) Q27.9
    brain Q28.3
    coronary Q24.5
    pulmonary Q25.79
    specified NEC Q27.8
    umbilical Q27.0
  auditory (canal) (external) Q16.1
  auricle (ear) Q16.0
  bile duct or passage Q44.5
  bladder Q64.5
  bone Q79.9
  brain Q00.0
    part of Q04.3
  breast (with nipple present) Q83.8
    with absent nipple Q83.0
  bronchus Q32.4
  canaliculus lacrimalis Q10.4
  carpus —*see* Agenesis, hand
  cartilage Q79.9
  cecum Q42.8
  cerebellum Q04.3
  cervix Q51.5
  chin Q18.8
  cilia Q10.3
  circulatory system, part NOS Q28.9
  clavicle Q74.0
  clitoris Q52.6
  coccyx Q76.49
  colon Q42.9
    specified NEC Q42.8
  corpus callosum Q04.0
  cricoid cartilage Q31.8
  diaphragm (with hernia) Q79.1
  digestive organ(s) or tract (complete) (partial)
    NEC Q45.8
    upper Q40.8

Agenesis *(Continued)*
  ductus arteriosus Q28.8
  duodenum Q41.0
  ear Q16.9
    auricle Q16.0
    lobe Q17.8
  ejaculatory duct Q55.4
  endocrine (gland) NEC Q89.2
  epiglottis Q31.8
  esophagus Q39.8
  eustachian tube Q16.2
  eye Q11.1
    adnexa Q15.8
  eyelid (fold) Q10.3
  face
    bones NEC Q75.8
    specified part NEC Q18.8
  fallopian tube Q50.6
  femur —*see* Defect, reduction, lower limb,
      longitudinal, femur
  fibula —*see* Defect, reduction, lower limb,
      longitudinal, fibula
  finger (complete) (partial) —*see* Agenesis,
      hand
  foot (and toes) (complete) (partial) Q72.3-●
  forearm (with hand present) —*see* Agenesis,
      arm, with hand present
    and hand Q71.2-●
  gallbladder Q44.0
  gastric Q40.2
  genitalia, genital (organ(s))
    female Q52.8
      external Q52.71
      internal NEC Q52.8
    male Q55.8
  glottis Q31.8
  hair Q84.0
  hand (and fingers) (complete) (partial) Q71.3-●
  heart Q24.8
    valve NEC Q24.8
      pulmonary Q22.0
  hepatic Q44.7
  humerus —*see* Defect, reduction, upper limb
  hymen Q52.4
  ileum Q41.2
  incus Q16.3
  intestine (small) Q41.9
    large Q42.9
      specified NEC Q42.8
  iris (dilator fibers) Q13.1
  jaw M26.09
  jejunum Q41.1
  kidney(s) (partial) Q60.2
    bilateral Q60.1
    unilateral Q60.0
  labium (majus) (minus) Q52.71
  labyrinth, membranous Q16.5
  lacrimal apparatus Q10.4
  larynx Q31.8
  leg (complete) Q72.0-●
    with foot present Q72.1-●
    lower leg (with foot present) —*see*
        Agenesis, leg, with foot present
      and foot Q72.2-●
  lens Q12.3
  limb (complete) Q73.0
    lower —*see* Agenesis, leg
    upper —*see* Agenesis, arm
  lip Q38.0
  liver Q44.7
  lung (fissure) (lobe) (bilateral) (unilateral)
      Q33.3
  mandible, maxilla M26.09
  metacarpus —*see* Agenesis, hand
  metatarsus —*see* Agenesis, foot
  muscle Q79.8
    eyelid Q10.3
    ocular Q15.8
  musculoskeletal system NEC Q79.8
  nail(s) Q84.3
  neck, part Q18.8

Agenesis *(Continued)*
  nerve Q07.8
  nervous system, part NEC Q07.8
  nipple Q83.2
  nose Q30.1
  nuclear Q07.8
  organ
    of Corti Q16.5
    or site not listed —*see* Anomaly, by site
  osseous meatus (ear) Q16.1
  ovary
    bilateral Q50.02
    unilateral Q50.01
  oviduct Q50.6
  pancreas Q45.0
  parathyroid (gland) Q89.2
  parotid gland(s) Q38.4
  patella Q74.1
  pelvic girdle (complete) (partial) Q74.2
  penis Q55.5
  pericardium Q24.8
  pituitary (gland) Q89.2
  prostate Q55.4
  punctum lacrimale Q10.4
  radioulnar —*see* Defect, reduction, upper limb
  radius —*see* Defect, reduction, upper limb,
      longitudinal, radius
  rectum Q42.1
    with fistula Q42.0
  renal Q60.2
    bilateral Q60.1
    unilateral Q60.0
  respiratory organ NEC Q34.8
  rib Q76.6
  roof of orbit Q75.8
  round ligament Q52.8
  sacrum Q76.49
  salivary gland Q38.4
  scapula Q74.0
  scrotum Q55.29
  seminal vesicles Q55.4
  septum
    atrial Q21.1
    between aorta and pulmonary artery Q21.4
    ventricular Q20.4
  shoulder girdle (complete) (partial) Q74.0
  skull (bone) Q75.8
    with
      anencephaly Q00.0
      encephalocele —*see* Encephalocele
      hydrocephalus Q03.9
        with spina bifida —*see* Spina bifida, by
            site, with hydrocephalus
      microcephaly Q02
  spermatic cord Q55.4
  spinal cord Q06.0
  spine Q76.49
  spleen Q89.01
  sternum Q76.7
  stomach Q40.2
  submaxillary gland(s) (congenital) Q38.4
  tarsus —*see* Agenesis, foot
  tendon Q79.8
  testicle Q55.0
  thymus (gland) Q89.2
  thyroid (gland) E03.1
    cartilage Q31.8
  tibia —*see* Defect, reduction, lower limb,
      longitudinal, tibia
  tibiofibular —*see* Defect, reduction, lower
      limb, specified type NEC
  toe (and foot) (complete) (partial) —*see*
      Agenesis, foot
  tongue Q38.3
  trachea (cartilage) Q32.1
  ulna —*see* Defect, reduction, upper limb,
      longitudinal, ulna
  upper limb —*see* Agenesis, arm
  ureter Q62.4
  urethra Q64.5
  urinary tract NEC Q64.8

Agenesis *(Continued)*
  uterus Q51.0
  uvula Q38.5
  vagina Q52.0
  vas deferens Q55.4
  vein(s) (peripheral) Q27.9
    brain Q28.3
    great NEC Q26.8
    portal Q26.5
  vena cava (inferior) (superior) Q26.8
  vermis of cerebellum Q04.3
  vertebra Q76.49
  vulva Q52.71
Ageusia R43.2
Agitated —*see* condition
Agitation R45.1
Aglossia (congenital) Q38.3
Aglossia-adactylia syndrome Q87.0
Aglycogenosis E74.00
Agnosia (body image) (other senses) (tactile)
    R48.1
  developmental F88
  verbal R48.1
    auditory R48.1
      developmental F80.2
    developmental F80.2
  visual (object) R48.3
Agoraphobia F40.00
  with panic disorder F40.01
  without panic disorder F40.02
Agrammatism R48.8
Agranulocytopenia —*see* Agranulocytosis
Agranulocytosis (chronic) (cyclical) (genetic)
    (infantile) (periodic) (pernicious) (*see also*
    Neutropenia) D70.9
  congenital D70.0
  cytoreductive cancer chemotherapy sequela
      D70.1
  drug-induced D70.2
    due to cytoreductive cancer chemotherapy
        D70.1
  due to infection D70.3
  secondary D70.4
    drug-induced D70.2
      due to cytoreductive cancer
          chemotherapy D70.1
Agraphia (absolute) R48.8
  with alexia R48.0
  developmental F81.81
Ague (dumb) —*see* Malaria
Agyria Q04.3
Ahumada-del Castillo syndrome E23.0
Aichmophobia F40.298
AIDS (related complex) B20
Ailment heart —*see* Disease, heart
Ailurophobia F40.218
Ainhum (disease) L94.6
AIN —*see* Neoplasia, intraepithelial, anal
AIPHI (acute idiopathic pulmonary hemorrhage
    in infants (over 28 days old)) R04.81
Air
  anterior mediastinum J98.2
  compressed, disease T70.3
  conditioner lung or pneumonitis J67.7
  embolism (artery) (cerebral) (any site) T79.0
    with ectopic or molar pregnancy O08.2
    due to implanted device NEC —*see*
        Complications, by site and type,
        specified NEC
    following
      abortion —*see* Abortion by type,
          complicated by, embolism
      ectopic or molar pregnancy O08.2
    infusion, therapeutic injection or
        transfusion T80.0
    in pregnancy, childbirth or puerperium —
        see Embolism, obstetric
    traumatic T79.0
  hunger, psychogenic F45.8
  rarefied, effects of —*see* Effect, adverse, high
      altitude
  sickness T75.3

▶ New   ⇒ Revised   ~~deleted~~ Deleted   ● Use Additional Character(s)

Airplane sickness T75.3
Akathisia (drug-induced) (treatment- induced)
 G25.71
 neuroleptic induced (acute) G25.71
▶tardive G25.71
Akinesia R29.898
Akinetic mutism R41.89
Akureyri's disease G93.3
Alactasia, congenital E73.0
Alagille's syndrome Q44.7
Alastrim B03
Albers-Schönberg syndrome Q78.2
Albert's syndrome —see Tendinitis, Achilles
Albinism, albino E70.30
 with hematologic abnormality E70.339
  Chédiak-Higashi syndrome E70.330
  Hermansky-Pudlak syndrome E70.331
  other specified E70.338
 I E70.320
 II E70.321
 ocular E70.319
  autosomal recessive E70.311
  other specified E70.318
  X-linked E70.310
 oculocutaneous E70.329
  other specified E70.328
  tyrosinase (ty) negative E70.320
  tyrosinase (ty) positive E70.321
 other specified E70.39
Albinismus E70.30
Albright (-McCune)(-Sternberg) syndrome
 Q78.1
Albuminous —see condition
Albuminuria, albuminuric (acute) (chronic)
 (subacute) —see also Proteinuria R80.9
 complicating pregnancy —see Proteinuria,
  gestational
  with
   gestational hypertension —see
    Pre-eclampsia
   pre-existing hypertension —see
    Hypertension, complicating
    pregnancy, pre-existing, with,
    pre-eclampsia
 gestational —see Proteinuria, gestational
  with
   gestational hypertension —see
    Pre-eclampsia
   pre-existing hypertension —see
    Hypertension, complicating
    pregnancy, pre-existing, with,
    pre-eclampsia
 orthostatic R80.2
 postural R80.2
 pre-eclamptic —see Pre-eclampsia
 scarlatinal A38.8
Albuminurophobia F40.298
Alcaptonuria E70.29
Alcohol, alcoholic, alcohol-induced
 addiction (without remission) F10.20
  with remission F10.21
 amnestic disorder, persisting F10.96
  with dependence F10.26
 anxiety disorder F10.980
 bipolar and related disorder F10.94
 brain syndrome, chronic F10.97
  with dependence F10.27
 cardiopathy I42.6
 counseling and surveillance Z71.41
  family member Z71.42
 delirium (acute) (tremens) (withdrawal)
  F10.231
  with intoxication F10.921
  in
   abuse F10.121
   dependence F10.221
 dementia F10.97
  with dependence F10.27
 depressive disorder F10.94
 deterioration F10.97
  with dependence F10.27

Alcohol, alcoholic, alcohol-induced *(Continued)*
 hallucinosis (acute) F10.951
  in
   abuse F10.151
   dependence F10.251
 insanity F10.959
 intoxication (acute) (without dependence)
  F10.129
  with
   delirium F10.121
   dependence F10.229
    with delirium F10.221
    uncomplicated F10.220
   uncomplicated F10.120
 jealousy F10.988
 Korsakoff's, Korsakov's, Korsakow's
  F10.26
 liver K70.9
  acute —see Disease, liver, alcoholic,
   hepatitis
 major neurocognitive disorder, amnestic-
  confabulatory type F10.96
 major neurocognitive disorder, nonamnestic-
  confabulatory type F10.97
 mania (acute) (chronic) F10.959
 mild neurocognitive disorder F10.988
 paranoia, paranoid (type) psychosis F10.950
 pellagra E52
 poisoning, accidental (acute) NEC —see
  Table of Drugs and Chemicals, alcohol,
  poisoning
 psychosis —see Psychosis, alcoholic
 psychotic disorder F10.959
 sexual dysfunction F10.981
 sleep disorder F10.982
 withdrawal (without convulsions) F10.239
  with delirium F10.231
Alcoholism (chronic) (without remission)
 F10.20
 with
  psychosis —see Psychosis, alcoholic
  remission F10.21
 Korsakov's F10.96
  with dependence F10.26
Alder (-Reilly) anomaly or syndrome
 (leukocyte granulation) D72.0
Aldosteronism E26.9
 familial (type I) E26.02
 glucocorticoid-remediable E26.02
 primary (due to (bilateral) adrenal
  hyperplasia) E26.09
 primary NEC E26.09
 secondary E26.1
 specified NEC E26.89
Aldosteronoma D44.10
Aldrich(-Wiskott) syndrome (eczema-
 thrombocytopenia) D82.0
Alektorophobia F40.218
Aleppo boil B55.1
Aleukemic —see condition Aleukia
 congenital D70.0
 hemorrhagica D61.9
  congenital D61.09
 splenica D73.1
Alexia R48.0
 developmental F81.0
 secondary to organic lesion R48.0
Algoneurodystrophy M89.00
 ankle M89.07-●
 foot M89.07-●
 forearm M89.03-●
 hand M89.04-●
 lower leg M89.06-●
 multiple sites M89.0-●
 shoulder M89.01-●
 specified site NEC M89.08
 thigh M89.05-●
 upper arm M89.02-●
Algophobia F40.298
Alienation, mental —see Psychosis
Alkalemia E87.3

Alkalosis E87.3
 metabolic E87.3
  with respiratory acidosis E87.4
 respiratory E87.3
Alkaptonuria E70.29
Allen-Masters syndrome N83.8
Allergy, allergic (reaction) (to) T78.40
 air-borne substance NEC (rhinitis) J30.89
 alveolitis (extrinsic) J67.9
  due to
   Aspergillus clavatus J67.4
   Cryptostroma corticale J67.6
   organisms (fungal, thermophilic
    actinomycete) growing in
    ventilation (air conditioning)
    systems J67.7
  specified type NEC J67.8
 anaphylactic reaction or shock T78.2
 angioneurotic edema T78.3
 animal (dander) (epidermal) (hair) (rhinitis)
  J30.81
 bee sting (anaphylactic shock) —see Toxicity,
  venom, arthropod, bee
 biological —see Allergy, drug
 colitis —see also Colitis, allergic K52.29
 dander (animal) (rhinitis) J30.81
 dandruff (rhinitis) J30.81
 dental restorative material (existing) K08.55
 dermatitis —see Dermatitis, contact, allergic
 diathesis —see History, allergy
 drug, medicament & biological (any)
  (external) (internal) T78.40
  correct substance properly administered —
   see Table of Drugs and Chemicals, by
   drug, adverse effect
  wrong substance given or taken NEC (by
   accident) —see Table of Drugs and
   Chemicals, by drug, poisoning
 due to pollen J30.1
 dust (house) (stock) (rhinitis) J30.89
  with asthma —see Asthma, allergic extrinsic
 eczema —see Dermatitis, contact, allergic
 epidermal (animal) (rhinitis) J30.81
 feathers (rhinitis) J30.89
 food (any) (ingested) NEC T78.1
  anaphylactic shock —see Shock,
   anaphylactic, due to food
  dermatitis —see Dermatitis, due to, food
  dietary counseling and surveillance Z71.3
  in contact with skin L23.6
  rhinitis J30.5
  status (without reaction) Z91.018
   eggs Z91.012
   milk products Z91.011
   peanuts Z91.010
   seafood Z91.013
   specified NEC Z91.018
 gastrointestinal —see also specific type of
  allergic reaction
  meaning colitis —see also Colitis, allergic)
   K52.29
  meaning gastroenteritis —see also
   Gastroenteritis, allergic) K52.29
  meaning other adverse food reaction not
   elsewhere classified T78.1
 grain J30.1
 grass (hay fever) (pollen) J30.1
  asthma —see Asthma, allergic extrinsic
 hair (animal) (rhinitis) J30.81
 history (of) —see History, allergy
 horse serum —see Allergy, serum
 inhalant (rhinitis) J30.89
  pollen J30.1
 kapok (rhinitis) J30.89
 medicine —see Allergy, drug
 milk protein —see also Allergy, food Z91.011
  anaphylactic reaction T78.07
  dermatitis L27.2
  enterocolitis syndrome K52.21
  enteropathy K52.22
  gastroenteritis K52.29

Allergy, allergic (Continued)
  milk protein (Continued)
    gastroesophageal reflux —see also Reaction,
      adverse, food) K21.9
      with esophagitis K21.0
    proctocolitis K52.82   ]
  nasal, seasonal due to pollen J30.1
  pneumonia J82
  pollen (any) (hay fever) J30.1
    asthma —see Asthma, allergic extrinsic
  primrose J30.1
  primula J30.1
  proctocolitis K52.82
  purpura D69.0
  ragweed (hay fever) (pollen) J30.1
    asthma —see Asthma, allergic extrinsic
  rose (pollen) J30.1
  seasonal NEC J30.2
  Senecio jacobae (pollen) J30.1
  serum —see also Reaction, serum T80.69
    anaphylactic shock T80.59
  shock (anaphylactic) T78.2
    due to
      administration of blood and blood
        products T80.51
      adverse effect of correct medicinal
        substance properly administered
        T88.6
      immunization T80.52
      serum NEC T80.59
      vaccination T80.52
  specific NEC T78.49
  tree (any) (hay fever) (pollen) J30.1
    asthma —see Asthma, allergic extrinsic
  upper respiratory J30.9
  urticaria L50.0
  vaccine —see Allergy, serum
  wheat —see Allergy, food
Allescheriasis B48.2
Alligator skin disease Q80.9
Allocheiria, allochiria R20.8
Almeida's disease —see
  Paracoccidioidomycosis
Alopecia (hereditaria) (seborrheica)
  L65.9
  androgenic L64.9
    drug-induced L64.0
    specified NEC L64.8
  areata L63.9
    ophiasis L63.2
    specified NEC L63.8
    totalis L63.0
    universalis L63.1
  cicatricial L66.9
    specified NEC L66.8
  circumscripta L63.9
  congenital, congenitalis Q84.0
  due to cytotoxic drugs NEC L65.8
  mucinosa L65.2
  postinfective NEC L65.8
  postpartum L65.0
  premature L64.8
  specific (syphilitic) A51.32
  specified NEC L65.8
  syphilitic (secondary) A51.32
  totalis (capitis) L63.0
  universalis (entire body) L63.1
  X-ray L58.1
Alpers' disease G31.81
Alpine sickness T70.29
Alport syndrome Q87.81
ALTE (apparent life threatening event) in
  newborn and infant R68.13
Alteration (of), **Altered**
  awareness
    transient R40.4
    unintended under general anesthesia,
      during procedure T88.53
  mental status R41.82
  pattern of family relationships affecting child
    Z62.898

Alteration (of), **Altered** (Continued)
  sensation
    following
      cerebrovascular disease I69.998
        cerebral infarction I69.398
        intracerebral hemorrhage I69.198
        nontraumatic intracranial hemorrhage
          NEC I69.298
        specified disease NEC I69.898
        subarachnoid hemorrhage I69.098
Alternating —see condition
Altitude, high (effects) —see Effect, adverse,
  high altitude
Aluminosis (of lung) J63.0
Alveolitis
  allergic (extrinsic) —see Pneumonitis,
    hypersensitivity
  due to
    Aspergillus clavatus J67.4
    Cryptostroma corticale J67.6
  fibrosing (cryptogenic) (idiopathic) J84.112
  jaw M27.3
  sicca dolorosa M27.3
Alveolus, alveolar —see condition
Alymphocytosis D72.810
  thymic (with immunodeficiency) D82.1
Alymphoplasia, thymic D82.1
Alzheimer's disease or sclerosis —see Disease,
  Alzheimer's
Amastia (with nipple present) Q83.8
  with absent nipple Q83.0
Amathophobia F40.228
Amaurosis (acquired) (congenital) —see also
  Blindness
  fugax G45.3
  hysterical F44.6
  Leber's congenital H35.50
  uremic —see Uremia
Amaurotic idiocy (infantile) (juvenile) (late) E75.4
Amaxophobia F40.248
Ambiguous genitalia Q56.4
Amblyopia (congenital) (ex anopsia) (partial)
  (suppression) H53.00-●
  anisometropic —see Amblyopia, refractive
  deprivation H53.01-●
  hysterical F44.6
  nocturnal —see also Blindness, night
    vitamin A deficiency E50.5
  refractive H53.02-●
  strabismic H53.03-●
  suspect H53.04-●
  tobacco H53.8
  toxic NEC H53.8
  uremic —see Uremia
Ameba, amebic (histolytica) —see also Amebiasis
  abscess (liver) A06.4
Amebiasis A06.9
  with abscess —see Abscess, amebic
  acute A06.0
  chronic (intestine) A06.1
    with abscess —see Abscess, amebic
  cutaneous A06.7
  cutis A06.7
  cystitis A06.81
  genitourinary tract NEC A06.82
  hepatic —see Abscess, liver, amebic
  intestine A06.0
  nondysenteric colitis A06.2
  skin A06.7
  specified site NEC A06.89
Ameboma (of intestine) A06.3
Amelia Q73.0
  lower limb —see Agenesis, leg
  upper limb —see Agenesis, arm
Ameloblastoma —see also Cyst, calcifying
  odontogenic
  long bones C40.9-●
    lower limb C40.2-●
    upper limb C40.0-●
  malignant C41.1
    jaw (bone) (lower) C41.1
      upper C41.0
  tibial C40.2-●

Amelogenesis imperfecta K00.5
  nonhereditaria (segmentalis) K00.4
Amenorrhea N91.2
  hyperhormonal E28.8
  primary N91.0
  secondary N91.1
Amentia —see Disability, intellectual
  Meynert's (nonalcoholic) F04
American
  leishmaniasis B55.2
  mountain tick fever A93.2
Ametropia —see Disorder, refraction
AMH (asymptomatic microscopic hematuria)
  R31.21
Amianthosis J61
Amimia R48.8
Amino-acid disorder E72.9
  anemia D53.0
Aminoacidopathy E72.9
Aminoaciduria E72.9
Amnes (t)ic **syndrome** (post-traumatic) F04
  induced by
    alcohol F10.96
      with dependence F10.26
    psychoactive NEC F19.96
      with
        abuse F19.16
        dependence F19.26
    sedative F13.96
      with dependence F13.26
Amnesia R41.3
  anterograde R41.1
  auditory R48.8
  dissociative F44.0
    with dissociative fugue F44.1
  hysterical F44.0
  postictal in epilepsy —see Epilepsy
  psychogenic F44.0
  retrograde R41.2
  transient global G45.4
Amnion, amniotic —see condition
Amnionitis —see Pregnancy, complicated by
Amok F68.8
Amoral traits F60.89
Amphetamine (or other stimulant) —
  induced
    anxiety disorder F15.980
    bipolar and related disorder F15.94
    delirium F15.921
    depressive disorder F15.94
    obsessive-compulsive and related disorder
      F15.988
    psychotic disorder F15.959
    sexual dysfunction F15.981
    sleep disorder F15.982
    stimulant withdrawal F15.23
Ampulla
  lower esophagus K22.8
  phrenic K22.8
Amputation —see also Absence, by site,
  acquired
  neuroma (postoperative) (traumatic) —see
    Complications, amputation stump,
    neuroma
  stump (surgical)
    abnormal, painful, or with complication
      (late) —see Complications, amputation
      stump
    healed or old NOS Z89.9
  traumatic (complete) (partial)
    arm (upper) (complete) S48.91-●
      at
        elbow S58.01-●
          partial S58.02-●
        shoulder joint (complete) S48.01-●
          partial S48.02-●
      between
        elbow and wrist (complete) S58.11-●
          partial S58.12-●
        shoulder and elbow (complete)
          S48.11-●
          partial S48.12-●
      partial S48.92-●

▶ New   ➡ Revised   ~~deleted~~ Deleted   ● Use Additional Character(s)

Amputation *(Continued)*
  traumatic *(Continued)*
    breast (complete) S28.21-●
      partial S28.22-●
    clitoris (complete) S38.211
      partial S38.212
    ear (complete) S08.11-●
      partial S08.12-●
    finger (complete) (metacarpophalangeal)
      S68.11-●
      index S68.11-●
      little S68.11-●
      middle S68.11-●
      partial S68.12-●
        index S68.12-●
        little S68.12-●
        middle S68.12-●
        ring S68.12-●
      ring S68.11-●
      thumb —*see* Amputation, traumatic,
        thumb
      transphalangeal (complete) S68.61-●
        index S68.61-●
        little S68.61-●
        middle S68.61-●
        partial S68.62-●
          index S68.62-●
          little S68.62-●
          middle S68.62-●
          ring S68.62-●
        ring S68.61-●
    foot (complete) S98.91-●
      at ankle level S98.01-●
        partial S98.02-●
      midfoot S98.31-●
        partial S98.32-●
      partial S98.92-●
    forearm (complete) S58.91-●
      at elbow level (complete) S58.01-●
        partial S58.02-●
      between elbow and wrist (complete)
        S58.11-●
        partial S58.12-●
      partial S58.92-●
    genital organ(s) (external)
      female (complete) S38.211
        partial S38.212
      male
        penis (complete) S38.221
          partial S38.222
        scrotum (complete) S38.231
          partial S38.232
        testes (complete) S38.231
          partial S38.232
    hand (complete) (wrist level) S68.41-●
      finger(s) alone —*see* Amputation,
        traumatic, finger
      partial S68.42-●
      thumb alone —*see* Amputation,
        traumatic, thumb
      transmetacarpal (complete) S68.71-●
        partial S68.72-●
    head
      ear —*see* Amputation, traumatic, ear
      nose (partial) S08.812
        complete S08.811
      part S08.89
        scalp S08.0
    hip (and thigh) (complete) S78.91-●
      at hip joint (complete) S78.01-●
        partial S78.02-●
      between hip and knee (complete) S78.11-●
        partial S78.12-●
      partial S78.92-●
    labium (majus) (minus) (complete) S38.21-●
      partial S38.21-●
    leg (lower) S88.91-●
      at knee level S88.01-●
        partial S88.02-●
      between knee and ankle S88.11-●
        partial S88.12-●
      partial S88.92-●

Amputation *(Continued)*
  traumatic *(Continued)*
    nose (partial) S08.812
      complete S08.811
    penis (complete) S38.221
      partial S38.222
    scrotum (complete) S38.231
      partial S38.232
    shoulder —*see* Amputation, traumatic, arm
      at shoulder joint —*see* Amputation,
        traumatic, arm, at shoulder joint
    testes (complete) S38.231
      partial S38.232
    thigh —*see* Amputation, traumatic, hip
    thorax, part of S28.1
      breast —*see* Amputation, traumatic,
        breast
    thumb (complete) (metacarpophalangeal)
      S68.01-●
      partial S68.02-●
      transphalangeal (complete) S68.51-●
        partial S68.52-●
    toe (lesser) S98.13-●
      great S98.11-●
        partial S98.12-●
      more than one S98.21-●
        partial S98.22-●
      partial S98.14-●
    vulva (complete) S38.211
      partial S38.212
Amputee (bilateral) (old) Z89.9
Amsterdam dwarfism Q87.1
Amusia R48.8
  developmental F80.89
Amyelencephalus, amyelencephaly Q00.0
Amyelia Q06.0
Amygdalitis —*see* Tonsillitis
Amygdalolith J35.8
Amyloid heart (disease) E85.4 *[I43]*
Amyloidosis (generalized) (primary) E85.9
  with lung involvement E85.4 *[J99]*
  familial E85.2
  genetic E85.2
  heart E85.4 *[I43]*
  hemodialysis-associated E85.3
  ▶light chain (AL) E85.81
  liver E85.4 *[K77]*
  localized E85.4
  neuropathic heredofamilial E85.1
  non-neuropathic heredofamilial E85.0
  organ limited E85.4
  Portuguese E85.1
  pulmonary E85.4 *[J99]*
  secondary systemic E85.3
  ▶senile systemic (SSA) E85.82
  skin (lichen) (macular) E85.4 *[L99]*
  ⟱specified NEC E85.89
  subglottic E85.4 *[J99]*
  ▶wild-type transthyretin-related (ATTR)
    E85.82
Amylopectinosis (brancher enzyme deficiency)
  E74.03
Amylophagia —*see* Pica
Amyoplasia congenita Q79.8
Amyotonia M62.89
  congenita G70.2
Amyotrophia, amyotrophy, amyotrophic G71.8
  congenita Q79.8
  diabetic —*see* Diabetes, amyotrophy
  lateral sclerosis G12.21
  neuralgic G54.5
  ⟱spinal progressive G12.25
Anacidity, gastric K31.83
  psychogenic F45.8
Anaerosis of newborn P28.89
Analbuminemia E88.09
Analgesia —*see* Anesthesia
Analphalipoproteinemia E78.6
Anaphylactic
  purpura D69.0
  shock or reaction —*see* Shock, anaphylactic

Anaphylactoid shock or reaction —*see* Shock,
  anaphylactic
Anaphylactoid syndrome of pregnancy O88.01-●
Anaphylaxis —*see* Shock, anaphylactic
Anaplasia cervix —*see also* Dysplasia, cervix
  N87.9
Anaplasmosis, human A77.49
Anarthria R47.1
Anasarca R60.1
  cardiac —*see* Failure, heart, congestive
  lung J18.2
  newborn P83.2
  nutritional E43
  pulmonary J18.2
  renal N04.9
Anastomosis
  aneurysmal —*see* Aneurysm
  arteriovenous ruptured brain I60.8
  intestinal K63.89
    complicated NEC K91.89
      involving urinary tract N99.89
  retinal and choroidal vessels (congenital) Q14.8
Anatomical narrow angle H40.03-●
Ancylostoma, ancylostomiasis (braziliense)
  (caninum) (ceylanicum) (duodenale) B76.0
  Necator americanus B76.1
Andersen's disease (glycogen storage) E74.09
Anderson-Fabry disease E75.21
Andes disease T70.29
Andrews' disease (bacterid) L08.89
Androblastoma
  benign
    specified site —*see* Neoplasm, benign, by
      site
    unspecified site
      female D27.9
      male D29.20
  malignant
    specified site —*see* Neoplasm, malignant,
      by site
    unspecified site
      female C56.9
      male C62.90
  specified site —*see* Neoplasm, uncertain
    behavior, by site
  tubular
    with lipid storage
      specified site —*see* Neoplasm, benign,
        by site
      unspecified site
        female D27.9
        male D29.20
    specified site —*see* Neoplasm, benign,
      by site
    unspecified site
      female D27.9
      male D29.20
  unspecified site
    female D39.10
    male D40.10
Androgen insensitivity syndrome —*see also*
  Syndrome, androgen insensitivity E34.50
Androgen resistance syndrome —*see also*
  Syndrome, androgen insensitivity E34.50
Android pelvis Q74.2
  with disproportion (fetopelvic) O33.3
    causing obstructed labor O65.3
Androphobia F40.290
Anectasis, pulmonary (newborn) —*see*
  Atelectasis
Anemia (essential) (general) (hemoglobin
  deficiency) (infantile) (primary) (profound)
  D64.9
  with (due to) (in)
    disorder of
      anaerobic glycolysis D55.2
      pentose phosphate pathway D55.1
    koilonychia D50.9
  achlorhydric D50.8
  achrestic D53.1
  Addison (-Biermer) (pernicious) D51.0

Anemia *(Continued)*
  agranulocytic —*see* Agranulocytosis
  amino-acid-deficiency D53.0
  aplastic D61.9
    congenital D61.09
    drug-induced D61.1
    due to
      drugs D61.1
      external agents NEC D61.2
      infection D61.2
      radiation D61.2
    idiopathic D61.3
    red cell (pure) D60.9
      chronic D60.0
      congenital D61.01
      specified type NEC D60.8
      transient D60.1
    specified type NEC D61.89
    toxic D61.2
  aregenerative
    congenital D61.09
  asiderotic D50.9
  atypical (primary) D64.9
  Baghdad spring D55.0
  Balantidium coli A07.0
  Biermer's (pernicious) D51.0
  blood loss (chronic) D50.0
    acute D62
  bothriocephalus B70.0 *[D63.8]*
  brickmaker's B76.9 *[D63.8]*
  cerebral I67.89
  childhood D58.9
  chlorotic D50.8
  chronic
    blood loss D50.0
    hemolytic D58.9
      idiopathic D59.9
    simple D53.9
  chronica congenita aregenerativa D61.09
  combined system disease NEC D51.0 *[G32.0]*
    due to dietary vitamin B12 deficiency
      D51.3 *[G32.0]*
  complicating pregnancy, childbirth
      or puerperium —*see* Pregnancy,
      complicated by (management affected
      by), anemia
  congenital P61.4
    aplastic D61.09
    due to isoimmunization NOS P55.9
    dyserythropoietic, dyshematopoietic D64.4
    following fetal blood loss P61.3
    Heinz body D58.2
    hereditary hemolytic NOS D58.9
    pernicious D51.0
    spherocytic D58.0
  Cooley's (erythroblastic) D56.1
  cytogenic D51.0
  deficiency D53.9
    2, 3 diphosphoglycurate mutase D55.2
    2, 3 PG D55.2
    6 phosphogluconate dehydrogenase D55.1
    6-PGD D55.1
    amino-acid D53.0
    combined B12 and folate D53.1
    enzyme D55.9
      drug-induced (hemolytic) D59.2
      glucose-6-phosphate dehydrogenase
        (G6PD) D55.0
      glycolytic D55.2
      nucleotide metabolism D55.3
      related to hexose monophosphate
        (HMP) shunt pathway NEC D55.1
      specified type NEC D55.8
    erythrocytic glutathione D55.1
    folate D52.9
      dietary D52.0
      drug-induced D52.1
    folic acid D52.9
      dietary D52.0
      drug-induced D52.1
    G SH D55.1

Anemia *(Continued)*
  deficiency *(Continued)*
    G6PD D55.0
    GGS-R D55.1
    glucose-6-phosphate dehydrogenase D55.0
    glutathione reductase D55.1
    glyceraldehyde phosphate dehydrogenase
      D55.2
    hexokinase D55.2
    iron D50.9
      secondary to blood loss (chronic) D50.0
    nutritional D53.9
      with
        poor iron absorption D50.8
        specified deficiency NEC D53.8
    phosphofructo-aldolase D55.2
    phosphoglycerate kinase D55.2
    PK D55.2
    protein D53.0
    pyruvate kinase D55.2
    transcobalamin II D51.2
    triose-phosphate isomerase D55.2
    vitamin B12 NOS D51.9
      dietary D51.3
      due to
        intrinsic factor deficiency D51.0
        selective vitamin B12 malabsorption
          with proteinuria D51.1
      pernicious D51.0
      specified type NEC D51.8
  Diamond-Blackfan (congenital hypoplastic)
    D61.01
  dibothriocephalus B70.0 *[D63.8]*
  dimorphic D53.1
  diphasic D53.1
  Diphyllobothrium (Dibothriocephalus) B70.0
    [D63.8]
  due to (in) (with)
    antineoplastic chemotherapy D64.81
    blood loss (chronic) D50.0
      acute D62
    chemotherapy, antineoplastic D64.81
    chronic disease classified elsewhere NEC
      D63.8
    chronic kidney disease D63.1
    deficiency
      amino-acid D53.0
      copper D53.8
      folate (folic acid) D52.9
        dietary D52.0
        drug-induced D52.1
      molybdenum D53.8
      protein D53.0
      zinc D53.8
    dietary vitamin B12 deficiency D51.3
    disorder of
      glutathione metabolism D55.1
      nucleotide metabolism D55.3
    drug —*see* Anemia, by type —*see also* Table
      of Drugs and Chemicals
    end stage renal disease D63.1
    enzyme disorder D55.9
    fetal blood loss P61.3
    fish tapeworm (D latum) infestation B70.0
      [D63.8]
    hemorrhage (chronic) D50.0
      acute D62
    impaired absorption D50.9
    loss of blood (chronic) D50.0
      acute D62
    myxedema E03.9 *[D63.8]*
    Necator americanus B76.1 *[D63.8]*
    prematurity P61.2
    selective vitamin B12 malabsorption with
      proteinuria D51.1
    transcobalamin II deficiency D51.2
  Dyke-Young type (secondary) (symptomatic)
    D59.1
  dyserythropoietic (congenital) D64.4
  dyshematopoietic (congenital) D64.4
  Egyptian B76.9 *[D63.8]*

Anemia *(Continued)*
  elliptocytosis —*see* Elliptocytosis
  enzyme-deficiency, drug-induced D59.2
  epidemic —*see also* Ancylostomiasis B76.9
    [D63.8]
  erythroblastic
    familial D56.1
    newborn —*see also* Disease, hemolytic P55.9
    of childhood D56.1
  erythrocytic glutathione deficiency D55.1
  erythropoietin-resistant anemia (EPO
    resistant anemia) D63.1
  Faber's (achlorhydric anemia) D50.9
  factitious (self-induced blood letting) D50.0
  familial erythroblastic D56.1
  Fanconi's (congenital pancytopenia) D61.09
  favism D55.0
  fish tapeworm (D. latum) infestation B70.0
    [D63.8]
  folate (folic acid) deficiency D52.9
  glucose-6-phosphate dehydrogenase (G6PD)
    deficiency D55.0
  glutathione-reductase deficiency D55.1
  goat's milk D52.0
  granulocytic —*see* Agranulocytosis
  Heinz body, congenital D58.2
  hemolytic D58.9
    acquired D59.9
      with hemoglobinuria NEC D59.6
      autoimmune NEC D59.1
      infectious D59.4
      specified type NEC D59.8
      toxic D59.4
    acute D59.9
      due to enzyme deficiency specified type
        NEC D55.8
      Lederer's D59.1
    autoimmune D59.1
      drug-induced D59.0
    chronic D58.9
      idiopathic D59.9
    cold type (secondary) (symptomatic) D59.1
    congenital (spherocytic) —*see* Spherocytosis
    due to
      cardiac conditions D59.4
      drugs (nonautoimmune) D59.2
        autoimmune D59.0
      enzyme disorder D55.9
        drug-induced D59.2
      presence of shunt or other internal
        prosthetic device D59.4
    familial D58.9
    hereditary D58.9
      due to enzyme disorder D55.9
        specified type NEC D55.8
      specified type NEC D58.8
    idiopathic (chronic) D59.9
    mechanical D59.4
    microangiopathic D59.4
    nonautoimmune D59.4
      drug-induced D59.2
    nonspherocytic
      congenital or hereditary NEC D55.8
        glucose-6-phosphate dehydrogenase
          deficiency D55.0
        pyruvate kinase deficiency D55.2
        type
          I D55.1
          II D55.2
      type
        I D55.1
        II D55.2
    secondary D59.4
      autoimmune D59.1
    specified (hereditary) type NEC D58.8
    Stransky-Regala type —*see also*
      Hemoglobinopathy D58.8
    symptomatic D59.4
      autoimmune D59.1
    toxic D59.4
    warm type (secondary) (symptomatic) D59.1

▶ New   ⇒ Revised   ~~deleted~~ Deleted   ● Use Additional Character(s)

Anemia *(Continued)*
 hemorrhagic (chronic) D50.0
  acute D62
 Herrick's D57.1
 hexokinase deficiency D55.2
 hookworm B76.9 *[D63.8]*
 hypochromic (idiopathic) (microcytic)
   (normoblastic) D50.9
  due to blood loss (chronic) D50.0
   acute D62
  familial sex-linked D64.0
  pyridoxine-responsive D64.3
  sideroblastic, sex-linked D64.0
 hypoplasia, red blood cells D61.9
  congenital or familial D61.01
 hypoplastic (idiopathic) D61.9
  congenital or familial (of childhood)
    D61.01
 hypoproliferative (refractive) D61.9
 idiopathic D64.9
  aplastic D61.3
  hemolytic, chronic D59.9
 in (due to) (with)
  chronic kidney disease D63.1
  end stage renal disease D63.1
  failure, kidney (renal) D63.1
  neoplastic disease —*see also* Neoplasm
    D63.0
 intertropical —*see also* Ancylostomiasis D63.8
 iron deficiency D50.9
  secondary to blood loss (chronic) D50.0
   acute D62
  specified type NEC D50.8
 Joseph-Diamond-Blackfan (congenital
   hypoplastic) D61.01
 Lederer's (hemolytic) D59.1
 leukoerythroblastic D61.82
 macrocytic D53.9
  nutritional D52.0
  tropical D52.8
 malarial *(see also* Malaria) B54 *[D63.8]*
 malignant (progressive) D51.0
 malnutrition D53.9
 marsh *(see also* Malaria) B54 *[D63.8]*
 Mediterranean (with other
   hemoglobinopathy) D56.9
 megaloblastic D53.1
  combined B12 and folate deficiency
    D53.1
  hereditary D51.1
  nutritional D52.0
  orotic aciduria D53.0
  refractory D53.1
  specified type NEC D53.1
 megalocytic D53.1
 microcytic (hypochromic) D50.9
  due to blood loss (chronic) D50.0
   acute D62
  familial D56.8
 microdrepanocytosis D57.40
 microelliptopoikilocytic (Rietti-Greppi-
   Micheli) D56.9
 miner's B76.9 *[D63.8]*
 myelodysplastic D46.9
 myelofibrosis D75.81
 myelogenous D64.89
 myelopathic D64.89
 myelophthisic D61.82
 myeloproliferative D47.Z9
 newborn P61.4
  due to
   ABO (antibodies, isoimmunization,
     maternal/fetal incompatibility)
     P55.1
   Rh (antibodies, isoimmunization,
     maternal/fetal incompatibility)
     P55.0
  following fetal blood loss P61.3
  posthemorrhagic (fetal) P61.3
 nonspherocytic hemolytic —*see* Anemia,
   hemolytic, nonspherocytic

Anemia *(Continued)*
 normocytic (infectional) D64.9
  due to blood loss (chronic) D50.0
   acute D62
  myelophthisic D61.82
 nutritional (deficiency) D53.9
  with
   poor iron absorption D50.8
   specified deficiency NEC D53.8
  megaloblastic D52.0
 of prematurity P61.2
 orotaciduric (congenital) (hereditary) D53.0
 osteosclerotic D64.89
 ovalocytosis (hereditary) —*see* Elliptocytosis
 paludal —*see also* Malaria B54 *[D63.8]*
 pernicious (congenital) (malignant)
   (progressive) D51.0
 pleochromic D64.89
  of sprue D52.8
 posthemorrhagic (chronic) D50.0
  acute D62
  newborn P61.3
 postoperative (postprocedural)
  due to (acute) blood loss D62
   chronic blood loss D50.0
  specified NEC D64.9
 postpartum O90.81
 pressure D64.89
 progressive D64.9
  malignant D51.0
  pernicious D51.0
 protein-deficiency D53.0
 pseudoleukemica infantum D64.89
 pure red cell D60.9
  congenital D61.01
 pyridoxine-responsive D64.3
 pyruvate kinase deficiency D55.2
 refractory D46.4
  with
   excess of blasts D46.20
    1 (RAEB 1) D46.21
    2 (RAEB 2) D46.22
    in transformation (RAEB T) —*see*
      Leukemia, acute myeloblastic
   hemochromatosis D46.1
   sideroblasts (ring) (RARS) D46.1
  without ring sideroblasts, so stated D46.0
  without sideroblasts without excess of
    blasts D46.0
  megaloblastic D53.1
  sideroblastic D46.1
  sideropenic D50.9
 Rietti-Greppi-Micheli D56.9
 scorbutic D53.2
 secondary to
  blood loss (chronic) D50.0
   acute D62
  hemorrhage (chronic) D50.0
   acute D62
 semiplastic D61.89
 sickle-cell —*see* Disease, sickle-cell
 sideroblastic D64.3
  hereditary D64.0
  hypochromic, sex-linked D64.0
  pyridoxine-responsive NEC D64.3
  refractory D46.1
  secondary (due to)
   disease D64.1
   drugs and toxins D64.2
  specified type NEC D64.3
 sideropenic (refractory) D50.9
  due to blood loss (chronic) D50.0
   acute D62
 simple chronic D53.9
 specified type NEC D64.89
 spherocytic (hereditary) —*see* Spherocytosis
 splenic D64.89
 splenomegalic D64.89
 stomatocytosis D58.8
 syphilitic (acquired) (late) A52.79 *[D63.8]*
 target cell D64.89

Anemia *(Continued)*
 thalassemia D56.9
 thrombocytopenic —*see* Thrombocytopenia
 toxic D61.2
 tropical B76.9 *[D63.8]*
  macrocytic D52.8
 tuberculous A18.89 *[D63.8]*
 vegan D51.3
 vitamin
  B6-responsive D64.3
  B12 deficiency (dietary) pernicious D51.0
 von Jaksch's D64.89
 Witts' (achlorhydric anemia) D50.8
Anemophobia F40.228
Anencephalus, anencephaly Q00.0
Anergasia —*see* Psychosis, organic
Anesthesia, anesthetic R20.0
 complication or reaction NEC —*see also*
   Complications, anesthesia T88.59
  due to
   correct substance properly
     administered —*see* Table of Drugs
     and Chemicals, by drug, adverse
     effect
   overdose or wrong substance given —*see*
     Table of Drugs and Chemicals, by
     drug, poisoning
   unintended awareness under general
     anesthesia during procedure
     T88.53
   personal history of Z92.84
 cornea H18.81-●
 dissociative F44.6
 functional (hysterical) F44.6
 hyperesthetic, thalamic G89.0
 hysterical F44.6
 local skin lesion R20.0
 sexual (psychogenic) F52.1
 shock (due to) T88.2
 skin R20.0
 testicular N50.9
Anetoderma (maculosum) (of) L90.8
 Jadassohn-Pellizzari L90.2
 Schweniger-Buzzi L90.1
Aneurin deficiency E51.9
Aneurysm (anastomotic) (artery) (cirsoid)
   (diffuse) (false) (fusiform) (multiple)
   (saccular) I72.9
 abdominal (aorta) I71.4
  ruptured I71.3
  syphilitic A52.01
 aorta, aortic (nonsyphilitic) I71.9
  abdominal I71.4
   ruptured I71.3
  arch I71.2
   ruptured I71.1
  arteriosclerotic I71.9
   ruptured I71.8
  ascending I71.2
   ruptured I71.1
  congenital Q25.43
  descending I71.9
   abdominal I71.4
    ruptured I71.3
   ruptured I71.8
   thoracic I71.2
    ruptured I71.1
  root Q25.43
  ruptured I71.8
  sinus, congenital Q25.43
  syphilitic A52.01
  thoracic I71.2
   ruptured I71.1
  thoracoabdominal I71.6
   ruptured I71.5
  thorax, thoracic (arch) I71.2
   ruptured I71.1
  transverse I71.2
   ruptured I71.1
  valve (heart) —*see also* Endocarditis, aortic
    I35.8

Aneurysm *(Continued)*
  arteriosclerotic I72.9
    cerebral I67.1
      ruptured —*see* Hemorrhage, intracranial,
        subarachnoid
  arteriovenous (congenital) —*see also*
    Malformation, arteriovenous
    acquired I77.0
      brain I67.1
      coronary I25.41
      pulmonary I28.0
    brain Q28.2
      ruptured I60.8
    peripheral —*see* Malformation,
      arteriovenous, peripheral
    precerebral vessels Q28.0
    specified site NEC —*see also* Malformation,
      arteriovenous
      acquired I77.0
  basal —*see* Aneurysm, brain
  basilar (trunk) I72.5
  berry (congenital) (nonruptured) I67.1
    ruptured I60.7
  brain I67.1
    arteriosclerotic I67.1
      ruptured —*see* Hemorrhage, intracranial,
        subarachnoid
    arteriovenous (congenital) (nonruptured)
      Q28.2
      acquired I67.1
        ruptured I60.8
      ruptured I60.8
    berry (congenital) (nonruptured) I67.1
      ruptured —*see also* Hemorrhage,
        intracranial, subarachnoid I60.7
    congenital Q28.3
      aorta (root) (sinus) Q25.43
      ruptured I60.7
    meninges I67.1
      ruptured I60.8
    miliary (congenital) (nonruptured) I67.1
      ruptured —*see also* Hemorrhage,
        intracranial, subarachnoid I60.7
    mycotic I33.0
    ruptured —*see* Hemorrhage, intracranial,
      subarachnoid
    syphilitic (hemorrhage) A52.05
  cardiac (false) —*see also* Aneurysm, heart
    I25.3
  carotid artery (common) (external) I72.0
    internal (intracranial) I67.1
      extracranial portion I72.0
    ruptured into brain I60.0-•
    syphilitic A52.09
      intracranial A52.05
  cavernous sinus I67.1
    arteriovenous (congenital) (nonruptured)
      Q28.3
      ruptured I60.8
  celiac I72.8
  central nervous system, syphilitic A52.05
  cerebral —*see* Aneurysm, brain
  chest —*see* Aneurysm, thorax
  circle of Willis I67.1
    congenital Q28.3
      ruptured I60.6
    ruptured I60.6
  common iliac artery I72.3
  congenital (peripheral) Q27.8
    aorta (root) (sinus) Q25.43
    brain Q28.3
      ruptured I60.7
    coronary Q24.5
    digestive system Q27.8
    lower limb Q27.8
    pulmonary Q25.79
    retina Q14.1
    specified site NEC Q27.8
    upper limb Q27.8
  conjunctiva —*see* Abnormality, conjunctiva,
    vascular

Aneurysm *(Continued)*
  conus arteriosus —*see* Aneurysm, heart
  coronary (arteriosclerotic) (artery) I25.41
    arteriovenous, congenital Q24.5
    congenital Q24.5
    ruptured —*see* Infarct, myocardium
    syphilitic A52.06
    vein I25.89
  cylindroid (aorta) I71.9
    ruptured I71.8
    syphilitic A52.01
  ductus arteriosus Q25.0
  endocardial, infective (any valve) I33.0
  femoral (artery) (ruptured) I72.4
  gastroduodenal I72.8
  gastroepiploic I72.8
  heart (wall) (chronic or with a stated duration
    of over 4 weeks) I25.3
    valve —*see* Endocarditis
  hepatic I72.8
  iliac (common) (artery) (ruptured) I72.3
  infective I72.9
    endocardial (any valve) I33.0
  innominate (nonsyphilitic) I72.8
    syphilitic A52.09
  interauricular septum —*see* Aneurysm,
    heart
  interventricular septum —*see* Aneurysm,
    heart
  intrathoracic (nonsyphilitic) I71.2
    ruptured I71.1
    syphilitic A52.01
  lower limb I72.4
  lung (pulmonary artery) I28.1
  mediastinal (nonsyphilitic) I72.8
    syphilitic A52.09
  miliary (congenital) I67.1
    ruptured —*see* Hemorrhage, intracerebral,
      subarachnoid, intracranial
  mitral (heart) (valve) I34.8
  mural —*see* Aneurysm, heart
  mycotic I72.9
    endocardial (any valve) I33.0
    ruptured, brain —*see* Hemorrhage,
      intracerebral, subarachnoid
  myocardium —*see* Aneurysm, heart
  neck I72.0
  pancreaticoduodenal I72.8
  patent ductus arteriosus Q25.0
  peripheral NEC I72.8
    congenital Q27.8
      digestive system Q27.8
      lower limb Q27.8
      specified site NEC Q27.8
      upper limb Q27.8
  popliteal (artery) (ruptured) I72.4
  precerebral
    congenital (nonruptured) Q28.1
    specified site, NEC I72.5
  pulmonary I28.1
    arteriovenous Q25.72
      acquired I28.0
    syphilitic A52.09
    valve (heart) —*see* Endocarditis,
      pulmonary
  racemose (peripheral) I72.9
    congenital —*see* Aneurysm,
      congenital
  radial I72.1
  Rasmussen NEC A15.0
  renal (artery) I72.2
  retina —*see also* Disorder, retina,
    microaneurysms
    congenital Q14.1
    diabetic —*see* Diabetes, microaneurysms,
      retinal
  sinus of Valsalva Q25.49
  specified NEC I72.8
  spinal (cord) I72.8
    syphilitic (hemorrhage) A52.09
  splenic I72.8

Aneurysm *(Continued)*
  subclavian (artery) (ruptured) I72.8
    syphilitic A52.09
  superior mesenteric I72.8
  syphilitic (aorta) A52.01
    central nervous system A52.05
    congenital (late) A50.54 *[I79.0]*
    spine, spinal A52.09
  thoracoabdominal (aorta) I71.6
    ruptured I71.5
    syphilitic A52.01
  thorax, thoracic (aorta) (arch) (nonsyphilitic)
    I71.2
    ruptured I71.1
    syphilitic A52.01
  traumatic (complication) (early), specified
    site —*see* Injury, blood vessel
  tricuspid (heart) (valve) I07.8
  ulnar I72.1
  upper limb (ruptured) I72.1
  valve, valvular —*see* Endocarditis
  visceral NEC I72.8
  venous —*see also* Varix I86.8
    congenital Q27.8
      digestive system Q27.8
      lower limb Q27.8
      specified site NEC Q27.8
      upper limb Q27.8
  ventricle —*see* Aneurysm, heart
  vertebral artery I72.6
  visceral NEC I72.8
Angelman syndrome Q93.5
Anger R45.4
Angiectasis, angiectopia I99.8
Angiitis I77.6
  allergic granulomatous M30.1
  hypersensitivity M31.0
  necrotizing M31.9
    specified NEC M31.8
  nervous system, granulomatous I67.7
Angina (attack) (cardiac) (chest) (heart)
  (pectoris) (syndrome) (vasomotor) I20.9
  with
    atherosclerotic heart disease —*see*
      Arteriosclerosis, coronary (artery)
    documented spasm I20.1
  abdominal K55.1
  accelerated —*see* Angina, unstable
  agranulocytic —*see* Agranulocytosis
  angiospastic —*see* Angina, with documented
    spasm
  aphthous B08.5
  crescendo —*see* Angina, unstable
  croupous J05.0
  cruris I73.9
  de novo effort —*see* Angina, unstable
  diphtheritic, membranous A36.0
  equivalent I20.8
  exudative, chronic J37.0
  following acute myocardial infarction
    I23.7
  gangrenous diphtheritic A36.0
  intestinal K55.1
  Ludovici K12.2
  Ludwig's K12.2
  malignant diphtheritic A36.0
  membranous J05.0
    diphtheritic A36.0
    Vincent's A69.1
  mesenteric K55.1
  monocytic —*see* Mononucleosis, infectious
  of effort —*see* Angina, specified NEC
  phlegmonous J36
    diphtheritic A36.0
  post-infarctional I23.7
  pre-infarctional —*see* Angina, unstable
  Prinzmetal —*see* Angina, with documented
    spasm
  progressive —*see* Angina, unstable
  pseudomembranous A69.1
  pultaceous, diphtheritic A36.0

▶ New   ➡ Revised   ~~deleted~~ Deleted   • Use Additional Character(s)

Angina *(Continued)*
  spasm-induced —*see* Angina, with
    documented spasm
  specified NEC I20.8
  stable I20.8
  stenocardia —*see* Angina, specified NEC
  stridulous, diphtheritic A36.2
  tonsil J36
  trachealis J05.0
  unstable I20.0
  variant —*see* Angina, with documented
    spasm
  Vincent's A69.1
  worsening effort —*see* Angina, unstable
Angioblastoma —*see* Neoplasm, connective
  tissue, uncertain behavior
Angiocholecystitis —*see* Cholecystitis, acute
Angiocholitis —*see also* Cholecystitis, acute
  K83.0
Angiodysgenesis spinalis G95.19
Angiodysplasia (cecum) (colon) K55.20
  with bleeding K55.21
  duodenum (and stomach) K31.819
    with bleeding K31.811
  stomach (and duodenum) K31.819
    with bleeding K31.811
Angioedema (allergic) (any site) (with urticaria)
  T78.3
  hereditary D84.1
Angioendothelioma —*see* Neoplasm, uncertain
  behavior, by site
  benign D18.00
    intra-abdominal D18.03
    intracranial D18.02
    skin D18.01
    specified site NEC D18.09
  bone —*see* Neoplasm, bone, malignant
  Ewing's —*see* Neoplasm, bone, malignant
Angioendotheliomatosis C85.8-•
Angiofibroma —*see also* Neoplasm, benign, by
  site
  juvenile
    specified site —*see* Neoplasm, benign, by
      site
    unspecified site D10.6
Angiohemophilia (A) (B) D68.0
Angioid streaks (choroid) (macula) (retina)
  H35.33
Angiokeratoma —*see* Neoplasm, skin,
  benign
  corporis diffusum E75.21
Angioleiomyoma —*see* Neoplasm, connective
  tissue, benign
Angiolipoma —*see also* Lipoma
  infiltrating —*see* Lipoma
Angioma —*see also* Hemangioma, by site
  capillary I78.1
  hemorrhagicum hereditaria I78.0
  intra-abdominal D18.03
  intracranial D18.02
  malignant —*see* Neoplasm, connective tissue,
    malignant
  plexiform D18.00
    intra-abdominal D18.03
    intracranial D18.02
    skin D18.01
    specified site NEC D18.09
  senile I78.1
  serpiginosum L81.7
  skin D18.01
  specified site NEC D18.09
  spider I78.1
  stellate I78.1
  venous Q28.3
Angiomatosis Q82.8
  bacillary A79.89
  encephalotrigeminal Q85.8
  hemorrhagic familial I78.0
  hereditary familial I78.0
  liver K76.4
Angiomyolipoma —*see* Lipoma

Angiomyoliposarcoma —*see* Neoplasm,
  connective tissue, malignant
Angiomyoma —*see* Neoplasm, connective
  tissue, benign
Angiomyosarcoma —*see* Neoplasm, connective
  tissue, malignant
Angiomyxoma —*see* Neoplasm, connective
  tissue, uncertain behavior
Angioneurosis F45.8
Angioneurotic edema (allergic) (any site) (with
  urticaria) T78.3
  hereditary D84.1
Angiopathia, angiopathy I99.9
  cerebral I67.9
    amyloid E85.4 *[I68.0]*
  diabetic (peripheral) —*see* Diabetes,
    angiopathy
  peripheral I73.9
    diabetic —*see* Diabetes, angiopathy
    specified type NEC I73.89
  retinae syphilitica A52.05
  retinalis (juvenilis)
    diabetic —*see* Diabetes, retinopathy
    proliferative —*see* Retinopathy,
      proliferative
Angiosarcoma —*see also* Neoplasm, connective
  tissue, malignant
  liver C22.3
Angiosclerosis —*see* Arteriosclerosis
Angiospasm (peripheral) (traumatic) (vessel)
  I73.9
  brachial plexus G54.0
  cerebral G45.9
  cervical plexus G54.2
  nerve
    arm —*see* Mononeuropathy, upper limb
      axillary G54.0
      median —*see* Lesion, nerve, median
      ulnar —*see* Lesion, nerve, ulnar
    axillary G54.0
    leg —*see* Mononeuropathy, lower limb
    median —*see* Lesion, nerve, median
    plantar —*see* Lesion, nerve, plantar
    ulnar —*see* Lesion, nerve, ulnar
Angiospastic disease or edema I73.9
Angiostrongyliasis
  due to
    Parastrongylus
      cantonensis B83.2
      costaricensis B81.3
    intestinal B81.3
Anguillulosis —*see* Strongyloidiasis
Angulation
  cecum —*see* Obstruction, intestine
  coccyx (acquired) —*see also* subcategory
    M43.8
    congenital NEC Q76.49
  femur (acquired) —*see also* Deformity, limb,
    specified type NEC, thigh
    congenital Q74.2
  intestine (large) (small) —*see* Obstruction,
    intestine
  sacrum (acquired) —*see also* subcategory
    M43.8
    congenital NEC Q76.49
  sigmoid (flexure) —*see* Obstruction,
    intestine
  spine —*see* Dorsopathy, deforming,
    specified NEC
  tibia (acquired) —*see also* Deformity, limb,
    specified type NEC, lower leg
    congenital Q74.2
  ureter N13.5
    with infection N13.6
  wrist (acquired) —*see also* Deformity,
    limb, specified type NEC, forearm
    congenital Q74.0
Angulus infectiosus (lips) K13.0
Anhedonia R45.84
  sexual F52.0
Anhidrosis L74.4

Anhydration E86.0
Anhydremia E86.0
Anidrosis L74.4
Aniridia (congenital) Q13.1
Anisakiasis (infection) (infestation) B81.0
Anisakis larvae infestation B81.0
Aniseikonia H52.32
Anisocoria (pupil) H57.02
  congenital Q13.2
Anisocytosis R71.8
Anisometropia (congenital) H52.31
Ankle —*see* condition
Ankyloblepharon (eyelid) (acquired) —*see also*
  Blepharophimosis
  filiforme (adnatum) (congenital) Q10.3
  total Q10.3
Ankyloglossia Q38.1
Ankylosis (fibrous) (osseous) (joint) M24.60
  ankle M24.67-•
  arthrodesis status Z98.1
  cricoarytenoid (cartilage) (joint) (larynx)
    J38.7
  dental K03.5
  ear ossicles H74.31-•
  elbow M24.62-•
  foot M24.67-•
  hand M24.64-•
  hip M24.65-•
  incostapedial joint (infectional) —*see*
    Ankylosis, ear ossicles
  jaw (temporomandibular) M26.61-•
  knee M24.66-•
  lumbosacral (joint) M43.27
  postoperative (status) Z98.1
  produced by surgical fusion, status Z98.1
  sacro-iliac (joint) M43.28
  shoulder M24.61-•
  spine (joint) —*see also* Fusion, spine
    spondylitic —*see* Spondylitis, ankylosing
  surgical Z98.1
  temporomandibular M26.61-•
  tooth, teeth (hard tissues) K03.5
  wrist M24.63-•
Ankylostoma —*see* Ancylostoma
Ankylostomiasis —*see* Ancylostomiasis
Ankylurethria —*see* Stricture, urethra
Annular —*see also* condition
  detachment, cervix N88.8
  organ or site, congenital NEC —*see* Distortion
  pancreas (congenital) Q45.1
Anodontia (complete) (partial) (vera) K00.0
  acquired K08.10
Anomaly, anomalous (congenital) (unspecified
  type) Q89.9
  abdominal wall NEC Q79.59
  acoustic nerve Q07.8
  adrenal (gland) Q89.1
  Alder (-Reilly) (leukocyte granulation)
    D72.0
  alimentary tract Q45.9
    upper Q40.9
  alveolar M26.70
    hyperplasia M26.79
      mandibular M26.72
      maxillary M26.71
    hypoplasia M26.79
      mandibular M26.74
      maxillary M26.73
    ridge (process) M26.79
    specified NEC M26.79
  ankle (joint) Q74.2
  anus Q43.9
  aorta (arch) NEC Q25.40
    coarctation (preductal) (postductal)
      Q25.1
  aortic cusp or valve Q23.9
  appendix Q43.8
  apple peel syndrome Q41.1
  aqueduct of Sylvius Q03.0
    with spina bifida —*see* Spina bifida, with
      hydrocephalus

Anomaly, anomalous *(Continued)*
arm Q74.0
arteriovenous NEC
    coronary Q24.5
    gastrointestinal Q27.33
        acquired —*see* Angiodysplasia
artery (peripheral) Q27.9
    basilar NEC Q28.1
    cerebral Q28.3
    coronary Q24.5
    digestive system Q27.8
    eye Q15.8
    great Q25.9
        specified NEC Q25.8
    lower limb Q27.8
    peripheral Q27.9
        specified NEC Q27.8
    pulmonary NEC Q25.79
    renal Q27.2
    retina Q14.1
    specified site NEC Q27.8
    subclavian Q27.8
        origin Q25.48
    umbilical Q27.0
    upper limb Q27.8
    vertebral NEC Q28.1
aryteno-epiglottic folds Q31.8
atrial
    bands or folds Q20.8
    septa Q21.1
atrioventricular
    excitation I45.6
    septum Q21.0
auditory canal Q17.8
auricle
    ear Q17.8
        causing impairment of hearing
            Q16.9
    heart Q20.8
Axenfeld's Q15.0
back Q89.9
band
    atrial Q20.8
    heart Q24.8
    ventricular Q24.8
Bartholin's duct Q38.4
biliary duct or passage Q44.5
bladder Q64.70
    absence Q64.5
    diverticulum Q64.6
    exstrophy Q64.10
        cloacal Q64.12
        extroversion Q64.19
        specified type NEC Q64.19
        supravesical fissure Q64.11
    neck obstruction Q64.31
    specified type NEC Q64.79
bone Q79.9
    arm Q74.0
    face Q75.9
    leg Q74.2
    pelvic girdle Q74.2
    shoulder girdle Q74.0
    skull Q75.9
        with
            anencephaly Q00.0
            encephalocele —*see* Encephalocele
            hydrocephalus Q03.9
                with spina bifida —*see* Spina bifida,
                    by site, with hydrocephalus
            microcephaly Q02
brain (multiple) Q04.9
    vessel Q28.3
breast Q83.9
broad ligament Q50.6
bronchus Q32.4
bulbus cordis Q21.9
bursa Q79.9
canal of Nuck Q52.4
canthus Q10.3
capillary Q27.9

Anomaly, anomalous *(Continued)*
cardiac Q24.9
    chambers Q20.9
        specified NEC Q20.8
    septal closure Q21.9
        specified NEC Q21.8
    valve NEC Q24.8
        pulmonary Q22.3
cardiovascular system Q28.8
carpus Q74.0
caruncle, lacrimal Q10.6
cascade stomach Q40.2
cauda equina Q06.3
cecum Q43.9
cerebral Q04.9
    vessels Q28.3
cervix Q51.9
Chédiak-Higashi(-Steinbrinck) (congenital
    gigantism of peroxidase granules)
    E70.330
cheek Q18.9
chest wall Q67.8
    bones Q76.9
chin Q18.9
chordae tendineae Q24.8
choroid Q14.3
    plexus Q07.8
chromosomes, chromosomal Q99.9
    D (1) —*see* condition, chromosome 13
    E (3) —*see* condition, chromosome 18
    G —*see* condition, chromosome 21
    sex
        female phenotype Q97.8
        gonadal dysgenesis (pure) Q99.1
        Klinefelter's Q98.4
        male phenotype Q98.9
        Turner's Q96.9
    specified NEC Q99.8
cilia Q10.3
circulatory system Q28.9
clavicle Q74.0
clitoris Q52.6
coccyx Q76.49
colon Q43.9
common duct Q44.5
communication
    coronary artery Q24.5
    left ventricle with right atrium Q21.0
concha (ear) Q17.3
connection
    portal vein Q26.5
    pulmonary venous Q26.4
        partial Q26.3
        total Q26.2
    renal artery with kidney Q27.2
cornea (shape) Q13.4
coronary artery or vein Q24.5
cranium —*see* Anomaly, skull
cricoid cartilage Q31.8
cystic duct Q44.5
dental
    alveolar —*see* Anomaly, alveolar
    arch relationship M26.20
        specified NEC M26.29
dentofacial M26.9
    alveolar —*see* Anomaly, alveolar
    dental arch relationship M26.20
        specified NEC M26.29
    functional M26.50
        specified NEC M26.59
    jaw-cranial base relationship M26.10
        asymmetry M26.12
            maxillary M26.11
        specified type NEC M26.19
    jaw size M26.00
        macrogenia M26.05
        mandibular
            hyperplasia M26.03
            hypoplasia M26.04
        maxillary
            hyperplasia M26.01
            hypoplasia M26.02

Anomaly, anomalous *(Continued)*
dentofacial *(Continued)*
    jaw size *(Continued)*
        microgenia M26.06
        specified type NEC M26.09
    malocclusion M26.4
        dental arch relationship NEC M26.29
        jaw-cranial base relationship —*see*
            Anomaly, dentofacial, jaw-cranial
            base relationship
        jaw size —*see* Anomaly, dentofacial, jaw
            size
    specified type NEC M26.89
    temporomandibular joint M26.60-●
        adhesions M26.61-●
        ankylosis M26.61-●
        arthralgia M26.62-●
        articular disc M26.63-●
        specified type NEC M26.69
    tooth position, fully erupted M26.30
        specified NEC M26.39
dermatoglyphic Q82.8
diaphragm (apertures) NEC Q79.1
digestive organ(s) or tract Q45.9
    lower Q43.9
    upper Q40.9
distance, interarch (excessive) (inadequate)
    M26.25
distribution, coronary artery Q24.5
ductus
    arteriosus Q25.0
    botalli Q25.0
duodenum Q43.9
dura (brain) Q04.9
    spinal cord Q06.9
ear (external) Q17.9
    causing impairment of hearing Q16.9
    inner Q16.5
    middle (causing impairment of hearing)
        Q16.4
        ossicles Q16.3
Ebstein's (heart) (tricuspid valve) Q22.5
ectodermal Q82.9
Eisenmenger's (ventricular septal defect)
    Q21.8
ejaculatory duct Q55.4
elbow Q74.0
endocrine gland NEC Q89.2
epididymis Q55.4
epiglottis Q31.8
esophagus Q39.9
eustachian tube Q17.8
eye Q15.9
    anterior segment Q13.9
        specified NEC Q13.89
    posterior segment Q14.9
        specified NEC Q14.8
    ptosis (eyelid) Q10.0
    specified NEC Q15.8
eyebrow Q18.8
eyelid Q10.3
    ptosis Q10.0
face Q18.9
    bone(s) Q75.9
fallopian tube Q50.6
fascia Q79.9
femur NEC Q74.2
fibula NEC Q74.2
finger Q74.0
fixation, intestine Q43.3
flexion (joint) NOS Q74.9
    hip or thigh Q65.89
foot NEC Q74.2
    varus (congenital) Q66.3
foramen
    Botalli Q21.1
    ovale Q21.1
forearm Q74.0
forehead Q75.8
form, teeth K00.2
fovea centralis Q14.1

Anomaly, anomalous *(Continued)*
- frontal bone —*see* Anomaly, skull
- gallbladder (position) (shape) (size) Q44.1
- Gartner's duct Q52.4
- gastrointestinal tract Q45.9
- genitalia, genital organ(s) or system
  - female Q52.9
    - external Q52.70
    - internal NOS Q52.9
  - male Q55.9
    - hydrocele P83.5
    - specified NEC Q55.8
- genitourinary NEC
  - female Q52.9
  - male Q55.9
- Gerbode Q21.0
- glottis Q31.8
- granulation or granulocyte, genetic (constitutional) (leukocyte) D72.0
- gum Q38.6
- gyri Q07.9
- hair Q84.2
- hand Q74.0
- hard tissue formation in pulp K04.3
- head —*see* Anomaly, skull
- heart Q24.9
  - auricle Q20.8
  - bands or folds Q24.8
  - fibroelastosis cordis I42.4
  - obstructive NEC Q22.6
  - patent ductus arteriosus (Botalli) Q25.0
  - septum Q21.9
    - auricular Q21.1
    - interatrial Q21.1
    - interventricular Q21.0
      - with pulmonary stenosis or atresia, dextraposition of aorta and hypertrophy of right ventricle Q21.3
    - specified NEC Q21.8
    - ventricular Q21.0
      - with pulmonary stenosis or atresia, dextraposition of aorta and hypertrophy of right ventricle Q21.3
  - tetralogy of Fallot Q21.3
  - valve NEC Q24.8
    - aortic
      - bicuspid valve Q23.1
      - insufficiency Q23.1
      - stenosis Q23.0
        - subaortic Q24.4
    - mitral
      - insufficiency Q23.3
      - stenosis Q23.2
    - pulmonary Q22.3
      - atresia Q22.0
      - insufficiency Q22.2
      - stenosis Q22.1
        - infundibular Q24.3
        - subvalvular Q24.3
    - tricuspid
      - atresia Q22.4
      - stenosis Q22.4
  - ventricle Q20.8
- heel NEC Q74.2
- Hegglin's D72.0
- hemianencephaly Q00.0
- hemicephaly Q00.0
- hemicrania Q00.0
- hepatic duct Q44.5
- hip NEC Q74.2
- hourglass stomach Q40.2
- humerus Q74.0
- hydatid of Morgagni
  - female Q50.5
  - male (epididymal) Q55.4
    - testicular Q55.29
- hymen Q52.4
- hypersegmentation of neutrophils, hereditary D72.0

Anomaly, anomalous *(Continued)*
- hypophyseal Q89.2
- ileocecal (coil) (valve) Q43.9
- ileum Q43.9
- ilium NEC Q74.2
- integument Q84.9
  - specified NEC Q84.8
- interarch distance (excessive) (inadequate) M26.25
- intervertebral cartilage or disc Q76.49
- intestine (large) (small) Q43.9
  - with anomalous adhesions, fixation or malrotation Q43.3
- iris Q13.2
- ischium NEC Q74.2
- jaw —*see* Anomaly, dentofacial
  - alveolar —*see* Anomaly, alveolar
- jaw-cranial base relationship —*see* Anomaly, dentofacial, jaw-cranial base relationship
- jejunum Q43.8
- joint Q74.9
  - specified NEC Q74.8
- Jordan's D72.0
- kidney(s) (calyx) (pelvis) Q63.9
  - artery Q27.2
  - specified NEC Q63.8
- Klippel-Feil (brevicollis) Q76.1
- knee Q74.1
- labium (majus) (minus) Q52.70
- labyrinth, membranous Q16.5
- lacrimal apparatus or duct Q10.6
- larynx, laryngeal (muscle) Q31.9
  - web (bed) Q31.0
- lens Q12.9
- leukocytes, genetic D72.0
  - granulation (constitutional) D72.0
- lid (fold) Q10.3
- ligament Q79.9
  - broad Q50.6
  - round Q52.8
- limb Q74.9
  - lower NEC Q74.2
    - reduction deformity —*see* Defect, reduction, lower limb
  - upper Q74.0
- lip Q38.0
- liver Q44.7
  - duct Q44.5
- lower limb NEC Q74.2
- lumbosacral (joint) (region) Q76.49
  - kyphosis —*see* Kyphosis, congenital
  - lordosis —*see* Lordosis, congenital
- lung (fissure) (lobe) Q33.9
- mandible —*see* Anomaly, dentofacial
- maxilla —*see* Anomaly, dentofacial
- May (-Hegglin) D72.0
- meatus urinarius NEC Q64.79
- meningeal bands or folds Q07.9
  - constriction of Q07.8
  - spinal Q06.9
- meninges Q07.9
  - cerebral Q04.8
  - spinal Q06.9
- meningocele Q05.9
- mesentery Q45.9
- metacarpus Q74.0
- metatarsus NEC Q74.2
- middle ear Q16.4
  - ossicles Q16.3
- mitral (leaflets) (valve) Q23.9
  - insufficiency Q23.3
  - specified NEC Q23.8
  - stenosis Q23.2
- mouth Q38.6
- Müllerian —*see also* Anomaly, by site
  - uterus NEC Q51.818
- multiple NEC Q89.7
- muscle Q79.9
  - eyelid Q10.3
- musculoskeletal system, except limbs Q79.9

Anomaly, anomalous *(Continued)*
- myocardium Q24.8
- nail Q84.6
- narrowness, eyelid Q10.3
- nasal sinus (wall) Q30.8
- neck (any part) Q18.9
- nerve Q07.9
  - acoustic Q07.8
  - optic Q07.8
- nervous system (central) Q07.9
- nipple Q83.9
- nose, nasal (bones) (cartilage) (septum) (sinus) Q30.9
  - specified NEC Q30.8
- ocular muscle Q15.8
- omphalomesenteric duct Q43.0
- opening, pulmonary veins Q26.4
- optic
  - disc Q14.2
  - nerve Q07.8
- opticociliary vessels Q13.2
- orbit (eye) Q10.7
- organ Q89.9
  - of Corti Q16.5
- origin
  - artery
    - innominate Q25.8
    - pulmonary Q25.79
    - renal Q27.2
    - subclavian Q25.48
  - osseous meatus (ear) Q16.1
- ovary Q50.39
- oviduct Q50.6
- palate (hard) (soft) NEC Q38.5
- pancreas or pancreatic duct Q45.3
- papillary muscles Q24.8
- parathyroid gland Q89.2
- paraurethral ducts Q64.79
- parotid (gland) Q38.4
- patella Q74.1
- Pelger-Huët (hereditary hyposegmentation) D72.0
- pelvic girdle NEC Q74.2
- pelvis (bony) NEC Q74.2
  - rachitic E64.3
- penis (glans) Q55.69
- pericardium Q24.8
- peripheral vascular system Q27.9
- Peter's Q13.4
- pharynx Q38.8
- pigmentation L81.9
  - congenital Q82.8
- pituitary (gland) Q89.2
- pleural (folds) Q34.0
- portal vein Q26.5
  - connection Q26.5
- position, tooth, teeth, fully erupted M26.30
  - specified NEC M26.39
- precerebral vessel Q28.1
- prepuce Q55.69
- prostate Q55.4
- pulmonary Q33.9
  - artery NEC Q25.79
  - valve Q22.3
    - atresia Q22.0
    - insufficiency Q22.2
    - specified type NEC Q22.3
    - stenosis Q22.1
      - infundibular Q24.3
      - subvalvular Q24.3
  - venous connection Q26.4
    - partial Q26.3
    - total Q26.2
- pupil Q13.2
  - function H57.00
    - anisocoria H57.02
    - Argyll Robertson pupil H57.01
    - miosis H57.03
    - mydriasis H57.04
    - specified type NEC H57.09
    - tonic pupil H57.05-●

Anomaly, anomalous *(Continued)*
  pylorus Q40.3
  radius Q74.0
  rectum Q43.9
  reduction (extremity) (limb)
    femur (longitudinal) —*see* Defect,
        reduction, lower limb, longitudinal,
        femur
    fibula (longitudinal) —*see* Defect,
        reduction, lower limb, longitudinal,
        fibula
    lower limb —*see* Defect, reduction, lower
        limb
    radius (longitudinal) —*see* Defect,
        reduction, upper limb, longitudinal,
        radius
    tibia (longitudinal) —*see* Defect, reduction,
        lower limb, longitudinal, tibia
    ulna (longitudinal) —*see* Defect, reduction,
        upper limb, longitudinal, ulna
    upper limb —*see* Defect, reduction, upper
        limb
  refraction —*see* Disorder, refraction
  renal Q63.9
    artery Q27.2
    pelvis Q63.9
      specified NEC Q63.8
  respiratory system Q34.9
    specified NEC Q34.8
  retina Q14.1
  rib Q76.6
    cervical Q76.5
  Rieger's Q13.81
  rotation —*see* Malrotation
    hip or thigh Q65.89
  round ligament Q52.8
  sacroiliac (joint) NEC Q74.2
  sacrum NEC Q76.49
    kyphosis —*see* Kyphosis, congenital
    lordosis —*see* Lordosis, congenital
  saddle nose, syphilitic A50.57
  salivary duct or gland Q38.4
  scapula Q74.0
  scrotum —*see* Malformation, testis and
      scrotum
  sebaceous gland Q82.9
  seminal vesicles Q55.4
  sense organs NEC Q07.8
  sex chromosomes NEC —*see also* Anomaly,
      chromosomes
    female phenotype Q97.8
    male phenotype Q98.9
  shoulder (girdle) (joint) Q74.0
  sigmoid (flexure) Q43.9
  simian crease Q82.8
  sinus of Valsalva Q25.49
  skeleton generalized Q78.9
  skin (appendage) Q82.9
  skull Q75.9
    with
      anencephaly Q00.0
      encephalocele —*see* Encephalocele
      hydrocephalus Q03.9
        with spina bifida —*see* Spina bifida, by
            site, with hydrocephalus
      microcephaly Q02
  specified organ or site NEC Q89.8
  spermatic cord Q55.4
  spine, spinal NEC Q76.49
    column NEC Q76.49
      kyphosis —*see* Kyphosis, congenital
      lordosis —*see* Lordosis, congenital
    cord Q06.9
    nerve root Q07.8
  spleen Q89.09
    agenesis Q89.01
  stenonian duct Q38.4
  sternum NEC Q76.7
  stomach Q40.3
  submaxillary gland Q38.4
  tarsus NEC Q74.2

Anomaly, anomalous *(Continued)*
  tendon Q79.9
  testis —*see* Malformation, testis and
      scrotum
  thigh NEC Q74.2
  thorax (wall) Q67.8
    bony Q76.9
  throat Q38.8
  thumb Q74.0
  thymus gland Q89.2
  thyroid (gland) Q89.2
    cartilage Q31.8
  tibia NEC Q74.2
    saber A50.56
  toe Q74.2
  tongue Q38.3
  tooth, teeth K00.9
    eruption K00.6
    position, fully erupted M26.30
    spacing, fully erupted M26.30
  trachea (cartilage) Q32.1
  tragus Q17.9
  tricuspid (leaflet) (valve) Q22.9
    atresia or stenosis Q22.4
    Ebstein's Q22.5
  Uhl's (hypoplasia of myocardium, right
      ventricle) Q24.8
  ulna Q74.0
  umbilical artery Q27.0
  union
    cricoid cartilage and thyroid cartilage
        Q31.8
    thyroid cartilage and hyoid bone
        Q31.8
    trachea with larynx Q31.8
  upper limb Q74.0
  urachus Q64.4
  ureter Q62.8
    obstructive NEC Q62.39
      cecoureterocele Q62.32
      orthotopic ureterocele Q62.31
  urethra Q64.70
    absence Q64.5
    double Q64.74
    fistula to rectum Q64.73
    obstructive Q64.39
      stricture Q64.32
    prolapse Q64.71
    specified type NEC Q64.79
  urinary tract Q64.9
  uterus Q51.9
    with only one functioning horn Q51.4
  uvula Q38.5
  vagina Q52.4
  valleculae Q31.8
  valve (heart) NEC Q24.8
    coronary sinus Q24.5
    inferior vena cava Q24.8
    pulmonary Q22.3
    sinus coronario Q24.5
    venae cavae inferioris Q24.8
  vas deferens Q55.4
  vascular Q27.9
    brain Q28.3
    ring Q25.45
  vein(s) (peripheral) Q27.9
    brain Q28.3
    cerebral Q28.3
    coronary Q24.5
    developmental Q28.3
    great Q26.9
      specified NEC Q26.8
  vena cava (inferior) (superior) Q26.9
  venous —*see* Anomaly, vein(s)
  venous return Q26.8
  ventricular
    bands or folds Q24.8
    septa Q21.0
  vertebra Q76.49
    kyphosis —*see* Kyphosis, congenital
    lordosis —*see* Lordosis, congenital

Anomaly, anomalous *(Continued)*
  vesicourethral orifice Q64.79
  vessel(s) Q27.9
    optic papilla Q14.2
    precerebral Q28.1
  vitelline duct Q43.0
  vitreous body or humor Q14.0
  vulva Q52.70
  wrist (joint) Q74.0
Anomia R48.8
Anonychia (congenital) Q84.3
  acquired L60.8
Anophthalmos, anophthalmus (congenital)
    (globe) Q11.1
  acquired Z90.01
Anopia, anopsia H53.46-●
  quadrant H53.46-●
Anorchia, anorchism, anorchidism Q55.0
Anorexia R63.0
  hysterical F44.89
  nervosa F50.00
    atypical F50.9
    binge-eating type F50.2
      with purging F50.02
    restricting type F50.01
Anorgasmy, psychogenic (female)
    F52.31
  male F52.32
Anosmia R43.0
  hysterical F44.6
  postinfectional J39.8
Anosognosia R41.89
Anosteoplasia Q78.9
Anovulatory cycle N97.0
Anoxemia R09.02
  newborn P84
Anoxia (pathological) R09.02
  altitude T70.29
  cerebral G93.1
    complicating
      anesthesia (general) (local) or other
          sedation T88.59
        in labor and delivery O74.3
        in pregnancy O29.21-●
        postpartum, puerperal O89.2
      delivery (cesarean) (instrumental)
          O75.4
    during a procedure G97.81
    newborn P84
    resulting from a procedure G97.82
  due to
    drowning T75.1
    high altitude T70.29
  heart —*see* Insufficiency, coronary
  intrauterine P84
  myocardial —*see* Insufficiency, coronary
  newborn P84
  spinal cord G95.11
  systemic (by suffocation) (low content in
      atmosphere) —*see* Asphyxia,
      traumatic
Anteflexion —*see* Anteversion
Antenatal
  care (normal pregnancy) Z34.90
  ⇒screening (encounter for) of mother —*see also*
      Encounter, antenatal screening Z36.9
Antepartum —*see* condition
Anterior —*see* condition
Antero-occlusion M26.220
Anteversion
  cervix —*see* Anteversion, uterus
  femur (neck), congenital Q65.89
  uterus, uterine (cervix) (postinfectional)
      (postpartal, old) N85.4
    congenital Q51.818
    in pregnancy or childbirth —*see* Pregnancy,
        complicated by
Anthophobia F40.228
Anthracosilicosis J60
Anthracosis (lung) (occupational) J60
  lingua K14.3

▶ New ⇒ Revised ~~deleted~~ Deleted ● Use Additional Character(s)

Anthrax A22.9
  with pneumonia A22.1
  cerebral A22.8
  colitis A22.2
  cutaneous A22.0
  gastrointestinal A22.2
  inhalation A22.1
  intestinal A22.2
  meningitis A22.8
  pulmonary A22.1
  respiratory A22.1
  sepsis A22.7
  specified manifestation NEC A22.8
Anthropoid pelvis Q74.2
  with disproportion (fetopelvic) O33.0
Anthropophobia F40.10
  generalized F40.11
Antibodies, maternal (blood group) —see
    Isoimmunization, affecting management of
    pregnancy
  anti-D —see Isoimmunization, affecting
    management of pregnancy, Rh
    newborn P55.0
Antibody
  anticardiolipin R76.0
    with
      hemorrhagic disorder D68.312
      hypercoagulable state D68.61
  antiphosphatidylglycerol R76.0
    with
      hemorrhagic disorder D68.312
      hypercoagulable state D68.61
  antiphosphatidylinositol R76.0
    with
      hemorrhagic disorder D68.312
      hypercoagulable state D68.61
  antiphosphatidylserine R76.0
    with
      hemorrhagic disorder D68.312
      hypercoagulable state D68.61
  antiphospholipid R76.0
    with
      hemorrhagic disorder D68.312
      hypercoagulable state D68.61
Anticardiolipin syndrome D68.61
Anticoagulant, circulating (intrinsic) —see also -
    Disorder, hemorrhagic D68.318
  drug-induced (extrinsic) —see also - Disorder,
    hemorrhagic D68.32
  iatrogenic D68.32
Antidiuretic hormone syndrome E22.2
Antimonial cholera —see Poisoning,
    antimony
Antiphospholipid
  antibody
    with hemorrhagic disorder D68.312
    syndrome D68.61
Antisocial personality F60.2
Antithrombinemia —see Circulating
    anticoagulants
Antithromboplastinemia D68.318
Antithromboplastinogenemia D68.318
Antitoxin complication or reaction —see
    Complications, vaccination
Antlophobia F40.228
Antritis J32.0
  maxilla J32.0
    acute J01.00
      recurrent J01.01
  stomach K29.60
    with bleeding K29.61
Antrum, antral —see condition
Anuria R34
  calculous (impacted) (recurrent) —see also
      Calculus, urinary N20.9
  following
    abortion —see Abortion by type
      complicated by, renal failure
    ectopic or molar pregnancy O08.4
  newborn P96.0
  postprocedural N99.0

Anuria (Continued)
  postrenal N13.8
  traumatic (following crushing) T79.5
Anus, anal —see condition
Anusitis K62.89
Anxiety F41.9
  depression F41.8
  episodic paroxysmal F41.0
  generalized F41.1
  hysteria F41.8
  neurosis F41.1
  panic type F41.0
  reaction F41.1
  separation, abnormal (of childhood) F93.0
  specified NEC F41.8
  state F41.1
Aorta, aortic —see condition
Aortectasia —see Ectasia, aorta
  with aneurysm —see Aneurysm, aorta
Aortitis (nonsyphilitic) (calcific) I77.6
  arteriosclerotic I70.0
  Doehle-Heller A52.02
  luetic A52.02
  rheumatic —see Endocarditis, acute,
    rheumatic
  specific (syphilitic) A52.02
  syphilitic A52.02
    congenital A50.54 [I79.1]
Apathetic thyroid storm —see Thyrotoxicosis
Apathy R45.3
Apeirophobia F40.228
Apepsia K30
  psychogenic F45.8
Aperistalsis, esophagus K22.0
Apertognathia M26.29
Apert's syndrome Q87.0
Aphagia R13.0
  psychogenic F50.9
Aphakia (acquired) (postoperative) H27.0-●
  congenital Q12.3
Aphasia (amnestic) (global) (nominal)
    (semantic) (syntactic) R47.01
  acquired, with epilepsy (Landau-Kleffner
    syndrome) —see Epilepsy, specified
    NEC
  auditory (developmental) F80.2
  developmental (receptive type) F80.2
    expressive type F80.1
    Wernicke's F80.2
  following
    cerebrovascular disease I69.920
      cerebral infarction I69.320
      intracerebral hemorrhage I69.120
      nontraumatic intracranial hemorrhage
        NEC I69.220
      specified disease NEC I69.820
      subarachnoid hemorrhage I69.020
  primary progressive G31.01 [F02.80]
    with behavioral disturbance G31.01
      [F02.81]
  progressive isolated G31.01 [F02.80]
    with behavioral disturbance G31.01
      [F02.81]
  sensory F80.2
  syphilis, tertiary A52.19
  Wernicke's (developmental) F80.2
Aphonia (organic) R49.1
  hysterical F44.4
  psychogenic F44.4
Aphthae, aphthous —see also condition
  Bednar's K12.0
  cachectic K14.0
  epizootic B08.8
  fever B08.8
  oral (recurrent) K12.0
  stomatitis (major) (minor) K12.0
  thrush B37.0
  ulcer (oral) (recurrent) K12.0
    genital organ(s) NEC
      female N76.6
      male N50.89
    larynx J38.7

Apical —see condition
Apiphobia F40.218
Aplasia —see also Agenesis
  abdominal muscle syndrome Q79.4
  alveolar process (acquired) —see Anomaly,
    alveolar
    congenital Q38.6
  aorta (congenital) Q25.41
  axialis extracorticalis (congenita) E75.29
  bone marrow (myeloid) D61.9
    congenital D61.01
  brain Q00.0
    part of Q04.3
  bronchus Q32.4
  cementum K00.4
  cerebellum Q04.3
  cervix (congenital) Q51.5
  congenital pure red cell D61.01
  corpus callosum Q04.0
  cutis congenita Q84.8
  erythrocyte congenital D61.01
  extracortical axial E75.29
  eye Q11.1
  fovea centralis (congenital) Q14.1
  gallbladder, congenital Q44.0
  iris Q13.1
  labyrinth, membranous Q16.5
  limb (congenital) Q73.8
    lower —see Defect, reduction, lower limb
    upper —see Agenesis, arm
  lung, congenital (bilateral) (unilateral) Q33.3
  pancreas Q45.0
  parathyroid-thymic D82.1
  Pelizaeus-Merzbacher E75.29
  penis Q55.5
  prostate Q55.4
  red cell (with thymoma) D60.9
    acquired D60.9
      due to drugs D60.9
    adult D60.9
    chronic D60.0
    congenital D61.01
    constitutional D61.01
    due to drugs D60.9
    hereditary D61.01
    of infants D61.01
    primary D61.01
    pure D61.01
      due to drugs D60.9
    specified type NEC D60.8
    transient D60.1
  round ligament Q52.8
  skin Q84.8
  spermatic cord Q55.4
  spleen Q89.01
  testicle Q55.0
  thymic, with immunodeficiency D82.1
  thyroid (congenital) (with myxedema) E03.1
  uterus Q51.0
  ventral horn cell Q06.1
Apnea, apneic (of) (spells) R06.81
  newborn NEC P28.4
    obstructive P28.4
    sleep (central) (obstructive) (primary) P28.3
  prematurity P28.4
  sleep G47.30
    central (primary) G47.31
    ▶idiopathic G47.31
      in conditions classified elsewhere
        G47.37
    obstructive (adult) (pediatric) G47.33
    ▶hypopnea G47.33
    primary central G47.31
    specified NEC G47.39
Apneumatosis, newborn P28.0
Apocrine metaplasia (breast) —see Dysplasia,
    mammary, specified type NEC
Apophysitis (bone) —see also
    Osteochondropathy
  calcaneus M92.8
  juvenile M92.9

Apoplectiform convulsions (cerebral ischemia) I67.82
Apoplexia, apoplexy, apoplectic
 adrenal A39.1
 heart (auricle) (ventricle) —see Infarct, myocardium
 heat T67.0
 hemorrhagic (stroke) —see Hemorrhage, intracranial
 meninges, hemorrhagic —see Hemorrhage, intracranial, subarachnoid
 uremic N18.9 [I68.8]
Appearance
 bizarre R46.1
 specified NEC R46.89
 very low level of personal hygiene R46.0
Appendage
 epididymal (organ of Morgagni) Q55.4
 intestine (epiploic) Q43.8
 preauricular Q17.0
 testicular (organ of Morgagni) Q55.29
Appendicitis (pneumococcal) (retrocecal) K37
 with
  perforation or rupture K35.2
  peritoneal abscess K35.3
  peritonitis NEC K35.3
   generalized (with perforation or rupture) K35.2
   localized (with perforation or rupture) K35.3
 acute (catarrhal) (fulminating) (gangrenous) (obstructive) (retrocecal) (suppurative) K35.80
  with
   peritoneal abscess K35.3
   peritonitis NEC K35.3
    generalized (with perforation or rupture) K35.2
    localized (with perforation or rupture) K35.3
   specified NEC K35.89
 amebic A06.89
 chronic (recurrent) K36
  exacerbation —see Appendicitis, acute
 gangrenous —see Appendicitis, acute
 healed (obliterative) K36
 interval K36
 neurogenic K36
 obstructive K36
 recurrent K36
 relapsing K36
 subacute (adhesive) K36
 subsiding K36
 suppurative —see Appendicitis, acute
 tuberculous A18.32
Appendicopathia oxyurica B80
Appendix, appendicular —see also condition
 epididymis Q55.4
 Morgagni
  female Q50.5
  male (epididymal) Q55.4
   testicular Q55.29
 testis Q55.29
Appetite
 depraved —see Pica
 excessive R63.2
 lack or loss —see also Anorexia R63.0
  nonorganic origin F50.89
  psychogenic F50.89
 perverted (hysterical) —see Pica
Apple peel syndrome Q41.1
Apprehension state F41.1
Apprehensiveness, abnormal F41.9
Approximal wear K03.0
Apraxia (classic) (ideational) (ideokinetic) (ideomotor) (motor) (verbal) R48.2
 following
  cerebrovascular disease I69.990
   cerebral infarction I69.390
   intracerebral hemorrhage I69.190

Apraxia (Continued)
 following (Continued)
  cerebrovascular disease (Continued)
   nontraumatic intracranial hemorrhage NEC I69.290
   specified disease NEC I69.890
   subarachnoid hemorrhage I69.090
 oculomotor, congenital H51.8
Aptyalism K11.7
Apudoma —see Neoplasm, uncertain behavior, by site
Aqueous misdirection H40.83-●
Arabicum elephantiasis —see Infestation, filarial
Arachnitis —see Meningitis
Arachnodactyly —see Syndrome, Marfan's
Arachnoiditis (acute) (adhesive) (basal) (brain) (cerebrospinal) —see Meningitis
Arachnophobia F40.210
Arboencephalitis, Australian A83.4
Arborization block (heart) I45.5
ARC (AIDS-related complex) B20
▶Arch
 ▶aortic Q25.49
 ▶bovine Q25.49
Arches —see condition
Arcuate uterus Q51.810
Arcuatus uterus Q51.810
Arcus (cornea) senilis —see Degeneration, cornea, senile
Arc-welder's lung J63.4
Areflexia R29.2
Areola —see condition
Argentaffinoma —see also Neoplasm, uncertain behavior, by site
 malignant —see Neoplasm, malignant, by site
 syndrome E34.0
Argininemia E72.21
Arginosuccinic aciduria E72.22
Argyll Robertson phenomenon, pupil or syndrome (syphilitic) A52.19
 atypical H57.09
 nonsyphilitic H57.09
Argyria, argyriasis
 conjunctival H11.13-●
 from drug or medicament —see Table of Drugs and Chemicals, by substance
Argyrosis, conjunctival H11.13-●
Arhinencephaly Q04.1
Ariboflavinosis E53.0
Arm —see condition
Arnold-Chiari disease, obstruction or syndrome (type II) Q07.00
 with
  hydrocephalus Q07.02
   with spina bifida Q07.03
  spina bifida Q07.01
   with hydrocephalus Q07.03
 type III —see Encephalocele
 type IV Q04.8
Aromatic amino-acid metabolism disorder E70.9
 specified NEC E70.8
Arousals, confusional G47.51
Arrest, arrested
 cardiac I46.9
  complicating
   abortion —see Abortion, by type, complicated by, cardiac arrest
   anesthesia (general) (local) or other sedation —see Table of Drugs and Chemicals, by drug
    in labor and delivery O74.2
    in pregnancy O29.11-●
    postpartum, puerperal O89.1
   delivery (cesarean) (instrumental) O75.4
  due to
   cardiac condition I46.2
   specified condition NEC I46.8
  intraoperative I97.71-●
  newborn P29.81
 ▶personal history, successfully resuscitated Z86.74

Arrest, arrested (Continued)
 cardiac (Continued)
  postprocedural I97.12-●
   obstetric procedure O75.4
 cardiorespiratory —see Arrest, cardiac
 circulatory —see Arrest, cardiac
 deep transverse O64.0
 development or growth
  bone —see Disorder, bone, development or growth
  child R62.50
  tracheal rings Q32.1
 epiphyseal
  complete
   femur M89.15-●
   humerus M89.12-●
   tibia M89.16-●
   ulna M89.13-●
  forearm M89.13-●
   specified NEC M89.13-●
   ulna —see Arrest, epiphyseal, by type, ulna
  lower leg M89.16-●
   specified NEC M89.168
   tibia —see Arrest, epiphyseal, by type, tibia
  partial
   femur M89.15-●
   humerus M89.12-●
   tibia M89.16-●
   ulna M89.13-●
  specified NEC M89.18
 granulopoiesis —see Agranulocytosis
 growth plate —see Arrest, epiphyseal
 heart —see Arrest, cardiac
 legal, anxiety concerning Z65.3
 physeal —see Arrest, epiphyseal
 respiratory R09.2
  newborn P28.81
 sinus I45.5
 spermatogenesis (complete) —see Azoospermia
  incomplete —see Oligospermia
 transverse (deep) O64.0
Arrhenoblastoma
 benign
  specified site —see Neoplasm, benign, by site
  unspecified site
   female D27.9
   male D29.20
 malignant
  specified site —see Neoplasm, malignant, by site
  unspecified site
   female C56.9
   male C62.90
 specified site —see Neoplasm, uncertain behavior, by site
 unspecified site
  female D39.10
  male D40.10
Arrhythmia (auricle)(cardiac) (juvenile)(nodal) (reflex)(sinus)(supraventricular)(transitory) (ventricle) I49.9
 block I45.9
 extrasystolic I49.49
 newborn
  bradycardia P29.12
  occurring before birth P03.819
   before onset of labor P03.810
   during labor P03.811
  tachycardia P29.11
 psychogenic F45.8
 specified NEC I49.8
 vagal R55
 ventricular re-entry I47.0
Arrillaga-Ayerza syndrome (pulmonary sclerosis with pulmonary hypertension) I27.0
Arsenical pigmentation L81.8
 from drug or medicament —see Table of Drugs and Chemicals
Arsenism —see Poisoning, arsenic

▶ New   ⇒ Revised   ~~deleted~~ Deleted   ● Use Additional Character(s)

Arterial —see condition
Arteriofibrosis —see Arteriosclerosis
Arteriolar sclerosis —see Arteriosclerosis
Arteriolith —see Arteriosclerosis
Arteriolitis I77.6
  necrotizing, kidney I77.5
  renal —see Hypertension, kidney
Arteriolosclerosis —see Arteriosclerosis
Arterionephrosclerosis —see Hypertension,
    kidney
Arteriopathy I77.9
Arteriosclerosis, arteriosclerotic (diffuse)
    (obliterans) (of) (senile) (with calcification)
    I70.90
  aorta I70.0
  arteries of extremities —see Arteriosclerosis,
    extremities
  brain I67.2
  bypass graft
    coronary —see Arteriosclerosis, coronary,
      bypass graft
    extremities —see Arteriosclerosis,
      extremities, bypass graft
  cardiac —see Disease, heart, ischemic,
    atherosclerotic
  cardiopathy —see Disease, heart, ischemic,
    atherosclerotic
  cardiorenal —see Hypertension, cardiorenal
  cardiovascular —see Disease, heart, ischemic,
    atherosclerotic
  carotid —see also Occlusion, artery, carotid
    I65.2-•
  central nervous system I67.2
  cerebral I67.2
  cerebrovascular I67.2
  coronary (artery) I25.10
    bypass graft I25.810
      with
        angina pectoris I25.709
          with documented spasm I25.701
          specified type NEC I25.708
          unstable I25.700
        ischemic chest pain I25.709
      autologous artery I25.810
        with
          angina pectoris I25.729
            with documented spasm I25.721
            specified type I25.728
            unstable I25.720
          ischemic chest pain I25.729
      autologous vein I25.810
        with
          angina pectoris I25.719
            with documented spasm I25.711
            specified type I25.718
            unstable I25.710
          ischemic chest pain I25.719
      nonautologous biological I25.810
        with
          angina pectoris I25.739
            with documented spasm I25.731
            specified type I25.738
            unstable I25.730
          ischemic chest pain I25.739
      specified type NEC I25.810
        with
          angina pectoris I25.799
            with documented spasm I25.791
            specified type I25.798
            unstable I25.790
          ischemic chest pain I25.799
    due to
      calcified coronary lesion (severely) I25.84
      lipid rich plaque I25.83
    native vessel
      with
        angina pectoris I25.119
          with documented spasm I25.111
          specified type NEC I25.118
          unstable I25.110
        ischemic chest pain I25.119

Arteriosclerosis, arteriosclerotic (Continued)
  coronary (Continued)
    transplanted heart I25.811
    bypass graft I25.812
      with
        angina pectoris I25.769
          with documented spasm
            I25.761
          specified type I25.768
          unstable I25.760
        ischemic chest pain I25.769
    native coronary artery I25.811
      with
        angina pectoris I25.759
          with documented spasm I25.751
          specified type I25.758
          unstable I25.750
        ischemic chest pain I25.759
  extremities (native arteries) I70.209
    bypass graft I70.309
      autologous vein graft I70.409
        leg I70.409
          with
            gangrene (and intermittent
              claudication, rest pain and
              ulcer) I70.469
            intermittent claudication
              I70.419
            rest pain (and intermittent
              claudication) I70.429
          bilateral I70.403
            with
              gangrene (and intermittent
                claudication, rest pain and
                ulcer) I70.463
              intermittent claudication
                I70.413
              rest pain (and intermittent
                claudication) I70.423
            specified type NEC I70.493
          left I70.402
            with
              gangrene (and intermittent
                claudication, rest pain and
                ulcer) I70.462
              intermittent claudication
                I70.412
              rest pain (and intermittent
                claudication) I70.422
              ulceration (and intermittent
                claudication and rest
                pain) I70.449
              ankle I70.443
              calf I70.442
              foot site NEC I70.445
              heel I70.444
              lower leg NEC I70.448
              midfoot I70.444
              thigh I70.441
            specified type NEC I70.492
          right I70.401
            with
              gangrene (and intermittent
                claudication, rest pain and
                ulcer) I70.461
              intermittent claudication
                I70.411
              rest pain (and intermittent
                claudication) I70.421
              ulceration (and intermittent
                claudication and rest
                pain) I70.439
              ankle I70.433
              calf I70.432
              foot site NEC I70.435
              heel I70.434
              lower leg NEC I70.438
              midfoot I70.434
              thigh I70.431
            specified type NEC I70.491
        specified type NEC I70.499

Arteriosclerosis, arteriosclerotic (Continued)
  extremities (Continued)
    bypass graft (Continued)
      autologous vein graft (Continued)
        specified NEC I70.408
          with
            gangrene (and intermittent
              claudication, rest pain and
              ulcer) I70.468
            intermittent claudication I70.418
            rest pain (and intermittent
              claudication) I70.428
            ulceration (and intermittent
              claudication and rest pain)
              I70.45
          specified type NEC I70.498
      leg I70.309
        with
          gangrene (and intermittent
            claudication, rest pain and
            ulcer) I70.369
          intermittent claudication I70.319
          rest pain (and intermittent
            claudication) I70.329
        bilateral I70.303
          with
            gangrene (and intermittent
              claudication, rest pain and
              ulcer) I70.363
            intermittent claudication I70.313
            rest pain (and intermittent
              claudication) I70.323
          specified type NEC I70.393
        left I70.302
          with
            gangrene (and intermittent
              claudication, rest pain and
              ulcer) I70.362
            intermittent claudication I70.312
            rest pain (and intermittent
              claudication) I70.322
            ulceration (and intermittent
              claudication and rest pain)
              I70.349
            ankle I70.343
            calf I70.342
            foot site NEC I70.345
            heel I70.344
            lower leg NEC I70.348
            midfoot I70.344
            thigh I70.341
          specified type NEC I70.392
        right I70.301
          with
            gangrene (and intermittent
              claudication, rest pain and
              ulcer) I70.361
            intermittent claudication I70.311
            rest pain (and intermittent
              claudication) I70.321
            ulceration (and intermittent
              claudication and rest pain)
              I70.339
            ankle I70.333
            calf I70.332
            foot site NEC I70.335
            heel I70.334
            lower leg NEC I70.338
            midfoot I70.334
            thigh I70.331
          specified type NEC I70.391
      specified type NEC I70.399
    nonautologous biological graft I70.509
      leg I70.509
        with
          gangrene (and intermittent
            claudication, rest pain and
            ulcer) I70.569
          intermittent claudication I70.519
          rest pain (and intermittent
            claudication) I70.529

A

Arteriosclerosis, arteriosclerotic *(Continued)*
  extremities *(Continued)*
    bypass graft *(Continued)*
      nonautologous biological graft
        (Continued)
        leg *(Continued)*
          bilateral I70.503
            with
              gangrene (and intermittent
                claudication, rest pain and
                ulcer) I70.563
              intermittent claudication
                I70.513
              rest pain (and intermittent
                claudication) I70.523
            specified type NEC I70.593
          left I70.502
            with
              gangrene (and intermittent
                claudication, rest pain and
                ulcer) I70.562
              intermittent claudication
                I70.512
              rest pain (and intermittent
                claudication)
                I70.522
              ulceration (and intermittent
                claudication and rest
                pain) I70.549
                ankle I70.543
                calf I70.542
                foot site NEC I70.545
                heel I70.544
                lower leg NEC I70.548
                midfoot I70.544
                thigh I70.541
            specified type NEC I70.592
          right I70.501
            with
              gangrene (and intermittent
                claudication, rest pain and
                ulcer) I70.561
              intermittent claudication
                I70.511
              rest pain (and intermittent
                claudication) I70.521
              ulceration (and intermittent
                claudication and rest
                pain) I70.539
                ankle I70.533
                calf I70.532
                foot site NEC I70.535
                heel I70.534
                lower leg NEC I70.538
                midfoot I70.534
                thigh I70.531
            specified type NEC I70.591
          specified type NEC I70.599
        specified NEC I70.508
          with
            gangrene (and intermittent
              claudication, rest pain and
              ulcer) I70.568
            intermittent claudication
              I70.518
            rest pain (and intermittent
              claudication) I70.528
            ulceration (and intermittent
              claudication and rest pain)
              I70.55
          specified type NEC I70.598
      nonbiological graft I70.609
        leg I70.609
          with
            gangrene (and intermittent
              claudication, rest pain and
              ulcer) I70.669
            intermittent claudication
              I70.619
            rest pain (and intermittent
              claudication) I70.629

Arteriosclerosis, arteriosclerotic *(Continued)*
  extremities *(Continued)*
    bypass graft *(Continued)*
      nonbiological graft *(Continued)*
        leg *(Continued)*
          bilateral I70.603
            with
              gangrene (and intermittent
                claudication, rest
                pain and ulcer)
                I70.663
              intermittent claudication
                I70.613
              rest pain (and intermittent
                claudication) I70.623
            specified type NEC I70.693
          left I70.602
            with
              gangrene (and intermittent
                claudication, rest
                pain and ulcer)
                I70.662
              intermittent claudication
                I70.612
              rest pain (and intermittent
                claudication) I70.622
              ulceration (and intermittent
                claudication and rest
                pain) I70.649
                ankle I70.643
                calf I70.642
                foot site NEC I70.645
                heel I70.644
                lower leg NEC I70.648
                midfoot I70.644
                thigh I70.641
            specified type NEC I70.692
          right I70.601
            with
              gangrene (and intermittent
                claudication, rest pain and
                ulcer) I70.661
              intermittent claudication
                I70.611
              rest pain (and intermittent
                claudication) I70.621
              ulceration (and intermittent
                claudication and rest
                pain) I70.639
                ankle I70.633
                calf I70.632
                foot site NEC I70.635
                heel I70.634
                lower leg NEC I70.638
                midfoot I70.634
                thigh I70.631
            specified type NEC I70.691
        specified type NEC I70.699
        specified NEC I70.608
          with
            gangrene (and intermittent
              claudication, rest pain and
              ulcer) I70.668
            intermittent claudication
              I70.618
            rest pain (and intermittent
              claudication) I70.628
            ulceration (and intermittent
              claudication and rest pain)
              I70.65
          specified type NEC I70.698
      specified graft NEC I70.709
        leg I70.709
          with
            gangrene (and intermittent
              claudication, rest pain and
              ulcer) I70.769
            intermittent claudication
              I70.719
            rest pain (and intermittent
              claudication) I70.729

Arteriosclerosis, arteriosclerotic *(Continued)*
  extremities *(Continued)*
    bypass graft *(Continued)*
      specified graft NEC *(Continued)*
        leg *(Continued)*
          bilateral I70.703
            with
              gangrene (and intermittent
                claudication, rest pain and
                ulcer) I70.763
              intermittent claudication
                I70.713
              rest pain (and intermittent
                claudication) I70.723
            specified type NEC I70.793
          left I70.702
            with
              gangrene (and intermittent
                claudication, rest pain and
                ulcer) I70.762
              intermittent claudication
                I70.712
              rest pain (and intermittent
                claudication) I70.722
              ulceration (and intermittent
                claudication and rest
                pain) I70.749
                ankle I70.743
                calf I70.742
                foot site NEC I70.745
                heel I70.744
                lower leg NEC I70.748
                midfoot I70.744
                thigh I70.741
            specified type NEC I70.792
          right I70.701
            with
              gangrene (and intermittent
                claudication, rest pain and
                ulcer) I70.761
              intermittent claudication
                I70.711
              rest pain (and intermittent
                claudication) I70.721
              ulceration (and intermittent
                claudication and rest
                pain) I70.739
                ankle I70.733
                calf I70.732
                foot site NEC I70.735
                heel I70.734
                lower leg NEC I70.738
                midfoot I70.734
                thigh I70.731
            specified type NEC I70.791
        specified type NEC I70.799
        specified NEC I70.708
          with
            gangrene (and intermittent
              claudication, rest pain and
              ulcer) I70.768
            intermittent claudication
              I70.718
            rest pain (and intermittent
              claudication) I70.728
            ulceration (and intermittent
              claudication and rest pain)
              I70.75
          specified type NEC I70.798
      specified NEC I70.308
        with
          gangrene (and intermittent
            claudication, rest pain and
            ulcer) I70.368
         intermittent claudication I70.318
         rest pain (and intermittent
           claudication) I70.328
         ulceration (and intermittent
           claudication and rest pain)
           I70.35
        specified type NEC I70.398

▶ New   ⇒ Revised   ~~deleted~~ Deleted   ● Use Additional Character(s)

Arteriosclerosis, arteriosclerotic (*Continued*)
  extremities (*Continued*)
    leg I70.209
      with
        gangrene (and intermittent
          claudication, rest pain and ulcer)
          I70.269
        intermittent claudication I70.219
        rest pain (and intermittent
          claudication) I70.229
      bilateral I70.203
        with
          gangrene (and intermittent
            claudication, rest pain and
            ulcer) I70.263
          intermittent claudication I70.213
          rest pain (and intermittent
            claudication) I70.223
        specified type NEC I70.293
      left I70.202
        with
          gangrene (and intermittent
            claudication, rest pain and
            ulcer) I70.262
          intermittent claudication I70.212
          rest pain (and intermittent
            claudication) I70.222
          ulceration (and intermittent
            claudication and rest pain)
            I70.249
            ankle I70.243
            calf I70.242
            foot site NEC I70.245
            heel I70.244
            lower leg NEC I70.248
            midfoot I70.244
            thigh I70.241
        specified type NEC I70.292
      right I70.201
        with
          gangrene (and intermittent
            claudication, rest pain and
            ulcer) I70.261
          intermittent claudication I70.211
          rest pain (and intermittent
            claudication) I70.221
          ulceration (and intermittent
            claudication and rest pain)
            I70.239
            ankle I70.233
            calf I70.232
            foot site NEC I70.235
            heel I70.234
            lower leg NEC I70.238
            midfoot I70.234
            thigh I70.231
        specified type NEC I70.291
      specified type NEC I70.299
    specified site NEC I70.208
      with
        gangrene (and intermittent
          claudication, rest pain and ulcer)
          I70.268
        intermittent claudication I70.218
        rest pain (and intermittent
          claudication) I70.228
        ulceration (and intermittent
          claudication and rest pain) I70.25
      specified type NEC I70.298
  generalized I70.91
  heart (disease) —*see* Arteriosclerosis,
    coronary (artery)
  kidney —*see* Hypertension, kidney
  medial —*see* Arteriosclerosis, extremities
  mesenteric (artery) K55.1
  Mönckeberg's —*see* Arteriosclerosis,
    extremities
  myocarditis I51.4
  peripheral (of extremities) —*see*
    Arteriosclerosis, extremities
  pulmonary (idiopathic) I27.0

Arteriosclerosis, arteriosclerotic (*Continued*)
  renal (arterioles) —*see also* Hypertension,
    kidney
    artery I70.1
  retina (vascular) I70.8 [*H35.0-●*]
  specified artery NEC I70.8
  spinal (cord) G95.19
  vertebral (artery) I67.2
Arteriospasm I73.9
Arteriovenous —*see* condition
Arteritis I77.6
  allergic M31.0
  aorta (nonsyphilitic) I77.6
    syphilitic A52.02
  aortic arch M31.4
  brachiocephalic M31.4
  brain I67.7
    syphilitic A52.04
  cerebral I67.7
    in
      diseases classified elsewhere I68.2
      systemic lupus erythematosus M32.19
    listerial A32.89
    syphilitic A52.04
    tuberculous A18.89
  coronary (artery) I25.89
    rheumatic I01.8
      chronic I09.89
    syphilitic A52.06
  cranial (left) (right), giant cell M31.6
  deformans —*see* Arteriosclerosis
  giant cell NEC M31.6
    with polymyalgia rheumatica M31.5
  necrosing or necrotizing M31.9
    specified NEC M31.8
  nodosa M30.0
  obliterans —*see* Arteriosclerosis
  pulmonary I28.8
  rheumatic —*see* Fever, rheumatic
  senile —*see* Arteriosclerosis
  suppurative I77.2
  syphilitic (general) A52.09
    brain A52.04
    coronary A52.06
    spinal A52.09
  temporal, giant cell M31.6
  young female aortic arch syndrome M31.4
Artery, arterial —*see also* condition
  abscess I77.89
  single umbilical Q27.0
Arthralgia (allergic) —*see also* Pain, joint
  in caisson disease T70.3
  temporomandibular M26.62
Arthritis, arthritic (acute) (chronic)
  (nonpyogenic) (subacute) M19.90
  allergic —*see* Arthritis, specified form NEC
  ankylosing (crippling) (spine) —*see also*
    Spondylitis, ankylosing
    sites other than spine —*see* Arthritis,
      specified form NEC
  atrophic —*see* Osteoarthritis
    spine —*see* Spondylitis, ankylosing
  back —*see* Spondylopathy, inflammatory
  blennorrhagic (gonococcal) A54.42
  Charcot's —*see* Arthropathy, neuropathic
    diabetic —*see* Diabetes, arthropathy,
      neuropathic
    syringomyelic G95.0
  chylous (filarial) —*see also* category M01
    B74.9
  climacteric (any site) NEC —*see* Arthritis,
    specified form NEC
  crystal (-induced) —*see* Arthritis, in, crystals
  deformans —*see* Osteoarthritis
  degenerative —*see* Osteoarthritis
  due to or associated with
    acromegaly E22.0
    brucellosis —*see* Brucellosis
    caisson disease T70.3
    diabetes —*see* Diabetes, arthropathy
    dracontiasis —*see also* category M01 B72

Arthritis, arthritic (*Continued*)
  due to or associated with (*Continued*)
    enteritis NEC
      regional —*see* Enteritis, regional
    erysipelas —*see also* category M01 A46
    erythema
      epidemic A25.1
      nodosum L52
    filariasis NOS B74.9
    glanders A24.0
    helminthiasis —*see also* category M01 B83.9
    hemophilia D66 [*M36.2*]
    Henoch-(Schönlein) purpura D69.0 [*M36.4*]
    human parvovirus —*see also* category M01
      B97.6
    infectious disease NEC —*see* category M01
    leprosy (*see also* category M01) —*see also*
      Leprosy A30.9
    Lyme disease A69.23
    mycobacteria —*see also* category M01
      A31.8
    parasitic disease NEC —*see also* category
      M01 B89
    paratyphoid fever (*see also* category M01)
      —*see also* Fever, paratyphoid A01.4
    rat bite fever —*see also* category M01
      A25.1
    regional enteritis —*see* Enteritis, regional
    respiratory disorder NOS J98.9
    serum sickness —*see also* Reaction, serum
      T80.69
    syringomyelia G95.0
    typhoid fever A01.04
  epidemic erythema A25.1
  febrile —*see* Fever, rheumatic
  gonococcal A54.42
  gouty (acute) —*see* Gout
  in (due to)
    acromegaly —*see also* subcategory
      M14.8-● E22.0
    amyloidosis —*see also* subcategory
      M14.8-● E85.4
    bacterial disease —*see also* subcategory
      M01 A49.9
    Behçet's syndrome M35.2
    caisson disease —*see also* subcategory
      M14.8-● T70.3
    coliform bacilli (Escherichia coli) —*see*
      Arthritis, in, pyogenic organism NEC
    crystals M11.9
      dicalcium phosphate —*see* Arthritis, in,
        crystals, specified type NEC
      hydroxyapatite M11.0-●
      pyrophosphate —*see* Arthritis, in,
        crystals, specified type NEC
      specified type NEC M11.80
        ankle M11.87-●
        elbow M11.82-●
        foot joint M11.87-●
        hand joint M11.84-●
        hip M11.85-●
        knee M11.86-●
        multiple sites M11.8-●
        shoulder M11.81-●
        vertebrae M11.88
        wrist M11.83-●
    dermatoarthritis, lipoid E78.81
    dracontiasis (dracunculiasis) —*see also*
      category M01 B72
    endocrine disorder NEC —*see also*
      subcategory M14.8-● E34.9
    enteritis, infectious NEC —*see also* category
      M01 A09
      specified organism NEC —*see also*
        category M01 A08.8
    erythema
      multiforme —*see also* subcategory
        M14.8-● L51.9
      nodosum —*see also* subcategory M14.8-●
        L52
    gout —*see* Gout

Arthritis, arthritic *(Continued)*
  in *(Continued)*
    helminthiasis NEC —*see also* category M01
      B83.9
    hemochromatosis —*see also* subcategory
      M14.8-● E83.118
    hemoglobinopathy NEC D58.2 *[M36.3]*
    hemophilia NEC D66 *[M36.2]*
    Hemophilus influenzae M00.8-● *[B96.3]*
    Henoch(-Schönlein) purpura D69.0 *[M36.4]*
    hyperparathyroidism NEC —*see also*
      subcategory M14.8-● E21.3
    hypersensitivity reaction NEC T78.49
      [M36.4]
    hypogammaglobulinemia —*see also*
      subcategory M14.8-● D80.1
    hypothyroidism NEC —*see also*
      subcategory M14.8-● E03.9
    infection —*see* Arthritis, pyogenic or
      pyemic
      spine —*see* Spondylopathy, infective
    infectious disease NEC —*see* category M01
    leprosy —*see also* category M01 A30.9
    leukemia NEC C95.9-● *[M36.1]*
    lipoid dermatoarthritis E78.81
    Lyme disease A69.23
    Mediterranean fever, familial —*see also*
      subcategory M14.8-● M04.1
    Meningococcus A39.83
    metabolic disorder NEC —*see also*
      subcategory M14.8-● E88.9
    multiple myelomatosis C90.0-● *[M36.1]*
    mumps B26.85
    mycosis NEC —*see also* category M01 B49
    myelomatosis (multiple) C90.0-● *[M36.1]*
    neurological disorder NEC G98.0
    ochronosis —*see also* subcategory M14.8-●
      E70.29
    O'nyong-nyong —*see also* category M01
      A92.1
    parasitic disease NEC —*see also* category
      M01 B89
    paratyphoid fever —*see also* category M01
      A01.4
    Pseudomonas —*see* Arthritis, pyogenic,
      bacterial NEC
    psoriasis L40.50
    pyogenic organism NEC —*see* Arthritis,
      pyogenic, bacterial NEC
    Reiter's disease —*see* Reiter's disease
    respiratory disorder NEC —*see also*
      subcategory M14.8-● J98.9
    reticulosis, malignant —*see also*
      subcategory M14.8-● C86.0
    rubella B06.82
    Salmonella (arizonae) (cholerae-suis)
      (enteritidis) (typhimurium)
      A02.23
    sarcoidosis D86.86
    specified bacteria NEC —*see* Arthritis,
      pyogenic, bacterial NEC
    sporotrichosis B42.82
    syringomyelia G95.0
    thalassemia NEC D56.9 *[M36.3]*
    tuberculosis —*see* Tuberculosis, arthritis
    typhoid fever A01.04
    urethritis, Reiter's —*see* Reiter's disease
    viral disease NEC —*see also* category M01
      B34.9
  infectious or infective —*see also* Arthritis,
    pyogenic or pyemic
    spine —*see* Spondylopathy, infective
  juvenile M08.90
    with systemic onset —*see* Still's disease
    ankle M08.97-●
    elbow M08.92-●
    foot joint M08.97-●
    hand joint M08.94-●
    hip M08.95-●
    knee M08.96-●
    multiple site M08.99

Arthritis, arthritic *(Continued)*
  juvenile *(Continued)*
    pauciarticular M08.40
      ankle M08.47-●
      elbow M08.42-●
      foot joint M08.47-●
      hand joint M08.44-●
      hip M08.45-●
      knee M08.46-●
      shoulder M08.41-●
      vertebrae M08.48
      wrist M08.43-●
    psoriatic L40.54
    rheumatoid —*see* Arthritis, rheumatoid,
      juvenile
    shoulder M08.91-●
    specified type NEC M08.80
      ankle M08.87-●
      elbow M08.82-●
      foot joint M08.87-●
      hand joint M08.84-●
      hip M08.85-●
      knee M08.86-●
      multiple site M08.89
      shoulder M08.81-●
      specified joint NEC M08.88
      vertebrae M08.88
      wrist M08.83-●
    vertebra M08.98
    wrist M08.93-●
  meaning osteoarthritis —*see* Osteoarthritis
  meningococcal A39.83
  menopausal (any site) NEC —*see* Arthritis,
    specified form NEC
  mutilans (psoriatic) L40.52
  mycotic NEC —*see also* category M01 B49
  neuropathic (Charcot) —*see* Arthropathy,
    neuropathic
    diabetic —*see* Diabetes, arthropathy,
      neuropathic
    nonsyphilitic NEC G98.0
    syringomyelic G95.0
  ochronotic —*see also* subcategory M14.8-●
    E70.29
  palindromic (any site) —*see* Rheumatism,
    palindromic
  pneumococcal M00.10
    ankle M00.17-●
    elbow M00.12-●
    foot joint —*see* Arthritis, pneumococcal,
      ankle
    hand joint M00.14-●
    hip M00.15-●
    knee M00.16-●
    multiple site M00.19
    shoulder M00.11-●
    vertebra M00.18
    wrist M00.13-●
  postdysenteric —*see* Arthropathy,
    postdysenteric
  postmeningococcal A39.84
  postrheumatic, chronic —*see* Arthropathy,
    postrheumatic, chronic
  primary progressive —*see also* Arthritis,
    specified form NEC
    spine —*see* Spondylitis, ankylosing
  psoriatic L40.50
  purulent (any site except spine) —*see*
    Arthritis, pyogenic or pyemic
    spine —*see* Spondylopathy, infective
  pyogenic or pyemic (any site except spine)
    M00.9
    bacterial NEC M00.80
      ankle M00.87-●
      elbow M00.82-●
      foot joint —*see* Arthritis, pyogenic,
        bacterial NEC, ankle
      hand joint M00.84-●
      hip M00.85-●
      knee M00.86-●
      multiple site M00.89

Arthritis, arthritic *(Continued)*
  pyogenic or pyemic *(Continued)*
    bacterial NEC *(Continued)*
      shoulder M00.81-●
      vertebra M00.88
      wrist M00.83-●
    pneumococcal —*see* Arthritis,
      pneumococcal
    spine —*see* Spondylopathy, infective
    staphylococcal —*see* Arthritis,
      staphylococcal
    streptococcal —*see* Arthritis, streptococcal
      NEC
    pneumococcal —*see* Arthritis,
      pneumococcal
  reactive —*see* Reiter's disease
  rheumatic —*see also* Arthritis, rheumatoid
    acute or subacute —*see* Fever, rheumatic
  rheumatoid M06.9
    with
      carditis —*see* Rheumatoid, carditis
      endocarditis —*see* Rheumatoid, carditis
      heart involvement NEC —*see*
        Rheumatoid, carditis
      lung involvement —*see* Rheumatoid,
        lung
      myocarditis —*see* Rheumatoid, carditis
      myopathy —*see* Rheumatoid, myopathy
      pericarditis —*see* Rheumatoid, carditis
      polyneuropathy —*see* Rheumatoid,
        polyneuropathy
      rheumatoid factor —*see* Arthritis,
        rheumatoid, seropositive
      splenoadenomegaly and leukopenia —
        see Felty's syndrome
      vasculitis —*see* Rheumatoid, vasculitis
      visceral involvement NEC —*see*
        Rheumatoid, arthritis, with
        involvement of organs NEC
    juvenile (with or without rheumatoid
      factor) M08.00
      ankle M08.07-●
      elbow M08.02-●
      foot joint M08.07-●
      hand joint M08.04-●
      hip M08.05-●
      knee M08.06-●
      multiple site M08.09
      shoulder M08.01-●
      vertebra M08.08
      wrist M08.03-●
    seronegative M06.00
      ankle M06.07-●
      elbow M06.02-●
      foot joint M06.07-●
      hand joint M06.04-●
      hip M06.05-●
      knee M06.06-●
      multiple sites M06.09
      shoulder M06.01-●
      vertebra M06.08
      wrist M06.03-●
    seropositive M05.9
      without organ involvement M05.70
        ankle M05.77-●
        elbow M05.72-●
        foot joint M05.77-●
        hand joint M05.74-●
        hip M05.75-●
        knee M05.76-●
        multiple sites M05.79
        shoulder M05.71-●
        vertebra —*see* Spondylitis, ankylosing
        wrist M05.73-●
    specified NEC M05.80
      ankle M05.87-●
      elbow M05.82-●
      foot joint M05.87-●
      hand joint M05.84-●
      hip M05.85-●
      knee M05.86-●

▶ New   ⇒ Revised   ~~deleted~~ Deleted   ● Use Additional Character(s)

A

Arthritis, arthritic *(Continued)*
  rheumatoid *(Continued)*
    specified NEC *(Continued)*
      multiple sites M05.89
      shoulder M05.81-●
      vertebra —*see* Spondylitis, ankylosing
      wrist M05.83-●
    specified type NEC M06.80
      ankle M06.87-●
      elbow M06.82-●
      foot joint M06.87-●
      hand joint M06.84-●
      hip M06.85-●
      knee M06.86-●
      multiple site M06.89
      shoulder M06.81-●
      vertebra M06.88
      wrist M06.83-●
    spine —*see* Spondylitis, ankylosing
  rubella B06.82
  scorbutic —*see also* subcategory M14.8-● E54
  senile or senescent —*see* Osteoarthritis
  septic (any site except spine) —*see* Arthritis,
    pyogenic or pyemic
  spine —*see* Spondylopathy, infective
  serum (nontherapeutic) (therapeutic) —*see*
    Arthropathy, postimmunization
  specified form NEC M13.80
    ankle M13.87-●
    elbow M13.82-●
    foot joint M13.87-●
    hand joint M13.84-●
    hip M13.85-●
    knee M13.86-●
    multiple site M13.89
    shoulder M13.81-●
    specified joint NEC M13.88
    wrist M13.83-●
  spine —*see also* Spondylopathy,
    inflammatory
    infectious or infective NEC —*see*
      Spondylopathy, infective
    Marie-Strümpell —*see* Spondylitis,
      ankylosing
    pyogenic —*see* Spondylopathy, infective
    rheumatoid —*see* Spondylitis, ankylosing
    traumatic (old) —*see* Spondylopathy,
      traumatic
    tuberculous A18.01
  staphylococcal M00.00
    ankle M00.07-●
    elbow M00.02-●
    foot joint —*see* Arthritis, staphylococcal,
      ankle
    hand joint M00.04-●
    hip M00.05-●
    knee M00.06-●
    multiple site M00.09
    shoulder M00.01-●
    vertebra M00.08
    wrist M00.03-●
  streptococcal NEC M00.20
    ankle M00.27-●
    elbow M00.22-●
    foot joint —*see* Arthritis, streptococcal,
      ankle
    hand joint M00.24-●
    hip M00.25-●
    knee M00.26-●
    multiple site M00.29
    shoulder M00.21-●
    vertebra M00.28
    wrist M00.23-●
  suppurative —*see* Arthritis, pyogenic or
    pyemic
  syphilitic (late) A52.16
    congenital A50.55 *[M12.80]*
  syphilitica deformans (Charcot) A52.16
  temporomandibular M26.69
  toxic of menopause (any site) —*see* Arthritis,
    specified form NEC

Arthritis, arthritic *(Continued)*
  transient —*see* Arthropathy, specified form
    NEC
  traumatic (chronic) —*see* Arthropathy,
    traumatic
  tuberculous A18.02
    spine A18.01
  uratic —*see* Gout
  urethritica (Reiter's) —*see* Reiter's disease
  vertebral —*see* Spondylopathy, inflammatory
  villous (any site) —*see* Arthropathy, specified
    form NEC
Arthrocele —*see* Effusion, joint
Arthrodesis status Z98.1
Arthrodynia —*see also* Pain, joint
Arthrodysplasia Q74.9
Arthrofibrosis, joint —*see* Ankylosis
Arthrogryposis (congenital) Q68.8
  multiplex congenita Q74.3
Arthrokatadysis M24.7
Arthropathy *(see also* Arthritis) M12.9
  Charcot's —*see* Arthropathy, neuropathic
    diabetic —*see* Diabetes, arthropathy,
      neuropathic
    syringomyelic G95.0
  cricoarytenoid J38.7
  crystal(-induced) —*see* Arthritis, in, crystals
  diabetic NEC —*see* Diabetes, arthropathy
  distal interphalangeal, psoriatic L40.51
  enteropathic M07.60
    ankle M07.67-●
    elbow M07.62-●
    foot joint M07.67-●
    hand joint M07.64-●
    hip M07.65-●
    knee M07.66-●
    multiple site M07.69
    shoulder M07.61-●
    vertebra M07.68
    wrist M07.63-●
  following intestinal bypass M02.00
    ankle M02.07-●
    elbow M02.02-●
    foot joint M02.07-●
    hand joint M02.04-●
    hip M02.05-●
    knee M02.06-●
    multiple site M02.09
    shoulder M02.01-●
    vertebra M02.08
    wrist M02.03-●
  gouty —*see also* Gout
    in (due to)
      Lesch-Nyhan syndrome E79.1 *[M14.8-●]*
      sickle-cell disorders D57-● *[M14.8-●]*
  hemophilic NEC D66 *[M36.2]*
    in (due to)
      hyperparathyroidism NEC E21.3
        [M14.8-●]
      metabolic disease NOS E88.9 *[M14.8-●]*
  in (due to)
    acromegaly E22.0 *[M14.8-●]*
    amyloidosis E85.4 *[M14.8-●]*
    blood disorder NOS D75.9 *[M36.3]*
    diabetes —*see* Diabetes, arthropathy
    endocrine disease NOS E34.9 *[M14.8-●]*
    erythema
      multiforme L51.9 *[M14.8-●]*
      nodosum L52 *[M14.8-●]*
    hemochromatosis E83.118 *[M14.8-●]*
    hemoglobinopathy NEC D58.2 *[M36.3]*
    hemophilia NEC D66 *[M36.2]*
    Henoch-Schönlein purpura D69.0 *[M36.4]*
    hyperthyroidism E05.90 *[M14.8-●]*
    hypothyroidism E03.9 *[M14.8-●]*
    infective endocarditis I33.0 *[M12.80]*
    leukemia NEC C95.9-● *[M36.1]*
    malignant histiocytosis C96.A *[M36.1]*
    metabolic disease NOS E88.9 *[M14.8-●]*
    multiple myeloma C90.0-● *[M36.1]*
    neoplastic disease NOS *(see also* Neoplasm)
      D49.9 *[M36.1]*

Arthropathy *(Continued)*
  hemochromatosis *(Continued)*
    nutritional deficiency —*see also*
      subcategory M14.8-● E63.9
    psoriasis NOS L40.50
    sarcoidosis D86.86
    syphilis (late) A52.77
      congenital A50.55 *[M12.80]*
    thyrotoxicosis —*see also* subcategory
      M14.8-● E05.90
    ulcerative colitis K51.90 *[M07.60]*
    viral hepatitis (postinfectious) NEC B19.9
      [M12.80]
    Whipple's disease —*see also* subcategory
      M14.8-● K90.81
  Jaccoud —*see* Arthropathy, postrheumatic,
    chronic
  juvenile —*see* Arthritis, juvenile
    psoriatic L40.54
  mutilans (psoriatic) L40.52
  neuropathic (Charcot) M14.60
    ankle M14.67-●
    diabetic —*see* Diabetes, arthropathy,
      neuropathic
    elbow M14.62-●
    foot joint M14.67-●
    hand joint M14.64-●
    hip M14.65-●
    knee M14.66-●
    multiple site M14.69
    nonsyphilitic NEC G98.0
    shoulder M14.61-●
    syringomyelic G95.0
    vertebra M14.68
    wrist M14.63-●
  osteopulmonary —*see* Osteoarthropathy,
    hypertrophic, specified NEC
  postdysenteric M02.10
    ankle M02.17-●
    elbow M02.12-●
    foot joint M02.17-●
    hand joint M02.14-●
    hip M02.15-●
    knee M02.16-●
    multiple site M02.19
    shoulder M02.11-●
    vertebra M02.18
    wrist M02.13-●
  postimmunization M02.20
    ankle M02.27-●
    elbow M02.22-●
    foot joint M02.27-●
    hand joint M02.24-●
    hip M02.25-●
    knee M02.26-●
    multiple site M02.29
    shoulder M02.21-●
    vertebra M02.28
    wrist M02.23-●
  postinfectious NEC B99 *[M12.80]*
    in (due to)
      enteritis due to Yersinia enterocolitica
        A04.6 *[M12.80]*
      syphilis A52.77
      viral hepatitis NEC B19.9
        [M12.80]
  postrheumatic, chronic (Jaccoud)
    M12.00
    ankle M12.07-●
    elbow M12.02-●
    foot joint M12.07-●
    hand joint M12.04-●
    hip M12.05-●
    knee M12.06-●
    multiple site M12.09
    shoulder M12.01-●
    specified joint NEC M12.08
    vertebrae M12.08
    wrist M12.03-●
  psoriatic NEC L40.59
    interphalangeal, distal L40.51

Arthropathy *(Continued)*
  reactive M02.9
    in (due to)
      infective endocarditis I33.0 *[M02.9]*
      specified type NEC M02.80
        ankle M02.87-●
        elbow M02.82-●
        foot joint M02.87-●
        hand joint M02.84-●
        hip M02.85-●
        knee M02.86-●
        multiple site M02.89
        shoulder M02.81-●
        vertebra M02.88
        wrist M02.83-●
  specified form NEC M12.80
    ankle M12.87-●
    elbow M12.82-●
    foot joint M12.87-●
    hand joint M12.84-●
    hip M12.85-●
    knee M12.86-●
    multiple site M12.89
    shoulder M12.81-●
    specified joint NEC M12.88
    vertebrae M12.88
    wrist M12.83-●
  syringomyelic G95.0
  tabes dorsalis A52.16
  tabetic A52.16
  transient —*see* Arthropathy, specified form
      NEC
  traumatic M12.50
    ankle M12.57-●
    elbow M12.52-●
    foot joint M12.57-●
    hand joint M12.54-●
    hip M12.55-●
    knee M12.56-●
    multiple site M12.59
    shoulder M12.51-●
    specified joint NEC M12.58
    vertebrae M12.58
    wrist M12.53-●
Arthropyosis —*see* Arthritis, pyogenic or pyemic
Arthrosis (deformans) (degenerative)
    (localized) —*see also* Osteoarthritis
    M19.90
  spine —*see* Spondylosis
Arthus' phenomenon or reaction T78.41
  due to
    drug —*see* Table of Drugs and Chemicals,
        by drug
Articular —*see* condition
Articulation, reverse (teeth) M26.24
Artificial
  insemination complication —*see*
      Complications, artificial, fertilization
  opening status (functioning) (without
      complication) Z93.9
    anus (colostomy) Z93.3
    colostomy Z93.3
    cystostomy Z93.50
      appendico-vesicostomy Z93.52
      cutaneous Z93.51
      specified NEC Z93.59
    enterostomy Z93.4
    gastrostomy Z93.1
    ileostomy Z93.2
    intestinal tract NEC Z93.4
    jejunostomy Z93.4
    nephrostomy Z93.6
    specified site NEC Z93.8
    tracheostomy Z93.0
    ureterostomy Z93.6
    urethrostomy Z93.6
    urinary tract NEC Z93.6
    vagina Z93.8
  vagina status Z93.8
Arytenoid —*see* condition
Asbestosis (occupational) J61

ASC-H (atypical squamous cells cannot exclude
    high grade squamous intraepithelial lesion
    on cytologic smear)
  anus R85.611
  cervix R87.611
  vagina R87.621
ASC-US (atypical squamous cells of
    undetermined significance on cytologic
    smear)
  anus R85.610
  cervix R87.610
  vagina R87.620
Ascariasis B77.9
  with
    complications NEC B77.89
    intestinal complications B77.0
    pneumonia, pneumonitis B77.81
Ascaridosis, ascariasis —*see* Ascariasis
Ascaris (infection) (infestation)
    (lumbricoides) —*see* Ascariasis
Ascending —*see* condition
Aschoff's bodies —*see* Myocarditis,
    rheumatic
Ascites (abdominal) R18.8
  ➡cardiac —*see also* Failure, heart, right
      I50.810
    chylous (nonfilarial) I89.8
      filarial —*see* Infestation, filarial
    due to
      cirrhosis, alcoholic K70.31
      hepatitis
        alcoholic K70.11
        chronic active K71.51
      S. japonicum B65.2
  ➡heart —*see also* Failure, heart, right I50.810
    malignant R18.0
    pseudochylous R18.8
    syphilitic A52.74
    tuberculous A18.31
Aseptic —*see* condition
Asherman's syndrome N85.6
Asialia K11.7
Asiatic cholera —*see* Cholera
Asimultagnosia (simultanagnosia) R48.3
Askin's tumor —*see* Neoplasm, connective
    tissue, malignant
Asocial personality F60.2
Asomatognosia R41.4
Aspartylglucosaminuria E77.1
Asperger's disease or syndrome F84.5
Aspergilloma —*see* Aspergillosis
Aspergillosis (with pneumonia) B44.9
  bronchopulmonary, allergic B44.81
  disseminated B44.7
  generalized B44.7
  pulmonary NEC B44.1
    allergic B44.81
    invasive B44.0
  specified NEC B44.89
  tonsillar B44.2
Aspergillus (flavus) (fumigatus) (infection)
    (terreus) —*see* Aspergillosis
Aspermatogenesis —*see* Azoospermia
Aspermia (testis) —*see* Azoospermia
Asphyxia, asphyxiation (by) R09.01
  antenatal P84
  birth P84
  bunny bag —*see* Asphyxia, due to,
      mechanical threat to breathing, trapped
      in bed clothes
  crushing S28.0
  drowning T75.1
  gas, fumes, or vapor —*see* Table of Drugs and
      Chemicals
  inhalation —*see* Inhalation
  intrauterine P84
  local I73.00
    with gangrene I73.01
  mucus —*see also* Foreign body, respiratory
      tract, causing asphyxia
  newborn P84

Asphyxia, asphyxiation *(Continued)*
  pathological R09.01
  postnatal P84
    mechanical —*see* Asphyxia, due to,
        mechanical threat to breathing
  prenatal P84
  reticularis R23.1
  strangulation —*see* Asphyxia, due to,
      mechanical threat to breathing
  submersion T75.1
  traumatic T71.9
    due to
      crushed chest S28.0
      foreign body (in) —*see* Foreign body,
          respiratory tract, causing asphyxia
      low oxygen content of ambient air T71.20
        due to
          being trapped in
            low oxygen environment T71.29
              in car trunk T71.221
                circumstances undetermined
                    T71.224
                done with intent to harm by
                    another person T71.223
                self T71.222
              in refrigerator T71.231
                circumstances undetermined
                    T71.234
                done with intent to harm by
                    another person T71.233
                self T71.232
          cave-in T71.21
    mechanical threat to breathing
        (accidental) T71.191
      circumstances undetermined T71.194
      done with intent to harm by
          another person T71.193
      self T71.192
      hanging T71.161
        circumstances undetermined
            T71.164
        done with intent to harm by
            another person T71.163
        self T71.162
      plastic bag T71.121
        circumstances undetermined
            T71.124
        done with intent to harm by
            another person T71.123
        self T71.122
      smothering
        in furniture T71.151
          circumstances undetermined
              T71.154
          done with intent to harm by
              another person T71.153
          self T71.152
        under
          another person's body T71.141
            circumstances undetermined
                T71.144
            done with intent to harm
                T71.143
          pillow T71.111
            circumstances undetermined
                T71.114
            done with intent to harm by
                another person T71.113
            self T71.112
        trapped in bed clothes T71.131
          circumstances undetermined
              T71.134
          done with intent to harm by
              another person T71.133
          self T71.132
  vomiting, vomitus —*see* Foreign body,
      respiratory tract, causing asphyxia
Aspiration
  amniotic (clear) fluid (newborn) P24.10
    with
      pneumonia (pneumonitis) P24.11
      respiratory symptoms P24.11

▶ New   ➡ Revised   ~~deleted~~ Deleted   ● Use Additional Character(s)

Aspiration (*Continued*)
  blood
    newborn (without respiratory symptoms)
      P24.20
      with
        pneumonia (pneumonitis) P24.21
        respiratory symptoms P24.21
    specified age NEC —*see* Foreign body,
      respiratory tract
  bronchitis J69.0
  food or foreign body (with asphyxiation) —
    see Asphyxia, food
  liquor (amnii) (newborn) P24.10
    with
      pneumonia (pneumonitis) P24.11
      respiratory symptoms P24.11
  meconium (newborn) (without respiratory
    symptoms) P24.00
    with
      pneumonitis (pneumonitis) P24.01
      respiratory symptoms P24.01
  milk (newborn) (without respiratory
    symptoms) P24.30
    with
      pneumonia (pneumonitis) P24.31
      respiratory symptoms P24.31
    specified age NEC —*see* Foreign body,
      respiratory tract
  mucus —*see also* Foreign body, by site,
    causing asphyxia
    newborn P24.10
      with
        pneumonia (pneumonitis) P24.11
        respiratory symptoms P24.11
  neonatal P24.9
    specific NEC (without respiratory
      symptoms) P24.80
      with
        pneumonia (pneumonitis) P24.81
        respiratory symptoms P24.81
  newborn P24.9
    specific NEC (without respiratory
      symptoms) P24.80
      with
        pneumonia (pneumonitis) P24.81
        respiratory symptoms P24.81
  pneumonia J69.0
  pneumonitis J69.0
  syndrome of newborn —*see* Aspiration, by
    substance, with pneumonia
  vernix caseosa (newborn) P24.80
    with
      pneumonia (pneumonitis) P24.81
      respiratory symptoms P24.81
  vomitus —*see also* Foreign body, respiratory
    tract
    newborn (without respiratory symptoms)
      P24.30
      with
        pneumonia (pneumonitis) P24.31
        respiratory symptoms P24.31
Asplenia (congenital) Q89.01
  postsurgical Z90.81
Assam fever B55.0
Assault, sexual —*see* Maltreatment
Assmann's focus NEC A15.0
Astasia (-abasia) (hysterical) F44.4
Asteatosis cutis L85.3
Astereognosia, astereognosis R48.1
Asterixis R27.8
  in liver disease K71.3
Asteroid hyalitis —*see* Deposit, crystalline
Asthenia, asthenic R53.1
  cardiac —*see also* Failure, heart I50.9
    psychogenic F45.8
  cardiovascular —*see also* Failure, heart
    I50.9
    psychogenic F45.8
  heart —*see also* Failure, heart I50.9
    psychogenic F45.8
  hysterical F44.4

Asthenia, asthenic (*Continued*)
  myocardial —*see also* Failure, heart I50.9
    psychogenic F45.8
  nervous F48.8
  neurocirculatory F45.8
  neurotic F48.8
  psychogenic F48.8
  psychoneurotic F48.8
  psychophysiologic F48.8
  reaction (psychophysiologic) F48.8
  senile R54
Asthenopia —*see also* Discomfort, visual
  hysterical F44.6
  psychogenic F44.6
Asthenospermia —*see* Abnormal, specimen,
  male genital organs
Asthma, asthmatic (bronchial) (catarrh)
    (spasmodic) J45.909
  with
    chronic obstructive bronchitis J44.9
      with
        acute lower respiratory infection J44.0
        exacerbation (acute) J44.1
    chronic obstructive pulmonary disease
      J44.9
      with
        acute lower respiratory infection J44.0
        exacerbation (acute) J44.1
    exacerbation (acute) J45.901
    hay fever —*see* Asthma, allergic extrinsic
    rhinitis, allergic —*see* Asthma, allergic
      extrinsic
    status asthmaticus J45.902
  allergic extrinsic J45.909
    with
      exacerbation (acute) J45.901
      status asthmaticus J45.902
  atopic —*see* Asthma, allergic extrinsic
  cardiac —*see* Failure, ventricular, left
  cardiobronchial I50.1
  childhood J45.909
    with
      exacerbation (acute) J45.901
      status asthmaticus J45.902
  chronic obstructive J44.9
    with
      acute lower respiratory infection J44.0
      exacerbation (acute) J44.1
  collier's J60
  cough variant J45.991
  detergent J69.8
  due to
    detergent J69.8
    inhalation of fumes J68.3
  eosinophilic J82
  extrinsic, allergic —*see* Asthma, allergic
    extrinsic
  grinder's J62.8
  hay —*see* Asthma, allergic extrinsic
  heart I50.1
  idiosyncratic —*see* Asthma, nonallergic
  intermittent (mild) J45.20
    with
      exacerbation (acute) J45.21
      status asthmaticus J45.22
  intrinsic, nonallergic —*see* Asthma, nonallergic
  Kopp's E32.8
  late-onset J45.909
    with
      exacerbation (acute) J45.901
      status asthmaticus J45.902
  mild intermittent J45.20
    with
      exacerbation (acute) J45.21
      status asthmaticus J45.22
  mild persistent J45.30
    with
      exacerbation (acute) J45.31
      status asthmaticus J45.32
  Millar's (laryngismus stridulus) J38.5
  miner's J60

Asthma, asthmatic (*Continued*)
  mixed J45.909
    with
      exacerbation (acute) J45.901
      status asthmaticus J45.902
  moderate persistent J45.40
    with
      exacerbation (acute) J45.41
      status asthmaticus J45.42
  nervous —*see* Asthma, nonallergic
  nonallergic (intrinsic) J45.909
    with
      exacerbation (acute) J45.901
      status asthmaticus J45.902
  persistent
    mild J45.30
      with
        exacerbation (acute) J45.31
        status asthmaticus J45.32
    moderate J45.40
      with
        exacerbation (acute) J45.41
        status asthmaticus J45.42
    severe J45.50
      with
        exacerbation (acute) J45.51
        status asthmaticus J45.52
  platinum J45.998
  pneumoconiotic NEC J64
  potter's J62.8
  predominantly allergic J45.909
  psychogenic F54
  pulmonary eosinophilic J82
  red cedar J67.8
  Rostan's I50.1
  sandblaster's J62.8
  sequoiosis J67.8
  severe persistent J45.50
    with
      exacerbation (acute) J45.51
      status asthmaticus J45.52
  specified NEC J45.998
  stonemason's J62.8
  thymic E32.8
  tuberculous —*see* Tuberculosis, pulmonary
  Wichmann's (laryngismus stridulus) J38.5
  wood J67.8
Astigmatism (compound) (congenital)
    H52.20-●
  irregular H52.21-●
  regular H52.22-●
Astraphobia F40.220
Astroblastoma
  specified site —*see* Neoplasm, malignant, by
    site
  unspecified site C71.9
Astrocytoma (cystic)
  anaplastic
    specified site —*see* Neoplasm, malignant,
      by site
    unspecified site C71.9
  fibrillary
    specified site —*see* Neoplasm, malignant,
      by site
    unspecified site C71.9
  fibrous
    specified site —*see* Neoplasm, malignant,
      by site
    unspecified site C71.9
  gemistocytic
    specified site —*see* Neoplasm, malignant,
      by site
    unspecified site C71.9
  juvenile
    specified site —*see* Neoplasm, malignant,
      by site
    unspecified site C71.9
  pilocytic
    specified site —*see* Neoplasm, malignant,
      by site
    unspecified site C71.9

Astrocytoma *(Continued)*
  piloid
    specified site —*see* Neoplasm, malignant,
      by site
    unspecified site C71.9
  protoplasmic
    specified site —*see* Neoplasm, malignant,
      by site
    unspecified site C71.9
  specified site NEC —*see* Neoplasm,
    malignant, by site
  subependymal D43.2
    giant cell
      specified site —*see* Neoplasm, uncertain
        behavior, by site
      unspecified site D43.2
    specified site —*see* Neoplasm, uncertain
      behavior, by site
    unspecified site D43.2
  unspecified site C71.9
Astroglioma
  specified site —*see* Neoplasm, malignant, by
    site
  unspecified site C71.9
Asymbolia R48.8
Asymmetry —*see also* Distortion
  between native and reconstructed breast N65.1
  face Q67.0
  jaw (lower) —*see* Anomaly, dentofacial, jaw-
    cranial base relationship, asymmetry
Asynergia, asynergy R27.8
  ventricular I51.89
Asystole (heart) —*see* Arrest, cardiac
At risk
  ~~for falling Z91.81~~
  ▶for
    ▶dental caries Z91.849
      ▶high Z91.843
      ▶low Z91.841
      ▶moderate Z91.842
    ▶falling Z91.81
Ataxia, ataxy, ataxic R27.0
  acute R27.8
  brain (hereditary) G11.9
  cerebellar (hereditary) G11.9
    with defective DNA repair G11.3
    alcoholic G31.2
    early-onset G11.1
    in
      alcoholism G31.2
      myxedema E03.9 *[G13.2]*
      neoplastic disease —*see also* Neoplasm
        D49.9 *[G32.81]*
      specified disease NEC G32.81
    late-onset (Marie's) G11.2
  cerebral (hereditary) G11.9
  congenital nonprogressive G11.0
  family, familial —*see* Ataxia, hereditary
  following
    cerebrovascular disease I69.993
      cerebral infarction I69.393
      intracerebral hemorrhage I69.193
      nontraumatic intracranial hemorrhage
        NEC I69.293
      specified disease NEC I69.893
      subarachnoid hemorrhage I69.093
  Friedreich's (heredofamilial) (cerebellar)
    (spinal) G11.1
  gait R26.0
    hysterical F44.4
  general R27.8
  gluten M35.9 *[G32.81]*
    with celiac disease K90.0 *[G32.81]*
  hereditary G11.9
    with neuropathy G60.2
    cerebellar —*see* Ataxia, cerebellar
    spastic G11.4
    specified NEC G11.8
    spinal (Friedreich's) G11.1
  heredofamilial —*see* Ataxia, hereditary
  Hunt's G11.1

Ataxia, ataxy, ataxic *(Continued)*
  hysterical F44.4
  locomotor (progressive) (syphilitic) (partial)
    (spastic) A52.11
    diabetic —*see* Diabetes, ataxia
  Marie's (cerebellar) (heredofamilial)
    (late- onset) G11.2
  nonorganic origin F44.4
  nonprogressive, congenital G11.0
  psychogenic F44.4
  Roussy-Lévy G60.0
  Sanger-Brown's (hereditary) G11.2
  spastic hereditary G11.4
  spinal
    hereditary (Friedreich's) G11.1
    progressive (syphilitic) A52.11
  spinocerebellar, X-linked recessive G11.1
  telangiectasia (Louis-Bar) G11.3
Ataxia-telangiectasia (Louis-Bar) G11.3
Atelectasis (massive) (partial) (pressure)
  (pulmonary) J98.11
  newborn P28.10
    due to resorption P28.11
    partial P28.19
    primary P28.0
    secondary P28.19
  primary (newborn) P28.0
  tuberculous —*see* Tuberculosis, pulmonary
Atelocardia Q24.9
Atelomyelia Q06.1
Atheroembolism
  of
    extremities
      lower I75.02-●
      upper I75.01-●
    kidney I75.81
    specified NEC I75.89
Atheroma, atheromatous —*see also*
  Arteriosclerosis I70.90
  aorta, aortic I70.0
    valve —*see also* Endocarditis, aortic I35.8
  aorto-iliac I70.0
  artery —*see* Arteriosclerosis
  basilar (artery) I67.2
  carotid (artery) (common) (internal) I67.2
  cerebral (arteries) I67.2
  coronary (artery) I25.10
    with angina pectoris —*see* Arteriosclerosis,
      coronary (artery)
  degeneration —*see* Arteriosclerosis
  heart, cardiac —*see* Disease, heart, ischemic,
    atherosclerotic
  mitral (valve) I34.8
  myocardium, myocardial —*see* Disease, heart,
    ischemic, atherosclerotic
  pulmonary valve (heart) —*see also*
    Endocarditis, pulmonary I37.8
  tricuspid (heart) (valve) I36.8
  valve, valvular —*see* Endocarditis
  vertebral (artery) I67.2
Atheromatosis —*see* Arteriosclerosis
Atherosclerosis —*see also* Arteriosclerosis
  coronary
    artery I25.10
      with angina pectoris —*see*
        Arteriosclerosis, coronary (artery),
      due to
        calcified coronary lesion (severely)
          I25.84
        lipid rich plaque I25.83
    transplanted heart I25.811
      bypass graft I25.812
        with angina pectoris —*see*
          Arteriosclerosis, coronary (artery)
      native coronary artery I25.811
        with angina pectoris —*see*
          Arteriosclerosis, coronary (artery)
Athetosis (acquired) R25.8
  bilateral (congenital) G80.3
  congenital (bilateral) (double) G80.3
  double (congenital) G80.3
  unilateral R25.8

Athlete's
  foot B35.3
  heart I51.7
Athrepsia E41
Athyrea (acquired) —*see also* Hypothyroidism
  congenital E03.1
Atonia, atony, atonic
  bladder (sphincter) (neurogenic) N31.2
  capillary I78.8
  cecum K59.8
    psychogenic F45.8
  colon —*see* Atony, intestine
  congenital P94.2
  esophagus K22.8
  intestine K59.8
    psychogenic F45.8
  stomach K31.89
    neurotic or psychogenic F45.8
  uterus (during labor) O62.2
    with hemorrhage (postpartum) O72.1
    postpartum (with hemorrhage) O72.1
      without hemorrhage O75.89
Atopy —*see* History, allergy
Atransferrinemia, congenital E88.09
Atresia, atretic
  alimentary organ or tract NEC Q45.8
    upper Q40.8
  ani, anus, anal (canal) Q42.3
    with fistula Q42.2
  aorta (ring) Q25.29
  aortic (orifice) (valve) Q23.0
    arch Q25.21
    congenital with hypoplasia of ascending
      aorta and defective development of
      left ventricle (with mitral stenosis)
      Q23.4
    in hypoplastic left heart syndrome Q23.4
  aqueduct of Sylvius Q03.0
    with spina bifida —*see* Spina bifida, with
      hydrocephalus
  artery NEC Q27.8
    cerebral Q28.3
    coronary Q24.5
    digestive system Q27.8
    eye Q15.8
    lower limb Q27.8
    pulmonary Q25.5
    specified site NEC Q27.8
    umbilical Q27.0
    upper limb Q27.8
  auditory canal (external) Q16.1
  bile duct (common) (congenital) (hepatic)
    Q44.2
    acquired —*see* Obstruction, bile duct
  bladder (neck) Q64.39
    obstruction Q64.31
  bronchus Q32.4
  cecum Q42.8
  cervix (acquired) N88.2
    congenital Q51.828
    in pregnancy or childbirth —*see* Anomaly,
      cervix, in pregnancy or childbirth
      causing obstructed labor O65.5
  choana Q30.0
  colon Q42.9
    specified NEC Q42.8
  common duct Q44.2
  cricoid cartilage Q31.8
  cystic duct Q44.2
    acquired K82.8
      with obstruction K82.0
  digestive organs NEC Q45.8
  duodenum Q41.0
  ear canal Q16.1
  ejaculatory duct Q55.4
  epiglottis Q31.8
  esophagus Q39.0
    with tracheoesophageal fistula Q39.1
  eustachian tube Q17.8
  fallopian tube (congenital) Q50.6
    acquired N97.1

▶ New   ⟹ Revised   ~~deleted~~ Deleted   ● Use Additional Character(s)

Atresia, atretic *(Continued)*
follicular cyst N83.0-•
foramen of
Luschka Q03.1
with spina bifida —*see* Spina bifida, with hydrocephalus
Magendie Q03.1
with spina bifida —*see* Spina bifida, with hydrocephalus
gallbladder Q44.1
genital organ
external
female Q52.79
male Q55.8
internal
female Q52.8
male Q55.8
glottis Q31.8
gullet Q39.0
with tracheoesophageal fistula Q39.1
heart valve NEC Q24.8
pulmonary Q22.0
tricuspid Q22.4
hymen Q52.3
acquired (postinfective) N89.6
ileum Q41.2
intestine (small) Q41.9
large Q42.9
specified NEC Q42.8
iris, filtration angle Q15.0
jejunum Q41.1
lacrimal apparatus Q10.4
larynx Q31.8
meatus urinarius Q64.33
mitral valve Q23.2
in hypoplastic left heart syndrome Q23.4
nares (anterior) (posterior) Q30.0
nasopharynx Q34.8
nose, nostril Q30.0
acquired J34.89
organ or site NEC Q89.8
osseous meatus (ear) Q16.1
oviduct (congenital) Q50.6
acquired N97.1
parotid duct Q38.4
acquired K11.8
pulmonary (artery) Q25.5
valve Q22.0
pulmonic Q22.0
pupil Q13.2
rectum Q42.1
with fistula Q42.0
salivary duct Q38.4
acquired K11.8
sublingual duct Q38.4
acquired K11.8
submandibular duct Q38.4
acquired K11.8
submaxillary duct Q38.4
acquired K11.8
thyroid cartilage Q31.8
trachea Q32.1
tricuspid valve Q22.4
ureter Q62.10
pelvic junction Q62.11
vesical orifice Q62.12
ureteropelvic junction Q62.11
ureterovesical orifice Q62.12
urethra (valvular) Q64.39
stricture Q64.32
urinary tract NEC Q64.8
uterus Q51.818
acquired N85.8
vagina (congenital) Q52.4
acquired (postinfectional) (senile) N89.5
vas deferens Q55.3
vascular NEC Q27.8
cerebral Q28.3
digestive system Q27.8

Atresia, atretic *(Continued)*
vascular NEC *(Continued)*
lower limb Q27.8
specified site NEC Q27.8
upper limb Q27.8
vein NEC Q27.8
digestive system Q27.8
great Q26.8
lower limb Q27.8
portal Q26.5
➡pulmonary Q26.4
▶partial Q26.3
▶total Q26.2
specified site NEC Q27.8
upper limb Q27.8
vena cava (inferior) (superior) Q26.8
vesicourethral orifice Q64.31
vulva Q52.79
acquired N90.5
Atrichia, atrichosis —*see* Alopecia
Atrophia —*see also* Atrophy
cutis senilis L90.8
due to radiation L57.8
gyrata of choroid and retina H31.23
senilis R54
dermatological L90.8
due to radiation (nonionizing) (solar) L57.8
unguium L60.3
congenita Q84.6
Atrophie blanche (en plaque) (de Milian) L95.0
Atrophoderma, atrophodermia (of) L90.9
diffusum (idiopathic) L90.4
maculatum L90.8
et striatum L90.8
due to syphilis A52.79
syphilitic A51.39
neuriticum L90.8
Pasini and Pierini L90.3
pigmentosum Q82.1
reticulatum symmetricum faciei L66.4
senile L90.8
due to radiation (nonionizing) (solar) L57.8
vermiculata (cheeks) L66.4
Atrophy, atrophic (of)
adrenal (capsule) (gland) E27.49
primary (autoimmune) E27.1
alveolar process or ridge (edentulous) K08.20
anal sphincter (disuse) N81.84
appendix K38.8
arteriosclerotic —*see* Arteriosclerosis
bile duct (common) (hepatic) K83.8
bladder N32.89
neurogenic N31.8
blanche (en plaque) (of Milian) L95.0
bone (senile) NEC —*see also* Disorder, bone, specified type NEC
due to
tabes dorsalis (neurogenic) A52.11
brain (cortex) (progressive) G31.9
frontotemporal circumscribed G31.01
[F02.80]
with behavioral disturbance G31.01
[F02.81]
senile NEC G31.1
breast N64.2
obstetric —*see* Disorder, breast, specified type NEC
buccal cavity K13.79
cardiac —*see* Degeneration, myocardial
cartilage (infectional) (joint) —*see* Disorder, cartilage, specified NEC
cerebellar —*see* Atrophy, brain
cerebral —*see* Atrophy, brain
cervix (mucosa) (senile) (uteri) N88.8
menopausal N95.8
Charcot-Marie-Tooth G60.0
choroid (central) (macular) (myopic) (retina) H31.10-•
diffuse secondary H31.12-•
gyrate H31.23
senile H31.11-•

Atrophy, atrophic *(Continued)*
ciliary body —*see* Atrophy, iris
conjunctiva (senile) H11.89
corpus cavernosum N48.89
cortical —*see* Atrophy, brain
cystic duct K82.8
Déjérine-Thomas G23.8
disuse NEC —*see* Atrophy, muscle
Duchenne-Aran G12.21
ear H93.8-•
edentulous alveolar ridge K08.20
endometrium (senile) N85.8
cervix N88.8
enteric K63.89
epididymis N50.89
eyeball —*see* Disorder, globe, degenerated condition, atrophy
eyelid (senile) —*see* Disorder, eyelid, degenerative
facial (skin) L90.9
fallopian tube (senile) N83.32-•
with ovary N83.33-•
fascioscapulohumeral (Landouzy-Déjérine) G71.0
fatty, thymus (gland) E32.8
gallbladder K82.8
gastric K29.40
with bleeding K29.41
gastrointestinal K63.89
glandular I89.8
globe H44.52-•
➡gum —*see* Recession, gingival
hair L67.8
heart (brown) —*see* Degeneration, myocardial
hemifacial Q67.4
Romberg G51.8
infantile E41
paralysis, acute —*see* Poliomyelitis, paralytic
intestine K63.89
iris (essential) (progressive) H21.26-•
specified NEC H21.29
kidney (senile) (terminal) —*see also* Sclerosis, renal N26.1
congenital or infantile Q60.5
bilateral Q60.4
unilateral Q60.3
hydronephrotic —*see* Hydronephrosis
lacrimal gland (primary) H04.14-•
secondary H04.15-•
Landouzy-Déjérine G71.0
laryngitis, infective J37.0
larynx J38.7
Leber's optic (hereditary) H47.22
lip K13.0
liver (yellow) K72.90
with coma K72.91
acute, subacute K72.00
with coma K72.01
chronic K72.10
with coma K72.11
lung (senile) J98.4
macular (dermatological) L90.8
syphilitic, skin A51.39
striated A52.79
mandible (edentulous) K08.20
minimal K08.21
moderate K08.22
severe K08.23
maxilla K08.20
minimal K08.24
moderate K08.25
severe K08.26
muscle, muscular (diffuse) (general) (idiopathic) (primary) M62.50
ankle M62.57-•
Duchenne-Aran G12.21
foot M62.57-•
forearm M62.53-•
hand M62.54-•
infantile spinal G12.0
lower leg M62.56-•

Atrophy, atrophic *(Continued)*
  muscle, muscular *(Continued)*
    multiple sites M62.59
    myelopathic —*see* Atrophy, muscle,
      spinal
    myotonic G71.11
    neuritic G58.9
    neuropathic (peroneal) (progressive)
      G60.0
    pelvic (disuse) N81.84
    peroneal G60.0
    progressive (bulbar) G12.21
      adult G12.1
      infantile (spinal) G12.0
    ⟹spinal G12.25
      adult G12.1
      infantile G12.0
    pseudohypertrophic G71.0
    shoulder region M62.51-●
    specified site NEC M62.58
    spinal G12.9
      adult form G12.1
      Aran-Duchenne G12.21
      childhood form, type II G12.1
      distal G12.1
      hereditary NEC G12.1
      infantile, type I (Werdnig-Hoffmann)
        G12.0
      juvenile form, type III (Kugelberg-
        Welander) G12.1
    ⟹progressive G12.25
      scapuloperoneal form G12.1
      specified NEC G12.8
    syphilitic A52.78
    thigh M62.55-●
    upper arm M62.52-●
  myocardium —*see* Degeneration,
    myocardial
  myometrium (senile) N85.8
    cervix N88.8
  myopathic NEC —*see* Atrophy, muscle
  myotonia G71.11
  nail L60.3
  nasopharynx J31.1
  nerve —*see also* Disorder, nerve
    abducens —*see* Strabismus, paralytic, sixth
      nerve
    accessory G52.8
    acoustic or auditory —*see* subcategory
      H93.3
    cranial G52.9
      eighth (auditory) —*see* subcategory
        H93.3
      eleventh (accessory) G52.8
      fifth (trigeminal) G50.8
      first (olfactory) G52.0
      fourth (trochlear) —*see* Strabismus,
        paralytic, fourth nerve
      second (optic) H47.20
      sixth (abducens) —*see* Strabismus,
        paralytic, sixth nerve
      tenth (pneumogastric) (vagus) G52.2
      third (oculomotor) —*see* Strabismus,
        paralytic, third nerve
      twelfth (hypoglossal) G52.3
    hypoglossal G52.3
    oculomotor —*see* Strabismus, paralytic,
      third nerve
    olfactory G52.0
    optic (papillomacular bundle)
      syphilitic (late) A52.15
      congenital A50.44
    pneumogastric G52.2
    trigeminal G50.8
    trochlear —*see* Strabismus, paralytic,
      fourth nerve
    vagus (pneumogastric) G52.2
  neurogenic, bone, tabetic A52.11
  nutritional E41
  old age R54
  olivopontocerebellar G23.8

Atrophy, atrophic *(Continued)*
  optic (nerve) H47.20
    glaucomatous H47.23-●
    hereditary H47.22
    primary H47.21-●
    specified type NEC H47.29-●
    syphilitic (late) A52.15
      congenital A50.44
  orbit H05.31-●
  ovary (senile) N83.31-●
    with fallopian tube N83.33-●
  oviduct (senile) —*see* Atrophy, fallopian tube
  palsy, diffuse (progressive) G12.22
  pancreas (duct) (senile) K86.89
  parotid gland K11.0
  pelvic muscle N81.84
  penis N48.89
  pharynx J39.2
  pluriglandular E31.8
    autoimmune E31.0
  polyarthritis M15.9
  prostate N42.89
  pseudohypertrophic (muscle) G71.0
  renal —*see also* Sclerosis, renal N26.1
  retina, retinal (postinfectional) H35.89
  rhinitis J31.0
  salivary gland K11.0
  scar L90.5
  sclerosis, lobar (of brain) G31.09 *[F02.80]*
    with behavioral disturbance G31.09
      [F02.81]
  scrotum N50.89
  seminal vesicle N50.89
  senile R54
    due to radiation (nonionizing) (solar) L57.8
  skin (patches) (spots) L90.9
    degenerative (senile) L90.8
    due to radiation (nonionizing) (solar) L57.8
    senile L90.8
  spermatic cord N50.89
  spinal (acute) (cord) G95.89
    muscular —*see* Atrophy, muscle, spinal
    paralysis G12.20
      acute —*see* Poliomyelitis, paralytic
      meaning progressive muscular atrophy
        G12.21
  spine (column) —*see* Spondylopathy,
    specified NEC
  spleen (senile) D73.0
  stomach K29.40
    with bleeding K29.41
  striate (skin) L90.6
    syphilitic A52.79
  subcutaneous L90.9
  sublingual gland K11.0
  submandibular gland K11.0
  submaxillary gland K11.0
  Sudeck's —*see* Algoneurodystrophy
  suprarenal (capsule) (gland) E27.49
    primary E27.1
  systemic affecting central nervous system
    in
      myxedema E03.9 *[G13.2]*
      neoplastic disease —*see also* Neoplasm
        D49.9 *[G13.1]*
      specified disease NEC G13.8
  tarso-orbital fascia, congenital Q10.3
  testis N50.0
  thenar, partial —*see* Syndrome, carpal tunnel
  thymus (fatty) E32.8
  thyroid (gland) (acquired) E03.4
    with cretinism E03.1
    congenital (with myxedema) E03.1
  tongue (senile) K14.8
    papillae K14.4
  trachea J39.8
  tunica vaginalis N50.89
  turbinate J34.89
  tympanic membrane (nonflaccid) H73.82-●
    flaccid H73.81-●
  upper respiratory tract J39.8

Atrophy, atrophic *(Continued)*
  uterus, uterine (senile) N85.8
    cervix N88.8
    due to radiation (intended effect)
      N85.8
      adverse effect or misadventure
        N99.89
  vagina (senile) N95.2
  vas deferens N50.89
  vascular I99.8
  vertebra (senile) —*see* Spondylopathy,
    specified NEC
  vulva (senile) N90.5
  Werdnig-Hoffmann G12.0
  yellow —*see* Failure, hepatic
Attack, attacks
  with alteration of consciousness (with
      automatisms) —*see* Epilepsy,
      localization-related, symptomatic, with
      complex partial seizures
  without alteration of consciousness —
      see Epilepsy, localization-related,
      symptomatic, with simple partial seizures
  Adams-Stokes I45.9
  akinetic —*see* Epilepsy, generalized, specified
      NEC
  angina —*see* Angina
  atonic —*see* Epilepsy, generalized, specified
      NEC
  benign shuddering G25.83
  cataleptic —*see* Catalepsy
  coronary —*see* Infarct, myocardium
  cyanotic, newborn P28.2
  drop NEC R55
  epileptic —*see* Epilepsy
  heart —*see* infarct, myocardium
  hysterical F44.9
  jacksonian —*see* Epilepsy, localization-
      related, symptomatic, with simple
      partial seizures
  myocardium, myocardial —*see* Infarct,
      myocardium
  myoclonic —*see* Epilepsy, generalized,
      specified NEC
  panic F41.0
  psychomotor —*see* Epilepsy, localization-
      related, symptomatic, with complex
      partial seizures
  salaam —*see* Epilepsy, spasms
  schizophreniform, brief F23
  shuddering, benign G25.83
  Stokes-Adams I45.9
  syncope R55
  transient ischemic (TIA) G45.9
    specified NEC G45.8
  unconsciousness R55
    hysterical F44.89
  vasomotor R55
  vasovagal (paroxysmal) (idiopathic) R55
Attention (to)
  artificial
    opening (of) Z43.9
      digestive tract NEC Z43.4
        colon Z43.3
        ilium Z43.2
        stomach Z43.1
      specified NEC Z43.8
      trachea Z43.0
      urinary tract NEC Z43.6
        cystostomy Z43.5
        nephrostomy Z43.6
        ureterostomy Z43.6
        urethrostomy Z43.6
      vagina Z43.7
  colostomy Z43.3
  cystostomy Z43.5
  deficit disorder or syndrome F98.8
    with hyperactivity —*see* Disorder,
        attention-deficit hyperactivity
  gastrostomy Z43.1
  ileostomy Z43.2

▶ New   ⟹ Revised   ~~deleted~~ Deleted   ● Use Additional Character(s)

Attention *(Continued)*
  jejunostomy Z43.4
  nephrostomy Z43.6
  surgical dressings Z48.01
  sutures Z48.02
  tracheostomy Z43.0
  ureterostomy Z43.6
  urethrostomy Z43.6
Attrition
  ➡gum —*see* Recession, gingival
  tooth, teeth (excessive) (hard tissues) K03.0
Atypical, atypism —*see also* condition
  cells (on cytolgocial smear) (endocervical)
      (endometrial) (glandular)
    cervix R87.619
    vagina R87.629
  cervical N87.9
  endometrium N85.9
    hyperplasia N85.00
  parenting situation Z62.9
Auditory —*see* condition
Aujeszky's disease B33.8
Aurantiasis, cutis E67.1
Auricle, auricular —*see also* condition
  cervical Q18.2
Auriculotemporal syndrome G50.8
Austin Flint murmur (aortic insufficiency)
    I35.1
Australian
  Q fever A78
  X disease A83.4
Autism, autistic (childhood) (infantile) F84.0
  atypical F84.9
  spectrum disorder F84.0
Autodigestion R68.89
Autoerythrocyte sensitization (syndrome)
    D69.2
Autographism L50.3
Autoimmune
  disease (systemic) M35.9
  inhibitors to clotting factors D68.311
  lymphoproliferative syndrome [ALPS]
      D89.82
  thyroiditis E06.3
Autointoxication R68.89
Automatism G93.89
  with temporal sclerosis G93.81
  epileptic —*see* Epilepsy, localization- related,
      symptomatic, with complex partial
      seizures

Automatism *(Continued)*
  paroxysmal, idiopathic —*see* Epilepsy,
      localization-related, symptomatic, with
      complex partial seizures
Autonomic, autonomous
  bladder (neurogenic) N31.2
  hysteria seizure F44.5
Autosensitivity, erythrocyte D69.2
Autosensitization, cutaneous L30.2
Autosome —*see* condition by chromosome
    involved
Autotopagnosia R48.1
Autotoxemia R68.89
Autumn —*see* condition
Avellis' syndrome G46.8
Aversion
  oral R63.3
    newborn P92.-●
    nonorganic origin F98.2
  sexual F52.1
Aviator's
  disease or sickness —*see* Effect, adverse, high
      altitude
  ear T70.0
Avitaminosis (multiple) —*see also* Deficiency,
      vitamin E56.9
  B E53.9
    with
      beriberi E51.11
      pellagra E52
  B2 E53.0
  B6 E53.1
  B12 E53.8
  D E55.9
    with rickets E55.0
  G E53.0
  K E56.1
  nicotinic acid E52
AVNRT (atrioventricular nodal re-entrant
    tachycardia) I47.1
AVRT (atrioventricular nodal re-entrant
    tachycardia) I47.1
Avulsion (traumatic)
  blood vessel —*see* Injury, blood vessel
  bone —*see* Fracture, by site
  cartilage —*see also* Dislocation, by site
    symphyseal (inner), complicating delivery
        O71.6
  external site other than limb —*see* Wound,
      open, by site

Avulsion *(Continued)*
  eye S05.7-●
  head (intracranial)
    external site NEC S08.89
    scalp S08.0
  internal organ or site —*see* Injury, by site
  joint —*see also* Dislocation, by site
    capsule —*see* Sprain, by site
  kidney S37.06-●
  ligament —*see* Sprain, by site
  limb —*see also* Amputation, traumatic,
      by site
    skin and subcutaneous tissue —*see* Wound,
        open, by site
  muscle —*see* Injury, muscle
  nerve (root) —*see* Injury, nerve
  scalp S08.0
  skin and subcutaneous tissue —*see* Wound,
      open, by site
  spleen S36.032
  symphyseal cartilage (inner), complicating
      delivery O71.6
  tendon —*see* Injury, muscle
  tooth S03.2
Awareness of heart beat R00.2
Axenfeld's
  anomaly or syndrome Q15.0
  degeneration (calcareous) Q13.4
Axilla, axillary —*see also* condition
  breast Q83.1
Axonotmesis —*see* Injury, nerve
Ayerza's disease or syndrome (pulmonary
    artery sclerosis with pulmonary
    hypertension) I27.0
Azoospermia (organic) N46.01
  due to
    drug therapy N46.021
    efferent duct obstruction N46.023
    infection N46.022
    radiation N46.024
    specified cause NEC N46.029
    systemic disease N46.025
Azotemia R79.89
  meaning uremia N19
Aztec ear Q17.3
Azygos
  continuation inferior vena cava Q26.8
  lobe (lung) Q33.1

A

B

Baastrup's disease —see Kissing spine
Babesiosis B60.0
Babington's disease (familial hemorrhagic telangiectasia) I78.0
Babinski's syndrome A52.79
Baby
  crying constantly R68.11
  floppy (syndrome) P94.2
Bacillary —see condition
Bacilluria R82.71
Bacillus —see also Infection, bacillus
  abortus infection A23.1
  anthracis infection A22.9
  coli infection —see also Escherichia coli B96.20
  Flexner's A03.1
  mallei infection A24.0
  Shiga's A03.0
  suipestifer infection —see Infection, salmonella
Back —see condition
Backache (postural) M54.9
  sacroiliac M53.3
  specified NEC M54.89
Backflow —see Reflux
Backward reading (dyslexia) F81.0
Bacteremia R78.81
  with sepsis —see Sepsis
Bactericholia —see Cholecystitis, acute
Bacterid, bacteride (pustular) L40.3
Bacterium, bacteria, bacterial
  agent NEC, as cause of disease classified elsewhere B96.89
  in blood —see Bacteremia
  in urine —see Bacteriuria
Bacteriuria, bacteruria R82.71
  asymptomatic R82.71
Bacteroides
  fragilis, as cause of disease classified elsewhere B96.6
Bad
  heart —see Disease, heart
  trip
    due to drug abuse —see Abuse, drug, hallucinogen
    due to drug dependence —see Dependence, drug, hallucinogen
Baelz's disease (cheilitis glandularis apostematosa) K13.0
Baerensprung's disease (eczema marginatum) B35.6
Bagasse disease or pneumonitis J67.1
Bagassosis J67.1
Baker's cyst —see Cyst, Baker's
Bakwin-Krida syndrome (metaphyseal dysplasia) Q78.5
Balancing side interference M26.56
Balanitis (circinata) (erosiva) (gangrenosa) (phagedenic) (vulgaris) N48.1
  amebic A06.82
  candidal B37.42
  due to Haemophilus ducreyi A57
  gonococcal (acute) (chronic) A54.09
  xerotica obliterans N48.0
Balanoposthitis N47.6
  gonococcal (acute) (chronic) A54.09
  ulcerative (specific) A63.8
Balanorrhagia —see Balanitis
Balantidiasis, balantidiosis A07.0
Bald tongue K14.4
Baldness —see also Alopecia
  male-pattern —see Alopecia, androgenic
Balkan grippe A78
Balloon disease —see Effect, adverse, high altitude
Balo's disease (concentric sclerosis) G37.5
Bamberger-Marie disease —see Osteoarthropathy, hypertrophic, specified type NEC
Bancroft's filariasis B74.0

Band(s)
  adhesive —see Adhesions, peritoneum
  anomalous or congenital —see also Anomaly, by site
    heart (atrial) (ventricular) Q24.8
    intestine Q43.3
    omentum Q43.3
  cervix N88.1
  constricting, congenital Q79.8
  gallbladder (congenital) Q44.1
  intestinal (adhesive) —see Adhesions, peritoneum
  obstructive
    intestine K56.50
      complete K56.52
      incomplete K56.51
      partial K56.51
    peritoneum K56.50
      complete K56.52
      incomplete K56.51
      partial K56.51
  periappendiceal, congenital Q43.3
  peritoneal (adhesive) —see Adhesions, peritoneum
  uterus N73.6
    internal N85.6
  vagina N89.5
Bandemia D72.825
Bandl's ring (contraction), complicating delivery O62.4
Bangkok hemorrhagic fever A91
Bang's disease (brucella abortus) A23.1
Bankruptcy, anxiety concerning Z59.8
Bannister's disease T78.3
  hereditary D84.1
Banti's disease or syndrome (with cirrhosis) (with portal hypertension) K76.6
Bar, median, prostate —see Enlargement, enlarged, prostate
Barcoo disease or rot —see Ulcer, skin
Barlow's disease E54
Barodontalgia T70.29
Baron Münchausen syndrome —see Disorder, factitious
Barosinusitis T70.1
Barotitis T70.0
Barotrauma T70.29
  odontalgia T70.29
  otitic T70.0
  sinus T70.1
Barraquer (-Simons) disease or syndrome (progressive lipodystrophy) E88.1
Barré-Guillain disease or syndrome G61.0
Barré-Liéou syndrome (posterior cervical sympathetic) M53.0
Barrel chest M95.4
Barrett's
  disease —see Barrett's, esophagus
  esophagus K22.70
    with dysplasia K22.719
      high grade K22.711
      low grade K22.710
    without dysplasia K22.70
  syndrome —see Barrett's, esophagus
  ulcer K22.10
    with bleeding K22.11
    without bleeding K22.10
Barth syndrome E78.71
Bársony (-Polgár) (-Teschendorf) syndrome (corkscrew esophagus) K22.4
Bartholinitis (suppurating) N75.8
  gonococcal (acute) (chronic) (with abscess) A54.1
Bartonellosis A44.9
  cutaneous A44.1
  mucocutaneous A44.1
  specified NEC A44.8
  systemic A44.0
Barton's fracture S52.56-
Bartter's syndrome E26.81
Basal —see condition

Basan's (hidrotic) ectodermal dysplasia Q82.4
Baseball finger —see Dislocation, finger
Basedow's disease (exophthalmic goiter) —see Hyperthyroidism, with, goiter
Basic —see condition
Basilar —see condition
Bason's (hidrotic) ectodermal dysplasia Q82.4
Basopenia —see Agranulocytosis
Basophilia D72.824
Basophilism (cortico-adrenal) (Cushing's) (pituitary) E24.0
Bassen-Kornzweig disease or syndrome E78.6
Bat ear Q17.5
Bateman's
  disease B08.1
  purpura (senile) D69.2
Bathing cramp T75.1
Bathophobia F40.248
Batten (-Mayou) disease E75.4
  retina E75.4 [H36]
Batten-Steinert syndrome G71.11
Battered —see Maltreatment
Battey Mycobacterium infection A31.0
Battle exhaustion F43.0
Battledore placenta O43.19-
Baumgarten-Cruveilhier cirrhosis, disease or syndrome K74.69
Bauxite fibrosis (of lung) J63.1
Bayle's disease (general paresis) A52.17
Bazin's disease (primary) (tuberculous) A18.4
Beach ear —see Swimmer's, ear
Beaded hair (congenital) Q84.1
Béal conjunctivitis or syndrome B30.2
Beard's disease (neurasthenia) F48.8
Beat(s)
  atrial, premature I49.1
  ectopic I49.49
  elbow —see Bursitis, elbow
  escaped, heart I49.49
  hand —see Bursitis, hand
  knee —see Bursitis, knee
  premature I49.40
    atrial I49.1
    auricular I49.1
    supraventricular I49.1
Beau's
  disease or syndrome —see Degeneration, myocardial
  lines (transverse furrows on fingernails) L60.4
Bechterev's syndrome —see Spondylitis, ankylosing
Beck's syndrome (anterior spinal artery occlusion) I65.8
Becker's
  cardiomyopathy I42.8
  disease
    idiopathic mural endomyocardial disease I42.3
    myotonia congenita, recessive form G71.12
  dystrophy G71.0
  pigmented hairy nevus D22.5
Beckwith-Wiedemann syndrome Q87.3
Bed confinement status Z74.01
Bed sore —see Ulcer, pressure, by site
Bedbug bite(s) —see Bite(s), by site, superficial, insect
Bedclothes, asphyxiation or suffocation by —see Asphyxia, traumatic, due to, mechanical, trapped
Bednar's
  aphthae K12.0
  tumor —see Neoplasm, malignant, by site
Bedridden Z74.01
Bedsore —see Ulcer, pressure, by site
Bedwetting —see Enuresis
Bee sting (with allergic or anaphylactic shock) —see Toxicity, venom, arthropod, bee
Beer drinker's heart (disease) I42.6
Begbie's disease (exophthalmic goiter) —see Hyperthyroidism, with, goiter

▶ New ⇒ Revised deleted Deleted ● Use Additional Character(s)

Behavior
  antisocial
    adult Z72.811
    child or adolescent Z72.810
  disorder, disturbance —see Disorder, conduct
  disruptive —see Disorder, conduct
  drug seeking Z76.5
  inexplicable R46.2
  marked evasiveness R46.5
  obsessive-compulsive R46.81
  overactivity R46.3
  poor responsiveness R46.4
  self-damaging (life-style) Z72.89
  sleep-incompatible Z72.821
  slowness R46.4
  specified NEC R46.89
  strange (and inexplicable) R46.2
  suspiciousness R46.5
  type A pattern Z73.1
  undue concern or preoccupation with
    stressful events R46.6
  verbosity and circumstantial detail obscuring
    reason for contact R46.7
Behcet's disease or syndrome M35.2
Behr's disease —see Degeneration, macula
Beigel's disease or morbus (white piedra)
  B36.2
Bejel A65
Bekhterev's syndrome —see Spondylitis,
  ankylosing
Belching —see Eructation
Bell's
  mania F30.8
  palsy, paralysis G51.0
    infant or newborn P11.3
  spasm G51.3
Bence Jones albuminuria or proteinuria NEC
  R80.3
Bends T70.3
Benedikt's paralysis or syndrome G46.3
Benign (see also condition)
  prostatic hyperplasia —see Hyperplasia,
    prostate
Bennett's fracture (displaced) S62.21-●
Benson's disease —see Deposit, crystalline
Bent
  back (hysterical) F44.4
  nose M95.0
    congenital Q67.4
Bereavement (uncomplicated) Z63.4
Bergeron's disease (hysterical chorea) F44.4
Berger's disease —see Nephropathy, IgA
Beriberi (dry) E51.11
  heart (disease) E51.12
  polyneuropathy E51.11
  wet E51.12
    involving circulatory system E51.11
Berlin's disease or edema (traumatic) S05.8X-●
Berlock (berloque) dermatitis L56.2
Bernard-Horner syndrome G90.2
Bernard-Soulier disease or thrombopathia
  D69.1
Bernhardt (-Roth) disease —see
  Mononeuropathy, lower limb, meralgia
  paresthetica
Bernheim's syndrome —see Failure, heart,
  right
Bertielliasis B71.8
Berylliosis (lung) J63.2
Besnier-Boeck (-Schaumann) disease —see
  Sarcoidosis
Besnier's
  lupus pernio D86.3
  prurigo L20.0
Bestiality F65.89
Best's disease H35.50
Beta-mercaptolactate-cysteine disulfiduria
  E72.09
Betalipoproteinemia, broad or floating E78.2
Betting and gambling Z72.6
  pathological (compulsive) F63.0

Bezoar T18.9
  intestine T18.3
  stomach T18.2
Bezold's abscess —see Mastoiditis, acute
Bianchi's syndrome R48.8
Bicornate or bicornis uterus Q51.3
  in pregnancy or childbirth O34.00
    causing obstructed labor O65.5
Bicuspid aortic valve Q23.1
Biedl-Bardet syndrome Q87.89
Bielschowsky (-Jansky) disease E75.4
Biermer's (pernicious) anemia or disease D51.0
Biett's disease L93.0
Bifid (congenital)
  apex, heart Q24.8
  clitoris Q52.6
  kidney Q63.8
  nose Q30.2
  patella Q74.1
  scrotum Q55.29
  toe NEC Q74.2
  tongue Q38.3
  ureter Q62.8
  uterus Q51.3
  uvula Q35.7
Biforis uterus (suprasimplex) Q51.3
Bifurcation (congenital)
  gallbladder Q44.1
  kidney pelvis Q63.8
  renal pelvis Q63.8
  rib Q76.6
  tongue, congenital Q38.3
  trachea Q32.1
  ureter Q62.8
  urethra Q64.74
  vertebra Q76.49
Big spleen syndrome D73.1
Bigeminal pulse R00.8
Bilateral —see condition
Bile
  duct —see condition
  pigments in urine R82.2
Bilharziasis —see also Schistosomiasis
  chyluria B65.0
  cutaneous B65.3
  galacturia B65.0
  hematochyluria B65.0
  intestinal B65.1
  lipemia B65.9
  lipuria B65.0
  oriental B65.2
  piarhemia B65.9
  pulmonary NOS B65.9 [J99]
    pneumonia B65.9 [J17]
  tropical hematuria B65.0
  vesical B65.0
Biliary —see condition
Bilirubin metabolism disorder E80.7
  specified NEC E80.6
Bilirubinemia, familial nonhemolytic E80.4
Bilirubinuria R82.2
Biliuria R82.2
Bilocular stomach K31.2
Binswanger's disease I67.3
Biparta, bipartite
  carpal scaphoid Q74.0
  patella Q74.1
  vagina Q52.10
Bird
  face Q75.8
  fancier's disease or lung J67.2
Birt-Hogg-Dube syndrome Q87.89
Birth
  complications in mother —see Delivery,
    complicated
  compression during NOS P15.9
  defect —see Anomaly
  immature (less than 37 completed weeks) —
    see Preterm, newborn
  extremely (less than 28 completed
    weeks) —see Immaturity, extreme

Birth (Continued)
  inattention, at or after —see Maltreatment,
    child, neglect
  injury NOS P15.9
    basal ganglia P11.1
    brachial plexus NEC P14.3
    brain (compression) (pressure) P11.2
    central nervous system NOS P11.9
    cerebellum P11.1
    cerebral hemorrhage P10.1
    external genitalia P15.5
    eye P15.3
    face P15.4
    fracture
      bone P13.9
        specified NEC P13.8
      clavicle P13.4
      femur P13.2
      humerus P13.3
      long bone, except femur P13.3
      radius and ulna P13.3
      skull P13.0
      spine P11.5
      tibia and fibula P13.3
    intracranial P11.2
      laceration or hemorrhage P10.9
        specified NEC P10.8
    intraventricular hemorrhage P10.2
    laceration
      brain P10.1
      by scalpel P15.8
      peripheral nerve P14.9
    liver P15.0
    meninges
      brain P11.1
      spinal cord P11.5
    nerve
      brachial plexus P14.3
      cranial NEC (except facial) P11.4
      facial P11.3
      peripheral P14.9
      phrenic (paralysis) P14.2
    paralysis
      facial nerve P11.3
      spinal P11.5
    penis P15.5
    rupture
      spinal cord P11.5
    scalp P12.9
    scalpel wound P15.8
    scrotum P15.5
    skull NEC P13.1
      fracture P13.0
    specified type NEC P15.8
    spinal cord P11.5
    spine P11.5
    spleen P15.1
    sternomastoid (hematoma) P15.2
    subarachnoid hemorrhage P10.3
    subcutaneous fat necrosis P15.6
    subdural hemorrhage P10.0
    tentorial tear P10.4
    testes P15.5
    vulva P15.5
  lack of care, at or after —see Maltreatment,
    child, neglect
  neglect, at or after —see Maltreatment, child,
    neglect
  palsy or paralysis, newborn, NOS (birth
    injury) P14.9
  premature (infant) —see Preterm, newborn
  shock, newborn P96.89
  trauma —see Birth, injury
  weight
    4000 grams to 4499 grams P08.1
    4500 grams or more P08.0
    low (2499 grams or less) —see Low,
      birthweight
      extremely (999 grams or less) —see Low,
        birthweight, extreme
Birthmark Q82.5

Bisalbuminemia E88.09
Biskra's button B55.1
Bite(s) (animal) (human)
  abdomen, abdominal
    wall S31.159
      with penetration into peritoneal cavity
        S31.659
      epigastric region S31.152
        with penetration into peritoneal cavity
          S31.652
      left
        lower quadrant S31.154
          with penetration into peritoneal
            cavity S31.654
        upper quadrant S31.151
          with penetration into peritoneal
            cavity S31.651
      periumbilic region S31.155
        with penetration into peritoneal cavity
          S31.655
      right
        lower quadrant S31.153
          with penetration into peritoneal
            cavity S31.653
        upper quadrant S31.150
          with penetration into peritoneal
            cavity S31.650
      superficial NEC S30.871
        insect S30.861
  alveolar (process) —see Bite, oral cavity
  amphibian (venomous) —see Venom, bite,
    amphibian
  animal —see also Bite, by site
    venomous —see Venom
  ankle S91.05-●
    superficial NEC S90.57-●
      insect S90.56-●
  antecubital space —see Bite, elbow
  anus S31.835
    superficial NEC S30.877
      insect S30.867
  arm (upper) S41.15-●
    lower —see Bite, forearm
    superficial NEC S40.87-●
      insect S40.86-●
  arthropod NEC —see Venom, bite, arthropod
  auditory canal (external) (meatus) —
    see Bite, ear
  auricle, ear —see Bite, ear
  axilla —see Bite, arm
  back —see also Bite, thorax, back
    lower S31.050
      with penetration into retroperitoneal
        space S31.051
      superficial NEC S30.870
        insect S30.860
  bedbug —see Bite(s), by site, superficial,
    insect
  breast S21.05-●
    superficial NEC S20.17-●
      insect S20.16-●
  brow —see Bite, head, specified site NEC
  buttock S31.805
    left S31.825
    right S31.815
    superficial NEC S30.870
      insect S30.860
  calf —see Bite, leg
  canaliculus lacrimalis —see Bite, eyelid
  canthus, eye —see Bite, eyelid
  centipede —see Toxicity, venom, arthropod,
    centipede
  cheek (external) S01.45-●
    internal —see Bite, oral cavity
    superficial NEC S00.87
      insect S00.86
  chest wall —see Bite, thorax
  chigger B88.0
  chin —see Bite, head, specified site NEC
  clitoris —see Bite, vulva
  costal region —see Bite, thorax

Bite (Continued)
  digit(s)
    hand —see Bite, finger
    toe —see Bite, toe
  ear (canal) (external) S01.35-●
    superficial NEC S00.47-●
      insect S00.46-●
  elbow S51.05-●
    superficial NEC S50.37-●
      insect S50.36-●
  epididymis —see Bite, testis
  epigastric region —see Bite, abdomen
  epiglottis —see Bite, neck, specified site
    NEC
  esophagus, cervical S11.25
    superficial NEC S10.17
      insect S10.16
  eyebrow —see Bite, eyelid
  eyelid S01.15-●
    superficial NEC S00.27-●
      insect S00.26-●
  face NEC —see Bite, head, specified site
    NEC
  finger(s) S61.259
    with
      damage to nail S61.359
    index S61.258
      with
        damage to nail S61.358
      left S61.251
        with
          damage to nail S61.351
      right S61.250
        with
          damage to nail S61.350
      superficial NEC S60.478
        insect S60.46-●
    little S61.25-●
      with
        damage to nail S61.35-●
      superficial NEC S60.47-●
        insect S60.46-●
    middle S61.25-●
      with
        damage to nail S61.35-●
      superficial NEC S60.47-●
        insect S60.46-●
    ring S61.25-●
      with
        damage to nail S61.35-●
      superficial NEC S60.47-●
        insect S60.46-●
    superficial NEC S60.479
      insect S60.469
    thumb —see Bite, thumb
  flank —see Bite, abdomen, wall
  flea —see Bite, by site, superficial,
    insect
  foot (except toe(s) alone) S91.35-●
    superficial NEC S90.87-●
      insect S90.86-●
    toe —see Bite, toe
  forearm S51.85-●
    elbow only —see Bite, elbow
    superficial NEC S50.87-●
      insect S50.86-●
  forehead —see Bite, head, specified site
    NEC
  genital organs, external
    female S31.552
      superficial NEC S30.876
        insect S30.866
      vagina and vulva —see Bite, vulva
    male S31.551
      penis —see Bite, penis
      scrotum —see Bite, scrotum
      superficial NEC S30.875
        insect S30.865
      testes —see Bite, testis
  groin —see Bite, abdomen, wall
  gum —see Bite, oral cavity

Bite (Continued)
  hand S61.45-●
    finger —see Bite, finger
    superficial NEC S60.57-●
      insect S60.56-●
    thumb —see Bite, thumb
  head S01.95
    cheek —see Bite, cheek
    ear —see Bite, ear
    eyelid —see Bite, eyelid
    lip —see Bite, lip
    nose —see Bite, nose
    oral cavity —see Bite, oral cavity
    scalp —see Bite, scalp
    specified site NEC S01.85
      superficial NEC S00.87
        insect S00.86
    superficial NEC S00.97
      insect S00.96
    temporomandibular area —see Bite, cheek
  heel —see Bite, foot
  hip S71.05-●
    superficial NEC S70.27-●
      insect S70.26-●
  hymen S31.45
  hypochondrium —see Bite, abdomen, wall
  hypogastric region —see Bite, abdomen, wall
  inguinal region —see Bite, abdomen, wall
  insect —see Bite, by site, superficial, insect
  instep —see Bite, foot
  interscapular region —see Bite, thorax, back
  jaw —see Bite, head, specified site NEC
  knee S81.05-●
    superficial NEC S80.27-●
      insect S80.26-●
  labium (majus) (minus) —see Bite, vulva
  lacrimal duct —see Bite, eyelid
  larynx S11.015
    superficial NEC S10.17
      insect S10.16
  leg (lower) S81.85-●
    ankle —see Bite, ankle
    foot —see Bite, foot
    knee —see Bite, knee
    superficial NEC S80.87-●
      insect S80.86-●
    toe —see Bite, toe
    upper —see Bite, thigh
  lip S01.551
    superficial NEC S00.571
      insect S00.561
  lizard (venomous) —see Venom, bite, reptile
  loin —see Bite, abdomen, wall
  lower back —see Bite, back, lower
  lumbar region —see Bite, back, lower
  malar region —see Bite, head, specified site
    NEC
  mammary —see Bite, breast
  marine animals (venomous) —see Toxicity,
    venom, marine animal
  mastoid region —see Bite, head, specified site
    NEC
  mouth —see Bite, oral cavity
  nail
    finger —see Bite, finger
    toe —see Bite, toe
  nape —see Bite, neck, specified site NEC
  nasal (septum) (sinus) —see Bite, nose
  nasopharynx —see Bite, head, specified site
    NEC
  neck S11.95
    involving
      cervical esophagus —see Bite,
        esophagus, cervical
      larynx —see Bite, larynx
      pharynx —see Bite, pharynx
      thyroid gland S11.15
      trachea —see Bite, trachea
    specified site NEC S11.85
      superficial NEC S10.87
        insect S10.86

▶ New   ➡ Revised   ~~deleted~~ Deleted   ● Use Additional Character(s)

Bite *(Continued)*
  neck *(Continued)*
    superficial NEC S10.97
      insect S10.96
    throat S11.85
      superficial NEC S10.17
        insect S10.16
  nose (septum) (sinus) S01.25
    superficial NEC S00.37
      insect S00.36
  occipital region —*see* Bite, scalp
  oral cavity S01.552
    superficial NEC S00.572
      insect S00.562
  orbital region —*see* Bite, eyelid
  palate —*see* Bite, oral cavity
  palm —*see* Bite, hand
  parietal region —*see* Bite, scalp
  pelvis S31.050
    with penetration into retroperitoneal space
      S31.051
    superficial NEC S30.870
      insect S30.860
  penis S31.25
    superficial NEC S30.872
      insect S30.862
  perineum
    female —*see* Bite, vulva
    male —*see* Bite, pelvis
  periocular area (with or without lacrimal
    passages) —*see* Bite, eyelid
  phalanges
    finger —*see* Bite, finger
    toe —*see* Bite, toe
  pharynx S11.25
    superficial NEC S10.17
      insect S10.16
  pinna —*see* Bite, ear
  poisonous —*see* Venom
  popliteal space —*see* Bite, knee
  prepuce —*see* Bite, penis
  pubic region —*see* Bite, abdomen, wall
  rectovaginal septum —*see* Bite, vulva
  red bug B88.0
  reptile NEC —*see also* Venom, bite,
    reptile
    nonvenomous —*see* Bite, by site
    snake —*see* Venom, bite, snake
  sacral region —*see* Bite, back, lower
  sacroiliac region —*see* Bite, back, lower
  salivary gland —*see* Bite, oral cavity
  scalp S01.05
    superficial NEC S00.07
      insect S00.06
  scapular region —*see* Bite, shoulder
  scrotum S31.35
    superficial NEC S30.873
      insect S30.863
  sea-snake (venomous) —*see* Toxicity, venom,
    snake, sea snake
  shin —*see* Bite, leg
  shoulder S41.05-●
    superficial NEC S40.27-●
      insect S40.26-●
  snake —*see also* Venom, bite, snake
    nonvenomous —*see* Bite, by site
  spermatic cord —*see* Bite, testis
  spider (venomous) —*see* Toxicity, venom,
    spider
    nonvenomous —*see* Bite, by site,
      superficial, insect
  sternal region —*see* Bite, thorax, front
  submaxillary region —*see* Bite, head,
    specified site NEC
  submental region —*see* Bite, head, specified
    site NEC
  subungual
    finger(s) —*see* Bite, finger
    toe —*see* Bite, toe
  superficial —*see* Bite, by site, superficial
  supraclavicular fossa S11.85

Bite *(Continued)*
  supraorbital —*see* Bite, head, specified site
    NEC
  temple, temporal region —*see* Bite, head,
    specified site NEC
  temporomandibular area —*see* Bite, cheek
  testis S31.35
    superficial NEC S30.873
      insect S30.863
  thigh S71.15-●
    superficial NEC S70.37-●
      insect S70.36-●
  thorax, thoracic (wall) S21.95
    back S21.25-●
      with penetration into thoracic cavity
        S21.45-●
    breast —*see* Bite, breast
    front S21.15-●
      with penetration into thoracic cavity
        S21.35-●
    superficial NEC S20.97
      back S20.47-●
      front S20.37-●
      insect S20.96
        back S20.46-●
        front S20.36-●
  throat —*see* Bite, neck, throat
  thumb S61.05-●
    with
      damage to nail S61.15-●
    superficial NEC S60.37-●
      insect S60.36-●
  thyroid S11.15
    superficial NEC S10.87
      insect S10.86
  toe(s) S91.15-●
    with
      damage to nail S91.25-●
    great S91.15-●
      with
        damage to nail S91.25-●
    lesser S91.15-●
      with
        damage to nail S91.25-●
    superficial NEC S90.47-●
      great S90.47-●
      insect S90.46-●
        great S90.46-●
  tongue S01.552
  trachea S11.025
    superficial NEC S10.17
      insect S10.16
  tunica vaginalis —*see* Bite, testis
  tympanum, tympanic membrane —*see* Bite,
    ear
  umbilical region S31.155
  uvula —*see* Bite, oral cavity
  vagina —*see* Bite, vulva
  venomous —*see* Venom
  vocal cords S11.035
    superficial NEC S10.17
      insect S10.16
  vulva S31.45
    superficial NEC S30.874
      insect S30.864
  wrist S61.55-●
    superficial NEC S60.87-●
      insect S60.86-●
Biting, cheek or lip K13.1
➡ Biventricular failure (heart) I50.82
Björck (-Thorson) syndrome (malignant
  carcinoid) E34.0
Black
  death A20.9
  eye S00.1-●
  hairy tongue K14.3
  heel (foot) S90.3-●
  lung (disease) J60
  palm (hand) S60.22-●
Blackfan-Diamond anemia or syndrome
  (congenital hypoplastic anemia) D61.01

Blackhead L70.0
Blackout R55
Bladder —*see* condition
Blast (air) (hydraulic) (immersion) (underwater)
  blindness S05.8X-●
  injury
    abdomen or thorax —*see* Injury, by site
    ear (acoustic nerve trauma) —*see* Injury,
      nerve, acoustic, specified type NEC
    syndrome NEC T70.8
Blastoma —*see* Neoplasm, malignant, by site
  pulmonary —*see* Neoplasm, lung, malignant
Blastomycosis, blastomycotic B40.9
  Brazilian —*see* Paracoccidioidomycosis
  cutaneous B40.3
  disseminated B40.7
  European —*see* Cryptococcosis
  generalized B40.7
  keloidal B48.0
  North American B40.9
  primary pulmonary B40.0
  pulmonary B40.2
    acute B40.0
    chronic B40.1
  skin B40.3
  South American —*see*
    Paracoccidioidomycosis
  specified NEC B40.89
Bleb(s) R23.8
  emphysematous (lung) (solitary) J43.9
  endophthalmitis H59.43
  filtering (vitreous), after glaucoma surgery
    Z98.83
  inflamed (infected), postprocedural H59.40
    stage 1 H59.41
    stage 2 H59.42
    stage 3 H59.43
  lung (ruptured) J43.9
    congenital —*see* Atelectasis
    newborn P25.8
  subpleural (emphysematous) J43.9
Blebitis, postprocedural H59.40
  stage 1 H59.41
  stage 2 H59.42
  stage 3 H59.43
Bleeder (familial) (hereditary) —*see* Hemophilia
Bleeding —*see also* Hemorrhage
  anal K62.5
  anovulatory N97.0
  atonic, following delivery O72.1
  capillary I78.8
    puerperal O72.2
  contact (postcoital) N93.0
  due to uterine subinvolution N85.3
  ear —*see* Otorrhagia
  excessive, associated with menopausal onset
    N92.4
  familial —*see* Defect, coagulation
  following intercourse N93.0
  gastrointestinal K92.2
  hemorrhoids —*see* Hemorrhoids
  intermenstrual (regular) N92.3
    irregular N92.1
  intraoperative —*see* Complication,
    intraoperative, hemorrhage
  irregular N92.6
  menopausal N92.4
  newborn, intraventricular —*see* Newborn,
    affected by, hemorrhage, intraventricular
  nipple N64.59
  nose R04.0
  ovulation N92.3
  postclimacteric N95.0
  postcoital N93.0
  postmenopausal N95.0
  postoperative —*see* Complication,
    postprocedural, hemorrhage
  preclimacteric N92.4
  pre-pubertal vaginal N93.1
  puberty (excessive, with onset of menstrual
    periods) N92.2

Bleeding *(Continued)*
rectum, rectal K62.5
newborn P54.2
tendencies —*see* Defect, coagulation
throat R04.1
tooth socket (post-extraction) K91.840
umbilical stump P51.9
uterus, uterine NEC N93.9
climacteric N92.4
dysfunctional or functional N93.8
menopausal N92.4
preclimacteric or premenopausal N92.4
unrelated to menstrual cycle N93.9
vagina, vaginal (abnormal) N93.9
dysfunctional or functional N93.8
newborn P54.6
pre-pubertal N93.1
vicarious N94.89
Blennorrhagia, blennorrhagic —*see* Gonorrhea
Blennorrhea (acute) (chronic) —*see also*
Gonorrhea
inclusion (neonatal) (newborn) P39.1
lower genitourinary tract (gonococcal)
A54.00
neonatorum (gonococcal ophthalmia)
A54.31
Blepharelosis —*see* Entropion
Blepharitis (angularis) (ciliaris) (eyelid)
(marginal) (nonulcerative) H01.009
herpes zoster B02.39
left H01.006
lower H01.005
upper H01.004
right H01.003
lower H01.002
upper H01.001
squamous H01.029
left H01.026
lower H01.025
upper H01.024
right H01.023
lower H01.022
upper H01.021
ulcerative H01.019
left H01.016
lower H01.015
upper H01.014
right H01.013
lower H01.012
upper H01.011
Blepharochalasis H02.30
congenital Q10.0
left H02.36
lower H02.35
upper H02.34
right H02.33
lower H02.32
upper H02.31
Blepharoclonus H02.59
Blepharoconjunctivitis H10.50-●
angular H10.52-●
contact H10.53-●
ligneous H10.51-●
Blepharophimosis (eyelid) H02.529
congenital Q10.3
left H02.526
lower H02.525
upper H02.524
right H02.523
lower H02.522
upper H02.521
Blepharoptosis H02.40-●
congenital Q10.0
mechanical H02.41-●
myogenic H02.42-●
neurogenic H02.43-●
paralytic H02.43-●
Blepharopyorrhea, gonococcal A54.39
Blepharospasm G24.5
drug induced G24.01
Blighted ovum O02.0

Blind —*see also* Blindness
bronchus (congenital) Q32.4
loop syndrome K90.2
congenital Q43.8
sac, fallopian tube (congenital) Q50.6
spot, enlarged —*see* Defect, visual field,
localized, scotoma, blind spot area
tract or tube, congenital NEC —*see* Atresia,
by site
▶**Blindness** (acquired) (congenital) (both eyes)
H54.0X-●
blast S05.8X-●
color —*see* Deficiency, color vision
concussion S05.8X-●
cortical H47.619
left brain H47.612
right brain H47.611
day H53.11
due to injury (current episode) S05.9-●
sequelae — code to injury with seventh
character S
eclipse (total) —*see* Retinopathy, solar
emotional (hysterical) F44.6
face H53.16
hysterical F44.6
legal (both eyes) (USA definition) H54.8
mind R48.8
night H53.60
abnormal dark adaptation curve H53.61
acquired H53.62
congenital H53.63
specified type NEC H53.69
vitamin A deficiency E50.5
one eye (other eye normal) H54.40
▶left (normal vision on right) H54.42-●
▶low vision on right H54.12-●
low vision, other eye H54.10
▶right (normal vision on left) H54.41-●
▶low vision on left H54.11-●
psychic R48.8
river B73.01
snow —*see* Photokeratitis
sun, solar —*see* Retinopathy, solar
transient —*see* Disturbance, vision, subjective,
loss, transient
traumatic (current episode) S05.9-●
word (developmental) F81.0
acquired R48.0
secondary to organic lesion R48.0
Blister (nonthermal)
abdominal wall S30.821
alveolar process S00.522
ankle S90.52-●
antecubital space —*see* Blister, elbow
anus S30.827
arm (upper) S40.82-●
auditory canal —*see* Blister, ear
auricle —*see* Blister, ear
axilla —*see* Blister, arm
back, lower S30.820
beetle dermatitis L24.89
breast S20.12-●
brow S00.82
calf —*see* Blister, leg
canthus —*see* Blister, eyelid
cheek S00.82
internal S00.522
chest wall —*see* Blister, thorax
chin S00.82
costal region —*see* Blister, thorax
digit(s)
foot —*see* Blister, toe
hand —*see* Blister, finger
due to burn —*see* Burn, by site, second degree
ear S00.42-●
elbow S50.32-●
epiglottis S10.12
esophagus, cervical S10.12
eyebrow —*see* Blister, eyelid
eyelid S00.22-●
face S00.82

Blister *(Continued)*
fever B00.1
finger(s) S60.429
index S60.42-●
little S60.42-●
middle S60.42-●
ring S60.42-●
foot (except toe(s) alone) S90.82-●
toe —*see* Blister, toe
forearm S50.82-●
elbow only —*see* Blister, elbow
forehead S00.82
fracture - omit code
genital organ
female S30.826
male S30.825
gum S00.522
hand S60.52-●
head S00.92
ear —*see* Blister, ear
eyelid —*see* Blister, eyelid
lip S00.521
nose S00.32
oral cavity S00.522
scalp S00.02
specified site NEC S00.82
heel —*see* Blister, foot
hip S70.22-●
interscapular region S20.429
jaw S00.82
knee S80.22-●
larynx S10.12
leg (lower) S80.82-●
knee —*see* Blister, knee
upper —*see* Blister, thigh
lip S00.521
malar region S00.82
mammary —*see* Blister, breast
mastoid region S00.82
mouth S00.522
multiple, skin, nontraumatic R23.8
nail
finger —*see* Blister, finger
toe —*see* Blister, toe
nasal S00.32
neck S10.92
specified site NEC S10.82
throat S10.12
nose S00.32
occipital region S00.02
oral cavity S00.522
orbital region —*see* Blister, eyelid
palate S00.522
palm —*see* Blister, hand
parietal region S00.02
pelvis S30.820
penis S30.822
periocular area —*see* Blister, eyelid
phalanges
finger —*see* Blister, finger
toe —*see* Blister, toe
pharynx S10.12
pinna —*see* Blister, ear
popliteal space —*see* Blister, knee
scalp S00.02
scapular region —*see* Blister, shoulder
scrotum S30.823
shin —*see* Blister, leg
shoulder S40.22-●
sternal region S20.329
submaxillary region S00.82
submental region S00.82
subungual
finger(s) —*see* Blister, finger
toe(s) —*see* Blister, toe
supraclavicular fossa S10.82
supraorbital S00.82
temple S00.82
temporal region S00.82
testis S30.823
thermal —*see* Burn, second degree, by site

▶ New   ➡ Revised   ~~deleted~~ Deleted   ● Use Additional Character(s)

Blister (Continued)
  thigh S70.32-●
  thorax, thoracic (wall) S20.92
    back S20.42-●
    front S20.32-●
  throat S10.12
  thumb S60.32-●
  toe(s) S90.42-●
    great S90.42-●
  tongue S00.522
  trachea S10.12
  tympanum, tympanic membrane —see Blister,
    ear
  upper arm —see Blister, arm (upper)
  uvula S00.522
  vagina S30.824
  vocal cords S10.12
  vulva S30.824
  wrist S60.82-●
Bloating R14.0
Bloch-Sulzberger disease or syndrome Q82.3
Block, blocked
  alveolocapillary J84.10
  arborization (heart) I45.5
  arrhythmic I45.9
  atrioventricular (incomplete) (partial) I44.30
    with atrioventricular dissociation I44.2
    complete I44.2
      congenital Q24.6
    congenital Q24.6
    first degree I44.0
    second degree (types I and II) I44.1
    specified NEC I44.39
    third degree I44.2
    types I and II I44.1
  auriculoventricular —see Block,
    atrioventricular
  bifascicular (cardiac) I45.2
  bundle-branch (complete) (false) (incomplete)
    I45.4
    bilateral I45.2
    left I44.7
      with right bundle branch block I45.2
      hemiblock I44.60
        anterior I44.4
        posterior I44.5
      incomplete I44.7
        with right bundle branch block I45.2
    right I45.10
      with
        left bundle branch block I45.2
        left fascicular block I45.2
      specified NEC I45.19
    Wilson's type I45.19
  cardiac I45.9
  conduction I45.9
    complete I44.2
  fascicular (left) I44.60
    anterior I44.4
    posterior I44.5
    right I45.0
    specified NEC I44.69
  foramen Magendie (acquired) G91.1
    congenital Q03.1
      with spina bifida —see Spina bifida, by
        site, with hydrocephalus
  heart I45.9
    bundle branch I45.4
      bilateral I45.2
    complete (atrioventricular) I44.2
    congenital Q24.6
    first degree (atrioventricular) I44.0
    second degree (atrioventricular) I44.1
    specified type NEC I45.5
    third degree (atrioventricular) I44.2
  hepatic vein I82.0
  intraventricular (nonspecific) I45.4
    bundle branch
      bilateral I45.2
  kidney N28.9
    postcystoscopic or postprocedural N99.0

Block, blocked (Continued)
  Mobitz (types I and II) I44.1
  myocardial —see Block, heart
  nodal I45.5
  organ or site, congenital NEC —see Atresia,
    by site
  portal (vein) I81
  second degree (types I and II) I44.1
  sinoatrial I45.5
  sinoauricular I45.5
  third degree I44.2
  trifascicular I45.3
  tubal N97.1
  vein NOS I82.90
  Wenckebach (types I and II) I44.1
Blockage —see Obstruction
Blocq's disease F44.4
Blood
  constituents, abnormal R78.9
  disease D75.9
  donor —see Donor, blood
  dyscrasia D75.9
    with
      abortion —see Abortion, by type,
        complicated by, hemorrhage
      ectopic pregnancy O08.1
      molar pregnancy O08.1
    following ectopic or molar pregnancy
      O08.1
    newborn P61.9
    puerperal, postpartum O72.3
  flukes NEC —see Schistosomiasis
  in
    feces K92.1
      occult R19.5
    urine —see Hematuria
  mole O02.0
  occult in feces R19.5
  pressure
    decreased, due to shock following injury
      T79.4
    examination only Z01.30
    fluctuating I99.8
    high —see Hypertension
      borderline R03.0
      incidental reading, without diagnosis of
        hypertension R03.0
    low —see also Hypotension
      incidental reading, without diagnosis of
        hypotension R03.1
  spitting —see Hemoptysis
  staining cornea —see Pigmentation, cornea,
    stromal
  transfusion
    reaction or complication —see
      Complications, transfusion
  type
    A (Rh positive) Z67.10
      Rh negative Z67.11
    AB (Rh positive) Z67.30
      Rh negative Z67.31
    B (Rh positive) Z67.20
      Rh negative Z67.21
    O (Rh positive) Z67.40
      Rh negative Z67.41
    Rh (positive) Z67.90
      negative Z67.91
  vessel rupture —see Hemorrhage
  vomiting —see Hematemesis
Blood-forming organs, disease D75.9
Bloodgood's disease —see Mastopathy,
  cystic
Bloom (-Machacek)(-Torre) syndrome Q82.8
Blount's disease or osteochondrosis —see
  Osteochondrosis, juvenile, tibia
Blue
  baby Q24.9
  diaper syndrome E72.09
  dome cyst (breast) —see Cyst, breast
  dot cataract Q12.0
  nevus D22.9

Blue (Continued)
  sclera Q13.5
    with fragility of bone and deafness Q78.0
  toe syndrome I75.02-●
Blueness —see Cyanosis
Blues, postpartal O90.6
  baby O90.6
Blurring, visual H53.8
Blushing (abnormal) (excessive) R23.2
BMI —see Body, mass index
Boarder, hospital NEC Z76.4
  accompanying sick person Z76.3
  healthy infant or child Z76.2
    foundling Z76.1
Bockhart's impetigo L01.02
Bodechtel-Guttman disease (subacute
  sclerosing panencephalitis) A81.1
Boder-Sedgwick syndrome (ataxia-
  telangiectasia) G11.3
Body, bodies
  Aschoff's —see Myocarditis, rheumatic
  asteroid, vitreous —see Deposit, crystalline
  cytoid (retina) —see Occlusion, artery, retina
  drusen (degenerative) (macula) (retinal) —see
    also Degeneration, macula, drusen
    optic disc —see Drusen, optic disc
  foreign —see Foreign body
  loose
    joint, except knee —see Loose, body, joint
    knee M23.4-●
    sheath, tendon —see Disorder, tendon,
      specified type NEC
  mass index (BMI)
    adult
      ~~19 or less Z68.1~~
    ▶ 19.9 or less Z68.1
      20.0-20.9 Z68.20
      21.0-21.9 Z68.21
      22.0-22.9 Z68.22
      23.0-23.9 Z68.23
      24.0-24.9 Z68.24
      25.0-25.9 Z68.25
      26.0-26.9 Z68.26
      27.0-27.9 Z68.27
      28.0-28.9 Z68.28
      29.0-29.9 Z68.29
      30.0-30.9 Z68.30
      31.0-31.9 Z68.31
      32.0-32.9 Z68.32
      33.0-33.9 Z68.33
      34.0-34.9 Z68.34
      35.0-35.9 Z68.35
      36.0-36.9 Z68.36
      37.0-37.9 Z68.37
      38.0-38.9 Z68.38
      39.0-39.9 Z68.39
      40.0-44.9 Z68.41
      45.0-49.9 Z68.42
      50.0-59.9 Z68.43
      60.0-69.9 Z68.44
      70 and over Z68.45
    pediatric
      5th percentile to less than 85th percentile
        for age Z68.52
      85th percentile to less than 95th
        percentile for age Z68.53
      greater than or equal to ninety-fifth
        percentile for age Z68.54
      less than fifth percentile for age Z68.51
  Mooser's A75.2
  rice —see also Loose, body, joint
    knee M23.4-●
  rocking F98.4
Boeck's
  disease or sarcoid —see Sarcoidosis
  lupoid (miliary) D86.3
Boerhaave's syndrome (spontaneous
  esophageal rupture) K22.3
Boggy
  cervix N88.8
  uterus N85.8

Boil —*see also* Furuncle, by site
  Aleppo B55.1
  Baghdad B55.1
  Delhi B55.1
  lacrimal
    gland —*see* Dacryoadenitis
    passages (duct) (sac) —*see* Inflammation,
      lacrimal, passages, acute
  Natal B55.1
  orbit, orbital —*see* Abscess, orbit
  tropical B55.1
Bold hives —*see* Urticaria
Bombé, iris —*see* Membrane, pupillary
Bone —*see* condition
Bonnevie-Ullrich syndrome —*see also* Turner's
  syndrome Q87.1
Bonnier's syndrome —*see* subcategory H81.8
Bonvale dam fever T73.3
Bony block of joint —*see* Ankylosis
BOOP (bronchiolitis obliterans organized
  pneumonia) J84.89
Borderline
  diabetes mellitus R73.03
  hypertension R03.0
  osteopenia M85.8-•
  pelvis, with obstruction during labor O65.1
  personality F60.3
Borna disease A83.9
Bornholm disease B33.0
Boston exanthem A88.0
Botalli, ductus (patent) (persistent) Q25.0
Bothriocephalus latus infestation B70.0
Botulism (foodborne intoxication) A05.1
  infant A48.51
  non-foodborne A48.52
  wound A48.52
Bouba —*see* Yaws
Bouchard's nodes (with arthropathy) M15.2
Bouffée délirante F23
Bouillaud's disease or syndrome (rheumatic
  heart disease) I01.9
Bourneville's disease Q85.1
Boutonniere deformity (finger) —*see*
  Deformity, finger, boutonniere
Bouveret (-Hoffmann) syndrome (paroxysmal
  tachycardia) I47.9
Bovine heart —*see* Hypertrophy, cardiac
Bowel —*see* condition
Bowen's
  dermatosis (precancerous) —*see* Neoplasm,
    skin, in situ
  disease —*see* Neoplasm, skin, in situ
  epithelioma —*see* Neoplasm, skin, in situ
  type
    epidermoid carcinoma-in-situ —*see*
      Neoplasm, skin, in situ
    intraepidermal squamous cell carcinoma —
      see Neoplasm, skin, in situ
Bowing
  femur —*see also* Deformity, limb, specified
    type NEC, thigh
    congenital Q68.3
  fibula —*see also* Deformity, limb, specified
    type NEC, lower leg
    congenital Q68.4
  forearm —*see* Deformity, limb, specified type
    NEC, forearm
  leg(s), long bones, congenital Q68.5
  radius —*see* Deformity, limb, specified type
    NEC, forearm
  tibia —*see also* Deformity, limb, specified type
    NEC, lower leg
    congenital Q68.4
Bowleg(s) (acquired) M21.16-•
  congenital Q68.5
  rachitic E64.3
Boyd's dysentery A03.2
Brachial —*see* condition
Brachycardia R00.1
Brachycephaly Q75.0
Bradley's disease A08.19

Bradyarrhythmia, cardiac I49.8
Bradycardia (sinoatrial) (sinus) (vagal) R00.1
  neonatal P29.12
  reflex G90.09
  tachycardia syndrome I49.5
Bradykinesia R25.8
Bradypnea R06.89
Bradytachycardia I49.5
Brailsford's disease or osteochondrosis —*see*
  Osteochondrosis, juvenile, radius
Brain —*see also* condition
  death G93.82
  syndrome —*see* Syndrome, brain
Branched-chain amino-acid disorder E71.2
Branchial —*see* condition
  cartilage, congenital Q18.2
Branchiogenic remnant (in neck) Q18.0
Brandt's syndrome (acrodermatitis
  enteropathica) E83.2
Brash (water) R12
Bravais-jacksonian epilepsy —*see* Epilepsy,
  localization-related, symptomatic, with
  simple partial seizures
Braxton Hicks contractions —*see* False, labor
Brazilian leishmaniasis B55.2
BRBPR K62.5
Break, retina (without detachment) H33.30-•
  with retinal detachment —*see* Detachment,
    retina
  horseshoe tear H33.31-•
  multiple H33.33-•
  round hole H33.32-•
Breakdown
  device, graft or implant —*see also*
    Complications, by site and type,
    mechanical T85.618
    arterial graft NEC —*see* Complication,
      cardiovascular device, mechanical,
      vascular
    breast (implant) T85.41
    catheter NEC T85.618
      cystostomy T83.010
      dialysis (renal) T82.41
        intraperitoneal T85.611
      Hopkins T83.018
      ileostomy T83.018
      infusion NEC T82.514
        cranial T85.610
        epidural T85.610
        intrathecal T85.610
        spinal T85.610
        subarachnoid T85.610
        subdural T85.610
      nephrostomy T83.012
      urethral indwelling T83.011
      urinary NEC T83.018
      urostomy T83.018
    electronic (electrode) (pulse generator)
      (stimulator)
      bone T84.310
      cardiac T82.119
        electrode T82.110
        pulse generator T82.111
        specified type NEC T82.118
      nervous system —*see* Complication,
        prosthetic device, mechanical,
        electronic nervous system stimulator
      urinary —*see* Complication,
        genitourinary, device, urinary,
        mechanical
    fixation, internal (orthopedic) NEC —
      see Complication, fixation device,
      mechanical
    gastrointestinal —*see* Complications,
      prosthetic device, mechanical,
      gastrointestinal device
    genital NEC T83.418
      intrauterine contraceptive device T83.31
      penile prosthesis (cylinder) (implanted)
        (pump) (resevoir) T83.410
      testicular prosthesis T83.411

Breakdown (*Continued*)
  device, graft or implant (*Continued*)
    heart NEC —*see* Complication,
      cardiovascular device, mechanical
    intrathecal infusion pump T85.615
    joint prosthesis —*see* Complications..., joint
      prosthesis,internal, mechanical, by site
    nervous system, specified device NEC
      T85.615
    ocular NEC —*see* Complications, prosthetic
      device, mechanical, ocular device
    orthopedic NEC —*see* Complication,
      orthopedic, device, mechanical
    specified NEC T85.618
    subcutaneous device pocket
      nervous system prosthetic device,
        implant, or graft T85.890
      other internal prosthetic device, implant,
        or graft T85.898
    sutures, permanent T85.612
      used in bone repair —*see* Complications,
        fixation device, internal
        (orthopedic), mechanical
    urinary NEC T83.118
      graft T83.21
      sphincter, implanted T83.111
      stent (ileal conduit) (nephroureteral)
        T83.113
      ureteral indwelling T83.112
    vascular NEC —*see* Complication,
      cardiovascular device, mechanical
    ventricular intracranial shunt T85.01
  nervous F48.8
  perineum O90.1
  respirator J95.850
    specified NEC J95.859
  ventilator J95.850
    specified NEC J95.859
Breast —*see also* condition
  buds E30.1
    in newborn P96.89
  dense R92.2
➡️nodule —*see also* Lump, breast N63.0
Breath
  foul R19.6
  holder, child R06.89
  holding spell R06.89
  shortness R06.02
Breathing
  labored —*see* Hyperventilation
  mouth R06.5
    causing malocclusion M26.5
  periodic R06.3
    high altitude G47.32
Breathlessness R06.81
Breda's disease —*see* Yaws
Breech presentation (mother) O32.1
  causing obstructed labor O64.1
  footling O32.8
    causing obstructed labor O64.8
  incomplete O32.8
    causing obstructed labor O64.8
Breisky's disease N90.4
Brennemann's syndrome I88.0
Brenner
  tumor (benign) D27.9
    borderline malignancy D39.1-•
    malignant C56
    proliferating D39.1
Bretonneau's disease or angina A36.0
Breus' mole O02.0
Brevicollis Q76.49
Brickmakers' anemia B76.9 [D63.8]
Bridge, myocardial Q24.5
Bright red blood per rectum (BRBPR) K62.5
Bright's disease —*see also* Nephritis
  arteriosclerotic —*see* Hypertension, kidney
Brill (-Zinsser) disease (recrudescent typhus)
  A75.1
  flea-borne A75.2
  louse-borne A75.1

▶ New   ➡ Revised   ~~deleted~~ Deleted   • Use Additional Character(s)

Brill-Symmers' disease C82.90
Brion-Kayser disease —*see* Fever, parathyroid
Briquet's disorder or syndrome F45.0
Brissaud's
  infantilism or dwarfism E23.0
  motor-verbal tic F95.2
Brittle
  bones disease Q78.0
  nails L60.3
    congenital Q84.6
Broad —*see also* condition
  beta disease E78.2
  ligament laceration syndrome N83.8
Broad- or floating-betalipoproteinemia E78.2
Brock's syndrome (atelectasis due to enlarged
  lymph nodes) J98.19
Brocq-Duhring disease (dermatitis
  herpetiformis) L13.0
Brodie's abscess or disease M86.8X-●
Broken
  arches —*see also* Deformity, limb, flat foot
  arm (meaning upper limb) —*see* Fracture, arm
  back —*see* Fracture, vertebra
  bone —*see* Fracture
  implant or internal device —*see*
    Complications, by site and type,
    mechanical
  leg (meaning lower limb) —*see* Fracture, leg
  nose S02.2
  tooth, teeth —*see* Fracture, tooth
Bromhidrosis, bromidrosis L75.0
Bromidism, bromism G92
  chronic (dependence) F13.20
  due to
    correct substance properly administered —
      see Table of Drugs and Chemicals, by
      drug, adverse effect
    overdose or wrong substance given
      or taken —*see* Table of Drugs and
      Chemicals, by drug, poisoning
Bromidrosiphobia F40.298
Bronchi, bronchial —*see* condition
Bronchiectasis (cylindrical) (diffuse) (fusiform)
  (localized) (saccular) J47.9
  with
    acute
      bronchitis J47.0
      lower respiratory infection J47.0
    exacerbation (acute) J47.1
  congenital Q33.4
  tuberculous NEC —*see* Tuberculosis,
    pulmonary
Bronchiolectasis —*see* Bronchiectasis
Bronchiolitis (acute) (infective) (subacute) J21.9
  with
    bronchospasm or obstruction J21.9
    influenza, flu or grippe —*see* Influenza,
      with, respiratory manifestations NEC
  chemical (chronic) J68.4
    acute J68.0
  chronic (fibrosing) (obliterative) J44.9
  due to
    external agent —*see* Bronchitis, acute, due to
    human metapneumovirus J21.1
    respiratory syncytial virus J21.0
    specified organism NEC J21.8
  fibrosa obliterans J44.9
  influenzal —*see* Influenza, with, respiratory
    manifestations NEC
  obliterans J42
    with organizing pneumonia (BOOP) J84.89
  obliterative (chronic) (subacute) J44.9
    due to chemicals, gases, fumes or vapors
      (inhalation) J68.4
    due to fumes or vapors J68.4
  respiratory, interstitial lung disease J84.115
Bronchitis (diffuse) (fibrinous) (hypostatic)
  (infective) (membranous) J40
  with
    influenza, flu or grippe —*see* Influenza,
      with, respiratory manifestations NEC

Bronchitis (*Continued*)
  with (*Continued*)
    obstruction (airway) (lung) J44.9
    tracheitis (15 years of age and above) J40
      acute or subacute J20.9
      chronic J42
      under 15 years of age J20.9
  acute or subacute (with bronchospasm or
    obstruction) J20.9
    with
      bronchiectasis J47.0
      chronic obstructive pulmonary disease
        J44.0
      chemical (due to gases, fumes or vapors)
        J68.0
    due to
      fumes or vapors J68.0
      Haemophilus influenzae J20.1
      Mycoplasma pneumoniae J20.0
      radiation J70.0
      specified organism NEC J20.8
      Streptococcus J20.2
      virus
        coxsackie J20.3
        echovirus J20.7
        parainfluenzae J20.4
        respiratory syncytial J20.5
        rhinovirus J20.6
    viral NEC J20.8
  allergic (acute) J45.909
    with
      exacerbation (acute) J45.901
      status asthmaticus J45.902
  arachidic T17.528
  aspiration (due to fumes or vapors) J68.0
  asthmatic J45.9
    chronic J44.9
    with
      acute lower respiratory infection J44.0
      exacerbation (acute) J44.1
  capillary —*see* Pneumonia, broncho
  caseous (tuberculous) A15.5
  Castellani's A69.8
  catarrhal (15 years of age and above) J40
    acute —*see* Bronchitis, acute
    chronic J41.0
    under 15 years of age J20.9
  chemical (acute) (subacute) J68.0
    chronic J68.4
    due to fumes or vapors J68.0
      chronic J68.4
  chronic J42
    with
      airways obstruction J44.9
      tracheitis (chronic) J42
    asthmatic (obstructive) J44.9
    catarrhal J41.0
    chemical (due to fumes or vapors) J68.4
    due to
      chemicals, gases, fumes or vapors
        (inhalation) J68.4
      radiation J70.1
      tobacco smoking J41.0
    emphysematous J44.9
    mucopurulent J41.1
    non-obstructive J41.0
    obliterans J44.9
    obstructive J44.9
    purulent J41.1
    simple J41.0
  croupous —*see* Bronchitis, acute
  due to gases, fumes or vapors (chemical)
    J68.0
  emphysematous (obstructive) J44.9
  exudative —*see* Bronchitis, acute
  fetid J41.1
  grippal —*see* Influenza, with, respiratory
    manifestations NEC
  in those under 15 years age —*see* Bronchitis,
    acute
    chronic —*see* Bronchitis, chronic

Bronchitis (*Continued*)
  influenzal —*see* Influenza, with, respiratory
    manifestations NEC
  mixed simple and mucopurulent J41.8
  moulder's J62.8
  mucopurulent (chronic) (recurrent) J41.1
    acute or subacute J20.9
    simple (mixed) J41.8
  obliterans (chronic) J44.9
  obstructive (chronic) (diffuse) J44.9
  pituitous J41.1
  pneumococcal, acute or subacute J20.2
  pseudomembranous, acute or subacute —*see*
    Bronchitis, acute
  purulent (chronic) (recurrent) J41.1
    acute or subacute —*see* Bronchitis, acute
  putrid J41.1
  senile (chronic) J42
  simple and mucopurulent (mixed) J41.8
  smokers' J41.0
  spirochetal NEC A69.8
  subacute —*see* Bronchitis, acute
  suppurative (chronic) J41.1
    acute or subacute —*see* Bronchitis, acute
  tuberculous A15.5
  under 15 years of age —*see* Bronchitis, acute
    chronic —*see* Bronchitis, chronic
  viral NEC, acute or subacute —*see also*
    Bronchitis, acute J20.8
Bronchoalveolitis J18.0
Bronchoaspergillosis B44.1
Bronchocele meaning goiter E04.0
Broncholithiasis J98.09
  tuberculous NEC A15.5
Bronchomalacia J98.09
  congenital Q32.2
Bronchomycosis NOS B49 [J99]
  candidal B37.1
Bronchopleuropneumonia —*see* Pneumonia,
  broncho
Bronchopneumonia —*see* Pneumonia, broncho
Bronchopneumonitis —*see* Pneumonia,
  broncho
Bronchopulmonary —*see* condition
Bronchopulmonitis —*see* Pneumonia, broncho
Bronchorrhagia (*see* Hemoptysis)
Bronchorrhea J98.09
  acute J20.9
  chronic (infective) (purulent) J42
Bronchospasm (acute) J98.01
  with
    bronchiolitis, acute J21.9
    bronchitis, acute (conditions in J20) —*see*
      Bronchitis, acute
  due to external agent —*see* condition,
    respiratory, acute, due to
  exercise induced J45.990
Bronchospirochetosis A69.8
  Castellani A69.8
Bronchostenosis J98.09
Bronchus —*see* condition
Brontophobia F40.220
➡ Bronze baby syndrome P83.88
Brooke's tumor —*see* Neoplasm, skin, benign
Brown enamel of teeth (hereditary) K00.5
Brown's sheath syndrome H50.61-●
Brown-Séquard disease, paralysis or
  syndrome G83.81
Bruce sepsis A23.0
Brucellosis (infection) A23.9
  abortus A23.1
  canis A23.3
  dermatitis A23.9
  melitensis A23.0
  mixed A23.8
  sepsis A23.9
    melitensis A23.0
    specified NEC A23.8
  suis A23.2
Bruck-de Lange disease Q87.1
Bruck's disease —*see* Deformity, limb

▶ New   ⇒ Revised   ~~deleted~~ Deleted   ● Use Additional Character(s)

B

▶BRUE (brief resolved unexplained event) R68.13
Brugsch's syndrome Q82.8
Bruise (skin surface intact) —see also Contusion
    with
        ▶open wound —see Wound, open
    internal organ —see Injury, by site
    newborn P54.5
    scalp, due to birth injury, newborn P12.3
    umbilical cord O69.5
Bruit (arterial) R09.89
    cardiac R01.1
Brush burn —see Abrasion, by site
Bruton's X-linked agammaglobulinemia D80.0
Bruxism
    psychogenic F45.8
    sleep related G47.63
Bubbly lung syndrome P27.0
Bubo I88.8
    blennorrhagic (gonococcal) A54.89
    chancroidal A57
    climatic A55
    due to Haemophilus ducreyi A57
    gonococcal A54.89
    indolent (nonspecific) I88.8
    inguinal (nonspecific) I88.8
        chancroidal A57
        climatic A55
        due to H. ducreyi A57
        infective I88.8
    scrofulous (tuberculous) A18.2
    soft chancre A57
    suppurating —see Lymphadenitis, acute
    syphilitic (primary) A51.0
        congenital A50.07
    tropical A55
    virulent (chancroidal) A57
Bubonic plague A20.0
Bubonocele —see Hernia, inguinal
Buccal —see condition
Buchanan's disease or osteochondrosis M91.0
Buchem's syndrome (hyperostosis corticalis)
    M85.2
Bucket-handle fracture or tear (semilunar
    cartilage) —see Tear, meniscus
Budd-Chiari syndrome (hepatic vein
    thrombosis) I82.0
Budgerigar fancier's disease or lung
    J67.2
Buds
    breast E30.1
        in newborn P96.89
Buerger's disease (thromboangiitis obliterans)
    I73.1
Bulbar —see condition
Bulbus cordis (left ventricle) (persistent) Q21.8
Bulimia (nervosa) F50.2
    atypical F50.9
    normal weight F50.9
Bulky
    stools R19.5
    uterus N85.2
Bulla (e) R23.8
    lung (emphysematous) (solitary) J43.9
        newborn P25.8
Bullet wound —see also Wound, open
    fracture - code as Fracture, by site
    internal organ —see Injury, by site
Bundle
    branch block (complete) (false)
        (incomplete) —see Block, bundle-branch
    of His —see condition
Bunion M21.61-●
    tailor's M21.62-●
Bunionette M21.62-●
Buphthalmia, buphthalmos (congenital) Q15.0
Burdwan fever B55.0
Bürger-Grütz disease or syndrome E78.3
Buried
    penis (congenital) Q55.64
        acquired N48.83
    roots K08.3

Burke's syndrome K86.89
Burkitt
    cell leukemia C91.0-●
    lymphoma (malignant) C83.7-●
        small noncleaved, diffuse C83.7-●
        spleen C83.77
        undifferentiated C83.7-●
    tumor C83.7-●
    type
        acute lymphoblastic leukemia C91.0-●
        undifferentiated C83.7-●
Burn (electricity) (flame) (hot gas, liquid or hot
    object) (radiation) (steam) (thermal) T30.0
    abdomen, abdominal (muscle) (wall)
        T21.02
        first degree T21.12
        second degree T21.22
        third degree T21.32
    above elbow T22.039
        first degree T22.139
        left T22.032
            first degree T22.132
            second degree T22.232
            third degree T22.332
        right T22.031
            first degree T22.131
            second degree T22.231
            third degree T22.331
        second degree T22.239
        third degree T22.339
    acid (caustic) (external) (internal) —see
        Corrosion, by site
    alimentary tract NEC T28.2
        esophagus T28.1
        mouth T28.0
        pharynx T28.0
    alkaline (caustic) (external) (internal) —see
        Corrosion, by site
    ankle T25.019
        first degree T25.119
        left T25.012
            first degree T25.112
            second degree T25.212
            third degree T25.312
        multiple with foot —see Burn, lower, limb,
            multiple, ankle and foot
        right T25.011
            first degree T25.111
            second degree T25.211
            third degree T25.311
        second degree T25.219
        third degree T25.319
    anus —see Burn, buttock
    arm (lower) (upper) —see Burn, upper,
        limb
    axilla T22.049
        first degree T22.149
        left T22.042
            first degree T22.142
            second degree T22.242
            third degree T22.342
        right T22.041
            first degree T22.141
            second degree T22.241
            third degree T22.341
        second degree T22.249
        third degree T22.349
    back (lower) T21.04
        first degree T21.14
        second degree T21.24
        third degree T21.34
        upper T21.03
            first degree T21.13
            second degree T21.23
            third degree T21.33
    blisters - code as Burn, second degree, by site
    breast(s) —see Burn, chest wall
    buttock(s) T21.05
        first degree T21.15
        second degree T21.25
        third degree T21.35

Burn (Continued)
    calf T24.039
        first degree T24.139
        left T24.032
            first degree T24.132
            second degree T24.232
            third degree T24.332
        right T24.031
            first degree T24.131
            second degree T24.231
            third degree T24.331
        second degree T24.239
        third degree T24.339
    canthus (eye) —see Burn, eyelid
    caustic acid or alkaline —see Corrosion, by
        site
    cervix T28.3
    cheek T20.06
        first degree T20.16
        second degree T20.26
        third degree T20.36
    chemical (acids) (alkalines) (caustics) (external)
        (internal) —see Corrosion, by site
    chest wall T21.01
        first degree T21.11
        second degree T21.21
        third degree T21.31
    chin T20.03
        first degree T20.13
        second degree T20.23
        third degree T20.33
    colon T28.2
    conjunctiva (and cornea) —see Burn, cornea
    cornea (and conjunctiva) T26.1-●
        chemical —see Corrosion, cornea
    corrosion (external) (internal) —see
        Corrosion, by site
    deep necrosis of underlying tissue - code as
        Burn, third degree, by site
    dorsum of hand T23.069
        first degree T23.169
        left T23.062
            first degree T23.162
            second degree T23.262
            third degree T23.362
        right T23.061
            first degree T23.161
            second degree T23.261
            third degree T23.361
        second degree T23.269
        third degree T23.369
    due to ingested chemical agent —see
        Corrosion, by site
    ear (auricle) (external) (canal) T20.01
        first degree T20.11
        second degree T20.21
        third degree T20.31
    elbow T22.029
        first degree T22.129
        left T22.022
            first degree T22.122
            second degree T22.222
            third degree T22.322
        right T22.021
            first degree T22.121
            second degree T22.221
            third degree T22.321
        second degree T22.229
        third degree T22.329
    epidermal loss - code as Burn, second degree,
        by site
    erythema, erythematous - code as Burn, first
        degree, by site
    esophagus T28.1
    extent (percentage of body surface)
        less than 10 percent T31.0
        10-19 percent T31.10
            with 0-9 percent third degree burns
                T31.10
            with 10-19 percent third degree burns
                T31.11

Burn *(Continued)*
  extent *(Continued)*
    20-29 percent T31.20
      with 0-9 percent third degree burns T31.20
      with 10-19 percent third degree burns T31.21
      with 20-29 percent third degree burns T31.22
    30-39 percent T31.30
      with 0-9 percent third degree burns T31.30
      with 10-19 percent third degree burns T31.31
      with 20-29 percent third degree burns T31.32
      with 30-39 percent third degree burns T31.33
    40-49 percent T31.40
      with 0-9 percent third degree burns T31.40
      with 10-19 percent third degree burns T31.41
      with 20-29 percent third degree burns T31.42
      with 30-39 percent third degree burns T31.43
      with 40-49 percent third degree burns T31.44
    50-59 percent T31.50
      with 0-9 percent third degree burns T31.50
      with 10-19 percent third degree burns T31.51
      with 20-29 percent third degree burns T31.52
      with 30-39 percent third degree burns T31.53
      with 40-49 percent third degree burns T31.54
      with 50-59 percent third degree burns T31.55
    60-69 percent T31.60
      with 0-9 percent third degree burns T31.60
      with 10-19 percent third degree burns T31.61
      with 20-29 percent third degree burns T31.62
      with 30-39 percent third degree burns T31.63
      with 40-49 percent third degree burns T31.64
      with 50-59 percent third degree burns T31.65
      with 60-69 percent third degree burns T31.66
    70-79 percent T31.70
      with 0-9 percent third degree burns T31.70
      with 10-19 percent third degree burns T31.71
      with 20-29 percent third degree burns T31.72
      with 30-39 percent third degree burns T31.73
      with 40-49 percent third degree burns T31.74
      with 50-59 percent third degree burns T31.75
      with 60-69 percent third degree burns T31.76
      with 70-79 percent third degree burns T31.77
    80-89 percent T31.80
      with 0-9 percent third degree burns T31.80
      with 10-19 percent third degree burns T31.81
      with 20-29 percent third degree burns T31.82
      with 30-39 percent third degree burns T31.83
      with 40-49 percent third degree burns T31.84

Burn *(Continued)*
  extent *(Continued)*
    80-89 percent T31.80 *(Continued)*
      with 50-59 percent third degree burns T31.85
      with 60-69 percent third degree burns T31.86
      with 70-79 percent third degree burns T31.87
      with 80-89 percent third degree burns T31.88
    90 percent or more T31.90
      with 0-9 percent third degree burns T31.90
      with 10-19 percent third degree burns T31.91
      with 20-29 percent third degree burns T31.92
      with 30-39 percent third degree burns T31.93
      with 40-49 percent third degree burns T31.94
      with 50-59 percent third degree burns T31.95
      with 60-69 percent third degree burns T31.96
      with 70-79 percent third degree burns T31.97
      with 80-89 percent third degree burns T31.98
      with 90 percent or more third degree burns T31.99
  extremity —*see* Burn, limb
  eye(s) and adnexa T26.4-•
    with resulting rupture and destruction of eyeball T26.2-•
    conjunctival sac —*see* Burn, cornea
    cornea —*see* Burn, cornea
    lid —*see* Burn, eyelid
    periocular area —*see* Burn, eyelid
    specified site NEC T26.3-•
  eyeball —*see* Burn, eye
  eyelid(s) T26.0-•
    chemical —*see* Corrosion, eyelid
  face —*see* Burn, head
  finger T23.029
    first degree T23.129
    left T23.022
      first degree T23.122
      second degree T23.222
      third degree T23.322
    multiple sites (without thumb) T23.039
      with thumb T23.049
        first degree T23.149
        left T23.042
          first degree T23.142
          second degree T23.242
          third degree T23.342
        right T23.041
          first degree T23.141
          second degree T23.241
          third degree T23.341
        second degree T23.249
        third degree T23.349
      first degree T23.139
      left T23.032
        first degree T23.132
        second degree T23.232
        third degree T23.332
      right T23.031
        first degree T23.131
        second degree T23.231
        third degree T23.331
      second degree T23.239
      third degree T23.339
    right T23.021
      first degree T23.121
      second degree T23.221
      third degree T23.321
    second degree T23.229
    third degree T23.329
  flank —*see* Burn, abdominal wall

Burn *(Continued)*
  foot T25.029
    first degree T25.129
    left T25.022
      first degree T25.122
      second degree T25.222
      third degree T25.322
    multiple with ankle —*see* Burn, lower, limb, multiple, ankle and foot
    right T25.021
      first degree T25.121
      second degree T25.221
      third degree T25.321
    second degree T25.229
    third degree T25.329
  forearm T22.019
    first degree T22.119
    left T22.012
      first degree T22.112
      second degree T22.212
      third degree T22.312
    right T22.011
      first degree T22.111
      second degree T22.211
      third degree T22.311
    second degree T22.219
    third degree T22.319
  forehead T20.06
    first degree T20.16
    second degree T20.26
    third degree T20.36
  fourth degree - code as Burn, third degree, by site
  friction —*see* Burn, by site
  from swallowing caustic or corrosive substance NEC —*see* Corrosion, by site
  full thickness skin loss - code as Burn, third degree, by site
  gastrointestinal tract NEC T28.2
    from swallowing caustic or corrosive substance T28.7
  genital organs
    external
      female T21.07
        first degree T21.17
        second degree T21.27
        third degree T21.37
      male T21.06
        first degree T21.16
        second degree T21.26
        third degree T21.36
    internal T28.3
      from caustic or corrosive substance T28.8
  groin —*see* Burn, abdominal wall
  hand(s) T23.009
    back —*see* Burn, dorsum of hand
    finger —*see* Burn, finger
    first degree T23.109
    left T23.002
      first degree T23.102
      second degree T23.202
      third degree T23.302
    multiple sites with wrist T23.099
      first degree T23.199
      left T23.092
        first degree T23.192
        second degree T23.292
        third degree T23.392
      right T23.091
        first degree T23.191
        second degree T23.291
        third degree T23.391
      second degree T23.299
      third degree T23.399
    palm —*see* Burn, palm
    right T23.001
      first degree T23.101
      second degree T23.201
      third degree T23.301

Burn *(Continued)*
  hand *(Continued)*
    second degree T23.209
    third degree T23.309
    thumb —*see* Burn, thumb
  head (and face) (and neck) T20.00
    cheek —*see* Burn, cheek
    chin —*see* Burn, chin
    ear —*see* Burn, ear
    eye(s) only —*see* Burn, eye
    first degree T20.10
    forehead —*see* Burn, forehead
    lip —*see* Burn, lip
    multiple sites T20.09
      first degree T20.19
      second degree T20.29
      third degree T20.39
    neck —*see* Burn, neck
    nose —*see* Burn, nose
    scalp —*see* Burn, scalp
    second degree T20.20
    third degree T20.30
  hip(s) —*see* Burn, thigh
  inhalation —*see* Burn, respiratory tract
    caustic or corrosive substance (fumes) —*see*
      Corrosion, respiratory tract
  internal organ(s) T28.40
    alimentary tract T28.2
      esophagus T28.1
    eardrum T28.41
    esophagus T28.1
    from caustic or corrosive substance
      (swallowing) NEC —*see* Corrosion,
      by site
    genitourinary T28.3
    mouth T28.0
    pharynx T28.0
    respiratory tract —*see* Burn, respiratory
      tract
    specified organ NEC T28.49
  interscapular region —*see* Burn, back,
    upper
  intestine (large) (small) T28.2
  knee T24.029
    first degree T24.129
    left T24.022
      first degree T24.122
      second degree T24.222
      third degree T24.322
    right T24.021
      first degree T24.121
      second degree T24.221
      third degree T24.321
    second degree T24.229
    third degree T24.329
  labium (majus) (minus) —*see* Burn, genital
    organs, external, female
  lacrimal apparatus, duct, gland or sac —*see*
    Burn, eye, specified site NEC
  larynx T27.0
    with lung T27.1
  leg(s) (lower) (upper) —*see* Burn, lower,
    limb
  lightning —*see* Burn, by site
  limb(s)
    lower (except ankle or foot alone) —*see*
      Burn, lower, limb
    upper —*see* Burn, upper limb
  lip(s) T20.02
    first degree T20.12
    second degree T20.22
    third degree T20.32
  lower
    back —*see* Burn, back
    limb T24.009
      ankle —*see* Burn, ankle
      calf —*see* Burn, calf
      first degree T24.109
      foot —*see* Burn, foot
      hip —*see* Burn, thigh
      knee —*see* Burn, knee

Burn *(Continued)*
  lower *(Continued)*
    limb *(Continued)*
      left T24.002
        first degree T24.102
        second degree T24.202
        third degree T24.302
      multiple sites, except ankle and foot
        T24.099
      ankle and foot T25.099
        first degree T25.199
        left T25.092
          first degree T25.192
          second degree T25.292
          third degree T25.392
        right T25.091
          first degree T25.191
          second degree T25.291
          third degree T25.391
        second degree T25.299
        third degree T25.399
      first degree T24.199
      left T24.092
        first degree T24.192
        second degree T24.292
        third degree T24.392
      right T24.091
        first degree T24.191
        second degree T24.291
        third degree T24.391
      second degree T24.299
      third degree T24.399
      right T24.001
        first degree T24.101
        second degree T24.201
        third degree T24.301
      second degree T24.209
      thigh —*see* Burn, thigh
      third degree T24.309
      toe —*see* Burn, toe
  lung (with larynx and trachea) T27.1
  mouth T28.0
  neck T20.07
    first degree T20.17
    second degree T20.27
    third degree T20.37
  nose (septum) T20.04
    first degree T20.14
    second degree T20.24
    third degree T20.34
  ocular adnexa —*see* Burn, eye
  orbit region —*see* Burn, eyelid
  palm T23.059
    first degree T23.159
    left T23.052
      first degree T23.152
      second degree T23.252
      third degree T23.352
    right T23.051
      first degree T23.151
      second degree T23.251
      third degree T23.351
    second degree T23.259
    third degree T23.359
  partial thickness - code as Burn, unspecified
    degree, by site
  pelvis —*see* Burn, trunk
  penis —*see* Burn, genital organs, external,
    male
  perineum
    female —*see* Burn, genital organs, external,
      female
    male —*see* Burn, genital organs, external,
      male
  periocular area —*see* Burn, eyelid
  pharynx T28.0
  rectum T28.2
  respiratory tract T27.3
    larynx —*see* Burn, larynx
    specified part NEC T27.2
    trachea —*see* Burn, trachea

Burn *(Continued)*
  sac, lacrimal —*see* Burn, eye, specified site
    NEC
  scalp T20.05
    first degree T20.15
    second degree T20.25
    third degree T20.35
  scapular region T22.069
    first degree T22.169
    left T22.062
      first degree T22.162
      second degree T22.262
      third degree T22.362
    right T22.061
      first degree T22.161
      second degree T22.261
      third degree T22.361
    second degree T22.269
    third degree T22.369
  sclera —*see* Burn, eye, specified site NEC
  scrotum —*see* Burn, genital organs, external,
    male
  shoulder T22.059
    first degree T22.159
    left T22.052
      first degree T22.152
      second degree T22.252
      third degree T22.352
    right T22.051
      first degree T22.151
      second degree T22.251
      third degree T22.351
    second degree T22.259
    third degree T22.359
  stomach T28.2
  temple —*see* Burn, head
  testis —*see* Burn, genital organs, external, male
  thigh T24.019
    first degree T24.119
    left T24.012
      first degree T24.112
      second degree T24.212
      third degree T24.312
    right T24.011
      first degree T24.111
      second degree T24.211
      third degree T24.311
    second degree T24.219
    third degree T24.319
  thorax (external) —*see* Burn, trunk
  throat (meaning pharynx) T28.0
  thumb(s) T23.019
    first degree T23.119
    left T23.012
      first degree T23.112
      second degree T23.212
      third degree T23.312
    multiple sites with fingers T23.049
      first degree T23.149
      left T23.042
        first degree T23.142
        second degree T23.242
        third degree T23.342
      right T23.041
        first degree T23.141
        second degree T23.241
        third degree T23.341
      second degree T23.249
      third degree T23.349
    right T23.011
      first degree T23.111
      second degree T23.211
      third degree T23.311
    second degree T23.219
    third degree T23.319
  toe T25.039
    first degree T25.139
    left T25.032
      first degree T25.132
      second degree T25.232
      third degree T25.332

▶ New   ➡ Revised   ~~deleted~~ Deleted   ● Use Additional Character(s)

Burn *(Continued)*
 toe *(Continued)*
  right T25.031
   first degree T25.131
   second degree T25.231
   third degree T25.331
  second degree T25.239
  third degree T25.339
 tongue T28.0
 tonsil(s) T28.0
 trachea T27.0
  with lung T27.1
 trunk T21.00
  abdominal wall —*see* Burn, abdominal wall
  anus —*see* Burn, buttock
  axilla —*see* Burn, upper limb
  back —*see* Burn, back
  breast —*see* Burn, chest wall
  buttock —*see* Burn, buttock
  chest wall —*see* Burn, chest wall
  first degree T21.10
  flank —*see* Burn, abdominal wall
  genital
   female —*see* Burn, genital organs, external, female
   male —*see* Burn, genital organs, external, male
  groin —*see* Burn, abdominal wall
  interscapular region —*see* Burn, back, upper
  labia —*see* Burn, genital organs, external, female
  lower back —*see* Burn, back
  penis —*see* Burn, genital organs, external, male
  perineum
   female —*see* Burn, genital organs, external, female
   male —*see* Burn, genital organs, external, male
  scapula region —*see* Burn, scapular region
  scrotum —*see* Burn, genital organs, external, male
  second degree T21.20
  specified site NEC T21.09
   first degree T21.19
   second degree T21.29
   third degree T21.39
  testes —*see* Burn, genital organs, external, male
  third degree T21.30
  upper back —*see* Burn, back, upper
  vulva —*see* Burn, genital organs, external, female
 unspecified site with extent of body surface involved specified
  ⇒less than 10 percent T31.0
  ⇒10-19 percent (0-9 percent third degree) T31.10
   with 10-19 percent third degree T31.11
  ⇒20-29 percent (0-9 percent third degree) T31.20
   with
    10-19 percent third degree T31.21
    20-29 percent third degree T31.22
  ⇒30-39 percent (0-9 percent third degree) T31.30
   with
    10-19 percent third degree T31.31
    20-29 percent third degree T31.32
    30-39 percent third degree T31.33
  ⇒40-49 percent (0-9 percent third degree) T31.40
   with
    10-19 percent third degree T31.41
    20-29 percent third degree T31.42
    30-39 percent third degree T31.43
    40-49 percent third degree T31.44

Burn *(Continued)*
 unspecified site with extent of body surface involved specified *(Continued)*
  ⇒50-59 percent (0-9 percent third degree) T31.50
   with
    10-19 percent third degree T31.51
    20-29 percent third degree T31.52
    30-39 percent third degree T31.53
    40-49 percent third degree T31.54
    50-59 percent third degree T31.55
  ⇒60-69 percent (0-9 percent third degree) T31.60
   with
    10-19 percent third degree T31.61
    20-29 percent third degree T31.62
    30-39 percent third degree T31.63
    40-49 percent third degree T31.64
    50-59 percent third degree T31.65
    60-69 percent third degree T31.66
  ⇒70-79 percent (0-9 percent third degree) T31.70
   with
    10-19 percent third degree T31.71
    20-29 percent third degree T31.72
    30-39 percent third degree T31.73
    40-49 percent third degree T31.74
    50-59 percent third degree T31.75
    60-69 percent third degree T31.76
    70-79 percent third degree T31.77
  ⇒80-89 percent (0-9 percent third degree) T31.80
   with
    10-19 percent third degree T31.81
    20-29 percent third degree T31.82
    30-39 percent third degree T31.83
    40-49 percent third degree T31.84
    50-59 percent third degree T31.85
    60-69 percent third degree T31.86
    70-79 percent third degree T31.87
    80-89 percent third degree T31.88
  ⇒90 percent or more (0-9 percent third degree) T31.90
   with
    10-19 percent third degree T31.91
    20-29 percent third degree T31.92
    30-39 percent third degree T31.93
    40-49 percent third degree T31.94
    50-59 percent third degree T31.95
    60-69 percent third degree T31.96
    70-79 percent third degree T31.97
    80-89 percent third degree T31.98
    90-99 percent third degree T31.99
 upper limb T22.00
  above elbow —*see* Burn, above elbow
  axilla —*see* Burn, axilla
  elbow —*see* Burn, elbow
  first degree T22.10
  forearm —*see* Burn, forearm
  hand —*see* Burn, hand
  interscapular region —*see* Burn, back, upper
  multiple sites T22.099
   first degree T22.199
   left T22.092
    first degree T22.192
    second degree T22.292
    third degree T22.392
   right T22.091
    first degree T22.191
    second degree T22.291
    third degree T22.391
   second degree T22.299
   third degree T22.399
  scapular region —*see* Burn, scapular region
  second degree T22.20
  shoulder —*see* Burn, shoulder
  third degree T22.30
  wrist —*see* Burn, wrist
 uterus T28.3
 vagina T28.3

Burn *(Continued)*
 vulva —*see* Burn, genital organs, external, female
 wrist T23.079
  first degree T23.179
  left T23.072
   first degree T23.172
   second degree T23.272
   third degree T23.372
  multiple sites with hand T23.099
   first degree T23.199
   left T23.092
    first degree T23.192
    second degree T23.292
    third degree T23.392
   right T23.091
    first degree T23.191
    second degree T23.291
    third degree T23.391
   second degree T23.299
   third degree T23.399
  right T23.071
   first degree T23.171
   second degree T23.271
   third degree T23.371
  second degree T23.279
  third degree T23.379
Burnett's syndrome E83.52
Burning
 feet syndrome E53.9
 sensation R20.8
 tongue K14.6
Burn-out (state) Z73.0
Burns' disease or osteochondrosis —*see* Osteochondrosis, juvenile, ulna
Bursa —*see* condition
Bursitis M71.9
 Achilles —*see* Tendinitis, Achilles
 adhesive —*see* Bursitis, specified NEC
 ankle —*see* Enthesopathy, lower limb, ankle, specified type NEC
 calcaneal —*see* Enthesopathy, foot, specified type NEC
 collateral ligament, tibial —*see* Bursitis, tibial collateral
 due to use, overuse, pressure —*see also* Disorder, soft tissue, due to use, specified type NEC
  specified NEC —*see* Disorder, soft tissue, due to use, specified NEC
 Duplay's M75.0
 elbow NEC M70.3-●
  olecranon M70.2-●
 finger —*see* Disorder, soft tissue, due to use, specified type NEC, hand
 foot —*see* Enthesopathy, foot, specified type NEC
 gonococcal A54.49
 gouty —*see* Gout
 hand M70.1-●
 hip NEC M70.7-●
  trochanteric M70.6-●
 infective NEC M71.10
  abscess —*see* Abscess, bursa
  ankle M71.17-●
  elbow M71.12-●
  foot M71.17-●
  hand M71.14-●
  hip M71.15-●
  knee M71.16-●
  multiple sites M71.19
  shoulder M71.11-●
  specified site NEC M71.18
  wrist M71.13-●
 ischial —*see* Bursitis, hip
 knee NEC M70.5-●
  prepatellar M70.4-●
 occupational NEC —*see also* Disorder, soft tissue, due to, use
 olecranon —*see* Bursitis, elbow, olecranon
 pharyngeal J39.1

Bursitis (*Continued*)
  popliteal —*see* Bursitis, knee
  prepatellar M70.4-●
  radiohumeral M77.8
  rheumatoid M06.20
    ankle M06.27-●
    elbow M06.22-●
    foot joint M06.27-●
    hand joint M06.24-●
    hip M06.25-●
    knee M06.26-●
    multiple site M06.29
    shoulder M06.21-●
    vertebra M06.28
    wrist M06.23-●
  scapulohumeral —*see* Bursitis, shoulder
  semimembranous muscle (knee) —*see*
      Bursitis, knee
  shoulder M75.5-●
    adhesive —*see* Capsulitis, adhesive
  specified NEC M71.50
    ankle M71.57-●
    due to use, overuse or pressure —*see*
        Disorder, soft tissue, due to, use
    elbow M71.52-●
    foot M71.57-●
    hand M71.54-●

Bursitis (*Continued*)
  specified NEC (*Continued*)
    hip M71.55-●
    knee M71.56-●
    shoulder —*see* Bursitis, shoulder
    specified site NEC M71.58
    tibial collateral M76.4-●
    wrist M71.53-●
  subacromial —*see* Bursitis, shoulder
  subcoracoid —*see* Bursitis, shoulder
  subdeltoid —*see* Bursitis, shoulder
  syphilitic A52.78
  Thornwaldt, Tornwaldt J39.2
  tibial collateral M76.4-●
  toe —*see* Enthesopathy, foot, specified type
      NEC
  trochanteric (area) —*see* Bursitis, hip,
      trochanteric
  wrist —*see* Bursitis, hand
Bursopathy M71.9
  specified type NEC M71.80
    ankle M71.87-●
    elbow M71.82-●
    foot M71.87-●
    hand M71.84-●
    hip M71.85-●
    knee M71.86-●

Bursopathy (*Continued*)
  specified type NEC (*Continued*)
    multiple sites M71.89
    shoulder M71.81-●
    specified site NEC M71.88
    wrist M71.83-●
Burst stitches or sutures (complication of
    surgery) T81.31
  external operation wound T81.31
  internal operation wound T81.32
Buruli ulcer A31.1
Bury's disease L95.1
Buschke's
  disease B45.3
  scleredema —*see* Sclerosis, systemic
Busse-Buschke disease B45.3
Buttock —*see* condition
Button
  Biskra B55.1
  Delhi B55.1
  oriental B55.1
Buttonhole deformity (finger) —*see* Deformity,
    finger, boutonniere
Bwamba fever A92.8
Byssinosis J66.0
Bywaters' syndrome T79.5

C

Cachexia R64
  cancerous R64
  cardiac —see Disease, heart
  dehydration E86.0
  due to malnutrition R64
  exophthalmic —see Hyperthyroidism
  heart —see Disease, heart
  hypophyseal E23.0
  hypopituitary E23.0
  lead —see Poisoning, lead
  malignant R64
  marsh —see Malaria
  nervous F48.8
  old age R54
  paludal —see Malaria
  pituitary E23.0
  renal N28.9
  saturnine —see Poisoning, lead
  senile R54
  Simmonds' E23.0
  splenica D73.0
  strumipriva E03.4
  tuberculous NEC —see Tuberculosis
Café au lait spots L81.3
Caffeine-induced
  anxiety disorder F15.980
  sleep disorder F15.982
Caffey's syndrome Q78.8
Caisson disease T70.3
Cake kidney Q63.1
Caked breast (puerperal, postpartum) O92.79
Calabar swelling B74.3
Calcaneal spur —see Spur, bone, calcaneal
Calcaneo-apophysitis M92.8
Calcareous —see condition
Calcicosis J62.8
Calciferol (vitamin D) deficiency E55.9
  with rickets E55.0
Calcification
  adrenal (capsule) (gland) E27.49
    tuberculous E35 [B90.8]
  aorta I70.0
  artery (annular) —see Arteriosclerosis
  auricle (ear) —see Disorder, pinna, specified type NEC
  basal ganglia G23.8
  bladder N32.89
    due to Schistosoma hematobium B65.0
  brain (cortex) —see Calcification, cerebral
  bronchus J98.09
  bursa M71.40
    ankle M71.47-●
    elbow M71.42-●
    foot M71.47-●
    hand M71.44-●
    hip M71.45-●
    knee M71.46-●
    multiple sites M71.49
    shoulder M75.3-●
    specified site NEC M71.48
    wrist M71.43-●
  cardiac —see Degeneration, myocardial
  cerebral (cortex) G93.89
    artery I67.2
  cervix (uteri) N88.8
  choroid plexus G93.89
  conjunctiva —see Concretion, conjunctiva
  corpora cavernosa (penis) N48.89
  cortex (brain) —see Calcification, cerebral
  dental pulp (nodular) K04.2
  dentinal papilla K00.4
  fallopian tube N83.8
  falx cerebri G96.19
  gallbladder K82.8
  general E83.59
  heart —see also Degeneration, myocardial
    valve —see Endocarditis

Calcification (Continued)
  idiopathic infantile arterial (IIAC) Q28.8
  intervertebral cartilage or disc
    (postinfective) —see Disorder, disc, specified NEC
  intracranial —see Calcification, cerebral
  joint —see Disorder, joint, specified type NEC
  kidney N28.89
    tuberculous N29 [B90.1]
  larynx (senile) J38.7
  lens —see Cataract, specified NEC
  lung (active) (postinfectional) J98.4
    tuberculous B90.9
  lymph gland or node (postinfectional) I89.8
    tuberculous —see also Tuberculosis, lymph gland B90.8
  mammographic R92.1
  massive (paraplegic) —see Myositis, ossificans, in, quadriplegia
  medial —see Arteriosclerosis, extremities
  meninges (cerebral) (spinal) G96.19
  metastatic E83.59
  Mönckeberg's —see Arteriosclerosis, extremities
  muscle M61.9
    due to burns —see Myositis, ossificans, in, burns
    paralytic —see Myositis, ossificans, in, quadriplegia
    specified type NEC M61.40
      ankle M61.47-●
      foot M61.47-●
      forearm M61.43-●
      hand M61.44-●
      lower leg M61.46-●
      multiple sites M61.49
      pelvic region M61.45-●
      shoulder region M61.41-●
      specified site NEC M61.48
      thigh M61.45-●
      upper arm M61.42-●
  myocardium, myocardial —see Degeneration, myocardial
  ovary N83.8
  pancreas K86.89
  penis N48.89
  periarticular —see Disorder, joint, specified type NEC
  pericardium —see also Pericarditis I31.1
  pineal gland E34.8
  pleura J94.8
    postinfectional J94.8
    tuberculous NEC B90.9
  pulpal (dental) (nodular) K04.2
  sclera H15.89
  spleen D73.89
  subcutaneous L94.2
  suprarenal (capsule) (gland) E27.49
  tendon (sheath) —see also Tenosynovitis, specified type NEC
    with bursitis, synovitis or tenosynovitis —see Tendinitis, calcific
  trachea J39.8
  ureter N28.89
  vitreous —see Deposit, crystalline
Calcified —see Calcification
Calcinosis (interstitial) (tumoral) (universalis) E83.59
  with Raynaud's phenomenon, esophageal dysfunction, sclerodactyly, telangiectasia (CREST syndrome) M34.1
  circumscripta (skin) L94.2
  cutis L94.2
Calciphylaxis —see also Calcification, by site E83.59
Calcium
  deposits —see Calcification, by site
  metabolism disorder E83.50
  salts or soaps in vitreous —see Deposit, crystalline

Calciuria R82.99
Calculi —see Calculus
Calculosis, intrahepatic —see Calculus, bile duct
Calculus, calculi, calculous
  ampulla of Vater —see Calculus, bile duct
  anuria (impacted) (recurrent) —see also Calculus, urinary N20.9
  appendix K38.1
  bile duct (common) (hepatic) K80.50
    with
      calculus of gallbladder —see Calculus, gallbladder and bile duct
      cholangitis K80.30
        with
          cholecystitis —see Calculus, bile duct, with cholecystitis
          obstruction K80.31
        acute K80.32
          with
            chronic cholangitis K80.36
              with obstruction K80.37
            obstruction K80.33
        chronic K80.34
          with
            acute cholangitis K80.36
              with obstruction K80.37
            obstruction K80.35
      cholecystitis (with cholangitis) K80.40
        with obstruction K80.41
        acute K80.42
          with
            chronic cholecystitis K80.46
              with obstruction K80.47
            obstruction K80.43
        chronic K80.44
          with
            acute cholecystitis K80.46
              with obstruction K80.47
            obstruction K80.45
      obstruction K80.51
  biliary —see also Calculus, gallbladder
    specified NEC K80.80
      with obstruction K80.81
  bilirubin, multiple —see Calculus, gallbladder
  bladder (encysted) (impacted) (urinary) (diverticulum) N21.0
  bronchus J98.09
  calyx (kidney) (renal) —see Calculus, kidney
  cholesterol (pure) (solitary) —see Calculus, gallbladder
  common duct (bile) —see Calculus, bile duct
  conjunctiva —see Concretion, conjunctiva
  cystic N21.0
    duct —see Calculus, gallbladder
  dental (subgingival) (supragingival) K03.6
  diverticulum
    bladder N21.0
    kidney N20.0
  epididymis N50.89
  gallbladder K80.20
    with
      bile duct calculus —see Calculus, gallbladder and bile duct
      cholecystitis K80.10
        with obstruction K80.11
        acute K80.00
          with
            chronic cholecystitis K80.12
              with obstruction K80.13
            obstruction K80.01
        chronic K80.10
          with
            acute cholecystitis K80.12
              with obstruction K80.13
            obstruction K80.11
      specified NEC K80.18
        with obstruction K80.19
      obstruction K80.21

Calculus, calculi, calculous (Continued)
  gallbladder and bile duct K80.70
    with
      cholecystitis K80.60
        with obstruction K80.61
        acute K80.62
          with
            chronic cholecystitis K80.66
              with obstruction K80.67
            obstruction K80.63
          chronic K80.64
            with
              acute cholecystitis K80.66
                with obstruction K80.67
              obstruction K80.65
          obstruction K80.71
  hepatic (duct) —see Calculus, bile duct
  hepatobiliary K80.80
    with obstruction K80.81
  ileal conduit N21.8
  intestinal (impaction) (obstruction) K56.49
  kidney (impacted) (multiple) (pelvis)
      (recurrent) (staghorn) N20.0
    with calculus, ureter N20.2
    congenital Q63.8
  lacrimal passages —see Dacryolith
  liver (impacted) —see Calculus, bile duct
  lung J98.4
  mammographic R92.1
  nephritic (impacted) (recurrent) —see
      Calculus, kidney
  nose J34.89
  pancreas (duct) K86.89
  parotid duct or gland K11.5
  pelvis, encysted —see Calculus, kidney
  prostate N42.0
  pulmonary J98.4
  pyelitis (impacted) (recurrent) N20.0
    with hydronephrosis N13.2
  pyelonephritis (impacted) (recurrent) —see
      category N20
    with hydronephrosis N13.2
  renal (impacted) (recurrent) —see Calculus,
      kidney
  salivary (duct) (gland) K11.5
  seminal vesicle N50.89
  staghorn —see Calculus, kidney
  Stensen's duct K11.5
  stomach K31.89
  sublingual duct or gland K11.5
    congenital Q38.4
  submandibular duct, gland or region K11.5
  submaxillary duct, gland or region K11.5
  suburethral N21.8
  tonsil J35.8
  tooth, teeth (subgingival) (supragingival)
      K03.6
  tunica vaginalis N50.89
  ureter (impacted) (recurrent) N20.1
    with calculus, kidney N20.2
      with hydronephrosis N13.2
        with infection N13.6
  urethra (impacted) N21.1
  urinary (duct) (impacted) (passage) (tract)
      N20.9
    with hydronephrosis N13.2
      with infection N13.6
    in (due to)
      lower N21.9
        specified NEC N21.8
  vagina N89.8
  vesical (impacted) N21.0
  Wharton's duct K11.5
  xanthine E79.8 [N22]
Calicectasis N28.89
Caliectasis N28.89
California
  disease B38.9
  encephalitis A83.5
Caligo cornea —see Opacity, cornea, central
Callositas, callosity (infected) L84

Callus (infected) L84
  bone —see Osteophyte
    excessive, following fracture - code as
        Sequelae of fracture
CALME (childhood asymmetric labium majus
    enlargement) N90.61
Calorie deficiency or malnutrition —see also
    Malnutrition E46
Calvé-Perthes disease —see Legg-Calve-Perthes
    disease
Calvé's disease —see Osteochondrosis, juvenile,
    spine
Calvities —see Alopecia, androgenic
Cameroon fever —see Malaria
Camptocormia (hysterical) F44.4
Camurati-Engelmann syndrome Q78.3
Canal —see also condition
  atrioventricular common Q21.2
Canaliculitis (lacrimal) (acute) (subacute)
    H04.33-●
  Actinomyces A42.89
  chronic H04.42-●
Canavan's disease E75.29
Canceled procedure (surgical) Z53.9
  because of
    contraindication Z53.09
      smoking Z53.01
    left against medical advice (AMA) Z53.21
    patient's decision Z53.20
      for reasons of belief or group pressure
          Z53.1
      specified reason NEC Z53.29
    specified reason NEC Z53.8
Cancer —see also Neoplasm, by site, malignant
  bile duct type, liver C22.1
  blood —see Leukemia
  breast —see also Neoplasm, breast, malignant
      C50.91-●
  hepatocellular C22.0
  lung —see also Neoplasm, lung, malignant
      C34.90-●
  ovarian —see also Neoplasm, ovary,
      malignant C56.9-●
  unspecified site (primary) C80.1
Cancer (o)phobia F45.29
Cancerous —see Neoplasm, malignant, by site
Cancrum oris A69.0
Candidiasis, candidal B37.9
  balanitis B37.42
  bronchitis B37.1
  cheilitis B37.83
  congenital P37.5
  cystitis B37.41
  disseminated B37.7
  endocarditis B37.6
  enteritis B37.82
  esophagitis B37.81
  intertrigo B37.2
  lung B37.1
  meningitis B37.5
  mouth B37.0
  nails B37.2
  neonatal P37.5
  onychia B37.2
  oral B37.0
  osteomyelitis B37.89
  otitis externa B37.84
  paronychia B37.2
  perionyxis B37.2
  pneumonia B37.1
  proctitis B37.82
  pulmonary B37.1
  pyelonephritis B37.49
  sepsis B37.7
  skin B37.2
  specified site NEC B37.89
  stomatitis B37.0
  systemic B37.7
  urethritis B37.41
  urogenital site NEC B37.49
  vagina B37.3
  vulva B37.3
  vulvovaginitis B37.3

Candidid L30.2
Candidosis —see Candidiasis
Candiru infection or infestation B88.8
Canities (premature) L67.1
  congenital Q84.2
Canker (mouth) (sore) K12.0
  rash A38.9
Cannabinosis J66.2
Cannabis induced
  anxiety disorder F12.980
  psychotic disorder F12.959
  sleep disorder F12.988
Canton fever A75.9
Cantrell's syndrome Q87.89
Capillariasis (intestinal) B81.1
  hepatic B83.8
Capillary —see condition
Caplan's syndrome —see Rheumatoid, lung
Capsule —see condition
Capsulitis (joint) —see also Enthesopathy
  adhesive (shoulder) M75.0-●
  hepatic K65.8
  labyrinthine —see Otosclerosis, specified NEC
  thyroid E06.9
Caput
  crepitus Q75.8
  medusae I86.8
  succedaneum P12.81
Car sickness T75.3
Carapata (disease) A68.0
Carate —see Pinta
Carbon lung J60
Carbuncle L02.93
  abdominal wall L02.231
  anus K61.0
  auditory canal, external —see Abscess, ear,
      external
  auricle ear —see Abscess, ear, external
  axilla L02.43-●
  back (any part) L02.232
  breast N61.1
  buttock L02.33
  cheek (external) L02.03
  chest wall L02.233
  chin L02.03
  corpus cavernosum N48.21
  ear (any part) (external) (middle) —see
      Abscess, ear, external
  external auditory canal —see Abscess, ear,
      external
  eyelid —see Abscess, eyelid
  face NEC L02.03
  femoral (region) —see Carbuncle, lower limb
  finger —see Carbuncle, hand
  flank L02.231
  foot L02.63-●
  forehead L02.03
  genital —see Abscess, genital
  gluteal (region) L02.33
  groin L02.234
  hand L02.53-●
  head NEC L02.831
  heel —see Carbuncle, foot
  hip —see Carbuncle, lower limb
  kidney —see Abscess, kidney
  knee —see Carbuncle, lower limb
  labium (majus) (minus) N76.4
  lacrimal
    gland —see Dacryoadenitis
    passages (duct) (sac) —see Inflammation,
        lacrimal, passages, acute
  leg —see Carbuncle, lower limb
  lower limb L02.43-●
  malignant A22.0
  navel L02.236
  neck L02.13
  nose (external) (septum) J34.0
  orbit, orbital —see Abscess, orbit
  palmar (space) —see Carbuncle, hand
  partes posteriores L02.33
  pectoral region L02.233
  penis N48.21

▶ New   ⇒ Revised   deleted Deleted   ● Use Additional Character(s)

Carbuncle *(Continued)*
  perineum L02.235
  pinna —*see* Abscess, ear, external
  popliteal —*see* Carbuncle, lower limb
  scalp L02.831
  seminal vesicle N49.0
  shoulder —*see* Carbuncle, upper limb
  specified site NEC L02.838
  temple (region) L02.03
  thumb —*see* Carbuncle, hand
  toe —*see* Carbuncle, foot
  trunk L02.239
    abdominal wall L02.231
    back L02.232
    chest wall L02.233
    groin L02.234
    perineum L02.235
    umbilicus L02.236
  umbilicus L02.236
  upper limb L02.43-●
  urethra N34.0
  vulva N76.4
Carbunculus —*see* Carbuncle
Carcinoid (tumor) —*see* Tumor, carcinoid
Carcinoidosis E34.0
Carcinoma (malignant) —*see also* Neoplasm,
    by site, malignant
  acidophil
    specified site —*see* Neoplasm, malignant,
      by site
    unspecified site C75.1
  acidophil-basophil, mixed
    specified site —*see* Neoplasm, malignant,
      by site
    unspecified site C75.1
  adnexal (skin) —*see* Neoplasm, skin, malignant
  adrenal cortical C74.0-●
  alveolar —*see* Neoplasm, lung, malignant
    cell —*see* Neoplasm, lung, malignant
  ameloblastic C41.1
    upper jaw (bone) C41.0
  apocrine
    breast —*see* Neoplasm, breast, malignant
    specified site NEC —*see* Neoplasm, skin,
      malignant
    unspecified site C44.99
  basal cell (pigmented) (*see also* Neoplasm,
    skin, malignant) C44.91
    fibro-epithelial —*see* Neoplasm, skin,
      malignant
    morphea —*see* Neoplasm, skin, malignant
    multicentric —*see* Neoplasm, skin,
      malignant
  basaloid
  basal-squamous cell, mixed —*see* Neoplasm,
    skin, malignant
  basophil
    specified site —*see* Neoplasm, malignant,
      by site
    unspecified site C75.1
  basophil-acidophil, mixed
    specified site —*see* Neoplasm, malignant,
      by site
    unspecified site C75.1
  basosquamous —*see* Neoplasm, skin, malignant
  bile duct
    with hepatocellular, mixed C22.0
    liver C22.1
    specified site NEC —*see* Neoplasm,
      malignant, by site
    unspecified site C22.1
  branchial or branchiogenic C10.4
  bronchial or bronchogenic —*see* Neoplasm,
    lung, malignant
  bronchiolar —*see* Neoplasm, lung, malignant
  bronchioloalveolar —*see* Neoplasm, lung,
    malignant
  C cell
    specified site —*see* Neoplasm, malignant,
      by site
    unspecified site C73
  ceruminous C44.29-●

Carcinoma *(Continued)*
  cervix uteri
    in situ D06.9
      endocervix D06.0
      exocervix D06.1
      specified site NEC D06.7
  chorionic
    specified site —*see* Neoplasm, malignant,
      by site
    unspecified site
      female C58
      male C62.90
  chromophobe
    specified site —*see* Neoplasm, malignant,
      by site
    unspecified site C75.1
  cloacogenic
    specified site —*see* Neoplasm, malignant,
      by site
    unspecified site C21.2
  diffuse type
    specified site —*see* Neoplasm, malignant,
      by site
    unspecified site C16.9
  duct (cell)
    with Paget's disease —*see* Neoplasm,
      breast, malignant
    infiltrating
      with lobular carcinoma (in situ)
        specified site —*see* Neoplasm,
          malignant, by site
        unspecified site (female) C50.91-●
          male C50.92-●
      specified site —*see* Neoplasm,
        malignant, by site
      unspecified site (female) C50.91-●
        male C50.92-●
  ductal
    with lobular
      specified site —*see* Neoplasm,
        malignant, by site
      unspecified site (female) C50.91-●
        male C50.92-●
  ductular, infiltrating
    specified site —*see* Neoplasm, malignant,
      by site
    unspecified site (female) C50.91-●
      male C50.92-●
  embryonal
    liver C22.7
  endometrioid
    specified site —*see* Neoplasm, malignant,
      by site
    unspecified site
      female C56.9
      male C61
  eosinophil
    specified site —*see* Neoplasm, malignant,
      by site
    unspecified site C75.1
  epidermoid —*see also* Neoplasm, skin
    malignant
    in situ, Bowen's type —*see* Neoplasm, skin,
      in situ
  fibroepithelial, basal cell —*see* Neoplasm,
    skin, malignant
  follicular
    with papillary (mixed) C73
    moderately differentiated C73
    pure follicle C73
    specified site —*see* Neoplasm, malignant,
      by site
    trabecular C73
    unspecified site C73
    well differentiated C73
  generalized, with unspecified primary site
    C80.0
  glycogen-rich —*see* Neoplasm, breast,
    malignant
  granulosa cell C56-●
  hepatic cell C22.0

Carcinoma *(Continued)*
  hepatocellular C22.0
    with bile duct, mixed C22.0
    fibrolamellar C22.0
  hepatocholangiolitic C22.0
  Hurthle cell C73
  in
    adenomatous
      polyposis coli C18.9
    pleomorphic adenoma —*see* Neoplasm,
      salivary glands, malignant
    situ —*see* Carcinoma-in-situ
  infiltrating
    duct
      with lobular
        specified site —*see* Neoplasm,
          malignant, by site
        unspecified site (female) C50.91-●
          male C50.92-●
      with Paget's disease —*see* Neoplasm,
        breast, malignant
      specified site —*see* Neoplasm,
        malignant
      unspecified site (female) C50.91-●
        male C50.92-●
    ductular
      specified site —*see* Neoplasm,
        malignant
      unspecified site (female) C50.91-●
        male C50.92-●
    lobular
      specified site —*see* Neoplasm,
        malignant
      unspecified site (female) C50.91-●
        male C50.92-●
  inflammatory
    specified site —*see* Neoplasm, malignant
    unspecified site (female) C50.91-●
      male C50.92-●
  intestinal type
    specified site —*see* Neoplasm, malignant,
      by site
    unspecified site C16.9
  intracystic
    noninfiltrating —*see* Neoplasm, in situ,
      by site
  intraductal (noninfiltrating)
    with Paget's disease —*see* Neoplasm,
      breast, malignant
    breast D05.1-●
    papillary
      with invasion
        specified site —*see* Neoplasm,
          malignant, by site
        unspecified site (female) C50.91-●
          male C50.92-●
      breast D05.1-●
      specified site NEC —*see* Neoplasm,
        in situ, by site
      unspecified site (female) D05.1-●
    specified site NEC —*see* Neoplasm,
      in situ, by site
    unspecified site (female) D05.1-●
  intraepidermal —*see* Neoplasm, in situ
    squamous cell, Bowen's type —*see*
      Neoplasm, skin, in situ
  intraepithelial —*see* Neoplasm, in situ,
      by site
    squamous cell —*see* Neoplasm, in situ,
      by site
  intraosseous C41.1
    upper jaw (bone) C41.0
  islet cell
    with exocrine, mixed
      specified site —*see* Neoplasm,
        malignant, by site
      unspecified site C25.9
    pancreas C25.4
    specified site NEC —*see* Neoplasm,
      malignant, by site
    unspecified site C25.4

Carcinoma *(Continued)*
  juvenile, breast —*see* Neoplasm, breast,
    malignant
  large cell
    small cell
      specified site —*see* Neoplasm,
        malignant, by site
      unspecified site C34.90
  Leydig cell (testis)
    specified site —*see* Neoplasm, malignant,
      by site
    unspecified site
      female C56.9
      male C62.90
  lipid-rich (female) C50.91-•
    male C50.92-•
  liver cell C22.0
  liver NEC C22.7
  lobular (infiltrating)
    with intraductal
      specified site —*see* Neoplasm,
        malignant, by site
      unspecified site (female) C50.91-•
        male C50.92-•
    noninfiltrating
      breast D05.0-•
      specified site NEC —*see* Neoplasm, in
        situ, by site
      unspecified site D05.0-•
    specified site —*see* Neoplasm, malignant,
      by site
    unspecified site (female) C50.91-•
      male C50.92-•
  medullary
    with
      amyloid stroma
        specified site —*see* Neoplasm,
          malignant, by site
        unspecified site C73
      lymphoid stroma
        specified site —*see* Neoplasm,
          malignant, by site
        unspecified site (female) C50.91-•
          male C50.92-•
  Merkel cell C4A.9
    anal margin C4A.51
    anal skin C4A.51
    canthus C4A.1-•
    ear and external auricular canal C4A.2-•
    external auricular canal C4A.2-•
    eyelid, including canthus C4A.1-•
    face C4A.30
      specified NEC C4A.39
    hip C4A.7-•
    lip C4A.0
    lower limb, including hip C4A.7-•
    neck C4A.4
    nodal presentation C7B.1
    nose C4A.31
    overlapping sites C4A.8
    perianal skin C4A.51
    scalp C4A.4
    secondary C7B.1
    shoulder C4A.6-•
    skin of breast C4A.52
    trunk NEC C4A.59
    upper limb, including shoulder C4A.6-•
    visceral metastatic C7B.1
  metastatic —*see* Neoplasm, secondary
  metatypical —*see* Neoplasm, skin, malignant
  morphea, basal cell —*see* Neoplasm, skin,
    malignant
  mucoid
    cell
      specified site —*see* Neoplasm,
        malignant, by site
      unspecified site C75.1
  neuroendocrine —*see also* Tumor,
      neuroendocrine
    high grade, any site C7A.1
    poorly differentiated, any site C7A.1

Carcinoma *(Continued)*
  nonencapsulated sclerosing C73
  noninfiltrating
    intracystic —*see* Neoplasm, in situ, by site
    intraductal
      breast D05.1-•
      papillary
        breast D05.1-•
        specified site NEC —*see* Neoplasm, in
          situ, by site
        unspecified site D05.1-•
      specified site —*see* Neoplasm, in situ,
        by site
      unspecified site D05.1-•
    lobular
      breast D05.0-•
      specified site NEC —*see* Neoplasm, in
        situ, by site
      unspecified site (female) D05.0-•
  oat cell
    specified site —*see* Neoplasm, malignant,
      by site
    unspecified site C34.90
  odontogenic C41.1
    upper jaw (bone) C41.0
  papillary
    with follicular (mixed) C73
    follicular variant C73
    intraductal (noninfiltrating)
      with invasion
        specified site —*see* Neoplasm,
          malignant, by site
        unspecified site (female) C50.91-•
          male C50.92-•
      breast D05.1-•
      specified site NEC —*see* Neoplasm, in
        situ, by site
      unspecified site D05.1-•
    serous
      specified site —*see* Neoplasm,
        malignant, by site
      surface
        specified site —*see* Neoplasm,
          malignant, by site
        unspecified site C56.9
      unspecified site C56.9
  papillocystic
    specified site —*see* Neoplasm, malignant,
      by site
    unspecified site C56.9
  parafollicular cell
    specified site —*see* Neoplasm, malignant,
      by site
    unspecified site C73
  pilomatrix —*see* Neoplasm, skin, malignant
  pseudomucinous
    specified site —*see* Neoplasm, malignant,
      by site
    unspecified site C56.9
  renal cell C64-•
  Schmincke —*see* Neoplasm, nasopharynx,
    malignant
  Schneiderian
    specified site —*see* Neoplasm, malignant,
      by site
    unspecified site C30.0
  sebaceous —*see* Neoplasm, skin, malignant
  secondary —*see also* Neoplasm, secondary,
      by site
    Merkel cell C7B.1
  secretory, breast —*see* Neoplasm, breast,
    malignant
  serous
    papillary
      specified site —*see* Neoplasm,
        malignant, by site
      unspecified site C56.9
    surface, papillary
      specified site —*see* Neoplasm,
        malignant, by site
      unspecified site C56.9

Carcinoma *(Continued)*
  Sertoli cell
    specified site —*see* Neoplasm, malignant,
      by site
    unspecified site C62.90
      female C56.9
      male C62.90
  skin appendage —*see* Neoplasm, skin,
    malignant
  small cell
    fusiform cell
      specified site —*see* Neoplasm,
        malignant, by site
      unspecified site C34.90
    intermediate cell
      specified site —*see* Neoplasm,
        malignant, by site
      unspecified site C34.90
    large cell
      specified site —*see* Neoplasm,
        malignant, by site
      unspecified site C34.90
  solid
    with amyloid stroma
      specified site —*see* Neoplasm,
        malignant, by site
      unspecified site C73
    microinvasive
      specified site —*see* Neoplasm,
        malignant, by site
      unspecified site C53.9
  sweat gland —*see* Neoplasm, skin,
    malignant
  theca cell C56.-•
  thymic C37
  unspecified site (primary) C80.1
  water-clear cell C75.0
Carcinoma-in-situ —*see also* Neoplasm, in situ,
    by site
  breast NOS D05.9-•
    specified type NEC D05.8-•
  epidermoid —*see also* Neoplasm, in situ, by
    site
    with questionable stromal invasion
      cervix D06.9
      specified site NEC —*see* Neoplasm, in
        situ, by site
      unspecified site D06.9
    Bowen's type —*see* Neoplasm, skin,
      in situ
  intraductal
    breast D05.1-•
    specified site NEC —*see* Neoplasm, in situ,
      by site
    unspecified site D05.1-•
  lobular
    with
      infiltrating duct
        breast (female) C50.91-•
          male C50.92-•
        specified site NEC —*see* Neoplasm,
          malignant
        unspecified site (female) C50.91-•
          male C50.92-•
      intraductal
        breast D05.8-•
        specified site NEC —*see* Neoplasm, in
          situ, by site
        unspecified site (female) D05.8-•
    breast D05.0-•
    specified site NEC —*see* Neoplasm, in situ,
      by site
    unspecified site D05.0-•
  squamous cell —*see also* Neoplasm, in situ,
    by site
    with questionable stromal invasion
      cervix D06.9
      specified site NEC —*see* Neoplasm, in
        situ, by site
      unspecified site D06.9
Carcinomaphobia F45.29

▶ New   ➡ Revised   ~~deleted~~ Deleted   • Use Additional Character(s)

Carcinomatosis C80.0
  peritonei C78.6
  unspecified site (primary) (secondary) C80.0
Carcinosarcoma —see Neoplasm, malignant,
    by site
  embryonal —see Neoplasm, malignant, by
    site
Cardia, cardial —see condition
Cardiac —see also condition
  death, sudden —see Arrest, cardiac
  pacemaker
    in situ Z95.0
      management or adjustment Z45.018
  tamponade I31.4
Cardialgia —see Pain, precordial
Cardiectasis —see Hypertrophy, cardiac
Cardiochalasia K21.9
Cardiomalacia I51.5
Cardiomegalia glycogenica diffusa E74.02 [143]
Cardiomegaly —see also Hypertrophy, cardiac
  congenital Q24.8
  glycogen E74.02 [143]
  idiopathic I51.7
Cardiomyoliposis I51.5
Cardiomyopathy (familial) (idiopathic) I42.9
  alcoholic I42.6
  amyloid E85.4 [143]
  ▶transthyretin-related (ATTR) familial E85.4
  arteriosclerotic —see Disease, heart, ischemic,
    atherosclerotic
  beriberi E51.12
  cobalt-beer I42.6
  congenital I42.4
  congestive I42.0
  constrictive NOS I42.5
  dilated I42.0
  due to
    alcohol I42.6
    beriberi E51.12
    cardiac glycogenosis E74.02 [143]
    drugs I42.7
    external agents NEC I42.7
    Friedreich's ataxia G11.1
    myotonia atrophica G71.11 [143]
  ⇒progressive muscular dystrophy G71.0 [143]
  glycogen storage E74.02 [143]
  hypertensive —see Hypertension, heart
  hypertrophic (nonobstructive) I42.2
    obstructive I42.1
      congenital Q24.8
  in
    Chagas' disease (chronic) B57.2
      acute B57.0
    sarcoidosis D86.85
  ischemic I25.5
  metabolic E88.9 [143]
    thyrotoxic E05.90 [143]
      with thyroid storm E05.91 [143]
  newborn I42.8
    congenital I42.4
  nutritional E63.9 [143]
    beriberi E51.12
  obscure of Africa I42.8
  peripartum O90.3
  postpartum O90.3
  restrictive NEC I42.5
  rheumatic I09.0
  secondary I42.9
  stress induced I51.81
  takotsubo I51.81
  thyrotoxic E05.90 [143]
    with thyroid storm E05.91 [143]
  toxic NEC I42.7
  ▶transthyretin-related (ATTR) familial amyloid
    E85.4
  tuberculous A18.84
  viral B33.24
Cardionephritis —see Hypertension,
    cardiorenal
Cardionephropathy —see Hypertension,
    cardiorenal

Cardionephrosis —see Hypertension, cardiorenal
Cardiopathia nigra I27.0
Cardiopathy —see also Disease, heart I51.9
  idiopathic I42.9
  mucopolysaccharidosis E76.3 [152]
Cardiopericarditis —see Pericarditis
Cardiophobia F45.29
Cardiorenal —see condition
Cardiorrhexis —see Infarct, myocardium
Cardiosclerosis —see Disease, heart, ischemic,
    atherosclerotic
Cardiosis —see Disease, heart
Cardiospasm (esophagus) (reflex) (stomach)
    K22.0
  congenital Q39.5
    with megaesophagus Q39.5
Cardiostenosis —see Disease, heart
Cardiosymphysis I31.0
Cardiovascular —see condition
Carditis (acute) (bacterial) (chronic) (subacute)
    I51.89
  meningococcal A39.50
  rheumatic —see Disease, heart, rheumatic
  rheumatoid —see Rheumatoid, carditis
  viral B33.20
Care (of) (for) (following)
  child (routine) Z76.2
  family member (handicapped) (sick)
    creating problem for family Z63.6
    provided away from home for holiday
      relief Z75.5
    unavailable, due to
      absence (person rendering care)
        (sufferer) Z74.2
      inability (any reason) of person
        rendering care Z74.2
  foundling Z76.1
  holiday relief Z75.5
  improper —see Maltreatment
  lack of (at or after birth) (infant) —see
      Maltreatment, child, neglect
  lactating mother Z39.1
  palliative Z51.5
  postpartum
    immediately after delivery Z39.0
    routine follow-up Z39.2
  respite Z75.5
  unavailable, due to
    absence of person rendering care Z74.2
    inability (any reason) of person rendering
      care Z74.2
  well-baby Z76.2
Caries
  bone NEC A18.03
  dental (dentino enamel junction) (early
      childhood) (of dentine) (pre-eruptive)
      (recurrent) (to the pulp) K02.9
    arrested (coronal) (root) K02.3
    chewing surface
      limited to enamel K02.51
      penetrating into dentin K02.52
      penetrating into pulp K02.53
    coronal surface
      chewing surface
        limited to enamel K02.51
        penetrating into dentin K02.52
        penetrating into pulp K02.53
      pit and fissure surface
        limited to enamel K02.51
        penetrating into dentin K02.52
        penetrating into pulp K02.53
      smooth surface
        limited to enamel K02.61
        penetrating into dentin K02.62
        penetrating into pulp K02.63
    pit and fissure surface
      limited to enamel K02.51
      penetrating into dentin K02.52
      penetrating into pulp K02.53
    primary, cervical origin K02.52
    root K02.7

Caries (Continued)
  dental (Continued)
    smooth surface
      limited to enamel K02.61
      penetrating into dentin K02.62
      penetrating into pulp K02.63
    external meatus —see Disorder, ear, external,
      specified type NEC
  hip (tuberculous) A18.02
  initial (tooth)
    chewing surface K02.51
    pit and fissure surface K02.51
    smooth surface K02.61
  knee (tuberculous) A18.02
  labyrinth —see subcategory H83.8
  limb NEC (tuberculous) A18.03
  mastoid process (chronic) —see Mastoiditis,
    chronic
    tuberculous A18.03
  middle ear —see subcategory H74.8
  nose (tuberculous) A18.03
  orbit (tuberculous) A18.03
  ossicles, ear —see Abnormal, ear ossicles
  petrous bone —see Petrositis
  root (dental) (tooth) K02.7
  sacrum (tuberculous) A18.01
  spine, spinal (column) (tuberculous) A18.01
  syphilitic A52.77
    congenital (early) A50.02 [M90.80]
  tooth, teeth —see Caries, dental
  tuberculous A18.03
  vertebra (column) (tuberculous) A18.01
Carious teeth —see Caries, dental
Carneous mole O02.0
Carnitine insufficiency E71.40
Carotid body or sinus syndrome G90.01
Carotidynia G90.01
Carotinemia (dietary) E67.1
Carotinosis (cutis) (skin) E67.1
Carpal tunnel syndrome —see Syndrome,
    carpal tunnel
Carpenter's syndrome Q87.0
Carpopedal spasm —see Tetany
Carr-Barr-Plunkett syndrome Q97.1
Carrier (suspected) of
  amebiasis Z22.1
  bacterial disease NEC Z22.39
    diphtheria Z22.2
    intestinal infectious NEC Z22.1
      typhoid Z22.0
    meningococcal Z22.31
    sexually transmitted Z22.4
    specified NEC Z22.39
    staphylococcal (Methicillin susceptible)
      Z22.321
      Methicillin resistant Z22.322
    streptococcal Z22.338
      group B Z22.330
        complicating pregnancy or delivery
          O99.82-●
    typhoid Z22.0
  cholera Z22.1
  diphtheria Z22.2
  gastrointestinal pathogens NEC Z22.1
  genetic Z14.8
    cystic fibrosis Z14.1
    hemophilia A (asymptomatic) Z14.01
      symptomatic Z14.02
  gestational, pregnant Z33.1
  gonorrhea Z22.4
  HAA (hepatitis Australian-antigen) B18.8
  HB (c)(s)-AG B18.1
  hepatitis (viral) B18.9
    Australia-antigen (HAA) B18.8
    B surface antigen (HBsAg) B18.1
      with acute delta- (super)infection
        B17.0
    C B18.2
    specified NEC B18.8
  human T-cell lymphotropic virus type-1
    (HTLV-1) infection Z22.6

Carrier of *(Continued)*
infectious organism Z22.9
specified NEC Z22.8
meningococci Z22.31
Salmonella typhosa Z22.0
serum hepatitis —*see* Carrier, hepatitis
staphylococci (Methicillin susceptible) Z22.321
Methicillin resistant Z22.322
streptococci Z22.338
group B Z22.330
complicating pregnancy or delivery
O99.82-●
syphilis Z22.4
typhoid Z22.0
venereal disease NEC Z22.4
Carrion's disease A44.0
Carter's relapsing fever (Asiatic) A68.1
Cartilage —*see* condition
Caruncle (inflamed)
conjunctiva (acute) —*see* Conjunctivitis, acute
labium (majus) (minus) N90.89
lacrimal —*see* Inflammation, lacrimal,
passages
myrtiform N89.8
urethral (benign) N36.2
Cascade stomach K31.2
Caseation lymphatic gland (tuberculous) A18.2
Cassidy (-Scholte) syndrome (malignant
carcinoid) E34.0
Castellani's disease A69.8
Castration, traumatic, male S38.231
Casts in urine R82.99
Cat
cry syndrome Q93.4
ear Q17.3
eye syndrome Q92.8
Catabolism, senile R54
Catalepsy (hysterical) F44.2
schizophrenic F20.2
Cataplexy (idiopathic) —*see* - Narcolepsy
Cataract (cortical) (immature) (incipient) H26.9
with
neovascularization —*see* Cataract,
complicated
age-related —*see* Cataract, senile
anterior
and posterior axial embryonal Q12.0
pyramidal Q12.0
associated with
galactosemia E74.21 *[H28]*
myotonic disorders G71.19 *[H28]*
blue Q12.0
central Q12.0
cerulean Q12.0
complicated H26.20
with
neovascularization H26.21-●
ocular disorder H26.22-●
glaucomatous flecks H26.23-●
congenital Q12.0
coraliform Q12.0
coronary Q12.0
crystalline Q12.0
diabetic —*see* Diabetes, cataract
drug-induced H26.3-●
due to
ocular disorder —*see* Cataract, complicated
radiation H26.8
electric H26.8
extraction status Z98.4-●
glass-blower's H26.8
heat ray H26.8
heterochromic —*see* Cataract, complicated
hypermature —*see* Cataract, senile,
morgagnian type
in (due to)
chronic iridocyclitis —*see* Cataract,
complicated
diabetes —*see* Diabetes, cataract
endocrine disease E34.9 *[H28]*
eye disease —*see* Cataract, complicated

Cataract *(Continued)*
in (due to) *(Continued)*
hypoparathyroidism E20.9 *[H28]*
malnutrition-dehydration E46 *[H28]*
metabolic disease E88.9 *[H28]*
myotonic disorders G71.19 *[H28]*
nutritional disease E63.9 *[H28]*
infantile —*see* Cataract, presenile
irradiational —*see* Cataract, specified NEC
juvenile —*see* Cataract, presenile
malnutrition-dehydration E46 *[H28]*
morgagnian —*see* Cataract, senile,
morgagnian type
myotonic G71.19 *[H28]*
myxedema E03.9 *[H28]*
nuclear
embryonal Q12.0
sclerosis —*see* Cataract, senile, nuclear
presenile H26.00-●
combined forms H26.06-●
cortical H26.01-●
lamellar —*see* Cataract, presenile, cortical
nuclear H26.03-●
specified NEC H26.09
subcapsular polar (anterior) H26.04-●
posterior H26.05-●
zonular —*see* Cataract, presenile, cortical
secondary H26.40
Soemmering's ring H26.41-●
specified NEC H26.49-●
to eye disease —*see* Cataract, complicated
senile H25.9
brunescens —*see* Cataract, senile, nuclear
combined forms H25.81-●
coronary —*see* Cataract, senile, incipient
cortical H25.01-●
hypermature —*see* Cataract, senile,
morgagnian type
incipient (mature) (total) H25.09-●
cortical —*see* Cataract, senile, cortical
subcapsular —*see* Cataract, senile,
subcapsular
morgagnian type (hypermature) H25.2-●
nuclear (sclerosis) H25.1-●
polar subcapsular (anterior) (posterior) —
see Cataract, senile, incipient
punctate —*see* Cataract, senile, incipient
specified NEC H25.89
subcapsular polar (anterior) H25.03-●
posterior H25.04-●
snowflake —*see* Diabetes, cataract
specified NEC H26.8
toxic —*see* Cataract, drug-induced
traumatic H26.10-●
localized H26.11-●
partially resolved H26.12-●
total H26.13-●
zonular (perinuclear) Q12.0
Cataracta —*see also* Cataract
brunescens —*see* Cataract, senile, nuclear
centralis pulverulenta Q12.0
cerulea Q12.0
complicata —*see* Cataract, complicated
congenita Q12.0
coralliformis Q12.0
coronaria Q12.0
diabetic —*see* Diabetes, cataract
membranacea
accreta —*see* Cataract, secondary
congenita Q12.0
nigra —*see* Cataract, senile, nuclear
sunflower —*see* Cataract, complicated
Catarrh, catarrhal (acute) (febrile) (infectious)
(inflammation) *(see also* condition) J00
bronchial —*see* Bronchitis
chest —*see* Bronchitis
chronic J31.0
due to congenital syphilis A50.03
enteric —*see* Enteritis
eustachian H68.009
fauces —*see* Pharyngitis

Catarrh, catarrhal *(Continued)*
gastrointestinal —*see* Enteritis
gingivitis K05.00
nonplaque induced K05.01
plaque induced K05.00
hay —*see* Fever, hay
intestinal —*see* Enteritis
larynx, chronic J37.0
liver B15.9
with hepatic coma B15.0
lung —*see* Bronchitis
middle ear, chronic —*see* Otitis, media,
nonsuppurative, chronic, serous
mouth K12.1
nasal (chronic) —*see* Rhinitis
nasobronchial J31.1
nasopharyngeal (chronic) J31.1
acute J00
pulmonary —*see* Bronchitis
spring (eye) (vernal) —*see* Conjunctivitis,
acute, atopic
summer (hay) —*see* Fever, hay
throat J31.2
tubotympanal —*see also* Otitis, media,
nonsuppurative
chronic —*see* Otitis, media,
nonsuppurative, chronic, serous
Catatonia (schizophrenic) F20.2
Catatonic
disorder due to known physiologic condition
F06.1
schizophrenia F20.2
stupor R40.1
Cat-scratch —*see also* Abrasion
disease or fever A28.1
Cauda equina —*see* condition
Cauliflower ear M95.1-●
Causalgia (upper limb) G56.4-●
lower limb G57.7-●
Cause
external, general effects T75.89
Caustic burn —*see* Corrosion, by site
Cavare's disease (familial periodic paralysis)
G72.3
Cave-in, injury
crushing (severe) —*see* Crush
suffocation —*see* Asphyxia, traumatic, due to
low oxygen, due to cave-in
Cavernitis (penis) N48.29
Cavernositis N48.29
Cavernous —*see* condition
Cavitation of lung —*see also* Tuberculosis,
pulmonary
nontuberculous J98.4
Cavities, dental —*see* Caries, dental
Cavity
lung —*see* Cavitation of lung
optic papilla Q14.2
pulmonary —*see* Cavitation of lung
Cavovarus foot, congenital Q66.1
Cavus foot (congenital) Q66.7
acquired —*see* Deformity, limb, foot, specified
NEC
Cazenave's disease L10.2
Cecitis K52.9
with perforation, peritonitis, or rupture K65.8
Cecum —*see* condition
Celiac
artery compression syndrome I77.4
disease (with steatorrhea) K90.0
infantilism K90.0
Cell(s), cellular —*see also* condition
in urine R82.99
Cellulitis (diffuse) (phlegmonous) (septic)
(suppurative) L03.90
abdominal wall L03.311
anaerobic A48.0
ankle —*see* Cellulitis, lower limb
anus K61.0
arm —*see* Cellulitis, upper limb
auricle (ear) —*see* Cellulitis, ear

Cellulitis (Continued)
  axilla L03.11-•
  back (any part) L03.312
  breast (acute) (nonpuerperal) (subacute)
      N61.0
    nipple N61.0
  broad ligament
    acute N73.0
  buttock L03.317
  cervical (meaning neck) L03.221
  cervix (uteri) —see Cervicitis
  cheek (external) L03.211
    internal K12.2
  chest wall L03.313
  chronic L03.90
  clostridial A48.0
  corpus cavernosum N48.22
  digit
    finger —see Cellulitis, finger
    toe —see Cellulitis, toe
  Douglas' cul-de-sac or pouch
    acute N73.0
  drainage site (following operation) T81.4
  ear (external) H60.1-•
  eosinophilic (granulomatous) L98.3
  erysipelatous —see Erysipelas
  external auditory canal —see Cellulitis, ear
  eyelid —see Abscess, eyelid
  face NEC L03.211
  finger (intrathecal) (periosteal)
      (subcutaneous) (subcuticular) L03.01-•
  foot —see Cellulitis, lower limb
  gangrenous —see Gangrene
  genital organ NEC
    female (external) N76.4
    male N49.9
      multiple sites N49.8
      specified NEC N49.8
  gluteal (region) L03.317
  gonococcal A54.89
  groin L03.314
  hand —see Cellulitis, upper limb
  head NEC L03.811
    face (any part, except ear, eye and nose)
        L03.211
  heel —see Cellulitis, lower limb
  hip —see Cellulitis, lower limb
  jaw (region) L03.211
  knee —see Cellulitis, lower limb
  labium (majus) (minus) —see Vulvitis
  lacrimal passages —see Inflammation,
      lacrimal, passages
  larynx J38.7
  leg —see Cellulitis, lower limb
  lip K13.0
  lower limb L03.11-•
    toe —see Cellulitis, toe
  mouth (floor) K12.2
  multiple sites, so stated L03.90
  nasopharynx J39.1
  navel L03.316
    newborn P38.9
      with mild hemorrhage P38.1
      without hemorrhage P38.9
  neck (region) L03.221
  nipple (acute) (nonpuerperal) (subacute)
      N61.0
  nose (septum) (external) J34.0
  orbit, orbital H05.01-•
  palate (soft) K12.2
  pectoral (region) L03.313
  pelvis, pelvic (chronic)
    female —see also Disease, pelvis,
        inflammatory N73.2
      acute N73.0
    following ectopic or molar pregnancy
        O08.0
    male K65.0
  penis N48.22
  perineal, perineum L03.315
  periorbital L03.213

Cellulitis (Continued)
  perirectal K61.1
  peritonsillar J36
  periurethral N34.0
  periuterine —see also Disease, pelvis,
      inflammatory N73.2
    acute N73.0
  pharynx J39.1
  preseptal L03.213
  rectum K61.1
  retroperitoneal K68.9
  round ligament
    acute N73.0
  scalp (any part) L03.811
  scrotum N49.2
  seminal vesicle N49.0
  shoulder —see Cellulitis, upper limb
  specified site NEC L03.818
  submandibular (region) (space) (triangle)
      K12.2
    gland K11.3
  submaxillary (region) K12.2
    gland K11.3
  thigh —see Cellulitis, lower limb
  thumb (intrathecal) (periosteal)
      (subcutaneous) (subcuticular) —see
      Cellulitis, finger
  toe (intrathecal) (periosteal) (subcutaneous)
      (subcuticular) L03.03-•
  tonsil J36
  trunk L03.319
    abdominal wall L03.311
    back (any part) L03.312
    buttock L03.317
    chest wall L03.313
    groin L03.314
    perineal, perineum L03.315
    umbilicus L03.316
  tuberculous (primary) A18.4
  umbilicus L03.316
  upper limb L03.11-•
    axilla —see Cellulitis, axilla
    finger —see Cellulitis, finger
    thumb —see Cellulitis, finger
  vaccinal T88.0
  vocal cord J38.3
  vulva —see Vulvitis
  wrist —see Cellulitis, upper limb
Cementoblastoma, benign —see Cyst,
    calcifying odontogenic
Cementoma —see Cyst, calcifying odontogenic
Cementoperiostitis —see Periodontitis
Cementosis K03.4
Central auditory processing disorder H93.25
Central pain syndrome G89.0
Cephalematocele, cephal (o)hematocele
  newborn P52.8
    birth injury P10.8
    traumatic —see Hematoma, brain
Cephalematoma, cephalhematoma (calcified)
  newborn (birth injury) P12.0
  traumatic —see Hematoma, brain
Cephalgia, cephalalgia —see also Headache
  histamine G44.009
    intractable G44.001
    not intractable G44.009
  trigeminal autonomic (TAC) NEC G44.099
    intractable G44.091
    not intractable G44.099
Cephalic —see condition
Cephalitis —see Encephalitis
Cephalocele —see Encephalocele
Cephalomenia N94.89
Cephalopelvic —see condition
Cerclage (with cervical incompetence) in
    pregnancy —see Incompetence, cervix, in
    pregnancy
Cerebellitis —see Encephalitis
Cerebellum, cerebellar —see condition
Cerebral —see condition
Cerebritis —see Encephalitis

Cerebro-hepato-renal syndrome Q87.89
Cerebromalacia —see Softening, brain
  sequelae of cerebrovascular disease I69.398
Cerebroside lipidosis E75.22
Cerebrospasticity (congenital) G80.1
Cerebrospinal —see condition
Cerebrum —see condition
Ceroid-lipofuscinosis, neuronal E75.4
Cerumen (accumulation) (impacted) H61.2-•
Cervical —see also condition
  auricle Q18.2
  dysplasia in pregnancy —see Abnormal,
      cervix, in pregnancy or childbirth
  erosion in pregnancy —see Abnormal, cervix,
      in pregnancy or childbirth
  fibrosis in pregnancy —see Abnormal, cervix,
      in pregnancy or childbirth
  fusion syndrome Q76.1
  rib Q76.5
  shortening (complicating pregnancy)
      O26.87-•
Cervicalgia M54.2
Cervicitis (acute) (chronic) (nonvenereal)
    (senile (atrophic)) (subacute) (with
    ulceration) N72
  with
    abortion —see Abortion, by type
        complicated by genital tract and
        pelvic infection
    ectopic pregnancy O08.0
    molar pregnancy O08.0
  chlamydial A56.09
  gonococcal A54.03
  herpesviral A60.03
  puerperal (postpartum) O86.11
  syphilitic A52.76
  trichomonal A59.09
  tuberculous A18.16
Cervicocolpitis (emphysematosa) (see also
    Cervicitis) N72
Cervix —see condition
Cesarean delivery, previous, affecting
    management of pregnancy O34.219
  classical (vertical) scar O34.212
  low transverse scar O34.211
Céstan (-Chenais) paralysis or syndrome G46.3
Céstan-Raymond syndrome I65.8
Cestode infestation B71.9
  specified type NEC B71.8
Cestodiasis B71.9
Chabert's disease A22.9
Chacaleh E53.8
Chafing L30.4
Chagas' (-Mazza) disease (chronic) B57.2
  with
    cardiovascular involvement NEC B57.2
    digestive system involvement B57.30
      megacolon B57.32
      megaesophagus B57.31
      other specified B57.39
    megacolon B57.32
    megaesophagus B57.31
    myocarditis B57.2
    nervous system involvement B57.40
      meningitis B57.41
      meningoencephalitis B57.42
      other specified B57.49
    specified organ involvement NEC B57.5
  acute (with) B57.1
    cardiovascular NEC B57.0
    myocarditis B57.0
Chagres fever B50.9
Chairridden Z74.09
Chalasia (cardiac sphincter) K21.9
Chalazion H00.19
  left H00.16
    lower H00.15
    upper H00.14
  right H00.13
    lower H00.12
    upper H00.11

▶ New   ⇒ Revised   ~~deleted~~ Deleted   • Use Additional Character(s)

Chalcosis —see also Disorder, globe, degenerative, chalcosis
  cornea —see Deposit, cornea
  crystalline lens —see Cataract, complicated
  retina H35.89
Chalicosis (pulmonum) J62.8
Chancre (any genital site) (hard) (hunterian) (mixed) (primary) (seronegative) (seropositive) (syphilitic) A51.0
  congenital A50.07
  conjunctiva NEC A51.2
  Ducrey's A57
  extragenital A51.2
  eyelid A51.2
  lip A51.2
  nipple A51.2
  Nisbet's A57
  of
    carate A67.0
    pinta A67.0
    yaws A66.0
  palate, soft A51.2
  phagedenic A57
  simple A57
  soft A57
    bubo A57
    palate A51.2
  urethra A51.0
  yaws A66.0
Chancroid (anus) (genital) (penis) (perineum) (rectum) (urethra) (vulva) A57
Chandler's disease (osteochondritis dissecans, hip) —see Osteochondritis, dissecans, hip
Change(s) (in) (of) —see also Removal
  arteriosclerotic —see Arteriosclerosis
  bone —see also Disorder, bone
    diabetic —see Diabetes, bone change
  bowel habit R19.4
  cardiorenal (vascular) —see Hypertension, cardiorenal
  cardiovascular —see Disease, cardiovascular
  circulatory I99.9
  cognitive (mild) (organic) R41.89
  color, tooth, teeth
    during formation K00.8
    posteruptive K03.7
  contraceptive device Z30.433
  corneal membrane H18.30
    Bowman's membrane fold or rupture H18.31-●
    Descemet's membrane
      fold H18.32-●
      rupture H18.33-●
  coronary —see Disease, heart, ischemic
  degenerative, spine or vertebra —see Spondylosis
  dental pulp, regressive K04.2
  dressing (nonsurgical) Z48.00
    surgical Z48.01
  heart —see Disease, heart
  hip joint —see Derangement, joint, hip
  hyperplastic larynx J38.7
  hypertrophic
    nasal sinus J34.89
    turbinate, nasal J34.3
    upper respiratory tract J39.8
  indwelling catheter Z46.6
  inflammatory —see also Inflammation
    sacroiliac M46.1
  job, anxiety concerning Z56.1
  joint —see Derangement, joint
  life —see Menopause
  mental status R41.82
  minimal (glomerular) —see also N00-N07
    with fourth character .0 N05.0
  myocardium, myocardial —see
    Degeneration, myocardial - of life —see Menopause
  pacemaker Z45.018
    pulse generator Z45.010

Change (Continued)
  personality (enduring) F68.8
    due to (secondary to)
      general medical condition F07.0
    secondary (nonspecific) F60.89
  regressive, dental pulp K04.2
  renal —see Disease, renal
  retina H35.9
    myopic —see also Myopia, degenerative H44.2-●
  sacroiliac joint M53.3
  senile —see also condition R54
  sensory R20.8
  skin R23.9
    acute, due to ultraviolet radiation L56.9
      specified NEC L56.8
    chronic, due to nonionizing radiation L57.9
      specified NEC L57.8
    cyanosis R23.0
    flushing R23.2
    pallor R23.1
    petechiae R23.3
    specified change NEC R23.8
    swelling —see Mass, localized
    texture R23.4
  trophic
    arm —see Mononeuropathy, upper limb
    leg —see Mononeuropathy, lower limb
  vascular I99.9
  vasomotor I73.9
  voice R49.9
    psychogenic F44.4
    specified NEC R49.8
Changing sleep-work schedule, affecting sleep G47.26
Changuinola fever A93.1
Chapping skin T69.8
Charcot-Marie-Tooth disease, paralysis or syndrome G60.0
Charcot's
  arthropathy —see Arthropathy, neuropathic
  cirrhosis K74.3
  disease (tabetic arthropathy) A52.16
  joint (disease) (tabetic) A52.16
    diabetic —see Diabetes, with, arthropathy
    syringomyelic G95.0
  syndrome (intermittent claudication) I73.9
CHARGE association Q89.8
Charley-horse (quadriceps) M62.831
  traumatic (quadriceps) S76.11-●
Charlouis' disease —see Yaws
Cheadle's disease E54
Checking (of)
  cardiac pacemaker (battery) (electrode(s)) Z45.018
    pulse generator Z45.010
  implantable subdermal contraceptive Z30.46
  intrauterine contraceptive device Z30.431
  ▶wound Z48.0-●
    ▶due to injury - code to Injury, by site, using appropriate seventh character for subsequent encounter
Check-up —see Examination
Chédiak-Higashi (-Steinbrinck) syndrome (congenital gigantism of peroxidase granules) E70.330
Cheek —see condition
Cheese itch B88.0
Cheese-washer's lung J67.8
Cheese-worker's lung J67.8
Cheilitis (acute) (angular) (catarrhal) (chronic) (exfoliative) (gangrenous) (glandular) (infectional) (suppurative) (ulcerative) (vesicular) K13.0
  actinic (due to sun) L56.8
    other than from sun L59.8
  candidal B37.83
Cheilodynia K13.0
Cheiloschisis —see Cleft, lip
Cheilosis (angular) K13.0
  with pellagra E52
  due to
    vitamin B2 (riboflavin) deficiency E53.0

Cheiromegaly M79.89
Cheiropompholyx L30.1
Cheloid —see Keloid
Chemical burn —see Corrosion, by site
Chemodectoma —see Paraganglioma, nonchromaffin
Chemosis, conjunctiva —see Edema, conjunctiva
Chemotherapy (session) (for)
  cancer Z51.11
  neoplasm Z51.11
Cherubism M27.8
Chest —see condition
Cheyne-Stokes breathing (respiration) R06.3
Chiari's
  disease or syndrome (hepatic vein thrombosis) I82.0
  malformation
    type I G93.5
    type II —see Spina bifida
  net Q24.8
Chicago disease B40.9
Chickenpox —see Varicella
Chiclero ulcer or sore B55.1
Chigger (infestation) B88.0
Chignon (disease) B36.8
  newborn (from vacuum extraction) (birth injury) P12.1
Chilaiditi's syndrome (subphrenic displacement, colon) Q43.3
Chilblain(s) (lupus) T69.1
Child
  custody dispute Z65.3
Childbirth —see Delivery
Childhood
  cerebral X-linked adrenoleukodystrophy E71.520
  period of rapid growth Z00.2
Chill(s) R68.83
  with fever R50.9
  without fever R68.83
  congestive in malarial regions B54
Chilomastigiasis A07.8
Chimera 46,XX/46,XY Q99.0
Chin —see condition
Chinese dysentery A03.9
Chionophobia F40.228
Chitral fever A93.1
Chlamydia, chlamydial A74.9
  cervicitis A56.09
  conjunctivitis A74.0
  cystitis A56.01
  endometritis A56.11
  epididymitis A56.19
  female
    pelvic inflammatory disease A56.11
    pelviperitonitis A56.11
  orchitis A56.19
  peritonitis A74.81
  pharyngitis A56.4
  proctitis A56.3
  psittaci (infection) A70
  salpingitis A56.11
  sexually-transmitted infection NEC A56.8
  specified NEC A74.89
  urethritis A56.01
  vulvovaginitis A56.02
Chlamydiosis —see Chlamydia
Chloasma (skin) (idiopathic) (symptomatic) L81.1
  eyelid H02.719
    hyperthyroid E05.90 [H02.719]
      with thyroid storm E05.91 [H02.719]
    left H02.716
      lower H02.715
      upper H02.714
    right H02.713
      lower H02.712
      upper H02.711
Chloroma C92.3-●
Chlorosis D50.9
  Egyptian B76.9 [D63.8]
  miner's B76.9 [D63.8]

▶ New   ⟾ Revised   ~~deleted~~ Deleted   ● Use Additional Character(s)

Chlorotic anemia D50.8
Chocolate cyst (ovary) N80.1
Choked
   disc or disk —see Papilledema
   on food, phlegm, or vomitus NOS —see
      Foreign body, by site
   while vomiting NOS —see Foreign body, by
      site
Chokes (resulting from bends) T70.3
Choking sensation R09.89
Cholangiectasis K83.8
Cholangiocarcinoma
   with hepatocellular carcinoma, combined
      C22.0
   liver C22.1
   specified site NEC —see Neoplasm,
      malignant, by site
   unspecified site C22.1
Cholangiohepatitis K83.8
   due to fluke infestation B66.1
Cholangiohepatoma C22.0
Cholangiolitis (acute) (chronic) (extrahepatic)
      (gangrenous) (intrahepatic) K83.0
   paratyphoidal —see Fever, paratyphoid
   typhoidal A01.09
Cholangioma D13.4
   malignant —see Cholangiocarcinoma
Cholangitis (ascending) (primary) (recurrent)
      (sclerosing) (secondary) (stenosing)
      (suppurative) K83.0
   with calculus, bile duct —see Calculus, bile
      duct, with cholangitis
   chronic nonsuppurative destructive K74.3
Cholecystectasia K82.8
Cholecystitis K81.9
   with
      calculus, stones in
         bile duct (common) (hepatic) —
            see Calculus, bile duct, with
            cholecystitis
         cystic duct —see Calculus, gallbladder,
            with cholecystitis
         gallbladder —see Calculus, gallbladder,
            with cholecystitis
      choledocholithiasis —see Calculus, bile
         duct, with cholecystitis
      cholelithiasis —see Calculus, gallbladder,
         with cholecystitis
      acute (emphysematous) (gangrenous)
         (suppurative) K81.0
         with
            calculus, stones in
               cystic duct —see Calculus, gallbladder,
                  with cholecystitis, acute
               gallbladder —see Calculus,
                  gallbladder, with cholecystitis,
                  acute
            choledocholithiasis —see Calculus, bile
               duct, with cholecystitis, acute
            cholelithiasis —see Calculus, gallbladder,
               with cholecystitis, acute
         chronic cholecystitis K81.2
            with gallbladder calculus K80.12
               with obstruction K80.13
      chronic K81.1
         with acute cholecystitis K81.2
            with gallbladder calculus K80.12
               with obstruction K80.13
      emphysematous (acute) —see Cholecystitis,
         acute
      gangrenous —see Cholecystitis, acute
      paratyphoidal, current A01.4
      suppurative —see Cholecystitis, acute
      typhoidal A01.09
Cholecystolithiasis —see Calculus, gallbladder
Choledochitis (suppurative) K83.0
Choledocholith —see Calculus, bile duct
Choledocholithiasis (common duct) (hepatic
      duct) —see Calculus, bile duct
   cystic —see Calculus, gallbladder
   typhoidal A01.09

Cholelithiasis (cystic duct) (gallbladder)
      (impacted) (multiple) —see Calculus,
      gallbladder
   bile duct (common) (hepatic) —see Calculus,
      bile duct
   hepatic duct —see Calculus, bile duct
   specified NEC K80.80
      with obstruction K80.81
Cholemia —see also Jaundice
   familial (simple) (congenital) E80.4
   Gilbert's E80.4
Choleperitoneum, choleperitonitis K65.3
Cholera (Asiatic) (epidemic) (malignant) A00.9
   antimonial —see Poisoning, antimony
   classical A00.0
   due to Vibrio cholerae 01 A00.9
      biovar cholerae A00.0
      biovar eltor A00.1
      el tor A00.1
   el tor A00.1
Cholerine —see Cholera
Cholestasis NEC K83.1
   with hepatocyte injury K71.0
   due to total parenteral nutrition (TPN) K76.89
   pure K71.0
Cholesteatoma (ear) (middle) (with reaction)
      H71.9-●
   attic H71.0-●
   external ear (canal) H60.4-●
   mastoid H71.2-●
   postmastoidectomy cavity (recurrent) —see
      Complications, postmastoidectomy,
      recurrent cholesteatoma
   recurrent (postmastoidectomy) —see
      Complications, postmastoidectomy,
      recurrent cholesteatoma
   tympanum H71.1-●
Cholesteatosis, diffuse H71.3-●
Cholesteremia E78.00
Cholesterin in vitreous —see Deposit, crystalline
Cholesterol
   deposit
      retina H35.89
      vitreous —see Deposit, crystalline
   elevated (high) E78.00
      with elevated (high) triglycerides E78.2
      screening for Z13.220
   imbibition of gallbladder K82.4
Cholesterolemia (essential) (pure) E78.00
   familial E78.01
   hereditary E78.01
Cholesterolosis, cholesterosis (gallbladder)
      K82.4
   cerebrotendinous E75.5
Cholocolic fistula K82.3
Choluria R82.2
Chondritis M94.8X9
   aurical H61.03-●
   costal (Tietze's) M94.0
   external ear H61.03-●
   patella, posttraumatic —see Chondromalacia,
      patella
   pinna H61.03-●
   purulent M94.8X-●
   tuberculous NEC A18.02
      intervertebral A18.01
Chondroblastoma —see also Neoplasm, bone,
      benign
   malignant —see Neoplasm, bone, malignant
Chondrocalcinosis M11.20
   ankle M11.27-●
   elbow M11.22-●
   familial M11.10
      ankle M11.17-●
      elbow M11.12-●
      foot joint M11.17-●
      hand joint M11.14-●
      hip M11.15-●
      knee M11.16-●
      multiple site M11.19
      shoulder M11.11-●

Chondrocalcinosis (Continued)
   familial (Continued)
      vertebrae M11.18
      wrist M11.13-●
   foot joint M11.27-●
   hand joint M11.24-●
   hip M11.25-●
   knee M11.26-●
   multiple site M11.29
   shoulder M11.21-●
   specified type NEC M11.20
      ankle M11.27-●
      elbow M11.22-●
      foot joint M11.27-●
      hand joint M11.24-●
      hip M11.25-●
      knee M11.26-●
      multiple site M11.29
      shoulder M11.21-●
      vertebrae M11.28
      wrist M11.23-●
   vertebrae M11.28
   wrist M11.23-●
Chondrodermatitis nodularis helicis or
      anthelicis —see Perichondritis, ear
Chondrodysplasia Q78.9
   with hemangioma Q78.4
   calcificans congenita Q77.3
   fetalis Q77.4
   metaphyseal (Jansen's) (McKusick's)
      (Schmid's) Q78.8
   punctata Q77.3
Chondrodystrophy, chondrodystrophia
      (familial) (fetalis) (hypoplastic) Q78.9
   calcificans congenita Q77.3
   myotonic (congenital) G71.13
   punctata Q77.3
Chondroectodermal dysplasia Q77.6
Chondrogenesis imperfecta Q77.4
Chondrolysis M94.35-●
Chondroma —see also Neoplasm, cartilage,
      benign
   juxtacortical —see Neoplasm, bone, benign
   periosteal —see Neoplasm, bone, benign
Chondromalacia (systemic) M94.20
   acromioclavicular joint M94.21-●
   ankle M94.27-●
   elbow M94.22-●
   foot joint M94.27-●
   glenohumeral joint M94.21-●
   hand joint M94.24-●
   hip M94.25-●
   knee M94.26-●
      patella M22.4-●
   multiple sites M94.29
   patella M22.4-●
   rib M94.28
   sacroiliac joint M94.259
   shoulder M94.21-●
   sternoclavicular joint M94.21-●
   vertebral joint M94.28
   wrist M94.23-●
Chondromatosis —see also Neoplasm, cartilage,
      uncertain behavior
   internal Q78.4
Chondromyxosarcoma —see Neoplasm,
      cartilage, malignant
Chondro-osteodysplasia (Morquio-Brailsford
      type) E76.219
Chondro-osteodystrophy E76.29
Chondro-osteoma —see Neoplasm, bone, benign
Chondropathia tuberosa M94.0
Chondrosarcoma —see Neoplasm, cartilage,
      malignant
   juxtacortical —see Neoplasm, bone, malignant
   mesenchymal —see Neoplasm, connective
      tissue, malignant
   myxoid —see Neoplasm, cartilage, malignant
Chordee (nonvenereal) N48.89
   congenital Q54.4
   gonococcal A54.09

Chorditis (fibrinous) (nodosa) (tuberosa) J38.2
Chordoma —*see* Neoplasm, vertebral (column), malignant
Chorea (chronic) (gravis) (posthemiplegic) (senile) (spasmodic) G25.5
  with
    heart involvement I02.0
      active or acute (conditions in I01-•) I02.0
      rheumatic I02.9
        with valvular disorder I02.0
      rheumatic heart disease (chronic) (inactive) (quiescent) — code to rheumatic heart condition involved
  drug-induced G25.4
  habit F95.8
  hereditary G10
  Huntington's G10
  hysterical F44.4
  minor I02.9
    with heart involvement I02.0
  progressive G25.5
    hereditary G10
  rheumatic (chronic) I02.9
    with heart involvement I02.0
  Sydenham's I02.9
    with heart involvement —*see* Chorea, with rheumatic heart disease
    nonrheumatic G25.5
Choreoathetosis (paroxysmal) G25.5
Chorioadenoma (destruens) D39.2
Chorioamnionitis O41.12-•
Chorioangioma D26.7
Choriocarcinoma —*see* Neoplasm, malignant, by site
  combined with
    embryonal carcinoma —*see* Neoplasm, malignant, by site
    other germ cell elements —*see* Neoplasm, malignant, by site
    teratoma —*see* Neoplasm, malignant, by site
  specified site —*see* Neoplasm, malignant, by site
  unspecified site
    female C58
    male C62.90
Chorioencephalitis (acute) (lymphocytic) (serous) A87.2
Chorioepithelioma —*see* Choriocarcinoma
Choriomeningitis (acute) (lymphocytic) (serous) A87.2
Chorionepithelioma —*see* Choriocarcinoma
Chorioretinitis —*see also* Inflammation, chorioretinal
  disseminated —*see also* Inflammation, chorioretinal, disseminated
    in neurosyphilis A52.19
  Egyptian B76.9 [D63.8]
  focal —*see also* Inflammation, chorioretinal, focal
  histoplasmic B39.9 [H32]
  in (due to)
    histoplasmosis B39.9 [H32]
    syphilis (secondary) A51.43
      late A52.71
    toxoplasmosis (acquired) B58.01
      congenital (active) P37.1 [H32]
    tuberculosis A18.53
  juxtapapillary, juxtapapillaris —*see* Inflammation, chorioretinal, focal, juxtapapillary
  leprous A30.9 [H32]
  miner's B76.9 [D63.8]
  progressive myopia (degeneration) —*see also* Myopia, degenerative H44.2-•
  syphilitic (secondary) A51.43
    congenital (early) A50.01 [H32]
      late A50.32
    late A52.71
  tuberculous A18.53
Chorioretinopathy, central serous H35.71-•

Choroid —*see* condition
Choroideremia H31.21
Choroiditis —*see* Chorioretinitis
Choroidopathy —*see* Disorder, choroid
Choroidoretinitis —*see* Chorioretinitis
Choroidoretinopathy, central serous —*see* Chorioretinopathy, central serous
Christian-Weber disease M35.6
Christmas disease D67
Chromaffinoma —*see also* Neoplasm, benign, by site
  malignant —*see* Neoplasm, malignant, by site
Chromatopsia —*see* Deficiency, color vision
Chromhidrosis, chromidrosis L75.1
Chromoblastomycosis —*see* Chromomycosis
Chromoconversion R82.91
Chromomycosis B43.9
  brain abscess B43.1
  cerebral B43.1
  cutaneous B43.0
  skin B43.0
  specified NEC B43.8
  subcutaneous abscess or cyst B43.2
Chromophytosis B36.0
Chromosome —*see* condition by chromosome involved
  D (1) —*see* condition, chromosome 13
  E (3) —*see* condition, chromosome 18
  G —*see* condition, chromosome 21
Chromotrichomycosis B36.8
Chronic —*see* condition
  fracture —*see* Fracture, pathological
Churg-Strauss syndrome M30.1
Chyle cyst, mesentery I89.8
Chylocele (nonfilarial) I89.8
  filarial —*see also* Infestation, filarial B74.9 [N51]
  tunica vaginalis N50.89
    filarial —*see also* Infestation, filarial B74.9 [N51]
Chylomicronemia (fasting) (with hyperprebetalipoproteinemia) E78.3
Chylopericardium I31.3
  acute I30.9
Chylothorax (nonfilarial) I89.8
  filarial —*see also* Infestation, filarial B74.9 [J91.8]
Chylous —*see* condition
Chyluria (nonfilarial) R82.0
  due to
    bilharziasis B65.0
    Brugia (malayi) B74.1
      timori B74.2
    schistosomiasis (bilharziasis) B65.0
    Wuchereria (bancrofti) B74.0
  filarial —*see* Infestation, filarial
Cicatricial (deformity) —*see* Cicatrix
Cicatrix (adherent) (contracted) (painful) (vicious) —*see also* Scar L90.5
  adenoid (and tonsil) J35.8
  alveolar process M26.79
  anus K62.89
  auricle —*see* Disorder, pinna, specified type NEC
  bile duct (common) (hepatic) K83.8
  bladder N32.89
  bone —*see* Disorder, bone, specified type NEC
  brain G93.89
  cervix (postoperative) (postpartal) N88.1
  common duct K83.8
  cornea H17.9
    tuberculous A18.59
  duodenum (bulb), obstructive K31.5
  esophagus K22.2
  eyelid —*see* Disorder, eyelid function
  hypopharynx J39.2
  lacrimal passages —*see* Obstruction, lacrimal
  larynx J38.7
  lung J98.4
  middle ear —*see* subcategory H74.8
  mouth K13.79

Cicatrix (*Continued*)
  muscle M62.89
    with contracture —*see* Contraction, muscle NEC
  nasopharynx J39.2
  palate (soft) K13.79
  penis N48.89
  pharynx J39.2
  prostate N42.89
  rectum K62.89
  retina —*see* Scar, chorioretinal
  semilunar cartilage —*see* Derangement, meniscus
  seminal vesicle N50.89
  skin L90.5
    infected L08.89
    postinfective L90.5
    tuberculous B90.8
  specified site NEC L90.5
  throat J39.2
  tongue K14.8
  tonsil (and adenoid) J35.8
  trachea J39.8
  tuberculous NEC B90.9
  urethra N36.8
  uterus N85.8
  vagina N89.8
    postoperative N99.2
  vocal cord J38.3
  wrist, constricting (annular) L90.5
CIDP (chronic inflammatory demyelinating polyneuropathy) G61.81
CIN —*see* Neoplasia, intraepithelial, cervix
CINCA (chronic infantile neurological, cutaneous and articular syndrome) M04.2
Cinchonism —*see* Deafness, ototoxic
  correct substance properly administered —*see* Table of Drugs and Chemicals, by drug, adverse effect
  overdose or wrong substance given or taken —*see* Table of Drugs and Chemicals, by drug, poisoning
Circle of Willis —*see* condition
Circular —*see* condition
Circulating anticoagulants —*see also* - Disorder, hemorrhagic D68.318
  due to drugs —*see also* - Disorder, hemorrhagic D68.32
  following childbirth O72.3
Circulation
  collateral, any site I99.8
  defective (lower extremity) I99.9
    congenital Q28.9
  embryonic Q28.9
  failure (peripheral) R57.9
    newborn P29.89
  fetal, persistent P29.38
  heart, incomplete Q28.9
Circulatory system —*see* condition
Circulus senilis (cornea) —*see* Degeneration, cornea, senile
Circumcision (in absence of medical indication) (ritual) (routine) Z41.2
Circumscribed —*see* condition
Circumvallate placenta O43.11-•
Cirrhosis, cirrhotic (hepatic) (liver) K74.60
  alcoholic K70.30
    with ascites K70.31
  atrophic —*see* Cirrhosis, liver
  Baumgarten-Cruveilhier K74.69
  biliary (cholangiolitic) (cholangitic) (hypertrophic) (obstructive) (pericholangiolitic) K74.5
  due to
    Clonorchiasis B66.1
    flukes B66.3
    primary K74.3
    secondary K74.4
  cardiac (of liver) K76.1
  Charcot's K74.3

▶ New   ⇶ Revised   ~~deleted~~ Deleted   • Use Additional Character(s)

Cirrhosis, cirrhotic (Continued)
 cholangiolitic, cholangitic, cholostatic
  (primary) K74.3
 congestive K76.1
 Cruveilhier-Baumgarten K74.69
 cryptogenic (liver) K74.69
 due to
  hepatolenticular degeneration E83.01
  Wilson's disease E83.01
  xanthomatosis E78.2
 fatty K76.0
  alcoholic K70.0
 Hanot's (hypertrophic) K74.3
 hepatic —see Cirrhosis, liver
 hypertrophic K74.3
 Indian childhood K74.69
 kidney —see Sclerosis, renal
 Laennec's K70.30
  with ascites K70.31
  alcoholic K70.30
   with ascites K70.31
  nonalcoholic K74.69
 liver K74.60
  alcoholic K70.30
   with ascites K70.31
   fatty K70.0
  congenital P78.81
  syphilitic A52.74
 lung (chronic) J84.10
 macronodular K74.69
  alcoholic K70.30
   with ascites K70.31
 micronodular K74.69
  alcoholic K70.30
   with ascites K70.31
 mixed type K74.69
 monolobular K74.3
 nephritis —see Sclerosis, renal
 nutritional K74.69
  alcoholic K70.30
   with ascites K70.31
 obstructive —see Cirrhosis, biliary
 ovarian N83.8
 pancreas (duct) K86.89
 pigmentary E83.110
 portal K74.69
  alcoholic K70.30
   with ascites K70.31
 postnecrotic K74.69
  alcoholic K70.30
   with ascites K70.31
 pulmonary J84.10
 renal —see Sclerosis, renal
 spleen D73.2
 stasis K76.1
 Todd's K74.3
 unilobar K74.3
 xanthomatous (biliary) K74.5
  due to xanthomatosis (familial) (metabolic)
   (primary) E78.2
Cistern, subarachnoid R93.0
Citrullinemia E72.23
Citrullinuria E72.23
Civatte's disease or poikiloderma L57.3
Clam digger's itch B65.3
Clammy skin R23.1
Clap —see Gonorrhea
Clarke-Hadfield syndrome (pancreatic
   infantilism) K86.89
Clark's paralysis G80.9
Clastothrix L67.8
Claude Bernard-Horner syndrome G90.2
 traumatic —see Injury, nerve, cervical
  sympathetic
Claude's disease or syndrome G46.3
Claudicatio venosa intermittens I87.8
Claudication (intermittent) I73.9
 cerebral (artery) G45.9
 spinal cord (arteriosclerotic) G95.19
  syphilitic A52.09
 venous (axillary) I87.8

Claustrophobia F40.240
Clavus (infected) L84
Clawfoot (congenital) Q66.89
 acquired —see Deformity, limb, clawfoot
Clawhand (acquired) —see also Deformity, limb,
  clawhand
 congenital Q68.1
Clawtoe (congenital) Q66.89
 acquired —see Deformity, toe, specified NEC
Clay eating —see Pica
Cleansing of artificial opening —see Attention
  to, artificial, opening
Cleft (congenital) —see also Imperfect, closure
 alveolar process M26.79
⟹branchial (persistent) Q18.2
▶cyst Q18.0
 ▶fistula Q18.0
 ▶sinus Q18.0
 cricoid cartilage, posterior Q31.8
 foot Q72.7
 hand Q71.6
 lip (unilateral) Q36.9
  with cleft palate Q37.9
   hard Q37.1
    with soft Q37.5
   soft Q37.3
    with hard Q37.5
  bilateral Q36.0
   with cleft palate Q37.8
    hard Q37.0
     with soft Q37.4
    soft Q37.2
     with hard Q37.4
  median Q36.1
 nose Q30.2
 palate Q35.9
  with cleft lip (unilateral) Q37.9
   bilateral Q37.8
  hard Q35.1
   with
    cleft lip (unilateral) Q37.1
     bilateral Q37.0
    soft Q35.5
     with cleft lip (unilateral) Q37.5
      bilateral Q37.4
  medial Q35.5
  soft Q35.3
   with
    cleft lip (unilateral) Q37.3
     bilateral Q37.2
    hard Q35.5
     with cleft lip (unilateral) Q37.5
      bilateral Q37.4
  penis Q55.69
  scrotum Q55.29
  thyroid cartilage Q31.8
  uvula Q35.7
Cleidocranial dysostosis Q74.0
Cleptomania F63.2
Clicking hip (newborn) R29.4
Climacteric (female) —see also Menopause
 arthritis (any site) NEC —see Arthritis,
  specified form NEC
 depression (single episode) F32.89
  recurrent episode F33.8
 male (symptoms) (syndrome) NEC N50.89
 melancholia (single episode) F32.89
  recurrent episode F33.8
 paranoid state F22
 polyarthritis NEC —see Arthritis, specified
  form NEC
 symptoms (female) N95.1
Clinical research investigation (clinical trial)
   (control subject) (normal comparison)
   (participant) Z00.6
Clitoris —see condition Cloaca (persistent)
   Q43.7
Clonorchiasis, clonorchis infection (liver)
   B66.1
Clonus R25.8
Closed bite M26.29

Clostridium (C.) perfringens, as cause of
  disease classified elsewhere B96.7
Closure
 congenital, nose Q30.0
 cranial sutures, premature Q75.0
 defective or imperfect NEC —see Imperfect,
  closure
 fistula, delayed —see Fistula
 foramen ovale, imperfect Q21.1
 hymen N89.6
 interauricular septum, defective Q21.1
 interventricular septum, defective Q21.0
 lacrimal duct —see also Stenosis, lacrimal,
  duct
   congenital Q10.5
 nose (congenital) Q30.0
  acquired M95.0
 of artificial opening —see Attention to,
  artificial, opening
 primary angle, without glaucoma damage
  H40.06-●
 vagina N89.5
 valve —see Endocarditis
 vulva N90.5
Clot (blood) —see also Embolism
 artery (obstruction) (occlusion) —see
  Embolism
 bladder N32.89
 brain (intradural or extradural) —see
  Occlusion, artery, cerebral
 circulation I74.9
 heart —see also Infarct, myocardium
  not resulting in infarction I51.3
 vein —see Thrombosis
Clouded state R40.1
 epileptic —see Epilepsy, specified NEC
 paroxysmal —see Epilepsy, specified NEC
Cloudy antrum, antra J32.0
Clouston's (hidrotic) ectodermal dysplasia
   Q82.4
Clubbed nail pachydermoperiostosis M89.40
   [L62]
Clubbing of finger(s) (nails) R68.3
Clubfinger R68.3
 congenital Q68.1
Clubfoot (congenital) Q66.89
 acquired —see Deformity, limb, clubfoot
 equinovarus Q66.0
 paralytic —see Deformity, limb, clubfoot
Clubhand (congenital) (radial) Q71.4-●
 acquired —see Deformity, limb, clubhand
Clubnail R68.3
 congenital Q84.6
Clump, kidney Q63.1
Clumsiness, clumsy child syndrome F82
Cluttering F98.81
Clutton's joints A50.51 [M12.80]
Coagulation, intravascular (diffuse)
   (disseminated) —see also Defibrination
   syndrome
 complicating abortion —see Abortion, by
  type, complicated by, intravascular
  coagulation
 following ectopic or molar pregnancy
  O08.1
Coagulopathy —see also Defect, coagulation
 consumption D65
 intravascular D65
  newborn P60
Coalition
 calcaneo-scaphoid Q66.89
 tarsal Q66.89
Coalminer's
 elbow —see Bursitis, elbow, olecranon
 lung or pneumoconiosis J60
Coalworker's lung or pneumoconiosis
   J60
Coarctation
 aorta (preductal) (postductal) Q25.1
 pulmonary artery Q25.71
Coated tongue K14.3

Coats' disease (exudative retinopathy) —see Retinopathy, exudative
Cocaine-induced
  anxiety disorder F14.980
  bipolar and related disorder F14.94
  depressive disorder F14.94
  obsessive-compulsive and related disorder F14.988
  psychotic disorder F14.959
  sleep disorder F14.982
  sexual dysfunction F14.981
Cocainism —see Disorder, cocaine use
Coccidioidomycosis B38.9
  cutaneous B38.3
  disseminated B38.7
  generalized B38.7
  meninges B38.4
  prostate B38.81
  pulmonary B38.2
    acute B38.0
    chronic B38.1
  skin B38.3
  specified NEC B38.89
Coccidioidosis —see Coccidioidomycosis
Coccidiosis (intestinal) A07.3
Coccydynia, coccygodynia M53.3
Coccyx —see condition
Cochin-China diarrhea K90.1
Cockayne's syndrome Q87.1
Cocked up toe —see Deformity, toe, specified NEC
Cock's peculiar tumor L72.3
Codman's tumor —see Neoplasm, bone, benign
Coenurosis B71.8
Coffee-worker's lung J67.8
Cogan's syndrome H16.32-•
  oculomotor apraxia H51.8
Coitus, painful (female) N94.10
  male N53.12
  psychogenic F52.6
Cold J00
  with influenza, flu, or grippe —see Influenza, with, respiratory manifestations NEC
  agglutinin disease or hemoglobinuria (chronic) D59.1
  bronchial —see Bronchitis
  chest —see Bronchitis
  common (head) J00
  effects of T69.9
    specified effect NEC T69.8
  excessive, effects of T69.9
    specified effect NEC T69.8
  exhaustion from T69.8
  exposure to T69.9
    specified effect NEC T69.8
  head J00
  injury syndrome (newborn) P80.0
  on lung —see Bronchitis
  rose J30.1
  sensitivity, auto-immune D59.1
  ▶symptoms J00
  virus J00
Coldsore B00.1
Colibacillosis A49.8
  as the cause of other disease (see also Escherichia coli) B96.20
  generalized A41.50
Colic (bilious) (infantile) (intestinal) (recurrent) (spasmodic) R10.83
  abdomen R10.83
    psychogenic F45.8
  appendix, appendicular K38.8
  bile duct —see Calculus, bile duct
  biliary —see Calculus, bile duct
  common duct —see Calculus, bile duct
  cystic duct —see Calculus, gallbladder
  Devonshire NEC —see Poisoning, lead
  gallbladder —see Calculus, gallbladder
  gallstone —see Calculus, gallbladder
    gallbladder or cystic duct —see Calculus, gallbladder

Colic (Continued)
  hepatic (duct) —see Calculus, bile duct
  hysterical F45.8
  kidney N23
  lead NEC —see Poisoning, lead
  mucous K58.9
    with diarrhea K58.0
    psychogenic F54
  nephritic N23
  painter's NEC —see Poisoning, lead
  pancreas K86.89
  psychogenic F45.8
  renal N23
  saturnine NEC —see Poisoning, lead
  ureter N23
  urethral N36.8
    due to calculus N21.1
  uterus NEC N94.89
    menstrual —see Dysmenorrhea
  worm NOS B83.9
Colicystitis —see Cystitis
Colitis (acute) (catarrhal) (chronic) (noninfective) (hemorrhagic) (see also Enteritis) K52.9
  allergic K52.29
    with
      food protein-induced enterocolitis syndrome K52.21
      proctocolitis K52.82
  amebic (acute) —see also Amebiasis A06.0
    nondysenteric A06.2
  anthrax A22.2
  bacillary —see Infection, Shigella
  balantidial A07.0
  ▶Clostridium difficile
    ▶not specified as recurrent A04.72
    ▶recurrent A04.71
  coccidial A07.3
  collagenous K52.831
  cystica superficialis K52.89
  dietary counseling and surveillance (for) Z71.3
  dietetic —see also Colitis, allergic K52.29
  drug-induced K52.1
  due to radiation K52.0
  eosinophilic K52.82
  food hypersensitivity —see also Colitis, allergic K52.29
  giardial A07.1
  granulomatous —see Enteritis, regional, large intestine
  infectious —see Enteritis, infectious
  indeterminate, so stated K52.3
  ischemic K55.9
    acute (subacute) —see also Ischemia, intestine, acute K55.039
    chronic K55.1
    due to mesenteric artery insufficiency K55.1
    fulminant (acute) —see also Ischemia, intestine, acute K55.039
  left sided K51.50
    with
      abscess K51.514
      complication K51.519
        specified NEC K51.518
      fistula K51.513
      obstruction K51.512
      rectal bleeding K51.511
  lymphocytic K52.832
  membranous
    psychogenic F54
  microscopic K52.839
    specified NEC K52.838
  mucous —see Syndrome, irritable, bowel
    psychogenic F54
  noninfective K52.9
    specified NEC K52.89
  polyposa —see Polyp, colon, inflammatory
  protozoal A07.9
  ▶pseudomembranous
    ▶not specified as recurrent A04.72
    ▶recurrent A04.71

Colitis (Continued)
  pseudomucinous —see Syndrome, irritable, bowel
  regional —see Enteritis, regional, large intestine
    ▶infectious A09
  segmental —see Enteritis, regional, large intestine
  septic —see Enteritis, infectious
  spastic K58.9
    with diarrhea K58.0
    psychogenic F54
  staphylococcal A04.8
    foodborne A05.0
  subacute ischemic —see also Ischemia, intestine, acute K55.039
  thromboulcerative —see also Ischemia, intestine, acute K55.039
  toxic NEC K52.1
  ▶due to Clostridium difficile
    ▶not specified as recurrent A04.72
    ▶recurrent A04.71
  transmural —see Enteritis, regional, large intestine
  trichomonal A07.8
  tuberculous (ulcerative) A18.32
  ulcerative (chronic) K51.90
    with
      complication K51.919
        abscess K51.914
        fistula K51.913
        obstruction K51.912
        rectal bleeding K51.911
        specified complication NEC K51.918
    enterocolitis —see Enterocolitis, ulcerative
    ileocolitis —see Ileocolitis, ulcerative
    mucosal proctocolitis —see Proctocolitis, mucosal
    proctitis —see Proctitis, ulcerative
    pseudopolyposis —see Polyp, colon, inflammatory
    psychogenic F54
    rectosigmoiditis —see Rectosigmoiditis, ulcerative
    specified type NEC K51.80
      with
        complication K51.819
          abscess K51.814
          fistula K51.813
          obstruction K51.812
          rectal bleeding K51.811
          specified complication NEC K51.818
Collagenosis, collagen disease (nonvascular) (vascular) M35.9
  cardiovascular I42.8
  reactive perforating L87.1
  specified NEC M35.8
Collapse R55
  adrenal E27.2
  cardiorespiratory R57.0
  cardiovascular R57.0
    newborn P29.89
  circulatory (peripheral) R57.9
    during or after labor and delivery O75.1
    following ectopic or molar pregnancy O08.3
    newborn P29.89
  during or
    after labor and delivery O75.1
    resulting from a procedure, not elsewhere classified T81.10
  external ear canal —see Stenosis, external ear canal
  general R55
  heart —see Disease, heart
  heat T67.1
  hysterical F44.89
  labyrinth, membranous (congenital) Q16.5
  lung (massive) —see also Atelectasis J98.19
    pressure due to anesthesia (general) (local) or other sedation T88.2
      during labor and delivery O74.1
    in pregnancy O29.02-•
    postpartum, puerperal O89.09

Collapse *(Continued)*
 myocardial —*see* Disease, heart
 nervous F48.8
 neurocirculatory F45.8
 nose M95.0
 postoperative T81.10
 pulmonary —*see also* Atelectasis J98.19
  newborn —*see* Atelectasis
 trachea J39.8
 tracheobronchial J98.09
 valvular —*see* Endocarditis
 vascular (peripheral) R57.9
  during or after labor and delivery O75.1
  following ectopic or molar pregnancy O08.3
  newborn P29.89
 vertebra M48.50-●
  cervical region M48.52-●
  cervicothoracic region M48.53-●
  in (due to)
   metastasis —*see* Collapse, vertebra, in,
    specified disease NEC
   osteoporosis —*see also* Osteoporosis
    M80.88
    cervical region M80.88
    cervicothoracic region M80.88
    lumbar region M80.88
    lumbosacral region M80.88
    multiple sites M80.88
    occipito-atlanto-axial region M80.88
    sacrococcygeal region M80.88
    thoracic region M80.88
    thoracolumbar region M80.88
   specified disease NEC M48.50-●
    cervical region M48.52-●
    cervicothoracic region M48.53-●
    lumbar region M48.56-●
    lumbosacral region M48.57-●
    occipito-atlanto-axial region M48.51-●
    sacrococcygeal region M48.58-●
    thoracic region M48.54-●
    thoracolumbar region M48.55-●
  lumbar region M48.56-●
  lumbosacral region M48.57-●
  occipito-atlanto-axial region M48.51-●
  sacrococcygeal region M48.58-●
  thoracic region M48.54-●
  thoracolumbar region M48.55-●
Collateral —*see also* condition
 circulation (venous) I87.8
 dilation, veins I87.8
Colles' fracture S52.53-●
Collet (-Sicard) syndrome G52.7
Collier's asthma or lung J60
Collodion baby Q80.2
Colloid nodule (of thyroid) (cystic) E04.1
Coloboma (iris) Q13.0
 eyelid Q10.3
 fundus Q14.8
 lens Q12.2
 optic disc (congenital) Q14.2
  acquired H47.31-●
Coloenteritis —*see* Enteritis
Colon —*see* condition
Colonization
 MRSA (Methicillin resistant Staphylococcus
  aureus) Z22.322
 MSSA (Methicillin susceptible
  Staphylococcus aureus) Z22.321
 status —*see* Carrier (suspected) of
Coloptosis K63.4
Color blindness —*see* Deficiency, color vision
Colostomy
 attention to Z43.3
 fitting or adjustment Z46.89
 malfunctioning K94.03
 status Z93.3
Colpitis (acute) —*see* Vaginitis
Colpocele N81.5
Colpocystitis —*see* Vaginitis
Colpospasm N94.2
Column, spinal, vertebral —*see* condition

Coma R40.20
 with
  motor response (none) R40.231
   abnormal R40.233
  ▶abnormal extensor posturing to pain or
    noxious stimuli (<2 years of age)
    R40.232
  ▶abnormal flexure posturing to pain or
    noxious stimuli (0-5 years of age)
    R40.233
   extension R40.232
  ▶extensor posturing to pain or noxious
    stimuli (2-5 years of age) R40.232
  ▶flexion/decorticate posturing
    (<2 years of age) R40.233
   flexion withdrawal R40.234
  ⇒localizes pain (2-5 years of age) R40.235
  ▶normal or spontaneous movement
    (<2 years of age) R40.236
  ⇒obeys commands (2-5 years of age)
    R40.236
  ▶withdraws from pain or noxious stimuli
    (0-5 years of age) R40.234
  ▶withdraws to touch (<2 years of age)
    R40.235
  opening of eyes (never) R40.211
   in response to
    pain R40.212
    sound R40.213
   spontaneous R40.214
  verbal response (none) R40.221
   confused conversation R40.224
  ▶cooing or babbling or crying
    appropriately (<2 years of age)
    R40.225
  ▶inappropriate crying or screaming
    (<2 years of age) R40.223
   inappropriate words R40.223
  ⇒inappropriate words (2-5 years of age)
    R40.224
  ▶incomprehensible sounds (2-5 years of
    age) R40.222
   incomprehensible words R40.222
  ▶irritable cries (<2 years of age) R40.224
  ▶moans/grunts to pain; restless
    (<2 years old) R40.222
   oriented R40.225
  ▶screaming (2-5 years of age) R40.223
  ▶uses appropriate words (2-5 years of
    age) R40.225
 eclamptic —*see* Eclampsia
 epileptic —*see* Epilepsy
 Glasgow, scale score —*see* Glasgow coma scale
 hepatic —*see* Failure, hepatic, by type, with
  coma
 hyperglycemic (diabetic) —*see* Diabetes, by
  type, with hyperosmolarity, with coma
 hyperosmolar (diabetic) —*see* Diabetes, by
  type, with hyperosmolarity, with coma
 hypoglycemic (diabetic) —*see* Diabetes, by
  type, with hypoglycemia, with coma
 nondiabetic E15
 in diabetes —*see* Diabetes, coma
 insulin-induced —*see* Coma, hypoglycemic
 ▶ketoacidotic (diabetic) —*see* Diabetes, by
  type, with ketoacidosis, with coma
 myxedematous E03.5
 newborn P91.5
 persistent vegetative state R40.3
 specified NEC, without documented
  Glasgow coma scale score, or with
  partial Glasgow coma scale score
  reported R40.244
Comatose —*see* Coma
Combat fatigue F43.0
Combined —*see* condition
Comedo, comedones (giant) L70.0
Comedocarcinoma —*see also* Neoplasm, breast,
 malignant
 noninfiltrating
  breast D05.8-●
  specified site —*see* Neoplasm, in situ, by site
  unspecified site D05.8-●

Comedomastitis —*see* Ectasia, mammary duct
Comminuted fracture - code as Fracture, closed
Common
 arterial trunk Q20.0
 atrioventricular canal Q21.2
 atrium Q21.1
 cold (head) J00
 truncus (arteriosus) Q20.0
 variable immunodeficiency —*see*
  Immunodeficiency, common variable
 ventricle Q20.4
Commotio, commotion (current)
 brain —*see* Injury, intracranial, concussion
 cerebri —*see* Injury, intracranial, concussion
 retinae S05.8X-●
 spinal cord —*see* Injury, spinal cord,
  by region
 spinalis —*see* Injury, spinal cord, by region
Communication
 between
  base of aorta and pulmonary artery
   Q21.4
  left ventricle and right atrium Q20.5
  pericardial sac and pleural sac Q34.8
  pulmonary artery and pulmonary vein,
   congenital Q25.72
 congenital between uterus and digestive or
  urinary tract Q51.7
Compartment syndrome (deep) (posterior)
 (traumatic) T79.A0
 abdomen T79.A3
 lower extremity (hip, buttock, thigh, leg, foot,
  toes) T79.A2
 nontraumatic
  abdomen M79.A3
  lower extremity (hip, buttock, thigh, leg,
   foot, toes) M79.A2-●
  specified site NEC M79.A9
  upper extremity (shoulder, arm, forearm,
   wrist, hand, fingers) M79.A1-●
 specified site NEC T79.A9
 upper extremity (shoulder, arm, forearm,
  wrist, hand, fingers) T79.A1
Compensation
 failure —*see* Disease, heart
 neurosis, psychoneurosis —*see* Disorder,
  factitious
Complaint —*see also* Disease
 bowel, functional K59.9
  psychogenic F45.8
 intestine, functional K59.9
  psychogenic F45.8
 kidney —*see* Disease, renal
 miners' J60
Complete —*see* condition
Complex
 Addison-Schilder E71.528
 cardiorenal —*see* Hypertension, cardiorenal
 Costen's M26.69
 disseminated mycobacterium avium-
  intracellulare (DMAC) A31.2
 ⇒Eisenmenger's (ventricular septal defect)
  I27.83
 hypersexual F52.8
 jumped process, spine —*see* Dislocation,
  vertebra
 primary, tuberculous A15.7
 Schilder-Addison E71.528
 subluxation (vertebral) M99.19
  abdomen M99.19
  acromioclavicular M99.17
  cervical region M99.11
  cervicothoracic M99.11
  costochondral M99.18
  costovertebral M99.18
  head region M99.10
  hip M99.15
  lower extremity M99.16
  lumbar region M99.13
  lumbosacral M99.13
  occipitocervical M99.10
  pelvic region M99.15
  pubic M99.15

Complex *(Continued)*
   subluxation (vertebral) *(Continued)*
      rib cage M99.18
      sacral region M99.14
      sacrococcygeal M99.14
      sacroiliac M99.14
      specified NEC M99.19
      sternochondral M99.18
      sternoclavicular M99.17
      thoracic region M99.12
      thoracolumbar M99.12
      upper extremity M99.17
   Taussig-Bing (transposition, aorta and overriding pulmonary artery) Q20.1
Complication(s) (from) (of)
   accidental puncture or laceration during a procedure (of) —see Complications, intraoperative (intraprocedural), puncture or laceration
   amputation stump (surgical) (late) NEC T87.9
      dehiscence T87.81
      infection or inflammation T87.40
         lower limb T87.4-●
         upper limb T87.4-●
      necrosis T87.50
         lower limb T87.5-●
         upper limb T87.5-●
      neuroma T87.30
         lower limb T87.3-●
         upper limb T87.3-●
      specified type NEC T87.89
   anastomosis (and bypass) —see also Complications, prosthetic device or implant
      intestinal (internal) NEC K91.89
         involving urinary tract N99.89
      urinary tract (involving intestinal tract) N99.89
      vascular —see Complications, cardiovascular device or implant
   anesthesia, anesthetic —see also Anesthesia, complication T88.59
      brain, postpartum, puerperal O89.2
      cardiac
         in
            labor and delivery O74.2
            pregnancy O29.19-●
         postpartum, puerperal O89.1
      central nervous system
         in
            labor and delivery O74.3
            pregnancy O29.29-●
         postpartum, puerperal O89.2
      difficult or failed intubation T88.4
         in pregnancy O29.6-●
      failed sedation (conscious) (moderate) during procedure T88.52
      general, unintended awareness during procedure T88.53
      hyperthermia, malignant T88.3
      hypothermia T88.51
      intubation failure T88.4
      malignant hyperthermia T88.3
      pulmonary
         in
            labor and delivery O74.1
            pregnancy NEC O29.09-●
         postpartum, puerperal O89.09
      shock T88.2
      spinal and epidural
         in
            labor and delivery NEC O74.6
               headache O74.5
            pregnancy NEC O29.5X-●
         postpartum, puerperal NEC O89.5
            headache O89.4
      unintended awareness under general anesthesia during procedure T88.53
   anti-reflux device —see Complications, esophageal anti-reflux device
   aortic (bifurcation) graft —see Complications, graft, vascular

Complication *(Continued)*
   aortocoronary (bypass) graft —see Complications, coronary artery (bypass) graft
   aortofemoral (bypass) graft —see Complications, extremity artery (bypass) graft
   arteriovenous
      fistula, surgically created T82.9
         embolism T82.818
         fibrosis T82.828
         hemorrhage T82.838
         infection or inflammation T82.7
         mechanical
            breakdown T82.510
            displacement T82.520
            leakage T82.530
            malposition T82.520
            obstruction T82.590
            perforation T82.590
            protrusion T82.590
         pain T82.848
         specified type NEC T82.898
         stenosis T82.858
         thrombosis T82.868
      shunt, surgically created T82.9
         embolism T82.818
         fibrosis T82.828
         hemorrhage T82.838
         infection or inflammation T82.7
         mechanical
            breakdown T82.511
            displacement T82.521
            leakage T82.531
            malposition T82.521
            obstruction T82.591
            perforation T82.591
            protrusion T82.591
         pain T82.848
         specified type NEC T82.898
         stenosis T82.858
         thrombosis T82.868
   arthroplasty —see Complications, joint prosthesis
   artificial
      fertilization or insemination N98.9
         attempted introduction (of)
            embryo in embryo transfer N98.3
            ovum following in vitro fertilization N98.2
         hyperstimulation of ovaries N98.1
         infection N98.0
         specified NEC N98.8
      heart T82.9
         embolism T82.817
         fibrosis T82.827
         hemorrhage T82.837
         infection or inflammation T82.7
         mechanical
            breakdown T82.512
            displacement T82.522
            leakage T82.532
            malposition T82.522
            obstruction T82.592
            perforation T82.592
            protrusion T82.592
         pain T82.847
         specified type NEC T82.897
         stenosis T82.857
         thrombosis T82.867
      opening
         cecostomy —see Complications, colostomy
         colostomy —see Complications, colostomy
         cystostomy —see Complications, cystostomy
         enterostomy —see Complications, enterostomy
         gastrostomy —see Complications, gastrostomy
         ileostomy —see Complications, enterostomy

Complication *(Continued)*
   artificial *(Continued)*
      opening *(Continued)*
         jejunostomy —see Complications, enterostomy
         nephrostomy —see Complications, stoma, urinary tract
         tracheostomy —see Complications, tracheostomy
         ureterostomy —see Complications, stoma, urinary tract
         urethrostomy —see Complications, stoma, urinary tract
   balloon implant or device
      gastrointestinal T85.9
         embolism T85.818
         fibrosis T85.828
         hemorrhage T85.838
         infection and inflammation T85.79
         pain T85.848
         specified type NEC T85.898
         stenosis T85.858
         thrombosis T85.868
      vascular (counterpulsation) T82.9
         embolism T82.818
         fibrosis T82.828
         hemorrhage T82.838
         infection or inflammation T82.7
         mechanical
            breakdown T82.513
            displacement T82.523
            leakage T82.533
            malposition T82.523
            obstruction T82.593
            perforation T82.593
            protrusion T82.593
         pain T82.848
         specified type NEC T82.898
         stenosis T82.858
         thrombosis T82.868
   bariatric procedure
      gastric band procedure K95.09
         infection K95.01
      specified procedure NEC K95.89
         infection K95.81
   bile duct implant (prosthetic) T85.9
      embolism T85.818
      fibrosis T85.828
      hemorrhage T85.838
      infection and inflammation T85.79
      mechanical
         breakdown T85.510
         displacement T85.520
         malfunction T85.510
         malposition T85.520
         obstruction T85.590
         perforation T85.590
         protrusion T85.590
         specified NEC T85.590
      pain T85.848
      specified type NEC T85.898
      stenosis T85.858
      thrombosis T85.868
   bladder device (auxiliary) —see Complications, genitourinary, device or implant, urinary system
   bleeding (postoperative) —see Complication, postoperative, hemorrhage
      intraoperative —see Complication, intraoperative, hemorrhage
   blood vessel graft —see Complications, graft, vascular
   bone
      device NEC T84.9
         embolism T84.81
         fibrosis T84.82
         hemorrhage T84.83
         infection or inflammation T84.7
         mechanical
            breakdown T84.318
            displacement T84.328
            malposition T84.328

Complication *(Continued)*
  bone *(Continued)*
    device *(Continued)*
      mechanical *(Continued)*
        obstruction T84.398
        perforation T84.398
        protrusion T84.398
      pain T84.84
      specified type NEC T84.89
      stenosis T84.85
      thrombosis T84.86
    graft —*see* Complications, graft, bone
    growth stimulator (electrode) —*see*
      Complications, electronic stimulator
      device, bone
    marrow transplant —*see* Complications,
      transplant, bone, marrow
  brain neurostimulator (electrode) —*see*
    Complications, electronic stimulator
    device, brain
  breast implant (prosthetic) T85.9
    capsular contracture T85.44
    embolism T85.818
    fibrosis T85.828
    hemorrhage T85.838
    infection and inflammation T85.79
    mechanical
      breakdown T85.41
      displacement T85.42
      leakage T85.43
      malposition T85.42
      obstruction T85.49
      perforation T85.49
      protrusion T85.49
      specified NEC T85.49
    pain T85.848
    specified type NEC T85.898
    stenosis T85.858
    thrombosis T85.868
  bypass —*see also* Complications, prosthetic
    device or implant
    aortocoronary —*see* Complications,
      coronary artery (bypass) graft
    arterial —*see also* Complications, graft,
      vascular
      extremity —*see* Complications, extremity
        artery (bypass) graft
  cardiac —*see also* Disease, heart
    device, implant or graft T82.9
      embolism T82.817
      fibrosis T82.827
      hemorrhage T82.837
      infection or inflammation T82.7
        valve prosthesis T82.6
      mechanical
        breakdown T82.519
          specified device NEC T82.518
        displacement T82.529
          specified device NEC T82.528
        leakage T82.539
          specified device NEC T82.538
        malposition T82.529
          specified device NEC T82.528
        obstruction T82.599
          specified device NEC T82.598
        perforation T82.599
          specified device NEC T82.598
        protrusion T82.599
          specified device NEC T82.598
      pain T82.847
      specified type NEC T82.897
      stenosis T82.857
      thrombosis T82.867
  cardiovascular device, graft or implant T82.9
    aortic graft —*see* Complications, graft,
      vascular
    arteriovenous
      fistula, artificial —*see* Complication,
        arteriovenous, fistula, surgically
        created
      shunt —*see* Complication, arteriovenous,
        shunt, surgically created

Complication *(Continued)*
  cardiovascular device, graft or implant
    (Continued)
    artificial heart —*see* Complication,
      artificial, heart
    balloon (counterpulsation) device —*see*
      Complication, balloon implant,
      vascular
    carotid artery graft —*see* Complications,
      graft, vascular
    coronary bypass graft —*see* Complication,
      coronary artery (bypass) graft
    dialysis catheter (vascular) —*see*
      Complication, catheter, dialysis
    electronic T82.9
      electrode T82.9
        embolism T82.817
        fibrosis T82.827
        hemorrhage T82.837
        infection T82.7
        mechanical
          breakdown T82.110
          displacement T82.120
          leakage T82.190
          obstruction T82.190
          perforation T82.190
          protrusion T82.190
          specified type NEC T82.190
        pain T82.847
        specified NEC T82.897
        stenosis T82.857
        thrombosis T82.867
      embolism T82.817
      fibrosis T82.827
      hemorrhage T82.837
      infection T82.7
      mechanical
        breakdown T82.119
        displacement T82.129
        leakage T82.199
        obstruction T82.199
        perforation T82.199
        protrusion T82.199
        specified type NEC T82.199
      pain T82.847
      pulse generator T82.9
        embolism T82.817
        fibrosis T82.827
        hemorrhage T82.837
        infection T82.7
        mechanical
          breakdown T82.111
          displacement T82.121
          leakage T82.191
          obstruction T82.191
          perforation T82.191
          protrusion T82.191
          specified type NEC T82.191
        pain T82.847
        specified NEC T82.897
        stenosis T82.857
        thrombosis T82.867
      specified condition NEC T82.897
      specified device NEC T82.9
        embolism T82.817
        fibrosis T82.827
        hemorrhage T82.837
        infection T82.7
        mechanical
          breakdown T82.118
          displacement T82.128
          leakage T82.198
          obstruction T82.198
          perforation T82.198
          protrusion T82.198
          specified type NEC T82.198
        pain T82.847
        specified NEC T82.897
        stenosis T82.857
        thrombosis T82.867
      stenosis T82.857
      thrombosis T82.867

Complication *(Continued)*
  cardiovascular device, graft or implant
    (Continued)
    extremity artery graft —*see* Complication,
      extremity artery (bypass) graft
    femoral artery graft —*see* Complication,
      extremity artery (bypass) graft
    heart
      transplant —*see* Complication,
        transplant, heart
      valve —*see* Complication, prosthetic
        device, heart valve
        graft —*see* Complication, heart, valve,
          graft
    heart-lung transplant —*see* Complication,
      transplant, heart, with lung
    infection or inflammation T82.7
    umbrella device —*see* Complication,
      umbrella device, vascular
    vascular graft (or anastomosis) —*see*
      Complication, graft, vascular
  carotid artery (bypass) graft —*see*
    Complications, graft, vascular
  catheter (device) NEC —*see also*
    Complications, prosthetic device or
    implant
    cranial infusion
      infection and inflammation T85.735
      mechanical
        breakdown T85.610
        displacement T85.620
        leakage T85.630
        malfunction T85.690
        malposition T85.620
        obstruction T85.690
        perforation T85.690
        protrusion T85.690
        specified NEC T85.690
    cystostomy T83.9
      embolism T83.81
      fibrosis T83.82
      hemorrhage T83.83
      infection and inflammation T83.510
      mechanical
        breakdown T83.010
        displacement T83.020
        leakage T83.030
        malposition T83.020
        obstruction T83.090
        perforation T83.090
        protrusion T83.090
        specified NEC T83.090
      pain T83.84
      specified type NEC T83.89
      stenosis T83.85
      thrombosis T83.86
    dialysis (vascular) T82.9
      embolism T82.818
      fibrosis T82.828
      hemorrhage T82.838
      infection and inflammation T82.7
      intraperitoneal —*see* Complications,
        catheter, intraperitoneal
      mechanical
        breakdown T82.41
        displacement T82.42
        leakage T82.43
        malposition T82.42
        obstruction T82.49
        perforation T82.49
        protrusion T82.49
      pain T82.848
      specified type NEC T82.898
      stenosis T82.858
      thrombosis T82.868
    epidural infusion T85.9
      embolism T85.810
      fibrosis T85.820
      hemorrhage T85.830
      infection and inflammation T85.735
      mechanical
        breakdown T85.610
        displacement T85.620

Complication *(Continued)*
  catheter NEC *(Continued)*
    epidural infusion *(Continued)*
      mechanical *(Continued)*
        leakage T85.63Ø
        malfunction T85.61Ø
        malposition T85.62Ø
        obstruction T85.69Ø
        perforation T85.69Ø
        protrusion T85.69Ø
        specified NEC T85.69Ø
      pain T85.84Ø
      specified type NEC T85.89Ø
      stenosis T85.85Ø
      thrombosis T85.86Ø
    intraperitoneal dialysis T85.9
      embolism T85.818
      fibrosis T85.828
      hemorrhage T85.838
      infection and inflammation T85.71
      mechanical
        breakdown T85.611
        displacement T85.621
        leakage T85.631
        malfunction T85.611
        malposition T85.621
        obstruction T85.691
        perforation T85.691
        protrusion T85.691
        specified NEC T85.691
      pain T85.848
      specified type NEC T85.898
      stenosis T85.858
      thrombosis T85.868
    intrathecal infusion
      infection and inflammation T85.735
      mechanical
        breakdown T85.61Ø
        displacement T85.62Ø
        leakage T85.63Ø
        malfunction T85.69Ø
        malposition T85.62Ø
        obstruction T85.69Ø
        perforation T85.69Ø
        protrusion T85.69Ø
        specified NEC T85.69Ø
    intravenous infusion T82.9
      embolism T82.818
      fibrosis T82.828
      hemorrhage T82.838
      infection or inflammation T82.7
      mechanical
        breakdown T82.514
        displacement T82.524
        leakage T82.534
        malposition T82.524
        obstruction T82.594
        perforation T82.594
        protrusion T82.594
      pain T82.848
      specified type NEC T82.898
      stenosis T82.858
      thrombosis T82.868
    spinal infusion
      infection and inflammation T85.735
      mechanical
        breakdown T85.61Ø
        displacement T85.62Ø
        leakage T85.63Ø
        malfunction T85.69Ø
        malposition T85.62Ø
        obstruction T85.69Ø
        perforation T85.69Ø
        protrusion T85.69Ø
        specified NEC T85.69Ø
    subarachnoid infusion
      infection and inflammation
          T85.735
      mechanical
        breakdown T85.61Ø
        displacement T85.62Ø

Complication *(Continued)*
  catheter NEC *(Continued)*
    subarachnoid infusion *(Continued)*
      mechanical *(Continued)*
        leakage T85.63Ø
        malfunction T85.69Ø
        malposition T85.62Ø
        obstruction T85.69Ø
        perforation T85.69Ø
        protrusion T85.69Ø
        specified NEC T85.69Ø
    subdural infusion T85.9
      embolism T85.81Ø
      fibrosis T85.82Ø
      hemorrhage T85.83Ø
      infection and inflammation T85.735
      mechanical
        breakdown T85.61Ø
        displacement T85.62Ø
        leakage T85.63Ø
        malfunction T85.61Ø
        malposition T85.62Ø
        obstruction T85.69Ø
        perforation T85.69Ø
        protrusion T85.69Ø
        specified NEC T85.69Ø
      pain T85.84Ø
      specified type NEC T85.89Ø
      stenosis T85.85Ø
      thrombosis T85.86Ø
    urethral T83.9
      displacement T83.Ø28
      embolism T83.81
      fibrosis T83.82
      hemorrhage T83.83
      indwelling
        breakdown T83.Ø11
        displacement T83.Ø21
        infection and inflammation
            T83.511
        leakage T83.Ø31
        specified complication NEC
            T83.Ø91
      infection and inflammation
          T83.511
      leakage T83.Ø38
      malposition T83.Ø28
      mechanical
        breakdown T83.Ø11
      obstruction (mechanical) T83.Ø91
      pain T83.84
      perforation T83.Ø91
      protrusion T83.Ø91
      specified type NEC T83.Ø91
      stenosis T83.85
      thrombosis T83.86
    urinary NEC
      breakdown T83.Ø18
      displacement T83.Ø28
      infection and inflammation T83.518
      leakage T83.Ø38
      specified complication NEC T83.Ø98
  cecostomy (stoma) —*see* Complications,
      colostomy
  cesarean delivery wound NEC O9Ø.89
    disruption O9Ø.Ø
    hematoma O9Ø.2
    infection (following delivery) O86.Ø
  chemotherapy (antineoplastic) NEC T88.7
  chin implant (prosthetic) —*see* Complication,
      prosthetic device or implant, specified
      NEC
  circulatory system I99.8
    intraoperative I97.88
    postprocedural I97.89
    ➠following cardiac surgery —*see also*
        Infarct, myocardium, associated
        with revascularization procedure
        I97.19-●
        postcardiotomy syndrome I97.Ø
    hypertension I97.3
    lymphedema after mastectomy I97.2

Complication *(Continued)*
  circulatory system *(Continued)*
    postprocedural *(Continued)*
      postcardiotomy syndrome I97.Ø
      specified NEC I97.89
  colostomy (stoma) K94.ØØ
    hemorrhage K94.Ø1
    infection K94.Ø2
    malfunction K94.Ø3
    mechanical K94.Ø3
    specified complication NEC K94.Ø9
  contraceptive device, intrauterine —
      see Complications, intrauterine,
      contraceptive device
  cord (umbilical) —*see* Complications,
      umbilical cord
  corneal graft —*see* Complications, graft, cornea
  coronary artery (bypass) graft T82.9
    atherosclerosis —*see* Arteriosclerosis,
        coronary (artery)
    embolism T82.818
    fibrosis T82.828
    hemorrhage T82.838
    infection and inflammation T82.7
    mechanical
      breakdown T82.211
      displacement T82.212
      leakage T82.213
      malposition T82.212
      obstruction T82.218
      perforation T82.218
      protrusion T82.218
      specified NEC T82.218
    pain T82.848
    specified type NEC T82.898
    stenosis T82.858
    thrombosis T82.868
  counterpulsation device (balloon), intra-
      aortic —*see* Complications, balloon
      implant, vascular
  cystostomy (stoma) N99.518
    catheter —*see* Complications, catheter,
        cystostomy
    hemorrhage N99.51Ø
    infection N99.511
    malfunction N99.512
    specified type NEC N99.518
  delivery —*see also* Complications, obstetric
      O75.9
    procedure (instrumental) (manual)
        (surgical) O75.4
    specified NEC O75.89
  dialysis (peritoneal) (renal) —*see also*
      Complications, infusion
    catheter (vascular) —*see* Complication,
        catheter, dialysis
    peritoneal, intraperitoneal —*see*
        Complications, catheter,
        intraperitoneal
  dorsal column (spinal) neurostimulator —*see*
      Complications, electronic stimulator
      device, spinal cord
  drug NEC T88.7
  ear procedure —*see also* Disorder, ear
    intraoperative H95.88-●
      hematoma —*see* Complications,
          intraoperative, hematoma (of), ear
      hemorrhage —*see* Complications,
          intraoperative, hemorrhage (of), ear
      laceration —*see* Complications,
          intraoperative, puncture or
          laceration..., ear
      seroma —*see* Complications,
          postprocedural, seroma (of),
          mastoid process
      specified NEC H95.88-●
    postoperative H95.89-●
      external ear canal stenosis H95.81-●
      hematoma —*see* Complications,
          postprocedural, hemorrhage
          (hematoma) (of), ear

▶ New   ⇒ Revised   ~~deleted~~ Deleted   ● Use Additional Character(s)

Complication *(Continued)*
  ear procedure *(Continued)*
    postoperative *(Continued)*
      hemorrhage —*see* Complications,
        postprocedural, hemorrhage
        (hematoma) (of), ear
      postmastoidectomy —*see* Complications,
        postmastoidectomy
      specified NEC H95.89-●
  ectopic pregnancy O08.9
    damage to pelvic organs O08.6
    embolism O08.2
    genital infection O08.0
    hemorrhage (delayed) (excessive) O08.1
    metabolic disorder O08.5
    renal failure O08.4
    shock O08.3
    specified type NEC O08.0
    venous complication NEC O08.7
  electronic stimulator device
    bladder (urinary) —*see* Complications,
      electronic stimulator device, urinary
    bone T84.9
      breakdown T84.310
      displacement T84.320
      embolism T84.81
      fibrosis T84.82
      hemorrhage T84.83
      infection or inflammation T84.7
      malfunction T84.310
      malposition T84.320
      mechanical NEC T84.390
      obstruction T84.390
      pain T84.84
      perforation T84.390
      protrusion T84.390
      specified type NEC T84.89
      stenosis T84.85
      thrombosis T84.86
    brain T85.9
      embolism T85.810
      fibrosis T85.820
      hemorrhage T85.830
      infection and inflammation T85.731
      mechanical
        breakdown T85.110
        displacement T85.120
        leakage T85.190
        malposition T85.120
        obstruction T85.190
        perforation T85.190
        protrusion T85.190
        specified NEC T85.190
      pain T85.840
      specified type NEC T85.890
      stenosis T85.850
      thrombosis T85.860
    cardiac (defibrillator) (pacemaker) —*see*
      Complications, cardiovascular device
      or implant, electronic
    generator (brain) (gastric) (peripheral)
      (sacral) (spinal)
      breakdown T85.113
      displacement T85.123
      leakage T85.193
      malposition T85.123
      obstruction T85.193
      perforation T85.193
      protrusion T85.193
      specified type NEC T85.193
    muscle T84.9
      breakdown T84.418
      displacement T84.428
      embolism T84.81
      fibrosis T84.82
      hemorrhage T84.83
      infection or inflammation T84.7
      mechanical NEC T84.498
      pain T84.84
      specified type NEC T84.89
      stenosis T84.85
      thrombosis T84.86

Complication *(Continued)*
  electronic stimulator device *(Continued)*
    nervous system T85.9
      brain —*see* Complications, electronic
        stimulator device, brain
      cranial nerve —*see* Complications,
        electronic stimulator device,
        peripheral nerve
      embolism T85.810
      fibrosis T85.820
      gastric nerve —*see* Complications,
        electronic stimulator device,
        peripheral nerve
      hemorrhage T85.830
      infection and inflammation T85.738
      mechanical
        breakdown T85.118
        displacement T85.128
        leakage T85.199
        malposition T85.128
        obstruction T85.199
        perforation T85.199
        protrusion T85.199
        specified NEC T85.199
      pain T85.840
      peripheral nerve —*see* Complications,
        electronic stimulator device,
        peripheral nerve
      sacral nerve —*see* Complications,
        electronic stimulator device,
        peripheral nerve
      specified type NEC T85.890
      spinal cord —*see* Complications,
        electronic stimulator device, spinal
        cord
      stenosis T85.850
      thrombosis T85.860
      vagal nerve —*see* Complications,
        electronic stimulator device,
        peripheral nerve
    peripheral nerve T85.9
      embolism T85.810
      fibrosis T85.820
      hemorrhage T85.830
      infection and inflammation T85.732
      mechanical
        breakdown T85.111
        displacement T85.121
        leakage T85.191
        malposition T85.121
        obstruction T85.191
        perforation T85.191
        protrusion T85.191
        specified NEC T85.191
      pain T85.840
      specified type NEC T85.890
      stenosis T85.850
      thrombosis T85.860
    spinal cord T85.9
      embolism T85.810
      fibrosis T85.820
      hemorrhage T85.830
      infection and inflammation T85.733
      mechanical
        breakdown T85.112
        displacement T85.122
        leakage T85.192
        malposition T85.122
        obstruction T85.192
        perforation T85.192
        protrusion T85.192
        specified NEC T85.192
      pain T85.840
      specified type NEC T85.890
      stenosis T85.850
      thrombosis T85.860
    urinary T83.9
      embolism T83.81
      fibrosis T83.82
      hemorrhage T83.83
      infection and inflammation T83.598

Complication *(Continued)*
  electronic stimulator device *(Continued)*
    urinary *(Continued)*
      mechanical
        breakdown T83.110
        displacement T83.120
        malposition T83.120
        perforation T83.190
        protrusion T83.190
        specified NEC T83.190
      pain T83.84
      specified type NEC T83.89
      stenosis T83.85
      thrombosis T83.86
  electroshock therapy T88.9
    specified NEC T88.8
  endocrine E34.9
    postprocedural
      adrenal hypofunction E89.6
      hypoinsulinemia E89.1
      hypoparathyroidism E89.2
      hypopituitarism E89.3
      hypothyroidism E89.0
      ovarian failure E89.40
        asymptomatic E89.40
        symptomatic E89.41
      specified NEC E89.89
      testicular hypofunction E89.5
  endodontic treatment NEC M27.59
  enterostomy (stoma) K94.10
    hemorrhage K94.11
    infection K94.12
    malfunction K94.13
    mechanical K94.13
    specified complication NEC K94.19
  episiotomy, disruption O90.1
  esophageal anti-reflux device T85.9
    embolism T85.818
    fibrosis T85.828
    hemorrhage T85.838
    infection and inflammation T85.79
    mechanical
      breakdown T85.511
      displacement T85.521
      malfunction T85.511
      malposition T85.521
      obstruction T85.591
      perforation T85.591
      protrusion T85.591
      specified NEC T85.591
    pain T85.848
    specified type NEC T85.898
    stenosis T85.858
    thrombosis T85.868
  esophagostomy K94.30
    hemorrhage K94.31
    infection K94.32
    malfunction K94.33
    mechanical K94.33
    specified complication NEC K94.39
  extracorporeal circulation T80.90
  extremity artery (bypass) graft T82.9
    arteriosclerosis —*see* Arteriosclerosis,
      extremities, bypass graft
    embolism T82.818
    fibrosis T82.828
    hemorrhage T82.838
    infection and inflammation T82.7
    mechanical
      breakdown T82.318
        femoral artery T82.312
      displacement T82.328
        femoral artery T82.322
      leakage T82.338
        femoral artery T82.332
      malposition T82.328
        femoral artery T82.322
      obstruction T82.398
        femoral artery T82.392
      perforation T82.398
        femoral artery T82.392
      protrusion T82.398
        femoral artery T82.392

Complication *(Continued)*
  extremity artery (bypass) graft *(Continued)*
    pain T82.848
    specified type NEC T82.898
    stenosis T82.858
    thrombosis T82.868
  eye H57.9
    corneal graft —*see* Complications, graft,
      cornea
    implant (prosthetic) T85.9
      embolism T85.818
      fibrosis T85.828
      hemorrhage T85.838
      infection and inflammation T85.79
      mechanical
        breakdown T85.318
        displacement T85.328
        leakage T85.398
        malposition T85.328
        obstruction T85.398
        perforation T85.398
        protrusion T85.398
        specified NEC T85.398
      pain T85.848
      specified type NEC T85.898
      stenosis T85.858
      thrombosis T85.868
    intraocular lens —*see* Complications,
      intraocular lens
    orbital prosthesis —*see* Complications,
      orbital prosthesis
  female genital N94.9
    device, implant or graft NEC —*see*
      Complications, genitourinary, device
      or implant, genital tract
  femoral artery (bypass) graft —*see*
    Complication, extremity artery (bypass)
    graft
  fixation device, internal (orthopedic) T84.9
    infection and inflammation T84.60
      arm T84.61-●
        humerus T84.61-●
        radius T84.61-●
        ulna T84.61-●
      leg T84.629
        femur T84.62-●
        fibula T84.62-●
        tibia T84.62-●
      specified site NEC T84.69
      spine T84.63
    mechanical
      breakdown
        limb T84.119
          carpal T84.210
          femur T84.11-●
          fibula T84.11-●
          humerus T84.11-●
          metacarpal T84.210
          metatarsal T84.213
          phalanx
            foot T84.213
            hand T84.210
          radius T84.11-●
          tarsal T84.213
          tibia T84.11-●
          ulna T84.11-●
        specified bone NEC T84.218
        spine T84.216
      displacement
        limb T84.129
          carpal T84.220
          femur T84.12-●
          fibula T84.12-●
          humerus T84.12-●
          metacarpal T84.220
          metatarsal T84.223
          phalanx
            foot T84.223
            hand T84.220
          radius T84.12-●
          tarsal T84.223

Complication *(Continued)*
  fixation device, internal *(Continued)*
    mechanical *(Continued)*
      displacement *(Continued)*
        limb *(Continued)*
          tibia T84.12-●
          ulna T84.12-●
        specified bone NEC T84.228
        spine T84.226
      malposition —*see* Complications,
        fixation device, internal,
        mechanical, displacement
      obstruction —*see* Complications, fixation
        device, internal, mechanical,
        specified type NEC
      perforation —*see* Complications, fixation
        device, internal, mechanical,
        specified type NEC
      protrusion —*see* Complications, fixation
        device, internal, mechanical,
        specified type NEC
      specified type NEC
        limb T84.199
          carpal T84.290
          femur T84.19-●
          fibula T84.19-●
          humerus T84.19-●
          metacarpal T84.290
          metatarsal T84.293
          phalanx
            foot T84.293
            hand T84.290
          radius T84.19-●
          tarsal T84.293
          tibia T84.19-●
          ulna T84.19-●
        specified bone NEC T84.298
        vertebra T84.296
    specified type NEC T84.89
      embolism T84.81
      fibrosis T84.82
      hemorrhage T84.83
      pain T84.84
      specified complication NEC T84.89
      stenosis T84.85
      thrombosis T84.86
  following
    acute myocardial infarction NEC I23.8
      aneurysm (false) (of cardiac wall)
        (of heart wall) (ruptured) I23.3
      angina I23.7
      atrial
        septal defect I23.1
        thrombosis I23.6
      cardiac wall rupture I23.3
      chordae tendinae rupture I23.4
      defect
        septal
          atrial (heart) I23.1
          ventricular (heart) I23.2
      hemopericardium I23.0
      papillary muscle rupture I23.5
      rupture
        cardiac wall I23.3
          with hemopericardium I23.0
        chordae tendineae I23.4
        papillary muscle I23.5
      specified NEC I23.8
      thrombosis
        atrium I23.6
        auricular appendage I23.6
        ventricle (heart) I23.6
      ventricular
        septal defect I23.2
        thrombosis I23.6
    ectopic or molar pregnancy O08.9
      cardiac arrest O08.81
      sepsis O08.82
      specified type NEC O08.89
      urinary tract infection O08.83
    termination of pregnancy —*see* Abortion

Complication *(Continued)*
  gastrointestinal K92.9
    bile duct prosthesis —*see* Complications,
      bile duct implant
    esophageal anti-reflux device —*see*
      Complications, esophageal
      anti-reflux device
    postoperative
      colostomy —*see* Complications, colostomy
      dumping syndrome K91.1
      enterostomy —*see* Complications,
        enterostomy
      gastrostomy —*see* Complications,
        gastrostomy
      malabsorption NEC K91.2
    ➠ obstruction —*see also* Obstruction,
        intestine, postoperative K91.30
      postcholecystectomy syndrome K91.5
      specified NEC K91.89
      vomiting after GI surgery K91.0
    prosthetic device or implant
      bile duct prosthesis —*see* Complications,
        bile duct implant
      esophageal anti-reflux device —*see*
        Complications, esophageal anti-
        reflux device
      specified type NEC
        embolism T85.818
        fibrosis T85.828
        hemorrhage T85.838
        mechanical
          breakdown T85.518
          displacement T85.528
          malfunction T85.518
          malposition T85.528
          obstruction T85.598
          perforation T85.598
          protrusion T85.598
          specified NEC T85.598
        pain T85.848
        specified complication NEC T85.898
        stenosis T85.858
        thrombosis T85.868
  gastrostomy (stoma) K94.20
    hemorrhage K94.21
    infection K94.22
    malfunction K94.23
    mechanical K94.23
    specified complication NEC K94.29
  genitourinary
    device or implant T83.9
      genital tract T83.9
        infection or inflammation T83.69
        intrauterine contraceptive device —*see*
          Complications, intrauterine,
          contraceptive device
        mechanical —*see* Complications, by
          device, mechanical
        mesh —*see* Complications, mesh
        penile prosthesis —*see* Complications,
          prosthetic device, penile
        specified type NEC T83.89
          embolism T83.81
          fibrosis T83.82
          hemorrhage T83.83
          pain T83.84
          specified complication NEC T83.89
          stenosis T83.85
          thrombosis T83.86
        vaginal mesh —*see* Complications,
          mesh
      urinary system T83.9
        cystostomy catheter —*see*
          Complication, catheter,
          cystostomy
        electronic stimulator —*see*
          Complications, electronic
          stimulator device, urinary
        indwelling urethral catheter —*see*
          Complications, catheter, urethral,
          indwelling

▶ New   ➠ Revised   ~~deleted~~ Deleted   ● Use Additional Character(s)

Complication (Continued)
 genitourinary (Continued)
  device or implant (Continued)
   urinary system (Continued)
    infection or inflammation T83.598
     indwelling urethral catheter T83.511
    kidney transplant —see Complication, transplant, kidney
    organ graft —see Complication, graft, urinary organ
    specified type NEC T83.89
     embolism T83.81
     fibrosis T83.82
     hemorrhage T83.83
     mechanical T83.198
      breakdown T83.118
      displacement T83.128
      malfunction T83.118
      malposition T83.128
      obstruction T83.198
      perforation T83.198
      protrusion T83.198
      specified NEC T83.198
     sphincter, implanted T83.191
     stent (ileal conduit) (nephroureteral) T83.193
     ureteral indwelling T83.192
     pain T83.84
     specified complication NEC T83.89
     stenosis T83.85
     thrombosis T83.86
    sphincter implant —see Complications, implant, urinary sphincter
  postprocedural
   pelvic peritoneal adhesions N99.4
   renal failure N99.0
   specified NEC N99.89
   stoma —see Complications, stoma, urinary tract
   urethral stricture —see Stricture, urethra, postprocedural
   vaginal
    adhesions N99.2
    vault prolapse N99.3
 graft (bypass) (patch) —see also Complications, prosthetic device or implant
  aorta —see Complications, graft, vascular
  arterial —see Complication, graft, vascular
  bone T86.839
   failure T86.831
   infection T86.832
   mechanical T84.318
    breakdown T84.318
    displacement T84.328
    protrusion T84.398
    specified type NEC T84.398
   rejection T86.830
   specified type NEC T86.838
  carotid artery —see Complications, graft, vascular
  cornea T86.849
   failure T86.841
   infection T86.842
   mechanical T85.398
    breakdown T85.318
    displacement T85.328
    protrusion T85.398
    specified type NEC T85.398
   rejection T86.840
   retroprosthetic membrane T85.398
   specified type NEC T86.848
  femoral artery (bypass) —see Complication, extremity artery (bypass) graft
  genital organ or tract —see Complications, genitourinary, device or implant, genital tract

Complication (Continued)
 graft (Continued)
  muscle T84.9
   breakdown T84.410
   displacement T84.420
   embolism T84.81
   fibrosis T84.82
   hemorrhage T84.83
   infection and inflammation T84.7
   mechanical NEC T84.490
   pain T84.84
   specified type NEC T84.89
   stenosis T84.85
   thrombosis T84.86
  nerve —see Complication, prosthetic device or implant, specified NEC
  skin —see Complications, prosthetic device or implant, skin graft
  tendon T84.9
   breakdown T84.410
   displacement T84.420
   embolism T84.81
   fibrosis T84.82
   hemorrhage T84.83
   infection and inflammation T84.7
   mechanical NEC T84.490
   pain T84.84
   specified type NEC T84.89
   stenosis T84.85
   thrombosis T84.86
  urinary organ T83.9
   embolism T83.81
   fibrosis T83.82
   hemorrhage T83.83
   infection and inflammation T83.598
    indwelling urethral catheter T83.511
   mechanical
    breakdown T83.21
    displacement T83.22
    erosion T83.24
    exposure T83.25
    leakage T83.23
    malposition T83.22
    obstruction T83.29
    perforation T83.29
    protrusion T83.29
    specified NEC T83.29
   pain T83.84
   specified type NEC T83.89
   stenosis T83.85
   thrombosis T83.86
  vascular T82.9
   embolism T82.818
   femoral artery —see Complication, extremity artery (bypass) graft
   fibrosis T82.828
   hemorrhage T82.838
   mechanical
    breakdown T82.319
     aorta (bifurcation) T82.310
     carotid artery T82.311
     specified vessel NEC T82.318
    displacement T82.329
     aorta (bifurcation) T82.320
     carotid artery T82.321
     specified vessel NEC T82.328
    leakage T82.339
     aorta (bifurcation) T82.330
     carotid artery T82.331
     specified vessel NEC T82.338
    malposition T82.329
     aorta (bifurcation) T82.320
     carotid artery T82.321
     specified vessel NEC T82.328
    obstruction T82.399
     aorta (bifurcation) T82.390
     carotid artery T82.391
     specified vessel NEC T82.398

Complication (Continued)
 graft (Continued)
  vascular (Continued)
   mechanical (Continued)
    perforation T82.399
     aorta (bifurcation) T82.390
     carotid artery T82.391
     specified vessel NEC T82.398
    protrusion T82.399
     aorta (bifurcation) T82.390
     carotid artery T82.391
     specified vessel NEC T82.398
   pain T82.848
   specified complication NEC T82.898
   stenosis T82.858
   thrombosis T82.868
 heart I51.9
  assist device
   infection and inflammation T82.7
  following acute myocardial infarction —see Complications, following, acute myocardial infarction
  postoperative —see Complications, circulatory system
  transplant —see Complication, transplant, heart
   and lung(s) —see Complications, transplant, heart, with lung
  valve
   graft (biological) T82.9
    embolism T82.817
    fibrosis T82.827
    hemorrhage T82.837
    infection and inflammation T82.7
    mechanical T82.228
     breakdown T82.221
     displacement T82.222
     leakage T82.223
     malposition T82.222
     obstruction T82.228
     perforation T82.228
     protrusion T82.228
    pain T82.847
    specified type NEC T82.897
    stenosis T82.857
    thrombosis T82.867
   prosthesis T82.9
    embolism T82.817
    fibrosis T82.827
    hemorrhage T82.837
    infection or inflammation T82.6
    mechanical T82.09
     breakdown T82.01
     displacement T82.02
     leakage T82.03
     malposition T82.02
     obstruction T82.09
     perforation T82.09
     protrusion T82.09
    pain T82.847
    specified type NEC T82.897
     mechanical T82.09
    stenosis T82.857
    thrombosis T82.867
 hematoma
  intraoperative —see Complication, intraoperative, hemorrhage
  postprocedural —see Complication, postprocedural, hematoma
 hemodialysis —see Complications, dialysis
 hemorrhage
  intraoperative —see Complication, intraoperative, hemorrhage
  postprocedural —see Complication, postprocedural, hemorrhage
 ileostomy (stoma) —see Complications, enterostomy
 immunization (procedure) —see Complications, vaccination

Complication *(Continued)*
  implant —*see also* Complications, by site and
    type
    urinary sphincter T83.9
      embolism T83.81
      fibrosis T83.82
      hemorrhage T83.83
      infection and inflammation T83.591
      mechanical
        breakdown T83.111
        displacement T83.121
        leakage T83.191
        malposition T83.121
        obstruction T83.191
        perforation T83.191
        protrusion T83.191
        specified NEC T83.191
      pain T83.84
      specified type NEC T83.89
      stenosis T83.85
      thrombosis T83.86
  infusion (procedure) T80.90
    air embolism T80.0
    blood —*see* Complications, transfusion
    catheter —*see* Complications, catheter
    infection T80.29
    pump —*see* Complications, cardiovascular,
      device or implant
    sepsis T80.29
    serum reaction —*see also* Reaction, serum
      T80.69
      anaphylactic shock —*see also* Shock,
        anaphylactic T80.59
    specified type NEC T80.89
  inhalation therapy NEC T81.81
  injection (procedure) T80.90
    drug reaction —*see* Reaction, drug
    infection T80.29
    sepsis T80.29
    serum (prophylactic) (therapeutic) —*see*
      Complications, vaccination
    specified type NEC T80.89
    vaccine (any) —*see* Complications,
      vaccination
  inoculation (any) —*see* Complications,
    vaccination
  insulin pump
    infection and inflammation T85.72
    mechanical
      breakdown T85.614
      displacement T85.624
      leakage T85.633
      malposition T85.624
      obstruction T85.694
      perforation T85.694
      protrusion T85.694
      specified NEC T85.694
  intestinal pouch NEC K91.858
  intraocular lens (prosthetic) T85.9
    embolism T85.818
    fibrosis T85.828
    hemorrhage T85.838
    infection and inflammation T85.79
    mechanical
      breakdown T85.21
      displacement T85.22
      malposition T85.22
      obstruction T85.29
      perforation T85.29
      protrusion T85.29
      specified NEC T85.29
    pain T85.848
    specified type NEC T85.898
    stenosis T85.858
    thrombosis T85.868
  intraoperative (intraprocedural)
  ➠cardiac arrest —*see also* Infarct,
    myocardium, associated with
    revascularization procedure
    during cardiac surgery I97.710
    during other surgery I97.711

Complication *(Continued)*
  intraoperative (intraprocedural) *(Continued)*
  ➠cardiac functional disturbance NEC —*see*
    also Infarct, myocardium, associated
    with revascularization procedure
    during cardiac surgery I97.790
    during other surgery I97.791
    hemorrhage (hematoma) (of)
      circulatory system organ or structure
        during cardiac bypass I97.411
        during cardiac catheterization I97.410
        during other circulatory system
          procedure I97.418
        during other procedure I97.42
      digestive system organ
        during procedure on digestive system
          K91.61
        during procedure on other organ
          K91.62
      ear
        during procedure on ear and mastoid
          process H95.21
        during procedure on other organ
          H95.22
      endocrine system organ or structure
        during procedure on endocrine
          system organ or structure E36.01
        during procedure on other organ
          E36.02
      eye and adnexa
        during ophthalmic procedure H59.11-●
        during other procedure H59.12-●
      genitourinary organ or structure
        during procedure on genitourinary
          organ or structure N99.61
        during procedure on other organ
          N99.62
      mastoid process
        during procedure on ear and mastoid
          process H95.21
        during procedure on other organ
          H95.22
      musculoskeletal structure
        during musculoskeletal surgery
          M96.810
        during non-orthopedic surgery
          M96.811
        during orthopedic surgery M96.810
      nervous system
        during a nervous system procedure
          G97.31
        during other procedure G97.32
      respiratory system
        during other procedure J95.62
        during procedure on respiratory
          system organ or structure J95.61
      skin and subcutaneous tissue
        during a dermatologic procedure
          L76.01
        during a procedure on other organ
          L76.02
      spleen
        during a procedure on other organ
          D78.02
        during a procedure on the spleen
          D78.01
    puncture or laceration (accidental)
      (unintentional) (of)
    brain
      during a nervous system procedure
        G97.48
      during other procedure G97.49
    circulatory system organ or structure
      during circulatory system procedure
        I97.51
      during other procedure I97.52
    digestive system
      during procedure on digestive system
        K91.71
      during procedure on other organ
        K91.72

Complication *(Continued)*
  intraoperative *(Continued)*
    puncture or laceration *(Continued)*
      ear
        during procedure on ear and mastoid
          process H95.31
        during procedure on other organ
          H95.32
      endocrine system organ or structure
        during procedure on endocrine
          system organ or structure
          E36.11
        during procedure on other organ
          E36.12
      eye and adnexa
        during ophthalmic procedure
          H59.21-●
        during other procedure H59.22-●
      genitourinary organ or structure
        during procedure on genitourinary
          organ or structure N99.71
        during procedure on other organ
          N99.72
      mastoid process
        during procedure on ear and mastoid
          process H95.31
        during procedure on other organ
          H95.32
      musculoskeletal structure
        during musculoskeletal surgery
          M96.820
        during non-orthopedic surgery
          M96.821
        during orthopedic surgery M96.820
      nervous system
        during a nervous system procedure
          G97.48
        during other procedure G97.49
      respiratory system
        during other procedure J95.72
        during procedure on respiratory
          system organ or structure
          J95.71
      skin and subcutaneous tissue
        during a dermatologic procedure
          L76.11
        during a procedure on other organ
          L76.12
      spleen
        during a procedure on other organ
          D78.12
        during a procedure on the spleen
          D78.11
    specified NEC
      circulatory system I97.88
      digestive system K91.81
      ear H95.88
      endocrine system E36.8
      eye and adnexa H59.88
      genitourinary system N99.81
      mastoid process H95.88
      musculoskeletal structure M96.89
      nervous system G97.81
      respiratory system J95.88
      skin and subcutaneous tissue L76.81
      spleen D78.81
  intraperitoneal catheter (dialysis)
    (infusion) —*see* Complications, catheter,
    intraperitoneal
  intrathecal infusion pump
    infection and inflammation T85.738
    mechanical
      breakdown T85.615
      displacement T85.625
      leakage T85.635
      malfunction T85.695
      malposition T85.625
      obstruction T85.695
      perforation T85.695
      protrusion T85.695
      specified NEC T85.695

Complication (Continued)
  intrauterine
    contraceptive device
      embolism T83.81
      fibrosis T83.82
      hemorrhage T83.83
      infection and inflammation T83.69
      mechanical
        breakdown T83.31
        displacement T83.32
        malposition T83.32
        obstruction T83.39
        perforation T83.39
        protrusion T83.39
        specified NEC T83.39
      pain T83.84
      specified type NEC T83.89
      stenosis T83.85
      thrombosis T83.86
    procedure (fetal), to newborn P96.5
  jejunostomy (stoma) —see Complications,
    enterostomy
  joint prosthesis, internal T84.9
    breakage (fracture) T84.01-●
    dislocation T84.02-●
    fracture T84.01-●
    infection or inflammation T84.50
      hip T84.5-●
      knee T84.5-●
      specified joint NEC T84.59
    instability T84.02-●
    malposition —see Complications, joint
      prosthesis, mechanical, displacement
    mechanical
      breakage, broken T84.01-●
      dislocation T84.02-●
      fracture T84.01-●
      instability T84.02-●
      leakage —see Complications, joint
        prosthesis, mechanical, specified
        NEC
      loosening T84.039
        hip T84.03-●
        knee T84.03-●
        specified joint NEC T84.038
      obstruction —see Complications, joint
        prosthesis, mechanical, specified
        NEC
      perforation —see Complications, joint
        prosthesis, mechanical, specified
        NEC
      osteolysis T84.059
        hip T84.05-●
        knee T84.05-●
        other specified joint T84.058
      protrusion —see Complications, joint
        prosthesis, mechanical, specified
        NEC
      specified complication NEC T84.099
        hip T84.09-●
        knee T84.09-●
        other specified joint T84.098
      subluxation T84.02-●
      wear of articular bearing surface
        T84.069
        hip T84.06-●
        knee T84.06-●
        other specified joint T84.068
    specified joint NEC T84.89
      embolism T84.81
      fibrosis T84.82
      hemorrhage T84.83
      pain T84.84
      specified complication NEC T84.89
      stenosis T84.85
      thrombosis T84.86
    subluxation T84.02-●
  kidney transplant —see Complications,
    transplant, kidney
  labor O75.9
    specified NEC O75.89

Complication (Continued)
  liver transplant (immune or nonimmune) —
    see Complications, transplant,
    liver
  lumbar puncture G97.1
    cerebrospinal fluid leak G97.0
    headache or reaction G97.1
  lung transplant —see Complications,
    transplant, lung
    and heart —see Complications, transplant,
      lung, with heart
  male genital N50.9
    device, implant or graft —see
      Complications, genitourinary,
      device or implant, genital tract
    postprocedural or postoperative —see
      Complications, genitourinary,
      postprocedural
    specified NEC N99.89
  mastoid (process) procedure
    intraoperative H95.88-●
      hematoma —see Complications,
        intraoperative, hemorrhage
        (hematoma) (of), mastoid
        process
      hemorrhage —see Complications,
        intraoperative, hemorrhage
        (hematoma) (of), mastoid
        process
      laceration —see Complications,
        intraoperative, puncture or
        laceration..., mastoid
        process
      specified NEC H95.88-●
    postmastoidectomy —see Complications,
      postmastoidectomy
    postoperative H95.89-●
      external ear canal stenosis H95.81-●
      hematoma —see Complications...,
        postprocedural, hematoma (of),
        mastoid process
      hemorrhage —see Complications...,
        postprocedural, hemorrhage (of),
        mastoid process
      postmastoidectomy —see Complications,
        postmastoidectomy
      seroma —see Complications,
        postprocedural, seroma (of),
        mastoid process
      specified NEC H95.89-●
  mastoidectomy cavity —see Complications,
    postmastoidectomy
  mechanical —see Complications, by site and
    type, mechanical
  medical procedures (see also Complication(s),
    intraoperative) T88.9
  metabolic E88.9
    postoperative E89.89
      specified NEC E89.89
  molar pregnancy NOS O08.9
    damage to pelvic organs O08.6
    embolism O08.2
    genital infection O08.0
    hemorrhage (delayed) (excessive)
      O08.1
    metabolic disorder O08.5
    renal failure O08.4
    shock O08.3
    specified type NEC O08.0
    venous complication NEC O08.7
  musculoskeletal system —see also
    Complication, intraoperative
    (intraprocedural), by site
    device, implant or graft NEC —see
      Complications, orthopedic, device or
      implant
    internal fixation (nail) (plate) (rod) —see
      Complications, fixation device,
      internal
    joint prosthesis —see Complications, joint
      prosthesis

Complication (Continued)
  musculoskeletal system (Continued)
    postoperative (postprocedural) M96.89
      with osteoporosis —see Osteoporosis
      fracture following insertion of device —
        see Fracture, following insertion of
        orthopedic implant, joint prosthesis
        or bone plate
      joint instability after prosthesis removal
        M96.89
      lordosis M96.4
      postlaminectomy syndrome NEC M96.1
        kyphosis M96.2
      pseudarthrosis M96.0
      specified complication NEC M96.89
    post radiation M96.89
      kyphosis M96.3
      scoliosis M96.5
      specified complication NEC M96.89
  nephrostomy (stoma) —see Complications,
    stoma, urinary tract, external NEC
  nervous system G98.8
    central G96.9
      device, implant or graft —see also
        Complication, prosthetic device or
        implant, specified NEC
      electronic stimulator (electrode(s)) —see
        Complications, electronic stimulator
        device
      specified NEC
        infection and inflammation T85.738
        mechanical T85.695
          breakdown T85.615
          displacement T85.625
          leakage T85.635
          malfunction T85.695
          malposition T85.625
          obstruction T85.695
          perforation T85.695
          protrusion T85.695
          specified NEC T85.695
      ventricular shunt —see Complications,
        ventricular shunt
    electronic stimulator (electrode(s)) —see
      Complications, electronic stimulator
      device
    postprocedural G97.82
      intracranial hypotension G97.2
      specified NEC G97.82
      spinal fluid leak G97.0
  newborn, due to intrauterine (fetal)
    procedure P96.5
  nonabsorbable (permanent) sutures —see
    Complication, sutures, permanent
  obstetric O75.9
    procedure (instrumental) (manual)
      (surgical) specified NEC O75.4
    specified NEC O75.89
    surgical wound NEC O90.89
      hematoma O90.2
      infection O86.0
  ocular lens implant —see Complications,
    intraocular lens
  ophthalmologic
    postprocedural bleb —see Blebitis
  orbital prosthesis T85.9
    embolism T85.818
    fibrosis T85.828
    hemorrhage T85.838
    infection and inflammation T85.79
    mechanical
      breakdown T85.31-●
      displacement T85.32-●
      malposition T85.32-●
      obstruction T85.39-●
      perforation T85.39-●
      protrusion T85.39-●
      specified NEC T85.39-●
    pain T85.848
    specified type NEC T85.898
    stenosis T85.858
    thrombosis T85.868

Complication *(Continued)*
  organ or tissue transplant (partial) (total) —
      see Complications, transplant
  orthopedic —*see also* Disorder, soft tissue
      device or implant T84.9
          bone
              device or implant —*see* Complication,
                  bone, device NEC
              graft —*see* Complication, graft, bone
          breakdown T84.418
          displacement T84.428
          electronic bone stimulator —*see*
              Complications, electronic stimulator
              device, bone
          embolism T84.81
          fibrosis T84.82
          fixation device —*see* Complication,
              fixation device, internal
          hemorrhage T84.83
          infection or inflammation T84.7
          joint prosthesis —*see* Complication, joint
              prosthesis, internal
          malfunction T84.418
          malposition T84.428
          mechanical NEC T84.498
          muscle graft —*see* Complications, graft,
              muscle
          obstruction T84.498
          pain T84.84
          perforation T84.498
          protrusion T84.498
          specified complication NEC T84.89
          stenosis T84.85
          tendon graft —*see* Complications, graft,
              tendon
          thrombosis T84.86
      fracture (following insertion of device) —
          see Fracture, following insertion of
          orthopedic implant, joint prosthesis or
          bone plate
      postprocedural M96.89
          fracture —*see* Fracture, following
              insertion of orthopedic implant,
              joint prosthesis or bone plate
          postlaminectomy syndrome NEC M96.1
              kyphosis M96.3
              lordosis M96.4
          postradiation
              kyphosis M96.2
              scoliosis M96.5
          pseudarthrosis post-fusion M96.0
          specified type NEC M96.89
  pacemaker (cardiac) —*see* Complications,
      cardiovascular device or implant,
      electronic
  pancreas transplant —*see* Complications,
      transplant, pancreas
  penile prosthesis (implant) —*see*
      Complications, prosthetic device, penile
  perfusion NEC T80.90
  perineal repair (obstetrical) NEC O90.89
      disruption O90.1
      hematoma O90.2
      infection (following delivery) O86.0
  phototherapy T88.9
      specified NEC T88.8
  postmastoidectomy NEC H95.19-●
      cyst, mucosal H95.13-●
      granulation H95.12-●
      inflammation, chronic H95.11-●
      recurrent cholesteatoma H95.0-●
  postoperative —*see* Complications,
      postprocedural
      circulatory —*see* Complications, circulatory
          system
      ear —*see* Complications, ear
      endocrine —*see* Complications,
          endocrine
      eye —*see* Complications, eye
      lumbar puncture G97.1
          cerebrospinal fluid leak G97.0

Complication *(Continued)*
  postoperative *(Continued)*
      nervous system (central) (peripheral) —*see*
          Complications, nervous system
      respiratory system —*see* Complications,
          respiratory system
  postprocedural —*see also* Complications,
      surgical procedure
      ⇒cardiac arrest —*see also* Infarct,
          myocardium, associated with
          revascularization procedure
          following cardiac surgery I97.120
          following other surgery I97.121
      ⇒cardiac functional disturbance NEC —*see
          also* Infarct, myocardium, associated
          with revascularization procedure
          following cardiac surgery I97.190
          following other surgery I97.191
      cardiac insufficiency
          following cardiac surgery I97.110
          following other surgery I97.111
      chorioretinal scars following retinal
          surgery H59.81-●
      following cataract surgery
          cataract (lens) fragments H59.02-●
          cystoid macular edema H59.03-●
          specified NEC H59.09-●
          vitreous (touch) syndrome H59.01-●
      heart failure
          following cardiac surgery I97.130
          following other surgery I97.131
      hematoma (of)
          circulatory system organ or structure
              following cardiac bypass I97.631
              following cardiac catheterization
                  I97.630
              following other circulatory system
                  procedure I97.638
              following other procedure I97.621
          digestive system
              following procedure on digestive
                  system K91.870
              following procedure on other organ
                  K91.871
          ear
              following other procedure H95.52
              following procedure on ear and
                  mastoid process H95.51
          endocrine system
              following endocrine system procedure
                  E89.820
              following other procedure E89.821
          eye and adnexa
              following ophthalmic procedure
                  H59.33-●
              following other procedure H59.34-●
          genitourinary organ or structure
              following procedure on genitourinary
                  organ or structure N99.840
              following procedure on other organ
                  N99.841
          mastoid process
              following other procedure H95.52
              following procedure on ear and
                  mastoid process H95.51
          musculoskeletal structure
              following musculoskeletal surgery
                  M96.840
              following non-orthopedic surgery
                  M96.841
              following orthopedic surgery M96.840
          nervous system
              following nervous system procedure
                  G97.61
              following other procedure G97.62
          respiratory system
              following other procedure J95.861
              following procedure on respiratory
                  system organ or structure J95.860
          skin and subcutaneous tissue
              following dermatologic procedure
                  L76.31

Complication *(Continued)*
  postprocedural *(Continued)*
      hematoma *(Continued)*
          skin and subcutaneous tissue *(Continued)*
              following procedure on other organ
                  L76.32
          spleen
              following procedure on other organ
                  D78.32
              following procedure on the spleen
                  D78.31
      hemorrhage (of)
          circulatory system organ or structure
              following cardiac bypass I97.611
              following cardiac catheterization
                  I97.610
              following other circulatory system
                  procedure I97.618
              following other procedure I97.620
          digestive system
              following procedure on digestive
                  system K91.840
              following procedure on other organ
                  K91.841
          ear
              following other procedure H95.42
              following procedure on ear and
                  mastoid process H95.41
          endocrine system
              following endocrine system procedure
                  E89.810
              following other procedure E89.811
          eye and adnexa
              following ophthalmic procedure
                  H59.31-●
              following other procedure H59.32-●
          genitourinary organ or structure
              following procedure on genitourinary
                  organ or structure N99.820
              following procedure on other organ
                  N99.821
          mastoid process
              following other procedure H95.42
              following procedure on ear and
                  mastoid process H95.41
          musculoskeletal structure
              following musculoskeletal surgery
                  M96.830
              following non-orthopedic surgery
                  M96.831
              following orthopedic surgery M96.830
          nervous system
              following nervous system procedure
                  G97.51
              following other procedure G97.52
          respiratory system
              following other procedure J95.831
              following procedure on respiratory
                  system organ or structure J95.830
          skin and subcutaneous tissue
              following dermatologic procedure
                  L76.21
              following a procedure on other organ
                  L76.22
          spleen
              following procedure on other organ
                  D78.22
              following procedure on the spleen
                  D78.21
      seroma (of)
          circulatory system organ or structure
              following cardiac bypass I97.641
              following cardiac catheterization
                  I97.640
              following other circulatory system
                  procedure I97.648
              following other procedure I97.622
          digestive system
              following procedure on digestive
                  system K91.872
              following procedure on other organ
                  K91.873

▶ New   ⇒ Revised   ~~deleted~~ Deleted   ● Use Additional Character(s)

Complication *(Continued)*
  postprocedural *(Continued)*
    seroma *(Continued)*
      ear
        following other procedure H95.54
        following procedure on ear and
          mastoid process H95.53
      endocrine system
        following endocrine system procedure
          E89.822
        following other procedure E89.823
      eye and adnexa
        following ophthalmic procedure
          H59.35-●
        following other procedure H59.36-●
      genitourinary organ or structure
        following procedure on genitourinary
          organ or structure N99.842
        following procedure on other organ
          N99.843
      mastoid process
        following other procedure H95.54
        following procedure on ear and
          mastoid process H95.53
      musculoskeletal structure
        following musculoskeletal surgery
          M96.842
        following non-orthopedic surgery
          M96.843
        following orthopedic surgery M96.842
      nervous system
        following nervous system procedure
          G97.63
        following other procedure G97.64
      respiratory system
        following other procedure J95.863
        following procedure on respiratory
          system organ or structure J95.862
      skin and subcutaneous tissue
        following dermatologic procedure
          L76.33
        following procedure on other organ
          L76.34
      spleen
        following procedure on other organ
          D78.34
        following procedure on the spleen
          D78.33
    specified NEC
      circulatory system I97.89
      digestive K91.89
      ear H95.89
      endocrine E89.89
      eye and adnexa H59.89
      genitourinary N99.89
      mastoid process H95.89
      metabolic E89.89
      musculoskeletal structure M96.89
      nervous system G97.82
      respiratory system J95.89
      skin and subcutaneous tissue L76.82
      spleen D78.89
  pregnancy NEC —*see* Pregnancy,
    complicated by
  prosthetic device or implant T85.9
    bile duct —*see* Complications, bile duct
      implant
    breast —*see* Complications, breast
      implant
    bulking agent
      ureteral
        erosion T83.714
        exposure T83.724
      urethral
        erosion T83.713
        exposure T83.723
    cardiac and vascular NEC —*see*
      Complications, cardiovascular device
      or implant
    corneal transplant —*see* Complications,
      graft, cornea

Complication *(Continued)*
  prosthetic device or implant *(Continued)*
    electronic nervous system stimulator —*see*
      Complications, electronic stimulator
      device
    epidural infusion catheter —*see*
      Complications, catheter, epidural
    esophageal anti-reflux device —*see*
      Complications, esophageal anti-reflux
      device
    genital organ or tract —*see* Complications,
      genitourinary, device or implant,
      genital tract
      specified NEC T83.79
    heart valve —*see* Complications, heart,
      valve, prosthesis
    infection or inflammation T85.79
      intestine transplant T86.892
      liver transplant T86.43
      lung transplant T86.812
      pancreas transplant T86.892
      skin graft T86.822
    intraocular lens —*see* Complications,
      intraocular lens
    intraperitoneal (dialysis) catheter —
      see Complications, catheter,
      intraperitoneal
    joint —*see* Complications, joint prosthesis,
      internal
    mechanical NEC T85.698
      dialysis catheter (vascular) —*see also*
        Complication, catheter, dialysis,
        mechanical
        peritoneal —*see* Complication, catheter,
          intraperitoneal, mechanical
      gastrointestinal device T85.598
      ocular device T85.398
      subdural (infusion) catheter T85.690
      suture, permanent T85.692
        that for bone repair —*see*
          Complications, fixation device,
          internal (orthopedic), mechanical
      ventricular shunt
        breakdown T85.01
        displacement T85.02
        leakage T85.03
        malposition T85.02
        obstruction T85.09
        perforation T85.09
        protrusion T85.09
        specified NEC T85.09
    mesh
    ▥erosion (to surrounding organ or tissue)
        T83.718
        urethral (into pelvic floor muscles)
          T83.712
        vaginal (into pelvic floor muscles)
          T83.711
    ▥exposure (into surrounding organ or
        tissue) T83.728
        urethral (through urethral wall)
          T83.722
        vaginal (into vagina) (through vaginal
          wall) T83.721
    orbital —*see* Complications, orbital
      prosthesis
    penile T83.9
      embolism T83.81
      fibrosis T83.82
      hemorrhage T83.83
      infection and inflammation T83.61
      mechanical
        breakdown T83.410
        displacement T83.420
        leakage T83.490
        malposition T83.420
        obstruction T83.490
        perforation T83.490
        protrusion T83.490
        specified NEC T83.490
      pain T83.84

Complication *(Continued)*
  prosthetic device or implant *(Continued)*
    penile *(Continued)*
      specified type NEC T83.89
      stenosis T83.85
      thrombosis T83.86
    prosthetic materials NEC
      erosion (to surrounding organ or tissue)
        T83.718
      exposure (into surrounding organ or
        tissue) T83.728
    skin graft T86.829
      artificial skin or decellularized
        allodermis
        embolism T85.818
        fibrosis T85.828
        hemorrhage T85.838
        infection and inflammation T85.79
        mechanical
          breakdown T85.613
          displacement T85.623
          malfunction T85.613
          malposition T85.623
          obstruction T85.693
          perforation T85.693
          protrusion T85.693
          specified NEC T85.693
        pain T85.848
        specified type NEC T85.898
        stenosis T85.858
        thrombosis T85.868
      failure T86.821
      infection T86.822
      rejection T86.820
      specified NEC T86.828
    sling
      urethral (female) (male)
        erosion T83.712
        exposure T83.722
    specified NEC T85.9
      embolism T85.818
      fibrosis T85.828
      hemorrhage T85.838
      infection and inflammation T85.79
      mechanical
        breakdown T85.618
        displacement T85.628
        leakage T85.638
        malfunction T85.618
        malposition T85.628
        obstruction T85.698
        perforation T85.698
        protrusion T85.698
        specified NEC T85.698
      pain T85.848
      specified type NEC T85.898
      stenosis T85.858
      thrombosis T85.868
    subdural infusion catheter —*see*
      Complications, catheter, subdural
    sutures —*see* Complications, sutures
    urinary organ or tract NEC —*see*
      Complications, genitourinary, device
      or implant, urinary system
    vascular —*see* Complications,
      cardiovascular device or implant
    ventricular shunt —*see* Complications,
      ventricular shunt (device)
  puerperium —*see* Puerperal
  puncture, spinal G97.1
    cerebrospinal fluid leak G97.0
    headache or reaction G97.1
  pyelogram N99.89
  radiation
    kyphosis M96.2
    scoliosis M96.5
  reattached
    extremity (infection) (rejection)
      lower T87.1X-●
      upper T87.0X-●
    specified body part NEC T87.2

Complication (*Continued*)
  reconstructed breast
    asymmetry between native and
        reconstructed breast N65.1
    deformity N65.0
    disproportion between native and
        reconstructed breast N65.1
    excess tissue N65.0
    misshappen N65.0
  reimplant NEC —*see also* Complications,
      prosthetic device or implant
    limb (infection) (rejection) —*see*
        Complications, reattached,
        extremity
    organ (partial) (total) —*see* Complications,
        transplant
    prosthetic device NEC —*see* Complications,
        prosthetic device
  renal N28.9
    allograft —*see* Complications, transplant,
        kidney
    dialysis —*see* Complications, dialysis
  respirator
    mechancial J95.850
      specified NEC J95.859
  respiratory system J98.9
    device, implant or graft —*see*
        Complication, prosthetic device or
        implant, specified NEC
    lung transplant —*see* Complications,
        prosthetic device or implant, lung
        transplant
    postoperative J95.89
      air leak J95.812
      Mendelson's syndrome (chemical
          pneumonitis) J95.4
      pneumothorax J95.811
      pulmonary insufficiency (acute) (after
          nonthoracic surgery) J95.2
        chronic J95.3
        following thoracic surgery J95.1
      respiratory failure (acute) J95.821
        acute and chronic J95.822
      specified NEC J95.89
      subglottic stenosis J95.5
      tracheostomy complication —*see*
          Complications, tracheostomy
    therapy T81.89
  sedation during labor and delivery O74.9
    cardiac O74.2
    central nervous system O74.3
    pulmonary NEC O74.1
  shunt —*see also* Complications, prosthetic
      device or implant
    arteriovenous —*see* Complications,
        arteriovenous, shunt
    ventricular (communicating) —*see*
        Complications, ventricular shunt
  skin
    graft T86.829
      failure T86.821
      infection T86.822
      rejection T86.820
      specified type NEC T86.828
  spinal
    anesthesia —*see* Complications, anesthesia,
        spinal
    catheter (epidural) (subdural) —*see*
        Complications, catheter
    puncture or tap G97.1
      cerebrospinal fluid leak G97.0
      headache or reaction G97.1
  stent
    bile duct —*see* Complications, bile duct
        prosthesis
    ureteral indwelling
      breakdown T83.112
      displacement T83.122
      leakage T83.192
      malposition T83.122

Complication (*Continued*)
  stent (*Continued*)
    ureteral indwelling (*Continued*)
      obstruction T83.192
      perforation T83.192
      protrusion T83.192
      specified NEC T83.192
    urinary (ileal conduit) (nephroureteral)
        T83.193
      embolism T83.81
      fibrosis T83.82
      hemorrhage T83.83
      infection and inflammation T83.593
      mechanical
        breakdown T83.113
        displacement T83.123
        leakage T83.193
        malposition T83.123
        obstruction T83.193
        perforation T83.193
        protrusion T83.193
        specified NEC T83.193
      pain T83.84
      specified type NEC T83.89
      stenosis T83.85
      thrombosis T83.86
    vascular
      end stent stenosis —*see* Restenosis,
          stent
      in stent stenosis —*see* Restenosis, stent
  stoma
    digestive tract
      colostomy —*see* Complications,
          colostomy
      enterostomy —*see* Complications,
          enterostomy
      esophagostomy —*see* Complications,
          esophagostomy
      gastrostomy —*see* Complications,
          gastrostomy
    urinary tract N99.528
      continent N99.538
        hemorrhage N99.530
        herniation N99.533
        infection N99.531
        malfunction N99.532
        specified type NEC N99.538
        stenosis N99.534
      cystostomy —*see* Complications,
          cystostomy
      external NOS N99.528
      hemorrhage N99.520
      herniation N99.523
      incontinent N99.528
        hemorrhage N99.520
        herniation N99.523
        infection N99.521
        malfunction N99.522
        specified type NEC N99.528
        stenosis N99.524
      infection N99.521
      malfunction N99.522
      specified type NEC N99.528
      stenosis N99.524
  stomach banding —*see* Complication(s),
      bariatric procedure
  stomach stapling —*see* Complication(s),
      bariatric procedure
  surgical material, nonabsorbable —*see*
      Complication, suture, permanent
  surgical procedure (on) T81.9
    amputation stump (late) —*see*
        Complications, amputation stump
    cardiac —*see* Complications, circulatory
        system
    cholesteatoma, recurrent —*see*
        Complications, postmastoidectomy,
        recurrent cholesteatoma
    circulatory (early) —*see* Complications,
        circulatory system

Complication (*Continued*)
  surgical procedure (*Continued*)
    digestive system —*see* Complications,
        gastrointestinal
    dumping syndrome (postgastrectomy)
        K91.1
    ear —*see* Complications, ear
    elephantiasis or lymphedema I97.89
      postmastectomy I97.2
    emphysema (surgical) T81.82
    endocrine —*see* Complications, endocrine
    eye —*see* Complications, eye
    fistula (persistent postoperative) T81.83
    foreign body inadvertently left in wound
        (sponge) (suture) (swab) —*see* Foreign
        body, accidentally left during a
        procedure
    gastrointestinal —*see* Complications,
        gastrointestinal
    genitourinary NEC N99.89
    hematoma
      intraoperative —*see* Complication,
          intraoperative, hemorrhage
      postprocedural —*see* Complication,
          postprocedural, hematoma
    hemorrhage
      intraoperative —*see* Complication,
          intraoperative, hemorrhage
      postprocedural —*see* Complication,
          postprocedural, hemorrhage
    hepatic failure K91.82
    hyperglycemia (postpancreatectomy) E89.1
    hypoinsulinemia (postpancreatectomy)
        E89.1
    hypoparathyroidism
        (postparathyroidectomy) E89.2
    hypopituitarism (posthypophysectomy)
        E89.3
    hypothyroidism (post-thyroidectomy)
        E89.0
  ➡ intestinal obstruction —*see also*
        Obstruction, intestine, postoperative
        K91.30
    intracranial hypotension following
        ventricular shunting
        (ventriculostomy) G97.2
    lymphedema I97.89
      postmastectomy I97.2
    malabsorption (postsurgical) NEC K91.2
      osteoporosis —*see* Osteoporosis,
          postsurgical malabsorption
    mastoidectomy cavity NEC —*see*
        Complications, postmastoidectomy
    metabolic E89.89
      specified NEC E89.89
    musculoskeletal —*see* Complications,
        musculoskeletal system
    nervous system (central) (peripheral) —*see*
        Complications, nervous system
    ovarian failure E89.40
      asymptomatic E89.40
      symptomatic E89.41
    peripheral vascular —*see* Complications,
        surgical procedure, vascular
    postcardiotomy syndrome I97.0
    postcholecystectomy syndrome K91.5
    postcommissurotomy syndrome I97.0
    postgastrectomy dumping syndrome K91.1
    postlaminectomy syndrome NEC M96.1
      kyphosis M96.3
    postmastectomy lymphedema syndrome
        I97.2
    postmastoidectomy cholesteatoma —*see*
        Complications, postmastoidectomy,
        recurrent cholesteatoma
    postvagotomy syndrome K91.1
    postvalvulotomy syndrome I97.0
    pulmonary insufficiency (acute) J95.2
      chronic J95.3
      following thoracic surgery J95.1

Complication (Continued)
  surgical procedure (Continued)
    reattached body part —see Complications, reattached
    respiratory —see Complications, respiratory system
    shock (hypovolemic) T81.19
    spleen (postoperative) D78.89
      intraoperative D78.81
    ⇒ stitch abscess T81.4
    subglottic stenosis (postsurgical) J95.5
    testicular hypofunction E89.5
    transplant —see Complications, organ or tissue transplant
    urinary NEC N99.89
    vaginal vault prolapse (posthysterectomy) N99.3
    vascular (peripheral)
      artery T81.719
        mesenteric T81.710
        renal T81.711
        specified NEC T81.718
      vein T81.72
    ⇒ wound infection T81.4
  suture, permanent (wire) NEC T85.9
    with repair of bone —see Complications, fixation device, internal
    embolism T85.818
    fibrosis T85.828
    hemorrhage T85.838
    infection and inflammation T85.79
    mechanical
      breakdown T85.612
      displacement T85.622
      malfunction T85.612
      malposition T85.622
      obstruction T85.692
      perforation T85.692
      protrusion T85.692
      specified NEC T85.692
    pain T85.848
    specified type NEC T85.898
    stenosis T85.858
    thrombosis T85.868
  tracheostomy J95.00
    granuloma J95.09
    hemorrhage J95.01
    infection J95.02
    malfunction J95.03
    mechanical J95.03
    obstruction J95.03
    specified type NEC J95.09
    tracheo-esophageal fistula J95.04
  transfusion (blood) (lymphocytes) (plasma) T80.92
    air embolism T80.0
    circulatory overload E87.71
    febrile nonhemolytic transfusion reaction R50.84
    hemochromatosis E83.111
    hemolysis T80.89
    hemolytic reaction (antigen unspecified) T80.919
    incompatibility reaction (antigen unspecified) T80.919
      ABO T80.30
        delayed serologic (DSTR) T80.39
        hemolytic transfusion reaction (HTR) (unspecified time after transfusion) T80.319
          acute (AHTR) (less than 24 hours after transfusion) T80.310
          delayed (DHTR) (24 hours or more after transfusion) T80.311
        specified NEC T80.39
      acute (antigen unspecified) T80.910
      delayed (antigen unspecified) T80.911
        delayed serologic (DSTR) T80.89

Complication (Continued)
  transfusion (Continued)
    incompatibility reaction (Continued)
      Non-ABO (minor antigens (Duffy) (Kell) (Kidd) (Lewis) (M) (N) (P) (S)) T80.A0
        delayed serologic (DSTR) T80.A9
        hemolytic transfusion reaction (HTR) (unspecified time after transfusion) T80.A19
          acute (AHTR) (less than 24 hours after transfusion) T80.A10
          delayed (DHTR) (24 hours or more after transfusion) T80.A11
        specified NEC T80.A9
      Rh (antigens (C) (c) (D) (E) (e)) (factor) T80.40
        delayed serologic (DSTR) T80.49
        hemolytic transfusion reaction (HTR) (unspecified time after transfusion) T80.419
          acute (AHTR) (less than 24 hours after transfusion) T80.410
          delayed (DHTR) (24 hours or more after transfusion) T80.411
        specified NEC T80.49
    infection T80.29
      acute T80.22
    reaction NEC T80.89
    sepsis T80.29
    shock T80.89
  transplant T86.90
    bone T86.839
      failure T86.831
      infection T86.832
      rejection T86.830
      specified type NEC T86.838
    bone marrow T86.00
      failure T86.02
      infection T86.03
      rejection T86.01
      specified type NEC T86.09
    cornea T86.849
      failure T86.841
      infection T86.842
      rejection T86.840
      specified type NEC T86.848
    failure T86.92
    heart T86.20
      with lung T86.30
        cardiac allograft vasculopathy T86.290
        failure T86.32
        infection T86.33
        rejection T86.31
        specified type NEC T86.39
      failure T86.22
      infection T86.23
      rejection T86.21
      specified type NEC T86.298
    infection T86.93
    intestine T86.859
      failure T86.851
      infection T86.852
      rejection T86.850
      specified type NEC T86.858
    kidney T86.10
      failure T86.12
      infection T86.13
      rejection T86.11
      specified type NEC T86.19
    liver T86.40
      failure T86.42
      infection T86.43
      rejection T86.41
      specified type NEC T86.49
    lung T86.819
      with heart T86.30
        failure T86.32
        infection T86.33
        rejection T86.31
        specified type NEC T86.39

Complication (Continued)
  transplant (Continued)
    lung (Continued)
      failure T86.811
      infection T86.812
      rejection T86.810
      specified type NEC T86.818
    malignant neoplasm C80.2
    pancreas T86.899
      failure T86.891
      infection T86.892
      rejection T86.890
      specified type NEC T86.898
    peripheral blood stem cells T86.5
    post-transplant lymphoproliferative disorder (PTLD) D47.Z1
    rejection T86.91
    skin T86.829
      failure T86.821
      infection T86.822
      rejection T86.820
      specified type NEC T86.828
    specified
      tissue T86.899
        failure T86.891
        infection T86.892
        rejection T86.890
        specified type NEC T86.898
      type NEC T86.99
    stem cell (from peripheral blood) (from umbilical cord) T86.5
    umbilical cord stem cells T86.5
  trauma (early) T79.9
    specified NEC T79.8
  ultrasound therapy NEC T88.9
  umbilical cord NEC
    complicating delivery O69.9
      specified NEC O69.89
  umbrella device, vascular T82.9
    embolism T82.818
    fibrosis T82.828
    hemorrhage T82.838
    infection or inflammation T82.7
    mechanical
      breakdown T82.515
      displacement T82.525
      leakage T82.535
      malposition T82.525
      obstruction T82.595
      perforation T82.595
      protrusion T82.595
    pain T82.848
    specified type NEC T82.898
    stenosis T82.858
    thrombosis T82.868
  urethral catheter —see Complications, catheter, urethral, indwelling
  vaccination T88.1
    anaphylaxis NEC T80.52
    arthropathy —see Arthropathy, postimmunization
    cellulitis T88.0
    encephalitis or encephalomyelitis G04.02
    infection (general) (local) NEC T88.0
    meningitis G03.8
    myelitis G04.02
    protein sickness T80.62
    rash T88.1
    reaction (allergic) T88.1
      serum T80.62
    sepsis T88.0
    serum intoxication, sickness, rash, or other serum reaction NEC T80.62
      anaphylactic shock T80.52
    shock (allergic) (anaphylactic) T80.52
    vaccinia (generalized) (localized) T88.1
  vas deferens device or implant —see Complications, genitourinary, device or implant, genital tract

Complication *(Continued)*
 vascular I99.9
  device or implant T82.9
   embolism T82.818
   fibrosis T82.828
   hemorrhage T82.838
   infection or inflammation T82.7
   mechanical
    breakdown T82.519
     specified device NEC T82.518
    displacement T82.529
     specified device NEC T82.528
    leakage T82.539
     specified device NEC T82.538
    malposition T82.529
     specified device NEC T82.528
    obstruction T82.599
     specified device NEC T82.598
    perforation T82.599
     specified device NEC T82.598
    protrusion T82.599
     specified device NEC T82.598
   pain T82.848
   specified type NEC T82.898
   stenosis T82.858
   thrombosis T82.868
  dialysis catheter —*see* Complication,
    catheter, dialysis
  following infusion, therapeutic injection or
    transfusion T80.1
  graft T82.9
   embolism T82.818
   fibrosis T82.828
   hemorrhage T82.838
   mechanical
    breakdown T82.319
     aorta (bifurcation) T82.310
     carotid artery T82.311
     specified vessel NEC T82.318
    displacement T82.329
     aorta (bifurcation) T82.320
     carotid artery T82.321
     specified vessel NEC T82.328
    leakage T82.339
     aorta (bifurcation) T82.330
     carotid artery T82.331
     specified vessel NEC T82.338
    malposition T82.329
     aorta (bifurcation) T82.320
     carotid artery T82.321
     specified vessel NEC T82.328
    obstruction T82.399
     aorta (bifurcation) T82.390
     carotid artery T82.391
     specified vessel NEC T82.398
    perforation T82.399
     aorta (bifurcation) T82.390
     carotid artery T82.391
     specified vessel NEC T82.398
    protrusion T82.399
     aorta (bifurcation) T82.390
     carotid artery T82.391
     specified vessel NEC T82.398
   pain T82.848
   specified complication NEC T82.898
   stenosis T82.858
   thrombosis T82.868
  postoperative —*see* Complications,
    postoperative, circulatory
  vena cava device (filter) (sieve) (umbrella) —
    see Complications, umbrella device,
    vascular
 ventilation therapy NEC T81.81
 ventilator
  mechanical J95.850
   specified NEC J95.859
 ventricular (communicating) shunt (device)
    T85.9
  embolism T85.810
  fibrosis T85.820
  hemorrhage T85.830

Complication *(Continued)*
 ventricular shunt *(Continued)*
  infection and inflammation T85.730
  mechanical
   breakdown T85.01
   displacement T85.02
   leakage T85.03
   malposition T85.02
   obstruction T85.09
   perforation T85.09
   protrusion T85.09
   specified NEC T85.09
  pain T85.840
  specified type NEC T85.890
  stenosis T85.850
  thrombosis T85.860
 wire suture, permanent (implanted) —*see*
    Complications, suture, permanent
Compressed air disease T70.3
Compression
 with injury - code by Nature of injury
 artery I77.1
  celiac, syndrome I77.4
 brachial plexus G54.0
 brain (stem) G93.5
  due to
   contusion (diffuse) —*see* Injury,
     intracranial, diffuse
    focal —*see* Injury, intracranial, focal
   injury NEC —*see* Injury, intracranial,
     diffuse
   traumatic —*see* Injury, intracranial, diffuse
 bronchus J98.09
 cauda equina G83.4
 celiac (artery) (axis) I77.4
 cerebral —*see* Compression, brain
 cervical plexus G54.2
 cord
  spinal —*see* Compression, spinal
  umbilical —*see* Compression, umbilical
    cord
 cranial nerve G52.9
  eighth —*see* subcategory H93.3
  eleventh G52.8
  fifth G50.8
  first G52.0
  fourth —*see* Strabismus, paralytic, fourth
    nerve
  ninth G52.1
  second —*see* Disorder, nerve, optic
  seventh G51.8
  sixth —*see* Strabismus, paralytic, sixth
    nerve
  tenth G52.2
  third —*see* Strabismus, paralytic, third
    nerve
  twelfth G52.3
 diver's squeeze T70.3
 during birth (newborn) P15.9
 esophagus K22.2
 eustachian tube —*see* Obstruction, eustachian
    tube, cartilaginous
 facies Q67.1
 fracture
  nontraumatic NOS —*see* Collapse, vertebra
  pathological —*see* Fracture, pathological
  traumatic —*see* Fracture, traumatic
 heart —*see* Disease, heart
 intestine —*see* Obstruction, intestine
 laryngeal nerve, recurrent G52.2
  with paralysis of vocal cords and larynx
    J38.00
   bilateral J38.02
   unilateral J38.01
 lumbosacral plexus G54.1
 lung J98.4
 lymphatic vessel I89.0
 medulla —*see* Compression, brain
 nerve —*see also* Disorder, nerve G58.9
  arm NEC —*see* Mononeuropathy, upper
    limb

Compression *(Continued)*
 nerve *(Continued)*
  axillary G54.0
  cranial —*see* Compression, cranial nerve
  leg NEC —*see* Mononeuropathy, lower
    limb
  median (in carpal tunnel) —*see* Syndrome,
    carpal tunnel
  optic —*see* Disorder, nerve, optic
  plantar —*see* Lesion, nerve, plantar
  posterior tibial (in tarsal tunnel) —*see*
    Syndrome, tarsal tunnel
  root or plexus NOS (in) G54.9
   intervertebral disc disorder NEC —
     see Disorder, disc, with,
     radiculopathy
    with myelopathy —*see* Disorder, disc,
      with, myelopathy
   neoplastic disease —*see also* Neoplasm
     D49.9 *[G55]*
   spondylosis —*see* Spondylosis, with
     radiculopathy
  sciatic (acute) —*see* Lesion, nerve, sciatic
  sympathetic G90.8
  traumatic —*see* Injury, nerve
  ulnar —*see* Lesion, nerve, ulnar
  upper extremity NEC —*see*
    Mononeuropathy, upper limb
 spinal (cord) G95.20
  by displacement of intervertebral disc
    NEC —*see also* Disorder, disc, with,
    myelopathy
  nerve root NOS G54.9
   due to displacement of intervertebral
     disc NEC —*see* Disorder, disc, with,
     radiculopathy
    with myelopathy —*see* Disorder, disc,
      with, myelopathy
  specified NEC G95.29
  spondylogenic (cervical) (lumbar,
    lumbosacral) (thoracic) —*see*
    Spondylosis, with myelopathy NEC
  anterior —*see* Syndrome, anterior, spinal
    artery, compression
  traumatic —*see* Injury, spinal cord, by
    region
 subcostal nerve (syndrome) —*see*
    Mononeuropathy, upper limb, specified
    NEC
 sympathetic nerve NEC G90.8
 syndrome T79.5
 trachea J39.8
 ulnar nerve (by scar tissue) —*see* Lesion,
    nerve, ulnar
 umbilical cord
  complicating delivery O69.2
   cord around neck O69.1
   prolapse O69.0
   specified NEC O69.2
 ureter N13.5
 vein I87.1
 vena cava (inferior) (superior) I87.1
Compulsion, compulsive
 gambling F63.0
 neurosis F42.8
 personality F60.5
 states F42.8
 swearing F42.8
  in Gilles de la Tourette's syndrome F95.2
 tics and spasms F95.9
Concato's disease (pericardial polyserositis)
    A19.9
 nontubercular I31.1
 pleural —*see* Pleurisy, with effusion
Concavity chest wall M95.4
Concealed penis Q55.69
Concern (normal) **about sick person in family**
    Z63.6
Concrescence (teeth) K00.2
Concretio cordis I31.1
 rheumatic I09.2

▶ New ⇒ Revised ~~deleted~~ Deleted • Use Additional Character(s)

Concretion —*see also* Calculus
  appendicular K38.1
  canaliculus —*see* Dacryolith
  clitoris N90.89
  conjunctiva H11.12-●
  eyelid —*see* Disorder, eyelid, specified type NEC
  lacrimal passages —*see* Dacryolith
  prepuce (male) N47.8
  salivary gland (any) K11.5
  seminal vesicle N50.89
  tonsil J35.8
Concussion (brain) (cerebral) (current) S06.0X9
  with
    loss of consciousness of 30 minutes or less S06.0X1
    loss of consciousness of unspecified duration S06.0X9
  blast (air) (hydraulic) (immersion) (underwater)
    abdomen or thorax —*see* Injury, blast, by site
    ear with acoustic nerve injury —*see* Injury, nerve, acoustic, specified type NEC
  cauda equina S34.3
  conus medullaris S34.02
  ocular S05.8X-●
  spinal (cord)
    cervical S14.0
    lumbar S34.01
    sacral S34.02
    thoracic S24.0
  syndrome F07.81
  Without loss of consciousness S06.0X0
Condition —*see* Disease
Conditions arising in the perinatal period —*see* Newborn, affected by
Conduct disorder —*see* Disorder, conduct
Condyloma A63.0
  acuminatum A63.0
  gonorrheal A54.09
  latum A51.31
  syphilitic A51.31
    congenital A50.07
  venereal, syphilitic A51.31
Conflagration —*see also* Burn
  asphyxia (by inhalation of gases, fumes or vapors) —*see also* Table of Drugs and Chemicals T59.9-●
Conflict (with) —*see also* Discord
  family Z73.9
  marital Z63.0
    involving divorce or estrangement Z63.5
  parent-child Z62.820
    parent-adopted child Z62.821
    parent-biological child Z62.820
    parent-foster child Z62.822
  social role NEC Z73.5
Confluent —*see* condition
Confusion, confused R41.0
  epileptic F05
  mental state (psychogenic) F44.89
  psychogenic F44.89
  reactive (from emotional stress, psychological trauma) F44.89
Confusional arousals G47.51
Congelation T69.9
Congenital —*see also* condition
  aortic septum Q25.49
  intrinsic factor deficiency D51.0
  malformation —*see* Anomaly
Congestion, congestive
  bladder N32.89
  bowel K63.89
  brain G93.89
  breast N64.59
  bronchial J98.09
  catarrhal J31.0
  chest R09.89
  chill, malarial —*see* Malaria

Congestion, congestive *(Continued)*
  circulatory NEC I99.8
  duodenum K31.89
  eye —*see* Hyperemia, conjunctiva
  facial, due to birth injury P15.4
  general R68.89
  glottis J37.0
  heart —*see* Failure, heart, congestive
  hepatic K76.1
  hypostatic (lung) —*see* Edema, lung
  intestine K63.89
  kidney N28.89
  labyrinth —*see* subcategory H83.8
  larynx J37.0
  liver K76.1
  lung R09.89
    active or acute —*see* Pneumonia
  malaria, malarial —*see* Malaria
  nasal R09.81
  nose R09.81
  orbit, orbital —*see also* Exophthalmos
    inflammatory (chronic) —*see* Inflammation, orbit
  ovary N83.8
  pancreas K86.89
  pelvic, female N94.89
  pleural J94.8
  prostate (active) N42.1
  pulmonary —*see* Congestion, lung
  renal N28.89
  retina H35.81
  seminal vesicle N50.1
  spinal cord G95.19
  spleen (chronic) D73.2
  stomach K31.89
  trachea —*see* Tracheitis
  urethra N36.8
  uterus N85.8
    with subinvolution N85.3
  venous (passive) I87.8
  viscera R68.89
Congestive —*see* Congestion
Conical
  cervix (hypertrophic elongation) N88.4
  cornea —*see* Keratoconus
  teeth K00.2
Conjoined twins Q89.4
Conjugal maladjustment Z63.0
  involving divorce or estrangement Z63.5
Conjunctiva —*see* condition
Conjunctivitis (staphylococcal) (streptococcal) NOS H10.9
  Acanthamoeba B60.12
  acute H10.3-●
    atopic H10.1-●
    chemical —*see also* Corrosion, cornea H10.21-●
    mucopurulent H10.02-●
      follicular H10.01-●
    pseudomembranous H10.22-●
    serous except viral H10.23-●
      viral —*see* Conjunctivitis, viral
    toxic H10.21-●
  adenoviral (acute) (follicular) B30.1
  allergic (acute) —*see* Conjunctivitis, acute, atopic
    chronic H10.45
    vernal H10.44
  anaphylactic —*see* Conjunctivitis, acute, atopic
  Apollo B30.3
  atopic (acute) —*see* Conjunctivitis, acute, atopic
  Béal's B30.2
  blennorrhagic (gonococcal) (neonatorum) A54.31
  chemical (acute) —*see also* Corrosion, cornea H10.21-●
  chlamydial A74.0
    due to trachoma A71.1
    neonatal P39.1

Conjunctivitis *(Continued)*
  chronic (nodosa) (petrificans) (phlyctenular) H10.40-●
    allergic H10.45
      vernal H10.44
    follicular H10.43-●
    giant papillary H10.41-●
    simple H10.42-●
    vernal H10.44
  coxsackievirus 24 B30.3
  diphtheritic A36.86
  due to
    dust —*see* Conjunctivitis, acute, atopic
    filariasis B74.9
    mucocutaneous leishmaniasis B55.2
  enterovirus type 70 (hemorrhagic) B30.3
  epidemic (viral) B30.9
    hemorrhagic B30.3
  gonococcal (neonatorum) A54.31
  granular (trachomatous) A71.1
    sequelae (late effect) B94.0
  hemorrhagic (acute) (epidemic) B30.3
  herpes zoster B02.31
  in (due to)
    Acanthamoeba B60.12
    adenovirus (acute) (follicular) B30.1
    Chlamydia A74.0
    coxsackievirus 24 B30.3
    diphtheria A36.86
    enterovirus type 70 (hemorrhagic) B30.3
    filariasis B74.9
    gonococci A54.31
    herpes (simplex) virus B00.53
      zoster B02.31
    infectious disease NEC B99
    meningococci A39.89
    mucocutaneous leishmaniasis B55.2
    rosacea L71.9
    syphilis (late) A52.71
    zoster B02.31
  inclusion A74.0
  infantile P39.1
    gonococcal A54.31
  Koch-Weeks' —*see* Conjunctivitis, acute, mucopurulent
  light —*see* Conjunctivitis, acute, atopic
  ligneous —*see* Blepharoconjunctivitis, ligneous
  meningococcal A39.89
  mucopurulent —*see* Conjunctivitis, acute, mucopurulent
  neonatal P39.1
    gonococcal A54.31
  Newcastle B30.8
  of Béal B30.2
  parasitic
    filariasis B74.9
    mucocutaneous leishmaniasis B55.2
  Parinaud's H10.89
  petrificans H10.89
  rosacea L71.9
  specified NEC H10.89
  swimming-pool B30.1
  trachomatous A71.1
    acute A71.0
    sequelae (late effect) B94.0
  traumatic NEC H10.89
  tuberculous A18.59
  tularemic A21.1
  tularensis A21.1
  viral B30.9
    due to
      adenovirus B30.1
      enterovirus B30.3
    specified NEC B30.8
Conjunctivochalasis H11.82-●
Connective tissue —*see* condition
Conn's syndrome E26.01
Conradi (-Hunermann) disease Q77.3
Consanguinity Z84.3
  counseling Z71.89

Conscious simulation (of illness) Z76.5
Consecutive —see condition
Consolidation lung (base) —see Pneumonia,
   lobar
Constipation (atonic) (neurogenic) (simple)
   (spastic) K59.00
   chronic K59.09
      idiopathic K59.04
   drug-induced K59.03
   functional K59.04
   outlet dysfunction K59.02
   psychogenic F45.8
   slow transit K59.01
   specified NEC K59.09
Constitutional —see also condition
   substandard F60.7
Constitutionally substandard F60.7
Constriction —see also Stricture
   auditory canal —see Stenosis, external ear
      canal
   bronchial J98.09
   duodenum K31.5
   esophagus K22.2
   external
      abdomen, abdominal (wall) S30.841
      alveolar process S00.542
      ankle S90.54-●
      antecubital space —see Constriction,
         external, forearm
      arm (upper) S40.84-●
      auricle —see Constriction, external, ear
      axilla —see Constriction, external, arm
      back, lower S30.840
      breast S20.14-●
      brow S00.84
      buttock S30.840
      calf —see Constriction, external, leg
      canthus —see Constriction, external, eyelid
      cheek S00.84
         internal S00.542
      chest wall —see Constriction, external,
         thorax
      chin S00.84
      clitoris S30.844
      costal region —see Constriction, external,
         thorax
      digit(s)
         foot —see Constriction, external, toe
         hand —see Constriction, external, finger
      ear S00.44-●
      elbow S50.34-●
      epididymis S30.843
      epigastric region S30.841
      esophagus, cervical S10.14
      eyebrow —see Constriction, external, eyelid
      eyelid S00.24-●
      face S00.84
      finger(s) S60.44-●
         index S60.44-●
         little S60.44-●
         middle S60.44-●
         ring S60.44-●
      flank S30.841
      foot (except toe(s) alone) S90.84-●
         toe —see Constriction, external, toe
      forearm S50.84-●
         elbow only —see Constriction, external,
            elbow
      forehead S00.84
      genital organs, external
         female S30.846
         male S30.845
      groin S30.841
      gum S00.542
      hand S60.54-●
      head S00.94
         ear —see Constriction, external, ear
         eyelid —see Constriction, external, eyelid
         lip S00.541
         nose S00.34
         oral cavity S00.542

Constriction (Continued)
   external (Continued)
      head (Continued)
         scalp S00.04
         specified site NEC S00.84
      heel —see Constriction, external, foot
      hip S70.24-●
      inguinal region S30.841
      interscapular region S20.449
      jaw S00.84
      knee S80.24-●
      labium (majus) (minus) S30.844
      larynx S10.14
      leg (lower) S80.84-●
         knee —see Constriction, external, knee
         upper —see Constriction, external, thigh
      lip S00.541
      lower back S30.840
      lumbar region S30.840
      malar region S00.84
      mammary —see Constriction, external,
         breast
      mastoid region S00.84
      mouth S00.542
      nail
         finger —see Constriction, external, finger
         toe —see Constriction, external, toe
      nasal S00.34
      neck S10.94
         specified site NEC S10.84
         throat S10.14
      nose S00.34
      occipital region S00.04
      oral cavity S00.542
      orbital region —see Constriction, external,
         eyelid
      palate S00.542
      palm —see Constriction, external, hand
      parietal region S00.04
      pelvis S30.840
      penis S30.842
      perineum
         female S30.844
         male S30.840
      periocular area —see Constriction, external,
         eyelid
      phalanges
         finger —see Constriction, external, finger
         toe —see Constriction, external, toe
      pharynx S10.14
      pinna —see Constriction, external, ear
      popliteal space —see Constriction, external,
         knee
      prepuce S30.842
      pubic region S30.840
      pudendum
         female S30.846
         male S30.845
      sacral region S30.840
      scalp S00.04
      scapular region —see Constriction,
         external, shoulder
      scrotum S30.843
      shin —see Constriction, external, leg
      shoulder S40.24-●
      sternal region S20.349
      submaxillary region S00.84
      submental region S00.84
      subungual
         finger(s) —see Constriction, external,
            finger
         toe(s) —see Constriction, external, toe
      supraclavicular fossa S10.84
      supraorbital S00.84
      temple S00.84
      temporal region S00.84
      testis S30.843
      thigh S70.34-●
      thorax, thoracic (wall) S20.94
         back S20.44-●
         front S20.34-●

Constriction (Continued)
   external (Continued)
      throat S10.14
      thumb S60.34-●
      toe(s) (lesser) S90.44-●
         great S90.44-●
      tongue S00.542
      trachea S10.14
      tunica vaginalis S30.843
      uvula S00.542
      vagina S30.844
      vulva S30.844
      wrist S60.84-●
   gallbladder —see Obstruction, gallbladder
   intestine —see Obstruction, intestine
   larynx J38.6
      congenital Q31.8
         specified NEC Q31.8
         subglottic Q31.1
   organ or site, congenital NEC —see Atresia,
      by site
   prepuce (acquired) (congenital) N47.1
   pylorus (adult hypertrophic) K31.1
      congenital or infantile Q40.0
      newborn Q40.0
   ring dystocia (uterus) O62.4
   spastic —see also Spasm
      ureter N13.5
   ureter N13.5
      with infection N13.6
   urethra —see Stricture, urethra
   visual field (peripheral) (functional) —see
      Defect, visual field
Constrictive —see condition
Consultation
   without complaint or sickness Z71.9
      feared complaint unfounded Z71.1
      specified reason NEC Z71.89
   medical —see Counseling, medical
   religious Z71.81
   specified reason NEC Z71.89
   spiritual Z71.81
Consumption —see Tuberculosis
Contact (with) —see also Exposure (to)
   acariasis Z20.7
   AIDS virus Z20.6
   air pollution Z77.110
   algae and algae toxins Z77.121
   algae bloom Z77.121
   anthrax Z20.810
   aromatic (hazardous) compounds NEC
      Z77.028
   aromatic amines Z77.020
   aromatic dyes NOS Z77.028
   arsenic Z77.010
   asbestos Z77.090
   bacterial disease NEC Z20.818
   benzene Z77.021
   blue-green algae bloom Z77.121
   body fluids (potentially hazardous) Z77.21
   brown tide Z77.121
   chemicals (chiefly nonmedicinal) (hazardous)
      NEC Z77.098
   cholera Z20.09
   chromium compounds Z77.018
   communicable disease Z20.9
      bacterial NEC Z20.818
      specified NEC Z20.89
      viral NEC Z20.828
   cyanobacteria bloom Z77.121
   dyes Z77.098
   Escherichia coli (E. coli) Z20.01
   fiberglass —see Table of Drugs and
      Chemicals, fiberglass
   German measles Z20.4
   gonorrhea Z20.2
   hazardous metals NEC Z77.018
   hazardous substances NEC Z77.29
   hazards in the physical environment NEC
      Z77.128
   hazards to health NEC Z77.9

▶ New   ⇒ Revised   ~~deleted~~ Deleted   ● Use Additional Character(s)

Contact *(Continued)*
  HIV Z20.6
  HTLV-III/LAV Z20.6
  human immunodeficiency virus (HIV) Z20.6
  infection Z20.9
    specified NEC Z20.89
  infestation (parasitic) NEC Z20.7
  intestinal infectious disease NEC Z20.09
    Escherichia coli (E. coli) Z20.01
  lead Z77.011
  meningococcus Z20.811
  mold (toxic) Z77.120
  nickel dust Z77.018
  noise Z77.122
  parasitic disease Z20.7
  pediculosis Z20.7
  pfiesteria piscicida Z77.121
  poliomyelitis Z20.89
  pollution
    air Z77.110
    environmental NEC Z77.118
    soil Z77.112
    water Z77.111
  polycyclic aromatic hydrocarbons Z77.028
  rabies Z20.3
  radiation, naturally occurring NEC Z77.123
  radon Z77.123
  red tide (Florida) Z77.121
  rubella Z20.4
  sexually-transmitted disease Z20.2
  smallpox (laboratory) Z20.89
  syphilis Z20.2
  tuberculosis Z20.1
  uranium Z77.012
  varicella Z20.820
  venereal disease Z20.2
  viral disease NEC Z20.828
  viral hepatitis Z20.5
  water pollution Z77.111
Contamination, food —*see* Intoxication,
  foodborne
Contraception, contraceptive
  advice Z30.09
  counseling Z30.09
  device (intrauterine) (in situ) Z97.5
    causing menorrhagia T83.83
    checking Z30.431
    complications —*see* Complications,
      intrauterine, contraceptive device
    in place Z97.5
    initial prescription Z30.014
    reinsertion Z30.433
    removal Z30.432
    replacement Z30.433
  emergency (postcoital) Z30.012
  initial prescription Z30.019
    barrier Z30.018
    diaphragm Z30.018
    injectable Z30.013
    intrauterine device Z30.014
    pills Z30.011
    postcoital (emergency) Z30.012
    specified type NEC Z30.018
    subdermal implantable Z30.017
    transdermal patch hormonal Z30.016
    vaginal ring hormonal Z30.015
  maintenance Z30.40
    barrier Z30.49
    diaphragm Z30.49
    examination Z30.8
    injectable Z30.42
    intrauterine device Z30.431
    pills Z30.41
    specified type NEC Z30.49
    subdermal implantable Z30.46
    transdermal patch hormonal Z30.45
    vaginal ring hormonal Z30.44
  management Z30.9
    specified NEC Z30.8
  postcoital (emergency) Z30.012
  prescription Z30.019
    repeat Z30.40

Contraception, contraceptive *(Continued)*
    sterilization Z30.2
    surveillance (drug) —*see* Contraception,
      maintenance
Contraction(s), contracture, contracted
  Achilles tendon —*see also* Short, tendon,
    Achilles
    congenital Q66.89
  amputation stump (surgical) (flexion) (late)
    next proximal joint T87.89
  anus K59.8
  bile duct (common) (hepatic) K83.8
  bladder N32.89
    neck or sphincter N32.0
  bowel, cecum, colon or intestine, any part —
    see Obstruction, intestine
  Braxton Hicks —*see* False, labor
  breast implant, capsular T85.44
  bronchial J98.09
  burn (old) —*see* Cicatrix
  cervix —*see* Stricture, cervix
  cicatricial —*see* Cicatrix
  conjunctiva, trachomatous, active A71.1
    sequelae (late effect) B94.0
  Dupuytren's M72.0
  eyelid —*see* Disorder, eyelid function
  fascia (lata) (postural) M72.8
    Dupuytren's M72.0
    palmar M72.0
    plantar M72.2
  finger NEC —*see also* Deformity, finger
    congenital Q68.1
    joint —*see* Contraction, joint, hand
  flaccid —*see* Contraction, paralytic
  gallbladder K82.0
  heart valve —*see* Endocarditis
  hip —*see* Contraction, joint, hip
  hourglass
    bladder N32.89
      congenital Q64.79
    gallbladder K82.0
      congenital Q44.1
    stomach K31.89
      congenital Q40.2
      psychogenic F45.8
    uterus (complicating delivery) O62.4
  hysterical F44.4
  internal os —*see* Stricture, cervix
  joint (abduction) (acquired) (adduction)
    (flexion) (rotation) M24.50
    ankle M24.57-●
    congenital NEC Q68.8
      hip Q65.89
    elbow M24.52-●
    foot joint M24.57-●
    hand joint M24.54-●
    hip M24.55-●
      congenital Q65.89
    hysterical F44.4
    knee M24.56-●
    shoulder M24.51-●
    wrist M24.53-●
  kidney (granular) (secondary) N26.9
    congenital Q63.8
    hydronephritic —*see* Hydronephrosis
    Page N26.2
    pyelonephritic —*see* Pyelitis, chronic
    tuberculous A18.11
  ligament —*see also* Disorder, ligament
    congenital Q79.8
  muscle (postinfective) (postural) NEC M62.40
    with contracture of joint —*see* Contraction,
      joint
    ankle M62.47-●
    congenital Q79.8
      sternocleidomastoid Q68.0
    extraocular —*see* Strabismus
    eye (extrinsic) —*see* Strabismus
    foot M62.47-●
    forearm M62.43-●
    hand M62.44-●

Contraction, contracture, contracted
  (Continued)
  muscle *(Continued)*
    hysterical F44.4
    ischemic (Volkmann's) T79.6
    lower leg M62.46-●
    multiple sites M62.49
    pelvic region M62.45-●
    posttraumatic —*see* Strabismus, paralytic
    psychogenic F45.8
      conversion reaction F44.4
    shoulder region M62.41-●
    specified site NEC M62.48
    thigh M62.45-●
    upper arm M62.42-●
  neck —*see* Torticollis
  ocular muscle —*see* Strabismus
  organ or site, congenital NEC —*see* Atresia,
    by site
  outlet (pelvis) —*see* Contraction, pelvis
  palmar fascia M72.0
  paralytic
    joint —*see* Contraction, joint
    muscle —*see also* Contraction, muscle NEC
      ocular —*see* Strabismus, paralytic
  pelvis (acquired) (general) M95.5
    with disproportion (fetopelvic) O33.1
      causing obstructed labor O65.1
    inlet O33.2
    mid-cavity O33.3
    outlet O33.3
  plantar fascia M72.2
  premature
    atrium I49.1
    auriculoventricular I49.49
    heart I49.49
    junctional I49.2
    supraventricular I49.1
    ventricular I49.3
  prostate N42.89
  pylorus NEC —*see also* Pylorospasm
    psychogenic F45.8
  rectum, rectal (sphincter) K59.8
  ring (Bandl's) (complicating delivery) O62.4
  scar —*see* Cicatrix
  spine —*see* Dorsopathy, deforming
  sternocleidomastoid (muscle), congenital
    Q68.0
  stomach K31.89
    hourglass K31.89
      congenital Q40.2
      psychogenic F45.8
    psychogenic F45.8
  tendon (sheath) M62.40
    with contracture of joint —*see* Contraction,
      joint
    Achilles —*see* Short, tendon, Achilles
    ankle M62.47-●
      Achilles —*see* Short, tendon, Achilles
    foot M62.47-●
    forearm M62.43-●
    hand M62.44-●
    lower leg M62.46-●
    multiple sites M62.49
    neck M62.48
    pelvic region M62.45-●
    shoulder region M62.41-●
    specified site NEC M62.48
    thigh M62.45-●
    thorax M62.48
    trunk M62.48
    upper arm M62.42-●
  toe —*see* Deformity, toe, specified NEC
  ureterovesical orifice (postinfectional) N13.5
    with infection N13.6
  urethra —*see also* Stricture, urethra
    orifice N32.0
  uterus N85.8
    abnormal NEC O62.9
    clonic (complicating delivery) O62.4
    dyscoordinate (complicating delivery) O62.4

Contraction, contracture, contracted
(Continued)
  uterus *(Continued)*
    hourglass (complicating delivery) O62.4
    hypertonic O62.4
    hypotonic NEC O62.2
    inadequate
      primary O62.0
      secondary O62.1
    incoordinate (complicating delivery) O62.4
    poor O62.2
    tetanic (complicating delivery) O62.4
  vagina (outlet) N89.5
  vesical N32.89
    neck or urethral orifice N32.0
  visual field —*see* Defect, visual field,
    generalized
  Volkmann's (ischemic) T79.6
Contusion (skin surface intact) T14.8
  abdomen, abdominal (muscle) (wall) S30.1
  adnexa, eye NEC S05.8X-●
  adrenal gland S37.812
  alveolar process S00.532
  ankle S90.0-●
  antecubital space —*see* Contusion, forearm
  anus S30.3
  arm (upper) S40.02-●
    lower (with elbow) —*see* Contusion,
      forearm
  auditory canal —*see* Contusion, ear
  auricle —*see* Contusion, ear
  axilla —*see* Contusion, arm, upper
  back —*see also* Contusion, thorax, back
    lower S30.0
  bile duct S36.13
  bladder S37.22
  bone NEC T14.8
  brain (diffuse) —*see* Injury, intracranial, diffuse
    focal —*see* Injury, intracranial, focal
  brainstem S06.38-●
  breast S20.0-●
  broad ligament S37.892
  brow S00.83
  buttock S30.0
  canthus, eye S00.1-●
  cauda equina S34.3
  cerebellar, traumatic S06.37-●
  cerebral S06.33-●
    left side S06.32-●
    right side S06.31-●
  cheek S00.83
    internal S00.532
  chest (wall) —*see* Contusion, thorax
  chin S00.83
  clitoris S30.23
  colon —*see* Injury, intestine, large, contusion
  common bile duct S36.13
  conjunctiva S05.1-●
    with foreign body (in conjunctival sac) —
      see Foreign body, conjunctival sac
  conus medullaris (spine) S34.139
  cornea —*see* Contusion, eyeball
    with foreign body —*see* Foreign body,
      cornea
  corpus cavernosum S30.21
  cortex (brain) (cerebral) —*see* Injury,
    intracranial, diffuse
    focal —*see* Injury, intracranial, focal
  costal region —*see* Contusion, thorax
  cystic duct S36.13
  diaphragm S27.802
  duodenum S36.420
  ear S00.43-●
  elbow S50.0-●
    with forearm —*see* Contusion, forearm
  epididymis S30.22
  epigastric region S30.1
  epiglottis S10.0
  esophagus (thoracic) S27.812
    cervical S10.0
  eyeball S05.1-●

Contusion *(Continued)*
  eyebrow S00.1-●
  eyelid (and periocular area) S00.1-●
  face NEC S00.83
  fallopian tube S37.529
    bilateral S37.522
    unilateral S37.521
  femoral triangle S30.1
  finger(s) S60.00
    with damage to nail (matrix) S60.10
    index S60.02-●
      with damage to nail S60.12-●
    little S60.05-●
      with damage to nail S60.15-●
    middle S60.03-●
      with damage to nail S60.13-●
    ring S60.04-●
      with damage to nail S60.14-●
    thumb —*see* Contusion, thumb
  flank S30.1
  foot (except toe(s) alone) S90.3-●
    toe —*see* Contusion, toe
  forearm S50.1-●
    elbow only —*see* Contusion, elbow
  forehead S00.83
  gallbladder S36.122
  genital organs, external
    female S30.202
    male S30.201
  globe (eye) —*see* Contusion, eyeball
  groin S30.1
  gum S00.532
  hand S60.22-●
    finger(s) —*see* Contusion, finger
    wrist —*see* Contusion, wrist
  head S00.93
    ear —*see* Contusion, ear
    eyelid —*see* Contusion, eyelid
    lip S00.531
    nose S00.33
    oral cavity S00.532
    scalp S00.03
    specified part NEC S00.83
  heart —*see also* Injury, heart S26.91
  heel —*see* Contusion, foot
  hepatic duct S36.13
  hip S70.0-●
  ileum S36.428
  iliac region S30.1
  inguinal region S30.1
  interscapular region S20.229
  intra-abdominal organ S36.92
    colon —*see* Injury, intestine, large, contusion
    liver S36.112
    pancreas —*see* Contusion, pancreas
    rectum S36.62
    small intestine —*see* Injury, intestine, small,
      contusion
    specified organ NEC S36.892
    spleen —*see* Contusion, spleen
    stomach S36.32
  iris (eye) —*see* Contusion, eyeball
  jaw S00.83
  jejunum S36.428
  kidney S37.01-●
    major (greater than 2 cm) S37.02-●
    minor (less than 2 cm) S37.01-●
  knee S80.0-●
  labium (majus) (minus) S30.23
  lacrimal apparatus, gland or sac S05.8X-●
  larynx S10.0
  leg (lower) S80.1-●
    knee —*see* Contusion, knee
  lens —*see* Contusion, eyeball
  lip S00.531
  liver S36.112
  lower back S30.0
  lumbar region S30.0
  lung S27.329
    bilateral S27.322
    unilateral S27.321

Contusion *(Continued)*
  malar region S00.83
  mastoid region S00.83
  membrane, brain —*see* Injury, intracranial,
    diffuse
    focal —*see* Injury, intracranial, focal
  mesentery S36.892
  mesosalpinx S37.892
  mouth S00.532
  muscle —*see* Contusion, by site
  nail
    finger —*see* Contusion, finger, with
      damage to nail
    toe —*see* Contusion, toe, with damage to
      nail
  nasal S00.33
  neck S10.93
    specified site NEC S10.83
    throat S10.0
  nerve —*see* Injury, nerve
  newborn P54.5
  nose S00.33
  occipital
    lobe (brain) —*see* Injury, intracranial,
      diffuse
      focal —*see* Injury, intracranial,
        focal
    region (scalp) S00.03
  orbit (region) (tissues) S05.1-●
  ovary S37.429
    bilateral S37.422
    unilateral S37.421
  palate S00.532
  pancreas S36.229
    body S36.221
    head S36.220
    tail S36.222
  parietal
    lobe (brain) —*see* Injury, intracranial,
      diffuse
      focal —*see* Injury, intracranial, focal
    region (scalp) S00.03
  pelvic organ S37.92
    adrenal gland S37.812
    bladder S37.22
    fallopian tube —*see* Contusion, fallopian
      tube
    kidney —*see* Contusion, kidney
    ovary —*see* Contusion, ovary
    prostate S37.822
    specified organ NEC S37.892
    ureter S37.12
    urethra S37.32
    uterus S37.62
  pelvis S30.0
  penis S30.21
  perineum
    female S30.23
    male S30.0
  periocular area S00.1-●
  peritoneum S36.81
  periurethral tissue —*see* Contusion,
    urethra
  pharynx S10.0
  pinna —*see* Contusion, ear
  popliteal space —*see* Contusion, knee
  prepuce S30.21
  prostate S37.822
  pubic region S30.1
  pudendum
    female S30.202
    male S30.201
  quadriceps femoris —*see* Contusion, thigh
  rectum S36.62
  retroperitoneum S36.892
  round ligament S37.892
  sacral region S30.0
  scalp S00.03
    due to birth injury P12.3
  scapular region —*see* Contusion, shoulder
  sclera —*see* Contusion, eyeball

▶ New   ⇨ Revised   ~~deleted~~ Deleted   ● Use Additional Character(s)

Contusion *(Continued)*
scrotum S30.22
seminal vesicle S37.892
shoulder S40.01-•
skin NEC T14.8
small intestine —*see* Injury, intestine, small, contusion
spermatic cord S30.22
spinal cord —*see* Injury, spinal cord, by region
cauda equina S34.3
conus medullaris S34.139
spleen S36.029
major S36.021
minor S36.020
sternal region S20.219
stomach S36.32
subconjunctival S05.1-•
subcutaneous NEC T14.8
submaxillary region S00.83
submental region S00.83
subperiosteal NEC T14.8
subungual
finger —*see* Contusion, finger, with damage to nail
toe —*see* Contusion, toe, with damage to nail
supraclavicular fossa S10.83
supraorbital S00.83
suprarenal gland S37.812
temple (region) S00.83
temporal
lobe (brain) —*see* Injury, intracranial, diffuse
focal —*see* Injury, intracranial, focal
region S00.83
testis S30.22
thigh S70.1-•
thorax (wall) S20.20
back S20.22-•
front S20.21-•
throat S10.0
thumb S60.01-•
with damage to nail S60.11-•
toe(s) (lesser) S90.12-•
with damage to nail S90.22-•
great S90.11-•
with damage to nail S90.21-•
specified type NEC S90.221
tongue S00.532
trachea (cervical) S10.0
thoracic S27.52
tunica vaginalis S30.22
tympanum, tympanic membrane —*see* Contusion, ear
ureter S37.12
urethra S37.32
urinary organ NEC S37.892
uterus S37.62
uvula S00.532
vagina S30.23
vas deferens S37.892
vesical S37.22
vocal cord(s) S10.0
vulva S30.23
wrist S60.21-•
Conus (congenital) (any type) Q14.8
cornea —*see* Keratoconus
medullaris syndrome G95.81
Conversion hysteria, neurosis or reaction F44.9
Converter, tuberculosis (test reaction) R76.11
Conviction (legal), anxiety concerning Z65.0
with imprisonment Z65.1
Convulsions (idiopathic) —*see also* Seizure(s) R56.9
apoplectiform (cerebral ischemia) I67.82
dissociative F44.5
epileptic —*see* Epilepsy
epileptiform, epileptoid —*see* Seizure, epileptiform

Convulsions *(Continued)*
ether (anesthetic) —*see* Table of Drugs and Chemicals, by drug
febrile R56.00
with status epilepticus G40.901
complex R56.01
with status epilepticus G40.901
simple R56.00
hysterical F44.5
infantile P90
epilepsy —*see* Epilepsy
jacksonian —*see* Epilepsy, localization-related, symptomatic, with simple partial seizures
myoclonic G25.3
newborn P90
obstetrical (nephritic) (uremic) —*see* Eclampsia
paretic A52.17
post traumatic R56.1
psychomotor —*see* Epilepsy, localization-related, symptomatic, with complex partial seizures
recurrent R56.9
reflex R25.8
scarlatinal A38.8
tetanus, tetanic —*see* Tetanus
thymic E32.8
Convulsive —*see also* Convulsions
Cooley's anemia D56.1
Coolie itch B76.9
Cooper's
disease —*see* Mastopathy, cystic
hernia —*see* Hernia, abdomen, specified site NEC
Copra itch B88.0
Coprophagy F50.89
Coprophobia F40.298
Coproporphyria, hereditary E80.29
Cor
biloculare Q20.8
bovis, bovinum —*see* Hypertrophy, cardiac
pulmonale (chronic) I27.81
acute I26.09
triatriatum, triatrium Q24.2
triloculare Q20.8
biatrium Q20.4
biventriculare Q21.1
Corbus' disease (gangrenous balanitis) N48.1
Cord —*see also* condition
around neck
complicating delivery O69.81
with compression O69.1
bladder G95.89
tabetic A52.19
Cordis ectopia Q24.8
Corditis (spermatic) N49.1
Corectopia Q13.2
Cori's disease (glycogen storage) E74.03
Corkhandler's disease or lung J67.3
Corkscrew esophagus K22.4
Corkworker's disease or lung J67.3
Corn (infected) L84
Cornea —*see also* condition
donor Z52.5
plana Q13.4
Cornelia de Lange syndrome Q87.1
Cornu cutaneum L85.8
Cornual gestation or pregnancy O00.80
with intrauterine pregnancy O00.81
Coronary (artery) —*see* condition
Coronavirus, as cause of disease classified elsewhere B97.29
SARS-associated B97.21
Corpora —*see also* condition
amylacea, prostate N42.89
cavernosa —*see* condition
Corpulence —*see* Obesity
Corpus —*see* condition
Corrected transposition Q20.5

Corrosion (injury) (acid) (caustic) (chemical) (lime) (external) (internal) T30.4
abdomen, abdominal (muscle) (wall) T21.42
first degree T21.52
second degree T21.62
third degree T21.72
above elbow T22.439
first degree T22.539
left T22.432
first degree T22.532
second degree T22.632
third degree T22.732
right T22.431
first degree T22.531
second degree T22.631
third degree T22.731
second degree T22.639
third degree T22.739
alimentary tract NEC T28.7
ankle T25.419
first degree T25.519
left T25.412
first degree T25.512
second degree T25.612
third degree T25.712
multiple with foot —*see* Corrosion, lower, limb, multiple, ankle and foot
right T25.411
first degree T25.511
second degree T25.611
third degree T25.711
second degree T25.619
third degree T25.719
anus —*see* Corrosion, buttock
arm(s) (meaning upper limb(s)) —*see* Corrosion, upper limb
axilla T22.449
first degree T22.549
left T22.442
first degree T22.542
second degree T22.642
third degree T22.742
right T22.441
first degree T22.541
second degree T22.641
third degree T22.741
second degree T22.649
third degree T22.749
back (lower) T21.44
first degree T21.54
second degree T21.64
third degree T21.74
upper T21.43
first degree T21.53
second degree T21.63
third degree T21.73
blisters - code as Corrosion, second degree, by site
breast(s) —*see* Corrosion, chest wall
buttock(s) T21.45
first degree T21.55
second degree T21.65
third degree T21.75
calf T24.439
first degree T24.539
left T24.432
first degree T24.532
second degree T24.632
third degree T24.732
right T24.431
first degree T24.531
second degree T24.631
third degree T24.731
second degree T24.639
third degree T24.739
canthus (eye) —*see* Corrosion, eyelid
cervix T28.8
cheek T20.46
first degree T20.56
second degree T20.66
third degree T20.76

Corrosion *(Continued)*
  chest wall T21.41
    first degree T21.51
    second degree T21.61
    third degree T21.71
  chin T20.43
    first degree T20.53
    second degree T20.63
    third degree T20.73
  colon T28.7
  conjunctiva (and cornea) —*see* Corrosion,
    cornea
  cornea (and conjunctiva) T26.6-●
  deep necrosis of underlying tissue - code as
    Corrosion, third degree, by site
  dorsum of hand T23.469
    first degree T23.569
    left T23.462
      first degree T23.562
      second degree T23.662
      third degree T23.762
    right T23.461
      first degree T23.561
      second degree T23.661
      third degree T23.761
    second degree T23.669
    third degree T23.769
  ear (auricle) (external) (canal) T20.41
    drum T28.91
    first degree T20.51
    second degree T20.61
    third degree T20.71
  elbow T22.429
    first degree T22.529
    left T22.422
      first degree T22.522
      second degree T22.622
      third degree T22.722
    right T22.421
      first degree T22.521
      second degree T22.621
      third degree T22.721
    second degree T22.629
    third degree T22.729
  entire body —*see* Corrosion, multiple body
    regions
  epidermal loss - code as Corrosion, second
    degree, by site
  epiglottis T27.4
  erythema, erythematous - code as Corrosion,
    first degree, by site
  esophagus T28.6
  extent (percentage of body surface)
  ➡ less than 10 percent T32.0
  ➡ 10-19 percent (0-9 percent third degree)
      T32.10
    with 10-19 percent third degree
        T32.11
  ➡ 20-29 percent (0-9 percent third degree)
      T32.20
    with
      10-19 percent third degree T32.21
      20-29 percent third degree T32.22
  ➡ 30-39 percent (0-9 percent third degree)
      T32.30
    with
      10-19 percent third degree T32.31
      20-29 percent third degree T32.32
      30-39 percent third degree T32.33
  ➡ 40-49 percent (0-9 percent third degree)
      T32.40
    with
      10-19 percent third degree T32.41
      20-29 percent third degree T32.42
      30-39 percent third degree T32.43
      40-49 percent third degree T32.44
  ➡ 50-59 percent (0-9 percent third degree)
      T32.50
    with
      10-19 percent third degree T32.51
      20-29 percent third degree T32.52

Corrosion *(Continued)*
  extent *(Continued)*
    50-59 percent *(Continued)*
      with *(Continued)*
        30-39 percent third degree T32.53
        40-49 percent third degree T32.54
        50-59 percent third degree T32.55
  ➡ 60-69 percent (0-9 percent third degree)
      T32.60
    with
      10-19 percent third degree T32.61
      20-29 percent third degree T32.62
      30-39 percent third degree T32.63
      40-49 percent third degree T32.64
      50-59 percent third degree T32.65
      60-69 percent third degree T32.66
  ➡ 70-79 percent (0-9 percent third degree)
      T32.70
    with
      10-19 percent third degree T32.71
      20-29 percent third degree T32.72
      30-39 percent third degree T32.73
      40-49 percent third degree T32.74
      50-59 percent third degree T32.75
      60-69 percent third degree T32.76
      70-79 percent third degree T32.77
  ➡ 80-89 percent (0-9 percent third degree)
      T32.80
    with
      10-19 percent third degree T32.81
      20-29 percent third degree T32.82
      30-39 percent third degree T32.83
      40-49 percent third degree T32.84
      50-59 percent third degree T32.85
      60-69 percent third degree T32.86
      70-79 percent third degree T32.87
      80-89 percent third degree T32.88
  ➡ 90 percent or more (0-9 percent third
      degree) T32.90
    with
      10-19 percent third degree T32.91
      20-29 percent third degree T32.92
      30-39 percent third degree T32.93
      40-49 percent third degree T32.94
      50-59 percent third degree T32.95
      60-69 percent third degree T32.96
      70-79 percent third degree T32.97
      80-89 percent third degree T32.98
      90-99 percent third degree T32.99
  extremity —*see* Corrosion, limb
  eye(s) and adnexa T26.9-●
    with resulting rupture and destruction of
      eyeball T26.7-●
    conjunctival sac —*see* Corrosion, cornea
    cornea —*see* Corrosion, cornea
    lid —*see* Corrosion, eyelid
    periocular area —*see* Corrosion eyelid
    specified site NEC T26.8-●
  eyeball —*see* Corrosion, eye
  eyelid(s) T26.5-●
  face —*see* Corrosion, head
  finger T23.429
    first degree T23.529
    left T23.422
      first degree T23.522
      second degree T23.622
      third degree T23.722
    multiple sites (without thumb)
      T23.439
      with thumb T23.449
        first degree T23.549
        left T23.442
          first degree T23.542
          second degree T23.642
          third degree T23.742
        right T23.441
          first degree T23.541
          second degree T23.641
          third degree T23.741
      second degree T23.649
      third degree T23.749

Corrosion *(Continued)*
  finger *(Continued)*
    multiple sites *(Continued)*
      first degree T23.539
      left T23.432
        first degree T23.532
        second degree T23.632
        third degree T23.732
      right T23.431
        first degree T23.531
        second degree T23.631
        third degree T23.731
      second degree T23.639
      third degree T23.739
    right T23.421
      first degree T23.521
      second degree T23.621
      third degree T23.721
    second degree T23.629
    third degree T23.729
  flank —*see* Corrosion, abdomen
  foot T25.429
    first degree T25.529
    left T25.422
      first degree T25.522
      second degree T25.622
      third degree T25.722
    multiple with ankle —*see* Corrosion, lower,
      limb, multiple, ankle and foot
    right T25.421
      first degree T25.521
      second degree T25.621
      third degree T25.721
    second degree T25.629
    third degree T25.729
  forearm T22.419
    first degree T22.519
    left T22.412
      first degree T22.512
      second degree T22.612
      third degree T22.712
    right T22.411
      first degree T22.511
      second degree T22.611
      third degree T22.711
    second degree T22.619
    third degree T22.719
  forehead T20.46
    first degree T20.56
    second degree T20.66
    third degree T20.76
  fourth degree - code as Corrosion, third
    degree, by site
  full thickness skin loss - code as Corrosion,
    third degree, by site
  gastrointestinal tract NEC T28.7
  genital organs
    external
      female T21.47
        first degree T21.57
        second degree T21.67
        third degree T21.77
      male T21.46
        first degree T21.56
        second degree T21.66
        third degree T21.76
    internal T28.8
  groin —*see* Corrosion, abdominal wall
  hand(s) T23.409
    back —*see* Corrosion, dorsum of hand
    finger —*see* Corrosion, finger
    first degree T23.509
    left T23.402
      first degree T23.502
      second degree T23.602
      third degree T23.702
    multiple sites with wrist T23.499
      first degree T23.599
      left T23.492
        first degree T23.592
        second degree T23.692
        third degree T23.792

▶ New   ➡ Revised   ~~deleted~~ Deleted   ● Use Additional Character(s)

Corrosion *(Continued)*
  hand(s) *(Continued)*
    multiple sites *(Continued)*
      right T23.491
        first degree T23.591
        second degree T23.691
        third degree T23.791
      second degree T23.699
      third degree T23.799
    palm —*see* Corrosion, palm
    right T23.401
      first degree T23.501
      second degree T23.601
      third degree T23.701
    second degree T23.609
    third degree T23.709
    thumb —*see* Corrosion, thumb
  head (and face) (and neck) T20.40
    cheek —*see* Corrosion, cheek
    chin —*see* Corrosion, chin
    ear —*see* Corrosion, ear
    eye(s) only —*see* Corrosion, eye
    first degree T20.50
    forehead —*see* Corrosion, forehead
    lip —*see* Corrosion, lip
    multiple sites T20.49
      first degree T20.59
      second degree T20.69
      third degree T20.79
    neck —*see* Corrosion, neck
    nose —*see* Corrosion, nose
    scalp —*see* Corrosion, scalp
    second degree T20.60
    third degree T20.70
  hip(s) —*see* Corrosion, lower, limb
  inhalation —*see* Corrosion, respiratory
    tract
  internal organ(s) (*see also* Corrosion, by site)
    T28.90
    alimentary tract T28.7
      esophagus T28.6
    esophagus T28.6
    genitourinary T28.8
    mouth T28.5
    pharynx T28.5
    specified organ NEC T28.99
  interscapular region —*see* Corrosion, back,
    upper
  intestine (large) (small) T28.7
  knee T24.429
    first degree T24.529
    left T24.422
      first degree T24.522
      second degree T24.622
      third degree T24.722
    right T24.421
      first degree T24.521
      second degree T24.621
      third degree T24.721
    second degree T24.629
    third degree T24.729
  labium (majus) (minus) —*see* Corrosion,
    genital organs, external, female
  lacrimal apparatus, duct, gland or sac —*see*
    Corrosion, eye, specified site NEC
  larynx T27.4
    with lung T27.5
  leg(s) (meaning lower limb(s)) —*see*
    Corrosion, lower limb
  limb(s)
    lower —*see* Corrosion, lower, limb
    upper —*see* Corrosion, upper limb
  lip(s) T20.42
    first degree T20.52
    second degree T20.62
    third degree T20.72
  lower
    back —*see* Corrosion, back
    limb T24.409
      ankle —*see* Corrosion, ankle
      calf —*see* Corrosion, calf

Corrosion *(Continued)*
  lower *(Continued)*
    limb *(Continued)*
      first degree T24.509
      foot —*see* Corrosion, foot
      hip —*see* Corrosion, thigh
      knee —*see* Corrosion, knee
      left T24.402
        first degree T24.502
        second degree T24.602
        third degree T24.702
      multiple sites, except ankle and foot
        T24.499
        ankle and foot T25.499
          first degree T25.599
          left T25.492
            first degree T25.592
            second degree T25.692
            third degree T25.792
          right T25.491
            first degree T25.591
            second degree T25.691
            third degree T25.791
          second degree T25.699
          third degree T25.799
        first degree T24.599
        left T24.492
          first degree T24.592
          second degree T24.692
          third degree T24.792
        right T24.491
          first degree T24.591
          second degree T24.691
          third degree T24.791
        second degree T24.699
        third degree T24.799
      right T24.401
        first degree T24.501
        second degree T24.601
        third degree T24.701
      second degree T24.609
      thigh —*see* Corrosion, thigh
      third degree T24.709
  lung (with larynx and trachea)
    T27.5
  mouth T28.5
  neck T20.47
    first degree T20.57
    second degree T20.67
    third degree T20.77
  nose (septum) T20.44
    first degree T20.54
    second degree T20.64
    third degree T20.74
  ocular adnexa —*see* Corrosion, eye
  orbit region —*see* Corrosion, eyelid
  palm T23.459
    first degree T23.559
    left T23.452
      first degree T23.552
      second degree T23.652
      third degree T23.752
    right T23.451
      first degree T23.551
      second degree T23.651
      third degree T23.751
    second degree T23.659
    third degree T23.759
  partial thickness - code as Corrosion,
    unspecified degree, by site
  pelvis —*see* Corrosion, trunk
  penis —*see* Corrosion, genital organs,
    external, male
  perineum
    female —*see* Corrosion, genital organs,
      external, female
    male —*see* Corrosion, genital organs,
      external, male
  periocular area —*see* Corrosion, eyelid
  pharynx T28.5
  rectum T28.7

Corrosion *(Continued)*
  respiratory tract T27.7
    larynx —*see* Corrosion, larynx
    specified part NEC T27.6
    trachea —*see* Corrosion, larynx
  sac, lacrimal —*see* Corrosion, eye,
    specified site NEC
  scalp T20.45
    first degree T20.55
    second degree T20.65
    third degree T20.75
  scapular region T22.469
    first degree T22.569
    left T22.462
      first degree T22.562
      second degree T22.662
      third degree T22.762
    right T22.461
      first degree T22.561
      second degree T22.661
      third degree T22.761
    second degree T22.669
    third degree T22.769
  sclera —*see* Corrosion, eye, specified site
    NEC
  scrotum —*see* Corrosion, genital organs,
    external, male
  shoulder T22.459
    first degree T22.559
    left T22.452
      first degree T22.552
      second degree T22.652
      third degree T22.752
    right T22.451
      first degree T22.551
      second degree T22.651
      third degree T22.751
    second degree T22.659
    third degree T22.759
  stomach T28.7
  temple —*see* Corrosion, head
  testis —*see* Corrosion, genital organs,
    external, male
  thigh T24.419
    first degree T24.519
    left T24.412
      first degree T24.512
      second degree T24.612
      third degree T24.712
    right T24.411
      first degree T24.511
      second degree T24.611
      third degree T24.711
    second degree T24.619
    third degree T24.719
  thorax (external) —*see* Corrosion, trunk
  throat (meaning pharynx) T28.5
  thumb(s) T23.419
    first degree T23.519
    left T23.412
      first degree T23.512
      second degree T23.612
      third degree T23.712
    multiple sites with fingers T23.449
      first degree T23.549
      left T23.442
        first degree T23.542
        second degree T23.642
        third degree T23.742
      right T23.441
        first degree T23.541
        second degree T23.641
        third degree T23.741
      second degree T23.649
      third degree T23.749
    right T23.411
      first degree T23.511
      second degree T23.611
      third degree T23.711
    second degree T23.619
    third degree T23.719

Corrosion *(Continued)*
 toe T25.439
  first degree T25.539
  left T25.432
   first degree T25.532
   second degree T25.632
   third degree T25.732
  right T25.431
   first degree T25.531
   second degree T25.631
   third degree T25.731
  second degree T25.639
  third degree T25.739
 tongue T28.5
 tonsil(s) T28.5
 total body —*see* Corrosion, multiple body
   regions
 trachea T27.4
  with lung T27.5
 trunk T21.40
  abdominal wall —*see* Corrosion,
    abdominal wall
  anus —*see* Corrosion, buttock
  axilla —*see* Corrosion, upper limb
  back —*see* Corrosion, back
  breast —*see* Corrosion, chest wall
  buttock —*see* Corrosion, buttock
  chest wall —*see* Corrosion, chest wall
  first degree T21.50
  flank —*see* Corrosion, abdominal wall
  genital
   female —*see* Corrosion, genital organs,
     external, female
   male —*see* Corrosion, genital organs,
     external, male
  groin —*see* Corrosion, abdominal wall
  interscapular region —*see* Corrosion, back,
    upper
  labia —*see* Corrosion, genital organs,
    external, female
  lower back —*see* Corrosion, back
  penis —*see* Corrosion, genital organs,
    external, male
  perineum
   female —*see* Corrosion, genital organs,
     external, female
   male —*see* Corrosion, genital organs,
     external, male
  scapular region —*see* Corrosion, upper
    limb
  scrotum —*see* Corrosion, genital organs,
    external, male
  second degree T21.60
  shoulder —*see* Corrosion, upper limb
  specified site NEC T21.49
   first degree T21.59
   second degree T21.69
   third degree T21.79
  testes —*see* Corrosion, genital organs,
    external, male
  third degree T21.70
  upper back —*see* Corrosion, back, upper
  vagina T28.8
  vulva —*see* Corrosion, genital organs,
    external, female
 unspecified site with extent of body surface
   involved specified
  ➠less than 10 percent T32.0
  ➠10-19 percent (0-9 percent third degree)
    T32.10
   with 10-19 percent third degree T32.11
  ➠20-29 percent (0-9 percent third degree)
    T32.20
   with
    10-19 percent third degree T32.21
    20-29 percent third degree T32.22
  ➠30-39 percent (0-9 percent third degree)
    T32.30
   with
    10-19 percent third degree T32.31
    20-29 percent third degree T32.32
    30-39 percent third degree T32.33

Corrosion *(Continued)*
 unspecified site with extent of body surface
   involved specified *(Continued)*
  ➠40-49 percent (0-9 percent third degree)
    T32.40
   with
    10-19 percent third degree T32.41
    20-29 percent third degree T32.42
    30-39 percent third degree T32.43
    40-49 percent third degree T32.44
  ➠50-59 percent (0-9 percent third degree)
    T32.50
   with
    10-19 percent third degree T32.51
    20-29 percent third degree T32.52
    30-39 percent third degree T32.53
    40-49 percent third degree T32.54
    50-59 percent third degree T32.55
  ➠60-69 percent (0-9 percent third degree)
    T32.60
   with
    10-19 percent third degree T32.61
    20-29 percent third degree T32.62
    30-39 percent third degree T32.63
    40-49 percent third degree T32.64
    50-59 percent third degree T32.65
    60-69 percent third degree T32.66
  ➠70-79 percent (0-9 percent third degree)
    T32.70
   with
    10-19 percent third degree T32.71
    20-29 percent third degree T32.72
    30-39 percent third degree T32.73
    40-49 percent third degree T32.74
    50-59 percent third degree T32.75
    60-69 percent third degree T32.76
    70-79 percent third degree T32.77
  ➠80-89 percent (0-9 percent third degree)
    T32.80
   with
    10-19 percent third degree T32.81
    20-29 percent third degree T32.82
    30-39 percent third degree T32.83
    40-49 percent third degree T32.84
    50-59 percent third degree T32.85
    60-69 percent third degree T32.86
    70-79 percent third degree T32.87
    80-89 percent third degree T32.88
  ➠90 percent or more (0-9 percent third
    degree) T32.90
   with
    10-19 percent third degree T32.91
    20-29 percent third degree T32.92
    30-39 percent third degree T32.93
    40-49 percent third degree T32.94
    50-59 percent third degree T32.95
    60-69 percent third degree T32.96
    70-79 percent third degree T32.97
    80-89 percent third degree T32.98
    90-99 percent third degree T32.99
 upper limb (axilla) (scapular region) T22.40
  above elbow —*see* Corrosion, above elbow
  axilla —*see* Corrosion, axilla
  elbow —*see* Corrosion, elbow
  first degree T22.50
  forearm —*see* Corrosion, forearm
  hand —*see* Corrosion, hand
  interscapular region —*see* Corrosion, back,
    upper
  multiple sites T22.499
   first degree T22.599
   left T22.492
    first degree T22.592
    second degree T22.692
    third degree T22.792
   right T22.491
    first degree T22.591
    second degree T22.691
    third degree T22.791
   second degree T22.699
   third degree T22.799

Corrosion *(Continued)*
 upper limb (axilla) (scapular region)
   (Continued)
  scapular region —*see* Corrosion, scapular
    region
  second degree T22.60
  shoulder —*see* Corrosion, shoulder
  third degree T22.70
  wrist —*see* Corrosion, hand
 uterus T28.8
 vagina T28.8
 vulva —*see* Corrosion, genital organs,
   external, female
 wrist T23.479
  first degree T23.579
  left T23.472
   first degree T23.572
   second degree T23.672
   third degree T23.772
  multiple sites with hand T23.499
   first degree T23.599
   left T23.492
    first degree T23.592
    second degree T23.692
    third degree T23.792
   right T23.491
    first degree T23.591
    second degree T23.691
    third degree T23.791
   second degree T23.699
   third degree T23.799
  right T23.471
   first degree T23.571
   second degree T23.671
   third degree T23.771
  second degree T23.679
  third degree T23.779
Corrosive burn —*see* Corrosion
Corsican fever —*see* Malaria
Cortical —*see* condition
Cortico-adrenal —*see* condition
Coryza (acute) J00
 with grippe or influenza —*see* Influenza,
   with, respiratory manifestations
   NEC
 syphilitic
  congenital (chronic) A50.05
Costen's syndrome or complex M26.69
Costiveness —*see* Constipation
Costochondritis M94.0
Cot death R99
Cotard's syndrome F22
Cotia virus B08.8
Cotton wool spots (retinal) H35.81
Cotungo's disease —*see* Sciatica
Cough (affected) (chronic) (epidemic) (nervous)
  R05
 with hemorrhage —*see* Hemoptysis
 bronchial R05
  with grippe or influenza —*see* Influenza,
    with, respiratory manifestations
    NEC
 functional F45.8
 hysterical F45.8
 laryngeal, spasmodic R05
 psychogenic F45.8
 smokers' J41.0
 tea taster's B49
Counseling (for) Z71.9
 abuse NEC
  perpetrator Z69.82
  victim Z69.81
 alcohol abuser Z71.41
  family Z71.42
 child abuse
  nonparental
   perpetrator Z69.021
   victim Z69.020
  parental
   perpetrator Z69.011
   victim Z69.010

Counseling *(Continued)*
  consanguinity Z71.89
  contraceptive Z30.09
  dietary Z71.3
  drug abuser Z71.51
    family member Z71.52
▶exercise Z71.82
  family Z71.89
  fertility preservation (prior to cancer therapy)
    (prior to removal of gonads) Z31.62
  for non-attending third party Z71.0
    related to sexual behavior or orientation
      Z70.2
  genetic NEC Z31.5
▶genetic
  ▶nonprocreative Z71.83
  ▶procreative NEC Z31.5
  gestational carrier Z31.7
  health (advice) (education) (instruction) —*see*
    Counseling, medical
  human immunodeficiency virus (HIV) Z71.7
  impotence Z70.1
  insulin pump use Z46.81
  medical (for) Z71.9
    boarding school resident Z59.3
    consanguinity Z71.89
    feared complaint and no disease found Z71.1
    human immunodeficiency virus (HIV) Z71.7
    institutional resident Z59.3
    on behalf of another Z71.0
      related to sexual behavior or orientation
        Z70.2
    person living alone Z60.2
    specified reason NEC Z71.89
  natural family planning
    procreative Z31.61
    to avoid pregnancy Z30.02
  perpetrator (of)
    abuse NEC Z69.82
    child abuse
      non-parental Z69.021
      parental Z69.011
    rape NEC Z69.82
    spousal abuse Z69.12
  procreative NEC Z31.69
    fertility preservation (prior to cancer
      therapy) (prior to removal of
      gonads) Z31.62
    using natural family planning Z31.61
  promiscuity Z70.1
  rape victim Z69.81
  religious Z71.81
  sex, sexual (related to) Z70.9
    attitude(s) Z70.0
    behavior or orientation Z70.1
    combined concerns Z70.3
    non-responsiveness Z70.1
    on behalf of third party Z70.2
    specified reason NEC Z70.8
  specified reason NEC Z71.89
  spiritual Z71.81
  spousal abuse (perpetrator) Z69.12
    victim Z69.11
  substance abuse Z71.89
    alcohol Z71.41
    drug Z71.51
    tobacco Z71.6
  tobacco use Z71.6
  use (of)
    insulin pump Z46.81
  victim (of)
    abuse Z69.81
    child abuse
      by parent Z69.010
      non-parental Z69.020
    rape NEC Z69.81
Coupled rhythm R00.8
Couvelaire syndrome or uterus (complicating
  delivery) O45.8X-●
Cowperitis —*see* Urethritis
Cowper's gland —*see* condition

Cowpox B08.010
  due to vaccination T88.1
Coxa
  magna M91.4-●
  plana M91.2-●
  valga (acquired) —*see also* Deformity, limb,
    specified type NEC, thigh
    congenital Q65.81
    sequelae (late effect) of rickets E64.3
  vara (acquired) —*see also* Deformity, limb,
    specified type NEC, thigh
    congenital Q65.82
    sequelae (late effect) of rickets E64.3
Coxalgia, coxalgic (nontuberculous) —*see also*
  Pain, joint, hip
  tuberculous A18.02
Coxitis —*see* Monoarthritis, hip
Coxsackie (virus) (infection) B34.1
  as cause of disease classified elsewhere B97.11
  carditis B33.20
  central nervous system NEC A88.8
  endocarditis B33.21
  enteritis A08.39
  meningitis (aseptic) A87.0
  myocarditis B33.22
  pericarditis B33.23
  pharyngitis B08.5
  pleurodynia B33.0
  specific disease NEC B33.8
Crabs, meaning pubic lice B85.3
Crack baby P04.41
Cracked nipple N64.0
  associated with
    lactation O92.13
      pregnancy O92.11-●
    puerperium O92.12
Cracked tooth K03.81
Cradle cap L21.0
Craft neurosis F48.8
Cramp(s) R25.2
  abdominal —*see* Pain, abdominal
  bathing T75.1
  colic R10.83
    psychogenic F45.8
  due to immersion T75.1
  fireman T67.2
  heat T67.2
  immersion T75.1
  intestinal —*see* Pain, abdominal
    psychogenic F45.8
  leg, sleep related G47.62
  limb (lower) (upper) NEC R25.2
    sleep related G47.62
  linotypist's F48.8
    organic G25.89
  muscle (limb) (general) R25.2
    due to immersion T75.1
    psychogenic F45.8
  occupational (hand) F48.8
    organic G25.89
  salt-depletion E87.1
  sleep related, leg G47.62
  stoker's T67.2
  swimmer's T75.1
  telegrapher's F48.8
    organic G25.89
  typist's F48.8
    organic G25.89
  uterus N94.89
    menstrual —*see* Dysmenorrhea
  writer's F48.8
    organic G25.89
Cranial —*see* condition
Craniocleidodysostosis Q74.0
Craniofenestria (skull) Q75.8
Craniolacunia (skull) Q75.8
Craniopagus Q89.4
Craniopathy, metabolic M85.2
Craniopharyngeal —*see* condition
Craniopharyngioma D44.4
Craniorachischisis (totalis) Q00.1

Cranioschisis Q75.8
Craniostenosis Q75.0
Craniosynostosis Q75.0
Craniotabes (cause unknown) M83.8
  neonatal P96.3
  rachitic E64.3
  syphilitic A50.56
Cranium —*see* condition
Craw-craw —*see* Onchocerciasis
Creaking joint —*see* Derangement, joint,
  specified type NEC
Creeping
  eruption B76.9
  palsy or paralysis G12.22
Crenated tongue K14.8
Creotoxism A05.9
Crepitus
  caput Q75.8
  joint —*see* Derangement, joint, specified type
    NEC
Crescent or conus choroid, congenital Q14.3
CREST syndrome M34.1
Cretin, cretinism (congenital) (endemic)
  (nongoitrous) (sporadic) E00.9
  pelvis
    with disproportion (fetopelvic) O33.0
      causing obstructed labor O65.0
  type
    hypothyroid E00.1
    mixed E00.2
    myxedematous E00.1
    neurological E00.0
Creutzfeldt-Jakob disease or syndrome (with
  dementia) A81.00
  familial A81.09
  iatrogenic A81.09
  specified NEC A81.09
  sporadic A81.09
  variant (vCJD) A81.01
Crib death R99
Cribriform hymen Q52.3
Cri-du-chat syndrome Q93.4
Crigler-Najjar disease or syndrome E80.5
Crime, victim of Z65.4
Crimean hemorrhagic fever A98.0
Criminalism F60.2
Crisis
  abdomen R10.0
  acute reaction F43.0
  addisonian E27.2
  adrenal (cortical) E27.2
  celiac K90.0
  Dietl's N13.8
  emotional —*see also* Disorder, adjustment
    acute reaction to stress F43.0
    specific to childhood and adolescence F93.8
  glaucomatocyclitic —*see* Glaucoma,
    secondary, inflammation
  heart —*see* Failure, heart
  nitritoid I95.2
    correct substance properly administered —
      see Table of Drugs and Chemicals, by
      drug, adverse effect
    overdose or wrong substance given
      or taken —*see* Table of Drugs and
      Chemicals, by drug, poisoning
  oculogyric H51.8
    psychogenic F45.8
  Pel's (tabetic) A52.11
  psychosexual identity F64.2
  renal N28.0
  sickle-cell D57.00
    with
      acute chest syndrome D57.01
      splenic sequestration D57.02
  state (acute reaction) F43.0
  tabetic A52.11
  thyroid —*see* Thyrotoxicosis with thyroid
    storm
  thyrotoxic —*see* Thyrotoxicosis with thyroid
    storm

Crocq's disease (acrocyanosis) I73.89
Crohn's disease —see Enteritis, regional
Crooked septum, nasal J34.2
Cross syndrome E70.328
Crossbite (anterior) (posterior) M26.24
Cross-eye —see Strabismus, convergent
    concomitant
Croup, croupous (catarrhal) (infectious)
        (inflammatory) (nondiphtheritic) J05.0
    bronchial J20.9
    diphtheritic A36.2
    false J38.5
    spasmodic J38.5
        diphtheritic A36.2
    stridulous J38.5
        diphtheritic A36.2
Crouzon's disease Q75.1
Crowding, tooth, teeth, fully erupted M26.31
CRST syndrome M34.1
Cruchet's disease A85.8
Cruelty in children —see also Disorder, conduct
Crural ulcer —see Ulcer, lower limb
Crush, crushed, crushing T14.8
    abdomen S38.1
    ankle S97.0-•
    arm (upper) (and shoulder) S47.-•
    axilla —see Crush, arm
    back, lower S38.1
    buttock S38.1
    cheek S07.0-•
    chest S28.0
    cranium S07.1
    ear S07.0
    elbow S57.0-•
    extremity
        lower
            ankle —see Crush, ankle
            below knee —see Crush, leg
            foot —see Crush, foot
            hip —see Crush, hip
            knee —see Crush, knee
            thigh —see Crush, thigh
            toe —see Crush, toe
        upper
            below elbow S67.9-•
            elbow —see Crush, elbow
            finger —see Crush, finger
            forearm —see Crush, forearm
            hand —see Crush, hand
            thumb —see Crush, thumb
            upper arm —see Crush, arm
            wrist —see Crush, wrist
    face S07.0
    finger(s) S67.1-•
        with hand (and wrist) —see Crush, hand,
            specified site NEC
        index S67.19-•
        little S67.19-•
        middle S67.19-•
        ring S67.19-•
        thumb —see Crush, thumb
    foot S97.8-•
        toe —see Crush, toe
    forearm S57.8-•
    genitalia, external
        female S38.002
            vagina S38.03
            vulva S38.03
        male S38.001
            penis S38.01
            scrotum S38.02
            testis S38.02
    hand (except fingers alone) S67.2-•
        with wrist S67.4-•
    head S07.9
        specified NEC S07.8
    heel —see Crush, foot
    hip S77.0-•
        with thigh S77.2-•
    internal organ (abdomen, chest, or pelvis)
        NEC T14.8

Crush, crushed, crushing (Continued)
    knee S87.0-•
    labium (majus) (minus) S38.03
    larynx S17.0
    leg (lower) S87.8-•
        knee —see Crush, knee
    lip S07.0
    lower
        back S38.1
        leg —see Crush, leg
    neck S17.9
    nerve —see Injury, nerve
    nose S07.0
    pelvis S38.1
    penis S38.01
    scalp S07.8
    scapular region —see Crush, arm
    scrotum S38.02
    severe, unspecified site T14.8
    shoulder (and upper arm) —see Crush, arm
    skull S07.1
    syndrome (complication of trauma) T79.5
    testis S38.02
    thigh S77.1-•
        with hip S77.2-•
    throat S17.8
    thumb S67.0-•
        with hand (and wrist) —see Crush, hand,
            specified site NEC
    toe(s) S97.10-•
        great S97.11-•
        lesser S97.12-•
    trachea S17.0
    vagina S38.03
    vulva S38.03
    wrist S67.3-•
        with hand S67.4-•
Crusta lactea L21.0
Crusts R23.4
Crutch paralysis —see Injury, brachial plexus
Cruveilhier-Baumgarten cirrhosis, disease or
        syndrome K74.69
Cruveilhier's atrophy or disease G12.8
Crying (constant) (continuous) (excessive)
    child, adolescent, or adult R45.83
    infant (baby) (newborn) R68.11
Cryofibrinogenemia D89.2
Cryoglobulinemia (essential) (idiopathic)
        (mixed) (primary) (purpura) (secondary)
        (vasculitis) D89.1
    with lung involvement D89.1 [J99]
Cryptitis (anal) (rectal) K62.89
Cryptococcosis, cryptococcus (infection)
        (neoformans) B45.9
    bone B45.3
    cerebral B45.1
    cutaneous B45.2
    disseminated B45.7
    generalized B45.7
    meningitis B45.1
    meningocerebralis B45.1
    osseous B45.3
    pulmonary B45.0
    skin B45.2
    specified NEC B45.8
Cryptopapillitis (anus) K62.89
Cryptophthalmos Q11.2
    syndrome Q87.0
Cryptorchid, cryptorchism, cryptorchidism
        Q53.9
    bilateral Q53.20
        ➧abdominal Q53.211
        perineal Q53.22
    unilateral Q53.10
        ➧abdominal Q53.111
        perineal Q53.12
Cryptosporidiosis A07.2
    hepatobiliary B88.8
    respiratory B88.8
Cryptostromosis J67.6
Crystalluria R82.99

Cubitus
    congenital Q68.8
    valgus (acquired) M21.0-•
        congenital Q68.8
        sequelae (late effect) of rickets E64.3
    varus (acquired) M21.1-•
        congenital Q68.8
        sequelae (late effect) of rickets E64.3
Cultural deprivation or shock Z60.3
Curling esophagus K22.4
Curling's ulcer —see Ulcer, peptic, acute
Curschmann (-Batten) (-Steinert) disease or
        syndrome G71.11
Curse, Ondine's —see Apnea, sleep
Curvature
    organ or site, congenital NEC —see Distortion
    penis (lateral) Q55.61
    Pott's (spinal) A18.01
    radius, idiopathic, progressive (congenital)
        Q74.0
    spine (acquired) (angular) (idiopathic)
        (incorrect) (postural) —see Dorsopathy,
        deforming
        congenital Q67.5
        due to or associated with
            Charcot-Marie-Tooth disease —see also
                subcategory M49.8 G60.0
            osteitis
                deformans M88.88
                fibrosa cystica —see also subcategory
                    M49.8 E21.0
            tuberculosis (Pott's curvature) A18.01
        sequelae (late effect) of rickets E64.3
        tuberculous A18.01
Cushingoid due to steroid therapy E24.2
    correct substance properly administered —see
        Table of Drugs and Chemicals, by drug,
        adverse effect
    overdose or wrong substance given
        or taken —see Table of Drugs and
        Chemicals, by drug, poisoning
Cushing's
    syndrome or disease E24.9
        drug-induced E24.2
        iatrogenic E24.2
        pituitary-dependent E24.0
        specified NEC E24.8
    ulcer —see Ulcer, peptic, acute
Cusp, Carabelli - omit code
Cut (external) —see also Laceration
    muscle —see Injury, muscle
Cutaneous —see also condition
    hemorrhage R23.3
    larva migrans B76.9
Cutis —see also condition
    hyperelastica Q82.8
        acquired L57.4
    laxa (hyperelastica) —see Dermatolysis
    marmorata R23.8
    osteosis L94.2
    pendula —see Dermatolysis
    rhomboidalis nuchae L57.2
    verticis gyrata Q82.8
        acquired L91.8
Cyanosis R23.0
    due to
        patent foramen botalli Q21.1
        persistent foramen ovale Q21.1
    enterogenous D74.8
    paroxysmal digital —see Raynaud's disease
        with gangrene I73.01
    retina, retinal H35.89
Cyanotic heart disease I24.9
    congenital Q24.9
Cycle
    anovulatory N97.0
    menstrual, irregular N92.6
Cyclencephaly Q04.9
Cyclical vomiting (see also Vomiting, cyclical)
        G43.A0
    psychogenic F50.89

Cyclitis —see also Iridocyclitis H20.9
  chronic —see Iridocyclitis, chronic
  Fuchs' heterochromic H20.81-●
  granulomatous —see Iridocyclitis, chronic
  lens-induced —see Iridocyclitis,
    lens-induced
  posterior H30.2-●
Cycloid personality F34.0
Cyclophoria H50.54
Cyclopia, cyclops Q87.0
Cyclopism Q87.0
Cyclosporiasis A07.4
Cyclothymia F34.0
Cyclothymic personality F34.0
Cyclotropia H50.41-●
Cylindroma —see also Neoplasm, malignant,
  by site
  eccrine dermal —see Neoplasm, skin,
    benign
  skin —see Neoplasm, skin, benign
Cylindruria R82.99
Cynanche
  diphtheritic A36.2
  tonsillaris J36
Cynophobia F40.218
Cynorexia R63.2
Cyphosis —see Kyphosis
Cyprus fever —see Brucellosis
Cyst (colloid) (mucous) (simple) (retention)
  adenoid (infected) J35.8
  adrenal gland E27.8
    congenital Q89.1
  air, lung J98.4
  allantoic Q64.4
  alveolar process (jaw bone) M27.40
  amnion, amniotic O41.8X-●
  aneurysmal M27.49
  anterior
    chamber (eye) —see Cyst, iris
    nasopalatine K09.1
  antrum J34.1
  anus K62.89
  apical (tooth) (periodontal) K04.8
  appendix K38.8
  arachnoid, brain (acquired) G93.0
    congenital Q04.6
  arytenoid J38.7
  Baker's M71.2-●
    ruptured M66.0
    tuberculous A18.02
  Bartholin's gland N75.0
  bile duct (common) (hepatic) K83.5
  bladder (multiple) (trigone) N32.89
  blue dome (breast) —see Cyst, breast
  bone (local) NEC M85.60
    aneurysmal M85.50
      ankle M85.57-●
      foot M85.57-●
      forearm M85.53-●
      hand M85.54-●
      jaw M27.49
      lower leg M85.56-●
      multiple site M85.59
      neck M85.58
      rib M85.58
      shoulder M85.51-●
      skull M85.58
      specified site NEC M85.58
      thigh M85.55-●
      toe M85.57-●
      upper arm M85.52-●
      vertebra M85.58
    solitary M85.40
      ankle M85.47-●
      fibula M85.46-●
      foot M85.47-●
      hand M85.44-●
      humerus M85.42-●
      jaw M27.49
      neck M85.48
      pelvis M85.45-●

Cyst (Continued)
  bone NEC (Continued)
    solitary (Continued)
      radius M85.43-●
      rib M85.48
      shoulder M85.41-●
      skull M85.48
      specified site NEC M85.48
      tibia M85.46-●
      toe M85.47-●
      ulna M85.43-●
      vertebra M85.48
    specified type NEC M85.60
      ankle M85.67-●
      foot M85.67-●
      forearm M85.63-●
      hand M85.64-●
      jaw M27.40
        developmental (nonodontogenic) K09.1
          odontogenic K09.0
        latent M27.0
      lower leg M85.66-●
      multiple site M85.69
      neck M85.68
      rib M85.68
      shoulder M85.61-●
      skull M85.68
      specified site NEC M85.68
      thigh M85.65-●
      toe M85.67-●
      upper arm M85.62-●
      vertebra M85.68
  brain (acquired) G93.0
    congenital Q04.6
    hydatid B67.99 [G94]
    third ventricle (colloid), congenital
      Q04.6
  branchial (cleft) Q18.0
  branchiogenic Q18.0
  breast (benign) (blue dome) (pedunculated)
    (solitary) N60.0-●
    involution —see Dysplasia, mammary,
      specified type NEC
    sebaceous —see Dysplasia, mammary,
      specified type NEC
  broad ligament (benign) N83.8
  bronchogenic (mediastinal) (sequestration)
    J98.4
    congenital Q33.0
  buccal K09.8
  bulbourethral gland N36.8
  bursa, bursal NEC M71.30
    with rupture —see Rupture, synovium
    ankle M71.37-●
    elbow M71.32-●
    foot M71.37-●
    hand M71.34-●
    hip M71.35-●
    multiple sites M71.39
    pharyngeal J39.2
    popliteal space —see Cyst, Baker's
    shoulder M71.31-●
    specified site NEC M71.38
    wrist M71.33-●
  calcifying odontogenic D16.5
    upper jaw (bone) (maxilla) D16.4
  canal of Nuck (female) N94.89
    congenital Q52.4
  canthus —see Cyst, conjunctiva
  carcinomatous —see Neoplasm, malignant,
    by site
  cauda equina G95.89
  cavum septi pellucidi —see Cyst, brain
  celomic (pericardium) Q24.8
  cerebellopontine (angle) —see Cyst, brain
  cerebellum —see Cyst, brain
  cerebral —see Cyst, brain
  cervical lateral Q18.0
  cervix NEC N88.8
    embryonic Q51.6
    nabothian N88.8

Cyst (Continued)
  chiasmal optic NEC —see Disorder, optic,
    chiasm
  chocolate (ovary) N80.1
  choledochus, congenital Q44.4
  chorion O41.8X-●
  choroid plexus G93.0
  ciliary body —see Cyst, iris
  clitoris N90.7
  colon K63.89
  common (bile) duct K83.5
  congenital NEC Q89.8
    adrenal gland Q89.1
    epiglottis Q31.8
    esophagus Q39.8
    fallopian tube Q50.4
    kidney Q61.00
      more than one (multiple) Q61.02
        specified as polycystic Q61.3
          adult type Q61.2
          infantile type NEC Q61.19
            collecting duct dilation Q61.11
      solitary Q61.01
    larynx Q31.8
    liver Q44.6
    lung Q33.0
    mediastinum Q34.1
    ovary Q50.1
    oviduct Q50.4
    periurethral (tissue) Q64.79
    prepuce Q55.69
    salivary gland (any) Q38.4
    sublingual Q38.6
    submaxillary gland Q38.6
    thymus (gland) Q89.2
    tongue Q38.3
    ureterovesical orifice Q62.8
    vulva Q52.79
  conjunctiva H11.44-●
  cornea H18.89-●
  corpora quadrigemina G93.0
  corpus
    albicans N83.29-●
    luteum (hemorrhagic) (ruptured) N83.1-●
  Cowper's gland (benign) (infected) N36.8
  cranial meninges G93.0
  craniobuccal pouch E23.6
  craniopharyngeal pouch E23.6
  cystic duct K82.8
  Cysticercus —see Cysticercosis
  Dandy-Walker Q03.1
    with spina bifida —see Spina bifida
  dental (root) K04.8
    developmental K09.0
    eruption K09.0
    primordial K09.0
  dentigerous (mandible) (maxilla) K09.0
  dermoid —see Neoplasm, benign, by site
    with malignant transformation C56.-●
    implantation
      external area or site (skin) NEC L72.0
      iris —see Cyst, iris, implantation
      vagina N89.8
      vulva N90.7
    mouth K09.8
    oral soft tissue K09.8
    sacrococcygeal —see Cyst, pilonidal
  developmental K09.1
    odontogenic K09.0
    oral region (nonodontogenic) K09.1
    ovary, ovarian Q50.1
  dura (cerebral) G93.0
    spinal G96.19
  ear (external) Q18.1
  echinococcal —see Echinococcus
  embryonic
    cervix uteri Q51.6
    fallopian tube Q50.4
  ➡ vagina Q52.4
  endometrium, endometrial (uterus) N85.8
    ectopic —see Endometriosis

Cyst (Continued)
  enterogenous Q43.8
  epidermal, epidermoid (inclusion) (see also
      Cyst, skin) L72.0
    mouth K09.8
      oral soft tissue K09.8
  epididymis N50.3
  epiglottis J38.7
  epiphysis cerebri E34.8
  epithelial (inclusion) L72.0
  epoophoron Q50.5
  eruption K09.0
  esophagus K22.8
  ethmoid sinus J34.1
  external female genital organs NEC N90.7
  eye NEC H57.8
    congenital Q15.8
  eyelid (sebaceous) H02.829
    infected —see Hordeolum
    left H02.826
      lower H02.825
      upper H02.824
    right H02.823
      lower H02.822
      upper H02.821
  fallopian tube N83.8
    congenital Q50.4
  fimbrial (twisted) Q50.4
  fissural (oral region) K09.1
  follicle (graafian) (hemorrhagic) N83.0-•
    nabothian N88.8
  follicular (atretic) (hemorrhagic) (ovarian)
      N83.0-•
    dentigerous K09.0
    odontogenic K09.0
    skin L72.9
      specified NEC L72.8
  frontal sinus J34.1
  gallbladder K82.8
  ganglion —see Ganglion
  Gartner's duct Q52.4
  gingiva K09.0
  gland of Moll —see Cyst, eyelid
  globulomaxillary K09.1
  graafian follicle (hemorrhagic) N83.0-•
  granulosal lutein (hemorrhagic) N83.1-•
  hemangiomatous D18.00
    intra-abdominal D18.03
    intracranial D18.02
    skin D18.01
    specified site NEC D18.09
  hemorrhagic M27.49
  hydatid —see also Echinococcus B67.90
    brain B67.99 [G94]
    liver —see also Cyst, liver, hydatid B67.8
    lung NEC B67.99 [J99]
    Morgagni
      female Q50.5
      male (epididymal) Q55.4
        testicular Q55.29
    specified site NEC B67.99
  hymen N89.8
    embryonic Q52.4
  hypopharynx J39.2
  hypophysis, hypophyseal (duct) (recurrent)
      E23.6
    cerebri E23.6
  implantation (dermoid)
    external area or site (skin) NEC L72.0
    iris —see Cyst, iris, implantation
    vagina N89.8
    vulva N90.7
  incisive canal K09.1
  inclusion (epidermal) (epithelial)
      (epidermoid) (squamous) L72.0
    not of skin - code under Cyst, by site
  intestine (large) (small) K63.89
  intracranial —see Cyst, brain
  intraligamentous —see also Disorder,
      ligament
    knee —see Derangement, knee

Cyst (Continued)
  intrasellar E23.6
  iris H21.309
    exudative H21.31-•
    idiopathic H21.30-•
    implantation H21.32-•
    parasitic H21.33-•
    pars plana (primary) H21.34-•
      exudative H21.35-•
  jaw (bone) M27.40
    aneurysmal M27.49
    developmental (odontogenic) K09.0
    fissural K09.1
    hemorrhagic M27.49
    traumatic M27.49
  joint NEC —see Disorder, joint, specified type
      NEC
  kidney (acquired) N28.1
    calyceal —see Hydronephrosis
    congenital Q61.00
    more than one (multiple) Q61.02
      specified as polycystic Q61.3
        adult type (autosomal dominant)
            Q61.2
        infantile type (autosomal recessive)
            NEC Q61.19
          collecting duct dilation Q61.11
    pyelogenic —see Hydronephrosis
    simple N28.1
    solitary (single) Q61.01
      acquired N28.1
  labium (majus) (minus) N90.7
    sebaceous N90.7
  lacrimal —see also Disorder, lacrimal system,
      specified NEC
    gland H04.13-•
    passages or sac —see Disorder, lacrimal
        system, specified NEC
  larynx J38.7
  lateral periodontal K09.0
  lens H27.8
    congenital Q12.8
  lip (gland) K13.0
  liver (idiopathic) (simple) K76.89
    congenital Q44.6
    hydatid B67.8
      granulosus B67.0
      multilocularis B67.5
  lung J98.4
    congenital Q33.0
    giant bullous J43.9
  lutein N83.1-•
  lymphangiomatous D18.1
  lymphoepithelial, oral soft tissue K09.8
  macula —see Degeneration, macula, hole
  malignant —see Neoplasm, malignant, by site
  mammary gland —see Cyst, breast
  mandible M27.40
    dentigerous K09.0
    radicular K04.8
  maxilla M27.40
    dentigerous K09.0
    radicular K04.8
  medial, face and neck Q18.8
  median
    anterior maxillary K09.1
    palatal K09.1
  mediastinum, congenital Q34.1
  meibomian (gland) —see Chalazion
    infected —see Hordeolum
  membrane, brain G93.0
  meninges (cerebral) G93.0
    spinal G96.19
  meniscus, knee —see Derangement, knee,
      meniscus, cystic
  mesentery, mesenteric K66.8
    chyle I89.8
  mesonephric duct
    female Q50.5
    male Q55.4
  milk N64.89

Cyst (Continued)
  Morgagni (hydatid)
    female Q50.5
    male (epididymal) Q55.4
      testicular Q55.29
  mouth K09.8
  Müllerian duct Q50.4
    appendix testis Q55.29
    cervix Q51.6
    fallopian tube Q50.4
    female Q50.4
    male Q55.29
    prostatic utricle Q55.4
    vagina (embryonal) Q52.4
  multilocular (ovary) D39.10
    benign —see Neoplasm, benign, by site
  myometrium N85.8
  nabothian (follicle) (ruptured) N88.8
  nasoalveolar K09.1
  nasolabial K09.1
  nasopalatine (anterior) (duct) K09.1
  nasopharynx J39.2
  neoplastic —see Neoplasm, uncertain
        behavior, by site
    benign —see Neoplasm, benign, by site
  nervous system NEC G96.8
  neuroenteric (congenital) Q06.8
  nipple —see Cyst, breast
  nose (turbinates) J34.1
    sinus J34.1
  odontogenic, developmental K09.0
  omentum (lesser) K66.8
    congenital Q45.8
  ora serrata —see Cyst, retina, ora serrata
  oral
    region K09.9
      developmental (nonodontogenic) K09.1
      specified NEC K09.8
    soft tissue K09.9
      specified NEC K09.8
  orbit H05.81-•
  ovary, ovarian (twisted) N83.20-•
    adherent N83.20-•
    chocolate N80.1
    corpus
      albicans N83.29-•
      luteum (hemorrhagic) N83.1-•
    dermoid D27.9
    developmental Q50.1
    due to failure of involution NEC N83.20-•
    endometrial N80.1
    follicular (graafian) (hemorrhagic) N83.0-•
    hemorrhagic N83.20-•
    in pregnancy or childbirth O34.8-•
      with obstructed labor O65.5
    multilocular D39.10
    pseudomucinous D27.9
    retention N83.29-•
    serous N83.20-•
    specified NEC N83.29-•
    theca lutein (hemorrhagic) N83.1-•
    tuberculous A18.18
  oviduct N83.8
  palate (median) (fissural) K09.1
  palatine papilla (jaw) K09.1
  pancreas, pancreatic (hemorrhagic) (true) K86.2
    congenital Q45.2
    false K86.3
  paralabral
    hip M24.85-•
    shoulder S43.43-•
  paramesonephric duct Q50.4
    female Q50.4
    male Q55.29
  paranephric N28.1
  paraphysis, cerebri, congenital Q04.6
  parasitic B89
  parathyroid (gland) E21.4
  paratubal N83.8
  paraurethral duct N36.8
  paroophoron Q50.5

▶ New   ⇒ Revised   ~~deleted~~ Deleted   • Use Additional Character(s)

Cyst *(Continued)*
  parotid gland K11.6
  parovarian Q50.5
  pelvis, female N94.89
    in pregnancy or childbirth O34.8-●
      causing obstructed labor O65.5
  penis (sebaceous) N48.89
  periapical K04.8
  pericardial (congenital) Q24.8
    acquired (secondary) I31.8
  pericoronal K09.0
  periodontal K04.8
    lateral K09.0
  peripelvic (lymphatic) N28.1
  peritoneum K66.8
    chylous I89.8
  periventricular, acquired, newborn P91.1
  pharynx (wall) J39.2
  pilar L72.11
  pilonidal (infected) (rectum) L05.91
    with abscess L05.01
    malignant C44.59-●
  pituitary (duct) (gland) E23.6
  placenta O43.19-●
  pleura J94.8
  popliteal —*see* Cyst, Baker's
  porencephalic Q04.6
    acquired G93.0
  postanal (infected) —*see* Cyst, pilonidal
  postmastoidectomy cavity (mucosal) —*see*
      Complications, postmastoidectomy, cyst
  preauricular Q18.1
  prepuce N47.4
    congenital Q55.69
  primordial (jaw) K09.0
  prostate N42.83
  pseudomucinous (ovary) D27.9
  pupillary, miotic H21.27-●
  radicular (residual) K04.8
  radiculodental K04.8
  ranular K11.8
  Rathke's pouch E23.6
  rectum (epithelium) (mucous) K62.89
  renal —*see* Cyst, kidney
  residual (radicular) K04.8
  retention (ovary) N83.29-●
    salivary gland K11.6
  retina H33.19-●
    ora serrata H33.11-●
    parasitic H33.12-●
  retroperitoneal K68.9
  sacrococcygeal (dermoid) —*see* Cyst,
      pilonidal
  salivary gland or duct (mucous extravasation
      or retention) K11.6
  Sampson's N80.1
  sclera H15.89
  scrotum L72.9
    sebaceous L72.3
  sebaceous (duct) (gland) L72.3
    breast —*see* Dysplasia, mammary, specified
        type NEC
    eyelid —*see* Cyst, eyelid
    genital organ NEC
      female N94.89
      male N50.89
    scrotum L72.3
  semilunar cartilage (knee) (multiple) —*see*
      Derangement, knee, meniscus, cystic
  seminal vesicle N50.89
  serous (ovary) N83.20-●
  sinus (accessory) (nasal) J34.1
  Skene's gland N36.8
  skin L72.9
    breast —*see* Dysplasia, mammary, specified
        type NEC
    epidermal, epidermoid L72.0
    epithelial L72.0
    eyelid —*see* Cyst, eyelid
    genital organ NEC
      female N90.7
      male N50.89

Cyst *(Continued)*
  skin *(Continued)*
    inclusion L72.0
    scrotum L72.9
    sebaceous L72.3
    sweat gland or duct L74.8
  solitary
    bone —*see* Cyst, bone, solitary
    jaw M27.40
    kidney N28.1
  spermatic cord N50.89
  sphenoid sinus J34.1
  spinal meninges G96.19
  spleen NEC D73.4
    congenital Q89.09
    hydatid —*see also* Echinococcus B67.99 [D77]
  Stafne's M27.0
  subarachnoid intrasellar R93.0
  subcutaneous, pheomycotic (chromomycotic)
      B43.2
  subdural (cerebral) G93.0
    spinal cord G96.19
  sublingual gland K11.6
  submandibular gland K11.6
  submaxillary gland K11.6
  suburethral N36.8
  suprarenal gland E27.8
  suprasellar —*see* Cyst, brain
  sweat gland or duct L74.8
  synovial —*see also* Cyst, bursa
    ruptured —*see* Rupture, synovium
  tarsal —*see* Chalazion
  tendon (sheath) —*see* Disorder, tendon,
      specified type NEC
  testis N44.2
    tunica albuginea N44.1
  theca lutein (ovary) N83.1-●
  Thornwaldt's J39.2
  thymus (gland) E32.8
  thyroglossal duct (infected) (persistent)
      Q89.2
  thyroid (gland) E04.1
  thyrolingual duct (infected) (persistent)
      Q89.2
  tongue K14.8
  tonsil J35.8
  tooth —*see* Cyst, dental
  Tornwaldt's J39.2
  trichilemmal (proliferating) L72.12
  trichodermal L72.12
  tubal (fallopian) N83.8
    inflammatory —*see* Salpingitis, chronic
  tubo-ovarian N83.8
    inflammatory N70.13
  tunica
    albuginea testis N44.1
    vaginalis N50.89
  turbinate (nose) J34.1
  Tyson's gland N48.89
  urachus, congenital Q64.4
  ureter N28.89
  ureterovesical orifice N28.89
  urethra, urethral (gland) N36.8
  uterine ligament N83.8
  uterus (body) (corpus) (recurrent)
      N85.8
    embryonic Q51.818
      cervix Q51.6
  vagina, vaginal (implantation) (inclusion)
      (squamous cell) (wall) N89.8
    embryonic Q52.4
  vallecula, vallecular (epiglottis) J38.7
  vesical (orifice) N32.89
  vitreous body H43.89
  vulva (implantation) (inclusion) N90.7
    congenital Q52.79
    sebaceous gland N90.7
  vulvovaginal gland N90.7
  wolffian
    female Q50.5
    male Q55.4

Cystadenocarcinoma —*see* Neoplasm,
    malignant, by site
  bile duct C22.1
  endometrioid —*see* Neoplasm, malignant,
      by site
    specified site —*see* Neoplasm, malignant,
        by site
    unspecified site
      female C56.9
      male C61
  mucinous
    papillary
      specified site —*see* Neoplasm,
          malignant, by site
      unspecified site C56.9
    specified site —*see* Neoplasm, malignant,
        by site
    unspecified site C56.9
  papillary
    mucinous
      specified site —*see* Neoplasm,
          malignant, by site
      unspecified site C56.9
    pseudomucinous
      specified site —*see* Neoplasm,
          malignant, by site
      unspecified site C56.9
    serous
      specified site —*see* Neoplasm,
          malignant, by site
      unspecified site C56.9
    specified site —*see* Neoplasm, malignant,
        by site
    unspecified site C56.9
  pseudomucinous
    papillary
      specified site —*see* Neoplasm,
          malignant, by site
      unspecified site C56.9
    specified site —*see* Neoplasm, malignant,
        by site
    unspecified site C56.9
  serous
    papillary
      specified site —*see* Neoplasm,
          malignant, by site
      unspecified site C56.9
    specified site —*see* Neoplasm, malignant,
        by site
    unspecified site C56.9
Cystadenofibroma
  clear cell —*see* Neoplasm, benign, by site
  endometrioid D27.9
    borderline malignancy D39.1-●
    malignant C56.-●
  mucinous
    specified site —*see* Neoplasm, benign, by site
    unspecified site D27.9
  serous
    specified site —*see* Neoplasm, benign, by site
    unspecified site D27.9
  specified site —*see* Neoplasm, benign, by site
  unspecified site D27.9
Cystadenoma —*see also* Neoplasm, benign, by
    site
  bile duct D13.4
  endometrioid —*see* Neoplasm, benign, by site
    borderline malignancy —*see* Neoplasm,
        uncertain behavior, by site
  malignant —*see* Neoplasm, malignant, by site
  mucinous
    borderline malignancy
      ovary C56.-●
      specified site NEC —*see* Neoplasm,
          uncertain behavior, by site
      unspecified site C56.9
    papillary
      borderline malignancy
        ovary C56.-●
        specified site NEC —*see* Neoplasm,
            uncertain behavior, by site
        unspecified site C56.9

Cystadenoma *(Continued)*
 mucinous *(Continued)*
  papillary *(Continued)*
   specified site —*see* Neoplasm, benign,
     by site
   unspecified site D27.9
  specified site —*see* Neoplasm, benign, by site
  unspecified site D27.9
 papillary
  borderline malignancy
   ovary C56-•
   specified site NEC —*see* Neoplasm,
     uncertain behavior, by site
   unspecified site C56.9
  lymphomatosum
   specified site —*see* Neoplasm, benign,
     by site
   unspecified site D11.9
  mucinous
   borderline malignancy
    ovary C56.-•
    specified site NEC —*see* Neoplasm,
      uncertain behavior, by site
    unspecified site C56.9
   specified site —*see* Neoplasm, benign,
     by site
   unspecified site D27.9
  pseudomucinous
   borderline malignancy
    ovary C56.-•
    specified site NEC —*see* Neoplasm,
      uncertain behavior, by site
    unspecified site C56.9
   specified site —*see* Neoplasm, benign,
     by site
   unspecified site D27.9
  serous
   borderline malignancy
    ovary C56.-•
    specified site NEC —*see* Neoplasm,
      uncertain behavior, by site
    unspecified site C56.9
   specified site —*see* Neoplasm, benign,
     by site
   unspecified site D27.9
  specified site —*see* Neoplasm, benign, by site
  unspecified site D27.9
 pseudomucinous
  borderline malignancy
   ovary C56.-•
   specified site NEC —*see* Neoplasm,
     uncertain behavior, by site
   unspecified site C56.9
  papillary
   borderline malignancy
    ovary C56.-•
    specified site NEC —*see* Neoplasm,
      uncertain behavior, by site
    unspecified site C56.9
   specified site —*see* Neoplasm, benign,
     by site
   unspecified site D27.9
  specified site —*see* Neoplasm, benign, by site
  unspecified site D27.9
 serous
  borderline malignancy
   ovary C56.-•
   specified site NEC —*see* Neoplasm,
     uncertain behavior, by site
   unspecified site C56.9
  papillary
   borderline malignancy
    ovary C56.-•
    specified site NEC —*see* Neoplasm,
      uncertain behavior, by site
    unspecified site C56.9
   specified site —*see* Neoplasm, benign,
     by site
   unspecified site D27.9
  specified site —*see* Neoplasm, benign, by site
  unspecified site D27.9

Cystathionine synthase deficiency E72.11
Cystathioninemia E72.19
Cystathioninuria E72.19
Cystic —*see also* condition
 breast (chronic) —*see* Mastopathy, cystic
 corpora lutea (hemorrhagic) N83.1-•
 duct —*see* condition
 eyeball (congenital) Q11.0
 fibrosis —*see* Fibrosis, cystic
 kidney (congenital) Q61.9
  adult type Q61.2
  infantile type NEC Q61.19
   collecting duct dilatation Q61.11
  medullary Q61.5
 liver, congenital Q44.6
 lung disease J98.4
  congenital Q33.0
 mastitis, chronic —*see* Mastopathy, cystic
 medullary, kidney Q61.5
 meniscus —*see* Derangement, knee,
   meniscus, cystic
 ovary N83.20-•
Cysticercosis, cysticerciasis B69.9
 with
  epileptiform fits B69.0
  myositis B69.81
 brain B69.0
 central nervous system B69.0
 cerebral B69.0
 ocular B69.1
 specified NEC B69.89
Cysticercus cellulose infestation —*see*
  Cysticercosis
Cystinosis (malignant) E72.04
Cystinuria E72.01
Cystitis (exudative) (hemorrhagic) (septic)
  (suppurative) N30.90
 with
  fibrosis —*see* Cystitis, chronic, interstitial
  hematuria N30.91
  leukoplakia —*see* Cystitis, chronic,
    interstitial
  malakoplakia —*see* Cystitis, chronic,
    interstitial
  metaplasia —*see* Cystitis, chronic, interstitial
  prostatitis N41.3
 acute N30.00
  with hematuria N30.01
  of trigone N30.30
   with hematuria N30.31
 allergic —*see* Cystitis, specified type NEC
 amebic A06.81
 bilharzial B65.9 [N33]
 blennorrhagic (gonococcal) A54.01
 bullous —*see* Cystitis, specified type NEC
 calculous N21.0
 chlamydial A56.01
 chronic N30.20
  with hematuria N30.21
  interstitial N30.10
   with hematuria N30.11
  of trigone N30.30
   with hematuria N30.31
  specified NEC N30.20
   with hematuria N30.21
 cystic (a) —*see* Cystitis, specified type NEC
 diphtheritic A36.85
 echinococcal
  granulosus B67.39
  multilocularis B67.69
 emphysematous —*see* Cystitis, specified type
   NEC
 encysted —*see* Cystitis, specified type NEC
 eosinophilic —*see* Cystitis, specified type
   NEC
 follicular —*see* Cystitis, of trigone
 gangrenous —*see* Cystitis, specified type
   NEC
 glandularis —*see* Cystitis, specified type
   NEC

Cystitis *(Continued)*
 gonococcal A54.01
 incrusted —*see* Cystitis, specified type
   NEC
 interstitial (chronic) —*see* Cystitis, chronic,
   interstitial
 irradiation N30.40
  with hematuria N30.41
 irritation —*see* Cystitis, specified type
   NEC
 malignant —*see* Cystitis, specified type
   NEC
 of trigone N30.30
  with hematuria N30.31
 panmural —*see* Cystitis, chronic, interstitial
 polyposa —*see* Cystitis, specified type NEC
 prostatic N41.3
 puerperal (postpartum) O86.22
 radiation —*see* Cystitis, irradiation
 specified type NEC N30.80
  with hematuria N30.81
 subacute —*see* Cystitis, chronic
 submucous —*see* Cystitis, chronic, interstitial
 syphilitic (late) A52.76
 trichomonal A59.03
 tuberculous A18.12
 ulcerative —*see* Cystitis, chronic, interstitial
Cystocele (-urethrocele)
 female N81.10
  with prolapse of uterus —*see* Prolapse,
    uterus
  lateral N81.12
  midline N81.11
  paravaginal N81.12
 in pregnancy or childbirth O34.8-•
  causing obstructed labor O65.5
 male N32.89
Cystolithiasis N21.0
Cystoma —*see also* Neoplasm, benign, by site
 endometrial, ovary N80.1
 mucinous
  specified site —*see* Neoplasm, benign, by site
  unspecified site D27.9
 serous
  specified site —*see* Neoplasm, benign, by site
  unspecified site D27.9
 simple (ovary) N83.29-•
Cystoplegia N31.2
Cystoptosis N32.89
Cystopyelitis —*see* Pyelonephritis
Cystorrhagia N32.89
Cystosarcoma phyllodes D48.6-•
 benign D24-•
 malignant —*see* Neoplasm, breast, malignant
Cystostomy
 attention to Z43.5
 complication —*see* Complications, cystostomy
 status Z93.50
  appendico-vesicostomy Z93.52
  cutaneous Z93.51
  specified NEC Z93.59
Cystourethritis —*see* Urethritis
Cystourethrocele —*see also* Cystocele
 female N81.10
  with uterine prolapse —*see* Prolapse,
    uterus
  lateral N81.12
  midline N81.11
  paravaginal N81.12
 male N32.89
Cytomegalic inclusion disease
 congenital P35.1
Cytomegalovirus infection B25.9
Cytomycosis (reticuloendothelial) B39.4
Cytopenia D75.9
 refractory
  with multilineage dysplasia D46.A
   and ring sideroblasts (RCMD RS) D46.B
Czerny's disease (periodic hydrarthrosis of the
  knee) —*see* Effusion, joint, knee

▶ New ⇒ Revised ~~deleted~~ Deleted • Use Additional Character(s)

D

Daae (-Finsen) disease (epidemic pleurodynia) B33.0
Dabney's grip B33.0
Da Costa's syndrome F45.8
Dacryoadenitis, dacryadenitis H04.00-●
  acute H04.01-●
  chronic H04.02-●
Dacryocystitis H04.30-●
  acute H04.32-●
  chronic H04.41-●
  neonatal P39.1
  phlegmonous H04.31-●
  syphilitic A52.71
    congenital (early) A50.01
  trachomatous, active A71.1
    sequelae (late effect) B94.0
Dacryocystoblenorrhea —see Inflammation, lacrimal, passages, chronic
Dacryocystocele —see Disorder, lacrimal system, changes
Dacryolith, dacryolithiasis H04.51-●
Dacryoma —see Disorder, lacrimal system, changes
Dacryopericystitis —see Dacryocystitis
Dacryops H04.11-●
Dacryostenosis —see also Stenosis, lacrimal
  congenital Q10.5
Dactylitis
  bone —see Osteomyelitis
  sickle-cell D57.00
    Hb C D57.219
    Hb SS D57.00
    specified NEC D57.819
  skin L08.9
  syphilitic A52.77
  tuberculous A18.03
Dactylolysis spontanea (ainhum) L94.6
Dactylosymphysis Q70.9
  fingers —see Syndactylism, complex, fingers
  toes —see Syndactylism, complex, toes
Damage
  arteriosclerotic —see Arteriosclerosis
  brain (nontraumatic) G93.9
    anoxic, hypoxic G93.1
      resulting from a procedure G97.82
    child NEC G80.9
    due to birth injury P11.2
  cardiorenal (vascular) —see Hypertension, cardiorenal
  cerebral NEC —see Damage, brain
  coccyx, complicating delivery O71.6
  coronary —see Disease, heart, ischemic
  eye, birth injury P15.3
  liver (nontraumatic) K76.9
    alcoholic K70.9
    due to drugs —see Disease, liver, toxic
    toxic —see Disease, liver, toxic
  medication T88.7
  pelvic
    joint or ligament, during delivery O71.6
    organ NEC
      during delivery O71.5
      following ectopic or molar pregnancy O08.6
  renal —see Disease, renal
  subendocardium, subendocardial —see Degeneration, myocardial
  vascular I99.9
Dana-Putnam syndrome (subacute combined sclerosis with pernicious anemia) —see Degeneration, combined
Danbolt (-Cross) syndrome (acrodermatitis enteropathica) E83.2
Dandruff L21.0
Dandy-Walker syndrome Q03.1
  with spina bifida —see Spina bifida
Danlos' syndrome Q79.6

Darier (-White) disease (congenital) Q82.8
  meaning erythema annulare centrifugum L53.1
Darier-Roussy sarcoid D86.3
Darling's disease or histoplasmosis B39.4
Darwin's tubercle Q17.8
Dawson's (inclusion body) encephalitis A81.1
De Beurmann (-Gougerot) disease B42.1
De la Tourette's syndrome F95.2
De Lange's syndrome Q87.1
De Morgan's spots (senile angiomas) I78.1
De Quervain's
  disease (tendon sheath) M65.4
  syndrome E34.51
  thyroiditis (subacute granulomatous thyroiditis) E06.1
De Toni-Fanconi (-Debré) syndrome E72.09
  with cystinosis E72.04
Dead
  fetus, retained (mother) O36.4
    early pregnancy O02.1
  labyrinth —see subcategory H83.2
  ovum, retained O02.0
Deaf nonspeaking NEC H91.3
Deafmutism (acquired) (congenital) NEC H91.3
  hysterical F44.6
  syphilitic, congenital —see also subcategory H94.8 A50.09
Deafness (acquired) (complete) (hereditary) (partial) H91.9-●
  with blue sclera and fragility of bone Q78.0
  auditory fatigue —see Deafness, specified type NEC
  aviation T70.0
    nerve injury —see Injury, nerve, acoustic, specified type NEC
  boilermaker's —see subcategory H83.3
  central —see Deafness, sensorineural
  conductive H90.2
    and sensorineural
      mixed H90.8
        bilateral H90.6
      bilateral H90.0
      unilateral H90.1-●
        with restricted hearing on the contralateral side H90.A-●
  congenital H90.5
    with blue sclera and fragility of bone Q78.0
  due to toxic agents —see Deafness, ototoxic
  emotional (hysterical) F44.6
  functional (hysterical) F44.6
  high frequency H91.9-●
  hysterical F44.6
  low frequency H91.9-●
  mental R48.8
  mixed conductive and sensorineural H90.8
    bilateral H90.6
    unilateral H90.7-●
  nerve —see Deafness, sensorineural
  neural —see Deafness, sensorineural
  noise-induced —see also subcategory H83.3
    nerve injury —see Injury, nerve, acoustic, specified type NEC
  nonspeaking H91.3
  ototoxic —see subcategory H91.0
  perceptive —see Deafness, sensorineural
  psychogenic (hysterical) F44.6
  sensorineural H90.5
    and conductive
      mixed H90.8
        bilateral H90.6
      bilateral H90.3
      unilateral H90.4-●
        with restricted hearing on the contralateral side H90.A-●
  sensory —see Deafness, sensorineural
  specified type NEC —see subcategory H91.8
  sudden (idiopathic) H91.2-●

Deafness (Continued)
  syphilitic A52.15
  transient ischemic H93.01-●
  traumatic —see Injury, nerve, acoustic, specified type NEC
  word (developmental) H93.25
Death (cause unknown) (of) (unexplained) (unspecified cause) R99
  brain G93.82
  cardiac (sudden) (with successful resuscitation) — code to underlying disease
    family history of Z82.41
    personal history of Z86.74
  family member (assumed) Z63.4
Debility (chronic) (general) (nervous) R53.81
  congenital or neonatal NOS P96.9
  nervous R53.81
  old age R54
  senile R54
Débove's disease (splenomegaly) R16.1
Decalcification
  bone —see Osteoporosis
  teeth K03.89
Decapsulation, kidney N28.89
Decay
  dental —see Caries, dental
  senile R54
  tooth, teeth —see Caries, dental
Deciduitis (acute)
  following ectopic or molar pregnancy O08.0
Decline (general) —see Debility
  cognitive, age-associated R41.81
Decompensation
  cardiac (acute) (chronic) —see Disease, heart
  cardiovascular —see Disease, cardiovascular
  heart —see Disease, heart
  hepatic —see Failure, hepatic
  myocardial (acute) (chronic) —see Disease, heart
  respiratory J98.8
Decompression sickness T70.3
Decrease (d)
  absolute neutrophile count —see Neutropenia
  blood
    platelets —see Thrombocytopenia
    pressure R03.1
      due to shock following
        injury T79.4
        operation T81.19
  estrogen E28.39
    postablative E89.40
      asymptomatic E89.40
      symptomatic E89.41
  fragility of erythrocytes D58.8
  function
    lipase (pancreatic) K90.3
    ovary in hypopituitarism E23.0
    parenchyma of pancreas K86.89
    pituitary (gland) (anterior) (lobe) E23.0
      posterior (lobe) E23.0
  functional activity R68.89
  glucose R73.09
  hematocrit R71.0
  hemoglobin R71.0
  leukocytes D72.819
    specified NEC D72.818
  libido R68.82
  lymphocytes D72.810
  platelets D69.6
  respiration, due to shock following injury T79.4
  sexual desire R68.82
  tear secretion NEC —see Syndrome, dry eye
  tolerance
    fat K90.49
    glucose R73.09
    pancreatic K90.3
    salt and water E87.8
  vision NEC H54.7
  white blood cell count D72.819
    specified NEC D72.818

Decubitus (ulcer) —see Ulcer, pressure, by site
  cervix N86
Deepening acetabulum —see Derangement,
  joint, specified type NEC, hip
Defect, defective Q89.9
  3-beta-hydroxysteroid dehydrogenase E25.0
  11-hydroxylase E25.0
  21-hydroxylase E25.0
  abdominal wall, congenital Q79.59
  antibody immunodeficiency D80.9
  aorticopulmonary septum Q21.4
  atrial septal (ostium secundum type) Q21.1
    following acute myocardial infarction
      (current complication) I23.1
    ostium primum type Q21.2
  atrioventricular
    canal Q21.2
    septum Q21.2
  auricular septal Q21.1
  bilirubin excretion NEC E80.6
  biosynthesis, androgen (testicular) E29.1
  bulbar septum Q21.0
  catalase E80.3
  cell membrane receptor complex (CR3) D71
  circulation I99.9
    congenital Q28.9
    newborn Q28.9
  coagulation (factor) —see also Deficiency,
    factor D68.9
    with
      ectopic pregnancy O08.1
      molar pregnancy O08.1
    acquired D68.4
    antepartum with hemorrhage —see
      Hemorrhage, antepartum, with
      coagulation defect
    due to
      liver disease D68.4
      vitamin K deficiency D68.4
    hereditary NEC D68.2
    intrapartum O67.0
    newborn, transient P61.6
    ➡ postpartum O99.13
      ▶ with hemorrhage O72.3
    specified type NEC D68.8
  complement system D84.1
  conduction (heart) I45.9
    bone —see Deafness, conductive
  congenital, organ or site not listed —see
    Anomaly, by site
  coronary sinus Q21.1
  cushion, endocardial Q21.2
  degradation, glycoprotein E77.1
  dental bridge, crown, fillings —see Defect,
    dental restoration
  dental restoration K08.50
    specified NEC K08.59
  dentin (hereditary) K00.5
  Descemet's membrane, congenital Q13.89
  developmental —see also Anomaly
    cauda equina Q06.3
  diaphragm
    with elevation, eventration or hernia —see
      Hernia, diaphragm
    congenital Q79.1
      with hernia Q79.0
      gross (with hernia) Q79.0
  ectodermal, congenital Q82.9
  Eisenmenger's Q21.8
  enzyme
    catalase E80.3
    peroxidase E80.3
  esophagus, congenital Q39.9
  extensor retinaculum M62.89
  fibrin polymerization D68.2
  filling
    bladder R93.41
    kidney R93.42-●
    renal pelvis R93.41
    stomach R93.3
    ureter R93.41
    urinary organs, specified NEC R93.49

Defect, defective (Continued)
  Gerbode Q21.0
  glycoprotein degradation E77.1
  Hageman (factor) D68.2
  hearing —see Deafness
  high grade F70
  interatrial septal Q21.1
  interauricular septal Q21.1
  interventricular septal Q21.0
    with dextroposition of aorta, pulmonary
      stenosis and hypertrophy of right
      ventricle Q21.3
    in tetralogy of Fallot Q21.3
  learning (specific) —see Disorder, learning
  lymphocyte function antigen-1 (LFA-1) D84.0
  lysosomal enzyme, post-translational
    modification E77.0
  major osseous M89.70
    ankle M89.77-●
    carpus M89.74-●
    clavicle M89.71-●
    femur M89.75-●
    fibula M89.76-●
    fingers M89.74-●
    foot M89.77-●
    forearm M89.73-●
    hand M89.74-●
    humerus M89.72-●
    lower leg M89.76-●
    metacarpus M89.74-●
    metatarsus M89.77-●
    multiple sites M89.79
    pelvic region M89.75-●
    pelvis M89.75-●
    radius M89.73-●
    scapula M89.71-●
    shoulder region M89.71-●
    specified NEC M89.78
    tarsus M89.77-●
    thigh M89.75-●
    tibia M89.76-●
    toes M89.77-●
    ulna M89.73-●
  mental —see Disability, intellectual
  modification, lysosomal enzymes, post-
    translational E77.0
  obstructive, congenital
    renal pelvis Q62.39
    ureter Q62.39
      atresia —see Atresia, ureter
      cecoureterocele Q62.32
      megaureter Q62.2
      orthotopic ureterocele Q62.31
  osseous, major M89.70
    ankle M89.77-●
    carpus M89.74-●
    clavicle M89.71-●
    femur M89.75-●
    fibula M89.76-●
    fingers M89.74-●
    foot M89.77-●
    forearm M89.73-●
    hand M89.74-●
    humerus M89.72-●
    lower leg M89.76-●
    metacarpus M89.74-●
    metatarsus M89.77-●
    multiple sites M89.9
    pelvic region M89.75-●
    pelvis M89.75-●
    radius M89.73-●
    scapula M89.71-●
    shoulder region M89.71-●
    specified NEC M89.78
    tarsus M89.77-●
    thigh M89.75-●
    tibia M89.76-●
    toes M89.77-●
    ulna M89.73-●
  osteochondral NEC —see also Deformity
    M95.8-●

Defect, defective (Continued)
  ostium
    primum Q21.2
    secundum Q21.1
  peroxidase E80.3
  placental blood supply —see Insufficiency,
    placental
  platelets, qualitative D69.1
    constitutional D68.0
  postural NEC, spine —see Dorsopathy,
    deforming
  reduction
    limb Q73.8
      lower Q72.9-●
        absence —see Agenesis, leg
          foot —see Agenesis, foot
        longitudinal
          femur Q72.4-●
          fibula Q72.6-●
          tibia Q72.5-●
        specified type NEC Q72.89-●
        split foot Q72.7-●
      specified type NEC Q73.8
      upper Q71.9-●
        absence —see Agenesis, arm
          forearm —see Agenesis, forearm
          hand —see Agenesis, hand
        lobster-claw hand Q71.6-●
        longitudinal
          radius Q71.4-●
          ulna Q71.5-●
        specified type NEC Q71.89-●
  renal pelvis Q63.8
    obstructive Q62.39
  respiratory system, congenital Q34.9
  restoration, dental K08.50
    specified NEC K08.59
  retinal nerve bundle fibers H35.89
  septal (heart) NOS Q21.9
    acquired (atrial) (auricular) (ventricular)
      (old) I51.0
    atrial Q21.1
      concurrent with acute myocardial
        infarction —see Infarct,
        myocardium
      following acute myocardial infarction
        (current complication) I23.1
    ventricular —see also Defect, ventricular
      septal Q21.0
  sinus venosus Q21.1
  speech R47.9
    developmental F80.9
    specified NEC R47.89
  Taussig-Bing (aortic transposition and
    overriding pulmonary artery) Q20.1
  teeth, wedge K03.1
  vascular (local) I99.9
    congenital Q27.9
  ventricular septal Q21.0
    concurrent with acute myocardial
      infarction —see Infarct, myocardium
    following acute myocardial infarction
      (current complication) I23.2
    in tetralogy of Fallot Q21.3
  vision NEC H54.7
  visual field H53.40
    bilateral
      heteronymous H53.47
      homonymous H53.46-●
    generalized contraction H53.48-●
    localized
      arcuate H53.43-●
      scotoma (central area) H53.41-●
        blind spot area H53.42-●
      sector H53.43-●
      specified type NEC H53.45-●
  voice R49.9
    specified NEC R49.8
  wedge, tooth, teeth (abrasion) K03.1
Deferentitis N49.1
  gonorrheal (acute) (chronic) A54.23

▶ New   ⇒ Revised   ~~deleted~~ Deleted   ● Use Additional Character(s)

Defibrination (syndrome) D65
  antepartum —see Hemorrhage, antepartum,
      with coagulation defect, disseminated
      intravascular coagulation
  following ectopic or molar pregnancy O08.1
  intrapartum O67.0
  newborn P60
  postpartum O72.3
Deficiency, deficient
  3-beta hydroxysteroid dehydrogenase E25.0
  11-hydroxylase E25.0
  21-hydroxylase E25.0
  5-alpha reductase (with male
      pseudohermaphroditism) E29.1
  abdominal muscle syndrome Q79.4
  AC globulin (congenital) (hereditary) D68.2
    acquired D68.4
  accelerator globulin (Ac G) (blood) D68.2
  acid phosphatase E83.39
  activating factor (blood) D68.2
  adenosine deaminase (ADA) D81.3
  aldolase (hereditary) E74.19
  alpha-1-antitrypsin E88.01
  amino-acids E72.9
  anemia —see Anemia
  aneurin E51.9
  antibody with
    hyperimmunoglobulinemia D80.6
    near-normal immunoglobins D80.6
  antidiuretic hormone E23.2
  anti-hemophilic
    factor (A) D66
      B D67
      C D68.1
    globulin (AHG) NEC D66
  antithrombin (antithrombin III) D68.59
  ascorbic acid E54
  attention (disorder) (syndrome) F98.8
    with hyperactivity —see Disorder,
        attention-deficit hyperactivity
  autoprothrombin
    I D68.2
    II D67
    C D68.2
  beta-glucuronidase E76.29
  biotin E53.8
  biotin-dependent carboxylase D81.819
  biotinidase D81.810
  brancher enzyme (amylopectinosis) E74.03
  C1 esterase inhibitor (C1-INH) D84.1
  calciferol E55.9
    with
      adult osteomalacia M83.8
      rickets —see Rickets
  calcium (dietary) E58
  calorie, severe E43
    with marasmus E41
      and kwashiorkor E42
  cardiac —see Insufficiency, myocardial
  carnitine E71.40
    due to
      hemodialysis E71.43
      inborn errors of metabolism E71.42
      Valproic acid therapy E71.43
    iatrogenic E71.43
    muscle palmityltransferase E71.314
    primary E71.41
    secondary E71.448
  carotene E50.9
  central nervous system G96.8
  ceruloplasmin (Wilson) E83.01
  choline E53.8
  Christmas factor D67
  chromium E61.4
  clotting (blood) —see also Deficiency,
      coagulation factor D68.9
  clotting factor NEC (hereditary) —see also
      Deficiency, factor D68.2
  coagulation NOS D68.9
    with
      ectopic pregnancy O08.1
      molar pregnancy O08.1

Deficiency, deficient (Continued)
  coagulation NOS (Continued)
    acquired (any) D68.4
      antepartum hemorrhage —see
          Hemorrhage, antepartum, with
          coagulation defect
      clotting factor NEC —see also Deficiency,
          factor D68.2
      due to
        hyperprothrombinemia D68.4
        liver disease D68.4
        vitamin K deficiency D68.4
      newborn, transient P61.6
      postpartum O72.3
      specified NEC D68.8
  cognitive F09
  color vision H53.50
    achromatopsia H53.51
    acquired H53.52
    deuteranomaly H53.53
    protanomaly H53.54
    specified type NEC H53.59
    tritanomaly H53.55
  combined glucocorticoid and
      mineralocorticoid E27.49
  contact factor D68.2
  copper (nutritional) E61.0
  corticoadrenal E27.40
    primary E27.1
  craniofacial axis Q75.0
  cyanocobalamin E53.8
  debrancher enzyme (limit dextrinosis) E74.03
  dehydrogenase
    long chain/very long chain acyl CoA
        E71.310
    medium chain acyl CoA E71.311
    short chain acyl CoA E71.312
  diet E63.9
  dihydropyrimidine dehydrogenase (DPD)
      E88.89
  disaccharidase E73.9
  edema —see Malnutrition, severe
  endocrine E34.9
  energy-supply —see Malnutrition
  enzymes, circulating NEC E88.09
  ergosterol E55.9
    with
      adult osteomalacia M83.8
      rickets —see Rickets
  essential fatty acid (EFA) E63.0
  factor —see also Deficiency, coagulation
    Hageman D68.2
    I (congenital) (hereditary) D68.2
    II (congenital) (hereditary) D68.2
    IX (congenital) (functional) (hereditary)
        (with functional defect) D67
    multiple (congenital) D68.8
      acquired D68.4
    V (congenital) (hereditary) D68.2
    VII (congenital) (hereditary) D68.2
    VIII (congenital) (functional) (hereditary)
        (with functional defect) D66
      with vascular defect D68.0
    X (congenital) (hereditary) D68.2
    XI (congenital) (hereditary) D68.1
    XII (congenital) (hereditary) D68.2
    XIII (congenital) (hereditary) D68.2
  femoral, proximal focal (congenital) —
      see Defect, reduction, lower limb,
      longitudinal, femur
  fibrin-stabilizing factor (congenital)
      (hereditary) D68.2
    acquired D68.4
  fibrinase D68.2
  fibrinogen (congenital) (hereditary) D68.2
    acquired D65
  folate E53.8
  folic acid E53.8
  foreskin N47.3
  fructokinase E74.11
  fructose 1,6-diphosphatase E74.19

Deficiency, deficient (Continued)
  fructose-1-phosphate aldolase E74.19
  galactokinase E74.29
  galactose-1-phosphate uridyl transferase
      E74.29
  gammaglobulin in blood D80.1
    hereditary D80.0
  glass factor D68.2
  glucocorticoid E27.49
    mineralocorticoid E27.49
  glucose-6-phosphatase E74.01
  glucose-6-phosphate dehydrogenase anemia
      D55.0
  glucuronyl transferase E80.5
  glycogen synthetase E74.09
  gonadotropin (isolated) E23.0
  growth hormone (idiopathic) (isolated) E23.0
  Hageman factor D68.2
  hemoglobin D64.9
  hepatophosphorylase E74.09
  homogentisate 1,2-dioxygenase E70.29
  hormone
    anterior pituitary (partial) NEC E23.0
      growth E23.0
    growth (isolated) E23.0
    pituitary E23.0
    testicular E29.1
  hypoxanthine-(guanine)-
      phosphoribosyltransferase (HG-PRT)
      (total HG-PRT) E79.1
  immunity D84.9
    cell-mediated D84.8
      with thrombocytopenia and eczema
          D82.0
    combined D81.9
    humoral D80.9
    IgA (secretory) D80.2
    IgG D80.3
    IgM D80.4
  immuno —see Immunodeficiency
  immunoglobulin, selective
    A (IgA) D80.2
    G (IgG) (subclasses) D80.3
    M (IgM) D80.4
  inositol (B complex) E53.8
  intrinsic
    factor (congenital) D51.0
    sphincter N36.42
      with urethral hypermobility N36.43
  iodine E61.8
    congenital syndrome —see Syndrome,
        iodine-deficiency, congenital
  iron E61.1
    anemia D50.9
  kalium E87.6
  kappa-light chain D80.8
  labile factor (congenital) (hereditary) D68.2
    acquired D68.4
  lacrimal fluid (acquired) —see also Syndrome,
      dry eye
    congenital Q10.6
  lactase
    congenital E73.0
    secondary E73.1
  Laki-Lorand factor D68.2
  lecithin cholesterol acyltransferase E78.6
  lipocaic K86.89
  lipoprotein (familial) (high density) E78.6
  liver phosphorylase E74.09
  lysosomal alpha-1, 4 glucosidase E74.02
  magnesium E61.2
  major histocompatibility complex
    class I D81.6
    class II D81.7
  manganese E61.3
  menadione (vitamin K) E56.1
    newborn P53
  mental (familial) (hereditary) —see Disability,
      intellectual
  methylenetetrahydrofolate reductase
      (MTHFR) E72.12

Deficiency, deficient *(Continued)*
  mevalonate kinase M04.1
  mineral NEC E61.8
  mineralocorticoid E27.49
    with glucocorticoid E27.49
  molybdenum (nutritional) E61.5
  moral F60.2
  multiple nutrient elements E61.7
  muscle
    carnitine (palmityltransferase) E71.314
    phosphofructokinase E74.09
  myoadenylate deaminase E79.2
  myocardial —*see* Insufficiency, myocardial
  myophosphorylase E74.04
  NADH diaphorase or reductase (congenital) D74.0
  NADH-methemoglobin reductase (congenital) D74.0
  natrium E87.1
  niacin (amide) (-tryptophan) E52
  nicotinamide E52
  nicotinic acid E52
  number of teeth —*see* Anodontia
  nutrient element E61.9
    multiple E61.7
    specified NEC E61.8
  nutrition, nutritional E63.9
    sequelae —*see* Sequelae, nutritional deficiency
    specified NEC E63.8
  of interleukin 1 receptor antagonist [DIRA] M04.8
  ornithine transcarbamylase E72.4
  ovarian E28.39
  oxygen —*see* Anoxia
  pantothenic acid E53.8
  parathyroid (gland) E20.9
  perineum (female) N81.89
  phenylalanine hydroxylase E70.1
  phosphoenolpyruvate carboxykinase E74.4
  phosphofructokinase E74.19
  phosphomannomutase E74.8
  phosphomannose isomerase E74.8
  phosphomannosyl mutase E74.8
  phosphorylase kinase, liver E74.09
  pituitary hormone (isolated) E23.0
  plasma thromboplastin
    antecedent (PTA) D68.1
    component (PTC) D67
  platelet NEC D69.1
    constitutional D68.0
  polyglandular E31.8
    autoimmune E31.0
  potassium (K) E87.6
  prepuce N47.3
  proaccelerin (congenital) (hereditary) D68.2
    acquired D68.4
  proconvertin factor (congenital) (hereditary) D68.2
    acquired D68.4
  protein —*see also* Malnutrition E46
    anemia D53.0
    C D68.59
    S D68.59
  prothrombin (congenital) (heredItary) D68.2
    acquired D68.4
  Prower factor D68.2
  pseudocholinesterase E88.09
  PTA (plasma thromboplastin antecedent) D68.1
  PTC (plasma thromboplastin component) D67
  purine nucleoside phosphorylase (PNP) D81.5
  pyracin (alpha) (beta) E53.1
  pyridoxal E53.1
  pyridoxamine E53.1
  pyridoxine (derivatives) E53.1
  pyruvate
    carboxylase E74.4
    dehydrogenase E74.4
  riboflavin (vitamin B2) E53.0

Deficiency, deficient *(Continued)*
  salt E87.1
  secretion
    ovary E28.39
    salivary gland (any) K11.7
    urine R34
  selenium (dietary) E59
  serum antitrypsin, familial E88.01
  short stature homeobox gene (SHOX)
    with
      dyschondrosteosis Q78.8
      short stature (idiopathic) E34.3
      Turner's syndrome Q96.9
  sodium (Na) E87.1
  SPCA (factor VII) D68.2
  sphincter, intrinsic N36.42
    with urethral hypermobility N36.43
  stable factor (congenital) (hereditary) D68.2
    acquired D68.4
  Stuart-Prower (factor X) D68.2
  sucrase E74.39
  sulfatase E75.29
  sulfite oxidase E72.19
  thiamin, thiaminic (chloride) E51.9
    beriberi (dry) E51.11
      wet E51.12
  thrombokinase D68.2
    newborn P53
  thyroid (gland) —*see* Hypothyroidism
  tocopherol E56.0
  tooth bud K00.0
  transcobalamine II (anemia) D51.2
  vanadium E61.6
  vascular I99.9
  vasopressin E23.2
  vertical ridge K06.8
  viosterol —*see* Deficiency, calciferol
  vitamin (multiple) NOS E56.9
    A E50.9
      with
        Bitot's spot (corneal) E50.1
        follicular keratosis E50.8
        keratomalacia E50.4
        manifestations NEC E50.8
        night blindness E50.5
        scar of cornea, xerophthalmic E50.6
        xeroderma E50.8
        xerophthalmia E50.7
        xerosis
          conjunctival E50.0
            and Bitot's spot E50.1
          cornea E50.2
            and ulceration E50.3
      sequelae E64.1
    B (complex) NOS E53.9
      with
        beriberi (dry) E51.11
          wet E51.12
        pellagra E52
    B1 NOS E51.9
      beriberi (dry) E51.11
        with circulatory system manifestations E51.11
        wet E51.12
    B12 E53.8
    B2 (riboflavin) E53.0
    B6 E53.1
    C E54
      sequelae E64.2
    D E55.9
      with
        adult osteomalacia M83.8
        rickets —*see* Rickets
      25-hydroxylase E83.32
    E E56.0
    folic acid E53.8
    G E53.0
    group B E53.9
      specified NEC E53.8

Deficiency, deficient *(Continued)*
  vitamin *(Continued)*
    H (biotin) E53.8
    K E56.1
      of newborn P53
    nicotinic E52
    P E56.8
    PP (pellagra-preventing) E52
    specified NEC E56.8
    thiamin E51.9
      beriberi —*see* Beriberi
  zinc, dietary E60
Deficit —*see also* Deficiency
  attention and concentration R41.840
    following
      cerebral infarction I69.310
      cerebrovascular disease I69.910
        specified disease NEC I69.810
      nontraumatic
        intracerebral hemorrhage I69.110
        specified intracranial hemorrhage NEC I69.210
        subarachnoid hemorrhage I69.010
    disorder —*see* Attention, deficit
  cognitive
    communication R41.841
    emotional
      following
        cerebral infarction I69.315
        cerebrovascular disease I69.915
          specified disease NEC I69.815
        nontraumatic
          intracerebral hemorrhage I69.115
          specified intracranial hemorrhage NEC I69.215
          subarachnoid hemorrhage I69.015
      following
        cerebral infarction I69.319
        cerebrovascular disease I69.919
          specified disease NEC I69.819
        nontraumatic
          intracerebral hemorrhage I69.119
          specified intracranial hemorrhage NEC I69.219
          subarachnoid hemorrhage I69.019
    social
      following
        cerebral infarction I69.315
        cerebrovascular disease I69.915
          specified disease NEC I69.815
        nontraumatic
          intracerebral hemorrhage I69.115
          specified intracranial hemorrhage NEC I69.215
          subarachnoid hemorrhage I69.015
  cognitive NEC R41.89
    following
      cerebral infarction I69.318
      cerebrovascular disease I69.918
        specified disease NEC I69.818
      nontraumatic
        intracerebral hemorrhage I69.118
        specified intracranial hemorrhage NEC I69.218
        subarachnoid hemorrhage I69.018
  concentration R41.840
  executive function R41.844
    following
      cerebral infarction I69.314
      cerebrovascular disease I69.914
        specified disease NEC I69.814
      nontraumatic
        intracerebral hemorrhage I69.114
        specified intracranial hemorrhage NEC I69.214
        subarachnoid hemorrhage I69.014
  frontal lobe R41.844
    following
      cerebral infarction I69.314
      cerebrovascular disease I69.914
        specified disease NEC I69.814

▶ New   ➡ Revised   ~~deleted~~ Deleted   ● Use Additional Character(s)

Deficit *(Continued)*
  frontal lobe *(Continued)*
    following *(Continued)*
      nontraumatic
        intracerebral hemorrhage I69.114
        specified intracranial hemorrhage
          NEC I69.214
        subarachnoid hemorrhage I69.014
  memory
    following
      cerebral infarction I69.311
      cerebrovascular disease I69.911
        specified disease NEC I69.811
      nontraumatic
        intracerebral hemorrhage I69.111
        specified intracranial hemorrhage
          NEC I69.211
        subarachnoid hemorrhage I69.011
  neurologic NEC R29.818
    ischemic
      reversible (RIND) I63.9
        prolonged (PRIND) I63.9
  oxygen R09.02
  prolonged reversible ischemic neurologic
    (PRIND) I63.9
  psychomotor R41.843
    following
      cerebral infarction I69.313
      cerebrovascular disease I69.913
        specified disease NEC I69.813
      nontraumatic
        intracerebral hemorrhage I69.113
        specified intracranial hemorrhage
          NEC I69.213
        subarachnoid hemorrhage
          I69.013
  visuospatial R41.842
    following
      cerebral infarction I69.312
      cerebrovascular disease I69.912
        specified disease NEC I69.812
      nontraumatic
        intracerebral hemorrhage I69.112
        specified intracranial hemorrhage
          NEC I69.212
        subarachnoid hemorrhage I69.012

Deflection
  radius —*see* Deformity, limb, specified type
    NEC, forearm
  septum (acquired) (nasal) (nose) J34.2
  spine —*see* Curvature, spine
  turbinate (nose) J34.2

Defluvium
  capillorum —*see* Alopecia
  ciliorum —*see* Madarosis
  unguium L60.8

Deformity Q89.9
  abdomen, congenital Q89.9
  abdominal wall
    acquired M95.8
    congenital Q79.59
  acquired (unspecified site) M95.9
  adrenal gland Q89.1
  alimentary tract, congenital Q45.9
    upper Q40.9
  ankle (joint) (acquired) —*see also* Deformity,
    limb, lower leg
    abduction —*see* Contraction, joint, ankle
    congenital Q68.8
    contraction —*see* Contraction, joint, ankle
    specified type NEC —*see* Deformity, limb,
      foot, specified NEC
  anus (acquired) K62.89
    congenital Q43.9
  aorta (arch) (congenital) Q25.40
    acquired I77.89
  aortic
    arch, acquired I77.89
    cusp or valve (congenital) Q23.8
      acquired —*see also* Endocarditis, aortic
        I35.8

Deformity *(Continued)*
  arm (acquired) (upper) —*see also* Deformity,
    limb, upper arm
    congenital Q68.8
    forearm —*see* Deformity, limb, forearm
  artery (congenital) (peripheral) NOS Q27.9
    acquired I77.89
    coronary (acquired) I25.9
      congenital Q24.5
    umbilical Q27.0
  atrial septal Q21.1
  auditory canal (external) (congenital) —*see
    also* Malformation, ear, external
    acquired —*see* Disorder, ear, external,
      specified type NEC
  auricle
    ear (congenital) —*see also* Malformation,
      ear, external
      acquired —*see* Disorder, pinna,
        deformity
  back —*see* Dorsopathy, deforming
  bile duct (common) (congenital) (hepatic)
    Q44.5
    acquired K83.8
  biliary duct or passage (congenital) Q44.5
    acquired K83.8
  bladder (neck) (trigone) (sphincter)
    (acquired) N32.89
    congenital Q64.79
  bone (acquired) NOS M95.9
    congenital Q79.9
    turbinate M95.0
  brain (congenital) Q04.9
    acquired G93.89
    reduction Q04.3
  breast (acquired) N64.89
    congenital Q83.9
    reconstructed N65.0
  bronchus (congenital) Q32.4
    acquired NEC J98.09
  bursa, congenital Q79.9
  canaliculi (lacrimalis) (acquired) —*see also*
    Disorder, lacrimal system, changes
    congenital Q10.6
  canthus, acquired —*see* Disorder, eyelid,
    specified type NEC
  capillary (acquired) I78.8
  cardiovascular system, congenital Q28.9
  caruncle, lacrimal (acquired) —*see also*
    Disorder, lacrimal system, changes
    congenital Q10.6
  cascade, stomach K31.2
  cecum (congenital) Q43.9
    acquired K63.89
  cerebral, acquired G93.89
    congenital Q04.9
  cervix (uterus) (acquired) NEC N88.8
    congenital Q51.9
  cheek (acquired) M95.2
    congenital Q18.9
  chest (acquired) (wall) M95.4
    congenital Q67.8
    sequelae (late effect) of rickets E64.3
  chin (acquired) M95.2
    congenital Q18.9
  choroid (congenital) Q14.3
    acquired H31.8
    plexus Q07.8
      acquired G96.19
  cicatricial —*see* Cicatrix
  cilia, acquired —*see* Disorder, eyelid,
    specified type NEC
  clavicle (acquired) M95.8
    congenital Q68.8
  clitoris (congenital) Q52.6
    acquired N90.89
  clubfoot —*see* Clubfoot
  coccyx (acquired) —*see* subcategory
    M43.8
  colon (congenital) Q43.9
    acquired K63.89

Deformity *(Continued)*
  concha (ear), congenital —*see also*
    Malformation, ear, external
    acquired —*see* Disorder, pinna, deformity
  cornea (acquired) H18.70
    congenital Q13.4
    descemetocele —*see* Descemetocele
    ectasia —*see* Ectasia, cornea
    specified NEC H18.79-●
    staphyloma —*see* Staphyloma, cornea
  coronary artery (acquired) I25.9
    congenital Q24.5
  cranium (acquired) —*see* Deformity,
    skull
  cricoid cartilage (congenital) Q31.8
    acquired J38.7
  cystic duct (congenital) Q44.5
    acquired K82.8
  Dandy-Walker Q03.1
    with spina bifida —*see* Spina bifida
  diaphragm (congenital) Q79.1
    acquired J98.6
  digestive organ NOS Q45.9
  ductus arteriosus Q25.0
  duodenal bulb K31.89
  duodenum (congenital) Q43.9
    acquired K31.89
  dura —*see* Deformity, meninges
  ear (acquired) —*see also* Disorder, pinna,
    deformity
    congenital (external) Q17.9
      internal Q16.5
      middle Q16.4
        ossicles Q16.3
      ossicles Q16.3
  ectodermal (congenital) NEC Q84.9
  ejaculatory duct (congenital) Q55.4
    acquired N50.89
  elbow (joint) (acquired) —*see also* Deformity,
    limb, upper arm
    congenital Q68.8
    contraction —*see* Contraction, joint,
      elbow
  endocrine gland NEC Q89.2
  epididymis (congenital) Q55.4
    acquired N50.89
  epiglottis (congenital) Q31.8
    acquired J38.7
  esophagus (congenital) Q39.9
    acquired K22.8
  eustachian tube (congenital) NEC Q17.8
  eye, congenital Q15.9
  eyebrow (congenital) Q18.8
  eyelid (acquired) —*see also* Disorder, eyelid,
    specified type NEC
    congenital Q10.3
  face (acquired) M95.2
    congenital Q18.9
  fallopian tube, acquired N83.8
  femur (acquired) —*see* Deformity, limb,
    specified type NEC, thigh
  fetal
    with fetopelvic disproportion O33.7
    causing obstructed labor O66.3
  finger (acquired) M20.00-●
    boutonniere M20.02-●
    congenital Q68.1
    flexion contracture —*see* Contraction, joint,
      hand
    mallet finger M20.01-●
    specified NEC M20.09-●
    swan-neck M20.03-●
  flexion (joint) (acquired) —*see also* Deformity,
    limb, flexion M21.20
    congenital NOS Q74.9
      hip Q65.89
  foot (acquired) —*see also* Deformity, limb,
    lower leg
    cavovarus (congenital) Q66.1
    congenital NOS Q66.9
      specified type NEC Q66.89

Deformity *(Continued)*
  foot *(Continued)*
    specified type NEC —*see* Deformity, limb, foot, specified NEC
    valgus (congenital) Q66.6
      acquired —*see* Deformity, valgus, ankle
    varus (congenital) NEC Q66.3
      acquired —*see* Deformity, varus, ankle
  forearm (acquired) —*see also* Deformity, forearm
    congenital Q68.8
  forehead (acquired) M95.2
    congenital Q75.8
  frontal bone (acquired) M95.2
    congenital Q75.8
  gallbladder (congenital) Q44.1
    acquired K82.8
  gastrointestinal tract (congenital) NOS Q45.9
    acquired K63.89
  genitalia, genital organ(s) or system NEC
    female (congenital) Q52.9
      acquired N94.89
      external Q52.70
    male (congenital) Q55.9
      acquired N50.89
  globe (eye) (congenital) Q15.8
    acquired H44.89
  gum, acquired NEC K06.8
  hand (acquired) —*see* Deformity, limb, hand
    congenital Q68.1
  head (acquired) M95.2
    congenital Q75.8
  heart (congenital) Q24.9
    septum Q21.9
      auricular Q21.1
      ventricular Q21.0
    valve (congenital) NEC Q24.8
      acquired —*see* Endocarditis
  heel (acquired) —*see* Deformity, foot
  hepatic duct (congenital) Q44.5
    acquired K83.8
  hip (joint) (acquired) —*see also* Deformity, limb, thigh
    congenital Q65.9
    due to (previous) juvenile osteochondrosis —*see* Coxa, plana
    flexion —*see* Contraction, joint, hip
  hourglass —*see* Contraction, hourglass
  humerus (acquired) M21.82-●
    congenital Q74.0
  hypophyseal (congenital) Q89.2
  ileocecal (coil) (valve) (acquired) K63.89
    congenital Q43.9
  ileum (congenital) Q43.9
    acquired K63.89
  ilium (acquired) M95.5
    congenital Q74.2
  integument (congenital) Q84.9
  intervertebral cartilage or disc (acquired) — *see* Disorder, disc, specified NEC
  intestine (large) (small) (congenital) NOS Q43.9
    acquired K63.89
  intrinsic minus or plus (hand) —*see* Deformity, limb, specified type NEC, forearm
  iris (acquired) H21.89
    congenital Q13.2
  ischium (acquired) M95.5
    congenital Q74.2
  jaw (acquired) (congenital) M26.9
  joint (acquired) NEC M21.90
    congenital Q68.8
    elbow M21.92-●
    hand M21.94-●
    hip M21.95-●
    knee M21.96-●
    shoulder M21.92-●
    wrist M21.93-●

Deformity *(Continued)*
  kidney(s) (calyx) (pelvis) (congenital) Q63.9
    acquired N28.89
    artery (congenital) Q27.2
      acquired I77.89
  Klippel-Feil (brevicollis) Q76.1
  knee (acquired) NEC —*see also* Deformity, limb, lower leg
    congenital Q68.2
  labium (majus) (minus) (congenital) Q52.79
    acquired N90.89
  lacrimal passages or duct (congenital) NEC Q10.6
    acquired —*see* Disorder, lacrimal system, changes
  larynx (muscle) (congenital) Q31.8
    acquired J38.7
    web (glottic) Q31.0
  leg (upper) (acquired) NEC —*see also* Deformity, limb, thigh
    congenital Q68.8
    lower leg —*see* Deformity, limb, lower leg
  lens (acquired) H27.8
    congenital Q12.9
  lid (fold) (acquired) —*see also* Disorder, eyelid, specified type NEC
    congenital Q10.3
  ligament (acquired) —*see* Disorder, ligament
    congenital Q79.9
  limb (acquired) M21.90
    clawfoot M21.53-●
    clawhand M21.51-●
    clubfoot M21.54-●
    clubhand M21.52-●
    congenital, except reduction deformity Q74.9
    flat foot M21.4-●
    flexion M21.20
      ankle M21.27-●
      elbow M21.22-●
      finger M21.24-●
      hip M21.25-●
      knee M21.26-●
      shoulder M21.21-●
      toe M21.27-●
      wrist M21.23-●
    foot
      claw —*see* Deformity, limb, clawfoot
      club —*see* Deformity, limb, clubfoot
      drop M21.37-●
      flat —*see* Deformity, limb, flat foot
      specified NEC M21.6X-●
    forearm M21.93-●
    hand M21.94-●
    lower leg M21.96-●
    specified type NEC M21.80
      forearm M21.83-●
      lower leg M21.86-●
      thigh M21.85-●
      upper arm M21.82-●
    thigh M21.95-●
    unequal length M21.70
      short site is
        femur M21.75-●
        fibula M21.76-●
        humerus M21.72-●
        radius M21.73-●
        tibia M21.76-●
        ulna M21.73-●
    upper arm M21.92-●
    valgus —*see* Deformity, valgus
    varus —*see* Deformity, varus
    wrist drop M21.33-●
  lip (acquired) NEC K13.0
    congenital Q38.0
  liver (congenital) Q44.7
    acquired K76.89
  lumbosacral (congenital) (joint) (region) Q76.49
    acquired —*see* subcategory M43.8
    kyphosis —*see* Kyphosis, congenital
    lordosis —*see* Lordosis, congenital

Deformity *(Continued)*
  lung (congenital) Q33.9
    acquired J98.4
  lymphatic system, congenital Q89.9
  Madelung's (radius) Q74.0
  mandible (acquired) (congenital) M26.9
  maxilla (acquired) (congenital) M26.9
  meninges or membrane (congenital) Q07.9
    cerebral Q04.8
      acquired G96.19
    spinal cord (congenital) G96.19
      acquired G96.19
  metacarpus (acquired) —*see* Deformity, limb, forearm
    congenital Q74.0
  metatarsus (acquired) —*see* Deformity, foot
    congenital Q66.9
  middle ear (congenital) Q16.4
    ossicles Q16.3
  mitral (leaflets) (valve) I05.8
    parachute Q23.2
    stenosis, congenital Q23.2
  mouth (acquired) K13.79
    congenital Q38.6
  multiple, congenital NEC Q89.7
  muscle (acquired) M62.89
    congenital Q79.9
      sternocleidomastoid Q68.0
  musculoskeletal system (acquired) M95.9
    congenital Q79.9
    specified NEC M95.8
  nail (acquired) L60.8
    congenital Q84.6
  nasal —*see* Deformity, nose
  neck (acquired) M95.3
    congenital Q18.9
    sternocleidomastoid Q68.0
  nervous system (congenital) Q07.9
  nipple (congenital) Q83.9
    acquired N64.89
  nose (acquired) (cartilage) M95.0
    bone (turbinate) M95.0
    congenital Q30.9
      bent or squashed Q67.4
    saddle M95.0
      syphilitic A50.57
    septum (acquired) J34.2
      congenital Q30.8
    sinus (wall) (congenital) Q30.8
      acquired M95.0
    syphilitic (congenital) A50.57
      late A52.73
  ocular muscle (congenital) Q10.3
    acquired —*see* Strabismus, mechanical
  opticociliary vessels (congenital) Q13.2
  orbit (eye) (acquired) H05.30
    atrophy —*see* Atrophy, orbit
    congenital Q10.7
    due to
      bone disease NEC H05.32-●
      trauma or surgery H05.33-●
    enlargement —*see* Enlargement, orbit
    exostosis —*see* Exostosis, orbit
  organ of Corti (congenital) Q16.5
  ovary (congenital) Q50.39
    acquired N83.8
  oviduct, acquired N83.8
  palate (congenital) Q38.5
    acquired M27.8
    cleft (congenital) —*see* Cleft, palate
  pancreas (congenital) Q45.3
    acquired K86.89
  parathyroid (gland) Q89.2
  parotid (gland) (congenital) Q38.4
    acquired K11.8
  patella (acquired) —*see* Disorder, patella, specified NEC
  pelvis, pelvic (acquired) (bony) M95.5
    with disproportion (fetopelvic) O33.0
      causing obstructed labor O65.0

▶ New   ⇒ Revised   ~~deleted~~ Deleted   ● Use Additional Character(s)

Deformity (Continued)
  pelvis, pelvic (Continued)
    congenital Q74.2
    rachitic sequelae (late effect) E64.3
  penis (glans) (congenital) Q55.69
    acquired N48.89
  pericardium (congenital) Q24.8
    acquired —see Pericarditis
  pharynx (congenital) Q38.8
    acquired J39.2
  pinna, acquired —see also Disorder, pinna,
      deformity
    congenital Q17.9
  pituitary (congenital) Q89.2
  posture —see Dorsopathy, deforming
  prepuce (congenital) Q55.69
    acquired N47.8
  prostate (congenital) Q55.4
    acquired N42.89
  pupil (congenital) Q13.2
    acquired —see Abnormality, pupillary
  pylorus (congenital) Q40.3
    acquired K31.89
  rachitic (acquired), old or healed E64.3
  radius (acquired) —see also Deformity, limb,
      forearm
    congenital Q68.8
  rectum (congenital) Q43.9
    acquired K62.89
  reduction (extremity) (limb), congenital (see
      also condition and site) Q73.8
    brain Q04.3
    lower —see Defect, reduction, lower limb
    upper —see Defect, reduction, upper
      limb
  renal —see Deformity, kidney
  respiratory system (congenital) Q34.9
  rib (acquired) M95.4
    congenital Q76.6
    cervical Q76.5
  rotation (joint) (acquired) —see Deformity,
      limb, specified site NEC
    congenital Q74.9
    hip —see Deformity, limb, specified type
      NEC, thigh
    congenital Q65.89
  sacroiliac joint (congenital) Q74.2
    acquired —see subcategory M43.8
  sacrum (acquired) —see subcategory
      M43.8
  saddle
    back —see Lordosis
    nose M95.0
      syphilitic A50.57
  salivary gland or duct (congenital) Q38.4
    acquired K11.8
  scapula (acquired) M95.8
    congenital Q68.8
  scrotum (congenital) —see also Malformation,
      testis and scrotum
    acquired N50.89
  seminal vesicles (congenital) Q55.4
    acquired N50.89
  septum, nasal (acquired) J34.2
  shoulder (joint) (acquired) —see Deformity,
      limb, upper arm
    congenital Q74.0
    contraction —see Contraction, joint,
      shoulder
  sigmoid (flexure) (congenital) Q43.9
    acquired K63.89
  skin (congenital) Q82.9
  skull (acquired) M95.2
    congenital Q75.8
      with
        anencephaly Q00.0
        encephalocele —see Encephalocele
        hydrocephalus Q03.9
          with spina bifida —see Spina bifida,
            by site, with hydrocephalus
        microcephaly Q02

Deformity (Continued)
  soft parts, organs or tissues (of pelvis)
    in pregnancy or childbirth NEC O34.8-●
      causing obstructed labor O65.5
  spermatic cord (congenital) Q55.4
    acquired N50.89
    torsion —see Torsion, spermatic cord
  spinal —see Dorsopathy, deforming
    column (acquired) —see Dorsopathy,
      deforming
    congenital Q67.5
    cord (congenital) Q06.9
      acquired G95.89
    nerve root (congenital) Q07.9
  spine (acquired) —see also Dorsopathy,
      deforming
    congenital Q67.5
    rachitic E64.3
    specified NEC —see Dorsopathy,
      deforming, specified NEC
  spleen
    acquired D73.89
    congenital Q89.09
  Sprengel's (congenital) Q74.0
  sternocleidomastoid (muscle), congenital
      Q68.0
  sternum (acquired) M95.4
    congenital NEC Q76.7
  stomach (congenital) Q40.3
    acquired K31.89
  submandibular gland (congenital) Q38.4
  submaxillary gland (congenital) Q38.4
    acquired K11.8
  talipes —see Talipes
  testis (congenital) —see also Malformation,
      testis and scrotum
    acquired N44.8
    torsion —see Torsion, testis
  thigh (acquired) —see also Deformity, limb,
      thigh
    congenital NEC Q68.8
  thorax (acquired) (wall) M95.4
    congenital Q67.8
    sequelae of rickets E64.3
  thumb (acquired) —see also Deformity, finger
    congenital NEC Q68.1
  thymus (tissue) (congenital) Q89.2
  thyroid (gland) (congenital) Q89.2
    cartilage Q31.8
      acquired J38.7
  tibia (acquired) —see also Deformity, limb,
      specified type NEC, lower leg
    congenital NEC Q68.8
    saber (syphilitic) A50.56
  toe (acquired) M20.6-●
    congenital Q66.9
    hallux rigidus M20.2-●
    hallux valgus M20.1-●
    hallux varus M20.3-●
    hammer toe M20.4-●
    specified NEC M20.5X-●
  tongue (congenital) Q38.3
    acquired K14.8
  tooth, teeth K00.2
  trachea (rings) (congenital) Q32.1
    acquired J39.8
  transverse aortic arch (congenital)
      Q25.49
  tricuspid (leaflets) (valve) I07.8
    atresia or stenosis Q22.4
    Ebstein's Q22.5
  trunk (acquired) M95.8
    congenital Q89.9
  ulna (acquired) —see also Deformity, limb,
      forearm
    congenital NEC Q68.8
  urachus, congenital Q64.4
  ureter (opening) (congenital) Q62.8
    acquired N28.89
  urethra (congenital) Q64.79
    acquired N36.8

Deformity (Continued)
  urinary tract (congenital) Q64.9
    urachus Q64.4
  uterus (congenital) Q51.9
    acquired N85.8
  uvula (congenital) Q38.5
  vagina (acquired) N89.8
    congenital Q52.4
  valgus NEC M21.00
    ankle M21.07-●
    elbow M21.02-●
    hip M21.05-●
    knee M21.06-●
  valve, valvular (congenital) (heart) Q24.8
    acquired —see Endocarditis
  varus NEC M21.10
    ankle M21.17-●
    elbow M21.12-●
    hip M21.15
    knee M21.16-●
    tibia —see Osteochondrosis, juvenile, tibia
  vas deferens (congenital) Q55.4
    acquired N50.89
  vein (congenital) Q27.9
    great Q26.9
  vertebra —see Dorsopathy, deforming
  vertical talus (congenital) Q66.80
    left foot Q66.82
    right foot Q66.81
  vesicourethral orifice (acquired) N32.89
    congenital NEC Q64.79
  vessels of optic papilla (congenital) Q14.2
  visual field (contraction) —see Defect, visual
      field
  vitreous body, acquired H43.89
  vulva (congenital) Q52.79
    acquired N90.89
  wrist (joint) (acquired) —see also Deformity,
      limb, forearm
    congenital Q68.8
    contraction —see Contraction, joint, wrist
Degeneration, degenerative
  adrenal (capsule) (fatty) (gland) (hyaline)
      (infectional) E27.8
  amyloid —see also Amyloidosis E85.9
  anterior cornua, spinal cord G12.29
  anterior labral S43.49-●
  aorta, aortic I70.0
    fatty I77.89
  aortic valve (heart) —see Endocarditis,
      aortic
  arteriovascular —see Arteriosclerosis
  artery, arterial (atheromatous) (calcareous) —
      see also Arteriosclerosis
    cerebral, amyloid E85.4 [168.0]
    medial —see Arteriosclerosis, extremities
  articular cartilage NEC —see Derangement,
      joint, articular cartilage, by site
  atheromatous —see Arteriosclerosis
  basal nuclei or ganglia G23.9
    specified NEC G23.8
  bone NEC —see Disorder, bone, specified
      type NEC
  brachial plexus G54.0
  brain (cortical) (progressive) G31.9
    alcoholic G31.2
    arteriosclerotic I67.2
    childhood G31.9
      specified NEC G31.89
    cystic G31.89
      congenital Q04.6
    in
      alcoholism G31.2
      beriberi E51.2
      cerebrovascular disease I67.9
      congenital hydrocephalus Q03.9
        with spina bifida —see also Spina
          bifida
      Fabry-Anderson disease E75.21
      Gaucher's disease E75.22
      Hunter's syndrome E76.1

Degeneration, degenerative *(Continued)*
  brain *(Continued)*
    in *(Continued)*
      lipidosis
        cerebral E75.4
        generalized E75.6
      mucopolysaccharidosis —*see*
        Mucopolysaccharidosis
      myxedema E03.9 *[G32.89]*
      neoplastic disease —*see also* Neoplasm
        D49.6 *[G32.89]*
      Niemann-Pick disease E75.249 *[G32.89]*
      sphingolipidosis E75.3 *[G32.89]*
      vitamin B12 deficiency E53.8 *[G32.89]*
    senile NEC G31.1
  breast N64.89
  Bruch's membrane —*see* Degeneration,
    choroid
  capillaries (fatty) I78.8
  ➡amyloid E85.89 *[I79.8]*
  cardiac —*see also* Degeneration, myocardial
    valve, valvular —*see* Endocarditis
  cardiorenal —*see* Hypertension, cardiorenal
  cardiovascular —*see also* Disease,
    cardiovascular
    renal —*see* Hypertension, cardiorenal
  cerebellar NOS G31.9
    alcoholic G31.2
    primary (hereditary) (sporadic) G11.9
  cerebral —*see* Degeneration, brain
  cerebrovascular I67.9
    due to hypertension I67.4
  cervical plexus G54.2
  cervix N88.8
    due to radiation (intended effect) N88.8
      adverse effect or misadventure N99.89
  chamber angle H21.21-●
  changes, spine or vertebra —*see* Spondylosis
  chorioretinal —*see also* Degeneration, choroid
    hereditary H31.20
  choroid (colloid) (drusen) H31.10-●
    atrophy —*see* Atrophy, choroidal
    hereditary —*see* Dystrophy, choroidal,
      hereditary
  ciliary body H21.22-●
  cochlear —*see* subcategory H83.8
  combined (spinal cord) (subacute) E53.8
    [G32.0]
    with anemia (pernicious) D51.0 *[G32.0]*
      due to dietary vitamin B12 deficiency
        D51.3 *[G32.0]*
    in (due to)
      vitamin B12 deficiency E53.8 *[G32.0]*
        anemia D51.9 *[G32.0]*
  conjunctiva H11.10
    concretions —*see* Concretion, conjunctiva
    deposits —*see* Deposit, conjunctiva
    pigmentations —*see* Pigmentation,
      conjunctiva
    pinguecula —*see* Pinguecula
    xerosis —*see* Xerosis, conjunctiva
  cornea H18.40
    calcerous H18.43
      band keratopathy H18.42-●
    familial, hereditary —*see* Dystrophy, cornea
    hyaline (of old scars) H18.49
    keratomalacia —*see* Keratomalacia
    nodular H18.45-●
    peripheral H18.46-●
    senile H18.41-●
    specified type NEC H18.49
  cortical (cerebellar) (parenchymatous)
    G31.89
    alcoholic G31.2
    diffuse, due to arteriopathy I67.2
  corticobasal G31.85
  cutis L98.8
    amyloid E85.4 *[L99]*
  dental pulp K04.2
  disc disease —*see* Degeneration,
    intervertebral disc NEC

Degeneration, degenerative *(Continued)*
  dorsolateral (spinal cord) —*see* Degeneration,
    combined
  extrapyramidal G25.9
  eye, macular —*see also* Degeneration, macula
    congenital or hereditary —*see* Dystrophy,
      retina
  facet joints —*see* Spondylosis
  fatty
    liver NEC K76.0
      alcoholic K70.0
  grey matter (brain) (Alpers') G31.81
  heart —*see also* Degeneration, myocardial
    amyloid E85.4 *[I43]*
    atheromatous —*see* Disease, heart,
      ischemic, atherosclerotic
    ischemic —*see* Disease, heart, ischemic
  hepatolenticular (Wilson's) E83.01
  hepatorenal K76.7
  hyaline (diffuse) (generalized)
    localized —*see* Degeneration, by site
  infrapatellar fat pad M79.4
  intervertebral disc NOS
    with
      myelopathy —*see* Disorder, disc, with,
        myelopathy
      radiculitis or radiculopathy —*see*
        Disorder, disc, with, radiculopathy
    cervical, cervicothoracic —*see* Disorder,
      disc, cervical, degeneration
      with
        myelopathy —*see* Disorder, disc,
          cervical, with myelopathy
        neuritis, radiculitis or
          radiculopathy —*see* Disorder,
          disc, cervical, with neuritis
    lumbar region M51.36
      with
        myelopathy M51.06
        neuritis, radiculitis, radiculopathy or
          sciatica M51.16
    lumbosacral region M51.37
      with
        neuritis, radiculitis, radiculopathy or
          sciatica M51.17
    sacrococcygeal region M53.3
    thoracic region M51.34
      with
        myelopathy M51.04
        neuritis, radiculitis, radiculopathy
          M51.14
    thoracolumbar region M51.35
      with
        myelopathy M51.05
        neuritis, radiculitis, radiculopathy
          M51.15
  intestine, amyloid E85.4
  iris (pigmentary) H21.23-●
  ischemic —*see* Ischemia
  joint disease —*see* Osteoarthritis
  kidney N28.89
    amyloid E85.4 *[N29]*
    cystic, congenital Q61.9
    fatty N28.89
    polycystic Q61.3
      adult type (autosomal dominant)
        Q61.2
      infantile type (autosomal recessive) NEC
        Q61.19
        collecting duct dilatation Q61.11
  Kuhnt-Junius —*see also* Degeneration, macula
    H35.32-●
  lens —*see* Cataract
  lenticular (familial) (progressive) (Wilson's)
    (with cirrhosis of liver) E83.01
  liver (diffuse) NEC K76.89
    amyloid E85.4 *[K77]*
    cystic K76.89
      congenital Q44.6
    fatty NEC K76.0
      alcoholic K70.0

Degeneration, degenerative *(Continued)*
  liver *(Continued)*
    hypertrophic K76.89
    parenchymatous, acute or subacute
      K72.00
      with coma K72.01
    pigmentary K76.89
    toxic (acute) K71.9
  lung J98.4
  lymph gland I89.8
    hyaline I89.8
  macula, macular (acquired) (age-related)
    (senile) H35.30
    angioid streaks H35.33
    atrophic age-related H35.31-●
    congenital or hereditary —*see* Dystrophy,
      retina
    cystoid H35.35-●
    drusen H35.36-●
    dry age-related H35.31-●
    exudative H35.32-●
    hole H35.34-●
    nonexudative H35.31-●
    puckering H35.37-●
    toxic H35.38-●
    wet age-related H35.32-●
  membranous labyrinth, congenital (causing
    impairment of hearing) Q16.5
  meniscus —*see* Derangement, meniscus
  mitral —*see* Insufficiency, mitral
  Mönckeberg's —*see* Arteriosclerosis,
    extremities
  motor centers, senile G31.1
  multi-system G90.3
  mural —*see* Degeneration, myocardial
  muscle (fatty) (fibrous) (hyaline)
    (progressive) M62.89
    heart —*see* Degeneration, myocardial
  myelin, central nervous system G37.9
  myocardial, myocardium (fatty) (hyaline)
    (senile) I51.5
    with rheumatic fever (conditions in I00)
      I09.0
      active, acute or subacute I01.2
        with chorea I02.0
      inactive or quiescent (with chorea) I09.0
    hypertensive —*see* Hypertension, heart
    rheumatic —*see* Degeneration, myocardial,
      with rheumatic fever
    syphilitic A52.06
  nasal sinus (mucosa) J32.9
    frontal J32.1
    maxillary J32.0
  nerve —*see* Disorder, nerve
  nervous system G31.9
    alcoholic G31.2
    amyloid E85.4 *[G99.8]*
    autonomic G90.9
    fatty G31.89
    specified NEC G31.89
  nipple N64.89
  olivopontocerebellar (hereditary) (familial)
    G23.8
  osseous labyrinth —*see* subcategory H83.8
  ovary N83.8
    cystic N83.20-●
    microcystic N83.20-●
  pallidal pigmentary (progressive) G23.0
  pancreas K86.89
    tuberculous A18.83
  penis N48.89
  pigmentary (diffuse) (general)
    localized —*see* Degeneration, by site
    pallidal (progressive) G23.0
  pineal gland E34.8
  pituitary (gland) E23.6
  popliteal fat pad M79.4
  posterolateral (spinal cord) —*see*
    Degeneration, combined
  pulmonary valve (heart) I37.8
  pulp (tooth) K04.2

▶ New   ⇒ Revised   ~~deleted~~ Deleted   ● Use Additional Character(s)

Degeneration, degenerative (Continued)
pupillary margin H21.24-●
renal —see Degeneration, kidney
retina H35.9
 hereditary (cerebroretinal) (congenital)
  (juvenile) (macula) (peripheral)
  (pigmentary) —see Dystrophy, retina
 Kuhnt-Junius —see also Degeneration,
  macula H35.32-●
 macula (cystic) (exudative) (hole)
  (nonexudative) (pseudohole) (senile)
  (toxic) —see Degeneration, macula
 peripheral H35.40
  lattice H35.41-●
  microcystoid H35.42-●
  paving stone H35.43-●
  secondary
   pigmentary H35.45-●
   vitreoretinal H35.46-●
  senile reticular H35.44-●
 pigmentary (primary) —see also Dystrophy,
  retina
  secondary —see Degeneration, retina,
   peripheral, secondary
 posterior pole —see Degeneration, macula
saccule, congenital (causing impairment of
 hearing) Q16.5
senile R54
 brain G31.1
 cardiac, heart or myocardium —see
  Degeneration, myocardial
 motor centers G31.1
 vascular —see Arteriosclerosis
sinus (cystic) —see also Sinusitis
 polypoid J33.1
skin L98.8
 amyloid E85.4 [L99]
 colloid L98.8
spinal (cord) G31.89
 amyloid E85.4 [G32.89]
 combined (subacute) —see Degeneration,
  combined
 dorsolateral —see Degeneration, combined
 familial NEC G31.89
 fatty G31.89
 funicular —see Degeneration, combined
 posterolateral —see Degeneration,
  combined
 subacute combined —see Degeneration,
  combined
 tuberculous A17.81
spleen D73.0
 amyloid E85.4 [D77]
stomach K31.89
striatonigral G23.2
suprarenal (capsule) (gland) E27.8
synovial membrane (pulpy) —see Disorder,
 synovium, specified type NEC
tapetoretinal —see Dystrophy, retina
thymus (gland) E32.8
 fatty E32.8
thyroid (gland) E07.89
tricuspid (heart) (valve) I07.9
tuberculous NEC —see Tuberculosis
turbinate J34.89
uterus (cystic) N85.8
vascular (senile) —see Arteriosclerosis
 hypertensive —see Hypertension
vitreoretinal, secondary —see Degeneration,
 retina, peripheral, secondary, vitreoretinal
vitreous (body) H43.81-●
Wallerian —see Disorder, nerve
Wilson's hepatolenticular E83.01
Deglutition
paralysis R13.0
 hysterical F44.4
pneumonia J69.0
Degos' disease I77.89
Dehiscence (of)
amputation stump T87.81
cesarean wound O90.0

Dehiscence (Continued)
closure of
 cornea T81.31
 craniotomy T81.32
 fascia (muscular) (superficial) T81.32
 internal organ or tissue T81.32
 laceration (external) (internal) T81.33
 ligament T81.32
 mucosa T81.31
 muscle or muscle flap T81.32
 ribs or rib cage T81.32
 skin and subcutaneous tissue (full-
  thickness) (superficial) T81.31
 skull T81.32
 sternum (sternotomy) T81.32
 tendon T81.32
 traumatic laceration (external) (internal)
  T81.33
episiotomy O90.1
operation wound NEC T81.31
 external operation wound (superficial)
  T81.31
 internal operation wound (deep)
  T81.32
perineal wound (postpartum) O90.1
traumatic injury wound repair T81.33
wound T81.30
 traumatic repair T81.33
Dehydration E86.0
newborn P74.1
Déjérine-Roussy syndrome G93.89
Déjérine-Sottas disease or neuropathy
 (hypertrophic) G60.0
Déjérine-Thomas atrophy G23.8
Delay, delayed
any plane in pelvis
 complicating delivery O66.9
birth or delivery NOS O63.9
➠closure, ductus arteriosus (Botalli) P29.38
coagulation —see Defect, coagulation
conduction (cardiac) (ventricular) I45.9
delivery, second twin, triplet, etc O63.2
development R62.50
 global F88
 intellectual (specific) F81.9
 language F80.9
  due to hearing loss F80.4
 learning F81.9
 pervasive F84.9
 physiological R62.50
  specified stage NEC R62.0
 reading F81.0
 sexual E30.0
 speech F80.9
  due to hearing loss F80.4
 spelling F81.81
ejaculation F52.32
gastric emptying K30
menarche E30.0
menstruation (cause unknown) N91.0
milestone R62.0
passage of meconium (newborn)
 P76.0
primary respiration P28.9
puberty (constitutional) E30.0
separation of umbilical cord P96.82
sexual maturation, female E30.0
sleep phase syndrome G47.21
union, fracture —see Fracture, by site
vaccination Z28.9
Deletion(s)
autosome Q93.9
 identified by fluorescence in situ
  hybridization (FISH) Q93.89
 identified by in situ hybridization (ISH)
  Q93.89
chromosome
 with complex rearrangements NEC
  Q93.7
 part of NEC Q93.5
 seen only at prometaphase Q93.89

Deletion (Continued)
chromosome (Continued)
 short arm
  4 Q93.3
  5p Q93.4
  22q11.2 Q93.81
  specified NEC Q93.89
 long arm chromosome 18 or 21 Q93.89
  with complex rearrangements NEC
   Q93.7
 microdeletions NEC Q93.88
Delhi boil or button B55.1
Delinquency (juvenile) (neurotic) F91.8
group Z72.810
Delinquent immunization status Z28.3
Delirium, delirious (acute or subacute) (not
 alcohol or drug-induced) (with dementia)
 R41.0
alcoholic (acute) (tremens) (withdrawal)
 F10.921
 with intoxication F10.921
 in
  abuse F10.121
  dependence F10.221
due to (secondary to)
 alcohol
  intoxication F10.921
  in
   abuse F10.121
   dependence F10.221
  withdrawal F10.231
 amphetamine intoxication F15.921
  in
   abuse F15.121
   dependence F15.221
 anxiolytic
  intoxication F13.921
  in
   abuse F13.121
   dependence F13.221
  withdrawal F13.231
 cannabis intoxication (acute) F12.921
  in
   abuse F12.121
   dependence F12.221
 cocaine intoxication (acute) F14.921
  in
   abuse F14.121
   dependence F14.221
 general medical condition F05
 hallucinogen intoxication F16.921
  in
   abuse F16.121
   dependence F16.221
 hypnotic
  intoxication F13.921
  in
   abuse F13.121
   dependence F13.221
  withdrawal F13.231
 inhalant intoxication (acute) F18.921
  in
   abuse F18.121
   dependence F18.221
 multiple etiologies F05
 opioid intoxication (acute) F11.921
  in
   abuse F11.121
   dependence F11.221
 other (or unknown) substance
  F19.921
 phencyclidine intoxication (acute)
  F16.921
  in
   abuse F16.121
   dependence F16.221
 psychoactive substance NEC intoxication
  (acute) F19.921
  in
   abuse F19.121
   dependence F19.221

Delirium, delirious *(Continued)*
  due to *(Continued)*
    sedative
      intoxication F13.921
        in
          abuse F13.121
          dependence F13.221
      withdrawal F13.231
    unknown etiology F05
  exhaustion F43.0
  hysterical F44.89
  postprocedural (postoperative) F05
  puerperal F05
  thyroid —*see* Thyrotoxicosis with thyroid
    storm
  traumatic —*see* Injury, intracranial
  tremens (alcohol-induced) F10.231
    sedative-induced F13.231
Delivery (childbirth) (labor)
  arrested active phase O62.1
  cesarean (for)
    without indication O82
    abnormal
      pelvis (bony) (deformity) (major) NEC
        with disproportion (fetopelvic)
        O33.0
        with obstructed labor O65.0
      presentation or position O32.9
    abruptio placentae —*see also* Abruptio
      placentae O45.9-●
    acromion presentation O32.2
    atony, uterus O62.2
    breech presentation O32.1
      incomplete O32.8
    brow presentation O32.3
    cephalopelvic disproportion O33.9
    cerclage O34.3-●
    chin presentation O32.3
    cicatrix of cervix O34.4-●
    contracted pelvis (general)
      inlet O33.2
      outlet O33.3
    cord presentation or prolapse O69.0
    cystocele O34.8-●
    deformity (acquired) (congenital)
      pelvic organs or tissues NEC O34.8-●
      pelvis (bony) NEC O33.0
    disproportion NOS O33.9
    eclampsia —*see* Eclampsia
    face presentation O32.3
    failed
      forceps O66.5
      induction of labor O61.9
        instrumental O61.1
        mechanical O61.1
        medical O61.0
        specified NEC O61.8
        surgical O61.1
      trial of labor NOS O66.40
        following previous cesarean delivery
        O66.41
      vacuum extraction O66.5
      ventouse O66.5
    fetal-maternal hemorrhage O43.01-●
    hemorrhage (intrapartum) O67.9
      with coagulation defect O67.0
      specified cause NEC O67.8
    high head at term O32.4
    hydrocephalic fetus O33.6
    incarceration of uterus O34.51-●
    incoordinate uterine action O62.4
    increased size, fetus O33.5
    inertia, uterus O62.2
      primary O62.0
      secondary O62.1
    lateroversion, uterus O34.59-●
    mal lie O32.9
    malposition
      fetus O32.9
      pelvic organs or tissues NEC O34.8-●
      uterus NEC O34.59-●

Delivery *(Continued)*
  cesarean *(Continued)*
    malpresentation NOS O32.9
    oblique presentation O32.2
    occurring after 37 completed weeks of
      gestation but before 39 completed
      weeks gestation due to (spontaneous)
      onset of labor O75.82
    oversize fetus O33.5
    pelvic tumor NEC O34.8-●
    placenta previa O44.0-●
      complete O44.0-●
        with hemorrhage O44.1-●
    placental insufficiency O36.51-●
    planned, occurring after 37 completed
      weeks of gestation but before 39
      completed weeks gestation due to
      (spontaneous) onset of labor O75.82
    polyp, cervix O34.4-●
      causing obstructed labor O65.5
    poor dilatation, cervix O62.0
    pre-eclampsia O14.94
      mild O14.04
      moderate O14.04
      severe O14.14
        with hemolysis, elevated liver
          enzymes and low platelet count
          (HELLP) O14.24
    previous
      cesarean delivery O34.219
        classical (vertical) scar O34.212
        low transverse scar O34.211
      surgery (to)
        cervix O34.4-●
        gynecological NEC O34.8-●
        rectum O34.7-●
        uterus O34.29
        vagina O34.6-●
    prolapse
      arm or hand O32.2
      uterus O34.52-●
    prolonged labor NOS O63.9
    rectocele O34.8-●
    retroversion
      uterus O34.53-●
    rigid
      cervix O34.4-●
      pelvic floor O34.8-●
      perineum O34.7-●
      vagina O34.6-●
      vulva O34.7-●
    sacculation, pregnant uterus O34.59-●
    scar(s)
      cervix O34.4-●
      cesarean delivery O34.219
        classical (vertical) O34.212
        low transverse O34.211
      transmural uterine O34.29
      uterus O34.29
    Shirodkar suture in situ O34.3-●
    shoulder presentation O32.2
    stenosis or stricture, cervix O34.4-●
    streptococcus group B (GBS) carrier state
      O99.824
    transmural uterine scar O34.29
    transverse presentation or lie O32.2
    tumor, pelvic organs or tissues NEC
      O34.8-●
      cervix O34.4-●
    umbilical cord presentation or prolapse
      O69.0
  completely normal case O80
  complicated O75.9
    by
      abnormal, abnormality (of)
        forces of labor O62.9
          specified type NEC O62.8
        glucose O99.814
        uterine contractions NOS O62.9
      abruptio placentae —*see also* Abruptio
        placentae O45.9-●

Delivery *(Continued)*
  complicated *(Continued)*
    by *(Continued)*
      abuse
        physical O9A.32
        psychological O9A.52
        sexual O9A.42
      adherent placenta O72.0
        without hemorrhage O73.0
      alcohol use O99.314
      anemia (pre-existing) O99.02
      anesthetic death O74.8
      annular detachment of cervix O71.3
      atony, uterus O62.2
      attempted vacuum extraction and
        forceps O66.5
      Bandl's ring O62.4
      bariatric surgery status O99.844
      biliary tract disorder O26.62
      bleeding —*see* Delivery, complicated by,
        hemorrhage
      blood disorder NEC O99.12
      cervical dystocia (hypotonic) O62.2
        primary O62.0
        secondary O62.1
      circulatory system disorder O99.42
      compression of cord (umbilical) NEC
        O69.2
      condition NEC O99.89
      contraction, contracted ring O62.4
      cord (umbilical)
        around neck
          with compression O69.1
          without compression O69.81
        bruising O69.5
        complication O69.9
          specified NEC O69.89
        compression NEC O69.2
        entanglement O69.2
          without compression O69.82
        hematoma O69.5
        presentation O69.0
        prolapse O69.0
        short O69.3
        thrombosis (vessels) O69.5
        vascular lesion O69.5
      Couvelaire uterus O45.8X-●
      damage to (injury to) NEC
        perineum O71.82
        periurethral tissue O71.82
        vulva O71.82
      delay following rupture of membranes
        (spontaneous) —*see* Pregnancy,
        complicated by, premature rupture
        of membranes
      depressed fetal heart tones O76
      diabetes O24.92
        gestational O24.429
          diet controlled O24.420
          insulin controlled O24.424
          oral drug controlled (antidiabetic)
            (hypoglycemic) O24.425
        pre-existing O24.32
          specified NEC O24.82
          type 1 O24.02
          type 2 O24.12
      diastasis recti (abdominis) O71.89
      dilatation
        bladder O66.8
        cervix incomplete, poor or slow O62.0
      disease NEC O99.89
      disruptio uteri —*see* Delivery,
        complicated by, rupture, uterus
      drug use O99.324
      dysfunction, uterus NOS O62.9
        hypertonic O62.4
        hypotonic O62.2
          primary O62.0
          secondary O62.1
        incoordinate O62.4
      eclampsia O15.1

▶ New   ⇒ Revised   ~~deleted~~ Deleted   ● Use Additional Character(s)

Delivery *(Continued)*
  complicated *(Continued)*
    by *(Continued)*
      embolism (pulmonary) —*see* Embolism,
          obstetric
      endocrine, nutritional or metabolic
          disease NEC O99.284
      failed
        attempted vaginal birth after
            previous cesarean delivery
            O66.41
        induction of labor O61.9
          instrumental O61.1
          mechanical O61.1
          medical O61.0
          specified NEC O61.8
          surgical O61.1
        trial of labor O66.40
      female genital mutilation O65.5
      fetal
        abnormal acid-base balance O68
        acidemia O68
        acidosis O68
        alkalosis O68
        death, early O02.1
        deformity O66.3
        heart rate or rhythm (abnormal) (non-
            reassuring) O76
        hypoxia O77.8
        stress O77.9
          due to drug administration O77.1
          electrocardiographic evidence of
              O77.8
          specified NEC O77.8
          ultrasound evidence of O77.8
      fever during labor O75.2
      gastric banding status O99.844
      gastric bypass status O99.844
      gastrointestinal disease NEC O99.62
      gestational
        diabetes O24.429
          diet controlled O24.420
          insulin (and diet) controlled
              O24.424
          oral drug controlled (antidiabetic)
              (hypoglycemic) O24.425
        edema O12.04
          with proteinuria O12.24
          proteinuria O12.14
      gonorrhea O98.22
      hematoma O71.7
        ischial spine O71.7
        pelvic O71.7
        vagina O71.7
        vulva or perineum O71.7
      hemorrhage (uterine) O67.9
        associated with
          afibrinogenemia O67.0
          coagulation defect O67.0
          hyperfibrinolysis O67.0
          hypofibrinogenemia O67.0
        due to
          low implantation of placenta
              O44.5-●
          low-lying placenta O44.5-●
          placenta previa O44.1-●
            marginal O44.3-●
            partial O44.3-●
          premature separation of placenta
              (normally implanted) *(see also*
              Abruptio placentae) O45.9-●
          retained placenta O72.0
          uterine leiomyoma O67.8
        placenta NEC O67.8
        postpartum NEC (atonic) (immediate)
            O72.1
          with retained or trapped placenta
              O72.0
          delayed O72.2
          secondary O72.2
          third stage O72.0

Delivery *(Continued)*
  complicated *(Continued)*
    by *(Continued)*
      hourglass contraction, uterus O62.4
      hypertension, hypertensive (pre-
          existing) —*see* Hypertension,
          complicated by, childbirth (labor)
      hypotension O26.5-●
      incomplete dilatation (cervix) O62.0
      incoordinate uterus contractions O62.4
      inertia, uterus O62.2
        during latent phase of labor O62.0
        primary O62.0
        secondary O62.1
      infection (maternal) O98.92
        carrier state NEC O99.834
        gonorrhea O98.22
        human immunodeficiency virus (HIV)
            O98.72
        sexually transmitted NEC O98.32
        specified NEC O98.82
        syphilis O98.12
        tuberculosis O98.02
        viral hepatitis O98.42
        viral NEC O98.52
      injury (to mother) *(see also* Delivery,
          complicated, by, damage to)
          O71.9
        nonobstetric O9A.22
          caused by abuse —*see* Delivery,
              complicated by, abuse
      intrauterine fetal death, early O02.1
      inversion, uterus O71.2
      laceration (perineal) O70.9
        anus (sphincter) O70.4
          with third degree laceration —*see*
              also Delivery, complicated, by,
              laceration, perineum, third
              degree O70.20
            with mucosa O70.3
          without third degree laceration
              O70.4
        bladder (urinary) O71.5
        bowel O71.5
        cervix (uteri) O71.3
        fourchette O70.0
        hymen O70.0
        labia O70.0
        pelvic
          floor O70.1
          organ NEC O71.5
        perineum, perineal O70.9
          first degree O70.0
          fourth degree O70.3
          muscles O70.1
          second degree O70.1
          skin O70.0
          slight O70.0
          third degree O70.20
            with
              both external anal sphincter
                  (EAS) and internal anal
                  sphincter (IAS) torn (IIIc)
                  O70.23
              less than 50% of external anal
                  sphincter (EAS) thickness
                  torn (IIIa) O70.21
              more than 50% external anal
                  sphincter (EAS) thickness
                  torn (IIIb) O70.22
            IIIa O70.21
            IIIb O70.22
            IIIc O70.23
          peritoneum (pelvic) O71.5
          rectovaginal (septum) (without
              perineal laceration) O71.4
            with perineum —*see also* Delivery,
                complicated, by, laceration,
                perineum, third degree
                O70.20
              with anal or rectal mucosa O70.3

Delivery *(Continued)*
  complicated *(Continued)*
    by *(Continued)*
      laceration *(Continued)*
        specified NEC O71.89
        sphincter ani —*see* Delivery,
            complicated, by, laceration, anus
            (sphincter)
        urethra O71.5
        uterus O71.81
          before labor O71.81
        vagina, vaginal (deep) (high)
            (without perineal laceration)
            O71.4
          with perineum O70.0
            muscles, with perineum O70.1
        vulva O70.0
      liver disorder O26.62
      malignancy O9A.12
      malnutrition O25.2
      malposition, malpresentation
        without obstruction O32.9 —*see*
            also Delivery, complicated by,
            obstruction
          breech O32.1
          compound O32.6
          face (brow) (chin) O32.3
          footling O38.8
          high head O32.4
          oblique O32.2
          specified NEC O32.8
          transverse O32.2
          unstable lie O32.0
        placenta O44.0-●
          with hemorrhage O44.1-●
        uterus or cervix O65.5
      meconium in amniotic fluid O77.0
      mental disorder NEC O99.344
      metrorrhexis —*see* Delivery, complicated
          by, rupture, uterus
      nervous system disorder O99.354
      obesity (pre-existing) O99.214
      obesity surgery status O99.844
      obstetric trauma O71.9
        specified NEC O71.89
      obstructed labor
        due to
          breech (complete) (frank)
              presentation O64.1
            incomplete O64.8
          brow presenation O64.3
          buttock presentation O64.1
          chin presentation O64.2
          compound presentation O64.5
          contracted pelvis O65.1
          deep transverse arrest O64.0
          deformed pelvis O65.0
          dystocia (fetal) O66.9
            due to
              conjoined twins O66.3
              fetal
                abnormality NEC O66.3
                ascites O66.3
                hydrops O66.3
                meningomyelocele O66.3
                sacral teratoma O66.3
                tumor O66.3
              hydrocephalic fetus O66.3
            shoulder O66.0
          face presentation O64.2
          fetopelvic disproportion O65.4
          footling presentation O64.8
          impacted shoulders O66.0
          incomplete rotation of fetal head
              O64.0
          large fetus O66.2
          locked twins O66.1
          malposition O64.9
            specified NEC O64.8
          malpresentation O64.9
            specified NEC O64.8

Delivery *(Continued)*
  complicated *(Continued)*
    by *(Continued)*
      obstructed labor *(Continued)*
        due to *(Continued)*
          multiple fetuses NEC O66.6
          pelvic
            abnormality (maternal) O65.9
              organ O65.5
              specified NEC O65.8
            contraction
              inlet O65.2
              mid-cavity O65.3
              outlet O65.3
          persistent (position)
            occipitoiliac O64.0
            occipitoposterior O64.0
            occipitosacral O64.0
            occipitotransverse O64.0
          prolapsed arm O64.4
          shoulder presentation O64.4
        specified NEC O66.8
      pathological retraction ring, uterus
        O62.4
      penetration, pregnant uterus by
        instrument O71.1
      perforation —*see* Delivery, complicated
        by, laceration
      placenta, placental
        ablatio —*see also* Abruptio placentae
          O45.9-•
        abnormality O43.9-•
          specified NEC O43.89-•
        abruptio —*see also* Abruptio placentae
          O45.9-•
        accreta O43.21-•
        adherent (with hemorrhage) O72.0
          without hemorrhage O73.0
        detachment (premature) —*see also*
          Abruptio placentae O45.9-•
        disorder O43.9-•
          specified NEC O43.89-•
        hemorrhage NEC O67.8
        increta O43.22-•
        low (implantation) (lying) O44.4-•
          with hemorrhage O44.5-•
        malformation O43.10-•
        malposition O44.0-•
          without hemorrhage O44.1-•
        percreta O43.23-•
        previa (central) (complete) (lateral)
          (total) O44.0-•
          with hemorrhage O44.1-•
            marginal O44.2-•
              with hemorrhage O44.3-•
            partial O44.2-•
              with hemorrhage O44.3-•
        retained (with hemorrhage) O72.0
          without hemorrhage O73.0
        separation (premature) O45.9-•
          specified NEC O45.8X-•
        vicious insertion O44.1-•
      precipitate labor O62.3
      premature rupture, membranes *(see
        also* Pregnancy, complicated by,
        premature rupture of membranes)
        O42.90
      prolapse
        arm or hand O32.2
        cord (umbilical) O69.0
        foot or leg O32.8
        uterus O34.52-•
      prolonged labor O63.9
        first stage O63.0
        second stage O63.1
      protozoal disease (maternal) O98.62
      respiratory disease NEC O99.52
      retained membranes or portions of
        placenta O72.2
        without hemorrhage O73.1
      retarded birth O63.9

Delivery *(Continued)*
  complicated *(Continued)*
    by *(Continued)*
      retention of secundines (with
        hemorrhage) O72.0
        without hemorrhage O73.0
        partial O72.2
          without hemorrhage O73.1
      rupture
        bladder (urinary) O71.5
        cervix O71.3
        pelvic organ NEC O71.5
        urethra O71.5
        uterus (during or after labor) O71.1
          before labor O71.0-•
      separation, pubic bone (symphysis
        pubis) O71.6
      shock O75.1
      shoulder presentation O64.4
      skin disorder NEC O99.72
      spasm, cervix O62.4
      stenosis or stricture, cervix O65.5
      streptococcus group B (GBS) carrier state
        O99.824
      subluxation of symphysis (pubis)
        O26.72
      syphilis (maternal) O98.12
      tear —*see* Delivery, complicated by,
        laceration
      tetanic uterus O62.4
      trauma (obstetrical) —*see also* Delivery,
        complicated, by, damage to O71.9
        non-obstetric O9A.22
        periurethral O71.82
        specified NEC O71.89
      tuberculosis (maternal) O98.02
      tumor, pelvic organs or tissues NEC
        O65.5
      umbilical cord around neck
        with compression O69.1
        without compression O69.81
      uterine inertia O62.2
        during latent phase of labor O62.0
        primary O62.0
        secondary O62.1
      vasa previa O69.4
      velamentous insertion of cord O43.12-•
    specified complication NEC O75.89
  delayed NOS O63.9
    following rupture of membranes
      artificial O75.5
    second twin, triplet, etc. O63.2
  forceps, low following failed vacuum
    extraction O66.5
  missed (at or near term) O36.4
  normal O80
➡ obstructed —*see* Delivery, complicated by,
    obstructed labor
  precipitate O62.3
  preterm —*see also* Pregnancy, complicated by,
    preterm labor O60.10
  spontaneous O80
  term pregnancy NOS O80
  uncomplicated O80
  vaginal, following previous cesarean delivery
    O34.219
    classical (vertical) scar O34.212
    low transverse scar O34.211
Delusions (paranoid) —*see* Disorder, delusional
Dementia (degenerative (primary)) (old age)
    (persisting) F03.90
  with
    aggressive behavior F03.91
    behavioral disturbance F03.91
    combative behavior F03.91
    Lewy bodies G31.83 *[F02.80]*
      with behavioral disturbance G31.83
        [F02.81]
    Parkinson's disease G20 *[F02.80]*
      with behavioral disturbance G20
        [F02.81]

Dementia *(Continued)*
  with *(Continued)*
    Parkinsonism G31.83 *[F02.80]*
      with behavioral disturbance G31.83
        [F02.81]
    violent behavior F03.91
  alcoholic F10.97
    with dependence F10.27
  Alzheimer's type —*see* Disease, Alzheimer's
  arteriosclerotic —*see* Dementia, vascular
  atypical, Alzheimer's type —*see* Disease,
    Alzheimer's, specified NEC
  congenital —*see* Disability, intellectual
  frontal (lobe) G31.09 *[F02.80]*
    with behavioral disturbance G31.09
      [F02.81]
  frontotemporal G31.09 *[F02.80]*
    with behavioral disturbance G31.09 *[F02.81]*
    specified NEC G31.09 *[F02.80]*
      with behavioral disturbance G31.09
        [F02.81]
  in (due to)
    alcohol F10.97
      with dependence F10.27
    Alzheimer's disease —*see* Disease,
      Alzheimer's
    arteriosclerotic brain disease —*see*
      Dementia, vascular
    cerebral lipidoses E75.- • *[F02.80]*
      with behavioral disturbance
        E75.- • *[F02.81]*
    Creutzfeldt-Jakob disease —*see also*
      Creutzfeldt-Jakob disease or
      syndrome (with dementia) A81.00
    epilepsy G40.- • *[F02.80]*
      with behavioral disturbance
        G40.- • *[F02.81]*
    hepatolenticular degeneration E83.01
      [F02.80]
      with behavioral disturbance E83.01
        [F02.81]
    human immunodeficiency virus (HIV)
      disease B20 *[F02.80]*
      with behavioral disturbance B20 *[F02.81]*
➡ Huntington's disease or chorea G10 *[F02.80]*
    ▶ with behavioral disturbance G10 *[F02.81]*
    hypercalcemia E83.52 *[F02.80]*
      with behavioral disturbance E83.52
        [F02.81]
    hypothyroidism, acquired E03.9 *[F02.80]*
      with behavioral disturbance E03.9
        [F02.81]
    due to iodine deficiency E01.8 *[F02.80]*
      with behavioral disturbance E01.8
        [F02.81]
    inhalants F18.97
      with dependence F18.27
    multiple
      etiologies F03
    sclerosis G35 *[F02.80]*
      with behavioral disturbance G35
        [F02.81]
    neurosyphilis A52.17 *[F02.80]*
      with behavioral disturbance A52.17
        [F02.81]
    juvenile A50.49 *[F02.80]*
      with behavioral disturbance A50.49
        [F02.81]
    niacin deficiency E52 *[F02.80]*
      with behavioral disturbance E52 *[F02.81]*
    paralysis agitans G20 *[F02.80]*
      with behavioral disturbance G20 *[F02.81]*
    Parkinson's disease G20 *[F02.80]*
    pellagra E52 *[F02.80]*
      with behavioral disturbance E52 *[F02.81]*
    Pick's G31.01 *[F02.80]*
      with behavioral disturbance G31.01
        [F02.81]
    polyarteritis nodosa M30.0 *[F02.80]*
      with behavioral disturbance M30.0
        [F02.81]

▶ New   ➡ Revised   ~~deleted~~ Deleted   • Use Additional Character(s)

Dementia (Continued)
  in (Continued)
    psychoactive drug F19.97
      with dependence F19.27
      inhalants F18.97
        with dependence F18.27
      sedatives, hypnotics or anxiolytics
        F13.97
        with dependence F13.27
    sedatives, hypnotics or anxiolytics F13.97
      with dependence F13.27
    systemic lupus erythematosus
      M32.- ● [F02.80]
      with behavioral disturbance
        M32.- ● [F02.81]
    trypanosomiasis
      African B56.9 [F02.80]
      with behavioral disturbance B56.9
        [F02.81]
    unknown etiology F03
    vitamin B12 deficiency E53.8 [F02.80]
      with behavioral disturbance E53.8
        [F02.81]
    volatile solvents F18.97
      with dependence F18.27
  infantile, infantilis F84.3
  Lewy body G31.83 [F02.80]
    with behavioral disturbance G31.83
      [F02.81]
  multi-infarct —see Dementia, vascular
  paralytica, paralytic (syphilitic) A52.17
    [F02.80]
    with behavioral disturbance A52.17
      [F02.81]
    juvenilis A50.45
  paretic A52.17
  praecox —see Schizophrenia
  presenile F03
    Alzheimer's type —see Disease,
      Alzheimer's, early onset
  primary degenerative F03
  progressive, syphilitic A52.17
  senile F03
    with acute confusional state F05
    Alzheimer's type —see Disease,
      Alzheimer's, late onset
    depressed or paranoid type F03
  vascular (acute onset) (mixed) (multi-infarct)
    (subcortical) F01.50
    with behavioral disturbance F01.51
Demineralization, bone —see Osteoporosis
Demodex folliculorum (infestation) B88.0
Demophobia F40.248
Demoralization R45.3
Demyelination, demyelinization
  central nervous system G37.9
    specified NEC G37.8
  corpus callosum (central) G37.1
  disseminated, acute G36.9
    specified NEC G36.8
  global G35
  in optic neuritis G36.0
Dengue (classical) (fever) A90
  hemorrhagic A91
  sandfly A93.1
Dennie-Marfan syphilitic syndrome
  A50.45
Dens evaginatus, in dente or invaginatus
  K00.2
Dense breasts R92.2
Density
  increased, bone (disseminated) (generalized)
    (spotted) —see Disorder, bone, density
    and structure, specified type NEC
  lung (nodular) J98.4
Dental —see also condition
  examination Z01.20
    with abnormal findings Z01.21
  restoration
    aesthetically inadequate or displeasing
      K08.56

Dental (Continued)
  restoration (Continued)
    defective K08.50
      specified NEC K08.59
    failure of marginal integrity K08.51
    failure of periodontal anatomical integrity
      K08.54
Dentia praecox K00.6
Denticles (pulp) K04.2
Dentigerous cyst K09.0
Dentin
  irregular (in pulp) K04.3
  opalescent K00.5
  secondary (in pulp) K04.3
  sensitive K03.89
Dentinogenesis imperfecta K00.5
Dentinoma —see Cyst, calcifying odontogenic
Dentition (syndrome) K00.7
  delayed K00.6
  difficult K00.7
  precocious K00.6
  premature K00.6
  retarded K00.6
Dependence (on) (syndrome) F19.20
  with remission F19.21
  alcohol (ethyl) (methyl) (without remission)
    F10.20
    with
      amnestic disorder, persisting F10.26
      anxiety disorder F10.280
      dementia, persisting F10.27
      intoxication F10.229
        with delirium F10.221
        uncomplicated F10.220
      mood disorder F10.24
      psychotic disorder F10.259
        with
          delusions F10.250
          hallucinations F10.251
      remission F10.21
      sexual dysfunction F10.281
      sleep disorder F10.282
      specified disorder NEC F10.288
      withdrawal F10.239
        with
          delirium F10.231
          perceptual disturbance F10.232
        uncomplicated F10.230
    counseling and surveillance Z71.41
  amobarbital —see Dependence, drug,
    sedative
  amphetamine(s) (type) —see Dependence,
    drug, stimulant NEC
  amytal (sodium) —see Dependence, drug,
    sedative
  analgesic NEC F55.8
  anesthetic (agent) (gas) (general) (local)
    NEC —see Dependence, drug,
    psychoactive NEC
  anxiolytic NEC —see Dependence, drug,
    sedative
  barbital(s) —see Dependence, drug, sedative
  barbiturate(s) (compounds) (drugs
    classifiable to T42) —see Dependence,
    drug, sedative
  benzedrine —see Dependence, drug,
    stimulant NEC
  bhang —see Dependence, drug, cannabis
  bromide(s) NEC —see Dependence, drug,
    sedative
  caffeine —see Dependence, drug, stimulant
    NEC
  cannabis (sativa) (indica) (resin) (derivatives)
    (type) —see Dependence, drug, cannabis
  chloral (betaine) (hydrate) —see Dependence,
    drug, sedative
  chlordiazepoxide —see Dependence, drug,
    sedative
  coca (leaf) (derivatives) —see Dependence,
    drug, cocaine
  cocaine —see Dependence, drug, cocaine

Dependence (Continued)
  codeine —see Dependence, drug, opioid
  combinations of drugs F19.20
  dagga —see Dependence, drug, cannabis
  demerol —see Dependence, drug, opioid
  dexamphetamine —see Dependence, drug,
    stimulant NEC
  dexedrine —see Dependence, drug, stimulant
    NEC
  dextromethorphan —see Dependence, drug,
    opioid
  dextromoramide —see Dependence, drug,
    opioid
  dextro-nor-pseudo-ephedrine —see
    Dependence, drug, stimulant NEC
  dextrorphan —see Dependence, drug, opioid
  diazepam —see Dependence, drug, sedative
  dilaudid —see Dependence, drug, opioid
  D-lysergic acid diethylamide —see
    Dependence, drug, hallucinogen
  drug NEC F19.20
    with sleep disorder F19.282
    cannabis F12.20
      with
        anxiety disorder F12.280
        intoxication F12.229
          with
            delirium F12.221
            perceptual disturbance F12.222
          uncomplicated F12.220
        other specified disorder F12.288
        psychosis F12.259
          delusions F12.250
          hallucinations F12.251
        unspecified disorder F12.29
      in remission F12.21
    cocaine F14.20
      with
        anxiety disorder F14.280
        intoxication F14.229
          with
            delirium F14.221
            perceptual disturbance F14.222
          uncomplicated F14.220
        mood disorder F14.24
        other specified disorder F14.288
        psychosis F14.259
          delusions F14.250
          hallucinations F14.251
        sexual dysfunction F14.281
        sleep disorder F14.282
        unspecified disorder F14.29
        withdrawal F14.23
      in remission F14.21
      withdrawal symptoms in newborn P96.1
    counseling and surveillance Z71.51
    hallucinogen F16.20
      with
        anxiety disorder F16.280
        flashbacks F16.283
        intoxication F16.229
          with delirium F16.221
          uncomplicated F16.220
        mood disorder F16.24
        other specified disorder F16.288
        perception disorder, persisting F16.283
        psychosis F16.259
          delusions F16.250
          hallucinations F16.251
        unspecified disorder F16.29
      in remission F16.21
    in remission F19.21
    inhalant F18.20
      with
        anxiety disorder F18.280
        dementia, persisting F18.27
        intoxication F18.229
          with delirium F18.221
          uncomplicated F18.220
        mood disorder F18.24
        other specified disorder F18.288

Dependence *(Continued)*
  drug NEC *(Continued)*
    inhalant *(Continued)*
      with *(Continued)*
        psychosis F18.259
          delusions F18.250
          hallucinations F18.251
        unspecified disorder F18.29
      in remission F18.21
    nicotine F17.200
      with disorder F17.209
        remission F17.201
      ▶in remission F17.201
        specified disorder NEC F17.208
        withdrawal F17.203
      chewing tobacco F17.220
        with disorder F17.229
          remission F17.221
        ▶in remission F17.221
          specified disorder NEC F17.228
          withdrawal F17.223
      cigarettes F17.210
        with disorder F17.219
          remission F17.211
        ▶in remission F17.211
          specified disorder NEC F17.218
          withdrawal F17.213
      specified product NEC F17.290
        with disorder F17.299
          remission F17.291
          specified disorder NEC F17.298
          withdrawal F17.293
    opioid F11.20
      with
        intoxication F11.229
          with
            delirium F11.221
            perceptual disturbance F11.222
          uncomplicated F11.220
        mood disorder F11.24
        other specified disorder F11.288
        psychosis F11.259
          delusions F11.250
          hallucinations F11.251
        sexual dysfunction F11.281
        sleep disorder F11.282
        unspecified disorder F11.29
        withdrawal F11.23
      in remission F11.21
    psychoactive NEC F19.20
      with
        amnestic disorder F19.26
        anxiety disorder F19.280
        dementia F19.27
        intoxication F19.229
          with
            delirium F19.221
            perceptual disturbance F19.222
          uncomplicated F19.220
        mood disorder F19.24
        other specified disorder F19.288
        psychosis F19.259
          delusions F19.250
          hallucinations F19.251
        sexual dysfunction F19.281
        sleep disorder F19.282
        unspecified disorder F19.29
        withdrawal F19.239
          with
            delirium F19.231
            perceptual disturbance F19.232
          uncomplicated F19.230
    sedative, hypnotic or anxiolytic F13.20
      with
        amnestic disorder F13.26
        anxiety disorder F13.280
        dementia, persisting F13.27
        intoxication F13.229
          with delirium F13.221
          uncomplicated F13.220
        mood disorder F13.24
        other specified disorder F13.288

Dependence *(Continued)*
  drug NEC *(Continued)*
    sedative, hypnotic or anxiolytic *(Continued)*
      with *(Continued)*
        psychosis F13.259
          delusions F13.250
          hallucinations F13.251
        sexual dysfunction F13.281
        sleep disorder F13.282
        unspecified disorder F13.29
        withdrawal F13.239
          with
            delirium F13.231
            perceptual disturbance F13.232
          uncomplicated F13.230
      in remission F13.21
    stimulant NEC F15.20
      with
        anxiety disorder F15.280
        intoxication F15.229
          with
            delirium F15.221
            perceptual disturbance F15.222
          uncomplicated F15.220
        mood disorder F15.24
        other specified disorder F15.288
        psychosis F15.259
          delusions F15.250
          hallucinations F15.251
        sexual dysfunction F15.281
        sleep disorder F15.282
        unspecified disorder F15.29
        withdrawal F15.23
      in remission F15.21
  ethyl
    alcohol (without remission) F10.20
      with remission F10.21
    bromide —*see* Dependence, drug, sedative
    carbamate F19.20
    chloride F19.20
    morphine —*see* Dependence, drug, opioid
  ganja —*see* Dependence, drug, cannabis
  glue (airplane) (sniffing) —*see* Dependence, drug, inhalant
  glutethimide —*see* Dependence, drug, sedative
  hallucinogenics —*see* Dependence, drug, hallucinogen
  hashish —*see* Dependence, drug, cannabis
  hemp —*see* Dependence, drug, cannabis
  heroin (salt) (any) —*see* Dependence, drug, opioid
  hypnotic NEC —*see* Dependence, drug, sedative
  Indian hemp —*see* Dependence, drug, cannabis
  inhalants —*see* Dependence, drug, inhalant
  khat —*see* Dependence, drug, stimulant NEC
  laudanum —*see* Dependence, drug, opioid
  LSD (-25) (derivatives) —*see* Dependence, drug, hallucinogen
  luminal —*see* Dependence, drug, sedative
  lysergic acid —*see* Dependence, drug, hallucinogen
  maconha —*see* Dependence, drug, cannabis
  marihuana —*see* Dependence, drug, cannabis
  meprobamate —*see* Dependence, drug, sedative
  mescaline —*see* Dependence, drug, hallucinogen
  methadone —*see* Dependence, drug, opioid
  methamphetamine(s) —*see* Dependence, drug, stimulant NEC
  methaqualone —*see* Dependence, drug, sedative
  methyl
    alcohol (without remission) F10.20
      with remission F10.21
    bromide —*see* Dependence, drug, sedative
    morphine —*see* Dependence, drug, opioid

Dependence *(Continued)*
  methyl *(Continued)*
    phenidate —*see* Dependence, drug, stimulant NEC
    sulfonal —*see* Dependence, drug, sedative
  morphine (sulfate) (sulfite) (type) —*see* Dependence, drug, opioid
  narcotic (drug) NEC —*see* Dependence, drug, opioid
  nembutal —*see* Dependence, drug, sedative
  neraval —*see* Dependence, drug, sedative
  neravan —*see* Dependence, drug, sedative
  neurobarb —*see* Dependence, drug, sedative
  nicotine —*see* Dependence, drug, nicotine
  nitrous oxide F19.20
  nonbarbiturate sedatives and tranquilizers with similar effect —*see* Dependence, drug, sedative
  on
    artificial heart (fully implantable) (mechanical) Z95.812
    aspirator Z99.0
    care provider (because of) Z74.9
      impaired mobility Z74.09
      need for
        assistance with personal care Z74.1
        continuous supervision Z74.3
      no other household member able to render care Z74.2
      specified reason NEC Z74.8
    machine Z99.89
      enabling NEC Z99.89
      specified type NEC Z99.89
    renal dialysis (hemodialysis) (peritoneal) Z99.2
    respirator Z99.11
    ventilator Z99.11
    wheelchair Z99.3
  opiate —*see* Dependence, drug, opioid
  opioids —*see* Dependence, drug, opioid
  opium (alkaloids) (derivatives) (tincture) —*see* Dependence, drug, opioid
  oxygen (long-term) (supplemental) Z99.81
  paraldehyde —*see* Dependence, drug, sedative
  paregoric —*see* Dependence, drug, opioid
  PCP (phencyclidine) (or related substance) —*see* Dependence, drug, hallucinogen
  pentobarbital —*see* Dependence, drug, sedative
  pentobarbitone (sodium) —*see* Dependence, drug, sedative
  pentothal —*see* Dependence, drug, sedative
  peyote —*see* Dependence, drug, hallucinogen
  phencyclidine (PCP) (or related substance) —*see* Dependence, drug, hallucinogen
  phenmetrazine —*see* Dependence, drug, stimulant NEC
  phenobarbital —*see* Dependence, drug, sedative
  polysubstance F19.20
  psilocibin, psilocin, psilocyn, psilocyline —*see* Dependence, drug, hallucinogen
  psychostimulant NEC —*see* Dependence, drug, stimulant NEC
  secobarbital —*see* Dependence, drug, sedative
  seconal —*see* Dependence, drug, sedative
  sedative NEC —*see* Dependence, drug, sedative
  specified drug NEC —*see* Dependence, drug
  stimulant NEC —*see* Dependence, drug, stimulant NEC
  substance NEC —*see* Dependence, drug
  supplemental oxygen Z99.81
  tobacco —*see* Dependence, drug, nicotine
    counseling and surveillance Z71.6
  tranquilizer NEC —*see* Dependence, drug, sedative
  vitamin B6 E53.1
  volatile solvents —*see* Dependence, drug, inhalant

▶ New   ⇒ Revised   ~~deleted~~ Deleted   • Use Additional Character(s)

Dependency
　care-provider Z74.9
　passive F60.7
　reactions (persistent) F60.7
Depersonalization (in neurotic state) (neurotic)
　　(syndrome) F48.1
Depletion
　extracellular fluid E86.9
　plasma E86.1
　potassium E87.6
　　nephropathy N25.89
　salt or sodium E87.1
　　causing heat exhaustion or prostration T67.4
　　nephropathy N28.9
　volume NOS E86.9
Deployment (current) (military) status Z56.82
　in theater or in support of military war,
　　peacekeeping and humanitarian
　　operations Z56.82
　personal history of Z91.82
　　military war, peacekeeping and
　　　humanitarian deployment (current or
　　　past conflict) Z91.82
　returned from Z91.82
Depolarization, premature I49.40
　atrial I49.1
　junctional I49.2
　specified NEC I49.49
　ventricular I49.3
Deposit
　bone in Boeck's sarcoid D86.89
　calcareous, calcium —see Calcification
　cholesterol
　　retina H35.89
　　vitreous (body) (humor) —see Deposit,
　　　crystalline
　conjunctiva H11.11-●
　cornea H18.00-●
　　argentous H18.02-●
　　due to metabolic disorder H18.03-●
　　Kayser-Fleischer ring H18.04-●
　　pigmentation —see Pigmentation, cornea
　crystalline, vitreous (body) (humor) H43.2-●
　hemosiderin in old scars of cornea —see
　　　Pigmentation, cornea, stromal
　metallic in lens —see Cataract, specified NEC
　skin R23.8
　tooth, teeth (betel) (black) (green) (materia
　　　alba) (orange) (tobacco) K03.6
　urate, kidney —see Calculus, kidney
Depraved appetite —see Pica
Depressed
　HDL cholesterol E78.6
Depression (acute) (mental) F32.9
　agitated (single episode) F32.2
　anaclitic —see Disorder, adjustment
　anxiety F41.8
　　persistent F34.1
　arches —see also Deformity, limb, flat foot
　atypical (single episode) F32.89
　　recurrent episode F33.8
　basal metabolic rate R94.8
　bone marrow D75.89
　central nervous system R09.2
　cerebral R29.818
　　newborn P91.4
　cerebrovascular I67.9
　chest wall M95.4
　climacteric (single episode) F32.89
　　recurrent episode F33.8
　endogenous (without psychotic symptoms)
　　　F33.2
　　with psychotic symptoms F33.3
　functional activity R68.89
　hysterical F44.89
　involutional (single episode) F32.89
　　recurrent episode F33.8
　major F32.9
　　with psychotic symptoms F32.3
　　recurrent —see Disorder, depressive,
　　　recurrent

Depression *(Continued)*
　manic-depressive —see Disorder, depressive,
　　　recurrent
　masked (single episode) F32.89
　medullary G93.89
　menopausal (single episode) F32.89
　　recurrent episode F33.8
　metatarsus —see Depression, arches
　monopolar F33.9
　nervous F34.1
　neurotic F34.1
　nose M95.0
　postnatal F53
　postpartum F53
　post-psychotic of schizophrenia F32.89
　post-schizophrenic F32.89
　psychogenic (reactive) (single episode) F32.9
　psychoneurotic F34.1
　psychotic (single episode) F32.3
　　recurrent F33.3
　reactive (psychogenic) (single episode) F32.9
　　psychotic (single episode) F32.3
　recurrent —see Disorder, depressive,
　　　recurrent
　respiratory center G93.89
　seasonal —see Disorder, depressive, recurrent
　senile F03
　severe, single episode F32.2
　situational F43.21
　skull Q67.4
　specified NEC (single episode) F32.89
　sternum M95.4
　visual field —see Defect, visual field
　vital (recurrent) (without psychotic
　　　symptoms) F33.2
　　with psychotic symptoms F33.3
　　single episode F32.2
Deprivation
　cultural Z60.3
　effects NOS T73.9
　　specified NEC T73.8
　emotional NEC Z65.8
　　affecting infant or child —see
　　　Maltreatment, child, psychological
　food T73.0
　protein —see Malnutrition
　sleep Z72.820
　social Z60.4
　　affecting infant or child —see
　　　Maltreatment, child, psychological
　specified NEC T73.8
　vitamins —see Deficiency, vitamin
　water T73.1
Derangement
　ankle (internal) —see Derangement, joint,
　　　ankle
　cartilage (articular) NEC —see Derangement,
　　　joint, articular cartilage, by site
　　recurrent —see Dislocation, recurrent
　cruciate ligament, anterior, current injury —
　　　see Sprain, knee, cruciate, anterior
　elbow (internal) —see Derangement, joint,
　　　elbow
　hip (joint) (internal) (old) —see Derangement,
　　　joint, hip
　joint (internal) M24.9
　　ankylosis —see Ankylosis
　　articular cartilage M24.10
　　　ankle M24.17-●
　　　elbow M24.12-●
　　　foot M24.17-●
　　　hand M24.14-●
　　　hip M24.15-●
　　　knee NEC M23.9-●
　　　loose body —see Loose, body
　　　shoulder M24.11-●
　　　wrist M24.13-●
　　contracture —see Contraction, joint
　　current injury —see also Dislocation
　　　knee, meniscus or cartilage —see Tear,
　　　　meniscus

Derangement *(Continued)*
　joint *(Continued)*
　　dislocation
　　　pathological —see Dislocation,
　　　　pathological
　　　recurrent —see Dislocation, recurrent
　　knee —see Derangement, knee
　　ligament —see Disorder, ligament
　　loose body —see Loose, body
　　recurrent —see Dislocation, recurrent
　　specified type NEC M24.80
　　　ankle M24.87-●
　　　elbow M24.82-●
　　　foot joint M24.87-●
　　　hand joint M24.84-●
　　　hip M24.85-●
　　　shoulder M24.81-●
　　　wrist M24.83-●
　　temporomandibular M26.69
　knee (recurrent) M23.9-●
　　ligament disruption, spontaneous
　　　M23.60-●
　　　anterior cruciate M23.61-●
　　　capsular M23.67-●
　　　instability, chronic M23.5-●
　　　lateral collateral M23.64-●
　　　medial collateral M23.63-●
　　　posterior cruciate M23.62-●
　　loose body M23.4-●
　　meniscus M23.30-●
　　　cystic M23.00-●
　　　　lateral M23.002
　　　　　anterior horn M23.04-●
　　　　　posterior horn M23.05-●
　　　　　specified NEC M23.06-●
　　　　medial M23.005
　　　　　anterior horn M23.01-●
　　　　　posterior horn M23.02-●
　　　　　specified NEC M23.03-●
　　　degenerate —see Derangement, knee,
　　　　meniscus, specified NEC
　　　detached —see Derangement, knee,
　　　　meniscus, specified NEC
　　　due to old tear or injury M23.20-●
　　　　lateral M23.20-●
　　　　　anterior horn M23.24-●
　　　　　posterior horn M23.25-●
　　　　　specified NEC M23.26-●
　　　　medial M23.20-●
　　　　　anterior horn M23.21-●
　　　　　posterior horn M23.22-●
　　　　　specified NEC M23.23-●
　　　retained —see Derangement, knee,
　　　　meniscus, specified NEC
　　　specified NEC M23.30-●
　　　　lateral M23.30-●
　　　　　anterior horn M23.34-●
　　　　　posterior horn M23.35-●
　　　　　specified NEC M23.36-●
　　　　medial M23.30-●
　　　　　anterior horn M23.31-●
　　　　　posterior horn M23.32-●
　　　　　specified NEC M23.33-●
　　old M23.8X-●
　　specified NEC —see subcategory M23.8
　　low back NEC —see Dorsopathy, specified
　　　NEC
　　meniscus —see Derangement, knee,
　　　meniscus
　　mental —see Psychosis
　　patella, specified NEC —see Disorder,
　　　patella, derangement NEC
　　semilunar cartilage (knee) —see
　　　Derangement, knee, meniscus,
　　　specified NEC
　　shoulder (internal) —see Derangement,
　　　joint, shoulder
Dercum's disease E88.2
Derealization (neurotic) F48.1
Dermal —see condition
Dermaphytid —see Dermatophytosis

Dermatitis (eczematous) L30.9
- ab igne L59.0
- acarine B88.0
- actinic (due to sun) L57.8
  - other than from sun L59.8
- allergic —*see* Dermatitis, contact, allergic
- ambustionis, due to burn or scald —*see* Burn
- amebic A06.7
- ammonia L22
- arsenical (ingested) L27.8
- artefacta L98.1
  - psychogenic F54
- atopic L20.9
  - psychogenic F54
  - specified NEC L20.89
- autoimmune progesterone L30.8
- berlock, berloque L56.2
- blastomycotic B40.3
- blister beetle L24.89
- bullous, bullosa L13.9
  - mucosynechial, atrophic L12.1
  - seasonal L30.8
  - specified NEC L13.8
- calorica L59.0
  - due to burn or scald —*see* Burn
- caterpillar L24.89
- cercarial B65.3
- combustionis L59.0
  - due to burn or scald —*see* Burn
- congelationis T69.1
- contact (occupational) L25.9
  - allergic L23.9
    - due to
      - adhesives L23.1
      - cement L23.5
      - chemical products NEC L23.5
      - chromium L23.0
      - cosmetics L23.2
      - dander (cat) (dog) L23.81
      - drugs in contact with skin L23.3
      - dyes L23.4
      - food in contact with skin L23.6
      - hair (cat) (dog) L23.81
      - insecticide L23.5
      - metals L23.0
      - nickel L23.0
      - plants, non-food L23.7
      - plastic L23.5
      - rubber L23.5
      - specified agent NEC L23.89
  - due to
    - cement L25.3
    - chemical products NEC L25.3
    - cosmetics L25.0
    - dander (cat) (dog) L23.81
    - drugs in contact with skin L25.1
    - dyes L25.2
    - food in contact with skin L25.4
    - hair (cat) (dog) L23.81
    - plants, non-food L25.5
    - specified agent NEC L25.8
  - irritant L24.9
    - due to
      - cement L24.5
      - chemical products NEC L24.5
      - cosmetics L24.3
      - detergents L24.0
      - drugs in contact with skin L24.4
      - food in contact with skin L24.6
      - oils and greases L24.1
      - plants, non-food L24.7
      - solvents L24.2
      - specified agent NEC L24.89
- contusiformis L52
- diabetic —*see* E08-E13 with .620
- diaper L22
- diphtheritica A36.3
- dry skin L85.3
- due to
  - acetone (contact) (irritant) L24.2
  - acids (contact) (irritant) L24.5

Dermatitis (*Continued*)
- due to (*Continued*)
  - adhesive(s) (allergic) (contact) (plaster) L23.1
    - irritant L24.5
  - alcohol (irritant) (skin contact) (substances in category T51) L24.2
    - taken internally L27.8
  - alkalis (contact) (irritant) L24.5
  - arsenic (ingested) L27.8
  - carbon disulfide (contact) (irritant) L24.2
  - caustics (contact) (irritant) L24.5
  - cement (contact) L25.3
  - cereal (ingested) L27.2
  - chemical(s) NEC L25.3
    - taken internally L27.8
  - chlorocompounds L24.2
  - chromium (contact) (irritant) L24.81
  - coffee (ingested) L27.2
  - cold weather L30.8
  - cosmetics (contact) L25.0
    - allergic L23.2
    - irritant L24.3
  - cyclohexanes L24.2
  - dander (cat) (dog) L23.81
  - Demodex species B88.0
  - Dermanyssus gallinae B88.0
  - detergents (contact) (irritant) L24.0
  - dichromate L24.81
  - drugs and medicaments (generalized) (internal use) L27.0
    - external —*see* Dermatitis, due to, drugs, in contact with skin
    - in contact with skin L25.1
      - allergic L23.3
      - irritant L24.4
    - localized skin eruption L27.1
    - specified substance —*see* Table of Drugs and Chemicals
  - dyes (contact) L25.2
    - allergic L23.3
    - irritant L24.89
  - epidermophytosis —*see* Dermatophytosis
  - esters L24.2
  - external irritant NEC L24.9
  - fish (ingested) L27.2
  - flour (ingested) L27.2
  - food (ingested) L27.2
    - in contact with skin L25.4
  - fruit (ingested) L27.2
  - furs (allergic) (contact) L23.81
  - glues —*see* Dermatitis, due to, adhesives
  - glycols L24.2
  - greases NEC (contact) (irritant) L24.1
  - hair (cat) (dog) L23.81
  - hot
    - objects and materials —*see* Burn
    - weather or places L59.0
  - hydrocarbons L24.2
  - infrared rays L59.8
  - ingestion, ingested substance L27.9
    - chemical NEC L27.8
    - drugs and medicaments —*see* Dermatitis, due to, drugs
    - food L27.2
    - specified NEC L27.8
  - insecticide in contact with skin L24.5
  - internal agent L27.9
    - drugs and medicaments (generalized) —*see* Dermatitis, due to, drugs
    - food L27.2
  - irradiation —*see* Dermatitis, due to, radioactive substance
  - ketones L24.2
  - lacquer tree (allergic) (contact) L23.7
  - light (sun) NEC L57.8
    - acute L56.8
    - other L59.8
  - Liponyssoides sanguineus B88.0
  - low temperature L30.8
  - meat (ingested) L27.2

Dermatitis (*Continued*)
- due to (*Continued*)
  - metals, metal salts (contact) (irritant) L24.81
  - milk (ingested) L27.2
  - nickel (contact) (irritant) L24.81
  - nylon (contact) (irritant) L24.5
  - oils NEC (contact) (irritant) L24.1
  - paint solvent (contact) (irritant) L24.2
  - petroleum products (contact) (irritant) (substances in T52) L24.2
  - plants NEC (contact) L25.5
    - allergic L23.7
    - irritant L24.7
  - plasters (adhesive) (any) (allergic) (contact) L23.1
    - irritant L24.5
  - plastic (contact) L25.3
  - preservatives (contact) —*see* Dermatitis, due to, chemical, in contact with skin
  - primrose (allergic) (contact) L23.7
  - primula (allergic) (contact) L23.7
  - radiation L59.8
    - nonionizing (chronic exposure) L57.8
    - sun NEC L57.8
      - acute L56.8
  - radioactive substance L58.9
    - acute L58.0
    - chronic L58.1
  - radium L58.9
    - acute L58.0
    - chronic L58.1
  - ragweed (allergic) (contact) L23.7
  - Rhus (allergic) (contact) (diversiloba) (radicans) (toxicodendron) (venenata) (verniciflua) L23.7
  - rubber (contact) L24.5
  - Senecio jacobaea (allergic) (contact) L23.7
  - solvents (contact) (irritant) (substances in categories T52) L24.2
  - specified agent NEC (contact) L25.8
    - allergic L23.89
    - irritant L24.89
  - sunshine NEC L57.8
    - acute L56.8
  - tetrachlorethylene (contact) (irritant) L24.2
  - toluene (contact) (irritant) L24.2
  - turpentine (contact) L24.2
  - ultraviolet rays (sun NEC) (chronic exposure) L57.8
    - acute L56.8
  - vaccine or vaccination L27.0
    - specified substance —*see* Table of Drugs and Chemicals
  - varicose veins —*see* Varix, leg, with, inflammation
  - X-rays L58.9
    - acute L58.0
    - chronic L58.1
- dyshydrotic L30.1
- dysmenorrheica N94.6
- escharotica —*see* Burn
- exfoliative, exfoliativa (generalized) L26
  - neonatorum L00
- eyelid —*see also* Dermatosis, eyelid
  - allergic H01.119
    - left H01.116
      - lower H01.115
      - upper H01.114
    - right H01.113
      - lower H01.112
      - upper H01.111
  - contact —*see* Dermatitis, eyelid, allergic
  - due to
    - Demodex species B88.0
    - herpes (zoster) B02.39
      - simplex B00.59

▶ New   ⇒ Revised   ~~deleted~~ Deleted   ● Use Additional Character(s)

Dermatitis *(Continued)*
  eyelid *(Continued)*
    eczematous H01.139
      left H01.136
        lower H01.135
        upper H01.134
      right H01.133
        lower H01.132
        upper H01.131
  facta, factitia, factitial L98.1
    psychogenic F54
  flexural NEC L20.82
  friction L30.4
  fungus B36.9
    specified type NEC B36.8
  gangrenosa, gangrenous infantum L08.0
  harvest mite B88.0
  heat L59.0
  herpesviral, vesicular (ear) (lip) B00.1
  herpetiformis (bullous) (erythematous)
      (pustular) (vesicular) L13.0
    juvenile L12.2
    senile L12.0
  hiemalis L30.8
  hypostatic, hypostatica —*see* Varix, leg, with,
      inflammation
  infectious eczematoid L30.3
  infective L30.3
  irritant —*see* Dermatitis, contact, irritant
  Jacquet's (diaper dermatitis) L22
  Leptus B88.0
  lichenified NEC L28.0
  medicamentosa (generalized) (internal
      use) —*see* Dermatitis, due to drugs
  mite B88.0
  multiformis L13.0
    juvenile L12.2
  napkin L22
  neurotica L13.0
  nummular L30.0
  papillaris capillitii L73.0
  pellagrous E52
  perioral L71.0
  photocontact L56.2
  polymorpha dolorosa L13.0
  pruriginosa L13.0
  pruritic NEC L30.8
  psychogenic F54
  purulent L08.0
  pustular
    contagious B08.02
    subcorneal L13.1
  pyococcal L08.0
  pyogenica L08.0
  repens L40.2
  Ritter's (exfoliativa) L00
  Schamberg's L81.7
  schistosome B65.3
  seasonal bullous L30.8
  seborrheic L21.9
    infantile L21.1
    specified NEC L21.8
  sensitization NOS L23.9
  septic L08.0
  solare L57.8
  specified NEC L30.8
  stasis I87.2
    with
      varicose ulcer —*see* Varix, leg, with ulcer,
        with inflammation
      varicose veins —*see* Varix, leg, with,
        inflammation
    due to postthrombotic syndrome —*see*
      Syndrome, postthrombotic
  suppurative L08.0
  traumatic NEC L30.4
  trophoneurotica L13.0
  ultraviolet (sun) (chronic exposure) L57.8
    acute L56.8
  varicose —*see* Varix, leg, with, inflammation
  vegetans L10.1

Dermatitis *(Continued)*
  verrucosa B43.0
  vesicular, herpesviral B00.1
Dermatoarthritis, lipoid E78.81
Dermatochalasis, eyelid H02.839
  left H02.836
    lower H02.835
    upper H02.834
  right H02.833
    lower H02.832
    upper H02.831
Dermatofibroma (lenticulare) —*see* Neoplasm,
    skin, benign
  protuberans —*see* Neoplasm, skin, uncertain
    behavior
Dermatofibrosarcoma (pigmented)
    (protuberans) —*see* Neoplasm, skin,
    malignant
Dermatographia L50.3
Dermatolysis (exfoliativa) (congenital) Q82.8
  acquired L57.4
  eyelids —*see* Blepharochalasis
  palpebrarum —*see* Blepharochalasis
  senile L57.4
Dermatomegaly NEC Q82.8
Dermatomucosomyositis M33.10
  with
    myopathy M33.12
    respiratory involvement M33.11
    specified organ involvement NEC M33.19
Dermatomycosis B36.9
  furfuracea B36.0
  specified type NEC B36.8
Dermatomyositis (acute) (chronic) —*see also*
    Dermatopolymyositis
▶adult —*see also* Dermatomyositis, specified
    NEC M33.10
  in (due to) neoplastic disease —*see also*
    Neoplasm D49.9 *[M36.0]*
▶juvenile M33.00
  ▶with
    ▶myopathy M33.02
    ▶respiratory involvement M33.01
    ▶specified organ involvement NEC
      M33.09
  ▶without myopathy M33.03
▶specified NEC M33.10
  ▶with
    ▶myopathy M33.12
    ▶respiratory involvement M33.11
    ▶specified organ involvement NEC M33.19
  ▶without myopathy M33.13
Dermatoneuritis of children —*see* Poisoning,
    mercury
Dermatophilosis A48.8
Dermatophytid L30.2
Dermatophytide —*see* Dermatophytosis
Dermatophytosis (epidermophyton) (infection)
    (Microsporum) (tinea) (Trichophyton)
    B35.9
  beard B35.0
  body B35.4
  capitis B35.0
  corporis B35.4
  deep-seated B35.8
  disseminated B35.8
  foot B35.3
  granulomatous B35.8
  groin B35.6
  hand B35.2
  nail B35.1
  perianal (area) B35.6
  scalp B35.0
  specified NEC B35.8
Dermatopolymyositis M33.90
  with
    myopathy M33.92
    respiratory involvement M33.91
    specified organ involvement NEC M33.99
  in neoplastic disease (*see also* Neoplasm)
    D49.9 *[M36.0]*

Dermatopolymyositis *(Continued)*
  juvenile M33.00
    with
      myopathy M33.02
      respiratory involvement M33.01
      specified organ involvement NEC M33.09
  specified NEC M33.10
    myopathy M33.12
    respiratory involvement M33.11
    specified organ involvement NEC M33.19
  ▶without myopathy M33.93
Dermatopolyneuritis —*see* Poisoning, mercury
Dermatorrhexis Q79.6
  acquired L57.4
Dermatosclerosis —*see also* Scleroderma
  localized L94.0
Dermatosis L98.9
  Andrews' L08.89
  Bowen's —*see* Neoplasm, skin, in situ
  bullous L13.9
    specified NEC L13.8
  exfoliativa L26
  eyelid (noninfectious)
    dermatitis —*see* Dermatitis, eyelid
    discoid lupus erythematosus —*see* Lupus,
      erythematosus, eyelid
    xeroderma —*see* Xeroderma, acquired,
      eyelid
  factitial L98.1
  febrile neutrophilic L98.2
  gonococcal A54.89
  herpetiformis L13.0
    juvenile L12.2
  linear IgA L13.8
  menstrual NEC L98.8
  neutrophilic, febrile L98.2
  occupational —*see* Dermatitis, contact
  papulosa nigra L82.1
  pigmentary L81.9
    progressive L81.7
    Schamberg's L81.7
  psychogenic F54
  purpuric, pigmented L81.7
  pustular, subcorneal L13.1
  transient acantholytic L11.1
Dermographia, dermographism L50.3
Dermoid (cyst) —*see also* Neoplasm, benign,
    by site
  with malignant transformation C56-●
  due to radiation (nonionizing) L57.8
Dermopathy
  infiltrative with thyrotoxicosis —*see*
    Thyrotoxicosis
  nephrogenic fibrosing L90.8
Dermophytosis —*see* Dermatophytosis
Descemetocele H18.73-●
Descemet's membrane —*see* condition
Descending —*see* condition
Descensus uteri —*see* Prolapse, uterus
Desert
  rheumatism B38.0
  sore —*see* Ulcer, skin
Desertion (newborn) —*see* Maltreatment
Desmoid (extra-abdominal) (tumor) —*see*
    Neoplasm, connective tissue, uncertain
    behavior
  abdominal D48.1
Despondency F32.9
Desquamation, skin R23.4
Destruction, destructive —*see also* Damage
  articular facet —*see also* Derangement, joint,
      specified type NEC
    knee M23.8X-●
    vertebra —*see* Spondylosis
  bone —*see also* Disorder, bone, specified type
      NEC
    syphilitic A52.77
  joint —*see also* Derangement, joint, specified
      type NEC
    sacroiliac M53.3
  rectal sphincter K62.89

Destruction, destructive *(Continued)*
  septum (nasal) J34.89
  tuberculous NEC —*see* Tuberculosis
  tympanum, tympanic membrane
    (nontraumatic) —*see* Disorder, tympanic
    membrane, specified NEC
  vertebral disc —*see* Degeneration,
    intervertebral disc
Destructiveness —*see also* Disorder, conduct
  adjustment reaction —*see* Disorder,
    adjustment
Desultory labor O62.2
Detachment
  cartilage —*see* Sprain
  cervix, annular N88.8
    complicating delivery O71.3
  choroid (old) (postinfectional) (simple)
    (spontaneous) H31.40-●
    hemorrhagic H31.41-●
    serous H31.42-●
  ligament —*see* Sprain
  meniscus (knee) —*see also* Derangement,
    knee, meniscus, specified NEC
    current injury —*see* Tear, meniscus
    due to old tear or injury —*see*
      Derangement, knee, meniscus, due to
      old tear
  retina (without retinal break) (serous)
    H33.2-●
    with retinal:
      break H33.00-●
        giant H33.03-●
        multiple H33.02-●
        single H33.01-●
      dialysis H33.04-●
    pigment epithelium —*see* Degeneration,
      retina, separation of layers, pigment
      epithelium detachment
    rhegmatogenous —*see* Detachment, retina,
      with retinal, break
    specified NEC H33.8
    total H33.05-●
    traction H33.4-●
  vitreous (body) H43.81
Detergent asthma J69.8
Deterioration
  epileptic F06.8
  general physical R53.81
  heart, cardiac —*see* Degeneration,
    myocardial
  mental —*see* Psychosis
  myocardial, myocardium —*see* Degeneration,
    myocardial
  senile (simple) R54
Deuteranomaly (anomalous trichromat) H53.53
Deuteranopia (complete) (incomplete) H53.53
Development
  abnormal, bone Q79.9
  arrested R62.50
    bone —*see* Arrest, development or growth,
      bone
    child R62.50
    due to malnutrition E45
  defective, congenital —*see also* Anomaly, by
    site
    cauda equina Q06.3
    left ventricle Q24.8
      in hypoplastic left heart syndrome Q23.4
    valve Q24.8
    pulmonary Q22.3
  delayed (*see also* Delay, development) R62.50
    arithmetical skills F81.2
    language (skills) (expressive) F80.1
    learning skill F81.9
    mixed skills F88
    motor coordination F82
    reading F81.0
    specified learning skill NEC F81.89
    speech F80.9
    spelling F81.81
    written expression F81.81

Development *(Continued)*
  imperfect, congenital —*see also* Anomaly, by
    site
    heart Q24.9
    lungs Q33.6
  incomplete
    bronchial tree Q32.4
    organ or site not listed —*see* Hypoplasia,
      by site
    respiratory system Q34.9
  sexual, precocious NEC E30.1
  tardy, mental (*see also* Disability, intellectual)
    F79
Developmental —*see* condition
  testing, infant or child —*see* Examination,
    child
Devergie's disease (pityriasis rubra pilaris)
  L44.0
Deviation (in)
  conjugate palsy (eye) (spastic) H51.0
  esophagus (acquired) K22.8
  eye, skew H51.8
  midline (jaw) (teeth) (dental arch) M26.29
    specified site NEC —*see* Malposition
  nasal septum J34.2
    congenital Q67.4
  opening and closing of the mandible M26.53
  organ or site, congenital NEC —*see*
    Malposition, congenital
  septum (nasal) (acquired) J34.2
    congenital Q67.4
  sexual F65.9
    bestiality F65.89
    erotomania F52.8
    exhibitionism F65.2
    fetishism, fetishistic F65.0
      transvestism F65.1
    frotteurism F65.81
    masochism F65.51
    multiple F65.89
    necrophilia F65.89
    nymphomania F52.8
    pederosis F65.4
    pedophilia F65.4
    sadism, sadomasochism F65.52
    satyriasis F52.8
    specified type NEC F65.89
    transvestism F64.1
    voyeurism F65.3
  teeth, midline M26.29
  trachea J39.8
  ureter, congenital Q62.61
Device
  cerebral ventricle (communicating) in situ
    Z98.2
  contraceptive —*see* Contraceptive, device
  drainage, cerebrospinal fluid, in situ Z98.2
Devic's disease G36.0
Devil's
  grip B33.0
  pinches (purpura simplex) D69.2
Devitalized tooth K04.99
Devonshire colic —*see* Poisoning, lead
Dextraposition, aorta Q20.3
  in tetralogy of Fallot Q21.3
Dextrinosis, limit (debrancher enzyme
  deficiency) E74.03
Dextrocardia (true) Q24.0
  with
    complete transposition of viscera Q89.3
    situs inversus Q89.3
Dextrotransposition, aorta Q20.3
d-glycericacidemia E72.59
Dhat syndrome F48.8
Dhobi itch B35.6
Di George's syndrome D82.1
Di Guglielmo's disease C94.0-●
Diabetes, diabetic (mellitus) (sugar) E11.9
  with
    amyotrophy E11.44
    arthropathy NEC E11.618

Diabetes, diabetic *(Continued)*
  with *(Continued)*
    autonomic (poly)neuropathy E11.43
    cataract E11.36
    Charcot's joints E11.610
    chronic kidney disease E11.22
    circulatory complication NEC E11.59
    complication E11.8
      specified NEC E11.69
    dermatitis E11.620
    foot ulcer E11.621
    gangrene E11.52
    gastroparalysis E11.43
    gastroparesis E11.43
    glomerulonephrosis, intracapillary E11.21
    glomerulosclerosis, intercapillary E11.21
    hyperglycemia E11.65
    hyperosmolarity E11.00
      with coma E11.01
    hypoglycemia E11.649
      with coma E11.641
  ▶ ketoacidosis E11.10
    ▶with coma E11.11
    kidney complications NEC E11.29
    Kimmelstiel-Wilson disease E11.21
    loss of protective sensation (LOPS) —*see*
      Diabetes, by type, with neuropathy
    mononeuropathy E11.41
    myasthenia E11.44
    necrobiosis lipoidica E11.620
    nephropathy E11.21
    neuralgia E11.42
    neurologic complication NEC E11.49
    neuropathic arthropathy E11.610
    neuropathy E11.40
    ophthalmic complication NEC E11.39
    oral complication NEC E11.638
    osteomyelitis E11.69
    periodontal disease E11.630
    peripheral angiopathy E11.51
      with gangrene E11.52
    polyneuropathy E11.42
    renal complication NEC E11.29
    renal tubular degeneration E11.29
    retinopathy E11.319
      with macular edema E11.311
        resolved following treatment
          E11.37
      nonproliferative E11.329
        with macular edema E11.321
        mild E11.329
          with macular edema E11.321
        moderate E11.339
          with macular edema E11.331
        severe E11.349
          with macular edema E11.341
      proliferative E11.359
        with
          combined traction retinal
            detachment and
            rhegmatogenous retinal
            detachment E11.354
          macular edema E11.351
          stable proliferative diabetic
            retinopathy E11.355
          traction retinal detachment
            involving the macula E11.352
          traction retinal detachment not
            involving the macula E11.353
    skin complication NEC E11.628
    skin ulcer NEC E11.622
  brittle —*see* Diabetes, type 1
  bronzed E83.110
  complicating pregnancy —*see* Pregnancy,
    complicated by, diabetes
  dietary counseling and surveillance Z71.3
  due to
    autoimmune process —*see* Diabetes, type 1
    immune mediated pancreatic islet
      beta-cell destruction —*see* Diabetes,
        type 1

Diabetes, diabetic *(Continued)*
  due to drug or chemical E09.9
    with
      amyotrophy E09.44
      arthropathy NEC E09.618
      autonomic (poly)neuropathy E09.43
      cataract E09.36
      Charcot's joints E09.610
      chronic kidney disease E09.22
      circulatory complication NEC E09.59
      complication E09.8
        specified NEC E09.69
      dermatitis E09.620
      foot ulcer E09.621
      gangrene E09.52
      gastroparalysis E09.43
      gastroparesis E09.43
      glomerulonephrosis, intracapillary E09.21
      glomerulosclerosis, intercapillary E09.21
      hyperglycemia E09.65
      hyperosmolarity E09.00
        with coma E09.01
      hypoglycemia E09.649
        with coma E09.641
      ketoacidosis E09.10
        with coma E09.11
      kidney complications NEC E09.29
      Kimmelsteil-Wilson disease E09.21
      mononeuropathy E09.41
      myasthenia E09.44
      necrobiosis lipoidica E09.620
      nephropathy E09.21
      neuralgia E09.42
      neurologic complication NEC E09.49
      neuropathic arthropathy E09.610
      neuropathy E09.40
      ophthalmic complication NEC E09.39
      oral complication NEC E09.638
      periodontal disease E09.630
      peripheral angiopathy E09.51
        with gangrene E09.52
      polyneuropathy E09.42
      renal complication NEC E09.29
      renal tubular degeneration E09.29
      retinopathy E09.319
        with macular edema E09.311
          resolved following treatment E09.37
        nonproliferative E09.329
          with macular edema E09.321
          mild E09.329
            with macular edema E09.321
          moderate E09.339
            with macular edema E09.331
          severe E09.349
            with macular edema E09.341
        proliferative E09.359
          with
            combined traction retinal detachment and rhegmatogenous retinal detachment E09.354
            macular edema E09.351
            stable proliferative diabetic retinopathy E09.355
            traction retinal detachment involving the macula E09.352
            traction retinal detachment not involving the macula E09.353
      skin complication NEC E09.628
      skin ulcer NEC E09.622
  due to underlying condition E08.9
    with
      amyotrophy E08.44
      arthropathy NEC E08.618
      autonomic (poly)neuropathy E08.43
      cataract E08.36
      Charcot's joints E08.610

Diabetes, diabetic *(Continued)*
  due to underlying condition *(Continued)*
    with *(Continued)*
      chronic kidney disease E08.22
      circulatory complication NEC E08.59
      complication E08.8
        specified NEC E08.69
      dermatitis E08.620
      foot ulcer E08.621
      gangrene E08.52
      gastroparalysis E08.43
      gastroparesis E08.43
      glomerulonephrosis, intracapillary E08.21
      glomerulosclerosis, intercapillary E08.21
      hyperglycemia E08.69
      hyperosmolarity E08.00
        with coma E08.01
      hypoglycemia E08.649
        with coma E08.641
      ketoacidosis E08.10
        with coma E08.11
      kidney complications NEC E08.29
      Kimmelsteil-WIlson disease E08.21
      mononeuropathy E08.41
      myasthenia E08.44
      necrobiosis lipoidica E08.620
      nephropathy E08.21
      neuralgia E08.42
      neurologic complication NEC E08.49
      neuropathic arthropathy E08.610
      neuropathy E08.40
      ophthalmic complication NEC E08.39
      oral complication NEC E08.638
      periodontal disease E08.630
      peripheral angiopathy E08.51
        with gangrene E08.52
      polyneuropathy E08.42
      renal complication NEC E08.29
      renal tubular degeneration E08.29
      retinopathy E08.319
        with macular edema E08.311
          resolved following treatment E08.37
        nonproliferative E08.329
          with macular edema E08.321
          mild E08.329
            with macular edema E08.321
          moderate E08.339
            with macular edema E08.331
          severe E08.349
            with macular edema E08.341
        proliferative E08.359
          with
            combined traction retinal detachment and rhegmatogenous retinal detachment E08.354
            macular edema E08.351
            stable proliferative diabetic retinopathy E08.355
            traction retinal detachment involving the macula E08.352
            traction retinal detachment not involving the macula E08.353
      skin complication NEC E08.628
      skin ulcer NEC E08.622
  gestational (in pregnancy) O24.419
    affecting newborn P70.0
    diet-controlled O24.410
    in childbirth O24.429
      diet-controlled O24.420
      insulin (and diet) controlled O24.424
      oral drug controlled (antidiabetic) (hypoglycemic) O24.425
    insulin (and diet) controlled O24.414
    oral drug controlled (antidiabetic) (hypoglycemic) O24.415

Diabetes, diabetic *(Continued)*
  gestational (in pregnancy) *(Continued)*
    puerperal O24.439
      diet-controlled O24.430
      insulin (and diet) controlled O24.434
      oral drug controlled (antidiabetic) (hypoglycemic) O24.435
  hepatogenous E13.9
  idiopathic —*see* Diabetes, type 1
  inadequately controlled — code to Diabetes, by type, with hyperglycemia
  insipidus E23.2
    nephrogenic N25.1
    pituitary E23.2
    vasopressin resistant N25.1
  insulin dependent — code to type of diabetes
  juvenile-onset —*see* Diabetes, type 1
  ketosis-prone —*see* Diabetes, type 1
  latent R73.03
  neonatal (transient) P70.2
  non-insulin dependent — code to type of diabetes
  out of control — code to Diabetes, by type, with hyperglycemia
  phosphate E83.39
  poorly controlled — code to Diabetes, by type, with hyperglycemia
  postpancreatectomy —*see* Diabetes, specified type NEC
  postprocedural —*see* Diabetes, specified type NEC
  secondary diabetes mellitus NEC —*see* Diabetes, specified type NEC
  specified type NEC E13.9
    with
      amyotrophy E13.44
      arthropathy NEC E13.618
      autonomic (poly)neuropathy E13.43
      cataract E13.36
      Charcot's joints E13.610
      chronic kidney disease E13.22
      circulatory complication NEC E13.59
      complication E13.8
        specified NEC E13.69
      dermatitis E13.620
      foot ulcer E13.621
      gangrene E13.52
      gastroparalysis E13.43
      gastroparesis E13.43
      glomerulonephrosis, intracapillary E13.21
      glomerulosclerosis, intercapillary E13.21
      hyperglycemia E13.65
      hyperosmolarity E13.00
        with coma E13.01
      hypoglycemia E13.649
        with coma E13.641
      ketoacidosis E13.10
        with coma E13.11
      kidney complications NEC E13.29
      Kimmelstein-Wilson disease E13.21
      mononeuropathy E13.41
      myasthenia E13.44
      necrobiosis lipoidica E13.620
      nephropathy E13.21
      neuralgia E13.42
      neurologic complication NEC E13.49
      neuropathic arthropathy E13.610
      neuropathy E13.40
      ophthalmic complication NEC E13.39
      oral complication NEC E13.638
      periodontal disease E13.630
      peripheral angiopathy E13.51
        with gangrene E13.52
      polyneuropathy E13.42
      renal complication NEC E13.29
      renal tubular degeneration E13.29
      retinopathy E13.319
        with macular edema E13.311
          resolved following treatment E13.37

Diabetes, diabetic *(Continued)*
  specified type NEC *(Continued)*
    with *(Continued)*
      retinopathy *(Continued)*
        nonproliferative E13.329
          with macular edema E13.321
          mild E13.329
            with macular edema E13.321
          moderate E13.339
            with macular edema E13.331
          severe E13.349
            with macular edema E13.341
        proliferative E13.359
          with
            combined traction retinal
              detachment and
              rhegmatogenous retinal
              detachment E13.354
            macular edema E13.351
            stable proliferative diabetic
              retinopathy E13.355
            traction retinal detachment
              involving the macula
              E13.352
            traction retinal detachment not
              involving the macula
              E13.353
      skin complication NEC E13.628
      skin ulcer NEC E13.622
  steroid-induced —*see* Diabetes, due to, drug
    or chemical
  type 1 E10.9
    with
      amyotrophy E10.44
      arthropathy NEC E10.618
      autonomic (poly)neuropathy E10.43
      cataract E10.36
      Charcot's joints E10.610
      chronic kidney disease E10.22
      circulatory complication NEC E10.59
      complication E10.8
        specified NEC E10.69
      dermatitis E10.620
      foot ulcer E10.621
      gangrene E10.52
      gastroparalysis E10.43
      gastroparesis E10.43
      glomerulonephrosis, intracapillary E10.21
      glomerulosclerosis, intercapillary E10.21
      hyperglycemia E10.65
      hypoglycemia E10.649
        with coma E10.641
      ketoacidosis E10.10
        with coma E10.11
      kidney complications NEC E10.29
      Kimmelstiel-Wilson disease E10.21
      mononeuropathy E10.41
      myasthenia E10.44
      necrobiosis lipoidica E10.620
      nephropathy E10.21
      neuralgia E10.42
      neurologic complication NEC E10.49
      neuropathic arthropathy E10.610
      neuropathy E10.40
      ophthalmic complication NEC E10.39
      oral complication NEC E10.638
    ▶osteomyelitis E10.69
      periodontal disease E10.630
      peripheral angiopathy E10.51
        with gangrene E10.52
      polyneuropathy E10.42
      renal complication NEC E10.29
      renal tubular degeneration E10.29
      retinopathy E10.319
        with macular edema E10.311
          resolved following treatment E10.37
        nonproliferative E10.329
          with macular edema E10.321
          mild E10.329
            with macular edema E10.321
          moderate E10.339
            with macular edema E10.331

Diabetes, diabetic *(Continued)*
  type 1 *(Continued)*
    with *(Continued)*
      retinopathy *(Continued)*
        nonproliferative *(Continued)*
          severe E10.349
            with macular edema E10.341
        proliferative E10.359
          with
            combined traction retinal
              detachment and
              rhegmatogenous retinal
              detachment E13.354
            macular edema E13.351
            stable proliferative diabetic
              retinopathy E13.355
            traction retinal detachment
              involving the macula E13.352
            traction retinal detachment not
              involving the macula E13.353
      skin complication NEC E10.628
      skin ulcer NEC E10.622
  type 2 E11.9
    with
      amyotrophy E11.44
      arthropathy NEC E11.618
      autonomic (poly)neuropathy E11.43
      cataract E11.36
      Charcot's joints E11.610
      chronic kidney disease E11.22
      circulatory complication NEC E11.59
      complication E11.8
        specified NEC E11.69
      dermatitis E11.620
      foot ulcer E11.621
      gangrene E11.52
      gastroparalysis E11.43
      gastroparesis E11.43
      glomerulonephrosis, intracapillary E11.21
      glomerulosclerosis, intercapillary E11.21
      hyperglycemia E11.65
      hyperosmolarity E11.00
        with coma E11.01
      hypoglycemia E11.649
        with coma E11.641
    ▶ketoacidosis E11.10
      ▶with coma E11.11
      kidney complications NEC E11.29
      Kimmelsteil-Wilson disease E11.21
      mononeuropathy E11.41
      myasthenia E11.44
      necrobiosis lipoidica E11.620
      nephropathy E11.21
      neuralgia E11.42
      neurologic complication NEC E11.49
      neuropathic arthropathy E11.610
      neuropathy E11.40
      ophthalmic complication NEC E11.39
      oral complication NEC E11.638
    ▶osteomyelitis E11.69
      periodontal disease E11.630
      peripheral angiopathy E11.51
        with gangrene E11.52
      polyneuropathy E11.42
      renal complication NEC E11.29
      renal tubular degeneration E11.29
      retinopathy E11.319
        with macular edema E11.311
          resolved following treatment E11.37
        nonproliferative E11.329
          with macular edema E11.321
          mild E11.329
            with macular edema E11.321
          moderate E11.339
            with macular edema E11.331
          severe E11.349
            with macular edema E11.341
        proliferative E11.359
          with
            combined traction retinal
              detachment and
              rhegmatogenous retinal
              detachment E11.354

Diabetes, diabetic *(Continued)*
  type 2 *(Continued)*
    with *(Continued)*
      retinopathy *(Continued)*
        proliferative *(Continued)*
          with *(Continued)*
            macular edema E11.351
            stable proliferative diabetic
              retinopathy E11.355
            traction retinal detachment
              involving the macula E11.352
            traction retinal detachment not
              involving the macula E11.353
      skin complication NEC E11.628
      skin ulcer NEC E11.622
  uncontrolled
    meaning
      hyperglycemia —*see* Diabetes, by type,
        with, hyperglycemia
      hypoglycemia —*see* Diabetes, by type,
        with, hypoglycemia
Diacyclothrombopathia D69.1
Diagnosis deferred R69
Dialysis (intermittent) (treatment)
  noncompliance (with) Z91.15
  renal (hemodialysis) (peritoneal), status Z99.2
  retina, retinal —*see* Detachment, retina, with
    retinal, dialysis
Diamond-Blackfan anemia (congenital
  hypoplastic) D61.01
Diamond-Gardener syndrome
  (autoerythrocyte sensitization) D69.2
Diaper rash L22
Diaphoresis (excessive) R61
Diaphragm —*see* condition
Diaphragmalgia R07.1
Diaphragmatitis, diaphragmitis J98.6
Diaphysial aclasis Q78.6
Diaphysitis —*see* Osteomyelitis, specified type
  NEC
Diarrhea, diarrheal (disease) (infantile)
  (inflammatory) R19.7
  achlorhydric K31.83
  allergic K52.29
    due to
      colitis —*see* Colitis, allergic
      enteritis —*see* Enteritis, allergic
  amebic —*see also* Amebiasis A06.0
    with abscess —*see* Abscess, amebic
    acute A06.0
    chronic A06.1
    nondysenteric A06.2
  bacillary —*see* Dysentery, bacillary
  balantidial A07.0
  cachectic NEC K52.89
  Chilomastix A07.8
  choleriformis A00.1
  chronic (noninfectious) K52.9
  coccidial A07.3
  Cochin-China K90.1
    strongyloidiasis B78.0
  Dientamoeba A07.8
  dietetic —*see also* Diarrhea, allergic K52.29
  drug-induced K52.1
  due to
    bacteria A04.9
      specified NEC A04.8
    Campylobacter A04.5
    Capillaria philippinensis B81.1
  ➧Clostridium difficile
    ▶not specified as recurrent A04.72
    ▶recurrent A04.71
    Clostridium perfringens (C) (F) A04.8
    Cryptosporidium A07.2
    drugs K52.1
    Escherichia coli A04.4
      enteroaggregative A04.4
      enterohemorrhagic A04.3
      enteroinvasive A04.2
      enteropathogenic A04.0
      enterotoxigenic A04.1
      specified NEC A04.4

▶ New   ➧ Revised   ~~deleted~~ Deleted   • Use Additional Character(s)

Diarrhea, diarrheal (Continued)
  due to (Continued)
    food hypersensitivity —see also Diarrhea,
      allergic K52.29
    Necator americanus B76.1
    S. japonicum B65.2
    specified organism NEC A08.8
      bacterial A04.8
      viral A08.39
    Staphylococcus A04.8
    Trichuris trichiuria B79
    virus —see Enteritis, viral
    Yersinia enterocolitica A04.6
  dysenteric A09
  endemic A09
  epidemic A09
  flagellate A07.9
  Flexner's (ulcerative) A03.1
  functional K59.1
    following gastrointestinal surgery
      K91.89
    psychogenic F45.8
  Giardia lamblia A07.1
  giardial A07.1
  hill K90.1
  infectious A09
  malarial —see Malaria
  mite B88.0
  mycotic NEC B49
  neonatal (noninfectious) P78.3
  nervous F45.8
  neurogenic K59.1
  noninfectious K52.9
  postgastrectomy K91.1
  postvagotomy K91.1
  protozoal A07.9
    specified NEC A07.8
  psychogenic F45.8
  specified
    bacterium NEC A04.8
    virus NEC A08.39
  strongyloidiasis B78.0
  toxic K52.1
  trichomonal A07.8
  tropical K90.1
  tuberculous A18.32
  viral —see Enteritis, viral
Diastasis
  cranial bones M84.88
    congenital NEC Q75.8
  joint (traumatic) —see Dislocation
  muscle M62.00
    ankle M62.07-●
    congenital Q79.8
    foot M62.07-●
    forearm M62.03-●
    hand M62.04-●
    lower leg M62.06-●
    pelvic region M62.05-●
    shoulder region M62.01-●
    specified site NEC M62.08
    thigh M62.05-●
    upper arm M62.02-●
  recti (abdomen)
    complicating delivery O71.89
    congenital Q79.59
Diastema, tooth, teeth, fully erupted
  M26.32
Diastematomyelia Q06.2
Diataxia, cerebral G80.4
Diathesis
  allergic —see History, allergy
  bleeding (familial) D69.9
  cystine (familial) E72.00
  gouty —see Gout
  hemorrhagic (familial) D69.9
    newborn NEC P53
  spasmophilic R29.0
Diaz's disease or osteochondrosis (juvenile)
    (talus) —see Osteochondrosis, juvenile,
    tarsus

Dibothriocephalus, dibothriocephaliasis
    (latus) (infection) (infestation) B70.0
  larval B70.1
Dicephalus, dicephaly Q89.4
Dichotomy, teeth K00.2
Dichromat, dichromatopsia (congenital) —see
    Deficiency, color vision
Dichuchwa A65
Dicroceliasis B66.2
Didelphia, didelphys —see Double uterus
Didymytis N45.1
  with orchitis N45.3
Dietary
  inadequacy or deficiency E63.9
  surveillance and counseling Z71.3
Dietl's crisis N13.8
Dieulafoy lesion (hemorrhagic)
  duodenum K31.82
  esophagus K22.8
  intestine (colon) K63.81
  stomach K31.82
Difficult, difficulty (in)
  acculturation Z60.3
  feeding R63.3
    newborn P92.9
      breast P92.5
      specified NEC P92.8
    nonorganic (infant or child) F98.29
  intubation, in anesthesia T88.4
  mechanical, gastroduodenal stoma K91.89
  ➠causing obstruction —see also Obstruction,
      intestine, postoperative K91.30
  micturition
    need to immediately re-void R39.191
    position dependent R39.192
    specified NEC R39.198
  reading (developmental) F81.0
    secondary to emotional disorders F93.9
  spelling (specific) F81.81
    with reading disorder F81.89
    due to inadequate teaching Z55.8
  swallowing —see Dysphagia
  walking R26.2
  work
    conditions NEC Z56.5
    schedule Z56.3
Diffuse —see condition
DiGeorge's syndrome (thymic hypoplasia)
    D82.1
Digestive —see condition
Dihydropyrimidine dehydrogenase disease
    (DPD) E88.89
Diktyoma —see Neoplasm, malignant, by site
Dilaceration, tooth K00.4
Dilatation
  anus K59.8
    venule —see Hemorrhoids
  aorta (focal) (general) —see Ectasia, aorta
    with aneurysm —see Aneurysm, aorta
    congenital Q25.44
  artery —see Aneurysm
  bladder (sphincter) N32.89
    congenital Q64.79
  blood vessel I99.8
  bronchial J47.9
    with
      exacerbation (acute) J47.1
      lower respiratory infection J47.0
  calyx (due to obstruction) —see
      Hydronephrosis
  capillaries I78.8
  cardiac (acute) (chronic) —see also
      Hypertrophy, cardiac
    congenital Q24.8
      valve NEC Q24.8
        pulmonary Q22.3
    valve —see Endocarditis
  cavum septi pellucidi Q06.8
  cervix (uteri) —see also Incompetency, cervix
    incomplete, poor, slow complicating
      delivery O62.0

Dilatation (Continued)
  colon K59.39
    congenital Q43.1
    psychogenic F45.8
    toxic K59.31
  common duct (acquired) K83.8
    congenital Q44.5
  cystic duct (acquired) K82.8
    congenital Q44.5
  duct, mammary —see Ectasia, mammary duct
  duodenum K59.8
  esophagus K22.8
    congenital Q39.5
    due to achalasia K22.0
  eustachian tube, congenital Q17.8
  gallbladder K82.8
  gastric —see Dilatation, stomach
  heart (acute) (chronic) —see also Hypertrophy,
      cardiac
    congenital Q24.8
    valve —see Endocarditis
  ileum K59.8
    psychogenic F45.8
  jejunum K59.8
    psychogenic F45.8
  kidney (calyx) (collecting structures) (cystic)
      (parenchyma) (pelvis) (idiopathic)
      N28.89
  lacrimal passages or duct —see Disorder,
      lacrimal system, changes
  lymphatic vessel I89.0
  mammary duct —see Ectasia, mammary
      duct
  Meckel's diverticulum (congenital) Q43.0
    malignant —see Table of Neoplasms, small
      intestine, malignant
  myocardium (acute) (chronic) —see
      Hypertrophy, cardiac organ or site,
      congenital NEC —see Distortion
  pancreatic duct K86.89
  pericardium —see Pericarditis
  pharynx J39.2
  prostate N42.89
  pulmonary
    artery (idiopathic) I28.8
    valve, congenital Q22.3
  pupil H57.04
  rectum K59.39
  saccule, congenital Q16.5
  salivary gland (duct) K11.8
  sphincter ani K62.89
  stomach K31.89
    acute K31.0
    psychogenic F45.8
  submaxillary duct K11.8
  trachea, congenital Q32.1
  ureter (idiopathic) N28.82
    congenital Q62.2
    due to obstruction N13.4
  urethra (acquired) N36.8
  vasomotor I73.9
  vein I86.8
  ventricular, ventricle (acute) (chronic) —see
      also Hypertrophy, cardiac
    cerebral, congenital Q04.8
  venule NEC I86.8
  vesical orifice N32.89
Dilated, dilation —see Dilatation
Diminished, diminution
  hearing (acuity) —see Deafness
  sense or sensation (cold) (heat) (tactile)
      (vibratory) R20.8
  vision NEC H54.7
  vital capacity R94.2
Diminuta taenia B71.0
Dimitri-Sturge-Weber disease Q85.8
Dimple
  congenital sacral Q82.6
  parasacral Q82.6
  pilonidal or postanal —see Cyst,
      pilonidal

Dioctophyme renalis (infection) (infestation) B83.8
Dipetalonemiasis B74.4
Diphallus Q55.69
Diphtheria, diphtheritic (gangrenous) (hemorrhagic) A36.9
  carrier (suspected) Z22.2
  cutaneous A36.3
  faucial A36.0
  infection of wound A36.3
  laryngeal A36.2
  myocarditis A36.81
  nasal, anterior A36.89
  nasopharyngeal A36.1
  neurological complication A36.89
  pharyngeal A36.0
  specified site NEC A36.89
  tonsillar A36.0
Diphyllobothriasis (intestine) B70.0
  larval B70.1
Diplacusis H93.22-●
Diplegia (upper limbs) G83.0
  congenital (cerebral) G80.8
  facial G51.0
  lower limbs G82.20
  spastic G80.1
Diplococcus, diplococcal —see condition
Diplopia H53.2
Dipsomania F10.20
  with
    psychosis —see Psychosis, alcoholic
    remission F10.21
Dipylidiasis B71.1
DIRA (deficiency of interleukin 1 receptor antagonist) M04.8
Direction, teeth, abnormal, fully erupted M26.30
Dirofilariasis B74.8
Dirt-eating child F98.3
Disability, disabilities
  heart —see Disease, heart
  intellectual F79
    with
      autistic features F84.9
    mild (I.Q. 50-69) F70
    moderate (I.Q. 35-49) F71
    profound (I.Q. under 20) F73
    severe (I.Q. 20-34) F72
    specified level NEC F78
  knowledge acquisition F81.9
  learning F81.9
  limiting activities Z73.6
  spelling, specific F81.81
Disappearance of family member Z63.4
Disarticulation —see Amputation
  meaning traumatic amputation —see Amputation, traumatic
Discharge (from)
  abnormal finding in —see Abnormal, specimen
  breast (female) (male) N64.52
  diencephalic autonomic idiopathic —see Epilepsy, specified NEC
  ear —see also Otorrhea
    blood —see Otorrhagia
  excessive urine R35.8
  nipple N64.52
  penile R36.9
  postnasal R09.82
  prison, anxiety concerning Z65.2
  urethral R36.9
    without blood R36.0
    hematospermia R36.1
  vaginal N89.8
Discitis, diskitis M46.40
  cervical region M46.42
  cervicothoracic region M46.43
  lumbar region M46.46
  lumbosacral region M46.47
  multiple sites M46.49
  occipito-atlanto-axial region M46.41

Discitis, diskitis (Continued)
  pyogenic —see Infection, intervertebral disc, pyogenic
  sacrococcygeal region M46.48
  thoracic region M46.44
  thoracolumbar region M46.45
Discoid
  meniscus (congenital) Q68.6
  semilunar cartilage (congenital) —see Derangement, knee, meniscus, specified NEC
Discoloration
  nails L60.8
  teeth (posteruptive) K03.7
    during formation K00.8
Discomfort
  chest R07.89
  visual H53.14-●
Discontinuity, ossicles, ear H74.2-●
Discord (with)
  boss Z56.4
  classmates Z55.4
  counselor Z64.4
  employer Z56.4
  family Z63.8
  fellow employees Z56.4
  in-laws Z63.1
  landlord Z59.2
  lodgers Z59.2
  neighbors Z59.2
  probation officer Z64.4
  social worker Z64.4
  teachers Z55.4
  workmates Z56.4
Discordant connection
  atrioventricular (congenital) Q20.5
  ventriculoarterial Q20.3
Discrepancy
  centric occlusion maximum intercuspation M26.55
  leg length (acquired) —see Deformity, limb, unequal length
    congenital —see Defect, reduction, lower limb
  uterine size date O26.84-●
Discrimination
  ethnic Z60.5
  political Z60.5
  racial Z60.5
  religious Z60.5
  sex Z60.5
Disease, diseased —see also Syndrome
  absorbent system I87.8
  acid-peptic K30
  Acosta's T70.29
  Adams-Stokes (-Morgagni) (syncope with heart block) I45.9
  Addison's anemia (pernicious) D51.0
  adenoids (and tonsils) J35.9
  adrenal (capsule) (cortex) (gland) (medullary) E27.9
    hyperfunction E27.0
    specified NEC E27.8
  ainhum L94.6
  airway
    obstructive, chronic J44.9
      due to
        cotton dust J66.0
        specific organic dusts NEC J66.8
    reactive —see Asthma
  akamushi (scrub typhus) A75.3
  Albers-Schönberg (marble bones) Q78.2
  Albert's —see Tendinitis, Achilles
  alimentary canal K63.9
  alligator-skin Q80.9
    acquired L85.0
  alpha heavy chain C88.3
  alpine T70.29
  altitude T70.20

Disease, diseased (Continued)
  alveolar ridge
    edentulous K06.9
      specified NEC K06.8
  alveoli, teeth K08.9
  Alzheimer's G30.9 [F02.80]
    with behavioral disturbance G30.9 [F02.81]
    early onset G30.0 [F02.80]
      with behavioral disturbance G30.0 [F02.81]
    late onset G30.1 [F02.80]
      with behavioral disturbance G30.1 [F02.81]
    specified NEC G30.8 [F02.80]
      with behavioral disturbance G30.8 [F02.81]
  amyloid —see Amyloidosis
  Andersen's (glycogenosis IV) E74.09
  Andes T70.29
  Andrews' (bacterid) L08.89
  angiospastic I73.9
    cerebral G45.9
    vein I87.8
  anterior
    chamber H21.9
    horn cell G12.29
  antiglomerular basement membrane (anti-GBM) antibody M31.0
    tubulo-interstitial nephritis N12
  antral —see Sinusitis, maxillary
  anus K62.9
    specified NEC K62.89
  aorta (nonsyphilitic) I77.9
    syphilitic NEC A52.02
  aortic (heart) (valve) I35.9
    rheumatic I06.9
  Apollo B30.3
  aponeuroses —see Enthesopathy
  appendix K38.9
    specified NEC K38.8
  aqueous (chamber) H21.9
  Arnold-Chiari —see Arnold-Chiari disease
  arterial I77.9
    occlusive —see Occlusion, by site
      due to stricture or stenosis I77.1
  arteriocardiorenal —see Hypertension, cardiorenal
  arteriolar (generalized) (obliterative) I77.9
  arteriorenal —see Hypertension, kidney
  arteriosclerotic —see also Arteriosclerosis
    cardiovascular —see Disease, heart, ischemic, atherosclerotic
    coronary (artery) —see Disease, heart, ischemic, atherosclerotic
    heart —see Disease, heart, ischemic, atherosclerotic
  artery I77.9
    cerebral I67.9
    coronary I25.10
      with angina pectoris —see Arteriosclerosis, coronary (artery),
  arthropod-borne NOS (viral) A94
    specified type NEC A93.8
  atticoantral, chronic H66.20
    left H66.22
      with right H66.23
    right H66.21
      with left H66.23
  auditory canal —see Disorder, ear, external
  auricle, ear NEC —see Disorder, pinna
  Australian X A83.4
  autoimmune (systemic) NOS M35.9
    hemolytic (cold type) (warm type) D59.1
      drug-induced D59.0
    thyroid E06.3
  aviator's —see Effect, adverse, high altitude
  Ayerza's (pulmonary artery sclerosis with pulmonary hypertension) I27.0

Disease, diseased *(Continued)*
  Babington's (familial hemorrhagic
    telangiectasia) I78.0
  bacterial A49.9
    specified NEC A48.8
    zoonotic A28.9
      specified type NEC A28.8
  Baelz's (cheilitis glandularis apostematosa)
    K13.0
  bagasse J67.1
  balloon —*see* Effect, adverse, high altitude
  Bang's (brucella abortus) A23.1
  Bannister's T78.3
  barometer makers' —*see* Poisoning, mercury
  Barraquer (-Simons') (progressive
    lipodystrophy) E88.1
  Barrett's —*see* Barrett's, esophagus
  Bartholin's gland N75.9
  basal ganglia G25.9
    degenerative G23.9
      specified NEC G23.8
    specified NEC G25.89
  Basedow's (exophthalmic goiter) —*see*
    Hyperthyroidism, with, goiter (diffuse)
  Bateman's B08.1
  Batten-Steinert G71.11
  Battey A31.0
  Beard's (neurasthenia) F48.8
  Becker
    idiopathic mural endomyocardial I42.3
    myotonia congenita G71.12
  Begbie's (exophthalmic goiter) —*see*
    Hyperthyroidism, with, goiter (diffuse)
  behavioral, organic F07.9
  Beigel's (white piedra) B36.2
  Benson's —*see* Deposit, crystalline
  Bernard-Soulier (thrombopathy) D69.1
  Bernhardt (-Roth) —*see* Mononeuropathy,
    lower limb, meralgia paresthetica
  Biermer's (pernicious anemia) D51.0
  bile duct (common) (hepatic) K83.9
    with calculus, stones —*see* Calculus, bile
      duct
    specified NEC K83.8
  biliary (tract) K83.9
    specified NEC K83.8
  Billroth's —*see* Spina bifida
  bird fancier's J67.2
  black lung J60
  bladder N32.9
    in (due to)
      schistosomiasis (bilharziasis) B65.0 *[N33]*
    specified NEC N32.89
  bleeder's D66
  blood D75.9
    forming organs D75.9
    vessel I99.9
  Bloodgood's —*see* Mastopathy, cystic
  Bodechtel-Guttmann (subacute sclerosing
    panencephalitis) A81.1
  bone —*see also* Disorder, bone
    aluminum M83.4
    fibrocystic NEC
      jaw M27.49
  bone-marrow D75.9
  Borna A83.9
  Bornholm (epidemic pleurodynia) B33.0
  Bouchard's (myopathic dilatation of the
    stomach) K31.0
  Bouillaud's (rheumatic heart disease) I01.9
  Bourneville (-Brissaud) (tuberous sclerosis)
    Q85.1
  Bouveret (-Hoffmann) (paroxysmal
    tachycardia) I47.9
  bowel K63.9
    functional K59.9
      psychogenic F45.8
  brain G93.9
    arterial, artery I67.9
    arteriosclerotic I67.2
    congenital Q04.9

Disease, diseased *(Continued)*
  brain *(Continued)*
    degenerative —*see* Degeneration, brain
    inflammatory —*see* Encephalitis
    organic G93.9
      arteriosclerotic I67.2
    parasitic NEC B71.9 *[G94]*
    senile NEC G31.1
    specified NEC G93.89
  breast (*see also* Disorder, breast) N64.9
    cystic (chronic) —*see* Mastopathy, cystic
    fibrocystic —*see* Mastopathy, cystic
    Paget's
      female, unspecified side C50.91-●
      male, unspecified side C50.92-●
    specified NEC N64.89
  Breda's —*see* Yaws
  Bretonneau's (diphtheritic malignant angina)
    A36.0
  Bright's —*see* Nephritis
    arteriosclerotic —*see* Hypertension, kidney
  Brill's (recrudescent typhus) A75.1
  Brill-Zinsser (recrudescent typhus) A75.1
  Brion-Kayser —*see* Fever, paratyphoid
  broad
    beta E78.2
    ligament (noninflammatory) N83.9
      inflammatory —*see* Disease, pelvis,
        inflammatory
      specified NEC N83.8
  Brocq-Duhring (dermatitis herpetiformis)
    L13.0
  Brocq's
    meaning
      dermatitis herpetiformis L13.0
      prurigo L28.2
  bronchopulmonary J98.4
  bronchus NEC J98.09
  bronze Addison's E27.1
    tuberculous A18.7
  budgerigar fancier's J67.2
  Buerger's (thromboangiitis obliterans)
    I73.1
  bullous L13.9
    chronic of childhood L12.2
    specified NEC L13.8
  Bürger-Grütz (essential familial
    hyperlipemia) E78.3
  bursa —*see* Bursopathy
  caisson T70.3
  California —*see* Coccidioidomycosis
  capillaries I78.9
    specified NEC I78.8
  Carapata A68.0
  cardiac —*see* Disease, heart
  cardiopulmonary, chronic I27.9
  cardiorenal (hepatic) (hypertensive)
    (vascular) —*see* Hypertension,
    cardiorenal
  cardiovascular (atherosclerotic) I25.10
    with angina pectoris —*see* Arteriosclerosis,
      coronary (artery),
    congenital Q28.9
    hypertensive —*see* Hypertension, heart
    newborn P29.9
      specified NEC P29.89
    renal (hypertensive) —*see* Hypertension,
      cardiorenal
    syphilitic (asymptomatic) A52.00
  cartilage —*see* Disorder, cartilage
  Castellani's A69.8
  Castleman (unicentric) (multicentric)
    D47.Z2
    HHV-8-associated —*see also* Herpesvirus,
      human, 8 D47.Z2
  cat-scratch A28.1
  Cavare's (familial periodic paralysis) G72.3
  cecum K63.9
  celiac (adult) (infantile) (with steatorrhea)
    K90.0
  cellular tissue L98.9

Disease, diseased *(Continued)*
  central core G71.2
  cerebellar, cerebellum —*see* Disease, brain
  cerebral —*see also* Disease, brain
    degenerative —*see* Degeneration, brain
  cerebrospinal G96.9
  cerebrovascular I67.9
    acute I67.89
      embolic I63.4-●
      thrombotic I63.3-●
    arteriosclerotic I67.2
    specified NEC I67.89
  cervix (uteri) (noninflammatory) N88.9
    inflammatory —*see* Cervicitis
    specified NEC N88.8
  Chabert's A22.9
  Chandler's (osteochondritis dissecans, hip) —
    see Osteochondritis, dissecans, hip
  Charlouis —*see* Yaws
  Chédiak-Steinbrinck (-Higashi) (congenital
    gigantism of peroxidase granules)
    E70.330
  chest J98.9
  Chiari's (hepatic vein thrombosis) I82.0
  Chicago B40.9
  Chignon B36.8
  chigo, chigoe B88.1
  childhood granulomatous D71
  Chinese liver fluke B66.1
  chlamydial A74.9
    specified NEC A74.89
  cholecystic K82.9
  choroid H31.9
    specified NEC H31.8
  Christmas D67
  chronic bullous of childhood L12.2
  chylomicron retention E78.3
  ciliary body H21.9
    specified NEC H21.89
  circulatory (system) NEC I99.8
    newborn P29.9
    syphilitic A52.00
      congenital A50.54
  coagulation factor deficiency (congenital) —
    see Defect, coagulation
  coccidioidal —*see* Coccidioidomycosis
  cold
    agglutinin or hemoglobinuria D59.1
      paroxysmal D59.6
    hemagglutinin (chronic) D59.1
  collagen NOS (nonvascular) (vascular) M35.9
    specified NEC M35.8
  colon K63.9
    functional K59.9
      congenital Q43.2
    ischemic —*see also* Ischemia, intestine,
      acute K55.039
  colonic inflammatory bowel, unclassified
    (IBDU) K52.3
  combined system —*see* Degeneration,
    combined
  compressed air T70.3
  Concato's (pericardial polyserositis) A19.9
    nontubercular I31.1
    pleural —*see* Pleurisy, with effusion
  conjunctiva H11.9
    chlamydial A74.0
    specified NEC H11.89
    viral B30.9
      specified NEC B30.8
  connective tissue, systemic (diffuse) M35.9
    in (due to)
      hypogammaglobulinemia D80.1 *[M36.8]*
      ochronosis E70.29 *[M36.8]*
    specified NEC M35.8
  Conor and Bruch's (boutonneuse fever) A77.1
  Cooper's —*see* Mastopathy, cystic
  Cori's (glycogenosis III) E74.03
  corkhandler's or corkworker's J67.3
  cornea H18.9
    specified NEC H18.89-●

Disease, diseased (Continued)
coronary (artery) —see Disease, heart, ischemic, atherosclerotic
   congenital Q24.5
   ostial, syphilitic (aortic) (mitral) (pulmonary) A52.03
corpus cavernosum N48.9
   specified NEC N48.89
Cotugno's —see Sciatica
coxsackie (virus) NEC B34.1
cranial nerve NOS G52.9
Creutzfeldt-Jakob —see Creutzfeldt-Jakob disease or syndrome
Crocq's (acrocyanosis) I73.89
Crohn's —see Enteritis, regional
Curschmann G71.11
cystic
   breast (chronic) —see Mastopathy, cystic
   kidney, congenital Q61.9
   liver, congenital Q44.6
   lung J98.4
      congenital Q33.0
cytomegalic inclusion (generalized) B25.9
   with pneumonia B25.0
   congenital P35.1
cytomegaloviral B25.9
   specified NEC B25.8
Czerny's (periodic hydrarthrosis of the knee) —see Effusion, joint, knee
Daae (-Finsen) (epidemic pleurodynia) B33.0
Darling's —see Histoplasmosis capsulati
Débove's (splenomegaly) R16.1
deer fly —see Tularemia
Degos' I77.8
demyelinating, demyelinizating (nervous system) G37.9
   multiple sclerosis G35
   specified NEC G37.8
dense deposit —see also N00-N07 with fourth character .6 N05.6
deposition, hydroxyapatite —see Disease, hydroxyapatite deposition
de Quervain's (tendon sheath) M65.4
   thyroid (subacute granulomatous thyroiditis) E06.1
Devergie's (pityriasis rubra pilaris) L44.0
Devic's G36.0
diaphorase deficiency D74.0
diaphragm J98.6
diarrheal, infectious NEC A09
digestive system K92.9
   specified NEC K92.89
disc, degenerative —see Degeneration, intervertebral disc
discogenic —see also Displacement, intervertebral disc NEC
   with myelopathy —see Disorder, disc, with, myelopathy
diverticular —see Diverticula
Dubois (thymus) A50.59 [E35]
Duchenne-Griesinger G71.0
Duchenne's
   muscular dystrophy G71.0
   pseudohypertrophy, muscles G71.0
ductless glands E34.9
Duhring's (dermatitis herpetiformis) L13.0
duodenum K31.9
   specified NEC K31.89
Dupré's (meningism) R29.1
Dupuytren's (muscle contracture) M72.0
Durand-Nicholas-Favre (climatic bubo) A55
Duroziez's (congenital mitral stenosis) Q23.2
ear —see Disorder, ear
Eberth's —see Fever, typhoid
Ebola (virus) A98.4
Ebstein's heart Q22.5
Echinococcus —see Echinococcus
echovirus NEC B34.1
Eddowes' (brittle bones and blue sclera) Q78.0
edentulous (alveolar) ridge K06.9
   specified NEC K06.8

Disease, diseased (Continued)
Edsall's T67.2
Eichstedt's (pityriasis versicolor) B36.0
▶ Eisenmenger's (irreversible) I27.83
Ellis-van Creveld (chondroectodermal dysplasia) Q77.6
end stage renal (ESRD) N18.6
   due to hypertension I12.0
endocrine glands or system NEC E34.9
endomyocardial (eosinophilic) I42.3
English (rickets) E55.0
enteroviral, enterovirus NEC B34.1
   central nervous system NEC A88.8
epidemic B99.9
   specified NEC B99.8
epididymis N50.9
Erb (-Landouzy) G71.0
Erdheim-Chester (ECD) E88.89
esophagus K22.9
   functional K22.4
   psychogenic F45.8
   specified NEC K22.8
Eulenburg's (congenital paramyotonia) G71.19
eustachian tube —see Disorder, eustachian tube
external
   auditory canal —see Disorder, ear, external
   ear —see Disorder, ear, external
extrapyramidal G25.9
   specified NEC G25.89
eye H57.9
   anterior chamber H21.9
   inflammatory NEC H57.8
   muscle (external) —see Strabismus
   specified NEC H57.8
   syphilitic —see Oculopathy, syphilitic
eyeball H44.9
   specified NEC H44.89
eyelid —see Disorder, eyelid
   specified NEC —see Disorder, eyelid, specified type NEC
eyeworm of Africa B74.3
facial nerve (seventh) G51.9
   newborn (birth injury) P11.3
Fahr (of brain) G23.8
Fahr Volhard (of kidney) I12.-●
fallopian tube (noninflammatory) N83.9
   inflammatory —see Salpingo-oophoritis
   specified NEC N83.8
familial periodic paralysis G72.3
Fanconi's (congenital pancytopenia) D61.09
fascia NEC —see also Disorder, muscle
   inflammatory —see Myositis
   specified NEC M62.89
Fauchard's (periodontitis) —see Periodontitis
Favre-Durand-Nicolas (climatic bubo) A55
Fede's K14.0
Feer's —see Poisoning, mercury
female pelvic inflammatory —see also Disease, pelvis, inflammatory N73.9
   syphilitic (secondary) A51.42
   tuberculous A18.17
Fernels' (aortic aneurysm) I71.9
fibrocaseous of lung —see Tuberculosis, pulmonary
fibrocystic —see Fibrocystic disease
Fiedler's (leptospiral jaundice) A27.0
fifth B08.3
file-cutter's —see Poisoning, lead
fish-skin Q80.9
   acquired L85.0
Flajani (-Basedow) (exophthalmic goiter) —see Hyperthyroidism, with, goiter (diffuse)
flax-dresser's J66.1
fluke —see Infestation, fluke
foot and mouth B08.8
foot process N04.9
Forbes' (glycogenosis III) E74.03
Fordyce-Fox (apocrine miliaria) L75.2
Fordyce's (ectopic sebaceous glands) (mouth) Q38.6

Disease, diseased (Continued)
Forestier's (rhizomelic pseudopolyarthritis) M35.3
   meaning ankylosing hyperostosis —see Hyperostosis, ankylosing
Fothergill's
   neuralgia —see Neuralgia, trigeminal
   scarlatina anginosa A38.9
Fournier (gangrene) N49.3
   female N76.89
fourth B08.8
Fox (-Fordyce) (apocrine miliaria) L75.2
Francis' —see Tularemia
Franklin C88.2
Frei's (climatic bubo) A55
Friedreich's
   combined systemic or ataxia G11.1
   myoclonia G25.3
frontal sinus —see Sinusitis, frontal
fungus NEC B49
Gaisböck's (polycythemia hypertonica) D75.1
gallbladder K82.9
   calculus —see Calculus, gallbladder
   cholecystitis —see Cholecystitis
   cholesterolosis K82.4
   fistula —see Fistula, gallbladder
   hydrops K82.1
   obstruction —see Obstruction, gallbladder
   perforation K82.2
   specified NEC K82.8
gamma heavy chain C88.2
Gamna's (siderotic splenomegaly) D73.2
Gamstorp's (adynamia episodica hereditaria) G72.3
Gandy-Nanta (siderotic splenomegaly) D73.2
ganister J62.8
gastric —see Disease, stomach
gastroesophageal reflux (GERD) K21.9
   with esophagitis K21.0
gastrointestinal (tract) K92.9
   amyloid E85.4
   functional K59.9
      psychogenic F45.8
   specified NEC K92.89
Gee (-Herter) (-Heubner) (-Thaysen) (nontropical sprue) K90.0
genital organs
   female N94.9
   male N50.9
Gerhardt's (erythromelalgia) I73.81
Gibert's (pityriasis rosea) L42
Gierke's (glycogenosis I) E74.01
Gilles de la Tourette's (motor-verbal tic) F95.2
gingiva K06.9
   plaque induced K05.00
   specified NEC K06.8
gland (lymph) I89.9
Glanzmann's (hereditary hemorrhagic thrombasthenia) D69.1
glass-blower's (cataract) —see Cataract, specified NEC
   salivary gland hypertrophy K11.1
Glisson's —see Rickets
globe H44.9
   specified NEC H44.89
glomerular —see also Glomerulonephritis
   with edema —see Nephrosis
   acute —see Nephritis, acute
   chronic —see Nephritis, chronic
   minimal change N05.0
   rapidly progressive N01.9
glycogen storage E74.00
   Andersen's E74.09
   Cori's E74.03
   Forbes' E74.03
   generalized E74.00
   glucose-6-phosphatase deficiency E74.01
   heart E74.02 [I43]
   hepatorenal E74.09
   Hers' E74.09
   liver and kidney E74.09

Disease, diseased *(Continued)*
  glycogen storage *(Continued)*
    McArdle's E74.04
    muscle phosphofructokinase E74.09
    myocardium E74.02 *[143]*
    Pompe's E74.02
    Tauri's E74.09
    type Ø E74.09
    type I E74.01
    type II E74.02
    type III E74.03
    type IV E74.09
    type V E74.04
    type VI-XI E74.09
    Von Gierke's E74.01
  Goldstein's (familial hemorrhagic
      telangiectasia) I78.0
  gonococcal NOS A54.9
  graft-versus-host (GVH) D89.813
    acute D89.810
    acute on chronic D89.812
    chronic D89.811
  grainhandler's J67.8
  granulomatous (childhood) (chronic) D71
  Graves' (exophthalmic goiter) —*see*
      Hyperthyroidism, with, goiter
      (diffuse)
  Griesinger's —*see* Ancylostomiasis
  Grisel's M43.6
  Gruby's (tinea tonsurans) B35.0
  Guillain-Barré G61.0
  Guinon's (motor-verbal tic) F95.2
  gum K06.9
  gynecological N94.9
  H (Hartnup's) E72.02
  Haff —*see* Poisoning, mercury
  Hageman (congenital factor XII deficiency)
      D68.2
  hair (color) (shaft) L67.9
    follicles L73.9
    specified NEC L73.8
  Hamman's (spontaneous mediastinal
      emphysema) J98.2
  hand, foot and mouth B08.4
  Hansen's —*see* Leprosy
  Hantavirus, with pulmonary manifestations
      B33.4
    with renal manifestations A98.5
  Harada's H30.81-●
  Hartnup (pellagra-cerebellar ataxia-renal
      aminoaciduria) E72.02
  Hart's (pellagra-cerebellar ataxia-renal
      aminoaciduria) E72.02
  Hashimoto's (struma lymphomatosa) E06.3
  Hb —*see* Disease, hemoglobin
  heart (organic) I51.9
    with
      pulmonary edema (acute) —*see also*
          Failure, ventricular, left I50.1
      rheumatic fever (conditions in I00)
        active I01.9
          with chorea I02.0
          specified NEC I01.8
        inactive or quiescent (with chorea)
            I09.9
          specified NEC I09.89
    amyloid E85.4 *[143]*
    aortic (valve) I35.9
    arteriosclerotic or sclerotic (senile) —
        see Disease, heart, ischemic,
        atherosclerotic
    artery, arterial —*see* Disease, heart,
        ischemic, atherosclerotic
    beer drinkers' I42.6
    beriberi (wet) E51.12
    black I27.0
    congenital Q24.9
      cyanotic Q24.9
      specified NEC Q24.8
    coronary —*see* Disease, heart, ischemic
    cryptogenic I51.9

Disease, diseased *(Continued)*
  heart *(Continued)*
    fibroid —*see* Myocarditis
    functional I51.89
      psychogenic F45.8
    glycogen storage E74.02 *[143]*
    gonococcal A54.83
    hypertensive —*see* Hypertension, heart
    hyperthyroid —*see also* Hyperthyroidism
        E05.90 *[143]*
      with thyroid storm E05.91 *[143]*
    ischemic (chronic or with a stated duration
        of over 4 weeks) I25.9
      atherosclerotic (of) I25.10
        with angina pectoris —*see*
            Arteriosclerosis, coronary (artery)
        coronary artery bypass graft —*see*
            Arteriosclerosis, coronary
            (artery),
      cardiomyopathy I25.5
      diagnosed on ECG or other special
          investigation, but currently
          presenting no symptoms I25.6
      silent I25.6
      specified form NEC I25.89
    kyphoscoliotic I27.1
    meningococcal A39.50
      endocarditis A39.51
      myocarditis A39.52
      pericarditis A39.53
    mitral I05.9
      specified NEC I05.8
    muscular —*see* Degeneration, myocardial
    psychogenic (functional) F45.8
    pulmonary (chronic) I27.9
      in schistosomiasis B65.9 *[152]*
      specified NEC I27.89
    rheumatic (chronic) (inactive) (old)
        (quiescent) (with chorea) I09.9
      active or acute I01.9
        with chorea (acute) (rheumatic)
            (Sydenham's) I02.0
      specified NEC I09.89
    senile —*see* Myocarditis
    syphilitic A52.06
      aortic A52.03
        aneurysm A52.01
      congenital A50.54 *[152]*
    thyrotoxic —*see also* Thyrotoxicosis E05.90
        [143]
      with thyroid storm E05.91 *[143]*
    valve, valvular (obstructive)
        (regurgitant) —*see also* Endocarditis
      congenital NEC Q24.8
        pulmonary Q22.3
    vascular —*see* Disease, cardiovascular
  heavy chain NEC C88.2
    alpha C88.3
    gamma C88.2
    mu C88.2
  Hebra's
    pityriasis
      maculata et circinata L42
      rubra pilaris L44.0
    prurigo L28.2
  hematopoietic organs D75.9
  hemoglobin or Hb
    abnormal (mixed) NEC D58.2
      with thalassemia D56.9
    AS genotype D57.3
    Bart's D56.0
    C (Hb-C) D58.2
      with other abnormal hemoglobin NEC
          D58.2
      elliptocytosis D58.1
      Hb-S D57.2-●
      sickle-cell D57.2-●
      thalassemia D56.8
    Constant Spring D58.2
    D (Hb-D) D58.2
    E (Hb-E) D58.2

Disease, diseased *(Continued)*
  hemoglobin or Hb *(Continued)*
    E-beta thalassemia D56.5
    elliptocytosis D58.1
    H (Hb-H) (thalassemia) D56.0
      with other abnormal hemoglobin NEC
          D56.9
      Constant Spring D56.0
    I thalassemia D56.9
    M D74.0
    S or SS D57.1
    SC D57.2-●
    SD D57.8-●
    SE D57.8-●
    spherocytosis D58.0
    unstable, hemolytic D58.2
  hemolytic (newborn) P55.9
    autoimmune (cold type) (warm type) D59.1
    drug-induced D59.0
    due to or with
      incompatibility
        ABO (blood group) P55.1
        blood (group) (Duffy) (K(ell)) (Kidd)
            (Lewis) (M) (S) NEC P55.8
        Rh (blood group) (factor) P55.0
    Rh negative mother P55.0
    specified type NEC P55.8
    unstable hemoglobin D58.2
  hemorrhagic D69.9
    newborn P53
  Henoch (-Schönlein) (purpura nervosa) D69.0
  hepatic —*see* Disease, liver
  hepatobiliary K83.9
    toxic K71.9
  hepatolenticular E83.01
  heredodegenerative NEC
    spinal cord G95.89
  herpesviral, disseminated B00.7
  Hers' (glycogenosis VI) E74.09
  Herter (-Gee) (-Heubner) (nontropical sprue)
      K90.0
  Heubner-Herter (nontropical sprue) K90.0
  high fetal gene or hemoglobin thalassemia
      D56.9
  Hildenbrand's —*see* Typhus
  hip (joint) M25.9
    congenital Q65.89
    suppurative M00.9
    tuberculous A18.02
  His (-Werner) (trench fever) A79.0
  Hodgson's I71.2
    ruptured I71.1
  Holla —*see* Spherocytosis
  hookworm B76.9
    specified NEC B76.8
  host-versus-graft D89.813
    acute D89.810
    acute on chronic D89.812
    chronic D89.811
  human immunodeficiency virus (HIV) B20
  Huntington's G10
  ▶with dementia G10 *[F02.80]*
  Hutchinson's (cheiropompholyx) —*see*
      Hutchinson's disease
  hyaline (diffuse) (generalized)
    membrane (lung) (newborn) P22.0
      adult J80
  hydatid —*see* Echinococcus
  hydroxyapatite deposition M11.00
    ankle M11.07-●
    elbow M11.02-●
    foot joint M11.07-●
    hand joint M11.04-●
    hip M11.05-●
    knee M11.06-●
    multiple site M11.09
    shoulder M11.01-●
    vertebra M11.08
    wrist M11.03-●
  hyperkinetic —*see* Hyperkinesia
  hypertensive —*see* Hypertension

Disease, diseased *(Continued)*
  hypophysis E23.7
  Iceland G93.3
  I-cell E77.0
  immune D89.9
  immunoproliferative (malignant) C88.9
    small intestinal C88.3
    specified NEC C88.8
  inclusion B25.9
    salivary gland B25.9
  infectious, infective B99.9
    congenital P37.9
      specified NEC P37.8
      viral P35.9
        specified type NEC P35.8
    specified NEC B99.8
  inflammatory
    penis N48.29
      abscess N48.21
      cellulitis N48.22
    prepuce N47.7
      balanoposthitis N47.6
    tubo-ovarian —*see* Salpingo-oophoritis
  intervertebral disc —*see also* Disorder, disc
    with myelopathy —*see* Disorder, disc, with, myelopathy
    cervical, cervicothoracic —*see* Disorder, disc, cervical
      with
        myelopathy —*see* Disorder, disc, cervical, with myelopathy
        neuritis, radiculitis or radiculopathy —*see* Disorder, disc, cervical, with neuritis
        specified NEC —*see* Disorder, disc, cervical, specified type NEC
    lumbar (with)
      myelopathy M51.06
      neuritis, radiculitis, radiculopathy or sciatica M51.16
      specified NEC M51.86
    lumbosacral (with)
      neuritis, radiculitis, radiculopathy or sciatica M51.17
      specified NEC M51.87
    specified NEC —*see* Disorder, disc, specified NEC
    thoracic (with)
      myelopathy M51.04
      neuritis, radiculitis or radiculopathy M51.14
      specified NEC M51.84
    thoracolumbar (with)
      myelopathy M51.05
      neuritis, radiculitis or radiculopathy M51.15
      specified NEC M51.85
  intestine K63.9
    functional K59.9
      psychogenic F45.8
      specified NEC K59.8
    organic K63.9
    protozoal A07.9
    specified NEC K63.89
  iris H21.9
    specified NEC H21.89
  iron metabolism or storage E83.10
  island (scrub typhus) A75.3
  itai-itai —*see* Poisoning, cadmium
  Jakob-Creutzfeldt —*see* Creutzfeldt-Jakob disease or syndrome
  jaw M27.9
    fibrocystic M27.49
    specified NEC M27.8
  jigger B88.1
  joint —*see also* Disorder, joint
    Charcot's —*see* Arthropathy, neuropathic (Charcot)
    degenerative —*see* Osteoarthritis
      multiple M15.9
      spine —*see* Spondylosis

Disease, diseased *(Continued)*
  joint *(Continued)*
    hypertrophic —*see* Osteoarthritis
    sacroiliac M53.3
    specified NEC —*see* Disorder, joint, specified type NEC
    spine NEC —*see* Dorsopathy
    suppurative —*see* Arthritis, pyogenic or pyemic
  Jourdain's (acute gingivitis) K05.00
    nonplaque induced K05.01
    plaque induced K05.00
  Kaschin-Beck (endemic polyarthritis) M12.10
    ankle M12.17-●
    elbow M12.12-●
    foot joint M12.17-●
    hand joint M12.14-●
    hip M12.15-●
    knee M12.16-●
    multiple site M12.19
    shoulder M12.11-●
    vertebra M12.18
    wrist M12.13-●
  Katayama B65.2
  Kedani (scrub typhus) A75.3
  Keshan E59
  kidney (functional) (pelvis) N28.9
    chronic N18.9
      hypertensive —*see* Hypertension, kidney
      stage 1 N18.1
      stage 2 (mild) N18.2
      stage 3 (moderate) N18.3
      stage 4 (severe) N18.4
      stage 5 N18.5
    complicating pregnancy —*see* Pregnancy, complicated by, renal disease
    cystic (congenital) Q61.9
    diabetic —*see* E08-E13 with .22
    fibrocystic (congenital) Q61.8
    hypertensive —*see* Hypertension, kidney
    in (due to)
      schistosomiasis (bilharziasis) B65.9 *[N29]*
    multicystic Q61.4
    polycystic Q61.3
      adult type Q61.2
      childhood type NEC Q61.19
        collecting duct dilatation Q61.11
  Kimmelstiel (-Wilson) (intercapillary polycystic (congenital) glomerulosclerosis) —*see* E08-E13 with .21
  Kimura D21.9
    specified site (see Neoplasm, connective tissue benign)
  Kinnier Wilson's (hepatolenticular degeneration) E83.01
  kissing —*see* Mononucleosis, infectious
  Klebs' —*see also* Glomerulonephritis N05.-●
  Klippel-Feil (brevicollis) Q76.1
  Köhler-Pellegrini-Stieda (calcification, knee joint) —*see* Bursitis, tibial collateral
  Kok Q89.8
  König's (osteochondritis dissecans) —*see* Osteochondritis, dissecans
  Korsakoff's (nonalcoholic) F04
    alcoholic F10.96
      with dependence F10.26
  Kostmann's (infantile genetic agranulocytosis) D70.0
  kuru A81.81
  Kyasanur Forest A98.2
  labyrinth, ear —*see* Disorder, ear, inner
  lacrimal system —*see* Disorder, lacrimal system
  Lafora's —*see* Epilepsy, generalized, idiopathic
  Lancereaux-Mathieu (leptospiral jaundice) A27.0
  Landry's G61.0
  Larrey-Weil (leptospiral jaundice) A27.0
  larynx J38.7

Disease, diseased *(Continued)*
  legionnaires' A48.1
    nonpneumonic A48.2
  Lenegre's I44.2
  lens H27.9
    specified NEC H27.8
  Lev's (acquired complete heart block) I44.2
  Lewy body (dementia) G31.83 *[F02.80]*
    with behavioral disturbance G31.83 *[F02.81]*
  Lichtheim's (subacute combined sclerosis with pernicious anemia) D51.0
  Lightwood's (renal tubular acidosis) N25.89
  Lignac's (cystinosis) E72.04
  lip K13.0
  lipid-storage E75.6
    specified NEC E75.5
  Lipschütz's N76.6
  liver (chronic) (organic) K76.9
    alcoholic (chronic) K70.9
      acute —*see* Disease, liver, alcoholic, hepatitis
      cirrhosis K70.30
        with ascites K70.31
      failure K70.40
        with coma K70.41
      fatty liver K70.0
      fibrosis K70.2
      hepatitis K70.10
        with ascites K70.11
      sclerosis K70.2
    cystic, congenital Q44.6
    drug-induced (idiosyncratic) (toxic) (predictable) (unpredictable) —*see* Disease, liver, toxic
    end stage K72.90
      due to hepatitis —*see* Hepatitis
    fatty, nonalcoholic (NAFLD) K76.0
      alcoholic K70.0
    fibrocystic (congenital) Q44.6
    fluke
      Chinese B66.1
      oriental B66.1
      sheep B66.3
    ▶ gestational alloimmune (GALD) P78.84
    glycogen storage E74.09 *[K77]*
    in (due to)
      schistosomiasis (bilharziasis) B65.9 *[K77]*
    inflammatory K75.9
      alcoholic K70.1
      specified NEC K75.89
    polycystic (congenital) Q44.6
    toxic K71.9
      with
        cholestasis K71.0
        cirrhosis (liver) K71.7
        fibrosis (liver) K71.7
        focal nodular hyperplasia K71.8
        hepatic granuloma K71.8
        hepatic necrosis K71.10
          with coma K71.11
        hepatitis NEC K71.6
          acute K71.2
          chronic
            active K71.50
              with ascites K71.51
            lobular K71.4
            persistent K71.3
          lupoid K71.50
            with ascites K71.51
        peliosis hepatis K71.8
        veno-occlusive disease (VOD) of liver K71.8
    veno-occlusive K76.5
  Lobo's (keloid blastomycosis) B48.0
  Lobstein's (brittle bones and blue sclera) Q78.0
  Ludwig's (submaxillary cellulitis) K12.2
  lumbosacral region M53.87
  lung J98.4
    black J60
    congenital Q33.9
    cystic J98.4
      congenital Q33.0

▶ New   ⇒ Revised   ~~deleted~~ Deleted   ● Use Additional Character(s)

Disease, diseased *(Continued)*
  lung *(Continued)*
    fibroid (chronic) —*see* Fibrosis, lung
    fluke B66.4
      oriental B66.4
    in
      amyloidosis E85.4 *[J99]*
      sarcoidosis D86.0
      Sjögren's syndrome M35.02
      systemic
        lupus erythematosus M32.13
        sclerosis M34.81
    interstitial J84.9
      of childhood, specified NEC J84.848
      respiratory bronchiolitis J84.115
      specified NEC J84.89
    obstructive (chronic) J44.9
      with
        acute
          bronchitis J44.0
          exacerbation NEC J44.1
          lower respiratory infection J44.0
        alveolitis, allergic J67.9
        asthma J44.9
        bronchiectasis J47.9
          with
            exacerbation (acute) J47.1
            lower respiratory infection J47.0
        bronchitis J44.9
          with
            exacerbation (acute) J44.1
            lower respiratory infection J44.0
        emphysema J43.9
        hypersensitivity pneumonitis J67.9
      decompensated J44.1
        with
          exacerbation (acute) J44.1
    polycystic J98.4
      congenital Q33.0
    rheumatoid (diffuse) (interstitial) —*see*
        Rheumatoid, lung
  Lutembacher's (atrial septal defect with
      mitral stenosis) Q21.1
  Lyme A69.20
  lymphatic (gland) (system) (channel) (vessel)
      I89.9
  lymphoproliferative D47.9
    specified NEC D47.Z9
    T-gamma D47.Z9
    X-linked D82.3
  Magitot's M27.2
  malarial —*see* Malaria
  malignant —*see also* Neoplasm, malignant,
      by site
  Manson's B65.1
  maple bark J67.6
  maple-syrup-urine E71.0
  Marburg (virus) A98.3
  Marion's (bladder neck obstruction) N32.0
  Marsh's (exophthalmic goiter) —*see*
      Hyperthyroidism, with, goiter (diffuse)
  mastoid (process) —*see* Disorder, ear, middle
  Mathieu's (leptospiral jaundice) A27.0
  Maxcy's A75.2
  McArdle (-Schmid-Pearson) (glycogenosis
      V) E74.04
  mediastinum J98.59
  medullary center (idiopathic) (respiratory)
      G93.89
  Meige's (chronic hereditary edema) Q82.0
  meningococcal —*see* Infection, meningococcal
  mental F99
    organic F09
  mesenchymal M35.9
  mesenteric embolic —*see also* Ischemia,
      intestine, acute K55.039
  metabolic, metabolism E88.9
    bilirubin E80.7
  metal-polisher's J62.8
  metastatic —*see also* Neoplasm, secondary, by
      site C79.9

Disease, diseased *(Continued)*
  microvascular — code to condition
  microvillus
    atrophy Q43.8
    inclusion (MVD) Q43.8
  middle ear —*see* Disorder, ear, middle
  Mikulicz' (dryness of mouth, absent or
      decreased lacrimation) K11.8
  Milroy's (chronic hereditary edema) Q82.0
  Minamata —*see* Poisoning, mercury
  minicore G71.2
  Minor's G95.19
  Minot's (hemorrhagic disease, newborn) P53
  Minot-von Willebrand-Jürgens
      (angiohemophilia) D68.0
  Mitchell's (erythromelalgia) I73.81
  mitral (valve) I05.9
    nonrheumatic I34.9
  mixed connective tissue M35.1
  moldy hay J67.0
  Monge's T70.29
  Morgagni-Adams-Stokes (syncope with heart
      block) I45.9
  Morgagni's (syndrome) (hyperostosis
      frontalis interna) M85.2
  Morton's (with metatarsalgia) —*see* Lesion,
      nerve, plantar
  Morvan's G60.8
  motor neuron (bulbar) (mixed type) (spinal)
      G12.20
    amyotrophic lateral sclerosis G12.21
    familial G12.24
    progressive bulbar palsy G12.22
    specified NEC G12.29
  moyamoya I67.5
  mu heavy chain disease C88.2
  multicore G71.2
  muscle —*see also* Disorder, muscle
    inflammatory —*see* Myositis
    ocular (external) —*see* Strabismus
  musculoskeletal system, soft tissue —*see also*
      Disorder, soft tissue
    specified NEC —*see* Disorder, soft tissue,
        specified type NEC
  mushroom workers' J67.5
  mycotic B49
  myelodysplastic, not classified C94.6
  myeloproliferative, not classified C94.6
    chronic D47.1
  myocardium, myocardial —*see also*
      Degeneration, myocardial I51.5
    primary (idiopathic) I42.9
  myoneural G70.9
  Naegeli's D69.1
  nails L60.9
    specified NEC L60.8
  Nairobi (sheep virus) A93.8
  nasal J34.9
  nemaline body G71.2
  nerve —*see* Disorder, nerve
  nervous system G98.8
    autonomic G90.9
    central G96.9
      specified NEC G96.8
    congenital Q07.9
    parasympathetic G90.9
    specified NEC G98.8
    sympathetic G90.9
    vegetative G90.9
  neuromuscular system G70.9
  Newcastle B30.8
  Nicolas (-Durand)-Favre (climatic bubo) A55
  nipple N64.9
    Paget's C50.01-●
      female C50.01-●
      male C50.02-●
  Nishimoto (-Takeuchi) I67.5
  nonarthropod-borne NOS (viral) B34.9
    enterovirus NEC B34.1
  nonautoimmune hemolytic D59.4
    drug-induced D59.2

Disease, diseased *(Continued)*
  Nonne-Milroy-Meige (chronic hereditary
      edema) Q82.0
  nose J34.9
  nucleus pulposus —*see* Disorder, disc
  nutritional E63.9
  oast-house-urine E72.19
    ocular
      herpesviral B00.50
      zoster B02.30
  obliterative vascular I77.1
  Ohara's —*see* Tularemia
  Opitz's (congestive splenomegaly)
      D73.2
  Oppenheim-Urbach (necrobiosis lipoidica
      diabeticorum) —*see* E08-E13 with .620
  optic nerve NEC —*see* Disorder, nerve, optic
    orbit —*see* Disorder, orbit
  Oriental liver fluke B66.1
  Oriental lung fluke B66.4
  Ormond's N13.5
  Oropouche virus A93.0
  Osler-Rendu (familial hemorrhagic
      telangiectasia) I78.0
  osteofibrocystic E21.0
  Otto's M24.7
  outer ear —*see* Disorder, ear, external
  ovary (noninflammatory) N83.9
    cystic N83.20-●
    inflammatory —*see* Salpingo-oophoritis
    polycystic E28.2
    specified NEC N83.8
  Owren's (congenital) —*see* Defect,
      coagulation
  pancreas K86.9
    cystic K86.2
    fibrocystic E84.9
    specified NEC K86.89
  panvalvular I08.9
    specified NEC I08.8
  parametrium (noninflammatory) N83.9
  parasitic B89
    cerebral NEC B71.9 *[G94]*
    intestinal NOS B82.9
    mouth B37.0
    skin NOS B88.9
    specified type —*see* Infestation
    tongue B37.0
  parathyroid (gland) E21.5
    specified NEC E21.4
  Parkinson's G20
  parodontal K05.6
  Parrot's (syphilitic osteochondritis) A50.02
  Parry's (exophthalmic goiter) —*see*
      Hyperthyroidism, with, goiter (diffuse)
  Parson's (exophthalmic goiter) —*see*
      Hyperthyroidism, with, goiter (diffuse)
  Paxton's (white piedra) B36.2
  pearl-worker's —*see* Osteomyelitis, specified
      type NEC
  Pellegrini-Stieda (calcification, knee joint) —
      see Bursitis, tibial collateral
  pelvis, pelvic
    female NOS N94.9
      specified NEC N94.89
    gonococcal (acute) (chronic) A54.24
    inflammatory (female) N73.9
      acute N73.0
      chlamydial A56.11
      chronic N73.1
      specified NEC N73.8
      syphilitic (secondary) A51.42
        late A52.76
      tuberculous A18.17
    organ, female N94.9
    peritoneum, female NEC N94.89
  penis N48.9
    inflammatory N48.29
      abscess N48.21
      cellulitis N48.22
    specified NEC N48.89

Disease, diseased (*Continued*)

periapical tissues NOS K04.90
periodontal K05.6
 specified NEC K05.5
periosteum —*see* Disorder, bone, specified
 type NEC
peripheral
 arterial I73.9
 autonomic nervous system G90.9
 nerves —*see* Polyneuropathy
 vascular NOS I73.9
peritoneum K66.9
 pelvic, female NEC N94.89
 specified NEC K66.8
persistent mucosal (middle ear) H66.20
 left H66.22
  with right H66.23
 right H66.21
  with left H66.23
Petit's —*see* Hernia, abdomen, specified site
 NEC
pharynx J39.2
 specified NEC J39.2
Phocas' —*see* Mastopathy, cystic
photochromogenic (acid-fast bacilli)
 (pulmonary) A31.0
 nonpulmonary A31.9
Pick's G31.01 [F02.80]
 with behavioral disturbance G31.01
  [F02.81]
 brain G31.01 [F02.80]
  with behavioral disturbance G31.01
   [F02.81]
 of pericardium (pericardial pseudocirrhosis
  of liver) I31.1
pigeon fancier's J67.2
pineal gland E34.8
pink —*see* Poisoning, mercury
Pinkus' (lichen nitidus) L44.1
pinworm B80
Piry virus A93.8
pituitary (gland) E23.7
pituitary-snuff-taker's J67.8
pleura (cavity) J94.9
 specified NEC J94.8
pneumatic drill (hammer) T75.21
Pollitzer's (hidradenitis suppurativa)
 L73.2
polycystic
 kidney or renal Q61.3
  adult type Q61.2
  childhood type NEC Q61.19
   collecting duct dilatation Q61.11
 liver or hepatic Q44.6
 lung or pulmonary J98.4
  congenital Q33.0
 ovary, ovaries E28.2
 spleen Q89.09
polyethylene T84.05-●
Pompe's (glycogenosis II) E74.02
Posadas-Wernicke B38.9
Potain's (pulmonary edema) —*see* Edema,
 lung
prepuce N47.8
 inflammatory N47.7
  balanoposthitis N47.6
Pringle's (tuberous sclerosis) Q85.1
prion, central nervous system A81.9
 specified NEC A81.89
prostate N42.9
 specified NEC N42.89
protozoal B64
 acanthamebiasis —*see* Acanthamebiasis
 African trypanosomiasis —*see* African
  trypanosomiasis
 babesiosis B60.0
 Chagas disease —*see* Chagas disease
 intestine, intestinal A07.9
 leishmaniasis —*see* Leishmaniasis
 malaria —*see* Malaria
 naegleriasis B60.2

Disease, diseased (*Continued*)

protozoal (*Continued*)
 pneumocystosis B59
 specified organism NEC B60.8
 toxoplasmosis —*see* Toxoplasmosis
pseudo-Hurler's E77.0
psychiatric F99
psychotic —*see* Psychosis
Puente's (simple glandular cheilitis) K13.0
puerperal —*see also* Puerperal O90.89
pulmonary —*see also* Disease, lung
 artery I28.9
 chronic obstructive J44.9
  with
   acute bronchitis J44.0
   exacerbation (acute) J44.1
   lower respiratory infection (acute)
    J44.0
  decompensated J44.1
   with
    exacerbation (acute) J44.1
 heart I27.9
  specified NEC I27.89
 ⟹hypertensive (vascular) —*see also*
  Hypertension, pulmonary I27.20
  ▶primary (idiopathic) I27.0
 valve I37.9
  rheumatic I09.89
pulp (dental) NOS K04.90
pulseless M31.4
Putnam's (subacute combined sclerosis with
 pernicious anemia) D51.0
Pyle (-Cohn) (metaphyseal dysplasia) Q78.5
ragpicker's or ragsorter's A22.1
Raynaud's —*see* Raynaud's disease
reactive airway —*see* Asthma
Reclus' (cystic) —*see* Mastopathy, cystic
rectum K62.9
 specified NEC K62.89
Refsum's (heredopathia atactica
 polyneuritiformis) G60.1
renal (functional) (pelvis) —*see also* Disease,
 kidney N28.9
 with
  edema —*see* Nephrosis
  glomerular lesion —*see*
   Glomerulonephritis
   with edema —*see* Nephrosis
  interstitial nephritis N12
 acute N28.9
 chronic —*see also* Disease, kidney, chronic
  N18.9
 cystic, congenital Q61.9
 diabetic —*see* E08-E13 with .22
 end-stage (failure) N18.6
  due to hypertension I12.0
 fibrocystic (congenital) Q61.8
 hypertensive —*see* Hypertension,
  kidney
 lupus M32.14
 phosphate-losing (tubular) N25.0
 polycystic (congenital) Q61.3
  adult type Q61.2
  childhood type NEC Q61.19
   collecting duct dilatation Q61.11
 rapidly progressive N01.9
 subacute N01.9
Rendu-Osler-Weber (familial hemorrhagic
 telangiectasia) I78.0
renovascular (arteriosclerotic) —*see*
 Hypertension, kidney
respiratory (tract) J98.9
 acute or subacute NOS J06.9
  due to
   chemicals, gases, fumes or vapors
    (inhalation) J68.3
   external agent J70.9
    specified NEC J70.8
   radiation J70.0
   smoke inhalation J70.5
  noninfectious J39.8

Disease, diseased (*Continued*)

respiratory (*Continued*)
 chronic NOS J98.9
  due to
   chemicals, gases, fumes or vapors
    J68.4
   external agent J70.9
    specified NEC J70.8
   radiation J70.1
  newborn P27.9
   specified NEC P27.8
 due to
  chemicals, gases, fumes or vapors J68.9
   acute or subacute NEC J68.3
   chronic J68.4
  external agent J70.9
   specified NEC J70.8
  newborn P28.9
   specified type NEC P28.89
 upper J39.9
  acute or subacute J06.9
  noninfectious NEC J39.8
  specified NEC J39.8
  streptococcal J06.9
retina, retinal H35.9
 Batten's or Batten-Mayou E75.4 [H36]
 specified NEC H35.89
rheumatoid —*see* Arthritis, rheumatoid
rickettsial NOS A79.9
 specified type NEC A79.89
Riga (-Fede) (cachectic aphthae) K14.0
Riggs' (compound periodontitis) —*see*
 Periodontitis
Ritter's L00
Rivalta's (cervicofacial actinomycosis)
 A42.2
Robles' (onchocerciasis) B73.01
Roger's (congenital interventricular septal
 defect) Q21.0
Rosenthal's (factor XI deficiency) D68.1
Ross River B33.1
Rossbach's (hyperchlorhydria) K30
Rotes Quérol —*see* Hyperostosis, ankylosing
Roth (-Bernhardt) —*see* Mononeuropathy,
 lower limb, meralgia paresthetica
Runeberg's (progressive pernicious anemia)
 D51.0
sacroiliac NEC M53.3
salivary gland or duct K11.9
 inclusion B25.9
 specified NEC K11.8
 virus B25.9
sandworm B76.9
Schimmelbusch's —*see* Mastopathy, cystic
Schmorl's —*see* Schmorl's disease or nodes
Schönlein (-Henoch) (purpura rheumatica)
 D69.0
Schottmüller's —*see* Fever, paratyphoid
Schultz's (agranulocytosis) —*see*
 Agranulocytosis
Schwalbe-Ziehen-Oppenheim G24.1
Schwartz-Jampel G71.13
sclera H15.9
 specified NEC H15.89
scrofulous (tuberculous) A18.2
scrotum N50.9
sebaceous glands L73.9
semilunar cartilage, cystic —*see also*
 Derangement, knee, meniscus, cystic
seminal vesicle N50.9
serum NEC —*see also* Reaction, serum T80.69
sexually transmitted A64
 anogenital
  herpesviral infection —*see* Herpes,
   anogenital
  warts A63.0
 chancroid A57
 chlamydial infection —*see* Chlamydia
 gonorrhea —*see* Gonorrhea
 granuloma inguinale A58
 specified organism NEC A63.8

 ▶ New ⟹ Revised ~~deleted~~ Deleted ● Use Additional Character(s)

Disease, diseased *(Continued)*

sexually transmitted *(Continued)*
  syphilis —*see* Syphilis
  trichomoniasis —*see* Trichomoniasis
Sézary C84.1-●
shimamushi (scrub typhus) A75.3
shipyard B30.0
sickle-cell D57.1
  with crisis (vasoocclusive pain) D57.00
    with
      acute chest syndrome D57.01
      splenic sequestration D57.02
  elliptocytosis D57.8-●
  Hb-C D57.20
    with crisis (vasoocclusive pain) D57.219
      with
        acute chest syndrome D57.211
        splenic sequestration D57.212
    without crisis D57.20
  Hb-SD D57.80
    with crisis D57.819
      with
        acute chest syndrome D57.811
        splenic sequestration D57.812
  Hb-SE D57.80
    with crisis D57.819
      with
        acute chest syndrome D57.811
        splenic sequestration D57.812
  specified NEC D57.80
    with crisis D57.819
      with
        acute chest syndrome D57.811
        splenic sequestration D57.812
  spherocytosis D57.80
    with crisis D57.819
      with
        acute chest syndrome D57.811
        splenic sequestration D57.812
  thalassemia D57.40
    with crisis (vasoocclusive pain) D57.419
      with
        acute chest syndrome D57.411
        splenic sequestration D57.412
    without crisis D57.40
silo-filler's J68.8
  bronchitis J68.0
  pneumonitis J68.0
  pulmonary edema J68.1
simian B B00.4
Simons' (progressive lipodystrophy) E88.1
sin nombre virus B33.4
sinus —*see* Sinusitis
Sirkari's B55.0
sixth B08.20
  due to human herpesvirus 6 B08.21
  due to human herpesvirus 7 B08.22
skin L98.9
  due to metabolic disorder NEC E88.9
    [L99]
  specified NEC L98.8
slim (HIV) B20
small vessel I73.9
Sneddon-Wilkinson (subcorneal pustular
  dermatosis) L13.1
South African creeping B88.0
spinal (cord) G95.9
  congenital Q06.9
  specified NEC G95.89
spine —*see also* Spondylopathy
  joint —*see* Dorsopathy
  tuberculous A18.01
spinocerebellar (hereditary) G11.9
  specified NEC G11.8
spleen D73.9
  amyloid E85.4 [D77]
  organic D73.9
  polycystic Q89.09
  postinfectional D73.89
sponge-diver's —*see* Toxicity, venom, marine
  animal, sea anemone

Disease, diseased *(Continued)*

Startle Q89.8
Steinert's G71.11
Sticker's (erythema infectiosum) B08.3
Stieda's (calcification, knee joint) —*see*
  Bursitis, tibial collateral
Stokes' (exophthalmic goiter) —*see*
  Hyperthyroidism, with, goiter (diffuse)
Stokes-Adams (syncope with heart block)
  I45.9
stomach K31.9
  functional, psychogenic F45.8
  specified NEC K31.89
stonemason's J62.8
storage
  glycogen —*see* Disease, glycogen storage
  mucopolysaccharide —*see*
    Mucopolysaccharidosis
striatopallidal system NEC G25.89
Stuart-Prower (congenital factor X deficiency)
  D68.2
Stuart's (congenital factor X deficiency) D68.2
subcutaneous tissue —*see* Disease, skin
supporting structures of teeth K08.9
  specified NEC K08.89
suprarenal (capsule) (gland) E27.9
  hyperfunction E27.0
  specified NEC E27.8
sweat glands L74.9
  specified NEC L74.8
Sweeley-Klionsky E75.21
Swift (-Feer) —*see* Poisoning, mercury
swimming-pool granuloma A31.1
Sylvest's (epidemic pleurodynia) B33.0
sympathetic nervous system G90.9
synovium —*see* Disorder, synovium
syphilitic —*see* Syphilis
systemic tissue mast cell C96.20
tanapox (virus) B08.71
Tangier E78.6
Tarral-Besnier (pityriasis rubra pilaris) L44.0
Tauri's E74.09
tear duct —*see* Disorder, lacrimal system
tendon, tendinous —*see also* Disorder, tendon
  nodular —*see* Trigger finger
terminal vessel I73.9
testis N50.9
thalassemia Hb-S —*see* Disease, sickle-cell,
  thalassemia
Thaysen-Gee (nontropical sprue) K90.0
Thomsen G71.12
throat J39.2
  septic J02.0
thromboembolic —*see* Embolism
thymus (gland) E32.9
  specified NEC E32.8
thyroid (gland) E07.9
  heart —*see also* Hyperthyroidism E05.90
    [I43]
    with thyroid storm E05.91 [I43]
  specified NEC E07.8
Tietze's M94.0
tongue K14.9
  specified NEC K14.89
tonsils, tonsillar (and adenoids) J35.9
tooth, teeth K08.9
  hard tissues K03.9
    specified NEC K03.89
  pulp NEC K04.99
  specified NEC K08.89
Tourette's F95.2
trachea NEC J39.8
tricuspid I07.9
  nonrheumatic I36.9
triglyceride-storage E75.5
trophoblastic —*see* Mole, hydatidiform
tsutsugamushi A75.3
tube (fallopian) (noninflammatory) N83.9
  inflammatory —*see* Salpingitis
  specified NEC N83.8
tuberculous NEC —*see* Tuberculosis

Disease, diseased *(Continued)*

tubo-ovarian (noninflammatory) N83.9
  inflammatory —*see* Salpingo-oophoritis
  specified NEC N83.8
tubotympanic, chronic —*see* Otitis, media,
  suppurative, chronic, tubotympanic
tubulo-interstitial N15.9
  specified NEC N15.8
tympanum —*see* Disorder, tympanic
  membrane
Uhl's Q24.8
Underwood's (sclerema neonatorum) P83.0
Unverricht (-Lundborg) —*see* Epilepsy,
  generalized, idiopathic
Urbach-Oppenheim (necrobiosis lipoidica
  diabeticorum) —*see* E08-E13 with .620
ureter N28.9
  in (due to)
    schistosomiasis (bilharziasis) B65.0 [N29]
urethra N36.9
  specified NEC N36.8
urinary (tract) N39.9
  bladder N32.9
    specified NEC N32.89
  specified NEC N39.8
uterus (noninflammatory) N85.9
  infective —*see* Endometritis
  inflammatory —*see* Endometritis
  specified NEC N85.8
uveal tract (anterior) H21.9
  posterior H31.9
vagabond's B85.1
vagina, vaginal (noninflammatory) N89.9
  inflammatory NEC N76.89
  specified NEC N89.8
valve, valvular I38
  multiple I08.9
    specified NEC I08.8
van Creveld-von Gierke (glycogenosis I)
  E74.01
vas deferens N50.9
vascular I99.9
  arteriosclerotic —*see* Arteriosclerosis
  ciliary body NEC —*see* Disorder, iris,
    vascular
  hypertensive —*see* Hypertension
  iris NEC —*see* Disorder, iris, vascular
  obliterative I77.1
    peripheral I73.9
  occlusive I99.8
  peripheral (occlusive) I73.9
    in diabetes mellitus —*see* E08-E13 with .51
vasomotor I73.9
vasospastic I73.9
vein I87.9
venereal —*see also* Disease, sexually
  transmitted A64
  chlamydial NEC A56.8
    anus A56.3
    genitourinary NOS A56.2
    pharynx A56.4
    rectum A56.3
  fifth A55
  sixth A55
  specified nature or type NEC A63.8
vertebra, vertebral —*see also* Spondylopathy
  disc —*see* Disorder, disc
vibration —*see* Vibration, adverse effects
viral, virus —*see also* Disease, by type of virus
  B34.9
  arbovirus NOS A94
  arthropod-borne NOS A94
  congenital P35.9
    specified NEC P35.8
  Hanta (with renal manifestations)
    (Dobrava) (Puumala) (Seoul) A98.5
    with pulmonary manifestations (Andes)
      (Bayou) (Bermejo) (Black Creek
      Canal) (Choclo) (Juquitiba) (Laguna
      negra) (Lechiguanas) (New York)
      (Oran) (Sin nombre) B33.4

▶ New   ⇒ Revised   ~~deleted~~ Deleted   ● Use Additional Character(s)

Disease, diseased *(Continued)*
  viral, virus *(Continued)*
    Hantaan (Korean hemorrhagic fever) A98.5
    human immunodeficiency (HIV) B20
    Kunjin A83.4
    nonarthropod-borne NOS B34.9
    Powassan A84.8
    Rocio (encephalitis) A83.6
    Sin nombre (Hantavirus) (cardio)-
      pulmonary syndrome B33.4
    Tahyna B33.8
    vesicular stomatitis A93.8
  vitreous H43.9
    specified NEC H43.89
  vocal cord J38.3
  Volkmann's, acquired T79.6
  von Eulenburg's (congenital paramyotonia)
    G71.19
  von Gierke's (glycogenosis I) E74.01
  von Graefe's —*see* Strabismus, paralytic,
    ophthalmoplegia, progressive
  von Willebrand (-Jürgens) (angiohemophilia)
    D68.0
  Vrolik's (osteogenesis imperfecta) Q78.0
  vulva (noninflammatory) N90.9
    inflammatory NEC N76.89
    specified NEC N90.89
  Wallgren's (obstruction of splenic vein with
    collateral circulation) I87.8
  Wassilieff's (leptospiral jaundice) A27.0
  wasting NEC R64
    due to malnutrition E41
  Waterhouse-Friderichsen A39.1
  Wegner's (syphilitic osteochondritis) A50.02
  Weil's (leptospiral jaundice of lung) A27.0
  Weir Mitchell's (erythromelalgia) I73.81
  Werdnig-Hoffmann G12.0
  Wermer's E31.21
  Werner-His (trench fever) A79.0
  Werner-Schultz (neutropenic splenomegaly)
    D73.81
  Wernicke-Posadas B38.9
  whipworm B79
  white blood cells D72.9
    specified NEC D72.89
  white matter R90.82
  white-spot, meaning lichen sclerosus et
    atrophicus L90.0
    penis N48.0
    vulva N90.4
  Wilkie's K55.1
  Wilkinson-Sneddon (subcorneal pustular
    dermatosis) L13.1
  Willis' —*see* Diabetes
  Wilson's (hepatolenticular degeneration)
    E83.01
  woolsorter's A22.1
  yaba monkey tumor B08.72
  yaba pox (virus) B08.72
  Zika virus A92.5
  zoonotic, bacterial A28.9
    specified type NEC A28.8
Disfigurement (due to scar) L90.5
Disgerminoma —*see* Dysgerminoma
DISH (diffuse idiopathic skeletal
    hyperostosis) —*see* Hyperostosis,
    ankylosing
Disinsertion, retina —*see* Detachment, retina
Dislocatable hip, congenital Q65.6
Dislocation (articular)
  with fracture —*see* Fracture
  acromioclavicular (joint) S43.10-●
    with displacement
      100%-200% S43.12-●
      more than 200% S43.13-●
    inferior S43.14-●
    posterior S43.15-●
  ankle S93.0-●
  astragalus —*see* Dislocation, ankle
  atlantoaxial S13.121
  atlantooccipital S13.111

Dislocation *(Continued)*
  atloidooccipital S13.111
  breast bone S23.29
  capsule, joint code by site under Dislocation
  carpal (bone) —*see* Dislocation, wrist
  carpometacarpal (joint) NEC S63.05-●
    thumb S63.04-●
  cartilage (joint) - code by site under
    Dislocation
  cervical spine (vertebra) —*see* Dislocation,
    vertebra, cervical
  chronic —*see* Dislocation, recurrent
  clavicle —*see* Dislocation, acromioclavicular
    joint
  coccyx S33.2
  congenital NEC Q68.8
  coracoid —*see* Dislocation, shoulder
  costal cartilage S23.29
  costochondral S23.29
  cricoarytenoid articulation S13.29
  cricothyroid articulation S13.29
  dorsal vertebra —*see* Dislocation, vertebra,
    thoracic
  ear ossicle —*see* Discontinuity, ossicles, ear
  elbow S53.10-●
    congenital Q68.8
    pathological —*see* Dislocation, pathological
      NEC, elbow
    radial head alone —*see* Dislocation, radial
      head
    recurrent —*see* Dislocation, recurrent,
      elbow
    traumatic S53.10-●
      anterior S53.11-●
      lateral S53.14-●
      medial S53.13-●
      posterior S53.12-●
      specified type NEC S53.19-●
  eye, nontraumatic —*see* Luxation, globe
  eyeball, nontraumatic —*see* Luxation, globe
  femur
    distal end —*see* Dislocation, knee
    proximal end —*see* Dislocation, hip
  fibula
    distal end —*see* Dislocation, ankle
    proximal end —*see* Dislocation, knee
  finger S63.25-●
    index S63.25-●
    interphalangeal S63.27-●
      distal S63.29-●
        index S63.29-●
        little S63.29-●
        middle S63.29-●
        ring S63.29-●
      index S63.27-●
      little S63.27-●
      middle S63.27-●
      proximal S63.28-●
        index S63.28-●
        little S63.28-●
        middle S63.28-●
        ring S63.28-●
      ring S63.27-●
    little S63.25-●
    metacarpophalangeal S63.26-●
      index S63.26-●
      little S63.26-●
      middle S63.26-●
      ring S63.26-●
    middle S63.25-●
    recurrent —*see* Dislocation, recurrent,
      finger
    ring S63.25-●
    thumb —*see* Dislocation, thumb
  foot S93.30-●
    recurrent —*see* Dislocation, recurrent,
      foot
    specified site NEC S93.33-●
    tarsal joint S93.31-●
    tarsometatarsal joint S93.32-●
    toe —*see* Dislocation, toe

Dislocation *(Continued)*
  fracture —*see* Fracture
  glenohumeral (joint) —*see* Dislocation,
    shoulder
  glenoid —*see* Dislocation, shoulder
  habitual —*see* Dislocation, recurrent
  hip S73.00-●
    anterior S73.03-●
      obturator S73.02-●
    central S73.04-●
    congenital (total) Q65.2
      bilateral Q65.1
      partial Q65.5
        bilateral Q65.4
        unilateral Q65.3-●
      unilateral Q65.0-●
    developmental M24.85-●
    pathological —*see* Dislocation, pathological
      NEC, hip
    posterior S73.01-●
    recurrent —*see* Dislocation, recurrent,
      hip
  humerus, proximal end —*see* Dislocation,
    shoulder
  incomplete —*see* Subluxation, by site
  incus —*see* Discontinuity, ossicles, ear
  infracoracoid —*see* Dislocation, shoulder
  innominate (pubic junction) (sacral junction)
    S33.39
    acetabulum —*see* Dislocation, hip
  interphalangeal (joint(s))
    finger S63.279
      distal S63.29-●
        index S63.29-●
        little S63.29-●
        middle S63.29-●
        ring S63.29-●
      index S63.27-●
      little S63.27-●
      middle S63.27-●
      proximal S63.28-●
        index S63.28-●
        little S63.28-●
        middle S63.28-●
        ring S63.28-●
      ring S63.27-●
    foot or toe —*see* Dislocation, toe
    thumb S63.12-●
      distal joint S63.14-●
      proximal joint S63.13-●
  jaw (cartilage) (meniscus) S03.0-●
  joint prosthesis —*see* Complications, joint
    prosthesis, mechanical, displacement,
    by site
  knee S83.106
    cap —*see* Dislocation, patella
    congenital Q68.2
    old M23.8X-●
    patella —*see* Dislocation, patella
    pathological —*see* Dislocation, pathological
      NEC, knee
    proximal tibia
      anteriorly S83.11-●
      laterally S83.14-●
      medially S83.13-●
      posteriorly S83.12-●
    recurrent —*see also* Derangement, knee,
      specified NEC
    specified type NEC S83.19-●
  lacrimal gland H04.16-●
  lens (complete) H27.10-●
    anterior H27.12-●
    congenital Q12.1
    ocular implant —*see* Complications,
      intraocular lens
    partial H27.11-●
    posterior H27.13-●
    traumatic S05.8X-●
  ligament code by site under Dislocation
  lumbar (vertebra) —*see* Dislocation, vertebra,
    lumbar

▶ New ⇒ Revised ~~deleted~~ Deleted ● Use Additional Character(s)

Dislocation *(Continued)*
  lumbosacral (vertebra) —*see also* Dislocation,
    vertebra, lumbar
    congenital Q76.49
  mandible S03.0-●
  meniscus (knee) —*see* Tear, meniscus
    other sites code by site under Dislocation
  metacarpal (bone)
    distal end —*see* Dislocation, finger
    proximal end S63.06-●
  metacarpophalangeal (joint)
    finger S63.26-●
      index S63.26-●
      little S63.26-●
      middle S63.26-●
      ring S63.26-●
      thumb S63.11-●
  metatarsal (bone) —*see* Dislocation, foot
  metatarsophalangeal (joint(s)) —*see*
    Dislocation, toe
  midcarpal (joint) S63.03-●
  midtarsal (joint) —*see* Dislocation, foot
  neck S13.20
    specified site NEC S13.29
    vertebra —*see* Dislocation, vertebra,
      cervical
  nose (septal cartilage) S03.1
  occipitoatloid S13.111
  old —*see* Derangement, joint, specified type
    NEC
  ossicles, ear —*see* Discontinuity, ossicles, ear
  partial —*see* Subluxation, by site
  patella S83.006
    congenital Q74.1
    lateral S83.01-●
    recurrent (nontraumatic) M22.0-●
      incomplete M22.1-●
    specified type NEC S83.09-●
  pathological NEC M24.30
    ankle M24.37-●
    elbow M24.32-●
    foot joint M24.37-●
    hand joint M24.34-●
    hip M24.35-●
    knee M24.36-●
    lumbosacral joint —*see* subcategory M53.2
    pelvic region —*see* Dislocation,
      pathological, hip
    sacroiliac —*see* subcategory M53.2
    shoulder M24.31-●
    wrist M24.33-●
  pelvis NEC S33.30
    specified NEC S33.39
  phalanx
    finger or hand —*see* Dislocation, finger
    foot or toe —*see* Dislocation, toe
  prosthesis, internal —*see* Complications,
    prosthetic device, by site, mechanical
  radial head S53.006
    anterior S53.01-●
    posterior S53.02-●
    specified type NEC S53.09-●
  radiocarpal (joint) S63.02-●
  radiohumeral (joint) —*see* Dislocation, radial
    head
  radioulnar (joint)
    distal S63.01-●
    proximal —*see* Dislocation, elbow
  radius
    distal end —*see* Dislocation, wrist
    proximal end —*see* Dislocation, radial head
  recurrent M24.40
    ankle M24.47-●
    elbow M24.42-●
    finger M24.44-●
    foot joint M24.47-●
    hand joint M24.44-●
    hip M24.45-●
    knee M24.46-●
      patella —*see* Dislocation, patella,
        recurrent

Dislocation *(Continued)*
  recurrent *(Continued)*
    patella —*see* Dislocation, patella, recurrent
    sacroiliac —*see* subcategory M53.2
    shoulder M24.41-●
    toe M24.47-●
    vertebra —*see also* subcategory M43.5
      atlantoaxial M43.4
        with myelopathy M43.3
    wrist M24.43-●
  rib (cartilage) S23.29
  sacrococcygeal S33.2
  sacroiliac (joint) (ligament) S33.2
    congenital Q74.2
    recurrent —*see* subcategory M53.2
  sacrum S33.2
  scaphoid (bone) (hand) (wrist) —*see*
    Dislocation, wrist
    foot —*see* Dislocation, foot
  scapula —*see* Dislocation, shoulder, girdle,
    scapula
  semilunar cartilage, knee —*see* Tear, meniscus
  septal cartilage (nose) S03.1
  septum (nasal) (old) J34.2
  sesamoid bone code by site under Dislocation
  shoulder (blade) (ligament) (joint) (traumatic)
    S43.006
    acromioclavicular —*see* Dislocation,
      acromioclavicular
    chronic —*see* Dislocation, recurrent,
      shoulder
    congenital Q68.8
    girdle S43.30-●
      scapula S43.31-●
      specified site NEC S43.39-●
    humerus S43.00-●
      anterior S43.01-●
      inferior S43.03-●
      posterior S43.02-●
    pathological —*see* Dislocation, pathological
      NEC, shoulder
    recurrent —*see* Dislocation, recurrent,
      shoulder
    specified type NEC S43.08-●
  spine
    cervical —*see* Dislocation, vertebra, cervical
    congenital Q76.49
    due to birth trauma P11.5
    lumbar —*see* Dislocation, vertebra, lumbar
    thoracic —*see* Dislocation, vertebra,
      thoracic
  spontaneous —*see* Dislocation, pathological
  sternoclavicular (joint) S43.206
    anterior S43.21-●
    posterior S43.22-●
  sternum S23.29
  subglenoid —*see* Dislocation, shoulder
  symphysis pubis S33.4
  talus —*see* Dislocation, ankle
  tarsal (bone(s)) (joint(s)) —*see* Dislocation,
    foot
  tarsometatarsal (joint(s)) —*see* Dislocation,
    foot
  temporomandibular (joint) S03.0-●
  thigh, proximal end —*see* Dislocation, hip
  thorax S23.20
    specified site NEC S23.29
    vertebra —*see* Dislocation, vertebra
  thumb S63.10-●
    interphalangeal joint —*see* Dislocation,
      interphalangeal (joint), thumb
    metacarpophalangeal joint —*see*
      Dislocation, metacarpophalangeal
      (joint), thumb
  thyroid cartilage S13.29
  tibia
    distal end —*see* Dislocation, ankle
    proximal end —*see* Dislocation, knee
  tibiofibular (joint)
    distal —*see* Dislocation, ankle
    superior —*see* Dislocation, knee

Dislocation *(Continued)*
  toe(s) S93.106
    great S93.10-●
      interphalangeal joint S93.11-●
      metatarsophalangeal joint S93.12-●
    interphalangeal joint S93.119
    lesser S93.106
      interphalangeal joint S93.11-●
      metatarsophalangeal joint S93.12-●
    metatarsophalangeal joint S93.12-●
  tooth S03.2
  trachea S23.29
  ulna
    distal end S63.07-●
    proximal end —*see* Dislocation, elbow
  ulnohumeral (joint) —*see* Dislocation, elbow
  vertebra (articular process) (body)
    (traumatic)
    cervical S13.101
      atlantoaxial joint S13.121
      atlantooccipital joint S13.111
      atloidooccipital joint S13.111
      joint between
        C0 and C1 S13.111
        C1 and C2 S13.121
        C2 and C3 S13.131
        C3 and C4 S13.141
        C4 and C5 S13.151
        C5 and C6 S13.161
        C6 and C7 S13.171
        C7 and T1 S13.181
      occipitoatloid joint S13.111
    congenital Q76.49
    lumbar S33.101
      joint between
        L1 and L2 S33.111
        L2 and L3 S33.121
        L3 and L4 S33.131
        L4 and L5 S33.141
    nontraumatic —*see* Displacement,
      intervertebral disc
    partial —*see* Subluxation, by site
    recurrent NEC —*see* subcategory
      M43.5
    thoracic S23.101
      joint between
        T1 and T2 S23.111
        T2 and T3 S23.121
        T3 and T4 S23.123
        T4 and T5 S23.131
        T5 and T6 S23.133
        T6 and T7 S23.141
        T7 and T8 S23.143
        T8 and T9 S23.151
        T9 and T10 S23.153
        T10 and T11 S23.161
        T11 and T12 S23.163
        T12 and L1 S23.171
  wrist (carpal bone) S63.006
    carpometacarpal joint —*see* Dislocation,
      carpometacarpal (joint)
    distal radioulnar joint —*see* Dislocation,
      radioulnar (joint), distal
    metacarpal bone, proximal —*see*
      Dislocation, metacarpal (bone),
      proximal end
    midcarpal —*see* Dislocation, midcarpal
      (joint)
    radiocarpal joint —*see* Dislocation,
      radiocarpal (joint)
    recurrent —*see* Dislocation, recurrent,
      wrist
    specified site NEC S63.09-●
    ulna —*see* Dislocation, ulna, distal end
  xiphoid cartilage S23.29
Disorder (of) —*see also* Disease
  acantholytic L11.9
    specified NEC L11.8
  acute
    psychotic —*see* Psychosis, acute
    stress F43.0

Disorder *(Continued)*
  adjustment (grief) F43.20
    with
      anxiety F43.22
        with depressed mood F43.23
      conduct disturbance F43.24
        with emotional disturbance F43.25
      depressed mood F43.21
        with anxiety F43.23
      other specified symptom F43.29
  adrenal (capsule) (gland) (medullary) E27.9
    specified NEC E27.8
  adrenogenital E25.9
    drug-induced E25.8
    iatrogenic E25.8
    idiopathic E25.8
  adult personality (and behavior) F69
    specified NEC F68.8
  affective (mood) —*see* Disorder, mood
  aggressive, unsocialized F91.1
  alcohol-related F10.99
    with
      amnestic disorder, persisting F10.96
      anxiety disorder F10.980
      dementia, persisting F10.97
      intoxication F10.929
        with delirium F10.921
        uncomplicated F10.920
      mood disorder F10.94
      other specified F10.988
      psychotic disorder F10.959
        with
          delusions F10.950
          hallucinations F10.951
      sexual dysfunction F10.981
      sleep disorder F10.982
  alcohol use
    mild F10.10
      with
        alcohol-induced
          anxiety disorder F10.180
          bipolar and related disorder
            F10.14
          depressive disorder F10.14
          psychotic disorder F10.159
          sexual dysfunction F10.181
          sleep disorder F10.182
        alcohol intoxication F10.129
          delirium F10.121
      ▶in remission (early) (sustained) F10.11
    moderate or severe F10.20
      with
        alcohol-induced
          anxiety disorder F10.280
          bipolar and related disorder F10.24
          depressive disorder F10.24
          major neurocognitive disorder,
            amnestic-confabulatory type
            F10.26
          major neurocognitive disorder,
            nonamnestic-confabulatory
            type F10.27
          mild neurocognitive disorder
            F10.288
          psychotic disorder F10.259
          sexual dysfunction F10.281
          sleep disorder F10.282
        alcohol intoxication F10.229
          delirium F10.221
      ▶in remission (early) (sustained) F10.21
  allergic —*see* Allergy
  alveolar NEC J84.09
  amino-acid
    cystathioninuria E72.19
    cystinosis E72.04
    cystinuria E72.01
    glycinuria E72.09
    homocystinuria E72.11
    metabolism —*see* Disturbance,
      metabolism, amino-acid
      specified NEC E72.8
    neonatal, transitory P74.8

Disorder *(Continued)*
  amino-acid *(Continued)*
    renal transport NEC E72.09
    transport NEC E72.09
  amnesic, amnestic
    alcohol-induced F10.96
      with dependence F10.26
    due to (secondary to) general medical
      condition F04
    psychoactive NEC-induced F19.96
      with
        abuse F19.16
        dependence F19.26
    sedative, hypnotic or anxiolytic-●
      induced F13.96
      with dependence F13.26
  amphetamine-type substance use
    mild F15.10
      ▶in remission (early) (sustained) F15.11
    moderate F15.20
      ▶in remission (early) (sustained) F15.21
    severe F15.20
      ▶in remission (early) (sustained) F15.21
  amphetamine (or other stimulant) use
    mild
      with
        amphetamine (or other stimulant)
          -induced
          anxiety disorder F15.180
          bipolar and related disorder
            F15.14
          depressive disorder F15.14
          obsessive-compulsive and related
            disorder F15.188
          psychotic disorder F15.159
          sexual dysfunction F15.181
        amphetamine, cocaine, or other
          stimulant intoxication
          with perceptual disturbances
            F15.122
          without perceptual disturbances
            F15.129
          intoxication delirium F15.121
    moderate or severe
      with
        amphetamine (or other stimulant)
          -induced
          anxiety disorder F15.280
          obsessive-compulsive and related
            disorder F15.288
          sexual dysfunction F15.281
          bipolar and related disorder
            F15.24
          depressive disorder F15.24
          psychotic disorder F15.259
        amphetamine, cocaine, or other
          stimulant intoxication
          with perceptual disturbances
            F15.222
          without perceptual disturbances
            F15.229
          intoxication delirium F15.221
  anaerobic glycolysis with anemia D55.2
  anxiety F41.9
    due to (secondary to)
      alcohol F10.980
        ▶in
          ▶abuse F10.180
          ▶dependence F10.280
      amphetamine F15.980
        in
          abuse F15.180
          dependence F15.280
      anxiolytic F13.980
        in
          abuse F13.180
          dependence F13.280
      caffeine F15.980
        in
          abuse F15.180
          dependence F15.280

Disorder *(Continued)*
  anxiety *(Continued)*
    due to *(Continued)*
      cannabis F12.980
        in
          abuse F12.180
          dependence F12.280
      cocaine F14.980
        in
          abuse F14.180
          dependence F14.180
      general medical condition F06.4
      hallucinogen F16.980
        in
          abuse F16.180
          dependence F16.280
      hypnotic F13.980
        in
          abuse F13.180
          dependence F13.280
      inhalant F18.980
        in
          abuse F18.180
          dependence F18.280
      phencyclidine F16.980
        in
          abuse F16.180
          dependence F16.280
      psychoactive substance NEC F19.980
        in
          abuse F19.180
          dependence F19.280
      sedative F13.980
        in
          abuse F13.180
          dependence F13.280
      volatile solvents F18.980
        in
          abuse F18.180
          dependence F18.280
    generalized F41.1
    illness F45.21
    mixed
      with depression (mild) F41.8
      specified NEC F41.3
    organic F06.4
    phobic F40.9
      of childhood F40.8
      specified NEC F41.8
  aortic valve —*see* Endocarditis, aortic
  aromatic amino-acid metabolism E70.9
    specified NEC E70.8
  arteriole NEC I77.89
  artery NEC I77.89
  articulation —*see* Disorder, joint
  attachment (childhood)
    disinhibited F94.2
    reactive F94.1
  attention-deficit hyperactivity (adolescent)
    (adult) (child) F98.8
    ~~combined type F90.2~~
    ~~hyperactive F90.1~~
    ~~inattentive type F90.0~~
    ▶combined
      ▶presentation F90.2
      ▶type F90.2
    ▶hyperactive
      ▶impulsive presentation F90.1
      ▶type F90.1
    ▶inattentive
      ▶presentation F90.0
      ▶type F90.0
    specified type NEC F90.8
  attention-deficit without hyperactivity
    (adolescent) (adult) (child) F90.0
  auditory processing (central) H93.25
  autism spectrum F84.0
  autistic F84.0
  ▶autoimmune D89.89
  autonomic nervous system G90.9
    specified NEC G90.8

Disorder *(Continued)*
  avoidant
    child or adolescent F40.10
    ⮞ restrictive food intake F50.82
  balance
    acid-base E87.8
      mixed E87.4
    electrolyte E87.8
    fluid NEC E87.8
  behavioral (disruptive) —*see* Disorder,
    conduct
  beta-amino-acid metabolism E72.8
  bile acid and cholesterol metabolism E78.70
    Barth syndrome E78.71
    other specified E78.79
    Smith-Lemli-Opitz syndrome E78.72
  bilirubin excretion E80.6
  binge eating F50.81
  binocular
    movement H51.9
      convergence
        excess H51.12
        insufficiency H51.11
      internuclear ophthalmoplegia —*see*
        Ophthalmoplegia, internuclear
      palsy of conjugate gaze H51.0
      specified type NEC H51.8
    vision NEC —*see* Disorder, vision, binocular
  ⮞ bipolar (I) (type 1) F31.9
    ~~current episode~~
      ~~depressed F31.9~~
        ~~with psychotic features F31.5~~
        ~~without psychotic features~~
          ~~F31.30~~
          ~~mild F31.31~~
          ~~moderate F31.32~~
          ~~severe (without psychotic features)~~
            ~~F31.4~~
            ~~with psychotic features F31.5~~
      ~~hypomanic F31.0~~
      ~~manic F31.9~~
        ~~with psychotic features F31.2~~
        ~~without psychotic features F31.10~~
          ~~mild F31.11~~
          ~~moderate F31.12~~
          ~~severe (without psychotic features)~~
            ~~F31.13~~
            ~~with psychotic features F31.2~~
      ~~mixed F31.60~~
        ~~mild F31.61~~
        ~~moderate F31.62~~
        ~~severe (without psychotic features)~~
          ~~F31.63~~
          ~~with psychotic features F31.64~~
      ~~severe depression (without psychotic~~
        ~~features) F31.4~~
        ~~with psychotic features F31.5~~
    ⮞ and related due to a known physiological
      condition
      ⮞ with
        ⮞ manic features F06.33
        ⮞ manic- or hypomanic-like episodes
          F06.33
        ⮞ mixed features F06.34
    ⮞ current (or most recent) episode
      ⮞ depressed F31.9
        ⮞ with psychotic features F31.5
        ⮞ without psychotic features F31.30
          ⮞ mild F31.31
          ⮞ moderate F31.32
          ⮞ severe (without psychotic features)
            F31.4
            ⮞ with psychotic features F31.5
      ⮞ hypomanic F31.0
      ⮞ manic F31.9
        ⮞ with psychotic features F31.2
        ⮞ without psychotic features F31.10
          ⮞ mild F31.11
          ⮞ moderate F31.12
          ⮞ severe (without psychotic features)
            F31.13
            ⮞ with psychotic features F31.2

Disorder *(Continued)*
  bipolar (I) (type 1) *(Continued)*
    current (or most recent) episode *(Continued)*
      ⮞ mixed F31.60
        ⮞ mild F31.61
        ⮞ moderate F31.62
        ⮞ severe (without psychotic features)
          F31.63
          ⮞ with psychotic features F31.64
        ⮞ severe depression (without psychotic
          features) F31.4
          ⮞ with psychotic features F31.5
    ⮞ II (type 2) F31.81
    in remission (currently) F31.70
      in full remission
        most recent episode
          depressed F31.76
          hypomanic F31.72
          manic F31.74
          mixed F31.78
      in partial remission
        most recent episode
          depressed F31.75
          hypomanic F31.71
          manic F31.73
          mixed F31.77
    organic F06.30
    single manic episode F30.9
      mild F30.11
      moderate F30.12
      hhsevere (without psychotic symptoms)
        F30.13
      with psychotic symptoms F30.2
    specified NEC F31.89
  bladder N32.9
    functional NEC N31.9
    in schistosomiasis B65.0 *[N33]*
    specified NEC N32.89
  bleeding D68.9
  blood D75.9
    in congenital early syphilis A50.09 *[D77]*
  body dysmorphic F45.22
  bone M89.9
    continuity M84.9
      specified type NEC M84.80
        ankle M84.87-●
        fibula M84.86-●
        foot M84.87-●
        hand M84.84-●
        humerus M84.82-●
        neck M84.88
        pelvis M84.859
        radius M84.83-●
        rib M84.88
        shoulder M84.81-●
        skull M84.88
        thigh M84.85-●
        tibia M84.86-●
        ulna M84.83-●
        vertebra M84.88
    density and structure M85.9
      cyst —*see also* Cyst, bone, specified type
        NEC
        aneurysmal —*see* Cyst, bone,
          aneurysmal
        solitary —*see* Cyst, bone, solitary
      diffuse idiopathic skeletal
        hyperostosis —*see* Hyperostosis,
          ankylosing
      fibrous dysplasia (monostotic) —*see*
        Dysplasia, fibrous, bone
      fluorosis —*see* Fluorosis, skeletal
      hyperostosis of skull M85.2
      osteitis condensans —*see* Osteitis,
        condensans
      specified type NEC M85.8-●
        ankle M85.87-●
        foot M85.87-●
        forearm M85.83-●
        hand M85.84-●
        lower leg M85.86-●

Disorder *(Continued)*
  bone *(Continued)*
    density and structure *(Continued)*
      specified type NEC *(Continued)*
        multiple sites M85.89
        neck M85.88
        rib M85.88
        shoulder M85.81-●
        skull M85.88
        thigh M85.85-●
        upper arm M85.82-●
        vertebra M85.88
    development and growth NEC M89.20
      carpus M89.24-●
      clavicle M89.21-●
      femur M89.25-●
      fibula M89.26-●
      finger M89.24-●
      humerus M89.22-●
      ilium M89.259
      ischium M89.259
      metacarpus M89.24-●
      metatarsus M89.27-●
      multiple sites M89.29
      neck M89.28
      radius M89.23-●
      rib M89.28
      scapula M89.21-●
      skull M89.28
      tarsus M89.27-●
      tibia M89.26-●
      toe M89.27-●
      ulna M89.23-●
      vertebra M89.28
    specified type NEC M89.8X-●
  brachial plexus G54.0
  branched-chain amino-acid metabolism E71.2
    specified NEC E71.19
  breast N64.9
    agalactia —*see* Agalactia
    associated with
      lactation O92.70
        specified NEC O92.79
      pregnancy O92.20
        specified NEC O92.29
      puerperium O92.20
        specified NEC O92.29
    cracked nipple —*see* Cracked nipple
    galactorrhea —*see* Galactorrhea
    hypogalactia O92.4
    lactation disorder NEC O92.79
    mastitis —*see* Mastitis
    nipple infection —*see* Infection, nipple
    retracted nipple —*see* Retraction, nipple
    specified type NEC N64.89
  Briquet's F45.0
  bullous, in diseases classified elsewhere L14
  caffeine use
    mild
      with
        caffeine-induced
          anxiety disorder F15.180
          sleep disorder F15.182
    moderate or severe
      with
        caffeine-induced
          anxiety disorder F15.280
          sleep disorder F15.282
  cannabis use
    mild F12.10
      with
        cannabis-induced
          anxiety disorder F12.180
          psychotic disorder F12.159
          sleep disorder F12.188
        cannabis intoxication delirium F12.121
          with perceptual disturbances
            F12.122
          without perceptual disturbances
            F12.129
    ⮞ in remission (early) (sustained) F12.11

Disorder *(Continued)*
  cannabis use *(Continued)*
    moderate or severe F12.20
      with
        cannabis-induced
          anxiety disorder F12.280
          psychotic disorder F12.259
          sleep disorder F12.288
        cannabis intoxication
          with perceptual disturbances
            F12.222
          without perceptual disturbances
            F12.229
        delirium F12.221
    ▶in remission (early) (sustained) F12.21
  carbohydrate
    absorption, intestinal NEC E74.39
    metabolism (congenital) E74.9
      specified NEC E74.8
  cardiac, functional I51.89
  carnitine metabolism E71.40
  cartilage M94.9
    articular NEC —*see* Derangement, joint,
      articular cartilage
    chondrocalcinosis —*see*
      Chondrocalcinosis
    specified type NEC M94.8X-●
      articular —*see* Derangement, joint,
        articular cartilage
      multiple sites M94.8X0
  catatonia (due to known physiological
    condition) (with another mental
    disorder) F06.1
  catatonic
    due to (secondary to) known physiological
      condition F06.1
    organic F06.1
  central auditory processing H93.25
  cervical
    region NEC M53.82
    root (nerve) NEC G54.2
  character NOS F60.9
  childhood disintegrative NEC F84.3
  cholesterol and bile acid metabolism E78.70
    Barth syndrome E78.71
    other specified E78.79
    Smith-Lemli-Opitz syndrome E78.72
  choroid H31.9
    atrophy —*see* Atrophy, choroid
    degeneration —*see* Degeneration, choroid
    detachment —*see* Detachment, choroid
    dystrophy —*see* Dystrophy, choroid
    hemorrhage —*see* Hemorrhage, choroid
    rupture —*see* Rupture, choroid
    scar —*see* Scar, chorioretinal
    solar retinopathy —*see* Retinopathy, solar
    specified type NEC H31.8
  ciliary body —*see* Disorder, iris
    degeneration —*see* Degeneration, ciliary
      body
  coagulation (factor) (*see also* Defect,
    coagulation) D68.9
    newborn, transient P61.6
  cocaine use
    mild F14.10
      with
        amphetamine, cocaine, or other
          stimulant intoxication
          with perceptual disturbances F14.122
          without perceptual disturbances
            F14.129
        cocaine-induced
          anxiety disorder F14.180
          bipolar and related disorder F14.14
          depressive disorder F14.14
          obsessive-compulsive and related
            disorder F14.188
          psychotic disorder F14.159
          sexual dysfunction F14.181
          sleep disorder F14.182
        cocaine intoxication delirium F14.121
    ▶in remission (early) (sustained) F14.11

Disorder *(Continued)*
  cocaine use *(Continued)*
    moderate or severe F14.20
      with
        amphetamine, cocaine, or other
          stimulant intoxication
          with perceptual disturbances F14.222
          without perceptual disturbances
            F14.229
        cocaine-induced
          anxiety disorder F14.280
          bipolar and related disorder F14.24
          depressive disorder F14.24
          obsessive-compulsive and related
            disorder F14.288
          psychotic disorder F14.259
          sexual dysfunction F14.281
          sleep disorder F14.282
        cocaine intoxication delirium F14.221
    ▶in remission (early) (sustained) F14.21
  coccyx NEC M53.3
  cognitive F09
    due to (secondary to) general medical
      condition F09
    persisting R41.89
      due to
        alcohol F10.97
          with dependence F10.27
        anxiolytics F13.97
          with dependence F13.27
        hypnotics F13.97
          with dependence F13.27
        sedatives F13.97
          with dependence F13.27
        specified substance NEC
          F19.97
          with
            abuse F19.17
            dependence F19.27
  communication F80.9
    social pragmatic F80.82
  conduct (childhood) F91.9
    adjustment reaction —*see* Disorder,
      adjustment
    adolescent onset type F91.2
    childhood onset type F91.1
    compulsive F63.9
    confined to family context F91.0
    depressive F91.8
    group type F91.2
    hyperkinetic —*see* Disorder, attention-
      deficit hyperactivity
    oppositional defiance F91.3
    socialized F91.2
    solitary aggressive type F91.1
    specified NEC F91.8
    unsocialized (aggressive) F91.1
  conduction, heart I45.9
  congenital glycosylation (CDG) E74.8
  conjunctiva H11.9
    infection —*see* Conjunctivitis
  connective tissue, localized L94.9
    specified NEC L94.8
  conversion (functional neurological symptom
    disorder)
    with
      abnormal movement F44.4
      anesthesia or sensory loss F44.6
      attacks or seizures F44.5
      mixed symptoms F44.7
      special sensory symptoms F44.6
      speech symptoms F44.4
      swallowing symptoms F44.4
      weakness or paralysis F44.4
  convulsive (secondary) —*see* Convulsions
  cornea H18.9
    deformity —*see* Deformity, cornea
    degeneration —*see* Degeneration, cornea
    deposits —*see* Deposit, cornea
    due to contact lens H18.82-●
      specified as edema —*see* Edema, cornea
    edema —*see* Edema, cornea

Disorder *(Continued)*
  cornea *(Continued)*
    keratitis —*see* Keratitis
    keratoconjunctivitis —*see*
      Keratoconjunctivitis
    membrane change —*see* Change, corneal
      membrane
    neovascularization —*see*
      Neovascularization, cornea
    scar —*see* Opacity, cornea
    specified type NEC H18.89-●
    ulcer —*see* Ulcer, cornea
  corpus cavernosum N48.9
  cranial nerve —*see* Disorder, nerve, cranial
  cyclothymic F34.0
  defiant oppositional F91.3
  delusional (persistent) (systematized) F22
    induced F24
  depersonalization F48.1
  depressive F32.9
  ▶due to known physiological condition
    ▶with
      ▶depressive features F06.31
      ▶major depressive-like episode F06.32
      ▶mixed features F06.34
    major F32.9
      with psychotic symptoms F32.3
      in remission (full) F32.5
        partial F32.4
      recurrent F33.9
      ▶with psychotic features F33.3
      single episode F32.9
        mild F32.0
        moderate F32.1
        severe (without psychotic symptoms)
          F32.2
          with psychotic symptoms F32.3
    organic F06.31
    persistent F34.1
    recurrent F33.9
      current episode
        mild F33.0
        moderate F33.1
        severe (without psychotic symptoms)
          F33.2
          with psychotic symptoms F33.3
      in remission F33.40
        full F33.42
        partial F33.41
      specified NEC F33.8
    single episode —*see* Episode,
      depressive
    specified NEC F32.89
  developmental F89
    arithmetical skills F81.2
    coordination (motor) F82
    expressive writing F81.81
    language F80.9
      expressive F80.1
      mixed receptive and expressive
        F80.2
      receptive type F80.2
      specified NEC F80.89
    learning F81.9
      arithmetical F81.2
      reading F81.0
    mixed F88
    motor coordination or function F82
    pervasive F84.9
      specified NEC F84.8
    phonological F80.0
    reading F81.0
    scholastic skills —*see also* Disorder,
      learning
      mixed F81.89
    specified NEC F88
    speech F80.9
      articulation F80.0
      specified NEC F80.89
    written expression F81.81
  diaphragm J98.6

▶ New   ⇨ Revised   ~~deleted~~ Deleted   ● Use Additional Character(s)

Disorder *(Continued)*
  digestive (system) K92.9
    newborn P78.9
      specified NEC P78.89
    postprocedural —*see* Complication,
      gastrointestinal
    psychogenic F45.8
  disc (intervertebral) M51.9
    with
      myelopathy
        cervical region M50.00
        cervicothoracic region M50.03
        high cervical region M50.01
        lumbar region M51.06
        mid-cervical region M50.020
        sacrococcygeal region M53.3
        thoracic region M51.04
        thoracolumbar region M51.05
      radiculopathy
        cervical region M50.10
        cervicothoracic region M50.13
        high cervical region M50.11
        lumbar region M51.16
        lumbosacral region M51.17
        mid-cervical region M50.120
        sacrococcygeal region M53.3
        thoracic region M51.14
        thoracolumbar region M51.15
    cervical M50.90
      with
        myelopathy M50.00
          C2-C3 M50.01
          C3-C4 M50.01
          C4-C5 M50.021
          C5-C6 M50.022
          C6-C7 M50.023
          C7-T1 M50.03
          cervicothoracic region M50.03
          high cervical region M50.01
          mid-cervical region M50.020
        neuritis, radiculitis or radiculopathy
          M50.10
          C2-C3 M50.11
          C3-C4 M50.11
          C4-C5 M50.121
          C5-C6 M50.122
          C6-C7 M50.123
          C7-T1 M50.13
          cervicothoracic region M50.13
          high cervical region M50.11
          mid-cervical region M50.120
        C2-C3 M50.91
        C3-C4 M50.91
        C4-C5 M50.921
        C5-C6 M50.922
        C6-C7 M50.923
        C7-T1 M50.93
        cervicothoracic region M50.93
        degeneration M50.30
          C2-C3 M50.31
          C3-C4 M50.31
          C4-C5 M50.321
          C5-C6 M50.322
          C6-C7 M50.323
          C7-T1 M50.33
          cervicothoracic region M50.33
          high cervical region M50.31
          mid-cervical region M50.320
        displacement M50.20
          C2-C3 M50.21
          C3-C4 M50.21
          C4-C5 M50.221
          C5-C6 M50.222
          C6-C7 M50.223
          C7-T1 M50.23
          cervicothoracic region M50.23
          high cervical region M50.21
          mid-cervical region M50.220
        high cervical region M50.91
        mid-cervical region M50.920
        specified type NEC M50.80
          C2-C3 M50.81
          C3-C4 M50.81

Disorder *(Continued)*
  disc (intervertebral) *(Continued)*
    cervical *(Continued)*
      specified type NEC *(Continued)*
        C4-C5 M50.821
        C5-C6 M50.822
        C6-C7 M50.823
        C7-T1 M50.83
        cervicothoracic region M50.83
        high cervical region M50.81
        mid-cervical region M50.820
      specified NEC
        lumbar region M51.86
        lumbosacral region M51.87
        sacrococcygeal region M53.3
        thoracic region M51.84
        thoracolumbar region M51.85
  disinhibited attachment (childhood) F94.2
  disintegrative, childhood NEC F84.3
  disruptive F91.9
    mood dysregulation F34.81
    specified NEC F91.8
  disruptive behavior —*see* Disorder, conduct
  dissocial personality F60.2
  dissociative F44.9
    affecting
      motor function F44.4
        and sensation F44.7
      sensation F44.6
        and motor function F44.7
    brief reactive F43.0
    due to (secondary to) general medical
      condition F06.8
    mixed F44.7
    organic F06.8
    other specified NEC F44.89
  double heterozygous sickling —*see* Disease,
    sickle-cell
  dream anxiety F51.5
  drug induced hemorrhagic D68.32
  drug related F19.99
    abuse —*see* Abuse, drug
    dependence —*see* Dependence, drug
  dysmorphic body F45.22
  dysthymic F34.1
  ear H93.9-•
    bleeding —*see* Otorrhagia
    deafness —*see* Deafness
    degenerative H93.09-•
    discharge —*see* Otorrhea
    external H61.9-•
      auditory canal stenosis —*see* Stenosis,
        external ear canal
      exostosis —*see* Exostosis, external ear canal
      impacted cerumen —*see* Impaction,
        cerumen
      otitis —*see* Otitis, externa
      perichondritis —*see* Perichondritis, ear
      pinna —*see* Disorder, pinna
      specified type NEC H61.89-•
        in diseases classified elsewhere
          H62.8X-•
    inner H83.9-•
      vestibular dysfunction —*see* Disorder,
        vestibular function
    middle H74.9-•
      adhesive H74.1-•
      ossicle —*see* Abnormal, ear ossicles
      polyp —*see* Polyp, ear (middle)
      specified NEC, in diseases classified
        elsewhere H75.8-•
    postprocedural —*see* Complications, ear,
      procedure
    specified NEC, in diseases classified
      elsewhere H94.8-•
  eating (adult) (psychogenic) F50.9
    anorexia —*see* Anorexia
    binge F50.81
    bulimia F50.2
    child F98.29
      pica F98.3
      rumination disorder F98.21

Disorder *(Continued)*
  eating *(Continued)*
    pica F50.89
      childhood F98.3
  electrolyte (balance) NEC E87.8
    with
      abortion —*see* Abortion by type
        complicated by specified condition
        NEC
      ectopic pregnancy O08.5
      molar pregnancy O08.5
    acidosis (metabolic) (respiratory) E87.2
    alkalosis (metabolic) (respiratory) E87.3
  elimination, transepidermal L87.9
    specified NEC L87.8
  emotional (persistent) F34.9
    of childhood F93.9
      specified NEC F93.8
  endocrine E34.9
    postprocedural E89.89
      specified NEC E89.89
  erectile (male) (organic) —*see also*
    Dysfunction, sexual, male, erectile N52.9
    nonorganic F52.21
  erythematous —*see* Erythema
  esophagus K22.9
    functional K22.4
    psychogenic F45.8
  eustachian tube H69.9-•
    infection —*see* Salpingitis, eustachian
    obstruction —*see* Obstruction, eustachian
      tube
    patulous —*see* Patulous, eustachian tube
    specified NEC H69.8-•
  ▶exhibitionistic F65.2
  extrapyramidal G25.9
    in diseases classified elsewhere —*see*
      category G26
    specified type NEC G25.89
  eye H57.9
    postprocedural —*see* Complication,
      postprocedural, eye
  eyelid H02.9
    cyst —*see* Cyst, eyelid
    degenerative H02.70
      chloasma —*see* Chloasma, eyelid
      madarosis —*see* Madarosis
      specified type NEC H02.79
      vitiligo —*see* Vitiligo, eyelid
      xanthelasma —*see* Xanthelasma
    dermatochalasis —*see* Dermato-chalasis
    edema —*see* Edema, eyelid
    elephantiasis —*see* Elephantiasis, eyelid
    foreign body, retained —*see* Foreign body,
      retained, eyelid
    function H02.59
      abnormal innervation syndrome —*see*
        Syndrome, abnormal innervation
      blepharochalasis —*see* Blepharochalasis
      blepharoclonus —*see* Blepharoclonus
      blepharophimosis —*see*
        Blepharophimosis
      blepharoptosis —*see* Blepharoptosis
      lagophthalmos —*see* Lagophthalmos
      lid retraction —*see* Retraction, lid
      hypertrichosis —*see* Hypertrichosis, eyelid
      specified type NEC H02.89
    vascular H02.879
      left H02.876
        lower H02.875
        upper H02.874
      right H02.873
        lower H02.872
        upper H02.871
  factitious F68.10
    with predominantly
      physical symptoms F68.12
        with psychological symptoms F68.13
      psychological symptoms F68.11
        with physical symptoms F68.13
  factor, coagulation —*see* Defect, coagulation

Disorder *(Continued)*
  fatty acid
    metabolism E71.30
      specified NEC E71.39
    oxidation
      LCAD E71.310
      MCAD E71.311
      SCAD E71.312
      specified deficiency NEC E71.318
  feeding (infant or child) —*see also* Disorder,
      eating R63.3-●
  ▶or eating disorder F50.9
  ▶specified NEC F50.9
  feigned (with obvious motivation) Z76.5
    without obvious motivation —*see* Disorder,
        factitious
  female
    hypoactive sexual desire F52.0
    orgasmic F52.31
    sexual arousal F52.22
  ▶sexual interest/arousal F52.22
  ▶fetishistic F65.0
  fibroblastic M72.9
    specified NEC M72.8
  fluency
    adult onset F98.5
    childhood onset F80.81
    following
      cerebral infarction I69.323
      cerebrovascular disease I69.923
        specified disease NEC I69.823
      intracerebral hemorrhage I69.123
      nontraumatic intracranial hemorrhage
          NEC I69.223
      subarachnoid hemorrhage I69.023
    in conditions classified elsewhere R47.82
  fluid balance E87.8
  follicular (skin) L73.9
    specified NEC L73.8
  ▶frotteuristic F65.81
  fructose metabolism E74.10
    essential fructosuria E74.11
    fructokinase deficiency E74.11
    fructose-1, 6-diphosphatase deficiency
        E74.19
    hereditary fructose intolerance E74.12
    other specified E74.19
  functional polymorphonuclear neutrophils D71
  gallbladder, biliary tract and pancreas in
      diseases classified elsewhere K87
  ▶gambling F63.0
  gamma-glutamyl cycle E72.8
  gastric (functional) K31.9
    motility K30
    psychogenic F45.8
    secretion K30
  gastrointestinal (functional) NOS K92.9
    newborn P78.9
    psychogenic F45.8
  gender-identity or -role F64.9
    childhood F64.2
    effect on relationship F66
    of adolescence or adulthood F64.0
      nontranssexual F64.8
    specified NEC F64.8
    uncertainty F66
  genito-pelvic pain penetration F52.6
  genitourinary system
    female N94.9
    male N50.9
    psychogenic F45.8
  globe H44.9
    degenerated condition H44.50
      absolute glaucoma H44.51-●
      atrophy H44.52-●
      leucocoria H44.53-●
    degenerative H44.30
      chalcosis H44.31-●
    ➡myopia —*see also* Myopia, degenerative
        H44.2-●
      siderosis H44.32-●
      specified type NEC H44.39-●

Disorder *(Continued)*
  globe *(Continued)*
    endophthalmitis —*see* Endophthalmitis
    foreign body, retained —*see* Foreign body,
        intraocular, old, retained
    hemophthalmos —*see* Hemophthalmos
    hypotony H44.40
      due to
        ocular fistula H44.42-●
        specified disorder NEC H44.43-●
      flat anterior chamber H44.41-●
      primary H44.44-●
    luxation —*see* Luxation, globe
    specified type NEC H44.89
  glomerular (in) N05.9
    amyloidosis E85.4 *[N08]*
    cryoglobulinemia D89.1 *[N08]*
    disseminated intravascular coagulation
        D65 *[N08]*
    Fabry's disease E75.21 *[N08]*
    familial lecithin cholesterol acyltransferase
        deficiency E78.6 *[N08]*
    Goodpasture's syndrome M31.0
    hemolytic-uremic syndrome D59.3
    Henoch (-Schönlein) purpura D69.0 *[N08]*
    malariae malaria B52.0
    microscopic polyangiitis M31.7 *[N08]*
    multiple myeloma C90.0-● *[N08]*
    mumps B26.83
    schistosomiasis B65.9 *[N08]*
    sepsis NEC A41.-● *[N08]*
      streptococcal A40.-● *[N08]*
    sickle-cell disorders D57.-● *[N08]*
    strongyloidiasis B78.9 *[N08]*
    subacute bacterial endocarditis I33.0 *[N08]*
    syphilis A52.75
    systemic lupus erythematosus M32.14
    thrombotic thrombocytopenic purpura
        M31.1 *[N08]*
    Waldenström macroglobulinemia C88.0
        [N08]
    Wegener's granulomatosis M31.31
  gluconeogenesis E74.4
  glucosaminoglycan metabolism —
      see Disorder, metabolism,
      glucosaminoglycan
  glycine metabolism E72.50
    d-glycericacidemia E72.59
    hyperhydroxyprolinemia E72.59
    hyperoxaluria E72.53
    hyperprolinemia E72.59
    non-ketotic hyperglycinemia E72.51
    oxalosis E72.53
    oxaluria E72.53
    sarcosinemia E72.59
    trimethylaminuria E72.52
  glycoprotein metabolism E77.9
    specified NEC E77.8
  habit (and impulse) F63.9
    involving sexual behavior NEC F65.9
    specified NEC F63.89
  hallucinogen use
    mild F16.10
      with
        hallucinogen-induced
          anxiety disorder F16.180
          bipolar and related disorder F16.14
          depressive disorder F16.14
          psychotic disorder F16.159
        hallucinogen intoxication delirium
            F16.121
        other hallucinogen intoxication
            F16.129
      ▶in remission (early) (sustained) F16.11
    moderate or severe F16.20
      with
        hallucinogen-induced
          anxiety disorder F16.280
          bipolar and related disorder F16.24
          depressive disorder F16.24
          psychotic disorder F16.259

Disorder *(Continued)*
  hallucinogen use *(Continued)*
    moderate or severe *(Continued)*
      with *(Continued)*
        hallucinogen intoxication delirium
            F16.221
        other hallucinogen intoxication F16.229
      ▶in remission (early) (sustained) F16.21
  heart action I49.9
  hematological D75.9
    newborn (transient) P61.9
      specified NEC P61.8
  hematopoietic organs D75.9
  hemorrhagic NEC D69.9
    drug-induced D68.32
    due to
      extrinsic circulating anticoagulants
          D68.32
      increase in
        anti-IIa D68.32
        anti-Xa D68.32
      intrinsic
        circulating anticoagulants D68.318
        increase in
          antithrombin D68.318
          anti-VIIIa D68.318
          anti-IXa D68.318
          anti-XIa D68.318
    following childbirth O72.3
  hemostasis —*see* Defect, coagulation
  histidine metabolism E70.40
    histidinemia E70.41
    other specified E70.49
  hoarding F42.3
  hyperkinetic —*see* Disorder, attention-deficit
      hyperactivity
  hyperleucine-isoleucinemia E71.19
  hypervalinemia E71.19
  hypoactive sexual desire F52.0
  hypochondriacal F45.20
    body dysmorphic F45.22
    neurosis F45.21
    other specified F45.29
  identity
    dissociative F44.81
    illness anxiety F45.21
    of childhood F93.8
  immune mechanism (immunity) D89.9
    specified type NEC D89.89
  impaired renal tubular function N25.9
    specified NEC N25.89
  impulse (control) F63.9
  inflammatory
    pelvic, in diseases classified elsewhere —
        see category N74
    penis N48.29
      abscess N48.21
      cellulitis N48.22
  inhalant use
    mild F18.10
      with
        inhalant-induced
          anxiety disorder F18.180
          depressive disorder F18.14
          major neurocognitive disorder
              F18.17
          mild neurocognitive disorder
              F18.188
          psychotic disorder F18.159
        inhalant intoxication F18.129
        inhalant intoxication delirium F18.121
      ▶in remission (early) (sustained) F18.11
    moderate or severe F18.20
      with
        inhalant-induced
          anxiety disorder F18.280
          depressive disorder F18.24
          major neurocognitive disorder F18.27
          mild neurocognitive disorder F18.288
          psychotic disorder F18.259
        inhalant intoxication F18.229
        inhalant intoxication delirium F18.221
      ▶in remission (early) (sustained) F18.21

Disorder *(Continued)*
  integument, newborn P83.9
    ⏩specified NEC P83.88
  intermittent explosive F63.81
  internal secretion pancreas —*see* Increased,
    secretion, pancreas, endocrine
  intestine, intestinal
    carbohydrate absorption NEC E74.39
      postoperative K91.2
    functional NEC K59.9
      postoperative K91.89
    psychogenic F45.8
    vascular K55.9
      chronic K55.1
      specified NEC K55.8
  intraoperative (intraprocedural) —*see*
    Complications, intraoperative
  involuntary emotional expression (IEED) F48.2
  iris H21.9
    adhesions —*see* Adhesions, iris
    atrophy —*see* Atrophy, iris
    chamber angle recession —*see* Recession,
      chamber angle
    cyst —*see* Cyst, iris
    degeneration —*see* Degeneration, iris
    in diseases classified elsewhere H22
    iridodialysis —*see* Iridodialysis
    iridoschisis —*see* Iridoschisis
    miotic pupillary cyst —*see* Cyst, pupillary
    pupillary
      abnormality —*see* Abnormality,
        pupillary
      membrane —*see* Membrane, pupillary
    specified type NEC H21.89
    vascular NEC H21.1X-•
  iron metabolism E83.10
    specified NEC E83.19
  isovaleric acidemia E71.110
  jaw, developmental M27.0
    temporomandibular —*see also* Anomaly,
      dentofacial, temporomandibular joint
      M26.60-•
  joint M25.9
    derangement —*see* Derangement, joint
    effusion —*see* Effusion, joint
    fistula —*see* Fistula, joint
    hemarthrosis —*see* Hemarthrosis
    instability —*see* Instability, joint
    osteophyte —*see* Osteophyte
    pain —*see* Pain, joint
    psychogenic F45.8
    specified type NEC M25.80
      ankle M25.87-•
      elbow M25.82-•
      foot joint M25.87-•
      hand joint M25.84-•
      hip M25.85-•
      knee M25.86-•
      shoulder M25.81-•
      wrist M25.83-•
    stiffness —*see* Stiffness, joint
  ketone metabolism E71.32
  kidney N28.9
    functional (tubular) N25.9
    in
      schistosomiasis B65.9 *[N29]*
    tubular function N25.9
      specified NEC N25.89
  lacrimal system H04.9
    changes H04.69
      fistula —*see* Fistula, lacrimal
    gland H04.19
      atrophy —*see* Atrophy, lacrimal gland
      cyst —*see* Cyst, lacrimal, gland
      dacryops —*see* Dacryops
      dislocation —*see* Dislocation, lacrimal
        gland
      dry eye syndrome —*see* Syndrome, dry
        eye
      infection —*see* Dacryoadenitis
      granuloma —*see* Granuloma, lacrimal

Disorder *(Continued)*
  lacrimal system *(Continued)*
    inflammation —*see* Inflammation, lacrimal
    obstruction —*see* Obstruction, lacrimal
    specified NEC H04.89
  lactation NEC O92.79
  language (developmental) F80.9
    expressive F80.1
    mixed receptive and expressive F80.2
    receptive F80.2
  late luteal phase dysphoric N94.89
  learning (specific) F81.9
    acalculia R48.8
    alexia R48.0
    mathematics F81.2
    reading F81.0
    ▶specified
      ▶with impairment in
        ▶mathematics F81.2
        ▶reading F81.0
        ▶written expression F81.81
    specified NEC F81.89
    spelling F81.81
    written expression F81.81
  lens H27.9
    aphakia —*see* Aphakia
    cataract —*see* Cataract
    dislocation —*see* Dislocation, lens
    specified type NEC H27.8
  ligament M24.20
    ankle M24.27-•
    attachment, spine —*see* Enthesopathy,
      spinal
    elbow M24.22-•
    foot joint M24.27-•
    hand joint M24.24-•
    hip M24.25-•
    knee —*see* Derangement, knee, specified
      NEC
    shoulder M24.21-•
    vertebra M24.28
    wrist M24.23-•
  ligamentous attachments —*see also*
    Enthesopathy
    spine —*see* Enthesopathy, spinal
  lipid
    metabolism, congenital E78.9
    storage E75.6
      specified NEC E75.5
  lipoprotein
    deficiency (familial) E78.6
    metabolism E78.9
      specified NEC E78.89
  liver K76.9
    malarial B54 *[K77]*
  low back —*see also* Dorsopathy, specified NEC
  lumbosacral
    plexus G54.1
    root (nerve) NEC G54.4
  lung, interstitial, drug-induced J70.4
    acute J70.2
    chronic J70.3
  lymphoproliferative, post-transplant (PTLD)
    D47.Z1
  lysine and hydroxylysine metabolism E72.3
  major neurocognitive —*see* Dementia, in (due
    to)
  male
    erectile (organic) —*see also* Dysfunction,
      sexual, male, erectile N52.9
      nonorganic F52.21
    hypoactive sexual desire F52.0
    orgasmic F52.32
  manic F30.9
    organic F06.33
  mast cell activation —*see* Activation, mast
    cell
  mastoid —*see also* Disorder, ear, middle
    postprocedural —*see* Complications, ear,
      procedure
  meniscus —*see* Derangement, knee, meniscus

Disorder *(Continued)*
  menopausal N95.9
    specified NEC N95.8
  menstrual N92.6
    psychogenic F45.8
    specified NEC N92.5
  mental (or behavioral) (nonpsychotic) F99
    due to (secondary to)
      amphetamine
        due to drug abuse —*see* Abuse, drug,
          stimulant
        due to drug dependence —*see*
          Dependence, drug, stimulant
      brain disease, damage and dysfunction
        F09
      caffeine use
        due to drug abuse —*see* Abuse, drug,
          stimulant
        due to drug dependence —*see*
          Dependence, drug, stimulant
      cannabis use
        due to drug abuse —*see* Abuse, drug,
          cannabis
        due to drug dependence —*see*
          Dependence, drug, cannabis
      general medical condition F09
      sedative or hypnotic use
        due to drug abuse —*see* Abuse, drug,
          sedative
        due to drug dependence —*see*
          Dependence, drug, sedative
      tobacco (nicotine) use —*see* Dependence,
        drug, nicotine
    following organic brain damage F07.9
      frontal lobe syndrome F07.0
      personality change F07.0
      postconcussional syndrome F07.81
      specified NEC F07.89
    infancy, childhood or adolescence F98.9
    neurotic —*see* Neurosis
    organic or symptomatic F09
    presenile, psychotic F03
    problem NEC
    psychoneurotic —*see* Neurosis
    psychotic —*see* Psychosis
    puerperal F53
    senile, psychotic NEC F03
  metabolic, amino acid, transitory, newborn
    P74.8
  metabolism NOS E88.9
    amino-acid E72.9
      aromatic E70.9
        albinism —*see* Albinism
        histidine E70.40
          histidinemia E70.41
          other specified E70.49
        hyperphenylalaninemia E70.1
          classical phenylketonuria E70.0
        other specified E70.8
        tryptophan E70.5
        tyrosine E70.20
          hypertyrosinemia E70.21
          other specified E70.29
      branched chain E71.2
        3-methylglutaconic aciduria E71.111
        hyperleucine-isoleucinemia E71.19
        hypervalinemia E71.19
        isovaleric acidemia E71.110
        maple syrup urine disease E71.0
        methylmalonic acidemia E71.120
        organic aciduria NEC E71.118
        other specified E71.19
        proprionate NEC E71.128
        proprionic acidemia E71.121
      glycine E72.50
        d-glycericacidemia E72.59
        hyperhydroxyprolinemia E72.59
        hyperoxaluria E72.53
        hyperprolinemia E72.59
        non-ketotic hyperglycinemia E72.51
        other specified E72.59
        sarcosinemia E72.59
        trimethylaminuria E72.52

Disorder *(Continued)*
  metabolism *(Continued)*
    amino-acid *(Continued)*
      hydroxylysine E72.3
      lysine E72.3
      ornithine E72.4
      other specified E72.8
        beta-amino acid E72.8
        gamma-glutamyl cycle E72.8
      straight-chain E72.8
      sulfur-bearing E72.10
        homocystinuria E72.11
        methylenetetrahydrofolate reductase
          deficiency E72.12
        other specified E72.19
    bile acid and cholesterol metabolism E78.70
    bilirubin E80.7
      specified NEC E80.6
    calcium E83.50
      hypercalcemia E83.52
      hypocalcemia E83.51
      other specified E83.59
    carbohydrate E74.9
      specified NEC E74.8
    cholesterol and bile acid metabolism
      E78.70
    congenital E88.9
    copper E83.00
      specified type NEC E83.09
      Wilson's disease E83.01
    cystinuria E72.01
    fructose E74.10
    galactose E74.20
    glucosaminoglycan E76.9
      mucopolysaccharidosis —*see*
        Mucopolysaccharidosis
      specified NEC E76.8
    glutamine E72.8
    glycine E72.50
    glycogen storage (hepatorenal) E74.09
    glycoprotein E77.9
      specified NEC E77.8
    glycosaminoglycan E76.9
      specified NEC E76.8
    in labor and delivery O75.89
    iron E83.10
    isoleucine E71.19
    leucine E71.19
    lipoid E78.9
    lipoprotein E78.9
      specified NEC E78.89
    magnesium E83.40
      hypermagnesemia E83.41
      hypomagnesemia E83.42
      other specified E83.49
    mineral E83.9
      specified NEC E83.89
    mitochondrial E88.40
      MELAS syndrome E88.41
      MERRF syndrome (myoclonic epilepsy
        associated with ragged-red fibers)
        E88.42
      other specified E88.49
    ornithine E72.4
    phosphatases E83.30
    phosphorus E83.30
      acid phosphatase deficiency E83.39
      hypophosphatasia E83.39
      hypophosphatemia E83.39
        familial E83.31
      other specified E83.39
      pseudovitamin D deficiency E83.32
    plasma protein NEC E88.09
    porphyrin —*see* Porphyria
    postprocedural E89.89
      specified NEC E89.89
    purine E79.9
      specified NEC E79.8
    pyrimidine E79.9
      specified NEC E79.8
    pyruvate E74.4

Disorder *(Continued)*
  metabolism *(Continued)*
    serine E72.8
    sodium E87.8
    specified NEC E88.89
    threonine E72.8
    valine E71.19
    zinc E83.2
  methylmalonic acidemia E71.120
  micturition NEC —*see also* Difficulty,
    micturition R39.198
    feeling of incomplete emptying R39.14
    hesitancy R39.11
    poor stream R39.12
    psychogenic F45.8
    split stream R39.13
    straining R39.16
    urgency R39.15
  mild neurocognitive G31.84
  mitochondrial metabolism E88.40
  mitral (valve) —*see* Endocarditis, mitral
  mixed
    anxiety and depressive F41.8
    of scholastic skills (developmental) F81.89
    receptive expressive language F80.2
  mood F39
    bipolar —*see* Disorder, bipolar
    depressive —*see* Disorder, depressive
    due to (secondary to)
      alcohol F10.94
      amphetamine F15.94
        in
          abuse F15.14
          dependence F15.24
      anxiolytic F13.94
        in
          abuse F13.14
          dependence F13.24
      cocaine F14.94
        in
          abuse F14.14
          dependence F14.24
      general medical condition F06.30
      hallucinogen F16.94
        in
          abuse F16.14
          dependence F16.24
      hypnotic F13.94
        in
          abuse F13.14
          dependence F13.24
      inhalant F18.94
        in
          abuse F18.14
          dependence F18.24
      opioid F11.94
        in
          abuse F11.14
          dependence F11.24
      phencyclidine (PCP) F16.94
        in
          abuse F16.14
          dependence F16.24
      physiological condition F06.30
        with
          depressive features F06.31
          major depressive-like episode
            F06.32
          manic features F06.33
          mixed features F06.34
      psychoactive substance NEC F19.94
        in
          abuse F19.14
          dependence F19.24
      sedative F13.94
        in
          abuse F13.14
          dependence F13.24
      volatile solvents F18.94
        in
          abuse F18.14
          dependence F18.24

Disorder *(Continued)*
  mood *(Continued)*
    manic episode F30.9
      with psychotic symptoms F30.2
      without psychotic symptoms F30.10
        mild F30.11
        moderate F30.12
        severe F30.13
      in remission (full) F30.4
        partial F30.3
      specified type NEC F30.8
    organic F06.30
      right hemisphere F07.89
    persistent F34.9
      cyclothymia F34.0
      dysthymia F34.1
      specified type NEC F34.89
    recurrent F39
    right hemisphere organic F07.89
  movement G25.9
    drug-induced G25.70
      akathisia G25.71
      specified NEC G25.79
    hysterical F44.4
    in diseases classified elsewhere —*see*
      category G26
    periodic limb G47.61
      sleep related G47.61
    sleep related NEC G47.69
    specified NEC G25.89
    stereotyped F98.4
    treatment-induced G25.9
  multiple personality F44.81
  muscle M62.9
    attachment, spine —*see* Enthesopathy,
      spinal
    in trichinellosis —*see* Trichinellosis, with
      muscle disorder
    psychogenic F45.8
    specified type NEC M62.89
    tone, newborn P94.9
      specified NEC P94.8
  muscular
    attachments —*see also* Enthesopathy
      spine —*see* Enthesopathy, spinal
    urethra N36.44
  musculoskeletal system, soft tissue —*see*
    Disorder, soft tissue
    postprocedural M96.89
    psychogenic F45.8
  myoneural G70.9
    due to lead G70.1
    specified NEC G70.89
    toxic G70.1
  myotonic NEC G71.19
  nail, in diseases classified elsewhere L62
  neck region NEC —*see* Dorsopathy, specified
    NEC
  neonatal onset multisystemic inflammatory
    (NOMID) M04.2
  nerve G58.9
    abducent NEC —*see* Strabismus, paralytic,
      sixth nerve
    accessory G52.8
    acoustic —*see* subcategory H93.3
    auditory —*see* subcategory H93.3
    auriculotemporal G50.8
    axillary G54.0
    cerebral —*see* Disorder, nerve, cranial
    cranial G52.9
      eighth —*see* subcategory H93.3
      eleventh G52.8
      fifth G50.9
      first G52.0
      fourth NEC —*see* Strabismus, paralytic,
        fourth nerve
      multiple G52.7
      ninth G52.1
      second NEC —*see* Disorder, nerve, optic
      seventh NEC G51.8
      sixth NEC —*see* Strabismus, paralytic,
        sixth nerve

Disorder *(Continued)*
　nerve *(Continued)*
　　cranial *(Continued)*
　　　specified NEC G52.8
　　　tenth G52.2
　　　third NEC —*see* Strabismus, paralytic,
　　　　third nerve
　　　twelfth G52.3
　　entrapment —*see* Neuropathy, entrapment
　　facial G51.9
　　　specified NEC G51.8
　　femoral —*see* Lesion, nerve, femoral
　　glossopharyngeal NEC G52.1
　　hypoglossal G52.3
　　intercostal G58.0
　　lateral
　　　cutaneous of thigh —*see*
　　　　Mononeuropathy, lower limb,
　　　　meralgia paresthetica
　　　popliteal —*see* Lesion, nerve, popliteal
　　lower limb —*see* Mononeuropathy, lower
　　　limb
　　medial popliteal —*see* Lesion, nerve,
　　　popliteal, medial
　　median NEC —*see* Lesion, nerve, median
　　multiple G58.7
　　oculomotor NEC —*see* Strabismus,
　　　paralytic, third nerve
　　olfactory G52.0
　　optic NEC H47.09-●
　　　hemorrhage into sheath —*see*
　　　　Hemorrhage, optic nerve
　　　ischemic H47.01-●
　　peroneal —*see* Lesion, nerve, popliteal
　　phrenic G58.8
　　plantar —*see* Lesion, nerve, plantar
　　pneumogastric G52.2
　　posterior tibial —*see* Syndrome, tarsal
　　　tunnel
　　radial —*see* Lesion, nerve, radial
　　recurrent laryngeal G52.2
　　root G54.9
　　　cervical G54.2
　　　lumbosacral G54.1
　　　specified NEC G54.8
　　　thoracic G54.3
　　sciatic NEC —*see* Lesion, nerve, sciatic
　　specified NEC G58.8
　　　lower limb —*see* Mononeuropathy,
　　　　lower limb, specified NEC
　　　upper limb —*see* Mononeuropathy,
　　　　upper limb, specified NEC
　　sympathetic G90.9
　　tibial —*see* Lesion, nerve, popliteal, medial
　　trigeminal G50.9
　　　specified NEC G50.8
　　trochlear NEC —*see* Strabismus, paralytic,
　　　fourth nerve
　　ulnar —*see* Lesion, nerve, ulnar
　　upper limb —*see* Mononeuropathy, upper
　　　limb
　　vagus G52.2
　nervous system G98.8
　　autonomic (peripheral) G90.9
　　　specified NEC G90.8
　　central G96.9
　　　specified NEC G96.8
　　parasympathetic G90.9
　　specified NEC G98.8
　　sympathetic G90.9
　　vegetative G90.9
➠neurocognitive R41.9
　major
　　with
　　　aggressive behavior F01.51
　　　combative behavior F01.51
　　　violent behavior F01.51
　　due to vascular disease, with behavioral
　　　disturbance F01.51
　　in (due to) (other diseases classified
　　　elsewhere) —*see also* Dementia, in
　　　(due to) F02.80

Disorder *(Continued)*
　neurocognitive *(Continued)*
　　major *(Continued)*
　　　in *(Continued)*
　　　　with
　　　　　aggressive behavior F02.81
　　　　　combative behavior F02.81
　　　　　violent behavior F02.81
　　　　without behavioral disturbance F01.50
　　　mild G31.84
　　neurodevelopmental F89
　　　specified NEC F88
　　neurohypophysis NEC E23.3
　　neurological NEC R29.818
　　neuromuscular G70.9
　　　hereditary NEC G71.9
　　　specified NEC G70.89
　　　toxic G70.1
　　neurotic F48.9
　　　specified NEC F48.8
　　neutrophil, polymorphonuclear D71
　　nicotine use —*see* Dependence, drug, nicotine
　　nightmare F51.5
▶non-rapid eye movement sleep arousal
　▶sleep terror type F51.4
　▶sleepwalking type F51.3
　nose J34.9
　　specified NEC J34.89
　obsessive-compulsive F42.9
▶and related disorder due to a known
　　physiological condition F06.8
　odontogenesis NOS K00.9
　opioid use
　　with
　　　opioid-induced psychotic disorder F11.959
　　　　with
　　　　　delusions F11.950
　　　　　hallucinations F11.951
　　due to drug abuse —*see* Abuse, drug,
　　　opioid
　　due to drug dependence —*see* Dependence,
　　　drug, opioid
　　mild F11.10
　　　with
　　　　opioid-induced
　　　　　anxiety disorder F11.188
　　　　　depressive disorder F11.14
　　　　　sexual dysfunction F11.181
　　　　opioid intoxication
　　　　　with perceptual disturbances F11.122
　　　　　delirium F11.121
　　　　　without perceptual disturbances
　　　　　　F11.129
　　▶in remission (early) (sustained) F11.11
　　moderate or severe F11.20
　　　with
　　　　opioid-induced
　　　　　anxiety disorder F11.288
　　　　　anxiety disorder F11.988
　　　　　depressive disorder F11.24
　　　　　depressive disorder F11.94
　　　　　sexual dysfunction F11.281
　　　　　sexual dysfunction F11.981
　　　　opioid intoxication
　　　　　with perceptual disturbances F11.222
　　　　　delirium F11.221
　　　　　without perceptual disturbances
　　　　　　F11.229
　　▶in remission (early) (sustained) F11.21
　oppositional defiant F91.3
　optic
　　chiasm H47.49
　　　due to
　　　　inflammatory disorder H47.41
　　　　neoplasm H47.42
　　　　vascular disorder H47.43
　　disc H47.39-●
　　　coloboma —*see* Coloboma, optic disc
　　　drusen —*see* Drusen, optic disc
　　　pseudopapilledema —*see*
　　　　Pseudopapilledema

Disorder *(Continued)*
　optic *(Continued)*
　　radiations —*see* Disorder, visual, pathway
　　tracts —*see* Disorder, visual, pathway
　orbit H05.9
　　cyst —*see* Cyst, orbit
　　deformity —*see* Deformity, orbit
　　edema —*see* Edema, orbit
　　enophthalmos —*see* Enophthalmos
　　exophthalmos —*see* Exophthalmos
　　hemorrhage —*see* Hemorrhage, orbit
　　inflammation —*see* Inflammation, orbit
　　myopathy —*see* Myopathy, extraocular
　　　muscles
　　retained foreign body —*see* Foreign body,
　　　orbit, old
　　specified type NEC H05.89
　organic
　　anxiety F06.4
　　catatonic F06.1
　　delusional F06.2
　　dissociative F06.8
　　emotionally labile (asthenic) F06.8
　　mood (affective) F06.30
　　schizophrenia-like F06.2
　orgasmic (female) F52.31
　　male F52.32
　ornithine metabolism E72.4
　overanxious F41.1
　　of childhood F93.8
　pain
　　with related psychological factors F45.42
　　exclusively related to psychological factors
　　　F45.41
　　genito-pelvic penetration disorder F52.6
　pancreatic internal secretion E16.9
　　specified NEC E16.8
　panic F41.0
　　with agoraphobia F40.01
　papulosquamous L44.9
　　in diseases classified elsewhere L45
　　specified NEC L44.8
　paranoid F22
　　induced F24
　　shared F24
▶paraphilic F65.9
　▶specified NEC F65.89
　parathyroid (gland) E21.5
　　specified NEC E21.4
　parietoalveolar NEC J84.09
　paroxysmal, mixed R56.9
　patella M22.9-●
　　chondromalacia —*see* Chondromalacia,
　　　patella
　　derangement NEC M22.3X-●
　　recurrent
　　　dislocation —*see* Dislocation, patella,
　　　　recurrent
　　　subluxation —*see* Dislocation, patella,
　　　　recurrent, incomplete
　　specified NEC M22.8X-●
　patellofemoral M22.2X-●
▶pedophilic F65.4
　pentose phosphate pathway with anemia
　　D55.1
　perception, due to hallucinogens F16.983
　　in
　　　abuse F16.183
　　　dependence F16.283
　peripheral nervous system NEC G64
　peroxisomal E71.50
　　biogenesis
　　　neonatal adrenoleukodystrophy E71.511
　　　specified disorder NEC E71.518
　　　Zellweger syndrome E71.510
　　rhizomelic chondrodysplasia punctata
　　　E71.540
　　specified form NEC E71.548
　　　group 1 E71.518
　　　group 2 E71.53
　　　group 3 E71.542

Disorder *(Continued)*
  peroxisomal *(Continued)*
    X-linked adrenoleukodystrophy E71.529
      adolescent E71.521
      adrenomyeloneuropathy E71.522
      childhood E71.520
      specified form NEC E71.528
    Zellweger-like syndrome E71.541
  persistent
    (somatoform) pain F45.41
    affective (mood) F34.9
  personality —*see also* Personality F60.9
    affective F34.0
    aggressive F60.3
    amoral F60.2
    anankastic F60.5
    antisocial F60.2
    anxious F60.6
    asocial F60.2
    asthenic F60.7
    avoidant F60.6
    borderline F60.3
    change (secondary) due to general medical
        condition F07.0
    compulsive F60.5
    cyclothymic F34.0
    dependent (passive) F60.7
    depressive F34.1
    dissocial F60.2
    emotional instability F60.3
    expansive paranoid F60.0
    explosive F60.3
    following organic brain damage F07.9
    histrionic F60.4
    hyperthymic F34.0
    hypothymic F34.1
    hysterical F60.4
    immature F60.89
    inadequate F60.7
    labile F60.3
    mixed (nonspecific) F60.89
    moral deficiency F60.2
    narcissistic F60.81
    negativistic F60.89
    obsessional F60.5
    obsessive (-compulsive) F60.5
    organic F07.9
    overconscientious F60.5
    paranoid F60.0
    passive (-dependent) F60.7
    passive-aggressive F60.89
    pathological NEC F60.9
    pseudosocial F60.2
    psychopathic F60.2
    schizoid F60.1
    schizotypal F21
    self-defeating F60.7
    specified NEC F60.89
    type A F60.5
    unstable (emotional) F60.3
  pervasive, developmental F84.9
  phencyclidine use
    mild F16.10
      with
        phencyclidine-induced
          anxiety disorder F16.180
          bipolar and related disorder F16.14
          depressive disorder F16.14
          psychotic disorder F16.159
        phencyclidine intoxication F16.129
        phencyclidine intoxication delirium
            F16.121
      ▶in remission (early) (sustained) F16.11
    moderate or severe F16.20
      with
        phencyclidine-induced
          anxiety disorder F16.280
          bipolar and related disorder F16.24
          depressive disorder F16.24
          psychotic disorder F16.259
        phencyclidine intoxication F16.229

Disorder *(Continued)*
  phencyclidine use *(Continued)*
    moderate or severe *(Continued)*
      with *(Continued)*
        phencyclidine intoxication delirium
            F16.221
      ▶in remission (early) (sustained) F16.21
  phobic anxiety, childhood F40.8
  phosphate-losing tubular N25.0
  pigmentation L81.9
    choroid, congenital Q14.3
    diminished melanin formation L81.6
    iron L81.8
    specified NEC L81.8
  pinna (noninfective) H61.10-●
    deformity, acquired H61.11-●
    hematoma H61.12-●
    perichondritis —*see* Perichondritis, ear
    specified type NEC H61.19-●
  pituitary gland E23.7
    iatrogenic (postprocedural) E89.3
    specified NEC E23.6
  platelets D69.1
  plexus G54.9
    specified NEC G54.8
  polymorphonuclear neutrophils D71
  porphyrin metabolism —*see* Porphyria
  postconcussional F07.81
  posthallucinogen perception F16.983
    in
      abuse F16.183
      dependence F16.283
  postmenopausal N95.9
    specified NEC N95.8
  postprocedural (postoperative) —*see*
      Complications, postprocedural
  post-transplant lymphoproliferative D47.z1
  post-traumatic stress (PTSD) F43.10
    acute F43.11
    chronic F43.12
  premenstrual dysphoric (PMDD) F32.81
  prepuce N47.8
  propionic acidemia E71.121
  prostate N42.9
    specified NEC N42.89
  psychogenic NOS —*see also* condition F45.9
    anxiety F41.8
    appetite F50.9
    asthenic F48.8
    cardiovascular (system) F45.8
    compulsive F42.8
    cutaneous F54
    depressive F32.9
    digestive (system) F45.8
    dysmenorrheic F45.8
    dyspneic F45.8
    endocrine (system) F54
    eye NEC F45.8
    feeding —*see* Disorder, eating
    functional NEC F45.8
    gastric F45.8
    gastrointestinal (system) F45.8
    genitourinary (system) F45.8
    heart (function) (rhythm) F45.8
    hyperventilatory F45.8
    hypochondriacal —*see* Disorder,
        hypochondriacal
    intestinal F45.8
    joint F45.8
    learning F81.9
    limb F45.8
    lymphatic (system) F45.8
    menstrual F45.8
    micturition F45.8
    monoplegic NEC F44.4
    motor F44.4
    muscle F45.8
    musculoskeletal F45.8
    neurocirculatory F45.8
    obsessive F42.8
    occupational F48.8
    organ or part of body NEC F45.8

Disorder *(Continued)*
  psychogenic NOS *(Continued)*
    paralytic NEC F44.4
    phobic F40.9
    physical NEC F45.8
    rectal F45.8
    respiratory (system) F45.8
    rheumatic F45.8
    sexual (function) F52.9
    skin (allergic) (eczematous) F54
    sleep F51.9
    specified part of body NEC F45.8
    stomach F45.8
  psychological F99
    associated with
      disease classified elsewhere F54
      sexual
        development F66
        relationship F66
      uncertainty about gender identity F64.9
  psychomotor NEC F44.4
    hysterical F44.4
  psychoneurotic —*see also* Neurosis
    mixed NEC F48.8
  psychophysiologic —*see* Disorder,
      somatoform
  psychosexual F65.9
    development F66
    identity of childhood F64.2
  psychosomatic NOS —*see* Disorder,
      somatoform
    multiple F45.0
    undifferentiated F45.1
  psychotic —*see* Psychosis
    transient (acute) F23
  puberty E30.9
    specified NEC E30.8
  pulmonary (valve) —*see* Endocarditis,
      pulmonary
  purine metabolism E79.9
  pyrimidine metabolism E79.9
  pyruvate metabolism E74.4
  reactive attachment (childhood) F94.1
  reading R48.0
    developmental (specific) F81.0
  receptive language F80.2
  receptor, hormonal, peripheral —*see also*
      Syndrome, androgen insensitivity E34.50
  recurrent brief depressive F33.8
  reflex R29.2
  refraction H52.7
    aniseikonia H52.32
    anisometropia H52.31
    astigmatism —*see* Astigmatism
    hypermetropia —*see* Hypermetropia
    myopia —*see* Myopia
    presbyopia H52.4
    specified NEC H52.6
  relationship F68.8
    due to sexual orientation F66
  REM sleep behavior G47.52
  renal function, impaired (tubular) N25.9
  resonance R49.9
    specified NEC R49.8
  respiratory function, impaired —*see also*
      Failure, respiration
    postprocedural —*see* Complication,
        postoperative, respiratory system
    psychogenic F45.8
  retina H35.9
    angioid streaks H35.33
    changes in vascular appearance H35.01-●
    degeneration —*see* Degeneration, retina
    dystrophy (hereditary) —*see* Dystrophy,
        retina
    edema H35.81
    hemorrhage —*see* Hemorrhage, retina
    ischemia H35.82
    macular degeneration —*see* Degeneration,
        macula
    microaneurysms H35.04-●
    microvascular abnormality NEC H35.09

▶ New   ⇒ Revised   ~~deleted~~ Deleted   ● Use Additional Character(s)

Disorder *(Continued)*
  retina *(Continued)*
    neovascularization —*see*
      Neovascularization, retina
    retinopathy —*see* Retinopathy
    separation of layers H35.70
      central serous chorioretinopathy H35.71-●
      pigment epithelium detachment (serous) H35.72-●
      hemorrhagic H35.73-●
    specified type NEC H35.89
    telangiectasis —*see* Telangiectasis, retina
    vasculitis —*see* Vasculitis, retina
  retroperitoneal K68.9
  right hemisphere organic affective F07.89
  rumination (infant or child) F98.21
  sacrum, sacrococcygeal NEC M53.3
  schizoaffective F25.9
    bipolar type F25.0
    depressive type F25.1
    manic type F25.0
    mixed type F25.0
    specified NEC F25.8
  schizoid of childhood F84.5
  ▶schizophrenia spectrum and other psychotic disorder F29
    ▶specified NEC F28
  schizophreniform F20.81
    brief F23
  schizotypal (personality) F21
  secretion, thyrocalcitonin E07.0
  sedative, hypnotic, or anxiolytic use
    mild F13.10
      with
        sedative, hypnotic, or anxiolytic-induced
          anxiety disorder F13.180
          bipolar and related disorder F13.14
          depressive disorder F13.14
          psychotic disorder F13.159
          sexual dysfunction F13.181
        sedative, hypnotic, or anxiolytic intoxication F13.129
        sedative, hypnotic, or anxiolytic intoxication delirium F13.121
      ▶in remission (early) (sustained) F13.11
    moderate or severe F13.20
      with
        sedative, hypnotic, or anxiolytic-induced
          anxiety disorder F13.280
          bipolar and related disorder F13.24
          depressive disorder F13.24
          major neurocognitive disorder F13.27
          mild neurocognitive disorder F13.288
          psychotic disorder F13.259
          sexual dysfunction F13.281
        sedative, hypnotic, or anxiolytic intoxication F13.229
        sedative, hypnotic, or anxiolytic intoxication delirium F13.221
      ▶in remission (early) (sustained) F13.21
  seizure —*see also* Epilepsy G40.909
    intractable G40.919
      with status epilepticus G40.911
  semantic pragmatic F80.89
    with autism F84.0
  sense of smell R43.1
    psychogenic F45.8
  separation anxiety, of childhood F93.0
  sexual
    arousal, female F52.22
    aversion F52.1
    function, psychogenic F52.9
    ▶interest/arousal, female F52.22
    ▶masochism F65.51
    maturation F66
    nonorganic F52.9
    preference —*see also* Deviation, sexual F65.9
      fetishistic transvestism F65.1
    relationship F66
    ▶sadism F65.52

Disorder *(Continued)*
  shyness, of childhood and adolescence F40.10
  sibling rivalry F93.8
  sickle-cell (sickling) (homozygous) —*see* Disease, sickle-cell
    heterozygous D57.3
    specified type NEC D57.8-●
    trait D57.3
  sinus (nasal) J34.9
    specified NEC J34.89
  skin L98.9
    atrophic L90.9
      specified NEC L90.8
    granulomatous L92.9
      specified NEC L92.8
    hypertrophic L91.9
      specified NEC L91.8
    infiltrative NEC L98.6
    newborn P83.9
    ⫸specified NEC P83.88
    picking F42.4
    psychogenic (allergic) (eczematous) F54
  sleep G47.9
    breathing-related —*see* Apnea, sleep
    circadian rhythm G47.20
      advance sleep phase type G47.22
      delayed sleep phase type G47.21
      due to
        alcohol
          abuse F10.182
          dependence F10.282
          use F10.982
        amphetamines
          abuse F15.182
          dependence F15.282
          use F15.982
        caffeine
          abuse F15.182
          dependence F15.282
          use F15.982
        cocaine
          abuse F14.182
          dependence F14.282
          use F14.982
        drug NEC
          abuse F19.182
          dependence F19.282
          use F19.982
        opioid
          abuse F11.182
          dependence F11.282
          use F11.982
        psychoactive substance NEC
          abuse F19.182
          dependence F19.282
          use F19.982
        sedative, hypnotic, or anxiolytic
          abuse F13.182
          dependence F13.282
          use F13.982
        stimulant NEC
          abuse F15.182
          dependence F15.282
          use F15.982
      free running type G47.24
      in conditions classified elsewhere G47.27
      irregular sleep wake type G47.23
      jet lag type G47.25
      ▶non-24-hour sleep-wake type G47.24
      shift work type G47.26
      specified NEC G47.29
    due to
      alcohol
        abuse F10.182
        dependence F10.282
        use F10.982
      amphetamine
        abuse F15.182
        dependence F15.282
        use F15.982

Disorder *(Continued)*
  sleep *(Continued)*
    due to *(Continued)*
      anxiolytic
        abuse F13.182
        dependence F13.282
        use F13.982
      caffeine
        abuse F15.182
        dependence F15.282
        use F15.982
      cocaine
        abuse F14.182
        dependence F14.282
        use F14.982
      drug NEC
        abuse F19.182
        dependence F19.282
        use F19.982
      hypnotic
        abuse F13.182
        dependence F13.282
        use F13.982
      opioid
        abuse F11.182
        dependence F11.282
        use F11.982
      psychoactive substance NEC
        abuse F19.182
        dependence F19.282
        use F19.982
      sedative
        abuse F13.182
        dependence F13.282
        use F13.982
      stimulant NEC
        abuse F15.182
        dependence F15.282
        use F15.982
    emotional F51.9
    excessive somnolence —*see* Hypersomnia
    hypersomnia type —*see* Hypersomnia
    initiating or maintaining —*see* Insomnia
    nightmares F51.5
    nonorganic F51.9
      specified NEC F51.8
    parasomnia type G47.50
    specified NEC G47.8
    terrors F51.4
    walking F51.3
  ⫸sleep-wake pattern or schedule —*see also* Disorder, sleep, circadian rhythm G47.9
    ▶specified NEC G47.8
  social
    ~~anxiety of childhood F40.10~~
    ▶anxiety (of childhood) F40.10
      ▶generalized F40.11
    functioning in childhood F94.9
      specified NEC F94.8
    pragmatic F80.82
  soft tissue M79.9
    ankle M79.9
    due to use, overuse and pressure M70.90
      ankle M70.97-●
      bursitis —*see* Bursitis
      foot M70.97-●
      forearm M70.93-●
      hand M70.94-●
      lower leg M70.96-●
      multiple sites M70.99
      pelvic region M70.95-●
      shoulder region M70.91-●
      specified site NEC M70.98
      specified type NEC M70.80
        ankle M70.87-●
        foot M70.87-●
        forearm M70.83-●
        hand M70.84-●
        lower leg M70.86-●
        multiple sites M70.89
        pelvic region M70.85-●

Disorder *(Continued)*
  soft tissue *(Continued)*
    due to use, overuse and pressure
      (Continued)
      specified type NEC *(Continued)*
        shoulder region M70.81-●
        specified site NEC M70.88
        thigh M70.85-●
        upper arm M70.82-●
      thigh M70.95-●
      upper arm M70.92-●
    foot M79.9
    forearm M79.9
    hand M79.9
    lower leg M79.9
    multiple sites M79.9
    occupational —*see* Disorder, soft tissue,
      due to use, overuse and pressure
    pelvic region M79.9
    shoulder region M79.9
    specified type NEC M79.89
    thigh M79.9
    upper arm M79.9
  somatic symptom F45.1
  somatization F45.0
  somatoform F45.9
    pain (persistent) F45.41
    somatization (multiple) (long-lasting) F45.0
    specified NEC F45.8
    undifferentiated F45.1
  somnolence, excessive —*see* Hypersomnia
  specific
    arithmetical F81.2
    developmental, of motor F82
    reading F81.0
    speech and language F80.9
    spelling F81.81
    written expression F81.81
  speech R47.9
    articulation (functional) (specific) F80.0
    developmental F80.9
    specified NEC R47.89
  speech-sound F80.0
  spelling (specific) F81.81
  spine —*see also* Dorsopathy
    ligamentous or muscular attachments,
      peripheral —*see* Enthesopathy, spinal
    specified NEC —*see* Dorsopathy, specified
      NEC
  stereotyped, habit or movement F98.4
  stimulant use (other) (unspecified)
    mild F15.10
    ▶in remission (early) (sustained) F15.11
    moderate or severe F15.20
    ▶in remission (early) (sustained) F15.21
  stomach (functional) —*see* Disorder, gastric
  stress F43.9
    acute F43.0
    post-traumatic F43.10
      acute F43.11
      chronic F43.12
  substance use (other) (unknown)
    mild F19.10
      with substance-induced
        anxiety disorder F19.180
        bipolar and related disorder F19.14
        depressive disorder F19.14
        major neurocognitive disorder F19.17
        mild neurocognitive disorder F19.188
        obsessive-compulsive and related
          disorder F19.188
        sexual dysfunction F19.181
      substance intoxication F19.129
      substance intoxication delirium F19.121
    moderate or severe F19.20
      with substance-induced
        anxiety disorder F19.280
        bipolar and related disorder F19.24
        depressive disorder F19.24
        major neurocognitive disorder F19.27
        mild neurocognitive disorder F19.288

Disorder *(Continued)*
  substance use (other) (unknown) *(Continued)*
    moderate or severe *(Continued)*
      with substance-induced anxiety disorder
        (Continued)
        obsessive-compulsive and related
          disorder F19.288
        sexual dysfunction F19.281
    ▶in remission (early) (sustained) F19.21
    substance intoxication F19.229
    substance intoxication delirium F19.221
  sulfur-bearing amino-acid metabolism E72.10
  sweat gland (eccrine) L74.9
    apocrine L75.9
      specified NEC L75.8
    specified NEC L74.8
  synovium M67.90
    acromioclavicular M67.91-●
    ankle M67.97-●
    elbow M67.92-●
    foot M67.97-●
    forearm M67.93-●
    hand M67.94-●
    hip M67.95-●
    knee M67.96-●
    multiple sites M67.99
    rupture —*see* Rupture, synovium
    shoulder M67.91-●
    specified type NEC M67.80
      acromioclavicular M67.81-●
      ankle M67.87-●
      elbow M67.82-●
      foot M67.87-●
      hand M67.84-●
      hip M67.85-●
      knee M67.86-●
      multiple sites M67.89
      wrist M67.83-●
    synovitis —*see* Synovitis
    upper arm M67.92-●
    wrist M67.93-●
  temperature regulation, newborn P81.9
    specified NEC P81.8
  temporomandibular joint M26.60-●
  tendon M67.90
    acromioclavicular M67.91-●
    ankle M67.97-●
    contracture —*see* Contracture, tendon
    elbow M67.92-●
    foot M67.97-●
    forearm M67.93-●
    hand M67.94-●
    hip M67.95-●
    knee M67.96-●
    multiple sites M67.99
    rupture —*see* Rupture, tendon
    shoulder M67.91-●
    specified type NEC M67.80
      acromioclavicular M67.81-●
      ankle M67.87-●
      elbow M67.82-●
      foot M67.87-●
      hand M67.84-●
      hip M67.85-●
      knee M67.86-●
      multiple sites M67.89
      trunk M67.88
      wrist M67.83-●
    synovitis —*see* Synovitis
    tendinitis —*see* Tendinitis
    tenosynovitis —*see* Tenosynovitis
    trunk M67.98
    upper arm M67.92-●
    wrist M67.93-●
  thoracic root (nerve) NEC G54.3
  thyrocalcitonin hypersecretion E07.0
  thyroid (gland) E07.9
    function NEC, neonatal, transitory P72.2
    iodine-deficiency related E01.8
    specified NEC E07.89
  tic —*see* Tic

Disorder *(Continued)*
  tobacco use
    ▶chewing tobacco (mild) (moderate) (severe)
      ▶in remission (early) (sustained) F17.221
    ▶cigarettes (mild) (moderate) (severe)
      ▶in remission (early) (sustained) F17.211
    mild Z72.0
      ▶in remission (early) (sustained) F17.201
    moderate F17.200
      ▶in remission (early) (sustained) F17.201
    severe F17.200
      ▶in remission (early) (sustained) F17.201
    ▶specified product NEC (mild) (moderate)
      (severe)
      ▶in remission (early) (sustained) F17.291
  tooth K08.9
    development K00.9
      specified NEC K00.8
    eruption K00.6
  Tourette's F95.2
  trance and possession F44.89
  ▶transvestic F65.1
  trauma and stressor-related F43.9
    other specified F43.8
  tricuspid (valve) —*see* Endocarditis, tricuspid
  tryptophan metabolism E70.5
  tubular, phosphate-losing N25.0
  tubulo-interstitial (in)
    brucellosis A23.9 *[N16]*
    cystinosis E72.04
    diphtheria A36.84
    glycogen storage disease E74.00 *[N16]*
    leukemia NEC C95.9-● *[N16]*
    lymphoma NEC C85.9-● *[N16]*
    mixed cryoglobulinemia D89.1 *[N16]*
    multiple myeloma C90.0-● *[N16]*
    Salmonella infection A02.25
    sarcoidosis D86.84
    sepsis A41.9 *[N16]*
      streptococcal A40.9 *[N16]*
    systemic lupus erythematosus M32.15
    toxoplasmosis B58.83
    transplant rejection T86.91 *[N16]*
    Wilson's disease E83.01 *[N16]*
  tubulo-renal function, impaired N25.9
    specified NEC N25.89
  tympanic membrane H73.9-●
    atrophy —*see* Atrophy, tympanic membrane
    infection —*see* Myringitis
    perforation —*see* Perforation, tympanum
    specified NEC H73.89-●
  unsocialized aggressive F91.1
  urea cycle metabolism E72.20
    argininemia E72.21
    arginosuccinic aciduria E72.22
    citrullinemia E72.23
    ornithine transcarbamylase deficiency E72.4
    other specified E72.29
  ureter (in) N28.9
    schistosomiasis B65.0 *[N29]*
    tuberculosis A18.11
  urethra N36.9
    specified NEC N36.8
  urinary system N39.9
    specified NEC N39.8
  valve, heart
    aortic —*see* Endocarditis, aortic
    mitral —*see* Endocarditis, mitral
    pulmonary —*see* Endocarditis, pulmonary
    rheumatic
      aortic —*see* Endocarditis, aortic,
        rheumatic
      mitral —*see* Endocarditis, mitral
      pulmonary —*see* Endocarditis,
        pulmonary, rheumatic
      tricuspid —*see* Endocarditis, tricuspid
    tricuspid —*see* Endocarditis, tricuspid
  vestibular function H81.9-●
    specified NEC —*see* subcategory H81.8
      in diseases classified elsewhere H82.-●
  vertigo —*see* Vertigo

Disorder *(Continued)*
vision, binocular H53.30
  abnormal retinal correspondence H53.31
  diplopia H53.2
  fusion with defective stereopsis H53.32
  simultaneous perception H53.33
  suppression H53.34
visual
  cortex
    blindness H47.619
      left brain H47.612
      right brain H47.611
    due to
      inflammatory disorder H47.629
        left brain H47.622
        right brain H47.621
      neoplasm H47.639
        left brain H47.632
        right brain H47.631
      vascular disorder H47.649
        left brain H47.642
        right brain H47.641
  pathway H47.9
    due to
      inflammatory disorder H47.51-•
      neoplasm H47.52-•
      vascular disorder H47.53-•
  optic chiasm —*see* Disorder, optic, chiasm
vitreous body H43.9
  crystalline deposits —*see* Deposit,
    crystalline
  degeneration —*see* Degeneration, vitreous
  hemorrhage —*see* Hemorrhage, vitreous
  opacities —*see* Opacity, vitreous
  prolapse —*see* Prolapse, vitreous
  specified type NEC H43.89
voice R49.9
  specified type NEC R49.8
volatile solvent use
  due to drug abuse —*see* Abuse, drug,
    inhalant
  due to drug dependence —*see* Dependence,
    drug, inhalant
▶voyeuristic F65.3
white blood cells D72.9
  specified NEC D72.89
withdrawing, child or adolescent
  F40.10
Disorientation R41.0
Displacement, displaced
acquired traumatic of bone, cartilage, joint,
  tendon NEC —*see* Dislocation
adrenal gland (congenital) Q89.1
appendix, retrocecal (congenital) Q43.8
auricle (congenital) Q17.4
bladder (acquired) N32.89
  congenital Q64.19
brachial plexus (congenital) Q07.8
brain stem, caudal (congenital) Q04.8
canaliculus (lacrimalis), congenital Q10.6
cardia through esophageal hiatus (congenital)
  Q40.1
cerebellum, caudal (congenital) Q04.8
cervix —*see* Malposition, uterus
colon (congenital) Q43.3
device, implant or graft —*see also*
  Complications, by site and type,
  mechanical T85.628
  arterial graft NEC —*see* Complication,
    cardiovascular device, mechanical,
    vascular
  breast (implant) T85.42
  catheter NEC T85.628
    dialysis (renal) T82.42
      intraperitoneal T85.621
    infusion NEC T82.524
      spinal (epidural) (subdural) T85.620
    urinary
      cystostomy T83.020
      Hopkins T83.028
      ileostomy T83.028

Displacement, displaced *(Continued)*
device, implant or graft *(Continued)*
  catheter NEC *(Continued)*
    urinary *(Continued)*
      indwelling T83.021
      nephrostomy T83.022
      specified NEC T83.028
      urostomy T83.028
  electronic (electrode) (pulse generator)
    (stimulator) —*see* Complication,
    electronic stimulator
  fixation, internal (orthopedic) NEC —
    see Complication, fixation device,
    mechanical
  gastrointestinal —*see* Complications,
    prosthetic device, mechanical,
    gastrointestinal device
  genital NEC T83.428
    intrauterine contraceptive device (string)
      T83.32
    penile prosthesis (cylinder) (implanted)
      (pump) (resevoir) T83.420
    testicular prosthesis T83.421
  heart NEC —*see* Complication,
    cardiovascular device, mechanical
  joint prosthesis —*see* Complications, joint
    prosthesis, mechanical
  ocular —*see* Complications, prosthetic
    device, mechanical, ocular device
  orthopedic NEC —*see* Complication,
    orthopedic, device or graft,
    mechanical
  specified NEC T85.628
  urinary NEC T83.128
    graft T83.22
    sphincter, implanted T83.121
    stent (ileal conduit) (nephroureteral)
      T83.123
    ureteral indwelling T83.122
  vascular NEC —*see* Complication,
    cardiovascular device, mechanical
  ventricular intracranial shunt T85.02
electronic stimulator
  bone T84.320
  cardiac —*see* Complications, cardiac
    device, electronic
  nervous system —*see* Complication,
    prosthetic device, mechanical,
    electronic nervous system
    stimulator
  urinary —*see* Complications, electronic
    stimulator, urinary
esophageal mucosa into cardia of stomach,
  congenital Q39.8
esophagus (acquired) K22.8
  congenital Q39.8
eyeball (acquired) (lateral) (old) —*see*
    Displacement, globe
  congenital Q15.8
  current —*see* Avulsion, eye
fallopian tube (acquired) N83.4-•
  congenital Q50.6
  opening (congenital) Q50.6
gallbladder (congenital) Q44.1
gastric mucosa (congenital) Q40.2
globe (acquired) (old) (lateral) H05.21-•
  current —*see* Avulsion, eye
heart (congenital) Q24.8
  acquired I51.89
hymen (upward) (congenital) Q52.4
intervertebral disc NEC
  with myelopathy —*see* Disorder, disc, with,
    myelopathy
  cervical, cervicothoracic (with)
    M50.20
    myelopathy —*see* Disorder, disc,
      cervical, with myelopathy
    neuritis, radiculitis or radiculopathy —
      see Disorder, disc, cervical, with
      neuritis
  due to trauma —*see* Dislocation, vertebra

Displacement, displaced *(Continued)*
intervertebral disc NEC *(Continued)*
  lumbar region M51.26
    with
      neuritis, radiculitis, radiculopathy or
        sciatica M51.16
  lumbosacral region M51.27
    with
      myelopathy M51.07
      neuritis, radiculitis, radiculopathy or
        sciatica M51.17
  sacrococcygeal region M53.3
  thoracic region M51.24
    with
      myelopathy M51.04
      neuritis, radiculitis, radiculopathy
        M51.14
  thoracolumbar region M51.25
    with
      myelopathy M51.05
      neuritis, radiculitis, radiculopathy
        M51.15
intrauterine device (string) T83.32
kidney (acquired) N28.83
  congenital Q63.2
lachrymal, lacrimal apparatus or duct
  (congenital) Q10.6
lens, congenital Q12.1
macula (congenital) Q14.1
Meckel's diverticulum Q43.0
  malignant —*see* Table of Neoplasms, small
    intestine, malignant
nail (congenital) Q84.6
  acquired L60.8
opening of Wharton's duct in mouth Q38.4
organ or site, congenital NEC —*see*
  Malposition, congenital
ovary (acquired) N83.4-•
  congenital Q50.39
  free in peritoneal cavity (congenital)
    Q50.39
  into hernial sac N83.4-•
oviduct (acquired) N83.4-•
  congenital Q50.6
parathyroid (gland) E21.4
parotid gland (congenital) Q38.4
punctum lacrimale (congenital) Q10.6
sacro-iliac (joint) (congenital) Q74.2
  current injury S33.2
  old —*see* subcategory M53.2
salivary gland (any) (congenital) Q38.4
spleen (congenital) Q89.09
stomach, congenital Q40.2
sublingual duct Q38.4
tongue (downward) (congenital) Q38.3
tooth, teeth, fully erupted M26.30
  horizontal M26.33
  vertical M26.34
trachea (congenital) Q32.1
ureter or ureteric opening or orifice
  (congenital) Q62.62
uterine opening of oviducts or fallopian tubes
  Q50.6
uterus, uterine —*see* Malposition, uterus
ventricular septum Q21.0
  with rudimentary ventricle Q20.4
Disproportion
between native and reconstructed breast N65.1
fiber-type G71.2
Disruptio uteri —*see* Rupture, uterus
Disruption (of)
ciliary body NEC H21.89
closure of
  cornea T81.31
  craniotomy T81.32
  fascia (muscular) (superficial) T81.32
  internal organ or tissue T81.32
  laceration (external) (internal) T81.33
  ligament T81.32
  mucosa T81.31
  muscle or muscle flap T81.32

Disruption *(Continued)*
  closure of *(Continued)*
    ribs or rib cage T81.32
    skin and subcutaneous tissue (full-
      thickness) (superficial) T81.31
    skull T81.32
    sternum (sternotomy) T81.32
    tendon T81.32
    traumatic laceration (external) (internal)
      T81.33
  family Z63.8
    due to
      absence of family member due to
        military deployment Z63.31
      absence of family member NEC Z63.32
      alcoholism and drug addiction in family
        Z63.72
      bereavement Z63.4
      death (assumed) or disappearance of
        family member Z63.4
      divorce or separation Z63.5
      drug addiction in family Z63.72
      return of family member from military
        deployment (current or past
        conflict) Z63.71
      stressful life events NEC Z63.79
  iris NEC H21.89
  ligament(s) —*see also* Sprain
    knee
      current injury —*see* Dislocation, knee
      old (chronic) —*see* Derangement, knee,
        ligament, instability, chronic
      spontaneous NEC —*see* Derangement,
        knee, disruption ligament
  ossicular chain —*see* Discontinuity, ossicles,
    ear
  pelvic ring (stable) S32.810
    unstable S32.811
  traumatic injury wound repair T81.33
  wound T81.30
    episiotomy O90.1
    operation T81.31
      cesarean O90.0
      external operation wound (superficial)
        T81.31
      internal operation wound (deep) T81.32
      perineal (obstetric) O90.1
    traumatic injury repair T81.33
Dissatisfaction with
  employment Z56.9
  school environment Z55.4
Dissecting —*see* condition
Dissection
  aorta I71.00
    abdominal I71.02
    thoracic I71.01
    thoracoabdominal I71.03
  artery I77.70
    basilar (trunk) I77.75
    carotid I77.71
    cerebral (nonruptured) I67.0
      ruptured —*see* Hemorrhage, intracranial,
        subarachnoid
    coronary I25.42
    extremity
      lower I77.77
      upper I77.76
    iliac I77.72
    precerebral
      congenital (nonruptured) Q28.1
      specified site NEC I77.75
    renal I77.73
    specified NEC I77.79
    vertebral I77.74
  ▶precerebral artery, congenital (nonruptured)
    Q28.1
    ▶Heartland A93.8
  traumatic —*see* Wound, open, by site
  vascular I99.8
  wound —*see* Wound, open
Disseminated —*see* condition

Dissociation
  auriculoventricular or atrioventricular (AV)
    (any degree) (isorhythmic) I45.89
    with heart block I44.2
    interference I45.89
Dissociative reaction, state F44.9
Dissolution, vertebra —*see* Osteoporosis
Distension, distention
  abdomen R14.0
  bladder N32.89
  cecum K63.89
  colon K63.89
  gallbladder K82.8
  intestine K63.89
  kidney N28.89
  liver K76.89
  seminal vesicle N50.89
  stomach K31.89
    acute K31.0
    psychogenic F45.8
  ureter —*see* Dilatation, ureter
  uterus N85.8
Distoma hepaticum infestation B66.3
Distomiasis B66.9
  bile passages B66.3
  hemic B65.9
  hepatic B66.3
    due to Clonorchis sinensis B66.1
  intestinal B66.5
  liver B66.3
    due to Clonorchis sinensis B66.1
  lung B66.4
  pulmonary B66.4
Distomolar (fourth molar) K00.1
Disto-occlusion (Division I) (Division II)
  M26.212
Distortion(s) (congenital)
  adrenal (gland) Q89.1
  arm NEC Q68.8
  bile duct or passage Q44.5
  bladder Q64.79
  brain Q04.9
  cervix (uteri) Q51.9
  chest (wall) Q67.8
    bones Q76.8
  clavicle Q74.0
  clitoris Q52.6
  coccyx Q76.49
  common duct Q44.5
  coronary Q24.5
  cystic duct Q44.5
  ear (auricle) (external) Q17.3
    inner Q16.5
    middle Q16.4
      ossicles Q16.3
  endocrine NEC Q89.2
  eustachian tube Q17.8
  eye (adnexa) Q15.8
  face bone(s) NEC Q75.8
  fallopian tube Q50.6
  femur NEC Q68.8
  fibula NEC Q68.8
  finger(s) Q68.1
  foot Q66.9
  genitalia, genital organ(s)
    female Q52.8
      external Q52.79
      internal NEC Q52.8
  gyri Q04.8
  hand bone(s) Q68.1
  heart (auricle) (ventricle) Q24.8
    valve (cusp) Q24.8
  hepatic duct Q44.5
  humerus NEC Q68.8
  hymen Q52.4
  intrafamilial communications Z63.8
  jaw NEC M26.89
  labium (majus) (minus) Q52.79
  leg NEC Q68.8
  lens Q12.8
  liver Q44.7

Distortion *(Continued)*
  lumbar spine Q76.49
    with disproportion O33.8
      causing obstructed labor O65.0
  lumbosacral (joint) (region) Q76.49
    kyphosis —*see* Kyphosis, congenital
    lordosis —*see* Lordosis, congenital
  nerve Q07.8
  nose Q30.8
  organ
    of Corti Q16.5
    or site not listed —*see* Anomaly, by site
      ossicles, ear Q16.3
  oviduct Q50.6
  pancreas Q45.3
  parathyroid (gland) Q89.2
  pituitary (gland) Q89.2
  radius NEC Q68.8
  sacroiliac joint Q74.2
  sacrum Q76.49
  scapula Q74.0
  shoulder girdle Q74.0
  skull bone(s) NEC Q75.8
    with
      anencephalus Q00.0
      encephalocele —*see* Encephalocele
      hydrocephalus Q03.9
        with spina bifida —*see* Spina bifida,
          with hydrocephalus
      microcephaly Q02
  spinal cord Q06.8
  spine Q76.49
    kyphosis —*see* Kyphosis, congenital
    lordosis —*see* Lordosis, congenital
  spleen Q89.09
  sternum NEC Q76.7
  thorax (wall) Q67.8
    bony Q76.8
  thymus (gland) Q89.2
  thyroid (gland) Q89.2
  tibia NEC Q68.8
  toe(s) Q66.9
  tongue Q38.3
  trachea (cartilage) Q32.1
  ulna NEC Q68.8
  ureter Q62.8
  urethra Q64.79
    causing obstruction Q64.39
  uterus Q51.9
  vagina Q52.4
  vertebra Q76.49
    kyphosis —*see* Kyphosis, congenital
    lordosis —*see* Lordosis, congenital
  visual —*see also* Disturbance, vision
    shape and size H53.15
  vulva Q52.79
  wrist (bones) (joint) Q68.8
Distress
  abdomen —*see* Pain, abdominal
  ▶acute respiratory R06.03
    syndrome (adult) (child) J80
  epigastric R10.13
  fetal P84
    complicating pregnancy —*see* Stress, fetal
  gastrointestinal (functional) K30
    psychogenic F45.8
  intestinal (functional) NOS K59.9
    psychogenic F45.8
  maternal, during labor and delivery O75.0
  ▶relationship, with spouse or intimate partner
    Z63.0
  ▶respiratory (adult) (child) R06.03
    newborn P22.9
      specified NEC P22.8
    orthopnea R06.01
    psychogenic F45.8
    shortness of breath R06.02
    specified type NEC R06.09
Distribution vessel, atypical Q27.9
  coronary artery Q24.5
  precerebral Q28.1

▶ New   ⇒ Revised   ~~deleted~~ Deleted   ● Use Additional Character(s)

Districhiasis L68.8
Disturbance(s) —see also Disease
  absorption K90.9
    calcium E58
    carbohydrate K90.49
    fat K90.49
      pancreatic K90.3
    protein K90.49
    starch K90.49
    vitamin —see Deficiency, vitamin
  acid-base equilibrium E87.8
    mixed E87.4
  activity and attention (with hyperkinesis) —
    see Disorder, attention-deficit
    hyperactivity
  amino acid transport E72.00
  assimilation, food K90.9
  auditory nerve, except deafness —see
    subcategory H93.3
  behavior —see Disorder, conduct
  blood clotting (mechanism) —see also Defect,
    coagulation D68.9
  cerebral
    nerve —see Disorder, nerve, cranial
    status, newborn P91.9
    ⟱specified NEC P91.88
  circulatory I99.9
  conduct —see also Disorder, conduct F91.9
    adjustment reaction —see Disorder,
      adjustment
    compulsive F63.9
    disruptive F91.9
    hyperkinetic —see Disorder, attention-
      deficit hyperactivity
    socialized F91.2
    specified NEC F91.8
    unsocialized F91.1
  coordination R27.8
  cranial nerve —see Disorder, nerve, cranial
  deep sensibility —see Disturbance, sensation
  digestive K30
    psychogenic F45.8
  electrolyte —see also Imbalance, electrolyte
    newborn, transitory P74.4
      hyperammonemia P74.6
      potassium balance P74.3
      sodium balance P74.2
      specified type NEC P74.4
  emotions specific to childhood and
    adolescence F93.9
    with
      anxiety and fearfulness NEC F93.8
      elective mutism F94.0
      oppositional disorder F91.3
      sensitivity (withdrawal) F40.10
      shyness F40.10
      social withdrawal F40.10
      involving relationship problems
        F93.8
      mixed F93.8
      specified NEC F93.8
  endocrine (gland) E34.9
    neonatal, transitory P72.9
      specified NEC P72.8
  equilibrium R42
  fructose metabolism E74.10
  gait —see Gait
    hysterical F44.4
    psychogenic F44.4
  gastrointestinal (functional) K30
    psychogenic F45.8
  habit, child F98.9
  hearing, except deafness and tinnitus —see
    Abnormal, auditory perception
  heart, functional (conditions in I44-I50)
    due to presence of (cardiac) prosthesis
      I97.19-●
    postoperative I97.89
    ⟱cardiac surgery —see also Infarct,
      myocardium, associated with
      revascularization procedure I97.19-●

Disturbance (Continued)
  hormones E34.9
  innervation uterus (parasympathetic)
    (sympathetic) N85.8
  keratinization NEC
    gingiva K05.10
      nonplaque induced K05.11
      plaque induced K05.10
    lip K13.0
    oral (mucosa) (soft tissue) K13.29
    tongue K13.29
  learning (specific) —see Disorder, learning
  memory —see Amnesia
    mild, following organic brain damage
      F06.8
  mental F99
    associated with diseases classified
      elsewhere F54
  metabolism E88.9
    with
      abortion —see Abortion, by type with
        other specified complication
      ectopic pregnancy O08.5
      molar pregnancy O08.5
    amino-acid E72.9
      aromatic E70.9
      branched-chain E71.2
      straight-chain E72.8
      sulfur-bearing E72.10
    ammonia E72.20
    arginine E72.21
    arginosuccinic acid E72.22
    carbohydrate E74.9
    cholesterol E78.9
    citrulline E72.23
    cystathionine E72.19
    general E88.9
    glutamine E72.8
    histidine E70.40
    homocystine E72.19
    hydroxylysine E72.3
    in labor or delivery O75.89
    iron E83.10
    lipoid E78.9
    lysine E72.3
    methionine E72.19
    neonatal, transitory P74.9
      calcium and magnesium P71.9
        specified type NEC P71.8
      carbohydrate metabolism P70.9
        specified type NEC P70.8
      specified NEC P74.8
    ornithine E72.4
    phosphate E83.39
    sodium NEC E87.8
    threonine E72.8
    tryptophan E70.5
    tyrosine E70.20
    urea cycle E72.20
  motor R29.2
  nervous, functional R45.0
  neuromuscular mechanism (eye), due to
    syphilis A52.15
  nutritional E63.9
    nail L60.3
  ocular motion H51.9
    psychogenic F45.8
  oculogyric H51.8
    psychogenic F45.8
  oculomotor H51.9
    psychogenic F45.8
  olfactory nerve R43.1
  optic nerve NEC —see Disorder, nerve, optic
  oral epithelium, including tongue NEC
    K13.29
  perceptual due to
    alcohol withdrawal F10.232
    amphetamine intoxication F15.922
      in
        abuse F15.122
        dependence F15.222

Disturbance (Continued)
  perceptual due to (Continued)
    anxiolytic withdrawal F13.232
    cannabis intoxication (acute) F12.922
      in
        abuse F12.122
        dependence F12.222
    cocaine intoxication (acute) F14.922
      in
        abuse F14.122
        dependence F14.222
    hypnotic withdrawal F13.232
    opioid intoxication (acute) F11.922
      in
        abuse F11.122
        dependence F11.222
    phencyclidine intoxication (acute)
      F16.122
    sedative withdrawal F13.232
  personality (pattern) (trait) —see also
    Disorder, personality F60.9
    following organic brain damage
      F07.9
  polyglandular E31.9
    specified NEC E31.8
  potassium balance, newborn P74.3
  psychogenic F45.9
  psychomotor F44.4
  psychophysical visual H53.16
  pupillary —see Anomaly, pupil, function
  reflex R29.2
  rhythm, heart I49.9
  salivary secretion K11.7
  sensation (cold) (heat) (localization) (tactile
    discrimination) (texture) (vibratory)
    NEC R20.9
    hysterical F44.6
    skin R20.9
      anesthesia R20.0
      hyperesthesia R20.3
      hypoesthesia R20.1
      paresthesia R20.2
      specified type NEC R20.8
    smell R43.9
      and taste (mixed) R43.8
      anosmia R43.0
      parosmia R43.1
      specified NEC R43.8
    taste R43.9
      and smell (mixed) R43.8
      parageusia R43.2
      specified NEC R43.8
  sensory —see Disturbance, sensation
  situational (transient) —see also Disorder,
    adjustment
    acute F43.0
  sleep G47.9
    nonorganic origin F51.9
  smell —see Disturbance, sensation, smell
  sociopathic F60.2
  sodium balance, newborn P74.2
  speech R47.9
    developmental F80.9
    specified NEC R47.89
  stomach (functional) K31.9
  sympathetic (nerve) G90.9
  taste —see Disturbance, sensation, taste
  temperature
    regulation, newborn P81.9
      specified NEC P81.8
    sense R20.8
      hysterical F44.6
  tooth
    eruption K00.6
    formation K00.4
    structure, hereditary NEC K00.5
  touch —see Disturbance, sensation
  vascular I99.9
    arteriosclerotic —see Arteriosclerosis
  vasomotor I73.9
  vasospastic I73.9

Disturbance *(Continued)*
  vision, visual H53.9
    following
      cerebral infarction I69.398
      cerebrovascular disease I69.998
        specified NEC I69.898
      intracerebral hemorrhage I69.198
      nontraumatic intracranial hemorrhage
        NEC I69.298
      specified disease NEC I69.898
      subarachnoid hemorrhage I69.098
    psychophysical H53.16
    specified NEC H53.8
    subjective H53.10
      day blindness H53.11
      discomfort H53.14-●
      distortions of shape and size H53.15
      loss
        sudden H53.13-●
        transient H53.12-●
      specified type NEC H53.19
  voice R49.9
    psychogenic F44.4
    specified NEC R49.8
Diuresis R35.8
Diver's palsy, paralysis or squeeze T70.3
Diverticulitis (acute) K57.92
  bladder —*see* Cystitis
  ileum —*see* Diverticulitis, intestine, small
  intestine K57.92
    with
      abscess, perforation or peritonitis K57.80
        with bleeding K57.81
      bleeding K57.93
    congenital Q43.8
    large K57.32
      with
        abscess, perforation or peritonitis
          K57.20
          with bleeding K57.21
        bleeding K57.33
        small intestine K57.52
          with
            abscess, perforation or peritonitis
              K57.40
              with bleeding K57.41
            bleeding K57.53
    small K57.12
      with
        abscess, perforation or peritonitis
          K57.00
          with bleeding K57.01
        bleeding K57.13
        large intestine K57.52
          with
            abscess, perforation or peritonitis
              K57.40
              with bleeding K57.41
            bleeding K57.53
Diverticulosis K57.90
  with bleeding K57.91
  large intestine K57.30
    with
      bleeding K57.31
      small intestine K57.50
        with bleeding K57.51
  small intestine K57.10
    with
      bleeding K57.11
      large intestine K57.50
        with bleeding K57.51
Diverticulum, diverticula (multiple) K57.90
  appendix (noninflammatory) K38.2
  bladder (sphincter) N32.3
    congenital Q64.6
  bronchus (congenital) Q32.4
    acquired J98.09
  calyx, calyceal (kidney) N28.89
  cardia (stomach) K31.4
  cecum —*see* Diverticulosis, intestine, large
    congenital Q43.8

Diverticulum, diverticula *(Continued)*
  colon —*see* Diverticulosis, intestine, large
    congenital Q43.8
  duodenum —*see* Diverticulosis, intestine,
    small
    congenital Q43.8
  epiphrenic (esophagus) K22.5
  esophagus (congenital) Q39.6
    acquired (epiphrenic) (pulsion) (traction)
      K22.5
  eustachian tube —*see* Disorder, eustachian
    tube, specified NEC
  fallopian tube N83.8
  gastric K31.4
  heart (congenital) Q24.8
  ileum —*see* Diverticulosis, intestine, small
  jejunum —*see* Diverticulosis, intestine, small
  kidney (pelvis) (calyces) N28.89
    with calculus —*see* Calculus, kidney
  Meckel's (displaced) (hypertrophic) Q43.0
    malignant —*see* Table of Neoplasms, small
      intestine, malignant
  midthoracic K22.5
  organ or site, congenital NEC —*see* Distortion
  pericardium (congenital) (cyst) Q24.8
    acquired I31.8
  pharyngoesophageal (congenital) Q39.6
    acquired K22.5
  pharynx (congenital) Q38.7
  rectosigmoid —*see* Diverticulosis, intestine,
    large
    congenital Q43.8
  rectum —*see* Diverticulosis, intestine, large
  Rokitansky's K22.5
  seminal vesicle N50.89
  sigmoid —*see* Diverticulosis, intestine, large
    congenital Q43.8
  stomach (acquired) K31.4
    congenital Q40.2
  trachea (acquired) J39.8
  ureter (acquired) N28.89
    congenital Q62.8
  ureterovesical orifice N28.89
  urethra (acquired) N36.1
    congenital Q64.79
  ventricle, left (congenital) Q24.8
  vesical N32.3
    congenital Q64.6
  Zenker's (esophagus) K22.5
Division
  cervix uteri (acquired) N88.8
  glans penis Q55.69
  labia minora (congenital) Q52.79
  ligament (partial or complete) (current) —*see
    also* Sprain
    with open wound —*see* Wound, open
  muscle (partial or complete) (current) —*see
    also* Injury, muscle
    with open wound —*see* Wound, open
  nerve (traumatic) —*see* Injury, nerve
  spinal cord —*see* Injury, spinal cord,
    by region
  vein I87.8
Divorce, causing family disruption Z63.5
Dix-Hallpike neurolabyrinthitis —*see*
  Neuronitis, vestibular
Dizziness R42
  hysterical F44.89
  psychogenic F45.8
DMAC (disseminated mycobacterium avium-
  intracellulare complex) A31.2
DNR (do not resuscitate) Z66
Doan-Wiseman syndrome (primary splenic
  neutropenia) —*see* Agranulocytosis
Doehle-Heller aortitis A52.02
Dog bite —*see* Bite
Dohle body panmyelopathic syndrome D72.0
Dolichocephaly Q67.2
Dolichocolon Q43.8
Dolichostenomelia —*see* Syndrome, Marfan's
Donohue's syndrome E34.8

Donor (organ or tissue) Z52.9
  blood (whole) Z52.000
    autologous Z52.010
    specified component (lymphocytes)
      (platelets) NEC Z52.008
      autologous Z52.018
      specified donor NEC Z52.098
    specified donor NEC Z52.090
    stem cells Z52.001
      autologous Z52.011
      specified donor NEC Z52.091
  bone Z52.20
    autologous Z52.21
    marrow Z52.3
    specified type NEC Z52.29
  cornea Z52.5
  egg (Oocyte) Z52.819
    age 35 and over Z52.812
      anonymous recipient Z52.812
      designated recipient Z52.813
    under age 35 Z52.810
      anonymous recipient Z52.810
      designated recipient Z52.811
  kidney Z52.4
  liver Z52.6
  lung Z52.89
  lymphocyte —*see* Donor, blood, specified
    components NEC
  Oocyte —*see* Donor, egg
  platelets Z52.008
  potential, examination of Z00.5
  semen Z52.89
  skin Z52.10
    autologous Z52.11
    specified type NEC Z52.19
  specified organ or tissue NEC Z52.89
  sperm Z52.89
Donovanosis A58
Dorsalgia M54.9
  psychogenic F45.41
  specified NEC M54.89
Dorsopathy M53.9
  deforming M43.9
    specified NEC —*see* subcategory M43.8
  specified NEC M53.80
    cervical region M53.82
    cervicothoracic region M53.83
    lumbar region M53.86
    lumbosacral region M53.87
    occipito-atlanto-axial region M53.81
    sacrococcygeal region M53.88
    thoracic region M53.84
    thoracolumbar region M53.85
Double
  albumin E88.09
  aortic arch Q25.45
  auditory canal Q17.8
  auricle (heart) Q20.8
  bladder Q64.79
  cervix Q51.820
    with doubling of uterus (and vagina) Q51.10
      with obstruction Q51.11
  inlet ventricle Q20.4
  kidney with double pelvis (renal) Q63.0
  meatus urinarius Q64.75
  monster Q89.4
  outlet
    left ventricle Q20.2
    right ventricle Q20.1
  pelvis (renal) with double ureter Q62.5
  tongue Q38.3
  ureter (one or both sides) Q62.5
    with double pelvis (renal) Q62.5
  urethra Q64.74
  urinary meatus Q64.75
  uterus Q51.2
    with
      doubling of cervix (and vagina) Q51.10
        with obstruction Q51.11
      in pregnancy or childbirth O34.59-●
        causing obstructed labor O65.5

▶ New   ⇒ Revised   ~~deleted~~ Deleted   ● Use Additional Character(s)

Double (Continued)
  vagina Q52.10
    with doubling of uterus (and cervix)
      Q51.10
      with obstruction Q51.11
  vision H53.2
  vulva Q52.79
Douglas' pouch, cul-de-sac —see condition
Down syndrome Q90.9
  meiotic nondisjunction Q90.0
  mitotic nondisjunction Q90.1
  mosaicism Q90.1
  translocation Q90.2
DPD (dihydropyrimidine dehydrogenase
  deficiency) E88.89
Dracontiasis B72
Dracunculiasis, dracunculosis B72
Dream state, hysterical F44.89
Drepanocytic anemia —see Disease, sickle-cell
Dresbach's syndrome (elliptocytosis) D58.1
Dreschlera (hawaiiensis) (infection) B43.8
Dressler's syndrome I24.1
Drift, ulnar —see Deformity, limb, specified
  type NEC, forearm
Drinking (alcohol)
  excessive, to excess NEC (without
    dependence) F10.10
    habitual (continual) (without remission)
      F10.20
      with remission F10.21
Drip, postnasal (chronic) R09.82
  due to
    allergic rhinitis —see Rhinitis, allergic
    common cold J00
    gastroesophageal reflux —see Reflux,
      gastroesophageal
    nasopharyngitis —see Nasopharyngitis
    other known condition — code to
      condition
    sinusitis —see Sinusitis
Droop
  facial R29.810
    cerebrovascular disease I69.992
      cerebral infarction I69.392
      intracerebral hemorrhage I69.192
      nontraumatic intracranial hemorrhage
        NEC I69.292
      specified disease NEC I69.892
      subarachnoid hemorrhage I69.092
Drop (in)
  attack NEC R55
  finger —see Deformity, finger
  foot —see Deformity, limb, foot, drop
  hematocrit (precipitous) R71.0
  hemoglobin R71.0
  toe —see Deformity, toe, specified NEC
  wrist —see Deformity, limb, wrist drop
Dropped heart beats I45.9
Dropsy, dropsical —see also Hydrops
  abdomen R18.8
  brain —see Hydrocephalus
  cardiac, heart —see Failure, heart, congestive
  gangrenous —see Gangrene
  heart —see Failure, heart, congestive
  kidney —see Nephrosis
  lung —see Edema, lung
  newborn due to isoimmunization P56.0
  pericardium —see Pericarditis
Drowned, drowning (near) T75.1
Drowsiness R40.0
Drug
  abuse counseling and surveillance Z71.51
  addiction —see Dependence
  dependence —see Dependence
  habit —see Dependence
  harmful use —see Abuse, drug
  induced fever R50.2
  overdose —see Table of Drugs and Chemicals,
    by drug, poisoning
  poisoning —see Table of Drugs and
    Chemicals, by drug, poisoning

Drug (Continued)
  resistant organism infection —see also
    Resistant, organism, to, drug Z16.30
  therapy
    long term (current) (prophylactic) —see
      Therapy, drug long-term (current)
      (prophylactic)
    short term - omit code
  wrong substance given or taken in error —see
    Table of Drugs and Chemicals, by drug,
    poisoning
Drunkenness (without dependence) F10.129
  acute in alcoholism F10.229
  chronic (without remission) F10.20
    with remission F10.21
  pathological (without dependence) F10.129
    with dependence F10.229
  sleep F51.9
Drusen
  macula (degenerative) (retina) —see
    Degeneration, macula, drusen
  optic disc H47.32-●
Dry, dryness —see also condition
  larynx J38.7
  mouth R68.2
    due to dehydration E86.0
  nose J34.89
  socket (teeth) M27.3
  throat J39.2
DSAP L56.5
Duane's syndrome H50.81-●
Dubin-Johnson disease or syndrome E80.6
Dubois' disease (thymus gland) A50.59 [E35]
Dubowitz' syndrome Q87.1
Duchenne-Aran muscular atrophy G12.21
Duchenne-Griesinger disease G71.0
Duchenne's
  disease or syndrome
    motor neuron disease G12.22
    muscular dystrophy G71.0
    locomotor ataxia (syphilitic) A52.11
  paralysis
    birth injury P14.0
    due to or associated with
      motor neuron disease G12.22
      muscular dystrophy G71.0
Ducrey's chancre A57
Duct, ductus —see condition
Duhring's disease (dermatitis herpetiformis)
  L13.0
Dullness, cardiac (decreased) (increased) R01.2
Dumb ague —see Malaria
Dumbness —see Aphasia
Dumdum fever B55.0
Dumping syndrome (postgastrectomy) K91.1
Duodenitis (nonspecific) (peptic) K29.80
  with bleeding K29.81
Duodenocholangitis —see Cholangitis
Duodenum, duodenal —see condition
Duplay's bursitis or periarthritis —see
  Tendinitis, calcific, shoulder
Duplication, duplex —see also Accessory
  alimentary tract Q45.8
  anus Q43.4
  appendix (and cecum) Q43.4
  biliary duct (any) Q44.5
  bladder Q64.79
  cecum (and appendix) Q43.4
  cervix Q51.820
  chromosome NEC
    with complex rearrangements NEC
      Q92.5
    seen only at prometaphase Q92.8
  cystic duct Q44.5
  digestive organs Q45.8
  esophagus Q39.8
  frontonasal process Q75.8
  intestine (large) (small) Q43.4
  kidney Q63.0
  liver Q44.7
  pancreas Q45.3

Duplication, duplex (Continued)
  penis Q55.69
  respiratory organs NEC Q34.8
  salivary duct Q38.4
  spinal cord (incomplete) Q06.2
  stomach Q40.2
Dupré's disease (meningism) R29.1
Dupuytren's contraction or disease M72.0
Durand-Nicolas-Favre disease A55
Durotomy (inadvertent) (incidental) G97.41
Duroziez's disease (congenital mitral stenosis)
  Q23.2
Dutton's relapsing fever (West African) A68.1
Dwarfism E34.3
  achondroplastic Q77.4
  congenital E34.3
  constitutional E34.3
  hypochondroplastic Q77.4
  hypophyseal E23.0
  infantile E34.3
  Laron-type E34.3
  Lorain (-Levi) type E23.0
  metatropic Q77.8
  nephrotic-glycosuric (with
    hypophosphatemic rickets) E72.09
  nutritional E45
  pancreatic K86.89
  pituitary E23.0
  renal N25.0
  thanatophoric Q77.1
Dyke-Young anemia (secondary)
  (symptomatic) D59.1
Dysacusis —see Abnormal, auditory
  perception
Dysadrenocortism E27.9
  hyperfunction E27.0
Dysarthria R47.1
  following
    cerebral infarction I69.322
    cerebrovascular disease I69.922
      specified disease NEC I69.822
    intracerebral hemorrhage I69.122
    nontraumatic intracranial hemorrhage
      NEC I69.222
    subarachnoid hemorrhage I69.022
Dysautonomia (familial) G90.1
Dysbarism T70.3
Dysbasia R26.2
  angiosclerotica intermittens I73.9
  hysterical F44.4
  lordotica (progressiva) G24.1
  nonorganic origin F44.4
  psychogenic F44.4
Dysbetalipoproteinemia (familial) E78.2
Dyscalculia R48.8
  developmental F81.2
Dyschezia K59.00
Dyschondroplasia (with hemangiomata) Q78.4
Dyschromia (skin) L81.9
Dyscollagenosis M35.9
Dyscranio-pygo-phalangy Q87.0
Dyscrasia
  blood (with) D75.9
    antepartum hemorrhage —see
      Hemorrhage, antepartum, with
      coagulation defect
    intrapartum hemorrhage O67.0
    newborn P61.9
      specified type NEC P61.8
    puerperal, postpartum O72.3
  polyglandular, pluriglandular E31.9
Dysendocrinism E34.9
Dysentery, dysenteric (catarrhal) (diarrhea)
  (epidemic) (hemorrhagic) (infectious)
  (sporadic) (tropical) A09
  abscess, liver A06.4
  amebic —see also Amebiasis A06.0
    with abscess —see Abscess, amebic
    acute A06.0
    chronic A06.1
  arthritis —see also category M01 A09
    bacillary —see also category M01 A03.9

Dysentery, dysenteric (Continued)
  bacillary A03.9
    arthritis —see also category M01 A03.9
    Boyd A03.2
    Flexner A03.1
    Schmitz (-Stutzer) A03.0
    Shiga (-Kruse) A03.0
    Shigella A03.9
      boydii A03.2
      dysenteriae A03.0
      flexneri A03.1
      group A A03.0
      group B A03.1
      group C A03.2
      group D A03.3
      sonnei A03.3
      specified type NEC A03.8
    Sonne A03.3
    specified type NEC A03.8
  balantidial A07.0
  Balantidium coli A07.0
  Boyd's A03.2
  candidal B37.82
  Chilomastix A07.8
  Chinese A03.9
  coccidial A07.3
  Dientamoeba (fragilis) A07.8
  Embadomonas A07.8
  Entamoeba, entamebic —see Dysentery,
      amebic
  Flexner-Boyd A03.2
  Flexner's A03.1
  Giardia lamblia A07.1
  Hiss-Russell A03.1
  Lamblia A07.1
  leishmanial B55.0
  malarial —see Malaria
  metazoal B82.0
  monilial B37.82
  protozoal A07.9
  Salmonella A02.0
  schistosomal B65.1
  Schmitz (-Stutzer) A03.0
  Shiga (-Kruse) A03.0
  Shigella NOS —see Dysentery, bacillary
  Sonne A03.3
  strongyloidiasis B78.0
  trichomonal A07.8
  viral —see also Enteritis, viral A08.4
Dysequilibrium R42
Dysesthesia R20.8
  hysterical F44.6
Dysfibrinogenemia (congenital) D68.2
Dysfunction
  adrenal E27.9
    hyperfunction E27.0
  autonomic
    due to alcohol G31.2
    somatoform F45.8
  bladder N31.9
    neurogenic NOS —see Dysfunction,
        bladder, neuromuscular
    neuromuscular NOS N31.9
      atonic (motor) (sensory) N31.2
      autonomous N31.2
      flaccid N31.2
      nonreflex N31.2
      reflex N31.1
      specified NEC N31.8
      uninhibited N31.0
  bleeding, uterus N93.8
  cerebral G93.89
  colon K59.9
    psychogenic F45.8
  colostomy K94.03
  cystic duct K82.8
  cystostomy (stoma) —see Complications,
      cystostomy
  ejaculatory N53.19
    anejaculatory orgasm N53.13
    painful N53.12

Dysfunction (Continued)
  ejaculatory (Continued)
    premature F52.4
    retarded N53.11
  endocrine NOS E34.9
  endometrium N85.8
  enterostomy K94.13
  erectile —see Dysfunction, sexual, male, erectile
  gallbladder K82.8
  gastrostomy (stoma) K94.23
  gland, glandular NOS E34.9
  heart I51.89
  hemoglobin D75.89
  hepatic K76.89
  hypophysis E23.7
  hypothalamic NEC E23.3
  ileostomy (stoma) K94.13
  jejunostomy (stoma) K94.13
  kidney —see Disease, renal
  labyrinthine —see subcategory H83.2
  left ventricular, following sudden emotional
      stress I51.81
  liver K76.89
  male —see Dysfunction, sexual, male
  orgasmic (female) F52.31
    male F52.32
  ovary E28.9
    specified NEC E28.8
  papillary muscle I51.89
  parathyroid E21.4
  physiological NEC R68.89
    psychogenic F59
  pineal gland E34.8
  pituitary (gland) E23.3
  platelets D69.1
  polyglandular E31.9
    specified NEC E31.8
  psychophysiologic F59
  psychosexual F52.9
    with
      dyspareunia F52.6
      premature ejaculation F52.4
      vaginismus F52.5
  pylorus K31.9
  rectum K59.9
    psychogenic F45.8
  reflex (sympathetic) —see Syndrome, pain,
      complex regional I
  segmental —see Dysfunction, somatic
  senile R54
  sexual (due to) R37
    alcohol F10.981
    amphetamine F15.981
      in
        abuse F15.181
        dependence F15.281
    anxiolytic F13.981
      in
        abuse F13.181
        dependence F13.281
    cocaine F14.981
      in
        abuse F14.181
        dependence F14.281
    excessive sexual drive F52.8
    failure of genital response (male) F52.21
      female F52.22
    female N94.9
      aversion F52.1
      dyspareunia N94.10
        psychogenic F52.6
      frigidity F52.22
      nymphomania F52.8
      orgasmic F52.31
      psychogenic F52.9
        aversion F52.1
        dyspareunia F52.6
        frigidity F52.22
        nymphomania F52.8
        orgasmic F52.31
        vaginismus F52.5

Dysfunction (Continued)
  sexual (Continued)
    female (Continued)
      vaginismus N94.2
        psychogenic F52.5
    hypnotic F13.981
      in
        abuse F13.181
        dependence F13.281
    inhibited orgasm (female) F52.31
      male F52.32
    lack
      of sexual enjoyment F52.1
      or loss of sexual desire F52.0
    male N53.9
      anejaculatory orgasm N53.13
      ejaculatory N53.19
        painful N53.12
        premature F52.4
        retarded N53.11
      erectile N52.9
        drug induced N52.2
        due to
          disease classified elsewhere N52.1
          drug N52.2
          postoperative (postprocedural) N52.39
            following
              cryotherapy N52.37
              interstitial seed therapy N52.36
              prostate ablative therapy N52.37
              prostatectomy N52.34
                radical N52.31
              radiation therapy N52.35
              radical cystectomy N52.32
              ultrasound ablative therapy
                  N52.37
              urethral surgery N52.33
        psychogenic F52.21
        specified cause NEC N52.8
        vasculogenic
          arterial insufficiency N52.01
            with corporo-venous occlusive
                N52.03
          corporo-venous occlusive N52.02
            with arterial insufficiency N52.03
      impotence —see Dysfunction, sexual,
          male, erectile
      psychogenic F52.9
        aversion F52.1
        erectile F52.21
        orgasmic F52.32
        premature ejaculation F52.4
        satyriasis F52.8
        specified type NEC F52.8
      specified type NEC N53.8
    nonorganic F52.9
      specified NEC F52.8
    opioid F11.981
      in
        abuse F11.181
        dependence F11.281
    orgasmic dysfunction (female) F52.31
      male F52.32
    premature ejaculation F52.4
    psychoactive substances NEC F19.981
      in
        abuse F19.181
        dependence F19.281
    psychogenic F52.9
    sedative F13.981
      in
        abuse F13.181
        dependence F13.281
    sexual aversion F52.1
    vaginismus (nonorganic) (psychogenic)
        F52.5
  sinoatrial node I49.5
  somatic M99.09
    abdomen M99.09
    acromioclavicular M99.07
    cervical region M99.01

▶ New   ⇒ Revised   ~~deleted~~ Deleted   ● Use Additional Character(s)

Dysfunction *(Continued)*
  somatic *(Continued)*
    cervicothoracic M99.01
    costochondral M99.08
    costovertebral M99.08
    head region M99.00
    hip M99.05
    lower extremity M99.06
    lumbar region M99.03
    lumbosacral M99.03
    occipitocervical M99.00
    pelvic region M99.05
    pubic M99.05
    rib cage M99.08
    sacral region M99.04
    sacrococcygeal M99.04
    sacroiliac M99.04
    specified NEC M99.09
    sternochondral M99.08
    sternoclavicular M99.07
    thoracic region M99.02
    thoracolumbar M99.02
    upper extremity M99.07
  somatoform autonomic F45.8
  stomach K31.89
    psychogenic F45.8
  suprarenal E27.9
    hyperfunction E27.0
  symbolic R48.9
    specified type NEC R48.8
  temporomandibular (joint) M26.69
    joint-pain syndrome M26.62-•
  testicular (endocrine) E29.9
    specified NEC E29.8
  thymus E32.9
  thyroid E07.9
  ureterostomy (stoma) —see Complications,
      stoma, urinary tract
  urethrostomy (stoma) —see Complications,
      stoma, urinary tract
  uterus, complicating delivery O62.9
    hypertonic O62.4
    hypotonic O62.2
      primary O62.0
      secondary O62.1
  ventricular I51.9
    ~~with congestive heart failure I50.9-•~~
    ~~left, reversible, following sudden~~
        ~~emotional stress I51.81~~
    ▶with congestive heart failure —see also
        Failure, heart I50.9
    ▶left, reversible, following sudden
        emotional stress I51.81
Dysgenesis
  gonadal (due to chromosomal anomaly)
      Q96.9
    pure Q99.1
  renal Q60.5
    bilateral Q60.4
    unilateral Q60.3
  reticular D72.0
  tidal platelet D69.3
Dysgerminoma
  specified site —see Neoplasm, malignant,
      by site
  unspecified site
    female C56.9
    male C62.90
Dysgeusia R43.2
Dysgraphia R27.8
Dyshidrosis, dysidrosis L30.1
Dyskaryotic cervical smear R87.619
Dyskeratosis L85.8
  cervix —see Dysplasia, cervix
  congenital Q82.8
  uterus NEC N85.8
Dyskinesia G24.9
  biliary (cystic duct or gallbladder) K82.8
  drug induced
    orofacial G24.01
  esophagus K22.4

Dyskinesia *(Continued)*
  hysterical F44.4
  intestinal K59.8
  nonorganic origin F44.4
  orofacial (idiopathic) G24.4
    drug induced G24.01
  psychogenic F44.4
  subacute, drug induced G24.01
  tardive G24.01
    neuroleptic induced G24.01
  trachea J39.8
  tracheobronchial J98.09
Dyslalia (developmental) F80.0
Dyslexia R48.0
  developmental F81.0
Dyslipidemia E78.5
  depressed HDL cholesterol E78.6
  elevated fasting triglycerides E78.1
Dysmaturity —see also Light for dates
  pulmonary (newborn) (Wilson-Mikity) P27.0
Dysmenorrhea (essential) (exfoliative) N94.6
  congestive (syndrome) N94.6
  primary N94.4
  psychogenic F45.8
  secondary N94.5
Dysmetabolic syndrome X E88.81
Dysmetria R27.8
Dysmorphism (due to)
  alcohol Q86.0
  exogenous cause NEC Q86.8
  hydantoin Q86.1
  warfarin Q86.2
Dysmorphophobia (nondelusional) F45.22
  delusional F22
Dysnomia R47.01
Dysorexia R63.0
  psychogenic F50.89
Dysostosis
  cleidocranial, cleidocranialis Q74.0
  craniofacial Q75.1
  Fairbank's (idiopathic familial generalized
      osteophytosis) Q78.9
  mandibulofacial (incomplete) Q75.4
  multiplex E76.01
  oculomandibular Q75.5
Dyspareunia (female) N94.10
  deep N94.12
  male N53.12
  nonorganic F52.6
  psychogenic F52.6
  secondary N94.19
  specified NEC N94.19
  superficial (introital) N94.11
Dyspepsia R10.13
  atonic K30
  functional (allergic) (congenital)
      (gastrointestinal) (occupational) (reflex)
      K30
  intestinal K59.8
  nervous F45.8
  neurotic F45.8
  psychogenic F45.8
Dysphagia R13.10
  cervical R13.19
  following
    cerebral infarction I69.391
    cerebrovascular disease I69.991
      specified NEC I69.891
    intracerebral hemorrhage I69.191
    nontraumatic intracranial hemorrhage
        NEC I69.291
    specified disease NEC I69.891
    subarachnoid hemorrhage I69.091
  functional (hysterical) F45.8
  hysterical F45.8
  nervous (hysterical) F45.8
  neurogenic R13.19
  oral phase R13.11
  oropharyngeal phase R13.12
  ~~pharyngeal phase R13.13~~
  ▶pharyngeal phase R13.13

Dysphagia *(Continued)*
  pharyngoesophageal phase R13.14
  psychogenic F45.8
  sideropenic D50.1
  spastica K22.4
  specified NEC R13.19
Dysphagocytosis, congenital D71
Dysphasia R47.02
  developmental
    expressive type F80.1
    receptive type F80.2
  following
    cerebrovascular disease I69.921
      cerebral infarction I69.321
      intracerebral hemorrhage I69.121
    nontraumatic intracranial hemorrhage NEC
        I69.221
      specified disease NEC I69.821
      subarachnoid hemorrhage I69.021
Dysphonia R49.0
  functional F44.4
  hysterical F44.4
  psychogenic F44.4
  spastica J38.3
Dysphoria
  ⇒gender F64.9
    in
        adolescence and adulthood F64.0
        children F64.2
    ▶specified NEC F64.8
    postpartal O90.6
Dyspituitarism E23.3
Dysplasia —see also Anomaly
  acetabular, congenital Q65.89
  alveolar capillary, with vein misalignment
      J84.843
  anus (histologically confirmed) (mild)
      (moderate) K62.82
    severe D01.3
  arrhythmogenic right ventricular I42.8
  arterial, fibromuscular I77.3
  asphyxiating thoracic (congenital) Q77.2
  brain Q07.9
  bronchopulmonary, perinatal P27.1
  cervix (uteri) N87.9
    mild N87.0
    moderate N87.1
    severe D06.9
  chondroectodermal Q77.6
  colon D12.6
  craniometaphyseal Q78.58
  dentinal K00.5
  diaphyseal, progressive Q78.3
  dystrophic Q77.5
  ectodermal (anhidrotic) (congenital)
      (hereditary) Q82.4
    hydrotic Q82.8
  epithelial, uterine cervix —see Dysplasia, cervix
  eye (congenital) Q11.2
  fibrous
    bone NEC (monostotic) M85.00
      ankle M85.07-•
      foot M85.07-•
      forearm M85.03-•
      hand M85.04-•
      lower leg M85.06-•
      multiple site M85.09
      neck M85.08
      rib M85.08
      shoulder M85.01-•
      skull M85.08
      specified site NEC M85.08
      thigh M85.05-•
      toe M85.07-•
      upper arm M85.02-•
      vertebra M85.08
    diaphyseal, progressive Q78.3
    jaw M27.8
    polyostotic Q78.1
  florid osseous —see also Cyst, calcifying
      odontogenic

Dysplasia *(Continued)*
  high grade, focal D12.6
  hip, congenital Q65.89
  joint, congenital Q74.8
  kidney Q61.4
    multicystic Q61.4
  leg Q74.2
  lung, congenital (not associated with short gestation) Q33.6
  mammary (gland) (benign) N60.9-●
    cyst (solitary) —*see* Cyst, breast
    cystic —*see* Mastopathy, cystic
    duct ectasia —*see* Ectasia, mammary duct
    fibroadenosis —*see* Fibroadenosis, breast
    fibrosclerosis —*see* Fibrosclerosis, breast
    specified type NEC N60.8-●
  metaphyseal Q78.5
  muscle Q79.8
  oculodentodigital Q87.0
  periapical (cemental) (cemento-osseous) —*see* Cyst, calcifying odontogenic
  periosteum —*see* Disorder, bone, specified type NEC
  polyostotic fibrous Q78.1
  prostate —*see also* Neoplasia, intraepithelial, prostate N42.30
    severe D07.5
    specified NEC N42.39
  renal Q61.4
    multicystic Q61.4
  retinal, congenital Q14.1
  right ventricular, arrhythmogenic I42.8
  septo-optic Q04.4
  skin L98.8
  spinal cord Q06.1
  spondyloepiphyseal Q77.7
  thymic, with immunodeficiency D82.1
  vagina N89.3
    mild N89.0
    moderate N89.1
    severe NEC D07.2
  vulva N90.3
    mild N90.0
    moderate N90.1
    severe NEC D07.1
Dyspnea (nocturnal) (paroxysmal) R06.00
  asthmatic (bronchial) J45.909
    with
      bronchitis J45.909
        with
          exacerbation (acute) J45.901
          status asthmaticus J45.902
        chronic J44.9
      exacerbation (acute) J45.901
      status asthmaticus J45.902
    cardiac —*see* Failure, ventricular, left
  cardiac —*see* Failure, ventricular, left
  functional F45.8
  hyperventilation R06.4
  hysterical F45.8
  newborn P28.89
  psychogenic F45.8
  shortness of breath R06.02
  specified type NEC R06.09
Dyspraxia R27.8
  developmental (syndrome) F82
Dysproteinemia E88.09
Dysreflexia, autonomic G90.4

Dysrhythmia
  cardiac I49.9
    newborn
      bradycardia P29.12
        occurring before birth P03.819
          before onset of labor P03.810
          during labor P03.811
      tachycardia P29.11
    postoperative I97.89
  cerebral or cortical —*see* Epilepsy
Dyssomnia —*see* Disorder, sleep
Dyssynergia
  biliary K83.8
  bladder sphincter N36.44
  cerebellaris myoclonica (Hunt's ataxia) G11.1
Dysthymia F34.1
Dysthyroidism E07.9
Dystocia O66.9
  affecting newborn P03.1
  cervical (hypotonic) O62.2
    affecting newborn P03.6
    primary O62.0
    secondary O62.1
  contraction ring O62.4
  fetal O66.9
    abnormality NEC O66.3
    conjoined twins O66.3
    oversize O66.2
  maternal O66.9
  positional O64.9
  shoulder (girdle) O66.0
    causing obstructed labor O66.0
  uterine NEC O62.4
Dystonia G24.9
  deformans progressiva G24.1
  drug induced NEC G24.09
    acute G24.02
    specified NEC G24.09
  familial G24.1
  idiopathic G24.1
    familial G24.1
    nonfamilial G24.2
    orofacial G24.4
  lenticularis G24.8
  musculorum deformans G24.1
  neuroleptic induced (acute) G24.02
  orofacial (idiopathic) G24.4
  oromandibular G24.4
    due to drug G24.01
  specified NEC G24.8
  torsion (familial) (idiopathic) G24.1
    acquired G24.8
    genetic G24.1
  symptomatic (nonfamilial) G24.2
Dystonic movements R25.8
Dystrophy, dystrophia
  adiposogenital E23.6
  Becker's type G71.0
  cervical sympathetic G90.2
  choroid (hereditary) H31.20
    central areolar H31.22
    choroideremia H31.21
    gyrate atrophy H31.23
    specified type NEC H31.29
  cornea (hereditary) H18.50
    endothelial H18.51
    epithelial H18.52
    granular H18.53

Dystrophy, dystrophia *(Continued)*
  cornea *(Continued)*
    lattice H18.54
    macular H18.55
    specified type NEC H18.59
  Duchenne's type G71.0
  due to malnutrition E45
  Erb's G71.0
  Fuchs' H18.51
  Gower's muscular G71.0
  hair L67.8
  infantile neuraxonal G31.89
  Landouzy-Déjérine G71.0
  Leyden-Möbius G71.0
  muscular G71.0
    benign (Becker type) G71.0
    congenital (hereditary) (progressive) (with specific morphological abnormalities of the muscle fiber) G71.0
      myotonic G71.11
    distal G71.0
    Duchenne type G71.0
    Emery-Dreifuss G71.0
    Erb type G71.0
    facioscapulohumeral G71.0
    Gower's G71.0
    hereditary (progressive) G71.0
    Landouzy-Déjérine type G71.0
    limb-girdle G71.0
    myotonic G71.11
    progressive (hereditary) G71.0
      Charcot-Marie (-Tooth) type G60.0
    pseudohypertrophic (infantile) G71.0
    severe (Duchenne type) G71.0
  myocardium, myocardial —*see* Degeneration, myocardial
  nail L60.3
    congenital Q84.6
  nutritional E45
  ocular G71.0
  oculocerebrorenal E72.03
  oculopharyngeal G71.0
  ovarian N83.8
  polyglandular E31.8
  reflex (neuromuscular) (sympathetic) — *see* Syndrome, pain, complex regional I
  retinal (hereditary) H35.50
    in
      lipid storage disorders E75.6 *[H36]*
      systemic lipidoses E75.6 *[H36]*
    involving
      pigment epithelium H35.54
      sensory area H35.53
    pigmentary H35.52
    vitreoretinal H35.51
  Salzmann's nodular —*see* Degeneration, cornea, nodular
  scapuloperoneal G71.0
  skin NEC L98.8
  sympathetic (reflex) —*see* Syndrome, pain, complex regional I
    cervical G90.2
  tapetoretinal H35.54
  thoracic, asphyxiating Q77.2
  unguium L60.3
    congenital Q84.6
  vitreoretinal H35.51
  vulva N90.4
  yellow (liver) —*see* Failure, hepatic
Dysuria R30.0
  psychogenic F45.8

E

Eales' disease H35.06-•
Ear —*see also* condition
  piercing Z41.3
  tropical NEC B36.9 *[H62.40]*
    in
      aspergillosis B44.89
      candidiasis B37.84
      moniliasis B37.84
  wax (impacted) H61.20
    left H61.22
      with right H61.23
    right H61.21
      with left H61.23
Earache —*see* subcategory H92.0
Early satiety R68.81
Eaton-Lambert syndrome—*see* Syndrome,
  Lambert-Eaton
Eberth's disease (typhoid fever) A01.00
Ebola virus disease A98.4
Ebstein's anomaly or syndrome (heart) Q22.5
Eccentro-osteochondrodysplasia E76.29
Ecchondroma —*see* Neoplasm, bone, benign
Ecchondrosis D48.0
Ecchymosis R58
  conjunctiva —*see* Hemorrhage, conjunctiva
  eye (traumatic) —*see* Contusion, eyeball
  eyelid (traumatic) —*see* Contusion, eyelid
  newborn P54.5
  spontaneous R23.3
  traumatic —*see* Contusion
Echinococciasis —*see* Echinococcus
Echinococcosis —*see* Echinococcus
Echinococcus (infection) B67.90
  granulosus B67.4
    bone B67.2
    liver B67.0
    lung B67.1
    multiple sites B67.32
    specified site NEC B67.39
    thyroid B67.31
  liver NOS B67.8
    granulosus B67.0
    multilocularis B67.5
  lung NEC B67.99
    granulosus B67.1
    multilocularis B67.69
  multilocularis B67.7
    liver B67.5
    multiple sites B67.61
    specified site NEC B67.69
  specified site NEC B67.99
    granulosus B67.39
    multilocularis B67.69
  thyroid NEC B67.99
    granulosus B67.31
    multilocularis B67.69 *[E35]*
Echinorhynchiasis B83.8
Echinostomiasis B66.8
Echolalia R48.8
Echovirus, as cause of disease classified
  elsewhere B97.12
Eclampsia, eclamptic (coma) (convulsions)
  (delirium) (with hypertension) NEC O15.9
  complicating
    labor and delivery O15.1
    postpartum O15.2
    pregnancy O15.0-•
    puerperium O15.2
Economic circumstances affecting care Z59.9
Economo's disease A85.8
Ectasia, ectasis
  annuloaortic I35.8
  aorta I77.819
    with aneurysm —*see* Aneurysm, aorta
    abdominal I77.811
    thoracic I77.810
    thoracoabdominal I77.812
  breast —*see* Ectasia, mammary duct

Ectasia, ectasis *(Continued)*
  capillary I78.8
  cornea H18.71-•
  gastric antral vascular (GAVE) K31.819
    with hemorrhage K31.811
    without hemorrhage K31.819
  mammary duct N60.4-•
  salivary gland (duct) K11.8
  sclera —*see* Sclerectasia
Ecthyma L08.0
  contagiosum B08.02
  gangrenosum L08.0
  infectiosum B08.02
Ectocardia Q24.8
Ectodermal dysplasia (anhidrotic) Q82.4
Ectodermosis erosiva pluriorificialis
  L51.1
Ectopic, ectopia (congenital)
  abdominal viscera Q45.8
    due to defect in anterior abdominal wall
      Q79.59
  ACTH syndrome E24.3
  adrenal gland Q89.1
  anus Q43.5
  atrial beats I49.1
  beats I49.49
    atrial I49.1
    ventricular I49.3
  bladder Q64.10
  bone and cartilage in lung Q33.5
  brain Q04.8
  breast tissue Q83.8
  cardiac Q24.8
  cerebral Q04.8
  cordis Q24.8
  endometrium —*see* Endometriosis
  gastric mucosa Q40.2
  gestation —*see* Pregnancy, by site
  heart Q24.8
  hormone secretion NEC E34.2
  kidney (crossed) (pelvis) Q63.2
  lens, lentis Q12.1
  mole —*see* Pregnancy, by site
  organ or site NEC —*see* Malposition,
    congenital
  pancreas Q45.3
  pregnancy —*see* Pregnancy, ectopic
  pupil —*see* Abnormality, pupillary
  renal Q63.2
  sebaceous glands of mouth Q38.6
  spleen Q89.09
  testis Q53.00
    bilateral Q53.02
    unilateral Q53.01
  thyroid Q89.2
  tissue in lung Q33.5
  ureter Q62.63
  ventricular beats I49.3
  vesicae Q64.10
Ectromelia Q73.8
  lower limb —*see* Defect, reduction, limb,
    lower, specified type NEC
  upper limb —*see* Defect, reduction, limb,
    upper, specified type NEC
Ectropion H02.109
  cervix N86
    with cervicitis N72
  congenital Q10.1
  eyelid (paralytic) H02.109
    cicatricial H02.119
      left H02.116
        lower H02.115
        upper H02.114
      right H02.113
        lower H02.112
        upper H02.111
    congenital Q10.1
    left H02.106
      lower H02.105
      upper H02.104

Ectropion *(Continued)*
  eyelid *(Continued)*
    mechanical H02.129
      left H02.126
        lower H02.125
        upper H02.124
      right H02.123
        lower H02.122
        upper H02.121
    right H02.103
      lower H02.102
      upper H02.101
    senile H02.139
      left H02.136
        lower H02.135
        upper H02.134
      right H02.133
        lower H02.132
        upper H02.131
    spastic H02.149
      left H02.146
        lower H02.145
        upper H02.144
      right H02.143
        lower H02.142
        upper H02.141
  iris H21.89
  lip (acquired) K13.0
    congenital Q38.0
  urethra N36.8
  uvea H21.89
Eczema (acute) (chronic) (erythematous)
  (fissum) (rubrum) (squamous) (*see also*
  Dermatitis) L30.9
  contact —*see* Dermatitis, contact
  dyshydrotic L30.1
  external ear —*see* Otitis, externa, acute,
    eczematoid
  flexural L20.82
  herpeticum B00.0
  hypertrophicum L28.0
  hypostatic —*see* Varix, leg, with,
    inflammation
  impetiginous L01.1
  infantile (due to any substance) L20.83
    intertriginous L21.1
    seborrheic L21.1
  intertriginous NEC L30.4
    infantile L21.1
  intrinsic (allergic) L20.84
  lichenified NEC L28.0
  marginatum (hebrae) B35.6
  pustular L30.3
  stasis I87.2
    with varicose veins —*see* Varix, leg, with,
      inflammation
  vaccination, vaccinatum T88.1
  varicose —*see* Varix, leg, with, inflammation
Eczematid L30.2
Eddowes (-Spurway) syndrome Q78.0
Edema, edematous (infectious) (pitting)
  (toxic) R60.9
  with nephritis —*see* Nephrosis
  allergic T78.3
  amputation stump (surgical) (sequelae
    (late effect)) T87.89
  angioneurotic (allergic) (any site) (with
    urticaria) T78.3
    hereditary D84.1
  angiospastic I73.9
  Berlin's (traumatic) S05.8X-•
  brain (cytotoxic) (vasogenic) G93.6
    due to birth injury P11.0
    newborn (anoxia or hypoxia) P52.4
      birth injury P11.0
    traumatic —*see* Injury, intracranial,
      cerebral edema
  cardiac —*see* Failure, heart, congestive
  cardiovascular —*see* Failure, heart, congestive
  cerebral —*see* Edema, brain

Edema, edematous *(Continued)*
 cerebrospinal —*see* Edema, brain
 cervix (uteri) (acute) N88.8
  puerperal, postpartum O90.89
 chronic hereditary Q82.0
 circumscribed, acute T78.3
  hereditary D84.1
 conjunctiva H11.42-●
 cornea H18.2-●
  idiopathic H18.22-●
  secondary H18.23-●
   due to contact lens H18.21-●
 due to
  lymphatic obstruction I89.0
  salt retention E87.0
 epiglottis —*see* Edema, glottis
 essential, acute T78.3
  hereditary D84.1
 extremities, lower —*see* Edema, legs
 eyelid NEC H02.849
  left H02.846
   lower H02.845
   upper H02.844
  right H02.843
   lower H02.842
   upper H02.841
 familial, hereditary Q82.0
 famine —*see* Malnutrition, severe
 generalized R60.1
 glottis, glottic, glottidis (obstructive) (passive)
  J38.4
  allergic T78.3
   hereditary D84.1
 heart —*see* Failure, heart, congestive
 heat T67.7
 hereditary Q82.0
 inanition —*see* Malnutrition, severe
 intracranial G93.6
 iris H21.89
 joint —*see* Effusion, joint
 larynx —*see* Edema, glottis
 legs R60.0
  due to venous obstruction I87.1
  hereditary Q82.0
 localized R60.0
  due to venous obstruction I87.1
 lower limbs —*see* Edema, legs
 lung J81.1
  with heart condition or failure —*see*
   Failure, ventricular, left
  acute J81.0
  chemical (acute) J68.1
   chronic J68.1
  chronic J81.1
   due to
    chemicals, gases, fumes or vapors
     (inhalation) J68.1
    external agent J70.9
     specified NEC J70.8
    radiation J70.1
  due to
   chemicals, fumes or vapors (inhalation)
    J68.1
   external agent J70.9
    specified NEC J70.8
   high altitude T70.29
   near drowning T75.1
   radiation J70.0
  meaning failure, left ventricle
   I50.1
 lymphatic I89.0
  due to mastectomy I97.2
 macula H35.81
  cystoid, following cataract surgery —*see*
   Complications, postprocedural,
   following cataract surgery
  diabetic —*see* Diabetes, by type,
   with, retinopathy, with macular
   edema
 malignant —*see* Gangrene, gas
 Milroy's Q82.0

Edema, edematous *(Continued)*
 nasopharynx J39.2
 newborn P83.30
  hydrops fetalis —*see* Hydrops, fetalis
  specified NEC P83.39
 nutritional —*see also* Malnutrition, severe
  with dyspigmentation, skin and hair E40
 optic disc or nerve —*see* Papilledema
 orbit H05.22-●
 pancreas K86.89
 papilla, optic —*see* Papilledema
 penis N48.89
 periodic T78.3
  hereditary D84.1
 pharynx J39.2
 pulmonary —*see* Edema, lung
 Quincke's T78.3
  hereditary D84.1
 renal —*see* Nephrosis
 retina H35.81
  diabetic —*see* Diabetes, by type, with,
   retinopathy, with macular edema
 salt E87.0
 scrotum N50.89
 seminal vesicle N50.89
 spermatic cord N50.89
 spinal (cord) (vascular) (nontraumatic) G95.19
 starvation —*see* Malnutrition, severe
 stasis —*see* Hypertension, venous, (chronic)
 subglottic —*see* Edema, glottis
 supraglottic —*see* Edema, glottis
 testis N44.8
 tunica vaginalis N50.89
 vas deferens N50.89
 vulva (acute) N90.89
Edentulism —*see* Absence, teeth, acquired
Edsall's disease T67.2
Educational handicap Z55.9
 specified NEC Z55.8
Edward's syndrome —*see* Trisomy, 18
Effect, adverse
 abnormal gravitational (G) forces or states
  T75.81
 abuse —*see* Maltreatment
 air pressure T70.9
  specified NEC T70.8
 altitude (high) —*see* Effect, adverse, high
  altitude
 anesthesia —*see also* Anesthesia T88.59
  in labor and delivery O74.9
  local, toxic
   in labor and delivery O74.4-●
   in pregnancy NEC O29.3-●
   postpartum, puerperal O89.3
  postpartum, puerperal O89.9
  specified NEC T88.59
   in labor and delivery O74.8
   postpartum, puerperal O89.8
  spinal and epidural T88.59
   headache T88.59
    in labor and delivery O74.5
    postpartum, puerperal O89.4
   specified NEC
    in labor and delivery O74.6
    postpartum, puerperal O89.5
 antitoxin —*see* Complications, vaccination
 atmospheric pressure T70.9
  due to explosion T70.8
  high T70.3
  low —*see* Effect, adverse, high altitude
  specified effect NEC T70.8
 biological, correct substance properly
  administered —*see* Effect, adverse, drug
 blood (derivatives) (serum) (transfusion) —
  see Complications, transfusion
 chemical substance —*see* Table of Drugs and
  Chemicals
 cold (temperature) (weather) T69.9
  chilblains T69.1
  frostbite —*see* Frostbite
  specified effect NEC T69.8

Effect, adverse *(Continued)*
 drugs and medicaments T88.7
  specified drug —*see* Table of Drugs and
   Chemicals, by drug, adverse effect
  specified effect — code to condition
 electric current, electricity (shock) T75.4
  burn —*see* Burn
 exertion (excessive) T73.3
 exposure —*see* Exposure
 external cause NEC T75.89
 foodstuffs T78.1
  allergic reaction —*see* Allergy, food
   causing anaphylaxis —*see* Shock,
    anaphylactic, due to food
  noxious —*see* Poisoning, food, noxious
 gases, fumes, or vapors T59.9-●
  specified agent —*see* Table of Drugs and
   Chemicals
 glue (airplane) sniffing
  due to drug abuse —*see* Abuse, drug,
   inhalant
  due to drug dependence —*see* Dependence,
   drug, inhalant
 heat —*see* Heat
 high altitude NEC T70.29
  anoxia T70.29
  on
   ears T70.0
   sinuses T70.1
  polycythemia D75.1
 high pressure fluids T70.4
 hot weather —*see* Heat
 hunger T73.0
 immersion, foot —*see* Immersion
 immunization —*see* Complications,
  vaccination
 immunological agents —*see* Complications,
  vaccination
 infrared (radiation) (rays) NOS T66
  dermatitis or eczema L59.8
 infusion —*see* Complications, infusion
 lack of care of infants —*see* Maltreatment,
  child
 lightning —*see* Lightning
 medical care T88.9
  specified NEC T88.8
 medicinal substance, correct, properly
  administered —*see* Effect, adverse, drug
 motion T75.3
 noise, on inner ear —*see* subcategory H83.3
 overheated places —*see* Heat
 psychosocial, of work environment Z56.5
 radiation (diagnostic) (infrared) (natural
  source) (therapeutic) (ultraviolet) (X-ray)
  NOS T66
  dermatitis or eczema —*see* Dermatitis, due
   to, radiation
  fibrosis of lung J70.1
  pneumonitis J70.0
  pulmonary manifestations
   acute J70.0
   chronic J70.1
  skin L59.9
 radioactive substance NOS
  dermatitis or eczema —*see* Radiodermatitis
 reduced temperature T69.9
  immersion foot or hand —*see* Immersion
  specified effect NEC T69.8
 serum NEC (*see also* Reaction, serum) T80.69
 specified NEC T78.8
  external cause NEC T75.89
 strangulation —*see* Asphyxia, traumatic
 submersion T75.1
 thirst T73.1
 toxic —*see* Toxicity
 transfusion —*see* Complications, transfusion
 ultraviolet (radiation) (rays) NOS T66
  burn —*see* Burn
  dermatitis or eczema —*see* Dermatitis, due
   to, ultraviolet rays
   acute L56.8

▶ New   ⇒ Revised   ~~deleted~~ Deleted   ● Use Additional Character(s)

Effect, adverse (Continued)
  vaccine (any) —see Complications, vaccination
  vibration —see Vibration, adverse effects
  water pressure NEC T70.9
    specified NEC T70.8
  weightlessness T75.82
  whole blood —see Complications, transfusion
  work environment Z56.5
Effect(s) (of) (from) —see Effect, adverse NEC
Effects, late —see Sequelae
Effluvium
  anagen L65.1
  telogen L65.0
Effort syndrome (psychogenic) F45.8
Effusion
  amniotic fluid —see Pregnancy, complicated
    by, prematue rupture of membranes
  brain (serous) G93.6
  bronchial —see Bronchitis
  cerebral G93.6
  cerebrospinal —see also Meningitis
    vessel G93.6
  chest —see Effusion, pleura
  chylous, chyliform (pleura) J94.0
  intracranial G93.6
  joint M25.40
    ankle M25.47-●
    elbow M25.42-●
    foot joint M25.47-●
    hand joint M25.44-●
    hip M25.45-●
    knee M25.46-●
    shoulder M25.41-●
    specified joint NEC M25.48
    wrist M25.43-●
  malignant pleural J91.0
  meninges —see Meningitis
  pericardium, pericardial (noninflammatory)
    I31.3
    acute —see Pericarditis, acute
  peritoneal (chronic) R18.8
  pleura, pleurisy, pleuritic, pleuropericardial
    J90
    chylous, chyliform J94.0
    due to systemic lupus erythematosis
      M32.13
  ▶ in conditions classified elsewhere J91.8
    influenzal —see Influenza, with, respiratory
      manifestations NEC
    malignant J91.0
    newborn P28.89
    tuberculous NEC A15.6
      primary (progressive) A15.7
  spinal —see Meningitis
  thorax, thoracic —see Effusion, pleura
Egg shell nails L60.3
  congenital Q84.6
Egyptian splenomegaly B65.1
Ehlers-Danlos syndrome Q79.6
Ehrlichiosis A77.40
  due to
    E. chafeensis A77.41
    E. sennetsu A79.81
    specified organism NEC A77.49
Eichstedt's disease B36.0
Eisenmenger's
  ⟹ complex or syndrome I27.83
  defect Q21.8
Ejaculation
  delayed F52.32
  painful N53.12
  premature F52.4
  retarded N53.11
  retrograde N53.14
  semen, painful N53.12
    psychogenic F52.6
Ekbom's syndrome (restless legs) G25.81
Ekman's syndrome (brittle bones and blue
  sclera) Q78.0
Elastic skin Q82.8
  acquired L57.4

Elastofibroma —see Neoplasm, connective
  tissue, benign
Elastoma (juvenile) Q82.8
  Miescher's L87.2
Elastomyofibrosis I42.4
Elastosis
  actinic, solar L57.8
  atrophicans (senile) L57.4
  perforans serpiginosa L87.2
  senilis L57.4
Elbow —see condition
Electric current, electricity, effects (concussion)
    (fatal) (nonfatal) (shock) T75.4
  burn —see Burn
Electric feet syndrome E53.8
Electrocution T75.4
  from electroshock gun (taser) T75.4
Electrolyte imbalance E87.8
  with
    abortion —see Abortion by type,
      complicated by, electrolyte imbalance
    ectopic pregnancy O08.5
    molar pregnancy O08.5
Elephantiasis (nonfilarial) I89.0
  arabicum —see Infestation, filarial
  bancroftian B74.0
  congenital (any site) (hereditary) Q82.0
  due to
    Brugia (malayi) B74.1
      timori B74.2
    mastectomy I97.2
    Wuchereria (bancrofti) B74.0
  eyelid H02.859
    left H02.856
      lower H02.855
      upper H02.854
    right H02.853
      lower H02.852
      upper H02.851
  filarial, filariensis —see Infestation, filarial
  glandular I89.0
  graecorum A30.9
  lymphangiectatic I89.0
  lymphatic vessel I89.0
    due to mastectomy I97.2
  scrotum (nonfilarial) I89.0
  streptococcal I89.0
  surgical I97.89
    postmastectomy I97.2
  telangiectodes I89.0
  vulva (nonfilarial) N90.89
Elevated, elevation
  antibody titer R76.0
  basal metabolic rate R94.8
  blood pressure —see also Hypertension
    reading (incidental) (isolated) (nonspecific),
      no diagnosis of hypertension R03.0
  blood sugar R73.9
  body temperature (of unknown origin) R50.9
  C-reactive protein (CRP) R79.82
  cancer antigen 125 [CA 125] R97.1
  carcinoembryonic antigen [CEA] R97.0
  cholesterol E78.00
    with high triglycerides E78.2
  conjugate, eye H51.0
  diaphragm, congenital Q79.1
  erythrocyte sedimentation rate R70.0
  fasting glucose R73.01
  fasting triglycerides E78.1
  finding on laboratory examination —see
    Findings, abnormal, inconclusive,
      without diagnosis, by type of exam
  GFR (glomerular filtration rate) —see
    Findings, abnormal, inconclusive,
      without diagnosis, by type of exam
  glucose tolerance (oral) R73.02
  immunoglobulin level R76.8
  indoleacetic acid R82.5
  lactic acid dehydrogenase (LDH) level R74.0
  leukocytes D72.829
  lipoprotein a level E78.8

Elevated, elevation (Continued)
  liver function
    study R94.5
    test R79.89
      alkaline phosphatase R74.8
      aminotransferase R74.0
      bilirubin R17
      hepatic enzyme R74.8
      lactate dehydrogenase R74.0
  lymphocytes D72.820
  prostate specific antigen [PSA] R97.20
  Rh titer —see Complication(s), transfusion,
    incompatibility reaction, Rh (factor)
  scapula, congenital Q74.0
  sedimentation rate R70.0
  SGOT R74.0
  SGPT R74.0
  transaminase level R74.0
  triglycerides E78.1
    with high cholesterol E78.2
  tumor associated antigens [TAA] NEC R97.8
  tumor specific antigens [TSA] NEC R97.8
  urine level of
    17-ketosteroids R82.5
    catecholamine R82.5
    indoleacetic acid R82.5
    steroids R82.5
    vanillylmandelic acid (VMA) R82.5
  venous pressure I87.8
  white blood cell count D72.829
    specified NEC D72.828
Elliptocytosis (congenital) (hereditary) D58.1
  Hb C (disease) D58.1
  hemoglobin disease D58.1
  sickle-cell (disease) D57.8-●
    trait D57.3
Ellison-Zollinger syndrome E16.4
Ellis-van Creveld syndrome
  (chondroectodermal dysplasia) Q77.6
Elongated, elongation (congenital) —see also
    Distortion
  bone Q79.9
  cervix (uteri) Q51.828
    acquired N88.4
    hypertrophic N88.4
  colon Q43.8
  common bile duct Q44.5
  cystic duct Q44.5
  frenulum, penis Q55.69
  labia minora (acquired) N90.69
  ligamentum patellae Q74.1
  petiolus (epiglottidis) Q31.8
  tooth, teeth K00.2
  uvula Q38.6
Eltor cholera A00.1
Emaciation (due to malnutrition) E41
Embadomoniasis A07.8
Embedded tooth, teeth K01.0
  root only K08.3
Embolic —see condition
Embolism (multiple) (paradoxical) I74.9
  air (any site) (traumatic) T79.0
    following
      abortion —see Abortion by type
        complicated by embolism
      ectopic pregnancy O08.2
      infusion, therapeutic injection or
        transfusion T80.0
      molar pregnancy O08.2
      procedure NEC
        artery T81.719
          mesenteric T81.710
          renal T81.711
          specified NEC T81.718
        vein T81.72
    in pregnancy, childbirth or puerperium —
      see Embolism, obstetric
  amniotic fluid (pulmonary) —see also
    Embolism, obstetric
    following
      abortion —see Abortion by type
        complicated by embolism

Embolism *(Continued)*
  amniotic fluid *(Continued)*
    following *(Continued)*
      ectopic pregnancy O08.2
      molar pregnancy O08.2
  aorta, aortic I74.10
    abdominal I74.09
      saddle I74.01
    bifurcation I74.09
    saddle I74.01
    thoracic I74.11
  artery I74.9
    auditory, internal I65.8
    basilar —*see* Occlusion, artery, basilar
    carotid (common) (internal) —*see*
      Occlusion, artery, carotid
    cerebellar (anterior inferior) (posterior
      inferior) (superior) I66.3
    cerebral —*see* Occlusion, artery, cerebral
    ⇒choroidal (anterior) I65.8
    ⇒communicating posterior I65.8
    coronary —*see also* Infarct, myocardium
      not resulting in infarction I24.0
    extremity I74.4
      lower I74.3
      upper I74.2
    ⇒hypophyseal I65.8
    iliac I74.5
    limb I74.4
      lower I74.3
      upper I74.2
    mesenteric (with gangrene) —*see also*
      Ischemia, intestine, acute K55.09
    ophthalmic —*see* Occlusion, artery, retina
    peripheral I74.4
    ⇒pontine I65.8
    precerebral —*see* Occlusion, artery,
      precerebral
    pulmonary —*see* Embolism, pulmonary
    renal N28.0
    retinal —*see* Occlusion, artery, retina
    septic I76
    specified NEC I74.8
    vertebral —*see* Occlusion, artery, vertebral
  basilar (artery) I65.1
  blood clot
    following
      abortion —*see* Abortion by type
        complicated by embolism
      ectopic or molar pregnancy O08.2
    in pregnancy, childbirth or puerperium —
      see Embolism, obstetric
  brain —*see also* Occlusion, artery, cerebral
    following
      abortion —*see* Abortion by type
        complicated by embolism
      ectopic or molar pregnancy O08.2
    puerperal, postpartum, childbirth —*see*
      Embolism, obstetric
  capillary I78.8
  cardiac —*see also* Infarct, myocardium
    not resulting in infarction I51.3
  carotid (artery) (common) (internal) —*see*
    Occlusion, artery, carotid
  cavernous sinus (venous) —*see* Embolism,
    intracranial venous sinus
  cerebral —*see* Occlusion, artery, cerebral
  cholesterol —*see* Atheroembolism
  coronary (artery or vein) (systemic) —*see*
    Occlusion, coronary
  due to device, implant or graft —*see also*
    Complications, by site and type,
    specified NEC
    arterial graft NEC T82.818
    breast (implant) T85.818
    catheter NEC T85.818
      dialysis (renal) T82.818
        intraperitoneal T85.818
      infusion NEC T82.818
        spinal (epidural) (subdural) T85.810
      urinary (indwelling) T83.81

Embolism *(Continued)*
  due to device, implant or graft *(Continued)*
    electronic (electrode) (pulse generator)
      (stimulator)
      bone T84.81
      cardiac T82.817
      nervous system (brain) (peripheral
        nerve) (spinal) T85.810
      urinary T83.81
    fixation, internal (orthopedic) NEC T84.81
    gastrointestinal (bile duct) (esophagus)
      T85.818
    genital NEC T83.81
    heart (graft) (valve) T82.817
    joint prosthesis T84.81
    ocular (corneal graft) (orbital implant)
      T85.818
    orthopedic (bone graft) NEC T86.838
    specified NEC T85.818
    urinary (graft) NEC T83.81
    vascular NEC T82.818
    ventricular intracranial shunt T85.810
  extremities
    lower —*see* Embolism, vein, lower
      extremity
    arterial I74.3
    upper I74.2
  eye H34.9
  fat (cerebral) (pulmonary) (systemic) T79.1
    complicating delivery —*see* Embolism,
      obstetric
    following
      abortion —*see* Abortion by type
        complicated by embolism
      ectopic or molar pregnancy O08.2
  following
    abortion —*see* Abortion by type
      complicated by embolism
    ectopic or molar pregnancy O08.2
    infusion, therapeutic injection or
      transfusion
      air T80.0
  heart (fatty) —*see also* Infarct, myocardium
    not resulting in infarction I51.3
  hepatic (vein) I82.0
  in pregnancy, childbirth or puerperium —*see*
    Embolism, obstetric
  intestine (artery) (vein) (with gangrene) —*see
    also* Ischemia, intestine, acute K55.039
  intracranial —*see also* Occlusion, artery,
    cerebral
    venous sinus (any) G08
      nonpyogenic I67.6
  intraspinal venous sinuses or veins G08
    nonpyogenic G95.19
  kidney (artery) N28.0
  lateral sinus (venous) —*see* Embolism,
    intracranial, venous sinus
  leg —*see* Embolism, vein, lower extremity
    arterial I74.3
  longitudinal sinus (venous) —*see* Embolism,
    intracranial, venous sinus
  lung (massive) —*see* Embolism, pulmonary
  meninges I66.8
  mesenteric (artery) (vein) (with gangrene) —
    see also Ischemia, intestine, acute
    K55.059
  obstetric (in) (pulmonary)
    childbirth O88.22
      air O88.02
      amniotic fluid O88.12
      blood clot O88.22
      fat O88.82
      pyemic O88.32
      septic O88.32
      specified type NEC O88.82
    pregnancy O88.21-●
      air O88.01-●
      amniotic fluid O88.11-●
      blood clot O88.21-●
      fat O88.81-●

Embolism *(Continued)*
  obstetric *(Continued)*
    pregnancy *(Continued)*
      pyemic O88.31-●
      septic O88.31-●
      specified type NEC O88.81-●
    puerperal O88.23
      air O88.03
      amniotic fluid O88.13
      blood clot O88.23
      fat O88.83
      pyemic O88.33
      septic O88.33
      specified type NEC O88.83
  ophthalmic —*see* Occlusion, artery, retina
  penis N48.81
  peripheral artery NOS I74.4
  pituitary E23.6
  popliteal (artery) I74.3
  portal (vein) I81
  postoperative, postprocedural
    artery T81.719
      mesenteric T81.710
      renal T81.711
      specified NEC T81.718
    vein T81.72
  precerebral artery —*see* Occlusion, artery,
    precerebral
  puerperal —*see* Embolism, obstetric
  pulmonary (acute) (artery) (vein) I26.99
    with acute cor pulmonale I26.09
      chronic I27.82
    following
      abortion —*see* Abortion by type
        complicated by embolism
      ectopic or molar pregnancy O08.2
    healed or old Z86.711
    in pregnancy, childbirth or puerperium —
      see Embolism, obstetric
    personal history of Z86.711
    saddle I26.92
      with acute cor pulmonale I26.02
    septic I26.90
      with acute cor pulmonale I26.01
  pyemic (multiple) I76
    following
      abortion —*see* Abortion by type
        complicated by embolism
      ectopic or molar pregnancy O08.2
    Hemophilus influenzae A41.3
    pneumococcal A40.3
      with pneumonia J13
    puerperal, postpartum, childbirth (any
      organism) —*see* Embolism, obstetric
    specified organism NEC A41.89
    staphylococcal A41.2
    streptococcal A40.9
  renal (artery) N28.0
    vein I82.3
  retina, retinal —*see* Occlusion, artery,
    retina
  saddle
    abdominal aorta I74.01
    pulmonary artery I26.92
      with acute cor pulmonale I26.02
  septic (arterial) I76
    complicating abortion —*see* Abortion, by
      type, complicated by, embolism
  sinus —*see* Embolism, intracranial, venous
    sinus
  soap complicating abortion —*see* Abortion,
    by type, complicated by, embolism
  spinal cord G95.19
    pyogenic origin G06.1
  spleen, splenic (artery) I74.8
  upper extremity I74.2
  vein (acute) I82.90
    antecubital I82.61-●
      chronic I82.71-●
    axillary I82.A1-●
      chronic I82.A2-●

Embolism *(Continued)*
  vein *(Continued)*
    basilic I82.61-●
      chronic I82.71-●
    brachial I82.62-●
      chronic I82.72-●
    brachiocephalic (innominate) I82.290
      chronic I82.291
    cephalic I82.61-●
      chronic I82.71-●
    chronic I82.91
    deep (DVT) I82.40-●
      calf I82.4Z-●
        chronic I82.5Z-●
      lower leg I82.4Z-●
        chronic I82.5Z-●
      thigh I82.4Y-●
        chronic I82.5Y-●
      upper leg I82.4Y
        chronic I82.5y--●
    femoral I82.41-●
      chronic I82.51-●
    iliac (iliofemoral) I82.42-●
      chronic I82.52-●
    innominate I82.290
      chronic I82.291
    internal jugular I82.C1-●
      chronic I82.C2-●
    lower extremity
      deep I82.40-●
        chronic I82.50-●
      specified NEC I82.49-●
        chronic NEC I82.59-●
      distal
        deep I82.4Z-●
      proximal
        deep I82.4Y-●
          chronic I82.5Y-●
      superficial I82.81-●
    popliteal I82.43-●
      chronic I82.53-●
    radial I82.62-●
      chronic I82.72-●
    renal I82.3
    saphenous (greater) (lesser) I82.81-●
    specified NEC I82.890
      chronic NEC I82.891
    subclavian I82.B1-●
      chronic I82.B2-●
    thoracic NEC I82.290
      chronic I82.291
    tibial I82.44-●
      chronic I82.54-●
    ulnar I82.62-●
      chronic I82.72-●
    upper extremity I82.60-●
      chronic I82.70-●
      deep I82.62-●
        chronic I82.72-●
      superficial I82.61-●
        chronic I82.71-●
  vena cava
    inferior (acute) I82.220
      chronic I82.221
    superior (acute) I82.210
      chronic I82.211
  venous sinus G08
  vessels of brain —*see* Occlusion, artery,
    cerebral
Embolus —*see* Embolism
Embryoma —*see also* Neoplasm, uncertain
  behavior, by site
  benign —*see* Neoplasm, benign, by site
  kidney C64.-●
  liver C22.0
  malignant —*see also* Neoplasm, malignant,
    by site
    kidney C64.-●
    liver C22.0
    testis C62.9-●
      descended (scrotal) C62.1-●
      undescended C62.0-●

Embryoma *(Continued)*
  testis C62.9-●
    descended (scrotal) C62.1-●
    undescended C62.0-●
Embryonic
  circulation Q28.9
  heart Q28.9
  vas deferens Q55.4
Embryopathia NOS Q89.9
Embryotoxon Q13.4
Emesis —*see* Vomiting
Emotional lability R45.86
Emotionality, pathological F60.3
Emotogenic disease —*see* Disorder,
  psychogenic
Emphysema (atrophic) (bullous) (chronic)
  (interlobular) (lung) (obstructive)
  (pulmonary) (senile) (vesicular)
  J43.9
  cellular tissue (traumatic) T79.7
    surgical T81.82
  centrilobular J43.2
  compensatory J98.3
  congenital (interstitial) P25.0
  conjunctiva H11.89
  connective tissue (traumatic) T79.7
    surgical T81.82
  due to chemicals, gases, fumes or vapors
    J68.4
  eyelid(s) —*see* Disorder, eyelid, specified type
    NEC
    surgical T81.82
    traumatic T79.7
  interstitial J98.2
    congenital P25.0
    perinatal period P25.0
  laminated tissue T79.7
    surgical T81.82
  mediastinal J98.2
    newborn P25.2
  orbit, orbital —*see* Disorder, orbit, specified
    type NEC
  panacinar J43.1
  panlobular J43.1
  specified NEC J43.8
  subcutaneous (traumatic) T79.7
    nontraumatic J98.2
    postprocedural T81.82
    surgical T81.82
  surgical T81.82
  thymus (gland) (congenital) E32.8
  traumatic (subcutaneous) T79.7
  unilateral J43.0
Empty nest syndrome Z60.0
Empyema (acute) (chest) (double) (pleura)
  (supradiaphragmatic) (thorax) J86.9
  with fistula J86.0
  accessory sinus (chronic) —*see* Sinusitis
  antrum (chronic) —*see* Sinusitis, maxillary
  brain (any part) —*see* Abscess, brain
  ethmoidal (chronic) (sinus) —*see* Sinusitis,
    ethmoidal
  extradural —*see* Abscess, extradural
  frontal (chronic) (sinus) —*see* Sinusitis,
    frontal
  gallbladder K81.0
  mastoid (process) (acute) —*see* Mastoiditis,
    acute
  maxilla, maxillary M27.2
    sinus (chronic) —*see* Sinusitis,
      maxillary
  nasal sinus (chronic) —*see* Sinusitis
  sinus (accessory) (chronic) (nasal) —*see*
    Sinusitis
  sphenoidal (sinus) (chronic) —*see* Sinusitis,
    sphenoidal
  subarachnoid —*see* Abscess, extradural
  subdural —*see* Abscess, subdural
  tuberculous A15.6
  ureter —*see* Ureteritis
  ventricular —*see* Abscess, brain

En coup de sabre lesion L94.1
Enamel pearls K00.2
Enameloma K00.2
Enanthema, viral B09
Encephalitis (chronic) (hemorrhagic)
  (idiopathic) (nonepidemic) (spurious)
  (subacute) G04.90
  acute —*see also* Encephalitis, viral A86
    disseminated G04.00
      infectious G04.01
      noninfectious G04.81
      postimmunization (postvaccination)
        G04.02
      postinfectious G04.01
    inclusion body A85.8
    necrotizing hemorrhagic G04.30
      postimmunization G04.32
      postinfectious G04.31
      specified NEC G04.39
  arboviral, arbovirus NEC A85.2
  arthropod-borne NEC (viral) A85.2
  Australian A83.4
  California (virus) A83.5
  Central European (tick-borne) A84.1
  Czechoslovakian A84.1
  Dawson's (inclusion body) A81.1
  diffuse sclerosing A81.1
  disseminated, acute G04.00
  due to
    cat scratch disease A28.1
    human immunodeficiency virus (HIV)
      disease B20 *[G05.3]*
    malaria —*see* Malaria
    rickettsiosis —*see* Rickettsiosis
    smallpox inoculation G04.02
    typhus —*see* Typhus
  Eastern equine A83.2
  endemic (viral) A86
  epidemic NEC (viral) A86
  equine (acute) (infectious) (viral) A83.9
    Eastern A83.2
    Venezuelan A92.2
    Western A83.1
  Far Eastern (tick-borne) A84.0
  following vaccination or other immunization
    procedure G04.02
  herpes zoster B02.0
  herpesviral B00.4
    due to herpesvirus 6 B10.01
    due to herpesvirus 7 B10.09
    specified NEC B10.09
  Ilheus (virus) A83.8
  in (due to)
    actinomycosis A42.82
    adenovirus A85.1
    African trypanosomiasis B56.9 *[G05.3]*
    Chagas' disease (chronic) B57.42
    cytomegalovirus B25.8
    enterovirus A85.0
    herpes (simplex) virus B00.4
      due to herpesvirus 6 B10.01
      due to herpesvirus 7 B10.09
      specified NEC B10.09
    infectious disease NEC B99 *[G05.3]*
    influenza —*see* Influenza, with,
      encephalopathy
    listeriosis A32.12
    measles B05.0
    mumps B26.2
    naegleriasis B60.2
    parasitic disease NEC B89 *[G05.3]*
    poliovirus A80.9 *[G05.3]*
    rubella B06.01
    syphilis
      congenital A50.42
      late A52.14
    systemic lupus erythematosus M32.19
    toxoplasmosis (acquired) B58.2
      congenital P37.1
    tuberculosis A17.82
    zoster B02.0

Encephalitis *(Continued)*
inclusion body A81.1
infectious (acute) (virus) NEC A86
Japanese (B type) A83.0
La Crosse A83.5
lead —*see* Poisoning, lead
lethargica (acute) (infectious) A85.8
louping ill A84.8
lupus erythematosus, systemic M32.19
lymphatica A87.2
Mengo A85.8
meningococcal A39.81
Murray Valley A83.4
otitic NEC H66.40 *[G05.3]*
parasitic NOS B71.9
periaxial G37.0
periaxialis (concentrica) (diffuse) G37.5
postchickenpox B01.11
postexanthematous NEC B09
postimmunization G04.02
postinfectious NEC G04.01
postmeasles B05.0
postvaccinal G04.02
postvaricella B01.11
postviral NEC A86
Powassan A84.8
Rasmussen G04.81
Rio Bravo A85.8
Russian
    autumnal A83.0
    spring-summer (taiga) A84.0
saturnine —*see* Poisoning, lead
specified NEC G04.81
St. Louis A83.3
subacute sclerosing A81.1
summer A83.0
suppurative G04.81
tick-borne A84.9
Torula, torular (cryptococcal) B45.1
toxic NEC G92
trichinosis B75 *[G05.3]*
type
    B A83.0
    C A83.3
van Bogaert's A81.1
Venezuelan equine A92.2
Vienna A85.8
viral, virus A86
    arthropod-borne NEC A85.2
        mosquito-borne A83.9
            Australian X disease A83.4
            California virus A83.5
            Eastern equine A83.2
            Japanese (B type) A83.0
            Murray Valley A83.4
            specified NEC A83.8
            St. Louis A83.3
            type B A83.0
            type C A83.3
            Western equine A83.1
        tick-borne A84.9
            biundulant A84.1
            central European A84.1
            Czechoslovakian A84.1
            diphasic meningoencephalitis A84.1
            Far Eastern A84.0
            Russian spring-summer (taiga)
                A84.0
            specified NEC A84.8
        specified type NEC A85.8
    Western equine A83.1
Encephalocele Q01.9
frontal Q01.0
nasofrontal Q01.1
occipital Q01.2
specified NEC Q01.8
Encephalocystocele —*see* Encephalocele
Encephaloduroarteriomyosynangiosis
    (EDAMS) I67.5
Encephalomalacia (brain) (cerebellar)
    (cerebral) —*see* Softening, brain

Encephalomeningitis —*see*
    Meningoencephalitis
Encephalomeningocele —*see* Encephalocele
Encephalomeningomyelitis —*see*
    Meningoencephalitis
Encephalomyelitis —*see also* Encephalitis
    G04.90
acute disseminated G04.00
    infectious G04.01
    noninfectious G04.81
    postimmunization G04.02
    postinfectious G04.01
acute necrotizing hemorrhagic G04.30
    postimmunization G04.32
    postinfectious G04.31
    specified NEC G04.39
benign myalgic G93.3
equine A83.9
    Eastern A83.2
    Venezuelan A92.2
    Western A83.1
in diseases classified elsewhere G05.3
myalgic, benign G93.3
postchickenpox B01.11
postinfectious NEC G04.01
postmeasles B05.0
postvaccinal G04.02
postvaricella B01.11
rubella B06.01
specified NEC G04.81
Venezuelan equine A92.2
Encephalomyelocele —*see* Encephalocele
Encephalomyelomeningitis —*see*
    Meningoencephalitis
Encephalomyelopathy G96.9
Encephalomyeloradiculitis (acute) G61.0
Encephalomyeloradiculoneuritis (acute)
    (Guillain-Barré) G61.0
Encephalomyeloradiculopathy G96.9
Encephalopathia hyperbilirubinemica,
    newborn P57.9
due to isoimmunization (conditions in P55)
    P57.0
Encephalopathy (acute) G93.40
acute necrotizing hemorrhagic G04.30
    postimmunization G04.32
    postinfectious G04.31
    specified NEC G04.39
alcoholic G31.2
anoxic —*see* Damage, brain, anoxic
arteriosclerotic I67.2
centrolobar progressive (Schilder) G37.0
congenital Q07.9
degenerative, in specified disease NEC
    G32.89
due to
    drugs (*see also* Table of Drugs and
        Chemicals) G92
demyelinating callosal G37.1
hepatic —*see* Failure, hepatic
hyperbilirubinemic, newborn P57.9
    due to isoimmunization (conditions in P55)
        P57.0
hypertensive I67.4
hypoglycemic E16.2
hypoxic —*see* Damage, brain, anoxic
hypoxic ischemic P91.60
    mild P91.61
    moderate P91.62
    severe P91.63
in (due to) (with)
    birth injury P11.1
    hyperinsulinism E16.1 *[G94]*
    influenza —*see* Influenza, with,
        encephalopathy
    lack of vitamin (*see also* Deficiency, vitamin)
        E56.9 *[G32.89]*
    neoplastic disease (*see also* Neoplasm)
        D49.9 *[G13.1]*
    serum (*see also* Reaction, serum) T80.69
    syphilis A52.17

Encephalopathy *(Continued)*
in *(Continued)*
    trauma (postconcussional) F07.81
        current injury —*see* Injury, intracranial
    vaccination G04.02
lead —*see* Poisoning, lead
metabolic G93.41
    drug induced G92
    toxic G92
myoclonic, early, symptomatic —*see* Epilepsy,
    generalized, specified NEC
necrotizing, subacute (Leigh) G31.82
▶neonatal P91.819
    ▶in diseases classified elsewhere P91.811
pellagrous E52 *[G32.89]*
portosystemic —*see* Failure, hepatic
postcontusional F07.81
    current injury —*see* Injury, intracranial,
        diffuse
posthypoglycemic (coma) E16.1 *[G94]*
postradiation G93.89
saturnine —*see* Poisoning, lead
septic G93.41
specified NEC G93.49
spongiform, subacute (viral) A81.09
toxic G92
    metabolic G92
traumatic (postconcussional) F07.81
    current injury —*see* Injury, intracranial
vitamin B deficiency NEC E53.9 *[G32.89]*
    vitamin B1 E51.2
Wernicke's E51.2
Encephalorrhagia —*see* Hemorrhage,
    intracranial, intracerebral
Encephalosis, posttraumatic F07.81
Enchondroma —*see also* Neoplasm, bone,
    benign
Enchondromatosis (cartilaginous) (multiple)
    Q78.4
Encopresis R15.9
functional F98.1
nonorganic origin F98.1
psychogenic F98.1
Encounter (with health service) (for) Z76.89
adjustment and management (of)
    breast implant Z45.81
    implanted device NEC Z45.89
    myringotomy device (stent) (tube) Z45.82
administrative purpose only Z02.9
    examination for
        adoption Z02.82
        armed forces Z02.3
        disability determination Z02.71
        driving license Z02.4
        employment Z02.1
        insurance Z02.6
        medical certificate NEC Z02.79
        paternity testing Z02.81
        residential institution admission Z02.2
        school admission Z02.0
        sports Z02.5
    specified reason NEC Z02.89
aftercare —*see* Aftercare
▶antenatal screening Z36.9
    ▶cervical length Z36.86
    ▶chromosomal anomalies Z36.0
    ▶congenital cardiac abnormalities Z36.83
    ▶elevated maternal serum alphafetoprotein
        level Z36.1
    ▶fetal growth retardation Z36.4
    ▶fetal lung maturity Z36.84
    ▶fetal macrosomia Z36.88
    ▶hydrops fetalis Z36.88
    ▶intrauterine growth restriction (IUGR)/
        small-for-dates Z36.4
    ▶isoimmunization Z36.5
    ▶large-for-dates Z36.88
    ▶malformations Z36.3
    ▶non-visualized anatomy on a previous scan
        Z36.2
    ▶nuchal translucency Z36.82

▶ New   ⇒ Revised   ~~deleted~~ Deleted   ● Use Additional Character(s)

Encounter *(Continued)*
 antenatal screening *(Continued)*
  ▶raised alphafetoprotein level Z36.1
  ▶risk of pre-term labor Z36.86
  ▶specified type NEC Z36.89
  ▶specified follow-up NEC Z36.2
  ▶specified genetic defects NEC Z36.8A
  ▶Streptococcus B Z36.85
  ▶suspected anomaly Z36.3
  ▶uncertain dates Z36.87
 assisted reproductive fertility procedure cycle Z31.83
 blood typing Z01.83
  Rh typing Z01.83
 breast augmentation or reduction Z41.1
 breast implant exchange (different material) (different size) Z45.81
 breast reconstruction following mastectomy Z42.1
 check-up —*see* Examination
 chemotherapy for neoplasm Z51.11
 colonoscopy, screening Z12.11
 counseling —*see* Counseling
 delivery, full-term, uncomplicated O80
  cesarean, without indication O82
 desensitization to allergens Z51.6
 ear piercing Z41.3
 examination —*see* Examination
 expectant parent(s) (adoptive) pre-birth pediatrician visit Z76.81
 fertility preservation procedure (prior to cancer therapy) (prior to removal of gonads) Z31.84
 fitting (of) —*see* Fitting (and adjustment) (of)
 genetic
  ⊯counseling
   ▶nonprocreative Z71.83
   ▶procreative Z31.5
  testing —*see* Test, genetic
 hearing conservation and treatment Z01.12
 immunotherapy for neoplasm Z51.12
 in vitro fertilization cycle Z31.83
 instruction (in)
  child care (postpartal) (prenatal) Z32.3
  childbirth Z32.2
  natural family planning
   procreative Z31.61
   to avoid pregnancy Z30.02
 insulin pump titration Z46.81
 joint prosthesis insertion following prior explantation of joint prosthesis (staged procedure)
  hip Z47.32
  knee Z47.33
  shoulder Z47.31
 laboratory (as part of a general medical examination) Z00.00
  with abnormal findings Z00.01
 mental health services (for)
  abuse NEC
   perpetrator Z69.82
   victim Z69.81
  child abuse
   nonparental
    perpetrator Z69.021
    victim Z69.020
   parental
    perpetrator Z69.011
    victim Z69.010
  ~~spousal or partner abuse~~
   ~~perpetrator Z69.12~~
   ~~victim Z69.11~~
  ▶child neglect
   ▶nonparental
    ▶perpetrator Z69.021
    ▶victim Z69.020
   ▶parental
    ▶perpetrator Z69.011
    ▶victim Z69.010
  ▶child psychological abuse
   ▶nonparental
    ▶perpetrator Z69.021
    ▶victim Z69.020

Encounter *(Continued)*
 mental health services *(Continued)*
  child psychological abuse *(Continued)*
   ▶parental
    ▶perpetrator Z69.011
    ▶victim Z69.010
  ▶child sexual abuse
   ▶nonparental
    ▶perpetrator Z69.021
    ▶victim Z69.020
   ▶parental
    ▶perpetrator Z69.011
    ▶victim Z69.010
  ▶non-spousal adult abuse (perpetrator) (victim) Z69.81
  ▶spousal or partner
   ▶abuse
    ▶perpetrator Z69.12
    ▶victim Z69.11
   ▶neglect
    ▶perpetrator Z69.12
    ▶victim Z69.11
   ▶psychological abuse
    ▶perpetrator Z69.12
    ▶victim Z69.11
   ▶violence
    ▶perpetrator (physical) (sexual) Z69.12
    ▶victim (physical) Z69.11
     ▶sexual Z69.81
 observation (for) (ruled out)
  exposure to (suspected)
   anthrax Z03.810
   biological agent NEC Z03.818
 pediatrician visit, by expectant parent(s) (adoptive) Z76.81
 ▶placental sample (taken vaginally) —*see also* Encounter, antenatal screening Z36.9
 plastic and reconstructive surgery following medical procedure or healed injury NEC Z42.8
 pregnancy
  supervision of —*see* Pregnancy, supervision of
  test Z32.00
   result negative Z32.02
   result positive Z32.01
 procreative management and counseling for gestational carrier Z31.7
 prophylactic measures Z29.9
  antivenin Z29.12
  fluoride administration Z29.3
  immunotherapy for respiratory syncytial virus (RSV) Z29.11
  rabies immune globin Z29.14
  Rho (D) immune globulin Z29.13
  specified NEC Z29.8
 radiation therapy (antineoplastic) Z51.0
 radiological (as part of a general medical examination) Z00.00
  with abnormal findings Z00.01
 reconstructive surgery following medical procedure or healed injury NEC Z42.8
 removal (of) —*see also* Removal
  artificial
   arm Z44.00-●
    complete Z44.01-●
    partial Z44.02-●
   eye Z44.2-●
   leg Z44.10-●
    complete Z44.11-●
    partial Z44.12-●
  breast implant Z45.81
   tissue expander (without synchronous insertion of permanent implant) Z45.81
  device Z46.9
   specified NEC Z46.89
  external
   fixation device — code to fracture with seventh character D

Encounter *(Continued)*
 removal *(Continued)*
  external *(Continued)*
   prosthesis, prosthetic device Z44.9
    breast Z44.3-●
    specified NEC Z44.8
  implanted device NEC Z45.89
  insulin pump Z46.81
  internal fixation device Z47.2
  myringotomy device (stent) (tube) Z45.82
  nervous system device NEC Z46.2
   brain neuropacemaker Z46.2
   visual substitution device Z46.2
    implanted Z45.31
  non-vascular catheter Z46.82
  orthodontic device Z46.4
  stent
   ureteral Z46.6
  urinary device Z46.6
 repeat cervical smear to confirm findings of recent normal smear following initial abnormal smear Z01.42
 respirator [ventilator] use during power failure (Z99.12)
 Rh typing Z01.83
 screening —*see* Screening
 specified NEC Z76.89
 sterilization Z30.2
 suspected condition, ruled out
  amniotic cavity and membrane Z03.71
  cervical shortening Z03.75
  fetal anomaly Z03.73
  fetal growth Z03.74
  maternal and fetal conditions NEC Z03.79
  oligohydramnios Z03.71
  placental problem Z03.72
  polyhydramnios Z03.71
 suspected exposure (to), ruled out
  anthrax Z03.810
  biological agents NEC Z03.818
 termination of pregnancy, elective Z33.2
 testing —*see* Test
 therapeutic drug level monitoring Z51.81
 titration, insulin pump Z46.81
 to determine fetal viability of pregnancy O36.80
 training
  insulin pump Z46.81
 X-ray of chest (as part of a general medical examination Z00.00)
  with abnormal findings Z00.01
Encystment —*see* Cyst
Endarteritis (bacterial, subacute) (infective) I77.6
 brain I67.7
 cerebral or cerebrospinal I67.7
 deformans —*see* Arteriosclerosis
 embolic —*see* Embolism
 obliterans —*see also* Arteriosclerosis
  pulmonary I28.8
 pulmonary I28.8
 retina —*see* Vasculitis, retina
 senile —*see* Arteriosclerosis
 syphilitic A52.09
  brain or cerebral A52.04
  congenital A50.54 *[I79.8]*
 tuberculous A18.89
Endemic —*see* condition
Endocarditis (chronic) (marantic) (nonbacterial) (thrombotic) (valvular) I38
 with rheumatic fever (conditions in I00)
  active —*see* Endocarditis, acute, rheumatic
  inactive or quiescent (with chorea) I09.1
 acute or subacute I33.9
  infective I33.0
  rheumatic (aortic) (mitral) (pulmonary) (tricuspid) I01.1
   with chorea (acute) (rheumatic) (Sydenham's) I02.0

Endocarditis *(Continued)*
　aortic (heart) (nonrheumatic) (valve) I35.8
　　with
　　　mitral disease I08.0
　　　　with tricuspid (valve) disease I08.3
　　　　active or acute I01.1
　　　　　with chorea (acute) (rheumatic)
　　　　　　(Sydenham's) I02.0
　　　　rheumatic fever (conditions in I00)
　　　　　active —*see* Endocarditis, acute,
　　　　　　rheumatic
　　　　　inactive or quiescent (with chorea)
　　　　　　I06.9
　　　　tricuspid (valve) disease I08.2
　　　　　with mitral (valve) disease I08.3
　　acute or subacute I33.9
　　arteriosclerotic I35.8
　　rheumatic I06.9
　　　with mitral disease I08.0
　　　　with tricuspid (valve) disease I08.3
　　　　active or acute I01.1
　　　　　with chorea (acute) (rheumatic)
　　　　　　(Sydenham's) I02.0
　　　active or acute I01.1
　　　　with chorea (acute) (rheumatic)
　　　　　(Sydenham's) I02.0
　　　specified NEC I06.8
　　specified cause NEC I35.8
　　syphilitic A52.03
　arteriosclerotic I38
　atypical verrucous (Libman-Sacks) M32.11
　bacterial (acute) (any valve) (subacute) I33.0
　candidal B37.6
　congenital Q24.8
　constrictive I33.0
　Coxiella burnetii A78 [I39]
　Coxsackie B33.21
　due to
　　prosthetic cardiac valve T82.6
　　Q fever A78 [I39]
　　Serratia marcescens I33.0
　　typhoid (fever) A01.02
　gonococcal A54.83
　infectious or infective (acute) (any valve)
　　(subacute) I33.0
　lenta (acute) (any valve) (subacute) I33.0
　Libman-Sacks M32.11
　listerial A32.82
　Löffler's I42.3
　malignant (acute) (any valve) (subacute) I33.0
　meningococcal A39.51
　mitral (chronic) (double) (fibroid) (heart)
　　(inactive) (valve) (with chorea) I05.9
　　with
　　　aortic (valve) disease I08.0
　　　　with tricuspid (valve) disease I08.3
　　　　active or acute I01.1
　　　　　with chorea (acute) (rheumatic)
　　　　　　(Sydenham's) I02.0
　　　rheumatic fever (conditions in I00)
　　　　active —*see* Endocarditis, acute,
　　　　　rheumatic
　　　　inactive or quiescent (with chorea)
　　　　　I05.9
　　　tricuspid (valve) disease I08.1
　　　　with aortic (valve) disease I08.3
　　active or acute I01.1
　　　with chorea (acute) (rheumatic)
　　　　(Sydenham's) I02.0
　　　bacterial I33.0
　　arteriosclerotic I34.8
　　nonrheumatic I34.8
　　　acute or subacute I33.9
　　specified NEC I05.8
　monilial B37.6
　multiple valves I08.9
　　specified disorders I08.8
　mycotic (acute) (any valve) (subacute) I33.0
　pneumococcal (acute) (any valve) (subacute)
　　I33.0
　pulmonary (chronic) (heart) (valve) I37.8

Endocarditis *(Continued)*
　pulmonary *(Continued)*
　　with rheumatic fever (conditions in I00)
　　　active —*see* Endocarditis, acute,
　　　　rheumatic
　　　inactive or quiescent (with chorea) I09.89
　　　　with aortic, mitral or tricuspid disease
　　　　　I08.8
　　acute or subacute I33.9
　　　rheumatic I01.1
　　　　with chorea (acute) (rheumatic)
　　　　　(Sydenham's) I02.0
　　arteriosclerotic I37.8
　　congenital Q22.2
　　rheumatic (chronic) (inactive) (with chorea)
　　　I09.89
　　　active or acute I01.1
　　　　with chorea (acute) (rheumatic)
　　　　　(Sydenham's) I02.0
　　syphilitic A52.03
　purulent (acute) (any valve) (subacute) I33.0
　Q fever A78 [I39]
　rheumatic (chronic) (inactive) (with chorea)
　　I09.1
　　active or acute (aortic) (mitral)
　　　(pulmonary) (tricuspid) I01.1
　　　with chorea (acute) (rheumatic)
　　　　(Sydenham's) I02.0
　rheumatoid —*see* Rheumatoid, carditis
　septic (acute) (any valve) (subacute) I33.0
　streptococcal (acute) (any valve) (subacute)
　　I33.0
　subacute —*see* Endocarditis, acute
　suppurative (acute) (any valve) (subacute)
　　I33.0
　syphilitic A52.03
　toxic I33.9
　tricuspid (chronic) (heart) (inactive)
　　(rheumatic) (valve) (with chorea) I07.9
　　with
　　　aortic (valve) disease I08.2
　　　　mitral (valve) disease I08.3
　　　mitral (valve) disease I08.1
　　　　aortic (valve) disease I08.3
　　　rheumatic fever (conditions in I00)
　　　　active —*see* Endocarditis, acute,
　　　　　rheumatic
　　　　inactive or quiescent (with chorea)
　　　　　I07.8
　　active or acute I01.1
　　　with chorea (acute) (rheumatic)
　　　　(Sydenham's) I02.0
　　arteriosclerotic I36.8
　　nonrheumatic I36.8
　　　acute or subacute I33.9
　　specified cause, except rheumatic I36.8
　tuberculous —*see* Tuberculosis, endocarditis
　typhoid A01.02
　ulcerative (acute) (any valve) (subacute) I33.0
　vegetative (acute) (any valve) (subacute) I33.0
　verrucous (atypical) (nonbacterial)
　　(nonrheumatic) M32.11
Endocardium, endocardial —*see also* condition
　cushion defect Q21.2
Endocervicitis —*see also* Cervicitis
　due to intrauterine (contraceptive) device
　　T83.69
　hyperplastic N72
Endocrine —*see* condition
Endocrinopathy, pluriglandular E31.9
Endodontic
　overfill M27.52
　underfill M27.53
Endodontitis K04.01
　irreversible K04.02
　reversible K04.01
Endomastoiditis —*see* Mastoiditis
Endometrioma N80.9
Endometriosis N80.9
　appendix N80.5
　bladder N80.8

Endometriosis *(Continued)*
　bowel N80.5
　broad ligament N80.3
　cervix N80.0
　colon N80.5
　cul-de-sac (Douglas') N80.3
　exocervix N80.0
　fallopian tube N80.2
　female genital organ NEC N80.8
　gallbladder N80.8
　in scar of skin N80.6
　internal N80.0
　intestine N80.5
　lung N80.8
　myometrium N80.0
　ovary N80.1
　parametrium N80.3
　pelvic peritoneum N80.3
　peritoneal (pelvic) N80.3
　rectovaginal septum N80.4
　rectum N80.5
　round ligament N80.3
　skin (scar) N80.6
　specified site NEC N80.8
　stromal D39.0
▶　thorax N80.8
　umbilicus N80.8
　uterus (internal) N80.0
　vagina N80.4
　vulva N80.8
Endometritis (decidual) (nonspecific) (purulent)
　　(senile (atrophic)) (suppurative) N71.9
　with ectopic pregnancy O08.0
　acute N71.0
　blenorrhagic (gonococcal) (acute) (chronic)
　　A54.24
　cervix, cervical (with erosion or ectropion) —
　　see also Cervicitis
　　hyperplastic N72
　chlamydial A56.11
　chronic N71.1
　following
　　abortion —*see* Abortion by type
　　　complicated by genital infection
　　ectopic or molar pregnancy O08.0
　gonococcal, gonorrheal (acute) (chronic) A54.24
　hyperplastic —*see also* Hyperplasia,
　　endometrial N85.00-●
　　cervix N72
　puerperal, postpartum, childbirth O86.12
　subacute N71.0
　tuberculous A18.17
Endometrium —*see* condition
Endomyocardiopathy, South African I42.3
Endomyocarditis —*see* Endocarditis
Endomyofibrosis I42.3
Endomyometritis —*see* Endometritis
Endopericarditis —*see* Endocarditis
Endoperineuritis —*see* Disorder, nerve
Endophlebitis —*see* Phlebitis
Endophthalmia —*see* Endophthalmitis,
　purulent
Endophthalmitis (acute) (infective) (metastatic)
　　(subacute) H44.009
　bleb associated H59.4 —*see also* Bleb,
　　inflamed (infected), postprocedural
　gonorrheal A54.39
　in (due to)
　　cysticercosis B69.1
　　onchocerciasis B73.01
　　toxocariasis B83.0
　panuveitis —*see* Panuveitis
　parasitic H44.12-●
　purulent H44.00-●
　　panophthalmitis —*see* Panophthalmitis
　　vitreous abscess H44.02-●
　specified NEC H44.19
　sympathetic —*see* Uveitis, sympathetic
Endosalpingioma D28.2
Endosalpingiosis N94.89
Endosteitis —*see* Osteomyelitis

Endothelioma, bone —*see* Neoplasm, bone, malignant
Endotheliosis (hemorrhagic infectional) D69.8
Endotoxemia — code to condition
Endotrachelitis —*see* Cervicitis
Engelmann (-Camurati) syndrome Q78.3
English disease —*see* Rickets
Engman's disease L30.3
Engorgement
　breast N64.59
　　newborn P83.4
　　puerperal, postpartum O92.79
　lung (passive) —*see* Edema, lung
　pulmonary (passive) —*see* Edema, lung
　stomach K31.89
　venous, retina —*see* Occlusion, retina, vein, engorgement
Enlargement, enlarged —*see also* Hypertrophy
　adenoids J35.2
　　with tonsils J35.3
　alveolar ridge K08.89
　　congenital —*see* Anomaly, alveolar
　apertures of diaphragm (congenital) Q79.1
　gingival K06.1
　heart, cardiac —*see* Hypertrophy, cardiac
　labium majus, childhood asymmetric (CALME) N90.61
　lacrimal gland, chronic H04.03-●
　liver —*see* Hypertrophy, liver
　lymph gland or node R59.9
　　generalized R59.1
　　localized R59.0
　orbit H05.34-●
　organ or site, congenital NEC —*see* Anomaly, by site
　parathyroid (gland) E21.0
　pituitary fossa R93.0
　prostate N40.0
　　with lower urinary tract symptoms (LUTS) N40.1
　　without lower urinary tract symptoms (LUTS) N40.0
　sella turcica R93.0
　spleen —*see* Splenomegaly
　thymus (gland) (congenital) E32.0
　thyroid (gland) —*see* Goiter
　tongue K14.8
　tonsils J35.1
　　with adenoids J35.3
　uterus N85.2
　▶vestibular aqueduct Q16.5
Enophthalmos H05.40-●
　due to
　　orbital tissue atrophy H05.41-●
　　trauma or surgery H05.42-●
Enostosis M27.8
Entamebic, entamebiasis —*see* Amebiasis
Entanglement
　⇒umbilical cord(s) O69.82
　　with compression O69.2
　　~~without compression O69.82~~
　⇒around neck (with compression) O69.81
　　▶with compression O69.1
　　without compression O69.81
　　of twins in monoamniotic sac O69.2
　　▶without compression O69.82
Enteralgia —*see* Pain, abdominal
Enteric —*see* condition
Enteritis (acute) (diarrheal) (hemorrhagic) (noninfective) K52.9
　adenovirus A08.2
　aertrycke infection A02.0
　allergic K52.29
　　with
　　　eosinophilic gastritis or gastroenteritis K52.81
　　　food protein-induced enterocolitis syndrome K52.21
　　　food protein-induced enteropathy K52.22

Enteritis (Continued)
　amebic (acute) A06.0
　　with abscess —*see* Abscess, amebic
　　chronic A06.1
　　　with abscess —*see* Abscess, amebic
　　　nondysenteric A06.2
　　nondysenteric A06.2
　astrovirus A08.32
　bacillary NOS A03.9
　bacterial A04.9
　　specified NEC A04.8
　calicivirus A08.31
　candidal B37.82
　Chilomastix A07.8
　choleriformis A00.1
　chronic (noninfectious) K52.9
　　ulcerative —*see* Colitis, ulcerative
　cicatrizing (chronic) —*see* Enteritis, regional, small intestine
　Clostridium
　　botulinum (food poisoning) A05.1
　　⇒difficile
　　　▶not specified as recurrent A04.72
　　　▶recurrent A04.71
　coccidial A07.3
　coxsackie virus A08.39
　dietetic —*see also* Enteritis, allergic K52.29
　drug-induced K52.1
　due to
　　astrovirus A08.32
　　calicivirus A08.31
　　coxsackie virus A08.39
　　drugs K52.1
　　echovirus A08.39
　　enterovirus NEC A08.39
　　food hypersensitivity —*see also* Enteritis, allergic K52.29
　　infectious organism (bacterial) (viral) —*see* Enteritis, infectious
　　torovirus A08.39
　　Yersinia enterocolitica A04.6
　echovirus A08.39
　eltor A00.1
　enterovirus NEC A08.39
　eosinophilic K52.81
　epidemic (infectious) A09
　fulminant —*see also* Ischemia, intestine, acute K55.019
　gangrenous —*see* Enteritis, infectious
　giardial A07.1
　infectious NOS A09
　　due to
　　　adenovirus A08.2
　　　Aerobacter aerogenes A04.8
　　　Arizona (bacillus) A02.0
　　　bacteria NOS A04.9
　　　　specified NEC A04.8
　　　Campylobacter A04.5
　　⇒Clostridium difficile
　　　▶not specified as recurrent A04.72
　　　▶recurrent A04.71
　　　Clostridium perfringens A04.8
　　　Enterobacter aerogenes A04.8
　　　enterovirus A08.39
　　　Escherichia coli A04.4
　　　　enteroaggregative A04.4
　　　　enterohemorrhagic A04.3
　　　　enteroinvasive A04.4
　　　　enteropathogenic A04.0
　　　　enterotoxigenic A04.1
　　　　specified NEC A04.4
　　　specified
　　　　bacteria NEC A04.8
　　　　virus NEC A08.39
　　　Staphylococcus A04.8
　　　virus NEC A08.4
　　　　specified type NEC A08.39
　　　Yersinia enterocolitica A04.6
　　　specified organism NEC A08.8
　influenzal —*see* Influenza, with, digestive manifestations

Enteritis (Continued)
　ischemic K55.9
　　acute —*see also* Ischemia, intestine, acute K55.019
　　chronic K55.1
　microsporidial A07.8
　mucomembranous, myxomembranous —*see* Syndrome, irritable bowel
　mucous —*see* Syndrome, irritable bowel
　necroticans A05.2
　necrotizing of newborn —*see* Enterocolitis, necrotizing, in newborn
　neurogenic —*see* Syndrome, irritable bowel
　newborn necrotizing —*see* Enterocolitis, necrotizing, in newborn
　noninfectious K52.9
　norovirus A08.11
　parasitic NEC B82.9
　paratyphoid (fever) —*see* Fever, paratyphoid
　protozoal A07.9
　　specified NEC A07.8
　radiation K52.0
　regional (of) K50.90
　　with
　　　complication K50.919
　　　　abscess K50.914
　　　　fistula K50.913
　　　　intestinal obstruction K50.912
　　　　rectal bleeding K50.911
　　　　specified complication NEC K50.918
　　colon —*see* Enteritis, regional, large intestine
　　duodenum —*see* Enteritis, regional, small intestine
　　ileum —*see* Enteritis, regional, small intestine
　　jejunum —*see* Enteritis, regional, small intestine
　　large bowel —*see* Enteritis, regional, large intestine
　　large intestine (colon) (rectum) K50.10
　　　with
　　　　complication K50.119
　　　　　abscess K50.114
　　　　　fistula K50.113
　　　　　intestinal obstruction K50.112
　　　　　rectal bleeding K50.111
　　　　　small intestine (duodenum) (ileum) (jejunum) involvement K50.80
　　　　　　with
　　　　　　　complication K50.819
　　　　　　　　abscess K50.814
　　　　　　　　fistula K50.813
　　　　　　　　intestinal obstruction K50.812
　　　　　　　　rectal bleeding K50.811
　　　　　　　　specified complication NEC K50.818
　　　　　specified complication NEC K50.118
　　rectum —*see* Enteritis, regional, large intestine
　　small intestine (duodenum) (ileum) (jejunum) K50.00
　　　with
　　　　complication K50.019
　　　　　abscess K50.014
　　　　　fistula K50.013
　　　　　intestinal obstruction K50.012
　　　　　large intestine (colon) (rectum) involvement K50.80
　　　　　　with
　　　　　　　complication K50.819
　　　　　　　　abscess K50.814
　　　　　　　　fistula K50.813
　　　　　　　　intestinal obstruction K50.812
　　　　　　　　rectal bleeding K50.811
　　　　　　　　specified complication NEC K50.818
　　　　　rectal bleeding K50.011
　　　　　specified complication NEC K50.018
　rotaviral A08.0

Enteritis (Continued)
  Salmonella, salmonellosis (arizonae)
    (cholerae-suis) (enteritidis)
    (typhimurium) A02.0
  segmental —see Enteritis, regional
  septic A09
  Shigella —see Infection, Shigella
  small round structured NEC A08.19
  spasmodic, spastic —see Syndrome, irritable
    bowel
  staphylococcal A04.8
    due to food A05.0
  torovirus A08.39
  toxic NEC K52.1
  ⟹ due to Clostridium difficile
    ▶ not specified as recurrent A04.72
    ▶ recurrent A04.71
  trichomonal A07.8
  tuberculous A18.32
  typhosa A01.00
  ulcerative (chronic) —see Colitis, ulcerative
  viral A08.4
    adenovirus A08.2
    enterovirus A08.39
    Rotavirus A08.0
    small round structured NEC A08.19
    specified NEC A08.39
    virus specified NEC A08.39
Enterobiasis B80
Enterobius vermicularis (infection) (infestation)
  B80
Enterocele —see also Hernia, abdomen
  pelvic, pelvis (acquired) (congenital) N81.5
  vagina, vaginal (acquired) (congenital)
    NEC N81.5
Enterocolitis —see also Enteritis K52.9
⟹ due to Clostridium difficile
  ▶ not specified as recurrent A04.72
  ▶ recurrent A04.71
  fulminant ischemic —see also Ischemia,
    intestine, acute K55.059
  granulomatous —see Enteritis, regional
  hemorrhagic (acute) —see also Ischemia,
    intestine, acute K55.059
    chronic K55.1
  infectious NEC A09
  ischemic K55.9
  necrotizing K55.30
    with
      perforation K55.33
      pneumatosis K55.32
      and perforation K55.33
    ⟹ due to Clostridium difficile
    ▶ not specified as recurrent A04.72
    ▶ recurrent A04.71
    in non-newborn K55.30
      stage 1 (without pneumatosis, without
        perforation) K55.31
      stage 2 (with pneumatosis, without
        perforation) K55.32
      stage 3 (with pneumatosis, with
        perforation) K55.33
    in newborn P77.9
      stage 1 (without pneumatosis, without
        perforation) P77.1
      stage 2 (with pneumatosis, without
        perforation) P77.2
      stage 3 (with pneumatosis, with
        perforation) P77.3
    without pneumatosis or perforation K55.31
  noninfectious K52.9
    newborn —see Enterocolitis, necrotizing, in
      newborn
  ⟹ pseudomembranous (newborn)
    ▶ not specified as recurrent A04.72
    ▶ recurrent A04.71
  radiation K52.0
    newborn —see Enterocolitis, necrotizing, in
      newborn
  ulcerative (chronic) —see Pancolitis,
    ulcerative (chronic)

Enterogastritis —see Enteritis
Enteropathy K63.9
▶ celiac-gluten-sensitive K90.0
  ▶ non-celiac K90.41
  food protein-induced enterocolitis K52.22
  gluten-sensitive K90.0
  non-celiac K90.41
  hemorrhagic, terminal —see also Ischemia,
    intestine, acute K55.059
  protein-losing K90.49
Enteroperitonitis —see Peritonitis
Enteroptosis K63.4
Enterorrhagia K92.2
Enterospasm —see also Syndrome, irritable,
  bowel
  psychogenic F45.8
⟹ Enterostenosis —see also Obstruction, intestine,
  specified NEC K56.699
Enterostomy
  complication —see Complication,
    enterostomy
  status Z93.4
Enterovirus, as cause of disease classified
  elsewhere B97.10
  coxsackievirus B97.11
  echovirus B97.12
  other specified B97.19
Enthesopathy (peripheral) M77.9
  Achilles tendinitis —see Tendinitis, Achilles
  ankle and tarsus M77.9
    specified type NEC —see Enthesopathy,
      foot, specified type NEC
  anterior tibial syndrome M76.81-●
  calcaneal spur —see Spur, bone, calcaneal
  elbow region M77.8
    lateral epicondylitis —see Epicondylitis,
      lateral
    medial epicondylitis —see Epicondylitis,
      medial
  foot NEC M77.9
    metatarsalgia —see Metatarsalgia
    specified type NEC M77.5-●
  forearm M77.9
  gluteal tendinitis —see Tendinitis, gluteal
  hand M77.9
  hip —see Enthesopathy, lower limb, specified
    type NEC
  iliac crest spur —see Spur, bone, iliac crest
  iliotibial band syndrome —see Syndrome,
    iliotibial band
  knee —see Enthesopathy, lower limb, lower
    leg, specified type NEC
  lateral epicondylitis —see Epicondylitis,
    lateral
  lower limb (excluding foot) M76.9
    Achilles tendinitis —see Tendinitis, Achilles
    anterior tibial syndrome M76.81-●
    gluteal tendinitis —see Tendinitis, gluteal
    iliac crest spur —see Spur, bone, iliac crest
    iliotibial band syndrome —see Syndrome,
      iliotibial band
    patellar tendinitis —see Tendinitis, patellar
    pelvic region —see Enthesopathy, lower
      limb, specified type NEC
    peroneal tendinitis —see Tendinitis,
      peroneal
    posterior tibial syndrome M76.82-●
    psoas tendinitis —see Tendinitis, psoas
    shoulder M77.9
    specified type NEC M76.89-●
    tibial collateral bursitis —see Bursitis, tibial
      collateral
  medial epicondylitis —see Epicondylitis,
    medial
  multiple sites M77.9
  patellar tendinitis —see Tendinitis, patellar
  pelvis M77.9
  periarthritis of wrist —see Periarthritis, wrist
  peroneal tendinitis —see Tendinitis, peroneal
  posterior tibial syndrome M76.82-●
  psoas tendinitis —see Tendinitis, psoas

Enthesopathy (Continued)
  shoulder region —see Lesion, shoulder
  specified site NEC M77.9
  specified type NEC M77.8
  spinal M46.00
    cervical region M46.02
    cervicothoracic region M46.03
    lumbar region M46.06
    lumbosacral region M46.07
    multiple sites M46.09
    occipito-atlanto-axial region M46.01
    sacrococcygeal region M46.08
    thoracic region M46.04
    thoracolumbar region M46.05
  tibial collateral bursitis —see Bursitis, tibial
    collateral
  upper arm M77.9
  wrist and carpus NEC M77.8
    calcaneal spur —see Spur, bone, calcaneal
    periarthritis of wrist —see Periarthritis,
      wrist
Entomophobia F40.218
Entomophthoromycosis B46.8
Entrance, air into vein —see Embolism, air
Entrapment, nerve —see Neuropathy,
  entrapment
Entropion (eyelid) (paralytic) H02.009
  cicatricial H02.019
    left H02.016
      lower H02.015
      upper H02.014
    right H02.013
      lower H02.012
      upper H02.011
  congenital Q10.2
  left H02.006
    lower H02.005
    upper H02.004
  mechanical H02.029
    left H02.026
      lower H02.025
      upper H02.024
    right H02.023
      lower H02.022
      upper H02.021
  right H02.003
    lower H02.002
    upper H02.001
  senile H02.039
    left H02.036
      lower H02.035
      upper H02.034
    right H02.033
      lower H02.032
      upper H02.031
  spastic H02.049
    left H02.046
      lower H02.045
      upper H02.044
    right H02.043
      lower H02.042
      upper H02.041
Enucleated eye (traumatic, current) S05.7-●
Enuresis R32
  functional F98.0
  habit disturbance F98.0
  nocturnal N39.44
    psychogenic F98.0
  nonorganic origin F98.0
  psychogenic F98.0
Eosinopenia —see Agranulocytosis
Eosinophilia (allergic) (hereditary) (idiopathic)
  (secondary) D72.1
  with
    angiolymphoid hyperplasia (ALHE)
      D18.01
  infiltrative J82
  Löffler's J82
  peritoneal —see Peritonitis, eosinophilic
  pulmonary NEC J82
  tropical (pulmonary) J82

▶ New   ⟹ Revised   deleted Deleted   ● Use Additional Character(s)

Eosinophilia-myalgia syndrome M35.8
Ependymitis (acute) (cerebral) (chronic)
 (granular) —see Encephalomyelitis
Ependymoblastoma
 specified site —see Neoplasm, malignant, by
  site
 unspecified site C71.9
Ependymoma (epithelial) (malignant)
 anaplastic
  specified site —see Neoplasm, malignant,
   by site
  unspecified site C71.9
 benign
  specified site —see Neoplasm, benign, by
   site
  unspecified site D33.2
 myxopapillary D43.2
  specified site —see Neoplasm, uncertain
   behavior, by site
  unspecified site D43.2
 papillary D43.2
  specified site —see Neoplasm, uncertain
   behavior, by site
  unspecified site D43.2
 specified site —see Neoplasm, malignant, by
  site
 unspecified site C71.9
Ependymopathy G93.89
Ephelis, ephelides L81.2
Epiblepharon (congenital) Q10.3
Epicanthus, epicanthic fold (eyelid)
 (congenital) Q10.3
Epicondylitis (elbow)
 lateral M77.1-●
 medial M77.0-●
Epicystitis —see Cystitis
Epidemic —see condition
Epidermidalization, cervix —see Dysplasia,
 cervix
Epidermis, epidermal —see condition
Epidermodysplasia verruciformis B07.8
Epidermolysis
 bullosa (congenital) Q81.9
  acquired L12.30
   drug-induced L12.31
   specified cause NEC L12.35
  dystrophica Q81.2
  letalis Q81.1
  simplex Q81.0
  specified NEC Q81.8
 necroticans combustiformis L51.2
  due to drug —see Table of Drugs and
   Chemicals, by drug
Epidermophytid —see Dermatophytosis
Epidermophytosis (infected) —see
 Dermatophytosis
Epididymis —see condition
Epididymitis (acute) (nonvenereal) (recurrent)
 (residual) N45.1
 with orchitis N45.3
 blennorrhagic (gonococcal) A54.23
 caseous (tuberculous) A18.15
 chlamydial A56.19
 filarial —see also Infestation, filarial B74.9
  [N51]
 gonococcal A54.23
 syphilitic A52.76
 tuberculous A18.15
Epididymo-orchitis —see also Epididymitis
 N45.3
Epidural —see condition
Epigastrium, epigastric —see condition
Epigastrocele —see Hernia, ventral
Epiglottis —see condition
Epiglottitis, epiglottiditis (acute) J05.10
 with obstruction J05.11
 chronic J37.0
Epignathus Q89.4
Epilepsia partialis continua —see also
 Kozhevnikof's epilepsy G40.1-●

Epilepsy, epileptic, epilepsia (attack) (cerebral)
 (convulsion) (fit) (seizure) G40.909

> Note: the following terms are to be
> considered equivalent to intractable:
> pharmacoresistant (pharmacologically
> resistant), treatment resistant, refractory
> (medically) and poorly controlled

with
 complex partial seizures —see Epilepsy,
  localization-related, symptomatic,
  with complex partial seizures
 grand mal seizures on awakening —
  see Epilepsy, generalized, specified
  NEC
 myoclonic absences —see Epilepsy,
  generalized, specified NEC
 myoclonic-astatic seizures —see Epilepsy,
  generalized, specified NEC
 simple partial seizures —see Epilepsy,
  localization-related, symptomatic,
  with simple partial seizures
akinetic —see Epilepsy, generalized, specified
 NEC
benign childhood with centrotemporal EEG
 spikes —see Epilepsy, localization-
 related, idiopathic
benign myoclonic in infancy G40.80-●
Bravais-jacksonian —see Epilepsy,
 localization-related, symptomatic,
 with simple partial seizures
childhood
 with occipital EEG paroxysms —see
  Epilepsy, localization-related,
  idiopathic
 absence G40.A09
  intractable G40.A19
   with status epilepticus G40.A11
   without status epilepticus G40.A19
  not intractable G40.A09
   with status epilepticus G40.A01
   without status epilepticus G40.A09
climacteric —see Epilepsy, specified NEC
cysticercosis B69.0
deterioration (mental) F06.8
due to syphilis A52.19
focal —see Epilepsy, localization-related,
 symptomatic, with simple partial
 seizures
generalized
 idiopathic G40.309
  intractable G40.319
   with status epilepticus G40.311
   without status epilepticus G40.319
  not intractable G40.309
   with status epilepticus G40.301
   without status epilepticus G40.309
 specified NEC G40.409
  intractable G40.419
   with status epilepticus G40.411
   without status epilepticus G40.419
  not intractable G40.409
   with status epilepticus G40.401
   without status epilepticus G40.409
impulsive petit mal —see Epilepsy, juvenile
 myoclonic
intractable G40.919
 with status epilepticus G40.911
 without status epilepticus G40.919
juvenile absence G40.A09
 intractable G40.A19
  with status epilepticus G40.A11
  without status epilepticus G40.A19
 not intractable G40.A09
  with status epilepticus G40.A01
  without status epilepticus G40.A09
juvenile myoclonic G40.B11
 intractable G40.B19
  with status epilepticus G40.B11
  without status epilepticus G40.B19

Epilepsy, epileptic, epilepsia (Continued)
 juvenile myoclonic (Continued)
  not intractable G40.B09
   with status epilepticus G40.B01
   without status epilepticus G40.B09
 localization-related (focal) (partial)
  idiopathic G40.009
   with seizures of localized onset G40.009
    intractable G40.019
     with status epilepticus G40.011
     without status epilepticus G40.019
    not intractable G40.009
     with status epilepticus G40.001
     without status epilepticus G40.009
  symptomatic
   with complex partial seizures G40.209
    intractable G40.219
     with status epilepticus G40.211
     without status epilepticus G40.219
    not intractable G40.209
     with status epilepticus G40.201
     without status epilepticus
      G40.209
   with simple partial seizures G40.109
    intractable G40.119
     with status epilepticus G40.111
     without status epilepticus
      G40.119
    not intractable G40.109
     with status epilepticus G40.101
     without status epilepticus G40.109
 myoclonus, myoclonic —see Epilepsy,
  generalized, specified NEC
 progressive —see Epilepsy, generalized,
  idiopathic
 not intractable G40.909
  with status epilepticus G40.901
  without status epilepticus G40.909
 on awakening —see Epilepsy, generalized,
  specified NEC
 parasitic NOS B71.9 [G94]
 partialis continua —see also Kozhevnikof's
  epilepsy G40.1-●
 peripheral —see Epilepsy, specified NEC
 procursiva —see Epilepsy, localization-
  related, symptomatic, with simple
  partial seizures
 progressive (familial) myoclonic —see
  Epilepsy, generalized, idiopathic
 reflex —see Epilepsy, specified NEC
 related to
  alcohol G40.509
   not intractable G40.509
    with status epilepticus G40.501
    without status epliepticus G40.509
  drugs G40.509
   not intractable G40.509
    with status epilepticus G40.501
    without status epliepticus G40.509
  external causes G40.509
   not intractable G40.509
    with status epilepticus G40.501
    without status epilepticus G40.509
  hormonal changes G40.509
   not intractable G40.509
    with status epilepticus G40.501
    without status epliepticus G40.509
  sleep deprivation G40.509
   not intractable G40.509
    with status epilepticus G40.501
    without status epliepticus G40.509
  stress G40.509
   not intractable G40.509
    with status epilepticus G40.501
    without status epilepticus G40.509
 somatomotor —see Epilepsy, localization-
  related, symptomatic, with simple
  partial seizures
 somatosensory —see Epilepsy, localization-
  related, symptomatic, with simple
  partial seizures

▶ New   ➡ Revised   d̶e̶l̶e̶t̶e̶d̶ Deleted   ● Use Additional Character(s)

Epilepsy, epileptic, epilepsia (Continued)
  spasms G40.822
    intractable G40.824
      with status epilepticus G40.823
      without status epilepticus G40.824
    not intractable G40.822
      with status epilepticus G40.821
      without status epilepticus G40.822
    specified NEC G40.802
      intractable G40.804
        with status epilepticus G40.803
        without status epilepticus G40.804
      not intractable G40.802
        with status epilepticus G40.801
        without status epilepticus G40.802
  syndromes
    generalized
      idiopathic G40.309
        intractable G40.319
          with status epilepticus G40.311
          without status epilepticus G40.319
        not intractable G40.309
          with status epilepticus G40.301
          without status epilepticus G40.309
      specified NEC G40.409
        intractable G40.419
          with status epilepticus G40.411
          without status epilepticus G40.419
        not intractable G40.409
          with status epilepticus G40.401
          without status epilepticus G40.409
    localization-related (focal) (partial)
      idiopathic G40.009
        with seizures of localized onset
          G40.009
          intractable G40.019
            with status epilepticus G40.011
            without status epilepticus
              G40.019
          not intractable G40.009
            with status epilepticus G40.001
            without status epilepticus
              G40.009
      symptomatic
        with complex partial seizures G40.209
          intractable G40.219
            with status epilepticus G40.211
            without status epilepticus G40.219
          not intractable G40.209
            with status epilepticus G40.201
            without status epilepticus G40.209
        with simple partial seizures G40.109
          intractable G40.119
            with status epilepticus G40.111
            without status epilepticus G40.119
          not intractable G40.109
            with status epilepticus G40.101
            without status epilepticus G40.109
    specified NEC G40.802
      intractable G40.804
        with status epilepticus G40.803
        without status epilepticus G40.804
      not intractable G40.802
        with status epilepticus G40.801
        without status epilepticus G40.802
  tonic (-clonic) —see Epilepsy, generalized,
    specified NEC
  twilight F05
  uncinate (gyrus) —see Epilepsy, localization-
    related, symptomatic, with complex
    partial seizures
  Unverricht (-Lundborg) (familial myoclonic) —
    see Epilepsy, generalized, idiopathic
  visceral —see Epilepsy, specified NEC
  visual —see Epilepsy, specified NEC
Epiloia Q85.1
Epimenorrhea N92.0
Epipharyngitis —see Nasopharyngitis
Epiphora H04.20-•
  due to
    excess lacrimation H04.21-•
    insufficient drainage H04.22-•

Epiphyseal arrest —see Arrest, epiphyseal
Epiphyseolysis, epiphysiolysis —see
  Osteochondropathy
Epiphysitis —see also Osteochondropathy
  juvenile M92.9
  syphilitic (congenital) A50.02
Epiplocele —see Hernia, abdomen
Epiploitis —see Peritonitis
Epiplosarcomphalocele —see Hernia, umbilicus
Episcleritis (suppurative) H15.10-•
  in (due to)
    syphilis A52.71
    tuberculosis A18.51
  nodular H15.12-•
  periodica fugax H15.11-•
    angioneurotic —see Edema, angioneurotic
  syphilitic (late) A52.71
  tuberculous A18.51
Episode
  affective, mixed F39
  depersonalization (in neurotic state) F48.1
  depressive F32.9
    major F32.9
      mild F32.0
      moderate F32.1
      severe (without psychotic symptoms)
        F32.2
        with psychotic symptoms F32.3
    recurrent F33.9
      brief F33.8
    specified NEC F32.89
  hypomanic F30.8
  manic F30.9
    with
      psychotic symptoms F30.2
      remission (full) F30.4
        partial F30.3
    without psychotic symptoms F30.10
      mild F30.11
      moderate F30.12
      severe (without psychotic symptoms)
        F30.13
        with psychotic symptoms F30.2
    other specified F30.8
    recurrent F31.89
  psychotic F23
    organic F06.8
  schizophrenic (acute) NEC, brief F23
Epispadias (female) (male) Q64.0
Episplenitis D73.89
Epistaxis (multiple) R04.0
  hereditary I78.0
  vicarious menstruation N94.89
Epithelioma (malignant) —see also Neoplasm,
  malignant, by site
  adenoides cysticum —see Neoplasm, skin,
    benign
  basal cell —see Neoplasm, skin, malignant
  benign —see Neoplasm, benign, by site
  Bowen's —see Neoplasm, skin, in situ
  calcifying, of Malherbe —see Neoplasm, skin,
    benign
  external site —see Neoplasm, skin, malignant
  intraepidermal, Jadassohn —see Neoplasm,
    skin, benign
  squamous cell —see Neoplasm, malignant,
    by site
Epitheliomatosis pigmented Q82.1
Epitheliopathy, multifocal placoid pigment
  H30.14-•
Epithelium, epithelial —see condition
Epituberculosis (with atelectasis) (allergic)
  A15.7
Eponychia Q84.6
Epstein's
  nephrosis or syndrome —see Nephrosis
  pearl K09.8
Epulis (gingiva) (fibrous) (giant cell) K06.8
Equinia A24.0
Equinovarus (congenital) (talipes) Q66.0
  acquired —see Deformity, limb, clubfoot

Equivalent
  convulsive (abdominal) —see Epilepsy,
    specified NEC
  epileptic (psychic) —see Epilepsy,
    localization-related, symptomatic, with
    complex partial seizures
Erb (-Duchenne) paralysis (birth injury)
  (newborn) P14.0
Erb's
  disease G71.0
  palsy, paralysis (brachial) (birth) (newborn)
    P14.0
    spinal (spastic) syphilitic A52.17
  pseudohypertrophic muscular dystrophy
    G71.0
Erb-Goldflam disease or syndrome G70.00
  with exacerbation (acute) G70.01
  in crisis G70.01
Erdheim's syndrome (acromegalic
  macrospondylitis) E22.0
Erection, painful (persistent) —see Priapism
Ergosterol deficiency (vitamin D) E55.9
  with
    adult osteomalacia M83.8
    rickets —see Rickets
Ergotism —see also Poisoning, food, noxious,
  plant
  from ergot used as drug (migraine
    therapy) —see Table of Drugs and
    Chemicals
Erosio interdigitalis blastomycetica B37.2
Erosion
  artery I77.2
    without rupture I77.89
  bone —see Disorder, bone, density and
    structure, specified NEC
  bronchus J98.09
  cartilage (joint) —see Disorder, cartilage,
    specified type NEC
  cervix (uteri) (acquired) (chronic) (congenital)
    N86
    with cervicitis N72
  cornea (nontraumatic) —see Ulcer, cornea
    recurrent H18.83-•
    traumatic —see Abrasion, cornea
  dental (idiopathic) (occupational) (due to
    diet, drugs or vomiting) K03.2
  duodenum, postpyloric —see Ulcer,
    duodenum
  esophagus K22.10
    with bleeding K22.11
  gastric —see Ulcer, stomach
  gastrojejunal —see Ulcer, gastrojejunal
  implanted mesh —see Complications, mesh
  intestine K63.3
  lymphatic vessel I89.8
  pylorus, pyloric (ulcer) —see Ulcer, stomach
  spine, aneurysmal A52.09
  stomach —see Ulcer, stomach
  subcutaneous device pocket
    nervous system prosthetic device, implant,
      or graft T85.890
    other internal prosthetic device, implant, or
      graft T85.898
  teeth (idiopathic) (occupational) (due to diet,
    drugs or vomiting) K03.2
  urethra N36.8
  uterus N85.8
Erotomania F52.8
Error
  metabolism, inborn —see Disorder, metabolism
  refractive —see Disorder, refraction
Eructation R14.2
  nervous or psychogenic F45.8
Eruption
  creeping B76.9
  drug (generalized) (taken internally) L27.0
    fixed L27.1
    in contact with skin —see Dermatitis, due
      to drugs
    localized L27.1

▶ New   ➡ Revised   ~~deleted~~ Deleted   • Use Additional Character(s)

Eruption *(Continued)*
    Hutchinson, summer L56.4
    Kaposi's varicelliform B00.0
    napkin L22
    polymorphous light (sun) L56.4
    recalcitrant pustular L13.8
    ringed R23.8
    skin (nonspecific) R21
        creeping (meaning hookworm) B76.9
        due to inoculation/vaccination
            (generalized) —*see also* Dermatitis,
            due to, vaccine L27.0
            localized L27.1
        erysipeloid A26.0
        feigned L98.1
        Kaposi's varicelliform B00.0
        lichenoid L28.0
        meaning dermatitis —*see* Dermatitis
        toxic NEC L53.0
    tooth, teeth, abnormal (incomplete) (late)
        (premature) (sequence) K00.6
    vesicular R23.8
Erysipelas (gangrenous) (infantile) (newborn)
    (phlegmonous) (suppurative) A46
    external ear A46 [H62.40]
    puerperal, postpartum O86.89
Erysipeloid A26.9
    cutaneous (Rosenbach's) A26.0
    disseminated A26.8
    sepsis A26.7
    specified NEC A26.8
Erythema, erythematous (infectional)
    (inflammation) L53.9
    ab igne L59.0
    annulare (centrifugum) (rheumaticum) L53.1
    arthriticum epidemicum A25.1
    brucellum —*see* Brucellosis
    chronic figurate NEC L53.3
    chronicum migrans (Borrelia burgdorferi)
        A69.20
    diaper L22
    due to
        chemical NEC L53.0
            in contact with skin L24.5
        drug (internal use) —*see* Dermatitis, due
            to, drugs
    elevatum diutinum L95.1
    endemic E52
    epidemic, arthritic A25.1
    figuratum perstans L53.3
    gluteal L22
    heat - code by site under Burn, first degree
    ichthyosiforme congenitum bullous Q80.3
    in diseases classified elsewhere L54
    induratum (nontuberculous) L52
        tuberculous A18.4
    infectiosum B08.3
    intertrigo L30.4
    iris L51.9
    marginatum L53.2
        in (due to) acute rheumatic fever I00
    medicamentosum —*see* Dermatitis, due to,
        drugs
    migrans A26.0
        chronicum A69.20
        tongue K14.1
    multiforme (major) (minor) L51.9
        bullous, bullosum L51.1
        conjunctiva L51.1
        nonbullous L51.0
        pemphigoides L12.0
        specified NEC L51.8
    napkin L22
    ⊯neonatorum P83.88
        toxic P83.1
    nodosum L52
        tuberculous A18.4
    palmar L53.8
    pernio T69.1
    ⊯rash, newborn P83.88
    scarlatiniform (recurrent) (exfoliative) L53.8

Erythema, erythematous *(Continued)*
    solare L55.0
    specified NEC L53.8
    toxic, toxicum NEC L53.0
        newborn P83.1
    tuberculous (primary) A18.4
Erythematous, erythematosus —*see* condition
Erythermalgia (primary) I73.81
Erythralgia I73.81
Erythrasma L08.1
Erythredema (polyneuropathy) —*see* Poisoning,
    mercury
Erythremia (acute) C94.0-●
    chronic D45
    secondary D75.1
Erythroblastopenia —*see also* Aplasia, red cell
    D60.9
    congenital D61.01
Erythroblastophthisis D61.09
Erythroblastosis (fetalis) (newborn) P55.9
    due to
        ABO (antibodies) (incompatibility)
            (isoimmunization) P55.1
        Rh (antibodies) (incompatibility)
            (isoimmunization) P55.0
Erythrocyanosis (crurum) I73.89
Erythrocythemia —*see* Erythremia
Erythrocytosis (megalosplenic) (secondary)
    D75.1
    familial D75.0
    oval, hereditary —*see* Elliptocytosis
    secondary D75.1
    stress D75.1
Erythroderma (secondary) —*see also* Erythema
    L53.9
    bullous ichthyosiform, congenital Q80.3
    desquamativum L21.1
    ichthyosiform, congenital (bullous) Q80.3
    ⊯neonatorum P83.88
    psoriaticum L40.8
Erythrodysesthesia, palmar plantar (PPE) L27.1
Erythrogenesis imperfecta D61.09
Erythroleukemia C94.0-●
Erythromelalgia I73.81
Erythrophagocytosis D75.89
Erythrophobia F40.298
Erythroplakia, oral epithelium, and tongue
    K13.29
Erythroplasia (Queyrat) D07.4
    specified site —*see* Neoplasm, skin, in situ
    unspecified site D07.4
Escherichia coli (E. coli), as cause of disease
    classified elsewhere B96.20
    non-O157 Shiga toxin-producing (with
        known O group) B96.22
    non-Shiga toxin-producing B96.29
    O157 with confirmation of Shiga toxin when
        H antigen is unknown, or is not H7
        B96.21
    O157:H- (nonmotile) with confirmation of
        Shiga toxin B96.21
    O157:H7 with or without confirmation of
        Shiga toxin-production B96.21
    Shiga toxin-producing (with unspecified O
        group) (STEC) B96.23
    O157 B96.21
    O157:H7 with or without confirmation of
        Shiga toxin-production B96.21
        specified NEC B96.22
    specified NEC B96.29
Esophagismus K22.4
Esophagitis (acute) (alkaline) (chemical)
    (chronic) (infectional) (necrotic) (peptic)
    (postoperative) K20.9
    candidal B37.81
    due to gastrointestinal reflux disease K21.0
    eosinophilic K20.0
    reflux K21.0
    specified NEC K20.8
    tuberculous A18.83
    ulcerative K22.10
        with bleeding K22.11

Esophagocele K22.5
Esophagomalacia K22.8
Esophagospasm K22.4
Esophagostenosis K22.2
Esophagostomiasis B81.8
Esophagotracheal —*see* condition
Esophagus —*see* condition
Esophoria H50.51
    convergence, excess H51.12
    divergence, insufficiency H51.8
Esotropia —*see* Strabismus, convergent
    concomitant
Espundia B55.2
Essential —*see* condition
Esthesioneuroblastoma C30.0
Esthesioneurocytoma C30.0
Esthesioneuroepithelioma C30.0
Esthiomene A55
Estivo-autumnal malaria (fever) B50.9
Estrangement (marital) Z63.5
    parent-child NEC Z62.890
Estriasis —*see* Myiasis
Ethanolism —*see* Alcoholism
Etherism —*see* Dependence, drug, inhalant
Ethmoid, ethmoidal —*see* condition
Ethmoiditis (chronic) (nonpurulent)
    (purulent) —*see also* Sinusitis, ethmoidal
    influenzal —*see* Influenza, with, respiratory
        manifestations NEC
    Woakes' J33.1
Ethylism —*see* Alcoholism
Eulenburg's disease (congenital paramyotonia)
    G71.19
Eumycetoma B47.0
Eunuchoidism E29.1
    hypogonadotropic E23.0
European blastomycosis —*see* Cryptococcosis
Eustachian —*see* condition
Evaluation (for) (of)
    development state
        adolescent Z00.3
        period of
            delayed growth in childhood Z00.70
                with abnormal findings Z00.71
            rapid growth in childhood Z00.2
            puberty Z00.3
    growth and developmental state (period of
        rapid growth) Z00.2
        delayed growth Z00.70
            with abnormal findings Z00.71
    mental health (status) Z00.8
        requested by authority Z04.6
    period of
        delayed growth in childhood Z00.70
            with abnormal findings Z00.71
        rapid growth in childhood Z00.2
    suspected condition —*see* Observation
Evans syndrome D69.41
~~Event, apparent life threatening in newborn and infant (ALTE) R68.13~~
▶Event
    ▶apparent life threatening in newborn and
        infant (ALTE) R68.13
    ▶brief resolved unexplained event (BRUE)
        R68.13
Eventration —*see also* Hernia, ventral
    colon into chest —*see* Hernia, diaphragm
    diaphragm (congenital) Q79.1
Eversion
    bladder N32.89
    cervix (uteri) N86
        with cervicitis N72
    foot NEC —*see also* Deformity, valgus, ankle
        congenital Q66.6
    punctum lacrimale (postinfectional) (senile)
        H04.52-●
    ureter (meatus) N28.89
    urethra (meatus) N36.8
    uterus N81.4
Evidence
    cytologic
        of malignancy on anal smear R85.614

Evidence *(Continued)*
  cytologic *(Continued)*
    of malignancy on cervical smear R87.614
    of malignancy on vaginal smear R87.624
Evisceration
  birth injury P15.8
  traumatic NEC
    eye —*see* Enucleated eye
Evulsion —*see* Avulsion
Ewing's sarcoma or tumor —*see* Neoplasm, bone, malignant
Examination (for) (following) (general) (of) (routine) Z00.00
  with abnormal findings Z00.01
  abuse, physical (alleged), ruled out
    adult Z04.71
    child Z04.72
  adolescent (development state) Z00.3
  alleged rape or sexual assault (victim), ruled out
    adult Z04.41
    child Z04.42
  allergy Z01.82
  annual (adult) (periodic) (physical) Z00.00
    with abnormal findings Z00.01
    gynecological Z01.419
      with abnormal findings Z01.411
  antibody response Z01.84
  blood —*see* Examination, laboratory
  blood pressure Z01.30
    with abnormal findings Z01.31
  cancer staging —*see* Neoplasm, malignant, by site
  cervical Papanicolaou smear Z12.4
    as part of routine gynecological examination Z01.419
      with abnormal findings Z01.411
  child (over 28 days old) Z00.129
    with abnormal findings Z00.121
    under 28 days old —*see* Newborn, examination
  clinical research control or normal comparison (control) (participant) Z00.6
  contraceptive (drug) maintenance (routine) Z30.8
    device (intrauterine) Z30.431
  dental Z01.20
    with abnormal findings Z01.21
  developmental —*see* Examination, child
  donor (potential) Z00.5
  ear Z01.10
    with abnormal findings NEC Z01.118
  eye Z01.00
    with abnormal findings Z01.01
  following
    accident NEC Z04.3
      transport Z04.1
      work Z04.2
    assault, alleged, ruled out
      adult Z04.71
      child Z04.72
    motor vehicle accident Z04.1
    treatment (for) Z09
      combined NEC Z09
        fracture Z09
        malignant neoplasm Z08
      malignant neoplasm Z08
      mental disorder Z09
      specified condition NEC Z09
  follow-up (routine) (following) Z09
    chemotherapy NEC Z09
      malignant neoplasm Z08
    fracture Z09
    malignant neoplasm Z08
    postpartum Z39.2
    psychotherapy Z09
    radiotherapy NEC Z09
      malignant neoplasm Z08
    surgery NEC Z09
      malignant neoplasm Z08

Examination *(Continued)*
  gynecological Z01.419
    with abnormal findings Z01.411
    for contraceptive maintenance Z30.8
  health —*see* Examination, medical
  hearing Z01.10
    with abnormal findings NEC Z01.118
    following failed hearing screening Z01.110
  immunity status testing Z01.84
  laboratory (as part of a general medical examination) Z00.00
    with abnormal findings Z00.01
    preprocedural Z01.812
  lactating mother Z39.1
  medical (adult) (for) (of) Z00.00
    with abnormal findings Z00.01
    administrative purpose only Z02.9
      specified NEC Z02.89
    admission to
      armed forces Z02.3
      old age home Z02.2
      prison Z02.89
      residential institution Z02.2
      school Z02.0
        following illness or medical treatment Z02.0
      summer camp Z02.89
    adoption Z02.82
    blood alcohol or drug level Z02.83
    camp (summer) Z02.89
    clinical research, normal subject (control) (participant) Z00.6
    control subject in clinical research (normal comparison) (participant) Z00.6
    donor (potential) Z00.5
    driving license Z02.4
    general (adult) Z00.00
      with abnormal findings Z00.01
    immigration Z02.89
    insurance purposes Z02.6
    marriage Z02.89
    medicolegal reasons NEC Z04.8
    naturalization Z02.89
    participation in sport Z02.5
    paternity testing Z02.81
    population survey Z00.8
    pre-employment Z02.1
    pre-operative —*see* Examination, pre-procedural
    pre-procedural
      cardiovascular Z01.810
      respiratory Z01.811
      specified NEC Z01.818
    preschool children
      for admission to school Z02.0
    prisoners
      for entrance into prison Z02.89
    recruitment for armed forces Z02.3
    specified NEC Z00.8
    sport competition Z02.5
  medicolegal reason NEC Z04.8
  newborn —*see* Newborn, examination
  pelvic (annual) (periodic) Z01.419
    with abnormal findings Z01.411
  period of rapid growth in childhood Z00.2
  periodic (adult) (annual) (routine) Z00.00
    with abnormal findings Z00.01
  physical (adult) —*see also* Examination, medical Z00.00
    sports Z02.5
  postpartum
    immediately after delivery Z39.0
    routine follow-up Z39.2
  pre-chemotherapy (antineoplastic) Z01.818
  prenatal (normal pregnancy) —*see also* Pregnancy, normal Z34.9-•
  pre-procedural (pre-operative)
    cardiovascular Z01.810
    laboratory Z01.812
    respiratory Z01.811
    specified NEC Z01.818

Examination *(Continued)*
  prior to chemotherapy (antineoplastic) Z01.818
  psychiatric NEC Z00.8
    follow-up not needing further care Z09
    requested by authority Z04.6
  radiological (as part of a general medical examination) Z00.00
    with abnormal findings Z00.01
  repeat cervical smear to confirm findings of recent normal smear following initial abnormal smear Z01.42
  skin (hypersensitivity) Z01.82
  special —*see also* Examination, by type Z01.89
    specified type NEC Z01.89
  specified type or reason NEC Z04.8
  teeth Z01.20
    with abnormal findings Z01.21
  urine —*see* Examination, laboratory
  vision Z01.00
    with abnormal findings Z01.01
Exanthem, exanthema —*see also* Rash
  with enteroviral vesicular stomatitis B08.4
  Boston A88.0
  epidemic with meningitis A88.0 *[G02]*
  subitum B08.20
    due to human herpesvirus 6 B08.21
    due to human herpesvirus 7 B08.22
  viral, virus B09
    specified type NEC B08.8
Excess, excessive, excessively
  alcohol level in blood R78.0
  androgen (ovarian) E28.1
  attrition, tooth, teeth K03.0
  carotene, carotin (dietary) E67.1
  cold, effects of T69.9
    specified effect NEC T69.8
  convergence H51.12
  crying
    in child, adolescent, or adult R45.83
    in infant R68.11
  development, breast N62
  divergence H51.8
  drinking (alcohol) NEC (without dependence) F10.10
    habitual (continual) (without remission) F10.20
  eating R63.2
  estrogen E28.0
  fat —*see also* Obesity
    in heart —*see* Degeneration, myocardial
    localized E65
  foreskin N47.8
  gas R14.0
  glucagon E16.3
  heat —*see* Heat
  intermaxillary vertical dimension of fully erupted teeth M26.37
  interocclusal distance of fully erupted teeth M26.37
  kalium E87.5
  large
    colon K59.39
      congenital Q43.8
    infant P08.0
    organ or site, congenital NEC —*see* Anomaly, by site
  long
    organ or site, congenital NEC —*see* Anomaly, by site
  menstruation (with regular cycle) N92.0
    with irregular cycle N92.1
  napping Z72.821
  natrium E87.0
  number of teeth K00.1
  nutrient (dietary) NEC R63.2
  potassium (K) E87.5
  salivation K11.7
  secretion —*see also* Hypersecretion
    milk O92.6
    sputum R09.3
    sweat R61

Excess, excessive, excessively *(Continued)*
   sexual drive F52.8
   short
      organ or site, congenital NEC —*see*
         Anomaly, by site
      umbilical cord in labor or delivery O69.3
   skin L98.7
      and subcutaneous tissue L98.7
      eyelid (acquired) —*see* Blepharochalasis
         congenital Q10.3
   sodium (Na) E87.0
   spacing of fully erupted teeth M26.32
   sputum R09.3
   sweating R61
   thirst R63.1
      due to deprivation of water T73.1
   tuberosity of jaw M26.07
   vitamin
      A (dietary) E67.0
         administered as drug (prolonged
            intake) —*see* Table of Drugs and
            Chemicals, vitamins, adverse
            effect
         overdose or wrong substance given
            or taken —*see* Table of Drugs and
            Chemicals, vitamins, poisoning
      D (dietary) E67.3
         administered as drug (prolonged
            intake) —*see* Table of Drugs and
            Chemicals, vitamins, adverse
            effect
         overdose or wrong substance given
            or taken —*see* Table of Drugs and
            Chemicals, vitamins, poisoning
   weight
      gain R63.5
      loss R63.4
Excitability, abnormal, under minor stress
      (personality disorder) F60.3
Excitation
   anomalous atrioventricular I45.6
   psychogenic F30.8
   reactive (from emotional stress, psychological
      trauma) F30.8
Excitement
   hypomanic F30.8
   manic F30.9
   mental, reactive (from emotional stress,
      psychological trauma) F30.8
   state, reactive (from emotional stress,
      psychological trauma) F30.8
Excoriation (traumatic) —*see also* Abrasion
   neurotic L98.1
   skin picking disorder F42.4
Exfoliation
   due to erythematous conditions according
      to extent of body surface involved
      L49.0
      10-19 percent of body surface L49.1
      20-29 percent of body surface L49.2
      30-39 percent of body surface L49.3
      40-49 percent of body surface L49.4
      50-59 percent of body surface L49.5
      60-69 percent of body surface L49.6
      70-79 percent of body surface L49.7
      80-89 percent of body surface L49.8
      90-99 percent of body surface L49.9
      less than 10 percent of body surface L49.0
   teeth, due to systemic causes K08.0
Exfoliative —*see* condition
Exhaustion, exhaustive (physical NEC) R53.83
   battle F43.0
   cardiac —*see* Failure, heart
   delirium F43.0
   due to
      cold T69.8
      excessive exertion T73.3
      exposure T73.2
      neurasthenia F48.8
   heart —*see* Failure, heart
   heat —*see also* Heat, exhaustion T67.5

Exhaustion, exhaustive *(Continued)*
   heat *(Continued)*
      due to
         salt depletion T67.4
         water depletion T67.3
   maternal, complicating delivery O75.81
   mental F48.8
   myocardium, myocardial —*see* Failure, heart
   nervous F48.8
   old age R54
   psychogenic F48.8
   psychosis F43.0
   senile R54
   vital NEC Z73.0
Exhibitionism F65.2
Exocervicitis —*see* Cervicitis
Exomphalos Q79.2
   meaning hernia —*see* Hernia, umbilicus
Exophoria H50.52
   convergence, insufficiency H51.11
   divergence, excess H51.8
Exophthalmos H05.2-●
   congenital Q15.8
   constant NEC H05.24-●
   displacement, globe —*see* Displacement,
      globe
   due to thyrotoxicosis (hyperthyroidism) —*see*
      Hyperthyroidism, with, goiter (diffuse)
   dysthyroid —*see* Hyperthyroidism, with,
      goiter (diffuse)
   goiter —*see* Hyperthyroidism, with, goiter
      (diffuse)
   intermittent NEC H05.25-●
   malignant —*see* Hyperthyroidism, with,
      goiter (diffuse)
   orbital
      edema —*see* Edema, orbit
      hemorrhage —*see* Hemorrhage, orbit
   pulsating NEC H05.26-●
   thyrotoxic, thyrotropic —*see*
      Hyperthyroidism, with, goiter (diffuse)
Exostosis —*see also* Disorder, bone
   cartilaginous —*see* Neoplasm, bone, benign
   congenital (multiple) Q78.6
   external ear canal H61.81-●
   gonococcal A54.49
   jaw (bone) M27.8
   multiple, congenital Q78.6
   orbit H05.35-●
   osteocartilaginous —*see* Neoplasm, bone,
      benign
   syphilitic A52.77
Exotropia —*see* Strabismus, divergent
      concomitant
Explanation of
   investigation finding Z71.2
   medication Z71.89
Exposure (to) —*see also* Contact, with T75.89
   acariasis Z20.7
   AIDS virus Z20.6
   air pollution Z77.110
   algae and algae toxins Z77.121
   algae bloom Z77.121
   anthrax Z20.810
   aromatic amines Z77.020
   aromatic (hazardous) compounds NEC
      Z77.028
   aromatic dyes NOS Z77.028
   arsenic Z77.010
   asbestos Z77.090
   bacterial disease NEC Z20.818
   benzene Z77.021
   blue-green algae bloom Z77.121
   body fluids (potentially hazardous) Z77.21
   brown tide Z77.121
   chemicals (chiefly nonmedicinal) (hazardous)
      NEC Z77.098
   cholera Z20.09
   chromium compounds Z77.018
   cold, effects of T69.9
      specified effect NEC T69.8

Exposure *(Continued)*
   communicable disease Z20.9
      bacterial NEC Z20.818
      specified NEC Z20.89
      viral NEC Z20.828
   cyanobacteria bloom Z77.121
   disaster Z65.5
   discrimination Z60.5
   dyes Z77.098
   effects of T73.9
   environmental tobacco smoke (acute)
      (chronic) Z77.22
   Escherichia coli (E. coli) Z20.01
   exhaustion due to T73.2
   fiberglass —*see* Table of Drugs and
      Chemicals, fiberglass
   German measles Z20.4
   gonorrhea Z20.2
   hazardous metals NEC Z77.018
   hazardous substances NEC Z77.29
   hazards in the physical environment NEC
      Z77.128
   hazards to health NEC Z77.9
   human immunodeficiency virus (HIV) Z20.6
   human T-lymphotropic virus type-1 (HTLV-1)
      Z20.89
   implanted
      mesh —*see* Complications, mesh
      prosthetic materials NEC —*see*
         Complications, prosthetic materials
         NEC
   infestation (parasitic) NEC Z20.7
   intestinal infectious disease NEC Z20.09
      Escherichia coli (E. coli) Z20.01
   lead Z77.011
   meningococcus Z20.811
   mold (toxic) Z77.120
   nickel dust Z77.018
   noise Z77.122
   occupational
      air contaminants NEC Z57.39
      dust Z57.2
      environmental tobacco smoke Z57.31
      extreme temperature Z57.6
      noise Z57.0
      radiation Z57.1
      risk factors Z57.9
         specified NEC Z57.8
      toxic agents (gases) (liquids) (solids)
         (vapors) in agriculture Z57.4
      toxic agents (gases) (liquids) (solids)
         (vapors) in industry NEC Z57.5
      vibration Z57.7
   parasitic disease NEC Z20.7
   pediculosis Z20.7
   persecution Z60.5
   pfiesteria piscicida Z77.121
   poliomyelitis Z20.89
   pollution
      air Z77.110
      environmental NEC Z77.118
      soil Z77.112
      water Z77.111
   polycyclic aromatic hydrocarbons
      Z77.028
   prenatal (drugs) (toxic chemicals) —*see*
      Newborn, affected by, noxious
      substances transmitted via placenta or
      breast milk
   rabies Z20.3
   radiation, naturally occurring NEC Z77.123
   radon Z77.123
   red tide (Florida) Z77.121
   rubella Z20.4
   second hand tobacco smoke (acute) (chronic)
      Z77.22
      in the perinatal period P96.81
   sexually-transmitted disease Z20.2
   smallpox (laboratory) Z20.89
   syphilis Z20.2
   terrorism Z65.4

Exposure *(Continued)*
  torture Z65.4
  tuberculosis Z20.1
  uranium Z77.012
  varicella Z20.820
  venereal disease Z20.2
  viral disease NEC Z20.828
  war Z65.5
  water pollution Z77.111
Exsanguination —*see* Hemorrhage
Exstrophy
  abdominal contents Q45.8
  bladder Q64.10
    cloacal Q64.12
    specified type NEC Q64.19
    supravesical fissure Q64.11
Extensive —*see* condition
Extra —*see also* Accessory
  marker chromosomes (normal individual)
      Q92.61
    in abnormal individual Q92.62

Extra *(Continued)*
  rib Q76.6
    cervical Q76.5
Extrasystoles (supraventricular) I49.49
  atrial I49.1
  auricular I49.1
  junctional I49.2
  ventricular I49.3
Extrauterine gestation or pregnancy —*see*
    Pregnancy, by site
Extravasation
  blood R58
  chyle into mesentery I89.8
  pelvicalyceal N13.8
  pyelosinus N13.8
  urine (from ureter) R39.0
  vesicant agent
    antineoplastic chemotherapy T80.810
    other agent NEC T80.818
Extremity —*see* condition, limb
Extrophy —*see* Exstrophy

Extroversion
  bladder Q64.19
  uterus N81.4
    complicating delivery O71.2
    postpartal (old) N81.4
Extruded tooth (teeth) M26.34
Extrusion
  breast implant (prosthetic) T85.42
  eye implant (globe) (ball) T85.328
  intervertebral disc —*see* Displacement,
      intervertebral disc
  ocular lens implant (prosthetic) —*see*
      Complications, intraocular lens
  vitreous —*see* Prolapse, vitreous
Exudate
  pleural —*see* Effusion, pleura
  retina H35.89
Exudative —*see* condition
Eye, eyeball, eyelid —*see* condition
Eyestrain —*see* Disturbance, vision, subjective
Eyeworm disease of Africa B74.3

▶ New   ⇒ Revised   ~~deleted~~ Deleted   • Use Additional Character(s)

F

Faber's syndrome (achlorhydric anemia) D50.9
Fabry (-Anderson) disease E75.21
Faciocephalalgia, autonomic —*see also*
  Neuropathy, peripheral, autonomic G90.09
Factor(s)
  psychic, associated with diseases classified
    elsewhere F54
  psychological
    affecting physical conditions F54
    or behavioral
      affecting general medical condition F54
      associated with disorders or diseases
        classified elsewhere F54
Fahr disease (of brain) G23.8
Fahr Volhard disease (of kidney) I12.-•
Failure, failed
  abortion —*see* Abortion, attempted
  aortic (valve) I35.8
    rheumatic I06.8
  attempted abortion —*see* Abortion, attempted
  biventricular I50.82
    due to left heart failure I50.814
  bone marrow —*see* Anemia, aplastic
  cardiac —*see* Failure, heart
  cardiorenal (chronic) —*see also* Failure, renal,
    and Failure, heart I50.9
    hypertensive I13.2
  cardiorespiratory (*see also* Failure, heart) R09.2
  cardiovascular (chronic) —*see* Failure, heart
  cerebrovascular I67.9
  cervical dilatation in labor O62.0
  circulation, circulatory (peripheral) R57.9
    newborn P29.89
  compensation —*see* Disease, heart
  compliance with medical treatment or
    regimen —*see* Noncompliance
  congestive —*see* Failure, heart, congestive
  dental implant (endosseous) M27.69
    due to
      failure of dental prosthesis M27.63
      lack of attached gingiva M27.62
      occlusal trauma (poor prosthetic design)
        M27.62
      parafunctional habits M27.62
      periodontal infection (peri-implantitis)
        M27.62
      poor oral hygiene M27.62
    osseointegration M27.61
      due to
        complications of systemic disease
          M27.61
        poor bone quality M27.61
      iatrogenic M27.61
    post-osseointegration
      biological M27.62
      due to complications of systemic disease
        M27.62
      iatrogenic M27.62
      mechanical M27.63
    pre-integration M27.61
    pre-osseointegration M27.61
    specified NEC M27.69
  descent of head (at term) of pregnancy
    (mother) O32.4
  endosseous dental implant —*see* Failure,
    dental implant
  engagement of head (term of pregnancy)
    (mother) O32.4
  erection (penile) —*see also* Dysfunction,
    sexual, male, erectile N52.9
    nonorganic F52.21
  examination(s), anxiety concerning Z55.2
  expansion terminal respiratory units
    (newborn) (primary) P28.0
  forceps NOS (with subsequent cesarean
    delivery) O66.5
  gain weight (child over 28 days old) R62.51
    adult R62.7
    newborn P92.6

Failure, failed (*Continued*)
  genital response (male) F52.21
    female F52.22
  heart (acute) (senile) (sudden) I50.9
    with
      acute pulmonary edema —*see* Failure,
        ventricular, left
      decompensation —*see also* Failure, heart,
        by type as diastolic or systolic,
        acute and chronic I50.9
      dilatation —*see* Disease, heart
      normal ejection fraction —*see* Failure,
        heart, diastolic
      preserved ejection fraction —*see* Failure,
        heart, diastolic
      reduced ejection fraction —*see* Failure,
        heart, systolic
    arteriosclerotic I70.90
    biventricular I50.82
      due to left heart failure I50.814
    combined left-right sided I50.82
      due to left heart failure I50.814
    compensated —*see also* Failure, heart, by
      type as diastolic or systolic, chronic
      I50.9
    complicating
      anesthesia (general) (local) or other
        sedation
        in labor and delivery O74.2
        in pregnancy O29.12-•
        postpartum, puerperal O89.1
      delivery (cesarean) (instrumental) O75.4
    congestive I50.9
      with rheumatic fever (conditions in I00)
        active I01.8
        inactive or quiescent (with chorea)
          I09.81
      newborn P29.0
      rheumatic (chronic) (inactive) (with
        chorea) I09.81
        active or acute I01.8
        with chorea I02.0
    decompensated —*see also* Failure, heart, by
      type as diastolic or systolic, acute and
      chronic I50.9
    degenerative —*see* Degeneration,
      myocardial
    diastolic (congestive) (left ventricular)
      I50.30
      acute (congestive) I50.31
        and (on) chronic (congestive) I50.33
      chronic (congestive) I50.32
        and (on) acute (congestive) I50.33
      combined with systolic (congestive)
        I50.40
        acute (congestive) I50.41
          and (on) chronic (congestive) I50.43
        chronic (congestive) I50.42
          and (on) acute (congestive) I50.43
      due to presence of cardiac prosthesis I97.13-•
    end stage —*see also* Failure, heart, by type
      as diastolic or systolic, chronic I50.84
    following cardiac surgery I97.13-•
    high output NOS I50.83
    hypertensive —*see* Hypertension, heart
    left (ventricular) —*see also* Failure,
      ventricular, left
      combined diastolic and systolic —*see*
        Failure, heart, diastolic, combined
        with systolic
      diastolic —*see* Failure, heart, diastolic
      systolic —*see* Failure, heart, systolic
    low output (syndrome) NOS I50.9
    newborn P29.0
    organic —*see* Disease, heart
    peripartum O90.3
    postprocedural I97.13-•
    rheumatic (chronic) (inactive) I09.9
    right (isolated) (ventricular) I50.810
      acute I50.811
        and (on) chronic I50.813

Failure, failed (*Continued*)
  heart (*Continued*)
    right (*Continued*)
      chronic I50.812
        and acute I50.813
      secondary to left heart failure I50.814
    ~~systolic (congestive) I50.20~~
    ~~acute (congestive) I50.21~~
      ~~and (on) chronic (congestive)~~
        ~~I50.23~~
    ~~chronic (congestive) I50.22~~
      ~~and (on) acute (congestive) I50.23~~
    ~~combined with diastolic (congestive)~~
      ~~I50.40~~
    ~~acute (congestive) I50.41~~
      ~~and (on) chronic (congestive)~~
        ~~I50.43~~
    ~~chronic (congestive) I50.42~~
      ~~and (on) acute (congestive)~~
        ~~I50.43~~
    ~~thyrotoxic —*see also* Thyrotoxicosis~~
      ~~E05.90 [I43]~~
      ~~with thyroid storm E05.91 [I43]~~
    ~~valvular —*see* Endocarditis~~
    specified NEC I50.89

> Note: heart failure stages A, B, C, and
> D are based on the American College of
> Cardiology and American Heart Association
> stages of heart failure, which complement
> and should not be confused with the New
> York Heart Association Classification of
> Heart Failure, into Class I, Class II, Class III,
> and Class IV

    stage A Z91.89
    stage B (see also Failure, heart, by type as
      diastolic or systolic) I50.9
    stage C (see also Failure, heart, by type as
      diastolic or systolic) I50.9
    stage D (see also Failure, heart, by type as
      diastolic or systolic, chronic) I50.84
    systolic (congestive) (left ventricular) I50.20
      acute (congestive) I50.21
        and (on) chronic (congestive) I50.23
      chronic (congestive) I50.22
        and (on) acute (congestive) I50.23
      combined with diastolic (congestive)
        I50.40
        acute (congestive) I50.41
          and (on) chronic (congestive) I50.43
        chronic (congestive) I50.42
          and (on) acute (congestive) I50.43
    thyrotoxic (see also Thyrotoxicosis) E05.90
      [I43]
    with
      high output (see also Thyrotoxicosis)
        I50.83
      thyroid storm E05.91 [I43]
        high output (see also
          Thyrotoxicosis) I50.83
    valvular —*see* Endocarditis
  hepatic K72.90
    with coma K72.91
    acute or subacute K72.00
      with coma K72.01
      due to drugs K71.10
        with coma K71.11
    alcoholic (acute) (chronic) (subacute)
      K70.40
      with coma K70.41
    chronic K72.10
      with coma K72.11
      due to drugs (acute) (subacute) (chronic)
        K71.10
        with coma K71.11
    due to drugs (acute) (subacute) (chronic)
      K71.10
      with coma K71.11
    postprocedural K91.82

Failure, failed (Continued)
hepatorenal K76.7
induction (of labor) O61.9
   abortion —see Abortion, attempted
   by
      oxytocic drugs O61.0
      prostaglandins O61.0
   instrumental O61.1
   mechanical O61.1
   medical O61.0
   specified NEC O61.8
   surgical O61.1
intubation during anesthesia T88.4
   in pregnancy O29.6-●
   labor and delivery O74.7
   postpartum, puerperal O89.6
involution, thymus (gland) E32.0
kidney —see also Disease, kidney, chronic N19
   acute —see also Failure, renal, acute
      N17.9-●
   diabetic —see E08-E13 with .22
lactation (complete) O92.3
   partial O92.4
Leydig's cell, adult E29.1
liver —see Failure, hepatic
menstruation at puberty N91.0
mitral I05.8
myocardial, myocardium —see also Failure,
      heart I50.9
   chronic —see also Failure, heart, congestive
      I50.9
   congestive —see also Failure, heart,
      congestive I50.9
orgasm (female) (psychogenic) F52.31
   male F52.32
ovarian (primary) E28.39
   iatrogenic E89.40
      asymptomatic E89.40
      symptomatic E89.41
   postprocedural (postablative)
      (postirradiation) (postsurgical) E89.40
      asymptomatic E89.40
      symptomatic E89.41
ovulation causing infertility N97.0
polyglandular, autoimmune E31.0
prosthetic joint implant —see Complications,
      joint prosthesis, mechanical, breakdown,
      by site
renal N19
   with
      tubular necrosis (acute) N17.0
   acute N17.9
      with
         cortical necrosis N17.1
         medullary necrosis N17.2
         tubular necrosis N17.0
      specified NEC N17.8
   chronic N18.9
      hypertensive —see Hypertension, kidney
   congenital P96.0
   end stage (chronic) N18.6
      due to hypertension I12.0
   following
      abortion —see Abortion by type
         complicated by specified
            condition NEC
      crushing T79.5
      ectopic or molar pregnancy O08.4
      labor and delivery (acute) O90.4
   hypertensive —see Hypertension, kidney
   postprocedural N99.0
respiration, respiratory J96.9
   with
      hypercapnia J96.92
      ▶hypercarbia J96.02
      hypoxia J96.91
   acute J96.00
      with
         hypercapnia J96.02
         ▶hypercarbia J96.02
         hypoxia J96.01

Failure, failed (Continued)
respiration, respiratory (Continued)
   acute and (on) chronic J96.20
      with
         hypercapnia J96.22
         ▶hypercarbia J96.22
         hypoxia J96.21
   center G93.89
   chronic J96.10
      with
         hypercapnia J96.12
         ▶hypercarbia J96.12
         hypoxia J96.11
   newborn P28.5
   postprocedural (acute) J95.821
      acute and chronic J95.822
rotation
   cecum Q43.3
   colon Q43.3
   intestine Q43.3
   kidney Q63.2
sedation (conscious) (moderate) during
      procedure T88.52
   history of Z92.83
segmentation —see also Fusion
   fingers —see Syndactylism, complex,
      fingers
   vertebra Q76.49
      with scoliosis Q76.3
seminiferous tubule, adult E29.1
senile (general) R54
sexual arousal (male) F52.21
   female F52.22
testicular endocrine function E29.1
to thrive (child over 28 days old) R62.51
   adult R62.7
   newborn P92.6
transplant T86.92
   bone T86.831
      marrow T86.02
   cornea T86.841
   heart T86.22
      with lung(s) T86.32
   intestine T86.851
   kidney T86.12
   liver T86.42
   lung(s) T86.811
      with heart T86.32
   pancreas T86.891
   skin (allograft) (autograft) T86.821
   specified organ or tissue NEC T86.891
   stem cell (peripheral blood) (umbilical
      cord) T86.5
trial of labor (with subsequent cesarean
      delivery) O66.40
   following previous cesarean delivery
      O66.41
tubal ligation N99.89
urinary —see Disease, kidney, chronic
vacuum extraction NOS (with subsequent
      cesarean delivery) O66.5
vasectomy N99.89
ventouse NOS (with subsequent cesarean
      delivery) O66.5
ventricular —see also Failure, heart I50.9
   ▬▶left —see also Failure, heart, left I50.1
      with rheumatic fever (conditions in I00)
         active I01.8
            with chorea I02.0
         inactive or quiescent (with chorea)
            I09.81
      rheumatic (chronic) (inactive) (with
         chorea) I09.81
         active or acute I01.8
            with chorea I02.0
   ▬▶right —see Failure, heart, right
▬▶vital centers, newborn P91.88
Fainting (fit) R55
Fallen arches —see Deformity, limb, flat foot
Falling, falls (repeated) R29.6
   any organ or part —see Prolapse

Fallopian
   insufflation Z31.41
   tube —see condition
Fallot's
   pentalogy Q21.8
   tetrad or tetralogy Q21.3
   triad or trilogy Q22.3
False —see also condition
   croup J38.5
   joint —see Nonunion, fracture
   labor (pains) O47.9
      at or after 37 completed weeks of gestation
         O47.1
      before 37 completed weeks of gestation
         O47.0-●
   passage, urethra (prostatic) N36.5
   pregnancy F45.8
Family, familial —see also condition
   disruption Z63.8
      involving divorce or separation Z63.5
   Li-Fraumeni (syndrome) Z15.01
   planning advice Z30.09
   problem Z63.9
      specified NEC Z63.8
   retinoblastoma C69.2-●
Famine (effects of) T73.0
   edema —see Malnutrition, severe
Fanconi (-de Toni)(-Debré) syndrome E72.09
   with cystinosis E72.04
Fanconi's anemia (congenital pancytopenia)
      D61.09
Farber's disease or syndrome E75.29
Farcy A24.0
Farmer's
   lung J67.0
   skin L57.8
Farsightedness —see Hypermetropia
Fascia —see condition
Fasciculation R25.3
Fasciitis M72.9
   diffuse (eosinophilic) M35.4
   infective M72.8
      necrotizing M72.6
   necrotizing M72.6
   nodular M72.4
   perirenal (with ureteral obstruction) N13.5
      with infection N13.6
   plantar M72.2
   specified NEC M72.8
   traumatic (old) M72.8
      current - code by site under Sprain
Fascioliasis B66.3
Fasciolopsis, fasciolopsiasis (intestinal) B66.5
Fascioscapulohumeral myopathy G71.0
Fast pulse R00.0
Fat
   embolism —see Embolism, fat
   excessive —see also Obesity
      in heart —see Degeneration, myocardial
   in stool R19.5
   localized (pad) E65
      heart —see Degeneration, myocardial
      knee M79.4
      retropatellar M79.4
   necrosis
      breast N64.1
      mesentery K65.4
      omentum K65.4
   pad E65
      knee M79.4
Fatigue R53.83
   auditory deafness —see Deafness
   chronic R53.82
   combat F43.0
   general R53.83
      psychogenic F48.8
   heat (transient) T67.6
   muscle M62.89
   myocardium —see Failure, heart
   neoplasm-related R53.0
   nervous, neurosis F48.8

▶ New ▬▶ Revised ~~deleted~~ Deleted ● Use Additional Character(s)

Fatigue (Continued)
    operational F48.8
    psychogenic (general) F48.8
    senile R54
    voice R49.8
Fatness —see Obesity
Fatty —see also condition
    apron E65
    degeneration —see Degeneration, fatty
    heart (enlarged) —see Degeneration,
        myocardial
    liver NEC K76.0
        alcoholic K70.0
        nonalcoholic K76.0
    necrosis —see Degeneration, fatty
Fauces —see condition
Fauchard's disease (periodontitis) —see
    Periodontitis
Faucitis J02.9
Favism (anemia) D55.0
Favus —see Dermatophytosis
Fazio-Londe disease or syndrome G12.1
Fear complex or reaction F40.9
Fear of —see Phobia
Feared complaint unfounded Z71.1
Febris, febrile —see also Fever
    flava —see also Fever, yellow A95.9
    melitensis A23.0
    pestis —see Plague
    recurrens —see Fever, relapsing
    rubra A38.9
Fecal
    incontinence R15.9
    smearing R15.1
    soiling R15.1
    urgency R15.2
Fecalith (impaction) K56.41
    appendix K38.1
    congenital P76.8
Fede's disease K14.0
Feeble rapid pulse due to shock following
    injury T79.4
Feeble-minded F70
Feeding
    difficulties R63.3
    problem R63.3
        newborn P92.9
            specified NEC P92.8
        nonorganic (adult) —see Disorder, eating
Feeling (of)
    foreign body in throat R09.89
Feer's disease —see Poisoning, mercury
Feet —see condition
Feigned illness Z76.5
Feil-Klippel syndrome (brevicollis) Q76.1
Feinmesser's (hidrotic) ectodermal dysplasia
    Q82.4
Felinophobia F40.218
Felon —see also Cellulitis, digit
    with lymphangitis —see Lymphangitis, acute,
        digit
Felty's syndrome M05.00
    ankle M05.07-●
    elbow M05.02-●
    foot joint M05.07-●
    hand joint M05.04-●
    hip M05.05-●
    knee M05.06-●
    multiple site M05.09
    shoulder M05.01-●
    vertebra —see Spondylitis, ankylosing
    wrist M05.03-●
Female genital cutting status —see Female
    genital mutilation status (FGM)
Female genital mutilation status (FGM) N90.810
    specified NEC N90.818
    type I (clitorectomy status) N90.811
    type II (clitorectomy with excision of labia
        minora status) N90.812
    type III (infibulation status) N90.813
    type IV N90.818

Femur, femoral —see condition
Fenestration, fenestrated —see also Imperfect,
    closure
    aortico-pulmonary Q21.4
    cusps, heart valve NEC Q24.8
        pulmonary Q22.3
    pulmonic cusps Q22.3
Fernell's disease (aortic aneurysm) I71.9
Fertile eunuch syndrome E23.0
Fetid
    breath R19.6
    sweat L75.0
Fetishism F65.0
    transvestic F65.1
Fetus, fetal —see also condition
    alcohol syndrome (dysmorphic) Q86.0
    compressus O31.0-●
    hydantoin syndrome Q86.1
    lung tissue P28.0
    papyraceous O31.0-●
Fever (inanition) (of unknown origin)
    (persistent) (with chills) (with rigor) R50.9
    abortus A23.1
    Aden (dengue) A90
    African tick-borne A68.1
    American
        mountain (tick) A93.2
        spotted A77.0
    aphthous B08.8
    arbovirus, arboviral A94
        hemorrhagic A94
        specified NEC A93.8
    Argentinian hemorrhagic A96.0
    Assam B55.0
    Australian Q A78
    Bangkok hemorrhagic A91
    Barmah forest A92.8
    Bartonella A44.0
    bilious, hemoglobinuric B50.8
    blackwater B50.8
    blister B00.1
    Bolivian hemorrhagic A96.1
    Bonvale dam T73.3
    boutonneuse A77.1
    brain —see Encephalitis
    Brazilian purpuric A48.4
    breakbone A90
    Bullis A77.0
    Bunyamwera A92.8
    Burdwan B55.0
    Bwamba A92.8
    Cameroon —see Malaria
    Canton A75.9
    catarrhal (acute) J00
        chronic J31.0
    cat-scratch A28.1
    Central Asian hemorrhagic A98.0
    cerebral —see Encephalitis
    cerebrospinal meningococcal A39.0
    Chagres B50.9
    Chandipura A92.8
    Changuinola A93.1
    Charcot's (biliary) (hepatic) (intermittent) —
        see Calculus, bile duct
    Chikungunya (viral) (hemorrhagic) A92.0
    Chitral A93.1
    Colombo —see Fever, paratyphoid
    Colorado tick (virus) A93.2
    congestive (remittent) —see Malaria
    Congo virus A98.0
    continued malarial B50.9
    Corsican —see Malaria
    Crimean-Congo hemorrhagic A98.0
    Cyprus —see Brucellosis
    dandy A90
    deer fly —see Tularemia
    dengue (virus) A90
        hemorrhagic A91
        sandfly A93.1
    desert B38.0
    drug induced R50.2

Fever (Continued)
    due to
        conditions classified elsewhere
            R50.81
        heat T67.0
    enteric A01.00
    enteroviral exanthematous (Boston
        exanthem) A88.0
    ephemeral (of unknown origin) R50.9
    epidemic hemorrhagic A98.5
    erysipelatous —see Erysipelas
    estivo-autumnal (malarial) B50.9
    famine A75.0
    five day A79.0
    following delivery O86.4
    Fort Bragg A27.89
    gastroenteric A01.00
    gastromalarial —see Malaria
    Gibraltar —see Brucellosis
    glandular —see Mononucleosis, infectious
    Guama (viral) A92.8
    Haverhill A25.1
    hay (allergic) J30.1
        with asthma (bronchial) J45.909
            with
                exacerbation (acute) J45.901
                status asthmaticus J45.902
        due to
            allergen other than pollen J30.89
            pollen, any plant or tree J30.1
    heat (effects) T67.0
    hematuric, bilious B50.8
    hemoglobinuric (malarial) (bilious) B50.8
    hemorrhagic (arthropod-borne) NOS A94
        with renal syndrome A98.5
        arenaviral A96.9
            specified NEC A96.8
        Argentinian A96.0
        Bangkok A91
        Bolivian A96.1
        Central Asian A98.0
        Chikungunya A92.0
        Crimean-Congo A98.0
        dengue (virus) A91
        epidemic A98.5
        Junin (virus) A96.0
        Korean A98.5
        Kyasanur forest A98.2
        Machupo (virus) A96.1
        mite-borne A93.8
        mosquito-borne A92.8
        Omsk A98.1
        Philippine A91
        Russian A98.5
        Singapore A91
        Southeast Asia A91
        Thailand A91
        tick-borne NEC A93.8
        viral A99
            specified NEC A98.8
    hepatic —see Cholecystitis
    herpetic —see Herpes
    icterohemorrhagic A27.0
    Indiana A93.8
    infective B99.9
        specified NEC B99.8
    intermittent (bilious) —see also Malaria
        of unknown origin R50.9
        pernicious B50.9
    iodide R50.2
    Japanese river A75.3
    jungle —see also Malaria
        yellow A95.0
    Junin (virus) hemorrhagic A96.0
    Katayama B65.2
    kedani A75.3
    Kenya (tick) A77.1
    Kew Garden A79.1
    Korean hemorrhagic A98.5
    Lassa A96.2
    Lone Star A77.0

Fever *(Continued)*
 Machupo (virus) hemorrhagic A96.1
 malaria, malarial —*see* Malaria
 Malta A23.9
 Marseilles A77.1
 marsh —*see* Malaria
 Mayaro (viral) A92.8
 Mediterranean —*see also* Brucellosis A23.9
  familial M04.1
  tick A77.1
 meningeal —*see* Meningitis
 Meuse A79.0
 Mexican A75.2
 mianeh A68.1
 miasmatic —*see* Malaria
 mosquito-borne (viral) A92.9
  hemorrhagic A92.8
 mountain —*see also* Brucellosis
  meaning Rocky Mountain spotted fever
   A77.0
  tick (American) (Colorado) (viral) A93.2
 Mucambo (viral) A92.8
 mud A27.9
 Neapolitan —*see* Brucellosis
 neutropenic D70.9
 newborn P81.9
  environmental P81.0
 Nine-Mile A78
 non-exanthematous tick A93.2
 North Asian tick-borne A77.2
 Omsk hemorrhagic A98.1
 O'nyong-nyong (viral) A92.1
 Oropouche (viral) A93.0
 Oroya A44.0
 paludal —*see* Malaria
 Panama (malarial) B50.9
 Pappataci A93.1
 paratyphoid A01.4
  A A01.1
  B A01.2
  C A01.3
 parrot A70
 periodic (Mediterranean) M04.1
 persistent (of unknown origin) R50.9
 petechial A39.0
 pharyngoconjunctival B30.2
 Philippine hemorrhagic A91
 phlebotomus A93.1
 Piry (virus) A93.8
 Pixuna (viral) A92.8
 Plasmodium ovale B53.0
 polioviral (nonparalytic) A80.4
 Pontiac A48.2
 postimmunization R50.83
 postoperative R50.82
 ➡ due to infection T81.4
 posttransfusion R50.84
 postvaccination R50.83
 presenting with conditions classified
   elsewhere R50.81
 pretibial A27.89
 puerperal O86.4
 Q A78
 quadrilateral A78
 quartan (malaria) B52.9
 Queensland (coastal) (tick) A77.3
 quintan A79.0
 rabbit —*see* Tularemia
 rat-bite A25.9
  due to
   Spirillum A25.0
   Streptobacillus moniliformis A25.1
 recurrent —*see* Fever, relapsing
 relapsing (Borrelia) A68.9
  Carter's (Asiatic) A68.1
  Dutton's (West African) A68.1
  Koch's A68.9
  louse-borne A68.0
  Novy's
   louse-borne A68.0
   tick-borne A68.1

Fever *(Continued)*
 relapsing (Borrelia) *(Continued)*
  Obermeyer's (European) A68.0
  tick-borne A68.1
 remittent (bilious) (congestive) (gastric) —*see*
   Malaria
 rheumatic (active) (acute) (chronic) (subacute)
   I00
  with central nervous system involvement
   I02.9
  active with heart involvement —*see*
    category I01
  inactive or quiescent with
   cardiac hypertrophy I09.89
   carditis I09.9
   endocarditis I09.1
    aortic (valve) I06.9
     with mitral (valve) disease I08.0
    mitral (valve) I05.9
     with aortic (valve) disease I08.0
    pulmonary (valve) I09.89
    tricuspid (valve) I07.8
   heart disease NEC I09.89
  ➡ heart failure (congestive) (conditions in
    I50.) I09.81
  ➡ left ventricular failure (conditions in
    I50.- I50.4-) I09.81
   myocarditis, myocardial degeneration
    (conditions in I51.4) I09.0
   pancarditis I09.9
   pericarditis I09.2
 Rift Valley (viral) A92.4
 Rocky Mountain spotted A77.0
 rose J30.1
 Ross River B33.1
 Russian hemorrhagic A98.5
 San Joaquin (Valley) B38.0
 sandfly A93.1
 Sao Paulo A77.0
 scarlet A38.9
 seven day (leptospirosis) (autumnal)
   (Japanese) A27.89
  dengue A90
 shin-bone A79.0
 Singapore hemorrhagic A91
 solar A90
 Songo A98.5
 sore B00.1
 South African tick-bite A68.1
 Southeast Asia hemorrhagic A91
 spinal —*see* Meningitis
 spirillary A25.0
 splenic —*see* Anthrax
 spotted A77.9
  American A77.0
  Brazilian A77.0
  cerebrospinal meningitis A39.0
  Colombian A77.0
  due to Rickettsia
   australis A77.3
   conorii A77.1
   rickettsii A77.0
   sibirica A77.2
   specified type NEC A77.8
  Ehrlichiosis A77.40
   due to
    E. chafeensis A77.41
    specified organism NEC A77.49
  Rocky Mountain A77.0
 steroid R50.2
 streptobacillary A25.1
 subtertian B50.9
 Sumatran mite A75.3
 sun A90
 swamp A27.9
 swine A02.8
 sylvatic, yellow A95.0
 Tahyna B33.8
 tertian —*see* Malaria, tertian
 Thailand hemorrhagic A91
 thermic T67.0

Fever *(Continued)*
 three-day A93.1
 tick
  American mountain A93.2
  Colorado A93.2
  Kemerovo A93.8
  Mediterranean A77.1
  mountain A93.2
  nonexanthematous A93.2
  Quaranfil A93.8
 tick-bite NEC A93.8
 tick-borne (hemorrhagic) NEC A93.8
 trench A79.0
 tsutsugamushi A75.3
 typhogastric A01.00
 typhoid (abortive) (hemorrhagic)
   (intermittent) (malignant) A01.00
  complicated by
   arthritis A01.04
   heart involvement A01.02
   meningitis A01.01
   osteomyelitis A01.05
   pneumonia A01.03
   specified NEC A01.09
 typhomalarial —*see* Malaria
 typhus —*see* Typhus (fever)
 undulant —*see* Brucellosis
 unknown origin R50.9
 uveoparotid D86.89
 valley B38.0
 Venezuelan equine A92.2
 vesicular stomatitis A93.8
 viral hemorrhagic —*see* Fever, hemorrhagic,
   by type of virus
 Volhynian A79.0
 Wesselsbron (viral) A92.8
 West
  African B50.8
  Nile (viral) A92.30
   with
    complications NEC A92.39
    cranial nerve disorders A92.32
    encephalitis A92.31
    encephalomyelitis A92.31
    neurologic manifestation NEC
     A92.32
    optic neuritis A92.32
    polyradiculitis A92.32
 Whitmore's —*see* Melioidosis
 Wolhynian A79.0
 worm B83.9
 yellow A95.9
  jungle A95.0
  sylvatic A95.0
  urban A95.1
 Zika virus A92.5
Fibrillation
 atrial or auricular (established) I48.91
  chronic I48.2
  paroxysmal I48.0
  permanent I48.2
  persistent I48.1
 cardiac I49.8
 heart I49.8
 muscular M62.89
 ventricular I49.01
Fibrin
 ball or bodies, pleural (sac) J94.1
 chamber, anterior (eye) (gelatinous
   exudate) —*see* Iridocyclitis, acute
Fibrinogenolysis —*see* Fibrinolysis
Fibrinogenopenia D68.8
 acquired D65
 congenital D68.2
Fibrinolysis (hemorrhagic) (acquired) D65
 antepartum hemorrhage —*see* Hemorrhage,
   antepartum, with coagulation defect
 following
  abortion —*see* Abortion by type
    complicated by hemorrhage
  ectopic or molar pregnancy O08.1

▶ New   ➡ Revised   ~~deleted~~ Deleted   ● Use Additional Character(s)

Fibrinolysis *(Continued)*
  intrapartum O67.0
  newborn, transient P60
  postpartum O72.3
Fibrinopenia (hereditary) D68.2
  acquired D68.4
Fibrinopurulent —*see* condition
Fibrinous —*see* condition
Fibroadenoma
  cellular intracanalicular D24-●
  giant D24-●
  intracanalicular
    cellular D24-●
    giant D24-●
    specified site —*see* Neoplasm, benign, by site
    unspecified site D24-●
  juvenile D24-●
  pericanalicular
    specified site —*see* Neoplasm, benign, by site
    unspecified site D24-●
  phyllodes D24-●
  prostate D29.1
  specified site NEC —*see* Neoplasm, benign, by site
  unspecified site D24-●
Fibroadenosis, breast (chronic) (cystic) (diffuse) (periodic) (segmental) N60.2-●
Fibroangioma —*see also* Neoplasm, benign, by site
  juvenile
    specified site —*see* Neoplasm, benign, by site
    unspecified site D10.6
Fibrochondrosarcoma —*see* Neoplasm, cartilage, malignant
Fibrocystic
  disease —*see also* Fibrosis, cystic
    breast —*see* Mastopathy, cystic
    jaw M27.49
    kidney (congenital) Q61.8
    liver Q44.6
    pancreas E84.9
  kidney (congenital) Q61.8
Fibrodysplasia ossificans progressiva —*see* Myositis, ossificans, progressiva
Fibroelastosis (cordis) (endocardial) (endomyocardial) I42.4
Fibroid (tumor) —*see also* Neoplasm, connective tissue, benign
  disease, lung (chronic) —*see* Fibrosis, lung
  heart (disease) —*see* Myocarditis
  in pregnancy or childbirth O34.1-●
    causing obstructed labor O65.5
  induration, lung (chronic) —*see* Fibrosis, lung
  lung —*see* Fibrosis, lung
  pneumonia (chronic) —*see* Fibrosis, lung
  uterus —*see also* Leiomyoma, uterus D25.9
Fibrolipoma —*see* Lipoma
Fibroliposarcoma —*see* Neoplasm, connective tissue, malignant
Fibroma —*see also* Neoplasm, connective tissue, benign
  ameloblastic —*see* Cyst, calcifying odontogenic
  bone (nonossifying) —*see* Disorder, bone, specified type NEC
    ossifying —*see* Neoplasm, bone, benign
  cementifying —*see* Neoplasm, bone, benign
  chondromyxoid —*see* Neoplasm, bone, benign
  desmoplastic —*see* Neoplasm, connective tissue, uncertain behavior
  durum —*see* Neoplasm, connective tissue, benign
  fascial —*see* Neoplasm, connective tissue, benign
  invasive —*see* Neoplasm, connective tissue, uncertain behavior
  molle —*see* Lipoma

Fibroma *(Continued)*
  myxoid —*see* Neoplasm, connective tissue, benign
  nasopharynx, nasopharyngeal (juvenile) D10.6
  nonosteogenic (nonossifying) —*see* Dysplasia, fibrous
  odontogenic (central) —*see* Cyst, calcifying odontogenic
  ossifying —*see* Neoplasm, bone, benign
  periosteal —*see* Neoplasm, bone, benign
  soft —*see* Lipoma
Fibromatosis M72.9
  abdominal —*see* Neoplasm, connective tissue, uncertain behavior
  aggressive —*see* Neoplasm, connective tissue, uncertain behavior
  congenital generalized —*see* Neoplasm, connective tissue, uncertain behavior
  Dupuytren's M72.0
  gingival K06.1
  palmar (fascial) M72.0
  plantar (fascial) M72.2
  pseudosarcomatous (proliferative) (subcutaneous) M72.4
  retroperitoneal D48.3
  specified NEC M72.8
Fibromyalgia M79.7
Fibromyoma —*see also* Neoplasm, connective tissue, benign
  uterus (corpus) —*see also* Leiomyoma, uterus
    in pregnancy or childbirth —*see* Fibroid, in pregnancy or childbirth
    causing obstructed labor O65.5
Fibromyositis M79.7
Fibromyxolipoma D17.9
Fibromyxoma —*see* Neoplasm, connective tissue, benign
Fibromyxosarcoma —*see* Neoplasm, connective tissue, malignant
Fibro-odontoma, ameloblastic —*see* Cyst, calcifying odontogenic
Fibro-osteoma —*see* Neoplasm, bone, benign
Fibroplasia, retrolental H35.17
Fibropurulent —*see* condition
Fibrosarcoma —*see also* Neoplasm, connective tissue, malignant
  ameloblastic C41.1
    upper jaw (bone) C41.0
  congenital —*see* Neoplasm, connective tissue, malignant
  fascial —*see* Neoplasm, connective tissue, malignant
  infantile —*see* Neoplasm, connective tissue, malignant
  odontogenic C41.1
    upper jaw (bone) C41.0
  periosteal —*see* Neoplasm, bone, malignant
Fibrosclerosis
  breast N60.3-●
  multifocal M35.5
  penis (corpora cavernosa) N48.6
Fibrosis, fibrotic
  adrenal (gland) E27.8
  amnion O41.8X-●
  anal papillae K62.89
  arteriocapillary —*see* Arteriosclerosis
  bladder N32.89
    interstitial —*see* Cystitis, chronic, interstitial
    localized submucosal —*see* Cystitis, chronic, interstitial
    panmural —*see* Cystitis, chronic, interstitial
  breast —*see* Fibrosclerosis, breast
  capillary —*see also* Arteriosclerosis I70.90
    lung (chronic) —*see* Fibrosis, lung
  cardiac —*see* Myocarditis
  cervix N88.8
  chorion O41.8X-●
  corpus cavernosum (sclerosing) N48.6
  cystic (of pancreas) E84.9

Fibrosis, fibrotic *(Continued)*
  cystic *(Continued)*
    with
      distal intestinal obstruction syndrome E84.19
      fecal impaction E84.19
      intestinal manifestations NEC E84.19
      pulmonary manifestations E84.0
      specified manifestations NEC E84.8
  due to device, implant or graft —*see also* Complications, by site and type, specified NEC T85.828
    arterial graft NEC T82.828
    breast (implant) T85.828
    catheter NEC T85.828
      dialysis (renal) T82.828
        intraperitoneal T85.828
      infusion NEC T82.828
        spinal (epidural) (subdural) T85.820
      urinary (indwelling) T83.82
    electronic (electrode) (pulse generator) (stimulator)
      bone T84.82
      cardiac T82.827
      nervous system (brain) (peripheral nerve) (spinal) T85.820
      urinary T83.82
    fixation, internal (orthopedic) NEC T84.82
    gastrointestinal (bile duct) (esophagus) T85.828
    genital NEC T83.82
    heart NEC T82.827
    joint prosthesis T84.82
    ocular (corneal graft) (orbital implant) NEC T85.828
    orthopedic NEC T84.82
    specified NEC T85.828
    urinary NEC T83.82
    vascular NEC T82.828
    ventricular intracranial shunt T85.820
  ejaculatory duct N50.89
  endocardium —*see* Endocarditis
  endomyocardial (tropical) I42.3
  epididymis N50.89
  eye muscle —*see* Strabismus, mechanical
  heart —*see* Myocarditis
  hepatic —*see* Fibrosis, liver
  hepatolienal (portal hypertension) K76.6
  hepatosplenic (portal hypertension) K76.6
  infrapatellar fat pad M79.4
  intrascrotal N50.89
  kidney N26.9
  liver K74.0
    with sclerosis K74.2
    alcoholic K70.2
  lung (atrophic) (chronic) (confluent) (massive) (perialveolar) (peribronchial) J84.10
    with
      anthracosilicosis J60
      anthracosis J60
      asbestosis J61
      bagassosis J67.1
      bauxite J63.1
      berylliosis J63.2
      byssinosis J66.0
      calcicosis J62.8
      chalicosis J62.8
      dust reticulation J64
      farmer's lung J67.0
      ganister disease J62.8
      graphite J63.3
      pneumoconiosis NOS J64
      siderosis J63.4
      silicosis J62.8
    capillary J84.10
    congenital P27.8
    diffuse (idiopathic) J84.10
      chemicals, gases, fumes or vapors (inhalation) J68.4

► New   ⇒ Revised   ~~deleted~~ Deleted   ● Use Additional Character(s)

Findings, abnormal, inconclusive, without diagnosis *(Continued)*
  transaminase (level) R74.0
  triglycerides E78.9
    high E78.1
      with high cholesterol E78.2
  tuberculin skin test (without active
      tuberculosis) R76.11
  urine R82.90
    acetone R82.4
    bacteria R82.71
    bile R82.2
    casts or cells R82.99
    chyle R82.0
    culture positive R82.79
    glucose R81
    hemoglobin R82.3
    ketone R82.4
    sugar R81
  vanillylmandelic acid (VMA), elevated
      R82.5
  vectorcardiogram (VCG) R94.39
  ventriculogram R93.0
  white blood cell (count) (differential)
      (morphology) D72.9
  xerography R92.8
Finger —*see* condition
Fire, Saint Anthony's —*see* Erysipelas
Fire-setting
  pathological (compulsive) F63.1
Fish hook stomach K31.89
Fishmeal-worker's lung J67.8
Fissure, fissured
  anus, anal K60.2
    acute K60.0
    chronic K60.1
    congenital Q43.8
  ear, lobule, congenital Q17.8
  epiglottis (congenital) Q31.8
  larynx J38.7
    congenital Q31.8
  lip K13.0
    congenital —*see* Cleft, lip
  nipple N64.0
    associated with
      lactation O92.13
      pregnancy O92.11- •
      puerperium O92.12
  nose Q30.2
  palate (congenital) —*see* Cleft, palate
  skin R23.4
  spine (congenital) —*see also* Spina bifida
    with hydrocephalus —*see* Spina bifida, by
        site, with hydrocephalus
  tongue (acquired) K14.5
    congenital Q38.3
Fistula (cutaneous) L98.8
  abdomen (wall) K63.2
    bladder N32.2
    intestine NEC K63.2
    ureter N28.89
    uterus N82.5
  abdominorectal K63.2
  abdominosigmoidal K63.2
  abdominothoracic J86.0
  abdominouterine N82.5
    congenital Q51.7
  abdominovesical N32.2
  accessory sinuses —*see* Sinusitis
  actinomycotic —*see* Actinomycosis
  alveolar antrum —*see* Sinusitis, maxillary
  alveolar process K04.6
  anorectal K60.5
  antrobuccal —*see* Sinusitis, maxillary
  antrum —*see* Sinusitis, maxillary
  anus, anal (recurrent) (infectional) K60.3
    congenital Q43.6
      with absence, atresia and stenosis Q42.2
    tuberculous A18.32
  aorta-duodenal I77.2
  appendix, appendicular K38.3

Fistula *(Continued)*
  arteriovenous (acquired) (nonruptured) I77.0
    brain I67.1
      congenital Q28.2
        ruptured I60.8
      ruptured I60.8
    cerebral —*see* Fistula, arteriovenous, brain
    congenital (peripheral) —*see also*
        Malformation, arteriovenous
      brain Q28.2
        ruptured I60.8
      coronary Q24.5
      pulmonary Q25.72
    coronary I25.41
      congenital Q24.5
    pulmonary I28.0
      congenital Q25.72
    surgically created (for dialysis) Z99.2
      complication —*see* Complication,
          arteriovenous, fistula, surgically
          created
    traumatic —*see* Injury, blood vessel
  artery I77.2
  aural (mastoid) —*see* Mastoiditis, chronic
  auricle —*see also* Disorder, pinna, specified
      type NEC
    congenital Q18.1
  Bartholin's gland N82.8
  bile duct (common) (hepatic) K83.3
    with calculus, stones —*see* Calculus, bile
        duct
  biliary (tract) —*see* Fistula, bile duct
  bladder (sphincter) NEC —*see also* Fistula,
      vesico- N32.2
    into seminal vesicle N32.2
  bone —*see also* Disorder, bone, specified type
      NEC
    with osteomyelitis, chronic —*see*
        Osteomyelitis, chronic, with draining
        sinus
  brain G93.89
    arteriovenous (acquired) I67.1
    congenital Q28.2
  branchial (cleft) Q18.0
  branchiogenous Q18.0
  breast N61.0
    puerperal, postpartum or gestational, due
        to mastitis (purulent) —*see* Mastitis,
        obstetric, purulent
  bronchial J86.0
  bronchocutaneous, bronchomediastinal,
      bronchopleural,
      bronchopleuromediastinal (infective)
      J86.0
    tuberculous NEC A15.5
  bronchoesophageal J86.0
    congenital Q39.2
      with atresia of esophagus Q39.1
  bronchovisceral J86.0
  buccal cavity (infective) K12.2
  cecosigmoidal K63.2
  cecum K63.2
  cerebrospinal (fluid) G96.0
  cervical, lateral Q18.1
  cervicoaural Q18.1
  cervicosigmoidal N82.4
  cervicovesical N82.1
  cervix N82.8
  chest (wall) J86.0
  cholecystenteric —*see* Fistula, gallbladder
  cholecystocolic —*see* Fistula, gallbladder
  cholecystocolonic —*see* Fistula, gallbladder
  cholecystoduodenal —*see* Fistula, gallbladder
  cholecystogastric —*see* Fistula, gallbladder
  cholecystointestinal —*see* Fistula, gallbladder
  choledochoduodenal —*see* Fistula, bile duct
  cholocolic K82.3
  coccyx —*see* Sinus, pilonidal
  colon K63.2
  colostomy K94.09
  common duct —*see* Fistula, bile duct

Fistula *(Continued)*
  congenital, site not listed —*see* Anomaly, by
      site
  coronary, arteriovenous I25.41
    congenital Q24.5
  costal region J86.0
  cul-de-sac, Douglas' N82.8
  cystic duct —*see also* Fistula, gallbladder
    congenital Q44.5
  dental K04.6
  diaphragm J86.0
  duodenum K31.6
  ear (external) (canal) —*see* Disorder, ear,
      external, specified type NEC
  enterocolic K63.2
  enterocutaneous K63.2
  enterouterine N82.4
    congenital Q51.7
  enterovaginal N82.4
    congenital Q52.2
    large intestine N82.3
    small intestine N82.2
  enterovesical N32.1
  epididymis N50.89
    tuberculous A18.15
  esophagobronchial J86.0
    congenital Q39.2
      with atresia of esophagus Q39.1
  esophagocutaneous K22.8
  esophagopleural-cutaneous J86.0
  esophagotracheal J86.0
    congenital Q39.2
      with atresia of esophagus Q39.1
  esophagus K22.8
    congenital Q39.2
      with atresia of esophagus Q39.1
  ethmoid —*see* Sinusitis, ethmoidal
  eyeball (cornea) (sclera) —*see* Disorder, globe,
      hypotony
  eyelid H01.8
  fallopian tube, external N82.5
  fecal K63.2
    congenital Q43.6
  from periapical abscess K04.6
  frontal sinus —*see* Sinusitis, frontal
  gallbladder K82.3
    with calculus, cholelithiasis, stones —*see*
        Calculus, gallbladder
  gastric K31.6
  gastrocolic K31.6
    congenital Q40.2
    tuberculous A18.32
  gastroenterocolic K31.6
  gastroesophageal K31.6
  gastrojejunal K31.6
  gastrojejunocolic K31.6
  genital tract (female) N82.9
    specified NEC N82.8
    to intestine NEC N82.4
    to skin N82.5
  hepatic artery-portal vein, congenital Q26.6
  hepatopleural J86.0
  hepatopulmonary J86.0
  ileorectal or ileosigmoidal K63.2
  ileovaginal N82.2
  ileovesical N32.1
  ileum K63.2
  in ano K60.3
    tuberculous A18.32
  inner ear (labyrinth) —*see* subcategory
      H83.1
  intestine NEC K63.2
  intestinocolonic (abdominal) K63.2
  intestinoureteral N28.89
  intestinouterine N82.4
  intestinovaginal N82.4
    large intestine N82.3
    small intestine N82.2
  intestinovesical N32.1
  ischiorectal (fossa) K61.3
  jejunum K63.2

Fistula *(Continued)*
joint M25.10
ankle M25.17-●
elbow M25.12-●
foot joint M25.17-●
hand joint M25.14-●
hip M25.15-●
knee M25.16-●
shoulder M25.11-●
specified joint NEC M25.18
tuberculous —*see* Tuberculosis, joint
vertebrae M25.18
wrist M25.13-●
kidney N28.89
labium (majus) (minus) N82.8
labyrinth —*see* subcategory H83.1
lacrimal (gland) (sac) H04.61-●
lacrimonasal duct —*see* Fistula, lacrimal
laryngotracheal, congenital Q34.8
larynx J38.7
lip K13.0
congenital Q38.0
lumbar, tuberculous A18.01
lung J86.0
lymphatic I89.8
mammary (gland) N61.0
mastoid (process) (region) —*see* Mastoiditis,
chronic
maxillary J32.0
medial, face and neck Q18.8
mediastinal J86.0
mediastinobronchial J86.0
mediastinocutaneous J86.0
middle ear —*see* subcategory H74.8
mouth K12.2
nasal J34.89
sinus —*see* Sinusitis
nasopharynx J39.2
nipple N64.0
nose J34.89
oral (cutaneous) K12.2
maxillary J32.0
nasal (with cleft palate) —*see* Cleft, palate
orbit, orbital —*see* Disorder, orbit, specified
type NEC
oroantral J32.0
oviduct, external N82.5
palate (hard) M27.8
pancreatic K86.89
pancreaticoduodenal K86.89
parotid (gland) K11.4
region K12.2
penis N48.89
perianal K60.3
pericardium (pleura) (sac) —*see* Pericarditis
pericecal K63.2
perineorectal K60.4 perineosigmoidal K63.2
perineosigmoidal K63.2
perineum, perineal (with urethral
involvement) NEC N36.0
tuberculous A18.13
ureter N28.89
perirectal K60.4
tuberculous A18.32
peritoneum K65.9
pharyngoesophageal J39.2
pharynx J39.2
branchial cleft (congenital) Q18.0
pilonidal (infected) (rectum) —*see* Sinus,
pilonidal
pleura, pleural, pleurocutaneous,
pleuroperitoneal J86.0
tuberculous NEC A15.6
pleuropericardial I31.8
portal vein-hepatic artery, congenital
Q26.6
postauricular H70.81-●
postoperative, persistent T81.83
specified site —*see* Fistula, by site
preauricular (congenital) Q18.1
prostate N42.89

Fistula *(Continued)*
pulmonary J86.0
arteriovenous I28.0
congenital Q25.72
tuberculous —*see* Tuberculosis, pulmonary
pulmonoperitoneal J86.0
rectolabial N82.4
rectosigmoid (intercommunicating) K63.2
rectoureteral N28.89
rectourethral N36.0
congenital Q64.73
rectouterine N82.4
congenital Q51.7
rectovaginal N82.3
congenital Q52.2
tuberculous A18.18
rectovesical N32.1
congenital Q64.79
rectovesicovaginal N82.3
rectovulval N82.4
congenital Q52.79
rectum (to skin) K60.4
congenital Q43.6
with absence, atresia and stenosis Q42.0
tuberculous A18.32
renal N28.89
retroauricular —*see* Fistula, postauricular
salivary duct or gland (any) K11.4
congenital Q38.4
scrotum (urinary) N50.89
tuberculous A18.15
semicircular canals —*see* subcategory H83.1
sigmoid K63.2
to bladder N32.1
sinus —*see* Sinusitis
skin L98.8
to genital tract (female) N82.5
splenocolic D73.89
stercoral K63.2
stomach K31.6
sublingual gland K11.4
submandibular gland K11.4
submaxillary (gland) K11.4
region K12.2
thoracic J86.0
duct I89.8
thoracoabdominal J86.0
thoracogastric J86.0
thoracointestinal J86.0
thorax J86.0
thyroglossal duct Q89.2
thyroid E07.89
trachea, congenital (external) (internal) Q32.1
tracheoesophageal J86.0
congenital Q39.2
with atresia of esophagus Q39.1
following tracheostomy J95.04
traumatic arteriovenous —*see* Injury, blood
vessel, by site
tuberculous - code by site under Tuberculosis
typhoid A01.09
umbilicourinary Q64.8
urachus, congenital Q64.4
ureter (persistent) N28.89
ureteroabdominal N28.89
ureterorectal N28.89
ureterosigmoido-abdominal N28.89
ureterovaginal N82.1
ureterovesical N32.2
urethra N36.0
congenital Q64.79
tuberculous A18.13
urethroperineal N36.0
urethroperineovesical N32.2
urethrorectal N36.0
congenital Q64.73
urethroscrotal N50.89
urethrovaginal N82.1
urethrovesical N32.2
urinary (tract) (persistent) (recurrent)
N36.0

Fistula *(Continued)*
uteroabdominal N82.5
congenital Q51.7
uteroenteric, uterointestinal N82.4
congenital Q51.7
uterorectal N82.4
congenital Q51.7
uteroureteric N82.1
uterourethral Q51.7
uterovaginal N82.8
uterovesical N82.1
congenital Q51.7
uterus N82.8
vagina (postpartal) (wall) N82.8
vaginocutaneous (postpartal) N82.5
vaginointestinal NEC N82.4
large intestine N82.3
small intestine N82.2
vaginoperineal N82.5
vasocutaneous, congenital Q55.7
vesical NEC N32.2
vesicoabdominal N32.2
vesicocervicovaginal N82.1
vesicocolic N32.1
vesicocutaneous N32.2
vesicoenteric N32.1
vesicointestinal N32.1
vesicometrorectal N82.4
vesicoperineal N32.2
vesicorectal N32.1
congenital Q64.79
vesicosigmoidal N32.1
vesicosigmoidovaginal N82.3
vesicoureteral N32.2
vesicoureterovaginal N82.1
vesicourethral N32.2
vesicourethrorectal N32.1
vesicouterine N82.1
congenital Q51.7
vesicovaginal N82.0
vulvorectal N82.4
congenital Q52.79
Fit R56.9
epileptic —*see* Epilepsy
fainting R55
hysterical F44.5
newborn P90
Fitting (and adjustment) (of)
artificial
arm —*see* Admission, adjustment, artificial,
arm
breast Z44.3
eye Z44.2
leg —*see* Admission, adjustment, artificial,
leg
automatic implantable cardiac defibrillator
(with synchronous cardiac pacemaker)
Z45.02
brain neuropacemaker Z46.2
implanted Z45.42
cardiac defibrillator —*see* Fitting (and
adjustment) (of), automatic implantable
cardiac defibrillator
catheter, non-vascular Z46.82
colostomy belt Z46.89
contact lenses Z46.0
CRT-D (resynchronization therapy
defibrillator) Z45.02
CRT-P (cardiac resynchronization therapy
pacemaker) Z45.018
pulse generator Z45.010
cystostomy device Z46.6
defibrillator, cardiac —*see* Fitting (and
adjustment) (of), automatic implantable
cardiac defibrillator
dentures Z46.3
device NOS Z46.9
abdominal Z46.89
gastrointestinal NEC Z46.59
implanted NEC Z45.89
nervous system Z46.2
implanted —*see* Admission, adjustment,
device, implanted, nervous system

Fitting (Continued)
  device NOS (Continued)
    orthodontic Z46.4
    orthoptic Z46.0
    orthotic Z46.89
    prosthetic (external) Z44.9
      breast Z44.3
      dental Z46.3
      eye Z44.2
      specified NEC Z44.8
    specified NEC Z46.89
    substitution
      auditory Z46.2
        implanted —see Admission,
          adjustment, device, implanted,
          hearing device
      nervous system Z46.2
        implanted —see Admission,
          adjustment, device, implanted,
          nervous system
      visual Z46.2
        implanted Z45.31
    urinary Z46.6
  gastric lap band Z46.51
  gastrointestinal appliance NEC Z46.59
  glasses (reading) Z46.0
  hearing aid Z46.1
  ileostomy device Z46.89
  insulin pump Z46.81
  intestinal appliance NEC Z46.89
  myringotomy device (stent) (tube) Z45.82
  neuropacemaker Z46.2
    implanted Z45.42
  non-vascular catheter Z46.82
  orthodontic device Z46.4
  orthopedic device (brace) (cast) (corset)
    (shoes) Z46.89
  pacemaker (cardiac) (cardiac
    resynchronization therapy (CRT-P))
    Z45.018
    nervous system (brain) (peripheral nerve)
      (spinal cord) Z46.2
      implanted Z45.42
    pulse generator Z45.010
  portacath (port-a-cath) Z45.2
  prosthesis (external) Z44.9
    arm —see Admission, adjustment, artificial,
      arm
    breast Z44.3
    dental Z46.3
    eye Z44.2
    leg —see Admission, adjustment, artificial,
      leg
    specified NEC Z44.8
  spectacles Z46.0
  wheelchair Z46.89
Fitzhugh-Curtis syndrome
  due to
    Chlamydia trachomatis A74.81
    Neisseria gonorrhorea (gonococcal
      peritonitis) A54.85
Fitz's syndrome (acute hemorrhagic
  pancreatitis) —see also Pancreatitis,
  acute K85.80
Fixation
  joint —see Ankylosis
  larynx J38.7
  stapes —see Ankylosis, ear ossicles
    deafness —see Deafness, conductive
  uterus (acquired) —see Malposition, uterus
  vocal cord J38.3
Flabby ridge K06.8
Flaccid —see also condition
  palate, congenital Q38.5
Flail
  chest S22.5-●
    newborn (birth injury) P13.8
  joint (paralytic) M25.20
    ankle M25.27-●
    elbow M25.22-●
    foot joint M25.27-●

Flail (Continued)
  joint (Continued)
    hand joint M25.24-●
    hip M25.25-●
    knee M25.26-●
    shoulder M25.21-●
    specified joint NEC M25.28
    wrist M25.23-●
Flajani's disease —see Hyperthyroidism, with,
  goiter (diffuse)
Flap, liver K71.3
Flashbacks (residual to hallucinogen use) F16.283
Flat
  chamber (eye) —see Disorder, globe,
    hypotony, flat anterior chamber
  chest, congenital Q67.8
  foot (acquired) (fixed type) (painful)
    (postural) —see also Deformity, limb,
    flat foot
    congenital (rigid) (spastic (everted)) Q66.5-●
    rachitic sequelae (late effect) E64.3
  organ or site, congenital NEC —see Anomaly,
    by site
  pelvis M95.5
    with disproportion (fetopelvic) O33.0
      causing obstructed labor O65.0
    congenital Q74.2
Flatau-Schilder disease G37.0
Flatback syndrome M40.30
  lumbar region M40.36
  lumbosacral region M40.37
  thoracolumbar region M40.35
Flattening
  head, femur M89.8X5
  hip —see Coxa, plana
  lip (congenital) Q18.8
  nose (congenital) Q67.4
    acquired M95.0
Flatulence R14.3
  psychogenic F45.8
Flatus R14.3
  vaginalis N89.8
Flax-dresser's disease J66.1
Flea bite —see Injury, bite, by site, superficial,
  insect
Flecks, glaucomatous (subcapsular) —see
  Cataract, complicated
Fleischer (-Kayser) ring (cornea) H18.04-●
Fleshy mole O02.0
Flexibilitas cerea —see Catalepsy
Flexion
  amputation stump (surgical) T87.89
  cervix —see Malposition, uterus
  contracture, joint —see Contraction, joint
  deformity, joint —see also Deformity, limb,
    flexion M21.20
    hip, congenital Q65.89
  uterus —see also Malposition, uterus
    lateral —see Lateroversion, uterus
Flexner-Boyd dysentery A03.2
Flexner's dysentery A03.1
Flexure —see Flexion
Flint murmur (aortic insufficiency) I35.1
Floater, vitreous —see Opacity, vitreous
Floating
  cartilage (joint) —see also Loose, body, joint
    knee —see Derangement, knee, loose body
  gallbladder, congenital Q44.1
  kidney N28.89
    congenital Q63.8
  spleen D73.89
Flooding N92.0
Floor —see condition
Floppy
  baby syndrome (nonspecific) P94.2
  iris syndrome (intraoperative) (IFIS) H21.81
  nonrheumatic mitral valve syndrome I34.1
Flu —see also Influenza
  avian —see also Influenza, due to, identified
    novel influenza A virus J09.X2
  bird —see also Influenza, due to, identified
    novel influenza A virus J09.X2

Flu (Continued)
  intestinal NEC A08.4
  swine (viruses that normally cause infections
    in pigs) —see also Influenza, due to,
    identified novel influenza A virus J09.X2
Fluctuating blood pressure I99.8
Fluid
  abdomen R18.8
  chest J94.8
  heart —see Failure, heart, congestive
  joint —see Effusion, joint
  loss (acute) E86.9
  lung —see Edema, lung
  overload E87.70
    specified NEC E87.79
  peritoneal cavity R18.8
  pleural cavity J94.8
  retention R60.9
Flukes NEC —see also Infestation, fluke
  blood NEC —see Schistosomiasis
  liver B66.3
Fluor (vaginalis) N89.8
  trichomonal or due to Trichomonas
    (vaginalis) A59.00
Fluorosis
  dental K00.3
  skeletal M85.10
    ankle M85.17-●
    foot M85.17-●
    forearm M85.13-●
    hand M85.14-●
    lower leg M85.16-●
    multiple site M85.19
    neck M85.18
    rib M85.18
    shoulder M85.11-●
    skull M85.18
    specified site NEC M85.18
    thigh M85.15-●
    toe M85.17-●
    upper arm M85.12-●
    vertebra M85.18
Flush syndrome E34.0
Flushing R23.2
  menopausal N95.1
Flutter
  atrial or auricular I48.92
    atypical I48.4
    type I I48.3
    type II I48.4
    typical I48.3
  heart I49.8
    atrial or auricular I48.92
      atypical I48.4
      type I I48.3
      type II I48.4
      typical I48.3
    ventricular I49.02
  ventricular I49.02
FNHTR (febrile nonhemolytic transfusion
  reaction) R50.84
Fochier's abscess - code by site under Abscess
Focus, Assmann's —see Tuberculosis,
  pulmonary
Fogo selvagem L10.3
Foix-Alajouanine syndrome G95.19
Fold, folds (anomalous) —see also Anomaly,
  by site
  Descemet's membrane —see Change, corneal
    membrane, Descemet's, fold
  epicanthic Q10.3
  heart Q24.8
Folie à deux F24
Follicle
  cervix (nabothian) (ruptured) N88.8
  graafian, ruptured, with hemorrhage N83.0-●
  nabothian N88.8
Follicular —see condition
Folliculitis (superficial) L73.9
  abscedens et suffodiens L66.3
  cyst N83.0-●

Folliculitis (*Continued*)
  decalvans L66.2
  deep —*see* Furuncle, by site
  gonococcal (acute) (chronic) A54.01
  keloid, keloidalis L73.0
  pustular L01.02
  ulerythematosa reticulata L66.4
Folliculome lipidique
  specified site —*see* Neoplasm, benign, by site
  unspecified site
    female D27.9
    male D29.20
Følling's disease E70.0
Follow-up —*see* Examination, follow-up
Fong's syndrome (hereditary osteo-
  onychodysplasia) Q87.2
Food
  allergy L27.2
  asphyxia (from aspiration or inhalation) —*see*
    Foreign body, by site
  choked on —*see* Foreign body, by site
  deprivation T73.0
    specified kind of food NEC E63.8
  intoxication —*see* Poisoning, food
  lack of T73.0
  poisoning —*see* Poisoning, food
  rejection NEC —*see* Disorder, eating
  strangulation or suffocation —*see* Foreign
    body, by site
  toxemia —*see* Poisoning, food
Foot —*see* condition
Foramen ovale (nonclosure) (patent)
  (persistent) Q21.1
Forbes' glycogen storage disease E74.03
Fordyce-Fox disease L75.2
Fordyce's disease (mouth) Q38.6
Forearm —*see* condition
Foreign body
  with
    laceration —*see* Laceration, by site, with
      foreign body
    puncture wound —*see* Puncture, by site,
      with foreign body
  accidentally left following a procedure
    T81.509
    aspiration T81.506
      resulting in
        adhesions T81.516
        obstruction T81.526
        perforation T81.536
        specified complication NEC T81.596
    cardiac catheterization T81.505
      resulting in
        acute reaction T81.60
          aseptic peritonitis T81.61
          specified NEC T81.69
        adhesions T81.515
        obstruction T81.525
        perforation T81.535
        specified complication NEC T81.595
    causing
      acute reaction T81.60
        aseptic peritonitis T81.61
        specified complication NEC T81.69
      adhesions T81.519
      aseptic peritonitis T81.61
      obstruction T81.529
      perforation T81.539
      specified complication NEC T81.599
    endoscopy T81.504
      resulting in
        adhesions T81.514
        obstruction T81.524
        perforation T81.534
        specified complication NEC T81.594
    immunization T81.503
      resulting in
        adhesions T81.513
        obstruction T81.523
        perforation T81.533
        specified complication NEC T81.593

Foreign body (*Continued*)
  accidentally left following a procedure
    (*Continued*)
    infusion T81.501
      resulting in
        adhesions T81.511
        obstruction T81.521
        perforation T81.531
        specified complication NEC T81.591
    injection T81.503
      resulting in
        adhesions T81.513
        obstruction T81.523
        perforation T81.533
        specified complication NEC T81.593
    kidney dialysis T81.502
      resulting in
        adhesions T81.512
        obstruction T81.522
        perforation T81.532
        specified complication NEC T81.592
    packing removal T81.507
      resulting in
        acute reaction T81.60
          aseptic peritonitis T81.61
          specified NEC T81.69
        adhesions T81.517
        obstruction T81.527
        perforation T81.537
        specified complication NEC T81.597
    puncture T81.506
      resulting in
        adhesions T81.516
        obstruction T81.526
        perforation T81.536
        specified complication NEC T81.596
    specified procedure NEC T81.508
      resulting in
        acute reaction T81.60
          aseptic peritonitis T81.61
          specified NEC T81.69
        adhesions T81.518
        obstruction T81.528
        perforation T81.538
        specified complication NEC
          T81.598
    surgical operation T81.500
      resulting in
        acute reaction T81.60
          aseptic peritonitis T81.61
          specified NEC T81.69
        adhesions T81.510
        obstruction T81.520
        perforation T81.530
        specified complication NEC T81.590
    transfusion T81.501
      resulting in
        adhesions T81.511
        obstruction T81.521
        perforation T81.531
        specified complication NEC T81.591
  alimentary tract T18.9
    anus T18.5
    colon T18.4
    esophagus —*see* Foreign body, esophagus
    mouth T18.0
    multiple sites T18.8
    rectosigmoid (junction) T18.5
    rectum T18.5
    small intestine T18.3
    specified site NEC T18.8
    stomach T18.2
  anterior chamber (eye) S05.5-●
  auditory canal —*see* Foreign body, entering
    through orifice, ear
  bronchus T17.508
    causing
      asphyxiation T17.500
        food (bone) (seed) T17.520
        gastric contents (vomitus) T17.510
        specified type NEC T17.590

Foreign body (*Continued*)
  bronchus (*Continued*)
    causing (*Continued*)
      injury NEC T17.508
        food (bone) (seed) T17.528
        gastric contents (vomitus) T17.518
        specified type NEC T17.598
  canthus —*see* Foreign body, conjunctival sac
  ciliary body (eye) S05.5-●
  conjunctival sac T15.1-●
  cornea T15.0-●
  entering through orifice
    accessory sinus T17.0
    alimentary canal T18.9
      multiple parts T18.8
      specified part NEC T18.8
    alveolar process T18.0
    antrum (Highmore's) T17.0
    anus T18.5
    appendix T18.4
    auditory canal —*see* Foreign body, entering
      through orifice, ear
    auricle —*see* Foreign body, entering
      through orifice, ear
    bladder T19.1
    bronchioles —*see* Foreign body, respiratory
      tract, specified site NEC
    bronchus (main) —*see* Foreign body,
      bronchus
    buccal cavity T18.0
    canthus (inner) —*see* Foreign body,
      conjunctival sac
    cecum T18.4
    cervix (canal) (uteri) T19.3
    colon T18.4
    conjunctival sac —*see* Foreign body,
      conjunctival sac
    cornea —*see* Foreign body, cornea
    digestive organ or tract NOS T18.9
      multiple parts T18.8
      specified part NEC T18.8
    duodenum T18.3
    ear (external) T16.-●
    esophagus —*see* Foreign body, esophagus
    eye (external) NOS T15.9-●
      conjunctival sac —*see* Foreign body,
        conjunctival sac
      cornea —*see* Foreign body, cornea
      specified part NEC T15.8-●
    eyeball —*see also* Foreign body, entering
      through orifice, eye, specified part
      NEC
      with penetrating wound —*see* Puncture,
        eyeball
    eyelid —*see also* Foreign body, conjunctival
      sac
      with
        laceration —*see* Laceration, eyelid,
          with foreign body
        puncture —*see* Puncture, eyelid, with
          foreign body
        superficial injury —*see* Foreign body,
          superficial, eyelid
    gastrointestinal tract T18.9
      multiple parts T18.8
      specified part NEC T18.8
    genitourinary tract T19.9
      multiple parts T19.8
      specified part NEC T19.8
    globe —*see* Foreign body, entering through
      orifice, eyeball
    gum T18.0
    Highmore's antrum T17.0
    hypopharynx —*see* Foreign body, pharynx
    ileum T18.3
    intestine (small) T18.3
      large T18.4
    lacrimal apparatus (punctum) —*see*
      Foreign body, entering through orifice,
      eye, specified part NEC
    large intestine T18.4

► New   ⇒ Revised   ~~deleted~~ Deleted   ● Use Additional Character(s)

Foreign body (Continued)
  entering through orifice (Continued)
    larynx —see Foreign body, larynx
    lung —see Foreign body, respiratory tract,
        specified site NEC
    maxillary sinus T17.0
    mouth T18.0
    nasal sinus T17.0
    nasopharynx —see Foreign body, pharynx
    nose (passage) T17.1
    nostril T17.1
    oral cavity T18.0
    palate T18.0
    penis T19.4
    pharynx —see Foreign body, pharynx
    piriform sinus —see Foreign body, pharynx
    rectosigmoid (junction) T18.5
    rectum T18.5
    respiratory tract —see Foreign body,
        respiratory tract
    sinus (accessory) (frontal) (maxillary)
        (nasal) T17.0
      piriform —see Foreign body, pharynx
    small intestine T18.3
    stomach T18.2
    suffocation by —see Foreign body, by site
    tear ducts or glands —see Foreign body,
        entering through orifice, eye, specified
        part NEC
    throat —see Foreign body, pharynx
    tongue T18.0
    tonsil, tonsillar (fossa) —see Foreign body,
        pharynx
    trachea —see Foreign body, trachea
    ureter T19.8
    urethra T19.0
    uterus (any part) T19.3
    vagina T19.2
    vulva T19.2
  esophagus T18.108
    causing
      injury NEC T18.108
        food (bone) (seed) T18.128
        gastric contents (vomitus) T18.118
        specified type NEC T18.198
      tracheal compression T18.100
        food (bone) (seed) T18.120
        gastric contents (vomitus) T18.110
        specified type NEC T18.190
  feeling of, in throat R09.89
▶ feeling of, in throat R09.89
  fragment —see Retained, foreign body
      fragments (type of)
  genitourinary tract T19.9
    bladder T19.1
    multiple parts T19.8
    penis T19.4
    specified site NEC T19.8
    urethra T19.0
    uterus T19.3
      IUD Z97.5
    vagina T19.2
      contraceptive device Z97.5
    vulva T19.2
  granuloma (old) (soft tissue) —see also
      Granuloma, foreign body
    skin L92.3
  in
    laceration —see Laceration, by site, with
        foreign body
    puncture wound —see Puncture, by site,
        with foreign body
    soft tissue (residual) M79.5
  inadvertently left in operation wound —see
      Foreign body, accidentally left during a
      procedure
  ingestion, ingested NOS T18.9
  inhalation or inspiration —see Foreign body,
      by site
  internal organ, not entering through a natural
      orifice - code as specific injury with
      foreign body

Foreign body (Continued)
  intraocular S05.5-●
    old, retained (nonmagnetic) H44.70-●
      anterior chamber H44.71-●
      ciliary body H44.72-●
      iris H44.72-●
      lens H44.73-●
      magnetic H44.60-●
        anterior chamber H44.61-●
        ciliary body H44.62-●
        iris H44.62-●
        lens H44.63-●
        posterior wall H44.64-●
        specified site NEC H44.69-●
        vitreous body H44.65-●
      posterior wall H44.74-●
      specified site NEC H44.79-●
      vitreous body H44.75-●
  iris —see Foreign body, intraocular
  lacrimal punctum —see Foreign body,
      entering through orifice, eye, specified
      part NEC
  larynx T17.308
    causing
      asphyxiation T17.300
        food (bone) (seed) T17.320
        gastric contents (vomitus) T17.310
        specified type NEC T17.390
      injury NEC T17.308
        food (bone) (seed) T17.328
        gastric contents (vomitus) T17.318
        specified type NEC T17.398
  lens —see Foreign body, intraocular
  ocular muscle S05.4-●
    old, retained —see Foreign body, orbit, old
  old or residual
    soft tissue (residual) M79.5
  operation wound, left accidentally —see
      Foreign body, accidentally left during a
      procedure
  orbit S05.4-●
    old, retained H05.5-●
  pharynx T17.208
    causing
      asphyxiation T17.200
        food (bone) (seed) T17.220
        gastric contents (vomitus)
            T17.210
        specified type NEC T17.290
      injury NEC T17.208
        food (bone) (seed) T17.228
        gastric contents (vomitus) T17.218
        specified type NEC T17.298
  respiratory tract T17.908
    bronchioles —see Foreign body, respiratory
        tract, specified site NEC
    bronchus —see Foreign body, bronchus
    causing
      asphyxiation T17.900
        food (bone) (seed) T17.920
        gastric contents (vomitus) T17.910
        specified type NEC T17.990
      injury NEC T17.908
        food (bone) (seed) T17.928
        gastric contents (vomitus) T17.918
        specified type NEC T17.998
    larynx —see Foreign body, larynx
    lung —see Foreign body, respiratory tract,
        specified site NEC
    multiple parts —see Foreign body,
        respiratory tract, specified site NEC
    nasal sinus T17.0
    nasopharynx —see Foreign body, pharynx
    nose T17.1
    nostril T17.1
    pharynx —see Foreign body, pharynx
    specified site NEC T17.808
      causing
        asphyxiation T17.800
          food (bone) (seed) T17.820
          gastric contents (vomitus) T17.810
          specified type NEC T17.890

Foreign body (Continued)
  respiratory tract (Continued)
    specified site NEC (Continued)
      causing (Continued)
        injury NEC T17.808
          food (bone) (seed) T17.828
          gastric contents (vomitus) T17.818
          specified type NEC T17.898
    throat —see Foreign body, pharynx
    trachea —see Foreign body, trachea
  retained (old) (nonmagnetic) (in)
    anterior chamber (eye) —see Foreign body,
        intraocular, old, retained, anterior
        chamber
      magnetic —see Foreign body, intraocular,
          old, retained, magnetic, anterior
          chamber
    ciliary body —see Foreign body,
        intraocular, old, retained, ciliary body
      magnetic —see Foreign body, intraocular,
          old, retained, magnetic, ciliary
          body
    eyelid H02.819
      left H02.816
        lower H02.815
        upper H02.814
      right H02.813
        lower H02.812
        upper H02.811
    fragments —see Retained, foreign body
        fragments (type of)
    globe —see Foreign body, intraocular, old,
        retained
      magnetic —see Foreign body, intraocular,
          old, retained, magnetic
    intraocular —see Foreign body, intraocular,
        old, retained
      magnetic —see Foreign body, intraocular,
          old, retained, magnetic
    iris —see Foreign body, intraocular, old,
        retained, iris
      magnetic —see Foreign body, intraocular,
          old, retained, magnetic, iris
    lens —see Foreign body, intraocular, old,
        retained, lens
      magnetic —see Foreign body, intraocular,
          old, retained, magnetic, lens
    muscle —see Foreign body, retained, soft
        tissue
    orbit —see Foreign body, orbit, old
    posterior wall of globe —see Foreign body,
        intraocular, old, retained, posterior
        wall
      magnetic —see Foreign body, intraocular,
          old, retained, magnetic, posterior
          wall
    retrobulbar —see Foreign body, orbit, old,
        retrobulbar
    soft tissue M79.5
    vitreous —see Foreign body, intraocular,
        old, retained, vitreous body
      magnetic —see Foreign body, intraocular,
          old, retained, magnetic, vitreous
          body
  retina S05.5-●
  superficial, without open wound
    abdomen, abdominal (wall) S30.851
    alveolar process S00.552
    ankle S90.55-●
    antecubital space —see Foreign body,
        superficial, forearm
    anus S30.857
    arm (upper) S40.85-●
    auditory canal —see Foreign body,
        superficial, ear
    auricle —see Foreign body, superficial, ear
    axilla —see Foreign body, superficial, arm
    back, lower S30.850
    breast S20.15-●
    brow S00.85
    buttock S30.850

Foreign body *(Continued)*
superficial, without open wound *(Continued)*
calf —*see* Foreign body, superficial, leg
canthus —*see* Foreign body, superficial, eyelid
cheek S00.85
internal S00.552
chest wall —*see* Foreign body, superficial, thorax
chin S00.85
clitoris S30.854
costal region —*see* Foreign body, superficial, thorax
digit(s)
foot —*see* Foreign body, superficial, toe
hand —*see* Foreign body, superficial, finger
ear S00.45-•
elbow S50.35-•
epididymis S30.853
epigastric region S30.851
epiglottis S10.15
esophagus, cervical S10.15
eyebrow —*see* Foreign body, superficial, eyelid
eyelid S00.25-•
face S00.85
finger(s) S60.459
index S60.45-•
little S60.45-•
middle S60.45-•
ring S60.45-•
flank S30.851
foot (except toe(s) alone) S90.85-•
toe —*see* Foreign body, superficial, toe
forearm S50.85-•
elbow only —*see* Foreign body, superficial, elbow
forehead S00.85
genital organs, external
female S30.856
male S30.855
groin S30.851
gum S00.552
hand S60.55-•
head S00.95
ear —*see* Foreign body, superficial, ear
eyelid —*see* Foreign body, superficial, eyelid
lip S00.551
nose S00.35
oral cavity S00.552
scalp S00.05
specified site NEC S00.85
heel —*see* Foreign body, superficial, foot
hip S70.25-•
inguinal region S30.851
interscapular region S20.459
jaw S00.85
knee S80.25-•
labium (majus) (minus) S30.854
larynx S10.15
leg (lower) S80.85-•
knee —*see* Foreign body, superficial, knee
upper —*see* Foreign body, superficial, thigh
lip S00.551
lower back S30.850
lumbar region S30.850
malar region S00.85
mammary —*see* Foreign body, superficial, breast
mastoid region S00.85
mouth S00.552
nail
finger —*see* Foreign body, superficial, finger
toe —*see* Foreign body, superficial, toe
nape S10.85
nasal S00.35

neck S10.95
specified site NEC S10.85
throat S10.15
nose S00.35
occipital region S00.05
oral cavity S00.552
orbital region —*see* Foreign body, superficial, eyelid
palate S00.552
palm —*see* Foreign body, superficial, hand
parietal region S00.05
pelvis S30.850
penis S30.852
perineum
female S30.854
male S30.850
periocular area —*see* Foreign body, superficial, eyelid
phalanges
finger —*see* Foreign body, superficial, finger
toe —*see* Foreign body, superficial, toe
pharynx S10.15
pinna —*see* Foreign body, superficial, ear
popliteal space —*see* Foreign body, superficial, knee
prepuce S30.852
pubic region S30.850
pudendum
female S30.856
male S30.855
sacral region S30.850
scalp S00.05
scapular region —*see* Foreign body, superficial, shoulder
scrotum S30.853
shin —*see* Foreign body, superficial, leg
shoulder S40.25-•
sternal region S20.359
submaxillary region S00.85
submental region S00.85
subungual
finger(s) —*see* Foreign body, superficial, finger
toe(s) —*see* Foreign body, superficial, toe
supraclavicular fossa S10.85
supraorbital S00.85
temple S00.85
temporal region S00.85
testis S30.853
thigh S70.35-•
thorax, thoracic (wall) S20.95
back S20.45-•
front S20.35-•
throat S10.15
thumb S60.35-•
toe(s) (lesser) S90.456
great S90.45-•
tongue S00.552
trachea S10.15
tunica vaginalis S30.853
tympanum, tympanic membrane —*see* Foreign body, superficial, ear
uvula S00.552
vagina S30.854
vocal cords S10.15
vulva S30.854
wrist S60.85-•
swallowed T18.9
trachea T17.408
causing
asphyxiation T17.400
food (bone) (seed) T17.420
gastric contents (vomitus) T17.410
specified type NEC T17.490
injury NEC T17.408
food (bone) (seed) T17.428
gastric contents (vomitus) T17.418
specified type NEC T17.498

Foreign body *(Continued)*
type of fragment —*see* Retained, foreign body fragments (type of)
vitreous (humor) S05.5-•
Forestier's disease (rhizomelic pseudopolyarthritis) M35.3-•
meaning ankylosing hyperostosis —*see* Hyperostosis, ankylosing
Formation
hyalin in cornea —*see* Degeneration, cornea
sequestrum in bone (due to infection) —*see* Osteomyelitis, chronic
valve
colon, congenital Q43.8
ureter (congenital) Q62.39
Formication R20.2
Fort Bragg fever A27.89
Fossa —*see also* condition
pyriform —*see* condition
Foster-Kennedy syndrome H47.14-•
Fothergill's
disease (trigeminal neuralgia) —*see also* Neuralgia, trigeminal
scarlatina anginosa A38.9
Foul breath R19.6
Foundling Z76.1
Fournier disease or gangrene N49.3
female N76.89
Fourth
cranial nerve —*see* condition
molar K00.1
Foville's (peduncular) **disease or syndrome** G46.3
Fox (-Fordyce) **disease** (apocrine miliaria) L75.2
Fracture, burst —*see* Fracture, traumatic, by site
➡ **Fracture, chronic** —*see* Fracture, pathological, by site
➡ **Fracture, insufficiency** —*see* Fracture, pathological, by site
Fracture, nontraumatic, NEC
atypical
femur M84.750-•
complete
oblique M84.759
left side M84.758
right side M84.757
transverse M84.756
left side M84.755
right side M84.754
incomplete M84.753
left side M84.752
right side M84.751
Fracture, pathological (pathologic) —*see also* Fracture, traumatic M84.40
ankle M84.47-•
carpus M84.44-•
clavicle M84.41-•
compression (not due to trauma) —*see also* Collapse, vertebra M48.50-•
dental implant M27.63
dental restorative material K08.539
with loss of material K08.531
without loss of material K08.530
due to
neoplastic disease NEC —*see also* Neoplasm M84.50
ankle M84.57-•
carpus M84.54-•
clavicle M84.51-•
femur M84.55-•
fibula M84.56-•
finger M84.54-•
hip M84.559
humerus M84.52-•
ilium M84.550
ischium M84.550
metacarpus M84.54-•
metatarsus M84.57-•
neck M84.58
pelvis M84.550
radius M84.53-•

▶ New   ⇒ Revised   ~~deleted~~ Deleted   • Use Additional Character(s)

Fracture, pathological *(Continued)*
  due to *(Continued)*
    neoplastic disease NEC *(Continued)*
      rib M84.58
      scapula M84.51-•
      skull M84.58
      specified site NEC M84.58
      tarsus M84.57-•
      tibia M84.56-•
      toe M84.57-•
      ulna M84.53-•
      vertebra M84.58
    osteoporosis M80.00
      disuse —*see* Osteoporosis, specified type NEC, with pathological fracture
      drug-induced —*see* Osteoporosis, drug induced, with pathological fracture
      idiopathic —*see* Osteoporosis, specified type NEC, with pathological fracture
      postmenopausal —*see* Osteoporosis, postmenopausal, with pathological fracture
      postoophorectomy —*see* Osteoporosis, postoophorectomy, with pathological fracture
      postsurgical malabsorption —*see* Osteoporosis, specified type NEC, with pathological fracture
      specified cause NEC —*see* Osteoporosis, specified type NEC, with pathological fracture
    specified disease NEC M84.60
      ankle M84.67-•
      carpus M84.64-•
      clavicle M84.61-•
      femur M84.65-•
      fibula M84.66-•
      finger M84.64-•
      hip M84.65-•
      humerus M84.62-•
      ilium M84.650
      ischium M84.650
      metacarpus M84.64-•
      metatarsus M84.67-•
      neck M84.68
      radius M84.63-•
      rib M84.68
      scapula M84.61-•
      skull M84.68
      tarsus M84.67-•
      tibia M84.66-•
      toe M84.67-•
      ulna M84.63-•
      vertebra M84.68
  femur M84.45-•
  fibula M84.46-•
  finger M84.44-•
  hip M84.459
  humerus M84.42-•
  ilium M84.454
  ischium M84.454
  joint prosthesis —*see* Complications, joint prosthesis, mechanical, breakdown, by site
    periprosthetic —*see* Fracture, pathological, periprosthetic
  metacarpus M84.44-•
  metatarsus M84.47-•
  neck M84.48
  pelvis M84.454
  periprosthetic M97.9
    ankle M97.2-•
    elbow M97.4-•
    finger M97.8
    hip M97.0-•
    knee M97.1-•
    other specified joint M97.8
    shoulder M97.3-•
    spinal joint M97.8
    toe joint M97.8
    wrist joint M97.8

Fracture, pathological *(Continued)*
  radius M84.43-•
  restorative material (dental) K08.539
    with loss of material K08.531
    without loss of material K08.530
  rib M84.48
  scapula M84.41-•
  skull M84.48
  tarsus M84.47-•
  tibia M84.46-•
  toe M84.47-•
  ulna M84.43-•
  vertebra M84.48
Fracture, traumatic (abduction) (adduction) (separation) —*see also* Fracture, pathological T14.8
  acetabulum S32.40-•
    column
      anterior (displaced) (iliopubic) S32.43-•
        nondisplaced S32.436
      posterior (displaced) (ilioischial) S32.443
        nondisplaced S32.44-•
    dome (displaced) S32.48-•
      nondisplaced S32.48
    specified NEC S32.49-•
    transverse (displaced) S32.45-•
      with associated posterior wall fracture (displaced) S32.46-•
        nondisplaced S32.46-•
      nondisplaced S32.45-•
    wall
      anterior (displaced) S32.41-•
        nondisplaced S32.41-•
      medial (displaced) S32.47-•
        nondisplaced S32.47-•
      posterior (displaced) S32.42-•
        with associated transverse fracture (displaced) S32.46-•
          nondisplaced S32.46-•
        nondisplaced S32.42-•
  acromion —*see* Fracture, scapula, acromial process
  ankle S82.899
    bimalleolar (displaced) S82.84-•
      nondisplaced S82.84-•
    lateral malleolus only (displaced) S82.6-•
      nondisplaced S82.6-•
    medial malleolus (displaced) S82.5-•
      associated with Maisonneuve's fracture —*see* Fracture, Maisonneuve's
      nondisplaced S82.5-•
    talus —*see* Fracture, tarsal, talus
    trimalleolar (displaced) S82.85-•
      nondisplaced S82.85-•
  arm (upper) —*see also* Fracture, humerus, shaft
    humerus —*see* Fracture, humerus
    radius —*see* Fracture, radius
    ulna —*see* Fracture, ulna
  astragalus —*see* Fracture, tarsal, talus
  atlas —*see* Fracture, neck, cervical vertebra, first
  axis —*see* Fracture, neck, cervical vertebra, second
  back —*see* Fracture, vertebra
  Barton's —*see* Barton's fracture
  base of skull —*see* Fracture, skull, base
  basicervical (basal) (femoral) S72.0
  Bennett's —*see* Bennett's fracture
  bimalleolar —*see* Fracture, ankle, bimalleolar
  blow-out S02.3-•
  bone NEC T14.8
    birth injury P13.9
    following insertion of orthopedic implant, joint prosthesis or bone plate —*see* Fracture, following insertion of orthopedic implant, joint prosthesis or bone plate

Fracture, traumatic *(Continued)*
  bone NEC *(Continued)*
    in (due to) neoplastic disease NEC — *see* Fracture, pathological, due to, neoplastic disease
    pathological (cause unknown) —*see* Fracture, pathological
  breast bone —*see* Fracture, sternum
  bucket handle (semilunar cartilage) —*see* Tear, meniscus
  burst —*see* Fracture, traumatic, by site
  calcaneus —*see* Fracture, tarsal, calcaneus
  carpal bone(s) S62.10-•
    capitate (displaced) S62.13-•
      nondisplaced S62.13-•
    cuneiform —*see* Fracture, carpal bone, triquetrum
    hamate (body) (displaced) S62.143
      hook process (displaced) S62.15-•
        nondisplaced S62.15-•
      nondisplaced S62.14-•
    larger multangular —*see* Fracture, carpal bones, trapezium
    lunate (displaced) S62.12-•
      nondisplaced S62.12-•
    navicular S62.00-•
      distal pole (displaced) S62.01-•
        nondisplaced S62.01-•
      middle third (displaced) S62.02-•
        nondisplaced S62.02-•
      proximal third (displaced) S62.03-•
        nondisplaced S62.03-•
      volar tuberosity —*see* Fracture, carpal bones, navicular, distal pole
    os magnum —*see* Fracture, carpal bones, capitate
    pisiform (displaced) S62.16-•
      nondisplaced S62.16-•
    semilunar —*see* Fracture, carpal bones, lunate
    smaller multangular —*see* Fracture, carpal bones, trapezoid
    trapezium (displaced) S62.17-•
      nondisplaced S62.17-•
    trapezoid (displaced) S62.18-•
      nondisplaced S62.18-•
    triquetrum (displaced) S62.11-•
      nondisplaced S62.11-•
    unciform —*see* Fracture, carpal bones, hamate
  cervical —*see* Fracture, vertebra, cervical
  clavicle S42.00-•
    acromial end (displaced) S42.03-•
      nondisplaced S42.03-•
    birth injury P13.4
    lateral end —*see* Fracture, clavicle, acromial end
    shaft (displaced) S42.02-•
      nondisplaced S42.02-•
    sternal end (anterior) (displaced) S42.01-•
      nondisplaced S42.01-•
      posterior S42.01-•
  coccyx S32.2
  collapsed —*see* Collapse, vertebra
  collar bone —*see* Fracture, clavicle
  Colles' —*see* Colles' fracture
  coronoid process —*see* Fracture, ulna, upper end, coronoid process
  corpus cavernosum penis S39.840
  costochondral cartilage S23.41
  costochondral, costosternal junction —*see* Fracture, rib
  cranium —*see* Fracture, skull
  cricoid cartilage S12.8
  cuboid (ankle) —*see* Fracture, tarsal, cuboid
  cuneiform
    foot —*see* Fracture, tarsal, cuneiform
    wrist —*see* Fracture, carpal, triquetrum
  delayed union —*see* Delay, union, fracture
  dental restorative material K08.539
    with loss of material K08.531
    without loss of material K08.530

Fracture, traumatic (*Continued*)
- due to
  - birth injury —*see* Birth, injury, fracture
  - osteoporosis —*see* Osteoporosis, with fracture
- Dupuytren's —*see* Fracture, ankle, lateral malleolus
- elbow S42.40-●
- ethmoid (bone) (sinus) —*see* Fracture, skull, base
- face bone S02.92
- fatigue —*see also* Fracture, stress
  - vertebra M48.40
    - cervical region M48.42
    - cervicothoracic region M48.43
    - lumbar region M48.46
    - lumbosacral region M48.47
    - occipito-atlanto-axial region M48.41
    - sacrococcygeal region M48.48
    - thoracic region M48.44
    - thoracolumbar region M48.45
- femur, femoral S72.9-●
  - basicervical (basal) S72.0
  - birth injury P13.2
  - capital epiphyseal S79.01-●
  - condyles, epicondyles —*see* Fracture, femur, lower end
  - distal end —*see* Fracture, femur, lower end
  - epiphysis
    - head —*see* Fracture, femur, upper end, epiphysis
    - lower —*see* Fracture, femur, lower end, epiphysis
    - upper —*see* Fracture, femur, upper end, epiphysis
  - following insertion of implant, prosthesis or plate M96.66-●
  - head —*see* Fracture, femur, upper end, head
  - intertrochanteric —*see* Fracture, femur, trochanteric
  - intratrochanteric —*see* Fracture, femur, trochanteric
  - lower end S72.40-●
    - condyle (displaced) S72.41-●
      - lateral (displaced) S72.42-●
        - nondisplaced S72.42-●
      - medial (displaced) S72.43-●
        - nondisplaced S72.43-●
      - nondisplaced S72.41-●
    - epiphysis (displaced) S72.44-●
      - nondisplaced S72.44-●
    - physeal S79.10-●
      - Salter-Harris
        - Type I S79.11-●
        - Type II S79.12-●
        - Type III S79.13-●
        - Type IV S79.14-●
        - specified NEC S79.19-●
    - specified NEC S72.49-●
    - supracondylar (displaced) S72.45-●
      - with intracondylar extension (displaced) S72.46-●
        - nondisplaced S72.46-●
      - nondisplaced S72.45-●
    - torus S72.47-●
  - neck —*see* Fracture, femur, upper end, neck
  - pertrochanteric —*see* Fracture, femur, trochanteric
  - shaft (lower third) (middle third) (upper third) S72.30-●
    - comminuted (displaced) S72.35-●
      - nondisplaced S72.35-●
    - oblique (displaced) S72.33-●
      - nondisplaced S72.33-●
    - segmental (displaced) S72.36-●
      - nondisplaced S72.36-●
    - specified NEC S72.39-●
    - spiral (displaced) S72.34-●
      - nondisplaced S72.34-●
    - transverse (displaced) S72.32-●
      - nondisplaced S72.32-●

Fracture, traumatic (*Continued*)
- femur, femoral (*Continued*)
  - specified site NEC —*see* subcategory S72.8
  - subcapital (displaced) S72.01-●
  - subtrochanteric (region) (section) (displaced) S72.2-●
    - nondisplaced S72.2-●
  - transcervical —*see* Fracture, femur, upper end, neck
  - transtrochanteric —*see* Fracture, femur, trochanteric
  - trochanteric S72.10-●
    - apophyseal (displaced) S72.13-●
      - nondisplaced S72.13-●
    - greater trochanter (displaced) S72.11-●
      - nondisplaced S72.11-●
    - intertrochanteric (displaced) S72.14-●
      - nondisplaced S72.14-●
    - lesser trochanter (displaced) S72.12-●
      - nondisplaced S72.12-●
  - upper end S72.00-●
    - apophyseal (displaced) S72.13-●
      - nondisplaced S72.13-●
    - cervicotrochanteric —*see* Fracture, femur, upper end, neck, base
    - epiphysis (displaced) S72.02-●
      - nondisplaced S72.02-●
    - head S72.05-●
      - articular (displaced) S72.06-●
        - nondisplaced S72.06-●
      - specified NEC S72.09-●
    - intertrochanteric (displaced) S72.14-●
      - nondisplaced S72.14-●
    - intracapsular S72.01-●
    - midcervical (displaced) S72.03-●
      - nondisplaced S72.03-●
    - neck S72.00-●
      - base (displaced) S72.04-●
        - nondisplaced S72.04-●
      - specified NEC S72.09-●
    - pertrochanteric —*see* Fracture, femur, upper end, trochanteric
    - physeal S79.00-●
      - Salter-Harris type I S79.01-●
      - specified NEC S79.09-●
    - subcapital (displaced) S72.01-●
    - subtrochanteric (displaced) S72.2-●
      - nondisplaced S72.2-●
    - transcervical —*see* Fracture, femur, upper end, midcervical
    - trochanteric S72.10-●
      - greater (displaced) S72.11-●
        - nondisplaced S72.11-●
      - lesser (displaced) S72.12-●
        - nondisplaced S72.12-●
- fibula (shaft) (styloid) S82.40-●
  - comminuted (displaced) S82.45-●
    - nondisplaced S82.45-●
  - following insertion of implant, prosthesis or plate M96.67-●
  - involving ankle or malleolus —*see* Fracture, fibula, lateral malleolus
  - lateral malleolus (displaced) S82.6-●
    - nondisplaced S82.6-●
  - lower end
    - physeal S89.30-●
      - Salter-Harris
        - Type I S89.31-●
        - Type II S89.32-●
        - specified NEC S89.39-●
    - specified NEC S82.83-●
    - torus S82.82-●
  - oblique (displaced) S82.43-●
    - nondisplaced S82.43-●
  - segmental (displaced) S82.46-●
    - nondisplaced S82.46-●
  - specified NEC S82.49-●
  - spiral (displaced) S82.44-●
    - nondisplaced S82.44-●
  - transverse (displaced) S82.42-●
    - nondisplaced S82.42-●

Fracture, traumatic (*Continued*)
- fibula (shaft) (styloid) (*Continued*)
  - upper end
    - physeal S89.20-●
      - Salter-Harris
        - Type I S89.21-●
        - Type II S89.22-●
        - specified NEC S89.29-●
    - specified NEC S82.83-●
    - torus S82.81-●
- finger (except thumb) S62.60-●
  - distal phalanx (displaced) S62.63-●
    - nondisplaced S62.66-●
  - index S62.60-●
    - distal phalanx (displaced) S62.63-●
      - nondisplaced S62.66-●
    - medial phalanx (displaced) S62.62-●
      - nondisplaced S62.65-●
    - proximal phalanx (displaced) S62.61-●
      - nondisplaced S62.64-●
  - little S62.60-●
    - distal phalanx (displaced) S62.63-●
      - nondisplaced S62.66-●
    - medial phalanx (displaced) S62.62-●
      - nondisplaced S62.65-●
    - proximal phalanx (displaced) S62.61-●
      - nondisplaced S62.64-●
  - medial phalanx (displaced) S62.62-●
    - nondisplaced S62.65-●
  - middle S62.60-●
    - distal phalanx (displaced) S62.63-●
      - nondisplaced S62.66-●
    - medial phalanx (displaced) S62.62-●
      - nondisplaced S62.65-●
    - proximal phalanx (displaced) S62.61-●
      - nondisplaced S62.64-●
  - proximal phalanx (displaced) S62.61-●
    - nondisplaced S62.64-●
  - ring S62.60-●
    - distal phalanx (displaced) S62.63-●
      - nondisplaced S62.66-●
    - medial phalanx (displaced) S62.62-●
      - nondisplaced S62.65-●
    - proximal phalanx (displaced) S62.61-●
      - nondisplaced S62.64-●
  - thumb —*see* Fracture, thumb
- following insertion (intraoperative) (postoperative) of orthopedic implant, joint prosthesis or bone plate M96.69
  - femur M96.66-●
  - fibula M96.67-●
  - humerus M96.62-●
  - pelvis M96.65
  - radius M96.63-●
  - specified bone NEC M96.69
  - tibia M96.67-●
  - ulna M96.63-●
- foot S92.90-●
  - astragalus —*see* Fracture, tarsal, talus
  - calcaneus —*see* Fracture, tarsal, calcaneus
  - cuboid —*see* Fracture, tarsal, cuboid
  - cuneiform —*see* Fracture, tarsal, cuneiform
  - metatarsal —*see* Fracture, metatarsal
  - navicular —*see* Fracture, tarsal, navicular
  - sesamoid S92.81-●
  - specified NEC S92.81-●
  - talus —*see* Fracture, tarsal, talus
  - tarsal —*see* Fracture, tarsal
  - toe —*see* Fracture, toe
- forearm S52.9-●
  - radius —*see* Fracture, radius
  - ulna —*see* Fracture, ulna
- fossa (anterior) (middle) (posterior) S02.19
- frontal (bone) (skull) S02.0
  - sinus S02.19
- glenoid (cavity) (scapula) —*see* Fracture, scapula, glenoid cavity
- greenstick —*see* Fracture, by site
- hallux —*see* Fracture, toe, great
- hand S62.9-●
  - carpal —*see* Fracture, carpal bone

Fracture, traumatic *(Continued)*
  hand *(Continued)*
    finger (except thumb) —*see* Fracture, finger
    metacarpal —*see* Fracture, metacarpal
    navicular (scaphoid) (hand) —*see* Fracture, carpal bone, navicular
    thumb —*see* Fracture, thumb
  healed or old
    with complications - code by Nature of the complication
  heel bone —*see* Fracture, tarsal, calcaneus
  Hill-Sachs S42.29-●
  hip —*see* Fracture, femur, neck
  humerus S42.30-●
    anatomical neck —*see* Fracture, humerus, upper end
    articular process —*see* Fracture, humerus, lower end
    capitellum —*see* Fracture, humerus, lower end, condyle, lateral
    distal end —*see* Fracture, humerus, lower end
    epiphysis
      lower —*see* Fracture, humerus, lower end, physeal
      upper —*see* Fracture, humerus, upper end, physeal
    external condyle —*see* Fracture, humerus, lower end, condyle, lateral
    following insertion of implant, prosthesis or plate M96.62-●
    great tuberosity —*see* Fracture, humerus, upper end, greater tuberosity
    intercondylar —*see* Fracture, humerus, lower end
    internal epicondyle —*see* Fracture, humerus, lower end, epicondyle, medial
    lesser tuberosity —*see* Fracture, humerus, upper end, lesser tuberosity
    lower end S42.40-●
      condyle
        lateral (displaced) S42.45-●
          nondisplaced S42.45-●
        medial (displaced) S42.46-●
          nondisplaced S42.46-●
      epicondyle
        lateral (displaced) S42.43-●
          nondisplaced S42.43-●
        medial (displaced) S42.44-●
          incarcerated S42.44-●
          nondisplaced S42.44-●
      physeal S49.10-●
        Salter-Harris
          Type I S49.11-●
          Type II S49.12-●
          Type III S49.13-●
          Type IV S49.14-●
        specified NEC S49.19-●
      specified NEC (displaced) S42.49-●
        nondisplaced S42.49-●
      supracondylar (simple) (displaced) S42.41-●
        with intercondylar fracture —*see* Fracture, humerus, lower end
        comminuted (displaced) S42.42-●
          nondisplaced S42.42-●
        nondisplaced S42.41-●
      torus S42.48-●
      transcondylar (displaced) S42.47-●
        nondisplaced S42.47-●
    proximal end —*see* Fracture, humerus, upper end
    shaft S42.30-●
      comminuted (displaced) S42.35-●
        nondisplaced S42.35-●
      greenstick S42.31-●
      oblique (displaced) S42.33-●
        nondisplaced S42.33-●
      segmental (displaced) S42.36-●
        nondisplaced S42.36-●
      specified NEC S42.39-●

Fracture, traumatic *(Continued)*
  humerus *(Continued)*
    shaft *(Continued)*
      spiral (displaced) S42.34-●
        nondisplaced S42.34-●
      transverse (displaced) S42.32-●
        nondisplaced S42.32-●
    supracondylar —*see* Fracture, humerus, lower end
    surgical neck —*see* Fracture, humerus, upper end, surgical neck
    trochlea —*see* Fracture, humerus, lower end, condyle, medial
    tuberosity —*see* Fracture, humerus, upper end
    upper end S42.20-●
      anatomical neck —*see* Fracture, humerus, upper end, specified NEC
      articular head —*see* Fracture, humerus, upper end, specified NEC
      epiphysis —*see* Fracture, humerus, upper end, physeal
      greater tuberosity (displaced) S42.25-●
        nondisplaced S42.25-●
      lesser tuberosity (displaced) S42.26-●
        nondisplaced S42.26-●
      physeal S49.00-●
        Salter-Harris
          Type I S49.01-●
          Type II S49.02-●
          Type III S49.03-●
          Type IV S49.04-●
        specified NEC S49.09-●
      specified NEC (displaced) S42.29-●
        nondisplaced S42.29-●
      surgical neck (displaced) S42.21-●
        four-part S42.24-●
        nondisplaced S42.21-●
        three-part S42.23-●
        two-part (displaced) S42.22-●
          nondisplaced S42.22-●
      torus S42.27-●
      transepiphyseal —*see* Fracture, humerus, upper end, physeal
  hyoid bone S12.8
  ilium S32.30-●
    with disruption of pelvic ring —*see* Disruption, pelvic ring
    avulsion (displaced) S32.31-●
      nondisplaced S32.31-●
    specified NEC S32.39-●
  impaction, impacted - code as Fracture, by site
  innominate bone —*see* Fracture, ilium
  instep —*see* Fracture, foot
  ischium S32.60-●
    with disruption of pelvic ring —*see* Disruption, pelvic ring
    avulsion (displaced) S32.61-●
      nondisplaced S32.61-●
    specified NEC S32.69-●
  jaw (bone) (lower) —*see* Fracture, mandible
    upper —*see* Fracture, maxilla
  joint prosthesis —*see* Complications, joint prosthesis, mechanical, breakdown, by site
    periprosthetic —*see* Fracture, traumatic, periprosthetic
  knee cap —*see* Fracture, patella
  larynx S12.8
  late effects —*see* Sequelae, fracture
  leg (lower) S82.9-●
    ankle —*see* Fracture, ankle
    femur —*see* Fracture, femur
    fibula —*see* Fracture, fibula
    malleolus —*see* Fracture, ankle
    patella —*see* Fracture, patella
    specified site NEC S82.89-●
    tibia —*see* Fracture, tibia
  lumbar spine —*see* Fracture, vertebra, lumbar
  lumbosacral spine S32.9

Fracture, traumatic *(Continued)*
  Maisonneuve's (displaced) S82.86-●
    nondisplaced S82.86-●
  malar bone —*see also* Fracture, maxilla S02.400
    left side S02.40B
    right side S02.40A
  malleolus —*see* Fracture, ankle
  malunion —*see* Fracture, by site
  mandible (lower jawbone) S02.609
    alveolus S02.67-●
    angle (of jaw) S02.65-●
    body, unspecified S02.600-●
      left side S02.602
      right side S02.601
    condylar process S02.61-●
    coronoid process S02.63-●
    ramus, unspecified S02.64-●
    specified site NEC S02.69
    subcondylar process S02.62-●
    symphysis S02.66
  manubrium (sterni) S22.21
    dissociation from sternum S22.23
  march —*see* Fracture, traumatic, stress, by site
  maxilla, maxillary (bone) (sinus) (superior) (upper jaw) S02.401
    alveolus S02.42
    inferior —*see* Fracture, mandible
    LeFort I S02.411
    LeFort II S02.412
    LeFort III S02.413
    left side S02.40D
    right side S02.40C
  metacarpal S62.309
    base (displaced) S62.319
      nondisplaced S62.349
    fifth S62.30-●
      base (displaced) S62.31-●
        nondisplaced S62.34-●
      neck (displaced) S62.33-●
        nondisplaced S62.36-●
      shaft (displaced) S62.32-●
        nondisplaced S62.35-●
      specified NEC S62.398
    first S62.20-●
      base NEC (displaced) S62.23-●
        nondisplaced S62.23-●
      Bennett's —*see* Bennett's fracture
      neck (displaced) S62.25-●
        nondisplaced S62.25-●
      shaft (displaced) S62.24-●
        nondisplaced S62.24-●
      specified NEC S62.29-●
    fourth S62.30-●
      base (displaced) S62.31-●
        nondisplaced S62.34-●
      neck (displaced) S62.33-●
        nondisplaced S62.36-●
      shaft (displaced) S62.32-●
        nondisplaced S62.35-●
      specified NEC S62.39-●
    neck (displaced) S62.33-●
      nondisplaced S62.36-●
    Rolando's —*see* Rolando's fracture
    second S62.30-●
      base (displaced) S62.31-●
        nondisplaced S62.34-●
      neck (displaced) S62.33-●
        nondisplaced S62.36-●
      shaft (displaced) S62.32-●
        nondisplaced S62.35-●
      specified NEC S62.39-●
    shaft (displaced) S62.32-●
      nondisplaced S62.35-●
    specified NEC S62.399
    third S62.30-●
      base (displaced) S62.31-●
        nondisplaced S62.34-●
      neck (displaced) S62.33-●
        nondisplaced S62.36-●
      shaft (displaced) S62.32-●
        nondisplaced S62.35-●
      specified NEC S62.39-●

▶ New   ⇒ Revised   ~~deleted~~ Deleted   ● Use Additional Character(s)

Fracture, traumatic *(Continued)*
  metastatic —*see* Fracture, pathological,
    due to, neoplastic disease —*see also*
    Neoplasm
  metatarsal bone S92.30-●
    fifth (displaced) S92.35-●
      nondisplaced S92.35-●
    first (displaced) S92.31-●
      nondisplaced S92.31-●
    fourth (displaced) S92.34-●
      nondisplaced S92.34-●
    physeal S99.10-●
      Salter-Harris
        Type I S99.11-●
        Type II S99.12-●
        Type III S99.13-●
        Type IV S99.14-●
      specified NEC S99.19-●
    second (displaced) S92.32-●
      nondisplaced S92.32-●
    third (displaced) S92.33-●
      nondisplaced S92.33-●
  Monteggia's —*see* Monteggia's
    fracture
  multiple
    hand (and wrist) NEC —*see* Fracture, by
      site
    ribs —*see* Fracture, rib, multiple
  nasal (bone(s)) S02.2
  navicular (scaphoid) (foot) —*see also* Fracture,
    tarsal, navicular
    hand —*see* Fracture, carpal, navicular
  neck S12.9
    cervical vertebra S12.9
      fifth (displaced) S12.400
        nondisplaced S12.401
        specified type NEC (displaced)
          S12.490
          nondisplaced S12.491
      first (displaced) S12.000
        burst (stable) S12.01
          unstable S12.02
        lateral mass (displaced) S12.040
          nondisplaced S12.041
        nondisplaced S12.001
        posterior arch (displaced) S12.030
          nondisplaced S12.031
        specified type NEC (displaced)
          S12.090
          nondisplaced S12.091
      fourth (displaced) S12.300
        nondisplaced S12.301
        specified type NEC (displaced)
          S12.390
          nondisplaced S12.391
      second (displaced) S12.100
        dens (anterior) (displaced) (type II)
          S12.110
          nondisplaced S12.112
          posterior S12.111
        specified type NEC (displaced)
          S12.120
          nondisplaced S12.121
        nondisplaced S12.101
        specified type NEC (displaced)
          S12.190
          nondisplaced S12.191
      seventh (displaced) S12.600
        nondisplaced S12.601
        specified type NEC (displaced) S12.690
          nondisplaced S12.691
      sixth (displaced) S12.500
        nondisplaced S12.501
        specified type NEC (displaced)
          S12.590
          nondisplaced S12.591
      third (displaced) S12.200
        nondisplaced S12.201
        specified type NEC (displaced)
          S12.290
          nondisplaced S12.291

Fracture, traumatic *(Continued)*
  neck *(Continued)*
    hyoid bone S12.8
    larynx S12.8
    specified site NEC S12.8
    thyroid cartilage S12.8
    trachea S12.8
  neoplastic NEC —*see* Fracture, pathological,
    due to, neoplastic disease
  neural arch —*see* Fracture, vertebra
  newborn —*see* Birth, injury, fracture
  nontraumatic —*see* Fracture, pathological
  nonunion —*see* Nonunion, fracture
  nose, nasal (bone) (septum) S02.2
  occiput —*see* Fracture, skull, base, occiput
  odontoid process —*see* Fracture, neck,
    cervical vertebra, second
  olecranon (process) (ulna) —*see* Fracture,
    ulna, upper end, olecranon process
  orbit, orbital (bone) (region) S02.8-●
    floor (blow-out) S02.3-●
    roof S02.19
  os
    calcis —*see* Fracture, tarsal, calcaneus
    magnum —*see* Fracture, carpal, capitate
    pubis —*see* Fracture, pubis
  palate S02.8-●
  parietal bone (skull) S02.0
  patella S82.00-●
    comminuted (displaced) S82.04-●
      nondisplaced S82.04-●
    longitudinal (displaced) S82.02-●
      nondisplaced S82.02-●
    osteochondral (displaced) S82.01-●
      nondisplaced S82.01-●
    specified NEC S82.09-●
    transverse (displaced) S82.03-●
      nondisplaced S82.03-●
  pedicle (of vertebral arch) —*see* Fracture,
    vertebra
  pelvis, pelvic (bone) S32.9
    acetabulum —*see* Fracture, acetabulum
    circle —*see* Disruption, pelvic ring
    following insertion of implant, prosthesis
      or plate M96.65
    ilium —*see* Fracture, ilium
    ischium —*see* Fracture, ischium
    multiple
      with disruption of pelvic ring (circle) —
        see Disruption, pelvic ring
      without disruption of pelvic ring (circle)
        S32.82
    pubis —*see* Fracture, pubis
    sacrum —*see* Fracture, sacrum
    specified site NEC S32.89
  periprosthetic, around internal prosthetic
    joint M97.9
    ankle M97.2-●
    elbow M97.4-●
    finger M97.8
    hip M97.0-●
    knee M97.1-●
    shoulder M97.3-●
    specified joint NEC M97.8
    spine M97.8
    toe M97.8
    wrist M97.8
  phalanx
    foot —*see* Fracture, toe
    hand —*see* Fracture, finger
  pisiform —*see* Fracture, carpal, pisiform
  pond —*see* Fracture, skull
  prosthetic device, internal —*see*
    Complications, prosthetic device, by site,
    mechanical
  pubis S32.50-●
    with disruption of pelvic ring —*see*
      Disruption, pelvic ring
    specified site NEC S32.59-●
    superior rim S32.59-●

Fracture, traumatic *(Continued)*
  radius S52.9-●
    distal end —*see* Fracture, radius,
      lower end
    following insertion of implant, prosthesis
      or plate M96.63-●
    head —*see* Fracture, radius, upper end,
      head
    lower end S52.50-●
      Barton's —*see* Barton's fracture
      Colles' —*see* Colles' fracture
      extraarticular NEC S52.55-●
      intraarticular NEC S52.57-●
      physeal S59.20-●
        Salter-Harris
          Type I S59.21-●
          Type II S59.22-●
          Type III S59.23-●
          Type IV S59.24-●
        specified NEC S59.29-●
      Smith's —*see* Smith's fracture
      specified NEC S52.59-●
      styloid process (displaced) S52.51-●
        nondisplaced S52.51-●
      torus S52.52-●
    neck —*see* Fracture, radius, upper end
    proximal end —*see* Fracture, radius, upper
      end
    shaft S52.30-●
      bent bone S52.38-●
      comminuted (displaced) S52.35-●
        nondisplaced S52.35-●
      Galeazzi's —*see* Galeazzi's fracture
      greenstick S52.31-●
      oblique (displaced) S52.33-●
        nondisplaced S52.33-●
      segmental (displaced) S52.36-●
        nondisplaced S52.36-●
      specified NEC S52.39-●
      spiral (displaced) S52.34-●
        nondisplaced S52.34-●
      transverse (displaced) S52.32-●
        nondisplaced S52.32-●
    upper end S52.10-●
      head (displaced) S52.12-●
        nondisplaced S52.12-●
      neck (displaced) S52.13-●
        nondisplaced S52.13-●
      physeal S59.10-●
        Salter-Harris
          Type I S59.11-●
          Type II S59.12-●
          Type III S59.13-●
          Type IV S59.14-●
        specified NEC S59.19-●
      specified NEC S52.18-●
      torus S52.11-●
  ramus
    inferior or superior, pubis —*see* Fracture,
      pubis
    mandible —*see* Fracture, mandible
  restorative material (dental) K08.539
    with loss of material K08.531
    without loss of material K08.530
  rib S22.3-●
    with flail chest —*see* Flail, chest
    multiple S22.4-●
      with flail chest —*see* Flail, chest
  root, tooth —*see* Fracture, tooth
  sacrum S32.10
    specified NEC S32.19
    Type
      1 S32.14
      2 S32.15
      3 S32.16
      4 S32.17
    Zone
      I S32.119
        displaced (minimally) S32.111
          severely S32.112
        nondisplaced S32.110

▶ New   ⇒ Revised   ~~deleted~~ Deleted   ● Use Additional Character(s)

Fracture, traumatic *(Continued)*
 sacrum *(Continued)*
  Zone *(Continued)*
   II S32.129
    displaced (minimally) S32.121
     severely S32.122
    nondisplaced S32.120
   III S32.139
    displaced (minimally) S32.131
     severely S32.132
    nondisplaced S32.130
 scaphoid (hand) —*see also* Fracture, carpal, navicular
  foot —*see* Fracture, tarsal, navicular
 scapula S42.10-●
  acromial process (displaced) S42.12-●
   nondisplaced S42.12-●
  body (displaced) S42.11-●
   nondisplaced S42.11-●
  coracoid process (displaced) S42.13-●
   nondisplaced S42.13-●
  glenoid cavity (displaced) S42.14-●
   nondisplaced S42.14-●
  neck (displaced) S42.15-●
   nondisplaced S42.15-●
  specified NEC S42.19-●
 semilunar bone, wrist —*see* Fracture, carpal, lunate
 sequelae —*see* Sequelae, fracture
 sesamoid bone
  foot S92.81-●
  hand —*see* Fracture, carpal
  other —*see* Fracture, traumatic, by site
 shepherd's —*see* Fracture, tarsal, talus
 shoulder (girdle) S42.9-●
  blade —*see* Fracture, scapula
 sinus (ethmoid) (frontal) S02.19
 skull S02.91
  base S02.10-●
   occiput S02.119
    condyle S02.113
     type I S02.110
      left side S02.11B
      right side S02.11A
     type II S02.111
      left side S02.11D
      right side S02.11C
     type III S02.112
      left side S02.11F
      right side S02.11E
     specified NEC S02.118
      left side S02.11H
      right side S02.11G
   specified NEC S02.19-●
  birth injury P13.0
  frontal bone S02.0
  parietal bone S02.0
  specified site NEC S02.8
  temporal bone S02.19
  vault S02.0
 Smith's —*see* Smith's fracture
 sphenoid (bone) (sinus) S02.19
 spine —*see* Fracture, vertebra
 spinous process —*see* Fracture, vertebra
 spontaneous (cause unknown) —*see* Fracture, pathological
 stave (of thumb) —*see* Fracture, metacarpal, first
 sternum S22.20
  with flail chest —*see* Flail, chest
  body S22.22
  manubrium S22.21
  xiphoid (process) S22.24
 stress M84.30
  ankle M84.37-●
  carpus M84.34-●
  clavicle M84.31-●
  femoral neck M84.359
  femur M84.35-●
  fibula M84.36-●
  finger M84.34-●

Fracture, traumatic *(Continued)*
 stress *(Continued)*
  hip M84.359
  humerus M84.32-●
  ilium M84.350
  ischium M84.350
  metacarpus M84.34-●
  metatarsus M84.37-●
  neck —*see* Fracture, fatigue, vertebra
  pelvis M84.350
  radius M84.33-●
  rib M84.38
  scapula M84.31-●
  skull M84.38
  tarsus M84.37-●
  tibia M84.36-●
  toe M84.37-●
  ulna M84.33-●
  vertebra —*see* Fracture, fatigue, vertebra
 supracondylar, elbow —*see* Fracture, humerus, lower end, supracondylar
 symphysis pubis —*see* Fracture, pubis
 talus (ankle bone) —*see* Fracture, tarsal, talus
 tarsal bone(s) S92.20-●
  astragalus —*see* Fracture, tarsal, talus
  calcaneus S92.00-●
   anterior process (displaced) S92.02-●
    nondisplaced S92.02-●
   body (displaced) S92.01-●
    nondisplaced S92.01-●
   extraarticular NEC (displaced) S92.05-●
    nondisplaced S92.05-●
   intraarticular (displaced) S92.06-●
    nondisplaced S92.06-●
   physeal S99.00-●
    Salter-Harris
     Type I S99.01-●
     Type II S99.02-●
     Type III S99.03-●
     Type IV S99.04-●
    specified NEC S99.09-●
   tuberosity (displaced) S92.04-●
    avulsion (displaced) S92.03-●
     nondisplaced S92.03-●
    nondisplaced S92.04-●
  cuboid (displaced) S92.21-●
   nondisplaced S92.21-●
  cuneiform
   intermediate (displaced) S92.23-●
    nondisplaced S92.23-●
   lateral (displaced) S92.22-●
    nondisplaced S92.22-●
   medial (displaced) S92.24-●
    nondisplaced S92.24-●
  navicular (displaced) S92.25-●
   nondisplaced S92.25-●
  scaphoid —*see* Fracture, tarsal, navicular
  talus S92.10-●
   avulsion (displaced) S92.15-●
    nondisplaced S92.15-●
   body (displaced) S92.12-●
    nondisplaced S92.12-●
   dome (displaced) S92.14-●
    nondisplaced S92.14-●
   head (displaced) S92.12-●
    nondisplaced S92.12-●
   lateral process (displaced) S92.14-●
    nondisplaced S92.14-●
   neck (displaced) S92.11-●
    nondisplaced S92.11-●
   posterior process (displaced) S92.13-●
    nondisplaced S92.13-●
   specified NEC S92.19-●
  temporal bone (styloid) S02.19
 thorax (bony) S22.9
  with flail chest —*see* Flail, chest
  rib S22.3-●
   multiple S22.4-●
    with flail chest —*see* Flail, chest

Fracture, traumatic *(Continued)*
 thorax *(Continued)*
  sternum S22.20
   body S22.22
   manubrium S22.21
   xiphoid process S22.24
  vertebra (displaced) S22.009
   burst (stable) S22.001
    unstable S22.002
   eighth S22.069
    burst (stable) S22.061
     unstable S22.062
    specified type NEC S22.068
    wedge compression S22.060
   eleventh S22.089
    burst (stable) S22.081
     unstable S22.082
    specified type NEC S22.088
    wedge compression S22.080
   fifth S22.059
    burst (stable) S22.051
     unstable S22.052
    specified type NEC S22.058
    wedge compression S22.050
   first S22.019
    burst (stable) S22.011
     unstable S22.012
    specified type NEC S22.018
    wedge compression S22.010
   fourth S22.049
    burst (stable) S22.041
     unstable S22.042
    specified type NEC S22.048
    wedge compression S22.040
   ninth S22.079
    burst (stable) S22.071
     unstable S22.072
    specified type NEC S22.078
    wedge compression S22.070
   nondisplaced S22.001
   second S22.029
    burst (stable) S22.021
     unstable S22.022
    specified type NEC S22.028
    wedge compression S22.020
   seventh S22.069
    burst (stable) S22.061
     unstable S22.062
    specified type NEC S22.068
    wedge compression S22.060
   sixth S22.059
    burst (stable) S22.051
     unstable S22.052
    specified type NEC S22.058
    wedge compression S22.050
   specified type NEC S22.008
   tenth S22.079
    burst (stable) S22.071
     unstable S22.072
    specified type NEC S22.078
    wedge compression S22.070
   third S22.039
    burst (stable) S22.031
     unstable S22.032
    specified type NEC S22.038
    wedge compression S22.030
   twelfth S22.089
    burst (stable) S22.081
     unstable S22.082
    specified type NEC S22.088
    wedge compression S22.080
   wedge compression S22.000
  thumb S62.50-●
   distal phalanx (displaced) S62.52-●
    nondisplaced S62.52-●
   proximal phalanx (displaced) S62.51-●
    nondisplaced S62.51-●
  thyroid cartilage S12.8
  tibia (shaft) S82.20-●
   comminuted (displaced) S82.25-●
    nondisplaced S82.25-●

▶ New   ➡ Revised   ~~deleted~~ Deleted   ● Use Additional Character(s)

Fracture, traumatic *(Continued)*
  tibia *(Continued)*
    condyles —*see* Fracture, tibia, upper end
    distal end —*see* Fracture, tibia, lower end
    epiphysis
      lower —*see* Fracture, tibia, lower end
      upper —*see* Fracture, tibia, upper end
    following insertion of implant, prosthesis
        or plate M96.67-●
    head (involving knee joint) —*see* Fracture,
        tibia, upper end
    intercondyloid eminence —*see* Fracture,
        tibia, upper end
    involving ankle or malleolus —*see*
        Fracture, ankle, medial malleolus
    lower end S82.30-●
      physeal S89.10-●
        Salter-Harris
          Type I S89.11-●
          Type II S89.12-●
          Type III S89.13-●
          Type IV S89.14-●
          specified NEC S89.19-●
      pilon (displaced) S82.87-●
        nondisplaced S82.87-●
      specified NEC S82.39-●
      torus S82.31-●
    malleolus —*see* Fracture, ankle, medial
        malleolus
    oblique (displaced) S82.23-●
      nondisplaced S82.23-●
    pilon —*see* Fracture, tibia, lower end, pilon
    proximal end —*see* Fracture, tibia, upper
        end
    segmental (displaced) S82.26-●
      nondisplaced S82.26-●
    specified NEC S82.29-●
    ⇒spine —*see* Fracture, tibia, upper end, spine
    spiral (displaced) S82.24-●
      nondisplaced S82.24-●
    transverse (displaced) S82.22-●
      nondisplaced S82.22-●
    tuberosity —*see* Fracture, tibia, upper end,
        tuberosity
    upper end S82.10-●
      bicondylar (displaced) S82.14-●
        nondisplaced S82.14-●
      lateral condyle (displaced) S82.12-●
        nondisplaced S82.12-●
      medial condyle (displaced) S82.13-●
        nondisplaced S82.13-●
      physeal S89.00-●
        Salter-Harris
          Type I S89.01-●
          Type II S89.02-●
          Type III S89.03-●
          Type IV S89.04-●
          specified NEC S89.09-●
      plateau —*see* Fracture, tibia, upper end,
          bicondylar
      specified NEC S82.19-●
      spine (displaced) S82.11-●
        nondisplaced S82.11-●
      torus S82.16-●
      tuberosity (displaced) S82.15-●
        nondisplaced S82.15-●
  toe S92.91-●
    great (displaced) S92.40-●
      distal phalanx (displaced) S92.42-●
        nondisplaced S92.42-●
      nondisplaced S92.40-●
      proximal phalanx (displaced)
          S92.41-●
        nondisplaced S92.41-●
      specified NEC S92.49-●
    lesser (displaced) S92.50-●
      distal phalanx (displaced) S92.53-●
        nondisplaced S92.53-●
      medial phalanx (displaced) S92.52-●
        nondisplaced S92.52-●
      nondisplaced S92.50-●

Fracture, traumatic *(Continued)*
  toe *(Continued)*
    lesser *(Continued)*
      proximal phalanx (displaced) S92.51-●
        nondisplaced S92.51-●
      specified NEC S92.59-●
    physeal
      phalanx S99.20-●
        Salter-Harris
          Type I S99.21-●
          Type II S99.22-●
          Type III S99.23-●
          Type IV S99.24-●
          specified NEC S99.29-●
  tooth (root) S02.5
  trachea (cartilage) S12.8
  transverse process —*see* Fracture, vertebra
  trapezium or trapezoid bone —*see* Fracture,
      carpal
  trimalleolar —*see* Fracture, ankle, trimalleolar
  triquetrum (cuneiform of carpus) —*see*
      Fracture, carpal, triquetrum
  trochanter —*see* Fracture, femur, trochanteric
  tuberosity (external) —*see* Fracture,
      traumatic, by site
  ulna (shaft) S52.20-●
    bent bone S52.28-●
    coronoid process —*see* Fracture, ulna,
        upper end, coronoid process
    distal end —*see* Fracture, ulna, lower end
    following insertion of implant, prosthesis
        or plate M96.63-●
    ⇒head S52.60-●
    lower end S52.60-●
      physeal S59.00-●
        Salter-Harris
          Type I S59.01-●
          Type II S59.02-●
          Type III S59.03-●
          Type IV S59.04-●
          specified NEC S59.09-●
      specified NEC S52.69-●
      styloid process (displaced) S52.61-●
        nondisplaced S52.61-●
      torus S52.62-●
    proximal end —*see* Fracture, ulna, upper
        end
    shaft S52.20-●
      comminuted (displaced) S52.25-●
        nondisplaced S52.25-●
      greenstick S52.21-●
      Monteggia's —*see* Monteggia's fracture
      oblique (displaced) S52.23-●
        nondisplaced S52.23-●
      segmental (displaced) S52.26-●
        nondisplaced S52.26-●
      specified NEC S52.29-●
      spiral (displaced) S52.24-●
        nondisplaced S52.24-●
      transverse (displaced) S52.22-●
        nondisplaced S52.22-●
    upper end S52.00-●
      coronoid process (displaced) S52.04-●
        nondisplaced S52.04-●
      olecranon process (displaced) S52.02-●
        with intraarticular extension S52.03-●
        nondisplaced S52.02-●
          with intraarticular extension S52.03-●
      specified NEC S52.09-●
      torus S52.01-●
  unciform —*see* Fracture, carpal, hamate
  vault of skull S02.0
  vertebra, vertebral (arch) (body) (column)
      (neural arch) (pedicle) (spinous process)
      (transverse process)
    atlas —*see* Fracture, neck, cervical vertebra,
        first
    axis —*see* Fracture, neck, cervical vertebra,
        second
    cervical (teardrop) S12.9
      axis —*see* Fracture, neck, cervical
          vertebra, second

Fracture, traumatic *(Continued)*
  vertebra, vertebral *(Continued)*
    cervical *(Continued)*
      first (atlas) —*see* Fracture, neck, cervical
          vertebra, first
      second (axis) —*see* Fracture, neck,
          cervical vertebra, second
    chronic M84.48
    coccyx S32.2
    dorsal —*see* Fracture, thorax, vertebra
    lumbar S32.009
      burst (stable) S32.001
        unstable S32.002
      fifth S32.059
        burst (stable) S32.051
          unstable S32.052
        specified type NEC S32.058
        wedge compression S32.050
      first S32.019
        burst (stable) S32.011
          unstable S32.012
        specified type NEC S32.018
        wedge compression S32.010
      fourth S32.049
        burst (stable) S32.041
          unstable S32.042
        specified type NEC S32.048
        wedge compression S32.040
      second S32.029
        burst (stable) S32.021
          unstable S32.022
        specified type NEC S32.028
        wedge compression S32.020
      specified type NEC S32.008
      third S32.039
        burst (stable) S32.031
          unstable S32.032
        specified type NEC S32.038
        wedge compression S32.030
      wedge compression S32.000
    metastatic —*see* Collapse, vertebra, in,
        specified disease NEC —*see also*
        Neoplasm
    newborn (birth injury) P11.5
    sacrum S32.10
      specified NEC S32.19
      Type
        1 S32.14
        2 S32.15
        3 S32.16
        4 S32.17
      Zone
        I S32.119
          displaced (minimally) S32.111
            severely S32.112
          nondisplaced S32.110
        II S32.129
          displaced (minimally) S32.121
            severely S32.122
          nondisplaced S32.120
        III S32.139
          displaced (minimally) S32.131
            severely S32.132
          nondisplaced S32.130
    thoracic —*see* Fracture, thorax, vertebra
  vertex S02.0
  vomer (bone) S02.2
  wrist S62.10-●
    carpal —*see* Fracture, carpal bone
    navicular (scaphoid) (hand) —*see* Fracture,
        carpal, navicular
  xiphisternum, xiphoid (process) S22.24
  zygoma S02.442
    left side S02.40F
    right side S02.40E
Fragile, fragility
  autosomal site Q95.5
  bone, congenital (with blue sclera) Q78.0
  capillary (hereditary) D69.8
  hair L67.8
  nails L60.3
  non-sex chromosome site Q95.5
  X chromosome Q99.2

Fragilitas
  crinium L67.8
  ossium (with blue sclerae) (hereditary) Q78.0
  unguium L60.3
    congenital Q84.6
Fragments, cataract (lens), following cataract
    surgery H59.02-●
  retained foreign body —see Retained, foreign
      body fragments (type of)
Frailty (frail) R54
  mental R41.81
Frambesia, frambesial (tropica) —see also Yaws
  initial lesion or ulcer A66.0
  primary A66.0
Frambeside
  gummatous A66.4
  of early yaws A66.2
Frambesioma A66.1
Franceschetti-Klein (-Wildervanck) disease or
    syndrome Q75.4
Francis' disease —see Tularemia
Franklin disease C88.2
Frank's essential thrombocytopenia D69.3
Fraser's syndrome Q87.0
Freckle(s) L81.2
  malignant melanoma in —see Melanoma
  melanotic (Hutchinson's) —see Melanoma,
      in situ
  retinal D49.81
Frederickson's hyperlipoproteinemia, type
  I and V E78.3
  IIA E78.00
  IIB and III E78.2
  IV E78.1
Freeman Sheldon syndrome Q87.0
Freezing —see also Effect, adverse, cold T69.9
Freiberg's disease (infraction of metatarsal head
    or osteochondrosis) —see Osteochondrosis,
    juvenile, metatarsus
Frei's disease A55
Fremitus, friction, cardiac R01.2
Frenum, frenulum
  external os Q51.828
  tongue (shortening) (congenital) Q38.1
Frequency micturition (nocturnal) R35.0
  psychogenic F45.8
Frey's syndrome
  auriculotemporal G50.8
  hyperhidrosis L74.52
Friction
  burn —see Burn, by site
  fremitus, cardiac R01.2
  precordial R01.2
  sounds, chest R09.89
Friderichsen-Waterhouse syndrome or disease
    A39.1
Friedländer's B (bacillus) NEC —see also
    condition A49.8
Friedreich's
  ataxia G11.1
  combined systemic disease G11.1
  facial hemihypertrophy Q67.4
  sclerosis (cerebellum) (spinal cord) G11.1
Frigidity F52.22
Fröhlich's syndrome E23.6
Frontal —see also condition
  lobe syndrome F07.0
Frostbite (superficial) T33.90
  with
    partial thickness skin loss —see Frostbite
        (superficial), by site
    tissue necrosis T34.90
  abdominal wall T33.3
    with tissue necrosis T34.3
  ankle T33.81-●
    with tissue necrosis T34.81-●
  arm T33.4-●
    with tissue necrosis T34.4-●
    finger(s) —see Frostbite, finger
    hand —see Frostbite, hand
    wrist —see Frostbite, wrist

Frostbite (Continued)
  ear T33.01-●
    with tissue necrosis T34.01-●
  face T33.09
    with tissue necrosis T34.09
  finger T33.53-●
    with tissue necrosis T34.53-●
  foot T33.82-●
    with tissue necrosis T34.82-●
  hand T33.52-●
    with tissue necrosis T34.52-●
  head T33.09
    with tissue necrosis T34.09
    ear —see Frostbite, ear
    nose —see Frostbite, nose
  hip (and thigh) T33.6-●
    with tissue necrosis T34.6-●
  knee T33.7-●
    with tissue necrosis T34.7-●
  leg T33.9-●
    with tissue necrosis T34.9-●
    ankle —see Frostbite, ankle
    foot —see Frostbite, foot
    knee —see Frostbite, knee
    lower T33.7-●
      with tissue necrosis T34.7-●
    thigh —see Frostbite, hip
    toe —see Frostbite, toe
  limb
    lower T33.99
      with tissue necrosis T34.99
    upper —see Frostbite, arm
  neck T33.1
    with tissue necrosis T34.1
  nose T33.02
    with tissue necrosis T34.02
  pelvis T33.3
    with tissue necrosis T34.3
  specified site NEC T33.99
    with tissue necrosis T34.99
  thigh —see Frostbite, hip
  thorax T33.2
    with tissue necrosis T34.2
  toes T33.83-●
    with tissue necrosis T34.83-●
  trunk T33.99
    with tissue necrosis T34.99
  wrist T33.51-●
    with tissue necrosis T34.51-●
Frotteurism F65.81
Frozen —see also Effect, adverse, cold T69.9
  pelvis (female) N94.89
    male K66.8
  shoulder —see Capsulitis, adhesive
Fructokinase deficiency E74.11
Fructose 1,6 diphosphatase deficiency E74.19
Fructosemia (benign) (essential) E74.12
Fructosuria (benign) (essential) E74.11
Fuchs'
  black spot (myopic) —see also Myopia,
      degenerative H44.2-●
  dystrophy (corneal endothelium) H18.51
  heterochromic cyclitis —see Cyclitis, Fuchs'
      heterochromic
Fucosidosis E77.1
Fugue R68.89
  dissociative F44.1
  hysterical (dissociative) F44.1
  postictal in epilepsy —see Epilepsy
  reaction to exceptional stress (transient)
      F43.0
Fulminant, fulminating —see condition
Functional —see also condition
  bleeding (uterus) N93.8
Functioning, intellectual, borderline R41.83
Fundus —see condition
Fungemia NOS B49
Fungus, fungous
  cerebral G93.89
  disease NOS B49
  infection —see Infection, fungus

Funiculitis (acute) (chronic) (endemic)
    N49.1
  gonococcal (acute) (chronic) A54.23
  tuberculous A18.15
Funnel
  breast (acquired) M95.4
    congenital Q67.6
    sequelae (late effect) of rickets E64.3
  chest (acquired) M95.4
    congenital Q67.6
    sequelae (late effect) of rickets E64.3
  pelvis (acquired) M95.5
    with disproportion (fetopelvic) O33.3
      causing obstructed labor O65.3
    congenital Q74.2
FUO (fever of unknown origin) R50.9
Furfur L21.0
  microsporon B36.0
Furrier's lung J67.8
Furrowed K14.5
  nail(s) (transverse) L60.4
    congenital Q84.6
  tongue K14.5
    congenital Q38.3
Furuncle L02.92
  abdominal wall L02.221
  ankle —see Furuncle, lower limb
  antecubital space —see Furuncle, upper
      limb
  anus K61.0
  arm —see Furuncle, upper limb
  auditory canal, external —see Abscess, ear,
      external
  auricle (ear) —see Abscess, ear, external
  axilla (region) L02.42-●
  back (any part) L02.222
  breast N61.1
  buttock L02.32
  cheek (external) L02.02
  chest wall L02.223
  chin L02.02
  corpus cavernosum N48.21
  ear, external —see Abscess, ear, external
  external auditory canal —see Abscess, ear,
      external
  eyelid —see Abscess, eyelid
  face L02.02
  femoral (region) —see Furuncle, lower
      limb
  finger —see Furuncle, hand
  flank L02.221
  foot L02.62-●
  forehead L02.02
  gluteal (region) L02.32
  groin L02.224
  hand L02.52-●
  head L02.821
    face L02.02
  hip —see Furuncle, lower limb
  kidney —see Abscess, kidney
  knee —see Furuncle, lower limb
  labium (majus) (minus) N76.4
  lacrimal
    gland —see Dacryoadenitis
    passages (duct) (sac) —see Inflammation,
        lacrimal, passages, acute
  leg (any part) —see Furuncle, lower limb
  lower limb L02.42-●
  malignant A22.0
  mouth K12.2
  navel L02.226
  neck L02.12
  nose J34.0
  orbit, orbital —see Abscess, orbit
  palmar (space) —see Furuncle, hand
  partes posteriores L02.32
  pectoral region L02.223
  penis N48.21
  perineum L02.225
  pinna —see Abscess, ear, external
  popliteal —see Furuncle, lower limb

Furuncle (Continued)
prepatellar —see Furuncle, lower limb
scalp L02.821
seminal vesicle N49.0
shoulder —see Furuncle, upper limb
specified site NEC L02.828
submandibular K12.2
temple (region) L02.02
thumb —see Furuncle, hand
toe —see Furuncle, foot
trunk L02.229
abdominal wall L02.221
back L02.222
chest wall L02.223
groin L02.224
perineum L02.225
umbilicus L02.226
umbilicus L02.226
upper limb L02.42-•
vulva N76.4
Furunculosis —see Furuncle
Fused —see Fusion, fused
Fusion, fused (congenital)
astragaloscaphoid Q74.2
atria Q21.1
auditory canal Q16.1
auricles, heart Q21.1
binocular with defective stereopsis H53.32
bone Q79.8
cervical spine M43.22

Fusion, fused (Continued)
choanal Q30.0
commissure, mitral valve Q23.2
cusps, heart valve NEC Q24.8
mitral Q23.2
pulmonary Q22.1
tricuspid Q22.4
ear ossicles Q16.3
fingers Q70.0-•
hymen Q52.3
joint (acquired) —see also Ankylosis
congenital Q74.8
kidneys (incomplete) Q63.1
labium (majus) (minus) Q52.5
larynx and trachea Q34.8
limb, congenital Q74.8
lower Q74.2
upper Q74.0
lobes, lung Q33.8
lumbosacral (acquired) M43.27
arthrodesis status Z98.1
congenital Q76.49
postprocedural status Z98.1
nares, nose, nasal, nostril(s) Q30.0
organ or site not listed —see Anomaly,
by site
ossicles Q79.9
auditory Q16.3
pulmonic cusps Q22.1
ribs Q76.6

Fusion, fused (Continued)
sacroiliac (joint) (acquired) M43.28
arthrodesis status Z98.1
congenital Q74.2
postprocedural status Z98.1
spine (acquired) NEC M43.20
arthrodesis status Z98.1
cervical region M43.22
cervicothoracic region M43.23
congenital Q76.49
lumbar M43.26
lumbosacral region M43.27
occipito-atlanto-axial region M43.21
postoperative status Z98.1
sacrococcygeal region M43.28
thoracic region M43.24
thoracolumbar region M43.25
sublingual duct with submaxillary duct at
opening in mouth Q38.4
testes Q55.1
toes Q70.2
tooth, teeth K00.2
trachea and esophagus Q39.8
twins Q89.4
vagina Q52.4
ventricles, heart Q21.0
vertebra (arch) —see Fusion, spine
vulva Q52.5
Fusospirillosis (mouth) (tongue) (tonsil) A69.1
Fussy baby R68.12

▶ New   ⇒ Revised   ~~deleted~~ Deleted   • Use Additional Character(s)

G

Gain in weight (abnormal) (excessive) —see also
Weight, gain
Gaisböck's disease (polycythemia hypertonica)
D75.1
Gait abnormality R26.9
ataxic R26.0
falling R29.6
hysterical (ataxic) (staggering) F44.4
paralytic R26.1
spastic R26.1
specified type NEC R26.89
staggering R26.0
unsteadiness R26.81
walking difficulty NEC R26.2
Galactocele (breast) N64.89
puerperal, postpartum O92.79
Galactokinase deficiency E74.29
Galactophoritis N61.0
gestational, puerperal, postpartum O91.2-•
Galactorrhea O92.6
not associated with childbirth N64.3
Galactosemia (classic) (congenital) E74.21
Galactosuria E74.29
Galacturia R82.0
schistosomiasis (bilharziasis) B65.0
▶GALD (gestational alloimmune liver disease)
P78.84
Galeazzi's fracture S52.37-•
Galen's vein —see condition
Galeophobia F40.218
Gall duct —see condition
Gallbladder —see also condition
acute K81.0
Gallop rhythm R00.8
Gallstone (colic) (cystic duct) (gallbladder)
(impacted) (multiple) —see also Calculus,
gallbladder
with
cholecystitis —see Calculus, gallbladder,
with cholecystitis
bile duct (common) (hepatic) —see Calculus,
bile duct
causing intestinal obstruction K56.3
specified NEC K80.80
with obstruction K80.81
Gambling Z72.6
pathological (compulsive) F63.0
Gammopathy (of undetermined significance
[MGUS]) D47.2
associated with lymphoplasmacytic dyscrasia
D47.2
monoclonal D47.2
polyclonal D89.0
Gamna's disease (siderotic splenomegaly) D73.1
Gamophobia F40.298
Gampsodactylia (congenital) Q66.7
Gamstorp's disease (adynamia episodica
hereditaria) G72.3
Gandy-Nanta disease (siderotic splenomegaly)
D73.1
Gang
membership offenses Z72.810
Gangliocytoma D36.10
Ganglioglioma —see Neoplasm, uncertain
behavior, by site
Ganglion (compound) (diffuse) (joint) (tendon
(sheath)) M67.40
ankle M67.47-•
foot M67.47-•
forearm M67.43-•
hand M67.44-•
lower leg M67.46-•
multiple sites M67.49
of yaws (early) (late) A66.6
pelvic region M67.45-•
periosteal —see Periostitis
shoulder region M67.41-•
specified site NEC M67.48
thigh region M67.45-•

Ganglion (Continued)
tuberculous A18.09
upper arm M67.42-•
wrist M67.43-•
Ganglioneuroblastoma —see Neoplasm, nerve,
malignant
Ganglioneuroma D36.10
malignant —see Neoplasm, nerve, malignant
Ganglioneuromatosis D36.10
Ganglionitis
fifth nerve —see Neuralgia, trigeminal
gasserian (postherpetic) (postzoster) B02.21
geniculate G51.1
newborn (birth injury) P11.3
postherpetic, postzoster B02.21
herpes zoster B02.21
postherpetic geniculate B02.21
Gangliosidosis E75.10
GM1 E75.19
GM2 E75.00
other specified E75.09
Sandhoff disease E75.01
Tay-Sachs disease E75.02
GM3 E75.19
mucolipidosis IV E75.11
Gangosa A66.5
Gangrene, gangrenous (connective tissue)
(dropsical) (dry) (moist) (skin) (ulcer) —see
also Necrosis I96
with diabetes (mellitus) —see Diabetes,
gangrene
abdomen (wall) I96
alveolar M27.3
appendix K35.80
with
perforation or rupture K35.2
peritoneal abscess K35.3
peritonitis NEC K35.3
generalized (with perforation or
rupture) K35.2
localized (with perforation or rupture)
K35.3
arteriosclerotic (general) (senile) —see
Arteriosclerosis, extremities, with,
gangrene
auricle I96
Bacillus welchii A48.0
bladder (infectious) —see Cystitis, specified
type NEC
bowel, cecum, or colon —see Gangrene,
intestine
Clostridium perfringens or welchii A48.0
cornea H18.89-•
corpora cavernosa N48.29
noninfective N48.89
cutaneous, spreading I96
decubital —see Ulcer, pressure, by site
diabetic (any site) —see Diabetes, gangrene
emphysematous —see Gangrene, gas
epidemic —see Poisoning, food, noxious,
plant
epididymis (infectional) N45.1
erysipelas —see Erysipelas
extremity (lower) (upper) I96
Fournier N49.3
female N76.89
fusospirochetal A69.0
gallbladder —see Cholecystitis, acute
gas (bacillus) A48.0
following
abortion —see Abortion by type
complicated by infection
ectopic or molar pregnancy O08.0
glossitis K14.0
hernia —see Hernia, by site, with gangrene
intestine, intestinal (hemorrhagic) (massive) —
see also Infarct, intestine K55.069
with
mesenteric embolism —see also Infarct,
intestine K55.069
obstruction —see Obstruction, intestine

Gangrene, gangrenous (Continued)
laryngitis J04.0
limb (lower) (upper) I96
lung J85.0
spirochetal A69.8
lymphangitis I89.1
Meleney's (synergistic) —see Ulcer, skin
mesentery —see also Infarct, intestine K55.069
with
embolism —see also Infarct, intestine
K55.069
intestinal obstruction —see Obstruction,
intestine
mouth A69.0
ovary —see Oophoritis
pancreas —see Pancreatitis, acute
penis N48.29
noninfective N48.89
perineum I96
pharynx —see also Pharyngitis
Vincent's A69.1
presenile I73.1
progressive synergistic —see Ulcer, skin
pulmonary J85.0
pulpal (dental) K04.1
quinsy J36
Raynaud's (symmetric gangrene) I73.01
retropharyngeal J39.2
scrotum N49.3
noninfective N50.89
senile (atherosclerotic) —see Arteriosclerosis,
extremities, with, gangrene
spermatic cord N49.1
noninfective N50.89
spine I96
spirochetal NEC A69.8
spreading cutaneous I96
stomatitis A69.0
symmetrical I73.01
testis (infectional) N45.2
noninfective N44.8
throat —see also Pharyngitis
diphtheritic A36.0
Vincent's A69.1
thyroid (gland) E07.89
tooth (pulp) K04.1
tuberculous NEC —see Tuberculosis
tunica vaginalis N49.1
noninfective N50.89
umbilicus I96
uterus —see Endometritis
uvulitis K12.2
vas deferens N49.1
noninfective N50.89
vulva N76.89
Ganister disease J62.8
Ganser's syndrome (hysterical) F44.89
Gardner-Diamond syndrome (autoerythrocyte
sensitization) D69.2
Gargoylism E76.01
Garré's disease, osteitis (sclerosing),
osteomyelitis —see Osteomyelitis,
specified type NEC
Garrod's pad, knuckle M72.1
Gartner's duct
cyst Q52.4
persistent Q50.6
Gas R14.3
asphyxiation, inhalation, poisoning, suffocation
NEC —see Table of Drugs and Chemicals
excessive R14.0
gangrene A48.0
following
abortion —see Abortion by type
complicated by infection
ectopic or molar pregnancy O08.0
on stomach R14.0
pains R14.1
Gastralgia —see also Pain, abdominal
Gastrectasis K31.0
psychogenic F45.8

Gastric —see condition
Gastrinoma
  malignant
    pancreas C25.4
    specified site NEC —see Neoplasm,
      malignant, by site
    unspecified site C25.4
  specified site —see Neoplasm, uncertain
    behavior
  unspecified site D37.9
Gastritis (simple) K29.70
  with bleeding K29.71
  acute (erosive) K29.00
    with bleeding K29.01
  alcoholic K29.20
    with bleeding K29.21
  allergic K29.60
    with bleeding K29.61
  atrophic (chronic) K29.40
    with bleeding K29.41
  chronic (antral) (fundal) K29.50
    with bleeding K29.51
    atrophic K29.40
      with bleeding K29.41
    superficial K29.30
      with bleeding K29.31
  dietary counseling and surveillance Z71.3
  due to diet deficiency E63.9
  eosinophilic K52.81
  giant hypertrophic K29.60
    with bleeding K29.61
  granulomatous K29.60
    with bleeding K29.61
  hypertrophic (mucosa) K29.60
    with bleeding K29.61
  nervous F54
  spastic K29.60
    with bleeding K29.61
  specified NEC K29.60
    with bleeding K29.61
  superficial chronic K29.30
    with bleeding K29.31
  tuberculous A18.83
  viral NEC A08.4
Gastrocarcinoma —see Neoplasm, malignant,
  stomach
Gastrocolic —see condition
Gastrodisciasis, gastrodiscoidiasis B66.8
Gastroduodenitis K29.90
  with bleeding K29.91
  virus, viral A08.4
    specified type NEC A08.39
Gastrodynia —see Pain, abdominal
Gastroenteritis (acute) (chronic) (noninfectious)
  (see also Enteritis) K52.9
  allergic K52.29
  with
    eosinophilic gastritis or gastroenteritis
      K52.81
    food protein-induced enterocolitis
      syndrome K52.21
    food protein-induced enteropathy K52.22
  dietetic —see also Gastroenteritis, allergic
    K52.29
  drug-induced K52.1
  due to
    Cryptosporidium A07.2
    drugs K52.1
    food poisoning —see Intoxication,
      foodborne
    radiation K52.0
  eosinophilic K52.81
  epidemic (infectious) A09
  food hypersensitivity —see also
    Gastroenteritis, allergic K52.29
  infectious —see Enteritis, infectious
  influenzal —see Influenza, with
    gastroenteritis
  noninfectious K52.9
    specified NEC K52.89
  rotaviral A08.0

Gastroenteritis (Continued)
  Salmonella A02.0
  toxic K52.1
  viral NEC A08.4
    acute infectious A08.39
      type Norwalk A08.11
    infantile (acute) A08.39
    Norwalk agent A08.11
    rotaviral A08.0
    severe of infants A08.39
    specified type NEC A08.39
Gastroenteropathy —see also Gastroenteritis
  K52.9
  acute, due to Norovirus A08.11
  acute, due to Norwalk agent A08.11
  infectious A09
Gastroenteroptosis K63.4
Gastroesophageal laceration-hemorrhage
  syndrome K22.6
Gastrointestinal —see condition
Gastrojejunal —see condition
Gastrojejunitis —see also Enteritis K52.9
Gastrojejunocolic —see condition
Gastroliths K31.89
Gastromalacia K31.89
Gastroparalysis K31.84
  diabetic —see Diabetes, gastroparalysis
Gastroparesis K31.84
  diabetic —see Diabetes, by type, with
    gastroparesis
Gastropathy K31.9
  congestive portal K31.89
  erythematous K29.70
  exudative K90.89
  portal hypertensive K31.89
Gastroptosis K31.89
Gastrorrhagia K92.2
  psychogenic F45.8
Gastroschisis (congenital) Q79.3
Gastrospasm (neurogenic) (reflex) K31.89
  neurotic F45.8
  psychogenic F45.8
Gastrostaxis —see Gastritis, with bleeding
Gastrostenosis K31.89
Gastrostomy
  attention to Z43.1
  status Z93.1
Gastrosuccorrhea (continuous) (intermittent)
  K31.89
  neurotic F45.8
  psychogenic F45.8
Gatophobia F40.218
Gaucher's disease or splenomegaly (adult)
  (infantile) E75.22
Gee (-Herter)(-Thaysen) disease (nontropical
  sprue) K90.0
Gélineau's syndrome G47.419
  with cataplexy G47.411
Gemination, tooth, teeth K00.2
Gemistocytoma
  specified site —see Neoplasm, malignant, by
    site
  unspecified site C71.9
General, generalized —see condition
Genetic
  carrier (status)
    cystic fibrosis Z14.1
    hemophilia A (asymptomatic) Z14.01
      symptomatic Z14.02
    specified NEC Z14.8
  susceptibility to disease NEC Z15.89
    malignant neoplasm Z15.09
      breast Z15.01
      endometrium Z15.04
      ovary Z15.02
      prostate Z15.03
      specified NEC Z15.09
    multiple endocrine neoplasia Z15.81
Genital —see condition
Genito-anorectal syndrome A55
Genitourinary system —see condition

Genu
  congenital Q74.1
  extrorsum (acquired) —see also Deformity,
    varus, knee
    congenital Q74.1
    sequelae (late effect) of rickets E64.3
  introrsum (acquired) —see also Deformity,
    valgus, knee
    congenital Q74.1
    sequelae (late effect) of rickets E64.3
  rachitic (old) E64.3
  recurvatum (acquired) —see also Deformity,
    limb, specified type NEC, lower leg
    congenital Q68.2
    sequelae (late effect) of rickets E64.3
  valgum (acquired) (knock-knee) M21.06-•
    congenital Q74.1
    sequelae (late effect) of rickets E64.3
  varum (acquired) (bowleg) M21.16-•
    congenital Q74.1
    sequelae (late effect) of rickets E64.3
Geographic tongue K14.1
Geophagia —see Pica
Geotrichosis B48.3
  stomatitis B48.3
Gephyrophobia F40.242
Gerbode defect Q21.0
GERD (gastroesophageal reflux disease) K21.9
Gerhardt's
  disease (erythromelalgia) I73.81
  syndrome (vocal cord paralysis)
    J38.00
    bilateral J38.02
    unilateral J38.01
German measles —see also Rubella
  exposure to Z20.4
Germinoblastoma (diffuse) C85.9-•
  follicular C82.9-•
Germinoma —see Neoplasm, malignant, by site
Gerontoxon —see Degeneration, cornea, senile
Gerstmann-Sträussler-Scheinker syndrome
  (GSS) A81.82
Gerstmann's syndrome R48.8
  developmental F81.2
Gestation (period) —see also Pregnancy
  ectopic —see Pregnancy, by site
  multiple O30.9-•
    greater than quadruplets —see Pregnancy,
      multiple (gestation), specified NEC
    specified NEC —see Pregnancy, multiple
      (gestation), specified NEC
Gestational
  mammary abscess O91.11-•
  purulent mastitis O91.11-•
  subareolar abscess O91.11-•
Ghon tubercle, primary infection A15.7
Ghost
  teeth K00.4
  vessels (cornea) H16.41-•
Ghoul hand A66.3
Gianotti-Crosti disease L44.4
Giant
  cell
    epulis K06.8
    peripheral granuloma K06.8
  esophagus, congenital Q39.5
  kidney, congenital Q63.3
  urticaria T78.3
    hereditary D84.1
Giardiasis A07.1
Gibert's disease or pityriasis L42
Giddiness R42
  hysterical F44.89
  psychogenic F45.8
Gierke's disease (glycogenosis I) E74.01
Gigantism (cerebral) (hypophyseal) (pituitary)
  E22.0
  constitutional E34.4
Gilbert's disease or syndrome E80.4
Gilchrist's disease B40.9
Gilford-Hutchinson disease E34.8

▶ New   ➡ Revised   ~~deleted~~ Deleted   • Use Additional Character(s)

Gilles de la Tourette's disease or syndrome (motor-verbal tic) F95.2
Gingivitis K05.10
  acute (catarrhal) K05.00
    necrotizing A69.1
    nonplaque induced K05.01
    plaque induced K05.00
  chronic (desquamative) (hyperplastic) (simple marginal) (pregnancy associated) (ulcerative) K05.10
    nonplaque induced K05.11
    plaque induced K05.10
  expulsiva —see Periodontitis
  necrotizing ulcerative (acute) A69.1
  pellagrous E52
    acute necrotizing A69.1
  Vincent's A69.1
Gingivoglossitis K14.0
Gingivopericementitis —see Periodontitis
Gingivosis —see Gingivitis, chronic
Gingivostomatitis K05.10
  herpesviral B00.2
  necrotizing ulcerative (acute) A69.1
Gland, glandular —see condition
Glanders A24.0
Glanzmann (-Naegeli) disease or thrombasthenia D69.1
Glasgow coma scale
  total score
    3-8 R40.243
    9-12 R40.242
    13-15 R40.241
Glass-blower's disease (cataract) —see Cataract, specified NEC
Glaucoma H40.9
  with
    increased episcleral venous pressure H40.81-•
    pseudoexfoliation of lens —see Glaucoma, open angle, primary, capsular
  absolute H44.51-•
  angle-closure (primary) H40.20-•
    acute (attack) (crisis) H40.21-•
    chronic H40.22-•
    intermittent H40.23-•
    residual stage H40.24-•
  borderline H40.00-•
  capsular (with pseudoexfoliation of lens) —see Glaucoma, open angle, primary, capsular
  childhood Q15.0
  closed angle —see Glaucoma, angle-closure
  congenital Q15.0
  corticosteroid-induced —see Glaucoma, secondary, drugs
  hypersecretion H40.82-•
  in (due to)
    amyloidosis E85.4 [H42]
    aniridia Q13.1 [H42]
    concussion of globe —see Glaucoma, secondary, trauma
    dislocation of lens —see Glaucoma, secondary
    disorder of lens NEC —see Glaucoma, secondary
    drugs —see Glaucoma, secondary, drugs
    endocrine disease NOS E34.9 [H42]
    eye
      inflammation —see Glaucoma, secondary, inflammation
      trauma —see Glaucoma, secondary, trauma
    hypermature cataract —see Glaucoma, secondary
    iridocyclitis —see Glaucoma, secondary, inflammation
    lens disorder —see Glaucoma, secondary, Lowe's syndrome E72.03 [H42]
    metabolic disease NOS E88.9 [H42]
    ocular disorders NEC —see Glaucoma, secondary

Glaucoma (Continued)
  in (due to) (Continued)
    onchocerciasis B73.02
    pupillary block —see Glaucoma, secondary
    retinal vein occlusion —see Glaucoma, secondary
    Rieger's anomaly Q13.81 [H42]
    rubeosis of iris —see Glaucoma, secondary
    tumor of globe —see Glaucoma, secondary
  infantile Q15.0
  low tension —see Glaucoma, open angle, primary, low-tension
  malignant H40.83-•
  narrow angle —see Glaucoma, angle-closure
  newborn Q15.0
  noncongestive (chronic) —see Glaucoma, open angle
  nonobstructive —see Glaucoma, open angle
  obstructive —see also Glaucoma, angle-closure
    due to lens changes —see Glaucoma, secondary
  open angle H40.10-•
    primary H40.11-•
      capsular (with pseudoexfoliation of lens) H40.14-•
      low-tension H40.12-•
      pigmentary H40.13-•
      residual stage H40.15-•
  phacolytic —see Glaucoma, secondary
  pigmentary —see Glaucoma, open angle, primary, pigmentary
  postinfectious —see Glaucoma, secondary, inflammation
  secondary (to) H40.5-•
    drugs H40.6-•
    inflammation H40.4-•
    trauma H40.3-•
  simple (chronic) H40.11-•
  simplex H40.11-•
  specified type NEC H40.89
  suspect H40.00-•
  syphilitic A52.71
  traumatic —see also Glaucoma, secondary, trauma
    newborn (birth injury) P15.3
  tuberculous A18.59
Glaucomatous flecks (subcapsular) —see Cataract, complicated
Glazed tongue K14.4
Gleet (gonococcal) A54.01
Glénard's disease K63.4
Glioblastoma (multiforme)
  with sarcomatous component
    specified site —see Neoplasm, malignant, by site
    unspecified site C71.9
  giant cell
    specified site —see Neoplasm, malignant, by site
    unspecified site C71.9
  specified site —see Neoplasm, malignant, by site
  unspecified site C71.9
Glioma (malignant)
  astrocytic
    specified site —see Neoplasm, malignant, by site
    unspecified site C71.9
  mixed
    specified site —see Neoplasm, malignant, by site
    unspecified site C71.9
  nose Q30.8
  specified site NEC —see Neoplasm, malignant, by site
  subependymal D43.2
    specified site —see Neoplasm, uncertain behavior, by site
    unspecified site D43.2
  unspecified site C71.9

Gliomatosis cerebri C71.0
Glioneuroma —see Neoplasm, uncertain behavior, by site
Gliosarcoma
  specified site —see Neoplasm, malignant, by site
  unspecified site C71.9
Gliosis (cerebral) G93.89
  spinal G95.89
Glisson's disease —see Rickets
Globinuria R82.3
Globus (hystericus) F45.8
Glomangioma D18.00
  intra-abdominal D18.03
  intracranial D18.02
  skin D18.01
  specified site NEC D18.09
Glomangiomyoma D18.00
  intra-abdominal D18.03
  intracranial D18.02
  skin D18.01
  specified site NEC D18.09
Glomangiosarcoma —see Neoplasm, connective tissue, malignant
Glomerular
  disease in syphilis A52.75
  nephritis —see Glomerulonephritis
Glomerulitis —see Glomerulonephritis
Glomerulonephritis —see also Nephritis N05.9
  with
    edema —see Nephrosis
    minimal change N05.0
    minor glomerular abnormality N05.0
  acute N00.9
  chronic N03.9
  crescentic (diffuse) NEC —see also N00-N07 with fourth character .7 N05.7
  dense deposit —see also N00-N07 with fourth character .6 N05.6
  diffuse
    crescentic —see also N00-N07 with fourth character .7 N05.7
    endocapillary proliferative —see also N00N07 with fourth character .4 N05.4
    membranous —see also N00-N07 with fourth character .2 N05.2
    mesangial proliferative —see also N00-N07 with fourth character .3 N05.3
    mesangiocapillary —see also N00-N07 with fourth character .5 N05.5
  ⮕sclerosing N18.9
  endocapillary proliferative (diffuse) NEC —see also N00-N07 with fourth character .4 N05.4
  extracapillary NEC —see also N00-N07 with fourth character .7 N05.7
  focal (and segmental) —see also N00-N07 with fourth character .1 N05.1
  hypocomplementemic —see Glomerulonephritis, membranoproliferative
  IgA —see Nephropathy, IgA
  immune complex (circulating) NEC N05.8
  in (due to)
    amyloidosis E85.4 [N08]
    bilharziasis B65.9 [N08]
    cryoglobulinemia D89.1 [N08]
    defibrination syndrome D65 [N08]
    diabetes mellitus —see Diabetes, glomerulosclerosis
    disseminated intravascular coagulation D65 [N08]
    Fabry (-Anderson) disease E75.21 [N08]
    Goodpasture's syndrome M31.0
    hemolytic-uremic syndrome D59.3
    Henoch (-Schönlein) purpura D69.0 [N08]
    lecithin cholesterol acyltransferase deficiency E78.6 [N08]

Glomerulonephritis (Continued)
in (Continued)
microscopic polyangiitis M31.7 [N08]
multiple myeloma C90.0-● [N08]
Plasmodium malariae B52.0
schistosomiasis B65.9 [N08]
sepsis A41.9-● [N08]
streptococcal A40-● [N08]
sickle-cell disorders D57.-● [N08]
strongyloidiasis B78.9 [N08]
subacute bacterial endocarditis I33.0
[N08]
syphilis (late) congenital A50.59 [N08]
systemic lupus erythematosus M32.14
thrombotic thrombocytopenic purpura
M31.1 [N08]
typhoid fever A01.09
Waldenström macroglobulinemia C88.0
[N08]
Wegener's granulomatosis M31.31
latent or quiescent N03.9
lobular, lobulonodular —
see Glomerulonephritis,
membranoproliferative
membranoproliferative (diffuse) (type 1
or 3) —see also N00-N07 with fourth
character .5 N05.5
dense deposit (type 2) NEC —see also
N00-N07 with fourth character .6
N05.6
membranous (diffuse) NEC —see also
N00-N07 with fourth character .2 N05.2
mesangial
IgA/IgG —see Nephropathy, IgA
proliferative (diffuse) NEC —see also
N00-N07 with fourth character .3
N05.3
mesangiocapillary (diffuse) NEC —see also
N00-N07 with fourth character .5 N05.5
necrotic, necrotizing NEC —see also N00-N07
with fourth character .8 N05.8
nodular —see Glomerulonephritis,
membranoproliferative
poststreptococcal NEC N05.9
acute N00.9
chronic N03.9
rapidly progressive N01.9
proliferative NEC —see also N00-N07 with
fourth character .8 N05.8
diffuse (lupus) M32.14
rapidly progressive N01.9
sclerosing, diffuse N18.9
specified pathology NEC —see also N00-N07
with fourth character .8 N05.8
subacute N01.9
Glomerulopathy —see Glomerulonephritis
Glomerulosclerosis —see also Sclerosis, renal
intercapillary (nodular) (with diabetes) —see
Diabetes, glomerulosclerosis
intracapillary —see Diabetes,
glomerulosclerosis
Glossagra K14.6
Glossalgia K14.6
Glossitis (chronic superficial) (gangrenous)
(Moeller's) K14.0
areata exfoliativa K14.1
atrophic K14.4
benign migratory K14.1
cortical superficial, sclerotic K14.0
Hunter's D51.0
interstitial, sclerous K14.0
median rhomboid K14.2
pellagrous E52
superficial, chronic K14.0
Glossocele K14.8
Glossodynia K14.6
exfoliativa K14.4
Glossoncus K14.8
Glossopathy K14.9
Glossophytia K14.3
Glossoplegia K14.8

Glossoptosis K14.8
Glossopyrosis K14.6
Glossotrichia K14.3
Glossy skin L90.8
Glottis —see condition
Glottitis —see also Laryngitis J04.0
Glucagonoma
pancreas
benign D13.7
malignant C25.4
uncertain behavior D37.8
specified site NEC
benign —see Neoplasm, benign, by site
malignant —see Neoplasm, malignant, by
site
uncertain behavior —see Neoplasm,
uncertain behavior, by site
unspecified site
benign D13.7
malignant C25.4
uncertain behavior D37.8
Glucoglycinuria E72.51
Glucose-galactose malabsorption E74.39
Glue
ear —see Otitis, media, nonsuppurative,
chronic, mucoid
sniffing (airplane) —see Abuse, drug,
inhalant
dependence —see Dependence, drug,
inhalant
Glutaric aciduria E72.3
Glycinemia E72.51
Glycinuria (renal) (with ketosis) E72.09
Glycogen
infiltration —see Disease, glycogen storage
storage disease —see Disease, glycogen
storage
Glycogenosis (diffuse) (generalized) —see also
Disease, glycogen storage
cardiac E74.02 [I43]
diabetic, secondary —see Diabetes,
glycogenosis, secondary
pulmonary interstitial J84.842
Glycopenia E16.2
Glycosuria R81
renal E74.8
Gnathostoma spinigerum (infection)
(infestation), gnathostomiasis (wandering
swelling) B83.1
Goiter (plunging) (substernal) E04.9
with
hyperthyroidism (recurrent) —see
Hyperthyroidism, with, goiter
thyrotoxicosis —see Hyperthyroidism,
with, goiter
adenomatous —see Goiter, nodular
cancerous C73
congenital (nontoxic) E03.0
diffuse E03.0
parenchymatous E03.0
transitory, with normal functioning
P72.0
cystic E04.2
due to iodine-deficiency E01.1
due to
enzyme defect in synthesis of thyroid
hormone E07.1
iodine-deficiency (endemic) E01.2
dyshormonogenetic (familial) E07.1
endemic (iodine-deficiency) E01.2
diffuse E01.0
multinodular E01.1
exophthalmic —see Hyperthyroidism, with,
goiter
iodine-deficiency (endemic) E01.2
diffuse E01.0
multinodular E01.1
nodular E01.1
lingual Q89.2
lymphadenoid E06.3
malignant C73

Goiter (Continued)
multinodular (cystic) (nontoxic) E04.2
toxic or with hyperthyroidism E05.20
with thyroid storm E05.21
neonatal NEC P72.0
nodular (nontoxic) (due to) E04.9
with
hyperthyroidism E05.20
with thyroid storm E05.21
thyrotoxicosis E05.20
with thyroid storm E05.21
endemic E01.1
iodine-deficiency E01.1
sporadic E04.9
toxic E05.20
with thyroid storm E05.21
nontoxic E04.9
diffuse (colloid) E04.0
multinodular E04.2
simple E04.0
specified NEC E04.8
uninodular E04.1
simple E04.0
toxic —see Hyperthyroidism, with, goiter
uninodular (nontoxic) E04.1
toxic or with hyperthyroidism E05.10
with thyroid storm E05.11
Goiter-deafness syndrome E07.1
Goldberg syndrome Q89.8
Goldberg-Maxwell syndrome E34.51
Goldblatt's hypertension or kidney I70.1
Goldenhar (-Gorlin) syndrome Q87.0
Goldflam-Erb disease or syndrome G70.00
with exacerbation (acute) G70.01
in crisis G70.01
Goldscheider's disease Q81.8
Goldstein's disease (familial hemorrhagic
telangiectasia) I78.0
Golfer's elbow —see Epicondylitis, medial
Gonadoblastoma
specified site —see Neoplasm, uncertain
behavior, by site
unspecified site
female D39.10
male D40.10
Gonecystitis —see Vesiculitis
Gongylonemiasis B83.8
Goniosynechiae —see Adhesions, iris,
goniosynechiae
Gonococcemia A54.86
Gonococcus, gonococcal (disease) (infection)
—see also condition A54.9
anus A54.6
bursa, bursitis A54.49
conjunctiva, conjunctivitis (neonatorum)
A54.31
endocardium A54.83
eye A54.30
conjunctivitis A54.31
iridocyclitis A54.32
keratitis A54.33
newborn A54.31
other specified A54.39
fallopian tubes (acute) (chronic) A54.24
genitourinary (organ) (system) (tract) (acute)
A54.00
lower A54.00
with abscess (accessory gland)
(periurethral) A54.1
upper —see also condition A54.29
heart A54.83
iridocyclitis A54.32
joint A54.42
lymphatic (gland) (node) A54.89
meninges, meningitis A54.81
musculoskeletal A54.40
arthritis A54.42
osteomyelitis A54.43
other specified A54.49
spondylopathy A54.41
pelviperitonitis A54.24
pelvis (acute) (chronic) A54.24

Gonococcus, gonococcal *(Continued)*
pharynx A54.5
proctitis A54.6
pyosalpinx (acute) (chronic) A54.24
rectum A54.6
skin A54.89
specified site NEC A54.89
tendon sheath A54.49
throat A54.5
urethra (acute) (chronic) A54.01
with abscess (accessory gland)
(periurethral) A54.1
vulva (acute) (chronic) A54.02
Gonocytoma
specified site —*see* Neoplasm, uncertain
behavior, by site
unspecified site
female D39.10
male D40.10
Gonorrhea (acute) (chronic) A54.9
Bartholin's gland (acute) (chronic) (purulent)
A54.02
with abscess (accessory gland)
(periurethral) A54.1
bladder A54.01
cervix A54.03
conjunctiva, conjunctivitis (neonatorum)
A54.31
contact Z20.2
Cowper's gland (with abscess) A54.1
exposure to Z20.2
fallopian tube (acute) (chronic) A54.24
kidney (acute) (chronic) A54.21
lower genitourinary tract A54.00
with abscess (accessory gland)
(periurethral) A54.1
ovary (acute) (chronic) A54.24
pelvis (acute) (chronic) A54.24
female pelvic inflammatory disease A54.24
penis A54.09
prostate (acute) (chronic) A54.22
seminal vesicle (acute) (chronic) A54.23
specified site not listed —*see also* Gonococcus
A54.89
spermatic cord (acute) (chronic) A54.23
urethra A54.01
with abscess (accessory gland)
(periurethral) A54.1
vagina A54.02
vas deferens (acute) (chronic) A54.23
vulva A54.02
Goodall's disease A08.19
Goodpasture's syndrome M31.0
Gopalan's syndrome (burning feet) E53.0
Gorlin-Chaudry-Moss syndrome Q87.0
Gottron's papules L94.4
Gougerot's syndrome (trisymptomatic) L81.7
Gougerot-Blum syndrome (pigmented
purpuric lichenoid dermatitis) L81.7
Gougerot-Carteaud disease or syndrome
(confluent reticulate papillomatosis) L83
Gouley's syndrome (constrictive pericarditis)
I31.1
Goundou A66.6
Gout, chronic (*see also* Gout, gouty) M1A.9-●
drug-induced M1A.20
ankle M1A.27-●
elbow M1A.22-●
foot joint M1A.27-●
hand joint M1A.24-●
hip M1A.25-●
knee M1A.26-●
multiple site M1A.29-●
shoulder M1A.21-●
vertebrae M1A.28
wrist M1A.23-●
idiopathic M1A.00
ankle M1A.07-●
elbow M1A.02-●
foot joint M1A.07-●
hand joint M1A.04-●

Gout, chronic *(Continued)*
idiopathic *(Continued)*
hip M1A.05-●
knee M1A.06-●
multiple site M1A.09
shoulder M1A.01-●
vertebrae M1A.08
wrist M1A.03-●
in (due to) renal impairment M1A.30
ankle M1A.37-●
elbow M1A.32-●
foot joint M1A.37-●
hand joint M1A.34-●
hip M1A.35-●
knee M1A.36-●
multiple site M1A.39
shoulder M1A.31-●
vertebrae M1A.38
wrist M1A.33-●
lead-induced M1A.10
ankle M1A.17-●
elbow M1A.12-●
foot joint M1A.17-●
hand joint M1A.14-●
hip M1A.15-●
knee M1A.16-●
multiple site M1A.19
shoulder M1A.11-●
vertebrae M1A.18
wrist M1A.13-●
primary —*see* Gout, chronic, idiopathic
saturnine —*see* Gout, chronic, lead-induced
secondary NEC M1A.40
ankle M1A.47-●
elbow M1A.42-●
foot joint M1A.47-●
hand joint M1A.44-●
hip M1A.45-●
knee M1A.46-●
multiple site M1A.49
shoulder M1A.41-●
vertebrae M1A.48
wrist M1A.43-●
syphilitic —*see also* subcategory M14.8-●
A52.77
tophi M1A.9
Gout, gouty (acute) (attack) (flare) —*see also*
Gout, chronic M10.9-●
drug-induced M10.20
ankle M10.27-●
elbow M10.22-●
foot joint M10.27-●
hand joint M10.24-●
hip M10.25-●
knee M10.26-●
multiple site M10.29
shoulder M10.21-●
vertebrae M10.28
wrist M10.23-●
idiopathic M10.00
ankle M10.07-●
elbow M10.02-●
foot joint M10.07-●
hand joint M10.04-●
hip M10.05-●
knee M10.06-●
multiple site M10.09
shoulder M10.01-●
vertebrae M10.08
wrist M10.03-●
in (due to) renal impairment M10.30
ankle M10.37-●
elbow M10.32-●
foot joint M10.37-●
hand joint M10.34-●
hip M10.35-●
knee M10.36-●
multiple site M10.39
shoulder M10.31-●
vertebrae M10.38
wrist M10.33-●

Gout, gouty *(Continued)*
lead-induced M10.10
ankle M10.17-●
elbow M10.12-●
foot joint M10.17-●
hand joint M10.14-●
hip M10.15-●
knee M10.16-●
multiple site M10.19
shoulder M10.11-●
vertebrae M10.18
wrist M10.13-●
primary —*see* Gout, idiopathic
saturnine —*see* Gout, lead-induced
secondary NEC M10.40
ankle M10.47-●
elbow M10.42-●
foot joint M10.47-●
hand joint M10.44-●
hip M10.45-●
knee M10.46-●
multiple site M10.49
shoulder M10.41-●
vertebrae M10.48
wrist M10.43-●
syphilitic —*see also* subcategory M14.8-●
A52.77
tophi NEC —*see* Gout, chronic
Gower's
muscular dystrophy G71.0
syndrome (vasovagal attack) R55
Gradenigo's syndrome —*see* Otitis, media,
suppurative, acute
Graefe's disease —*see* Strabismus, paralytic,
ophthalmoplegia, progressive
Graft-versus-host disease D89.813
acute D89.810
acute on chronic D89.812
chronic D89.811
Grain mite (itch) B88.0
Grainhandler's disease or lung J67.8
Grand mal —*see* Epilepsy, generalized,
specified NEC
Grand multipara status only (not pregnant)
Z64.1
pregnant —*see* Pregnancy, complicated by,
grand multiparity
Granite worker's lung J62.8
Granular —*see also* condition
inflammation, pharynx J31.2
kidney (contracting) —*see* Sclerosis, renal
liver K74.69
Granulation tissue (abnormal) (excessive) L92.9
postmastoidectomy cavity —*see*
Complications, postmastoidectomy,
granulation
Granulocytopenia (primary) (malignant) —*see*
Agranulocytosis
Granuloma L92.9
abdomen K66.8
from residual foreign body L92.3
pyogenicum L98.0
actinic L57.5
annulare (perforating) L92.0
apical K04.5
aural —*see* Otitis, externa, specified NEC
beryllium (skin) L92.3
bone
eosinophilic C96.6
from residual foreign body —*see*
Osteomyelitis, specified type NEC
lung C96.6
brain (any site) G06.0
schistosomiasis B65.9 [G07]
canaliculus lacrimalis —*see* Granuloma,
lacrimal
candidal (cutaneous) B37.2
cerebral (any site) G06.0
coccidioidal (primary) (progressive) B38.7
lung B38.1
meninges B38.4

Granuloma (Continued)
  colon K63.89
  conjunctiva H11.22-•
  dental K04.5
  ear, middle —see Cholesteatoma
  eosinophilic C96.6
    bone C96.6
    lung C96.6
    oral mucosa K13.4
    skin L92.2
  eyelid H01.8
  facial (e) L92.2
  foreign body (in soft tissue) NEC M60.20
    ankle M60.27-•
    foot M60.27-•
    forearm M60.23-•
    hand M60.24-•
    in operation wound —see Foreign body,
      accidentally left during a procedure
    lower leg M60.26-•
    pelvic region M60.25-•
    shoulder region M60.21-•
    skin L92.3
    specified site NEC M60.28
    subcutaneous tissue L92.3
    thigh M60.25-•
    upper arm M60.22-•
  gangraenescens M31.2
  genito-inguinale A58
  giant cell (central) (reparative) (jaw) M27.1
    gingiva (peripheral) K06.8
  gland (lymph) I88.8
  hepatic NEC K75.3
    in (due to)
      berylliosis J63.2 [K77]
      sarcoidosis D86.89
  Hodgkin C81.9
  ileum K63.89
  infectious B99.9
    specified NEC B99.8
  inguinale (Donovan) (venereal) A58
  intestine NEC K63.89
  intracranial (any site) G06.0
  intraspinal (any part) G06.1
  iridocyclitis —see Iridocyclitis, chronic
  jaw (bone) (central) M27.1
    reparative giant cell M27.1
  kidney —see also Infection, kidney N15.8
  lacrimal H04.81-•
  larynx J38.7
  lethal midline (faciale (e)) M31.2
  liver NEC —see Granuloma, hepatic
  lung (infectious) —see also Fibrosis, lung
    coccidioidal B38.1
    eosinophilic C96.6
  Majocchi's B35.8
  malignant (facial (e)) M31.2
  mandible (central) M27.1
  midline (lethal) M31.2
  monilial (cutaneous) B37.2
  nasal sinus —see Sinusitis
  operation wound T81.89
    foreign body —see Foreign body,
      accidentally left during a procedure
    stitch T81.89
    talc —see Foreign body, accidentally left
      during a procedure
  oral mucosa K13.4
  orbit, orbital H05.11-•
  paracoccidioidal B41.8
  penis, venereal A58
  periapical K04.5
  peritoneum K66.8
    due to ova of helminths NOS —see also
      Helminthiasis B83.9 [K67]
  postmastoidectomy cavity —see
    Complications, postmastoidectomy,
    recurrent cholesteatoma
  prostate N42.89
  pudendi (ulcerating) A58
  pulp, internal (tooth) K03.3

Granuloma (Continued)
  pyogenic, pyogenicum (of) (skin) L98.0
    gingiva K06.8
      maxillary alveolar ridge K04.5
      oral mucosa K13.4
  rectum K62.89
  reticulohistiocytic D76.3
  rubrum nasi L74.8
  Schistosoma —see Schistosomiasis
  septic (skin) L98.0
  silica (skin) L92.3
  sinus (accessory) (infective) (nasal) —see
    Sinusitis
  skin L92.9
    from residual foreign body L92.3
    pyogenicum L98.0
  spine
    syphilitic (epidural) A52.19
    tuberculous A18.01
  stitch (postoperative) T81.89
  suppurative (skin) L98.0
  swimming pool A31.1
  talc —see also Granuloma, foreign body
    in operation wound —see Foreign body,
      accidentally left during a procedure
  telangiectaticum (skin) L98.0
  tracheostomy J95.09
  trichophyticum B35.8
  tropicum A66.4
  ▶umbilical P83.81
  ⇒umbilicus P83.81
  urethra N36.8
  uveitis —see Iridocyclitis, chronic
  vagina A58
  venereum A58
  vocal cord J38.3
Granulomatosis L92.9
  lymphoid C83.8-•
  miliary (listerial) A32.89
  necrotizing, respiratory M31.30
  progressive septic D71
  specified NEC L92.8
  Wegener's M31.30
    with renal involvement M31.31
Granulomatous tissue (abnormal) (excessive)
  L92.9
Granulosis rubra nasi L74.8
Graphite fibrosis (of lung) J63.3
Graphospasm F48.8
  organic G25.89
Grating scapula M89.8X1
Gravel (urinary) —see Calculus, urinary
Graves' disease —see Hyperthyroidism, with,
  goiter
Gravis —see condition
Grawitz tumor C64.-•
Gray syndrome (newborn) P93.0
Grayness, hair (premature) L67.1
  congenital Q84.2
Green sickness D50.8
Greenfield's disease
  meaning
    concentric sclerosis (encephalitis periaxialis
      concentrica) G37.5
    metachromatic leukodystrophy E75.25
Greenstick fracture - code as Fracture, by site
Grey syndrome (newborn) P93.0
Grief F43.21
  prolonged F43.29
  reaction —see also Disorder, adjustment F43.20
Griesinger's disease B76.9
Grinder's lung or pneumoconiosis J62.8
Grinding, teeth
  psychogenic F45.8
  sleep related G47.63
Grip
  Dabney's B33.0
  devil's B33.0
Grippe, grippal —see also Influenza
  Balkan A78
  summer, of Italy A93.1
Grisel's disease M43.6

Groin —see condition
Grooved tongue K14.5
Ground itch B76.9
Grover's disease or syndrome L11.1
Growing pains, children R29.898
Growth (fungoid) (neoplastic) (new) —see also
  Neoplasm
  adenoid (vegetative) J35.8
  benign —see Neoplasm, benign, by site
  malignant —see Neoplasm, malignant, by site
  rapid, childhood Z00.2
  secondary —see Neoplasm, secondary, by site
Gruby's disease B35.0
Gubler-Millard paralysis or syndrome G46.3
Guerin-Stern syndrome Q74.3
Guidance, insufficient anterior (occlusal) M26.54
Guillain-Barré disease or syndrome G61.0
  sequelae G65.0
Guinea worms (infection) (infestation) B72
Guinon's disease (motor-verbal tic) F95.2
Gull's disease E03.4
Gum —see condition
Gumboil K04.7
  with sinus K04.6
Gumma (syphilitic) A52.79
  artery A52.09
    cerebral A52.04
  bone A52.77
    of yaws (late) A66.6
  brain A52.19
  cauda equina A52.19
  central nervous system A52.3
  ciliary body A52.71
  congenital A50.59
  eyelid A52.71
  heart A52.06
  intracranial A52.19
  iris A52.71
  kidney A52.75
  larynx A52.73
  leptomeninges A52.19
  liver A52.74
  meninges A52.19
  myocardium A52.06
  nasopharynx A52.73
  neurosyphilitic A52.3
  nose A52.73
  orbit A52.71
  palate (soft) A52.79
  penis A52.76
  pericardium A52.06
  pharynx A52.73
  pituitary A52.79
  scrofulous (tuberculous) A18.4
  skin A52.79
  specified site NEC A52.79
  spinal cord A52.19
  tongue A52.79
  tonsil A52.73
  trachea A52.73
  tuberculous A18.4
  ulcerative due to yaws A66.4
  ureter A52.75
  yaws A66.4
    bone A66.6
Gunn's syndrome Q07.8
Gunshot wound —see also Wound, open
  fracture - code as Fracture, by site
  internal organs —see Injury, by site
Gynandrism Q56.0
Gynandroblastoma
  specified site —see Neoplasm, uncertain
    behavior, by site
  unspecified site
    female D39.10
    male D40.10
Gynecological examination (periodic) (routine)
  Z01.419
  with abnormal findings Z01.411
Gynecomastia N62
Gynephobia F40.291
Gyrate scalp Q82.8

H

H (Hartnup's) disease E72.02
Haas' disease or osteochondrosis (juvenile)
    (head of humerus) —see Osteochondrosis,
    juvenile, humerus
Habit, habituation
  bad sleep Z72.821
  chorea F95.8
  disturbance, child F98.9
  drug —see Dependence, drug
  irregular sleep Z72.821
  laxative F55.2
  spasm —see Tic
  tic —see Tic
Haemophilus (H.) influenzae, as cause of
    disease classified elsewhere B96.3
Haff disease —see Poisoning, mercury
Hageman's factor defect, deficiency or disease
    D68.2
Haglund's disease or osteochondrosis
    (juvenile) (os tibiale externum) —see
    Osteochondrosis, juvenile, tarsus
Hailey-Hailey disease Q82.8
Hair —see also condition
  plucking F63.3
    in stereotyped movement disorder F98.4
  tourniquet syndrome —see also Constriction,
    external, by site
    finger S60.44-●
    penis S30.842
    thumb S60.34-●
    toe S90.44-●
Hairball in stomach T18.2
Hair-pulling, pathological (compulsive) F63.3
Hairy black tongue K14.3
Half vertebra Q76.49
Halitosis R19.6
Hallerman-Streiff syndrome Q87.0
Hallervorden-Spatz disease G23.0
Hallopeau's acrodermatitis or disease L40.2
Hallucination R44.3
  auditory R44.0
  gustatory R44.2
  olfactory R44.2
  specified NEC R44.2
  tactile R44.2
  visual R44.1
Hallucinosis (chronic) F28
  alcoholic (acute) F10.951
    in
      abuse F10.151
      dependence F10.251
  drug-induced F19.951
    cannabis F12.951
    cocaine F14.951
    hallucinogen F16.151
    in
      abuse F19.151
        cannabis F12.151
        cocaine F14.151
        hallucinogen F16.151
        inhalant F18.151
        opioid F11.151
        sedative, anxiolytic or hypnotic
          F13.151
        stimulant NEC F15.151
      dependence F19.251
        cannabis F12.251
        cocaine F14.251
        hallucinogen F16.251
        inhalant F18.251
        opioid F11.251
        sedative, anxiolytic or hypnotic
          F13.251
        stimulant NEC F15.251
    inhalant F18.951
    opioid F11.951
    sedative, anxiolytic or hypnotic F13.951
    stimulant NEC F15.951
  organic F06.0

Hallux
  deformity (acquired) NEC M20.5X-●
  limitus M20.5X-●
  malleus (acquired) NEC M20.3-●
  rigidus (acquired) M20.2-●
    congenital Q74.2
    sequelae (late effect) of rickets E64.3
  valgus (acquired) M20.1-●
    congenital Q66.6
  varus (acquired) M20.3-●
    congenital Q66.3
Halo, visual H53.19
Hamartoma, hamartoblastoma Q85.9
  epithelial (gingival), odontogenic, central
    or peripheral —see Cyst, calcifying
    odontogenic
Hamartosis Q85.9
Hamman-Rich syndrome J84.114
Hammer toe (acquired) NEC —see also
    Deformity, toe, hammer toe
  congenital Q66.89
  sequelae (late effect) of rickets E64.3
Hand —see condition
Hand-foot syndrome L27.1
Handicap, handicapped
  educational Z55.9
    specified NEC Z55.8
Hand-Schüller-Christian disease or syndrome
    C96.5
Hanging (asphyxia) (strangulation)
    (suffocation) —see Asphyxia, traumatic,
    due to mechanical threat
Hangnail —see also Cellulitis, digit
  with lymphangitis —see Lymphangitis, acute,
    digit
Hangover (alcohol) F10.129
Hanhart's syndrome Q87.0
Hanot-Chauffard (-Troisier) syndrome E83.19
Hanot's cirrhosis or disease K74.3
Hansen's disease —see Leprosy
Hantaan virus disease (Korean hemorrhagic
    fever) A98.5
Hantavirus disease (with renal manifestations)
    (Dobrava) (Puumala) (Seoul) A98.5
  with pulmonary manifestations (Andes)
    (Bayou) (Bermejo) (Black Creek Canal)
    (Choclo) (Juquitiba) (Laguna negra)
    (Lechiguanas) (New York) (Oran) (Sin
    nombre) B33.4
Happy puppet syndrome Q93.5
Harada's disease or syndrome H30.81-●
Hardening
  artery —see Arteriosclerosis
  brain G93.89
Harelip (complete) (incomplete) —see Cleft, lip
Harlequin (newborn) Q80.4
Harley's disease D59.6
Harmful use (of)
  alcohol F10.10
  anxiolytics —see Abuse, drug, sedative
  cannabinoids —see Abuse, drug, cannabis
  cocaine —see Abuse, drug, cocaine
  drug —see Abuse, drug
  hallucinogens —see Abuse, drug,
    hallucinogen
  hypnotics —see Abuse, drug, sedative -
    opioids —see Abuse, drug, opioid
  PCP (phencyclidine) —see Abuse, drug,
    hallucinogen
  sedatives —see Abuse, drug, sedative
  stimulants NEC —see Abuse, drug, stimulant
Harris' lines —see Arrest, epiphyseal
Hartnup's disease E72.02
Harvester's lung J67.0
Harvesting ovum for in vitro fertilization
    Z31.83
Hashimoto's disease or thyroiditis E06.3
Hashitoxicosis (transient) E06.3
Hassal-Henle bodies or warts (cornea) H18.49
Haut mal —see Epilepsy, generalized, specified
    NEC

Haverhill fever A25.1
Hay fever —see also Fever, hay J30.1
Hayem-Widal syndrome D59.8
Haygarth's nodes M15.8
Haymaker's lung J67.0
Hb (abnormal)
  Bart's disease D56.0
  disease —see Disease, hemoglobin
  trait —see Trait
Head —see condition
Headache R51
  allergic NEC G44.89
  associated with sexual activity
    G44.82
  chronic daily R51
  cluster G44.009
    chronic G44.029
      intractable G44.021
      not intractable G44.029
    episodic G44.019
      intractable G44.011
      not intractable G44.019
    intractable G44.001
    not intractable G44.009
  cough (primary) G44.83
  daily chronic R51
  drug-induced NEC G44.40
    intractable G44.41
    not intractable G44.40
  exertional (primary) G44.84
  histamine G44.009
    intractable G44.001
    not intractable G44.009
  hypnic G44.81
  lumbar puncture G97.1
  medication overuse G44.40
    intractable G44.41
    not intractable G44.40
  menstrual —see Migraine, menstrual
  migraine (type) —see also Migraine
    G43.909
  nasal septum R51
  neuralgiform, short lasting unilateral, with
    conjunctival injection and tearing
    (SUNCT) G44.059
    intractable G44.051
    not intractable G44.059
  new daily persistent (NDPH) G44.52
  orgasmic G44.82
  periodic syndromes in adults and children
    G43.C0
    with refractory migraine G43.C1
    intractable G43.C1
    not intractable G43.C0
    without refractory migraine G43.C0
  postspinal puncture G97.1
  post-traumatic G44.309
    acute G44.319
      intractable G44.311
      not intractable G44.319
    chronic G44.329
      intractable G44.321
      not intractable G44.329
    intractable G44.301
    not intractable G44.309
  pre-menstrual —see Migraine, menstrual
  preorgasmic G44.82
  primary
    cough G44.83
    exertional G44.84
    stabbing G44.85
    thunderclap G44.53
  rebound G44.40
    intractable G44.41
    not intractable G44.40
  short lasting unilateral neuralgiform, with
    conjunctival injection and tearing
    (SUNCT) G44.059
    intractable G44.051
    not intractable G44.059
  specified syndrome NEC G44.89

▶ New   ⟹ Revised   ~~deleted~~ Deleted   ● Use Additional Character(s)

Headache (Continued)
spinal and epidural anesthesia - induced T88.59
in labor and delivery O74.5
in pregnancy O29.4-●
postpartum, puerperal O89.4
spinal fluid loss (from puncture) G97.1
stabbing (primary) G44.85
tension (-type) G44.209
chronic G44.229
intractable G44.221
not intractable G44.229
episodic G44.219
intractable G44.211
not intractable G44.219
intractable G44.201
not intractable G44.209
thunderclap (primary) G44.53
vascular NEC G44.1
Healthy
infant
accompanying sick mother Z76.3
receiving care Z76.2
person accompanying sick person Z76.3
Hearing examination Z01.10
with abnormal findings NEC Z01.118
following failed hearing screening Z01.110
for hearing conservation and treatment Z01.12
Heart —see condition
Heart beat
abnormality R00.9
specified NEC R00.8
awareness R00.2
rapid R00.0
slow R00.1
Heartburn R12
psychogenic F45.8
▶**Heartland virus disease** A93.8
Heat (effects) T67.9
apoplexy T67.0
burn —see also Burn L55.9
collapse T67.1
cramps T67.2
dermatitis or eczema L59.0
edema T67.7
erythema - code by site under Burn, first degree
excessive T67.9
specified effect NEC T67.8
exhaustion T67.5
anhydrotic T67.3
due to
salt (and water) depletion T67.4
water depletion T67.3
with salt depletion T67.4
fatigue (transient) T67.6
fever T67.0
hyperpyrexia T67.0
prickly L74.0
prostration —see Heat, exhaustion
pyrexia T67.0
rash L74.0
specified effect NEC T67.8
stroke T67.0
sunburn —see Sunburn
syncope T67.1
Heavy-for-dates NEC (infant) (4000g to 4499g) P08.1
exceptionally (4500g or more) P08.0
Hebephrenia, hebephrenic (schizophrenia) F20.1
Heberden's disease or nodes (with arthropathy) M15.1
Hebra's
pityriasis L26
prurigo L28.2
Heel —see condition
Heerfordt's disease D86.89
Hegglin's anomaly or syndrome D72.0
Heilmeyer-Schoner disease D45
Heine-Medin disease A80.9

Heinz body anemia, congenital D58.2
Heliophobia F40.228
Heller's disease or syndrome F84.3
HELLP syndrome (hemolysis, elevated liver enzymes and low platelet count) O14.2-●
complicating
childbirth O14.24
puerperium O14.25
Helminthiasis —see also Infestation, helminth
Ancylostoma B76.0
intestinal B82.0
mixed types (types classifiable to more than one of the titles B65.0-B81.3 and B81.8) B81.4
specified type NEC B81.8
mixed types (intestinal) (types classifiable to more than one of the titles B65.0-B81.3 and B81.8) B81.4
Necator (americanus) B76.1
specified type NEC B83.8
Heloma L84
Hemangioblastoma —see Neoplasm, connective tissue, uncertain behavior
malignant —see Neoplasm, connective tissue, malignant
Hemangioendothelioma —see also Neoplasm, uncertain behavior, by site
benign D18.00
intra-abdominal D18.03
intracranial D18.02
skin D18.01
specified site NEC D18.09
bone (diffuse) —see Neoplasm, bone, malignant
epithelioid —see also Neoplasm, uncertain behavior, by site
malignant —see Neoplasm, malignant, by site
malignant —see Neoplasm, connective tissue, malignant
Hemangiofibroma —see Neoplasm, benign, by site
Hemangiolipoma —see Lipoma
Hemangioma D18.00
arteriovenous D18.00
intra-abdominal D18.03
intracranial D18.02
skin D18.01
specified site NEC D18.09
capillary D18.00
intra-abdominal D18.03
intracranial D18.02
skin D18.01
specified site NEC D18.09
cavernous D18.00
intra-abdominal D18.03
intracranial D18.02
skin D18.01
specified site NEC D18.09
epithelioid D18.00
intra-abdominal D18.03
intracranial D18.02
skin D18.01
specified site NEC D18.09
histiocytoid D18.00
intra-abdominal D18.03
intracranial D18.02
skin D18.01
specified site NEC D18.09
infantile D18.00
intra-abdominal D18.03
intracranial D18.02
skin D18.01
specified site NEC D18.09
intra-abdominal D18.03
intracranial D18.02
intramuscular D18.00
intra-abdominal D18.03
intracranial D18.02
skin D18.01
specified site NEC D18.09

Hemangioma (Continued)
intrathoracic structures D18.09
juvenile D18.00
malignant —see Neoplasm, connective tissue, malignant
plexiform D18.00
intra-abdominal D18.03
intracranial D18.02
skin D18.01
specified site NEC D18.09
racemose D18.00
intra-abdominal D18.03
intracranial D18.02
skin D18.01
specified site NEC D18.09
sclerosing —see Neoplasm, skin, benign
simplex D18.00
intra-abdominal D18.03
intracranial D18.02
skin D18.01
specified site NEC D18.09
skin D18.01
specified site NEC D18.09
venous D18.00
intra-abdominal D18.03
intracranial D18.02
skin D18.01
specified site NEC D18.09
verrucous keratotic D18.00
intra-abdominal D18.03
intracranial D18.02
skin D18.01
specified site NEC D18.09
Hemangiomatosis (systemic) I78.8
involving single site —see Hemangioma
Hemangiopericytoma —see also Neoplasm, connective tissue, uncertain behavior
benign —see Neoplasm, connective tissue, benign
malignant —see Neoplasm, connective tissue, malignant
Hemangiosarcoma —see Neoplasm, connective tissue, malignant
Hemarthrosis (nontraumatic) M25.00
ankle M25.07-●
elbow M25.02-●
foot joint M25.07-●
hand joint M25.04-●
hip M25.05-●
in hemophilic arthropathy —see Arthropathy, hemophilic
knee M25.06-●
shoulder M25.01-●
specified joint NEC M25.08
traumatic —see Sprain, by site
vertebrae M25.08
wrist M25.03-●
Hematemesis K92.0
with ulcer - code by site under Ulcer, with hemorrhage K27.4
newborn, neonatal P54.0
due to swallowed maternal blood P78.2
Hematidrosis L74.8
Hematinuria —see also Hemoglobinuria
malarial B50.8
Hematobilia K83.8
Hematocele
female NEC N94.89
with ectopic pregnancy O00.90
with intrauterine pregnancy O00.91
ovary N83.8
male N50.1
Hematochezia —see also Melena K92.1
Hematochyluria —see also Infestation, filarial
schistosomiasis (bilharziasis) B65.0
Hematocolpos (with hematometra or hematosalpinx) N89.7
Hematocornea —see Pigmentation, cornea, stromal
Hematogenous —see condition

▶ New   ⇒ Revised   ~~deleted~~ Deleted   ● Use Additional Character(s)

Hematoma (traumatic) (skin surface intact) —
  see also Contusion
  with
    injury of internal organs —*see* Injury, by site
    open wound —*see* Wound, open
  amputation stump (surgical) (late) T87.89
  aorta, dissecting I71.00
    abdominal I71.02
    thoracic I71.01
    thoracoabdominal I71.03
  aortic intramural —*see* Dissection, aorta
  arterial (complicating trauma) —*see* Injury,
    blood vessel, by site
  auricle —*see* Contusion, ear
    nontraumatic —*see* Disorder, pinna,
      hematoma
  birth injury NEC P15.8
  brain (traumatic)
    with
      cerebral laceration or contusion
        (diffuse) —*see* Injury, intracranial,
          diffuse
        focal —*see* Injury, intracranial, focal
    cerebellar, traumatic S06.37-●
    intracerebral, traumatic —*see* Injury,
      intracranial, intracerebral hemorrhage
    newborn NEC P52.4
      birth injury P10.1
    nontraumatic —*see* Hemorrhage,
      intracranial
    subarachnoid, arachnoid, traumatic —*see*
      Injury, intracranial, subarachnoid
      hemorrhage
    subdural, traumatic —*see* Injury,
      intracranial, subdural hemorrhage
  breast (nontraumatic) N64.89
  broad ligament (nontraumatic) N83.7
    traumatic S37.892
  cerebellar, traumatic S06.37-●
  cerebral —*see* Hematoma, brain
  cerebrum S06.36-●
    left S06.35-●
    right S06.34-●
  cesarean delivery wound O90.2
  complicating delivery (perineal) (pelvic)
    (vagina) (vulva) O71.7
  corpus cavernosum (nontraumatic) N48.89
  epididymis (nontraumatic) N50.1
  epidural (traumatic) —*see* Injury, intracranial,
    epidural hemorrhage
    spinal —*see* Injury, spinal cord, by region
  episiotomy O90.2
  face, birth injury P15.4
  genital organ NEC (nontraumatic)
    female (nonobstetric) N94.89
      traumatic S30.202
    male N50.1
      traumatic S30.201
  internal organs —*see* Injury, by site
  intracerebral, traumatic —*see* Injury,
    intracranial, intracerebral hemorrhage
  intraoperative —*see* Complications,
    intraoperative, hemorrhage
  labia (nontraumatic) (nonobstetric) N90.8
  liver (subcapsular) (nontraumatic) K76.89
    birth injury P15.0
  mediastinum —*see* Injury, intrathoracic
  mesosalpinx (nontraumatic) N83.7
    traumatic S37.898
  muscle - code by site under Contusion
  nontraumatic
    muscle M79.81
    soft tissue M79.81
  obstetrical surgical wound O90.2
  orbit, orbital (nontraumatic) —*see also*
    Hemorrhage, orbit
    traumatic —*see* Contusion, orbit
  pelvis (female) (nontraumatic) (nonobstetric)
    N94.89
    obstetric O71.7
    traumatic —*see* Injury, by site

Hematoma (*Continued*)
  penis (nontraumatic) N48.89
    birth injury P15.5
  perianal (nontraumatic) K64.5
  perineal S30.23
    complicating delivery O71.7
  perirenal —*see* Injury, kidney
  pinna —*see* Contusion, ear
    nontraumatic —*see* Disorder, pinna,
      hematoma
  placenta O43.89-●
  postoperative (postprocedural) —*see*
    Complication, postprocedural,
    hematoma
  retroperitoneal (nontraumatic) K66.1
    traumatic S36.892
  scrotum, superficial S30.22
    birth injury P15.5
  seminal vesicle (nontraumatic) N50.1
    traumatic S37.892
  spermatic cord (traumatic) S37.892
    nontraumatic N50.1
  spinal (cord) (meninges) —*see also* Injury,
    spinal cord, by region
    newborn (birth injury) P11.5
  spleen D73.5
    intraoperative —*see* Complications,
      intraoperative, hemorrhage, spleen
    postprocedural (postoperative) —*see*
      Complications, postprocedural,
      hemorrhage, spleen
  sternocleidomastoid, birth injury P15.2
  sternomastoid, birth injury P15.2
  subarachnoid (traumatic) —*see* Injury,
    intracranial, subarachnoid hemorrhage
    newborn (nontraumatic) P52.5
      due to birth injury P10.3
    nontraumatic —*see* Hemorrhage,
      intracranial, subarachnoid
  subdural (traumatic) —*see* Injury, intracranial,
    subdural hemorrhage
    newborn (localized) P52.8
      birth injury P10.0
    nontraumatic —*see* Hemorrhage,
      intracranial, subdural
  superficial, newborn P54.5
  testis (nontraumatic) N50.1
    birth injury P15.5
  tunica vaginalis (nontraumatic) N50.1
  umbilical cord, complicating delivery O69.5
  uterine ligament (broad) (nontraumatic)
    N83.7
    traumatic S37.892
  vagina (ruptured) (nontraumatic) N89.8
    complicating delivery O71.7
  vas deferens (nontraumatic) N50.1
    traumatic S37.892
  vitreous —*see* Hemorrhage, vitreous
  vulva (nontraumatic) (nonobstetric) N90.89
    complicating delivery O71.7
    newborn (birth injury) P15.5
Hematometra N85.7
  with hematocolpos N89.7
Hematomyelia (central) G95.19
  newborn (birth injury) P11.5
  traumatic T14.8
Hematomyelitis G04.90
Hematoperitoneum —*see* Hemoperitoneum
Hematophobia F40.230
Hematopneumothorax (*see* Hemothorax)
Hematopoiesis, cyclic D70.4
Hematoporphyria —*see* Porphyria
Hematorachis, hematorrhachis G95.19
  newborn (birth injury) P11.5
Hematosalpinx N83.6
  with
    hematocolpos N89.7
    hematometra N85.7
      with hematocolpos N89.7
    infectional —*see* Salpingitis
Hematospermia R36.1

Hematothorax (*see* Hemothorax)
Hematuria R31.9
  benign (familial) (of childhood) —*see also*
    Hematuria, idiopathic
    essential microscopic R31.1
  due to sulphonamide, sulfonamide —*see* Table
    of Drugs and Chemicals, by drug
  endemic —*see also* Schistosomiasis B65.0
  gross R31.0
  idiopathic N02.9
    with glomerular lesion
      crescentic (diffuse) glomerulonephritis
        N02.7
      dense deposit disease N02.6
      endocapillary proliferative
        glomerulonephritis N02.4
      focal and segmental hyalinosis or
        sclerosis N02.1
      membranoproliferative (diffuse) N02.5
      membranous (diffuse) N02.2
      mesangial proliferative (diffuse) N02.3
      mesangiocapillary (diffuse) N02.5
      minor abnormality N02.0
      proliferative NEC N02.8
      specified pathology NEC N02.8
  intermittent —*see* Hematuria, idiopathic
  malarial B50.8
  microscopic NEC (with symptoms) R31.29
    asymptomatic R31.21
    benign essential R31.1
  paroxysmal —*see also* Hematuria, idiopathic
    nocturnal D59.5
  persistent —*see* Hematuria, idiopathic
  recurrent —*see* Hematuria, idiopathic
  tropical —*see also* Schistosomiasis B65.0
  tuberculous A18.13
Hemeralopia (day blindness) H53.11
  vitamin A deficiency E50.5
Hemi-akinesia R41.4
Hemianalgesia R20.0
Hemianencephaly Q00.0
Hemianesthesia R20.0
Hemianopia, hemianopsia (heteronymous)
  H53.47
  homonymous H53.46-●
  syphilitic A52.71
Hemiathetosis R25.8
Hemiatrophy R68.89
  cerebellar G31.9
  face, facial, progressive (Romberg) G51.8
  tongue K14.8
Hemiballism (us) G25.5
Hemicardia Q24.8
Hemicephalus, hemicephaly Q00.0
Hemichorea G25.5
Hemicolitis, left —*see* Colitis, left sided
Hemicrania
  congenital malformation Q00.0
  continua G44.51
  meaning migraine —*see also* Migraine G43.909
  paroxysmal G44.039
    chronic G44.049
      intractable G44.041
      not intractable G44.049
    episodic G44.039
      intractable G44.031
      not intractable G44.039
    intractable G44.031
    not intractable G44.039
Hemidystrophy —*see* Hemiatrophy
Hemiectromelia Q73.8
Hemihypalgesia R20.8
Hemihypesthesia R20.1
Hemi-inattention R41.4
Hemimelia Q73.8
  lower limb —*see* Defect, reduction, lower
    limb, specified type NEC
  upper limb —*see* Defect, reduction, upper
    limb, specified type NEC
Hemiparalysis —*see* Hemiplegia
Hemiparesis —*see* Hemiplegia

Hemiparesthesia R20.2
Hemiparkinsonism G20
Hemiplegia G81.9-●
   alternans facialis G83.89
   ascending NEC G81.90
      spinal G95.89
   congenital (cerebral) G80.8
      spastic G80.2
   embolic (current episode) I63.4-●
   flaccid G81.0-●
   following
      cerebrovascular disease I69.959
         cerebral infarction I69.35-●
         intracerebral hemorrhage I69.15-●
         nontraumatic intracranial hemorrhage
            NEC I69.25-●
         specified disease NEC I69.85-●
         stroke NOS I69.35-●
         subarachnoid hemorrhage I69.05-●
   hysterical F44.4
   newborn NEC P91.88
      birth injury P11.9
   spastic G81.1-●
      congenital G80.2
   thrombotic (current episode) I63.3-●
Hemisection, spinal cord —see Injury, spinal
   cord, by region
Hemispasm (facial) R25.2
Hemisporosis B48.8
Hemitremor R25.1
Hemivertebra Q76.49
   failure of segmentation with scoliosis Q76.3
   fusion with scoliosis Q76.3
Hemochromatosis E83.119
   with refractory anemia D46.1
   due to repeated red blood cell transfusion
      E83.111
   hereditary (primary) E83.110
   neonatal P78.84
   primary E83.110
   specified NEC E83.118
Hemoglobin —see also condition
   abnormal (disease) —see Disease, hemoglobin
   AS genotype D57.3
   Constant Spring D58.2
   E-beta thalassemia D56.5
   fetal, hereditary persistence (HPFH) D56.4
   H Constant Spring D56.0
   low NOS D64.9
   S (Hb S), heterozygous D57.3
Hemoglobinemia D59.9
   due to blood transfusion T80.89
   paroxysmal D59.6
      nocturnal D59.5
Hemoglobinopathy (mixed) D58.2
   with thalassemia D56.8
   sickle-cell D57.1
      with thalassemia D57.40
         with crisis (vasoocclusive pain) D57.419
            with
               acute chest syndrome D57.411
               splenic sequestration D57.412
         without crisis D57.40
Hemoglobinuria R82.3
   with anemia, hemolytic, acquired (chronic)
      NEC D59.6
   cold (agglutinin) (paroxysmal) (with
      Raynaud's syndrome) D59.6
   due to exertion or hemolysis NEC D59.6
   intermittent D59.6
   malarial B50.8
   march D59.6
   nocturnal (paroxysmal) D59.5
   paroxysmal (cold) D59.6
      nocturnal D59.5
Hemolymphangioma D18.1
Hemolysis
   intravascular
      with
         abortion —see Abortion, by type,
            complicated by, hemorrhage
         ectopic or molar pregnancy O08.1

Hemolysis (Continued)
   intravascular (Continued)
      with (Continued)
         hemorrhage
            antepartum —see Hemorrhage,
               antepartum, with coagulation
               defect
            intrapartum —see also Hemorrhage,
               complicating, delivery O67.0
         postpartum O72.3
   neonatal (excessive) P58.9
      specified NEC P58.8
Hemolytic —see condition
Hemopericardium I31.2
   following acute myocardial infarction
      (current complication) I23.0
   newborn P54.8
   traumatic —see Injury, heart, with
      hemopericardium
Hemoperitoneum K66.1
   infectional K65.9
   traumatic S36.899
      with open wound —see Wound, open, with
         penetration into peritoneal cavity
Hemophilia (classical) (familial) (hereditary)
   D66
   A D66
   B D67
   C D68.1
   acquired D68.311
   autoimmune D68.311
   calcipriva —see also Defect, coagulation D68.4
   nonfamilial —see also Defect, coagulation
      D68.4
   secondary D68.311
   vascular D68.0
Hemophthalmos H44.81-●
Hemopneumothorax —see also Hemothorax
   traumatic S27.2
Hemoptysis R04.2
   newborn P26.9
   tuberculous —see Tuberculosis, pulmonary
Hemorrhage, hemorrhagic (concealed) R58
   abdomen R58
   accidental antepartum —see Hemorrhage,
      antepartum
   acute idiopathic pulmonary, in infants
      R04.81
   adenoid J35.8
   adrenal (capsule) (gland) E27.49
      medulla E27.8
      newborn P54.4
   after delivery —see Hemorrhage, postpartum
   alveolar
      lung, newborn P26.8
      process K08.89
   alveolus K08.89
   amputation stump (surgical) T87.89
   anemia (chronic) D50.0
      acute D62
   antepartum (with) O46.90
      with coagulation defect O46.00-●
         afibrinogenemia O46.01-●
         disseminated intravascular coagulation
            O46.02-●
         hypofibrinogenemia O46.01-●
         specified defect NEC O46.09-●
      before 20 weeks gestation O20.9
         specified type NEC O20.8
         threatened abortion O20.0
      due to
         abruptio placenta —see also Abruptio
            placentae O45.9-●
         leiomyoma, uterus —see Hemorrhage,
            antepartum, specified cause NEC
         placenta previa O44.1-●
      specified cause NEC —see subcategory
         O46.8X-●
   anus (sphincter) K62.5
   apoplexy (stroke) —see Hemorrhage,
      intracranial, intracerebral

Hemorrhage, hemorrhagic (Continued)
   arachnoid —see Hemorrhage, intracranial,
      subarachnoid
   artery R58
      brain —see Hemorrhage, intracranial,
         intracerebral
   basilar (ganglion) I61.0
   bladder N32.89
   bowel K92.2
      newborn P54.3
   brain (miliary) (nontraumatic) —see
      Hemorrhage, intracranial, intracerebral
      due to
         birth injury P10.1
         syphilis A52.05
      epidural or extradural (traumatic) —
         see Injury, intracranial, epidural
         hemorrhage
      newborn P52.4
         birth injury P10.1
      subarachnoid —see Hemorrhage,
         intracranial, subarachnoid
      subdural —see Hemorrhage, intracranial,
         subdural
   brainstem (nontraumatic) I61.3
      traumatic S06.38-●
   breast N64.59
   bronchial tube —see Hemorrhage, lung
   bronchopulmonary —see Hemorrhage, lung
   bronchus —see Hemorrhage, lung
   bulbar I61.5
   capillary I78.8
      primary D69.8
   cecum K92.2
   cerebellar, cerebellum (nontraumatic) I61.4
      newborn P52.6
      traumatic S06.37-●
   cerebral, cerebrum —see also Hemorrhage,
      intracranial, intracerebral
      lobe I61.1
      newborn (anoxic) P52.4
         birth injury P10.1
   cerebromeningeal I61.8
   cerebrospinal —see Hemorrhage, intracranial,
      intracerebral
   cervix (uteri) (stump) NEC N88.8
   chamber, anterior (eye) —see Hyphema
   childbirth —see Hemorrhage, complicating,
      delivery
   choroid H31.30-●
      expulsive H31.31-●
   ciliary body —see Hyphema
   cochlea —see subcategory H83.8
   colon K92.2
   complicating
      abortion —see Abortion, by type,
         complicated by, hemorrhage
      delivery O67.9
         associated with coagulation defect
            (afibrinogenemia) (DIC)
            (hyperfibrinolysis) O67.0
         specified cause NEC O67.8
      surgical procedure —see Hemorrhage,
         intraoperative
   conjunctiva H11.3-●
      newborn P54.8
   cord, newborn (stump) P51.9
   corpus luteum (ruptured) cyst N83.1-●
   cortical (brain) I61.1
   cranial —see Hemorrhage, intracranial
   cutaneous R23.3
      due to autosensitivity, erythrocyte D69.2
      newborn P54.5
   delayed
      following ectopic or molar pregnancy
         O08.1
      postpartum O72.2
   diathesis (familial) D69.9
   disease D69.9
      newborn P53
      specified type NEC D69.8

Hemorrhage, hemorrhagic *(Continued)*
  due to or associated with
    afibrinogenemia or other coagulation defect
        (conditions in categories D65-D69)
      antepartum —*see* Hemorrhage,
          antepartum, with coagulation
          defect
      intrapartum O67.0
    dental implant M27.61
    device, implant or graft —*see also*
        Complications, by site and type,
        specified NEC T85.838
      arterial graft NEC T82.838
      breast T85.838
      catheter NEC T85.838
        dialysis (renal) T82.838
          intraperitoneal T85.838
        infusion NEC T82.838
          spinal (epidural) (subdural)
              T85.830
        urinary (indwelling) T83.83
      electronic (electrode) (pulse generator)
          (stimulator)
        bone T84.83
        cardiac T82.837
        nervous system (brain) (peripheral
            nerve) (spinal) T85.830
        urinary T83.83
      fixation, internal (orthopedic) NEC T84.83
      gastrointestinal (bile duct) (esophagus)
          T85.838
      genital NEC T83.83
      heart NEC T82.837
      joint prosthesis T84.83
      ocular (corneal graft) (orbital implant)
          NEC T85.838
      orthopedic NEC T84.83
        bone graft T86.838
      specified NEC T85.838
      urinary NEC T83.83
      vascular NEC T82.838
      ventricular intracranial shunt T85.838
  duodenum, duodenal K92.2
    ulcer —*see* Ulcer, duodenum, with
        hemorrhage
  dura mater —*see* Hemorrhage, intracranial,
      subdural
  endotracheal —*see* Hemorrhage, lung
  epicranial subaponeurotic (massive), birth
      injury P12.2
  epidural (traumatic) —*see also* Injury,
      intracranial, epidural hemorrhage
    nontraumatic I62.1
  esophagus K22.8
    varix I85.01
      secondary I85.11
  excessive, following ectopic gestation
      (subsequent episode) O08.1
  extradural (traumatic) —*see* Injury,
      intracranial, epidural hemorrhage
    birth injury P10.8
    newborn (anoxic) (nontraumatic) P52.8
    nontraumatic I62.1
  eye NEC H57.8
    fundus —*see* Hemorrhage, retina
    lid —*see* Disorder, eyelid, specified type
        NEC
  fallopian tube N83.6
  fibrinogenolysis —*see* Fibrinolysis
  fibrinolytic (acquired) —*see* Fibrinolysis
  from
    ear (nontraumatic) —*see* Otorrhagia
    tracheostomy stoma J95.01
  fundus, eye —*see* Hemorrhage, retina
  funis —*see* Hemorrhage, umbilicus, cord
  gastric —*see* Hemorrhage, stomach
  gastroenteric K92.2
    newborn P54.3
  gastrointestinal (tract) K92.2
    newborn P54.3
  genital organ, male N50.1

Hemorrhage, hemorrhagic *(Continued)*
  genitourinary (tract) NOS R31.9
  gingiva K06.8
  globe (eye) —*see* Hemophthalmos
  graafian follicle cyst (ruptured) N83.0-•
  gum K06.8
  heart I51.89
  hypopharyngeal (throat) R04.1
  intermenstrual (regular) N92.3
    irregular N92.1
  internal (organs) NEC R58
    capsule I61.0
    ear —*see* subcategory H83.8
    newborn P54.8
  intestine K92.2
    newborn P54.3
  intra-abdominal R58
  intra-alveolar (lung), newborn P26.8
  intracerebral (nontraumatic) —*see*
      Hemorrhage, intracranial,
      intracerebral
  intracranial (nontraumatic) I62.9
    birth injury P10.9
    epidural, nontraumatic I62.1
    extradural, nontraumatic I62.1
    intracerebral (nontraumatic) (in) I61.9
      brain stem I61.3
      cerebellum I61.4
      hemisphere I61.2
        cortical (superficial) I61.1
        subcortical (deep) I61.0
      intraoperative
        during a nervous system procedure
            G97.31
        during other procedure G97.32
      intraventricular I61.5
      multiple localized I61.6
      newborn P52.4
        birth injury P10.1
      postprocedural
        following a nervous system procedure
            G97.51
        following other procedure
            G97.52
      specified NEC I61.8
      superficial I61.1
      traumatic (diffuse) —*see* Injury,
          intracranial, diffuse
        focal —*see* Injury, intracranial, focal
    newborn P52.9
    specified NEC P52.8
    subarachnoid (nontraumatic) (from) I60.9
      intracranial (cerebral) artery I60.7
        anterior communicating I60.2
        basilar I60.4
        carotid siphon and bifurcation
            I60.0-•
        communicating I60.7
          anterior I60.2
          posterior I60.3-•
        middle cerebral I60.1-•
        posterior communicating I60.3-•
        specified artery NEC I60.6
        vertebral I60.5-•
      newborn P52.5
        birth injury P10.3
      specified NEC I60.8
      traumatic S06.6X-•
    subdural (nontraumatic) I62.00
      acute I62.01
      birth injury P10.0
      chronic I62.03
      newborn (anoxic) (hypoxic) P52.8
        birth injury P10.0
      spinal G95.19
      subacute I62.02
      traumatic —*see* Injury, intracranial,
          subdural hemorrhage
    traumatic —*see* Injury, intracranial, focal
        brain injury
  intramedullary NEC G95.19

Hemorrhage, hemorrhagic *(Continued)*
  intraocular —*see* Hemophthalmos
  intraoperative, intraprocedural —*see*
      Complication, hemorrhage (hematoma),
      intraoperative (intraprocedural), by site
  intrapartum —*see* Hemorrhage, complicating,
      delivery
  intrapelvic
    female N94.89
    male K66.1
  intraperitoneal K66.1
  intrapontine I61.3
  intraprocedural —*see* Complication,
      hemorrhage (hematoma), intraoperative
      (intraprocedural), by site
  intrauterine N85.7
    complicating delivery —*see also* Hemorrhage,
        complicating, delivery O67.9
    postpartum —*see* Hemorrhage, postpartum
  intraventricular I61.5
    newborn (nontraumatic) —*see also* Newborn,
        affected by, hemorrhage P52.3
      due to birth injury P10.2
      grade
        1 P52.0
        2 P52.1
        3 P52.21
        4 P52.22
  intravesical N32.89
  iris (postinfectional) (postinflammatory)
      (toxic) —*see* Hyphema
  joint (nontraumatic) —*see* Hemarthrosis
  kidney N28.89
  knee (joint) (nontraumatic) —*see*
      Hemarthrosis, knee
  labyrinth —*see* subcategory H83.8
  lenticular striate artery I61.0
  ligature, vessel —*see* Hemorrhage,
      postoperative
  liver K76.89
  lung R04.89
    newborn P26.9
      massive P26.1
      specified NEC P26.8
    tuberculous —*see* Tuberculosis, pulmonary
  massive umbilical, newborn P51.0
  mediastinum —*see* Hemorrhage, lung
  medulla I61.3
  membrane (brain) I60.8
    spinal cord —*see* Hemorrhage, spinal cord
  meninges, meningeal (brain) (middle) I60.8
    spinal cord —*see* Hemorrhage, spinal cord
  mesentery K66.1
  metritis —*see* Endometritis
  mouth K13.79
  mucous membrane NEC R58
    newborn P54.8
  muscle M62.89
  nail (subungual) L60.8
  nasal turbinate R04.0
    newborn P54.8
  navel, newborn P51.9
  newborn P54.9
    specified NEC P54.8
  nipple N64.59
  nose R04.0
    newborn P54.8
  omentum K66.1
  optic nerve (sheath) H47.02-•
  orbit, orbital H05.23-•
  ovary NEC N83.8
  oviduct N83.6
  pancreas K86.89
  parathyroid (gland) (spontaneous) E21.4
  parturition —*see* Hemorrhage, complicating,
      delivery
  penis N48.89
  pericardium, pericarditis I31.2
  peritoneum, peritoneal K66.1
  peritonsillar tissue J35.8
    due to infection J36

Hemorrhage, hemorrhagic *(Continued)*
  petechial R23.3
    due to autosensitivity, erythrocyte D69.2
  pituitary (gland) E23.6
  pleura —*see* Hemorrhage, lung
  polioencephalitis, superior E51.2
  polymyositis —*see* Polymyositis
  pons, pontine I61.3
  posterior fossa (nontraumatic) I61.8
    newborn P52.6
  postmenopausal N95.0
  postnasal R04.0
  postoperative —*see* Complications,
      postprocedural, hemorrhage, by site
  postpartum NEC (following delivery of
      placenta) O72.1
    delayed or secondary O72.2
    retained placenta O72.0
    third stage O72.0
  pregnancy —*see* Hemorrhage, antepartum
  preretinal —*see* Hemorrhage, retina
  prostate N42.1
  puerperal —*see* Hemorrhage, postpartum
    delayed or secondary O72.2
  pulmonary R04.89
    newborn P26.9
      massive P26.1
      specified NEC P26.8
    tuberculous —*see* Tuberculosis, pulmonary
  purpura (primary) D69.3
  rectum (sphincter) K62.5
    newborn P54.2
  recurring, following initial hemorrhage at
      time of injury T79.2
  renal N28.89
  respiratory passage or tract R04.9
    specified NEC R04.89
  retina, retinal (vessels) H35.6-●
    diabetic —*see* Diabetes, retinal, hemorrhage
  retroperitoneal R58
  scalp R58
  scrotum N50.1
  secondary (nontraumatic) R58
    following initial hemorrhage at time of
        injury T79.2
  seminal vesicle N50.1
  skin R23.3
    newborn P54.5
  slipped umbilical ligature P51.8
  spermatic cord N50.1
  spinal (cord) G95.19
    newborn (birth injury) P11.5
  spleen D73.5
    intraoperative —*see* Complications,
        intraoperative, hemorrhage, spleen
    postprocedural —*see* Complications,
        postprocedural, hemorrhage, spleen
  stomach K92.2
    newborn P54.3
    ulcer —*see* Ulcer, stomach, with
        hemorrhage
  subarachnoid (nontraumatic) —*see*
      Hemorrhage, intracranial, subarachnoid
  subconjunctival —*see also* Hemorrhage,
      conjunctiva
    birth injury P15.3
  subcortical (brain) I61.0
  subcutaneous R23.3
  subdiaphragmatic R58
  subdural (acute) (nontraumatic) —*see*
      Hemorrhage, intracranial, subdural
  subependymal
    newborn P52.0
      with intraventricular extension P52.1
        and intracerebral extension P52.22
  subgaleal P12.2
  subhyaloid —*see* Hemorrhage, retina
  subperiosteal —*see* Disorder, bone, specified
      type NEC
  subretinal —*see* Hemorrhage, retina
  subtentorial —*see* Hemorrhage, intracranial,
      subdural

Hemorrhage, hemorrhagic *(Continued)*
  subungual L60.8
  suprarenal (capsule) (gland) E27.49
    newborn P54.4
  tentorium (traumatic) NEC —*see*
      Hemorrhage, brain
    newborn (birth injury) P10.4
  testis N50.1
  third stage (postpartum) O72.0
  thorax —*see* Hemorrhage, lung
  throat R04.1
  thymus (gland) E32.8
  thyroid (cyst) (gland) E07.89
  tongue K14.8
  tonsil J35.8
  trachea —*see* Hemorrhage, lung
  tracheobronchial R04.89
    newborn P26.0
  traumatic — code to specific injury
    cerebellar —*see* Hemorrhage, brain
    intracranial —*see* Hemorrhage, brain
    recurring or secondary (following initial
        hemorrhage at time of injury)
        T79.2
  tuberculous NEC —*see also* Tuberculosis,
      pulmonary A15.0
  tunica vaginalis N50.1
  ulcer - code by site under Ulcer, with
      hemorrhage K27.4
  umbilicus, umbilical
    cord
      after birth, newborn P51.9
      complicating delivery O69.5
    newborn P51.9
      massive P51.0
      slipped ligature P51.8
    stump P51.9
  urethra (idiopathic) N36.8
  uterus, uterine (abnormal) N93.9
    climacteric N92.4
    complicating delivery —*see* Hemorrhage,
        complicating, delivery
    dysfunctional or functional N93.8
    intermenstrual (regular) N92.3
      irregular N92.1
    postmenopausal N95.0
    postpartum —*see* Hemorrhage,
        postpartum
    preclimacteric or premenopausal N92.4
    prepubertal N93.8
    pubertal N92.2
  vagina (abnormal) N93.9
    newborn P54.6
  vas deferens N50.1
  vasa previa O69.4
  ventricular I61.5
  vesical N32.89
  viscera NEC R58
    newborn P54.8
  vitreous (humor) (intraocular) H43.1-●
  vulva N90.89
Hemorrhoids (bleeding) (without mention of
    degree) K64.9
  1st degree (grade/stage I) (without prolapse
      outside of anal canal) K64.0
  2nd degree (grade/stage II) (that prolapse
      with straining but retract spontaneously)
      K64.1
  3rd degree (grade/stage III) (that prolapse
      with straining and require manual
      replacement back inside anal canal)
      K64.2
  4th degree (grade/stage IV) (with prolapsed
      tissue that cannot be manually replaced)
      K64.3
  complicating
    pregnancy O22.4
    puerperium O87.2
  external K64.4
    with
      thrombosis K64.5

Hemorrhoids *(Continued)*
  internal (without mention of degree) K64.8
  prolapsed K64.8
  skin tags
    anus K64.4
    residual K64.4
  specified NEC K64.8
  strangulated —*see also* Hemorrhoids, by
      degree K64.8
  thrombosed —*see also* Hemorrhoids, by
      degree K64.5
  ulcerated —*see also* Hemorrhoids, by degree
      K64.8
Hemosalpinx N83.6
  with
    hematocolpos N89.7
    hematometra N85.7
      with hematocolpos N89.7
Hemosiderosis (dietary) E83.19
  pulmonary, idiopathic E83.1 *[J84.03]*
  transfusion T80.89
Hemothorax (bacterial) (nontuberculous) J94.2
  newborn P54.8
  traumatic S27.1
    with pneumothorax S27.2
  tuberculous NEC A15.6
Henoch (-Schönlein) disease or syndrome
    (purpura) D69.0
Henpue, henpuye A66.6
Hepar lobatum (syphilitic) A52.74
Hepatalgia K76.89
Hepatitis K75.9
  acute B17.9
    with coma K72.01
    with hepatic failure —*see* Failure, hepatic
    alcoholic —*see* Hepatitis, alcoholic
    infectious B15.9
    non-viral K72.0
    viral B17.9
  alcoholic (acute) (chronic) K70.10
    with ascites K70.11
  amebic —*see* Abscess, liver, amebic
  anicteric (viral) —*see* Hepatitis, viral
  antigen-associated (HAA) —*see* Hepatitis, B
  Australia-antigen (positive) —*see* Hepatitis, B
  autoimmune K75.4
  B B19.10
    with hepatic coma B19.11
    acute B16.9
      with
        delta-agent (coinfection) (without
            hepatic coma) B16.1
          with hepatic coma B16.0
        hepatic coma (without delta-agent
            coinfection) B16.2
    chronic B18.1
      with delta-agent B18.0
  bacterial NEC K75.89
  C (viral) B19.20
    with hepatic coma B19.21
    acute B17.10
      with hepatic coma B17.11
    chronic B18.2
  catarrhal (acute) B15.9
    with hepatic coma B15.0
  cholangiolitic K75.89
  cholestatic K75.89
  chronic K73.9
    active NEC K73.2
    lobular NEC K73.1
    persistent NEC K73.0
    specified NEC K73.8
  cytomegaloviral B25.1
  due to ethanol (acute) (chronic) —*see*
      Hepatitis, alcoholic
  epidemic B15.9
    with hepatic coma B15.0
  fulminant NEC (viral) —*see* Hepatitis,
      viral
  granulomatous NEC K75.3
  herpesviral B00.81

▶ New　　➡ Revised　　~~deleted~~ Deleted　　● Use Additional Character(s)

Hepatitis *(Continued)*
  history of
    B Z86.19
    C Z86.19
  homologous serum —*see* Hepatitis, viral,
    type B
  in (due to)
    mumps B26.81
    toxoplasmosis (acquired) B58.1
      congenital (active) P37.1 *[K77]*
  infectious, infective B15.9
    acute (subacute) B17.9
    chronic B18.9
  inoculation —*see* Hepatitis, viral, type B
  interstitial (chronic) K74.69
  lupoid NEC K75.2
  malignant NEC (with hepatic failure)
    K72.90
    with coma K72.91
  neonatal giant cell P59.29
  neonatal (idiopathic) (toxic) P59.29
  newborn P59.29
  postimmunization —*see* Hepatitis, viral,
    type B
  post-transfusion —*see* Hepatitis, viral, type B
  reactive, nonspecific K75.2
  serum —*see* Hepatitis, viral, type B
  specified type NEC
    with hepatic failure —*see* Failure, hepatic
  syphilitic (late) A52.74
    congenital (early) A50.08 *[K77]*
      late A50.59 *[K77]*
    secondary A51.45
  toxic —*see also* Disease, liver, toxic K71.6
  tuberculous A18.83
  viral, virus B19.9
    with hepatic coma B19.0
    acute B17.9
    chronic B18.9
      specified NEC B18.8
      type
        B B18.1
          with delta-agent B18.0
        C B18.2
    congenital P35.3
    coxsackie B33.8 *[K77]*
    cytomegalic inclusion B25.1
    in remission, any type — code to Hepatitis,
      chronic, by type
    non-A, non-B B17.8
    specified type NEC (with or without coma)
      B17.8
    type
      A B15.9
        with hepatic coma B15.0
      B B19.10
        with hepatic coma B19.11
        acute B16.9
          with
            delta-agent (coinfection) (without
              hepatic coma) B16.1
              with hepatic coma B16.0
            hepatic coma (without delta-
              agent coinfection) B16.2
        chronic B18.1
          with delta-agent B18.0
      C B19.20
        with hepatic coma B19.21
        acute B17.10
          with hepatic coma B17.11
        chronic B18.2
      E B17.2
      non-A, non-B B17.8
Hepatization lung (acute) —*see* Pneumonia,
  lobar
Hepatoblastoma C22.2
Hepatocarcinoma C22.0
Hepatocholangiocarcinoma C22.0
Hepatocholangioma, benign D13.4
Hepatocholangitis K75.89
Hepatolenticular degeneration E83.01

Hepatoma (malignant) C22.0
  benign D13.4
  embryonal C22.0
Hepatomegaly —*see also* Hypertrophy, liver
  with splenomegaly R16.2
  congenital Q44.7
  in mononucleosis
    gammaherpesviral B27.09
    infectious specified NEC B27.89
Hepatoptosis K76.89
Hepatorenal syndrome following labor and
  delivery O90.4
Hepatosis K76.89
Hepatosplenomegaly R16.2
  hyperlipemic (Bürger-Grütz type) E78.3 *[K77]*
Hereditary —*see* condition
Heredodegeneration, macular —*see* Dystrophy,
  retina
Heredopathia atactica polyneuritiformis G60.1
Heredosyphilis —*see* Syphilis, congenital
Herlitz' syndrome Q81.1
Hermansky-Pudlak syndrome E70.331
Hermaphrodite, hermaphroditism (true)
  Q56.0
  46,XX with streak gonads Q99.1
  46,XX/46,XY Q99.0
  46,XY with streak gonads Q99.1
  chimera 46,XX/46,XY Q99.0
Hernia, hernial (acquired) (recurrent) K46.9
  with
    gangrene —*see* Hernia, by site, with,
      gangrene
    incarceration —*see* Hernia, by site, with,
      obstruction
    irreducible —*see* Hernia, by site, with,
      obstruction
    obstruction —*see* Hernia, by site, with,
      obstruction
    strangulation —*see* Hernia, by site, with,
      obstruction
  abdomen, abdominal K46.9
    with
      gangrene (and obstruction) K46.1
      obstruction K46.0
    femoral —*see* Hernia, femoral
    incisional —*see* Hernia, incisional
    inguinal —*see* Hernia, inguinal
    specified site NEC K45.8
      with
        gangrene (and obstruction) K45.1
        obstruction K45.0
    umbilical —*see* Hernia, umbilical
    wall —*see* Hernia, ventral
  appendix —*see* Hernia, abdomen
  bladder (mucosa) (sphincter)
    congenital (female) (male) Q79.51
    female —*see* Cystocele
    male N32.89
  brain, congenital —*see* Encephalocele
  cartilage, vertebra —*see* Displacement,
    intervertebral disc
  cerebral, congenital —*see also* Encephalocele
    endaural Q01.8
  ciliary body (traumatic) S05.2-●
  colon —*see* Hernia, abdomen
  Cooper's —*see* Hernia, abdomen, specified
    site NEC
  crural —*see* Hernia, femoral
  diaphragm, diaphragmatic K44.9
    with
      gangrene (and obstruction) K44.1
      obstruction K44.0
    congenital Q79.0
  direct (inguinal) —*see* Hernia, inguinal
  diverticulum, intestine —*see* Hernia,
    abdomen
  double (inguinal) —*see* Hernia, inguinal,
    bilateral
⇒due to adhesions (with obstruction) K56.50
  epigastric —*see also* Hernia, ventral K43.9
  esophageal hiatus —*see* Hernia, hiatal

Hernia, hernial *(Continued)*
  external (inguinal) —*see* Hernia, inguinal
  fallopian tube N83.4-●
  fascia M62.89
  femoral K41.90
    with
      gangrene (and obstruction) K41.40
        not specified as recurrent K41.40
        recurrent K41.41
      obstruction K41.30
        not specified as recurrent K41.30
        recurrent K41.31
    bilateral K41.20
      with
        gangrene (and obstruction) K41.10
          not specified as recurrent K41.10
          recurrent K41.11
        obstruction K41.00
          not specified as recurrent K41.00
          recurrent K41.01
      not specified as recurrent K41.20
      recurrent K41.21
    not specified as recurrent K41.90
    recurrent K41.91
    unilateral K41.90
      with
        gangrene (and obstruction) K41.40
          not specified as recurrent K41.40
          recurrent K41.41
        obstruction K41.30
          not specified as recurrent K41.30
          recurrent K41.31
      not specified as recurrent K41.90
      recurrent K41.91
  foramen magnum G93.5
    congenital Q01.8
  funicular (umbilical) —*see also* Hernia,
    umbilicus
    spermatic (cord) —*see* Hernia, inguinal
  gastrointestinal tract —*see* Hernia, abdomen
  Hesselbach's —*see* Hernia, femoral, specified
    site NEC
  hiatal (esophageal) (sliding) K44.9
    with
      gangrene (and obstruction) K44.1
      obstruction K44.0
    congenital Q40.1
  hypogastric —*see* Hernia, ventral
  incarcerated —*see also* Hernia, by site, with
    obstruction
    with gangrene —*see* Hernia, by site, with
      gangrene
  incisional K43.92
    with
      gangrene (and obstruction) K43.1
      obstruction K43.0
  indirect (inguinal) —*see* Hernia, inguinal
  inguinal (direct) (external) (funicular)
    (indirect) (internal) (oblique) (scrotal)
    (sliding) K40.90
    with
      gangrene (and obstruction) K40.40
        not specified as recurrent K40.40
        recurrent K40.41
      obstruction K40.30
        not specified as recurrent K40.30
        recurrent K40.31
    bilateral K40.20
      with
        gangrene (and obstruction)
          K40.10
          not specified as recurrent
            K40.10
          recurrent K40.11
        obstruction K40.00
          not specified as recurrent K40.00
          recurrent K40.01
      not specified as recurrent K40.20
      recurrent K40.21
    not specified as recurrent K40.90
    recurrent K40.91

Hernia, hernial (Continued)
inguinal (Continued)
unilateral K40.90
with
gangrene (and obstruction) K40.40
not specified as recurrent K40.40
recurrent K40.41
obstruction K40.30
not specified as recurrent K40.30
recurrent K40.31
not specified as recurrent K40.90
recurrent K40.91
internal —see also Hernia, abdomen
inguinal —see Hernia, inguinal
interstitial —see Hernia, abdomen
intervertebral cartilage or disc —see
Displacement, intervertebral disc
intestine, intestinal —see Hernia, by site
intra-abdominal —see Hernia, abdomen
iris (traumatic) S05.2-●
irreducible —see also Hernia, by site, with
obstruction
with gangrene —see Hernia, by site, with
gangrene
ischiatic —see Hernia, abdomen, specified
site NEC
ischiorectal —see Hernia, abdomen, specified
site NEC
lens (traumatic) S05.2-●
linea (alba) (semilunaris) —see Hernia,
ventral
Littre's —see Hernia, abdomen
lumbar —see Hernia, abdomen, specified site
NEC
lung (subcutaneous) J98.4
mediastinum J98.59
mesenteric (internal) —see Hernia, abdomen
midline —see Hernia, ventral
muscle (sheath) M62.89
nucleus pulposus —see Displacement,
intervertebral disc
oblique (inguinal) —see Hernia, inguinal
obstructive —see also Hernia, by site, with
obstruction
with gangrene —see Hernia, by site, with
gangrene
obturator —see Hernia, abdomen, specified
site NEC
omental —see Hernia, abdomen
ovary N83.4-●
oviduct N83.4-●
paraesophageal —see also Hernia, diaphragm
congenital Q40.1
parastomal K43.5
with
gangrene (and obstruction) K43.4
obstruction K43.3
paraumbilical —see Hernia, umbilicus
perineal —see Hernia, abdomen, specified
site NEC
Petit's —see Hernia, abdomen, specified site
NEC
postoperative —see Hernia, incisional
pregnant uterus —see Abnormal, uterus in
pregnancy or childbirth
prevesical N32.89
properitoneal —see Hernia, abdomen,
specified site NEC
pudendal —see Hernia, abdomen, specified
site NEC
rectovaginal N81.6
retroperitoneal —see Hernia, abdomen,
specified site NEC
Richter's —see Hernia, abdomen, with
obstruction
Rieux's, Riex's —see Hernia, abdomen,
specified site NEC
sac condition (adhesion) (dropsy)
(inflammation) (laceration)
(suppuration) - code by site under
Hernia

Hernia, hernial (Continued)
sciatic —see Hernia, abdomen, specified site
NEC
scrotum, scrotal —see Hernia, inguinal
sliding (inguinal) —see also Hernia,
inguinal
hiatus —see Hernia, hiatal
spigelian —see Hernia, ventral
spinal —see Spina bifida
strangulated —see also Hernia, by site, with
obstruction
with gangrene —see Hernia, by site, with
gangrene
subxiphoid —see Hernia, ventral
supra-umbilicus —see Hernia, ventral
tendon —see Disorder, tendon, specified type
NEC
Treitz's (fossa) —see Hernia, abdomen,
specified site NEC
tunica vaginalis Q55.29
umbilicus, umbilical K42.9
with
gangrene (and obstruction) K42.1
obstruction K42.0
ureter N28.89
urethra, congenital Q64.79
urinary meatus, congenital Q64.79
uterus N81.4
pregnant —see Abnormal, uterus in
pregnancy or childbirth
vaginal (anterior) (wall) —see Cystocele
Velpeau's —see Hernia, femoral
ventral K43.9
with
gangrene (and obstruction) K43.7
obstruction K43.6
incisional K43.2
with
gangrene (and obstruction) K43.1
obstruction K43.0
recurrent —see Hernia, incisional
specified NEC K43.9
with
gangrene (and obstruction) K43.7
obstruction K43.6
vesical
congenital (female) (male) Q79.51
female —see Cystocele
male N32.89
vitreous (into wound) S05.2-●
into anterior chamber —see Prolapse,
vitreous
Herniation —see also Hernia
brain (stem) G93.5
cerebral G93.5
mediastinum J98.59
nucleus pulposus —see Displacement,
intervertebral disc
Herpangina B08.5
Herpes, herpesvirus, herpetic B00.9
anogenital A60.9
perianal skin A60.1
rectum A60.1
urogenital tract A60.00
cervix A60.03
male genital organ NEC A60.02
penis A60.01
specified site NEC A60.09
vagina A60.04
vulva A60.04
blepharitis (zoster) B02.39
simplex B00.59
circinatus B35.4
bullosus L12.0
conjunctivitis (simplex) B00.53
zoster B02.31
cornea B02.33
encephalitis B00.4
due to herpesvirus 6 B10.01
due to herpesvirus 7 B10.09
specified NEC B10.09

Herpes, herpesvirus, herpetic (Continued)
eye (zoster) B02.30
simplex B00.50
eyelid (zoster) B02.39
simplex B00.59
facialis B00.1
febrilis B00.1
geniculate ganglionitis B02.21
genital, genitalis A60.00
female A60.09
male A60.02
gestational, gestationis O26.4-●
gingivostomatitis B00.2
human B00.9
1 —see Herpes, simplex
2 —see Herpes, simplex
3 —see Varicella
4 —see Mononucleosis, Epstein-Barr (virus)
5 —see Disease, cytomegalic inclusion
(generalized)
6
encephalitis B10.01
specified NEC B10.81
7
encephalitis B10.09
specified NEC B10.82
8 B10.89
infection NEC B10.89
Kaposi's sarcoma associated B10.89
iridocyclitis (simplex) B00.51
zoster B02.32
iris (vesicular erythema multiforme) L51.9
iritis (simplex) B00.51
Kaposi's sarcoma associated B10.89
keratitis (simplex) (dendritic) (disciform)
(interstitial) B00.52
zoster (interstitial) B02.33
keratoconjunctivitis (simplex) B00.52
zoster B02.33
labialis B00.1
lip B00.1
meningitis (simplex) B00.3
zoster B02.1
ophthalmicus (zoster) NEC B02.30
simplex B00.50
penis A60.01
perianal skin A60.1
pharyngitis, pharyngotonsillitis B00.2
rectum A60.1
scrotum A60.02
sepsis B00.7
simplex B00.9
complicated NEC B00.89
congenital P35.2
conjunctivitis B00.53
external ear B00.1
eyelid B00.59
hepatitis B00.81
keratitis (interstitial) B00.52
myelitis B00.82
specified complication NEC B00.89
visceral B00.89
stomatitis B00.2
tonsurans B35.0
visceral B00.89
vulva A60.04
whitlow B00.89
zoster —see also condition B02.9
auricularis B02.21
complicated NEC B02.8
conjunctivitis B02.31
disseminated B02.7
encephalitis B02.0
eye(lid) B02.39
geniculate ganglionitis B02.21
keratitis (interstitial) B02.33
meningitis B02.1
myelitis B02.24
neuritis, neuralgia B02.29
ophthalmicus NEC B02.30
oticus B02.21

▶ New   ⇒ Revised   ~~deleted~~ Deleted   ● Use Additional Character(s)

Herpes, herpesvirus, herpetic *(Continued)*
  zoster *(Continued)*
    polyneuropathy B02.23
    specified complication NEC B02.8
    trigeminal neuralgia B02.22
Herpesvirus (human) —*see* Herpes
Herpetophobia F40.218
Herrick's anemia —*see* Disease, sickle-cell
Hers' disease E74.09
Herter-Gee syndrome K90.0
Herxheimer's reaction R68.89
Hesitancy
  of micturition R39.11
  urinary R39.11
Hesselbach's hernia —*see* Hernia, femoral,
    specified site NEC
Heterochromia (congenital) Q13.2
  cataract —*see* Cataract, complicated
  cyclitis (Fuchs) —*see* Cyclitis, Fuchs'
      heterochromic
  hair L67.1
  iritis —*see* Cyclitis, Fuchs' heterochromic
  retained metallic foreign body
      (nonmagnetic) —*see* Foreign body,
      intraocular, old, retained
    magnetic —*see* Foreign body, intraocular,
        old, retained, magnetic
  uveitis —*see* Cyclitis, Fuchs' heterochromic
Heterophoria —*see* Strabismus, heterophoria
Heterophyes, heterophyiasis (small intestine)
    B66.8
Heterotopia, heterotopic —*see also* Malposition,
    congenital
  cerebralis Q04.8
Heterotropia —*see* Strabismus
Heubner-Herter disease K90.0
Hexadactylism Q69.9
HGSIL (cytology finding) (high grade
    squamous intraepithelial lesion on
    cytologic smear) (Pap smear finding)
  anus R85.613
  cervix R87.613
    biopsy (histology) finding — *see* Neoplasia,
        intraepithelial, cervix, grade II or
        grade III
  vagina R87.623
    biopsy (histology) finding — *see* Neoplasia,
        intraepithelial, vagina, grade II or
        grade III
Hibernoma —*see* Lipoma
Hiccup, hiccough R06.6
  epidemic B33.0
  psychogenic F45.8
Hidden penis (congenital) Q55.64
  acquired N48.83
Hidradenitis (axillaris) (suppurative) L73.2
Hidradenoma (nodular) —*see also* Neoplasm,
    skin, benign
  clear cell —*see* Neoplasm, skin, benign
  papillary —*see* Neoplasm, skin, benign
Hidrocystoma —*see* Neoplasm, skin, benign
High
  altitude effects T70.20
    anoxia T70.29
    on
      ears T70.0
      sinuses T70.1
    polycythemia D75.1
  arch
    foot Q66.7
    palate, congenital Q38.5
  arterial tension —*see* Hypertension
  basal metabolic rate R94.8
  blood pressure —*see also* Hypertension
    borderline R03.0
    reading (incidental) (isolated)
        (nonspecific), without diagnosis of
        hypertension R03.0
  cholesterol E78.00
    with high triglycerides E78.2
  diaphragm (congenital) Q79.1

High *(Continued)*
  expressed emotional level within family Z63.8
  head at term O32.4
  palate, congenital Q38.5
  risk
    infant NEC Z76.2
    sexual behavior (heterosexual) Z72.51
      bisexual Z72.53
      homosexual Z72.52
  ▶scrotal testis, testes
    ▶bilateral Q53.23
    ▶unilateral Q53.13
  temperature (of unknown origin) R50.9
  thoracic rib Q76.6
  triglycerides E78.1
    with high cholesterol E78.2
Hildenbrand's disease A75.0
Hilum —*see* condition
Hip —*see* condition
Hippel's disease Q85.8
Hippophobia F40.218
Hippus H57.09
Hirschsprung's disease or megacolon Q43.1
Hirsutism, hirsuties L68.0
Hirudiniasis
  external B88.3
  internal B83.4
Hiss-Russell dysentery A03.1
Histidinemia, histidinuria E70.41
Histiocytoma —*see also* Neoplasm, skin, benign
  fibrous —*see also* Neoplasm, skin, benign
    atypical —*see* Neoplasm, connective tissue,
        uncertain behavior
    malignant —*see* Neoplasm, connective
        tissue, malignant
Histiocytosis D76.3
  acute differentiated progressive C96.0
  Langerhans' cell NEC C96.6
    multifocal X
      multisystemic (disseminated) C96.0
      unisystemic C96.5
    pulmonary, adult (adult PLCH) J84.82
    unifocal (X) C96.6
  lipid, lipoid D76.3
    essential E75.29
  malignant C96.A
  mononuclear phagocytes NEC D76.1
    Langerhans' cells C96.6
  non-Langerhans cell D76.3
  polyostotic sclerosing D76.3
  sinus, with massive lymphadenopathy D76.3
  syndrome NEC D76.3
  X NEC C96.6
    acute (progressive) C96.0
    chronic C96.6
    multifocal C96.5
    multisystemic C96.0
    unifocal C96.6
Histoplasmosis B39.9
  with pneumonia NEC B39.2
  African B39.5
  American —*see* Histoplasmosis, capsulati
  capsulati B39.4
    disseminated B39.3
    generalized B39.3
    pulmonary B39.2
      acute B39.0
      chronic B39.1
  Darling's B39.4
  duboisii B39.5
  lung NEC B39.2
History
  family (of) —*see also* History, personal (of)
    alcohol abuse Z81.1
    allergy NEC Z84.89
    anemia Z83.2
    arthritis Z82.61
    asthma Z82.5
    blindness Z82.1
    cardiac death (sudden) Z82.41
    carrier of genetic disease Z84.81
    chromosomal anomaly Z82.79

History *(Continued)*
  family *(Continued)*
    chronic
      disabling disease NEC Z82.8
      lower respiratory disease Z82.5
    colonic polyps Z83.71
    congenital malformations and
        deformations Z82.79
      polycystic kidney Z82.71
    consanguinity Z84.3
    deafness Z82.2
    diabetes mellitus Z83.3
    disability NEC Z82.8
    disease or disorder (of)
      allergic NEC Z84.89
      behavioral NEC Z81.8
      blood and blood-forming organs Z83.2
      cardiovascular NEC Z82.49
      chronic disabling NEC Z82.8
      digestive Z83.79
      ear NEC Z83.52
      endocrine NEC Z83.49
      eye NEC Z83.518
        glaucoma Z83.511
      familial hypercholesterolemia Z83.42
      genitourinary NEC Z84.2
      glaucoma Z83.511
      hematological Z83.2
      immune mechanism Z83.2
      infectious NEC Z83.1
      ischemic heart Z82.49
      kidney Z84.1
      mental NEC Z81.8
      metabolic Z83.49
      musculoskeletal NEC Z82.69
      neurological NEC Z82.0
      nutritional Z83.49
      parasitic NEC Z83.1
      psychiatric NEC Z81.8
      respiratory NEC Z83.6
      skin and subcutaneous tissue NEC Z84.0
      specified NEC Z84.89
    drug abuse NEC Z81.3
    epilepsy Z82.0
    familial hypercholesterolemia Z83.42
    genetic disease carrier Z84.81
    glaucoma Z83.511
    hearing loss Z82.2
    human immunodeficiency virus (HIV)
        infection Z83.0
    Huntington's chorea Z82.0
    intellectual disability Z81.0
    leukemia Z80.6
    malignant neoplasm (of) NOS Z80.9
      bladder Z80.52
      breast Z80.3
      bronchus Z80.1
      digestive organ Z80.0
      gastrointestinal tract Z80.0
      genital organ Z80.49
        ovary Z80.41
        prostate Z80.42
        specified organ NEC Z80.49
        testis Z80.43
      hematopoietic NEC Z80.7
      intrathoracic organ NEC Z80.2
      kidney Z80.51
      lung Z80.1
      lymphatic NEC Z80.7
      ovary Z80.41
      prostate Z80.42
      respiratory organ NEC Z80.2
      specified site NEC Z80.8
      testis Z80.43
      trachea Z80.1
      urinary organ or tract Z80.59
        bladder Z80.52
        kidney Z80.51
    mental
      disorder NEC Z81.8
    multiple endocrine neoplasia (MEN)
        syndrome Z83.41

H

History *(Continued)*
  family *(Continued)*
    osteoporosis Z82.62
    polycystic kidney Z82.71
    polyps (colon) Z83.71
    psychiatric disorder Z81.8
    psychoactive substance abuse NEC Z81.3
    respiratory condition NEC Z83.6
      asthma and other lower respiratory
        conditions Z82.5
    self-harmful behavior Z81.8
    SIDS (sudden infant death syndrome)
      Z84.82
    skin condition Z84.0
    specified condition NEC Z84.89
    stroke (cerebrovascular) Z82.3
    substance abuse NEC Z81.4
      alcohol Z81.1
      drug NEC Z81.3
      psychoactive NEC Z81.3
      tobacco Z81.2
    sudden
      cardiac death Z82.41
      infant death syndrome (SIDS)
        Z84.82
    tobacco abuse Z81.2
    violence, violent behavior Z81.8
    visual loss Z82.1
  personal (of) —*see also* History, family (of)
    abuse
      adult Z91.419
        physical and sexual Z91.410
        psychological Z91.411
      childhood Z62.819
        physical Z62.810
        psychological Z62.811
        sexual Z62.810
    alcohol dependence F10.21
    allergy (to) Z88.9
      analgesic agent NEC Z88.6
      anesthetic Z88.4
      antibiotic agent NEC Z88.1
      anti-infective agent NEC Z88.3
      contrast media Z91.041
      drugs, medicaments and biological
        substances Z88.9
        specified NEC Z88.8
      food Z91.018
        additives Z91.02
        eggs Z91.012
        milk products Z91.011
        peanuts Z91.010
        seafood Z91.013
        specified food NEC Z91.018
      insect Z91.038
        bee Z91.030
      latex Z91.040
      medicinal agents Z88.9
        specified NEC Z88.8
      narcotic agent NEC Z88.5
      nonmedicinal agents Z91.048
      penicillin Z88.0
      serum Z88.7
      specified NEC Z91.09
      sulfonamides Z88.2
      vaccine Z88.7
    anaphylactic shock Z87.892
    anaphylaxis Z87.892
    behavioral disorders Z86.59
    benign carcinoid tumor Z86.012
    benign neoplasm Z86.018
      brain Z86.011
      carcinoid Z86.012
      colonic polyps Z86.010
    brain injury (traumatic) Z87.820
    breast implant removal Z98.86
    calculi, renal Z87.442
    cancer —*see* History, personal (of),
      malignant neoplasm (of)
    cardiac arrest (death), successfully
      resuscitated Z86.74

History *(Continued)*
  personal *(Continued)*
    cerebral infarction without residual deficit
      Z86.73
    cervical dysplasia Z87.410
    chemotherapy for neoplastic condition
      Z92.21
    childhood abuse —*see* History, personal
      (of), abuse
    cleft lip (corrected) Z87.730
    cleft palate (corrected) Z87.730
    collapsed vertebra (healed) Z87.311
      due to osteoporosis Z87.310
    combat and operational stress reaction
      Z86.51
    congenital malformation (corrected)
      Z87.798
      circulatory system (corrected) Z87.74
      digestive system (corrected) NEC
        Z87.738
➡ ear (corrected) Z87.721
➡ eye (corrected) Z87.720
      face and neck (corrected) Z87.790
      genitourinary system (corrected) NEC
        Z87.718
      heart (corrected) Z87.74
      integument (corrected) Z87.76
      limb(s) (corrected) Z87.76
      musculoskeletal system (corrected)
        Z87.76
      neck (corrected) Z87.790
      nervous system (corrected) NEC
        Z87.728
      respiratory system (corrected) Z87.75
      sense organs (corrected) NEC Z87.728
      specified NEC Z87.798
    contraception Z92.0
    deployment (military) Z91.82
    diabetic foot ulcer Z86.31
    disease or disorder (of) Z87.898
      blood and blood-forming organs Z86.2
      circulatory system Z86.79
        specified condition NEC Z86.79
      connective tissue NEC Z87.39
      digestive system Z87.19
        colonic polyp Z86.010
        peptic ulcer disease Z87.11
        specified condition NEC Z87.19
      ear Z86.69
      endocrine Z86.39
        diabetic foot ulcer Z86.31
        gestational diabetes Z86.32
        specified type NEC Z86.39
      eye Z86.69
      genital (track) system NEC
        female Z87.42
        male Z87.438
      hematological Z86.2
      Hodgkin Z85.71
      immune mechanism Z86.2
      infectious Z86.19
        malaria Z86.13
        Methicillin resistant Staphylococcus
          aureus (MRSA) Z86.14
        poliomyelitis Z86.12
        specified NEC Z86.19
        tuberculosis Z86.11
      mental NEC Z86.59
      metabolic Z86.39
        diabetic foot ulcer Z86.31
        gestational diabetes Z86.32
        specified type NEC Z86.39
      musculoskeletal NEC Z87.39
      nervous system Z86.69
      nutritional Z86.39
      parasitic Z86.19
      respiratory system NEC Z87.09
      sense organs Z86.69
      skin Z87.2
      specified site or type NEC Z87.898
      subcutaneous tissue Z87.2

History *(Continued)*
  personal *(Continued)*
    disease or disorder (of) *(Continued)*
      trophoblastic Z87.59
      urinary system NEC Z87.448
    drug dependence —*see* Dependence, drug,
      by type, in remission
    drug therapy
      antineoplastic chemotherapy Z92.21
      estrogen Z92.23
      immunosupression Z92.25
      inhaled steroids Z92.240
      monoclonal drug Z92.22
      specified NEC Z92.29
      steroid Z92.241
      systemic steroids Z92.241
    dysplasia
      cervical (mild) (moderate) Z87.410
        severe (grade III) Z86.001
      prostatic Z87.430
      vaginal Z87.411
      vulvar (mild) (moderate) Z87.412
        severe (grade III) Z86.008
    embolism (venous) Z86.718
      pulmonary Z86.711
    encephalitis Z86.61
    estrogen therapy Z92.23
    extracorporeal membrane oxygenation
      (ECMO) Z92.81
    failed conscious sedation Z92.83
    failed moderate sedation Z92.83
    fall, falling Z91.81
    fracture (healed)
      fatigue Z87.312
      fragility Z87.310
      osteoporosis Z87.310
      pathological NEC Z87.311
      stress Z87.312
      traumatic Z87.81
    gestational diabetes Z86.32
    hepatitis
      B Z86.19
      C Z86.19
    Hodgkin disease Z85.71
    hyperthermia, malignant Z88.4
    hypospadias (corrected) Z87.710
    hysterectomy Z90.710
    immunosupression therapy Z92.25
    in situ neoplasm
      breast Z86.000
      cervix uteri Z86.001
      specified NEC Z86.008
    infection NEC Z86.19
      central nervous system Z86.61
      Methicillin resistant Staphylococcus
        aureus (MRSA) Z86.14
      urinary (tract) Z87.41
    injury NEC Z87.828
    in utero procedure during pregnancy
      Z98.870
    in utero procedure while a fetus Z98.871
    irradiation Z92.3
    kidney stones Z87.442
    leukemia Z85.6
    lymphoma (non-Hodgkin) Z85.72
    malignant melanoma (skin) Z85.820
    malignant neoplasm (of) Z85.9
      accessory sinuses Z85.22
      anus NEC Z85.048
        carcinoid Z85.040
      bladder Z85.51
      bone Z85.830
      brain Z85.841
      breast Z85.3
      bronchus NEC Z85.118
        carcinoid Z85.110
      carcinoid —*see* History, personal (of),
        malignant neoplasm, by site,
        carcinoid
      cervix Z85.41
      colon NEC Z85.038
        carcinoid Z85.030

▶ New　　⟹ Revised　　~~deleted~~ Deleted　　● Use Additional Character(s)

History *(Continued)*
  personal *(Continued)*
    malignant neoplasm *(Continued)*
      digestive organ Z85.00
        specified NEC Z85.09
      endocrine gland NEC Z85.858
      epididymis Z85.48
      esophagus Z85.01
      eye Z85.840
      gastrointestinal tract —*see* History,
        malignant neoplasm, digestive
        organ
      genital organ
        female Z85.40
          specified NEC Z85.44
        male Z85.45
          specified NEC Z85.49
      hematopoietic NEC Z85.79
      intrathoracic organ Z85.20-●
      kidney NEC Z85.528
        carcinoid Z85.520
      large intestine NEC Z85.038
        carcinoid Z85.030
      larynx Z85.21
      liver Z85.05
      lung NEC Z85.118
        carcinoid Z85.110
      mediastinum Z85.29
      Merkel cell Z85.821
      middle ear Z85.22
      nasal cavities Z85.22
      nervous system NEC Z85.848
      oral cavity Z85.819
        specified site NEC Z85.818
      ovary Z85.43
      pancreas Z85.07
      pelvis Z85.53
      pharynx Z85.819
        specified site NEC Z85.818
      pleura Z85.29
      prostate Z85.46
      rectosigmoid junction NEC Z85.048
        carcinoid Z85.040
      rectum NEC Z85.048
        carcinoid Z85.040
      respiratory organ Z85.20
      sinuses, accessory Z85.22
      skin NEC Z85.828
        melanoma Z85.820
        Merkel cell Z85.821
      small intestine NEC Z85.068
        carcinoid Z85.060
      soft tissue Z85.831
      specified site NEC Z85.89
      stomach NEC Z85.028
        carcinoid Z85.020
      testis Z85.47
      thymus NEC Z85.238
        carcinoid Z85.230
      thyroid Z85.850
      tongue Z85.810
      trachea Z85.12
      ureter Z85.54
      urinary organ or tract Z85.50
        specified NEC Z85.59
      uterus Z85.42
    maltreatment Z91.89
    medical treatment NEC Z92.89
    melanoma (malignant) (skin) Z85.820
    meningitis Z86.61
    mental disorder Z86.59
    Merkel cell carcinoma (skin) Z85.821
    Methicillin resistant Staphylococcus aureus
      (MRSA) Z86.14
    military deployment Z91.82
    military war, peacekeeping and
      humanitarian deployment (current or
      past conflict) Z91.82
    myocardial infarction (old) I25.2
    neglect (in)
      adult Z91.412
      childhood Z62.812

History *(Continued)*
  personal *(Continued)*
    neoplasm
      benign Z86.018
        brain Z86.011
        colon polyp Z86.010
      in situ
        breast Z86.000
        cervix uteri Z86.001
        specified NEC Z86.008
      malignant —*see* History of, malignant
        neoplasm
      uncertain behavior Z86.03
    nephrotic syndrome Z87.441
    nicotine dependence Z87.891
    noncompliance with medical treatment or
      regimen —*see* Noncompliance
    nutritional deficiency Z86.39
    obstetric complications Z87.59
      childbirth Z87.59
      pregnancy Z87.59
      pre-term labor Z87.51
      puerperium Z87.59
    osteoporosis fractures Z87.31
    parasuicide (attempt) Z91.5
    physical trauma NEC Z87.828
      self-harm or suicide attempt Z91.5
    pneumonia (recurrent) Z87.01
    poisoning NEC Z91.89
      self-harm or suicide attempt Z91.5
    poor personal hygiene Z91.89
    preterm labor Z87.51
    procedure during pregnancy Z98.870
    procedure while a fetus Z98.871
    prolonged reversible ischemic neurologic
      deficit (PRINO) Z86.73
    prostatic dysplasia Z87.430
    psychiatric disorder NEC Z87.89
    psychological
      abuse
        adult Z91.411
        child Z62.811
      trauma, specified NEC Z91.49
    radiation therapy Z92.3
    removal
      implant
        breast Z98.86
    renal calculi Z87.442
    respiratory condition NEC Z87.09
    retained foreign body fully removed
      Z87.821
    risk factors NEC Z91.89
    self-harm Z91.5
    self-poisoning attempt Z91.5
    sex reassignment Z87.890
    sleep-wake cycle problem Z72.821
    specified NEC Z87.898
    steroid therapy (systemic) Z92.241
      inhaled Z92.240
    stroke without residual deficits Z86.73
    ~~substance abuse NEC F10-F19 with~~
      ~~fifth character 1~~
    ▶ substance abuse NEC F10-F19
    sudden cardiac arrest Z86.74
    sudden cardiac death successfully
      resuscitated Z86.74
    suicide attempt Z91.5
    surgery NEC Z98.890
      with uterine scar Z98.891
      sex reassignment Z87.890
      transplant —*see* Transplant
    thrombophlebitis Z86.72
    thrombosis (venous) Z86.718
      pulmonary Z86.711
    tobacco dependence Z87.891
    transient ischemic attack (TIA) without
      residual deficits Z86.73
    trauma (physical) NEC Z87.828
      psychological NEC Z91.49
      self-harm Z91.5
    traumatic brain injury Z87.820
    unhealthy sleep-wake cycle Z72.821

History *(Continued)*
  personal *(Continued)*
    unintended awareness under general
      anesthesia Z92.84
    urinary (recurrent) (tract) infection(s)
      Z87.440
    urinary calculi Z87.42
    uterine scar from previous surgery
      Z98.891
    vaginal dysplasia Z87.411
    venous thrombosis or embolism Z86.718
      pulmonary Z86.711
    vulvar dysplasia Z87.412
His-Werner disease A79.0
HIV —*see also* Human, immunodeficiency virus
  B20
  laboratory evidence (nonconclusive) R75
  nonconclusive test (in infants) R75
  positive, seropositive Z21
Hives (bold) —*see* Urticaria
Hoarseness R49.0
Hobo Z59.0
Hodgkin disease —*see* Lymphoma,
  Hodgkin
Hodgson's disease I71.2
  ruptured I71.1
Hoffa-Kastert disease E88.89
Hoffa's disease E88.89
Hoffmann-Bouveret syndrome I47.9
Hoffmann's syndrome E03.9 *[G73.7]*
Hole (round)
  macula H35.34-●
  retina (without detachment) —*see* Break,
    retina, round hole
    with detachment —*see* Detachment, retina,
      with retinal, break
Holiday relief care Z75.5
Hollenhorst's plaque —*see* Occlusion, artery,
  retina
Hollow foot (congenital) Q66.7
  acquired —*see* Deformity, limb, foot, specified
    NEC
Holoprosencephaly Q04.2
Holt-Oram syndrome Q87.2
Homelessness Z59.0
Homesickness —*see* Disorder, adjustment
Homocystinemia, homocystinuria E72.11
Homogentisate 1,2-dioxygenase deficiency
  E70.29
Homologous serum hepatitis (prophylactic)
  (therapeutic) —*see* Hepatitis, viral, type B
Honeycomb lung J98.4
  congenital Q33.0
Hooded
  clitoris Q52.6
  penis Q55.69
Hookworm (anemia) (disease) (infection)
  (infestation) B76.9
  specified NEC B76.8
Hordeolum (eyelid) (externum) (recurrent)
  H00.019
  internum H00.029
    left H00.026
      lower H00.025
      upper H00.024
    right H00.023
      lower H00.022
      upper H00.021
  left H00.016
    lower H00.015
    upper H00.014
  right H00.013
    lower H00.012
    upper H00.011
Horn
  cutaneous L85.8
  nail L60.2
    congenital Q84.6
Horner (-Claude Bernard) syndrome G90.2
  traumatic —*see* Injury, nerve, cervical
    sympathetic

Horseshoe kidney (congenital) Q63.1
Horton's headache or neuralgia G44.099
  intractable G44.091
  not intractable G44.099
Hospital hopper syndrome —see Disorder,
    factitious
Hospitalism in children —see Disorder,
    adjustment
Hostility R45.5
  towards child Z62.3
Hot flashes
  menopausal N95.1
Hourglass (contracture) —see also Contraction,
    hourglass
  stomach K31.89
    congenital Q40.2
    stricture K31.2
Household, housing circumstance affecting
    care Z59.9
  specified NEC Z59.8
Housemaid's knee —see Bursitis, prepatellar
Hudson (-Stähli) line (cornea) —see
    Pigmentation, cornea, anterior
Human
  bite (open wound) —see also Bite
    intact skin surface —see Bite, superficial
  herpesvirus —see Herpes
  immunodeficiency virus (HIV) disease
      (infection) B20
    asymptomatic status Z21
    contact Z20.6
    counseling Z71.7
    dementia B20 [F02.80]
      with behavioral disturbance B20 [F02.81]
    exposure to Z20.6
    laboratory evidence R75
    type-2 (HIV 2) as cause of disease classified
        elsewhere B97.35
  papillomavirus (HPV)
    DNA test positive
      high risk
        cervix R87.810
        vagina R87.811
      low risk
        cervix R87.820
        vagina R87.821
    screening for Z11.51
  T-cell lymphotropic virus
    type-1 (HTLV-I) infection B33.3
      as cause of disease classified elsewhere
          B97.33
      carrier Z22.6
    type-2 (HTLV-II) as cause of disease
        classified elsewhere B97.34
Humidifier lung or pneumonitis J67.7
Humiliation (experience) in childhood Z62.898
Humpback (acquired) —see Kyphosis
Hunchback (acquired) —see Kyphosis
Hunger T73.0
  air, psychogenic F45.8
Hungry bone syndrome E83.81
Hunner's ulcer —see Cystitis, chronic,
    interstitial
Hunter's
  glossitis D51.0
  syndrome E76.1
Huntington's disease or chorea G10
  with dementia G10 [F02.80]
    with behavioral disturbance G10 [F02.81]
Hunt's
  disease or syndrome (herpetic geniculate
      ganglionitis) B02.21
  dyssynergia cerebellaris myoclonica G11.1
  neuralgia B02.21
Hurler (-Scheie) disease or syndrome E76.02
Hurst's disease G36.1
Hurthle cell
  adenocarcinoma C73
  adenoma D34
  carcinoma C73
  tumor D34

Hutchinson-Boeck disease or syndrome —see
    Sarcoidosis
Hutchinson-Gilford disease or syndrome E34.8
Hutchinson's
  disease, meaning
    angioma serpiginosum L81.7
    pompholyx (cheiropompholyx) L30.1
    prurigo estivalis L56.4
    summer eruption or summer prurigo L56.4
  melanotic freckle —see Melanoma, in situ
    malignant melanoma in —see Melanoma
  teeth or incisors (congenital syphilis) A50.52
  triad (congenital syphilis) A50.53
Hyalin plaque, sclera, senile H15.89
Hyaline membrane (disease) (lung)
    (pulmonary) (newborn) P22.0
Hyalinosis
  cutis (et mucosae) E78.89
  focal and segmental (glomerular) —see also
      N00-N07 with fourth character .1 N05.1
Hyalitis, hyalosis, asteroid —see also Deposit,
    crystalline
  syphilitic (late) A52.71
Hydatid
  cyst or tumor —see Echinococcus
  mole —see Hydatidiform mole
  Morgagni
    female Q50.5
    male (epididymal) Q55.4
      testicular Q55.29
Hydatidiform mole (benign) (complicating
    pregnancy) (delivered) (undelivered) O01.9
  classical O01.0
  complete O01.0
  incomplete O01.1
  invasive D39.2
  malignant D39.2
  partial O01.1
Hydatidosis —see Echinococcus
Hydradenitis (axillaris) (suppurative) L73.2
Hydradenoma —see Hidradenoma
Hydramnios O40.-●
Hydrancephaly, hydranencephaly Q04.3
  with spina bifida —see Spina bifida, with
      hydrocephalus
Hydrargyrism NEC —see Poisoning, mercury
Hydrarthrosis —see also Effusion, joint
  gonococcal A54.42
  intermittent M12.40
    ankle M12.47-●
    elbow M12.42-●
    foot joint M12.47-●
    hand joint M12.44-●
    hip M12.45-●
    knee M12.46-●
    multiple site M12.49
    shoulder M12.41-●
    specified joint NEC M12.48
    wrist M12.43-●
  of yaws (early) (late) —see also subcategory
      M14.8-● A66.6
  syphilitic (late) A52.77
    congenital A50.55 [M12.80]
Hydremia D64.89
Hydrencephalocele (congenital) —see
    Encephalocele
Hydrencephalomeningocele (congenital) —see
    Encephalocele
Hydroa R23.8
  aestivale L56.4
  vacciniforme L56.4
Hydroadenitis (axillaris) (suppurative)
    L73.2
Hydrocalycosis —see Hydronephrosis
Hydrocele (spermatic cord) (testis) (tunica
    vaginalis) N43.3
  canal of Nuck N94.89
  communicating N43.2
    congenital P83.5
  congenital P83.5
  encysted N43.0

Hydrocele (Continued)
  female NEC N94.89
  infected N43.1
  newborn P83.5
  round ligament N94.89
  specified NEC N43.2
  spinalis —see Spina bifida
  vulva N90.89
Hydrocephalus (acquired) (external) (internal)
    (malignant) (recurrent) G91.9
  aqueduct Sylvius stricture Q03.0
  causing disproportion O33.6
    with obstructed labor O66.3
  communicating G91.0
  congenital (external) (internal) Q03.9
    with spina bifida Q05.4
      cervical Q05.0
      dorsal Q05.1
      lumbar Q05.2
      lumbosacral Q05.2
      sacral Q05.3
      thoracic Q05.1
      thoracolumbar Q05.1
    specified NEC Q03.8
  due to toxoplasmosis (congenital) P37.1
  foramen Magendie block (acquired) G91.1
    congenital —see also Hydrocephalus,
        congenital Q03.1
  in (due to)
    infectious disease NEC B89 [G91.4]
    neoplastic disease NEC (see also Neoplasm)
        G91.4
    parasitic disease B89 [G91.4]
  newborn Q03.9
    with spina bifida —see Spina bifida, with
        hydrocephalus
  noncommunicating G91.1
  normal pressure G91.2
    secondary G91.0
  obstructive G91.1
  otitic G93.2
  post-traumatic NEC G91.3
  secondary G91.4
    post-traumatic G91.3
  specified NEC G91.8
  syphilitic, congenital A50.49
Hydrocolpos (congenital) N89.8
Hydrocystoma —see Neoplasm, skin, benign
Hydroencephalocele (congenital) —see
    Encephalocele
Hydroencephalomeningocele (congenital) —
    see Encephalocele
Hydrohematopneumothorax —see Hemothorax
Hydromeningitis —see Meningitis
Hydromeningocele (spinal) —see also Spina
    bifida
  cranial —see Encephalocele
Hydrometra N85.8
Hydrometrocolpos N89.8
Hydromicrocephaly Q02
Hydromphalos (since birth) Q45.8
Hydromyelia Q06.4
Hydromyelocele —see Spina bifida
Hydronephrosis (atrophic) (early)
    (functionless) (intermittent) (primary)
    (secondary) NEC N13.30
  with
    infection N13.6
    obstruction (by) (of)
      renal calculus N13.2
        with infection N13.6
      ureteral NEC N13.1
        with infection N13.6
        calculus N13.2
          with infection N13.6
      ➡ureteropelvic junction (congenital)
          Q62.11
        acquired N13.0
          with infection N13.6
      ureteral stricture NEC N13.1
        with infection N13.6

Hydronephrosis NEC *(Continued)*
  congenital Q62.0
    due to acquired occlusion of ureteropelvic
      junction N13.0
    specified type NEC N13.39
    tuberculous A18.11
Hydropericarditis —*see* Pericarditis
Hydropericardium —*see* Pericarditis
Hydroperitoneum R18.8
Hydrophobia —*see* Rabies
Hydrophthalmos Q15.0
Hydropneumohemothorax —*see* Hemothorax
Hydropneumopericarditis —*see* Pericarditis
Hydropneumopericardium —*see* Pericarditis
Hydropneumothorax J94.8
  traumatic —*see* Injury, intrathoracic, lung
  tuberculous NEC A15.6
Hydrops R60.9
  abdominis R18.8
  articulorum intermittens —*see* Hydrarthrosis,
    intermittent
  cardiac —*see* Failure, heart, congestive
  causing obstructed labor (mother) O66.3
  endolymphatic H81.0-●
  fetal —*see* Pregnancy, complicated by,
    hydrops, fetalis
  fetalis P83.2
    due to
      ABO isoimmunization P56.0
      alpha thalassemia D56.0
      hemolytic disease P56.90
        specified NEC P56.99
      isoimmunization (ABO) (Rh) P56.0
      other specified nonhemolytic disease
        NEC P83.2
      Rh incompatibility P56.0
    during pregnancy —*see* Pregnancy,
      complicated by, hydrops, fetalis
  gallbladder K82.1
  joint —*see* Effusion, joint
  labyrinth H81.0
  newborn (idiopathic) P83.2
    due to
      ABO isoimmunization P56.0
      alpha thalassemia D56.0
      hemolytic disease P56.90
        specified NEC P56.99
      isoimmunization (ABO) (Rh) P56.0
      Rh incompatibility P56.0
  nutritional —*see* Malnutrition, severe
  pericardium —*see* Pericarditis
  pleura —*see* Hydrothorax
  spermatic cord —*see* Hydrocele
Hydropyonephrosis N13.6
Hydrorachis Q06.4
Hydrorrhea (nasal) J34.89
  pregnancy —*see* Rupture, membranes,
    premature
Hydrosadenitis (axillaris) (suppurative) L73.2
Hydrosalpinx (fallopian tube) (follicularis) N70.11
Hydrothorax (double) (pleura) J94.8
  chylous (nonfilarial) I89.8
    filarial —*see also* Infestation, filarial B74.9
      [J91.8]
  traumatic —*see* Injury, intrathoracic
  tuberculous NEC (non primary) A15.6
Hydroureter —*see also* Hydronephrosis N13.4
  with infection N13.6
  congenital Q62.39
Hydroureteronephrosis —*see* Hydronephrosis
Hydrourethra N36.8
Hydroxykynureninuria E70.8
Hydroxylysinemia E72.3
Hydroxyprolinemia E72.59
Hygiene, sleep
  abuse Z72.821
  inadequate Z72.821
  poor Z72.821
Hygroma (congenital) (cystic) D18.1
  praepatellare, prepatellar —*see* Bursitis,
    prepatellar

Hymen —*see* condition
Hymenolepis, hymenolepiasis (diminuta)
  (infection) (infestation) (nana) B71.0
Hypalgesia R20.8
Hyperacidity (gastric) K31.89
  psychogenic F45.8
Hyperactive, hyperactivity F90.9
  basal cell, uterine cervix —*see* Dysplasia,
    cervix
  bowel sounds R19.12
  cervix epithelial (basal) —*see* Dysplasia,
    cervix
  child F90.9
    attention deficit —*see* Disorder, attention-
      deficit hyperactivity
  detrusor muscle N32.81
  gastrointestinal K31.89
    psychogenic F45.8
  nasal mucous membrane J34.3
  stomach K31.89
  thyroid (gland) —*see* Hyperthyroidism
Hyperacusis H93.23-●
Hyperadrenalism E27.5
Hyperadrenocorticism E24.9
  congenital E25.0
  iatrogenic E24.2
    correct substance properly administered —
      see Table of Drugs and Chemicals, by
      drug, adverse effect
    overdose or wrong substance given
      or taken —*see* Table of Drugs and
      Chemicals, by drug, poisoning
  not associated with Cushing's syndrome E27.0
  pituitary-dependent E24.0
Hyperaldosteronism E26.9
  familial (type I) E26.02
  glucocorticoid-remediable E26.02
  primary (due to (bilateral) adrenal
    hyperplasia) E26.09
  primary NEC E26.09
  secondary E26.1
  specified NEC E26.89
Hyperalgesia R20.8
Hyperalimentation R63.2
  carotene, carotin E67.1
  specified NEC E67.8
  vitamin
    A E67.0
    D E67.3
Hyperaminoaciduria
  arginine E72.21
  cystine E72.01
  lysine E72.3
  ornithine E72.4
Hyperammonemia (congenital) E72.20
Hyperazotemia —*see* Uremia
Hyperbetalipoproteinemia (familial) E78.00
  with prebetalipoproteinemia E78.2
Hyperbilirubinemia
  constitutional E80.6
  familial conjugated E80.6
  neonatal (transient) —*see* Jaundice, newborn
Hypercalcemia, hypocalciuric, familial E83.52
Hypercalciuria, idiopathic E83.52
Hypercapnia R06.89
  newborn P84
Hypercarotenemia, hypercarotinemia (dietary)
  E67.1
Hypercementosis K03.4
Hyperchloremia E87.8
Hyperchlorhydria K31.89
  neurotic F45.8
  psychogenic F45.8
Hypercholesterinemia —*see*
  Hypercholesterolemia
Hypercholesterolemia (essential) (primary)
  (pure) E78.00
  with hyperglyceridemia, endogenous E78.2
  dietary counseling and surveillance Z71.3
  familial E78.01
  hereditary E78.01

Hyperchylia gastrica, psychogenic F45.8
Hyperchylomicronemia (familial) (primary)
  E78.3
  with hyperbetalipoproteinemia E78.3
Hypercoagulable (state) D68.59
  activated protein C resistance D68.51
  antithrombin (III) deficiency D68.59
  factor V Leiden mutation D68.51
  primary NEC D68.59
  protein C deficiency D68.59
  protein S deficiency D68.59
  prothrombin gene mutation D68.52
  secondary D68.69
  specified NEC D68.69
Hypercoagulation (state) D68.59
Hypercorticalism, pituitary-dependent E24.0
Hypercorticosolism —*see* Cushing's, syndrome
Hypercorticosteronism E24.2
  correct substance properly administered —*see*
    Table of Drugs and Chemicals, by drug,
    adverse effect
  overdose or wrong substance given
    or taken —*see* Table of Drugs and
    Chemicals, by drug, poisoning
Hypercortisonism E24.2
  correct substance properly administered —*see*
    Table of Drugs and Chemicals, by drug,
    adverse effect
  overdose or wrong substance given
    or taken —*see* Table of Drugs and
    Chemicals, by drug, poisoning
Hyperekplexia Q89.8
Hyperelectrolytemia E87.8
Hyperemesis R11.10
  with nausea R11.2
  gravidarum (mild) O21.0
    with
      carbohydrate depletion O21.1
      dehydration O21.1
      electrolyte imbalance O21.1
      metabolic disturbance O21.1
    severe (with metabolic disturbance) O21.1
  projectile R11.12
  psychogenic F45.8
Hyperemia (acute) (passive) R68.89
  anal mucosa K62.89
  bladder N32.89
  cerebral I67.89
  conjunctiva H11.43-●
  ear internal, acute —*see* subcategory H83.0
  enteric K59.8
  eye —*see* Hyperemia, conjunctiva
  eyelid (active) (passive) —*see* Disorder,
    eyelid, specified type NEC
  intestine K59.8
  iris —*see* Disorder, iris, vascular
  kidney N28.89
  labyrinth —*see* subcategory H83.0
  liver (active) K76.89
  lung (passive) —*see* Edema, lung
  pulmonary (passive) —*see* Edema, lung
  renal N28.89
  retina H35.89
  stomach K31.89
Hyperesthesia (body surface) R20.3
  larynx (reflex) J38.7
    hysterical F44.89
  pharynx (reflex) J39.2
    hysterical F44.89
Hyperestrogenism (drug-induced) (iatrogenic)
  E28.0
Hyperexplexia Q89.8
Hyperfibrinolysis —*see* Fibrinolysis
Hyperfructosemia E74.19
Hyperfunction
  adrenal cortex, not associated with Cushing's
    syndrome E27.0
    medulla E27.5
      adrenomedullary E27.5
    virilism E25.9
      congenital E25.0

Hyperfunction (Continued)
ovarian E28.8
pancreas K86.89
parathyroid (gland) E21.3
pituitary (gland) (anterior) E22.9
specified NEC E22.8
polyglandular E31.1
testicular E29.0
Hypergammaglobulinemia D89.2
polyclonal D89.0
Waldenström D89.0
Hypergastrinemia E16.4
Hyperglobulinemia R77.1
Hyperglycemia, hyperglycemic (transient) R73.9
coma —see Diabetes, by type, with coma
postpancreatectomy E89.1
Hyperglyceridemia (endogenous) (essential)
(familial) (hereditary) (pure) E78.1
mixed E78.3
Hyperglycinemia (non-ketotic) E72.51
Hypergonadism
ovarian E28.8
testicular (primary) (infantile) E29.0
Hyperheparinemia D68.32
Hyperhidrosis, hyperidrosis R61
focal
primary L74.519
axilla L74.510
face L74.511
palms L74.512
soles L74.513
secondary L74.52
generalized R61
localized
primary L74.519
axilla L74.510
face L74.511
palms L74.512
soles L74.513
secondary L74.52
psychogenic F45.8
secondary R61
focal L74.52
Hyperhistidinemia E70.41
Hyperhomocysteinemia E72.11
Hyperhydroxyprolinemia E72.59
Hyperinsulinism (functional) E16.1
with
coma (hypoglycemic) E15
encephalopathy E16.1 [G94]
ectopic E16.1
therapeutic misadventure (from
administration of insulin) —see
subcategory T38.3
Hyperkalemia E87.5
Hyperkeratosis —see also Keratosis L85.9
cervix N88.0
due to yaws (early) (late) (palmar or plantar)
A66.3
follicularis Q82.8
penetrans (in cutem) L87.0
palmoplantaris climacterica L85.1
pinta A67.1
senile (with pruritus) L57.0
universalis congenita Q80.8
vocal cord J38.3
vulva N90.4
Hyperkinesia, hyperkinetic (disease) (reaction)
(syndrome) (childhood) (adolescence) —see
also Disorder, attention-deficit hyperactivity
heart I51.89
Hyperleucine-isoleucinemia E71.19
Hyperlipemia, hyperlipidemia E78.5
combined E78.2
familial E78.4
group
A E78.00
B E78.1
C E78.2
D E78.3
mixed E78.2
specified NEC E78.4

Hyperlipidosis E75.6
hereditary NEC E75.5
Hyperlipoproteinemia E78.5
Fredrickson's type
I E78.3
IIa E78.00
IIb E78.2
III E78.2
IV E78.1
V E78.3
low-density-lipoprotein-type (LDL) E78.00
very-low-density-lipoprotein-type (VLDL)
E78.1
Hyperlucent lung, unilateral J43.0
Hyperlysinemia E72.3
Hypermagnesemia E83.41
neonatal P71.8
Hypermenorrhea N92.0
Hypermethioninemia E72.19
Hypermetropia (congenital) H52.0-●
Hypermobility, hypermotility
cecum —see Syndrome, irritable bowel
coccyx —see subcategory M53.2
colon —see Syndrome, irritable bowel
psychogenic F45.8
ileum K58.9
intestine —see also Syndrome, irritable bowel
K58.9
psychogenic F45.8
meniscus (knee) —see Derangement, knee,
meniscus
scapula —see Instability, joint, shoulder
stomach K31.89
psychogenic F45.8
syndrome M35.7
urethra N36.41
with intrinsic sphincter deficiency N36.43
Hypernasality R49.21
Hypernatremia E87.0
Hypernephroma C64.-●
Hyperopia —see Hypermetropia
Hyperorexia nervosa F50.2
Hyperornithinemia E72.4
Hyperosmia R43.1
Hyperosmolality E87.0
Hyperostosis (monomelic) —see also Disorder,
bone, density and structure, specified NEC
ankylosing (spine) M48.10
cervical region M48.12
cervicothoracic region M48.13
lumbar region M48.16
lumbosacral region M48.17
multiple sites M48.19
occipito-atlanto-axial region M48.11
sacrococcygeal region M48.18
thoracic region M48.14
thoracolumbar region M48.15
cortical (skull) M85.2
infantile M89.8X-●
frontal, internal of skull M85.2
interna frontalis M85.2
skeletal, diffuse idiopathic —see
Hyperostosis, ankylosing
skull M85.2
congenital Q75.8
vertebral, ankylosing —see Hyperostosis,
ankylosing
Hyperovarism E28.8
Hyperoxaluria (primary) E72.53
Hyperparathyroidism E21.3
primary E21.0
secondary (renal) N25.81
non-renal E21.1
specified NEC E21.2
tertiary E21.2
Hyperpathia R20.8
Hyperperistalsis R19.2
psychogenic F45.8
Hyperpermeability, capillary I78.8
Hyperphagia R63.2
Hyperphenylalaninemia NEC E70.1

Hyperphoria (alternating) H50.53
Hyperphosphatemia E83.39
Hyperpiesis, hyperpiesia —see Hypertension
Hyperpigmentation —see also Pigmentation
melanin NEC L81.4
postinflammatory L81.0
Hyperpinealism E34.8
Hyperpituitarism E22.9
Hyperplasia, hyperplastic
adenoids J35.2
adrenal (capsule) (cortex) (gland) E27.8
with
sexual precocity (male) E25.9
congenital E25.0
virilism, adrenal E25.9
congenital E25.0
virilization (female) E25.9
congenital E25.0
congenital E25.0
salt-losing E25.0
adrenomedullary E27.5
angiolymphoid, eosinophilia (ALHE) D18.01
appendix (lymphoid) K38.0
artery, fibromuscular I77.3
bone —see also Hypertrophy, bone
marrow D75.89
breast —see also Hypertrophy, breast
ductal (atypical) N60.9-●
C-cell, thyroid E07.0
cementation (tooth) (teeth) K03.4
cervical gland R59.0
cervix (uteri) (basal cell) (endometrium)
(polypoid) —see also Dysplasia, cervix
congenital Q51.828
clitoris, congenital Q52.6
denture K06.2
endocervicitis N72
endometrium, endometrial (adenomatous)
(benign) (cystic) (glandular) (glandular-
cystic) (polypoid) N85.00
with atypia N85.02
cervix —see Dysplasia, cervix
complex (without atypia) N85.01
simple (without atypia) N85.01
epithelial L85.9
focal, oral, including tongue K13.29
nipple N62
skin L85.9
tongue K13.29
vaginal wall N89.3
erythroid D75.89
fibromuscular of artery (carotid) (renal)
I77.3
genital
female NEC N94.89
male N50.89
gingiva K06.1
glandularis cystica uteri (interstitialis) —see
also Hyperplasia, endometrial N85.00-●
gum K06.1
hymen, congenital Q52.4
irritative, edentulous (alveolar) K06.2
jaw M26.09
alveolar M26.79
lower M26.03
alveolar M26.72
upper M26.01
alveolar M26.71
kidney (congenital) Q63.3
labia N90.69
epithelial N90.3
liver (congenital) Q44.7
nodular, focal K76.89
lymph gland or node R59.9
mandible, mandibular M26.03
alveolar M26.72
unilateral condylar M27.8
maxilla, maxillary M26.01
alveolar M26.71
myometrium, myometrial N85.2
neuroendocrine cell, of infancy J84.841

▶ New ⇒ Revised ~~deleted~~ Deleted ● Use Additional Character(s)

Hyperplasia, hyperplastic *(Continued)*
  nose
    lymphoid J34.89
    polypoid J33.9
  oral mucosa (irritative) K13.6
  organ or site, congenital NEC —*see* Anomaly, by site
  ovary N83.8
  palate, papillary (irritative) K13.6
  pancreatic islet cells E16.9
    alpha E16.8
      with excess
        gastrin E16.4
        glucagon E16.3
    beta E16.1
  parathyroid (gland) E21.0
  pharynx (lymphoid) J39.2
  prostate (adenofibromatous) (nodular) N40.0
    with lower urinary tract symptoms (LUTS) N40.1
    without lower urinary tract symptoms (LUTS) N40.0
  renal artery I77.89
  reticulo-endothelial (cell) D75.89
  salivary gland (any) K11.1
  Schimmelbusch's —*see* Mastopathy, cystic
  suprarenal capsule (gland) E27.8
  thymus (gland) (persistent) E32.0
  thyroid (gland) —*see* Goiter
  tonsils (faucial) (infective) (lingual) (lymphoid) J35.1
    with adenoids J35.3
  unilateral condylar M27.8
  uterus, uterine N85.2
    endometrium (glandular) —*see also* Hyperplasia, endometrial N85.00-●
  vulva N90.69
    epithelial N90.3
Hyperpnea —*see* Hyperventilation
Hyperpotassemia E87.5
Hyperprebetalipoproteinemia (familial) E78.1
Hyperprolactinemia E22.1
Hyperprolinemia (type I) (type II) E72.59
Hyperproteinemia E88.09
Hyperprothrombinemia, causing coagulation factor deficiency D68.4
Hyperpyrexia R50.9
  heat (effects) T67.0
  malignant, due to anesthetic T88.3
  rheumatic —*see* Fever, rheumatic
  unknown origin R50.9
Hyper-reflexia R29.2
Hypersalivation K11.7
Hypersecretion
  ACTH (not associated with Cushing's syndrome) E27.0
    pituitary E24.0
  adrenaline E27.5
  adrenomedullary E27.5
  androgen (testicular) E29.0
    ovarian (drug-induced) (iatrogenic) E28.1
  calcitonin E07.0
  catecholamine E27.5
  corticoadrenal E24.9
  cortisol E24.9
  epinephrine E27.5
  estrogen E28.0
  gastric K31.89
    psychogenic F45.8
  gastrin E16.4
  glucagon E16.3
  hormone(s)
    ACTH (not associated with Cushing's syndrome) E27.0
      pituitary E24.0
    antidiuretic E22.2
    growth E22.0
    intestinal NEC E34.1
    ovarian androgen E28.1
    pituitary E22.9
    testicular E29.0

Hypersecretion *(Continued)*
  hormone *(Continued)*
    thyroid stimulating E05.80
      with thyroid storm E05.81
  insulin —*see* Hyperinsulinism
  lacrimal glands —*see* Epiphora
  medulloadrenal E27.5
  milk O92.6
  ovarian androgens E28.1
  salivary gland (any) K11.7
  thyrocalcitonin E07.0
  upper respiratory J39.8
Hypersegmentation, leukocytic, hereditary D72.0
Hypersensitive, hypersensitiveness, hypersensitivity —*see also* Allergy
  carotid sinus G90.01
  colon —*see* Irritable, colon
  drug T88.7
  gastrointestinal K52.29
    immediate K52.29
    psychogenic F45.8
  labyrinth —*see* subcategory H83.2
  pain R20.8
  pneumonitis —*see* Pneumonitis, allergic
  reaction T78.40
    upper respiratory tract NEC J39.3
Hypersomnia (organic) G47.10
  due to
    alcohol
      abuse F10.182
      dependence F10.282
      use F10.982
    amphetamines
      abuse F15.182
      dependence F15.282
      use F15.982
    caffeine
      abuse F15.182
      dependence F15.282
      use F15.982
    cocaine
      abuse F14.182
      dependence F14.282
      use F14.982
    drug NEC
      abuse F19.182
      dependence F19.282
      use F19.982
    medical condition G47.14
    mental disorder F51.13
    opioid
      abuse F11.182
      dependence F11.282
      use F11.982
    psychoactive substance NEC
      abuse F19.182
      dependence F19.282
      use F19.982
    sedative, hypnotic, or anxiolytic
      abuse F13.182
      dependence F13.282
      use F13.982
    stimulant NEC
      abuse F15.182
      dependence F15.282
      use F15.982
  idiopathic G47.11
    with long sleep time G47.11
    without long sleep time G47.12
  menstrual related G47.13
  nonorganic origin F51.11
    specified NEC F51.19
  not due to a substance or known physiological condition F51.11
    specified NEC F51.19
  primary F51.11
  recurrent G47.13
  specified NEC G47.19
Hypersplenia, hypersplenism D73.1
Hyperstimulation, ovaries (associated with induced ovulation) N98.1

Hypersusceptibility —*see* Allergy
Hypertelorism (ocular) (orbital) Q75.2
Hypertension, hypertensive (accelerated) (benign) (essential) (idiopathic) (malignant) (systemic) I10
  with
    ▶heart failure (congestive) I11.0
    ⇒heart involvement (conditions in I50.-, I51.4-I51.9 due to hypertension) —*see* Hypertension, heart
    kidney involvement —*see* Hypertension, kidney
  benign, intracranial G93.2
  borderline R03.0
  cardiorenal (disease) I13.10
    with heart failure I13.0
      with stage 1 through stage 4 chronic kidney disease I13.0
      with stage 5 or end stage renal disease I13.2
    without heart failure I13.10
      with stage 1 through stage 4 chronic kidney disease I13.10
      with stage 5 or end stage renal disease I13.11
  cardiovascular
    disease (arteriosclerotic) (sclerotic) —*see* Hypertension, heart
    renal (disease) —*see* Hypertension, cardiorenal
  chronic venous —*see* Hypertension, venous (chronic)
  complicating
    childbirth (labor) O16.4
    pre-existing O10.92
      with
        heart disease O10.12
          with renal disease O10.32
        pre-eclampsia O11.4
        renal disease O10.22
          with heart disease O10.32
      essential O10.02
      secondary O10.42
    pregnancy O16.-●
      with edema —*see also* Pre-eclampsia O14.9-●
      gestational (pregnancy induced) (without proteinuria) O13.-●
        with proteinuria O14.9-●
          mild pre-eclampsia O14.0-●
          moderate pre-eclampsia O14.0-●
          severe pre-eclampsia O14.1-●
            with hemolysis, elevated liver enzymes and low platelet count (HELLP) O14.2-●
      pre-existing O10.91-●
        with
          heart disease O10.11-●
            with renal disease O10.31-●
          pre-eclampsia —*see* category O11
          renal disease O10.21-●
            with heart disease O10.31-●
        essential O10.01-●
        secondary O10.41-●
      transient O13.-●
    puerperium pre-existing O16.5
      pre-existing
        with
          heart disease O10.13
            with renal disease O10.33
          pre-eclampsia O11.5
          renal disease O10.23
            with heart disease O10.33
        essential O10.03
      pregnancy-induced O13.9
      secondary O10.43
  crisis I16.9
  due to
    endocrine disorders I15.2
    pheochromocytoma I15.2

Hypertension, hypertensive *(Continued)*
  due to *(Continued)*
    renal disorders NEC I15.1
      arterial I15.0
    renovascular disorders I15.0
    specified disease NEC I15.8
  ⇒emergency I16.1
  encephalopathy I67.4
  gestational (without significant proteinuria)
    (pregnancy-induced) (transient) O13.-●
    with significant proteinuria —*see*
      Pre-eclampsia
  complicating
    delivery O13.4
    puerperium O13.5
  Goldblatt's I70.1
  heart (disease) (conditions in I51.4-I51.9 due
    to hypertension) I11.9
    with
      heart failure (congestive) I11.0
      kidney disease (chronic) —*see*
        Hypertension, cardiorenal
  intracranial (benign) G93.2
  kidney I12.9
    with
      heart disease —*see* Hypertension,
        cardiorenal
      stage 1 through stage 4 chronic kidney
        disease I12.9
      stage 5 chronic kidney disease (CKD) or
        end stage renal disease (ESRD) I12.0
  lesser circulation I27.0
  maternal O16.-●
  newborn P29.2
  ⇒pulmonary (persistent) P29.30
  ocular H40.05-●
  pancreatic duct — code to underlying condition
    with chronic pancreatitis K86.1
  portal (due to chronic liver disease)
    (idiopathic) K76.6
    gastropathy K31.89
    in (due to) schistosomiasis (bilharziasis)
      B65.9 *[K77]*
  postoperative I97.3
  psychogenic F45.8
  ⇒pulmonary NEC I27.20
    with
      ⇒cor pulmonale (chronic) I27.29
        acute I26.09
      ⇒right heart ventricular strain/failure
        I27.29
        acute I26.09
    ▶right to left shunt related to congenital
      heart disease I27.83
    ▶unclear multifactorial mechanisms I27.29
    ▶arterial (associated) (drug-induced)
      (toxin-induced) I27.21
    ▶chronic thromboembolic I27.24
    ▶due to
      ▶hematologic disorders I27.29
      ▶left heart disease I27.22
      ▶lung diseases and hypoxia I27.23
      ▶metabolic disorders I27.29
      ▶specified systemic disorders NEC I27.29
    ▶group 1 (associated) (drug-induced)
      (toxin-induced) I27.21
    ▶group 2 I27.22
    ▶group 3 I27.23
    ▶group 4 I27.24
    ▶group 5 I27.29
    ⇒of newborn (persistent) P29.30
    ▶secondary
      ▶arterial I27.21
      ▶specified NEC I27.29
    primary (idiopathic) I27.0
  renal —*see* Hypertension, kidney
  renovascular I15.0
  secondary NEC I15.9
    due to
      endocrine disorders I15.2
      pheochromocytoma I15.2

Hypertension, hypertensive *(Continued)*
  secondary NEC *(Continued)*
    due to *(Continued)*
      renal disorders NEC I15.1
        arterial I15.0
        renovascular disorders I15.0
      specified NEC I15.8
  transient, of pregnancy O13.-●
  urgency I16.0
  venous (chronic)
    due to
      deep vein thrombosis —*see* Syndrome,
        postthrombotic
    idiopathic I87.309
      with
        inflammation I87.32-●
          with ulcer I87.33-●
        specified complication NEC I87.39-●
        ulcer I87.31-●
          with inflammation I87.33-●
      asymptomatic I87.30-●
Hypertensive urgency —*see* Hypertension
Hyperthecosis ovary E28.8
Hyperthermia (of unknown origin) —*see also*
  Hyperpyrexia
  malignant, due to anesthesia T88.3
  newborn P81.9
    environmental P81.0
Hyperthyroid (recurrent) —*see*
  Hyperthyroidism
Hyperthyroidism (latent) (pre-adult)
  (recurrent) E05.90
  with
    goiter (diffuse) E05.00
      with thyroid storm E05.01
      nodular (multinodular) E05.20
        with thyroid storm E05.21
        uninodular E05.10
          with thyroid storm E05.11
    storm E05.91
  due to ectopic thyroid tissue E05.30
    with thyroid storm E05.31
  neonatal, transitory P72.1
  specified NEC E05.80
    with thyroid storm E05.81
Hypertony, hypertonia, hypertonicity
  bladder N31.8
  congenital P94.1
  stomach K31.89
    psychogenic F45.8
  uterus, uterine (contractions) (complicating
    delivery) O62.4
Hypertrichosis L68.9
  congenital Q84.2
  eyelid H02.869
    left H02.866
      lower H02.865
      upper H02.864
    right H02.863
      lower H02.862
      upper H02.861
  lanuginosa Q84.2
    acquired L68.1
  localized L68.2
  specified NEC L68.8
Hypertriglyceridemia, essential E78.1
Hypertrophy, hypertrophic
  adenofibromatous, prostate —*see*
    Enlargement, enlarged, prostate
  adenoids (infective) J35.2
    with tonsils J35.3
  adrenal cortex E27.8
  alveolar process or ridge —*see* Anomaly,
    alveolar
  anal papillae K62.89
  artery I77.89
    congenital NEC Q27.8
      digestive system Q27.8
      lower limb Q27.8
      specified site NEC Q27.8
      upper limb Q27.8

Hypertrophy, hypertrophic *(Continued)*
  auricular —*see* Hypertrophy, cardiac
  Bartholin's gland N75.8
  bile duct (common) (hepatic) K83.8
  bladder (sphincter) (trigone) N32.89
  bone M89.30
    carpus M89.34-●
    clavicle M89.31-●
    femur M89.35-●
    fibula M89.36-●
    finger M89.34-●
    humerus M89.32-●
    ilium M89.359
    ischium M89.359
    metacarpus M89.34-●
    metatarsus M89.37-●
    multiple sites M89.39
    neck M89.38
    radius M89.33-●
    rib M89.38
    scapula M89.31-●
    skull M89.38
    tarsus M89.37-●
    tibia M89.36-●
    toe M89.37-●
    ulna M89.33-●
    vertebra M89.38
  brain G93.89
  breast N62
    cystic —*see* Mastopathy, cystic
    newborn P83.4
    pubertal, massive N62
    puerperal, postpartum —*see* Disorder,
      breast, specified type NEC
    senile (parenchymatous) N62
  cardiac (chronic) (idiopathic) I51.7
    with rheumatic fever (conditions in I00)
      active I01.8
      inactive or quiescent (with chorea) I09.89
    congenital NEC Q24.8
    fatty —*see* Degeneration, myocardial
    hypertensive —*see* Hypertension, heart
    rheumatic (with chorea) I09.89
      active or acute I01.8
        with chorea I02.0
    valve —*see* Endocarditis
  cartilage —*see* Disorder, cartilage, specified
    type NEC
  cecum —*see* Megacolon
  cervix (uteri) N88.8
    congenital Q51.828
    elongation N88.4
  clitoris (cirrhotic) N90.89
    congenital Q52.6
  colon —*see also* Megacolon
    congenital Q43.2
  conjunctiva, lymphoid H11.89
  corpora cavernosa N48.89
  cystic duct K82.8
  duodenum K31.89
  endometrium (glandular) —*see also*
    Hyperplasia, endometrial N85.00-●
    cervix N88.8
  epididymis N50.89
  esophageal hiatus (congenital) Q79.1
    with hernia —*see* Hernia, hiatal
  eyelid —*see* Disorder, eyelid, specified type
    NEC
  fat pad E65
    knee (infrapatellar) (popliteal) (prepatellar)
      (retropatellar) M79.4
  foot (congenital) Q74.2
  frenulum, frenum (tongue) K14.8
    lip K13.0
  gallbladder K82.8
  gastric mucosa K29.60
    with bleeding K29.61
  gland, glandular R59.9
    generalized R59.1
    localized R59.0
  gum (mucous membrane) K06.1

Hypertrophy, hypertrophic *(Continued)*
heart (idiopathic) —*see also* Hypertrophy, cardiac
 valve —*see also* Endocarditis I38
hemifacial Q67.4
hepatic —*see* Hypertrophy, liver
hiatus (esophageal) Q79.1
hilus gland R59.0
hymen, congenital Q52.4
ileum K63.89
intestine NEC K63.89
jejunum K63.89
kidney (compensatory) N28.81
 congenital Q63.3
labium (majus) (minus) N90.60
ligament —*see* Disorder, ligament
lingual tonsil (infective) J35.1
 with adenoids J35.3
lip K13.0
 congenital Q18.6
liver R16.0
 acute K76.89
 cirrhotic —*see* Cirrhosis, liver
 congenital Q44.7
 fatty —*see* Fatty, liver
lymph, lymphatic gland R59.9
 generalized R59.1
 localized R59.0
 tuberculous —*see* Tuberculosis, lymph gland
mammary gland —*see* Hypertrophy, breast
Meckel's diverticulum (congenital) Q43.0
 malignant —*see* Table of Neoplasms, small intestine, malignant
median bar —*see* Hyperplasia, prostate
meibomian gland —*see* Chalazion
meniscus, knee, congenital Q74.1
metatarsal head —*see* Hypertrophy, bone, metatarsus
metatarsus —*see* Hypertrophy, bone, metatarsus
mucous membrane
 alveolar ridge K06.2
 gum K06.1
 nose (turbinate) J34.3
muscle M62.89
muscular coat, artery I77.89
myocardium —*see also* Hypertrophy, cardiac
 idiopathic I42.2
myometrium N85.2
nail L60.2
 congenital Q84.5
nasal J34.89
 alae J34.89
 bone J34.89
 cartilage J34.89
 mucous membrane (septum) J34.3
 sinus J34.89
 turbinate J34.3
nasopharynx, lymphoid (infectional) (tissue) (wall) J35.2
nipple N62
organ or site, congenital NEC —*see* Anomaly, by site - ovary N83.8
palate (hard) M27.8
 soft K13.79
pancreas, congenital Q45.3
parathyroid (gland) E21.0
parotid gland K11.1
penis N48.89
pharyngeal tonsil J35.2
pharynx J39.2
 lymphoid (infectional) (tissue) (wall) J35.2
pituitary (anterior) (fossa) (gland) E23.6
prepuce (congenital) N47.8
 female N90.89

Hypertrophy, hypertrophic *(Continued)*
prostate —*see* Enlargement, enlarged, prostate
 congenital Q55.4
pseudomuscular G71.0
pylorus (adult) (muscle) (sphincter) K31.1
 congenital or infantile Q40.0
rectal, rectum (sphincter) K62.89
rhinitis (turbinate) J31.0
salivary gland (any) K11.1
 congenital Q38.4
scaphoid (tarsal) —*see* Hypertrophy, bone, tarsus
scar L91.0
scrotum N50.89
seminal vesicle N50.89
sigmoid —*see* Megacolon
skin L91.9
 specified NEC L91.8
spermatic cord N50.89
spleen —*see* Splenomegaly
spondylitis —*see* Spondylosis
stomach K31.89
sublingual gland K11.1
submandibular gland K11.1
suprarenal cortex (gland) E27.8
synovial NEC M67.20
 acromioclavicular M67.21-●
 ankle M67.27-●
 elbow M67.22-●
 foot M67.27-●
 hand M67.24-●
 hip M67.25-●
 knee M67.26-●
 multiple sites M67.29
 specified site NEC M67.28
 wrist M67.23-●
tendon —*see* Disorder, tendon, specified type NEC
testis N44.8
 congenital Q55.29
thymic, thymus (gland) (congenital) E32.0
thyroid (gland) —*see* Goiter
toe (congenital) Q74.2
 acquired —*see also* Deformity, toe, specified NEC
tongue K14.8
 congenital Q38.2
 papillae (foliate) K14.3
tonsils (faucial) (infective) (lingual) (lymphoid) J35.1
 with adenoids J35.3
tunica vaginalis N50.89
ureter N28.89
urethra N36.8
uterus N85.2
 neck (with elongation) N88.4
 puerperal O90.89
uvula K13.79
vagina N89.8
vas deferens N50.89
vein I87.8
ventricle, ventricular (heart) —*see also* Hypertrophy, cardiac
 congenital Q24.8
 in tetralogy of Fallot Q21.3
verumontanum N36.8
vocal cord J38.3
vulva N90.60
 stasis (nonfilarial) N90.69
Hypertropia H50.2-●
Hypertyrosinemia E70.21
Hyperuricemia (asymptomatic) E79.0
Hypervalinemia E71.19
Hyperventilation (tetany) R06.4
 hysterical F45.8
 psychogenic F45.8
 syndrome F45.8

Hypervitaminosis (dietary) NEC E67.8
 A E67.0
  administered as drug (prolonged intake) —*see* Table of Drugs and Chemicals, vitamins, adverse effect
  overdose or wrong substance given or taken —*see* Table of Drugs and Chemicals, vitamins, poisoning
 B6 E67.2
 D E67.3
  administered as drug (prolonged intake) —*see* Table of Drugs and Chemicals, vitamins, adverse effect
  overdose or wrong substance given or taken —*see* Table of Drugs and Chemicals, vitamins, poisoning
 K E67.8
  administered as drug (prolonged intake) —*see* Table of Drugs and Chemicals, vitamins, adverse effect
  overdose or wrong substance given or taken —*see* Table of Drugs and Chemicals, vitamins, poisoning
Hypervolemia E87.70
 specified NEC E87.79
Hypesthesia R20.1
 cornea —*see* Anesthesia, cornea
Hyphema H21.0-●
 traumatic S05.1-●
Hypoacidity, gastric K31.89
 psychogenic F45.8
Hypoadrenalism, hypoadrenia E27.40
 primary E27.1
 tuberculous A18.7
Hypoadrenocorticism E27.40
 pituitary E23.0
 primary E27.1
Hypoalbuminemia E88.09
Hypoaldosteronism E27.40
Hypoalphalipoproteinemia E78.6
Hypobarism T70.29
Hypobaropathy T70.29
Hypobetalipoproteinemia (familial) E78.6
Hypocalcemia E83.51
 dietary E58
 neonatal P71.1
  due to cow's milk P71.0
 phosphate-loading (newborn) P71.1
Hypochloremia E87.8
Hypochlorhydria K31.89
 neurotic F45.8
 psychogenic F45.8
Hypochondria, hypochondriac, hypochondriasis (reaction) F45.21
 sleep F51.03
Hypochondrogenesis Q77.0
Hypochondroplasia Q77.4
Hypochromasia, blood cells D50.8
Hypodontia —*see* Anodontia
Hypoeosinophilia D72.89
Hypoesthesia R20.1
Hypofibrinogenemia D68.8
 acquired D65
 congenital (hereditary) D68.2
Hypofunction
 adrenocortical E27.40
  drug-induced E27.3
  postprocedural E89.6
  primary E27.1
 adrenomedullary, postprocedural E89.6
 cerebral R29.818
 corticoadrenal NEC E27.40
 intestinal K59.8
 labyrinth —*see* subcategory H83.2
 ovary E28.39
 pituitary (gland) (anterior) E23.0
 testicular E29.1
  postprocedural (postsurgical) (postirradiation) (iatrogenic) E89.5
Hypogalactia O92.4

Hypogammaglobulinemia —*see also*
   Agammaglobulinemia D80.1
   hereditary D80.0
   nonfamilial D80.1
   transient, of infancy D80.7
Hypogenitalism (congenital) —*see*
   Hypogonadism
Hypoglossia Q38.3
Hypoglycemia (spontaneous) E16.2
   coma E15
   ⟹diabetic —*see* Diabetes, by type, with
      hypoglycemia, with coma
   diabetic —*see* Diabetes, hypoglycemia
   dietary counseling and surveillance Z71.3
   drug-induced E16.0
      with coma (nondiabetic) E15
   due to insulin E16.0
      with coma (nondiabetic) E15
      therapeutic misadventure —*see*
         subcategory T38.3
   functional, nonhyperinsulinemic E16.1
   iatrogenic E16.0
      with coma (nondiabetic) E15
   in infant of diabetic mother P70.1
      gestational diabetes P70.0
   infantile E16.1
   leucine-induced E71.19
   neonatal (transitory) P70.4
      iatrogenic P70.3
   reactive (not drug-induced) E16.1
   transitory neonatal P70.4
Hypogonadism
   female E28.39
   hypogonadotropic E23.0
   male E29.1
   ovarian (primary) E28.39
   pituitary E23.0
   testicular (primary) E29.1
Hypohidrosis, hypoidrosis L74.4
Hypoinsulinemia, postprocedural E89.1
Hypokalemia E87.6
Hypoleukocytosis —*see* Agranulocytosis
Hypolipoproteinemia (alpha) (beta) E78.6
Hypomagnesemia E83.42
   neonatal P71.2
Hypomania, hypomanic reaction F30.8
Hypomenorrhea —*see* Oligomenorrhea
Hypometabolism R63.8
Hypomotility
   gastrointestinal (tract) K31.89
      psychogenic F45.8
   intestine K59.8
      psychogenic F45.8
   stomach K31.89
      psychogenic F45.8
Hyponasality R49.22
Hyponatremia E87.1
Hypo-osmolality E87.1
Hypo-ovarianism, hypo-ovarism E28.39
Hypoparathyroidism E20.9
   familial E20.8
   idiopathic E20.0
   neonatal, transitory P71.4
   postprocedural E89.2
   specified NEC E20.8
Hypoperfusion (in)
   newborn P96.89
Hypopharyngitis —*see* Laryngopharyngitis
Hypophoria H50.53
Hypophosphatemia, hypophosphatasia
   (acquired) (congenital) (renal) E83.39
   familial E83.31
Hypophyseal, hypophysis —*see also* condition
   dwarfism E23.0
   gigantism E22.0
Hypopiesis —*see* Hypotension
Hypopinealism E34.8
Hypopituitarism (juvenile) E23.0
   drug-induced E23.1
   due to
      hypophysectomy E89.3
      radiotherapy E89.3

Hypopituitarism (Continued)
   iatrogenic NEC E23.1
   postirradiation E89.3
   postpartum O99.285
   postprocedural E89.3
Hypoplasia, hypoplastic
   adrenal (gland), congenital Q89.1
   alimentary tract, congenital Q45.8
      upper Q40.8
   anus, anal (canal) Q42.3
      with fistula Q42.2
   aorta, aortic Q25.42
      ascending, in hypoplastic left heart
         syndrome Q23.4
      valve Q23.1
         in hypoplastic left heart syndrome
            Q23.4
   areola, congenital Q83.8
   arm (congenital) —*see* Defect, reduction,
      upper limb
   artery (peripheral) Q27.8
      brain (congenital) Q28.3
      coronary Q24.5
      digestive system Q27.8
      lower limb Q27.8
      pulmonary Q25.79
         functional, unilateral J43.0
      retinal (congenital) Q14.1
      specified site NEC Q27.8
      umbilical Q27.0
      upper limb Q27.8
   auditory canal Q17.8
      causing impairment of hearing Q16.9
   biliary duct or passage Q44.5
   bone NOS Q79.9
      face Q75.8
      marrow D61.9
         megakaryocytic D69.49
      skull —*see* Hypoplasia, skull
   brain Q02
      gyri Q04.3
      part of Q04.3
   breast (areola) N64.82
   bronchus Q32.4
   cardiac Q24.8
   carpus —*see* Defect, reduction, upper limb,
      specified type NEC
   cartilage hair Q78.8
   cecum Q42.8
   cementum K00.4
   cephalic Q02
   cerebellum Q04.3
   cervix (uteri), congenital Q51.821
   clavicle (congenital) Q74.0
   coccyx Q76.49
   colon Q42.9
      specified NEC Q42.8
   corpus callosum Q04.0
   cricoid cartilage Q31.2
   digestive organ(s) or tract NEC Q45.8
      upper (congenital) Q40.8
   ear (auricle) (lobe) Q17.2
      middle Q16.4
   enamel of teeth (neonatal) (postnatal)
      (prenatal) K00.4
   endocrine (gland) NEC Q89.2
   endometrium N85.8
   epididymis (congenital) Q55.4
   epiglottis Q31.2
   erythroid, congenital D61.01
   esophagus (congenital) Q39.8
   eustachian tube Q17.8
   eye Q11.2
   eyelid (congenital) Q10.3
   face Q18.8
      bone(s) Q75.8
   femur (congenital) —*see* Defect,
      reduction, lower limb, specified
      type NEC
   fibula (congenital) —*see* Defect, reduction,
      lower limb, specified type NEC

Hypoplasia, hypoplastic (Continued)
   finger (congenital) —*see* Defect, reduction,
      upper limb, specified type NEC
   focal dermal Q82.8
   foot —*see* Defect, reduction, lower limb,
      specified type NEC
   gallbladder Q44.0
   genitalia, genital organ(s)
      female, congenital Q52.8
         external Q52.79
         internal NEC Q52.8
      in adiposogenital dystrophy E23.6
   glottis Q31.2
   hair Q84.2
   hand (congenital) —*see* Defect, reduction,
      upper limb, specified type NEC
   heart Q24.8
   humerus (congenital) —*see* Defect, reduction,
      upper limb, specified type NEC
   intestine (small) Q41.9
      large Q42.9
         specified NEC Q42.8
   jaw M26.09
      alveolar M26.79
      lower M26.04
         alveolar M26.74
      upper M26.02
         alveolar M26.73
   kidney(s) Q60.5
      bilateral Q60.4
      unilateral Q60.3
   labium (majus) (minus), congenital Q52.79
   larynx Q31.2
   left heart syndrome Q23.4
   leg (congenital) —*see* Defect, reduction, lower
      limb
   limb Q73.8
      lower (congenital) —*see* Defect, reduction,
         lower limb
      upper (congenital) —*see* Defect, reduction,
         upper limb
   liver Q44.7
   lung (lobe) (not associated with short
      gestation) Q33.6
      associated with immaturity, low birth
         weight, prematurity, or short gestation
         P28.0
   mammary (areola), congenital Q83.8
   mandible, mandibular M26.04
      alveolar M26.74
      unilateral condylar M27.8
   maxillary M26.02
      alveolar M26.73
   medullary D61.9
   megakaryocytic D69.49
   metacarpus —*see* Defect, reduction, upper
      limb, specified type NEC
   metatarsus —*see* Defect, reduction, lower
      limb, specified type NEC
   muscle Q79.8
   nail(s) Q84.6
   nose, nasal Q30.1
   optic nerve H47.03-●
   osseous meatus (ear) Q17.8
   ovary, congenital Q50.39
   pancreas Q45.0
   parathyroid (gland) Q89.2
   parotid gland Q38.4
   patella Q74.1
   pelvis, pelvic girdle Q74.2
   penis (congenital) Q55.62
   peripheral vascular system Q27.8
      digestive system Q27.8
      lower limb Q27.8
      specified site NEC Q27.8
      upper limb Q27.8
   pituitary (gland) (congenital) Q89.2
   pulmonary (not associated with short
      gestation) Q33.6
      artery, functional J43.0
      associated with short gestation P28.0

Hypoplasia, hypoplastic *(Continued)*
  radioulnar —*see* Defect, reduction, upper
      limb, specified type NEC
  radius —*see* Defect, reduction, upper limb
  rectum Q42.1
    with fistula Q42.0
  respiratory system NEC Q34.8
  rib Q76.6
  right heart syndrome Q22.6
  sacrum Q76.49
  scapula Q74.0
  scrotum Q55.1
  shoulder girdle Q74.0
  skin Q82.8
  skull (bone) Q75.8
    with
        anencephaly Q00.0
        encephalocele —*see* Encephalocele
        hydrocephalus Q03.9
            with spina bifida —*see* Spina bifida, by
                site, with hydrocephalus
        microcephaly Q02
  spinal (cord) (ventral horn cell)
      Q06.1
  spine Q76.49
  sternum Q76.7
  tarsus —*see* Defect, reduction, lower limb,
      specified type NEC
  testis Q55.1
  thymic, with immunodeficiency D82.1
  thymus (gland) Q89.2
    with immunodeficiency D82.1
  thyroid (gland) E03.1
    cartilage Q31.2
  tibiofibular (congenital) —*see* Defect,
      reduction, lower limb, specified type
      NEC
  toe —*see* Defect, reduction, lower limb,
      specified type NEC
  tongue Q38.3
  Turner's K00.4
  ulna (congenital) —*see* Defect, reduction,
      upper limb
  umbilical artery Q27.0
  unilateral condylar M27.8
  ureter Q62.8
  uterus, congenital Q51.811
  vagina Q52.4
  vascular NEC peripheral Q27.8
    brain Q28.3
    digestive system Q27.8
    lower limb Q27.8
    specified site NEC Q27.8
    upper limb Q27.8
  vein(s) (peripheral) Q27.8
    brain Q28.3
    digestive system Q27.8
    great Q26.8
    lower limb Q27.8
    specified site NEC Q27.8
    upper limb Q27.8
  vena cava (inferior) (superior) Q26.8
  vertebra Q76.49
  vulva, congenital Q52.79
  zonule (ciliary) Q12.8
▶**Hypopnea, obstructive sleep apnea** G47.33

Hypopotassemia E87.6
Hypoproconvertinemia, congenital
    (hereditary) D68.2
Hypoproteinemia E77.8
Hypoprothrombinemia (congenital)
    (hereditary) (idiopathic) D68.2
  acquired D68.4
  newborn, transient P61.6
Hypoptyalism K11.7
Hypopyon (eye) (anterior chamber) —*see*
    Iridocyclitis, acute, hypopyon
Hypopyrexia R68.0
Hyporeflexia R29.2
Hyposecretion
  ACTH E23.0
  antidiuretic hormone E23.2
  ovary E28.39
  salivary gland (any) K11.7
  vasopressin E23.2
Hyposegmentation, leukocytic, hereditary
    D72.0
Hyposiderinemia D50.9
Hypospadias Q54.9
  balanic Q54.0
  coronal Q54.0
  glandular Q54.0
  penile Q54.1
  penoscrotal Q54.2
  perineal Q54.3
  specified NEC Q54.8
Hypospermatogenesis —*see* Oligospermia
Hyposplenism D73.0
Hypostasis pulmonary, passive —*see* Edema,
    lung
Hypostatic —*see* condition
Hyposthenuria N28.89
Hypotension (arterial) (constitutional)
    I95.9
  chronic I95.89
  drug-induced I95.2
  due to (of) hemodialysis I95.3
  iatrogenic I95.89
  idiopathic (permanent) I95.0
  intracranial, following ventricular shunting
      (ventriculostomy) G97.2
  intra-dialytic I95.3
  maternal, syndrome (following labor and
      delivery) O26.5-●
  neurogenic, orthostatic G90.3
  orthostatic (chronic) I95.1
      due to drugs I95.2
      neurogenic G90.3
  postoperative I95.81
  postural I95.1
  specified NEC I95.89
Hypothermia (accidental) T68
  due to anesthesia, anesthetic T88.51
  low environmental temperature T68
  neonatal P80.9
    environmental (mild) NEC P80.8
    mild P80.8
    severe (chronic) (cold injury syndrome)
        P80.0
    specified NEC P80.8
  not associated with low environmental
      temperature R68.0

Hypothyroidism (acquired) E03.9
▶autoimmune —*see* Thyroiditis, autoimmune
  congenital (without goiter) E03.1
    with goiter (diffuse) E03.0
  due to
    exogenous substance NEC E03.2
    iodine-deficiency, acquired E01.8
      subclinical E02
    irradiation therapy E89.0
    medicament NEC E03.2
    P-aminosalicylic acid (PAS) E03.2
    phenylbutazone E03.2
    resorcinol E03.2
 ' sulfonamide E03.2
    surgery E89.0
    thiourea group drugs E03.2
  iatrogenic NEC E03.2
  iodine-deficiency (acquired) E01.8
    congenital —*see* Syndrome, iodine-
        deficiency, congenital
    subclinical E02
  neonatal, transitory P72.2
  postinfectious E03.3
  postirradiation E89.0
  postprocedural E89.0
  postsurgical E89.0
  specified NEC E03.8
  subclinical, iodine-deficiency related
      E02
Hypotonia, hypotonicity, hypotony
  bladder N31.2
  congenital (benign) P94.2
  eye —*see* Disorder, globe, hypotony
Hypotrichosis —*see* Alopecia
Hypotropia H50.2-●
Hypoventilation R06.89
  congenital central alveolar G47.35
  sleep related
    idiopathic nonobstructive alveolar
        G47.34
    in conditions classified elsewhere
        G47.36
Hypovitaminosis —*see* Deficiency, vitamin
Hypovolemia E86.1
  surgical shock T81.19
  traumatic (shock) T79.4
Hypoxemia R09.02
  newborn P84
  sleep related, in conditions classified
      elsewhere G47.36
Hypoxia —*see also* Anoxia R09.02
  cerebral, during a procedure NEC G97.81
      postprocedural NEC G97.82
  intrauterine P84
  myocardial —*see* Insufficiency, coronary
  newborn P84
  sleep-related G47.34
Hypsarhythmia —*see* Epilepsy, generalized,
    specified NEC
Hysteralgia, pregnant uterus O26.89-●
Hysteria, hysterical (conversion) (dissociative
    state) F44.9
  anxiety F41.8
  convulsions F44.5
  psychosis, acute F44.9
Hysteroepilepsy F44.5

I

IBDU (colonic inflammatory bowel dissease unclassified) K52.3

Ichthyoparasitism due to Vandellia cirrhosa B88.8

Ichthyosis (congenital) Q80.9
  acquired L85.0
  fetalis Q80.4
  hystrix Q80.8
  lamellar Q80.2
  lingual K13.29
  palmaris and plantaris Q82.8
  simplex Q80.0
  vera Q80.8
  vulgaris Q80.0
  X-linked Q80.1

Ichthyotoxism —see Poisoning, fish
  bacterial —see Intoxication, foodborne

Icteroanemia, hemolytic (acquired) D59.9
  congenital —see Spherocytosis

Icterus —see also Jaundice
  conjunctiva R17
  gravis, newborn P55.0
  hematogenous (acquired) D59.9
  hemolytic (acquired) D59.9
    congenital —see Spherocytosis
  hemorrhagic (acute) (leptospiral) (spirochetal) A27.0
    newborn P53
  infectious B15.9
    with hepatic coma B15.0
    leptospiral A27.0
    spirochetal A27.0
  neonatorum —see Jaundice, newborn
  newborn P59.9
  spirochetal A27.0

Ictus solaris, solis T67.0

Ideation
  homicidal R45.850
  suicidal R45.851

Identity disorder (child) F64.9
  gender role F64.2
  psychosexual F64.2

Idioglossia F80.0

Idiopathic —see condition

Idiot, idiocy (congenital) F73
  amaurotic (Bielschowsky(-Jansky)) (family) (infantile (late)) (juvenile (late)) (Vogt-Spielmeyer) E75.4
  microcephalic Q02

Id reaction (due to bacteria) L30.2

IgE asthma J45.909

IIAC (idiopathic infantile arterial calcification) Q28.8

Ileitis (chronic) (noninfectious) —see also Enteritis K52.9
  backwash —see Pancolitis, ulcerative (chronic)
  infectious A09
  regional (ulcerative) —see Enteritis, regional, small intestine
  segmental —see Enteritis, regional
  terminal (ulcerative) —see Enteritis, regional, small intestine

Ileocolitis —see also Enteritis K52.9
  infectious A09
  regional —see Enteritis, regional
  ▶ulcerative K51.0-●

Ileostomy
  attention to Z43.2
  malfunctioning K94.13
  status Z93.2
    with complication —see Complications, enterostomy

Ileotyphus —see Typhoid

Ileum —see condition

Ileus (bowel) (colon) (inhibitory) (intestine) K56.7
  adynamic K56.0
  due to gallstone (in intestine) K56.3
  duodenal (chronic) K31.5

Ileus (Continued)
  gallstone K56.3
  ▶mechanical NEC —see also Obstruction, intestine, specified K56.699
  meconium P76.0
    in cystic fibrosis E84.11
    meaning meconium plug (without cystic fibrosis) P76.0
  myxedema K59.8
  neurogenic K56.0
    Hirschsprung's disease or megacolon Q43.1
  newborn
    due to meconium P76.0
      in cystic fibrosis E84.11
      meaning meconium plug (without cystic fibrosis) P76.0
    transitory P76.1
  ▶obstructive —see also Obstruction, intestine, specified K56.699
  paralytic K56.0
  ▶postoperative K91.89

Iliac —see condition

Iliotibial band syndrome M76.3-●

Illiteracy Z55.0

Illness —see also Disease R69
  manic-depressive —see Disorder, bipolar

Imbalance R26.89
  autonomic G90.8
  constituents of food intake E63.1
  electrolyte E87.8
    with
      abortion —see Abortion by type, complicated by, electrolyte imbalance
      molar pregnancy O08.5
    due to hyperemesis gravidarum O21.1
    following ectopic or molar pregnancy O08.5
    neonatal, transitory NEC P74.4
      potassium P74.3
      sodium P74.2
  endocrine E34.9
  eye muscle NOS H50.9
  hormone E34.9
  hysterical F44.4
  labyrinth —see subcategory H83.2
  posture R29.3
  protein-energy —see Malnutrition
  sympathetic G90.8

Imbecile, imbecility (I.Q. 35-49) F71

Imbedding, intrauterine device T83.39

Imbibition, cholesterol (gallbladder) K82.4

Imbrication, teeth, fully erupted M26.30

Imerslund (-Gräsbeck) syndrome D51.1

Immature —see also Immaturity
  birth (less than 37 completed weeks) —see Preterm, newborn
    extremely (less than 28 completed weeks) —see Immaturity, extreme
  personality F60.89

Immaturity (less than 37 completed weeks) —see also Preterm, newborn
  extreme of newborn (less than 28 completed weeks of gestation) (less than 196 completed days of gestation) (unspecified weeks of gestation) P07.20
    gestational age
      23 completed weeks (23 weeks, 0 days through 23 weeks, 6 days) P07.22
      24 completed weeks (24 weeks, 0 days through 24 weeks, 6 days) P07.23
      25 completed weeks (25 weeks, 0 days through 25 weeks, 6 days) P07.24
      26 completed weeks (26 weeks, 0 days through 26 weeks, 6 days) P07.25
      27 completed weeks (27 weeks, 0 days through 27 weeks, 6 days) P07.26
      less than 23 completed weeks P07.21
  fetus or infant light-for-dates —see Light-for-dates
  lung, newborn P28.0
  organ or site NEC —see Hypoplasia

Immaturity (Continued)
  pulmonary, newborn P28.0
  reaction F60.89
  sexual (female) (male), after puberty E30.0

Immersion T75.1
  foot T69.02-●
  hand T69.01-●

Immobile, immobility
  complete, due to severe physical disability or frailty R53.2
  intestine K59.8
  syndrome (paraplegic) M62.3

Immune reconstitution (inflammatory) syndrome [IRIS] D89.3

Immunization —see also Vaccination
  ABO —see Incompatibility, ABO
    in newborn P55.1
  complication —see Complications, vaccination
  encounter for Z23
  not done (not carried out) Z28.9
    because (of)
      acute illness of patient Z28.01
      allergy to vaccine (or component) Z28.04
      caregiver refusal Z28.82
      chronic illness of patient Z28.02
      contraindication NEC Z28.09
      group pressure Z28.1
      guardian refusal Z28.82
      immune compromised state of patient Z28.03
      parent refusal Z28.82
      patient's belief Z28.1
      patient had disease being vaccinated against Z28.81
      patient refusal Z28.21
      religious beliefs of patient Z28.1
      specified reason NEC Z28.89
        of patient Z28.29
      unspecified patient reason Z28.20
  Rh factor
    affecting management of pregnancy NEC O36.09-●
      anti-D antibody O36.01-●
    from transfusion —see Complication(s), transfusion, incompatibility reaction, Rh (factor)

Immunocytoma C83.0-●

Immunodeficiency D84.9
  with
    adenosine-deaminase deficiency D81.3
    antibody defects D80.9
      specified type NEC D80.8
    hyperimmunoglobulinemia D80.6
    increased immunoglobulin M (IgM) D80.5
    major defect D82.9
      specified type NEC D82.8
    partial albinism D82.8
    short-limbed stature D82.2
    thrombocytopenia and eczema D82.0
  antibody with
    hyperimmunoglobulinemia D80.6
    near-normal immunoglobulins D80.6
  autosomal recessive, Swiss type D80.0
  combined D81.9
    biotin-dependent carboxylase D81.819
      biotinidase D81.810
      holocarboxylase synthetase D81.818
      specified type NEC D81.818
    severe (SCID) D81.9
      with
        low or normal B-cell numbers D81.2
        low T- and B-cell numbers D81.1
        reticular dysgenesis D81.0
    specified type NEC D81.89
  common variable D83.9
    with
      abnormalities of B-cell numbers and function D83.0
      autoantibodies to B- or T-cells D83.2
      immunoregulatory T-cell disorders D83.1
    specified type NEC D83.8

▶ New   ⇒ Revised   ~~deleted~~ Deleted   ● Use Additional Character(s)

Immunodeficiency *(Continued)*
  following hereditary defective response to
      Epstein-Barr virus (EBV) D82.3
  selective, immunoglobulin
      A (IgA) D80.2
      G (IgG) (subclasses) D80.3
      M (IgM) D80.4
  severe combined (SCID) D81.9
  specified type NEC D84.8
  X-linked, with increased IgM D80.5
Immunotherapy (encounter for)
  antineoplastic Z51.12
Impaction, impacted
  bowel, colon, rectum —*see also* Impaction,
      fecal K56.49
      by gallstone K56.3
  calculus —*see* Calculus
  cerumen (ear) (external) H61.2-●
  cuspid —*see* Impaction, tooth
  dental (same or adjacent tooth) K01.1
  fecal, feces K56.41
  fracture —*see* Fracture, by site
  gallbladder —*see* Calculus, gallbladder
  gallstone(s) —*see* Calculus, gallbladder
      bile duct (common) (hepatic) —*see*
          Calculus, bile duct
      cystic duct —*see* Calculus, gallbladder
      in intestine, with obstruction (any part) K56.3
  intestine (calculous) NEC —*see also*
      Impaction, fecal K56.49
      gallstone, with ileus K56.3
  intrauterine device (IUD) T83.39
  molar —*see* Impaction, tooth
  shoulder, causing obstructed labor O66.0
  tooth, teeth K01.1
  turbinate J34.89
Impaired, impairment (function)
  auditory discrimination —*see* Abnormal,
      auditory perception
  cognitive, mild, so stated G31.84
  dual sensory Z73.82
  fasting glucose R73.01
  glucose tolerance (oral) R73.02
  hearing —*see* Deafness
  heart —*see* Disease, heart
  kidney N28.9
      disorder resulting from N25.9
          specified NEC N25.89
  liver K72.90
      with coma K72.91
  mastication K08.89
  mild cognitive, so stated G31.84
  mobility
      ear ossicles —*see* Ankylosis, ear ossicles
      requiring care provider Z74.09
  myocardium, myocardial —*see* Insufficiency,
      myocardial
  rectal sphincter R19.8
  renal (acute) (chronic) N28.9
      disorder resulting from N25.9
          specified NEC N25.89
  vision NEC H54.7
      both eyes H54.3
Impediment, speech R47.9
  psychogenic (childhood) F98.8
  slurring R47.81
  specified NEC R47.89
Impending
  coronary syndrome I20.0
  delirium tremens F10.239
  myocardial infarction I20.0
Imperception auditory (acquired) —*see also*
      Deafness
  congenital H93.25
Imperfect
  aeration, lung (newborn) NEC —*see* Atelectasis
  closure (congenital)
      alimentary tract NEC Q45.8
          lower Q43.8
          upper Q40.8
      atrioventricular ostium Q21.2

Imperfect *(Continued)*
  closure *(Continued)*
      atrium (secundum) Q21.1
      ~~branchial cleft or sinus Q18.0~~
      ▶branchial cleft NOS Q18.2
      ▶cyst Q18.0
      ▶fistula Q18.0
      ▶sinus Q18.0
      choroid Q14.3
      cricoid cartilage Q31.8
      cusps, heart valve NEC Q24.8
          pulmonary Q22.3
      ductus
          arteriosus Q25.0
          Botalli Q25.0
      ear drum (causing impairment of hearing)
          Q16.4
      esophagus with communication to
          bronchus or trachea Q39.1
      eyelid Q10.3
      foramen
          botalli Q21.1
          ovale Q21.1
      genitalia, genital organ(s) or system
          female Q52.8
              external Q52.79
              internal NEC Q52.8
          male Q55.8
      glottis Q31.8
      interatrial ostium or septum Q21.1
      interauricular ostium or septum Q21.1
      interventricular ostium or septum Q21.0
      larynx Q31.8
      lip —*see* Cleft, lip
      nasal septum Q30.3
      nose Q30.2
      omphalomesenteric duct Q43.0
      optic nerve entry Q14.2
      organ or site not listed —*see* Anomaly, by
          site
      ostium
          interatrial Q21.1
          interauricular Q21.1
          interventricular Q21.0
      palate —*see* Cleft, palate
      preauricular sinus Q18.1
      retina Q14.1
      roof of orbit Q75.8
      sclera Q13.5
      septum
          aorticopulmonary Q21.4
          atrial (secundum) Q21.1
          between aorta and pulmonary artery
              Q21.4
          heart Q21.9
          interatrial (secundum) Q21.1
          interauricular (secundum) Q21.1
          interventricular Q21.0
              in tetralogy of Fallot Q21.3
          nasal Q30.3
          ventricular Q21.0
              with pulmonary stenosis or atresia,
                  dextraposition of aorta, and
                  hypertrophy of right ventricle
                  Q21.3
              in tetralogy of Fallot Q21.3
      skull Q75.0
          with
              anencephaly Q00.0
              encephalocele —*see* Encephalocele
              hydrocephalus Q03.9
                  with spina bifida —*see* Spina bifida,
                      by site, with hydrocephalus
              microcephaly Q02
      spine (with meningocele) —*see* Spina bifida
      trachea Q32.1
      tympanic membrane (causing impairment
          of hearing) Q16.4
      uterus Q51.818
      vitelline duct Q43.0
  erection —*see* Dysfunction, sexual, male,
      erectile

Imperfect *(Continued)*
  fusion —*see* Imperfect, closure
  inflation, lung (newborn) —*see* Atelectasis
  posture R29.3
  rotation, intestine Q43.3
  septum, ventricular Q21.0
Imperfectly descended testis —*see* Cryptorchid
Imperforate (congenital) —*see also* Atresia
  anus Q42.3
      with fistula Q42.2
  cervix (uteri) Q51.828
  esophagus Q39.0
      with tracheoesophageal fistula Q39.1
  hymen Q52.3
  jejunum Q41.1
  pharynx Q38.8
  rectum Q42.1
      with fistula Q42.0
  urethra Q64.39
  vagina Q52.4
Impervious (congenital) —*see also* Atresia
  anus Q42.3
      with fistula Q42.2
  bile duct Q44.2
  esophagus Q39.0
      with tracheoesophageal fistula Q39.1
  intestine (small) Q41.9
      large Q42.9
          specified NEC Q42.8
  rectum Q42.1
      with fistula Q42.0
  ureter —*see* Atresia, ureter
  urethra Q64.39
Impetiginization of dermatoses L01.1
Impetigo (any organism) (any site) (circinate)
      (contagiosa) (simplex) (vulgaris) L01.00
  Bockhart's L01.02
  bullous, bullosa L01.03
  external ear L01.00 *[H62.40]*
  follicularis L01.02
  furfuracea L30.5
  herpetiformis L40.1
      nonobstetrical L40.1
  neonatorum L01.03
  nonbullous L01.01
  specified type NEC L01.09
  ulcerative L01.09
Impingement (on teeth)
  soft tissue
      anterior M26.81
      posterior M26.82
Implant, endometrial N80.9
Implantation
  anomalous —*see* Anomaly, by site
      ureter Q62.63
  cyst
      external area or site (skin) NEC L72.0
      iris —*see* Cyst, iris, implantation
      vagina N89.8
      vulva N90.7
  dermoid (cyst) —*see* Implantation, cyst
Impotence (sexual) N52.9
  counseling Z70.1
  organic origin —*see also* Dysfunction, sexual,
      male, erectile N52.9
  psychogenic F52.21
Impression, basilar Q75.8
Imprisonment, anxiety concerning Z65.1
Improper care (child) (newborn) —*see*
      Maltreatment
Improperly tied umbilical cord (causing
      hemorrhage) P51.8
Impulsiveness (impulsive) R45.87
Inability to swallow —*see* Aphagia
Inaccessible, inaccessibility
  health care NEC Z75.3
      due to
          waiting period Z75.2
              for admission to facility elsewhere
                  Z75.1
      other helping agencies Z75.4
Inactive —*see* condition

Inadequate, inadequacy
aesthetics of dental restoration K08.56
biologic, constitutional, functional, or social
    F60.7
development
    child R62.50
    genitalia
        after puberty NEC E30.0
        congenital
            female Q52.8
                external Q52.79
                internal Q52.8
            male Q55.8
    lungs Q33.6
        associated with short gestation P28.0
    organ or site not listed —see Anomaly, by
        site
diet (causing nutritional deficiency) E63.9
eating habits Z72.4
environment, household Z59.1
family support Z63.8
food (supply) NEC Z59.4
    hunger effects T73.0
functional F60.7
household care, due to
    family member
        handicapped or ill Z74.2
        on vacation Z75.5
        temporarily away from home Z74.2
    technical defects in home Z59.1
    temporary absence from home of person
        rendering care Z74.2
housing (heating) (space) Z59.1
income (financial) Z59.6
intrafamilial communication Z63.8
material resources Z59.9
mental —see Disability, intellectual
parental supervision or control of child
    Z62.0
personality F60.7
pulmonary
    function R06.89
        newborn P28.5
    ventilation, newborn P28.5
sample of cytologic smear
    anus R85.615
    cervix R87.615
    vagina R87.625
social F60.7
    insurance Z59.7
    skills NEC Z73.4
supervision of child by parent Z62.0
teaching affecting education Z55.8
welfare support Z59.7
Inanition R64
with edema —see Malnutrition, severe
due to
    deprivation of food T73.0
    malnutrition —see Malnutrition
fever R50.9
Inappropriate
change in quantitative human chorionic
    gonadotropin (hCG) in early pregnancy
    O02.81
diet or eating habits Z72.4
level of quantitative human chorionic
    gonadotropin (hCG) for gestational age
    in early pregnancy O02.81
secretion
    antidiuretic hormone (ADH) (excessive)
        E22.2
    deficiency E23.2
    pituitary (posterior) E22.2
Inattention at or after birth —see Neglect
Incarceration, incarcerated
enterocele K46.0
    gangrenous K46.1
epiplocele K46.0
    gangrenous K46.1
exomphalos K42.0
    gangrenous K42.1

Incarceration, incarcerated *(Continued)*
hernia —see also Hernia, by site, with
    obstruction
    with gangrene —see Hernia, by site, with
        gangrene
iris, in wound —see Injury, eye, laceration,
    with prolapse
lens, in wound —see Injury, eye, laceration,
    with prolapse
omphalocele K42.0
prison, anxiety concerning Z65.1
rupture —see Hernia, by site
sarcoepiplocele K46.0
    gangrenous K46.1
sarcoepiplomphalocele K42.0
    with gangrene K42.1
uterus N85.8
    gravid O34.51-•
        causing obstructed labor O65.5
Incised wound
external —see Laceration
internal organs —see Injury, by site
Incision, incisional
hernia K43.2
    with
        gangrene (and obstruction) K43.1
        obstruction K43.0
    surgical, complication —see Complications,
        surgical procedure
    traumatic
        external —see Laceration
        internal organs —see Injury, by site
Inclusion
azurophilic leukocytic D72.0
blennorrhea (neonatal) (newborn) P39.1
gallbladder in liver (congenital) Q44.1
Incompatibility
ABO
    affecting management of pregnancy
        O36.11-•
        anti-A sensitization O36.11-•
        anti-B sensitization O36.19-•
        specified NEC O36.19-•
    infusion or transfusion reaction —see
        Complication(s), transfusion,
        incompatibility reaction, ABO
    newborn P55.1
blood (group) (Duffy) (K(ell)) (Kidd) (Lewis)
    (M) (S) NEC
    affecting management of pregnancy
        O36.11-•
        anti-A sensitization O36.11-•
        anti-B sensitization O36.19-•
    infusion or transfusion reaction T80.89
    newborn P55.8
divorce or estrangement Z63.5
Rh (blood group) (factor) Z31.82
    affecting management of pregnancy NEC
        O36.09-•
        anti-D antibody O36.01-•
    infusion or transfusion reaction —see
        Complication(s), transfusion,
        incompatibility reaction, Rh (factor)
    newborn P55.0
rhesus —see Incompatibility, Rh
Incompetency, incompetent, incompetence
annular
    aortic (valve) —see Insufficiency, aortic
    mitral (valve) I34.0
    pulmonary valve (heart) I37.1
aortic (valve) —see Insufficiency, aortic
cardiac valve —see Endocarditis
cervix, cervical (os) N88.3
    in pregnancy O34.3-•
chronotropic I45.89
    with
        autonomic dysfunction G90.8
        ischemic heart disease I25.89
        left ventricular dysfunction I51.89
        sinus node dysfunction I49.8
esophagogastric (junction) (sphincter) K22.0

Incompetency, incompetent, incompetence
    (Continued)
mitral (valve) —see Insufficiency, mitral
pelvic fundus N81.89
pubocervical tissue N81.82
pulmonary valve (heart) I37.1
    congenital Q22.3
rectovaginal tissue N81.83
tricuspid (annular) (valve) —see Insufficiency,
    tricuspid
valvular —see Endocarditis
    congenital Q24.8
vein, venous (saphenous) (varicose) —see
    Varix, leg
Incomplete —see also condition
bladder, emptying R33.9
defecation R15.0
expansion lungs (newborn) NEC —see
    Atelectasis
rotation, intestine Q43.3
Inconclusive
diagnostic imaging due to excess body fat of
    patient R93.9
findings on diagnostic imaging of breast NEC
    R92.8
mammogram (due to dense breasts) R92.2
Incontinence R32
anal sphincter R15.9
coital N39.491
feces R15.9
    nonorganic origin F98.1
insensible (urinary) N39.42
overflow N39.490
postural (urinary) N39.492
psychogenic F45.8
rectal R15.9
reflex N39.498
stress (female) (male) N39.3
    and urge N39.46
urethral sphincter R32
urge N39.41
    and stress (female) (male) N39.46
urine (urinary) R32
    continuous N39.45
    due to cognitive impairment, or severe
        physical disability or immobility R39.81
    functional R39.81
    insensible N39.42
    mixed (stress and urge) N39.46
    nocturnal N39.44
    nonorganic origin F98.0
    overflow N39.490
    post dribbling N39.43
    postural N39.492
    reflex N39.498
    specified NEC N39.498
    stress (female) (male) N39.3
        and urge N39.46
    total N39.498
    unaware N39.42
    urge N39.41
        and stress (female) (male) N39.46
Incontinentia pigmenti Q82.3
Incoordinate, incoordination
esophageal-pharyngeal (newborn) —see
    Dysphagia
muscular R27.8
uterus (action) (contractions) (complicating
    delivery) O62.4
Increase, increased
abnormal, in development R63.8
androgens (ovarian) E28.1
anticoagulants (antithrombin) (anti-VIIIa)
    (anti-IXa) (anti-Xa) (anti-XIa) —see
    Circulating anticoagulants
cold sense R20.8
estrogen E28.0
function
    adrenal
        cortex —see Cushing's, syndrome
        medulla E27.5

▶ New   ⇒ Revised   ~~deleted~~ Deleted   • Use Additional Character(s)

Increase, increased *(Continued)*
  function *(Continued)*
    pituitary (gland) (anterior) (lobe) E22.9
      posterior E22.2
  heat sense R20.8
  intracranial pressure (benign) G93.2
  permeability, capillaries I78.8
  pressure, intracranial G93.2
  secretion
    gastrin E16.4
    glucagon E16.3
    pancreas, endocrine E16.9
      growth hormone-releasing hormone E16.8
      pancreatic polypeptide E16.8
      somatostatin E16.8
      vasoactive-intestinal polypeptide E16.8
  sphericity, lens Q12.4
  splenic activity D73.1
  venous pressure I87.8
    portal K76.6
Increta placenta O43.22-•
Incrustation, cornea, foreign body (lead)
  (zinc) —*see* Foreign body, cornea
Incyclophoria H50.54
Incyclotropia —*see* Cyclotropia
Indeterminate sex Q56.4
India rubber skin Q82.8
Indigestion (acid) (bilious) (functional) K30
  catarrhal K31.89
  due to decomposed food NOS A05.9
  nervous F45.8
  psychogenic F45.8
Indirect —*see* condition
Induratio penis plastica N48.6
Induration, indurated
  brain G93.89
  breast (fibrous) N64.51
    puerperal, postpartum O92.29
  broad ligament N83.8
  chancre
    anus A51.1
    congenital A50.07
    extragenital NEC A51.2
  corpora cavernosa (penis) (plastic) N48.6
  liver (chronic) K76.89
  lung (black) (chronic) (fibroid) —*see also*
    Fibrosis, lung J84.10
    essential brown J84.03
  penile (plastic) N48.6
  phlebitic —*see* Phlebitis
  skin R23.4
Inebriety (without dependence) —*see* Alcohol,
  intoxication
Inefficiency, kidney N28.9
Inelasticity, skin R23.4
Inequality, leg (length) (acquired) —*see also*
  Deformity, limb, unequal length
  congenital —*see* Defect, reduction, lower limb
  lower leg —*see* Deformity, limb, unequal
    length
Inertia
  bladder (neurogenic) N31.2
  stomach K31.89
    psychogenic F45.8
  uterus, uterine during labor O62.2
    during latent phase of labor O62.0
    primary O62.0
    secondary O62.1
  vesical (neurogenic) N31.2
Infancy, infantile, infantilism —*see also*
  condition
  celiac K90.0
  genitalia, genitals (after puberty) E30.0
  Herter's (nontropical sprue) K90.0
  intestinal K90.0
  Lorain E23.0
  pancreatic K86.89
  pelvis M95.5
    with disproportion (fetopelvic) O33.1
      causing obstructed labor O65.1
  pituitary E23.0

Infancy, infantile, infantilism *(Continued)*
  renal N25.0
  uterus —*see* Infantile, genitalia
Infant(s) —*see also* Infancy
  excessive crying R68.11
  irritable child R68.12
  lack of care —*see* Neglect
  liveborn (singleton) Z38.2
    born in hospital Z38.00
      by cesarean Z38.01
    born outside hospital Z38.1
    multiple NEC Z38.8
      born in hospital Z38.68
        by cesarean Z38.69
      born outside hospital Z38.7
    quadruplet Z38.8
      born in hospital Z38.63
        by cesarean Z38.64
      born outside hospital Z38.7
    quintuplet Z38.8
      born in hospital Z38.65
        by cesarean Z38.66
      born outside hospital Z38.7
    triplet Z38.8
      born in hospital Z38.61
        by cesarean Z38.62
      born outside hospital Z38.7
    twin Z38.5
      born in hospital Z38.30
        by cesarean Z38.31
      born outside hospital Z38.4
  of diabetic mother (syndrome of) P70.1
    gestational diabetes P70.0
Infantile —*see also* condition
  genitalia, genitals E30.0
  os, uterine E30.0
  penis E30.0
  testis E29.1
  uterus E30.0
Infantilism —*see* Infancy
Infarct, infarction
  adrenal (capsule) (gland) E27.49
  appendices epiploicae —*see also* Infarct,
    intestine K55.069
  bowel —*see also* Infarct, intestine K55.069
  brain (stem) —*see* Infarct, cerebral
  breast N64.89
  brewer's (kidney) N28.0
  cardiac —*see* Infarct, myocardium
  cerebellar —*see* Infarct, cerebral
  cerebral —*see also* Occlusion, artery cerebral
    or precerebral, with infarction I63.9-•
    aborted I63.9
    cortical I63.9
    due to
      cerebral venous thrombosis,
        nonpyogenic I63.6
      embolism
        cerebral arteries I63.4-•
        precerebral arteries I63.1-•
      occlusion NEC
        cerebral arteries I63.5-•
        precerebral arteries I63.2-•
      stenosis NEC
        cerebral arteries I63.5-•
        precerebral arteries I63.2-•
      thrombosis
        cerebral artery I63.3-•
        precerebral artery I63.0-•
    intraoperative
      during cardiac surgery I97.810
      during other surgery I97.811
    postprocedural
      following cardiac surgery I97.820
      following other surgery I97.821
    specified NEC I63.8
  colon (acute) (agnogenic) (embolic)
    (hemorrhagic) (nonocclusive)
    (nonthrombotic) (occlusive) (segmental)
    (thrombotic) (with gangrene) —*see also*
    Infarct, intestine K55.049

Infarct, infarction *(Continued)*
  coronary artery —*see* Infarct, myocardium
  embolic —*see* Embolism
  fallopian tube N83.8
  gallbladder K82.8
  heart —*see* Infarct, myocardium
  hepatic K76.3
  hypophysis (anterior lobe) E23.6
  impending (myocardium) I20.0
  intestine (acute) (agnogenic) (embolic)
    (hemorrhagic) (nonocclusive)
    (nonthrombotic) (occlusive) (thrombotic)
    (with gangrene) K55.069
    diffuse K55.062
    focal K55.061
    large K55.049
      diffuse K55.042
      focal K55.041
    small K55.029
      diffuse K55.022
      focal K55.021
  kidney N28.0
  liver K76.3
  lung (embolic) (thrombotic) —*see* Embolism,
    pulmonary
  lymph node I89.8
  mesentery, mesenteric (embolic) (thrombotic)
    (with gangrene) —*see also* Infarct,
    intestine K55.069
  muscle (ischemic) M62.20
    ankle M62.27-•
    foot M62.27-•
    forearm M62.23-•
    hand M62.24-•
    lower leg M62.26-•
    pelvic region M62.25-•
    shoulder region M62.21-•
    specified site NEC M62.28
    thigh M62.25-•
    upper arm M62.22-•
➡ myocardium, myocardial (acute) (with stated
    duration of 4 weeks or less) I21.9
▶ associated with revascularization
    procedure I21.A9
  diagnosed on ECG, but presenting no
    symptoms I25.2
▶ due to
  ▶ demand ischemia I21.A1
  ▶ ischemic imbalance I21.A1
  healed or old I25.2
➡ intraoperative —*see also* Infarct,
    myocardium, associated with
    revascularization procedure
    during cardiac surgery I97.790
    during other surgery I97.791
  non-Q wave I21.4
  non-ST elevation (NSTEMI) I21.4
    subsequent I22.2
  nontransmural I21.4
  past (diagnosed on ECG or other
    investigation, but currently presenting
    no symptoms) I25.2
➡ postprocedural —*see also* Infarct,
    myocardium, associated with
    revascularization procedure
    ~~following cardiac surgery I97.190~~
  ▶ following cardiac surgery —*see also*
    Infarct, myocardium, type 4 or
    type 5 I97.190
    following other surgery I97.191
  Q wave —*see also* Infarct, myocardium, by
    site I21.3
▶ secondary to
  ▶ demand ischemia I21.A1
  ▶ ischemic imbalance I21.A1
  ST elevation (STEMI) I21.3
    anterior (anteroapical) (anterolateral)
      (anteroseptal) (Q wave) (wall) I21.09
      subsequent I22.0
    inferior (diaphragmatic) (inferolateral)
      (inferoposterior) (wall) NEC I21.19
      subsequent I22.1
    inferoposterior transmural (Q wave) I21.11

Infarct, infarction (Continued)
    myocardium, myocardial (Continued)
        ST elevation (Continued)
            involving
                coronary artery of anterior wall NEC
                    I21.09
                coronary artery of inferior wall NEC
                    I21.19
                diagonal coronary artery I21.02
                left anterior descending coronary
                    artery I21.02
                left circumflex coronary artery I21.21
                left main coronary artery I21.01
                oblique marginal coronary artery
                    I21.21
                right coronary artery I21.11
            lateral (apical-lateral) (basal-lateral)
                (high) I21.29
                subsequent I22.8
            posterior (posterobasal) (posterolateral)
                (posteroseptal) (true) I21.29
                subsequent I22.8
            septal I21.29
                subsequent I22.8
            specified NEC I21.29
                subsequent I22.8
            subsequent I22.9
        subsequent (recurrent) (reinfarction) I22.9
            anterior (anteroapical) (anterolateral)
                (anteroseptal) (wall) I22.0
            diaphragmatic (wall) I22.1
            inferior (diaphragmatic) (inferolateral)
                (inferoposterior) (wall) I22.1
            lateral (apical-lateral) (basal-lateral)
                (high) I22.8
            non-ST elevation (NSTEMI) I22.2
            posterior (posterobasal) (posterolateral)
                (posteroseptal) (true) I22.8
            septal I22.8
            specified NEC I22.8
            ST elevation I22.9
                anterior (anteroapical) (anterolateral)
                    (anteroseptal) (wall) I22.0
                inferior (diaphragmatic) (inferolateral)
                    (inferoposterior) (wall) I22.1
                specified NEC I22.8
            subendocardial I22.2
            transmural I22.9
                anterior (anteroapical) (anterolateral)
                    (anteroseptal) (wall) I22.0
                diaphragmatic (wall) I22.1
                inferior (diaphragmatic) (inferolateral)
                    (inferoposterior) (wall) I22.1
                lateral (apical-lateral) (basal-lateral)
                    (high) I22.8
                posterior (posterobasal)
                    (posterolateral) (posteroseptal)
                    (true) I22.8
                specified NEC I22.8
        ▶type 1 —see also Infarction, myocardial,
            subsequent, by site, or by ST
            elevation or non-ST elevation I22.9
        ▶type 2 I21.A1
        ▶type 3 I21.A9
        ▶type 4 I21.A9
        ▶type 5 I21.A9
        syphilitic A52.06
        ⇒transmural I21.9
            anterior (anteroapical) (anterolateral)
                (anteroseptal) (Q wave) (wall) NEC
                I21.09
            inferior (diaphragmatic) (inferolateral)
                (inferoposterior) (Q wave) (wall)
                NEC I21.19
            inferoposterior (Q wave) I21.11
            lateral (apical-lateral) (basal-lateral)
                (high) NEC I21.29
            posterior (posterobasal) (posterolateral)
                (posteroseptal) (true) NEC I21.29
            septal NEC I21.29
            specified NEC I21.29

Infarct, infarction (Continued)
    myocardium, myocardial (Continued)
        ▶type 1 —see also Infarction, myocardial, by
            site, or by ST elevation or non-ST
            elevation I21.9
        ▶type 2 I21.A1
        ▶type 3 I21.A9
        ▶type 4 (a) (b) (c) I21.A9
        ▶type 5 I21.A9
    nontransmural I21.4
    omentum —see also Infarct, intestine K55.069
    ovary N83.8
    pancreas K86.89
    papillary muscle —see Infarct, myocardium
    parathyroid gland E21.4
    pituitary (gland) E23.6
    placenta O43.81-•
    prostate N42.89
    pulmonary (artery) (vein) (hemorrhagic) —
        see Embolism, pulmonary
    renal (embolic) (thrombotic) N28.0
    retina, retinal (artery) —see Occlusion, artery,
        retina
    spinal (cord) (acute) (embolic) (nonembolic)
        G95.11
    spleen D73.5
        embolic or thrombotic I74.8
    subendocardial (acute) (nontransmural) I21.4
    suprarenal (capsule) (gland) E27.49
    testis N50.1
    thrombotic —see also Thrombosis
        artery, arterial —see Embolism
    thyroid (gland) E07.89
    ventricle (heart) —see Infarct, myocardium
Infecting —see condition
Infection, infected, infective (opportunistic)
    B99.9
    with
        drug resistant organism —see Resistance
            (to), drug —see also specific organism
        lymphangitis —see Lymphangitis
        organ dysfunction (acute) R65.20
            with septic shock R65.21
    abscess (skin) - code by site under Abscess
    Absidia —see Mucormycosis
    Acanthamoeba —see Acanthamebiasis
    Acanthocheilonema (perstans) (streptocerca)
        B74.4
    accessory sinus (chronic) —see Sinusitis
    achorion —see Dermatophytosis
    Acremonium falciforme B47.0
    acromioclavicular M00.9
    Actinobacillus (actinomycetem-comitans)
        A28.8
        mallei A24.0
        muris A25.1
    Actinomadura B47.1
    Actinomyces (israelii) —see also
        Actinomycosis A42.9
    Actinomycetales —see Actinomycosis
    actinomycotic NOS —see Actinomycosis
    adenoid (and tonsil) J03.90
        chronic J35.02
    adenovirus NEC
        as cause of disease classified elsewhere
            B97.0
        unspecified nature or site B34.0
    aerogenes capsulatus A48.0
    aertrycke —see Infection, salmonella
    alimentary canal NOS —see Enteritis,
        infectious
    Allescheria boydii B48.2
    Alternaria B48.8
    alveolus, alveolar (process) K04.7
    Ameba, amebic (histolytica) —see Amebiasis
    amniotic fluid, sac or cavity O41.10-•
        chorioamnionitis O41.12-•
        placentitis O41.14-•
    amputation stump (surgical) —see
        Complication, amputation stump,
        infection

Infection, infected, infective (Continued)
    Ancylostoma (duodenalis) B76.0
    Anisakiasis, Anisakis larvae B81.0
    anthrax —see Anthrax
    antrum (chronic) —see Sinusitis, maxillary
    anus, anal (papillae) (sphincter) K62.89
    arbovirus (arbor virus) A94
        specified type NEC A93.8
    artificial insemination N98.0
    Ascaris lumbricoides —see Ascariasis
    Ascomycetes B47.0
    Aspergillus (flavus) (fumigatus) (terreus) —
        see Aspergillosis
    atypical
        acid-fast (bacilli) —see Mycobacterium,
            atypical
        mycobacteria —see Mycobacterium,
            atypical
        virus A81.9
            specified type NEC A81.89
    auditory meatus (external) —see Otitis,
        externa, infective
    auricle (ear) —see Otitis, externa, infective
    axillary gland (lymph) L04.2
    Bacillus A49.9
        abortus A23.1
        anthracis —see Anthrax
        Ducrey's (any location) A57
        Flexner's A03.1
        Friedländer's NEC A49.8
        gas (gangrene) A48.0
        mallei A24.0
        melitensis A23.0
        paratyphoid, paratyphosus A01.4
            A A01.1
            B A01.2
            C A01.3
        Shiga (-Kruse) A03.0
        suipestifer —see Infection, salmonella
        swimming pool A31.1
        typhosa A01.00
        welchii —see Gangrene, gas
    bacterial NOS A49.9
        as cause of disease classified elsewhere
            B96.89
            Bacteroides fragilis [B. fragilis] B96.6
            Clostridium perfringens [C. perfringens]
                B96.7
            Enterobacter sakazakii B96.89
            Enterococcus B95.2
            Escherichia coli [E. coli] (see also
                Escherichia coli) B96.20
            Helicobacter pylori [H.pylori] B96.81
            Hemophilus influenzae [H. influenzae]
                B96.3
            Klebsiella pneumoniae [K. pneumoniae]
                B96.1
            Mycoplasma pneumoniae [M.
                pneumoniae] B96.0
            Proteus (mirabilis) (morganii) B96.4
            Pseudomonas (aeruginosa) (mallei)
                (pseudomallei) B96.5
            Staphylococcus B95.8
                aureus (methicillin susceptible)
                    (MSSA) B95.61
                    methicillin resistant (MRSA)
                        B95.62
                specified NEC B95.7
            Streptococcus B95.5
                group A B95.0
                group B B95.1
                pneumoniae B95.3
                specified NEC B95.4
            Vibrio vulnificus B96.82
        specified NEC A48.8
    Bacterium
        paratyphosum A01.4
            A A01.1
            B A01.2
            C A01.3
        typhosum A01.00

▶ New   ⇒ Revised   ~~deleted~~ Deleted   • Use Additional Character(s)

Infection, infected, infective (*Continued*)
 Bacteroides NEC A49.8
  fragilis, as cause of disease classified
    elsewhere B96.6
 Balantidium coli A07.0
 Bartholin's gland N75.8
 Basidiobolus B46.8
 bile duct (common) (hepatic) —*see*
    Cholangitis
 bladder —*see* Cystitis
 Blastomyces, blastomycotic —*see also*
    Blastomycosis
  brasiliensis —*see* Paracoccidioidomycosis
  dermatitidis —*see* Blastomycosis
  European —*see* Cryptococcosis
  Loboi B48.0
  North American B40.9
  South American —*see*
    Paracoccidioidomycosis
 bleb, postprocedure —*see* Blebitis
 bone —*see* Osteomyelitis
 Bordetella —*see* Whooping cough
 Borrelia bergdorfi A69.20
 brain —*see also* Encephalitis G04.90
  membranes —*see* Meningitis
  septic G06.0
   meninges —*see* Meningitis, bacterial
 branchial cyst Q18.0
 breast —*see* Mastitis
 bronchus —*see* Bronchitis
 Brucella A23.9
  abortus A23.1
  canis A23.3
  melitensis A23.0
  mixed A23.8
  specified NEC A23.8
  suis A23.2
 Brugia (malayi) B74.1
  timori B74.2
 bursa —*see* Bursitis, infective
 buttocks (skin) L08.9
 Campylobacter, intestinal A04.5
  as cause of disease classified elsewhere
    B96.81
 Candida (albicans) (tropicalis) —*see*
    Candidiasis
 candiru B88.8
 Capillaria (intestinal) B81.1
  hepatica B83.8
  philippinensis B81.1
 cartilage —*see* Disorder, cartilage, specified
    type NEC
 catheter-related bloodstream (CRBSI) T80.211
 cat liver fluke B66.0
 cellulitis - code by site under Cellulitis
 central line-associated T80.219
  bloodstream (CLABSI) T80.211
  specified NEC T80.218
 Cephalosporium falciforme B47.0
 cerebrospinal —*see* Meningitis
 cervical gland (lymph) L04.0
 cervix —*see* Cervicitis
 cesarean delivery wound (puerperal) O86.0
 cestodes —*see* Infestation, cestodes
 chest J22
 Chilomastix (intestinal) A07.8
 Chlamydia, chlamydial A74.9
  anus A56.3
  genitourinary tract A56.2
   lower A56.00
   specified NEC A56.19
  lymphogranuloma A55
  pharynx A56.4
  psittaci A70
  rectum A56.3
  sexually transmitted NEC A56.8
 cholera —*see* Cholera
 Cladosporium
  bantianum (brain abscess) B43.1
  carrionii B43.0
  castellanii B36.1

Infection, infected, infective (*Continued*)
 Cladosporium (*Continued*)
  trichoides (brain abscess) B43.1
  werneckii B36.1
 Clonorchis (sinensis) (liver) B66.1
 Clostridium NEC
  bifermentans A48.0
  botulinum (food poisoning) A05.1
   infant A48.51
   wound A48.52
  difficile
   as cause of disease classified elsewhere
     B96.89
   ▸foodborne (disease)
     ▶not specified as recurrent
       A04.72
     ▶recurrent A04.71
    gas gangrene A48.0
   ▸necrotizing enterocolitis
     ▶not specified as recurrent
       A04.72
     ▶recurrent A04.71
    sepsis A41.4
  gas-forming NEC A48.0
  histolyticum A48.0
  novyi, causing gas gangrene A48.0
  oedematiens A48.0
  perfringens
   as cause of disease classified elsewhere
     B96.7
   due to food A05.2
   foodborne (disease) A05.2
   gas gangrene A48.0
   sepsis A41.4
  septicum, causing gas gangrene A48.0
  sordellii, causing gas gangrene A48.0
  welchii
   as cause of disease classified elsewhere
     B96.7
   foodborne (disease) A05.2
   gas gangrene A48.0
   necrotizing enteritis A05.2
   sepsis A41.4
 Coccidioides (immitis) —*see*
    Coccidioidomycosis
 colon —*see* Enteritis, infectious
 colostomy K94.02
 common duct —*see* Cholangitis
 congenital P39.9
  Candida (albicans) P37.5
  cytomegalovirus P35.1
  hepatitis, viral P35.3
  herpes simplex P35.2
  infectious or parasitic disease P37.9
   specified NEC P37.8
  listeriosis (disseminated) P37.2
  malaria NEC P37.4
   falciparum P37.3
  Plasmodium falciparum P37.3
  poliomyelitis P35.8
  rubella P35.0
  skin P39.4
  toxoplasmosis (acute) (subacute) (chronic)
    P37.1
  tuberculosis P37.0
  urinary (tract) P39.3
  vaccinia P35.8
  virus P35.9
   specified type NEC P35.8
 Conidiobolus B46.8
 coronavirus NEC B34.2
  as cause of disease classified elsewhere
    B97.29
  severe acute respiratory syndrome (SARS
    associated) B97.21
 corpus luteum —*see* Salpingo-oophoritis
 Corynebacterium diphtheriae —*see*
    Diphtheria
 cotia virus B08.8
 Coxiella burnetii A78
 coxsackie —*see* Coxsackie

Infection, infected, infective (*Continued*)
 Cryptococcus neoformans —*see*
    Cryptococcosis
 Cryptosporidium A07.2
 Cunninghamella —*see* Mucormycosis
 cyst —*see* Cyst
 cystic duct —*see also* Cholecystitis K81.9
 Cysticercus cellulosae —*see* Cysticercosis
 cytomegalovirus, cytomegaloviral B25.9
  congenital P35.1
  maternal, maternal care for (suspected)
    damage to fetus O35.3
  mononucleosis B27.10
   with
    complication NEC B27.19
    meningitis B27.12
    polyneuropathy B27.11
 delta-agent (acute), in hepatitis B carrier
    B17.0
 dental (pulpal origin) K04.7
 Deuteromycetes B47.0
 Dicrocoelium dendriticum B66.2
 Dipetalonema (perstans) (streptocerca) B74.4
 diphtherial —*see* Diphtheria
 Diphyllobothrium (adult) (latum) (pacificum)
    B70.0
  larval B70.1
 Diplogonoporus (grandis) B71.8
 Dipylidium caninum B67.4
 Dirofilaria B74.8
 Dracunculus medinensis B72
 Drechslera (hawaiiensis) B43.8
 Ducrey Haemophilus (any location) A57
 due to or resulting from
  artificial insemination N98.0
  central venous catheter T80.219
   bloodstream T80.211
   exit or insertion site T80.212
   localized T80.212
   port or reservoir T80.212
   specified NEC T80.218
   tunnel T80.212
  device, implant or graft —*see also*
    Complications, by site and type,
    infection or inflammation
    T85.79
   arterial graft NEC T82.7
   breast (implant) T85.79
   catheter NEC T85.79
    dialysis (renal) T82.7
     intraperitoneal T85.71
    infusion NEC T82.7
     cranial T85.735
     intrathecal T85.735
     spinal (epidural) (subdural)
       T85.735
     subarachnoid T85.735
    urinary T83.518
     cystostomy T83.510
     Hopkins T83.518
     ileostomy T83.518
     nephrostomy T83.512
     specified NEC T83.518
     urethral indwelling T83.511
     urostomy T83.518
   electronic (electrode) (pulse generator)
     (stimulator)
    bone T84.7
    cardiac T82.7
    nervous system T85.738
     brain T85.731
     cranial nerve T85.732
     gastric nerve T85.732
     generator pocket T85.734
     neurostimulator generator
       T85.734
     peripheral nerve T85.732
     sacral nerve T85.732
     spinal cord T85.733
     vagal nerve T85.732
    urinary T83.590

Infection, infected, infective *(Continued)*
  due to or resulting from *(Continued)*
    device, implant or graft *(Continued)*
      fixation, internal (orthopedic) NEC —
          see Complication, fixation device,
          infection
      gastrointestinal (bile duct) (esophagus)
          T85.79
        neurostimulator electrode (lead)
          T85.732
      genital NEC T83.69
      heart NEC T82.7
        valve (prosthesis) T82.6
        graft T82.7
      joint prosthesis —*see* Complication, joint
          prosthesis, infection
      ocular (corneal graft) (orbital implant)
          NEC T85.79
      orthopedic NEC T84.7
      penile (cylinder) (pump) (resevoir)
          T83.61
      specified NEC T85.79
      testicular T83.62
      urinary NEC T83.598
        ileal conduit stent T83.593
        implanted neurostimulation
          T83.590
        implanted sphincter T83.591
        indwelling ureteral stent T83.592
        nephroureteral stent T83.593
        specified stent NEC T83.593
      vascular NEC T82.7
      ventricular intracranial (communicating)
          shunt T85.730
    Hickman catheter T80.219
      bloodstream T80.211
      localized T80.212
      specified NEC T80.218
    immunization or vaccination T88.0
    infusion, injection or transfusion NEC
        T80.29
      acute T80.22
    injury NEC - code by site under Wound,
        open
    peripherally inserted central catheter
        (PICC) T80.219
      bloodstream T80.211
      localized T80.212
      specified NEC T80.218
    portacath (port-a-cath) T80.219
      bloodstream T80.211
      localized T80.212
      specified NEC T80.218
    pulmonary artery catheter —*see* Infection,
        due to or resulting from, central
        venous catheter
    ⇒surgery T81.4
    Swan Ganz catheter —*see* Infection, due to
        or resulting from, central venous
        catheter
    triple lumen catheter T80.219
      bloodstream T80.211
      localized T80.212
      specified NEC T80.218
    umbilical venous catheter T80.219
      bloodstream T80.211
      localized T80.212
      specified NEC T80.218
  during labor NEC O75.3
  ear (middle) —*see also* Otitis media
    external —*see* Otitis, externa, infective
    inner —*see* subcategory H83.0
  Eberthella typhosa A01.00
  Echinococcus —*see* Echinococcus
  echovirus
    as cause of disease classified elsewhere
        B97.12
    unspecified nature or site B34.1
  endocardium I33.0
  endocervix —*see* Cervicitis
  Entamoeba —*see* Amebiasis

Infection, infected, infective *(Continued)*
  enteric —*see* Enteritis, infectious
  Enterobacter sakazakii B96.89
  Enterobius vermicularis B80
  enterostomy K94.12
  enterovirus B34.1
    as cause of disease classified elsewhere
        B97.10
      coxsackievirus B97.11
      echovirus B97.12
      specified NEC B97.19
  Entomophthora B46.8
  Epidermophyton —*see* Dermatophytosis
  epididymis —*see* Epididymitis
  episiotomy (puerperal) O86.0
  Erysipelothrix (insidiosa) (rhusiopathiae) —
      see Erysipeloid
  erythema infectiosum B08.3
  Escherichia (E.) coli NEC A49.8
    as cause of disease classified elsewhere
        —*see also* Escherichia coli B96.20
    congenital P39.8
      sepsis P36.4
    generalized A41.51
    intestinal —*see* Enteritis, infectious, due to,
        Escherichia coli
  ethmoidal (chronic) (sinus) —*see* Sinusitis,
      ethmoidal
  eustachian tube (ear) —*see* Salpingitis,
      eustachian
  external auditory canal (meatus) NEC —*see*
      Otitis, externa, infective
  eye (purulent) —*see* Endophthalmitis, purulent
  eyelid —*see* Inflammation, eyelid
  fallopian tube —*see* Salpingo-oophoritis
  Fasciola (gigantica) (hepatica) (indica) B66.3
  Fasciolopsis (buski) B66.5
  filarial —*see* Infestation, filarial
  finger (skin) L08.9
    nail L03.01-●
      fungus B35.1
  fish tapeworm B70.0
    larval B70.1
  flagellate, intestinal A07.9
  fluke —*see* Infestation, fluke
  focal
    teeth (pulpal origin) K04.7
    tonsils J35.01
  Fonsecaea (compactum) (pedrosoi) B43.0
  food —*see* Intoxication, foodborne
  foot (skin) L08.9
    dermatophytic fungus B35.3
  Francisella tularensis —*see* Tularemia
  frontal (sinus) (chronic) —*see* Sinusitis, frontal
  fungus NOS B49
    beard B35.0
    dermatophytic —*see* Dermatophytosis
    foot B35.3
    groin B35.6
    hand B35.2
    nail B35.1
    pathogenic to compromised host only B48.8
    perianal (area) B35.6
    scalp B35.0
    skin B36.9
      foot B35.3
      hand B35.2
      toenails B35.1
  Fusarium B48.8
  gallbladder —*see* Cholecystitis
  gas bacillus —*see* Gangrene, gas
  gastrointestinal —*see* Enteritis, infectious
  generalized NEC —*see* Sepsis
  generator pocket, implanted electronic
      neurostimulator T85.734
  genital organ or tract
    female —*see* Disease, pelvis, inflammatory
    male N49.9
      multiple sites N49.8
      specified NEC N49.8
  Ghon tubercle, primary A15.7

Infection, infected, infective *(Continued)*
  Giardia lamblia A07.1
  gingiva (chronic) K05.10
    acute K05.00
      nonplaque induced K05.01
      plaque induced K05.00
    nonplaque induced K05.11
    plaque induced K05.10
  glanders A24.0
  glenosporopsis B48.0
  Gnathostoma (spinigerum) B83.1
  Gongylonema B83.8
  gonococcal —*see* Gonococcus
  gram-negative bacilli NOS A49.9
  guinea worm B72
  gum (chronic) K05.10
    acute K05.00
      nonplaque induced K05.01
      plaque induced K05.00
    nonplaque induced K05.11
    plaque induced K05.10
  Haemophilus —*see* Infection, Hemophilus
  heart —*see* Carditis
  Helicobacter pylori A04.8
    as cause of disease classified elsewhere
        B96.81
  helminths B83.9
    intestinal B82.0
      mixed (types classifiable to more than
          one of the titles B65.0-B81.3 and
          B81.8) B81.4
      specified type NEC B81.8
    specified type NEC B83.8
  Hemophilus
    aegyptius, systemic A48.4
    ducrey (any location) A57
    generalized A41.3
    influenzae NEC A49.2
      as cause of disease classified elsewhere
          B96.3
  herpes (simplex) —*see also* Herpes
    congenital P35.2
    disseminated B00.7
    zoster B02.9
  herpesvirus, herpesviral —*see* Herpes
  Heterophyes (heterophyes) B66.8
  hip (joint) NEC M00.9
    due to internal joint prosthesis
      left T84.52
      right T84.51
    skin NEC L08.9
  Histoplasma —*see* Histoplasmosis
    American B39.4
    capsulatum B39.4
  hookworm B76.9
  human
    papilloma virus A63.0
    T-cell lymphotropic virus type-1 (HTLV-1)
        B33.3
  hydrocele N43.0
  Hymenolepis B71.0
  hypopharynx —*see* Pharyngitis
  inguinal (lymph) glands L04.1
    due to soft chancre A57
  intervertebral disc, pyogenic M46.30
    cervical region M46.32
    cervicothoracic region M46.33
    lumbar region M46.36
    lumbosacral region M46.37
    multiple sites M46.39
    occipito-atlanto-axial region M46.31
    sacrococcygeal region M46.38
    thoracic region M46.34
    thoracolumbar region M46.35
  intestine, intestinal —*see* Enteritis, infectious
    specified NEC A08.8
  intra-amniotic affecting newborn NEC P39.2
  Isospora belli or hominis A07.3
  Japanese B encephalitis A83.0
  jaw (bone) (lower) (upper) M27.2
  joint NEC M00.9
    due to internal joint prosthesis T84.50

Infection, infected, infective *(Continued)*
  kidney (cortex) (hematogenous) N15.9
    with calculus N20.0
      with hydronephrosis N13.6
    following ectopic gestation O08.83
    pelvis and ureter (cystic) N28.85
    puerperal (postpartum) O86.21
    specified NEC N15.8
  Klebsiella (K.) pneumoniae NEC A49.8
    as cause of disease classified elsewhere B96.1
  knee (joint) NEC M00.9
    due to internal joint prosthesis
      left T84.54
      right T84.53
    joint M00.9
    skin L08.9
  Koch's —*see* Tuberculosis
  labia (majora) (minora) (acute) —*see* Vulvitis
  lacrimal
    gland —*see* Dacryoadenitis
    passages (duct) (sac) —*see* Inflammation,
      lacrimal, passages
  lancet fluke B66.2
  larynx NEC J38.7
  leg (skin) NOS L08.9
  Legionella pneumophila A48.1
    nonpneumonic A48.2
  Leishmania —*see also* Leishmaniasis
    aethiopica B55.1
    braziliensis B55.2
    chagasi B55.0
    donovani B55.0
    infantum B55.0
    major B55.1
    mexicana B55.1
    tropica B55.1
  lentivirus, as cause of disease classified
    elsewhere B97.31
  Leptosphaeria senegalensis B47.0
  Leptospira interrogans A27.9
    autumnalis A27.89
    canicola A27.89
    hebdomadis A27.89
    icterohaemorrhagiae A27.0
    pomona A27.89
    specified type NEC A27.89
  leptospirochetal NEC —*see* Leptospirosis
  Listeria monocytogenes —*see also* Listeriosis
    congenital P37.2
  Loa loa B74.3
    with conjunctival infestation B74.3
    eyelid B74.3
  Loboa loboi B48.0
  local, skin (staphylococcal) (streptococcal)
    L08.9
    abscess - code by site under Abscess
    cellulitis - code by site under Cellulitis
    specified NEC L08.89
    ulcer —*see* Ulcer, skin
  Loefflerella mallei A24.0
  lung —*see also* Pneumonia J18.9
    atypical Mycobacterium A31.0
    spirochetal A69.8
    tuberculous —*see* Tuberculosis, pulmonary
    virus —*see* Pneumonia, viral
  lymph gland —*see also* Lymphadenitis, acute
    mesenteric I88.0
  lymphoid tissue, base of tongue or posterior
    pharynx, NEC (chronic) J35.03
  Madurella (grisea) (mycetomii) B47.0
  major
    following ectopic or molar pregnancy O08.0
    puerperal, postpartum, childbirth O85
  Malassezia furfur B36.0
  Malleomyces
    mallei A24.0
    pseudomallei (whitmori) —*see* Melioidosis
    mammary gland N61.0
  Mansonella (ozzardi) (perstans) (streptocerca)
    B74.4
  mastoid —*see* Mastoiditis

Infection, infected, infective *(Continued)*
  maxilla, maxillary M27.2
    sinus (chronic) —*see* Sinusitis, maxillary
  mediastinum J98.51
  Medina (worm) B72
  meibomian cyst or gland —*see* Hordeolum
  meninges —*see* Meningitis, bacterial
  meningococcal —*see also* condition A39.9
    adrenals A39.1
    brain A39.81
    cerebrospinal A39.0
    conjunctiva A39.89
    endocardium A39.51
    heart A39.50
      endocardium A39.51
      myocardium A39.52
      pericardium A39.53
    joint A39.83
    meninges A39.0
    meningococcemia A39.4
      acute A39.2
      chronic A39.3
    myocardium A39.52
    pericardium A39.53
    retrobulbar neuritis A39.82
    specified site NEC A39.89
  mesenteric lymph nodes or glands NEC I88.0
  Metagonimus B66.8
  metatarsophalangeal M00.9
  methicillin
    resistant Staphylococcus aureus (MRSA)
      A49.02
    susceptible Staphylococcus aureus (MSSA)
      A49.01
  Microsporum, microsporic —*see*
    Dermatophytosis
  mixed flora (bacterial) NEC A49.8
  Monilia —*see* Candidiasis
  Monosporium apiospermum B48.2
  mouth, parasitic B37.0
  Mucor —*see* Mucormycosis
  muscle NEC —*see* Myositis, infective
  mycelium NOS B49
  mycetoma B47.9
    actinomycotic NEC B47.1
    mycotic NEC B47.0
  Mycobacterium, mycobacterial —*see*
    Mycobacterium
  Mycoplasma NEC A49.3
    pneumoniae, as cause of disease classified
      elsewhere B96.0
  mycotic NOS B49
    pathogenic to compromised host only B48.8
    skin NOS B36.9
  myocardium NEC I40.0
  nail (chronic)
    with lymphangitis —*see* Lymphangitis,
      acute, digit
    finger L03.01-●
      fungus B35.1
    ingrowing L60.0
    toe L03.03-●
      fungus B35.1
  nasal sinus (chronic) —*see* Sinusitis
  nasopharynx —*see* Nasopharyngitis
  navel L08.82
  Necator americanus B76.1
  Neisseria —*see* Gonococcus
  Neotestudina rosatii B47.0
  newborn P39.9
    intra-amniotic NEC P39.2
    skin P39.4
    specified type NEC P39.8
  nipple N61.0
    associated with
      lactation O91.03
      pregnancy O91.01-●
      puerperium O91.02
  Nocardia —*see* Nocardiosis
  obstetrical surgical wound (puerperal) O86.0
  Oesophagostomum (apiostomum) B81.8

Infection, infected, infective *(Continued)*
  Oestrus ovis —*see* Myiasis
  Oidium albicans B37.9
  Onchocerca (volvulus) —*see* Onchocerciasis -
    oncovirus, as cause of disease classified
      elsewhere B97.32
  operation wound T81.4
  Opisthorchis (felineus) (viverrini) B66.0
  orbit, orbital —*see* Inflammation, orbit
  orthopoxvirus NEC B08.09
  ovary —*see* Salpingo-oophoritis
  Oxyuris vermicularis B80
  pancreas (acute) —*see* Pancreatitis, acute
    abscess —*see* Pancreatitis, acute
      specified NEC —*see also* Pancreatitis, acute
        K85.80
  papillomavirus, as cause of disease classified
    elsewhere B97.7
  papovavirus NEC B34.4
  Paracoccidioides brasiliensis —*see*
    Paracoccidioidomycosis
  Paragonimus (westermani) B66.4
  parainfluenza virus B34.8
  parameningococcus NOS A39.9
  paramyxovirus NEC B34.3
  parapoxvirus B08.60
    specified NEC B08.69
  parasitic B89
  Parastrongylus
    cantonensis B83.2
    costaricensis B81.3
    paratyphoid A01.4
      Type A A01.1
      Type B A01.2
      Type C A01.3
  paraurethral ducts N34.2
  parotid gland —*see* Sialoadenitis
  parvovirus NEC B34.3
    as cause of disease classified elsewhere B97.6
  Pasteurella NEC A28.0
    multocida A28.0
    pestis —*see* Plague
    pseudotuberculosis A28.0
    septica (cat bite) (dog bite) A28.0
    tularensis —*see* Tularemia
  pelvic, female —*see* Disease, pelvis,
    inflammatory
  Penicillium (marneffei) B48.4
  penis (glans) (retention) NEC N48.29
  periapical K04.5
  peridental, periodontal K05.20
    generalized —*see* Peridontitis, aggressive,
      generalized
    localized —*see* Peridontitis, aggressive,
      localized
  perinatal period P39.9
    specified type NEC P39.8
  perineal repair (puerperal) O86.0
  periorbital —*see* Inflammation, orbit
  perirectal K62.89
  perirenal —*see* Infection, kidney
  peritoneal —*see* Peritonitis
  periureteral N28.89
  Petriellidium boydii B48.2
  pharynx —*see also* Pharyngitis
    coxsackievirus B08.5
    posterior, lymphoid (chronic) J35.03
  Phialophora
    gougerotii (subcutaneous abscess or cyst)
      B43.2
    jeanselmei (subcutaneous abscess or cyst)
      B43.2
    verrucosa (skin) B43.0
  Piedraia hortae B36.3
  pinta A67.9
    intermediate A67.1
    late A67.2
    mixed A67.3
    primary A67.0
  pinworm B80
  pityrosporum furfur B36.0
  pleuro-pneumonia-like organism (PPLO)
    NEC A49.3
    as cause of disease classified elsewhere B96.0

Infection, infected, infective (Continued)
  pneumococcus, pneumococcal NEC A49.1
    as cause of disease classified elsewhere B95.3
    generalized (purulent) A40.3
      with pneumonia J13
  Pneumocystis carinii (pneumonia) B59
  Pneumocystis jiroveci (pneumonia) B59
  port or reservoir T80.212
  ➡postoperative T81.4
  ➡postoperative wound T81.4
  ➡postprocedural T81.4
    ~~deep incisional surgical site T81.42~~
    ~~organ and space surgical site T81.43~~
    ~~sepsis T81.49~~
    ~~specified surgical site NEC T81.48~~
    ~~superficial incisional surgical site T81.41~~
  postvaccinal T88.0
  prepuce NEC N47.7
    with penile inflammation N47.6
  prion —see Disease, prion, central nervous system
  prostate (capsule) —see Prostatitis
  Proteus (mirabilis) (morganii) (vulgaris) NEC A49.8
    as cause of disease classified elsewhere B96.4
  protozoal NEC B64
    intestinal A07.9
      specified NEC A07.8
    specified NEC B60.8
  Pseudoallescheria boydii B48.2
  Pseudomonas NEC A49.8
    as cause of disease classified elsewhere B96.5
    mallei A24.0
    pneumonia J15.1
    pseudomallei —see Melioidosis
  puerperal O86.4
    genitourinary tract NEC O86.89
    major or generalized O85
    minor O86.4
    specified NEC O86.89
  pulmonary —see Infection, lung
  purulent —see Abscess
  Pyrenochaeta romeroi B47.0
  Q fever A78
  rectum (sphincter) K62.89
  renal —see also Infection, kidney
    pelvis and ureter (cystic) N28.85
  reovirus, as cause of disease classified elsewhere B97.5
  respiratory (tract) NEC J98.8
    acute J22
    chronic J98.8
    influenzal (upper) (acute) —see Influenza, with, respiratory manifestations NEC
    lower (acute) J22
      chronic —see Bronchitis, chronic
    rhinovirus J00
    syncytial virus, as cause of disease classified elsewhere B97.4
    upper (acute) NOS J06.9
      chronic J39.8
      streptococcal J06.9
      viral NOS J06.9
  resulting from
    presence of internal prosthesis, implant, graft —see Complications, by site and type, infection
  retortamoniasis A07.8
  retroperitoneal NEC K68.9
  retrovirus B33.3
    as cause of disease classified elsewhere B97.30
    human
      immunodeficiency, type 2 (HIV 2) B97.35
      T-cell lymphotropic
        type I (HTLV-I) B97.33
        type II (HTLV-II) B97.34
    lentivirus B97.31
    oncovirus B97.32
    specified NEC B97.39
  Rhinosporidium (seeberi) B48.1

Infection, infected, infective (Continued)
  rhinovirus
    as cause of disease classified elsewhere B97.89
    unspecified nature or site B34.8
  Rhizopus —see Mucormycosis
  rickettsial NOS A79.9
  roundworm (large) NEC B82.0
    Ascariasis —see also Ascariasis B77.9
  rubella —see Rubella
  Saccharomyces —see Candidiasis
  salivary duct or gland (any) —see Sialoadenitis
  Salmonella (aertrycke) (arizonae) (callinarum) (cholerae-suis) (enteritidis) (suipestifer) (typhimurium) A02.9
    with
      (gastro) enteritis A02.0
      sepsis A02.1
      specified manifestation NEC A02.8
    due to food (poisoning) A02.9
    hirschfeldii A01.3
    localized A02.20
      arthritis A02.23
      meningitis A02.21
      osteomyelitis A02.24
      pneumonia A02.22
      pyelonephritis A02.25
      specified NEC A02.29
    paratyphi A01.4
      A A01.1
      B A01.2
      C A01.3
    schottmuelleri A01.2
    typhi, typhosa —see Typhoid
  Sarcocystis A07.8
  scabies B86
  Schistosoma —see Infestation, Schistosoma
  scrotum (acute) NEC N49.2
  seminal vesicle —see Vesiculitis
  septic
    localized, skin —see Abscess
  sheep liver fluke B66.3
  Shigella A03.9
    boydii A03.2
    dysenteriae A03.0
    flexneri A03.1
    group
      A A03.0
      B A03.1
      C A03.2
      D A03.3
    Schmitz (-Stutzer) A03.0
    schmitzii A03.0
    shigae A03.0
    sonnei A03.3
    specified NEC A03.8
  shoulder (joint) NEC M00.9
    due to internal joint prosthesis T84.59
    skin NEC L08.9
  sinus (accessory) (chronic) (nasal) —see also Sinusitis
    pilonidal —see Sinus, pilonidal
    skin NEC L08.89
  Skene's duct or gland —see Urethritis
  skin (local) (staphylococcal) (streptococcal) L08.9
    abscess - code by site under Abscess
    cellulitis - code by site under Cellulitis
    due to fungus B36.9
      specified type NEC B36.8
    mycotic B36.9
      specified type NEC B36.8
    newborn P39.4
    ulcer —see Ulcer, skin
  slow virus A81.9
    specified NEC A81.89
  Sparganum (mansoni) (proliferum) (baxteri) B70.1
  specific —see also Syphilis
    to perinatal period —see Infection, congenital

Infection, infected, infective (Continued)
  specified NEC B99.8
  spermatic cord NEC N49.1
  sphenoidal (sinus) —see Sinusitis, sphenoidal
  spinal cord NOS —see also Myelitis G04.91
    abscess G06.1
    meninges —see Meningitis
    streptococcal G04.89
  Spirillum A25.0
  spirochetal NOS A69.9
    lung A69.8
    specified NEC A69.8
  Spirometra larvae B70.1
  spleen D73.89
  Sporotrichum, Sporothrix (schenckii) —see Sporotrichosis
  staphylococcal, unspecified site
    aureus (methicillin susceptible) (MSSA) A49.01
      methicillin resistant (MRSA) A49.02
    as cause of disease classified elsewhere B95.8
      aureus (methicillin susceptible) (MSSA) B95.61
        methicillin resistant (MRSA) B95.62
      specified NEC B95.7
    food poisoning A05.0
    generalized (purulent) A41.2
    pneumonia —see Pneumonia, staphylococcal
  Stellantchasmus falcatus B66.8
  streptobacillus moniliformis A25.1
  streptococcal NEC A49.1
    as cause of disease classified elsewhere B95.5
    B genitourinary complicating
      childbirth O98.82
      pregnancy O98.81-●
      puerperium O98.83
    congenital
      sepsis P36.10
        group B P36.0
        specified NEC P36.19
    generalized (purulent) A40.9
  Streptomyces B47.1
  Strongyloides (stercoralis) —see Strongyloidiasis
  stump (amputation) (surgical) —see Complication, amputation stump, infection
  subcutaneous tissue, local L08.9
  suipestifer —see Infection, salmonella
  swimming pool bacillus A31.1
  Taenia —see Infestation, Taenia
  Taeniarhynchus saginatus B68.1
  tapeworm —see Infestation, tapeworm
  tendon (sheath) —see Tenosynovitis, infective NEC
  Ternidens diminutus B81.8
  testis —see Orchitis
  threadworm B80
  throat —see Pharyngitis
  thyroglossal duct K14.8
  toe (skin) L08.9
    cellulitis L03.03-●
      fungus B35.1
    nail L03.03-●
      fungus B35.1
  tongue NEC K14.0
    parasitic B37.0
  tonsil (and adenoid) (faucial) (lingual) (pharyngeal) —see Tonsillitis
  tooth, teeth K04.7
    irreversible K04.02
    periapical K04.7
    peridental, periodontal K05.20
      generalized —see Peridontitis, aggressive, generalized
      localized —see Peridontitis, aggressive, localized

Infection, infected, infective (Continued)
  tooth, teeth (Continued)
    pulp K04.01
      ▶irreversible K04.02
      ▶reversible K04.01
      ~~reversible K04.01~~
      ~~socket M27.3~~
  TORCH —see Infection, congenital
    without active infection P00.2
  Torula histolytica —see Cryptococcosis
  Toxocara (canis) (cati) (felis) B83.0
  Toxoplasma gondii —see Toxoplasma
  trachea, chronic J42
  trematode NEC —see Infestation, fluke
  trench fever A79.0
  Treponema pallidum —see Syphilis
  Trichinella (spiralis) B75
  Trichomonas A59.9
    cervix A59.09
    intestine A07.8
    prostate A59.02
    specified site NEC A59.8
    urethra A59.03
    urogenitalis A59.00
    vagina A59.01
    vulva A59.01
  Trichophyton, trichophytic —see
    Dermatophytosis
  Trichosporon (beigelii) cutaneum B36.2
  Trichostrongylus B81.2
  Trichuris (trichiura) B79
  Trombicula (irritans) B88.0
  Trypanosoma
    brucei
      gambiense B56.0
      rhodesiense B56.1
    cruzi —see Chagas' disease
  tubal —see Salpingo-oophoritis
  tuberculous NEC —see Tuberculosis
  tubo-ovarian —see Salpingo-oophoritis
  tunica vaginalis N49.1
  tunnel T80.212
  tympanic membrane NEC —see Myringitis
  typhoid (abortive) (ambulant) (bacillus) —see
    Typhoid
  typhus A75.9
    flea-borne A75.2
    mite-borne A75.3
    recrudescent A75.1
    tick-borne A77.9
      African A77.1
      North Asian A77.2
  umbilicus L08.82
  ureter N28.86
  urethra —see Urethritis
  urinary (tract) N39.0
    bladder —see Cystitis
    complicating
      pregnancy O23.4-●
        specified type NEC O23.3-●
    kidney —see Infection, kidney
    newborn P39.3
    puerperal (postpartum) O86.20
    tuberculous A18.13
    urethra —see Urethritis
  uterus, uterine —see Endometritis
  vaccination T88.0
  vaccinia not from vaccination B08.011
  vagina (acute) —see Vaginitis
  varicella B01.9
  varicose veins —see Varix
  vas deferens NEC N49.1
  vesical —see Cystitis
  Vibrio
    cholerae A00.0
      El Tor A00.1
    parahaemolyticus (food poisoning) A05.3
    vulnificus
      as cause of disease classified elsewhere
        B96.82
      foodborne intoxication A05.5
  Vincent's (gum) (mouth) (tonsil) A69.1

Infection, infected, infective (Continued)
  virus, viral NOS B34.9
    adenovirus
      as cause of disease classified elsewhere
        B97.0
      unspecified nature or site B34.0
    arbovirus, arbovirus arthropod-borne A94
    as cause of disease classified elsewhere
      B97.89
      adenovirus B97.0
      coronavirus B97.29
        SARS-associated B97.21
      coxsackievirus B97.11
      echovirus B97.12
      enterovirus B97.10
        coxsackievirus B97.11
        echovirus B97.12
        specified NEC B97.19
      human
        immunodeficiency, type 2 (HIV 2)
          B97.35
        metapneumovirus B97.81
        T-cell lymphotropic,
          type I (HTLV-I) B97.33
          type II (HTLV-II) B97.34
      papillomavirus B97.7
      parvovirus B97.6
      reovirus B97.5
      respiratory syncytial B97.4
      retrovirus B97.30
        human
          immunodeficiency, type 2 (HIV 2)
            B97.35
          T-cell lymphotropic,
            type I (HTLV-I) B97.33
            type II (HTLV-II) B97.34
        lentivirus B97.31
        oncovirus B97.32
        specified NEC B97.39
      specified NEC B97.89
    central nervous system A89
      atypical A81.9
        specified NEC A81.89
      enterovirus NEC A88.8
        meningitis A87.0
      slow virus A81.9
        specified NEC A81.89
      specified NEC A88.8
    chest J98.8
    cotia B08.8
    coxsackie —see also Infection, coxsackie B34.1
      as cause of disease classified elsewhere
        B97.11
    ECHO
      as cause of disease classified elsewhere
        B97.12
      unspecified nature or site B34.1
    encephalitis, tick-borne A84.9
    enterovirus, as cause of disease classified
      elsewhere B97.10
      coxsackievirus B97.11
      echovirus B97.12
      specified NEC B97.19
    exanthem NOS B09
    human metapneumovirus as cause of
      disease classified elsewhere B97.81
    human papilloma as cause of disease
      classified elsewhere B97.7
    intestine —see Enteritis, viral
    respiratory syncytial
      as cause of disease classified elsewhere
        B97.4
      bronchopneumonia J12.1
      common cold syndrome J00
      nasopharyngitis (acute) J00
    rhinovirus
      as cause of disease classified elsewhere
        B97.89
      unspecified nature or site B34.8
    slow A81.9
      specified NEC A81.89

Infection, infected, infective (Continued)
  virus, viral NOS (Continued)
    specified type NEC B33.8
      as cause of disease classified elsewhere
        B97.89
      unspecified nature or site B34.8
    unspecified nature or site B34.9
    West Nile —see Virus, West Nile
  vulva (acute) —see Vulvitis
  West Nile —see Virus, West Nile
  whipworm B79
  worms B83.9
    specified type NEC B83.8
  Wuchereria (bancrofti) B74.0
    malayi B74.1
    yatapoxvirus B08.70
      specified NEC B08.79
  yeast (see also Candidiasis) B37.9
  yellow fever —see Fever, yellow
  Yersinia
    enterocolitica (intestinal) A04.6
    pestis —see Plague
    pseudotuberculosis A28.2
  Zeis' gland —see Hordeolum
  Zika virus A92.5
  zoonotic bacterial NOS A28.9
  Zopfia senegalensis B47.0
Infective, infectious —see condition
Infertility
  female N97.9
    age-related N97.8
    associated with
      anovulation N97.0
      cervical (mucus) disease or anomaly
        N88.3
      congenital anomaly
        cervix N88.3
        fallopian tube N97.1
        uterus N97.2
        vagina N97.8
      dysmucorrhea N88.3
      fallopian tube disease or anomaly N97.1
      pituitary-hypothalamic origin E23.0
      specified origin NEC N97.8
      Stein-Leventhal syndrome E28.2
      uterine disease or anomaly N97.2
      vaginal disease or anomaly N97.8
    due to
      cervical anomaly N88.3
      fallopian tube anomaly N97.1
      ovarian failure E28.39
      Stein-Leventhal syndrome E28.2
      uterine anomaly N97.2
      vaginal anomaly N97.8
    nonimplantation N97.2
    origin
      cervical N88.3
      tubal (block) (occlusion) (stenosis) N97.1
      uterine N97.2
      vaginal N97.8
  male N46.9
    azoospermia N46.01
      extratesticular cause N46.029
        drug therapy N46.021
        efferent duct obstruction N46.023
        infection N46.022
        radiation N46.024
        specified cause NEC N46.029
        systemic disease N46.025
    oligospermia N46.11
      extratesticular cause N46.129
        drug therapy N46.121
        efferent duct obstruction N46.123
        infection N46.122
        radiation N46.124
        specified cause NEC N46.129
        systemic disease N46.125
    specified type NEC N46.8
Infestation B88.9
  Acanthocheilonema (perstans) (streptocerca)
    B74.4

▶ New   ⟹ Revised   ~~deleted~~ Deleted   ● Use Additional Character(s)

Infestation *(Continued)*
  Acariasis B88.Ø
    demodex folliculorum B88.Ø
    sarcoptes scabiei B86
    trombiculae B88.Ø
  Agamofilaria streptocerca B74.4
  Ancylostoma, ankylostoma (braziliense)
      (caninum) (ceylanicum) (duodenale)
      B76.Ø
    americanum B76.1
    new world B76.1
  Anisakis larvae, anisakiasis B81.Ø
  arthropod NEC B88.2
  Ascaris lumbricoides —*see* Ascariasis
  Balantidium coli AØ7.Ø
  beef tapeworm B68.1
  Bothriocephalus (latus) B7Ø.Ø
    larval B7Ø.1
  broad tapeworm B7Ø.Ø
    larval B7Ø.1
  Brugia (malayi) B74.1
    timori B74.2
  candiru B88.8
  Capillaria
    hepatica B83.8
    philippinensis B81.1
  cat liver fluke B66.Ø
  cestodes B71.9
    diphyllobothrium —*see* Infestation,
        diphyllobothrium
    dipylidiasis B71.1
    hymenolepiasis B71.Ø
    specified type NEC B71.8
  chigger B88.Ø
  chigo, chigoe B88.1
  Clonorchis (sinensis) (liver) B66.1
  coccidial AØ7.3
  crab-lice B85.3
  Cysticercus cellulosae —*see* Cysticercosis
  Demodex (folliculorum) B88.Ø
  Dermanyssus gallinae B88.Ø
  Dermatobia (hominis) —*see* Myiasis
  Dibothriocephalus (latus) B7Ø.Ø
    larval B7Ø.1
  Dicrocoelium dendriticum B66.2
  Diphyllobothrium (adult) (latum) (intestinal)
      (pacificum) B7Ø.Ø
    larval B7Ø.1
  Diplogonoporus (grandis) B71.8
  Dipylidium caninum B67.4
  Distoma hepaticum B66.3
  dog tapeworm B67.4
  Dracunculus medinensis B72
  dragon worm B72
  dwarf tapeworm B71.Ø
  Echinococcus —*see* Echinococcus
  Echinostomum ilocanum B66.8
  Entamoeba (histolytica) —*see* Infection,
      Ameba
  Enterobius vermicularis B8Ø
  eyelid
    in (due to)
      leishmaniasis B55.1
      loiasis B74.3
      onchocerciasis B73.Ø9
      phthiriasis B85.3
      parasitic NOS B89
  eyeworm B74.3
  Fasciola (gigantica) (hepatica) (indica) B66.3
  Fasciolopsis (buski) (intestine) B66.5
  filarial B74.9
    bancroftian B74.Ø
    conjunctiva B74.9
    due to
      Acanthocheilonema (perstans)
          (streptocerca) B74.4
      Brugia (malayi) B74.1
        timori B74.2
      Dracunculus medinensis B72
      guinea worm B72
      loa loa B74.3

Infestation *(Continued)*
  filarial *(Continued)*
    due to *(Continued)*
      Mansonella (ozzardi) (perstans)
          (streptocerca) B74.4
      Onchocerca volvulus B73.ØØ
        eye B73.ØØ
        eyelid B73.Ø9
      Wuchereria (bancrofti) B74.Ø
    Malayan B74.1
    ozzardi B74.4
    specified type NEC B74.8
  fish tapeworm B7Ø.Ø
    larval B7Ø.1
  fluke B66.9
    blood NOS —*see* Schistosomiasis
    cat liver B66.Ø
    intestinal B66.5
    lancet B66.2
    liver (sheep) B66.3
      cat B66.Ø
      Chinese B66.1
      due to clonorchiasis B66.1
      oriental B66.1
    lung (oriental) B66.4
    sheep liver B66.3
    specified type NEC B66.8
  fly larvae —*see* Myiasis
  Gasterophilus (intestinalis) —*see* Myiasis
  Gastrodiscoides hominis B66.8
  Giardia lamblia AØ7.1
  Gnathostoma (spinigerum) B83.1
  Gongylonema B83.8
  guinea worm B72
  helminth B83.9
    angiostrongyliasis B83.2
      intestinal B81.3
    gnathostomiasis B83.1
    hirudiniasis, internal B83.4
    intestinal B82.Ø
      angiostrongyliasis B81.3
      anisakiasis B81.Ø
      ascariasis —*see* Ascariasis
      capillariasis B81.1
      cysticercosis —*see* Cysticercosis
      diphyllobothriasis —*see* Infestation,
          diphyllobothriasis
      dracunculiasis B72
      echinococcus —*see* Echinococcosis
      enterobiasis B8Ø
      filariasis —*see* Infestation, filarial
      fluke —*see* Infestation, fluke
      hookworm —*see* Infestation, hookworm
      mixed (types classifiable to more than
          one of the titles B65.Ø-B81.3 and
          B81.8) B81.4
      onchocerciasis —*see* Onchocerciasis
      schistosomiasis —*see* Infestation,
          schistosoma
      specified
        cestode NEC —*see* Infestation, cestode
            type NEC B81.8
        strongyloidiasis —*see* Strongyloidiasis
        taenia —*see* Infestation, taenia
      trichinellosis B75
      trichostrongyliasis B81.2
      trichuriasis B79
    specified type NEC B83.8
    syngamiasis B83.3
    visceral larva migrans B83.Ø
  Heterophyes (heterophyes) B66.8
  hookworm B76.9
    ancylostomiasis B76.Ø
    necatoriasis B76.1
    specified type NEC B76.8
  Hymenolepis (diminuta) (nana) B71.Ø
  intestinal NEC B82.9
  leeches (aquatic) (land) —*see* Hirudiniasis
  Leishmania —*see* Leishmaniasis
  lice, louse —*see* Infestation, Pediculus
  Linguatula B88.8

Infestation *(Continued)*
  Liponyssoides sanguineus B88.Ø
  Loa loa B74.3
    conjunctival B74.3
    eyelid B74.3
  louse —*see* Infestation, Pediculus
  maggots —*see* Myiasis
  Mansonella (ozzardi) (perstans) (streptocerca)
      B74.4
  Medina (worm) B72
  Metagonimus (yokogawai) B66.8
  microfilaria streptocerca —*see* Onchocerciasis
    eye B73.ØØ
    eyelid B73.Ø9
  mites B88.9
    scabic B86
  Monilia (albicans) —*see* Candidiasis
  mouth B37.Ø
  Necator americanus B76.1
  nematode NEC (intestinal) B82.Ø
    Ancylostoma B76.Ø
    conjunctiva NEC B83.9
    Enterobius vermicularis B8Ø
    Gnathostoma spinigerum B83.1
    physaloptera B8Ø
    specified NEC B81.8
    trichostrongylus B81.2
    trichuris (trichuria) B79
  Oesophagostomum (apiostomum) B81.8
  Oestrus ovis —*see also* Myiasis B87.9
  Onchocerca (volvulus) —*see* Onchocerciasis
  Opisthorchis (felineus) (viverrini) B66.Ø
  orbit, parasitic NOS B89
  Oxyuris vermicularis B8Ø
  Paragonimus (westermani) B66.4
  parasite, parasitic B89
    eyelid B89
    intestinal NOS B82.9
    mouth B37.Ø
    skin B88.9
    tongue B37.Ø
  Parastrongylus
    cantonensis B83.2
    costaricensis B81.3
  Pediculus B85.2
    body B85.1
    capitis (humanus) (any site) B85.Ø
    corporis (humanus) (any site) B85.1
    head B85.Ø
    mixed (classifiable to more than one of the
        titles B85.Ø-B85.3) B85.4
    pubis (any site) B85.3
  Pentastoma B88.8
  Phthirus (pubis) (any site) B85.3
    with any infestation classifiable to
        B85.Ø-B85.2 B85.4
  pinworm B8Ø
  pork tapeworm (adult) B68.Ø
  protozoal NEC B64
    intestinal AØ7.9
      specified NEC AØ7.8
    specified NEC B6Ø.8
  pubic, louse B85.3
  rat tapeworm B71.Ø
  red bug B88.Ø
  roundworm (large) NEC B82.Ø
    Ascariasis —*see also* Ascariasis B77.9
  sandflea B88.1
  Sarcoptes scabiei B86
  scabies B86
  Schistosoma B65.9
    bovis B65.8
    cercariae B65.3
    haematobium B65.Ø
    intercalatum B65.8
    japonicum B65.2
    mansoni B65.1
    mattheei B65.8
    mekongi B65.8
    specified type NEC B65.8
    spindale B65.8

▶ New   ⇒ Revised   ~~deleted~~ Deleted   ● Use Additional Character(s)

Infestation (Continued)
  screw worms —see Myiasis
  skin NOS B88.9
  Sparganum (mansoni) (proliferum) (baxteri) B70.1
    larval B70.1
  specified type NEC B88.8
  Spirometra larvae B70.1
  Stellantchasmus falcatus B66.8
  Strongyloides stercoralis —see Strongyloidiasis
  Taenia B68.9
    diminuta B71.0
    echinococcus —see Echinococcus
    mediocanellata B68.1
    nana B71.0
    saginata B68.1
    solium (intestinal form) B68.0
      larval form —see Cysticercosis
  Taeniarhynchus saginatus B68.1
  tapeworm B71.9
    beef B68.1
    broad B70.0
      larval B70.1
    dog B67.4
    dwarf B71.0
    fish B70.0
      larval B70.1
    pork B68.0
    rat B71.0
  Ternidens diminutus B81.8
  Tetranychus molestissimus B88.0
  threadworm B80
  tongue B37.0
  Toxocara (canis) (cati) (felis) B83.0
  trematode(s) NEC —see Infestation, fluke
  Trichinella (spiralis) B75
  Trichocephalus B79
  Trichomonas —see Trichomoniasis
  Trichostrongylus B81.2
  Trichuris (trichiura) B79
  Trombicula (irritans) B88.0
  Tunga penetrans B88.1
  Uncinaria americana B76.1
  Vandellia cirrhosa B88.8
  whipworm B79
  worms B83.9
    intestinal B82.0
  Wuchereria (bancrofti) B74.0
Infiltrate, infiltration
  amyloid (generalized) (localized) —see Amyloidosis
  calcareous NEC R89.7
    localized —see Degeneration, by site
  calcium salt R89.7
  cardiac
    fatty —see Degeneration, myocardial
    glycogenic E74.02 [I43]
  corneal —see Edema, cornea
  eyelid —see Inflammation, eyelid
  glycogen, glycogenic —see Disease, glycogen storage
  heart, cardiac
    fatty —see Degeneration, myocardial
    glycogenic E74.02 [I43]
  inflammatory in vitreous H43.89
  kidney N28.89
  leukemic —see Leukemia
  liver K76.89
    fatty —see Fatty, liver NEC
    glycogen —see also Disease, glycogen storage E74.03 [K77]
  lung R91.8
    eosinophilic J82
  lymphatic —see also Leukemia, lymphatic C91.9-●
    gland I88.9
  muscle, fatty M62.89
  myocardium, myocardial
    fatty —see Degeneration, myocardial
    glycogenic E74.02 [I43]

Infiltrate, infiltration (Continued)
  on chest x-ray R91.8
  pulmonary R91.8
    with eosinophilia J82
  skin (lymphocytic) L98.6
  thymus (gland) (fatty) E32.8
  urine R39.0
  vesicant agent
    antineoplastic chemotherapy T80.810
    other agent NEC T80.818
  vitreous body H43.89
Infirmity R68.89
  senile R54
Inflammation, inflamed, inflammatory (with exudation)
  abducent (nerve) —see Strabismus, paralytic, sixth nerve
  accessory sinus (chronic) —see Sinusitis
  adrenal (gland) E27.8
  alveoli, teeth M27.3
    scorbutic E54
  anal canal, anus K62.89
  antrum (chronic) —see Sinusitis, maxillary
  appendix —see Appendicitis
  arachnoid —see Meningitis
  areola N61.0
    puerperal, postpartum or gestational —see Infection, nipple
  areolar tissue NOS L08.9
  artery —see Arteritis
  auditory meatus (external) —see Otitis, externa
  Bartholin's gland N75.8
  bile duct (common) (hepatic) or passage —see Cholangitis
  bladder —see Cystitis
  bone —see Osteomyelitis
  brain —see also Encephalitis
    membrane —see Meningitis
  breast N61.0
    puerperal, postpartum, gestational —see Mastitis, obstetric
  broad ligament —see Disease, pelvis, inflammatory
  bronchi —see Bronchitis
  catarrhal J00
  cecum —see Appendicitis
  cerebral —see also Encephalitis
    membrane —see Meningitis
  cerebrospinal
    meningococcal A39.0
  cervix (uteri) —see Cervicitis
  chest J98.8
  chorioretinal H30.9-●
    cyclitis —see Cyclitis
    disseminated H30.10-●
      generalized H30.13-●
      peripheral H30.12-●
      posterior pole H30.11-●
    epitheliopathy —see Epitheliopathy
    focal H30.00-●
      juxtapapillary H30.01-●
      macular H30.04-●
      paramacular —see Inflammation, chorioretinal, focal, macular
      peripheral H30.03-●
      posterior pole H30.02-●
    specified type NEC H30.89-●
  choroid —see Inflammation, chorioretinal
  chronic, postmastoidectomy cavity —see Complications, postmastoidectomy, inflammation
  colon —see Enteritis
  connective tissue (diffuse) NEC —see Disorder, soft tissue, specified type NEC
  cornea —see Keratitis
  corpora cavernosa N48.29
  cranial nerve —see Disorder, nerve, cranial
  Douglas' cul-de-sac or pouch (chronic) N73.0

Inflammation, inflamed, inflammatory (Continued)
  due to device, implant or graft —see also Complications, by site and type, infection or inflammation
    arterial graft T82.7
    breast (implant) T85.79
    catheter T85.79
      dialysis (renal) T82.7
        intraperitoneal T85.71
      infusion T82.7
        cranial T85.735
        intrathecal T85.735
        spinal (epidural) (subdural) T85.735
        subarachnoid T85.735
      urinary T83.518
        cystostomy T83.510
        Hopkins T83.518
        ileostomy T83.518
        nephrostomy T83.512
        specified NEC T83.518
        urethral indwelling T83.511
        urostomy T83.518
    electronic (electrode) (pulse generator) (stimulator)
      bone T84.7
      cardiac T82.7
      nervous system T85.738
        brain T85.731
        cranial nerve T85.732
        gastric nerve T85.732
        neurostimulator generator T85.734
        peripheral nerve T85.732
        sacral nerve T85.732
        spinal cord T85.733
        vagal nerve T85.732
      urinary T83.590
    fixation, internal (orthopedic) NEC — see Complication, fixation device, infection
    gastrointestinal (bile duct) (esophagus) T85.79
      neurostimulator electrode (lead) T85.732
    genital NEC T83.69
    heart NEC T82.7
      valve (prosthesis) T82.6
        graft T82.7
    joint prosthesis —see Complication, joint prosthesis, infection
    ocular (corneal graft) (orbital implant) NEC T85.79
    orthopedic NEC T84.7
    penile (cylinder) (pump) (resevoir) T83.61
    specified NEC T85.79
    testicular T83.62
    urinary NEC T83.598
      ileal conduit stent T83.593
      implanted neurostimulation T83.590
      implanted sphincter T83.591
      indwelling ureteral stent T83.592
      nephroureteral stent T83.593
      specified stent NEC T83.593
    vascular NEC T82.7
    ventricular intracranial (communicating) shunt T85.730
  duodenum K29.80
    with bleeding K29.81
  dura mater —see Meningitis
  ear (middle) —see also Otitis, media
    external —see Otitis, externa
    inner —see subcategory H83.0
  epididymis —see Epididymitis
  esophagus K20.9
  ethmoidal (sinus) (chronic) —see Sinusitis, ethmoidal
  eustachian tube (catarrhal) —see Salpingitis, eustachian

Inflammation, inflamed, inflammatory
(Continued)
eyelid H01.9
    abscess —see Abscess, eyelid
    blepharitis —see Blepharitis
    chalazion —see Chalazion
    dermatosis (noninfectious) —see
        Dermatosis, eyelid
    hordeolum —see Hordeolum
    specified NEC H01.8
fallopian tube —see Salpingo-oophoritis
fascia —see Myositis
follicular, pharynx J31.2
frontal (sinus) (chronic) —see Sinusitis, frontal
gallbladder —see Cholecystitis
gastric —see Gastritis
gastrointestinal —see Enteritis
genital organ (internal) (diffuse)
    female —see Disease, pelvis, inflammatory
    male N49.9
        multiple sites N49.8
        specified NEC N49.8
gland (lymph) —see Lymphadenitis
glottis —see Laryngitis
granular, pharynx J31.2
gum K05.10
    nonplaque induced K05.11
    plaque induced K05.10
heart —see Carditis
hepatic duct —see Cholangitis
ileoanal (internal) pouch K91.850
ileum —see also Enteritis
    regional or terminal —see Enteritis, regional
intestinal pouch K91.850
intestine (any part) —see Enteritis
jaw (acute) (bone) (chronic) (lower)
    (suppurative) (upper) M27.2
joint NEC —see Arthritis
    sacroiliac M46.1
kidney —see Nephritis
knee (joint) M13.169
    tuberculous A18.02
labium (majus) (minus) —see Vulvitis
lacrimal
    gland —see Dacryoadenitis
    passages (duct) (sac) —see also
        Dacryocystitis
        canaliculitis —see Canaliculitis, lacrimal
larynx —see Laryngitis
leg NOS L08.9
lip K13.0
liver (capsule) —see also Hepatitis
    chronic K73.9
    suppurative K75.0
lung (acute) —see also Pneumonia
    chronic J98.4
lymphatic vessel —see Lymphangitis
lymph gland or node —see Lymphadenitis
maxilla, maxillary M27.2
    sinus (chronic) —see Sinusitis, maxillary
membranes of brain or spinal cord —see
        Meningitis
meninges —see Meningitis
mouth K12.1
muscle —see Myositis
myocardium —see Myocarditis
nasal sinus (chronic) —see Sinusitis
nasopharynx —see Nasopharyngitis
navel L08.82
nerve NEC —see Neuralgia
nipple N61.0
    puerperal, postpartum or gestational —see
        Infection, nipple
nose —see Rhinitis
oculomotor (nerve) —see Strabismus,
    paralytic, third nerve
optic nerve —see Neuritis, optic
orbit (chronic) H05.10
    acute H05.00
        abscess —see Abscess, orbit
        cellulitis —see Cellulitis, orbit

Inflammation, inflamed, inflammatory
(Continued)
orbit (chronic) (Continued)
    acute (Continued)
        osteomyelitis —see Osteomyelitis,
            orbit
        periostitis —see Periostitis, orbital
        tenonitis —see Tenonitis, eye
    granuloma —see Granuloma, orbit
    myositis —see Myositis, orbital
ovary —see Salpingo-oophoritis
oviduct —see Salpingo-oophoritis
pancreas (acute) —see Pancreatitis
parametrium N73.0
parotid region L08.9
pelvis, female —see Disease, pelvis,
    inflammatory
penis (corpora cavernosa) N48.29
perianal K62.89
pericardium —see Pericarditis
perineum (female) (male) L08.9
perirectal K62.89
peritoneum —see Peritonitis
periuterine —see Disease, pelvis,
    inflammatory
perivesical —see Cystitis
petrous bone (acute) (chronic) —see Petrositis
pharynx (acute) —see Pharyngitis
pia mater —see Meningitis
pleura —see Pleurisy
polyp, colon —see also Polyp, colon,
    inflammatory K51.40
prostate —see also Prostatitis
    specified type NEC N41.8
rectosigmoid —see Rectosigmoiditis
rectum —see also Proctitis K62.89
respiratory, upper —see also Infection,
    respiratory, upper J06.9
    acute, due to radiation J70.0
    chronic, due to external agent —see
        condition, respiratory, chronic, due to
    due to
        chemicals, gases, fumes or vapors
            (inhalation) J68.2
        radiation J70.1
retina —see Chorioretinitis
retrocecal —see Appendicitis
retroperitoneal —see Peritonitis
salivary duct or gland (any) (suppurative) —
    see Sialoadenitis
scorbutic, alveoli, teeth E54
scrotum N49.2
seminal vesicle —see Vesiculitis
sigmoid —see Enteritis
sinus —see Sinusitis
Skene's duct or gland —see Urethritis
skin L08.9
spermatic cord N49.1
sphenoidal (sinus) —see Sinusitis, sphenoidal
spinal
    cord —see Encephalitis
    membrane —see Meningitis
    nerve —see Disorder, nerve
spine —see Spondylopathy, inflammatory
spleen (capsule) D73.89
stomach —see Gastritis
subcutaneous tissue L08.9
suprarenal (gland) E27.8
synovial —see Tenosynovitis
tendon (sheath) NEC —see Tenosynovitis
testis —see Orchitis
throat (acute) —see Pharyngitis
thymus (gland) E32.8
thyroid (gland) —see Thyroiditis
tongue K14.0
tonsil —see Tonsillitis
trachea —see Tracheitis
trochlear (nerve) —see Strabismus, paralytic,
    fourth nerve
tubal —see Salpingo-oophoritis
tuberculous NEC —see Tuberculosis

Inflammation, inflamed, inflammatory
(Continued)
tubo-ovarian —see Salpingo-oophoritis
tunica vaginalis N49.1
tympanic membrane —see Tympanitis
umbilicus, umbilical L08.82
uterine ligament —see Disease, pelvis,
    inflammatory
uterus (catarrhal) —see Endometritis
uveal tract (anterior) NOS —see also
        Iridocyclitis
    posterior —see Chorioretinitis
vagina —see Vaginitis
vas deferens N49.1
vein —see also Phlebitis
    intracranial or intraspinal (septic) G08
    thrombotic I80.9
        leg —see Phlebitis, leg
        lower extremity —see Phlebitis, leg
vocal cord J38.3
vulva —see Vulvitis
Wharton's duct (suppurative) —see
        Sialoadenitis
Inflation, lung, imperfect (newborn) —see
    Atelectasis
Influenza (bronchial) (epidemic) (respiratory
    (upper)) (unidentified influenza virus)
    J11.1
with
    digestive manifestations J11.2
    encephalopathy J11.81
    enteritis J11.2
    gastroenteritis J11.2
    gastrointestinal manifestations J11.2
    laryngitis J11.1
    myocarditis J11.82
    otitis media J11.83
    pharyngitis J11.1
    pneumonia J11.00
        specified type J11.08
    respiratory manifestations NEC J11.1
    specified manifestation NEC J11.89
A/H5N1 —see also Influenza, due to,
    identified novel influenza A virus J09.X2
avian —see also Influenza, due to, identified
    novel influenza A virus J09.X2
bird —see also Influenza, due to, identified
    novel influenza A virus J09.X2
novel (2009) H1N1 influenza —see also
    Influenza, due to, identified influenza
    virus NEC J10.1
novel influenza A/H1N1 —see also Influenza,
    due to, identified influenza virus NEC
    J10.1
due to
    avian (see also Influenza, due to, identified
        novel influenza A virus) J09.X2
    identified influenza virus NEC J10.1
        with
            digestive manifestations J10.2
            encephalopathy J10.81
            enteritis J10.2
            gastroenteritis J10.2
            gastrointestinal manifestations J10.2
            laryngitis J10.1
            myocarditis J10.82
            otitis media J10.83
            pharyngitis J10.1
            pneumonia (unspecified type) J10.00
                with same identified influenza virus
                    J10.01
                specified type NEC J10.08
            respiratory manifestations NEC J10.1
            specified manifestation NEC J10.89
    identified novel influenza A virus J09.X2
        with
            digestive manifestations J09.X3
            encephalopathy J09.X9
            enteritis J09.X3
            gastroenteritis J09.X3
            gastrointestinal manifestations J09.X3

▶ New   ⇒ Revised   ~~deleted~~ Deleted   • Use Additional Character(s)

Influenza *(Continued)*
  due to *(Continued)*
    identified novel influenza A virus
      (Continued)
      with *(Continued)*
        laryngitis J09.X2
        myocarditis J09.X9
        otitis media J09.X9
        pharyngitis J09.X2
        pneumonia J09.X1
        respiratory manifestations NEC J09.X2
        specified manifestation NEC J09.X9
        upper respiratory symptoms J09.X2
    of other animal origin, not bird or swine *(see also* Influenza, due to, identified novel influenza A virus) J09.X2
    swine (viruses that normally cause infections in pigs) *—see also* Influenza, due to, identified novel influenza A virus J09.X2
Influenza-like disease *—see* Influenza
Influenzal *—see* Influenza
Infraction, Freiberg's (metatarsal head) *—see* Osteochondrosis, juvenile, metatarsus
Infraeruption of tooth (teeth) M26.34
Infusion complication, misadventure, or reaction *—see* Complications, infusion
Ingestion
  chemical *—see* Table of Drugs and Chemicals, by substance, poisoning
  drug or medicament
    correct substance properly administered *—see* Table of Drugs and Chemicals, by drug, adverse effect
    overdose or wrong substance given or taken *—see* Table of Drugs and Chemicals, by drug, poisoning
  foreign body *—see* Foreign body, alimentary tract
  tularemia A21.3
Ingrowing
  hair (beard) L73.1
  nail (finger) (toe) L60.0
Inguinal *—see also* condition
  testicle Q53.9
  ⟩bilateral Q53.212
  ⟩unilateral Q53.112
Inhalant-induced
  anxiety disorder F18.980
  depressive disorder F18.94
  major neurocognitive disorder F18.97
  mild neurocognitive disorder F18.988
  psychotic disorder F18.959
Inhalation
  anthrax A22.1
  flame T27.3
  food or foreign body *—see* Foreign body, by site
  gases, fumes, or vapors NEC T59.9-●
    specified agent *—see* Table of Drugs and Chemicals, by substance
  liquid or vomitus *—see* Asphyxia
  meconium (newborn) P24.00
    with
      with respiratory symptoms P24.01
      pneumonia (pneumonitis) P24.01
  mucus *—see* Asphyxia, mucus
  oil or gasoline (causing suffocation) *—see* Foreign body, by site
  smoke J70.5
    due to chemicals, gases, fumes and vapors J68.9
  steam *—see* Toxicity, vapors
  stomach contents or secretions *—see* Foreign body, by site
    due to anesthesia (general) (local) or other sedation T88.59
    in labor and delivery O74.0
    in pregnancy O29.01-●
    postpartum, puerperal O89.01

Inhibition, orgasm
  female F52.31
  male F52.32
Inhibitor, systemic lupus erythematosus (presence of) D68.62
Iniencephalus, iniencephaly Q00.2
Injection, traumatic jet (air) (industrial) (water) (paint or dye) T70.4
Injury *—see also* specified injury type
  T14.90
  abdomen, abdominal S39.91
    blood vessel *—see* Injury, blood vessel, abdomen
    cavity *—see* Injury, intra-abdominal
    contusion S30.1
    internal *—see* Injury, intra-abdominal
    intra-abdominal organ *—see* Injury, intra-abdominal
    nerve *—see* Injury, nerve, abdomen
    open *—see* Wound, open, abdomen
    specified NEC S39.81
    superficial *—see* Injury, superficial, abdomen
  Achilles tendon S86.00-●
    laceration S86.02-●
    specified type NEC S86.09-●
    strain S86.01-●
  acoustic, resulting in deafness *—see* Injury, nerve, acoustic
  adrenal (gland) S37.819
    contusion S37.812
    laceration S37.813
    specified type NEC S37.818
  alveolar (process) S09.93
  ankle S99.91-●
    contusion *—see* Contusion, ankle
    dislocation *—see* Dislocation, ankle
    fracture *—see* Fracture, ankle
    nerve *—see* Injury, nerve, ankle
    open *—see* Wound, open, ankle
    specified type NEC S99.81-●
    sprain *—see* Sprain, ankle
    superficial *—see* Injury, superficial, ankle
  anterior chamber, eye *—see* Injury, eye, specified site NEC
  anus *—see* Injury, abdomen
  aorta (thoracic) S25.00
    abdominal S35.00
      laceration (minor) (superficial) S35.01
        major S35.02
      specified type NEC S35.09
    laceration (minor) (superficial) S25.01
      major S25.02
    specified type NEC S25.09
  arm (upper) S49.9-●
    blood vessel *—see* Injury, blood vessel, arm
    contusion *—see* Contusion, arm, upper
    fracture *—see* Fracture, humerus
    lower *—see* Injury, forearm
    muscle *—see* Injury, muscle, shoulder
    nerve *—see* Injury, nerve, arm
    open *—see* Wound, open, arm
    specified type NEC S49.8-●
    superficial *—see* Injury, superficial, arm
  artery (complicating trauma) *—see also* Injury, blood vessel, by site
    cerebral or meningeal *—see* Injury, intracranial
  auditory canal (external) (meatus) S09.91
  auricle, auris, ear S09.91
  axilla *—see* Injury, shoulder
  back *—see* Injury, back, lower
  bile duct S36.13
  birth *—see also* Birth, injury P15.9
  bladder (sphincter) S37.20
    at delivery O71.5
    contusion S37.22
    laceration S37.23
    obstetrical trauma O71.5
    specified type NEC S37.29

Injury *(Continued)*
  blast (air) (hydraulic) (immersion) (underwater) NEC T14.8
    acoustic nerve trauma *—see* Injury, nerve, acoustic
    bladder *—see* Injury, bladder
    brain *—see* Concussion
    colon *—see* Injury, intestine, large, blast injury
    ear (primary) S09.31-●
      secondary S09.39-●
    generalized T70.8
    lung *—see* Injury, intrathoracic, lung, blast injury
    multiple body organs T70.8
    peritoneum S36.81
    rectum S36.61
    retroperitoneum S36.898
    small intestine S36.419
      duodenum S36.410
      specified site NEC S36.418
    specified
      intra-abdominal organ NEC S36.898
      pelvic organ NEC S37.899
  blood vessel NEC T14.8
    abdomen S35.9-●
      aorta *—see* Injury, aorta, abdominal
      celiac artery *—see* Injury, blood vessel, celiac artery
      iliac vessel *—see* Injury, blood vessel, iliac
      laceration S35.91
      mesenteric vessel *—see* Injury, mesenteric
      portal vein *—see* Injury, blood vessel, portal vein
      renal vessel *—see* Injury, blood vessel, renal
      specified vessel NEC S35.8X-●
      splenic vessel *—see* Injury, blood vessel, splenic
      vena cava *—see* Injury, vena cava, inferior
    ankle *—see* Injury, blood vessel, foot
    aorta (abdominal) (thoracic) *—see* Injury, aorta
    arm (upper) NEC S45.90-●
      forearm *—see* Injury, blood vessel, forearm
      laceration S45.91-●
      specified
        site NEC S45.80-●
          laceration S45.81-●
          specified type NEC S45.89-●
        type NEC S45.99-●
      superficial vein S45.30-●
        laceration S45.31-●
        specified type NEC S45.39-●
    axillary
      artery S45.00-●
        laceration S45.01-●
        specified type NEC S45.09-●
      vein S45.20-●
        laceration S45.21-●
        specified type NEC S45.29-●
    azygos vein *—see* Injury, blood vessel, thoracic, specified site NEC
    brachial
      artery S45.10-●
        laceration S45.11-●
        specified type NEC S45.19-●
      vein S45.20-●
        laceration S45.219
        specified type NEC S45.29-●
    carotid artery (common) (external) (internal, extracranial) S15.00-●
      internal, intracranial S06.8-●
      laceration (minor) (superficial) S15.01-●
        major S15.02-●
      specified type NEC S15.09-●

Injury *(Continued)*
  blood vessel NEC *(Continued)*
    celiac artery S35.219
      branch S35.299
        laceration (minor) (superficial) S35.291
          major S35.292
        specified NEC S35.298
      laceration (minor) (superficial) S35.211
        major S35.212
      specified type NEC S35.218
    cerebral —*see* Injury, intracranial
    deep plantar —*see* Injury, blood vessel,
      plantar artery
    digital (hand) —*see* Injury, blood vessel,
      finger
    dorsal
      artery (foot) S95.00-●
        laceration S95.01-●
        specified type NEC S95.09-●
      vein (foot) S95.20-●
        laceration S95.21-●
        specified type NEC S95.29-●
    due to accidental laceration during
      procedure —*see* Laceration, accidental
      complicating surgery
    extremity —*see* Injury, blood vessel, limb
    femoral
      artery (common) (superficial) S75.00-●
        laceration (minor) (superficial)
          S75.01-●
          major S75.02-●
        specified type NEC S75.09-●
      vein (hip level) (thigh level) S75.10-●
        laceration (minor) (superficial) S75.11-●
          major S75.12-●
        specified type NEC S75.19-●
    finger S65.50-●
      index S65.50-●
        laceration S65.51-●
        specified type NEC S65.59-●
      laceration S65.51-●
      little S65.50-●
        laceration S65.51-●
        specified type NEC S65.59-●
      middle S65.50-●
        laceration S65.51-●
        specified type NEC S65.59-●
      specified type NEC S65.59-●
      thumb —*see* Injury, blood vessel, thumb
    foot S95.90-●
      dorsal
        artery —*see* Injury, blood vessel,
          dorsal, artery
        vein —*see* Injury, blood vessel, dorsal,
          vein
      laceration S95.91-●
      plantar artery —*see* Injury, blood vessel,
        plantar artery
      specified
        site NEC S95.80-●
          laceration S95.81-●
          specified type NEC S95.89-●
        specified type NEC S95.99-●
    forearm S55.90-●
      laceration S55.91-●
      radial artery —*see* Injury, blood vessel,
        radial artery
      specified
        site NEC S55.80-●
          laceration S55.81-●
          specified type NEC S55.89-●
        type NEC S55.99-●
      ulnar artery —*see* Injury, blood vessel,
        ulnar artery
      vein S55.20-●
        laceration S55.21-●
        specified type NEC S55.29-●
    gastric
      artery —*see* Injury, mesenteric, artery,
        branch
      vein —*see* Injury, blood vessel, abdomen

Injury *(Continued)*
  blood vessel NEC *(Continued)*
    gastroduodenal artery —*see* Injury,
      mesenteric, artery, branch
    greater saphenous vein (lower leg level)
      S85.30-●
      hip (and thigh) level S75.20-●
        laceration (minor) (superficial) S75.21-●
          major S75.22-●
        specified type NEC S75.29-●
      laceration S85.31-●
      specified type NEC S85.39-●
    hand (level) S65.90-●
      finger —*see* Injury, blood vessel, finger
      laceration S65.91-●
      palmar arch —*see* Injury, blood vessel,
        palmar arch
      radial artery —*see* Injury, blood vessel,
        radial artery, hand
      specified
        site NEC S65.80-●
          laceration S65.81-●
          specified type NEC S65.89-●
        type NEC S65.99-●
      thumb —*see* Injury, blood vessel,
        thumb
      ulnar artery —*see* Injury, blood vessel,
        ulnar artery, hand
    head S09.0
      intracranial —*see* Injury, intracranial
      multiple S09.0
    hepatic
      artery —*see* Injury, mesenteric, artery
      vein —*see* Injury, vena cava, inferior
    hip S75.90-●
      femoral artery —*see* Injury, blood vessel,
        femoral, artery
      femoral vein —*see* Injury, blood vessel,
        femoral, vein
      greater saphenous vein —*see* Injury,
        blood vessel, greater saphenous,
        hip level
      laceration S75.91-●
      specified
        site NEC S75.80-●
          laceration S75.81-●
          specified type NEC S75.89-●
        type NEC S75.99-●
    hypogastric (artery) (vein) —*see* Injury,
      blood vessel, iliac
    iliac S35.5-
      artery S35.51-●
      specified vessel NEC S35.5-●
      uterine vessel —*see* Injury, blood vessel,
        uterine
      vein S35.51-●
    innominate —*see* Injury, blood vessel,
      thoracic, innominate
    intercostal (artery) (vein) —*see* Injury,
      blood vessel, thoracic, intercostal
    jugular vein (external) S15.20-●
      internal S15.30-●
        laceration (minor) (superficial) S15.31-●
          major S15.32-●
        specified type NEC S15.39-●
      laceration (minor) (superficial) S15.21-●
        major S15.22-●
      specified type NEC S15.29-●
    leg (level) (lower) S85.90-●
      greater saphenous —*see* Injury, blood
        vessel, greater saphenous
      laceration S85.91-●
      lesser saphenous —*see* Injury, blood
        vessel, lesser saphenous
      peroneal artery —*see* Injury, blood
        vessel, peroneal artery
      popliteal
        artery —*see* Injury, blood vessel,
          popliteal, artery
        vein —*see* Injury, blood vessel,
          popliteal, vein

Injury *(Continued)*
  blood vessel NEC *(Continued)*
    leg (level) (lower) *(Continued)*
      specified
        site NEC S85.80-●
          laceration S85.81-●
          specified type NEC S85.89-●
        type NEC S85.99-●
      thigh —*see* Injury, blood vessel, hip
      tibial artery —*see* Injury, blood vessel,
        tibial artery
    lesser saphenous vein (lower leg level)
      S85.40-●
      laceration S85.41-●
      specified type NEC S85.49-●
    limb
      lower —*see* Injury, blood vessel, leg
      upper —*see* Injury, blood vessel, arm
    lower back —*see* Injury, blood vessel,
      abdomen
      specified NEC —*see* Injury, blood
        vessel, abdomen, specified, site
        NEC
    mammary (artery) (vein) —*see* Injury,
      blood vessel, thoracic, specified site
      NEC
    mesenteric (inferior) (superior)
      artery —*see* Injury, mesenteric, artery
      vein —*see* Injury, mesenteric, vein
    neck S15.9
      specified site NEC S15.8
    ovarian (artery) (vein) —*see* subcategory
      S35.8
    palmar arch (superficial) S65.20-●
      deep S65.30-●
        laceration S65.31-●
        specified type NEC S65.39-●
      laceration S65.21-●
      specified type NEC S65.29-●
    pelvis —*see* Injury, blood vessel, abdomen
      specified NEC —*see* Injury, blood vessel,
        abdomen, specified, site NEC
    peroneal artery S85.20-●
      laceration S85.21-●
      specified type NEC S85.29-●
    plantar artery (deep) (foot) S95.10-●
      laceration S95.11-●
      specified type NEC S95.19-●
    popliteal
      artery S85.00-●
        laceration S85.01-●
        specified type NEC S85.09-●
      vein S85.50-●
        laceration S85.51-●
        specified type NEC S85.59-●
    portal vein S35.319
      laceration S35.311
      specified type NEC S35.318
    precerebral —*see* Injury, blood vessel, neck
    pulmonary (artery) (vein) —*see* Injury,
      blood vessel, thoracic, pulmonary
    radial artery (forearm level) S55.10-●
      hand and wrist (level) S65.10-●
        laceration S65.11-●
        specified type NEC S65.19-●
      laceration S55.11-●
      specified type NEC S55.19-●
    renal
      artery S35.40-●
        laceration S35.41-●
        specified NEC S35.49-●
      vein S35.40-●
        laceration S35.41-●
        specified NEC S35.49-●
    saphenous vein (greater) (lower leg
      level) —*see* Injury, blood vessel,
      greater saphenous
      hip and thigh level —*see* Injury, blood
        vessel, greater saphenous, hip level
      lesser —*see* Injury, blood vessel, lesser
        saphenous

Injury *(Continued)*
  blood vessel NEC *(Continued)*
    shoulder
      specified NEC —*see* Injury, blood vessel, arm, specified site NEC
      superficial vein —*see* Injury, blood vessel, arm, superficial vein
    specified NEC T14.8
    splenic
      artery —*see* Injury, blood vessel, celiac artery, branch
      vein S35.329
        laceration S35.321
        specified NEC S35.328
    subclavian —*see* Injury, blood vessel, thoracic, innominate
    thigh —*see* Injury, blood vessel, hip
    thoracic S25.90
      aorta S25.00
        laceration (minor) (superficial) S25.01
          major S25.02
        specified type NEC S25.09
      azygos vein —*see* Injury, blood vessel, thoracic, specified, site NEC
      innominate
        artery S25.10-●
          laceration (minor) (superficial) S25.11-●
            major S25.12-●
          specified type NEC S25.19-●
        vein S25.30-●
          laceration (minor) (superficial) S25.31-●
            major S25.32-●
          specified type NEC S25.39-●
      intercostal S25.50-●
        laceration S25.51-●
        specified type NEC S25.59-●
      laceration S25.91
      mammary vessel —*see* Injury, blood vessel, thoracic, specified, site NEC
      pulmonary S25.40-●
        laceration (minor) (superficial) S25.41-●
          major S25.42-●
        specified type NEC S25.49-●
      specified
        site NEC S25.80-●
          laceration S25.81-●
          specified type NEC S25.89-●
        type NEC S25.99
      subclavian —*see* Injury, blood vessel, thoracic, innominate
      vena cava (superior) S25.20
        laceration (minor) (superficial) S25.21
          major S25.22
        specified type NEC S25.29
    thumb S65.40-●
      laceration S65.41-●
      specified type NEC S65.49-●
    tibial artery S85.10-●
      anterior S85.13-●
        laceration S85.14-●
        specified injury NEC S85.15-●
      laceration S85.11-●
      posterior S85.16-●
        laceration S85.17-●
        specified injury NEC S85.18-●
      specified injury NEC S85.12-●
    ulnar artery (forearm level) S55.00-●
      hand and wrist (level) S65.00-●
        laceration S65.01-●
        specified type NEC S65.09-●
      laceration S55.01-●
      specified type NEC S55.09-●
    upper arm (level) —*see* Injury, blood vessel, arm
    superficial vein —*see* Injury, blood vessel, arm, superficial vein
    uterine S35.5-●
      artery S35.53-●
      vein S35.53-●

  blood vessel NEC *(Continued)*
    vena cava —*see* Injury, vena cava
    vertebral artery S15.10-●
      laceration (minor) (superficial) S15.11-●
        major S15.12-●
      specified type NEC S15.19-●
    wrist (level) —*see* Injury, blood vessel, hand
  brachial plexus S14.3
    newborn P14.3
  brain (traumatic) S06.9-●
    diffuse (axonal) S06.2X-●
    focal S06.30-●
  brainstem S06.38-●
  breast NOS S29.9
  broad ligament —*see* Injury, pelvic organ, specified site NEC
  bronchus, bronchi —*see* Injury, intrathoracic, bronchus
  brow S09.90
  buttock S39.92
  canthus, eye S05.90
  cardiac plexus —*see* Injury, nerve, thorax, sympathetic
  cauda equina S34.3
  cavernous sinus —*see* Injury, intracranial
  cecum —*see* Injury, colon
  celiac ganglion or plexus —*see* Injury, nerve, lumbosacral, sympathetic
  cerebellum —*see* Injury, intracranial
  cerebral —*see* Injury, intracranial
  cervix (uteri) —*see* Injury, uterus
  cheek (wall) S09.93
  chest —*see* Injury, thorax
  childbirth (newborn) —*see also* Birth, injury
    maternal NEC O71.9
  chin S09.93
  choroid (eye) —*see* Injury, eye, specified site NEC
  clitoris S39.94
  coccyx —*see also* Injury, back, lower
    complicating delivery O71.6
  colon —*see* Injury, intestine, large
  common bile duct —*see* Injury, liver
  conjunctiva (superficial) —*see* Injury, eye, conjunctiva
  conus medullaris —*see* Injury, spinal, sacral cord
    spermatic (pelvic region) S37.898
      scrotal region S39.848
    spinal —*see* Injury, spinal cord, by region
  cornea —*see* Injury, eye, specified site NEC
    abrasion —*see* Injury, eye, cornea, abrasion
  cortex (cerebral) —*see also* Injury, intracranial
    visual —*see* Injury, nerve, optic
  costal region NEC S29.9
  costochondral NEC S29.9
  cranial
    cavity —*see* Injury, intracranial
    nerve —*see* Injury, nerve, cranial
  crushing —*see* Crush
  cutaneous sensory nerve
  cystic duct —*see* Injury, liver
  deep tissue —*see* Contusion, by site
    meaning pressure ulcer —*see* Ulcer, pressure, unstageable, by site
  delivery (newborn) P15.9
    maternal NEC O71.9
  Descemet's membrane —*see* Injury, eyeball, penetrating
  diaphragm —*see* Injury, intrathoracic, diaphragm
  duodenum —*see* Injury, intestine, small, duodenum
  ear (auricle) (external) (canal) S09.91
    abrasion —*see* Abrasion, ear
    bite —*see* Bite, ear
    blister —*see* Blister, ear
    bruise —*see* Contusion, ear

Injury *(Continued)*
  ear *(Continued)*
    contusion —*see* Contusion, ear
    external constriction —*see* Constriction, external, ear
    hematoma —*see* Hematoma, ear
    inner —*see* Injury, ear, middle
    laceration —*see* Laceration, ear
    middle S09.30-●
      blast —*see* Injury, blast, ear
      specified NEC S09.39-●
    puncture —*see* Puncture, ear
    superficial —*see* Injury, superficial, ear
  eighth cranial nerve (acoustic or auditory) —*see* Injury, nerve, acoustic
  elbow S59.90-●
    contusion —*see* Contusion, elbow
    dislocation —*see* Dislocation, elbow
    fracture —*see* Fracture, ulna, upper end
    open —*see* Wound, open, elbow
    specified NEC S59.80-●
    sprain —*see* Sprain, elbow
    superficial —*see* Injury, superficial, elbow
  eleventh cranial nerve (accessory) —*see* Injury, nerve, accessory
  epididymis S39.94
  epigastric region S39.91
  epiglottis NEC S19.89
  esophageal plexus —*see* Injury, nerve, thorax, sympathetic
  esophagus (thoracic part) —*see also* Injury, intrathoracic, esophagus
    cervical NEC S19.85
  eustachian tube S09.30-●
  eye S05.9-●
    avulsion S05.7-●
    ball —*see* Injury, eyeball
    conjunctiva S05.0-●
    cornea
      abrasion S05.0-●
      laceration S05.3-●
        with prolapse S05.2-●
    lacrimal apparatus S05.8X-●
    orbit penetration S05.4-●
    specified site NEC S05.8X-●
  eyeball S05.8X-●
    contusion S05.1-●
    penetrating S05.6-●
      with
        foreign body S05.5-●
        prolapse or loss of intraocular tissue S05.2-●
        without prolapse or loss of intraocular tissue S05.3-●
    specified type NEC S05.8-●
  eyebrow S09.93
  eyelid S09.93
    abrasion —*see* Abrasion, eyelid
    contusion —*see* Contusion, eyelid
    open —*see* Wound, open, eyelid
  face S09.93
  fallopian tube S37.509
    bilateral S37.502
      blast injury S37.512
      contusion S37.522
      laceration S37.532
      specified type NEC S37.592
    blast injury (primary) S37.519
      bilateral S37.512
      secondary —*see* Injury, fallopian tube, specified type NEC
      unilateral S37.511
    contusion S37.529
      bilateral S37.522
      unilateral S37.521
    laceration S37.539
      bilateral S37.532
      unilateral S37.531
    specified type NEC S37.599
      bilateral S37.592
      unilateral S37.591

Injury *(Continued)*
  fallopian tube *(Continued)*
    unilateral S37.501
      blast injury S37.511
      contusion S37.521
      laceration S37.531
      specified type NEC S37.591
  fascia —*see* Injury, muscle
  fifth cranial nerve (trigeminal) —*see* Injury,
      nerve, trigeminal
  finger (nail) S69.9-●
    blood vessel —*see* Injury, blood vessel,
        finger
    contusion —*see* Contusion, finger
    dislocation —*see* Dislocation, finger
    fracture —*see* Fracture, finger
    muscle —*see* Injury, muscle, finger
    nerve —*see* Injury, nerve, digital, finger
    open —*see* Wound, open, finger
    specified NEC S69.8-●
    sprain —*see* Sprain, finger
    superficial —*see* Injury, superficial, finger
  first cranial nerve (olfactory) —*see* Injury,
      nerve, olfactory
  flank —*see* Injury, abdomen
  foot S99.92-●
    blood vessel —*see* Injury, blood vessel, foot
    contusion —*see* Contusion, foot
    dislocation —*see* Dislocation, foot
    fracture —*see* Fracture, foot
    muscle —*see* Injury, muscle, foot
    open —*see* Wound, open, foot
    specified type NEC S99.82-●
    sprain —*see* Sprain, foot
    superficial —*see* Injury, superficial, foot
  forceps NOS P15.9
  forearm S59.91-●
    blood vessel —*see* Injury, blood vessel,
        forearm
    contusion —*see* Contusion, forearm
    fracture —*see* Fracture, forearm
    muscle —*see* Injury, muscle, forearm
    nerve —*see* Injury, nerve, forearm
    open —*see* Wound, open, forearm
    specified NEC S59.81-●
    superficial —*see* Injury, superficial,
        forearm
  forehead S09.90
  fourth cranial nerve (trochlear) —*see* Injury,
      nerve, trochlear
  gallbladder S36.129
    contusion S36.122
    laceration S36.123
    specified NEC S36.128
  ganglion
    celiac, coeliac —*see* Injury, nerve,
        lumbosacral, sympathetic
    gasserian —*see* Injury, nerve, trigeminal
    stellate —*see* Injury, nerve, thorax,
        sympathetic
    thoracic sympathetic —*see* Injury, nerve,
        thorax, sympathetic
  gasserian ganglion —*see* Injury, nerve,
      trigeminal
  gastric artery —*see* Injury, blood vessel, celiac
      artery, branch
  gastroduodenal artery —*see* Injury, blood
      vessel, celiac artery, branch
  gastrointestinal tract —*see* Injury,
      intra-abdominal
    with open wound into abdominal cavity —
        see Wound, open, with penetration
        into peritoneal cavity
    colon —*see* Injury, intestine, large
    rectum —*see* Injury, intestine, large, rectum
        with open wound into abdominal cavity
        S36.61
    small intestine —*see* Injury, intestine, small
    specified site NEC —*see* Injury, intra-
        abdominal, specified, site NEC
    stomach —*see* Injury, stomach

Injury *(Continued)*
  genital organ(s)
    external S39.94
      specified NEC S39.848
    internal S37.90
      fallopian tube —*see* Injury, fallopian tube
      ovary —*see* Injury, ovary
      prostate —*see* Injury, prostate
      seminal vesicle —*see* Injury, pelvis,
          organ, specified site NEC
      uterus —*see* Injury, uterus
      vas deferens —*see* Injury, pelvis, organ,
          specified site NEC
    obstetrical trauma O71.9
  gland
    lacrimal laceration —*see* Injury, eye,
        specified site NEC
    salivary S09.93
    thyroid NEC S19.84
  globe (eye) S05.90
    specified NEC S05.8X-●
  groin —*see* Injury, abdomen
  gum S09.90
  hand S69.9-●
    blood vessel —*see* Injury, blood vessel,
        hand
    contusion —*see* Contusion, hand
    fracture —*see* Fracture, hand
    muscle —*see* Injury, muscle, hand
    nerve —*see* Injury, nerve, hand
    open —*see* Wound, open, hand
    specified NEC S69.8-●
    sprain —*see* Sprain, hand
    superficial —*see* Injury, superficial, hand
  head S09.90
    with loss of consciousness S06.9-●
    specified NEC S09.8-●
  heart S26.90
    with hemopericardium S26.00
      contusion S26.01
      laceration (mild) S26.020
        major S26.022
        moderate S26.021
      specified type NEC S26.09
    without hemopericardium S26.10
      contusion S26.11
      laceration S26.12
      specified type NEC S26.19
    contusion S26.91
    laceration S26.92
    specified type NEC S26.99
  heel —*see* Injury, foot
  hepatic
    artery —*see* Injury, blood vessel, celiac
        artery, branch
    duct —*see* Injury, liver
    vein —*see* Injury, vena cava, inferior
  hip S79.91-●
    blood vessel —*see* Injury, blood vessel,
        hip
    contusion —*see* Contusion, hip
    dislocation —*see* Dislocation, hip
    fracture —*see* Fracture, femur, neck
    muscle —*see* Injury, muscle, hip
    nerve —*see* Injury, nerve, hip
    open —*see* Wound, open, hip
    specified NEC S79.81-●
    sprain —*see* Sprain, hip
    superficial —*see* Injury, superficial, hip
  hymen S39.94
  hypogastric
    blood vessel —*see* Injury, blood vessel, iliac
    plexus —*see* Injury, nerve, lumbosacral,
        sympathetic
  ileum —*see* Injury, intestine, small
  iliac region S39.91
  instrumental (during surgery) —*see*
      Laceration, accidental complicating
      surgery
    birth injury —*see* Birth, injury
    nonsurgical —*see* Injury, by site

Injury *(Continued)*
  instrumental *(Continued)*
    obstetrical O71.9
      bladder O71.5
      cervix O71.3
      high vaginal O71.4
      perineal NOS O70.9
      urethra O71.5
      uterus O71.5
        with rupture or perforation O71.1
  internal T14.8
    aorta —*see* Injury, aorta
    bladder (sphincter) —*see* Injury, bladder
    with
        ectopic or molar pregnancy O08.6
        following ectopic or molar pregnancy
            O08.6
      obstetrical trauma O71.5
    bronchus, bronchi —*see* Injury,
        intrathoracic, bronchus
    cecum —*see* Injury, intestine, large
    cervix (uteri) —*see also* Injury, uterus
      with ectopic or molar pregnancy O08.6
      following ectopic or molar pregnancy
          O08.6
      obstetrical trauma O71.3
    chest —*see* Injury, intrathoracic
    gastrointestinal tract —*see* Injury,
        intra-abdominal
    heart —*see* Injury, heart
    intestine NEC —*see* Injury, intestine
    intrauterine —*see* Injury, uterus
    mesentery —*see* Injury, intra-abdominal,
        specified, site NEC
    pelvis, pelvic (organ) S37.90
      following ectopic or molar pregnancy
          (subsequent episode) O08.6
      obstetrical trauma NEC O71.5
        rupture or perforation O71.1
      specified NEC S39.83
    rectum —*see* Injury, intestine, large,
        rectum
    stomach —*see* Injury, stomach
    ureter —*see* Injury, ureter
    urethra (sphincter) following ectopic or
        molar pregnancy O08.6
    uterus —*see* Injury, uterus
  interscapular area —*see* Injury, thorax
  intestine
    large S36.509
      ascending (right) S36.500
        blast injury (primary) S36.510
          secondary S36.590
        contusion S36.520
        laceration S36.530
        specified type NEC S36.590
      blast injury (primary) S36.519
        ascending (right) S36.510
        descending (left) S36.512
        rectum S36.61
        sigmoid S36.513
        specified site NEC S36.518
        transverse S36.511
      contusion S36.529
        ascending (right) S36.520
        descending (left) S36.522
        rectum S36.62
        sigmoid S36.523
        specified site NEC S36.528
        transverse S36.521
      descending (left) S36.502
        blast injury (primary) S36.512
          secondary S36.592
        contusion S36.522
        laceration S36.532
        specified type NEC S36.592
      laceration S36.539
        ascending (right) S36.530
        descending (left) S36.532
        rectum S36.63
        sigmoid S36.533

▶ New ➡ Revised ~~deleted~~ Deleted ● Use Additional Character(s)

Injury (Continued)
  intestine (Continued)
    large (Continued)
      laceration (Continued)
        specified site NEC S36.538
        transverse S36.531
      rectum S36.60
        blast injury (primary) S36.61
          secondary S36.69
        contusion S36.62
        laceration S36.63
        specified type NEC S36.69
      sigmoid S36.503
        blast injury (primary) S36.513
          secondary S36.593
        contusion S36.523
        laceration S36.533
        specified type NEC S36.593
      specified
        site NEC S36.508
          blast injury (primary) S36.518
            secondary S36.598
          contusion S36.528
          laceration S36.538
          specified type NEC S36.598
        type NEC S36.599
          ascending (right) S36.590
          descending (left) S36.592
          rectum S36.69
          sigmoid S36.593
          specified site NEC S36.598
          transverse S36.591
      transverse S36.501
        blast injury (primary) S36.511
          secondary S36.591
        contusion S36.521
        laceration S36.531
        specified type NEC S36.591
    small S36.409
      blast injury (primary) S36.419
        duodenum S36.410
        secondary S36.499
          duodenum S36.490
          specified site NEC S36.498
        specified site NEC S36.418
      contusion S36.429
        duodenum S36.420
        specified site NEC S36.428
      duodenum S36.400
        blast injury (primary) S36.410
          secondary S36.490
        contusion S36.420
        laceration S36.430
        specified NEC S36.490
      laceration S36.439
        duodenum S36.430
        specified site NEC S36.438
      specified
        site NEC S36.408
        type NEC S36.499
          duodenum S36.490
          specified site NEC S36.498
  intra-abdominal S36.90
    adrenal gland —see Injury, adrenal gland
    bladder —see Injury, bladder
    colon —see Injury, intestine, large
    contusion S36.92
    fallopian tube —see Injury, fallopian tube
    gallbladder —see Injury, gallbladder
    intestine —see Injury, intestine
    kidney —see Injury, kidney
    laceration S36.93
    liver —see Injury, liver
    ovary —see Injury, ovary
    pancreas —see Injury, pancreas
    pelvic NOS S37.90
    peritoneum —see Injury, intra-abdominal, specified, site NEC
    prostate —see Injury, prostate
    rectum —see Injury, intestine, large, rectum

Injury (Continued)
  intra-abdominal (Continued)
    retroperitoneum —see Injury, intra-abdominal, specified, site NEC
    seminal vesicle —see Injury, pelvis, organ, specified site NEC
    small intestine —see Injury, intestine, small
    specified
      pelvic S37.90
        specified
          site NEC S37.899
            specified type NEC S37.898
          type NEC S37.99
      site NEC S36.899
        contusion S36.892
        laceration S36.893
        specified type NEC S36.898
      type NEC S36.99
    spleen —see Injury, spleen
    stomach —see Injury, stomach
    ureter —see Injury, ureter
    urethra —see Injury, urethra
    uterus —see Injury, uterus
    vas deferens —see Injury, pelvis, organ, specified site NEC
  intracranial (traumatic) S06.9-●
    cerebellar hemorrhage, traumatic —see Injury, intracranial, focal
    cerebral edema, traumatic S06.1X-●
      diffuse S06.1X-●
      focal S06.1X-●
    diffuse (axonal) S06.2X-●
    epidural hemorrhage (traumatic) S06.4X-●
    focal brain injury S06.30-●
      contusion —see Contusion, cerebral
      laceration —see Laceration, cerebral
      intracerebral hemorrhage, traumatic S06.36-●
        left side S06.35-●
        right side S06.34-●
    subarachnoid hemorrhage, traumatic S06.6X-●
    subdural hemorrhage, traumatic S06.5X-●
  intraocular —see Injury, eyeball, penetrating
  intrathoracic S27.9
    bronchus S27.409
      bilateral S27.402
      blast injury (primary) S27.419
        bilateral S27.412
        secondary —see Injury, intrathoracic, bronchus, specified type NEC
        unilateral S27.411
      contusion S27.429
        bilateral S27.422
        unilateral S27.421
      laceration S27.439
        bilateral S27.432
        unilateral S27.431
      specified type NEC S27.499
        bilateral S27.492
        unilateral S27.491
      unilateral S27.401
    diaphragm S27.809
      contusion S27.802
      laceration S27.803
      specified type NEC S27.808
    esophagus (thoracic) S27.819
      contusion S27.812
      laceration S27.813
      specified type NEC S27.818
    heart —see Injury, heart
    hemopneumothorax S27.2
    hemothorax S27.1
    lung S27.309
      aspiration J69.0
      bilateral S27.302
      blast injury (primary) S27.319
        bilateral S27.312
        secondary —see Injury, intrathoracic, lung, specified type NEC
        unilateral S27.311

Injury (Continued)
  intrathoracic (Continued)
    bronchus (Continued)
      contusion S27.329
        bilateral S27.322
        unilateral S27.321
      laceration S27.339
        bilateral S27.332
        unilateral S27.331
      specified type NEC S27.399
        bilateral S27.392
        unilateral S27.391
      unilateral S27.301
    pleura S27.60
      laceration S27.63
      specified type NEC S27.69
    pneumothorax S27.0
    specified organ NEC S27.899
      contusion S27.892
      laceration S27.893
      specified type NEC S27.898
    thoracic duct —see Injury, intrathoracic, specified organ NEC
    thymus gland —see Injury, intrathoracic, specified organ NEC
    trachea, thoracic S27.50
      blast (primary) S27.51
      contusion S27.52
      laceration S27.53
      specified type NEC S27.59
  iris —see Injury, eye, specified site NEC
    penetrating —see Injury, eyeball, penetrating
  jaw S09.93
  jejunum —see Injury, intestine, small
  joint NOS T14.8
    old or residual —see Disorder, joint, specified type NEC
  kidney S37.00-●
    acute (nontraumatic) N17.9
    contusion —see Contusion, kidney
    laceration —see Laceration, kidney
    specified NEC S37.09-●
  knee S89.9-●
    contusion —see Contusion, knee
    dislocation —see Dislocation, knee
    meniscus (lateral) (medial) —see Sprain, knee, specified site NEC
      old injury or tear —see Derangement, knee, meniscus, due to old injury
    open —see Wound, open, knee
    specified NEC S89.8-●
    sprain —see Sprain, knee
    superficial —see Injury, superficial, knee
  labium (majus) (minus) S39.94
  labyrinth, ear S09.30-●
  lacrimal apparatus, duct, gland, or sac —see Injury, eye, specified site NEC
  larynx NEC S19.81
  leg (lower) S89.9-●
    blood vessel —see Injury, blood vessel, leg
    contusion —see Contusion, leg
    fracture —see Fracture, leg
    muscle —see Injury, muscle, leg
    nerve —see Injury, nerve, leg
    open —see Wound, open, leg
    specified NEC S89.8-●
    superficial —see Injury, superficial, leg
  lens, eye —see Injury, eye, specified site NEC
    penetrating —see Injury, eyeball, penetrating
  limb NEC T14.8
  lip S09.93
  liver S36.119
    contusion S36.112
    laceration S36.113
      major (stellate) S36.116
      minor S36.114
      moderate S36.115
    specified NEC S36.118
  lower back S39.92
    specified NEC S39.82

▶ New   ⟹ Revised   ~~deleted~~ Deleted   ● Use Additional Character(s)

Injury *(Continued)*
  muscle *(Continued)*
    hand (level) S66.90-●
      laceration S66.92-●
      specified
        site NEC S66.80-●
          laceration S66.82-●
          specified type NEC S66.89-●
          strain S66.81-●
          type NEC S66.99-●
      strain S66.91-●
    head S09.10
      laceration S09.12
      specified type NEC S09.19
      strain S09.11
    hip NEC S76.00-●
      laceration S76.02-●
      specified type NEC S76.09-●
      strain S76.01-●
    intrinsic
      ankle and foot level —*see* Injury, muscle, foot, intrinsic
      finger (other than thumb) —*see* Injury, muscle, finger by site, intrinsic
      foot (level) —*see* Injury, muscle, foot, intrinsic
      thumb —*see* Injury, muscle, thumb, intrinsic
    leg (level) (lower) S86.90-●
      Achilles tendon —*see* Injury, Achilles tendon
      anterior muscle group —*see* Injury, muscle, anterior muscle group
      laceration S86.92-●
      peroneal muscle group —*see* Injury, muscle, peroneal muscle group
      posterior muscle group —*see* Injury, muscle, posterior muscle group, leg level
      specified
        site NEC S86.80-●
          laceration S86.82-●
          specified type NEC S86.89-●
          strain S86.81-●
          type NEC S86.99-●
      strain S86.91-●
    long
      extensor toe, at ankle and foot level —*see* Injury, muscle, toe, extensor
      flexor, toe, at ankle and foot level —*see* Injury, muscle, toe, flexor
      head, biceps —*see* Injury, muscle, biceps, long head
    lower back S39.002
      laceration S39.022
      specified type NEC S39.092
      strain S39.012
    neck (level) S16.9
      laceration S16.2
      specified type NEC S16.8
      strain S16.1
    pelvis S39.003
      laceration S39.023
      specified type NEC S39.093
      strain S39.013
    peroneal muscle group, at leg level (lower) S86.30-●
      laceration S86.32-●
      specified type NEC S86.39-●
      strain S86.31-●
    posterior muscle (group)
      leg level (lower) S86.10-●
        laceration S86.12-●
        specified type NEC S86.19-●
        strain S86.11-●
      thigh level S76.30-●
        laceration S76.32-●
        specified type NEC S76.39-●
        strain S76.31-●

Injury *(Continued)*
  muscle *(Continued)*
    quadriceps (thigh) S76.10-●
      laceration S76.12-●
      specified type NEC S76.19-●
      strain S76.11-●
    shoulder S46.90-●
      laceration S46.92-●
      rotator cuff —*see* Injury, rotator cuff
      specified site NEC S46.80-●
        laceration S46.82-●
        specified type NEC S46.89-●
        strain S46.81-●
      specified type NEC S46.99-●
      strain S46.91-●
    thigh NEC (level) S76.90-●
      adductor —*see* Injury, muscle, adductor, thigh
      laceration S76.92-●
      posterior muscle (group) —*see* Injury, muscle, posterior muscle, thigh level
      quadriceps —*see* Injury, muscle, quadriceps
      specified
        site NEC S76.80-●
          laceration S76.82-●
          specified type NEC S76.89-●
          strain S76.81-●
        type NEC S76.99-●
      strain S76.91-●
    thorax (level) S29.009
      back wall S29.002
      front wall S29.001
      laceration S29.029
        back wall S29.022
        front wall S29.021
      specified type NEC S29.099
        back wall S29.092
        front wall S29.091
      strain S29.019
        back wall S29.012
        front wall S29.011
    thumb
      abductor (forearm level) S56.30-●
        laceration S56.32-●
        specified type NEC S56.39-●
        strain S56.31-●
      extensor (forearm level) S56.30-●
        hand level S66.20-●
          laceration S66.22-●
          specified type NEC S66.29-●
          strain S66.21-●
        laceration S56.32-●
        specified type NEC S56.39-●
        strain S56.31-●
      flexor (forearm level) S56.00-●
        hand level S66.00-●
          laceration S66.02-●
          specified type NEC S66.09-●
          strain S66.01-●
        laceration S56.02-●
        specified type NEC S56.09-●
        strain S56.01-●
        wrist level —*see* Injury, muscle, thumb, flexor, hand level
      intrinsic S66.40-●
        laceration S66.42-●
        specified type NEC S66.49-●
        strain S66.41-●
    toe —*see also* Injury, muscle, foot
      extensor, long S96.10-●
        laceration S96.12-●
        specified type NEC S96.19-●
        strain S96.11-●
      flexor, long S96.00-●
        laceration S96.02-●
        specified type NEC S96.09-●
        strain S96.01-●

Injury *(Continued)*
  muscle *(Continued)*
    triceps S46.30-●
      laceration S46.32-●
      specified type NEC S46.39-●
      strain S46.31-●
    wrist (and hand) level —*see* Injury, muscle, hand
  musculocutaneous nerve —*see* Injury, nerve, musculocutaneous
  myocardium —*see* Injury, heart
  nape —*see* Injury, neck
  nasal (septum) (sinus) S09.92
  nasopharynx S09.92
  neck S19.9
    specified NEC S19.80
      specified site NEC S19.89
  nerve NEC T14.8
    abdomen S34.9
      peripheral S34.6
      specified site NEC S34.8
    abducens S04.4-●
      contusion S04.4-●
      laceration S04.4-●
      specified type NEC S04.4-●
    abducent —*see* Injury, nerve, abducens
    accessory S04.7-●
      contusion S04.7-●
      laceration S04.7-●
      specified type NEC S04.7-●
    acoustic S04.6-●
      contusion S04.6-●
      laceration S04.6-●
      specified type NEC S04.6-●
    ankle S94.9-●
      cutaneous sensory S94.3-●
      specified site NEC —*see* subcategory S94.8
    anterior crural, femoral —*see* Injury, nerve, femoral
    arm (upper) S44.9-●
      axillary —*see* Injury, nerve, axillary
      cutaneous —*see* Injury, nerve, cutaneous, arm
      median —*see* Injury, nerve, median, upper arm
      musculocutaneous —*see* Injury, nerve, musculocutaneous
      radial —*see* Injury, nerve, radial, upper arm
      specified site NEC —*see* subcategory S44.8
      ulnar —*see* Injury, nerve, ulnar, arm
    auditory —*see* Injury, nerve, acoustic
    axillary S44.3-●
    brachial plexus —*see* Injury, brachial plexus
    cervical sympathetic S14.5
    cranial S04.9
      contusion S04.9
      eighth (acoustic or auditory) —*see* Injury, nerve, acoustic
      eleventh (accessory) —*see* Injury, nerve, accessory
      fifth (trigeminal) —*see* Injury, nerve, trigeminal
      first (olfactory) —*see* Injury, nerve, olfactory
      fourth (trochlear) —*see* Injury, nerve, trochlear
      laceration S04.9
      ninth (glossopharyngeal) —*see* Injury, nerve, glossopharyngeal
      second (optic) —*see* Injury, nerve, optic
      seventh (facial) —*see* Injury, nerve, facial
      sixth (abducent) —*see* Injury, nerve, abducens
      specified
        nerve NEC S04.89-●
          contusion S04.89-●
          laceration S04.89-●
          specified type NEC S04.89-●
        type NEC S04.9

Injury *(Continued)*
  nerve NEC *(Continued)*
    cranial *(Continued)*
      tenth (pneumogastric or vagus) —*see*
        Injury, nerve, vagus
      third (oculomotor) —*see* Injury, nerve,
        oculomotor
      twelfth (hypoglossal) —*see* Injury, nerve,
        hypoglossal
    cutaneous sensory
      ankle (level) S94.3-●
      arm (upper) (level) S44.5-●
      foot (level) —*see* Injury, nerve, cutaneous
        sensory, ankle
      forearm (level) S54.3-●
      hip (level) S74.2-●
      leg (lower level) S84.2-●
      shoulder (level) —*see* Injury, nerve,
        cutaneous sensory, arm
      thigh (level) —*see* Injury, nerve,
        cutaneous sensory, hip
    deep peroneal —*see* Injury, nerve, peroneal,
      foot
    digital
      finger S64.4-●
        index S64.49-●
        little S64.49-●
        middle S64.49-●
        ring S64.49-●
      thumb S64.3-●
      toe —*see* Injury, nerve, ankle, specified
        site NEC
    eighth cranial (acoustic or auditory) —*see*
      Injury, nerve, acoustic
    eleventh cranial (accessory) —*see* Injury,
      nerve, accessory
    facial S04.5-●
      contusion S04.5-●
      laceration S04.5-●
      newborn P11.3
      specified type NEC S04.5-●
    femoral (hip level) (thigh level) S74.1-●
    fifth cranial (trigeminal) —*see* Injury, nerve,
      trigeminal
    finger (digital) —*see* Injury, nerve, digital,
      finger
    first cranial (olfactory) —*see* Injury, nerve,
      olfactory
    foot S94.9-●
      cutaneous sensory S94.3-●
      deep peroneal S94.2-●
      lateral plantar S94.0-●
      medial plantar S94.1-●
      specified site NEC —*see* subcategory
        S94.8
    forearm (level) S54.9-●
      cutaneous sensory —*see* Injury, nerve,
        cutaneous sensory, forearm
      median —*see* Injury, nerve, median
      radial —*see* Injury, nerve, radial
      specified site NEC —*see* subcategory
        S54.8
      ulnar —*see* Injury, nerve, ulnar
    fourth cranial (trochlear) —*see* Injury,
      nerve, trochlear
    glossopharyngeal S04.89-●
      specified type NEC S04.89-●
    hand S64.9-●
      median —*see* Injury, nerve, median,
        hand
      radial —*see* Injury, nerve, radial, hand
      specified NEC —*see* subcategory
        S64.8
      ulnar —*see* Injury, nerve, ulnar, hand
    hip (level) S74.9-●
      cutaneous sensory —*see* Injury, nerve,
        cutaneous sensory, hip
      femoral —*see* Injury, nerve, femoral
      sciatic —*see* Injury, nerve, sciatic
      specified site NEC —*see* subcategory
        S74.8

Injury *(Continued)*
  nerve NEC *(Continued)*
    hypoglossal S04.89-●
      specified type NEC S04.89-●
    lateral plantar S94.0-●
    leg (lower) S84.9-●
      cutaneous sensory —*see* Injury, nerve,
        cutaneous sensory, leg
      peroneal —*see* Injury, nerve, peroneal
      specified site NEC —*see* subcategory
        S84.8
      tibial —*see* Injury, nerve, tibial
      upper —*see* Injury, nerve, thigh
    lower
      back —*see* Injury, nerve, abdomen,
        specified site NEC
        peripheral —*see* Injury, nerve,
          abdomen, peripheral
      limb —*see* Injury, nerve, leg
    lumbar plexus —*see* Injury, nerve,
      lumbosacral, sympathetic
    lumbar spinal —*see* Injury, nerve, spinal,
      lumbar
    lumbosacral
      plexus —*see* Injury, nerve, lumbosacral,
        sympathetic
      sympathetic S34.5
    medial plantar S94.1-●
    median (forearm level) S54.1-●
      hand (level) S64.1-●
      upper arm (level) S44.1-●
      wrist (level) —*see* Injury, nerve, median,
        hand
    musculocutaneous S44.4-●
    musculospiral (upper arm level) —*see*
      Injury, nerve, radial, upper arm
    neck S14.9
      peripheral S14.4
      specified site NEC S14.8
      sympathetic S14.5
    ninth cranial (glossopharyngeal) —*see*
      Injury, nerve, glossopharyngeal
    oculomotor S04.1-●
      contusion S04.1-●
      laceration S04.1-●
      specified type NEC S04.1-●
    olfactory S04.81-●
      specified type NEC S04.81-●
    optic S04.01-●
      contusion S04.01-●
      laceration S04.01-●
      specified type NEC S04.01-●
    pelvic girdle —*see* Injury, nerve, hip
    pelvis —*see* Injury, nerve, abdomen,
      specified site NEC
      peripheral —*see* Injury, nerve, abdomen,
        peripheral
    peripheral NEC T14.8
      abdomen —*see* Injury, nerve, abdomen,
        peripheral
      lower back —*see* Injury, nerve, abdomen,
        peripheral
      neck —*see* Injury, nerve, neck, peripheral
      pelvis —*see* Injury, nerve, abdomen,
        peripheral
      specified NEC T14.8
    peroneal (lower leg level) S84.1-●
      foot S94.2-●
    plexus
      brachial —*see* Injury, brachial plexus
      celiac, coeliac —*see* Injury, nerve,
        lumbosacral, sympathetic
      mesenteric, inferior —*see* Injury, nerve,
        lumbosacral, sympathetic
      sacral —*see* Injury, lumbosacral
        plexus
      spinal
        brachial —*see* Injury, brachial
          plexus
        lumbosacral —*see* Injury, lumbosacral
          plexus

Injury *(Continued)*
  nerve NEC *(Continued)*
    pneumogastric —*see* Injury, nerve, vagus
    radial (forearm level) S54.2-●
      hand (level) S64.2-●
      upper arm (level) S44.2-●
      wrist (level) —*see* Injury, nerve, radial,
        hand
    root —*see* Injury, nerve, spinal, root
    sacral plexus —*see* Injury, lumbosacral
      plexus
    sacral spinal —*see* Injury, nerve, spinal,
      sacral
    sciatic (hip level) (thigh level) S74.0-●
    second cranial (optic) —*see* Injury, nerve,
      optic
    seventh cranial (facial) —*see* Injury, nerve,
      facial
    shoulder —*see* Injury, nerve, arm
    sixth cranial (abducent) —*see* Injury, nerve,
      abducens
    spinal
      plexus —*see* Injury, nerve, plexus, spinal
      root
        cervical S14.2
        dorsal S24.2
        lumbar S34.21
        sacral S34.22
        thoracic —*see* Injury, nerve, spinal,
          root, dorsal
    splanchnic —*see* Injury, nerve, lumbosacral,
      sympathetic
    sympathetic NEC —*see* Injury, nerve,
      lumbosacral, sympathetic
      cervical —*see* Injury, nerve, cervical
        sympathetic
    tenth cranial (pneumogastric or vagus) —
      see Injury, nerve, vagus
    thigh (level) —*see* Injury, nerve, hip
      cutaneous sensory —*see* Injury, nerve,
        cutaneous sensory, hip
      femoral —*see* Injury, nerve, femoral
      sciatic —*see* Injury, nerve, sciatic
      specified NEC —*see* Injury, nerve, hip
    third cranial (oculomotor) —*see* Injury,
      nerve, oculomotor
    thorax S24.9
      peripheral S24.3
      specified site NEC S24.8
      sympathetic S24.4
    thumb, digital —*see* Injury, nerve, digital,
      thumb
    tibial (lower leg level) (posterior) S84.0-●
    toe —*see* Injury, nerve, ankle
    trigeminal S04.3-●
      contusion S04.3-●
      laceration S04.3-●
      specified type NEC S04.3-●
    trochlear S04.2-●
      contusion S04.2-●
      laceration S04.2-●
      specified type NEC S04.2-●
    twelfth cranial (hypoglossal) —*see* Injury,
      nerve, hypoglossal
    ulnar (forearm level) S54.0-●
      arm (upper) (level) S44.0-●
      hand (level) S64.0-●
      wrist (level) —*see* Injury, nerve, ulnar,
        hand
    vagus S04.89-●
      specified type NEC S04.89-●
    wrist (level) —*see* Injury, nerve, hand
  ninth cranial nerve (glossopharyngeal) —*see*
    Injury, nerve, glossopharyngeal
  nose (septum) S09.92
  obstetrical O71.9
    specified NEC O71.89
  occipital (region) (scalp) S09.90
    lobe —*see* Injury, intracranial
  optic chiasm S04.02
  optic radiation S04.03-●

▶ New   ⇒ Revised   ~~deleted~~ Deleted   ● Use Additional Character(s)

Injury *(Continued)*
　optic tract and pathways S04.03-●
　orbit, orbital (region) —*see* Injury, eye
　　penetrating (with foreign body) —*see*
　　　Injury, eye, orbit, penetrating
　　specified NEC —*see* Injury, eye, specified
　　　site NEC
　ovary, ovarian S37.409
　　bilateral S37.402
　　　contusion S37.422
　　　laceration S37.432
　　　specified type NEC S37.492
　　blood vessel —*see* Injury, blood vessel,
　　　ovarian
　　contusion S37.429
　　　bilateral S37.422
　　　unilateral S37.421
　　laceration S37.439
　　　bilateral S37.432
　　　unilateral S37.431
　　specified type NEC S37.499
　　　bilateral S37.492
　　　unilateral S37.491
　　unilateral S37.401
　　　contusion S37.421
　　　laceration S37.431
　　　specified type NEC S37.491
　palate (hard) (soft) S09.93
　pancreas S36.209
　　body S36.201
　　　contusion S36.221
　　　laceration S36.231
　　　　major S36.261
　　　　minor S36.241
　　　　moderate S36.251
　　　specified type NEC S36.291
　　contusion S36.229
　　head S36.200
　　　contusion S36.220
　　　laceration S36.230
　　　　major S36.260
　　　　minor S36.240
　　　　moderate S36.250
　　　specified type NEC S36.290
　　laceration S36.239
　　　major S36.269
　　　minor S36.249
　　　moderate S36.259
　　specified type NEC S36.299
　　tail S36.202
　　　contusion S36.222
　　　laceration S36.232
　　　　major S36.262
　　　　minor S36.242
　　　　moderate S36.252
　　　specified type NEC S36.292
　parietal (region) (scalp) S09.90
　　lobe —*see* Injury, intracranial
　patellar ligament (tendon) S76.10-●
　　laceration S76.12-●
　　specified NEC S76.19-●
　　strain S76.11-●
　pelvis, pelvic (floor) S39.93
　　complicating delivery O70.1
　　joint or ligament, complicating delivery
　　　O71.6
　　organ S37.90
　　　with ectopic or molar pregnancy O08.6
　　　complication of abortion —*see* Abortion
　　　contusion S37.92
　　　following ectopic or molar pregnancy
　　　　O08.6
　　　laceration S37.93
　　　obstetrical trauma NEC O71.5
　　　specified
　　　　site NEC S37.899
　　　　　contusion S37.892
　　　　　laceration S37.893
　　　　　specified type NEC S37.898
　　　　type NEC S37.99
　　　specified NEC S39.83

Injury *(Continued)*
　penis S39.94
　perineum S39.94
　peritoneum S36.81
　　laceration S36.893
　periurethral tissue —*see* Injury, urethra
　　complicating delivery O71.82
　phalanges
　　foot —*see* Injury, foot
　　hand —*see* Injury, hand
　pharynx NEC S19.85
　pleura —*see* Injury, intrathoracic, pleura
　plexus
　　brachial —*see* Injury, brachial plexus
　　cardiac —*see* Injury, nerve, thorax,
　　　sympathetic
　　celiac, coeliac —*see* Injury, nerve,
　　　lumbosacral, sympathetic
　　esophageal —*see* Injury, nerve, thorax,
　　　sympathetic
　　hypogastric —*see* Injury, nerve,
　　　lumbosacral, sympathetic
　　lumbar, lumbosacral —*see* Injury,
　　　lumbosacral plexus
　　mesenteric —*see* Injury, nerve, lumbosacral,
　　　sympathetic
　　pulmonary —*see* Injury, nerve, thorax,
　　　sympathetic
　postcardiac surgery (syndrome) I97.0
　prepuce S39.94
　prostate S37.829
　　contusion S37.822
　　laceration S37.823
　　specified type NEC S37.828
　pubic region S39.94
　pudendum S39.94
　pulmonary plexus —*see* Injury, nerve, thorax,
　　sympathetic
　rectovaginal septum NEC S39.83
　rectum —*see* Injury, intestine, large, rectum
　retina —*see* Injury, eye, specified site NEC
　　penetrating —*see* Injury, eyeball,
　　　penetrating
　retroperitoneal —*see* Injury, intra-abdominal,
　　specified site NEC
　rotator cuff (muscle(s)) (tendon(s)) S46.00-●
　　laceration S46.02-●
　　specified type NEC S46.09-●
　　strain S46.01-●
　round ligament —*see* Injury, pelvic organ,
　　specified site NEC
　sacral plexus —*see* Injury, lumbosacral
　　plexus
　salivary duct or gland S09.93
　scalp S09.90
　　newborn (birth injury) P12.9
　　　due to monitoring (electrode) (sampling
　　　　incision) P12.4
　　　specified NEC P12.89
　　　　caput succedaneum P12.81
　scapular region —*see* Injury, shoulder
　sclera —*see* Injury, eye, specified site NEC
　　penetrating —*see* Injury, eyeball,
　　　penetrating
　scrotum S39.94
　second cranial nerve (optic) —*see* Injury,
　　nerve, optic
　seminal vesicle —*see* Injury, pelvic organ,
　　specified site NEC
　seventh cranial nerve (facial) —*see* Injury,
　　nerve, facial
　shoulder S49.9-●
　　blood vessel —*see* Injury, blood vessel,
　　　arm
　　contusion —*see* Contusion, shoulder
　　dislocation —*see* Dislocation, shoulder
　　fracture —*see* Fracture, shoulder
　　muscle —*see* Injury, muscle, shoulder
　　nerve —*see* Injury, nerve, shoulder
　　open —*see* Wound, open, shoulder
　　specified type NEC S49.8-●

Injury *(Continued)*
　shoulder *(Continued)*
　　sprain —*see* Sprain, shoulder girdle
　　superficial —*see* Injury, superficial,
　　　shoulder
　sinus
　　cavernous —*see* Injury, intracranial
　　nasal S09.92
　sixth cranial nerve (abducent) —*see* Injury,
　　nerve, abducens
　skeleton, birth injury P13.9
　　specified part NEC P13.8
　skin NEC T14.8
　　surface intact —*see* Injury, superficial
　skull NEC S09.90
　specified NEC T14.8
　spermatic cord (pelvic region) S37.898
　　scrotal region S39.848
　spinal (cord)
　　cervical (neck) S14.109
　　　anterior cord syndrome S14.139
　　　　C1 level S14.131
　　　　C2 level S14.132
　　　　C3 level S14.133
　　　　C4 level S14.134
　　　　C5 level S14.135
　　　　C6 level S14.136
　　　　C7 level S14.137
　　　　C8 level S14.138
　　　Brown-Séquard syndrome S14.149
　　　　C1 level S14.141
　　　　C2 level S14.142
　　　　C3 level S14.143
　　　　C4 level S14.144
　　　　C5 level S14.145
　　　　C6 level S14.146
　　　　C7 level S14.147
　　　　C8 level S14.148
　　　C1 level S14.101
　　　C2 level S14.102
　　　C3 level S14.103
　　　C4 level S14.104
　　　C5 level S14.105
　　　C6 level S14.106
　　　C7 level S14.107
　　　C8 level S14.108
　　　central cord syndrome S14.129
　　　　C1 level S14.121
　　　　C2 level S14.122
　　　　C3 level S14.123
　　　　C4 level S14.124
　　　　C5 level S14.125
　　　　C6 level S14.126
　　　　C7 level S14.127
　　　　C8 level S14.128
　　　complete lesion S14.119
　　　　C1 level S14.111
　　　　C2 level S14.112
　　　　C3 level S14.113
　　　　C4 level S14.114
　　　　C5 level S14.115
　　　　C6 level S14.116
　　　　C7 level S14.117
　　　　C8 level S14.118
　　　concussion S14.0
　　　edema S14.0
　　　incomplete lesion specified NEC S14.159
　　　　C1 level S14.151
　　　　C2 level S14.152
　　　　C3 level S14.153
　　　　C4 level S14.154
　　　　C5 level S14.155
　　　　C6 level S14.156
　　　　C7 level S14.157
　　　　C8 level S14.158
　　　posterior cord syndrome S14.159
　　　　C1 level S14.151
　　　　C2 level S14.152
　　　　C3 level S14.153
　　　　C4 level S14.154
　　　　C5 level S14.155

Injury *(Continued)*
  spinal *(Continued)*
    cervical *(Continued)*
      posterior cord syndrome *(Continued)*
        C6 level S14.156
        C7 level S14.157
        C8 level S14.158
    dorsal —*see* Injury, spinal, thoracic
    lumbar S34.109
      complete lesion S34.119
        L1 level S34.111
        L2 level S34.112
        L3 level S34.113
        L4 level S34.114
        L5 level S34.115
      concussion S34.01
      edema S34.01
      incomplete lesion S34.129
        L1 level S34.121
        L2 level S34.122
        L3 level S34.123
        L4 level S34.124
        L5 level S34.125
      L1 level S34.101
      L2 level S34.102
      L3 level S34.103
      L4 level S34.104
      L5 level S34.105
    nerve root NEC
      cervical —*see* Injury, nerve, spinal, root,
        cervical
      dorsal —*see* Injury, nerve, spinal, root,
        dorsal
      lumbar S34.21
      sacral S34.22
      thoracic —*see* Injury, nerve, spinal, root,
        dorsal
    plexus
      brachial —*see* Injury, brachial plexus
      lumbosacral —*see* Injury, lumbosacral
        plexus
    sacral S34.139
      complete lesion S34.131
      incomplete lesion S34.132
    thoracic S24.109
      anterior cord syndrome S24.139
        T1 level S24.131
        T2-T6 level S24.132
        T7-T10 level S24.133
        T11-T12 level S24.134
      Brown-Séquard syndrome
        S24.149
        T1 level S24.141
        T2-T6 level S24.142
        T7-T10 level S24.143
        T11-T12 level S24.144
      complete lesion S24.119
        T1 level S24.111
        T2-T6 level S24.112
        T7-T10 level S24.113
        T11-T12 level S24.114
      concussion S24.0
      edema S24.0
      incomplete lesion specified NEC
        S24.159
        T1 level S24.151
        T2-T6 level S24.152
        T7-T10 level S24.153
        T11-T12 level S24.154
      posterior cord syndrome
        S24.159
        T1 level S24.151
        T2-T6 level S24.152
        T7-T10 level S24.153
        T11-T12 level S24.154
      T1 level S24.101
      T2-T6 level S24.102
      T7-T10 level S24.103
      T11-T12 level S24.104
  splanchnic nerve —*see* Injury, nerve,
    lumbosacral, sympathetic

Injury *(Continued)*
  spleen S36.00
    contusion S36.029
      major S36.021
      minor S36.020
    laceration S36.039
      major (massive) (stellate) S36.032
      moderate S36.031
      superficial (capsular) (minor) S36.030
    specified type NEC S36.09
  splenic artery —*see* Injury, blood vessel, celiac
    artery, branch
  stellate ganglion —*see* Injury, nerve, thorax,
    sympathetic
  sternal region S29.9
  stomach S36.30
    contusion S36.32
    laceration S36.33
    specified type NEC S36.39
  subconjunctival —*see* Injury, eye, conjunctiva
  subcutaneous NEC T14.8
  submaxillary region S09.93
  submental region S09.93
  subungual
    fingers —*see* Injury, hand
    toes —*see* Injury, foot
  superficial NEC T14.8
    abdomen, abdominal (wall) S30.92
      abrasion S30.811
      bite S30.871
        insect S30.861
      contusion S30.1
      external constriction S30.841
      foreign body S30.851
    abrasion —*see* Abrasion, by site
    adnexa, eye NEC —*see* Injury, eye,
      specified site NEC
    alveolar process —*see* Injury, superficial,
      oral cavity
    ankle S90.91-●
      abrasion —*see* Abrasion, ankle
      bite —*see* Bite, ankle
      blister —*see* Blister, ankle
      contusion —*see* Contusion, ankle
      external constriction —*see* Constriction,
        external, ankle
      foreign body —*see* Foreign body,
        superficial, ankle
    anus S30.98
    arm (upper) S40.92-●
      abrasion —*see* Abrasion, arm
      bite —*see* Bite, superficial, arm
      blister —*see* Blister, arm (upper)
      contusion —*see* Contusion, arm
      external constriction —*see* Constriction,
        external, arm
      foreign body —*see* Foreign body,
        superficial, arm
    auditory canal (external) (meatus) —*see*
      Injury, superficial, ear
    auricle —*see* Injury, superficial, ear
    axilla —*see* Injury, superficial, arm
    back —*see also* Injury, superficial, thorax,
      back
      lower S30.91
        abrasion S30.810
        contusion S30.0
        external constriction S30.840
        superficial
          bite NEC S30.870
            insect S30.860
          foreign body S30.850
    bite NEC —*see* Bite, superficial NEC, by site
    blister —*see* Blister, by site
    breast S20.10-●
      abrasion —*see* Abrasion, breast
      bite —*see* Bite, superficial, breast
      contusion —*see* Contusion, breast
      external constriction —*see* Constriction,
        external, breast
      foreign body —*see* Foreign body,
        superficial, breast

Injury *(Continued)*
  superficial NEC *(Continued)*
    brow —*see* Injury, superficial, head,
      specified NEC
    buttock S30.91
    calf —*see* Injury, superficial, leg
    canthus, eye —*see* Injury, superficial,
      periocular area
    cheek (external) —*see* Injury, superficial,
      head, specified NEC
      internal —*see* Injury, superficial, oral
        cavity
    chest wall —*see* Injury, superficial, thorax
    chin —*see* Injury, superficial, head NEC
    clitoris S30.95
    conjunctiva —*see* Injury, eye, conjunctiva
      with foreign body (in conjunctival
        sac) —*see* Foreign body,
        conjunctival sac
    contusion —*see* Contusion, by site
    costal region —*see* Injury, superficial, thorax
    digit(s)
      hand —*see* Injury, superficial, finger
    ear (auricle) (canal) (external) S00.40-●
      abrasion —*see* Abrasion, ear
      bite —*see* Bite, superficial, ear
      contusion —*see* Contusion, ear
      external constriction —*see* Constriction,
        external, ear
      foreign body —*see* Foreign body,
        superficial, ear
    elbow S50.90-●
      abrasion —*see* Abrasion, elbow
      bite —*see* Bite, superficial, elbow
      blister —*see* Blister, elbow
      contusion —*see* Contusion, elbow
      external constriction —*see* Constriction,
        external, elbow
      foreign body —*see* Foreign body,
        superficial, elbow
    epididymis S30.94
    epigastric region S30.92
    epiglottis —*see* Injury, superficial, throat
    esophagus
      cervical —*see* Injury, superficial, throat
    external constriction —*see* Constriction,
      external, by site
    extremity NEC T14.8
    eyeball NEC —*see* Injury, eye, specified
      site NEC
    eyebrow —*see* Injury, superficial,
      periocular area
    eyelid S00.20-●
      abrasion —*see* Abrasion, eyelid
      bite —*see* Bite, superficial, eyelid
      contusion —*see* Contusion, eyelid
      external constriction —*see* Constriction,
        external, eyelid
      foreign body —*see* Foreign body,
        superficial, eyelid
    face NEC —*see* Injury, superficial, head,
      specified NEC
    finger(s) S60.949
      abrasion —*see* Abrasion, finger
      bite —*see* Bite, superficial, finger
      blister —*see* Blister, finger
      contusion —*see* Contusion, finger
      external constriction —*see* Constriction,
        external, finger
      foreign body —*see* Foreign body,
        superficial, finger
      index S60.94-●
      insect bite —*see* Bite, by site, superficial,
        insect
      little S60.94-●
      middle S60.94-●
      ring S60.94-●
    flank S30.92
    foot S90.92-●
      abrasion —*see* Abrasion, foot
      bite —*see* Bite, foot

▶ New   ⮕ Revised   ~~deleted~~ Deleted   ● Use Additional Character(s)

Injury *(Continued)*
    superficial NEC *(Continued)*
        foot *(Continued)*
            blister —*see* Blister, foot
            contusion —*see* Contusion, foot
            external constriction —*see* Constriction, external, foot
            foreign body —*see* Foreign body, superficial, foot
        forearm S50.91-●
            abrasion —*see* Abrasion, forearm
            bite —*see* Bite, forearm, superficial
            blister —*see* Blister, forearm
            contusion —*see* Contusion, forearm
            elbow only —*see* Injury, superficial, elbow
            external constriction —*see* Constriction, external, forearm
            foreign body —*see* Foreign body, superficial, forearm
        forehead —*see* Injury, superficial, head NEC
        foreign body —*see* Foreign body, superficial
        genital organs, external
            female S30.97
            male S30.96
        globe (eye) —*see* Injury, eye, specified site NEC
        groin S30.92
        gum —*see* Injury, superficial, oral cavity
        hand S60.92-●
            abrasion —*see* Abrasion, hand
            bite —*see* Bite, superficial, hand
            contusion —*see* Contusion, hand
            external constriction —*see* Constriction, external, hand
            foreign body —*see* Foreign body, superficial, hand
        head S00.90
            ear —*see* Injury, superficial, ear
            eyelid —*see* Injury, superficial, eyelid
            nose S00.30
            oral cavity S00.502
            scalp S00.00
            specified site NEC S00.80
        heel —*see* Injury, superficial, foot
        hip S70.91-●
            abrasion —*see* Abrasion, hip
            bite —*see* Bite, superficial, hip
            blister —*see* Blister, hip
            contusion —*see* Contusion, hip
            external constriction —*see* Constriction, external, hip
            foreign body —*see* Foreign body, superficial, hip
        iliac region —*see* Injury, superficial, abdomen
        inguinal region —*see* Injury, superficial, abdomen
        insect bite —*see* Bite, by site, superficial, insect
        interscapular region —*see* Injury, superficial, thorax, back
        jaw —*see* Injury, superficial, head, specified NEC
        knee S80.91-●
            abrasion —*see* Abrasion, knee
            bite —*see* Bite, superficial, knee
            blister —*see* Blister, knee
            contusion —*see* Contusion, knee
            external constriction —*see* Constriction, external, knee
            foreign body —*see* Foreign body, superficial, knee
        labium (majus) (minus) S30.95
        lacrimal (apparatus) (gland) (sac) —*see* Injury, eye, specified site NEC
        larynx —*see* Injury, superficial, throat
        leg (lower) S80.92-●
            abrasion —*see* Abrasion, leg
            bite —*see* Bite, superficial, leg

Injury *(Continued)*
    superficial NEC *(Continued)*
        leg *(Continued)*
            contusion —*see* Contusion, leg
            external constriction —*see* Constriction, external, leg
            foreign body —*see* Foreign body, superficial, leg
            knee —*see* Injury, superficial, knee
        limb NEC T14.8
        lip S00.501
        lower back S30.91
        lumbar region S30.91
        malar region —*see* Injury, superficial, head, specified NEC
        mammary —*see* Injury, superficial, breast
        mastoid region —*see* Injury, superficial, head, specified NEC
        mouth —*see* Injury, superficial, oral cavity
        muscle NEC T14.8
        nail NEC T14.8
            finger —*see* Injury, superficial, finger
            toe —*see* Injury, superficial, toe
        nasal (septum) —*see* Injury, superficial, nose
        neck S10.90
            specified site NEC S10.80
        nose (septum) S00.30
        occipital region —*see* Injury, superficial, scalp
        oral cavity S00.502
        orbital region —*see* Injury, superficial, periocular area
        palate —*see* Injury, superficial, oral cavity
        palm —*see* Injury, superficial, hand
        parietal region —*see* Injury, superficial, scalp
        pelvis S30.91
            girdle —*see* Injury, superficial, hip
        penis S30.93
        perineum
            female S30.95
            male S30.91
        periocular area S00.20-●
            abrasion —*see* Abrasion, eyelid
            bite —*see* Bite, superficial, eyelid
            contusion —*see* Contusion, eyelid
            external constriction —*see* Constriction, external, eyelid
            foreign body —*see* Foreign body, superficial, eyelid
        phalanges
            finger —*see* Injury, superficial, finger
            toe —*see* Injury, superficial, toe
        pharynx —*see* Injury, superficial, throat
        pinna —*see* Injury, superficial, ear
        popliteal space —*see* Injury, superficial, knee
        prepuce S30.93
        pubic region S30.91
        pudendum
            female S30.97
            male S30.96
        sacral region S30.91
        scalp S00.00
        scapular region —*see* Injury, superficial, shoulder
        sclera —*see* Injury, eye, specified site NEC
        scrotum S30.94
        shin —*see* Injury, superficial, leg
        shoulder S40.91-●
            abrasion —*see* Abrasion, shoulder
            bite —*see* Bite, superficial, shoulder
            blister —*see* Blister, shoulder
            contusion —*see* Contusion, shoulder
            external constriction —*see* Constriction, external, shoulder
            foreign body —*see* Foreign body, superficial, shoulder

Injury *(Continued)*
    superficial NEC *(Continued)*
        skin NEC T14.8
        sternal region —*see* Injury, superficial, thorax, front
        subconjunctival —*see* Injury, eye, specified site NEC
        subcutaneous NEC T14.8
        submaxillary region —*see* Injury, superficial, head, specified NEC
        submental region —*see* Injury, superficial, head, specified NEC
        subungual
            finger(s) —*see* Injury, superficial, finger
            toe(s) —*see* Injury, superficial, toe
        supraclavicular fossa —*see* Injury, superficial, neck
        supraorbital —*see* Injury, superficial, head, specified NEC
        temple —*see* Injury, superficial, head, specified NEC
        temporal region —*see* Injury, superficial, head, specified NEC
        testis S30.94
        thigh S70.92-●
            abrasion —*see* Abrasion, thigh
            bite —*see* Bite, superficial, thigh
            blister —*see* Blister, thigh
            contusion —*see* Contusion, thigh
            external constriction —*see* Constriction, external, thigh
            foreign body —*see* Foreign body, superficial, thigh
        thorax, thoracic (wall) S20.90
            abrasion —*see* Abrasion, thorax
            back S20.40-●
            bite —*see* Bite, thorax, superficial
            blister —*see* Blister, thorax
            contusion —*see* Contusion, thorax
            external constriction —*see* Constriction, external, thorax
            foreign body —*see* Foreign body, superficial, thorax
            front S20.30-●
        throat S10.10
            abrasion S10.11
            bite S10.17
                insect S10.16
            blister S10.12
            contusion S10.0
            external constriction S10.14
            foreign body S10.15
        thumb S60.93-●
            abrasion —*see* Abrasion, thumb
            bite —*see* Bite, superficial, thumb
            blister —*see* Blister, thumb
            contusion —*see* Contusion, thumb
            external constriction —*see* Constriction, external, thumb
            foreign body —*see* Foreign body, superficial, thumb
            insect bite —*see* Bite, by site, superficial, insect
            specified type NEC S60.39-●
        toe(s) S90.93-●
            abrasion —*see* Abrasion, toe
            bite —*see* Bite, toe
            blister —*see* Blister, toe
            contusion —*see* Contusion, toe
            external constriction —*see* Constriction, external, toe
            foreign body —*see* Foreign body, superficial, toe
            great S90.93-●
        tongue —*see* Injury, superficial, oral cavity
        tooth, teeth —*see* Injury, superficial, oral cavity
        trachea S10.10
        tunica vaginalis S30.94
        tympanum, tympanic membrane —*see* Injury, superficial, ear

Injury (Continued)
  superficial NEC (Continued)
    uvula —see Injury, superficial, oral cavity
    vagina S30.95
    vocal cords —see Injury, superficial, throat
    vulva S30.95
    wrist S60.91-●
  supraclavicular region —see Injury, neck
  supraorbital S09.93
  suprarenal gland (multiple) —see Injury,
      adrenal
  surgical complication (external or internal
      site) —see Laceration, accidental
      complicating surgery
  temple S09.90
  temporal region S09.90
  tendon —see also Injury, muscle, by site
    abdomen —see Injury, muscle, abdomen
    Achilles —see Injury, Achilles tendon
    lower back —see Injury, muscle, lower back
    pelvic organs —see Injury, muscle, pelvis
  tenth cranial nerve (pneumogastric or
      vagus) —see Injury, nerve, vagus
  testis S39.94
  thigh S79.92-●
    blood vessel —see Injury, blood vessel, hip
    contusion —see Contusion, thigh
    fracture —see Fracture, femur
    muscle —see Injury, muscle, thigh
    nerve —see Injury, nerve, thigh
    open —see Wound, open, thigh
    specified NEC S79.82-●
    superficial —see Injury, superficial, thigh
  third cranial nerve (oculomotor) —see Injury,
      nerve, oculomotor
  thorax, thoracic S29.9
    blood vessel —see Injury, blood vessel,
        thorax
    cavity —see Injury, intrathoracic
    dislocation —see Dislocation, thorax
    external (wall) S29.9
      contusion —see Contusion, thorax
      nerve —see Injury, nerve, thorax
      open —see Wound, open, thorax
      specified NEC S29.8
      sprain —see Sprain, thorax
      superficial —see Injury, superficial,
          thorax
    fracture —see Fracture, thorax
    internal —see Injury, intrathoracic
    intrathoracic organ —see Injury,
        intrathoracic
    sympathetic ganglion —see Injury, nerve,
        thorax, sympathetic
  throat —see also Injury, neck S19.9
  thumb S69.9-●
    blood vessel —see Injury, blood vessel,
        thumb
    contusion —see Contusion, thumb
    dislocation —see Dislocation, thumb
    fracture —see Fracture, thumb
    muscle —see Injury, muscle, thumb
    nerve —see Injury, nerve, digital, thumb
    open —see Wound, open, thumb
    specified NEC S69.8-●
    sprain —see Sprain, thumb
    superficial —see Injury, superficial, thumb
  thymus (gland) —see Injury, intrathoracic,
      specified organ NEC
  thyroid (gland) NEC S19.84
  toe S99.92-●
    contusion —see Contusion, toe
    dislocation —see Dislocation, toe
    fracture —see Fracture, toe
    muscle —see Injury, muscle, toe
    open —see Wound, open, toe
    specified type NEC S99.82-●
    sprain —see Sprain, toe
    superficial —see Injury, superficial, toe
  tongue S09.93
  tonsil S09.93

Injury (Continued)
  tooth S09.93
  trachea (cervical) NEC S19.82
    thoracic —see Injury, intrathoracic, trachea,
        thoracic
  transfusion-related acute lung (TRALI) J95.84
  tunica vaginalis S39.94
  twelfth cranial nerve (hypoglossal) —see
      Injury, nerve, hypoglossal
  ureter S37.10
    contusion S37.12
    laceration S37.13
    specified type NEC S37.19
  urethra (sphincter) S37.30
    at delivery O71.5
    contusion S37.32
    laceration S37.33
    specified type NEC S37.38
  urinary organ S37.899
    contusion S37.92
    laceration S37.93
    specified
      site NEC S37.899
        contusion S37.892
        laceration S37.893
        specified type NEC S37.898
      type NEC S37.99
  uterus, uterine S37.60
    with ectopic or molar pregnancy O08.6
    blood vessel —see Injury, blood vessel, iliac
    contusion S37.62
    laceration S37.63
      cervix at delivery O71.3
    rupture associated with obstetrics —see
        Rupture, uterus
    specified type NEC S37.69
  uvula S09.93
  vagina S39.93
    abrasion S30.814
    bite S31.45
      insect S30.864
      superficial NEC S30.874
    contusion S30.23
    crush S38.03
    during delivery —see Laceration, vagina,
        during delivery
    external constriction S30.844
    insect bite S30.864
    laceration S31.41
      with foreign body S31.42
    open wound S31.40
    puncture S31.43
      with foreign body S31.44
    superficial S30.95
      foreign body S30.854
  vas deferens —see Injury, pelvic organ,
      specified site NEC
  vascular NEC T14.8
  vein —see Injury, blood vessel
  vena cava (superior) S25.20
    inferior S35.10
      laceration (minor) (superficial) S35.11
        major S35.12
      specified type NEC S35.19
    laceration (minor) (superficial) S25.21
      major S25.22
    specified type NEC S25.29
  vesical (sphincter) —see Injury, bladder
  visual cortex S04.04-●
  vitreous (humor) S05.90
    specified NEC S05.8X-●
  vocal cord NEC S19.83
  vulva S39.94
    abrasion S30.814
    bite S31.45
      insect S30.864
      superficial NEC S30.874
    contusion S30.23
    crush S38.03
    during delivery —see Laceration,
        perineum, female, during delivery

Injury (Continued)
  vulva (Continued)
    external constriction S30.844
    insect bite S30.864
    laceration S31.41
      with foreign body S31.42
    open wound S31.40
    puncture S31.43
      with foreign body S31.44
    superficial S30.95
      foreign body S30.854
  whiplash (cervical spine) S13.4
  wrist S69.9-●
    blood vessel —see Injury, blood vessel,
        hand
    contusion —see Contusion, wrist
    dislocation —see Dislocation, wrist
    fracture —see Fracture, wrist
    muscle —see Injury, muscle, hand
    nerve —see Injury, nerve, hand
    open —see Wound, open, wrist
    specified NEC S69.8-●
    sprain —see Sprain, wrist
    superficial —see Injury, superficial, wrist
Inoculation —see also Vaccination
  complication or reaction —see Complications,
      vaccination
Insanity, insane —see also Psychosis
  adolescent —see Schizophrenia
  confusional F28
    acute or subacute F05
  delusional F22
  senile F03
Insect
  bite —see Bite, by site, superficial, insect
  venomous, poisoning NEC (by) —see Venom,
      arthropod
Insensitivity
  adrenocorticotropin hormone (ACTH)
      E27.49
  androgen E34.50
    complete E34.51
    partial E34.52
Insertion
  cord (umbilical) lateral or velamentous
      O43.12-●
  intrauterine contraceptive device (encounter
      for) —see Intrauterine contraceptive
      device
Insolation (sunstroke) T67.0
Insomnia (organic) G47.00
  without objective findings F51.02
  adjustment F51.02
  adjustment disorder F51.02
  behavioral, of childhood Z73.819
    combined type Z73.812
    limit setting type Z73.811
    sleep-onset association type Z73.810
  childhood Z73.819
  chronic F51.04
    somatized tension F51.04
  conditioned F51.04
  due to
    alcohol
      abuse F10.182
      dependence F10.282
      use F10.982
    amphetamines
      abuse F15.182
      dependence F15.282
      use F15.982
    anxiety disorder F51.05
    caffeine
      abuse F15.182
      dependence F15.282
      use F15.982
    cocaine
      abuse F14.182
      dependence F14.282
      use F14.982
    depression F51.05

▶ New   ⇒ Revised   ~~deleted~~ Deleted   ● Use Additional Character(s)

Insomnia *(Continued)*
  due to *(Continued)*
    drug NEC
      abuse F19.182
      dependence F19.282
      use F19.982
    medical condition G47.01
    mental disorder NEC F51.05
    opioid
      abuse F11.182
      dependence F11.282
      use F11.982
    psychoactive substance NEC
      abuse F19.182
      dependence F19.282
      use F19.982
    sedative, hypnotic, or anxiolytic
      abuse F13.182
      dependence F13.282
      use F13.982
    stimulant NEC
      abuse F15.182
      dependence F15.282
      use F15.982
  fatal familial (FFI) A81.83
  idiopathic F51.01
  learned F51.3
  nonorganic origin F51.01
  not due to a substance or known
    physiological condition F51.01
    specified NEC F51.09
  paradoxical F51.03
  primary F51.01
  psychiatric F51.05
  psychophysiologic F51.04
  related to psychopathology F51.05
  short-term F51.02
  specified NEC G47.09
  stress-related F51.02
  transient F51.02
Inspiration
  food or foreign body —*see* Foreign body, by site
  mucus —*see* Asphyxia, mucus
Inspissated bile syndrome (newborn) P59.1
Instability
  emotional (excessive) F60.3
  joint (post-traumatic) M25.30
    ankle M25.37-●
    due to old ligament injury —*see* Disorder, ligament
    elbow M25.32-●
    flail —*see* Flail, joint
    foot M25.37-●
    hand M25.34-●
    hip M25.35-●
    knee M25.36-●
    lumbosacral —*see* subcategory M53.2
    prosthesis —*see* Complications, joint prosthesis, mechanical, displacement, by site
    sacroiliac —*see* subcategory M53.2
    secondary to
      old ligament injury —*see* Disorder, ligament
      removal of joint prosthesis M96.89
    shoulder (region) M25.31-●
    spine —*see* subcategory M53.2
    wrist M25.33-●
  knee (chronic) M23.5-●
  lumbosacral —*see* subcategory M53.2
  nervous F48.8
  personality (emotional) F60.3
  spine —*see* Instability, joint, spine
  vasomotor R55
Institutional syndrome (childhood) F94.2
Institutionalization, affecting child Z62.22
  disinhibited attachment F94.2

Insufficiency, insufficient
  accommodation, old age H52.4
  adrenal (gland) E27.40
    primary E27.1
  adrenocortical E27.40
    drug-induced E27.3
    iatrogenic E27.3
    primary E27.1
  anatomic crown height K08.89
  anterior (occlusal) guidance M26.54
  anus K62.89
  aortic (valve) I35.1
    with
      mitral (valve) disease I08.0
        with tricuspid (valve) disease I08.3
      stenosis I35.2
      tricuspid (valve) disease I08.2
        with mitral (valve) disease I08.3
    congenital Q23.1
    rheumatic I06.1
      with
        mitral (valve) disease I08.0
          with tricuspid (valve) disease I08.3
        stenosis I06.2
          with mitral (valve) disease I08.0
            with tricuspid (valve) disease I08.3
        tricuspid (valve) disease I08.2
          with mitral (valve) disease I08.3
    specified cause NEC I35.1
    syphilitic A52.03
  arterial I77.1
    basilar G45.0
    carotid (hemispheric) G45.1
    cerebral I67.81
    coronary (acute or subacute) I24.8
    mesenteric K55.1
    peripheral I73.9
    precerebral (multiple) (bilateral) G45.2
    vertebral G45.0
  arteriovenous I99.8
  biliary K83.8
  cardiac —*see also* Insufficiency, myocardial
    due to presence of (cardiac) prosthesis I97.11-●
    postprocedural I97.11-●
  cardiorenal, hypertensive I13.2
  cardiovascular —*see* Disease, cardiovascular
  cerebrovascular (acute) I67.81
    with transient focal neurological signs and symptoms G45.8
  circulatory NEC I99.8
    newborn P29.89
  clinical crown length K08.89
  convergence H51.11
  coronary (acute or subacute) I24.8
    chronic or with a stated duration of over 4 weeks I25.89
  corticoadrenal E27.40
    primary E27.1
  dietary E63.9
  divergence H51.8
  food T73.0
  gastroesophageal K22.8
  gonadal
    ovary E28.39
    testis E29.1
  heart —*see also* Insufficiency, myocardial
    newborn P29.0
    valve —*see* Endocarditis
  hepatic —*see* Failure, hepatic
  idiopathic autonomic G90.09
  interocclusal distance of fully erupted teeth (ridge) M26.36
  kidney N28.9
    acute N28.9
    chronic N18.9
  lacrimal (secretion) H04.12-●
    passages —*see* Stenosis, lacrimal
  liver —*see* Failure, hepatic

Insufficiency, insufficient *(Continued)*
  lung —*see* Insufficiency, pulmonary
  mental (congenital) —*see* Disability, intellectual
  mesenteric K55.1
  mitral (valve) I34.0
    with
      aortic valve disease I08.0
        with tricuspid (valve) disease I08.3
      obstruction or stenosis I05.2
        with aortic valve disease I08.0
      tricuspid (valve) disease I08.1
        with aortic (valve) disease I08.3
    congenital Q23.3
    rheumatic I05.1
      with
        aortic valve disease I08.0
          with tricuspid (valve) disease I08.3
        obstruction or stenosis I05.2
          with aortic valve disease I08.0
            with tricuspid (valve) disease I08.3
        tricuspid (valve) disease I08.1
          with aortic (valve) disease I08.3
      active or acute I01.1
        with chorea, rheumatic (Sydenham's) I02.0
    specified cause, except rheumatic I34.0
  muscle —*see also* Disease, muscle
    heart —*see* Insufficiency, myocardial
    ocular NEC H50.9
➡ myocardial, myocardium (with arteriosclerosis) —*see also* Failure, heart I50.9
    with
      rheumatic fever (conditions in I00) I09.0
        active, acute or subacute I01.2
          with chorea I02.0
        inactive or quiescent (with chorea) I09.0
    congenital Q24.8
    hypertensive —*see* Hypertension, heart
    newborn P29.0
    rheumatic I09.0
      active, acute, or subacute I01.2
    syphilitic A52.06
  nourishment T73.0
  pancreatic K86.89
    exocrine K86.81
  parathyroid (gland) E20.9
  peripheral vascular (arterial) I73.9
  pituitary E23.0
  placental (mother) O36.51-●
  platelets D69.6
  prenatal care affecting management of pregnancy O09.3-●
  progressive pluriglandular E31.0
  pulmonary J98.4
    acute, following surgery (nonthoracic) J95.2
      thoracic J95.1
    chronic, following surgery J95.3
    following
      shock J98.4
      trauma J98.4
    newborn P28.5
    valve I37.1
      with stenosis I37.2
      congenital Q22.2
      rheumatic I09.89
        with aortic, mitral or tricuspid (valve) disease I08.8
  pyloric K31.89
  renal (acute) N28.9
    chronic N18.9
  respiratory R06.89
    newborn P28.5
  rotation —*see* Malrotation
  sleep syndrome F51.12

Insufficiency, insufficient (Continued)
  social insurance Z59.7
  suprarenal E27.40
    primary E27.1
  tarso-orbital fascia, congenital Q10.3
  testis E29.1
  thyroid (gland) (acquired) E03.9
    congenital E03.1
  tricuspid (valve) (rheumatic) I07.1
    with
      aortic (valve) disease I08.2
        with mitral (valve) disease I08.3
      mitral (valve) disease I08.1
        with aortic (valve) disease I08.3
      obstruction or stenosis I07.2
        with aortic (valve) disease I08.2
          with mitral (valve) disease I08.3
    congenital Q22.8
    nonrheumatic I36.1
      with stenosis I36.2
  urethral sphincter R32
➡️valve, valvular (heart) I38
  ▶aortic —see Insufficiency, aortic (valve)
  ▶mitral —see Insufficiency, mitral (valve)
  ▶pulmonary —see Insufficiency, pulmonary, valve
  ▶tricuspid —see Insufficiency, tricuspid (valve)
    congenital Q24.8
  vascular I99.8
    intestine K55.9
      acute —see also Ischemia, intestine, acute K55.059
    mesenteric K55.1
    peripheral I73.9
    renal —see Hypertension, kidney
  velopharyngeal
    acquired K13.79
    congenital Q38.8
  venous (chronic) (peripheral) I87.2
  ventricular —see Insufficiency, myocardial
  welfare support Z59.7
Insufflation, fallopian Z31.41
Insular —see condition
Insulinoma
  pancreas
    benign D13.7
    malignant C25.4
    uncertain behavior D37.8
  specified site
    benign —see Neoplasm, by site, benign
    malignant —see Neoplasm, by site, malignant
    uncertain behavior —see Neoplasm, by site, uncertain behavior
  unspecified site
    benign D13.7
    malignant C25.4
    uncertain behavior D37.8
Insuloma —see Insulinoma
Interference
  balancing side M26.56
  non-working side M26.56
Intermenstrual —see condition
Intermittent —see condition
Internal —see condition
Interrogation
  cardiac defibrillator (automatic) (implantable) Z45.02
  cardiac pacemaker Z45.018
  cardiac (event) (loop) recorder Z45.09
  infusion pump (implanted) (intrathecal) Z45.1
  neurostimulator Z46.2
Interruption
  aortic arch Q25.21
  phase-shift, sleep cycle —see Disorder, sleep, circadian rhythm
  sleep phase-shift, or 24 hour sleep-wake cycle —see Disorder, sleep, circadian rhythm

Interstitial —see condition
Intertrigo L30.4
  labialis K13.0
Intervertebral disc —see condition
Intestine, intestinal —see condition
Intolerance
  carbohydrate K90.49
  disaccharide, hereditary E73.0
  fat NEC K90.49
    pancreatic K90.3
  food K90.49
    dietary counseling and surveillance Z71.3
  fructose E74.10
    hereditary E74.12
  glucose(-galactose) E74.39
  gluten K90.01
  lactose E73.9
    specified NEC E73.8
  lysine E72.3
  milk NEC K90.49
    lactose E73.9
  protein K90.49
  starch NEC K90.49
  sucrose (-isomaltose) E74.31
Intoxicated NEC (without dependence) —see Alcohol, intoxication
Intoxication
  acid E87.2
  alcoholic (acute) (without dependence) —see Alcohol, intoxication
  alimentary canal K52.1
  amphetamine (without dependence) — see Abuse, drug, stimulant, with intoxication
    with dependence —see Dependence, drug, stimulant, with intoxication
  anxiolytic (acute) (without dependence) —see Abuse, drug, sedative, with intoxication
    with dependence —see Dependence, drug, sedative, with intoxication
  caffeine F15.929
    with dependence —see Dependence, drug, stimulant, with intoxication
  cannabinoids (acute) (without dependence) —see Use, cannabis, with intoxication
    with
      abuse —see Abuse, drug, cannabis, with intoxication
      dependence —see Dependence, drug, cannabis, with intoxication
  chemical —see Table of Drugs and Chemicals
    via placenta or breast milk —see - Absorption, chemical, through placenta
  cocaine (acute) (without dependence) —see Abuse, drug, cocaine, with intoxication
    with dependence —see Dependence, drug, cocaine, with intoxication
  drug
    acute (without dependence) —see Abuse, drug, by type with intoxication
      with dependence —see Dependence, drug, by type with intoxication
    addictive
      via placenta or breast milk —see Absorption, drug, addictive, through placenta
    newborn P93.8
      gray baby syndrome P93.0
    overdose or wrong substance given or taken —see Table of Drugs and Chemicals, by drug, poisoning
  enteric K52.1
  foodborne A05.9
    bacterial A05.9
    classical (Clostridium botulinum) A05.1
    due to
      Bacillus cereus A05.4
      bacterium A05.9
        specified NEC A05.8

Intoxication (Continued)
  foodborne (Continued)
    due to (Continued)
      Clostridium
        botulinum A05.1
        perfringens A05.2
        welchii A05.2
      Salmonella A02.9
        with
          (gastro) enteritis A02.0
          localized infection(s) A02.20
            arthritis A02.23
            meningitis A02.21
            osteomyelitis A02.24
            pneumonia A02.22
            pyelonephritis A02.25
            specified NEC A02.29
          sepsis A02.1
          specified manifestation NEC A02.8
      Staphylococcus A05.0
      Vibrio
        parahaemolyticus A05.3
        vulnificus A05.5
    enterotoxin, staphylococcal A05.0
    noxious —see Poisoning, food, noxious
  gastrointestinal K52.1
  hallucinogenic (without dependence) — see Abuse, drug, hallucinogen, with intoxication
    with dependence —see Dependence, drug, hallucinogen, with intoxication
  hypnotic (acute) (without dependence) —see Abuse, drug, sedative, with intoxication
    with dependence —see Dependence, drug, sedative, with intoxication
  inhalant (acute) (without dependence) —see Abuse, drug, inhalant, with intoxication
    with dependence —see Dependence, drug, inhalant, with intoxication
  meaning
    inebriation —see category F10
    poisoning —see Table of Drugs and Chemicals
  methyl alcohol (acute) (without dependence) —see Alcohol, intoxication
  opioid (acute) (without dependence) —see Abuse, drug, opioid, with intoxication
    with dependence —see Dependence, drug, opioid, with intoxication
  pathologic NEC (without dependence) —see Alcohol, intoxication
  phencyclidine (without dependence) —see Abuse, drug, hallucinogen, with intoxication
    with dependence —see Dependence, drug, hallucinogen, with intoxication
  potassium (K) E87.5
  psychoactive substance NEC (without dependence) —see Abuse, drug, psychoactive NEC, with intoxication
    with dependence —see Dependence, drug, psychoactive NEC, with intoxication
  sedative (acute) (without dependence) —see Abuse, drug, sedative, with intoxication
    with dependence —see Dependence, drug, sedative, with intoxication
  serum —see also Reaction, serum T80.69
  uremic —see Uremia
  volatile solvents (acute) (without dependence) —see Abuse, drug, inhalant, with intoxication
    with dependence —see Dependence, drug, inhalant, with intoxication
  water E87.79
▶**Intraabdominal testis, testes**
▶ bilateral Q53.211
▶ unilateral Q53.111
Intracranial —see condition
Intrahepatic gallbladder Q44.1
Intraligamentous —see condition

▶ New   ➡️ Revised   ~~deleted~~ Deleted   ● Use Additional Character(s)

Intrathoracic —*see also* condition
  kidney Q63.2
Intrauterine contraceptive device
  checking Z30.431
  in situ Z97.5
  insertion Z30.430
    immediately following removal Z30.433
  management Z30.431
  reinsertion Z30.433
  removal Z30.432
  replacement Z30.433
  retention in pregnancy O26.3-•
Intraventricular —*see* condition
Intrinsic deformity —*see* Deformity
Intubation, difficult or failed T88.4
Intumescence, lens (eye) (cataract) —*see*
  Cataract
Intussusception (bowel) (colon) (enteric)
  (ileocecal) (ileocolic) (intestine) (rectum)
  K56.1
  appendix K38.8
  congenital Q43.8
  ureter (with obstruction) N13.5
Invagination (bowel, colon, intestine or rectum)
  K56.1
Inversion
  albumin-globulin (A-G) ratio E88.09
  bladder N32.89
  cecum —*see* Intussusception
  cervix N88.8
  chromosome in normal individual Q95.1
  circadian rhythm —*see* Disorder, sleep,
    circadian rhythm
  nipple N64.59
    congenital Q83.8
    gestational —*see* Retraction, nipple
    puerperal, postpartum —*see* Retraction,
      nipple
  nyctohemeral rhythm —*see* Disorder, sleep,
    circadian rhythm
  optic papilla Q14.2
  organ or site, congenital NEC —*see* Anomaly,
    by site
  sleep rhythm —*see* Disorder, sleep, circadian
    rhythm
  testis (congenital) Q55.29
  uterus (chronic) (postinfectional) (postpartal,
    old) N85.5
    postpartum O71.2
  vagina (posthysterectomy) N99.3
  ventricular Q20.5
Investigation —*see also* Examination Z04.9
  clinical research subject (control) (normal
    comparison) (participant) Z00.6
Involuntary movement, abnormal R25.9
Involution, involutional —*see also* condition
  breast, cystic —*see* Dysplasia, mammary,
    specified type NEC
  depression (single episode) F32.89
    recurrent episode F33.9
  melancholia (single episode) F32.89
    recurrent episode F33.8
  ovary, senile —*see* Atrophy, ovary
  thymus failure E32.8
I.Q.
  under 20 F73
  20-34 F72
  35-49 F71
  50-69 F70
IRDS (type I) P22.0
  type II P22.1
Irideremia Q13.1
Iridis rubeosis —*see* Disorder, iris, vascular
Iridochoroiditis (panuveitis) —*see* Panuveitis
Iridocyclitis H20.9-•
  acute H20.0-•
    hypopyon H20.05-•
    primary H20.01-•
    recurrent H20.02-•
    secondary (noninfectious) H20.04-•
      infectious H20.03-•

Iridocyclitis (*Continued*)
  chronic H20.1-•
  due to allergy —*see* Iridocyclitis, acute,
    secondary
  endogenous —*see* Iridocyclitis, acute, primary
  Fuchs' —*see* Cyclitis, Fuchs' heterochromic
  gonococcal A54.32
  granulomatous —*see* Iridocyclitis, chronic
  herpes, herpetic (simplex) B00.51
    zoster B02.32
  hypopyon —*see* Iridocyclitis, acute,
    hypopyon
  in (due to)
    ankylosing spondylitis M45.9
    gonococcal infection A54.32
    herpes (simplex) virus B00.51
      zoster B02.32
    infectious disease NOS B99
    parasitic disease NOS B89 *[H22]*
    sarcoidosis D86.83
    syphilis A51.43
    tuberculosis A18.54
    zoster B02.32
  lens-induced H20.2-•
  nongranulomatous —*see* Iridocyclitis, acute
  recurrent —*see* Iridocyclitis, acute, recurrent
  rheumatic —*see* Iridocyclitis, chronic
  subacute —*see* Iridocyclitis, acute
  sympathetic —*see* Uveitis, sympathetic
  syphilitic (secondary) A51.43
  tuberculous (chronic) A18.54
  Vogt-Koyanagi H20.82-•
Iridocyclochoroiditis (panuveitis) —*see*
  Panuveitis
Iridodialysis H21.53-•
Iridodonesis H21.89
Iridoplegia (complete) (partial) (reflex) H57.09
Iridoschisis H21.25-•
Iris —*see also* condition
  bombé —*see* Membrane, pupillary
Iritis —*see also* Iridocyclitis
  chronic —*see* Iridocyclitis, chronic
  diabetic —*see* E08-E13 with .39
  due to
    herpes simplex B00.51
    leprosy A30.9 *[H22]*
  gonococcal A54.32
  gouty —*see also* Gout, by type M10.9 *[H22]*
  granulomatous —*see* Iridocyclitis, chronic
  lens induced —*see* Iridocyclitis, lens-induced
  papulosa (syphilitic) A52.71
  rheumatic —*see* Iridocyclitis, chronic
  syphilitic (secondary) A51.43
    congenital (early) A50.01
    late A52.71
  tuberculous A18.54
Iron —*see* condition
Iron-miner's lung J63.4
Irradiated enamel (tooth, teeth) K03.89
Irradiation effects, adverse T66
Irreducible, irreducibility —*see* condition
Irregular, irregularity
  action, heart I49.9
  alveolar process K08.89
  bleeding N92.6
  breathing R06.89
  contour of cornea (acquired) —*see* Deformity,
    cornea
    congenital Q13.4
  contour, reconstructed breast N65.0
  dentin (in pulp) K04.3
  eye movements H55.89
    nystagmus —*see* Nystagmus
    saccadic H55.81
  labor O62.2
  menstruation (cause unknown) N92.6
  periods N92.6
  prostate N42.9
  pupil —*see* Abnormality, pupillary
  reconstructed breast N65.0
  respiratory R06.89

Irregular, irregularity (*Continued*)
  septum (nasal) J34.2
  shape, organ or site, congenital NEC —*see*
    Distortion
  sleep-wake pattern (rhythm) G47.23
Irritable, irritability R45.4
  bladder N32.89
  bowel (syndrome) K58.9
    with
      constipation K58.1
      diarrhea K58.0
    mixed K58.2
    psychogenic F45.8
    specified NEC K58.8
  bronchial —*see* Bronchitis
  cerebral, in newborn P91.3
  colon —*see also* Irritable, bowel K58.9
    with diarrhea K58.0
    psychogenic F45.8
  duodenum K59.8
  heart (psychogenic) F45.8
  hip —*see* Derangement, joint, specified type
    NEC, hip
  ileum K59.8
  infant R68.12
  jejunum K59.8
  rectum K59.8
  stomach K31.89
    psychogenic F45.8
  sympathetic G90.8
  urethra N36.8
Irritation
  anus K62.89
  axillary nerve G54.0
  bladder N32.89
  brachial plexus G54.0
  bronchial —*see* Bronchitis
  cervical plexus G54.2
  cervix —*see* Cervicitis
  choroid, sympathetic —*see* Endophthalmitis
  cranial nerve —*see* Disorder, nerve, cranial
  gastric K31.89
    psychogenic F45.8
  globe, sympathetic —*see* Uveitis,
    sympathetic
  labyrinth —*see* subcategory H83.2
  lumbosacral plexus G54.1
  meninges (traumatic) —*see* Injury, intracranial
    nontraumatic —*see* Meningismus
  nerve —*see* Disorder, nerve
  nervous R45.0
  penis N48.89
  perineum NEC L29.3
  peripheral autonomic nervous system
    G90.8
  peritoneum —*see* Peritonitis
  pharynx J39.2
  plantar nerve —*see* Lesion, nerve, plantar
  spinal (cord) (traumatic) —*see also* Injury,
    spinal cord, by region
    nerve G58.9
      root NEC —*see* Radiculopathy
      nontraumatic —*see* Myelopathy
  stomach K31.89
    psychogenic F45.8
  sympathetic nerve NEC G90.8
  ulnar nerve —*see* Lesion, nerve, ulnar
  vagina N89.8
Ischemia, ischemic I99.8
  bowel (transient)
    acute —*see also* Ischemia, intestine, acute
      K55.059
    chronic K55.1
    due to mesenteric artery insufficiency
      K55.1
  brain —*see* Ischemia, cerebral
  cardiac (*see* Disease, heart, ischemic)
  cardiomyopathy I25.5
  cerebral (chronic) (generalized) I67.82
    arteriosclerotic I67.2
    intermittent G45.9

Ischemia, ischemic *(Continued)*
  cerebral (chronic) (generalized) *(Continued)*
    newborn P91.0
    recurrent focal G45.8
    transient G45.9
  colon chronic (due to mesenteric artery
      insufficiency) K55.1
  coronary —*see* Disease, heart, ischemic
  demand (coronary) —*see also* Angina I24.8
  ▶with myocardial infarction I21.A1
  ▶resulting in myocardial infarction I21.A1
  heart (chronic or with a stated duration of
      over 4 weeks) I25.9
    acute or with a stated duration of 4 weeks
        or less I24.9
    subacute I24.9
  infarction, muscle —*see* Infarct, muscle
  intestine (large) (small) (transient) K55.9
    acute K55.059
      diffuse K55.052
      focal K55.051
      large K55.039
        diffuse K55.032
        focal K55.031
      small K55.019
        diffuse K55.012
        focal K55.011
    chronic K55.1
    due to mesenteric artery insufficiency K55.1
  kidney N28.0
  mesenteric, acute —*see also* Ischemia,
      intestine, acute K55.059
  muscle, traumatic T79.6
  myocardium, myocardial (chronic or with a
      stated duration of over 4 weeks) I25.9
    acute, without myocardial infarction
        I51.3
    silent (asymptomatic) I25.6
    transient of newborn P29.4
  renal N28.0
  retina, retinal —*see* Occlusion, artery, retina
  small bowel
    acute K55.019
      diffuse K55.012
      focal K55.011
    chronic K55.1
    due to mesenteric artery insufficiency K55.1

Ischemia, ischemic *(Continued)*
  spinal cord G95.11
  subendocardial —*see* Insufficiency, coronary
  supply (coronary) —*see also* Angina I25.9
    due to vasospasm I20.1
Ischial spine —*see* condition
Ischialgia —*see* Sciatica
Ischiopagus Q89.4
Ischium, ischial —*see* condition
Ischuria R34
Iselin's disease or osteochondrosis —*see*
    Osteochondrosis, juvenile, metatarsus
Islands of
  parotid tissue in
    lymph nodes Q38.6
    neck structures Q38.6
  submaxillary glands in
    fascia Q38.6
    lymph nodes Q38.6
    neck muscles Q38.6
Islet cell tumor, pancreas D13.7
Isoimmunization NEC —*see also*
    Incompatibility
  affecting management of pregnancy (ABO)
      (with hydrops fetalis) O36.11-●
    anti-A sensitization O36.11-●
    anti-B sensitization O36.19-●
    anti-c sensitization O36.09-●
    anti-C sensitization O36.09-●
    anti-e sensitization O36.09-●
    anti-E sensitization O36.09-●
    Rh NEC O36.09-●
      anti-D antibody O36.01-●
    specified NEC O36.19-●
  newborn P55.9
    with
      hydrops fetalis P56.0
      kernicterus P57.0
    ABO (blood groups) P55.1
    Rhesus (Rh) factor P55.0
    specified type NEC P55.8
Isolation, isolated
  dwelling Z59.8
  family Z63.79
  social Z60.4
Isoleucinosis E71.19

Isomerism atrial appendages (with asplenia or
    polysplenia) Q20.6
Isosporiasis, isosporosis A07.3
Isovaleric acidemia E71.110
Issue of
  medical certificate Z02.79
    for disability determination Z02.71
  repeat prescription (appliance) (glasses)
      (medicinal substance, medicament,
      medicine) Z76.0
    contraception —*see* Contraception
Itch, itching —*see also* Pruritus
  baker's L23.6
  barber's B35.0
  bricklayer's L24.5
  cheese B88.0
  clam digger's B65.3
  coolie B76.9
  copra B88.0
  dew B76.9
  dhobi B35.6
  filarial —*see* Infestation, filarial
  grain B88.0
  grocer's B88.0
  ground B76.9
  harvest B88.0
  jock B35.6
  Malabar B35.5
    beard B35.0
    foot B35.3
    scalp B35.0
  meaning scabies B86
  Norwegian B86
  perianal L29.0
  poultrymen's B88.0
  sarcoptic B86
  scabies B86
  scrub B88.0
  straw B88.0
  swimmer's B65.3
  water B76.9
  winter L29.8
Ivemark's syndrome (asplenia with congenital
    heart disease) Q89.01
Ivory bones Q78.2
Ixodiasis NEC B88.8

▶ New   ⇒ Revised   ~~deleted~~ Deleted   ● Use Additional Character(s)

J

Jaccoud's syndrome —*see* Arthropathy, postrheumatic, chronic

Jackson's
- membrane Q43.3
- paralysis or syndrome G83.89
- veil Q43.3

Jacquet's dermatitis (diaper dermatitis) L22

Jadassohn-Pellizari's disease or anetoderma L90.2

Jadassohn's
- blue nevus —*see* Nevus
- intraepidermal epithelioma —*see* Neoplasm, skin, benign

Jaffe-Lichtenstein (-Uehlinger) syndrome —*see* Dysplasia, fibrous, bone NEC

Jakob-Creutzfeldt disease or syndrome —*see* Creutzfeldt-Jakob disease or syndrome

Jaksch-Luzet disease D64.89

Jamaican
- neuropathy G92
- paraplegic tropical ataxic-spastic syndrome G92

Janet's disease F48.8

Janiceps Q89.4

Jansky-Bielschowsky amaurotic idiocy E75.4

Japanese
- B-type encephalitis A83.0
- river fever A75.3

Jaundice (yellow) R17
- acholuric (familial) (splenomegalic) —*see also* Spherocytosis
  - acquired D59.8
- breast-milk (inhibitor) P59.3
- catarrhal (acute) B15.9
  - with hepatic coma B15.0
- cholestatic (benign) R17
- due to or associated with
  - delayed conjugation P59.8
    - associated with (due to) preterm delivery P59.0
  - preterm delivery P59.0
- epidemic (catarrhal) B15.9
  - with hepatic coma B15.0
  - leptospiral A27.0
  - spirochetal A27.0
- familial nonhemolytic (congenital) (Gilbert) E80.4
  - Crigler-Najjar E80.5
- febrile (acute) B15.9
  - with hepatic coma B15.0
  - leptospiral A27.0
  - spirochetal A27.0
- hematogenous D59.9
- hemolytic (acquired) D59.9
  - congenital —*see* Spherocytosis

Jaundice (*Continued*)
- hemorrhagic (acute) (leptospiral) (spirochetal) A27.0
- infectious (acute) (subacute) B15.9
  - with hepatic coma B15.0
  - leptospiral A27.0
  - spirochetal A27.0
- leptospiral (hemorrhagic) A27.0
- malignant (without coma) K72.90
  - with coma K72.91
- neonatal —*see* Jaundice, newborn
- newborn P59.9
  - due to or associated with
    - ABO
      - antibodies P55.1
      - incompatibility, maternal/fetal P55.1
      - isoimmunization P55.1
    - absence or deficiency of enzyme system for bilirubin conjugation (congenital) P59.8
    - bleeding P58.1
    - breast milk inhibitors to conjugation P59.3
      - associated with preterm delivery P59.0
    - bruising P58.0
    - Crigler-Najjar syndrome E80.5
    - delayed conjugation P59.8
      - associated with preterm delivery P59.0
    - drugs or toxins
      - given to newborn P58.42
      - transmitted from mother P58.41
    - excessive hemolysis P58.9
      - due to
        - bleeding P58.1
        - bruising P58.0
        - drugs or toxins
          - given to newborn P58.42
          - transmitted from mother P58.41
        - infection P58.2
        - polycythemia P58.3
        - swallowed maternal blood P58.5
      - specified type NEC P58.8
    - galactosemia E74.21
    - Gilbert syndrome E80.4
    - hemolytic disease P55.9
      - ABO isoimmunization P55.1
      - Rh isoimmunization P55.0
      - specified NEC P55.8
    - hepatocellular damage P59.20
      - specified NEC P59.29
    - hereditary hemolytic anemia P58.8
    - hypothyroidism, congenital E03.1
    - incompatibility, maternal/fetal NOS P55.9
    - infection P58.2

Jaundice (*Continued*)
- newborn (*Continued*)
  - due to or associated with (*Continued*)
    - inspissated bile syndrome P59.1
    - isoimmunization NOS P55.9
    - mucoviscidosis E84.9
    - polycythemia P58.3
    - preterm delivery P59.0
    - Rh
      - antibodies P55.0
      - incompatibility, maternal/fetal P55.0
      - isoimmunization P55.0
    - specified cause NEC P59.8
    - swallowed maternal blood P58.5
  - spherocytosis (congenital) D58.0
  - nonhemolytic congenital familial (Gilbert) E80.4
  - nuclear, newborn —*see also* Kernicterus of newborn P57.9
  - obstructive —*see also* Obstruction, bile duct K83.1
  - post-immunization —*see* Hepatitis, viral, type, B
  - post-transfusion —*see* Hepatitis, viral, type, B
  - regurgitation —*see also* Obstruction, bile duct K83.1
  - serum (homologous) (prophylactic) (therapeutic) —*see* Hepatitis, viral, type, B
  - spirochetal (hemorrhagic) A27.0
  - symptomatic R17
    - newborn P59.9

Jaw —*see* condition

Jaw-winking phenomenon or syndrome Q07.8

Jealousy
- alcoholic F10.988
- childhood F93.8
- sibling F93.8

Jejunitis —*see* Enteritis

Jejunostomy status Z93.4

Jejunum, jejunal —*see* condition

Jensen's disease —*see* Inflammation, chorioretinal, focal, juxtapapillary

Jerks, myoclonic G25.3

Jervell-Lange-Nielsen syndrome I45.81

Jeune's disease Q77.2

Jigger disease B88.1

Job's syndrome (chronic granulomatous disease) D71

Joint —*see also* condition
- mice —*see* Loose, body, joint
  - knee M23.4-●

Jordan's anomaly or syndrome D72.0

Joseph-Diamond-Blackfan anemia (congenital hypoplastic) D61.01

Jungle yellow fever A95.0

Jüngling's disease —*see* Sarcoidosis

Juvenile —*see* condition

K

Kahler's disease C90.0-●
Kakke E51.11
Kala-azar B55.0
Kallmann's syndrome E23.0
Kanner's syndrome (autism) —see Psychosis,
    childhood
Kaposi's
  dermatosis (xeroderma pigmentosum) Q82.1
  lichen ruber L44.0
    acuminatus L44.0
  sarcoma
    colon C46.4
    connective tissue C46.1
    gastrointestinal organ C46.4
    lung C46.5-●
    lymph node (multiple) C46.3
    palate (hard) (soft) C46.2
    rectum C46.4
    skin (multiple sites) C46.0
    specified site NEC C46.7
    stomach C46.4
    unspecified site C46.9
  varicelliform eruption B00.0
    vaccinia T88.1
Kartagener's syndrome or triad (sinusitis,
    bronchiectasis, situs inversus) Q89.3
Karyotype
  with abnormality except iso (Xq) Q96.2
  45,X Q96.0
  46,X
    iso (Xq) Q96.1
  46,XX Q98.3
    with streak gonads Q50.32
    hermaphrodite (true) Q99.1
    male Q98.3
  46,XY
    with streak gonads Q56.1
    female Q97.3
    hermaphrodite (true) Q99.1
  47,XXX Q97.0
  47,XXY Q98.0
  47,XYY Q98.5
Kaschin-Beck disease —see Disease,
    Kaschin-Beck
Katayama's disease or fever B65.2
Kawasaki's syndrome M30.3
Kayser-Fleischer ring (cornea)
    (pseudosclerosis) H18.04-●
Kaznelson's syndrome (congenital hypoplastic
    anemia) D61.01
Kearns-Sayre syndrome H49.81-●
Kedani fever A75.3
Kelis L91.0
Kelly (-Patterson) syndrome (sideropenic
    dysphagia) D50.1
Keloid, cheloid L91.0
  acne L73.0
  Addison's L94.0
  cornea —see Opacity, cornea
  Hawkin's L91.0
  scar L91.0
Keloma L91.0
Kenya fever A77.1
Keratectasia —see also Ectasia, cornea
  congenital Q13.4
Keratinization of alveolar ridge mucosa
  excessive K13.23
  minimal K13.22
Keratinized residual ridge mucosa
  excessive K13.23
  minimal K13.22
Keratitis (nodular) (nonulcerative) (simple)
    (zonular) H16.9
  with ulceration (central) (marginal)
    (perforated) (ring) —see Ulcer, cornea
  actinic —see Photokeratitis
  arborescens (herpes simplex) B00.52
  areolar H16.11-●
  bullosa H16.8

Keratitis (Continued)
  deep H16.309
    specified type NEC H16.399
  dendritic (a) (herpes simplex) B00.52
  disciform (is) (herpes simplex) B00.52
    varicella B01.81
  filamentary H16.12-●
  gonococcal (congenital or prenatal) A54.33
  herpes, herpetic (simplex) B00.52
    zoster B02.33
  in (due to)
    acanthamebiasis B60.13
    adenovirus B30.0
    exanthema —see also Exanthem B09
    herpes (simplex) virus B00.52
    measles B05.81
    syphilis A50.31
    tuberculosis A18.52
    zoster B02.33
  interstitial (nonsyphilitic) H16.30-●
    diffuse H16.32-●
    herpes, herpetic (simplex) B00.52
      zoster B02.33
    sclerosing H16.33-●
    specified type NEC H16.39-●
    syphilitic (congenital) (late) A50.31
    tuberculous A18.52
  macular H16.11-●
  nummular H16.11-●
  oyster shuckers' H16.8
  parenchymatous —see Keratitis, interstitial
  petrificans H16.8
  postmeasles B05.81
  punctata
    leprosa A30.9 [H16.14-●]
    syphilitic (profunda) A50.31
  punctate H16.14-●
  purulent H16.8
  rosacea L71.8
  sclerosing H16.33-●
  specified type NEC H16.8
  stellate H16.11-●
  striate H16.11-●
  superficial H16.10-●
    with conjunctivitis —see
      Keratoconjunctivitis
    due to light —see Photokeratitis
  suppurative H16.8
  syphilitic (congenital) (prenatal) A50.31
  trachomatous A71.1
    sequelae B94.0
  tuberculous A18.52
  vesicular H16.8
  xerotic —see also Keratomalacia H16.8
    vitamin A deficiency E50.4
Keratoacanthoma L85.8
Keratocele —see Descemetocele
Keratoconjunctivitis H16.20-●
  Acanthamoeba B60.13
  adenoviral B30.0
  epidemic B30.0
  exposure H16.21-●
  herpes, herpetic (simplex) B00.52
    zoster B02.33
  in exanthema —see also Exanthem B09
  infectious B30.0
  lagophthalmic —see Keratoconjunctivitis,
    specified type NEC
  neurotrophic H16.23-●
  phlyctenular H16.25-●
  postmeasles B05.81
  shipyard B30.0
  sicca (Sjogren's) M35.0-●
    not Sjogren's H16.22-●
  specified type NEC H16.29-●
  tuberculous (phlyctenular) A18.52
  vernal H16.26-●
Keratoconus H18.60-●
  congenital Q13.4
  stable H18.61-●
  unstable H18.62-●

Keratocyst (dental) (odontogenic) —see Cyst,
    calcifying odontogenic
Keratoderma, keratodermia (congenital)
    (palmaris et plantaris) (symmetrical) Q82.8
  acquired L85.1
    in diseases classified elsewhere L86
  climactericum L85.1
  gonococcal A54.89
  gonorrheal A54.89
  punctata L85.2
  Reiter's —see Reiter's disease
Keratodermatocele —see Descemetocele
Keratoglobus H18.79
  congenital Q15.8
    with glaucoma Q15.0
Keratohemia —see Pigmentation, cornea,
    stromal
Keratoiritis —see also Iridocyclitis
  syphilitic A50.39
  tuberculous A18.54
Keratoma L57.0
  palmaris and plantaris hereditarium Q82.8
  senile L57.0
Keratomalacia H18.44-●
  vitamin A deficiency E50.4
Keratomegaly Q13.4
Keratomycosis B49
  nigrans, nigricans (palmaris) B36.1
Keratopathy H18.9
  band H18.42-●
  bullous H18.1-●
  bullous (aphakic), following cataract surgery
    H59.01-●
Keratoscleritis, tuberculous A18.52
Keratosis L57.0
  actinic L57.0
  arsenical L85.8
  congenital, specified NEC Q80.8
  female genital NEC N94.89
  follicularis Q82.8
    acquired L11.0
    congenita Q82.8
    et parafollicularis in cutem penetrans
      L87.0
    spinulosa (decalvans) Q82.8
    vitamin A deficiency E50.8
  gonococcal A54.89
  male genital (external) N50.89
  nigricans L83
  obturans, external ear (canal) —see
    Cholesteatoma, external ear
  palmaris et plantaris (inherited)
    (symmetrical) Q82.8
    acquired L85.1
  penile N48.89
  pharynx J39.2
  pilaris, acquired L85.8
  punctata (palmaris et plantaris) L85.2
  scrotal N50.89
  seborrheic L82.1
    inflamed L82.0
  senile L57.0
  solar L57.0
  tonsillaris J35.8
  vagina N89.4
  vegetans Q82.8
  vitamin A deficiency E50.8
  vocal cord J38.3
Kerato-uveitis —see Iridocyclitis
Kerion (celsi) B35.0
Kernicterus of newborn (not due to
    isoimmunization) P57.9
  due to isoimmunization (conditions in
    P55.0-P55.9) P57.0
  specified type NEC P57.8
Kerunoparalysis T75.09
Keshan disease E59
Ketoacidosis E87.2
  diabetic —see Diabetes, by type, with
    ketoacidosis
Ketonuria R82.4

▶ New   ➡ Revised   ~~deleted~~ Deleted   ● Use Additional Character(s)

Ketosis NEC E88.89
   diabetic —see Diabetes, by type, with
      ketoacidosis
Kew Garden fever A79.1
Kidney —see condition
Kienböck's disease —see also Osteochondrosis,
   juvenile, hand, carpal lunate
   adult M93.1
Kimmelstiel (-Wilson) disease —see Diabetes,
   Kimmelstiel (-Wilson) disease
Kimura disease D21.9
   specified site (see Neoplasm, connective
      tissue benign)
Kink, kinking
   artery I77.1
   hair (acquired) L67.8
   ileum or intestine —see Obstruction,
      intestine
   Lane's —see Obstruction, intestine
   organ or site, congenital NEC —see Anomaly,
      by site
   ureter (pelvic junction) N13.5
     with
       hydronephrosis N13.1
         with infection N13.6
       pyelonephritis (chronic) N11.1
     congenital Q62.39
   vein(s) I87.8
     caval I87.1
     peripheral I87.1
Kinnier Wilson's disease (hepatolenticular
   degeneration) E83.01
Kissing spine M48.20
   cervical region M48.22
   cervicothoracic region M48.23
   lumbar region M48.26
   lumbosacral region M48.27
   occipito-atlanto-axial region M48.21
   thoracic region M48.24
   thoracolumbar region M48.25
Klatskin's tumor C24.0
Klauder's disease A26.8
Klebs' disease —see also Glomerulonephritis
   N05.-●
Klebsiella (K.) pneumoniae, as cause of
   disease classified elsewhere B96.1
Klein (e)-Levin syndrome G47.13
Kleptomania F63.2
Klinefelter's syndrome Q98.4
   karyotype 47,XXY Q98.0
   male with more than two X chromosomes
      Q98.1
Klippel-Feil deficiency, disease, or syndrome
   (brevicollis) Q76.1
Klippel's disease I67.2
Klippel-Trenaunay (-Weber) syndrome
   Q87.2
Klumpke (-Déjerine) palsy, paralysis (birth)
   (newborn) P14.1
Knee —see condition
Knock knee (acquired) M21.06-●
   congenital Q74.1

Knot(s)
   intestinal, syndrome (volvulus) K56.2
   surfer S89.8-●
   umbilical cord (true) O69.2
Knotting (of)
   hair L67.8
   intestine K56.2
Knuckle pad (Garrod's) M72.1
Koch's
   infection —see Tuberculosis
   relapsing fever A68.9
Koch-Weeks' conjunctivitis —see
   Conjunctivitis, acute, mucopurulent
Köebner's syndrome Q81.8
Köenig's disease (osteochondritis dissecans) —
   see Osteochondritis, dissecans
Köhler-Pellegrini-Steida disease or syndrome
   (calcification, knee joint) —see Bursitis,
   tibial collateral
Köhler's disease
   patellar —see Osteochondrosis, juvenile,
      patella
   tarsal navicular —see Osteochondrosis,
      juvenile, tarsus
Koilonychia L60.3
   congenital Q84.6
Kojevnikov's, epilepsy —see Kozhevnikof's
   epilepsy
Koplik's spots B05.9
Kopp's asthma E32.8
Korsakoff's (Wernicke) disease, psychosis or
   syndrome (alcoholic) F10.96
   with dependence F10.26
   drug-induced
     due to drug abuse —see Abuse, drug, by
       type, with amnestic disorder
     due to drug dependence —see Dependence,
       drug, by type, with amnestic disorder
   nonalcoholic F04
Korsakov's disease, psychosis or syndrome —
   see Korsakoff's disease
Korsakow's disease, psychosis or syndrome —
   see Korsakoff's disease
Kostmann's disease or syndrome (infantile
   genetic agranulocytosis) —see
   Agranulocytosis
Kozhevnikof's epilepsy G40.109
   intractable G40.119
     with status epilepticus G40.111
     without status epilepticus G40.119
   not intractable G40.109
     with status epilepticus G40.101
     without status epilepticus G40.109
Krabbe's
   disease E75.23
   syndrome, congenital muscle hypoplasia
      Q79.8
Kraepelin-Morel disease —see Schizophrenia
Kraft-Weber-Dimitri disease Q85.8
Kraurosis
   ani K62.89
   penis N48.0

Kraurosis (Continued)
   vagina N89.8
   vulva N90.4
Kreotoxism A05.9
Krukenberg's
   spindle —see Pigmentation, cornea, posterior
   tumor C79.6-●
Kufs' disease E75.4
Kugelberg-Welander disease G12.1
Kuhnt-Junius degeneration —see also
   Degeneration, macula H35.32-●
Kümmell's disease or spondylitis —see
   Spondylopathy, traumatic
Kupffer cell sarcoma C22.3
Kuru A81.81
Kussmaul's
   disease M30.0
   respiration E87.2
     in diabetic acidosis —see Diabetes, by type,
      with ketoacidosis
Kwashiorkor E40
   marasmic, marasmus type E42
Kyasanur Forest disease A98.2
Kyphoscoliosis, kyphoscoliotic (acquired) —
   see also Scoliosis M41.9
   congenital Q67.5
   heart (disease) I27.1
   sequelae of rickets E64.3
   tuberculous A18.01
Kyphosis, kyphotic (acquired) M40.209
   cervical region M40.202
   cervicothoracic region M40.203
   congenital Q76.419
     cervical region Q76.412
     cervicothoracic region Q76.413
     occipito-atlanto-axial region Q76.411
     thoracic region Q76.414
     thoracolumbar region Q76.415
   Morquio-Brailsford type (spinal) —see also
     subcategory M49.8 E76.219
   postlaminectomy M96.3
   postradiation therapy M96.2
   postural (adolescent) M40.00
     cervicothoracic region M40.03
     thoracic region M40.04
     thoracolumbar region M40.05
   secondary NEC M40.10
     cervical region M40.12
     cervicothoracic region M40.13
     thoracic region M40.14
     thoracolumbar region M40.15
   sequelae of rickets E64.3
   specified type NEC M40.299
     cervical region M40.292
     cervicothoracic region M40.293
     thoracic region M40.294
     thoracolumbar region M40.295
   syphilitic, congenital A50.56
   thoracic region M40.204
   thoracolumbar region M40.205
   tuberculous A18.01
Kyrle disease L87.0

L

Labia, labium —*see* condition
Labile
  blood pressure R09.89
  vasomotor system I73.9
Labioglossal paralysis G12.29
Labium leporinum —*see* Cleft, lip
Labor —*see* Delivery
Labored breathing —*see* Hyperventilation
Labyrinthitis (circumscribed) (destructive)
  (diffuse) (inner ear) (latent) (purulent)
  (suppurative) (*see also* subcategory)
  H83.0
  syphilitic A52.79
Laceration
  with abortion —*see* Abortion, by type,
    complicated by laceration of pelvic
    organs
  abdomen, abdominal
    wall S31.119
      with
        foreign body S31.129
        penetration into peritoneal cavity
          S31.619
          with foreign body S31.629
      epigastric region S31.112
        with
          foreign body S31.122
          penetration into peritoneal cavity
            S31.612
            with foreign body S31.622
      left
        lower quadrant S31.114
          with
            foreign body S31.124
            penetration into peritoneal cavity
              S31.614
              with foreign body S31.624
        upper quadrant S31.111
          with
            foreign body S31.121
            penetration into peritoneal cavity
              S31.611
              with foreign body S31.621
      periumbilic region S31.115
        with
          foreign body S31.125
          penetration into peritoneal cavity
            S31.615
            with foreign body S31.625
      right
        lower quadrant S31.113
          with
            foreign body S31.123
            penetration into peritoneal cavity
              S31.613
              with foreign body S31.623
        upper quadrant S31.110
          with
            foreign body S31.120
            penetration into peritoneal cavity
              S31.610
              with foreign body S31.620
  accidental, complicating surgery —*see*
    Complications, surgical, accidental
    puncture or laceration
  Achilles tendon S86.02-•
  adrenal gland S37.813
  alveolar (process) —*see* Laceration, oral cavity
  ankle S91.01-•
    with
      foreign body S91.02-•
  antecubital space —*see* Laceration, elbow
  anus (sphincter) S31.831
    with
      ectopic or molar pregnancy O08.6
      foreign body S31.832
    complicating delivery —*see* Delivery,
      complicated, by, laceration, anus
      (sphincter)

Laceration *(Continued)*
  anus *(Continued)*
    following ectopic or molar pregnancy
      O08.6
    nontraumatic, nonpuerperal —*see* Fissure,
      anus
  arm (upper) S41.11-•
    with foreign body S41.12-•
    lower —*see* Laceration, forearm
  auditory canal (external) (meatus) —*see*
    Laceration, ear
  auricle, ear —*see* Laceration, ear
  axilla —*see* Laceration, arm
  back —*see also* Laceration, thorax, back
    lower S31.010
      with
        foreign body S31.020
          with penetration into
            retroperitoneal space S31.021
        penetration into retroperitoneal space
          S31.011
  bile duct S36.13
  bladder S37.23
    with ectopic or molar pregnancy O08.6
    following ectopic or molar pregnancy
      O08.6
    obstetrical trauma O71.5
  blood vessel —*see* Injury, blood vessel
  bowel —*see also* Laceration, intestine
    with ectopic or molar pregnancy O08.6
    complicating abortion —*see* Abortion,
      by type, complicated by, specified
      condition NEC
    following ectopic or molar pregnancy
      O08.6
    obstetrical trauma O71.5
  brain (any part) (cortex) (diffuse)
    (membrane) —*see also* Injury,
    intracranial, diffuse
    during birth P10.8
      with hemorrhage P10.1
    focal —*see* Injury, intracranial, focal brain
      injury
  brainstem S06.38-•
  breast S21.01-•
    with foreign body S21.02-•
  broad ligament S37.893
    with ectopic or molar pregnancy O08.6
    following ectopic or molar pregnancy
      O08.6
    laceration syndrome N83.8
    obstetrical trauma O71.6
    syndrome (laceration) N83.8
  buttock S31.801
    with foreign body S31.802
    left S31.821
      with foreign body S31.822
    right S31.811
      with foreign body S31.812
  calf —*see* Laceration, leg
  canaliculus lacrimalis —*see* Laceration,
    eyelid
  canthus, eye —*see* Laceration, eyelid
  capsule, joint —*see* Sprain
  causing eversion of cervix uteri (old) N86
  central (perineal), complicating delivery
    O70.9
  cerebellum, traumatic S06.37-•
  cerebral S06.33-•
    during birth P10.8
      with hemorrhage P10.1
    left side S06.32-•
    right side S06.31-•
  cervix (uteri)
    with ectopic or molar pregnancy O08.6
    following ectopic or molar pregnancy
      O08.6
    nonpuerperal, nontraumatic N88.1
    obstetrical trauma (current) O71.3
    old (postpartal) N88.1
    traumatic S37.63

Laceration *(Continued)*
  cheek (external) S01.41-•
    with foreign body S01.42-•
    internal —*see* Laceration, oral cavity
  chest wall —*see* Laceration, thorax
  chin —*see* Laceration, head, specified site
    NEC
  chordae tendinae NEC I51.1
    concurrent with acute myocardial
      infarction —*see* Infarct, myocardium
    following acute myocardial infarction
      (current complication) I23.4
  clitoris —*see* Laceration, vulva
  colon —*see* Laceration, intestine, large,
    colon
  common bile duct S36.13
  cortex (cerebral) —*see* Injury, intracranial,
    diffuse
  costal region —*see* Laceration, thorax
  cystic duct S36.13
  diaphragm S27.803
  digit(s)
    foot —*see* Laceration, toe
    hand —*see* Laceration, finger
  duodenum S36.430
  ear (canal) (external) S01.31-•
    with foreign body S01.32-•
    drum S09.2-•
  elbow S51.01-•
    with
      foreign body S51.02-•
  epididymis —*see* Laceration, testis
  epigastric region —*see* Laceration, abdomen,
    wall, epigastric region
  esophagus K22.8
    traumatic
      cervical S11.21
        with foreign body S11.22
      thoracic S27.813
  eye (ball) S05.3-•
    with prolapse or loss of intraocular tissue
      S05.2-•
    penetrating S05.6-•
  eyebrow —*see* Laceration, eyelid
  eyelid S01.11-•
    with foreign body S01.12-•
  face NEC —*see* Laceration, head, specified
    site NEC
  fallopian tube S37.539
    bilateral S37.532
    unilateral S37.531
  finger(s) S61.219
    with
      damage to nail S61.319
        with
          foreign body S61.329
      foreign body S61.229
    index S61.218
      with
        damage to nail S61.318
          with
            foreign body S61.328
        foreign body S61.228
    left S61.211
      with
        damage to nail S61.311
          with
            foreign body S61.321
        foreign body S61.221
    right S61.210
      with
        damage to nail S61.310
          with
            foreign body S61.320
        foreign body S61.220
    little S61.218
      with
        damage to nail S61.318
          with
            foreign body S61.328
        foreign body S61.228

▶ New   ⇒ Revised   ~~deleted~~ Deleted   • Use Additional Character(s)

Laceration *(Continued)*
  finger *(Continued)*
    little *(Continued)*
      left S61.217
        with
          damage to nail S61.317
            with
              foreign body S61.327
          foreign body S61.227
      right S61.216
        with
          damage to nail S61.316
            with
              foreign body S61.326
          foreign body S61.226
    middle S61.218
      with
        damage to nail S61.318
          with
            foreign body S61.328
        foreign body S61.228
      left S61.213
        with
          damage to nail S61.313
            with
              foreign body S61.323
          foreign body S61.223
      right S61.212
        with
          damage to nail S61.312
            with
              foreign body S61.322
          foreign body S61.222
    ring S61.218
      with
        damage to nail S61.318
          with
            foreign body S61.328
        foreign body S61.228
      left S61.215
        with
          damage to nail S61.315
            with
              foreign body S61.325
          foreign body S61.225
      right S61.214
        with
          damage to nail S61.314
            with
              foreign body S61.324
          foreign body S61.224
  flank S31.119
    with foreign body S31.129
  foot (except toe(s) alone) S91.319
    with foreign body S91.329
    left S91.312
      with foreign body S91.322
    right S91.311
      with foreign body S91.321
    toe —*see* Laceration, toe
  forearm S51.819
    with
      foreign body S51.829
    elbow only —*see* Laceration,
      elbow
    left S51.812
      with
        foreign body S51.822
    right S51.811
      with
        foreign body S51.821
  forehead S01.81
    with foreign body S01.82
  fourchette O70.0
    with ectopic or molar pregnancy
      O08.6
    complicating delivery O70.0
    following ectopic or molar pregnancy
      O08.6
  gallbladder S36.123

Laceration *(Continued)*
  genital organs, external
    female S31.512
      with foreign body S31.522
      vagina —*see* Laceration, vagina
      vulva —*see* Laceration, vulva
    male S31.511
      with foreign body S31.521
      penis —*see* Laceration, penis
      scrotum —*see* Laceration, scrotum
      testis —*see* Laceration, testis
  groin —*see* Laceration, abdomen, wall
  gum —*see* Laceration, oral cavity
  hand S61.419
    with
      foreign body S61.429
    finger —*see* Laceration, finger
    left S61.412
      with
        foreign body S61.422
    right S61.411
      with
        foreign body S61.421
    thumb —*see* Laceration, thumb
  head S01.91
    with foreign body S01.92
    cheek —*see* Laceration, cheek
    ear —*see* Laceration, ear
    eyelid —*see* Laceration, eyelid
    lip —*see* Laceration, lip
    nose —*see* Laceration, nose
    oral cavity —*see* Laceration, oral
      cavity
    scalp S01.01
      with foreign body S01.02
    specified site NEC S01.81
      with foreign body S01.82
    temporomandibular area —*see* Laceration,
      cheek
  heart —*see* Injury, heart, laceration
  heel —*see* Laceration, foot
  hepatic duct S36.13
  hip S71.019
    with foreign body S71.029
    left S71.012
      with foreign body S71.022
    right S71.011
      with foreign body S71.021
  hymen —*see* Laceration, vagina
  hypochondrium —*see* Laceration, abdomen,
    wall
  hypogastric region —*see* Laceration,
    abdomen, wall
  ileum S36.438
  inguinal region —*see* Laceration, abdomen,
    wall
  instep —*see* Laceration, foot
  internal organ —*see* Injury, by site
  interscapular region —*see* Laceration, thorax,
    back
  intestine
    large
      colon S36.539
        ascending S36.530
        descending S36.532
        sigmoid S36.533
        specified site NEC S36.538
      rectum S36.63
        transverse S36.531
    small S36.439
      duodenum S36.430
      specified site NEC S36.438
  intra-abdominal organ S36.93
    intestine —*see* Laceration, intestine
    liver —*see* Laceration, liver
    pancreas —*see* Laceration, pancreas
    peritoneum S36.81
    specified site NEC S36.893
    spleen —*see* Laceration, spleen
    stomach —*see* Laceration, stomach

Laceration *(Continued)*
  intracranial NEC —*see also* Injury,
    intracranial, diffuse
    birth injury P10.9
  jaw —*see* Laceration, head, specified site NEC
  jejunum S36.438
  joint capsule —*see* Sprain, by site
  kidney S37.03-●
    major (greater than 3 cm) (massive)
      (stellate) S37.06-●
    minor (less than 1 cm) S37.04-●
    moderate (1 to 3 cm) S37.05-●
    multiple S37.06-●
  knee S81.01-●
    with foreign body S81.02-●
  labium (majus) (minus) —*see* Laceration,
    vulva
  lacrimal duct —*see* Laceration, eyelid
  large intestine —*see* Laceration, intestine,
    large
  larynx S11.011
    with foreign body S11.012
  leg (lower) S81.819
    with foreign body S81.829
    foot —*see* Laceration, foot
    knee —*see* Laceration, knee
    left S81.812
      with foreign body S81.822
    right S81.811
      with foreign body S81.821
    upper —*see* Laceration, thigh
  ligament —*see* Sprain
  lip S01.511
    with foreign body S01.521
  liver S36.113
    major (stellate) S36.116
    minor S36.114
    moderate S36.115
  loin —*see* Laceration, abdomen, wall
  lower back —*see* Laceration, back, lower
  lumbar region —*see* Laceration, back, lower
  lung S27.339
    bilateral S27.332
    unilateral S27.331
  malar region —*see* Laceration, head, specified
    site NEC
  mammary —*see* Laceration, breast
  mastoid region —*see* Laceration, head,
    specified site NEC
  meninges —*see* Injury, intracranial, diffuse
  meniscus —*see* Tear, meniscus
  mesentery S36.893
  mesosalpinx S37.893
  mouth —*see* Laceration, oral cavity
  muscle —*see* Injury, muscle, by site,
    laceration
  nail
    finger —*see* Laceration, finger, with
      damage to nail
    toe —*see* Laceration, toe, with damage to nail
  nasal (septum) (sinus) —*see* Laceration, nose
  nasopharynx —*see* Laceration, head, specified
    site NEC
  neck S11.91
    with foreign body S11.92
    involving
      cervical esophagus S11.21
        with foreign body S11.22
      larynx —*see* Laceration, larynx
      pharynx —*see* Laceration, pharynx
      thyroid gland —*see* Laceration, thyroid
        gland
      trachea —*see* Laceration, trachea
    specified site NEC S11.81
      with foreign body S11.82
  nerve —*see* Injury, nerve
  nose (septum) (sinus) S01.21
    with foreign body S01.22
  ocular NOS S05.3-●
    adnexa NOS S01.11-●

Laceration *(Continued)*
  oral cavity S01.512
    with foreign body S01.522
  orbit (eye) —*see* Wound, open, ocular, orbit
  ovary S37.439
    bilateral S37.432
    unilateral S37.431
  palate —*see* Laceration, oral cavity
  palm —*see* Laceration, hand
  pancreas S36.239
    body S36.231
      major S36.261
      minor S36.241
      moderate S36.251
    head S36.230
      major S36.260
      minor S36.240
      moderate S36.250
    major S36.269
    minor S36.249
    moderate S36.259
    tail S36.232
      major S36.262
      minor S36.242
      moderate S36.252
  pelvic S31.010
    with
      foreign body S31.020
        penetration into retroperitoneal cavity S31.021
      penetration into retroperitoneal cavity S31.011
  floor —*see also* Laceration, back, lower
    with ectopic or molar pregnancy O08.6
    complicating delivery O70.1
    following ectopic or molar pregnancy O08.6
    old (postpartal) N81.89
  organ S37.93
    with ectopic or molar pregnancy O08.6
    adrenal gland S37.813
    bladder S37.23
    fallopian tube —*see* Laceration, fallopian tube
    following ectopic or molar pregnancy O08.6
    kidney —*see* Laceration, kidney
    obstetrical trauma O71.5
    ovary —*see* Laceration, ovary
    prostate S37.823
    specified site NEC S37.893
    ureter S37.13
    urethra S37.33
    uterus S37.63
  penis S31.21
    with foreign body S31.22
  perineum
    female S31.41
      with
        ectopic or molar pregnancy O08.6
        foreign body S31.42
      during delivery O70.9
        first degree O70.0
        fourth degree O70.3
        second degree O70.1
        third degree —*see also* Delivery, complicated, by, laceration, perineum, third degree O70.20
      old (postpartal) N81.89
      postpartal N81.89
      secondary (postpartal) O90.1
    male S31.119
      with foreign body S31.129
  periocular area (with or without lacrimal passages) —*see* Laceration, eyelid
  peritoneum S36.893
  periumbilic region —*see* Laceration, abdomen, wall, periumbilic

periurethral tissue —*see* Laceration, urethra
phalanges
  finger —*see* Laceration, finger
  toe —*see* Laceration, toe
pharynx S11.21
  with foreign body S11.22
pinna —*see* Laceration, ear
popliteal space —*see* Laceration, knee
prepuce —*see* Laceration, penis
prostate S37.823
pubic region S31.119
  with foreign body S31.129
pudendum —*see* Laceration, genital organs, external
rectovaginal septum —*see* Laceration, vagina
rectum S36.63
retroperitoneum S36.893
round ligament S37.893
sacral region —*see* Laceration, back, lower
sacroiliac region —*see* Laceration, back, lower
salivary gland —*see* Laceration, oral cavity
scalp S01.01
  with foreign body S01.02
scapular region —*see* Laceration, shoulder
scrotum S31.31
  with foreign body S31.32
seminal vesicle S37.893
shin —*see* Laceration, leg
shoulder S41.019
  with foreign body S41.029
  left S41.012
    with foreign body S41.022
  right S41.011
    with foreign body S41.021
small intestine —*see* Laceration, intestine, small
spermatic cord —*see* Laceration, testis
spinal cord (meninges) —*see also* Injury, spinal cord, by region
  due to injury at birth P11.5
  newborn (birth injury) P11.5
spleen S36.039
  major (massive) (stellate) S36.032
  moderate S36.031
  superficial (minor) S36.030
sternal region —*see* Laceration, thorax, front
stomach S36.33
submaxillary region —*see* Laceration, head, specified site NEC
submental region —*see* Laceration, head, specified site NEC
subungual
  finger(s) —*see* Laceration, finger, with damage to nail
  toe(s) —*see* Laceration, toe, with damage to nail
suprarenal gland —*see* Laceration, adrenal gland
temple, temporal region —*see* Laceration, head, specified site NEC
temporomandibular area —*see* Laceration, cheek
tendon —*see* Injury, muscle, by site, laceration
  Achilles S86.02-●
tentorium cerebelli —*see* Injury, intracranial, diffuse
testis S31.31
  with foreign body S31.32
thigh S71.11-●
  with foreign body S71.12-●
thorax, thoracic (wall) S21.91
  with foreign body S21.92
    back S21.22-●
      with penetration into thoracic cavity S21.42-●
    front S21.12-●
      with penetration into thoracic cavity S21.32-●

Laceration *(Continued)*
  thorax, thoracic *(Continued)*
    back S21.21-●
      with
        foreign body S21.22-●
          with penetration into thoracic cavity S21.42-●
        penetration into thoracic cavity S21.41-●
    breast —*see* Laceration, breast
    front S21.11-●
      with
        foreign body S21.12-●
          with penetration into thoracic cavity S21.32-●
        penetration into thoracic cavity S21.31-●
  thumb S61.019
    with
      damage to nail S61.119
        with
          foreign body S61.129
      foreign body S61.029
    left S61.012
      with
        damage to nail S61.112
          with
            foreign body S61.122
        foreign body S61.022
    right S61.011
      with
        damage to nail S61.111
          with
            foreign body S61.121
        foreign body S61.021
  thyroid gland S11.11
    with foreign body S11.12
  toe(s) S91.119
    with
      damage to nail S91.219
        with
          foreign body S91.229
      foreign body S91.129
    great S91.113
      with
        damage to nail S91.213
          with
            foreign body S91.223
        foreign body S91.123
    left S91.112
      with
        damage to nail S91.212
          with
            foreign body S91.222
        foreign body S91.122
    right S91.111
      with
        damage to nail S91.211
          with
            foreign body S91.221
        foreign body S91.121
    lesser S91.116
      with
        damage to nail S91.216
          with
            foreign body S91.226
        foreign body S91.126
    left S91.115
      with
        damage to nail S91.215
          with
            foreign body S91.225
        foreign body S91.125
    right S91.114
      with
        damage to nail S91.214
          with
            foreign body S91.224
        foreign body S91.124
  tongue —*see* Laceration, oral cavity

▶ New   ⇒ Revised   ~~deleted~~ Deleted   ● Use Additional Character(s)

Laceration *(Continued)*
trachea S11.021
  with foreign body S11.022
tunica vaginalis —*see* Laceration, testis
tympanum, tympanic membrane —*see*
    Laceration, ear, drum
umbilical region S31.115
  with foreign body S31.125
ureter S37.13
urethra S37.33
  with or following ectopic or molar
    pregnancy O08.6
  obstetrical trauma O71.5
urinary organ NEC S37.893
uterus S37.63
  with ectopic or molar pregnancy O08.6
  following ectopic or molar pregnancy O08.6
  nonpuerperal, nontraumatic N85.8
  obstetrical trauma NEC O71.81
  old (postpartal) N85.8
uvula —*see* Laceration, oral cavity
vagina S31.41
  with
    ectopic or molar pregnancy O08.6
    foreign body S31.42
  during delivery O71.4
    with perineal laceration —*see* Laceration,
      perineum, female, during delivery
  following ectopic or molar pregnancy
    O08.6
  nonpuerperal, nontraumatic N89.8
  old (postpartal) N89.8
vas deferens S37.893
vesical —*see* Laceration, bladder
vocal cords S11.031
  with foreign body S11.032
vulva S31.41
  with
    ectopic or molar pregnancy O08.6
    foreign body S31.42
  complicating delivery O70.0
  following ectopic or molar pregnancy
    O08.6
  nonpuerperal, nontraumatic N90.89
  old (postpartal) N90.89
wrist S61.519
  with
    foreign body S61.529
  left S61.512
    with
      foreign body S61.522
  right S61.511
    with
      foreign body S61.521
Lack of
achievement in school Z55.3
adequate
  food Z59.4
  intermaxillary vertical dimension of fully
    erupted teeth M26.36
  sleep Z72.820
appetite (*see* Anorexia) R63.0
awareness R41.9
care
  in home Z74.2
  of infant (at or after birth) T76.02
    confirmed T74.02
cognitive functions R41.9
coordination R27.9
  ataxia R27.0
  specified type NEC R27.8
development (physiological) R62.50
  failure to thrive (child over 28 days old)
    R62.51
    adult R62.7
    newborn P92.6
  short stature R62.52
  specified type NEC R62.59
energy R53.83
financial resources Z59.6

Lack of *(Continued)*
food T73.0
growth R62.52
heating Z59.1
housing (permanent) (temporary) Z59.0
  adequate Z59.1
learning experiences in childhood Z62.898
leisure time (affecting life-style) Z73.2
material resources Z59.9
memory —*see also* Amnesia
  mild, following organic brain damage
    F06.8
ovulation N97.0
parental supervision or control of child Z62.0
person able to render necessary care Z74.2
physical exercise Z72.3
play experience in childhood Z62.898
posterior occlusal support M26.57
relaxation (affecting life-style) Z73.2
sexual
  desire F52.0
  enjoyment F52.1
shelter Z59.0
sleep (adequate) Z72.820
supervision of child by parent Z62.0
support, posterior occlusal M26.57
water T73.1
Lacrimal —*see* condition
Lacrimation, abnormal —*see* Epiphora
Lacrimonasal duct —*see* condition
Lactation, lactating (breast) (puerperal,
  postpartum)
associated
  cracked nipple O92.13
  retracted nipple O92.03
defective O92.4
disorder NEC O92.79
excessive O92.6
failed (complete) O92.3
  partial O92.4
mastitis NEC —*see* Mastitis, obstetric
mother (care and/or examination) Z39.1
nonpuerperal N64.3
Lacticemia, excessive E87.2
Lacunar skull Q75.8
Laennec's cirrhosis K70.30
  with ascites K70.31
  nonalcoholic K74.69
Lafora's disease —*see* Epilepsy, generalized,
  idiopathic
Lag, lid (nervous) —*see* Retraction, lid
Lagophthalmos (eyelid) (nervous) H02.209
cicatricial H02.219
  left H02.216
    lower H02.215
    upper H02.214
  right H02.213
    lower H02.212
    upper H02.211
keratoconjunctivitis —*see* Keratoconjunctivitis
left H02.206
  lower H02.205
  upper H02.204
mechanical H02.229
  left H02.226
    lower H02.225
    upper H02.224
  right H02.223
    lower H02.222
    upper H02.221
paralytic H02.239
  left H02.236
    lower H02.235
    upper H02.234
  right H02.233
    lower H02.232
    upper H02.231
right H02.203
  lower H02.202
  upper H02.201

Laki-Lorand factor deficiency —*see* Defect,
  coagulation, specified type NEC
Lalling F80.0
Lambert-Eaton syndrome —*see* Syndrome,
  Lambert-Eaton
Lambliasis, lambliosis A07.1
Landau-Kleffner syndrome —*see* Epilepsy,
  specified NEC
Landouzy-Déjérine dystrophy or
  facioscapulohumeral atrophy G71.0
Landouzy's disease (icterohemorrhagic
  leptospirosis) A27.0
Landry-Guillain-Barré, syndrome or paralysis
  G61.0
Landry's disease or paralysis G61.0
Lane's
band Q43.3
kink —*see* Obstruction, intestine
syndrome K90.2
Langdon Down's syndrome —*see* Trisomy, 21
Lapsed immunization schedule status Z28.3
Large
baby (regardless of gestational age) (4000g to
  4499g) P08.1
ear, congenital Q17.1
physiological cup Q14.2
stature R68.89
Large-for-dates NEC (infant) (4000g to 4499g)
  P08.1
  affecting management of pregnancy O36.6- ●
  exceptionally (4500g or more) P08.0
Larsen-Johansson disease
  orosteochondrosis —*see* Osteochondrosis,
    juvenile, patella
Larsen's syndrome (flattened facies and
  multiple congenital dislocations) Q74.8
Larva migrans
cutaneous B76.9
  Ancylostoma B76.0
visceral B83.0
Laryngeal —*see* condition
Laryngismus (stridulus) J38.5
congenital P28.89
diphtheritic A36.2
Laryngitis (acute) (edematous) (fibrinous)
  (infective) (infiltrative) (malignant)
  (membranous) (phlegmonous)
  (pneumococcal) (pseudomembranous)
  (septic) (subglottic) (suppurative)
  (ulcerative) J04.0
with
  influenza, flu, or grippe —*see* Influenza,
    with, laryngitis
  tracheitis (acute) —*see* Laryngotracheitis
atrophic J37.0
catarrhal J37.0
chronic J37.0
  with tracheitis (chronic) J37.1
diphtheritic A36.2
due to external agent —*see* Inflammation,
  respiratory, upper, due to
Hemophilus influenzae J04.0
H. influenzae J04.0
hypertrophic J37.0
influenzal —*see* Influenza, with, respiratory
  manifestations NEC
obstructive J05.0
sicca J37.0
spasmodic J05.0
  acute J04.0
streptococcal J04.0
stridulous J05.0
syphilitic (late) A52.73
  congenital A50.59 *[J99]*
    early A50.03 *[J99]*
tuberculous A15.5
Vincent's A69.1
Laryngocele (congenital) (ventricular) Q31.3
Laryngofissure J38.7
congenital Q31.8
Laryngomalacia (congenital) Q31.5

▶ New   ⇒ Revised   ~~deleted~~ Deleted   ● Use Additional Character(s)

Laryngopharyngitis (acute) J06.0
  chronic J37.0
  due to external agent —see Inflammation,
    respiratory, upper, due to
Laryngoplegia J38.00
  bilateral J38.02
  unilateral J38.01
Laryngoptosis J38.7
Laryngospasm J38.5
Laryngostenosis J38.6
Laryngotracheitis (acute) (Infectional)
    (infective) (viral) J04.2
  atrophic J37.1
  catarrhal J37.1
  chronic J37.1
  diphtheritic A36.2
  due to external agent —see Inflammation,
    respiratory, upper, due to
  Hemophilus influenzae J04.2
  hypertrophic J37.1
  influenzal —see Influenza, with, respiratory
    manifestations NEC
  pachydermic J38.7
  sicca J37.1
  spasmodic J38.5
    acute J05.0
  streptococcal J04.2
  stridulous J38.5
  syphilitic (late) A52.73
    congenital A50.59 [J99]
    early A50.03 [J99]
  tuberculous A15.5
  Vincent's A69.1
Laryngotracheobronchitis —see Bronchitis
Larynx, laryngeal —see condition
Lassa fever A96.2
Lassitude —see Weakness
Late
  talker R62.0
  walker R62.0
Late effect(s) —see Sequelae
Latent —see condition
Laterocession —see Lateroversion
Lateroflexion —see Lateroversion
Lateroversion
  cervix —see Lateroversion, uterus
  uterus, uterine (cervix) (postinfectional)
    (postpartal, old) N85.4
    congenital Q51.818
    in pregnancy or childbirth O34.59-●
Lathyrism —see Poisoning, food, noxious, plant
Launois' syndrome (pituitary gigantism) E22.0
Launois-Bensaude adenolipomatosis E88.89
Laurence-Moon (-Bardet)-Biedl syndrome
  Q87.89
Lax, laxity —see also Relaxation
  ligament (ous) —see also Disorder, ligament
    familial M35.7
    knee —see Derangement, knee
  skin (acquired) L57.4
    congenital Q82.8
Laxative habit F55.2
Lazy leukocyte syndrome D70.8
Lead miner's lung J63.6
Leak, leakage
  air NEC J93.82
    postprocedural J95.812
  amniotic fluid —see Rupture, membranes,
    premature
  blood (microscopic), fetal, into maternal
    circulation affecting management of
    pregnancy —see Pregnancy, complicated
    by
  cerebrospinal fluid G96.0
    from spinal (lumbar) puncture G97.0
  device, implant or graft —see also
    Complications, by site and type,
    mechanical
    arterial graft NEC —see Complication,
     cardiovascular device, mechanical,
     vascular

Leak, leakage (Continued)
  device, implant or graft (Continued)
    breast (implant) T85.43
    catheter NEC T85.638
     dialysis (renal) T82.43
      intraperitoneal T85.631
     infusion NEC T82.534
      spinal (epidural) (subdural)
       T85.630
     urinary T83.038
      cystostomy T83.030
      Hopkins T83.038
      ileostomy T83.038
      indwelling T83.031
      nephrostomy T83.032
      specified NEC T83.038
      urostomy T83.038
    gastrointestinal —see Complications,
     prosthetic device, mechanical,
     gastrointestinal device
    genital NEC T83.498
     penile prosthesis (cylinder) (implanted)
      (pump) (resevoir) T83.490
     testicular prosthesis T83.491
    heart NEC —see Complication,
     cardiovascular device, mechanical
    joint prosthesis —see Complications, joint
     prosthesis, mechanical, specified NEC,
     by site
    ocular NEC —see Complications,
     prosthetic device, mechanical,
     ocular device
    orthopedic NEC —see Complication,
     orthopedic, device, mechanical
    persistent air J93.82
    specified NEC T85.638
    urinary NEC —see also Complication,
     genitourinary, device, urinary,
     mechanical
     graft T83.23
    vascular NEC —see Complication,
     cardiovascular device, mechanical
    ventricular intracranial shunt T85.03
  urine —see Incontinence
Leaky heart —see Endocarditis
Learning defect (specific) F81.9
Leather bottle stomach C16.9
Leber's
  congenital amaurosis H35.50
  optic atrophy (hereditary) H47.22
Lederer's anemia D59.1
Leeches (external) —see Hirudiniasis
Leg —see condition
Legg (-Calvé)-Perthes disease, syndrome or
  osteochondrosis M91.1-●
Legionellosis A48.1
  nonpneumonic A48.2
Legionnaires'
  disease A48.1
    nonpneumonic A48.2
    pneumonia A48.1
Leigh's disease G31.82
Leiner's disease L21.1
Leiofibromyoma —see Leiomyoma
Leiomyoblastoma —see Neoplasm, connective
  tissue, benign
Leiomyofibroma —see also Neoplasm,
  connective tissue, benign
  uterus (cervix) (corpus) D25.9
Leiomyoma —see also Neoplasm, connective
  tissue, benign
  bizarre —see Neoplasm, connective tissue,
    benign
  cellular —see Neoplasm, connective tissue,
    benign
  epithelioid —see Neoplasm, connective
    tissue, benign
  uterus (cervix) (corpus) D25.9
    intramural D25.1
    submucous D25.0
    subserosal D25.2

Leiomyoma (Continued)
  vascular —see Neoplasm, connective tissue,
    benign
Leiomyoma, leiomyomatosis (intravascular) —
    see Neoplasm, connective tissue, uncertain
    behavior
Leiomyosarcoma —see also Neoplasm,
    connective tissue, malignant
  epithelioid —see Neoplasm, connective
    tissue, malignant
  myxoid —see Neoplasm, connective tissue,
    malignant
Leishmaniasis B55.9
  American (mucocutaneous) B55.2
    cutaneous B55.1
  Asian Desert B55.1
  Brazilian B55.2
  cutaneous (any type) B55.1
  dermal —see also Leishmaniasis, cutaneous
    post-kala-azar B55.0
  eyelid B55.1
  infantile B55.0
  Mediterranean B55.0
  mucocutaneous (American) (New World)
    B55.2
  naso-oral B55.2
  nasopharyngeal B55.2
  old world B55.1
  tegumentaria diffusa B55.1
  visceral B55.0
Leishmanoid, dermal —see also Leishmaniasis,
    cutaneous
  post-kala-azar B55.0
Lenegre's disease I44.2
Lengthening, leg —see Deformity, limb,
  unequal length
Lennert's lymphoma —see Lymphoma,
    Lennert's
Lennox-Gastaut syndrome G40.812
  intractable G40.814
    with status epilepticus G40.813
    without status epilepticus G40.814
  not intractable G40.812
    with status epilepticus G40.811
    without status epilepticus G40.812
Lens —see condition
Lenticonus (anterior) (posterior) (congenital)
  Q12.8
Lenticular degeneration, progressive E83.01
Lentiglobus (posterior) (congenital) Q12.8
Lentigo (congenital) L81.4
  maligna —see also Melanoma, in situ
    melanoma —see Melanoma
Lentivirus, as cause of disease classified
    elsewhere B97.31
Leontiasis
  ossium M85.2
  syphilitic (late) A52.78
    congenital A50.59
Lepothrix A48.8
Lepra —see Leprosy
Leprechaunism E34.8
Leprosy A30.-●
  with muscle disorder A30.9 [M63.80]
    ankle A30.9 [M63.87-●]
    foot A30.9 [M63.87-●]
    forearm A30.9 [M63.83-●]
    hand A30.9 [M63.84-●]
    lower leg A30.9 [M63.86-●]
    multiple sites A30.9 [M63.89]
    pelvic region A30.9 [M63.85-●]
    shoulder region A30.9 [M63.81-●]
    specified site NEC A30.9 [M63.88]
    thigh A30.9 [M63.85-●]
    upper arm A30.9 [M63.82-●]
  anesthetic A30.9
  BB A30.3
  BL A30.4
  borderline (infiltrated) (neuritic) A30.3
    lepromatous A30.4
    tuberculoid A30.2

▶ New   ➡ Revised   ~~deleted~~ Deleted   ● Use Additional Character(s)

Leprosy (Continued)
BT A30.2
dimorphous (infiltrated) (neuritic) A30.3
I A30.0
indeterminate (macular) (neuritic) A30.0
lepromatous (diffuse) (infiltrated) (macular)
   (neuritic) (nodular) A30.5
LL A30.5
macular (early) (neuritic) (simple)
   A30.9
maculoanesthetic A30.9
mixed A30.3
neural A30.9
nodular A30.5
primary neuritic A30.3
specified type NEC A30.8
TT A30.1
tuberculoid (major) (minor) A30.1
Leptocytosis, hereditary D56.9
Leptomeningitis (chronic) (circumscribed)
   (hemorrhagic) (nonsuppurative) —*see*
   Meningitis
Leptomeningopathy G96.19
Leptospiral —*see* condition
Leptospirochetal —*see* condition
Leptospirosis A27.9
canicola A27.89
due to Leptospira interrogans serovar
   icterohaemorrhagiae A27.0
icterohemorrhagica A27.0
pomona A27.89
Weil's disease A27.0
Leptus dermatitis B88.0
Leriche's syndrome (aortic bifurcation
   occlusion) I74.09
Leri's pleonosteosis Q78.8
Leri-Weill syndrome Q77.8
Lermoyez' syndrome —*see* Vertigo, peripheral
   NEC
Lesch-Nyhan syndrome E79.1
Leser-Trélat disease L82.1
inflamed L82.0
Lesion(s) (nontraumatic)
abducens nerve —*see* Strabismus, paralytic,
   sixth nerve
alveolar process K08.9
angiocentric immunoproliferative D47.Z9
anorectal K62.9
aortic (valve) I35.9
auditory nerve —*see* subcategory H93.3
basal ganglion G25.9
bile duct —*see* Disease, bile duct
biomechanical M99.9
   specified type NEC M99.89
      abdomen M99.89
      acromioclavicular M99.87
      cervical region M99.81
      cervicothoracic M99.81
      costochondral M99.88
      costovertebral M99.88
      head region M99.80
      hip M99.85
      lower extremity M99.86
      lumbar region M99.83
      lumbosacral M99.83
      occipitocervical M99.80
      pelvic region M99.85
      pubic M99.85
      rib cage M99.88
      sacral region M99.84
      sacrococcygeal M99.84
      sacroiliac M99.84
      specified NEC M99.89
      sternochondral M99.88
      sternoclavicular M99.87
      thoracic region M99.82
      thoracolumbar M99.82
      upper extremity M99.87
bladder N32.9
bone —*see* Disorder, bone
brachial plexus G54.0

Lesion (Continued)
brain G93.9
   congenital Q04.9
   vascular I67.9
      degenerative I67.9
      hypertensive I67.4
buccal cavity K13.79
calcified —*see* Calcification
canthus —*see* Disorder, eyelid
carate —*see* Pinta, lesions
cardia K31.9
cardiac —*see also* Disease, heart I51.9
   congenital Q24.9
   valvular —*see* Endocarditis
cauda equina G83.4
cecum K63.9
cerebral —*see* Lesion, brain
cerebrovascular I67.9
   degenerative I67.9
   hypertensive I67.4
cervical (nerve) root NEC G54.2
chiasmal —*see* Disorder, optic, chiasm
chorda tympani G51.8
coin, lung R91.1
colon K63.9
combined periodontic - endodontic K05.5
congenital —*see* Anomaly, by site
conjunctiva H11.9
conus medullaris —*see* Injury, conus
   medullaris
coronary artery —*see* Ischemia, heart
cranial nerve G52.9
   eighth —*see* Disorder, ear
   eleventh G52.9
   fifth G50.9
   first G52.0
   fourth —*see* Strabismus, paralytic, fourth
      nerve
   seventh G51.9
   sixth —*see* Strabismus, paralytic, sixth
      nerve
   tenth G52.2
   twelfth G52.3
cystic —*see* Cyst
degenerative —*see* Degeneration
duodenum K31.9
edentulous (alveolar) ridge, associated with
   trauma, due to traumatic occlusion
   K06.2
en coup de sabre L94.1
eyelid —*see* Disorder, eyelid
gasserian ganglion G50.8
gastric K31.9
gastroduodenal K31.9
gastrointestinal K63.9
gingiva, associated with trauma K06.2
glomerular
   focal and segmental —*see also* N00-N07
      with fourth character .1 N05.1
   minimal change —*see also* N00-N07 with
      fourth character .0 N05.0
heart (organic) —*see* Disease, heart
hyperchromic, due to pinta (carate)
   A67.1
hyperkeratotic —*see* Hyperkeratosis
hypothalamic E23.7
ileocecal K63.9
ileum K63.9
iliohypogastric nerve G57.8-●
inflammatory —*see* Inflammation
intestine K63.9
intracerebral —*see* Lesion, brain
intrachiasmal (optic) —*see* Disorder, optic,
   chiasm
intracranial, space-occupying R90.0
joint —*see* Disorder, joint
   sacroiliac (old) M53.3
keratotic —*see* Keratosis
kidney —*see* Disease, renal
laryngeal nerve (recurrent) G52.2
lip K13.0

Lesion (Continued)
liver K76.9
lumbosacral
   plexus G54.1
   root (nerve) NEC G54.4
lung (coin) R91.1
maxillary sinus J32.0
mitral I05.9
Morel-Lavallée —*see* Hematoma,
   by site
motor cortex NEC G93.89
mouth K13.79
nerve G58.9
   femoral G57.2-●
   median G56.1-●
      carpal tunnel syndrome —*see* Syndrome,
         carpal tunnel
   plantar G57.6-●
   popliteal (lateral) G57.3-●
      medial G57.4-●
   radial G56.3-●
   sciatic G57.0-●
   spinal —*see* Injury, nerve, spinal
   ulnar G56.2-●
nervous system, congenital Q07.9
nonallopathic —*see* Lesion, biomechanical
nose (internal) J34.89
obstructive —*see* Obstruction
obturator nerve G57.8-●
oral mucosa K13.70
organ or site NEC —*see* Disease, by site
osteolytic —*see* Osteolysis
peptic K27.9
periodontal, due to traumatic occlusion
   K05.5
pharynx J39.2
pigment, pigmented (skin) L81.9
pinta —*see* Pinta, lesions
polypoid —*see* Polyp
prechiasmal (optic) —*see* Disorder, optic,
   chiasm
primary —*see also* Syphilis, primary A51.0
   carate A67.0
   pinta A67.0
   yaws A66.0
pulmonary J98.4
   valve I37.9
pylorus K31.9
rectosigmoid K63.9
retina, retinal H35.9
sacroiliac (joint) (old) M53.3
salivary gland K11.9
   benign lymphoepithelial K11.8
saphenous nerve G57.8-●
sciatic nerve G57.0-●
secondary —*see* Syphilis, secondary
shoulder (region) M75.9-●
   specified NEC M75.8-●
sigmoid K63.9
sinus (accessory) (nasal) J34.89
skin L98.9
   suppurative L08.0
SLAP S43.43-●
spinal cord G95.9
   congenital Q06.9
spleen D73.89
stomach K31.9
superior glenoid labrum S43.43-●
syphilitic —*see* Syphilis
tertiary —*see* Syphilis, tertiary
thoracic root (nerve) NEC G54.3
tonsillar fossa J35.9
tooth, teeth K08.9
   white spot
      chewing surface K02.51
      pit and fissure surface K02.51
      smooth surface K02.61
traumatic —*see* specific type of injury by site
tricuspid (valve) I07.9
   nonrheumatic I36.9
trigeminal nerve G50.9

Lesion *(Continued)*
    ulcerated or ulcerative —*see* Ulcer, skin
    uterus N85.9
    vagus nerve G52.2
    valvular —*see* Endocarditis
    vascular I99.9
        affecting central nervous system I67.9
        following trauma NEC T14.8
        umbilical cord, complicating delivery
            O69.5
    warty —*see* Verruca
    white spot (tooth)
        chewing surface K02.51
        pit and fissure surface K02.51
        smooth surface K02.61
Lethargic —*see* condition
Lethargy R53.83
Letterer-Siwe's disease C96.0
Leukemia, leukemic C95.9-●
    acute basophilic C94.8-●
    acute bilineal C95.0-●
    acute erythroid C94.0-●
    acute lymphoblastic C91.0-●
    acute megakaryoblastic C94.2-●
    acute megakaryocytic C94.2-●
    acute mixed lineage C95.0-●
    acute monoblastic (monoblastic/monocytic)
        C93.0-●
    acute monocytic (monoblastic/monocytic)
        C93.0-●
    acute myeloblastic (minimal differentiation)
        (with maturation) C92.0-●
    acute myeloid
        with
            11q23-abnormality C92.6-●
            dysplasia of remaining hematopoesis
                and/or myelodysplastic disease in
                its history C92.A-●
            multilineage dysplasia C92.A-●
            variation of MLL-gene C92.6-●
        M6 (a)(b) C94.0-●
        M7 C94.2-●
    acute myelomonocytic C92.5-●
    acute promyelocytic C92.4-●
    adult T-cell (HTLV-1-associated) (acute
        variant) (chronic variant)
        (lymphomatoid variant) (smouldering
        variant) C91.5-●
    aggressive NK-cell C94.8-●
    AML (1/ETO) (M0) (M1) (M2) (without a
        FAB classification) C92.0-●
    AML M3 C92.4-●
    AML M4 (Eo with inv(16) or t(16;16))
        C92.5-●
    AML M5 C93.0-●
    AML M5a C93.0-●
    AML M5b C93.0-●
    AML Me with t (15;17) and variants C92.4-●
    atypical chronic myeloid, BCR/ABL-negative
        C92.2-●
    biphenotypic acute C95.0-●
    blast cell C95.0-●
    Burkitt-type, mature B-cell C91.A-●
    chronic lymphocytic, of B-cell type C91.1-●
    chronic monocytic C93.1-●
    chronic myelogenous (Philadelphia
        chromosome (Ph1) positive) (t(9;22))
        (q34;q11) (with crisis of blast cells)
        C92.1-●
    chronic myeloid, BCR/ABL-positive C92.1-●
        atypical, BCR/ABL-negative C92.2-●
    chronic myelomonocytic C93.1-●
    chronic neutrophilic D47.1
    CMML (-1) (-2) (with eosinophilia) C93.1-●
    granulocytic —*see also* Category C92 C92.9-●
    hairy-cell C91.4-●
    juvenile myelomonocytic C93.3-●
    lymphoid C91.9-●
        specified NEC C91.Z-●
    mast cell C94.3-●
    mature B-cell, Burkitt-type C91.A-●

Leukemia, leukemic *(Continued)*
    monocytic (subacute) C93.9-●
        specified NEC C93.Z-●
    myelogenous —*see also* Category C92 C92.9-●
    myeloid C92.9-●
        specified NEC C92.Z-●
    plasma cell C90.1-●
    plasmacytic C90.1-●
    prolymphocytic
        of B-cell type C91.3-●
        of T-cell type C91.6-●
        specified NEC C94.8-●
    stem cell, of unclear lineage C95.0-●
    subacute lymphocytic C91.9-●
    T-cell large granular lymphocytic C91.Z-●
    unspecified cell type C95.9-●
        acute C95.0-●
        chronic C95.1-●
Leukemoid reaction —*see also* Reaction,
        leukemoid D72.823-●
Leukoaraiosis (hypertensive) I67.81
Leukoariosis —*see* Leukoaraiosis
Leukocoria —*see* Disorder, globe, degenerated
        condition, leucocoria
Leukocytopenia D72.819
Leukocytosis D72.829
    eosinophilic D72.1
Leukoderma, leukodermia NEC L81.5
    syphilitic A51.39
        late A52.79
Leukodystrophy E75.29
Leukoedema, oral epithelium K13.29
Leukoencephalitis G04.81
    acute (subacute) hemorrhagic G36.1
        postimmunization or postvaccinal G04.02
    postinfectious G04.01
    subacute sclerosing A81.1
    van Bogaert's (sclerosing) A81.1
Leukoencephalopathy —*see also*
        Encephalopathy G93.49
    Binswanger's I67.3
    heroin vapor G92
    metachromatic E75.25
    multifocal (progressive) A81.2
    postimmunization and postvaccinal G04.02
    progressive multifocal A81.2
    reversible, posterior G93.6
    van Bogaert's (sclerosing) A81.1
    vascular, progressive I67.3
Leukoerythroblastosis D75.9
Leukokeratosis —*see also* Leukoplakia
    mouth K13.21
    nicotina palati K13.24
    oral mucosa K13.21
    tongue K13.21
    vocal cord J38.3
Leukokraurosis vulva (e) N90.4
Leukoma (cornea) —*see also* Opacity, cornea
    adherent H17.0-●
    interfering with central vision —*see* Opacity,
        cornea, central
Leukomalacia, cerebral, newborn P91.2
    periventricular P91.2
Leukomelanopathy, hereditary D72.0
Leukonychia (punctata) (striata) L60.8
    congenital Q84.4
Leukopathia unguium L60.8
    congenital Q84.4
Leukopenia D72.819
    basophilic D72.818
    chemotherapy (cancer) induced D70.1
    congenital D70.0
    cyclic D70.0
    drug induced NEC D70.2
        due to cytoreductive cancer chemotherapy
            D70.1
    eosinophilic D72.818
    familial D70.0
    infantile genetic D70.0
    malignant D70.9
    periodic D70.0
    transitory neonatal P61.5

Leukopenic —*see* condition
Leukoplakia
    anus K62.89
    bladder (postinfectional) N32.89
    buccal K13.21
    cervix (uteri) N88.0
    esophagus K22.8
    gingiva K13.21
    hairy (oral mucosa) (tongue) K13.3
    kidney (pelvis) N28.89
    larynx J38.7
    lip K13.21
    mouth K13.21
    oral epithelium, including tongue (mucosa)
        K13.21
    palate K13.21
    pelvis (kidney) N28.89
    penis (infectional) N48.0
    rectum K62.89
    syphilitic (late) A52.79
    tongue K13.21
    ureter (postinfectional) N28.89
    urethra (postinfectional) N36.8
    uterus N85.8
    vagina N89.4
    vocal cord J38.3
    vulva N90.4
Leukorrhea N89.8
    due to Trichomonas (vaginalis)
        A59.00
    trichomonal A59.00
Leukosarcoma C85.9
Levocardia (isolated) Q24.1
    with situs inversus Q89.3
Levotransposition Q20.5
Lev's disease or syndrome (acquired complete
        heart block) I44.2
Levulosuria —*see* Fructosuria
Levurid L30.2
Lewy body (ies) (dementia) (disease)
        G31.83
Leyden-Moebius dystrophy G71.0
Leydig cell
    carcinoma
        specified site —*see* Neoplasm, malignant,
            by site
        unspecified site
            female C56.9-●
            male C62.9-●
    tumor
        benign
            specified site —*see* Neoplasm, benign,
                by site
            unspecified site
                female D27.-●
                male D29.2-●
        malignant
            specified site —*see* Neoplasm,
                malignant, by site
            unspecified site
                female C56.-●
                male C62.9-●
        specified site —*see* Neoplasm, uncertain
            behavior, by site
        unspecified site
            female D39.1-●
            male D40.1-●
Leydig-Sertoli cell tumor
    specified site —*see* Neoplasm, benign,
        by site
    unspecified site
        female D27.-●
        male D29.2-●
LGSIL (Low grade squamous intraepithelial
        lesion on cytologic smear of)
    anus R85.612
    cervix R87.612
    vagina R87.622
Liar, pathologic F60.2
Libido
    decreased R68.82

▶ New   ⇒ Revised   ~~deleted~~ Deleted   ● Use Additional Character(s)

Libman-Sacks disease M32.11
Lice (infestation) B85.2
  body (Pediculus corporis) B85.1
  crab B85.3
  head (Pediculus capitis) B85.0
  mixed (classifiable to more than one of the
      titles B85.0-B85.3) B85.4
  pubic (Phthirus pubis) B85.3
Lichen L28.0
  albus L90.0
    penis N48.0
    vulva N90.4
  amyloidosis E85.4 [L99]
  atrophicus L90.0
    penis N48.0
    vulva N90.4
  congenital Q82.8
  myxedematosus L98.5
  nitidus L44.1
  pilaris Q82.8
    acquired L85.8
  planopilaris L66.1
  planus (chronicus) L43.9
    annularis L43.8
    bullous L43.1
    follicular L66.1
    hypertrophic L43.0
    moniliformis L44.3
    of Wilson L43.9
    specified NEC L43.8
    subacute (active) L43.3
    tropicus L43.3
  ruber
    acuminatus L44.0
    moniliformis L44.3
    planus L43.9
  sclerosus (et atrophicus) L90.0
    penis N48.0
    vulva N90.4
  scrofulosus (primary) (tuberculous) A18.4
  simplex (chronicus) (circumscriptus) L28.0
  striatus L44.2
  urticatus L28.2
Lichenification L28.0
Lichenoides tuberculosis (primary) A18.4
Lichtheim's disease or syndrome —see
      Degeneration, combined
Lien migrans D73.89
Ligament —see condition
Light
  for gestational age —see Light for dates
  headedness R42
Light-for-dates (infant) P05.00
  with weight of
    499 grams or less P05.01
    500-749 grams P05.02
    750-999 grams P05.03
    1000-1249 grams P05.04
    1250-1499 grams P05.05
    1500-1749 grams P05.06
    1750-1999 grams P05.07
    2000-2499 grams P05.08
    2500 grams and over P05.09
  affecting management of pregnancy O36.59-•
  and small-for-dates —see Small for dates
  specified NEC P05.09
Lightning (effects) (stroke) (struck by) T75.00
  burn —see Burn
  foot E53.8
  shock T75.01
  specified effect NEC T75.09
Lightwood-Albright syndrome N25.89
Lightwood's disease or syndrome (renal
      tubular acidosis) N25.89
Lignac (-de Toni) (-Fanconi) (-Debré) disease or
      syndrome E72.09
  with cystinosis E72.04
Ligneous thyroiditis E06.5
Likoff's syndrome I20.8
Limb —see condition
Limbic epilepsy personality syndrome F07.0

Limitation, limited
  activities due to disability Z73.6
  cardiac reserve —see Disease, heart
  eye muscle duction, traumatic —see
      Strabismus, mechanical
  mandibular range of motion M26.52
Lindau (-von Hippel) disease Q85.8
Line(s)
  Beau's L60.4
  Harris' —see Arrest, epiphyseal
  Hudson's (cornea) —see Pigmentation,
      cornea, anterior
  Stähli's (cornea) —see Pigmentation, cornea,
      anterior
Linea corneae senilis —see Change, cornea,
  senile
Lingua
  geographica K14.1
  nigra (villosa) K14.3
  plicata K14.5
  tylosis K13.29
Lingual —see condition
Linguatulosis B88.8
Linitis (gastric) plastica C16.9
Lip —see condition
Lipedema —see Edema
Lipemia —see also Hyperlipidemia
  retina, retinalis E78.3
Lipidosis E75.6
  cerebral (infantile) (juvenile) (late) E75.4
  cerebroretinal E75.4
  cerebroside E75.22
  cholesterol (cerebral) E75.5
  glycolipid E75.21
  hepatosplenomegalic E78.3
  sphingomyelin —see Niemann-Pick disease
      or syndrome
  sulfatide E75.29
Lipoadenoma —see Neoplasm, benign, by site
Lipoblastoma —see Lipoma
Lipoblastomatosis —see Lipoma
Lipochondrodystrophy E76.01
Lipochrome histiocytosis (familial) D71
Lipodermatosclerosis —see Varix, leg, with,
      inflammation
  ulcerated —see Varix, leg, with, ulcer, with
      inflammation by site
Lipodystrophia progressiva E88.1
Lipodystrophy (progressive) E88.1
  insulin E88.1
  intestinal K90.81
  mesenteric K65.4
Lipofibroma —see Lipoma
Lipofuscinosis, neuronal (with ceroidosis)
  E75.4
Lipogranuloma, sclerosing L92.8
Lipogranulomatosis E78.89
Lipoid —see also condition
  histiocytosis D76.3
    essential E75.29
  nephrosis N04.9
  proteinosis of Urbach E78.89
Lipoidemia —see Hyperlipidemia
Lipoidosis —see Lipidosis
Lipoma D17.9
  fetal D17.9
  fat cell D17.9
  infiltrating D17.9
  intramuscular D17.9
  pleomorphic D17.9
  site classification
    arms (skin) (subcutaneous) D17.2-•
    connective tissue D17.30
      intra-abdominal D17.5
      intrathoracic D17.4
      peritoneum D17.79
      retroperitoneum D17.79
      specified site NEC D17.39
      spermatic cord D17.6
    face (skin) (subcutaneous) D17.0
    genitourinary organ NEC D17.72

Lipoma (Continued)
  site classification (Continued)
    head (skin) (subcutaneous) D17.0
    intra-abdominal D17.5
    intrathoracic D17.4
    kidney D17.71
    legs (skin) (subcutaneous) D17.2-•
    neck (skin) (subcutaneous) D17.0
    peritoneum D17.79
    retroperitoneum D17.79
    skin D17.30
      specified site NEC D17.39
    specified site NEC D17.79
    spermatic cord D17.6
    subcutaneous D17.30
      specified site NEC D17.39
    trunk (skin) (subcutaneous) D17.1
    unspecified D17.9
  spindle cell D17.9
Lipomatosis E88.2
  dolorosa (Dercum) E88.2
  fetal —see Lipoma
  Launois-Bensaude E88.89
Lipomyoma —see Lipoma
Lipomyxoma —see Lipoma
Lipomyxosarcoma —see Neoplasm, connective
      tissue, malignant
Lipoprotein metabolism disorder E78.9
Lipoproteinemia E78.5
  broad-beta E78.2
  floating-beta E78.2
  hyper-pre-beta E78.1
Liposarcoma —see also Neoplasm, connective
      tissue, malignant
  dedifferentiated —see Neoplasm, connective
      tissue, malignant
  differentiated type —see Neoplasm,
      connective tissue, malignant
  embryonal —see Neoplasm, connective tissue,
      malignant
  mixed type —see Neoplasm, connective
      tissue, malignant
  myxoid —see Neoplasm, connective tissue,
      malignant
  pleomorphic —see Neoplasm, connective
      tissue, malignant
  round cell —see Neoplasm, connective tissue,
      malignant
  well differentiated type —see Neoplasm,
      connective tissue, malignant
Liposynovitis prepatellaris E88.89
Lipping, cervix N86
Lipschütz disease or ulcer N76.6
Lipuria R82.0
  schistosomiasis (bilharziasis) B65.0
Lisping F80.0
Lissauer's paralysis A52.17
Lissencephalia, lissencephaly Q04.3
Listeriosis, listerellosis A32.9
  congenital (disseminated) P37.2
  cutaneous A32.0
  neonatal, newborn (disseminated) P37.2
  oculoglandular A32.81
  specified NEC A32.89
Lithemia E79.0
Lithiasis —see Calculus
Lithosis J62.8
Lithuria R82.99
Litigation, anxiety concerning Z65.3
Little leaguer's elbow —see Epicondylitis,
      medial
Little's disease G80.9
Littre's
  gland —see condition
  hernia —see Hernia, abdomen
Littritis —see Urethritis
Livedo (annularis) (racemosa) (reticularis)
  R23.1
Liver —see condition
Living alone (problems with) Z60.2
  with handicapped person Z74.2

▶ New   ⇒ Revised   ~~deleted~~ Deleted   • Use Additional Character(s)

Louis-Bar syndrome (ataxia-telangiectasia)
    G11.3
Louping ill (encephalitis) A84.8
Louse, lousiness —see Lice
Low
    achiever, school Z55.3
    back syndrome M54.5
    basal metabolic rate R94.8
    birthweight (2499 grams or less) P07.10
        with weight of
            1000-1249 grams P07.14
            1250-1499 grams P07.15
            1500-1749 grams P07.16
            1750-1999 grams P07.17
            2000-2499 grams P07.18
        extreme (999 grams or less) P07.00
            with weight of
                499 grams or less P07.01
                500-749 grams P07.02
                750-999 grams P07.03
        for gestational age —see Light for dates
    blood pressure —see also Hypotension
        reading (incidental) (isolated) (nonspecific)
            R03.1
    cardiac reserve —see Disease, heart
    function —see also Hypofunction
        kidney N28.9
    hematocrit D64.9
    hemoglobin D64.9
    income Z59.6
    level of literacy Z55.0
    lying
        kidney N28.89
        organ or site, congenital —see Malposition,
            congenital
    output syndrome (cardiac) —see Failure,
        heart
    platelets (blood) —see Thrombocytopenia
    reserve, kidney N28.89
    salt syndrome E87.1
    self esteem R45.81
    set ears Q17.4
    vision H54.2X-
        one eye (other eye normal) H54.50
            left (normal vision on right) H54.52A-
                other eye blind —see Blindness
            right (normal vision on left) H54.511-
Low-density-lipoprotein-type (LDL)
    hyperlipoproteinemia E78.00
Lowe's syndrome E72.03
Lown-Ganong-Levine syndrome I45.6
LSD reaction (acute) (without dependence)
    F16.90
    with dependence F16.20
L-shaped kidney Q63.8
Ludwig's angina or disease K12.2
Lues (venerea), luetic —see Syphilis
Luetscher's syndrome (dehydration) E86.0
Lumbago, lumbalgia M54.5
    with sciatica M54.4-•
        due to intervertebral disc disorder M51.17
    due to displacement, intervertebral disc
        M51.27
        with sciatica M51.17
Lumbar —see condition
Lumbarization, vertebra, congenital Q76.49
Lumbermen's itch B88.0
Lump —see also Mass
    breast N63.0
        axillary tail
            left N63.32
            right N63.31
        left
            lower inner quadrant N63.24
            lower outer quadrant N63.23
            unspecified quadrant N63.20
            upper inner quadrant N63.22
            upper outer quadrant N63.21
        right
            lower inner quadrant N63.14
            lower outer quadrant N63.13

Lump (Continued)
    breast (Continued)
        right (Continued)
            unspecified quadrant N63.10
            upper inner quadrant N63.12
            upper outer quadrant N63.11
        subareolar
            left N63.42
            right N63.41
Lunacy —see Psychosis
Lung —see condition
Lupoid (miliary) of Boeck D86.3
Lupus
    anticoagulant D68.62
        with
            hemorrhagic disorder D68.312
            hypercoagulable state D68.62
        finding without diagnosis R76.0
    discoid (local) L93.0
    erythematosus (discoid) (local) L93.0
        disseminated —see Lupus, erythematosus,
            systemic
        eyelid H01.129
            left H01.126
                lower H01.125
                upper H01.124
            right H01.123
                lower H01.122
                upper H01.121
        profundus L93.2
        specified NEC L93.2
        subacute cutaneous L93.1
        systemic M32.9
            with organ or system involvement
                M32.10
                endocarditis M32.11
                lung M32.13
                pericarditis M32.12
                renal (glomerular) M32.14
                    tubulo-interstitial M32.15
                specified organ or system NEC
                    M32.19
            drug-induced M32.0
            inhibitor (presence of) D68.62
                with
                    hemorrhagic disorder D68.312
                    hypercoagulable state D68.62
                finding without diagnosis R76.0
            specified NEC M32.8
    exedens A18.4
    hydralazine M32.0
        correct substance properly administered —
            see Table of Drugs and Chemicals, by
            drug, adverse effect
        overdose or wrong substance given
            or taken —see Table of Drugs and
            Chemicals, by drug, poisoning
    nephritis (chronic) M32.14
    nontuberculous, not disseminated L93.0
    panniculitis L93.2
    pernio (Besnier) D86.3
    systemic —see Lupus, erythematosus,
        systemic
    tuberculous A18.4
        eyelid A18.4
    vulgaris A18.4
        eyelid A18.4
Luteinoma D27.-•
Lutembacher's disease or syndrome (atrial
    septal defect with mitral stenosis) Q21.1
Luteoma D27.-•
Lutz (-Splendore-de Almeida) disease —see
    Paracoccidioidomycosis
Luxation —see also Dislocation
    eyeball (nontraumatic) —see Luxation, globe
        birth injury P15.3
    globe, nontraumatic H44.82-•
    lacrimal gland —see Dislocation, lacrimal
        gland
    lens (old) (partial) (spontaneous)
        congenital Q12.1
        syphilitic A50.39

Lycanthropy F22
Lyell's syndrome L51.2
    due to drug L51.2
        correct substance properly administered —
            see Table of Drugs and Chemicals, by
            drug, adverse effect
        overdose or wrong substance given
            or taken —see Table of Drugs and
            Chemicals, by drug, poisoning
Lyme disease A69.20
Lymph
    gland or node —see condition
    scrotum —see Infestation, filarial
Lymphadenitis I88.9
    with ectopic or molar pregnancy O08.0
    acute L04.9
        axilla L04.2
        face L04.0
        head L04.0
        hip L04.3
        limb
            lower L04.3
            upper L04.2
        neck L04.0
        shoulder L04.2
        specified site NEC L04.8
        trunk L04.1
    anthracosis (occupational) J60
    any site, except mesenteric I88.9
        chronic I88.1
        subacute I88.1
    breast
        gestational —see Mastitis, obstetric
        puerperal, postpartum (nonpurulent) O91.22
    chancroidal (congenital) A57
    chronic I88.1
        mesenteric I88.0
    due to
        Brugia (malayi) B74.1
            timori B74.2
        chlamydial lymphogranuloma A55
        diphtheria (toxin) A36.89
        lymphogranuloma venereum A55
        Wuchereria bancrofti B74.0
    following ectopic or molar pregnancy O08.0
    gonorrheal A54.89
    infective —see Lymphadenitis, acute
    mesenteric (acute) (chronic) (nonspecific)
        (subacute) I88.0
        due to Salmonella typhi A01.09
        tuberculous A18.39
    mycobacterial A31.8
    purulent —see Lymphadenitis, acute
    pyogenic —see Lymphadenitis, acute
    regional, nonbacterial I88.8
    septic —see Lymphadenitis, acute
    subacute, unspecified site I88.1
    suppurative —see Lymphadenitis, acute
    syphilitic (early) (secondary) A51.49
        late A52.79
    tuberculous —see Tuberculosis, lymph gland
    venereal (chlamydial) A55
Lymphadenoid goiter E06.3
Lymphadenopathy (generalized) R59.1
    angioimmunoblastic, with dysproteinemia
        (AILD) C86.5
    due to toxoplasmosis (acquired) B58.89
        congenital (acute) (subacute) (chronic) P37.1
    localized R59.0
    syphilitic (early) (secondary) A51.49
Lymphadenosis R59.1
Lymphangiectasis I89.0
    conjunctiva H11.89
    postinfectional I89.0
    scrotum I89.0
Lymphangiectatic elephantiasis, nonfilarial
    I89.0
Lymphangioendothelioma D18.1
    malignant —see Neoplasm, connective tissue,
        malignant
Lymphangioleiomyomatosis J84.81

▶ New   ⇒ Revised   ~~deleted~~ Deleted   ● Use Additional Character(s)

Lymphoma *(Continued)*
    SALT C88.4
    skin-associated lymphoid tissue
        [SALT-lymphoma] C88.4
    small cell B-cell C83.0-•
    splenic marginal zone C83.0-•
    subcutaneous panniculitis-like T-cell C86.3
    T-precursor C83.5-•
    true histiocytic C96.A

Lymphomatosis —*see* Lymphoma
Lymphopathia venereum, veneris A55
Lymphopenia D72.810
Lymphoplasmacytic leukemia —*see* Leukemia,
    chronic lymphocytic, B-cell type
Lymphoproliferation, X-linked disease D82.3
Lymphoreticulosis, benign (of inoculation)
    A28.1

Lymphorrhea I89.8
Lymphosarcoma (diffuse) —*see also* Lymphoma
    C85.9-•
Lymphostasis I89.8
Lypemania —*see* Melancholia
Lysine and hydroxylysine metabolism
    disorder E72.3
Lyssa —*see* Rabies

M

Macacus ear Q17.3
Maceration, wet feet, tropical (syndrome)
  T69.02-•
MacLeod's syndrome J43.0
Macrocephalia, macrocephaly Q75.3
Macrocheilia, macrochilia (congenital)Q18.6
Macrocolon —see also Megacolon Q43.1
Macrocornea Q15.8
  with glaucoma Q15.0
Macrocytic —see condition
Macrocytosis D75.89
Macrodactylia, macrodactylism (fingers)
    (thumbs) Q74.0
  toes Q74.2
Macrodontia K00.2
Macrogenia M26.05
Macrogenitosomia (adrenal) (male) (praecox)
    E25.9
  congenital E25.0
Macroglobulinemia (idiopathic) (primary)
    C88.0
  monoclonal (essential) D47.2
  Waldenström C88.0
Macroglossia (congenital) Q38.2
  acquired K14.8
Macrognathia, macrognathism (congenital)
    (mandibular) (maxillary) M26.09
Macrogyria (congenital) Q04.8
Macrohydrocephalus —see Hydrocephalus
Macromastia —see Hypertrophy, breast
Macrophthalmos Q11.3
  in congenital glaucoma Q15.0
Macropsia H53.15
Macrosigmoid K59.39
  congenital Q43.2
Macrospondylitis, acromegalic E22.0
Macrostomia (congenital) Q18.4
Macrotia (external ear) (congenital) Q17.1
Macula
  cornea, corneal —see Opacity, cornea
  degeneration (atrophic) (exudative)
      (senile) —see also Degeneration, macula
    hereditary —see Dystrophy, retina
Maculae ceruleae — B85.1
Maculopathy, toxic —see Degeneration, macula,
    toxic
Madarosis (eyelid) H02.729
  left H02.726
    lower H02.725
    upper H02.724
  right H02.723
    lower H02.722
    upper H02.721
Madelung's
  deformity (radius) Q74.0
  disease
    radial deformity Q74.0
    symmetrical lipomas, neck E88.89
Madness —see Psychosis
Madura
  foot B47.9
    actinomycotic B47.1
    mycotic B47.0
Maduromycosis B47.0
Maffucci's syndrome Q78.4
Magnesium metabolism disorder —see
    Disorder, metabolism, magnesium
Main en griffe (acquired) —see also Deformity,
    limb, clawhand
  congenital Q74.0
Maintenance (encounter for)
  antineoplastic chemotherapy Z51.11
  antineoplastic radiation therapy Z51.0
  methadone F11.20
Majocchi's
  disease L81.7
  granuloma B35.8
Major —see condition
Malabar itch (any site) B35.5

Malabsorption K90.9
  calcium K90.89
  carbohydrate K90.49
  disaccharide E73.9
  fat K90.49
  galactose E74.20
  glucose(-galactose) E74.39
  intestinal K90.9
    specified NEC K90.89
  isomaltose E74.31
  lactose E73.9
  methionine E72.19
  monosaccharide E74.39
  postgastrectomy K91.2
  postsurgical K91.2
  protein K90.49
  starch K90.49
  sucrose E74.39
  syndrome K90.9
    postsurgical K91.2
Malacia, bone (adult) M83.9
  juvenile —see Rickets
Malacoplakia
  bladder N32.89
  pelvis (kidney) N28.89
  ureter N28.89
  urethra N36.8
Malacosteon, juvenile —see Rickets
Maladaptation —see Maladjustment
Maladie de Roger Q21.0
Maladjustment
  conjugal Z63.0
    involving divorce or estrangement Z63.5
  educational Z55.4
  family Z63.9
  marital Z63.0
    involving divorce or estrangement Z63.5
  occupational NEC Z56.89
  simple, adult —see Disorder, adjustment
  situational —see Disorder, adjustment
  social Z60.9
    due to
      acculturation difficulty Z60.3
      discrimination and persecution
          (perceived) Z60.5
      exclusion and isolation Z60.4
      life-cycle (phase of life) transition Z60.0
      rejection Z60.4
      specified reason NEC Z60.8
Malaise R53.81
Malakoplakia —see Malacoplakia
Malaria, malarial (fever) B54
  with
    blackwater fever B50.8
      hemoglobinuric (bilious) B50.8
      hemoglobinuria B50.8
    accidentally induced (therapeutically) - code
        by type under Malaria
  algid B50.9
  cerebral B50.0 [G94]
  clinically diagnosed (without parasitological
      confirmation) B54
  congenital NEC P37.4
    falciparum P37.3
  congestion, congestive B54
  continued (fever) B50.9
  estivo-autumnal B50.9
  falciparum B50.9
    with complications NEC B50.8
      cerebral B50.0 [G94]
    severe B50.8
  hemorrhagic B54
  malariae B52.9
    with
      complications NEC B52.8
      glomerular disorder B52.0
  malignant (tertian) —see Malaria, falciparum
  mixed infections — code to first listed type
      in B50-B53
  ovale B53.0
  parasitologically confirmed NEC B53.8

Malaria, malarial (Continued)
  pernicious, acute —see Malaria, falciparum
  Plasmodium (P.)
    falciparum NEC —see Malaria, falciparum
    malariae NEC B52.9
      with Plasmodium
        falciparum (and or vivax) —see
            Malaria, falciparum
        vivax —see also Malaria, vivax
            and falciparum —see Malaria,
              falciparum
    ovale B53.0
      with Plasmodium malariae —see also
          Malaria, malariae
        and vivax —see also Malaria, vivax
            and falciparum —see Malaria,
              falciparum
    simian B53.1
      with Plasmodium malariae —see also
          Malaria, malariae
        and vivax —see also Malaria, vivax
            and falciparum —see Malaria,
              falciparum
    vivax NEC B51.9
      with Plasmodium falciparum —see
          Malaria, falciparum
  quartan —see Malaria, malariae
  quotidian —see Malaria, falciparum
  recurrent B54
  remittent B54
  specified type NEC (parasitologically
      confirmed) B53.8
  spleen B54
  subtertian (fever) —see Malaria, falciparum
  tertian (benign) —see also Malaria, vivax
    malignant B50.9
  tropical B50.9
  typhoid B54
  vivax B51.9
    with
      complications NEC B51.8
      ruptured spleen B51.0
Malassez's disease (cystic) N50.89
Malassimilation K90.9
Mal de los pintos —see Pinta
Mal de mer T75.3
Maldescent, testis Q53.9
  bilateral Q53.20
    ▸abdominal Q53.211
    perineal Q53.22
  unilateral Q53.10
    ▸abdominal Q53.111
    perineal Q53.12
Maldevelopment —see also Anomaly
  brain Q07.9
  colon Q43.9
  hip Q74.2
    congenital dislocation Q65.2
      bilateral Q65.1
      unilateral Q65.0-•
  mastoid process Q75.8
  middle ear Q16.4
    except ossicles Q16.4
    ossicles Q16.3
  ossicles Q16.3
  spine Q76.49
  toe Q74.2
Male type pelvis Q74.2
  with disproportion (fetopelvic) O33.3
    causing obstructed labor O65.3
Malformation (congenital) —see also Anomaly
  adrenal gland Q89.1
  affecting multiple systems with skeletal
      changes NEC Q87.5
  alimentary tract Q45.9
    specified type NEC Q45.8
    upper Q40.9
      specified type NEC Q40.8
  aorta Q25.40
    absence Q25.41
    aneurysm, congenital Q25.43

▶ New   ⟹ Revised   ~~deleted~~ Deleted   • Use Additional Character(s)

Malformation (Continued)
  aorta (Continued)
    aplasia Q25.41
    atresia Q25.29
      aortic arch Q25.21
    coarctation (preductal) (postductal) Q25.1
    dilatation, congenital Q25.44
    hypoplasia Q25.42
    patent ductus arteriosus Q25.0
    specified type NEC Q25.49
    stenosis Q25.1
      supravalvular Q25.3
  aortic valve Q23.9
    specified NEC Q23.8
  arteriovenous, aneurysmatic (congenital)
    Q27.30
    brain Q28.2
    cerebral Q28.2
    peripheral Q27.30
      digestive system Q27.33
      lower limb Q27.32
      other specified site Q27.39
      renal vessel Q27.34
      upper limb Q27.31
    precerebral vessels (nonruptured)
      Q28.0
  auricle
    ear (congenital) Q17.3
      acquired H61.119
        left H61.112
          with right H61.113
        right H61.111
          with left H61.113
  bile duct Q44.5
  bladder Q64.79
    aplasia Q64.5
    diverticulum Q64.6
    exstrophy —see Exstrophy, bladder
    neck obstruction Q64.31
  bone Q79.9
    face Q75.9
      specified type NEC Q75.8
    skull Q75.9
      specified type NEC Q75.8
  brain (multiple) Q04.9
    arteriovenous Q28.2
    specified type NEC Q04.8
  branchial cleft Q18.2
  breast Q83.9
    specified type NEC Q83.8
  broad ligament Q50.6
  bronchus Q32.4
  bursa Q79.9
  cardiac
    chambers Q20.9
      specified type NEC Q20.8
    septum Q21.9
      specified type NEC Q21.8
  cerebral Q04.9
    vessels Q28.3
  cervix uteri Q51.9
    specified type NEC Q51.828
  Chiari
    Type I G93.5
    Type II Q07.01
  choroid (congenital) Q14.3
    plexus Q07.8
  circulatory system Q28.9
  cochlea Q16.5
  cornea Q13.4
  coronary vessels Q24.5
  corpus callosum (congenital) Q04.0
  diaphragm Q79.1
  digestive system NEC, specified type NEC
    Q45.8
  dura Q07.9
    brain Q04.9
    spinal Q06.9
  ear Q17.9
    causing impairment of hearing
      Q16.9

Malformation (Continued)
  ear (Continued)
    external Q17.9
      accessory auricle Q17.0
      causing impairment of hearing Q16.9
        absence of
          auditory canal Q16.1
          auricle Q16.0
      macrotia Q17.1
      microtia Q17.2
      misplacement Q17.4
      misshapen NEC Q17.3
      prominence Q17.5
      specified type NEC Q17.8
    inner Q16.5
    middle Q16.4
      absence of eustachian tube Q16.2
      ossicles (fusion) Q16.3
    ossicles Q16.3
    specified type NEC Q17.8
  epididymis Q55.4
  esophagus Q39.9
    specified type NEC Q39.8
  eye Q15.9
    lid Q10.3
    specified NEC Q15.8
  fallopian tube Q50.6
  genital organ —see Anomaly, genitalia
  great
    artery Q25.9
      aorta —see Malformation, aorta
      pulmonary artery —see Malformation,
        pulmonary, artery
      specified type NEC Q25.8
    vein Q26.9
      anomalous
        portal venous connection Q26.5
        pulmonary venous connection Q26.4
          partial Q26.3
          total Q26.2
      persistent left superior vena cava Q26.1
      portal vein-hepatic artery fistula Q26.6
      specified type NEC Q26.8
      vena cava stenosis, congenital Q26.0
  gum Q38.6
  hair Q84.2
  heart Q24.9
    specified type NEC Q24.8
  integument Q84.9
    specified type NEC Q84.8
  internal ear Q16.5
  intestine Q43.9
    specified type NEC Q43.8
  iris Q13.2
  joint Q74.9
    ankle Q74.2
    lumbosacral Q76.49
    sacroiliac Q74.2
    specified type NEC Q74.8
  kidney Q63.9
    accessory Q63.0
    giant Q63.3
    horseshoe Q63.1
    hydronephrosis Q62.0
    malposition Q63.2
    specified type NEC Q63.8
  lacrimal apparatus Q10.6
  lingual Q38.3
  lip Q38.0
  liver Q44.7
  lung Q33.9
  meninges or membrane (congenital)
    Q07.9
    cerebral Q04.8
    spinal (cord) Q06.9
  middle ear Q16.4
    ossicles Q16.3
  mitral valve Q23.9
    specified NEC Q23.8
  Mondini's (congenital) (malformation,
    cochlea) Q16.5

Malformation (Continued)
  mouth (congenital) Q38.6
  multiple types NEC Q89.7
  musculoskeletal system Q79.9
  myocardium Q24.8
  nail Q84.6
  nervous system (central) Q07.9
  nose Q30.9
    specified type NEC Q30.8
  optic disc Q14.2
  orbit Q10.7
  ovary Q50.39
  palate Q38.5
  parathyroid gland Q89.2
  pelvic organs or tissues NEC
    in pregnancy or childbirth O34.8- •
      causing obstructed labor O65.5
  penis Q55.69
    aplasia Q55.5
    curvature (lateral) Q55.61
    hypoplasia Q55.62
  pericardium Q24.8
  peripheral vascular system Q27.9
    specified type NEC Q27.8
  pharynx Q38.8
  precerebral vessels Q28.1
  prostate Q55.4
  pulmonary
    arteriovenous Q25.72
    artery Q25.9
      atresia Q25.5
      specified type NEC Q25.79
      stenosis Q25.6
    valve Q22.3
  renal artery Q27.2
  respiratory system Q34.9
  retina Q14.1
  scrotum —see Malformation, testis and
    scrotum
  seminal vesicles Q55.4
  sense organs NEC Q07.9
  skin Q82.9
  specified NEC Q89.8
  spinal
    cord Q06.9
    nerve root Q07.8
  spine Q76.49
    kyphosis —see Kyphosis, congenital
    lordosis —see Lordosis, congenital
  spleen Q89.09
  stomach Q40.3
    specified type NEC Q40.2
  teeth, tooth K00.9
  tendon Q79.9
  testis and scrotum Q55.20
    aplasia Q55.0
    hypoplasia Q55.1
    polyorchism Q55.21
    retractile testis Q55.22
    scrotal transposition Q55.23
    specified NEC Q55.29
  thorax, bony Q76.9
  throat Q38.8
  thyroid gland Q89.2
  tongue (congenital) Q38.3
    hypertrophy Q38.2
    tie Q38.1
  trachea Q32.1
  tricuspid valve Q22.9
    specified type NEC Q22.8
  umbilical cord NEC (complicating delivery)
    O69.89
  umbilicus Q89.9
  ureter Q62.8
    agenesis Q62.4
    duplication Q62.5
    malposition —see Malposition, congenital,
      ureter
    obstructive defect —see Defect, obstructive,
      ureter
    vesico-uretero-renal reflux Q62.7

M

M

Malformation (Continued)
  urethra Q64.79
    aplasia Q64.5
    duplication Q64.74
    posterior valves Q64.2
    prolapse Q64.71
    stricture Q64.32
  urinary system Q64.9
  uterus Q51.9
    specified type NEC Q51.818
  vagina Q52.4
  vascular system, peripheral Q27.9
  vas deferens Q55.4
    atresia Q55.3
  venous —see Anomaly, vein(s)
  vulva Q52.70
Malfunction —see also Dysfunction
  cardiac electronic device T82.119
    electrode T82.110
    pulse generator T82.111
    specified type NEC T82.118
  catheter device NEC T85.618
    cystostomy T83.010
    dialysis (renal) (vascular) T82.41
      intraperitoneal T85.611
    infusion NEC T82.514
      cranial T85.610
      epidural T85.610
      intrathecal T85.610
      spinal T85.610
      subarachnoid T85.610
      subdural T85.610
    urinary —see also Breakdown, device,
        catheter T83.018
  colostomy K94.03
    valve K94.03
  cystostomy (stoma) N99.512
    catheter T83.010
  enteric stoma K94.13
  enterostomy K94.13
  esophagostomy K94.33
  gastroenteric K31.89
  gastrostomy K94.23
  ileostomy K94.13
    valve K94.13
  intrathecal infusion pump T85.615
  jejunostomy K94.13
  nervous system device, implant or graft,
      specified NEC T85.615
  pacemaker —see Malfunction, cardiac
      electronic device
  prosthetic device, internal —see
      Complications, prosthetic device, by site,
      mechanical
  tracheostomy J95.03
  urinary device NEC —see Complication,
      genitourinary, device, urinary,
      mechanical
  valve
    colostomy K94.03
    heart T82.09
    ileostomy K94.13
  vascular graft or shunt NEC —see
      Complication, cardiovascular device,
      mechanical, vascular
  ventricular (communicating shunt) T85.01
Malherbe's tumor —see Neoplasm, skin,
    benign
Malibu disease L98.8-●
Malignancy —see also Neoplasm, malignant,
    by site
  unspecified site (primary) C80.1
Malignant —see condition
Malingerer, malingering Z76.5
Mallet finger (acquired) —see Deformity, finger,
    mallet finger
  congenital Q74.0
  sequelae of rickets E64.3
Malleus A24.0
Mallory's bodies R89.7
Mallory-Weiss syndrome K22.6

Malnutrition E46
  degree
    first E44.1
    mild (protein) E44.1
    moderate (protein) E44.0
    second E44.0
    severe (protein-energy) E43
      intermediate form E42
        with
          kwashiorkor (and marasmus) E42
          marasmus E41
    third E43
  following gastrointestinal surgery K91.2
  intrauterine
    light-for-dates —see Light for dates
    small-for-dates —see Small for dates
  lack of care, or neglect (child) (infant) T76.02
    confirmed T74.02
  malignant E40
  protein E46
    calorie E46
      mild E44.1
      moderate E44.0
      severe E43
        intermediate form E42
          with
            kwashiorkor (and marasmus)
                E42
            marasmus E41
    energy E46
      mild E44.1
      moderate E44.0
      severe E43
        intermediate form E42
          with
            kwashiorkor (and marasmus)
                E42
            marasmus E41
    severe (protein-energy) E43
      with
        kwashiorkor (and marasmus) E42
        marasmus E41
Malocclusion (teeth) M26.4
  Angle's M26.219
    class I M26.211
    class II M26.212
    class III M26.213
  due to
    abnormal swallowing M26.59
    mouth breathing M26.59
    tongue, lip or finger habits M26.59
  temporomandibular (joint) M26.69
Malposition
  cervix —see Malposition, uterus
  congenital
    adrenal (gland) Q89.1
    alimentary tract Q45.8
      lower Q43.8
      upper Q40.8
    aorta Q25.49
    appendix Q43.8
    arterial trunk Q20.0
    artery (peripheral) Q27.8
      coronary Q24.5
      digestive system Q27.8
      lower limb Q27.8
      pulmonary Q25.79
      specified site NEC Q27.8
      upper limb Q27.8
    auditory canal Q17.8
      causing impairment of hearing Q16.9
    auricle (ear) Q17.4
      causing impairment of hearing Q16.9
    cervical Q18.2
    biliary duct or passage Q44.5
    bladder (mucosa) —see Exstrophy,
        bladder
    brachial plexus Q07.8
    brain tissue Q04.8
    breast Q83.8
    bronchus Q32.4

Malposition (Continued)
  congenital (Continued)
    cecum Q43.8
    clavicle Q74.0
    colon Q43.8
    digestive organ or tract NEC Q45.8
      lower Q43.8
      upper Q40.8
    ear (auricle) (external) Q17.4
      ossicles Q16.3
    endocrine (gland) NEC Q89.2
    epiglottis Q31.8
    eustachian tube Q17.8
    eye Q15.8
    facial features Q18.8
    fallopian tube Q50.6
    finger(s) Q68.1
      supernumerary Q69.0
    foot Q66.9
    gallbladder Q44.1
    gastrointestinal tract Q45.8
    genitalia, genital organ(s) or tract
      female Q52.8
        external Q52.79
        internal NEC Q52.8
      male Q55.8
    glottis Q31.8
    hand Q68.1
    heart Q24.8
      dextrocardia Q24.0
        with complete transposition of viscera
            Q89.3
    hepatic duct Q44.5
    hip (joint) Q65.89
    intestine (large) (small) Q43.8
      with anomalous adhesions, fixation or
          malrotation Q43.3
    joint NEC Q68.8
    kidney Q63.2
    larynx Q31.8
    limb Q68.8
      lower Q68.8
      upper Q68.8
    liver Q44.7
    lung (lobe) Q33.8
    nail(s) Q84.6
    nerve Q07.8
    nervous system NEC Q07.8
    nose, nasal (septum) Q30.8
    organ or site not listed —see Anomaly,
        by site
    ovary Q50.39
    pancreas Q45.3
    parathyroid (gland) Q89.2
    patella Q74.1
    peripheral vascular system Q27.8
    pituitary (gland) Q89.2
    respiratory organ or system NEC
        Q34.8
    rib (cage) Q76.6
      supernumerary in cervical region
          Q76.5
    scapula Q74.0
    shoulder Q74.0
    spinal cord Q06.8
    spleen Q89.09
    sternum NEC Q76.7
    stomach Q40.2
    symphysis pubis Q74.2
    thymus (gland) Q89.2
    thyroid (gland) (tissue) Q89.2
      cartilage Q31.8
    toe(s) Q66.9
      supernumerary Q69.2
    tongue Q38.3
    trachea Q32.1
    ureter Q62.60
      deviation Q62.61
      displacement Q62.62
      ectopia Q62.63
      specified type NEC Q62.69

Malposition (Continued)
congenital (Continued)
uterus Q51.818
vein(s) (peripheral) Q27.8
great Q26.8
vena cava (inferior) (superior) Q26.8
device, implant or graft —see also
Complications, by site and type,
mechanical T85.628
arterial graft NEC —see Complication,
cardiovascular device, mechanical,
vascular
breast (implant) T85.42
catheter NEC T85.628
cystostomy T83.020
dialysis (renal) T82.42
intraperitoneal T85.621
infusion NEC T82.524
spinal (epidural) (subdural) T85.620
urinary —see also Displacement, device,
catheter, urinary T83.028
electronic (electrode) (pulse generator)
(stimulator)
bone T84.320
cardiac T82.129
electrode T82.120
pulse generator T82.121
specified type NEC T82.128
nervous system —see Complication,
prosthetic device, mechanical,
electronic nervous system
stimulator
urinary —see Complication,
genitourinary, device, urinary,
mechanical
fixation, internal (orthopedic) NEC —
see Complication, fixation device,
mechanical
gastrointestinal —see Complications,
prosthetic device, mechanical,
gastrointestinal device
genital NEC T83.428
intrauterine contraceptive device (string)
T83.32
penile prosthesis (cylinder) (implanted)
(pump) (resevoir) T83.420
testicular prosthesis T83.421
heart NEC —see Complication,
cardiovascular device, mechanical
joint prosthesis —see Complication, joint
prosthesis, mechanical
ocular NEC —see Complications,
prosthetic device, mechanical,
ocular device
orthopedic NEC —see Complication,
orthopedic, device, mechanical
specified NEC T85.628
urinary NEC —see also Complication,
genitourinary, device, urinary,
mechanical
graft T83.22
vascular NEC —see Complication,
cardiovascular device, mechanical
ventricular intracranial shunt T85.02
fetus —see Pregnancy, complicated by
(management affected by), presentation,
fetal
gallbladder K82.8
gastrointestinal tract, congenital Q45.8
heart, congenital NEC Q24.8
joint prosthesis —see Complications, joint
prosthesis, mechanical, displacement,
by site
stomach K31.89
congenital Q40.2
tooth, teeth, fully erupted M26.30
uterus (acute) (acquired) (adherent)
(asymptomatic) (postinfectional)
(postpartal, old) N85.4
anteflexion or anteversion N85.4
congenital Q51.818

Malposition (Continued)
uterus (Continued)
flexion N85.4
lateral —see Lateroversion, uterus
inversion N85.5
lateral (flexion) (version) —see
Lateroversion, uterus
in pregnancy or childbirth —see
subcategory O34.5
retroflexion or retroversion —see
Retroversion, uterus
Malposture R29.3
Malrotation
cecum Q43.3
colon Q43.3
intestine Q43.3
kidney Q63.2
Malta fever —see Brucellosis
Maltreatment
adult
abandonment
confirmed T74.01
suspected T76.01
confirmed T74.91
history of Z91.419
neglect
confirmed T74.01
suspected T76.01
physical abuse
confirmed T74.11
suspected T76.11
psychological abuse
confirmed T74.31
history of Z91.411
suspected T76.31
sexual abuse
confirmed T74.21
suspected T76.21
suspected T76.91
child
abandonment
confirmed T74.02
suspected T76.02
confirmed T74.92
history of —see History, personal (of),
abuse
neglect
confirmed T74.02
history of —see History, personal (of),
abuse
suspected T76.02
physical abuse
confirmed T74.12
history of —see History, personal (of),
abuse
suspected T76.12
psychological abuse
confirmed T74.32
history of —see History, personal (of),
abuse
suspected T76.32
sexual abuse
confirmed T74.22
history of —see History, personal (of),
abuse
suspected T76.22
suspected T76.92
personal history of Z91.89
Maltworker's lung J67.4
Malunion, fracture —see Fracture, by site
Mammillitis N61.0
puerperal, postpartum O91.02
Mammitis —see Mastitis
Mammogram (examination) Z12.39
routine Z12.31
Mammoplasia N62
Management (of)
bone conduction hearing device (implanted)
Z45.320
cardiac pacemaker NEC Z45.018
cerebrospinal fluid drainage device Z45.41

Management (Continued)
cochlear device (implanted) Z45.321
contraceptive Z30.9
specified NEC Z30.8
implanted device Z45.9
specified NEC Z45.89
infusion pump Z45.1
procreative Z31.9
male factor infertility in female Z31.81
specified NEC Z31.89
prosthesis (external) —see also Fitting Z44.9
implanted Z45.9
specified NEC Z45.89
renal dialysis catheter Z49.01
vascular access device Z45.2
Mangled —see specified injury by site
Mania (monopolar) —see also Disorder, mood,
manic episode
with psychotic symptoms F30.2
without psychotic symptoms F30.10
mild F30.11
moderate F30.12
severe F30.13
Bell's F30.8
chronic (recurrent) F31.89
hysterical F44.89
puerperal F30.8
recurrent F31.89
▶ **Manic depression** F31.9
Manic-depressive insanity, psychosis, or
syndrome —see Disorder, bipolar
Mannosidosis E77.1
Mansonelliasis, mansonellosis B74.4
Manson's
disease B65.1
schistosomiasis B65.1
Manual —see condition
Maple-bark-stripper's lung (disease) J67.6
Maple-syrup-urine disease E71.0
Marable's syndrome (celiac artery
compression) I77.4
Marasmus E41
due to malnutrition E41
intestinal E41
nutritional E41
senile R54
tuberculous NEC —see Tuberculosis
Marble
bones Q78.2
skin R23.8
Marburg virus disease A98.3
March
fracture —see Fracture, traumatic, stress, by
site
hemoglobinuria D59.6
Marchesani (-Weill) syndrome Q87.0
Marchiafava (-Bignami) syndrome or disease
G37.1
Marchiafava-Micheli syndrome D59.5
Marcus Gunn's syndrome Q07.8
Marfan's syndrome —see Syndrome, Marfan's
Marie-Bamberger disease —see
Osteoarthropathy, hypertrophic, specified
NEC
Marie-Charcot-Tooth neuropathic muscular
atrophy G60.0
Marie's
cerebellar ataxia (late-onset) G11.2
disease or syndrome (acromegaly) E22.0
Marie-Strümpell arthritis, disease or
spondylitis —see Spondylitis, ankylosing
Marion's disease (bladder neck obstruction)
N32.0
Marital conflict Z63.0
Mark
port wine Q82.5
raspberry Q82.5
strawberry Q82.5
stretch L90.6
tattoo L81.8
Marker heterochromatin —see Extra, marker
chromosomes

Maroteaux-Lamy syndrome (mild) (severe)
E76.29
Marrow (bone)
  arrest D61.9
  poor function D75.89
Marseilles fever A77.1
Marsh fever —see Malaria
Marshall's (hidrotic) ectodermal dysplasia
  Q82.4
Marsh's disease (exophthalmic goiter) E05.00
  with storm E05.01
Masculinization (female) with adrenal
  hyperplasia E25.9
  congenital E25.0
Masculinovoblastoma D27.-●
Masochism (sexual) F65.51
Mason's lung J62.8
Mass
  abdominal R19.00
    epigastric R19.06
    generalized R19.07
    left lower quadrant R19.04
    left upper quadrant R19.02
    periumbilic R19.05
    right lower quadrant R19.03
    right upper quadrant R19.01
    specified site NEC R19.09
  breast —see also Lump, breast N63.0
  chest R22.2
  cystic —see Cyst
  ear H93.8-●
  head R22.0
  intra-abdominal (diffuse) (generalized) —see
    Mass, abdominal
  kidney N28.89
  liver R16.0
  localized (skin) R22.9
    chest R22.2
    head R22.0
    limb
      lower R22.4-●
      upper R22.3-●
    neck R22.1
    trunk R22.2
  lung R91.8
  malignant —see Neoplasm, malignant,
    by site
  neck R22.1
  pelvic (diffuse) (generalized) —see Mass,
    abdominal
  specified organ NEC —see Disease, by site
  splenic R16.1
  substernal thyroid —see Goiter
  superficial (localized) R22.9
  umbilical (diffuse) (generalized) R19.09
Massive —see condition
Mast cell
  disease, systemic tissue D47.02
  leukemia C94.3-●
  neoplasm
    malignant C96.20
      specified type NEC C96.29
    of uncertain behavior NEC D47.09
  sarcoma C96.22
  tumor D47.09
    malignant C96.2
Mastalgia N64.4
Masters-Allen syndrome N83.8
Mastitis (acute) (diffuse) (nonpuerperal)
  (subacute) N61.0
  with abscess N61.1
  chronic (cystic) —see Mastopathy, cystic
  cystic (Schimmelbusch's type) —see
    Mastopathy, cystic
  fibrocystic —see Mastopathy, cystic
  infective N61.0
    newborn P39.0
  interstitial, gestational or puerperal —see
    Mastitis, obstetric
  neonatal (noninfective) P83.4
    infective P39.0

Mastitis (Continued)
  obstetric (interstitial) (nonpurulent)
    associated with
      lactation O91.23
      pregnancy O91.21-●
      puerperium O91.22
    purulent
      associated with
        lactation O91.13
        pregnancy O91.11-●
        puerperium O91.12
  periductal —see Ectasia, mammary duct
  phlegmonous —see Mastopathy, cystic
  plasma cell —see Ectasia, mammary duct
  without abscess N61.0
Mastocytoma (extracutaneous) D47.09
  malignant C96.29
  solitary D47.01
Mastocytosis D47.09
  aggressive systemic C96.21
  cutaneous (diffuse) (maculopapular) D47.01
    congenital Q82.2
    of neonatal onset Q82.2
    of newborn onset Q82.2
  indolent systemic D47.02
  isolated bone marrow D47.02
  malignant C96.29
  systemic, associated with clonal hematopoetic
    non-mast-cell disease (SM-AHNMD)
    D47.0
  systemic (indolent) (smoldering)
    with an associated hematological non-mast
      cell lineage disease (SM-AHNMD)
      D47.02
Mastodynia N64.4
Mastoid —see condition
Mastoidalgia —see subcategory H92.0
Mastoiditis (coalescent) (hemorrhagic)
  (suppurative) H70.9-●
  acute, subacute H70.00-●
    complicated NEC H70.09-●
    subperiosteal H70.01-●
  chronic (necrotic) (recurrent) H70.1-●
  in (due to)
    infectious disease NEC B99 [H75.0-●]
    parasitic disease NEC B89 [H75.0-●]
    tuberculosis A18.03
  petrositis —see Petrositis
  postauricular fistula —see Fistula, postauricular
  specified NEC H70.89-●
  tuberculous A18.03
Mastopathy, mastopathia N64.9
  chronica cystica —see Mastopathy, cystic
  cystic (chronic) (diffuse) N60.1
    with epithelial proliferation N60.3-●
  diffuse cystic —see Mastopathy, cystic
  estrogenic, oestrogenica N64.89
  ovarian origin N64.89
Mastoplasia, mastoplastia N62
Masturbation (excessive) F98.8
Maternal care (for) —see Pregnancy
  (complicated by) (management affected by)
Matheiu's disease (leptospiral jaundice) A27.0
Mauclaire's disease or osteochondrosis —
  see Osteochondrosis, juvenile, hand,
  metacarpal
Maxcy's disease A75.2
Maxilla, maxillary —see condition
May (-Hegglin) anomaly or syndrome D72.0
McArdle (-Schmid)(-Pearson) disease
  (glycogen storage) E74.04
McCune-Albright syndrome Q78.1
McQuarrie's syndrome (idiopathic familial
  hypoglycemia) E16.2
Meadow's syndrome Q86.1
Measles (black) (hemorrhagic) (suppressed)
  B05.9
  with
    complications NEC B05.89
    encephalitis B05.0
    intestinal complications B05.4

Measles (Continued)
  with (Continued)
    keratitis (keratoconjunctivitis) B05.81
    meningitis B05.1
    otitis media B05.3
    pneumonia B05.2
  French —see Rubella
  German —see Rubella
  Liberty —see Rubella
Meatitis, urethral —see Urethritis
Meatus, meatal —see condition
Meat-wrappers' asthma J68.9
Meckel-Gruber syndrome Q61.9
Meckel's diverticulitis, diverticulum
  (displaced) (hypertrophic) Q43.0
Meconium
  ileus, newborn P76.0
    in cystic fibrosis E84.11
    meaning meconium plug (without cystic
      fibrosis) P76.0
  obstruction, newborn P76.0
    due to fecaliths P76.0
    in mucoviscidosis E84.11
  peritonitis P78.0
  plug syndrome (newborn) NEC P76.0
Median —see also condition
  arcuate ligament syndrome I77.4
  bar (prostate) (vesical orifice) —see
    Hyperplasia, prostate
  rhomboid glossitis K14.2
Mediastinal shift R93.8
Mediastinitis (acute) (chronic) J98.51
  syphilitic A52.73
  tuberculous A15.8
Mediastinopericarditis —see also Pericarditis
  acute I30.9
  adhesive I31.0
  chronic I31.8
    rheumatic I09.2
Mediastinum, mediastinal —see condition
Medicine poisoning —see Table of Drugs and
  Chemicals, by drug, poisoning
Mediterranean
  fever —see Brucellosis
    familial M04.1
    tick A77.1
  kala-azar B55.0
  leishmaniasis B55.0
  tick fever A77.1
Medulla —see condition
Medullary cystic kidney Q61.5
Medullated fibers
  optic (nerve) Q14.8
  retina Q14.1
Medulloblastoma
  desmoplastic C71.6
  specified site —see Neoplasm, malignant, by
    site
  unspecified site C71.6
Medulloepithelioma —see also Neoplasm,
  malignant, by site
  teratoid —see Neoplasm, malignant, by site
Medullomyoblastoma
  specified site —see Neoplasm, malignant, by
    site
  unspecified site C71.6
Meekeren-Ehlers-Danlos syndrome Q79.6
Megacolon (acquired) (functional) (not
  Hirschsprung's disease) (in) K59.39
  Chagas' disease B57.32
  congenital, congenitum (aganglionic) Q43.1
  Hirschsprung's (disease) Q43.1
  toxic NEC K59.31
    due to Clostridium difficile
      not specified as recurrent A04.72
      recurrent A04.71
Megaesophagus (functional) K22.0
  congenital Q39.5
  in (due to) Chagas' disease B57.31
Megalencephaly Q04.5
Megalerythema (epidemic) B08.3

▶ New   ⟹ Revised   deleted Deleted   ● Use Additional Character(s)

Megaloappendix Q43.8
Megalocephalus, megalocephaly NEC Q75.3
Megalocornea Q15.8
  with glaucoma Q15.0
Megalocytic anemia D53.1
Megalodactylia (fingers) (thumbs) (congenital)
  Q74.0
  toes Q74.2
Megaloduodenum Q43.8
Megaloesophagus (functional) K22.0
  congenital Q39.5
Megalogastria (acquired) K31.89
  congenital Q40.2
Megalophthalmos Q11.3
Megalopsia H53.15
Megalosplenia —see Splenomegaly
Megaloureter N28.82
  congenital Q62.2
Megarectum K62.89
Megasigmoid K59.39
  congenital Q43.2
Megaureter N28.82
  congenital Q62.2
Megavitamin-B6 syndrome E67.2
Megrim —see Migraine
Meibomian
  cyst, infected —see Hordeolum
  gland —see condition
  sty, stye —see Hordeolum
Meibomitis —see Hordeolum
Meige-Milroy disease (chronic hereditary
  edema) Q82.0
Meige's syndrome Q82.0
Melalgia, nutritional E53.8
Melancholia F32.9
  climacteric (single episode) F32.89
    recurrent episode F33.8
  hypochondriac F45.29
  intermittent (single episode) F32.89
    recurrent episode F33.8
  involutional (single episode) F32.89
    recurrent episode F33.8
  menopausal (single episode) F32.89
    recurrent episode F33.8
  puerperal F32.89
  reactive (emotional stress or trauma) F32.3
  recurrent F33.9
  senile F03
  stuporous (single episode) F32.89
    recurrent episode F33.8
Melanemia R79.89
Melanoameloblastoma —see Neoplasm, bone,
  benign
Melanoblastoma —see Melanoma
Melanocarcinoma —see Melanoma
Melanocytoma, eyeball D31.9-●
Melanocytosis, neurocutaneous Q82.8
Melanoderma, melanodermia L81.4
Melanodontia, infantile K03.89
Melanodontoclasia K03.89
Melanoepithelioma —see Melanoma
Melanoma (malignant) C43.9
  acral lentiginous, malignant —see Melanoma,
    skin, by site
  amelanotic —see Melanoma, skin, by site
  balloon cell —see Melanoma, skin, by site
  benign —see Nevus
  desmoplastic, malignant —see Melanoma,
    skin, by site
  epithelioid cell —see Melanoma, skin, by site
    with spindle cell, mixed —see Melanoma,
      skin, by site
  in
    giant pigmented nevus —see Melanoma,
      skin, by site
    Hutchinson's melanotic freckle —see
      Melanoma, skin, by site
    junctional nevus —see Melanoma, skin,
      by site
    precancerous melanosis —see Melanoma,
      skin, by site

Melanoma (Continued)
  in situ D03.9
    abdominal wall D03.59
    ala nasi D03.39
    ankle D03.7-●
    anus, anal (margin) (skin) D03.51
    arm D03.6-●
    auditory canal D03.2-●
    auricle (ear) D03.2-●
    auricular canal (external) D03.2-●
    axilla, axillary fold D03.59
    back D03.59
    breast D03.52
    brow D03.39
    buttock D03.59
    canthus (eye) D03.1-●
    cheek (external) D03.39
    chest wall D03.59
    chin D03.39
    choroid D03.8
    conjunctiva D03.8
    ear (external) D03.2-●
    external meatus (ear) D03.2-●
    eye D03.8
    eyebrow D03.39
    eyelid (lower) (upper) D03.1-●
    face D03.30
      specified NEC D03.39
    female genital organ (external) NEC D03.8
    finger D03.6-●
    flank D03.59
    foot D03.7-●
    forearm D03.6-●
    forehead D03.39
    foreskin D03.8
    gluteal region D03.59
    groin D03.59
    hand D03.6-●
    heel D03.7-●
    helix D03.2-●
    hip D03.7-●
    interscapular region D03.59
    iris D03.8
    jaw D03.39
    knee D03.7-●
    labium (majus) (minus) D03.8
    lacrimal gland D03.8
    leg D03.7-●
    lip (lower) (upper) D03.0
    lower limb NEC D03.7-●
    male genital organ (external) NEC D03.8
    nail D03.9
      finger D03.6-●
      toe D03.7-●
    neck D03.4
    nose (external) D03.39
    orbit D03.8
    penis D03.8
    perianal skin D03.51
    perineum D03.51
    pinna D03.2-●
    popliteal fossa or space D03.7-●
    prepuce D03.8
    pudendum D03.8
    retina D03.8
    retrobulbar D03.8
    scalp D03.4
    scrotum D03.8
    shoulder D03.6-●
    specified site NEC D03.8
    submammary fold D03.52
    temple D03.39
    thigh D03.7-●
    toe D03.7-●
    trunk NEC D03.59
    umbilicus D03.59
    upper limb NEC D03.6-●
    vulva D03.8
  juvenile —see Nevus
  malignant, of soft parts except skin —see
    Neoplasm, connective tissue, malignant

Melanoma (Continued)
  metastatic
    breast C79.81
    genital organ C79.82
    specified site NEC C79.89
  neurotropic, malignant —see Melanoma, skin,
    by site
  nodular —see Melanoma, skin, by site
  regressing, malignant —see Melanoma, skin,
    by site
  skin C43.9
    abdominal wall C43.59
    ala nasi C43.31
    ankle C43.7-●
    anus, anal (skin) C43.51
    arm C43.6-●
    auditory canal (external) C43.2-●
    auricle (ear) C43.2-●
    auricular canal (external) C43.2-●
    axilla, axillary fold C43.59
    back C43.59
    breast (female) (male) C43.52
    brow C43.39
    buttock C43.59
    canthus (eye) C43.1-●
    cheek (external) C43.39
    chest wall C43.59
    chin C43.39
    ear (external) C43.2-●
    elbow C43.6-●
    external meatus (ear) C43.2-●
    eyebrow C43.39
    eyelid (lower) (upper) C43.1-●
    face C43.30
      specified NEC C43.39
    female genital organ (external) NEC C51.9
    finger C43.6-●
    flank C43.59
    foot C43.7-●
    forearm C43.6-●
    forehead C43.39
    foreskin C60.0
    glabella C43.39
    gluteal region C43.59
    groin C43.59
    hand C43.6-●
    heel C43.7-●
    helix C43.2-●
    hip C43.7-●
    interscapular region C43.59
    jaw (external) C43.39
    knee C43.7-●
    labium C51.9
      majus C51.0
      minus C51.1
    leg C43.7-●
    lip (lower) (upper) C43.0
    lower limb NEC C43.7-●
    male genital organ (external) NEC C63.9
    nail
      finger C43.6-●
      toe C43.7-●
    nasolabial groove C43.39
    nates C43.59
    neck C43.4
    nose (external) C43.31
    overlapping site C43.8
    palpebra C43.1-●
    penis C60.9
    perianal skin C43.51
    perineum C43.51
    pinna C43.2-●
    popliteal fossa or space C43.7-●
    prepuce C60.0
    pudendum C51.9
    scalp C43.4
    scrotum C63.2
    shoulder C43.6-●
    skin NEC C43.9
    submammary fold C43.52
    temple C43.39

M

Melanoma *(Continued)*
  skin *(Continued)*
    thigh C43.7-•
    toe C43.7-•
    trunk NEC C43.59
    umbilicus C43.59
    upper limb NEC C43.6-•
    vulva C51.9
      overlapping sites C51.8
  spindle cell
    with epithelioid, mixed —*see* Melanoma,
      skin, by site
    type A C69.4-•
    type B C69.4-•
  superficial spreading —*see* Melanoma, skin,
    by site
Melanosarcoma —*see also* Melanoma
  epithelioid cell —*see* Melanoma
Melanosis L81.4
  addisonian E27.1
    tuberculous A18.7
  adrenal E27.1
  colon K63.89
  conjunctiva —*see* Pigmentation, conjunctiva
    congenital Q13.89
  cornea (presenile) (senile) —*see also*
      Pigmentation, cornea
    congenital Q13.4
  eye NEC H57.8
    congenital Q15.8
  lenticularis progressiva Q82.1
  liver K76.89
  precancerous —*see also* Melanoma, in situ
    malignant melanoma in —*see* Melanoma
  Riehl's L81.4
  sclera H15.89
    congenital Q13.89
  suprarenal E27.1
  tar L81.4
  toxic L81.4
Melanuria R82.99
MELAS syndrome E88.41
Melasma L81.1
  adrenal (gland) E27.1
  suprarenal (gland) E27.1
Melena K92.1
  with ulcer - code by site under Ulcer, with
      hemorrhage K27.4
  due to swallowed maternal blood P78.2
  newborn, neonatal P54.1
    due to swallowed maternal blood P78.2
Meleney's
  gangrene (cutaneous) —*see* Ulcer, skin
  ulcer (chronic undermining) —*see* Ulcer, skin
Melioidosis A24.9
  acute A24.1
  chronic A24.2
  fulminating A24.1
  pneumonia A24.1
  pulmonary (chronic) A24.2
    acute A24.1
    subacute A24.2
  sepsis A24.1
  specified NEC A24.3
  subacute A24.2
Melitensis, febris A23.0
Melkersson (-Rosenthal) syndrome G51.2
Mellitus, diabetes —*see* Diabetes
Melorheostosis (bone) —*see* Disorder, bone,
    density and structure, specified NEC
Meloschisis Q18.4
Melotia Q17.4
Membrana
  capsularis lentis posterior Q13.89
  epipapillaris Q14.2
Membranacea placenta O43.19-•
Membranaceous uterus N85.8
Membrane(s), membranous —*see also* condition
  cyclitic —*see* Membrane, pupillary
  folds, congenital —*see* Web
  Jackson's Q43.3

Membrane(s), membranous *(Continued)*
  over face of newborn P28.9
  premature rupture —*see* Rupture,
      membranes, premature
  pupillary H21.4-•
    persistent Q13.89
  retained (with hemorrhage) (complicating
      delivery) O72.2
    without hemorrhage O73.1
  secondary cataract —*see* Cataract, secondary
  unruptured (causing asphyxia) —*see*
      Asphyxia, newborn
  vitreous —*see* Opacity, vitreous, membranes
      and strands
Membranitis —*see* Chorioamnionitis
Memory disturbance, lack or loss —*see also*
    Amnesia
  mild, following organic brain damage F06.8
Menadione deficiency E56.1
Menarche
  delayed E30.0
  precocious E30.1
Mendacity, pathologic F60.2
Mendelson's syndrome (due to anesthesia)
    J95.4
  in labor and delivery O74.0
  in pregnancy O29.01-•
  obstetric O74.0
  postpartum, puerperal O89.01
Ménétrier's disease or syndrome K29.60
  with bleeding K29.61
Ménière's disease, syndrome or vertigo H81.0-•
Meninges, meningeal —*see* condition
Meningioma —*see also* Neoplasm, meninges,
    benign
  angioblastic —*see* Neoplasm, meninges, benign
  angiomatous —*see* Neoplasm, meninges,
      benign
  endotheliomatous —*see* Neoplasm, meninges,
      benign
  fibroblastic —*see* Neoplasm, meninges, benign
  fibrous —*see* Neoplasm, meninges, benign
  hemangioblastic —*see* Neoplasm, meninges,
      benign
  hemangiopericytic —*see* Neoplasm,
      meninges, benign
  malignant —*see* Neoplasm, meninges,
      malignant
  meningiothelial —*see* Neoplasm, meninges,
      benign
  meningotheliomatous —*see* Neoplasm,
      meninges, benign
  mixed —*see* Neoplasm, meninges, benign
  multiple —*see* Neoplasm, meninges,
      uncertain behavior
  papillary —*see* Neoplasm, meninges,
      uncertain behavior
  psammomatous —*see* Neoplasm, meninges,
      benign
  syncytial —*see* Neoplasm, meninges, benign
  transitional —*see* Neoplasm, meninges,
      benign
Meningiomatosis (diffuse) —*see* Neoplasm,
    meninges, uncertain behavior
Meningism —*see* Meningismus
Meningismus (infectional) (pneumococcal)
    R29.1
  due to serum or vaccine R29.1
  influenzal —*see* Influenza, with,
      manifestations NEC
Meningitis (basal) (basic) (brain) (cerebral)
    (cervical) (congestive) (diffuse)
    (hemorrhagic) infantile) (membranous)
    (metastatic) (nonspecific) (pontine)
    (progressive) (simple) (spinal) (subacute)
    (sympathetic) (toxic) G03.9
  abacterial G03.0
  actinomycotic A42.81
  adenoviral A87.1
  arbovirus A87.8
  aseptic (acute) G03.0

Meningitis *(Continued)*
  bacterial G00.9
    Escherichia coli (E. coli) G00.8
    Friedländer (bacillus) G00.8
    gram-negative G00.9
    H. influenzae G00.0
    Klebsiella G00.8
    pneumococcal G00.1
    specified organism NEC G00.8
    staphylococcal G00.3
    streptococcal (acute) G00.2
  benign recurrent (Mollaret) G03.2
  candidal B37.5
  caseous (tuberculous) A17.0
  cerebrospinal A39.0
  chronic NEC G03.1
  clear cerebrospinal fluid NEC G03.0
  coxsackievirus A87.0
  cryptococcal B45.1
  diplococcal (gram positive) A39.0
  echovirus A87.0
  enteroviral A87.0
  eosinophilic B83.2
  epidemic NEC A39.0
  Escherichia coli (E. coli) G00.8
  fibrinopurulent G00.9
    specified organism NEC G00.8
  Friedländer (bacillus) G00.8
  gonococcal A54.81
  gram-negative cocci G00.9
  gram-positive cocci G00.9
  Haemophilus (influenzae) G00.0
  H. influenzae G00.0
  in (due to)
    adenovirus A87.1
    African trypanosomiasis B56.9 *[G02]*
    anthrax A22.8
    bacterial disease NEC A48.8 *[G01]*
    Chagas' disease (chronic) B57.41
    chickenpox B01.0
    coccidioidomycosis B38.4
    Diplococcus pneumoniae G00.1
    enterovirus A87.0
    herpes (simplex) virus B00.3
      zoster B02.1
    infectious mononucleosis B27.92
    leptospirosis A27.81
    Listeria monocytogenes A32.11
    Lyme disease A69.21
    measles B05.1
    mumps (virus) B26.1
    neurosyphilis (late) A52.13
    parasitic disease NEC B89 *[G02]*
    poliovirus A80.9 *[G02]*
    preventive immunization, inoculation or
        vaccination G03.8
    rubella B06.02
    Salmonella infection A02.21
    specified cause NEC G03.8
    Streptococcal pneumoniae G00.1
    typhoid fever A01.01
    varicella B01.0
    viral disease NEC A87.8
    whooping cough A37.90
    zoster B02.1
  infectious G00.9
  influenzal (H. influenzae) G00.0
  Klebsiella G00.8
  leptospiral (aseptic) A27.81
  lymphocytic (acute) (benign) (serous) A87.2
  meningococcal A39.0
  Mima polymorpha G00.8
  Mollaret (benign recurrent) G03.2
  monilial B37.5
  mycotic NEC B49 *[G02]*
  Neisseria A39.0
  nonbacterial G03.0
  nonpyogenic NEC G03.0
  ossificans G96.19
  pneumococcal streptococcus pneumoniae
      G00.1

▶ New   ⇒ Revised   ~~deleted~~ Deleted   • Use Additional Character(s)

Meningitis *(Continued)*
poliovirus A80.9 *[G02]*
postmeasles B05.1
purulent G00.9
    specified organism NEC G00.8
pyogenic G00.9
    specified organism NEC G00.8
Salmonella (arizonae) (Cholerae-Suis)
        (enteritidis) (typhimurium) A02.21
septic G00.9
    specified organism NEC G00.8
serosa circumscripta NEC G03.0
serous NEC G93.2
specified organism NEC G00.8
sporotrichosis B42.81
staphylococcal G00.3
sterile G03.0
Streptococcal (acute) G00.2
    pneumoniae G00.1
suppurative G00.9
    specified organism NEC G00.8
syphilitic (late) (tertiary) A52.13
    acute A51.41
    congenital A50.41
    secondary A51.41
Torula histolytica (cryptococcal) B45.1
traumatic (complication of injury) T79.8
tuberculous A17.0
typhoid A01.01
viral NEC A87.9
Yersinia pestis A20.3
Meningocele (spinal) —*see also* Spina bifida
with hydrocephalus —*see* Spina bifida, by
    site, with hydrocephalus
acquired (traumatic) G96.19
cerebral —*see* Encephalocele
Meningocerebritis —*see* Meningoencephalitis
Meningococcemia A39.4
acute A39.2
chronic A39.3
Meningococcus, meningococcal —*see also*
    condition A39.9
adrenalitis, hemorrhagic A39.1
carrier (suspected) of Z22.31
meningitis (cerebrospinal) A39.0
Meningoencephalitis —*see also* Encephalitis
    G04.90
acute NEC —*see also* Encephalitis, viral A86
bacterial NEC G04.2
California A83.5
diphasic A84.1
eosinophilic B83.2
epidemic A39.81
herpesviral, herpetic B00.4
    due to herpesvirus 6 B10.01
    due to herpesvirus 7 B10.09
    specified NEC B10.09
in (due to)
    blastomycosis NEC B40.81
    diseases classified elsewhere G05.3
    free-living amebae B60.2
    Hemophilus influenzae (H. influenzae)
        G00.0
    herpes B00.4
        due to herpesvirus 6 B10.01
        due to herpesvirus 7 B10.09
        specified NEC B10.09
    H. influenzae G00.0
    Lyme disease A69.22
    mercury —*see* subcategory T56.1
    mumps B26.2
    Naegleria (amebae) (organisms) (fowleri)
        B60.2
    Parastrongylus cantonensis B83.2
    toxoplasmosis (acquired) B58.2
        congenital P37.1
infectious (acute) (viral) A86
influenzal (H. influenzae) G00.0
Listeria monocytogenes A32.12
lymphocytic (serous) A87.2
mumps B26.2

Meningoencephalitis *(Continued)*
parasitic NEC B89 *[G05.3]*
pneumococcal G04.2
primary amebic B60.2
specific (syphilitic) A52.14
specified organism NEC G04.81
staphylococcal G04.2
streptococcal G04.2
syphilitic A52.14
toxic NEC G92
    due to mercury —*see* subcategory T56.1
tuberculous A17.82
virus NEC A86
Meningoencephalocele —*see also*
    Encephalocele
syphilitic A52.19
    congenital A50.49
Meningoencephalomyelitis —*see also*
    Meningoencephalitis
acute NEC (viral) A86
    disseminated G04.00
        postimmunization or postvaccination
            G04.02
        postinfectious G04.01
due to
    actinomycosis A42.82
    Torula B45.1
    Toxoplasma or toxoplasmosis (acquired)
        B58.2
        congenital P37.1
postimmunization or postvaccination G04.02
Meningoencephalomyelopathy G96.9
Meningoencephalopathy G96.9
Meningomyelitis —*see also*
    Meningoencephalitis
bacterial NEC G04.2
blastomycotic NEC B40.81
cryptococcal B45.1
in diseases classified elsewhere G05.4
meningococcal A39.81
syphilitic A52.14
tuberculous A17.82
Meningomyelocele —*see also* Spina bifida
syphilitic A52.19
Meningomyeloneuritis —*see*
    Meningoencephalitis
Meningoradiculitis —*see* Meningitis
Meningovascular —*see* condition
Menkes' disease or syndrome E83.09
    meaning maple-syrup-urine disease E71.0
Menometrorrhagia N92.1
Menopause, menopausal (asymptomatic)
        (state) Z78.0
arthritis (any site) NEC —*see* Arthritis,
        specified form NEC
bleeding N92.4
depression (single episode) F32.89
    agitated (single episode) F32.2
        recurrent episode F33.9
    psychotic (single episode) F32.89
        recurrent episode F33.8
    recurrent episode F33.9
melancholia (single episode) F32.89
    recurrent episode F33.8
paranoid state F22
premature E28.319
    asymptomatic E28.319
        postirradiation E89.40
        postsurgical E89.40
    symptomatic E28.310
        postirradiation E89.41
        postsurgical E89.41
psychosis NEC F28
symptomatic N95.1
toxic polyarthritis NEC —*see* Arthritis,
        specified form NEC
Menorrhagia (primary) N92.0
climacteric N92.4
    menopausal N92.4
menopausal N92.4
postclimacteric N95.0

Menorrhagia *(Continued)*
postmenopausal N95.0
preclimacteric or premenopausal N92.4
pubertal (menses retained) N92.2
Menostaxis N92.0
Menses, retention N94.89
Menstrual —*see* Menstruation
Menstruation
absent —*see* Amenorrhea
anovulatory N97.0
cycle, irregular N92.6
delayed N91.0
disorder N93.9
    psychogenic F45.8
during pregnancy O20.8
excessive (with regular cycle) N92.0
    with irregular cycle N92.1
    at puberty N92.2
frequent N92.0
infrequent —*see* Oligomenorrhea
irregular N92.6
    specified NEC N92.5
latent N92.5
membranous N92.5
painful —*see also* Dysmenorrhea N94.6
    primary N94.4
    psychogenic F45.8
    secondary N94.5
passage of clots N92.0
precocious E30.1
protracted N92.5
rare —*see* Oligomenorrhea
retained N94.89
retrograde N92.5
scanty —*see* Oligomenorrhea
suppression N94.89
vicarious (nasal) N94.89
Mental —*see also* condition
deficiency —*see* Disability, intellectual
deterioration —*see* Psychosis
disorder —*see* Disorder, mental
exhaustion F48.8
insufficiency (congenital) —*see* Disability,
        intellectual
observation without need for further medical
        care Z03.89
retardation —*see* Disability, intellectual
subnormality —*see* Disability, intellectual
upset —*see* Disorder, mental
Meralgia paresthetica G57.1-●
Mercurial —*see* condition
Mercurialism —*see* subcategory T56.1
MERRF syndrome (myoclonic epilepsy
        associated with ragged-red fiber) E88.42
Merkel cell tumor —*see* Carcinoma, Merkel cell
Merocele —*see* Hernia, femoral
Meromelia
lower limb —*see* Defect, reduction, lower limb
    intercalary
        femur —*see* Defect, reduction, lower
            limb, specified type NEC
        tibiofibular (complete) (incomplete) —
            see Defect, reduction, lower limb
upper limb —*see* Defect, reduction, upper
        limb
    intercalary, humeral, radioulnar —*see*
        Agenesis, arm, with hand present
Merzbacher-Pelizaeus disease E75.29
Mesaortitis —*see* Aortitis
Mesarteritis —*see* Arteritis
Mesencephalitis —*see* Encephalitis
Mesenchymoma —*see also* Neoplasm,
        connective tissue, uncertain behavior
benign —*see* Neoplasm, connective tissue,
        benign
malignant —*see* Neoplasm, connective tissue,
        malignant
Mesenteritis
retractile K65.4
sclerosing K65.4
Mesentery, mesenteric —*see* condition

M

Mesiodens, mesiodentes K00.1
Mesio-occlusion M26.213
Mesocolon —see condition
Mesonephroma (malignant) —see Neoplasm, malignant, by site
benign —see Neoplasm, benign, by site
Mesophlebitis —see Phlebitis
Mesostromal dysgenesis Q13.89
Mesothelioma (malignant) C45.9
  benign
    mesentery D19.1
    mesocolon D19.1
    omentum D19.1
    peritoneum D19.1
    pleura D19.0
    specified site NEC D19.7
    unspecified site D19.9
  biphasic C45.9
    benign
      mesentery D19.1
      mesocolon D19.1
      omentum D19.1
      peritoneum D19.1
      pleura D19.0
      specified site NEC D19.7
      unspecified site D19.9
  cystic D48.4
  epithelioid C45.9
    benign
      mesentery D19.1
      mesocolon D19.1
      omentum D19.1
      peritoneum D19.1
      pleura D19.0
      specified site NEC D19.7
      unspecified site D19.9
  fibrous C45.9
    benign
      mesentery D19.1
      mesocolon D19.1
      omentum D19.1
      peritoneum D19.1
      pleura D19.0
      specified site NEC D19.7
      unspecified site D19.9
  site classification
    liver C45.7
    lung C45.7
    mediastinum C45.7
    mesentery C45.1
    mesocolon C45.1
    omentum C45.1
    pericardium C45.2
    peritoneum C45.1
    pleura C45.0
      parietal C45.0
    retroperitoneum C45.7
    specified site NEC C45.7
    unspecified C45.9
Metabolic syndrome E88.81
Metagonimiasis B66.8
Metagonimus infestation (intestine) B66.8
Metal
  pigmentation L81.8
  polisher's disease J62.8
Metamorphopsia H53.15
Metaplasia
  apocrine (breast) —see Dysplasia, mammary, specified type NEC
  cervix (squamous) —see Dysplasia, cervix
  endometrium (squamous) (uterus) N85.8
  esophagus K22.7-•
  kidney (pelvis) (squamous) N28.89
  myelogenous D73.1
  myeloid (agnogenic) (megakaryocytic) D73.1
  spleen D73.1
  squamous cell, bladder N32.89
Metastasis, metastatic
  abscess —see Abscess
  calcification E83.59

Metastasis, metastatic (Continued)
  cancer
    from specified site —see Neoplasm, malignant, by site
    to specified site —see Neoplasm, secondary, by site
    deposits (in) —see Neoplasm, secondary, by site
    disease (see also Neoplasm, secondary, by site) C79.9
    spread (to) —see Neoplasm, secondary, by site
Metastrongyliasis B83.8
Metatarsalgia M77.4-•
  anterior G57.6-•
  Morton's G57.6-•
Metatarsus, metatarsal —see also condition
  adductus, congenital Q66.22
  valgus (abductus), congenital Q66.6
  varus (congenital) Q66.22
    primus Q66.21
Methadone use —see Use, opioid
Methemoglobinemia D74.9
  acquired (with sulfhemoglobinemia) D74.8
  congenital D74.0
  enzymatic (congenital) D74.0
  Hb M disease D74.0
  hereditary D74.0
  toxic D74.8
Methemoglobinuria —see Hemoglobinuria
Methioninemia E72.19
Methylmalonic acidemia E71.120
Metritis (catarrhal) (hemorrhagic) (septic) (suppurative) —see also Endometritis
  cervical —see Cervicitis
Metropathia hemorrhagica N93.8
Metroperitonitis —see Peritonitis, pelvic, female
Metrorrhagia N92.1
  climacteric N92.4
  menopausal N92.4
  postpartum NEC (atonic) (following delivery of placenta) O72.1
    delayed or secondary O72.2
  preclimacteric or premenopausal N92.4
  psychogenic F45.8
Metrorrhexis —see Rupture, uterus
Metrosalpingitis N70.91
Metrostaxis N93.8
Metrovaginitis —see Endometritis
Meyer-Schwickerath and Weyers syndrome Q87.0
Meynert's amentia (nonalcoholic) F04
  alcoholic F10.96
    with dependence F10.26
Mibelli's disease (porokeratosis) Q82.8
Mice, joint —see Loose, body, joint
  knee M23.4
Micrencephalon, micrencephaly Q02
Microalbuminuria R80.9
Microaneurysm, retinal —see also Disorder, retina, microaneurysms
  diabetic —see E08-E13 with .31
Microangiopathy (peripheral) I73.9
  thrombotic M31.1
Microcalcifications, breast R92.0
Microcephalus, microcephalic, microcephaly Q02
  due to toxoplasmosis (congenital) P37.1
Microcheilia Q18.7
Microcolon (congenital) Q43.8
Microcornea (congenital) Q13.4
Microcytic —see condition D57.40
Microdeletions NEC Q93.88
Microdontia K00.2
Microdrepanocytosis D57.40
  with crisis (vasoocclusive pain) D57.419
  with
    acute chest syndrome D57.411
    splenic sequestration D57.412
Microembolism
  atherothrombotic —see Atheroembolism
  retinal —see Occlusion, artery, retina

Microencephalon Q02
Microfilaria streptocerca infestation —see Onchocerciasis
Microgastria (congenital) Q40.2
Microgenia M26.06
Microgenitalia, congenital
  female Q52.8
  male Q55.8
Microglioma —see Lymphoma, non-Hodgkin, specified NEC
Microglossia (congenital) Q38.3
Micrognathia, micrognathism (congenital) (mandibular) (maxillary) M26.09
Microgyria (congenital) Q04.3
Microinfarct of heart —see Insufficiency, coronary
Microlentia (congenital) Q12.8
Microlithiasis, alveolar, pulmonary J84.02
Micromastia N64.82
Micromyelia (congenital) Q06.8
Micropenis Q55.62
Microphakia (congenital) Q12.8
Microphthalmos, microphthalmia (congenital) Q11.2
  due to toxoplasmosis P37.1
Micropsia H53.15
Microscopic polyangiitis (polyarteritis) M31.7
Microsporidiosis B60.8
  intestinal A07.8
Microsporon furfur infestation B36.0
Microsporosis —see also Dermatophytosis
  nigra B36.1
Microstomia (congenital) Q18.5
Microtia (congenital) (external ear) Q17.2
Microtropia H50.40
Microvillus inclusion disease (MVD) (MVID) Q43.8
Micturition
  disorder NEC —see also Difficulty, micturition R39.198
    psychogenic F45.8
  frequency R35.0
    psychogenic F45.8
  hesitancy R39.11
  incomplete emptying R39.14
  nocturnal R35.1
  painful R30.9
    dysuria R30.0
    psychogenic F45.8
    tenesmus R30.1
  poor stream R39.12
  position dependent R39.192
  split stream R39.13
  straining R39.16
  urgency R39.15
Mid plane —see condition
Middle
  ear —see condition
  lobe (right) syndrome J98.19
Miescher's elastoma L87.2
Mietens' syndrome Q87.2
Migraine (idiopathic) G43.909
  with refractory migraine G43.919
    with status migrainosus G43.911
    without status migrainosus G43.919
  with aura (acute-onset) (prolonged) (typical) (without headache) G43.109
    with refractory migraine G43.119
      with status migrainosus G43.111
      without status migrainosus G43.119
    intractable G43.119
      with status migrainosus G43.111
      without status migrainosus G43.119
    not intractable G43.109
      with status migrainosus G43.101
      without status migrainosus G43.109
    persistent G43.509
      with cerebral infarction G43.609
        with refractory migraine G43.619
          with status migrainosus G43.611
          without status migrainosus G43.619

▶ New   ⟹ Revised   ~~deleted~~ Deleted   • Use Additional Character(s)

Migraine (Continued)
  with aura (Continued)
    persistent (Continued)
      with cerebral infarction (Continued)
        intractable G43.619
          with status migrainosus G43.611
          without status migrainosus G43.619
        not intractable G43.609
          with status migrainosus G43.601
          without status migrainosus G43.609
        without refractory migraine G43.609
          with status migrainosus G43.601
          without status migrainosus G43.609
      without cerebral infarction G43.509
        with refractory migraine G43.519
          with status migrainosus G43.511
          without status migrainosus G43.519
        intractable G43.519
          with status migrainosus G43.511
          without status migrainosus G43.519
        not intractable G43.509
          with status migrainosus G43.501
          without status migrainosus G43.509
        without refractory migraine G43.509
          with status migrainosus G43.501
          without status migrainosus G43.509
    without mention of refractory migraine G43.109
      with status migrainosus G43.101
      without status migrainosus G43.109
  abdominal G43.D0
    with refractory migraine G43.D1
    intractable G43.D1
    not intractable G43.D0
    without refractory migraine G43.D0
  basilar —see Migraine, with aura
  classical —see Migraine, with aura
  common —see Migraine, without aura
  complicated G43.109
  equivalents —see Migraine, with aura
  familiar —see Migraine, hemiplegic
  hemiplegic G43.409
    with refractory migraine G43.419
      with status migrainosus G43.411
      without status migrainosus G43.419
    intractable G43.419
      with status migrainosus G43.411
      without status migrainosus G43.419
    not intractable G43.409
      with status migrainosus G43.401
      without status migrainosus G43.409
    without refractory migraine G43.409
      with status migrainosus G43.401
      without status migrainosus G43.409
  intractable G43.919
    with status migrainosus G43.911
    without status migrainosus G43.919
  menstrual G43.829
    with refractory migraine G43.839
      with status migrainosus G43.831
      without status migrainosus G43.839
    intractable G43.839
      with status migrainosus G43.831
      without status migrainosus G43.839
    not intractable G43.829
      with status migrainosus G43.821
      without status migrainosus G43.829
    without refractory migraine G43.829
      with status migrainosus G43.821
      without status migrainosus G43.829
  menstrually related —see Migraine, menstrual
  not intractable G43.909
    with status migrainosus G43.901
    without status migrainosus G43.919
  ophthalmoplegic G43.B0
    with refractory migraine G43.B1
    intractable G43.B1
    not intractable G43.B0
    without refractory migraine G43.B0

Migraine (Continued)
  persistent aura (with, without) cerebral infarction —see Migraine, with aura, persistent
  preceded or accompanied by transient focal neurological phenomena —see Migraine, with aura
  pre-menstrual —see Migraine, menstrual
  pure menstrual —see Migraine, menstrual
  retinal —see Migraine, with aura
  specified NEC G43.809
    intractable G43.819
      with status migrainosus G43.811
      without status migrainosus G43.819
    not intractable G43.809
      with status migrainosus G43.801
      without status migrainosus G43.809
  sporadic —see Migraine, hemiplegic
  transformed —see Migraine, without aura, chronic
  triggered seizures —see Migraine, with aura
  without aura G43.009
    with refractory migraine G43.019
      with status migrainosus G43.011
      without status migrainosus G43.019
    chronic G43.709
      with refractory migraine G43.719
        with status migrainosus G43.711
        without status migrainosus G43.719
      intractable
        with status migrainosus G43.711
        without status migrainosus G43.719
      not intractable
        with status migrainosus G43.701
        without status migrainosus G43.709
      without refractory migraine G43.709
        with status migrainosus G43.701
        without status migrainosus G43.709
    intractable
      with status migrainosus G43.011
      without status migrainosus G43.019
    not intractable
      with status migrainosus G43.001
      without status migrainosus G43.009
    without mention of refractory migraine G43.009
      with status migrainosus G43.001
      without status migrainosus G43.009
  without refractory migraine G43.909
    with status migrainosus G43.901
    without status migrainosus G43.919
Migrant, social Z59.0
Migration, anxiety concerning Z60.3
Migratory, migrating —see also condition
  person Z59.0
  testis Q55.29
Mikity-Wilson disease or syndrome P27.0
Mikulicz' disease or syndrome K11.8
Miliaria L74.3
  alba L74.1
  apocrine L75.2
  crystallina L74.1
  profunda L74.2
  rubra L74.0
  tropicalis L74.2
Miliary —see condition
Milium L72.0
  colloid L57.8
Milk
  crust L21.0
  excessive secretion O92.6
  poisoning —see Poisoning, food, noxious
  retention O92.79
  sickness —see Poisoning, food, noxious
  spots I31.0
Milk-alkali disease or syndrome E83.52
Milk-leg (deep vessels) (nonpuerperal) —see Embolism, vein, lower extremity
  complicating pregnancy O22.3-•
  puerperal, postpartum, childbirth O87.1

Milkman's disease or syndrome M83.8
Milky urine —see Chyluria
Millard-Gubler (-Foville) paralysis or syndrome G46.3
Millar's asthma J38.5
Miller-Fisher syndrome G61.0
Mills' disease —see Hemiplegia
Millstone maker's pneumoconiosis J62.8
Milroy's disease (chronic hereditary edema) Q82.0
Minamata disease T56.1-•
Miners' asthma or lung J60
Minkowski-Chauffard syndrome —see Spherocytosis
Minor —see condition
Minor's disease (hematomyelia) G95.19
Minot's disease (hemorrhagic disease), newborn P53
Minot-von Willebrand-Jurgens disease or syndrome (angiohemophilia) D68.0
Minus (and plus) hand (intrinsic) —see Deformity, limb, specified type NEC, forearm
Miosis (pupil) H57.03
Mirizzi's syndrome (hepatic duct stenosis) K83.1
Mirror writing F81.0
Misadventure (of) (prophylactic) (therapeutic) —see also Complications T88.9
  administration of insulin (by accident) —see subcategory T38.3
  infusion —see Complications, infusion
  local applications (of fomentations, plasters, etc.) T88.9
    burn or scald —see Burn
    specified NEC T88.8
  medical care (early) (late) T88.9
    adverse effect of drugs or chemicals —see Table of Drugs and Chemicals
  medical care (early) (late)
    burn or scald —see Burn
    specified NEC T88.8
  specified NEC T88.8
  surgical procedure (early) (late) —see Complications, surgical procedure
  transfusion —see Complications, transfusion
  vaccination or other immunological procedure —see Complications, vaccination
Miscarriage O03.9
Misdirection, aqueous H40.83-•
Misperception, sleep state F51.02
Misplaced, misplacement
  ear Q17.4
  kidney (acquired) N28.89
    congenital Q63.2
  organ or site, congenital NEC —see Malposition, congenital
Missed
  abortion O02.1
  delivery O36.4
Missing —see also Absence
  string of intrauterine contraceptive device T83.32
Misuse of drugs F19.99
Mitchell's disease (erythromelalgia) I73.81
Mite(s) (infestation) B88.9
  diarrhea B88.0
  grain (itch) B88.0
  hair follicle (itch) B88.0
  in sputum B88.0
Mitral —see condition
Mittelschmerz N94.0
Mixed —see condition
MMN (multifocal motor neuropathy) G61.82
MNGIE (Mitochondrial Neurogastrointestinal Encephalopathy) syndrome E88.49
Mobile, mobility
  cecum Q43.3
  excessive —see Hypermobility
  gallbladder, congenital Q44.1

Mobile, mobility (Continued)
  kidney N28.89
  organ or site, congenital NEC —see
      Malposition, congenital
Mobitz heart block (atrioventricular) I44.1
Moebius, Möbius
  disease (ophthalmoplegic migraine) —see
      Migraine, ophthalmoplegic
  syndrome Q87.0
      congenital oculofacial paralysis (with other
          anomalies) Q87.0
      ophthalmoplegic migraine —see Migraine,
          ophthalmoplegic
Moeller's glossitis K14.0
Mohr's syndrome (Types I and II) Q87.0
Mola destruens D39.2
Molar pregnancy O02.0
Molarization of premolars K00.2
Molding, head (during birth) - omit code
Mole (pigmented) —see also Nevus
  blood O02.0
  Breus' O02.0
  cancerous —see Melanoma
  carneous O02.0
  destructive D39.2
  fleshy O02.0
  hydatid, hydatidiform (benign) (complicating
      pregnancy) (delivered) (undelivered)
      O01.9
      classical O01.0
      complete O01.0
      incomplete O01.1
      invasive D39.2
      malignant D39.2
      partial O01.1
  intrauterine O02.0
  invasive (hydatidiform) D39.2
  malignant
      meaning
          malignant hydatidiform mole D39.2
          melanoma —see Melanoma
  nonhydatidiform O02.0
  nonpigmented —see Nevus
  pregnancy NEC O02.0
  skin —see Nevus
  ⇛tubal O00.10-
      ⇛with intrauterine pregnancy O00.11-
  vesicular —see Mole, hydatidiform
Molimen, molimina (menstrual) N94.3
Molluscum contagiosum (epitheliale) B08.1
Mönckeberg's arteriosclerosis, disease, or
      sclerosis —see Arteriosclerosis, extremities
Mondini's malformation (cochlea) Q16.5
Mondor's disease I80.8
Monge's disease T70.29
Monilethrix (congenital) Q84.1
Moniliasis —see also Candidiasis B37.9
  neonatal P37.5
Monitoring (encounter for)
  therapeutic drug level Z51.81
Monkey malaria B53.1
Monkeypox B04
Monoarthritis M13.10
  ankle M13.17-●
  elbow M13.12-●
  foot joint M13.17-●
  hand joint M13.14-●
  hip M13.15-●
  knee M13.16-●
  shoulder M13.11-●
  wrist M13.13-●
Monoblastic —see condition
Monochromat (ism), monochromatopsia
      (acquired) (congenital) H53.51
Monocytic —see condition
Monocytopenia D72.818
Monocytosis (symptomatic) D72.821
Monomania —see Psychosis
Mononeuritis G58.9
  cranial nerve —see Disorder, nerve,
      cranial

Mononeuritis (Continued)
  femoral nerve G57.2-●
  lateral
      cutaneous nerve of thigh G57.1-●
      popliteal nerve G57.3-●
  lower limb G57.9-●
      specified nerve NEC G57.8-●
  medial popliteal nerve G57.4-●
  median nerve G56.1-●
  multiplex G58.7
  plantar nerve G57.6-●
  posterior tibial nerve G57.5-●
  radial nerve G56.3-●
  sciatic nerve G57.0-●
  specified NEC G58.8
  tibial nerve G57.4-●
  ulnar nerve G56.2-●
  upper limb G56.9-●
      specified nerve NEC G56.8-●
  vestibular —see subcategory H93.3
Mononeuropathy G58.9
  carpal tunnel syndrome —see Syndrome,
      carpal tunnel
  diabetic NEC —see E08-E13 with .41
  femoral nerve —see Lesion, nerve, femoral
  ilioinguinal nerve G57.8-●
  in diseases classified elsewhere —see category
      G59
  intercostal G58.0
  lower limb G57.9-●
      causalgia —see Causalgia, lower limb
      femoral nerve —see Lesion, nerve,
          femoral
      meralgia paresthetica G57.1-●
      plantar nerve —see Lesion, nerve, plantar
      popliteal nerve —see Lesion, nerve,
          popliteal
      sciatic nerve —see Lesion, nerve, sciatic
      specified NEC G57.8-●
      tarsal tunnel syndrome —see Syndrome,
          tarsal tunnel
  median nerve —see Lesion, nerve, median
  multiplex G58.7
  obturator nerve G57.8-●
  popliteal nerve —see Lesion, nerve,
      popliteal
  radial nerve —see Lesion, nerve, radial
  saphenous nerve G57.8-●
  specified NEC G58.8
  tarsal tunnel syndrome —see Syndrome,
      tarsal tunnel
  tuberculous A17.83
  ulnar nerve —see Lesion, nerve, ulnar
  upper limb G56.9-●
      carpal tunnel syndrome —see Syndrome,
          carpal tunnel
      causalgia —see Causalgia
      median nerve —see Lesion, nerve, median
      radial nerve —see Lesion, nerve, radial
      specified site NEC G56.8-●
      ulnar nerve —see Lesion, nerve, ulnar
Mononucleosis, infectious B27.90
  with
      complication NEC B27.99
      meningitis B27.92
      polyneuropathy B27.91
  cytomegaloviral B27.10
      with
          complication NEC B27.19
          meningitis B27.12
          polyneuropathy B27.11
  Epstein-Barr (virus) B27.00
      with
          complication NEC B27.09
          meningitis B27.02
          polyneuropathy B27.01
  gammaherpesviral B27.00
      with
          complication NEC B27.09
          meningitis B27.02
          polyneuropathy B27.01

Mononucleosis, infectious (Continued)
  specified NEC B27.80
      with
          complication NEC B27.89
          meningitis B27.82
          polyneuropathy B27.81
Monoplegia G83.3-●
  congenital (cerebral) G80.8
      spastic G80.1
  embolic (current episode) I63.4-●
  following
      cerebrovascular disease
          cerebral infarction
              lower limb I69.34-●
              upper limb I69.33-●
          intracerebral hemorrhage
              lower limb I69.14-●
              upper limb I69.13-●
          lower limb I69.94-●
          nontraumatic intracranial hemorrhage
              NEC
              lower limb I69.24-●
              upper limb I69.23-●
          specified disease NEC
              lower limb I69.84-●
              upper limb I69.83-●
          stroke NOS
              lower limb I69.34-●
              upper limb I69.33-●
          subarachnoid hemorrhage
              lower limb I69.04-●
              upper limb I69.03-●
          upper limb I69.93-●
  hysterical (transient) F44.4
  lower limb G83.1-●
  psychogenic (conversion reaction) F44.4
  thrombotic (current episode) I63.3-●
  transient R29.818
  upper limb G83.2-●
Monorchism, monorchidism Q55.0
Monosomy —see also Deletion, chromosome
      Q93.9
  specified NEC Q93.89
  whole chromosome
      meiotic nondisjunction Q93.0
      mitotic nondisjunction Q93.1
      mosaicism Q93.1
  X Q96.9
Monster, monstrosity (single) Q89.7
  acephalic Q00.0
  twin Q89.4
Monteggia's fracture (-dislocation) S52.27-●
Mooren's ulcer (cornea) —see Ulcer, cornea,
      Mooren's
Moore's syndrome —see Epilepsy, specified NEC
Mooser-Neill reaction A75.2
Mooser's bodies A75.2
Morbidity not stated or unknown R69
Morbilli —see Measles
Morbus —see also Disease
  angelicus, anglorum E55.0
  Beigel B36.2
  caducus —see Epilepsy
  celiacus K90.0
  comitialis —see Epilepsy
  cordis —see also Disease, heart I51.9
      valvulorum —see Endocarditis
  coxae senilis M16.9
      tuberculous A18.02
  hemorrhagicus neonatorum P53
  maculosus neonatorum P54.5
Morel (-Stewart)(-Morgagni) syndrome M85.2
Morel-Kraepelin disease —see Schizophrenia
Morel-Moore syndrome M85.2
Morgagni's
  cyst, organ, hydatid, or appendage
      female Q50.5
      male (epididymal) Q55.4
          testicular Q55.29
  syndrome M85.2
Morgagni-Stewart-Morel syndrome M85.2

▶ New   ⇛ Revised   ~~deleted~~ Deleted   ● Use Additional Character(s)

Morgagni-Stokes-Adams syndrome I45.9
Morgagni-Turner (-Albright) syndrome Q96.9
Moria F07.0
Moron (I.Q. 50-69) F70
Morphea L94.0
Morphinism (without remission) F11.20
  with remission F11.21
Morphinomania (without remission) F11.20
  with remission F11.21
Morquio (-Ullrich)(-Brailsford) disease or
  syndrome —see Mucopolysaccharidosis
Mortification (dry) (moist) —see Gangrene
Morton's metatarsalgia (neuralgia)(neuroma)
  (syndrome) G57.6
Morvan's disease or syndrome G60.8
Mosaicism, mosaic (autosomal) (chromosomal)
  45,X/46,XX Q96.3
  45,X/other cell lines NEC with abnormal sex
    chromosome Q96.4
  sex chromosome
    female Q97.8
    lines with various numbers of
      X chromosomes Q97.2
    male Q98.7
    XY Q96.3
Moschowitz' disease M31.1
Mother yaw A66.0
Motion sickness (from travel, any vehicle)
  (from roundabouts or swings) T75.3
Mottled, mottling, teeth (enamel) (endemic)
  (nonendemic) K00.3
Mounier-Kuhn syndrome Q32.4
  with bronchiectasis J47.9
    exacerbation (acute) J47.1
    lower respiratory infection J47.0
  acquired J98.09
    with bronchiectasis J47.9
      with
        exacerbation (acute) J47.1
        lower respiratory infection J47.0
Mountain
  sickness T70.29
    with polycythemia , acquired (acute) D75.1
  tick fever A93.2
Mouse, joint —see Loose, body, joint
  knee M23.4- •
Mouth —see condition
Movable
  coccyx —see subcategory M53.2
  kidney N28.89
    congenital Q63.8
  spleen D73.89
Movements, dystonic R25.8
Moyamoya disease I67.5
MRSA (Methicillin resistant Staphylococcus
  aureus)
  infection A49.02
    as the cause of diseases classified
      elsewhere B95.62
  sepsis A41.02
MSSA (Methicillin susceptible Staphylococcus
  aureus)
  infection A49.01
    as the cause of diseases classified
      elsewhere B95.61
  sepsis A41.01
Mucha-Habermann disease L41.0
Mucinosis (cutaneous) (focal) (papular)
  (reticular erythematous) (skin) L98.5
  oral K13.79
Mucocele
  appendix K38.8
  buccal cavity K13.79
  gallbladder K82.1
  lacrimal sac, chronic H04.43- •
  nasal sinus J34.1
  nose J34.1
  salivary gland (any) K11.6
  sinus (accessory) (nasal) J34.1
  turbinate (bone) (middle) (nasal) J34.1
  uterus N85.8

Mucolipidosis
  I E77.1
  II, III E77.0
  IV E75.11
Mucopolysaccharidosis E76.3
  beta-gluduronidase deficiency E76.29
  cardiopathy E76.3 [I52]
  Hunter's syndrome E76.1
  Hurler's syndrome E76.01
  Hurler-Scheie syndrome E76.02
  Maroteaux-Lamy syndrome E76.29
  Morquio syndrome E76.219
    A E76.210
    B E76.211
    classic E76.210
  Sanfilippo syndrome E76.22
  Scheie's syndrome E76.03
  specified NEC E76.29
  type
    I
      Hurler's syndrome E76.01
      Hurler-Scheie syndrome E76.02
      Scheie's syndrome E76.03
    II E76.1
    III E76.22
    IV E76.219
    IVA E76.210
    IVB E76.211
    VI E76.29
    VII E76.29
Mucormycosis B46.5
  cutaneous B46.3
  disseminated B46.4
  gastrointestinal B46.2
  generalized B46.4
  pulmonary B46.0
  rhinocerebral B46.1
  skin B46.3
  subcutaneous B46.3
Mucositis (ulcerative) K12.30
  due to drugs NEC K12.32
  gastrointestinal K92.81
  mouth (oral) (oropharyngeal) K12.30
    due to antineoplastic therapy K12.31
    due to drugs NEC K12.32
    due to radiation K12.33
    specified NEC K12.39
    viral K12.39
  nasal J34.81
  oral cavity —see Mucositis, mouth
  oral soft tissues —see Mucositis, mouth
  vagina and vulva N76.81
Mucositis necroticans agranulocytica —see
  Agranulocytosis
Mucous —see also condition
  patches (syphilitic) A51.39
    congenital A50.07
Mucoviscidosis E84.9
  with meconium obstruction E84.11
Mucus
  asphyxia or suffocation —see Asphyxia,
    mucus
  in stool R19.5
  plug —see Asphyxia, mucus
Muguet B37.0
Mulberry molars (congenital syphilis)
  A50.52
Müllerian mixed tumor
  specified site —see Neoplasm, malignant, by
    site
  unspecified site C54.9
Multicystic kidney (development) Q61.4
Multiparity (grand) Z64.1
  affecting management of pregnancy, labor
    and delivery (supervision only)
    O09.4- •
  requiring contraceptive management —see
    Contraception
Multipartita placenta O43.19- •
Multiple, multiplex —see also condition
  digits (congenital) Q69.9

Multiple, multiplex (Continued)
  endocrine neoplasia —see Neoplasia,
    endocrine, multiple [MEN]
  personality F44.81
Mumps B26.9
  arthritis B26.85
  complication NEC B26.89
  encephalitis B26.2
  hepatitis B26.81
  meningitis (aseptic) B26.1
  meningoencephalitis B26.2
  myocarditis B26.82
  oophoritis B26.89
  orchitis B26.0
  pancreatitis B26.3
  polyneuropathy B26.84
Mumu —see also Infestation, filarial B74.9
  [N51]
Münchhausen's syndrome —see Disorder,
  factitious
Münchmeyer's syndrome —see Myositis,
  ossificans, progressiva
Mural —see condition
Murmur (cardiac) (heart) (organic) R01.1
  abdominal R19.15
  aortic (valve) —see Endocarditis, aortic
  benign R01.0
  diastolic —see Endocarditis
  Flint I35.1
  functional R01.0
  Graham Steell I37.1
  innocent R01.0
  mitral (valve) —see Insufficiency, mitral
  nonorganic R01.0
  presystolic, mitral —see Insufficiency, mitral
  pulmonic (valve) I37.8
  systolic R01.1
  tricuspid (valve) I07.9
  valvular —see Endocarditis
Murri's disease (intermittent hemoglobinuria)
  D59.6
Muscle, muscular —see also condition
  carnitine (palmityltransferase) deficiency
    E71.314
Musculoneuralgia —see Neuralgia
Mushroom-workers' (pickers') disease or lung
  J67.5
Mushrooming hip —see Derangement, joint,
  specified NEC, hip
Mutation(s)
  factor V Leiden D68.51
  surfactant, of lung J84.83
  prothrombin gene D68.52
Mutism —see also Aphasia
  deaf (acquired) (congenital) NEC H91.3
  elective (adjustment reaction) (childhood)
    F94.0
  hysterical F44.4
  selective (childhood) F94.0
MVD (microvillus inclusion disease) Q43.8
MVID (microvillus inclusion disease) Q43.8
Myalgia M79.1
  epidemic (cervical) B33.0
  traumatic NEC T14.8
Myasthenia G70.9
  congenital G70.2
  cordis —see Failure, heart
  developmental G70.2
  gravis G70.00
    with exacerbation (acute) G70.01
    in crisis G70.01
    neonatal, transient P94.0
    pseudoparalytica G70.00
      with exacerbation (acute) G70.01
      in crisis G70.01
  stomach, psychogenic F45.8
  syndrome
    in
      diabetes mellitus —see E08-E13 with .44
      neoplastic disease —see also Neoplasm
        D49.9 [G73.3]

▶ New   ⟹ Revised   ~~deleted~~ Deleted   • Use Additional Character(s)

Myasthenia *(Continued)*
  syndrome *(Continued)*
    in *(Continued)*
      pernicious anemia D51.0 *[G73.3]*
      thyrotoxicosis E05.90 *[G73.3]*
        with thyroid storm E05.91 *[G73.3]*
Myasthenic M62.81
Mycelium infection B49
Mycetismus —*see* Poisoning, food, noxious, mushroom
Mycetoma B47.9
  actinomycotic B47.1
  bone (mycotic) B47.9 *[M90.80]*
  eumycotic B47.0
  foot B47.9
    actinomycotic B47.1
    mycotic B47.0
  madurae NEC B47.9
    mycotic B47.0
  maduromycotic B47.0
  mycotic B47.0
  nocardial B47.1
Mycobacteriosis —*see* Mycobacterium
Mycobacterium, mycobacterial (infection) A31.9
  anonymous A31.9
  atypical A31.9
    cutaneous A31.1
    pulmonary A31.0
      tuberculous —*see* Tuberculosis, pulmonary
    specified site NEC A31.8
  avium (intracellulare complex) A31.0
  balnei A31.1
  Battey A31.0
  chelonei A31.8
  cutaneous A31.1
  extrapulmonary systemic A31.8
  fortuitum A31.8
  intracellulare (Battey bacillus) A31.0
  kakaferifu A31.8
  kansasii (yellow bacillus) A31.0
  kasongo A31.8
  leprae —*see also* Leprosy A30.9
  luciflavum A31.1
  marinum (M. balnei) A31.1
  nonspecific —*see* Mycobacterium, atypical
  pulmonary (atypical) A31.0
    tuberculous —*see* Tuberculosis, pulmonary
  scrofulaceum A31.8
  simiae A31.8
  systemic, extrapulmonary A31.8
  szulgai A31.8
  terrae A31.8
  triviale A31.8
  tuberculosis (human, bovine) —*see* Tuberculosis
  ulcerans A31.1
  xenopi A31.8
Mycoplasma (M.) pneumoniae, as cause of disease classified elsewhere B96.0
Mycosis, mycotic B49
  cutaneous NEC B36.9
  ear B36.9
    in
      aspergillosis B44.89
      candidiasis B37.84
      moniliasis B37.84
  fungoides (extranodal) (solid organ) C84.0-●
  mouth B37.0
  nails B35.1
  opportunistic B48.8
  skin NEC B36.9
  specified NEC B48.8
  stomatitis B37.0
  vagina, vaginitis (candidal) B37.3
Mydriasis (pupil) H57.04
Myelatelia Q06.1
Myelinolysis, pontine, central G37.2

Myelitis (acute) (ascending) (childhood) (chronic) (descending) (diffuse) (disseminated) (idiopathic) (pressure) (progressive) (spinal cord) (subacute) —*see also* Encephalitis G04.91
  herpes simplex B00.82
  herpes zoster B02.24
  in diseases classified elsewhere G05.4
  necrotizing, subacute G37.4
  optic neuritis in G36.0
  postchickenpox B01.12
  postherpetic B02.24
  postimmunization G04.02
  postinfectious NEC G04.89
  postvaccinal G04.02
  specified NEC G04.89
  syphilitic (transverse) A52.14
  toxic G92
  transverse (in demyelinating diseases of central nervous system) G37.3
  tuberculous A17.82
  varicella B01.12
Myeloblastic —*see* condition
Myeloblastoma
  granular cell —*see also* Neoplasm, connective tissue
    malignant —*see* Neoplasm, connective tissue, malignant
    tongue D10.1
Myelocele —*see* Spina bifida
Myelocystocele —*see* Spina bifida
Myelocytic —*see* condition
Myelodysplasia D46.9
  specified NEC D46.Z
  spinal cord (congenital) Q06.1
Myelodysplastic syndrome D46.9
  with
    5q deletion D46.C
    isolated del (5q) chromosomal abnormality C46.C
    specified NEC D46.Z
Myeloencephalitis —*see* Encephalitis
Myelofibrosis D75.81
  with myeloid metaplasia D47.4
  acute C94.4-●
  idiopathic (chronic) D47.4
  primary D47.1
  secondary D75.81
    in myeloproliferative disease D47.4
Myelogenous —*see* condition
Myeloid —*see* condition
Myelokathexis D70.9
Myeloleukodystrophy E75.29
Myelolipoma —*see* Lipoma
Myeloma (multiple) C90.0-●
  monostotic C90.3
    plasma cell C90.0-●
  plasma cell C90.0-●
  solitary —*see also* Plasmacytoma, solitary C90.3-●
Myelomalacia G95.89
Myelomatosis C90.0-●
Myelomeningitis —*see* Meningoencephalitis
Myelomeningocele (spinal cord) —*see* Spina bifida
Myelo-osteo-musculodysplasia hereditaria Q79.8
Myelopathic
  anemia D64.89
  muscle atrophy —*see* Atrophy, muscle, spinal
  pain syndrome G89.0
Myelopathy (spinal cord) G95.9
  drug-induced G95.89
  in (due to)
    degeneration or displacement, intervertebral disc NEC —*see* Disorder, disc, with, myelopathy
    infection —*see* Encephalitis
    intervertebral disc disorder —*see also* Disorder, disc, with, myelopathy
    mercury —*see* subcategory T56.1

Myelopathy *(Continued)*
  in (due to) *(Continued)*
    neoplastic disease —*see also* Neoplasm D49.9 *[G99.2]*
    pernicious anemia D51.0 *[G99.2]*
    spondylosis —*see* Spondylosis, with myelopathy NEC
  necrotic (subacute) (vascular) G95.19
  radiation-induced G95.89
  spondylogenic NEC —*see* Spondylosis, with myelopathy NEC
  toxic G95.89
  transverse, acute G37.3
  vascular G95.19
  vitamin B12 E53.8 *[G32.0]*
Myelophthisis D61.82
Myeloradiculitis G04.91
Myeloradiculodysplasia (spinal) Q06.1
Myelosarcoma C92.3-●
Myelosclerosis D75.89
  with myeloid metaplasia D47.4
  disseminated, of nervous system G35
  megakaryocytic D47.4
    with myeloid metaplasia D47.4
Myelosis
  acute C92.0-●
  aleukemic C92.9-●
  chronic D47.1
  erythremic (acute) C94.0-●
  megakaryocytic C94.2-●
  nonleukemic D72.828
  subacute C92.9-●
Myiasis (cavernous) B87.9
  aural B87.4
  creeping B87.0
  cutaneous B87.0
  dermal B87.0
  ear (external) (middle) B87.4
  eye B87.2
  genitourinary B87.81
  intestinal B87.82
  laryngeal B87.3
  nasopharyngeal B87.3
  ocular B87.2
  orbit B87.2
  skin B87.0
  specified site NEC B87.89
  traumatic B87.1
  wound B87.1
Myoadenoma, prostate —*see* Hyperplasia, prostate
Myoblastoma
  granular cell —*see also* Neoplasm, connective tissue, benign
    malignant —*see* Neoplasm, connective tissue, malignant
  tongue D10.1
Myocardial —*see* condition
Myocardiopathy (congestive) (constrictive) (familial) (hypertrophic nonobstructive) (idiopathic) (infiltrative) (obstructive) (primary) (restrictive) (sporadic) —*see also* Cardiomyopathy I42.9
  alcoholic I42.6
  cobalt-beer I42.6
  glycogen storage E74.02 *[I43]*
  hypertrophic obstructive I42.1
  in (due to)
    beriberi E51.12
    cardiac glycogenosis E74.02 *[I43]*
    Friedreich's ataxia G11.1 *[I43]*
    myotonia atrophica G71.11 *[I43]*
    progressive muscular dystrophy G71.0 *[I43]*
  obscure (African) I42.8
  secondary I42.9
  thyrotoxic E05.90 *[I43]*
    with storm E05.91 *[I43]*
  toxic NEC I42.7

Myocarditis (with arteriosclerosis) (chronic)
    (fibroid) (interstitial) (old) (progressive)
    (senile) I51.4
with
    rheumatic fever (conditions in I00) I09.0
        active —see Myocarditis, acute,
            rheumatic
        inactive or quiescent (with chorea) I09.0
active I40.9
    rheumatic I01.2
        with chorea (acute) (rheumatic)
            (Sydenham's) I02.0
acute or subacute (interstitial) I40.9
    due to
        streptococcus (beta-hemolytic) I01.2
    idiopathic I40.1
    rheumatic I01.2
        with chorea (acute) (rheumatic)
            (Sydenham's) I02.0
    specified NEC I40.8
aseptic of newborn B33.22
bacterial (acute) I40.0
Coxsackie (virus) B33.22
diphtheritic A36.81
eosinophilic I40.1
epidemic of newborn (Coxsackie) B33.22
Fiedler's (acute) (isolated) I40.1
giant cell (acute) (subacute) I40.1
gonococcal A54.83
granulomatous (idiopathic) (isolated)
    (nonspecific) I40.1
hypertensive —see Hypertension, heart
idiopathic (granulomatous) I40.1
in (due to)
    diphtheria A36.81
    epidemic louse-borne typhus A75.0 [I41]
    Lyme disease A69.29
    sarcoidosis D86.85
    scarlet fever A38.1
    toxoplasmosis (acquired) B58.81
    typhoid A01.02
    typhus NEC A75.9 [I41]
infective I40.0
influenzal —see Influenza, with, myocarditis
isolated (acute) I40.1
meningococcal A39.52
mumps B26.82
nonrheumatic, active I40.9
parenchymatous I40.9
pneumococcal I40.0
rheumatic (chronic) (inactive) (with chorea)
    I09.0
    active or acute I01.2
        with chorea (acute) (rheumatic)
            (Sydenham's) I02.0
rheumatoid —see Rheumatoid, carditis
septic I40.0
staphylococcal I40.0
suppurative I40.0
syphilitic (chronic) A52.06
toxic I40.8
    rheumatic —see Myocarditis, acute,
        rheumatic
tuberculous A18.84
typhoid A01.02
valvular —see Endocarditis
virus, viral I40.0
    of newborn (Coxsackie) B33.22
Myocardium, myocardial —see condition
Myocardosis —see Cardiomyopathy
Myoclonus, myoclonic, myoclonia (familial)
    (essential) (multifocal) (simplex) G25.3
drug-induced G25.3
epilepsy —see also Epilepsy, generalized,
    specified NEC G40.4-●
    familial (progressive) G25.3
epileptica G40.409
    with status epilepticus G40.401
facial G51.3
familial progressive G25.3
Friedreich's G25.3

Myoclonus, myoclonic, myoclonia (Continued)
    jerks G25.3
    massive G25.3
    palatal G25.3
    pharyngeal G25.3
Myocytolysis I51.5
Myodiastasis —see Diastasis, muscle
Myoendocarditis —see Endocarditis
Myoepithelioma —see Neoplasm, benign, by
    site
Myofasciitis (acute) —see Myositis
Myofibroma —see also Neoplasm, connective
    tissue, benign
    uterus (cervix) (corpus) —see Leiomyoma
Myofibromatosis D48.1
    infantile Q89.8
Myofibrosis M62.89
    heart —see Myocarditis
    scapulohumeral —see Lesion, shoulder,
        specified NEC
Myofibrositis M79.7
    scapulohumeral —see Lesion, shoulder,
        specified NEC
Myoglobulinuria, myoglobinuria (primary)
    R82.1
Myokymia, facial G51.4
Myolipoma —see Lipoma
Myoma —see also Neoplasm, connective tissue,
    benign
    malignant —see Neoplasm, connective tissue,
        malignant
    prostate D29.1
    uterus (cervix) (corpus) —see Leiomyoma
Myomalacia M62.89
Myometritis —see Endometritis
Myometrium —see condition
Myonecrosis, clostridial A48.0
Myopathy G72.9
    acute
        necrotizing G72.81
        quadriplegic G72.81
    alcoholic G72.1
    benign congenital G71.2
    central core G71.2
    centronuclear G71.2
    congenital (benign) G71.2
    critical illness G72.81
    distal G71.0
    drug-induced G72.0
    endocrine NEC E34.9 [G73.7]
    extraocular muscles H05.82-●
    facioscapulohumeral G71.0
    hereditary G71.9
        specified NEC G71.8
    immune NEC G72.49
    in (due to)
        Addison's disease E27.1 [G73.7]
        alcohol G72.1
        amyloidosis E85.0 [G73.7]
        cretinism E00.9 [G73.7]
        Cushing's syndrome E24.9 [G73.7]
        drugs G72.0
        endocrine disease NEC E34.9 [G73.7]
        giant cell arteritis M31.6 [G73.7]
        glycogen storage disease E74.00 [G73.7]
        hyperadrenocorticism E24.9 [G73.7]
        hyperparathyroidism NEC E21.3 [G73.7]
        hypoparathyroidism E20.9 [G73.7]
        hypopituitarism E23.0 [G73.7]
        hypothyroidism E03.9 [G73.7]
        infectious disease NEC B99 [G73.7]
        lipid storage disease E75.6 [G73.7]
        metabolic disease NEC E88.9 [G73.7]
        myxedema E03.9 [G73.7]
        parasitic disease NEC B89 [G73.7]
        polyarteritis nodosa M30.0 [G73.7]
        rheumatoid arthritis —see Rheumatoid,
            myopathy
        sarcoidosis D86.87
        scleroderma M34.82
        sicca syndrome M35.03

Myopathy (Continued)
    in (due to) (Continued)
        Sjögren's syndrome M35.03
        systemic lupus erythematosus M32.19
        thyrotoxicosis (hyperthyroidism) E05.90
            [G73.7]
            with thyroid storm E05.91 [G73.7]
        toxic agent NEC G72.2
    inflammatory NEC G72.49
    intensive care (ICU) G72.81
    limb-girdle G71.0
    mitochondrial NEC G71.3
    myotubular G71.2
    mytonic, proximal (PROMM) G71.11
    nemaline G71.2
    ocular G71.0
    oculopharyngeal G71.0
    of critical illness G72.81
    primary G71.9
        specified NEC G71.8
    progressive NEC G72.89
    proximal myotonic (PROMM) G71.11
    rod G71.2
    scapulohumeral G71.0
    specified NEC G72.89
    toxic G72.2
Myopericarditis —see also Pericarditis
    chronic rheumatic I09.2
Myopia (axial) (congenital) H52.1-●
    degenerative (malignant) H44.20
        with
            choroidal neovascularization H44.2A-●
            foveoschisis H44.2D-●
            macular hole H44.2B-●
            retinal detachment H44.2C-●
            specified maculopathy NEC H44.2E-●
        bilateral H44.23
        left eye H44.22
        right eye H44.21
    malignant —see also Myopia, degenerative
        H44.2-●
    pernicious —see also Myopia, degenerative
        H44.2-●
    progressive high (degenerative) —see also
        Myopia, degenerative H44.2-●
Myosarcoma —see Neoplasm, connective tissue,
    malignant
Myosis (pupil) H57.03
    stromal (endolymphatic) D39.0
Myositis M60.9
    clostridial A48.0
    due to posture —see Myositis, specified type
        NEC
    epidemic B33.0
    fibrosa or fibrous (chronic), Volkmann's T79.6
    foreign body granuloma —see Granuloma,
        foreign body
    in (due to)
        bilharziasis B65.9 [M63.8-●]
        cysticercosis B69.81
        leprosy A30.9 [M63.8-●]
        mycosis B49 [M63.8-●]
        sarcoidosis D86.87
        schistosomiasis B65.9 [M63.8-●]
        syphilis
            late A52.78
            secondary A51.49
        toxoplasmosis (acquired) B58.82
        trichinellosis B75 [M63.8-●]
        tuberculosis A18.09
    inclusion body [IBM] G72.41
    infective M60.009
        arm M60.002
            left M60.001
            right M60.000
        leg M60.005
            left M60.004
            right M60.003
        lower limb M60.005
            ankle M60.07-●
            foot M60.07-●
            lower leg M60.06-●

Myositis (Continued)
  infective (Continued)
    lower limb (Continued)
      thigh M60.05-●
      toe M60.07-●
    multiple sites M60.09
    specified site NEC M60.08
    upper limb M60.002
      finger M60.04-●
      forearm M60.03-●
      hand M60.04-●
      shoulder region M60.01-●
      upper arm M60.02-●
  interstitial M60.10
    ankle M60.17-●
    foot M60.17-●
    forearm M60.13-●
    hand M60.14-●
    lower leg M60.16-●
    multiple sites M60.19
    shoulder region M60.11-●
    specified site NEC M60.18
    thigh M60.15-●
    upper arm M60.12-●
  mycotic B49 [M63.8-●]
  ossificans or ossifying (circumscripta) —see
      also Ossification, muscle, specified NEC
    in (due to)
      burns M61.30
        ankle M61.37-●
        foot M61.37-●
        forearm M61.33-●
        hand M61.34-●
        lower leg M61.36-●
        multiple sites M61.39
        pelvic region M61.35-●
        shoulder region M61.31-●
        specified site NEC M61.38
        thigh M61.35-●
        upper arm M61.32-●
      quadriplegia or paraplegia M61.20
        ankle M61.27-●
        foot M61.27-●
        forearm M61.23-●
        hand M61.24-●
        lower leg M61.26-●
        multiple sites M61.29
        pelvic region M61.25-●
        shoulder region M61.21-●
        specified site NEC M61.28
        thigh M61.25-●
        upper arm M61.22-●

Myositis (Continued)
  ossificans or ossifying (Continued)
    progressiva M61.10
      ankle M61.17-●
      finger M61.14-●
      foot M61.17-●
      forearm M61.13-●
      hand M61.14-●
      lower leg M61.16-●
      multiple sites M61.19
      pelvic region M61.15-●
      shoulder region M61.11-●
      specified site NEC M61.18
      thigh M61.15-●
      toe M61.17-●
      upper arm M61.12-●
    traumatica M61.00
      ankle M61.07-●
      foot M61.07-●
      forearm M61.03-●
      hand M61.04-●
      lower leg M61.06-●
      multiple sites M61.09
      pelvic region M61.05-●
      shoulder region M61.01-●
      specified site NEC M61.08
      thigh M61.05-●
      upper arm M61.02-●
  purulent —see Myositis, infective
  specified type NEC M60.80
    ankle M60.87-●
    foot M60.87-●
    forearm M60.83-●
    hand M60.84-●
    lower leg M60.86-●
    multiple sites M60.89
    pelvic region M60.85-●
    shoulder region M60.81-●
    specified site NEC M60.88
    thigh M60.85-●
    upper arm M60.82-●
  suppurative —see Myositis, infective
  traumatic (old) —see Myositis, specified type
      NEC
Myospasia impulsiva F95.2
Myotonia (acquisita) (intermittens) M62.89
  atrophica G71.11
  chondrodystrophic G71.13
  congenita (acetazolamide responsive)
      (dominant) (recessive) G71.12

Myotonia (Continued)
  drug-induced G71.14
  dystrophica G71.11
  fluctuans G71.19
  levior G71.12
  permanens G71.19
  symptomatic G71.19
Myotonic pupil —see Anomaly, pupil, function,
    tonic pupil
Myriapodiasis B88.2
Myringitis H73.2-●
  with otitis media —see Otitis, media
  acute H73.00-●
    bullous H73.01-●
    specified NEC H73.09-●
  bullous —see Myringitis, acute, bullous
  chronic H73.1-●
Mysophobia F40.228
Mytilotoxism —see Poisoning, fish
Myxadenitis labialis K13.0
Myxedema (adult) (idiocy) (infantile)
    (juvenile) —see also Hypothyroidism
    E03.9
  circumscribed E05.90
    with storm E05.91
  coma E03.5
  congenital E00.1
  cutis L98.5
  localized (pretibial) E05.90
    with storm E05.91
  papular L98.5
Myxochondrosarcoma —see Neoplasm,
    cartilage, malignant
Myxofibroma —see Neoplasm, connective
    tissue, benign
  odontogenic —see Cyst, calcifying
    odontogenic
Myxofibrosarcoma —see Neoplasm, connective
    tissue, malignant
Myxolipoma D17.9
Myxoliposarcoma —see Neoplasm, connective
    tissue, malignant
Myxoma —see also Neoplasm, connective tissue,
    benign
  nerve sheath —see Neoplasm, nerve,
    benign
  odontogenic —see Cyst, calcifying
    odontogenic
Myxosarcoma —see Neoplasm, connective
    tissue, malignant

▶ New   ⇒ Revised   ~~deleted~~ Deleted   ● Use Additional Character(s)

N

Naegeli's
  disease Q82.8
  leukemia, monocytic C93.1-●
Naegleriasis (with meningoencephalitis)
    B60.2
Naffziger's syndrome G54.0
Naga sore —see Ulcer, skin
Nägele's pelvis M95.5
  with disproportion (fetopelvic) O33.0
    causing obstructed labor O65.0
Nail —see also condition
  biting F98.8
  patella syndrome Q87.2
Nanism, nanosomia —see Dwarfism
Nanophyetiasis B66.8
Nanukayami A27.89
Napkin rash L22
Narcolepsy G47.419
  with cataplexy G47.411
  in conditions classified elsewhere
      G47.429
    with cataplexy G47.421
Narcosis R06.89
Narcotism —see Dependence
NARP (Neuropathy, Ataxia and Retinitis
    pigmentosa) syndrome E88.49
Narrow
  anterior chamber angle H40.03-●
  gingival width (of periodontal soft tissue)
      K05.5
  pelvis —see Contraction, pelvis
Narrowing —see also Stenosis
  artery I77.1
    auditory, internal I65.8
    basilar —see Occlusion, artery, basilar
    carotid —see Occlusion, artery, carotid
    cerebellar —see Occlusion, artery, cerebellar
    cerebral —see Occlusion artery, cerebral
    choroidal —see Occlusion, artery, cerebral,
        specified NEC
    communicating posterior —see Occlusion,
        artery, cerebral, specified NEC
    coronary —see also Disease, heart, ischemic,
        atherosclerotic
      congenital Q24.5
        syphilitic A50.54 [I52]
        due to syphilis NEC A52.06
    hypophyseal —see Occlusion, artery,
        cerebral, specified NEC
    pontine —see Occlusion, artery, cerebral,
        specified NEC
    precerebral —see Occlusion, artery,
        precerebral
    vertebral —see Occlusion, artery, vertebral
  auditory canal (external) —see Stenosis,
      external ear canal
  eustachian tube —see Obstruction, eustachian
      tube
  eyelid —see Disorder, eyelid function
  larynx J38.6
  mesenteric artery —see also Ischemia,
      intestine, acute K55.059
  palate M26.89
  palpebral fissure —see Disorder, eyelid
      function
  ureter N13.5
    with infection N13.6
  urethra —see Stricture, urethra
Narrowness, abnormal, eyelid Q10.3
Nasal —see condition
Nasolachrymal, nasolacrimal —see condition
Nasopharyngeal —see also condition
  pituitary gland Q89.2
  torticollis M43.6
Nasopharyngitis (acute) (infective)
    (streptococcal) (subacute) J00
  chronic (suppurative) (ulcerative) J31.1
Nasopharynx, nasopharyngeal —see condition
Natal tooth, teeth K00.6

Nausea (without vomiting) R11.0
  with vomiting R11.2
  gravidarum —see Hyperemesis, gravidarum
  marina T75.3
  navalis T75.3
Navel —see condition
Neapolitan fever —see Brucellosis
Near drowning T75.1
Nearsightedness —see Myopia
Near-syncope R55
Nebula, cornea —see Opacity, cornea
Necator americanus infestation B76.1
Necatoriasis B76.1
Neck —see condition
Necrobiosis R68.89
  lipoidica NEC L92.1
    with diabetes —see E08-E13 with .620
Necrolysis, toxic epidermal L51.2
  due to drug
    correct substance properly administered —
        see Table of Drugs and Chemicals, by
        drug, adverse effect
    overdose or wrong substance given
        or taken —see Table of Drugs and
        Chemicals, by drug, poisoning
Necrophilia F65.89
Necrosis, necrotic (ischemic) —see also
    Gangrene
  adrenal (capsule) (gland) E27.49
  amputation stump (surgical) (late) T87.50
    arm T87.5-●
    leg T87.5-●
  antrum J32.0
  aorta (hyaline) —see also Aneurysm, aorta
    cystic medial —see Dissection, aorta
  artery I77.5
  bladder (aseptic) (sphincter) N32.89
  bone —see also Osteonecrosis M87.9
    aseptic or avascular —see Osteonecrosis
      idiopathic M87.00
    ethmoid J32.2
    jaw M27.2
    tuberculous —see Tuberculosis, bone
  brain I67.89
  breast (aseptic) (fat) (segmental) N64.1
  bronchus J98.09
  central nervous system NEC I67.89
  cerebellar I67.89
  cerebral I67.89
  colon —see also Infarct, intestine K55.049
  cornea H18.89-●
  cortical (acute) (renal) N17.1
  cystic medial (aorta) —see Dissection, aorta
  dental pulp K04.1
  esophagus K22.8
  ethmoid (bone) J32.2
  eyelid —see Disorder, eyelid, degenerative
  fat, fatty (generalized) —see also Disorder, soft
      tissue, specified type NEC
    abdominal wall K65.4
    breast (aseptic) (segmental) N64.1
    localized —see Degeneration, by site, fatty
    mesentery K65.4
    omentum K65.4
    pancreas K86.89
    peritoneum K65.4
    skin (subcutaneous), newborn P83.0
    subcutaneous, due to birth injury P15.6
  gallbladder —see Cholecystitis, acute
  heart —see Infarct, myocardium
  hip, aseptic or avascular —see Osteonecrosis,
      by type, femur
  intestine (acute) (hemorrhagic) (massive) —
      see also Infarct, intestine K55.069
  jaw M27.2
  kidney (bilateral) N28.0
    acute N17.9
    cortical (acute) (bilateral) N17.1
      with ectopic or molar pregnancy O08.4
    medullary (bilateral) (in acute renal failure)
        (papillary) N17.2

Necrosis, necrotic (Continued)
  kidney (Continued)
    papillary (bilateral) (in acute renal
        failure) N17.2
    tubular N17.0
      with ectopic or molar pregnancy
          O08.4
      complicating
        abortion —see Abortion, by type,
            complicated by, tubular necrosis
        ectopic or molar pregnancy O08.4
        pregnancy —see Pregnancy,
            complicated by, diseases of,
            specified type or system NEC
      following ectopic or molar pregnancy
          O08.4
  traumatic T79.5
  larynx J38.7
  liver (with hepatic failure) (cell) —see Failure,
      hepatic
    hemorrhagic, central K76.2
  lung J85.0
  lymphatic gland —see Lymphadenitis, acute
  mammary gland (fat) (segmental) N64.1
  mastoid (chronic) —see Mastoiditis, chronic
  medullary (acute) (renal) N17.2
  mesentery —see also Infarct, intestine
      K55.069
    fat K65.4
  mitral valve —see Insufficiency, mitral
  myocardium, myocardial —see Infarct,
      myocardium
  nose J34.0
  omentum (with mesenteric infarction) —see
      also Infarct, intestine K55.069
    fat K65.4
  orbit, orbital —see Osteomyelitis, orbit
  ossicles, ear —see Abnormal, ear ossicles
  ovary N70.92
  pancreas (aseptic) (duct) (fat) K86.89
    acute (infective) —see Pancreatitis, acute
    infective —see Pancreatitis, acute
  papillary (acute) (renal) N17.2
  perineum N90.89
  peritoneum (with mesenteric infarction) —see
      also Infarct, intestine K55.069
    fat K65.4
  pharynx J02.9
    in granulocytopenia —see Neutropenia
    Vincent's A69.1
  phosphorus —see subcategory T54.2
  pituitary (gland) E23.0
    postpartum O99.285
    Sheehan O99.285
  pressure —see Ulcer, pressure, by site
  pulmonary J85.0
  pulp (dental) K04.1
  radiation —see Necrosis, by site
  radium —see Necrosis, by site
  renal —see Necrosis, kidney
  sclera H15.89
  scrotum N50.89
  skin or subcutaneous tissue NEC I96
  spine, spinal (column) —see also
      Osteonecrosis, by type, vertebra
    cord G95.19
  spleen D73.5
  stomach K31.89
  stomatitis (ulcerative) A69.0
➡subcutaneous fat, newborn P83.88
  subendocardial (acute) I21.4
    chronic I25.89
  suprarenal (capsule) (gland) E27.49
  testis N50.89
  thymus (gland) E32.8
  tonsil J35.8
  trachea J39.8
  tuberculous NEC —see Tuberculosis
  tubular (acute) (anoxic) (renal) (toxic)
      N17.0
    postprocedural N99.0

Necrosis, necrotic (Continued)
  vagina N89.8
  vertebra —see also Osteonecrosis, by type,
      vertebra
    tuberculous A18.01
  vulva N90.89
  X-ray —see Necrosis, by site
Necrospermia —see Infertility, male
Need (for)
  care provider because (of)
    assistance with personal care Z74.1
    continuous supervision required Z74.3
    impaired mobility Z74.09
    no other household member able to render
        care Z74.2
    specified reason NEC Z74.8
  immunization —see Vaccination
  vaccination —see Vaccination
Neglect
  adult
    confirmed T74.01
    history of Z91.412
    suspected T76.01
  child (childhood)
    confirmed T74.02
    history of Z62.812
    suspected T76.02
  emotional, in childhood Z62.898
  hemispatial R41.4
  left-sided R41.4
  sensory R41.4
  visuospatial R41.4
Neisserian infection NEC —see Gonococcus
Nelaton's syndrome G60.8
Nelson's syndrome E24.1
Nematodiasis (intestinal) B82.0
  Ancylostoma B76.0
Neonatal —see also Newborn
  acne L70.4
  bradycardia P29.12
  screening, abnormal findings on P09
  tachycardia P29.11
  tooth, teeth K00.6
Neonatorum —see condition
Neoplasia
  endocrine, multiple (MEN) E31.20
    type I E31.21
    type IIA E31.22
    type IIB E31.23
  intraepithelial (histologically confirmed)
    anal (AIN) (histologically confirmed)
        K62.82
      grade I K62.82
      grade II K62.82
      severe D01.3
    cervical glandular (histologically
        confirmed) D06.9
    cervix (uteri) (CIN) (histologically
        confirmed) N87.9
      glandular D06.9
      grade I N87.0
      grade II N87.1
      grade III (severe dysplasia) —see also
          Carcinoma, cervix uteri, in situ
          D06.9
    prostate (histologically confirmed) (PIN)
        N42.31
      grade I N42.31
      grade II N42.31
      grade III (severe dysplasia) D07.5
    vagina (histologically confirmed) (VAIN)
        N89.3
      grade I N89.0
      grade II N89.1
      grade III (severe dysplasia) D07.2
    vulva (histologically confirmed) (VIN)
        N90.3
      grade I N90.0
      grade II N90.1
      grade III (severe dysplasia)
          D07.1

Neoplasm, neoplastic —see also Table of
    Neoplasms
  lipomatous, benign —see Lipoma
▶malignant mast cell C96.20
    ▶specified type NEC C96.29
▶mast cell, of uncertain behavior NEC D47.09
Neovascularization
  ciliary body —see Disorder, iris, vascular
  cornea H16.40-●
    deep H16.44-●
    ghost vessels —see Ghost, vessels
    localized H16.43-●
    pannus —see Pannus
  iris —see Disorder, iris, vascular
  retina H35.05-●
Nephralgia N23
Nephritis, nephritic (albuminuric) (azotemic)
    (congenital) (disseminated) (epithelial)
    (familial) (focal) (granulomatous)
    (hemorrhagic) (infantile) (nonsuppurative,
    excretory) (uremic) N05.9
  with
    dense deposit disease N05.6
    diffuse
      crescentic glomerulonephritis N05.7
      endocapillary proliferative
          glomerulonephritis N05.4
      membranous glomerulonephritis N05.2
      mesangial proliferative
          glomerulonephritis N05.3
      mesangiocapillary glomerulonephritis
          N05.5
    edema —see Nephrosis
    focal and segmental glomerular lesions
        N05.1
    foot process disease N04.9
    glomerular lesion
      diffuse sclerosing N05.8
      hypocomplementemic —see Nephritis,
          membranoproliferative
      IgA —see Nephropathy, IgA
      lobular, lobulonodular —see Nephritis,
          membranoproliferative
      nodular —see Nephritis,
          membranoproliferative
    lesion of
      glomerulonephritis, proliferative N05.8
      renal necrosis N05.9
    minor glomerular abnormality N05.0
    specified morphological changes NEC
        N05.8
  acute N00.9
    with
      dense deposit disease N00.6
      diffuse
        crescentic glomerulonephritis
            N00.7
        endocapillary proliferative
            glomerulonephritis N00.4
        membranous glomerulonephritis
            N00.2
        mesangial proliferative
            glomerulonephritis N00.3
        mesangiocapillary glomerulonephritis
            N00.5
      focal and segmental glomerular lesions
          N00.1
      minor glomerular abnormality N00.0
      specified morphological changes NEC
          N00.8
  amyloid E85.4 [N08]
  antiglomerular basement membrane (anti-
      GBM) antibody NEC
    in Goodpasture's syndrome M31.0
  antitubular basement membrane (tubulo-
      interstitial) NEC N12
    toxic —see Nephropathy, toxic
  arteriolar —see Hypertension, kidney
  arteriosclerotic —see Hypertension, kidney
  ascending —see Nephritis, tubulo-interstitial
  atrophic N03.9

Nephritis, nephritic (Continued)
  Balkan (endemic) N15.0
  calculous, calculus —see Calculus,
      kidney
  cardiac —see Hypertension, kidney
  cardiovascular —see Hypertension,
      kidney
  chronic N03.9
    with
      dense deposit disease N03.6
      diffuse
        crescentic glomerulonephritis
            N03.7
        endocapillary proliferative
            glomerulonephritis N03.4
        membranous glomerulonephritis
            N03.2
        mesangial proliferative
            glomerulonephritis N03.3
        mesangiocapillary glomerulonephritis
            N03.5
      focal and segmental glomerular lesions
          N03.1
      minor glomerular abnormality
          N03.0
      specified morphological changes
          NEC N03.8
    arteriosclerotic —see Hypertension,
        kidney
  cirrhotic N26.9
  complicating pregnancy O26.83-●
  croupous N00.9
  degenerative —see Nephrosis
  diffuse sclerosing N05.8
  due to
    diabetes mellitus —see E08-E13 with .21
    subacute bacterial endocarditis I33.0
    systemic lupus erythematosus (chronic)
        M32.14
    typhoid fever A01.09
  gonococcal (acute) (chronic) A54.21
  hypocomplementemic —see Nephritis,
      membranoproliferative
  IgA —see Nephropathy, IgA
  immune complex (circulating) NEC N05.8
  infective —see Nephritis, tubulo-interstitial
  interstitial —see Nephritis, tubulo-interstitial
  lead N14.3
  membranoproliferative (diffuse) (type 1
      or 3) —see also N00-N07 with fourth
      character .5 N05.5
    type 2 —see also N00-N07 with fourth
        character .6 N05.6
  minimal change N05.0
  necrotic, necrotizing NEC —see also
      N00-N07 with fourth character .8
      N05.8
  nephrotic —see Nephrosis
  nodular —see Nephritis,
      membranoproliferative
  polycystic Q61.3
    adult type Q61.2
    autosomal
      dominant Q61.2
      recessive NEC Q61.19
    childhood type NEC Q61.19
    infantile type NEC Q61.19
  poststreptococcal N05.9
    acute N00.9
    chronic N03.9
    rapidly progressive N01.9
  proliferative NEC —see also N00-N07 with
      fourth character .8 N05.8
  purulent —see Nephritis, tubulo-interstitial
  rapidly progressive N01.9
    with
      dense deposit disease N01.6
      diffuse
        crescentic glomerulonephritis N01.7
        endocapillary proliferative
            glomerulonephritis N01.4

Nephritis, nephritic (*Continued*)
  rapidly progressive (*Continued*)
    with (*Continued*)
      diffuse (*Continued*)
        membranous glomerulonephritis
          N01.2
        mesangial proliferative
          glomerulonephritis N01.3
        mesangiocapillary glomerulonephritis
          N01.5
        focal and segmental glomerular lesions
          N01.1
        minor glomerular abnormality N01.0
        specified morphological changes NEC
          N01.8
  salt losing or wasting NEC N28.89
  saturnine N14.3
  sclerosing, diffuse N05.8
  septic —*see* Nephritis, tubulo-interstitial
  specified pathology NEC —*see also* N00-N07
    with fourth character .8 N05.8
  subacute N01.9
  suppurative —*see* Nephritis,
    tubulo-interstitial
  syphilitic (late) A52.75
    congenital A50.59 [N08]
    early (secondary) A51.44
  toxic —*see* Nephropathy, toxic
  tubal, tubular —*see* Nephritis,
    tubulo-interstitial
  tuberculous A18.11
  tubulo-interstitial (in) N12
    acute (infectious) N10
    chronic (infectious) N11.9
      nonobstructive N11.8
        reflux-associated N11.0
      obstructive N11.1
      specified NEC N11.8
    due to
      brucellosis A23.9 [N16]
      cryoglobulinemia D89.1 [N16]
      glycogen storage disease E74.00
        [N16]
      Sjögren's syndrome M35.04
  vascular —*see* Hypertension, kidney
  war N00.9
Nephroblastoma (epithelial) (mesenchymal)
  C64-●
Nephrocalcinosis E83.59 [N29]
Nephrocystitis, pustular —*see* Nephritis,
  tubulo-interstitial
Nephrolithiasis (congenital) (pelvis)
  (recurrent) —*see also* Calculus, kidney
Nephroma C64-●
  mesoblastic D41.0-●
Nephronephritis —*see* Nephrosis
Nephronophthisis Q61.5
Nephropathia epidemica A98.5
Nephropathy —*see also* Nephritis N28.9
  with
    edema —*see* Nephrosis
    glomerular lesion —*see*
      Glomerulonephritis
  amyloid, hereditary E85.0
  analgesic N14.0
    with medullary necrosis, acute N17.2
  Balkan (endemic) N15.0
  chemical —*see* Nephropathy, toxic
  diabetic —*see* E08-E13 with .21
  drug-induced N14.2
    specified NEC N14.1
  focal and segmental hyalinosis or sclerosis
    N02.1
  heavy metal-induced N14.3
  hereditary NEC N07.9
    with
      dense deposit disease N07.6
      diffuse
        crescentic glomerulonephritis N07.7
        endocapillary proliferative
          glomerulonephritis N07.4

Nephropathy (*Continued*)
  hereditary NEC (*Continued*)
    with (*Continued*)
      diffuse (*Continued*)
        membranous glomerulonephritis
          N07.2
        mesangial proliferative
          glomerulonephritis N07.3
        mesangiocapillary glomerulonephritis
          N07.5
        focal and segmental glomerular lesions
          N07.1
        minor glomerular abnormality N07.0
        specified morphological changes NEC
          N07.8
  hypercalcemic N25.89
  hypertensive —*see* Hypertension, kidney
  hypokalemic (vacuolar) N25.89
  IgA N02.8
    with glomerular lesion N02.9
      focal and segmental hyalinosis or
        sclerosis N02.1
      membranoproliferative (diffuse) N02.5
      membranous (diffuse) N02.2
      mesangial proliferative (diffuse) N02.3
      mesangiocapillary (diffuse) N02.5
      proliferative NEC N02.8
      specified pathology NEC N02.8
  lead N14.3
  membranoproliferative (diffuse) N02.5
  membranous (diffuse) N02.2
  mesangial (IgA/IgG) —*see* Nephropathy, IgA
    proliferative (diffuse) N02.3
  mesangiocapillary (diffuse) N02.5
  obstructive N13.8
  phenacetin N17.2
  phosphate-losing N25.0
  potassium depletion N25.89
  pregnancy-related O26.83-●
  proliferative NEC (*see also* N00-N07 with
    fourth character .8) N05.8
  protein-losing N25.89
  saturnine N14.3
  sickle-cell D57.-● [N08]
  toxic NEC N14.4
    due to
      drugs N14.2
        analgesic N14.0
        specified NEC N14.1
      heavy metals N14.3
  vasomotor N17.0
  water-losing N25.89
Nephroptosis N28.83
Nephropyosis —*see* Abscess, kidney
Nephrorrhagia N28.89
Nephrosclerosis (arteriolar) (arteriosclerotic)
  (chronic) (hyaline) —*see also* Hypertension,
  kidney
  hyperplastic —*see* Hypertension, kidney
  senile N26.9
Nephrosis, nephrotic (Epstein's) (syndrome)
  (congenital) N04.9
  with
    foot process disease N04.9
    glomerular lesion N04.1
    hypocomplementemic N04.5
  acute N04.9
  anoxic —*see* Nephrosis, tubular
  chemical —*see* Nephrosis, tubular
  cholemic K76.7
  diabetic —*see* E08-E13 with .21
  Finnish type (congenital) Q89.8
  hemoglobin N10
  hemoglobinuric —*see* Nephrosis, tubular
  in
    amyloidosis E85.4 [N08]
    diabetes mellitus —*see* E08-E13 with .21
    epidemic hemorrhagic fever A98.5
    malaria (malariae) B52.0
  ischemic —*see* Nephrosis, tubular
  lipoid N04.9

Nephrosis, nephrotic (*Continued*)
  lower nephron —*see* Nephrosis, tubular
  malarial (malariae) B52.0
  minimal change N04.0
  myoglobin N10
  necrotizing —*see* Nephrosis, tubular
  osmotic (sucrose) N25.89
  radiation N04.9
  syphilitic (late) A52.75
  toxic —*see* Nephrosis, tubular
  tubular (acute) N17.0
    postprocedural N99.0
    radiation N04.9
Nephrosonephritis, hemorrhagic (endemic)
  A98.5
Nephrostomy
  attention to Z43.6
  status Z93.6
Nerve —*see also* condition
  injury —*see* Injury, nerve, by body site
Nerves R45.0
Nervous —*see also* condition R45.0
  heart F45.8
  stomach F45.8
  tension R45.0
Nervousness R45.0
Nesidioblastoma
  pancreas D13.7
  specified site NEC —*see* Neoplasm, benign,
    by site
  unspecified site D13.7
⇒ **Nettleship's syndrome** —*see* Urticaria
  pigmentosa
Neumann's disease or syndrome L10.1
Neuralgia, neuralgic (acute) M79.2
  accessory (nerve) G52.8
  acoustic (nerve) —*see* subcategory H93.3
  auditory (nerve) —*see* subcategory H93.3
  ciliary G44.009
    intractable G44.001
    not intractable G44.009
  cranial
    nerve —*see also* Disorder, nerve, cranial
      fifth or trigeminal —*see* Neuralgia,
        trigeminal
    postherpetic, postzoster B02.29
  ear —*see* subcategory H92.0
  facialis vera G51.1
  Fothergill's —*see* Neuralgia, trigeminal
  glossopharyngeal (nerve) G52.1
  Horton's G44.099
    intractable G44.091
    not intractable G44.099
  Hunt's B02.21
  hypoglossal (nerve) G52.3
  infraorbital —*see* Neuralgia, trigeminal
  malarial —*see* Malaria
  migrainous G44.009
    intractable G44.001
    not intractable G44.009
  Morton's G57.6-●
  nerve, cranial —*see* Disorder, nerve, cranial
  nose G52.0
  occipital M54.81
  olfactory G52.0
  penis N48.9
  perineum R10.2
  postherpetic NEC B02.29
    trigeminal B02.22
  pubic region R10.2
  scrotum R10.2
  Sluder's G44.89
  specified nerve NEC G58.8
  spermatic cord R10.2
  sphenopalatine (ganglion) G90.09
  trifacial —*see* Neuralgia, trigeminal
  trigeminal G50.0
    postherpetic, postzoster B02.22
  vagus (nerve) G52.2
  writer's F48.8
    organic G25.89

Neurapraxia —see Injury, nerve
Neurasthenia F48.8
  cardiac F45.8
  gastric F45.8
  heart F45.8
Neurilemmoma —see also Neoplasm, nerve,
    benign
  acoustic (nerve) D33.3
  malignant —see also Neoplasm, nerve,
      malignant
    acoustic (nerve) C72.4
Neurilemmosarcoma —see Neoplasm, nerve,
    malignant
Neurinoma —see Neoplasm, nerve, benign
Neurinomatosis —see Neoplasm, nerve,
    uncertain behavior
Neuritis (rheumatoid) M79.2
  abducens (nerve) —see Strabismus, paralytic,
      sixth nerve
  accessory (nerve) G52.8
  acoustic (nerve) —see also subcategory H93.3
    in (due to)
      infectious disease NEC B99 [H94.0-●]
      parasitic disease NEC B89 [H94.0-●]
      syphilitic A52.15
  alcoholic G62.1
    with psychosis —see Psychosis, alcoholic
  amyloid, any site E85.4 [G63]
  auditory (nerve) —see also subcategory H93.3
  brachial —see Radiculopathy
    due to displacement, intervertebral
        disc —see Disorder, disc, cervical, with
        neuritis
  cranial nerve
    due to Lyme disease A69.22
    eighth or acoustic or auditory —see
        subcategory H93.3
    eleventh or accessory G52.8
    fifth or trigeminal G51.0
    first or olfactory G52.0
    fourth or trochlear —see Strabismus,
        paralytic, fourth nerve
    second or optic —see Neuritis, optic
    seventh or facial G51.8
      newborn (birth injury) P11.3
    sixth or abducent —see Strabismus,
        paralytic, sixth nerve
    tenth or vagus G52.2
    third or oculomotor —see Strabismus,
        paralytic, third nerve
    twelfth or hypoglossal G52.3
  Déjérine-Sottas G60.0
  diabetic (mononeuropathy) —see E08-E13
      with .41
    polyneuropathy —see E08-E13 with .42
  due to
    beriberi E51.11
    displacement, prolapse or rupture,
        intervertebral disc —see Disorder, disc,
        with, radiculopathy
    herniation, nucleus pulposus M51.9 [G55]
  endemic E51.11
  facial G51.8
    newborn (birth injury) P11.3
  general —see Polyneuropathy
  geniculate ganglion G51.1
    due to herpes (zoster) B02.21
  gouty —see also Gout, by type M10.9 [G63]
  hypoglossal (nerve) G52.3
  ilioinguinal (nerve) G57.9-●
  infectious (multiple) NEC G61.0
  interstitial hypertrophic progressive G60.0
  lumbar M54.16
  lumbosacral M54.17
  multiple —see also Polyneuropathy
    endemic E51.11
    infective, acute G61.0
  multiplex endemica E51.11
  nerve root —see Radiculopathy
  oculomotor (nerve) —see Strabismus,
      paralytic, third nerve

Neuritis (Continued)
  olfactory nerve G52.0
  optic (nerve) (hereditary) (sympathetic) H46.9
    with demyelination G36.0
    in myelitis G36.0
    nutritional H46.2
    papillitis —see Papillitis, optic
    retrobulbar H46.1-●
    specified type NEC H46.8
    toxic H46.3
  peripheral (nerve) G62.9
    multiple —see Polyneuropathy
    single —see Mononeuritis
  pneumogastric (nerve) G52.2
  postherpetic, postzoster B02.29
  progressive hypertrophic interstitial G60.0
  retrobulbar —see also Neuritis, optic,
      retrobulbar
    in (due to)
      late syphilis A52.15
      meningococcal infection A39.82
    meningococcal A39.82
    syphilitic A52.15
  sciatic (nerve) —see also Sciatica
    due to displacement of intervertebral
        disc —see Disorder, disc, with,
        radiculopathy
  serum —see also Reaction, serum T80.69
  shoulder-girdle G54.5
  specified nerve NEC G58.8
  spinal (nerve) root —see Radiculopathy
  syphilitic A52.15
  thenar (median) G56.1-●
  thoracic M54.14
  toxic NEC G62.2
  trochlear (nerve) —see Strabismus, paralytic,
      fourth nerve
  vagus (nerve) G52.2
Neuroastrocytoma —see Neoplasm, uncertain
    behavior, by site
Neuroavitaminosis E56.9 [G99.8]
Neuroblastoma
  olfactory C30.0
  specified site —see Neoplasm, malignant, by
      site
  unspecified site C74.90
Neurochorioretinitis —see Chorioretinitis
Neurocirculatory asthenia F45.8
Neurocysticercosis B69.0
Neurocytoma —see Neoplasm, benign, by site
Neurodermatitis (circumscribed)
    (circumscripta) (local) L28.0
  atopic L20.81
  diffuse (Brocq) L20.81
  disseminated L20.81
Neuroencephalomyelopathy, optic G36.0
Neuroepithelioma —see also Neoplasm,
    malignant, by site
  olfactory C30.0
Neurofibroma —see also Neoplasm, nerve,
    benign
  melanotic —see Neoplasm, nerve, benign
  multiple —see Neurofibromatosis
  plexiform —see Neoplasm, nerve, benign
Neurofibromatosis (multiple) (nonmalignant)
    Q85.00
  acoustic Q85.02
  malignant —see Neoplasm, nerve, malignant
  specified NEC Q85.09
  type 1 (von Recklinghausen) Q85.01
  type 2 Q85.02
Neurofibrosarcoma —see Neoplasm, nerve,
    malignant
Neurogenic —see also condition
  bladder (see also Dysfunction, bladder,
      neuromuscular) N31.9
    cauda equina syndrome G83.4
  bowel NEC K59.2
  heart F45.8
Neuroglioma —see Neoplasm, uncertain
    behavior, by site

Neurolabyrinthitis (of Dix and Hallpike) —see
    Neuronitis, vestibular
Neurolathyrism —see Poisoning, food, noxious,
    plant
Neuroleprosy A30.9
Neuroma —see also Neoplasm, nerve, benign
  acoustic (nerve) D33.3
  amputation (stump) (traumatic) (surgical
      complication) (late) T87.3-●
    arm T87.3-●
    leg T87.3-●
  digital (toe) G57.6-●
  interdigital G58.8
    lower limb toe G57.8-●
    upper limb G56.8-●
  intermetatarsal G57.8-●
  Morton's G57.6-●
  nonneoplastic
    arm G56.9-●
    leg G57.9-●
    lower extremity G57.9-●
    upper extremity G56.9-●
  optic (nerve) D33.3
  plantar G57.6-●
  plexiform —see Neoplasm, nerve,
      benign
  surgical (nonneoplastic)
    arm G56.9-●
    leg G57.9-●
    lower extremity G57.9-●
    upper extremity G56.9-●
Neuromyalgia —see Neuralgia
Neuromyasthenia (epidemic) (postinfectious)
    G93.3
Neuromyelitis G36.9
  ascending G61.0
  optica G36.0
Neuromyopathy G70.9
  paraneoplastic D49.9 [G13.0]
Neuromyotonia (Isaacs) G71.19
Neuronevus —see Nevus
Neuronitis G58.9
  ascending (acute) G57.2-●
  vestibular H81.2-●
Neuroparalytic —see condition
Neuropathy, neuropathic G62.9
  acute motor G62.81
  alcoholic G62.1
    with psychosis —see Psychosis, alcoholic
  arm G56.9-●
  autonomic, peripheral —see Neuropathy,
      peripheral, autonomic
  axillary G56.9-●
  bladder N31.9
    atonic (motor) (sensory) N31.2
    autonomous N31.2
    flaccid N31.2
    nonreflex N31.2
    reflex N31.1
    uninhibited N31.0
  brachial plexus G54.0
  cervical plexus G54.2
  chronic
    progressive segmentally demyelinating
        G62.89
    relapsing demyelinating G62.89
  Déjérine-Sottas G60.0
  diabetic —see E08-E13 with .40
    mononeuropathy —see E08-E13 with .41
    polyneuropathy —see E08-E13 with .42
  entrapment G58.9
    iliohypogastric nerve G57.8-●
    ilioinguinal nerve G57.8-●
    lateral cutaneous nerve of thigh
        G57.1-●
    median nerve G56.0-●
    obturator nerve G57.8-●
    peroneal nerve G57.3-●
    posterior tibial nerve G57.5-●
    saphenous nerve G57.8-●
    ulnar nerve G56.2-●

▶ New   ⮕ Revised   ~~deleted~~ Deleted   ● Use Additional Character(s)

Neuropathy, neuropathic *(Continued)*
facial nerve G51.9
hereditary G60.9
   motor and sensory (types I-IV) G60.0
   sensory G60.8
   specified NEC G60.8
hypertrophic G60.0
   Charcot-Marie-Tooth G60.0
   Déjérine-Sottas G60.0
   interstitial progressive G60.0
   of infancy G60.0
   Refsum G60.1
idiopathic G60.9
   progressive G60.3
   specified NEC G60.8
in association with hereditary ataxia G60.2
intercostal G58.0
ischemic —*see* Disorder, nerve
Jamaica (ginger) G62.2
leg NEC G57.9-●
lower extremity G57.9-●
lumbar plexus G54.1
median nerve G56.1-●
motor and sensory —*see also* Polyneuropathy
   hereditary (types I-IV) G60.0
multifocal motor (MMN) G61.82
multiple (acute) (chronic) —*see*
   Polyneuropathy
optic (nerve) —*see also* Neuritis, optic
   ischemic H47.01-●
paraneoplastic (sensorial) (Denny Brown)
   D49.9 *[G13.0]*
peripheral (nerve) —*see also* Polyneuropathy
   G62.9
   autonomic G90.9
      idiopathic G90.09
      in (due to)
         amyloidosis E85.4 *[G99.0]*
         diabetes mellitus —*see* E08-E13 with
            .43
         endocrine disease NEC E34.9 *[G99.0]*
         gout M10.00 *[G99.0]*
         hyperthyroidism E05.90 *[G99.0]*
           with thyroid storm E05.91 *[G99.0]*
         metabolic disease NEC E88.9 *[G99.0]*
   idiopathic G60.9
   progressive G60.3
   in (due to)
      antitetanus serum G62.0
      arsenic G62.2
      drugs NEC G62.0
      lead G62.2
      organophosphate compounds G62.2
      toxic agent NEC G62.2
plantar nerves G57.6-●
progressive
   hypertrophic interstitial G60.0
   inflammatory G62.81
radicular NEC —*see* Radiculopathy
sacral plexus G54.1
sciatic G57.0-●
serum G61.1
toxic NEC G62.2
trigeminal sensory G50.8
ulnar nerve G56.2-●
uremic N18.9 *[G63]*
vitamin B12 E53.8 *[G63]*
   with anemia (pernicious) D51.0 *[G63]*
      due to dietary deficiency D51.3 *[G63]*
Neurophthisis —*see also* Disorder, nerve
peripheral, diabetic —*see* E08-E13 with .42
Neuroretinitis —*see* Chorioretinitis
Neuroretinopathy, hereditary optic H47.22
Neurosarcoma —*see* Neoplasm, nerve, malignant
Neurosclerosis —*see* Disorder, nerve
Neurosis, neurotic F48.9
anankastic F42.8
anxiety (state) F41.1
   panic type F41.0
asthenic F48.8
bladder F45.8

Neurosis, neurotic *(Continued)*
cardiac (reflex) F45.8
cardiovascular F45.8
character F60.9
colon F45.8
compensation F68.1
compulsive, compulsion F42.8
conversion F44.9
craft F48.8
cutaneous F45.8
depersonalization F48.1
depressive (reaction) (type) F34.1
environmental F48.8
excoriation L98.1
fatigue F48.8
functional —*see* Disorder, somatoform
gastric F45.8
gastrointestinal F45.8
heart F45.8
hypochondriacal F45.21
hysterical F44.9
incoordination F45.8
   larynx F45.8
   vocal cord F45.8
intestine F45.8
larynx (sensory) F45.8
   hysterical F44.4
mixed NEC F48.8
musculoskeletal F45.8
obsessional F42.8
obsessive-compulsive F42.8
occupational F48.8
ocular NEC F45.8
organ —*see* Disorder, somatoform
pharynx F45.8
phobic F40.9
posttraumatic (situational) F43.10
   acute F43.11
   chronic F43.12
psychasthenic (type) F48.8
railroad F48.8
rectum F45.8
respiratory F45.8
rumination F45.8
sexual F65.9
situational F48.8
social F40.10
   generalized F40.11
specified type NEC F48.8
state F48.9
   with depersonalization episode F48.1
stomach F45.8
traumatic F43.10
   acute F43.11
   chronic F43.12
vasomotor F45.8
visceral F45.8
war F48.8
Neurospongioblastosis diffusa Q85.1
Neurosyphilis (arrested) (early) (gumma) (late)
   (latent) (recurrent) (relapse) A52.3
with ataxia (cerebellar) (locomotor) (spastic)
   (spinal) A52.19
aneurysm (cerebral) A52.05
arachnoid (adhesive) A52.13
arteritis (any artery) (cerebral) A52.04
asymptomatic A52.2
congenital A50.40
dura (mater) A52.13
general paresis A52.17
hemorrhagic A52.05
juvenile (asymptomatic) (meningeal)
   A50.40
leptomeninges (aseptic) A52.13
meningeal, meninges (adhesive) A52.13
meningitis A52.13
meningovascular (diffuse) A52.13
optic atrophy A52.15
parenchymatous (degenerative) A52.19
paresis, paretic A52.17
   juvenile A50.45

Neurosyphilis *(Continued)*
remission in (sustained) A52.3
serological (without symptoms) A52.2
specified nature or site NEC A52.19
tabes, tabetic (dorsalis) A52.11
   juvenile A50.45
taboparesis A52.17
   juvenile A50.45
thrombosis (cerebral) A52.05
vascular (cerebral) NEC A52.05
Neurothekeoma —*see* Neoplasm, nerve, benign
Neurotic —*see* Neurosis
Neurotoxemia —*see* Toxemia
Neutroclusion M26.211
Neutropenia, neutropenic (chronic) (genetic)
   (idiopathic) (immune) (infantile)
   (malignant) (pernicious) (splenic) D70.9
congenital (primary) D70.0
cyclic D70.4
cytoreductive cancer chemotherapy sequela
   D70.1
drug-induced D70.2
   due to cytoreductive cancer chemotherapy
      D70.1
due to infection D70.3
fever D70.9
neonatal, transitory (isoimmune) (maternal
   transfer) P61.5
periodic D70.4
secondary (cyclic) (periodic) (splenic) D70.4
   drug-induced D70.2
      due to cytoreductive cancer
         chemotherapy D70.1
toxic D70.8
Neutrophilia, hereditary giant D72.0
Nevocarcinoma —*see* Melanoma
Nevus D22.9
achromic —*see* Neoplasm, skin, benign
amelanotic —*see* Neoplasm, skin, benign
angiomatous D18.00
   intra-abdominal D18.03
   intracranial D18.02
   skin D18.01
   specified site NEC D18.09
araneus I78.1
balloon cell —*see* Neoplasm, skin, benign
bathing trunk D48.5
blue —*see* Neoplasm, skin, benign
   cellular —*see* Neoplasm, skin, benign
   giant —*see* Neoplasm, skin, benign
   Jadassohn's —*see* Neoplasm, skin, benign
   malignant —*see* Melanoma
capillary D18.00
   intra-abdominal D18.03
   intracranial D18.02
   skin D18.01
   specified site NEC D18.09
cavernous D18.00
   intra-abdominal D18.03
   intracranial D18.02
   skin D18.01
   specified site NEC D18.09
cellular —*see* Neoplasm, skin, benign
   blue —*see* Neoplasm, skin, benign
choroid D31.3-●
comedonicus Q82.5
conjunctiva D31.0-●
dermal —*see* Neoplasm, skin, benign
   with epidermal nevus —*see* Neoplasm,
      skin, benign
dysplastic —*see* Neoplasm, skin, benign
eye D31.9-●
flammeus Q82.5
hemangiomatous D18.00
   intra-abdominal D18.03
   intracranial D18.02
   skin D18.01
   specified site NEC D18.09
iris D31.4-●
lacrimal gland D31.5-●
lymphatic D18.1

Nevus *(Continued)*
  magnocellular
    specified site —*see* Neoplasm, benign, by
      site
    unspecified site D31.40
  malignant —*see* Melanoma
  meaning hemangioma D18.00
    intra-abdominal D18.03
    intracranial D18.02
    skin D18.01
    specified site NEC D18.09
  mouth (mucosa) D10.30
    specified site NEC D10.39
    white sponge Q38.6
  multiplex Q85.1
  non-neoplastic I78.1
  oral mucosa D10.30
    specified site NEC D10.39
    white sponge Q38.6
  orbit D31.6-●
  pigmented
    giant —*see also* Neoplasm, skin, uncertain
      behavior D48.5
      malignant melanoma in —*see* Melanoma
  portwine Q82.5
  retina D31.2-●
  retrobulbar D31.6-●
  sanguineous Q82.5
  senile I78.1
  skin D22.9
    abdominal wall D22.5
    ala nasi D22.39
    ankle D22.7-●
    anus, anal D22.5
    arm D22.6-●
    auditory canal (external) D22.2-●
    auricle (ear) D22.2-●
    auricular canal (external) D22.2-●
    axilla, axillary fold D22.5
    back D22.5
    breast D22.5
    brow D22.39
    buttock D22.5
    canthus (eye) D22.1-●
    cheek (external) D22.39
    chest wall D22.5
    chin D22.39
    ear (external) D22.2-●
    external meatus (ear) D22.2-●
    eyebrow D22.39
    eyelid (lower) (upper) D22.1-●
    face D22.30
      specified NEC D22.39
    female genital organ (external) NEC D28.0
    finger D22.6-●
    flank D22.5
    foot D22.7-●
    forearm D22.6-●
    forehead D22.39
    foreskin D29.0
    genital organ (external) NEC
      female D28.0
      male D29.9
    gluteal region D22.5
    groin D22.5
    hand D22.6-●
    heel D22.7-●
    helix D22.2-●
    hip D22.7-●
    interscapular region D22.5
    jaw D22.39
    knee D22.7-●
    labium (majus) (minus) D28.0
    leg D22.7-●
    lip (lower) (upper) D22.0
    lower limb D22.7-●
    male genital organ (external) D29.9
    nail D22.9
      finger D22.6-●
      toe D22.7-●
    nasolabial groove D22.39
    nates D22.5

Nevus *(Continued)*
  skin *(Continued)*
    neck D22.4
    nose (external) D22.39
    palpebra D22.1-●
    penis D29.0
    perianal skin D22.5
    perineum D22.5
    pinna D22.2-●
    popliteal fossa or space D22.7-●
    prepuce D29.0
    pudendum D28.0
    scalp D22.4
    scrotum D29.4
    shoulder D22.6-●
    submammary fold D22.5
    temple D22.39
    thigh D22.7-●
    toe D22.7-●
    trunk NEC D22.5
    umbilicus D22.5
    upper limb D22.6-●
    vulva D28.0
  specified site NEC —*see* Neoplasm, benign,
    by site
  spider I78.1
  stellar I78.1
  strawberry Q82.5
  ~~Sutton's —see Neoplasm, skin, benign~~
▶ Sutton's benign D22.9
  unius lateris Q82.5
  Unna's Q82.5
  vascular Q82.5
  verrucous Q82.5
Newborn (infant) (liveborn) (singleton) Z38.2
  abstinence syndrome P96.1
  acne L70.4
  affected by
    abnormalities of membranes P02.9
      specified NEC P02.8
    abruptio placenta P02.1
    amino-acid metabolic disorder, transitory
      P74.8
    amniocentesis (while in utero) P00.6
    amnionitis P02.7
    apparent life threatening event (ALTE)
      R68.13
    bleeding (into)
      cerebral cortex P52.22
      germinal matrix P52.0
      ventricles P52.1
    breech delivery P03.0
    cardiac arrest P29.81
    cardiomyopathy I42.8
      congenital I42.4
    cerebral ischemia P91.0
    Cesarean delivery P03.4
    chemotherapy agents P04.1
    chorioamnionitis P02.7
    cocaine (crack) P04.41
    complications of labor and delivery P03.9
      specified NEC P03.89
    compression of umbilical cord NEC P02.5
    contracted pelvis P03.1
    delivery P03.9
      Cesarean P03.4
      forceps P03.2
      vacuum extractor P03.3
    entanglement (knot) in umbilical cord P02.5
    environmental chemicals P04.6
    fetal (intrauterine)
      growth retardation P05.9
      malnutrition not light or small for
        gestational age P05.2
    forceps delivery P03.2
    heart rate abnormalities
      bradycardia P29.12
      intrauterine P03.819
        before onset of labor P03.810
        during labor P03.811
    tachycardia P29.11

Newborn *(Continued)*
  affected by *(Continued)*
    hemorrhage (antepartum) P02.1
      cerebellar (nontraumatic) P52.6
      intracerebral (nontraumatic) P52.4
      intracranial (nontraumatic) P52.9
        specified NEC P52.8
      intraventricular (nontraumatic) P52.3
        grade 1 P52.0
        grade 2 P52.1
        grade 3 P52.21
        grade 4 P52.22
      posterior fossa (nontraumatic) P52.6
      subarachnoid (nontraumatic) P52.5
      subependymal P52.0
        with intracerebral extension P52.22
        with intraventricular extension P52.1
          with enlargment of ventricles
            P52.21
          without intraventricular extension
            P52.0
    hypoxic ischemic encephalopathy [HIE]
      P91.60
      mild P91.61
      moderate P91.62
      severe P91.63
    induction of labor P03.89
    intestinal perforation P78.0
    intrauterine (fetal) blood loss P50.9
      due to (from)
        cut end of co-twin cord P50.5
        hemorrhage into
          co-twin P50.3
          maternal circulation P50.4
        placenta P50.2
        ruptured cord blood P50.1
        vasa previa P50.0
      specified NEC P50.8
    intrauterine (fetal) hemorrhage P50.9
    intrauterine (in utero) procedure P96.5
    malpresentation (malposition) NEC P03.1
    maternal (complication of) (use of)
      alcohol P04.3
      analgesia (maternal) P04.0
      anesthesia (maternal) P04.0
      blood loss P02.1
      circulatory disease P00.3
      condition P00.9
        specified NEC P00.89
      delivery P03.9
        Cesarean P03.4
        forceps P03.2
        vacuum extractor P03.3
      diabetes mellitus (pre-existing) P70.1
      disorder P00.9
        specified NEC P00.89
      drugs (addictive) (illegal) NEC P04.49
      ectopic pregnancy P01.4
      gestational diabetes P70.0
      hemorrhage P02.1
      hypertensive disorder P00.0
      incompetent cervix P01.0
      infectious disease P00.2
      injury P00.5
      labor and delivery P03.9
      malpresentation before labor P01.7
      maternal death P01.6
      medical procedure P00.7
      medication P04.1
      multiple pregnancy P01.5
      nutritional disorder P00.4
      oligohydramnios P01.2
      parasitic disease P00.2
      periodontal disease P00.81
      placenta previa P02.0
      polyhydramnios P01.3
      precipitate delivery P03.5
      pregnancy P01.9
        specified P01.8
      premature rupture of membranes P01.1
      renal disease P00.1

▶ New ⇒ Revised ~~deleted~~ Deleted ● Use Additional Character(s)

Newborn *(Continued)*
  affected by *(Continued)*
    maternal *(Continued)*
      respiratory disease P00.3
      surgical procedure P00.6
      urinary tract disease P00.1
      uterine contraction (abnormal) P03.6
    meconium peritonitis P78.0
    medication (legal) (maternal use)
      (prescribed) P04.1
    membrane abnormalities P02.9
      specified NEC P02.8
    membranitis P02.7
    methamphetamine(s) P04.49
    mixed metabolic and respiratory acidosis
      P84
    neonatal abstinence syndrome P96.1
    noxious substances transmitted via
      placenta or breast milk P04.9
      specified NEC P04.8
    nutritional supplements P04.5
    placenta previa P02.0
    placental
      abnormality (functional)
        (morphological) P02.20
        specified NEC P02.29
      dysfunction P02.29
      infarction P02.29
      insufficiency P02.29
      separation NEC P02.1
      transfusion syndromes P02.3
    placentitis P02.7
    precipitate delivery P03.5
    prolapsed cord P02.4
    respiratory arrest P28.81
    slow intrauterine growth P05.9
    tobacco P04.2
    twin to twin transplacental transfusion
      P02.3
    umbilical cord (tightly) around neck
      P02.5
    umbilical cord condition P02.60
      short cord P02.69
      specified NEC P02.69
    uterine contractions (abnormal) P03.6
    vasa previa P02.69
      from intrauterine blood loss P50.0
  apnea P28.4
    obstructive P28.4
    primary P28.3
    sleep (central) (obstructive) (primary)
      P28.3
  born in hospital Z38.00
    by cesarean Z38.01
  born outside hospital Z38.1
  breast buds P96.89
  breast engorgement P83.4
  check-up —*see* Newborn, examination
  convulsion P90
  dehydration P74.1
  examination
    8 to 28 days old Z00.111
    under 8 days old Z00.110
  fever P81.9
    environmentally-induced P81.0
  hyperbilirubinemia P59.9
    of prematurity P59.0
  hypernatremia P74.2
  hyponatremia P74.2
  infection P39.9
    candidal P37.5
    specified NEC P39.8
    urinary tract P39.3
  jaundice P59.9
    due to
      breast milk inhibitor P59.3
      hepatocellular damage P59.20
        specified NEC P59.29
      preterm delivery P59.0
    of prematurity P59.0
    specified NEC P59.8

Newborn *(Continued)*
  late metabolic acidosis P74.0
  mastitis P39.0
    infective P39.0
    noninfective P83.4
  multiple born NEC Z38.8
    born in hospital Z38.68
      by cesarean Z38.69
    born outside hospital Z38.7
  omphalitis P38.9
    with mild hemorrhage P38.1
    without hemorrhage P38.9
  post-term P08.21
  prolonged gestation (over 42 completed
    weeks) P08.22
  quadruplet Z38.8
    born in hospital Z38.63
      by cesarean Z38.64
    born outside hospital Z38.7
  quintuplet Z38.8
    born in hospital Z38.65
      by cesarean Z38.66
    born outside hospital Z38.7
  seizure P90
  sepsis (congenital) P36.9
    due to
      anaerobes NEC P36.5
      Escherichia coli P36.4
      Staphylococcus P36.30
        aureus P36.2
        specified NEC P36.39
      Streptococcus P36.10
        group B P36.0
        specified NEC P36.19
      specified NEC P36.8
  triplet Z38.8
    born in hospital Z38.61
      by cesarean Z38.62
    born outside hospital Z38.7
  twin Z38.5
    born in hospital Z38.30
      by cesarean Z38.31
    born outside hospital Z38.4
  vomiting P92.09
    bilious P92.01
  weight check Z00.111
Newcastle conjunctivitis or disease B30.8
Nezelof's syndrome (pure alymphocytosis)
  D81.4
Niacin (amide) deficiency E52
Nicolas (-Durand)-Favre disease A55
Nicotine —*see* Tobacco
Nicotinic acid deficiency E52
Niemann-Pick disease or syndrome E75.249
  specified NEC E75.248
  type
    A E75.240
    B E75.241
    C E75.242
    D E75.243
Night
  blindness —*see* Blindness, night
  sweats R61
  terrors (child) F51.4
Nightmares (REM sleep type) F51.5
NIHSS (National Institutes of Health Stroke
  Scale) score R29.7-●
Nipple —*see* condition
Nisbet's chancre A57
Nishimoto (-Takeuchi) disease I67.5
Nitritoid crisis or reaction —*see* Crisis, nitritoid
Nitrosohemoglobinemia D74.8
Njovera A65
Nocardiosis, nocardiasis A43.9
  cutaneous A43.1
  lung A43.0
  pneumonia A43.0
  pulmonary A43.0
  specified site NEC A43.8
Nocturia R35.1
  psychogenic F45.8

Nocturnal —*see* condition
Nodal rhythm I49.8
Node(s) —*see also* Nodule
  Bouchard's (with arthropathy) M15.2
  Haygarth's M15.8
  Heberden's (with arthropathy) M15.1
  larynx J38.7
  lymph —*see* condition
  milker's B08.03
  Osler's I33.0
  Schmorl's —*see* Schmorl's disease
  singer's J38.2
  teacher's J38.2
  tuberculous —*see* Tuberculosis, lymph
    gland
  vocal cord J38.2
Nodule(s), nodular
  actinomycotic —*see* Actinomycosis
  ▶breast NEC —*see also* Lump, breast N63.0
  colloid (cystic), thyroid E04.1
  cutaneous —*see* Swelling, localized
  endometrial (stromal) D26.1
  Haygarth's M15.8
  inflammatory —*see* Inflammation
  juxta-articular
    syphilitic A52.77
    yaws A66.7
  larynx J38.7
  lung, solitary (subsegmental branch of the
    bronchial tree) R91.1
    multiple R91.8
  milker's B08.03
  prostate N40.2
    with lower urinary tract symptoms (LUTS)
      N40.3
    without lower urinary tract symptoms
      (LUTS) N40.2
  pulmonary, solitary (subsegmental branch of
    the bronchial tree) R91.1
  retrocardiac R09.89
  rheumatoid M06.30
    ankle M06.37-●
    elbow M06.32-●
    foot joint M06.37-●
    hand joint M06.34-●
    hip M06.35-●
    knee M06.36-●
    multiple site M06.39
    shoulder M06.31-●
    vertebra M06.38
    wrist M06.33-●
  scrotum (inflammatory) N49.2
  singer's J38.2
  solitary, lung (subsegmental branch of the
    bronchial tree) R91.1
    multiple R91.8
  subcutaneous —*see* Swelling, localized
  teacher's J38.2
  thyroid (cold) (gland) (nontoxic) E04.1
    with thyrotoxicosis E05.20
      with thyroid storm E05.21
    toxic or with hyperthyroidism E05.20
      with thyroid storm E05.21
  vocal cord J38.2
Noma (gangrenous) (hospital) (infective)
  A69.0
  auricle I96
  mouth A69.0
  pudendi N76.89
  vulvae N76.89
Nomad, nomadism Z59.0
NOMID (neonatal onset multisystemic
  inflammatory disorder) M04.2
▶Nonadherence to medical treatment Z91.19
Nonautoimmune hemolytic anemia D59.4
  drug-induced D59.2
Nonclosure —*see also* Imperfect, closure
  ductus arteriosus (Botallo's) Q25.0
  foramen
    botalli Q21.1
    ovale Q21.1

Noncompliance Z91.19
  with
    dialysis Z91.15
    dietary regimen Z91.11
    medical treatment Z91.19
    medication regimen NEC Z91.14
      underdosing —*see also* Table of Drugs
        and Chemicals, categories T36-T50,
        with final character 6 Z91.14
      intentional NEC Z91.128
        due to financial hardship of patient
          Z91.120
      unintentional NEC Z91.138
        due to patient's age related debility
          Z91.130
    renal dialysis Z91.15
Nondescent (congenital) —*see also* Malposition,
  congenital
  cecum Q43.3
  colon Q43.3
  testicle Q53.9
    bilateral Q53.20
      abdominal Q53.211
      perineal Q53.22
    unilateral Q53.10
      abdominal Q53.111
      perineal Q53.12
Nondevelopment
  brain Q02
    part of Q04.3
  heart Q24.8
  organ or site, congenital NEC —*see*
    Hypoplasia
Nonengagement
  head NEC O32.4
    in labor, causing obstructed labor O64.8
Nonexanthematous tick fever A93.2
Nonexpansion, lung (newborn) P28.0
Nonfunctioning
  cystic duct —*see also* Disease, gallbladder
    K82.8
  gallbladder —*see also* Disease, gallbladder
    K82.8
  kidney N28.9
  labyrinth —*see* subcategory H83.2

Non-Hodgkin lymphoma NEC —*see*
  Lymphoma, non-Hodgkin
Nonimplantation, ovum N97.2
Noninsufflation, fallopian tube N97.1
Non-ketotic hyperglycinemia E72.51
Nonne-Milroy syndrome Q82.0
Nonovulation N97.0
Non-palpable testicle(s)
  bilateral R39.84
  unilateral R39.83
Nonpatent fallopian tube N97.1
Nonpneumatization, lung NEC P28.0
Nonrotation —*see* Malrotation
Nonsecretion, urine —*see* Anuria
Nonunion
  fracture —*see* Fracture, by site
  joint, following fusion or arthrodesis
    M96.0
  organ or site, congenital NEC —*see* Imperfect,
    closure
  symphysis pubis, congenital Q74.2
Nonvisualization, gallbladder R93.2
Nonvital, nonvitalized tooth K04.99
Non-working side interference
  M26.56
Noonan's syndrome Q87.1
Normocytic anemia (infectional) due to blood
  loss (chronic) D50.0
  acute D62
Norrie's disease (congenital) Q15.8
North American blastomycosis B40.9
Norwegian itch B86
Nose, nasal —*see* condition
Nosebleed R04.0
Nose-picking F98.8
Nosomania F45.21
Nosophobia F45.22
Nostalgia F43.20
Notch of iris Q13.2
Notching nose, congenital (tip)
  Q30.2
Nothnagel's
  syndrome —*see* Strabismus, paralytic, third
    nerve
  vasomotor acroparesthesia I73.89

Novy's relapsing fever A68.9
  louse-borne A68.0
  tick-borne A68.1
Noxious
  foodstuffs, poisoning by —*see* Poisoning,
    food, noxious, plant
  substances transmitted through placenta or
    breast milk P04.9
Nucleus pulposus —*see* condition
Numbness R20.0
Nuns' knee —*see* Bursitis, prepatellar
Nursemaid's elbow S53.03-•
Nutcracker esophagus K22.4
Nutmeg liver K76.1
Nutrient element deficiency E61.9
  specified NEC E61.8
Nutrition deficient or insufficient —*see also*
  Malnutrition E46
  due to
    insufficient food T73.0
    lack of
      care (child) T76.02
        adult T76.01
      food T73.0
Nutritional stunting E45
Nyctalopia (night blindness) —*see* Blindness,
  night
Nycturia R35.1
  psychogenic F45.8
Nymphomania F52.8
Nystagmus H55.00
  benign paroxysmal —*see* Vertigo, benign
    paroxysmal
  central positional H81.4-•
  congenital H55.01
  dissociated H55.04
  latent H55.02
  miners' H55.09
  positional
    benign paroxysmal H81.4-•
    central H81.4-•
  specified form NEC H55.09
  visual deprivation H55.03

▶ New   ⇒ Revised   ~~deleted~~ Deleted   • Use Additional Character(s)

O

Obermeyer's relapsing fever (European)
A68.0
Obesity E66.9
with alveolar hypoventilation E66.2
adrenal E27.8
complicating
childbirth O99.214
pregnancy O99.21-●
puerperium O99.215
constitutional E66.8
dietary counseling and surveillance
Z71.3
drug-induced E66.1
due to
drug E66.1
excess calories E66.09
morbid E66.01
severe E66.01
endocrine E66.8
endogenous E66.8
exogenous E66.09
familial E66.8
glandular E66.8
hypothyroid —see Hypothyroidism
hypoventilation syndrome (OHS)
E66.2
morbid E66.01
with
alveolar hypoventilation E66.2
obesity hypoventilation syndrome
(OHS) E66.2
due to excess calories E66.01
nutritional E66.09
pituitary E23.6
severe E66.01
specified type NEC E66.8
Oblique —see condition
Obliteration
appendix (lumen) K38.8
artery I77.1
bile duct (noncalculous) K83.1
common duct (noncalculous) K83.1
cystic duct —see Obstruction, gallbladder
disease, arteriolar I77.1
endometrium N85.8
eye, anterior chamber —see Disorder, globe,
hypotony
fallopian tube N97.1
lymphatic vessel I89.0
due to mastectomy I97.2
organ or site, congenital NEC —see Atresia,
by site
ureter N13.5
with infection N13.6
urethra —see Stricture, urethra
vein I87.8
vestibule (oral) K08.89
Observation (following) (for) (without need for
further medical care) Z04.9
accident NEC Z04.3
at work Z04.2
transport Z04.1
adverse effect of drug Z03.6
alleged rape or sexual assault (victim),
ruled out
adult Z04.41
child Z04.42
criminal assault Z04.8
development state
adolescent Z00.3
period of rapid growth in childhood
Z00.2
puberty Z00.3
disease, specified NEC Z03.89
following work accident Z04.2
growth and development state —see
Observation, development state
injuries (accidental) NEC —see also
Observation, accident

Observation (Continued)
newborn (for)
suspected condition, related to exposure
from the mother or birth process —
see Newborn, affected by,
maternal
ruled out Z05.9
cardiac Z05.0
connective tissue Z05.73
gastrointestinal Z05.5
genetic Z05.41
genitourinary Z05.6
immunologic Z05.43
infectious Z05.1
metabolic Z05.42
musculoskeletal Z05.72
neurological Z05.2
respiratory Z05.3
skin and subcutaneous tissue
Z05.71
specified condition NEC
Z05.8
postpartum
immediately after delivery Z39.0
routine follow-up Z39.2
pregnancy (normal) (without complication)
Z34.9-●
high risk O09.9-●
suicide attempt, alleged NEC Z03.89
self-poisoning Z03.6
suspected, ruled out —see also Suspected
condition, ruled out
abuse, physical
adult Z04.71
child Z04.72
accident at work Z04.2
adult battering victim Z04.71
child battering victim Z04.72
condition NEC Z03.89
newborn —see also Observation,
newborn (for), suspected condition,
ruled out Z05.9
drug poisoning or adverse effect
Z03.6
exposure (to)
anthrax Z03.810
biological agent NEC Z03.818
inflicted injury NEC Z04.8
suicide attempt, alleged Z03.89
self-poisoning Z03.6
toxic effects from ingested substance (drug)
(poison) Z03.6
toxic effects from ingested substance (drug)
(poison) Z03.6
Obsession, obsessional state F42.8
mixed thoughts and acts F42.2
Obsessive-compulsive neurosis or reaction
F42.8
Obstetric embolism, septic —see Embolism,
obstetric, septic
Obstetrical trauma (complicating delivery)
O71.9
with or following ectopic or molar pregnancy
O08.6
specified type NEC O71.89
Obstipation —see Constipation
Obstruction, obstructed, obstructive
airway J98.8
with
allergic alveolitis J67.9
asthma J45.909
with
exacerbation (acute) J45.901
status asthmaticus J45.902
bronchiectasis J47.9
with
exacerbation (acute) J47.1
lower respiratory infection
J47.0
bronchitis (chronic) J44.9
emphysema J43.9

Obstruction, obstructed, obstructive
(Continued)
airway (Continued)
chronic J44.9
with
allergic alveolitis —see Pneumonitis,
hypersensitivity
bronchiectasis J47.9
with
exacerbation (acute) J47.1
lower respiratory infection J47.0
due to
foreign body —see Foreign body, by site,
causing asphyxia
inhalation of fumes or vapors J68.9
laryngospasm J38.5
ampulla of Vater K83.1
aortic (heart) (valve) —see Stenosis, aortic
aortoiliac I74.09
aqueduct of Sylvius G91.1
congenital Q03.0
with spina bifida —see Spina bifida, by
site, with hydrocephalus
Arnold-Chiari —see Arnold-Chiari disease
⇒ artery (see also Atherosclerosis, artery) I70.9
basilar (complete) (partial) —see Occlusion,
artery, basilar
carotid (complete) (partial) —see Occlusion,
artery, carotid
cerebellar —see Occlusion, artery, cerebellar
cerebral (anterior) (middle) (posterior) —
see Occlusion, artery, cerebral
precerebral —see Occlusion, artery,
precerebral
renal N28.0
retinal NEC —see Occlusion, artery, retina
stent —see Restenosis, stent
vertebral (complete) (partial) —see
Occlusion, artery, vertebral
⇒ band (intestinal) —see also Obstruction,
intestine, specified NEC K56.699
bile duct or passage (common) (hepatic)
(noncalculous) K83.1
with calculus K80.51
congenital (causing jaundice) Q44.3
biliary (duct) (tract) K83.1
gallbladder K82.0
bladder-neck (acquired) N32.0
congenital Q64.31
due to hyperplasia (hypertrophy) of
prostate —see Hyperplasia, prostate
bowel —see Obstruction, intestine
bronchus J98.09
canal, ear —see Stenosis, external ear canal
cardia K22.2
caval veins (inferior) (superior) I87.1
cecum —see Obstruction, intestine
circulatory I99.8
colon —see Obstruction, intestine
common duct (noncalculous) K83.1
coronary (artery) —see Occlusion, coronary
cystic duct —see also Obstruction, gallbladder
with calculus K80.21
device, implant or graft —see also
Complications, by site and type,
mechanical T85.698
arterial graft NEC —see Complication,
cardiovascular device, mechanical,
vascular
catheter NEC T85.628
cystostomy T83.090
dialysis (renal) T82.49
intraperitoneal T85.691
Hopkins T83.098
ileostomy T83.098
infusion NEC T82.594
spinal (epidural) (subdural) T85.690
nephrostomy T83.092
urethral indwelling T83.091
urinary T83.098
urostomy T83.098

Obstruction, obstructed, obstructive
   (Continued)
   device, implant or graft (Continued)
      due to infection T85.79
      gastrointestinal —see Complications,
         prosthetic device, mechanical,
         gastrointestinal device
      genital NEC T83.498
         intrauterine contraceptive device T83.39
         penile prosthesis (cylinder) (implanted)
            (pump) (resevoir) T83.490
         testicular prosthesis T83.491
      heart NEC —see Complication,
         cardiovascular device, mechanical
      joint prosthesis —see Complications, joint
         prosthesis, mechanical, specified NEC,
         by site
      orthopedic NEC —see Complication,
         orthopedic, device, mechanical
      specified NEC T85.628
      urinary NEC —see also Complication,
         genitourinary, device, urinary,
         mechanical
         graft T83.29
      vascular NEC —see Complication,
         cardiovascular device, mechanical
      ventricular intracranial shunt T85.09
   device to foreign body accidentally left in
      operative wound T81.529
   duodenum K31.5
   ejaculatory duct N50.89
   esophagus K22.2
   eustachian tube (complete) (partial) H68.10-•
      cartilagenous (extrinsic) H68.13-•
         intrinsic H68.12-•
      osseous H68.11-•
   fallopian tube (bilateral) N97.1
   fecal K56.41
      with hernia —see Hernia, by site, with
         obstruction
   foramen of Monro (congenital) Q03.8
      with spina bifida —see Spina bifida,
         by site, with hydrocephalus
   foreign body —see Foreign body
   gallbladder K82.0
      with calculus, stones K80.21
      congenital Q44.1
   gastric outlet K31.1
   gastrointestinal —see Obstruction, intestine
   hepatic K76.89
      duct (noncalculous) K83.1
   hepatobiliary K83.1
   ileum —see Obstruction, intestine
   iliofemoral (artery) I74.5
   ⇒intestine K56.609
     ▶complete K56.601
     ▶incomplete K56.600
     ▶partial K56.600
     with
       ⇒adhesions (intestinal) (peritoneal) K56.50
         ▶complete K56.52
         ▶incomplete K56.51
         ▶partial K56.51
     adynamic K56.0
     by gallstone K56.3
     congenital (small) Q41.9
       large Q42.9
         specified part NEC Q42.8
     neurogenic K56.0
       Hirschsprung's disease or megacolon
         Q43.1
     newborn P76.9
       due to
         fecaliths P76.8
         inspissated milk P76.2
         meconium (plug) P76.0
           in mucoviscidosis E84.11
       specified NEC P76.8
   ⇒postoperative K91.30
     ▶complete K91.32
     ▶incomplete K91.31
     ▶partial K91.31

Obstruction, obstructed, obstructive
   (Continued)
   intestine (Continued)
      reflex K56.0
     ⇒specified NEC K56.699
       ▶complete K56.691
       ▶incomplete K56.690
       ▶partial K56.690
      volvulus K56.2
   intracardiac ball valve prosthesis T82.09
   jejunum —see Obstruction, intestine
   joint prosthesis —see Complications, joint
      prosthesis, mechanical, specified NEC,
      by site
   kidney (calices) N28.89
   labor —see Delivery
   lacrimal (passages) (duct)
      by
        dacryolith —see Dacryolith
        stenosis —see Stenosis, lacrimal
      congenital Q10.5
      neonatal H04.53-•
   lacrimonasal duct —see Obstruction, lacrimal
   lacteal, with steatorrhea K90.2
   laryngitis —see Laryngitis
   larynx NEC J38.6
      congenital Q31.8
   lung J98.4
      disease, chronic J44.9
   lymphatic I89.0
   meconium (plug)
      newborn P76.0
        due to fecaliths P76.0
        in mucoviscidosis E84.11
   mitral —see Stenosis, mitral
   nasal J34.89
   nasolacrimal duct —see also Obstruction,
      lacrimal
      congenital Q10.5
   nasopharynx J39.2
   nose J34.89
   organ or site, congenital NEC —see Atresia,
      by site
   pancreatic duct K86.89
   parotid duct or gland K11.8
   pelviureteral junction N13.5
      with hydronephrosis N13.0
      congenital Q62.39
   pharynx J39.2
   portal (circulation) (vein) I81
   prostate —see also Hyperplasia, prostate
      valve (urinary) N32.0
   pulmonary valve (heart) I37.0
   pyelonephritis (chronic) N11.1
   pylorus
      adult K31.1
      congenital or infantile Q40.0
   rectosigmoid —see Obstruction,
      intestine
   rectum K62.4
   renal N28.89
      outflow N13.8
      pelvis, congenital Q62.39
   respiratory J98.8
      chronic J44.9
   retinal (vessels) H34.9
   salivary duct (any) K11.8
      with calculus K11.5
   sigmoid —see Obstruction, intestine
   sinus (accessory) (nasal) J34.89
   Stensen's duct K11.8
   stomach NEC K31.89
      acute K31.0
      congenital Q40.2
      due to pylorospasm K31.3
   submandibular duct K11.8
   submaxillary gland K11.8
      with calculus K11.5
   thoracic duct I89.0
   thrombotic —see Thrombosis
   trachea J39.8

Obstruction, obstructed, obstructive
   (Continued)
   tracheostomy airway J95.03
   tricuspid (valve) —see Stenosis, tricuspid
   upper respiratory, congenital Q34.8
   ureter (functional) (pelvic junction) NEC N13.5
      with
        hydronephrosis N13.1
         with infection N13.6
        pyelonephritis (chronic) N11.1
      congenital Q62.39
      due to calculus —see Calculus, ureter
   urethra NEC N36.8
      congenital Q64.39
   urinary (moderate) N13.9
      due to hyperplasia (hypertrophy) of
         prostate —see Hyperplasia, prostate
      organ or tract (lower) N13.9
      prostatic valve N32.0
      specified NEC N13.8
   uropathy N13.9
   uterus N85.8
   vagina N89.5
   valvular —see Endocarditis
   vein, venous I87.1
      caval (inferior) (superior) I87.1
      thrombotic —see Thrombosis
   vena cava (inferior) (superior) I87.1
   vesical NEC N32.0
   vesicourethral orifice N32.0
      congenital Q64.31
   vessel NEC I99.8
      stent —see Restenosis, stent
Obturator —see condition
Occlusal wear, teeth K03.0
Occlusio pupillae —see Membrane, pupillary
Occlusion, occluded
   anus K62.4
      congenital Q42.3
        with fistula Q42.2
   aortoiliac (chronic) I74.09
   aqueduct of Sylvius G91.1
      congenital Q03.0
        with spina bifida —see Spina bifida, by
         site, with hydrocephalus
   ⇒artery —see also Atherosclerosis, artery I70.9
      auditory, internal I65.8
      basilar I65.1
        with
         infarction I63.22
          due to
           embolism I63.12
           thrombosis I63.02
      brain or cerebral I66.9
        with infarction (due to) I63.5-•
         embolism I63.4-•
         thrombosis I63.3-•
      carotid I65.2-•
        with
         infarction I63.23-•
          due to
           embolism I63.13-•
           thrombosis I63.03-•
      cerebellar (anterior inferior) (posterior
        inferior) (superior) I66.3
        with infarction I63.54-•
         due to
          embolism I63.44-•
          thrombosis I63.34-•
      cerebral I66.9
        with infarction I63.50
         due to
          embolism I63.40
           specified NEC I63.49
          thrombosis I63.30
           specified NEC I63.39
      anterior I66.1-•
        with infarction I63.52-•
         due to
          embolism I63.42-•
          thrombosis I63.32-•

▶ New   ⇒ Revised   ~~deleted~~ Deleted   • Use Additional Character(s)

Occlusion, occluded *(Continued)*
  artery *(Continued)*
    cerebral *(Continued)*
      middle I66.0-•
        with infarction I63.51-•
          due to
            embolism I63.41-•
            thrombosis I63.31-•
      posterior I66.2-•
        with infarction I63.53-•
          due to
            embolism I63.43-•
            thrombosis I63.33-•
      specified NEC I66.8
        with infarction I63.59
          due to
            embolism I63.4-•
            thrombosis I63.3-•
      choroidal (anterior) —*see* Occlusion,
        artery, cerebral, specified NEC
    ➠communicating posterior —*see* Occlusion,
        artery, precerebral, specified NEC
    complete
      coronary I25.82
      extremities I70.92
    coronary (acute) (thrombotic) (without
      myocardial infarction) I24.0
      with myocardial infarction —*see*
        Infarction, myocardium
      chronic total I25.82
      complete I25.82
      healed or old I25.2
      total (chronic) I25.82
    hypophyseal —*see* Occlusion, artery,
      precerebral, specified NEC
    iliac I74.5
    lower extremities due to stenosis or
      stricture I77.1
    mesenteric (embolic) (thrombotic) —*see also*
      Infarct, intestine K55.069
    perforating —*see* Occlusion, artery,
      cerebral, specified NEC
    peripheral I77.9
      thrombotic or embolic I74.4
  ➠pontine —*see* Occlusion, artery, precerebral,
      specified NEC
    precerebral I65.9
      with infarction I63.20
        due to
          embolism I63.10
            specified NEC I63.19
          thrombosis I63.00
            specified NEC I63.09
          specified NEC I63.29
      basilar —*see* Occlusion, artery, basilar
      carotid —*see* Occlusion, artery, carotid
      puerperal O88.23
      specified NEC I65.8
        with infarction I63.29
          due to
            embolism I63.19
           ➠thrombosis I63.09
      vertebral —*see* Occlusion, artery,
        vertebral
    renal N28.0
    retinal
      branch H34.23-•
      central H34.1-•
      partial H34.21-•
      transient H34.0-•
    spinal —*see* Occlusion, artery, precerebral,
      vertebral
    total (chronic)
      coronary I25.82
      extremities I70.92
    vertebral I65.0-•
      with
        infarction I63.21-•
          due to
            embolism I63.11-•
            thrombosis I63.01-•

Occlusion, occluded *(Continued)*
  basilar artery —*see* Occlusion, artery, basilar
  bile duct (common) (hepatic) (noncalculous)
    K83.1
  bowel —*see* Obstruction, intestine
  carotid (artery) (common) (internal) —*see*
    Occlusion, artery, carotid
  centric (of teeth) M26.59
    maximum intercuspation discrepancy
      M26.55
  cerebellar (artery) —*see* Occlusion, artery,
    cerebellar
  cerebral (artery) —*see* Occlusion, artery,
    cerebral
  cerebrovascular —*see also* Occlusion, artery,
    cerebral
    with infarction I63.5-•
  cervical canal —*see* Stricture, cervix
  cervix (uteri) —*see* Stricture, cervix
  choanal Q30.0
  choroidal (artery) —*see* Occlusion, artery,
    precerebral, specified NEC
  colon —*see* Obstruction, intestine
  communicating posterior artery —*see*
    Occlusion, artery, precerebral, specified
    NEC
  coronary (artery) (vein) (thrombotic) —*see*
    also Infarct, myocardium
    chronic total I25.82
    healed or old I25.2
    not resulting in infarction I24.0
    total (chronic) I25.82
  cystic duct —*see* Obstruction, gallbladder
  embolic —*see* Embolism
  fallopian tube N97.1
    congenital Q50.6
  gallbladder —*see also* Obstruction,
    gallbladder
    congenital (causing jaundice) Q44.1
  gingiva, traumatic K06.2
  hymen N89.6
    congenital Q52.3
  hypophyseal (artery) —*see* Occlusion, artery,
    precerebral, specified NEC
  iliac artery I74.5
  intestine —*see* Obstruction, intestine
  lacrimal passages —*see* Obstruction, lacrimal
  lung J98.4
  lymph or lymphatic channel I89.0
  mammary duct N64.89
  mesenteric artery (embolic) (thrombotic) —
    see also Infarct, intestine K55.069
  nose J34.89
    congenital Q30.0
  organ or site, congenital NEC —*see* Atresia,
    by site
  oviduct N97.1
    congenital Q50.6
  peripheral arteries
    due to stricture or stenosis I77.1
    upper extremity I74.2
  pontine (artery) —*see* Occlusion, artery,
    precerebral, specified NEC
  posterior lingual, of mandibular teeth M26.29
  precerebral artery —*see* Occlusion, artery,
    precerebral
  punctum lacrimale —*see* Obstruction,
    lacrimal
  pupil —*see* Membrane, pupillary
  pylorus, adult —*see also* Stricture, pylorus
    K31.1
  renal artery N28.0
  retina, retinal
    artery —*see* Occlusion, artery, retinal
    vein (central) H34.81-•
      engorgement H34.82-•
      tributary H34.83-•
    vessels H34.9
  spinal artery —*see* Occlusion, artery,
    precerebral, vertebral
  teeth (mandibular) (posterior lingual) M26.29

Occlusion, occluded *(Continued)*
  thoracic duct I89.0
  thrombotic —*see* Thrombosis, artery
  traumatic
    edentulous (alveolar) ridge K06.2
    gingiva K06.2
    periodontal K05.5
  tubal N97.1
  ureter (complete) (partial) N13.5
    congenital Q62.10
  ureteropelvic junction N13.5
    congenital Q62.11
  ureterovesical orifice N13.5
    congenital Q62.12
  urethra —*see* Stricture, urethra
  uterus N85.8
  vagina N89.5
  vascular NEC I99.8
  vein —*see* Thrombosis
    retinal —*see* Occlusion, retinal, vein
  vena cava (inferior) (superior) —*see*
    Embolism, vena cava
  ventricle (brain) NEC G91.1
  vertebral (artery) —*see* Occlusion, artery,
    vertebral
  vessel (blood) I99.8
  vulva N90.5
Occult
  blood in feces (stools) R19.5
Occupational
  problems NEC Z56.89
Ochlophobia —*see* Agoraphobia
Ochronosis (endogenous) E70.29
Ocular muscle —*see* condition
Oculogyric crisis or disturbance H51.8
  psychogenic F45.8
Oculomotor syndrome H51.9
Oculopathy
  syphilitic NEC A52.71
    congenital
      early A50.01
      late A50.30
    early (secondary) A51.43
    late A52.71
Oddi's sphincter spasm K83.4
Odontalgia K08.89
Odontoameloblastoma —*see* Cyst, calcifying
  odontogenic
Odontoclasia K03.89
Odontodysplasia, regional K00.4
Odontogenesis imperfecta K00.5
Odontoma (ameloblastic) (complex)
  (compound) (fibroameloblastic) —*see* Cyst,
  calcifying odontogenic
Odontomyelitis (closed) (open) K04.01
  irreversible K04.02
  reversible K04.01
Odontorrhagia K08.89
Odontosarcoma, ameloblastic C41.1
  upper jaw (bone) C41.0
Oestriasis —*see* Myiasis
Oguchi's disease H53.63
Ohara's disease —*see* Tularemia
OHS (obesity hypoventilation syndrome) E66.2

Oidiomycosis —*see* Candidiasis
Oidium albicans infection —*see* Candidiasis
Old (previous) myocardial infarction
  I25.2
Old age (without mention of debility) R54-•
  dementia F03
Olfactory —*see* condition
Oligemia —*see* Anemia
Oligoastrocytoma
  specified site —*see* Neoplasm, malignant,
    by site
  unspecified site C71.9
Oligocythemia D64.9
Oligodendroblastoma
  specified site —*see* Neoplasm, malignant
  unspecified site C71.9

Oligodendroglioma
 anaplastic type
  specified site —see Neoplasm, malignant,
   by site
  unspecified site C71.9
 specified site —see Neoplasm, malignant,
  by site
 unspecified site C71.9
Oligodontia —see Anodontia
Oligoencephalon Q02
Oligohidrosis L74.4
Oligohydramnios O41.0-●
Oligohydrosis L74.4
Oligomenorrhea N91.5
 primary N91.3
 secondary N91.4
Oligophrenia —see also Disability, intellectual
 phenylpyruvic E70.0
Oligospermia N46.11
 due to
  drug therapy N46.121
  efferent duct obstruction N46.123
  infection N46.122
  radiation N46.124
  specified cause NEC N46.129
  systemic disease N46.125
Oligotrichia —see Alopecia
Oliguria R34
 with, complicating or following ectopic or
  molar pregnancy O08.4
 postprocedural N99.0
Ollier's disease Q78.4
Omenotocele —see Hernia, abdomen, specified
 site NEC
Omentitis —see Peritonitis
Omentum, omental —see condition
Omphalitis (congenital) (newborn) P38.9
 with mild hemorrhage P38.1
 without hemorrhage P38.9
 not of newborn L08.82
 tetanus A33
Omphalocele Q79.2
Omphalomesenteric duct, persistent Q43.0
Omphalorrhagia, newborn P51.9
Omsk hemorrhagic fever A98.1
Onanism (excessive) F98.8
Onchocerciasis, onchocercosis B73.1
 with
  eye disease B73.00
   endophthalmitis B73.01
   eyelid B73.09
   glaucoma B73.02
   specified NEC B73.09
  eye NEC B73.00
  eyelid B73.09
Oncocytoma —see Neoplasm, benign, by site
Oncovirus, as cause of disease classified
 elsewhere B97.32
Ondine's curse —see Apnea, sleep
Oneirophrenia F23
Onychauxis L60.2
 congenital Q84.5
Onychia —see also Cellulitis, digit
 with lymphangitis —see Lymphangitis, acute,
  digit
 candidal B37.2
 dermatophytic B35.1
Onychitis —see also Cellulitis, digit
 with lymphangitis —see Lymphangitis, acute,
  digit
Onychocryptosis L60.0
Onychodystrophy L60.3
 congenital Q84.6
Onychogryphosis, onychogryposis L60.2
Onycholysis L60.1
Onychomadesis L60.8
Onychomalacia L60.3
Onychomycosis (finger) (toe) B35.1
Onycho-osteodysplasia Q87.2
Onychophagia F98.8
Onychophosis L60.8

Onychoptosis L60.8
Onychorrhexis L60.3
 congenital Q84.6
Onychoschizia L60.3
Onyxis (finger) (toe) L60.0
Onyxitis —see also Cellulitis, digit
 with lymphangitis —see Lymphangitis, acute,
  digit
Oophoritis (cystic) (infectional) (interstitial)
  N70.92
 with salpingitis N70.93
 acute N70.02
  with salpingitis N70.03
 chronic N70.12
  with salpingitis N70.13
 complicating abortion —see Abortion, by
  type, complicated by, oophoritis
Oophorocele N83.4-●
Opacity, opacities
 cornea H17.-●
  central H17.1-●
  congenital Q13.3
  degenerative —see Degeneration, cornea
  hereditary —see Dystrophy, cornea
  inflammatory —see Keratitis
  minor H17.81-●
  peripheral H17.82-●
  sequelae of trachoma (healed) B94.0
  specified NEC H17.89
 enamel (teeth) (fluoride) (nonfluoride) K00.3
 lens —see Cataract
 snowball —see Deposit, crystalline
 vitreous (humor) NEC H43.39-●
  congenital Q14.0
  membranes and strands H43.31-●
Opalescent dentin (hereditary) K00.5
Open, opening
 abnormal, organ or site, congenital —see
  Imperfect, closure
 angle with
  borderline
   findings
    high risk H40.02-●
    low risk H40.01-●
   intraocular pressure H40.00-●
  cupping of discs H40.01-●
  glaucoma (primary) —see Glaucoma, open
   angle
 bite
  anterior M26.220
  posterior M26.221
 false —see Imperfect, closure
 margin on tooth restoration K08.51
 restoration margins of tooth K08.51
 wound —see Wound, open
Operational fatigue F48.8
Operative —see condition
Operculitis —see Periodontitis
Operculum —see Break, retina
Ophiasis L63.2
Ophthalmia —see also Conjunctivitis H10.9
 actinic rays —see Photokeratitis
 allergic (acute) —see Conjunctivitis, acute,
  atopic
 blennorrhagic (gonococcal) (neonatorum)
  A54.31
 diphtheritic A36.86
 Egyptian A71.1
 electrica —see Photokeratitis
 gonococcal (neonatorum) A54.31
 metastatic —see Endophthalmitis, purulent
 migraine —see Migraine, ophthalmoplegic
 neonatorum, newborn P39.1
  gonococcal A54.31
 nodosa H16.24-●
 purulent —see Conjunctivitis, acute,
  mucopurulent
 spring —see Conjunctivitis, acute, atopic
 sympathetic —see Uveitis, sympathetic
Ophthalmitis —see Ophthalmia
Ophthalmocele (congenital) Q15.8

Ophthalmoneuromyelitis G36.0
Ophthalmoplegia —see also Strabismus,
  paralytic
 anterior internuclear —see Ophthalmoplegia,
  internuclear
 ataxia-areflexia G61.0
 diabetic —see E08-E13 with .39
 exophthalmic E05.00
  with thyroid storm E05.01
 external H49.88-●
  progressive H49.4-●
   with pigmentary retinopathy —see
    Kearns-Sayre syndrome
  total H49.3-●
 internal (complete) (total) H52.51-●
 internuclear H51.2-●
 migraine —see Migraine, ophthalmoplegic
 Parinaud's H49.88-●
 progressive external —see Ophthalmoplegia,
  external, progressive
 supranuclear, progressive G23.1
 total (external) —see Ophthalmoplegia,
  external, total
Opioid(s)
 abuse —see Abuse, drug, opioids
 dependence —see Dependence, drug, opioids
 induced, without use disorder
  anxiety disorder F11.988
  delirium F11.921
  depressive disorder F11.94
  sexual dysfunction F11.981
  sleep disorder F11.982
Opisthognathism M26.09
Opisthorchiasis (felineus) (viverrini) B66.0
Opitz' disease D73.2
Opiumism —see Dependence, drug, opioid
Oppenheim's disease G70.2
Oppenheim-Urbach disease (necrobiosis
  lipoidica diabeticorum) —see E08-E13 with
  .620
Optic nerve —see condition
Orbit —see condition
Orchioblastoma C62.9-●
Orchitis (gangrenous) (nonspecific) (septic)
  (suppurative) N45.2
 blennorrhagic (gonococcal) (acute) (chronic)
  A54.23
 chlamydial A56.19
 filarial —see also Infestation, filarial B74.9
  [N51]
 gonococcal (acute) (chronic) A54.23
 mumps B26.0
 syphilitic A52.76
 tuberculous A18.15
Orf (virus disease) B08.02
Organic —see also condition
 brain syndrome F09
 heart —see Disease, heart
 mental disorder F09
 psychosis F09
Orgasm
 anejaculatory N53.13
Oriental
 bilharziasis B65.2
 schistosomiasis B65.2
Orifice —see condition
Origin of both great vessels from right
  ventricle Q20.1
Ormond's disease (with ureteral obstruction)
  N13.5
 with infection N13.6
Ornithine metabolism disorder E72.4
Ornithinemia (Type I) (Type II) E72.4
Ornithosis A70
Orotaciduria, oroticaciduria (congenital)
  (hereditary) (pyrimidine deficiency) E79.8
 anemia D53.0
Orthodontics
 adjustment Z46.4
 fitting Z46.4
Orthopnea R06.01

▶ New   ⇒ Revised   ~~deleted~~ Deleted   ● Use Additional Character(s)

Orthopoxvirus B08.09
    specified NEC B08.09
Os, uterus —see condition
Osgood-Schlatter disease or
        osteochondrosis —see Osteochondrosis,
        juvenile, tibia
Osler (-Weber)-Rendu disease I78.0
Osler's nodes I33.0
Osmidrosis L75.0
Osseous —see condition
Ossification
    artery —see Arteriosclerosis
    auricle (ear) —see Disorder, pinna, specified
        type NEC
    bronchial J98.09
    cardiac —see Degeneration, myocardial
    cartilage (senile) —see Disorder, cartilage,
        specified type NEC
    coronary (artery) —see Disease, heart,
        ischemic, atherosclerotic
    diaphragm J98.6
    ear, middle —see Otosclerosis
    falx cerebri G96.19
    fontanel, premature Q75.0
    heart —see also Degeneration, myocardial
        valve —see Endocarditis
    larynx J38.7
    ligament —see Disorder, tendon, specified
        type NEC
        posterior longitudinal —see
            Spondylopathy, specified NEC
    meninges (cerebral) (spinal) G96.19
    multiple, eccentric centers —see Disorder,
        bone, development or growth
    muscle —see also Calcification, muscle
        due to burns —see Myositis, ossificans, in,
            burns
        paralytic —see Myositis, ossificans, in,
            quadriplegia
        progressive —see Myositis, ossificans,
            progressiva
        specified NEC M61.50
            ankle M61.57-●
            foot M61.57-●
            forearm M61.53-●
            hand M61.54-●
            lower leg M61.56-●
            multiple sites M61.59
            pelvic region M61.55-●
            shoulder region M61.51-●
            specified site NEC M61.58
            thigh M61.55-●
            upper arm M61.52-●
        traumatic —see Myositis, ossificans,
            traumatica
    myocardium, myocardial —see Degeneration,
        myocardial
    penis N48.89
    periarticular —see Disorder, joint, specified
        type NEC
    pinna —see Disorder, pinna, specified type
        NEC
    rider's bone —see Ossification, muscle,
        specified NEC
    sclera H15.89
    subperiosteal, post-traumatic M89.8X-●
    tendon —see Disorder, tendon, specified
        type NEC
    trachea J39.8
    tympanic membrane —see Disorder,
        tympanic membrane, specified NEC
    vitreous (humor) —see Deposit, crystalline
Osteitis —see also Osteomyelitis
    alveolar M27.3
    condensans M85.30
        ankle M85.37-●
        foot M85.37-●
        forearm M85.33-●
        hand M85.34-●
        lower leg M85.36-●
        multiple site M85.39

Osteitis (Continued)
    condensans (Continued)
        neck M85.38
        rib M85.38
        shoulder M85.31-●
        skull M85.38
        specified site NEC M85.38
        thigh M85.35-●
        toe M85.37-●
        upper arm M85.32-●
        vertebra M85.38
    deformans M88.9
        in (due to)
            malignant neoplasm of bone
                C41.9 [M90.60]
            neoplastic disease —see also Neoplasm
                D49.9 [M90.60]
            carpus D49.9 [M90.64-●]
            clavicle D49.9 [M90.61-●]
            femur D49.9 [M90.65-●]
            fibula D49.9 [M90.66-●]
            finger D49.9 [M90.64-●]
            humerus D49.9 [M90.62-●]
            ilium D49.9 [M90.65-●]
            ischium D49.9 [M90.65-●]
            metacarpus D49.9 [M90.64-●]
            metatarsus D49.9 [M90.67-●]
            multiple sites D49.9 [M90.69]
            neck D49.9 [M90.68]
            radius D49.9 [M90.63-●]
            rib D49.9 [M90.68]
            scapula D49.9 [M90.61-●]
            skull D49.9 [M90.68]
            tarsus D49.9 [M90.67-●]
            tibia D49.9 [M90.66-●]
            toe D49.9 [M90.67-●]
            ulna D49.9 [M90.63-●]
            vertebra D49.9 [M90.68]
        skull M88.0
        specified NEC —see Paget's disease, bone,
            by site
        vertebra M88.1
    due to yaws A66.6
    fibrosa NEC —see Cyst, bone, by site
        circumscripta —see Dysplasia, fibrous,
            bone NEC
        cystica (generalisata) E21.0
        disseminata Q78.1
        osteoplastica E21.0
    fragilitans Q78.0
    Garr's (sclerosing) —see Osteomyelitis,
        specified type NEC
    jaw (acute) (chronic) (lower) (suppurative)
        (upper) M27.2
    parathyroid E21.0
    petrous bone (acute) (chronic) —see Petrositis
    sclerotic, nonsuppurative —see Osteomyelitis,
        specified type NEC
    tuberculosa A18.09
        cystica D86.89
        multiplex cystoides D86.89
Osteoarthritis M19.90
    ankle M19.07-●
    elbow M19.02-●
    foot joint M19.07-●
    generalized M15.9
        erosive M15.4
        primary M15.0
        specified NEC M15.8
    hand joint M19.04-●
        first carpometacarpal joint M18.9-●
    hip M16.1-●
        bilateral M16.0
        due to hip dysplasia (unilateral)
            M16.3-●
            bilateral M16.2
    interphalangeal
        distal (Heberden) M15.1
        proximal (Bouchard) M15.2
    ⇒ knee M17.1-●
        bilateral M17.0

Osteoarthritis (Continued)
    post-traumatic NEC M19.92
        ankle M19.17-●
        elbow M19.12-●
        foot joint M19.17-●
        hand joint M19.14-●
            first carpometacarpal joint M18.3-●
                bilateral M18.2
        hip M16.5-●
            bilateral M16.4
        knee M17.3-●
            bilateral M17.2
        shoulder M19.11-●
        wrist M19.13-●
    primary M19.91
        ankle M19.07-●
        elbow M19.02-●
        foot joint M19.07-●
        hand joint M19.04-●
            first carpometacarpal joint M18.1-●
                bilateral M18.0
        hip M16.1-●
            bilateral M16.0
        knee M17.1-●
            bilateral M17.0
        shoulder M19.01-●
        spine —see Spondylosis
        wrist M19.03-●
    secondary M19.93
        ankle M19.27-●
        elbow M19.22-●
        foot joint M19.27-●
        hand joint M19.24-●
            first carpometacarpal joint M18.5-●
                bilateral M18.4
        hip M16.7
            bilateral M16.6
        knee M17.5
            bilateral M17.4
        multiple M15.3
        shoulder M19.21-●
        spine —see Spondylosis
        wrist M19.23-●
    shoulder M19.01-●
    spine —see Spondylosis
    wrist M19.03-●
Osteoarthropathy (hypertrophic) M19.90
    ankle —see Osteoarthritis, primary, ankle
    elbow —see Osteoarthritis, primary, elbow
    foot joint —see Osteoarthritis, primary, foot
    hand joint —see Osteoarthritis, primary, hand
        joint
    knee joint —see Osteoarthritis, primary, knee
    multiple site —see Osteoarthritis, primary,
        multiple joint
    pulmonary —see also Osteoarthropathy,
        specified type NEC
        hypertrophic —see Osteoarthropathy,
            hypertrophic, specified type NEC
    secondary —see Osteoarthropathy, specified
        type NEC
    secondary hypertrophic —see
        Osteoarthropathy, specified type NEC
    shoulder —see Osteoarthritis, primary,
        shoulder
    specified joint NEC —see Osteoarthritis,
        primary, specified joint NEC
    specified type NEC M89.40
        carpus M89.44-●
        clavicle M89.41-●
        femur M89.45-●
        fibula M89.46-●
        finger M89.44-●
        humerus M89.42-●
        ilium M89.459
        ischium M89.459
        metacarpus M89.44-●
        metatarsus M89.47-●
        multiple sites M89.49
        neck M89.48
        radius M89.43-●

Osteoarthropathy *(Continued)*
  specified type NEC *(Continued)*
    rib M89.48
    scapula M89.41-•
    skull M89.48
    tarsus M89.47-•
    tibia M89.46-•
    toe M89.47-•
    ulna M89.43-•
    vertebra M89.48
  spine —*see* Spondylosis
  wrist —*see* Osteoarthritis, primary, wrist
Osteoarthrosis (degenerative) (hypertrophic)
    (joint) —*see also* Osteoarthritis
  deformans alkaptonurica E70.29 *[M36.8]*
  erosive M15.4
  generalized M15.9
    primary M15.0
  polyarticular M15.9
  spine —*see* Spondylosis
Osteoblastoma —*see* Neoplasm, bone, benign
  aggressive —*see* Neoplasm, bone, uncertain
    behavior
Osteochondroarthrosis deformans
    endemica —*see* Disease, Kaschin-Beck
Osteochondritis —*see also* Osteochondropathy,
    by site
  Brailsford's —*see* Osteochondrosis, juvenile,
    radius
  dissecans M93.20
    ankle M93.27-•
    elbow M93.22-•
    foot M93.27-•
    hand M93.24-•
    hip M93.25-•
    knee M93.26-•
    multiple sites M93.29
    shoulder joint M93.21-•
    specified site NEC M93.28
    wrist M93.23-•
  juvenile M92.9
    patellar —*see* Osteochondrosis, juvenile,
      patella
  syphilitic (congenital) (early) A50.02
    [M90.80]
    ankle A50.02 *[M90.87-•]*
    elbow A50.02 *[M90.82-•]*
    foot A50.02 *[M90.87-•]*
    forearm A50.02 *[M90.83-•]*
    hand A50.02 *[M90.84-•]*
    hip A50.02 *[M90.85-•]*
    knee A50.02 *[M90.86•-]*
    multiple sites A50.02 *[M90.89]*
    shoulder joint A50.02 *[M90.81-•]*
    specified site NEC A50.02 *[M90.88]*
Osteochondrodysplasia Q78.9
  with defects of growth of tubular bones and
    spine Q77.9
    specified NEC Q77.8
  specified NEC Q78.8
Osteochondrodystrophy E78.9
Osteochondrolysis —*see* Osteochondritis,
    dissecans
Osteochondroma —*see* Neoplasm, bone, benign
Osteochondromatosis D48.0
  syndrome Q78.4
Osteochondromyxosarcoma —*see* Neoplasm,
    bone, malignant
Osteochondropathy M93.90
  ankle M93.97-•
  elbow M93.92-•
  foot M93.97-•
  hand M93.94-•
  hip M93.95-•
  Kienböck's disease of adults M93.1
  knee M93.96-•
  multiple joints M93.99
  osteochondritis dissecans —*see*
    Osteochondritis, dissecans
  osteochondrosis —*see* Osteochondrosis
  shoulder region M93.91-•

Osteochondropathy *(Continued)*
  slipped upper femoral epiphysis —*see*
    Slipped, epiphysis, upper femoral
  specified joint NEC M93.98
  specified type NEC M93.80
    ankle M93.87-•
    elbow M93.82-•
    foot M93.87-•
    hand M93.84-•
    hip M93.85-•
    knee M93.86-•
    multiple joints M93.89
    shoulder region M93.81-•
    specified joint NEC M93.88
    wrist M93.83-•
  syphilitic, congenital
    early A50.02 *[M90.80]*
    late A50.56 *[M90.80]*
  wrist M93.93-•
Osteochondrosarcoma —*see* Neoplasm, bone,
    malignant
Osteochondrosis —*see also* Osteochondropathy,
    by site
  acetabulum (juvenile) M91.0
  adult —*see* Osteochondropathy, specified
    type NEC, by site
  astragalus (juvenile) —*see* Osteochondrosis,
    juvenile, tarsus
  Blount's —*see* Osteochondrosis, juvenile, tibia
  Buchanan's M91.0
  Burns' —*see* Osteochondrosis, juvenile, ulna
  calcaneus (juvenile) —*see* Osteochondrosis,
    juvenile, tarsus
  capitular epiphysis (femur) (juvenile) —*see*
    Legg-Calvé-Perthes disease
  carpal (juvenile) (lunate) (scaphoid) —*see*
    Osteochondrosis, juvenile, hand, carpal
    lunate
    adult M93.1
  coxae juvenilis —*see* Legg-Calvé-Perthes
    disease
  deformans juvenilis, coxae —*see* Legg-Calvé-
    Perthes disease
  Diaz's —*see* Osteochondrosis, juvenile, tarsus
  dissecans (knee) (shoulder) —*see*
    Osteochondritis, dissecans
  femoral capital epiphysis (juvenile) —*see*
    Legg-Calvé-Perthes disease
  femur (head), juvenile —*see* Legg-Calvé-
    Perthes disease
  fibula (juvenile) —*see* Osteochondrosis,
    juvenile, fibula
  foot NEC (juvenile) M92.8
  Freiberg's —*see* Osteochondrosis, juvenile,
    metatarsus
  Haas' (juvenile) —*see* Osteochondrosis,
    juvenile, humerus
  Haglund's —*see* Osteochondrosis, juvenile,
    tarsus
  hip (juvenile) —*see* Legg-Calvé-Perthes disease
  humerus (capitulum) (head) (juvenile) —*see*
    Osteochondrosis, juvenile, humerus
  ilium, iliac crest (juvenile) M91.0
  ischiopubic synchondrosis M91.0
  Iselin's —*see* Osteochondrosis, juvenile,
    metatarsus
  juvenile, juvenilis M92.9
    after congenital dislocation of hip
      reduction —*see* Osteochondrosis,
      juvenile, hip, specified NEC
    arm —*see* Osteochondrosis, juvenile, upper
      limb NEC
    capitular epiphysis (femur) —*see* Legg-
      Calvé-Perthes disease
    clavicle, sternal epiphysis —*see*
      Osteochondrosis, juvenile, upper limb
      NEC
    coxae —*see* Legg-Calvé-Perthes disease
    deformans M92.9
    fibula M92.5-•
    foot NEC M92.8

Osteochondrosis *(Continued)*
  juvenile, juvenilis *(Continued)*
    hand M92.20-•
      carpal lunate M92.21-•
      metacarpal head M92.22-•
      specified site NEC M92.29-•
    head of femur —*see* Legg-Calvé-Perthes
      disease
    hip and pelvis M91.9-•
      coxa plana —*see* Coxa, plana
      femoral head —*see* Legg-Calvé-Perthes
        disease
      pelvis M91.0
      pseudocoxalgia —*see* Pseudocoxalgia
      specified NEC M91.8-•
    humerus M92.0-•
    limb
      lower NEC M92.8
      upper NEC —*see* Osteochondrosis,
        juvenile, upper limb NEC
    medial cuneiform bone —*see*
      Osteochondrosis, juvenile, tarsus
    metatarsus M92.7-•
    patella M92.4-•
    radius M92.1-•
    specified site NEC M92.8
    spine M42.00
      cervical region M42.02
      cervicothoracic region M42.03
      lumbar region M42.06
      lumbosacral region M42.07
      multiple sites M42.09
      occipito-atlanto-axial region M42.01
      sacrococcygeal region M42.08
      thoracic region M42.04
      thoracolumbar region M42.05
    tarsus M92.6-•
    tibia M92.5-•
    ulna M92.1-•
    upper limb NEC M92.3-•
    vertebra (body) (epiphyseal plates)
      (Calvé's) (Scheuermann's) —*see*
      Osteochondrosis, juvenile, spine
  Kienböck's —*see* Osteochondrosis, juvenile,
    hand, carpal lunate
    adult M93.1
  Köhler's
    patellar —*see* Osteochondrosis, juvenile,
      patella
    tarsal navicular —*see* Osteochondrosis,
      juvenile, tarsus
  Legg-Perthes (-Calvé's) (-Waldenström) —*see*
    Legg-Calvé-Perthes disease
  limb
    lower NEC (juvenile) M92.8
    upper NEC (juvenile) —*see*
      Osteochondrosis, juvenile, upper limb
      NEC
  lunate bone (carpal) (juvenile) —*see also*
    Osteochondrosis, juvenile, hand, carpal
    lunate
    adult M93.1
  Mauclaire's —*see* Osteochondrosis, juvenile,
    hand, metacarpal
  metacarpal (head) (juvenile) —*see*
    Osteochondrosis, juvenile, hand,
    metacarpal
  metatarsus (fifth) (head) (juvenile)
    (second) —*see* Osteochondrosis, juvenile,
    metatarsus
  navicular (juvenile) —*see* Osteochondrosis,
    juvenile, tarsus
  os
    calcis (juvenile) —*see* Osteochondrosis,
      juvenile, tarsus
    tibiale externum (juvenile) —*see*
      Osteochondrosis, juvenile, tarsus
  Osgood-Schlatter —*see* Osteochondrosis,
    juvenile, tibia
  Panner's —*see* Osteochondrosis, juvenile,
    humerus

Osteochondrosis *(Continued)*
  patellar center (juvenile) (primary)
      (secondary) —*see* Osteochondrosis,
      juvenile, patella
  pelvis (juvenile) M91.0
  Pierson's M91.0
  radius (head) (juvenile) —*see*
      Osteochondrosis, juvenile, radius
  Scheuermann's —*see* Osteochondrosis,
      juvenile, spine
  Sever's —*see* Osteochondrosis, juvenile,
      tarsus
  Sinding-Larsen —*see* Osteochondrosis,
      juvenile, patella
  spine M42.9
    adult M42.10
      cervical region M42.12
      cervicothoracic region M42.13
      lumbar region M42.16
      lumbosacral region M42.17
      multiple sites M42.19
      occipito-atlanto-axial region M42.11
      sacrococcygeal region M42.18
      thoracic region M42.14
      thoracolumbar region M42.15
    juvenile —*see* Osteochondrosis, juvenile,
        spine
  symphysis pubis (juvenile) M91.0
  syphilitic (congenital) A50.02
  talus (juvenile) —*see* Osteochondrosis,
      juvenile, tarsus
  tarsus (navicular) (juvenile) —*see*
      Osteochondrosis, juvenile, tarsus
  tibia (proximal) (tubercle) (juvenile) —*see*
      Osteochondrosis, juvenile, tibia
  tuberculous —*see* Tuberculosis, bone
  ulna (lower) (juvenile) —*see* Osteochondrosis,
      juvenile, ulna
  van Neck's M91.0
  vertebral —*see* Osteochondrosis,
      spine
Osteoclastoma D48.0
  malignant —*see* Neoplasm, bone,
      malignant
Osteodynia —*see* Disorder, bone,
    specified type NEC
Osteodystrophy Q78.9
  azotemic N25.0
  congenital Q78.9
  parathyroid, secondary E21.1
  renal N25.0
Osteofibroma —*see* Neoplasm, bone,
    benign
Osteofibrosarcoma —*see* Neoplasm,
    bone, malignant
Osteogenesis imperfecta Q78.0
Osteogenic —*see* condition
Osteolysis M89.50
  carpus M89.54-●
  clavicle M89.51-●
  femur M89.55-●
  fibula M89.56-●
  finger M89.54-●
  humerus M89.52-●
  ilium M89.559
  ischium M89.559
  joint prosthesis (periprosthetic) —*see*
      Complications, joint prosthesis,
      mechanical, periprosthetic, osteolysis,
      by site
  metacarpus M89.54-●
  metatarsus M89.57-●
  multiple sites M89.59
  neck M89.58
  periprosthetic —*see* Complications, joint
      prosthesis, mechanical, periprosthetic,
      osteolysis, by site
  radius M89.53-●
  rib M89.58
  scapula M89.51-●
  skull M89.58

Osteolysis *(Continued)*
  tarsus M89.57-●
  tibia M89.56-●
  toe M89.57-●
  ulna M89.53-●
  vertebra M89.58
Osteoma —*see also* Neoplasm, bone, benign
  osteoid —*see also* Neoplasm, bone, benign
    giant —*see* Neoplasm, bone, benign
Osteomalacia M83.9
  adult M83.9
    drug-induced NEC M83.5
    due to
      malabsorption (postsurgical) M83.2
      malnutrition M83.3
    specified NEC M83.8
  aluminium-induced M83.4
  infantile —*see* Rickets
  juvenile —*see* Rickets
  oncogenic E83.89
  pelvis M83.8
  puerperal M83.0
  senile M83.1
  vitamin-D-resistant in adults E83.31
      [M90.8-●]
    carpus E83.31 [M90.84-●]
    clavicle E83.31 [M90.81-●]
    femur E83.31 [M90.85-●]
    fibula E83.31 [M90.86-●]
    finger E83.31 [M90.84-●]
    humerus E83.31 [M90.82-●]
    ilium E83.31 [M90.859]
    ischium E83.31 [M90.859]
    metacarpus E83.31 [M90.84-●]
    metatarsus E83.31 [M90.87-●]
    multiple sites E83.31 [M90.89]
    neck E83.31 [M90.88]
    radius E83.31 [M90.83-●]
    rib E83.31 [M90.88]
    scapula E83.31 [M90.819]
    skull E83.31 [M90.88]
    tarsus E83.31 [M90.879]
    tibia E83.31 [M90.869]
    toe E83.31 [M90.879]
    ulna E83.31 [M90.839]
    vertebra E83.31 [M90.88]
Osteomyelitis (general) (infective)
    (localized) (neonatal) (purulent)
    (septic) (staphylococcal) (streptococcal)
    (suppurative) (with periostitis) M86.9
  acute M86.10
    carpus M86.14-●
    clavicle M86.11-●
    femur M86.15-●
    fibula M86.16-●
    finger M86.14-●
    hematogenous M86.00
      carpus M86.04-●
      clavicle M86.01-●
      femur M86.05-●
      fibula M86.06-●
      finger M86.04-●
      humerus M86.02-●
      ilium M86.059
      ischium M86.059
      mandible M27.2
      metacarpus M86.04-●
      metatarsus M86.07-●
      multiple sites M86.09
      neck M86.08
      orbit H05.02-●
      petrous bone —*see* Petrositis
      radius M86.03-●
      rib M86.08
      scapula M86.01-●
      skull M86.08
      tarsus M86.07-●
      tibia M86.06-●
      toe M86.07-●
      ulna M86.03-●
      vertebra —*see* Osteomyelitis, vertebra

Osteomyelitis *(Continued)*
  acute *(Continued)*
    humerus M86.12-●
    ilium M86.159
    ischium M86.159
    mandible M27.2
    metacarpus M86.14-●
    metatarsus M86.17-●
    multiple sites M86.19
    neck M86.18
    orbit H05.02-●
    petrous bone —*see* Petrositis
    radius M86.13-●
    rib M86.18
    scapula M86.11-●
    skull M86.18
    tarsus M86.17-●
    tibia M86.16-●
    toe M86.17-●
    ulna M86.13-●
    vertebra —*see* Osteomyelitis, vertebra
  chronic (or old) M86.60
    with draining sinus M86.40
      carpus M86.44-●
      clavicle M86.41-●
      femur M86.45-●
      fibula M86.46-●
      finger M86.44-●
      humerus M86.42-●
      ilium M86.459
      ischium M86.459
      mandible M27.2
      metacarpus M86.44-●
      metatarsus M86.47-●
      multiple sites M86.49
      neck M86.48
      orbit H05.02-●
      petrous bone —*see* Petrositis
      radius M86.43-●
      rib M86.48
      scapula M86.41-●
      skull M86.48
      tarsus M86.47-●
      tibia M86.46-●
      toe M86.47-●
      ulna M86.43-●
      vertebra —*see* Osteomyelitis,
          vertebra
    carpus M86.64-●
    clavicle M86.61-●
    femur M86.65-●
    fibula M86.66-●
    finger M86.64-●
    hematogenous NEC M86.50
      carpus M86.54-●
      clavicle M86.51-●
      femur M86.55-●
      fibula M86.56-●
      finger M86.54-●
      humerus M86.52-●
      ilium M86.559
      ischium M86.559
      mandible M27.2
      metacarpus M86.54-●
      metatarsus M86.57-●
      multifocal M86.30
        carpus M86.34-●
        clavicle M86.31-●
        femur M86.35-●
        fibula M86.36-●
        finger M86.34-●
        humerus M86.32-●
        ilium M86.359
        ischium M86.359
        metacarpus M86.34-●
        metatarsus M86.37-●
        multiple sites M86.39
        neck M86.38
        radius M86.33-●
        rib M86.38
        scapula M86.31-●

Osteomyelitis *(Continued)*
  chronic *(Continued)*
    hematogenous NEC *(Continued)*
      multifocal *(Continued)*
        skull M86.38
        tarsus M86.37-•
        tibia M86.36-•
        toe M86.37-•
        ulna M86.33-•
        vertebra —*see* Osteomyelitis, vertebra
      multiple sites M86.59
      neck M86.58
      orbit H05.02-•
      petrous bone —*see* Petrositis
      radius M86.53-•
      rib M86.58
      scapula M86.51-•
      skull M86.58
      tarsus M86.57-•
      tibia M86.56-•
      toe M86.57-•
      ulna M86.53-•
      vertebra —*see* Osteomyelitis, vertebra
    humerus M86.62-•
    ilium M86.659
    ischium M86.659
    mandible M27.2
    metacarpus M86.64-•
    metatarsus M86.67-•
    multifocal —*see* Osteomyelitis, chronic, hematogenous, multifocal
    multiple sites M86.69
    neck M86.68
    orbit H05.02-•
    petrous bone —*see* Petrositis
    radius M86.63-•
    rib M86.68
    scapula M86.61-•
    skull M86.68
    tarsus M86.67-•
    tibia M86.66-•
    toe M86.67-•
    ulna M86.63-•
    vertebra —*see* Osteomyelitis, vertebra
  echinococcal B67.2
  Garr's —*see* Osteomyelitis, specified type NEC
  in diabetes mellitus —*see* E08-E13 with .69
  jaw (acute) (chronic) (lower) (neonatal) (suppurative) (upper) M27.2
  nonsuppurating —*see* Osteomyelitis, specified type NEC
  orbit H05.02-•
  petrous bone —*see* Petrositis
  Salmonella (arizonae) (cholerae-suis) (enteritidis) (typhimurium) A02.24
  sclerosing, nonsuppurative —*see* Osteomyelitis, specified type NEC
  specified type NEC —*see also* subcategory M86.8X-•
    mandible M27.2
    orbit H05.02-•
    petrous bone —*see* Petrositis
    vertebra —*see* Osteomyelitis, vertebra
  subacute M86.20
    carpus M86.24-•
    clavicle M86.21-•
    femur M86.25-•
    fibula M86.26-•
    finger M86.24-•
    humerus M86.22-•
    mandible M27.2
    metacarpus M86.24-•
    metatarsus M86.27-•
    multiple sites M86.29
    neck M86.28
    orbit H05.02-•
    petrous bone —*see* Petrositis
    radius M86.23-•
    rib M86.28
    scapula M86.21-•

Osteomyelitis *(Continued)*
  subacute *(Continued)*
    skull M86.28
    tarsus M86.27-•
    tibia M86.26-•
    toe M86.27-•
    ulna M86.23-•
    vertebra —*see* Osteomyelitis, vertebra
  syphilitic A52.77
    congenital (early) A50.02 *[M90.80]*
  tuberculous —*see* Tuberculosis, bone
  typhoid A01.05
  vertebra M46.20
    cervical region M46.22
    cervicothoracic region M46.23
    lumbar region M46.26
    lumbosacral region M46.27
    occipito-atlanto-axial region M46.21
    sacrococcygeal region M46.28
    thoracic region M46.24
    thoracolumbar region M46.25
Osteomyelofibrosis D47.4
Osteomyelosclerosis D75.89
Osteonecrosis M87.9
  due to
    drugs —*see* Osteonecrosis, secondary, due to, drugs
    trauma —*see* Osteonecrosis, secondary, due to, trauma
  idiopathic aseptic M87.00
    ankle M87.07-•
    carpus M87.03-•
    clavicle M87.01-•
    femur M87.05-•
    fibula M87.06-•
    finger M87.04-•
    humerus M87.02-•
    ilium M87.050
    ischium M87.050
    metacarpus M87.04-•
    metatarsus M87.07-•
    multiple sites M87.09
    neck M87.08
    pelvis M87.050
    radius M87.03-•
    rib M87.08
    scapula M87.01-•
    skull M87.08
    tarsus M87.07-•
    tibia M87.06-•
    toe M87.07-•
    ulna M87.03-•
    vertebra M87.08
  secondary NEC M87.30
    carpus M87.33-•
    clavicle M87.31-•
    due to
      drugs M87.10
        carpus M87.13-•
        clavicle M87.11-•
        femur M87.15-•
        fibula M87.16-•
        finger M87.14-•
        humerus M87.12-•
        ilium M87.159
        ischium M87.159
        jaw M87.180
        metacarpus M87.14-•
        metatarsus M87.17-•
        multiple sites M87.19
        neck M87.18
        radius M87.13-•
        rib M87.18
        scapula M87.11-•
        skull M87.18
        tarsus M87.17-•
        tibia M87.16-•
        toe M87.17-•
        ulna M87.13-•
        vertebra M87.18

Osteonecrosis *(Continued)*
  secondary NEC *(Continued)*
    due to *(Continued)*
      hemoglobinopathy NEC D58.2 *[M90.50]*
        carpus D58.2 *[M90.54-•]*
        clavicle D58.2 *[M90.51-•]*
        femur D58.2 *[M90.55-•]*
        fibula D58.2 *[M90.56-•]*
        finger D58.2 *[M90.54-•]*
        humerus D58.2 *[M90.52-•]*
        ilium D58.2 *[M90.55-•]*
        ischium D58.2 *[M90.55-•]*
        metacarpus D58.2 *[M90.54-•]*
        metatarsus D58.2 *[M90.57-•]*
        multiple sites D58.2 *[M90.58]*
        neck D58.2 *[M90.58]*
        radius D58.2 *[M90.53-•]*
        rib D58.2 *[M90.58]*
        scapula D58.2 *[M90.51-•]*
        skull D58.2 *[M90.58]*
        tarsus D58.2 *[M90.57-•]*
        tibia D58.2 *[M90.56-•]*
        toe D58.2 *[M90.57-•]*
        ulna D58.2 *[M90.53-•]*
        vertebra D58.2 *[M90.58]*
      trauma (previous) M87.20
        carpus M87.23-•
        clavicle M87.21-•
        femur M87.25-•
        fibula M87.26-•
        finger M87.24-•
        humerus M87.22-•
        ilium M87.25-•
        ischium M87.25-•
        metacarpus M87.24-•
        metatarsus M87.27-•
        multiple sites M87.29
        neck M87.28
        radius M87.23-•
        rib M87.28
        scapula M87.21-•
        skull M87.28
        tarsus M87.27-•
        tibia M87.26-•
        toe M87.27-•
        ulna M87.23-•
        vertebra M87.28
    femur M87.35-•
    fibula M87.36-•
    finger M87.34-•
    humerus M87.32
    ilium M87.350
    in
      caisson disease T70.3 *[M90.50]*
        carpus T70.3 *[M90.54-•]*
        clavicle T70.3 *[M90.51-•]*
        femur T70.3 *[M90.55-•]*
        fibula T70.3 *[M90.56-•]*
        finger T70.3 *[M90.54-•]*
        humerus T70.3 *[M90.52-•]*
        ilium T70.3 *[M90.55-•]*
        ischium T70.3 *[M90.55-•]*
        metacarpus T70.3 *[M90.54-•]*
        metatarsus T70.3 *[M90.57-•]*
        multiple sites T70.3 *[M90.59]*
        neck T70.3 *[M90.58]*
        radius T70.3 *[M90.53-•]*
        rib T70.3 *[M90.58]*
        scapula T70.3 *[M90.51-•]*
        skull T70.3 *[M90.58]*
        tarsus T70.3 *[M90.57-•]*
        tibia T70.3 *[M90.56-•]*
        toe T70.3 *[M90.57-•]*
        ulna T70.3 *[M90.53-•]*
        vertebra T70.3 *[M90.58]*
    ischium M87.350
    metacarpus M87.34-•
    metatarsus M87.37-•
    multiple site M87.39
    neck M87.38

▶ New   ⇛ Revised   ~~deleted~~ Deleted   • Use Additional Character(s)

Osteonecrosis (Continued)
  secondary NEC (Continued)
    radius M87.33-●
    rib M87.38
    scapula M87.319
    skull M87.38
    tarsus M87.379
    tibia M87.366
    toe M87.379
    ulna M87.33-●
    vertebra M87.38
  specified type NEC M87.80
    carpus M87.83-●
    clavicle M87.81-●
    femur M87.85-●
    fibula M87.86-●
    finger M87.84-●
    humerus M87.82-●
    ilium M87.85-●
    ischium M87.85-●
    metacarpus M87.84-●
    metatarsus M87.87-●
    multiple sites M87.89
    neck M87.88
    radius M87.83-●
    rib M87.88-●
    scapula M87.81-●
    skull M87.88
    tarsus M87.87-●
    tibia M87.86-●
    toe M87.87-●
    ulna M87.83-●
    vertebra M87.88
Osteo-onycho-arthro-dysplasia Q87.2
Osteo-onychodysplasia, hereditary Q87.2
Osteopathia condensans disseminata Q78.8
Osteopathy —see also Osteomyelitis,
  Osteonecrosis, Osteoporosis
  after poliomyelitis M89.60
    carpus M89.64-●
    clavicle M89.61-●
    femur M89.65-●
    fibula M89.66-●
    finger M89.64-●
    humerus M89.62-●
    ilium M89.659
    ischium M89.659
    metacarpus M89.64-●
    metatarsus M89.67-●
    multiple sites M89.69
    neck M89.68
    radius M89.63-●
    rib M89.68
    scapula M89.61-●
    skull M89.68
    tarsus M89.67-●
    tibia M89.66-●
    toe M89.67-●
    ulna M89.63-●
    vertebra M89.68
  in (due to)
    renal osteodystrophy N25.0
    specified diseases classified elsewhere —
      see subcategory M90.8
Osteopenia M85.8-●
  borderline M85.8-●
Osteoperiostitis —see Osteomyelitis, specified
  type NEC
Osteopetrosis (familial) Q78.2
Osteophyte M25.70
  ankle M25.77-●
  elbow M25.72-●
  foot joint M25.77-●
  hand joint M25.74-●
  hip M25.75-●
  knee M25.76-●
  shoulder M25.71-●
  spine M25.78
  vertebrae M25.78
  wrist M25.73-●
Osteopoikilosis Q78.8

Osteoporosis (female) (male) M81.0
  with current pathological fracture M80.00
  age-related M81.0
    with current pathologic fracture M80.00
      carpus M80.04-●
      clavicle M80.01-●
      fibula M80.06-●
      finger M80.04-●
      humerus M80.02-●
      ilium M80.05-●
      ischium M80.05-●
      metacarpus M80.04-●
      metatarsus M80.07-●
      pelvis M80.05-●
      radius M80.03-●
      scapula M80.01-●
      tarsus M80.07-●
      tibia M80.06-●
      toe M80.07-●
      ulna M80.03-●
      vertebra M80.08
  disuse M81.8
    with current pathological fracture M80.80
      carpus M80.84-●
      clavicle M80.81-●
      fibula M80.86-●
      finger M80.84-●
      humerus M80.82-●
      ilium M80.85-●
      ischium M80.85-●
      metacarpus M80.84-●
      metatarsus M80.87-●
      pelvis M80.85-●
      radius M80.83-●
      scapula M80.81-●
      tarsus M80.87-●
      tibia M80.86-●
      toe M80.87-●
      ulna M80.83-●
      vertebra M80.88
  drug-induced —see Osteoporosis, specified
    type NEC
  idiopathic —see Osteoporosis, specified type
    NEC
  involutional —see Osteoporosis, age-related
  Lequesne M81.6
  localized M81.6
  postmenopausal M81.0
    with pathological fracture M80.00
      carpus M80.04-●
      clavicle M80.01-●
      fibula M80.06-●
      finger M80.04-●
      humerus M80.02-●
      ilium M80.05-●
      ischium M80.05-●
      metacarpus M80.04-●
      metatarsus M80.07-●
      pelvis M80.05-●
      radius M80.03-●
      scapula M80.01-●
      tarsus M80.07-●
      tibia M80.06-●
      toe M80.07-●
      ulna M80.03-●
      vertebra M80.08
  postoophorectomy —see Osteoporosis,
    specified type NEC
  postsurgical malabsorption —see
    Osteoporosis, specified type NEC
  post-traumatic —see Osteoporosis, specified
    type NEC
  senile —see Osteoporosis, age-related
  specified type NEC M81.8
    with pathological fracture M80.80
      carpus M80.84-●
      clavicle M80.81-●
      fibula M80.86-●
      finger M80.84-●
      humerus M80.82-●
      ilium M80.85-●

Osteoporosis (Continued)
  specified type NEC (Continued)
    with pathological fracture (Continued)
      ischium M80.85-●
      metacarpus M80.84-●
      metatarsus M80.87-●
      pelvis M80.85-●
      radius M80.83-●
      scapula M80.81-●
      tarsus M80.87-●
      tibia M80.86-●
      toe M80.87-●
      ulna M80.83-●
      vertebra M80.88
Osteopsathyrosis (idiopathica) Q78.0
Osteoradionecrosis, jaw (acute) (chronic)
  (lower) (suppurative) (upper)
  M27.2
Osteosarcoma (any form) —see Neoplasm,
  bone, malignant
Osteosclerosis Q78.2
  acquired M85.8-●
  congenita Q77.4
  fragilitas (generalisata) Q78.2
  myelofibrosis D75.81
Osteosclerotic anemia D64.89
Osteosis
  cutis L94.2
  renal fibrocystic N25.0
Österreicher-Turner syndrome Q87.2
Ostium
  atrioventriculare commune Q21.2
  primum (arteriosum) (defect) (persistent)
    Q21.2
  secundum (arteriosum) (defect) (patent)
    (persistent) Q21.1
Ostrum-Furst syndrome Q75.8
Otalgia —see subcategory H92.0
Otitis (acute) H66.90
  with effusion —see also Otitis, media,
    nonsuppurative
    purulent —see Otitis, media, suppurative
  adhesive —see subcategory H74.1
  chronic —see also Otitis, media, chronic
    with effusion —see also Otitis, media,
      nonsuppurative, chronic
  externa H60.9-●
    abscess —see Abscess, ear, external
    acute (noninfective) H60.50-●
      actinic H60.51-●
      chemical H60.52-●
      contact H60.53-●
      eczematoid H60.54-●
      infective —see Otitis, externa, infective
      reactive H60.55-●
      specified NEC H60.59-●
    cellulitis —see Cellulitis, ear
    chronic H60.6-●
    diffuse —see Otitis, externa, infective,
      diffuse
    hemorrhagic —see Otitis, externa, infective,
      hemorrhagic
    in (due to)
      aspergillosis B44.89
      candidiasis B37.84
      erysipelas A46 [H62.40]
      herpes (simplex) virus infection B00.1
        zoster B02.8
      impetigo L01.00 [H62.40]
      infectious disease NEC B99 [H62.4-●]
      mycosis NEC B36.9 [H62.40]
      parasitic disease NEC B89 [H62.40]
      viral disease NEC B34.9 [H62.40]
      zoster B02.8
    infective NEC H60.39-●
      abscess —see Abscess, ear, external
      cellulitis —see Cellulitis, ear
      diffuse H60.31-●
      hemorrhagic H60.32-●
      swimmer's ear —see Swimmer's, ear
    malignant H60.2-●

Otitis *(Continued)*
  externa *(Continued)*
    mycotic NEC B36.9 *[H62.40]*
      in
        aspergillosis B44.89
        candidiasis B37.84
        moniliasis B37.84
    necrotizing —*see* Otitis, externa,
        malignant
    Pseudomonas aeruginosa —*see* Otitis,
        externa, malignant
    reactive —*see* Otitis, externa, acute,
        reactive
    specified NEC —*see* subcategory H60.8
    tropical NEC B36.9 *[H62.40]*
      in
        aspergillosis B44.89
        candidiasis B37.84
        moniliasis B37.84
  insidiosa —*see* Otosclerosis
  interna —*see* subcategory H83.0
  media (hemorrhagic) (staphylococcal)
      (streptococcal) H66.9-●
    with effusion (nonpurulent) —*see* Otitis,
        media, nonsuppurative
    acute, subacute H66.90
      allergic —*see* Otitis, media,
          nonsuppurative, acute, allergic
      exudative —*see* Otitis, media,
          suppurative, acute
      mucoid —*see* Otitis, media,
          nonsuppurative, acute
      necrotizing —*see also* Otitis, media,
          suppurative, acute
        in
          measles B05.3
          scarlet fever A38.0
      nonsuppurative NEC —*see* Otitis, media,
          nonsuppurative, acute
      purulent —*see* Otitis, media,
          suppurative, acute
      sanguinous —*see* Otitis, media,
          nonsuppurative, acute
      secretory —*see* Otitis, media,
          nonsuppurative, acute, serous
      seromucinous —*see* Otitis, media,
          nonsuppurative, acute
      serous —*see* Otitis, media,
          nonsuppurative, acute, serous
      suppurative —*see* Otitis, media,
          suppurative, acute
    allergic —*see* Otitis, media, nonsuppurative
    catarrhal —*see* Otitis, media,
        nonsuppurative
    chronic H66.90
      with effusion (nonpurulent) —*see* Otitis,
          media, nonsuppurative, chronic
      allergic —*see* Otitis, media,
          nonsuppurative, chronic, allergic
      benign suppurative —*see* Otitis, media,
          suppurative, chronic, tubotympanic
      catarrhal —*see* Otitis, media,
          nonsuppurative, chronic, serous
      exudative —*see* Otitis, media,
          suppurative, chronic
      mucinous —*see* Otitis, media,
          suppurative, chronic, mucoid
      mucoid —*see* Otitis, media,
          nonsuppurative, chronic, mucoid
      nonsuppurative NEC —*see* Otitis, media,
          nonsuppurative, chronic
      purulent —*see* Otitis, media,
          suppurative, chronic
      secretory —*see* Otitis, media,
          nonsuppurative, chronic, mucoid
      seromucinous —*see* Otitis, media,
          nonsuppurative, chronic
      serous —*see* Otitis, media,
          nonsuppurative, chronic, serous
      suppurative —*see* Otitis, media,
          suppurative, chronic

Otitis *(Continued)*
  media *(Continued)*
    chronic *(Continued)*
      transudative —*see* Otitis, media,
          nonsuppurative, chronic, mucoid
      exudative —*see* Otitis, media,
          nonsuppurative
    in (due to) (with)
      influenza —*see* Influenza, with, otitis
          media
      measles B05.3
      scarlet fever A38.0
      tuberculosis A18.6
      viral disease NEC B34.-● *[H67.-●]*
    mucoid —*see* Otitis, media, nonsuppurative
    nonsuppurative H65.9-●
      acute or subacute NEC H65.19-●
        allergic H65.11-●
          recurrent H65.11-●
        recurrent H65.19-●
        secretory —*see* Otitis, media,
            nonsuppurative, serous
        serous H65.0-●
          recurrent H65.0-●
      chronic H65.49-●
        allergic H65.41-●
        mucoid H65.3-●
        serous H65.2-●
    postmeasles B05.3
    purulent —*see* Otitis, media, suppurative
    secretory —*see* Otitis, media,
        nonsuppurative
    seromucinous —*see* Otitis, media,
        nonsuppurative
    serous —*see* Otitis, media, nonsuppurative
    suppurative H66.4-●
      acute H66.00-●
        with rupture of ear drum H66.01-●
        recurrent H66.00-●
          with rupture of ear drum H66.01-●
      chronic —*see also* subcategory H66.3
        atticoantral H66.2-●
        benign —*see* Otitis, media,
            suppurative, chronic,
            tubotympanic
        tubotympanic H66.1-●
      transudative —*see* Otitis, media,
          nonsuppurative
    tuberculous A18.6
  Otocephaly Q18.2
  Otolith syndrome —*see* subcategory H81.8
  Otomycosis (diffuse) NEC B36.9 *[H62.40]*
    in
      aspergillosis B44.89
      candidiasis B37.84
      moniliasis B37.84
  Otoporosis —*see* Otosclerosis
  Otorrhagia (nontraumatic) H92.2-●
    traumatic - code by Type of injury
  Otorrhea H92.1-●
    cerebrospinal G96.0
  Otosclerosis (general) H80.9-●
    cochlear (endosteal) H80.2-●
    involving
      otic capsule —*see* Otosclerosis, cochlear
      oval window
        nonobliterative H80.0-●
        obliterative H80.1-●
      round window —*see* Otosclerosis, cochlear
    nonobliterative —*see* Otosclerosis, involving,
        oval window, nonobliterative
    obliterative —*see* Otosclerosis, involving, oval
        window, obliterative
    specified NEC H80.8-●
  Otospongiosis —*see* Otosclerosis
  Otto's disease or pelvis M24.7
  Outcome of delivery Z37.9
    multiple births Z37.9
      all liveborn Z37.50
        quadruplets Z37.52
        quintuplets Z37.53

Outcome of delivery *(Continued)*
  multiple births *(Continued)*
    all liveborn *(Continued)*
      sextuplets Z37.54
      specified number NEC Z37.59
      triplets Z37.51
    all stillborn Z37.7
    some liveborn Z37.60
      quadruplets Z37.62
      quintuplets Z37.63
      sextuplets Z37.64
      specified number NEC Z37.69
      triplets Z37.61
  single NEC Z37.9
    liveborn Z37.0
    stillborn Z37.1
  twins NEC Z37.9
    both liveborn Z37.2
    both stillborn Z37.4
    one liveborn, one stillborn Z37.3
Outlet —*see* condition
Ovalocytosis (congenital) (hereditary) —*see*
    Elliptocytosis
Ovarian —*see* Condition
Ovariocele N83.4-●
Ovaritis (cystic) —*see* Oophoritis
Ovary, ovarian —*see also* condition
  resistant syndrome E28.39
  vein syndrome N13.8
Overactive —*see also* Hyperfunction
  adrenal cortex NEC E27.0
  bladder N32.81
  hypothalamus E23.3
  thyroid —*see* Hyperthyroidism
Overactivity R46.3
  child —*see* Disorder, attention-deficit
      hyperactivity
Overbite (deep) (excessive) (horizontal)
    (vertical) M26.29
Overbreathing —*see* Hyperventilation
Overconscientious personality F60.5
Overdevelopment —*see* Hypertrophy
Overdistension —*see* Distension
Overdose, overdosage (drug) —*see* Table of
    Drugs and Chemicals, by drug, poisoning
Overeating R63.2
  nonorganic origin F50.89
  psychogenic F50.89
Overexertion (effects) (exhaustion) T73.3
Overexposure (effects) T73.9
  exhaustion T73.2
Overfeeding —*see* Overeating
  newborn P92.4
Overfill, endodontic M27.52
Overgrowth, bone —*see* Hypertrophy, bone
Overhanging of dental restorative material
    (unrepairable) K08.52
Overheated (places) (effects) —*see* Heat
Overjet (excessive horizontal) M26.23
Overlaid, overlying (suffocation) —*see* Asphyxia,
    traumatic, due to mechanical threat
Overlap, excessive horizontal (teeth) M26.23
Overlapping toe (acquired) —*see also*
    Deformity, toe, specified NEC
  congenital (fifth toe) Q66.89
Overload
  circulatory, due to transfusion (blood) (blood
      components) (TACO) E87.71
  fluid E87.70
    due to transfusion (blood) (blood
        components) E87.71
    specified NEC E87.79
  iron, due to repeated red blood cell
      transfusions E83.111
  potassium (K) E87.5
  sodium (Na) E87.0
Overnutrition —*see* Hyperalimentation
Overproduction —*see also* Hypersecretion
  ACTH E27.0
  catecholamine E27.5
  growth hormone E22.0

▶ New   ⇒ Revised   ~~deleted~~ Deleted   ● Use Additional Character(s)

Overprotection, child by parent Z62.1
Overriding
    aorta Q25.49
    finger (acquired) —*see* Deformity, finger
       congenital Q68.1
    toe (acquired) —*see also* Deformity, toe,
       specified NEC
       congenital Q66.89
Overstrained R53.83
    heart —*see* Hypertrophy, cardiac

Overuse, muscle NEC
    M70.8-●
Overweight E66.3
Overworked R53.83
Oviduct —*see* condition
Ovotestis Q56.0
Ovulation (cycle)
    failure or lack of N97.0
    pain N94.0
Ovum —*see* condition

Owren's disease or syndrome (parahemophilia)
    D68.2
Ox heart —*see* Hypertrophy, cardiac
Oxalosis E72.53
Oxaluria E72.53
Oxycephaly, oxycephalic Q75.0
    syphilitic, congenital A50.02
Oxyuriasis B80
Oxyuris vermicularis (infestation) B80
Ozena J31.0

P

Pachyderma, pachydermia L85.9
  larynx (verrucosa) J38.7
Pachydermatocele (congenital) Q82.8
Pachydermoperiostosis —see also
    Osteoarthropathy, hypertrophic, specified
    type NEC
  clubbed nail M89.40 [L62]
Pachygyria Q04.3
Pachymeningitis (adhesive) (basal) (brain)
    (cervical) (chronic) (circumscribed)
    (external) (fibrous) (hemorrhagic)
    (hypertrophic) (internal) (purulent) (spinal)
    (suppurative) —see Meningitis
Pachyonychia (congenital) Q84.5
Pacinian tumor —see Neoplasm, skin, benign
Pad, knuckle or Garrod's M72.1
Paget-Schroetter syndrome I82.890
Paget's disease
  with infiltrating duct carcinoma —see
    Neoplasm, breast, malignant
  bone M88.9
    carpus M88.84-●
    clavicle M88.81-●
    femur M88.85-●
    fibula M88.86-●
    finger M88.84-●
    humerus M88.82-●
    ilium M88.85-●
    in neoplastic disease —see Osteitis,
      deformans, in neoplastic disease
    ischium M88.85-●
    metacarpus M88.84-●
    metatarsus M88.87-●
    multiple sites M88.89
    neck M88.88
    radius M88.83-●
    rib M88.88
    scapula M88.81-●
    skull M88.0
    tarsus M88.87-●
    tibia M88.86-●
    toe M88.87-●
    ulna M88.83-●
    vertebra M88.88
  breast (female) C50.01-●
    male C50.02-●
  extramammary —see also Neoplasm, skin,
    malignant
    anus C21.0
      margin C44.590
      skin C44.590
  intraductal carcinoma —see Neoplasm,
    breast, malignant
  malignant —see Neoplasm, skin, malignant
    breast (female) C50.01-●
      male C50.02-●
    unspecified site (female) C50.01-●
      male C50.02-●
  mammary —see Paget's disease, breast
  nipple —see Paget's disease, breast
  osteitis deformans —see Paget's disease, bone
Pain(s) —see also Painful R52
  abdominal R10.9
    colic R10.83
    generalized R10.84
      with acute abdomen R10.0
    lower R10.30
      left quadrant R10.32
      pelvic or perineal R10.2
      periumbilical R10.33
      right quadrant R10.31
    rebound —see Tenderness, abdominal,
      rebound
    severe with abdominal rigidity R10.0
    tenderness —see Tenderness, abdominal
    upper R10.10
      epigastric R10.13
      left quadrant R10.12
      right quadrant R10.11

Pain (Continued)
  acute R52
    due to trauma G89.11
    neoplasm related G89.3
    postprocedural NEC G89.18
    post-thoracotomy G89.12
    specified by site — code to Pain, by site
  adnexa (uteri) R10.2
  anginoid —see Pain, precordial
  anus K62.89
  arm —see Pain, limb, upper
  axillary (axilla) M79.62-●
  back (postural) M54.9
  bladder R39.89
    associated with micturition —see
      Micturition, painful
    chronic R39.82
  bone —see Disorder, bone, specified type
    NEC
  breast N64.4
  broad ligament R10.2
  cancer associated (acute) (chronic) G89.3
  cecum —see Pain, abdominal
  cervicobrachial M53.1
  chest (central) R07.9
    anterior wall R07.89
    atypical R07.89
    ischemic I20.9
    musculoskeletal R07.89
    non-cardiac R07.89
    on breathing R07.1
    pleurodynia R07.81
    precordial R07.2
    wall (anterior) R07.89
  chronic G89.29
    associated with significant psychosocial
      dysfunction G89.4
    due to trauma G89.21
    neoplasm related G89.3
    postoperative NEC G89.28
    postprocedural NEC G89.28
    post-thoracotomy G89.22
    specified NEC G89.29
  coccyx M53.3
  colon —see Pain, abdominal
  coronary —see Angina
  costochondral R07.1
  diaphragm R07.1
  due to cancer G89.3
  due to device, implant or graft —see also
    Complications, by site and type,
      specified NEC T85.848
    arterial graft NEC T82.848
    breast (implant) T85.848
    catheter NEC T85.848
      dialysis (renal) T82.848
        intraperitoneal T85.848
      infusion NEC T82.848
        spinal (epidural) (subdural) T85.840
      urinary (indwelling) T83.84
    electronic (electrode) (pulse generator)
      (stimulator)
      bone T84.84
      cardiac T82.847
      nervous system (brain) (peripheral
        nerve) (spinal) T85.840
      urinary T83.84
    fixation, internal (orthopedic) NEC T84.84
    gastrointestinal (bile duct) (esophagus)
      T85.848
    genital NEC T83.84
    heart NEC T82.847
    infusion NEC T85.848
    joint prosthesis T84.84
    ocular (corneal graft) (orbital implant)
      NEC T85.848
    orthopedic NEC T84.84
    specified NEC T85.848
    urinary NEC T83.84
    vascular NEC T82.848
    ventricular intracranial shunt T85.840

Pain (Continued)
  due to malignancy (primary) (secondary)
    G89.3
  ear —see subcategory H92.0
  epigastric, epigastrium R10.13
  eye —see Pain, ocular
  face, facial R51
    atypical G50.1
  female genital organs NEC N94.89
  finger —see Pain, limb, upper
  flank —see Pain, abdominal
  foot —see Pain, limb, lower
  gallbladder K82.9
  gas (intestinal) R14.1
  gastric —see Pain, abdominal
  generalized NOS R52
  genital organ
    female N94.89
    male N50.89
  groin —see Pain, abdominal, lower
  hand —see Pain, limb, upper
  head —see Headache
  heart —see Pain, precordial
  infra-orbital —see Neuralgia, trigeminal
  intercostal R07.82
  intermenstrual N94.0
  jaw R68.84
  joint M25.50
    ankle M25.57-●
    elbow M25.52-●
    finger M25.54-●
    foot M25.57-●
    hand M25.54-●
    hip M25.55-●
    knee M25.56-●
    shoulder M25.51-●
    toe M25.57-●
    wrist M25.53-●
  kidney N23
  laryngeal R07.0
  leg —see Pain, limb, lower
  limb M79.609
    lower M79.60-●
      foot M79.67-●
      lower leg M79.66-●
      thigh M79.65-●
      toe M79.67-●
    upper M79.60-●
      axilla M79.62-●
      finger M79.64-●
      forearm M79.63-●
      hand M79.64-●
      upper arm M79.62-●
  loin M54.5
  low back M54.5
  lumbar region M54.5
  mandibular R68.84
  mastoid —see subcategory H92.0
  maxilla R68.84
  menstrual —see also Dysmenorrhea N94.6
  metacarpophalangeal (joint) —see Pain, joint,
    hand
  metatarsophalangeal (joint) —see Pain, joint,
    foot
  mouth K13.79
  muscle —see Myalgia
  musculoskeletal —see also Pain, by site M79.1
  myofascial M79.1
  nasal J34.89
  nasopharynx J39.2
  neck NEC M54.2
  nerve NEC —see Neuralgia
  neuromuscular —see Neuralgia
  nose J34.89
  ocular H57.1-●
  ophthalmic —see Pain, ocular
  orbital region —see Pain, ocular
  ovary N94.89
  over heart —see Pain, precordial
  ovulation N94.0
  pelvic (female) R10.2

▶ New   ⟹ Revised   deleted Deleted   ● Use Additional Character(s)

Pain *(Continued)*
  penis N48.89
  pericardial —*see* Pain, precordial
  perineal, perineum R10.2
  pharynx J39.2
  pleura, pleural, pleuritic R07.81
  postoperative NOS G89.18
  postprocedural NOS G89.18
  post-thoracotomy G89.12
  precordial (region) R07.2
  premenstrual N94.3
  psychogenic (persistent) (any site) F45.41
  radicular (spinal) —*see* Radiculopathy
  rectum K62.89
  respiration R07.1
  retrosternal R07.2
  rheumatoid, muscular —*see* Myalgia
  rib R07.81
  root (spinal) —*see* Radiculopathy
  round ligament (stretch) R10.2
  sacroiliac M53.3
  sciatic —*see* Sciatica
  scrotum N50.82
  seminal vesicle N50.89
  shoulder M25.51-●
  spermatic cord N50.89
  spinal root —*see* Radiculopathy
  spine M54.9
   cervical M54.2
   low back M54.5
    with sciatica M54.4-●
   thoracic M54.6
  stomach —*see* Pain, abdominal
  substernal R07.2
  temporomandibular (joint) M26.62-●
  testis N50.81-●
  thoracic spine M54.6
   with radicular and visceral pain M54.14
  throat R07.0
  tibia —*see* Pain, limb, lower
  toe —*see* Pain, limb, lower
  tongue K14.6
  tooth K08.89
  trigeminal —*see* Neuralgia, trigeminal
  tumor associated G89.3
  ureter N23
  urinary (organ) (system) N23
  uterus NEC N94.89
  vagina R10.2
  vertebrogenic (syndrome) M54.89
  vesical R39.89
   associated with micturition —*see* Micturition, painful
  vulva R10.2
Painful —*see also* Pain
  coitus
   female N94.10
   male N53.12
   psychogenic F52.6
  ejaculation (semen) N53.12
   psychogenic F52.6
  erection —*see* Priapism
  feet syndrome E53.8
  joint replacement (hip) (knee) T84.84
  menstruation —*see* Dysmenorrhea
   psychogenic F45.8
  micturition —*see* Micturition, painful
  respiration R07.1
  scar NEC L90.5
  wire sutures T81.89
Painter's colic —*see* subcategory T56.0
Palate —*see* condition
Palatoplegia K13.79
Palatoschisis —*see* Cleft, palate
Palilalia R48.8
Palliative care Z51.5
Pallor R23.1
  optic disc, temporal —*see* Atrophy, optic
Palmar —*see also* condition
  fascia —*see* condition

Palpable
  cecum K63.89
  kidney N28.89
  ovary N83.8
  prostate N42.9
  spleen —*see* Splenomegaly
Palpitations (heart) R00.2
  psychogenic F45.8
Palsy —*see also* Paralysis G83.9
  atrophic diffuse (progressive) G12.22
  Bell's —*see also* Palsy, facial
   newborn P11.3
  brachial plexus NEC G54.0
   newborn (birth injury) P14.3
  brain —*see* Palsy, cerebral
  bulbar (progressive) (chronic) G12.22
   of childhood (Fazio-Londe) G12.1
   pseudo NEC G12.29
   supranuclear (progressive) G23.1
  cerebral (congenital) G80.9
   ataxic G80.4
   athetoid G80.3
   choreathetoid G80.3
   diplegic G80.8
    spastic G80.1
   dyskinetic G80.3
    athetoid G80.3
    choreathetoid G80.3
    distonic G80.3
   dystonic G80.3
   hemiplegic G80.8
    spastic G80.2
   mixed G80.8
   monoplegic G80.8
    spastic G80.1
   paraplegic G80.8
    spastic G80.1
   quadriplegic G80.8
    spastic G80.0
   spastic G80.1
    diplegic G80.1
    hemiplegic G80.2
    monoplegic G80.1
    quadriplegic G80.0
    specified NEC G80.1
    tetrapelgic G80.0
   specified NEC G80.8
   syphilitic A52.12
    congenital A50.49
   tetraplegic G80.8
    spastic G80.0
  cranial nerve —*see also* Disorder, nerve, cranial
   multiple G52.7
    in
     infectious disease B99 *[G53]*
     neoplastic disease —*see also* Neoplasm D49.9 *[G53]*
     parasitic disease B89 *[G53]*
     sarcoidosis D86.82
  creeping G12.22
  diver's T70.3
  Erb's P14.0
  facial G51.0
   newborn (birth injury) P11.3
  glossopharyngeal G52.1
  Klumpke (-Déjérine) P14.1
  lead —*see* subcategory T56.0
  median nerve (tardy) G56.1-●
  nerve G58.9
   specified NEC G58.8
  peroneal nerve (acute) (tardy) G57.3-●
  progressive supranuclear G23.1
  pseudobulbar NEC G12.29
  radial nerve (acute) G56.3-●
  seventh nerve —*see also* Palsy, facial
   newborn P11.3
  shaking —*see* Parkinsonism
  spastic (cerebral) (spinal) G80.1
  ulnar nerve (tardy) G56.2-●
  wasting G12.29

Paludism —*see* Malaria
Panangiitis M30.0
Panaris, panaritium —*see also* Cellulitis, digit
  with lymphangitis —*see* Lymphangitis, acute, digit
Panarteritis nodosa M30.0
  brain or cerebral I67.7
Pancake heart R93.1
  with cor pulmonale (chronic) I27.81
Pancarditis (acute) (chronic) I51.89
  rheumatic I09.89
   active or acute I01.8
Pancoast's syndrome or tumor C34.1-●
Pancolitis, ulcerative (chronic) K51.00
  with
   abscess K51.014
   complication K51.019
   fistula K51.013
   obstruction K51.012
   rectal bleeding K51.011
   specified complication NEC K51.018
Pancreas, pancreatic —*see* condition
Pancreatitis (annular) (apoplectic) (calcareous) (edematous) (hemorrhagic) (malignant) (recurrent) (subacute) (suppurative) K85.90
  with necrosis (uninfected) K85.91
   infected K85.92
  acute (without necrosis or infection) K85.90
   with necrosis (uninfected) K85.91
    infected K85.92
   alcohol induced (without necrosis or infection) K85.20
    with necrosis (uninfected) K85.21
     infected K85.22
   biliary (without necrosis or infection) K85.10
    with necrosis (uninfected) K85.11
     infected K85.12
   drug induced (without necrosis or infection) K85.30
    with necrosis (uninfected) K85.31
     infected K85.32
   gallstone (without necrosis or infection) K85.10
    with necrosis (uninfected) K85.11
     infected K85.12
   idiopathic (without necrosis or infection) K85.00
    with necrosis (uninfected) K85.01
     infected K85.02
   specified NEC (without necrosis or infection) K85.80
    with necrosis (uninfected) K85.81
     infected K85.82
  chronic (infectious) K86.1
   alcohol-induced K86.0
   recurrent K86.1
   relapsing K86.1
  cystic (chronic) K86.1
  cytomegaloviral B25.2
  fibrous (chronic) K86.1
  gallstone (without necrosis or infection) K85.10
   with necrosis (uninfected) K85.11
    infected K85.12
  gangrenous —*see* Pancreatitis, acute
  interstitial (chronic) K86.1
   acute —*see also* Pancreatitis, acute K85.80
  mumps B26.3
  recurrent (chronic) K86.1
  relapsing, chronic K86.1
  syphilitic A52.74
Pancreatoblastoma —*see* Neoplasm, pancreas, malignant
Pancreolithiasis K86.89
Pancytolysis D75.89

Pancytopenia (acquired) D61.818
  with
    malformations D61.09
    myelodysplastic syndrome —see
      Syndrome, myelodysplastic
  antineoplastic chemotherapy induced
    D61.810
  congenital D61.09
  drug-induced NEC D61.811
▶PANDAS (pediatric autoimmune
    neuropsychiatric disorders associated with
    streptococcal infections syndrome) D89.89
Panencephalitis, subacute, sclerosing
  A81.1
Panhematopenia D61.9
  congenital D61.09
  constitutional D61.09
  splenic, primary D73.1
Panhemocytopenia D61.9
  congenital D61.09
  constitutional D61.09
Panhypogonadism E29.1
Panhypopituitarism E23.0
  prepubertal E23.0
Panic (attack) (state) F41.0
  reaction to exceptional stress (transient) F43.0
Panmyelopathy, familial, constitutional D61.09
Panmyelophthisis D61.82
  congenital D61.09
Panmyelosis (acute) (with myelofibrosis)
  C94.4-●
Panner's disease —see Osteochondrosis,
  juvenile, humerus
Panneuritis endemica E51.11
Panniculitis (nodular) (nonsuppurative) M79.3
  back M54.00
    cervical region M54.02
    cervicothoracic region M54.03
    lumbar region M54.06
    lumbosacral region M54.07
    multiple sites M54.09
    occipito-atlanto-axial region M54.01
    sacrococcygeal region M54.08
    thoracic region M54.04
    thoracolumbar region M54.05
  lupus L93.2
  mesenteric K65.4
  neck M54.02
    cervicothoracic region M54.03
    occipito-atlanto-axial region M54.01
  relapsing M35.6
Panniculus adiposus (abdominal) E65
Pannus (allergic) (cornea) (degenerativus)
  (keratic) H16.42-●
  abdominal (symptomatic) E65
  trachomatosus, trachomatous (active) A71.1
Panophthalmitis H44.01-●
Pansinusitis (chronic) (hyperplastic)
  (nonpurulent) (purulent) J32.4
  acute J01.40
    recurrent J01.41
  tuberculous A15.8
Panuveitis (sympathetic) H44.11-●
Panvalvular disease I08.9
  specified NEC I08.8
PAPA (pyogenic arthritis, pyoderma
  gangrenosum, and acne syndrome) M04.8
Papanicolaou smear, cervix Z12.4
  as part of routine gynecological examination
    Z01.419
    with abnormal findings Z01.411
  for suspected neoplasm Z12.4
  nonspecific abnormal finding R87.619
  routine Z01.419
    with abnormal findings Z01.411
Papilledema (choked disc) H47.10
  associated with
    decreased ocular pressure H47.12
    increased intracranial pressure H47.11
    retinal disorder H47.13
  Foster-Kennedy syndrome H47.14-●

Papillitis H46.00
  anus K62.89
  chronic lingual K14.4
  necrotizing, kidney N17.2
  optic H46.0-●
  rectum K62.89
  renal, necrotizing N17.2
  tongue K14.0
Papilloma —see also Neoplasm, benign,
  by site
  acuminatum (female) (male) (anogenital)
    A63.0
  basal cell L82.1
    inflamed L82.0
  benign pinta (primary) A67.0
  bladder (urinary) (transitional cell) D41.4
  choroid plexus (lateral ventricle) (third
    ventricle) D33.0
    anaplastic C71.5
    fourth ventricle D33.1
    malignant C71.5
  renal pelvis (transitional cell) D41.1-●
    benign D30.1-●
  Schneiderian
    specified site —see Neoplasm, benign, by
      site
    unspecified site D14.0
  serous surface
    borderline malignancy
      specified site —see Neoplasm, uncertain
        behavior, by site
      unspecified site D39.10
    specified site —see Neoplasm, benign, by
      site
    unspecified site D27.9
  transitional (cell)
    bladder (urinary) D41.4
    inverted type —see Neoplasm, uncertain
      behavior, by site
    renal pelvis D41.1-●
    ureter D41.2-●
  ureter (transitional cell) D41.2-●
    benign D30.2-●
  urothelial —see Neoplasm, uncertain
    behavior, by site
  villous —see Neoplasm, uncertain behavior,
    by site
    adenocarcinoma in —see Neoplasm,
      malignant, by site
    in situ —see Neoplasm, in situ
  yaws, plantar or palmar A66.1
Papillomata, multiple, of yaws A66.1
Papillomatosis —see also Neoplasm, benign,
  by site
  confluent and reticulated L83
  cystic, breast —see Mastopathy, cystic
  ductal, breast —see Mastopathy, cystic
  intraductal (diffuse) —see Neoplasm, benign,
    by site
  subareolar duct D24-●
Papillomavirus, as cause of disease classified
  elsewhere B97.7
Papillon-Léage and Psaume syndrome
  Q87.0
Papule(s) R23.8
  carate (primary) A67.0
  fibrous, of nose D22.39
  Gottron's L94.4
  pinta (primary) A67.0
Papulosis
  lymphomatoid C86.6
  malignant I77.89
Papyraceous fetus O31.0-●
Para-albuminemia E88.09
Paracephalus Q89.7
Parachute mitral valve Q23.2
Paracoccidioidomycosis B41.9
  disseminated B41.7
  generalized B41.7
  mucocutaneous-lymphangitic B41.8
  pulmonary B41.0

Paracoccidioidomycosis (Continued)
  specified NEC B41.8
  visceral B41.8
Paradentosis K05.4
Paraffinoma T88.8
Paraganglioma D44.7
  adrenal D35.0-●
    malignant C74.1-●
  aortic body D44.7
    malignant C75.5
  carotid body D44.6
    malignant C75.4
  chromaffin —see also Neoplasm, benign, by
    site
    malignant —see Neoplasm, malignant, by
      site
  extra-adrenal D44.7
    malignant C75.5
      specified site —see Neoplasm,
        malignant, by site
      unspecified site C75.5
    specified site —see Neoplasm, uncertain
      behavior, by site
    unspecified site D44.7
  gangliocytic D13.2
    specified site —see Neoplasm, benign, by
      site
    unspecified site D13.2
  glomus jugulare D44.7
    malignant C75.5
  jugular D44.7
  malignant C75.5
    specified site —see Neoplasm, malignant,
      by site
    unspecified site C75.5
  nonchromaffin D44.7
    malignant C75.5
      specified site —see Neoplasm,
        malignant, by site
      unspecified site C75.5
    specified site —see Neoplasm, uncertain
      behavior, by site
    unspecified site D44.7
  parasympathetic D44.7
    specified site —see Neoplasm, uncertain
      behavior, by site
    unspecified site D44.7
  specified site —see Neoplasm, uncertain
    behavior, by site
  sympathetic D44.7
    specified site —see Neoplasm, uncertain
      behavior, by site
    unspecified site D44.7
  unspecified site D44.7
Parageusia R43.2
  psychogenic F45.8
Paragonimiasis B66.4
▶Paragranuloma, Hodgkin —see Lymphoma,
  Hodgkin, specified NEC
Parahemophilia —see also Defect, coagulation
  D68.2
Parakeratosis R23.4
  variegata L41.0
Paralysis, paralytic (complete) (incomplete)
  G83.9
  with
    syphilis A52.17
  abducens, abducent (nerve) —see Strabismus,
    paralytic, sixth nerve
  abductor, lower extremity G57.9-●
  accessory nerve G52.8
  accommodation —see also Paresis, of
    accommodation
    hysterical F44.89
  acoustic nerve (except Deafness) —see
    subcategory H93.3
  agitans —see also Parkinsonism G20
    arteriosclerotic G21.4
  alternating (oculomotor) G83.89
  amyotrophic G12.21

▶ New   ⇒ Revised   ~~deleted~~ Deleted   ● Use Additional Character(s)

Paralysis, paralytic (Continued)
ankle G57.9-●
anus (sphincter) K62.89
arm —see Monoplegia, upper limb
ascending (spinal), acute G61.0
association G12.29
asthenic bulbar G70.00
    with exacerbation (acute) G70.01
    in crisis G70.01
ataxic (hereditary) G11.9
    general (syphilitic) A52.17
atrophic G58.9
    infantile, acute —see Poliomyelitis, paralytic
    progressive G12.22
    spinal (acute) —see Poliomyelitis, paralytic
axillary G54.0
Babinski-Nageotte's G83.89
Bell's G51.0
    newborn P11.3
Benedikt's G46.3
birth injury P14.9
    spinal cord P11.5
bladder (neurogenic) (sphincter)
    N31.2
bowel, colon or intestine K56.0
brachial plexus G54.0
    birth injury P14.3
    newborn (birth injury) P14.3
brain G83.9
    diplegia G83.0
    triplegia G83.89
bronchial J98.09
Brown-Séquard G83.81
bulbar (chronic) (progressive) G12.22
    infantile —see Poliomyelitis, paralytic
    poliomyelitic —see Poliomyelitis, paralytic
    pseudo G12.29
bulbospinal G70.00
    with exacerbation (acute) G70.01
    in crisis G70.01
cardiac —see also Failure, heart I50.9
cerebrocerebellar, diplegic G80.1
cervical
    plexus G54.2
    sympathetic G90.09
Céstan-Chenais G46.3
Charcot-Marie-Tooth type G60.0
Clark's G80.9
colon K56.0
compressed air T70.3
compression
    arm G56.9-●
    leg G57.9-●
    lower extremity G57.9-●
    upper extremity G56.9-●
congenital (cerebral) —see Palsy, cerebral
conjugate movement (gaze) (of eye) H51.0
    cortical (nuclear) (supranuclear) H51.0
cordis —see Failure, heart
cranial or cerebral nerve G52.9
creeping G12.22
crossed leg G83.89
crutch —see Injury, brachial plexus
deglutition R13.0
    hysterical F44.4
dementia A52.17
descending (spinal) NEC G12.29
diaphragm (flaccid) J98.6
    due to accidental dissection of phrenic
        nerve during procedure —see
        Puncture, accidental complicating
        surgery
digestive organs NEC K59.8
diplegic —see Diplegia
divergence (nuclear) H51.8
diver's T70.3
Duchenne's
    birth injury P14.0
    due to or associated with
        motor neuron disease G12.22
        muscular dystrophy G71.0

Paralysis, paralytic (Continued)
due to intracranial or spinal birth injury —see
    Palsy, cerebral
embolic (current episode) I63.4-●
Erb (-Duchenne) (birth) (newborn) P14.0
Erb's syphilitic spastic spinal A52.17
esophagus K22.8
eye muscle (extrinsic) H49.9
    intrinsic —see also Paresis, of
        accommodation
facial (nerve) G51.0
    birth injury P11.3
    congenital P11.3
    following operation NEC —see Puncture,
        accidental complicating surgery
    newborn (birth injury) P11.3
familial (recurrent) (periodic) G72.3
    spastic G11.4
fauces J39.2
finger G56.9-●
gait R26.1
gastric nerve (nondiabetic) G52.2
gaze, conjugate H51.0
general (progressive) (syphilitic) A52.17
    juvenile A50.45
glottis J38.00
    bilateral J38.02
    unilateral J38.01
gluteal G54.1
Gubler (-Millard) G46.3
hand —see Monoplegia, upper limb
heart —see Arrest, cardiac
hemiplegic —see Hemiplegia
hyperkalemic periodic (familial) G72.3
hypoglossal (nerve) G52.3
hypokalemic periodic G72.3
hysterical F44.4
ileus K56.0
infantile —see also Poliomyelitis, paralytic
    A80.30
    bulbar —see Poliomyelitis, paralytic
    cerebral —see Palsy, cerebral
    spastic —see Palsy, cerebral, spastic
infective —see Poliomyelitis, paralytic
inferior nuclear G83.9
internuclear —see Ophthalmoplegia,
    internuclear
intestine K56.0
iris H57.09
    due to diphtheria (toxin) A36.89
ischemic, Volkmann's (complicating trauma)
    T79.6
Jackson's G83.89
jake —see Poisoning, food, noxious, plant
Jamaica ginger (jake) G62.2
juvenile general A50.45
Klumpke (-Déjérine) (birth) (newborn) P14.1
labioglossal (laryngeal) (pharyngeal) G12.29
Landry's G61.0
laryngeal nerve (recurrent) (superior)
    (unilateral) J38.00
    bilateral J38.02
    unilateral J38.01
larynx J38.00
    bilateral J38.02
    due to diphtheria (toxin) A36.2
    unilateral J38.01
lateral G12.23
lead —see subcategory T56.0
left side —see Hemiplegia
leg G83.1-●
    both —see Paraplegia
    crossed G83.89
    hysterical F44.4
    psychogenic F44.4
    transient or transitory R29.818
        traumatic NEC —see Injury, nerve, leg
levator palpebrae superioris —see
    Blepharoptosis, paralytic
limb —see Monoplegia
lip K13.0

Paralysis, paralytic (Continued)
Lissauer's A52.17
lower limb —see Monoplegia, lower
    limb
    both —see Paraplegia
lung J98.4
median nerve G56.1-●
medullary (tegmental) G83.89
mesencephalic NEC G83.89
    tegmental G83.89
middle alternating G83.89
Millard-Gubler-Foville G46.3
monoplegic —see Monoplegia
motor G83.9
muscle, muscular NEC G72.89
    due to nerve lesion G58.9
    eye (extrinsic) H49.9
        intrinsic —see Paresis, of
            accommodation
        oblique —see Strabismus, paralytic,
            fourth nerve
    iris sphincter H21.9
    ischemic (Volkmann's) (complicating
        trauma) T79.6
    progressive G12.21
    pseudohypertrophic G71.0
musculocutaneous nerve G56.9-●
musculospiral G56.9-●
nerve —see also Disorder, nerve
    abducent —see Strabismus, paralytic, sixth
        nerve
    accessory G52.8
    auditory (except Deafness) —see
        subcategory H93.3
    birth injury P14.9
    cranial or cerebral G52.9
    facial G51.0
        birth injury P11.3
        congenital P11.3
        newborn (birth injury) P11.3
    fourth or trochlear —see Strabismus,
        paralytic, fourth nerve
    newborn (birth injury) P14.9
    oculomotor —see Strabismus, paralytic,
        third nerve
    phrenic (birth injury) P14.2
    radial G56.3-●
    seventh or facial G51.0
        newborn (birth injury) P11.3
    sixth or abducent —see Strabismus,
        paralytic, sixth nerve
    syphilitic A52.15
    third or oculomotor —see Strabismus,
        paralytic, third nerve
    trigeminal G50.9
    trochlear —see Strabismus, paralytic,
        fourth nerve
    ulnar G56.2-●
normokalemic periodic G72.3
ocular H49.9
    alternating G83.89
oculofacial, congenital (Moebius) Q87.0
oculomotor (external bilateral) (nerve) —see
    Strabismus, paralytic, third nerve
palate (soft) K13.79
paratrigeminal G50.9
periodic (familial) (hyperkalemic)
    (hypokalemic) (myotonic)
    (normokalemic) (potassium sensitive)
    (secondary) G72.3
peripheral autonomic nervous system —see
    Neuropathy, peripheral, autonomic
peroneal (nerve) G57.3-●
pharynx J39.2
phrenic nerve G56.8-●
plantar nerve(s) G57.6-●
pneumogastric nerve G52.2
poliomyelitis (current) —see Poliomyelitis,
    paralytic
popliteal nerve G57.3-●
postepileptic transitory G83.84

Paralysis, paralytic (Continued)
  progressive (atrophic) (bulbar) (spinal)
      G12.22
    general A52.17
    infantile acute —see Poliomyelitis, paralytic
    supranuclear G23.1
  pseudobulbar G12.29
  pseudohypertrophic (muscle) G71.0
  psychogenic F44.4
  quadriceps G57.9-●
  quadriplegic —see Tetraplegia
  radial nerve G56.3-●
  rectus muscle (eye) H49.9
  recurrent isolated sleep G47.53
  respiratory (muscle) (system) (tract) R06.81
    center NEC G93.89
    congenital P28.89
    newborn P28.89
  right side —see Hemiplegia
  saturnine —see subcategory T56.0
  sciatic nerve G57.0-●
  senile G83.9
  shaking —see Parkinsonism
  shoulder G56.9-●
  sleep, recurrent isolated G47.53
  spastic G83.9
    cerebral —see Palsy, cerebral, spastic
    congenital (cerebral) —see Palsy, cerebral,
        spastic
    familial G11.4
    hereditary G11.4
    quadriplegic G80.0
    syphilitic (spinal) A52.17
  sphincter, bladder —see Paralysis, bladder
  spinal (cord) G83.9
    accessory nerve G52.8
    acute —see Poliomyelitis, paralytic
    ascending acute G61.0
    atrophic (acute) —see also Poliomyelitis,
        paralytic
      spastic, syphilitic A52.17
    congenital NEC —see Palsy, cerebral
    hereditary G95.89
    infantile —see Poliomyelitis, paralytic
    progressive G12.21
    sequelae NEC G83.89
  sternomastoid G52.8
  stomach K31.84
    diabetic —see Diabetes, by type, with
        gastroparesis
    nerve G52.2
      diabetic —see Diabetes, by type, with
          gastroparesis
  stroke —see Infarct, brain
  subcapsularis G56.8-●
  supranuclear (progressive) G23.1
  sympathetic G90.8
    cervical G90.09
    nervous system —see Neuropathy,
        peripheral, autonomic
  syndrome G83.9
    specified NEC G83.89
  syphilitic spastic spinal (Erb's) A52.17
  thigh G57.9-●
  throat J39.2
    diphtheritic A36.0
    muscle J39.2
  thrombotic (current episode) I63.3-●
  thumb G56.9-●
  tick —see Toxicity, venom, arthropod,
      specified NEC
  Todd's (postepileptic transitory paralysis)
      G83.84
  toe G57.6-●
  tongue K14.8
  transient R29.5
    arm or leg NEC R29.818
    traumatic NEC —see Injury, nerve
  trapezius G52.8
  traumatic, transient NEC —see Injury,
      nerve

Paralysis, paralytic (Continued)
  trembling —see Parkinsonism
  triceps brachii G56.9-●
  trigeminal nerve G50.9
  trochlear (nerve) —see Strabismus, paralytic,
      fourth nerve
  ulnar nerve G56.2-●
  upper limb —see Monoplegia, upper limb
  uremic N18.9 [G99.8]
  uveoparotitic D86.89
  uvula K13.79
    postdiphtheritic A36.0
  vagus nerve G52.2
  vasomotor NEC G90.8
  velum palati K13.79
  vesical —see Paralysis, bladder
  vestibular nerve (except Vertigo) —see
      subcategory H93.3
  vocal cords J38.00
    bilateral J38.02
    unilateral J38.01
  Volkmann's (complicating trauma)
      T79.6
  wasting G12.29
  Weber's G46.3
  wrist G56.9-●
Paramedial urethrovesical orifice
    Q64.79
Paramenia N92.6
Parametritis —see also Disease, pelvis,
    inflammatory N73.2
  acute N73.0
  complicating abortion —see Abortion, by
      type, complicated by, parametritis
Parametrium, parametric —see condition
Paramnesia —see Amnesia
Paramolar K00.1
Paramyloidosis E85.89
Paramyoclonus multiplex G25.3
Paramyotonia (congenita) G71.19
Parangi —see Yaws
Paranoia (querulans) F22
  senile F03
Paranoid
  dementia (senile) F03
    praecox —see Schizophrenia
  personality F60.0
  psychosis (climacteric) (involutional)
      (menopausal) F22
    psychogenic (acute) F23
    senile F03
  reaction (acute) F23
    chronic F22
  schizophrenia F20.0
  state (climacteric) (involutional)
      (menopausal) (simple) F22
    senile F03
  tendencies F60.0
  traits F60.0
  trends F60.0
  type, psychopathic personality F60.0
Paraparesis —see Paraplegia
Paraphasia R47.02
Paraphilia F65.9
Paraphimosis (congenital) N47.2
  chancroidal A57
Paraphrenia, paraphrenic (late) F22
  schizophrenia F20.0
Paraplegia (lower) G82.20
  ataxic —see Degeneration, combined, spinal
      cord
  complete G82.21
  congenital (cerebral) G80.8
    spastic G80.1
  familial spastic G11.4
  functional (hysterical) F44.4
  hereditary, spastic G11.4
  hysterical F44.4
  incomplete G82.22
  Pott's A18.01
  psychogenic F44.4

Paraplegia (Continued)
  spastic
    Erb's spinal, syphilitic A52.17
    hereditary G11.4
    tropical G04.1
  syphilitic (spastic) A52.17
  tropical spastic G04.1
Parapoxvirus B08.60
  specified NEC B08.69
Paraproteinemia D89.2
  benign (familial) D89.2
  monoclonal D47.2
  secondary to malignant disease D47.2
Parapsoriasis L41.9
  en plaques L41.4
  guttata L41.1
  large plaque L41.4
  retiform, retiformis L41.5
  small plaque L41.3
  specified NEC L41.8
  varioliformis (acuta) L41.0
Parasitic —see also condition
  disease NEC B89
  stomatitis B37.0
  sycosis (beard) (scalp) B35.0
  twin Q89.4
Parasitism B89
  intestinal B82.9
  skin B88.9
  specified —see Infestation
Parasitophobia F40.218
Parasomnia G47.50
  due to
    alcohol
      abuse F10.182
      dependence F10.282
      use F10.982
    amphetamines
      abuse F15.182
      dependence F15.282
      use F15.982
    caffeine
      abuse F15.182
      dependence F15.282
      use F15.982
    cocaine
      abuse F14.182
      dependence F14.282
      use F14.982
    drug NEC
      abuse F19.182
      dependence F19.282
      use F19.982
    opioid
      abuse F11.182
      dependence F11.282
      use F11.982
    psychoactive substance NEC
      abuse F19.182
      dependence F19.282
      use F19.982
    sedative, hypnotic, or anxiolytic
      abuse F13.182
      dependence F13.282
      use F13.982
    stimulant NEC
      abuse F15.182
      dependence F15.282
      use F15.982
  in conditions classified elsewhere G47.54
  nonorganic origin F51.8
  organic G47.50
  specified NEC G47.59
Paraspadias Q54.9
Paraspasmus facialis G51.8
Parasuicide (attempt)
  history of (personal) Z91.5
    in family Z81.8
Parathyroid gland —see condition
Parathyroid tetany E20.9
Paratrachoma A74.0

▶ New   ⟹ Revised   ~~deleted~~ Deleted   ● Use Additional Character(s)

Paratyphilitis —*see* Appendicitis
Paratyphoid (fever) —*see* Fever, paratyphoid
Paratyphus —*see* Fever, paratyphoid
Paraurethral duct Q64.79
 nonorganic origin F51.5
Paraurethritis —*see also* Urethritis
 gonococcal (acute) (chronic) (with abscess)
  A54.1
Paravaccinia NEC B08.04
Paravaginitis —*see* Vaginitis
Parencephalitis —*see also* Encephalitis
 sequelae G09
Parent-child conflict —*see* Conflict, parent-child
 estrangement NEC Z62.890
Paresis —*see also* Paralysis
 accommodation —*see* Paresis, of
  accommodation
 Bernhardt's G57.1-●
 bladder (sphincter) —*see also* Paralysis, bladder
  tabetic A52.17
 bowel, colon or intestine K56.0
 extrinsic muscle, eye H49.9
 general (progressive) (syphilitic) A52.17
  juvenile A50.45
 heart —*see* Failure, heart
 insane (syphilitic) A52.17
 juvenile (general) A50.45
 of accommodation H52.52-●
 peripheral progressive (idiopathic) G60.3
 pseudohypertrophic G71.0
 senile G83.9
 syphilitic (general) A52.17
  congenital A50.45
 vesical NEC N31.2
➡ Paresthesia —*see also* Disturbance, sensation,
  skin R20.2
 Bernhardt G57.1-●
Paretic —*see* condition
Parinaud's
 conjunctivitis H10.89
 oculoglandular syndrome H10.89
 ophthalmoplegia H49.88
Parkinsonism (idiopathic) (primary) G20
 with neurogenic orthostatic hypotension
  (symptomatic) G90.3
 arteriosclerotic G21.4
 dementia G31.83 *[F02.80]*
  with behavioral disturbance G31.83
   [F02.81]
 due to
  drugs NEC G21.19
   neuroleptic G21.11
 ▶ medication-induced NEC G21.19
 neuroleptic induced G21.11
 postencephalitic G21.3
 secondary G21.9
  due to
   arteriosclerosis G21.4
   drugs NEC G21.19
    neuroleptic G21.11
   encephalitis G21.3
   external agents NEC G21.2
   syphilis A52.19
  specified NEC G21.8
 syphilitic A52.19
 treatment-induced NEC G21.19
 vascular G21.4
Parkinson's disease, syndrome or tremor —*see*
 Parkinsonism
Parodontitis —*see* Periodontitis
Parodontosis K05.4
Paronychia —*see also* Cellulitis, digit
 with lymphangitis —*see* Lymphangitis, acute,
  digit
 candidal (chronic) B37.2
 tuberculous (primary) A18.4
Parorexia (psychogenic) F50.89
Parosmia R43.1
 psychogenic F45.8
Parotid gland —*see* condition
Parotitis, parotiditis (allergic) (nonspecific
 toxic) (purulent) (septic) (suppurative) —
 see also Sialoadenitis

Parotitis, parotiditis (Continued)
 epidemic —*see* Mumps
 infectious —*see* Mumps
 postoperative K91.89
 surgical K91.89
Parrot fever A70
Parrot's disease (early congenital syphilitic
 pseudoparalysis) A50.02
Parry-Romberg syndrome G51.8
Parry's disease or syndrome E05.00
 with thyroid storm E05.01
Pars planitis —*see* Cyclitis
Parsonage (-Aldren)-Turner syndrome G54.5
Parson's disease (exophthalmic goiter) E05.00
 with thyroid storm E05.01
Particolored infant Q82.8
Parturition —*see* Delivery
Parulis K04.7
 with sinus K04.6
Parvovirus, as cause of disease classified
 elsewhere B97.6
Pasini and Pierini's atrophoderma L90.3
Passage
 false, urethra N36.5
 meconium (newborn) during delivery
  P03.82
 of sounds or bougies —*see* Attention to,
  artificial, opening
Passive —*see* condition
 smoking Z77.22
Pasteurella septica A28.0
Pasteurellosis —*see* Infection, Pasteurella
PAT (paroxysmal atrial tachycardia) I47.1
Patau's syndrome —*see* Trisomy, 13
Patches
 mucous (syphilitic) A51.39
  congenital A50.07
 smokers' (mouth) K13.24
Patellar —*see* condition
Patent —*see also* Imperfect, closure
 canal of Nuck Q52.4
 cervix N88.3
 ductus arteriosus or Botallo's Q25.0
 foramen
  botalli Q21.1
  ovale Q21.1
 interauricular septum Q21.1
 interventricular septum Q21.0
 omphalomesenteric duct Q43.0
 os (uteri) —*see* Patent, cervix
 ostium secundum Q21.1
 urachus Q64.4
 vitelline duct Q43.0
Paterson (-Brown)(-Kelly) syndrome or web
 D50.1
Pathologic, pathological —*see also* condition
 asphyxia R09.01
 fire-setting F63.1
 gambling F63.0
 ovum O02.0
 resorption, tooth K03.3
 stealing F63.2
Pathology (of) —*see* Disease
 periradicular, associated with previous
  endodontic treatment NEC M27.59
Pattern, sleep-wake, irregular G47.23
Patulous —*see also* Imperfect, closure
 (congenital)
 alimentary tract Q45.8
  lower Q43.8
  upper Q40.8
 eustachian tube H69.0-●
Pause, sinoatrial I49.5
Paxton's disease B36.2
Pearl(s)
 enamel K00.2
 Epstein's K09.8
Pearl-worker's disease —*see* Osteomyelitis,
 specified type NEC
Pectenosis K62.4
Pectoral —*see* condition

Pectus
 carinatum (congenital) Q67.7
  acquired M95.4
  rachitic sequelae (late effect) E64.3
 excavatum (congenital) Q67.6
  acquired M95.4
  rachitic sequelae (late effect) E64.3
 recurvatum (congenital) Q67.6
Pedatrophia E41
Pederosis F65.4
Pediculosis (infestation) B85.2
 capitis (head-louse) (any site) B85.0
 corporis (body-louse) (any site) B85.1
 eyelid B85.0
 mixed (classifiable to more than one of the
  titles B85.0-B85.3) B85.4
 pubis (pubic louse) (any site) B85.3
 vestimenti B85.1
 vulvae B85.3
Pediculus (infestation) —*see* Pediculosis
Pedophilia F65.4
Peg-shaped teeth K00.2
Pelade —*see* Alopecia, areata
Pelger-Huët anomaly or syndrome D72.0
Peliosis (rheumatica) D69.0
 hepatis K76.4
  with toxic liver disease K71.8
Pelizaeus-Merzbacher disease E75.29
Pellagra (alcoholic) (with polyneuropathy) E52
Pellagra-cerebellar-ataxia-renal aminoaciduria
 syndrome E72.02
Pellegrini (-Stieda) disease or syndrome —*see*
 Bursitis, tibial collateral
Pellizzi's syndrome E34.8
Pel's crisis A52.11
Pelvic —*see also* condition
 examination (periodic) (routine) Z01.419
  with abnormal findings Z01.411
 kidney, congenital Q63.2
Pelviolithiasis —*see* Calculus, kidney
Pelviperitonitis —*see also* Peritonitis, pelvic
 gonococcal A54.24
 puerperal O85
Pelvis —*see* condition or type
Pemphigoid L12.9
 benign, mucous membrane L12.1
 bullous L12.0
 cicatricial L12.1
 juvenile L12.2
 ocular L12.1
 specified NEC L12.8
Pemphigus L10.9
 benign familial (chronic) Q82.8
 Brazilian L10.3
 circinatus L13.0
 conjunctiva L12.1
 drug-induced L10.5
 erythematosus L10.4
 foliaceous L10.2
 gangrenous —*see* Gangrene
 neonatorum L01.03
 ocular L12.1
 paraneoplastic L10.81
 specified NEC L10.89
 syphilitic (congenital) A50.06
 vegetans L10.1
 vulgaris L10.0
 wildfire L10.3
Pendred's syndrome E07.1
Pendulous
 abdomen, in pregnancy —*see* Pregnancy,
  complicated by, abnormal, pelvic organs
  or tissues NEC
 breast N64.89
Penetrating wound —*see also* Puncture
 with internal injury —*see* Injury, by site
 eyeball —*see* Puncture, eyeball
 orbit (with or without foreign body) —*see*
  Puncture, orbit
 uterus by instrument with or following
  ectopic or molar pregnancy O08.6

P

Penicillosis B48.4
Penis —*see* condition
Penitis N48.29
Pentalogy of Fallot Q21.8
Pentasomy X syndrome Q97.1
Pentosuria (essential) E74.8
Percreta placenta O43.23-●
Peregrinating patient —*see* Disorder, factitious
Perforation, perforated (nontraumatic) (of)
  accidental during procedure (blood vessel)
    (nerve) (organ) —*see* Complication,
    accidental puncture or laceration
  antrum —*see* Sinusitis, maxillary
  appendix K35.2
    with localized peritonitis K35.3
  atrial septum, multiple Q21.1
  attic, ear —*see* Perforation, tympanum, attic
  bile duct (common) (hepatic) K83.2
    cystic K82.2
  bladder (urinary)
    with or following ectopic or molar
      pregnancy O08.6
    obstetrical trauma O71.5
    traumatic S37.29
      at delivery O71.5
  bowel K63.1
    with or following ectopic or molar
      pregnancy O08.6
    newborn P78.0
    obstetrical trauma O71.5
    traumatic —*see* Laceration, intestine
  broad ligament N83.8
    with or following ectopic or molar
      pregnancy O08.6
    obstetrical trauma O71.6
  by
    device, implant or graft —*see also*
      Complications, by site and type,
      mechanical T85.628
      arterial graft NEC —*see* Complication,
        cardiovascular device, mechanical,
        vascular
      breast (implant) T85.49
      catheter NEC T85.698
        cystostomy T83.090
        dialysis (renal) T82.49
          intraperitoneal T85.691
        infusion NEC T82.594
          spinal (epidural) (subdural) T85.690
        urinary —*see also* Complications,
          catheter, urinary T83.098
      electronic (electrode) (pulse generator)
        (stimulator)
        bone T84.390
        cardiac T82.199
          electrode T82.190
          pulse generator T82.191
          specified type NEC T82.198
        nervous system —*see* Complication,
          prosthetic device, mechanical,
          electronic nervous system
          stimulator
        urinary —*see* Complication,
          genitourinary, device, urinary,
          mechanical
      fixation, internal (orthopedic) NEC —
        see Complication, fixation device,
        mechanical
      gastrointestinal —*see* Complications,
        prosthetic device, mechanical,
        gastrointestinal device
      genital NEC T83.498
        intrauterine contraceptive device
          T83.39
        penile prosthesis T83.490
      heart NEC —*see* Complication,
        cardiovascular device,
        mechanical
      joint prosthesis —*see* Complications,
        joint prosthesis, mechanical,
        specified NEC, by site

Perforation, perforated *(Continued)*
  by *(Continued)*
    urinary *(Continued)*
      ocular NEC —*see* Complications,
        prosthetic device, mechanical,
        ocular device
      orthopedic NEC —*see* Complication,
        orthopedic, device, mechanical
      specified NEC T85.628
      urinary NEC —*see also* Complication,
        genitourinary, device, urinary,
        mechanical
        graft T83.29
      vascular NEC —*see* Complication,
        cardiovascular device, mechanical
      ventricular intracranial shunt T85.09
    foreign body left accidentally in
      operative wound T81.539
    instrument (any) during a procedure,
      accidental —*see* Puncture, accidental
      complicating surgery
  cecum K35.2
    with localized peritonitis K35.3
  cervix (uteri) N88.8
    with or following ectopic or molar
      pregnancy O08.6
    obstetrical trauma O71.3
  colon K63.1
    newborn P78.0
    obstetrical trauma O71.5
    traumatic —*see* Laceration, intestine, large
  common duct (bile) K83.2
  cornea (due to ulceration) —*see* Ulcer,
    cornea, perforated
  cystic duct K82.2
  diverticulum (intestine) K57.80
    with bleeding K57.81
    large intestine K57.20
      with
        bleeding K57.21
        small intestine K57.40
          with bleeding K57.41
    small intestine K57.00
      with
        bleeding K57.01
        large intestine K57.40
          with bleeding K57.41
  ear drum —*see* Perforation, tympanum
  esophagus K22.3
  ethmoidal sinus —*see* Sinusitis, ethmoidal
  frontal sinus —*see* Sinusitis, frontal
  gallbladder K82.2
  heart valve —*see* Endocarditis
  ileum K63.1
    newborn P78.0
    obstetrical trauma O71.5
    traumatic —*see* Laceration, intestine, small
  instrumental, surgical (accidental) (blood
    vessel) (nerve) (organ) —*see* Puncture,
    accidental complicating surgery
  intestine NEC K63.1
    with ectopic or molar pregnancy O08.6
    newborn P78.0
    obstetrical trauma O71.5
    traumatic —*see* Laceration, intestine
    ulcerative NEC K63.1
      newborn P78.0
  jejunum, jejunal K63.1
    obstetrical trauma O71.5
    traumatic —*see* Laceration, intestine,
      small
    ulcer —*see* Ulcer, gastrojejunal, with
      perforation
  joint prosthesis —*see* Complications, joint
    prosthesis, mechanical, specified NEC,
    by site
  mastoid (antrum) (cell) —*see* Disorder,
    mastoid, specified NEC
  maxillary sinus —*see* Sinusitis, maxillary
  membrana tympani —*see* Perforation,
    tympanum

Perforation, perforated *(Continued)*
  nasal
    septum J34.89
      congenital Q30.3
      syphilitic A52.73
    sinus J34.89
      congenital Q30.8
      due to sinusitis —*see* Sinusitis
  palate —*see also* Cleft, palate Q35.9
    syphilitic A52.79
  palatine vault —*see also* Cleft, palate, hard Q35.1
    syphilitic A52.79
    congenital A50.59
  pars flaccida (ear drum) —*see* Perforation,
    tympanum, attic
  pelvic
    floor S31.030
      with
        ectopic or molar pregnancy O08.6
        penetration into retroperitoneal space
          S31.031
        retained foreign body S31.040
          with penetration into
            retroperitoneal space S31.041
      following ectopic or molar pregnancy
        O08.6
      obstetrical trauma O70.1
    organ S37.99
      adrenal gland S37.818
      bladder —*see* Perforation, bladder
      fallopian tube S37.599
        bilateral S37.592
        unilateral S37.591
      kidney S37.09-●
      obstetrical trauma O71.5
      ovary S37.499
        bilateral S37.492
        unilateral S37.491
      prostate S37.828
      specified organ NEC S37.898
      ureter —*see* Perforation, ureter
      urethra —*see* Perforation, urethra
      uterus —*see* Perforation, uterus
  perineum —*see* Laceration, perineum
  pharynx J39.2
  rectum K63.1
    newborn P78.0
    obstetrical trauma O71.5
    traumatic S36.63
  root canal space due to endodontic treatment
    M27.51
  sigmoid K63.1
    newborn P78.0
    obstetrical trauma O71.5
    traumatic S36.533
  sinus (accessory) (chronic) (nasal) J34.89
  sphenoidal sinus —*see* Sinusitis, sphenoidal
  surgical (accidental) (by instrument) (blood
    vessel) (nerve) (organ) —*see* Puncture,
    accidental complicating surgery
  traumatic
    external —*see* Puncture
    eye —*see* Puncture, eyeball
    internal organ —*see* Injury, by site
  tympanum, tympanic (membrane) (persistent
    post-traumatic) (postinflammatory)
    H72.9-●
    attic H72.1-●
      multiple —*see* Perforation, tympanum,
        multiple
      total —*see* Perforation, tympanum, total
    central H72.0-●
      multiple —*see* Perforation, tympanum,
        multiple
      total —*see* Perforation, tympanum, total
    marginal NEC —*see* subcategory H72.2
    multiple H72.81-●
    pars flaccida —*see* Perforation, tympanum,
      attic
    total H72.82-●
    traumatic, current episode S09.2-●

▶ New   ⇒ Revised   ~~deleted~~ Deleted   ● Use Additional Character(s)

Perforation, perforated (Continued)
  typhoid, gastrointestinal —see Typhoid
  ulcer —see Ulcer, by site, with perforation
  ureter N28.89
    traumatic S37.19
  urethra N36.8
    with ectopic or molar pregnancy O08.6
    following ectopic or molar pregnancy
      O08.6
    obstetrical trauma O71.5
    traumatic S37.39
      at delivery O71.5
  uterus
    with ectopic or molar pregnancy O08.6
    by intrauterine contraceptive device T83.39
    following ectopic or molar pregnancy
      O08.6
    obstetrical trauma O71.1
    traumatic S37.69
      obstetric O71.1
  uvula K13.79
    syphilitic A52.79
  vagina
    obstetrical trauma O71.4
    other trauma - see Puncture, vagina
Periadenitis mucosa necrotica recurrens K12.0
Periappendicitis (acute) —see Appendicitis
Periarteritis nodosa (disseminated) (infectious)
    (necrotizing) M30.0
Periarthritis (joint) —see also Enthesopathy
  Duplay's M75.0-●
  gonococcal A54.42
  humeroscapularis —see Capsulitis, adhesive
  scapulohumeral —see Capsulitis, adhesive
  shoulder —see Capsulitis, adhesive
  wrist M77.2-●
Periarthrosis (angioneural) —see
    Enthesopathy
Pericapsulitis, adhesive (shoulder) —see
    Capsulitis, adhesive
Pericarditis (with decompensation) (with
    effusion) I31.9
  with rheumatic fever (conditions in I00)
    active —see Pericarditis, rheumatic
    inactive or quiescent I09.2
  acute (hemorrhagic) (nonrheumatic) (Sicca)
    I30.9
    with chorea (acute) (rheumatic)
      (Sydenham's) I02.0
    benign I30.8
    nonspecific I30.0
    rheumatic I01.0
      with chorea (acute) (Sydenham's)
        I02.0
  adhesive or adherent (chronic) (external)
    (internal) I31.0
    acute —see Pericarditis, acute
    rheumatic I09.2
  bacterial (acute) (subacute) (with serous or
    seropurulent effusion) I30.1
  calcareous I31.1
  cholesterol (chronic) I31.8
    acute I30.9
  chronic (nonrheumatic) I31.9
    rheumatic I09.2
  constrictive (chronic) I31.1
  coxsackie B33.23
  fibrinocaseous (tuberculous) A18.84
  fibrinopurulent I30.1
  fibrinous I30.8
  fibrous I31.0
  gonococcal A54.83
  idiopathic I30.0
  in systemic lupus erythematosus M32.12
  infective I30.1
  meningococcal A39.53
  neoplastic (chronic) I31.8
    acute I30.9
  obliterans, obliterating I31.0
  plastic I31.0
  pneumococcal I30.1

Pericarditis (Continued)
  postinfarction I24.1
  purulent I30.1
  rheumatic (active) (acute) (with effusion)
    (with pneumonia) I01.0
    with chorea (acute) (rheumatic)
      (Sydenham's) I02.0
    chronic or inactive (with chorea) I09.2
  rheumatoid —see Rheumatoid, carditis
  septic I30.1
  serofibrinous I30.8
  staphylococcal I30.1
  streptococcal I30.1
  suppurative I30.1
  syphilitic A52.06
  tuberculous A18.84
  uremic N18.9 [132]
  viral I30.1
Pericardium, pericardial —see condition
Pericellulitis —see Cellulitis
Pericementitis (chronic) (suppurative) —see also
    Periodontitis
  acute K05.20
    generalized —see Peridontitis, aggressive,
      generalized
    localized —see Peridontitis, aggressive,
      localized
Perichondritis
  auricle —see Perichondritis, ear
  bronchus J98.09
  ear (external) H61.00-●
    acute H61.01-●
    chronic H61.02-●
  external auditory canal —see Perichondritis,
    ear
  larynx J38.7
    syphilitic A52.73
    typhoid A01.09
  nose J34.89
  pinna —see Perichondritis, ear
  trachea J39.8
Periclasia K05.4
Pericoronitis —see Periodontitis
Pericystitis N30.90
  with hematuria N30.91
Peridiverticulitis (intestine) K57.92
  cecum —see Diverticulitis, intestine, large
  colon —see Diverticulitis, intestine, large
  duodenum —see Diverticulitis, intestine,
    small
  intestine —see Diverticulitis, intestine
  jejunum —see Diverticulitis, intestine, small
  rectosigmoid —see Diverticulitis, intestine,
    large
  rectum —see Diverticulitis, intestine, large
  sigmoid —see Diverticulitis, intestine, large
Periendocarditis —see Endocarditis
Periepididymitis N45.1
Perifolliculitis L01.02
  abscedens, caput, scalp L66.3
  capitis, abscedens (et suffodiens) L66.3
  superficial pustular L01.02
Perihepatitis K65.8
Perilabyrinthitis (acute) —see subcategory H83.0
Perimeningitis —see Meningitis
Perimetritis —see Endometritis
Perimetrosalpingitis —see Salpingo-oophoritis
Perineocele N81.81
Perinephric, perinephritic —see condition
Perinephritis —see also Infection, kidney
  purulent —see Abscess, kidney
Perineum, perineal —see condition
Perineuritis NEC —see Neuralgia
Periodic —see condition
Periodontitis (chronic) (complex) (compound)
    (local) (simplex) K05.30
  acute K05.20
    generalized K05.229
      moderate K05.222
      severe K05.223
      slight K05.221

Periodontitis (Continued)
  acute (Continued)
    localized K05.219
      moderate K05.212
      severe K05.213
      slight K05.211
  apical K04.5
    acute (pulpal origin) K04.4
  generalized K05.329
    moderate K05.322
    severe K05.323
    slight K05.321
  localized K05.319
    moderate K05.312
    severe K05.313
    slight K05.311
Periodontoclasia K05.4
Periodontosis (juvenile) K05.4
Periods —see also Menstruation
  heavy N92.0
  irregular N92.6
  shortened intervals (irregular) N92.1
Perionychia —see also Cellulitis, digit
  with lymphangitis —see Lymphangitis, acute,
    digit
Perioophoritis —see Salpingo-oophoritis
Periorchitis N45.2
Periosteum, periosteal —see condition
Periostitis (albuminosa) (circumscribed)
    (diffuse) (infective) (monomelic) —see also
    Osteomyelitis
  alveolar M27.3
  alveolodental M27.3
  dental M27.3
  gonorrheal A54.43
  jaw (lower) (upper) M27.2
  orbit H05.03-●
  syphilitic A52.77
    congenital (early) A50.02 [M90.80]
    secondary A51.46
  tuberculous —see Tuberculosis, bone
  yaws (hypertrophic) (early) (late) A66.6
    [M90.80]
Periostosis (hyperplastic) —see also Disorder,
    bone, specified type NEC
  with osteomyelitis —see Osteomyelitis,
    specified type NEC
Peripartum
  cardiomyopathy O90.3
Periphlebitis —see Phlebitis
Periproctitis K62.89
Periprostatitis —see Prostatitis
Perirectal —see condition
Perirenal —see condition
Perisalpingitis —see Salpingo-oophoritis
Perisplenitis (infectional) D73.89
Peristalsis, visible or reversed R19.2
Peritendinitis —see Enthesopathy
Peritoneum, peritoneal —see condition
Peritonitis (adhesive) (bacterial) (fibrinous)
    (hemorrhagic) (idiopathic) (localized)
    (perforative) (primary) (with adhesions)
    (with effusion) K65.9
  with or following
    abscess K65.1
    appendicitis K35.3
      with perforation or rupture K35.2
        generalized K35.2
        localized K35.3
    diverticular disease (intestine) K57.80
      with bleeding K57.81
      ectopic or molar pregnancy O08.0
      large intestine K57.20
        with
          bleeding K57.21
          small intestine K57.40
            with bleeding K57.41
      small intestine K57.00
        with
          bleeding K57.01
          large intestine K57.40
            with bleeding K57.41

Peritonitis *(Continued)*
  acute (generalized) K65.Ø
  aseptic T81.61
  bile, biliary K65.3
  chemical T81.61
  chlamydial A74.81
  chronic proliferative K65.8
  complicating abortion —*see* Abortion, by
      type, complicated by, pelvic peritonitis
  congenital P78.1
  diaphragmatic K65.Ø
  diffuse K65.Ø
  diphtheritic A36.89
  disseminated K65.Ø
  due to
    bile K65.3
    foreign
      body or object accidentally left during
        a procedure (instrument) (sponge)
        (swab) T81.599
      substance accidentally left during a
        procedure (chemical) (powder)
        (talc) T81.61
    talc T81.61
    urine K65.8
  eosinophilic K65.8
    acute K65.Ø
  fibrocaseous (tuberculous) A18.31
  fibropurulent K65.Ø
  following ectopic or molar pregnancy
      OØ8.Ø
  general (ized) K65.Ø
  gonococcal A54.85
  meconium (newborn) P78.Ø
  neonatal P78.1
    meconium P78.Ø
  pancreatic K65.Ø
  paroxysmal, familial E85.Ø
    benign E85.Ø
  pelvic
    female N73.5
      acute N73.3
      chronic N73.4
        with adhesions N73.6
    male K65.Ø
  periodic, familial E85.Ø
  proliferative, chronic K65.8
  puerperal, postpartum, childbirth O85
  purulent K65.Ø
  septic K65.Ø
  specified NEC K65.8
  spontaneous bacterial K65.2
  subdiaphragmatic K65.Ø
  subphrenic K65.Ø
  suppurative K65.Ø
  syphilitic A52.74
    congenital (early) A5Ø.Ø8 [K67]
  talc T81.61
  tuberculous A18.31
  urine K65.8
Peritonsillar —*see* condition
Peritonsillitis J36
Perityphlitis K37
Periureteritis N28.89
Periurethral —*see* condition
Periurethritis (gangrenous) —*see* Urethritis
Periuterine —*see* condition
Perivaginitis —*see* Vaginitis
Perivasculitis, retinal H35.Ø6-●
Perivasitis (chronic) N49.1
Perivesiculitis (seminal) —*see* Vesiculitis
Perlèche NEC K13.Ø
  due to
    candidiasis B37.83
    moniliasis B37.83
    riboflavin deficiency E53.Ø
    vitamin B2 (riboflavin) deficiency E53.Ø
Pernicious —*see* condition
Pernio, perniosis T69.1
Perpetrator (of abuse) —*see* Index to External
    Causes of Injury, Perpetrator

Persecution
  delusion F22
  social Z6Ø.5
Perseveration (tonic) R48.8
Persistence, persistent (congenital)
  anal membrane Q42.3
    with fistula Q42.2
  arteria stapedia Q16.3
  atrioventricular canal Q21.2
  branchial cleft Q18.Ø
  ▶branchial cleft NOS Q18.2
    ▶cyst Q18.Ø
    ▶fistula Q18.Ø
    ▶sinus Q18.Ø
  bulbus cordis in left ventricle Q21.8
  canal of Cloquet Q14.Ø
  capsule (opaque) Q12.8
  cilioretinal artery or vein Q14.8
  cloaca Q43.7
  communication —*see* Fistula, congenital
  convolutions
    aortic arch Q25.46
    fallopian tube Q5Ø.6
    oviduct Q5Ø.6
    uterine tube Q5Ø.6
  double aortic arch Q25.45
  ductus arteriosus (Botalli) Q25.Ø
  fetal
    ⇒circulation P29.38
    form of cervix (uteri) Q51.828
    hemoglobin, hereditary (HPFH) D56.4
  foramen
    Botalli Q21.1
    ovale Q21.1
  Gartner's duct Q52.4
  hemoglobin, fetal (hereditary) (HPFH) D56.4
  hyaloid
    artery (generally incomplete) Q14.Ø
    system Q14.8
  hymen, in pregnancy or childbirth —*see*
      Pregnancy, complicated by, abnormal,
      vulva
  lanugo Q84.2
  left
    posterior cardinal vein Q26.8
    root with right arch of aorta Q25.49
    superior vena cava Q26.1
  Meckel's diverticulum Q43.Ø
    malignant —*see* Table of Neoplasms, small
        intestine, malignant
  mucosal disease (middle ear) —*see*
      Otitis, media, suppurative, chronic,
      tubotympanic
  nail(s), anomalous Q84.6
  omphalomesenteric duct Q43.Ø
  organ or site not listed —*see* Anomaly, by site
  ostium
    atrioventriculare commune Q21.2
    primum Q21.2
    secundum Q21.1
  ovarian rests in fallopian tube Q5Ø.6
  pancreatic tissue in intestinal tract Q43.8
  primary (deciduous)
    teeth KØØ.6
    vitreous hyperplasia Q14.Ø
  pupillary membrane Q13.89
  rhesus (Rh)titer —*see* Complication(s),
      transfusion, incompatibility reaction, Rh
      (factor)
  right aortic arch Q25.47
  sinus
    urogenitalis
      female Q52.8
      male Q55.8
    venosus with imperfect incorporation in
        right auricle Q26.8
  thymus (gland) (hyperplasia) E32.Ø
  thyroglossal duct Q89.2
  thyrolingual duct Q89.2
  truncus arteriosus or communis Q2Ø.Ø
  tunica vasculosa lentis Q12.2

Persistence, persistent *(Continued)*
  umbilical sinus Q64.4
  urachus Q64.4
  vitelline duct Q43.Ø
Person (with)
  admitted for clinical research, as a
      control subject (normal comparison)
      (participant) ZØØ.6
  awaiting admission to adequate facility
      elsewhere Z75.1
  concern (normal) about sick person in family
      Z63.6
  consulting on behalf of another Z71.Ø
  feigning illness Z76.5
  living (in)
    without
      adequate housing (heating) (space) Z59.1
      housing (permanent) (temporary) Z59.Ø
      person able to render necessary care
          Z74.2
      shelter Z59.Ø
    alone Z6Ø.2
    boarding school Z59.3
    residential institution Z59.3
  on waiting list Z75.1
  sick or handicapped in family Z63.6
Personality (disorder) F6Ø.9
  accentuation of traits (type A pattern) Z73.1
  affective F34.Ø
  aggressive F6Ø.3
  amoral F6Ø.2
  anacastic, anankastic F6Ø.5
  antisocial F6Ø.2
  anxious F6Ø.6
  asocial F6Ø.2
  asthenic F6Ø.7
  avoidant F6Ø.6
  borderline F6Ø.3
  change due to organic condition (enduring)
      FØ7.Ø
  compulsive F6Ø.5
  cycloid F34.Ø
  cyclothymic F34.Ø
  dependent F6Ø.7
  depressive F34.1
  dissocial F6Ø.2
  dual F44.81
  eccentric F6Ø.89
  emotionally unstable F6Ø.3
  expansive paranoid F6Ø.Ø
  explosive F6Ø.3
  fanatic F6Ø.Ø
  haltlose type F6Ø.89
  histrionic F6Ø.4
  hyperthymic F34.Ø
  hypothymic F34.1
  hysterical F6Ø.4
  immature F6Ø.89
  inadequate F6Ø.7
  labile (emotional) F6Ø.3
  mixed (nonspecific) F6Ø.89
  morally defective F6Ø.2
  multiple F44.81
  narcissistic F6Ø.81
  obsessional F6Ø.5
  obsessive (-compulsive) F6Ø.5
  organic FØ7.Ø
  overconscientious F6Ø.5
  paranoid F6Ø.Ø
  passive (-dependent) F6Ø.7
  passive-aggressive F6Ø.89
  pathologic F6Ø.9
  pattern defect or disturbance F6Ø.9
  pseudopsychopathic (organic) FØ7.Ø
  pseudoretarded (organic) FØ7.Ø
  psychoinfantile F6Ø.4
  psychoneurotic NEC F6Ø.89
  psychopathic F6Ø.2
  querulant F6Ø.Ø
  sadistic F6Ø.89
  schizoid F6Ø.1

▶ New   ⇒ Revised   ~~deleted~~ Deleted   ● Use Additional Character(s)

Personality *(Continued)*
  self-defeating F60.7
  sensitive paranoid F60.0
  sociopathic (amoral) (antisocial) (asocial)
    (dissocial) F60.2
  specified NEC F60.89
  type A Z73.1
  unstable (emotional) F60.3
Perthes' disease —*see* Legg-Calvé-Perthes
    disease
Pertussis *(see also* Whooping cough) A37.90
Perversion, perverted
  appetite F50.89
    psychogenic F50.89
  function
    pituitary gland E23.2
      posterior lobe E22.2
  sense of smell and taste R43.8
    psychogenic F45.8
  sexual —*see* Deviation, sexual
Pervious, congenital —*see also* Imperfect, closure
  ductus arteriosus Q25.0
Pes (congenital) —*see also* Talipes
  acquired —*see also* Deformity, limb, foot,
    specified NEC
    planus —*see* Deformity, limb, flat foot
  adductus Q66.89
  cavus Q66.7
  deformity NEC, acquired —*see* Deformity,
    limb, foot, specified NEC
  planus (acquired) (any degree) —*see also*
    Deformity, limb, flat foot
    rachitic sequelae (late effect) E64.3
  valgus Q66.6
Pest, pestis —*see* Plague
Petechia, petechiae R23.3
  newborn P54.5
Petechial typhus A75.9
Peter's anomaly Q13.4
Petit mal seizure —*see* Epilepsy, generalized,
    specified NEC
Petit's hernia —*see* Hernia, abdomen, specified
    site NEC
Petrellidosis B48.2
Petrositis H70.20-•
  acute H70.21-•
  chronic H70.22-•
Peutz-Jeghers disease or syndrome Q85.8
Peyronie's disease N48.6
PFAPA (periodic fever, aphthous stomatitis,
    pharyngitis, and adenopathy syndrome)
    M04.8
Pfeiffer's disease —*see* Mononucleosis,
    infectious
Phagedena (dry) (moist) (sloughing) —*see also*
    Gangrene
  geometric L88
  penis N48.29
  tropical —*see* Ulcer, skin
  vulva N76.6
Phagedenic —*see* condition
Phakoma H35.89
Phakomatosis —*see also* specific eponymous
    syndromes Q85.9
  Bourneville's Q85.1
  specified NEC Q85.8
Phantom limb syndrome (without pain) G54.7
  with pain G54.6
Pharyngeal pouch syndrome D82.1
Pharyngitis (acute) (catarrhal) (gangrenous)
    (infective) (malignant) (membranous)
    (phlegmonous) (pseudomembranous)
    (simple) (subacute) (suppurative)
    (ulcerative) (viral) J02.9
  with influenza, flu, or grippe —*see* Influenza,
    with, pharyngitis
  aphthous B08.5
  atrophic J31.2
  chlamydial A56.4
  chronic (atrophic) (granular) (hypertrophic)
    J31.2

Pharyngitis *(Continued)*
  coxsackievirus B08.5
  diphtheritic A36.0
  enteroviral vesicular B08.5
  follicular (chronic) J31.2
  fusospirochetal A69.1
  gonococcal A54.5
  granular (chronic) J31.2
  herpesviral B00.2
  hypertrophic J31.2
  infectional, chronic J31.2
  influenzal —*see* Influenza, with, respiratory
    manifestations NEC
  lymphonodular, acute (enteroviral) B08.8
  pneumococcal J02.8
  purulent J02.9
  putrid J02.9
  septic J02.0
  sicca J31.2
  specified organism NEC J02.8
  staphylococcal J02.8
  streptococcal J02.0
  syphilitic, congenital (early) A50.03
  tuberculous A15.8
  vesicular, enteroviral B08.5
  viral NEC J02.8
Pharyngoconjunctivitis, viral B30.2
Pharyngolaryngitis (acute) J06.0
  chronic J37.0
Pharyngoplegia J39.2
Pharyngotonsillitis, herpesviral B00.2
Pharyngotracheitis, chronic J42
Pharynx, pharyngeal —*see* condition
Phencyclidine-induced
  anxiety disorder F16.980
  bipolar and related disorder F16.94
  depressive disorder F16.94
  psychotic disorder F16.959
Phenomenon
  Arthus' —*see* Arthus' phenomenon
  jaw-winking Q07.8
  lupus erythematosus (LE) cell M32.9
  Raynaud's (secondary) I73.00
    with gangrene I73.01
  vasomotor R55
  vasospastic I73.9
  vasovagal R55
  Wenckebach's I44.1
Phenylketonuria E70.1
  classical E70.0
  maternal E70.1
Pheochromoblastoma
  specified site —*see* Neoplasm, malignant, by
    site
  unspecified site C74.10
Pheochromocytoma
  malignant
    specified site —*see* Neoplasm, malignant,
      by site
    unspecified site C74.10
  specified site —*see* Neoplasm, benign, by site
  unspecified site D35.00
Pheohyphomycosis —*see* Chromomycosis
Pheomycosis —*see* Chromomycosis
Phimosis (congenital) (due to infection) N47.1
  chancroidal A57
Phlebectasia —*see also* Varix
  congenital Q27.4
Phlebitis (infective) (pyemic) (septic)
    (suppurative) I80.9
  antepartum —*see* Thrombophlebitis,
    antepartum
  blue —*see* Phlebitis, leg, deep
  breast, superficial I80.8
  cavernous (venous) sinus —*see* Phlebitis,
    intracranial (venous) sinus
  cerebral (venous) sinus —*see* Phlebitis,
    intracranial (venous) sinus
  chest wall, superficial I80.8
  cranial (venous) sinus —*see* Phlebitis,
    intracranial (venous) sinus

Phlebitis *(Continued)*
  deep (vessels) —*see* Phlebitis, leg, deep
  due to implanted device —*see* Complications,
    by site and type, specified NEC
  during or resulting from a procedure
    T81.72
  femoral vein (superficial) I80.1-•
  femoropopliteal vein I80.0-•
  gestational —*see* Phlebopathy, gestational
  hepatic veins I80.8
  iliofemoral —*see* Phlebitis, femoral vein
  intracranial (venous) sinus (any) G08
    nonpyogenic I67.6
  intraspinal venous sinuses and veins G08
    nonpyogenic G95.19
  lateral (venous) sinus —*see* Phlebitis,
    intracranial (venous) sinus
  leg I80.3
    antepartum —*see* Thrombophlebitis,
      antepartum
    deep (vessels) NEC I80.20-•
      iliac I80.21-•
      popliteal vein I80.22-•
      specified vessel NEC I80.29-•
      tibial vein I80.23-•
    femoral vein (superficial) I80.1-•
    superficial (vessels) I80.0-•
  longitudinal sinus —*see* Phlebitis, intracranial
    (venous) sinus
  lower limb —*see* Phlebitis, leg
  migrans, migrating (superficial) I82.1
  pelvic
    with ectopic or molar pregnancy O08.0
    following ectopic or molar pregnancy
      O08.0
    puerperal, postpartum O87.1
  popliteal vein —*see* Phlebitis, leg, deep,
    popliteal
  portal (vein) K75.1
  postoperative T81.72
  pregnancy —*see* Thrombophlebitis,
    antepartum
  puerperal, postpartum, childbirth O87.0
    deep O87.1
    pelvic O87.1
    superficial O87.0
  retina —*see* Vasculitis, retina
  saphenous (accessory) (great) (long)
    (small) —*see* Phlebitis, leg, superficial
  sinus (meninges) —*see* Phlebitis, intracranial
    (venous) sinus
  specified site NEC I80.8
  syphilitic A52.09
  tibial vein —*see* Phlebitis, leg, deep, tibial
  ulcerative I80.9
    leg —*see* Phlebitis, leg
  umbilicus I80.8
  uterus (septic) —*see* Endometritis
  varicose (leg) (lower limb) —*see* Varix, leg,
    with, inflammation
Phlebofibrosis I87.8
Phleboliths I87.8
Phlebopathy
  gestational O22.9-•
  puerperal O87.9
Phlebosclerosis I87.8
Phlebothrombosis —*see also* Thrombosis
  antepartum —*see* Thrombophlebitis,
    antepartum
  pregnancy —*see* Thrombophlebitis,
    antepartum
  puerperal —*see* Thrombophlebitis,
    puerperal
Phlebotomus fever A93.1
Phlegmasia
  alba dolens O87.1
    nonpuerperal —*see* Phlebitis, femoral
      vein
  cerulea dolens —*see* Phlebitis, leg, deep
Phlegmon —*see* Abscess
Phlegmonous —*see* condition

Phlyctenulosis (allergic) (keratoconjunctivitis)
     (nontuberculous) —see also
     Keratoconjunctivitis
  cornea —see Keratoconjunctivitis
  tuberculous A18.52
Phobia, phobic F40.9
  animal F40.218
     spiders F40.210
  examination F40.298
  reaction F40.9
  simple F40.298
  social F40.10
     generalized F40.11
  specific (isolated) F40.298
     animal F40.218
        spiders F40.210
     blood F40.230
     injection F40.231
     injury F40.233
     men F40.290
     natural environment F40.228
        thunderstorms F40.220
     situational F40.248
        bridges F40.242
        closed in spaces F40.240
        flying F40.243
        heights F40.241
     specified focus NEC F40.298
     transfusion F40.231
     women F40.291
  specified NEC F40.8
     medical care NEC F40.232
  state F40.9
Phocas' disease —see Mastopathy, cystic
Phocomelia Q73.1
  lower limb —see Agenesis, leg, with foot
     present
  upper limb —see Agenesis, arm, with hand
     present
Phoria H50.50
Phosphate-losing tubular disorder N25.0
Phosphatemia E83.39
Phosphaturia E83.39
Photodermatitis (sun) L56.8
  chronic L57.8
  due to drug L56.8
  light other than sun L59.8
Photokeratitis H16.13-●
Photophobia H53.14-●
Photophthalmia —see Photokeratitis
Photopsia H53.19
Photoretinitis —see Retinopathy, solar
Photosensitivity, photosensitization (sun) skin
     L56.8
  light other than sun L59.8
Phrenitis —see Encephalitis
Phrynoderma (vitamin A deficiency)
     E50.8
Phthiriasis (pubis) B85.3
  with any infestation classifiable to
     B85.0-B85.2 B85.4
Phthirus infestation —see Phthiriasis
Phthisis —see also Tuberculosis
  bulbi (infectional) —see Disorder, globe,
     degenerated condition, atrophy
  eyeball (due to infection) —see Disorder,
     globe, degenerated condition, atrophy
Phycomycosis —see Zygomycosis
Physalopteriasis B81.8
Physical restraint status Z78.1
Phytobezoar T18.9
  intestine T18.3
  stomach T18.2
Pian —see Yaws
Pianoma A66.1
Pica F50.89
  in adults F50.89
  infant or child F98.3
Picking, nose F98.8
Pick-Niemann disease —see Niemann-Pick
  disease or syndrome

Pick's
  cerebral atrophy G31.01 [F02.80]
     with behavioral disturbance G31.01
        [F02.81]
  disease or syndrome (brain) G31.01 [F02.80]
     with behavioral disturbance G31.01
        [F02.81]
     brain G31.01 [F02.80]
        with behavioral disturbance G31.01
           [F02.81]
     pericardium (pericardial pseudocirrhosis
        of liver) I31.1
  syndrome
     brain G31.01 [F02.80]
        with behavioral disturbance G31.01
           [F02.81]
     of heart (pericardial pseudocirrhosis of
        liver) I31.1
Pickwickian syndrome E66.2
Piebaldism E70.39
Piedra (beard) (scalp) B36.8
  black B36.3
  white B36.2
Pierre Robin deformity or syndrome Q87.0
Pierson's disease or osteochondrosis M91.0
Pig-bel A05.2
Pigeon
  breast or chest (acquired) M95.4
     congenital Q67.7
        rachitic sequelae (late effect) E64.3
  breeder's disease or lung J67.2
  fancier's disease or lung J67.2
  toe —see Deformity, toe, specified NEC
Pigmentation (abnormal) (anomaly) L81.9
  conjunctiva H11.13-●
  cornea (anterior) H18.01-●
     posterior H18.05-●
     stromal H18.06-●
  diminished melanin formation NEC L81.6
  iron L81.8
  lids, congenital Q82.8
  limbus corneae —see Pigmentation, cornea
  metals L81.8
  optic papilla, congenital Q14.2
  retina, congenital (grouped) (nevoid) Q14.1
  scrotum, congenital Q82.8
  tattoo L81.8
Piles —see also Hemorrhoids K64.9
Pili
  annulati or torti (congenital) Q84.1
  incarnati L73.1
Pill roller hand (intrinsic) —see Parkinsonism
Pilomatrixoma —see Neoplasm, skin, benign
  malignant —see Neoplasm, skin, malignant
Pilonidal —see condition
Pimple R23.8
PIN —see Neoplasia, intraepithelial, prostate
Pinched nerve —see Neuropathy, entrapment
Pindborg tumor —see Cyst, calcifying
  odontogenic
Pineal body or gland —see condition
Pinealoblastoma C75.3
Pinealoma D44.5
  malignant C75.3
Pineoblastoma C75.3
Pineocytoma D44.5
Pinguecula H11.15-●
Pingueculitis H10.81-●
Pinhole meatus —see also Stricture, urethra
     N35.9
Pink
  disease —see subcategory T56.1
  eye —see Conjunctivitis, acute, mucopurulent
Pinkus' disease (lichen nitidus) L44.1
Pinpoint
  meatus —see Stricture, urethra
  os (uteri) —see Stricture, cervix
Pins and needles R20.2
Pinta A67.9
  cardiovascular lesions A67.2
  chancre (primary) A67.0

Pinta (Continued)
  erythematous plaques A67.1
  hyperchromic lesions A67.1
  hyperkeratosis A67.1
  lesions A67.9
     cardiovascular A67.2
     hyperchromic A67.1
     intermediate A67.1
     late A67.2
     mixed A67.3
     primary A67.0
     skin (achromic) (cicatricial) (dyschromic)
        A67.2
        hyperchromic A67.1
        mixed (achromic and hyperchromic)
           A67.3
  papule (primary) A67.0
  skin lesions (achromic) (cicatricial)
     (dyschromic) A67.2
     hyperchromic A67.1
     mixed (achromic and hyperchromic)
        A67.3
  vitiligo A67.2
Pintids A67.1
Pinworm (disease) (infection) (infestation) B80
Piroplasmosis B60.0
Pistol wound —see Gunshot wound
Pitchers' elbow —see Derangement, joint,
     specified type NEC, elbow
Pithecoid pelvis Q74.2
  with disproportion (fetopelvic) O33.0
     causing obstructed labor O65.0
Pithiatism F48.8
Pitted —see Pitting
Pitting —see also Edema R60.9
  lip R60.0
  nail L60.8
  teeth K00.4
Pituitary gland —see condition
Pituitary-snuff-taker's disease J67.8
Pityriasis (capitis) L21.0
  alba L30.5
  circinata (et maculata) L42
  furfuracea L21.0
  Hebra's L26
  lichenoides L41.0
     chronica L41.1
     et varioliformis (acuta) L41.0
  maculata (et circinata) L30.5
  nigra B36.1
  pilaris, Hebra's L44.0
  rosea L42
  rotunda L44.8
  rubra (Hebra) pilaris L44.0
  simplex L30.5
  specified type NEC L30.5
  streptogenes L30.5
  versicolor (scrotal) B36.0
Placenta, placental —see Pregnancy,
     complicated by (care of) (management
     affected by), specified condition
Placentitis O41.14-●
Plagiocephaly Q67.3
Plague A20.9
  abortive A20.8
  ambulatory A20.8
  asymptomatic A20.8
  bubonic A20.0
  cellulocutaneous A20.1
  cutaneobubonic A20.1
  lymphatic gland A20.0
  meningitis A20.3
  pharyngeal A20.8
  pneumonic (primary) (secondary) A20.2
  pulmonary, pulmonic A20.2
  septicemic A20.7
  tonsillar A20.8
     septicemic A20.7
Planning, family
  contraception Z30.9
  procreation Z31.69

Plaque(s)
    artery, arterial —see Arteriosclerosis
    calcareous —see Calcification
    coronary, lipid rich I25.83
    epicardial I31.8
    erythematous, of pinta A67.1
    Hollenhorst's —see Occlusion, artery,
        retina
    lipid rich, coronary I25.83
    pleural (without asbestos) J92.9
        with asbestos J92.0
    tongue K13.29
Plasmacytoma C90.3-●
    extramedullary C90.2-●
    medullary C90.0-●
    solitary C90.3-●
Plasmacytopenia D72.818
Plasmacytosis D72.822
Plaster ulcer —see Ulcer, pressure, by site
Plateau iris syndrome (post-iridectomy)
        (postprocedural) (without glaucoma)
        H21.82
    with glaucoma H40.22-●
Platybasia Q75.8
Platyonychia (congenital) Q84.6
    acquired L60.8
Platypelloid pelvis M95.5
    with disproportion (fetopelvic) O33.0
        causing obstructed labor O65.0
    congenital Q74.2
Platyspondylisis Q76.49
Plaut (-Vincent) disease —see also Vincent's
        A69.1
Plethora R23.2
    newborn P61.1
Pleura, pleural —see condition
Pleuralgia R07.81
Pleurisy (acute) (adhesive) (chronic) (costal)
        (diaphragmatic) (double) (dry) (fibrinous)
        (fibrous) (interlobar) (latent) (plastic)
        (primary) (residual) (sicca) (sterile)
        (subacute) (unresolved) R09.1
    with
        adherent pleura J86.0
        effusion J90
            chylous, chyliform J94.0
            tuberculous (non primary)
                A15.6
                primary (progressive) A15.7
            tuberculosis —see Pleurisy, tuberculous
                (non primary)
    encysted —see Pleurisy, with effusion
    exudative —see Pleurisy, with effusion
    fibrinopurulent, fibropurulent —see
        Pyothorax
    hemorrhagic —see Hemothorax
    pneumococcal J90
    purulent —see Pyothorax
    septic —see Pyothorax
    serofibrinous —see Pleurisy, with effusion
    seropurulent —see Pyothorax
    serous —see Pleurisy, with effusion
    staphylococcal J86.9
    streptococcal J90
    suppurative —see Pyothorax
    traumatic (post) (current) —see Injury,
        intrathoracic, pleura
    tuberculous (with effusion) (non primary)
        A15.6
        primary (progressive) A15.7
Pleuritis sicca —see Pleurisy
Pleurobronchopneumonia —see Pneumonia,
        broncho
Pleurodynia R07.81
    epidemic B33.0
    viral B33.0
Pleuropericarditis —see also Pericarditis
    acute I30.9
Pleuropneumonia (acute) (bilateral) (double)
        (septic) —see also Pneumonia J18.8
    chronic —see Fibrosis, lung

Pleuro-pneumonia-like-organism (PPLO),
        as cause of disease classified elsewhere
        B96.0
Pleurorrhea —see Pleurisy, with effusion
Plexitis, brachial G54.0
Plica
    polonica B85.0
    syndrome, knee M67.5
    tonsil J35.8
Plicated tongue K14.5
Plug
    bronchus NEC J98.09
    meconium (newborn) NEC syndrome P76.0
    mucus —see Asphyxia, mucus
Plumbism —see subcategory T56.0
Plummer's disease E05.20
    with thyroid storm E05.21
Plummer-Vinson syndrome D50.1
Pluricarential syndrome of infancy E40
Plus (and minus) hand (intrinsic) —see
        Deformity, limb, specified type NEC,
        forearm
Pneumathemia —see Air, embolism
Pneumatic hammer (drill) syndrome T75.21
Pneumatocele (lung) J98.4
    intracranial G93.89
    tension J44.9
Pneumatosis
    cystoides intestinalis K63.89
    intestinalis K63.89
    peritonei K66.8
Pneumaturia R39.89
Pneumoblastoma —see Neoplasm, lung,
        malignant
Pneumocephalus G93.89
Pneumococcemia A40.3
Pneumococcus, pneumococcal —see condition
Pneumoconiosis (due to) (inhalation of) J64
    with tuberculosis (any type in A15) J65
    aluminum J63.0
    asbestos J61
    bagasse, bagassosis J67.1
    bauxite J63.1
    beryllium J63.2
    coal miners' (simple) J60
    coalworkers' (simple) J60
    collier's J60
    cotton dust J66.0
    diatomite (diatomaceous earth) J62.8
    dust
        inorganic NEC J63.6
        lime J62.8
        marble J62.8
        organic NEC J66.8
    fumes or vapors (from silo) J68.9
    graphite J63.3
    grinder's J62.8
    kaolin J62.8
    mica J62.8
    millstone maker's J62.8
    mineral fibers NEC J61
    miner's J60
    moldy hay J67.0
    potter's J62.8
    rheumatoid —see Rheumatoid, lung
    sandblaster's J62.8
    silica, silicate NEC J62.8
        with carbon J60
    stonemason's J62.8
    talc (dust) J62.0
Pneumocystis carinii pneumonia B59
Pneumocystis jiroveci (pneumonia) B59
Pneumocystosis (with pneumonia) B59
Pneumohemopericardium I31.2
Pneumohemothorax J94.2
    traumatic S27.2
Pneumohydropericardium —see Pericarditis
Pneumohydrothorax —see Hydrothorax
Pneumomediastinum J98.2
    congenital or perinatal P25.2
Pneumomycosis B49 [J99]

Pneumonia (acute) (double) (migratory)
        (purulent) (septic) (unresolved) J18.9
    with
        influenza —see Influenza, with, pneumonia
        lung abscess J85.1
            due to specified organism —see
                Pneumonia, in (due to)
    adenoviral J12.0
    adynamic J18.2
    alba A50.04
    allergic (eosinophilic) J82
    alveolar —see Pneumonia, lobar
    anaerobes J15.8
    anthrax A22.1
    apex, apical —see Pneumonia, lobar
    Ascaris B77.81
    aspiration J69.0
        due to
            aspiration of microorganisms
                bacterial J15.9
                viral J12.9
            food (regurgitated) J69.0
            gastric secretions J69.0
            milk (regurgitated) J69.0
            oils, essences J69.1
            solids, liquids NEC J69.8
            vomitus J69.0
        newborn P24.81
            amniotic fluid (clear) P24.11
            blood P24.21
            food (regurgitated) P24.31
            liquor (amnii) P24.11
            meconium P24.01
            milk P24.31
            mucus P24.11
            specified NEC P24.81
            stomach contents P24.31
        postprocedural J95.4
    atypical NEC J18.9
    bacillus J15.9
        specified NEC J15.8
    bacterial J15.9
        specified NEC J15.8
    Bacteroides (fragilis) (oralis)
            (melaninogenicus) J15.8
    basal, basic, basilar —see Pneumonia, by type
    bronchiolitis obliterans organized (BOOP)
            J84.89
    broncho-, bronchial (confluent) (croupous)
            (diffuse) (disseminated) (hemorrhagic)
            (involving lobes) (lobar) (terminal) J18.0
        allergic (eosinophilic) J82
        aspiration —see Pneumonia, aspiration
        bacterial J15.9
            specified NEC J15.8
        chronic —see Fibrosis, lung
        diplococcal J13
        Eaton's agent J15.7
        Escherichia coli (E. coli) J15.5
        Friedländer's bacillus J15.0
        Hemophilus influenzae J14
        hypostatic J18.2
        inhalation —see also Pneumonia, aspiration
            due to fumes or vapors (chemical) J68.0
            of oils or essences J69.1
        Klebsiella (pneumoniae) J15.0
        lipid, lipoid J69.1
            endogenous J84.89
        Mycoplasma (pneumoniae) J15.7
        pleuro-pneumonia-like-organisms (PPLO)
            J15.7
        pneumococcal J13
        Proteus J15.6
        Pseudomonas J15.1
        Serratia marcescens J15.6
        specified organism NEC J16.8
        staphylococcal —see Pneumonia,
            staphylococcal
        streptococcal NEC J15.4
            group B J15.3
            pneumoniae J13
        viral, virus —see Pneumonia, viral

Pneumonia (*Continued*)
Butyrivibrio (fibriosolvens) J15.8
Candida B37.1
caseous —*see* Tuberculosis, pulmonary
catarrhal —*see* Pneumonia, broncho
chlamydial J16.0
  congenital P23.1
cholesterol J84.89
cirrhotic (chronic) —*see* Fibrosis, lung
Clostridium (haemolyticum) (novyi) J15.8
confluent —*see* Pneumonia, broncho
congenital (infective) P23.9
  due to
    bacterium NEC P23.6
    Chlamydia P23.1
    Escherichia coli P23.4
    Haemophilus influenzae P23.6
    infective organism NEC P23.8
    Klebsiella pneumoniae P23.6
    Mycoplasma P23.6
    Pseudomonas P23.5
    Staphylococcus P23.2
    Streptococcus (except group B) P23.6
      group B P23.3
    viral agent P23.0
  specified NEC P23.8
croupous —*see* Pneumonia, lobar
cryptogenic organizing J84.116
cytomegalic inclusion B25.0
cytomegaloviral B25.0
deglutition —*see* Pneumonia, aspiration
desquamative interstitial J84.117
diffuse —*see* Pneumonia, broncho
diplococcal, diplococcus (broncho-) (lobar)
  J13
disseminated (focal) —*see* Pneumonia,
  broncho
Eaton's agent J15.7
embolic, embolism —*see* Embolism,
  pulmonary
Enterobacter J15.6
eosinophilic J82
Escherichia coli (E. coli) J15.5
Eubacterium J15.8
fibrinous —*see* Pneumonia, lobar
fibroid, fibrous (chronic) —*see* Fibrosis, lung
Friedländer's bacillus J15.0
Fusobacterium (nucleatum) J15.8
gangrenous J85.0
giant cell (measles) B05.2
gonococcal A54.84
gram-negative bacteria NEC J15.6
  anaerobic J15.8
Hemophilus influenzae (broncho) (lobar) J14
human metapneumovirus J12.3
hypostatic (broncho) (lobar) J18.2
in (due to)
  actinomycosis A42.0
  adenovirus J12.0
  anthrax A22.1
  ascariasis B77.81
  aspergillosis B44.9
  Bacillus anthracis A22.1
  Bacterium anitratum J15.6
  candidiasis B37.1
  chickenpox B01.2
  Chlamydia J16.0
    neonatal P23.1
  coccidioidomycosis B38.2
    acute B38.0
    chronic B38.1
  cytomegalovirus disease B25.0
  Diplococcus (pneumoniae) J13
  Eaton's agent J15.7
  Enterobacter J15.6
  Escherichia coli (E. coli) J15.5
  Friedländer's bacillus J15.0
  fumes and vapors (chemical) (inhalation)
    J68.0
  gonorrhea A54.84
  Hemophilus influenzae (H. influenzae) J14

Pneumonia (*Continued*)
in (*Continued*)
  Herellea J15.6
  histoplasmosis B39.2
    acute B39.0
    chronic B39.1
  human metapneumovirus J12.3
  Klebsiella (pneumoniae) J15.0
  measles B05.2
  Mycoplasma (pneumoniae) J15.7
  nocardiosis, nocardiasis A43.0
  ornithosis A70
  parainfluenza virus J12.2
  pleuro-pneumonia-like-organism (PPLO)
    J15.7
  pneumococcus J13
  pneumocystosis (Pneumocystis carinii)
    (Pneumocystis jiroveci) B59
  Proteus J15.6
  Pseudomonas NEC J15.1
    pseudomallei A24.1
  psittacosis A70
  Q fever A78
  respiratory syncytial virus J12.1
  rheumatic fever I00 *[J17]*
  rubella B06.81
  Salmonella (infection) A02.22
    typhi A01.03
  schistosomiasis B65.9 *[J17]*
  Serratia marcescens J15.6
  specified
    bacterium NEC J15.8
    organism NEC J16.8
  spirochetal NEC A69.8
  Staphylococcus J15.20
    aureus (methicillin susceptible) (MSSA)
      J15.211
      methicillin resistant (MRSA)
        J15.212
    specified NEC J15.29
  Streptococcus J15.4
    group B J15.3
    pneumoniae J13
    specified NEC J15.4
  toxoplasmosis B58.3
  tularemia A21.2
  typhoid (fever) A01.03
  varicella B01.2
  virus —*see* Pneumonia, viral
  whooping cough A37.91
    due to
      Bordetella parapertussis A37.11
      Bordetella pertussis A37.01
      specified NEC A37.81
  Yersinia pestis A20.2
inhalation of food or vomit —*see* Pneumonia,
  aspiration
interstitial J84.9
  chronic J84.111
  desquamative J84.117
  due to
    collagen vascular disease J84.17
    known underlying cause J84.17
  idiopathic NOS J84.111
  in disease classified elsewhere J84.17
  lymphocytic (due to collagen vascular
    disease) (in diseases classified
    elsewhere) J84.17
  lymphoid J84.2
  non-specific J84.89
    due to
      collagen vascular disease J84.17
      known underlying cause J84.17
    idiopathic J84.113
    in diseases classified elsewhere J84.17
  plasma cell B59
  pseudomonas J15.1
  usual J84.112
    due to collagen vascular disease J84.17
    idiopathic J84.112
    in diseases classified elsewhere J84.17

Pneumonia (*Continued*)
  Klebsiella (pneumoniae) J15.0
  lipid, lipoid (exogenous) J69.1
    endogenous J84.89
  lobar (disseminated) (double) (interstitial)
    J18.1
    bacterial J15.9
      specified NEC J15.8
    chronic —*see* Fibrosis, lung
    Escherichia coli (E. coli) J15.5
    Friedländer's bacillus J15.0
    Hemophilus influenzae J14
    hypostatic J18.2
    Klebsiella (pneumoniae) J15.0
    pneumococcal J13
    Proteus J15.6
    Pseudomonas J15.1
    specified organism NEC J16.8
    staphylococcal —*see* Pneumonia,
      staphylococcal
    streptococcal NEC J15.4
    Streptococcus pneumoniae J13
    viral, virus —*see* Pneumonia, viral
  lobular —*see* Pneumonia, broncho
  Löffler's J82
  lymphoid interstitial J84.2
  massive —*see* Pneumonia, lobar
  meconium P24.01
  MRSA (Methicillin resistant Staphylococcus
    aureus) J15.212
  MSSA (methicillin susceptible Staphylococcus
    aureus) J15.211
  multilobar —*see* Pneumonia, by type
  Mycoplasma (pneumoniae) J15.7
  necrotic J85.0
  neonatal P23.9
    aspiration —*see* Aspiration, by substance,
      with pneumonia
  nitrogen dioxide J68.0
  organizing J84.89
    due to
      collagen vascular disease J84.17
      known underlying cause J84.17
    in diseases classified elsewhere
      J84.17
  orthostatic J18.2
  parainfluenza virus J12.2
  parenchymatous —*see* Fibrosis, lung
  passive J18.2
  patchy —*see* Pneumonia, broncho
  Peptococcus J15.8
  Peptostreptococcus J15.8
  plasma cell (of infants) B59
  pleurolobar —*see* Pneumonia, lobar
  pleuro-pneumonia-like organism (PPLO)
    J15.7
  pneumococcal (broncho) (lobar) J13
  Pneumocystis (carinii) (jiroveci) B59
  postinfectional NEC B99 *[J17]*
  postmeasles B05.2
  Proteus J15.6
  Pseudomonas J15.1
  psittacosis A70
  radiation J70.0
  respiratory syncytial virus J12.1
  resulting from a procedure J95.89
  rheumatic I00 *[J17]*
  Salmonella (arizonae) (cholerae-suis)
    (enteritidis) (typhimurium)
    A02.22
    typhi A01.03
    typhoid fever A01.03
  SARS-associated coronavirus J12.81
  segmented, segmental —*see* Pneumonia,
    broncho- •
  Serratia marcescens J15.6
  specified NEC J18.8
    bacterium NEC J15.8
    organism NEC J16.8
    virus NEC J12.89
  spirochetal NEC A69.8

▶ New   ⇒ Revised   ~~deleted~~ Deleted   • Use Additional Character(s)

Pneumonia *(Continued)*
  staphylococcal (broncho) (lobar) J15.20
    aureus (methicillin susceptible) (MSSA)
      J15.211
      methicillin resistant (MRSA) J15.212
    specified NEC J15.29
  static, stasis J18.2
  streptococcal NEC (broncho) (lobar) J15.4
    group
      A J15.4
      B J15.3
      specified NEC J15.4
  Streptococcus pneumoniae J13
  syphilitic, congenital (early) A50.04
  traumatic (complication) (early) (secondary)
    T79.8
  tuberculous (any) —*see* Tuberculosis,
    pulmonary
  tularemic A21.2
  varicella B01.2
  Veillonella J15.8
  ventilator associated J95.851
  viral, virus (broncho) (interstitial) (lobar) J12.9
    adenoviral J12.0
    congenital P23.0
    human metapneumovirus J12.3
    parainfluenza J12.2
    respiratory syncytial J12.1
    SARS-associated coronavirus J12.81
    specified NEC J12.89
  white (congenital) A50.04
Pneumonic —*see* condition
Pneumonitis (acute) (primary) —*see also*
    Pneumonia
  air-conditioner J67.7
  allergic (due to) J67.9
    organic dust NEC J67.8
    red cedar dust J67.8
    sequoiosis J67.8
    wood dust J67.8
  aspiration J69.0
    due to
      anesthesia J95.4
        during
          labor and delivery O74.0
          pregnancy O29.01-•
          puerperium O89.01
      fumes or gases J68.0
      obstetric O74.0
  chemical (due to gases, fumes or vapors)
    (inhalation) J68.0
    due to anesthesia J95.4
  cholesterol J84.89
  chronic —*see* Fibrosis, lung
  congenital rubella P35.0
  crack (cocaine) J68.0
  due to
    beryllium J68.0
    cadmium J68.0
    crack (cocaine) J68.0
    detergent J69.8
    fluorocarbon-polymer J68.0
    food, vomit (aspiration) J69.0
    fumes or vapors J68.0
    gases, fumes or vapors (inhalation) J68.0
    inhalation
      blood J69.8
      essences J69.1
      food (regurgitated), milk, vomit
        J69.0
      oils, essences J69.1
      saliva J69.0
      solids, liquids NEC J69.8
    manganese J68.0
    nitrogen dioxide J68.0
    oils, essences J69.1
    solids, liquids NEC J69.8
    toxoplasmosis (acquired) B58.3
      congenital P37.1
    vanadium J68.0
    ventilator J95.851

Pneumonitis *(Continued)*
  eosinophilic J82
  hypersensitivity J67.9
    air conditioner lung J67.7
    bagassosis J67.1
    bird fancier's lung J67.2
    farmer's lung J67.0
    maltworker's lung J67.4
    maple bark-stripper's lung J67.6
    mushroom worker's lung J67.5
    specified organic dust NEC J67.8
    suberosis J67.3
  interstitial (chronic) J84.89
    acute J84.114
    lymphoid J84.2
    non-specific J84.89
      idiopathic J84.113
  lymphoid, interstitial J84.2
  meconium P24.01
  postanesthetic J95.4
    correct substance properly administered —
      see Table of Drugs and Chemcials, by
      drug, adverse effect
    in labor and delivery O74.0
    in pregnancy O29.01-•
    obstetric O74.0
    overdose or wrong substance given or taken
      (by accident) —*see* Table of Drugs and
      Chemicals, by drug, poisoning
    postpartum, puerperal O89.01
  postoperative J95.4
    obstetric O74.0
  radiation J70.0
  rubella, congenital P35.0
  ventilation (air-conditioning) J67.7
  ventilator associated J95.851
  wood-dust J67.8
Pneumonoconiosis —*see* Pneumoconiosis
Pneumoparotid K11.8
Pneumopathy NEC J98.4
  alveolar J84.09
  due to organic dust NEC J66.8
  parietoalveolar J84.09
Pneumopericarditis —*see also* Pericarditis
  acute I30.9
Pneumopericardium —*see also* Pericarditis
  congenital P25.3
  newborn P25.3
  traumatic (post) —*see* Injury, heart
Pneumophagia (psychogenic) F45.8
Pneumopleurisy, pneumopleuritis —*see also*
    Pneumonia J18.8
Pneumopyopericardium I30.1
Pneumopyothorax —*see* Pyopneumothorax
  with fistula J86.0
Pneumorrhagia —*see also* Hemorrhage, lung
  tuberculous —*see* Tuberculosis, pulmonary
Pneumothorax NOS J93.9
  acute J93.83
  chronic J93.81
  congenital P25.1
  perinatal period P25.1
  postprocedural J95.811
  specified NEC J93.83
  spontaneous NOS J93.83
    newborn P25.1
    primary J93.11
    secondary J93.12
    tension J93.0
  tense valvular, infectional J93.0
  tension (spontaneous) J93.0
  traumatic S27.0
    with hemothorax S27.2
  tuberculous —*see* Tuberculosis, pulmonary
Podagra —*see also* Gout M10.9
Podencephalus Q01.9
Poikilocytosis R71.8
Poikiloderma L81.6
  Civatte's L57.3
  congenital Q82.8
  vasculare atrophicans L94.5

Poikilodermatomyositis M33.10
  with
    myopathy M33.12
    respiratory involvement M33.11
    specified organ involvement NEC M33.19
Pointed ear (congenital) Q17.3
Poison ivy, oak, sumac or other plant
  dermatitis (allergic) (contact) L23.7
Poisoning (acute) —*see also* Table of Drugs and
  Chemicals
  algae and toxins T65.82-•
  Bacillus B (aertrycke) (cholerae (suis))
    (paratyphosus) (suipestifer) A02.9
  botulinus A05.1
  bacterial toxins A05.9
  berries, noxious —*see* Poisoning, food,
    noxious, berries
  botulism A05.1
  ciguatera fish T61.0-•
  Clostridium botulinum A05.1
  death-cap (Amanita phalloides) (Amanita
    verna) —*see* Poisoning, food, noxious,
    mushrooms
  drug —*see* Table of Drugs and Chemicals, by
    drug, poisoning
  epidemic, fish (noxious) —*see* Poisoning,
    seafood
    bacterial A05.9
  fava bean D55.0
  fish (noxious) T61.9-•
    bacterial —*see* Intoxication, foodborne, by
      agent
    ciguatera fish —*see* Poisoning, ciguatera
      fish
    scombroid fish —*see* Poisoning, scombroid
      fish
    specified type NEC T61.77-•
  food (acute) (diseased) (infected) (noxious)
    NEC T62.9-•
    bacterial —*see* Intoxication, foodborne, by
      agent
    due to
      Bacillus (aertrycke) (choleraesuis)
        (paratyphosus) (suipestifer) A02.9
      botulinus A05.1
      Clostridium (perfringens) (Welchii)
        A05.2
      salmonella (aertrycke) (callinarum)
        (choleraesuis) (enteritidis)
        (paratyphi) (suipestifer) A02.9
      with
        gastroenteritis A02.0
        sepsis A02.1
      staphylococcus A05.0
      Vibrio
        parahaemolyticus A05.3
        vulnificus A05.5
    noxious or naturally toxic T62.9-•
      berries —*see* subcategory T62.1-•
      fish —*see* Poisoning, seafood
      mushrooms —*see* subcategory T62.0X-•
      plants NEC —*see* subcategory T62.2X-•
      seafood —*see* Poisoning, seafood
      specified NEC —*see* subcategory
        T62.8X-•
  ichthyotoxism —*see* Poisoning, seafood
  kreotoxism, food A05.9
  latex T65.81-•
  lead T56.0-•
  mushroom —*see* Poisoning, food, noxious,
    mushroom
  mussels —*see also* Poisoning, shellfish
    bacterial —*see* Intoxication, foodborne, by
      agent
  nicotine (tobacco) T65.2-•
  noxious foodstuffs —*see* Poisoning, food,
    noxious
  plants, noxious —*see* Poisoning, food,
    noxious, plants NEC
  ptomaine —*see* Poisoning, food
  radiation J70.0

Poisoning *(Continued)*
  Salmonella (arizonae) (cholerae-suis)
    (enteritidis) (typhimurium) A02.9
  scombroid fish T61.1-●
  seafood (noxious) T61.9-●
    bacterial —*see* Intoxication, foodborne, by
      agent
    fish —*see* Poisoning, fish
    shellfish —*see* Poisoning, shellfish
    specified NEC —*see* subcategory T61.8X-●
  shellfish (amnesic) (azaspiracid) (diarrheic)
    (neurotoxic) (noxious) (paralytic)
    T61.78-●
    bacterial —*see* Intoxication, foodborne, by
      agent
    ciguatera mollusk —*see* Poisoning,
      ciguatera fish
  specified substance NEC T65.891
  Staphylococcus, food A05.0
  tobacco (nicotine) T65.2-●
  water E87.79
Poker spine —*see* Spondylitis, ankylosing
Poland syndrome Q79.8
Polioencephalitis (acute) (bulbar) A80.9
  inferior G12.22
  influenzal —*see* Influenza, with,
    encephalopathy
  superior hemorrhagic (acute) (Wernicke's)
    E51.2
  Wernicke's E51.2
Polioencephalomyelitis (acute) (anterior) A80.9
  with beriberi E51.2
Polioencephalopathy, superior hemorrhagic
  E51.2
  with
    beriberi E51.11
    pellagra E52
Poliomeningoencephalitis —*see*
  Meningoencephalitis
Poliomyelitis (acute) (anterior) (epidemic)
  A80.9
  with paralysis (bulbar) —*see* Poliomyelitis,
    paralytic
  abortive A80.4
  ascending (progressive) —*see* Poliomyelitis,
    paralytic
  bulbar (paralytic) —*see* Poliomyelitis,
    paralytic
  congenital P35.8
  nonepidemic A80.9
  nonparalytic A80.4
  paralytic A80.30
    specified NEC A80.39
    vaccine-associated A80.0
    wild virus
      imported A80.1
      indigenous A80.2
  spinal, acute A80.9
Poliosis (eyebrow) (eyelashes) L67.1
  circumscripta, acquired L67.1
Pollakiuria R35.0
  psychogenic F45.8
Pollinosis J30.1
Pollitzer's disease L73.2
Polyadenitis —*see also* Lymphadenitis
  malignant A20.0
Polyalgia M79.89
Polyangiitis M30.0
  microscopic M31.7
  overlap syndrome M30.8
Polyarteritis
  microscopic M31.7
  nodosa M30.0
    with lung involvement M30.1
    juvenile M30.2
    related condition NEC M30.8
Polyarthralgia —*see* Pain, joint
Polyarthritis, polyarthropathy —*see also*
  Arthritis M13.0
  due to or associated with other specified
    conditions —*see* Arthritis

Polyarthritis, polyarthropathy *(Continued)*
  epidemic (Australian) (with exanthema)
    B33.1
  infective —*see* Arthritis, pyogenic or
    pyemic
  inflammatory M06.4
  juvenile (chronic) (seronegative)
    M08.3
  migratory —*see* Fever, rheumatic
  rheumatic, acute —*see* Fever, rheumatic
Polyarthrosis M15.9
  post-traumatic M15.3
  primary M15.0
  specified NEC M15.8
Polycarential syndrome of infancy E40
Polychondritis (atrophic) (chronic) —*see also*
  Disorder, cartilage, specified type
    NEC
  relapsing M94.1
Polycoria Q13.2
Polycystic (disease)
  degeneration, kidney Q61.3
    autosomal dominant (adult type) Q61.2
    autosomal recessive (infantile type) NEC
      Q61.19
  kidney Q61.3
    autosomal
      dominant Q61.2
      recessive NEC Q61.19
    autosomal dominant (adult type) Q61.2
    autosomal recessive (childhood type) NEC
      Q61.19
    infantile type NEC Q61.19
  liver Q44.6
  lung J98.4
    congenital Q33.0
  ovary, ovaries E28.2
  spleen Q89.09
Polycythemia (secondary) D75.1
  acquired D75.1
  benign (familial) D75.0
  due to
    donor twin P61.1
    erythropoietin D75.1
    fall in plasma volume D75.1
    high altitude D75.1
    maternal-fetal transfusion P61.1
    stress D75.1
  emotional D75.1
  erythropoietin D75.1
  familial (benign) D75.0
  Gaisböck's (hypertonica) D75.1
  high altitude D75.1
  hypertonica D75.1
  hypoxemic D75.1
  neonatorum P61.1
  nephrogenous D75.1
  relative D75.1
  secondary D75.1
  spurious D75.1
  stress D75.1
  vera D45
Polycytosis cryptogenica D75.1
Polydactylism, polydactyly Q69.9
  toes Q69.2
Polydipsia R63.1
Polydystrophy, pseudo-Hurler E77.0
Polyembryoma —*see* Neoplasm, malignant,
  by site
Polyglandular
  deficiency E31.0
  dyscrasia E31.9
  dysfunction E31.9
  syndrome E31.8
Polyhydramnios O40.-●
Polymastia Q83.1
Polymenorrhea N92.0
Polymyalgia M35.3
  arteritica, giant cell M31.5
  rheumatica M35.3
    with giant cell arteritis M31.5

Polymyositis (acute) (chronic) (hemorrhagic)
  M33.20
  with
    myopathy M33.22
    respiratory involvement M33.21
    skin involvement —*see*
      Dermatopolymyositis
    specified organ involvement NEC M33.29
  ossificans (generalisata) (progressiva) —*see*
    Myositis, ossificans, progressiva
Polyneuritis, polyneuritic —*see also*
  Polyneuropathy
  acute (post-)infective G61.0
  alcoholic G62.1
  cranialis G52.7
  demyelinating, chronic inflammatory (CIDP)
    G61.81
  diabetic —*see* Diabetes, polyneuropathy
  diphtheritic A36.83
  due to lack of vitamin NEC E56.9 *[G63]*
  endemic E51.11
  erythredema —*see* subcategory T56.1
  febrile, acute G61.0
  hereditary ataxic G60.1
  idiopathic, acute G61.0
  infective (acute) G61.0
  inflammatory, chronic demyelinating (CIDP)
    G61.81
  nutritional E63.9 *[G63]*
  postinfective (acute) G61.0
  specified NEC G62.89
Polyneuropathy (peripheral) G62.9
  alcoholic G62.1
  amyloid (Portuguese) E85.1 *[G63]*
  ▶transthyretin-related (ATTR) familial E85.1
  arsenical G62.2
  critical illness G62.81
  demyelinating, chronic inflammatory (CIDP)
    G61.81
  diabetic —*see* Diabetes, polyneuropathy
  drug-induced G62.0
  hereditary G60.9
    specified NEC G60.8
  idiopathic G60.9
    progressive G60.3
  in (due to)
    alcohol G62.1
      sequelae G65.2
    amyloidosis, familial (Portuguese) E85.1
      [G63]
    antitetanus serum G61.1
    arsenic G62.2
      sequelae G65.2
    avitaminosis NEC E56.9 *[G63]*
    beriberi E51.11
    collagen vascular disease NEC M35.9 *[G63]*
    deficiency (of)
      B (-complex) vitamins E53.9 *[G63]*
      vitamin B6 E53.1 *[G63]*
    diabetes —*see* Diabetes, polyneuropathy
    diphtheria A36.83
    drug or medicament G62.0
      correct substance properly
        administered —*see* Table of Drugs
        and Chemicals, by drug, adverse
        effect
      overdose or wrong substance given
        or taken —*see* Table of Drugs and
        Chemicals, by drug, poisoning
    endocrine disease NEC E34.9 *[G63]*
    herpes zoster B02.23
    hypoglycemia E16.2 *[G63]*
    infectious
      disease NEC B99 *[G63]*
      mononucleosis B27.91
    lack of vitamin NEC E56.9 *[G63]*
    lead G62.2
      sequelae G65.2
    leprosy A30.9 *[G63]*
    Lyme disease A69.22
    metabolic disease NEC E88.9 *[G63]*

▶ New   ⇒ Revised   ~~deleted~~ Deleted   ● Use Additional Character(s)

Polyneuropathy *(Continued)*
    in *(Continued)*
        microscopic polyangiitis M31.7 *[G63]*
        mumps B26.84
        neoplastic disease —*see also* Neoplasm
            D49.9 *[G63]*
        nutritional deficiency NEC E63.9 *[G63]*
        organophosphate compounds G62.2
            sequelae G65.2
        parasitic disease NEC B89 *[G63]*
        pellagra E52 *[G63]*
        polyarteritis nodosa M30.0
        porphyria E80.20 *[G63]*
        radiation G62.82
        rheumatoid arthritis —*see* Rheumatoid,
            polyneuropathy
        sarcoidosis D86.89
        serum G61.1
        syphilis (late) A52.15
            congenital A50.43
        systemic
            connective tissue disorder M35.9 *[G63]*
            lupus erythematosus M32.19
        toxic agent NEC G62.2
            sequelae G65.2
        ~~triorthocresyl phosphate G62.2~~
            ~~sequelae G65.2~~
        ~~tuberculosis A17.89~~
        ~~uremia N18.9 [G63]~~
        ~~vitamin B12 deficiency E53.8 [G63]~~
            ~~with anemia (pernicious) D51.0 [G63]~~
                ~~due to dietary deficiency D51.3 [G63]~~
        ~~zoster B02.23~~
        ▶transthyretin-related (ATTR) familial
            amyloid E85.1
        ▶triorthocresyl phosphate G62.2
            ▶sequelae G65.2
        ▶tuberculosis A17.89
        ▶uremia N18.9 [G63]
        ▶vitamin B12 deficiency E53.8 [G63]
            ▶with anemia (pernicious) D51.0 [G63]
                ▶due to dietary deficiency D51.3 [G63]
        ▶zoster B02.23
    inflammatory G61.9
        chronic demyelinating (CIDP) G61.81
        sequelae G65.1
        specified NEC G61.89
    lead G62.2
        sequelae G65.2
    nutritional NEC E63.9 *[G63]*
    postherpetic (zoster) B02.23
    progressive G60.3
    radiation-induced G62.82
    sensory (hereditary) (idiopathic) G60.8
    specified NEC G62.89
    syphilitic (late) A52.15
        congenital A50.43
Polyopia H53.8
Polyorchism, polyorchidism Q55.21
Polyosteoarthritis —*see also* Osteoarthritis,
    generalized M15.9-●
    post-traumatic M15.3
    specified NEC M15.8
Polyostotic fibrous dysplasia Q78.1
Polyotia Q17.0
Polyp, polypus
    accessory sinus J33.8
    adenocarcinoma in —*see* Neoplasm,
        malignant, by site
    adenocarcinoma in situ in —*see* Neoplasm, in
        situ, by site
    adenoid tissue J33.0
    adenomatous —*see also* Neoplasm, benign,
        by site
        adenocarcinoma in —*see* Neoplasm,
            malignant, by site
        adenocarcinoma in situ in —*see* Neoplasm,
            in situ, by site
        carcinoma in —*see* Neoplasm, malignant,
            by site
        carcinoma in situ in —*see* Neoplasm, in
            situ, by site

Polyp, polypus *(Continued)*
    adenomatous *(Continued)*
        multiple —*see* Neoplasm, benign
            adenocarcinoma in —*see* Neoplasm,
                malignant, by site
            adenocarcinoma in situ in —*see*
                Neoplasm, in situ, by site
    antrum J33.8
    anus, anal (canal) K62.0
    Bartholin's gland N84.3
    bladder D41.4
    carcinoma in —*see* Neoplasm, malignant, by
        site
    carcinoma in situ in —*see* Neoplasm, in situ,
        by site
    cecum D12.0
    cervix (uteri) N84.1
        in pregnancy or childbirth —*see* Pregnancy,
            complicated by, abnormal, cervix
        mucous N84.1
        nonneoplastic N84.1
    choanal J33.0
    cholesterol K82.4
    clitoris N84.3
    colon K63.5
        adenomatous D12.6
        ascending D12.2
        cecum D12.0
        descending D12.4
        inflammatory K51.40
            with
                abscess K51.414
                complication K51.419
                    specified NEC K51.418
                fistula K51.413
                intestinal obstruction K51.412
                rectal bleeding K51.411
        sigmoid D12.5
        transverse D12.3
    corpus uteri N84.0
    dental K04.01
        irreversible K04.02
        reversible K04.01
    duodenum K31.7
    ear (middle) H74.4-●
    endometrium N84.0
    ethmoidal (sinus) J33.8
    fallopian tube N84.8
    female genital tract N84.9
        specified NEC N84.8
    frontal (sinus) J33.8
    gallbladder K82.4
    gingiva, gum K06.8
    labia, labium (majus) (minus) N84.3
    larynx (mucous) J38.1
        adenomatous D14.1
    malignant —*see* Neoplasm, malignant, by site
    maxillary (sinus) J33.8
    middle ear —*see* Polyp, ear (middle)
    myometrium N84.0
    nares
        anterior J33.9
        posterior J33.0
    nasal (mucous) J33.9
        cavity J33.0
        septum J33.0
    nasopharyngeal J33.0
    nose (mucous) J33.9
    oviduct N84.8
    pharynx J39.2
    placenta O90.89
    prostate —*see* Enlargement, enlarged,
        prostate
    pudenda, pudendum N84.3
    pulpal (dental) K04.01
        irreversible K04.02
        reversible K04.01
    rectum (nonadenomatous) K62.1
        adenomatous —*see* Polyp, adenomatous
    septum (nasal) J33.0
    sinus (accessory) (ethmoidal) (frontal)
        (maxillary) (sphenoidal) J33.8

Polyp, polypus *(Continued)*
    sphenoidal (sinus) J33.8
    stomach K31.7
        adenomatous D13.1
    tube, fallopian N84.8
    turbinate, mucous membrane J33.8
    umbilical, newborn P83.6
    ureter N28.89
    urethra N36.2
    uterus (body) (corpus) (mucous) N84.0
        cervix N84.1
        in pregnancy or childbirth —*see* Pregnancy,
            complicated by, tumor, uterus
    vagina N84.2
    vocal cord (mucous) J38.1
    vulva N84.3
Polyphagia R63.2
Polyploidy Q92.7
Polypoid —*see* condition
Polyposis —*see also* Polyp
    coli (adenomatous) D12.6
        adenocarcinoma in C18.9
        adenocarcinoma in situ in —*see* Neoplasm,
            in situ, by site
        carcinoma in C18.9
    colon (adenomatous) D12.6
    familial D12.6
        adenocarcinoma in situ in —*see* Neoplasm,
            in situ, by site
    intestinal (adenomatous) D12.6
    malignant lymphomatous C83.1
    multiple, adenomatous —*see also* Neoplasm,
        benign D36.9
Polyradiculitis —*see* Polyneuropathy
Polyradiculoneuropathy (acute) (postinfective)
    (segmentally demyelinating) G61.0
Polyserositis
    due to pericarditis I31.1
    pericardial I31.1
    periodic, familial E85.0
    tuberculous A19.9
        acute A19.1
        chronic A19.8
Polysplenia syndrome Q89.09
Polysyndactyly —*see also* Syndactylism,
    syndactyly Q70.4
Polytrichia L68.3
Polyunguia Q84.6
Polyuria R35.8
    nocturnal R35.1
    psychogenic F45.8
Pompe's disease (glycogen storage) E74.02
Pompholyx L30.1
Poncet's disease (tuberculous rheumatism)
    A18.09
Pond fracture —*see* Fracture, skull
Ponos B55.0
Pons, pontine —*see* condition
Poor
    aesthetic of existing restoration of tooth
        K08.56
    contractions, labor O62.2
    gingival margin to tooth restoration K08.51
    personal hygiene R46.0
    prenatal care, affecting management of
        pregnancy —*see* Pregnancy, complicated
        by, insufficient, prenatal care
    sucking reflex (newborn) R29.2
    urinary stream R39.12
    vision NEC H54.7
Poradenitis, nostras inguinalis or venerea A55
Porencephaly (congenital) (developmental)
    (true) Q04.6
    acquired G93.0
    nondevelopmental G93.0
    traumatic (post) F07.89
Porocephaliasis B88.8
Porokeratosis Q82.8
Poroma, eccrine —*see* Neoplasm, skin, benign
Porphyria (South African) E80.20
    acquired E80.20
    acute intermittent (hepatic) (Swedish) E80.21

Porphyria *(Continued)*
cutanea tarda (hereditary) (symptomatic) E80.1
due to drugs E80.20
correct substance properly administered — *see* Table of Drugs and Chemicals, by drug, adverse effect
overdose or wrong substance given or taken — *see* Table of Drugs and Chemicals, by drug, poisoning
erythropoietic (congenital) (hereditary) E80.0
hepatocutaneous type E80.1
secondary E80.20
toxic NEC E80.20
variegata E80.20
Porphyrinuria — *see* Porphyria
Porphyruria — *see* Porphyria
Portal — *see* condition
Port wine nevus, mark, or stain Q82.5
Posadas-Wernicke disease B38.9
Positive
culture (nonspecific)
blood R78.81
bronchial washings R84.5
cerebrospinal fluid R83.5
cervix uteri R87.5
nasal secretions R84.5
nipple discharge R89.5
nose R84.5
staphylococcus (Methicillin susceptible) Z22.321
Methicillin resistant Z22.322
peritoneal fluid R85.5
pleural fluid R84.5
prostatic secretions R86.5
saliva R85.5
seminal fluid R86.5
sputum R84.5
synovial fluid R89.5
throat scrapings R84.5
urine R82.79
vagina R87.5
vulva R87.5
wound secretions R89.5
PPD (skin test) R76.11
serology for syphilis A53.0
with signs or symptoms - code as Syphilis, by site and stage
false R76.8
skin test, tuberculin (without active tuberculosis) R76.11
test, human immunodeficiency virus (HIV) R75
VDRL A53.0
with signs or symptoms - code by site and stage under Syphilis A53.9
Wassermann reaction A53.0
Postcardiotomy syndrome I97.0
Postcaval ureter Q62.62
Postcholecystectomy syndrome K91.5
Postclimacteric bleeding N95.0
Postcommissurotomy syndrome I97.0
Postconcussional syndrome F07.81
Postcontusional syndrome F07.81
Postcricoid region — *see* condition
Post-dates (40-42 weeks) (pregnancy) (mother) O48.0
more than 42 weeks gestation O48.1
Postencephalitic syndrome F07.89
Posterior — *see* condition
Posterolateral sclerosis (spinal cord) — *see* Degeneration, combined
Postexanthematous — *see* condition
Postfebrile — *see* condition
Postgastrectomy dumping syndrome K91.1
Posthemiplegic chorea — *see* Monoplegia
Posthemorrhagic anemia (chronic) D50.0
acute D62
newborn P61.3
Postherpetic neuralgia (zoster) B02.29
trigeminal B02.22
Posthitis N47.7

Postimmunization complication or reaction — *see* Complications, vaccination
Postinfectious — *see* condition
Postlaminectomy syndrome NEC M96.1
Postleukotomy syndrome F07.0
Postmastectomy lymphedema (syndrome) I97.2
Postmaturity, postmature (over 42 weeks)
maternal (over 42 weeks gestation) O48.1
newborn P08.22
Postmeasles complication NEC — *see also* condition B05.89
Postmenopausal
endometrium (atrophic) N95.8
suppurative — *see also* Endometritis N71.9
osteoporosis — *see* Osteoporosis, postmenopausal
Postnasal drip R09.82
due to
allergic rhinitis — *see* Rhinitis, allergic
common cold J00
gastroesophageal reflux — *see* Reflux, gastroesophageal
nasopharyngitis — *see* Nasopharyngitis
other know condition — code to condition
sinusitis — *see* Sinusitis
Postnatal — *see* condition
Postoperative (postprocedural) — *see* Complication, postoperative
pneumothorax, therapeutic Z98.3
state NEC Z98.890
Postpancreatectomy hyperglycemia E89.1
Postpartum — *see* Puerperal
Postphlebitic syndrome — *see* Syndrome, postthrombotic
Postpolio (myelitic) syndrome G14
Postpoliomyelitic — *see also* condition
osteopathy — *see* Osteopathy, after poliomyelitis
Postprocedural — *see also* Postoperative
hypoinsulinemia E89.1
Postschizophrenic depression F32.89
Postsurgery status — *see also* Status (post)
pneumothorax, therapeutic Z98.3
Post-term (40-42 weeks) (pregnancy) (mother) O48.0
infant P08.21
more than 42 weeks gestation (mother) O48.1
Post-traumatic brain syndrome, nonpsychotic F07.81
Post-typhoid abscess A01.09
Postures, hysterical F44.2
Postvaccinal reaction or complication — *see* Complications, vaccination
Postvalvulotomy syndrome I97.0
Potain's
disease (pulmonary edema) — *see* Edema, lung
syndrome (gastrectasis with dyspepsia) K31.0
Potter's
asthma J62.8
facies Q60.6
lung J62.8
syndrome (with renal agenesis) Q60.6
Pott's
curvature (spinal) A18.01
disease or paraplegia A18.01
spinal curvature A18.01
tumor, puffy — *see* Osteomyelitis, specified type NEC
Pouch
bronchus Q32.4
Douglas' — *see* condition
esophagus, esophageal, congenital Q39.6
acquired K22.5
gastric K31.4
Hartmann's K82.8
pharynx, pharyngeal (congenital) Q38.7
Pouchitis K91.850
Poultrymen's itch B88.0
Poverty NEC Z59.6
extreme Z59.5
Poxvirus NEC B08.8

Prader-Willi syndrome Q87.1
Preauricular appendage or tag Q17.0
Prebetalipoproteinemia (acquired) (essential) (familial) (hereditary) (primary) (secondary) E78.1
with chylomicronemia E78.3
Precipitate labor or delivery O62.3
Preclimacteric bleeding (menorrhagia) N92.4
Precocious
adrenarche E30.1
menarche E30.1
menstruation E30.1
pubarche E30.1
puberty E30.1
central E22.8
sexual development NEC E30.1
thelarche E30.8
Precocity, sexual (constitutional) (cryptogenic) (female) (idiopathic) (male) E30.1
with adrenal hyperplasia E25.9
congenital E25.0
Precordial pain R07.2
Predeciduous teeth K00.2
Prediabetes, prediabetic R73.03
complicating
pregnancy — *see* Pregnancy, complicated by, diseases of, specified type or system NEC
puerperium O99.89
Predislocation status of hip at birth Q65.6
Pre-eclampsia O14.9-•
with pre-existing hypertension — *see* Hypertension, complicating pregnancy, pre-existing, with, pre-eclampsia
complicating
childbirth O14.94
puerperium O14.95
mild O14.0-•
complicating
childbirth O14.04
puerperium O14.05
moderate O14.0-•
complicating
childbirth O14.04
puerperium O14.05
severe O14.1-•
with hemolysis, elevated liver enzymes and low platelet count (HELLP) O14.2-•
complicating
childbirth O14.24
puerperium O14.25
complicating
childbirth O14.14
puerperium O14.15
Pre-eruptive color change, teeth, tooth K00.8
Pre-excitation atrioventricular conduction I45.6
Preglaucoma H40.00-•
Pregnancy (single) (uterine) — *see also* Delivery and Puerperal

> Note: The Tabular must be reviewed for assignment of the appropriate character indicating the trimester of the pregnancy
>
> Note: The Tabular must be reviewed for assignment of appropriate seventh character for multiple gestation codes in Chapter 15

abdominal (ectopic) O00.00
with intrauterine pregnancy O00.01
with viable fetus O36.7-•
➠ampullar O00.10-•
➠with intrauterine pregnancy O00.11-•
biochemical O02.81
broad ligament O00.80
with intrauterine pregnancy O00.81
cervical O00.80
with intrauterine pregnancy O00.81

▶ New   ⇒ Revised   ~~deleted~~ Deleted   • Use Additional Character(s)

Pregnancy *(Continued)*
  chemical O02.81
  complicated NOS O26.9-●
  complicated by (care of) (management
      affected by)
    abnormal, abnormality
      cervix O34.4-●
        causing obstructed labor O65.5
      cord (umbilical) O69.9
      ▶fetal heart rate or rhythm O36.83-●
      findings on antenatal screening of
          mother O28.9
        biochemical O28.1
        chromosomal O28.5
        cytological O28.2
        genetic O28.5
        hematological O28.0
        radiological O28.4
        specified NEC O28.8
        ultrasonic O28.3
      glucose (tolerance) NEC O99.810
      pelvic organs O34.9-●
        specified NEC O34.8-●
          causing obstructed labor O65.5
      pelvis (bony) (major) NEC O33.0
      perineum O34.7-●
      position
        placenta O44.0-●
          with hemorrhage O44.1-●
        uterus O34.59-●
      uterus O34.59-●
        causing obstructed labor O65.5
        congenital O34.0-●
      vagina O34.6-●
        causing obstructed labor O65.5
      vulva O34.7-●
        causing obstructed labor O65.5
    abruptio placentae —*see* Abruptio
        placentae
    abscess or cellulitis
      bladder O23.1-●
      breast O91.11-●
      genital organ or tract O23.9-●
    abuse
      physical O9A.31-●
      psychological O9A.51-●
      sexual O9A.41-●
    adverse effect anesthesia O29.9-●
      aspiration pneumonitis O29.01-●
      cardiac arrest O29.11-●
      cardiac complication NEC O29.19-●
      cardiac failure O29.12-●
      central nervous system complication
          NEC O29.29-●
      cerebral anoxia O29.21-●
      failed or difficult intubation O29.6-●
      inhalation of stomach contents or
          secretions NOS O29.01-●
      local, toxic reaction O29.3X
      Mendelson's syndrome O29.01-●
      pressure collapse of lung O29.02-●
      pulmonary complications NEC O29.09-●
      specified NEC O29.8X
      spinal and epidural type NEC O29.5X
        induced headache O29.4-●
    albuminuria —*see also* Proteinuria,
        gestational O12.1-●
    alcohol use O99.31-●
    amnionitis O41.12-●
    anaphylactoid syndrome of pregnancy
        O88.01-●
    anemia (conditions in D50-D64) (pre-
        existing) O99.01-●
      complicating the puerperium O99.03
    antepartum hemorrhage O46.9-●
      with coagulation defect —*see*
          Hemorrhage, antepartum, with
          coagulation defect
      specified NEC O46.8X-●
    appendicitis O99.61-●
    atrophy (yellow) (acute) liver (subacute)
        O26.61-●

Pregnancy *(Continued)*
  complicated by *(Continued)*
    bariatric surgery status O99.84-●
    bicornis or bicornuate uterus O34.0-●
    biliary tract problems O26.61-●
    breech presentation O32.1
    cardiovascular diseases (conditions in
        I00-I09, I20-I52, I70-I99) O99.41-●
    cerebrovascular disorders (conditions in
        I60-I69) O99.41-●
    cervical shortening O26.87-●
    cervicitis O23.51-●
    chloasma (gravidarum) O26.89-●
    cholecystitis O99.61-●
    cholestasis (intrahepatic) O26.61-●
    chorioamnionitis O41.12-●
    circulatory system disorder (conditions in
        I00-I09, I20-I99, O99.41-●)
    compound presentation O32.6
    conjoined twins O30.02-●
    connective system disorders (conditions in
        M00-M99) O99.89
    contracted pelvis (general) O33.1
      inlet O33.2
      outlet O33.3
    convulsions (eclamptic) (uremic) —*see also*
        Eclampsia O15.9-●
    cracked nipple O92.11-●
    cystitis O23.1-●
    cystocele O34.8-●
    death of fetus (near term) O36.4
      early pregnancy O02.1
      of one fetus or more in multiple
          gestation O31.2-●
    deciduitis O41.14-●
    decreased fetal movement O36.81-●
    dental problems O99.61-●
    diabetes (mellitus) O24.91-●
      gestational (pregnancy induced) —*see*
          Diabetes, gestational
      pre-existing O24.31-●
        specified NEC O24.81-●
        type 1 O24.01-●
        type 2 O24.11-●
    digestive system disorders (conditions in
        K00-K93) O99.61-●
    diseases of —*see* Pregnancy, complicated
        by, specified body system disease
      biliary tract O26.61-●
      blood NEC (conditions in D65-D77)
          O99.11-●
      liver O26.61-●
      specified NEC O99.89
    disorders of —*see* Pregnancy, complicated
        by, specified body system disorder
      amniotic fluid and membranes
          O41.9-●
        specified NEC O41.8X-●
      biliary tract O26.61-●
      ear and mastoid process (conditions in
          H60-H95) O99.89
      eye and adnexa (conditions in H00-H59)
          O99.89
      liver O26.61-●
      skin (conditions in L00-L99) O99.71-●
      specified NEC O99.89
    displacement, uterus NEC O34.59-●
      causing obstructed labor O65.5
    disproportion (due to) O33.9
      fetal (ascites) (hydrops)
          (meningomyelocele) (sacral
          teratoma) (tumor) deformities NEC
          O33.7
      generally contracted pelvis O33.1
      hydrocephalic fetus O33.6
      inlet contraction of pelvis O33.2
      mixed maternal and fetal origin O33.4
      specified NEC O33.8
    double uterus O34.0-●
      causing obstructed labor O65.5
    drug use (conditions in F11-F19)
        O99.32-●

Pregnancy *(Continued)*
  complicated by *(Continued)*
    eclampsia, eclamptic (coma) (convulsions)
        (delirium) (nephritis) (uremia) *(see also*
        Eclampsia) O15-●
    ectopic pregnancy —*see* Pregnancy, ectopic
    edema O12.0-●
      with
        gestational hypertension, mild —*see
            also* Pre-eclampsia O14.0-●
        proteinuria O12.2-●
    effusion, amniotic fluid —*see* Pregnancy,
        complicated by, premature rupture of
        membranes
    elderly
      multigravida O09.52-●
      primigravida O09.51-●
    embolism —*see also* Embolism, obstetric,
        pregnancy O88.-●
    endocrine diseases NEC O99.28-●
    endometritis O86.12
    excessive weight gain O26.0-●
    exhaustion O26.81-●
      during labor and delivery O75.81
    face presentation O32.3
    failed induction of labor O61.9
    failed or difficult intubation for anesthesia
        O29.6-●
      instrumental O61.1
      mechanical O61.1
      medical O61.0
      specified NEC O61.8
      surgical O61.1
    false labor (pains) O47.9
      at or after 37 completed weeks of
          pregnancy O47.1
      before 37 completed weeks of pregnancy
          O47.0-●
    fatigue O26.81-●
      during labor and delivery O75.81
    fatty metamorphosis of liver O26.61-●
    female genital mutilation O34.8-● *[N90.81-●]*
    fetal (maternal care for)
      abnormality or damage O35.9
        acid-base balance O68
        specified type NEC O35.8
      acidemia O68
      acidosis O68
      alkalosis O68
      anemia and thrombocytopenia O36.82-●
      anencephaly O35.0
      chromosomal abnormality (conditions in
          Q90-Q99) O35.1
      conjoined twins O30.02-●
      damage from
        amniocentesis O35.7
        biopsy procedures O35.7
        drug addiction O35.5
        hematological investigation O35.7
        intrauterine contraceptive device
            O35.7
        maternal
          alcohol addiction O35.4
          cytomegalovirus infection O35.3
          disease NEC O35.8
          drug addiction O35.5
          listeriosis O35.8
          rubella O35.3
          toxoplasmosis O35.8
          viral infection O35.3
        medical procedure NEC O35.7
        radiation O35.6
      death (near term) O36.4
        early pregnancy O02.1
      decreased movement O36.81-●
      disproportion due to deformity (fetal)
          O33.7
      excessive growth (large for dates) O36.6-●
      growth retardation O36.59-●
        light for dates O36.59-●
        small for dates O36.59-●

Pregnancy *(Continued)*
  complicated by *(Continued)*
    fetal *(Continued)*
      heart rate irregularity (bradycardia)
        (decelerations) (tachycardia) O76
      hereditary disease O35.2
      hydrocephalus O35.0
      intrauterine death O36.4
      poor growth O36.59-●
        light for dates O36.59-●
        small for dates O36.59-●
      problem O36.9-●
        specified NEC O36.89-●
      reduction (elective) O31.3-●
      selective termination O31.3-●
      spina bifida O35.0
      thrombocytopenia O36.82-●
    fibroid (tumor) (uterus) O34.1-●
    fissure of nipple O92.11-●
    gallstones O99.61-●
    gastric banding status O99.84-●
    gastric bypass status O99.84-●
  ➠genital herpes (asymptomatic) (history of)
      (inactive) O98.3-●
    genital tract infection O23.9-●
    glomerular diseases (conditions in
      N00-N07) O26.83-●
      with hypertension, pre-existing —*see*
        Hypertension, complicating,
        pregnancy, pre-existing, with, renal
        disease
    gonorrhea O98.21-●
    grand multiparity O09.4
    habitual aborter —*see* Pregnancy,
      complicated by, recurrent pregnancy
      loss
    HELLP syndrome (hemolysis, elevated
      liver enzymes and low platelet count)
      O14.2-●
    hemorrhage
      antepartum —*see* Hemorrhage,
        antepartum
      before 20 completed weeks gestation
        O20.9
        specified NEC O20.8
      due to premature separation, placenta —
        see also Abruptio placentae O45.9-●
      early O20.9
        specified NEC O20.8
      threatened abortion O20.0
    hemorrhoids O22.4-●
    hepatitis (viral) O98.41-●
    herniation of uterus O34.59-●
    high
      head at term O32.4
      risk —*see* Supervision (of) (for), high-risk
    history of in utero procedure during
      previous pregnancy O09.82-●
    HIV O98.71-●
    human immunodeficiency virus (HIV)
      disease O98.71-●
    hydatidiform mole —*see also* Mole,
      hydatidiform O01.9-●
    hydramnios O40.-●
    hydrocephalic fetus (disproportion) O33.6
    hydrops
      amnii O40.-●
      fetalis O36.2-●
        associated with isoimmunization —*see*
         also Pregnancy, complicated by,
         isoimmunization O36.11-●
    hydrorrhea O42.90
    hyperemesis (gravidarum) (mild) —*see also*
      Hyperemesis, gravidarum O21.0-●
    hypertension —*see* Hypertension,
      complicating pregnancy
    hypertensive
      heart and renal disease, pre-existing —
        see Hypertension, complicating,
        pregnancy, pre-existing, with, heart
        disease, with renal disease

Pregnancy *(Continued)*
  complicated by *(Continued)*
    hypertensive *(Continued)*
      heart disease, pre-existing —*see*
        Hypertension, complicating,
        pregnancy, pre-existing, with, heart
        disease
      renal disease, pre-existing —*see*
        Hypertension, complicating,
        pregnancy, pre-existing, with, renal
        disease
    hypotension O26.5-●
    immune disorders NEC (conditions in
      D80-D89) O99.11-●
    incarceration, uterus O34.51-●
    incompetent cervix O34.3-●
    inconclusive fetal viability O36.80
    infection(s) O98.91-●
      amniotic fluid or sac O41.10-●
      bladder O23.1-●
      carrier state NEC O99.830
        streptococcus B O99.820
      genital organ or tract O23.9-●
        specified NEC O23.59-●
      genitourinary tract O23.9-●
      gonorrhea O98.21-●
      hepatitis (viral) O98.41-●
      HIV O98.71-●
      human immunodeficiency virus (HIV)
        O98.71-●
      kidney O23.0-●
      nipple O91.01-●
      parasitic disease O98.91-●
        specified NEC O98.81-●
      protozoal disease O98.61-●
      sexually transmitted NEC O98.31-●
      specified type NEC O98.81-●
      syphilis O98.11-●
      tuberculosis O98.01-●
      urethra O23.2-●
      urinary (tract) O23.4-●
        specified NEC O23.3-●
      viral disease O98.51-●
    injury or poisoning (conditions in S00-T88)
      O9A.21-●
      due to abuse
        physical O9A.31-●
        psychological O9A.51-●
        sexual O9A.41-●
    insufficient
      prenatal care O09.3-●
      weight gain O26.1-●
    insulin resistance O26.89
    intrauterine fetal death (near term) O36.4
      early pregnancy O02.1
      multiple gestation (one fetus or more)
        O31.2-●
    isoimmunization O36.11-●
      anti-A sensitization O36.11-●
      anti-B sensitization O36.19-●
      Rh O36.09-●
        anti-D antibody O36.01-●
      specified NEC O36.19-●
    laceration of uterus NEC O71.81
    malformation
      placenta, placental (vessel) O43.10-●
        specified NEC O43.19-●
      uterus (congenital) O34.0-●
    malnutrition (conditions in E40-E46)
      O25.1-●
    maternal hypotension syndrome O26.5-●
    mental disorders (conditions in F01-F09,
      F20-F99) O99.34-●
      alcohol use O99.31-●
      drug use O99.32-●
      smoking O99.33-●
    mentum presentation O32.3
    metabolic disorders O99.28-●
    missed
      abortion O02.1
      delivery O36.4

Pregnancy *(Continued)*
  complicated by *(Continued)*
    multiple gestations O30.9-●
      conjoined twins O30.02-●
      quadruplet —*see* Pregnancy, quadruplet
      specified complication NEC O31.8X-●
      specified number of multiples NEC —*see*
        Pregnancy, multiple (gestation),
        specified NEC
      triplet —*see* Pregnancy, triplet
      twin —*see* Pregnancy, twin
    musculoskeletal condition (conditions is
      M00-M99) O99.89
    necrosis, liver (conditions in K72)
      O26.61-●
    neoplasm
      benign
        cervix O34.4-●
        corpus uteri O34.1-●
        uterus O34.1-●
      malignant O9A.11-●
    nephropathy NEC O26.83-●
    nervous system condition (conditions in
      G00-G99) O99.35-●
    nutritional diseases NEC O99.28-●
    obesity (pre-existing) O99.21-●
    obesity surgery status O99.84-●
    oblique lie or presentation O32.2
    older mother —*see* Pregnancy, complicated
      by, elderly
    oligohydramnios O41.0-●
      with premature rupture of
        membranes —*see also* Pregnancy,
        complicated by, premature rupture
        of membranes O42-●
    onset (spontaneous) of labor after 37
      completed weeks of gestation but
      before 39 completed weeks gestation,
      with delivery by (planned) cesarean
      section O75.82
    oophoritis O23.52-●
    overdose, drug —*see also* Table of Drugs
      and Chemicals, by drug, poisoning
      O9A.21-●
    oversize fetus O33.5
    papyraceous fetus O31.0-●
    pelvic inflammatory disease O99.89
    periodontal disease O99.61-●
    peripheral neuritis O26.82-●
    peritoneal (pelvic) adhesions O99.89
    phlebitis O22.9-●
    phlebopathy O22.9-●
    phlebothrombosis (superficial) O22.2-●
      deep O22.3-●
    placenta accreta O43.21-●
    placenta increta O43.22-●
    placenta percreta O43.23-●
    placenta previa O44.0-●
      complete O44.0-●
        with hemorrhage O44.1-●
      marginal O44.2-●
        with hemorrhage O44.3-●
      partial O44.2-●
        with hemorrhage O44.3-●
    placental disorder O43.9-●
      specified NEC O43.89-●
    placental dysfunction O43.89-●
    placental infarction O43.81-●
    placental insufficiency O36.51-●
    placental transfusion syndromes
      fetomaternal O43.01-●
      fetus to fetus O43.02-●
      maternofetal O43.01-●
    placentitis O41.14-●
    pneumonia O99.51-●
    poisoning —*see also* Table of Drugs and
      Chemicals O9A.21-●
    polyhydramnios O40-●
    polymorphic eruption of pregnancy
      O26.86
    poor obstetric history NEC O09.29-●

  ▶ New   ➠ Revised   ~~deleted~~ Deleted   ● Use Additional Character(s)

Pregnancy *(Continued)*
  complicated by *(Continued)*
    postmaturity (post-term) (40 to 42 weeks) O48.0
      more than 42 completed weeks gestation (prolonged) O48.1
    pre-eclampsia O14.9-●
      mild O14.0-●
      moderate O14.0-●
      severe O14.1-●
        with hemolysis, elevated liver enzymes and low platelet count (HELLP) O14.2-●
    premature labor —*see* Pregnancy, complicated by, preterm labor
    premature rupture of membranes O42.90
      full-term, unspecified as to length of time between rupture and onset of labor O42.92
      with onset of labor
        within 24 hours O42.00
          at or after 37 weeks gestation, onset of labor within 24 hours of rupture O42.02
          pre-term (before 37 completed weeks of gestation) O42.01-●
        after 24 hours O42.10
          at or after 37 weeks gestation, onset of labor more than 24 hours following rupture O42.12
          pre-term (before 37 completed weeks of gestation) O42.11-●
      at or after 37 weeks gestation, unspecified as to length of time between rupture and onset of labor O42.92
      pre-term (before 37 completed weeks of gestation) O42.91-●
    premature separation of placenta —*see also* Abruptio placentae O45.9-●
    presentation, fetal —*see* Delivery, complicated by, malposition
    preterm delivery O60.10
    preterm labor
      with delivery O60.10
        preterm O60.10
        term O60.20
      second trimester
        with preterm delivery
          second trimester O60.12
          third trimester O60.13
        with term delivery O60.22
        without delivery O60.02
      third trimester
        with term delivery O60.23
        with third trimester preterm delivery O60.14
        without delivery O60.03
      without delivery O60.00
        second trimester O60.02
        third trimester O60.03
    previous history of —*see* Pregnancy, supervision of, high-risk
    prolapse, uterus O34.52-●
    proteinuria (gestational) —*see also* Proteinuria, gestational O12.1-●
      with edema O12.2-●
    pruritic urticarial papules and plaques of pregnancy (PUPPP) O26.86
    pruritus (neurogenic) O26.89-●
    psychosis or psychoneurosis (puerperal) F53
    ptyalism O26.89-●
    PUPPP (pruritic urticarial papules and plaques of pregnancy) O26.86
    pyelitis O23.0-●
    recurrent pregnancy loss O26.2-●

Pregnancy *(Continued)*
  complicated by *(Continued)*
    renal disease or failure NEC O26.83-●
      with secondary hypertension, pre-existing —*see* Hypertension, complicating, pregnancy, pre-existing, secondary
      hypertensive, pre-existing —*see* Hypertension, complicating, pregnancy, pre-existing, with, renal disease
    respiratory condition (conditions in J00-J99) O99.51-●
    retained, retention
      dead ovum O02.0
      intrauterine contraceptive device O26.3-●
    retroversion, uterus O34.53-●
    Rh immunization, incompatibility or sensitization NEC O36.09-●
      anti-D antibody O36.01-●
    rupture
      amnion (premature) —*see also* Pregnancy, complicated by, premature rupture of membranes O42-●
      membranes (premature) —*see also* Pregnancy, complicated by, premature rupture of membranes O42-●
      uterus (during labor) O71.1
        before onset of labor O71.0-●
    salivation (excessive) O26.89-●
    salpingitis O23.52-●
    salpingo-oophoritis O23.52-●
    sepsis (conditions in A40, A41) O98.81-●
    size date discrepancy (uterine) O26.84-●
    skin condition (conditions in L00-L99) O99.71-●
    smoking (tobacco) O99.33-●
    social problem O09.7-●
    specified condition NEC O26.89-●
    spotting O26.85-●
    streptococcus group B (GBS) carrier state O99.820
    subluxation of symphysis (pubis) O26.71-●
    syphilis (conditions in A50-A53) O98.11-●
    threatened
      abortion O20.0
      labor O47.9
        at or after 37 completed weeks of gestation O47.1
        before 37 completed weeks of gestation O47.0-●
    thrombophlebitis (superficial) O22.2-●
    thrombosis O22.9-●
      cerebral venous O22.5-●
      cerebrovenous sinus O22.5-●
      deep O22.3-●
    tobacco use disorder (smoking) O99.33-●
    torsion of uterus O34.59-●
    toxemia O14.9-●
    transverse lie or presentation O32.2
    tuberculosis (conditions in A15-A19) O98.01-●
    tumor (benign)
      cervix O34.4-●
      malignant O9A.11-●
      uterus O34.1-●
    unstable lie O32.0
    upper respiratory infection O99.51-●
    urethritis O23.2-●
    uterine size date discrepancy O26.84-●
    vaginitis or vulvitis O23.59-●
    varicose veins (lower extremities) O22.0-●
      genitals O22.1-●
      legs O22.0-●
      perineal O22.1-●
      vaginal or vulval O22.1-●
    venereal disease NEC (conditions in A63.8) O98.31-●

Pregnancy *(Continued)*
  complicated by *(Continued)*
    venous disorders O22.9-●
      specified NEC O22.8X-●
    very young mother —*see* Pregnancy, complicated by, young mother
    viral diseases (conditions in A80-B09, B25-B34) O98.51-●
    vomiting O21.9
      due to diseases classified elsewhere O21.8
      hyperemesis gravidarum (mild) —*see also* Hyperemesis, gravidarum O21.0-●
      late (occurring after 20 weeks of gestation) O21.2
    young mother
      multigravida O09.62-●
      primigravida O09.61-●
  concealed O09.3-●
  continuing following
    elective fetal reduction of one or more fetus O31.3-●
    intrauterine death of one or more fetus O31.2-●
    spontaneous abortion of one or more fetus O31.1-●
  cornual O00.80
    with intrauterine pregnancy O00.81
  ectopic (ruptured) O00.90
    with intrauterine pregnancy O00.91
    abdominal O00.00
      with
        intrauterine pregnancy O00.01
        viable fetus O36.7-●
    cervical O00.80
      with intrauterine pregnancy O00.81
    complicated (by) O08.9
      afibrinogenemia O08.1
      cardiac arrest O08.81
      chemical damage of pelvic organ(s) O08.6
      circulatory collapse O08.3
      defibrination syndrome O08.1
      electrolyte imbalance O08.5
      embolism (amniotic fluid) (blood clot) (pulmonary) (septic) O08.2
      endometritis O08.0
      genital tract and pelvic infection O08.0
      hemorrhage (delayed) (excessive) O08.1
      infection
        genital tract or pelvic O08.0
        kidney O08.83
        urinary tract O08.83
      intravascular coagulation O08.1
      laceration of pelvic organ(s) O08.6
      metabolic disorder O08.5
      oliguria O08.4
      oophoritis O08.0
      parametritis O08.0
      pelvic peritonitis O08.0
      perforation of pelvic organ(s) O08.6
      renal failure or shutdown O08.4
      salpingitis or salpingo-oophoritis O08.0
      sepsis O08.82
      shock O08.83
        septic O08.82
      specified condition NEC O08.89
      tubular necrosis (renal) O08.4
      uremia O08.4
      urinary infection O08.83
      venous complication NEC O08.7
        embolism O08.2
    cornual O00.80
      with intrauterine pregnancy O00.81
    intraligamentous O00.80
      with intrauterine pregnancy O00.81

Pregnancy *(Continued)*
  ectopic *(Continued)*
    mural O00.80
      with intrauterine pregnancy O00.81
    ⇒ovarian O00.20-●
      ⇒with intrauterine pregnancy O00.21-●
    specified site NEC O00.80
      with intrauterine pregnancy O00.81
    ⇒tubal (ruptured) O00.10-●
      ⇒with intrauterine pregnancy O00.11-●
  examination (normal) Z34.9-●
    first Z34.0-●
    high-risk —*see* Pregnancy, supervision of,
      high-risk
    specified Z34.8-●
  extrauterine —*see* Pregnancy, ectopic
  ⇒fallopian O00.10-●
    ⇒with intrauterine pregnancy O00.11-●
  false F45.8
  gestational carrier Z33.3
  hidden O09.3-●
  high-risk —*see* Pregnancy, supervision of,
    high-risk
  incidental finding Z33.1
  interstitial O00.80
    with intrauterine pregnancy O00.81
  intraligamentous O00.80
    with intrauterine pregnancy O00.81
  intramural O00.80
    with intrauterine pregnancy O00.81
  intraperitoneal O00.00
    with intrauterine pregnancy O00.01
  ⇒isthmian O00.10-●
    ⇒with intrauterine pregnancy O00.11-●
  mesometric (mural) O00.80
    with intrauterine pregnancy O00.81
  molar NEC O02.0
    complicated (by) O08.9
      afibrinogenemia O08.1
      cardiac arrest O08.81
      chemical damage of pelvic organ(s)
        O08.6
      circulatory collapse O08.3
      defibrination syndrome O08.1
      electrolyte imbalance O08.5
      embolism (amniotic fluid) (blood clot)
        (pulmonary) (septic) O08.2
      endometritis O08.0
      genital tract and pelvic infection
        O08.0
      hemorrhage (delayed) (excessive)
        O08.1
      infection
        genital tract or pelvic O08.0
        kidney O08.83
        urinary tract O08.83
      intravascular coagulation O08.1
      laceration of pelvic organ(s)
        O08.6
      metabolic disorder O08.5
      oliguria O08.4
      oophoritis O08.0
      parametritis O08.0
      pelvic peritonitis O08.0
      perforation of pelvic organ(s) O08.6
      renal failure or shutdown O08.4
      salpingitis or salpingo-oophoritis O08.0
      sepsis O08.82
      shock O08.3
        septic O08.82
      specified condition NEC O08.89
      tubular necrosis (renal) O08.4
      uremia O08.4
      urinary infection O08.83
      venous complication NEC O08.7
        embolism O08.2
  hydatidiform —*see also* Mole, hydatidiform
    O01.9-●
  multiple (gestation) O30.9-●
    greater than quadruplets —*see* Pregnancy,
      multiple (gestation), specified NEC

Pregnancy *(Continued)*
  multiple (gestation) *(Continued)*
    specified NEC O30.80-●
      with
        two or more monoamniotic fetuses
          O30.82-●
        two or more monochorionic fetuses
          O30.81-●
      two or more monoamniotic fetuses
        O30.82-●
      two or more monochorionic fetuses
        O30.81-●
      unable to determine number of placenta
        and number of amniotic sacs
        O30.89-●
      unspecified number of placenta and
        unspecified number of amniotic
        sacs O30.80-●
  mural O00.80
    with intrauterine pregnancy O00.81
  normal (supervision of) Z34.9-●
    first Z34.0-●
    high-risk —*see* Pregnancy, supervision of,
      high-risk
    specified Z34.8-●
  ⇒ovarian O00.20-●
    ⇒with intrauterine pregnancy O00.21-●
  postmature (40 to 42 weeks) O48.0
    more than 42 weeks gestation O48.1
  post-term (40 to 42 weeks) O48.0
  prenatal care only Z34.9-●
    first Z34.0-●
    high-risk —*see* Pregnancy, supervision of,
      high-risk
    specified Z34.8-●
  prolonged (more than 42 weeks gestation)
    O48.1
  quadruplet O30.20-●
    with
      two or more monoamniotic fetuses
        O30.22-●
      two or more monochorionic fetuses
        O30.21-●
    two or more monoamniotic fetuses O30.22-●
    two or more monochorionic fetuses
      O30.21-●
    unable to determine number of placenta
      and number of amniotic sacs O30.29-●
    unspecified number of placenta and
      unspecified number of amniotic sacs
      O30.20-●
  quintuplet —*see* Pregnancy, multiple
    (gestation), specified NEC
  sextuplet —*see* Pregnancy, multiple
    (gestation), specified NEC
  supervision of
    concealed pregnancy O09.3-●
    elderly mother
      multigravida O09.52-●
      primigravida O09.51-●
    hidden pregnancy O09.3-●
    high-risk O09.9-●
      due to (history of)
        ectopic pregnancy O09.1-●
        elderly —*see* Pregnancy, supervision,
          elderly mother
        grand multiparity O09.4
        infertility O09.0-●
        insufficient prenatal care O09.3-●
        in utero procedure during previous
          pregnancy O09.82-●
        in vitro fertilization O09.81-●
        molar pregnancy O09.A-●
        multiple previous pregnancies O09.4-●
        older mother —*see* Pregnancy,
          supervision of, elderly mother
        poor reproductive or obstetric history
          NEC O09.29-●
        pre-term labor O09.21-●
        previous
          neonatal death O09.29-●

Pregnancy *(Continued)*
  supervision of *(Continued)*
    high-risk *(Continued)*
      due to *(Continued)*
        social problems O09.7-●
        specified NEC O09.89-●
        very young mother —*see* Pregnancy,
          supervision, young mother
      resulting from in vitro fertilization
        O09.81-●
    normal Z34.9-●
      first Z34.0-●
      specified NEC Z34.8-●
    young mother
      multigravida O09.62-●
      primigravida O09.61-●
  triplet O30.10-●
    with
      two or more monoamniotic fetuses
        O30.12-●
      ~~two or more monochorionic fetuses~~
        ~~O30.11-●~~
      ▶two or more monochorionic fetuses
        O30.11-●
    two or more monoamniotic fetuses O30.12-●
    ~~two or more monochorionic fetuses~~
      ~~O30.11-●~~
    ▶two or more monochorionic fetuses O30.11-●
    unable to determine number of placenta
      and number of amniotic sacs O30.19-●
    unspecified number of placenta and
      unspecified number of amniotic sacs
      O30.10-●
  ⇒tubal (with abortion) (with rupture) O00.10-●
    ⇒with intrauterine pregnancy O00.11-●
  twin O30.00-●
    conjoined O30.02-●
    dichorionic/diamniotic (two placenta, two
      amniotic sacs) O30.04-●
    monochorionic/diamniotic (one placenta,
      two amniotic sacs) O30.03-●
    monochorionic/monoamniotic (one
      placenta, one amniotic sac) O30.01-●
    unable to determine number of placenta
      and number of amniotic sacs O30.09-●
    unspecified number of placenta and
      unspecified number of amniotic sacs
      O30.00-●
  unwanted Z64.0
  weeks of gestation
    8 weeks Z3A.08
    9 weeks Z3A.09
    10 weeks Z3A.10
    11 weeks Z3A.11
    12 weeks Z3A.12
    13 weeks Z3A.13
    14 weeks Z3A.14
    15 weeks Z3A.15
    16 weeks Z3A.16
    17 weeks Z3A.17
    18 weeks Z3A.18
    19 weeks Z3A.19
    20 weeks Z3A.20
    21 weeks Z3A.21
    22 weeks Z3A.22
    23 weeks Z3A.23
    24 weeks Z3A.24
    25 weeks Z3A.25
    26 weeks Z3A.26
    27 weeks Z3A.27
    28 weeks Z3A.28
    29 weeks Z3A.29
    30 weeks Z3A.30
    31 weeks Z3A.31
    32 weeks Z3A.32
    33 weeks Z3A.33
    34 weeks Z3A.34
    35 weeks Z3A.35
    36 weeks Z3A.36
    37 weeks Z3A.37
    38 weeks Z3A.38

▶ New   ⇒ Revised   ~~deleted~~ Deleted   ● Use Additional Character(s)

Pregnancy *(Continued)*
  weeks of gestation *(Continued)*
    39 weeks Z3A.39
    40 weeks Z3A.40
    41 weeks Z3A.41
    42 weeks Z3A.42
    greater than 42 weeks Z3A.49
    less than 8 weeks Z3A.01
    not specified Z3A.00
Preiser's disease —*see* Osteonecrosis,
  secondary, due to, trauma, metacarpus
Pre-kwashiorkor —*see* Malnutrition, severe
Preleukemia (syndrome) D46.9
Preluxation, hip, congenital Q65.6
Premature —*see also* condition
  adrenarche E27.0
  aging E34.8
  beats I49.40
    atrial I49.1
    auricular I49.1
    supraventricular I49.1
  birth NEC —*see* Preterm, newborn
  closure, foramen ovale Q21.8
  contraction
    atrial I49.1
    atrioventricular I49.49
    auricular I49.1
    auriculoventricular I49.2
    heart (extrasystole) I49.49
    junctional I49.2
    ventricular I49.3
  delivery —*see also* Pregnancy, complicated by,
    preterm labor O60.10
  ejaculation F52.4
  infant NEC —*see* Preterm, newborn
    light-for-dates —*see* Light for dates
  labor —*see* Pregnancy, complicated by,
    preterm labor
  lungs P28.0
  menopause E28.319
    asymptomatic E28.319
    symptomatic E28.310
  newborn
    extreme (less than 28 completed weeks) —
      see Immaturity, extreme
    less than 37 completed weeks —*see*
      Preterm, newborn
  puberty E30.1
  rupture membranes or amnion —*see*
    Pregnancy, complicated by, premature
    rupture of membranes
  senility E34.8
  thelarche E30.8
  ventricular systole I49.3
Prematurity NEC (less than 37 completed
  weeks) —*see* Preterm, newborn
  extreme (less than 28 completed weeks) —*see*
    Immaturity, extreme
Premenstrual
  dysphoric disorder (PMDD) F32.81
  tension (syndrome) N94.3
Premolarization, cuspids K00.2
Prenatal
  care, normal pregnancy —*see* Pregnancy,
    normal
  screening of mother —*see also* Encounter,
    antenatal Z36.9
  teeth K00.6
Preparatory care for subsequent treatment
  NEC
  for dialysis Z49.01
    peritoneal Z49.02
Prepartum —*see* condition
Preponderance, left or right ventricular I51.7
Prepuce —*see* condition
PRES (posterior reversible encephalopathy
  syndrome) I67.83
Presbycardia R54
Presbycusis, presbyacusia H91.1-•
Presbyesophagus K22.8
Presbyophrenia F03
Presbyopia H52.4

Prescription of contraceptives (initial) Z30.019
  barrier Z30.018
  diaphragm Z30.018
  emergency (postcoital) Z30.012
  implantable subdermal Z30.017
  injectable Z30.013
  intrauterine contraceptive device Z30.014
  pills Z30.011
  postcoital (emergency) Z30.012
  repeat Z30.40
    barrier Z30.49
    diaphragm Z30.49
    implantable subdermal Z30.46
    injectable Z30.42
    pills Z30.41
    specified type NEC Z30.49
    transdermal patch hormonal Z30.45
    vaginal ring hormonal Z30.44
  specified type NEC Z30.018
    transdermal patch hormonal Z30.016
    vaginal ring hormonal Z30.015
Presence (of)
  ankle-joint implant (functional) (prosthesis)
    Z96.66-•
  aortocoronary (bypass) graft Z95.1
  arterial-venous shunt (dialysis) Z99.2
  artificial
    eye (globe) Z97.0
    heart (fully implantable) (mechanical)
      Z95.812
      valve Z95.2
    larynx Z96.3
    lens (intraocular) Z96.1
    limb (complete) (partial) Z97.1-•
      arm Z97.1-•
        bilateral Z97.15
      leg Z97.1-•
        bilateral Z97.16
  audiological implant (functional) Z96.29
  bladder implant (functional) Z96.0
  bone
    conduction hearing device Z96.29
    implant (functional) NEC Z96.7
    joint (prosthesis) —*see* Presence, joint implant
  cardiac
    defibrillator (functional) (with synchronous
      cardiac pacemaker)Z95.810
    implant or graft Z95.9
      specified type NEC Z95.818
    pacemaker Z95.0
    resynchronization therapy
      defibrillator Z95.810
      pacemaker Z95.0
  cerebrospinal fluid drainage device Z98.2
  cochlear implant (functional) Z96.21
  contact lens (es) Z97.3
  coronary artery graft or prosthesis Z95.5
  CRT-D (cardiac resynchronization therapy
    defibrillator) Z95.810
  CRT-P (cardiac resynchronization therapy
    pacemaker) Z95.0
  cardioverter-defibrillator (ICD) Z95.810
  CSF shunt Z98.2
  dental prosthesis device Z97.2
  dentures Z97.2
  device (external) NEC Z97.8
    cardiac NEC Z95.818
    heart assist Z95.811
    implanted (functional) Z96.9
      specified NEC Z96.89
    prosthetic Z97.8
  ear implant Z96.20
    cochlear implant Z96.21
    myringotomy tube Z96.22
    specified type NEC Z96.29
  elbow-joint implant (functional) (prosthesis)
    Z96.62-•
  endocrine implant (functional) NEC Z96.49
  eustachian tube stent or device (functional)
    Z96.29
  external hearing-aid or device Z97.4
  finger-joint implant (functional) (prosthetic)
    Z96.69-•

Presence *(Continued)*
  functional implant Z96.9
    specified NEC Z96.89
  graft
    cardiac NEC Z95.818
    vascular NEC Z95.828
  hearing-aid or device (external) Z97.4
    implant (bone) (cochlear) (functional)
      Z96.21
  heart assist device Z95.811
  heart valve implant (functional) Z95.2
    prosthetic Z95.2
    specified type NEC Z95.4
    xenogenic Z95.3
  hip-joint implant (functional) (prosthesis)
    Z96.64-•
  ICD (cardioverter-defibrillator) Z95.810
  implanted device (artificial) (functional)
    (prosthetic) Z96.9
    automatic cardiac defibrillator (with
      synchronous cardiac pacemaker)
      Z95.810
    cardiac pacemaker Z95.0
    cochlear Z96.21
    dental Z96.5
    heart Z95.812
    heart valve Z95.2
      prosthetic Z95.2
      specified NEC Z95.4
      xenogenic Z95.3
    insulin pump Z96.41
    intraocular lens Z96.1
    joint Z96.60
      ankle Z96.66-•
      elbow Z96.62-•
      finger Z96.69-•
      hip Z96.64-•
      knee Z96.65-•
      shoulder Z96.61-•
      specified NEC Z96.698
      wrist Z96.63-•
    larynx Z96.3
    myringotomy tube Z96.22
    otological Z96.20
      cochlear Z96.21
      eustachian stent Z96.29
      myringotomy Z96.22
      specified NEC Z96.29
      stapes Z96.29
    skin Z96.81
    skull plate Z96.7
    specified NEC Z96.89
    urogenital Z96.0
  insulin pump (functional) Z96.41
  intestinal bypass or anastomosis Z98.0
  intraocular lens (functional) Z96.1
  intrauterine contraceptive device (IUD) Z97.5
  intravascular implant (functional) (prosthetic)
    NEC Z95.9
    coronary artery Z95.5
    defibrillator (with synchronous cardiac
      pacemaker) Z95.810
    peripheral vessel (with angioplasty)
      Z95.820
  joint implant (prosthetic) (any) Z96.60
    ankle —*see* Presence, ankle joint implant
    elbow —*see* Presence, elbow joint implant
    finger —*see* Presence, finger joint implant
    hip —*see* Presence, hip joint implant
    knee —*see* Presence, knee joint implant
    shoulder —*see* Presence, shoulder joint
      implant
    specified joint NEC Z96.698
    wrist —*see* Presence, wrist joint implant
  knee-joint implant (functional) (prosthesis)
    Z96.65-•
  laryngeal implant (functional) Z96.3
  mandibular implant (dental) Z96.5
  myringotomy tube(s) Z96.22
  orthopedic-joint implant (prosthetic) (any) —
    see Presence, joint implant

Presence *(Continued)*
otological implant (functional) Z96.29
shoulder-joint implant (functional)
(prosthesis) Z96.61-●
skull-plate implant Z96.7
spectacles Z97.3
stapes implant (functional) Z96.29
systemic lupus erythematosus [SLE] inhibitor
D68.62
tendon implant (functional) (graft) Z96.7
tooth root(s) implant Z96.5
ureteral stent Z96.0
urethral stent Z96.0
urogenital implant (functional) Z96.0
vascular implant or device Z95.9
access port device Z95.828
specified type NEC Z95.828
wrist-joint implant (functional) (prosthesis)
Z96.63-●
Presenile —*see also* condition
dementia F03
premature aging E34.8
Presentation, fetal —*see* Delivery, complicated
by, malposition
Prespondylolisthesis (congenital) Q76.2
Pressure
area, skin —*see* Ulcer, pressure, by site
brachial plexus G54.0
brain G93.5
injury at birth NEC P11.1
cerebral —*see* Pressure, brain
chest R07.89
cone, tentorial G93.5
hyposystolic —*see also* Hypotension
incidental reading, without diagnosis of
hypotension R03.1
increased
intracranial (benign) G93.2
injury at birth P11.0
intraocular H40.05-●
lumbosacral plexus G54.1
mediastinum J98.59
necrosis (chronic) —*see* Ulcer, pressure,
by site
parental, inappropriate (excessive)
Z62.6
sore (chronic) —*see* Ulcer, pressure,
by site
spinal cord G95.20
ulcer (chronic) —*see* Ulcer, pressure,
by site
venous, increased I87.8
Pre-syncope R55
Preterm
delivery (*see also* Pregnancy, complicated by,
preterm labor) O60.10
labor —*see* Pregnancy, complicated by,
preterm labor
newborn (infant) P07.30
gestational age
28 completed weeks (28 weeks, 0 days
through 28 weeks, 6 days) P07.31
29 completed weeks (29 weeks, 0 days
through 29 weeks, 6 days) P07.32
30 completed weeks (30 weeks, 0 days
through 30 weeks, 6 days) P07.33
31 completed weeks (31 weeks, 0 days
through 31 weeks, 6 days) P07.34
32 completed weeks (32 weeks, 0 days
through 32 weeks, 6 days) P07.35
33 completed weeks (33 weeks, 0 days
through 33 weeks, 6 days) P07.36
34 completed weeks (34 weeks, 0 days
through 34 weeks, 6 days) P07.37
35 completed weeks (35 weeks, 0 days
through 35 weeks, 6 days) P07.38
36 completed weeks (36 weeks, 0 days
through 36 weeks, 6 days) P07.39
Previa
placenta (total) (without hemorrhage)
O44.0-●

Previa *(Continued)*
placenta *(Continued)*
with hemorrhage O44.1-●
complete O44.0-●
with hemorrhage O44.1-●
low —*see also* Delivery, complicated, by,
placenta, low O44.4-●
with hemorrhage O44.5-●
marginal O44.2-●
with hemorrhage O44.3-●
partial O44.2-●
with hemorrhage O44.3-●
vasa O69.4
Priapism N48.30
due to
disease classified elsewhere N48.32
drug N48.33
specified cause NEC N48.39
trauma N48.31
Prickling sensation (skin) R20.2
Prickly heat L74.0
Primary —*see* condition
Primigravida
elderly, affecting management of pregnancy,
labor and delivery (supervision only) —
see Pregnancy, complicated by, elderly,
primigravida
older, affecting management of pregnancy,
labor and delivery (supervision only) —
see Pregnancy, complicated by, elderly,
primigravida
very young, affecting management of
pregnancy, labor and delivery (supervision
only) —*see* Pregnancy, complicated by,
young mother, primigravida
Primipara
elderly, affecting management of pregnancy,
labor and delivery (supervision only) —
see Pregnancy, complicated by, elderly,
primigravida
older, affecting management of pregnancy,
labor and delivery (supervision only) —
see Pregnancy, complicated by, elderly,
primigravida
very young, affecting management
of pregnancy, labor and delivery
(supervision only) —*see* Pregnancy,
complicated by, young mother,
primigravida
Primus varus (bilateral) Q66.2
PRIND (Prolonged reversible ischemic
neurologic deficit) I63.9
Pringle's disease (tuberous sclerosis) Q85.1
Prinzmetal angina I20.1
Prizefighter ear —*see* Cauliflower ear
Problem (with) (related to)
academic Z55.8
acculturation Z60.3
adjustment (to)
change of job Z56.1
life-cycle transition Z60.0
pension Z60.0
retirement Z60.0
adopted child Z62.821
alcoholism in family Z63.72
atypical parenting situation Z62.9
bankruptcy Z59.8
behavioral (adult) F69
drug seeking Z76.5
birth of sibling affecting child Z62.898
care (of)
provider dependency Z74.9
specified NEC Z74.8
sick or handicapped person in family or
household Z63.6
child
abuse (affecting the child) —*see*
Maltreatment, child
custody or support proceedings Z65.3
in care of non-parental family member
Z62.21

Problem *(Continued)*
child *(Continued)*
in foster care Z62.21
in welfare custody Z62.21
living in orphanage or group home Z62.22
child-rearing Z62.9
specified NEC Z62.898
communication (developmental) F80.9
conflict or discord (with)
boss Z56.4
classmates Z55.4
counselor Z64.4
employer Z56.4
family Z63.9
specified NEC Z63.8
probation officer Z64.4
social worker Z64.4
teachers Z55.4
workmates Z56.4
conviction in legal proceedings Z65.0
with imprisonment Z65.1
counselor Z64.4
creditors Z59.8
digestive K92.9
drug addict in family Z63.72
ear —*see* Disorder, ear
economic Z59.9
affecting care Z59.9
specified NEC Z59.8
education Z55.9
specified NEC Z55.8
employment Z56.9
change of job Z56.1
discord Z56.4
environment Z56.5
sexual harassment Z56.81
specified NEC Z56.89
stress NEC Z56.6
stressful schedule Z56.3
threat of job loss Z56.2
unemployment Z56.0
enuresis, child F98.0
eye H57.9
failed examinations (school) Z55.2
falling Z91.81
family —*see also* Disruption, family Z63.9-●
specified NEC Z63.8
feeding (elderly) (infant) R63.3
newborn P92.9
breast P92.5
overfeeding P92.4
slow P92.2
specified NEC P92.8
underfeeding P92.3
nonorganic F50.89
finance Z59.9
specified NEC Z59.8
foreclosure on loan Z59.8
foster child Z62.822
frightening experience(s) in childhood
Z62.898
genital NEC
female N94.9
male N50.9
health care Z75.9
specified NEC Z75.8
hearing —*see* Deafness
homelessness Z59.0
housing Z59.9
inadequate Z59.1
isolated Z59.8
specified NEC Z59.8
identity (of childhood) F93.8
illegitimate pregnancy (unwanted) Z64.0
illiteracy Z55.0
impaired mobility Z74.09
imprisonment or incarceration Z65.1
inadequate teaching affecting education
Z55.8
inappropriate (excessive) parental pressure
Z62.6

▶ New ⇒ Revised ~~deleted~~ Deleted ● Use Additional Character(s)

Problem *(Continued)*
  influencing health status NEC Z78.9
  in-law Z63.1
  institutionalization, affecting child
      Z62.22
  intrafamilial communication Z63.8
  jealousy, child F93.8
  landlord Z59.2
  language (developmental) F80.9
  learning (developmental) F81.9
  legal Z65.3
    conviction without imprisonment
        Z65.0
    imprisonment Z65.1
    release from prison Z65.2
  life-management Z73.9
    specified NEC Z73.89
  life-style Z72.9
    gambling Z72.6
    high-risk sexual behavior (heterosexual)
        Z72.51
      bisexual Z72.53
      homosexual Z72.52
    inappropriate eating habits Z72.4
    self-damaging behavior NEC Z72.89
    specified NEC Z72.89
    tobacco use Z72.0
  literacy Z55.9
    low level Z55.0
    specified NEC Z55.8
  living alone Z60.2
  lodgers Z59.2
  loss of love relationship in childhood
      Z62.898
  marital Z63.0
    involving
        divorce Z63.5
        estrangement Z63.5
        gender identity F66
  mastication K08.89
  medical
    care, within family Z63.6
    facilities Z75.9
      specified NEC Z75.8
  mental F48.9
  multiparity Z64.1
  negative life events in childhood Z62.9
    altered pattern of family relationships
        Z62.898
    frightening experience Z62.898
    loss of
        love relationship Z62.898
        self-esteem Z62.898
    physical abuse (alleged) —*see*
        Maltreatment, child
    removal from home Z62.29
    specified event NEC Z62.898
  neighbor Z59.2
  neurological NEC R29.818
  new step-parent affecting child Z62.898
  none (feared complaint unfounded) Z71.1
  occupational NEC Z56.89
  parent-child —*see* Conflict, parent-child
  personal hygiene Z91.89
  personality F69
  phase-of-life transition, adjustment Z60.0
  presence of sick or disabled person
      in family or household Z63.79
      needing care Z63.6
  primary support group (family) Z63.9
    specified NEC Z63.8
  probation officer Z64.4
  psychiatric F99
  psychosexual (development) F66
  psychosocial Z65.9
  ▶religious or spiritual Z65.8
    specified NEC Z65.8
  relationship Z63.9
    childhood F93.8
  release from prison Z65.2
  ▶religious or spiritual Z65.8

Problem *(Continued)*
  removal from home affecting child
      Z62.29
  seeking and accepting known hazardous and
      harmful
    behavioral or psychological interventions
        Z65.8
    chemical, nutritional or physical
        interventions Z65.8
  sexual function (nonorganic) F52.9
  sight H54.7
  sleep disorder, child F51.9
  smell —*see* Disturbance, sensation, smell
  social
    environment Z60.9
        specified NEC Z60.8
    exclusion and rejection Z60.4
    worker Z64.4
  speech R47.9
    developmental F80.9
    specified NEC R47.89
  swallowing —*see* Dysphagia
  taste —*see* Disturbance, sensation, taste
  tic, child F95.0
  underachievement in school Z55.3
  unemployment Z56.0
    threatened Z56.2
  unwanted pregnancy Z64.0
  upbringing Z62.9
    specified NEC Z62.898
  urinary N39.9
  voice production R47.89
  work schedule (stressful) Z56.3
Procedure (surgical)
  converted
    arthroscopic to open Z53.33
    laparoscopic to open Z53.31
    specified procedure NEC to open
        Z53.39
    thoracoscopic to open Z53.32
  for purpose other than remedying health
      state Z41.9
    specified NEC Z41.8
  not done Z53.9
    because of
        administrative reasons Z53.8
        contraindication Z53.09
          smoking Z53.01
        patient's decision Z53.20
          for reasons of belief or group pressure
              Z53.1
          left against medical advice (AMA)
              Z53.21
        specified reason NEC Z53.29
    specified reason NEC Z53.8
Procidentia (uteri) N81.3
Proctalgia K62.89
  fugax K59.4
  spasmodic K59.4
Proctitis K62.89
  amebic (acute) A06.0
  chlamydial A56.3
  gonococcal A54.6
  granulomatous —*see* Enteritis, regional, large
      intestine
  herpetic A60.1
  radiation K62.7
  tuberculous A18.32
  ulcerative (chronic) K51.20
    with
        complication K51.219
          abscess K51.214
          fistula K51.213
          obstruction K51.212
          rectal bleeding K51.211
          specified NEC K51.218
Proctocele
  female (without uterine prolapse) N81.6
    with uterine prolapse N81.2
        complete N81.3
  male K62.3

Proctocolitis
  food-induced eosinophilic K52.82
  food protein-induced K52.82
  milk protein-induced K52.82
  mucosal —*see* Rectosigmoiditis, ulcerative
Proctoptosis K62.3
Proctorrhagia K62.5
Proctosigmoiditis K63.89
  ulcerative (chronic) —*see* Rectosigmoiditis,
      ulcerative
Proctospasm K59.4
  psychogenic F45.8
Profichet's disease —*see* Disorder, soft tissue,
      specified type NEC
Progeria E34.8
Prognathism (mandibular) (maxillary) M26.19
Progonoma (melanotic) —*see* Neoplasm,
      benign, by site
Progressive —*see* condition
Prolactinoma
  specified site —*see* Neoplasm, benign,
      by site
  unspecified site D35.2
Prolapse, prolapsed
  anus, anal (canal) (sphincter) K62.2
  arm or hand O32.2
    causing obstructed labor O64.4
  bladder (mucosa) (sphincter) (acquired)
    congenital Q79.4
    female —*see* Cystocele
    male N32.89
  breast implant (prosthetic) T85.49
  cecostomy K94.09
  cecum K63.4
  cervix, cervical (hypertrophied) N81.2
    anterior lip, obstructing labor O65.5
    congenital Q51.828
    postpartal, old N81.2
    stump N81.85
  ciliary body (traumatic) —*see* Laceration,
      eye(ball), with prolapse or loss of
      interocular tissue
  colon (pedunculated) K63.4
  colostomy K94.09
  disc (intervertebral) —*see* Displacement,
      intervertebral disc
  eye implant (orbital) T85.398
    lens (ocular) —*see* Complications,
        intraocular lens
  fallopian tube N83.4-●
  gastric (mucosa) K31.89
  genital, female N81.9
    specified NEC N81.89
  globe, nontraumatic —*see* Luxation, globe
  ileostomy bud K94.19
  intervertebral disc —*see* Displacement,
      intervertebral disc
  intestine (small) K63.4
  iris (traumatic) —*see* Laceration, eye(ball),
      with prolapse or loss of interocular
      tissue
    nontraumatic H21.89
  kidney N28.83
    congenital Q63.2
  laryngeal muscles or ventricle J38.7
  liver K76.89
  meatus urinarius N36.8
  mitral (valve) I34.1
  ocular lens implant —*see* Complications,
      intraocular lens
  organ or site, congenital NEC —*see*
      Malposition, congenital
  ovary N83.4-●
  pelvic floor, female N81.89
  perineum, female N81.89
  rectum (mucosa) (sphincter) K62.3
    due to trichuris trichuria B79
  spleen D73.89
  stomach K31.89
  umbilical cord
    complicating delivery O69.0

Prolapse, prolapsed (Continued)
  urachus, congenital Q64.4
  ureter N28.89
    with obstruction N13.5
      with infection N13.6
  ureterovesical orifice N28.89
  urethra (acquired) (infected) (mucosa)
      N36.8
    congenital Q64.71
  urinary meatus N36.8
    congenital Q64.72
  uterovaginal N81.4
    complete N81.3
    incomplete N81.2
  uterus (with prolapse of vagina) N81.4
    complete N81.3
    congenital Q51.818
    first degree N81.2
    in pregnancy or childbirth —see
        Pregnancy, complicated by,
        abnormal, uterus
    incomplete N81.2
    postpartal (old) N81.4
    second degree N81.2
    third degree N81.3
  uveal (traumatic) —see Laceration, eye(ball),
      with prolapse or loss of interocular
      tissue
  vagina (anterior) (wall) —see Cystocele
    with prolapse of uterus N81.4
      complete N81.3
      incomplete N81.2
    posterior wall N81.6
    posthysterectomy N99.3
  vitreous (humor) H43.0-●
    in wound —see Laceration, eye(ball), with
        prolapse or loss of interocular tissue
  womb —see Prolapse, uterus
Prolapsus, female N81.9
  specified NEC N81.89
Proliferation(s)
  primary cutaneous CD30-positive large T-cell
      C86.6
  prostate, atypical small acinar N42.32
Proliferative —see condition
Prolonged, prolongation (of)
  bleeding (time) (idiopathic) R79.1
  coagulation (time) R79.1
  gestation (over 42 completed weeks)
    mother O48.1
    newborn P08.22
  interval I44.0
  labor O63.9
    first stage O63.0
    second stage O63.1
  partial thromboplastin time (PTT) R79.1
  pregnancy (more than 42 weeks gestation)
      O48.1
  prothrombin time R79.1
  QT interval I45.81
  uterine contractions in labor O62.4
Prominence, prominent
  with disproportion (fetopelvic) O33.0
    causing obstructed labor O65.0
  auricle (congenital) (ear) Q17.5
  ischial spine or sacral promontory
  nose (congenital) acquired M95.0
Promiscuity —see High, risk, sexual behavior
Pronation
  ankle —see Deformity, limb, foot, specified
      NEC
  foot —see also Deformity, limb, foot, specified
      NEC
    congenital Q74.2
Prophylactic
  administration of
    antibiotics, long-term Z79.2
      short-term use - omit code
    drug —see also Long-term (current) drug
        therapy (use of) Z79.899-●
  medication Z79.899

Prophylactic (Continued)
  organ removal (for neoplasia management)
      Z40.00
    breast Z40.01
    ▶fallopian tube(s) Z40.03
      ▶with ovary(s) Z40.02
    ⇒ovary(s) Z40.02
    specified site NEC Z40.09
  surgery Z40.9
    for risk factors related to malignant
        neoplasm —see Prophylactic, organ
        removal
    specified NEC Z40.8
  vaccination Z23
Propionic acidemia E71.121
Proptosis (ocular) —see also Exophthalmos
  thyroid —see Hyperthyroidism, with goiter
Prosecution, anxiety concerning Z65.3
Prosopagnosia R48.3
Prosopalgia R48.81
Prostate, prostatic —see condition
Prostatism —see Hyperplasia, prostate
Prostatitis (congestive) (suppurative) (with
    cystitis) N41.9
  acute N41.0
  cavitary N41.8
  chronic N41.1
  diverticular N41.8
  due to Trichomonas (vaginalis) A59.02
  fibrous N41.1
  gonococcal (acute) (chronic) A54.22
  granulomatous N41.4
  hypertrophic N41.1
  subacute N41.1
  trichomonal A59.02
  tuberculous A18.14
Prostatocystitis N41.3
Prostatorrhea N42.89
Prostatosis N42.82
Prostration R53.83
  heat —see also Heat, exhaustion
    anhydrotic T67.3
    due to
      salt (and water) depletion T67.4
      water depletion T67.3
  nervous F48.8
  senile R54
Protanomaly (anomalous trichromat) H53.54
Protanopia (complete) (incomplete) H53.54
Protection (against) (from) —see Prophylactic
Protein
  deficiency NEC —see Malnutrition
  malnutrition —see Malnutrition
  sickness —see also Reaction, serum T80.69
Proteinemia R77.9
Proteinosis
  alveolar (pulmonary) J84.01
  lipid or lipoid (of Urbach) E78.89
Proteinuria R80.9
  Bence Jones R80.3
  complicating pregnancy —see Proteinuria,
      gestational
  gestational
    complicating
      childbirth O12.14
      pregnancy O12.1-●
        with edema O12.2-●
      puerperium O12.15
  idiopathic R80.0
  isolated R80.0
    with glomerular lesion N06.9
      dense deposit disease N06.6
      diffuse
        crescentic glomerulonephritis N06.7
        endocapillary proliferative
            glomerulonephritis N06.4
        mesangiocapillary glomerulonephritis
            N06.5
      focal and segmental hyalinosis or
          sclerosis N06.1
      membranous (diffuse) N06.2

Proteinuria (Continued)
  isolated (Continued)
    with glomerular lesion (Continued)
      mesangial proliferative (diffuse)
          N06.3
      minimal change N06.0
      specified pathology NEC N06.8
  orthostatic R80.2
    with glomerular lesion —see Proteinuria,
        isolated, with glomerular lesion
  persistent R80.1
    with glomerular lesion —see Proteinuria,
        isolated, with glomerular lesion
  postural R80.2
    with glomerular lesion —see Proteinuria,
        isolated, with glomerular lesion
  pre-eclamptic —see Pre-eclampsia
  puerperal O12.15
  specified type NEC R80.8
Proteolysis, pathologic D65
Proteus (mirabilis) (morganii), as cause of
    disease classified elsewhere B96.4
Prothrombin gene mutation D68.52
Protoporphyria, erythropoietic E80.0
Protozoal —see also condition
  disease B64
    specified NEC B60.8
Protrusion, protrusio
  acetabuli M24.7
  acetabulum (into pelvis) M24.7
  device, implant or graft —see also
      Complications, by site and type,
      mechanical T85.698
    arterial graft NEC —see Complication,
        cardiovascular device, mechanical,
        vascular
    breast (implant) T85.49
    catheter NEC T85.698
      cystostomy T83.090
      dialysis (renal) T82.49
        intraperitoneal T85.691
      infusion NEC T82.594
        spinal (epidural) (subdural)
            T85.690
      urinary —see also Complications,
          catheter, urinary T83.098
    electronic (electrode) (pulse generator)
        (stimulator)
      bone T84.390
      nervous system —see Complication,
          prosthetic device, mechanical,
          electronic nervous system
          stimulator
    fixation, internal (orthopedic) NEC —
        see Complication, fixation device,
        mechanical
    gastrointestinal —see Complications,
        prosthetic device, mechanical,
        gastrointestinal device
    genital NEC T83.498
      intrauterine contraceptive device
          T83.39
      penile prosthesis (cylinder) (implanted)
          (pump) (resevoir) T83.490
      testicular prosthesis T83.491
    heart NEC —see Complication,
        cardiovascular device, mechanical
    joint prosthesis —see Complications, joint
        prosthesis, mechanical, specified NEC,
        by site
    ocular NEC —see Complications, prosthetic
        device, mechanical, ocular device
    orthopedic NEC —see Complication,
        orthopedic, device, mechanical
    specified NEC T85.628
    urinary NEC —see also Complication,
        genitourinary, device, urinary,
        mechanical
      graft T83.29
    vascular NEC —see Complication,
        cardiovascular device, mechanical

Protrusion, protrusio *(Continued)*
  device, implant or graft *(Continued)*
    ventricular intracranial shunt T85.09
  intervertebral disc —*see* Displacement,
    intervertebral disc
  joint prosthesis —*see* Complications, joint
    prosthesis, mechanical, specified NEC,
    by site
  nucleus pulposus —*see* Displacement,
    intervertebral disc
Prune belly (syndrome) Q79.4
Prurigo (ferox) (gravis) (Hebrae) (Hebra's)
  (mitis) (simplex) L28.2
  Besnier's L20.0
  estivalis L56.4
  nodularis L28.1
  psychogenic F45.8
Pruritus, pruritic (essential) L29.9
  ani, anus L29.0
    psychogenic F45.8
  anogenital L29.3
    psychogenic F45.8
  due to onchocerca volvulus B73.1
  gravidarum —*see* Pregnancy, complicated by,
    specified pregnancy-related condition
    NEC
  hiemalis L29.8
  neurogenic (any site) F45.8
  perianal L29.0
  psychogenic (any site) F45.8
  scroti, scrotum L29.1
    psychogenic F45.8
  senile, senilis L29.8
  specified NEC L29.8
    psychogenic F45.8
  Trichomonas A59.9
  vulva, vulvae L29.2
    psychogenic F45.8
Pseudarthrosis, pseudoarthrosis (bone) —*see*
  Nonunion, fracture
  clavicle, congenital Q74.0
  joint, following fusion or arthrodesis M96.0
Pseudoaneurysm —*see* Aneurysm
Pseudoangina (pectoris) —*see* Angina
Pseudoangioma I81
Pseudoarteriosus Q28.8
Pseudoarthrosis —*see* Pseudarthrosis
Pseudobulbar affect (PBA) F48.2
Pseudochromhidrosis L67.8
Pseudocirrhosis, liver, pericardial I31.1
Pseudocowpox B08.03
Pseudocoxalgia M91.3-●
Pseudocroup J38.5
Pseudo-Cushing's syndrome, alcohol-induced
  E24.4
Pseudocyesis F45.8
Pseudocyst
  lung J98.4
  pancreas K86.3
  retina —*see* Cyst, retina
Pseudoelephantiasis neuroarthritica Q82.0
Pseudoexfoliation, capsule (lens) —*see*
  Cataract, specified NEC
Pseudofolliculitis barbae L73.1
Pseudoglioma H44.89
Pseudohemophilia (Bernuth's) (hereditary)
  (type B) D68.0
  Type A D69.8
  vascular D69.8
Pseudohermaphroditism Q56.3
  adrenal E25.8
  female Q56.2
    with adrenocortical disorder E25.8
    without adrenocortical disorder
      Q56.2
    adrenal (congenital) E25.0
    ▶unspecified E25.9
  male Q56.1
    with
      adrenocortical disorder E25.8
      androgen resistance E34.51

Pseudohermaphroditism *(Continued)*
  male *(Continued)*
    with *(Continued)*
      cleft scrotum Q56.1
      feminizing testis E34.51
      5-alpha-reductase deficiency E29.1
    without gonadal disorder Q56.1
    adrenal E25.8
    ▶unspecified E25.9
Pseudo-Hurler's polydystrophy E77.0
Pseudohydrocephalus G93.2
Pseudohypertrophic muscular dystrophy
  (Erb's) G71.0
Pseudohypertrophy, muscle G71.0
Pseudohypoparathyroidism E20.1
Pseudoinsomnia F51.03
Pseudoleukemia, infantile D64.89
Pseudomembranous —*see* condition
Pseudomeningocele (cerebral) (infective) (post-
  traumatic) G96.19
  postprocedural (spinal) G97.82
Pseudomenses (newborn) P54.6
Pseudomenstruation (newborn) P54.6
Pseudomonas
  aeruginosa, as cause of disease classified
    elsewhere B96.5
  mallei infection A24.0
    as cause of disease classified elsewhere
      B96.5
  pseudomallei, as cause of disease classified
    elsewhere B96.5
Pseudomyotonia G71.19
Pseudomyxoma peritonei C78.6
Pseudoneuritis, optic (nerve) (disc) (papilla),
  congenital Q14.2
Pseudo-obstruction intestine (acute) (chronic)
  (idiopathic) (intermittent secondary)
  (primary) K59.8
Pseudopapilledema H47.33-●
  congenital Q14.2
Pseudoparalysis
  arm or leg R29.818
  atonic, congenital P94.2
Pseudopelade L66.0
Pseudophakia Z96.1
Pseudopolyarthritis, rhizomelic M35.3
Pseudopolycythemia D75.1
Pseudopseudohypoparathyroidism E20.1
Pseudopterygium H11.81-●
Pseudoptosis (eyelid) —*see* Blepharochalasis
Pseudopuberty, precocious
  female heterosexual E25.8
  male isosexual E25.8
Pseudorickets (renal) N25.0
Pseudorubella B08.20
➡**Pseudosclerema, newborn** P83.88
Pseudosclerosis (brain)
  Jakob's —*see* Creutzfeldt-Jakob disease or
    syndrome
  of Westphal (Strüümpell) E83.01
  spastic —*see* Creutzfeldt-Jakob disease or
    syndrome
Pseudotetanus —*see* Convulsions
Pseudotetany R29.0
  hysterical F44.5
Pseudotruncus arteriosus Q25.49
Pseudotuberculosis A28.2
  enterocolitis A04.8
  pasteurella (infection) A28.0
Pseudotumor
  cerebri G93.2
  orbital H05.11-●
Pseudoxanthoma elasticum Q82.8
Psilosis (sprue) (tropical) K90.1
  nontropical K90.0
Psittacosis A70
Psoitis M60.88
Psoriasis L40.9
  arthropathic L40.50
    arthritis mutilans L40.52
    distal interphalangeal L40.51

Psoriasis *(Continued)*
  arthropathic *(Continued)*
    juvenile L40.54
    other specified L40.59
    spondylitis L40.53
  buccal K13.29
  flexural L40.8
  guttate L40.4
  mouth K13.29
  nummular L40.0
  plaque L40.0
  psychogenic F54
  pustular (generalized) L40.1
    palmaris et plantaris L40.3
  specified NEC L40.8
  vulgaris L40.0
Psychasthenia F48.8
Psychiatric disorder or problem F99
Psychogenic —*see also* condition
  factors associated with physical conditions
    F54
Psychological and behavioral factors affecting
  medical condition F59
Psychoneurosis, psychoneurotic —*see also*
  Neurosis
  anxiety (state) F41.1
  depersonalization F48.1
  hypochondriacal F45.21
  hysteria F44.9
  neurasthenic F48.8
  personality NEC F60.89
Psychopathy, psychopathic
  affectionless F94.2
  autistic F84.5
  constitution, post-traumatic F07.81
  personality —*see* Disorder, personality
  sexual —*see* Deviation, sexual
  state F60.2
Psychosexual identity disorder of childhood
  F64.2
Psychosis, psychotic F29
  acute (transient) F23
    hysterical F44.9
  affective —*see* Disorder, mood
  alcoholic F10.959
    with
      abuse F10.159
      anxiety disorder F10.980
        with
          abuse F10.180
          dependence F10.280
      delirium tremens F10.231
      delusions F10.950
        with
          abuse F10.150
          dependence F10.250
      dementia F10.97
        with dependence F10.27
      dependence F10.259
      hallucinosis F10.951
        with
          abuse F10.151
          dependence F10.251
      mood disorder F10.94
        with
          abuse F10.14
          dependence F10.24
      paranoia F10.950
        with
          abuse F10.150
          dependence F10.250
      persisting amnesia F10.96
        with dependence F10.26
    amnestic confabulatory F10.96
      with dependence F10.26
    delirium tremens F10.231
    Korsakoff's, Korsakov's, Korsakow's F10.26
    paranoid type F10.950
      with
        abuse F10.150
        dependence F10.250

Psychosis, psychotic *(Continued)*
  anergastic —*see* Psychosis, organic
  arteriosclerotic (simple type) (uncomplicated)
    F01.50
    with behavioral disturbance F01.51
  childhood F84.0
    atypical F84.8
  climacteric —*see* Psychosis, involutional
  confusional F29
    acute or subacute F05
    reactive F23
  cycloid F23
  depressive —*see* Disorder, depressive
  disintegrative (childhood) F84.3
  drug-induced —*see* F11-F19 with .x59
    paranoid and hallucinatory states —*see*
      F11-F19 with .x50 or .x51
  due to or associated with
    addiction, drug —*see* F11-F19 with .X59
    dependence
      alcohol F10.259
      drug —*see* F11-F19 with .x59
    epilepsy F06.8
    Huntington's chorea F06.8
    ischemia, cerebrovascular (generalized)
      F06.8
    multiple sclerosis F06.8
    physical disease F06.8
    presenile dementia F03
    senile dementia F03
    vascular disease (arteriosclerotic) (cerebral)
      F01.50
      with behavioral disturbance F01.51
  epileptic F06.8
  episode F23
    due to or associated with physical
      condition F06.8
  exhaustive F43.0
  hallucinatory, chronic F28
  hypomanic F30.8
  hysterical (acute) F44.9
  induced F24
  infantile F84.0
    atypical F84.8
  infective (acute) (subacute) F05
  involutional F28
    depressive —*see* Disorder, depressive
    melancholic —*see* Disorder, depressive
    paranoid (state) F22
  Korsakoff's, Korsakov's, Korsakow's
    (nonalcoholic) F04
    alcoholic F10.96
      in dependence F10.26
    induced by other psychoactive
      substance —*see* categories F11-F19
      with .x5x
  mania, manic (single episode) F30.2
    recurrent type F31.89
  manic-depressive —*see* Disorder, bipolar
  menopausal —*see* Psychosis, involutional
  mixed schizophrenic and affective F25.8
  multi-infarct (cerebrovascular) F01.50
    with behavioral disturbance F01.51
  nonorganic F29
    specified NEC F28
  organic F09
    due to or associated with
      arteriosclerosis (cerebral) —*see*
        Psychosis, arteriosclerotic
      cerebrovascular disease,
        arteriosclerotic —*see* Psychosis,
        arteriosclerotic
      childbirth —*see* Psychosis, puerperal
      Creutzfeldt-Jakob disease or
        syndrome —*see* Creutzfeldt-Jakob
        disease or syndrome
      dependence, alcohol F10.259
      disease
        alcoholic liver F10.259
        brain, arteriosclerotic —*see* Psychosis,
          arteriosclerotic

Psychosis, psychotic *(Continued)*
  organic *(Continued)*
    due to or associated with *(Continued)*
      disease *(Continued)*
        cerebrovascular F01.50
          with behavioral disturbance
            F01.51
        Creutzfeldt-Jakob —*see* Creutzfeldt-
          Jakob disease or syndrome
        endocrine or metabolic F06.8
          acute or subacute F05
        liver, alcoholic F10.259
      epilepsy transient (acute) F05
      infection
        brain (intracranial) F06.8
          acute or subacute F05
      intoxication
        alcoholic (acute) F10.259
        drug F19 with .X59 F11-•
      ischemia, cerebrovascular (generalized) —
        see Psychosis, arteriosclerotic
      puerperium —*see* Psychosis, puerperal
      trauma, brain (birth) (from electric
        current) (surgical) F06.8
        acute or subacute F05
    infective F06.8
      acute or subacute F05
    post-traumatic F06.8
      acute or subacute F05
  paranoiac F22
  paranoid (climacteric) (involutional)
    (menopausal) F22
    psychogenic (acute) F23
    schizophrenic F20.0
    senile F03
  postpartum F53
  presbyophrenic (type) F03
  presenile F03
  psychogenic (paranoid) F23
    depressive F32.3
  puerperal F53
    specified type —*see* Psychosis, by type
  reactive (brief) (transient) (emotional stress)
    (psychological trauma) F23
    depressive F32.3
      recurrent F33.3
    excitative type F30.8
  schizoaffective F25.9
    depressive type F25.1
    manic type F25.0
  schizophrenia, schizophrenic —*see*
    Schizophrenia
  schizophrenia-like, in epilepsy F06.2
  schizophreniform F20.81
    affective type F25.9
    brief F23
    confusional type F23
    ~~depressive type F25.1~~
    ~~manic type F25.0~~
    mixed type F25.0
  senile NEC F03
    depressed or paranoid type F03
    simple deterioration F03
    specified type — code to condition
  shared F24
  situational (reactive) F23
  symbiotic (childhood) F84.3
  symptomatic F09
Psychosomatic —*see* Disorder, psychosomatic
Psychosyndrome, organic F07.9
Psychotic episode due to or associated with
  physical condition F06.8
Pterygium (eye) H11.00-•
  amyloid H11.01-•
  central H11.02-•
  colli Q18.3
  double H11.03-•
  peripheral
    progressive H11.05-•
    stationary H11.04-•
  recurrent H11.06-•

Ptilosis (eyelid) —*see* Madarosis
Ptomaine (poisoning) —*see* Poisoning, food
Ptosis —*see also* Blepharoptosis
  adiposa (false) —*see* Blepharoptosis
  breast N64.81
  cecum K63.4
  colon K63.4
  congenital (eyelid) Q10.0
    specified site NEC —*see* Anomaly, by site
  eyelid —*see* Blepharoptosis
    congenital Q10.0
  gastric K31.89
  intestine K63.4
  kidney N28.83
  liver K76.89
  renal N28.83
  splanchnic K63.4
  spleen D73.89
  stomach K31.89
  viscera K63.4
PTP D69.51
Ptyalism (periodic) K11.7
  hysterical F45.8
  pregnancy —*see* Pregnancy, complicated by,
    specified pregnancy-related condition
    NEC
  psychogenic F45.8
Ptyalolithiasis K11.5
Pubarche, precocious E30.1
Pubertas praecox E30.1
Puberty (development state) Z00.3
  bleeding (excessive) N92.2
  delayed E30.0
  precocious (constitutional) (cryptogenic)
    (idiopathic) E30.1
    central E22.8
    due to
      ovarian hyperfunction E28.1
        estrogen E28.0
      testicular hyperfunction E29.0
  premature E30.1
    due to
      adrenal cortical hyperfunction E25.8
      pineal tumor E34.8
      pituitary (anterior) hyperfunction E22.8
Puckering, macula —*see* Degeneration, macula,
  puckering
Pudenda, pudendum —*see* condition
Puente's disease (simple glandular cheilitis)
  K13.0
Puerperal, puerperium (complicated by,
  complications)
  abnormal glucose (tolerance test) O99.815
  abscess
    areola O91.02
      associated with lactation O91.03
    Bartholin's gland O86.19
    breast O91.12
      associated with lactation O91.13
    cervix (uteri) O86.11
    genital organ NEC O86.19
    kidney O86.21
    mammary O91.12
      associated with lactation O91.13
    nipple O91.02
      associated with lactation O91.03
    peritoneum O85
    subareolar O91.12
      associated with lactation O91.13
    urinary tract —*see* Puerperal, infection,
      urinary
    uterus O86.12
    vagina (wall) O86.13
    vaginorectal O86.13
    vulvovaginal gland O86.13
  adnexitis O86.19
  afibrinogenemia, or other coagulation defect
    O72.3
  albuminuria (acute) (subacute) —*see*
    Proteinuria, gestational
  alcohol use O99.315

▶ New   ⇒ Revised   ~~deleted~~ Deleted   • Use Additional Character(s)

Puerperal, puerperium *(Continued)*
anemia O90.81
  pre-existing (pre-pregnancy) O99.03
anesthetic death O89.8
apoplexy O99.43
bariatric surgery status O99.845
blood disorder NEC O99.13
blood dyscrasia O72.3
cardiomyopathy O90.3
cerebrovascular disorder (conditions in
    I60-I69) O99.43
cervicitis O86.11
circulatory system disorder O99.43
coagulopathy (any) O99.13
  with hemorrhage O72.3
complications O90.9
  specified NEC O90.89
convulsions —*see* Eclampsia
cystitis O86.22
cystopyelitis O86.29
delirium NEC F05
diabetes O24.93
  gestational —*see* Puerperal, gestational
    diabetes
  pre-existing O24.33
    specified NEC O24.83
    type 1 O24.03
    type 2 O24.13
digestive system disorder O99.63
disease O90.9
  breast NEC O92.29
  cerebrovascular (acute) O99.43
  nonobstetric NEC O99.89
  tubo-ovarian O86.19
  Valsuani's O99.03
disorder O90.9
  biliary tract O26.63
  lactation O92.70
  liver O26.63
  nonobstetric NEC O99.89
disruption
  cesarean wound O90.0
  episiotomy wound O90.1
  perineal laceration wound O90.1
drug use O99.325
eclampsia (with pre-existing hypertension)
    O15.2
embolism (pulmonary) (blood clot) —*see*
    Embolism, obstetric, puerperal
endocrine, nutritional or metabolic disease
    NEC O99.285
endophlebitis —*see* Puerperal, phlebitis
endotrachelitis O86.11
failure
  lactation (complete) O92.3
    partial O92.4
  renal, acute O90.4
fever (of unknown origin) O86.4
  septic O85
fissure, nipple O92.12
  associated with lactation O92.13
fistula
  breast (due to mastitis) O91.12
    associated with lactation O91.13
  nipple O91.02
    associated with lactation O91.03
galactophoritis O91.22
  associated with lactation O91.23
galactorrhea O92.6
gastric banding status O99.845
gastric bypass status O99.845
gastrointestinal disease NEC O99.63
gestational
  diabetes O24.439
    diet controlled O24.430
    insulin (and diet) controlled O24.434
    oral drug controlled (antidiabetic)
      (hypoglycemic) O24.435
  edema O12.05
    with proteinuria O12.25
  proteinuria O12.15

Puerperal, puerperium *(Continued)*
gonorrhea O98.23
hematoma, subdural O99.43
hemiplegia, cerebral O99.355-●
  due to cerebrovascular disorder
    O99.43
hemorrhage O72.1
  brain O99.43
  bulbar O99.43
  cerebellar O99.43
  cerebral O99.43
  cortical O99.43
  delayed or secondary O72.2
  extradural O99.43
  internal capsule O99.43
  intracranial O99.43
  intrapontine O99.43
  meningeal O99.43
  pontine O99.43
  retained placenta O72.0
  subarachnoid O99.43
  subcortical O99.43
  subdural O99.43
  third stage O72.0
  uterine, delayed O72.2
  ventricular O99.43
hemorrhoids O87.2
hepatorenal syndrome O90.4
hypertension —*see* Hypertension,
    complicating, puerperium
hypertrophy, breast O92.29
induration breast (fibrous) O92.29
infection O86.4
  cervix O86.11
  generalized O85
  genital tract NEC O86.19
    obstetric surgical wound O86.0
  kidney (bacillus coli) O86.21
  maternal O98.93
    carrier state NEC O99.835
    gonorrhea O98.23
    human immunodeficiency virus (HIV)
      O98.73
    protozoal O98.63
    sexually transmitted NEC O98.33
    specified NEC O98.83
    streptococcus group B (GBS) carrier state
      O99.825
    syphilis O98.13
    tuberculosis O98.03
    viral hepatitis O98.43
    viral NEC O98.53
  nipple O91.02
    associated with lactation O91.03
  peritoneum O85
  renal O86.21
  specified NEC O86.89
  urinary (asymptomatic) (tract) NEC
    O86.20
    bladder O86.22
    kidney O86.21
    specified site NEC O86.29
    urethra O86.22
  vagina O86.13
  vein —*see* Puerperal, phlebitis
ischemia, cerebral O99.43
lymphangitis O86.89
  breast O91.22
    associated with lactation
      O91.23
malignancy O9A.13
malnutrition O25.3
mammillitis O91.02
  associated with lactation O91.03
mammitis O91.22
  associated with lactation O91.23
mania F30.8
mastitis O91.22
  associated with lactation O91.23
  purulent O91.12
    associated with lactation O91.13

Puerperal, puerperium *(Continued)*
melancholia —*see* Disorder, depressive
mental disorder NEC O99.345
metroperitonitis O85
metrorrhagia —*see* Hemorrhage,
    postpartum
metrosalpingitis O86.19
metrovaginitis O86.13
milk leg O87.1
monoplegia, cerebral O99.43
mood disturbance O90.6
necrosis, liver (acute) (subacute)
    (conditions in subcategory K72.0)
    O26.63
  with renal failure O90.4
nervous system disorder O99.355
neuritis O90.89
obesity (pre-existing prior to pregnancy)
    O99.215
obesity surgery status O99.845
occlusion, precerebral artery O99.43
paralysis
  bladder (sphincter) O90.89
  cerebral O99.43
paralytic stroke O99.43
parametritis O85
paravaginitis O86.13
pelviperitonitis O85
perimetritis O86.12
perimetrosalpingitis O86.19
perinephritis O86.21
periphlebitis —*see* Puerperal phlebitis
peritoneal infection O85
peritonitis (pelvic) O85
perivaginitis O86.13
phlebitis O87.0
  deep O87.1
  pelvic O87.1
  superficial O87.0
phlebothrombosis, deep O87.1
phlegmasia alba dolens O87.1
placental polyp O90.89
pneumonia, embolic —*see* Embolism,
    obstetric, puerperal
pre-eclampsia —*see* Pre-eclampsia
psychosis F53
pyelitis O86.21
pyelocystitis O86.29
pyelonephritis O86.21
pyelonephrosis O86.21
pyemia O85
pyocystitis O86.29
pyohemia O85
pyometra O86.12
pyonephritis O86.21
pyosalpingitis O86.19
pyrexia (of unknown origin) O86.4
renal
  disease NEC O90.89
  failure O90.4
respiratory disease NEC O99.53
retention
  decidua —*see* Retention, decidua
  placenta O72.0
  secundines —*see* Retention,
    secundines
retrated nipple O92.02
salpingo-ovaritis O86.19
salpingoperitonitis O85
secondary perineal tear O90.1
sepsis O85
sepsis (pelvic) O85
septic thrombophlebitis O86.81
skin disorder NEC O99.73
specified condition NEC O99.89
stroke O99.43
subinvolution (uterus) O90.89
subluxation of symphysis (pubis)
    O26.73
suppuration —*see* Puerperal, abscess
tetanus A34

Puerperal, puerperium (Continued)
  thelitis O91.02
    associated with lactation O91.03
  thrombocytopenia O72.3
  thrombophlebitis (superficial) O87.0
    deep O87.1
    pelvic O87.1
    septic O86.81
  thrombosis (venous) —see Thrombosis,
      puerperal
  thyroiditis O90.5
  toxemia (eclamptic) (pre-eclamptic)
      (with convulsions) O15.2
  trauma, non-obstetric O9A.23
    caused by abuse (physical) (suspected)
        O9A.33
      confirmed O9A.33
      psychological (suspected)
          O9A.53
        confirmed O9A.53
      sexual (suspected) O9A.43
        confirmed O9A.43
  uremia (due to renal failure)
      O90.4
  urethritis O86.22
  vaginitis O86.13
  varicose veins (legs) O87.4
    vulva or perineum O87.8
  venous O87.9
  vulvitis O86.19
  vulvovaginitis O86.13
  white leg O87.1
Puerperium —see Puerperal
Pulmolithiasis J98.4
Pulmonary —see condition
Pulpitis (acute) (anachoretic) (chronic)
    (hyperplastic) (putrescent) (suppurative)
    (ulcerative) K04.01
  irreversible K04.02
  reversible K04.01
Pulpless tooth K04.99
Pulse
  alternating R00.8
  bigeminal R00.8
  fast R00.0
  feeble, rapid due to shock following injury
      T79.4
  rapid R00.0
  weak R09.89
Pulsus alternans or trigeminus R00.8
Punch drunk F07.81
Punctum lacrimale occlusion —see Obstruction,
    lacrimal
Puncture
  abdomen, abdominal
    wall S31.139
      with
        foreign body S31.149
        penetration into peritoneal cavity
            S31.639
          with foreign body S31.649
      epigastric region S31.132
        with
          foreign body S31.142
          penetration into peritoneal cavity
              S31.632
            with foreign body S31.642
      left
        lower quadrant S31.134
          with
            foreign body S31.144
            penetration into peritoneal cavity
                S31.634
              with foreign body S31.644
        upper quadrant S31.131
          with
            foreign body S31.141
            penetration into peritoneal cavity
                S31.631
              with foreign body S31.641

Puncture (Continued)
  abdomen, abdominal (Continued)
    wall (Continued)
      periumbilic region S31.135
        with
          foreign body S31.145
          penetration into peritoneal cavity
              S31.635
            with foreign body S31.645
      right
        lower quadrant S31.133
          with
            foreign body S31.143
            penetration into peritoneal cavity
                S31.633
              with foreign body S31.643
        upper quadrant S31.130
          with
            foreign body S31.140
            penetration into peritoneal cavity
                S31.630
              with foreign body S31.640
  accidental, complicating surgery —see
      Complication, accidental puncture or
      laceration
  alveolar (process) —see Puncture, oral cavity
  ankle S91.039
    with
      foreign body S91.049
    left S91.032
      with
        foreign body S91.042
    right S91.031
      with
        foreign body S91.041
  anus S31.833
    with foreign body S31.834
  arm (upper) S41.139
    with foreign body S41.149
    left S41.132
      with foreign body S41.142
    lower —see Puncture, forearm
    right S41.131
      with foreign body S41.141
  auditory canal (external) (meatus) —see
      Puncture, ear
  auricle, ear —see Puncture, ear
  axilla —see Puncture, arm
  back —see also Puncture, thorax, back
    lower S31.030
      with
        foreign body S31.040
          with penetration into
              retroperitoneal space S31.041
        penetration into retroperitoneal space
            S31.031
  bladder (traumatic) S37.29
    nontraumatic N32.89
  breast S21.039
    with foreign body S21.049
    left S21.032
      with foreign body S21.042
    right S21.031
      with foreign body S21.041
  buttock S31.803
    with foreign body S31.804
    left S31.823
      with foreign body S31.824
    right S31.813
      with foreign body S31.814
  by
    device, implant or graft —see
        Complications, by site and type,
        mechanical
    foreign body left accidentally in operative
        wound T81.539
    instrument (any) during a procedure,
        accidental —see Puncture, accidental
        complicating surgery
  calf —see Puncture, leg
  canaliculus lacrimalis —see Puncture, eyelid

Puncture (Continued)
  canthus, eye —see Puncture, eyelid
  cervical esophagus S11.23
    with foreign body S11.24
  cheek (external) S01.439
    with foreign body S01.449
    internal —see Puncture, oral cavity
    left S01.432
      with foreign body S01.442
    right S01.431
      with foreign body S01.441
  chest wall —see Puncture, thorax
  chin —see Puncture, head, specified site NEC
  clitoris —see Puncture, vulva
  costal region —see Puncture, thorax
  digit(s)
    foot —see Puncture, toe
    hand —see Puncture, finger
  ear (canal) (external) S01.339
    with foreign body S01.349
    drum S09.2-●
    left S01.332
      with foreign body S01.342
    right S01.331
      with foreign body S01.341
  elbow S51.039
    with
      foreign body S51.049
    left S51.032
      with
        foreign body S51.042
    right S51.031
      with
        foreign body S51.041
  epididymis —see Puncture, testis
  epigastric region —see Puncture, abdomen,
      wall, epigastric
  epiglottis S11.83
    with foreign body S11.84
  esophagus
    cervical S11.23
      with foreign body S11.24
    thoracic S27.818
  eyeball S05.6-●
    with foreign body S05.5-●
  eyebrow —see Puncture, eyelid
  eyelid S01.13-●
    with foreign body S01.14-●
    left S01.132
      with foreign body S01.142
    right S01.131
      with foreign body S01.141
  face NEC —see Puncture, head, specified site
      NEC
  finger(s) S61.239
    with
      damage to nail S61.339
        with
          foreign body S61.349
      foreign body S61.249
    index S61.238
      with
        damage to nail S61.338
          with
            foreign body S61.348
        foreign body S61.248
      left S61.231
        with
          damage to nail S61.331
            with
              foreign body S61.341
          foreign body S61.241
      right S61.230
        with
          damage to nail S61.330
            with
              foreign body S61.340
          foreign body S61.240
    little S61.238
      with
        damage to nail S61.338

▶ New   ⇨ Revised   ~~deleted~~ Deleted   ● Use Additional Character(s)

Puncture *(Continued)*
  finger *(Continued)*
    with *(Continued)*
      with *(Continued)*
        damage to nail *(Continued)*
          with
            foreign body S61.348
          foreign body S61.248
      left S61.237
        with
          damage to nail S61.337
            with
              foreign body S61.347
          foreign body S61.247
      right S61.236
        with
          damage to nail S61.336
            with
              foreign body S61.346
          foreign body S61.246
    middle S61.238
      with
        damage to nail S61.338
          with
            foreign body S61.348
        foreign body S61.248
      left S61.233
        with
          damage to nail S61.333
            with
              foreign body S61.343
          foreign body S61.243
      right S61.232
        with
          damage to nail S61.332
            with
              foreign body S61.342
          foreign body S61.242
    ring S61.238
      with
        damage to nail S61.338
          with
            foreign body S61.348
        foreign body S61.248
      left S61.235
        with
          damage to nail S61.335
            with
              foreign body S61.345
          foreign body S61.245
      right S61.234
        with
          damage to nail S61.334
            with
              foreign body S61.344
          foreign body S61.244
  flank S31.139
    with foreign body S31.149
  foot (except toe(s) alone) S91.339
    with foreign body S91.349
    left S91.332
      with foreign body S91.342
    right S91.331
      with foreign body S91.341
    toe —*see* Puncture, toe
  forearm S51.839
    with
      foreign body S51.849
    elbow only —*see* Puncture, elbow
    left S51.832
      with
        foreign body S51.842
    right S51.831
      with
        foreign body S51.841
  forehead —*see* Puncture, head, specified site
    NEC
  genital organs, external
    female S31.532
      with foreign body S31.542
      vagina —*see* Puncture, vagina
      vulva —*see* Puncture, vulva

Puncture *(Continued)*
  genital organs, external *(Continued)*
    male S31.531
      with foreign body S31.541
      penis —*see* Puncture, penis
      scrotum —*see* Puncture, scrotum
      testis —*see* Puncture, testis
  groin —*see* Puncture, abdomen, wall
  gum —*see* Puncture, oral cavity
  hand S61.439
    with
      foreign body S61.449
    finger —*see* Puncture, finger
    left S61.432
      with
        foreign body S61.442
    right S61.431
      with
        foreign body S61.441
    thumb —*see* Puncture, thumb
  head S01.93
    with foreign body S01.94
    cheek —*see* Puncture, cheek
    ear —*see* Puncture, ear
    eyelid —*see* Puncture, eyelid
    lip —*see* Puncture, oral cavity
    nose —*see* Puncture, nose
    oral cavity —*see* Puncture, oral cavity
    scalp S01.03
      with foreign body S01.04
    specified site NEC S01.83
      with foreign body S01.84
    temporomandibular area —*see* Puncture,
      cheek
  heart S26.99
    with hemopericardium S26.09
    without hemopericardium S26.19
  heel —*see* Puncture, foot
  hip S71.039
    with foreign body S71.049
    left S71.032
      with foreign body S71.042
    right S71.031
      with foreign body S71.041
  hymen —*see* Puncture, vagina
  hypochondrium —*see* Puncture, abdomen,
    wall
  hypogastric region —*see* Puncture, abdomen,
    wall
  inguinal region —*see* Puncture, abdomen,
    wall
  instep —*see* Puncture, foot
  internal organs —*see* Injury, by site
  interscapular region —*see* Puncture, thorax,
    back
  intestine
    large
      colon S36.599
        ascending S36.590
        descending S36.592
        sigmoid S36.593
        specified site NEC S36.598
        transverse S36.591
      rectum S36.69
    small S36.499
      duodenum S36.490
      specified site NEC S36.498
  intra-abdominal organ S36.99
    gallbladder S36.128
    intestine —*see* Puncture, intestine
    liver S36.118
    pancreas —*see* Puncture, pancreas
    peritoneum S36.81
    specified site NEC S36.898
    spleen S36.09
    stomach S36.39
  jaw —*see* Puncture, head, specified site NEC
  knee S81.039
    with foreign body S81.049
    left S81.032
      with foreign body S81.042

Puncture *(Continued)*
  knee *(Continued)*
    right S81.031
      with foreign body S81.041
  labium (majus) (minus) —*see* Puncture,
    vulva
  lacrimal duct —*see* Puncture, eyelid
  larynx S11.013
    with foreign body S11.014
  leg (lower) S81.839
    with foreign body S81.849
    foot —*see* Puncture, foot
    knee —*see* Puncture, knee
    left S81.832
      with foreign body S81.842
    right S81.831
      with foreign body S81.841
    upper —*see* Puncture, thigh
  lip S01.531
    with foreign body S01.541
  loin —*see* Puncture, abdomen, wall
  lower back —*see* Puncture, back, lower
  lumbar region —*see* Puncture, back, lower
  malar region —*see* Puncture, head, specified
    site NEC
  mammary —*see* Puncture, breast
  mastoid region —*see* Puncture, head,
    specified site NEC
  mouth —*see* Puncture, oral cavity
  nail
    finger —*see* Puncture, finger, with damage
      to nail
    toe —*see* Puncture, toe, with damage to
      nail
  nasal (septum) (sinus) —*see* Puncture, nose
  nasopharynx —*see* Puncture, head, specified
    site NEC
  neck S11.93
    with foreign body S11.94
    involving
      cervical esophagus —*see* Puncture,
        cervical esophagus
      larynx —*see* Puncture, larynx
      pharynx —*see* Puncture, pharynx
      thyroid gland —*see* Puncture, thyroid
        gland
      trachea —*see* Puncture, trachea
    specified site NEC S11.83
      with foreign body S11.84
  nose (septum) (sinus) S01.23
    with foreign body S01.24
  ocular —*see* Puncture, eyeball - oral cavity
    S01.532
    with foreign body S01.542
  orbit S05.4-●
  palate —*see* Puncture, oral cavity
  palm —*see* Puncture, hand
  pancreas S36.299
    body S36.291
    head S36.290
    tail S36.292
  pelvis —*see* Puncture, back, lower
  penis S31.23
    with foreign body S31.24
  perineum
    female S31.43
      with foreign body S31.44
    male S31.139
      with foreign body S31.149
  periocular area (with or without lacrimal
    passages) —*see* Puncture, eyelid
  phalanges
    finger —*see* Puncture, finger
    toe —*see* Puncture, toe
  pharynx S11.23
    with foreign body S11.24
  pinna —*see* Puncture, ear
  popliteal space —*see* Puncture, knee
  prepuce —*see* Puncture, penis
  pubic region S31.139
    with foreign body S31.149

Puncture *(Continued)*
  pudendum —*see* Puncture, genital organs,
    external
  rectovaginal septum —*see* Puncture,
    vagina
  sacral region —*see* Puncture, back,
    lower
  sacroiliac region —*see* Puncture, back,
    lower
  salivary gland —*see* Puncture, oral
    cavity
  scalp S01.03
    with foreign body S01.04
  scapular region —*see* Puncture,
    shoulder
  scrotum S31.33
    with foreign body S31.34
  shin —*see* Puncture, leg
  shoulder S41.039
    with foreign body S41.049
    left S41.032
      with foreign body S41.042
    right S41.031
      with foreign body S41.041
  spermatic cord —*see* Puncture, testis
  sternal region —*see* Puncture, thorax, front
  submaxillary region —*see* Puncture, head,
    specified site NEC
  submental region —*see* Puncture, head,
    specified site NEC
  subungual
    finger(s) —*see* Puncture, finger, with
      damage to nail
    toe —*see* Puncture, toe, with damage to
      nail
  supraclavicular fossa —*see* Puncture, neck,
    specified site NEC
  temple, temporal region —*see* Puncture, head,
    specified site NEC
  temporomandibular area —*see* Puncture,
    cheek
  testis S31.33
    with foreign body S31.34
  thigh S71.139
    with foreign body S71.149
    left S71.132
      with foreign body S71.142
    right S71.131
      with foreign body S71.141
  thorax, thoracic (wall) S21.93
    with foreign body S21.94
    back S21.23-●
      with
        foreign body S21.24-●
          with penetration S21.44
        penetration S21.43
    breast —*see* Puncture, breast
    front S21.13-●
      with
        foreign body S21.14-●
          with penetration S21.34
        penetration S21.33
  throat —*see* Puncture, neck
  thumb S61.039
    with
      damage to nail S61.139
        with
          foreign body S61.149
      foreign body S61.049
    left S61.032
      with
        damage to nail S61.132
          with
            foreign body S61.142
        foreign body S61.042
    right S61.031
      with
        damage to nail S61.131
          with
            foreign body S61.141
        foreign body S61.041

Puncture *(Continued)*
  thyroid gland S11.13
    with foreign body S11.14
  toe(s) S91.139
    with
      damage to nail S91.239
        with
          foreign body S91.249
      foreign body S91.149
    great S91.133
      with
        damage to nail S91.233
          with
            foreign body S91.243
        foreign body S91.143
      left S91.132
        with
          damage to nail S91.232
            with
              foreign body S91.242
          foreign body S91.142
      right S91.131
        with
          damage to nail S91.231
            with
              foreign body S91.241
          foreign body S91.141
    lesser S91.136
      with
        damage to nail S91.236
          with
            foreign body S91.246
        foreign body S91.146
      left S91.135
        with
          damage to nail S91.235
            with
              foreign body S91.245
          foreign body S91.145
      right S91.134
        with
          damage to nail S91.234
            with
              foreign body S91.244
          foreign body S91.144
  tongue —*see* Puncture, oral cavity
  trachea S11.023
    with foreign body S11.024
  tunica vaginalis —*see* Puncture, testis
  tympanum, tympanic membrane
    S09.2-●
  umbilical region S31.135
    with foreign body S31.145
  uvula —*see* Puncture, oral cavity
  vagina S31.43
    with foreign body S31.44
  vocal cords S11.033
    with foreign body S11.034
  vulva S31.43
    with foreign body S31.44
  wrist S61.539
    with
      foreign body S61.549
    left S61.532
      with
        foreign body S61.542
    right S61.531
      with
        foreign body S61.541
PUO (pyrexia of unknown origin) R50.9
Pupillary membrane (persistent) Q13.89
Pupillotonia —*see* Anomaly, pupil, function,
  tonic pupil
Purpura D69.2
  abdominal D69.0
  allergic D69.0
  anaphylactoid D69.0
  annularis telangiectodes L81.7
  arthritic D69.0
  autoerythrocyte sensitization D69.2
  autoimmune D69.0

Purpura *(Continued)*
  bacterial D69.0
  Bateman's (senile) D69.2
  capillary fragility (hereditary) (idiopathic)
    D69.8
  cryoglobulinemic D89.1
  Devil's pinches D69.2
  fibrinolytic —*see* Fibrinolysis
  fulminans, fulminous D65
  gangrenous D65
  hemorrhagic, hemorrhagica D69.3
    not due to thrombocytopenia D69.0
  Henoch (-Schönlein) (allergic) D69.0
  hypergammaglobulinemic (benign)
    (Waldenström's) D89.0
  idiopathic (thrombocytopenic) D69.3
    nonthrombocytopenic D69.0
  immune thrombocytopenic D69.3
  infectious D69.0
  malignant D69.0
  neonatorum P54.5
  nervosa D69.0
  newborn P54.5
  nonthrombocytopenic D69.2
    hemorrhagic D69.0
    idiopathic D69.0
  nonthrombopenic D69.2
  peliosis rheumatica D69.0
  posttransfusion (post-transfusion) (from
    (fresh) whole blood or blood products)
    D69.51
  primary D69.49
  red cell membrane sensitivity D69.2
  rheumatica D69.0
  Schönlein (-Henoch) (allergic) D69.0
  scorbutic E54 [D77]
  senile D69.2
  simplex D69.2
  symptomatica D69.0
  telangiectasia annularis L81.7
  thrombocytopenic D69.49
    congenital D69.42
    hemorrhagic D69.3
    hereditary D69.42
    idiopathic D69.3
    immune D69.3
    neonatal, transitory P61.0
    thrombotic M31.1
  thrombohemolytic —*see* Fibrinolysis
  thrombolytic —*see* Fibrinolysis
  thrombopenic D69.49
  thrombotic, thrombocytopenic
    M31.1
  toxic D69.0
  vascular D69.0
  visceral symptoms D69.0
Purpuric spots R23.3
Purulent —*see* condition
Pus
  in
    stool R19.5
    urine N39.0
  tube (rupture) —*see* Salpingo-oophoritis
Pustular rash L08.0
Pustule (nonmalignant) L08.9
  malignant A22.0
Pustulosis palmaris et plantaris
  L40.3
Putnam (-Dana) disease or syndrome —*see*
  Degeneration, combined
Putrescent pulp (dental) K04.1
Pyarthritis, pyarthrosis —*see* Arthritis,
  pyogenic or pyemic
  tuberculous —*see* Tuberculosis, joint
Pyelectasis —*see* Hydronephrosis
Pyelitis (congenital) (uremic) —*see also*
  Pyelonephritis
  with
    calculus —*see* category N20
      with hydronephrosis N13.2
    contracted kidney N11.9

▶ New   ⇒ Revised   ~~deleted~~ Deleted   ● Use Additional Character(s)

Pyelitis *(Continued)*
  acute N10
  chronic N11.9
    with calculus —*see* category N20
      with hydronephrosis N13.2
  cystica N28.84
  puerperal (postpartum) O86.21
  tuberculous A18.11
Pyelocystitis —*see* Pyelonephritis
Pyelonephritis —*see also* Nephritis,
    tubulo-interstitial
  with
    calculus —*see* category N20
      with hydronephrosis N13.2
    contracted kidney N11.9
  acute N10
    calculus —*see* category N20
      with hydronephrosis N13.2
  chronic N11.9
    with calculus —*see* category N20
      with hydronephrosis N13.2
    associated with ureteral obstruction or
        stricture N11.1
    nonobstructive N11.8
      with reflux (vesicoureteral) N11.0
    obstructive N11.1
    specified NEC N11.8
  in (due to)
    brucellosis A23.9 *[N16]*
    cryoglobulinemia (mixed) D89.1 *[N16]*
    cystinosis E72.04
    diphtheria A36.84
    glycogen storage disease E74.09 *[N16]*
    leukemia NEC C95.9-● *[N16]*
    lymphoma NEC C85.90 *[N16]*
    multiple myeloma C90.0-● *[N16]*
    obstruction N11.1
    Salmonella infection A02.25
    sarcoidosis D86.84
    sepsis A41.9 *[N16]*
    Sjögren's disease M35.04
    toxoplasmosis B58.83
    transplant rejection T86.91 *[N16]*
    Wilson's disease E83.01 *[N16]*
  nonobstructive N12
    with reflux (vesicoureteral) N11.0
    chronic N11.8
  syphilitic A52.75

Pyelonephrosis (obstructive) N11.1
  chronic N11.9
Pyelophlebitis I80.8
Pyeloureteritis cystica N28.85
Pyemia, pyemic (fever) (infection) (purulent) —
    see also Sepsis
  joint —*see* Arthritis, pyogenic or pyemic
  liver K75.1
  pneumococcal A40.3
  portal K75.1
  postvaccinal T88.0
  puerperal, postpartum, childbirth O85
  specified organism NEC A41.89
  tuberculous —*see* Tuberculosis, miliary
Pygopagus Q89.4
Pyknoepilepsy (idiopathic) —*see* Pyknolepsy
Pyknolepsy G40.A09
  intractable G40.A19
    with status epilepticus G40.A11
    without status epilepticus G40.A19
  not intractable G40.A09
    with status epilepticus G40.A01
    without status epilepticus G40.A09
Pylephlebitis K75.1
Pyle's syndrome Q78.5
Pylethrombophlebitis K75.1
Pylethrombosis K75.1
Pyloritis K29.90
  with bleeding K29.91
Pylorospasm (reflex) NEC K31.3
  congenital or infantile Q40.0
  neurotic F45.8
  newborn Q40.0
  psychogenic F45.8
Pylorus, pyloric —*see* condition
Pyoarthrosis —*see* Arthritis, pyogenic or
    pyemic
Pyocele
  mastoid —*see* Mastoiditis, acute
  sinus (accessory) —*see* Sinusitis
  turbinate (bone) J32.9
  urethra —*see also* Urethritis N34.0
Pyocolpos —*see* Vaginitis
Pyocystitis N30.80
  with hematuria N30.81
Pyoderma, pyodermia L08.0
  gangrenosum L88
  newborn P39.4

Pyoderma, pyodermia *(Continued)*
  phagedenic L88
  vegetans L08.81
Pyodermatitis L08.0
  vegetans L08.81
Pyogenic —*see* condition
Pyohydronephrosis N13.6
Pyometra, pyometrium, pyometritis —*see*
    Endometritis
Pyomyositis (tropical) —*see* Myositis,
    infective
Pyonephritis N12
Pyonephrosis N13.6
  tuberculous A18.11
Pyo-oophoritis —*see* Salpingo-oophoritis
Pyo-ovarium —*see* Salpingo-oophoritis
Pyopericarditis, pyopericardium
    I30.1
Pyophlebitis —*see* Phlebitis
Pyopneumopericardium I30.1
Pyopneumothorax (infective) J86.9
  with fistula J86.0
  tuberculous NEC A15.6
Pyosalpinx, pyosalpingitis —*see also*
    Salpingo-oophoritis
Pyothorax J86.9
  with fistula J86.0
  tuberculous NEC A15.6
Pyoureter N28.89
  tuberculous A18.11
Pyramidopallidonigral syndrome
    G20
Pyrexia (of unknown origin) R50.9
  atmospheric T67.0
  during labor NEC O75.2
  heat T67.0
  newborn P81.9
    environmentally-induced P81.0
  persistent R50.9
  puerperal O86.4
Pyroglobulinemia NEC E88.09
Pyromania F63.1
Pyrosis R12
Pyuria (bacterial) N39.0

P

Q

Q fever A78
   with pneumonia A78
Quadricuspid aortic valve Q23.8
Quadrilateral fever A78
Quadriparesis —*see* Quadriplegia
   meaning muscle weakness M62.81
Quadriplegia G82.50-●
   complete
      C1-C4 level G82.51
      C5-C7 level G82.53
   congenital (cerebral) (spinal) G80.8
      spastic G80.0

Quadriplegia (*Continued*)
   embolic (current episode) I63.4-●
   functional R53.2
   incomplete
      C1-C4 level G82.52
      C5-C7 level G82.54
   thrombotic (current episode) I63.3-●
   traumatic — code to injury with seventh
      character S
      current episode —*see* Injury, spinal (cord),
         cervical
Quadruplet, pregnancy —*see* Pregnancy,
   quadruplet
Quarrelsomeness F60.3

Queensland fever A77.3
Quervain's disease M65.4
   thyroid E06.1
Queyrat's erythroplasia D07.4
   penis D07.4
   specified site —*see* Neoplasm, skin,
      in situ
   unspecified site D07.4
Quincke's disease or edema T78.3
   hereditary D84.1
Quinsy (gangrenous) J36
Quintan fever A79.0
Quintuplet, pregnancy —*see* Pregnancy,
   quintuplet

R

Rabbit fever —see Tularemia
Rabies A82.9
  contact Z20.3
  exposure to Z20.3
  inoculation reaction —see Complications,
    vaccination
  sylvatic A82.0
  urban A82.1
Rachischisis —see Spina bifida
Rachitic —see also condition
  deformities of spine (late effect) (sequelae)
    E64.3
  pelvis (late effect) (sequelae) E64.3
    with disproportion (fetopelvic) O33.0
      causing obstructed labor O65.0
Rachitis, rachitism (acute) (tarda) —see also
    Rickets
  renalis N25.0
  sequelae E64.3
Radial nerve —see condition
Radiation
  burn —see Burn
  effects NOS T66
  sickness NOS T66
  therapy, encounter for Z51.0
Radiculitis (pressure) (vertebrogenic) —see
    Radiculopathy
Radiculomyelitis —see also Encephalitis
  toxic, due to
    Clostridium tetani A35
    Corynebacterium diphtheriae A36.82
Radiculopathy M54.10
  cervical region M54.12
  cervicothoracic region M54.13
  due to
    disc disorder
      C3 M50.11
      C4 M50.11
      C5 M50.121
      C6 M50.122
      C7 M50.123
      C8 M50.13
    displacement of intervertebral disc —see
      Disorder, disc, with, radiculopathy
  leg M54.1-●
  lumbar region M54.16
  lumbosacral region M54.17
  occipito-atlanto-axial region M54.11
  postherpetic B02.29
  sacrococcygeal region M54.18
  syphilitic A52.11
  thoracic region (with visceral pain)
    M54.14
  thoracolumbar region M54.15
Radiodermal burns (acute, chronic, or
    occupational) —see Burn
Radiodermatitis L58.9
  acute L58.0
  chronic L58.1
Radiotherapy session Z51.0
RAEB (refractory anemia with excess blasts)
    D46.2-●
Rage, meaning rabies —see Rabies
Ragpicker's disease A22.1
Ragsorter's disease A22.1
Raillietiniasis B71.8
Railroad neurosis F48.8
Railway spine F48.8
Raised —see also Elevated
  antibody titer R76.0
Rake teeth, tooth M26.39
Rales R09.89
Ramifying renal pelvis Q63.8
Ramsay-Hunt disease or syndrome —see also
    Hunt's disease B02.21
  meaning dyssynergia cerebellaris myoclonica
    G11.1
Ranula K11.6
  congenital Q38.4

Rape
  adult
    confirmed T74.21
    suspected T76.21
  alleged, observation or examination, ruled out
    adult Z04.41
    child Z04.42
  child
    confirmed T74.22
    suspected T76.22
Rapid
  feeble pulse, due to shock, following injury
    T79.4
  heart (beat) R00.0
    psychogenic F45.8
  second stage (delivery) O62.3
  time-zone change syndrome —see Disorder,
    sleep, circadian rhythm, psychogenic
Rarefaction, bone —see Disorder, bone, density
    and structure, specified NEC
Rash (toxic) R21
  canker A38.9
  diaper L22
  drug (internal use) L27.0
    contact —see also Dermatitis, due to, drugs,
      external L25.1
  following immunization T88.1
  food —see Dermatitis, due to, food
  heat L74.0
  napkin (psoriasiform) L22
  nettle —see Urticaria
  pustular L08.0
  rose R21
    epidemic B06.9
  scarlet A38.9
  serum —see also Reaction, serum T80.69
  wandering tongue K14.1
Rasmussen aneurysm —see Tuberculosis,
    pulmonary
Rasmussen encephalitis G04.81
Rat-bite fever A25.9
  due to Streptobacillus moniliformis A25.1
  spirochetal (morsus muris) A25.0
Rathke's pouch tumor D44.3
Raymond (-Céstan) syndrome I65.8
Raynaud's disease, phenomenon or syndrome
    (secondary) I73.00
  with gangrene (symmetric) I73.01
RDS (newborn) (type I) P22.0
  type II P22.1
Reaction —see also Disorder
  adaptation —see Disorder, adjustment
  adjustment (anxiety) (conduct disorder)
      (depressiveness) (distress) —see
      Disorder, adjustment
    with
      mutism, elective (child) (adolescent) F94.0
  adverse
    food (any) (ingested) NEC T78.1
      anaphylactic —see Shock, anaphylactic,
        due to food
  anaphylactoid —see Shock, anaphylactic
  affective —see Disorder, mood
  allergic —see Allergy
  anaphylactic —see Shock, anaphylactic
  anesthesia —see Anesthesia, complication
  antitoxin (prophylactic) (therapeutic) —see
      Complications, vaccination
  anxiety F41.1
  Arthus —see Arthus' phenomenon
  asthenic F48.8
  combat and operational stress F43.0
  compulsive F42.8
  conversion F44.9
  crisis, acute F43.0
  deoxyribonuclease (DNA) (DNase)
      hypersensitivity D69.2
  depressive (single episode) F32.9
    affective (single episode) F31.4
      recurrent episode F33.9
    neurotic F34.1
    psychoneurotic F34.1

Reaction (Continued)
  depressive (Continued)
    psychotic F32.3
    recurrent —see Disorder, depressive,
      recurrent
  dissociative F44.9
  drug NEC T88.7
    addictive —see Dependence, drug
      transmitted via placenta or breast
        milk —see Absorption, drug,
        addictive, through placenta
    allergic —see Allergy, drug
    lichenoid L43.2
    newborn P93.8
      gray baby syndrome P93.0
    overdose or poisoning (by accident) —see
      Table of Drugs and Chemicals, by
      drug, poisoning
    photoallergic L56.1
    phototoxic L56.0
    withdrawal —see Dependence, by drug,
      with, withdrawal
      infant of dependent mother P96.1
      newborn P96.1
    wrong substance given or taken (by
      accident) —see Table of Drugs and
      Chemicals, by drug, poisoning
  fear F40.9
    child (abnormal) F93.8
  febrile nonhemolytic transfusion (FNHTR)
      R50.84
  fluid loss, cerebrospinal G97.1
  foreign
    body NEC —see Granuloma, foreign body
      in operative wound (inadvertently
        left) —see Foreign body, accidentally
        left during a procedure
    substance accidentally left during a
      procedure (chemical) (powder) (talc)
      T81.60
      aseptic peritonitis T81.61
      body or object (instrument) (sponge)
        (swab) —see Foreign body,
        accidentally left during a
        procedure
      specified reaction NEC T81.69
  grief —see Disorder, adjustment
  Herxheimer's R68.89
  hyperkinetic —see Hyperkinesia
  hypochondriacal F45.20
  hypoglycemic, due to insulin E16.0
    with coma (diabetic) —see Diabetes, coma
      nondiabetic E15
    therapeutic misadventure —see
      subcategory T38.3
  hypomanic F30.8
  hysterical F44.9
  immunization —see Complications, vaccination
  incompatibility
    ABO blood group (infusion) (transfusion) —
      see Complication(s), transfusion,
      incompatibility reaction, ABO
    delayed serologic T80.39
    minor blood group (Duffy) (E) (K(ell))
      (Kidd) (Lewis) (M) (N) (P) (S)
      T80.89
    Rh (factor) (infusion) (transfusion) —
      see Complication(s), transfusion,
      incompatibility reaction, Rh (factor)
  inflammatory —see Infection
  infusion —see Complications, infusion
  inoculation (immune serum) —see
      Complications, vaccination
  insulin T38.3-●
  involutional psychotic —see Disorder,
      depressive
  leukemoid D72.823
    basophilic D72.823
    lymphocytic D72.823
    monocytic D72.823
    myelocytic D72.823
    neutrophilic D72.823

Reaction *(Continued)*
LSD (acute)
due to drug abuse —*see* Abuse, drug, hallucinogen
due to drug dependence —*see* Dependence, drug, hallucinogen
lumbar puncture G97.1
manic-depressive —*see* Disorder, bipolar
neurasthenic F48.8
neurogenic —*see* Neurosis
neurotic F48.9
neurotic-depressive F34.1
nitritoid —*see* Crisis, nitritoid - obsessive-compulsive F42
nonspecific
to
cell mediated immunity measurement of gamma interferon antigen response without active tuberculosis R76.12
QuantiFERON-TB test (QFT) without active tuberculosis R76.12
tuberculin test —*see also* Reaction, tuberculin skin test R76.11
obsessive-compulsive F42.8
organic, acute or subacute —*see* Delirium
paranoid (acute) F23
chronic F22
senile F03
passive dependency F60.7
phobic F40.9
post-traumatic stress, uncomplicated Z73.3
psychogenic F99
psychoneurotic —*see also* Neurosis
compulsive F42.8
depersonalization F48.1
depressive F34.1
hypochondriacal F45.20
neurasthenic F48.8
obsessive F42.8
psychophysiologic —*see* Disorder, somatoform
psychosomatic —*see* Disorder, somatoform
psychotic —*see* Psychosis
scarlet fever toxin —*see* Complications, vaccination
schizophrenic F23
acute (brief) (undifferentiated) F23
latent F21
undifferentiated (acute) (brief) F23
serological for syphilis —*see* Serology for syphilis
serum T80.69
anaphylactic (immediate) —*see also* Shock, anaphylactic T80.59
specified reaction NEC
due to
administration of blood and blood products T80.61
immunization T80.62
serum specified NEC T80.69
vaccination T80.62
situational —*see* Disorder, adjustment
somatization —*see* Disorder, somatoform
spinal puncture G97.1
stress (severe) F43.9
acute (agitation) ("daze") (disorientation) (disturbance of consciousness) (flight reaction) (fugue) F43.0
specified NEC F43.8
surgical procedure —*see* Complications, surgical procedure
tetanus antitoxin —*see* Complications, vaccination
toxic, to local anesthesia T81.59
in labor and delivery O74.4
in pregnancy O29.3X-●
postpartum, puerperal O89.3
toxin-antitoxin —*see* Complications, vaccination

Reaction *(Continued)*
transfusion (blood) (bone marrow) (lymphocytes) (allergic) —*see* Complications, transfusion
tuberculin skin test, abnormal R76.11
vaccination (any) —*see* Complications, vaccination
withdrawing, child or adolescent F93.8
Reactive airway disease —*see* Asthma
Reactive depression —*see* Reaction, depressive
Rearrangement
chromosomal
balanced (in) Q95.9
abnormal individual (autosomal) Q95.2
non-sex (autosomal) chromosomes Q95.2
sex/non-sex chromosomes Q95.3
specified NEC Q95.8
Recalcitrant patient —*see* Noncompliance
Recanalization, thrombus —*see* Thrombosis
Recession, receding
chamber angle (eye) H21.55-●
chin M26.09
gingival (postinfective) (postoperative)
▶generalized K06.020
▶minimal K06.021
▶moderate K06.022
▶severe K06.023
▶localized K06.010
▶minimal K06.011
▶moderate K06.012
▶severe K06.013
Miller Class I K06.01
Miller Class II K06.02
Miller Class III K06.03
Miller Class IV K06.04
Recklinghausen's disease Q85.01
bones E21.0
Reclus' disease (cystic) —*see* Mastopathy, cystic
Recrudescent typhus (fever) A75.1
Recruitment, auditory H93.21-●
Rectalgia K62.89
Rectitis K62.89
Rectocele
female (without uterine prolapse) N81.6
with uterine prolapse N81.4
incomplete N81.2
in pregnancy —*see* Pregnancy, complicated by, abnormal, pelvic organs or tissues NEC
male K62.3
Rectosigmoid junction —*see* condition
Rectosigmoiditis K63.89
ulcerative (chronic) K51.30
with
complication K51.319
abscess K51.314
fistula K51.313
obstruction K51.312
rectal bleeding K51.311
specified NEC K51.318
Rectourethral —*see* condition
Rectovaginal —*see* condition
Rectovesical —*see* condition
Rectum, rectal —*see* condition
Recurrent —*see* condition
pregnancy loss —*see* Loss (of), pregnancy, recurrent
Red bugs B88.0
Red-cedar lung or pneumonitis J67.8
Red tide —*see also* Table of Drugs and Chemicals T65.82-●
Reduced
mobility Z74.09
ventilatory or vital capacity R94.2
Redundant, redundancy
anus (congenital) Q43.8
clitoris N90.89
colon (congenital) Q43.8
foreskin (congenital) N47.8
intestine (congenital) Q43.8

Redundant, redundancy *(Continued)*
labia N90.69
organ or site, congenital NEC —*see* Accessory
panniculus (abdominal) E65
prepuce (congenital) N47.8
pylorus K31.89
rectum (congenital) Q43.8
scrotum N50.89
sigmoid (congenital) Q43.8
skin L98.7
and subcutaneous tissue L98.7
of face L57.4
eyelids —*see* Blepharochalasis
stomach K31.89
Reduplication —*see* Duplication
Reflex R29.2
hyperactive gag J39.2
pupillary, abnormal —*see* Anomaly, pupil, function
vasoconstriction I73.9
vasovagal R55
Reflux K21.9
acid K21.9
esophageal K21.9
with esophagitis K21.0
newborn P78.83
gastroesophageal K21.9
with esophagitis K21.0
mitral —*see* Insufficiency, mitral
ureteral —*see* Reflux, vesicoureteral
vesicoureteral (with scarring) N13.70
with
nephropathy N13.729
with hydroureter N13.739
bilateral N13.732
unilateral N13.731
without hydroureter N13.729
bilateral N13.722
unilateral N13.721
bilateral N13.722
unilateral N13.721
pyelonephritis (chronic) N11.0
without nephropathy N13.71
congenital Q62.7
Reforming, artificial openings —*see* Attention to, artificial, opening
Refractive error —*see* Disorder, refraction
Refsum's disease or syndrome G60.1
Refusal of
food, psychogenic F50.89
treatment (because of) Z53.20
left against medical advice (AMA) Z53.21
patient's decision NEC Z53.29
reasons of belief or group pressure Z53.1
Regional —*see* condition
Regurgitation R11.10
aortic (valve) —*see* Insufficiency, aortic
food —*see also* Vomiting
with reswallowing —*see* Rumination
newborn P92.1
gastric contents —*see* Vomiting
heart —*see* Endocarditis
mitral (valve) —*see* Insufficiency, mitral
congenital Q23.3
myocardial —*see* Endocarditis
pulmonary (valve) (heart) I37.1
congenital Q22.2
syphilitic A52.03
tricuspid —*see* Insufficiency, tricuspid
valve, valvular —*see* Endocarditis
congenital Q24.8
vesicoureteral —*see* Reflux, vesicoureteral
Reichmann's disease or syndrome K31.89
Reifenstein syndrome E34.52
Reinsertion
implantable subdermal contraceptive Z30.46
intrauterine contraceptive device Z30.433
Reiter's disease, syndrome, or urethritis M02.30
ankle M02.37-●
elbow M02.32-●

▶ New   ⇒ Revised   deleted Deleted   ● Use Additional Character(s)

Reiter's disease, syndrome, or urethritis
(Continued)
  foot joint M02.37-●
  hand joint M02.34-●
  hip M02.35-●
  knee M02.36-●
  multiple site M02.39
  shoulder M02.31-●
  vertebra M02.38
  wrist M02.33-●
Rejection
  food, psychogenic F50.89
  transplant T86.91
   bone T86.830
    marrow T86.01
   cornea T86.840
   heart T86.21
    with lung(s) T86.31
   intestine T86.850
   kidney T86.11
   liver T86.41
   lung(s) T86.810
    with heart T86.31
   organ (immune or nonimmune cause) T86.91
   pancreas T86.890
   skin (allograft) (autograft) T86.820
   specified NEC T86.890
   stem cell (peripheral blood) (umbilical cord) T86.5
Relapsing fever A68.9
  Carter's (Asiatic) A68.1
  Dutton's (West African) A68.1
  Koch's A68.9
  louse-borne (epidemic) A68.0
  Novy's (American) A68.1
  Obermeyers's (European) A68.0
  Spirillum A68.9
  tick-borne (endemic) A68.1
Relationship
  occlusal
   open anterior M26.220
   open posterior M26.221
Relaxation
  anus (sphincter) K62.89
   psychogenic F45.8
  arch (foot) —see also Deformity, limb, flat foot
  back ligaments —see Instability, joint, spine
  bladder (sphincter) N31.2
  cardioesophageal K21.9
  cervix —see Incompetency, cervix
  diaphragm J98.6
  joint (capsule) (ligament) (paralytic) —see Flail, joint
   congenital NEC Q74.8
  lumbosacral (joint) —see subcategory M53.2
  pelvic floor N81.89
  perineum N81.89
  posture R29.3
  rectum (sphincter) K62.89
  sacroiliac (joint) —see subcategory M53.2
  scrotum N50.89
  urethra (sphincter) N36.44
  vesical N31.2
Release from prison, anxiety concerning Z65.2
Remains
  canal of Cloquet Q14.0
  capsule (opaque) Q14.8
Remittent fever (malarial) B54
Remnant
  canal of Cloquet Q14.0
  capsule (opaque) Q14.8
  cervix, cervical stump (acquired) (postoperative) N88.8
  cystic duct, postcholecystectomy K91.5
  fingernail L60.8
   congenital Q84.6
  meniscus, knee —see Derangement, knee, meniscus, specified NEC
  thyroglossal duct Q89.2
  tonsil J35.8
   infected (chronic) J35.01
  urachus Q64.4

Removal (from) (of)
  artificial
   arm Z44.00-●
    complete Z44.01-●
    partial Z44.02-●
   eye Z44.2-●
   leg Z44.10-●
    complete Z44.11-●
    partial Z44.12-●
  breast implant Z45.81
  cardiac pulse generator (battery) (end-of-life) Z45.010
  catheter (urinary) (indwelling) Z46.6
   from artificial opening —see Attention to, artificial, opening
   non-vascular Z46.82
   vascular NEC Z45.2
  device Z46.9
   contraceptive Z30.432
    implantable subdermal Z30.46
   implanted NEC Z45.89
   specified NEC Z46.89
  drains Z48.03
  dressing (nonsurgical) Z48.00
   surgical Z48.01
  external
   fixation device — code to fracture with seventh character D
   prosthesis, prosthetic device Z44.9
    breast Z44.3-●
    specified NEC Z44.8
  home in childhood (to foster home or institution) Z62.29
  ileostomy Z43.2
  insulin pump Z46.81
  myringotomy device (stent) (tube) Z45.82
  nervous system device NEC Z46.2
   brain neuropacemaker Z46.2
   visual substitution device Z46.2
    implanted Z45.31
  non-vascular catheter Z46.82
  organ, prophylactic (for neoplasia management) —see Prophylactic, organ removal
  orthodontic device Z46.4
  staples Z48.02
  stent
   ureteral Z46.6
  suture Z48.02
  urinary device Z46.6
  vascular access device or catheter Z45.2
Ren
  arcuatus Q63.1
  mobile, mobilis N28.89
   congenital Q63.8
  unguliformis Q63.1
Renal —see condition
Rendu-Osler-Weber disease or syndrome I78.0
Reninoma D41.0-●
Renon-Delille syndrome E23.3
Reovirus, as cause of disease classified elsewhere B97.5
Repeated falls NEC R29.6
Replaced chromosome by dicentric ring Q93.2
Replacement by artificial or mechanical device or prosthesis of
  bladder Z96.0
  blood vessel NEC Z95.828
  bone NEC Z96.7
  cochlea Z96.21
  coronary artery Z95.5
  eustachian tube Z96.29
  eye globe Z97.0
  heart Z95.812
   valve Z95.2
    prosthetic Z95.2
    specified NEC Z95.4
    xenogenic Z95.3
  intestine Z96.89
  joint Z96.60
   hip —see Presence, hip joint implant
   knee —see Presence, knee joint implant
   specified site NEC Z96.698

Replacement by artificial or mechanical device or prosthesis of (Continued)
  larynx Z96.3
  lens Z96.1
  limb(s) —see Presence, artificial, limb
  mandible NEC (for tooth root implant(s)) Z96.5
  organ NEC Z96.89
  peripheral vessel NEC Z95.828
  stapes Z96.29
  teeth Z97.2
  tendon Z96.7
  tissue NEC Z96.89
  tooth root(s) Z96.5
  vessel NEC Z95.828
   coronary (artery) Z95.5
Request for expert evidence Z04.8
Reserve, decreased or low
  cardiac —see Disease, heart
  kidney N28.89
Residual —see also condition
  ovary syndrome N99.83
  state, schizophrenic F20.5
  urine R39.198
Resistance, resistant (to)
  activated protein C D68.51
  complicating pregnancy O26.89
  insulin E88.81
  organism(s)
   to
    drug Z16.30
     aminoglycosides Z16.29
     amoxicillin Z16.11
     ampicillin Z16.11
     antibiotic(s) Z16.20
      multiple Z16.24
      specified NEC Z16.29
     antifungal Z16.32
     antimicrobial (single) Z16.30
      multiple Z16.35
      specified NEC Z16.39
     antimycobacterial (single) Z16.341
      multiple Z16.342
     antiparasitic Z16.31
     antiviral Z16.33
     beta lactam antibiotics Z16.10
      specified NEC Z16.19
     cephalosporins Z16.19
     extended beta lactamase (ESBL) Z16.12
     fluoroquinolones Z16.23
     macrolides Z16.29
     methicillin —see MRSA
     multiple drugs (MDRO)
      antibiotics Z16.24
      antimicrobial Z16.35
      antimycobacterials Z16.342
     penicillins Z16.11
     quinine (and related compounds) Z16.31
     quinolones Z16.23
     sulfonamides Z16.29
     tetracyclines Z16.29
     tuberculostatics (single) Z16.341
      multiple Z16.342
     vancomycin Z16.21
      related antibiotics Z16.22
  thyroid hormone E07.89
Resorption
  dental (roots) K03.3
   alveoli M26.79
  teeth (external) (internal) (pathological) (roots) K03.3
Respiration
  Cheyne-Stokes R06.3
  decreased due to shock, following injury T79.4
  disorder of, psychogenic F45.8
  insufficient, or poor R06.89
   newborn P28.5
  painful R07.1
  sighing, psychogenic F45.8

Respiratory —see also condition
  distress syndrome (newborn) (type I)
      P22.0
    type II P22.1
  syncytial virus, as cause of disease classified
      elsewhere B97.4
Respite care Z75.5
Response (drug)
  photoallergic L56.1
  phototoxic L56.0
Restenosis
  stent
    vascular
      end stent
        adjacent to stent —see
            Arteriosclerosis
        within the stent
            coronary T82.855
            peripheral T82.856
      in stent
        coronary vessel T82.855
        peripheral vessel T82.856
Restless legs (syndrome) G25.81
Restlessness R45.1
Restoration (of)
  dental
    aesthetically inadequate or displeasing
        K08.56
    defective K08.50
      specified NEC K08.59
    failure of marginal integrity K08.51
    failure of periodontal anatomical intergrity
        K08.54
  organ continuity from previous sterilization
      (tuboplasty) (vasoplasty) Z31.0
    aftercare Z31.42
  tooth (existing)
    contours biologically incompatible with
        oral health K08.54
    open margins K08.51
    overhanging K08.52
    poor aesthetic K08.56
    poor gingival margins K08.51
  unsatisfactory, of tooth K08.50
    specified NEC K08.59
Restorative material (dental)
  allergy to K08.55
  fractured K08.539
    with loss of material K08.531
    without loss of material K08.530
  unrepairable overhanging of K08.52
Restriction of housing space Z59.1
Rests, ovarian, in fallopian tube Q50.6
Restzustand (schizophrenic) F20.5
Retained —see also Retention
  cholelithiasis following cholecystectomy
      K91.86
  foreign body fragments (type of) Z18.9
    acrylics Z18.2
    animal quill(s) or spines Z18.31
    cement Z18.83
    concrete Z18.83
    crystalline Z18.83
    depleted isotope Z18.09
    depleted uranium Z18.01
    diethylhexylphthalates Z18.2
    glass Z18.81
    isocyanate Z18.2
    magnetic metal Z18.11
    metal Z18.10
    nonmagnetic metal Z18.12
    nontherapeutic radioactive Z18.09
    organic NEC Z18.39
    plastic Z18.2
    quill(s) (animal) Z18.31
    radioactive (nontherapeutic) NEC Z18.09
    specified NEC Z18.89
    spine(s) (animal) Z18.31
    stone Z18.83
    tooth (teeth) Z18.32
    wood Z18.33

Retained (Continued)
  fragments (type of) Z18.9
    acrylics Z18.2
    animal quill(s) or spines Z18.31
    cement Z18.83
    concrete Z18.83
    crystalline Z18.83
    depleted isotope Z18.09
    depleted uranium Z18.01
    diethylhexylphthalates Z18.2
    glass Z18.81
    isocyanate Z18.2
    magnetic metal Z18.11
    metal Z18.10
    nonmagnectic metal Z18.12
    nontherapeutic radioactive Z18.09
    organic NEC Z18.39
    plastic Z18.2
    quill(s) (animal) Z18.31
    radioactive (nontherapeutic) NEC Z18.09
    specified NEC Z18.89
    spine(s) (animal) Z18.31
    stone Z18.83
    tooth (teeth) Z18.32
    wood Z18.33
  gallstones, following cholecystectomy K91.86
Retardation
  development, developmental, specific —see
      Disorder, developmental
  endochondral bone growth —see Disorder,
      bone, development or growth
  growth R62.50
    due to malnutrition E45
  mental —see Disability, intellectual
  motor function, specific F82
  physical (child) R62.52
    due to malnutrition E45
  reading (specific) F81.0
  spelling (specific) (without reading disorder)
      F81.81
Retching —see Vomiting
Retention —see also Retained
  bladder —see Retention, urine
  carbon dioxide E87.2
  cholelithiasis following cholecystectomy K91.86
  cyst —see Cyst
  dead
    fetus (at or near term) (mother) O36.4
      early fetal death O02.1
    ovum O02.0
  decidua (fragments) (following delivery)
      (with hemorrhage) O72.2
    without hemorrhage O73.1
  deciduous tooth K00.6
  dental root K08.3
  fecal —see Constipation
  fetus
    dead O36.4
    early O02.1
  fluid R60.9
  foreign body —see also Foreign body, retained
    current trauma - code as Foreign body, by
        site or type
  gallstones, following cholecystectomy K91.86
  gastric K31.89
  intrauterine contraceptive device, in
      pregnancy —see Pregnancy, complicated
      by, retention, intrauterine device
  membranes (complicating delivery) (with
      hemorrhage) O72.2
    with abortion —see Abortion, by type
    without hemorrhage O73.1
  meniscus —see Derangement, meniscus
  menses N94.89
  milk (puerperal, postpartum) O92.79
  nitrogen, extrarenal R39.2
  ovary syndrome N99.83
  placenta (total) (with hemorrhage) O72.0
    without hemorrhage O73.0
    portions or fragments (with hemorrhage)
        O72.2
      without hemorrhage O73.1

Retention (Continued)
  products of conception
    early pregnancy (dead fetus) O02.1
    following
        delivery (with hemorrhage) O72.2
          without hemorrhage O73.1
      secundines (following delivery) (with
          hemorrhage) O72.0
        without hemorrhage O73.0
      complicating puerperium (delayed
          hemorrhage) O72.2
      partial O72.2
        without hemorrhage O73.1
  smegma, clitoris N90.89
  urine R33.9
    drug-induced R33.0
    due to hyperplasia (hypertrophy) of
        prostate —see Hyperplasia, prostate
    organic R33.8
      drug-induced R33.0
    psychogenic F45.8
    specified NEC R33.8
  water (in tissues) —see Edema
Reticular erythematous mucinosis L98.5
Reticulation, dust —see Pneumoconiosis
Reticulocytosis R70.1
Reticuloendotheliosis
  acute infantile C96.0
  leukemic C91.4-●
  nonlipid C96.0
Reticulohistiocytoma (giant-cell) D76.3
Reticuloid, actinic L57.1
Reticulosis (skin)
  acute of infancy C96.0
  hemophagocytic, familial D76.1
  histiocytic medullary C96.A
  lipomelanotic I89.8
  malignant (midline) C86.0
  polymorphic C86.0
  Sézary —see Sézary disease
Retina, retinal —see also condition
  dark area D49.81
Retinitis —see also Inflammation,
    chorioretinal
  albuminurica N18.9 [H32]
  diabetic —see Diabetes, retinitis
  disciformis —see Degeneration, macula
  focal —see Inflammation, chorioretinal, focal
  gravidarum —see Pregnancy, complicated by,
      specified pregnancy-related condition
      NEC
  juxtapapillaris —see Inflammation,
      chorioretinal, focal, juxtapapillary
  luetic —see Retinitis, syphilitic
  pigmentosa H35.52
  proliferans —see Disorder, globe,
      degenerative, specified type NEC
  proliferating —see Disorder, globe,
      degenerative, specified type NEC
  renal N18.9 [H32]
  syphilitic (early) (secondary) A51.43
    central, recurrent A52.71
    congenital (early) A50.01 [H32]
    late A52.71
  tuberculous A18.53
Retinoblastoma C69.2-●
  differentiated C69.2-●
  undifferentiated C69.2-●
Retinochoroiditis —see also Inflammation,
    chorioretinal
  disseminated —see Inflammation,
      chorioretinal, disseminated
    syphilitic A52.71
  focal —see Inflammation, chorioretinal
  juxtapapillaris —see Inflammation,
      chorioretinal, focal, juxtapapillary
Retinopathy (background) H35.00
  arteriosclerotic I70.8 [H35.0-●]
  atherosclerotic I70.8 [H35.0-●]
  central serous —see Chorioretinopathy,
      central serous

▶ New   ⮕ Revised   ~~deleted~~ Deleted   ● Use Additional Character(s)

Retinopathy *(Continued)*
  Coats H35.02-●
  diabetic —*see* Diabetes, retinopathy
  exudative H35.02-●
  hypertensive H35.03-●
  in (due to)
    diabetes —*see* Diabetes, retinopathy
    sickle-cell disorders D57.- ● *[H36]*
  of prematurity H35.10-●
    stage Ø H35.11-●
    stage 1 H35.12-●
    stage 2 H35.13-●
    stage 3 H35.14-●
    stage 4 H35.15-●
    stage 5 H35.16-●
  pigmentary, congenital —*see* Dystrophy,
      retina
  proliferative NEC H35.2-●
    diabetic —*see* Diabetes, retinopathy,
        proliferative
    sickle-cell D57.-● *[H36]*
  solar H31.02-●
Retinoschisis H33.10-●
  congenital Q14.1
  specified type NEC H33.19-●
Retortamoniasis A07.8
Retractile testis Q55.22
Retraction
  cervix —*see* Retroversion, uterus
  drum (membrane) —*see* Disorder, tympanic
      membrane, specified NEC
  finger —*see* Deformity, finger
  lid H02.539
    left H02.536
      lower H02.535
      upper H02.534
    right H02.533
      lower H02.532
      upper H02.531
  lung J98.4
  mediastinum J98.59
  nipple N64.53
    associated with
      lactation O92.03
      pregnancy O92.01-●
      puerperium O92.02
    congenital Q83.8
  palmar fascia M72.0
  pleura —*see* Pleurisy
  ring, uterus (Bandl's) (pathological)
      O62.4
  sternum (congenital) Q76.7
    acquired M95.4
  uterus —*see* Retroversion, uterus
  valve (heart) —*see* Endocarditis
Retrobulbar —*see* condition
Retrocecal —*see* condition
Retrocession —*see* Retroversion
Retrodisplacement —*see* Retroversion
Retroflection, retroflexion —*see* Retroversion
Retrognathia, retrognathism (mandibular)
    (maxillary) M26.19
Retrograde menstruation N92.5
Retroperineal —*see* condition
Retroperitoneal —*see* condition
Retroperitonitis K68.9
Retropharyngeal —*see* condition
Retroplacental —*see* condition
Retroposition —*see* Retroversion
Retroprosthetic membrane T85.398
Retrosternal thyroid (congenital) Q89.2
Retroversion, retroverted
  cervix —*see* Retroversion, uterus
  female NEC —*see* Retroversion, uterus
  iris H21.89
  testis (congenital) Q55.29
  uterus (acquired) (acute) (any degree)
      (asymptomatic) (cervix) (postinfectional)
      (postpartal, old) N85.4
    congenital Q51.818
    in pregnancy O34.53-●

Retrovirus, as cause of disease classified
    elsewhere B97.30
  human
    immunodeficiency, type 2 (HIV 2) B97.35
    T-cell lymphotropic
      type I (HTLV-I) B97.33
      type II (HTLV-II) B97.34
  lentivirus B97.31
  oncovirus B97.32
  specified NEC B97.39
Retrusion, premaxilla (developmental) M26.09
Rett's disease or syndrome F84.2
Reverse peristalsis R19.2
Reye's syndrome G93.7
Rh (factor)
  hemolytic disease (newborn) P55.0
  incompatibility, immunization or
      sensitization
    affecting management of pregnancy NEC
        O36.09-●
      anti-D antibody O36.01-●
    newborn P55.0
    transfusion reaction —*see* Complication(s),
        transfusion, incompatibility reaction,
        Rh (factor)
  negative mother affecting newborn P55.0
  titer elevated —*see* Complication(s),
      transfusion, incompatibility reaction, Rh
      (factor)
  transfusion reaction —*see* Complication(s),
      transfusion, incompatibility reaction, Rh
      (factor)
Rhabdomyolysis (idiopathic) NEC M62.82
  traumatic T79.6
Rhabdomyoma —*see also* Neoplasm, connective
    tissue, benign
  adult —*see* Neoplasm, connective tissue,
      benign
  fetal —*see* Neoplasm, connective tissue, benign
  glycogenic —*see* Neoplasm, connective tissue,
      benign
Rhabdomyosarcoma (any type) —*see*
    Neoplasm, connective tissue, malignant
Rhabdosarcoma —*see* Rhabdomyosarcoma
Rhesus (factor) incompatibility —*see* Rh,
    incompatibility
Rheumatic (acute) (subacute) (chronic)
  adherent pericardium I09.2
  coronary arteritis I01.9
  degeneration, myocardium I09.0
  fever (acute) —*see* Fever, rheumatic
  heart —*see* Disease, heart, rheumatic
  myocardial degeneration —*see* Degeneration,
      myocardium
  myocarditis (chronic) (inactive) (with chorea)
      I09.0
    with chorea (acute) (rheumatic)
        (Sydenham's) I02.0
    active or acute I01.2
  pancarditis, acute I01.8
    with chorea (acute) (rheumatic)
        Sydenham's) I02.0
  pericarditis (active) (acute) (with effusion)
      (with pneumonia) I01.0
    with chorea (acute) (rheumatic)
        (Sydenham's) I02.0
    chronic or inactive I09.2
  pneumonia I00 *[J17]*
  torticollis M43.6
  typhoid fever A01.09
Rheumatism (articular) (neuralgic)
    (nonarticular) M79.0
  gout —*see* Arthritis, rheumatoid
  intercostal, meaning Tietze's disease M94.0
  palindromic (any site) M12.30
    ankle M12.37-●
    elbow M12.32-●
    foot joint M12.37-●
    hand joint M12.34-●
    hip M12.35-●
    knee M12.36-●

Rheumatism *(Continued)*
  palindromic *(Continued)*
    multiple site M12.39
    shoulder M12.31-●
    specified joint NEC M12.38
    vertebrae M12.38
    wrist M12.33-●
  sciatic M54.4-●
Rheumatoid —*see also* condition
  arthritis —*see also* Arthritis, rheumatoid
    with involvement of organs NEC M05.60
      ankle M05.67-●
      elbow M05.62-●
      foot joint M05.67-●
      hand joint M05.64-●
      hip M05.65-●
      knee M05.66-●
      multiple site M05.69
      shoulder M05.61-●
      vertebra —*see* Spondylitis, ankylosing
      wrist M05.63-●
    seronegative —*see* Arthritis, rheumatoid,
        seronegative
    seropositive —*see* Arthritis, rheumatoid,
        seropositive
  carditis M05.30
    ankle M05.37-●
    elbow M05.32-●
    foot joint M05.37-●
    hand joint M05.34-●
    hip M05.35-●
    knee M05.36-●
    multiple site M05.39
    shoulder M05.31-●
    vertebra —*see* Spondylitis, ankylosing
    wrist M05.33-●
  endocarditis —*see* Rheumatoid, carditis
  lung (disease) M05.10
    ankle M05.17-●
    elbow M05.12-●
    foot joint M05.17-●
    hand joint M05.14-●
    hip M05.15-●
    knee M05.16-●
    multiple site M05.19
    shoulder M05.11-●
    vertebra —*see* Spondylitis, ankylosing
    wrist M05.13-●
  myocarditis —*see* Rheumatoid, carditis
  myopathy M05.40
    ankle M05.47-●
    elbow M05.42-●
    foot joint M05.47-●
    hand joint M05.44-●
    hip M05.45-●
    knee M05.46-●
    multiple site M05.49
    shoulder M05.41-●
    vertebra —*see* Spondylitis, ankylosing
    wrist M05.43-●
  pericarditis —*see* Rheumatoid, carditis
  polyarthritis —*see* Arthritis, rheumatoid
  polyneuropathy M05.50
    ankle M05.57-●
    elbow M05.52-●
    foot joint M05.57-●
    hand joint M05.54-●
    hip M05.55-●
    knee M05.56-●
    multiple site M05.59
    shoulder M05.51-●
    vertebra —*see* Spondylitis, ankylosing
    wrist M05.53-●
  vasculitis M05.20
    ankle M05.27-●
    elbow M05.22-●
    foot joint M05.27-●
    hand joint M05.24-●
    hip M05.25-●
    knee M05.26-●
    multiple site M05.29

Rheumatoid *(Continued)*
 vasculitis *(Continued)*
  shoulder M05.21-•
  vertebra —*see* Spondylitis, ankylosing
  wrist M05.23-•
Rhinitis (atrophic) (catarrhal) (chronic)
  (croupous) (fibrinous) (granulomatous)
  (hyperplastic) (hypertrophic)
  (membranous) (obstructive) (purulent)
  (suppurative) (ulcerative) J31.0
 with
  sore throat —*see* Nasopharyngitis
 acute J00
 allergic J30.9
  with asthma J45.909
   with
    exacerbation (acute) J45.901
    status asthmaticus J45.902
  due to
   food J30.5
   pollen J30.1
  nonseasonal J30.89
  perennial J30.89
  seasonal NEC J30.2
  specified NEC J30.89
 infective J00
 pneumococcal J00
 syphilitic A52.73
  congenital A50.05 *[J99]*
 tuberculous A15.8
 vasomotor J30.0
Rhinoantritis (chronic) —*see* Sinusitis,
  maxillary
Rhinodacryolith —*see* Dacryolith
Rhinolith (nasal sinus) J34.89
Rhinomegaly J34.89
Rhinopharyngitis (acute) (subacute) —*see also*
  Nasopharyngitis
 chronic J31.1
 destructive ulcerating A66.5
 mutilans A66.5
Rhinophyma L71.1
Rhinorrhea J34.89
 cerebrospinal (fluid) G96.0
 paroxysmal —*see* Rhinitis, allergic
 spasmodic —*see* Rhinitis, allergic
Rhinosalpingitis —*see* Salpingitis, eustachian
Rhinoscleroma A48.8
Rhinosporidiosis B48.1
Rhinovirus infection NEC B34.8
Rhizomelic chondrodysplasia punctata E71.540
Rhythm
 atrioventricular nodal I49.8
 disorder I49.9
  coronary sinus I49.8
  ectopic I49.8
  nodal I49.8
 escape I49.9
 heart, abnormal I49.9
 idioventricular I44.2
 nodal I49.8
 sleep, inversion G47.2-•
  nonorganic origin —*see* Disorder, sleep,
   circadian rhythm, psychogenic
Rhytidosis facialis L98.8
Rib —*see also* condition
 cervical Q76.5
Riboflavin deficiency E53.0
Rice bodies —*see also* Loose, body, joint
 knee M23.4-•
Richter syndrome —*see* Leukemia, chronic
  lymphocytic, B-cell type
Richter's hernia —*see* Hernia, abdomen, with
  obstruction
Ricinism —*see* Poisoning, food, noxious, plant
Rickets (active) (acute) (adolescent) (chest wall)
  (congenital) (current) (infantile) (intestinal)
  E55.0
 adult —*see* Osteomalacia
 celiac K90.0
 hypophosphatemic with nephrotic-glycosuric
   dwarfism E72.09
 inactive E64.3

Rickets *(Continued)*
 kidney N25.0
 renal N25.0
 sequelae, any E64.3
 vitamin-D-resistant E83.31 *[M90.80]*
Rickettsial disease A79.9
 specified type NEC A79.89
Rickettsialpox (Rickettsia akari) A79.1
Rickettsiosis A79.9
 due to
  Ehrlichia sennetsu A79.81
  Rickettsia akari (rickettsialpox) A79.1
 specified type NEC A79.89
 tick-borne A77.9
 vesicular A79.1
Rider's bone —*see* Ossification, muscle,
  specified NEC
Ridge, alveolus —*see also* condition
 flabby K06.8
Ridged ear, congenital Q17.3
Riedel's
 lobe, liver Q44.7
 struma, thyroiditis or disease E06.5
Rieger's anomaly or syndrome Q13.81
Riehl's melanosis L81.4
Rietti-Greppi-Micheli anemia D56.9
Rieux's hernia —*see* Hernia, abdomen, specified
  site NEC
Riga (-Fede) disease K14.0
Riggs' disease —*see* Periodontitis
Right aortic arch Q25.47
Right middle lobe syndrome J98.11
Rigid, rigidity —*see also* condition
 abdominal R19.30
  with severe abdominal pain R10.0
  epigastric R19.36
  generalized R19.37
  left lower quadrant R19.34
  left upper quadrant R19.32
  periumbilic R19.35
  right lower quadrant R19.33
  right upper quadrant R19.31
 articular, multiple, congenital Q68.8
 cervix (uteri) in pregnancy —*see* Pregnancy,
   complicated by, abnormal, cervix
 hymen (acquired) (congenital) N89.6
 nuchal R29.1
 pelvic floor in pregnancy —*see* Pregnancy,
   complicated by, abnormal, pelvic organs
   or tissues NEC
 perineum or vulva in pregnancy —*see*
   Pregnancy, complicated by, abnormal,
   vulva
 spine —*see* Dorsopathy, specified NEC
 vagina in pregnancy —*see* Pregnancy,
   complicated by, abnormal, vagina
Rigors R68.89
 with fever R50.9
Riley-Day syndrome G90.1
RIND (reversible ischemic neurologic deficit)
  I63.9
Ring(s)
 aorta (vascular) Q25.45
 Bandl's O62.4
 contraction, complicating delivery O62.4
 esophageal, lower (muscular) K22.2
 Fleischer's (cornea) H18.04-•
 hymenal, tight (acquired) (congenital) N89.6
 Kayser-Fleischer (cornea) H18.04-•
 retraction, uterus, pathological O62.4
 Schatzki's (esophagus) (lower) K22.2
  congenital Q39.3
 Soemmerring's —*see* Cataract, secondary
 vascular (congenital) Q25.8
  aorta Q25.45
Ringed hair (congenital) Q84.1
Ringworm B35.9
 beard B35.0
 black dot B35.0
 body B35.4
 Burmese B35.5
 corporeal B35.4
 foot B35.3

Ringworm *(Continued)*
 groin B35.6
 hand B35.2
 honeycomb B35.0
 nails B35.1
 perianal (area) B35.6
 scalp B35.0
 specified NEC B35.8
 Tokelau B35.5
Rise, venous pressure I87.8
Rising, PSA following treatment for malignant
  neoplasm of prostate R97.21
~~**Risk, suicidal**~~
  ~~meaning personal history of attempted~~
   ~~suicide Z91.5~~
  ~~meaning suicidal ideation —*see* Ideation,~~
   ~~suicidal~~
►**Risk**
►for
  ►dental caries Z91.849
   ►high Z91.843
   ►low Z91.841
   ►moderate Z91.842
 ►suicidal
  ►meaning personal history of attempted
    suicide Z91.5
  ►meaning suicidal ideation —*see* Ideation,
    suicidal
Ritter's disease L00
Rivalry, sibling Z62.891
Rivalta's disease A42.2
River blindness B73.01
Robert's pelvis Q74.2
 with disproportion (fetopelvic) O33.0
  causing obstructed labor O65.0
Robin (-Pierre) syndrome Q87.0
Robinow-Silvermann-Smith syndrome Q87.1
Robinson's (hidrotic) ectodermal dysplasia or
  syndrome Q82.4
Robles' disease B73.01
Rocky Mountain (spotted) fever A77.0
Roetheln —*see* Rubella
Roger's disease Q21.0
Rokitansky-Aschoff sinuses (gallbladder) K82.8
Rolando's fracture (displaced) S62.22-•
 nondisplaced S62.22-•
Romano-Ward (prolonged QT interval)
  syndrome I45.81
Romberg's disease or syndrome G51.8
Roof, mouth —*see* condition
Rosacea L71.9
 acne L71.9
 keratitis L71.8
 specified NEC L71.8
Rosary, rachitic E55.0
Rose
 cold J30.1
 fever J30.1
 rash R21
  epidemic B06.9
Rosenbach's erysipeloid A26.0
Rosenthal's disease or syndrome D68.1
Roseola B09
 infantum B08.20
  due to human herpesvirus 6 B08.21
  due to human herpesvirus 7 B08.22
Ross River disease or fever B33.1
Rossbach's disease K31.89
 psychogenic F45.8
Rostan's asthma (cardiac) —*see* Failure,
  ventricular, left
Rotation
 anomalous, incomplete or insufficient,
   intestine Q43.3
 cecum (congenital) Q43.3
 colon (congenital) Q43.3
 spine, incomplete or insufficient —*see*
   Dorsopathy, deforming, specified NEC
 tooth, teeth, fully erupted M26.35
 vertebra, incomplete or insufficient —*see*
   Dorsopathy, deforming, specified NEC
Rotes Quérol disease or syndrome —*see*
  Hyperostosis, ankylosing

► New   ⇒ Revised   ~~deleted~~ Deleted   • Use Additional Character(s)

Roth (-Bernhardt) disease or syndrome —see
    Meralgia paraesthetica
Rothmund (-Thomson) syndrome Q82.8
Rotor's disease or syndrome E80.6
Round
    back (with wedging of vertebrae) —see
        Kyphosis
    sequelae (late effect) of rickets E64.3
    worms (large) (infestation) NEC B82.0
        Ascariasis —see also Ascariasis B77.9
Roussy-Lévy syndrome G60.0
Rubella (German measles) B06.9
    complication NEC B06.09
        neurological B06.00
    congenital P35.0
    contact Z20.4
    exposure to Z20.4
    maternal
        care for (suspected) damage to fetus O35.3
        manifest rubella in infant P35.0
        suspected damage to fetus affecting
            management of pregnancy O35.3
    specified complications NEC B06.89
Rubeola (meaning measles) —see Measles
    meaning rubella —see Rubella
Rubeosis, iris —see Disorder, iris, vascular
Rubinstein-Taybi syndrome Q87.2
Rudimentary (congenital) —see also Agenesis
    arm —see Defect, reduction, upper limb
    bone Q79.9
    cervix uteri Q51.828
    eye Q11.2
    lobule of ear Q17.3
    patella Q74.1
    respiratory organs in thoracopagus Q89.4
    tracheal bronchus Q32.4
    uterus Q51.818
        in male Q56.1
    vagina Q52.0
Ruled out condition —see Observation, suspected
Rumination R11.10
    with nausea R11.2
    disorder of infancy F98.21
    neurotic F42.8
    newborn P92.1
    obsessional F42.8
    psychogenic F42.8
Runeberg's disease D51.0
Runny nose R09.89
Rupia (syphilitic) A51.39
    congenital A50.06
    tertiary A52.79
Rupture, ruptured
    abscess (spontaneous) - code by site under
        Abscess
    aneurysm —see Aneurysm
    anus (sphincter) —see Laceration, anus
    aorta, aortic I71.8
        abdominal I71.3
        arch I71.1
        ascending I71.1
        descending I71.8
            abdominal I71.3
            thoracic I71.1
        syphilitic A52.01
        thoracoabdominal I71.5
        thorax, thoracic I71.1
        transverse I71.1
        traumatic —see Injury, aorta, laceration,
            major
        valve or cusp —see also Endocarditis, aortic
            I35.8
    appendix (with peritonitis) K35.2
        with localized peritonitis K35.3
    arteriovenous fistula, brain I60.8
    artery I77.2
        brain —see Hemorrhage, intracranial,
            intracerebral
        coronary —see Infarct, myocardium
        heart —see Infarct, myocardium
        pulmonary I28.8
        traumatic (complication) —see Injury,
            blood vessel

Rupture, ruptured (Continued)
    bile duct (common) (hepatic) K83.2
        cystic K82.2
    bladder (sphincter) (nontraumatic)
        (spontaneous) N32.89
        following ectopic or molar pregnancy O08.6
        obstetrical trauma O71.5
        traumatic S37.29
    blood vessel —see also Hemorrhage
        brain —see Hemorrhage, intracranial,
            intracerebral
        heart —see Infarct, myocardium
        traumatic (complication) —see Injury,
            blood vessel, laceration, major, by site
    bone —see Fracture
    bowel (nontraumatic) K63.1
    brain
        aneurysm (congenital) —see also
            Hemorrhage, intracranial,
            subarachnoid
            syphilitic A52.05
        hemorrhagic —see Hemorrhage,
            intracranial, intracerebral
    capillaries I78.8
    cardiac (auricle) (ventricle) (wall) I23.3
        with hemopericardium I23.0
        infectional I40.9
        traumatic —see Injury, heart
    cartilage (articular) (current) —see also Sprain
        knee S83.3-●
        semilunar —see Tear, meniscus
    cecum (with peritonitis) K65.0
        with peritoneal abscess K35.3
        traumatic S36.59●
    celiac artery, traumatic —see Injury, blood
        vessel, celiac artery, laceration, major
    cerebral aneurysm (congenital) (see
        Hemorrhage, intracranial, subarachnoid)
    cervix (uteri)
        with ectopic or molar pregnancy O08.6
        following ectopic or molar pregnancy O08.6
        obstetrical trauma O71.3
        traumatic S37.69
    chordae tendineae NEC I51.1
        concurrent with acute myocardial
            infarction —see Infarct, myocardium
        following acute myocardial infarction
            (current complication) I23.4
    choroid (direct) (indirect) (traumatic) H31.32-●
    circle of Willis I60.6
    colon (nontraumatic) K63.1
        traumatic —see Injury, intestine, large
    cornea (traumatic) —see Injury, eye, laceration
    coronary (artery) (thrombotic) —see Infarct,
        myocardium
    corpus luteum (infected) (ovary) N83.1-●
    cyst —see Cyst
    cystic duct K82.2
    Descemet's membrane —see Change, corneal
        membrane, Descemet's, rupture
        traumatic —see Injury, eye, laceration
    diaphragm, traumatic —see Injury,
        intrathoracic, diaphragm
    disc —see Rupture, intervertebral disc
    diverticulum (intestine) K57.80
        with bleeding K57.81
        bladder N32.3
        large intestine K57.20
            with
                bleeding K57.21
                small intestine K57.40
                    with bleeding K57.41
        small intestine K57.00
            with
                bleeding K57.01
                large intestine K57.40
                    with bleeding K57.41
    duodenal stump K31.89
    ear drum (nontraumatic) —see also
        Perforation, tympanum
        traumatic S09.2-●
            due to blast injury —see Injury, blast, ear
    esophagus K22.3

Rupture, ruptured (Continued)
    eye (without prolapse or loss of intraocular
        tissue) —see Injury, eye, laceration
    fallopian tube NEC (nonobstetric)
        (nontraumatic) N83.8
    ➜ due to pregnancy O00.10-●
        ➜ with intrauterine pregnancy O00.11-●
    fontanel P13.1
    gallbladder K82.2
        traumatic S36.128
    gastric —see also Rupture, stomach
        vessel K92.2
    globe (eye) (traumatic) —see Injury, eye,
        laceration
    graafian follicle (hematoma) N83.0-●
    heart —see Rupture, cardiac
    hymen (nontraumatic) (nonintentional) N89.8
    internal organ, traumatic —see Injury, by site
    intervertebral disc —see Displacement,
        intervertebral disc
        traumatic —see Rupture, traumatic,
            intervertebral disc
    intestine NEC (nontraumatic) K63.1
        traumatic —see Injury, intestine
    iris —see also Abnormality, pupillary
        traumatic —see Injury, eye, laceration
    joint capsule, traumatic —see Sprain
    kidney (traumatic) S37.06-●
        birth injury P15.8
        nontraumatic N28.89
    lacrimal duct (traumatic) —see Injury, eye,
        specified site NEC
    lens (cataract) (traumatic) —see Cataract,
        traumatic
    ligament, traumatic —see Rupture, traumatic,
        ligament, by site
    liver S36.116
        birth injury P15.0
    lymphatic vessel I89.8
    marginal sinus (placental) (with
        hemorrhage) —see Hemorrhage,
        antepartum, specified cause NEC
    membrana tympani (nontraumatic) —see
        Perforation, tympanum
    membranes (spontaneous)
        artificial
            delayed delivery following O75.5
        delayed delivery following —see
            Pregnancy, complicated by, premature
            rupture of membranes
    meningeal artery I60.8
    meniscus (knee) —see also Tear, meniscus
        old —see Derangement, meniscus
        site other than knee - code as Sprain
    mesenteric artery, traumatic —see Injury,
        mesenteric, artery, laceration, major
    mesentery (nontraumatic) K66.8
        traumatic —see Injury, intra-abdominal,
            specified, site NEC
    mitral (valve) I34.8
    muscle (traumatic) —see also Strain
        diastasis —see Diastasis, muscle
        nontraumatic M62.10
            ankle M62.17-●
            foot M62.17-●
            forearm M62.13-●
            hand M62.14-●
            lower leg M62.16-●
            pelvic region M62.15-●
            shoulder region M62.11-●
            specified site NEC M62.18
            thigh M62.15-●
            upper arm M62.12-●
        traumatic —see Strain, by site
    musculotendinous junction NEC,
        nontraumatic —see Rupture, tendon,
        spontaneous
    mycotic aneurysm causing cerebral
        hemorrhage —see Hemorrhage,
        intracranial, subarachnoid
    myocardium, myocardial —see Rupture,
        cardiac
        traumatic —see Injury, heart

Rupture, ruptured *(Continued)*
nontraumatic, meaning hernia —*see* Hernia
obstructed —*see* Hernia, by site, obstructed
operation wound —*see* Disruption, wound, operation
ovary, ovarian N83.8
  corpus luteum cyst N83.1-●
  follicle (graafian) N83.0-●
oviduct (nonobstetric) (nontraumatic) N83.8
➡due to pregnancy O00.10-●
  ➡with intrauterine pregnancy O00.11-●
pancreas (nontraumatic) K86.89
  traumatic S36.299
papillary muscle NEC I51.2
  following acute myocardial infarction (current complication) I23.5
pelvic
  floor, complicating delivery O70.1
  organ NEC, obstetrical trauma O71.5
perineum (nonobstetric) (nontraumatic) N90.89
  complicating delivery —*see* Delivery, complicated, by, laceration, anus (sphincter)
postoperative wound —*see* Disruption, wound, operation
prostate (traumatic) S37.828
pulmonary
  artery I28.8
  valve (heart) I37.8
  vein I28.8
  vessel I28.8
pus tube —*see* Salpingitis
pyosalpinx —*see* Salpingitis
rectum (nontraumatic) K63.1
  traumatic S36.69
retina, retinal (traumatic) (without detachment) —*see also* Break, retina
  with detachment —*see* Detachment, retina, with retinal, break
rotator cuff (nontraumatic) M75.10-●
  complete M75.12-●
  incomplete M75.11-●
sclera —*see* Injury, eye, laceration
sigmoid (nontraumatic) K63.1
  traumatic S36.593
spinal cord —*see also* Injury, spinal cord, by region
  due to injury at birth P11.5
  newborn (birth injury) P11.5
spleen (traumatic) S36.09
  birth injury P15.1
  congenital (birth injury) P15.1
  due to P. vivax malaria B51.0
  nontraumatic D73.5
  spontaneous D73.5
splenic vein R58
  traumatic —*see* Injury, blood vessel, splenic vein
stomach (nontraumatic) (spontaneous) K31.89
  traumatic S36.39
supraspinatus (complete) (incomplete) (nontraumatic) —*see* Tear, rotator cuff
symphysis pubis
  obstetric O71.6
  traumatic S33.4
synovium (cyst) M66.10
  ankle M66.17-●
  elbow M66.12-●
  finger M66.14-●
  foot M66.17-●
  forearm M66.13-●
  hand M66.14-●
  pelvic region M66.15-●
  shoulder region M66.11-●
  specified site NEC M66.18
  thigh M66.15-●
  toe M66.17-●
  upper arm M66.12-●
  wrist M66.13-●
tendon (traumatic) —*see* Strain
  nontraumatic (spontaneous) M66.9
    ankle M66.87-●

Rupture, ruptured *(Continued)*
tendon *(Continued)*
  nontraumatic *(Continued)*
    extensor M66.20
      ankle M66.27-●
      foot M66.27-●
      forearm M66.23-●
      hand M66.24-●
      lower leg M66.26-●
      multiple sites M66.29
      pelvic region M66.25-●
      shoulder region M66.21-●
      specified site NEC M66.28
      thigh M66.25-●
      upper arm M66.22-●
    flexor M66.30
      ankle M66.37-●
      foot M66.37-●
      forearm M66.33-●
      hand M66.34-●
      lower leg M66.36-●
      multiple sites M66.39
      pelvic region M66.35-●
      shoulder region M66.31-●
      specified site NEC M66.38
      thigh M66.35-●
      upper arm M66.32-●
    foot M66.87-●
    forearm M66.83-●
    hand M66.84-●
    lower leg M66.86-●
    multiple sites M66.89
    pelvic region M66.85-●
    shoulder region M66.81-●
    specified
      site NEC M66.88
      tendon M66.80
    thigh M66.85-●
    upper arm M66.82-●
thoracic duct I89.8
tonsil J35.8
traumatic
  aorta —*see* Injury, aorta, laceration, major
  diaphragm —*see* Injury, intrathoracic, diaphragm
  external site —*see* Wound, open, by site
  eye —*see* Injury, eye, laceration
  internal organ —*see* Injury, by site
  intervertebral disc
    cervical S13.0
    lumbar S33.0
    thoracic S23.0
  kidney S37.06-●
  ligament —*see also* Sprain
    ankle —*see* Sprain, ankle
    carpus —*see* Rupture, traumatic, ligament, wrist
    collateral (hand) —*see* Rupture, traumatic, ligament, finger, collateral
    finger (metacarpophalangeal) (interphalangeal) S63.40-●
      collateral S63.41-●
        index S63.41-●
        little S63.41-●
        middle S63.41-●
        ring S63.41-●
      index S63.40-●
      little S63.40-●
      middle S63.40-●
      palmar S63.42-●
        index S63.42-●
        little S63.42-●
        middle S63.42-●
        ring S63.42-●
      ring S63.40-●
      specified site NEC S63.499
        index S63.49-●
        little S63.49-●
        middle S63.49-●
        ring S63.49-●
      volar plate S63.43-●
        index S63.43-●
        little S63.43-●

Rupture, ruptured *(Continued)*
traumatic *(Continued)*
  ligament *(Continued)*
    finger *(Continued)*
      volar plate *(Continued)*
        middle S63.43-●
        ring S63.43-●
    foot —*see* Sprain, foot
    radial collateral S53.2-●
    radiocarpal —*see* Rupture, traumatic, ligament, wrist, radiocarpal
    ulnar collateral S53.3-●
    ulnocarpal —*see* Rupture, traumatic, ligament, wrist, ulnocarpal
    wrist S63.30-●
      collateral S63.31-●
      radiocarpal S63.32-●
      specified site NEC S63.39-●
      ulnocarpal (palmar) S63.33-●
  liver S36.116
  membrana tympani —*see* Rupture, ear drum, traumatic
  muscle or tendon —*see* Strain
  myocardium —*see* Injury, heart
  pancreas S36.299
  rectum S36.69
  sigmoid S36.593
  spleen S36.09
  stomach S36.39
  symphysis pubis S33.4
  tympanum, tympanic (membrane) —*see* Rupture, ear drum, traumatic
  ureter S37.19
  uterus S37.69
  vagina —*see* Injury, vagina
  vena cava —*see* Injury, vena cava, laceration, major
tricuspid (heart) (valve) I07.8
tube, tubal (nonobstetric) (nontraumatic) N83.8
  abscess —*see* Salpingitis
  ➡due to pregnancy O00.10-●
    ➡with intrauterine pregnancy O00.11-●
tympanum, tympanic (membrane) (nontraumatic) —*see also* Perforation, tympanic membrane H72.9-●
  traumatic —*see* Rupture, ear drum, traumatic
umbilical cord, complicating delivery O69.89
ureter (traumatic) S37.19
  nontraumatic N28.89
urethra (nontraumatic) N36.8
  with ectopic or molar pregnancy O08.6
  following ectopic or molar pregnancy O08.6
  obstetrical trauma O71.5
  traumatic S37.39
uterosacral ligament (nonobstetric) (nontraumatic) N83.8
uterus (traumatic) S37.69
  before labor O71.0-●
  during or after labor O71.1
  nonpuerperal, nontraumatic N85.8
  pregnant (during labor) O71.1
    before labor O71.0-●
vagina —*see* Injury, vagina
valve, valvular (heart) —*see* Endocarditis
varicose vein —*see* Varix
varix —*see* Varix
vena cava R58
  traumatic —*see* Injury, vena cava, laceration, major
vesical (urinary) N32.89
vessel (blood) R58
  pulmonary I28.8
  traumatic —*see* Injury, blood vessel
viscus R19.8
vulva complicating delivery O70.0
Russell-Silver syndrome Q87.1
Russian spring-summer type encephalitis A84.0
Rust's disease (tuberculous cervical spondylitis) A18.01
Ruvalcaba-Myhre-Smith syndrome E71.440
Rytand-Lipsitch syndrome I44.2

▶ New   ➡ Revised   ~~deleted~~ Deleted   ● Use Additional Character(s)

S

Saber, sabre shin or tibia (syphilitic) A50.56
　[M90.8-●]
Sac lacrimal —see condition
Saccharomyces infection B37.9
Saccharopinuria E72.3
Saccular —see condition
Sacculation
　aorta (nonsyphilitic) —see Aneurysm, aorta
　bladder N32.3
　intralaryngeal (congenital) (ventricular)
　　Q31.3
　larynx (congenital) (ventricular) Q31.3
　organ or site, congenital —see Distortion
　pregnant uterus —see Pregnancy, complicated
　　by, abnormal, uterus
　ureter N28.89
　urethra N36.1
　vesical N32.3
Sachs' amaurotic familial idiocy or disease
　E75.02
Sachs-Tay disease E75.02
Sacks-Libman disease M32.11
Sacralgia M53.3
Sacralization Q76.49
Sacrodynia M53.3
Sacroiliac joint —see condition
Sacroiliitis NEC M46.1
Sacrum —see condition
Saddle
　back —see Lordosis
　embolus
　　abdominal aorta I74.01
　　pulmonary artery I26.92
　　　with acute cor pulmonale I26.02
　injury — code to condition
　nose M95.0
　　due to syphilis A50.57
Sadism (sexual) F65.52
Sadness, postpartal O90.6
Sadomasochism F65.50
Saemisch's ulcer (cornea) —see Ulcer, cornea,
　central
Sagging
　skin and subcutaneous tissue (following
　　bariatric surgery weight loss) (following
　　dietary weight loss) L98.7
Sahib disease B55.0
Sailors' skin L57.8
Saint
　Anthony's fire —see Erysipelas
　triad —see Hernia, diaphragm
　Vitus' dance —see Chorea, Sydenham's
Salaam
　attack(s) —see Epilepsy, spasms
　tic R25.8
Salicylism
　abuse F55.8
　overdose or wrong substance given —see
　　Table of Drugs and Chemicals, by drug,
　　poisoning
Salivary duct or gland —see condition
Salivation, excessive K11.7
Salmonella —see Infection, Salmonella
Salmonellosis A02.0
Salpingitis (catarrhal) (fallopian tube) (nodular)
　(pseudofollicular) (purulent) (septic)
　N70.91
　with oophoritis N70.93
　acute N70.01
　　with oophoritis N70.03
　chlamydial A56.11
　chronic N70.11
　　with oophoritis N70.13
　complicating abortion —see Abortion, by
　　type, complicated by, salpingitis
　ear —see Salpingitis, eustachian
　eustachian (tube) H68.00-●
　　acute H68.01-●
　　chronic H68.02-●

Salpingitis (Continued)
　follicularis N70.11
　　with oophoritis N70.13
　gonococcal (acute) (chronic) A54.24
　interstitial, chronic N70.11
　　with oophoritis N70.13
　isthmica nodosa N70.11
　　with oophoritis N70.13
　specific (gonococcal) (acute) (chronic) A54.24
　tuberculous (acute) (chronic) A18.17
　venereal (gonococcal) (acute) (chronic) A54.24
Salpingocele N83.4-●
Salpingo-oophoritis (catarrhal) (purulent)
　(ruptured) (septic) (suppurative) N70.93
　acute N70.03
　　with ectopic or molar pregnancy O08.0
　　following ectopic or molar pregnancy
　　　O08.0
　　gonococcal A54.24
　chronic N70.13
　following ectopic or molar pregnancy O08.0
　gonococcal (acute) (chronic) A54.24
　puerperal O86.19
　specific (gonococcal) (acute) (chronic) A54.24
　subacute N70.03
　tuberculous (acute) (chronic) A18.17
　venereal (gonococcal) (acute) (chronic) A54.24
Salpingo-ovaritis —see Salpingo-oophoritis
Salpingoperitonitis —see Salpingo-oophoritis
Salzmann's nodular dystrophy —see
　Degeneration, cornea, nodular
Sampson's cyst or tumor N80.1
San Joaquin (Valley) fever B38.0
Sandblaster's asthma, lung or pneumoconiosis
　J62.8
Sander's disease (paranoia) F22
Sandfly fever A93.1
Sandhoff's disease E75.01
Sanfilippo (Type B) (Type C) (Type D)
　syndrome E76.22
Sanger-Brown ataxia G11.2
Sao Paulo fever or typhus A77.0
Saponification, mesenteric K65.8
Sarcocele (benign)
　syphilitic A52.76
　　congenital A50.59
Sarcocystosis A07.8
Sarcoepiplocele —see Hernia
Sarcoepiplomphalocele Q79.2
Sarcoid —see also Sarcoidosis
　arthropathy D86.86
　Boeck's D86.9
　Darier-Roussy D86.3
　iridocyclitis D86.83
　meningitis D86.81
　myocarditis D86.85
　myositis D86.87
　pyelonephritis D86.84
　Spiegler-Fendt L08.89
Sarcoidosis D86.9
　with
　　cranial nerve palsies D86.82
　　hepatic granuloma D86.89
　　polyarthritis D86.86
　　tubulo-interstitial nephropathy D86.84
　combined sites NEC D86.89
　lung D86.0
　　and lymph nodes D86.2
　lymph nodes D86.1
　　and lung D86.2
　meninges D86.81
　skin D86.3
　specified type NEC D86.89
Sarcoma (of) —see also Neoplasm, connective
　tissue, malignant
　alveolar soft part —see Neoplasm, connective
　　tissue, malignant
　ameloblastic C41.1
　　upper jaw (bone) C41.0
　botryoid —see Neoplasm, connective tissue,
　　malignant

Sarcoma (Continued)
　botryoides —see Neoplasm, connective tissue,
　　malignant
　cerebellar C71.6
　　circumscribed (arachnoidal) C71.6
　circumscribed (arachnoidal) cerebellar
　　C71.6
　clear cell —see also Neoplasm, connective
　　tissue, malignant
　　kidney C64.-●
　dendritic cells (accessory cells) C96.4
　embryonal —see Neoplasm, connective tissue,
　　malignant
　endometrial (stromal) C54.1
　　isthmus C54.0
　epithelioid (cell) —see Neoplasm, connective
　　tissue, malignant
　Ewing's —see Neoplasm, bone, malignant
　follicular dendritic cell C96.4
　germinoblastic (diffuse) —see Lymphoma,
　　diffuse, large cell
　　follicular —see Lymphoma, follicular,
　　　specified NEC
　giant cell (except of bone) —see also Neoplasm,
　　connective tissue, malignant
　　bone —see Neoplasm, bone, malignant
　glomoid —see Neoplasm, connective tissue,
　　malignant
　granulocytic C92.3-●
　hemangioendothelial —see Neoplasm,
　　connective tissue, malignant
　hemorrhagic, multiple —see Sarcoma,
　　Kaposi's
　histiocytic C96.A
　Hodgkin —see Lymphoma, Hodgkin
　immunoblastic (diffuse) —see Lymphoma,
　　diffuse large cell
　interdigitating dendritic cell C96.4
　Kaposi's
　　colon C46.4
　　connective tissue C46.1
　　gastrointestinal organ C46.4
　　lung C46.5-●
　　lymph node(s) C46.3
　　palate (hard) (soft) C46.2
　　rectum C46.4
　　skin C46.0
　　specified site NEC C46.7
　　stomach C46.4
　　unspecified site C46.9
　Kupffer cell C22.3
　Langerhans cell C96.4
　leptomeningeal —see Neoplasm, meninges,
　　malignant
　liver NEC C22.4
　lymphangioendothelial —see Neoplasm,
　　connective tissue, malignant
　lymphoblastic —see Lymphoma,
　　lymphoblastic (diffuse)
　lymphocytic —see Lymphoma, small cell
　　B-cell
　mast cell C96.22
　melanotic —see Melanoma
　meningeal —see Neoplasm, meninges,
　　malignant
　meningothelial —see Neoplasm, meninges,
　　malignant
　mesenchymal —see also Neoplasm,
　　connective tissue, malignant
　　mixed —see Neoplasm, connective tissue,
　　　malignant
　mesothelial —see Mesothelioma
　monstrocellular
　　specified site —see Neoplasm, malignant,
　　　by site
　　unspecified site C71.9
　myeloid C92.3-●
　neurogenic —see Neoplasm, nerve,
　　malignant
　odontogenic C41.1
　　upper jaw (bone) C41.0

Sarcoma *(Continued)*
 osteoblastic —*see* Neoplasm, bone,
  malignant
 osteogenic —*see also* Neoplasm, bone,
  malignant
  juxtacortical —*see* Neoplasm, bone,
   malignant
  periosteal —*see* Neoplasm, bone,
   malignant
 periosteal —*see also* Neoplasm, bone,
  malignant
  osteogenic —*see* Neoplasm, bone,
   malignant
 pleomorphic cell —*see* Neoplasm, connective
  tissue, malignant
 reticulum cell (diffuse) —*see* Lymphoma,
  diffuse large cell
  nodular —*see* Lymphoma, follicular
  pleomorphic cell type —*see* Lymphoma,
   diffuse large cell
 rhabdoid —*see* Neoplasm, malignant, by site
 round cell —*see* Neoplasm, connective tissue,
  malignant
 small cell —*see* Neoplasm, connective tissue,
  malignant
 soft tissue —*see* Neoplasm, connective tissue,
  malignant
 spindle cell —*see* Neoplasm, connective
  tissue, malignant
 stromal (endometrial) C54.1
  isthmus C54.0
 synovial —*see also* Neoplasm, connective
  tissue, malignant
  biphasic —*see* Neoplasm, connective tissue,
   malignant
  epithelioid cell —*see* Neoplasm, connective
   tissue, malignant
  spindle cell —*see* Neoplasm, connective
   tissue, malignant
Sarcomatosis
 meningeal —*see* Neoplasm, meninges,
  malignant
 specified site NEC —*see* Neoplasm,
  connective tissue, malignant
 unspecified site C80.1
Sarcopenia (age-related) M62.84
Sarcosinemia E72.59
Sarcosporidiosis (intestinal) A07.8
Satiety, early R68.81
Saturnine —*see* condition
Saturnism
 overdose or wrong substance given
  or taken —*see* Table of Drugs and
  Chemicals, by drug, poisoning
Satyriasis F52.8
Sauriasis —*see* Ichthyosis
SBE (subacute bacterial endocarditis) I33.0
Scabies (any site) B86
Scabs R23.4
Scaglietti-Dagnini syndrome E22.0
Scald —*see* Burn
Scalenus anticus (anterior) syndrome G54.0
Scales R23.4
Scaling, skin R23.4
Scalp —*see* condition
Scapegoating affecting child Z62.3
Scaphocephaly Q75.0
Scapulalgia M89.8X1
Scapulohumeral myopathy G71.0
Scar, scarring —*see also* Cicatrix L90.5
 adherent L90.5
 atrophic L90.5
 cervix
  in pregnancy or childbirth —*see* Pregnancy,
   complicated by, abnormal cervix
 cheloid L91.0
 chorioretinal H31.00-•
  posterior pole macula H31.01-•
  postsurgical H59.81-•
  solar retinopathy H31.02-•
  specified type NEC H31.09-•

Scar, scarring *(Continued)*
 choroid —*see* Scar, chorioretinal
 conjunctiva H11.24-•
 cornea H17.9
  xerophthalmic —*see also* Opacity, cornea
   vitamin A deficiency E50.6
 duodenum, obstructive K31.5
 hypertrophic L91.0
 keloid L91.0
 labia N90.89
 lung (base) J98.4
 macula —*see* Scar, chorioretinal, posterior
  pole
 muscle M62.89
 myocardium, myocardial I25.2
 painful L90.5
 posterior pole (eye) —*see* Scar, chorioretinal,
  posterior pole
 retina —*see* Scar, chorioretinal
 trachea J39.8
 transmural uterine, in pregnancy O34.29
 uterus N85.8
  in pregnancy O34.29
 vagina N89.8
  postoperative N99.2
 vulva N90.89
Scarabiasis B88.2
➠**Scarlatina** (anginosa) (maligna) A38.9
 myocarditis (acute) A38.1
  old —*see* Myocarditis
 otitis media A38.0
▶ulcerosa A38.8
Scarlet fever (albuminuria) (angina) A38.9
Schamberg's disease (progressive pigmentary
  dermatosis) L81.7
Schatzki's ring (acquired) (esophagus) (lower)
  K22.2
 congenital Q39.3
Schaufenster krankheit I20.8
Schaumann's
 benign lymphogranulomatosis D86.1
 disease or syndrome —*see* Sarcoidosis
Scheie's syndrome E76.03
Schenck's disease B42.1
Scheuermann's disease or osteochondrosis —
  see Osteochondrosis, juvenile, spine
Schilder (-Flatau) disease G37.0
Schilling-type monocytic leukemia C93.0-•
Schimmelbusch's disease, cystic mastitis, or
  hyperplasia —*see* Mastopathy, cystic
Schistosoma infestation —*see* Infestation,
  Schistosoma
Schistosomiasis B65.9
 with muscle disorder B65.9 [M63.80]
  ankle B65.9 [M63.87-•]
  foot B65.9 [M63.87-•]
  forearm B65.9 [M63.83-•]
  hand B65.9 [M63.84-•]
  lower leg B65.9 [M63.86-•]
  multiple sites B65.9 [M63.89]
  pelvic region B65.9 [M63.85-•]
  shoulder region B65.9 [M63.81-•]
  specified site NEC B65.9 [M63.88]
  thigh B65.9 [M63.85-•]
  upper arm B65.9 [M63.82-•]
 Asiatic B65.2
 bladder B65.0
 chestermani B65.8
 colon B65.1
 cutaneous B65.3
 due to
  S. haematobium B65.0
  S. japonicum B65.2
  S. mansoni B65.1
  S. mattheii B65.8
 Eastern B65.2
 genitourinary tract B65.0
 intestinal B65.1
 lung NEC B65.9 [J99]
  pneumonia B65.9 [J17]
 Manson's (intestinal) B65.1

Schistosomiasis *(Continued)*
 oriental B65.2
 pulmonary NEC B65.9 [J99]
  pneumonia B65.9
 Schistosoma
  haematobium B65.0
  japonicum B65.2
  mansoni B65.1
 specified type NEC B65.8
 urinary B65.0
 vesical B65.0
Schizencephaly Q04.6
Schizoaffective psychosis F25.9
Schizodontia K00.2
Schizoid personality F60.1
Schizophrenia, schizophrenic F20.9
 acute (brief) (undifferentiated) F23
 atypical (form) F20.3
 borderline F21
 catalepsy F20.2
 catatonic (type) (excited) (withdrawn) F20.2
 cenesthopathic, cenesthesiopathic F20.89
 childhood type F84.5
 chronic undifferentiated F20.5
 cyclic F25.0
 disorganized (type) F20.1
 flexibilitas cerea F20.2
 hebephrenic (type) F20.1
 incipient F21
 latent F21
 negative type F20.5
 paranoid (type) F20.0
 paraphrenic F20.0
 post-psychotic depression F32.89
 prepsychotic F21
 prodromal F21
 pseudoneurotic F21
 pseudopsychopathic F21
 reaction F23
 residual (state) (type) F20.5
 restzustand F20.5
 schizoaffective (type) —*see* Psychosis,
  schizoaffective
 simple (type) F20.89
 simplex F20.89
 specified type NEC F20.89
▶spectrum and other psychotic disorder F29
 ▶specified NEC F28
 stupor F20.2
 syndrome of childhood F84.5
 undifferentiated (type) F20.3
  chronic F20.5
Schizothymia (persistent) F60.1
Schlatter-Osgood disease or
  osteochondrosis —*see* Osteochondrosis,
  juvenile, tibia
Schlatter's tibia —*see* Osteochondrosis,
  juvenile, tibia
Schmidt's syndrome (polyglandular,
  autoimmune) E31.0
Schmincke's carcinoma or tumor —*see*
  Neoplasm, nasopharynx, malignant
Schmitz (-Stutzer) dysentery A03.0
Schmorl's disease or nodes
 lumbar region M51.46
 lumbosacral region M51.47
 sacrococcygeal region M53.3
 thoracic region M51.44
 thoracolumbar region M51.45
Schneiderian
 papilloma —*see* Neoplasm, nasopharynx
  benign
  specified site —*see* Neoplasm, benign, by
   site
  unspecified site D14.0
 specified site —*see* Neoplasm, malignant, by
  site
 unspecified site C30.0
Scholte's syndrome (malignant carcinoid) E34.0
Scholz (-Bielchowsky-Henneberg) disease or
  syndrome E75.25
Schönlein (-Henoch) disease or purpura
  (primary) (rheumatic) D69.0

Schottmuller's disease A01.4
Schroeder's syndrome (endocrine
    hypertensive) E27.0
Schüller-Christian disease or syndrome C96.5
Schultze's type acroparesthesia, simple I73.89
Schultz's disease or syndrome —*see*
    Agranulocytosis
Schwalbe-Ziehen-Oppenheim disease G24.1
Schwannoma —*see also* Neoplasm, nerve,
    benign
   malignant —*see also* Neoplasm, nerve,
     malignant
     with rhabdomyoblastic differentiation —
      see Neoplasm, nerve, malignant
   melanocytic —*see* Neoplasm, nerve, benign
   pigmented —*see* Neoplasm, nerve, benign
Schwannomatosis Q85.03
Schwartz (-Jampel) syndrome G71.13
Schwartz-Bartter syndrome E22.2
Schweniger-Buzzi anetoderma L90.1
Sciatic —*see* condition
Sciatica (infective)
   with lumbago M54.4-●
     due to intervertebral disc disorder —*see*
      Disorder, disc, with, radiculopathy
   due to displacement of intervertebral disc
     (with lumbago) —*see* Disorder, disc,
     with, radiculopathy
   wallet M54.3-●
Scimitar syndrome Q26.8
Sclera —*see* condition
Sclerectasia H15.84-●
Scleredema
   adultorum —*see* Sclerosis, systemic
   Buschke's —*see* Sclerosis, systemic
   newborn P83.0
Sclerema (adiposum) (edematosum)
    (neonatorum) (newborn) P83.0
   adultorum —*see* Sclerosis, systemic
Scleriasis —*see* Scleroderma
Scleritis H15.00-●
   with corneal involvement H15.04-●
   anterior H15.01-●
   brawny H15.02-●
   in (due to) zoster B02.34
   posterior H15.03-●
   specified type NEC H15.09-●
   syphilitic A52.71
   tuberculous (nodular) A18.51
Sclerochoroiditis H31.8
Scleroconjunctivitis —*see* Scleritis
Sclerocystic ovary syndrome E28.2
Sclerodactyly, sclerodactylia L94.3
Scleroderma, sclerodermia (acrosclerotic)
    (diffuse) (generalized) (progressive)
    (pulmonary) —*see also* Sclerosis, systemic
    M34.9-●
   circumscribed L94.0
   linear L94.1
   localized L94.0
➧ newborn P83.88
   systemic M34.9
Sclerokeratitis H16.8
   tuberculous A18.52
Scleroma nasi A48.8
Scleromalacia (perforans) H15.05-●
Scleromyxedema L98.5
Sclérose en plaques G35
Sclerosis, sclerotic
   adrenal (gland) E27.8
   Alzheimer's —*see* Disease, Alzheimer's
   amyotrophic (lateral) G12.21
   aorta, aortic I70.0
     valve —*see* Endocarditis, aortic
   artery, arterial, arteriolar, arteriovascular —
     see Arteriosclerosis
   ascending multiple G35
   brain (generalized) (lobular) G37.9
     artery, arterial I67.2
     diffuse G37.0
     disseminated G35

Sclerosis, sclerotic (*Continued*)
   brain (*Continued*)
     insular G35
     Krabbe's E75.23
     miliary G35
     multiple G35
     presenile (Alzheimer's) —*see* Disease,
      Alzheimer's, early onset
     senile (arteriosclerotic) I67.2
     stem, multiple G35
     tuberous Q85.1
   bulbar, multiple G35
   bundle of His I44.39
   cardiac —*see* Disease, heart, ischemic,
     atherosclerotic
   cardiorenal —*see* Hypertension, cardiorenal
   cardiovascular —*see also* Disease,
     cardiovascular
     renal —*see* Hypertension, cardiorenal
   cerebellar —*see* Sclerosis, brain
   cerebral —*see* Sclerosis, brain
   cerebrospinal (disseminated) (multiple) G35
   cerebrovascular I67.2
   choroid —*see* Degeneration, choroid
   combined (spinal cord) —*see also*
     Degeneration, combined
     multiple G35
   concentric (Balo) G37.5
   cornea —*see* Opacity, cornea
   coronary (artery) I25.10
     with angina pectoris —*see* Arteriosclerosis,
      coronary (artery),
   corpus cavernosum
     female N90.89
     male N48.6
   diffuse (brain) (spinal cord) G37.0
   disseminated G35
   dorsal G35
   dorsolateral (spinal cord) —*see* Degeneration,
     combined
   endometrium N85.5
   extrapyramidal G25.9
   eye, nuclear (senile) —*see* Cataract, senile,
     nuclear
   focal and segmental (glomerular) —*see also*
     N00-N07 with fourth character .1 N05.1
   Friedreich's (spinal cord) G11.1
   funicular (spermatic cord) N50.89
   general (vascular) —*see* Arteriosclerosis
   gland (lymphatic) I89.8
   hepatic K74.1
     alcoholic K70.2
   hereditary
     cerebellar G11.9
     spinal (Friedreich's ataxia) G11.1
   hippocampal G93.81
   insular G35
   kidney —*see* Sclerosis, renal
   larynx J38.7
➧ lateral (amyotrophic) (descending) (spinal)
     G12.21
   ▶ primary G12.23
   lens, senile nuclear —*see* Cataract, senile,
     nuclear
   liver K74.1
     with fibrosis K74.2
      alcoholic K70.2
     alcoholic K70.2
     cardiac K76.1
   lung —*see* Fibrosis, lung
   mastoid —*see* Mastoiditis, chronic
   mesial temporal G93.81
   mitral I05.8
   Mönckeberg's (medial) —*see* Arteriosclerosis,
     extremities
   multiple (brain stem) (cerebral) (generalized)
     (spinal cord) G35
   myocardium, myocardial —*see* Disease, heart,
     ischemic, atherosclerotic
   nuclear (senile), eye —*see* Cataract, senile,
     nuclear

Sclerosis, sclerotic (*Continued*)
   ovary N83.8
   pancreas K86.89
   penis N48.6
   peripheral arteries —*see* Arteriosclerosis,
     extremities
   plaques G35
   pluriglandular E31.8
   polyglandular E31.8
   posterolateral (spinal cord) —*see*
     Degeneration, combined
   presenile (Alzheimer's) —*see* Disease,
     Alzheimer's, early onset
➧ primary, lateral G12.23
   progressive, systemic M34.0
   pulmonary —*see* Fibrosis, lung
     artery I27.0
     valve (heart) —*see* Endocarditis,
      pulmonary
   renal N26.9
     with
      cystine storage disease E72.09
      hypertensive heart disease (conditions in
       I11) —*see* Hypertension, cardiorenal
     arteriolar (hyaline) (hyperplastic) —*see*
      Hypertension, kidney
   retina (senile) (vascular) H35.00
   senile (vascular) —*see* Arteriosclerosis
   spinal (cord) (progressive) G95.89
     ascending G61.0
     combined —*see also* Degeneration,
      combined
      multiple G35
      syphilitic A52.11
     disseminated G35
     dorsolateral —*see* Degeneration,
      combined
     hereditary (Friedreich's) (mixed form)
      G11.1
➧   lateral (amyotrophic) G12.23
     multiple G35
     posterior (syphilitic) A52.11
   stomach K31.89
   subendocardial, congenital I42.4
   systemic M34.9
     with
      lung involvement M34.81
      myopathy M34.82
      polyneuropathy M34.83
     drug-induced M34.2
     due to chemicals NEC M34.2
     progressive M34.0
     specified NEC M34.89
   temporal (mesial) G93.81
   tricuspid (heart) (valve) I07.8
   tuberous (brain) Q85.1
   tympanic membrane —*see* Disorder,
     tympanic membrane, specified NEC
   valve, valvular (heart) —*see* Endocarditis
   vascular —*see* Arteriosclerosis
   vein I87.8
Scoliosis (acquired) (postural) M41.9
   adolescent (idiopathic) —*see* Scoliosis,
     idiopathic, adolescent
   congenital Q67.5
     due to bony malformation Q76.3
     failure of segmentation (hemivertebra)
      Q76.3
     hemivertebra fusion Q76.3
     postural Q67.5
   idiopathic M41.20
     adolescent M41.129
      cervical region M41.122
      cervicothoracic region M41.123
      lumbar region M41.126
      lumbosacral region M41.127
      thoracic region M41.124
      thoracolumbar region
       M41.125
     cervical region M41.22
     cervicothoracic region M41.23

S

Scoliosis (Continued)
 idiopathic (Continued)
  infantile M41.00
   cervical region M41.02
   cervicothoracic region M41.03
   lumbar region M41.06
   lumbosacral region M41.07
   sacrococcygeal region M41.08
   thoracic region M41.04
   thoracolumbar region M41.05
  juvenile M41.119
   cervical region M41.112
   cervicothoracic region M41.113
   lumbar region M41.116
   lumbosacral region M41.117
   thoracic region M41.114
   thoracolumbar region M41.115
  lumbar region M41.26
  lumbosacral region M41.27
  thoracic region M41.24
  thoracolumbar region M41.25
 infantile —see Scoliosis, idiopathic,
   infantile
 neuromuscular M41.40
  cervical region M41.42
  cervicothoracic region M41.43
  lumbar region M41.46
  lumbosacral region M41.47
  occipito-atlanto-axial region M41.41
  thoracic region M41.44
  thoracolumbar region M41.45
 paralytic —see Scoliosis, neuromuscular
 postradiation therapy M96.5
 rachitic (late effect or sequelae) E64.3
   [M49.80]
  cervical region E64.3 [M49.82]
  cervicothoracic region E64.3 [M49.83]
  lumbar region E64.3 [M49.86]
  lumbosacral region E64.3 [M49.87]
  multiple sites E64.3 [M49.89]
  occipito-atlanto-axial region E64.3
   [M49.81]
  sacrococcygeal region E64.3 [M49.88]
  thoracic region E64.3 [M49.84]
  thoracolumbar region E64.3 [M49.85]
 sciatic M54.4-●
 secondary (to) NEC M41.50
  cerebral palsy, Friedreich's ataxia,
    poliomyelitis, neuromuscular
    disorders —see Scoliosis,
    neuromuscular
  cervical region M41.52
  cervicothoracic region M41.53
  lumbar region M41.56
  lumbosacral region M41.57
  thoracic region M41.54
  thoracolumbar region M41.55
 specified form NEC M41.80
  cervical region M41.82
  cervicothoracic region M41.83
  lumbar region M41.86
  lumbosacral region M41.87
  thoracic region M41.84
  thoracolumbar region M41.85
 thoracogenic M41.30
  thoracic region M41.34
  thoracolumbar region M41.35
 tuberculous A18.01
Scoliotic pelvis
 with disproportion (fetopelvic) O33.0
  causing obstructed labor O65.0
Scorbutus, scorbutic —see also Scurvy
 anemia D53.2
Score, NIHSS (National Institutes of Health
   Stroke Scale) R29.7-●
Scotoma (arcuate) (Bjerrum) (central) (ring) —
   see also Defect, visual field, localized,
   scotoma
 scintillating H53.19
Scratch —see Abrasion
Scratchy throat R09.89

Screening (for) Z13.9
 alcoholism Z13.89
 anemia Z13.0
 anomaly, congenital Z13.89
➥ antenatal, of mother —see also Encounter,
   antenatal Z36.9
 arterial hypertension Z13.6
 arthropod-borne viral disease NEC Z11.59
 bacteriuria, asymptomatic Z13.89
 behavioral disorder Z13.89
 brain injury, traumatic Z13.850
 bronchitis, chronic Z13.83
 brucellosis Z11.2
 cardiovascular disorder Z13.6
 cataract Z13.5
 chlamydial diseases Z11.8
 cholera Z11.0
 chromosomal abnormalities (nonprocreative)
   NEC Z13.79
 colonoscopy Z12.11
 congenital
  dislocation of hip Z13.89
  eye disorder Z13.5
  malformation or deformation Z13.89
 contamination NEC Z13.88
 cystic fibrosis Z13.228
 dengue fever Z11.59
 dental disorder Z13.84
 depression Z13.89
 developmental handicap Z13.42
  in early childhood Z13.42
  infant Z13.41
 diabetes mellitus Z13.1
 diphtheria Z11.2
 disability, intellectual Z13.42
  infant Z13.41
 disease or disorder Z13.9
  bacterial NEC Z11.2
   intestinal infectious Z11.0
   respiratory tuberculosis Z11.1
  blood or blood-forming organ Z13.0
  cardiovascular Z13.6
  Chagas' Z11.6
  chlamydial Z11.8
  dental Z13.89
  developmental Z13.42
   in child Z13.42
   infant Z13.41
  digestive tract NEC Z13.818
   lower GI Z13.811
   upper GI Z13.810
  ear Z13.5
  endocrine Z13.29
  eye Z13.5
  genitourinary Z13.89
  heart Z13.6
  human immunodeficiency virus (HIV)
    infection Z11.4
  immunity Z13.0
  infection
   intestinal Z11.0
    specified NEC Z11.6
  infectious Z11.9
  mental Z13.89
  metabolic Z13.228
  neurological Z13.89
  nutritional Z13.21
   metabolic Z13.228
    lipoid disorders Z13.220
  protozoal Z11.6
   intestinal Z11.0
  respiratory Z13.83
  rheumatic Z13.828
  rickettsial Z11.8
  sexually-transmitted NEC Z11.3
   human immunodeficiency virus (HIV)
    Z11.4
  sickle-cell (trait) Z13.0
  skin Z13.89
  specified NEC Z13.89
  spirochetal Z11.8

Screening (Continued)
 disease or disorder (Continued)
  thyroid Z13.29
  vascular Z13.6
  venereal Z11.3
  viral NEC Z11.59
   human immunodeficiency virus (HIV)
    Z11.4
   intestinal Z11.0
 elevated titer Z13.89
 emphysema Z13.83
 encephalitis, viral (mosquito- or tick-borne)
   Z11.59
 exposure to contaminants (toxic) Z13.88
 fever
  dengue Z11.59
  hemorrhagic Z11.59
  yellow Z11.59
 filariasis Z11.6
 galactosemia Z13.228
 gastrointestinal condition Z13.818
 genetic (nonprocreative)- for procreative
    management —see Testing, genetic, for
    procreative management
  disease carrier status (nonprocreative)
    Z13.71
  specified NEC (nonprocreative) Z13.79
 genitourinary condition Z13.89
 glaucoma Z13.5
 gonorrhea Z11.3
 gout Z13.89
 helminthiasis (intestinal) Z11.6
 hematopoietic malignancy Z12.89
 hemoglobinopathies NEC Z13.0
 hemorrhagic fever Z11.59
 Hodgkin disease Z12.89
 human immunodeficiency virus (HIV) Z11.4
 human papillomavirus Z11.51
 hypertension Z13.6
 immunity disorders Z13.0
 infection
  mycotic Z11.8
  parasitic Z11.8
 ingestion of radioactive substance Z13.88
 intellectual disability Z13.42
  infant Z13.41
 intestinal
  helminthiasis Z11.6
  infectious disease Z11.0
 leishmaniasis Z11.6
 leprosy Z11.2
 leptospirosis Z11.8
 leukemia Z12.89
 lymphoma Z12.89
 malaria Z11.6
 malnutrition Z13.29
  metabolic Z13.228
  nutritional Z13.21
 measles Z11.59
 mental disorder Z13.89
 metabolic errors, inborn Z13.228
 multiphasic Z13.89
 musculoskeletal disorder Z13.828
  osteoporosis Z13.820
 mycoses Z11.8
 myocardial infarction (acute) Z13.6
 neoplasm (malignant) (of) Z12.9
  bladder Z12.6
  blood Z12.89
  breast Z12.39
   routine mammogram Z12.31
  cervix Z12.4
  colon Z12.11
  genitourinary organs NEC Z12.79
   bladder Z12.6
   cervix Z12.4
   ovary Z12.73
   prostate Z12.5
   testis Z12.71
   vagina Z12.72
  hematopoietic system Z12.89

▶ New   ⇒ Revised   ~~deleted~~ Deleted   ● Use Additional Character(s)

Screening *(Continued)*
  neoplasm *(Continued)*
    intestinal tract Z12.10
      colon Z12.11
      rectum Z12.12
      small intestine Z12.13
    lung Z12.2
    lymph (glands) Z12.89
    nervous system Z12.82
    oral cavity Z12.81
    prostate Z12.5
    rectum Z12.12
    respiratory organs Z12.2
    skin Z12.83
    small intestine Z12.13
    specified site NEC Z12.89
    stomach Z12.0
  nephropathy Z13.89
  nervous system disorders NEC Z13.858
  neurological condition Z13.89
  osteoporosis Z13.820
  parasitic infestation Z11.9
    specified NEC Z11.8
  phenylketonuria Z13.228
  plague Z11.2
  poisoning (chemical) (heavy metal) Z13.88
  poliomyelitis Z11.59
  postnatal, chromosomal abnormalities
    Z13.89
  ▶ prenatal, of mother —*see also* Encounter,
    antenatal Z36.9
  protozoal disease Z11.6
    intestinal Z11.0
  pulmonary tuberculosis Z11.1
  radiation exposure Z13.88
  respiratory condition Z13.83
  respiratory tuberculosis Z11.1
  rheumatoid arthritis Z13.828
  rubella Z11.59
  schistosomiasis Z11.6
  sexually-transmitted disease NEC Z11.3
    human immunodeficiency virus (HIV)
      Z11.4
  sickle-cell disease or trait Z13.0
  skin condition Z13.89
  sleeping sickness Z11.6
  special Z13.9
    specified NEC Z13.89
  syphilis Z11.3
  tetanus Z11.2
  trachoma Z11.8
  traumatic brain injury Z13.850
  trypanosomiasis Z11.6
  tuberculosis, respiratory Z11.1
  venereal disease Z11.3
  viral encephalitis (mosquito- or tick-borne)
    Z11.59
  whooping cough Z11.2
  worms, intestinal Z11.6
  yaws Z11.8
  yellow fever Z11.59
Scrofula, scrofulosis (tuberculosis of cervical
  lymph glands) A18.2
Scrofulide (primary) (tuberculous) A18.4
Scrofuloderma, scrofulodermia (any site)
  (primary) A18.4
Scrofulosus lichen (primary) (tuberculous)
  A18.4
Scrofulous —*see* condition
Scrotal tongue K14.5
Scrotum —*see* condition
Scurvy, scorbutic E54
  anemia D53.2
  gum E54
  infantile E54
  rickets E55.0 *[M90.80]*
Sealpox B08.62
Seasickness T75.3
Seatworm (infection) (infestation) B80
Sebaceous —*see also* condition
  cyst —*see* Cyst, sebaceous

Seborrhea, seborrheic L21.9
  capillitii R23.8
  capitis L21.0
  dermatitis L21.9
    infantile L21.1
  eczema L21.9
    infantile L21.1
  sicca L21.0
Seckel's syndrome Q87.1
Seclusion, pupil —*see* Membrane, pupillary
Second hand tobacco smoke exposure (acute)
  (chronic) Z77.22
  in the perinatal period P96.81
Secondary
  dentin (in pulp) K04.3
  neoplasm, secondaries —*see* Table of
    Neoplasms, secondary
Secretion
  antidiuretic hormone, inappropriate E22.2
  catecholamine, by pheochromocytoma E27.5
  hormone
    antidiuretic, inappropriate (syndrome)
      E22.2
    by
      carcinoid tumor E34.0
      pheochromocytoma E27.5
    ectopic NEC E34.2
  urinary
    excessive R35.8
    suppression R34
Section
  nerve, traumatic —*see* Injury, nerve
Sedative, hypnotic, or anxiolytic-induced
  anxiety disorder F13.980
  bipolar and related disorder F13.94
  delirium F13.921
  depressive disorder F13.94
  major neurocognitive disorder F13.97
  mild neurocognitive disorder F13.988
  psychotic disorder F13.959
  sexual dysfunction F13.981
  sleep disorder F13.982
Segmentation, incomplete (congenital) —*see*
  also Fusion
  bone NEC Q78.8
  lumbosacral (joint) (vertebra) Q76.49
Seitelberger's syndrome (infantile neuraxonal
  dystrophy) G31.89
Seizure(s) —*see also* Convulsions R56.9
  akinetic —*see* Epilepsy, generalized, specified
    NEC
  atonic —*see* Epilepsy, generalized, specified
    NEC
  autonomic (hysterical) F44.5
  convulsive —*see* Convulsions
  cortical (focal) (motor) —*see* Epilepsy,
    localization-related, symptomatic, with
    simple partial seizures
  disorder —*see also* Epilepsy G40.909
  due to stroke —*see* Sequelae (of), disease,
    cerebrovascular, by type, specified NEC
  epileptic —*see* Epilepsy
  febrile (simple) R56.00
    with status epilepticus G40.901
    complex (atypical) (complicated) R56.01
      with status epilepticus G40.901
  grand mal G40.409
    intractable G40.419
      with status epilepticus G40.411
      without status epilepticus G40.419
    not intractable G40.409
      with status epilepticus G40.401
      without status epilepticus G40.409
  heart —*see* Disease, heart
  hysterical F44.5
  intractable G40.919
    with status epilepticus G40.911
  Jacksonian (focal) (motor type) (sensory
    type) —*see* Epilepsy, localization-related,
    symptomatic, with simple partial
    seizures

Seizure *(Continued)*
  newborn P90
  nonspecific epileptic
    atonic —*see* Epilepsy, generalized, specified
      NEC
    clonic —*see* Epilepsy, generalized, specified
      NEC
    myoclonic —*see* Epilepsy, generalized,
      specified NEC
    tonic —*see* Epilepsy, generalized, specified
      NEC
    tonic-clonic —*see* Epilepsy, generalized,
      specified NEC
  partial, developing into secondarily
    generalized seizures
    complex —*see* Epilepsy, localization-
      related, symptomatic, with complex
      partial seizures
    simple —*see* Epilepsy, localization-related,
      symptomatic, with simple partial
      seizures
  petit mal G40.409
    intractable G40.419
      with status epilepticus G40.411
      without status epilepticus G40.419
    not intractable G40.409
      with status epilepticus G40.401
      without status epilepticus G40.409
  post traumatic R56.1
  recurrent G40.909
  specified NEC G40.89
  uncinate —*see* Epilepsy, localization-related,
    symptomatic, with complex partial
    seizures
Selenium deficiency, dietary E59
Self-damaging behavior (life-style) Z72.89
Self-harm (attempted)
  history (personal) Z91.5
    in family Z81.8
Self-mutilation (attempted)
  history (personal) Z91.5
    in family Z81.8
Self-poisoning
  history (personal) Z91.5
    in family Z81.8
  observation following (alleged) attempt Z03.6
Semicoma R40.1
Seminal vesiculitis N49.0
Seminoma C62.9- ●
  specified site —*see* Neoplasm, malignant, by
    site
Senear-Usher disease or syndrome L10.4
Senectus R54
Senescence (without mention of psychosis)
  R54
Senile, senility —*see also* condition R41.81
  with
    acute confusional state F05
    mental changes NOS F03
    psychosis NEC —*see* Psychosis, senile
  asthenia R54
  cervix (atrophic) N88.8
  debility R54
  endometrium (atrophic) N85.8
  fallopian tube (atrophic) —*see* Atrophy,
    fallopian tube
  heart (failure) R54
  ovary (atrophic) —*see* Atrophy, ovary
  premature E34.8
  vagina, vaginitis (atrophic) N95.2
  wart L82.1
Sensation
  burning (skin) R20.8
    tongue K14.6
  loss of R20.8
  prickling (skin) R20.2
  tingling (skin) R20.2
Sense loss
  smell —*see* Disturbance, sensation, smell
  taste —*see* Disturbance, sensation, taste
  touch R20.8

Sensibility disturbance (cortical) (deep)
(vibratory) R20.9
Sensitive, sensitivity —see also Allergy
carotid sinus G90.01
child (excessive) F93.8
cold, autoimmune D59.1
dentin K03.89
gluten (non-celiac) K90.41
latex Z91.040
methemoglobin D74.8
tuberculin, without clinical or radiological
symptoms R76.11
visual
glare H53.71
impaired contrast H53.72
Sensitiver Beziehungswahn F22
Sensitization, auto-erythrocytic D69.2
Separation
anxiety, abnormal (of childhood) F93.0
apophysis, traumatic - code as Fracture, by
site
choroid —see Detachment, choroid
epiphysis, epiphyseal
nontraumatic —see also
Osteochondropathy, specified type
NEC
upper femoral —see Slipped, epiphysis,
upper femoral
traumatic - code as Fracture, by site
fracture —see Fracture
infundibulum cardiac from right ventricle by
a partition Q24.3
joint (traumatic) (current) - code by site under
Dislocation
pubic bone, obstetrical trauma O71.6
retina, retinal —see Detachment, retina
symphysis pubis, obstetrical trauma O71.6
tracheal ring, incomplete, congenital Q32.1
Sepsis (generalized) (unspecified organism)
A41.9
with
organ dysfunction (acute) (multiple) R65.20
with septic shock R65.21
actinomycotic A42.7
adrenal hemorrhage syndrome
(meningococcal) A39.1
anaerobic A41.4
Bacillus anthracis A22.7
Brucella —see also Brucellosis A23.9
candidal B37.7
cryptogenic A41.9
due to device, implant or graft T85.79
arterial graft NEC T82.7
breast (implant) T85.79
catheter NEC T85.79
dialysis (renal) T82.7
intraperitoneal T85.71
infusion NEC T82.7
spinal (cranial) (epidural) (intrathecal)
(spinal) (subarachnoid)
(subdural) T85.735
urethral indwelling T83.511
urinary T83.518
ectopic or molar pregnancy O08.82
electronic (electrode) (pulse generator)
(stimulator)
bone T84.7
cardiac T82.7
nervous system T85.738
brain T85.731
neurostimulator generator T85.734
peripheral nerve T85.732
spinal cord T85.733
urinary T83.590
fixation, internal (orthopedic) —see
Complication, fixation device,
infection
gastrointestinal (bile duct) (esophagus)
T85.79
neurostimulator electrode (lead)
T85.732

Sepsis (Continued)
due to device, implant or graft (Continued)
genital T83.69
heart NEC T82.7
valve (prosthesis) T82.6
graft T82.7
joint prosthesis —see Complication, joint
prosthesis, infection
ocular (corneal graft) (orbital implant)
T85.79
orthopedic NEC T84.7
fixation device, internal —see
Complication, fixation device,
infection
specified NEC T85.79
vascular T82.7
ventricular intracranial (communicating)
shunt T85.730
during labor O75.3
Enterococcus A41.81
Erysipelothrix (rhusiopathiae) (erysipeloid)
A26.7
Escherichia coli (E. coli) A41.5
extraintestinal yersiniosis A28.2
following
abortion (subsequent episode) O08.0
current episode —see Abortion
ectopic or molar pregnancy O08.82
immunization T88.0
infusion, therapeutic injection or
transfusion NEC T80.29
gangrenous A41.9
gonococcal A54.86
Gram-negative (organism) A41.5
anaerobic A41.4
Haemophilus influenzae A41.3
herpesviral B00.7
intra-abdominal K65.1
intraocular —see Endophthalmitis,
purulent
Listeria monocytogenes A32.7
localized — code to specific localized
infection
⇒in operation wound T81.4
skin —see Abscess
malleus A24.0
melioidosis A24.1
meningeal —see Meningitis
meningococcal A39.4
acute A39.2
chronic A39.3
MSSA (Methicillin susceptible
Staphylococcus aureus) A41.01
newborn P36.9
due to
anaerobes NEC P36.5
Escherichia coli P36.4
Staphylococcus P36.30
aureus P36.2
specified NEC P36.39
Streptococcus P36.10
group B P36.0
specified NEC P36.19
specified NEC P36.8
Pasteurella multocida A28.0
pelvic, puerperal, postpartum, childbirth O85
pneumococcal A40.3
⇒postprocedural T81.4
puerperal, postpartum, childbirth (pelvic)
O85
Salmonella (arizonae) (cholerae-suis)
(enteritidis) (typhimurium) A02.1
severe R65.20
with septic shock R65.21
Shigella (see also Dysentery, bacillary) A03.9
skin, localized —see Abscess
specified organism NEC A41.89
Staphylococcus, staphylococcal A41.2
aureus (methicillin susceptible) (MSSA)
A41.01
methicillin resistant (MRSA) A41.02

Sepsis (Continued)
Staphylococcus, staphylococcal (Continued)
coagulase-negative A41.1
specified NEC A41.1
Streptococcus, streptococcal A40.9
agalactiae A40.1
group
A A40.0
B A40.1
D A41.81
neonatal P36.10
group B P36.0
specified NEC P36.19
pneumoniae A40.3
pyogenes A40.0
specified NEC A40.8
tracheostomy stoma J95.02
tularemic A21.7
umbilical, umbilical cord (newborn) —see
Sepsis, newborn
Yersinia pestis A20.7
Septate —see Septum
Septic —see condition
arm —see Cellulitis, upper limb
with lymphangitis —see Lymphangitis,
acute, upper limb
embolus —see Embolism
finger —see Cellulitis, digit
with lymphangitis —see Lymphangitis,
acute, digit
foot —see Cellulitis, lower limb
with lymphangitis —see Lymphangitis,
acute, lower limb
gallbladder (acute) K81.0
hand —see Cellulitis, upper limb
with lymphangitis —see Lymphangitis,
acute, upper limb
joint —see Arthritis, pyogenic or pyemic
leg —see Cellulitis, lower limb
with lymphangitis —see Lymphangitis,
acute, lower limb
nail —see also Cellulitis, digit
with lymphangitis —see Lymphangitis,
acute, digit
sore —see also Abscess
throat J02.0
streptococcal J02.0
spleen (acute) D73.89
teeth, tooth (pulpal origin) K04.4
throat —see Pharyngitis
thrombus —see Thrombosis
toe —see Cellulitis, digit
with lymphangitis —see Lymphangitis,
acute, digit
tonsils, chronic J35.01
with adenoiditis J35.03
uterus —see Endometritis
Septicemia A41.9
meaning sepsis —see Sepsis
Septum, septate (congenital) —see also
Anomaly, by site
anal Q42.3
with fistula Q42.2
aqueduct of Sylvius Q03.0
with spina bifida —see Spina bifida, by site,
with hydrocephalus
uterus (complete) (partial) Q51.2
vagina Q52.10
in pregnancy —see Pregnancy,
complicated by, abnormal
vagina
causing obstructed labor O65.5
longitudinal Q52.129
microperforate
left side Q52.124
right side Q52.123
nonobstruction Q52.120
obstructing Q52.129
left side Q52.122
right side Q52.121
transverse Q52.11

Sequelae (of) —*see also* condition
  abscess, intracranial or intraspinal (conditions in G06) G09
  amputation — code to injury with seventh character S
  burn and corrosion — code to injury with seventh character S
  calcium deficiency E64.8
  cerebrovascular disease —*see* Sequelae, disease, cerebrovascular
  childbirth O94
  contusion — code to injury with seventh character S
  corrosion —*see* Sequelae, burn and corrosion
  crushing injury — code to injury with seventh character S
  disease
    cerebrovascular I69.90
      alteration of sensation I69.998
      aphasia I69.920
      apraxia I69.990
      ataxia I69.993
      cognitive deficits I69.91
      disturbance of vision I69.998
      dysarthria I69.922
      dysphagia I69.991
      dysphasia I69.921
      facial droop I69.992
      facial weakness I69.992
      fluency disorder I69.923
      hemiplegia I69.95-●
      hemorrhage
        intracerebral —*see* Sequelae, hemorrhage, intracerebral
        intracranial, nontraumatic NEC — *see* Sequelae, hemorrhage, intracranial, nontraumatic
        subarachnoid —*see* Sequelae, hemorrhage, subarachnoid
      language deficit I69.928
      monoplegia
        ⇒lower limb I69.94-●
        upper limb I69.93-●
      paralytic syndrome I69.96-●
      specified effect NEC I69.998
      specified type NEC I69.80
        alteration of sensation I69.898
        aphasia I69.820
        apraxia I69.890
        ataxia I69.893
        cognitive deficits I69.81
        disturbance of vision I69.898
        dysarthria I69.822
        dysphagia I69.891
        dysphasia I69.821
        facial droop I69.892
        facial weakness I69.892
        fluency disorder I69.823
        hemiplegia I69.85-●
        language deficit I69.828
        monoplegia
          lower limb I69.84-●
          upper limb I69.83-●
        paralytic syndrome I69.86-●
        specified effect NEC I69.898
      speech deficit I69.928
        speech deficit I69.828
      stroke NOS —*see* Sequelae, stroke NOS
  dislocation — code to injury with seventh character S
  encephalitis or encephalomyelitis (conditions in G04) G09
    in infectious disease NEC B94.8
    viral B94.1
  external cause — code to injury with seventh character S
  foreign body entering natural orifice — code to injury with seventh character S
  fracture — code to injury with seventh character S

Sequelae (*Continued*)
  frostbite — code to injury with seventh character S
  Hansen's disease B92
  hemorrhage
    intracerebral I69.10
      alteration of sensation I69.198
      aphasia I69.120
      apraxia I69.190
      ataxia I69.193
      cognitive deficits I69.11
      disturbance of vision I69.198
      dysarthria I69.122
      dysphagia I69.191
      dysphasia I69.121
      facial droop I69.192
      facial weakness I69.192
      fluency disorder I69.123
      hemiplegia I69.15-●
      language deficit NEC I69.128
      monoplegia
        lower limb I69.14-●
        upper limb I69.13-●
      paralytic syndrome I69.16-●
      specified effect NEC I69.198
      speech deficit NEC I69.128
    intracranial, nontraumatic NEC I69.20
      alteration of sensation I69.298
      aphasia I69.220
      apraxia I69.290
      ataxia I69.293
      cognitive deficits I69.21
      disturbance of vision I69.298
      dysarthria I69.222
      dysphagia I69.291
      dysphasia I69.221
      facial droop I69.292
      facial weakness I69.292
      fluency disorder I69.223
      hemiplegia I69.25-●
      language deficit NEC I69.228
      monoplegia
        lower limb I69.24-●
        upper limb I69.23-●
      paralytic syndrome I69.26-●
      specified effect NEC I69.298
      speech deficit NEC I69.228
    subarachnoid I69.00
      alteration of sensation I69.098
      aphasia I69.020
      apraxia I69.090
      ataxia I69.093
      cognitive deficits —*see* subcategory I69.01-●
      disturbance of vision I69.098
      dysarthria I69.022
      dysphagia I69.091
      dysphasia I69.021
      facial droop I69.092
      facial weakness I69.092
      fluency disorder I69.023
      hemiplegia I69.05-●
      language deficit NEC I69.028
      monoplegia
        lower limb I69.04-●
        upper limb I69.03-●
      paralytic syndrome I69.06-●
      specified effect NEC I69.098
      speech deficit NEC I69.028
  hepatitis, viral B94.2
  hyperalimentation E68
  infarction
    cerebral I69.30
      alteration of sensation I69.398
      aphasia I69.320
      apraxia I69.390
      ataxia I69.393
      cognitive deficits I69.31
      disturbance of vision I69.398
      dysarthria I69.322
      dysphagia I69.391

Sequelae (*Continued*)
  infarction (*Continued*)
    cerebral (*Continued*)
      dysphasia I69.321
      facial droop I69.392
      facial weakness I69.392
      fluency disorder I69.323
      hemiplegia I69.35-●
      language deficit NEC I69.328
      monoplegia
        lower limb I69.34-●
        upper limb I69.33-●
      paralytic syndrome I69.36-●
      specified effect NEC I69.398
      speech deficit NEC I69.328
  infection, pyogenic, intracranial or intraspinal G09
  infectious disease B94.9
    specified NEC B94.8
  injury — code to injury with seventh character S
  leprosy B92
  meningitis
    bacterial (conditions in G00) G09
    other or unspecified cause (conditions in G03) G09
  muscle (and tendon) injury — code to injury with seventh character S
  myelitis —*see* Sequelae, encephalitis
  niacin deficiency E64.8
  nutritional deficiency E64.9
    specified NEC E64.8
  obstetrical condition O94
  parasitic disease B94.9
  phlebitis or thrombophlebitis of intracranial or intraspinal venous sinuses and veins (conditions in G08) G09
  poisoning — code to poisoning with seventh character S
    nonmedicinal substance —*see* Sequelae, toxic effect, nonmedicinal substance
  poliomyelitis (acute) B91
  pregnancy O94
  protein-energy malnutrition E64.0
  puerperium O94
  rickets E64.3
  selenium deficiency E64.8
  sprain and strain — code to injury with seventh character S
  stroke NOS I69.30
    alteration in sensation I69.398
    aphasia I69.320
    apraxia I69.390
    ataxia I69.393
    cognitive deficits I69.31
    disturbance of vision I69.398
    dysarthria I69.322
    dysphagia I69.391
    dysphasia I69.321
    facial droop I69.392
    facial weakness I69.392
    hemiplegia I69.35-●
    language deficit NEC I69.328
    monoplegia
      lower limb I69.34-●
      upper limb I69.33-●
    paralytic syndrome I69.36-●
    specified effect NEC I69.398
    speech deficit NEC I69.328
  tendon and muscle injury — code to injury with seventh character S
  thiamine deficiency E64.8
  trachoma B94.0
  tuberculosis B90.9
    bones and joints B90.2
    central nervous system B90.0
    genitourinary B90.1
    pulmonary (respiratory) B90.9
    specified organs NEC B90.8

Sequelae *(Continued)*
viral
  encephalitis B94.1
  hepatitis B94.2
vitamin deficiency NEC E64.8
  A E64.1
  B E64.8
  C E64.2
wound, open — code to injury with seventh character S
Sequestration —*see also* Sequestrum
disk —*see* Displacement, intervertebral disk
lung, congenital Q33.2
Sequestrum
bone —*see* Osteomyelitis, chronic
dental M27.2
jaw bone M27.2
orbit —*see* Osteomyelitis, orbit
sinus (accessory) (nasal) —*see* Sinusitis
Sequoiosis lung or pneumonitis J67.8
Serology for syphilis
doubtful
  with signs or symptoms - code by site and stage under Syphilis
  follow-up of latent syphilis —*see* Syphilis, latent
negative, with signs or symptoms — code by site and stage under Syphilis
positive A53.0
  with signs or symptoms - code by site and stage under Syphilis
reactivated A53.0
Seroma —*see also* Hematoma
postprocedural —*see* Complication, postprocedural, seroma
traumatic, secondary and recurrent T79.2
Seropurulent —*see* condition
Serositis, multiple K65.8
pericardial I31.1
peritoneal K65.8
Serous —*see* condition
Sertoli cell
adenoma
  specified site —*see* Neoplasm, benign, by site
  unspecified site
    female D27.9
    male D29.20
carcinoma
  specified site —*see* Neoplasm, malignant, by site
  unspecified site (male) C62.9-●
    female C56.9
tumor
  with lipid storage
    specified site —*see* Neoplasm, benign, by site
    unspecified site
      female D27.9
      male D29.20
  specified site —*see* Neoplasm, benign, by site
  unspecified site
    female D27.9
    male D29.20
Sertoli-Leydig cell tumor —*see* Neoplasm, benign, by site
specified site —*see* Neoplasm, benign, by site
unspecified site
  female D27.9
  male D29.20
Serum
allergy, allergic reaction —*see also* Reaction, serum T80.69
  shock —*see also* Shock, anaphylactic T80.59
arthritis —*see also* Reaction, serum T80.69
complication or reaction NEC —*see also* Reaction, serum T80.69

Serum *(Continued)*
disease NEC —*see also* Reaction, serum T80.69
hepatitis —*see also* Hepatitis, viral, type B carrier (suspected) of B18.1
intoxication —*see also* Reaction, serum T80.69
neuritis —*see also* Reaction, serum T80.69
neuropathy G61.1
poisoning NEC —*see also* Reaction, serum T80.69
rash NEC —*see also* Reaction, serum T80.69
reaction NEC —*see also* Reaction, serum T80.69
sickness NEC —*see also* Reaction, serum T80.69
urticaria —*see also* Reaction, serum T80.69
Sesamoiditis M25.8-●
Sever's disease or osteochondrosis —*see* Osteochondrosis, juvenile, tarsus
Severe sepsis R65.20
with septic shock R65.21
Sex
chromosome mosaics Q97.8
  lines with various numbers of X chromosomes Q97.2
education Z70.8
reassignment surgery status Z87.890
Sextuplet pregnancy —*see* Pregnancy, sextuplet
Sexual
function, disorder of (psychogenic) F52.9
immaturity (female) (male) E30.0
impotence (psychogenic) organic origin NEC —*see* Dysfunction, sexual, male
precocity (constitutional) (cryptogenic) (female) (idiopathic) (male) E30.1
Sexuality, pathologic —*see* Deviation, sexual
Sézary disease C84.1-●
Shadow, lung R91.8
Shaking palsy or paralysis —*see* Parkinsonism
Shallowness, acetabulum —*see* Derangement, joint, specified type NEC, hip
Shaver's disease J63.1
Sheath (tendon) —*see* condition
Sheathing, retinal vessels H35.01-●
Shedding
nail L60.8
premature, primary (deciduous) teeth K00.6
Sheehan's disease or syndrome E23.0
Shelf, rectal K62.89
Shell teeth K00.5
Shellshock (current) F43.0
lasting state —*see* Disorder, post-traumatic stress
Shield kidney Q63.1
Shift
auditory threshold (temporary) H93.24-●
mediastinal R93.8
Shifting sleep-work schedule (affecting sleep) G47.26
Shiga (-Kruse) dysentery A03.0
Shiga's bacillus A03.0
Shigella (dysentery) —*see* Dysentery, bacillary
Shigellosis A03.9
Group A A03.0
Group B A03.1
Group C A03.2
Group D A03.3
Shin splints S86.89
Shingles —*see* Herpes, zoster
Shipyard disease or eye B30.0
Shirodkar suture, in pregnancy —*see* Pregnancy, complicated by, incompetent cervix
Shock R57.9
with ectopic or molar pregnancy O08.3
adrenal (cortical) (Addisonian) E27.2
adverse food reaction (anaphylactic) —*see* Shock, anaphylactic, due to food
allergic —*see* Shock, anaphylactic

Shock *(Continued)*
anaphylactic T78.2
  chemical —*see* Table of Drugs and Chemicals
  due to drug or medicinal substance
    correct substance properly administered T88.6
    overdose or wrong substance given or taken (by accident) —*see* Table of Drugs and Chemicals, by drug, poisoning
  due to food (nonpoisonous) T78.00
    additives T78.06
    dairy products T78.07
    eggs T78.08
    fish T78.03
      shellfish T78.02
    fruit T78.04
    milk T78.07
    nuts T78.05
      multiple types T78.05
      peanuts T78.01
    peanuts T78.01
    seeds T78.05
    specified type NEC T78.09
    vegetable T78.04
  following sting(s) —*see* Venom
  immunization T80.52
  serum T80.59
    blood and blood products T80.51
    immunization T80.52
    specified NEC T80.59
    vaccination T80.52
anaphylactoid —*see* Shock, anaphylactic
anesthetic
  correct substance properly administered T88.2
  overdose or wrong substance given or taken —*see* Table of Drugs and Chemicals, by drug, poisoning
  specified anesthetic —*see* Table of Drugs and Chemicals, by drug, poisoning
cardiogenic R57.0
chemical substance —*see* Table of Drugs and Chemicals
complicating ectopic or molar pregnancy O08.3
culture —*see* Disorder, adjustment
drug
  due to correct substance properly administered T88.6
  overdose or wrong substance given or taken (by accident) —*see* Table of Drugs and Chemicals, by drug, poisoning
during or after labor and delivery O75.1
electric T75.4
  (taser) T75.4
endotoxic R65.21
  postprocedural (resulting from a procedure, not elsewhere classified) T81.12
following
  ectopic or molar pregnancy O08.3
  injury (immediate) (delayed) T79.4
  labor and delivery O75.1
food (anaphylactic) —*see* Shock, anaphylactic, due to food
from electroshock gun (taser) T75.4
gram-negative R65.21
  postprocedural (resulting from a procedure, not elsewhere classified) T81.12
hematologic R57.8
➡hemorrhagic R57.8
  surgery (intraoperative) (postoperative) T81.19
  trauma T79.4
hypovolemic R57.1
  surgical T81.19
  traumatic T79.4

Shock *(Continued)*
insulin E15
  therapeutic misadventure —*see* subcategory T38.3
kidney N17.0
  traumatic (following crushing) T79.5
lightning T75.01
liver K72.00
lung J80
obstetric O75.1
  with ectopic or molar pregnancy O08.3
  following ectopic or molar pregnancy O08.3
pleural (surgical) T81.19
  due to trauma T79.4
postprocedural (postoperative) T81.10
  with ectopic or molar pregnancy O08.3
  cardiogenic T81.11
  endotoxic T81.12
  following ectopic or molar pregnancy O08.3
  gram-negative T81.12
  hypovolemic T81.19
  septic T81.12
  specified type NEC T81.19
psychic F43.0
septic (due to severe sepsis) R65.21
specified NEC R57.8
surgical T81.10
taser gun (taser) T75.4
therapeutic misadventure NEC T81.10
thyroxin
  overdose or wrong substance given or taken —*see* Table of Drugs and Chemicals, by drug, poisoning
toxic, syndrome A48.3
transfusion —*see* Complications, transfusion
traumatic (immediate) (delayed) T79.4
Shoemaker's chest M95.4
Short, shortening, shortness
arm (acquired) —*see also* Deformity, limb, unequal length
  congenital Q71.81-●
    forearm —*see* Deformity, limb, unequal length
bowel syndrome K91.2
breath R06.02
cervical (complicating pregnancy) O26.87-●
  non-gravid uterus N88.3
common bile duct, congenital Q44.5
cord (umbilical), complicating delivery O69.3
cystic duct, congenital Q44.5
esophagus (congenital) Q39.8
femur (acquired) —*see* Deformity, limb, unequal length, femur
  congenital —*see* Defect, reduction, lower limb, longitudinal, femur
frenum, frenulum, linguae (congenital) Q38.1
hip (acquired) —*see also* Deformity, limb, unequal length
  congenital Q65.89
leg (acquired) —*see also* Deformity, limb, unequal length
  congenital Q72.81-●
    lower leg —*see also* Deformity, limb, unequal length
limbed stature, with immunodeficiency D82.2
lower limb (acquired) —*see also* Deformity, limb, unequal length
  congenital Q72.81-●
organ or site, congenital NEC —*see* Distortion
palate, congenital Q38.5
radius (acquired) —*see also* Deformity, limb, unequal length
  congenital —*see* Defect, reduction, upper limb, longitudinal, radius
rib syndrome Q77.2
stature (child) (hereditary) (idiopathic) NEC R62.52
  constitutional E34.3
  due to endocrine disorder E34.3
  Laron-type E34.3

Short, shortening, shortness *(Continued)*
tendon —*see also* Contraction, tendon
  with contracture of joint —*see* Contraction, joint
    Achilles (acquired) M67.0-●
      congenital Q66.89
    congenital Q79.8
thigh (acquired) —*see also* Deformity, limb, unequal length, femur
  congenital —*see* Defect, reduction, lower limb, longitudinal, femur
tibialis anterior (tendon) —*see* Contraction, tendon
umbilical cord
  complicating delivery O69.3
upper limb, congenital —*see* Defect, reduction, upper limb, specified type NEC
urethra N36.8
uvula, congenital Q38.5
vagina (congenital) Q52.4
Shortsightedness —*see* Myopia
Shoshin (acute fulminating beriberi) E51.11
Shoulder —*see* condition
Shovel-shaped incisors K00.2
Shower, thromboembolic —*see* Embolism
Shunt
arterial-venous (dialysis) Z99.2
arteriovenous, pulmonary (acquired) I28.0
  congenital Q25.72
cerebral ventricle (communicating) in situ Z98.2
surgical, prosthetic, with complications —*see* Complications, cardiovascular, device or implant Shutdown, renal N28.9
Shutdown, renal N28.9
Shy-Drager syndrome G90.3
Sialadenitis, sialadenosis (any gland) (chronic) (periodic) (suppurative) —*see* Sialoadenitis
Sialectasia K11.8
Sialidosis E77.1
Sialitis, silitis (any gland) (chronic) (suppurative) —*see* Sialoadenitis
Sialoadenitis (any gland) (periodic) (suppurative) K11.20
acute K11.21
  recurrent K11.22
chronic K11.23
Sialoadenopathy K11.9
Sialoangitis —*see* Sialoadenitis
Sialodochitis (fibrinosa) —*see* Sialoadenitis
Sialodocholithiasis K11.5
Sialolithiasis K11.5
Sialometaplasia, necrotizing K11.8
Sialorrhea —*see also* Ptyalism
periodic —*see* Sialoadenitis
Sialosis K11.7
Siamese twin Q89.4
Sibling rivalry Z62.891
Sicard's syndrome G52.7
Sicca syndrome M35.00
with
  keratoconjunctivitis M35.01
  lung involvement M35.02
  myopathy M35.03
  renal tubulo-interstitial disorders M35.04
specified organ involvement NEC M35.09
Sick R69
or handicapped person in family Z63.79
  needing care at home Z63.6
sinus (syndrome) I49.5
Sick-euthyroid syndrome E07.81
Sickle-cell
anemia —*see* Disease, sickle-cell
trait D57.3
Sicklemia —*see also* Disease, sickle-cell
trait D57.3
Sickness
air (travel) T75.3
airplane T75.3
alpine T70.29

Sickness *(Continued)*
altitude T70.20
Andes T70.29
aviator's T70.29
balloon T70.29
car T75.3
compressed air T70.3
decompression T70.3
green D50.8
milk —*see* Poisoning, food, noxious
motion T75.3
mountain T70.29
  acute D75.1
protein —*see also* Reaction, serum T80.69
radiation T66
roundabout (motion) T75.3
sea T75.3
serum NEC —*see also* Reaction, serum T80.69
sleeping (African) B56.9
  by Trypanosoma B56.9
    brucei
      gambiense B56.0
      rhodesiense B56.1
    East African B56.1
    Gambian B56.0
    Rhodesian B56.1
    West African B56.0
swing (motion) T75.3
train (railway) (travel) T75.3
travel (any vehicle) T75.3
Sideropenia —*see* Anemia, iron deficiency
Siderosilicosis J62.8
Siderosis (lung) J63.4
eye (globe) —*see* Disorder, globe, degenerative, siderosis
Siemens' syndrome (ectodermal dysplasia) Q82.8
Sighing R06.89
psychogenic F45.8
Sigmoid —*see also* condition
flexure —*see* condition
kidney Q63.1
Sigmoiditis —*see also* Enteritis K52.9
infectious A09
noninfectious K52.9
Silfversköld's syndrome Q78.9
Silicosiderosis J62.8
Silicosis, silicotic (simple) (complicated) J62.8
with tuberculosis J65
Silicotuberculosis J65
Silo-fillers' disease J68.8
bronchitis J68.0
pneumonitis J68.0
pulmonary edema J68.1
Silver's syndrome Q87.1
Simian malaria B53.1
Simmonds' cachexia or disease E23.0
Simons' disease or syndrome (progressive lipodystrophy) E88.1
Simple, simplex —*see* condition
Simulation, conscious (of illness) Z76.5
Simultanagnosia (asimultagnosia) R48.3
Sin Nombre virus disease (Hantavirus) (cardio)-pulmonary syndrome B33.4
Sinding-Larsen disease or osteochondrosis —*see* Osteochondrosis, juvenile, patella
Singapore hemorrhagic fever A91
Singer's node or nodule J38.2
Single
atrium Q21.2
coronary artery Q24.5
umbilical artery Q27.0
ventricle Q20.4
Singultus R06.6
epidemicus B33.0
Sinus —*see also* Fistula
abdominal K63.89
arrest I45.5
arrhythmia I49.8
bradycardia R00.1
branchial cleft (internal) (external) Q18.0
coccygeal —*see* Sinus, pilonidal

Sinus *(Continued)*
dental K04.6
dermal (congenital) Q06.8
  with abscess Q06.8
  coccygeal, pilonidal —*see* Sinus,
    coccygeal
infected, skin NEC L08.89
marginal, ruptured or bleeding —*see*
  Hemorrhage, antepartum, specified
  cause NEC
medial, face and neck Q18.8
pause I45.5
pericranii Q01.9
pilonidal (infected) (rectum) L05.92
  with abscess L05.02
preauricular Q18.1
rectovaginal N82.3
Rokitansky-Aschoff (gallbladder) K82.8
sacrococcygeal (dermoid) (infected) —*see*
  Sinus, pilonidal
tachycardia R00.0
  paroxysmal I47.1
tarsi syndrome M25.57-●
testis N50.89
tract (postinfective) —*see* Fistula
urachus Q64.4
Sinusitis (accessory) (chronic) (hyperplastic)
(nasal) (nonpurulent) (purulent) J32.9
acute J01.90
  ethmoidal J01.20
    recurrent J01.21
  frontal J01.10
    recurrent J01.11
  involving more than one sinus, other than
    pansinusitis J01.80
    recurrent J01.81
  maxillary J01.00
    recurrent J01.01
  pansinusitis J01.40
    recurrent J01.41
  recurrent J01.91
  specified NEC J01.80
    recurrent J01.81
  sphenoidal J01.30
    recurrent J01.31
allergic —*see* Rhinitis, allergic
due to high altitude T70.1
ethmoidal J32.2
  acute J01.20
    recurrent J01.21
frontal J32.1
  acute J01.10
    recurrent J01.11
influenzal —*see* Influenza, with, respiratory
  manifestations NEC
involving more than one sinus but not
  pansinusitis J32.8
  acute J01.80
    recurrent J01.81
maxillary J32.0
  acute J01.00
    recurrent J01.01
sphenoidal J32.3
  acute J01.30
    recurrent J01.31
tuberculous, any sinus A15.8
Sinusitis-bronchiectasis-situs inversus
(syndrome) (triad) Q89.3
Sipple's syndrome E31.22
Sirenomelia (syndrome) Q87.2
Siriasis T67.0
Sirkari's disease B55.0
Siti A65
Situation, psychiatric F99
Situational
disturbance (transient) —*see* Disorder,
  adjustment
  acute F43.0
maladjustment —*see* Disorder, adjustment
reaction —*see* Disorder, adjustment
  acute F43.0

Situs inversus or transversus (abdominalis)
(thoracis) Q89.3
Sixth disease B08.20
due to human herpesvirus 6 B08.21
due to human herpesvirus 7 B08.22
Sjögren-Larsson syndrome Q87.1
Sjögren's syndrome or disease —*see* Sicca
syndrome
Skeletal —*see* condition
Skene's gland —*see* condition
Skenitis —*see* Urethritis
Skerljevo A65
Skevas-Zerfus disease —*see* Toxicity, venom,
marine animal, sea anemone
Skin —*see also* condition
clammy R23.1
donor —*see* Donor, skin
hidebound M35.9
Slate-dressers' or slate-miners' lung J62.8
Sleep
apnea —*see* Apnea, sleep
deprivation Z72.820
disorder or disturbance G47.9
  child F51.9
  nonorganic origin F51.9
  specified NEC G47.8
disturbance G47.9
  nonorganic origin F51.9
drunkenness F51.9
rhythm inversion G47.2-●
terrors F51.4
walking F51.3
  hysterical F44.89
Sleep hygiene
abuse Z72.821
inadequate Z72.821
poor Z72.821
Sleeping sickness —*see* Sickness, sleeping
Sleeplessness —*see* Insomnia
menopausal N95.11
Sleep-wake schedule disorder G47.20
Slim disease (in HIV infection) B20
Slipped, slipping
epiphysis (traumatic) —*see also*
  Osteochondropathy, specified type
  NEC
  capital femoral (traumatic)
    acute (on chronic) S79.01-●
  current traumatic - code as Fracture, by site
  upper femoral (nontraumatic) M93.00-●
    acute M93.01-●
      on chronic M93.03-●
    chronic M93.02-●
intervertebral disc —*see* Displacement,
  intervertebral disc
ligature, umbilical P51.8
patella —*see* Disorder, patella, derangement
  NEC
rib M89.8X8
sacroiliac joint —*see* subcategory M53.2
tendon —*see* Disorder, tendon
ulnar nerve, nontraumatic —*see* Lesion,
  nerve, ulnar
vertebra NEC —*see* Spondylolisthesis
Slocumb's syndrome E27.0
Sloughing (multiple) (phagedena) (skin) —*see*
also Gangrene
abscess —*see* Abscess
appendix K38.8
fascia —*see* Disorder, soft tissue, specified
  type NEC
scrotum N50.89
tendon —*see* Disorder, tendon
transplanted organ —*see* Rejection, transplant
ulcer —*see* Ulcer, skin
Slow
feeding, newborn P92.2
flow syndrome, coronary I20.8
heart(beat) R00.1
Slowing, urinary stream R39.198
Sluder's neuralgia (syndrome) G44.89

Slurred, slurring speech R47.81
Small (ness)
for gestational age —*see* Small for dates
introitus, vagina N89.6
kidney (unknown cause) N27.9
  bilateral N27.1
  unilateral N27.0
ovary (congenital) Q50.39
pelvis
  with disproportion (fetopelvic) O33.1
    causing obstructed labor O65.1
uterus N85.8
white kidney N03.9
Small-and-light-for-dates —*see* Small for
dates
Small-for-dates (infant) P05.10
with weight of
  499 grams or less P05.11
  500-749 grams P05.12
  750-999 grams P05.13
  1000-1249 grams P05.14
  1250-1499 grams P05.15
  1500-1749 grams P05.16
  1750-1999 grams P05.17
  2000-2499 grams P05.18
  2500 grams and over P05.19
specified NEC P05.19
Smallpox B03
Smearing, fecal R15.1
Smith-Lemli-Opitz syndrome E78.72
Smith's fracture S52.54-●
Smoker —*see* Dependence, drug, nicotine
Smoker's
bronchitis J41.0
cough J41.0
palate K13.24
throat J31.2
tongue K13.24
Smoking
passive Z77.22
Smothering spells R06.81
Snaggle teeth, tooth M26.39
Snapping
finger —*see* Trigger finger
hip —*see* Derangement, joint, specified type
  NEC, hip
  involving the iliotiblial band M76.3-●
knee —*see* Derangement, knee
  involving the iliotiblial band M76.3-●
Sneddon-Wilkinson disease or syndrome (subcorneal pustular dermatosis) L13.1
Sneezing (intractable) R06.7
Sniffing
cocaine
  abuse —*see* Abuse, drug, cocaine
  dependence —*see* Dependence, drug,
    cocaine
gasoline
  abuse —*see* Abuse, drug, inhalant
  dependence —*see* Dependence, drug,
    inhalant
glue (airplane)
  abuse —*see* Abuse, drug, inhalant
  drug dependence —*see* Dependence, drug,
    inhalant
Sniffles
newborn P28.89
Snoring R06.83
Snow blindness —*see* Photokeratitis
Snuffles (non-syphilitic) R06.5
newborn P28.89
syphilitic (infant) A50.05 *[J99]*
Social
exclusion Z60.4
  due to discrimination or persecution
    (perceived) Z60.5
migrant Z59.0
  acculturation difficulty Z60.3
rejection Z60.4
  due to discrimination or persecution
    Z60.5

Social *(Continued)*
  role conflict NEC Z73.5
  skills inadequacy NEC Z73.4
  transplantation Z60.3
Sodoku A25.0
Soemmerring's ring —*see* Cataract, secondary
Soft —*see also* condition
  nails L60.3
Softening
  bone —*see* Osteomalacia
  brain (necrotic) (progressive) G93.89
    congenital Q04.8
    embolic I63.4-•
    hemorrhagic —*see* Hemorrhage,
      intracranial, intracerebral
    occlusive I63.5-•
    thrombotic I63.3-•
  cartilage M94.2-•
    patella M22.4-•
  cerebellar —*see* Softening, brain
  cerebral —*see* Softening, brain
  cerebrospinal —*see* Softening, brain
  myocardial, heart —*see* Degeneration,
    myocardial
  spinal cord G95.89
  stomach K31.89
Soldier's
  heart F45.8
  patches I31.0
Solitary
  cyst, kidney N28.1
  kidney, congenital Q60.0
Solvent abuse —*see* Abuse, drug, inhalant
  dependence —*see* Dependence, drug,
    inhalant
Somatization reaction, somatic reaction —*see*
  Disorder, somatoform
Somnambulism F51.3
  hysterical F44.89
Somnolence R40.0
  nonorganic origin F51.11
Sonne dysentery A03.3
Soor B37.0
Sore
  bed —*see* Ulcer, pressure, by site
  chiclero B55.1
  Delhi B55.1
  desert —*see* Ulcer, skin
  eye H57.1-•
  Lahore B55.1
  mouth K13.79
    canker K12.0
  muscle M79.1
  Naga —*see* Ulcer, skin
  of skin —*see* Ulcer, skin - oriental B55.1
  pressure —*see* Ulcer, pressure, by site
  skin L98.9
  soft A57
  throat (acute) —*see also* Pharyngitis
    with influenza, flu, or grippe —*see*
      Influenza, with, respiratory
      manifestations NEC
    chronic J31.2
    coxsackie (virus) B08.5
    diphtheritic A36.0
    herpesviral B00.2
    influenzal —*see* Influenza, with, respiratory
      manifestations NEC
    septic J02.0
    streptococcal (ulcerative) J02.0
    viral NEC J02.8
      coxsackie B08.5
  tropical —*see* Ulcer, skin
  veldt —*see* Ulcer, skin
Soto's syndrome (cerebral gigantism) Q87.3
South African cardiomyopathy syndrome I42.8
Southeast Asian hemorrhagic fever A91
Spacing
  abnormal, tooth, teeth, fully erupted M26.30
  excessive, tooth, fully erupted M26.32
Spade-like hand (congenital) Q68.1

Spading nail L60.8
  congenital Q84.6
Spanish collar N47.1
Sparganosis B70.1
Spasm(s), spastic, spasticity —*see also* condition
  R25.2
  accommodation —*see* Spasm, of
    accommodation
  ampulla of Vater K83.4
  anus, ani (sphincter) (reflex) K59.4
    psychogenic F45.8
  artery I73.9
    cerebral G45.9
  Bell's G51.3
  bladder (sphincter, external or internal) N32.89
    psychogenic F45.8
  bronchus, bronchiole J98.01
  cardia K22.0
  cardiac I20.1
  carpopedal —*see* Tetany
  cerebral (arteries) (vascular) G45.9
  cervix, complicating delivery O62.4
  ciliary body (of accommodation) —*see* Spasm,
    of accommodation
  colon —*see also* Irritable, bowel K58.9
    with diarrhea K58.0
    psychogenic F45.8
  common duct K83.8
  compulsive —*see* Tic
  conjugate H51.8
  coronary (artery) I20.1
  diaphragm (reflex) R06.6
    epidemic B33.0
    psychogenic F45.8
  duodenum K59.8
  epidemic diaphragmatic (transient) B33.0
  esophagus (diffuse) K22.4
    psychogenic F45.8
  facial G51.3
  fallopian tube N83.8
  gastrointestinal (tract) K31.89
    psychogenic F45.8
  glottis J38.5
    hysterical F44.4
    psychogenic F45.8
      conversion reaction F44.4
    reflex through recurrent laryngeal nerve
      J38.5
  habit —*see* Tic
  heart I20.1
  hemifacial (clonic) G51.3
  hourglass —*see* Contraction, hourglass
  hysterical F44.4
  infantile —*see* Epilepsy, spasms
  inferior oblique, eye H51.8
  intestinal —*see also* Syndrome, irritable bowel
    K58.9
    psychogenic F45.8
  larynx, laryngeal J38.5
    hysterical F44.4
    psychogenic F45.8
      conversion reaction F44.4
  levator palpebrae superioris —*see* Disorder,
    eyelid function
  muscle NEC M62.838
    back M62.830
  nerve, trigeminal G51.0
  nervous F45.8
  nodding F98.4
  occupational F48.8
  oculogyric H51.8
    psychogenic F45.8
  of accommodation H52.53-•
  ophthalmic artery —*see* Occlusion, artery,
    retina
  perineal, female N94.89
  peroneo-extensor —*see also* Deformity, limb,
    flat foot
  pharynx (reflex) J39.2
    hysterical F45.8
    psychogenic F45.8

Spasm(s), spastic, spasticity *(Continued)*
  psychogenic F45.8
  pylorus NEC K31.3
    adult hypertrophic K31.89
    congenital or infantile Q40.0
    psychogenic F45.8
  rectum (sphincter) K59.4
    psychogenic F45.8
  retinal (artery) —*see* Occlusion, artery, retina
  sigmoid —*see also* Syndrome, irritable bowel
    K58.9
    psychogenic F45.8
  sphincter of Oddi K83.4
  stomach K31.89
    neurotic F45.8
  throat J39.2
    hysterical F45.8
    psychogenic F45.8
  tic F95.9
    chronic F95.1
    transient of childhood F95.0
  tongue K14.8
  torsion (progressive) G24.1
  trigeminal nerve —*see* Neuralgia, trigeminal
  ureter N13.5
  urethra (sphincter) N35.9
  uterus N85.8
    complicating labor O62.4
  vagina N94.2
    psychogenic F52.5
  vascular I73.9
  vasomotor I73.9
  vein NEC I87.8
  viscera —*see* Pain, abdominal
Spasmodic —*see* condition
Spasmophilia —*see* Tetany
Spasmus nutans F98.4
Spastic, spasticity —*see also* Spasm
  child (cerebral) (congenital) (paralysis) G80.1
Speaker's throat R49.8
Specific, specified —*see* condition
Speech
  defect, disorder, disturbance, impediment
    R47.9
    psychogenic, in childhood and adolescence
      F98.8
  slurring R47.81
  specified NEC R47.89
Spencer's disease A08.19
Spens' syndrome (syncope with heart block)
  I45.9
Sperm counts (fertility testing) Z31.41
  postvasectomy Z30.8
  reversal Z31.42
Spermatic cord —*see* condition
Spermatocele N43.40
  congenital Q55.4
  multiple N43.42
  single N43.41
Spermatocystitis N49.0
Spermatocytoma C62.9-•
  specified site —*see* Neoplasm, malignant, by
    site
Spermatorrhea N50.89
Sphacelus —*see* Gangrene
Sphenoidal —*see* condition
Sphenoiditis (chronic) —*see* Sinusitis,
  sphenoidal
Sphenopalatine ganglion neuralgia G90.09
Sphericity, increased, lens (congenital)
  Q12.4
Spherocytosis (congenital) (familial)
  (hereditary) D58.0
  hemoglobin disease D58.0
  sickle-cell (disease) D57.8-•
Spherophakia Q12.4
Sphincter —*see* condition
Sphincteritis, sphincter of Oddi —*see*
  Cholangitis
Sphingolipidosis E75.3
  specified NEC E75.29

Sphingomyelinosis E75.3
Spicule tooth K00.2
Spider
  bite —*see* Toxicity, venom, spider
  fingers —*see* Syndrome, Marfan's
  nevus I78.1
  toes —*see* Syndrome, Marfan's
  vascular I78.1
Spiegler-Fendt
  benign lymphocytoma L98.8
  sarcoid L08.89
Spielmeyer-Vogt disease E75.4
Spina bifida (aperta) Q05.9
  with hydrocephalus NEC Q05.4
  cervical Q05.5
    with hydrocephalus Q05.0
  dorsal Q05.6
    with hydrocephalus Q05.1
  lumbar Q05.7
    with hydrocephalus Q05.2
  lumbosacral Q05.7
    with hydrocephalus Q05.2
  occulta Q76.0
  sacral Q05.8
    with hydrocephalus Q05.3
  thoracic Q05.6
    with hydrocephalus Q05.1
  thoracolumbar Q05.6
    with hydrocephalus Q05.1
Spindle, Krukenberg's —*see* Pigmentation,
    cornea, posterior
Spine, spinal —*see* condition
Spiradenoma (eccrine) —*see* Neoplasm, skin,
    benign
Spirillosis A25.0
Spirillum
  minus A25.0
  obermeieri infection A68.0
Spirochetal —*see* condition
Spirochetosis A69.9
  arthritic, arthritica A69.9
  bronchopulmonary A69.8
  icterohemorrhagic A27.0
  lung A69.8
Spirometrosis B70.1
Spitting blood —*see* Hemoptysis
Splanchnoptosis K63.4
Spleen, splenic —*see* condition
Splenectasis —*see* Splenomegaly
Splenitis (interstitial) (malignant) (nonspecific)
    D73.89
  malarial —*see also* Malaria B54 *[D77]*
  tuberculous A18.85
Splenocele D73.89
Splenomegaly, splenomegalia (Bengal)
    (cryptogenic) (idiopathic) (tropical) R16.1
  with hepatomegaly R16.2
  cirrhotic D73.2
  congenital Q89.09
  congestive, chronic D73.2
  Egyptian B65.1
  Gaucher's E75.22
  malarial —*see also* Malaria B54 *[D77]*
  neutropenic D73.81
  Niemann-Pick —*see* Niemann-Pick disease or
      syndrome
  siderotic D73.2
  syphilitic A52.79
    congenital (early) A50.08 *[D77]*
Splenopathy D73.9
Splenoptosis D73.89
Splenosis D73.89
Splinter —*see* Foreign body, superficial, by site
Split, splitting
  foot Q72.7-●
  hand Q71.6
  heart sounds R01.2
  lip, congenital —*see* Cleft, lip
  nails L60.3
  urinary stream R39.13
Spondylarthrosis —*see* Spondylosis

Spondylitis (chronic) —*see also* Spondylopathy,
    inflammatory
  ankylopoietica —*see* Spondylitis, ankylosing
  ankylosing (chronic) M45.9
    with lung involvement M45.9 *[J99]*
    cervical region M45.2
    cervicothoracic region M45.3
    juvenile M08.1
    lumbar region M45.6
    lumbosacral region M45.7
    multiple sites M45.0
    occipito-atlanto-axial region M45.1
    sacrococcygeal region M45.8
    thoracic region M45.4
    thoracolumbar region M45.5
  atrophic (ligamentous) —*see* Spondylitis,
      ankylosing
  deformans (chronic) —*see* Spondylosis
  gonococcal A54.41
  gouty —*see also* Gout, by type, vertebrae
      M10.08
  in (due to)
    brucellosis A23.9 *[M49.80]*
      cervical region A23.9 *[M49.82]*
      cervicothoracic region A23.9 *[M49.83]*
      lumbar region A23.9 *[M49.86]*
      lumbosacral region A23.9 *[M49.87]*
      multiple sites A23.9 *[M49.89]*
      occipito-atlanto-axial region A23.9
          [M49.81]
      sacrococcygeal region A23.9 *[M49.88]*
      thoracic region A23.9 *[M49.84]*
      thoracolumbar region A23.9 *[M49.85]*
    enterobacteria —*see also* subcategory M49.8
        A04.9
    tuberculosis A18.01
  infectious NEC —*see* Spondylopathy,
      infective
  juvenile ankylosing (chronic) M08.1
  Kümmell's —*see* Spondylopathy, traumatic
  Marie-Strümpell —*see* Spondylitis,
      ankylosing
  muscularis —*see* Spondylopathy, specified
      NEC
  psoriatic L40.53
  rheumatoid —*see* Spondylitis, ankylosing
  rhizomelica —*see* Spondylitis, ankylosing
  sacroiliac NEC M46.1
  senescent, senile —*see* Spondylosis
  traumatic (chronic) or post-traumatic —*see*
      Spondylopathy, traumatic
  tuberculous A18.01
  typhosa A01.05
Spondylolisthesis (acquired) (degenerative)
    M43.10
  with disproportion (fetopelvic) O33.0
    causing obstructed labor O65.0
  cervical region M43.12
  cervicothoracic region M43.13
  congenital Q76.2
  lumbar region M43.16
  lumbosacral region M43.17
  multiple sites M43.19
  occipito-atlanto-axial region M43.11
  sacrococcygeal region M43.18
  thoracic region M43.14
  thoracolumbar region M43.15
  traumatic (old) M43.10
    acute
      fifth cervical (displaced) S12.430
        nondisplaced S12.431
        specified type NEC (displaced)
            S12.450
          nondisplaced S12.451
          type III S12.44
      fourth cervical (displaced) S12.330
        nondisplaced S12.331
        specified type NEC (displaced)
            S12.350
          nondisplaced S12.351
          type III S12.34

Spondylolisthesis (*Continued*)
  traumatic (*Continued*)
    acute (*Continued*)
      second cervical (displaced) S12.130
        nondisplaced S12.131
        specified type NEC (displaced)
            S12.150
          nondisplaced S12.151
          type III S12.14
      seventh cervical (displaced) S12.630
        nondisplaced S12.631
        specified type NEC (displaced)
            S12.650
          nondisplaced S12.651
          type III S12.64
      sixth cervical (displaced) S12.530
        nondisplaced S12.531
        specified type NEC (displaced)
            S12.550
          nondisplaced S12.551
          type III S12.54
      third cervical (displaced) S12.230
        nondisplaced S12.231
        specified type NEC (displaced)
            S12.250
          nondisplaced S12.251
          type III S12.24
Spondylolysis (acquired) M43.00
  cervical region M43.02
  cervicothoracic region M43.03
  congenital Q76.2
  lumbar region M43.06
  lumbosacral region M43.07
    with disproportion (fetopelvic) O33.0
      causing obstructed labor O65.8
  multiple sites M43.09
  occipito-atlanto-axial region M43.01
  sacrococcygeal region M43.08
  thoracic region M43.04
  thoracolumbar region M43.05
Spondylopathy M48.9
  infective NEC M46.50
    cervical region M46.52
    cervicothoracic region M46.53
    lumbar region M46.56
    lumbosacral region M46.57
    multiple sites M46.59
    occipito-atlanto-axial region M46.51
    sacrococcygeal region M46.58
    thoracic region M46.54
    thoracolumbar region M46.55
  inflammatory M46.90
    cervical region M46.92
    cervicothoracic region M46.93
    lumbar region M46.96
    lumbosacral region M46.97
    multiple sites M46.99
    occipito-atlanto-axial region M46.91
    sacrococcygeal region M46.98
    specified type NEC M46.80
      cervical region M46.82
      cervicothoracic region M46.83
      lumbar region M46.86
      lumbosacral region M46.87
      multiple sites M46.89
      occipito-atlanto-axial region M46.81
      sacrococcygeal region M46.88
      thoracic region M46.84
      thoracolumbar region M46.85
    thoracic region M46.94
    thoracolumbar region M46.95
  neuropathic, in
    syringomyelia and syringobulbia G95.0
    tabes dorsalis A52.11
  specified NEC —*see* subcategory M48.8
  traumatic M48.30
    cervical region M48.32
    cervicothoracic region M48.33
    lumbar region M48.36
    lumbosacral region M48.37
    occipito-atlanto-axial region M48.31

Spondylopathy (Continued)
  traumatic (Continued)
    sacrococcygeal region M48.38
    thoracic region M48.34
    thoracolumbar region M48.35
Spondylosis M47.9
  with
    disproportion (fetopelvic) O33.0
      causing obstructed labor O65.0
    myelopathy NEC M47.10
      cervical region M47.12
      cervicothoracic region M47.13
      lumbar region M47.16
      occipito-atlanto-axial region M47.11
      thoracic region M47.14
      thoracolumbar region M47.15
    radiculopathy M47.20
      cervical region M47.22
      cervicothoracic region M47.23
      lumbar region M47.26
      lumbosacral region M47.27
      occipito-atlanto-axial region M47.21
      sacrococcygeal region M47.28
      thoracic region M47.24
      thoracolumbar region M47.25
  without myelopathy or radiculopathy M47.819
    cervical region M47.812
    cervicothoracic region M47.813
    lumbar region M47.816
    lumbosacral region M47.817
    occipito-atlanto-axial region M47.811
    sacrococcygeal region M47.818
    thoracic region M47.814
    thoracolumbar region M47.815
  specified NEC M47.899
    cervical region M47.892
    cervicothoracic region M47.893
    lumbar region M47.896
    lumbosacral region M47.897
    occipito-atlanto-axial region M47.891
    sacrococcygeal region M47.898
    thoracic region M47.894
    thoracolumbar region M47.895
  traumatic —see Spondylopathy, traumatic
Sponge
  inadvertently left in operation wound —see Foreign body, accidentally left during a procedure
  kidney (medullary) Q61.5
Sponge-diver's disease —see Toxicity, venom, marine animal, sea anemone
Spongioblastoma (any type) —see Neoplasm, malignant, by site
  specified site —see Neoplasm, malignant, by site
  unspecified site C71.9
Spongioneuroblastoma —see Neoplasm, malignant, by site
Spontaneous —see also condition
  fracture (cause unknown) —see Fracture, pathological
Spoon nail L60.3
  congenital Q84.6
Sporadic —see condition
Sporothrix schenckii infection —see Sporotrichosis
Sporotrichosis B42.9
  arthritis B42.82
  disseminated B42.7
  generalized B42.7
  lymphocutaneous (fixed) (progressive) B42.1
  pulmonary B42.0
  specified NEC B42.89
Spots, spotting (in) (of)
  Bitot's —see also Pigmentation, conjunctiva
    in the young child E50.1
      vitamin A deficiency E50.1

Spots, spotting (Continued)
  café, au lait L81.3
  Cayenne pepper I78.1
  cotton wool, retina —see Occlusion, artery, retina
  de Morgan's (senile angiomas) I78.1
  Fuchs' black (myopic) —see also Myopia, degenerative H44.2-
  intermenstrual (regular) N92.0
    irregular N92.1
  Koplik's B05.9
  liver L81.4
  pregnancy O26.85-
  purpuric R23.3
  ruby I78.1
Spotted fever —see Fever, spotted N92.3
Sprain (joint) (ligament)
  acromioclavicular joint or ligament S43.5-
  ankle S93.40-
    calcaneofibular ligament S93.41-
    deltoid ligament S93.42-
    internal collateral ligament —see Sprain, ankle, specified ligament NEC
    specified ligament NEC S93.49-
    talofibular ligament —see Sprain, ankle, specified ligament NEC
    tibiofibular ligament S93.43-
  anterior longitudinal, cervical S13.4
  atlas, atlanto-axial, atlanto-occipital S13.4
  breast bone —see Sprain, sternum
  calcaneofibular —see Sprain, ankle
  carpal —see Sprain, wrist
  carpometacarpal —see Sprain, hand, specified site NEC
  cartilage
    costal S23.41
    semilunar (knee) —see Sprain, knee, specified site NEC
      with current tear —see Tear, meniscus
    thyroid region S13.5
    xiphoid —see Sprain, sternum
  cervical, cervicodorsal, cervicothoracic S13.4
  chondrosternal S23.421
  coracoclavicular S43.8-
  coracohumeral S43.41-
  coronary, knee —see Sprain, knee, specified site NEC
  costal cartilage S23.41
  cricoarytenoid articulation or ligament S13.5
  cricothyroid articulation S13.5
  cruciate, knee —see Sprain, knee, cruciate
  deltoid, ankle —see Sprain, ankle
  dorsal (spine) S23.3
  elbow S53.40-
    radial collateral ligament S53.43-
    radiohumeral S53.41-
    rupture
      radial collateral ligament —see Rupture, traumatic, ligament, radial collateral
      ulnar collateral ligament —see Rupture, traumatic, ligament, ulnar collateral
    specified type NEC S53.49-
    ulnar collateral ligament S53.44-
    ulnohumeral S53.42-
  femur, head —see Sprain, hip
  fibular collateral, knee —see Sprain, knee, collateral
  fibulocalcaneal —see Sprain, ankle
  finger(s) S63.61-
    index S63.61-
    interphalangeal (joint) S63.63-
      index S63.63-
      little S63.63-
      middle S63.63-
      ring S63.63-
    little S63.61-
    metacarpophalangeal (joint) S63.65-
    middle S63.61-
    ring S63.61-

Sprain (Continued)
  finger(s) (Continued)
    specified site NEC S63.69-
      index S63.69-
      little S63.69-
      middle S63.69-
      ring S63.69-
  foot S93.60-
    specified ligament NEC S93.69-
    tarsal ligament S93.61-
    tarsometatarsal ligament S93.62-
    toe —see Sprain, toe
  hand S63.9-
    finger —see Sprain, finger
    specified site NEC —see subcategory S63.8
    thumb —see Sprain, thumb
  head S03.9
  hip S73.10-
    iliofemoral ligament S73.11-
    ischiocapsular (ligament) S73.12-
    specified NEC S73.19-
  iliofemoral —see Sprain, hip
  innominate
    acetabulum —see Sprain, hip
    sacral junction S33.6
  internal
    collateral, ankle —see Sprain, ankle
    semilunar cartilage —see Sprain, knee, specified site NEC
  interphalangeal
    finger —see Sprain, finger, interphalangeal (joint)
    toe —see Sprain, toe, interphalangeal joint
  ischiocapsular —see Sprain, hip
  ischiofemoral —see Sprain, hip
  jaw (articular disc) (cartilage) (meniscus) S03.4-
    old M26.69
  knee S83.9-
    collateral ligament S83.40-
      lateral (fibular) S83.42-
      medial (tibial) S83.41-
    cruciate ligament S83.50-
      anterior S83.51-
      posterior S83.52-
    lateral (fibular) collateral ligament S83.42-
    medial (tibial) collateral ligament S83.41-
    patellar ligament S76.11-
    specified site NEC S83.8X-
    superior tibiofibular joint (ligament) S83.6-
  lateral collateral, knee —see Sprain, knee, collateral
  lumbar (spine) S33.5
  lumbosacral S33.9
  mandible (articular disc) S03.4-
    old M26.69
  medial collateral, knee —see Sprain, knee, collateral
  meniscus
    jaw S03.4-
      old M26.69
    knee —see Sprain, knee, specified site NEC
      with current tear —see Tear, meniscus
        old —see Derangement, knee, meniscus, due to old tear
    mandible S03.4-
      old M26.69
  metacarpal (distal) (proximal) —see Sprain, hand, specified site NEC
  metacarpophalangeal —see Sprain, finger, metacarpophalangeal (joint)
  metatarsophalangeal —see Sprain, toe, metatarsophalangeal joint
  midcarpal —see Sprain, hand, specified site NEC
  midtarsal —see Sprain, foot, specified site NEC
  neck S13.9
    anterior longitudinal cervical ligament S13.4
    atlanto-axial joint S13.4

Sprain *(Continued)*
  neck *(Continued)*
    atlanto-occipital joint S13.4
    cervical spine S13.4
    cricoarytenoid ligament S13.5
    cricothyroid ligament S13.5
    specified site NEC S13.8
    thyroid region (cartilage) S13.5
  nose S03.8
  orbicular, hip —*see* Sprain, hip
  patella —*see* Sprain, knee, specified site NEC
  patellar ligament S76.11-●
  pelvis NEC S33.8
  phalanx
    finger —*see* Sprain, finger
    toe —*see* Sprain, toe
  pubofemoral —*see* Sprain, hip
  radiocarpal —*see* Sprain, wrist
  radiohumeral —*see* Sprain, elbow
  radius, collateral —*see* Rupture, traumatic, ligament, radial collateral
  rib (cage) S23.41
  rotator cuff (capsule) S43.42-●
  sacroiliac (region)
    chronic or old —*see* subcategory M53.2
    joint S33.6
  scaphoid (hand) —*see* Sprain, hand, specified site NEC
  scapula (r) —*see* Sprain, shoulder girdle, specified site NEC
  semilunar cartilage (knee) —*see* Sprain, knee, specified site NEC
    with current tear —*see* Tear, meniscus
    old —*see* Derangement, knee, meniscus, due to old tear
  shoulder joint S43.40-●
    acromioclavicular joint (ligament) —*see* Sprain, acromioclavicular joint
    blade —*see* Sprain, shoulder, girdle, specified site NEC
    coracoclavicular joint (ligament) —*see* Sprain, coracoclavicular joint
    coracohumeral ligament —*see* Sprain, coracohumeral joint
    girdle S43.9-●
      specified site NEC S43.8-●
    rotator cuff —*see* Sprain, rotator cuff
    specified site NEC S43.49-●
    sternoclavicular joint (ligament) —*see* Sprain, sternoclavicular joint
  spine
    cervical S13.4
    lumbar S33.5
    thoracic S23.3
  sternoclavicular joint S43.6-●
  sternum S23.429
    chondrosternal joint S23.421
    specified site NEC S23.428
    sternoclavicular (joint) (ligament) S23.420
  symphysis
    jaw S03.4-●
      old M26.69
    mandibular S03.4-●
      old M26.69
  talofibular —*see* Sprain, ankle
  tarsal —*see* Sprain, foot, specified site NEC
  tarsometatarsal —*see* Sprain, foot, specified site NEC
  temporomandibular S03.4-●
    old M26.69
  thorax S23.9
    ribs S23.41
    specified site NEC S23.8
    spine S23.3
    sternum —*see* Sprain, sternum
  thumb S63.60-●
    interphalangeal (joint) S63.62-●
    metacarpophalangeal (joint) S63.64-●
    specified site NEC S63.68-●
  thyroid cartilage or region S13.5

Sprain *(Continued)*
  tibia (proximal end) —*see* Sprain, knee, specified site NEC
  tibial collateral, knee —*see* Sprain, knee, collateral
  tibiofibular
    distal —*see* Sprain, ankle
    superior —*see* Sprain, knee, specified site NEC
  toe(s) S93.50-●
    great S93.50-●
    interphalangeal joint S93.51-●
      great S93.51-●
      lesser S93.51-●
    lesser S93.50-●
    metatarsophalangeal joint S93.52-●
      great S93.52-●
      lesser S93.52-●
  ulna, collateral —*see* Rupture, traumatic, ligament, ulnar collateral
  ulnohumeral —*see* Sprain, elbow
  wrist S63.50-●
    carpal S63.51-●
    radiocarpal S63.52-●
    specified site NEC S63.59-●
  xiphoid cartilage —*see* Sprain, sternum
Sprengel's deformity (congenital) Q74.0
Sprue (tropical) K90.1
  celiac K90.0
  idiopathic K90.49
  meaning thrush B37.0
  nontropical K90.0
Spur, bone —*see also* Enthesopathy
  calcaneal M77.3-●
  iliac crest M76.2-●
  nose (septum) J34.89
Spurway's syndrome Q78.0
Sputum
  abnormal (amount) (color) (odor) (purulent) R09.3
  blood-stained R04.2
  excessive (cause unknown) R09.3
Squamous —*see also* condition
  epithelium in
    cervical canal (congenital) Q51.828
    uterine mucosa (congenital) Q51.818
Squashed nose M95.0
  congenital Q67.4
Squeeze, diver's T70.3
Squint —*see also* Strabismus
  accommodative —*see* Strabismus, convergent concomitant
St. Hubert's disease A82.9
Stab —*see also* Laceration
  internal organs —*see* Injury, by site
Stafne's cyst or cavity M27.0
Staggering gait R26.0
  hysterical F44.4
Staghorn calculus —*see* Calculus, kidney
Stähli's line (cornea) (pigment) —*see* Pigmentation, cornea, anterior
Stain, staining
  meconium (newborn) P96.83
  port wine Q82.5
  tooth, teeth (hard tissues) (extrinsic) K03.6
    due to
      accretions K03.6
      deposits (betel) (black) (green) (materia alba) (orange) (soft) (tobacco) K03.6
      metals (copper) (silver) K03.7
      nicotine K03.6
      pulpal bleeding K03.7
      tobacco K03.6
    intrinsic K00.8
Stammering —*see also* Disorder, fluency F80.81
Standstill
  auricular I45.5
  cardiac —*see* Arrest, cardiac
  sinoatrial I45.5
  ventricular —*see* Arrest, cardiac
Stannosis J63.5

Stanton's disease —*see* Melioidosis
Staphylitis (acute) (catarrhal) (chronic) (gangrenous) (membranous) (suppurative) (ulcerative) K12.2
Staphylococcal scalded skin syndrome L00
Staphylococcemia A41.2
Staphylococcus, staphylococcal —*see also* condition
  as cause of disease classified elsewhere B95.8
    aureus (methicillin susceptible) (MSSA) B95.61
    methicillin resistant (MRSA) B95.62
    specified NEC, as cause of disease classified elsewhere B95.7
Staphyloma (sclera)
  cornea H18.72-●
  equatorial H15.81-●
  localized (anterior) H15.82-●
  posticum H15.83-●
  ring H15.85-●
Stargardt's disease —*see* Dystrophy, retina
Starvation (inanition) (due to lack of food) T73.0
  edema —*see* Malnutrition, severe
Stasis
  bile (noncalculous) K83.1
  bronchus J98.09
    with infection —*see* Bronchitis
  cardiac —*see* Failure, heart, congestive
  cecum K59.8
  colon K59.8
  dermatitis I87.2
    with
      varicose ulcer —*see* Varix, leg, with ulcer, with inflammation
      varicose veins —*see* Varix, leg, with, inflammation
    due to postthrombotic syndrome —*see* Syndrome, postthrombotic
  duodenal K31.5
  eczema —*see* Varix, leg, with, inflammation
  edema —*see* Hypertension, venous (chronic), idiopathic
  foot T69.0-●
  ileocecal coil K59.8
  ileum K59.8
  intestinal K59.8
  jejunum K59.8
  kidney N19
  liver (cirrhotic) K76.1
  lymphatic I89.8
  pneumonia J18.2
  pulmonary —*see* Edema, lung
  rectal K59.8
  renal N19
    tubular N17.0
  ulcer —*see* Varix, leg, with, ulcer
    without varicose veins I87.2
  urine —*see* Retention, urine
  venous I87.8
State (of)
  affective and paranoid, mixed, organic psychotic F06.8
  agitated R45.1
    acute reaction to stress F43.0
  anxiety (neurotic) F41.1
  apprehension F41.1
  burn-out Z73.0
  climacteric, female Z78.0
    symptomatic N95.1
  compulsive F42.8
    mixed with obsessional thoughts F42.2
  confusional (psychogenic) F44.89
    acute —*see also* Delirium
      with
        arteriosclerotic dementia F01.50
          with behavioral disturbance F01.51
        senility or dementia F05
        alcoholic F10.231

▶ New   ⇒ Revised   ~~deleted~~ Deleted   ● Use Additional Character(s)

State *(Continued)*
  confusional (psychogenic) *(Continued)*
    epileptic F05
    reactive (from emotional stress,
        psychological trauma) F44.89
    subacute —*see* Delirium
  convulsive —*see* Convulsions
  crisis F43.0
  depressive F32.9
    neurotic F34.1
  dissociative F44.9
  emotional shock (stress) R45.7
  hypercoagulation —*see* Hypercoagulable
  locked-in G83.5
  menopausal Z78.0
    symptomatic N95.1
  neurotic F48.9
    with depersonalization F48.1
  obsessional F42.8
  oneiroid (schizophrenia-like) F23
  organic
    hallucinatory (nonalcoholic) F06.0
    paranoid (-hallucinatory) F06.2
  panic F41.0
  paranoid F22
    climacteric F22
    involutional F22
    menopausal F22
    organic F06.2
    senile F03
    simple F22
  persistent vegetative R40.3
  phobic F40.9
  postleukotomy F07.0
  pregnant
    gestational carrier Z33.3
    incidental Z33.1
  psychogenic, twilight F44.89
  psychopathic (constitutional) F60.2
  psychotic, organic —*see also* Psychosis,
      organic
    mixed paranoid and affective F06.8
    senile or presenile F03
    transient NEC F06.8
      with
        depression F06.31
        hallucinations F06.0
  residual schizophrenic F20.5
  restlessness R45.1
  stress (emotional) R45.7
  tension (mental) F48.9
    specified NEC F48.8
  transient organic psychotic NEC F06.8
    depressive type F06.31
    hallucinatory type F06.0
  twilight
    epileptic F05
    psychogenic F44.89
  vegetative, persistent R40.3
  vital exhaustion Z73.0
  withdrawal —*see* Withdrawal, state
Status (post) —*see also* Presence (of)
  absence, epileptic —*see* Epilepsy, by type,
      with status epilepticus
  administration of tPA (rtPA) in a different
      facility within the last 24 hours prior to
      admission to the current facility
      Z92.82
  adrenalectomy (unilateral) (bilateral)
      E89.6
  anastomosis Z98.0
  anginosus I20.9
  angioplasty (peripheral) Z98.62
    with implant Z95.820
    coronary artery Z98.61
      with implant Z95.5
  aortocoronary bypass Z95.1
  arthrodesis Z98.1
  artificial opening (of) Z93.9
    gastrointestinal tract Z93.4
    specified NEC Z93.8

Status *(Continued)*
  artificial opening (of) *(Continued)*
    urinary tract Z93.6
    vagina Z93.8
  asthmaticus —*see* Asthma, by type, with
      status asthmaticus
  awaiting organ transplant Z76.82
  bariatric surgery Z98.84
  bed confinement Z74.01
  bleb, filtering (vitreous), after glaucoma
      surgery Z98.83
  breast implant Z98.82
    removal Z98.86
  cataract extraction Z98.4- •
  cholecystectomy Z90.49
  clitorectomy N90.811
    with excision of labia minora N90.812
  colectomy (complete) (partial) Z90.49
  colonization —*see* Carrier (suspected) of
  colostomy Z93.3
  convulsivus idiopathicus —*see* Epilepsy, by
      type, with status epilepticus
  coronary artery angioplasty —*see* Status,
      angioplasty, coronary artery
  ▶coronary artery bypass graft Z95.1
  cystectomy (urinary bladder) Z90.6
  cystostomy Z93.50
    appendico-vesicostomy Z93.52
    cutaneous Z93.51
    specified NEC Z93.59
  delinquent immunization Z28.3
  dental Z98.818
    crown Z98.811
    fillings Z98.811
    restoration Z98.811
    sealant Z98.810
    specified NEC Z98.818
  deployment (current) (military) Z56.82
  dialysis (hemodialysis) (peritoneal) Z99.2
  do not resuscitate (DNR) Z66
  donor —*see* Donor
  embedded fragments —*see* Retained, foreign
      body fragments (type of)
  embedded splinter —*see* Retained, foreign
      body fragments (type of)
  enterostomy Z93.4
  epileptic, epilepticus —*see also* Epilepsy, by
      type, with status epilepticus G40.901
  estrogen receptor
    negative Z17.1
    positive Z17.0
  female genital cutting —*see* Female genital
      mutilation status
  female genital mutilation —*see* Female genital
      mutilation status
  filtering (vitreous) bleb after glaucoma
      surgery Z98.83
  gastrectomy (complete) (partial) Z90.3
  gastric banding Z98.84
  gastric bypass for obesity Z98.84
  gastrostomy Z93.1
  human immunodeficiency virus (HIV)
      infection, asymptomatic Z21
  hysterectomy (complete) (total) Z90.710
    partial (with remaining cervial stump)
      Z90.711
  ileostomy Z93.2
  implant
    breast Z98.82
  infibulation N90.813
  intestinal bypass Z98.0
  jejunostomy Z93.4
  lapsed immunization schedule Z28.3
  laryngectomy Z90.02
  lymphaticus E32.8
  malignancy
    castrate resistant prostate Z19.2
    hormone resistant Z19.2
    hormone sensitive Z19.1
  marmoratus G80.3
  mastectomy (unilateral) (bilateral)
      Z90.1- •

Status *(Continued)*
  military deployment status (current) Z56.82
    in theater or in support of military war,
        peacekeeping and humanitarian
        operations Z56.82
  nephrectomy (unilateral) (bilateral) Z90.5
  nephrostomy Z93.6
  obesity surgery Z98.84
  oophorectomy
    bilateral Z90.722
    unilateral Z90.721
  organ replacement
    by artificial or mechanical device or
        prosthesis of
      artery Z95.828
      bladder Z96.0
      blood vessel Z95.828
      breast Z97.8
      eye globe Z97.0
      heart Z95.812
        valve Z95.2
      intestine Z97.8
      joint Z96.60
        hip —*see* Presence, hip joint implant
        knee —*see* Presence, knee joint
            implant
        specified site NEC Z96.698
      kidney Z97.8
      larynx Z96.3
      lens Z96.1
      limbs —*see* Presence, artificial, limb
      liver Z97.8
      lung Z97.8
      pancreas Z97.8
    by organ transplant (heterologous)
        (homologous) —*see* Transplant
  pacemaker
    brain Z96.89
    cardiac Z95.0
    specified NEC Z96.89
  pancreatectomy Z90.410
    complete Z90.410
    partial Z90.411
    total Z90.410
  pneumonectomy (complete) (partial) Z90.2
  pneumothorax, therapeutic Z98.3
  postcommotio cerebri F07.81
  postoperative (postprocedural) NEC
      Z98.890
    breast implant Z98.82
    dental Z98.818
      crown Z98.811
      fillings Z98.811
      restoration Z98.811
      sealant Z98.810
      specified NEC Z98.818
    pneumothorax, therapeutic Z98.3
    uterine scar Z98.891
  postpartum (routine follow-up) Z39.2
    care immediately after delivery Z39.0
  postsurgical (postprocedural) NEC
      Z98.890
    pneumothorax, therapeutic Z98.3
  pregnancy, incidental Z33.1
  prosthesis coronary angioplasty Z95.5
  pseudophakia Z96.1
  renal dialysis (hemodialysis) (peritoneal)
      Z99.2
  retained foreign body —*see* Retained, foreign
      body fragments (type of)
  reversed jejunal transposition (for bypass)
      Z98.0
  salpingo-oophorectomy
    bilateral Z90.722
    unilateral Z90.721
  sex reassignment surgery status Z87.890
  shunt
    arteriovenous (for dialysis) Z99.2
    cerebrospinal fluid Z98.2
    ventricular (communicating) (for
        drainage) Z98.2

▶ New   ⇒ Revised   ~~deleted~~ Deleted   • Use Additional Character(s)

Status *(Continued)*
  splenectomy Z90.81
  thymicolymphaticus E32.8
  thymicus E32.8
  thymolymphaticus E32.8
  thyroidectomy (hypothyroidism) E89.0
  tooth (teeth) extraction —*see also* Absence,
    teeth, acquired K08.409
  tPA (rtPA) administration in a different
    facility within the last 24 hours prior to
    admission to current facility Z92.82
  tracheostomy Z93.0
  transplant —*see* Transplant
    organ removed Z98.85
  tubal ligation Z98.51
  underimmunization Z28.3
  ureterostomy Z93.6
  urethrostomy Z93.6
  vagina, artificial Z93.8
  vasectomy Z98.52
  wheelchair confinement Z99.3
Stealing
  child problem F91.8
    in company with others Z72.810
  pathological (compulsive) F63.2
Steam burn —*see* Burn
Steatocystoma multiplex L72.2
Steatohepatitis (nonalcoholic) (NASH)
  K75.81
Steatoma L72.3
  eyelid (cystic) —*see* Dermatosis, eyelid
    infected —*see* Hordeolum
Steatorrhea (chronic) K90.9
  with lacteal obstruction K90.2
  idiopathic (adult) (infantile) K90.9
  pancreatic K90.3
  primary K90.0
  tropical K90.1
Steatosis E88.89
  heart —*see* Degeneration, myocardial
  kidney N28.89
  liver NEC K76.0
Steele-Richardson-Olszewski disease or
  syndrome G23.1
Steinbrocker's syndrome G90.8
Steinert's disease G71.11
Stein-Leventhal syndrome E28.2
Stein's syndrome E28.2
STEMI —*see also* Infarct, myocardium, ST
  elevation I21.3
Stenocardia I20.8
Stenocephaly Q75.8
Stenosis, stenotic (cicatricial) —*see also*
  Stricture
  ampulla of Vater K83.1
  anus, anal (canal) (sphincter) K62.4
    and rectum K62.4
    congenital Q42.3
      with fistula Q42.2
  aorta (ascending) (supraventricular)
    (congenital) Q25.1
    arteriosclerotic I70.0
    calcified I70.0
    supravalvular Q25.3
  aortic (valve) I35.0
    with insufficiency I35.2
    congenital Q23.0
    rheumatic I06.0
      with
        incompetency, insufficiency or
          regurgitation I06.2
          with mitral (valve) disease I08.0
            with tricuspid (valve) disease
              I08.3
        mitral (valve) disease I08.0
          with tricuspid (valve) disease
            I08.3
        tricuspid (valve) disease I08.2
          with mitral (valve) disease I08.3
    specified cause NEC I35.0
    syphilitic A52.03

Stenosis, stenotic *(Continued)*
  aqueduct of Sylvius (congenital) Q03.0
    with spina bifida —*see* Spina bifida,
      by site, with hydrocephalus
    acquired G91.1
  artery NEC —*see also* Arteriosclerosis
    I77.1
    celiac I77.4
    cerebral —*see* Occlusion, artery, cerebral
    extremities —*see* Arteriosclerosis,
      extremities
    precerebral —*see* Occlusion, artery,
      precerebral
    pulmonary (congenital) Q25.6
      acquired I28.8
    renal I70.1
    stent
      coronary T82.855
      peripheral T82.856
  bile duct (common) (hepatic) K83.1
    congenital Q44.3
  bladder-neck (acquired) N32.0
    congenital Q64.31
  brain G93.89
  bronchus J98.09
    congenital Q32.3
    syphilitic A52.72
  cardia (stomach) K22.2
    congenital Q39.3
  cardiovascular —*see* Disease, cardiovascular
  caudal M48.08
  cervix, cervical (canal) N88.2
    congenital Q51.828
    in pregnancy or childbirth —*see* Pregnancy,
      complicated by, abnormal cervix
  colon —*see also* Obstruction, intestine
    congenital Q42.9
      specified NEC Q42.8
  colostomy K94.03
  common (bile) duct K83.1
    congenital Q44.3
  coronary (artery) —*see* Disease, heart,
    ischemic, atherosclerotic
  cystic duct —*see* Obstruction, gallbladder
  due to presence of device, implant or
    graft —*see also* Complications, by site
    and type, specified NEC T85.858
    arterial graft NEC T82.858
    breast (implant) T85.858
    catheter T85.858
      dialysis (renal) T82.858
        intraperitoneal T85.858
      infusion NEC T82.858
        spinal (epidural) (subdural)
          T85.850
      urinary (indwelling) T83.85
    fixation, internal (orthopedic) NEC
      T84.85
    gastrointestinal (bile duct) (esophagus)
      T85.858
    genital NEC T83.85
    heart NEC T82.857
    joint prosthesis T84.85
    ocular (corneal graft) (orbital implant)
      NEC T85.858
    orthopedic NEC T84.85
    specified NEC T85.858
    urinary NEC T83.85
    vascular NEC T82.858
    ventricular intracranial shunt T85.850
  duodenum K31.5
    congenital Q41.0
  ejaculatory duct NEC N50.89
  endocervical os —*see* Stenosis, cervix
  enterostomy K94.13
  esophagus K22.2
    congenital Q39.3
    syphilitic A52.79
      congenital A50.59 *[K23]*
  eustachian tube —*see* Obstruction, eustachian
    tube

Stenosis, stenotic *(Continued)*
  external ear canal (acquired) H61.30-●
    congenital Q16.1
    due to
      inflammation H61.32-●
      trauma H61.31-●
    postprocedural H95.81-●
    specified cause NEC H61.39-●
  gallbladder —*see* Obstruction, gallbladder
  glottis J38.6
  heart valve (congenital) Q24.8
    aortic Q23.0
    mitral Q23.2
    pulmonary Q22.1
    tricuspid Q22.4
  hepatic duct K83.1
  hymen N89.6
  hypertrophic subaortic (idiopathic) I42.1
➡ ileum —*see also* Obstruction, intestine,
    specified NEC K56.699
    congenital Q41.2
  infundibulum cardia Q24.3
  intervertebral foramina —*see also* Lesion,
    biomechanical, specified NEC
    connective tissue M99.79
      abdomen M99.79
      cervical region M99.71
      cervicothoracic M99.71
      head region M99.70
      lumbar region M99.73
      lumbosacral M99.73
      occipitocervical M99.70
      sacral region M99.74
      sacrococcygeal M99.74
      sacroiliac M99.74
      specified NEC M99.79
      thoracic region M99.72
      thoracolumbar M99.72
    disc M99.79
      abdomen M99.79
      cervical region M99.71
      cervicothoracic M99.71
      head region M99.70
      lower extremity M99.76
      lumbar region M99.73
      lumbosacral M99.73
      occipitocervical M99.70
      pelvic M99.75
      rib cage M99.78
      sacral region M99.74
      sacrococcygeal M99.74
      sacroiliac M99.74
      specified NEC M99.79
      thoracic region M99.72
      thoracolumbar M99.72
      upper extremity M99.77
    osseous M99.69
      abdomen M99.69
      cervical region M99.61
      cervicothoracic M99.61
      head region M99.60
      lower extremity M99.66
      lumbar region M99.63
      lumbosacral M99.63
      occipitocervical M99.60
      pelvic M99.65
      rib cage M99.68
      sacral region M99.64
      sacrococcygeal M99.64
      sacroiliac M99.64
      specified NEC M99.69
      thoracic region M99.62
      thoracolumbar M99.62
      upper extremity M99.67
    subluxation —*see* Stenosis, intervertebral
      foramina, osseous
  intestine —*see also* Obstruction, intestine
    congenital (small) Q41.9
      large Q42.9
        specified NEC Q42.8
      specified NEC Q41.8

▶ New   ⇒ Revised   ~~deleted~~ Deleted   ● Use Additional Character(s)

Stenosis, stenotic *(Continued)*
jejunum —*see also* Obstruction, intestine,
     specified NEC K56.699
  congenital Q41.1
 lacrimal (passage)
  canaliculi H04.54-•
  congenital Q10.5
  duct H04.55-•
  punctum H04.56-•
  sac H04.57-•
 lacrimonasal duct —*see* Stenosis, lacrimal, duct
  congenital Q10.5
 larynx J38.6
  congenital NEC Q31.8
   subglottic Q31.1
  syphilitic A52.73
   congenital A50.59 *[J99]*
 mitral (chronic) (inactive) (valve) I05.0
  with
   aortic valve disease I08.0
   incompetency, insufficiency or
        regurgitation I05.2
  active or acute I01.1
   with rheumatic or Sydenham's chorea
        I02.0
  congenital Q23.2
  specified cause, except rheumatic I34.2
  syphilitic A52.03
 myocardium, myocardial —*see also*
     Degeneration, myocardial
  hypertrophic subaortic (idiopathic) I42.1
 nares (anterior) (posterior) J34.89
  congenital Q30.0
 nasal duct —*see also* Stenosis, lacrimal, duct
  congenital Q10.5
 nasolacrimal duct —*see also* Stenosis, lacrimal,
     duct
  congenital Q10.5
 neural canal —*see also* Lesion, biomechanical,
     specified NEC
  connective tissue M99.49
   abdomen M99.49
   cervical region M99.41
   cervicothoracic M99.41
   head region M99.40
   lower extremity M99.46
   lumbar region M99.43
   lumbosacral M99.43
   occipitocervical M99.40
   pelvic M99.45
   rib cage M99.48
   sacral region M99.44
   sacrococcygeal M99.44
   sacroiliac M99.44
   specified NEC M99.49
   thoracic region M99.42
   thoracolumbar M99.42
   upper extremity M99.47
  intervertebral disc M99.59
   abdomen M99.59
   cervical region M99.51
   cervicothoracic M99.51
   head region M99.50
   lower extremity M99.56
   lumbar region M99.53
   lumbosacral M99.53
   occipitocervical M99.50
   pelvic M99.55
   rib cage M99.58
   sacral region M99.54
   sacrococcygeal M99.54
   sacroiliac M99.54
   specified NEC M99.59
   thoracic region M99.52
   thoracolumbar M99.52
   upper extremity M99.57
  osseous M99.39
   abdomen M99.39
   cervical region M99.31
   cervicothoracic M99.31
   head region M99.30

Stenosis, stenotic *(Continued)*
 neural canal *(Continued)*
  osseous *(Continued)*
   lower extremity M99.36
   lumbar region M99.33
   lumbosacral M99.33
   occipitocervical M99.30
   pelvic M99.35
   rib cage M99.38
   sacral region M99.34
   sacrococcygeal M99.34
   sacroiliac M99.34
   specified NEC M99.39
   thoracic region M99.32
   thoracolumbar M99.32
   upper extremity M99.37
  subluxation M99.29
   cervical region M99.21
   cervicothoracic M99.21
   head region M99.20
   lower extremity M99.26
   lumbar region M99.23
   lumbosacral M99.23
   occipitocervical M99.20
   pelvic M99.25
   rib cage M99.28
   sacral region M99.24
   sacrococcygeal M99.24
   sacroiliac M99.24
   specified NEC M99.29
   thoracic region M99.22
   thoracolumbar M99.22
   upper extremity M99.27
 organ or site, congenital NEC —*see* Atresia,
     by site
 papilla of Vater K83.1
 pulmonary (artery) (congenital) Q25.6
  with ventricular septal defect,
     transposition of aorta, and
     hypertrophy of right ventricle Q21.3
  acquired I28.8
  in tetralogy of Fallot Q21.3
  infundibular Q24.3
  subvalvular Q24.3
  supravalvular Q25.6
  valve I37.0
   with insufficiency I37.2
   congenital Q22.1
   rheumatic I09.89
    with aortic, mitral or tricuspid (valve)
         disease I08.8
  vein, acquired I28.8
  vessel NEC I28.8
 pulmonic (congenital) Q22.1
  infundibular Q24.3
  subvalvular Q24.3
 pylorus (hypertrophic) (acquired) K31.1
  adult K31.1
  congenital Q40.0
  infantile Q40.0
 rectum (sphincter) —*see* Stricture, rectum
 renal artery I70.1
  congenital Q27.1
 salivary duct (any) K11.8
 sphincter of Oddi K83.1
 spinal M48.00
  cervical region M48.02
  cervicothoracic region M48.03
  lumbar region (NOS) (without neurogenic
     claudication) M48.061
  with neurogenic claudication M48.062
  lumbosacral region M48.07
  occipito-atlanto-axial region M48.01
  sacrococcygeal region M48.08
  thoracic region M48.04
  thoracolumbar region M48.05
 stent
  vascular
   end stent
    adjacent to stent —*see*
         Arteriosclerosis

Stenosis, stenotic *(Continued)*
 stent *(Continued)*
  vascular *(Continued)*
   end stent *(Continued)*
    within the stent
     coronary T82.855
     peripheral T82.856
   in stent
    coronary vessel T82.855
    peripheral vessel T82.856
 stomach, hourglass K31.2
 subaortic (congenital) Q24.4
  hypertrophic (idiopathic) I42.1
 subglottic J38.6
  congenital Q31.1
  postprocedural J95.5
 trachea J39.8
  congenital Q32.1
  syphilitic A52.73
  tuberculous NEC A15.5
 tracheostomy J95.03
 tricuspid (valve) I07.0
  with
   aortic (valve) disease I08.2
   incompetency, insufficiency or
        regurgitation I07.2
    with aortic (valve) disease I08.2
     with mitral (valve) disease
          I08.3
   mitral (valve) disease I08.1
    with aortic (valve) disease I08.3
  congenital Q22.4
  nonrheumatic I36.0
   with insufficiency I36.2
 tubal N97.1
 ureter —*see* Atresia, ureter
 ureteropelvic junction, congenital
     Q62.11
 ureterovesical orifice, congenital Q62.12
 urethra (valve) —*see also* Stricture, urethra
  congenital Q64.32
 urinary meatus, congenital Q64.33
 vagina N89.5
  congenital Q52.4
  in pregnancy —*see* Pregnancy, complicated
     by, abnormal vagina
   causing obstructed labor O65.5
 valve (cardiac) (heart) —*see also* Endocarditis
     I38
  congenital Q24.8
   aortic Q23.0
   mitral Q23.2
   pulmonary Q22.1
   tricuspid Q22.4
 vena cava (inferior) (superior) I87.1
  congenital Q26.0
 vesicourethral orifice Q64.31
 vulva N90.5
Stent jail T82.897
Stercolith (impaction) K56.41
 appendix K38.1
Stercoraceous, stercoral ulcer K63.3
 anus or rectum K62.6
Stereotypies NEC F98.4
Sterility —*see* Infertility
Sterilization —*see* Encounter (for),
     sterilization
Sternalgia —*see* Angina
Sternopagus Q89.4
Sternum bifidum Q76.7
Steroid
 effects (adverse) (adrenocortical)
     (iatrogenic)
  cushingoid E24.2
   correct substance properly
        administered —*see* Table of Drugs
        and Chemicals, by drug, adverse
        effect
   overdose or wrong substance given
        or taken —*see* Table of Drugs and
        Chemicals, by drug, poisoning

Steroid *(Continued)*
  effects *(Continued)*
    diabetes —*see* category E09
      correct substance properly
        administered —*see* Table of Drugs
        and Chemicals, by drug, adverse
        effect
      overdose or wrong substance given
        or taken —*see* Table of Drugs and
        Chemicals, by drug, poisoning
    fever R50.2
    insufficiency E27.3
      correct substance properly
        administered —*see* Table of Drugs
        and Chemicals, by drug, adverse
        effect
      overdose or wrong substance given
        or taken —*see* Table of Drugs and
        Chemicals, by drug, poisoning
  responder H40.04-●
Stevens-Johnson disease or syndrome L51.1
  toxic epidermal necrolysis overlap L51.3
Stewart-Morel syndrome M85.2
Sticker's disease B08.3
Sticky eye —*see* Conjunctivitis, acute, mucopurulent
Stieda's disease —*see* Bursitis, tibial collateral
Stiff neck —*see* Torticollis
Stiff-man syndrome G25.82
Stiffness, joint NEC M25.60-●
  ankle M25.67-●
  ankylosis —*see* Ankylosis, joint
  contracture —*see* Contraction, joint
  elbow M25.62-●
  foot M25.67-●
  hand M25.64-●
  hip M25.65-●
  knee M25.66-●
  shoulder M25.61-●
  wrist M25.63-●
Stigmata congenital syphilis A50.59
Stillbirth P95
Still-Felty syndrome —*see* Felty's syndrome
Still's disease or syndrome (juvenile) M08.20
  adult-onset M06.1
  ankle M08.27-●
  elbow M08.22-●
  foot joint M08.27-●
  hand joint M08.24-●
  hip M08.25-●
  knee M08.26-●
  multiple site M08.29
  shoulder M08.21-●
  vertebra M08.28
  wrist M08.23-●
Stimulation, ovary E28.1
Sting (venomous) (with allergic or anaphylactic shock) —*see* Table of Drugs and Chemicals, by animal or substance, poisoning
Stippled epiphyses Q78.8
Stitch
  abscess T81.4
  burst (in operation wound) —*see* Disruption, wound, operation
Stokes-Adams disease or syndrome I45.9
Stokes' disease E05.00
  with thyroid storm E05.01
Stokvis (-Talma) disease D74.8
Stoma malfunction
  colostomy K94.03
  enterostomy K94.13
  gastrostomy K94.23
  ileostomy K94.13
  tracheostomy J95.03
Stomach —*see* condition
Stomatitis (denture) (ulcerative) K12.1
  angular K13.0
    due to dietary or vitamin deficiency E53.0
  aphthous K12.0
  bovine B08.61

Stomatitis *(Continued)*
  candidal B37.0
  catarrhal K12.1
  diphtheritic A36.89
  due to
    dietary deficiency E53.0
    thrush B37.0
    vitamin deficiency
      B group NEC E53.9
      B2 (riboflavin) E53.0
  epidemic B08.8
  epizootic B08.8
  follicular K12.1
  gangrenous A69.0
  Geotrichum B48.3
  herpesviral, herpetic B00.2
  herpetiformis K12.0
  malignant K12.1
  membranous acute K12.1
  monilial B37.0
  mycotic B37.0
  necrotizing ulcerative A69.0
  parasitic B37.0
  septic K12.1
  spirochetal A69.1
  suppurative (acute) K12.2
  ulceromembranous A69.1
  vesicular K12.1
    with exanthem (enteroviral) B08.4
    virus disease A93.8
  Vincent's A69.1
Stomatocytosis D58.8
Stomatomycosis B37.0
Stomatorrhagia K13.79
Stone(s) —*see also* Calculus
  bladder (diverticulum) N21.0
  cystine E72.09
  heart syndrome I50.1
  kidney N20.0
  prostate N42.0
  pulpal (dental) K04.2
  renal N20.0
  salivary gland or duct (any) K11.5
  urethra (impacted) N21.1
  urinary (duct) (impacted) (passage) N20.9
    bladder (diverticulum) N21.0
    lower tract N21.9
    specified NEC N21.8
  xanthine E79.8 *[N22]*
Stonecutter's lung J62.8
Stonemason's asthma, disease, lung or pneumoconiosis J62.8
Stoppage
  heart —*see* Arrest, cardiac
  urine —*see* Retention, urine
Storm, thyroid —*see* Thyrotoxicosis
Strabismus (congenital) (nonparalytic) H50.9
  concomitant H50.40
    convergent —*see* Strabismus, convergent concomitant
    divergent —*see* Strabismus, divergent concomitant
  convergent concomitant H50.00
    accommodative component H50.43
    alternating H50.05
      with
        A pattern H50.06
        specified nonconcomitances NEC H50.08
        V pattern H50.07
    monocular H50.01-●
      with
        A pattern H50.02-●
        specified nonconcomitances NEC H50.04-●
        V pattern H50.03-●
    intermittent H50.31-●
      alternating H50.32

Strabismus *(Continued)*
  cyclotropia H50.41
  divergent concomitant H50.10
    alternating H50.15
      with
        A pattern H50.16
        specified noncomitances NEC H50.18
        V pattern H50.17
    monocular H50.11-●
      with
        A pattern H50.12-●
        specified noncomitances NEC H50.14-●
        V pattern H50.13-●
    intermittent H50.33-●
      alternating H50.34
  Duane's syndrome H50.81-●
  due to adhesions, scars H50.69
  heterophoria H50.50
    alternating H50.55
    cyclophoria H50.54
    esophoria H50.51
    exophoria H50.52
    vertical H50.53
  heterotropia H50.40
    intermittent H50.30
  hypertropia H50.2-●
  hypotropia —*see* Hypertropia
  latent H50.50
  mechanical H50.60
    Brown's sheath syndrome H50.61-●
    specified type NEC H50.69
  monofixation syndrome H50.42
  paralytic H49.9
    abducens nerve H49.2-●
    fourth nerve H49.1-●
    Kearns-Sayre syndrome H49.81-●
    ophthalmoplegia (external)
      progressive H49.4-●
        with pigmentary retinopathy H49.81-●
      total H49.3-●
    sixth nerve H49.2-●
    specified type NEC H49.88-●
    third nerve H49.0-●
    trochlear nerve H49.1-●
  specified type NEC H50.89
  vertical H50.2-●
Strain
  back S39.012
  cervical S16.1
  eye NEC —*see* Disturbance, vision, subjective
  heart —*see* Disease, heart
  low back S39.012
  mental NOS Z73.3
    work-related Z56.6
  muscle (tendon) —*see* Injury, muscle, by site, strain
  neck S16.1
  physical NOS Z73.3
    work-related Z56.6
  postural —*see also* Disorder, soft tissue, due to use
  psychological NEC Z73.3
  tendon —*see* Injury, muscle, by site, strain
Straining, on urination R39.16
Strand, vitreous —*see* Opacity, vitreous, membranes and strands
Strangulation, strangulated —*see also* Asphyxia, traumatic
  appendix K38.8
  bladder-neck N32.0
  bowel or colon K56.2
  food or foreign body —*see* Foreign body, by site
  hemorrhoids —*see* Hemorrhoids, with complication
  hernia —*see also* Hernia, by site, with obstruction
    with gangrene —*see* Hernia, by site, with gangrene

► New   ⇒ Revised   ~~deleted~~ Deleted   ● Use Additional Character(s)

Strangulation, strangulated *(Continued)*
  intestine (large) (small) K56.2
    with hernia —*see also* Hernia, by site, with
      obstruction
      with gangrene —*see* Hernia, by site, with
        gangrene
  mesentery K56.2
  mucus —*see* Asphyxia, mucus
  omentum K56.2
  organ or site, congenital NEC —*see* Atresia,
    by site
  ovary —*see* Torsion, ovary
  penis N48.89
    foreign body T19.4
  rupture —*see* Hernia, by site, with obstruction
  stomach due to hernia —*see also* Hernia, by
    site, with obstruction
    with gangrene —*see* Hernia, by site, with
      gangrene
  vesicourethral orifice N32.0
Strangury R30.0
Straw itch B88.0
Strawberry
  gallbladder K82.4
  mark Q82.5
  tongue (red) (white) K14.3
Streak(s)
  macula, angioid H35.33
  ovarian Q50.32
Strephosymbolia F81.0
  secondary to organic lesion R48.8
Streptobacillary fever A25.1
Streptobacillosis A25.1
Streptobacillus moniliformis A25.1
Streptococcus, streptococcal —*see also*
  condition
  as cause of disease classified elsewhere B95.5
  group
    A, as cause of disease classified elsewhere
      B95.0
    B, as cause of disease classified elsewhere
      B95.1
    D, as cause of disease classified elsewhere
      B95.2
    pneumoniae, as cause of disease classified
      elsewhere B95.3
    specified NEC, as cause of disease classified
      elsewhere B95.4
Streptomycosis B47.1
Streptotrichosis A48.8
Stress F43.9
  family —*see* Disruption, family
  fetal P84
    complicating pregnancy O77.9
      due to drug administration O77.1
  mental NEC Z73.3
    work-related Z56.6
  physical NEC Z73.3
    work-related Z56.6
  polycythemia D75.1
  reaction —*see also* Reaction, stress F43.9
  work schedule Z56.3
Stretching, nerve —*see* Injury, nerve
Striae albicantes, atrophicae or distensae
  (cutis) L90.6
Stricture —*see also* Stenosis
  ampulla of Vater K83.1
  anus (sphincter) K62.4
    congenital Q42.3
      with fistula Q42.2
    infantile Q42.3
      with fistula Q42.2
  aorta (ascending) (congenital) Q25.1
    arteriosclerotic I70.0
    calcified I70.0
    supravalvular, congenital Q25.3
  aortic (valve) —*see* Stenosis, aortic
  aqueduct of Sylvius (congenital) Q03.0
    with spina bifida —*see* Spina bifida, by site,
      with hydrocephalus
    acquired G91.1

Stricture *(Continued)*
  artery I77.1
    basilar —*see* Occlusion, artery, basilar
    carotid —*see* Occlusion, artery, carotid
    celiac I77.4
    congenital (peripheral) Q27.8
      cerebral Q28.3
      coronary Q24.5
      digestive system Q27.8
      lower limb Q27.8
      retinal Q14.1
      specified site NEC Q27.8
      umbilical Q27.0
      upper limb Q27.8
    coronary —*see* Disease, heart, ischemic,
      atherosclerotic
      congenital Q24.5
    precerebral —*see* Occlusion, artery,
      precerebral
    pulmonary (congenital) Q25.6
      acquired I28.8
    renal I70.1
    vertebral —*see* Occlusion, artery, vertebral
  auditory canal (external) (congenital)
    acquired —*see* Stenosis, external ear canal
  bile duct (common) (hepatic) K83.1
    congenital Q44.3
    postoperative K91.89
  bladder N32.89
    neck N32.0
  bowel —*see* Obstruction, intestine
  brain G93.89
  bronchus J98.09
    congenital Q32.3
    syphilitic A52.72
  cardia (stomach) K22.2
    congenital Q39.3
  cardiac —*see also* Disease, heart
    orifice (stomach) K22.2
  cecum —*see* Obstruction, intestine
  cervix, cervical (canal) N88.2
    congenital Q51.828
    in pregnancy —*see* Pregnancy, complicated
      by, abnormal cervix
      causing obstructed labor O65.5
  colon —*see also* Obstruction, intestine
    congenital Q42.9
      specified NEC Q42.8
  colostomy K94.03
  common (bile) duct K83.1
  coronary (artery) —*see* Disease, heart,
    ischemic, atherosclerotic
  cystic duct —*see* Obstruction, gallbladder
  digestive organs NEC, congenital Q45.8
  duodenum K31.5
    congenital Q41.0
  ear canal (external) (congenital) Q16.1
    acquired —*see* Stricture, auditory canal,
      acquired
  ejaculatory duct N50.89
  enterostomy K94.13
  esophagus K22.2
    congenital Q39.3
    syphilitic A52.79
      congenital A50.59 *[K23]*
  eustachian tube —*see also* Obstruction,
    eustachian tube
    congenital Q17.8
  fallopian tube N97.1
    gonococcal A54.24
    tuberculous A18.17
  gallbladder —*see* Obstruction, gallbladder
  glottis J38.6
  heart —*see also* Disease, heart
    valve (*see also* Endocarditis) I38
      aortic Q23.0
      mitral Q23.2
      pulmonary Q22.1
      tricuspid Q22.4
  hepatic duct K83.1
  hourglass, of stomach K31.2

Stricture *(Continued)*
  hymen N89.6
  hypopharynx J39.2
  ileum —*see also* Obstruction, intestine,
    specified NEC K56.699
    congenital Q41.2
  intestine —*see also* Obstruction, intestine
    congenital (small) Q41.9
      large Q42.9
        specified NEC Q42.8
      specified NEC Q41.8
    ischemic K55.1
  jejunum —*see also* Obstruction, intestine,
    specified NEC K56.699
    congenital Q41.1
  lacrimal passages —*see also* Stenosis, lacrimal
    congenital Q10.5
  larynx J38.6
    congenital NEC Q31.8
      subglottic Q31.1
    syphilitic A52.73
      congenital A50.59 *[J99]*
  meatus
    ear (congenital) Q16.1
      acquired —*see* Stricture, auditory canal,
        acquired
    osseous (ear) (congenital) Q16.1
      acquired —*see* Stricture, auditory canal,
        acquired
    urinarius —*see also* Stricture, urethra
      congenital Q64.33
  mitral (valve) —*see* Stenosis, mitral
  myocardium, myocardial I51.5
    hypertrophic subaortic (idiopathic) I42.1
  nares (anterior) (posterior) J34.89
    congenital Q30.0
  nasal duct —*see also* Stenosis, lacrimal, duct
    congenital Q10.5
  nasolacrimal duct —*see also* Stenosis, lacrimal,
    duct
    congenital Q10.5
  nasopharynx J39.2
    syphilitic A52.73
  nose J34.89
    congenital Q30.0
  nostril (anterior) (posterior) J34.89
    congenital Q30.0
    syphilitic A52.73
      congenital A50.59 *[J99]*
  organ or site, congenital NEC —*see* Atresia,
    by site
  os uteri —*see* Stricture, cervix
  osseous meatus (ear) (congenital) Q16.1
    acquired —*see* Stricture, auditory canal,
      acquired
  oviduct —*see* Stricture, fallopian tube
  pelviureteric junction (congenital) Q62.11
    acquired, with hydronephrosis N13.0
  penis, by foreign body T19.4
  pharynx J39.2
  prostate N42.89
  pulmonary, pulmonic
    artery (congenital) Q25.6
      acquired I28.8
      noncongenital I28.8
    infundibulum (congenital) Q24.3
    valve I37.0
      congenital Q22.1
    vein, acquired I28.8
    vessel NEC I28.8
  punctum lacrimale —*see also* Stenosis,
    lacrimal, punctum
    congenital Q10.5
  pylorus (hypertrophic) K31.1
    adult K31.1
    congenital Q40.0
    infantile Q40.0
  rectosigmoid —*see also* Obstruction, intestine,
    specified NEC K56.699
  rectum (sphincter) K62.4
    congenital Q42.1
      with fistula Q42.0

Stricture *(Continued)*
  rectum *(Continued)*
    due to
      chlamydial lymphogranuloma A55
      irradiation K91.89
      lymphogranuloma venereum A55
    gonococcal A54.6
    inflammatory (chlamydial) A55
    syphilitic A52.74
    tuberculous A18.32
  renal artery I70.1
    congenital Q27.1
  salivary duct or gland (any) K11.8
  sigmoid (flexure) —*see* Obstruction, intestine
  spermatic cord N50.89
  stoma (following) (of)
    colostomy K94.03
    enterostomy K94.13
    gastrostomy K94.23
    ileostomy K94.13
    tracheostomy J95.03
  stomach K31.89
    congenital Q40.2
    hourglass K31.2
  subaortic Q24.4
    hypertrophic (acquired) (idiopathic) I42.1
  subglottic J38.6
  syphilitic NEC A52.79
  trachea J39.8
    congenital Q32.1
    syphilitic A52.73
    tuberculous NEC A15.5
  tracheostomy J95.03
  tricuspid (valve) —*see* Stenosis, tricuspid
  tunica vaginalis N50.89
  ureter (postoperative) N13.5
    with
      hydronephrosis N13.1
        with infection N13.6
      pyelonephritis (chronic) N11.1
    congenital —*see* Atresia, ureter
    tuberculous A18.11
  ureteropelvic junction (congenital) Q62.11
    acquired, with hydronephrosis N13.0
  ureterovesical orifice N13.5
    with infection N13.6
  urethra (organic) (spasmodic) N35.9
    associated with schistosomiasis
      B65.0 [N37]
    congenital Q64.39
      valvular (posterior) Q64.2
    due to
      infection —*see* Stricture, urethra,
        postinfective
      trauma —*see* Stricture, urethra,
        post-traumatic
    gonococcal, gonorrheal A54.01
    infective NEC —*see* Stricture, urethra,
      postinfective
    late effect (sequelae) of injury —*see*
      Stricture, urethra, post-traumatic
    postcatheterization —*see* Stricture, urethra,
      postprocedural
    postinfective NEC
      female N35.12
      male N35.119
        anterior urethra N35.114
        bulbous urethra N35.112
        meatal N35.111
        membranous urethra N35.113
    postobstetric N35.021
    postoperative —*see* Stricture, urethra,
      postprocedural
    postprocedural
      female N99.12
      male N99.114
        anterior bulbous urethra N99.113
        bulbous urethra N99.111
        fossa navicularis N99.115
        meatal N99.110
        membranous urethra N99.112

Stricture *(Continued)*
  urethra (organic) (spasmodic) *(Continued)*
    post-traumatic
      female N35.028
        due to childbirth N35.021
      male N35.014
        anterior urethra N35.013
        bulbous urethra N35.011
        meatal N35.010
        membranous urethra N35.012
    sequela (late effect) of
      childbirth N35.021
      injury —*see* Stricture, urethra,
        post-traumatic
    specified cause NEC N35.8
    syphilitic A52.76
    traumatic —*see* Stricture, urethra,
      post-traumatic
    valvular (posterior), congenital Q64.2
  urinary meatus —*see* Stricture, urethra
  uterus, uterine (synechiae) N85.6
    os (external) (internal) —*see* Stricture, cervix
  vagina (outlet) —*see* Stenosis, vagina
  valve (cardiac) (heart) —*see also* Endocarditis
    congenital
      aortic Q23.0
      mitral Q23.2
      pulmonary Q22.1
      tricuspid Q22.4
  vas deferens N50.89
    congenital Q55.4
  vein I87.1
  vena cava (inferior) (superior) NEC I87.1
    congenital Q26.0
  vesicourethral orifice N32.0
    congenital Q64.31
  vulva (acquired) N90.5
Stridor R06.1
  congenital (larynx) P28.89
Stridulous —*see* condition
Stroke (apoplectic) (brain) (embolic) (ischemic)
  (paralytic) (thrombotic) I63.9
▶cryptogenic —*see also* infarction, cerebral
    I63.9
  epileptic —*see* Epilepsy
  heat T67.0
  in evolution I63.9
  intraoperative
    during cardiac surgery I97.810
    during other surgery I97.811
  lightning —*see* Lightning
  meaning
    cerebral hemorrhage — code to
      Hemorrhage, intracranial
    cerebral infarction — code to Infarction,
      cerebral
  postprocedural
    following cardiac surgery I97.820
    following other surgery I97.821
  unspecified (NOS) I63.9
Stromatosis, endometrial D39.0
Strongyloidiasis, strongyloidosis B78.9
  cutaneous B78.1
  disseminated B78.7
  intestinal B78.0
Strophulus pruriginosus L28.2
Struck by lightning —*see* Lightning
Struma —*see also* Goiter
  Hashimoto E06.3
  lymphomatosa E06.3
  nodosa (simplex) E04.9
    endemic E01.2
      multinodular E01.1
    multinodular E04.2
      iodine-deficiency related E01.1
    toxic or with hyperthyroidism E05.20
      with thyroid storm E05.21
      multinodular E05.20
        with thyroid storm E05.21
      uninodular E05.10
        with thyroid storm E05.11

Struma *(Continued)*
  nodosa (simplex) *(Continued)*
    toxicosa E05.20
      with thyroid storm E05.21
      multinodular E05.20
        with thyroid storm E05.21
      uninodular E05.10
        with thyroid storm E05.11
    uninodular E04.1
  ovarii D27.-●
  Riedel's E06.5
Strumipriva cachexia E03.4
Strümpell-Marie spine —*see* Spondylitis,
  ankylosing
Strümpell-Westphal pseudosclerosis E83.01
Stuart deficiency disease (factor X) D68.2
Stuart-Prower factor deficiency (factor X)
  D68.2
Student's elbow —*see* Bursitis, elbow,
  olecranon
Stump —*see* Amputation
Stunting, nutritional E45
Stupor (catatonic) R40.1
  depressive (single episode) F32.89
    recurrent episode F33.8
  dissociative F44.2
  manic F30.2
  manic-depressive F31.89
  psychogenic (anergic) F44.2
  reaction to exceptional stress (transient)
    F43.0
Sturge (-Weber) (-Dimitri) (-Kalischer) disease
  or syndrome Q85.8
Stuttering F80.81
  adult onset F98.5
  childhood onset F80.81
  following cerebrovascular disease —
    see Disorder, fluency, following
    cerebrovascular disease
  in conditions classified elsewhere R47.82
Sty, stye (external) (internal) (meibomian)
  (zeisian) —*see* Hordeolum
Subacidity, gastric K31.89
  psychogenic F45.8
Subacute —*see* condition
Subarachnoid —*see* condition
Subcortical —*see* condition
Subcostal syndrome, nerve compression —*see*
  Mononeuropathy, upper limb, specified
  site NEC
Subcutaneous, subcuticular —*see* condition
Subdural —*see* condition
Subendocardium —*see* condition
Subependymoma
  specified site —*see* Neoplasm, uncertain
    behavior, by site
  unspecified site D43.2
Suberosis J67.3
Subglossitis —*see* Glossitis
Subhemophilia D66
Subinvolution
  breast (postlactational) (postpuerperal)
    N64.89
    puerperal O90.89
  uterus (chronic) (nonpuerperal) N85.3
    puerperal O90.89
Sublingual —*see* condition
Sublinguitis —*see* Sialoadenitis
Subluxatable hip Q65.6
Subluxation —*see also* Dislocation
  acromioclavicular S43.11-●
  ankle S93.0-●
  atlantoaxial, recurrent M43.4
    with myelopathy M43.3
  carpometacarpal (joint) NEC S63.05-●
    thumb S63.04-●
  complex, vertebral —*see* Complex,
    subluxation
  congenital —*see also* Malposition, congenital
    hip —*see* Dislocation, hip, congenital,
      partial

▶ New   ⇒ Revised   deleted Deleted   ● Use Additional Character(s)

Subluxation *(Continued)*
congenital *(Continued)*
joint (excluding hip)
lower limb Q68.8
shoulder Q68.8
upper limb Q68.8
elbow (traumatic) S53.10-●
anterior S53.11-●
lateral S53.14-●
medial S53.13-●
posterior S53.12-●
specified type NEC S53.19-●
finger S63.20-●
index S63.20-●
interphalangeal S63.22-●
distal S63.24-●
index S63.24-●
little S63.24-●
middle S63.24-●
ring S63.24-●
index S63.22-●
little S63.22-●
middle S63.22-●
proximal S63.23-●
index S63.23-●
little S63.23-●
middle S63.23-●
ring S63.23-●
ring S63.22-●
little S63.20-●
metacarpophalangeal S63.21-●
index S63.21-●
little S63.21-●
middle S63.21-●
ring S63.21-●
middle S63.20-●
ring S63.20-●
foot S93.30-●
specified site NEC S93.33-●
tarsal joint S93.31-●
tarsometatarsal joint S93.32-●
toe —*see* Subluxation, toe
hip S73.00-●
anterior S73.03-●
obturator S73.02-●
central S73.04-●
posterior S73.01-●
interphalangeal (joint)
finger S63.22-●
distal joint S63.24-●
index S63.24-●
little S63.24-●
middle S63.24-●
ring S63.24-●
index S63.22-●
little S63.22-●
middle S63.22-●
proximal joint S63.23-●
index S63.23-●
little S63.23-●
middle S63.23-●
ring S63.23-●
ring S63.22-●
thumb S63.12-●
distal joint S63.14-●
proximal joint S63.13-●
toe S93.13-●
great S93.13-●
lesser S93.13-●
joint prosthesis —*see* Complications, joint
prosthesis, mechanical, displacement,
by site
knee S83.10-●
cap —*see* Subluxation, patella
patella —*see* Subluxation, patella
proximal tibia
anteriorly S83.11-●
laterally S83.14-●
medially S83.13-●
posteriorly S83.12-●
specified type NEC S83.19-●

Subluxation *(Continued)*
lens —*see* Dislocation, lens, partial
ligament, traumatic —*see* Sprain, by site
metacarpal (bone)
proximal end S63.06-●
metacarpophalangeal (joint)
finger S63.21-●
index S63.21-●
little S63.21-●
middle S63.21-●
ring S63.21-●
thumb S63.11-●
metatarsophalangeal joint S93.14-●
great toe S93.14-●
lesser toe S93.14-●
midcarpal (joint) S63.03-●
patella S83.00-●
lateral S83.01-●
recurrent (nontraumatic) —*see* Dislocation,
patella, recurrent, incomplete
specified type NEC S83.09-●
pathological —*see* Dislocation, pathological
radial head S53.00-●
anterior S53.01-●
nursemaid's elbow S53.03-●
posterior S53.02-●
specified type NEC S53.09-●
radiocarpal (joint) S63.02-●
radioulnar (joint)
distal S63.01-●
proximal —*see* Subluxation, elbow
shoulder
congenital Q68.8
girdle S43.30-●
scapula S43.31-●
specified site NEC S43.39-●
traumatic S43.00-●
anterior S43.01-●
inferior S43.03-●
posterior S43.02-●
specified type NEC S43.08-●
sternoclavicular (joint) S43.20-●
anterior S43.21-●
posterior S43.22-●
symphysis (pubis)
thumb S63.103
interphalangeal joint —*see* Subluxation,
interphalangeal (joint), thumb
metacarpophalangeal joint —*see*
Subluxation, metacarpophalangeal
(joint), thumb
toe(s) S93.10-●
great S93.10-●
interphalangeal joint S93.13-●
metatarsophalangeal joint S93.14-●
interphalangeal joint S93.13-●
lesser S93.10-●
interphalangeal joint S93.13-●
metatarsophalangeal joint S93.14-●
metatarsophalangeal joint S93.149
ulnohumeral joint —*see* Subluxation,
elbow
vertebral
recurrent NEC —*see* subcategory
M43.5
traumatic
cervical S13.100
atlantoaxial joint S13.120
atlantooccipital joint S13.110
atloidooccipital joint S13.110
joint between
C0 and C1 S13.110
C1 and C2 S13.120
C2 and C3 S13.130
C3 and C4 S13.140
C4 and C5 S13.150
C5 and C6 S13.160
C6 and C7 S13.170
C7 and T1 S13.180
occipitoatloid joint
S13.110

Subluxation *(Continued)*
vertebral *(Continued)*
traumatic *(Continued)*
lumbar S33.100
joint between
L1 and L2 S33.110
L2 and L3 S33.120
L3 and L4 S33.130
L4 and L5 S33.140
thoracic S23.100
joint between
T1 and T2 S23.110
T2 and T3 S23.120
T3 and T4 S23.122
T4 and T5 S23.130
T5 and T6 S23.132
T6 and T7 S23.140
T7 and T8 S23.142
T8 and T9 S23.150
T9 and T10 S23.152
T10 and T11 S23.160
T11 and T12 S23.162
T12 and L1 S23.170
ulna
distal end S63.07-●
proximal end —*see* Subluxation, elbow
wrist (carpal bone) S63.00-●
carpometacarpal joint —*see* Subluxation,
carpometacarpal (joint)
distal radioulnar joint —*see* Subluxation,
radioulnar (joint), distal
metacarpal bone, proximal —*see*
Subluxation, metacarpal (bone),
proximal end
midcarpal —*see* Subluxation, midcarpal
(joint)
radiocarpal joint —*see* Subluxation,
radiocarpal (joint)
recurrent —*see* Dislocation, recurrent, wrist
specified site NEC S63.09-●
ulna —*see* Subluxation, ulna, distal end
Submaxillary —*see* condition
Submersion (fatal) (nonfatal) T75.1
Submucous —*see* condition
Subnormal, subnormality
accommodation (old age) H52.4
mental —*see* Disability, intellectual
temperature (accidental) T68
Subphrenic —*see* condition
Subscapular nerve —*see* condition
Subseptus uterus Q51.2
Subsiding appendicitis K36
Substance (other psychoactive) -induced
anxiety disorder F19.980
bipolar and related disorder F19.94
delirium F19.921
depressive disorder F19.94
major neurocognitive disorder F19.97
mild neurocognitive disorder F19.988
obsessive-compulsive and related disorder
F19.988
psychotic disorder F19.959
sexual dysfunction F19.981
sleep disorder F19.982
Substernal thyroid E04.9
congenital Q89.2
Substitution disorder F44.9
Subtentorial —*see* condition
Subthyroidism (acquired) —*see also*
Hypothyroidism
congenital E03.1
Succenturiate placenta O43.19-●
Sucking thumb, child (excessive) F98.8
Sudamen, sudamina L74.1
Sudanese kala-azar B55.0
Sudden
hearing loss —*see* Deafness, sudden
heart failure —*see* Failure, heart
Sudeck's atrophy, disease, or syndrome —*see*
Algoneurodystrophy
Suffocation —*see* Asphyxia, traumatic

S

S

Sugar
  blood
    high (transient) R73.9
    low (transient) E16.2
  in urine R81
Suicide, suicidal (attempted) T14.91
  by poisoning —*see* Table of Drugs and
      Chemicals
  history of (personal) Z91.5
    in family Z81.8
  ideation —*see* Ideation, suicidal
  risk
    meaning personal history of attempted
        suicide Z91.5
    meaning suicidal ideation —*see* Ideation,
        suicidal
  tendencies
    meaning personal history of attempted
        suicide Z91.5
    meaning suicidal ideation —*see* Ideation,
        suicidal
  trauma —*see* nature of injury by site
Suipestifer infection —*see* Infection, salmonella
Sulfhemoglobinemia, sulphemoglobinemia
      (acquired) (with methemoglobinemia)
      D74.8
Sumatran mite fever A75.3
Summer —*see* condition
Sunburn L55.9
  due to
    tanning bed (acute) L56.8
      chronic L57.8
    ultraviolet radiation (acute) L56.8
      chronic L57.8
  first degree L55.0
  second degree L55.1
  third degree L55.2
SUNCT (short lasting unilateral neuralgiform
      headache with conjunctival injection and
      tearing) G44.059
  intractable G44.051
  not intractable G44.059
▶ **Sundowning** F05
Sunken acetabulum —*see* Derangement, joint,
      specified type NEC, hip
Sunstroke T67.0
Superfecundation —*see* Pregnancy, multiple
Superfetation —*see* Pregnancy, multiple
Superinvolution (uterus) N85.8
Supernumerary (congenital)
  aortic cusps Q23.8
  auditory ossicles Q16.3
  bone Q79.8
  breast Q83.1
  carpal bones Q74.0
  cusps, heart valve NEC Q24.8
    aortic Q23.8
    mitral Q23.2
    pulmonary Q22.3
  digit(s) Q69.9
  ear (lobule) Q17.0
  fallopian tube Q50.6
  finger Q69.0
  hymen Q52.4
  kidney Q63.0
  lacrimonasal duct Q10.6
  lobule (ear) Q17.0
  mitral cusps Q23.2
  muscle Q79.8
  nipple(s) Q83.3
  organ or site not listed —*see* Accessory
  ossicles, auditory Q16.3
  ovary Q50.31
  oviduct Q50.6
  pulmonary, pulmonic cusps Q22.3
  rib Q76.6
    cervical or first (syndrome) Q76.5
  roots (of teeth) K00.2
  spleen Q89.09
  tarsal bones Q74.2
  teeth K00.1

Supernumerary (*Continued*)
  testis Q55.29
  thumb Q69.1
  toe Q69.2
  uterus Q51.2
  vagina Q52.1
  vertebra Q76.49
Supervision (of)
  contraceptive —*see* Prescription,
      contraceptives
  dietary (for) Z71.3
    allergy (food) Z71.3
    colitis Z71.3
    diabetes mellitus Z71.3
    food allergy or intolerance Z71.3
    gastritis Z71.3
    hypercholesterolemia Z71.3
    hypoglycemia Z71.3
    intolerance (food) Z71.3
    obesity Z71.3
    specified NEC Z71.3
  healthy infant or child Z76.2
    foundling Z76.1
  high-risk pregnancy —*see* Pregnancy,
      complicated by, high, risk
  lactation Z39.1
  pregnancy —*see* Pregnancy, supervision of
Supplemental teeth K00.1
Suppression
  binocular vision H53.34
  lactation O92.5
  menstruation N94.89
  ovarian secretion E28.39
  renal N28.9
  urine, urinary secretion R34
Suppuration, suppurative —*see also* condition
  accessory sinus (chronic) —*see* Sinusitis
  adrenal gland
  antrum (chronic) —*see* Sinusitis, maxillary
  bladder —*see* Cystitis
  brain G06.0
    sequelae G09
  breast N61.1
    puerperal, postpartum or gestational —*see*
        Mastitis, obstetric, purulent
  dental periosteum M27.3
  ear (middle) —*see also* Otitis, media
    external NEC —*see* Otitis, externa,
        infective
    internal —*see* subcategory H83.0
  ethmoidal (chronic) (sinus) —*see* Sinusitis,
      ethmoidal
  fallopian tube —*see* Salpingo-oophoritis
  frontal (chronic) (sinus) —*see* Sinusitis,
      frontal
  gallbladder (acute) K81.0
  gum K05.20
    generalized —*see* Peridontitis, aggressive,
        generalized
    localized —*see* Peridontitis, aggressive,
        localized
  intracranial G06.0
  joint —*see* Arthritis, pyogenic or pyemic
  labyrinthine —*see* subcategory H83.0
  lung —*see* Abscess, lung
  mammary gland N61.1
    puerperal, postpartum O91.12
      associated with lactation O91.13
  maxilla, maxillary M27.2
    sinus (chronic) —*see* Sinusitis, maxillary
  muscle —*see* Myositis, infective
  nasal sinus (chronic) —*see* Sinusitis
  pancreas, acute —*see also* Pancreatitis, acute
      K85.80
  parotid gland —*see* Sialoadenitis
  pelvis, pelvic
    female —*see* Disease, pelvis, inflammatory
    male K65.0
  pericranial —*see* Osteomyelitis
  salivary duct or gland (any) —*see*
      Sialoadenitis

Suppuration, suppurative (*Continued*)
  sinus (accessory) (chronic) (nasal) —*see*
      Sinusitis
  sphenoidal sinus (chronic) —*see* Sinusitis,
      sphenoidal
  thymus (gland) E32.1
  thyroid (gland) E06.0
  tonsil —*see* Tonsillitis
  uterus —*see* Endometritis
Supraeruption of tooth (teeth) M26.34
Supraglottitis J04.30
  with obstruction J04.31
Suprarenal (gland) —*see* condition
Suprascapular nerve —*see* condition
Suprasellar —*see* condition
Surfer's knots or nodules S89.8-●
Surgical
  emphysema T81.82
  procedures, complication or misadventure —
      see Complications, surgical procedures
  shock T81.10
Surveillance (of) (for) —*see also* Observation
  alcohol abuse Z71.41
  contraceptive —*see* Prescription,
      contraceptives
  dietary Z71.3
  drug abuse Z71.51
Susceptibility to disease, genetic Z15.89
  malignant neoplasm Z15.09
    breast Z15.01
    endometrium Z15.04
    ovary Z15.02
    prostate Z15.03
    specified NEC Z15.09
  multiple endocrine neoplasia Z15.81
Suspected condition, ruled out —*see also*
      Observation, suspected
  amniotic cavity and membrane Z03.71
  cervical shortening Z03.75
  fetal anomaly Z03.73
  fetal growth Z03.74
  maternal and fetal conditions NEC Z03.79
  newborn —*see also* Observation, newborn,
      suspected condition ruled out Z05.9
  oligohydramnios Z03.71
  placental problem Z03.72
  polyhydramnios Z03.71
Suspended uterus
  in pregnancy or childbirth —*see* Pregnancy,
      complicated by, abnormal uterus
Sutton's nevus D22.9
Suture
  burst (in operation wound) T81.31
    external operation wound T81.31
    internal operation wound T81.32
  inadvertently left in operation wound —*see*
      Foreign body, accidentally left during a
      procedure
  removal Z48.02
Swab inadvertently left in operation wound —
      see Foreign body, accidentally left during a
      procedure
Swallowed, swallowing
  difficulty —*see* Dysphagia
  foreign body —*see* Foreign body, alimentary
      tract
Swan-neck deformity (finger) —*see* Deformity,
      finger, swan-neck
Swearing, compulsive F42.8
  in Gilles de la Tourette's syndrome F95.2
Sweat, sweats
  fetid L75.0
  night R61
Sweating, excessive R61
Sweeley-Klionsky disease E75.21
Sweet's disease or dermatosis L98.2
Swelling (of) R60.9
  abdomen, abdominal (not referable to any
      particular organ) —*see* Mass,
      abdominal
  ankle —*see* Effusion, joint, ankle

▶ New   ⇒ Revised   ~~deleted~~ Deleted   ● Use Additional Character(s)

Swelling *(Continued)*
  arm M79.89
    forearm M79.89
  breast —*see also* Lump, breast N63.0
  Calabar B74.3
  cervical gland R59.0
  chest, localized R22.2
  ear H93.8-●
  extremity (lower) (upper) —*see* Disorder, soft
      tissue, specified type NEC
  finger M79.89
  foot M79.89
  glands R59.9
    generalized R59.1
    localized R59.0
  hand M79.89
  head (localized) R22.0
  inflammatory —*see* Inflammation
  intra-abdominal —*see* Mass, abdominal
  joint —*see* Effusion, joint
  leg M79.89
    lower M79.89
  limb —*see* Disorder, soft tissue, specified type
      NEC
  localized (skin) R22.9
    chest R22.2
    head R22.0
    limb
      lower —*see* Mass, localized, limb, lower
      upper —*see* Mass, localized, limb, upper
    neck R22.1
    trunk R22.2
  neck (localized) R22.1
  pelvic —*see* Mass, abdominal
  scrotum N50.89
  splenic —*see* Splenomegaly
  testis N50.89
  toe M79.89
  umbilical R19.09
  wandering, due to Gnathostoma
      (spinigerum) B83.1
  white —*see* Tuberculosis, arthritis
Swift (-Feer) disease
  overdose or wrong substance given
      or taken —*see* Table of Drugs and
      Chemicals, by drug, poisoning
Swimmer's
  cramp T75.1
  ear H60.33-●
  itch B65.3
Swimming in the head R42
Swollen —*see* Swelling
Swyer syndrome Q99.1
Sycosis L73.8
  barbae (not parasitic) L73.8
  contagiosa (mycotic) B35.0
  lupoides L73.8
  mycotic B35.0
  parasitic B35.0
  vulgaris L73.8
Sydenham's chorea —*see* Chorea, Sydenham's
Sylvatic yellow fever A95.0
Sylvest's disease B33.0
Symblepharon H11.23-●
  congenital Q10.3
Symond's syndrome G93.2
Sympathetic —*see* condition
Sympatheticotonia G90.8
Sympathicoblastoma
  specified site —*see* Neoplasm, malignant, by
      site
  unspecified site C74.90
Sympathogonioma —*see* Sympathicoblastoma
Symphalangy (fingers) (toes) Q70.9
Symptoms NEC R68.89
  breast NEC N64.59
▶ cold J00
  development NEC R63.8
  factitious, self-induced —*see* Disorder,
      factitious
  genital organs, female R10.2

Symptoms NEC *(Continued)*
  involving
    abdomen NEC R19.8
    appearance NEC R46.89
    awareness R41.9
      altered mental status R41.82
      amnesia —*see* Amnesia
      borderline intellectual functioning
          R41.83
      coma —*see* Coma
      disorientation R41.0
      neurologic neglect syndrome R41.4
      senile cognitive decline R41.81
      specified symptom NEC R41.89
    behavior NEC R46.89
    cardiovascular system NEC R09.89
    chest NEC R09.89
    circulatory system NEC R09.89
    cognitive functions R41.9
      altered mental status R41.82
      amnesia —*see* Amnesia
      borderline intellectual functioning
          R41.83
      coma —*see* Coma
      disorientation R41.0
      neurologic neglect syndrome R41.4
      senile cognitive decline R41.81
      specified symptom NEC R41.89
    development NEC R62.50
    digestive system NEC R19.8
    emotional state NEC R45.89
      emotional lability R45.86
    food and fluid intake R63.8
    general perceptions and sensations
        R44.9
      specified NEC R44.8
    musculoskeletal system R29.91
      specified NEC R29.898
    nervous system R29.90
      specified NEC R29.818
    pelvis NEC R19.8
    respiratory system NEC R09.89
    skin and integument R23.9
    urinary system R39.9
  menopausal N95.1
  metabolism NEC R63.8
  neurotic F48.8
  of infancy R68.19
  pelvis NEC, female R10.2
  skin and integument NEC R23.9
  subcutaneous tissue NEC R23.9
▶ viral cold J00
Sympus Q74.2
Syncephalus Q89.4
Synchondrosis
  abnormal (congenital) Q78.8
  ischiopubic M91.0
Synchysis (scintillans) (senile) (vitreous body)
    H43.89
Syncope (near) (pre-) R55
  anginosa I20.8
  bradycardia R00.1
  cardiac R55
  carotid sinus G90.01
  due to spinal (lumbar) puncture G97.1
  heart R55
  heat T67.1
  laryngeal R05
  psychogenic F48.8
  tussive R05
  vasoconstriction R55
  vasodepressor R55
  vasomotor R55
  vasovagal R55
Syndactylism, syndactyly Q70.9
  complex (with synostosis)
    fingers Q70.0-●
    toes Q70.2-●
  simple (without synostosis)
    fingers Q70.1-●
    toes Q70.3-●

Syndrome —*see also* Disease
  5q minus NOS D46.C
  48,XXXX Q97.1
  49,XXXXX Q97.1
  abdominal
    acute R10.0
    muscle deficiency Q79.4
  abnormal innervation H02.519
    left H02.516
      lower H02.515
      upper H02.514
    right H02.513
      lower H02.512
      upper H02.511
  abstinence, neonatal P96.1
  acid pulmonary aspiration, obstetric O74.0
  acquired immunodeficiency —*see* Human,
      immunodeficiency virus (HIV) disease
  acute abdominal R10.0
  acute respiratory distress (adult) (child) J80
    idiopathic J84.114
  Adair-Dighton Q78.0
  Adams-Stokes (-Morgagni) I45.9
  adiposogenital E23.6
  adrenal
    hemorrhage (meningococcal) A39.1
    meningococcic A39.1
  adrenocortical —*see* Cushing's, syndrome
  adrenogenital E25.9
    congenital, associated with enzyme
        deficiency E25.0
  afferent loop NEC K91.89
  Alagille's Q44.7
  alcohol withdrawal (without convulsions) —
      see Dependence, alcohol, with,
      withdrawal
  Alder's D72.0
  Aldrich (-Wiskott) D82.0
  alien hand R41.4
  Alport Q87.81
  alveolar hypoventilation E66.2
  alveolocapillary block J84.10
  amnesic, amnestic (confabulatory) (due to) —
      see Disorder, amnesic
  amyostatic (Wilson's disease) E83.01
  androgen insensitivity E34.50
    complete E34.51
    partial E34.52
  androgen resistance (*see also* Syndrome,
      androgen insensitivity) E34.50
  Angelman Q93.5
  anginal —*see* Angina
  ankyloglossia superior Q38.1
  anterior
    chest wall R07.89
    cord G83.82
    spinal artery G95.19
      compression M47.019
        cervical region M47.012
        cervicothoracic region M47.013
        lumbar region M47.016
        occipito-atlanto-axial region M47.011
        thoracic region M47.014
        thoracolumbar region M47.015
    tibial M76.81-●
  antibody deficiency D80.9
    agammaglobulinemic D80.1
      hereditary D80.0
    congenital D80.0
    hypogammaglobulinemic D80.1
      hereditary D80.0
  anticardiolipin (-antibody) D68.61
▶ antidepressant discontinuation T43.205
  antiphospholipid (-antibody) D68.61
  aortic
    arch M31.4
    bifurcation I74.09
  aortomesenteric duodenum occlusion K31.5
  apical ballooning (transient left ventricular)
      I51.81
  arcuate ligament I77.4

Syndrome *(Continued)*
　argentaffin, argintaffinoma E34.0
　Arnold-Chiari —*see* Arnold-Chiari disease
　Arrillaga-Ayerza I27.0
　arterial tortuosity Q87.82
　arteriovenous steal T82.898-●
　Asherman's N85.6
　aspiration, of newborn —*see* Aspiration, by
　　　substance, with pneumonia
　　meconium P24.01
　ataxia-telangiectasia G11.3
　auriculotemporal G50.8
　autoerythrocyte sensitization (Gardner-
　　Diamond) D69.2
　autoimmune lymphoproliferative [ALPS]
　　D89.82
　autoimmune polyglandular E31.0
　autoinflammatory M04.9
　　specified type NEC M04.8
　autosomal —*see* Abnormal, autosomes
　Avellis' G46.8
　Ayerza (-Arrillaga) I27.0
　Babinski-Nageotte G83.89
　Bakwin-Krida Q78.5
　bare lymphocyte D81.6
　Barré-Guillain G61.0
　Barré-Liéou M53.0
　Barrett's —*see* Barrett's, esophagus
　Barsony-Polgar K22.4
　Barsony-Teschendorf K22.4
　Barth E78.71
　Bartter's E26.81
　basal cell nevus Q87.89
　Basedow's E05.00
　　with thyroid storm E05.01
　basilar artery G45.0
　Batten-Steinert G71.11
　battered
　　baby or child —*see* Maltreatment, child,
　　　physical abuse
　　spouse —*see* Maltreatment, adult, physical
　　　abuse
　Beals Q87.40
　Beau's I51.5
　Beck's I65.8
　Benedikt's G46.3
　Béquez César (-Steinbrinck-Chédiak-Higashi)
　　D70.330
　Bernhardt-Roth —*see* Meralgia paresthetica
➠Bernheim's —*see* Failure, heart, right
　big spleen D73.1
　bilateral polycystic ovarian E28.2
　Bing-Horton's —*see* Horton's headache
　Birt-Hogg-Dube syndrome Q87.89
　Björck (-Thorsen) E34.0
　black
　　lung J60
　　widow spider bite —*see* Toxicity, venom,
　　　spider, black widow
　Blackfan-Diamond D61.01
　Blau M04.8
　blind loop K90.2
　　congenital Q43.8
　　postsurgical K91.2
　blue sclera Q78.0
　blue toe I75.02-●
　Boder-Sedgewick G11.3
　Boerhaave's K22.3
　Borjeson Forssman Lehmann Q89.8
　Bouillaud's I01.9
　Bourneville (-Pringle) Q85.1
　Bouveret (-Hoffman) I47.9
　brachial plexus G54.0
　bradycardia-tachycardia I49.5
　brain (nonpsychotic) F09
　　with psychosis, psychotic reaction F09
　　acute or subacute —*see* Delirium
　　congenital —*see* Disability, intellectual
　　organic F09
　　　post-traumatic (nonpsychotic) F07.81
　　　　psychotic F09

Syndrome *(Continued)*
　brain (nonpsychotic) *(Continued)*
　　personality change F07.0
　　postcontusional F07.81
　　post-traumatic, nonpsychotic F07.81
　　psycho-organic F09
　　psychotic F06.8
　brain stem stroke G46.3
　Brandt's (acrodermatitis enteropathica) E83.2
　broad ligament laceration N83.8
　Brock's J98.11
➠bronze baby P83.88
　Brown-Sequard G83.81
▶Brugada I49.8
　bubbly lung P27.0
　Buchem's M85.2
　Budd-Chiari I82.0
　Bürger-Grütz E78.3
　Burke's K86.89
　Burnett's (milk-alkali) E83.52
　burning feet E53.9
　Bywaters' T79.5
　Call-Fleming I67.841
　carbohydrate-deficient glycoprotein (CDGS)
　　E77.8
　carcinogenic thrombophlebitis I82.1
　carcinoid E34.0
　cardiac asthma I50.1
　cardiacos negros I27.0
　cardiofaciocutaneous Q87.89
　cardiopulmonary-obesity E66.2
　cardiorenal —*see* Hypertension, cardiorenal
　cardiorespiratory distress (idiopathic),
　　newborn P22.0
　cardiovascular renal —*see* Hypertension,
　　cardiorenal
　carotid
　　artery (hemispheric) (internal) G45.1
　　body G90.01
　　sinus G90.01
　carpal tunnel G56.0-●
　Cassidy (-Scholte) E34.0
　cat-cry Q93.4
　cat eye Q92.8
　cauda equina G83.4
　causalgia —*see* Causalgia
　celiac K90.0
　　artery compression I77.4
　　axis I77.4
　central pain G89.0
　cerebellar
　　hereditary G11.9
　　stroke G46.4
　cerebellomedullary malformation —*see* Spina
　　bifida
　cerebral
　　artery
　　　anterior G46.1
　　　middle G46.0
　　　posterior G46.2
　　gigantism E22.0
　cervical (root) M53.1
　　disc —*see* Disorder, disc, cervical, with
　　　neuritis
　　fusion Q76.1
　　posterior, sympathicus M53.0
　　rib Q76.5
　　sympathetic paralysis G90.2
　cervicobrachial (diffuse) M53.1
　cervicocranial M53.0
　cervicodorsal outlet G54.2
　cervicothoracic outlet G54.0
　Céstan (-Raymond) I65.8
　Charcot's (angina cruris) (intermittent
　　claudication) I73.9
　Charcot-Weiss-Baker G90.09
　CHARGE Q89.8
　Chédiak-Higashi (-Steinbrinck) E70.330
　chest wall R07.1
　Chiari's (hepatic vein thrombosis) I82.0

Syndrome *(Continued)*
　Chilaiditi's Q43.3
　child maltreatment —*see* Maltreatment, child
　chondrocostal junction M94.0
　chondroectodermal dysplasia Q77.6
　chromosome 4 short arm deletion Q93.3
　chromosome 5 short arm deletion Q93.4
　chronic
　　infantile neurological, cutaneous and
　　　articular (CINCA) M04.2
　　pain G89.4
　　　personality F68.8
　Clarke-Hadfield K86.89
　Clerambault's automatism G93.89
　Clouston's (hidrotic ectodermal dysplasia)
　　Q82.4
　clumsiness, clumsy child F82
　cluster headache G44.009
　　intractable G44.001
　　not intractable G44.009
　Coffin-Lowry Q89.8
　cold injury (newborn) P80.0
　combined immunity deficiency D81.9
　compartment (deep) (posterior) (traumatic)
　　T79.A0
　　abdomen T79.A3
　　lower extremity (hip, buttock, thigh, leg,
　　　foot, toes) T79.A2
　　nontraumatic
　　　abdomen M79.A3
　　　lower extremity (hip, buttock, thigh, leg,
　　　　foot, toes) M79.A2-●
　　　specified site NEC M79.A9
　　　upper extremity (shoulder, arm, forearm,
　　　　wrist, hand, fingers) M79.A1-●
　　postprocedural —*see* Syndrome
　　　compartment, nontraumatic
　　specified site NEC T79.A9
　　upper extremity (shoulder, arm, forearm,
　　　wrist, hand, fingers) T79.A1
　complex regional pain —*see* Syndrome, pain,
　　complex regional
　compression T79.5
　　anterior spinal —*see* Syndrome, anterior,
　　　spinal artery, compression
　　cauda equina G83.4
　　celiac artery I77.4
　　vertebral artery M47.029
　　　cervical region M47.022
　　　occipito-atlanto-axial region M47.021
　concussion F07.81
　congenital
　　affecting multiple systems NEC Q87.89
　　central alveolar hypoventilation G47.35
　　facial diplegia Q87.0
　　muscular hypertrophy-cerebral Q87.89
　　oculo-auriculovertebral Q87.0
　　oculofacial diplegia (Moebius) Q87.0
　　rubella (manifest) P35.0
　congestion-fibrosis (pelvic), female N94.89
　congestive dysmenorrhea N94.6
　Conn's E26.01
　connective tissue M35.9
　　overlap NEC M35.1
　conus medullaris G95.81
　cord
　　anterior G83.82
　　posterior G83.83
　coronary
　　acute NEC I24.9
　　insufficiency or intermediate I20.0
　　slow flow I20.8
　Costen's (complex) M26.69
　costochondral junction M94.0
　costoclavicular G54.0
　costovertebral E22.0
　Cowden Q85.8
　craniovertebral M53.0
　Creutzfeldt-Jakob —*see* Creutzfeldt-Jakob
　　disease or syndrome
　cri-du-chat Q93.4

Syndrome (Continued)
  crib death R99
  cricopharyngeal —see Dysphagia
  croup J05.0
  CRPS I —see Syndrome, pain, complex
      regional I
  crush T79.5
  cubital tunnel —see Lesion, nerve, ulnar
  Curschmann (-Batten) (-Steinert) G71.11
  Cushing's E24.9
    alcohol-induced E24.4
    drug-induced E24.2
    due to
      alcohol
        drugs E24.2
        ectopic ACTH E24.3
        overproduction of pituitary ACTH E24.0
      overdose or wrong substance given
          or taken —see Table of Drugs and
          Chemicals, by drug, poisoning
    pituitary-dependent E24.0
    specified type NEC E24.8
  cryopyrin-associated periodic M04.2
  cryptophthalmos Q87.0
  cystic duct stump K91.5
  Dana-Putnam D51.0
  Danbolt (-Cross) (acrodermatitis
      enteropathica) E83.2
  Dandy-Walker Q03.1
    with spina bifida Q07.01
  Danlos' Q79.6
  defibrination —see also Fibrinolysis
    with
      antepartum hemorrhage —see
          Hemorrhage, antepartum, with
          coagulation defect
      intrapartum hemorrhage —see
          Hemorrhage, complicating,
          delivery
    newborn P60
    postpartum O72.3
  Degos' I77.8
  Déjérine-Roussy G89.0
  delayed sleep phase G47.21
  demyelinating G37.9
  dependence —see F10-F19 with fourth
      character .2
  depersonalization (-derealization) F48.1
  De Quervain E34.51
  de Toni-Fanconi (-Debré) E72.09
    with cystinosis E72.04
  diabetes mellitus-hypertension-nephrosis —
      see Diabetes, nephrosis
  diabetes mellitus in newborn infant P70.2
  diabetes-nephrosis —see Diabetes, nephrosis
  diabetic amyotrophy —see Diabetes,
      amyotrophy
  dialysis associated steal T82.898-●
  Diamond-Blackfan D61.01
  Diamond-Gardner D69.2
  DIC (diffuse or disseminated intravascular
      coagulopathy) D65
  di George's D82.1
  Dighton's Q78.0
  disequilibrium E87.8
  Döhle body-panmyelopathic D72.0
  dorsolateral medullary G46.4
  double athetosis G80.3
  Down (see also Down syndrome) Q90.9
  Dresbach's (elliptocytosis) D58.1
  Dressler's (postmyocardial infarction) I24.1
    postcardiotomy I97.0
  drug withdrawal, infant of dependent mother
      P96.1
  dry eye H04.12-●
  due to abnormality
    chromosomal Q99.9
      sex
        female phenotype Q97.9
        male phenotype Q98.9
      specified NEC Q99.8

Syndrome (Continued)
  dumping (postgastrectomy) K91.1
    nonsurgical K31.89
  Dupré's (meningism) R29.1
  dysmetabolic X E88.81
  dyspraxia, developmental F82
  Eagle-Barrett Q79.4
  Eaton-Lambert —see Syndrome,
      Lambert-Eaton
  Ebstein's Q22.5
  ectopic ACTH E24.3
  eczema-thrombocytopenia D82.0
  Eddowes' Q78.0
  effort (psychogenic) F45.8
  Ehlers-Danlos Q79.6
  Eisenmenger's I27.83
  Ekman's Q78.0
  electric feet E53.8
  Ellis-van Creveld Q77.6
  empty nest Z60.0
  endocrine-hypertensive E27.0
  entrapment —see Neuropathy,
      entrapment
  eosinophilia-myalgia M35.8
  epileptic —see also Epilepsy, by type
    absence G40.A09
      intractable G40.A19
        with status epilepticus G40.A11
        without status epilepticus G40.A19
      not intractable G40.A09
        with status epilepticus G40.A01
        without status epilepticus G40.A09
  Erdheim-Chester (ECD) E88.89
  Erdheim's E22.0
  erythrocyte fragmentation D59.4
  Evans D69.41
  exhaustion F48.8
  extrapyramidal G25.9
    specified NEC G25.89
  eye retraction —see Strabismus
  eyelid-malar-mandible Q87.0
  Faber's D50.9
  facial pain, paroxysmal G50.0
  Fallot's Q21.3
  familial cold autoinflammatory M04.2
  familial eczema-thrombocytopenia (Wiskott-
      Aldrich) D82.0
  Fanconi (-de Toni) (-Debré) E72.09
    with cystinosis E72.04
  Fanconi's (anemia) (congenital pancytopenia)
      D61.09
  fatigue
    chronic R53.82
    psychogenic F48.8
  faulty bowel habit K59.39
  Feil-Klippel (brevicollis) Q76.1
  Felty's —see Felty's syndrome
  fertile eunuch E23.0
  fetal
    alcohol (dysmorphic) Q86.0
    hydantoin Q86.1
  Fiedler's I40.1
  first arch Q87.0
  fish odor E72.8
  Fisher's G61.0
  Fitzhugh-Curtis
    due to
      Chlamydia trachomatis A74.81
      Neisseria gonorrhoea (gonococcal
          peritonitis) A54.85
  Fitz's —see also Pancreatitis, acute K85.80
  Flajani (-Basedow) E05.00
    with thyroid storm E05.01
  flatback —see Flatback syndrome
  floppy
    baby P94.2
    iris (intraoperative) (IFIS) H21.81
    mitral valve I34.1
  flush E34.0
  Foix-Alajouanine G95.19
  Fong's Q87.2

Syndrome (Continued)
  food protein-induced enterocolitis K52.21
  foramen magnum G93.5
  Foster-Kennedy H47.14-●
  Foville's (peduncular) G46.3
  fragile X Q99.2
  Franceschetti Q75.4
  Frey's
    auriculotemporal G50.8
    hyperhidrosis L74.52
  Friderichsen-Waterhouse A39.1
  Froin's G95.89
  frontal lobe F07.0
  Fukuhara E88.49
  functional
    bowel K59.9
    prepubertal castrate E29.1
  Gaisböck's D75.1
  ganglion (basal ganglia brain) G25.9
    geniculi G51.1
  Gardner-Diamond D69.2
  gastroesophageal
    junction K22.0
    laceration-hemorrhage K22.6
  gastrojejunal loop obstruction K91.89
  Gee-Herter-Heubner K90.0
  Gelineau's G47.419
    with cataplexy G47.411
  genito-anorectal A55
  Gerstmann-Sträussler-Scheinker (GSS)
      A81.82
  Gianotti-Crosti L44.4
  giant platelet (Bernard-Soulier) D69.1
  Gilles de la Tourette's F95.2
  goiter-deafness E07.1
  Goldberg Q89.8
  Goldberg-Maxwell E34.51
  Good's D83.8
  Gopalan' (burning feet) E53.8
  Gorlin's Q87.89
  Gougerot-Blum L81.7
  Gouley's I31.1
  Gower's R55
  gray or grey (newborn) P93.0
    platelet D69.1
  Gubler-Millard G46.3
  Guillain-Barré (-Strohl) G61.0
  gustatory sweating G50.8
  Hadfield-Clarke K86.89
  hair tourniquet —see Constriction, external,
      by site
  Hamman's J98.19
  hand-foot L27.1
  hand-shoulder G90.8
  hantavirus (cardio)-pulmonary (HPS) (HCPS)
      B33.4
  happy puppet Q93.5
  Harada's H30.81-●
  Hayem-Faber D50.9
  headache NEC G44.89
    complicated NEC G44.59
  Heberden's I20.8
  Hedinger's E34.0
  Hegglin's D72.0
  HELLP (hemolysis, elevated liver enzymes
      and low platelet count) O14.2-●
    complicating
      childbirth O14.24
        puerperium O14.25
  hemolytic-uremic D59.3
  hemophagocytic, infection-associated
      D76.2
  Henoch-Schönlein D69.0
  hepatic flexure K59.8
  hepatopulmonary K76.81
  hepatorenal K76.7
    following delivery O90.4
    postoperative or postprocedural K91.83
    postpartum, puerperal O90.4
  hepatourologic K76.7
  Herter (-Gee) (nontropical sprue) K90.0

▶ New   ⟹ Revised   deleted Deleted   ● Use Additional Character(s)

Syndrome (Continued)

Heubner-Herter K90.0
Heyd's K76.7
Hilger's G90.09
histamine-like (fish poisoning) —see Poisoning, fish
histiocytic D76.3
histiocytosis NEC D76.3
HIV infection, acute B20
Hoffmann-Werdnig G12.0
Hollander-Simons E88.1
Hoppe-Goldflam G70.00
    with exacerbation (acute) G70.01
    in crisis G70.01
Horner's G90.2
hungry bone E83.81
hunterian glossitis D51.0
Hutchinson's triad A50.53
hyperabduction G54.0
hyperammonemia-hyperornithinemia-homocitrullinemia E72.4
hypereosinophilic (idiopathic) D72.1
hyperimmunoglobulin D M04.1
hyperimmunoglobulin E (IgE) D82.4
hyperkalemic E87.5
hyperkinetic —see Hyperkinesia
hypermobility M35.7
hypernatremia E87.0
hyperosmolarity E87.0
hyperperfusion G97.82
hypersplenic D73.1
hypertransfusion, newborn P61.1
hyperventilation F45.8
hyperviscosity (of serum)
    polycythemic D75.1
    sclerothymic D58.8
hypoglycemic (familial) (neonatal) E16.2
hypokalemic E87.6
hyponatremic E87.1
hypopituitarism E23.0
hypoplastic left-heart Q23.4
hypopotassemia E87.6
hyposmolality E87.1
hypotension, maternal O26.5-●
hypothenar hammer I73.89
hypoventilation, obesity (OHS) E66.2
ICF (intravascular coagulation-fibrinolysis) D65
idiopathic
    cardiorespiratory distress, newborn P22.0
    nephrotic (infantile) N04.9
iliotibial band M76.3-●
immobility, immobilization (paraplegic) M62.3
immune reconstitution D89.3
immune reconstitution inflammatory [IRIS] D89.3
immunity deficiency, combined D81.9
immunodeficiency
    acquired —see Human, immunodeficiency virus (HIV) disease
    combined D81.9
impending coronary I20.0
impingement, shoulder M75.4-●
inappropriate secretion of antidiuretic hormone E22.2
infant
    gestational diabetes P70.0
    of diabetic mother P70.1
infantilism (pituitary) E23.0
inferior vena cava I87.1
inspissated bile (newborn) P59.1
institutional (childhood) F94.2
insufficient sleep F51.12
intermediate coronary (artery) I20.0
interspinous ligament —see Spondylopathy, specified NEC
intestinal
    carcinoid E34.0
    knot K56.2

Syndrome (Continued)

intravascular coagulation-fibrinolysis (ICF) D65
iodine-deficiency, congenital E00.9
    type
        mixed E00.2
        myxedematous E00.1
        neurological E00.0
IRDS (idiopathic respiratory distress, newborn) P22.0
irritable
    bowel K58.9
        with
            constipation K58.1
            diarrhea K58.0
        mixed K58.2
        psychogenic F45.8
        specified NEC K58.8
    heart (psychogenic) F45.8
    weakness F48.8
ischemic
    bowel (transient) K55.9
        chronic K55.1
        due to mesenteric artery insufficiency K55.1
    steal T82.898
IVC (intravascular coagulopathy) D65
Ivemark's Q89.01
Jaccoud's —see Arthropathy, postrheumatic, chronic
Jackson's G83.89
Jakob-Creutzfeldt —see Creutzfeldt-Jakob disease or syndrome
jaw-winking Q07.8
Jervell-Lange-Nielsen I45.81
jet lag G47.25
Job's D71
Joseph-Diamond-Blackfan D61.01
jugular foramen G52.7
Kabuki Q89.8
Kanner's (autism) F84.0
Kartagener's Q89.3
Kelly's D50.1
Kimmelstiel-Wilson —see Diabetes, specified type, with Kimmelstiel-Wilson disease
Klein (e)-Levine G47.13
Klippel-Feil (brevicollis) Q76.1
Köhler-Pellegrini-Steida —see Bursitis, tibial collateral
König's K59.8
Korsakoff (-Wernicke) (nonalcoholic) F04
    alcoholic F10.26
Kostmann's D70.0
Krabbe's congenital muscle hypoplasia Q79.8
labyrinthine —see subcategory H83.2
lacunar NEC G46.7
Lambert-Eaton G70.80
    in
        neoplastic disease G73.1
        specified disease NEC G70.81
Landau-Kleffner —see Epilepsy, specified NEC
Larsen's Q74.8
lateral
    cutaneous nerve of thigh G57.1-●
    medullary G46.4
Launois' E22.0
lazy
    leukocyte D70.8
    posture M62.3
Lemiere I80.8
Lennox-Gastaut G40.812
    intractable G40.814
        with status epilepticus G40.813
        without status epilepticus G40.814
    not intractable G40.812
        with status epilepticus G40.811
        without status epilepticus G40.812

Syndrome (Continued)

lenticular, progressive E83.01
Leopold-Levi's E05.90
Lev's I44.2
Li-Fraumeni Z15.01
Lichtheim's D51.0
Lightwood's N25.89
Lignac (de Toni) (-Fanconi) (-Debré) E72.09
    with cystinosis E72.04
Likoff's I20.8
limbic epilepsy personality F07.0
liver-kidney K76.7
lobotomy F07.0
Loffler's J82
long arm 18 or 21 deletion Q93.89
long QT I45.81
Louis-Barré G11.3
low
    atmospheric pressure T70.29
    back M54.5
    output (cardiac) I50.9
lower radicular, newborn (birth injury) P14.8
Luetscher's (dehydration) E86.0
Lupus anticoagulant D68.62
Lutembacher's Q21.1
macrophage activation D76.1
    due to infection D76.2
magnesium-deficiency R29.0
Majeed M04.8
Mal de Debarquement R42
malabsorption K90.9
    postsurgical K91.2
malformation, congenital, due to
    alcohol Q86.0
    exogenous cause NEC Q86.8
    hydantoin Q86.1
    warfarin Q86.2
malignant
    carcinoid E34.0
    neuroleptic G21.0
Mallory-Weiss K22.6
mandibulofacial dysostosis Q75.4
manic-depressive —see Disorder, bipolar
maple-syrup-urine E71.0
Marable's I77.4
Marfan's Q87.40
    with
        cardiovascular manifestations Q87.418
            aortic dilation Q87.410
        ocular manifestations Q87.42
        skeletal manifestations Q87.43
Marie's (acromegaly) E22.0
mast cell activation —see Activation, mast cell
maternal hypotension —see Syndrome, hypotension, maternal
May (-Hegglin) D72.0
McArdle (-Schmidt) (-Pearson) E74.04
McQuarrie's E16.2
meconium plug (newborn) P76.0
median arcuate ligament I77.4
Meekeren-Ehlers-Danlos Q79.6
megavitamin-B6 E67.2
Meige G24.4
MELAS E88.41
Mendelson's O74.0
MERRF (myoclonic epilepsy associated with ragged-red fibers) E88.42
mesenteric
    artery (superior) K55.1
    vascular insufficiency K55.1
metabolic E88.81
metastatic carcinoid E34.0
micrognathia-glossoptosis Q87.0
midbrain NEC G93.89
middle lobe (lung) J98.19
middle radicular G54.0
migraine —see also Migraine G43.909-●
Mikulicz' K11.8
milk-alkali E83.52
Millard-Gubler G46.3

▶ New   ⇒ Revised   ~~deleted~~ Deleted   ● Use Additional Character(s)

Syndrome *(Continued)*
   Miller-Dieker Q93.88
   Miller-Fisher G61.0
   Minkowski-Chauffard D58.0
   Mirizzi's K83.1
   MNGIE (Mitochondrial Neurogastrointestinal
      Encephalopathy) E88.49
   Möbius, ophthalmoplegic migraine —*see*
      Migraine, ophthalmoplegic
   monofixation H50.42
   Morel-Moore M85.2
   Morel-Morgagni M85.2
   Morgagni (-Morel) (-Stewart) M85.2
   Morgagni-Adams-Stokes I45.9
   Mounier-Kuhn Q32.4
     with bronchiectasis J47.9
       with
          exacerbation (acute) J47.1
          lower respiratory infection J47.0
     acquired J98.09
       with bronchiectasis J47.9
         with
            exacerbation (acute) J47.1
            lower respiratory infection J47.0
   Muckle-Wells M04.2
   mucocutaneous lymph node (acute febrile)
      (MCLS) M30.3
   multiple endocrine neoplasia (MEN) —*see*
      Neoplasia, endocrine, multiple (MEN}
   multiple operations —*see* Disorder, factitious
   myasthenic G70.9
     in
       diabetes mellitus —*see* Diabetes,
         amyotrophy
       endocrine disease NEC E34.9 *[G73.3]*
       neoplastic disease —*see also* Neoplasm
         D49.9 *[G73.3]*
       thyrotoxicosis (hyperthyroidism) E05.90
         [G73.3]
         with thyroid storm E05.91 *[G73.3]*
   myelodysplastic D46.9
     with
       5q deletion D46.C
       isolated del (5q) chromosomal
         abnormality D46.C
       lesions, low grade D46.20
       specified NEC D46.Z
   myelopathic pain G89.0
   myeloproliferative (chronic) D47.1
   myofascial pain M79.1
   Naffziger's G54.0
   nail patella Q87.2
   NARP (Neuropathy, Ataxia and Retinitis
      pigmentosa) E88.49
   neonatal abstinence P96.1
   nephritic —*see also* Nephritis
     with edema —*see* Nephrosis
     acute N00.9
     chronic N03.9
     rapidly progressive N01.9
   nephrotic (congenital) —*see also* Nephrosis
      N04.9
     with
       dense deposit disease N04.6
       diffuse
         crescentic glomerulonephritis
           N04.7
         endocapillary proliferative
           glomerulonephritis N04.4
         membranous glomerulonephritis
           N04.2
         mesangial proliferative
           glomerulonephritis N04.3
         mesangiocapillary glomerulonephritis
           N04.5
       focal and segmental glomerular lesions
         N04.1
       minor glomerular abnormality N04.0
       specified morphological changes NEC
         N04.8
     diabetic —*see* Diabetes, nephrosis

Syndrome *(Continued)*
   neurologic neglect R41.4
   Nezelof's D81.4
   Nonne-Milroy-Meige Q82.0
   Nothnagel's vasomotor acroparesthesia I73.89
   obesity hypoventilation (OHS) E66.2
   oculomotor H51.9
   ophthalmoplegia-cerebellar ataxia —*see*
      Strabismus, paralytic, third nerve
   oral allergy T78.1
   oral-facial-digital Q87.0
   organic
     affective F06.30
     amnesic (not alcohol- or drug-induced) F04
     brain F09
     depressive F06.31
     hallucinosis F06.0
     personality F07.0
   Ormond's N13.5
   oro-facial-digital Q87.0
   os trigonum Q68.8
   Osler-Weber-Rendu I78.0
   osteoporosis-osteomalacia M83.8
   Osterreicher-Turner Q87.2
   otolith —*see* subcategory H81.8
   oto-palatal-digital Q87.0
   outlet (thoracic) G54.0
   ovary
     polycystic E28.2
     resistant E28.39
     sclerocystic E28.2
   Owren's D68.2
   Paget-Schroetter I82.890
   pain —*see also* Pain
     complex regional I G90.50
       lower limb G90.52-●
       specified site NEC G90.59
       upper limb G90.51-●
     complex regional II —*see* Causalgia
   painful
     bruising D69.2
     feet E53.8
     prostate N42.81
   paralysis agitans —*see* Parkinsonism
   paralytic G83.9
     specified NEC G83.89
   Parinaud's H51.0
   parkinsonian —*see* Parkinsonism
   Parkinson's —*see* Parkinsonism
   paroxysmal facial pain G50.0
   Parry's E05.00
     with thyroid storm E05.01
   Parsonage (-Aldren)-Turner G54.5
   patella clunk M25.86-●
   Paterson (-Brown) (-Kelly) D50.1
   pectoral girdle I77.89
   pectoralis minor I77.89
▶ pediatric autoimmune neuropsychiatric
      disorders associated with streptococcal
      infections (PANDAS) D89.89
   Pelger-Huet D72.0
   pellagra-cerebellar ataxia-renal
      aminoaciduria E72.02
   pellagroid E52
   Pellegrini-Stieda —*see* Bursitis, tibial collateral
   pelvic congestion-fibrosis, female N94.89
   penta X Q97.1
   peptic ulcer —*see* Ulcer, peptic
   perabduction I77.89
   periodic fever M04.1
   periodic fever, aphthous stomatitis, pharyngitis,
      and adenopathy [PFAPA] M04.8
   periodic headache, in adults and children —
      see Headache, periodic syndromes in
      adults and children
   periurethral fibrosis N13.5
   phantom limb (without pain) G54.7
     with pain G54.6
   pharyngeal pouch D82.1
   Pick's —*see* Disease, Pick's
   Pickwickian E66.2

Syndrome *(Continued)*
   PIE (pulmonary infiltration with
      eosinophilia) J82
   pigmentary pallidal degeneration
      (progressive) G23.0
   pineal E34.8
   pituitary E22.0
   placental transfusion —*see* Pregnancy,
      complicated by, placental transfusion
      syndromes
   plantar fascia M72.2
   plateau iris (post-iridectomy)
      (postprocedural) H21.82
   Plummer-Vinson D50.1
   pluricarential of infancy E40
   plurideficiency E40
   pluriglandular (compensatory) E31.8
     autoimmune E31.0
   pneumatic hammer T75.21
   polyangiitis overlap M30.8
   polycarential of infancy E40
   polyglandular E31.8
     autoimmune E31.0
   polysplenia Q89.09
   pontine NEC G93.89
   popliteal
     artery entrapment I77.89
     web Q87.89
   postcardiac injury
     postcardiotomy I97.0
     postmyocardial infarction I24.1
   postcardiotomy I97.0
   post chemoembolization — code to
      associated conditions
   postcholecystectomy K91.5
   postcommissurotomy I97.0
   postconcussional F07.81
   postcontusional F07.81
   postencephalitic F07.89
   posterior
     cervical sympathetic M53.0
     cord G83.83
     fossa compression G93.5
     reversible encephalopathy (PRES) I67.83
   postgastrectomy (dumping) K91.1
   postgastric surgery K91.1
   postinfarction I24.1
   postlaminectomy NEC M96.1
   postleukotomy F07.0
   postmastectomy lymphedema I97.2
   postmyocardial infarction I24.1
   postoperative NEC T81.9
     blind loop K90.2
   postpartum panhypopituitary (Sheehan)
      E23.0
   postpolio (myelitic) G14
   postthrombotic I87.009
     with
       inflammation I87.02-●
         with ulcer I87.03-●
       specified complication NEC I87.09-●
       ulcer I87.01-●
         with inflammation I87.03-●
     asymptomatic I87.00-●
   postvagotomy K91.1
   postvalvulotomy I97.0
   postviral NEC G93.3
     fatigue G93.3
   Potain's K31.0
   potassium intoxication E87.5
   precerebral artery (multiple) (bilateral)
      G45.2
   preinfarction I20.0
   preleukemic D46.9
   premature senility E34.8
   premenstrual dysphoric F32.89
   premenstrual tension N94.3
   Prinzmetal-Massumi R07.1
   prune belly Q79.4
   pseudocarpal tunnel (sublimis) —*see*
      Syndrome, carpal tunnel

Syndrome *(Continued)*
pseudoparalytica G70.00
  with exacerbation (acute) G70.01
  in crisis G70.01
pseudo-Turner's Q87.1
psycho-organic (nonpsychotic severity) F07.9
  acute or subacute F05
  depressive type F06.31
  hallucinatory type F06.0
  nonpsychotic severity F07.0
  specified NEC F07.89
pulmonary
  arteriosclerosis I27.0
  dysmaturity (Wilson-Mikity) P27.0
  hypoperfusion (idiopathic) P22.0
  renal (hemorrhagic) (Goodpasture's) M31.0
pure
  motor lacunar G46.5
  sensory lacunar G46.6
Putnam-Dana D51.0
pyogenic arthritis, pyoderma gangrenosum, and acne [PAPA] M04.8
pyramidopallidonigral G20
pyriformis —*see* Lesion, nerve, sciatic
QT interval prolongation I45.81
radicular NEC —*see* Radiculopathy
  upper limbs, newborn (birth injury) P14.3
rapid time-zone change G47.25
Rasmussen G04.81
Raymond (-Céstan) I65.8
Raynaud's I73.00
  with gangrene I73.01
RDS (respiratory distress syndrome, newborn) P22.0
reactive airways dysfunction J68.3
Refsum's G60.1
Reifenstein E34.52
renal glomerulohyalinosis-diabetic —*see* Diabetes, nephrosis
Rendu-Osler-Weber I78.0
residual ovary N99.83
resistant ovary E28.39
respiratory
  distress
    acute J80
      adult J80
      child J80
      idiopathic J84.114
    newborn (idiopathic) (type I) P22.0
      type II P22.1
restless legs G25.81
retinoblastoma (familial) C69.2
retroperitoneal fibrosis N13.5
retroviral seroconversion (acute) Z21
Reye's G93.7
Richter —*see* Leukemia, chronic lymphocytic, B-cell type
Ridley's I50.1
right
  heart, hypoplastic Q22.6
  ventricular obstruction —*see* Failure, heart, congestive
Romano-Ward (prolonged QT interval) I45.81
rotator cuff, shoulder —*see also* Tear, rotator cuff M75.10-●
Rotes Quérol —*see* Hyperostosis, ankylosing
Roth —*see* Meralgia paresthetica
rubella (congenital) P35.0
Ruvalcaba-Myhre-Smith E71.440
Rytand-Lipsitch I44.2
salt
  depletion E87.1
    due to heat NEC T67.8
      causing heat exhaustion or prostration T67.4
  low E87.1
salt-losing N28.89
Scaglietti-Dagnini E22.0
scalenus anticus (anterior) G54.0
scapulocostal —*see* Mononeuropathy, upper limb, specified site NEC

Syndrome *(Continued)*
scapuloperoneal G71.0
schizophrenic, of childhood NEC F84.5
Schnitzler D47.2
Scholte's E34.0
Schroeder's E27.0
Schüller-Christian C96.5
Schwachman's —*see* Syndrome, Shwachman's
Schwartz (-Jampel) G71.13
Schwartz-Bartter E22.2
scimitar Q26.8
sclerocystic ovary E28.2
Seitelberger's G31.89
septicemic adrenal hemorrhage A39.1
seroconversion, retroviral (acute) Z21
serous meningitis G93.2
severe acute respiratory (SARS) J12.81
shaken infant T74.4
shock (traumatic) T79.4
  kidney N17.0
    following crush injury T79.5
  toxic A48.3
shock-lung J80
Shone's — code to specific anomalies
short
  bowel K91.2
  rib Q77.2
shoulder-hand —*see* Algoneurodystrophy
Shwachman's D70.4
sicca —*see* Sicca syndrome
sick
  cell E87.1
  sinus I49.5
sick-euthyroid E07.81
sideropenic D50.1
Siemens' ectodermal dysplasia Q82.4
Silfversköld's Q78.9
Simons' E88.1
sinus tarsi M25.57-●
sinusitis-bronchiectasis-situs inversus Q89.3
Sipple's E31.22
sirenomelia Q87.2
Slocumb's E27.0
slow flow, coronary I20.8
Sluder's G44.89
Smith-Magenis Q93.88
Sneddon-Wilkinson L13.1
Sotos' Q87.3
South African cardiomyopathy I42.8
spasmodic
  upward movement, eyes H51.8
  winking F95.8
Spen's I45.9
splenic
  agenesis Q89.01
  flexure K59.8
  neutropenia D73.81
Spurway's Q78.0
staphylococcal scalded skin L00
steal
  arteriovenous T82.898-●
  ischemic T82.898-●
  subclavian G45.8
Stein-Leventhal E28.2
Stein's E28.2
Stevens-Johnson syndrome L51.1
  toxic epidermal necrolysis overlap L51.3
Stewart-Morel M85.2
Stickler Q89.8
stiff baby Q89.8
stiff man G25.82
Still-Felty —*see* Felty's syndrome
Stokes (-Adams) I45.9
stone heart I50.1
straight back, congenital Q76.49
subclavian steal G45.8
subcoracoid-pectoralis minor G54.0
subcostal nerve compression I77.89
subphrenic interposition Q43.3

Syndrome *(Continued)*
superior
  cerebellar artery I63.8
  mesenteric artery K55.1
  semi-circular canal dehiscence H83.8X-●
  vena cava I87.1
supine hypotensive (maternal) —*see* Syndrome, hypotension, maternal
suprarenal cortical E27.0
supraspinatus —*see also* Tear, rotator cuff M75.10-●
Susac G93.49
swallowed blood P78.2
sweat retention L74.0
Swyer Q99.1
Symond's G93.2
sympathetic
  cervical paralysis G90.2
  pelvic, female N94.89
systemic inflammatory response (SIRS), of non-infectious origin (without organ dysfunction) R65.10
  with acute organ dysfunction R65.11
tachycardia-bradycardia I49.5
takotsubo I51.81
TAR (thrombocytopenia with absent radius) Q87.2
tarsal tunnel G57.5-●
teething K00.7
tegmental G93.89
telangiectasic-pigmentation-cataract Q82.8
temporal pyramidal apex —*see* Otitis, media, suppurative, acute
temporomandibular joint-pain-dysfunction M26.62-●
Terry's —*see also* Myopia, degenerative H44.2-●
testicular feminization —*see also* Syndrome, androgen insensitivity E34.51
thalamic pain (hyperesthetic) G89.0
thoracic outlet (compression) G54.0
Thorson-Björck E34.0
thrombocytopenia with absent radius (TAR) Q87.2
thyroid-adrenocortical insufficiency E31.0
tibial
  anterior M76.81-●
  posterior M76.82-●
Tietze's M94.0
time-zone (rapid) G47.25
Toni-Fanconi E72.09
  with cystinosis E72.04
Touraine's Q79.8
tourniquet —*see* Constriction, external, by site
toxic shock A48.3
transient left ventricular apical ballooning I51.81
traumatic vasospastic T75.22
Treacher Collins Q75.4
triple X, female Q97.0
trisomy Q92.9
  13 Q91.7
    meiotic nondisjunction Q91.4
    mitotic nondisjunction Q91.5
    mosaicism Q91.5
    translocation Q91.6
  18 Q91.3
    meiotic nondisjunction Q91.0
    mitotic nondisjunction Q91.1
    mosaicism Q91.1
    translocation Q91.2
  20 (q)(p) Q92.8
  21 Q90.9
    meiotic nondisjunction Q90.0
    mitotic nondisjunction Q90.1
    mosaicism Q90.1
    translocation Q90.2
  22 Q92.8
tropical wet feet T69.0-●
Trousseau's I82.1

▶ New   ⇒ Revised   ~~deleted~~ Deleted   ● Use Additional Character(s)

Syndrome *(Continued)*
  tumor lysis (following antineoplastic chemotherapy) (spontaneous) NEC E88.3
  tumor necrosis factor receptor associated periodic (TRAPS) M04.1
  Twiddler's (due to)
    automatic implantable defibrillator T82.198
    cardiac pacemaker T82.198
  Unverricht (-Lundborg) —*see* Epilepsy, generalized, idiopathic
  upward gaze H51.8
  uremia, chronic —*see also* Disease, kidney, chronic N18.9
  urethral N34.3
  urethro-oculo-articular —*see* Reiter's disease
  urohepatic K76.7
  vago-hypoglossal G52.7
  van Buchem's M85.2
  van der Hoeve's Q78.0
  vascular NEC in cerebrovascular disease G46.8
  vasoconstriction, reversible cerebrovascular I67.841
  vasomotor I73.9
  vasospastic (traumatic) T75.22
  vasovagal R55
  VATER Q87.2
  velo-cardio-facial Q93.81
  vena cava (inferior) (superior) (obstruction) I87.1
  vertebral
    artery G45.0
      compression —*see* Syndrome, anterior, spinal artery, compression
    steal G45.0
  vertebro-basilar artery G45.0
  vertebrogenic (pain) M54.89
  vertiginous —*see* Disorder, vestibular function
  Vinson-Plummer D50.1
  virus B34.9
  visceral larva migrans B83.0
  visual disorientation H53.8
  vitamin B6 deficiency E53.1
  vitreal corneal H59.01-•
  vitreous (touch) H59.01-•
  Vogt-Koyanagi H20.82-•
  Volkmann's T79.6
  von Schroetter's I82.890
  von Willebrand (-Jürgen) D68.0
  Waldenström-Kjellberg D50.1
  Wallenberg's G46.3
  water retention E87.79
  Waterhouse (-Friderichsen) A39.1
  Weber-Gubler G46.3
  Weber-Leyden G46.3
  Weber's G46.3
  Wegener's M31.30
    with
      kidney involvement M31.31
      lung involvement M31.30
        with kidney involvement M31.31
  Weingarten's (tropical eosinophilia) J82
  Weiss-Baker G90.09
  Werdnig-Hoffman G12.0
  Wermer's E31.21
  Werner's E34.8
  Wernicke-Korsakoff (nonalcoholic) F04
    alcoholic F10.26
  West's —*see* Epilepsy, spasms
  Westphal-Strümpell E83.01
  wet
    feet (maceration) (tropical) T69.0-•
    lung, newborn P22.1
  whiplash S13.4
  whistling face Q87.0
  Wilkie's K55.1
  Wilkinson-Sneddon L13.1
  Willebrand (-Jürgens) D68.0

Syndrome *(Continued)*
  Wilson's (hepatolenticular degeneration) E83.01
  Wiskott-Aldrich D82.0
  withdrawal —*see* Withdrawal, state
    drug
      infant of dependent mother P96.1
      therapeutic use, newborn P96.2
  Woakes' (ethmoiditis) J33.1
  ➠Wright's (hyperabduction) G54.0
  X I20.9
  XXXX Q97.1
  XXXXX Q97.1
  XXXXY Q98.1
  XXY Q98.0
  yellow nail L60.5
  Zahorsky's B08.5
  Zellweger syndrome E71.510
  Zellweger-like syndrome E71.541
Synechia (anterior) (iris) (posterior) (pupil) — *see also* Adhesions, iris
  intra-uterine (traumatic) N85.6
Synesthesia R20.8
Syngamiasis, syngamosis B83.3
Synodontia K00.2
Synorchidism, synorchism Q55.1
Synostosis (congenital) Q78.8
  astragalo-scaphoid Q74.2
  radioulnar Q74.0
Synovial sarcoma —*see* Neoplasm, connective tissue, malignant
Synovioma (malignant) —*see also* Neoplasm, connective tissue, malignant
  benign —*see* Neoplasm, connective tissue, benign
Synoviosarcoma —*see* Neoplasm, connective tissue, malignant
Synovitis —*see also* Tenosynovitis M65.9
  crepitant
    hand M70.0-•
    wrist M70.03-•
  gonococcal A54.49
  gouty —*see* Gout
  in (due to)
    crystals M65.8-•
    gonorrhea A54.49
    syphilis (late) A52.78
    use, overuse, pressure —*see* Disorder, soft tissue, due to use
  infective NEC —*see* Tenosynovitis, infective NEC
  specified NEC —*see* Tenosynovitis, specified type NEC
  syphilitic A52.78
    congenital (early) A50.02
  toxic —*see* Synovitis, transient
  transient M67.3-•
    ankle M67.37-•
    elbow M67.32-•
    foot joint M67.37-•
    hand joint M67.34-•
    hip M67.35-•
    knee M67.36-•
    multiple site M67.39
    pelvic region M67.35-•
    shoulder M67.31-•
    specified joint NEC M67.38
    wrist M67.33-•
  traumatic, current —*see* Sprain
  tuberculous —*see* Tuberculosis, synovitis
  villonodular (pigmented) M12.2-•
    ankle M12.27-•
    elbow M12.22-•
    foot joint M12.27-•
    hand joint M12.24-•
    hip M12.25-•
    knee M12.26-•
    multiple site M12.29
    pelvic region M12.25-•
    shoulder M12.21-•
    specified joint NEC M12.28

Synovitis *(Continued)*
  villonodular (pigmented) *(Continued)*
    vertebrae M12.28
    wrist M12.23-•
Syphilid A51.39
  congenital A50.06
  newborn A50.06
  tubercular (late) A52.79
Syphilis, syphilitic (acquired) A53.9
  abdomen (late) A52.79
  acoustic nerve A52.15
  adenopathy (secondary) A51.49
  adrenal (gland) (with cortical hypofunction) A52.79
  age under 2 years NOS —*see also* Syphilis, congenital, early
    acquired A51.9
  alopecia (secondary) A51.32
  anemia (late) A52.79 [D63.8]
  aneurysm (aorta) (ruptured) A52.01
    central nervous system A52.05
    congenital A50.54 [I79.0]
  anus (late) A52.74
    primary A51.1
    secondary A51.39
  aorta (arch) (abdominal) (thoracic) A52.02
    aneurysm A52.01
  aortic (insufficiency) (regurgitation) (stenosis)A52.03
    aneurysm A52.01
  arachnoid (adhesive) (cerebral) (spinal) A52.13
  asymptomatic —*see* Syphilis, latent
  ataxia (locomotor) A52.11
  atrophoderma maculatum A51.39
  auricular fibrillation A52.06
  bladder (late) A52.76
  bone A52.77
    secondary A51.46
  brain A52.17
  breast (late) A52.79
  bronchus (late) A52.72
  bubo (primary) A51.0
  bulbar palsy A52.19
  bursa (late) A52.78
  cardiac decompensation A52.06
  cardiovascular A52.00
  central nervous system (late) (recurrent) (relapse) (tertiary) A52.3
    with
      ataxia A52.11
      general paralysis A52.17
        juvenile A50.45
      paresis (general) A52.17
        juvenile A50.45
      tabes (dorsalis) A52.11
        juvenile A50.45
      taboparesis A52.17
        juvenile A50.45
    aneurysm A52.05
    congenital A50.40
    juvenile A50.40
    remission in (sustained) A52.3
    serology doubtful, negative, or positive A52.3
    specified nature or site NEC A52.19
    vascular A52.05
  cerebral A52.17
    meningovascular A52.13
    nerves (multiple palsies) A52.15
    sclerosis A52.17
    thrombosis A52.05
  cerebrospinal (tabetic type) A52.12
  cerebrovascular A52.05
  cervix (late) A52.76
  chancre (multiple) A51.0
    extragenital A51.2
    Rollet's A51.0
  Charcot's joint A52.16
  chorioretinitis A51.43
    congenital A50.01
    late A52.71
    prenatal A50.01

▶ New   ⇒ Revised   ~~deleted~~ Deleted   ● Use Additional Character(s)

Syphilis, syphilitic *(Continued)*
  orbit (late) A52.71
  organic A53.9
  osseous (late) A52.77
  osteochondritis (congenital) (early) A50.02
    [M90.80]
  osteoporosis A52.77
  ovary (late) A52.76
  oviduct (late) A52.76
  palate (late) A52.79
  pancreas (late) A52.74
  paralysis A52.17
    general A52.17
      juvenile A50.45
  paresis (general) A52.17
    juvenile A50.45
  paresthesia A52.19
  Parkinson's disease or syndrome A52.19
  paroxysmal tachycardia A52.06
  pemphigus (congenital) A50.06
  penis (chancre) A51.0
    late A52.76
  pericardium A52.06
  perichondritis, larynx (late) A52.73
  periosteum (late) A52.77
    congenital (early) A50.02 *[M90.80]*
    early (secondary) A51.46
  peripheral nerve A52.79
  petrous bone (late) A52.77
  pharynx (late) A52.73
    secondary A51.39
  pituitary (gland) A52.79
  pleura (late) A52.73
  pneumonia, white A50.04
  pontine lesion A52.17
  portal vein A52.09
  primary A51.0
    anal A51.1
    and secondary —*see* Syphilis, secondary
    central nervous system A52.3
    extragenital chancre NEC A51.2
    fingers A51.2
    genital A51.0
    lip A51.2
    specified site NEC A51.2
    tonsils A51.2
  prostate (late) A52.76
  ptosis (eyelid) A52.71
  pulmonary (late) A52.72
    artery A52.09
  pyelonephritis (late) A52.75
  recently acquired, symptomatic A51.9
  rectum (late) A52.74
  respiratory tract (late) A52.73
  retina, late A52.71
  retrobulbar neuritis A52.15
  salpingitis A52.76
  sclera (late) A52.71
  sclerosis
    cerebral A52.17
    coronary A52.06
    multiple A52.11
  scotoma (central) A52.71
  scrotum (late) A52.76

Syphilis, syphilitic *(Continued)*
  secondary (and primary) A51.49
    adenopathy A51.49
    anus A51.39
    bone A51.46
    chorioretinitis, choroiditis A51.43
    hepatitis A51.45
    liver A51.45
    lymphadenitis A51.49
    meningitis (acute) A51.41
    mouth A51.39
    mucous membranes A51.39
    periosteum, periostitis A51.46
    pharynx A51.39
    relapse (treated, untreated) A51.49
    skin A51.39
    specified form NEC A51.49
    tonsil A51.39
    ulcer A51.39
    viscera NEC A51.49
    vulva A51.39
  seminal vesicle (late) A52.76
  seronegative with signs or symptoms - code
    by site and stage under Syphilis
  seropositive
    with signs or symptoms - code by site and
      stage under Syphilis
    follow-up of latent syphilis —*see* Syphilis,
      latent
    only finding —*see* Syphilis, latent
  seventh nerve (paralysis) A52.15
  sinus, sinusitis (late) A52.73
  skeletal system A52.77
  skin (with ulceration) (early) (secondary)
    A51.39
    late or tertiary A52.79
  small intestine A52.74
  spastic spinal paralysis A52.17
  spermatic cord (late) A52.76
  spinal (cord) A52.12
  spleen A52.79
  splenomegaly A52.79
  spondylitis A52.77
  staphyloma A52.71
  stigmata (congenital) A50.59
  stomach A52.74
  synovium A52.78
  tabes dorsalis (late) A52.11
    juvenile A50.45
  tabetic type A52.11
    juvenile A50.45
  taboparesis A52.17
    juvenile A50.45
  tachycardia A52.06
  tendon (late) A52.78
  tertiary A52.9
    with symptoms NEC A52.79
    cardiovascular A52.00
    central nervous system A52.3
    multiple NEC A52.79
    specified site NEC A52.79
  testis A52.76
  thorax A52.73
  throat A52.73

Syphilis, syphilitic *(Continued)*
  thymus (gland) (late) A52.79
  thyroid (late) A52.79
  tongue (late) A52.79
  tonsil (lingual) (late) A52.73
    primary A51.2
    secondary A51.39
  trachea (late) A52.73
  tunica vaginalis (late) A52.76
  ulcer (any site) (early) (secondary)
    A51.39
    late A52.79
    perforating A52.79
      foot A52.11
  urethra (late) A52.76
  urogenital (late) A52.76
  uterus (late) A52.76
  uveal tract (secondary) A51.43
    late A52.71
  uveitis (secondary) A51.43
    late A52.71
  uvula (late) (perforated) A52.79
  vagina A51.0
    late A52.76
  valvulitis NEC A52.03
  vascular A52.00
    brain (cerebral) A52.05
  ventriculi A52.74
  vesicae urinariae (late) A52.76
  viscera (abdominal) (late) A52.74
    secondary A51.49
  vitreous (opacities) (late) A52.71
    hemorrhage A52.71
  vulva A51.0
    late A52.76
    secondary A51.39
Syphiloma A52.79
  cardiovascular system A52.00
  central nervous system A52.3
  circulatory system A52.00
  congenital A50.59
Syphilophobia F45.29
Syringadenoma —*see also* Neoplasm, skin,
  benign
  papillary —*see* Neoplasm, skin, benign
Syringobulbia G95.0
Syringocystadenoma —*see* Neoplasm, skin,
  benign
  papillary —*see* Neoplasm, skin, benign
Syringoma —*see also* Neoplasm, skin, benign
  chondroid —*see* Neoplasm, skin, benign
Syringomyelia G95.0
Syringomyelitis —*see* Encephalitis
Syringomyelocele —*see* Spina bifida
Syringopontia G95.0
System, systemic —*see also* condition
  disease, combined —*see* Degeneration,
    combined
  inflammatory response syndrome (SIRS) of
    non-infectious origin (without organ
    dysfunction) R65.10
    with acute organ dysfunction R65.11
  lupus erythematosus M32.9
    inhibitor present D68.62

S

T

Tabacism, tabacosis, tabagism —*see also*
      Poisoning, tobacco
   meaning dependence (without remission)
      F17.200
      with
         disorder F17.299
         ~~remission F17.211~~
         ▶in remission F17.211
            specified disorder NEC F17.298
            withdrawal F17.203
Tabardillo A75.9
   flea-borne A75.2
   louse-borne A75.0
Tabes, tabetic A52.10
   with
      central nervous system syphilis A52.10
      Charcot's joint A52.16
      cord bladder A52.19
      crisis, viscera (any) A52.19
      paralysis, general A52.17
      paresis (general) A52.17
      perforating ulcer (foot) A52.19
   arthropathy (Charcot) A52.16
   bladder A52.19
   bone A52.11
   cerebrospinal A52.12
   congenital A50.45
   conjugal A52.10
   dorsalis A52.11
      juvenile A50.49
   juvenile A50.49
   latent A52.19
   mesenterica A18.39
   paralysis, insane, general A52.17
   spasmodic A52.17
   syphilis (cerebrospinal) A52.12
Taboparalysis A52.17
Taboparesis (remission) A52.17
   juvenile A50.45
TAC (trigeminal autonomic cephalgia) NEC
      G44.099
   intractable G44.091
   not intractable G44.099
Tache noir S60.22-●
Tachyalimentation K91.2
Tachyarrhythmia, tachyrhythmia —*see*
      Tachycardia
Tachycardia R00.0
   atrial (paroxysmal) I47.1
   auricular I47.1
   AV nodal re-entry (re-entrant) I47.1
   junctional (paroxysmal) I47.1
   newborn P29.11
   nodal (paroxysmal) I47.1
   non-paroxysmal AV nodal I45.89
   paroxysmal (sustained) (nonsustained) I47.9
      with sinus bradycardia I49.5
      atrial (PAT) I47.1
      atrioventricular (AV) (re-entrant) I47.1
         psychogenic F54
      junctional I47.1
         ectopic I47.1
      nodal I47.1
      psychogenic (atrial) (supraventricular)
         (ventricular) F54
      supraventricular (sustained) I47.1
         psychogenic F54
      ventricular I47.2
         psychogenic F54
   psychogenic F45.8
   sick sinus I49.5
   sinoauricular NOS R00.0
      paroxysmal I47.1
   sinus [sinusal] NOS R00.0
      paroxysmal I47.1
   supraventricular I47.1
   ventricular (paroxysmal) (sustained) I47.2
      psychogenic F54
Tachygastria K31.89

Tachypnea R06.82
   hysterical F45.8
   newborn (idiopathic) (transitory) P22.1
   psychogenic F45.8
   transitory, of newborn P22.1
TACO (transfusion associated circulatory
      overload) E87.71
Taenia (infection) (infestation) B68.9
   diminuta B71.0
   echinococcal infestation B67.90
   mediocanellata B68.1
   nana B71.0
   saginata B68.1
   solium (intestinal form) B68.0
      larval form —*see* Cysticercosis
Taeniasis (intestine) —*see* Taenia
Tag (hypertrophied skin) (infected) L91.8
   adenoid J35.8
   anus K64.4
   hemorrhoidal K64.4
   hymen N89.8
   perineal N90.89
   preauricular Q17.0
   sentinel K64.4
   skin L91.8
      accessory (congenital) Q82.8
      anus K64.4
      congenital Q82.8
      preauricular Q17.0
   tonsil J35.8
   urethra, urethral N36.8
   vulva N90.89
Tahyna fever B33.8
Takahara's disease E80.3
Takayasu's disease or syndrome M31.4
Talcosis (pulmonary) J62.0
Talipes (congenital) Q66.89
   acquired, planus —*see* Deformity, limb, flat
      foot
   asymmetric Q66.89
   calcaneovalgus Q66.4
   calcaneovarus Q66.1
   calcaneus Q66.89
   cavus Q66.7
   equinovalgus Q66.6
   equinovarus Q66.0
   equinus Q66.89
   percavus Q66.7
   planovalgus Q66.6
   planus (acquired) (any degree) —*see also*
      Deformity, limb, flat foot
      congenital Q66.5-●
      due to rickets (sequelae) E64.3
   valgus Q66.6
   varus Q66.3
Tall stature, constitutional E34.4
Talma's disease M62.89
Talon noir S90.3-●
   hand S60.22-●
   heel S90.3-●
   toe S90.1-●
Tamponade, heart I31.4
Tanapox (virus disease) B08.71
Tangier disease E78.6
Tantrum, child problem F91.8
Tapeworm (infection) (infestation) —*see*
      Infestation, tapeworm
Tapia's syndrome G52.7
TAR (thrombocytopenia with absent radius)
      syndrome Q87.2
Tarral-Besnier disease L44.0
Tarsal tunnel syndrome —*see* Syndrome, tarsal
      tunnel
Tarsalgia —*see* Pain, limb, lower
Tarsitis (eyelid) H01.8
   syphilitic A52.71
   tuberculous A18.4
Tartar (teeth) (dental calculus) K03.6
Tattoo (mark) L81.8
Tauri's disease E74.09
Taurodontism K00.2

Taussig-Bing syndrome Q20.1
Taybi's syndrome Q87.2
Tay-Sachs amaurotic familial idiocy or disease
      E75.02
TBI (traumatic brain injury) S06.9
Teacher's node or nodule J38.2
Tear, torn (traumatic) —*see also* Laceration
   with abortion —*see* Abortion
   annular fibrosis M51.35
   anus, anal (sphincter) S31.831
      complicating delivery
         with third degree perineal laceration —
            see also Delivery, complicated, by,
            laceration, perineum, third degree
            O70.20
            with mucosa O70.3
         without third degree perineal laceration
            O70.4
      nontraumatic (healed) (old) K62.81
   articular cartilage, old —*see* Derangement,
      joint, articular cartilage, by site
   bladder
      with ectopic or molar pregnancy O08.6
      following ectopic or molar pregnancy
         O08.6
      obstetrical O71.5
      traumatic —*see* Injury, bladder
   bowel
      with ectopic or molar pregnancy O08.6
      following ectopic or molar pregnancy
         O08.6
      obstetrical trauma O71.5
   broad ligament
      with ectopic or molar pregnancy O08.6
      following ectopic or molar pregnancy O08.6
      obstetrical trauma O71.6
   bucket handle (knee) (meniscus) —*see* Tear,
      meniscus
   capsule, joint —*see* Sprain
   cartilage —*see also* Sprain
      articular, old —*see* Derangement, joint,
         articular cartilage, by site
   cervix
      with ectopic or molar pregnancy O08.6
      following ectopic or molar pregnancy
         O08.6
      obstetrical trauma (current) O71.3
      old N88.1
      traumatic —*see* Injury, uterus
   dural G97.41
      nontraumatic G96.11
   internal organ —*see* Injury, by site
   knee cartilage
      articular (current) S83.3-●
      old —*see* Derangement, knee, meniscus,
         due to old tear
   ligament —*see* Sprain
   meniscus (knee) (current injury) S83.209
      bucket-handle S83.20-●
      lateral
         bucket-handle S83.25-●
         complex S83.27-●
         peripheral S83.26-●
         specified type NEC S83.28-●
      medial
         bucket-handle S83.21-●
         complex S83.23-●
         peripheral S83.22-●
         specified type NEC S83.24-●
      old —*see* Derangement, knee, meniscus,
         due to old tear
      site other than knee - code as Sprain
      specified type NEC S83.20-●
   muscle —*see* Strain
   pelvic
      floor, complicating delivery O70.1
      organ NEC, obstetrical trauma O71.5
         with ectopic or molar pregnancy O08.6
         following ectopic or molar pregnancy
            O08.6
   perineal, secondary O90.1

Tear, torn *(Continued)*
  periurethral tissue, obstetrical trauma O71.82
    with ectopic or molar pregnancy O08.6
    following ectopic or molar pregnancy O08.6
  rectovaginal septum —*see* Laceration, vagina
  retina, retinal (without detachment) (horseshoe) —*see also* Break, retina, horseshoe
    with detachment —*see* Detachment, retina, with retinal, break
  rotator cuff (nontraumatic) M75.10-●
    complete M75.12-●
    incomplete M75.11-●
    traumatic S46.01-●
      capsule S43.42-●
  semilunar cartilage, knee —*see* Tear, meniscus
  supraspinatus (complete) (incomplete) (nontraumatic) —*see also* Tear, rotator cuff M75.10-●
  tendon —*see* Strain
  tentorial, at birth P10.4
  umbilical cord
    complicating delivery O69.89
  urethra
    with ectopic or molar pregnancy O08.6
    following ectopic or molar pregnancy O08.6
    obstetrical trauma O71.5
  uterus —*see* Injury, uterus
  vagina —*see* Laceration, vagina
  vessel, from catheter —*see* Puncture, accidental complicating surgery
  vulva, complicating delivery O70.0
Tear-stone —*see* Dacryolith
Teeth —*see also* condition
  grinding
    psychogenic F45.8
    sleep related G47.63
Teething (syndrome) K00.7
Telangiectasia, telangiectasis (verrucous) I78.1
  ataxic (cerebellar) (Louis-Bar) G11.3
  familial I78.0
  hemorrhagic, hereditary (congenital) (senile) I78.0
  hereditary, hemorrhagic (congenital) (senile) I78.0
  juxtafoveal H35.07-●
  macular H35.07-●
  ▶macularis eruptiva perstans D47.01
  parafoveal H35.07-●
  retinal (idiopathic) (juxtafoveal) (macular) (parafoveal) H35.07-●
  spider I78.1
Telephone scatologia F65.89
Telescoped bowel or intestine K56.1
  congenital Q43.8
Temperature
  body, high (of unknown origin) R50.9
  cold, trauma from T69.9
    newborn P80.0
    specified effect NEC T69.8
Temple —*see* condition
Temporal —*see* condition
Temporomandibular joint pain-dysfunction syndrome M26.62-●
Temporosphenoidal —*see* condition
Tendency
  bleeding —*see* Defect, coagulation
  suicide
    meaning personal history of attempted suicide Z91.5
    meaning suicidal ideation —*see* Ideation, suicidal
  to fall R29.6
Tenderness, abdominal R10.819
  epigastric R10.816
  generalized R10.817
  left lower quadrant R10.814
  left upper quadrant R10.812
  periumbilic R10.815

Tenderness, abdominal *(Continued)*
  rebound R10.829
    epigastric R10.826
    generalized R10.827
    left lower quadrant R10.824
    left upper quadrant R10.822
    periumbilic R10.825
    right lower quadrant R10.823
    right upper quadrant R10.821
  right lower quadrant R10.813
  right upper quadrant R10.811
Tendinitis, tendonitis —*see also* Enthesopathy
  Achilles M76.6-●
  adhesive —*see* Tenosynovitis, specified type NEC
    shoulder —*see* Capsulitis, adhesive
  bicipital M75.2-●
  calcific M65.2-●
    ankle M65.27-●
    foot M65.27-●
    forearm M65.23-●
    hand M65.24-●
    lower leg M65.26-●
    multiple sites M65.29
    pelvic region M65.25-●
    shoulder M75.3-●
    specified site NEC M65.28
    thigh M65.25-●
    upper arm M65.22-●
  due to use, overuse, pressure —*see also* Disorder, soft tissue, due to use
    specified NEC —*see* Disorder, soft tissue, due to use, specified NEC
  gluteal M76.0-●
  patellar M76.5-●
  peroneal M76.7-●
  psoas M76.1-●
  tibial (posterior) M76.82-●
    anterior M76.81-●
  trochanteric —*see* Bursitis, hip, trochanteric
Tendon —*see* condition
Tendosynovitis —*see* Tenosynovitis
Tenesmus (rectal) R19.8
  vesical R30.1
Tennis elbow —*see* Epicondylitis, lateral
Tenonitis —*see also* Tenosynovitis
  eye (capsule) H05.04-●
Tenontosynovitis —*see* Tenosynovitis
Tenontothecitis —*see* Tenosynovitis
Tenophyte —*see* Disorder, synovium, specified type NEC
Tenosynovitis —*see also* Synovitis M65.9
  adhesive —*see* Tenosynovitis, specified type NEC
    shoulder —*see* Capsulitis, adhesive
  bicipital (calcifying) —*see* Tendinitis, bicipital
  gonococcal A54.49
  in (due to)
    crystals M65.8-●
    gonorrhea A54.49
    syphilis (late) A52.78
    use, overuse, pressure —*see also* Disorder, soft tissue, due to use
      specified NEC —*see* Disorder, soft tissue, due to use, specified NEC
  infective NEC M65.1-●
    ankle M65.17-●
    foot M65.17-●
    forearm M65.13-●
    hand M65.14-●
    lower leg M65.16-●
    multiple sites M65.19
    pelvic region M65.15-●
    shoulder region M65.11-●
    specified site NEC M65.18
    thigh M65.15-●
    upper arm M65.12-●
  radial styloid M65.4
  shoulder region M65.81-●
    adhesive —*see* Capsulitis, adhesive

Tenosynovitis *(Continued)*
  specified type NEC M65.88-●
    ankle M65.87-●
    foot M65.87-●
    forearm M65.83-●
    hand M65.84-●
    lower leg M65.86-●
    multiple sites M65.89
    pelvic region M65.85-●
    shoulder region M65.81-●
    specified site NEC M65.88
    thigh M65.85-●
    upper arm M65.82-●
  tuberculous —*see* Tuberculosis, tenosynovitis
Tenovaginitis —*see* Tenosynovitis
Tension
  arterial, high —*see also* Hypertension
    without diagnosis of hypertension R03.0
  headache G44.209
    intractable G44.201
    not intractable G44.209
  nervous R45.0
  pneumothorax J93.0
  premenstrual N94.3
  state (mental) F48.9
Tentorium —*see* condition
Teratencephalus Q89.8
Teratism Q89.7
Teratoblastoma (malignant) —*see* Neoplasm, malignant, by site
Teratocarcinoma —*see also* Neoplasm, malignant, by site
  liver C22.7
Teratoma (solid) —*see also* Neoplasm, uncertain behavior, by site
  with embryonal carcinoma, mixed —*see* Neoplasm, malignant, by site
  with malignant transformation —*see* Neoplasm, malignant, by site
  adult (cystic) —*see* Neoplasm, benign, by site
  benign —*see* Neoplasm, benign, by site
  combined with choriocarcinoma —*see* Neoplasm, malignant, by site
  cystic (adult) —*see* Neoplasm, benign, by site
  differentiated —*see* Neoplasm, benign, by site
  embryonal —*see also* Neoplasm, malignant, by site
    liver C22.7
  immature —*see* Neoplasm, malignant, by site
  liver C22.7
    adult, benign, cystic, differentiated type or mature D13.4
  malignant —*see also* Neoplasm, malignant, by site
    anaplastic —*see* Neoplasm, malignant, by site
    intermediate —*see* Neoplasm, malignant, by site
    specified site —*see* Neoplasm, malignant, by site
    unspecified site C62.90
    undifferentiated —*see* Neoplasm, malignant, by site
  mature —*see* Neoplasm, uncertain behavior, by site
  malignant —*see* Neoplasm, by site, malignant, by site
  ovary D27.-●
    embryonal, immature or malignant C56-●
  solid —*see* Neoplasm, uncertain behavior, by site
  testis C62.9-●
    adult, benign, cystic, differentiated type or mature D29.2-●
    scrotal C62.1-●
    undescended C62.0-●
Termination
  anomalous —*see also* Malposition, congenital
    right pulmonary vein Q26.3
  pregnancy, elective Z33.2

Ternidens diminutus infestation B81.8
Ternidensiasis B81.8
Terror(s) night (child) F51.4
Terrorism, victim of Z65.4
➠Terry's syndrome —see also Myopia,
    degenerative H44.2-●
Tertiary —see condition
Test, tests, testing (for)
    adequacy (for dialysis)
        hemodialysis Z49.31
        peritoneal Z49.32
    blood pressure Z01.30
        abnormal reading —see Blood, pressure
    blood typing Z01.83
        Rh typing Z01.83
    blood-alcohol Z04.8
        positive —see Findings, abnormal, in
            blood
    blood-drug Z04.8
        positive —see Findings, abnormal, in
            blood
    cardiac pulse generator (battery) Z45.010
    fertility Z31.41
    genetic
        disease carrier status for procreative
            management
            female Z31.430
            male Z31.440
        male partner of patient with recurrent
            pregnancy loss Z31.441
        procreative management NEC
            female Z31.438
            male Z31.448
    hearing Z01.10
        with abnormal findings NEC Z01.118
    HIV (human immunodeficiency virus)
        nonconclusive (in infants) R75
        positive Z21
        seropositive Z21
    immunity status Z01.84
    intelligence NEC Z01.89
    laboratory (as part of a general medical
        examination) Z00.00
        with abnormal finding Z00.01
        for medicolegal reason NEC Z04.8
    male partner of patient with recurrent
        pregnancy loss Z31.441
    Mantoux (for tuberculosis) Z11.1
        abnormal result R76.11
    pregnancy, positive first pregnancy —see
        Pregnancy, normal, first
    procreative Z31.49
        fertility Z31.41
    skin, diagnostic
        allergy Z01.82
        special screening examination —see
            Screening, by name of disease
        Mantoux Z11.1
        tuberculin Z11.1
    specified NEC Z01.89
    tuberculin Z11.1
        abnormal result R76.11
    vision Z01.00
        with abnormal findings Z01.01
    Wassermann Z11.3
        positive —see Serology for syphilis,
            positive
Testicle, testicular, testis —see also condition
    feminization syndrome —see also Syndrome,
        androgen insensitivity E34.51
    migrans Q55.29
Tetanus, tetanic (cephalic) (convulsions) A35
    with
        abortion A34
        ectopic or molar pregnancy O08.0
    following ectopic or molar pregnancy O08.0
    inoculation reaction (due to serum) —see
        Complications, vaccination
    neonatorum A33
    obstetrical A34
    puerperal, postpartum, childbirth A34

Tetany (due to) R29.0
    alkalosis E87.3
    associated with rickets E55.0
    convulsions R29.0
        hysterical F44.5
    functional (hysterical) F44.5
    hyperkinetic R29.0
        hysterical F44.5
    hyperpnea R06.4
        hysterical F44.5
        psychogenic F45.8
    hyperventilation —see also Hyperventilation
        R06.4
        hysterical F44.5
    neonatal (without calcium or magnesium
        deficiency) P71.3
    parathyroid (gland) E20.9
    parathyroprival E89.2
    post- (para)thyroidectomy E89.2
    postoperative E89.2
    pseudotetany R29.0
    psychogenic (conversion reaction) F44.5
Tetralogy of Fallot Q21.3
Tetraplegia (chronic) —see also Quadriplegia
    G82.50-●
Thailand hemorrhagic fever A91
Thalassanemia —see Thalassemia
Thalassemia (anemia) (disease) D56.9
    with other hemoglobinopathy D56.8
    alpha (major) (severe) (triple gene defect)
        D56.0
        minor D56.3
        silent carrier D56.3
        trait D56.3
    beta (severe) D56.1
        homozygous D56.1
        major D56.1
        minor D56.3
        trait D56.3
    delta-beta (homozygous) D56.2
        minor D56.3
        trait D56.3
    dominant D56.8
    hemoglobin
        C D56.8
        E-beta D56.5
    intermedia D56.1
    major D56.1
    minor D56.3
    mixed D56.8
    sickle-cell —see Disease, sickle-cell,
        thalassemia
    specified type NEC D56.8
    trait D56.3
    variants D56.8
Thanatophoric dwarfism or short stature Q77.1
Thaysen-Gee disease (nontropical sprue) K90.0
Thaysen's disease K90.0
Thecoma D27-●
    luteinized D27-●
    malignant C56-●
Thelarche, premature E30.8
Thelaziasis B83.8
Thelitis N61.0
    puerperal, postpartum or gestational —see
        Infection, nipple
Therapeutic —see condition
Therapy
    drug, long-term (current) (prophylactic)
        agents affecting estrogen receptors and
            estrogen levels NEC Z79.818
        anastrozole (Arimidex) Z79.811
        antibiotics Z79.2
            short-term use - omit code
        anticoagulants Z79.01
        anti-inflammatory Z79.1
        antiplatelet Z79.02
        antithrombotics Z79.02
        aromatase inhibitors Z79.811
        aspirin Z79.82
        birth control pill or patch Z79.3

Therapy (Continued)
    drug, long-term (Continued)
        bisphosphonates Z79.83
        contraceptive, oral Z79.3
        drug, specified NEC Z79.899
        estrogen receptor downregulators
            Z79.818
        Evista Z79.810
        exemestane (Aromasin) Z79.811
        Fareston Z79.810
        fulvestrant (Faslodex) Z79.818
        gonadotropin-releasing hormone (GnRH)
            agonist Z79.818
        goserelin acetate (Zoladex) Z79.818
    ➠   hormone replacement Z79.890
        insulin Z79.4
        letrozole (Femara) Z79.811
        leuprolide acetate (leuprorelin) (Lupron)
            Z79.818
        megestrol acetate (Megace) Z79.818
        methadone
            for pain management Z79.891
            maintenance therapy F11.20
        Nolvadex Z79.810
        opiate analgesic Z79.891
        oral contraceptive Z79.3
        raloxifene (Evista) Z79.810
        selective estrogen receptor modulators
            (SERMs) Z79.810
        short term - omit code
        steroids
            inhaled Z79.51
            systemic Z79.52
        tamoxifen (Nolvadex) Z79.810
        toremifene (Fareston) Z79.810
Thermic —see condition
Thermography (abnormal) —see also Abnormal,
    diagnostic imaging R93.8
    breast R92.8
Thermoplegia T67.0
Thesaurismosis, glycogen —see Disease,
    glycogen storage
Thiamin deficiency E51.9
    specified NEC E51.8
Thiaminic deficiency with beriberi E51.11
Thibierge-Weissenbach syndrome —see
    Sclerosis, systemic
Thickening
    bone —see Hypertrophy, bone
    breast N64.59
    endometrium R93.8
    epidermal L85.9
        specified NEC L85.8
    hymen N89.6
    larynx J38.7
    nail L60.2
        congenital Q84.5
    periosteal —see Hypertrophy, bone
    pleura J92.9
        with asbestos J92.0
    skin R23.4
    subepiglottic J38.7
    tongue K14.8
    valve, heart —see Endocarditis
Thigh —see condition
Thinning vertebra —see Spondylopathy,
    specified NEC
Thirst, excessive R63.1
    due to deprivation of water T73.1
Thomsen disease G71.12
Thoracic —see also condition
    kidney Q63.2
    outlet syndrome G54.0
Thoracogastroschisis (congenital)
    Q79.8
Thoracopagus Q89.4
Thorax —see condition
Thorn's syndrome N28.89
Thorson-Björck syndrome E34.0
Threadworm (infection) (infestation)
    B80

    ▶ New   ➠ Revised   ~~deleted~~ Deleted   ● Use Additional Character(s)

Threatened
- abortion O20.0
  - with subsequent abortion O03.9
- job loss, anxiety concerning Z56.2
- labor (without delivery) O47.9
  - at or after 37 completed weeks of gestation O47.1
  - before 37 completed weeks of gestation O47.0-●
- loss of job, anxiety concerning Z56.2
- miscarriage O20.0
- unemployment, anxiety concerning Z56.2

Three-day fever A93.1
Threshers' lung J67.0
Thrix annulata (congenital) Q84.1
Throat —see condition
Thrombasthenia (Glanzmann) (hemorrhagic) (hereditary) D69.1
Thromboangiitis I73.1
- obliterans (general) I73.1
  - cerebral I67.89
  - vessels
    - brain I67.89
    - spinal cord I67.89
Thromboarteritis —see Arteritis
Thromboasthenia (Glanzmann) (hemorrhagic) (hereditary) D69.1
Thrombocytasthenia (Glanzmann) D69.1
Thrombocythemia (essential) (hemorrhagic) (idiopathic) (primary) D47.3
Thrombocytopathy (dystrophic) (granulopenic) D69.1
Thrombocytopenia, thrombocytopenic D69.6
- with absent radius (TAR) Q87.2
- congenital D69.42
- dilutional D69.59
- due to
  - drugs D69.59
  - extracorporeal circulation of blood D69.59
  - (massive)blood transfusion D69.59
  - platelet alloimmunization D69.59
- essential D69.3
- heparin induced (HIT) D75.82
- hereditary D69.42
- idiopathic D69.3
- neonatal, transitory P61.0
  - due to
    - exchange transfusion P61.0
    - idiopathic maternal thrombocytopenia P61.0
    - isoimmunization P61.0
- primary NEC D69.49
  - idiopathic D69.3
- puerperal, postpartum O72.3
- secondary D69.59
- transient neonatal P61.0
Thrombocytosis, essential D47.3
- primary D47.3
Thromboembolism —see Embolism
Thrombopathy (Bernard-Soulier) D69.1
- constitutional D68.0
- Willebrand-Jurgens D68.0
Thrombopenia —see Thrombocytopenia
Thrombophilia D68.59
- primary NEC D68.59
- secondary NEC D68.69
- specified NEC D68.69
Thrombophlebitis I80.9
- antepartum O22.2-●
  - deep O22.3-●
  - superficial O22.2-●
- cavernous (venous) sinus G08
  - complicating pregnancy O22.5-●
  - nonpyogenic I67.6
- cerebral (sinus) (vein) G08
  - nonpyogenic I67.6
  - sequelae G09
- due to implanted device —see Complications, by site and type, specified NEC

Thrombophlebitis (Continued)
- during or resulting from a procedure NEC T81.72
- femoral vein (superficial) I80.1-●
- femoropopliteal vein I80.0-●
- hepatic (vein) I80.8
- idiopathic, recurrent I82.1
- iliofemoral I80.1-●
- intracranial venous sinus (any) G08
  - nonpyogenic I67.6
  - sequelae G09
- intraspinal venous sinuses and veins G08
  - nonpyogenic G95.19
- lateral (venous) sinus G08
  - nonpyogenic I67.6
- ⇒leg I80.3
  - superficial I80.0-●
- longitudinal (venous) sinus G08
  - nonpyogenic I67.6
- lower extremity I80.299
- migrans, migrating I82.1
- pelvic
  - with ectopic or molar pregnancy O08.0
  - following ectopic or molar pregnancy O08.0
  - puerperal O87.1
- popliteal vein —see Phlebitis, leg, deep, popliteal
- portal (vein) K75.1
- postoperative T81.72
- pregnancy —see Thrombophlebitis, antepartum
- puerperal, postpartum, childbirth O87.0
  - deep O87.1
  - pelvic O87.1
  - septic O86.81
  - superficial O87.0
- saphenous (greater) (lesser) I80.0-●
- sinus (intracranial) G08
  - nonpyogenic I67.6
- specified site NEC I80.8
- tibial vein I80.23-●
Thrombosis, thrombotic (bland) (multiple) (progressive) (silent) (vessel) I82.90
- anal K64.5
- antepartum —see Thrombophlebitis, antepartum
- aorta, aortic I74.10
  - abdominal I74.09
    - saddle I74.01
  - bifurcation I74.09
  - saddle I74.01
  - specified site NEC I74.19
  - terminal I74.09
  - thoracic I74.11
  - valve —see Endocarditis, aortic
- apoplexy I63.3-●
- artery, arteries (postinfectional) I74.9
  - auditory, internal —see Occlusion, artery, precerebral, specified NEC
  - basilar —see Occlusion, artery, basilar
  - carotid (common) (internal) —see Occlusion, artery, carotid
  - cerebellar (anterior inferior) (posterior inferior) (superior) —see Occlusion, artery, cerebellar
  - cerebral —see Occlusion, artery, cerebral
  - ⇒choroidal (anterior) —see Occlusion, artery, precerebral, specified NEC
  - ⇒communicating, posterior —see Occlusion, artery, precerebral, specified NEC
  - coronary —see also Infarct, myocardium
    - not resulting in infarction I24.0
  - hepatic I74.8
  - ⇒hypophyseal —see Occlusion, artery, precerebral, specified NEC
  - iliac I74.5
  - limb I74.4
    - lower I74.3
    - upper I74.2

Thrombosis, thrombotic (Continued)
- artery, arteries (Continued)
  - meningeal, anterior or posterior —see Occlusion, artery, cerebral, specified NEC
  - mesenteric (with gangrene) —see also Infarct, intestine K55.069
  - ophthalmic —see Occlusion, artery, retina
  - ⇒pontine —see Occlusion, artery, precerebral, specified NEC
  - precerebral —see Occlusion, artery, precerebral
  - pulmonary (iatrogenic) —see Embolism, pulmonary
  - renal N28.0
  - retinal —see Occlusion, artery, retina
  - spinal, anterior or posterior G95.11
  - traumatic NEC T14.8
  - vertebral —see Occlusion, artery, vertebral
- atrium, auricular —see also Infarct, myocardium
  - following acute myocardial infarction (current complication) I23.6
  - not resulting in infarction I51.3
  - ▶old I51.3
- basilar (artery) —see Occlusion, artery, basilar
- brain (artery) (stem) —see also Occlusion, artery, cerebral
  - due to syphilis A52.05
  - puerperal O99.43
  - sinus —see Thrombosis, intracranial venous sinus
- capillary I78.8
- cardiac —see also Infarct, myocardium
  - not resulting in infarction I51.3
  - valve —see Endocarditis
  - ▶old I51.3
- carotid (artery) (common) (internal) —see Occlusion, artery, carotid
- cavernous (venous) sinus —see Thrombosis, intracranial venous sinus
- cerebellar artery (anterior inferior) (posterior inferior) (superior) I66.3
- cerebral (artery) —see Occlusion, artery, cerebral
- cerebrovenous sinus —see also Thrombosis, intracranial venous sinus
  - puerperium O87.3
- chronic I82.91
- coronary (artery) (vein) —see also Infarct, myocardium
  - not resulting in infarction I24.0
- corpus cavernosum N48.89
- cortical I66.9
- deep —see Embolism, vein, lower extremity
- due to device, implant or graft —see also Complications, by site and type, specified NEC T85.868
  - arterial graft NEC T82.868
  - breast (implant) T85.868
  - catheter NEC T85.868
    - dialysis (renal) T82.868
      - intraperitoneal T85.868
    - infusion NEC T82.868
      - spinal (epidural) (subdural) T85.860
    - urinary (indwelling) T83.86
  - electronic (electrode) (pulse generator) (stimulator)
    - bone T84.86
    - cardiac T82.867
    - nervous system (brain) (peripheral nerve) (spinal) T85.860
    - urinary T83.86
  - fixation, internal (orthopedic) NEC T84.86
  - gastrointestinal (bile duct) (esophagus) T85.868
  - genital NEC T83.86
  - heart T82.867
  - joint prosthesis T84.86
  - ocular (corneal graft) (orbital implant) NEC T85.868
  - orthopedic NEC T84.86

Thrombosis, thrombotic (Continued)
   due to device, implant or graft (Continued)
      specified NEC T85.868
      urinary NEC T83.86
      vascular NEC T82.868
      ventricular intracranial shunt T85.860
   during the puerperium —see Thrombosis,
      puerperal
   endocardial —see also Infarct, myocardium
      not resulting in infarction I51.3
   eye —see Occlusion, retina
   genital organ
      female NEC N94.89
         pregnancy —see Thrombophlebitis,
            antepartum
      male N50.1
   gestational —see Phlebopathy, gestational
   heart (chamber) —see also Infarct, myocardium
      not resulting in infarction I51.3
      ▶old I51.3
   hepatic (vein) I82.0
      artery I74.8
   history (of) Z86.718
   intestine (with gangrene) —see also Infarct,
      intestine K55.069
   intracardiac NEC (apical) (atrial) (auricular)
      (ventricular) (old) I51.3
   intracranial (arterial) I66.9
      venous sinus (any) G08
         nonpyogenic origin I67.6
         puerperium O87.3
   intramural —see also Infarct, myocardium
      not resulting in infarction I51.3
      ▶old I51.3
   intraspinal venous sinuses and veins G08
      nonpyogenic G95.19
   kidney (artery) N28.0
   lateral (venous) sinus —see Thrombosis,
      intracranial venous sinus
   leg —see Thrombosis, vein, lower extremity
      arterial I74.3
   liver (venous) I82.0
      artery I74.8
      portal vein I81
   longitudinal (venous) sinus —see Thrombosis,
      intracranial venous sinus
   lower limb —see Thrombosis, vein, lower
      extremity
   lung (iatrogenic) (postoperative) —see
      Embolism, pulmonary
   meninges (brain) (arterial) I66.8
   mesenteric (artery) (with gangrene) —see also
      Infarct, intestine K55.069
      vein (inferior) (superior) I81
   mitral I34.8
   mural —see also Infarct, myocardium
      due to syphilis A52.06
      not resulting in infarction I51.3
      ▶old I51.3
   omentum (with gangrene) —see also Infarct,
      intestine K55.069
   ophthalmic —see Occlusion, retina
   pampiniform plexus (male) N50.1
   parietal —see also Infarct, myocardium
      not resulting in infarction I24.0
   penis, superficial vein N48.81
   perianal venous K64.5
   peripheral arteries I74.4
      upper I74.2
   personal history (of) Z86.718
   portal I81
      due to syphilis A52.09
   precerebral artery —see Occlusion, artery,
      precerebral
   puerperal, postpartum O87.0
      brain (artery) O99.43
         venous (sinus) O87.3
      cardiac O99.43
      cerebral (artery) O99.43
         venous (sinus) O87.3
      superficial O87.0

Thrombosis, thrombotic (Continued)
   pulmonary (artery) (iatrogenic)
      (postoperative) (vein) —see Embolism,
      pulmonary
   renal (artery) N28.0
      vein I82.3
   resulting from presence of device, implant or
      graft —see Complications, by site and
      type, specified NEC
   retina, retinal —see Occlusion, retina
   scrotum N50.1
   seminal vesicle N50.1
   sigmoid (venous) sinus —see Thrombosis,
      intracranial venous sinus
   sinus, intracranial (any) —see Thrombosis,
      intracranial venous sinus
   specified site NEC I82.890
      chronic I82.891
   spermatic cord N50.1
   spinal cord (arterial) G95.11
      due to syphilis A52.09
      pyogenic origin G06.1
   spleen, splenic D73.5
      artery I74.8
   testis N50.1
   traumatic NEC T14.8
   tricuspid I07.8
   tumor —see Neoplasm, by site
   tunica vaginalis N50.1
   umbilical cord (vessels), complicating
      delivery O69.5
   vas deferens N50.1
   vein (acute) I82.90
      antecubital I82.61-●
         chronic I82.71-●
      axillary I82.A1-●
         chronic I82.A2-●
      basilic I82.61-●
         chronic I82.71-●
      brachial I82.62-●
         chronic I82.72-●
      brachiocephalic (innominate) I82.290
         chronic I82.291
      cerebral, nonpyogenic I67.6
      cephalic I82.61-●
         chronic I82.71-●
      chronic I82.91
      deep (DVT) I82.40-●
         calf I82.4Z-●
            chronic I82.5Z-●
         lower leg I82.4Z-●
            chronic I82.5Z-●
         thigh I82.4Y-●
            chronic I82.5Y-●
         upper leg I82.4Y
            chronic I82.5y-●
      femoral I82.41-●
         chronic I82.51-●
      iliac (iliofemoral) I82.42-●
         chronic I82.52-●
      innominate I82.290
         chronic I82.291
      internal jugular I82.C1-●
         chronic I82.C2-●
      lower extremity
         deep I82.40-●
            chronic I82.50-●
            specified NEC I82.49-●
               chronic NEC I82.59-●
         distal
            deep I82.4Z-●
         proximal
            deep I82.4Y-●
               chronic I82.5Y-●
         superficial I82.81-●
      perianal K64.5
      popliteal I82.43-●
         chronic I82.53-●
      radial I82.62-●
         chronic I82.72-●
      renal I82.3

Thrombosis, thrombotic (Continued)
   vein (Continued)
      saphenous (greater) (lesser) I82.81-●
      specified NEC I82.890
         chronic NEC I82.891
      subclavian I82.B1-●
         chronic I82.B2-●
      thoracic NEC I82.290
         chronic I82.291
      tibial I82.44-●
         chronic I82.54-●
      ulnar I82.62-●
         chronic I82.72-●
      upper extremity I82.60-●
         chronic I82.70-●
         deep I82.62-●
            chronic I82.72-●
         superficial I82.61-●
            chronic I82.71-●
   vena cava
      inferior I82.220
         chronic I82.221
      superior I82.210
         chronic I82.211
   venous, perianal K64.5
   ventricle —see also Infarct, myocardium
      following acute myocardial infarction
         (current complication) I23.6
      not resulting in infarction I24.0
      ▶old I51.3
Thrombus —see Thrombosis
Thrush —see also Candidiasis
   newborn P37.5
   oral B37.0
   vaginal B37.3
Thumb —see also condition
   sucking (child problem) F98.8
Thymitis E32.8
Thymoma (benign) D15.0
   malignant C37
Thymus, thymic (gland) —see condition
Thyrocele —see Goiter
Thyroglossal —see also condition
   cyst Q89.2
   duct, persistent Q89.2
Thyroid (gland) (body) —see also condition
   hormone resistance E07.89
   lingual Q89.2
   nodule (cystic) (nontoxic) (single) E04.1
Thyroiditis E06.9
   acute (nonsuppurative) (pyogenic)
      (suppurative) E06.0
   autoimmune E06.3
   chronic (nonspecific) (sclerosing) E06.5
      with thyrotoxicosis, transient E06.2
      fibrous E06.5
      lymphadenoid E06.3
      lymphocytic E06.3
      lymphoid E06.3
   de Quervain's E06.1
   drug-induced E06.4
   fibrous (chronic) E06.5
   giant-cell (follicular) E06.1
   granulomatous (de Quervain) (subacute) E06.1
   Hashimoto's (struma lymphomatosa) E06.3
   iatrogenic E06.4
   ligneous E06.5
   lymphocytic (chronic) E06.3
   lymphoid E06.3
   lymphomatous E06.3
   nonsuppurative E06.1
   postpartum, puerperal O90.5
   pseudotuberculous E06.1
   pyogenic E06.0
   radiation E06.4
   Riedel's E06.5
   subacute (granulomatous) E06.1
   suppurative E06.0
   tuberculous A18.81
   viral E06.1
   woody E06.5

▶ New   ⇒ Revised   deleted Deleted   ● Use Additional Character(s)

Thyrolingual duct, persistent Q89.2
Thyromegaly E01.0
Thyrotoxic
  crisis —see Thyrotoxicosis
  heart disease or failure —see also
      Thyrotoxicosis E05.90 [I43]
    with thyroid storm E05.91 [I43]
  storm —see Thyrotoxicosis
Thyrotoxicosis (recurrent) E05.90
  with
    goiter (diffuse) E05.00
      with thyroid storm E05.01
      adenomatous uninodular E05.10
        with thyroid storm E05.11
      multinodular E05.20
        with thyroid storm E05.21
      nodular E05.20
        with thyroid storm E05.21
      uninodular E05.10
        with thyroid storm E05.11
    infiltrative
      dermopathy E05.00
        with thyroid storm E05.01
      ophthalmopathy E05.00
        with thyroid storm E05.01
    single thyroid nodule E05.10
      with thyroid storm E05.11
    thyroid storm E05.91
  due to
    ectopic thyroid nodule or tissue E05.30
      with thyroid storm E05.31
    ingestion of (excessive) thyroid material
        E05.40
      with thyroid storm E05.41
    overproduction of thyroid-stimulating
        hormone E05.80
      with thyroid storm E05.81
    specified cause NEC E05.80
      with thyroid storm E05.81
  factitia E05.40
    with thyroid storm E05.41
  ➡ heart —see also Failure, heart, high-output
      E05.90 [I43]
    ➡ with thyroid storm —see also Failure, heart,
        high-output E05.91 [I43]
    ➡ failure —see also Failure, heart, high-output
        E05.90 [I43]
  neonatal (transient) P72.1
  transient with chronic thyroiditis E06.2
Tibia vara —see Osteochondrosis, juvenile, tibia
Tic (disorder) F95.9
  breathing F95.8
  child problem F95.0
  compulsive F95.1
  de la Tourette F95.2
  degenerative (generalized) (localized) G25.69
    facial G25.69
  disorder
    chronic
      motor F95.1
      vocal F95.1
    combined vocal and multiple motor F95.2
    transient F95.0
  douloureux G50.0
    atypical G50.1
    postherpetic, postzoster B02.22
  drug-induced G25.61
  eyelid F95.8
  habit F95.9
    chronic F95.1
    transient of childhood F95.0
  lid, transient of childhood F95.0
  motor-verbal F95.2
  occupational F48.8
  orbicularis F95.8
    transient of childhood F95.0
  organic origin G25.69
  postchoreic G25.69
  provisional F95.0
  psychogenic, compulsive F95.1
  salaam R25.8

Tic (Continued)
  spasm (motor or vocal) F95.9
    chronic F95.1
    transient of childhood F95.0
  specified NEC F95.8
Tick-borne —see condition
Tietze's disease or syndrome M94.0
Tight, tightness
  anus K62.89
  chest R07.89
  fascia (lata) M62.89
  foreskin (congenital) N47.1
  hymen, hymenal ring N89.6
  introitus (acquired) (congenital) N89.6
  rectal sphincter K62.89
  tendon —see Short, tendon
  urethral sphincter N35.9
Tilting vertebra —see Dorsopathy, deforming,
    specified NEC
Timidity, child F93.8
Tin-miner's lung J63.5
Tinea (intersecta) (tarsi) B35.9
  amiantacea L44.8
  asbestina B35.0
  barbae B35.0
  beard B35.0
  black dot B35.0
  blanca B36.2
  capitis B35.0
  corporis B35.4
  cruris B35.6
  flava B36.0
  foot B35.3
  furfuracea B36.0
  imbricata (Tokelau) B35.5
  kerion B35.0
  manuum B35.2
  microsporic —see Dermatophytosis
  nigra B36.1
  nodosa —see Piedra
  pedis B35.3
  scalp B35.0
  ~~specified site NEC B35.8~~
  ▶ specified NEC B35.8
  sycosis B35.0
  tonsurans B35.0
  trichophytic —see Dermatophytosis
  unguium B35.1
  versicolor B36.0
Tingling sensation (skin) R20.2
Tinnitus NOS H93.1-●
  audible H93.1-●
  aurium H93.1-●
  pulsatile H93.A-●
  subjective H93.1-●
Tipped tooth (teeth) M26.33
Tipping
  pelvis M95.5
    with disproportion (fetopelvic) O33.0
      causing obstructed labor O65.0
  tooth (teeth), fully erupted M26.33
Tiredness R53.83
Tissue —see condition
Tobacco (nicotine)
  abuse —see Tobacco, use
  dependence —see Dependence, drug, nicotine
  harmful use Z72.0
  heart —see Tobacco, toxic effect
  maternal use, affecting newborn P04.2
  toxic effect —see Table of Drugs and
      Chemicals, by substance, poisoning
    chewing tobacco —see Table of Drugs
        and Chemicals, by substance, poisoning
    cigarettes —see Table of Drugs and
        Chemicals, by substance, poisoning
  use Z72.0
    complicating
      childbirth O99.334
      pregnancy O99.33-●
      puerperium O99.335
    counseling and surveillance Z71.6
    history Z87.891

Tobacco (Continued)
  withdrawal state —see also Dependence,
      drug, nicotine F17.203
Tocopherol deficiency E56.0
Todd's
  cirrhosis K74.3
  paralysis (postepileptic) (transitory) G83.84
Toe —see condition
Toilet, artificial opening —see Attention to,
    artificial, opening
Tokelau (ringworm) B35.5
Tollwut —see Rabies
Tommaselli's disease R31.9
  correct substance properly administered —see
      Table of Drugs and Chemicals, by drug,
      adverse effect
  overdose or wrong substance given
      or taken —see Table of Drugs and
      Chemicals, by drug, poisoning
Tongue —see also condition
  tie Q38.1
Tonic pupil —see Anomaly, pupil, function,
    tonic pupil
Toni-Fanconi syndrome (cystinosis) E72.09
  with cystinosis E72.04
Tonsil —see condition
Tonsillitis (acute) (catarrhal) (croupous)
    (follicular) (gangrenous) (infective)
    (lacunar) (lingual) (malignant)
    (membranous) (parenchymatous)
    (phlegmonous) (pseudomembranous)
    (purulent) (septic) (subacute) (suppurative)
    (toxic) (ulcerative) (vesicular) (viral) J03.90
  chronic J35.01
    with adenoiditis J35.03
  diphtheritic A36.0
  hypertrophic J35.01
    with adenoiditis J35.03
  recurrent J03.91
  specified organism NEC J03.80
    recurrent J03.81
  staphylococcal J03.80
    recurrent J03.81
  streptococcal J03.00
    recurrent J03.01
  tuberculous A15.8
  Vincent's A69.1
Tooth, teeth —see condition
Toothache K08.89
Topagnosis R20.8
Tophi —see Gout, chronic
TORCH infection —see Infection, congenital
    without active infection P00.2
Torn —see Tear
Tornwaldt's cyst or disease J39.2
Torsion
  accessory tube —see Torsion, fallopian tube
  adnexa (female) —see Torsion, fallopian tube
  aorta, acquired I77.1
  appendix epididymis N44.04
  appendix testis N44.03
  bile duct (common) (hepatic) K83.8
    congenital Q44.5
  bowel, colon or intestine K56.2
  cervix —see Malposition, uterus
  cystic duct K82.8
  dystonia —see Dystonia, torsion
  epididymis (appendix) N44.04
  fallopian tube N83.52-●
    with ovary N83.53
  gallbladder K82.8
    congenital Q44.1
  hydatid of Morgagni
    female N83.52-●
    male N44.03
  kidney (pedicle) (leading to infarction) N28.0
  Meckel's diverticulum (congenital) Q43.0
    malignant —see Table of Neoplasms, small
        intestine, malignant
  mesentery K56.2
  omentum K56.2

Torsion *(Continued)*
  organ or site, congenital NEC —*see* Anomaly,
      by site
  ovary (pedicle) N83.51-●
      with fallopian tube N83.53
      congenital Q50.2
  oviduct —*see* Torsion, fallopian tube
  penis (acquired) N48.82
      congenital Q55.63
  spasm —*see* Dystonia, torsion
  spermatic cord N44.02
      extravaginal N44.01
      intravaginal N44.02
  spleen D73.5
  testis, testicle N44.00
      appendix N44.03
  tibia —*see* Deformity, limb, specified type
      NEC, lower leg
  uterus —*see* Malposition, uterus
Torticollis (intermittent) (spastic) M43.6
  congenital (sternomastoid) Q68.0
  due to birth injury P15.8
  hysterical F44.4
  ocular R29.891
  psychogenic F45.8
      conversion reaction F44.4
  rheumatic M43.6
  rheumatoid M06.88
  spasmodic G24.3
  traumatic, current S13.4
Tortipelvis G24.1
Tortuous
  aortic arch Q25.46
  artery I77.1
  organ or site, congenital NEC —*see* Distortion
  retinal vessel, congenital Q14.1
  ureter N13.8
  urethra N36.8
  vein —*see* Varix
Torture, victim of Z65.4
Torula, torular (histolytica) (infection) —*see*
      Cryptococcosis
Torulosis —*see* Cryptococcosis
Torus (mandibularis) (palatinus) M27.0
  fracture —*see* Fracture, by site, torus
Touraine's syndrome Q79.8
Tourette's syndrome F95.2
Tourniquet syndrome —*see* Constriction,
      external, by site
Tower skull Q75.0
  with exophthalmos Q87.0
Toxemia R68.89
  bacterial —*see* Sepsis
  burn —*see* Burn
  eclamptic (with pre-existing hypertension) —
      see Eclampsia
  erysipelatous —*see* Erysipelas
  fatigue R68.89
  food —*see* Poisoning, food
  gastrointestinal K52.1
  intestinal K52.1
  kidney —*see* Uremia
  malarial —*see* Malaria
  myocardial —*see* Myocarditis, toxic
  of pregnancy —*see* Pre-eclampsia
  pre-eclamptic —*see* Pre-eclampsia
  small intestine K52.1
  staphylococcal, due to food A05.0
  stasis R68.89
  uremic —*see* Uremia
  urinary —*see* Uremia
Toxemica cerebropathia psychica
      (nonalcoholic) F04
  alcoholic —*see* Alcohol, amnestic disorder
Toxic (poisoning) —*see also* condition T65.91
  effect —*see* Table of Drugs and Chemicals, by
      substance, poisoning
  shock syndrome A48.3
  thyroid (gland) —*see* Thyrotoxicosis
Toxicemia —*see* Toxemia
Toxicity —*see* Table of Drugs and Chemicals, by
      substance, poisoning

Toxic *(Continued)*
  fava bean D55.0
  food, noxious —*see* Poisoning, food
  from drug or nonmedicinal substance —*see*
      Table of Drugs and Chemicals, by drug
Toxicosis —*see also* Toxemia
  capillary, hemorrhagic D69.0
Toxinfection, gastrointestinal K52.1
Toxocariasis B83.0
Toxoplasma, toxoplasmosis (acquired) B58.9
  with
      hepatitis B58.1
      meningoencephalitis B58.2
      ocular involvement B58.00
      other organ involvement B58.89
      pneumonia, pneumonitis B58.3
  congenital (acute) (subacute) (chronic) P37.1
  maternal, manifest toxoplasmosis in infant
      (acute) (subacute) (chronic) P37.1
tPA (rtPA) administation in a different facility
      within the last 24 hours prior to admission
      to current facility Z92.82
Trabeculation, bladder N32.89
Trachea —*see* condition
Tracheitis (catarrhal) (infantile) (membranous)
      (plastic) (septal) (suppurative) (viral) J04.10
  with
      bronchitis (15 years of age and above) J40
          acute or subacute —*see* Bronchitis, acute
          chronic J42
          tuberculous NEC A15.5
          under 15 years of age J20.9
      laryngitis (acute) J04.2
          chronic J37.1
          tuberculous NEC A15.5
  acute J04.10
      with obstruction J04.11
  chronic J42
      with
          bronchitis (chronic) J42
          laryngitis (chronic) J37.1
  diphtheritic (membranous) A36.89
  due to external agent —*see* Inflammation,
      respiratory, upper, due to
  syphilitic A52.73
  tuberculous A15.5
Trachelitis (nonvenereal) —*see* Cervicitis
Tracheobronchial —*see* condition
Tracheobronchitis (15 years of age and
      above) —*see also* Bronchitis
  due to
      Bordetella bronchiseptica A37.80
          with pneumonia A37.81
      Francisella tularensis A21.8
Tracheobronchomegaly Q32.4
  with bronchiectasis J47.9
      with
          exacerbation (acute) J47.1
          lower respiratory infection J47.0
  acquired J98.09
      with bronchiectasis J47.9
          with
              exacerbation (acute) J47.1
              lower respiratory infection J47.0
Tracheobronchopneumonitis —*see* Pneumonia,
      broncho-●
Tracheocele (external) (internal) J39.8
  congenital Q32.1
Tracheomalacia J39.8
  congenital Q32.0
Tracheopharyngitis (acute) J06.9
  chronic J42
  due to external agent —*see* Inflammation,
      respiratory, upper, due to
Tracheostenosis J39.8
Tracheostomy
  complication —*see* Complication,
      tracheostomy
  status Z93.0
      attention to Z43.0
      malfunctioning J95.03

Trachoma, trachomatous A71.9
  active (stage) A71.1
  contraction of conjunctiva A71.1
  dubium A71.0
  healed or sequelae B94.0
  initial (stage) A71.0
  pannus A71.1
  Türck's J37.0
Traction, vitreomacular H43.82-●
Train sickness T75.3
Trait(s)
  Hb-S D57.3
  hemoglobin
      abnormal NEC D58.2
          with thalassemia D56.3
      C —*see* Disease, hemoglobin C
      S (Hb-S) D57.3
  Lepore D56.3
  personality, accentuated Z73.1
  sickle-cell D57.3
      with elliptocytosis or spherocytosis D57.3
  type A personality Z73.1
Tramp Z59.0
Trance R41.89
  hysterical F44.89
Transaminasemia R74.0
Transection
  abdomen (partial) S38.3
  aorta (incomplete) —*see also* Injury, aorta
      complete —*see* Injury, aorta, laceration,
          major
  carotid artery (incomplete) —*see also* Injury,
      blood vessel, carotid, laceration
      complete —*see* Injury, blood vessel, carotid,
          laceration, major
  celiac artery (incomplete) S35.211
      branch (incomplete) S35.291
          complete S35.292
      complete S35.212
  innominate
      artery (incomplete) —*see also* Injury, blood
          vessel, thoracic, innominate, artery,
          laceration
          complete —*see* Injury, blood vessel,
              thoracic, innominate, artery,
              laceration, major
      vein (incomplete) —*see also* Injury, blood
          vessel, thoracic, innominate, vein,
          laceration
          complete —*see* Injury, blood vessel,
              thoracic, innominate, vein,
              laceration, major
  jugular vein (external) (incomplete) —*see
      also* Injury, blood vessel, jugular vein,
      laceration
      complete —*see* Injury, blood vessel, jugular
          vein, laceration, major
      internal (incomplete) —*see also* Injury,
          blood vessel, jugular vein, internal,
          laceration
          complete —*see* Injury, blood vessel,
              jugular vein, internal, laceration,
              major
  mesenteric artery (incomplete) —*see also*
      Injury, mesenteric, artery, laceration
      complete —*see* Injury, mesenteric artery,
          laceration, major
  pulmonary vessel (incomplete) —*see also*
      Injury, blood vessel, thoracic, pulmonary,
      laceration
      complete —*see* Injury, blood vessel,
          thoracic, pulmonary, laceration, major
  subclavian —*see* Transection, innominate
  vena cava (incomplete) —*see also* Injury, vena
      cava
      complete —*see* Injury, vena cava,
          laceration, major
  vertebral artery (incomplete) —*see also* Injury,
      blood vessel, vertebral, laceration
      complete —*see* Injury, blood vessel,
          vertebral, laceration, major

▶ New   ➡ Revised   ~~deleted~~ Deleted   ● Use Additional Character(s)

Transfusion
- associated (red blood cell) hemochromatosis E83.111
- blood
  - ABO incompatible —*see* Complication(s), transfusion, incompatibility reaction, ABO
  - minor blood group (Duffy) (E) (K(ell)) (Kidd) (Lewis) (M) (N) (P) (S) T80.89
  - reaction or complication —*see* Complications, transfusion
- fetomaternal (mother) —*see* Pregnancy, complicated by, placenta, transfusion syndrome
- maternofetal (mother) —*see* Pregnancy, complicated by, placenta, transfusion syndrome
- placental (syndrome) (mother) —*see* Pregnancy, complicated by, placenta, transfusion syndrome
- reaction (adverse) —*see* Complications, transfusion
- related acute lung injury (TRALI) J95.84
- twin-to-twin —*see* Pregnancy, complicated by, placenta, transfusion syndrome, fetus to fetus

Transient (meaning homeless) —*see also* condition Z59.0

Translocation
- balanced autosomal Q95.9
  - in normal individual Q95.0
- chromosomes NEC Q99.8
  - balanced and insertion in normal individual Q95.0
- Down's syndrome Q90.2
- trisomy
  - 13 Q91.6
  - 18 Q91.2
  - 21 Q90.2

Translucency, iris —*see* Degeneration, iris

Transmission of chemical substances through the placenta —*see* Absorption, chemical, through placenta

Transparency, lung, unilateral J43.0

Transplant (ed) (status) Z94.9
- awaiting organ Z76.82
- bone Z94.6
  - marrow Z94.81
- candidate Z76.82
- complication —*see* Complication, transplant
- cornea Z94.7
- heart Z94.1
  - and lung(s) Z94.3
  - valve Z95.2
    - prosthetic Z95.2
    - specified NEC Z95.4
    - xenogenic Z95.3
- intestine Z94.82
- kidney Z94.0
- liver Z94.4
- lung(s) Z94.2
  - and heart Z94.3
- organ (failure) (infection) (rejection)Z94.9
  - removal status Z98.85
- pancreas Z94.83
- skin Z94.5
- social Z60.3
- specified organ or tissue NEC Z94.89
- stem cells Z94.84
- tissue Z94.9

Transplants, ovarian, endometrial N80.1

Transposed —*see* Transposition

Transposition (congenital) —*see also* Malposition, congenital
- abdominal viscera Q89.3
- aorta (dextra) Q20.3
- appendix Q43.8
- colon Q43.8
- corrected Q20.5
- great vessels (complete) (partial) Q20.3

Transposition (*Continued*)
- heart Q24.0
  - with complete transposition of viscera Q89.3
- intestine (large) (small) Q43.8
- reversed jejunal (for bypass) (status) Z98.0
- scrotum Q55.23
- stomach Q40.2
  - with general transposition of viscera Q89.3
- tooth, teeth, fully erupted M26.30
- vessels, great (complete) (partial) Q20.3
- viscera (abdominal) (thoracic) Q89.3

Transsexualism F64.0

Transverse —*see also* condition
- arrest (deep), in labor O64.0
- lie (mother) O32.2
  - causing obstructed labor O64.8

Transvestism, transvestitism (dual-role) F64.1
- fetishistic F65.1

Trapped placenta (with hemorrhage) O72.0
- without hemorrhage O73.0

TRAPS (tumor necrosis factor receptor associated periodic syndrome) M04.1

Trauma, traumatism —*see also* Injury
- acoustic —*see* subcategory H83.3
- birth —*see* Birth, injury
- complicating ectopic or molar pregnancy O08.6
- during delivery O71.9
- following ectopic or molar pregnancy O08.6
- obstetric O71.9
  - specified NEC O71.89
- occlusal
  - primary K08.81
  - secondary K08.82

Traumatic —*see also* condition
- brain injury S06.9

Treacher Collins syndrome Q75.4

Treitz's hernia —*see* Hernia, abdomen, specified site NEC

Trematode infestation —*see* Infestation, fluke

Trematodiasis —*see* Infestation, fluke

Trembling paralysis —*see* Parkinsonism

Tremor(s) R25.1
- drug induced G25.1
- essential (benign) G25.0
- familial G25.0
- hereditary G25.0
- hysterical F44.4
- intention G25.2
- medication induced postural G25.1
- mercurial —*see* subcategory T56.1
- Parkinson's —*see* Parkinsonism
- psychogenic (conversion reaction) F44.4
- senilis R54
- specified type NEC G25.2

Trench
- fever A79.0
- foot —*see* Immersion, foot
- mouth A69.1

Treponema pallidum infection —*see* Syphilis

Treponematosis
- due to
  - T. pallidum —*see* Syphilis
  - T. pertenue —*see* Yaws

Triad
- Hutchinson's (congenital syphilis) A50.53
- Kartagener's Q89.3
- Saint's —*see* Hernia, diaphragm

Trichiasis (eyelid) H02.059
- with entropion —*see* Entropion
- left H02.056
  - lower H02.055
  - upper H02.054
- right H02.053
  - lower H02.052
  - upper H02.051

Trichinella spiralis (infection) (infestation) B75

Trichinellosis, trichiniasis, trichinelliasis, trichinosis B75
- with muscle disorder B75 [*M63.80*]
  - ankle B75 [*M63.87-●*]
  - foot B75 [*M63.87-●*]
  - forearm B75 [*M63.83-●*]
  - hand B75 [*M63.84-●*]
  - lower leg B75 [*M63.86-●*]
  - multiple sites B75 [*M63.89*]
  - pelvic region B75 [*M63.85-●*]
  - shoulder region B75 [*M63.81-●*]
  - specified site NEC B75 [*M63.88*]
  - thigh B75 [*M63.85-●*]
  - upper arm B75 [*M63.82-●*]

Trichobezoar T18.9
- intestine T18.3
- stomach T18.2

Trichocephaliasis, trichocephalosis B79

Trichocephalus infestation B79

Trichoclasis L67.8

Trichoepithelioma —*see also* Neoplasm, skin, benign
- malignant —*see* Neoplasm, skin, malignant

Trichofolliculoma —*see* Neoplasm, skin, benign

Tricholemmoma —*see* Neoplasm, skin, benign

Trichomoniasis A59.9
- bladder A59.03
- cervix A59.09
- intestinal A07.8
- prostate A59.02
- seminal vesicles A59.09
- specified site NEC A59.8
- urethra A59.03
- urogenitalis A59.00
- vagina A59.01
- vulva A59.01

Trichomycosis
- axillaris A48.8
- nodosa, nodularis B36.8

Trichonodosis L67.8

Trichophytid, trichophyton infection —*see* Dermatophytosis

Trichophytobezoar T18.9
- intestine T18.3
- stomach T18.2

Trichophytosis —*see* Dermatophytosis

Trichoptilosis L67.8

Trichorrhexis (nodosa) (invaginata) L67.0

Trichosis axillaris A48.8

Trichosporosis nodosa B36.2

Trichostasis spinulosa (congenital) Q84.1

Trichostrongyliasis, trichostrongylosis (small intestine) B81.2

Trichostrongylus infection B81.2

Trichotillomania F63.3

Trichromat, trichromatopsia, anomalous (congenital) H53.55

Trichuriasis B79

Trichuris trichiura (infection) (infestation) (any site) B79

Tricuspid (valve) —*see* condition

Trifid —*see also* Accessory
- kidney (pelvis) Q63.8
- tongue Q38.3

Trigeminal neuralgia —*see* Neuralgia, trigeminal

Trigeminy R00.8

Trigger finger (acquired) M65.30
- congenital Q74.0
- index finger M65.32-●
- little finger M65.35-●
- middle finger M65.33-●
- ring finger M65.34-●
- thumb M65.31-●

Trigonitis (bladder) (chronic) (pseudomembranous) N30.30
- with hematuria N30.31

Trigonocephaly Q75.0

Trilocular heart —*see* Cor triloculare

Trimethylaminuria E72.52
Tripartite placenta O43.19-●
Triphalangeal thumb Q74.0
Triple —see also Accessory
  kidneys Q63.0
  uteri Q51.818
  X, female Q97.0
Triplegia G83.89
  congenital G80.8
Triplet (newborn) —see also Newborn, triplet
  complicating pregnancy —see Pregnancy,
    triplet
Triplication —see Accessory
Triploidy Q92.7
Trismus R25.2
  neonatorum A33
  newborn A33
Trisomy (syndrome) Q92.9
  13 (partial) Q91.7
    meiotic nondisjunction Q91.4
    mitotic nondisjunction Q91.5
    mosaicism Q91.5
    translocation Q91.6
  18 (partial) Q91.3
    meiotic nondisjunction Q91.0
    mitotic nondisjunction Q91.1
    mosaicism Q91.1
    translocation Q91.2
  20 Q92.8
  21 (partial) Q90.9
    meiotic nondisjunction Q90.0
    mitotic nondisjunction Q90.1
    mosaicism Q90.1
    translocation Q90.2
  22 Q92.8
  autosomes Q92.9
  chromosome specified NEC Q92.8
    partial Q92.2
      due to unbalanced translocation Q92.5
    specified NEC Q92.8
    whole (nonsex chromosome)
      meiotic nondisjunction Q92.0
      mitotic nondisjunction Q92.1
      mosaicism Q92.1
  due to
    dicentrics —see Extra, marker
      chromosomes
    extra rings —see Extra, marker
      chromosomes
    isochromosomes —see Extra, marker
      chromosomes
  specified NEC Q92.8
  whole chromosome Q92.9
    meiotic nondisjunction Q92.0
    mitotic nondisjunction Q92.1
    mosaicism Q92.1
    partial Q92.9
    specified NEC Q92.8
Tritanomaly, tritanopia H53.55
Trombiculosis, trombiculiasis, trombidiosis
  B88.0
Trophedema (congenital) (hereditary) Q82.0
Trophoblastic disease —see also Mole,
  hydatidiform O01.9
Tropholymphedema Q82.0
Trophoneurosis NEC G96.8
  disseminated M34.9
Tropical —see condition
Trouble —see also Disease
  heart —see Disease, heart
  kidney —see Disease, renal
  nervous R45.0
  sinus —see Sinusitis
Trousseau's syndrome (thrombophlebitis
  migrans) I82.1
Truancy, childhood
  from school Z72.810
Truncus
  arteriosus (persistent) Q20.0
  communis Q20.0
Trunk —see condition

Trypanosomiasis
  African B56.9
    by Trypanosoma brucei
      gambiense B56.0
      rhodesiense B56.1
  American —see Chagas' disease
  Brazilian —see Chagas' disease
  by Trypanosoma
    brucei gambiense B56.0
    brucei rhodesiense B56.1
    cruzi —see Chagas' disease
  gambiensis, Gambian B56.0
  rhodesiensis, Rhodesian B56.1
  South American —see Chagas' disease
  where
    African trypanosomiasis is prevalent B56.9
    Chagas' disease is prevalent B57.2
T-shaped incisors K00.2
Tsutsugamushi (disease) (fever) A75.3
Tube, tubal, tubular —see condition
Tubercle —see also Tuberculosis
  brain, solitary A17.81
  Darwin's Q17.8
  Ghon, primary infection A15.7
Tuberculid, tuberculide (indurating,
  subcutaneous) (lichenoid) (miliary)
  (papulonecrotic) (primary) (skin) A18.4
Tuberculoma —see also Tuberculosis
  brain A17.81
  meninges (cerebral) (spinal) A17.1
  spinal cord A17.81
Tuberculosis, tubercular, tuberculous
  (calcification) (calcified) (caseous)
  (chromogenic acid-fast bacilli)
  (degeneration) (fibrocaseous) (fistula)
  (interstitial) (isolated circumscribed
  lesions) (necrosis) (parenchymatous)
  (ulcerative) A15.9
  with pneumoconiosis (any condition in
    J60-J64) J65
  abdomen (lymph gland) A18.39
  abscess (respiratory) A15.9
    bone A18.03
      hip A18.02
      knee A18.02
      sacrum A18.01
      specified site NEC A18.03
      spinal A18.01
      vertebra A18.01
    brain A17.81
    breast A18.89
    Cowper's gland A18.15
    dura (mater) (cerebral) (spinal) A17.81
    epidural (cerebral) (spinal) A17.81
    female pelvis A18.17
    frontal sinus A15.8
    genital organs NEC A18.10
    genitourinary A18.10
    gland (lymphatic) —see Tuberculosis,
      lymph gland
    hip A18.02
    intestine A18.32
    ischiorectal A18.32
    joint NEC A18.02
      hip A18.02
      knee A18.02
      specified NEC A18.02
      vertebral A18.01
    kidney A18.11
    knee A18.02
    latent R76.11
    lumbar (spine) A18.01
    lung —see Tuberculosis, pulmonary
    meninges (cerebral) (spinal) A17.0
    muscle A18.09
    perianal (fistula) A18.32
    perinephritic A18.11
    perirectal A18.32
    rectum A18.32
    retropharyngeal A15.8
    sacrum A18.01

Tuberculosis, tubercular, tuberculous
  (Continued)
  abscess (Continued)
    scrofulous A18.2
    scrotum A18.15
    skin (primary) A18.4
    spinal cord A17.81
    spine or vertebra (column) A18.01
    subdiaphragmatic A18.31
    testis A18.15
    urinary A18.13
    uterus A18.17
  accessory sinus —see Tuberculosis, sinus
  Addison's disease A18.7
  adenitis —see Tuberculosis, lymph gland
  adenoids A15.8
  adenopathy —see Tuberculosis, lymph gland
  adherent pericardium A18.84
  adnexa (uteri) A18.17
  adrenal (capsule) (gland) A18.7
  alimentary canal A18.32
  anemia A18.89
  ankle (joint) (bone) A18.02
  anus A18.32
  apex, apical —see Tuberculosis, pulmonary
  appendicitis, appendix A18.32
  arachnoid A17.0
  artery, arteritis A18.89
    cerebral A18.89
  arthritis (chronic) (synovial) A18.02
    spine or vertebra (column) A18.01
  articular —see Tuberculosis, joint
  ascites A18.31
  asthma —see Tuberculosis, pulmonary
  axilla, axillary (gland) A18.2
  bladder A18.12
  bone A18.03
    hip A18.02
    knee A18.02
    limb NEC A18.03
    sacrum A18.01
    spine or vertebral column A18.01
  bowel (miliary) A18.32
  brain A17.81
  breast A18.89
  broad ligament A18.17
  bronchi, bronchial, bronchus A15.5
    ectasia, ectasis (bronchiectasis) —see
      Tuberculosis, pulmonary
    fistula A15.5
      primary (progressive) A15.7
    gland or node A15.4
      primary (progressive) A15.7
    lymph gland or node A15.4
      primary (progressive) A15.7
  bronchiectasis —see Tuberculosis, pulmonary
  bronchitis A15.5
  bronchopleural A15.6
  bronchopneumonia, bronchopneumonic —see
    Tuberculosis, pulmonary
  bronchorrhagia A15.5
  bronchotracheal A15.5
  bronze disease A18.7
  buccal cavity A18.83
  bulbourethral gland A18.15
  bursa A18.09
  cachexia A15.9
  cardiomyopathy A18.84
  caries —see Tuberculosis, bone
  cartilage A18.02
    intervertebral A18.01
  catarrhal —see Tuberculosis, respiratory
  cecum A18.32
  cellulitis (primary) A18.4
  cerebellum A17.81
  cerebral, cerebrum A17.81
  cerebrospinal A17.81
    meninges A17.0
  cervical (lymph gland or node) A18.2
  cervicitis, cervix (uteri) A18.16
  chest —see Tuberculosis, respiratory

Tuberculosis, tubercular, tuberculous
(Continued)
chorioretinitis A18.53
choroid, choroiditis A18.53
ciliary body A18.54
colitis A18.32
collier's J65
colliquativa (primary) A18.4
colon A18.32
complex, primary A15.7
congenital P37.0
conjunctiva A18.59
connective tissue (systemic) A18.89
contact Z20.1
cornea (ulcer) A18.52
Cowper's gland A18.15
coxae A18.02
coxalgia A18.02
cul-de-sac of Douglas A18.17
curvature, spine A18.01
cutis (colliquativa) (primary) A18.4
cyst, ovary A18.18
cystitis A18.12
dactylitis A18.03
diarrhea A18.32
diffuse —see Tuberculosis, miliary
digestive tract A18.32
disseminated —see Tuberculosis, miliary
duodenum A18.32
dura (mater) (cerebral) (spinal) A17.0
abscess (cerebral) (spinal) A17.81
dysentery A18.32
ear (inner) (middle) A18.6
bone A18.03
external (primary) A18.4
skin (primary) A18.4
elbow A18.02
emphysema —see Tuberculosis, pulmonary
empyema A15.6
encephalitis A17.82
endarteritis A18.89
endocarditis A18.84
aortic A18.84
mitral A18.84
pulmonary A18.84
tricuspid A18.84
endocrine glands NEC A18.82
endometrium A18.17
enteric, enterica, enteritis A18.32
enterocolitis A18.32
epididymis, epididymitis A18.15
epidural abscess (cerebral) (spinal) A17.81
epiglottis A15.5
episcleritis A18.51
erythema (induratum) (nodosum) (primary) A18.4
esophagus A18.83
eustachian tube A18.6
exposure (to) Z20.1
exudative —see Tuberculosis, pulmonary
eye A18.50
eyelid (primary) (lupus) A18.4
fallopian tube (acute) (chronic) A18.17
fascia A18.09
fauces A15.8
female pelvic inflammatory disease A18.17
finger A18.03
first infection A15.7
gallbladder A18.83
ganglion A18.09
gastritis A18.83
gastrocolic fistula A18.32
gastroenteritis A18.32
gastrointestinal tract A18.32
general, generalized —see Tuberculosis, miliary
genital organs A18.10
genitourinary A18.10
genu A18.02
glandula suprarenalis A18.7
glandular, general A18.2

glottis A15.5
grinder's J65
gum A18.83
hand A18.03
heart A18.84
hematogenous —see Tuberculosis, miliary
hemoptysis —see Tuberculosis, pulmonary
hemorrhage NEC —see Tuberculosis, pulmonary
hemothorax A15.6
hepatitis A18.83
hilar lymph nodes A15.4
primary (progressive) A15.7
hip (joint) (disease) (bone) A18.02
hydropneumothorax A15.6
hydrothorax A15.6
hypoadrenalism A18.7
hypopharynx A15.8
ileocecal (hyperplastic) A18.32
ileocolitis A18.32
ileum A18.32
iliac spine (superior) A18.03
immunological findings only A15.7
indurativa (primary) A18.4
infantile A15.7
infection A15.9
without clinical manifestations A15.7
infraclavicular gland A18.2
inguinal gland A18.2
inguinalis A18.2
intestine (any part) A18.32
iridocyclitis A18.54
iris, iritis A18.54
ischiorectal A18.32
jaw A18.03
jejunum A18.32
joint A18.02
vertebral A18.01
keratitis (interstitial) A18.52
keratoconjunctivitis A18.52
kidney A18.11
knee (joint) A18.02
kyphosis, kyphoscoliosis A18.01
laryngitis A15.5
larynx A15.5
latent R76.11
leptomeninges, leptomeningitis (cerebral) (spinal) A17.0
lichenoides (primary) A18.4
linguae A18.83
lip A18.83
liver A18.83
lordosis A18.01
lung —see Tuberculosis, pulmonary
lupus vulgaris A18.4
lymph gland or node (peripheral) A18.2
abdomen A18.39
bronchial A15.4
primary (progressive) A15.7
cervical A18.2
hilar A15.4
primary (progressive) A15.7
intrathoracic A15.4
primary (progressive) A15.7
mediastinal A15.4
primary (progressive) A15.7
mesenteric A18.39
retroperitoneal A18.39
tracheobronchial A15.4
primary (progressive) A15.7
lymphadenitis —see Tuberculosis, lymph gland
lymphangitis —see Tuberculosis, lymph gland
lymphatic (gland) (vessel) —see Tuberculosis, lymph gland
mammary gland A18.89
marasmus A15.9
mastoiditis A18.03

mediastinal lymph gland or node A15.4
primary (progressive) A15.7
mediastinitis A15.8
primary (progressive) A15.7
mediastinum A15.8
primary (progressive) A15.7
medulla A17.81
melanosis, Addisonian A18.7
meninges, meningitis (basilar) (cerebral) (cerebrospinal) (spinal) A17.0
meningoencephalitis A17.82
mesentery, mesenteric (gland or node) A18.39
miliary A19.9
acute A19.2
multiple sites A19.1
single specified site A19.0
chronic A19.8
specified NEC A19.8
millstone makers' J65
miner's J65
molder's J65
mouth A18.83
multiple A19.9
acute A19.1
chronic A19.8
muscle A18.09
myelitis A17.82
myocardium, myocarditis A18.84
nasal (passage) (sinus) A15.8
nasopharynx A15.8
neck gland A18.2
nephritis A18.11
nerve (mononeuropathy) A17.83
nervous system A17.9
nose (septum) A15.8
ocular A18.50
omentum A18.31
oophoritis (acute) (chronic) A18.17
optic (nerve trunk) (papilla) A18.59
orbit A18.59
orchitis A18.15
organ, specified NEC A18.89
osseous —see Tuberculosis, bone
osteitis —see Tuberculosis, bone
osteomyelitis —see Tuberculosis, bone
otitis media A18.6
ovary, ovaritis (acute) (chronic) A18.17
oviduct (acute) (chronic) A18.17
pachymeningitis A17.0
palate (soft) A18.83
pancreas A18.83
papulonecrotic (a) (primary) A18.4
parathyroid glands A18.82
paronychia (primary) A18.4
parotid gland or region A18.83
pelvis (bony) A18.03
penis A18.15
peribronchitis A15.5
pericardium, pericarditis A18.84
perichondritis, larynx A15.5
periostitis —see Tuberculosis, bone
perirectal fistula A18.32
peritoneum NEC A18.31
peritonitis A18.31
pharynx, pharyngitis A15.8
phlyctenulosis (keratoconjunctivitis) A18.52
phthisis NEC —see Tuberculosis, pulmonary
pituitary gland A18.82
pleura, pleural, pleurisy, pleuritis (fibrinous) (obliterative) (purulent) (simple plastic) (with effusion) A15.6
primary (progressive) A15.7
pneumonia, pneumonic —see Tuberculosis, pulmonary
pneumothorax (spontaneous) (tense valvular) —see Tuberculosis, pulmonary
polyneuropathy A17.89

Tuberculosis, tubercular, tuberculous
(Continued)
polyserositis A19.9
  acute A19.1
  chronic A19.8
potter's J65
prepuce A18.15
primary (complex) A15.7
proctitis A18.32
prostate, prostatitis A18.14
pulmonalis —see Tuberculosis, pulmonary
pulmonary (cavitated) (fibrotic) (infiltrative)
  (nodular) A15.0
  childhood type or first infection A15.7
  primary (complex) A15.7
pyelitis A18.11
pyelonephritis A18.11
pyemia —see Tuberculosis, miliary
pyonephrosis A18.11
pyopneumothorax A15.6
pyothorax A15.6
rectum (fistula) (with abscess) A18.32
reinfection stage —see Tuberculosis,
  pulmonary
renal A18.11
renis A18.11
respiratory A15.9
  primary A15.7
  specified site NEC A15.8
retina, retinitis A18.53
retroperitoneal (lymph gland or node)
  A18.39
rheumatism NEC A18.09
rhinitis A15.8
sacroiliac (joint) A18.01
sacrum A18.01
salivary gland A18.83
salpingitis (acute) (chronic) A18.17
sandblaster's J65
sclera A18.51
scoliosis A18.01
scrofulous A18.2
scrotum A18.15
seminal tract or vesicle A18.15
senile A15.9
septic —see Tuberculosis, miliary
shoulder (joint) A18.02
  blade A18.03
sigmoid A18.32
sinus (any nasal) A15.8
  bone A18.03
  epididymis A18.15
skeletal NEC A18.03
skin (any site) (primary) A18.4
small intestine A18.32
soft palate A18.83
spermatic cord A18.15
spine, spinal (column) A18.01
  cord A17.81
  medulla A17.81
  membrane A17.0
  meninges A17.0
spleen, splenitis A18.85
spondylitis A18.01
sternoclavicular joint A18.02
stomach A18.83
stonemason's J65
subcutaneous tissue (cellular) (primary)
  A18.4
subcutis (primary) A18.4
subdeltoid bursa A18.83
submaxillary (region) A18.83
supraclavicular gland A18.2
suprarenal (capsule) (gland) A18.7
swelling, joint —see also category M01 (see also
  Tuberculosis, joint) A18.02
symphysis pubis A18.02
synovitis A18.09
  articular A18.02
  spine or vertebra A18.01
systemic —see Tuberculosis, miliary

Tuberculosis, tubercular, tuberculous
(Continued)
tarsitis A18.4
tendon (sheath) —see Tuberculosis,
  tenosynovitis
tenosynovitis A18.09
  spine or vertebra A18.01
testis A18.15
throat A15.8
thymus gland A18.82
thyroid gland A18.81
tongue A18.83
tonsil, tonsillitis A15.8
trachea, tracheal A15.5
  lymph gland or node A15.4
    primary (progressive) A15.7
tracheobronchial A15.5
  lymph gland or node A15.4
    primary (progressive) A15.7
tubal (acute) (chronic) A18.17
tunica vaginalis A18.15
ulcer (skin) (primary) A18.4
  bowel or intestine A18.32
  specified NEC - code under Tuberculosis,
    by site
unspecified site A15.9
ureter A18.11
urethra, urethral (gland) A18.13
urinary organ or tract A18.13
uterus A18.17
uveal tract A18.54
uvula A18.83
vagina A18.18
vas deferens A18.15
verruca, verrucosa (cutis) (primary) A18.4
vertebra (column) A18.01
vesiculitis A18.15
vulva A18.18
wrist (joint) A18.02
Tuberculum
  Carabelli —see Note at K00.2
  occlusal —see Note at K00.2
  paramolare K00.2
Tuberosity, enitre maxillary M26.07
Tuberous sclerosis (brain) Q85.1
Tubo-ovarian —see condition
Tuboplasty, after previous sterilization
  Z31.0
  aftercare Z31.42
Tubotympanitis, catarrhal (chronic) —see Otitis,
  media, nonsuppurative, chronic, serous
Tularemia A21.9
  with
    conjunctivitis A21.1
    pneumonia A21.2
  abdominal A21.3
  bronchopneumonic A21.2
  conjunctivitis A21.1
  cryptogenic A21.3
  enteric A21.3
  gastrointestinal A21.3
  generalized A21.7
  ingestion A21.3
  intestinal A21.3
  oculoglandular A21.1
  ophthalmic A21.1
  pneumonia (any), pneumonic A21.2
  pulmonary A21.2
  sepsis A21.7
  specified NEC A21.8
  typhoidal A21.7
  ulceroglandular A21.0
Tularensis conjunctivitis A21.1
Tumefaction —see also Swelling
  liver —see Hypertrophy, liver
Tumor —see also Neoplasm, unspecified
  behavior, by site
  acinar cell —see Neoplasm, uncertain
    behavior, by site
  acinic cell —see Neoplasm, uncertain
    behavior, by site

Tumor (Continued)
adenocarcinoid —see Neoplasm, malignant,
  by site
adenomatoid —see also Neoplasm, benign,
  by site
  odontogenic —see Cyst, calcifying
    odontogenic
adnexal (skin) —see Neoplasm, skin, benign,
  by site
adrenal
  cortical (benign) D35.0-●
    malignant C74.0-●
  rest —see Neoplasm, benign, by site
alpha-cell
  malignant
    pancreas C25.4
    specified site NEC —see Neoplasm,
      malignant, by site
    unspecified site C25.4
  pancreas D13.7
  specified site NEC —see Neoplasm, benign,
    by site
  unspecified site D13.7
aneurysmal —see Aneurysm
aortic body D44.7
  malignant C75.5
Askin's —see Neoplasm, connective tissue,
  malignant
basal cell —see also Neoplasm, skin, uncertain
  behavior D48.5
Bednar —see Neoplasm, skin, malignant
benign (unclassified) —see Neoplasm, benign,
  by site
beta-cell
  malignant
    pancreas C25.4
    specified site NEC —see Neoplasm,
      malignant, by site
    unspecified site C25.4
  pancreas D13.7
  specified site NEC —see Neoplasm, benign,
    by site
  unspecified site D13.7
Brenner D27.9
  borderline malignancy D39.1-●
  malignant C56-●
  proliferating D39.1
bronchial alveolar, intravascular D38.1
Brooke's —see Neoplasm, skin, benign
brown fat —see Lipoma
Burkitt —see Lymphoma, Burkitt
calcifying epithelial odontogenic —see Cyst,
  calcifying odontogenic
carcinoid
  benign D3A.00
    appendix D3A.020
    ascending colon D3A.022
    bronchus (lung) D3A.090
    cecum D3A.021
    colon D3A.029
    descending colon D3A.024
    duodenum D3A.010
    foregut NOS D3A.094
    hindgut NOS D3A.096
    ileum D3A.012
    jejunum D3A.011
    kidney D3A.093
    large intestine D3A.029
    lung (bronchus) D3A.090
    midgut NOS D3A.095
    rectum D3A.026
    sigmoid colon D3A.025
    small intestine D3A.019
    specified NEC D3A.098
    stomach D3A.092
    thymus D3A.091
    transverse colon D3A.023
  malignant C7A.00
    appendix C7A.020
    ascending colon C7A.022
    bronchus (lung) C7A.090

▶ New   ⇒ Revised   ~~deleted~~ Deleted   ● Use Additional Character(s)

Tumor *(Continued)*
  carcinoid *(Continued)*
    malignant *(Continued)*
      cecum C7A.021
      colon C7A.029
      descending colon C7A.024
      duodenum C7A.010
      foregut NOS C7A.094
      hindgut NOS C7A.096
      ileum C7A.012
      jejunum C7A.011
      kidney C7A.093
      large intestine C7A.029
      lung (bronchus) C7A.090
      midgut NOS C7A.095
      rectum C7A.026
      sigmoid colon C7A.025
      small intestine C7A.019
      specified NEC C7A.098
      stomach C7A.092
      thymus C7A.091
      transverse colon C7A.023
    mesentary metastasis C7B.04
    secondary C7B.00
      bone C7B.03
      distant lymph nodes C7B.01
      liver C7B.02
      peritoneum C7B.04
      specified NEC C7B.09
  carotid body D44.6
    malignant C75.4
  cells —*see also* Neoplasm, unspecified
    behavior, by site
    benign —*see* Neoplasm, benign,
      by site
    malignant —*see* Neoplasm, malignant,
      by site
    uncertain whether benign or malignant —
      see Neoplasm, uncertain behavior,
      by site
  cervix, in pregnancy or childbirth —*see*
    Pregnancy, complicated by, tumor,
    cervix
  chondromatous giant cell —*see* Neoplasm,
    bone, benign
  chromaffin —*see also* Neoplasm, benign, by
    site
    malignant —*see* Neoplasm, malignant, by
      site
  Cock's peculiar L72.3
  Codman's —*see* Neoplasm, bone, benign
  dentigerous, mixed —*see* Cyst, calcifying
    odontogenic
  dermoid —*see* Neoplasm, benign,
    by site
    with malignant transformation C56-●
  desmoid (extra-abdominal) —*see also*
    Neoplasm, connective tissue, uncertain
    behavior
    abdominal —*see* Neoplasm, connective
      tissue, uncertain behavior
  embolus —*see* Neoplasm, secondary,
    by site
  embryonal (mixed) —*see also* Neoplasm,
    uncertain behavior, by site
    liver C22.7
  endodermal sinus
    specified site —*see* Neoplasm, malignant,
      by site
    unspecified site
      female C56.-●
      male C62.90
  epithelial
    benign —*see* Neoplasm, benign,
      by site
    malignant —*see* Neoplasm, malignant, by
      site
  Ewing's —*see* Neoplasm, bone, malignant,
    by site
  fatty —*see* Lipoma
  fibroid —*see* Leiomyoma

Tumor *(Continued)*
  G cell
    malignant
      pancreas C25.4
      specified site NEC —*see* Neoplasm,
        malignant, by site
      unspecified site C25.4
    specified site —*see* Neoplasm, uncertain
      behavior, by site
    unspecified site D37.8
  germ cell —*see also* Neoplasm, malignant,
    by site
    mixed —*see* Neoplasm, malignant,
      by site
  ghost cell, odontogenic —*see* Cyst, calcifying
    odontogenic
  giant cell —*see also* Neoplasm, uncertain
    behavior, by site
    bone D48.0
      malignant —*see* Neoplasm, bone,
        malignant
      chondromatous —*see* Neoplasm, bone,
        benign
    malignant —*see* Neoplasm, malignant, by
      site
    soft parts —*see* Neoplasm, connective
      tissue, uncertain behavior
      malignant —*see* Neoplasm, connective
        tissue, malignant
  glomus D18.00
    intra-abdominal D18.03
    intracranial D18.02
    jugulare D44.7
      malignant C75.5
    skin D18.01
    specified site NEC D18.09
  gonadal stromal —*see* Neoplasm, uncertain
    behavior, by site
  granular cell —*see also* Neoplasm, connective
    tissue, benign
    malignant —*see* Neoplasm, connective
      tissue, malignant
  granulosa cell D39.1-●
    juvenile D39.1-●
    malignant C56-●
  granulosa cell-theca cell D39.1-●
    malignant C56-●
  Grawitz's C64-●
  hemorrhoidal —*see* Hemorrhoids
  hilar cell D27-●
  hilus cell D27-●
  Hurthle cell (benign) D34
    malignant C73
  hydatid —*see* Echinococcus
  hypernephroid —*see also* Neoplasm,
    uncertain behavior, by site
  interstitial cell —*see also* Neoplasm, uncertain
    behavior, by site
    benign —*see* Neoplasm, benign, by site
    malignant —*see* Neoplasm, malignant, by
      site
  intravascular bronchial alveolar D38.1
  islet cell —*see* Neoplasm, benign, by site
    malignant —*see* Neoplasm, malignant, by
      site
    pancreas C25.4
    specified site NEC —*see* Neoplasm,
      malignant, by site
    unspecified site C25.4
    pancreas D13.7
    specified site NEC —*see* Neoplasm, benign,
      by site
    unspecified site D13.7
  juxtaglomerular D41.0-●
  Klatskin's C24.0
  Krukenberg's C79.6-●
  Leydig cell —*see* Neoplasm, uncertain
    behavior, by site
    benign —*see* Neoplasm, benign, by site
      specified site —*see* Neoplasm, benign,
        by site

Tumor *(Continued)*
  Leydig cell *(Continued)*
    benign *(Continued)*
      unspecified site
        female D27.9
        male D29.20
    malignant —*see* Neoplasm, malignant, by
      site
      specified site —*see* Neoplasm,
        malignant, by site
      unspecified site
        female C56.9
        male C62.90
    specified site —*see* Neoplasm, uncertain
      behavior, by site
    unspecified site
      female D39.10
      male D40.10
  lipid cell, ovary D27-●
  lipoid cell, ovary D27-●
  malignant —*see also* Neoplasm, malignant, by
    site C80.1
    fusiform cell (type) C80.1
    giant cell (type) C80.1
    localized, plasma cell —*see* Plasmacytoma,
      solitary
    mixed NEC C80.1
    small cell (type) C80.1
    spindle cell (type) C80.1
    unclassified C80.1
  ⏩mast cell D47.09
    ~~malignant C96.2~~
  melanotic, neuroectodermal —*see* Neoplasm,
    benign, by site
  Merkel cell —*see* Carcinoma, Merkel cell
  mesenchymal
    malignant —*see* Neoplasm, connective
      tissue, malignant
    mixed —*see* Neoplasm, connective tissue,
      uncertain behavior
  mesodermal, mixed —*see also* Neoplasm,
    malignant, by site
    liver C22.4
  mesonephric —*see also* Neoplasm, uncertain
    behavior, by site
    malignant —*see* Neoplasm, malignant, by
      site
  metastatic
    from specified site —*see* Neoplasm,
      malignant, by site
    of specified site —*see* Neoplasm,
      malignant, by site
    to specified site —*see* Neoplasm, secondary,
      by site
  mixed NEC —*see also* Neoplasm, benign, by
    site
    malignant —*see* Neoplasm, malignant, by
      site
  mucinous of low malignant potential
    specified site —*see* Neoplasm, malignant,
      by site
    unspecified site C56.9
  mucocarcinoid
    specified site —*see* Neoplasm, malignant,
      by site
    unspecified site C18.1
  mucoepidermoid —*see* Neoplasm, uncertain
    behavior, by site
  Müllerian, mixed
    specified site —*see* Neoplasm, malignant,
      by site
    unspecified site C54.9
  myoepithelial —*see* Neoplasm, benign,
    by site
  neuroectodermal (peripheral) —*see*
    Neoplasm, malignant, by site
  primitive
    specified site —*see* Neoplasm,
      malignant,
      by site
    unspecified site C71.9

Tumor (Continued)
  neuroendocrine D3A.8
    malignant poorly differentiated C7A.1
    secondary NEC C7B.8
    specified NEC C7A.8
  neurogenic olfactory C30.0
  nonencapsulated sclerosing C73
  odontogenic (adenomatoid) (benign)
    (calcifying epithelial) (keratocystic)
    (squamous) —see Cyst, calcifying
    odontogenic
    malignant C41.1
      upper jaw (bone) C41.0
  ovarian stromal D39.1-●
  ovary, in pregnancy —see Pregnancy,
    complicated by
  pacinian —see Neoplasm, skin, benign
  Pancoast's —see Pancoast's syndrome
  papillary —see also Papilloma
    cystic D37.9
    mucinous of low malignant potential C56-●
      specified site —see Neoplasm,
        malignant, by site
      unspecified site C56.9
    serous of low malignant potential
      specified site —see Neoplasm,
        malignant, by site
      unspecified site C56.9
  pelvic, in pregnancy or childbirth —see
    Pregnancy, complicated by
  phantom F45.8
  phyllodes D48.6-●
    benign D24-●
    malignant —see Neoplasm, breast,
      malignant
  Pindborg —see Cyst, calcifying odontogenic
  placental site trophoblastic D39.2
  plasma cell (malignant) (localized) —see
    Plasmacytoma, solitary
  polyvesicular vitelline
    specified site —see Neoplasm, malignant,
      by site
    unspecified site
      female C56.9
      male C62.90
  Pott's puffy —see Osteomyelitis, specified NEC
  Rathke's pouch D44.3
  retinal anlage —see Neoplasm, benign, by site
  salivary gland type, mixed —see Neoplasm,
    salivary gland, benign
    malignant —see Neoplasm, salivary gland,
      malignant
  Sampson's N80.1
  Schmincke's —see Neoplasm, nasopharynx,
    malignant
  sclerosing stromal D27-●
  sebaceous —see Cyst, sebaceous
  secondary —see Neoplasm, secondary, by site
    carcinoid C7B.00
      bone C7B.03
      distant lymph nodes C7B.01
      liver C7B.02
      peritoneum C7B.04
      specified NEC C7B.09
    neuroendocrine NEC C7B.8
  serous of low malignant potential
    specified site —see Neoplasm, malignant,
      by site
    unspecified site C56.9
  Sertoli cell —see Neoplasm, benign, by site
    with lipid storage
      specified site —see Neoplasm, benign,
        by site
      unspecified site
        female D27.9
        male D29.20
    specified site —see Neoplasm, benign, by
      site
    unspecified site
      female D27.9
      male D29.20

Tumor (Continued)
  Sertoli-Leydig cell —see Neoplasm, benign,
    by site
    specified site —see Neoplasm, benign, by
      site
    unspecified site
      female D27.9
      male D29.20
  sex cord(-stromal) —see Neoplasm, uncertain
    behavior, by site
    with annular tubules D39.1-●
  skin appendage —see Neoplasm, skin,
    benign
  smooth muscle —see Neoplasm, connective
    tissue, uncertain behavior
  soft tissue
    benign —see Neoplasm, connective tissue,
      benign
    malignant —see Neoplasm, connective
      tissue, malignant
  sternomastoid (congenital) Q68.0
  stromal
    endometrial D39.0
    gastric D48.1
      benign D21.4
      malignant C16.9
      uncertain behavior D48.1
    gastrointestinal C49.A-●
      benign D21.4
      esophagus C49.A1
      large intestine C49.A4
      malignant C49.A0
        colon C49.A4
        duodenum C49.A3
        esophagus C49.A1
        ileum C49.A3
        jejunum C49.A3
        Meckel diverticulum C49.A3
        large intestine C49.A4
        omentum C49.A9
        peritoneum C49.A9
        rectum C49.A5
        small intestine C49.A3
        specified site NEC C49.A9
        stomach C49.A2
      ~~large intestine C49.A4~~
      rectum C49.A5
      small intestine C49.A3
      specified site NEC C49.A9
      stomach C49.A2
      uncertain behavior D48.1
    intestine
      benign D21.4
      malignant
        large C49.A4
        small C49.A3
      uncertain behavior D48.1
    ovarian D39.1-●
    stomach C49.A2
      benign D21.4
      malignant C49.A2
      uncertain behavior D48.1
  sweat gland —see also Neoplasm, skin,
    uncertain behavior
    benign —see Neoplasm, skin, benign
    malignant —see Neoplasm, skin, malignant
  syphilitic, brain A52.17
  testicular D40.10
  testicular stromal D40.1-●
  theca cell D27.-●
  theca cell-granulosa cell D39.1-●
  Triton, malignant —see Neoplasm, nerve,
    malignant
  trophoblastic, placental site D39.2
  turban D23.4
  uterus (body), in pregnancy or childbirth —
    see Pregnancy, complicated by, tumor,
    uterus
  vagina, in pregnancy or childbirth —see
    Pregnancy, complicated by
  varicose —see Varix

Tumor (Continued)
  von Recklinghausen's —see
    Neurofibromatosis
  vulva or perineum, in pregnancy or
    childbirth —see Pregnancy, complicated
    by
    causing obstructed labor O65.5
  Warthin's —see Neoplasm, salivary gland,
    benign
  Wilms' C64-●
  yolk sac —see Neoplasm, malignant, by site
    specified site —see Neoplasm, malignant,
      by site
    unspecified site
      female C56.9
      male C62.90
Tumor lysis syndrome (following
  antineoplastic chemotherapy)
  (spontaneous) NEC E88.3
Tumorlet —see Neoplasm, uncertain behavior,
  by site
Tungiasis B88.1
Tunica vasculosa lentis Q12.2
Turban tumor D23.4
Türck's trachoma J37.0
Turner-Kieser syndrome Q87.2
Turner-like syndrome Q87.1
Turner's
  hypoplasia (tooth) K00.4
  syndrome Q96.9
    specified NEC Q96.8
  tooth K00.4
Turner-Ullrich syndrome Q96.9
Tussis convulsiva —see Whooping cough
Twiddler's syndrome (due to)
  automatic implantable defibrillator T82.198
  cardiac pacemaker T82.198
Twilight state
  epileptic F05
  psychogenic F44.89
Twin (newborn) —see also Newborn, twin
  conjoined Q89.4
  pregnancy —see Pregnancy, twin
Twinning, teeth K00.2
Twist, twisted
  bowel, colon or intestine K56.2
  hair (congenital) Q84.1
  mesentery K56.2
  omentum K56.2
  organ or site, congenital NEC —see Anomaly,
    by site
  ovarian pedicle —see Torsion, ovary
Twitching R25.3
Tylosis (acquired) L84
  buccalis K13.29
  linguae K13.29
  palmaris et plantaris (congenital) (inherited)
    Q82.8
    acquired L85.1
Tympanism R14.0
Tympanites (abdominal) (intestinal) R14.0
Tympanitis —see Myringitis
Tympanosclerosis —see subcategory H74.0
Tympanum —see condition
Tympany
  abdomen R14.0
  chest R09.89
Type A behavior pattern Z73.1
Typhlitis —see Appendicitis
Typhoenteritis —see Typhoid
Typhoid (abortive) (ambulant) (any site)
  (clinical) (fever) (hemorrhagic) (infection)
  (intermittent) (malignant) (rheumatic)
  (Widal negative) A01.00
  with pneumonia A01.03
  abdominal A01.09
  arthritis A01.04
  carrier (suspected) of Z22.0
  cholecystitis (current) A01.09
  endocarditis A01.02
  heart involvement A01.02

▶ New   ⇒ Revised   ~~deleted~~ Deleted   ● Use Additional Character(s)

Typhoid *(Continued)*
    inoculation reaction —*see* Complications,
       vaccination
    meningitis A01.01
    mesenteric lymph nodes A01.09
    myocarditis A01.02
    osteomyelitis A01.05
    perichondritis, larynx A01.09
    pneumonia A01.03
    specified NEC A01.09
    spine A01.05
    ulcer (perforating) A01.09
Typhomalaria (fever) —*see* Malaria
Typhomania A01.00
Typhoperitonitis A01.09
Typhus (fever) A75.9
    abdominal, abdominalis —*see* Typhoid
    African tick A77.1
    amarillic A95.9
    brain A75.9 *[G94]*

Typhus *(Continued)*
    cerebral A75.9 *[G94]*
    classical A75.0
    due to Rickettsia
       prowazekii A75.0
         recrudescent A75.1
       tsutsugamushi A75.3
       typhi A75.2
    endemic (flea-borne) A75.2
    epidemic (louse-borne) A75.0
    exanthematic NEC A75.0
    exanthematicus SAI A75.0
       brillii SAI A75.1
       mexicanus SAI A75.2
       typhus murinus A75.2
    flea-borne A75.2
    India tick A77.1
    Kenya (tick) A77.1
    louse-borne A75.0
    Mexican A75.2

Typhus *(Continued)*
    mite-borne A75.3
    murine A75.2
    North Asian tick-borne A77.2
    petechial A75.9
    Queensland tick A77.3
    rat A75.2
    recrudescent A75.1
    recurrens —*see* Fever, relapsing
    Sao Paulo A77.0
    scrub (China) (India) (Malaysia) (New
       Guinea) A75.3
    shop (of Malaysia) A75.2
    Siberian tick A77.2
    tick-borne A77.9
    tropical (mite-borne) A75.3
Tyrosinemia E70.21
    newborn, transitory P74.5
Tyrosinosis E70.21
Tyrosinuria E70.29

U

Uhl's anomaly or disease Q24.8
Ulcer, ulcerated, ulcerating, ulceration, ulcerative
 alveolar process M27.3
 amebic (intestine) A06.1
  skin A06.7
 anastomotic —see Ulcer, gastrojejunal
 anorectal K62.6
 antral —see Ulcer, stomach
 anus (sphincter) (solitary) K62.6
 aorta —see Aneurysm
 aphthous (oral) (recurrent) K12.0
  genital organ(s)
   female N76.6
   male N50.89
 artery I77.2
 atrophic —see Ulcer, skin
  decubitus —see Ulcer, pressure, by site
 back L98.429
  with
   ▶bone involvement without evidence of
    necrosis L98.426
   bone necrosis L98.424
   exposed fat layer L98.422
   ▶muscle involvement without evidence of
    necrosis L98.425
   muscle necrosis L98.423
   skin breakdown only L98.421
   ▶specified severity NEC L98.428
 Barrett's (esophagus) K22.10
  with bleeding K22.11
 bile duct (common) (hepatic) K83.8
 bladder (solitary) (sphincter) NEC N32.89
  bilharzial B65.9 [N33]
  in schistosomiasis (bilharzial) B65.9 [N33]
  submucosal —see Cystitis, interstitial
  tuberculous A18.12
 bleeding K27.4
 bone —see Osteomyelitis, specified type NEC
 bowel —see Ulcer, intestine
 breast N61.1
 bronchus J98.09
 buccal (cavity) (traumatic) K12.1
 Buruli A31.1
 buttock L98.419
  with
   ▶bone involvement without evidence of
    necrosis L98.416
   bone necrosis L98.414
   exposed fat layer L98.412
   ▶muscle involvement without evidence of
    necrosis L98.415
   muscle necrosis L98.413
   skin breakdown only L98.411
   ▶specified severity NEC L98.418
 cancerous —see Neoplasm, malignant, by site
 cardia K22.10
  with bleeding K22.11
 cardioesophageal (peptic) K22.10
  with bleeding K22.11
 cecum —see Ulcer, intestine
 cervix (uteri) (decubitus) (trophic) N86
  with cervicitis N72
 chancroidal A57
 chiclero B55.1
 chronic (cause unknown) —see Ulcer, skin
 Cochin-China B55.1
 colon —see Ulcer, intestine
 conjunctiva H10.89
 cornea H16.00-•
  with hypopyon H16.03-•
  central H16.01-•
  dendritic (herpes simplex) B00.52
  marginal H16.04-•
  Mooren's H16.05-•
  mycotic H16.06-•
  perforated H16.07-•
  ring H16.02-•
  tuberculous (phlyctenular) A18.52

Ulcer, ulcerated, ulcerating, ulceration, ulcerative (Continued)
 corpus cavernosum (chronic) N48.5
 crural —see Ulcer, lower limb
 Curling's —see Ulcer, peptic, acute
 Cushing's —see Ulcer, peptic, acute
 cystic duct K82.8
 cystitis (interstitial) —see Cystitis, interstitial
 decubitus —see Ulcer, pressure, by site
 dendritic, cornea (herpes simplex) B00.52
 diabetes, diabetic —see Diabetes, ulcer
 Dieulafoy's K25.0
 due to
  infection NEC —see Ulcer, skin
  radiation NEC L59.8
  trophic disturbance (any region) —see
   Ulcer, skin
  X-ray L58.1
 duodenum, duodenal (eroded) (peptic) K26.9
  with
   hemorrhage K26.4
    and perforation K26.6
   perforation K26.5
  acute K26.3
   with
    hemorrhage K26.0
     and perforation K26.2
    perforation K26.1
  chronic K26.7
   with
    hemorrhage K26.4
     and perforation K26.6
    perforation K26.5
 dysenteric A09
 elusive —see Cystitis, interstitial
 endocarditis (acute) (chronic) (subacute) I28.8
 epiglottis J38.7
 esophagus (peptic) K22.10
  with bleeding K22.11
  due to
   aspirin K22.10
    with bleeding K22.11
   gastrointestinal reflux disease K21.0
   ingestion of chemical or medicament
    K22.10
    with bleeding K22.11
   fungal K22.10
    with bleeding K22.11
   infective K22.10
    with bleeding K22.11
  varicose —see Varix, esophagus
 eyelid (region) H01.8
 fauces J39.2
 Fenwick (-Hunner) (solitary) —see Cystitis,
  interstitial
 fistulous —see Ulcer, skin
 foot (indolent) (trophic) —see Ulcer, lower
  limb
 frambesial, initial A66.0
 frenum (tongue) K14.0
 gallbladder or duct K82.8
 gangrenous —see Gangrene
 gastric —see Ulcer, stomach
 gastrocolic —see Ulcer, gastrojejunal
 gastroduodenal —see Ulcer, peptic
 gastroesophageal —see Ulcer, stomach
 gastrointestinal —see Ulcer, gastrojejunal
 gastrojejunal (peptic) K28.9
  with
   hemorrhage K28.4
    and perforation K28.6
   perforation K28.5
  acute K28.3
   with
    hemorrhage K28.0
     and perforation K28.2
    perforation K28.1
  chronic K28.7
   with
    hemorrhage K28.4
     and perforation K28.6
    perforation K28.5

Ulcer, ulcerated, ulcerating, ulceration, ulcerative (Continued)
 gastrojejunocolic —see Ulcer,
  gastrojejunal
 gingiva K06.8
 gingivitis K05.10
  nonplaque induced K05.11
  plaque induced K05.10
 glottis J38.7
 granuloma of pudenda A58
 gum K06.8
 gumma, due to yaws A66.4
 heel —see Ulcer, lower limb
 hemorrhoid —see also Hemorrhoids, by
  degree K64.8
 Hunner's —see Cystitis, interstitial
 hypopharynx J39.2
 hypopyon (chronic) (subacute) —see Ulcer,
  cornea, with hypopyon
 hypostaticum —see Ulcer, varicose
 ileum —see Ulcer, intestine
 intestine, intestinal K63.3
  with perforation K63.1
  amebic A06.1
  duodenal —see Ulcer, duodenum
  granulocytopenic (with hemorrhage) —see
   Neutropenia
  marginal —see Ulcer, gastrojejunal
  perforating K63.1
   newborn P78.0
  primary, small intestine K63.3
  rectum K62.6
  stercoraceous, stercoral K63.3
  tuberculous A18.32
  typhoid (fever) —see Typhoid
  varicose I86.8
 jejunum, jejunal —see Ulcer, gastrojejunal
 keratitis —see Ulcer, cornea
 knee —see Ulcer, lower limb
 labium (majus) (minus) N76.6
 laryngitis —see Laryngitis
 larynx (aphthous) (contact) J38.7
  diphtheritic A36.2
 leg —see Ulcer, lower limb
 lip K13.0
 Lipschütz's N76.6
 lower limb (atrophic) (chronic) (neurogenic)
  (perforating) (pyogenic) (trophic)
  (tropical) L97.909
  with
   ▶bone involvement without evidence of
    necrosis L97.906
   bone necrosis L97.904
   exposed fat layer L97.902
   ▶muscle involvement without evidence of
    necrosis L97.905
   muscle necrosis L97.903
   skin breakdown only L97.901
   ▶specified severity NEC L97.908
  ankle L97.309
   with
    ▶bone involvement without evidence of
     necrosis L97.306
    bone necrosis L97.304
    exposed fat layer L97.302
    ▶muscle involvement without evidence
     of necrosis L97.305
    muscle necrosis L97.303
    skin breakdown only L97.301
    ▶specified severity NEC L97.308
  left L97.329
   with
    ▶bone involvement without evidence
     of necrosis L97.326
    bone necrosis L97.324
    exposed fat layer L97.322
    ▶muscle involvement without
     evidence of necrosis L97.325
    muscle necrosis L97.323
    skin breakdown only L97.321
    ▶specified severity NEC L97.328

▶ New   ⇒ Revised   ~~deleted~~ Deleted   • Use Additional Character(s)

Ulcer, ulcerated, ulcerating, ulceration, ulcerative *(Continued)*
  lower limb *(Continued)*
    ankle *(Continued)*
      right L97.319
        with
          bone involvement without evidence of necrosis L97.316
          bone necrosis L97.314
          exposed fat layer L97.312
          muscle involvement without evidence of necrosis L97.315
          muscle necrosis L97.313
          skin breakdown only L97.311
          specified severity NEC L97.318
      calf L97.209
        with
          bone involvement without evidence of necrosis L97.206
          bone necrosis L97.204
          exposed fat layer L97.202
          muscle involvement without evidence of necrosis L97.205
          muscle necrosis L97.203
          skin breakdown only L97.201
          specified severity NEC L97.208
      left L97.229
        with
          bone involvement without evidence of necrosis L97.226
          bone necrosis L97.224
          exposed fat layer L97.222
          muscle involvement without evidence of necrosis L97.225
          muscle necrosis L97.223
          skin breakdown only L97.221
          specified severity NEC L97.228
      right L97.219
        with
          bone involvement without evidence of necrosis L97.216
          bone necrosis L97.214
          exposed fat layer L97.212
          muscle involvement without evidence of necrosis L97.215
          muscle necrosis L97.213
          skin breakdown only L97.211
          specified severity NEC L97.218
    decubitus —*see* Ulcer, pressure, by site
    foot specified NEC L97.509
      with
        bone involvement without evidence of necrosis L97.506
        bone necrosis L97.504
        exposed fat layer L97.502
        muscle involvement without evidence of necrosis L97.505
        muscle necrosis L97.503
        skin breakdown only L97.501
        specified severity NEC L97.508
      left L97.529
        with
          bone involvement without evidence of necrosis L97.526
          bone necrosis L97.524
          exposed fat layer L97.522
          muscle involvement without evidence of necrosis L97.525
          muscle necrosis L97.523
          skin breakdown only L97.521
          specified severity NEC L97.528
      right L97.519
        with
          bone involvement without evidence of necrosis L97.516
          bone necrosis L97.514
          exposed fat layer L97.512
          muscle involvement without evidence of necrosis L97.515
          muscle necrosis L97.513
          skin breakdown only L97.511
          specified severity NEC L97.518

Ulcer, ulcerated, ulcerating, ulceration, ulcerative *(Continued)*
  lower limb *(Continued)*
    heel L97.409
      with
        bone involvement without evidence of necrosis L97.406
        bone necrosis L97.404
        exposed fat layer L97.402
        muscle involvement without evidence of necrosis L97.405
        muscle necrosis L97.403
        skin breakdown only L97.401
        specified severity NEC L97.408
      left L97.429
        with
          bone involvement without evidence of necrosis L97.426
          bone necrosis L97.424
          exposed fat layer L97.422
          muscle involvement without evidence of necrosis L97.425
          muscle necrosis L97.423
          skin breakdown only L97.421
          specified severity NEC L97.428
      right L97.419
        with
          bone involvement without evidence of necrosis L97.416
          bone necrosis L97.414
          exposed fat layer L97.412
          muscle involvement without evidence of necrosis L97.415
          muscle necrosis L97.413
          skin breakdown only L97.411
          specified severity NEC L97.418
    left L97.929
      with
        bone involvement without evidence of necrosis L97.926
        bone necrosis L97.924
        exposed fat layer L97.922
        muscle involvement without evidence of necrosis L97.925
        muscle necrosis L97.923
        skin breakdown only L97.921
        specified severity NEC L97.928
    lower leg NOS L97.909
      with
        bone involvement without evidence of necrosis L97.906
        bone necrosis L97.904
        exposed fat layer L97.902
        muscle involvement without evidence of necrosis L97.905
        muscle necrosis L97.903
        skin breakdown only L97.901
        specified severity NEC L97.908
      left L97.929
        with
          bone involvement without evidence of necrosis L97.926
          bone necrosis L97.924
          exposed fat layer L97.922
          muscle involvement without evidence of necrosis L97.925
          muscle necrosis L97.923
          skin breakdown only L97.921
          specified severity NEC L97.928
      right L97.919
        with
          bone involvement without evidence of necrosis L97.916
          bone necrosis L97.914
          exposed fat layer L97.912
          muscle involvement without evidence of necrosis L97.915
          muscle necrosis L97.913
          skin breakdown only L97.911
          specified severity NEC L97.918
      specified site NEC L97.809

Ulcer, ulcerated, ulcerating, ulceration, ulcerative *(Continued)*
  lower limb *(Continued)*
    lower leg NOS *(Continued)*
      specified site NEC *(Continued)*
        with
          bone involvement without evidence of necrosis L97.806
          bone necrosis L97.804
          exposed fat layer L97.802
          muscle involvement without evidence of necrosis L97.805
          muscle necrosis L97.803
          skin breakdown only L97.801
          specified severity NEC L97.808
        left L97.829
          with
            bone involvement without evidence of necrosis L97.826
            bone necrosis L97.824
            exposed fat layer L97.822
            muscle involvement without evidence of necrosis L97.825
            muscle necrosis L97.823
            skin breakdown only L97.821
            specified severity NEC L97.828
        right L97.819
          with
            bone involvement without evidence of necrosis L97.816
            bone necrosis L97.814
            exposed fat layer L97.812
            muscle involvement without evidence of necrosis L97.815
            muscle necrosis L97.813
            skin breakdown only L97.811
            specified severity NEC L97.818
    midfoot L97.409
      with
        bone involvement without evidence of necrosis L97.406
        bone necrosis L97.404
        exposed fat layer L97.402
        muscle involvement without evidence of necrosis L97.405
        muscle necrosis L97.403
        skin breakdown only L97.401
        specified severity NEC L97.408
      left L97.429
        with
          bone involvement without evidence of necrosis L97.426
          bone necrosis L97.424
          exposed fat layer L97.422
          muscle involvement without evidence of necrosis L97.425
          muscle necrosis L97.423
          skin breakdown only L97.421
          specified severity NEC L97.428
      right L97.419
        with
          bone involvement without evidence of necrosis L97.416
          bone necrosis L97.414
          exposed fat layer L97.412
          muscle involvement without evidence of necrosis L97.415
          muscle necrosis L97.413
          skin breakdown only L97.411
          specified severity NEC L97.418
      right L97.919
        with
          bone involvement without evidence of necrosis L97.916
          bone necrosis L97.914
          exposed fat layer L97.912
          muscle involvement without evidence of necrosis L97.915
          muscle necrosis L97.913
          skin breakdown only L97.911
          specified severity NEC L97.918

▶ New   ⇒ Revised   ~~deleted~~ Deleted   ● Use Additional Character(s)

Ulcer, ulcerated, ulcerating, ulceration, ulcerative *(Continued)*
 lower limb *(Continued)*
  thigh L97.109
   with
    ▶bone involvement without evidence of necrosis L97.106
    bone necrosis L97.104
    exposed fat layer L97.102
    ▶muscle involvement without evidence of necrosis L97.105
    muscle necrosis L97.103
    skin breakdown only L97.101
    ▶specified severity NEC L97.108
   left L97.129
    with
     ▶bone involvement without evidence of necrosis L97.126
     bone necrosis L97.124
     exposed fat layer L97.122
     ▶muscle involvement without evidence of necrosis L97.125
     muscle necrosis L97.123
     skin breakdown only L97.121
     ▶specified severity NEC L97.128
   right L97.119
    with
     ▶bone involvement without evidence of necrosis L97.116
     bone necrosis L97.114
     exposed fat layer L97.112
     ▶muscle involvement without evidence of necrosis L97.115
     muscle necrosis L97.113
     skin breakdown only L97.111
     ▶specified severity NEC L97.118
  toe L97.509
   with
    ▶bone involvement without evidence of necrosis L97.506
    bone necrosis L97.504
    exposed fat layer L97.502
    ▶muscle involvement without evidence of necrosis L97.505
    muscle necrosis L97.503
    skin breakdown only L97.501
    ▶specified severity NEC L97.508
   left L97.529
    with
     ▶bone involvement without evidence of necrosis L97.526
     bone necrosis L97.524
     exposed fat layer L97.522
     ▶muscle involvement without evidence of necrosis L97.525
     muscle necrosis L97.523
     skin breakdown only L97.521
     ▶specified severity NEC L97.528
   right L97.519
    with
     ▶bone involvement without evidence of necrosis L97.516
     bone necrosis L97.514
     exposed fat layer L97.512
     ▶muscle involvement without evidence of necrosis L97.515
     muscle necrosis L97.513
     skin breakdown only L97.511
     ▶specified severity NEC L97.518
 leprous A30.1
 syphilitic A52.19
 varicose —*see* Varix, leg, with, ulcer
luetic —*see* Ulcer, syphilitic
lung J98.4
 tuberculous —*see* Tuberculosis, pulmonary
malignant —*see* Neoplasm, malignant, by site
marginal NEC —*see* Ulcer, gastrojejunal
meatus (urinarius) N34.2
Meckel's diverticulum Q43.0
 malignant —*see* Table of Neoplasms, small intestine, malignant

Ulcer, ulcerated, ulcerating, ulceration, ulcerative *(Continued)*
Meleney's (chronic undermining) —*see* Ulcer, skin
Mooren's (cornea) —*see* Ulcer, cornea, Mooren's
mycobacterial (skin) A31.1
nasopharynx J39.2
neck, uterus N86
neurogenic NEC —*see* Ulcer, skin
nose, nasal (passage) (infective) (septum) J34.0
 skin —*see* Ulcer, skin
 spirochetal A69.8
 varicose (bleeding) I86.8
oral mucosa (traumatic) K12.1
palate (soft) K12.1
penis (chronic) N48.5
peptic (site unspecified) K27.9
 with
  hemorrhage K27.4
   and perforation K27.6
  perforation K27.5
 acute K27.3
  with
   hemorrhage K27.0
    and perforation K27.2
   perforation K27.1
 chronic K27.7
  with
   hemorrhage K27.4
    and perforation K27.6
   perforation K27.5
 esophagus K22.10
  with bleeding K22.11
 newborn P78.82
perforating K27.5
 skin —*see* Ulcer, skin
peritonsillar J35.8
phagedenic (tropical) —*see* Ulcer, skin
pharynx J39.2
phlebitis —*see* Phlebitis
plaster —*see* Ulcer, pressure, by site
popliteal space —*see* Ulcer, lower limb
postpyloric —*see* Ulcer, duodenum
prepuce N47.7
prepyloric —*see* Ulcer, stomach
pressure (pressure area) L89.9-●
 ankle L89.5-●
 back L89.1-●
 buttock L89.3-●
 coccyx L89.15-●
 contiguous site of back, buttock, hip L89.4-●
 elbow L89.0-●
 face L89.81-●
 head L89.81-●
 heel L89.6-●
 hip L89.2-●
 sacral region (tailbone) L89.15-●
 specified site NEC L89.89-●
 stage 1 (healing) (pre-ulcer skin changes limited to persistent focal edema)
  ankle L89.5-●
  back L89.1-●
  buttock L89.3-●
  coccyx L89.15-●
  contiguous site of back, buttock, hip L89.4-●
  elbow L89.0-●
  face L89.81-●
  head L89.81-●
  heel L89.6-●
  hip L89.2-●
  sacral region (tailbone) L89.15-●
  specified site NEC L89.89-●
 stage 2 (healing) (abrasion, blister, partial thickness skin loss involving epidermis and/or dermis)
  ankle L89.5-●
  back L89.1-●
  buttock L89.3-●

Ulcer, ulcerated, ulcerating, ulceration, ulcerative *(Continued)*
 pressure *(Continued)*
  stage 2 *(Continued)*
   coccyx L89.15-●
   contiguous site of back, buttock, hip L89.4-●
   elbow L89.0-●
   face L89.81-●
   head L89.81-●
   heel L89.6-●
   hip L89.2-●
   sacral region (tailbone) L89.15-●
   specified site NEC L89.89-●
  stage 3 (healing) (full thickness skin loss involving damage or necrosis of subcutaneous tissue)
   ankle L89.5-●
   back L89.1-●
   buttock L89.3-●
   coccyx L89.15-●
   contiguous site of back, buttock, hip L89.4-●
   elbow L89.0-●
   face L89.81-●
   head L89.81-●
   heel L89.6-●
   hip L89.2-●
   sacral region (tailbone) L89.15-●
   specified site NEC L89.89-●
  stage 4 (healing) (necrosis of soft tissues through to underlying muscle, tendon, or bone)
   ankle L89.5-●
   back L89.1-●
   buttock L89.3-●
   coccyx L89.15-●
   contiguous site of back, buttock, hip L89.4-●
   elbow L89.0-●
   face L89.81-●
   head L89.81-●
   heel L89.6-●
   hip L89.2-●
   sacral region (tailbone) L89.15-●
   specified site NEC L89.89-●
  unspecified stage
   ankle L89.5-●
   back L89.1-●
   buttock L89.3-●
   coccyx L89.15-●
   contiguous site of back, buttock, hip L89.4-●
   elbow L89.0-●
   face L89.81-●
   head L89.81-●
   heel L89.6-●
   hip L89.2-●
   sacral region (tailbone) L89.15-●
   specified site NEC L89.89-●
  unstageable
   ankle L89.5-●
   back L89.1-●
   buttock L89.3-●
   coccyx L89.15-●
   contiguous site of back, buttock, hip L89.4-●
   elbow L89.0-●
   face L89.81-●
   head L89.81-●
   heel L89.6-●
   hip L89.2-●
   sacral region (tailbone) L89.15-●
   specified site NEC L89.89-●
 primary of intestine K63.3
  with perforation K63.1
 prostate N41.9
 pyloric —*see* Ulcer, stomach
 rectosigmoid K63.3
  with perforation K63.1
 rectum (sphincter) (solitary) K62.6
  stercoraceous, stercoral K62.6

▶ New ⇒ Revised ~~deleted~~ Deleted ● Use Additional Character(s)

Ulcer, ulcerated, ulcerating, ulceration, ulcerative (Continued)
  retina —see Inflammation, chorioretinal
  rodent —see also Neoplasm, skin, malignant
  sclera —see Scleritis
  scrofulous (tuberculous) A18.2
  scrotum N50.89
    tuberculous A18.15
    varicose I86.1
  seminal vesicle N50.89
  sigmoid —see Ulcer, intestine
  skin (atrophic) (chronic) (neurogenic) (non-healing) (perforating) (pyogenic) (trophic) (tropical) L98.499
    with gangrene —see Gangrene
    amebic A06.7
    back —see Ulcer, back
    buttock —see Ulcer, buttock
    decubitus —see Ulcer, pressure
    lower limb —see Ulcer, lower limb
    mycobacterial A31.1
    specified site NEC L98.499
      with
        ▶bone involvement without evidence of necrosis L98.496
        bone necrosis L98.494
        exposed fat layer L98.492
        ▶muscle involvement without evidence of necrosis L98.495
        muscle necrosis L98.493
        skin breakdown only L98.491
        ▶specified severity NEC L98.498
    tuberculous (primary) A18.4
    varicose —see Ulcer, varicose
  sloughing —see Ulcer, skin
  solitary, anus or rectum (sphincter) K62.6
  sore throat J02.9
    streptococcal J02.0
  spermatic cord N50.89
  spine (tuberculous) A18.01
  stasis (venous) —see Varix, leg, with, ulcer
    without varicose veins I87.2
  stercoraceous, stercoral K63.3
    with perforation K63.1
    anus or rectum K62.6
  stoma, stomal —see Ulcer, gastrojejunal
  stomach (eroded) (peptic) (round) K25.9
    with
      hemorrhage K25.4
        and perforation K25.6
      perforation K25.5
    acute K25.3
      with
        hemorrhage K25.0
          and perforation K25.2
        perforation K25.1
    chronic K25.7
      with
        hemorrhage K25.4
          and perforation K25.6
        perforation K25.5
  stomal —see Ulcer, gastrojejunal
  stomatitis K12.1
  stress —see Ulcer, peptic
  strumous (tuberculous) A18.2
  submucosal, bladder —see Cystitis, interstitial
  syphilitic (any site) (early) (secondary) A51.39
    late A52.79
    perforating A52.79
      foot A52.11
  testis N50.89
  thigh —see Ulcer, lower limb
  throat J39.2
    diphtheritic A36.0
  toe —see Ulcer, lower limb
  tongue (traumatic) K14.0
  tonsil J35.8
    diphtheritic A36.0
  trachea J39.8
  trophic —see Ulcer, skin

Ulcer, ulcerated, ulcerating, ulceration, ulcerative (Continued)
  tropical —see Ulcer, skin
  tuberculous —see Tuberculosis, ulcer
  tunica vaginalis N50.89
  turbinate J34.89
  typhoid (perforating) —see Typhoid
  unspecified site —see Ulcer, skin
  urethra (meatus) —see Urethritis
  uterus N85.8
    cervix N86
      with cervicitis N72
    neck N86
      with cervicitis N72
  vagina N76.5
    in Behçet's disease M35.2 [N77.0]
    pessary N89.8
  valve, heart I33.0
  varicose (lower limb, any part) —see also Varix, leg, with, ulcer
    broad ligament I86.2
    esophagus —see Varix, esophagus
    inflamed or infected —see Varix, leg, with ulcer, with inflammation
    nasal septum I86.8
    perineum I86.3
    scrotum I86.1
    specified site NEC I86.8
    sublingual I86.0
    vulva I86.3
  vas deferens N50.89
  vulva (acute) (infectional) N76.6
    in (due to)
      Behçet's disease M35.2 [N77.0]
      herpesviral (herpes simplex) infection A60.04
      tuberculosis A18.18
  vulvobuccal, recurring N76.6
  X-ray L58.1
  yaws A66.4
Ulcerosa scarlatina A38.8
Ulcus —see also Ulcer
  cutis tuberculosum A18.4
  duodeni —see Ulcer, duodenum
  durum (syphilitic) A51.0
    extragenital A51.2
  gastrojejunale —see Ulcer, gastrojejunal
  hypostaticum —see Ulcer, varicose
  molle (cutis) (skin) A57
  serpens corneae —see Ulcer, cornea, central
  ventriculi —see Ulcer, stomach
Ulegyria Q04.8
Ulerythema
  ophryogenes, congenital Q84.2
  sycosiforme L73.8
Ullrich(-Bonnevie)(-Turner) syndrome —see also Turner's syndrome Q87.1
Ullrich-Feichtiger syndrome Q87.0
Ulnar —see condition
Ulorrhagia, ulorrhea K06.8
Umbilicus, umbilical —see condition
Unacceptable
  contours of tooth K08.54
  morphology of tooth K08.54
Unavailability (of)
  bed at medical facility Z75.1
  health service-related agencies Z75.4
  medical facilities (at) Z75.3
    due to
      investigation by social service agency Z75.2
      lack of services at home Z75.0
      remoteness from facility Z75.3
      waiting list Z75.1
      home Z75.0
      outpatient clinic Z75.3
    schooling Z55.1
    social service agencies Z75.4
Uncinaria americana infestation B76.1
Uncinariasis B76.9
Uncongenial work Z56.5

Unconscious (ness) —see Coma
Underachievement in school Z55.3
Underdevelopment —see also Undeveloped
  nose Q30.1
  sexual E30.0
Underdosing —see also Table of Drugs and Chemicals, categories T36-T50, with final character 6 Z91.14
  intentional NEC Z91.128
    due to financial hardship of patient Z91.120
  unintentional NEC Z91.138
    due to patient's age related debility Z91.130
Underfeeding, newborn P92.3
Underfill, endodontic M27.53
Underimmunization status Z28.3
Undernourishment —see Malnutrition
Undernutrition —see Malnutrition
Under observation —see Observation
Underweight R63.6
  for gestational age —see Light for dates
Underwood's disease P83.0
Undescended —see also Malposition, congenital
  cecum Q43.3
  colon Q43.3
  testicle —see Cryptorchid
Undeveloped, undevelopment —see also Hypoplasia
  brain (congenital) Q02
  cerebral (congenital) Q02
  heart Q24.8
  lung Q33.6
  testis E29.1
  uterus E30.0
Undiagnosed (disease) R69
Undulant fever —see Brucellosis
Unemployment, anxiety concerning Z56.0
  threatened Z56.2
Unequal length (acquired) (limb) —see also Deformity, limb, unequal length
  leg —see also Deformity, limb, unequal length
    congenital Q72.9-●
Unextracted dental root K08.3
Unguis incarnatus L60.0
Unhappiness R45.2
Unicornate uterus Q51.4
  ▶in pregnancy or childbirth O34.00
Unilateral —see also condition
  development, breast N64.89
  organ or site, congenital NEC —see Agenesis, by site
Unilocular heart Q20.8
Union, abnormal —see also Fusion
  larynx and trachea Q34.8
Universal mesentery Q43.3
Unrepairable overhanging of dental restorative materials K08.52
Unsatisfactory
  restoration of tooth K08.50
    specified NEC K08.59
  sample of cytologic smear
    anus R85.615
    cervix R87.615
    vagina R87.625
  surroundings Z59.1
  work Z56.5
Unsoundness of mind —see Psychosis
Unstable
  back NEC —see Instability, joint, spine
  hip (congenital) Q65.6
    acquired —see Derangement, joint, specified type NEC, hip
  joint —see Instability, joint
    secondary to removal of joint prosthesis M96.89
  lie (mother) O32.0
  lumbosacral joint (congenital)
    acquired —see subcategory M53.2
  sacroiliac —see subcategory M53.2
  spine NEC —see Instability, joint, spine
Unsteadiness on feet R26.81

Untruthfulness, child problem F91.8
Unverricht(-Lundborg) disease or epilepsy —
    see Epilepsy, generalized, idiopathic
Unwanted pregnancy Z64.0
Upbringing, institutional Z62.22
    away from parents NEC Z62.29
    in care of non-parental family member Z62.21
    in foster care Z62.21
    in orphanage or group home Z62.22
    in welfare custody Z62.21
Upper respiratory —see condition
Upset
    gastric K30
    gastrointestinal K30
        psychogenic F45.8
    intestinal (large) (small) K59.9
        psychogenic F45.8
    menstruation N93.9
    mental F48.9
    stomach K30
        psychogenic F45.8
Urachus —see also condition
    patent or persistent Q64.4
Urbach-Oppenheim disease (necrobiosis
        lipoidica diabeticorum) —see E08-E13 with
        .620
Urbach's lipoid proteinosis E78.89
Urbach-Wiethe disease E78.89
Urban yellow fever A95.1
Urea
    blood, high —see Uremia
    cycle metabolism disorder —see Disorder,
        urea cycle metabolism
Uremia, uremic N19
    with
        ectopic or molar pregnancy O08.4
        polyneuropathy N18.9 [G63]
    ~~chronic —see also Disease, kidney, chronic~~
        ~~N18.9~~
            ~~due to hypertension —see Hypertensive,~~
            ~~kidney~~
    ▶chronic NOS —see also Disease, kidney,
        chronic N18.9
            ▶due to hypertension —see Hypertensive,
            kidney
    complicating
        ectopic or molar pregnancy O08.4
    congenital P96.0
    extrarenal R39.2
    following ectopic or molar pregnancy O08.4
    newborn P96.0
    prerenal R39.2
Ureter, ureteral —see condition
Ureteralgia N23
Ureterectasis —see Hydroureter
Ureteritis N28.89
    cystica N28.86
    due to calculus N20.1
        with calculus, kidney N20.2
            with hydronephrosis N13.2
    gonococcal (acute) (chronic) A54.21
    nonspecific N28.89
Ureterocele N28.89
    congenital (orthotopic) Q62.31
        ectopic Q62.32
Ureterolith, ureterolithiasis —see Calculus,
    ureter
Ureterostomy
    attention to Z43.6
    status Z93.6
Urethra, urethral —see condition
Urethralgia R39.89
Urethritis (anterior) (posterior) N34.2
    calculous N21.1
    candidal B37.41
    chlamydial A56.01
    diplococcal (gonococcal) A54.01
        with abscess (accessory gland)
            (periurethral) A54.1
    gonococcal A54.01
        with abscess (accessory gland)
            (periurethral) A54.1

Urethritis (Continued)
    nongonococcal N34.1
        Reiter's —see Reiter's disease
    nonspecific N34.1
    nonvenereal N34.1
    postmenopausal N34.2
    puerperal O86.22
    Reiter's —see Reiter's disease
    specified NEC N34.2
    trichomonal or due to Trichomonas
        (vaginalis) A59.03
Urethrocele N81.0
    with
        cystocele —see Cystocele
        prolapse of uterus —see Prolapse, uterus
Urethrolithiasis (with colic or infection) N21.1
Urethrorectal —see condition
Urethrorrhagia N36.8
Urethrorrhea R36.9
Urethrostomy
    attention to Z43.6
    status Z93.6
Urethrotrigonitis —see Trigonitis
Urethrovaginal —see condition
Urgency
    fecal R15.2
    hypertensive —see Hypertension
    urinary N39.15
Urhidrosis, uridrosis L74.8
Uric acid in blood (increased) E79.0
Uricacidemia (asymptomatic) E79.0
Uricemia (asymptomatic) E79.0
Uricosuria R82.99
Urinary —see condition
Urination
    frequent R35.0
    painful R30.9
Urine
    blood in —see Hematuria
    discharge, excessive R35.8
    enuresis, nonorganic origin F98.0
    extravasation R39.0
    frequency R35.0
    incontinence R32
        nonorganic origin F98.0
    intermittent stream R39.198
    pus in N39.0
    retention or stasis R33.9
        organic R33.8
            drug-induced R33.0
        psychogenic F45.8
    secretion
        deficient R34
        excessive R35.8
        frequency R35.0
    stream
        intermittent R39.198
        slowing R39.198
        splitting R39.13
        weak R39.12
Urinemia —see Uremia
Urinoma, urethra N36.8
Uroarthritis, infectious (Reiter's) —see Reiter's
    disease
Urodialysis R34
Urolithiasis —see Calculus, urinary
Uronephrosis —see Hydronephrosis
Uropathy N39.9
    obstructive N13.9
        specified NEC N13.8
    reflux N13.9
        specified NEC N13.8
    vesicoureteral reflux-associated —see Reflux,
        vesicoureteral
Urosepsis — code to condition
Urticaria L50.9
    with angioneurotic edema T78.3
        hereditary D84.1
    allergic L50.0
    cholinergic L50.5
    chronic L50.8

Urticaria (Continued)
    cold, familial L50.2
    contact L50.6
    dermatographic L50.3
    due to
        cold or heat L50.2
        drugs L50.0
        food L50.0
        inhalants L50.0
        plants L50.6
        serum —see also Reaction, serum T80.69
    factitial L50.3
    familial cold M04.2
    giant T78.3
        hereditary D84.1
    gigantea T78.3
    idiopathic L50.1
    larynx T78.3
        hereditary D84.1
    ⇒neonatorum P83.88
    nonallergic L50.1
    papulosa (Hebra) L28.2
    ⇒pigmentosa D47.01
        ▶congenital Q82.2
        ▶of neonatal onset Q82.2
        ▶of newborn onset Q82.2
    recurrent periodic L50.8
    serum —see also Reaction, serum T80.69
    solar L56.3
    specified type NEC L50.8
    thermal (cold) (heat) L50.2
    vibratory L50.4
    ⇒xanthelasmoidea —see Urticaria pigmentosa
Use (of)
    alcohol Z72.89
        with
            intoxication F10.929
            sleep disorder F10.982
        harmful —see Abuse, alcohol
    amphetamines —see Use, stimulant NEC
    caffeine —see Use, stimulant NEC
    cannabis F12.90
        with
            anxiety disorder F12.980
            intoxication F12.929
                with
                    delirium F12.921
                    perceptual disturbance F12.922
                uncomplicated F12.920
            other specified disorder F12.988
            psychosis F12.959
                delusions F12.950
                hallucinations F12.951
            unspecified disorder F12.99
    cocaine F14.90
        with
            anxiety disorder F14.980
            intoxication F14.929
                with
                    delirium F14.921
                    perceptual disturbance F14.922
                uncomplicated F14.920
            other specified disorder F14.988
            psychosis F14.959
                delusions F14.950
                hallucinations F14.951
            sexual dysfunction F14.981
            sleep disorder F14.982
            unspecified disorder F14.99
        harmful —see Abuse, drug, cocaine
    drug(s) NEC F19.90
        with sleep disorder F19.982
        harmful —see Abuse, drug, by type
    hallucinogen NEC F16.90
        with
            anxiety disorder F16.980
            intoxication F16.929
                with
                    delirium F16.921
                uncomplicated F16.920
            mood disorder F16.94
            other specified disorder F16.988

▶ New   ⇒ Revised   ~~deleted~~ Deleted   ● Use Additional Character(s)

Use *(Continued)*
  hallucinogen NEC *(Continued)*
    with *(Continued)*
      perception disorder (flashbacks) F16.983
      psychosis F16.959
        delusions F16.950
        hallucinations F16.951
      unspecified disorder F16.99
    harmful —*see* Abuse, drug, hallucinogen NEC
  inhalants F18.90
    with
      anxiety disorder F18.980
      intoxication F18.929
        with delirium F18.921
        uncomplicated F18.920
      mood disorder F18.94
      other specified disorder F18.988
      persisting dementia F18.97
      psychosis F18.959
        delusions F18.950
        hallucinations F18.951
      unspecified disorder F18.99
    harmful —*see* Abuse, drug, inhalant
  methadone —*see* Use, opioid
  nonprescribed drugs F19.90
    harmful —*see* Abuse, non-psychoactive substance
  opioid F11.90
    with
      disorder F11.99
        mood F11.94
        sleep F11.982
        specified type NEC F11.988
      intoxication F11.929
        with
          delirium F11.921
          perceptual disturbance F11.922
        uncomplicated F11.920
      withdrawal F11.93
    harmful —*see* Abuse, drug, opioid
  patent medicines F19.90
    harmful —*see* Abuse, non-psychoactive substance
  psychoactive drug NEC F19.90
    with
      anxiety disorder F19.980
      intoxication F19.929
        with
          delirium F19.921
          perceptual disturbance F19.922
        uncomplicated F19.920

Use *(Continued)*
  psychoactive drug NEC *(Continued)*
    with *(Continued)*
      mood disorder F19.94
      other specified disorder F19.988
      persisting
        amnestic disorder F19.96
        dementia F19.97
      psychosis F19.959
        delusions F19.950
        hallucinations F19.951
      sexual dysfunction F19.981
      sleep disorder F19.982
      unspecified disorder F19.99
      withdrawal F19.939
        with
          delirium F19.931
          perceptual disturbance F19.932
        uncomplicated F19.930
    harmful —*see* Abuse, drug NEC, psychoactive NEC
  sedative, hypnotic, or anxiolytic F13.90
    with
      anxiety disorder F13.980
      intoxication F13.929
        with
          delirium F13.921
        uncomplicated F13.920
      other specified disorder F13.988
      persisting
        amnestic disorder F13.96
        dementia F13.97
      psychosis F13.959
        delusions F13.950
        hallucinations F13.951
      sexual dysfunction F13.981
      sleep disorder F13.982
      unspecified disorder F13.99
    harmful —*see* Abuse, drug, sedative, hypnotic, or anxiolytic
  stimulant NEC F15.90
    with
      anxiety disorder F15.980
      intoxication F15.929
        with
          delirium F15.921
          perceptual disturbance F15.922
        uncomplicated F15.920
      mood disorder F15.94
      other specified disorder F15.988

Use *(Continued)*
  stimulant NEC *(Continued)*
    with *(Continued)*
      psychosis F15.959
        delusions F15.950
        hallucinations F15.951
      sexual dysfunction F15.981
      sleep disorder F15.982
      unspecified disorder F15.99
      withdrawal F15.93
    harmful —*see* Abuse, drug, stimulant NEC
  tobacco Z72.0
    with dependence —*see* Dependence, drug, nicotine
  volatile solvents —*see also* Use, inhalant F18.90
    harmful —*see* Abuse, drug, inhalant
Usher-Senear disease or syndrome L10.4
Uta B55.1
Uteromegaly N85.2
Uterovaginal —*see* condition
Uterovesical —*see* condition
Uveal —*see* condition
Uveitis (anterior) —*see also* Iridocyclitis
  acute —*see* Iridocyclitis, acute
  chronic —*see* Iridocyclitis, chronic
  due to toxoplasmosis (acquired) B58.09
    congenital P37.1
  granulomatous —*see* Iridocyclitis, chronic
  heterochromic —*see* Cyclitis, Fuchs' heterochromic
  lens-induced —*see* Iridocyclitis, lens-induced
  posterior —*see* Chorioretinitis
  sympathetic H44.13-●
  syphilitic (secondary) A51.43
    congenital (early) A50.01
    late A52.71
  tuberculous A18.54
Uveoencephalitis —*see* Inflammation, chorioretinal
Uveokeratitis —*see* Iridocyclitis
Uveoparotitis D86.89
Uvula —*see* condition
Uvulitis (acute) (catarrhal) (chronic) (membranous) (suppurative) (ulcerative) K12.2

V

Vaccination (prophylactic)
  complication or reaction —see Complications, vaccination
  delayed Z28.9
  encounter for Z23
  not done —see Immunization, not done, because (of)
Vaccinia (generalized) (localized) T88.1
  without vaccination B08.011
  congenital P35.8
Vacuum, in sinus (accessory) (nasal) J34.89
Vagabond, vagabondage Z59.0
Vagabond's disease B85.1
Vagina, vaginal —see condition
Vaginalitis (tunica) (testis) N49.1
Vaginismus (reflex) N94.2
  functional F52.5
  nonorganic F52.5
  psychogenic F52.5
  secondary N94.2
Vaginitis (acute) (circumscribed) (diffuse) (emphysematous) (nonvenereal) (ulcerative) N76.0
  with ectopic or molar pregnancy O08.0
  amebic A06.82
  atrophic, postmenopausal N95.2
  bacterial N76.0
  blennorrhagic (gonococcal) A54.02
  candidal B37.3
  chlamydial A56.02
  chronic N76.1
  due to Trichomonas (vaginalis) A59.01
  following ectopic or molar pregnancy O08.0
  gonococcal A54.02
    with abscess (accessory gland) (periurethral) A54.1
  granuloma A58
  in (due to)
    candidiasis B37.3
    herpesviral (herpes simplex) infection A60.04
    pinworm infection B80 [N77.1]
  monilial B37.3
  mycotic (candidal) B37.3
  postmenopausal atrophic N95.2
  puerperal (postpartum) O86.13
  senile (atrophic) N95.2
  subacute or chronic N76.1
  syphilitic (early) A51.0
    late A52.76
  trichomonal A59.01
  tuberculous A18.18
Vaginosis —see Vaginitis
Vagotonia G52.2
Vagrancy Z59.0
VAIN —see Neoplasia, intraepithelial, vagina
Vallecula —see condition
Valley fever B38.0
Valsuani's disease —see Anemia, obstetric
Valve, valvular (formation) —see also condition
  cerebral ventricle (communicating) in situ Z98.2
  cervix, internal os Q51.828
  congenital NEC —see Atresia, by site
  ureter (pelvic junction) (vesical orifice) Q62.39
  urethra (congenital) (posterior) Q64.2
Valvulitis (chronic) —see Endocarditis
Valvulopathy —see Endocarditis
Van Bogaert's leukoencephalopathy (sclerosing) (subacute) A81.1
Van Bogaert-Scherer-Epstein disease or syndrome E75.5
Van Buchem's syndrome M85.2
Van Creveld-von Gierke disease E74.01
Van der Hoeve (-de Kleyn) syndrome Q78.0
Van der Woude's syndrome Q38.0
Van Neck's disease or osteochondrosis M91.0
Vanishing lung J44.9

Vapor asphyxia or suffocation T59.9
  specified agent —see Table of Drugs and Chemicals
Variance, lethal ball, prosthetic heart valve T82.09
Variants, thalassemic D56.8
Variations in hair color L67.1
Varicella B01.9
  with
    complications NEC B01.89
    encephalitis B01.11
    encephalomyelitis B01.11
    meningitis B01.0
    myelitis B01.12
    pneumonia B01.2
  congenital P35.8
Varices —see Varix
Varicocele (scrotum) (thrombosed) I86.1
  ovary I86.2
  perineum I86.3
  spermatic cord (ulcerated) I86.1
Varicose
  aneurysm (ruptured) I77.0
  dermatitis —see Varix, leg, with, inflammation
  eczema —see Varix, leg, with, inflammation
  phlebitis —see Varix, with, inflammation
  tumor —see Varix
  ulcer (lower limb, any part) —see also Varix, leg, with, ulcer
    anus —see also Hemorrhoids K64.8
    esophagus —see Varix, esophagus
    inflamed or infected —see Varix, leg, with ulcer, with inflammation
    nasal septum I86.8
    perineum I86.3
    scrotum I86.1
    specified site NEC I86.8
  vein —see Varix
  vessel —see Varix, leg
Varicosis, varicosities, varicosity —see Varix
Variola (major) (minor) B03
Varioloid B03
Varix (lower limb) (ruptured) I83.90
  with
    edema I83.899
    inflammation I83.10
      with ulcer (venous) I83.209
    pain I83.819
    specified complication NEC I83.899
    stasis dermatitis I83.10
      with ulcer (venous) I83.209
    swelling I83.899
    ulcer I83.009
      with inflammation I83.209
  aneurysmal I77.0
  asymptomatic I83.9-•
  bladder I86.2
  broad ligament I86.2
  complicating
    childbirth (lower extremity) O87.4
      anus or rectum O87.2
      genital (vagina, vulva or perineum) O87.8
    pregnancy (lower extremity) O22.0-•
      anus or rectum O22.4-•
      genital (vagina, vulva or perineum) O22.1-•
    puerperium (lower extremity) O87.4
      anus or rectum O87.2
      genital (vagina, vulva, perineum) O87.8
  congenital (any site) Q27.8
  esophagus (idiopathic) (primary) (ulcerated) I85.00
    bleeding I85.01
    congenital Q27.8
    in (due to)
      alcoholic liver disease I85.10
        bleeding I85.11
      cirrhosis of liver I85.10
        bleeding I85.11

Varix (Continued)
  esophagus (Continued)
    in (Continued)
      portal hypertension I85.10
        bleeding I85.11
      schistosomiasis I85.10
        bleeding I85.11
      toxic liver disease I85.10
        bleeding I85.11
    secondary I85.10
      bleeding I85.11
  gastric I86.4
  inflamed or infected I83.10
    ulcerated I83.209
  labia (majora) I86.3
  leg (asymptomatic) I83.90
    with
      edema I83.899
      inflammation I83.10
        with ulcer —see Varix, leg, with, ulcer, with inflammation by site
      pain I83.819
      specified complication NEC I83.899
      swelling I83.899
      ulcer I83.009
        with inflammation I83.209
        ankle I83.003
          with inflammation I83.203
        calf I83.002
          with inflammation I83.202
        foot NEC I83.005
          with inflammation I83.205
        heel I83.004
          with inflammation I83.204
        lower leg NEC I83.008
          with inflammation I83.208
        midfoot I83.004
          with inflammation I83.204
        thigh I83.001
          with inflammation I83.201
    bilateral (asymptomatic) I83.93
      with
        edema I83.893
        pain I83.813
        specified complication NEC I83.893
        swelling I83.893
        ulcer I83.0-•
          with inflammation I83.209
    left (asymptomatic) I83.92
      with
        edema I83.892
        inflammation I83.12
          with ulcer —see Varix, leg, with, ulcer, with inflammation by site
        pain I83.812
        specified complication NEC I83.892
        swelling I83.892
        ulcer I83.029
          with inflammation I83.229
          ankle I83.023
            with inflammation I83.223
          calf I83.022
            with inflammation I83.222
          foot NEC I83.025
            with inflammation I83.225
          heel I83.024
            with inflammation I83.224
          lower leg NEC I83.028
            with inflammation I83.228
          midfoot I83.024
            with inflammation I83.224
          thigh I83.021
            with inflammation I83.221
    right (asymptomatic) I83.91
      with
        edema I83.891
        inflammation I83.11
          with ulcer —see Varix, leg, with, ulcer, with inflammation by site

▶ New   ⟹ Revised   ~~deleted~~ Deleted   • Use Additional Character(s)

Varix *(Continued)*
  leg *(Continued)*
    right *(Continued)*
      with *(Continued)*
        pain I83.811
        specified complication NEC I83.891
        swelling I83.891
        ulcer I83.019
          with inflammation I83.219
          ankle I83.013
            with inflammation I83.213
          calf I83.012
            with inflammation I83.212
          foot NEC I83.015
            with inflammation I83.215
          heel I83.014
            with inflammation I83.214
          lower leg NEC I83.018
            with inflammation I83.218
          midfoot I83.014
            with inflammation I83.214
          thigh I83.011
            with inflammation I83.211
  nasal septum I86.8
  orbit I86.8
    congenital Q27.8
  ovary I86.2
  papillary I78.1
  pelvis I86.2
  perineum I86.3
  pharynx I86.8
  placenta O43.89-•
  renal papilla I86.8
  retina H35.09
  scrotum (ulcerated) I86.1
  sigmoid colon I86.8
  specified site NEC I86.8
  spinal (cord) (vessels) I86.8
  spleen, splenic (vein) (with phlebolith) I86.8
  stomach I86.4
  sublingual I86.0
  ulcerated I83.009
    inflamed or infected I83.209
  uterine ligament I86.2
  vagina I86.8
  vocal cord I86.8
  vulva I86.3
Vas deferens —*see* condition
Vas deferentitis N49.1
Vasa previa O69.4
  hemorrhage from, affecting newborn
    P50.0
Vascular —*see also* condition
  loop on optic papilla Q14.2
  spasm I73.9
  spider I78.1
Vascularization, cornea —*see*
  Neovascularization, cornea
Vasculitis I77.6
  allergic D69.0
  cryoglobulinemic D89.1
  disseminated I77.6
  hypocomplementemic M31.8
  kidney I77.89
  livedoid L95.0
  nodular L95.8
  retina H35.06-•
  rheumatic —*see* Fever, rheumatic
  rheumatoid —*see* Rheumatoid, vasculitis
  skin (limited to) L95.9
    specified NEC L95.8
▶ systemic M31.8
Vasculopathy, necrotizing M31.9
  cardiac allograft T86.290
  specified NEC M31.8
Vasitis (nodosa) N49.1
  tuberculous A18.15
Vasodilation I73.9
Vasomotor —*see* condition
Vasoplasty, after previous sterilization Z31.0
  aftercare Z31.42

Vasospasm (vasoconstriction) I73.9
  cerebral (cerebrovascular) (artery)
    I67.848
    reversible I67.841
  coronary I20.1
  nerve
    arm —*see* Mononeuropathy, upper limb
    brachial plexus G54.0
    cervical plexus G54.2
    leg —*see* Mononeuropathy, lower limb
  peripheral NOS I73.9
  retina (artery) —*see* Occlusion, artery,
    retina
Vasospastic —*see* condition
Vasovagal attack (paroxysmal) R55
  psychogenic F45.8
VATER syndrome Q87.2
Vater's ampulla —*see* condition
Vegetation, vegetative
  adenoid (nasal fossa) J35.8
  endocarditis (acute) (any valve) (subacute)
    I33.0
  heart (mycotic) (valve) I33.0
Veil
  Jackson's Q43.3
Vein, venous —*see* condition
Veldt sore —*see* Ulcer, skin
Velpeau's hernia —*see* Hernia, femoral
Venereal
  bubo A55
  disease A64
  granuloma inguinale A58
  lymphogranuloma (Durand-Nicolas-Favre)
    A55
Venofibrosis I87.8
Venom, venomous —*see* Table of Drugs and
  Chemicals, by animal or substance,
  poisoning
Venous —*see* condition
Ventilator lung, newborn P27.8
Ventral —*see* condition
Ventricle, ventricular —*see also* condition
  escape I49.3
  inversion Q20.5
Ventriculitis (cerebral) —*see also* Encephalitis
  G04.90
Ventriculostomy status Z98.2
Vernet's syndrome G52.7
Verneuil's disease (syphilitic bursitis) A52.78
Verruca (due to HPV) (filiformis) (simplex)
  (viral) (vulgaris) B07.9
  acuminata A63.0
  necrogenica (primary) (tuberculosa) A18.4
  plana B07.8
  plantaris B07.0
  seborrheica L82.1
    inflamed L82.0
  senile (seborrheic) L82.1
    inflamed L82.0
  tuberculosa (primary) A18.4
  venereal A63.0
Verrucosities —*see* Verruca
Verruga peruana, peruviana A44.1
Version
  with extraction
  cervix —*see* Malposition, uterus
  uterus (postinfectional) (postpartal, old) —*see*
    Malposition, uterus
Vertebra, vertebral —*see* condition
Vertical talus (congenital) Q66.80
  left foot Q66.82
  right foot Q66.81
Vertigo R42
  auditory —*see* Vertigo, aural
  aural H81.31-•
  benign paroxysmal (positional) H81.1-•
  central (origin) H81.4-•
  cerebral H81.4-•
  Dix and Hallpike (epidemic) —*see* Neuronitis,
    vestibular
  due to infrasound T75.23

Vertigo *(Continued)*
  epidemic A88.1
    Dix and Hallpike —*see* Neuronitis,
      vestibular
    Pedersen's —*see* Neuronitis, vestibular
    vestibular neuronitis —*see* Neuronitis,
      vestibular
  hysterical F44.89
  infrasound T75.23
  labyrinthine —*see* subcategory H81.0
  laryngeal R05
  malignant positional H81.4-•
  Ménière's —*see* subcategory H81.40
  menopausal N95.11
  otogenic —*see* Vertigo, aural
  paroxysmal positional, benign —*see* Vertigo,
    benign paroxysmal
  Pedersen's (epidemic) —*see* Neuronitis,
    vestibular
  peripheral NEC H81.39-•
  positional
    benign paroxysmal —*see* Vertigo, benign
      paroxysmal
    malignant H81.4-•
Very-low-density-lipoprotein-type (VLDL)
  hyperlipoproteinemia E78.1
Vesania —*see* Psychosis
Vesical —*see* condition
Vesicle
  cutaneous R23.8
  seminal —*see* condition
  skin R23.8
Vesicocolic —*see* condition
Vesicoperineal —*see* condition
Vesicorectal —*see* condition
Vesicourethrorectal —*see* condition
Vesicovaginal —*see* condition
Vesicular —*see* condition
Vesiculitis (seminal) N49.0
  amebic A06.82
  gonorrheal (acute) (chronic) A54.23
  trichomonal A59.09
  tuberculous A18.15
Vestibulitis (ear) —*see also* subcategory H83.0
  nose (external) J34.89
  vulvar N94.810
Vestibulopathy, acute peripheral (recurrent) —
  see Neuronitis, vestibular
Vestige, vestigial —*see also* Persistence
  branchial Q18.0
  structures in vitreous Q14.0
Vibration
  adverse effects T75.20
    pneumatic hammer syndrome T75.21
    specified effect NEC T75.29
    vasospastic syndrome T75.22
    vertigo from infrasound T75.23
  exposure (occupational) Z57.7
  vertigo T75.23
Vibriosis A28.9
Victim (of)
  crime Z65.4
  disaster Z65.5
  terrorism Z65.4
  torture Z65.4
  war Z65.5
Vidal's disease L28.0
Villaret's syndrome G52.7
Villous —*see* condition
VIN —*see* Neoplasia, intraepithelial, vulva
Vincent's infection (angina) (gingivitis) A69.1
  stomatitis NEC A69.1
Vinson-Plummer syndrome D50.1
Violence, physical R45.6
Viosterol deficiency —*see* Deficiency, calciferol
Vipoma —*see* Neoplasm, malignant, by site
Viremia B34.9
Virilism (adrenal) E25.9
  congenital E25.0
Virilization (female) (suprarenal) E25.9
  congenital E25.0
  isosexual E28.2

Virulent bubo A57
Virus, viral —*see also* condition
  as cause of disease classified elsewhere
    B97.89
  cytomegalovirus B25.9
  human immunodeficiency (HIV) —*see*
    Human, immunodeficiency virus (HIV)
    disease
  infection —*see* Infection, virus
  specified NEC B34.8
  swine influenza (viruses that normally cause
    infections in pigs) —*see also* Influenza,
    due to, identified novel influenza A virus
    J09.X2
  West Nile (fever) A92.30
    with
      complications NEC A92.39
      cranial nerve disorders A92.32
      encephalitis A92.31
      encephalomyelitis A92.31
      neurologic manifestation NEC A92.32
      optic neuritis A92.32
      polyradiculitis A92.32
Viscera, visceral —*see* condition
Visceroptosis K63.4
Visible peristalsis R19.2
Vision, visual
  binocular, suppression H53.34
  blurred, blurring H53.8
    hysterical F44.6
  defect, defective NEC H54.7
  disorientation (syndrome) H53.8
  disturbance H53.9
    hysterical F44.6
  double H53.2
  examination Z01.00
    with abnormal findings Z01.01
  field, limitation (defect) —*see* Defect, visual
    field
  hallucinations R44.1
  halos H53.19
  loss —*see* Loss, vision
    sudden —*see* Disturbance, vision,
      subjective, loss, sudden
  low (both eyes) —*see* Low, vision
  perception, simultaneous without fusion
    H53.33
Vitality, lack or want of R53.83
  newborn P96.89
Vitamin deficiency —*see* Deficiency, vitamin
Vitelline duct, persistent Q43.0
Vitiligo L80
  eyelid H02.739
    left H02.736
      lower H02.735
      upper H02.734
    right H02.733
      lower H02.732
      upper H02.731

Vitiligo (*Continued*)
  pinta A67.2
  vulva N90.89
Vitreal corneal syndrome H59.01-•
Vitreoretinopathy, proliferative —*see also*
  Retinopathy, proliferative
  with retinal detachment —*see* Detachment,
    retina, traction
Vitreous —*see also* condition
  touch syndrome —*see* Complication,
    postprocedural, following cataract
    surgery
Vocal cord —*see* condition
Vogt-Koyanagi syndrome H20.82-•
Vogt's disease or syndrome G80.3
Vogt-Spielmeyer amaurotic idiocy or disease
  E75.4
Voice
  change R49.9
    specified NEC R49.8
  loss —*see* Aphonia
Volhynian fever A79.0
Volkmann's ischemic contracture or paralysis
  (complicating trauma) T79.6
Volvulus (bowel) (colon) (intestine) K56.2
  with perforation K56.2
  congenital Q43.8
  duodenum K31.5
  fallopian tube —*see* Torsion, fallopian
    tube
  oviduct —*see* Torsion, fallopian tube
  stomach (due to absence of gastrocolic
    ligament) K31.89
Vomiting R11.10
  with nausea R11.2
  without nausea R11.11
  asphyxia —*see* Foreign body, by site, causing
    asphyxia, gastric contents
  bilious (cause unknown) R11.14
    following gastro-intestinal surgery
      K91.0
    in newborn P92.01
  blood —*see* Hematemesis
  causing asphyxia, choking, or suffocation —
    see Foreign body, by site
  cyclical G43.A0
    with refractory migraine G43.A1
    intractable G43.A1
    not intractable G43.A0
    psychogenic F50.89
    without refractory migraine G43.A0
  fecal mater R11.13
  following gastrointestinal surgery
    K91.0
    psychogenic F50.89
  functional K31.89
  hysterical F50.89

Vomiting (*Continued*)
  nervous F50.89
  neurotic F50.89
  newborn NEC P92.09
    bilious P92.01
  periodic R11.10
    psychogenic F50.89
  projectile R11.12
  psychogenic F50.89
  uremic —*see* Uremia
Vomito negro —*see* Fever, yellow
Von Bezold's abscess —*see* Mastoiditis,
  acute
Von Economo-Cruchet disease A85.8
Von Eulenburg's disease G71.19
Von Gierke's disease E74.01
Von Hippel (-Lindau) disease or syndrome
  Q85.8
Von Jaksch's anemia or disease D64.89
Von Recklinghausen
  disease (neurofibromatosis) Q85.01
    bones E21.0
Von Schroetter's syndrome I82.890
Von Willebrand (-Jurgens)(-Minot) disease or
  syndrome D68.0
Von Zumbusch's disease L40.1
Voyeurism F65.3
Vrolik's disease Q78.0
Vulva —*see* condition
Vulvismus N94.2
Vulvitis (acute) (allergic) (atrophic)
  (hypertrophic) (intertriginous) (senile)
  N76.2
  with ectopic or molar pregnancy O08.0
  adhesive, congenital Q52.79
  blennorrhagic (gonococcal) A54.02
  candidal B37.3
  chlamydial A56.02
  due to Haemophilus ducreyi A57
  following ectopic or molar pregnancy
    O08.0
  gonococcal A54.02
    with abscess (accessory gland)
      (periurethral) A54.1
  herpesviral A60.04
  leukoplakic N90.4
  monilial B37.3
  puerperal (postpartum) O86.19
  subacute or chronic N76.3
  syphilitic (early) A51.0
    late A52.76
  trichomonal A59.01
  tuberculous A18.18
Vulvodynia N94.819
  specified NEC N94.818
Vulvorectal —*see* condition
Vulvovaginitis (acute) —*see* Vaginitis

▶ New   ⇒ Revised   ~~deleted~~ Deleted   • Use Additional Character(s)

W

Waiting list, person on Z75.1
  for organ transplant Z76.82
  undergoing social agency investigation
      Z75.2
Waldenström
  hypergammaglobulinemia D89.0
  syndrome or macroglobulinemia
      C88.0
Waldenström-Kjellberg syndrome
      D50.1
Walking
  difficulty R26.2
    psychogenic F44.4
  sleep F51.3
    hysterical F44.89
Wall, abdominal —see condition
Wallenberg's disease or syndrome G46.3
Wallgren's disease I87.8
Wandering
  gallbladder, congenital Q44.1
  in diseases classified elsewhere Z91.83
  kidney, congenital Q63.8
  organ or site, congenital NEC —see
      Malposition, congenital, by site
  pacemaker (heart) I49.8
  spleen D73.89
War neurosis F48.8
Wart (due to HPV) (filiform) (infectious)
      (viral) B07.9
  anogenital region (venereal) A63.0
  common B07.8
  external genital organs (venereal)
      A63.0
  flat B07.8
  Hassal-Henle's (of cornea) H18.49
  Peruvian A44.1
  plantar B07.0
  prosector (tuberculous) A18.4
  seborrheic L82.1
    inflamed L82.0
  senile (seborrheic) L82.1
    inflamed L82.0
  tuberculous A18.4
  venereal A63.0
Warthin's tumor —see Neoplasm, salivary
      gland, benign
Wassilieff's disease A27.0
Wasting
  disease R64
    due to malnutrition E41
  extreme (due to malnutrition) E41
  muscle NEC —see Atrophy, muscle
Water
  clefts (senile cataract) —see Cataract, senile,
      incipient
  deprivation of T73.1
  intoxication E87.79
  itch B76.9
  lack of T73.1
  loading E87.70
  on
    brain —see Hydrocephalus
    chest J94.8
  poisoning E87.79
Waterbrash R12
Waterhouse(-Friderichsen) syndrome or
      disease (meningococcal) A39.1
Water-losing nephritis N25.89
Watermelon stomach K31.819
  with hemorrhage K31.811
  without hemorrhage K31.819
Watsoniasis B66.8
Wax in ear —see Impaction, cerumen
Weak, weakening, weakness (generalized)
      R53.1
  arches (acquired) —see also Deformity, limb,
      flat foot
  bladder (sphincter) R32

Weak, weakening, weakness (Continued)
  facial R29.810
    following
      cerebrovascular disease I69.992
        cerebral infarction I69.392
        intracerebral hemorrhage I69.192
        nontraumatic intracranial hemorrhage
            NEC I69.292
        specified disease NEC I69.892
        stroke I69.392
        subarachnoid hemorrhage I69.092
  foot (double) —see Weak, arches
  heart, cardiac —see Failure, heart
  mind F70
  muscle M62.81
  myocardium —see Failure, heart
  newborn P96.89
  pelvic fundus N81.89
  pubocervical tissue N81.82
  rectovaginal tissue N81.83
  senile R54
  urinary stream R39.12
  valvular —see Endocarditis
Wear, worn (with normal or routine use)
  articular bearing surface of internal joint
        prosthesis —see Complications, joint
        prosthesis, mechanical, wear of articular
        bearing surfaces, by site
  device, implant or graft —see Complications,
        by site, mechanical complication
  tooth, teeth (approximal) (hard tissues)
        (interproximal) (occlusal) K03.0
Weather, weathered
  effects of
    cold T69.9
      specified effect NEC T69.8
    hot —see Heat
  skin L57.8
Weaver's syndrome Q87.3
Web, webbed (congenital)
  duodenal Q43.8
  esophagus Q39.4
  fingers Q70.1
  larynx (glottic) (subglottic) Q31.0
  neck (pterygium colli) Q18.3
  Paterson-Kelly D50.1
  popliteal syndrome Q87.89
  toes Q70.3
Weber-Christian disease M35.6
Weber-Cockayne syndrome (epidermolysis
      bullosa) Q81.8
Weber-Gubler syndrome G46.3
Weber-Leyden syndrome G46.3
Weber-Osler syndrome I78.0
Weber's paralysis or syndrome G46.3
Wedge-shaped or wedging vertebra —see
      Collapse, vertebra NEC
Wegener's granulomatosis or syndrome
      M31.30
  with
    kidney involvement M31.31
    lung involvement M31.30
      with kidney involvement M31.31
Wegner's disease A50.02
Weight
  1000-2499 grams at birth (low) —see Low,
      birthweight
  999 grams or less at birth (extremely low) —
      see Low, birthweight, extreme
  and length below 10th percentile for
      gestational age P05.1-●
  below but length above 10th percentile for
      gestational age P05.0-●
  gain (abnormal) (excessive) R63.5
    in pregnancy —see Pregnancy, complicated
        by, excessive weight gain
    low —see Pregnancy, complicated by,
        insufficient, weight gain
  loss (abnormal) (cause unknown) R63.4
Weightlessness (effect of) T75.82

Weil (l)-Marchesani syndrome Q87.1
Weil's disease A27.0
Weingarten's syndrome J82
Weir Mitchell's disease I73.81
Weiss-Baker syndrome G90.09
Wells' disease L98.3
Wen —see Cyst, sebaceous
Wenckebach's block or phenomenon I44.1
Werdnig-Hoffmann syndrome (muscular
      atrophy) G12.0
Werlhof's disease D69.3
Werner-His disease A79.0
Werner's disease or syndrome E31.21
Werner's disease or syndrome E34.8
Wernicke-Korsakoff's syndrome or psychosis
      (alcoholic) F10.96
  with dependence F10.26
  drug-induced
    due to drug abuse —see Abuse, drug, by
        type, with amnestic disorder
    due to drug dependence —see
        Dependence, drug, by type, with
        amnestic disorder
  nonalcoholic F04
Wernicke-Posadas disease B38.9
Wernicke's
  developmental aphasia F80.2
  disease or syndrome E51.2
  encephalopathy E51.2
  polioencephalitis, superior E51.2
West African fever B50.8
Westphal-Strümpell syndrome E83.01
West's syndrome —see Epilepsy, spasms
Wet
  feet, tropical (maceration) (syndrome) —see
      Immersion, foot
  lung (syndrome), newborn P22.1
Wharton's duct —see condition
Wheal —see Urticaria
Wheezing R06.2
Whiplash injury S13.4
Whipple's disease —see also subcategory
      M14.8-● K90.81
Whipworm (disease) (infection) (infestation)
      B79
Whistling face Q87.0
White —see also condition
  kidney, small N03.9
  leg, puerperal, postpartum, childbirth O87.1
  mouth B37.0
  patches of mouth K13.29
  spot lesions, teeth
    chewing surface K02.51
    pit and fissure surface K02.51
    smooth surface K02.61
Whitehead L70.0
Whitlow —see also Cellulitis, digit
  with lymphangitis —see Lymphangitis, acute,
      digit
  herpesviral B00.89
Whitmore's disease or fever —see Melioidosis
Whooping cough A37.90
  with pneumonia A37.91
    due to Bordetella
      bronchiseptica A37.81
      parapertussis A37.11
      pertussis A37.01
      specified organism NEC A37.81
    due to
      Bordetella
        bronchiseptica A37.80
          with pneumonia A37.81
        parapertussis A37.10
          with pneumonia A37.11
        pertussis A37.00
          with pneumonia A37.01
        specified NEC A37.80
          with pneumonia A37.81
Wichman's asthma J38.5
Wide cranial sutures, newborn P96.3

Widening aorta —*see* Ectasia, aorta
  with aneurysm —*see* Aneurysm, aorta
Wilkie's disease or syndrome K55.1
Wilkinson-Sneddon disease or syndrome
  L13.1
Willebrand (-Jürgens) thrombopathy D68.0
Willige-Hunt disease or syndrome G23.1
Wilms' tumor C64-●
Wilson-Mikity syndrome P27.0
Wilson's
  disease or syndrome E83.01
  hepatolenticular degeneration E83.01
  lichen ruber L43.9
Window —*see also* Imperfect, closure
  aorticopulmonary Q21.4
Winter —*see* condition
Wiskott-Aldrich syndrome D82.0
Withdrawal state —*see also* Dependence, drug
  by type, with withdrawal
  alcohol
    with perceptual disturbances F10.232
    without perceptual disturbances
      F10.239
  caffeine F15.93
  cannabis F12.288
  newborn
    correct therapeutic substance properly
      administered P96.2
    infant of dependent mother P96.1
    therapeutic substance, neonatal P96.2
Witts' anemia D50.8
Witzelsucht F07.0
Woakes' ethmoiditis or syndrome J33.1
Wolff-Hirschhorn syndrome Q93.3
Wolff-Parkinson-White syndrome I45.6
Wolhynian fever A79.0
Wolman's disease E75.5
Wood lung or pneumonitis J67.8
Woolly, wooly hair (congenital) (nevus) Q84.1
Woolsorter's disease A22.1
Word
  blindness (congenital) (developmental)
    F81.0
  deafness (congenital) (developmental)
    H93.25
Worm(s) (infection) (infestation) —*see also*
  Infestation, helminth
  guinea B72
  in intestine NEC B82.0
Worm-eaten soles A66.3
Worn out —*see* Exhaustion
  cardiac
    defibrillator (with synchronous cardiac
      pacemaker) Z45.02
    pacemaker
      battery Z45.010
      lead Z45.018
  device, implant or graft —*see* Complications,
    by site, mechanical
Worried well Z71.1
Worries R45.82
▶Wound check Z48.0-●
  ▶due to injury - code to Injury, by site, using
    appropriate seventh character for
    subsequent encounter
⇒Wound, open T14.8-●
  abdomen, abdominal
    wall S31.109
      with penetration into peritoneal cavity
        S31.609
      bite —*see* Bite, abdomen, wall
      epigastric region S31.102
        with penetration into peritoneal cavity
          S31.602
        bite —*see* Bite, abdomen, wall,
          epigastric region
        laceration —*see* Laceration, abdomen,
          wall, epigastric region
        puncture —*see* Puncture, abdomen,
          wall, epigastric region

Wound, open *(Continued)*
  abdomen, abdominal *(Continued)*
    wall *(Continued)*
      laceration —*see* Laceration, abdomen, wall
      left
        lower quadrant S31.104
          with penetration into peritoneal
            cavity S31.604
          bite —*see* Bite, abdomen, wall, left,
            lower quadrant
          laceration —*see* Laceration, abdomen,
            wall, left, lower quadrant
          puncture —*see* Puncture, abdomen,
            wall, left, lower quadrant
        upper quadrant S31.101
          with penetration into peritoneal
            cavity S31.601
          bite —*see* Bite, abdomen, wall, left,
            upper quadrant
          laceration —*see* Laceration,
            abdomen, wall, left, upper
            quadrant
          puncture —*see* Puncture, abdomen,
            wall, left, upper quadrant
      periumbilic region S31.105
        with penetration into peritoneal cavity
          S31.605
        bite —*see* Bite, abdomen, wall,
          periumbilic region
        laceration —*see* Laceration, abdomen,
          wall, periumbilic region
        puncture —*see* Puncture, abdomen,
          wall, periumbilic region
      puncture —*see* Puncture, abdomen,
        wall
      right
        lower quadrant S31.103
          with penetration into peritoneal
            cavity S31.603
          bite —*see* Bite, abdomen, wall, right,
            lower quadrant
          laceration —*see* Laceration,
            abdomen, wall, right, lower
            quadrant
          puncture —*see* Puncture, abdomen,
            wall, right, lower quadrant
        upper quadrant S31.100
          with penetration into peritoneal
            cavity S31.600
          bite —*see* Bite, abdomen, wall, right,
            upper quadrant
          laceration —*see* Laceration,
            abdomen, wall, right, upper
            quadrant
          puncture —*see* Puncture, abdomen,
            wall, right, upper quadrant
    alveolar (process) —*see* Wound, open, oral
      cavity
  ankle S91.00-●
    bite —*see* Bite, ankle
    laceration —*see* Laceration, ankle
    puncture —*see* Puncture, ankle
  antecubital space —*see* Wound, open, elbow
  anterior chamber, eye —*see* Wound, open,
    ocular
  anus S31.839
    bite S31.835
    laceration —*see* Laceration, anus
    puncture —*see* Puncture, anus
  arm (upper) S41.10-●
    with amputation —*see* Amputation,
      traumatic, arm
    bite —*see* Bite, arm
    forearm —*see* Wound, open, forearm
    laceration —*see* Laceration, arm
    puncture —*see* Puncture, arm
  auditory canal (external) (meatus) —*see*
    Wound, open, ear
  auricle, ear —*see* Wound, open, ear
  axilla —*see* Wound, open, arm

Wound, open *(Continued)*
  back —*see also* Wound, open, thorax, back
    lower S31.000
      with penetration into retroperitoneal
        space S31.001
      bite —*see* Bite, back, lower
      laceration —*see* Laceration, back, lower
      puncture —*see* Puncture, back, lower
    bite —*see* Bite
  blood vessel —*see* Injury, blood vessel
  breast S21.00-●
    with amputation —*see* Amputation,
      traumatic, breast
    bite —*see* Bite, breast
    laceration —*see* Laceration, breast
    puncture —*see* Puncture, breast
  buttock S31.809
    bite —*see* Bite, buttock
    laceration —*see* Laceration, buttock
    left S31.829
    puncture —*see* Puncture, buttock
    right S31.819
  calf —*see* Wound, open, leg
  canaliculus lacrimalis —*see* Wound, open,
    eyelid
  canthus, eye —*see* Wound, open, eyelid
  cervical esophagus S11.20
    bite S11.25
    laceration —*see* Laceration, esophagus,
      traumatic, cervical
    puncture —*see* Puncture, cervical
      esophagus
  cheek (external) S01.40-●
    bite —*see* Bite, cheek
    internal —*see* Wound, open, oral cavity
    laceration —*see* Laceration, cheek
    puncture —*see* Puncture, cheek
  chest wall —*see* Wound, open, thorax
  chin —*see* Wound, open, head, specified site
    NEC
  choroid —*see* Wound, open, ocular
  ciliary body (eye) —*see* Wound, open,
    ocular
  clitoris S31.40
    with amputation —*see* Amputation,
      traumatic, clitoris
    bite S31.45
    laceration —*see* Laceration, vulva
    puncture —*see* Puncture, vulva
  conjunctiva —*see* Wound, open, ocular
  cornea —*see* Wound, open, ocular
  costal region —*see* Wound, open, thorax
  Descemet's membrane —*see* Wound, open,
    ocular
  digit(s)
    foot —*see* Wound, open, toe
    hand —*see* Wound, open, finger
  ear (canal) (external) S01.30-●
    with amputation —*see* Amputation,
      traumatic, ear
    bite —*see* Bite, ear
    drum S09.2-●
    laceration —*see* Laceration, ear
    puncture —*see* Puncture, ear
  elbow S51.00-●
    bite —*see* Bite, elbow
    laceration —*see* Laceration, elbow
    puncture —*see* Puncture, elbow
  epididymis —*see* Wound, open, testis
  epigastric region S31.102
    with penetration into peritoneal cavity
      S31.602
    bite —*see* Bite, abdomen, wall, epigastric
      region
    laceration —*see* Laceration, abdomen, wall,
      epigastric region
    puncture —*see* Puncture, abdomen, wall,
      epigastric region
  epiglottis —*see* Wound, open, neck, specified
    site NEC

▶ New   ⇒ Revised   ~~deleted~~ Deleted   ● Use Additional Character(s)

Wound, open *(Continued)*
  esophagus (thoracic) S27.819
    cervical —*see* Wound, open, cervical
      esophagus
    laceration S27.813
    specified type NEC S27.818
  eye —*see* Wound, open, ocular
  eyeball —*see* Wound, open, ocular
  eyebrow —*see* Wound, open, eyelid
  eyelid S01.10-●
    bite —*see* Bite, eyelid
    laceration —*see* Laceration, eyelid
    puncture —*see* Puncture, eyelid
  face NEC —*see* Wound, open, head, specified
    site NEC
  finger(s) S61.209
    with
      amputation —*see* Amputation,
        traumatic, finger
      damage to nail S61.309
    bite —*see* Bite, finger
    index S61.208
      with
        damage to nail S61.308
      left S61.201
        with
          damage to nail S61.301
      right S61.200
        with
          damage to nail S61.300
    laceration —*see* Laceration, finger
    little S61.208
      with
        damage to nail S61.308
      left S61.207
        with damage to nail S61.307
      right S61.206
        with damage to nail S61.306
    middle S61.208
      with
        damage to nail S61.308
      left S61.203
        with damage to nail S61.303
      right S61.202
        with damage to nail S61.302
    puncture —*see* Puncture, finger
    ring S61.208
      with
        damage to nail S61.308
      left S61.205
        with damage to nail S61.305
      right S61.204
        with damage to nail S61.304
  flank —*see* Wound, open, abdomen, wall
  foot (except toe(s) alone) S91.30-●
    with amputation —*see* Amputation,
      traumatic, foot
    bite —*see* Bite, foot
    laceration —*see* Laceration, foot
    puncture —*see* Puncture, foot
    toe —*see* Wound, open, toe
  forearm S51.80-●
    with
      amputation —*see* Amputation,
        traumatic, forearm
    bite —*see* Bite, forearm
    elbow only —*see* Wound, open, elbow
    laceration —*see* Laceration, forearm
    puncture —*see* Puncture, forearm
  forehead —*see* Wound, open, head, specified
    site NEC
  genital organs, external
    with amputation —*see* Amputation,
      traumatic, genital organs
    bite —*see* Bite, genital organ
    female S31.502
      vagina S31.40
      vulva S31.40
    laceration —*see* Laceration, genital
      organ

Wound, open *(Continued)*
  genital organs, external *(Continued)*
    male S31.501
      penis S31.20
      scrotum S31.30
      testes S31.30
    puncture —*see* Puncture, genital organ
  globe (eye) —*see* Wound, open, ocular
  groin —*see* Wound, open, abdomen, wall
  gum —*see* Wound, open, oral cavity
  hand S61.40-●
    with
      amputation —*see* Amputation,
        traumatic, hand
    bite —*see* Bite, hand
    finger(s) —*see* Wound, open, finger
    laceration —*see* Laceration, hand
    puncture —*see* Puncture, hand
    thumb —*see* Wound, open, thumb
  head S01.90
    bite —*see* Bite, head
    cheek —*see* Wound, open, cheek
    ear —*see* Wound, open, ear
    eyelid —*see* Wound, open, eyelid
    laceration —*see* Laceration, head
    lip —*see* Wound, open, lip
    nose S01.20
    oral cavity —*see* Wound, open, oral
      cavity
    puncture —*see* Puncture, head
    scalp —*see* Wound, open, scalp
    specified site NEC S01.80
    temporomandibular area —*see* Wound,
      open, cheek
  heel —*see* Wound, open, foot
  hip S71.00-●
    with amputation —*see* Amputation,
      traumatic, hip
    bite —*see* Bite, hip
    laceration —*see* Laceration, hip
    puncture —*see* Puncture, hip
  hymen S31.40
    bite —*see* Bite, vulva
    laceration —*see* Laceration, vagina
    puncture —*see* Puncture, vagina
  hypochondrium S31.109
    bite —*see* Bite, hypochondrium
    laceration —*see* Laceration,
      hypochondrium
    puncture —*see* Puncture, hypochondrium
  hypogastric region S31.109
    bite —*see* Bite, hypogastric region
    laceration —*see* Laceration, hypogastric
      region
    puncture —*see* Puncture, hypogastric
      region
  iliac (region) —*see* Wound, open, inguinal
    region
  inguinal region S31.109
    bite —*see* Bite, abdomen, wall, lower
      quadrant
    laceration —*see* Laceration, inguinal
      region
    puncture —*see* Puncture, inguinal
      region
  instep —*see* Wound, open, foot
  interscapular region —*see* Wound, open,
    thorax, back
  intraocular —*see* Wound, open, ocular
  iris —*see* Wound, open, ocular
  jaw —*see* Wound, open, head, specified site
    NEC
  knee S81.00-●
    bite —*see* Bite, knee
    laceration —*see* Laceration, knee
    puncture —*see* Puncture, knee
  labium (majus) (minus) —*see* Wound, open,
    vulva
  laceration —*see* Laceration, by site
  lacrimal duct —*see* Wound, open, eyelid

Wound, open *(Continued)*
  larynx S11.019
    bite —*see* Bite, larynx
    laceration —*see* Laceration, larynx
    puncture —*see* Puncture, larynx
  left
    lower quadrant S31.104
      with penetration into peritoneal cavity
        S31.604
      bite —*see* Bite, abdomen, wall, left, lower
        quadrant
      laceration —*see* Laceration, abdomen,
        wall, left, lower quadrant
      puncture —*see* Puncture, abdomen, wall,
        left, lower quadrant
    upper quadrant S31.101
      with penetration into peritoneal cavity
        S31.601
      bite —*see* Bite, abdomen, wall, left,
        upper quadrant
      laceration —*see* Laceration, abdomen,
        wall, left, upper quadrant
      puncture —*see* Puncture, abdomen, wall,
        left, upper quadrant
  leg (lower) S81.80-●
    with amputation —*see* Amputation,
      traumatic, leg
    ankle —*see* Wound, open, ankle
    bite —*see* Bite, leg
    foot —*see* Wound, open, foot
    knee —*see* Wound, open, knee
    laceration —*see* Laceration, leg
    puncture —*see* Puncture, leg
    toe —*see* Wound, open, toe
    upper —*see* Wound, open, thigh
  lip S01.501
    bite —*see* Bite, lip
    laceration —*see* Laceration, lip
    puncture —*see* Puncture, lip
  loin S31.109
    bite —*see* Bite, abdomen, wall
    laceration —*see* Laceration, loin
    puncture —*see* Puncture, loin
  lower back —*see* Wound, open, back,
    lower
  lumbar region —*see* Wound, open, back,
    lower
  malar region —*see* Wound, open, head,
    specified site NEC
  mammary —*see* Wound, open, breast
  mastoid region —*see* Wound, open, head,
    specified site NEC
  mouth —*see* Wound, open, oral cavity
  nail
    finger —*see* Wound, open, finger, with
      damage to nail
    toe —*see* Wound, open, toe, with damage
      to nail
  nape (neck) —*see* Wound, open, neck
  nasal (septum) (sinus) —*see* Wound, open,
    nose
  nasopharynx —*see* Wound, open, head,
    specified site NEC
  neck S11.90
    bite —*see* Bite, neck
    involving
      cervical esophagus S11.20
      larynx —*see* Wound, open, larynx
      pharynx S11.20
      thyroid S11.10
      trachea (cervical) S11.029
        bite —*see* Bite, trachea
        laceration S11.021
          with foreign body S11.022
        puncture S11.023
          with foreign body S11.024
    laceration —*see* Laceration, neck
    puncture —*see* Puncture, neck
    specified site NEC S11.80
      specified type NEC S11.89

▶ New   ⇒ Revised   ~~deleted~~ Deleted   ● Use Additional Character(s)

Wound, open *(Continued)*
nose (septum) (sinus) S01.20
   with amputation —*see* Amputation,
     traumatic, nose
   bite —*see* Bite, nose
   laceration —*see* Laceration, nose
   puncture —*see* Puncture, nose
ocular S05.90
   avulsion (traumatic enucleation) S05.7-●
   eyeball S05.6-●
     with foreign body S05.5-●
   eyelid —*see* Wound, open, eyelid
   laceration and rupture S05.3-●
     with prolapse or loss of intraocular
       tissue S05.2-●
   orbit (penetrating) (with or without foreign
     body) S05.4-●
   periocular area —*see* Wound, open, eyelid
   specified NEC S05.8X-●
oral cavity S01.502
   bite S01.552
   laceration —*see* Laceration, oral cavity
   puncture —*see* Puncture, oral cavity
orbit —*see* Wound, open, ocular, orbit
palate —*see* Wound, open, oral cavity
palm —*see* Wound, open, hand
pelvis, pelvic —*see also* Wound, open, back,
   lower
   girdle —*see* Wound, open, hip
penetrating —*see* Puncture, by site
penis S31.20
   with amputation —*see* Amputation,
     traumatic, penis
   bite S31.25
   laceration —*see* Laceration, penis
   puncture —*see* Puncture, penis
perineum
   bite —*see* Bite, perineum
   female S31.502
   laceration —*see* Laceration, perineum
   male S31.501
   puncture —*see* Puncture, perineum
periocular area (with or without lacrimal
   passages) —*see* Wound, open, eyelid
periumbilic region S31.105
   with penetration into peritoneal cavity
     S31.605
   bite —*see* Bite, abdomen, wall, periumbilic
     region
   laceration —*see* Laceration, abdomen, wall,
     periumbilic region
   puncture —*see* Puncture, abdomen, wall,
     periumbilic region
phalanges
   finger —*see* Wound, open, finger
   toe —*see* Wound, open, toe
pharynx S11.20
pinna —*see* Wound, open, ear
popliteal space —*see* Wound, open, knee
prepuce —*see* Wound, open, penis
pubic region —*see* Wound, open, back, lower
pudendum —*see* Wound, open, genital
   organs, external
puncture wound —*see* Puncture
rectovaginal septum —*see* Wound, open,
   vagina
right
   lower quadrant S31.103
     with penetration into peritoneal cavity
       S31.603
     bite —*see* Bite, abdomen, wall, right,
       lower quadrant
     laceration —*see* Laceration, abdomen,
       wall, right, lower quadrant
     puncture —*see* Puncture, abdomen, wall,
       right, lower quadrant
   upper quadrant S31.100
     with penetration into peritoneal cavity
       S31.600

Wound, open *(Continued)*
right *(Continued)*
   upper quadrant *(Continued)*
     bite —*see* Bite, abdomen, wall, right,
       upper quadrant
     laceration —*see* Laceration, abdomen,
       wall, right, upper quadrant
     puncture —*see* Puncture, abdomen, wall,
       right, upper quadrant
sacral region —*see* Wound, open, back, lower
sacroiliac region —*see* Wound, open, back,
   lower
salivary gland —*see* Wound, open, oral cavity
scalp S01.00
   bite S01.05
   laceration —*see* Laceration, scalp
   puncture —*see* Puncture, scalp
scalpel, newborn (birth injury) P15.8
scapular region —*see* Wound, open, shoulder
sclera —*see* Wound, open, ocular
scrotum S31.30
   with amputation —*see* Amputation,
     traumatic, scrotum
   bite S31.35
   laceration —*see* Laceration, scrotum
   puncture —*see* Puncture, scrotum
shin —*see* Wound, open, leg
shoulder S41.00-●
   with amputation —*see* Amputation,
     traumatic, arm
   bite —*see* Bite, shoulder
   laceration —*see* Laceration, shoulder
   puncture —*see* Puncture, shoulder
skin NOS T14.8
spermatic cord —*see* Wound, open, testis
sternal region —*see* Wound, open, thorax,
   front wall
submaxillary region —*see* Wound, open,
   head, specified site NEC
submental region —*see* Wound, open, head,
   specified site NEC
subungual
   finger(s) —*see* Wound, open, finger
   toe(s) —*see* Wound, open, toe
supraclavicular region —*see* Wound, open,
   neck, specified site NEC
temple, temporal region —*see* Wound, open,
   head, specified site NEC
temporomandibular area —*see* Wound, open,
   cheek
testis S31.30
   with amputation —*see* Amputation,
     traumatic, testes
   bite S31.35
   laceration —*see* Laceration, testis
   puncture —*see* Puncture, testis
thigh S71.10-●
   with amputation —*see* Amputation,
     traumatic, hip
   bite —*see* Bite, thigh
   laceration —*see* Laceration, thigh
   puncture —*see* Puncture, thigh
thorax, thoracic (wall) S21.90
   back S21.20-●
     with penetration S21.40
     bite —*see* Bite, thorax
   breast —*see* Wound, open, breast
   front S21.10-●
     with penetration S21.30
   laceration —*see* Laceration, thorax
   puncture —*see* Puncture, thorax
throat —*see* Wound, open, neck
thumb S61.009
   with
     amputation —*see* Amputation,
       traumatic, thumb
     damage to nail S61.109
   bite —*see* Bite, thumb
   laceration —*see* Laceration, thumb

Wound, open *(Continued)*
thumb *(Continued)*
   left S61.002
     with
       damage to nail S61.102
     puncture —*see* Puncture, thumb
   right S61.001
     with
       damage to nail S61.101
thyroid (gland) —*see* Wound, open, neck,
   thyroid
toe(s) S91.109
   with
     amputation —*see* Amputation,
       traumatic, toe
     damage to nail S91.209
   bite —*see* Bite, toe
   great S91.103
     with
       damage to nail S91.203
     left S91.102
       with
         damage to nail S91.202
     right S91.101
       with
         damage to nail S91.201
   laceration —*see* Laceration, toe
   lesser S91.106
     with
       damage to nail S91.206
     left S91.105
       with
         damage to nail S91.205
     right S91.104
       with
         damage to nail S91.204
   puncture —*see* Puncture, toe
tongue —*see* Wound, open, oral cavity
trachea (cervical region) —*see* Wound, open,
   neck, trachea
tunica vaginalis —*see* Wound, open, testis
tympanum, tympanic membrane S09.2-●
   laceration —*see* Laceration, ear, drum
   puncture —*see* Puncture, tympanum
umbilical region —*see* Wound, open,
   abdomen, wall, periumbilic region
uvula —*see* Wound, open, oral cavity
vagina S31.40
   bite S31.45
   laceration —*see* Laceration, vagina
   puncture —*see* Puncture, vagina
vitreous (humor) —*see* Wound, open, ocular
vocal cord S11.039
   bite —*see* Bite, vocal cord
   laceration S11.031
     with foreign body S11.032
   puncture S11.033
     with foreign body S11.034
vulva S31.40
   with amputation —*see* Amputation,
     traumatic, vulva
   bite S31.45
   laceration —*see* Laceration, vulva
   puncture —*see* Puncture, vulva
wrist S61.50-●
   bite —*see* Bite, wrist
   laceration —*see* Laceration, wrist
   puncture —*see* Puncture, wrist
Wound, superficial —*see* Injury (*see also*
   specified injury type)
Wright's syndrome G54.0
Wrist —*see* condition
Wrong drug (by accident) (given in error) —
   see Table of Drugs and Chemicals, by
   drug, poisoning
Wry neck —*see* Torticollis
Wuchereria (bancrofti) infestation B74.0
Wuchereriasis B74.0
Wuchernde Struma Langhans C73

▶ New   ⇒ Revised   ~~deleted~~ Deleted   ● Use Additional Character(s)

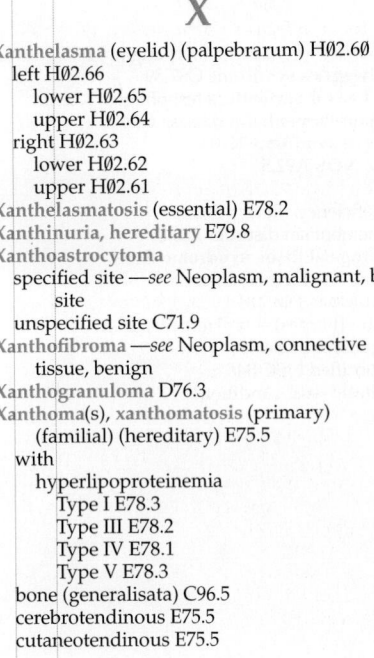

Xanthelasma (eyelid) (palpebrarum) H02.60
  left H02.66
    lower H02.65
    upper H02.64
  right H02.63
    lower H02.62
    upper H02.61
Xanthelasmatosis (essential) E78.2
Xanthinuria, hereditary E79.8
Xanthoastrocytoma
  specified site —*see* Neoplasm, malignant, by
    site
  unspecified site C71.9
Xanthofibroma —*see* Neoplasm, connective
  tissue, benign
Xanthogranuloma D76.3
Xanthoma(s), xanthomatosis (primary)
    (familial) (hereditary) E75.5
  with
    hyperlipoproteinemia
      Type I E78.3
      Type III E78.2
      Type IV E78.1
      Type V E78.3
  bone (generalisata) C96.5
  cerebrotendinous E75.5
  cutaneotendinous E75.5

Xanthoma(s), xanthomatosis *(Continued)*
  disseminatum (skin) E78.2
  eruptive E78.2
  hypercholesterinemic E78.00
  hypercholesterolemic E78.00
  hyperlipidemic E78.5
  joint E75.5
  multiple (skin) E78.2
  tendon (sheath) E75.5
  tuberosum E78.2
  tuberous E78.2
  tubo-eruptive E78.2
  verrucous, oral mucosa K13.4
Xanthosis R23.8
Xenophobia F40.10
Xeroderma —*see also* Ichthyosis
  acquired L85.0
    eyelid H01.149
      left H01.146
        lower H01.145
        upper H01.144
      right H01.143
        lower H01.142
        upper H01.141
  pigmentosum Q82.1
  vitamin A deficiency E50.8
Xerophthalmia (vitamin A deficiency) E50.7
  unrelated to vitamin A deficiency —*see*
    Keratoconjunctivitis

Xerosis
  conjunctiva H11.14-•
    with Bitot's spots —*see also* Pigmentation,
      conjunctiva
      vitamin A deficiency E50.1
    vitamin A deficiency E50.0
  cornea H18.89-•
    with ulceration —*see* Ulcer, cornea
      vitamin A deficiency E50.3
    vitamin A deficiency E50.2
  cutis L85.3
  skin L85.3
Xerostomia K11.7
Xiphopagus Q89.4
XO syndrome Q96.9
X-ray (of)
  abnormal findings —*see* Abnormal,
    diagnostic imaging
  breast (mammogram) (routine) Z12.31
  chest
    routine (as part of a general medical
      examination) Z00.00
      with abnormal findings Z00.01
  routine (as part of a general medical
    examination) Z00.00
    with abnormal findings Z00.01
XXXXY syndrome Q98.1
XXY syndrome Q98.0

Y

Yaba pox virus disease B08.72
Yatapoxvirus B08.70
  specified NEC B08.79
Yawning R06.89
  psychogenic F45.8
Yaws A66.9
  bone lesions A66.6
  butter A66.1
  chancre A66.0
  cutaneous, less than five years after infection
    A66.2
  early (cutaneous) (macular) (maculopapular)
    (micropapular) (papular) A66.2
    frambeside A66.2
    skin lesions NEC A66.2
  eyelid A66.2
  ganglion A66.6
  gangosis, gangosa A66.5
  gumma, gummata A66.4
    bone A66.6
  gummatous
    frambeside A66.4
    osteitis A66.6
    periostitis A66.6
  hydrarthrosis —*see also* subcategory
    M14.8-● A66.6
  hyperkeratosis (early) (late) A66.3

Yaws *(Continued)*
  initial lesions A66.0
  joint lesions —*see also* subcategory
    M14.8-● A66.6
  juxta-articular nodules A66.7
  late nodular (ulcerated) A66.4
  latent (without clinical manifestations) (with
    positive serology) A66.8
  mother A66.0
  mucosal A66.7
  multiple papillomata A66.1
  nodular, late (ulcerated) A66.4
  osteitis A66.6
  papilloma, plantar or palmar A66.1
  periostitis (hypertrophic) A66.6
  specified NEC A66.7
  ulcers A66.4
  wet crab A66.1
Yeast infection —*see also* Candidiasis B37.9
Yellow
  atrophy (liver) —*see* Failure, hepatic
  fever —*see* Fever, yellow
  jack —*see* Fever, yellow
  jaundice —*see* Jaundice
  nail syndrome L60.5
Yersiniosis —*see also* Infection, Yersinia
  extraintestinal A28.2
  intestinal A04.6

Z

Zahorsky's syndrome (herpangina) B08.5
Zellweger's syndrome Q87.89
Zenker's diverticulum (esophagus) K22.5
Ziehen-Oppenheim disease G24.1
Zieve's syndrome K70.0
Zika NOS A92.5
Zinc
  deficiency, dietary E60
  metabolism disorder E83.2
Zollinger-Ellison syndrome E16.4
Zona —*see* Herpes, zoster
Zoophobia F40.218
Zoster (herpes) —*see* Herpes, zoster
Zygomycosis B46.9
  specified NEC B46.8
Zymotic —*see* condition

▶ New   ⇒ Revised   ~~deleted~~ Deleted   ● Use Additional Character(s)

ICD-10-CM
Table of Neoplasms

ICD-10-CM
Table of Neoplasms

The list below gives the code numbers for neoplasms by anatomical site. For each site there are six possible code numbers according to whether the neoplasm in question is malignant, benign, in situ, of uncertain behavior, or of unspecified nature. The description of the neoplasm will often indicate which of the six columns is appropriate; e.g., malignant melanoma of skin, benign fibroadenoma of breast, carcinoma in situ of cervix uteri.

Where such descriptors are not present, the remainder of the Index should be consulted where guidance is given to the appropriate column for each morphological (histological) variety listed; e.g., Mesonephroma—*see Neoplasm, malignant;* Embryoma—*see also Neoplasm, uncertain behavior;* Disease, Bowen's—*see Neoplasm, skin, in situ.* However, the guidance in the Index can be overridden if one of the descriptors mentioned above is present; e.g., malignant adenoma of colon is coded to C18.9 and not to D12.6 as the adjective "Malignant" overrides the Index entry 'Adenoma—*see also Neoplasm, benign.*'

Codes listed with a dash -, following the code have a required additional character for laterality. The Tablular must be reviewed for the complete code.

	Malignant Primary	Malignant Secondary	Ca in situ	Benign	Uncertain Behavior	Unspecified Behavior
Neoplasm, neoplastic	C80.1	C79.9	D09.9	D36.9	D48.9	D49.9
abdomen, abdominal	C76.2	C79.8-●	D09.8	D36.7	D48.7	D49.89
cavity	C76.2	C79.8-●	D09.8	D36.7	D48.7	D49.89
organ	C76.2	C79.8-●	D09.8	D36.7	D48.7	D49.89
viscera	C76.2	C79.8-●	D09.8	D36.7	D48.7	D49.89
wall—*see also Neoplasm, abdomen, wall, skin*	C44.509	C79.2-●	D04.5	D23.5	D48.5	D49.2
connective tissue	C49.4	C79.8-●	—	D21.4	D48.1	D49.2
skin	C44.509					
basal cell carcinoma	C44.519	—	—	—	—	—
specified type NEC	C44.599	—	—	—	—	—
squamous cell carcinoma	C44.529	—	—	—	—	—
abdominopelvic	C76.8	C79.8-●	—	D36.7	D48.7	D49.89
accessory sinus—*see Neoplasm, sinus*						
acoustic nerve	C72.4-●	C79.49	—	D33.3	D43.3	D49.7
adenoid (pharynx) (tissue)	C11.1	C79.89	D00.08	D10.6	D37.05	D49.0
adipose tissue—*see also Neoplasm, connective tissue*	C49.4	C79.89	—	D21.9	D48.1	D49.2
adnexa (uterine)	C57.4	C79.89	D07.39	D28.7	D39.8	D49.59
adrenal	C74.9-●	C79.7-●	D09.3	D35.0-●	D44.1-●	D49.7
capsule	C74.9-●	C79.7-●	D09.3	D35.0-●	D44.1-●	D49.7
cortex	C74.0-●	C79.7-●	D09.3	D35.0-●	D44.1-●	D49.7
gland	C74.9-●	C79.7-●	D09.3	D35.0-●	D44.1-●	D49.7
medulla	C74.1-●	C79.7-●	D09.3	D35.0-●	D44.1-●	D49.7
ala nasi (external)—*see also Neoplasm, skin, nose*	C44.301	C79.2	D04.39	D23.39	D48.5	D49.2
alimentary canal or tract NEC	C26.9	C78.80	D01.9	D13.9	D37.9	D49.0
alveolar	C03.9	C79.89	D00.03	D10.39	D37.09	D49.0
mucosa	C03.9	C79.89	D00.03	D10.39	D37.09	D49.0
lower	C03.1	C79.89	D00.03	D10.39	D37.09	D49.0
upper	C03.0	C79.89	D00.03	D10.39	D37.09	D49.0
ridge or process	C41.1	C79.51	—	D16.5-●	D48.0	D49.2
carcinoma	C03.9	C79.8-●	—	—	—	—
lower	C03.1	C79.8-●	—	—	—	—
upper	C03.0	C79.8-●	—	—	—	—
lower	C41.1	C79.51	—	D16.5-●	D48.0	D49.2
mucosa	C03.9	C79.89	D00.03	D10.39	D37.09	D49.0
lower	C03.1	C79.89	D00.03	D10.39	D37.09	D49.0
upper	C03.0	C79.89	D00.03	D10.39	D37.09	D49.0
upper	C41.0	C79.51	—	D16.4-●	D48.0	D49.2
sulcus	C06.1	C79.89	D00.02	D10.39	D37.09	D49.0
alveolus	C03.9	C79.89	D00.03	D10.39	D37.09	D49.0
lower	C03.1	C79.89	D00.03	D10.39	D37.09	D49.0
upper	C03.0	C79.89	D00.03	D10.39	D37.09	D49.0
ampulla of Vater	C24.1	C78.89	D01.5	D13.5	D37.6	D49.0
ankle NEC	C76.5-●	C79.89	D04.7-●	D36.7	D48.7	D49.89
anorectum, anorectal (junction)	C21.8	C78.5	D01.3	D12.9	D37.8	D49.0
antecubital fossa or space	C76.4-●	C79.89	D04.6-●	D36.7	D48.7	D49.89
antrum (Highmore) (maxillary)	C31.0	C78.39	D02.3	D14.0	D38.5	D49.1
pyloric	C16.3	C78.89	D00.2	D13.1	D37.1	D49.0
tympanicum	C30.1	C78.39	D02.3	D14.0	D38.5	D49.1
anus, anal	C21.0	C78.5	D01.3	D12.9	D37.8	D49.0
canal	C21.1	C78.5	D01.3	D12.9	D37.8	D49.0
cloacogenic zone	C21.2	C78.5	D01.3	D12.9	D37.8	D49.0
margin—*see also Neoplasm, anus, skin*	C44.500	C79.2	D04.5	D23.5	D48.5	D49.2
overlapping lesion with rectosigmoid junction or rectum	C21.8	—	—	—	—	—
skin	C44.500	C79.2	D04.5	D23.5	D48.5	D49.2
basal cell carcinoma	C44.510	—	—	—	—	—
specified type NEC	C44.590	—	—	—	—	—
squamous cell carcinoma	C44.520	—	—	—	—	—
sphincter	C21.1	C78.5	D01.3	D12.9	D37.8	D49.0
aorta (thoracic)	C49.3	C79.89	—	D21.3	D48.1	D49.2
abdominal	C49.4	C79.89	—	D21.4	D48.1	D49.2
aortic body	C75.5	C79.89	—	D35.6	D44.7	D49.7
aponeurosis	C49.9	C79.89	—	D21.9	D48.1	D49.2
palmar	C49.1-●	C79.89	—	D21.1-●	D48.1	D49.2
plantar	C49.2-●	C79.89	—	D21.2-●	D48.1	D49.2

TABLE OF NEOPLASMS

	Malignant Primary	Malignant Secondary	Ca in situ	Benign	Uncertain Behavior	Unspecified Behavior
appendix	C18.1	C78.5	D01.0	D12.1	D37.3	D49.0
arachnoid	C70.9	C79.49	—	D32.9	D42.9	D49.7
cerebral	C70.0	C79.32	—	D32.0	D42.0	D49.7
spinal	C70.1	C79.49	—	D32.1	D42.1	D49.7
areola	C50.0-●	C79.81	D05.-●	D24.-●	D48.6-●	D49.3
arm NEC	C76.4-●	C79.89	D04.6-●	D36.7	D48.7	D49.89
artery — see Neoplasm, connective tissue						
aryepiglottic fold	C13.1	C79.89	D00.08	D10.7	D37.05	D49.0
hypopharyngeal aspect	C13.1	C79.89	D00.08	D10.7	D37.05	D49.0
laryngeal aspect	C32.1	C78.39	D02.0	D14.1	D38.0	D49.1
marginal zone	C13.1	C79.89	D00.08	D10.7	D37.05	D49.0
arytenoid (cartilage)	C32.3	C78.39	D02.0	D14.1	D38.0	D49.1
fold — see Neoplasm, aryepiglottic						
associated with transplanted organ	C80.2	—	—	—	—	—
atlas	C41.2	C79.51	—	D16.6	D48.0	D49.2
atrium, cardiac	C38.0	C79.89	—	D15.1	D48.7	D49.89
auditory						
canal (external) (skin)	C44.20-●	C79.2	D04.2-●	D23.2-●	D48.5	D49.2
internal	C30.1	C78.39	D02.3	D14.0	D38.5	D49.1
nerve	C72.4-●	C79.49	—	D33.3	D43.3	D49.7
tube	C30.1	C78.39	D02.3	D14.0	D38.5	D49.1
opening	C11.2	C79.89	D00.08	D10.6	D37.05	D49.0
auricle, ear — see also Neoplasm, skin, ear	C44.20-●	C79.2	D04.2-●	D23.2-●	D48.5	D49.2
auricular canal (external) — see also Neoplasm, skin, ear	C44.20-●	C79.2	D04.2-●	D23.2-●	D48.5	D49.2
internal	C30.1	C78.39	D02.3	D14.0	D38.5	D49.2
autonomic nerve or nervous system NEC (see Neoplasm, nerve, peripheral)						
axilla, axillary	C76.1	C79.89	D09.8	D36.7	D48.7	D49.89
fold — see also Neoplasm, skin, trunk	C44.509	C79.2	D04.5	D23.5	D48.5	D49.2
back NEC	C76.8	C79.89	D04.5	D36.7	D48.7	D49.89
Bartholin's gland	C51.0	C79.82	D07.1	D28.0	D39.8	D49.59
basal ganglia	C71.0	C79.31	—	D33.0	D43.0	D49.6
basis pedunculi	C71.7	C79.31	—	D33.1	D43.1	D49.6
bile or biliary (tract)	C24.9	C78.89	D01.5	D13.5	D37.6	D49.0
canaliculi (biliferi) (intrahepatic)	C22.1	C78.7	D01.5	D13.4	D37.6	D49.0
canals, interlobular	C22.1	C78.89	D01.5	D13.4	D37.6	D49.0

	Malignant Primary	Malignant Secondary	Ca in situ	Benign	Uncertain Behavior	Unspecified Behavior
bile or biliary (Continued)						
duct or passage (common) (cystic) (extrahepatic)	C24.0	C78.89	D01.5	D13.5	D37.6	D49.0
interlobular	C22.1	C78.89	D01.5	D13.4	D37.6	D49.0
intrahepatic	C22.1	C78.7	D01.5	D13.4	D37.6	D49.0
and extrahepatic	C24.8	C78.89	D01.5	D13.5	D37.6	D49.0
bladder (urinary)	C67.9	C79.11	D09.0	D30.3	D41.4	D49.4
dome	C67.1	C79.11	D09.0	D30.3	D41.4	D49.4
neck	C67.5	C79.11	D09.0	D30.3	D41.4	D49.4
orifice	C67.9	C79.11	D09.0	D30.3	D41.4	D49.4
ureteric	C67.6	C79.11	D09.0	D30.3	D41.4	D49.4
urethral	C67.5	C79.11	D09.0	D30.3	D41.4	D49.4
overlapping lesion	C67.8	—	—	—	—	—
sphincter	C67.8	C79.11	D09.0	D30.3	D41.4	D49.4
trigone	C67.0	C79.11	D09.0	D30.3	D41.4	D49.4
urachus	C67.7	C79.11	D09.0	D30.3	D41.4	D49.4
wall	C67.9	C79.11	D09.0	D30.3	D41.4	D49.4
anterior	C67.3	C79.11	D09.0	D30.3	D41.4	D49.4
lateral	C67.2	C79.11	D09.0	D30.3	D41.4	D49.4
posterior	C67.4	C79.11	D09.0	D30.3	D41.4	D49.4
blood vessel — see Neoplasm, connective tissue						
bone (periosteum)	C41.9	C79.51	—	D16.9-●	D48.0	D49.2
acetabulum	C41.4	C79.51	—	D16.8-●	D48.0	D49.2
ankle	C40.3-●	C79.51	—	D16.3-●	—	—
arm NEC	C40.0-●	C79.51	—	D16.0-●	—	—
astragalus	C40.3-●	C79.51	—	D16.3-●	—	—
atlas	C41.2	C79.51	—	D16.6-●	D48.0	D49.2
axis	C41.2	C79.51	—	D16.6-●	D48.0	D49.2
back NEC	C41.2	C79.51	—	D16.6-●	D48.0	D49.2
calcaneus	C40.3-●	C79.51	—	D16.3-●	—	—
calvarium	C41.0	C79.51	—	D16.4-●	D48.0	D49.2
carpus (any)	C40.1-●	C79.51	—	D16.1-●	—	—
cartilage NEC	C41.9	C79.51	—	D16.9-●	D48.0	D49.2
clavicle	C41.3	C79.51	—	D16.7-●	D48.0	D49.2
clivus	C41.0	C79.51	—	D16.4-●	D48.0	D49.2
coccygeal vertebra	C41.4	C79.51	—	D16.8-●	D48.0	D49.2
coccyx	C41.4	C79.51	—	D16.8-●	D48.0	D49.2
costal cartilage	C41.3	C79.51	—	D16.7-●	D48.0	D49.2
costovertebral joint	C41.3	C79.51	—	D16.7-●	D48.0	D49.2
cranial	C41.0	C79.51	—	D16.4-●	D48.0	D49.2
cuboid	C40.3-●	C79.51	—	D16.3-●	—	—
cuneiform	C41.9	C79.51	—	D16.9-●	D48.0	D49.2
elbow	C40.0-●	C79.51	—	D16.0-●	—	—

◀ New   ◀ Revised   ~~deleted~~ Deleted   ● Use Additional Character(s)

bone *(Continued)*	Malignant Primary	Malignant Secondary	Ca in situ	Benign	Uncertain Behavior	Unspecified Behavior
ethmoid (labyrinth)	C41.0	C79.51	—	D16.4-•	D48.0	D49.2
face	C41.0	C79.51	—	D16.4-•	D48.0	D49.2
femur (any part)	C40.2-•	C79.51	—	D16.2-•	—	—
fibula (any part)	C40.2-•	C79.51	—	D16.2-•	—	—
finger (any)	C40.1-•	C79.51	—	D16.1-•	—	—
foot	C40.3-•	C79.51	—	D16.3-•	—	—
forearm	C40.0-•	C79.51	—	D16.0-•	—	—
frontal	C41.0	C79.51	—	D16.4-•	D48.0	D49.2
hand	C40.1-•	C79.51	—	D16.1-•	—	—
heel	C40.3-•	C79.51	—	D16.3-•	—	—
hip	C41.4	C79.51	—	D16.8-•	D48.0	D49.2
humerus (any part)	C40.0-•	C79.51	—	D16.0-•	—	—
hyoid	C41.0	C79.51	—	D16.4-•	D48.0	D49.2
ilium	C41.4	C79.51	—	D16.8-•	D48.0	D49.2
innominate	C41.4	C79.51	—	D16.8-•	D48.0	D49.2
intervertebral cartilage or disc	C41.2	C79.51	—	D16.6-•	D48.0	D49.2
ischium	C41.4	C79.51	—	D16.8-•	D48.0	D49.2
jaw (lower)	C41.1	C79.51	—	D16.5-•	D48.0	D49.2
knee	C40.2-•	C79.51	—	D16.2-•	—	—
leg NEC	C40.2-•	C79.51	—	D16.2-•	—	—
limb NEC	C40.9-•	C79.51	—	D16.9-•	—	—
lower (long bones)	C40.2-•	C79.51	—	D16.2-•	—	—
short bones	C40.3-•	C79.51	—	D16.3-•	—	—
upper (long bones)	C40.0-•	C79.51	—	D16.0-•	—	—
short bones	C40.1-•	C79.51	—	D16.1-•	—	—
malar	C41.0	C79.51	—	D16.4-•	D48.0	D49.2
mandible	C41.1	C79.51	—	D16.5-•	D48.0	D49.2
marrow NEC (any bone)	C96.9	C79.52		—	D47.9	D49.89
mastoid	C41.0	C79.51	—	D16.4-•	D48.0	D49.2
maxilla, maxillary (superior)	C41.0	C79.51	—	D16.4-•	D48.0	D49.2
inferior	C41.1	C79.51	—	D16.5-•	D48.0	D49.2
metacarpus (any)	C40.1-•	C79.51	—	D16.1-•	—	—
metatarsus (any)	C40.3-•	C79.51	—	D16.3-•	—	—
overlapping sites	C40.8-•	—	—	—	—	—
navicular						
ankle	C40.3-•	C79.51	—	—	—	—
hand	C40.1-•	C79.51	—	—	—	—
nose, nasal	C41.0	C79.51	—	D16.4-•	D48.0	D49.2
occipital	C41.0	C79.51	—	D16.4-•	D48.0	D49.2
orbit	C41.0	C79.51	—	D16.4-•	D48.0	D49.2
parietal	C41.0	C79.51	—	D16.4-•	D48.0	D49.2
patella	C40.2-•	C79.51	—	—	—	—
pelvic	C41.4	C79.51	—	D16.8	D48.0	D49.2

bone *(Continued)*	Malignant Primary	Malignant Secondary	Ca in situ	Benign	Uncertain Behavior	Unspecified Behavior
phalanges						
foot	C40.3-•	C79.51	—	—	—	—
hand	C40.1-•	C79.51	—	—	—	—
pubic	C41.4	C79.51	—	D16.8	D48.0	D49.2
radius (any part)	C40.0-•	C79.51	—	D16.0-•	—	—
rib	C41.3	C79.51	—	D16.7	D48.0	D49.2
sacral vertebra	C41.4	C79.51	—	D16.8	D48.0	D49.2
sacrum	C41.4	C79.51	—	D16.8	D48.0	D49.2
scaphoid					—	—
of ankle	C40.3-•	C79.51	—	—	—	—
of hand	C40.1-•	C79.51	—	—	—	—
scapula (any part)	C40.0-•	C79.51	—	D16.0-•	—	—
sella turcica	C41.0	C79.51	—	D16.4-•	D48.0	D49.2
shoulder	C40.0-•	C79.51	—	D16.0-•	—	—
skull	C41.0	C79.51	—	D16.4-•	D48.0	D49.2
sphenoid	C41.0	C79.51	—	D16.4-•	D48.0	D49.2
spine, spinal (column)	C41.2	C79.51	—	D16.6	D48.0	D49.2
coccyx	C41.4	C79.51	—	D16.8	D48.0	D49.2
sacrum	C41.4	C79.51	—	D16.8	D48.0	D49.2
sternum	C41.3	C79.51	—	D16.7	D48.0	D49.2
tarsus (any)	C40.3-•	C79.51	—	—	—	—
temporal	C41.0	C79.51	—	D16.4-•	D48.0	D49.2
thumb	C40.1-•	C79.51	—	—	—	—
tibia (any part)	C40.2-•	C79.51	—	—	—	—
toe (any)	C40.3-•	C79.51	—	—	—	—
trapezium	C40.1-•	C79.51	—	—	—	—
trapezoid	C40.1-•	C79.51	—	—	—	—
turbinate	C41.0	C79.51	—	D16.4-•	D48.0	D49.2
ulna (any part)	C40.0-•	C79.51	—	D16.0-•	—	—
unciform	C40.1-•	C79.51	—	—	—	—
vertebra (column)	C41.2	C79.51	—	D16.6	D48.0	D49.2
coccyx	C41.4	C79.51	—	D16.8	D48.0	D49.2
sacrum	C41.4	C79.51	—	D16.8	D48.0	D49.2
vomer	C41.0	C79.51	—	D16.4-•	D48.0	D49.2
wrist	C40.1-•	C79.51				
xiphoid process	C41.3	C79.51	—	D16.7	D48.0	D49.2
zygomatic	C41.0	C79.51	—	D16.4-•	D48.0	D49.2
book-leaf (mouth)	C06.89	C79.89	D00.00	D10.39	D37.09	D49.0
bowel — *see Neoplasm, intestine*						
brachial plexus	C47.1-•	C79.89	—	D36.12	D48.2	D49.2
brain NEC	C71.9	C79.31	—	D33.2	D43.2	D49.6
basal ganglia	C71.0	C79.31	—	D33.0	D43.0	D49.6
cerebellopontine angle	C71.6	C79.31	—	D33.1	D43.1	D49.6

◀ New   ◀ Revised   ~~deleted~~ Deleted   • Use Additional Character(s)

469

TABLE OF NEOPLASMS

	Malignant Primary	Malignant Secondary	Ca in situ	Benign	Uncertain Behavior	Unspecified Behavior
brain NEC *(Continued)*						
cerebellum NOS	C71.6	C79.31	—	D33.1	D43.1	D49.6
cerebrum	C71.0	C79.31	—	D33.0	D43.0	D49.6
choroid plexus	C71.7	C79.31	—	D33.1	D43.1	D49.6
corpus callosum	C71.8	C79.31	—	D33.2	D43.2	D49.6
corpus striatum	C71.0	C79.31	—	D33.0	D43.0	D49.6
cortex (cerebral)	C71.0	C79.31	—	D33.0	D43.0	D49.6
frontal lobe	C71.1	C79.31	—	D33.0	D43.0	D49.6
globus pallidus	C71.0	C79.31	—	D33.0	D43.0	D49.6
hippocampus	C71.2	C79.31	—	D33.0	D43.0	D49.6
hypothalamus	C71.0	C79.31	—	D33.0	D43.0	D49.6
internal capsule	C71.0	C79.31	—	D33.0	D43.0	D49.6
medulla oblongata	C71.7	C79.31	—	D33.1	D43.1	D49.6
meninges	C70.0	C79.32	—	D32.0	D42.0	D49.7
midbrain	C71.7	C79.31	—	D33.1	D43.1	D49.6
occipital lobe	C71.4	C79.31	—	D33.0	D43.0	D49.6
overlapping lesion	C71.8	C79.31	—	—	—	—
parietal lobe	C71.3	C79.31	—	D33.0	D43.0	D49.6
peduncle	C71.7	C79.31	—	D33.1	D43.1	D49.6
pons	C71.7	C79.31	—	D33.1	D43.1	D49.6
stem	C71.7	C79.31	—	D33.1	D43.1	D49.6
tapetum	C71.8	C79.31	—	D33.2	D43.2	D49.6
temporal lobe	C71.2	C79.31	—	D33.0	D43.0	D49.6
thalamus	C71.0	C79.31	—	D33.0	D43.0	D49.6
uncus	C71.2	C79.31	—	D33.0	D43.0	D49.6
ventricle (floor)	C71.5	C79.31	—	D33.0	D43.0	D49.6
fourth	C71.7	C79.31	—	D33.1	D43.1	D49.6
branchial (cleft) (cyst) (vestiges)	C10.4	C79.89	D00.08	D10.5	D37.05	D49.0
breast (connective tissue) (glandular tissue) (soft parts)	C50.9-●	C79.81	D05.-●	D24.-●	D48.6-●	D49.3
areola	C50.0-●	C79.81	D05.-●	D24.-●	D48.6-●	D49.3
axillary tail	C50.6-●	C79.81	D05.-●	D24.-●	D48.6-●	D49.3
central portion	C50.1-●	C79.81	D05.-●	D24.-●	D48.6-●	D49.3
inner	C50.8-●	C79.81	D05.-●	D24.-●	D48.6-●	D49.3
lower	C50.8-●	C79.81	D05.-●	D24.-●	D48.6-●	D49.3
lower-inner quadrant	C50.3-●	C79.81	D05.-●	D24.-●	D48.6-●	D49.3
lower-outer quadrant	C50.5-●	C79.81	D05.-●	D24.-●	D48.6-●	D49.3
mastectomy site (skin) — *see also Neoplasm, breast, skin*	C44.501	C79.2	—	—	—	—
specified as breast tissue	C50.8-●	C79.81	—	—	—	—
midline	C50.8-●	C79.81	D05.-●	D24.-●	D48.6-●	D49.3
nipple	C50.0-●	C79.81	D05.-●	D24.-●	D48.6-●	D49.3
outer	C50.8-●	C79.81	D05.-●	D24.-●	D48.6-●	D49.3
overlapping lesion	C50.8-●	—	—	—	—	—

	Malignant Primary	Malignant Secondary	Ca in situ	Benign	Uncertain Behavior	Unspecified Behavior
breast *(Continued)*						
skin	C44.501	C79.2	D04.5	D23.5	D48.5	D49.2
basal cell carcinoma	C44.511	—	—	—	—	—
specified type NEC	C44.591	—	—	—	—	—
squamous cell carcinoma	C44.521	—	—	—	—	—
tail (axillary)	C50.6-●	C79.81	D05.-●	D24.-●	D48.6-●	D49.3
upper	C50.8-●	C79.81	D05.-●	D24.-●	D48.6-●	D49.3
upper-inner quadrant	C50.2-●	C79.81	D05.-●	D24.-●	D48.6-●	D49.3
upper-outer quadrant	C50.4-●	C79.81	D05.-●	D24.-●	D48.6-●	D49.3
broad ligament	C57.1	C79.82	D07.39	D28.2	D39.8	D49.59
bronchiogenic, bronchogenic (lung)	C34.9-●	C78.0-●	D02.2-●	D14.3-●	D38.1	D49.1
bronchiole	C34.9-●	C78.0-●	D02.2-●	D14.3-●	D38.1	D49.1
bronchus	C34.9-●	C78.0-●	D02.2-●	D14.3-●	D38.1	D49.1
carina	C34.0-●	C78.0-●	D02.2-●	D14.3-●	D38.1	D49.1
lower lobe of lung	C34.3-●	C78.0-●	D02.2-●	D14.3-●	D38.1	D49.1
main	C34.0-●	C78.0-●	D02.2-●	D14.3-●	D38.1	D49.1
middle lobe of lung	C34.2	C78.0-●	D02.21	D14.31	D38.1	D49.1
overlapping lesion	C34.8-●	—	—	—	—	—
upper lobe of lung	C34.1-●	C78.0-●	D02.2-●	D14.3-●	D38.1	D49.1
brow	C44.309	C79.2	D04.39	D23.39	D48.5	D49.2
basal cell carcinoma	C44.319	—	—	—	—	—
specified type NEC	C44.399	—	—	—	—	—
squamous cell carcinoma	C44.329	—	—	—	—	—
buccal (cavity)	C06.9	C79.89	D00.00	D10.39	D37.09	D49.0
commissure	C06.0	C79.89	D00.02	D10.39	D37.09	D49.0
groove (lower) (upper)	C06.1	C79.89	D00.02	D10.39	D37.09	D49.0
mucosa	C06.0	C79.89	D00.02	D10.39	D37.09	D49.0
sulcus (lower) (upper)	C06.1	C79.89	D00.02	D10.39	D37.09	D49.0
bulbourethral gland	C68.0	C79.19	D09.19	D30.4	D41.3	D49.59
bursa — *see Neoplasm, connective tissue*						
buttock NEC	C76.3	C79.89	D04.5	D36.7	D48.7	D49.89
calf	C76.5-●	C79.89	D04.7-●	D36.7	D48.7	D49.89
calvarium	C41.0	C79.51	—	D16.4-●	D48.0	D49.2
calyx, renal	C65.-●	C79.0-●	D09.19	D30.1-●	D41.1-●	D49.51-●
canal						
anal	C21.1	C78.5	D01.3	D12.9	D37.8	D49.0
auditory (external) — *see also Neoplasm, skin, ear*	C44.20-●	C79.2	D04.2-●	D23.2-●	D48.5	D49.2
auricular (external) — *see also Neoplasm, skin, ear*	C44.20-●	C79.2	D04.2-●	D23.2-●	D48.5	D49.2
canaliculi, biliary (biliferi) (intrahepatic)	C22.1	C78.7	D01.5	D13.4	D37.6	D49.0

◄ New ◄ Revised ~~deleted~~ Deleted ● Use Additional Character(s)

	Malignant Primary	Malignant Secondary	Ca in situ	Benign	Uncertain Behavior	Unspecified Behavior
canthus (eye) (inner) (outer)	C44.1Ø-●	C79.2	DØ4.1-●	D23.1-●	D48.5	D49.2
basal cell carcinoma	C44.11-●	—	—	—	—	—
specified type NEC	C44.19-●	—	—	—	—	—
squamous cell carcinoma	C44.12-●	—	—	—	—	—
capillary — see Neoplasm, connective tissue						
caput coli	C18.Ø	C78.5	DØ1.Ø	D12.Ø	D37.4	D49.Ø
carcinoid — see Tumor, carcinoid						
cardia (gastric)	C16.Ø	C78.89	DØØ.2	D13.1	D37.1	D49.Ø
cardiac orifice (stomach)	C16.Ø	C78.89	DØØ.2	D13.1	D37.1	D49.Ø
cardio-esophageal junction	C16.Ø	C78.89	DØØ.2	D13.1	D37.1	D49.Ø
cardio-esophagus	C16.Ø	C78.89	DØØ.2	D13.1	D37.1	D49.Ø
carina (bronchus)	C34.Ø-●	C78.Ø-●	DØ2.2-●	D14.3-●	D38.1	D49.1
carotid (artery)	C49.Ø	C79.89	—	D21.Ø	D48.1	D49.2
body	C75.4	C79.89	—	D35.5	D44.6	D49.7
carpus (any bone)	C4Ø.1-●	C79.51	—	D16.1-●	—	—
cartilage (articular) (joint) NEC — see also Neoplasm, bone	C41.9	C79.51	—	D16.9-●	D48.Ø	D49.2
arytenoid	C32.3	C78.39	DØ2.Ø	D14.1	D38.Ø	D49.1
auricular	C49.Ø	C79.89	—	D21.Ø	D48.1	D49.2
bronchi	C34.Ø-●	C78.39	—	D14.3-●	D38.1	D49.1
costal	C41.3	C79.51	—	D16.7	D48.Ø	D49.2
cricoid	C32.3	C78.39	DØ2.Ø	D14.1	D38.Ø	D49.1
cuneiform	C32.3	C78.39	DØ2.Ø	D14.1	D38.Ø	D49.1
ear (external)	C49.Ø	C79.89	—	D21.Ø	D48.1	D49.2
ensiform	C41.3	C79.51	—	D16.7	D48.Ø	D49.2
epiglottis	C32.1	C78.39	DØ2.Ø	D14.1	D38.Ø	D49.1
anterior surface	C1Ø.1	C79.89	DØØ.Ø8	D1Ø.5	D37.Ø5	D49.Ø
eyelid	C49.Ø	C79.89	—	D21.Ø	D48.1	D49.2
intervertebral	C41.2	C79.51	—	D16.6	D48.Ø	D49.2
larynx, laryngeal	C32.3	C78.39	DØ2.Ø	D14.1	D38.Ø	D49.1
nose, nasal	C3Ø.Ø	C78.39	DØ2.3	D14.Ø	D38.5	D49.1
pinna	C49.Ø	C79.89	—	D21.Ø	D48.1	D49.2
rib	C41.3	C79.51	—	D16.7	D48.Ø	D49.2
semilunar (knee)	C4Ø.2-●	C79.51	—	D16.2-●	D48.Ø	D49.2
thyroid	C32.3	C78.39	DØ2.Ø	D14.1	D38.Ø	D49.1
trachea	C33	C78.39	DØ2.1	D14.2	D38.1	D49.1
cauda equina	C72.1	C79.49	—	D33.4	D43.4	D49.7
cavity						
buccal	CØ6.9	C79.89	DØØ.ØØ	D1Ø.3Ø	D37.Ø9	D49.Ø
nasal	C3Ø.Ø	C78.39	DØ2.3	D14.Ø	D38.5	D49.1
oral	CØ6.9	C79.89	DØØ.ØØ	D1Ø.3Ø	D37.Ø9	D49.Ø
peritoneal	C48.2	C78.6	—	D2Ø.1	D48.4	D49.Ø
tympanic	C3Ø.1	C78.39	DØ2.3	D14.Ø	D38.5	D49.1

	Malignant Primary	Malignant Secondary	Ca in situ	Benign	Uncertain Behavior	Unspecified Behavior
cecum	C18.Ø	C78.5	DØ1.Ø	D12.Ø	D37.4	D49.Ø
central nervous system	C72.9	C79.4Ø	—	—	—	—
cerebellopontine (angle)	C71.6	C79.31	—	D33.1	D43.1	D49.6
cerebellum, cerebellar	C71.6	C79.31	—	D33.1	D43.1	D49.6
cerebrum, cerebral (cortex) (hemisphere) (white matter)	C71.Ø	C79.31	—	D33.Ø	D43.Ø	D49.6
meninges	C7Ø.Ø	C79.32	—	D32.Ø	D42.Ø	D49.7
peduncle	C71.7	C79.31	—	D33.1	D43.1	D49.6
ventricle	C71.5	C79.31	—	D33.Ø	D43.Ø	D49.6
fourth	C71.7	C79.31	—	D33.1	D43.1	D49.6
cervical region	C76.Ø	C79.89	DØ9.8	D36.7	D48.7	D49.89
cervix (cervical) (uteri) (uterus)	C53.9	C79.82	DØ6.9	D26.Ø	D39.Ø	D49.59
canal	C53.Ø	C79.82	DØ6.Ø	D26.Ø	D39.Ø	D49.59
endocervix (canal) (gland)	C53.Ø	C79.82	DØ6.Ø	D26.Ø	D39.Ø	D49.59
exocervix	C53.1	C79.82	DØ6.1	D26.Ø	D39.Ø	D49.59
external os	C53.1	C79.82	DØ6.1	D26.Ø	D39.Ø	D49.59
internal os	C53.Ø	C79.82	DØ6.Ø	D26.Ø	D39.Ø	D49.59
nabothian gland	C53.Ø	C79.82	DØ6.Ø	D26.Ø	D39.Ø	D49.59
overlapping lesion	C53.8	—	—	—	—	—
squamocolumnar junction	C53.8	C79.82	DØ6.7	D26.Ø	D39.Ø	D49.59
stump	C53.8	C79.82	DØ6.7	D26.Ø	D39.Ø	D49.59
cheek	C76.Ø	C79.89	DØ9.8	D36.7	D48.7	D49.89
external	C44.3Ø9	C79.2	DØ4.39	D23.39	D48.5	D49.2
basal cell carcinoma	C44.319	—	—	—	—	—
specified type NEC	C44.399	—	—	—	—	—
squamous cell carcinoma	C44.329	—	—	—	—	—
inner aspect	CØ6.Ø	C79.89	DØØ.Ø2	D1Ø.39	D37.Ø9	D49.Ø
internal	CØ6.Ø	C79.89	DØØ.Ø2	D1Ø.39	D37.Ø9	D49.Ø
mucosa	CØ6.Ø	C79.89	DØØ.Ø2	D1Ø.39	D37.Ø9	D49.Ø
chest (wall) NEC	C76.1	C79.89	DØ9.8	D36.7	D48.7	D49.89
chiasma opticum	C72.3-●	C79.49	—	D33.3	D43.3	D49.7
chin	C44.3Ø9	C79.2	DØ4.39	D23.39	D48.5	D49.2
basal cell carcinoma	C44.319	—	—	—	—	—
specified type NEC	C44.399	—	—	—	—	—
squamous cell carcinoma	C44.329	—	—	—	—	—
choana	C11.3	C79.89	DØØ.Ø8	D1Ø.6	D37.Ø5	D49.Ø
cholangiole	C22.1	C78.89	DØ1.5	D13.4	D37.6	D49.Ø
choledochal duct	C24.Ø	C78.89	DØ1.5	D13.5	D37.6	D49.Ø
choroid	C69.3-●	C79.49	DØ9.2-●	D31.3-●	D48.7	D49.81
plexus	C71.5	C79.31	—	D33.Ø	D43.Ø	D49.6
ciliary body	C69.4-●	C79.49	DØ9.2-●	D31.4-●	D48.7	D49.89
clavicle	C41.3	C79.51	—	D16.7	D48.Ø	D49.2
clitoris	C51.2	C79.82	DØ7.1	D28.Ø	D39.8	D49.59
clivus	C41.Ø	C79.51	—	D16.4-●	D48.Ø	D49.2

TABLE OF NEOPLASMS

	Malignant Primary	Malignant Secondary	Ca in situ	Benign	Uncertain Behavior	Unspecified Behavior
cloacogenic zone	C21.2	C78.5	D01.3	D12.9	D37.8	D49.0
coccygeal						
body or glomus	C49.5	C79.89	—	D21.5	D48.1	D49.2
vertebra	C41.4	C79.51	—	D16.8	D48.0	D49.2
coccyx	C41.4	C79.51	—	D16.8	D48.0	D49.2
colon — *see also Neoplasm, intestine, large*	C18.9	C78.5	—	—	—	—
with rectum	C19	C78.5	D01.1	D12.7	D37.5	D49.0
column, spinal — *see Neoplasm, spine*						
columnella — *see also Neoplasm, skin, face*	C44.390	C79.2	D04.39	D23.39	D48.5	D49.2
commissure						
labial, lip	C00.6	C79.89	D00.01	D10.39	D37.01	D49.0
laryngeal	C32.0	C78.39	D02.0	D14.1	D38.0	D49.1
common (bile) duct	C24.0	C78.89	D01.5	D13.5	D37.6	D49.0
concha — *see also Neoplasm, skin, ear*	C44.20-•	C79.2	D04.2-•	D23.2-•	D48.5	D49.2
nose	C30.0	C78.39	D02.3	D14.0	D38.5	D49.1
conjunctiva	C69.0-•	C79.49	D09.2-•	D31.0-•	D48.7	D49.89
connective tissue NEC	C49.9	C79.89	—	D21.9	D48.1	D49.2

Note: For neoplasms of connective tissue (blood vessel, bursa, fascia, ligament, muscle, peripheral nerves, sympathetic and parasympathetic nerves and ganglia, synovia, tendon, etc.) or of morphological types that indicate connective tissue, code according to the list under "Neoplasm, connective tissue". For sites that do not appear in this list, code to neoplasm of that site; e.g., fibrosarcoma, pancreas (C25.9)

Note: Morphological types that indicate connective tissue appear in their proper place in the alphabetic index with the instruction "*see Neoplasm, connective tissue ....*"

	Malignant Primary	Malignant Secondary	Ca in situ	Benign	Uncertain Behavior	Unspecified Behavior
abdomen	C49.4	C79.89	—	D21.4	D48.1	D49.2
abdominal wall	C49.4	C79.89	—	D21.4	D48.1	D49.2
ankle	C49.2-•	C79.89	—	D21.2-•	D48.1	D49.2
antecubital fossa or space	C49.1-•	C79.89	—	D21.1-•	D48.1	D49.2
arm	C49.1-•	C79.89	—	D21.1-•	D48.1	D49.2
auricle (ear)	C49.0	C79.89	—	D21.0	D48.1	D49.2
axilla	C49.3	C79.89	—	D21.3	D48.1	D49.2
back	C49.6	C79.89	—	D21.6	D48.1	D49.2
breast — *see Neoplasm, breast*						
buttock	C49.5	C79.89	—	D21.5	D48.1	D49.2
calf	C49.2-•	C79.89	—	D21.2-•	D48.1	D49.2
cervical region	C49.0	C79.89	—	D21.0	D48.1	D49.2
cheek	C49.0	C79.89	—	D21.0	D48.1	D49.2
chest (wall)	C49.3	C79.89	—	D21.3	D48.1	D49.2
chin	C49.0	C79.89	—	D21.0	D48.1	D49.2

	Malignant Primary	Malignant Secondary	Ca in situ	Benign	Uncertain Behavior	Unspecified Behavior
connective tissue NEC *(Continued)*						
diaphragm	C49.3	C79.89	—	D21.3	D48.1	D49.2
ear (external)	C49.0	C79.89	—	D21.0	D48.1	D49.2
elbow	C49.1-•	C79.89	—	D21.1-•	D48.1	D49.2
extrarectal	C49.5	C79.89	—	D21.5	D48.1	D49.2
extremity	C49.9	C79.89	—	D21.9	D48.1	D49.2
lower	C49.2-•	C79.89	—	D21.2-•	D48.1	D49.2
upper	C49.1-•	C79.89	—	D21.1-•	D48.1	D49.2
eyelid	C49.0	C79.89	—	D21.0	D48.1	D49.2
face	C49.0	C79.89	—	D21.0	D48.1	D49.2
finger	C49.1-•	C79.89	—	D21.1-•	D48.1	D49.2
flank	C49.6	C79.89	—	D21.6	D48.1	D49.2
foot	C49.2-•	C79.89	—	D21.2-•	D48.1	D49.2
forearm	C49.1-•	C79.89	—	D21.1-•	D48.1	D49.2
forehead	C49.0	C79.89	—	D21.0	D48.1	D49.2
gastric	C49.4	C79.89	—	D21.4	D48.1	D49.2
gastrointestinal	C49.4	C79.89	—	D21.4	D48.1	D49.2
gluteal region	C49.5	C79.89	—	D21.5	D48.1	D49.2
great vessels NEC	C49.3	C79.89	—	D21.3	D48.1	D49.2
groin	C49.5	C79.89	—	D21.5	D48.1	D49.2
hand	C49.1-•	C79.89	—	D21.1-•	D48.1	D49.2
head	C49.0	C79.89	—	D21.0	D48.1	D49.2
heel	C49.2-•	C79.89	—	D21.2-•	D48.1	D49.2
hip	C49.2-•	C79.89	—	D21.2-•	D48.1	D49.2
hypochondrium	C49.4	C79.89	—	D21.4	D48.1	D49.2
iliopsoas muscle	C49.5	C79.89	—	D21.5	D48.1	D49.2
infraclavicular region	C49.3	C79.89	—	D21.3	D48.1	D49.2
inguinal (canal) (region)	C49.5	C79.89	—	D21.5	D48.1	D49.2
intestinal	C49.4	C79.89	—	D21.4	D48.1	D49.2
intrathoracic	C49.3	C79.89	—	D21.3	D48.1	D49.2
ischiorectal fossa	C49.5	C79.89	—	D21.5	D48.1	D49.2
jaw	C03.9	C79.89	D00.03	D10.39	D48.1	D49.0
knee	C49.2-•	C79.89	—	D21.2-•	D48.1	D49.2
leg	C49.2-•	C79.89	—	D21.2-•	D48.1	D49.2
limb NEC	C49.9	C79.89	—	D21.9	D48.1	D49.2
lower	C49.2-•	C79.89	—	D21.2-•	D48.1	D49.2
upper	C49.1-•	C79.89	—	D21.1-•	D48.1	D49.2
nates	C49.5	C79.89	—	D21.5	D48.1	D49.2
neck	C49.0	C79.89	—	D21.0	D48.1	D49.2
orbit	C69.6-•	C79.49	D09.2-•	D31.6-•	D48.1	D49.89
overlapping lesion	C49.8	—	—	—	—	—
pararectal	C49.5	C79.89	—	D21.5	D48.1	D49.2
para-urethral	C49.5	C79.89	—	D21.5	D48.1	D49.2
paravaginal	C49.5	C79.89	—	D21.5	D48.1	D49.2

◀ New   ◀ Revised   ~~deleted~~ Deleted   • Use Additional Character(s)

TABLE OF NEOPLASMS

	Malignant Primary	Malignant Secondary	Ca in situ	Benign	Uncertain Behavior	Unspecified Behavior
connective tissue NEC (Continued)						
pelvis (floor)	C49.5	C79.89	—	D21.5	D48.1	D49.2
pelvo-abdominal	C49.8	C79.89	—	D21.6	D48.1	D49.2
perineum	C49.5	C79.89	—	D21.5	D48.1	D49.2
perirectal (tissue)	C49.5	C79.89	—	D21.5	D48.1	D49.2
periurethral (tissue)	C49.5	C79.89	—	D21.5	D48.1	D49.2
popliteal fossa or space	C49.2-•	C79.89	—	D21.2-•	D48.1	D49.2
presacral	C49.5	C79.89	—	D21.5	D48.1	D49.2
psoas muscle	C49.4	C79.89	—	D21.4	D48.1	D49.2
pterygoid fossa	C49.0	C79.89	—	D21.0	D48.1	D49.2
rectovaginal septum or wall	C49.5	C79.89	—	D21.5	D48.1	D49.2
rectovesical	C49.5	C79.89	—	D21.5	D48.1	D49.2
retroperitoneum	C48.0	C78.6	—	D20.0	D48.3	D49.0
sacrococcygeal region	C49.5	C79.89	—	D21.5	D48.1	D49.2
scalp	C49.0	C79.89	—	D21.0	D48.1	D49.2
scapular region	C49.3	C79.89	—	D21.3	D48.1	D49.2
shoulder	C49.1-•	C79.89	—	D21.1-•	D48.1	D49.2
skin (dermis) NEC—see also Neoplasm, skin, by site	C44.90	C79.2	D04.9	D23.9	D48.5	D49.2
stomach	C49.4	C79.89	—	D21.4	D48.1	D49.2
submental	C49.0	C79.89	—	D21.0	D48.1	D49.2
supraclavicular region	C49.0	C79.89	—	D21.0	D48.1	D49.2
temple	C49.0	C79.89	—	D21.0	D48.1	D49.2
temporal region	C49.0	C79.89	—	D21.0	D48.1	D49.2
thigh	C49.2-•	C79.89	—	D21.2-•	D48.1	D49.2
thoracic (duct) (wall)	C49.3	C79.89	—	D21.3	D48.1	D49.2
thorax	C49.3	C79.89	—	D21.3	D48.1	D49.2
thumb	C49.1-•	C79.89	—	D21.1-•	D48.1	D49.2
toe	C49.2-•	C79.89	—	D21.2-•	D48.1	D49.2
trunk	C49.6	C79.89	—	D21.6	D48.1	D49.2
umbilicus	C49.4	C79.89	—	D21.4	D48.1	D49.2
vesicorectal	C49.5	C79.89	—	D21.5	D48.1	D49.2
wrist	C49.1-•	C79.89	—	D21.1-•	D48.1	D49.2
conus medullaris	C72.0	C79.49	—	D33.4	D43.4	D49.7
cord (true) (vocal)	C32.0	C78.39	D02.0	D14.1	D38.0	D49.1
false	C32.1	C78.39	D02.0	D14.1	D38.0	D49.1
spermatic	C63.1-•	C79.82	D07.69	D29.8	D40.8	D49.59
spinal (cervical) (lumbar) (thoracic)	C72.0	C79.49	—	D33.4	D43.4	D49.7
cornea (limbus)	C69.1-•	C79.49	D09.2-•	D31.1-•	D48.7	D49.89
corpus						
albicans	C56.-•	C79.6-•	D07.39	D27.-•	D39.1-•	D49.59
callosum, brain	C71.0	C79.31	—	D33.2	D43.2	D49.6
cavernosum	C60.2	C79.82	D07.4	D29.0	D40.8	D49.59

	Malignant Primary	Malignant Secondary	Ca in situ	Benign	Uncertain Behavior	Unspecified Behavior
corpus (Continued)						
gastric	C16.2	C78.89	D00.2	D13.1	D37.1	D49.0
overlapping sites	C54.8	—	—	—	—	—
penis	C60.2	C79.82	D07.4	D29.0	D40.8	D49.59
striatum, cerebrum	C71.0	C79.31	—	D33.0	D43.0	D49.6
uteri	C54.9	C79.82	D07.0	D26.1	D39.0	D49.59
isthmus	C54.0	C79.82	D07.0	D26.1	D39.0	D49.59
cortex						
adrenal	C74.0-•	C79.7-•	D09.3	D35.0-•	D44.1-•	D49.7
cerebral	C71.0	C79.31	—	D33.0	D43.0	D49.6
costal cartilage	C41.3	C79.51	—	D16.7	D48.0	D49.2
costovertebral joint	C41.3	C79.51	—	D16.7	D48.0	D49.2
Cowper's gland	C68.0	C79.19	D09.19	D30.4	D41.3	D49.59
cranial (fossa, any)	C71.9	C79.31	—	D33.2	D43.2	D49.6
meninges	C70.0	C79.32	—	D32.0	D42.0	D49.7
nerve	C72.50	C79.49	—	D33.3	D43.3	D49.7
specified NEC	C72.59	C79.49	—	D33.3	D43.3	D49.7
craniobuccal pouch	C75.2	C79.89	D09.3	D35.2	D44.3	D49.7
craniopharyngeal (duct) (pouch)	C75.2	C79.89	D09.3	D35.3	D44.4	D49.7
cricoid	C13.0	C79.89	D00.08	D10.7	D37.05	D49.0
cartilage	C32.3	C78.39	D02.0	D14.1	D38.0	D49.1
cricopharynx	C13.0	C79.89	D00.08	D10.7	D37.05	D49.0
crypt of Morgagni	C21.8	C78.5	D01.3	D12.9	D37.8	D49.0
crystalline lens	C69.4-•	C79.49	D09.2-•	D31.4-•	D48.7	D49.89
cul-de-sac (Douglas')	C48.1	C78.6	—	D20.1	D48.4	D49.0
cuneiform cartilage	C32.3	C78.39	D02.0	D14.1	D38.0	D49.1
cutaneous—see Neoplasm, skin						
cutis—see Neoplasm, skin						
cystic (bile) duct (common)	C24.0	C78.89	D01.5	D13.5	D37.6	D49.0
dermis—see Neoplasm, skin						
diaphragm	C49.3	C79.89	—	D21.3	D48.1	D49.2
digestive organs, system, tube, or tract NEC	C26.9	C78.89	D01.9	D13.9	D37.9	D49.0
disc, intervertebral	C41.2	C79.51	—	D16.6	D48.0	D49.2
disease, generalized	C80.0					
disseminated	C80.0	—	—	—	—	—
Douglas' cul-de-sac or pouch	C48.1	C78.6	—	D20.1	D48.4	D49.0
duodenojejunal junction	C17.8	C78.4	D01.49	D13.39	D37.2	D49.0
duodenum	C17.0	C78.4	D01.49	D13.2	D37.2	D49.0
dura (cranial) (mater)	C70.9	C79.49	—	D32.9	D42.9	D49.7
cerebral	C70.0	C79.32	—	D32.0	D42.0	D49.7
spinal	C70.1	C79.49	—	D32.1	D42.1	D49.7

TABLE OF NEOPLASMS

	Malignant Primary	Malignant Secondary	Ca in situ	Benign	Uncertain Behavior	Unspecified Behavior
ear (external) — see also Neoplasm, skin, ear	C44.20-●	C79.2	D04.2-●	D23.2-●	D48.5	D49.2
auricle or auris — see also Neoplasm, skin, ear	C44.20-●	C79.2	D04.2-●	D23.2-●	D48.5	D49.2
canal, external — see also Neoplasm, skin, ear	C44.20-●	C79.2	D04.2-●	D23.2-●	D48.5	D49.2
cartilage	C49.0	C79.89	—	D21.0	D48.1	D49.2
external meatus — see also Neoplasm, skin, ear	C44.20-●	C79.2	D04.2-●	D23.2-●	D48.5	D49.2
inner	C30.1	C78.39	D02.3	D14.0	D38.5	D49.1
lobule — see also Neoplasm, skin, ear	C44.20-●	C79.2	D04.2-●	D23.2-●	D48.5	D49.2
middle	C30.1	C78.39	D02.3	D14.0	D38.5	D49.1
overlapping lesion with accessory sinuses	C31.8	—	—	—	—	—
skin	C44.20-●	C79.2	D04.2-●	D23.2-●	D48.5	D49.2
basal cell carcinoma	C44.21-●	—	—	—	—	—
specified type NEC	C44.29-●	—	—	—	—	—
squamous cell carcinoma	C44.22-●	—	—	—	—	—
earlobe	C44.20-●	C79.2	D04.2-●	D23.2-●	D48.5	D49.2
basal cell carcinoma	C44.21-●	—	—	—	—	—
specified type NEC	C44.29-●	—	—	—	—	—
squamous cell carcinoma	C44.22-●	—	—	—	—	—
ejaculatory duct	C63.7	C79.82	D07.69	D29.8	D40.8	D49.59
elbow NEC	C76.4-●	C79.89	D04.6-●	D36.7	D48.7	D49.89
endocardium	C38.0	C79.89	—	D15.1	D48.7	D49.89
endocervix (canal) (gland)	C53.0	C79.82	D06.0	D26.0	D39.0	D49.59
endocrine gland NEC	C75.9	C79.89	D09.3	D35.9	D44.9	D49.7
pluriglandular	C75.8	C79.89	D09.3	D35.7	D44.9	D49.7
endometrium (gland) (stroma)	C54.1	C79.82	D07.0	D26.1	D39.0	D49.59
ensiform cartilage	C41.3	C79.51		D16.7	D48.0	D49.2
enteric — see Neoplasm, intestine						
ependyma (brain)	C71.5	C79.31	—	D33.0	D43.0	D49.6
fourth ventricle	C71.7	C79.31	—	D33.1	D43.1	D49.6
epicardium	C38.0	C79.89	—	D15.1	D48.7	D49.89
epididymis	C63.0-●	C79.82	D07.69	D29.3-●	D40.8	D49.59
epidural	C72.9	C79.49		D33.9	D43.9	D49.7
epiglottis	C32.1	C78.39	D02.0	D14.1	D38.0	D49.1
anterior aspect or surface	C10.1	C79.89	D00.08	D10.5	D37.05	D49.0
cartilage	C32.3	C78.39	D02.0	D14.1	D38.0	D49.1
free border (margin)	C10.1	C79.89	D00.08	D10.5	D37.05	D49.0
junctional region	C10.8	C79.89	D00.08	D10.5	D37.05	D49.0
posterior (laryngeal) surface	C32.1	C78.39	D02.0	D14.1	D38.0	D49.1
suprahyoid portion	C32.1	C78.39	D02.0	D14.1	D38.0	D49.1

	Malignant Primary	Malignant Secondary	Ca in situ	Benign	Uncertain Behavior	Unspecified Behavior
esophagogastric junction	C16.0	C78.89	D00.2	D13.1	D37.1	D49.0
esophagus	C15.9	C78.89	D00.1	D13.0	D37.8	D49.0
abdominal	C15.5	C78.89	D00.1	D13.0	D37.8	D49.0
cervical	C15.3	C78.89	D00.1	D13.0	D37.8	D49.0
distal (third)	C15.5	C78.89	D00.1	D13.0	D37.8	D49.0
lower (third)	C15.5	C78.89	D00.1	D13.0	D37.8	D49.0
middle (third)	C15.4	C78.89	D00.1	D13.0	D37.8	D49.0
overlapping lesion	C15.8	—	—	—	—	—
proximal (third)	C15.3	C78.89	D00.1	D13.0	D37.8	D49.0
thoracic	C15.4	C78.89	D00.1	D13.0	D37.8	D49.0
upper (third)	C15.3	C78.89	D00.1	D13.0	D37.8	D49.0
ethmoid (sinus)	C31.1	C78.39	D02.3	D14.0	D38.5	D49.1
bone or labyrinth	C41.0	C79.51	—	D16.4-●	D48.0	D49.2
eustachian tube	C30.1	C78.39	D02.3	D14.0	D38.5	D49.1
exocervix	C53.1	C79.82	D06.1	D26.0	D39.0	D49.59
external						
meatus (ear) — see also Neoplasm, skin, ear	C44.20-●	C79.2	D04.2-●	D23.2-●	D48.5	D49.2
os, cervix uteri	C53.1	C79.82	D06.1	D26.0	D39.0	D49.59
extradural	C72.9	C79.49	—	D33.9	D43.9	D49.7
extrahepatic (bile) duct	C24.0	C78.89	D01.5	D13.5	D37.6	D49.0
overlapping lesion with gallbladder	C24.8	—	—	—	—	—
extraocular muscle	C69.6-●	C79.49	D09.2-●	D31.6-●	D48.7	D49.89
extrarectal	C76.3	C79.89	D09.8	D36.7	D48.7	D49.89
extremity	C76.8	C79.89	D04.8	D36.7	D48.7	D49.89
lower	C76.5-●	C79.89	D04.7-●	D36.7	D48.7	D49.89
upper	C76.4-●	C79.89	D04.6-●	D36.7	D48.7	D49.89
eye NEC	C69.9-●	C79.49	D09.2	D31.9	D48.7	D49.89
overlapping sites	C69.8	—	—	—	—	—
eyeball	C69.9-●	C79.49	D09.2-●	D31.9-●	D48.7	D49.89
eyebrow	C44.309	C79.2	D04.39	D23.39	D48.5	D49.2
basal cell carcinoma	C44.319	—	—	—	—	—
specified type NEC	C44.399	—	—	—	—	—
squamous cell carcinoma	C44.329	—	—	—	—	—
eyelid (lower) (skin) (upper)	C44.10-●					
basal cell carcinoma	C44.11-●					
cartilage	C49.0	C79.89	—	D21.0	D48.1	D49.2
specified type NEC	C44.19-●					
squamous cell carcinoma	C44.12-●					
face NEC	C76.0	C79.89	D04.39	D36.7	D48.7	D49.89
fallopian tube (accessory)	C57.0-●	C79.82	D07.39	D28.2	D39.8	D49.59
falx (cerebella) (cerebri)	C70.0	C79.32	—	D32.0	D42.0	D49.7

◀ New   ◀ Revised   ~~deleted~~ Deleted   ● Use Additional Character(s)

	Malignant Primary	Malignant Secondary	Ca in situ	Benign	Uncertain Behavior	Unspecified Behavior
fascia — *see also Neoplasm, connective tissue*						
palmar	C49.1-●	C79.89	—	D21.1-●	D48.1	D49.2
plantar	C49.2-●	C79.89	—	D21.2-●	D48.1	D49.2
fatty tissue — *see Neoplasm, connective tissue*						
fauces, faucial NEC	C10.9	C79.89	D00.08	D10.5	D37.05	D49.0
pillars	C09.1	C79.89	D00.08	D10.5	D37.05	D49.0
tonsil	C09.9	C79.89	D00.08	D10.4	D37.05	D49.0
femur (any part)	C40.2-●	—	—	D16.2-●	—	—
fetal membrane	C58	C79.82	D07.0	D26.7	D39.2	D49.59
fibrous tissue — *see Neoplasm, connective tissue*						
fibula (any part)	C40.2-●	C79.51	—	D16.2-●	—	—
filum terminale	C72.0	C79.49	—	D33.4	D43.4	D49.7
finger NEC	C76.4-●	C79.89	D04.6-●	D36.7	D48.7	D49.89
flank NEC	C76.8	C79.89	D04.5	D36.7	D48.7	D49.89
follicle, nabothian	C53.0	C79.82	D06.0	D26.0	D39.0	D49.59
foot NEC	C76.5-●	C79.89	D04.7-●	D36.7	D48.7	D49.89
forearm NEC	C76.4-●	C79.89	D04.6-●	D36.7	D48.7	D49.89
forehead (skin)	C44.309	C79.2	D04.39	D23.39	D48.5	D49.2
basal cell carcinoma	C44.319	—	—	—	—	—
specified type NEC	C44.399	—	—	—	—	—
squamous cell carcinoma	C44.329	—	—	—	—	—
foreskin	C60.0	C79.82	D07.4	D29.0	D40.8	D49.59
fornix						
pharyngeal	C11.3	C79.89	D00.08	D10.6	D37.05	D49.0
vagina	C52	C79.82	D07.2	D28.1	D39.8	D49.59
fossa (of)						
anterior (cranial)	C71.9	C79.31	—	D33.2	D43.2	D49.6
cranial	C71.9	C79.31	—	D33.2	D43.2	D49.6
ischiorectal	C76.3	C79.89	D09.8	D36.7	D48.7	D49.89
middle (cranial)	C71.9	C79.31	—	D33.2	D43.2	D49.6
piriform	C12	C79.89	D00.08	D10.7	D37.05	D49.0
pituitary	C75.1	C79.89	D09.3	D35.2	D44.3	D49.7
posterior (cranial)	C71.9	C79.31	—	D33.2	D43.2	D49.6
pterygoid	C49.0	C79.89	—	D21.0	D48.1	D49.2
pyriform	C12	C79.89	D00.08	D10.7	D37.05	D49.0
Rosenmuller	C11.2	C79.89	D00.08	D10.6	D37.05	D49.0
tonsillar	C09.0	C79.89	D00.08	D10.5	D37.05	D49.0
fourchette	C51.9	C79.82	D07.1	D28.0	D39.8	D49.59
frenulum						
labii — *see Neoplasm, lip, internal*						
linguae	C02.2	C79.89	D00.07	D10.1	D37.02	D49.0

	Malignant Primary	Malignant Secondary	Ca in situ	Benign	Uncertain Behavior	Unspecified Behavior
frontal						
bone	C41.0	C79.51	—	D16.4-●	D48.0	D49.2
lobe, brain	C71.1	C79.31	—	D33.0	D43.0	D49.6
pole	C71.1	C79.31	—	D33.0	D43.0	D49.6
sinus	C31.2	C78.39	D02.3	D14.0	D38.5	D49.1
fundus						
stomach	C16.1	C78.89	D00.2	D13.1	D37.1	D49.0
uterus	C54.3	C79.82	D07.0	D26.1	D39.0	D49.59
gall duct (extrahepatic)	C24.0	C78.89	D01.5	D13.5	D37.6	D49.0
intrahepatic	C22.1	C78.7	D01.5	D13.4	D37.6	D49.0
gallbladder	C23	C78.89	D01.5	D13.5	D37.6	D49.0
overlapping lesion with extrahepatic bile ducts	C24.8	—	—	—	—	—
ganglia — *see also Neoplasm, nerve, peripheral*	C47.9	C79.89	—	D36.10	D48.2	D49.2
basal	C71.0	C79.31	—	D33.0	D43.0	D49.6
cranial nerve	C72.50	C79.49	—	D33.3	D43.3	D49.7
Gartner's duct	C52	C79.82	D07.2	D28.1	D39.8	D49.59
gastric — *see Neoplasm, stomach*						
gastrocolic	C26.9	C78.89	D01.9	D13.9	D37.9	D49.0
gastroesophageal junction	C16.0	C78.89	D00.2	D13.1	D37.1	D49.0
gastrointestinal (tract) NEC	C26.9	C78.89	D01.9	D13.9	D37.9	D49.0
generalized	C80.0	—	—	—	—	—
genital organ or tract						
female NEC	C57.9	C79.82	D07.30	D28.9	D39.9	D49.59
overlapping lesion	C57.8	—	—	—	—	—
specified site NEC	C57.7	C79.82	D07.39	D28.7	D39.8	D49.59
male NEC	C63.9	C79.82	D07.60	D29.9	D40.9	D49.59
overlapping lesion	C63.8	—	—	—	—	—
specified site NEC	C63.7	C79.82	D07.69	D29.8	D40.8	D49.59
genitourinary tract						
female	C57.9	C79.82	D07.30	D28.9	D39.9	D49.59
male	C63.9	C79.82	D07.60	D29.9	D40.9	D49.59
gingiva (alveolar) (marginal)	C03.9	C79.89	D00.03	D10.39	D37.09	D49.0
lower	C03.1	C79.89	D00.03	D10.39	D37.09	D49.0
mandibular	C03.1	C79.89	D00.03	D10.39	D37.09	D49.0
maxillary	C03.0	C79.89	D00.03	D10.39	D37.09	D49.0
upper	C03.0	C79.89	D00.03	D10.39	D37.09	D49.0
gland, glandular (lymphatic) (system) — *see also Neoplasm, lymph gland*						
endocrine NEC	C75.9	C79.89	D09.3	D35.9	D44.9	D49.7
salivary — *see Neoplasm, salivary gland*						

	Malignant Primary	Malignant Secondary	Ca in situ	Benign	Uncertain Behavior	Unspecified Behavior
glans penis	C60.1	C79.82	D07.4	D29.0	D40.8	D49.59
globus pallidus	C71.0	C79.31	—	D33.0	D43.0	D49.6
glomus						
coccygeal	C49.5	C79.89	—	D21.5	D48.1	D49.2
jugularis	C75.5	C79.89	—	D35.6	D44.7	D49.7
glosso-epiglottic fold(s)	C10.1	C79.89	D00.08	D10.5	D37.05	D49.0
glossopalatine fold	C09.1	C79.89	D00.08	D10.5	D37.05	D49.0
glossopharyngeal sulcus	C09.0	C79.89	D00.08	D10.5	D37.05	D49.0
glottis	C32.0	C78.39	D02.0	D14.1	D38.0	D49.1
gluteal region	C76.3	C79.89	D04.5	D36.7	D48.7	D49.89
great vessels NEC	C49.3	C79.89	—	D21.3	D48.1	D49.2
groin NEC	C76.3	C79.89	D04.5	D36.7	D48.7	D49.89
gum	C03.9	C79.89	D00.03	D10.39	D37.09	D49.0
lower	C03.1	C79.89	D00.03	D10.39	D37.09	D49.0
upper	C03.0	C79.89	D00.03	D10.39	D37.09	D49.0
hand NEC	C76.4-●	C79.89	D04.6-●	D36.7	D48.7	D49.89
head NEC	C76.0	C79.89	D04.4	D36.7	D48.7	D49.89
heart	C38.0	C79.89	—	D15.1	D48.7	D49.89
heel NEC	C76.5-●	C79.89	D04.7-●	D36.7	D48.7	D49.89
helix — *see also Neoplasm, skin, ear*	C44.20-●	C79.2	D04.2-●	D23.2-●	D48.5	D49.2
hematopoietic, hemopoietic tissue NEC	C96.9	—	—	—	—	—
specified NEC	C96.Z	—	—	—	—	—
hemisphere, cerebral	C71.0	C79.31	—	D33.0	D43.0	D49.6
hemorrhoidal zone	C21.1	C78.5	D01.3	D12.9	D37.8	D49.0
hepatic — *see also Index to disease, by histology*	C22.9	C78.7	D01.5	D13.4	D37.6	D49.0
duct (bile)	C24.0	C78.89	D01.5	D13.5	D37.6	D49.0
flexure (colon)	C18.3	C78.5	D01.0	D12.3	D37.4	D49.0
primary	C22.8	C78.7	D01.5	D13.4	D37.6	D49.0
hepatobiliary	C24.9	C79.89	D01.5	D13.5	D37.6	D49.0
hepatoblastoma	C22.2	C78.7	D01.5	D13.4	D37.6	D49.0
hepatoma	C22.0	C78.7	D01.5	D13.4	D37.6	D49.0
hilus of lung	C34.0-●	C78.0-●	D02.2-●	D14.3-●	D38.1	D49.1
hip NEC	C76.5-●	C79.89	D04.7-●	D36.7	D48.7	D49.89
hippocampus, brain	C71.2	C79.31	—	D33.0	D43.0	D49.6
humerus (any part)	C40.0-●	C79.51	—	D16.0-●	—	—
hymen	C52	C79.82	D07.2	D28.1	D39.8	D49.59
hypopharynx, hypopharyngeal NEC	C13.9	C79.89	D00.08	D10.7	D37.05	D49.0
overlapping lesion	C13.8	—	—	—	—	—
postcricoid region	C13.0	C79.89	D00.08	D10.7	D37.05	D49.0
posterior wall	C13.2	C79.89	D00.08	D10.7	D37.05	D49.0
pyriform fossa (sinus)	C12	C79.89	D00.08	D10.7	D37.05	D49.0
hypophysis	C75.1	C79.89	D09.3	D35.2	D44.3	D49.7

	Malignant Primary	Malignant Secondary	Ca in situ	Benign	Uncertain Behavior	Unspecified Behavior
hypothalamus	C71.0	C79.31	—	D33.0	D43.0	D49.6
ileocecum, ileocecal (coil) (junction) (valve)	C18.0	C78.5	D01.0	D12.0	D37.4	D49.0
ileum	C17.2	C78.4	D01.49	D13.39	D37.2	D49.0
ilium	C41.4	C79.51	—	D16.8	D48.0	D49.2
immunoproliferative NEC	C88.9	—	—	—	—	—
infraclavicular (region)	C76.1	C79.89	D04.5	D36.7	D48.7	D49.89
inguinal (region)	C76.3	C79.89	D04.5	D36.7	D48.7	D49.89
insula	C71.0	C79.31	—	D33.0	D43.0	D49.6
insular tissue (pancreas)	C25.4	C78.89	D01.7	D13.7	D37.8	D49.0
brain	C71.0	C79.31	—	D33.0	D43.0	D49.6
interarytenoid fold	C13.1	C79.89	D00.08	D10.7	D37.05	D49.0
hypopharyngeal aspect	C13.1	C79.89	D00.08	D10.7	D37.05	D49.0
laryngeal aspect	C32.1	C78.39	D02.0	D14.1	D38.0	D49.1
marginal zone	C13.1	C79.89	D00.08	D10.7	D37.05	D49.0
interdental papillae	C03.9	C79.89	D00.03	D10.39	D37.09	D49.0
lower	C03.1	C79.89	D00.03	D10.39	D37.09	D49.0
upper	C03.0	C79.89	D00.03	D10.39	D37.09	D49.0
internal						
capsule	C71.0	C79.31	—	D33.0	D43.0	D49.6
os (cervix)	C53.0	C79.82	D06.0	D26.0	D39.0	D49.59
intervertebral cartilage or disc	C41.2	C79.51	—	D16.6	D48.0	D49.2
intestine, intestinal	C26.0	C78.80	D01.40	D13.9	D37.8	D49.0
large	C18.9	C78.5	D01.0	D12.6	D37.4	D49.0
appendix	C18.1	C78.5	D01.0	D12.1	D37.3	D49.0
caput coli	C18.0	C78.5	D01.0	D12.0	D37.4	D49.0
cecum	C18.0	C78.5	D01.0	D12.0	D37.4	D49.0
colon	C18.9	C78.5	D01.0	D12.6	D37.4	D49.0
and rectum	C19	C78.5	D01.1	D12.7	D37.5	D49.0
ascending	C18.2	C78.5	D01.0	D12.2	D37.4	D49.0
caput	C18.0	C78.5	D01.0	D12.0	D37.4	D49.0
descending	C18.6	C78.5	D01.0	D12.4	D37.4	D49.0
distal	C18.6	C78.5	D01.0	D12.4	D37.4	D49.0
left	C18.6	C78.5	D01.0	D12.4	D37.4	D49.0
overlapping lesion	C18.8	—	—	—	—	—
pelvic	C18.7	C78.5	D01.0	D12.5	D37.4	D49.0
right	C18.2	C78.5	D01.0	D12.2	D37.4	D49.0
sigmoid (flexure)	C18.7	C78.5	D01.0	D12.5	D37.4	D49.0
transverse	C18.4	C78.5	D01.0	D12.3	D37.4	D49.0
hepatic flexure	C18.3	C78.5	D01.0	D12.3	D37.4	D49.0
ileocecum, ileocecal (coil) (valve)	C18.0	C78.5	D01.0	D12.0	D37.4	D49.0
overlapping lesion	C18.8	—	—	—	—	—

◀ New   ◀◀ Revised   ~~deleted~~ Deleted   ● Use Additional Character(s)

	Malignant Primary	Malignant Secondary	Ca in situ	Benign	Uncertain Behavior	Unspecified Behavior
intestine, intestinal *(Continued)*						
large *(Continued)*						
sigmoid flexure (lower) (upper)	C18.7	C78.5	D01.0	D12.5	D37.4	D49.0
splenic flexure	C18.5	C78.5	D01.0	D12.3	D37.4	D49.0
small	C17.9	C78.4	D01.40	D13.30	D37.2	D49.0
duodenum	C17.0	C78.4	D01.49	D13.2	D37.2	D49.0
ileum	C17.2	C78.4	D01.49	D13.39	D37.2	D49.0
jejunum	C17.1	C78.4	D01.49	D13.39	D37.2	D49.0
overlapping lesion	C17.8	—	—	—	—	—
tract NEC	C26.0	C78.89	D01.40	D13.9	D37.8	D49.0
intra-abdominal	C76.2	C79.89	D09.8	D36.7	D48.7	D49.89
intracranial NEC	C71.9	C79.31	—	D33.2	D43.2	D49.6
intrahepatic (bile) duct	C22.1	C78.7	D01.5	D13.4	D37.6	D49.0
intraocular	C69.9-•	C79.49	D09.2-•	D31.9-•	D48.7	D49.89
intraorbital	C69.6-•	C79.49	D09.2-•	D31.6-•	D48.7	D49.89
intrasellar	C75.1	C79.89	D09.3	D35.2	D44.3	D49.7
intrathoracic (cavity) (organs)	C76.1	C79.89	D09.8	D15.9	D48.7	D49.89
specified NEC	C76.1	C79.89	D09.8	D15.7	—	—
iris	C69.4-•	C79.49	D09.2-•	D31.4-•	D48.7	D49.89
ischiorectal (fossa)	C76.3	C79.89	D09.8	D36.7	D48.7	D49.89
ischium	C41.4	C79.51	—	D16.8	D48.0	D49.2
island of Reil	C71.0	C79.31	—	D33.0	D43.0	D49.6
islands or islets of Langerhans	C25.4	C78.89	D01.7	D13.7	D37.8	D49.0
isthmus uteri	C54.0	C79.82	D07.0	D26.1	D39.0	D49.59
jaw	C76.0	C79.89	D09.8	D36.7	D48.7	D49.89
bone	C41.1	C79.51	—	D16.5-•	D48.0	D49.2
lower	C41.1	C79.51	—	D16.5-•	—	—
upper	C41.0	C79.51	—	D16.4-•	—	—
carcinoma (any type) (lower) (upper)	C76.0	C79.89	—	—	—	—
skin—*see also Neoplasm, skin, face*	C44.309	C79.2	D04.39	D23.39	D48.5	D49.2
soft tissues	C03.9	C79.89	D00.03	D10.39	D37.09	D49.0
lower	C03.1	C79.89	D00.03	D10.39	D37.09	D49.0
upper	C03.0	C79.89	D00.03	D10.39	D37.09	D49.0
jejunum	C17.1	C78.4	D01.49	D13.39	D37.2	D49.0
joint NEC—*see also Neoplasm, bone*	C41.9	C79.51	—	D16.9-•	D48.0	D49.2
acromioclavicular	C40.0-•	C79.51	—	D16.0-•	—	—
bursa or synovial membrane—*see Neoplasm, connective tissue*						
costovertebral	C41.3	C79.51	—	D16.7	D48.0	D49.2
sternocostal	C41.3	C79.51	—	D16.7	D48.0	D49.2
temporomandibular	C41.1	C79.51	—	D16.5-•	D48.0	D49.2

	Malignant Primary	Malignant Secondary	Ca in situ	Benign	Uncertain Behavior	Unspecified Behavior
junction						
anorectal	C21.8	C78.5	D01.3	D12.9	D37.8	D49.0
cardioesophageal	C16.0	C78.89	D00.2	D13.1	D37.1	D49.0
esophagogastric	C16.0	C78.89	D00.2	D13.1	D37.1	D49.0
gastroesophageal	C16.0	C78.89	D00.2	D13.1	D37.1	D49.0
hard and soft palate	C05.9	C79.89	D00.00	D10.39	D37.09	D49.0
ileocecal	C18.0	C78.5	D01.0	D12.0	D37.4	D49.0
pelvirectal	C19	C78.5	D01.1	D12.7	D37.5	D49.0
pelviureteric	C65.-•	C79.0-•	D09.19	D30.1-•	D41.1-•	D49.59
rectosigmoid	C19	C78.5	D01.1	D12.7	D37.5	D49.0
squamocolumnar, of cervix	C53.8	C79.82	D06.7	D26.0	D39.0	D49.59
Kaposi's sarcoma—*see Kaposi's, sarcoma*						
kidney (parenchymal)	C64.-•	C79.0-•	D09.19	D30.0-•	D41.0-•	D49.51-•
calyx	C65.-•	C79.0-•	D09.19	D30.1-•	D41.1-•	D49.51-•
hilus	C65.-•	C79.0-•	D09.19	D30.1-•	D41.1-•	D49.51-•
pelvis	C65.-•	C79.0-•	D09.19	D30.1-•	D41.1-•	D49.51-•
knee NEC	C76.5-•	C79.89	D04.7-•	D36.7	D48.7	D49.89
labia (skin)	C51.9	C79.82	D07.1	D28.0	D39.8	D49.59
majora	C51.0	C79.82	D07.1	D28.0	D39.8	D49.59
minora	C51.1	C79.82	D07.1	D28.0	D39.8	D49.59
labial—*see also Neoplasm, lip*	C00.9	C79.89	D00.01	D10.0	D37.01	D49.0
sulcus (lower) (upper)	C06.1	C79.89	D00.02	D10.39	D37.09	D49.0
labium (skin)	C51.9	C79.82	D07.1	D28.0	D39.8	D49.59
majus	C51.0	C79.82	D07.1	D28.0	D39.8	D49.59
minus	C51.1	C79.82	D07.1	D28.0	D39.8	D49.59
lacrimal						
canaliculi	C69.5-•	C79.49	D09.2-•	D31.5-•	D48.7	D49.89
duct (nasal)	C69.5-•	C79.49	D09.2-•	D31.5-•	D48.7	D49.89
gland	C69.5-•	C79.49	D09.2-•	D31.5-•	D48.7	D49.89
punctum	C69.5-•	C79.49	D09.2-•	D31.5-•	D48.7	D49.89
sac	C69.5-•	C79.49	D09.2-•	D31.5-•	D48.7	D49.89
Langerhans, islands or islets	C25.4	C78.89	D01.7	D13.7	D37.8	D49.0
laryngopharynx	C13.9	C79.89	D00.08	D10.7	D37.05	D49.0
larynx, laryngeal NEC	C32.9	C78.39	D02.0	D14.1	D38.0	D49.1
aryepiglottic fold	C32.1	C78.39	D02.0	D14.1	D38.0	D49.1
cartilage (arytenoid) (cricoid) (cuneiform) (thyroid)	C32.3	C78.39	D02.0	D14.1	D38.0	D49.1
commissure (anterior) (posterior)	C32.0	C78.39	D02.0	D14.1	D38.0	D49.1
extrinsic NEC	C32.1	C78.39	D02.0	D14.1	D38.0	D49.1
meaning hypopharynx	C13.9	C79.89	D00.08	D10.7	D37.05	D49.0
interarytenoid fold	C32.1	C78.39	D02.0	D14.1	D38.0	D49.1
intrinsic	C32.0	C78.39	D02.0	D14.1	D38.0	D49.1

◀ New   ◀ Revised   ~~deleted~~ Deleted   • Use Additional Character(s)

	Malignant Primary	Malignant Secondary	Ca in situ	Benign	Uncertain Behavior	Unspecified Behavior
larynx, laryngeal NEC *(Continued)*						
overlapping lesion	C32.8	—	—	—	—	—
ventricular band	C32.1	C78.39	D02.0	D14.1	D38.0	D49.1
leg NEC	C76.5-●	C79.89	D04.7-●	D36.7	D48.7	D49.89
lens, crystalline	C69.4-●	C79.49	D09.2-●	D31.4-●	D48.7	D49.89
lid (lower) (upper)	C44.10-●	C79.2	D04.1-●	D23.1-●	D48.5	D49.2
basal cell carcinoma	C44.11-●	—	—	—	—	—
specified type NEC	C44.19-●	—	—	—	—	—
squamous cell carcinoma	C44.12-●	—	—	—	—	—
ligament — *see also Neoplasm, connective tissue*						
broad	C57.1	C79.82	D07.39	D28.2	D39.8	D49.59
Mackenrodt's	C57.7	C79.82	D07.39	D28.7	D39.8	D49.59
non-uterine — *see Neoplasm, connective tissue*						
round	C57.2	C79.82	—	D28.2	D39.8	D49.59
sacro-uterine	C57.3	C79.82	—	D28.2	D39.8	D49.59
uterine	C57.3	C79.82	—	D28.2	D39.8	D49.59
utero-ovarian	C57.7	C79.82	D07.39	D28.2	D39.8	D49.59
uterosacral	C57.3	C79.82	—	D28.2	D39.8	D49.59
limb	C76.8	C79.89	D04.8	D36.7	D48.7	D49.89
lower	C76.5-●	C79.89	D04.7-●	D36.7	D48.7	D49.89
upper	C76.4-●	C79.89	D04.6-●	D36.7	D48.7	D49.89
limbus of cornea	C69.1-●	C79.49	D09.2-●	D31.1-●	D48.7	D49.89
lingual NEC — *see also Neoplasm, tongue*	C02.9	C79.89	D00.07	D10.1	D37.02	D49.0
lingula, lung	C34.1-●	C78.0-●	D02.2-●	D14.3-●	D38.1	D49.1
lip	C00.9	C79.89	D00.01	D10.0	D37.01	D49.0
buccal aspect — *see Neoplasm, lip, internal*						
commissure	C00.6	C79.89	D00.01	D10.0	D37.01	D49.0
external	C00.2	C79.89	D00.01	D10.0	D37.01	D49.0
lower	C00.1	C79.89	D00.01	D10.0	D37.01	D49.0
upper	C00.0	C79.89	D00.01	D10.0	D37.01	D49.0
frenulum — *see Neoplasm, lip, internal*						
inner aspect — *see Neoplasm, lip, internal*						
internal	C00.5	C79.89	D00.01	D10.0	D37.01	D49.0
lower	C00.4	C79.89	D00.01	D10.0	D37.01	D49.0
upper	C00.3	C79.89	D00.01	D10.0	D37.01	D49.0
lipstick area	C00.2	C79.89	D00.01	D10.0	D37.01	D49.0
lower	C00.1	C79.89	D00.01	D10.0	D37.01	D49.0
upper	C00.0	C79.89	D00.01	D10.0	D37.01	D49.0

	Malignant Primary	Malignant Secondary	Ca in situ	Benign	Uncertain Behavior	Unspecified Behavior
lip *(Continued)*						
lower	C00.1	C79.89	D00.01	D10.0	D37.01	D49.0
internal	C00.4	C79.89	D00.01	D10.0	D37.01	D49.0
mucosa — *see Neoplasm, lip, internal*						
oral aspect — *see Neoplasm, lip, internal*						
overlapping lesion	C00.8	—	—	—	—	—
with oral cavity or pharynx	C14.8	—	—	—	—	—
skin (commissure) (lower) (upper)	C44.00	C79.2	D04.0	D23.0	D48.5	D49.2
basal cell carcinoma	C44.01	—	—	—	—	—
specified type NEC	C44.09	—	—	—	—	—
squamous cell carcinoma	C44.02	—	—	—	—	—
upper	C00.0	C79.89	D00.01	D10.0	D37.01	D49.0
internal	C00.3	C79.89	D00.01	D10.0	D37.01	D49.0
vermilion border	C00.2	C79.89	D00.01	D10.0	D37.01	D49.0
lower	C00.1	C79.89	D00.01	D10.0	D37.01	D49.0
upper	C00.0	C79.89	D00.01	D10.0	D37.01	D49.0
lipomatous — *see Lipoma, by site*						
liver — *see also Index to disease, by histology*	C22.9	C78.7	D01.5	D13.4	D37.6	D49.0
primary	C22.8	C78.7	D01.5	D13.4	D37.6	D49.0
lumbosacral plexus	C47.5	C79.89	—	D36.16	D48.2	D49.2
lung	C34.9-●	C78.0-●	D02.2-●	D14.3-●	D38.1	D49.1
azygos lobe	C34.1-●	C78.0-●	D02.2-●	D14.3-●	D38.1	D49.1
carina	C34.0-●	C78.0-●	D02.2-●	D14.3-●	D38.1	D49.1
hilus	C34.0-●	C78.0-●	D02.2-●	D14.3-●	D38.1	D49.1
lingula	C34.1-●	C78.0-●	D02.2-●	D14.3-●	D38.1	D49.1
lobe NEC	C34.9-●	C78.0-●	D02.2-●	D14.3-●	D38.1	D49.1
lower lobe	C34.3-●	C78.0-●	D02.2-●	D14.3-●	D38.1	D49.1
main bronchus	C34.0-●	C78.0-●	D02.2-●	D14.3-●	D38.1	D49.1
mesothelioma — *see Mesothelioma*						
middle lobe	C34.2	C78.0-●	D02.21	D14.31	D38.1	D49.1
overlapping lesion	C34.8-●	—	—	—	—	—
upper lobe	C34.1-●	C78.0-●	D02.2-●	D14.3-●	D38.1	D49.1
lymph, lymphatic channel NEC	C49.9	C79.89	—	D21.9	D48.1	D49.2
gland (secondary)	—	C77.9	—	D36.0	D48.7	D49.89
abdominal	—	C77.2	—	D36.0	D48.7	D49.89
aortic	—	C77.2	—	D36.0	D48.7	D49.89
arm	—	C77.3	—	D36.0	D48.7	D49.89
auricular (anterior) (posterior)	—	C77.0	—	D36.0	D48.7	D49.89

◀ New ◀ Revised ~~deleted~~ Deleted ● Use Additional Character(s)

	Malignant Primary	Malignant Secondary	Ca in situ	Benign	Uncertain Behavior	Unspecified Behavior
lymph, lymphatic channel NEC *(Continued)*						
gland *(Continued)*						
axilla, axillary	—	C77.3	—	D36.0	D48.7	D49.89
brachial	—	C77.3	—	D36.0	D48.7	D49.89
bronchial	—	C77.1	—	D36.0	D48.7	D49.89
bronchopulmonary	—	C77.1	—	D36.0	D48.7	D49.89
celiac	—	C77.2	—	D36.0	D48.7	D49.89
cervical	—	C77.0	—	D36.0	D48.7	D49.89
cervicofacial	—	C77.0	—	D36.0	D48.7	D49.89
Cloquet	—	C77.4	—	D36.0	D48.7	D49.89
colic	—	C77.2	—	D36.0	D48.7	D49.89
common duct	—	C77.2	—	D36.0	D48.7	D49.89
cubital	—	C77.3	—	D36.0	D48.7	D49.89
diaphragmatic	—	C77.1	—	D36.0	D48.7	D49.89
epigastric, inferior	—	C77.1	—	D36.0	D48.7	D49.89
epitrochlear	—	C77.3	—	D36.0	D48.7	D49.89
esophageal	—	C77.1	—	D36.0	D48.7	D49.89
face	—	C77.0	—	D36.0	D48.7	D49.89
femoral	—	C77.4	—	D36.0	D48.7	D49.89
gastric	—	C77.2	—	D36.0	D48.7	D49.89
groin	—	C77.4	—	D36.0	D48.7	D49.89
head	—	C77.0	—	D36.0	D48.7	D49.89
hepatic	—	C77.2	—	D36.0	D48.7	D49.89
hilar (pulmonary)	—	C77.1	—	D36.0	D48.7	D49.89
splenic	—	C77.2	—	D36.0	D48.7	D49.89
hypogastric	—	C77.5	—	D36.0	D48.7	D49.89
ileocolic	—	C77.2	—	D36.0	D48.7	D49.89
iliac	—	C77.5	—	D36.0	D48.7	D49.89
infraclavicular	—	C77.3	—	D36.0	D48.7	D49.89
inguina, inguinal	—	C77.4	—	D36.0	D48.7	D49.89
innominate	—	C77.1	—	D36.0	D48.7	D49.89
intercostal	—	C77.1	—	D36.0	D48.7	D49.89
intestinal	—	C77.2	—	D36.0	D48.7	D49.89
intrabdominal	—	C77.2	—	D36.0	D48.7	D49.89
intrapelvic	—	C77.5	—	D36.0	D48.7	D49.89
intrathoracic	—	C77.1	—	D36.0	D48.7	D49.89
jugular	—	C77.0	—	D36.0	D48.7	D49.89
leg	—	C77.4	—	D36.0	D48.7	D49.89
limb						
lower	—	C77.4	—	D36.0	D48.7	D49.89
upper	—	C77.3	—	D36.0	D48.7	D49.89
lower limb	—	C77.4	—	D36.0	D48.7	D49.89
lumbar	—	C77.2	—	D36.0	D48.7	D49.89

	Malignant Primary	Malignant Secondary	Ca in situ	Benign	Uncertain Behavior	Unspecified Behavior
lymph, lymphatic channel NEC *(Continued)*						
gland *(Continued)*						
mandibular	—	C77.0	—	D36.0	D48.7	D49.89
mediastinal	—	C77.1	—	D36.0	D48.7	D49.89
mesenteric (inferior) (superior)	—	C77.2	—	D36.0	D48.7	D49.89
midcolic	—	C77.2	—	D36.0	D48.7	D49.89
multiple sites in categories C77.0 - C77.5	—	C77.8	—	D36.0	D48.7	D49.89
neck	—	C77.0	—	D36.0	D48.7	D49.89
obturator	—	C77.5	—	D36.0	D48.7	D49.89
occipital	—	C77.0	—	D36.0	D48.7	D49.89
pancreatic	—	C77.2	—	D36.0	D48.7	D49.89
para-aortic	—	C77.2	—	D36.0	D48.7	D49.89
paracervical	—	C77.5	—	D36.0	D48.7	D49.89
parametrial	—	C77.5	—	D36.0	D48.7	D49.89
parasternal	—	C77.1	—	D36.0	D48.7	D49.89
parotid	—	C77.0	—	D36.0	D48.7	D49.89
pectoral	—	C77.3	—	D36.0	D48.7	D49.89
pelvic	—	C77.5	—	D36.0	D48.7	D49.89
peri-aortic	—	C77.2	—	D36.0	D48.7	D49.89
peripancreatic	—	C77.2	—	D36.0	D48.7	D49.89
popliteal	—	C77.4	—	D36.0	D48.7	D49.89
porta hepatis	—	C77.2	—	D36.0	D48.7	D49.89
portal	—	C77.2	—	D36.0	D48.7	D49.89
preauricular	—	C77.0	—	D36.0	D48.7	D49.89
prelaryngeal	—	C77.0	—	D36.0	D48.7	D49.89
presymphysial	—	C77.5	—	D36.0	D48.7	D49.89
pretracheal	—	C77.0	—	D36.0	D48.7	D49.89
primary (any site) NEC	C96.9	—	—	—	—	—
pulmonary (hiler)	—	C77.1	—	D36.0	D48.7	D49.89
pyloric	—	C77.2	—	D36.0	D48.7	D49.89
retroperitoneal	—	C77.2	—	D36.0	D48.7	D49.89
retropharyngeal	—	C77.0	—	D36.0	D48.7	D49.89
Rosenmuller's	—	C77.4	—	D36.0	D48.7	D49.89
sacral	—	C77.5	—	D36.0	D48.7	D49.89
scalene	—	C77.0	—	D36.0	D48.7	D49.89
site NEC	—	C77.9	—	D36.0	D48.7	D49.89
splenic (hilar)	—	C77.2	—	D36.0	D48.7	D49.89
subclavicular	—	C77.3	—	D36.0	D48.7	D49.89
subinguinal	—	C77.4	—	D36.0	D48.7	D49.89
sublingual	—	C77.0	—	D36.0	D48.7	D49.89
submandibular	—	C77.0	—	D36.0	D48.7	D49.89

TABLE OF NEOPLASMS

	Malignant Primary	Malignant Secondary	Ca in situ	Benign	Uncertain Behavior	Unspecified Behavior
lymph, lymphatic channel NEC *(Continued)*						
gland *(Continued)*						
submaxillary	—	C77.0	—	D36.0	D48.7	D49.89
submental	—	C77.0	—	D36.0	D48.7	D49.89
subscapular	—	C77.3	—	D36.0	D48.7	D49.89
supraclavicular	—	C77.0	—	D36.0	D48.7	D49.89
thoracic	—	C77.1	—	D36.0	D48.7	D49.89
tibial	—	C77.4	—	D36.0	D48.7	D49.89
tracheal	—	C77.1	—	D36.0	D48.7	D49.89
tracheobronchial	—	C77.1	—	D36.0	D48.7	D49.89
upper limb	—	C77.3	—	D36.0	D48.7	D49.89
Virchow's	—	C77.0	—	D36.0	D48.7	D49.89
node — *see also Neoplasm, lymph gland*						
primary NEC	C96.9	—	—	—	—	—
vessel — *see also Neoplasm, connective tissue*	C49.9	C79.89	—	D21.9	D48.1	D49.2
Mackenrodt's ligament	C57.7	C79.82	D07.39	D28.7	D39.8	D49.59
malar	C41.0	C79.51	—	D16.4-•	D48.0	D49.2
region — *see Neoplasm, cheek*						
mammary gland — *see Neoplasm, breast*						
mandible	C41.1	C79.51	—	D16.5-•	D48.0	D49.2
alveolar						
mucosa (carcinoma)	C03.1	C79.89	D00.03	D10.39	D37.09	D49.0
ridge or process	C41.1	C79.51	—	D16.5-•	D48.0	D49.2
marrow (bone) NEC	C96.9	C79.52	—	—	D47.9	D49.89
mastectomy site (skin) — *see also Neoplasm, breast, skin*	C44.501	C79.2	—	—	—	—
specified as breast tissue	C50.8-•	C79.81	—	—	—	—
mastoid (air cells) (antrum) (cavity)	C30.1	C78.39	D02.3	D14.0	D38.5	D49.1
bone or process	C41.0	C79.51	—	D16.4-•	D48.0	D49.2
maxilla, maxillary (superior)	C41.0	C79.51	—	D16.4-•	D48.0	D49.2
alveolar						
mucosa	C03.0	C79.89	D00.03	D10.39	D37.09	D49.0
ridge or process (carcinoma)	C41.0	C79.51	—	D16.4-•	D48.0	D49.2
antrum	C31.0	C78.39	D02.3	D14.0	D38.5	D49.1
carcinoma	C03.0	C79.51	—	—	—	—
inferior — *see Neoplasm, mandible*						
sinus	C31.0	C78.39	D02.3	D14.0	D38.5	D49.1
meatus external (ear) — *see also Neoplasm, skin, ear*	C44.20-•	C79.2	D04.2-•	D23.2-•	D48.5	D49.2
Meckel diverticulum, malignant	C17.3	C78.4	D01.49	D13.39	D37.2	D49.0

	Malignant Primary	Malignant Secondary	Ca in situ	Benign	Uncertain Behavior	Unspecified Behavior
mediastinum, mediastinal	C38.3	C78.1	—	D15.2	D38.3	D49.89
anterior	C38.1	C78.1	—	D15.2	D38.3	D49.89
posterior	C38.2	C78.1	—	D15.2	D38.3	D49.89
medulla						
adrenal	C74.1-•	C79.7-•	D09.3	D35.0-•	D44.1-•	D49.7
oblongata	C71.7	C79.31	—	D33.1	D43.1	D49.6
meibomian gland	C44.10-•	C79.2	D04.1-•	D23.1-•	D48.5	D49.2
basal cell carcinoma	C44.11-•	—	—	—	—	—
specified type NEC	C44.19-•	—	—	—	—	—
squamous cell carcinoma	C44.12-•	—	—	—	—	—
melanoma — *see Melanoma*						
meninges	C70.9	C79.49	—	D32.9	D42.9	D49.7
brain	C70.0	C79.32	—	D32.0	D42.0	D49.7
cerebral	C70.0	C79.32	—	D32.0	D42.0	D49.7
crainial	C70.0	C79.32	—	D32.0	D42.0	D49.7
intracranial	C70.0	C79.32	—	D32.0	D42.0	D49.7
spinal (cord)	C70.1	C79.49	—	D32.1	D42.1	D49.7
meniscus, knee joint (lateral) (medial)	C40.2-•	C79.51	—	D16.2-•	D48.0	D49.2
Merkel cell — *see Carcinoma, Merkel cell*						
mesentery, mesenteric	C48.1	C78.6	—	D20.1	D48.4	D49.0
mesoappendix	C48.1	C78.6	—	D20.1	D48.4	D49.0
mesocolon	C48.1	C78.6	—	D20.1	D48.4	D49.0
mesopharynx — *see Neoplasm, oropharynx*						
mesosalpinx	C57.1	C79.82	D07.39	D28.2	D39.8	D49.59
mesothelial tissue — *see Mesothelioma*						
mesothelioma — *see Mesothelioma*						
mesovarium	C57.1	C79.82	D07.39	D28.2	D39.8	D49.59
metacarpus (any bone)	C40.1-•	C79.51	—	D16.1-•	—	—
metastatic NEC — *see also Neoplasm, by site, secondary*	—	C79.9	—	—	—	—
metatarsus (any bone)	C40.3-•	C79.51	—	D16.3-•	—	—
midbrain	C71.7	C79.31	—	D33.1	D43.1	D49.6
milk duct — *see Neoplasm, breast*						
mons						
pubis	C51.9	C79.82	D07.1	D28.0	D39.8	D49.59
veneris	C51.9	C79.82	D07.1	D28.0	D39.8	D49.59
motor tract	C72.9	C79.49	—	D33.9	D43.9	D49.7
brain	C71.9	C79.31	—	D33.2	D43.2	D49.6
cauda equina	C72.1	C79.49	—	D33.4	D43.4	D49.7
spinal	C72.0	C79.49	—	D33.4	D43.4	D49.7

◀ New ◀ Revised ~~deleted~~ Deleted • Use Additional Character(s)

TABLE OF NEOPLASMS

	Malignant Primary	Malignant Secondary	Ca in situ	Benign	Uncertain Behavior	Unspecified Behavior
mouth	CØ6.9	C79.89	DØØ.ØØ	D1Ø.3Ø	D37.Ø9	D49.Ø
book-leaf	CØ6.89	C79.89	—	—	—	—
floor	CØ4.9	C79.89	DØØ.Ø6	D1Ø.2	D37.Ø9	D49.Ø
anterior portion	CØ4.Ø	C79.89	DØØ.Ø6	D1Ø.2	D37.Ø9	D49.Ø
lateral portion	CØ4.1	C79.89	DØØ.Ø6	D1Ø.2	D37.Ø9	D49.Ø
overlapping lesion	CØ4.8	—	—	—	—	—
overlapping NEC	CØ6.8Ø	—	—	—	—	—
roof	CØ5.9	C79.89	DØØ.ØØ	D1Ø.39	D37.Ø9	D49.Ø
specified part NEC	CØ6.89	C79.89	DØØ.ØØ	D1Ø.39	D37.Ø9	D49.Ø
vestibule	CØ6.1	C79.89	DØØ.ØØ	D1Ø.39	D37.Ø9	D49.Ø
mucosa						
alveolar (ridge or process)	CØ3.9	C79.89	DØØ.Ø3	D1Ø.39	D37.Ø9	D49.Ø
lower	CØ3.1	C79.89	DØØ.Ø3	D1Ø.39	D37.Ø9	D49.Ø
upper	CØ3.Ø	C79.89	DØØ.Ø3	D1Ø.39	D37.Ø9	D49.Ø
buccal	CØ6.Ø	C79.89	DØØ.Ø2	D1Ø.39	D37.Ø9	D49.Ø
cheek	CØ6.Ø	C79.89	DØØ.Ø2	D1Ø.39	D37.Ø9	D49.Ø
lip — see Neoplasm, lip, internal						
nasal	C3Ø.Ø	C78.39	DØ2.3	D14.Ø	D38.5	D49.1
oral	CØ6.Ø	C79.89	DØØ.Ø2	D1Ø.39	D37.Ø9	D49.Ø
Mullerian duct						
female	C57.7	C79.82	DØ7.39	D28.7	D39.8	D49.59
male	C63.7	C79.82	DØ7.69	D29.8	D4Ø.8	D49.59
muscle — see also Neoplasm, connective tissue						
extraocular	C69.6-●	C79.49	DØ9.2-●	D31.6-●	D48.7	D49.89
myocardium	C38.Ø	C79.89	—	D15.1	D48.7	D49.89
myometrium	C54.2	C79.82	DØ7.Ø	D26.1	D39.Ø	D49.59
myopericardium	C38.Ø	C79.89	—	D15.1	D48.7	D49.89
nabothian gland (follicle)	C53.Ø	C79.82	DØ6.Ø	D26.Ø	D39.Ø	D49.59
nail — see also Neoplasm, skin, limb	C44.9Ø	C79.2	DØ4.9	D23.9	D48.5	D49.2
finger — see also Neoplasm, skin, limb, upper	C44.6Ø-●	C79.2	DØ4.6-●	D23.6-●	D48.5	D49.2
toe — see also Neoplasm, skin, limb, lower	C44.7Ø-●	C79.2	DØ4.7-●	D23.7-●	D48.5	D49.2
nares, naris (anterior) (posterior)	C3Ø.Ø	C78.39	DØ2.3	D14.Ø	D38.5	D49.1
nasal — see Neoplasm, nose						
nasolabial groove — see also Neoplasm, skin, face	C44.3Ø9	C79.2	DØ4.39	D23.39	D48.5	D49.2
nasolacrimal duct	C69.5-●	C79.49	DØ9.2-●	D31.5-●	D48.7	D49.89
nasopharynx, nasopharyngeal	C11.9	C79.89	DØØ.Ø8	D1Ø.6	D37.Ø5	D49.Ø
floor	C11.3	C79.89	DØØ.Ø8	D1Ø.6	D37.Ø5	D49.Ø
overlapping lesion	C11.8	—	—	—	—	—
roof	C11.Ø	C79.89	DØØ.Ø8	D1Ø.6	D37.Ø5	D49.Ø
nasopharynx, nasopharyngeal (Continued) wall	C11.9	C79.89	DØØ.Ø8	D1Ø.6	D37.Ø5	D49.Ø
anterior	C11.3	C79.89	DØØ.Ø8	D1Ø.6	D37.Ø5	D49.Ø
lateral	C11.2	C79.89	DØØ.Ø8	D1Ø.6	D37.Ø5	D49.Ø
posterior	C11.1	C79.89	DØØ.Ø8	D1Ø.6	D37.Ø5	D49.Ø
superior	C11.Ø	C79.89	DØØ.Ø8	D1Ø.6	D37.Ø5	D49.Ø
nates — see also Neoplasm, skin, trunk	C44.5Ø9	C79.2	DØ4.5	D23.5	D48.5	D49.2
neck NEC	C76.Ø	C79.89	DØ9.8	D36.7	D48.7	D49.89
skin	C44.4Ø	—	—	—	—	—
basal cell carcinoma	C44.41	—	—	—	—	—
specified type NEC	C44.49	—	—	—	—	—
squamous cell carcinoma	C44.42	—	—	—	—	—
nerve (ganglion)	C47.9	C79.89	—	D36.1Ø	D48.2	D49.2
abducens	C72.59	C79.49	—	D33.3	D43.3	D49.7
accessory (spinal)	C72.59	C79.49	—	D33.3	D43.3	D49.7
acoustic	C72.4-●	C79.49	—	D33.3	D43.3	D49.7
auditory	C72.4-●	C79.49	—	D33.3	D43.3	D49.7
autonomic NEC — see also Neoplasm, nerve, peripheral	C47.9	C79.89	—	D36.1Ø	D48.2	D49.2
brachial	C47.1-●	C79.89	—	D36.12	D48.2	D49.2
cranial	C72.5Ø	C79.49	—	D33.3	D43.3	D49.7
specified NEC	C72.59	C79.49	—	D33.3	D43.3	D49.7
facial	C72.59	C79.49	—	D33.3	D43.3	D49.7
femoral	C47.2-●	C79.89	—	D36.13	D48.2	D49.2
ganglion NEC — see also Neoplasm, nerve, peripheral	C47.9	C79.89	—	D36.1Ø	D48.2	D49.2
glossopharyngeal	C72.59	C79.49	—	D33.3	D43.3	D49.7
hypoglossal	C72.59	C79.49	—	D33.3	D43.3	D49.7
intercostal	C47.3	C79.89	—	D36.14	D48.2	D49.2
lumbar	C47.6	C79.89	—	D36.17	D48.2	D49.2
median	C47.1-●	C79.89	—	D36.12	D48.2	D49.2
obturator	C47.2-●	C79.89	—	D36.13	D48.2	D49.2
oculomotor	C72.59	C79.49	—	D33.3	D43.3	D49.7
olfactory	C47.2-●	C79.49	—	D33.3	D43.3	D49.7
optic	C72.3-●	C79.49	—	D33.3	D43.3	D49.7
parasympathetic NEC	C47.9	C79.89	—	D36.1Ø	D48.2	D49.2
peripheral NEC	C47.9	C79.89	—	D36.1Ø	D48.2	D49.2
abdomen	C47.4	C79.89	—	D36.15	D48.2	D49.2
abdominal wall	C47.4	C79.89	—	D36.15	D48.2	D49.2
ankle	C47.2-●	C79.89	—	D36.13	D48.2	D49.2

	Malignant Primary	Malignant Secondary	Ca in situ	Benign	Uncertain Behavior	Unspecified Behavior
nerve *(Continued)*						
peripheral NEC *(Continued)*						
antecubital fossa or space	C47.1-●	C79.89	—	D36.12	D48.2	D49.2
arm	C47.1-●	C79.89	—	D36.12	D48.2	D49.2
auricle (ear)	C47.0	C79.89	—	D36.11	D48.2	D49.2
axilla	C47.3	C79.89	—	D36.12	D48.2	D49.2
back	C47.6	C79.89	—	D36.17	D48.2	D49.2
buttock	C47.5	C79.89	—	D36.16	D48.2	D49.2
calf	C47.2-●	C79.89	—	D36.13	D48.2	D49.2
cervical region	C47.0	C79.89	—	D36.11	D48.2	D49.2
cheek	C47.0	C79.89	—	D36.11	D48.2	D49.2
chest (wall)	C47.3	C79.89	—	D36.14	D48.2	D49.2
chin	C47.0	C79.89	—	D36.11	D48.2	D49.2
ear (external)	C47.0	C79.89	—	D36.11	D48.2	D49.2
elbow	C47.1-●	C79.89	—	D36.12	D48.2	D49.2
extrarectal	C47.5	C79.89	—	D36.16	D48.2	D49.2
extremity	C47.9	C79.89	—	D36.10	D48.2	D49.2
lower	C47.2-●	C79.89	—	D36.13	D48.2	D49.2
upper	C47.1-●	C79.89	—	D36.12	D48.2	D49.2
eyelid	C47.0	C79.89	—	D36.11	D48.2	D49.2
face	C47.0	C79.89	—	D36.11	D48.2	D49.2
finger	C47.1-●	C79.89	—	D36.12	D48.2	D49.2
flank	C47.6	C79.89	—	D36.17	D48.2	D49.2
foot	C47.2-●	C79.89	—	D36.13	D48.2	D49.2
forearm	C47.1-●	C79.89	—	D36.12	D48.2	D49.2
forehead	C47.0	C79.89	—	D36.11	D48.2	D49.2
gluteal region	C47.5	C79.89	—	D36.16	D48.2	D49.2
groin	C47.5	C79.89	—	D36.16	D48.2	D49.2
hand	C47.1-●	C79.89	—	D36.12	D48.2	D49.2
head	C47.0	C79.89	—	D36.11	D48.2	D49.2
heel	C47.2-●	C79.89	—	D36.13	D48.2	D49.2
hip	C47.2-●	C79.89	—	D36.13	D48.2	D49.2
infraclavicular region	C47.3	C79.89	—	D36.14	D48.2	D49.2
inguinal (canal) (region)	C47.5	C79.89	—	D36.16	D48.2	D49.2
intrathoracic	C47.3	C79.89	—	D36.14	D48.2	D49.2
ischiorectal fossa	C47.5	C79.89	—	D36.16	D48.2	D49.2
knee	C47.2-●	C79.89	—	D36.13	D48.2	D49.2
leg	C47.2-●	C79.89	—	D36.13	D48.2	D49.2
limb NEC	C47.9	C79.89	—	D36.10	D48.2	D49.2
lower	C47.2-●	C79.89	—	D36.13	D48.2	D49.2
upper	C47.1-●	C79.89	—	D36.12	D48.2	D49.2
nates	C47.5	C79.89	—	D36.16	D48.2	D49.2
neck	C47.0	C79.89	—	D36.11	D48.2	D49.2
orbit	C69.6-●	C79.49	—	D31.6-●	D48.7	D49.2
nerve *(Continued)*						
peripheral NEC *(Continued)*						
pararectal	C47.5	C79.89	—	D36.16	D48.2	D49.2
paraurethral	C47.5	C79.89	—	D36.16	D48.2	D49.2
paravaginal	C47.5	C79.89	—	D36.16	D48.2	D49.2
pelvis (floor)	C47.5	C79.89	—	D36.16	D48.2	D49.2
pelvoabdominal	C47.8	C79.89	—	D36.17	D48.2	D49.2
perineum	C47.5	C79.89	—	D36.16	D48.2	D49.2
perirectal (tissue)	C47.5	C79.89	—	D36.16	D48.2	D49.2
periurethral (tissue)	C47.5	C79.89	—	D36.16	D48.2	D49.2
popliteal fossa or space	C47.2-●	C79.89	—	D36.13	D48.2	D49.2
presacral	C47.5	C79.89	—	D36.16	D48.2	D49.2
pterygoid fossa	C47.0	C79.89	—	D36.11	D48.2	D49.2
rectovaginal septum or wall	C47.5	C79.89	—	D36.16	D48.2	D49.2
rectovesical	C47.5	C79.89	—	D36.16	D48.2	D49.2
sacrococcygeal region	C47.5	C79.89	—	D36.16	D48.2	D49.2
scalp	C47.0	C79.89	—	D36.11	D48.2	D49.2
scapular region	C47.3	C79.89	—	D36.14	D48.2	D49.2
shoulder	C47.1-●	C79.89	—	D36.12	D48.2	D49.2
submental	C47.0	C79.89	—	D36.11	D48.2	D49.2
supraclavicular region	C47.0	C79.89	—	D36.11	D48.2	D49.2
temple	C47.0	C79.89	—	D36.11	D48.2	D49.2
temporal region	C47.0	C79.89	—	D36.11	D48.2	D49.2
thigh	C47.2-●	C79.89	—	D36.13	D48.2	D49.2
thoracic (duct) (wall)	C47.3	C79.89	—	D36.14	D48.2	D49.2
thorax	C47.3	C79.89	—	D36.14	D48.2	D49.2
thumb	C47.1-●	C79.89	—	D36.12	D48.2	D49.2
toe	C47.2-●	C79.89	—	D36.13	D48.2	D49.2
trunk	C47.6	C79.89	—	D36.17	D48.2	D49.2
umbilicus	C47.4	C79.89	—	D36.15	D48.2	D49.2
vesicorectal	C47.5	C79.89	—	D36.16	D48.2	D49.2
wrist	C47.1-●	C79.89	—	D36.12	D48.2	D49.2
radial	C47.1-●	C79.89	—	D36.12	D48.2	D49.2
sacral	C47.5	C79.89	—	D36.16	D48.2	D49.2
sciatic	C47.2-●	C79.89	—	D36.13	D48.2	D49.2
spinal NEC	C47.9	C79.89	—	D36.10	D48.2	D49.2
accessory	C72.59	C79.49	—	D33.3	D43.3	D49.7
sympathetic NEC—*see also* Neoplasm, nerve, peripheral	C47.9	C79.89	—	D36.10	D48.2	D49.2
trigeminal	C72.59	C79.49	—	D33.3	D43.3	D49.7
trochlear	C72.59	C79.49	—	D33.3	D43.3	D49.7
ulnar	C47.1-●	C79.89	—	D36.12	D48.2	D49.2
vagus	C72.59	C79.49	—	D33.3	D43.3	D49.7

◀ New　◀❙ Revised　deleted Deleted　● Use Additional Character(s)

	Malignant Primary	Malignant Secondary	Ca in situ	Benign	Uncertain Behavior	Unspecified Behavior
nervous system (central)	C72.9	C79.40	—	D33.9	D43.9	D49.7
autonomic — see Neoplasm, nerve, peripheral						
parasympathetic — see Neoplasm, nerve, peripheral						
specified site NEC	—	C79.49	—	D33.7	D43.8	—
sympathetic — see Neoplasm, nerve, peripheral						
nevus — see Nevus						
nipple	C50.0-●	C79.81	D05.-●	D24.-●	—	—
nose, nasal	C76.0	C79.89	D09.8	D36.7	D48.7	D49.89
ala (external) (nasi) — see also Neoplasm, nose, skin	C44.301	C79.2	D04.39	D23.39	D48.5	D49.2
bone	C41.0	C79.51	—	D16.4-●	D48.0	D49.2
cartilage	C30.0	C78.39	D02.3	D14.0	D38.5	D49.1
cavity	C30.0	C78.39	D02.3	D14.0	D38.5	D49.1
choana	C11.3	C79.89	D00.08	D10.6	D37.05	D49.0
external (skin) — see also Neoplasm, nose, skin	C44.301	C79.2	D04.39	D23.39	D48.5	D49.2
fossa	C30.0	C78.39	D02.3	D14.0	D38.5	D49.1
internal	C30.0	C78.39	D02.3	D14.0	D38.5	D49.1
mucosa	C30.0	C78.39	D02.3	D14.0	D38.5	D49.1
septum	C30.0	C78.39	D02.3	D14.0	D38.5	D49.1
posterior margin	C11.3	C79.89	D00.08	D10.6	D37.05	D49.0
sinus — see Neoplasm, sinus						
skin	C44.301	C79.2	D04.39	D23.39	D48.5	D49.2
basal cell carcinoma	C44.311	—	—	—	—	—
specified type NEC	C44.391	—	—	—	—	—
squamous cell carcinoma	C44.321	—	—	—	—	—
turbinate (mucosa)	C30.0	C78.39	D02.3	D14.0	D38.5	D49.1
bone	C41.0	C79.51	—	D16.4-●	D48.0	D49.2
vestibule	C30.0	C78.39	D02.3	D14.0	D38.5	D49.1
nostril	C30.0	C78.39	D02.3	D14.0	D38.5	D49.1
nucleus pulposus	C41.2	C79.51	—	D16.6	D48.0	D49.2
occipital						
bone	C41.0	C79.51	—	D16.4-●	D48.0	D49.2
lobe or pole, brain	C71.4	C79.31	—	D33.0	D43.0	D49.6
odontogenic — see Neoplasm, jaw bone						
olfactory nerve or bulb	C72.2-●	C79.49	—	D33.3	D43.3	D49.7
olive (brain)	C71.7	C79.31	—	D33.1	D43.1	D49.6
omentum	C48.1	C78.6	—	D20.1	D48.4	D49.0
operculum (brain)	C71.0	C79.31	—	D33.0	D43.0	D49.6

	Malignant Primary	Malignant Secondary	Ca in situ	Benign	Uncertain Behavior	Unspecified Behavior
optic nerve, chiasm, or tract	C72.3-●	C79.49	—	D33.3	D43.3	D49.7
oral (cavity)	C06.9	C79.89	D00.00	D10.30	D37.09	D49.0
ill-defined	C14.8	C79.89	D00.00	D10.30	D37.09	D49.0
mucosa	C06.0	C79.89	D00.02	D10.39	D37.09	D49.0
orbit	C69.6-●	C79.49	D09.2-●	D31.6-●	D48.7	D49.89
autonomic nerve	C69.6-●	C79.49	—	D31.6-●	D48.7	D49.2
bone	C41.0	C79.51	—	D16.4-●	D48.0	D49.2
eye	C69.6-●	C79.49	D09.2-●	D31.6-●	D48.7	D49.89
peripheral nerves	C69.6-●	C79.49	—	D31.6-●	D48.7	D49.2
soft parts	C69.6-●	C79.49	D09.2-●	D31.6-●	D48.7	D49.89
organ of Zuckerkandl	C75.5	C79.89	—	D35.6	D44.7	D49.7
oropharynx	C10.9	C79.89	D00.08	D10.5	D37.05	D49.0
branchial cleft (vestige)	C10.4	C79.89	D00.08	D10.5	D37.05	D49.0
junctional region	C10.8	C79.89	D00.08	D10.5	D37.05	D49.0
lateral wall	C10.2	C79.89	D00.08	D10.5	D37.05	D49.0
overlapping lesion	C10.8	—	—	—	—	—
pillars or fauces	C09.1	C79.89	D00.08	D10.5	D37.05	D49.0
posterior wall	C10.3	C79.89	D00.08	D10.5	D37.05	D49.0
vallecula	C10.0	C79.89	D00.08	D10.5	D37.05	D49.0
os						
external	C53.1	C79.82	D06.1	D26.0	D39.0	D49.59
internal	C53.0	C79.82	D06.0	D26.0	D39.0	D49.59
ovary	C56.-●	C79.6-●	D07.39	D27.-●	D39.1-●	D49.59
oviduct	C57.0-●	C79.82	D07.39	D28.2	D39.8	D49.59
palate	C05.9	C79.89	D00.00	D10.39	D37.09	D49.0
hard	C05.0	C79.89	D00.05	D10.39	D37.09	D49.0
junction of hard and soft palate	C05.9	C79.89	D00.00	D10.39	D37.09	D49.0
overlapping lesions	C05.8	—	—	—	—	—
soft	C05.1	C79.89	D00.04	D10.39	D37.09	D49.0
nasopharyngeal surface	C11.3	C79.89	D00.08	D10.6	D37.05	D49.0
posterior surface	C11.3	C79.89	D00.08	D10.6	D37.05	D49.0
superior surface	C11.3	C79.89	D00.08	D10.6	D37.05	D49.0
palatoglossal arch	C09.1	C79.89	D00.00	D10.5	D37.09	D49.0
palatopharyngeal arch	C09.1	C79.89	D00.00	D10.5	D37.09	D49.0
pallium	C71.0	C79.31	—	D33.0	D43.0	D49.6
palpebra	C44.10-●	C79.2	D04.1-●	D23.1-●	D48.5	D49.2
basal cell carcinoma	C44.11-●	—	—	—	—	—
specified type NEC	C44.19-●	—	—	—	—	—
squamous cell carcinoma	C44.12-●	—	—	—	—	—
pancreas	C25.9	C78.89	D01.7	D13.6	D37.8	D49.0
body	C25.1	C78.89	D01.7	D13.6	D37.8	D49.0
duct (of Santorini) (of Wirsung)	C25.3	C78.89	D01.7	D13.6	D37.8	D49.0
ectopic tissue	C25.7	C78.89	—	D13.6	D37.8	D49.0
head	C25.0	C78.89	D01.7	D13.6	D37.8	D49.0

◀ New ◀ Revised ~~deleted~~ Deleted ● Use Additional Character(s)

TABLE OF NEOPLASMS

	Malignant Primary	Malignant Secondary	Ca in situ	Benign	Uncertain Behavior	Unspecified Behavior
pancreas *(Continued)*						
islet cells	C25.4	C78.89	D01.7	D13.7	D37.8	D49.0
neck	C25.7	C78.89	D01.7	D13.6	D37.8	D49.0
overlapping lesion	C25.8	—	—	—	—	—
tail	C25.2	C78.89	D01.7	D13.6	D37.8	D49.0
para-aortic body	C75.5	C79.89	—	D35.6	D44.7	D49.7
paraganglion NEC	C75.5	C79.89	—	D35.6	D44.7	D49.7
parametrium	C57.3	C79.82	—	D28.2	D39.8	D49.59
paranephric	C48.0	C78.6	—	D20.0	D48.3	D49.0
pararectal	C76.3	C79.89	—	D36.7	D48.7	D49.89
parasagittal (region)	C76.0	C79.89	D09.8	D36.7	D48.7	D49.89
parasellar	C72.9	C79.49	—	D33.9	D43.8	D49.7
parathyroid (gland)	C75.0	C79.89	D09.3	D35.1	D44.2	D49.7
paraurethral	C76.3	C79.89	—	D36.7	D48.7	D49.89
gland	C68.1	C79.19	D09.19	D30.8	D41.8	D49.59
paravaginal	C76.3	C79.89	—	D36.7	D48.7	D49.89
parenchyma, kidney	C64.-●	C79.0-●	D09.19	D30.0-●	D41.0-●	D49.51-●
parietal						
bone	C41.0	C79.51	—	D16.4-●	D48.0	D49.2
lobe, brain	C71.3	C79.31	—	D33.0	D43.0	D49.6
paroophoron	C57.1	C79.82	D07.39	D28.2	D39.8	D49.59
parotid (duct) (gland)	C07	C79.89	D00.00	D11.0	D37.030	D49.0
parovarium	C57.1	C79.82	D07.39	D28.2	D39.8	D49.59
patella	C40.20	C79.51	—	—	—	—
peduncle, cerebral	C71.7	C79.31	—	D33.1	D43.1	D49.6
pelvirectal junction	C19	C78.5	D01.1	D12.7	D37.5	D49.0
pelvis, pelvic	C76.3	C79.89	D09.8	D36.7	D48.7	D49.89
bone	C41.4	C79.51	—	D16.8	D48.0	D49.2
floor	C76.3	C79.89	D09.8	D36.7	D48.7	D49.89
renal	C65.-●	C79.0-●	D09.19	D30.1-●	D41.1-●	D49.51-●
viscera	C76.3	C79.89	D09.8	D36.7	D48.7	D49.89
wall	C76.3	C79.89	D09.8	D36.7	D48.7	D49.89
pelvo-abdominal	C76.8	C79.89	D09.8	D36.7	D48.7	D49.89
penis	C60.9	C79.82	D07.4	D29.0	D40.8	D49.59
body	C60.2	C79.82	D07.4	D29.0	D40.8	D49.59
corpus (cavernosum)	C60.2	C79.82	D07.4	D29.0	D40.8	D49.59
glans	C60.1	C79.82	D07.4	D29.0	D40.8	D49.59
overlapping sites	C60.8	—	—	—	—	—
skin NEC	C60.9	C79.82	D07.4	D29.0	D40.8	D49.59
periadrenal (tissue)	C48.0	C78.6	—	D20.0	D48.3	D49.0
perianal (skin) — *see also* Neoplasm, anus, skin	C44.500	C79.2	D04.5	D23.5	D48.5	D49.2
pericardium	C38.0	C79.89	—	D15.1	D48.7	D49.89
perinephric	C48.0	C78.6	—	D20.0	D48.3	D49.0

	Malignant Primary	Malignant Secondary	Ca in situ	Benign	Uncertain Behavior	Unspecified Behavior
perineum	C76.3	C79.89	D09.8	D36.7	D48.7	D49.89
periodontal tissue NEC	C03.9	C79.89	D00.03	D10.39	D37.09	D49.0
periosteum — *see Neoplasm, bone*						
peripancreatic	C48.0	C78.6	—	D20.0	D48.3	D49.0
peripheral nerve NEC	C47.9	C79.89	—	D36.10	D48.2	D49.2
perirectal (tissue)	C76.3	C79.89	—	D36.7	D48.7	D49.89
perirenal (tissue)	C48.0	C78.6	—	D20.0	D48.3	D49.0
peritoneum, peritoneal (cavity)	C48.2	C78.6	—	D20.1	D48.4	D49.0
benign mesothelial tissue — *see* Mesothelioma, benign						
overlapping lesion	C48.8	—	—	—	—	—
with digestive organs	C26.9	—	—	—	—	—
parietal	C48.1	C78.6	—	D20.1	D48.4	D49.0
pelvic	C48.1	C78.6	—	D20.1	D48.4	D49.0
specified part NEC	C48.1	C78.6	—	D20.1	D48.4	D49.0
peritonsillar (tissue)	C76.0	C79.89	D09.8	D36.7	D48.7	D49.89
periurethral tissue	C76.3	C79.89	—	D36.7	D48.7	D49.89
phalanges						
foot	C40.3-●	C79.51	—	D16.3-●	—	—
hand	C40.1-●	C79.51	—	D16.1-●	—	—
pharynx, pharyngeal	C14.0	C79.89	D00.08	D10.9	D37.05	D49.0
bursa	C11.1	C79.89	D00.08	D10.6	D37.05	D49.0
fornix	C11.3	C79.89	D00.08	D10.6	D37.05	D49.0
recess	C11.2	C79.89	D00.08	D10.6	D37.05	D49.0
region	C14.0	C79.89	D00.08	D10.9	D37.05	D49.0
tonsil	C11.1	C79.89	D00.08	D10.6	D37.05	D49.0
wall (lateral) (posterior)	C14.0	C79.89	D00.08	D10.9	D37.05	D49.0
pia mater	C70.9	C79.40	—	D32.9	D42.9	D49.7
cerebral	C70.0	C79.32	—	D32.0	D42.0	D49.7
cranial	C70.0	C79.32	—	D32.0	D42.0	D49.7
spinal	C70.1	C79.49	—	D32.1	D42.1	D49.7
pillars of fauces	C09.1	C79.89	D00.08	D10.5	D37.05	D49.0
pineal (body) (gland)	C75.3	C79.89	D09.3	D35.4	D44.5	D49.7
pinna (ear) NEC — *see also* Neoplasm, skin, ear	C44.20-●	C79.2	D04.2-●	D23.2-●	D48.5	D49.2
piriform fossa or sinus	C12	C79.89	D00.08	D10.7	D37.05	D49.0
pituitary (body) (fossa) (gland) (lobe)	C75.1	C79.89	D09.3	D35.2	D44.3	D49.7
placenta	C58	C79.82	D07.0	D26.7	D39.2	D49.59
pleura, pleural (cavity)	C38.4	C78.2	—	D19.0	D38.2	D49.1
overlapping lesion with heart or mediastinum	C38.8	—	—	—	—	—
parietal	C38.4	C78.2	—	D19.0	D38.2	D49.1
visceral	C38.4	C78.2	—	D19.0	D38.2	D49.1

◀ New   ◀▮ Revised   ~~deleted~~ Deleted   ● Use Additional Character(s)

	Malignant Primary	Malignant Secondary	Ca in situ	Benign	Uncertain Behavior	Unspecified Behavior
plexus						
brachial	C47.1-●	C79.89	—	D36.12	D48.2	D49.2
cervical	C47.0	C79.89	—	D36.11	D48.2	D49.2
choroid	C71.5	C79.31	—	D33.0	D43.0	D49.6
lumbosacral	C47.5	C79.89	—	D36.16	D48.2	D49.2
sacral	C47.5	C79.89	—	D36.16	D48.2	D49.2
pluriendocrine	C75.8	C79.89	D09.3	D35.7	D44.9	D49.7
pole						
frontal	C71.1	C79.31	—	D33.0	D43.0	D49.6
occipital	C71.4	C79.31	—	D33.0	D43.0	D49.6
pons (varolii)	C71.7	C79.31	—	D33.1	D43.1	D49.6
popliteal fossa or space	C76.5-●	C79.89	D04.7-●	D36.7	D48.7	D49.89
postcricoid (region)	C13.0	C79.89	D00.08	D10.7	D37.05	D49.0
posterior fossa (cranial)	C71.9	C79.31	—	D33.2	D43.2	D49.6
postnasal space	C11.9	C79.89	D00.08	D10.6	D37.05	D49.0
prepuce	C60.0	C79.82	D07.4	D29.0	D40.8	D49.59
prepylorus	C16.4	C78.89	D00.2	D13.1	D37.1	D49.0
presacral (region)	C76.3	C79.89	—	D36.7	D48.7	D49.89
prostate (gland)	C61	C79.82	D07.5	D29.1	D40.0	D49.59
utricle	C68.0	C79.19	D09.19	D30.4	D41.3	D49.59
pterygoid fossa	C49.0	C79.89	—	D21.0	D48.1	D49.2
pubic bone	C41.4	C79.51	—	D16.8	D48.0	D49.2
pudenda, pudendum (female)	C51.9	C79.82	D07.1	D28.0	D39.8	D49.59
pulmonary—*see also Neoplasm,*						
lung	C34.9-●	C78.0-●	D02.2-●	D14.3-●	D38.1	D49.1
putamen	C71.0	C79.31	—	D33.0	D43.0	D49.6
pyloric						
antrum	C16.3	C78.89	D00.2	D13.1	D37.1	D49.0
canal	C16.4	C78.89	D00.2	D13.1	D37.1	D49.0
pylorus	C16.4	C78.89	D00.2	D13.1	D37.1	D49.0
pyramid (brain)	C71.7	C79.31	—	D33.1	D43.1	D49.6
pyriform fossa or sinus	C12	C79.89	D00.08	D10.7	D37.05	D49.0
radius (any part)	C40.0-●	C79.51	—	D16.0-●	—	—
Rathke's pouch	C75.1	C79.89	D09.3	D35.2	D44.3	D49.7
rectosigmoid (junction)	C19	C78.5	D01.1	D12.7	D37.5	D49.0
overlapping lesion with anus or						
rectum	C21.8	—	—	—	—	—
rectouterine pouch	C48.1	C78.6	—	D20.1	D48.4	D49.0
rectovaginal septum or wall	C76.3	C79.89	D09.8	D36.7	D48.7	D49.89
rectovesical septum	C76.3	C79.89	D09.8	D36.7	D48.7	D49.89
rectum (ampulla)	C20	C78.5	D01.2	D12.8	D37.5	D49.0
and colon	C19	C78.5	D01.1	D12.7	D37.5	D49.0
overlapping lesion with anus or						
rectosigmoid junction	C21.8	—	—	—	—	—

	Malignant Primary	Malignant Secondary	Ca in situ	Benign	Uncertain Behavior	Unspecified Behavior
renal	C64.-●	C79.0-●	D09.19	D30.0-●	D41.0-●	D49.51-●
calyx	C65.-●	C79.0-●	D09.19	D30.1-●	D41.1-●	D49.51-●
hilus	C65.-●	C79.0-●	D09.19	D30.1-●	D41.1-●	D49.51-●
parenchyma	C64.-●	C79.0-●	D09.19	D30.0-●	D41.0-●	D49.51-●
pelvis	C65.-●	C79.0-●	D09.19	D30.1-●	D41.1-●	D49.51-●
respiratory						
organs or system NEC	C39.9	C78.30	D02.4	D14.4	D38.6	D49.1
tract NEC	C39.9	C78.30	D02.4	D14.4	D38.5	D49.1
upper	C39.0	C78.30	D02.4	D14.4	D38.5	D49.1
retina	C69.2-●	C79.49	D09.2-●	D31.2-●	D48.7	D49.81
retrobulbar	C69.6-●	C79.49	—	D31.6-●	D48.7	D49.89
retrocecal	C48.0	C78.6	—	D20.0	D48.3	D49.0
retromolar (area) (triangle)						
(trigone)	C06.2	C79.89	D00.00	D10.39	D37.09	D49.0
retro-orbital	C76.0	C79.89	D09.8	D36.7	D48.7	D49.89
retroperitoneal (space)						
(tissue)	C48.0	C78.6	—	D20.0	D48.3	D49.0
retroperitoneum	C48.0	C78.6	—	D20.0	D48.3	D49.0
retropharyngeal	C14.0	C79.89	D00.08	D10.9	D37.05	D49.0
retrovesical (septum)	C76.3	C79.89	D09.8	D36.7	D48.7	D49.89
rhinencephalon	C71.0	C79.31	—	D33.0	D43.0	D49.6
rib	C41.3	C79.51	—	D16.7	D48.0	D49.2
Rosenmuller's fossa	C11.2	C79.89	D00.08	D10.6	D37.05	D49.0
round ligament	C57.2	C79.82	—	D28.2	D39.8	D49.59
sacrococcyx, sacrococcygeal	C41.4	C79.51	—	D16.8	D48.0	D49.2
region	C76.3	C79.89	D09.8	D36.7	D48.7	D49.89
sacrouterine ligament	C57.3	C79.82	—	D28.2	D39.8	D49.59
sacrum, sacral (vertebra)	C41.4	C79.51	—	D16.8	D48.0	D49.2
salivary gland or duct (major)	C08.9	C79.89	D00.00	D11.9	D37.039	D49.0
minor NEC	C06.9	C79.89	D00.00	D10.39	D37.04	D49.0
overlapping lesion	C08.9	—	—	—	—	—
parotid	C07	C79.89	D00.00	D11.0	D37.030	D49.0
pluriglandular	C08.9	C79.89	D00.00	D11.9	D37.039	D49.0
sublingual	C08.1	C79.89	D00.00	D11.7	D37.031	D49.0
submandibular	C08.0	C79.89	D00.00	D11.7	D37.032	D49.0
submaxillary	C08.0	C79.89	D00.00	D11.7	D37.032	D49.0
salpinx (uterine)	C57.0-●	C79.82	D07.39	D28.2	D39.8	D49.59
Santorini's duct	C25.3	C78.89	D01.7	D13.6	D37.8	D49.0
scalp	C44.40	C79.2	D04.4	D23.4	D48.5	D49.2
basal cell carcinoma	C44.41	—	—	—	—	—
specified type NEC	C44.49	—	—	—	—	—
squamous cell carcinoma	C44.42	—	—	—	—	—
scapula (any part)	C40.0-●	C79.51	—	D16.0-●	—	—
scapular region	C76.1	C79.89	D09.8	D36.7	D48.7	D49.89

◀ New   ◀ Revised   ~~deleted~~ Deleted   ● Use Additional Character(s)

TABLE OF NEOPLASMS

	Malignant Primary	Malignant Secondary	Ca in situ	Benign	Uncertain Behavior	Unspecified Behavior
scar NEC — see also Neoplasm, skin, by site	C44.90	C79.2	D04.9	D23.9	D48.5	D49.2
sciatic nerve	C47.2-●	C79.89	—	D36.13	D48.2	D49.2
sclera	C69.4-●	C79.49	D09.2-●	D31.4-●	D48.7	D49.89
scrotum (skin)	C63.2	C79.82	D07.61	D29.4	D40.8	D49.59
sebaceous gland — see Neoplasm, skin						
sella turcica	C75.1	C79.89	D09.3	D35.2	D44.3	D49.7
bone	C41.0	C79.51	—	D16.4-●	D48.0	D49.2
semilunar cartilage (knee)	C40.2-●	C79.51	—	D16.2-●	D48.0	D49.2
seminal vesicle	C63.7	C79.82	D07.69	D29.8	D40.8	D49.59
septum						
nasal	C30.0	C78.39	D02.3	D14.0	D38.5	D49.1
posterior margin	C11.3	C79.89	D00.08	D10.6	D37.05	D49.0
rectovaginal	C76.3	C79.89	D09.8	D36.7	D48.7	D49.89
rectovesical	C76.3	C79.89	D09.8	D36.7	D48.7	D49.89
urethrovaginal	C57.9	C79.82	D07.30	D28.9	D39.9	D49.59
vesicovaginal	C57.9	C79.82	D07.30	D28.9	D39.9	D49.59
shoulder NEC	C76.4-●	C79.89	D04.6-●	D36.7	D48.7	D49.89
sigmoid flexure (lower) (upper)	C18.7	C78.5	D01.0	D12.5	D37.4	D49.0
sinus (accessory)	C31.9	C78.39	D02.3	D14.0	D38.5	D49.1
bone (any)	C41.0	C79.51	—	D16.4-●	D48.0	D49.2
ethmoidal	C31.1	C78.39	D02.3	D14.0	D38.5	D49.1
frontal	C31.2	C78.39	D02.3	D14.0	D38.5	D49.1
maxillary	C31.0	C78.39	D02.3	D14.0	D38.5	D49.1
nasal, paranasal NEC	C31.9	C78.39	D02.3	D14.0	D38.5	D49.1
overlapping lesion	C31.8	—	—	—	—	—
pyriform	C12	C79.89	D00.08	D10.7	D37.05	D49.0
sphenoid	C31.3	C78.39	D02.3	D14.0	D38.5	D49.1
skeleton, skeletal NEC	C41.9	C79.51	—	D16.9-●	D48.0	D49.2
Skene's gland	C68.1	C79.19	D09.19	D30.8	D41.8	D49.59
skin NOS	C44.90	C79.2	D04.9	D23.9	D48.5	D49.2
abdominal wall	C44.509	C79.2	D04.5	D23.5	D48.5	D49.2
basal cell carcinoma	C44.519	—	—	—	—	—
specified type NEC	C44.599	—	—	—	—	—
squamous cell carcinoma	C44.529	—	—	—	—	—
ala nasi — see also Neoplasm, nose, skin	C44.301	C79.2	D04.39	D23.39	D48.5	D49.2
ankle — see also Neoplasm, skin, limb, lower	C44.70-●	C79.2	D04.7-●	D23.7-●	D48.5	D49.2
antecubital space — see also Neoplasm, skin, limb, upper	C44.60-●	C79.2	D04.6-●	D23.6-●	D48.5	D49.2

skin NOS (Continued)	Malignant Primary	Malignant Secondary	Ca in situ	Benign	Uncertain Behavior	Unspecified Behavior
anus	C44.500	C79.2	D04.5	D23.5	D48.5	D49.2
basal cell carcinoma	C44.510	—	—	—	—	—
specified type NEC	C44.590	—	—	—	—	—
squamous cell carcinoma	C44.520	—	—	—	—	—
arm — see also Neoplasm, skin, limb, upper	C44.60-●	C79.2	D04.6-●	D23.6-●	D48.5	D49.2
auditory canal (external) — see also Neoplasm, skin, ear	C44.20-●	C79.2	D04.2-●	D23.2-●	D48.5	D49.2
auricle (ear) — see also Neoplasm, skin, ear	C44.20-●	C79.2	D04.2-●	D23.2-●	D48.5	D49.2
auricular canal (external) — see also Neoplasm, skin, ear	C44.20-●	C79.2	D04.2-●	D23.2-●	D48.5	D49.2
axilla, axillary fold — see also Neoplasm, skin, trunk	C44.509	C79.2	D04.5	D23.5	D48.5	D49.2
back — see also Neoplasm, skin, trunk	C44.509	C79.2	D04.5	D23.5	D48.5	D49.2
basal cell carcinoma	C44.91					
breast	C44.501	C79.2	D04.5	D23.5	D48.5	D49.2
basal cell carcinoma	C44.511	—	—	—	—	—
specified type NEC	C44.591	—	—	—	—	—
squamous cell carcinoma	C44.521	—	—	—	—	—
brow — see also Neoplasm, skin, face	C44.309	C79.2	D04.39	D23.39	D48.5	D49.2
buttock — see also Neoplasm, skin, trunk	C44.509	C79.2	D04.5	D23.5	D48.5	D49.2
calf — see also Neoplasm, skin, limb, lower	C44.70-●	C79.2	D04.7-●	D23.7-●	D48.5	D49.2
canthus (eye) (inner) (outer)	C44.10-●	C79.2	D04.1-●	D23.1-●	D48.5	D49.2
basal cell carcinoma	C44.11-●	—	—	—	—	—
specified type NEC	C44.19-●	—	—	—	—	—
squamous cell carcinoma	C44.12-●	—	—	—	—	—
cervical region — see also Neoplasm, skin, neck	C44.40	C79.2	D04.4	D23.4	D48.5	D49.2
cheek (external) — see also Neoplasm, skin, face	C44.309	C79.2	D04.39	D23.39	D48.5	D49.2
chest (wall) — see also Neoplasm, skin, trunk	C44.509	C79.2	D04.5	D23.5	D48.5	D49.2
chin — see also Neoplasm, skin, face	C44.309	C79.2	D04.39	D23.39	D48.5	D49.2
clavicular area — see also Neoplasm, skin, trunk	C44.509	C79.2	D04.5	D23.5	D48.5	D49.2
clitoris	C51.2	C79.82	D07.1	D28.0	D39.8	D49.59
columnella — see also Neoplasm, skin, face	C44.309	C79.2	D04.39	D23.39	D48.5	D49.2

◀ New ◀ Revised ~~deleted~~ Deleted ● Use Additional Character(s)

	Malignant Primary	Malignant Secondary	Ca in situ	Benign	Uncertain Behavior	Unspecified Behavior
skin NOS *(Continued)*						
concha — *see also* Neoplasm, skin, ear	C44.20-•	C79.2	D04.2-•	D23.2-•	D48.5	D49.2
ear (external)	C44.20-•	C79.2	D04.2-•	D23.2-•	D48.5	D49.2
basal cell carcinoma	C44.21-•	—	—	—	—	—
specified type NEC	C44.29-•	—	—	—	—	—
squamous cell carcinoma	C44.22-•	—	—	—	—	—
elbow — *see also* Neoplasm, skin, limb, upper	C44.60-•	C79.2	D04.6-•	D23.6-•	D48.5	D49.2
eyebrow — *see also* Neoplasm, skin, face	C44.309	C79.2	D04.39	D23.39	D48.5	D49.2
eyelid	C44.10-•	C79.2	D04.1-•	D23.1-•	D48.5	D49.2
basal cell carcinoma	C44.11-•	—	—	—	—	—
specified type NEC	C44.19-•	—	—	—	—	—
squamous cell carcinoma	C44.12-•	—	—	—	—	—
face NOS	C44.300	C79.2	D04.30	D23.30	D48.5	D49.2
basal cell carcinoma	C44.310	—	—	—	—	—
specified type NEC	C44.390	—	—	—	—	—
squamous cell carcinoma	C44.320	—	—	—	—	—
female genital organs (external)	C51.9	C79.82	D07.1	D28.0	D39.8	D49.59
clitoris	C51.2	C79.82	D07.1	D28.0	D39.8	D49.59
labium NEC	C51.9	C79.82	D07.1	D28.0	D39.8	D49.59
majus	C51.0	C79.82	D07.1	D28.0	D39.8	D49.59
minus	C51.1	C79.82	D07.1	D28.0	D39.8	D49.59
pudendum	C51.9	C79.82	D07.1	D28.0	D39.8	D49.59
vulva	C51.9	C79.82	D07.1	D28.0	D39.8	D49.59
finger — *see also* Neoplasm, skin, limb, upper	C44.60-•	C79.2	D04.6-•	D23.6-•	D48.5	D49.2
flank — *see also* Neoplasm, skin, trunk	C44.509	C79.2	D04.5	D23.5	D48.5	D49.2
foot — *see also* Neoplasm, skin, limb, lower	C44.70-•	C79.2	D04.7-•	D23.7-•	D48.5	D49.2
forearm — *see also* Neoplasm, skin, limb, upper	C44.60-•	C79.2	D04.6-•	D23.6-•	D48.5	D49.2
forehead — *see also* Neoplasm, skin, face	C44.309	C79.2	D04.39	D23.39	D48.5	D49.2
glabella — *see also* Neoplasm, skin, face	C44.309	C79.2	D04.39	D23.39	D48.5	D49.2
gluteal region — *see also* Neoplasm, skin, trunk	C44.509	C79.2	D04.5	D23.5	D48.5	D49.2
groin — *see also* Neoplasm, skin, trunk	C44.509	C79.2	D04.5	D23.5	D48.5	D49.2
hand — *see also* Neoplasm, skin, limb, upper	C44.60-•	C79.2	D04.6-•	D23.6-•	D48.5	D49.2

	Malignant Primary	Malignant Secondary	Ca in situ	Benign	Uncertain Behavior	Unspecified Behavior
skin NOS *(Continued)*						
head NEC — *see also* Neoplasm, skin, scalp	C44.40	C79.2	D04.4	D23.4	D48.5	D49.2
heel — *see also* Neoplasm, skin, limb, lower	C44.70-•	C79.2	D04.7-•	D23.7-•	D48.5	D49.2
helix — *see also* Neoplasm, skin, ear	C44.20-•	C79.2	D04.2-•	D23.2-•	D48.5	D49.2
hip — *see also* Neoplasm, skin, limb, lower	C44.70-•	C79.2	D04.7-•	D23.7-•	D48.5	D49.2
infraclavicular region — *see also* Neoplasm, skin, trunk	C44.509	C79.2	D04.5	D23.5	D48.5	D49.2
inguinal region — *see also* Neoplasm, skin, trunk	C44.509	C79.2	D04.5	D23.5	D48.5	D49.2
jaw — *see also* Neoplasm, skin, face	C44.309	C79.2	D04.39	D23.39	D48.5	D49.2
Kaposi's sarcoma — *see* Kaposi's, sarcoma, skin						
knee — *see also* Neoplasm, skin, limb, lower	C44.70-•	C79.2	D04.7-•	D23.7-•	D48.5	D49.2
labia						
majora	C51.0	C79.82	D07.1	D28.0	D39.8	D49.59
minora	C51.1	C79.82	D07.1	D28.0	D39.8	D49.59
leg — *see also* Neoplasm, skin, limb, lower	C44.70-•	C79.2	D04.7-•	D23.7-•	D48.5	D49.2
lid (lower) (upper)	C44.10-•	C79.2	D04.1-•	D23.1-•	D48.5	D49.2
basal cell carcinoma	C44.11-•	—	—	—	—	—
specified type NEC	C44.19-•	—	—	—	—	—
squamous cell carcinoma	C44.12-•	—	—	—	—	—
limb NEC	C44.90	C79.2	D04.9	D23.9	D48.5	D49.2
basal cell carcinoma	C44.91					
lower	C44.70-•	C79.2	D04.7-•	D23.7-•	D48.5	D49.2
basal cell carcinoma	C44.71-•	—	—	—	—	—
specified type NEC	C44.79-•	—	—	—	—	—
squamous cell carcinoma	C44.72-•	—	—	—	—	—
upper	C44.60-•	C79.2	D04.6-•	D23.6-•	D48.5	D49.2
basal cell carcinoma	C44.61-•	—	—	—	—	—
specified type NEC	C44.69-•	—	—	—	—	—
squamous cell carcinoma	C44.62-•	—	—	—	—	—
lip (lower) (upper)	C44.00	C79.2	D04.0	D23.0	D48.5	D49.2
basal cell carcinoma	C44.01	—	—	—	—	—
specified type NEC	C44.09	—	—	—	—	—
squamous cell carcinoma	C44.02	—	—	—	—	—

◀ New   ◀ Revised   deleted Deleted   • Use Additional Character(s)

TABLE OF NEOPLASMS

	Malignant Primary	Malignant Secondary	Ca in situ	Benign	Uncertain Behavior	Unspecified Behavior
skin NOS *(Continued)*						
male genital organs	C63.9	C79.82	D07.60	D29.9	D40.8	D49.59
penis	C60.9	C79.82	D07.4	D29.0	D40.8	D49.59
prepuce	C60.0	C79.82	D07.4	D29.0	D40.8	D49.59
scrotum	C63.2	C79.82	D07.61	D29.4	D40.8	D49.59
mastectomy site (skin) — *see also Neoplasm, skin, breast*	C44.501	C79.2	—	—	—	—
specified as breast tissue	C50.8-●	C79.81	—	—	—	—
meatus, acoustic (external) — *see also Neoplasm, skin, ear*	C44.20-●	C79.2	D04.2-●	D23.2-●	D48.5	D49.2
melanotic — *see Melanoma*						
Merkel cell — *see Carcinoma, Merkel cell*						
nates — *see also Neoplasm, skin, trunk*	C44.509	C79.2	D04.5	D23.5	D48.5	D49.2
neck	C44.40	C79.2	D04.4	D23.4	D48.5	D49.2
basal cell carcinoma	C44.41	—	—	—	—	—
specified type NEC	C44.49	—	—	—	—	—
squamous cell carcinoma	C44.42	—	—	—	—	—
nevus — *see Nevus, skin*						
nose (external) — *see also Neoplasm, nose, skin*	C44.301	C79.2	D04.39	D23.39	D48.5	D49.2
overlapping lesion	C44.80	—	—	—	—	—
basal cell carcinoma	C44.81	—	—	—	—	—
specified type NEC	C44.89	—	—	—	—	—
squamous cell carcinoma	C44.82	—	—	—	—	—
palm — *see also Neoplasm, skin, limb, upper*	C44.60-●	C79.2	D04.6-●	D23.6-●	D48.5	D49.2
palpebra	C44.10-●	C79.2	D04.1-●	D23.1-●	D48.5	D49.2
basal cell carcinoma	C44.11-●	—	—	—	—	—
specified type NEC	C44.19-●	—	—	—	—	—
squamous cell carcinoma	C44.12-●	—	—	—	—	—
penis NEC	C60.9	C79.82	D07.4	D29.0	D40.8	D49.59
perianal — *see also Neoplasm, skin, anus*	C44.500	C79.2	D04.5	D23.5	D48.5	D49.2
perineum — *see also Neoplasm, skin, anus*	C44.500	C79.2	D04.5	D23.5	D48.5	D49.2
pinna — *see also Neoplasm, skin, ear*	C44.20-●	C79.2	D04.2-●	D23.2-●	D48.5	D49.2
plantar — *see also Neoplasm, skin, limb, lower*	C44.70-●	C79.2	D04.7-●	D23.7-●	D48.5	D49.2
popliteal fossa or space — *see also Neoplasm, skin, limb, lower*	C44.70-●	C79.2	D04.7-●	D23.7-●	D48.5	D49.2
prepuce	C60.0	C79.82	D07.4	D29.0	D40.8	D49.59

	Malignant Primary	Malignant Secondary	Ca in situ	Benign	Uncertain Behavior	Unspecified Behavior
skin NOS *(Continued)*						
pubes — *see also Neoplasm, skin, trunk*	C44.509	C79.2	D04.5	D23.5	D48.5	D49.2
sacrococcygeal region — *see also Neoplasm, skin, trunk*	C44.509	C79.2	D04.5	D23.5	D48.5	D49.2
scalp	C44.40	C79.2	D04.4	D23.4	D48.5	D49.2
basal cell carcinoma	C44.41	—	—	—	—	—
specified type NEC	C44.49	—	—	—	—	—
squamous cell carcinoma	C44.42	—	—	—	—	—
scapular region — *see also Neoplasm, skin, trunk*	C44.509	C79.2	D04.5	D23.5	D48.5	D49.2
scrotum	C63.2	C79.82	D07.61	D29.4	D40.8	D49.59
shoulder — *see also Neoplasm, skin, limb, upper*	C44.60-●	C79.2	D04.6-●	D23.6-●	D48.5	D49.2
sole (foot) — *see also Neoplasm, skin, limb, lower*	C44.70-●	C79.2	D04.7-●	D23.7-●	D48.5	D49.2
specified sites NEC	C44.80	C79.2	D04.8	D23.9	D48.5	D49.2
basal cell carcinoma	C44.81	—	—	—	—	—
specified type NEC	C44.89	—	—	—	—	—
squamous cell carcinoma	C44.82	—	—	—	—	—
specified type NEC	C44.99	—	—	—	—	—
squamous cell carcinoma	C44.92	—	—	—	—	—
submammary fold — *see also Neoplasm, skin, trunk*	C44.509	C79.2	D04.5	D23.5	D48.5	D49.2
supraclavicular region — *see also Neoplasm, skin, neck*	C44.40	C79.2	D04.4	D23.4	D48.5	D49.2
temple — *see also Neoplasm, skin, face*	C44.309	C79.2	D04.39	D23.39	D48.5	D49.2
thigh — *see also Neoplasm, skin, limb, lower*	C44.70-●	C79.2	D04.7-●	D23.7-●	D48.5	D49.2
thoracic wall — *see also Neoplasm, skin, trunk*	C44.509	C79.2	D04.5	D23.5	D48.5	D49.2
thumb — *see also Neoplasm, skin, limb, upper*	C44.60-●	C79.2	D04.6-●	D23.6-●	D48.5	D49.2
toe — *see also Neoplasm, skin, limb, lower*	C44.70-●	C79.2	D04.7-●	D23.7-●	D48.5	D49.2
tragus — *see also Neoplasm, skin, ear*	C44.20-●	C79.2	D04.2-●	D23.2-●	D48.5	D49.2
trunk	C44.509	C79.2	D04.5	D23.5	D48.5	D49.2
basal cell carcinoma	C44.519	—	—	—	—	—
specified type NEC	C44.599	—	—	—	—	—
squamous cell carcinoma	C44.529	—	—	—	—	—
umbilicus — *see also Neoplasm, skin, trunk*	C44.509	C79.2	D04.5	D23.5	D48.5	D49.2

◄ New   ◄ Revised   ~~deleted~~ Deleted   ● Use Additional Character(s)

	Malignant Primary	Malignant Secondary	Ca in situ	Benign	Uncertain Behavior	Unspecified Behavior
skin NOS *(Continued)*						
vulva	C51.9	C79.82	D07.1	D28.0	D39.8	D49.59
overlapping lesion	C51.8	—	—	—	—	—
wrist — *see also Neoplasm, skin, limb, upper*	C44.60-●	C79.2	D04.6-●	D23.6-●	D48.5	D49.2
skull	C41.0	C79.51	—	D16.4-●	D48.0	D49.2
soft parts or tissues — *see Neoplasm, connective tissue*						
specified site NEC	C76.8	C79.89	D09.8	D36.7	D48.7	D49.89
spermatic cord	C63.1-●	C79.82	D07.69	D29.8	D40.8	D49.59
sphenoid	C31.3	C78.39	D02.3	D14.0	D38.5	D49.1
bone	C41.0	C79.51	—	D16.4-●	D48.0	D49.2
sinus	C31.3	C78.39	D02.3	D14.0	D38.5	D49.1
sphincter						
anal	C21.1	C78.5	D01.3	D12.9	D37.8	D49.0
of Oddi	C24.0	C78.89	D01.5	D13.5	D37.6	D49.0
spine, spinal (column)	C41.2	C79.51	—	D16.6	D48.0	D49.2
bulb	C71.7	C79.31	—	D33.1	D43.1	D49.6
coccyx	C41.4	C79.51	—	D16.8	D48.0	D49.2
cord (cervical) (lumbar) (sacral) (thoracic)	C72.0	C79.49	—	D33.4	D43.4	D49.7
dura mater	C70.1	C79.49	—	D32.1	D42.1	D49.7
lumbosacral	C41.2	C79.51	—	D16.6	D48.0	D49.2
marrow NEC	C96.9	C79.52	—	—	D47.9	D49.89
membrane	C70.1	C79.49	—	D32.1	D42.1	D49.7
meninges	C70.1	C79.49	—	D32.1	D42.1	D49.7
nerve (root)	C47.9	C79.89	—	D36.10	D48.2	D49.2
pia mater	C70.1	C79.49	—	D32.1	D42.1	D49.7
root	C47.9	C79.89	—	D36.10	D48.2	D49.2
sacrum	C41.4	C79.51	—	D16.8	D48.0	D49.2
spleen, splenic NEC	C26.1	C78.89	D01.7	D13.9	D37.8	D49.0
flexure (colon)	C18.5	C78.5	D01.0	D12.3	D37.4	D49.0
stem, brain	C71.7	C79.31	—	D33.1	D43.1	D49.6
Stensen's duct	C07	C79.89	D00.00	D11.0	D37.030	D49.0
sternum	C41.3	C79.51	—	D16.7	D48.0	D49.2
stomach	C16.9	C78.89	D00.2	D13.1	D37.1	D49.0
antrum (pyloric)	C16.3	C78.89	D00.2	D13.1	D37.1	D49.0
body	C16.2	C78.89	D00.2	D13.1	D37.1	D49.0
cardia	C16.0	C78.89	D00.2	D13.1	D37.1	D49.0
cardiac orifice	C16.0	C78.89	D00.2	D13.1	D37.1	D49.0
corpus	C16.2	C78.89	D00.2	D13.1	D37.1	D49.0
fundus	C16.1	C78.89	D00.2	D13.1	D37.1	D49.0
greater curvature NEC	C16.6	C78.89	D00.2	D13.1	D37.1	D49.0
lesser curvature NEC	C16.5	C78.89	D00.2	D13.1	D37.1	D49.0

	Malignant Primary	Malignant Secondary	Ca in situ	Benign	Uncertain Behavior	Unspecified Behavior
stomach *(Continued)*						
overlapping lesion	C16.8	—	—	—	—	—
prepylorus	C16.4	C78.89	D00.2	D13.1	D37.1	D49.0
pylorus	C16.4	C78.89	D00.2	D13.1	D37.1	D49.0
wall NEC	C16.9	C78.89	D00.2	D13.1	D37.1	D49.0
anterior NEC	C16.8	C78.89	D00.2	D13.1	D37.1	D49.0
posterior NEC	C16.8	C78.89	D00.2	D13.1	D37.1	D49.0
stroma, endometrial	C54.1	C79.82	D07.0	D26.1	D39.0	D49.59
stump, cervical	C53.8	C79.82	D06.7	D26.0	D39.0	D49.59
subcutaneous (nodule) (tissue) NEC — *see Neoplasm, connective tissue*						
subdural	C70.9	C79.32	—	D32.9	D42.9	D49.7
subglottis, subglottic	C32.2	C78.39	D02.0	D14.1	D38.0	D49.1
sublingual	C04.9	C79.89	D00.06	D10.2	D37.09	D49.0
gland or duct	C08.1	C79.89	D00.00	D11.7	D37.031	D49.0
submandibular gland	C08.0	C79.89	D00.00	D11.7	D37.032	D49.0
submaxillary gland or duct	C08.0	C79.89	D00.00	D11.7	D37.032	D49.0
submental	C76.0	C79.89	D09.8	D36.7	D48.7	D49.89
subpleural	C34.9-●	C78.0-●	D02.2-●	D14.3-●	D38.1	D49.1
substernal	C38.1	C78.1	—	D15.2	D38.3	D49.89
sudoriferous, sudoriparous gland, site unspecified	C44.90	C79.2	D04.9	D23.9	D48.5	D49.2
specified site — *see Neoplasm, skin*						
supraclavicular region	C76.0	C79.89	D09.8	D36.7	D48.7	D49.89
supraglottis	C32.1	C78.39	D02.0	D14.1	D38.0	D49.1
suprarenal	C74.9-●	C79.7-●	D09.3	D35.0-●	D44.1-●	D49.7
capsule	C74.9-●	C79.7-●	D09.3	D35.0-●	D44.1-●	D49.7
cortex	C74.0-●	C79.7-●	D09.3	D35.0-●	D44.1-●	D49.7
gland	C74.9-●	C79.7-●	D09.3	D35.0-●	D44.1-●	D49.7
medulla	C74.1-●	C79.7-●	D09.3	D35.0-●	D44.1-●	D49.7
suprasellar (region)	C71.9	C79.31	—	D33.2	D43.2	D49.6
supratentorial (brain) NEC	C71.0	C79.31	—	D33.0	D43.0	D49.6
sweat gland (apocrine) (eccrine), site unspecified	C44.90	C79.2	D04.9	D23.9	D48.5	D49.2
specified site — *see Neoplasm, skin*						
sympathetic nerve or nervous system NEC	C47.9	C79.89	—	D36.10	D48.2	D49.2
symphysis pubis	C41.4	C79.51	—	D16.8	D48.0	D49.2
synovial membrane — *see Neoplasm, connective tissue*						
tapetum, brain	C71.8	C79.31	—	D33.2	D43.2	D49.6

TABLE OF NEOPLASMS

	Malignant Primary	Malignant Secondary	Ca in situ	Benign	Uncertain Behavior	Unspecified Behavior
tarsus (any bone)	C40.3-●	C79.51	—	D16.3-●	—	—
temple (skin) — see also Neoplasm, skin, face	C44.309	C79.2	D04.39	D23.39	D48.5	D49.2
temporal						
bone	C41.0	C79.51	—	D16.4-●	D48.0	D49.2
lobe or pole	C71.2	C79.31	—	D33.0	D43.0	D49.6
region	C76.0	C79.89	D09.8	D36.7	D48.7	D49.89
skin — see also Neoplasm, skin, face	C44.309	C79.2	D04.39	D23.39	D48.5	D49.2
tendon (sheath) — see Neoplasm, connective tissue						
tentorium (cerebelli)	C70.0	C79.32	—	D32.0	D42.0	D49.7
testis, testes	C62.9-●	C79.82	D07.69	D29.2-●	D40.1-●	D49.59
descended	C62.1-●	C79.82	D07.69	D29.2-●	D40.1-●	D49.59
ectopic	C62.0-●	C79.82	D07.69	D29.2-●	D40.1-●	D49.59
retained	C62.0-●	C79.82	D07.69	D29.2-●	D40.1-●	D49.59
scrotal	C62.1-●	C79.82	D07.69	D29.2-●	D40.1-●	D49.59
undescended	C62.0-●	C79.82	D07.69	D29.2-●	D40.1-●	D49.59
unspecified whether descended or undescended	C62.9-●	C79.82	D07.69	D29.2-●	D40.1-●	D49.59
thalamus	C71.0	C79.31	—	D33.0	D43.0	D49.6
thigh NEC	C76.5-●	C79.89	D04.7-●	D36.7	D48.7	D49.89
thorax, thoracic (cavity) (organs NEC)	C76.1	C79.89	D09.8	D36.7	D48.7	D49.89
duct	C49.3	C79.89	—	D21.3	D48.1	D49.2
wall NEC	C76.1	C79.89	D09.8	D36.7	D48.7	D49.89
throat	C14.0	C79.89	D00.08	D10.9	D37.05	D49.0
thumb NEC	C76.4-●	C79.89	D04.6-●	D36.7	D48.7	D49.89
thymus (gland)	C37	C79.89	D09.3	D15.0	D38.4	D49.89
thyroglossal duct	C73	C79.89	D09.3	D34	D44.0	D49.7
thyroid (gland)	C73	C79.89	D09.3	D34	D44.0	D49.7
cartilage	C32.3	C78.39	D02.0	D14.1	D38.0	D49.1
tibia (any part)	C40.2-●	C79.51	—	D16.2-●	—	—
toe NEC	C76.5-●	C79.89	D04.7-●	D36.7	D48.7	D49.89
tongue	C02.9	C79.89	D00.07	D10.1	D37.02	D49.0
anterior (two-thirds) NEC	C02.3	C79.89	D00.07	D10.1	D37.02	D49.0
dorsal surface	C02.0	C79.89	D00.07	D10.1	D37.02	D49.0
ventral surface	C02.2	C79.89	D00.07	D10.1	D37.02	D49.0
base (dorsal surface)	C01	C79.89	D00.07	D10.1	D37.02	D49.0
border (lateral)	C02.1	C79.89	D00.07	D10.1	D37.02	D49.0
dorsal surface NEC	C02.0	C79.89	D00.07	D10.1	D37.02	D49.0
fixed part NEC	C01	C79.89	D00.07	D10.1	D37.02	D49.0
foreamen cecum	C02.0	C79.89	D00.07	D10.1	D37.02	D49.0
frenulum linguae	C02.2	C79.89	D00.07	D10.1	D37.02	D49.0

	Malignant Primary	Malignant Secondary	Ca in situ	Benign	Uncertain Behavior	Unspecified Behavior
tongue (Continued)						
junctional zone	C02.8	C79.89	D00.07	D10.1	D37.02	D49.0
margin (lateral)	C02.1	C79.89	D00.07	D10.1	D37.02	D49.0
midline NEC	C02.0	C79.89	D00.07	D10.1	D37.02	D49.0
mobile part NEC	C02.3	C79.89	D00.07	D10.1	D37.02	D49.0
overlapping lesion	C02.8	—	—	—	—	—
posterior (third)	C01	C79.89	D00.07	D10.1	D37.02	D49.0
root	C01	C79.89	D00.07	D10.1	D37.02	D49.0
surface (dorsal)	C02.0	C79.89	D00.07	D10.1	D37.02	D49.0
base	C01	C79.89	D00.07	D10.1	D37.02	D49.0
ventral	C02.2	C79.89	D00.07	D10.1	D37.02	D49.0
tip	C02.1	C79.89	D00.07	D10.1	D37.02	D49.0
tonsil	C02.4	C79.89	D00.07	D10.1	D37.02	D49.0
tonsil	C09.9	C79.89	D00.08	D10.4	D37.05	D49.0
fauces, faucial	C09.9	C79.89	D00.08	D10.4	D37.05	D49.0
lingual	C02.4	C79.89	D00.07	D10.1	D37.02	D49.0
overlapping sites	C09.8	—	—	—	—	—
palatine	C09.9	C79.89	D00.08	D10.4	D37.05	D49.0
pharyngeal	C11.1	C79.89	D00.08	D10.6	D37.05	D49.0
pillar (anterior) (posterior)	C09.1	C79.89	D00.08	D10.5	D37.05	D49.0
tonsillar fossa	C09.0	C79.89	D00.08	D10.5	D37.05	D49.0
tooth socket NEC	C03.9	C79.89	D00.03	D10.39	D37.09	D49.0
trachea (cartilage) (mucosa)	C33	C78.39	D02.1	D14.2	D38.1	D49.1
overlapping lesion with bronchus or lung	C34.8-●	—	—	—	—	—
tracheobronchial	C34.8-●	C78.39	D02.1	D14.2	D38.1	D49.1
overlapping lesion with lung	C34.8-●	—	—	—	—	—
tragus — see also Neoplasm, skin, ear	C44.20-●	C79.2	D04.2-●	D23.2-●	D48.5	D49.2
trunk NEC	C76.8	C79.89	D04.5	D36.7	D48.7	D49.89
tubo-ovarian	C57.8	C79.82	D07.39	D28.7	D39.8	D49.59
tunica vaginalis	C63.7	C79.82	D07.69	D29.8	D40.8	D49.59
turbinate (bone)	C41.0	C79.51	—	D16.4-●	D48.0	D49.2
nasal	C30.0	C78.39	D02.3	D14.0	D38.5	D49.1
tympanic cavity	C30.1	C78.39	D02.3	D14.0	D38.5	D49.1
ulna (any part)	C40.0-●	C79.51	—	D16.0-●	—	—
umbilicus, umbilical — see also Neoplasm, skin, trunk	C44.509	C79.2	D04.5	D23.5	D48.5	D49.2
uncus, brain	C71.2	C79.31	—	D33.0	D43.0	D49.6
unknown site or unspecified	C80.1	C79.9	D09.9	D36.9	D48.9	D49.9
urachus	C67.7	C79.11	D09.0	D30.3	D41.4	D49.4
ureter, ureteral	C66.-●	C79.19	D09.19	D30.2-●	D41.2-●	D49.59
orifice (bladder)	C67.6	C79.11	D09.0	D30.3	D41.4	D49.4
ureter-bladder (junction)	C67.6	C79.11	D09.0	D30.3	D41.4	D49.4

◄ New ◀ Revised ~~deleted~~ Deleted ● Use Additional Character(s)

	Malignant Primary	Malignant Secondary	Ca in situ	Benign	Uncertain Behavior	Unspecified Behavior
urethra, urethral (gland)	C68.0	C79.19	D09.19	D30.4	D41.3	D49.59
orifice, internal	C67.5	C79.11	D09.0	D30.3	D41.4	D49.4
urethrovaginal (septum)	C57.9	C79.82	D07.30	D28.9	D39.8	D49.59
urinary organ or system	C68.9	C79.10	D09.10	D30.9	D41.9	D49.59
bladder — see Neoplasm, bladder						
overlapping lesion	C68.8	—	—	—	—	—
specified sites NEC	C68.8	C79.19	D09.19	D30.8	D41.8	D49.59
utero-ovarian	C57.8	C79.82	D07.39	D28.7	D39.8	D49.59
ligament	C57.1	C79.82	D07.39	D28.2	D39.8	D49.59
uterosacral ligament	C57.3	C79.82	—	D28.2	D39.8	D49.59
uterus, uteri, uterine	C55	C79.82	D07.0	D26.9	D39.0	D49.59
adnexa NEC	C57.4	C79.82	D07.39	D28.7	D39.8	D49.59
body	C54.9	C79.82	D07.0	D26.1	D39.0	D49.59
cervix	C53.9	C79.82	D06.9	D26.0	D39.0	D49.59
cornu	C54.9	C79.82	D07.0	D26.1	D39.0	D49.59
corpus	C54.9	C79.82	D07.0	D26.1	D39.0	D49.59
endocervix (canal) (gland)	C53.0	C79.82	D06.0	D26.0	D39.0	D49.59
endometrium	C54.1	C79.82	D07.0	D26.1	D39.0	D49.59
exocervix	C53.1	C79.82	D06.1	D26.0	D39.0	D49.59
external os	C53.1	C79.82	D06.1	D26.0	D39.0	D49.59
fundus	C54.3	C79.82	D07.0	D26.1	D39.0	D49.59
internal os	C53.0	C79.82	D06.0	D26.0	D39.0	D49.59
isthmus	C54.0	C79.82	D07.0	D26.1	D39.0	D49.59
ligament	C57.3	C79.82	—	D28.2	D39.8	D49.59
broad	C57.1	C79.82	D07.39	D28.2	D39.8	D49.59
round	C57.2	C79.82	—	D28.2	D39.8	D49.59
lower segment	C54.0	C79.82	D07.0	D26.1	D39.0	D49.59
myometrium	C54.2	C79.82	D07.0	D26.1	D39.0	D49.59
overlapping sites	C54.8	—	—	—	—	—
squamocolumnar junction	C53.8	C79.82	D06.7	D26.0	D39.0	D49.59
tube	C57.0-●	C79.82	D07.39	D28.2	D39.8	D49.59
utricle, prostatic	C68.0	C79.19	D09.19	D30.4	D41.3	D49.59
uveal tract	C69.4-●	C79.49	D09.2-●	D31.4-●	D48.7	D49.89
uvula	C05.2	C79.89	D00.04	D10.39	D37.09	D49.0
vagina, vaginal (fornix) (vault) (wall)	C52	C79.82	D07.2	D28.1	D39.8	D49.59
vaginovesical	C57.9	C79.82	D07.30	D28.9	D39.9	D49.59
septum	C57.9	C79.82	D07.30	D28.9	D39.9	D49.59
vallecula (epigiottis)	C10.0	C79.89	D00.08	D10.5	D37.05	D49.0
vas deferens	C63.1-●	C79.82	D07.69	D29.8	D40.8	D49.59
vascular — see Neoplasm, connective tissue						

	Malignant Primary	Malignant Secondary	Ca in situ	Benign	Uncertain Behavior	Unspecified Behavior
Vater's ampulla	C24.1	C78.89	D01.5	D13.5	D37.6	D49.0
vein, venous — see Neoplasm, connective tissue						
vena cava (abdominal) (inferior)	C49.4	C79.89	—	D21.4	D48.1	D49.2
superior	C49.3	C79.89	—	D21.3	D48.1	D49.2
ventricle (cerebral) (floor) (lateral) (third)	C71.5	C79.31	—	D33.0	D43.0	D49.6
cardiac (left) (right)	C38.0	C79.89	—	D15.1	D48.7	D49.89
fourth	C71.7	C79.31	—	D33.1	D43.1	D49.6
ventricular band of larynx	C32.1	C78.39	D02.0	D14.1	D38.0	D49.1
ventriculus — see Neoplasm, stomach						
vermillion border — see Neoplasm, lip						
vermis, cerebellum	C71.6	C79.31	—	D33.1	D43.1	D49.6
vertebra (column)	C41.2	C79.51	—	D16.6	D48.0	D49.2
coccyx	C41.4	C79.51	—	D16.8-●	D48.0	D49.2
marrow NEC	C96.9	C79.52	—	D47.9	D49.89
sacrum	C41.4	C79.51	—	D16.8-●	D48.0	D49.2
vesical — see Neoplasm, bladder						
vesicle, seminal	C63.7	C79.82	D07.69	D29.8	D40.8	D49.59
vesicocervical tissue	C57.9	C79.82	D07.30	D28.9	D39.9	D49.59
vesicorectal	C76.3	C79.82	D09.8	D36.7	D48.7	D49.89
vesicovaginal	C57.9	C79.82	D07.30	D28.9	D39.9	D49.59
septum	C57.9	C79.82	D07.30	D28.9	D39.8	D49.59
vessel (blood) — see Neoplasm, connective tissue						
vestibular gland, greater	C51.0	C79.82	D07.1	D28.0	D39.8	D49.59
vestibule						
mouth	C06.1	C79.89	D00.00	D10.39	D37.09	D49.0
nose	C30.0	C78.39	D02.3	D14.0	D38.5	D49.1
Virchow's gland	C77.0	C77.0	—	D36.0	D48.7	D49.89
viscera NEC	C76.8	C79.89	D09.8	D36.7	D48.7	D49.89
vocal cords (true)	C32.0	C78.39	D02.0	D14.1	D38.0	D49.1
false	C32.1	C78.39	D02.0	D14.1	D38.0	D49.1
vomer	C41.0	C79.51	—	D16.4-●	D48.0	D49.2
vulva	C51.9	C79.82	D07.1	D28.0	D39.8	D49.59
vulvovaginal gland	C51.0	C79.82	D07.1	D28.0	D39.8	D49.59
Waldeyer's ring	C14.2	C79.89	D00.08	D10.9	D37.05	D49.0
Wharton's duct	C08.0	C79.89	D00.00	D11.7	D37.032	D49.0
white matter (central) (cerebral)	C71.0	C79.31	—	D33.0	D43.0	D49.6
windpipe	C33	C78.39	D02.1	D14.2	D38.1	D49.1

TABLE OF NEOPLASMS

	Malignant Primary	Malignant Secondary	Ca in situ	Benign	Uncertain Behavior	Unspecified Behavior
Wirsung's duct	C25.3	C78.89	D01.7	D13.6	D37.8	D49.0
wolffian (body) (duct)						
female	C57.7	C79.82	D07.39	D28.7	D39.8	D49.59
male	C63.7	C79.82	D07.69	D29.8	D40.8	D49.59

	Malignant Primary	Malignant Secondary	Ca in situ	Benign	Uncertain Behavior	Unspecified Behavior
womb — *see Neoplasm, uterus*						
wrist NEC	C76.4-●	C79.89	D04.6-●	D36.7	D48.7	D49.89
xiphoid process	C41.3	C79.51	—	D16.7	D48.0	D49.2
Zuckerkandl organ	C75.5	C79.89	—	D35.6	D44.7	D49.7

◀ New　◀ Revised　deleted Deleted　● Use Additional Character(s)

ICD-10-CM
Table of Drugs and Chemicals

Substance	Poisoning, Accidental (Unintentional)	Poisoning, Intentional Self-Harm	Poisoning, Assault	Poisoning, Undetermined	Adverse Effect	Underdosing
			#			
1-propanol	T51.3X1	T51.3X2	T51.3X3	T51.3X4	—	—
2-propanol	T51.2X1	T51.2X2	T51.2X3	T51.2X4	—	—
2,4-D (dichlorophen-oxyacetic acid)	T60.3X1	T60.3X2	T60.3X3	T60.3X4	—	—
2,4-toluene diisocyanate	T65.0X1	T65.0X2	T65.0X3	T65.0X4	—	—
2,4,5-T (trichloro-phenoxyacetic acid)	T60.1X1	T60.1X2	T60.1X3	T60.1X4	—	—
14-hydroxydihydro-morphinone	T40.2X1	T40.2X2	T40.2X3	T40.2X4	T40.2X5	T40.2X6
			A			
ABOB	T37.5X1	T37.5X2	T37.5X3	T37.5X4	T37.5X5	T37.5X6
Abrine	T62.2X1	T62.2X2	T62.2X3	T62.2X4		
Abrus (seed)	T62.2X1	T62.2X2	T62.2X3	T62.2X4	—	—
Absinthe	T51.0X1	T51.0X2	T51.0X3	T51.0X4	—	—
beverage	T51.0X1	T51.0X2	T51.0X3	T51.0X4	—	—
Acaricide	T60.8X1	T60.8X2	T60.8X3	T60.8X4	—	—
Acebutolol	T44.7X1	T44.7X2	T44.7X3	T44.7X4	T44.7X5	T44.7X6
Acecarbromal	T42.6X1	T42.6X2	T42.6X3	T42.6X4	T42.6X5	T42.6X6
Aceclidine	T44.1X1	T44.1X2	T44.1X3	T44.1X4	T44.1X5	T44.1X6
Acedapsone	T37.0X1	T37.0X2	T37.0X3	T37.0X4	T37.0X5	T37.0X6
Acefylline piperazine	T48.6X1	T48.6X2	T48.6X3	T48.6X4	T48.6X5	T48.6X6
Acemorphan	T40.2X1	T40.2X2	T40.2X3	T40.2X4	T40.2X5	T40.2X6
Acenocoumarin	T45.511	T45.512	T45.513	T45.514	T45.515	T45.516
Acenocoumarol	T45.511	T45.512	T45.513	T45.514	T45.515	T45.516
Acepifylline	T48.6X1	T48.6X2	T48.6X3	T48.6X4	T48.6X5	T48.6X6
Acepromazine	T43.3X1	T43.3X2	T43.3X3	T43.3X4	T43.3X5	T43.3X6
Acesulfamethoxypyridazine	T37.0X1	T37.0X2	T37.0X3	T37.0X4	T37.0X5	T37.0X6
Acetal	T52.8X1	T52.8X2	T52.8X3	T52.8X4	—	—
Acetaldehyde (vapor)	T52.8X1	T52.8X2	T52.8X3	T52.8X4	—	—
liquid	T65.891	T65.892	T65.893	T65.894	—	—
P-Acetamidophenol	T39.1X1	T39.1X2	T39.1X3	T39.1X4	T39.1X5	T39.1X6
Acetaminophen	T39.1X1	T39.1X2	T39.1X3	T39.1X4	T39.1X5	T39.1X6
Acetaminosalol	T39.1X1	T39.1X2	T39.1X3	T39.1X4	T39.1X5	T39.1X6
Acetanilide	T39.1X1	T39.1X2	T39.1X3	T39.1X4	T39.1X5	T39.1X6
Acetarsol	T37.3X1	T37.3X2	T37.3X3	T37.3X4	T37.3X5	T37.3X6
Acetazolamide	T50.2X1	T50.2X2	T50.2X3	T50.2X4	T50.2X5	T50.2X6
Acetiamine	T45.2X1	T45.2X2	T45.2X3	T45.2X4	T45.2X5	T45.2X6
Acetic						
acid	T54.2X1	T54.2X2	T54.2X3	T54.2X4		
with sodium acetate (ointment)	T49.3X1	T49.3X2	T49.3X3	T49.3X4	T49.3X5	T49.3X6

Substance	Poisoning, Accidental (Unintentional)	Poisoning, Intentional Self-Harm	Poisoning, Assault	Poisoning, Undetermined	Adverse Effect	Underdosing
Acetic *(Continued)*						
acid *(Continued)*						
ester (solvent) (vapor)	T52.8X1	T52.8X2	T52.8X3	T52.8X4	—	—
irrigating solution	T50.3X1	T50.3X2	T50.3X3	T50.3X4	T50.3X5	T50.3X6
medicinal (lotion)	T49.2X1	T49.2X2	T49.2X3	T49.2X4	T49.2X5	T49.2X6
anhydride	T65.891	T65.892	T65.893	T65.894	—	—
ether (vapor)	T52.8X1	T52.8X2	T52.8X3	T52.8X4		
Acetohexamide	T38.3X1	T38.3X2	T38.3X3	T38.3X4	T38.3X5	T38.3X6
Acetohydroxamic acid	T50.991	T50.992	T50.993	T50.994	T50.995	T50.996
Acetomenaphthone	T45.7X1	T45.7X2	T45.7X3	T45.7X4	T45.7X5	T45.7X6
Acetomorphine	T40.1X1	T40.1X2	T40.1X3	T40.1X4		
Acetone (oils)	T52.4X1	T52.4X2	T52.4X3	T52.4X4	—	—
chlorinated	T52.4X1	T52.4X2	T52.4X3	T52.4X4	—	—
vapor	T52.4X1	T52.4X2	T52.4X3	T52.4X4		
Acetonitrile	T52.8X1	T52.8X2	T52.8X3	T52.8X4	—	—
Acetophenazine	T43.3X1	T43.3X2	T43.3X3	T43.3X4	T43.3X5	T43.3X6
Acetophenetedin	T39.1X1	T39.1X2	T39.1X3	T39.1X4	T39.1X5	T39.1X6
Acetophenone	T52.4X1	T52.4X2	T52.4X3	T52.4X4	—	—
Acetorphine	T40.2X1	T40.2X2	T40.2X3	T40.2X4		
Acetosulfone (sodium)	T37.1X1	T37.1X2	T37.1X3	T37.1X4	T37.1X5	T37.1X6
Acetrizoate (sodium)	T50.8X1	T50.8X2	T50.8X3	T50.8X4	T50.8X5	T50.8X6
Acetylcarbromal	T42.6X1	T42.6X2	T42.6X3	T42.6X4	T42.6X5	T42.6X6
Acetrizoic acid	T50.8X1	T50.8X2	T50.8X3	T50.8X4	T50.8X5	T50.8X6
Acetyl						
bromide	T53.6X1	T53.6X2	T53.6X3	T53.6X4	—	—
chloride	T53.6X1	T53.6X2	T53.6X3	T53.6X4	—	—
Acetylcholine						
chloride	T44.1X1	T44.1X2	T44.1X3	T44.1X4	T44.1X5	T44.1X6
derivative	T44.1X1	T44.1X2	T44.1X3	T44.1X4	T44.1X5	T44.1X6
Acetylcysteine	T48.4X1	T48.4X2	T48.4X3	T48.4X4	T48.4X5	T48.4X6
Acetyldigitoxin	T46.0X1	T46.0X2	T46.0X3	T46.0X4	T46.0X5	T46.0X6
Acetyldigoxin	T46.0X1	T46.0X2	T46.0X3	T46.0X4	T46.0X5	T46.0X6
Acetyldihydrocodeine	T40.2X1	T40.2X2	T40.2X3	T40.2X4	—	—
Acetyldihydrocodeinone	T40.2X1	T40.2X2	T40.2X3	T40.2X4	—	—
Acetylene (gas)	T59.891	T59.892	T59.893	T59.894	—	—
dichloride	T53.6X1	T53.6X2	T53.6X3	T53.6X4	—	—
incomplete combustion of	T58.11	T58.12	T58.13	T58.14	—	—
industrial	T59.891	T59.892	T59.893	T59.894	—	—
tetrachloride	T53.6X1	T53.6X2	T53.6X3	T53.6X4	—	—
vapor	T53.6X1	T53.6X2	T53.6X3	T53.6X4	—	—
Acetylphenylhydrazine	T39.8X1	T39.8X2	T39.8X3	T39.8X4	T39.8X5	T39.8X6
Acetylpheneturide	T42.6X1	T42.6X2	T42.6X3	T42.6X4	T42.6X5	T42.6X6

◄ New ◄ Revised ~~deleted~~ Deleted

TABLE OF DRUGS AND CHEMICALS

TABLE OF DRUGS AND CHEMICALS

Substance	External Cause (T-Code)					
	Poisoning, Accidental (Unintentional)	Poisoning, Intentional Self-Harm	Poisoning, Assault	Poisoning, Undetermined	Adverse Effect	Underdosing
Acetylsalicylic acid (salts)	T39.011	T39.012	T39.013	T39.014	T39.015	T39.016
enteric coated	T39.011	T39.012	T39.013	T39.014	T39.015	T39.016
Acetylsulfamethoxypyridazine	T37.0X1	T37.0X2	T37.0X3	T37.0X4	T37.0X5	T37.0X6
Achromycin	T36.4X1	T36.4X2	T36.4X3	T36.4X4	T36.4X5	T36.4X6
ophthalmic preparation	T49.5X1	T49.5X2	T49.5X3	T49.5X4	T49.5X5	T49.5X6
topical NEC	T49.0X1	T49.0X2	T49.0X3	T49.0X4	T49.0X5	T49.0X6
Aciclovir	T37.5X1	T37.5X2	T37.5X3	T37.5X4	T37.5X5	T37.5X6
Acid (corrosive) NEC	T54.2X1	T54.2X2	T54.2X3	T54.2X4	—	—
Acidifying agent NEC	T50.901	T50.902	T50.903	T50.904	T50.905	T50.906
Acipimox	T46.6X1	T46.6X2	T46.6X3	T46.6X4	T46.6X5	T46.6X6
Acitretin	T50.991	T50.992	T50.993	T50.994	T50.995	T50.996
Aclarubicin	T45.1X1	T45.1X2	T45.1X3	T45.1X4	T45.1X5	T45.1X6
Aclatonium napadisilate	T48.1X1	T48.1X2	T48.1X3	T48.1X4	T48.1X5	T48.1X6
Aconite (wild)	T46.991	T46.992	T46.993	T46.994	T46.995	T46.996
Aconitine	T46.991	T46.992	T46.993	T46.994	T46.995	T46.996
Aconitum ferox	T46.991	T46.992	T46.993	T46.994	T46.995	T46.996
Acridine	T65.6X1	T65.6X2	T65.6X3	T65.6X4	—	—
vapor	T59.891	T59.892	T59.893	T59.894	—	—
Acriflavine	T37.91	T37.92	T37.93	T37.94	T37.95	T37.96
Acriflavinium chloride	T49.0X1	T49.0X2	T49.0X3	T49.0X4	T49.0X5	T49.0X6
Acrinol	T49.0X1	T49.0X2	T49.0X3	T49.0X4	T49.0X5	T49.0X6
Acrisorcin	T49.0X1	T49.0X2	T49.0X3	T49.0X4	T49.0X5	T49.0X6
Acrivastine	T45.0X1	T45.0X2	T45.0X3	T45.0X4	T45.0X5	T45.0X6
Acrolein (gas)	T59.891	T59.892	T59.893	T59.894	—	—
liquid	T54.1X1	T54.1X2	T54.1X3	T54.1X4	—	—
Acrylamide	T65.891	T65.892	T65.893	T65.894	—	—
Acrylic resin	T49.3X1	T49.3X2	T49.3X3	T49.3X4	T49.3X5	T49.3X6
Acrylonitrile	T65.891	T65.892	T65.893	T65.894	—	—
Actaea spicata	T62.2X1	T62.2X2	T62.2X3	T62.2X4	—	—
berry	T62.1X1	T62.1X2	T62.1X3	T62.1X4	—	—
Acterol	T37.3X1	T37.3X2	T37.3X3	T37.3X4	T37.3X5	T37.3X6
ACTH	T38.811	T38.812	T38.813	T38.814	T38.815	T38.816
Actinomycin C	T45.1X1	T45.1X2	T45.1X3	T45.1X4	T45.1X5	T45.1X6
Actinomycin D	T45.1X1	T45.1X2	T45.1X3	T45.1X4	T45.1X5	T45.1X6
Activated charcoal — see also Charcoal, medicinal	T47.6X1	T47.6X2	T47.6X3	T47.6X4	T47.6X5	T47.6X6
Acyclovir	T37.5X1	T37.5X2	T37.5X3	T37.5X4	T37.5X5	T37.5X6
Adenine	T45.2X1	T45.2X2	T45.2X3	T45.2X4	T45.2X5	T45.2X6
arabinoside	T37.5X1	T37.5X2	T37.5X3	T37.5X4	T37.5X5	T37.5X6
Adenosine (phosphate)	T46.2X1	T46.2X2	T46.2X3	T46.2X4	T46.2X5	T46.2X6
ADH	T38.891	T38.892	T38.893	T38.894	T38.895	T38.896
Adhesive NEC	T65.891	T65.892	T65.893	T65.894	—	—

Substance	External Cause (T-Code)					
	Poisoning, Accidental (Unintentional)	Poisoning, Intentional Self-Harm	Poisoning, Assault	Poisoning, Undetermined	Adverse Effect	Underdosing
Adicillin	T36.0X1	T36.0X2	T36.0X3	T36.0X4	T36.0X5	T36.0X6
Adiphenine	T44.3X1	T44.3X2	T44.3X3	T44.3X4	T44.3X5	T44.3X6
Adipiodone	T50.8X1	T50.8X2	T50.8X3	T50.8X4	T50.8X5	T50.8X6
Adjunct, pharmaceutical	T50.901	T50.902	T50.903	T50.904	T50.905	T50.906
Adrenal (extract, cortex or medulla) (glucocorticoids) (hormones) (mineralo corticoids)	T38.0X1	T38.0X2	T38.0X3	T38.0X4	T38.0X5	T38.0X6
ENT agent	T49.6X1	T49.6X2	T49.6X3	T49.6X4	T49.6X5	T49.6X6
ophthalmic preparation	T49.5X1	T49.5X2	T49.5X3	T49.5X4	T49.5X5	T49.5X6
topical NEC	T49.0X1	T49.0X2	T49.0X3	T49.0X4	T49.0X5	T49.0X6
Adrenaline	T44.5X1	T44.5X2	T44.5X3	T44.5X4	T44.5X5	T44.5X6
Adrenalin — see Adrenaline						
Adrenergic NEC	T44.901	T44.902	T44.903	T44.904	T44.905	T44.906
blocking agent NEC	T44.8X1	T44.8X2	T44.8X3	T44.8X4	T44.8X5	T44.8X6
beta, heart	T44.7X1	T44.7X2	T44.7X3	T44.7X4	T44.7X5	T44.7X6
specified NEC	T44.991	T44.992	T44.993	T44.994	T44.995	T44.996
Adrenochrome						
(mono) semicarbazone	T46.991	T46.992	T46.993	T46.994	T46.995	T46.996
derivative	T46.991	T46.992	T46.993	T46.994	T46.995	T46.996
Adrenocorticotrophic hormone	T38.811	T38.812	T38.813	T38.814	T38.815	T38.816
Adrenocorticotrophin	T38.811	T38.812	T38.813	T38.814	T38.815	T38.816
Adriamycin	T45.1X1	T45.1X2	T45.1X3	T45.1X4	T45.1X5	T45.1X6
Aerosol spray NEC	T65.91	T65.92	T65.93	T65.94	—	—
Aerosporin	T36.8X1	T36.8X2	T36.8X3	T36.8X4	T36.8X5	T36.8X6
ENT agent	T49.6X1	T49.6X2	T49.6X3	T49.6X4	T49.6X5	T49.6X6
ophthalmic preparation	T49.5X1	T49.5X2	T49.5X3	T49.5X4	T49.5X5	T49.5X6
topical NEC	T49.0X1	T49.0X2	T49.0X3	T49.0X4	T49.0X5	T49.0X6
Aethusa cynapium	T62.2X1	T62.2X2	T62.2X3	T62.2X4	—	—
Afghanistan black	T40.7X1	T40.7X2	T40.7X3	T40.7X4	T40.7X5	T40.7X6
Aflatoxin	T64.01	T64.02	T64.03	T64.04	—	—
Afloqualone	T42.8X1	T42.8X2	T42.8X3	T42.8X4	T42.8X5	T42.8X6
African boxwood	T62.2X1	T62.2X2	T62.2X3	T62.2X4	—	—
Agar	T47.4X1	T47.4X2	T47.4X3	T47.4X4	T47.4X5	T47.4X6
Agonist						
predominantly						
alpha-adrenoreceptor	T44.4X1	T44.4X2	T44.4X3	T44.4X4	T44.4X5	T44.4X6
beta-adrenoreceptor	T44.5X1	T44.5X2	T44.5X3	T44.5X4	T44.5X5	T44.5X6
Agricultural agent NEC	T65.91	T65.92	T65.93	T65.94	—	—
Agrypnal	T42.3X1	T42.3X2	T42.3X3	T42.3X4	T42.3X5	T42.3X6
AHLG	T50.Z11	T50.Z12	T50.Z13	T50.Z14	T50.Z15	T50.Z16
Air contaminant(s), source/type NOS	T65.91	T65.92	T65.93	T65.94	—	—

◀ New   ◀ Revised   ~~deleted~~ Deleted

Substance	Poisoning, Accidental (Unintentional)	Poisoning, Intentional Self-Harm	Poisoning, Assault	Poisoning, Undetermined	Adverse Effect	Underdosing
Ajmaline	T46.2X1	T46.2X2	T46.2X3	T46.2X4	T46.2X5	T46.2X6
Akritoin	T37.8X1	T37.8X2	T37.8X3	T37.8X4	T37.8X5	T37.8X6
Akee	T62.1X1	T62.1X2	T62.1X3	T62.1X4	—	—
Akrinol	T49.0X1	T49.0X2	T49.0X3	T49.0X4	T49.0X5	T49.0X6
Alacepril	T46.4X1	T46.4X2	T46.4X3	T46.4X4	T46.4X5	T46.4X6
Alantolactone	T37.4X1	T37.4X2	T37.4X3	T37.4X4	T37.4X5	T37.4X6
Albamycin	T36.8X1	T36.8X2	T36.8X3	T36.8X4	T36.8X5	T36.8X6
Albendazole	T37.4X1	T37.4X2	T37.4X3	T37.4X4	T37.4X5	T37.4X6
Albumin						
bovine	T45.8X1	T45.8X2	T45.8X3	T45.8X4	T45.8X5	T45.8X6
human serum	T45.8X1	T45.8X2	T45.8X3	T45.8X4	T45.8X5	T45.8X6
salt-poor	T45.8X1	T45.8X2	T45.8X3	T45.8X4	T45.8X5	T45.8X6
normal human serum	T45.8X1	T45.8X2	T45.8X3	T45.8X4	T45.8X5	T45.8X6
Albuterol	T48.6X1	T48.6X2	T48.6X3	T48.6X4	T48.6X5	T48.6X6
Albutoin	T42.0X1	T42.0X2	T42.0X3	T42.0X4	T42.0X5	T42.0X6
Alclometasone	T49.0X1	T49.0X2	T49.0X3	T49.0X4	T49.0X5	T49.0X6
Alcohol	T51.91	T51.92	T51.93	T51.94	—	—
absolute	T51.0X1	T51.0X2	T51.0X3	T51.0X4	—	—
beverage	T51.0X1	T51.0X2	T51.0X3	T51.0X4	—	—
allyl	T51.8X1	T51.8X2	T51.8X3	T51.8X4	—	—
amyl	T51.3X1	T51.3X2	T51.3X3	T51.3X4	—	—
antifreeze	T51.1X1	T51.1X2	T51.1X3	T51.1X4	—	—
beverage	T51.0X1	T51.0X2	T51.0X3	T51.0X4	—	—
butyl	T51.3X1	T51.3X2	T51.3X3	T51.3X4	—	—
dehydrated	T51.0X1	T51.0X2	T51.0X3	T51.0X4	—	—
beverage	T51.0X1	T51.0X2	T51.0X3	T51.0X4	—	—
denatured	T51.0X1	T51.0X2	T51.0X3	T51.0X4	—	—
deterrent NEC	T50.6X1	T50.6X2	T50.6X3	T50.6X4	T50.6X5	T50.6X6
diagnostic (gastric function)	T50.8X1	T50.8X2	T50.8X3	T50.8X4	T50.8X5	T50.8X6
ethyl	T51.0X1	T51.0X2	T51.0X3	T51.0X4	—	—
beverage	T51.0X1	T51.0X2	T51.0X3	T51.0X4	—	—
grain	T51.0X1	T51.0X2	T51.0X3	T51.0X4	—	—
beverage	T51.0X1	T51.0X2	T51.0X3	T51.0X4	—	—
industrial	T51.0X1	T51.0X2	T51.0X3	T51.0X4	—	—
isopropyl	T51.2X1	T51.2X2	T51.2X3	T51.2X4	—	—
methyl	T51.1X1	T51.1X2	T51.1X3	T51.1X4	—	—
preparation for consumption	T51.0X1	T51.0X2	T51.0X3	T51.0X4	—	—
propyl	T51.3X1	T51.3X2	T51.3X3	T51.3X4	—	—
secondary	T51.2X1	T51.2X2	T51.2X3	T51.2X4	—	—
radiator	T51.1X1	T51.1X2	T51.1X3	T51.1X4	—	—
rubbing	T51.2X1	T51.2X2	T51.2X3	T51.2X4	—	—
specified type NEC	T51.8X1	T51.8X2	T51.8X3	T51.8X4	—	—

Substance	Poisoning, Accidental (Unintentional)	Poisoning, Intentional Self-Harm	Poisoning, Assault	Poisoning, Undetermined	Adverse Effect	Underdosing
Alcohol (Continued)						
surgical	T51.0X1	T51.0X2	T51.0X3	T51.0X4	—	—
vapor (from any type of Alcohol)	T59.891	T59.892	T59.893	T59.894	—	—
wood	T51.1X1	T51.1X2	T51.1X3	T51.1X4	—	—
Alcuronium (chloride)	T48.1X1	T48.1X2	T48.1X3	T48.1X4	T48.1X5	T48.1X6
Aldactone	T50.0X1	T50.0X2	T50.0X3	T50.0X4	T50.0X5	T50.0X6
Aldesulfone sodium	T37.1X1	T37.1X2	T37.1X3	T37.1X4	T37.1X5	T37.1X6
Aldicarb	T60.0X1	T60.0X2	T60.0X3	T60.0X4		
Aldomet	T46.5X1	T46.5X2	T46.5X3	T46.5X4	T46.5X5	T46.5X6
Aldosterone	T50.0X1	T50.0X2	T50.0X3	T50.0X4	T50.0X5	T50.0X6
Aldrin (dust)	T60.1X1	T60.1X2	T60.1X3	T60.1X4		
Aleve — see Naproxen						
Alexitol sodium	T47.1X1	T47.1X2	T47.1X3	T47.1X4	T47.1X5	T47.1X6
Alfacalcidol	T45.2X1	T45.2X2	T45.2X3	T45.2X4	T45.2X5	T45.2X6
Alfadolone	T41.1X1	T41.1X2	T41.1X3	T41.1X4	T41.1X5	T41.1X6
Alfaxalone	T41.1X1	T41.1X2	T41.1X3	T41.1X4	T41.1X5	T41.1X6
Alfentanil	T40.4X1	T40.4X2	T40.4X3	T40.4X4	T40.4X5	T40.4X6
Alfuzosin (hydrochloride)	T44.8X1	T44.8X2	T44.8X3	T44.8X4	T44.8X5	T44.8X6
Algae (harmful) (toxin)	T65.821	T65.822	T65.823	T65.824	—	—
Algeldrate	T47.1X1	T47.1X2	T47.1X3	T47.1X4	T47.1X5	T47.1X6
Algin	T47.8X1	T47.8X2	T47.8X3	T47.8X4	T47.8X5	T47.8X6
Alglucerase	T45.3X1	T45.3X2	T45.3X3	T45.3X4	T45.3X5	T45.3X6
Alidase	T45.3X1	T45.3X2	T45.3X3	T45.3X4	T45.3X5	T45.3X6
Alimemazine	T43.3X1	T43.3X2	T43.3X3	T43.3X4	T43.3X5	T43.3X6
Aliphatic thiocyanates	T65.0X1	T65.0X2	T65.0X3	T65.0X4	—	—
Alizapride	T45.0X1	T45.0X2	T45.0X3	T45.0X4	T45.0X5	T45.0X6
Alkali (caustic)	T54.3X1	T54.3X2	T54.3X3	T54.3X4	—	—
Alkalizing agent NEC	T50.901	T50.902	T50.903	T50.904	T50.905	T50.906
Alkaline antiseptic solution (aromatic)	T49.6X1	T49.6X2	T49.6X3	T49.6X4	T49.6X5	T49.6X6
Alkalinizing agents (medicinal)	T50.901	T50.902	T50.903	T50.904	T50.905	T50.906
Alka-seltzer	T39.011	T39.012	T39.013	T39.014	T39.015	T39.016
Alkavervir	T46.5X1	T46.5X2	T46.5X3	T46.5X4	T46.5X5	T46.5X6
Alkonium (bromide)	T49.0X1	T49.0X2	T49.0X3	T49.0X4	T49.0X5	T49.0X6
Alkylating drug NEC	T45.1X1	T45.1X2	T45.1X3	T45.1X4	T45.1X5	T45.1X6
antimyeloproliferative	T45.1X1	T45.1X2	T45.1X3	T45.1X4	T45.1X5	T45.1X6
lymphatic	T45.1X1	T45.1X2	T45.1X3	T45.1X4	T45.1X5	T45.1X6
Alkylisocyanate	T65.0X1	T65.0X2	T65.0X3	T65.0X4	—	—
Allantoin	T49.411	T49.412	T49.413	T49.414	T49.415	T49.416
Allegron	T43.0X1	T43.0X2	T43.0X3	T43.0X4	T43.0X5	T43.0X6
Allethrin	T49.0X1	T49.0X2	T49.0X3	T49.0X4	T49.0X5	T49.0X6
Allobarbital	T42.3X1	T42.3X2	T42.3X3	T42.3X4	T42.3X5	T42.3X6

TABLE OF DRUGS AND CHEMICALS

TABLE OF DRUGS AND CHEMICALS

Substance	Poisoning, Accidental (Unintentional)	Poisoning, Intentional Self-Harm	Poisoning, Assault	Poisoning, Undetermined	Adverse Effect	Underdosing
Allopurinol	T50.4X1	T50.4X2	T50.4X3	T50.4X4	T50.4X5	T50.4X6
Allyl						
alcohol	T51.8X1	T51.8X2	T51.8X3	T51.8X4	—	—
disulfide	T46.6X1	T46.6X2	T46.6X3	T46.6X4	T46.6X5	T46.6X6
Allylestrenol	T38.5X1	T38.5X2	T38.5X3	T38.5X4	T38.5X5	T38.5X6
Allylisopropylacetylurea	T42.6X1	T42.6X2	T42.6X3	T42.6X4	T42.6X5	T42.6X6
Allylisopropylmalonylurea	T42.3X1	T42.3X2	T42.3X3	T42.3X4	T42.3X5	T42.3X6
Allylthiourea	T49.3X1	T49.3X2	T49.3X3	T49.3X4	T49.3X5	T49.3X6
Allyltribromide	T42.6X1	T42.6X2	T42.6X3	T42.6X4	T42.6X5	T42.6X6
Allypropymal	T42.3X1	T42.3X2	T42.3X3	T42.3X4	T42.3X5	T42.3X6
Almagate	T47.1X1	T47.1X2	T47.1X3	T47.1X4	T47.1X5	T47.1X6
Almasilate	T47.1X1	T47.1X2	T47.1X3	T47.1X4	T47.1X5	T47.1X6
Almitrine	T50.7X1	T50.7X2	T50.7X3	T50.7X4	T50.7X5	T50.7X6
Aloes	T47.2X1	T47.2X2	T47.2X3	T47.2X4	T47.2X5	T47.2X6
Aloglutamol	T47.1X1	T47.1X2	T47.1X3	T47.1X4	T47.1X5	T47.1X6
Aloin	T47.2X1	T47.2X2	T47.2X3	T47.2X4	T47.2X5	T47.2X6
Aloxidone	T42.2X1	T42.2X2	T42.2X3	T42.2X4	T42.2X5	T42.2X6
Alpha						
acetyldigoxin	T46.0X1	T46.0X2	T46.0X3	T46.0X4	T46.0X5	T46.0X6
adrenergic blocking drug	T44.6X1	T44.6X2	T44.6X3	T44.6X4	T44.6X5	T44.6X6
amylase	T45.3X1	T45.3X2	T45.3X3	T45.3X4	T45.3X5	T45.3X6
tocoferol (acetate)	T45.2X1	T45.2X2	T45.2X3	T45.2X4	T45.2X5	T45.2X6
tocopherol	T45.2X1	T45.2X2	T45.2X3	T45.2X4	T45.2X5	T45.2X6
Alphadolone	T41.1X1	T41.1X2	T41.1X3	T41.1X4	T41.1X5	T41.1X6
Alphaprodine	T40.4X1	T40.4X2	T40.4X3	T40.4X4	T40.4X5	T40.4X6
Alphaxalone	T41.1X1	T41.1X2	T41.1X3	T41.1X4	T41.1X5	T41.1X6
Alprazolam	T42.4X1	T42.4X2	T42.4X3	T42.4X4	T42.4X5	T42.4X6
Alprenolol	T44.7X1	T44.7X2	T44.7X3	T44.7X4	T44.7X5	T44.7X6
Alprostadil	T46.7X1	T46.7X2	T46.7X3	T46.7X4	T46.7X5	T46.7X6
Alsactide	T38.811	T38.812	T38.813	T38.814	T38.815	T38.816
Alseroxylon	T46.5X1	T46.5X2	T46.5X3	T46.5X4	T46.5X5	T46.5X6
Alteplase	T45.611	T45.612	T45.613	T45.614	T45.615	T45.616
Altizide	T50.2X1	T50.2X2	T50.2X3	T50.2X4	T50.2X5	T50.2X6
Altretamine	T45.1X1	T45.1X2	T45.1X3	T45.1X4	T45.1X5	T45.1X6
Alum (medicinal)	T49.4X1	T49.4X2	T49.4X3	T49.4X4	T49.4X5	T49.4X6
nonmedicinal (ammonium) (potassium)	T56.891	T56.892	T56.893	T56.894	—	—
Aluminium, aluminum						
acetate	T49.2X1	T49.2X2	T49.2X3	T49.2X4	T49.2X5	T49.2X6
solution	T49.0X1	T49.0X2	T49.0X3	T49.0X4	T49.0X5	T49.0X6
aspirin	T39.011	T39.012	T39.013	T39.014	T39.015	T39.016
bis (acetylsalicylate)	T39.011	T39.012	T39.013	T39.014	T39.015	T39.016

Substance	Poisoning, Accidental (Unintentional)	Poisoning, Intentional Self-Harm	Poisoning, Assault	Poisoning, Undetermined	Adverse Effect	Underdosing
Aluminium, aluminum (Continued)						
carbonate (gel, basic)	T47.1X1	T47.1X2	T47.1X3	T47.1X4	T47.1X5	T47.1X6
chlorhydroxide-complex	T47.1X1	T47.1X2	T47.1X3	T47.1X4	T47.1X5	T47.1X6
chloride	T49.2X1	T49.2X2	T49.2X3	T49.2X4	T49.2X5	T49.2X6
clofibrate	T46.6X1	T46.6X2	T46.6X3	T46.6X4	T46.6X5	T46.6X6
diacetate	T49.2X1	T49.2X2	T49.2X3	T49.2X4	T49.2X5	T49.2X6
glycinate	T47.1X1	T47.1X2	T47.1X3	T47.1X4	T47.1X5	T47.1X6
hydroxide (gel)	T47.1X1	T47.1X2	T47.1X3	T47.1X4	T47.1X5	T47.1X6
hydroxide-magnesium carb. gel	T47.1X1	T47.1X2	T47.1X3	T47.1X4	T47.1X5	T47.1X6
magnesium silicate	T47.1X1	T47.1X2	T47.1X3	T47.1X4	T47.1X5	T47.1X6
nicotinate	T46.7X1	T46.7X2	T46.7X3	T46.7X4	T46.7X5	T46.7X6
ointment (surgical) (topical)	T49.3X1	T49.3X2	T49.3X3	T49.3X4	T49.3X5	T49.3X6
phosphate	T47.1X1	T47.1X2	T47.1X3	T47.1X4	T47.1X5	T47.1X6
salicylate	T39.091	T39.092	T39.093	T39.094	T39.095	T39.096
silicate	T47.1X1	T47.1X2	T47.1X3	T47.1X4	T47.1X5	T47.1X6
sodium silicate	T47.1X1	T47.1X2	T47.1X3	T47.1X4	T47.1X5	T47.1X6
subacetate	T49.2X1	T49.2X2	T49.2X3	T49.2X4	T49.2X5	T49.2X6
sulfate	T49.0X1	T49.0X2	T49.0X3	T49.0X4	T49.0X5	T49.0X6
tannate	T47.6X1	T47.6X2	T47.6X3	T47.6X4	T47.6X5	T47.6X6
topical NEC	T49.3X1	T49.3X2	T49.3X3	T49.3X4	T49.3X5	T49.3X6
Alurate	T42.3X1	T42.3X2	T42.3X3	T42.3X4	T42.3X5	T42.3X6
Alverine	T44.3X1	T44.3X2	T44.3X3	T44.3X4	T44.3X5	T44.3X6
Alvodine	T40.2X1	T40.2X2	T40.2X3	T40.2X4	T40.2X5	T40.2X6
Amanita phalloides	T62.0X1	T62.0X2	T62.0X3	T62.0X4	—	—
Amanitine	T62.0X1	T62.0X2	T62.0X3	T62.0X4	—	—
Amantadine	T42.8X1	T42.8X2	T42.8X3	T42.8X4	T42.8X5	T42.8X6
Ambazone	T49.6X1	T49.6X2	T49.6X3	T49.6X4	T49.6X5	T49.6X6
Ambenonium (chloride)	T44.0X1	T44.0X2	T44.0X3	T44.0X4	T44.0X5	T44.0X6
Ambroxol	T48.4X1	T48.4X2	T48.4X3	T48.4X4	T48.4X5	T48.4X6
Ambuphylline	T48.6X1	T48.6X2	T48.6X3	T48.6X4	T48.6X5	T48.6X6
Ambutonium bromide	T44.3X1	T44.3X2	T44.3X3	T44.3X4	T44.3X5	T44.3X6
Amcinonide	T49.0X1	T49.0X2	T49.0X3	T49.0X4	T49.0X5	T49.0X6
Amdinocilline	T36.0X1	T36.0X2	T36.0X3	T36.0X4	T36.0X5	T36.0X6
Ametazole	T50.8X1	T50.8X2	T50.8X3	T50.8X4	T50.8X5	T50.8X6
Amethocaine	T41.3X1	T41.3X2	T41.3X3	T41.3X4	T41.3X5	T41.3X6
regional	T41.3X1	T41.3X2	T41.3X3	T41.3X4	T41.3X5	T41.3X6
spinal	T41.3X1	T41.3X2	T41.3X3	T41.3X4	T41.3X5	T41.3X6
Amethopterin	T45.1X1	T45.1X2	T45.1X3	T45.1X4	T45.1X5	T45.1X6
Amezinium metilsulfate	T44.991	T44.992	T44.993	T44.994	T44.995	T44.996
Amfebutamone	T43.291	T43.292	T43.293	T43.294	T43.295	T43.296
Amfepramone	T50.5X1	T50.5X2	T50.5X3	T50.5X4	T50.5X5	T50.5X6

◀ New   ◀ Revised   ~~deleted~~ Deleted

Substance	External Cause (T-Code)					
	Poisoning, Accidental (Unintentional)	Poisoning, Intentional Self-Harm	Poisoning, Assault	Poisoning, Undetermined	Adverse Effect	Underdosing
Amfetamine	T43.621	T43.622	T43.623	T43.624	T43.625	T43.626
Amfetaminil	T43.621	T43.622	T43.623	T43.624	T43.625	T43.626
Amfomycin	T36.8X1	T36.8X2	T36.8X3	T36.8X4	T36.8X5	T36.8X6
Amidefrine mesilate	T48.5X1	T48.5X2	T48.5X3	T48.5X4	T48.5X5	T48.5X6
Amidone	T40.3X1	T40.3X2	T40.3X3	T40.3X4	T40.3X5	T40.3X6
Amidopyrine	T39.2X1	T39.2X2	T39.2X3	T39.2X4	T39.2X5	T39.2X6
Amidotrizoate	T50.8X1	T50.8X2	T50.8X3	T50.8X4	T50.8X5	T50.8X6
Amiflamine	T43.1X1	T43.1X2	T43.1X3	T43.1X4	T43.1X5	T43.1X6
Amikacin	T36.5X1	T36.5X2	T36.5X3	T36.5X4	T36.5X5	T36.5X6
Amikhelline	T46.3X1	T46.3X2	T46.3X3	T46.3X4	T46.3X5	T46.3X6
Amiloride	T50.2X1	T50.2X2	T50.2X3	T50.2X4	T50.2X5	T50.2X6
Aminacrine	T49.0X1	T49.0X2	T49.0X3	T49.0X4	T49.0X5	T49.0X6
Amineptine	T43.011	T43.012	T43.013	T43.014	T43.015	T43.016
Aminitrozole	T37.3X1	T37.3X2	T37.3X3	T37.3X4	T37.3X5	T37.3X6
Aminoacetic acid (derivatives)	T50.3X1	T50.3X2	T50.3X3	T50.3X4	T50.3X5	T50.3X6
Amino acids	T50.3X1	T50.3X2	T50.3X3	T50.3X4	T50.3X5	T50.3X6
Aminoacridine	T49.0X1	T49.0X2	T49.0X3	T49.0X4	T49.0X5	T49.0X6
Aminobenzoic acid (-p)	T49.3X1	T49.3X2	T49.3X3	T49.3X4	T49.3X5	T49.3X6
4-Aminobutyric acid	T43.8X1	T43.8X2	T43.8X3	T43.8X4	T43.8X5	T43.8X6
Aminocaproic acid	T45.621	T45.622	T45.623	T45.624	T45.625	T45.626
Aminofenazone	T39.2X1	T39.2X2	T39.2X3	T39.2X4	T39.2X5	T39.2X6
Aminoethylisothiourium	T45.8X1	T45.8X2	T45.8X3	T45.8X4	T45.8X5	T45.8X6
Aminoglutethimide	T45.1X1	T45.1X2	T45.1X3	T45.1X4	T45.1X5	T45.1X6
Aminohippuric acid	T50.8X1	T50.8X2	T50.8X3	T50.8X4	T50.8X5	T50.8X6
Aminomethylbenzoic acid	T45.691	T45.692	T45.693	T45.694	T45.695	T45.696
Aminometradine	T50.2X1	T50.2X2	T50.2X3	T50.2X4	T50.2X5	T50.2X6
Aminopentamide	T44.3X1	T44.3X2	T44.3X3	T44.3X4	T44.3X5	T44.3X6
Aminophenazone	T39.2X1	T39.2X2	T39.2X3	T39.2X4	T39.2X5	T39.2X6
Aminophenol	T54.0X1	T54.0X2	T54.0X3	T54.0X4	—	—
4-Aminophenol derivatives	T39.1X1	T39.1X2	T39.1X3	T39.1X4	T39.1X5	T39.1X6
Aminophenylpyridone	T43.591	T43.592	T43.593	T43.594	T43.595	T43.596
Aminophylline	T48.6X1	T48.6X2	T48.6X3	T48.6X4	T48.6X5	T48.6X6
Aminopterin sodium	T45.1X1	T45.1X2	T45.1X3	T45.1X4	T45.1X5	T45.1X6
Aminopyrine	T39.2X1	T39.2X2	T39.2X3	T39.2X4	T39.2X5	T39.2X6
8-Aminoquinoline drugs	T37.2X1	T37.2X2	T37.2X3	T37.2X4	T37.2X5	T37.2X6
Aminorex	T50.5X1	T50.5X2	T50.5X3	T50.5X4	T50.5X5	T50.5X6
Aminosalicylic acid	T37.1X1	T37.1X2	T37.1X3	T37.1X4	T37.1X5	T37.1X6
Aminosalylum	T37.1X1	T37.1X2	T37.1X3	T37.1X4	T37.1X5	T37.1X6
Amiodarone	T46.2X1	T46.2X2	T46.2X3	T46.2X4	T46.2X5	T46.2X6
Amiphenazole	T50.7X1	T50.7X2	T50.7X3	T50.7X4	T50.7X5	T50.7X6
Amiquinsin	T46.5X1	T46.5X2	T46.5X3	T46.5X4	T46.5X5	T46.5X6
Amisometradine	T50.2X1	T50.2X2	T50.2X3	T50.2X4	T50.2X5	T50.2X6

Substance	External Cause (T-Code)					
	Poisoning, Accidental (Unintentional)	Poisoning, Intentional Self-Harm	Poisoning, Assault	Poisoning, Undetermined	Adverse Effect	Underdosing
Amisulpride	T43.591	T43.592	T43.593	T43.594	T43.595	T43.596
Amitriptyline	T43.021	T43.022	T43.023	T43.024	T43.025	T43.026
Amitriptylinoxide	T43.021	T43.022	T43.023	T43.024	T43.025	T43.026
Amlexanox	T48.6X1	T48.6X2	T48.6X3	T48.6X4	T48.6X5	T48.6X6
Ammonia (fumes) (gas) (vapor)	T59.891	T59.892	T59.893	T59.894	—	—
aromatic spirit	T48.991	T48.992	T48.993	T48.994	T48.995	T48.996
liquid (household)	T54.3X1	T54.3X2	T54.3X3	T54.3X4	—	—
Ammoniated mercury	T49.0X1	T49.0X2	T49.0X3	T49.0X4	T49.0X5	T49.0X6
Ammonium						
acid tartrate	T49.5X1	T49.5X2	T49.5X3	T49.5X4	T49.5X5	T49.5X6
bromide	T42.6X1	T42.6X2	T42.6X3	T42.6X4	T42.6X5	T42.6X6
carbonate	T54.3X1	T54.3X2	T54.3X3	T54.3X4	—	—
chloride	T50.991	T50.992	T50.993	T50.994	T50.995	T50.996
expectorant	T48.4X1	T48.4X2	T48.4X3	T48.4X4	T48.4X5	T48.4X6
compounds (household) NEC	T54.3X1	T54.3X2	T54.3X3	T54.3X4	—	—
fumes (any usage)	T59.891	T59.892	T59.893	T59.894	—	—
industrial	T54.3X1	T54.3X2	T54.3X3	T54.3X4	—	—
ichthyosulronate	T49.4X1	T49.4X2	T49.4X3	T49.4X4	T49.4X5	T49.4X6
mandelate	T37.91	T37.92	T37.93	T37.94	T37.95	T37.96
sulfamate	T60.3X1	T60.3X2	T60.3X3	T60.3X4	—	—
sulfonate resin	T47.8X1	T47.8X2	T47.8X3	T47.8X4	T47.8X5	T47.8X6
Amobarbital (sodium)	T42.3X1	T42.3X2	T42.3X3	T42.3X4	T42.3X5	T42.3X6
Amodiaquine	T37.2X1	T37.2X2	T37.2X3	T37.2X4	T37.2X5	T37.2X6
Amopyroquin(e)	T37.2X1	T37.2X2	T37.2X3	T37.2X4	T37.2X5	T37.2X6
Amoxapine	T43.011	T43.012	T43.013	T43.014	T43.015	T43.016
Amoxicillin	T36.0X1	T36.0X2	T36.0X3	T36.0X4	T36.0X5	T36.0X6
Amperozide	T43.591	T43.592	T43.593	T43.594	T43.595	T43.596
Amphenidone	T43.591	T43.592	T43.593	T43.594	T43.595	T43.596
Amphetamine NEC	T43.621	T43.622	T43.623	T43.624	T43.625	T43.626
Amphomycin	T36.8X1	T36.8X2	T36.8X3	T36.8X4	T36.8X5	T36.8X6
Amphotalide	T37.4X1	T37.4X2	T37.4X3	T37.4X4	T37.4X5	T37.4X6
Amphotericin B	T36.7X1	T36.7X2	T36.7X3	T36.7X4	T36.7X5	T36.7X6
topical	T49.0X1	T49.0X2	T49.0X3	T49.0X4	T49.0X5	T49.0X6
Ampicillin	T36.0X1	T36.0X2	T36.0X3	T36.0X4	T36.0X5	T36.0X6
Amprotropine	T44.3X1	T44.3X2	T44.3X3	T44.3X4	T44.3X5	T44.3X6
Amsacrine	T45.1X1	T45.1X2	T45.1X3	T45.1X4	T45.1X5	T45.1X6
Amygdaline	T62.2X1	T62.2X2	T62.2X3	T62.2X4	—	—
Amyl						
acetate	T52.8X1	T52.8X2	T52.8X3	T52.8X4	—	—
vapor	T59.891	T59.892	T59.893	T59.894	—	—
alcohol	T51.3X1	T51.3X2	T51.3X3	T51.3X4	—	—
chloride	T53.6X1	T53.6X2	T53.6X3	T53.6X4	—	—

TABLE OF DRUGS AND CHEMICALS

◀ New ◀ Revised ~~deleted~~ Deleted

Substance	External Cause (T-Code)					
	Poisoning, Accidental (Unintentional)	Poisoning, Intentional Self-Harm	Poisoning, Assault	Poisoning, Undetermined	Adverse Effect	Underdosing
Amyl *(Continued)*						
formate	T52.8X1	T52.8X2	T52.8X3	T52.8X4	—	—
nitrite	T46.3X1	T46.3X2	T46.3X3	T46.3X4	T46.3X5	T46.3X6
propionate	T65.891	T65.892	T65.893	T65.894		
Amylase	T47.5X1	T47.5X2	T47.5X3	T47.5X4	T47.5X5	T47.5X6
Amyleine, regional	T41.3X1	T41.3X2	T41.3X3	T41.3X4	T41.3X5	T41.3X6
Amylene						
dichloride	T53.6X1	T53.6X2	T53.6X3	T53.6X4	—	—
hydrate	T51.3X1	T51.3X2	T51.3X3	T51.3X4	—	—
Amylmetacresol	T49.6X1	T49.6X2	T49.6X3	T49.6X4	T49.6X5	T49.6X6
Amylobarbitone	T42.3X1	T42.3X2	T42.3X3	T42.3X4	T42.3X5	T42.3X6
Amylocaine, regional	T41.3X1	T41.3X2	T41.3X3	T41.3X4	T41.3X5	T41.3X6
infiltration (subcutaneous)	T41.3X1	T41.3X2	T41.3X3	T41.3X4	T41.3X5	T41.3X6
nerve block (peripheral) (plexus)	T41.3X1	T41.3X2	T41.3X3	T41.3X4	T41.3X5	T41.3X6
spinal	T41.3X1	T41.3X2	T41.3X3	T41.3X4	T41.3X5	T41.3X6
topical (surface)	T41.3X1	T41.3X2	T41.3X3	T41.3X4	T41.3X5	T41.3X6
Amylopectin	T47.6X1	T47.6X2	T47.6X3	T47.6X4	T47.6X5	T47.6X6
Amytal (sodium)	T42.3X1	T42.3X2	T42.3X3	T42.3X4	T42.3X5	T42.3X6
Anabolic steroid	T38.7X1	T38.7X2	T38.7X3	T38.7X4	T38.7X5	T38.7X6
Analeptic NEC	T50.7X1	T50.7X2	T50.7X3	T50.7X4	T50.7X5	T50.7X6
Analgesic	T39.91	T39.92	T39.93	T39.94	T39.95	T39.96
anti-inflammatory NEC	T39.91	T39.92	T39.93	T39.94	T39.95	T39.96
propionic acid derivative	T39.311	T39.312	T39.313	T39.314	T39.315	T39.316
antirheumatic NEC	T39.4X1	T39.4X2	T39.4X3	T39.4X4	T39.4X5	T39.4X6
aromatic NEC	T39.1X1	T39.1X2	T39.1X3	T39.1X4	T39.1X5	T39.1X6
narcotic NEC	T40.601	T40.602	T40.603	T40.604	T40.605	T40.606
combination	T40.601	T40.602	T40.603	T40.604	T40.605	T40.606
obstetric	T40.601	T40.602	T40.603	T40.604	T40.605	T40.606
non-narcotic NEC	T39.91	T39.92	T39.93	T39.94	T39.95	T39.96
combination	T39.91	T39.92	T39.93	T39.94	T39.95	T39.96
pyrazole	T39.2X1	T39.2X2	T39.2X3	T39.2X4	T39.2X5	T39.2X6
specified NEC	T39.8X1	T39.8X2	T39.8X3	T39.8X4	T39.8X5	T39.8X6
Analgin	T39.2X1	T39.2X2	T39.2X3	T39.2X4	T39.2X5	T39.2X6
Anamirta cocculus	T62.1X1	T62.1X2	T62.1X3	T62.1X4	—	—
Ancillin	T36.0X1	T36.0X2	T36.0X3	T36.0X4	T36.0X5	T36.0X6
Ancrod	T45.691	T45.692	T45.693	T45.694	T45.695	T45.696
Androgen	T38.7X1	T38.7X2	T38.7X3	T38.7X4	T38.7X5	T38.7X6
Androgen-estrogen mixture	T38.7X1	T38.7X2	T38.7X3	T38.7X4	T38.7X5	T38.7X6
Androstalone	T38.7X1	T38.7X2	T38.7X3	T38.7X4	T38.7X5	T38.7X6
Androstanolone	T38.7X1	T38.7X2	T38.7X3	T38.7X4	T38.7X5	T38.7X6
Androsterone	T38.7X1	T38.7X2	T38.7X3	T38.7X4	T38.7X5	T38.7X6

Substance	External Cause (T-Code)					
	Poisoning, Accidental (Unintentional)	Poisoning, Intentional Self-Harm	Poisoning, Assault	Poisoning, Undetermined	Adverse Effect	Underdosing
Anemone pulsatilla	T62.2X1	T62.2X2	T62.2X3	T62.2X4	—	—
Anesthesia						
caudal	T41.3X1	T41.3X2	T41.3X3	T41.3X4	T41.3X5	T41.3X6
endotracheal	T41.0X1	T41.0X2	T41.0X3	T41.0X4	T41.0X5	T41.0X6
epidural	T41.3X1	T41.3X2	T41.3X3	T41.3X4	T41.3X5	T41.3X6
inhalation	T41.0X1	T41.0X2	T41.0X3	T41.0X4	T41.0X5	T41.0X6
local	T41.3X1	T41.3X2	T41.3X3	T41.3X4	T41.3X5	T41.3X6
mucosal	T41.3X1	T41.3X2	T41.3X3	T41.3X4	T41.3X5	T41.3X6
muscle relaxation	T48.1X1	T48.1X2	T48.1X3	T48.1X4	T48.1X5	T48.1X6
nerve blocking	T41.3X1	T41.3X2	T41.3X3	T41.3X4	T41.3X5	T41.3X6
plexus blocking	T41.3X1	T41.3X2	T41.3X3	T41.3X4	T41.3X5	T41.3X6
potentiated	T41.201	T41.202	T41.203	T41.204	T41.205	T41.206
rectal	T41.201	T41.202	T41.203	T41.204	T41.205	T41.206
general	T41.201	T41.202	T41.203	T41.204	T41.205	T41.206
local	T41.3X1	T41.3X2	T41.3X3	T41.3X4	T41.3X5	T41.3X6
regional	T41.3X1	T41.3X2	T41.3X3	T41.3X4	T41.3X5	T41.3X6
surface	T41.3X1	T41.3X2	T41.3X3	T41.3X4	T41.3X5	T41.3X6
Anesthetic NEC — *see also Anesthesia*	T41.41	T41.42	T41.43	T41.44	T41.45	T41.46
with muscle relaxant	T41.201	T41.202	T41.203	T41.204	T41.205	T41.206
general	T41.201	T41.202	T41.203	T41.204	T41.205	T41.206
local	T41.3X1	T41.3X2	T41.3X3	T41.3X4	T41.3X5	T41.3X6
gaseous NEC	T41.0X1	T41.0X2	T41.0X3	T41.0X4	T41.0X5	T41.0X6
general NEC	T41.201	T41.202	T41.203	T41.204	T41.205	T41.206
halogenated hydrocarbon derivatives NEC	T41.0X1	T41.0X2	T41.0X3	T41.0X4	T41.0X5	T41.0X6
infiltration NEC	T41.3X1	T41.3X2	T41.3X3	T41.3X4	T41.3X5	T41.3X6
intravenous NEC	T41.1X1	T41.1X2	T41.1X3	T41.1X4	T41.1X5	T41.1X6
local NEC	T41.3X1	T41.3X2	T41.3X3	T41.3X4	T41.3X5	T41.3X6
rectal	T41.201	T41.202	T41.203	T41.204	T41.205	T41.206
general	T41.201	T41.202	T41.203	T41.204	T41.205	T41.206
local	T41.3X1	T41.3X2	T41.3X3	T41.3X4	T41.3X5	T41.3X6
regional NEC	T41.3X1	T41.3X2	T41.3X3	T41.3X4	T41.3X5	T41.3X6
spinal NEC	T41.3X1	T41.3X2	T41.3X3	T41.3X4	T41.3X5	T41.3X6
thiobarbiturate	T41.1X1	T41.1X2	T41.1X3	T41.1X4	T41.1X5	T41.1X6
topical	T41.3X1	T41.3X2	T41.3X3	T41.3X4	T41.3X5	T41.3X6
Aneurine	T45.2X1	T45.2X2	T45.2X3	T45.2X4	T45.2X5	T45.2X6
Angio-Conray	T50.8X1	T50.8X2	T50.8X3	T50.8X4	T50.8X5	T50.8X6
Angiotensin	T44.5X1	T44.5X2	T44.5X3	T44.5X4	T44.5X5	T44.5X6
Angiotensinamide	T44.991	T44.992	T44.993	T44.994	T44.995	T44.996
Anhydrohydroxy-progesterone	T38.5X1	T38.5X2	T38.5X3	T38.5X4	T38.5X5	T38.5X6
Anhydron	T50.2X1	T50.2X2	T50.2X3	T50.2X4	T50.2X5	T50.2X6
Anileridine	T40.4X1	T40.4X2	T40.4X3	T40.4X4	T40.4X5	T40.4X6

◄ New   ◄ Revised   ~~deleted~~ Deleted

	External Cause (T-Code)					
Substance	Poisoning, Accidental (Unintentional)	Poisoning, Intentional Self-Harm	Poisoning, Assault	Poisoning, Undetermined	Adverse Effect	Underdosing
Aniline (dye) (liquid)	T65.3X1	T65.3X2	T65.3X3	T65.3X4	—	—
analgesic	T39.1X1	T39.1X2	T39.1X3	T39.1X4	T39.1X5	T39.1X6
derivatives, therapeutic NEC	T39.1X1	T39.1X2	T39.1X3	T39.1X4	T39.1X5	T39.1X6
vapor	T65.3X1	T65.3X2	T65.3X3	T65.3X4	—	—
Anise oil	T47.5X1	T47.5X2	T47.5X3	T47.5X4	T47.5X5	T47.5X6
Aniscoropine	T44.3X1	T44.3X2	T44.3X3	T44.3X4	T44.3X5	T44.3X6
Anisidine	T65.3X1	T65.3X2	T65.3X3	T65.3X4	—	—
Anisindione	T45.511	T45.512	T45.513	T45.514	T45.515	T45.516
Anisotropine methyl-bromide	T44.3X1	T44.3X2	T44.3X3	T44.3X4	T44.3X5	T44.3X6
Anistreplase	T45.611	T45.612	T45.613	T45.614	T45.615	T45.616
Anorexiant (central)	T50.5X1	T50.5X2	T50.5X3	T50.5X4	T50.5X5	T50.5X6
Anorexic agents	T50.5X1	T50.5X2	T50.5X3	T50.5X4	T50.5X5	T50.5X6
Ansamycin	T36.6X1	T36.6X2	T36.6X3	T36.6X4	T36.6X5	T36.6X6
Ant (bite) (sting)	T63.421	T63.422	T63.423	T63.424	—	—
Antabuse	T50.6X1	T50.6X2	T50.6X3	T50.6X4	T50.6X5	T50.6X6
Ant poison — see Insecticide						
Antacid NEC	T47.1X1	T47.1X2	T47.1X3	T47.1X4	T47.1X5	T47.1X6
Antagonist						
Aldosterone	T50.0X1	T50.0X2	T50.0X3	T50.0X4	T50.0X5	T50.0X6
alpha-adrenoreceptor	T44.6X1	T44.6X2	T44.6X3	T44.6X4	T44.6X5	T44.6X6
anticoagulant	T45.7X1	T45.7X2	T45.7X3	T45.7X4	T45.7X5	T45.7X6
beta-adrenoreceptor	T44.7X1	T44.7X2	T44.7X3	T44.7X4	T44.7X5	T44.7X6
extrapyramidal NEC	T44.3X1	T44.3X2	T44.3X3	T44.3X4	T44.3X5	T44.3X6
folic acid	T45.1X1	T45.1X2	T45.1X3	T45.1X4	T45.1X5	T45.1X6
H2 receptor	T47.0X1	T47.0X2	T47.0X3	T47.0X4	T47.0X5	T47.0X6
heavy metal	T45.8X1	T45.8X2	T45.8X3	T45.8X4	T45.8X5	T45.8X6
narcotic analgesic	T50.7X1	T50.7X2	T50.7X3	T50.7X4	T50.7X5	T50.7X6
opiate	T50.7X1	T50.7X2	T50.7X3	T50.7X4	T50.7X5	T50.7X6
pyrimidine	T45.1X1	T45.1X2	T45.1X3	T45.1X4	T45.1X5	T45.1X6
serotonin	T46.5X1	T46.5X2	T46.5X3	T46.5X4	T46.5X5	T46.5X6
Antazolin(e)	T45.0X1	T45.0X2	T45.0X3	T45.0X4	T45.0X5	T45.0X6
Anterior pituitary hormone NEC	T38.811	T38.812	T38.813	T38.814	T38.815	T38.816
Anthelmintic NEC	T37.4X1	T37.4X2	T37.4X3	T37.4X4	T37.4X5	T37.4X6
Anthiolimine	T37.4X1	T37.4X2	T37.4X3	T37.4X4	T37.4X5	T37.4X6
Anthralin	T49.4X1	T49.4X2	T49.4X3	T49.4X4	T49.4X5	T49.4X6
Anthramycin	T45.1X1	T45.1X2	T45.1X3	T45.1X4	T45.1X5	T45.1X6
Antiadrenergic NEC	T44.8X1	T44.8X2	T44.8X3	T44.8X4	T44.8X5	T44.8X6
Antiallergic NEC	T45.0X1	T45.0X2	T45.0X3	T45.0X4	T45.0X5	T45.0X6
Anti-anemic (drug) (preparation)	T45.8X1	T45.8X2	T45.8X3	T45.8X4	T45.8X5	T45.8X6
Antiandrogen NEC	T38.6X1	T38.6X2	T38.6X3	T38.6X4	T38.6X5	T38.6X6
Antianxiety drug NEC	T43.501	T43.502	T43.503	T43.504	T43.505	T43.506
Antiaris toxicaria	T65.891	T65.892	T65.893	T65.894	—	—

	External Cause (T-Code)					
Substance	Poisoning, Accidental (Unintentional)	Poisoning, Intentional Self-Harm	Poisoning, Assault	Poisoning, Undetermined	Adverse Effect	Underdosing
Antiarteriosclerotic drug	T46.6X1	T46.6X2	T46.6X3	T46.6X4	T46.6X5	T46.6X6
Antiasthmatic drug NEC	T48.6X1	T48.6X2	T48.6X3	T48.6X4	T48.6X5	T48.6X6
Antibiotic NEC	T36.91	T36.92	T36.93	T36.94	T36.95	T36.96
aminoglycoside	T36.5X1	T36.5X2	T36.5X3	T36.5X4	T36.5X5	T36.5X6
anticancer	T45.1X1	T45.1X2	T45.1X3	T45.1X4	T45.1X5	T45.1X6
antifungal	T36.7X1	T36.7X2	T36.7X3	T36.7X4	T36.7X5	T36.7X6
antimycobacterial	T36.5X1	T36.5X2	T36.5X3	T36.5X4	T36.5X5	T36.5X6
antineoplastic	T45.1X1	T45.1X2	T45.1X3	T45.1X4	T45.1X5	T45.1X6
cephalosporin (group)	T36.1X1	T36.1X2	T36.1X3	T36.1X4	T36.1X5	T36.1X6
chloramphenicol (group)	T36.2X1	T36.2X2	T36.2X3	T36.2X4	T36.2X5	T36.2X6
ENT	T49.6X1	T49.6X2	T49.6X3	T49.6X4	T49.6X5	T49.6X6
eye	T49.5X1	T49.5X2	T49.5X3	T49.5X4	T49.5X5	T49.5X6
fungicidal (local)	T49.0X1	T49.0X2	T49.0X3	T49.0X4	T49.0X5	T49.0X6
intestinal	T36.8X1	T36.8X2	T36.8X3	T36.8X4	T36.8X5	T36.8X6
b-lactam NEC	T36.1X1	T36.1X2	T36.1X3	T36.1X4	T36.1X5	T36.1X6
local	T49.0X1	T49.0X2	T49.0X3	T49.0X4	T49.0X5	T49.0X6
macrolides	T36.3X1	T36.3X2	T36.3X3	T36.3X4	T36.3X5	T36.3X6
polypeptide	T36.8X1	T36.8X2	T36.8X3	T36.8X4	T36.8X5	T36.8X6
specified NEC	T36.8X1	T36.8X2	T36.8X3	T36.8X4	T36.8X5	T36.8X6
tetracycline (group)	T36.4X1	T36.4X2	T36.4X3	T36.4X4	T36.4X5	T36.4X6
throat	T49.6X1	T49.6X2	T49.6X3	T49.6X4	T49.6X5	T49.6X6
Anticancer agents NEC	T45.1X1	T45.1X2	T45.1X3	T45.1X4	T45.1X5	T45.1X6
Anticholesterolemic drug NEC	T46.6X1	T46.6X2	T46.6X3	T46.6X4	T46.6X5	T46.6X6
Anticholinergic NEC	T44.3X1	T44.3X2	T44.3X3	T44.3X4	T44.3X5	T44.3X6
Anticholinesterase	T44.0X1	T44.0X2	T44.0X3	T44.0X4	T44.0X5	T44.0X6
organophosphorus	T44.0X1	T44.0X2	T44.0X3	T44.0X4	T44.0X5	T44.0X6
insecticide	T60.0X1	T60.0X2	T60.0X3	T60.0X4	—	—
nerve gas	T59.891	T59.892	T59.893	T59.894	—	—
reversible	T44.0X1	T44.0X2	T44.0X3	T44.0X4	T44.0X5	T44.0X6
ophthalmological	T49.5X1	T49.5X2	T49.5X3	T49.5X4	T49.5X5	T49.5X6
Anticoagulant NEC	T45.511	T45.512	T45.513	T45.514	T45.515	T45.516
Antagonist	T45.7X1	T45.7X2	T45.7X3	T45.7X4	T45.7X5	T45.7X6
Anti-common-cold drug NEC	T48.5X1	T48.5X2	T48.5X3	T48.5X4	T48.5X5	T48.5X6
Anticonvulsant	T42.71	T42.72	T42.73	T42.74	T42.75	T42.76
barbiturate	T42.3X1	T42.3X2	T42.3X3	T42.3X4	T42.3X5	T42.3X6
combination (with barbiturate)	T42.3X1	T42.3X2	T42.3X3	T42.3X4	T42.3X5	T42.3X6
hydantoin	T42.0X1	T42.0X2	T42.0X3	T42.0X4	T42.0X5	T42.0X6
hypnotic NEC	T42.6X1	T42.6X2	T42.6X3	T42.6X4	T42.6X5	T42.6X6
oxazolidinedione	T42.2X1	T42.2X2	T42.2X3	T42.2X4	T42.2X5	T42.2X6
pyrimidinedione	T42.6X1	T42.6X2	T42.6X3	T42.6X4	T42.6X5	T42.6X6
specified NEC	T42.6X1	T42.6X2	T42.6X3	T42.6X4	T42.6X5	T42.6X6
succinimide	T42.2X1	T42.2X2	T42.2X3	T42.2X4	T42.2X5	T42.2X6

◀ New ◀ Revised ~~deleted~~ Deleted

TABLE OF DRUGS AND CHEMICALS

Substance	External Cause (T-Code)					
	Poisoning, Accidental (Unintentional)	Poisoning, Intentional Self-Harm	Poisoning, Assault	Poisoning, Undetermined	Adverse Effect	Underdosing
Anti-D immunoglobulin (human)	T50.Z11	T50.Z12	T50.Z13	T50.Z14	T50.Z15	T50.Z16
Antidepressant NEC	T43.201	T43.202	T43.203	T43.204	T43.205	T43.206
monoamine oxidase inhibitor	T43.1X1	T43.1X2	T43.1X3	T43.1X4	T43.1X5	T43.1X6
selective serotonin norepinephrine reuptake inhibitor	T43.211	T43.212	T43.213	T43.214	T43.215	T43.216
selective serotonin reuptake inhibitor	T43.221	T43.222	T43.223	T43.224	T43.225	T43.226
specified NEC	T43.291	T43.292	T43.293	T43.294	T43.295	T43.296
tetracyclic	T43.021	T43.022	T43.023	T43.024	T43.025	T43.026
triazolopyridine	T43.221	T43.222	T43.223	T43.224	T43.225	T43.226
tricyclic	T43.011	T43.012	T43.013	T43.014	T43.015	T43.016
Antidiabetic NEC	T38.3X1	T38.3X2	T38.3X3	T38.3X4	T38.3X5	T38.3X6
biguanide	T38.3X1	T38.3X2	T38.3X3	T38.3X4	T38.3X5	T38.3X6
and sulfonyl combined	T38.3X1	T38.3X2	T38.3X3	T38.3X4	T38.3X5	T38.3X6
combined	T38.3X1	T38.3X2	T38.3X3	T38.3X4	T38.3X5	T38.3X6
sulfonylurea	T38.3X1	T38.3X2	T38.3X3	T38.3X4	T38.3X5	T38.3X6
Antidiarrheal drug NEC	T47.6X1	T47.6X2	T47.6X3	T47.6X4	T47.6X5	T47.6X6
absorbent	T47.6X1	T47.6X2	T47.6X3	T47.6X4	T47.6X5	T47.6X6
Antidiphtheria serum	T50.Z11	T50.Z12	T50.Z13	T50.Z14	T50.Z15	T50.Z16
Antidiuretic hormone	T38.891	T38.892	T38.893	T38.894	T38.895	T38.896
Antidote NEC	T50.6X1	T50.6X2	T50.6X3	T50.6X4	T50.6X5	T50.6X6
heavy metal	T45.8X1	T45.8X2	T45.8X3	T45.8X4	T45.8X5	T45.8X6
Antidysrhythmic NEC	T46.2X1	T46.2X2	T46.2X3	T46.2X4	T46.2X5	T46.2X6
Antiemetic drug	T45.0X1	T45.0X2	T45.0X3	T45.0X4	T45.0X5	T45.0X6
Antiepilepsy agent	T42.71	T42.72	T42.73	T42.74	T42.75	T42.76
combination	T42.5X1	T42.5X2	T42.5X3	T42.5X4	T42.5X5	T42.5X6
mixed	T42.5X1	T42.5X2	T42.5X3	T42.5X4	T42.5X5	T42.5X6
specified, NEC	T42.6X1	T42.6X2	T42.6X3	T42.6X4	T42.6X5	T42.6X6
Antiestrogen NEC	T38.6X1	T38.6X2	T38.6X3	T38.6X4	T38.6X5	T38.6X6
Antifertility pill	T38.4X1	T38.4X2	T38.4X3	T38.4X4	T38.4X5	T38.4X6
Antifibrinolytic drug	T45.621	T45.622	T45.623	T45.624	T45.625	T45.626
Antifilarial drug	T37.4X1	T37.4X2	T37.4X3	T37.4X4	T37.4X5	T37.4X6
Antiflatulent	T47.5X1	T47.5X2	T47.5X3	T47.5X4	T47.5X5	T47.5X6
Antifreeze	T65.91	T65.92	T65.93	T65.94	—	—
alcohol	T51.1X1	T51.1X2	T51.1X3	T51.1X4	—	—
ethylene glycol	T51.8X1	T51.8X2	T51.8X3	T51.8X4	—	—
Antifungal						
antibiotic (systemic)	T36.7X1	T36.7X2	T36.7X3	T36.7X4	T36.7X5	T36.7X6
anti-infective NEC	T37.91	T37.92	T37.93	T37.94	T37.95	T37.96
disinfectant, local	T49.0X1	T49.0X2	T49.0X3	T49.0X4	T49.0X5	T49.0X6
nonmedicinal (spray)	T60.3X1	T60.3X2	T60.3X3	T60.3X4	—	—
topical	T49.0X1	T49.0X2	T49.0X3	T49.0X4	T49.0X5	T49.0X6

Substance	External Cause (T-Code)					
	Poisoning, Accidental (Unintentional)	Poisoning, Intentional Self-Harm	Poisoning, Assault	Poisoning, Undetermined	Adverse Effect	Underdosing
Anti-gastric-secretion drug NEC	T47.1X1	T47.1X2	T47.1X3	T47.1X4	T47.1X5	T47.1X6
Antigonadotrophin NEC	T38.6X1	T38.6X2	T38.6X3	T38.6X4	T38.6X5	T38.6X6
Antihallucinogen	T43.501	T43.502	T43.503	T43.504	T43.505	T43.506
Antihelmintics	T37.4X1	T37.4X2	T37.4X3	T37.4X4	T37.4X5	T37.4X6
Antihemophilic						
factor	T45.8X1	T45.8X2	T45.8X3	T45.8X4	T45.8X5	T45.8X6
fraction	T45.8X1	T45.8X2	T45.8X3	T45.8X4	T45.8X5	T45.8X6
globulin concentrate	T45.7X1	T45.7X2	T45.7X3	T45.7X4	T45.7X5	T45.7X6
human plasma	T45.8X1	T45.8X2	T45.8X3	T45.8X4	T45.8X5	T45.8X6
plasma, dried	T45.7X1	T45.7X2	T45.7X3	T45.7X4	T45.7X5	T45.7X6
Antihemorrhoidal preparation	T49.2X1	T49.2X2	T49.2X3	T49.2X4	T49.2X5	T49.2X6
Antiheparin drug	T45.7X1	T45.7X2	T45.7X3	T45.7X4	T45.7X5	T45.7X6
Antihistamine	T45.0X1	T45.0X2	T45.0X3	T45.0X4	T45.0X5	T45.0X6
Antihookworm drug	T37.4X1	T37.4X2	T37.4X3	T37.4X4	T37.4X5	T37.4X6
Anti-human lymphocytic globulin	T50.Z11	T50.Z12	T50.Z13	T50.Z14	T50.Z15	T50.Z16
Antihyperlipidemic drug	T46.6X1	T46.6X2	T46.6X3	T46.6X4	T46.6X5	T46.6X6
Antihypertensive drug NEC	T46.5X1	T46.5X2	T46.5X3	T46.5X4	T46.5X5	T46.5X6
Anti-infective NEC	T37.91	T37.92	T37.93	T37.94	T37.95	T37.96
anthelmintic	T37.4X1	T37.4X2	T37.4X3	T37.4X4	T37.4X5	T37.4X6
antibiotics	T36.91	T36.92	T36.93	T36.94	T36.95	T36.96
specified NEC	T36.8X1	T36.8X2	T36.8X3	T36.8X4	T36.8X5	T36.8X6
antimalarial	T37.2X1	T37.2X2	T37.2X3	T37.2X4	T37.2X5	T37.2X6
antimycobacterial NEC	T37.1X1	T37.1X2	T37.1X3	T37.1X4	T37.1X5	T37.1X6
antibiotics	T36.5X1	T36.5X2	T36.5X3	T36.5X4	T36.5X5	T36.5X6
antiprotozoal NEC	T37.3X1	T37.3X2	T37.3X3	T37.3X4	T37.3X5	T37.3X6
blood	T37.2X1	T37.2X2	T37.2X3	T37.2X4	T37.2X5	T37.2X6
antiviral	T37.5X1	T37.5X2	T37.5X3	T37.5X4	T37.5X5	T37.5X6
arsenical	T37.8X1	T37.8X2	T37.8X3	T37.8X4	T37.8X5	T37.8X6
bismuth, local	T49.0X1	T49.0X2	T49.0X3	T49.0X4	T49.0X5	T49.0X6
ENT	T49.6X1	T49.6X2	T49.6X3	T49.6X4	T49.6X5	T49.6X6
eye NEC	T49.5X1	T49.5X2	T49.5X3	T49.5X4	T49.5X5	T49.5X6
heavy metals NEC	T37.8X1	T37.8X2	T37.8X3	T37.8X4	T37.8X5	T37.8X6
local NEC	T49.0X1	T49.0X2	T49.0X3	T49.0X4	T49.0X5	T49.0X6
specified NEC	T49.0X1	T49.0X2	T49.0X3	T49.0X4	T49.0X5	T49.0X6
mixed	T37.91	T37.92	T37.93	T37.94	T37.95	T37.96
ophthalmic preparation	T49.5X1	T49.5X2	T49.5X3	T49.5X4	T49.5X5	T49.5X6
topical NEC	T49.0X1	T49.0X2	T49.0X3	T49.0X4	T49.0X5	T49.0X6
Anti-inflammatory drug NEC	T49.0X1	T49.0X2	T49.0X3	T49.0X4	T49.0X5	T49.0X6
local	T49.0X1	T49.0X2	T49.0X3	T49.0X4	T49.0X5	T49.0X6
nonsteroidal NEC	T39.391	T39.392	T39.393	T39.394	T39.395	T39.396
propionic acid derivative	T39.311	T39.312	T39.313	T39.314	T39.315	T39.316
specified NEC	T39.391	T39.392	T39.393	T39.394	T39.395	T39.396

502

◀ New   ◀|| Revised   ~~deleted~~ Deleted

Substance	External Cause (T-Code)					
	Poisoning, Accidental (Unintentional)	Poisoning, Intentional Self-Harm	Poisoning, Assault	Poisoning, Undetermined	Adverse Effect	Underdosing
Antikaluretic	T5Ø.3X1	T5Ø.3X2	T5Ø.3X3	T5Ø.3X4	T5Ø.3X5	T5Ø.3X6
Antiknock (tetraethyl lead)	T56.ØX1	T56.ØX2	T56.ØX3	T56.ØX4	—	—
Antilipemic drug NEC	T46.6X1	T46.6X2	T46.6X3	T46.6X4	T46.6X5	T46.6X6
Antimalarial	T37.2X1	T37.2X2	T37.2X3	T37.2X4	T37.2X5	T37.2X6
prophylactic NEC	T37.2X1	T37.2X2	T37.2X3	T37.2X4	T37.2X5	T37.2X6
pyrimidine derivative	T37.2X1	T37.2X2	T37.2X3	T37.2X4	T37.2X5	T37.2X6
Antimetabolite	T45.1X1	T45.1X2	T45.1X3	T45.1X4	T45.1X5	T45.1X6
Antimitotic agent	T45.1X1	T45.1X2	T45.1X3	T45.1X4	T45.1X5	T45.1X6
Antimony (compounds) (vapor) NEC	T56.891	T56.892	T56.893	T56.894	—	—
anti-infectives	T37.8X1	T37.8X2	T37.8X3	T37.8X4	T37.8X5	T37.8X6
dimercaptosuccinate	T37.3X1	T37.3X2	T37.3X3	T37.3X4	T37.3X5	T37.3X6
hydride	T56.891	T56.892	T56.893	T56.894	—	—
pesticide (vapor)	T6Ø.8X1	T6Ø.8X2	T6Ø.8X3	T6Ø.8X4	—	—
potassium (sodium) tartrate	T37.8X1	T37.8X2	T37.8X3	T37.8X4	T37.8X5	T37.8X6
sodium dimercaptosuccinate	T37.3X1	T37.3X2	T37.3X3	T37.3X4	T37.3X5	T37.3X6
tartrated	T37.8X1	T37.8X2	T37.8X3	T37.8X4	T37.8X5	T37.8X6
Antimuscarinic NEC	T44.3X1	T44.3X2	T44.3X3	T44.3X4	T44.3X5	T44.3X6
Antimycobacterial drug NEC	T37.1X1	T37.1X2	T37.1X3	T37.1X4	T37.1X5	T37.1X6
antibiotics	T36.5X1	T36.5X2	T36.5X3	T36.5X4	T36.5X5	T36.5X6
combination	T37.1X1	T37.1X2	T37.1X3	T37.1X4	T37.1X5	T37.1X6
Antinausea drug	T45.ØX1	T45.ØX2	T45.ØX3	T45.ØX4	T45.ØX5	T45.ØX6
Antinematode drug	T37.4X1	T37.4X2	T37.4X3	T37.4X4	T37.4X5	T37.4X6
Antineoplastic NEC	T45.1X1	T45.1X2	T45.1X3	T45.1X4	T45.1X5	T45.1X6
alkaloidal	T45.1X1	T45.1X2	T45.1X3	T45.1X4	T45.1X5	T45.1X6
antibiotics	T45.1X1	T45.1X2	T45.1X3	T45.1X4	T45.1X5	T45.1X6
combination	T45.1X1	T45.1X2	T45.1X3	T45.1X4	T45.1X5	T45.1X6
estrogen	T38.5X1	T38.5X2	T38.5X3	T38.5X4	T38.5X5	T38.5X6
steroid	T38.7X1	T38.7X2	T38.7X3	T38.7X4	T38.7X5	T38.7X6
Antiparasitic drug (systemic)	T37.91	T37.92	T37.93	T37.94	T37.95	T37.96
local	T49.ØX1	T49.ØX2	T49.ØX3	T49.ØX4	T49.ØX5	T49.ØX6
specified NEC	T37.8X1	T37.8X2	T37.8X3	T37.8X4	T37.8X5	T37.8X6
Antiparkinsonism drug NEC	T42.8X1	T42.8X2	T42.8X3	T42.8X4	T42.8X5	T42.8X6
Antiperspirant NEC	T49.2X1	T49.2X2	T49.2X3	T49.2X4	T49.2X5	T49.2X6
Antiphlogistic NEC	T39.4X1	T39.4X2	T39.4X3	T39.4X4	T39.4X5	T39.4X6
Antiplatyhelmintic drug	T37.4X1	T37.4X2	T37.4X3	T37.4X4	T37.4X5	T37.4X6
Antiprotozoal drug NEC	T37.3X1	T37.3X2	T37.3X3	T37.3X4	T37.3X5	T37.3X6
blood	T37.2X1	T37.2X2	T37.2X3	T37.2X4	T37.2X5	T37.2X6
local	T49.ØX1	T49.ØX2	T49.ØX3	T49.ØX4	T49.ØX5	T49.ØX6
Antipruritic drug NEC	T49.1X1	T49.1X2	T49.1X3	T49.1X4	T49.1X5	T49.1X6
Antipsychotic drug	T43.5Ø1	T43.5Ø2	T43.5Ø3	T43.5Ø4	T43.5Ø5	T43.5Ø6
specified NEC	T43.591	T43.592	T43.593	T43.594	T43.595	T43.596

Substance	External Cause (T-Code)					
	Poisoning, Accidental (Unintentional)	Poisoning, Intentional Self-Harm	Poisoning, Assault	Poisoning, Undetermined	Adverse Effect	Underdosing
Antipyretic	T39.91	T39.92	T39.93	T39.94	T39.95	T39.96
specified NEC	T39.8X1	T39.8X2	T39.8X3	T39.8X4	T39.8X5	T39.8X6
Antipyrine	T39.2X1	T39.2X2	T39.2X3	T39.2X4	T39.2X5	T39.2X6
Antirabies hyperimmune serum	T5Ø.Z11	T5Ø.Z12	T5Ø.Z13	T5Ø.Z14	T5Ø.Z15	T5Ø.Z16
Antirheumatic NEC	T39.4X1	T39.4X2	T39.4X3	T39.4X4	T39.4X5	T39.4X6
Antirigidity drug NEC	T42.8X1	T42.8X2	T42.8X3	T42.8X4	T42.8X5	T42.8X6
Antischistosomal drug	T37.4X1	T37.4X2	T37.4X3	T37.4X4	T37.4X5	T37.4X6
Antiscorpion sera	T5Ø.Z11	T5Ø.Z12	T5Ø.Z13	T5Ø.Z14	T5Ø.Z15	T5Ø.Z16
Antiseborrheics	T49.4X1	T49.4X2	T49.4X3	T49.4X4	T49.4X5	T49.4X6
Antiseptics (external) (medicinal)	T49.ØX1	T49.ØX2	T49.ØX3	T49.ØX4	T49.ØX5	T49.ØX6
Antistine	T45.ØX1	T45.ØX2	T45.ØX3	T45.ØX4	T45.ØX5	T45.ØX6
Antitapeworm drug	T37.4X1	T37.4X2	T37.4X3	T37.4X4	T37.4X5	T37.4X6
Antitetanus immunoglobulin	T5Ø.Z11	T5Ø.Z12	T5Ø.Z13	T5Ø.Z14	T5Ø.Z15	T5Ø.Z16
Antithrombotic	T45.521	T45.522	T45.523	T45.524	T45.525	T45.526
Antithyroid drug NEC	T38.2X1	T38.2X2	T38.2X3	T38.2X4	T38.2X5	T38.2X6
Antitoxin	T5Ø.Z11	T5Ø.Z12	T5Ø.Z13	T5Ø.Z14	T5Ø.Z15	T5Ø.Z16
diphtheria	T5Ø.Z11	T5Ø.Z12	T5Ø.Z13	T5Ø.Z14	T5Ø.Z15	T5Ø.Z16
gas gangrene	T5Ø.Z11	T5Ø.Z12	T5Ø.Z13	T5Ø.Z14	T5Ø.Z15	T5Ø.Z16
tetanus	T5Ø.Z11	T5Ø.Z12	T5Ø.Z13	T5Ø.Z14	T5Ø.Z15	T5Ø.Z16
Antitoxin, any	T5Ø.9Ø1	T5Ø.9Ø2	T5Ø.9Ø3	T5Ø.9Ø4	T5Ø.9Ø5	T5Ø.9Ø6
Antitrichomonal drug	T37.3X1	T37.3X2	T37.3X3	T37.3X4	T37.3X5	T37.3X6
Antituberculars	T37.1X1	T37.1X2	T37.1X3	T37.1X4	T37.1X5	T37.1X6
antibiotics	T36.5X1	T36.5X2	T36.5X3	T36.5X4	T36.5X5	T36.5X6
Antitussive NEC	T48.3X1	T48.3X2	T48.3X3	T48.3X4	T48.3X5	T48.3X6
codeine mixture	T4Ø.2X1	T4Ø.2X2	T4Ø.2X3	T4Ø.2X4	T4Ø.2X5	T4Ø.2X6
opiate	T4Ø.2X1	T4Ø.2X2	T4Ø.2X3	T4Ø.2X4	T4Ø.2X5	T4Ø.2X6
Antivaricose drug	T46.8X1	T46.8X2	T46.8X3	T46.8X4	T46.8X5	T46.8X6
Antivenin, antivenom (sera)	T5Ø.Z11	T5Ø.Z12	T5Ø.Z13	T5Ø.Z14	T5Ø.Z15	T5Ø.Z16
crotaline	T5Ø.Z11	T5Ø.Z12	T5Ø.Z13	T5Ø.Z14	T5Ø.Z15	T5Ø.Z16
spider bite	T5Ø.Z11	T5Ø.Z12	T5Ø.Z13	T5Ø.Z14	T5Ø.Z15	T5Ø.Z16
Antivertigo drug	T45.ØX1	T45.ØX2	T45.ØX3	T45.ØX4	T45.ØX5	T45.ØX6
Antiviral drug NEC	T37.5X1	T37.5X2	T37.5X3	T37.5X4	T37.5X5	T37.5X6
eye	T49.5X1	T49.5X2	T49.5X3	T49.5X4	T49.5X5	T49.5X6
Antiwhipworm drug	T37.4X1	T37.4X2	T37.4X3	T37.4X4	T37.4X5	T37.4X6
Ant poisons — see Pesticides						
Antrol — see also by specific chemical substance	T6Ø.91	T6Ø.92	T6Ø.93	T6Ø.94	—	—
fungicide	T6Ø.91	T6Ø.92	T6Ø.93	T6Ø.94	—	—
ANTU (alpha naphthylthiourea)	T6Ø.4X1	T6Ø.4X2	T6Ø.4X3	T6Ø.4X4	—	—
Apalcillin	T36.ØX1	T36.ØX2	T36.ØX3	T36.ØX4	T36.ØX5	T36.ØX6
APC	T48.5X1	T48.5X2	T48.5X3	T48.5X4	T48.5X5	T48.5X6
Aplonidine	T44.4X1	T44.4X2	T44.4X3	T44.4X4	T44.4X5	T44.4X6
Apomorphine	T47.7X1	T47.7X2	T47.7X3	T47.7X4	T47.7X5	T47.7X6

TABLE OF DRUGS AND CHEMICALS

TABLE OF DRUGS AND CHEMICALS

Substance	External Cause (T-Code) Poisoning, Accidental (Unintentional)	Poisoning, Intentional Self-Harm	Poisoning, Assault	Poisoning, Undetermined	Adverse Effect	Underdosing
Appetite depressants, central	T50.5X1	T50.5X2	T50.5X3	T50.5X4	T50.5X5	T50.5X6
Apraclonidine (hydrochloride)	T44.4X1	T44.4X2	T44.4X3	T44.4X4	T44.4X5	T44.4X6
Apresoline	T46.5X1	T46.5X2	T46.5X3	T46.5X4	T46.5X5	T46.5X6
Aprindine	T46.2X1	T46.2X2	T46.2X3	T46.2X4	T46.2X5	T46.2X6
Aprobarbital	T42.3X1	T42.3X2	T42.3X3	T42.3X4	T42.3X5	T42.3X6
Apronalide	T42.6X1	T42.6X2	T42.6X3	T42.6X4	T42.6X5	T42.6X6
Aprotinin	T45.621	T45.622	T45.623	T45.624	T45.625	T45.626
Aptocaine	T41.3X1	T41.3X2	T41.3X3	T41.3X4	T41.3X5	T41.3X6
Aqua fortis	T54.2X1	T54.2X2	T54.2X3	T54.2X4	—	—
Ara-A	T37.5X1	T37.5X2	T37.5X3	T37.5X4	T37.5X5	T37.5X6
Ara-C	T45.1X1	T45.1X2	T45.1X3	T45.1X4	T45.1X5	T45.1X6
Arachis oil	T49.3X1	T49.3X2	T49.3X3	T49.3X4	T49.3X5	T49.3X6
cathartic	T47.4X1	T47.4X2	T47.4X3	T47.4X4	T47.4X5	T47.4X6
Aralen	T37.2X1	T37.2X2	T37.2X3	T37.2X4	T37.2X5	T37.2X6
Arecoline	T44.1X1	T44.1X2	T44.1X3	T44.1X4	T44.1X5	T44.1X6
Arginine	T50.991	T50.992	T50.993	T50.994	T50.995	T50.996
glutamate	T50.991	T50.992	T50.993	T50.994	T50.995	T50.996
Argyrol	T49.0X1	T49.0X2	T49.0X3	T49.0X4	T49.0X5	T49.0X6
ENT agent	T49.6X1	T49.6X2	T49.6X3	T49.6X4	T49.6X5	T49.6X6
ophthalmic preparation	T49.5X1	T49.5X2	T49.5X3	T49.5X4	T49.5X5	T49.5X6
Aristocort	T38.0X1	T38.0X2	T38.0X3	T38.0X4	T38.0X5	T38.0X6
ENT agent	T49.6X1	T49.6X2	T49.6X3	T49.6X4	T49.6X5	T49.6X6
ophthalmic preparation	T49.5X1	T49.5X2	T49.5X3	T49.5X4	T49.5X5	T49.5X6
topical NEC	T49.0X1	T49.0X2	T49.0X3	T49.0X4	T49.0X5	T49.0X6
Aromatics, corrosive	T54.1X1	T54.1X2	T54.1X3	T54.1X4	—	—
disinfectants	T54.1X1	T54.1X2	T54.1X3	T54.1X4	—	—
Arsenate of lead	T57.0X1	T57.0X2	T57.0X3	T57.0X4	—	—
herbicide	T57.0X1	T57.0X2	T57.0X3	T57.0X4	—	—
Arsenic, arsenicals (compounds) (dust) (vapor) NEC	T57.0X1	T57.0X2	T57.0X3	T57.0X4	—	—
anti-infectives	T37.8X1	T37.8X2	T37.8X3	T37.8X4	T37.8X5	T37.8X6
pesticide (dust) (fumes)	T57.0X1	T57.0X2	T57.0X3	T57.0X4	—	—
Arsine (gas)	T57.0X1	T57.0X2	T57.0X3	T57.0X4	—	—
Arsphenamine (silver)	T37.8X1	T37.8X2	T37.8X3	T37.8X4	T37.8X5	T37.8X6
Arsthinol	T37.3X1	T37.3X2	T37.3X3	T37.3X4	T37.3X5	T37.3X6
Artane	T44.3X1	T44.3X2	T44.3X3	T44.3X4	T44.3X5	T44.3X6
Arthropod (venomous) NEC	T63.481	T63.482	T63.483	T63.484	—	—
Articaine	T41.3X1	T41.3X2	T41.3X3	T41.3X4	T41.3X5	T41.3X6
Asbestos	T57.8X1	T57.8X2	T57.8X3	T57.8X4	—	—
Ascaridole	T37.4X1	T37.4X2	T37.4X3	T37.4X4	T37.4X5	T37.4X6
Ascorbic acid	T45.2X1	T45.2X2	T45.2X3	T45.2X4	T45.2X5	T45.2X6
Asiaticoside	T49.0X1	T49.0X2	T49.0X3	T49.0X4	T49.0X5	T49.0X6

Substance	External Cause (T-Code) Poisoning, Accidental (Unintentional)	Poisoning, Intentional Self-Harm	Poisoning, Assault	Poisoning, Undetermined	Adverse Effect	Underdosing
Asparaginase	T45.1X1	T45.1X2	T45.1X3	T45.1X4	T45.1X5	T45.1X6
Aspidium (oleoresin)	T37.4X1	T37.4X2	T37.4X3	T37.4X4	T37.4X5	T37.4X6
Aspirin (aluminum) (soluble)	T39.011	T39.012	T39.013	T39.014	T39.015	T39.016
Aspoxicillin	T36.0X1	T36.0X2	T36.0X3	T36.0X4	T36.0X5	T36.0X6
Astemizole	T45.0X1	T45.0X2	T45.0X3	T45.0X4	T45.0X5	T45.0X6
Astringent (local)	T49.2X1	T49.2X2	T49.2X3	T49.2X4	T49.2X5	T49.2X6
specified NEC	T49.2X1	T49.2X2	T49.2X3	T49.2X4	T49.2X5	T49.2X6
Astromicin	T36.5X1	T36.5X2	T36.5X3	T36.5X4	T36.5X5	T36.5X6
Ataractic drug NEC	T43.501	T43.502	T43.503	T43.504	T43.505	T43.506
Atenolol	T44.7X1	T44.7X2	T44.7X3	T44.7X4	T44.7X5	T44.7X6
Atonia drug, intestinal	T47.4X1	T47.4X2	T47.4X3	T47.4X4	T47.4X5	T47.4X6
Atophan	T50.4X1	T50.4X2	T50.4X3	T50.4X4	T50.4X5	T50.4X6
Atracurium besilate	T48.1X1	T48.1X2	T48.1X3	T48.1X4	T48.1X5	T48.1X6
Atropine	T44.3X1	T44.3X2	T44.3X3	T44.3X4	T44.3X5	T44.3X6
derivative	T44.3X1	T44.3X2	T44.3X3	T44.3X4	T44.3X5	T44.3X6
methonitrate	T44.3X1	T44.3X2	T44.3X3	T44.3X4	T44.3X5	T44.3X6
Attapulgite	T47.6X1	T47.6X2	T47.6X3	T47.6X4	T47.6X5	T47.6X6
Attenuvax	T50.991	T50.992	T50.993	T50.994	T50.995	T50.996
Auramine	T65.891	T65.892	T65.893	T65.894	—	—
dye	T65.6X1	T65.6X2	T65.6X3	T65.6X4	—	—
fungicide	T60.3X1	T60.3X2	T60.3X3	T60.3X4	—	—
Auranofin	T39.4X1	T39.4X2	T39.4X3	T39.4X4	T39.4X5	T39.4X6
Aurantiin	T46.991	T46.992	T46.993	T46.994	T46.995	T46.996
Aureomycin	T36.4X1	T36.4X2	T36.4X3	T36.4X4	T36.4X5	T36.4X6
ophthalmic preparation	T49.5X1	T49.5X2	T49.5X3	T49.5X4	T49.5X5	T49.5X6
topical NEC	T49.0X1	T49.0X2	T49.0X3	T49.0X4	T49.0X5	T49.0X6
Aurothioglucose	T39.4X1	T39.4X2	T39.4X3	T39.4X4	T39.4X5	T39.4X6
Aurothioglycanide	T39.4X1	T39.4X2	T39.4X3	T39.4X4	T39.4X5	T39.4X6
Aurothiomalate sodium	T39.4X1	T39.4X2	T39.4X3	T39.4X4	T39.4X5	T39.4X6
Aurotioprol	T39.4X1	T39.4X2	T39.4X3	T39.4X4	T39.4X5	T39.4X6
Automobile fuel	T52.0X1	T52.0X2	T52.0X3	T52.0X4	—	—
Autonomic nervous system agent NEC	T44.901	T44.902	T44.903	T44.904	T44.905	T44.906
Avlosulfon	T37.1X1	T37.1X2	T37.1X3	T37.1X4	T37.1X5	T37.1X6
Avomine	T42.6X1	T42.6X2	T42.6X3	T42.6X4	T42.6X5	T42.6X6
Axerophthol	T45.2X1	T45.2X2	T45.2X3	T45.2X4	T45.2X5	T45.2X6
Azacitidine	T45.1X1	T45.1X2	T45.1X3	T45.1X4	T45.1X5	T45.1X6
Azacyclonol	T43.591	T43.592	T43.593	T43.594	T43.595	T43.596
Azadirachta	T60.2X1	T60.2X2	T60.2X3	T60.2X4	—	—
Azanidazole	T37.3X1	T37.3X2	T37.3X3	T37.3X4	T37.3X5	T37.3X6
Azapetine	T46.7X1	T46.7X2	T46.7X3	T46.7X4	T46.7X5	T46.7X6
Azapropazone	T39.2X1	T39.2X2	T39.2X3	T39.2X4	T39.2X5	T39.2X6

◄ New   ◄ Revised   ~~deleted~~ Deleted

TABLE OF DRUGS AND CHEMICALS

Substance	Poisoning, Accidental (Unintentional)	Poisoning, Intentional Self-Harm	Poisoning, Assault	Poisoning, Undetermined	Adverse Effect	Underdosing
Azaribine	T45.1X1	T45.1X2	T45.1X3	T45.1X4	T45.1X5	T45.1X6
Azaserine	T45.1X1	T45.1X2	T45.1X3	T45.1X4	T45.1X5	T45.1X6
Azatadine	T45.0X1	T45.0X2	T45.0X3	T45.0X4	T45.0X5	T45.0X6
Azatepa	T45.1X1	T45.1X2	T45.1X3	T45.1X4	T45.1X5	T45.1X6
Azathioprine	T45.1X1	T45.1X2	T45.1X3	T45.1X4	T45.1X5	T45.1X6
Azelaic acid	T49.0X1	T49.0X2	T49.0X3	T49.0X4	T49.0X5	T49.0X6
Azelastine	T45.0X1	T45.0X2	T45.0X3	T45.0X4	T45.0X5	T45.0X6
Azidocillin	T36.0X1	T36.0X2	T36.0X3	T36.0X4	T36.0X5	T36.0X6
Azidothymidine	T37.5X1	T37.5X2	T37.5X3	T37.5X4	T37.5X5	T37.5X6
Azinphos (ethyl) (methyl)	T60.0X1	T60.0X2	T60.0X3	T60.0X4	—	—
Aziridine (chelating)	T54.1X1	T54.1X2	T54.1X3	T54.1X4	—	—
Azithromycin	T36.3X1	T36.3X2	T36.3X3	T36.3X4	T36.3X5	T36.3X6
Azlocillin	T36.01	T36.02	T36.03	T36.04	T36.05	T36.06
Azobenzene smoke	T65.3X1	T65.3X2	T65.3X3	T65.3X4	—	—
acaricide	T60.8X1	T60.8X2	T60.8X3	T60.8X4	—	—
Azosulfamide	T37.0X1	T37.0X2	T37.0X3	T37.0X4	T37.0X5	T37.0X6
AZT	T37.5X1	T37.5X2	T37.5X3	T37.5X4	T37.5X5	T37.5X6
Aztreonam	T36.1X1	T36.1X2	T36.1X3	T36.1X4	T36.1X5	T36.1X6
Azulfidine	T37.0X1	T37.0X2	T37.0X3	T37.0X4	T37.0X5	T37.0X6
Azuresin	T50.8X1	T50.8X2	T50.8X3	T50.8X4	T50.8X5	T50.8X6
B						
Bacampicillin	T36.0X1	T36.0X2	T36.0X3	T36.0X4	T36.0X5	T36.0X6
Bacillus						
lactobacillus	T47.8X1	T47.8X2	T47.8X3	T47.8X4	T47.8X5	T47.8X6
subtilis	T47.6X1	T47.6X2	T47.6X3	T47.6X4	T47.6X5	T47.6X6
Bacimycin	T49.0X1	T49.0X2	T49.0X3	T49.0X4	T49.0X5	T49.0X6
ophthalmic preparation	T49.5X1	T49.5X2	T49.5X3	T49.5X4	T49.5X5	T49.5X6
Bacitracin zinc	T49.0X1	T49.0X2	T49.0X3	T49.0X4	T49.0X5	T49.0X6
with neomycin	T49.0X1	T49.0X2	T49.0X3	T49.0X4	T49.0X5	T49.0X6
ENT agent	T49.6X1	T49.6X2	T49.6X3	T49.6X4	T49.6X5	T49.6X6
ophthalmic preparation	T49.5X1	T49.5X2	T49.5X3	T49.5X4	T49.5X5	T49.5X6
topical NEC	T49.0X1	T49.0X2	T49.0X3	T49.0X4	T49.0X5	T49.0X6
Baclofen	T42.8X1	T42.8X2	T42.8X3	T42.8X4	T42.8X5	T42.8X6
Baking soda	T50.991	T50.992	T50.993	T50.994	T50.995	T50.996
BAL	T45.8X1	T45.8X2	T45.8X3	T45.8X4	T45.8X5	T45.8X6
Bambuterol	T48.6X1	T48.6X2	T48.6X3	T48.6X4	T48.6X5	T48.6X6
Bamethan (sulfate)	T46.7X1	T46.7X2	T46.7X3	T46.7X4	T46.7X5	T46.7X6
Bamifylline	T48.6X1	T48.6X2	T48.6X3	T48.6X4	T48.6X5	T48.6X6
Bamipine	T45.0X1	T45.0X2		T45.0X4	T45.0X5	T45.0X6
Baneberry — see Actaea spicata						
Banewort — see Belladonna						

Substance	Poisoning, Accidental (Unintentional)	Poisoning, Intentional Self-Harm	Poisoning, Assault	Poisoning, Undetermined	Adverse Effect	Underdosing
Barbenyl	T42.3X1	T42.3X2	T42.3X3	T42.3X4	T42.3X5	T42.3X6
Barbexaclone	T42.6X1	T42.6X2	T42.6X3	T42.6X4	T42.6X5	T42.6X6
Barbital	T42.3X1	T42.3X2	T42.3X3	T42.3X4	T42.3X5	T42.3X6
sodium	T42.3X1	T42.3X2	T42.3X3	T42.3X4	T42.3X5	T42.3X6
Barbitone	T42.3X1	T42.3X2	T42.3X3	T42.3X4	T42.3X5	T42.3X6
Barbiturate NEC	T42.3X1	T42.3X2	T42.3X3	T42.3X4	T42.3X5	T42.3X6
with tranquilizer	T42.3X1	T42.3X2	T42.3X3	T42.3X4	T42.3X5	T42.3X6
anesthetic (intravenous)	T41.1X1	T41.1X2	T41.1X3	T41.1X4	T41.1X5	T41.1X6
Barium (carbonate) (chloride) (sulfite)	T57.8X1	T57.8X2	T57.8X3	T57.8X4	—	—
diagnostic agent	T50.8X1	T50.8X2	T50.8X3	T50.8X4	T50.8X5	T50.8X6
pesticide	T60.4X1	T60.4X2	T60.4X3	T60.4X4	—	—
rodenticide	T60.4X1	T60.4X2	T60.4X3	T60.4X4	—	—
sulfate (medicinal)	T50.8X1	T50.8X2	T50.8X3	T50.8X4	T50.8X5	T50.8X6
Barrier cream	T49.3X1	T49.3X2	T49.3X3	T49.3X4	T49.3X5	T49.3X6
Basic fuchsin	T49.0X1	T49.0X2	T49.0X3	T49.0X4	T49.0X5	T49.0X6
Battery acid or fluid	T54.2X1	T54.2X2	T54.2X3	T54.2X4	—	—
Bay rum	T51.8X1	T51.8X2	T51.8X3	T51.8X4	—	—
BCG (vaccine)	T50.A91	T50.A92	T50.A93	T50.A94	T50.A95	T50.A96
BCNU	T45.1X1	T45.1X2	T45.1X3	T45.1X4	T45.1X5	T45.1X6
Bearsfoot	T62.2X1	T62.2X2	T62.2X3	T62.2X4	—	—
Beclamide	T42.6X1	T42.6X2	T42.6X3	T42.6X4	T42.6X5	T42.6X6
Beclomethasone	T44.5X1	T44.5X2	T44.5X3	T44.5X4	T44.5X5	T44.5X6
Bee (sting) (venom)	T63.441	T63.442	T63.443	T63.444	—	—
Befunolol	T49.5X1	T49.5X2	T49.5X3	T49.5X4	T49.5X5	T49.5X6
Bekanamycin	T36.5X1	T36.5X2	T36.5X3	T36.5X4	T36.5X5	T36.5X6
Belladonna — see also Nightshade						
alkaloids	T44.3X1	T44.3X2	T44.3X3	T44.3X4	T44.3X5	T44.3X6
extract	T44.3X1	T44.3X2	T44.3X3	T44.3X4	T44.3X5	T44.3X6
herb	T44.3X1	T44.3X2	T44.3X3	T44.3X4	T44.3X5	T44.3X6
Bemegride	T50.7X1	T50.7X2	T50.7X3	T50.7X4	T50.7X5	T50.7X6
Benactyzine	T44.3X1	T44.3X2	T44.3X3	T44.3X4	T44.3X5	T44.3X6
Benadryl	T45.0X1	T45.0X2	T45.0X3	T45.0X4	T45.0X5	T45.0X6
Benaprizine	T44.3X1	T44.3X2	T44.3X3	T44.3X4	T44.3X5	T44.3X6
Benazepril	T46.4X1	T46.4X2	T46.4X3	T46.4X4	T46.4X5	T46.4X6
Bencyclane	T46.7X1	T46.7X2	T46.7X3	T46.7X4	T46.7X5	T46.7X6
Bendazol	T46.3X1	T46.3X2	T46.3X3	T46.3X4	T46.3X5	T46.3X6
Bendrofluazide	T50.2X1	T50.2X2	T50.2X3	T50.2X4	T50.2X5	T50.2X6
Bendroflumethiazide	T50.2X1	T50.2X2	T50.2X3	T50.2X4	T50.2X5	T50.2X6
Benemid	T50.4X1	T50.4X2	T50.4X3	T50.4X4	T50.4X5	T50.4X6
Benethamine penicillin	T36.0X1	T36.0X2	T36.0X3	T36.0X4	T36.0X5	T36.0X6
Benisone	T49.0X1	T49.0X2	T49.0X3	T49.0X4	T49.0X5	T49.0X6

TABLE OF DRUGS AND CHEMICALS

TABLE OF DRUGS AND CHEMICALS

Substance	External Cause (T-Code) Poisoning, Accidental (Unintentional)	Poisoning, Intentional Self-Harm	Poisoning, Assault	Poisoning, Undetermined	Adverse Effect	Underdosing
Benexate	T47.1X1	T47.1X2	T47.1X3	T47.1X4	T47.1X5	T47.1X6
Benfluorex	T46.6X1	T46.6X2	T46.6X3	T46.6X4	T46.6X5	T46.6X6
Benfotiamine	T45.2X1	T45.2X2	T45.2X3	T45.2X4	T45.2X5	T45.2X6
Benomyl	T60.0X1	T60.0X2	T60.0X3	T60.0X4	—	—
Benoquin	T49.8X1	T49.8X2	T49.8X3	T49.8X4	T49.8X5	T49.8X6
Benoxinate	T41.3X1	T41.3X2	T41.3X3	T41.3X4	T41.3X5	T41.3X6
Benperidol	T43.4X1	T43.4X2	T43.4X3	T43.4X4	T43.4X5	T43.4X6
Benproperine	T48.3X1	T48.3X2	T48.3X3	T48.3X4	T48.3X5	T48.3X6
Benserazide	T42.8X1	T42.8X2	T42.8X3	T42.8X4	T42.8X5	T42.8X6
Bentazepam	T42.4X1	T42.4X2	T42.4X3	T42.4X4	T42.4X5	T42.4X6
Bentiromide	T50.8X1	T50.8X2	T50.8X3	T50.8X4	T50.8X5	T50.8X6
Bentonite	T49.3X1	T49.3X2	T49.3X3	T49.3X4	T49.3X5	T49.3X6
Benzalbutyramide	T46.6X1	T46.6X2	T46.6X3	T46.6X4	T46.6X5	T46.6X6
Benzalkonium (chloride)	T49.0X1	T49.0X2	T49.0X3	T49.0X4	T49.0X5	T49.0X6
ophthalmic preparation	T49.5X1	T49.5X2	T49.5X3	T49.5X4	T49.5X5	T49.5X6
Benzamine	T41.3X1	T41.3X2	T41.3X3	T41.3X4	T41.3X5	T41.3X6
lactate	T49.1X1	T49.1X2	T49.1X3	T49.1X4	T49.1X5	T49.1X6
Benzamidosalicylate (calcium)	T37.1X1	T37.1X2	T37.1X3	T37.1X4	T37.1X5	T37.1X6
Benzamphetamine	T50.5X1	T50.5X2	T50.5X3	T50.5X4	T50.5X5	T50.5X6
Benzapril hydrochloride	T46.5X1	T46.5X2	T46.5X3	T46.5X4	T46.5X5	T46.5X6
Benzathine benzylpenicillin	T36.0X1	T36.0X2	T36.0X3	T36.0X4	T36.0X5	T36.0X6
Benzathine penicillin	T36.0X1	T36.0X2	T36.0X3	T36.0X4	T36.0X5	T36.0X6
Benzatropine	T42.8X1	T42.8X2	T42.8X3	T42.8X4	T42.8X5	T42.8X6
Benzbromarone	T50.4X1	T50.4X2	T50.4X3	T50.4X4	T50.4X5	T50.4X6
Benzcarbimine	T45.1X1	T45.1X2	T45.1X3	T45.1X4	T45.1X5	T45.1X6
Benzedrex	T44.991	T44.992	T44.993	T44.994	T44.995	T44.996
Benzedrine (amphetamine)	T43.621	T43.622	T43.623	T43.624	T43.625	T43.626
Benzenamine	T65.3X1	T65.3X2	T65.3X3	T65.3X4	—	—
Benzene	T52.1X1	T52.1X2	T52.1X3	T52.1X4	—	—
homologues (acetyl) (dimethyl) (methyl) (solvent)	T52.2X1	T52.2X2	T52.2X3	T52.2X4	—	—
Benzethonium (chloride)	T49.0X1	T49.0X2	T49.0X3	T49.0X4	T49.0X5	T49.0X6
Benzfetamine	T50.5X1	T50.5X2	T50.5X3	T50.5X4	T50.5X5	T50.5X6
Benzhexol	T44.3X1	T44.3X2	T44.3X3	T44.3X4	T44.3X5	T44.3X6
Benzhydramine (chloride)	T45.0X1	T45.0X2	T45.0X3	T45.0X4	T45.0X5	T45.0X6
Benzidine	T65.891	T65.892	T65.893	T65.894	—	—
Benzilonium bromide	T44.3X1	T44.3X2	T44.3X3	T44.3X4	T44.3X5	T44.3X6
Benzimidazole	T60.3X1	T60.3X2	T60.3X3	T60.3X4	—	—
Benzin(e) — see Ligroin						
Benziodarone	T46.3X1	T46.3X2	T46.3X3	T46.3X4	T46.3X5	T46.3X6
Benznidazole	T37.3X1	T37.3X2	T37.3X3	T37.3X4	T37.3X5	T37.3X6
Benzocaine	T41.3X1	T41.3X2	T41.3X3	T41.3X4	T41.3X5	T41.3X6

Substance	External Cause (T-Code) Poisoning, Accidental (Unintentional)	Poisoning, Intentional Self-Harm	Poisoning, Assault	Poisoning, Undetermined	Adverse Effect	Underdosing
Benzoctamine	T43.0X1	T43.0X2	T43.0X3	T43.0X4	T43.0X5	T43.0X6
Benzodiapin	T42.4X1	T42.4X2	T42.4X3	T42.4X4	T42.4X5	T42.4X6
Benzodiazepine NEC	T42.4X1	T42.4X2	T42.4X3	T42.4X4	T42.4X5	T42.4X6
Benzoic acid	T49.0X1	T49.0X2	T49.0X3	T49.0X4	T49.0X5	T49.0X6
with salicylic acid	T49.0X1	T49.0X2	T49.0X3	T49.0X4	T49.0X5	T49.0X6
Benzoin (tincture)	T48.5X1	T48.5X2	T48.5X3	T48.5X4	T48.5X5	T48.5X6
Benzol (benzene)	T52.1X1	T52.1X2	T52.1X3	T52.1X4	—	—
vapor	T52.0X1	T52.0X2	T52.0X3	T52.0X4	—	—
Benzomorphan	T40.2X1	T40.2X2	T40.2X3	T40.2X4	T40.2X5	T40.2X6
Benzonatate	T48.3X1	T48.3X2	T48.3X3	T48.3X4	T48.3X5	T48.3X6
Benzophenones	T49.3X1	T49.3X2	T49.3X3	T49.3X4	T49.3X5	T49.3X6
Benzopyrone	T46.991	T46.992	T46.993	T46.994	T46.995	T46.996
Benzothiadiazides	T50.2X1	T50.2X2	T50.2X3	T50.2X4	T50.2X5	T50.2X6
Benzoxonium chloride	T49.0X1	T49.0X2	T49.0X3	T49.0X4	T49.0X5	T49.0X6
Benzoyl peroxide	T49.0X1	T49.0X2	T49.0X3	T49.0X4	T49.0X5	T49.0X6
Benzoylpas calcium	T37.1X1	T37.1X2	T37.1X3	T37.1X4	T37.1X5	T37.1X6
Benzperidin	T43.591	T43.592	T43.593	T43.594	T43.595	T43.596
Benzperidol	T43.591	T43.592	T43.593	T43.594	T43.595	T43.596
Benzphetamine	T50.5X1	T50.5X2	T50.5X3	T50.5X4	T50.5X5	T50.5X6
Benzpyrinium bromide	T44.1X1	T44.1X2	T44.1X3	T44.1X4	T44.1X5	T44.1X6
Benzquinamide	T45.0X1	T45.0X2	T45.0X3	T45.0X4	T45.0X5	T45.0X6
Benzthiazide	T50.2X1	T50.2X2	T50.2X3	T50.2X4	T50.2X5	T50.2X6
Benztropine						
anticholinergic	T44.3X1	T44.3X2	T44.3X3	T44.3X4	T44.3X5	T44.3X6
antiparkinson	T42.8X1	T42.8X2	T42.8X3	T42.8X4	T42.8X5	T42.8X6
Benzydamine	T49.0X1	T49.0X2	T49.0X3	T49.0X4	T49.0X5	T49.0X6
Benzyl						
acetate	T52.8X1	T52.8X2	T52.8X3	T52.8X4	—	—
alcohol	T49.0X1	T49.0X2	T49.0X3	T49.0X4	T49.0X5	T49.0X6
benzoate	T49.0X1	T49.0X2	T49.0X3	T49.0X4	T49.0X5	T49.0X6
Benzoic acid	T49.0X1	T49.0X2	T49.0X3	T49.0X4	T49.0X5	T49.0X6
morphine	T40.2X1	T40.2X2	T40.2X3	T40.2X4	—	—
nicotinate	T46.6X1	T46.6X2	T46.6X3	T46.6X4	T46.6X5	T46.6X6
penicillin	T36.0X1	T36.0X2	T36.0X3	T36.0X4	T36.0X5	T36.0X6
Benzylhydrochlorthia-zide	T50.2X1	T50.2X2	T50.2X3	T50.2X4	T50.2X5	T50.2X6
Benzylpenicillin	T36.0X1	T36.0X2	T36.0X3	T36.0X4	T36.0X5	T36.0X6
Benzylthiouracil	T38.2X1	T38.2X2	T38.2X3	T38.2X4	T38.2X5	T38.2X6
Bephenium hydroxy-naphthoate	T37.4X1	T37.4X2	T37.4X3	T37.4X4	T37.4X5	T37.4X6
Bepridil	T46.1X1	T46.1X2	T46.1X3	T46.1X4	T46.1X5	T46.1X6
Bergamot oil	T65.891	T65.892	T65.893	T65.894	—	—
Bergapten	T50.991	T50.992	T50.993	T50.994	T50.995	T50.996
Berries, poisonous	T62.1X1	T62.1X2	T62.1X3	T62.1X4	—	—

◀ New ◀ Revised ~~deleted~~ Deleted

	External Cause (T-Code)					
Substance	Poisoning, Accidental (Unintentional)	Poisoning, Intentional Self-Harm	Poisoning, Assault	Poisoning, Undetermined	Adverse Effect	Underdosing
Beryllium (compounds)	T56.7X1	T56.7X2	T56.7X3	T56.7X4	—	—
b-acetyldigoxin	T46.0X1	T46.0X2	T46.0X3	T46.0X4	T46.0X5	T46.0X6
beta adrenergic blocking agent, heart	T44.7X1	T44.7X2	T44.7X3	T44.7X4	T44.7X5	T44.7X6
b-benzalbutyramide	T46.6X1	T46.6X2	T46.6X3	T46.6X4	T46.6X5	T46.6X6
Betacarotene	T45.2X1	T45.2X2	T45.2X3	T45.2X4	T45.2X5	T45.2X6
b-eucaine	T49.1X1	T49.1X2	T49.1X3	T49.1X4	T49.1X5	T49.1X6
Beta-Chlor	T42.6X1	T42.6X2	T42.6X3	T42.6X4	T42.6X5	T42.6X6
b-galactosidase	T47.5X1	T47.5X2	T47.5X3	T47.5X4	T47.5X5	T47.5X6
Betahistine	T46.7X1	T46.7X2	T46.7X3	T46.7X4	T46.7X5	T46.7X6
Betaine	T47.5X1	T47.5X2	T47.5X3	T47.5X4	T47.5X5	T47.5X6
Betamethasone	T49.0X1	T49.0X2	T49.0X3	T49.0X4	T49.0X5	T49.0X6
topical	T49.0X1	T49.0X2	T49.0X3	T49.0X4	T49.0X5	T49.0X6
Betamicin	T36.8X1	T36.8X2	T36.8X3	T36.8X4	T36.8X5	T36.8X6
Betanidine	T46.5X1	T46.5X2	T46.5X3	T46.5X4	T46.5X5	T46.5X6
b-sitosterol(s)	T46.6X1	T46.6X2	T46.6X3	T46.6X4	T46.6X5	T46.6X6
Betaxolol	T44.7X1	T44.7X2	T44.7X3	T44.7X4	T44.7X5	T44.7X6
Betazole	T50.8X1	T50.8X2	T50.8X3	T50.8X4	T50.8X5	T50.8X6
Bethanechol	T44.1X1	T44.1X2	T44.1X3	T44.1X4	T44.1X5	T44.1X6
chloride	T44.1X1	T44.1X2	T44.1X3	T44.1X4	T44.1X5	T44.1X6
Bethanidine	T46.5X1	T46.5X2	T46.5X3	T46.5X4	T46.5X5	T46.5X6
Betoxycaine	T41.3X1	T41.3X2	T41.3X3	T41.3X4	T41.3X5	T41.3X6
Betula oil	T49.3X1	T49.3X2	T49.3X3	T49.3X4	T49.3X5	T49.3X6
Bevantolol	T44.7X1	T44.7X2	T44.7X3	T44.7X4	T44.7X5	T44.7X6
Bevonium metilsulfate	T44.3X1	T44.3X2	T44.3X3	T44.3X4	T44.3X5	T44.3X6
Bezafibrate	T46.6X1	T46.6X2	T46.6X3	T46.6X4	T46.6X5	T46.6X6
Bezitramide	T40.4X1	T40.4X2	T40.4X3	T40.4X4	T40.4X5	T40.4X6
BHA	T50.991	T50.992	T50.993	T50.994	T50.995	T50.996
Bhang	T40.7X1	T40.7X2	T40.7X3	T40.7X4	T40.7X5	T40.7X6
BHC (medicinal)	T49.0X1	T49.0X2	T49.0X3	T49.0X4	T49.0X5	T49.0X6
nonmedicinal (vapor)	T53.6X1	T53.6X2	T53.6X3	T53.6X4	—	—
Bialamicol	T37.3X1	T37.3X2	T37.3X3	T37.3X4	T37.3X5	T37.3X6
Bibenzonium bromide	T48.3X1	T48.3X2	T48.3X3	T48.3X4	T48.3X5	T48.3X6
Bibrocathol	T49.5X1	T49.5X2	T49.5X3	T49.5X4	T49.5X5	T49.5X6
Bichloride of mercury — see Mercury, chloride						
Bichromates (calcium) (potassium) (sodium) (crystals)	T57.8X1	T57.8X2	T57.8X3	T57.8X4	—	—
fumes	T56.2X1	T56.2X2	T56.2X3	T56.2X4	—	—
Biclotymol	T49.6X1	T49.6X2	T49.6X3	T49.6X4	T49.6X5	T49.6X6
Bicuculline	T50.7X1	T50.7X2	T50.7X3	T50.7X4	T50.7X5	T50.7X6
Bifemelane	T43.291	T43.292	T43.293	T43.294	T43.295	T43.296
Biguanide derivatives, oral	T38.3X1	T38.3X2	T38.3X3	T38.3X4	T38.3X5	T38.3X6

	External Cause (T-Code)					
Substance	Poisoning, Accidental (Unintentional)	Poisoning, Intentional Self-Harm	Poisoning, Assault	Poisoning, Undetermined	Adverse Effect	Underdosing
Biligrafin	T50.8X1	T50.8X2	T50.8X3	T50.8X4	T50.8X5	T50.8X6
Bile salts	T47.5X1	T47.5X2	T47.5X3	T47.5X4	T47.5X5	T47.5X6
Bilopaque	T50.8X1	T50.8X2	T50.8X3	T50.8X4	T50.8X5	T50.8X6
Binifibrate	T46.6X1	T46.6X2	T46.6X3	T46.6X4	T46.6X5	T46.6X6
Binitrobenzol	T65.3X1	T65.3X2	T65.3X3	T65.3X4	—	—
Bioflavonoid(s)	T46.991	T46.992	T46.993	T46.994	T46.995	T46.996
Biological substance NEC	T50.901	T50.902	T50.903	T50.904	T50.905	T50.906
Biotin	T45.2X1	T45.2X2	T45.2X3	T45.2X4	T45.2X5	T45.2X6
Biperiden	T44.3X1	T44.3X2	T44.3X3	T44.3X4	T44.3X5	T44.3X6
Bisacodyl	T47.2X1	T47.2X2	T47.2X3	T47.2X4	T47.2X5	T47.2X6
Bisbentiamine	T45.2X1	T45.2X2	T45.2X3	T45.2X4	T45.2X5	T45.2X6
Bisbutiamine	T45.2X1	T45.2X2	T45.2X3	T45.2X4	T45.2X5	T45.2X6
Bisdequalinium (salts) (diacetate)	T49.6X1	T49.6X2	T49.6X3	T49.6X4	T49.6X5	T49.6X6
Bishydroxycoumarin	T45.511	T45.512	T45.513	T45.514	T45.515	T45.516
Bismarsen	T37.8X1	T37.8X2	T37.8X3	T37.8X4	T37.8X5	T37.8X6
Bismuth salts	T47.6X1	T47.6X2	T47.6X3	T47.6X4	T47.6X5	T47.6X6
aluminate	T47.1X1	T47.1X2	T47.1X3	T47.1X4	T47.1X5	T47.1X6
anti-infectives	T37.8X1	T37.8X2	T37.8X3	T37.8X4	T37.8X5	T37.8X6
formic iodide	T49.0X1	T49.0X2	T49.0X3	T49.0X4	T49.0X5	T49.0X6
glycolylarsenate	T49.0X1	T49.0X2	T49.0X3	T49.0X4	T49.0X5	T49.0X6
nonmedicinal (compounds) NEC	T65.91	T65.92	T65.93	T65.94	—	—
subcarbonate	T47.6X1	T47.6X2	T47.6X3	T47.6X4	T47.6X5	T47.6X6
subsalicylate	T37.8X1	T37.8X2	T37.8X3	T37.8X4	T37.8X5	T37.8X6
sulfarsphenamine	T37.8X1	T37.8X2	T37.8X3	T37.8X4	T37.8X5	T37.8X6
Bisoprolol	T44.7X1	T44.7X2	T44.7X3	T44.7X4	T44.7X5	T44.7X6
Bisoxatin	T47.2X1	T47.2X2	T47.2X3	T47.2X4	T47.2X5	T47.2X6
Bisulepin (hydrochloride)	T45.0X1	T45.0X2	T45.0X3	T45.0X4	T45.0X5	T45.0X6
Bithionol	T37.8X1	T37.8X2	T37.8X3	T37.8X4	T37.8X5	T37.8X6
anthelminthic	T37.4X1	T37.4X2	T37.4X3	T37.4X4	T37.4X5	T37.4X6
Bitolterol	T48.6X1	T48.6X2	T48.6X3	T48.6X4	T48.6X5	T48.6X6
Bitoscanate	T37.4X1	T37.4X2	T37.4X3	T37.4X4	T37.4X5	T37.4X6
Bitter almond oil	T62.8X1	T62.8X2	T62.8X3	T62.8X4	—	—
Bittersweet	T62.2X1	T62.2X2	T62.2X3	T62.2X4	—	—
Black						
flag	T60.91	T60.92	T60.93	T60.94	—	—
henbane	T62.2X1	T62.2X2	T62.2X3	T62.2X4	—	—
leaf (40)	T60.91	T60.92	T60.93	T60.94	—	—
widow spider (bite)	T63.311	T63.312	T63.313	T63.314		
antivenin	T50.Z11	T50.Z12	T50.Z13	T50.Z14	T50.Z15	T50.Z16
Blast furnace gas (carbon monoxide from)	T58.8X1	T58.8X2	T58.8X3	T58.8X4	—	—
Bleach	T54.91	T54.92	T54.93	T54.94		

TABLE OF DRUGS AND CHEMICALS

Substance	Poisoning, Accidental (Unintentional)	Poisoning, Intentional Self-Harm	Poisoning, Assault	Poisoning, Undetermined	Adverse Effect	Underdosing
Bleaching agent (medicinal)	T49.4X1	T49.4X2	T49.4X3	T49.4X4	T49.4X5	T49.4X6
Bleomycin	T45.1X1	T45.1X2	T45.1X3	T45.1X4	T45.1X5	T45.1X6
Blockain	T41.3X1	T41.3X2	T41.3X3	T41.3X4	T41.3X5	T41.3X6
infiltration (subcutaneous)	T41.3X1	T41.3X2	T41.3X3	T41.3X4	T41.3X5	T41.3X6
nerve block (peripheral) (plexus)	T41.3X1	T41.3X2	T41.3X3	T41.3X4	T41.3X5	T41.3X6
topical (surface)	T41.3X1	T41.3X2	T41.3X3	T41.3X4	T41.3X5	T41.3X6
Blockers, calcium channel	T46.1X1	T46.1X2	T46.1X3	T46.1X4	T46.1X5	T46.1X6
Blood (derivatives) (natural) (plasma) (whole)	T45.8X1	T45.8X2	T45.8X3	T45.8X4	T45.8X5	T45.8X6
dried	T45.8X1	T45.8X2	T45.8X3	T45.8X4	T45.8X5	T45.8X6
drug affecting NEC	T45.91	T45.92	T45.93	T45.94	T45.95	T45.96
expander NEC	T45.8X1	T45.8X2	T45.8X3	T45.8X4	T45.8X5	T45.8X6
fraction NEC	T45.8X1	T45.8X2	T45.8X3	T45.8X4	T45.8X5	T45.8X6
substitute (macromolecular)	T45.8X1	T45.8X2	T45.8X3	T45.8X4	T45.8X5	T45.8X6
Blue velvet	T40.2X1	T40.2X2	T40.2X3	T40.2X4	—	—
Bone meal	T62.8X1	T62.8X2	T62.8X3	T62.8X4	—	—
Bonine	T45.0X1	T45.0X2	T45.0X3	T45.0X4	T45.0X5	T45.0X6
Bopindolol	T44.7X1	T44.7X2	T44.7X3	T44.7X4	T44.7X5	T44.7X6
Boracic acid	T49.0X1	T49.0X2	T49.0X3	T49.0X4	T49.0X5	T49.0X6
ENT agent	T49.6X1	T49.6X2	T49.6X3	T49.6X4	T49.6X5	T49.6X6
ophthalmic preparation	T49.5X1	T49.5X2	T49.5X3	T49.5X4	T49.5X5	T49.5X6
Borane complex	T57.8X1	T57.8X2	T57.8X3	T57.8X4	—	—
Borate(s)	T57.8X1	T57.8X2	T57.8X3	T57.8X4	—	—
buffer	T50.991	T50.992	T50.993	T50.994	T50.995	T50.996
cleanser	T54.91	T54.92	T54.93	T54.94	—	—
sodium	T57.8X1	T57.8X2	T57.8X3	T57.8X4	—	—
Borax (cleanser)	T54.91	T54.92	T54.93	T54.94	—	—
Bordeaux mixture	T60.3X1	T60.3X2	T60.3X3	T60.3X4	—	—
Boric acid	T49.0X1	T49.0X2	T49.0X3	T49.0X4	T49.0X5	T49.0X6
ENT agent	T49.6X1	T49.6X2	T49.6X3	T49.6X4	T49.6X5	T49.6X6
ophthalmic preparation	T49.5X1	T49.5X2	T49.5X3	T49.5X4	T49.5X5	T49.5X6
Bornaprine	T44.3X1	T44.3X2	T44.3X3	T44.3X4	T44.3X5	T44.3X6
Boron	T57.8X1	T57.8X2	T57.8X3	T57.8X4	—	—
hydride NEC	T57.8X1	T57.8X2	T57.8X3	T57.8X4	—	—
fumes or gas	T57.8X1	T57.8X2	T57.8X3	T57.8X4	—	—
trifluoride	T59.891	T59.892	T59.893	T59.894	—	—
Botox	T48.291	T48.292	T48.293	T48.294	T48.295	T48.296
Botulinus anti-toxin (type A, B)	T50.Z11	T50.Z12	T50.Z13	T50.Z14	T50.Z15	T50.Z16
Brake fluid vapor	T59.891	T59.892	T59.893	T59.894	—	—
Brallobarbital	T42.3X1	T42.3X2	T42.3X3	T42.3X4	T42.3X5	T42.3X6
Bran (wheat)	T47.4X1	T47.4X2	T47.4X3	T47.4X4	T47.4X5	T47.4X6
Brass (fumes)	T56.891	T56.892	T56.893	T56.894	—	—

Substance	Poisoning, Accidental (Unintentional)	Poisoning, Intentional Self-Harm	Poisoning, Assault	Poisoning, Undetermined	Adverse Effect	Underdosing
Brasso	T52.0X1	T52.0X2	T52.0X3	T52.0X4	—	—
Bretylium tosilate	T46.2X1	T46.2X2	T46.2X3	T46.2X4	T46.2X5	T46.2X6
Brevital (sodium)	T41.1X1	T41.1X2	T41.1X3	T41.1X4	T41.1X5	T41.1X6
Brinase	T45.3X1	T45.3X2	T45.3X3	T45.3X4	T45.3X5	T45.3X6
British antilewisite	T45.8X1	T45.8X2	T45.8X3	T45.8X4	T45.8X5	T45.8X6
Brodifacoum	T60.4X1	T60.4X2	T60.4X3	T60.4X4	—	—
Bromal (hydrate)	T42.6X1	T42.6X2	T42.6X3	T42.6X4	T42.6X5	T42.6X6
Bromazepam	T42.4X1	T42.4X2	T42.4X3	T42.4X4	T42.4X5	T42.4X6
Bromazine	T45.0X1	T45.0X2	T45.0X3	T45.0X4	T45.0X5	T45.0X6
Brombenzylcyanide	T59.3X1	T59.3X2	T59.3X3	T59.3X4	—	—
Bromelains	T45.3X1	T45.3X2	T45.3X3	T45.3X4	T45.3X5	T45.3X6
Bromethalin	T60.4X1	T60.4X2	T60.4X3	T60.4X4	—	—
Bromhexine	T48.4X1	T48.4X2	T48.4X3	T48.4X4	T48.4X5	T48.4X6
Bromide salts	T42.6X1	T42.6X2	T42.6X3	T42.6X4	T42.6X5	T42.6X6
Bromindione	T45.511	T45.512	T45.513	T45.514	T45.515	T45.516
Bromine						
compounds (medicinal)	T42.6X1	T42.6X2	T42.6X3	T42.6X4	T42.6X5	T42.6X6
sedative	T42.6X1	T42.6X2	T42.6X3	T42.6X4	T42.6X5	T42.6X6
vapor	T59.891	T59.892	T59.893	T59.894	—	—
Bromisovalum	T42.6X1	T42.6X2	T42.6X3	T42.6X4	T42.6X5	T42.6X6
Bromisoval	T42.6X1	T42.6X2	T42.6X3	T42.6X4	T42.6X5	T42.6X6
Bromobenzylcyanide	T59.3X1	T59.3X2	T59.3X3	T59.3X4	—	—
Bromochlorosalicylani-lide	T49.0X1	T49.0X2	T49.0X3	T49.0X4	T49.0X5	T49.0X6
Bromocriptine	T42.8X1	T42.8X2	T42.8X3	T42.8X4	T42.8X5	T42.8X6
Bromodiphenhydramine	T45.0X1	T45.0X2	T45.0X3	T45.0X4	T45.0X5	T45.0X6
Bromoform	T42.6X1	T42.6X2	T42.6X3	T42.6X4	T42.6X5	T42.6X6
Bromophenol blue reagent	T50.991	T50.992	T50.993	T50.994	T50.995	T50.996
Bromopride	T47.8X1	T47.8X2	T47.8X3	T47.8X4	T47.8X5	T47.8X6
Bromosalicylchloranitide	T49.0X1	T49.0X2	T49.0X3	T49.0X4	T49.0X5	T49.0X6
Bromosalicylhydroxamic acid	T37.1X1	T37.1X2	T37.1X3	T37.1X4	T37.1X5	T37.1X6
Bromo-seltzer	T39.1X1	T39.1X2	T39.1X3	T39.1X4	T39.1X5	T39.1X6
Bromoxynil	T60.3X1	T60.3X2	T60.3X3	T60.3X4	—	—
Bromperidol	T43.4X1	T43.4X2	T43.4X3	T43.4X4	T43.4X5	T43.4X6
Brompheniramine	T45.0X1	T45.0X2	T45.0X3	T45.0X4	T45.0X5	T45.0X6
Bromsulfophthalein	T50.8X1	T50.8X2	T50.8X3	T50.8X4	T50.8X5	T50.8X6
Bromural	T42.6X1	T42.6X2	T42.6X3	T42.6X4	T42.6X5	T42.6X6
Bromvaletone	T42.6X1	T42.6X2	T42.6X3	T42.6X4	T42.6X5	T42.6X6
Bronchodilator NEC	T48.6X1	T48.6X2	T48.6X3	T48.6X4	T48.6X5	T48.6X6
Brotizolam	T42.4X1	T42.4X2	T42.4X3	T42.4X4	T42.4X5	T42.4X6
Brovincamine	T46.7X1	T46.7X2	T46.7X3	T46.7X4	T46.7X5	T46.7X6
Brown spider (bite) (venom)	T63.391	T63.392	T63.393	T63.394	—	—

◄ New ◄ Revised ~~deleted~~ Deleted

Substance	Poisoning, Accidental (Unintentional)	Poisoning, Intentional Self-Harm	Poisoning, Assault	Poisoning, Undetermined	Adverse Effect	Underdosing
Brown recluse spider (bite) (venom)	T63.331	T63.332	T63.333	T63.334	—	—
Broxaterol	T48.6X1	T48.6X2	T48.6X3	T48.6X4	T48.6X5	T48.6X6
Broxuridine	T45.1X1	T45.1X2	T45.1X3	T45.1X4	T45.1X5	T45.1X6
Broxyquinoline	T37.8X1	T37.8X2	T37.8X3	T37.8X4	T37.8X5	T37.8X6
Bruceine	T48.291	T48.292	T48.293	T48.294	T48.295	T48.296
Brucia	T62.2X1	T62.2X2	T62.2X3	T62.2X4	—	—
Brucine	T65.1X1	T65.1X2	T65.1X3	T65.1X4	—	—
Brunswick green — see Copper						
Bruten — see Ibuprofen						
Bryonia	T47.2X1	T47.2X2	T47.2X3	T47.2X4	T47.2X5	T47.2X6
Buclizine	T45.0X1	T45.0X2	T45.0X3	T45.0X4	T45.0X5	T45.0X6
Buclosamide	T49.0X1	T49.0X2	T49.0X3	T49.0X4	T49.0X5	T49.0X6
Budesonide	T44.5X1	T44.5X2	T44.5X3	T44.5X4	T44.5X5	T44.5X6
Budralazine	T46.5X1	T46.5X2	T46.5X3	T46.5X4	T46.5X5	T46.5X6
Bufferin	T39.011	T39.012	T39.013	T39.014	T39.015	T39.016
Buflomedil	T46.7X1	T46.7X2	T46.7X3	T46.7X4	T46.7X5	T46.7X6
Buformin	T38.3X1	T38.3X2	T38.3X3	T38.3X4	T38.3X5	T38.3X6
Bufotenine	T40.991	T40.992	T40.993	T40.994	—	—
Bufrolin	T48.6X1	T48.6X2	T48.6X3	T48.6X4	T48.6X5	T48.6X6
Bufylline	T48.6X1	T48.6X2	T48.6X3	T48.6X4	T48.6X5	T48.6X6
Bulk filler	T50.5X1	T50.5X2	T50.5X3	T50.5X4	T50.5X5	T50.5X6
cathartic	T47.4X1	T47.4X2	T47.4X3	T47.4X4	T47.4X5	T47.4X6
Bumetanide	T50.1X1	T50.1X2	T50.1X3	T50.1X4	T50.1X5	T50.1X6
Bunaftine	T46.2X1	T46.2X2	T46.2X3	T46.2X4	T46.2X5	T46.2X6
Bunamiodyl	T50.8X1	T50.8X2	T50.8X3	T50.8X4	T50.8X5	T50.8X6
Bunazosin	T44.6X1	T44.6X2	T44.6X3	T44.6X4	T44.6X5	T44.6X6
Bunitrolol	T44.7X1	T44.7X2	T44.7X3	T44.7X4	T44.7X5	T44.7X6
Buphenine	T46.7X1	T46.7X2	T46.7X3	T46.7X4	T46.7X5	T46.7X6
Bupivacaine	T41.3X1	T41.3X2	T41.3X3	T41.3X4	T41.3X5	T41.3X6
infiltration (subcutaneous)	T41.3X1	T41.3X2	T41.3X3	T41.3X4	T41.3X5	T41.3X6
nerve block (peripheral) (plexus)	T41.3X1	T41.3X2	T41.3X3	T41.3X4	T41.3X5	T41.3X6
spinal	T41.3X1	T41.3X2	T41.3X3	T41.3X4	T41.3X5	T41.3X6
Bupranolol	T44.7X1	T44.7X2	T44.7X3	T44.7X4	T44.7X5	T44.7X6
Buprenorphine	T40.4X1	T40.4X2	T40.4X3	T40.4X4	T40.4X5	T40.4X6
Bupropion	T43.291	T43.292	T43.293	T43.294	T43.295	T43.296
Burimamide	T47.1X1	T47.1X2	T47.1X3	T47.1X4	T47.1X5	T47.1X6
Buserelin	T38.891	T38.892	T38.893	T38.894	T38.895	T38.896
Buspirone	T43.591	T43.592	T43.593	T43.594	T43.595	T43.596
Busulfan, busulphan	T45.1X1	T45.1X2	T45.1X3	T45.1X4	T45.1X5	T45.1X6
Butabarbital (sodium)	T42.3X1	T42.3X2	T42.3X3	T42.3X4	T42.3X5	T42.3X6
Butabarbitone	T42.3X1	T42.3X2	T42.3X3	T42.3X4	T42.3X5	T42.3X6

Substance	Poisoning, Accidental (Unintentional)	Poisoning, Intentional Self-Harm	Poisoning, Assault	Poisoning, Undetermined	Adverse Effect	Underdosing
Butabarpal	T42.3X1	T42.3X2	T42.3X3	T42.3X4	T42.3X5	T42.3X6
Butacaine	T41.3X1	T41.3X2	T41.3X3	T41.3X4	T41.3X5	T41.3X6
Butalamine	T46.7X1	T46.7X2	T46.7X3	T46.7X4	T46.7X5	T46.7X6
Butalbital	T42.3X1	T42.3X2	T42.3X3	T42.3X4	T42.3X5	T42.3X6
Butallylonal	T42.3X1	T42.3X2	T42.3X3	T42.3X4	T42.3X5	T42.3X6
Butamben	T41.3X1	T41.3X2	T41.3X3	T41.3X4	T41.3X5	T41.3X6
Butamirate	T48.3X1	T48.3X2	T48.3X3	T48.3X4	T48.3X5	T48.3X6
Butane (distributed in mobile container)	T59.891	T59.892	T59.893	T59.894	—	—
distributed through pipes	T59.891	T59.892	T59.893	T59.894	—	—
incomplete combustion	T58.11	T58.12	T58.13	T58.14	—	—
Butanilicaine	T41.3X1	T41.3X2	T41.3X3	T41.3X4	T41.3X5	T41.3X6
Butanol	T51.3X1	T51.3X2	T51.3X3	T51.3X4	—	—
Butanone, 2-butanone	T52.4X1	T52.4X2	T52.4X3	T52.4X4	—	—
Butantrone	T49.4X1	T49.4X2	T49.4X3	T49.4X4	T49.4X5	T49.4X6
Butaperazine	T43.3X1	T43.3X2	T43.3X3	T43.3X4	T43.3X5	T43.3X6
Butazolidin	T39.2X1	T39.2X2	T39.2X3	T39.2X4	T39.2X5	T39.2X6
Butetamate	T48.6X1	T48.6X2	T48.6X3	T48.6X4	T48.6X5	T48.6X6
Butethal	T42.3X1	T42.3X2	T42.3X3	T42.3X4	T42.3X5	T42.3X6
Butethamate	T44.3X1	T44.3X2	T44.3X3	T44.3X4	T44.3X5	T44.3X6
Buthalitone (sodium)	T41.1X1	T41.1X2	T41.1X3	T41.1X4	T41.1X5	T41.1X6
Butisol (sodium)	T42.3X1	T42.3X2	T42.3X3	T42.3X4	T42.3X5	T42.3X6
Butizide	T50.2X1	T50.2X2	T50.2X3	T50.2X4	T50.2X5	T50.2X6
Butobarbital	T42.3X1	T42.3X2	T42.3X3	T42.3X4	T42.3X5	T42.3X6
sodium	T42.3X1	T42.3X2	T42.3X3	T42.3X4	T42.3X5	T42.3X6
Butobarbitone	T42.3X1	T42.3X2	T42.3X3	T42.3X4	T42.3X5	T42.3X6
Butoconazole (nitrate)	T49.0X1	T49.0X2	T49.0X3	T49.0X4	T49.0X5	T49.0X6
Butorphanol	T40.4X1	T40.4X2	T40.4X3	T40.4X4	T40.4X5	T40.4X6
Butriptyline	T43.011	T43.012	T43.013	T43.014	T43.015	T43.016
Butropium bromide	T44.3X1	T44.3X2	T44.3X3	T44.3X4	T44.3X5	T44.3X6
Buttercups	T62.2X1	T62.2X2	T62.2X3	T62.2X4	—	—
Butter of antimony — see Antimony						
Butyl						
acetate (secondary)	T52.8X1	T52.8X2	T52.8X3	T52.8X4	—	—
alcohol	T51.3X1	T51.3X2	T51.3X3	T51.3X4	—	—
aminobenzoate	T41.3X1	T41.3X2	T41.3X3	T41.3X4	T41.3X5	T41.3X6
butyrate	T52.8X1	T52.8X2	T52.8X3	T52.8X4	—	—
carbinol	T51.3X1	T51.3X2	T51.3X3	T51.3X4	—	—
carbitol	T52.3X1	T52.3X2	T52.3X3	T52.3X4	—	—
cellosolve	T52.3X1	T52.3X2	T52.3X3	T52.3X4	—	—
chloral (hydrate)	T42.6X1	T42.6X2	T42.6X3	T42.6X4	T42.6X5	T42.6X6
formate	T52.8X1	T52.8X2	T52.8X3	T52.8X4	—	—

◀ New ◀ Revised ~~deleted~~ Deleted

TABLE OF DRUGS AND CHEMICALS

Substance	External Cause (T-Code)					
	Poisoning, Accidental (Unintentional)	Poisoning, Intentional Self-Harm	Poisoning, Assault	Poisoning, Undetermined	Adverse Effect	Underdosing
Butyl (Continued)						
lactate	T52.8X1	T52.8X2	T52.8X3	T52.8X4	—	—
propionate	T52.8X1	T52.8X2	T52.8X3	T52.8X4	—	—
scopolamine bromide	T44.3X1	T44.3X2	T44.3X3	T44.3X4	T44.3X5	T44.3X6
thiobarbital sodium	T41.1X1	T41.1X2	T41.1X3	T41.1X4	T41.1X5	T41.1X6
Butylated hydroxy-anisole	T50.991	T50.992	T50.993	T50.994	T50.995	T50.996
Butylchloral hydrate	T42.6X1	T42.6X2	T42.6X3	T42.6X4	T42.6X5	T42.6X6
Butyltoluene	T52.2X1	T52.2X2	T52.2X3	T52.2X4	—	—
Butyn	T41.3X1	T41.3X2	T41.3X3	T41.3X4	T41.3X5	T41.3X6
Butyrophenone (-based tranquilizers)	T43.4X1	T43.4X2	T43.4X3	T43.4X4	T43.4X5	T43.4X6
C						
Cabergoline	T42.8X1	T42.8X2	T42.8X3	T42.8X4	T42.8X5	T42.8X6
Cacodyl, cacodylic acid	T57.0X1	T57.0X2	T57.0X3	T57.0X4	—	—
Cactinomycin	T45.1X1	T45.1X2	T45.1X3	T45.1X4	T45.1X5	T45.1X6
Cade oil	T49.4X1	T49.4X2	T49.4X3	T49.4X4	T49.4X5	T49.4X6
Cadexomer iodine	T49.0X1	T49.0X2	T49.0X3	T49.0X4	T49.0X5	T49.0X6
Cadmium (chloride) (fumes) (oxide)	T56.3X1	T56.3X2	T56.3X3	T56.3X4	—	—
sulfide (medicinal) NEC	T49.4X1	T49.4X2	T49.4X3	T49.4X4	T49.4X5	T49.4X6
Cadralazine	T46.5X1	T46.5X2	T46.5X3	T46.5X4	T46.5X5	T46.5X6
Caffeine	T43.611	T43.612	T43.613	T43.614	T43.615	T43.616
Calabar bean	T62.2X1	T62.2X2	T62.2X3	T62.2X4	—	—
Caladium seguinum	T62.2X1	T62.2X2	T62.2X3	T62.2X4	—	—
Calamine (lotion)	T49.3X1	T49.3X2	T49.3X3	T49.3X4	T49.3X5	T49.3X6
Calcifediol	T45.2X1	T45.2X2	T45.2X3	T45.2X4	T45.2X5	T45.2X6
Calciferol	T45.2X1	T45.2X2	T45.2X3	T45.2X4	T45.2X5	T45.2X6
Calcitonin	T50.991	T50.992	T50.993	T50.994	T50.995	T50.996
Calcitriol	T45.2X1	T45.2X2	T45.2X3	T45.2X4	T45.2X5	T45.2X6
Calcium	T50.3X1	T50.3X2	T50.3X3	T50.3X4	T50.3X5	T50.3X6
actylsalicylate	T39.011	T39.012	T39.013	T39.014	T39.015	T39.016
benzamidosalicylate	T37.1X1	T37.1X2	T37.1X3	T37.1X4	T37.1X5	T37.1X6
bromide	T42.6X1	T42.6X2	T42.6X3	T42.6X4	T42.6X5	T42.6X6
bromolactobionate	T42.6X1	T42.6X2	T42.6X3	T42.6X4	T42.6X5	T42.6X6
carbaspirin	T39.011	T39.012	T39.013	T39.014	T39.015	T39.016
carbimide	T50.6X1	T50.6X2	T50.6X3	T50.6X4	T50.6X5	T50.6X6
carbonate	T47.1X1	T47.1X2	T47.1X3	T47.1X4	T47.1X5	T47.1X6
chloride	T50.991	T50.992	T50.993	T50.994	T50.995	T50.996
anhydrous	T50.991	T50.992	T50.993	T50.994	T50.995	T50.996
cyanide	T57.8X1	T57.8X2	T57.8X3	T57.8X4	—	—
dioctyl sulfosuccinate	T47.4X1	T47.4X2	T47.4X3	T47.4X4	T47.4X5	T47.4X6
disodium edathamil	T45.8X1	T45.8X2	T45.8X3	T45.8X4	T45.8X5	T45.8X6

Substance	External Cause (T-Code)					
	Poisoning, Accidental (Unintentional)	Poisoning, Intentional Self-Harm	Poisoning, Assault	Poisoning, Undetermined	Adverse Effect	Underdosing
Calcium (Continued)						
disodium edetate	T45.8X1	T45.8X2	T45.8X3	T45.8X4	T45.8X5	T45.8X6
dobesilate	T46.991	T46.992	T46.993	T46.994	T46.995	T46.996
EDTA	T45.8X1	T45.8X2	T45.8X3	T45.8X4	T45.8X5	T45.8X6
ferrous citrate	T45.4X1	T45.4X2	T45.4X3	T45.4X4	T45.4X5	T45.4X6
folinate	T45.8X1	T45.8X2	T45.8X3	T45.8X4	T45.8X5	T45.8X6
glubionate	T50.3X1	T50.3X2	T50.3X3	T50.3X4	T50.3X5	T50.3X6
gluconate	T50.3X1	T50.3X2	T50.3X3	T50.3X4	T50.3X5	T50.3X6
gluconogalactogluconate	T50.3X1	T50.3X2	T50.3X3	T50.3X4	T50.3X5	T50.3X6
hydrate, hydroxide	T54.3X1	T54.3X2	T54.3X3	T54.3X4	—	—
hypochlorite	T54.3X1	T54.3X2	T54.3X3	T54.3X4	—	—
iodide	T48.4X1	T48.4X2	T48.4X3	T48.4X4	T48.4X5	T48.4X6
ipodate	T50.8X1	T50.8X2	T50.8X3	T50.8X4	T50.8X5	T50.8X6
lactate	T50.3X1	T50.3X2	T50.3X3	T50.3X4	T50.3X5	T50.3X6
leucovorin	T45.8X1	T45.8X2	T45.8X3	T45.8X4	T45.8X5	T45.8X6
mandelate	T37.91	T37.92	T37.93	T37.94	T37.95	T37.96
oxide	T54.3X1	T54.3X2	T54.3X3	T54.3X4	—	—
pantothenate	T45.2X1	T45.2X2	T45.2X3	T45.2X4	T45.2X5	T45.2X6
phosphate	T50.3X1	T50.3X2	T50.3X3	T50.3X4	T50.3X5	T50.3X6
salicylate	T39.091	T39.092	T39.093	T39.094	T39.095	T39.096
salts	T50.3X1	T50.3X2	T50.3X3	T50.3X4	T50.3X5	T50.3X6
Calculus-dissolving drug	T50.991	T50.992	T50.993	T50.994	T50.995	T50.996
Calomel	T49.0X1	T49.0X2	T49.0X3	T49.0X4	T49.0X5	T49.0X6
Caloric agent	T50.3X1	T50.3X2	T50.3X3	T50.3X4	T50.3X5	T50.3X6
Calusterone	T38.7X1	T38.7X2	T38.7X3	T38.7X4	T38.7X5	T38.7X6
Camazepam	T42.4X1	T42.4X2	T42.4X3	T42.4X4	T42.4X5	T42.4X6
Camomile	T49.0X1	T49.0X2	T49.0X3	T49.0X4	T49.0X5	T49.0X6
Camoquin	T37.2X1	T37.2X2	T37.2X3	T37.2X4	T37.2X5	T37.2X6
Camphor						
insecticide	T60.2X1	T60.2X2	T60.2X3	T60.2X4	—	—
medicinal	T49.8X1	T49.8X2	T49.8X3	T49.8X4	T49.8X5	T49.8X6
Camylofin	T44.3X1	T44.3X2	T44.3X3	T44.3X4	T44.3X5	T44.3X6
Cancer chemotherapy drug regimen	T45.1X1	T45.1X2	T45.1X3	T45.1X4	T45.1X5	T45.1X6
Candeptin	T49.0X1	T49.0X2	T49.0X3	T49.0X4	T49.0X5	T49.0X6
Candicidin	T49.0X1	T49.0X2	T49.0X3	T49.0X4	T49.0X5	T49.0X6
Cannabinol	T40.7X1	T40.7X2	T40.7X3	T40.7X4	T40.7X5	T40.7X6
Cannabis (derivatives)	T40.7X1	T40.7X2	T40.7X3	T40.7X4	T40.7X5	T40.7X6
Canned heat	T51.1X1	T51.1X2	T51.1X3	T51.1X4	—	—
Canrenoic acid	T50.0X1	T50.0X2	T50.0X3	T50.0X4	T50.0X5	T50.0X6
Canrenone	T50.0X1	T50.0X2	T50.0X3	T50.0X4	T50.0X5	T50.0X6
Cantharides, cantharidin, cantharis	T49.8X1	T49.8X2	T49.8X3	T49.8X4	T49.8X5	T49.8X6

◄ New   ◄ Revised   deleted Deleted

Substance	Poisoning, Accidental (Unintentional)	Poisoning, Intentional Self-Harm	Poisoning, Assault	Poisoning, Undetermined	Adverse Effect	Underdosing
Canthaxanthin	T50.991	T50.992	T50.993	T50.994	T50.995	T50.996
Capillary-active drug NEC	T46.901	T46.902	T46.903	T46.904	T46.905	T46.906
Capreomycin	T36.8X1	T36.8X2	T36.8X3	T36.8X4	T36.8X5	T36.8X6
Capsicum	T49.4X1	T49.4X2	T49.4X3	T49.4X4	T49.4X5	T49.4X6
Captafol	T60.3X1	T60.3X2	T60.3X3	T60.3X4	—	—
Captan	T60.3X1	T60.3X2	T60.3X3	T60.3X4	—	—
Captodiame, captodiamine	T43.591	T43.592	T43.593	T43.594	T43.595	T43.596
Captopril	T46.4X1	T46.4X2	T46.4X3	T46.4X4	T46.4X5	T46.4X6
Caramiphen	T44.3X1	T44.3X2	T44.3X3	T44.3X4	T44.3X5	T44.3X6
Carazolol	T44.7X1	T44.7X2	T44.7X3	T44.7X4	T44.7X5	T44.7X6
Carbachol	T44.1X1	T44.1X2	T44.1X3	T44.1X4	T44.1X5	T44.1X6
Carbacrylamine (resin)	T50.3X1	T50.3X2	T50.3X3	T50.3X4	T50.3X5	T50.3X6
Carbamate (insecticide)	T60.0X1	T60.0X2	T60.0X3	T60.0X4	—	—
Carbamate (sedative)	T42.6X1	T42.6X2	T42.6X3	T42.6X4	T42.6X5	T42.6X6
herbicide	T60.0X1	T60.0X2	T60.0X3	T60.0X4	—	—
insecticide	T60.0X1	T60.0X2	T60.0X3	T60.0X4	—	—
Carbamazepine	T42.1X1	T42.1X2	T42.1X3	T42.1X4	T42.1X5	T42.1X6
Carbamide	T47.3X1	T47.3X2	T47.3X3	T47.3X4	T47.3X5	T47.3X6
peroxide	T49.0X1	T49.0X2	T49.0X3	T49.0X4	T49.0X5	T49.0X6
topical	T49.8X1	T49.8X2	T49.8X3	T49.8X4	T49.8X5	T49.8X6
Carbamylcholine chloride	T44.1X1	T44.1X2	T44.1X3	T44.1X4	T44.1X5	T44.1X6
Carbaril	T60.0X1	T60.0X2	T60.0X3	T60.0X4	—	—
Carbarsone	T37.3X1	T37.3X2	T37.3X3	T37.3X4	T37.3X5	T37.3X6
Carbaryl	T60.0X1	T60.0X2	T60.0X3	T60.0X4	—	—
Carbaspirin	T39.011	T39.012	T39.013	T39.014	T39.015	T39.016
Carbazochrome (salicylate) (sodium sulfonate)	T49.4X1	T49.4X2	T49.4X3	T49.4X4	T49.4X5	T49.4X6
Carbenicillin	T36.0X1	T36.0X2	T36.0X3	T36.0X4	T36.0X5	T36.0X6
Carbenoxolone	T47.1X1	T47.1X2	T47.1X3	T47.1X4	T47.1X5	T47.1X6
Carbetapentane	T48.3X1	T48.3X2	T48.3X3	T48.3X4	T48.3X5	T48.3X6
Carbethyl salicylate	T39.091	T39.092	T39.093	T39.094	T39.095	T39.096
Carbidopa (with levodopa)	T42.8X1	T42.8X2	T42.8X3	T42.8X4	T42.8X5	T42.8X6
Carbimazole	T38.2X1	T38.2X2	T38.2X3	T38.2X4	T38.2X5	T38.2X6
Carbinol	T51.1X1	T51.1X2	T51.1X3	T51.1X4	—	—
Carbinoxamine	T45.0X1	T45.0X2	T45.0X3	T45.0X4	T45.0X5	T45.0X6
Carbiphene	T39.8X1	T39.8X2	T39.8X3	T39.8X4	T39.8X5	T39.8X6
Carbitol	T52.3X1	T52.3X2	T52.3X3	T52.3X4	—	—
Carbocaine	T41.3X1	T41.3X2	T41.3X3	T41.3X4	T41.3X5	T41.3X6
infiltration (subcutaneous)	T41.3X1	T41.3X2	T41.3X3	T41.3X4	T41.3X5	T41.3X6
nerve block (peripheral) (plexus)	T41.3X1	T41.3X2	T41.3X3	T41.3X4	T41.3X5	T41.3X6
topical (surface)	T41.3X1	T41.3X2	T41.3X3	T41.3X4	T41.3X5	T41.3X6
Carbo medicinalis	T47.6X1	T47.6X2	T47.6X3	T47.6X4	T47.6X5	T47.6X6

Substance	Poisoning, Accidental (Unintentional)	Poisoning, Intentional Self-Harm	Poisoning, Assault	Poisoning, Undetermined	Adverse Effect	Underdosing
Carbomycin	T36.8X1	T36.8X2	T36.8X3	T36.8X4	T36.8X5	T36.8X6
Carbocisteine	T48.4X1	T48.4X2	T48.4X3	T48.4X4	T48.4X5	T48.4X6
Carbocromen	T46.3X1	T46.3X2	T46.3X3	T46.3X4	T46.3X5	T46.3X6
Carbol fuchsin	T49.0X1	T49.0X2	T49.0X3	T49.0X4	T49.0X5	T49.0X6
Carbolic acid — see also Phenol	T54.0X1	T54.0X2	T54.0X3	T54.0X4	—	—
Carbolonium (bromide)	T48.1X1	T48.1X2	T48.1X3	T48.1X4	T48.1X5	T48.1X6
Carbon						
bisulfide (liquid)	T65.4X1	T65.4X2	T65.4X3	T65.4X4		
vapor	T65.4X1	T65.4X2	T65.4X3	T65.4X4	—	—
dioxide (gas)	T59.7X1	T59.7X2	T59.7X3	T59.7X4	—	—
medicinal	T41.5X1	T41.5X2	T41.5X3	T41.5X4	T41.5X5	T41.5X6
nonmedicinal	T59.7X1	T59.7X2	T59.7X3	T59.7X4	—	—
snow	T49.4X1	T49.4X2	T49.4X3	T49.4X4	T49.4X5	T49.4X6
disulfide (liquid)	T65.4X1	T65.4X2	T65.4X3	T65.4X4	—	—
vapor	T65.4X1	T65.4X2	T65.4X3	T65.4X4	—	—
monoxide (from incomplete combustion)	T58.91	T58.92	T58.93	T58.94	—	—
blast furnace gas	T58.8X1	T58.8X2	T58.8X3	T58.8X4	—	—
butane (distributed in mobile container)	T58.11	T58.12	T58.13	T58.14	—	—
distributed through pipes	T58.11	T58.12	T58.13	T58.14	—	—
charcoal fumes	T58.2X1	T58.2X2	T58.2X3	T58.2X4	—	—
coal	T58.2X1	T58.2X2	T58.2X3	T58.2X4		
coke (in domestic stoves, fireplaces)	T58.2X1	T58.2X2	T58.2X3	T58.2X4	—	—
gas (piped)	T58.11	T58.12	T58.13	T58.14	—	—
solid (in domestic stoves, fireplaces)	T58.2X1	T58.2X2	T58.2X3	T58.2X4	—	—
exhaust gas (motor) not in transit	T58.01	T58.02	T58.03	T58.04	—	—
combustion engine, any not in watercraft	T58.01	T58.02	T58.03	T58.04	—	—
farm tractor, not in transit	T58.01	T58.02	T58.03	T58.04	—	—
gas engine	T58.01	T58.02	T58.03	T58.04	—	—
motor pump	T58.01	T58.02	T58.03	T58.04	—	—
motor vehicle, not in transit	T58.01	T58.02	T58.03	T58.04	—	—
fuel (in domestic use)	T58.2X1	T58.2X2	T58.2X3	T58.2X4	—	—
gas (piped)	T58.11	T58.12	T58.13	T58.14	—	—
in mobile container	T58.11	T58.12	T58.13	T58.14	—	—
utility	T58.11	T58.12	T58.13	T58.14	—	—
in mobile container	T58.11	T58.12	T58.13	T58.14	—	—
piped (natural)	T58.11	T58.12	T58.13	T58.14	—	—

◀ New ◀ Revised ~~deleted~~ Deleted

Substance	Poisoning, Accidental (Unintentional)	Poisoning, Intentional Self-Harm	Poisoning, Assault	Poisoning, Undetermined	Adverse Effect	Underdosing
Carbon (Continued)						
monoxide (Continued)						
illuminating gas	T58.11	T58.12	T58.13	T58.14	—	—
industrial fuels or gases, any	T58.8X1	T58.8X2	T58.8X3	T58.8X4	—	—
kerosene (in domestic stoves, fireplaces)	T58.2X1	T58.2X2	T58.2X3	T58.2X4	—	—
kiln gas or vapor	T58.8X1	T58.8X2	T58.8X3	T58.8X4	—	—
motor exhaust gas, not in transit	T58.01	T58.02	T58.03	T58.04	—	—
piped gas (manufactured) (natural)	T58.11	T58.12	T58.13	T58.14	—	—
producer gas	T58.8X1	T58.8X2	T58.8X3	T58.8X4	—	—
propane (distributed in mobile container)	T58.11	T58.12	T58.13	T58.14	—	—
distributed through pipes	T58.11	T58.12	T58.13	T58.14	—	—
specified source NEC	T58.8X1	T58.8X2	T58.8X3	T58.8X4	—	—
stove gas	T58.11	T58.12	T58.13	T58.14	—	—
piped	T58.11	T58.12	T58.13	T58.14	—	—
utility gas	T58.11	T58.12	T58.13	T58.14	—	—
piped	T58.11	T58.12	T58.13	T58.14	—	—
water gas	T58.11	T58.12	T58.13	T58.14	—	—
wood (in domestic stoves, fireplaces)	T58.2X1	T58.2X2	T58.2X3	T58.2X4	—	—
tetrachloride (vapor) NEC	T53.0X1	T53.0X2	T53.0X3	T53.0X4	—	—
liquid (cleansing agent) NEC	T53.0X1	T53.0X2	T53.0X3	T53.0X4	—	—
solvent	T53.0X1	T53.0X2	T53.0X3	T53.0X4	—	—
Carbonic acid gas	T59.7X1	T59.7X2	T59.7X3	T59.7X4	—	—
anhydrase inhibitor NEC	T50.2X1	T50.2X2	T50.2X3	T50.2X4	T50.2X5	T50.2X6
Carbophenothion	T60.0X1	T60.0X2	T60.0X3	T60.0X4	—	—
Carboplatin	T45.1X1	T45.1X2	T45.1X3	T45.1X4	T45.1X5	T45.1X6
Carboprost	T48.0X1	T48.0X2	T48.0X3	T48.0X4	T48.0X5	T48.0X6
Carboquone	T45.1X1	T45.1X2	T45.1X3	T45.1X4	T45.1X5	T45.1X6
Carbowax	T49.3X1	T49.3X2	T49.3X3	T49.3X4	T49.3X5	T49.3X6
Carboxymethyl-cellulose	T47.4X1	T47.4X2	T47.4X3	T47.4X4	T47.4X5	T47.4X6
S-Carboxymethyl-cysteine	T48.4X1	T48.4X2	T48.4X3	T48.4X4	T48.4X5	T48.4X6
Carbrital	T42.3X1	T42.3X2	T42.3X3	T42.3X4	T42.3X5	T42.3X6
Carbromal	T42.6X1	T42.6X2	T42.6X3	T42.6X4	T42.6X5	T42.6X6
Carbutamide	T38.3X1	T38.3X2	T38.3X3	T38.3X4	T38.3X5	T38.3X6
Carbuterol	T48.6X1	T48.6X2	T48.6X3	T48.6X4	T48.6X5	T48.6X6
Cardiac						
depressants	T46.2X1	T46.2X2	T46.2X3	T46.2X4	T46.2X5	T46.2X6
rhythm regulator	T46.2X1	T46.2X2	T46.2X3	T46.2X4	T46.2X5	T46.2X6
specified NEC	T46.2X1	T46.2X2	T46.2X3	T46.2X4	T46.2X5	T46.2X6

Substance	Poisoning, Accidental (Unintentional)	Poisoning, Intentional Self-Harm	Poisoning, Assault	Poisoning, Undetermined	Adverse Effect	Underdosing
Cardiografin	T50.8X1	T50.8X2	T50.8X3	T50.8X4	T50.8X5	T50.8X6
Cardio-green	T50.8X1	T50.8X2	T50.8X3	T50.8X4	T50.8X5	T50.8X6
Cardiotonic (glycoside) NEC	T46.0X1	T46.0X2	T46.0X3	T46.0X4	T46.0X5	T46.0X6
Cardiovascular drug NEC	T46.901	T46.902	T46.903	T46.904	T46.905	T46.906
Cardrase	T50.2X1	T50.2X2	T50.2X3	T50.2X4	T50.2X5	T50.2X6
Carfusin	T49.0X1	T49.0X2	T49.0X3	T49.0X4	T49.0X5	T49.0X6
Carfecillin	T36.0X1	T36.0X2	T36.0X3	T36.0X4	T36.0X5	T36.0X6
Carfenazine	T43.3X1	T43.3X2	T43.3X3	T43.3X4	T43.3X5	T43.3X6
Carindacillin	T36.0X1	T36.0X2	T36.0X3	T36.0X4	T36.0X5	T36.0X6
Carisoprodol	T42.8X1	T42.8X2	T42.8X3	T42.8X4	T42.8X5	T42.8X6
Carmellose	T47.4X1	T47.4X2	T47.4X3	T47.4X4	T47.4X5	T47.4X6
Carminative	T47.5X1	T47.5X2	T47.5X3	T47.5X4	T47.5X5	T47.5X6
Carmofur	T45.1X1	T45.1X2	T45.1X3	T45.1X4	T45.1X5	T45.1X6
Carmustine	T45.1X1	T45.1X2	T45.1X3	T45.1X4	T45.1X5	T45.1X6
Carotene	T45.2X1	T45.2X2	T45.2X3	T45.2X4	T45.2X5	T45.2X6
Carphenazine	T43.3X1	T43.3X2	T43.3X3	T43.3X4	T43.3X5	T43.3X6
Carpipramine	T42.4X1	T42.4X2	T42.4X3	T42.4X4	T42.4X5	T42.4X6
Carprofen	T39.311	T39.312	T39.313	T39.314	T39.315	T39.316
Carpronium chloride	T44.3X1	T44.3X2	T44.3X3	T44.3X4	T44.3X5	T44.3X6
Carrageenan	T47.8X1	T47.8X2	T47.8X3	T47.8X4	T47.8X5	T47.8X6
Carteolol	T44.7X1	T44.7X2	T44.7X3	T44.7X4	T44.7X5	T44.7X6
Carter's Little Pills	T47.2X1	T47.2X2	T47.2X3	T47.2X4	T47.2X5	T47.2X6
Cascara (sagrada)	T47.2X1	T47.2X2	T47.2X3	T47.2X4	T47.2X5	T47.2X6
Cassava	T62.2X1	T62.2X2	T62.2X3	T62.2X4	—	—
Castellani's paint	T49.0X1	T49.0X2	T49.0X3	T49.0X4	T49.0X5	T49.0X6
Castor						
bean	T62.2X1	T62.2X2	T62.2X3	T62.2X4	—	—
oil	T47.2X1	T47.2X2	T47.2X3	T47.2X4	T47.2X5	T47.2X6
Catalase	T45.3X1	T45.3X2	T45.3X3	T45.3X4	T45.3X5	T45.3X6
Caterpillar (sting)	T63.431	T63.432	T63.433	T63.434	—	—
Catha (edulis) (tea)	T43.691	T43.692	T43.693	T43.694	—	—
Cathartic NEC	T47.4X1	T47.4X2	T47.4X3	T47.4X4	T47.4X5	T47.4X6
anthacene derivative	T47.2X1	T47.2X2	T47.2X3	T47.2X4	T47.2X5	T47.2X6
bulk	T47.4X1	T47.4X2	T47.4X3	T47.4X4	T47.4X5	T47.4X6
contact	T47.2X1	T47.2X2	T47.2X3	T47.2X4	T47.2X5	T47.2X6
emollient NEC	T47.4X1	T47.4X2	T47.4X3	T47.4X4	T47.4X5	T47.4X6
irritant NEC	T47.2X1	T47.2X2	T47.2X3	T47.2X4	T47.2X5	T47.2X6
mucilage	T47.4X1	T47.4X2	T47.4X3	T47.4X4	T47.4X5	T47.4X6
saline	T47.3X1	T47.3X2	T47.3X3	T47.3X4	T47.3X5	T47.3X6
vegetable	T47.2X1	T47.2X2	T47.2X3	T47.2X4	T47.2X5	T47.2X6
Cathine	T50.5X1	T50.5X2	T50.5X3	T50.5X4	T50.5X5	T50.5X6
Cathomycin	T36.8X1	T36.8X2	T36.8X3	T36.8X4	T36.8X5	T36.8X6

◀ New ◀ Revised ~~deleted~~ Deleted

Substance	External Cause (T-Code)					
	Poisoning, Accidental (Unintentional)	Poisoning, Intentional Self-Harm	Poisoning, Assault	Poisoning, Undetermined	Adverse Effect	Underdosing
Cation exchange resin	T50.3X1	T50.3X2	T50.3X3	T50.3X4	T50.3X5	T50.3X6
Caustic(s) NEC	T54.91	T54.92	T54.93	T54.94	—	—
alkali	T54.3X1	T54.3X2	T54.3X3	T54.3X4	—	—
hydroxide	T54.3X1	T54.3X2	T54.3X3	T54.3X4	—	—
potash	T54.3X1	T54.3X2	T54.3X3	T54.3X4	—	—
soda	T54.3X1	T54.3X2	T54.3X3	T54.3X4	—	—
specified NEC	T54.91	T54.92	T54.93	T54.94	—	—
Ceepryn	T49.0X1	T49.0X2	T49.0X3	T49.0X4	T49.0X5	T49.0X6
ENT agent	T49.6X1	T49.6X2	T49.6X3	T49.6X4	T49.6X5	T49.6X6
lozenges	T49.6X1	T49.6X2	T49.6X3	T49.6X4	T49.6X5	T49.6X6
Cefacetrile	T36.1X1	T36.1X2	T36.1X3	T36.1X4	T36.1X5	T36.1X6
Cefaclor	T36.1X1	T36.1X2	T36.1X3	T36.1X4	T36.1X5	T36.1X6
Cefadroxil	T36.1X1	T36.1X2	T36.1X3	T36.1X4	T36.1X5	T36.1X6
Cefalexin	T36.1X1	T36.1X2	T36.1X3	T36.1X4	T36.1X5	T36.1X6
Cefaloglycin	T36.1X1	T36.1X2	T36.1X3	T36.1X4	T36.1X5	T36.1X6
Cefaloridine	T36.1X1	T36.1X2	T36.1X3	T36.1X4	T36.1X5	T36.1X6
Cefalosporins	T36.1X1	T36.1X2	T36.1X3	T36.1X4	T36.1X5	T36.1X6
Cefalotin	T36.1X1	T36.1X2	T36.1X3	T36.1X4	T36.1X5	T36.1X6
Cefamandole	T36.1X1	T36.1X2	T36.1X3	T36.1X4	T36.1X5	T36.1X6
Cefamycin antibiotic	T36.1X1	T36.1X2	T36.1X3	T36.1X4	T36.1X5	T36.1X6
Cefapirin	T36.1X1	T36.1X2	T36.1X3	T36.1X4	T36.1X5	T36.1X6
Cefatrizine	T36.1X1	T36.1X2	T36.1X3	T36.1X4	T36.1X5	T36.1X6
Cefazedone	T36.1X1	T36.1X2	T36.1X3	T36.1X4	T36.1X5	T36.1X6
Cefazolin	T36.1X1	T36.1X2	T36.1X3	T36.1X4	T36.1X5	T36.1X6
Cefbuperazone	T36.1X1	T36.1X2	T36.1X3	T36.1X4	T36.1X5	T36.1X6
Cefetamet	T36.1X1	T36.1X2	T36.1X3	T36.1X4	T36.1X5	T36.1X6
Cefixime	T36.1X1	T36.1X2	T36.1X3	T36.1X4	T36.1X5	T36.1X6
Cefmenoxime	T36.1X1	T36.1X2	T36.1X3	T36.1X4	T36.1X5	T36.1X6
Cefmetazole	T36.1X1	T36.1X2	T36.1X3	T36.1X4	T36.1X5	T36.1X6
Cefminox	T36.1X1	T36.1X2	T36.1X3	T36.1X4	T36.1X5	T36.1X6
Cefonicid	T36.1X1	T36.1X2	T36.1X3	T36.1X4	T36.1X5	T36.1X6
Cefoperazone	T36.1X1	T36.1X2	T36.1X3	T36.1X4	T36.1X5	T36.1X6
Ceforanide	T36.1X1	T36.1X2	T36.1X3	T36.1X4	T36.1X5	T36.1X6
Cefotaxime	T36.1X1	T36.1X2	T36.1X3	T36.1X4	T36.1X5	T36.1X6
Cefotetan	T36.1X1	T36.1X2	T36.1X3	T36.1X4	T36.1X5	T36.1X6
Cefotiam	T36.1X1	T36.1X2	T36.1X3	T36.1X4	T36.1X5	T36.1X6
Cefoxitin	T36.1X1	T36.1X2	T36.1X3	T36.1X4	T36.1X5	T36.1X6
Cefpimizole	T36.1X1	T36.1X2	T36.1X3	T36.1X4	T36.1X5	T36.1X6
Cefpiramide	T36.1X1	T36.1X2	T36.1X3	T36.1X4	T36.1X5	T36.1X6
Cefradine	T36.1X1	T36.1X2	T36.1X3	T36.1X4	T36.1X5	T36.1X6
Cefroxadine	T36.1X1	T36.1X2	T36.1X3	T36.1X4	T36.1X5	T36.1X6
Cefsulodin	T36.1X1	T36.1X2	T36.1X3	T36.1X4	T36.1X5	T36.1X6

Substance	External Cause (T-Code)					
	Poisoning, Accidental (Unintentional)	Poisoning, Intentional Self-Harm	Poisoning, Assault	Poisoning, Undetermined	Adverse Effect	Underdosing
Ceftazidime	T36.1X1	T36.1X2	T36.1X3	T36.1X4	T36.1X5	T36.1X6
Cefteram	T36.1X1	T36.1X2	T36.1X3	T36.1X4	T36.1X5	T36.1X6
Ceftezole	T36.1X1	T36.1X2	T36.1X3	T36.1X4	T36.1X5	T36.1X6
Ceftizoxime	T36.1X1	T36.1X2	T36.1X3	T36.1X4	T36.1X5	T36.1X6
Ceftriaxone	T36.1X1	T36.1X2	T36.1X3	T36.1X4	T36.1X5	T36.1X6
Cefuroxime	T36.1X1	T36.1X2	T36.1X3	T36.1X4	T36.1X5	T36.1X6
Cefuzonam	T36.1X1	T36.1X2	T36.1X3	T36.1X4	T36.1X5	T36.1X6
Celestone	T38.0X1	T38.0X2	T38.0X3	T38.0X4	T38.0X5	T38.0X6
topical	T49.0X1	T49.0X2	T49.0X3	T49.0X4	T49.0X5	T49.0X6
Celiprolol	T44.7X1	T44.7X2	T44.7X3	T44.7X4	T44.7X5	T44.7X6
Cellosolve	T52.91	T52.92	T52.93	T52.94	—	—
Cell stimulants and proliferants	T49.8X1	T49.8X2	T49.8X3	T49.8X4	T49.8X5	T49.8X6
Cellulose						
cathartic	T47.4X1	T47.4X2	T47.4X3	T47.4X4	T47.4X5	T47.4X6
hydroxyethyl	T47.4X1	T47.4X2	T47.4X3	T47.4X4	T47.4X5	T47.4X6
nitrates (topical)	T49.3X1	T49.3X2	T49.3X3	T49.3X4	T49.3X5	T49.3X6
oxidized	T49.4X1	T49.4X2	T49.4X3	T49.4X4	T49.4X5	T49.4X6
Centipede (bite)	T63.411	T63.412	T63.413	T63.414	—	—
Central nervous system						
depressants	T42.71	T42.72	T42.73	T42.74	T42.75	T42.76
anesthetic (general) NEC	T41.201	T41.202	T41.203	T41.204	T41.205	T41.206
gases NEC	T41.0X1	T41.0X2	T41.0X3	T41.0X4	T41.0X5	T41.0X6
intravenous	T41.1X1	T41.1X2	T41.1X3	T41.1X4	T41.1X5	T41.1X6
barbiturates	T42.3X1	T42.3X2	T42.3X3	T42.3X4	T42.3X5	T42.3X6
benzodiazepines	T42.4X1	T42.4X2	T42.4X3	T42.4X4	T42.4X5	T42.4X6
bromides	T42.6X1	T42.6X2	T42.6X3	T42.6X4	T42.6X5	T42.6X6
cannabis sativa	T40.7X1	T40.7X2	T40.7X3	T40.7X4	T40.7X5	T40.7X6
chloral hydrate	T42.6X1	T42.6X2	T42.6X3	T42.6X4	T42.6X5	T42.6X6
ethanol	T51.0X1	T51.0X2	T51.0X3	T51.0X4	—	—
hallucinogenics	T40.901	T40.902	T40.903	T40.904	T40.905	T40.906
hypnotics	T42.71	T42.72	T42.73	T42.74	T42.75	T42.76
specified NEC	T42.6X1	T42.6X2	T42.6X3	T42.6X4	T42.6X5	T42.6X6
muscle relaxants	T42.8X1	T42.8X2	T42.8X3	T42.8X4	T42.8X5	T42.8X6
paraldehyde	T42.6X1	T42.6X2	T42.6X3	T42.6X4	T42.6X5	T42.6X6
sedatives; sedative-hypnotics	T42.71	T42.72	T42.73	T42.74	T42.75	T42.76
mixed NEC	T42.6X1	T42.6X2	T42.6X3	T42.6X4	T42.6X5	T42.6X6
specified NEC	T42.6X1	T42.6X2	T42.6X3	T42.6X4	T42.6X5	T42.6X6
muscle-tone depressants	T42.8X1	T42.8X2	T42.8X3	T42.8X4	T42.8X5	T42.8X6
stimulants	T43.601	T43.602	T43.603	T43.604	T43.605	T43.606
amphetamines	T43.621	T43.622	T43.623	T43.624	T43.625	T43.626
analeptics	T50.7X1	T50.7X2	T50.7X3	T50.7X4	T50.7X5	T50.7X6

◀ New　◀ Revised　deleted Deleted

Substance	Poisoning, Accidental (Unintentional)	Poisoning, Intentional Self-Harm	Poisoning, Assault	Poisoning, Undetermined	Adverse Effect	Underdosing
Central nervous system *(Continued)*						
stimulants *(Continued)*						
antidepressants	T43.201	T43.202	T43.203	T43.204	T43.205	T43.206
opiate antagonists	T50.7X1	T50.7X2	T50.7X3	T50.7X4	T50.7X5	T50.7X6
specified NEC	T43.691	T43.692	T43.693	T43.694	T43.695	T43.696
Cephalexin	T36.1X1	T36.1X2	T36.1X3	T36.1X4	T36.1X5	T36.1X6
Cephaloglycin	T36.1X1	T36.1X2	T36.1X3	T36.1X4	T36.1X5	T36.1X6
Cephaloridine	T36.1X1	T36.1X2	T36.1X3	T36.1X4	T36.1X5	T36.1X6
Cephalosporins	T36.1X1	T36.1X2	T36.1X3	T36.1X4	T36.1X5	T36.1X6
N (adicillin)	T36.0X1	T36.0X2	T36.0X3	T36.0X4	T36.0X5	T36.0X6
Cephalothin	T36.1X1	T36.1X2	T36.1X3	T36.1X4	T36.1X5	T36.1X6
Cephalotin	T36.1X1	T36.1X2	T36.1X3	T36.1X4	T36.1X5	T36.1X6
Cephradine	T36.1X1	T36.1X2	T36.1X3	T36.1X4	T36.1X5	T36.1X6
Cerbera (odallam)	T62.2X1	T62.2X2	T62.2X3	T62.2X4	—	—
Cerberin	T46.0X1	T46.0X2	T46.0X3	T46.0X4	T46.0X5	T46.0X6
Cerebral stimulants	T43.601	T43.602	T43.603	T43.604	T43.605	T43.606
psychotherapeutic	T43.601	T43.602	T43.603	T43.604	T43.605	T43.606
specified NEC	T43.691	T43.692	T43.693	T43.694	T43.695	T43.696
Cerium oxalate	T45.0X1	T45.0X2	T45.0X3	T45.0X4	T45.0X5	T45.0X6
Cerous oxalate	T45.0X1	T45.0X2	T45.0X3	T45.0X4	T45.0X5	T45.0X6
Ceruletide	T50.8X1	T50.8X2	T50.8X3	T50.8X4	T50.8X5	T50.8X6
Cetalkonium (chloride)	T49.0X1	T49.0X2	T49.0X3	T49.0X4	T49.0X5	T49.0X6
Cethexonium chloride	T49.0X1	T49.0X2	T49.0X3	T49.0X4	T49.0X5	T49.0X6
Cetiedil	T46.7X1	T46.7X2	T46.7X3	T46.7X4	T46.7X5	T46.7X6
Cetirizine	T45.0X1	T45.0X2	T45.0X3	T45.0X4	T45.0X5	T45.0X6
Cetomacrogol	T50.991	T50.992	T50.993	T50.994	T50.995	T50.996
Cetotiamine	T45.2X1	T45.2X2	T45.2X3	T45.2X4	T45.2X5	T45.2X6
Cetoxime	T45.0X1	T45.0X2	T45.0X3	T45.0X4	T45.0X5	T45.0X6
Cetraxate	T47.1X1	T47.1X2	T47.1X3	T47.1X4	T47.1X5	T47.1X6
Cetrimide	T49.0X1	T49.0X2	T49.0X3	T49.0X4	T49.0X5	T49.0X6
Cetrimonium (bromide)	T49.0X1	T49.0X2	T49.0X3	T49.0X4	T49.0X5	T49.0X6
Cetylpyridinium chloride	T49.0X1	T49.0X2	T49.0X3	T49.0X4	T49.0X5	T49.0X6
ENT agent	T49.6X1	T49.6X2	T49.6X3	T49.6X4	T49.6X5	T49.6X6
lozenges	T49.6X1	T49.6X2	T49.6X3	T49.6X4	T49.6X5	T49.6X6
Cevadillasee Sabadilla						
Cevitamic acid	T45.2X1	T45.2X2	T45.2X3	T45.2X4	T45.2X5	T45.2X6
Chalk, precipitated	T47.1X1	T47.1X2	T47.1X3	T47.1X4	T47.1X5	T47.1X6
Chamomile	T49.0X1	T49.0X2	T49.0X3	T49.0X4	T49.0X5	T49.0X6
Ch'an su	T46.0X1	T46.0X2	T46.0X3	T46.0X4	T46.0X5	T46.0X6
Charcoal	T47.6X1	T47.6X2	T47.6X3	T47.6X4	T47.6X5	T47.6X6
activated — *see also* Charcoal, medicinal	T47.6X1	T47.6X2	T47.6X3	T47.6X4	T47.6X5	T47.6X6

Substance	Poisoning, Accidental (Unintentional)	Poisoning, Intentional Self-Harm	Poisoning, Assault	Poisoning, Undetermined	Adverse Effect	Underdosing
Charcoal *(Continued)*						
fumes (Carbon monoxide)	T58.2X1	T58.2X2	T58.2X3	T58.2X4	—	—
industrial	T58.8X1	T58.8X2	T58.8X3	T58.8X4	—	—
medicinal (activated)	T47.6X1	T47.6X2	T47.6X3	T47.6X4	T47.6X5	T47.6X6
antidiarrheal	T47.6X1	T47.6X2	T47.6X3	T47.6X4	T47.6X5	T47.6X6
poison control	T47.8X1	T47.8X2	T47.8X3	T47.8X4	T47.8X5	T47.8X6
specified use other than for diarrhea	T47.8X1	T47.8X2	T47.8X3	T47.8X4	T47.8X5	T47.8X6
topical	T49.8X1	T49.8X2	T49.8X3	T49.8X4	T49.8X5	T49.8X6
Chaulmosulfone	T37.1X1	T37.1X2	T37.1X3	T37.1X4	T37.1X5	T37.1X6
Chelating agent NEC	T50.6X1	T50.6X2	T50.6X3	T50.6X4	T50.6X5	T50.6X6
Chelidonium majus	T62.2X1	T62.2X2	T62.2X3	T62.2X4	—	—
Chemical substance NEC	T65.91	T65.92	T65.93	T65.94	—	—
Chenodeoxycholic acid	T47.5X1	T47.5X2	T47.5X3	T47.5X4	T47.5X5	T47.5X6
Chenodiol	T47.5X1	T47.5X2	T47.5X3	T47.5X4	T47.5X5	T47.5X6
Chenopodium	T37.4X1	T37.4X2	T37.4X3	T37.4X4	T37.4X5	T37.4X6
Cherry laurel	T62.2X1	T62.2X2	T62.2X3	T62.2X4	—	—
Chinidin(e)	T46.2X1	T46.2X2	T46.2X3	T46.2X4	T46.2X5	T46.2X6
Chiniofon	T37.8X1	T37.8X2	T37.8X3	T37.8X4	T37.8X5	T37.8X6
Chlophedianol	T48.3X1	T48.3X2	T48.3X3	T48.3X4	T48.3X5	T48.3X6
Chloral	T42.6X1	T42.6X2	T42.6X3	T42.6X4	T42.6X5	T42.6X6
derivative	T42.6X1	T42.6X2	T42.6X3	T42.6X4	T42.6X5	T42.6X6
hydrate	T42.6X1	T42.6X2	T42.6X3	T42.6X4	T42.6X5	T42.6X6
Chloralamide	T42.6X1	T42.6X2	T42.6X3	T42.6X4	T42.6X5	T42.6X6
Chloralodol	T42.6X1	T42.6X2	T42.6X3	T42.6X4	T42.6X5	T42.6X6
Chloralose	T60.4X1	T60.4X2	T60.4X3	T60.4X4	—	—
Chlorambucil	T45.1X1	T45.1X2	T45.1X3	T45.1X4	T45.1X5	T45.1X6
Chloramine	T57.8X1	T57.8X2	T57.8X3	T57.8X4	—	—
T	T49.0X1	T49.0X2	T49.0X3	T49.0X4	T49.0X5	T49.0X6
topical	T49.0X1	T49.0X2	T49.0X3	T49.0X4	T49.0X5	T49.0X6
Chloramphenicol	T36.2X1	T36.2X2	T36.2X3	T36.2X4	T36.2X5	T36.2X6
ENT agent	T49.6X1	T49.6X2	T49.6X3	T49.6X4	T49.6X5	T49.6X6
ophthalmic preparation	T49.5X1	T49.5X2	T49.5X3	T49.5X4	T49.5X5	T49.5X6
topical NEC	T49.0X1	T49.0X2	T49.0X3	T49.0X4	T49.0X5	T49.0X6
Chlorate (potassium) (sodium) NEC	T60.3X1	T60.3X2	T60.3X3	T60.3X4	—	—
herbicide	T60.3X1	T60.3X2	T60.3X3	T60.3X4	—	—
Chlorazanil	T50.2X1	T50.2X2	T50.2X3	T50.2X4	T50.2X5	T50.2X6
Chlorbenzene, chlorbenzol	T53.7X1	T53.7X2	T53.7X3	T53.7X4	—	—
Chlorbenzoxamine	T44.3X1	T44.3X2	T44.3X3	T44.3X4	T44.3X5	T44.3X6
Chlorbutol	T42.6X1	T42.6X2	T42.6X3	T42.6X4	T42.6X5	T42.6X6
Chlorcyclizine	T45.0X1	T45.0X2	T45.0X3	T45.0X4	T45.0X5	T45.0X6

◀ New ◀ Revised ~~deleted~~ Deleted

Substance	External Cause (T-Code)					
	Poisoning, Accidental (Unintentional)	Poisoning, Intentional Self-Harm	Poisoning, Assault	Poisoning, Undetermined	Adverse Effect	Underdosing
Chlordan(e) (dust)	T60.1X1	T60.1X2	T60.1X3	T60.1X4	—	—
Chlordantoin	T49.0X1	T49.0X2	T49.0X3	T49.0X4	T49.0X5	T49.0X6
Chlordiazepoxide	T42.4X1	T42.4X2	T42.4X3	T42.4X4	T42.4X5	T42.4X6
Chlordiethyl benzamide	T49.3X1	T49.3X2	T49.3X3	T49.3X4	T49.3X5	T49.3X6
Chloresium	T49.8X1	T49.8X2	T49.8X3	T49.8X4	T49.8X5	T49.8X6
Chlorethiazol	T42.6X1	T42.6X2	T42.6X3	T42.6X4	T42.6X5	T42.6X6
Chlorethyl — see Ethyl chloride						
Chloretone	T42.6X1	T42.6X2	T42.6X3	T42.6X4	T42.6X5	T42.6X6
Chlorex	T53.6X1	T53.6X2	T53.6X3	T53.6X4	—	—
insecticide	T60.1X1	T60.1X2	T60.1X3	T60.1X4	—	—
Chlorfenvinphos	T60.0X1	T60.0X2	T60.0X3	T60.0X4	—	—
Chlorhexadol	T42.6X1	T42.6X2	T42.6X3	T42.6X4	T42.6X5	T42.6X6
Chlorhexamide	T45.1X1	T45.1X2	T45.1X3	T45.1X4	T45.1X5	T45.1X6
Chlorhexidine	T49.0X1	T49.0X2	T49.0X3	T49.0X4	T49.0X5	T49.0X6
Chlorhydroxyquinolin	T49.0X1	T49.0X2	T49.0X3	T49.0X4	T49.0X5	T49.0X6
Chloride of lime (bleach)	T54.3X1	T54.3X2	T54.3X3	T54.3X4	—	—
Chlorimipramine	T43.011	T43.012	T43.013	T43.014	T43.015	T43.016
Chlorinated						
camphene	T53.6X1	T53.6X2	T53.6X3	T53.6X4	—	—
diphenyl	T53.7X1	T53.7X2	T53.7X3	T53.7X4	—	—
hydrocarbons NEC	T53.91	T53.92	T53.93	T53.94	—	—
solvents	T53.91	T53.92	T53.93	T53.94	—	—
lime (bleach)	T54.3X1	T54.3X2	T54.3X3	T54.3X4	—	—
and boric acid solution	T49.0X1	T49.0X2	T49.0X3	T49.0X4	T49.0X5	T49.0X6
naphthalene (insecticide)	T60.1X1	T60.1X2	T60.1X3	T60.1X4	—	—
industrial (non-pesticide)	T53.7X1	T53.7X2	T53.7X3	T53.7X4	—	—
pesticide NEC	T60.8X1	T60.8X2	T60.8X3	T60.8X4	—	—
soda — see also sodium hypochlorite						
solution	T49.0X1	T49.0X2	T49.0X3	T49.0X4	T49.0X5	T49.0X6
Chlorine (fumes) (gas)	T59.4X1	T59.4X2	T59.4X3	T59.4X4	—	—
bleach	T54.3X1	T54.3X2	T54.3X3	T54.3X4	—	—
compound gas NEC	T59.4X1	T59.4X2	T59.4X3	T59.4X4	—	—
disinfectant	T59.4X1	T59.4X2	T59.4X3	T59.4X4	—	—
releasing agents NEC	T59.4X1	T59.4X2	T59.4X3	T59.4X4	—	—
Chlorisondamine chloride	T46.991	T46.992	T46.993	T46.994	T46.995	T46.996
Chlormadinone	T38.5X1	T38.5X2	T38.5X3	T38.5X4	T38.5X5	T38.5X6
Chlormephos	T60.0X1	T60.0X2	T60.0X3	T60.0X4	—	—
Chlormerodrin	T50.2X1	T50.2X2	T50.2X3	T50.2X4	T50.2X5	T50.2X6
Chlormethiazole	T42.6X1	T42.6X2	T42.6X3	T42.6X4	T42.6X5	T42.6X6
Chlormethine	T45.1X1	T45.1X2	T45.1X3	T45.1X4	T45.1X5	T45.1X6
Chlormethylenecycline	T36.4X1	T36.4X2	T36.4X3	T36.4X4	T36.4X5	T36.4X6

Substance	External Cause (T-Code)					
	Poisoning, Accidental (Unintentional)	Poisoning, Intentional Self-Harm	Poisoning, Assault	Poisoning, Undetermined	Adverse Effect	Underdosing
Chlormezanone	T42.6X1	T42.6X2	T42.6X3	T42.6X4	T42.6X5	T42.6X6
Chloroacetic acid	T60.3X1	T60.3X2	T60.3X3	T60.3X4	—	—
Chloroacetone	T59.3X1	T59.3X2	T59.3X3	T59.3X4	—	—
Chloroacetophenone	T59.3X1	T59.3X2	T59.3X3	T59.3X4	—	—
Chloroaniline	T53.7X1	T53.7X2	T53.7X3	T53.7X4	—	—
Chlorobenzene, chlorobenzol	T53.7X1	T53.7X2	T53.7X3	T53.7X4	—	—
Chlorobromomethane (fire extinguisher)	T53.6X1	T53.6X2	T53.6X3	T53.6X4	—	—
Chlorobutanol	T49.0X1	T49.0X2	T49.0X3	T49.0X4	T49.0X5	T49.0X6
Chlorocresol	T49.0X1	T49.0X2	T49.0X3	T49.0X4	T49.0X5	T49.0X6
Chlorodehydro-methyltestosterone	T38.7X1	T38.7X2	T38.7X3	T38.7X4	T38.7X5	T38.7X6
Chlorodinitrobenzene	T53.7X1	T53.7X2	T53.7X3	T53.7X4	—	—
dust or vapor	T53.7X1	T53.7X2	T53.7X3	T53.7X4	—	—
Chlorodiphenyl	T53.7X1	T53.7X2	T53.7X3	T53.7X4	—	—
Chloroethane — see Ethyl chloride						
Chloroethylene	T53.6X1	T53.6X2	T53.6X3	T53.6X4	—	—
Chlorofluorocarbons	T53.5X1	T53.5X2	T53.5X3	T53.5X4	—	—
Chloroform (fumes) (vapor)	T53.1X1	T53.1X2	T53.1X3	T53.1X4	—	—
anesthetic	T41.0X1	T41.0X2	T41.0X3	T41.0X4	T41.0X5	T41.0X6
solvent	T53.1X1	T53.1X2	T53.1X3	T53.1X4	—	—
water, concentrated	T41.0X1	T41.0X2	T41.0X3	T41.0X4	T41.0X5	T41.0X6
Chloroguanide	T37.2X1	T37.2X2	T37.2X3	T37.2X4	T37.2X5	T37.2X6
Chloromycetin	T36.2X1	T36.2X2	T36.2X3	T36.2X4	T36.2X5	T36.2X6
ENT agent	T49.6X1	T49.6X2	T49.6X3	T49.6X4	T49.6X5	T49.6X6
ophthalmic preparation	T49.5X1	T49.5X2	T49.5X3	T49.5X4	T49.5X5	T49.5X6
otic solution	T49.6X1	T49.6X2	T49.6X3	T49.6X4	T49.6X5	T49.6X6
topical NEC	T49.0X1	T49.0X2	T49.0X3	T49.0X4	T49.0X5	T49.0X6
Chloronitrobenzene	T53.7X1	T53.7X2	T53.7X3	T53.7X4	—	—
dust or vapor	T53.7X1	T53.7X2	T53.7X3	T53.7X4	—	—
Chlorophacinone	T60.4X1	T60.4X2	T60.4X3	T60.4X4	—	—
Chlorophenol	T53.7X1	T53.7X2	T53.7X3	T53.7X4	—	—
Chlorophenothane	T60.1X1	T60.1X2	T60.1X3	T60.1X4	—	—
Chlorophyll	T50.991	T50.992	T50.993	T50.994	T50.995	T50.996
Chloropicrin (fumes)	T53.6X1	T53.6X2	T53.6X3	T53.6X4	—	—
fumigant	T60.8X1	T60.8X2	T60.8X3	T60.8X4	—	—
fungicide	T60.3X1	T60.3X2	T60.3X3	T60.3X4	—	—
pesticide	T60.8X1	T60.8X2	T60.8X3	T60.8X4	—	—
Chloroprocaine	T41.3X1	T41.3X2	T41.3X3	T41.3X4	T41.3X5	T41.3X6
infiltration (subcutaneous)	T41.3X1	T41.3X2	T41.3X3	T41.3X4	T41.3X5	T41.3X6
nerve block (peripheral) (plexus)	T41.3X1	T41.3X2	T41.3X3	T41.3X4	T41.3X5	T41.3X6
spinal	T41.3X1	T41.3X2	T41.3X3	T41.3X4	T41.3X5	T41.3X6

◀ New ◀ Revised ~~deleted~~ Deleted

TABLE OF DRUGS AND CHEMICALS

TABLE OF DRUGS AND CHEMICALS

Substance	Poisoning, Accidental (Unintentional)	Poisoning, Intentional Self-Harm	Poisoning, Assault	Poisoning, Undetermined	Adverse Effect	Underdosing
Chloroptic	T49.5X1	T49.5X2	T49.5X3	T49.5X4	T49.5X5	T49.5X6
Chloropurine	T45.1X1	T45.1X2	T45.1X3	T45.1X4	T45.1X5	T45.1X6
Chloropyramine	T45.0X1	T45.0X2	T45.0X3	T45.0X4	T45.0X5	T45.0X6
Chloropyrifos	T60.0X1	T60.0X2	T60.0X3	T60.0X4	—	—
Chloropyrilene	T45.0X1	T45.0X2	T45.0X3	T45.0X4	T45.0X5	T45.0X6
Chloroquine	T37.2X1	T37.2X2	T37.2X3	T37.2X4	T37.2X5	T37.2X6
Chlorothalonil	T60.3X1	T60.3X2	T60.3X3	T60.3X4	—	—
Chlorothen	T45.0X1	T45.0X2	T45.0X3	T45.0X4	T45.0X5	T45.0X6
Chlorothiazide	T50.2X1	T50.2X2	T50.2X3	T50.2X4	T50.2X5	T50.2X6
Chlorothymol	T49.4X1	T49.4X2	T49.4X3	T49.4X4	T49.4X5	T49.4X6
Chlorotrianisene	T38.5X1	T38.5X2	T38.5X3	T38.5X4	T38.5X5	T38.5X6
Chlorovinyldichloro-arsine, not in war	T57.0X1	T57.0X2	T57.0X3	T57.0X4	—	—
Chloroxine	T49.4X1	T49.4X2	T49.4X3	T49.4X4	T49.4X5	T49.4X6
Chloroxylenol	T49.0X1	T49.0X2	T49.0X3	T49.0X4	T49.0X5	T49.0X6
Chlorphenamine	T45.0X1	T45.0X2	T45.0X3	T45.0X4	T45.0X5	T45.0X6
Chlorphenesin	T42.8X1	T42.8X2	T42.8X3	T42.8X4	T42.8X5	T42.8X6
topical (antifungal)	T49.0X1	T49.0X2	T49.0X3	T49.0X4	T49.0X5	T49.0X6
Chlorpheniramine	T45.0X1	T45.0X2	T45.0X3	T45.0X4	T45.0X5	T45.0X6
Chlorphenoxamine	T45.0X1	T45.0X2	T45.0X3	T45.0X4	T45.0X5	T45.0X6
Chlorphentermine	T50.5X1	T50.5X2	T50.5X3	T50.5X4	T50.5X5	T50.5X6
Chlorprocaine — see Chloroprocaine						
Chlorproguanil	T37.2X1	T37.2X2	T37.2X3	T37.2X4	T37.2X5	T37.2X6
Chlorpromazine	T43.3X1	T43.3X2	T43.3X3	T43.3X4	T43.3X5	T43.3X6
Chlorpropamide	T38.3X1	T38.3X2	T38.3X3	T38.3X4	T38.3X5	T38.3X6
Chlorprothixene	T43.4X1	T43.4X2	T43.4X3	T43.4X4	T43.4X5	T43.4X6
Chlorquinaldol	T49.0X1	T49.0X2	T49.0X3	T49.0X4	T49.0X5	T49.0X6
Chlorquinol	T49.0X1	T49.0X2	T49.0X3	T49.0X4	T49.0X5	T49.0X6
Chlortalidone	T50.2X1	T50.2X2	T50.2X3	T50.2X4	T50.2X5	T50.2X6
Chlortetracycline	T36.4X1	T36.4X2	T36.4X3	T36.4X4	T36.4X5	T36.4X6
Chlorthalidone	T50.2X1	T50.2X2	T50.2X3	T50.2X4	T50.2X5	T50.2X6
Chlorthiophos	T60.0X1	T60.0X2	T60.0X3	T60.0X4	—	—
Chlorotrianisene	T38.5X1	T38.5X2	T38.5X3	T38.5X4	T38.5X5	T38.5X6
Chlor-Trimeton	T45.0X1	T45.0X2	T45.0X3	T45.0X4	T45.0X5	T45.0X6
Chlorthion	T60.0X1	T60.0X2	T60.0X3	T60.0X4	—	—
Chlorzoxazone	T42.8X1	T42.8X2	T42.8X3	T42.8X4	T42.8X5	T42.8X6
Choke damp	T59.7X1	T59.7X2	T59.7X3	T59.7X4	—	—
Cholagogues	T47.5X1	T47.5X2	T47.5X3	T47.5X4	T47.5X5	T47.5X6
Cholebrine	T50.8X1	T50.8X2	T50.8X3	T50.8X4	T50.8X5	T50.8X6
Cholecalciferol	T45.2X1	T45.2X2	T45.2X3	T45.2X4	T45.2X5	T45.2X6
Cholecystokinin	T50.8X1	T50.8X2	T50.8X3	T50.8X4	T50.8X5	T50.8X6
Cholera vaccine	T50.A91	T50.A92	T50.A93	T50.A94	T50.A95	T50.A96

Substance	Poisoning, Accidental (Unintentional)	Poisoning, Intentional Self-Harm	Poisoning, Assault	Poisoning, Undetermined	Adverse Effect	Underdosing
Choleretic	T47.5X1	T47.5X2	T47.5X3	T47.5X4	T47.5X5	T47.5X6
Cholesterol-lowering agents	T46.6X1	T46.6X2	T46.6X3	T46.6X4	T46.6X5	T46.6X6
Cholestyramine (resin)	T46.6X1	T46.6X2	T46.6X3	T46.6X4	T46.6X5	T46.6X6
Cholic acid	T47.5X1	T47.5X2	T47.5X3	T47.5X4	T47.5X5	T47.5X6
Choline	T48.6X1	T48.6X2	T48.6X3	T48.6X4	T48.6X5	T48.6X6
chloride	T50.991	T50.992	T50.993	T50.994	T50.995	T50.996
dihydrogen citrate	T50.991	T50.992	T50.993	T50.994	T50.995	T50.996
salicylate	T39.091	T39.092	T39.093	T39.094	T39.095	T39.096
theophyllinate	T48.6X1	T48.6X2	T48.6X3	T48.6X4	T48.6X5	T48.6X6
Cholinergic (drug) NEC	T44.1X1	T44.1X2	T44.1X3	T44.1X4	T44.1X5	T44.1X6
muscle tone enhancer	T44.1X1	T44.1X2	T44.1X3	T44.1X4	T44.1X5	T44.1X6
organophosphorus	T44.0X1	T44.0X2	T44.0X3	T44.0X4	T44.0X5	T44.0X6
insecticide	T60.0X1	T60.0X2	T60.0X3	T60.0X4	—	—
nerve gas	T59.891	T59.892	T59.893	T59.894	—	—
trimethyl ammonium propanediol	T44.1X1	T44.1X2	T44.1X3	T44.1X4	T44.1X5	T44.1X6
Cholinesterase reactivator	T50.6X1	T50.6X2	T50.6X3	T50.6X4	T50.6X5	T50.6X6
Cholografin	T50.8X1	T50.8X2	T50.8X3	T50.8X4	T50.8X5	T50.8X6
Chorionic gonadotropin	T38.891	T38.892	T38.893	T38.894	T38.895	T38.896
Chromate	T56.2X1	T56.2X2	T56.2X3	T56.2X4	—	—
dust or mist	T56.2X1	T56.2X2	T56.2X3	T56.2X4	—	—
lead — see also lead	T56.0X1	T56.0X2	T56.0X3	T56.0X4	—	—
paint	T56.0X1	T56.0X2	T56.0X3	T56.0X4	—	—
Chromic						
acid	T56.2X1	T56.2X2	T56.2X3	T56.2X4	—	—
dust or mist	T56.2X1	T56.2X2	T56.2X3	T56.2X4	—	—
phosphate 32P	T45.1X1	T45.1X2	T45.1X3	T45.1X4	T45.1X5	T45.1X6
Chromium	T56.2X1	T56.2X2	T56.2X3	T56.2X4	—	—
compounds — see Chromate						
sesquioxide	T50.8X1	T50.8X2	T50.8X3	T50.8X4	T50.8X5	T50.8X6
Chromomycin A3	T45.1X1	T45.1X2	T45.1X3	T45.1X4	T45.1X5	T45.1X6
Chromonar	T46.3X1	T46.3X2	T46.3X3	T46.3X4	T46.3X5	T46.3X6
Chromyl chloride	T56.2X1	T56.2X2	T56.2X3	T56.2X4	—	—
Chrysarobin	T49.4X1	T49.4X2	T49.4X3	T49.4X4	T49.4X5	T49.4X6
Chrysazin	T47.2X1	T47.2X2	T47.2X3	T47.2X4	T47.2X5	T47.2X6
Chymar	T45.3X1	T45.3X2	T45.3X3	T45.3X4	T45.3X5	T45.3X6
ophthalmic preparation	T49.5X1	T49.5X2	T49.5X3	T49.5X4	T49.5X5	T49.5X6
Chymopapain	T45.3X1	T45.3X2	T45.3X3	T45.3X4	T45.3X5	T45.3X6
Chymotrypsin	T45.3X1	T45.3X2	T45.3X3	T45.3X4	T45.3X5	T45.3X6
ophthalmic preparation	T49.5X1	T49.5X2	T49.5X3	T49.5X4	T49.5X5	T49.5X6
Cianidanol	T50.991	T50.992	T50.993	T50.994	T50.995	T50.996
Cianopramine	T43.011	T43.012	T43.013	T43.014	T43.015	T43.016
Cibenzoline	T46.2X1	T46.2X2	T46.2X3	T46.2X4	T46.2X5	T46.2X6

◄ New ◄ Revised deleted Deleted

Substance	Poisoning, Accidental (Unintentional)	Poisoning, Intentional Self-Harm	Poisoning, Assault	Poisoning, Undetermined	Adverse Effect	Underdosing
Ciclacillin	T36.0X1	T36.0X2	T36.0X3	T36.0X4	T36.0X5	T36.0X6
Ciclobarbital — see Hexobarbital						
Ciclonicate	T46.7X1	T46.7X2	T46.7X3	T46.7X4	T46.7X5	T46.7X6
Ciclopirox (olamine)	T49.0X1	T49.0X2	T49.0X3	T49.0X4	T49.0X5	T49.0X6
Ciclosporin	T45.1X1	T45.1X2	T45.1X3	T45.1X4	T45.1X5	T45.1X6
Cicuta maculata or virosa	T62.2X1	T62.2X2	T62.2X3	T62.2X4	—	—
Cicutoxin	T62.2X1	T62.2X2	T62.2X3	T62.2X4	—	—
Cigarette lighter fluid	T52.0X1	T52.0X2	T52.0X3	T52.0X4	—	—
Cigarettes (tobacco)	T65.221	T65.222	T65.223	T65.224	—	—
Ciguatoxin	T61.01	T61.02	T61.03	T61.04	—	—
Cilazapril	T46.4X1	T46.4X2	T46.4X3	T46.4X4	T46.4X5	T46.4X6
Cimetidine	T47.0X1	T47.0X2	T47.0X3	T47.0X4	T47.0X5	T47.0X6
Cimetropium bromide	T44.3X1	T44.3X2	T44.3X3	T44.3X4	T44.3X5	T44.3X6
Cinchocaine	T41.3X1	T41.3X2	T41.3X3	T41.3X4	T41.3X5	T41.3X6
topical (surface)	T41.3X1	T41.3X2	T41.3X3	T41.3X4	T41.3X5	T41.3X6
Cinchona	T37.2X1	T37.2X2	T37.2X3	T37.2X4	T37.2X5	T37.2X6
Cinchonine alkaloids	T37.2X1	T37.2X2	T37.2X3	T37.2X4	T37.2X5	T37.2X6
Cinchophen	T50.4X1	T50.4X2	T50.4X3	T50.4X4	T50.4X5	T50.4X6
Cinepazide	T46.7X1	T46.7X2	T46.7X3	T46.7X4	T46.7X5	T46.7X6
Cinnamedrine	T48.5X1	T48.5X2	T48.5X3	T48.5X4	T48.5X5	T48.5X6
Cinnarizine	T45.0X1	T45.0X2	T45.0X3	T45.0X4	T45.0X5	T45.0X6
Cinoxacin	T37.8X1	T37.8X2	T37.8X3	T37.8X4	T37.8X5	T37.8X6
Ciprofibrate	T46.6X1	T46.6X2	T46.6X3	T46.6X4	T46.6X5	T46.6X6
Ciprofloxacin	T36.8X1	T36.8X2	T36.8X3	T36.8X4	T36.8X5	T36.8X6
Cisapride	T47.8X1	T47.8X2	T47.8X3	T47.8X4	T47.8X5	T47.8X6
Cisplatin	T45.1X1	T45.1X2	T45.1X3	T45.1X4	T45.1X5	T45.1X6
Citalopram	T43.221	T43.222	T43.223	T43.224	T43.225	T43.226
Citanest	T41.3X1	T41.3X2	T41.3X3	T41.3X4	T41.3X5	T41.3X6
infiltration (subcutaneous)	T41.3X1	T41.3X2	T41.3X3	T41.3X4	T41.3X5	T41.3X6
nerve block (peripheral) (plexus)	T41.3X1	T41.3X2	T41.3X3	T41.3X4	T41.3X5	T41.3X6
Citric acid	T47.5X1	T47.5X2	T47.5X3	T47.5X4	T47.5X5	T47.5X6
Citrovorum (factor)	T45.8X1	T45.8X2	T45.8X3	T45.8X4	T45.8X5	T45.8X6
Claviceps purpurea	T62.2X1	T62.2X2	T62.2X3	T62.2X4	—	—
Clavulanic acid	T36.1X1	T36.1X2	T36.1X3	T36.1X4	T36.1X5	T36.1X6
Cleaner, cleansing agent, type not specified	T65.891	T65.892	T65.893	T65.894	—	—
of paint or varnish	T52.91	T52.92	T52.93	T52.94	—	—
specified type NEC	T65.891	T65.892	T65.893	T65.894	—	—
Clebopride	T47.8X1	T47.8X2	T47.8X3	T47.8X4	T47.8X5	T47.8X6
Clefamide	T37.3X1	T37.3X2	T37.3X3	T37.3X4	T37.3X5	T37.3X6
Clemastine	T45.0X1	T45.0X2	T45.0X3	T45.0X4	T45.0X5	T45.0X6
Clematis vitalba	T62.2X1	T62.2X2	T62.2X3	T62.2X4	—	—

Substance	Poisoning, Accidental (Unintentional)	Poisoning, Intentional Self-Harm	Poisoning, Assault	Poisoning, Undetermined	Adverse Effect	Underdosing
Clemizole	T45.0X1	T45.0X2	T45.0X3	T45.0X4	T45.0X5	T45.0X6
penicillin	T36.0X1	T36.0X2	T36.0X3	T36.0X4	T36.0X5	T36.0X6
Clenbuterol	T48.6X1	T48.6X2	T48.6X3	T48.6X4	T48.6X5	T48.6X6
Clidinium bromide	T44.3X1	T44.3X2	T44.3X3	T44.3X4	T44.3X5	T44.3X6
Clindamycin	T36.8X1	T36.8X2	T36.8X3	T36.8X4	T36.8X5	T36.8X6
Clinofibrate	T46.6X1	T46.6X2	T46.6X3	T46.6X4	T46.6X5	T46.6X6
Clioquinol	T37.8X1	T37.8X2	T37.8X3	T37.8X4	T37.8X5	T37.8X6
Cliradon	T40.2X1	T40.2X2	T40.2X3	T40.2X4	—	—
Clobazam	T42.4X1	T42.4X2	T42.4X3	T42.4X4	T42.4X5	T42.4X6
Clobenzorex	T50.5X1	T50.5X2	T50.5X3	T50.5X4	T50.5X5	T50.5X6
Clobetasol	T49.0X1	T49.0X2	T49.0X3	T49.0X4	T49.0X5	T49.0X6
Clobetasone	T49.0X1	T49.0X2	T49.0X3	T49.0X4	T49.0X5	T49.0X6
Clobutinol	T48.3X1	T48.3X2	T48.3X3	T48.3X4	T48.3X5	T48.3X6
Clocapramine	T43.0X1	T43.0X2	T43.0X3	T43.0X4	T43.0X5	T43.0X6
Clocortolone	T38.0X1	T38.0X2	T38.0X3	T38.0X4	T38.0X5	T38.0X6
Clodantoin	T49.0X1	T49.0X2	T49.0X3	T49.0X4	T49.0X5	T49.0X6
Clodronic acid	T50.991	T50.992	T50.993	T50.994	T50.995	T50.996
Clofazimine	T37.1X1	T37.1X2	T37.1X3	T37.1X4	T37.1X5	T37.1X6
Clofedanol	T48.3X1	T48.3X2	T48.3X3	T48.3X4	T48.3X5	T48.3X6
Clofenamide	T50.2X1	T50.2X2	T50.2X3	T50.2X4	T50.2X5	T50.2X6
Clofenotane	T49.0X1	T49.0X2	T49.0X3	T49.0X4	T49.0X5	T49.0X6
Clofezone	T39.2X1	T39.2X2	T39.2X3	T39.2X4	T39.2X5	T39.2X6
Clofibrate	T46.6X1	T46.6X2	T46.6X3	T46.6X4	T46.6X5	T46.6X6
Clofibride	T46.6X1	T46.6X2	T46.6X3	T46.6X4	T46.6X5	T46.6X6
Cloforex	T50.5X1	T50.5X2	T50.5X3	T50.5X4	T50.5X5	T50.5X6
Clomacran	T43.0X1	T43.0X2	T43.0X3	T43.0X4	T43.0X5	T43.0X6
Clomethiazole	T42.6X1	T42.6X2	T42.6X3	T42.6X4	T42.6X5	T42.6X6
Clometocillin	T36.0X1	T36.0X2	T36.0X3	T36.0X4	T36.0X5	T36.0X6
Clomifene	T38.5X1	T38.5X2	T38.5X3	T38.5X4	T38.5X5	T38.5X6
Clomiphene	T38.5X1	T38.5X2	T38.5X3	T38.5X4	T38.5X5	T38.5X6
Clomipramine	T43.011	T43.012	T43.013	T43.014	T43.015	T43.016
Clomocycline	T36.4X1	T36.4X2	T36.4X3	T36.4X4	T36.4X5	T36.4X6
Clonazepam	T42.4X1	T42.4X2	T42.4X3	T42.4X4	T42.4X5	T42.4X6
Clonidine	T46.5X1	T46.5X2	T46.5X3	T46.5X4	T46.5X5	T46.5X6
Clonixin	T39.8X1	T39.8X2	T39.8X3	T39.8X4	T39.8X5	T39.8X6
Clopamide	T50.2X1	T50.2X2	T50.2X3	T50.2X4	T50.2X5	T50.2X6
Clopenthixol	T43.4X1	T43.4X2	T43.4X3	T43.4X4	T43.4X5	T43.4X6
Cloperastine	T48.3X1	T48.3X2	T48.3X3	T48.3X4	T48.3X5	T48.3X6
Clophedianol	T48.3X1	T48.3X2	T48.3X3	T48.3X4	T48.3X5	T48.3X6
Cloponone	T36.2X1	T36.2X2	T36.2X3	T36.2X4	T36.2X5	T36.2X6
Cloprednol	T38.0X1	T38.0X2	T38.0X3	T38.0X4	T38.0X5	T38.0X6
Cloral betaine	T42.6X1	T42.6X2	T42.6X3	T42.6X4	T42.6X5	T42.6X6

◀ New ◀ Revised ~~deleted~~ Deleted

Substance	External Cause (T-Code)					
	Poisoning, Accidental (Unintentional)	Poisoning, Intentional Self-Harm	Poisoning, Assault	Poisoning, Undetermined	Adverse Effect	Underdosing
Cloramfenicol	T36.2X1	T36.2X2	T36.2X3	T36.2X4	T36.2X5	T36.2X6
Clorazepate (dipotassium)	T42.4X1	T42.4X2	T42.4X3	T42.4X4	T42.4X5	T42.4X6
Clorexolone	T50.2X1	T50.2X2	T50.2X3	T50.2X4	T50.2X5	T50.2X6
Clorox (bleach)	T54.91	T54.92	T54.93	T54.94	—	—
Clorfenamine	T45.0X1	T45.0X2	T45.0X3	T45.0X4	T45.0X5	T45.0X6
Clorgiline	T43.1X1	T43.1X2	T43.1X3	T43.1X4	T43.1X5	T43.1X6
Clorotepine	T44.3X1	T44.3X2	T44.3X3	T44.3X4	T44.3X5	T44.3X6
Clorprenaline	T48.6X1	T48.6X2	T48.6X3	T48.6X4	T48.6X5	T48.6X6
Clortermine	T50.5X1	T50.5X2	T50.5X3	T50.5X4	T50.5X5	T50.5X6
Clotiapine	T43.591	T43.592	T43.593	T43.594	T43.595	T43.596
Clotiazepam	T42.4X1	T42.4X2	T42.4X3	T42.4X4	T42.4X5	T42.4X6
Clotibric acid	T46.6X1	T46.6X2	T46.6X3	T46.6X4	T46.6X5	T46.6X6
Clotrimazole	T49.0X1	T49.0X2	T49.0X3	T49.0X4	T49.0X5	T49.0X6
Cloxacillin	T36.0X1	T36.0X2	T36.0X3	T36.0X4	T36.0X5	T36.0X6
Cloxazolam	T42.4X1	T42.4X2	T42.4X3	T42.4X4	T42.4X5	T42.4X6
Cloxiquine	T49.0X1	T49.0X2	T49.0X3	T49.0X4	T49.0X5	T49.0X6
Clozapine	T42.4X1	T42.4X2	T42.4X3	T42.4X4	T42.4X5	T42.4X6
Coagulant NEC	T45.7X1	T45.7X2	T45.7X3	T45.7X4	T45.7X5	T45.7X6
Coal (carbon monoxide from) — see also Carbon, monoxide, coal	T58.2X1	T58.2X2	T58.2X3	T58.2X4	—	—
oil — see Kerosene						
tar	T49.1X1	T49.1X2	T49.1X3	T49.1X4	T49.1X5	T49.1X6
fumes	T59.891	T59.892	T59.893	T59.894	—	—
medicinal (ointment)	T49.4X1	T49.4X2	T49.4X3	T49.4X4	T49.4X5	T49.4X6
analgesics NEC	T39.2X1	T39.2X2	T39.2X3	T39.2X4	T39.2X5	T39.2X6
naphtha (solvent)	T52.0X1	T52.0X2	T52.0X3	T52.0X4		
Cobalamine	T45.2X1	T45.2X2	T45.2X3	T45.2X4	T45.2X5	T45.2X6
Cobalt (nonmedicinal) (fumes) (industrial)	T56.891	T56.892	T56.893	T56.894		
medicinal (trace) (chloride)	T45.8X1	T45.8X2	T45.8X3	T45.8X4	T45.8X5	T45.8X6
Cobra (venom)	T63.041	T63.042	T63.043	T63.044		
Coca (leaf)	T40.5X1	T40.5X2	T40.5X3	T40.5X4	T40.5X5	T40.5X6
Cocaine	T40.5X1	T40.5X2	T40.5X3	T40.5X4	T40.5X5	T40.5X6
topical anesthetic	T41.3X1	T41.3X2	T41.3X3	T41.3X4	T41.3X5	T41.3X6
Cocarboxylase	T45.3X1	T45.3X2	T45.3X3	T45.3X4	T45.3X5	T45.3X6
Coccidioidin	T50.8X1	T50.8X2	T50.8X3	T50.8X4	T50.8X5	T50.8X6
Cocculus indicus	T62.1X1	T62.1X2	T62.1X3	T62.1X4		
Cochineal	T65.6X1	T65.6X2	T65.6X3	T65.6X4		
medicinal products	T50.991	T50.992	T50.993	T50.994	T50.995	T50.996
Codeine	T40.2X1	T40.2X2	T40.2X3	T40.2X4	T40.2X5	T40.2X6
Cod-liver oil	T45.2X1	T45.2X2	T45.2X3	T45.2X4	T45.2X5	T45.2X6

Substance	External Cause (T-Code)					
	Poisoning, Accidental (Unintentional)	Poisoning, Intentional Self-Harm	Poisoning, Assault	Poisoning, Undetermined	Adverse Effect	Underdosing
Coenzyme A	T50.991	T50.992	T50.993	T50.994	T50.995	T50.996
Coffee	T62.8X1	T62.8X2	T62.8X3	T62.8X4	—	—
Cogalactoisomerase	T50.991	T50.992	T50.993	T50.994	T50.995	T50.996
Cogentin	T44.3X1	T44.3X2	T44.3X3	T44.3X4	T44.3X5	T44.3X6
Coke fumes or gas (carbon monoxide)	T58.2X1	T58.2X2	T58.2X3	T58.2X4	—	—
industrial use	T58.8X1	T58.8X2	T58.8X3	T58.8X4	—	—
Colace	T47.4X1	T47.4X2	T47.4X3	T47.4X4	T47.4X5	T47.4X6
Colaspase	T45.1X1	T45.1X2	T45.1X3	T45.1X4	T45.1X5	T45.1X6
Colchicine	T50.4X1	T50.4X2	T50.4X3	T50.4X4	T50.4X5	T50.4X6
Colchicum	T62.2X1	T62.2X2	T62.2X3	T62.2X4	—	—
Cold cream	T49.3X1	T49.3X2	T49.3X3	T49.3X4	T49.3X5	T49.3X6
Colecalciferol	T45.2X1	T45.2X2	T45.2X3	T45.2X4	T45.2X5	T45.2X6
Colestipol	T46.6X1	T46.6X2	T46.6X3	T46.6X4	T46.6X5	T46.6X6
Colestyramine	T46.6X1	T46.6X2	T46.6X3	T46.6X4	T46.6X5	T46.6X6
Colimycin	T36.8X1	T36.8X2	T36.8X3	T36.8X4	T36.8X5	T36.8X6
Colistimethate	T36.8X1	T36.8X2	T36.8X3	T36.8X4	T36.8X5	T36.8X6
Colistin	T36.8X1	T36.8X2	T36.8X3	T36.8X4	T36.8X5	T36.8X6
sulfate (eye preparation)	T49.5X1	T49.5X2	T49.5X3	T49.5X4	T49.5X5	T49.5X6
Collagen	T50.991	T50.992	T50.993	T50.994	T50.995	T50.996
Collagenase	T49.4X1	T49.4X2	T49.4X3	T49.4X4	T49.4X5	T49.4X6
Collodion	T49.3X1	T49.3X2	T49.3X3	T49.3X4	T49.3X5	T49.3X6
Colocynth	T47.2X1	T47.2X2	T47.2X3	T47.2X4	T47.2X5	T47.2X6
Colophony adhesive	T49.3X1	T49.3X2	T49.3X3	T49.3X4	T49.3X5	T49.3X6
Colorant — see also Dye	T50.991	T50.992	T50.993	T50.994	T50.995	T50.996
Coloring matter — see Dye(s)						
Combustion gas (after combustion) — see Carbon, monoxide						
prior to combustion	T59.891	T59.892	T59.893	T59.894	—	—
Compazine	T43.3X1	T43.3X2	T43.3X3	T43.3X4	T43.3X5	T43.3X6
Compound						
42 (warfarin)	T60.4X1	T60.4X2	T60.4X3	T60.4X4	—	—
269 (endrin)	T60.1X1	T60.1X2	T60.1X3	T60.1X4	—	—
497 (dieldrin)	T60.1X1	T60.1X2	T60.1X3	T60.1X4	—	—
1080 (sodium fluoroacetate)	T60.4X1	T60.4X2	T60.4X3	T60.4X4	—	—
3422 (parathion)	T60.0X1	T60.0X2	T60.0X3	T60.0X4	—	—
3911 (phorate)	T60.0X1	T60.0X2	T60.0X3	T60.0X4	—	—
3956 (toxaphene)	T60.1X1	T60.1X2	T60.1X3	T60.1X4	—	—
4049 (malathion)	T60.0X1	T60.0X2	T60.0X3	T60.0X4	—	—
4069 (malathion)	T60.0X1	T60.0X2	T60.0X3	T60.0X4	—	—
4124 (dicapthon)	T60.0X1	T60.0X2	T60.0X3	T60.0X4	—	—

◀ New ◀ Revised deleted Deleted

Substance	Poisoning, Accidental (Unintentional)	Poisoning, Intentional Self-Harm	Poisoning, Assault	Poisoning, Undetermined	Adverse Effect	Underdosing
Compound (Continued)						
E (cortisone)	T38.0X1	T38.0X2	T38.0X3	T38.0X4	T38.0X5	T38.0X6
F (hydrocortisone)	T38.0X1	T38.0X2	T38.0X3	T38.0X4	T38.0X5	T38.0X6
Congener, anabolic	T38.7X1	T38.7X2	T38.7X3	T38.7X4	T38.7X5	T38.7X6
Congo red	T50.8X1	T50.8X2	T50.8X3	T50.8X4	T50.8X5	T50.8X6
Coniine, conine	T62.2X1	T62.2X2	T62.2X3	T62.2X4	—	—
Conium (maculatum)	T62.2X1	T62.2X2	T62.2X3	T62.2X4	—	—
Conjugated estrogenic substances	T38.5X1	T38.5X2	T38.5X3	T38.5X4	T38.5X5	T38.5X6
Contac	T48.5X1	T48.5X2	T48.5X3	T48.5X4	T48.5X5	T48.5X6
Contact lens solution	T49.5X1	T49.5X2	T49.5X3	T49.5X4	T49.5X5	T49.5X6
Contraceptive (oral)	T38.4X1	T38.4X2	T38.4X3	T38.4X4	T38.4X5	T38.4X6
vaginal	T49.8X1	T49.8X2	T49.8X3	T49.8X4	T49.8X5	T49.8X6
Contrast medium, radiography	T50.8X1	T50.8X2	T50.8X3	T50.8X4	T50.8X5	T50.8X6
Convallaria glycosides	T46.0X1	T46.0X2	T46.0X3	T46.0X4	T46.0X5	T46.0X6
Convallaria majalis	T62.2X1	T62.2X2	T62.2X3	T62.2X4	—	—
berry	T62.1X1	T62.1X2	T62.1X3	T62.1X4	—	—
Copper (dust) (fumes) (nonmedicinal) NEC	T56.4X1	T56.4X2	T56.4X3	T56.4X4	—	—
arsenate, arsenite	T57.0X1	T57.0X2	T57.0X3	T57.0X4	—	—
insecticide	T60.2X1	T60.2X2	T60.2X3	T60.2X4	—	—
emetic	T47.7X1	T47.7X2	T47.7X3	T47.7X4	T47.7X5	T47.7X6
fungicide	T60.3X1	T60.3X2	T60.3X3	T60.3X4	—	—
gluconate	T49.0X1	T49.0X2	T49.0X3	T49.0X4	T49.0X5	T49.0X6
insecticide	T60.2X1	T60.2X2	T60.2X3	T60.2X4	—	—
medicinal (trace)	T45.8X1	T45.8X2	T45.8X3	T45.8X4	T45.8X5	T45.8X6
oleate	T49.0X1	T49.0X2	T49.0X3	T49.0X4	T49.0X5	T49.0X6
sulfate	T56.4X1	T56.4X2	T56.4X3	T56.4X4	—	—
cupric	T56.4X1	T56.4X2	T56.4X3	T56.4X4	—	—
fungicide	T60.3X1	T60.3X2	T60.3X3	T60.3X4	—	—
medicinal						
ear	T49.6X1	T49.6X2	T49.6X3	T49.6X4	T49.6X5	T49.6X6
emetic	T47.7X1	T47.7X2	T47.7X3	T47.7X4	T47.7X5	T47.7X6
eye	T49.5X1	T49.5X2	T49.5X3	T49.5X4	T49.5X5	T49.5X6
cuprous	T56.4X1	T56.4X2	T56.4X3	T56.4X4	—	—
fungicide	T60.3X1	T60.3X2	T60.3X3	T60.3X4	—	—
medicinal						
ear	T49.6X1	T49.6X2	T49.6X3	T49.6X4	T49.6X5	T49.6X6
emetic	T47.7X1	T47.7X2	T47.7X3	T47.7X4	T47.7X5	T47.7X6
eye	T49.5X1	T49.5X2	T49.5X3	T49.5X4	T49.5X5	T49.5X6
Copperhead snake (bite) (venom)	T63.061	T63.062	T63.063	T63.064	—	—
Coral (sting)	T63.691	T63.692	T63.693	T63.694	—	—
snake (bite) (venom)	T63.021	T63.022	T63.023	T63.024	—	—
Corbadrine	T49.6X1	T49.6X2	T49.6X3	T49.6X4	T49.6X5	T49.6X6
Cordran	T49.0X1	T49.0X2	T49.0X3	T49.0X4	T49.0X5	T49.0X6
Cordite	T65.891	T65.892	T65.893	T65.894	—	—
vapor	T59.891	T59.892	T59.893	T59.894	—	—
Corn cures	T49.4X1	T49.4X2	T49.4X3	T49.4X4	T49.4X5	T49.4X6
Cornhusker's lotion	T49.3X1	T49.3X2	T49.3X3	T49.3X4	T49.3X5	T49.3X6
Corn starch	T49.3X1	T49.3X2	T49.3X3	T49.3X4	T49.3X5	T49.3X6
Coronary vasodilator NEC	T46.3X1	T46.3X2	T46.3X3	T46.3X4	T46.3X5	T46.3X6
Corrosive NEC	T54.91	T54.92	T54.93	T54.94	—	—
acid NEC	T54.2X1	T54.2X2	T54.2X3	T54.2X4	—	—
aromatics	T54.1X1	T54.1X2	T54.1X3	T54.1X4	—	—
disinfectant	T54.1X1	T54.1X2	T54.1X3	T54.1X4	—	—
fumes NEC	T54.91	T54.92	T54.93	T54.94	—	—
specified NEC	T54.91	T54.92	T54.93	T54.94	—	—
sublimate	T56.1X1	T56.1X2	T56.1X3	T56.1X4	—	—
Cortate	T38.0X1	T38.0X2	T38.0X3	T38.0X4	T38.0X5	T38.0X6
Cort-Dome	T38.0X1	T38.0X2	T38.0X3	T38.0X4	T38.0X5	T38.0X6
ENT agent	T49.6X1	T49.6X2	T49.6X3	T49.6X4	T49.6X5	T49.6X6
ophthalmic preparation	T49.5X1	T49.5X2	T49.5X3	T49.5X4	T49.5X5	T49.5X6
topical NEC	T49.0X1	T49.0X2	T49.0X3	T49.0X4	T49.0X5	T49.0X6
Cortef	T38.0X1	T38.0X2	T38.0X3	T38.0X4	T38.0X5	T38.0X6
ENT agent	T49.6X1	T49.6X2	T49.6X3	T49.6X4	T49.6X5	T49.6X6
ophthalmic preparation	T49.5X1	T49.5X2	T49.5X3	T49.5X4	T49.5X5	T49.5X6
topical NEC	T49.0X1	T49.0X2	T49.0X3	T49.0X4	T49.0X5	T49.0X6
Corticosteroid	T38.0X1	T38.0X2	T38.0X3	T38.0X4	T38.0X5	T38.0X6
ENT agent	T49.6X1	T49.6X2	T49.6X3	T49.6X4	T49.6X5	T49.6X6
mineral	T50.0X1	T50.0X2	T50.0X3	T50.0X4	T50.0X5	T50.0X6
ophthalmic	T49.5X1	T49.5X2	T49.5X3	T49.5X4	T49.5X5	T49.5X6
topical NEC	T49.0X1	T49.0X2	T49.0X3	T49.0X4	T49.0X5	T49.0X6
Corticotropin	T38.811	T38.812	T38.813	T38.814	T38.815	T38.816
Cortisol	T49.0X1	T49.0X2	T49.0X3	T49.0X4	T49.0X5	T49.0X6
ENT agent	T49.6X1	T49.6X2	T49.6X3	T49.6X4	T49.6X5	T49.6X6
ophthalmic preparation	T49.5X1	T49.5X2	T49.5X3	T49.5X4	T49.5X5	T49.5X6
topical NEC	T49.0X1	T49.0X2	T49.0X3	T49.0X4	T49.0X5	T49.0X6
Cortisone (acetate)	T38.0X1	T38.0X2	T38.0X3	T38.0X4	T38.0X5	T38.0X6
ENT agent	T49.6X1	T49.6X2	T49.6X3	T49.6X4	T49.6X5	T49.6X6
ophthalmic preparation	T49.5X1	T49.5X2	T49.5X3	T49.5X4	T49.5X5	T49.5X6
topical NEC	T49.0X1	T49.0X2	T49.0X3	T49.0X4	T49.0X5	T49.0X6
Cortivazol	T38.0X1	T38.0X2	T38.0X3	T38.0X4	T38.0X5	T38.0X6
Cortogen	T38.0X1	T38.0X2	T38.0X3	T38.0X4	T38.0X5	T38.0X6
ENT agent	T49.6X1	T49.6X2	T49.6X3	T49.6X4	T49.6X5	T49.6X6
ophthalmic preparation	T49.5X1	T49.5X2	T49.5X3	T49.5X4	T49.5X5	T49.5X6

◀ New ◀◀ Revised ~~deleted~~ Deleted

TABLE OF DRUGS AND CHEMICALS

Substance	External Cause (T-Code)					
	Poisoning, Accidental (Unintentional)	Poisoning, Intentional Self-Harm	Poisoning, Assault	Poisoning, Undetermined	Adverse Effect	Underdosing
Cortone	T38.0X1	T38.0X2	T38.0X3	T38.0X4	T38.0X5	T38.0X6
ENT agent	T49.6X1	T49.6X2	T49.6X3	T49.6X4	T49.6X5	T49.6X6
ophthalmic preparation	T49.5X1	T49.5X2	T49.5X3	T49.5X4	T49.5X5	T49.5X6
Cortril	T38.0X1	T38.0X2	T38.0X3	T38.0X4	T38.0X5	T38.0X6
ENT agent	T49.6X1	T49.6X2	T49.6X3	T49.6X4	T49.6X5	T49.6X6
ophthalmic preparation	T49.5X1	T49.5X2	T49.5X3	T49.5X4	T49.5X5	T49.5X6
topical NEC	T49.0X1	T49.0X2	T49.0X3	T49.0X4	T49.0X5	T49.0X6
Corynebacterium parvum	T45.1X1	T45.1X2	T45.1X3	T45.1X4	T45.1X5	T45.1X6
Cosmetic preparation	T49.8X1	T49.8X2	T49.8X3	T49.8X4	T49.8X5	T49.8X6
Cosmetics	T49.8X1	T49.8X2	T49.8X3	T49.8X4	T49.8X5	T49.8X6
Cosyntropin	T38.811	T38.812	T38.813	T38.814	T38.815	T38.816
Cotarnine	T45.7X1	T45.7X2	T45.7X3	T45.7X4	T45.7X5	T45.7X6
Co-trimoxazole	T36.8X1	T36.8X2	T36.8X3	T36.8X4	T36.8X5	T36.8X6
Cottonseed oil	T49.3X1	T49.3X2	T49.3X3	T49.3X4	T49.3X5	T49.3X6
Cough mixture (syrup)	T48.4X1	T48.4X2	T48.4X3	T48.4X4	T48.4X5	T48.4X6
containing opiates	T40.2X1	T40.2X2	T40.2X3	T40.2X4	T40.2X5	T40.2X6
expectorants	T48.4X1	T48.4X2	T48.4X3	T48.4X4	T48.4X5	T48.4X6
Coumadin	T45.511	T45.512	T45.513	T45.514	T45.515	T45.516
rodenticide	T60.4X1	T60.4X2	T60.4X3	T60.4X4	—	—
Coumaphos	T60.0X1	T60.0X2	T60.0X3	T60.0X4	—	—
Coumarin	T45.511	T45.512	T45.513	T45.514	T45.515	T45.516
Coumetarol	T45.511	T45.512	T45.513	T45.514	T45.515	T45.516
Cowbane	T62.2X1	T62.2X2	T62.2X3	T62.2X4	—	—
Cozyme	T45.2X1	T45.2X2	T45.2X3	T45.2X4	T45.2X5	T45.2X6
Crack	T40.5X1	T40.5X2	T40.5X3	T40.5X4	—	—
Crataegus extract	T46.0X1	T46.0X2	T46.0X3	T46.0X4	T46.0X5	T46.0X6
Creolin	T54.1X1	T54.1X2	T54.1X3	T54.1X4	—	—
disinfectant	T54.1X1	T54.1X2	T54.1X3	T54.1X4	—	—
Creosol (compound)	T49.0X1	T49.0X2	T49.0X3	T49.0X4	T49.0X5	T49.0X6
Creosote (coal tar) (beechwood)	T49.0X1	T49.0X2	T49.0X3	T49.0X4	T49.0X5	T49.0X6
medicinal (expectorant)	T48.4X1	T48.4X2	T48.4X3	T48.4X4	T48.4X5	T48.4X6
syrup	T48.4X1	T48.4X2	T48.4X3	T48.4X4	T48.4X5	T48.4X6
Cresol(s)	T49.0X1	T49.0X2	T49.0X3	T49.0X4	T49.0X5	T49.0X6
and soap solution	T49.0X1	T49.0X2	T49.0X3	T49.0X4	T49.0X5	T49.0X6
Cresyl acetate	T49.0X1	T49.0X2	T49.0X3	T49.0X4	T49.0X5	T49.0X6
Cresylic acid	T49.0X1	T49.0X2	T49.0X3	T49.0X4	T49.0X5	T49.0X6
Crimidine	T60.4X1	T60.4X2	T60.4X3	T60.4X4	—	—
Croconazole	T37.8X1	T37.8X2	T37.8X3	T37.8X4	T37.8X5	T37.8X6
Cromoglicic acid	T48.6X1	T48.6X2	T48.6X3	T48.6X4	T48.6X5	T48.6X6
Cromolyn	T48.6X1	T48.6X2	T48.6X3	T48.6X4	T48.6X5	T48.6X6
Cromonar	T46.3X1	T46.3X2	T46.3X3	T46.3X4	T46.3X5	T46.3X6

Substance	External Cause (T-Code)					
	Poisoning, Accidental (Unintentional)	Poisoning, Intentional Self-Harm	Poisoning, Assault	Poisoning, Undetermined	Adverse Effect	Underdosing
Cropropamide	T39.8X1	T39.8X2	T39.8X3	T39.8X4	T39.8X5	T39.8X6
with crotethamide	T50.7X1	T50.7X2	T50.7X3	T50.7X4	T50.7X5	T50.7X6
Crotamiton	T49.0X1	T49.0X2	T49.0X3	T49.0X4	T49.0X5	T49.0X6
Crotethamide	T39.8X1	T39.8X2	T39.8X3	T39.8X4	T39.8X5	T39.8X6
with cropropamide	T50.7X1	T50.7X2	T50.7X3	T50.7X4	T50.7X5	T50.7X6
Croton (oil)	T47.2X1	T47.2X2	T47.2X3	T47.2X4	T47.2X5	T47.2X6
chloral	T42.6X1	T42.6X2	T42.6X3	T42.6X4	T42.6X5	T42.6X6
Crude oil	T52.0X1	T52.0X2	T52.0X3	T52.0X4	—	—
Cryogenine	T39.8X1	T39.8X2	T39.8X3	T39.8X4	T39.8X5	T39.8X6
Cryolite (vapor)	T60.1X1	T60.1X2	T60.1X3	T60.1X4	—	—
insecticide	T60.1X1	T60.1X2	T60.1X3	T60.1X4	—	—
Cryptenamine (tannates)	T46.5X1	T46.5X2	T46.5X3	T46.5X4	T46.5X5	T46.5X6
Crystal violet	T49.0X1	T49.0X2	T49.0X3	T49.0X4	T49.0X5	T49.0X6
Cuckoopint	T62.2X1	T62.2X2	T62.2X3	T62.2X4	—	—
Cumetharol	T45.511	T45.512	T45.513	T45.514	T45.515	T45.516
Cupric						
acetate	T60.3X1	T60.3X2	T60.3X3	T60.3X4	—	—
acetoarsenite	T57.0X1	T57.0X2	T57.0X3	T57.0X4	—	—
arsenate	T57.0X1	T57.0X2	T57.0X3	T57.0X4	—	—
gluconate	T49.0X1	T49.0X2	T49.0X3	T49.0X4	T49.0X5	T49.0X6
oleate	T49.0X1	T49.0X2	T49.0X3	T49.0X4	T49.0X5	T49.0X6
sulfate	T56.4X1	T56.4X2	T56.4X3	T56.4X4	—	—
Cuprous sulfate — see also Copper sulfate	T56.4X1	T56.4X2	T56.4X3	T56.4X4	—	—
Curare, curarine	T48.1X1	T48.1X2	T48.1X3	T48.1X4	T48.1X5	T48.1X6
Cyamemazine	T43.3X1	T43.3X2	T43.3X3	T43.3X4	T43.3X5	T43.3X6
Cyamopsis tetragono-loba	T46.6X1	T46.6X2	T46.6X3	T46.6X4	T46.6X5	T46.6X6
Cyanacetyl hydrazide	T37.1X1	T37.1X2	T37.1X3	T37.1X4	T37.1X5	T37.1X6
Cyanic acid (gas)	T59.891	T59.892	T59.893	T59.894	—	—
Cyanide(s) (compounds) (potassium) (sodium) NEC	T65.0X1	T65.0X2	T65.0X3	T65.0X4	—	—
dust or gas (inhalation) NEC	T57.3X1	T57.3X2	T57.3X3	T57.3X4	—	—
fumigant	T65.0X1	T65.0X2	T65.0X3	T65.0X4	—	—
hydrogen	T57.3X1	T57.3X2	T57.3X3	T57.3X4	—	—
mercuric — see Mercury						
pesticide (dust) (fumes)	T65.0X1	T65.0X2	T65.0X3	T65.0X4	—	—
Cyanoacrylate adhesive	T49.3X1	T49.3X2	T49.3X3	T49.3X4	T49.3X5	T49.3X6
Cyanocobalamin	T45.8X1	T45.8X2	T45.8X3	T45.8X4	T45.8X5	T45.8X6
Cyanogen (chloride) (gas) NEC	T59.891	T59.892	T59.893	T59.894	—	—
Cyclacillin	T36.0X1	T36.0X2	T36.0X3	T36.0X4	T36.0X5	T36.0X6
Cyclaine	T41.3X1	T41.3X2	T41.3X3	T41.3X4	T41.3X5	T41.3X6
Cyclamate	T50.991	T50.992	T50.993	T50.994	T50.995	T50.996

◄ New ◄ Revised deleted Deleted

Substance	External Cause (T-Code)					
	Poisoning, Accidental (Unintentional)	Poisoning, Intentional Self-Harm	Poisoning, Assault	Poisoning, Undetermined	Adverse Effect	Underdosing
Cyclamen europaeum	T62.2X1	T62.2X2	T62.2X3	T62.2X4	—	—
Cyclandelate	T46.7X1	T46.7X2	T46.7X3	T46.7X4	T46.7X5	T46.7X6
Cyclazocine	T50.7X1	T50.7X2	T50.7X3	T50.7X4	T50.7X5	T50.7X6
Cyclizine	T45.0X1	T45.0X2	T45.0X3	T45.0X4	T45.0X5	T45.0X6
Cyclobarbital	T42.3X1	T42.3X2	T42.3X3	T42.3X4	T42.3X5	T42.3X6
Cyclobarbitone	T42.3X1	T42.3X2	T42.3X3	T42.3X4	T42.3X5	T42.3X6
Cyclobenzaprine	T48.1X1	T48.1X2	T48.1X3	T48.1X4	T48.1X5	T48.1X6
Cyclodrine	T44.3X1	T44.3X2	T44.3X3	T44.3X4	T44.3X5	T44.3X6
Cycloguanil embonate	T37.2X1	T37.2X2	T37.2X3	T37.2X4	T37.2X5	T37.2X6
Cycloheptadiene	T43.291	T43.292	T43.293	T43.294	T43.295	T43.296
Cyclohexane	T52.8X1	T52.8X2	T52.8X3	T52.8X4	—	—
Cyclohexanol	T51.8X1	T51.8X2	T51.8X3	T51.8X4	—	—
Cyclohexanone	T52.4X1	T52.4X2	T52.4X3	T52.4X4	—	—
Cycloheximide	T60.3X1	T60.3X2	T60.3X3	T60.3X4	—	—
Cyclohexyl acetate	T52.8X1	T52.8X2	T52.8X3	T52.8X4	—	—
Cycloleucin	T45.1X1	T45.1X2	T45.1X3	T45.1X4	T45.1X5	T45.1X6
Cyclomethycaine	T41.3X1	T41.3X2	T41.3X3	T41.3X4	T41.3X5	T41.3X6
Cyclopentamine	T44.4X1	T44.4X2	T44.4X3	T44.4X4	T44.4X5	T44.4X6
Cyclopenthiazide	T50.2X1	T50.2X2	T50.2X3	T50.2X4	T50.2X5	T50.2X6
Cyclopentolate	T44.3X1	T44.3X2	T44.3X3	T44.3X4	T44.3X5	T44.3X6
Cyclophosphamide	T45.1X1	T45.1X2	T45.1X3	T45.1X4	T45.1X5	T45.1X6
Cycloplegic drug	T49.5X1	T49.5X2	T49.5X3	T49.5X4	T49.5X5	T49.5X6
Cyclopropane	T41.291	T41.292	T41.293	T41.294	T41.295	T41.296
Cyclopyrabital	T39.8X1	T39.8X2	T39.8X3	T39.8X4	T39.8X5	T39.8X6
Cycloserine	T37.1X1	T37.1X2	T37.1X3	T37.1X4	T37.1X5	T37.1X6
Cyclosporin	T45.1X1	T45.1X2	T45.1X3	T45.1X4	T45.1X5	T45.1X6
Cyclothiazide	T50.2X1	T50.2X2	T50.2X3	T50.2X4	T50.2X5	T50.2X6
Cycrimine	T44.3X1	T44.3X2	T44.3X3	T44.3X4	T44.3X5	T44.3X6
Cyhalothrin	T60.1X1	T60.1X2	T60.1X3	T60.1X4	—	—
Cymarin	T46.0X1	T46.0X2	T46.0X3	T46.0X4	T46.0X5	T46.0X6
Cypermethrin	T60.1X1	T60.1X2	T60.1X3	T60.1X4	—	—
Cyphenothrin	T60.2X1	T60.2X2	T60.2X3	T60.2X4	—	—
Cyproheptadine	T45.0X1	T45.0X2	T45.0X3	T45.0X4	T45.0X5	T45.0X6
Cyprolidol	T43.291	T43.292	T43.293	T43.294	T43.295	T43.296
Cyproterone	T38.6X1	T38.6X2	T38.6X3	T38.6X4	T38.6X5	T38.6X6
Cysteamine	T50.6X1	T50.6X2	T50.6X3	T50.6X4	T50.6X5	T50.6X6
Cytarabine	T45.1X1	T45.1X2	T45.1X3	T45.1X4	T45.1X5	T45.1X6
Cytisus						
laburnum	T62.2X1	T62.2X2	T62.2X3	T62.2X4	—	—
scoparius	T62.2X1	T62.2X2	T62.2X3	T62.2X4	—	—
Cytochrome C	T47.5X1	T47.5X2	T47.5X3	T47.5X4	T47.5X5	T47.5X6
Cytomel	T38.1X1	T38.1X2	T38.1X3	T38.1X4	T38.1X5	T38.1X6

Substance	External Cause (T-Code)					
	Poisoning, Accidental (Unintentional)	Poisoning, Intentional Self-Harm	Poisoning, Assault	Poisoning, Undetermined	Adverse Effect	Underdosing
Cytosine arabinoside	T45.1X1	T45.1X2	T45.1X3	T45.1X4	T45.1X5	T45.1X6
Cytoxan	T45.1X1	T45.1X2	T45.1X3	T45.1X4	T45.1X5	T45.1X6
Cytozyme	T45.7X1	T45.7X2	T45.7X3	T45.7X4	T45.7X5	T45.7X6
2,4-D	T60.3X1	T60.3X2	T60.3X3	T60.3X4	—	—
D						
Dacarbazine	T45.1X1	T45.1X2	T45.1X3	T45.1X4	T45.1X5	T45.1X6
Dactinomycin	T45.1X1	T45.1X2	T45.1X3	T45.1X4	T45.1X5	T45.1X6
DADPS	T37.1X1	T37.1X2	T37.1X3	T37.1X4	T37.1X5	T37.1X6
Dakin's solution	T49.0X1	T49.0X2	T49.0X3	T49.0X4	T49.0X5	T49.0X6
Dalapon (sodium)	T60.3X1	T60.3X2	T60.3X3	T60.3X4	—	—
Dalmane	T42.4X1	T42.4X2	T42.4X3	T42.4X4	T42.4X5	T42.4X6
Danazol	T38.6X1	T38.6X2	T38.6X3	T38.6X4	T38.6X5	T38.6X6
Danilone	T45.511	T45.512	T45.513	T45.514	T45.515	T45.516
Danthron	T47.2X1	T47.2X2	T47.2X3	T47.2X4	T47.2X5	T47.2X6
Dantrolene	T42.8X1	T42.8X2	T42.8X3	T42.8X4	T42.8X5	T42.8X6
Dantron	T47.2X1	T47.2X2	T47.2X3	T47.2X4	T47.2X5	T47.2X6
Daphne (gnidium) (mezereum)	T62.2X1	T62.2X2	T62.2X3	T62.2X4	—	—
berry	T62.1X1	T62.1X2	T62.1X3	T62.1X4	—	—
Dapsone	T37.1X1	T37.1X2	T37.1X3	T37.1X4	T37.1X5	T37.1X6
Daraprim	T37.2X1	T37.2X2	T37.2X3	T37.2X4	T37.2X5	T37.2X6
Darnel	T62.2X1	T62.2X2	T62.2X3	T62.2X4	—	—
Darvon	T39.8X1	T39.8X2	T39.8X3	T39.8X4	T39.8X5	T39.8X6
Daunomycin	T45.1X1	T45.1X2	T45.1X3	T45.1X4	T45.1X5	T45.1X6
Daunorubicin	T45.1X1	T45.1X2	T45.1X3	T45.1X4	T45.1X5	T45.1X6
DBI	T38.3X1	T38.3X2	T38.3X3	T38.3X4	T38.3X5	T38.3X6
D-Con	T60.91	T60.92	T60.93	T60.94	—	—
insecticide	T60.2X1	T60.2X2	T60.2X3	T60.2X4	—	—
rodenticide	T60.4X1	T60.4X2	T60.4X3	T60.4X4	—	—
DDAVP	T38.891	T38.892	T38.893	T38.894	T38.895	T38.896
DDE (bis(chlorophenyl)-dichloroethylene)	T60.2X1	T60.2X2	T60.2X3	T60.2X4	—	—
DDS	T37.1X1	T37.1X2	T37.1X3	T37.1X4	T37.1X5	T37.1X6
DDT (dust)	T60.1X1	T60.1X2	T60.1X3	T60.1X4	—	—
Deadly nightshade — see also Belladonna	T62.2X1	T62.2X2	T62.2X3	T62.2X4	—	—
berry	T62.1X1	T62.1X2	T62.1X3	T62.1X4	—	—
Deamino-D-arginine vasopressin	T38.891	T38.892	T38.893	T38.894	T38.895	T38.896
Deanol (aceglumate)	T50.991	T50.992	T50.993	T50.994	T50.995	T50.996
Debrisoquine	T46.5X1	T46.5X2	T46.5X3	T46.5X4	T46.5X5	T46.5X6
Decaborane	T57.8X1	T57.8X2	T57.8X3	T57.8X4	—	—
fumes	T59.891	T59.892	T59.893	T59.894	—	—

◀ New   ◀◀ Revised   ~~deleted~~ Deleted

TABLE OF DRUGS AND CHEMICALS

Substance	Poisoning, Accidental (Unintentional)	Poisoning, Intentional Self-Harm	Poisoning, Assault	Poisoning, Undetermined	Adverse Effect	Underdosing
Decadron	T38.0X1	T38.0X2	T38.0X3	T38.0X4	T38.0X5	T38.0X6
ENT agent	T49.6X1	T49.6X2	T49.6X3	T49.6X4	T49.6X5	T49.6X6
ophthalmic preparation	T49.5X1	T49.5X2	T49.5X3	T49.5X4	T49.5X5	T49.5X6
topical NEC	T49.0X1	T49.0X2	T49.0X3	T49.0X4	T49.0X5	T49.0X6
Decahydronaphthalene	T52.8X1	T52.8X2	T52.8X3	T52.8X4	—	—
Decalin	T52.8X1	T52.8X2	T52.8X3	T52.8X4	—	—
Decamethonium (bromide)	T48.1X1	T48.1X2	T48.1X3	T48.1X4	T48.1X5	T48.1X6
Decholin	T47.5X1	T47.5X2	T47.5X3	T47.5X4	T47.5X5	T47.5X6
Declomycin	T36.4X1	T36.4X2	T36.4X3	T36.4X4	T36.4X5	T36.4X6
Decongestant, nasal (mucosa)	T48.5X1	T48.5X2	T48.5X3	T48.5X4	T48.5X5	T48.5X6
combination	T48.5X1	T48.5X2	T48.5X3	T48.5X4	T48.5X5	T48.5X6
Deet	T60.8X1	T60.8X2	T60.8X3	T60.8X4	—	—
Deferoxamine	T45.8X1	T45.8X2	T45.8X3	T45.8X4	T45.8X5	T45.8X6
Deflazacort	T38.0X1	T38.0X2	T38.0X3	T38.0X4	T38.0X5	T38.0X6
Deglycyrrhizinized extract of licorice	T48.4X1	T48.4X2	T48.4X3	T48.4X4	T48.4X5	T48.4X6
Dehydrocholic acid	T47.5X1	T47.5X2	T47.5X3	T47.5X4	T47.5X5	T47.5X6
Dehydroemetine	T37.3X1	T37.3X2	T37.3X3	T37.3X4	T37.3X5	T37.3X6
Dekalin	T52.8X1	T52.8X2	T52.8X3	T52.8X4	—	—
Delalutin	T38.5X1	T38.5X2	T38.5X3	T38.5X4	T38.5X5	T38.5X6
Delphinium	T62.2X1	T62.2X2	T62.2X3	T62.2X4		
Deltasone	T38.0X1	T38.0X2	T38.0X3	T38.0X4	T38.0X5	T38.0X6
Deltra	T38.0X1	T38.0X2	T38.0X3	T38.0X4	T38.0X5	T38.0X6
Delvinal	T42.3X1	T42.3X2	T42.3X3	T42.3X4	T42.3X5	T42.3X6
Delorazepam	T42.4X1	T42.4X2	T42.4X3	T42.4X4	T42.4X5	T42.4X6
Deltamethrin	T60.1X1	T60.1X2	T60.1X3	T60.1X4	—	—
Demecarium (bromide)	T49.5X1	T49.5X2	T49.5X3	T49.5X4	T49.5X5	T49.5X6
Demeclocycline	T36.4X1	T36.4X2	T36.4X3	T36.4X4	T36.4X5	T36.4X6
Demecolcine	T45.1X1	T45.1X2	T45.1X3	T45.1X4	T45.1X5	T45.1X6
Demegestone	T38.5X1	T38.5X2	T38.5X3	T38.5X4	T38.5X5	T38.5X6
Demelanizing agents	T49.8X1	T49.8X2	T49.8X3	T49.8X4	T49.8X5	T49.8X6
Demephion -O and -S	T60.0X1	T60.0X2	T60.0X3	T60.0X4	—	—
Demerol	T40.2X1	T40.2X2	T40.2X3	T40.2X4	T40.2X5	T40.2X6
Demethylchlortetracycline	T36.4X1	T36.4X2	T36.4X3	T36.4X4	T36.4X5	T36.4X6
Demethyltetracycline	T36.4X1	T36.4X2	T36.4X3	T36.4X4	T36.4X5	T36.4X6
Demeton -O and -S	T60.0X1	T60.0X2	T60.0X3	T60.0X4	—	—
Demulcent (external)	T49.3X1	T49.3X2	T49.3X3	T49.3X4	T49.3X5	T49.3X6
specified NEC	T49.3X1	T49.3X2	T49.3X3	T49.3X4	T49.3X5	T49.3X6
Demulen	T38.4X1	T38.4X2	T38.4X3	T38.4X4	T38.4X5	T38.4X6
Denatured alcohol	T51.0X1	T51.0X2	T51.0X3	T51.0X4	—	—
Dendrid	T49.5X1	T49.5X2	T49.5X3	T49.5X4	T49.5X5	T49.5X6
Dental drug, topical application NEC	T49.7X1	T49.7X2	T49.7X3	T49.7X4	T49.7X5	T49.7X6

Substance	Poisoning, Accidental (Unintentional)	Poisoning, Intentional Self-Harm	Poisoning, Assault	Poisoning, Undetermined	Adverse Effect	Underdosing
Dentifrice	T49.7X1	T49.7X2	T49.7X3	T49.7X4	T49.7X5	T49.7X6
Deodorant spray (feminine hygiene)	T49.8X1	T49.8X2	T49.8X3	T49.8X4	T49.8X5	T49.8X6
Deoxycortone	T50.0X1	T50.0X2	T50.0X3	T50.0X4	T50.0X5	T50.0X6
2-Deoxy-5-fluorouridine	T45.1X1	T45.1X2	T45.1X3	T45.1X4	T45.1X5	T45.1X6
5-Deoxy-5-fluorouridine	T45.1X1	T45.1X2	T45.1X3	T45.1X4	T45.1X5	T45.1X6
Deoxyribonuclease (pancreatic)	T45.3X1	T45.3X2	T45.3X3	T45.3X4	T45.3X5	T45.3X6
Depilatory	T49.4X1	T49.4X2	T49.4X3	T49.4X4	T49.4X5	T49.4X6
Deprenalin	T42.8X1	T42.8X2	T42.8X3	T42.8X4	T42.8X5	T42.8X6
Deprenyl	T42.8X1	T42.8X2	T42.8X3	T42.8X4	T42.8X5	T42.8X6
Depressant, appetite	T50.5X1	T50.5X2	T50.5X3	T50.5X4	T50.5X5	T50.5X6
Depressant						
appetite, central	T50.5X1	T50.5X2	T50.5X3	T50.5X4	T50.5X5	T50.5X6
cardiac	T46.2X1	T46.2X2	T46.2X3	T46.2X4	T46.2X5	T46.2X6
central nervous system (anesthetic) — see also Central nervous system, depressants	T42.71	T42.72	T42.73	T42.74	T42.75	T42.76
general anesthetic	T41.201	T41.202	T41.203	T41.204	T41.205	T41.206
muscle tone	T42.8X1	T42.8X2	T42.8X3	T42.8X4	T42.8X5	T42.8X6
muscle tone, central	T42.8X1	T42.8X2	T42.8X3	T42.8X4	T42.8X5	T42.8X6
psychotherapeutic	T43.501	T43.502	T43.503	T43.504	T43.505	T43.506
Deptropine	T45.0X1	T45.0X2	T45.0X3	T45.0X4	T45.0X5	T45.0X6
Dequalinium (chloride)	T49.0X1	T49.0X2	T49.0X3	T49.0X4	T49.0X5	T49.0X6
Derris root	T60.2X1	T60.2X2	T60.2X3	T60.2X4	—	—
Deserpidine	T43.011	T43.012	T43.013	T43.014	T43.015	T43.016
Desferrioxamine	T45.8X1	T45.8X2	T45.8X3	T45.8X4	T45.8X5	T45.8X6
Desipramine	T43.0X1	T43.0X2	T43.0X3	T43.0X4	T43.0X5	T43.0X6
Deslanoside	T46.0X1	T46.0X2	T46.0X3	T46.0X4	T46.0X5	T46.0X6
Desloughing agent	T49.4X1	T49.4X2	T49.4X3	T49.4X4	T49.4X5	T49.4X6
Desmethylimipramine	T43.011	T43.012	T43.013	T43.014	T43.015	T43.016
Desmopressin	T38.891	T38.892	T38.893	T38.894	T38.895	T38.896
Desocodeine	T40.2X1	T40.2X2	T40.2X3	T40.2X4	T40.2X5	T40.2X6
Desogestrel	T38.5X1	T38.5X2	T38.5X3	T38.5X4	T38.5X5	T38.5X6
Desomorphine	T40.2X1	T40.2X2	T40.2X3	T40.2X4	—	—
Desonide	T49.0X1	T49.0X2	T49.0X3	T49.0X4	T49.0X5	T49.0X6
Desoximetasone	T49.0X1	T49.0X2	T49.0X3	T49.0X4	T49.0X5	T49.0X6
Desoxycorticosteroid	T50.0X1	T50.0X2	T50.0X3	T50.0X4	T50.0X5	T50.0X6
Desoxycortone	T50.0X1	T50.0X2	T50.0X3	T50.0X4	T50.0X5	T50.0X6
Desoxyephedrine	T43.621	T43.622	T43.623	T43.624	T43.625	T43.626
Detaxtran	T46.6X1	T46.6X2	T46.6X3	T46.6X4	T46.6X5	T46.6X6
Detergent	T49.2X1	T49.2X2	T49.2X3	T49.2X4	T49.2X5	T49.2X6
external medication	T49.2X1	T49.2X2	T49.2X3	T49.2X4	T49.2X5	T49.2X6
local	T49.2X1	T49.2X2	T49.2X3	T49.2X4	T49.2X5	T49.2X6

◄ New ◄ Revised ~~deleted~~ Deleted

	External Cause (T-Code)					
Substance	Poisoning, Accidental (Unintentional)	Poisoning, Intentional Self-Harm	Poisoning, Assault	Poisoning, Undetermined	Adverse Effect	Underdosing
Detergent *(Continued)*						
medicinal	T49.2X1	T49.2X2	T49.2X3	T49.2X4	T49.2X5	T49.2X6
nonmedicinal	T55.1X1	T55.1X2	T55.1X3	T55.1X4	—	—
specified NEC	T55.1X1	T55.1X2	T55.1X3	T55.1X4	T55.1X5	T55.1X6
Deterrent, alcohol	T50.6X1	T50.6X2	T50.6X3	T50.6X4	T50.6X5	T50.6X6
Detoxifying agent	T50.6X1	T50.6X2	T50.6X3	T50.6X4	T50.6X5	T50.6X6
Detrothyronine	T38.1X1	T38.1X2	T38.1X3	T38.1X4	T38.1X5	T38.1X6
Dettol (external medication)	T49.0X1	T49.0X2	T49.0X3	T49.0X4	T49.0X5	T49.0X6
Dexamethasone	T38.0X1	T38.0X2	T38.0X3	T38.0X4	T38.0X5	T38.0X6
ENT agent	T49.6X1	T49.6X2	T49.6X3	T49.6X4	T49.6X5	T49.6X6
ophthalmic preparation	T49.5X1	T49.5X2	T49.5X3	T49.5X4	T49.5X5	T49.5X6
topical NEC	T49.0X1	T49.0X2	T49.0X3	T49.0X4	T49.0X5	T49.0X6
Dexamfetamine	T43.621	T43.622	T43.623	T43.624	T43.625	T43.626
Dexamphetamine	T43.621	T43.622	T43.623	T43.624	T43.625	T43.626
Dexbrompheniramine	T45.0X1	T45.0X2	T45.0X3	T45.0X4	T45.0X5	T45.0X6
Dexchlorpheniramine	T45.0X1	T45.0X2	T45.0X3	T45.0X4	T45.0X5	T45.0X6
Dexedrine	T43.621	T43.622	T43.623	T43.624	T43.625	T43.626
Dexetimide	T44.3X1	T44.3X2	T44.3X3	T44.3X4	T44.3X5	T44.3X6
Dexfenfluramine	T50.5X1	T50.5X2	T50.5X3	T50.5X4	T50.5X5	T50.5X6
Dexpanthenol	T45.2X1	T45.2X2	T45.2X3	T45.2X4	T45.2X5	T45.2X6
Dextran (40) (70) (150)	T45.8X1	T45.8X2	T45.8X3	T45.8X4	T45.8X5	T45.8X6
Dextriferron	T45.4X1	T45.4X2	T45.4X3	T45.4X4	T45.4X5	T45.4X6
Dextroamphetamine	T43.621	T43.622	T43.623	T43.624	T43.625	T43.626
Dextro calcium pantothenate	T45.2X1	T45.2X2	T45.2X3	T45.2X4	T45.2X5	T45.2X6
Dextromethorphan	T48.3X1	T48.3X2	T48.3X3	T48.3X4	T48.3X5	T48.3X6
Dextromoramide	T40.4X1	T40.4X2	T40.4X3	T40.4X4	—	—
topical	T49.8X1	T49.8X2	T49.8X3	T49.8X4	T49.8X5	T49.8X6
Dextro pantothenyl alcohol	T45.2X1	T45.2X2	T45.2X3	T45.2X4	T45.2X5	T45.2X6
Dextropropoxyphene	T40.4X1	T40.4X2	T40.4X3	T40.4X4	T40.4X5	T40.4X6
Dextrorphan	T40.2X1	T40.2X2	T40.2X3	T40.2X4	T40.2X5	T40.2X6
Dextrose	T50.3X1	T50.3X2	T50.3X3	T50.3X4	T50.3X5	T50.3X6
concentrated solution, intravenous	T46.8X1	T46.8X2	T46.8X3	T46.8X4	T46.8X5	T46.8X6
Dextrothyroxin	T38.1X1	T38.1X2	T38.1X3	T38.1X4	T38.1X5	T38.1X6
Dextrothyroxine sodium	T38.1X1	T38.1X2	T38.1X3	T38.1X4	T38.1X5	T38.1X6
DFP	T44.0X1	T44.0X2	T44.0X3	T44.0X4	T44.0X5	T44.0X6
DHE	T37.3X1	T37.3X2	T37.3X3	T37.3X4	T37.3X5	T37.3X6
45	T46.5X1	T46.5X2	T46.5X3	T46.5X4	T46.5X5	T46.5X6
Diabinese	T38.3X1	T38.3X2	T38.3X3	T38.3X4	T38.3X5	T38.3X6
Diacetone alcohol	T52.4X1	T52.4X2	T52.4X3	T52.4X4	—	—
Diacetyl monoxime	T50.991	T50.992	T50.993	T50.994	—	—
Diacetylmorphine	T40.1X1	T40.1X2	T40.1X3	T40.1X4	—	—

	External Cause (T-Code)					
Substance	Poisoning, Accidental (Unintentional)	Poisoning, Intentional Self-Harm	Poisoning, Assault	Poisoning, Undetermined	Adverse Effect	Underdosing
Diachylon plaster	T49.4X1	T49.4X2	T49.4X3	T49.4X4	T49.4X5	T49.4X6
Diaethylstilboestrolum	T38.5X1	T38.5X2	T38.5X3	T38.5X4	T38.5X5	T38.5X6
Diagnostic agent NEC	T50.8X1	T50.8X2	T50.8X3	T50.8X4	T50.8X5	T50.8X6
Dial (soap)	T49.2X1	T49.2X2	T49.2X3	T49.2X4	T49.2X5	T49.2X6
sedative	T42.3X1	T42.3X2	T42.3X3	T42.3X4	T42.3X5	T42.3X6
Dialkyl carbonate	T52.91	T52.92	T52.93	T52.94	—	—
Diallylbarbituric acid	T42.3X1	T42.3X2	T42.3X3	T42.3X4	T42.3X5	T42.3X6
Diallymal	T42.3X1	T42.3X2	T42.3X3	T42.3X4	T42.3X5	T42.3X6
Dialysis solution (intraperitoneal)	T50.3X1	T50.3X2	T50.3X3	T50.3X4	T50.3X5	T50.3X6
Diaminodiphenylsulfone	T37.1X1	T37.1X2	T37.1X3	T37.1X4	T37.1X5	T37.1X6
Diamorphine	T40.1X1	T40.1X2	T40.1X3	T40.1X4	—	—
Diamox	T50.2X1	T50.2X2	T50.2X3	T50.2X4	T50.2X5	T50.2X6
Diamthazole	T49.0X1	T49.0X2	T49.0X3	T49.0X4	T49.0X5	T49.0X6
Dianthone	T47.2X1	T47.2X2	T47.2X3	T47.2X4	T47.2X5	T47.2X6
Diaphenylsulfone	T37.0X1	T37.0X2	T37.0X3	T37.0X4	T37.0X5	T37.0X6
Diasone (sodium)	T37.1X1	T37.1X2	T37.1X3	T37.1X4	T37.1X5	T37.1X6
Diastase	T47.5X1	T47.5X2	T47.5X3	T47.5X4	T47.5X5	T47.5X6
Diatrizoate	T50.8X1	T50.8X2	T50.8X3	T50.8X4	T50.8X5	T50.8X6
Diazepam	T42.4X1	T42.4X2	T42.4X3	T42.4X4	T42.4X5	T42.4X6
Diazinon	T60.0X1	T60.0X2	T60.0X3	T60.0X4	—	—
Diazomethane (gas)	T59.891	T59.892	T59.893	T59.894	—	—
Diazoxide	T46.5X1	T46.5X2	T46.5X3	T46.5X4	T46.5X5	T46.5X6
Dibekacin	T36.5X1	T36.5X2	T36.5X3	T36.5X4	T36.5X5	T36.5X6
Dibenamine	T44.6X1	T44.6X2	T44.6X3	T44.6X4	T44.6X5	T44.6X6
Dibenzepin	T43.011	T43.012	T43.013	T43.014	T43.015	T43.016
Dibenzheptropine	T45.0X1	T45.0X2	T45.0X3	T45.0X4	T45.0X5	T45.0X6
Dibenzyline	T44.6X1	T44.6X2	T44.6X3	T44.6X4	T44.6X5	T44.6X6
Diborane (gas)	T59.891	T59.892	T59.893	T59.894	—	—
Dibromochloropropane	T60.8X1	T60.8X2	T60.8X3	T60.8X4	—	—
Dibromodulcitol	T45.1X1	T45.1X2	T45.1X3	T45.1X4	T45.1X5	T45.1X6
Dibromoethane	T53.6X1	T53.6X2	T53.6X3	T53.6X4	—	—
Dibromomannitol	T45.1X1	T45.1X2	T45.1X3	T45.1X4	T45.1X5	T45.1X6
Dibromopropamidine isethionate	T49.0X1	T49.0X2	T49.0X3	T49.0X4	T49.0X5	T49.0X6
Dibrompropamidine	T49.0X1	T49.0X2	T49.0X3	T49.0X4	T49.0X5	T49.0X6
Dibucaine	T41.3X1	T41.3X2	T41.3X3	T41.3X4	T41.3X5	T41.3X6
topical (surface)	T41.3X1	T41.3X2	T41.3X3	T41.3X4	T41.3X5	T41.3X6
Dibunate sodium	T48.3X1	T48.3X2	T48.3X3	T48.3X4	T48.3X5	T48.3X6
Dibutoline sulfate	T44.3X1	T44.3X2	T44.3X3	T44.3X4	T44.3X5	T44.3X6
Dicamba	T60.3X1	T60.3X2	T60.3X3	T60.3X4	—	—
Dicapthon	T60.0X1	T60.0X2	T60.0X3	T60.0X4	—	—
Dichlobenil	T60.3X1	T60.3X2	T60.3X3	T60.3X4	—	—
Dichlone	T60.3X1	T60.3X2	T60.3X3	T60.3X4	—	—

TABLE OF DRUGS AND CHEMICALS

Substance	Poisoning, Accidental (Unintentional)	Poisoning, Intentional Self-Harm	Poisoning, Assault	Poisoning, Undetermined	Adverse Effect	Underdosing
Dichloralphenozone	T42.6X1	T42.6X2	T42.6X3	T42.6X4	T42.6X5	T42.6X6
Dichlorbenzidine	T65.3X1	T65.3X2	T65.3X3	T65.3X4	—	—
Dichlorhydrin	T52.8X1	T52.8X2	T52.8X3	T52.8X4	—	—
Dichlorhydroxyquinoline	T37.8X1	T37.8X2	T37.8X3	T37.8X4	T37.8X5	T37.8X6
Dichlorobenzene	T53.7X1	T53.7X2	T53.7X3	T53.7X4		
Dichlorobenzyl alcohol	T49.6X1	T49.6X2	T49.6X3	T49.6X4	T49.6X5	T49.6X6
Dichlorodifluoromethane	T53.5X1	T53.5X2	T53.5X3	T53.5X4	—	—
Dichloroethane	T52.8X1	T52.8X2	T52.8X3	T52.8X4		
Sym-Dichloroethyl ether	T53.6X1	T53.6X2	T53.6X3	T53.6X4		
Dichloroethyl sulfide, not in war	T59.891	T59.892	T59.893	T59.894	—	—
Dichloroethylene	T53.6X1	T53.6X2	T53.6X3	T53.6X4		
Dichloroformoxine, not in war	T59.891	T59.892	T59.893	T59.894		
Dichlorohydrin, alpha-dichlorohydrin	T52.8X1	T52.8X2	T52.8X3	T52.8X4	—	—
Dichloromethane (solvent)	T53.4X1	T53.4X2	T53.4X3	T53.4X4	—	—
vapor	T53.4X1	T53.4X2	T53.4X3	T53.4X4	—	—
Dichloronaphthoquinone	T60.3X1	T60.3X2	T60.3X3	T60.3X4	—	—
Dichlorophen	T37.4X1	T37.4X2	T37.4X3	T37.4X4	T37.4X5	T37.4X6
2,4-Dichlorophenoxy-acetic acid	T60.3X1	T60.3X2	T60.3X3	T60.3X4	—	—
Dichloropropene	T60.3X1	T60.3X2	T60.3X3	T60.3X4	—	—
Dichloropropionic acid	T60.3X1	T60.3X2	T60.3X3	T60.3X4	—	—
Dichlorphenamide	T50.2X1	T50.2X2	T50.2X3	T50.2X4	T50.2X5	T50.2X6
Dichlorvos	T60.0X1	T60.0X2	T60.0X3	T60.0X4	—	—
Diclofenac	T39.391	T39.392	T39.393	T39.394	T39.395	T39.396
Diclofenamide	T50.2X1	T50.2X2	T50.2X3	T50.2X4	T50.2X5	T50.2X6
Diclofensine	T43.291	T43.292	T43.293	T43.294	T43.295	T43.296
Diclonixine	T39.8X1	T39.8X2	T39.8X3	T39.8X4	T39.8X5	T39.8X6
Dicloxacillin	T36.0X1	T36.0X2	T36.0X3	T36.0X4	T36.0X5	T36.0X6
Dicophane	T49.0X1	T49.0X2	T49.0X3	T49.0X4	T49.0X5	T49.0X6
Dicoumarol, dicoumarin, dicumarol	T45.511	T45.512	T45.513	T45.514	T45.515	T45.516
Dicrotophos	T60.0X1	T60.0X2	T60.0X3	T60.0X4	—	—
Dicyanogen (gas)	T65.0X1	T65.0X2	T65.0X3	T65.0X4	—	—
Dicyclomine	T44.3X1	T44.3X2	T44.3X3	T44.3X4	T44.3X5	T44.3X6
Dicycloverine	T44.3X1	T44.3X2	T44.3X3	T44.3X4	T44.3X5	T44.3X6
Dideoxycytidine	T37.5X1	T37.5X2	T37.5X3	T37.5X4	T37.5X5	T37.5X6
Dideoxyinosine	T37.5X1	T37.5X2	T37.5X3	T37.5X4	T37.5X5	T37.5X6
Dieldrin (vapor)	T60.1X1	T60.1X2	T60.1X3	T60.1X4	—	—
Diemal	T42.3X1	T42.3X2	T42.3X3	T42.3X4	T42.3X5	T42.3X6
Dienestrol	T38.5X1	T38.5X2	T38.5X3	T38.5X4	T38.5X5	T38.5X6
Dienoestrol	T38.5X1	T38.5X2	T38.5X3	T38.5X4	T38.5X5	T38.5X6
Dietetic drug NEC	T50.901	T50.902	T50.903	T50.904	T50.905	T50.906
Diethazine	T42.8X1	T42.8X2	T42.8X3	T42.8X4	T42.8X5	T42.8X6

Substance	Poisoning, Accidental (Unintentional)	Poisoning, Intentional Self-Harm	Poisoning, Assault	Poisoning, Undetermined	Adverse Effect	Underdosing
Diethyl						
barbituric acid	T42.3X1	T42.3X2	T42.3X3	T42.3X4	T42.3X5	T42.3X6
carbamazine	T37.4X1	T37.4X2	T37.4X3	T37.4X4	T37.4X5	T37.4X6
carbinol	T51.3X1	T51.3X2	T51.3X3	T51.3X4	—	—
carbonate	T52.8X1	T52.8X2	T52.8X3	T52.8X4	—	—
ether (vapor) — see also ether	T41.0X1	T41.0X2	T41.0X3	T41.0X4	T41.0X5	T41.0X6
oxide	T52.8X1	T52.8X2	T52.8X3	T52.8X4	—	—
propion	T50.5X1	T50.5X2	T50.5X3	T50.5X4	T50.5X5	T50.5X6
stilbestrol	T38.5X1	T38.5X2	T38.5X3	T38.5X4	T38.5X5	T38.5X6
toluamide (nonmedicinal)	T60.8X1	T60.8X2	T60.8X3	T60.8X4	—	—
medicinal	T49.3X1	T49.3X2	T49.3X3	T49.3X4	T49.3X5	T49.3X6
Diethylcarbamazine	T37.4X1	T37.4X2	T37.4X3	T37.4X4	T37.4X5	T37.4X6
Diethylene						
dioxide	T52.8X1	T52.8X2	T52.8X3	T52.8X4	—	—
glycol (monoacetate) (monobutyl ether) (monoethyl ether)	T52.3X1	T52.3X2	T52.3X3	T52.3X4	—	—
Diethylhexylphthalate	T65.891	T65.892	T65.893	T65.894	—	—
Diethylpropion	T50.5X1	T50.5X2	T50.5X3	T50.5X4	T50.5X5	T50.5X6
Diethylstilbestrol	T38.5X1	T38.5X2	T38.5X3	T38.5X4	T38.5X5	T38.5X6
Diethylstilboestrol	T38.5X1	T38.5X2	T38.5X3	T38.5X4	T38.5X5	T38.5X6
Diethylsulfone-diethylmethane	T42.6X1	T42.6X2	T42.6X3	T42.6X4	T42.6X5	T42.6X6
Diethyltoluamide	T49.0X1	T49.0X2	T49.0X3	T49.0X4	T49.0X5	T49.0X6
Diethyltryptamine (DET)	T40.991	T40.992	T40.993	T40.994	—	—
Difebarbamate	T42.3X1	T42.3X2	T42.3X3	T42.3X4	T42.3X5	T42.3X6
Difencloxazine	T40.2X1	T40.2X2	T40.2X3	T40.2X4	T40.2X5	T40.2X6
Difenidol	T45.0X1	T45.0X2	T45.0X3	T45.0X4	T45.0X5	T45.0X6
Difenoxin	T47.6X1	T47.6X2	T47.6X3	T47.6X4	T47.6X5	T47.6X6
Difetarsone	T37.3X1	T37.3X2	T37.3X3	T37.3X4	T37.3X5	T37.3X6
Diffusin	T45.3X1	T45.3X2	T45.3X3	T45.3X4	T45.3X5	T45.3X6
Diflorasone	T49.0X1	T49.0X2	T49.0X3	T49.0X4	T49.0X5	T49.0X6
Diflubenzuron	T60.1X1	T60.1X2	T60.1X3	T60.1X4	—	—
Diflos	T44.0X1	T44.0X2	T44.0X3	T44.0X4	T44.0X5	T44.0X6
Diflucortolone	T49.0X1	T49.0X2	T49.0X3	T49.0X4	T49.0X5	T49.0X6
Diflunisal	T39.091	T39.092	T39.093	T39.094	T39.095	T39.096
Difluoromethyldopa	T42.8X1	T42.8X2	T42.8X3	T42.8X4	T42.8X5	T42.8X6
Difluorophate	T44.0X1	T44.0X2	T44.0X3	T44.0X4	T44.0X5	T44.0X6
Digestant NEC	T47.5X1	T47.5X2	T47.5X3	T47.5X4	T47.5X5	T47.5X6
Digitalin(e)	T46.0X1	T46.0X2	T46.0X3	T46.0X4	T46.0X5	T46.0X6
Digitalis (leaf) (glycoside)	T46.0X1	T46.0X2	T46.0X3	T46.0X4	T46.0X5	T46.0X6
lanata	T46.0X1	T46.0X2	T46.0X3	T46.0X4	T46.0X5	T46.0X6
purpurea	T46.0X1	T46.0X2	T46.0X3	T46.0X4	T46.0X5	T46.0X6
Digitoxin	T46.0X1	T46.0X2	T46.0X3	T46.0X4	T46.0X5	T46.0X6

◀ New   ◀◀ Revised   ~~deleted~~ Deleted

Substance	Poisoning, Accidental (Unintentional)	Poisoning, Intentional Self-Harm	Poisoning, Assault	Poisoning, Undetermined	Adverse Effect	Underdosing
Digitoxose	T46.0X1	T46.0X2	T46.0X3	T46.0X4	T46.0X5	T46.0X6
Digoxin	T46.0X1	T46.0X2	T46.0X3	T46.0X4	T46.0X5	T46.0X6
Digoxine	T46.0X1	T46.0X2	T46.0X3	T46.0X4	T46.0X5	T46.0X6
Dihydralazine	T46.5X1	T46.5X2	T46.5X3	T46.5X4	T46.5X5	T46.5X6
Dihydrazine	T46.5X1	T46.5X2	T46.5X3	T46.5X4	T46.5X5	T46.5X6
Dihydrocodeinone	T40.2X1	T40.2X2	T40.2X3	T40.2X4	T40.2X5	T40.2X6
Dihydroergocornine	T46.7X1	T46.7X2	T46.7X3	T46.7X4	T46.7X5	T46.7X6
Dihydroergocristine (mesilate)	T46.7X1	T46.7X2	T46.7X3	T46.7X4	T46.7X5	T46.7X6
Dihydroergokryptine	T46.7X1	T46.7X2	T46.7X3	T46.7X4	T46.7X5	T46.7X6
Dihydroergotamine	T46.5X1	T46.5X2	T46.5X3	T46.5X4	T46.5X5	T46.5X6
Dihydroergotoxine	T46.7X1	T46.7X2	T46.7X3	T46.7X4	T46.7X5	T46.7X6
mesilate	T46.7X1	T46.7X2	T46.7X3	T46.7X4	T46.7X5	T46.7X6
Dihydrohydroxycodein-one	T40.2X1	T40.2X2	T40.2X3	T40.2X4	T40.2X5	T40.2X6
Dihydrohydroxymorphinone	T40.2X1	T40.2X2	T40.2X3	T40.2X4	T40.2X5	T40.2X6
Dihydroisocodeine	T40.2X1	T40.2X2	T40.2X3	T40.2X4	T40.2X5	T40.2X6
Dihydromorphine	T40.2X1	T40.2X2	T40.2X3	T40.2X4	—	—
Dihydromorphinone	T40.2X1	T40.2X2	T40.2X3	T40.2X4	T40.2X5	T40.2X6
Dihydrostreptomycin	T36.5X1	T36.5X2	T36.5X3	T36.5X4	T36.5X5	T36.5X6
Dihydrotachysterol	T45.2X1	T45.2X2	T45.2X3	T45.2X4	T45.2X5	T45.2X6
Dihydroxyaluminum aminoacetate	T47.1X1	T47.1X2	T47.1X3	T47.1X4	T47.1X5	T47.1X6
Dihydroxyaluminum sodium carbonate	T47.1X1	T47.1X2	T47.1X3	T47.1X4	T47.1X5	T47.1X6
Dihydroxyanthraquinone	T47.2X1	T47.2X2	T47.2X3	T47.2X4	T47.2X5	T47.2X6
Dihydroxycodeinone	T40.2X1	T40.2X2	T40.2X3	T40.2X4	T40.2X5	T40.2X6
Dihydroxypropyl theophylline	T50.2X1	T50.2X2	T50.2X3	T50.2X4	T50.2X5	T50.2X6
Diiodohydroxyquin	T37.8X1	T37.8X2	T37.8X3	T37.8X4	T37.8X5	T37.8X6
topical	T49.0X1	T49.0X2	T49.0X3	T49.0X4	T49.0X5	T49.0X6
Diiodohydroxyquinoline	T37.8X1	T37.8X2	T37.8X3	T37.8X4	T37.8X5	T37.8X6
Diiodotyrosine	T38.2X1	T38.2X2	T38.2X3	T38.2X4	T38.2X5	T38.2X6
Diisopromine	T44.3X1	T44.3X2	T44.3X3	T44.3X4	T44.3X5	T44.3X6
Diisopropylamine	T46.3X1	T46.3X2	T46.3X3	T46.3X4	T46.3X5	T46.3X6
Diisopropylfluorophosphonate	T44.0X1	T44.0X2	T44.0X3	T44.0X4	T44.0X5	T44.0X6
Dilantin	T42.0X1	T42.0X2	T42.0X3	T42.0X4	T42.0X5	T42.0X6
Dilaudid	T40.2X1	T40.2X2	T40.2X3	T40.2X4	T40.2X5	T40.2X6
Dilazep	T46.3X1	T46.3X2	T46.3X3	T46.3X4	T46.3X5	T46.3X6
Dill	T47.5X1	T47.5X2	T47.5X3	T47.5X4	T47.5X5	T47.5X6
Diloxanide	T37.3X1	T37.3X2	T37.3X3	T37.3X4	T37.3X5	T37.3X6
Diltiazem	T46.1X1	T46.1X2	T46.1X3	T46.1X4	T46.1X5	T46.1X6
Dimazole	T49.0X1	T49.0X2	T49.0X3	T49.0X4	T49.0X5	T49.0X6
Dimefline	T50.7X1	T50.7X2	T50.7X3	T50.7X4	T50.7X5	T50.7X6
Dimefox	T60.0X1	T60.0X2	T60.0X3	T60.0X4	—	—
Dimemorfan	T48.3X1	T48.3X2	T48.3X3	T48.3X4	T48.3X5	T48.3X6
Dimenhydrinate	T45.0X1	T45.0X2	T45.0X3	T45.0X4	T45.0X5	T45.0X6
Dimercaprol (British anti-lewisite)	T45.8X1	T45.8X2	T45.8X3	T45.8X4	T45.8X5	T45.8X6
Dimercaptopropanol	T45.8X1	T45.8X2	T45.8X3	T45.8X4	T45.8X5	T45.8X6
Dimestrol	T38.5X1	T38.5X2	T38.5X3	T38.5X4	T38.5X5	T38.5X6
Dimetane	T45.0X1	T45.0X2	T45.0X3	T45.0X4	T45.0X5	T45.0X6
Dimethicone	T47.1X1	T47.1X2	T47.1X3	T47.1X4	T47.1X5	T47.1X6
Dimethindene	T45.0X1	T45.0X2	T45.0X3	T45.0X4	T45.0X5	T45.0X6
Dimethisoquin	T49.1X1	T49.1X2	T49.1X3	T49.1X4	T49.1X5	T49.1X6
Dimethisterone	T38.5X1	T38.5X2	T38.5X3	T38.5X4	T38.5X5	T38.5X6
Dimethoate	T60.0X1	T60.0X2	T60.0X3	T60.0X4	—	—
Dimethocaine	T41.3X1	T41.3X2	T41.3X3	T41.3X4	T41.3X5	T41.3X6
Dimethoxanate	T48.3X1	T48.3X2	T48.3X3	T48.3X4	T48.3X5	T48.3X6
Dimethyl						
arsine, arsinic acid	T57.0X1	T57.0X2	T57.0X3	T57.0X4		
carbinol	T51.2X1	T51.2X2	T51.2X3	T51.2X4	—	—
carbonate	T52.8X1	T52.8X2	T52.8X3	T52.8X4	—	—
diguanide	T38.3X1	T38.3X2	T38.3X3	T38.3X4	T38.3X5	T38.3X6
ketone	T52.4X1	T52.4X2	T52.4X3	T52.4X4	—	—
vapor	T52.4X1	T52.4X2	T52.4X3	T52.4X4	—	—
meperidine	T40.2X1	T40.2X2	T40.2X3	T40.2X4	T40.2X5	T40.2X6
parathion	T60.0X1	T60.0X2	T60.0X3	T60.0X4	—	—
phthlate	T49.3X1	T49.3X2	T49.3X3	T49.3X4	T49.3X5	T49.3X6
polysiloxane	T47.8X1	T47.8X2	T47.8X3	T47.8X4	T47.8X5	T47.8X6
sulfate (fumes)	T59.891	T59.892	T59.893	T59.894	—	—
liquid	T65.891	T65.892	T65.893	T65.894	—	—
sulfoxide (nonmedicinal)	T52.8X1	T52.8X2	T52.8X3	T52.8X4	—	—
medicinal	T49.4X1	T49.4X2	T49.4X3	T49.4X4	T49.4X5	T49.4X6
tryptamine	T40.991	T40.992	T40.993	T40.994	—	—
tubocurarine	T48.1X1	T48.1X2	T48.1X3	T48.1X4	T48.1X5	T48.1X6
Dimethylamine sulfate	T49.4X1	T49.4X2	T49.4X3	T49.4X4	T49.4X5	T49.4X6
Dimethylformamide	T52.8X1	T52.8X2	T52.8X3	T52.8X4	—	—
Dimethyltubocurarinium chloride	T48.1X1	T48.1X2	T48.1X3	T48.1X4	T48.1X5	T48.1X6
Dimeticone	T47.1X1	T47.1X2	T47.1X3	T47.1X4	T47.1X5	T47.1X6
Dimetilan	T60.0X1	T60.0X2	T60.0X3	T60.0X4	—	—
Dimetindene	T45.0X1	T45.0X2	T45.0X3	T45.0X4	T45.0X5	T45.0X6
Dimetotiazine	T43.3X1	T43.3X2	T43.3X3	T43.3X4	T43.3X5	T43.3X6
Dimorpholamine	T50.7X1	T50.7X2	T50.7X3	T50.7X4	T50.7X5	T50.7X6
Dimoxyline	T46.3X1	T46.3X2	T46.3X3	T46.3X4	T46.3X5	T46.3X6
Dinitrobenzene	T65.3X1	T65.3X2	T65.3X3	T65.3X4		
vapor	T59.891	T59.892	T59.893	T59.894	—	—

TABLE OF DRUGS AND CHEMICALS

Substance	Poisoning, Accidental (Unintentional)	Poisoning, Intentional Self-Harm	Poisoning, Assault	Poisoning, Undetermined	Adverse Effect	Underdosing
Dinitrobenzol	T65.3X1	T65.3X2	T65.3X3	T65.3X4	—	—
vapor	T59.891	T59.892	T59.893	T59.894	—	—
Dinitrobutylphenol	T65.3X1	T65.3X2	T65.3X3	T65.3X4		
Dinitro (-ortho-)cresol (pesticide) (spray)	T65.3X1	T65.3X2	T65.3X3	T65.3X4	—	—
Dinitrocyclohexylphenol	T65.3X1	T65.3X2	T65.3X3	T65.3X4		
Dinitrophenol	T65.3X1	T65.3X2	T65.3X3	T65.3X4		
Dinoprost	T48.0X1	T48.0X2	T48.0X3	T48.0X4	T48.0X5	T48.0X6
Dinoprostone	T48.0X1	T48.0X2	T48.0X3	T48.0X4	T48.0X5	T48.0X6
Dinoseb	T60.3X1	T60.3X2	T60.3X3	T60.3X4		
Dioctyl sulfosuccinate (calcium) (sodium)	T47.4X1	T47.4X2	T47.4X3	T47.4X4	T47.4X5	T47.4X6
Diodone	T50.8X1	T50.8X2	T50.8X3	T50.8X4	T50.8X5	T50.8X6
Diodoquin	T37.8X1	T37.8X2	T37.8X3	T37.8X4	T37.8X5	T37.8X6
Dionin	T40.2X1	T40.2X2	T40.2X3	T40.2X4	T40.2X5	T40.2X6
Diosmin	T46.991	T46.992	T46.993	T46.994	T46.995	T46.996
Dioxane	T52.8X1	T52.8X2	T52.8X3	T52.8X4		
Dioxathion	T60.0X1	T60.0X2	T60.0X3	T60.0X4		
Dioxin	T53.7X1	T53.7X2	T53.7X3	T53.7X4	—	
Dioxopromethazine	T43.3X1	T43.3X2	T43.3X3	T43.3X4	T43.3X5	T43.3X6
Dioxyline	T46.3X1	T46.3X2	T46.3X3	T46.3X4	T46.3X5	T46.3X6
Dipentene	T52.8X1	T52.8X2	T52.8X3	T52.8X4	—	—
Diperodon	T41.3X1	T41.3X2	T41.3X3	T41.3X4	T41.3X5	T41.3X6
Diphacinone	T60.4X1	T60.4X2	T60.4X3	T60.4X4		
Diphemanil	T44.3X1	T44.3X2	T44.3X3	T44.3X4	T44.3X5	T44.3X6
metilsulfate	T44.3X1	T44.3X2	T44.3X3	T44.3X4	T44.3X5	T44.3X6
Diphenadione	T45.511	T45.512	T45.513	T45.514	T45.515	T45.516
rodenticide	T60.4X1	T60.4X2	T60.4X3	T60.4X4	—	—
Diphenhydramine	T45.0X1	T45.0X2	T45.0X3	T45.0X4	T45.0X5	T45.0X6
Diphenidol	T45.0X1	T45.0X2	T45.0X3	T45.0X4	T45.0X5	T45.0X6
Diphenoxylate	T47.6X1	T47.6X2	T47.6X3	T47.6X4	T47.6X5	T47.6X6
Diphenylamine	T65.3X1	T65.3X2	T65.3X3	T65.3X4		
Diphenylbutazone	T39.2X1	T39.2X2	T39.2X3	T39.2X4	T39.2X5	T39.2X6
Diphenylchloroarsine, not in war	T57.0X1	T57.0X2	T57.0X3	T57.0X4	—	—
Diphenylhydantoin	T42.0X1	T42.0X2	T42.0X3	T42.0X4	T42.0X5	T42.0X6
Diphenylmethane dye	T52.1X1	T52.1X2	T52.1X3	T52.1X4	—	—
Diphenylpyraline	T45.0X1	T45.0X2	T45.0X3	T45.0X4	T45.0X5	T45.0X6
Diphtheria						
antitoxin	T50.Z11	T50.Z12	T50.Z13	T50.Z14	T50.Z15	T50.Z16
toxoid	T50.A91	T50.A92	T50.A93	T50.A94	T50.A95	T50.A96
with tetanus toxoid	T50.A21	T50.A22	T50.A23	T50.A24	T50.A25	T50.A26
with pertussis component	T50.A11	T50.A12	T50.A13	T50.A14	T50.A15	T50.A16

Substance	Poisoning, Accidental (Unintentional)	Poisoning, Intentional Self-Harm	Poisoning, Assault	Poisoning, Undetermined	Adverse Effect	Underdosing
Diphtheria (Continued)						
vaccine (combination)	T50.A91	T50.A92	T50.A93	T50.A94	T50.A95	T50.A96
combination						
including pertussis	T50.A11	T50.A12	T50.A13	T50.A14	T50.A15	T50.A16
without pertussis	T50.A21	T50.A22	T50.A23	T50.A24	T50.A25	T50.A26
Diphylline	T50.2X1	T50.2X2	T50.2X3	T50.2X4	T50.2X5	T50.2X6
Dipipanone	T40.4X1	T40.4X2	T40.4X3	T40.4X4	—	—
Dipivefrine	T49.5X1	T49.5X2	T49.5X3	T49.5X4	T49.5X5	T49.5X6
Diplovax	T50.B91	T50.B92	T50.B93	T50.B94	T50.B95	T50.B96
Diprophylline	T50.2X1	T50.2X2	T50.2X3	T50.2X4	T50.2X5	T50.2X6
Dipropyline	T48.291	T48.292	T48.293	T48.294	T48.295	T48.296
Dipyridamole	T46.3X1	T46.3X2	T46.3X3	T46.3X4	T46.3X5	T46.3X6
Dipyrone	T39.2X1	T39.2X2	T39.2X3	T39.2X4	T39.2X5	T39.2X6
Diquat (dibromide)	T60.3X1	T60.3X2	T60.3X3	T60.3X4	—	—
Disinfectant	T65.891	T65.892	T65.893	T65.894	—	—
alkaline	T54.3X1	T54.3X2	T54.3X3	T54.3X4	—	—
aromatic	T54.1X1	T54.1X2	T54.1X3	T54.1X4		
intestinal	T37.8X1	T37.8X2	T37.8X3	T37.8X4	T37.8X5	T37.8X6
Disipal	T42.8X1	T42.8X2	T42.8X3	T42.8X4	T42.8X5	T42.8X6
Disodium edetate	T50.6X1	T50.6X2	T50.6X3	T50.6X4	T50.6X5	T50.6X6
Disoprofol	T41.291	T41.292	T41.293	T41.294	T41.295	T41.296
Disopyramide	T46.2X1	T46.2X2	T46.2X3	T46.2X4	T46.2X5	T46.2X6
Distigmine (bromide)	T44.0X1	T44.0X2	T44.0X3	T44.0X4	T44.0X5	T44.0X6
Disulfamide	T50.2X1	T50.2X2	T50.2X3	T50.2X4	T50.2X5	T50.2X6
Disulfanilamide	T37.0X1	T37.0X2	T37.0X3	T37.0X4	T37.0X5	T37.0X6
Disulfiram	T50.6X1	T50.6X2	T50.6X3	T50.6X4	T50.6X5	T50.6X6
Disulfoton	T60.0X1	T60.0X2	T60.0X3	T60.0X4	—	—
Dithiazanine iodide	T37.4X1	T37.4X2	T37.4X3	T37.4X4	T37.4X5	T37.4X6
Dithiocarbamate	T60.0X1	T60.0X2	T60.0X3	T60.0X4	—	—
Dithranol	T49.4X1	T49.4X2	T49.4X3	T49.4X4	T49.4X5	T49.4X6
Diucardin	T50.2X1	T50.2X2	T50.2X3	T50.2X4	T50.2X5	T50.2X6
Diupres	T50.2X1	T50.2X2	T50.2X3	T50.2X4	T50.2X5	T50.2X6
Diuretic NEC	T50.2X1	T50.2X2	T50.2X3	T50.2X4	T50.2X5	T50.2X6
benzothiadiazine	T50.2X1	T50.2X2	T50.2X3	T50.2X4	T50.2X5	T50.2X6
carbonic acid anhydrase inhibitors	T50.2X1	T50.2X2	T50.2X3	T50.2X4	T50.2X5	T50.2X6
furfuryl NEC	T50.2X1	T50.2X2	T50.2X3	T50.2X4	T50.2X5	T50.2X6
loop (high-ceiling)	T50.1X1	T50.1X2	T50.1X3	T50.1X4	T50.1X5	T50.1X6
mercurial NEC	T50.2X1	T50.2X2	T50.2X3	T50.2X4	T50.2X5	T50.2X6
osmotic	T50.2X1	T50.2X2	T50.2X3	T50.2X4	T50.2X5	T50.2X6
purine NEC	T50.2X1	T50.2X2	T50.2X3	T50.2X4	T50.2X5	T50.2X6
saluretic NEC	T50.2X1	T50.2X2	T50.2X3	T50.2X4	T50.2X5	T50.2X6

◀ New ◀ Revised ~~deleted~~ Deleted

Substance	External Cause (T-Code)					
	Poisoning, Accidental (Unintentional)	Poisoning, Intentional Self-Harm	Poisoning, Assault	Poisoning, Undetermined	Adverse Effect	Underdosing
Diuretic NEC (Continued)						
sulfonamide	T50.2X1	T50.2X2	T50.2X3	T50.2X4	T50.2X5	T50.2X6
thiazide NEC	T50.2X1	T50.2X2	T50.2X3	T50.2X4	T50.2X5	T50.2X6
xanthine	T50.2X1	T50.2X2	T50.2X3	T50.2X4	T50.2X5	T50.2X6
Diurgin	T50.2X1	T50.2X2	T50.2X3	T50.2X4	T50.2X5	T50.2X6
Diuril	T50.2X1	T50.2X2	T50.2X3	T50.2X4	T50.2X5	T50.2X6
Diuron	T60.3X1	T60.3X2	T60.3X3	T60.3X4	—	—
Divalproex	T42.6X1	T42.6X2	T42.6X3	T42.6X4	T42.6X5	T42.6X6
Divinyl ether	T41.0X1	T41.0X2	T41.0X3	T41.0X4	T41.0X5	T41.0X6
Dixanthogen	T49.0X1	T49.0X2	T49.0X3	T49.0X4	T49.0X5	T49.0X6
Dixyrazine	T43.3X1	T43.3X2	T43.3X3	T43.3X4	T43.3X5	T43.3X6
D-lysergic acid diethylamide	T40.8X1	T40.8X2	T40.8X3	T40.8X4	—	—
DMCT	T36.4X1	T36.4X2	T36.4X3	T36.4X4	T36.4X5	T36.4X6
DMSO — see Dimethyl sulfoxide						
DNBP	T60.3X1	T60.3X2	T60.3X3	T60.3X4	—	—
DNOC	T65.3X1	T65.3X2	T65.3X3	T65.3X4	—	—
DOCA	T38.0X1	T38.0X2	T38.0X3	T38.0X4	T38.0X5	T38.0X6
Dobutamine	T44.5X1	T44.5X2	T44.5X3	T44.5X4	T44.5X5	T44.5X6
Docusate sodium	T47.4X1	T47.4X2	T47.4X3	T47.4X4	T47.4X5	T47.4X6
Dodicin	T49.0X1	T49.0X2	T49.0X3	T49.0X4	T49.0X5	T49.0X6
Dofamium chloride	T49.0X1	T49.0X2	T49.0X3	T49.0X4	T49.0X5	T49.0X6
Dolophine	T40.3X1	T40.3X2	T40.3X3	T40.3X4	T40.3X5	T40.3X6
Doloxene	T39.8X1	T39.8X2	T39.8X3	T39.8X4	T39.8X5	T39.8X6
Domestic gas (after combustion) — see Gas, utility						
prior to combustion	T59.891	T59.892	T59.893	T59.894	—	—
Domiodol	T48.4X1	T48.4X2	T48.4X3	T48.4X4	T48.4X5	T48.4X6
Domiphen (bromide)	T49.0X1	T49.0X2	T49.0X3	T49.0X4	T49.0X5	T49.0X6
Domperidone	T45.0X1	T45.0X2	T45.0X3	T45.0X4	T45.0X5	T45.0X6
Dopa	T42.8X1	T42.8X2	T42.8X3	T42.8X4	T42.8X5	T42.8X6
Dopamine	T44.991	T44.992	T44.993	T44.994	T44.995	T44.996
Doriden	T42.6X1	T42.6X2	T42.6X3	T42.6X4	T42.6X5	T42.6X6
Dormiral	T42.3X1	T42.3X2	T42.3X3	T42.3X4	T42.3X5	T42.3X6
Dormison	T42.6X1	T42.6X2	T42.6X3	T42.6X4	T42.6X5	T42.6X6
Dornase	T48.4X1	T48.4X2	T48.4X3	T48.4X4	T48.4X5	T48.4X6
Dorsacaine	T41.3X1	T41.3X2	T41.3X3	T41.3X4	T41.3X5	T41.3X6
Dosulepin	T43.011	T43.012	T43.013	T43.014	T43.015	T43.016
Dothiepin	T43.011	T43.012	T43.013	T43.014	T43.015	T43.016
Doxantrazole	T48.6X1	T48.6X2	T48.6X3	T48.6X4	T48.6X5	T48.6X6
Doxapram	T50.7X1	T50.7X2	T50.7X3	T50.7X4	T50.7X5	T50.7X6
Doxazosin	T44.6X1	T44.6X2	T44.6X3	T44.6X4	T44.6X5	T44.6X6
Doxepin	T43.011	T43.012	T43.013	T43.014	T43.015	T43.016

Substance	External Cause (T-Code)					
	Poisoning, Accidental (Unintentional)	Poisoning, Intentional Self-Harm	Poisoning, Assault	Poisoning, Undetermined	Adverse Effect	Underdosing
Doxifluridine	T45.1X1	T45.1X2	T45.1X3	T45.1X4	T45.1X5	T45.1X6
Doxorubicin	T45.1X1	T45.1X2	T45.1X3	T45.1X4	T45.1X5	T45.1X6
Doxycycline	T36.4X1	T36.4X2	T36.4X3	T36.4X4	T36.4X5	T36.4X6
Doxylamine	T45.0X1	T45.0X2	T45.0X3	T45.0X4	T45.0X5	T45.0X6
Dramamine	T45.0X1	T45.0X2	T45.0X3	T45.0X4	T45.0X5	T45.0X6
Drano (drain cleaner)	T54.3X1	T54.3X2	T54.3X3	T54.3X4	—	—
Dressing, live pulp	T49.7X1	T49.7X2	T49.7X3	T49.7X4	T49.7X5	T49.7X6
Drocode	T40.2X1	T40.2X2	T40.2X3	T40.2X4	T40.2X5	T40.2X6
Dromoran	T40.2X1	T40.2X2	T40.2X3	T40.2X4	T40.2X5	T40.2X6
Dromostanolone	T38.7X1	T38.7X2	T38.7X3	T38.7X4	T38.7X5	T38.7X6
Dronabinol	T40.7X1	T40.7X2	T40.7X3	T40.7X4	T40.7X5	T40.7X6
Droperidol	T43.591	T43.592	T43.593	T43.594	T43.595	T43.596
Dropropizine	T48.3X1	T48.3X2	T48.3X3	T48.3X4	T48.3X5	T48.3X6
Drostanolone	T38.7X1	T38.7X2	T38.7X3	T38.7X4	T38.7X5	T38.7X6
Drotaverine	T44.3X1	T44.3X2	T44.3X3	T44.3X4	T44.3X5	T44.3X6
Drotrecogin alfa	T45.511	T45.512	T45.513	T45.514	T45.515	T45.516
Drug NEC	T50.901	T50.902	T50.903	T50.904	T50.905	T50.906
specified NEC	T50.991	T50.992	T50.993	T50.994	T50.995	T50.996
DTIC	T45.1X1	T45.1X2	T45.1X3	T45.1X4	T45.1X5	T45.1X6
Duboisine	T44.3X1	T44.3X2	T44.3X3	T44.3X4	T44.3X5	T44.3X6
Dulcolax	T47.2X1	T47.2X2	T47.2X3	T47.2X4	T47.2X5	T47.2X6
Duponol (C) (EP)	T49.2X1	T49.2X2	T49.2X3	T49.2X4	T49.2X5	T49.2X6
Durabolin	T38.7X1	T38.7X2	T38.7X3	T38.7X4	T38.7X5	T38.7X6
Dyclone	T41.3X1	T41.3X2	T41.3X3	T41.3X4	T41.3X5	T41.3X6
Dyclonine	T41.3X1	T41.3X2	T41.3X3	T41.3X4	T41.3X5	T41.3X6
Dydrogesterone	T38.5X1	T38.5X2	T38.5X3	T38.5X4	T38.5X5	T38.5X6
Dye NEC	T65.6X1	T65.6X2	T65.6X3	T65.6X4	—	—
antiseptic	T49.0X1	T49.0X2	T49.0X3	T49.0X4	T49.0X5	T49.0X6
diagnostic agents	T50.8X1	T50.8X2	T50.8X3	T50.8X4	T50.8X5	T50.8X6
pharmaceutical NEC	T50.901	T50.902	T50.903	T50.904	T50.905	T50.906
Dyflos	T44.0X1	T44.0X2	T44.0X3	T44.0X4	T44.0X5	T44.0X6
Dymelor	T38.3X1	T38.3X2	T38.3X3	T38.3X4	T38.3X5	T38.3X6
Dynamite	T65.3X1	T65.3X2	T65.3X3	T65.3X4	—	—
fumes	T59.891	T59.892	T59.893	T59.894	—	—
Dyphylline	T44.3X1	T44.3X2	T44.3X3	T44.3X4	T44.3X5	T44.3X6
E						
Ear drug NEC	T49.6X1	T49.6X2	T49.6X3	T49.6X4	T49.6X5	T49.6X6
Ear preparations	T49.6X1	T49.6X2	T49.6X3	T49.6X4	T49.6X5	T49.6X6
Econazole	T49.0X1	T49.0X2	T49.0X3	T49.0X4	T49.0X5	T49.0X6
Ecothiopate iodide	T49.5X1	T49.5X2	T49.5X3	T49.5X4	T49.5X5	T49.5X6
Echothiophate, echothiopate, ecothiopate	T49.5X1	T49.5X2	T49.5X3	T49.5X4	T49.5X5	T49.5X6

TABLE OF DRUGS AND CHEMICALS

Substance	Poisoning, Accidental (Unintentional)	Poisoning, Intentional Self-Harm	Poisoning, Assault	Poisoning, Undetermined	Adverse Effect	Underdosing
Ecstasy	T43.621	T43.622	T43.623	T43.624	T43.625	T43.626
Ectylurea	T42.6X1	T42.6X2	T42.6X4	T42.6X4	T42.6X5	T42.6X6
Edathamil disodium	T45.8X1	T45.8X2	T45.8X3	T45.8X4	T45.8X5	T45.8X6
Edecrin	T50.1X1	T50.1X2	T50.1X3	T50.1X4	T50.1X5	T50.1X6
Edetate, disodium (calcium)	T45.8X1	T45.8X2	T45.8X3	T45.8X4	T45.8X5	T45.8X6
Edoxudine	T49.5X1	T49.5X2	T49.5X3	T49.5X4	T49.5X5	T49.5X6
Edrophonium	T44.0X1	T44.0X2	T44.0X3	T44.0X4	T44.0X5	T44.0X6
chloride	T44.0X1	T44.0X2	T44.0X3	T44.0X4	T44.0X5	T44.0X6
EDTA	T50.6X1	T50.6X2	T50.6X3	T50.6X4	T50.6X5	T50.6X6
Eflornithine	T37.2X1	T37.2X2	T37.2X3	T37.2X4	T37.2X5	T37.2X6
Efloxate	T46.3X1	T46.3X2	T46.3X3	T46.3X4	T46.3X5	T46.3X6
Elase	T49.8X1	T49.8X2	T49.8X3	T49.8X4	T49.8X5	T49.8X6
Elastase	T47.5X1	T47.5X2	T47.5X3	T47.5X4	T47.5X5	T47.5X6
Elaterium	T47.2X1	T47.2X2	T47.2X3	T47.2X4	T47.2X5	T47.2X6
Elcatonin	T50.991	T50.992	T50.993	T50.994	T50.995	T50.996
Elder	T62.2X1	T62.2X2	T62.2X3	T62.2X4	—	—
berry (unripe)	T62.1X1	T62.1X2	T62.1X3	T62.1X4	—	—
Electrolyte balance drug	T50.3X1	T50.3X2	T50.3X3	T50.3X4	T50.3X5	T50.3X6
Electrolytes NEC	T50.3X1	T50.3X2	T50.3X3	T50.3X4	T50.3X5	T50.3X6
Electrolytic agent NEC	T50.3X1	T50.3X2	T50.3X3	T50.3X4	T50.3X5	T50.3X6
Elemental diet	T50.901	T50.902	T50.903	T50.904	T50.905	T50.906
Elliptinium acetate	T45.1X1	T45.1X2	T45.1X3	T45.1X4	T45.1X5	T45.1X6
Embramine	T45.0X1	T45.0X2	T45.0X3	T45.0X4	T45.0X5	T45.0X6
Emepronium (salts)	T44.3X1	T44.3X2	T44.3X3	T44.3X4	T44.3X5	T44.3X6
bromide	T44.3X1	T44.3X2	T44.3X3	T44.3X4	T44.3X5	T44.3X6
Emetic NEC	T47.7X1	T47.7X2	T47.7X3	T47.7X4	T47.7X5	T47.7X6
Emetine	T37.3X1	T37.3X2	T37.3X3	T37.3X4	T37.3X5	T37.3X6
Emollient NEC	T49.3X1	T49.3X2	T49.3X3	T49.3X4	T49.3X5	T49.3X6
Emorfazone	T39.8X1	T39.8X2	T39.8X3	T39.8X4	T39.8X5	T39.8X6
Emylcamate	T43.591	T43.592	T43.593	T43.594	T43.595	T43.596
Enalapril	T46.4X1	T46.4X2	T46.4X3	T46.4X4	T46.4X5	T46.4X6
Enalaprilat	T46.4X1	T46.4X2	T46.4X3	T46.4X4	T46.4X5	T46.4X6
Encainide	T46.2X1	T46.2X2	T46.2X3	T46.2X4	T46.2X5	T46.2X6
Endocaine	T41.3X1	T41.3X2	T41.3X3	T41.3X4	T41.3X5	T41.3X6
Endosulfan	T60.2X1	T60.2X2	T60.2X3	T60.2X4	—	—
Endothall	T60.3X1	T60.3X2	T60.3X3	T60.3X4		
Endralazine	T46.5X1	T46.5X2	T46.5X3	T46.5X4	T46.5X5	T46.5X6
Endrin	T60.1X1	T60.1X2	T60.1X3	T60.1X4	—	—
Enflurane	T41.0X1	T41.0X2	T41.0X3	T41.0X4	T41.0X5	T41.0X6
Enhexymal	T42.3X1	T42.3X2	T42.3X3	T42.3X4	T42.3X5	T42.3X6
Enocitabine	T45.1X1	T45.1X2	T45.1X3	T45.1X4	T45.1X5	T45.1X6
Enovid	T38.4X1	T38.4X2	T38.4X3	T38.4X4	T38.4X5	T38.4X6

Substance	Poisoning, Accidental (Unintentional)	Poisoning, Intentional Self-Harm	Poisoning, Assault	Poisoning, Undetermined	Adverse Effect	Underdosing
Enoxacin	T36.8X1	T36.8X2	T36.8X3	T36.8X4	T36.8X5	T36.8X6
Enoxaparin (sodium)	T45.511	T45.512	T45.513	T45.514	T45.515	T45.516
Enpiprazole	T43.591	T43.592	T43.593	T43.594	T43.595	T43.596
Enprofylline	T48.6X1	T48.6X2	T48.6X3	T48.6X4	T48.6X5	T48.6X6
Enprostil	T47.1X1	T47.1X2	T47.1X3	T47.1X4	T47.1X5	T47.1X6
ENT preparations (anti-infectives)	T49.6X1	T49.6X2	T49.6X3	T49.6X4	T49.6X5	T49.6X6
Enviomycin	T36.8X1	T36.8X2	T36.8X3	T36.8X4	T36.8X5	T36.8X6
Enzodase	T45.3X1	T45.3X2	T45.3X3	T45.3X4	T45.3X5	T45.3X6
Enzyme NEC	T45.3X1	T45.3X2	T45.3X3	T45.3X4	T45.3X5	T45.3X6
depolymerizing	T49.8X1	T49.8X2	T49.8X3	T49.8X4	T49.8X5	T49.8X6
fibrolytic	T45.3X1	T45.3X2	T45.3X3	T45.3X4	T45.3X5	T45.3X6
gastric	T47.5X1	T47.5X2	T47.5X3	T47.5X4	T47.5X5	T47.5X6
intestinal	T47.5X1	T47.5X2	T47.5X3	T47.5X4	T47.5X5	T47.5X6
local action	T49.4X1	T49.4X2	T49.4X3	T49.4X4	T49.4X5	T49.4X6
proteolytic	T49.4X1	T49.4X2	T49.4X3	T49.4X4	T49.4X5	T49.4X6
thrombolytic	T45.3X1	T45.3X2	T45.3X3	T45.3X4	T45.3X5	T45.3X6
EPAB	T41.3X1	T41.3X2	T41.3X3	T41.3X4	T41.3X5	T41.3X6
Epanutin	T42.0X1	T42.0X2	T42.0X3	T42.0X4	T42.0X5	T42.0X6
Ephedra	T44.991	T44.992	T44.993	T44.994	T44.995	T44.996
Ephedrine	T44.991	T44.992	T44.993	T44.994	T44.995	T44.996
Epichlorhydrin, epichlorohydrin	T52.8X1	T52.8X2	T52.8X3	T52.8X4	—	—
Epicillin	T36.0X1	T36.0X2	T36.0X3	T36.0X4	T36.0X5	T36.0X6
Epiestriol	T38.5X1	T38.5X2	T38.5X3	T38.5X4	T38.5X5	T38.5X6
Epilim — see Sodium valproate						
Epimestrol	T38.5X1	T38.5X2	T38.5X3	T38.5X4	T38.5X5	T38.5X6
Epinephrine	T44.5X1	T44.5X2	T44.5X3	T44.5X4	T44.5X5	T44.5X6
Epirubicin	T45.1X1	T45.1X2	T45.1X3	T45.1X4	T45.1X5	T45.1X6
Epitiostanol	T38.7X1	T38.7X2	T38.7X3	T38.7X4	T38.7X5	T38.7X6
Epitizide	T50.2X1	T50.2X2	T50.2X3	T50.2X4	T50.2X5	T50.2X6
EPN	T60.0X1	T60.0X2	T60.0X3	T60.0X4	—	—
EPO	T45.8X1	T45.8X2	T45.8X3	T45.8X4	T45.8X5	T45.8X6
Epoetin alpha	T45.8X1	T45.8X2	T45.8X3	T45.8X4	T45.8X5	T45.8X6
Epomediol	T50.991	T50.992	T50.993	T50.994	T50.995	T50.996
Epoprostenol	T45.521	T45.522	T45.523	T45.524	T45.525	T45.526
Epoxy resin	T65.891	T65.892	T65.893	T65.894	—	—
Eprazinone	T48.4X1	T48.4X2	T48.4X3	T48.4X4	T48.4X5	T48.4X6
Epsilon amino-caproic acid	T45.621	T45.622	T45.623	T45.624	T45.625	T45.626
Epsom salt	T47.3X1	T47.3X2	T47.3X3	T47.3X4	T47.3X5	T47.3X6
Eptazocine	T40.4X1	T40.4X2	T40.4X3	T40.4X4	T40.4X5	T40.4X6
Equanil	T43.591	T43.592	T43.593	T43.594	T43.595	T43.596
Equisetum	T62.2X1	T62.2X2	T62.2X3	T62.2X4	—	—
diuretic	T50.2X1	T50.2X2	T50.2X3	T50.2X4	T50.2X5	T50.2X6

◀ New ◀ Revised deleted Deleted

Substance	Poisoning, Accidental (Unintentional)	Poisoning, Intentional Self-Harm	Poisoning, Assault	Poisoning, Undetermined	Adverse Effect	Underdosing
Ergobasine	T48.0X1	T48.0X2	T48.0X3	T48.0X4	T48.0X5	T48.0X6
Ergocalciferol	T45.2X1	T45.2X2	T45.2X3	T45.2X4	T45.2X5	T45.2X6
Ergoloid mesylates	T46.7X1	T46.7X2	T46.7X3	T46.7X4	T46.7X5	T46.7X6
Ergometrine	T48.0X1	T48.0X2	T48.0X3	T48.0X4	T48.0X5	T48.0X6
Ergonovine	T48.0X1	T48.0X2	T48.0X3	T48.0X4	T48.0X5	T48.0X6
Ergot NEC	T64.81	T64.82	T64.83	T64.84	—	—
derivative	T48.0X1	T48.0X2	T48.0X3	T48.0X4	T48.0X5	T48.0X6
medicinal (alkaloids)	T48.0X1	T48.0X2	T48.0X3	T48.0X4	T48.0X5	T48.0X6
prepared	T48.0X1	T48.0X2	T48.0X3	T48.0X4	T48.0X5	T48.0X6
Ergotamine	T46.5X1	T46.5X2	T46.5X3	T46.5X4	T46.5X5	T46.5X6
Ergotocine	T48.0X1	T48.0X2	T48.0X3	T48.0X4	T48.0X5	T48.0X6
Ergotrate	T48.0X1	T48.0X2	T48.0X3	T48.0X4	T48.0X5	T48.0X6
Eritrityl tetranitrate	T46.3X1	T46.3X2	T46.3X3	T46.3X4	T46.3X5	T46.3X6
Erythrityl tetranitrate	T46.3X1	T46.3X2	T46.3X3	T46.3X4	T46.3X5	T46.3X6
Erythrol tetranitrate	T46.3X1	T46.3X2	T46.3X3	T46.3X4	T46.3X5	T46.3X6
Erythromycin (salts)	T36.3X1	T36.3X2	T36.3X3	T36.3X4	T36.3X5	T36.3X6
ophthalmic preparation	T49.5X1	T49.5X2	T49.5X3	T49.5X4	T49.5X5	T49.5X6
topical NEC	T49.0X1	T49.0X2	T49.0X3	T49.0X4	T49.0X5	T49.0X6
Erythropoietin	T45.8X1	T45.8X2	T45.8X3	T45.8X4	T45.8X5	T45.8X6
human	T45.8X1	T45.8X2	T45.8X3	T45.8X4	T45.8X5	T45.8X6
Escin	T46.991	T46.992	T46.993	T46.994	T46.995	T46.996
Esculin	T45.2X1	T45.2X2	T45.2X3	T45.2X4	T45.2X5	T45.2X6
Esculoside	T45.2X1	T45.2X2	T45.2X3	T45.2X4	T45.2X5	T45.2X6
ESDT (ether-soluble tar distillate)	T49.1X1	T49.1X2	T49.1X3	T49.1X4	T49.1X5	T49.1X6
Eserine	T49.5X1	T49.5X2	T49.5X3	T49.5X4	T49.5X5	T49.5X6
Esflurbiprofen	T39.311	T39.312	T39.313	T39.314	T39.315	T39.316
Eskabarb	T42.3X1	T42.3X2	T42.3X3	T42.3X4	T42.3X5	T42.3X6
Eskalith	T43.8X1	T43.8X2	T43.8X3	T43.8X4	T43.8X5	T43.8X6
Esmolol	T44.7X1	T44.7X2	T44.7X3	T44.7X4	T44.7X5	T44.7X6
Estanozolol	T38.7X1	T38.7X2	T38.7X3	T38.7X4	T38.7X5	T38.7X6
Estazolam	T42.4X1	T42.4X2	T42.4X3	T42.4X4	T42.4X5	T42.4X6
Estradiol	T38.5X1	T38.5X2	T38.5X3	T38.5X4	T38.5X5	T38.5X6
with testosterone	T38.7X1	T38.7X2	T38.7X3	T38.7X4	T38.7X5	T38.7X6
benzoate	T38.5X1	T38.5X2	T38.5X3	T38.5X4	T38.5X5	T38.5X6
Estramustine	T45.1X1	T45.1X2	T45.1X3	T45.1X4	T45.1X5	T45.1X6
Estriol	T38.5X1	T38.5X2	T38.5X3	T38.5X4	T38.5X5	T38.5X6
Estrogen	T38.5X1	T38.5X2	T38.5X3	T38.5X4	T38.5X5	T38.5X6
with progesterone	T38.5X1	T38.5X2	T38.5X3	T38.5X4	T38.5X5	T38.5X6
conjugated	T38.5X1	T38.5X2	T38.5X3	T38.5X4	T38.5X5	T38.5X6
Estrone	T38.5X1	T38.5X2	T38.5X3	T38.5X4	T38.5X5	T38.5X6
Estropipate	T38.5X1	T38.5X2	T38.5X3	T38.5X4	T38.5X5	T38.5X6

Substance	Poisoning, Accidental (Unintentional)	Poisoning, Intentional Self-Harm	Poisoning, Assault	Poisoning, Undetermined	Adverse Effect	Underdosing
Etacrynate sodium	T50.1X1	T50.1X2	T50.1X3	T50.1X4	T50.1X5	T50.1X6
Etacrynic acid	T50.1X1	T50.1X2	T50.1X3	T50.1X4	T50.1X5	T50.1X6
Etafedrine	T48.6X1	T48.6X2	T48.6X3	T48.6X4	T48.6X5	T48.6X6
Etafenone	T46.3X1	T46.3X2	T46.3X3	T46.3X4	T46.3X5	T46.3X6
Etambutol	T37.1X1	T37.1X2	T37.1X3	T37.1X4	T37.1X5	T37.1X6
Etamiphyllin	T48.6X1	T48.6X2	T48.6X3	T48.6X4	T48.6X5	T48.6X6
Etamivan	T50.7X1	T50.7X2	T50.7X3	T50.7X4	T50.7X5	T50.7X6
Etamsylate	T45.7X1	T45.7X2	T45.7X3	T45.7X4	T45.7X5	T45.7X6
Etebenecid	T50.4X1	T50.4X2	T50.4X3	T50.4X4	T50.4X5	T50.4X6
Ethacridine	T49.0X1	T49.0X2	T49.0X3	T49.0X4	T49.0X5	T49.0X6
Ethacrynic acid	T50.1X1	T50.1X2	T50.1X3	T50.1X4	T50.1X5	T50.1X6
Ethadione	T42.2X1	T42.2X2	T42.2X3	T42.2X4	T42.2X5	T42.2X6
Ethambutol	T37.1X1	T37.1X2	T37.1X3	T37.1X4	T37.1X5	T37.1X6
Ethamide	T50.2X1	T50.2X2	T50.2X3	T50.2X4	T50.2X5	T50.2X6
Ethamivan	T50.7X1	T50.7X2	T50.7X3	T50.7X4	T50.7X5	T50.7X6
Ethamsylate	T45.7X1	T45.7X2	T45.7X3	T45.7X4	T45.7X5	T45.7X6
Ethanol	T51.0X1	T51.0X2	T51.0X3	T51.0X4	—	—
beverage	T51.0X1	T51.0X2	T51.0X3	T51.0X4	—	—
Ethanolamine oleate	T46.8X1	T46.8X2	T46.8X3	T46.8X4	T46.8X5	T46.8X6
Ethaverine	T44.3X1	T44.3X2	T44.3X3	T44.3X4	T44.3X5	T44.3X6
Ethchlorvynol	T42.6X1	T42.6X2	T42.6X3	T42.6X4	T42.6X5	T42.6X6
Ethebenecid	T50.4X1	T50.4X2	T50.4X3	T50.4X4	T50.4X5	T50.4X6
Ether (vapor)	T41.0X1	T41.0X2	T41.0X3	T41.0X4	T41.0X5	T41.0X6
anesthetic	T41.0X1	T41.0X2	T41.0X3	T41.0X4	T41.0X5	T41.0X6
divinyl	T41.0X1	T41.0X2	T41.0X3	T41.0X4	T41.0X5	T41.0X6
ethyl (medicinal)	T41.0X1	T41.0X2	T41.0X3	T41.0X4	T41.0X5	T41.0X6
nonmedicinal	T52.8X1	T52.8X2	T52.8X3	T52.8X4	—	—
petroleum—see Ligroin						
solvent	T52.8X1	T52.8X2	T52.8X3	T52.8X4	—	—
Ethiazide	T50.2X1	T50.2X2	T50.2X3	T50.2X4	T50.2X5	T50.2X6
Ethidium chloride (vapor)	T59.891	T59.892	T59.893	T59.894	—	—
Ethinamate	T42.6X1	T42.6X2	T42.6X3	T42.6X4	T42.6X5	T42.6X6
Ethinylestradiol, ethinyloestradiol	T38.5X1	T38.5X2	T38.5X3	T38.5X4	T38.5X5	T38.5X6
with						
levonorgestrel	T38.4X1	T38.4X2	T38.4X3	T38.4X4	T38.4X5	T38.4X6
norethisterone	T38.4X1	T38.4X2	T38.4X3	T38.4X4	T38.4X5	T38.4X6
Ethiodized oil (131 I)	T50.8X1	T50.8X2	T50.8X3	T50.8X4	T50.8X5	T50.8X6
Ethion	T60.0X1	T60.0X2	T60.0X3	T60.0X4	—	—
Ethionamide	T37.1X1	T37.1X2	T37.1X3	T37.1X4	T37.1X5	T37.1X6
Ethioniamide	T37.1X1	T37.1X2	T37.1X3	T37.1X4	T37.1X5	T37.1X6
Ethisterone	T38.5X1	T38.5X2	T38.5X3	T38.5X4	T38.5X5	T38.5X6
Ethobral	T42.3X1	T42.3X2	T42.3X3	T42.3X4	T42.3X5	T42.3X6

◀ New   ◀ Revised   ~~deleted~~ Deleted

TABLE OF DRUGS AND CHEMICALS

Substance	Poisoning, Accidental (Unintentional)	Poisoning, Intentional Self-Harm	Poisoning, Assault	Poisoning, Undetermined	Adverse Effect	Underdosing
Ethocaine (infiltration) (topical)	T41.3X1	T41.3X2	T41.3X3	T41.3X4	T41.3X5	T41.3X6
nerve block (peripheral) (plexus)	T41.3X1	T41.3X2	T41.3X3	T41.3X4	T41.3X5	T41.3X6
spinal	T41.3X1	T41.3X2	T41.3X3	T41.3X4	T41.3X5	T41.3X6
Ethoheptazine	T40.4X1	T40.4X2	T40.4X3	T40.4X4	T40.4X5	T40.4X6
Ethopropazine	T44.3X1	T44.3X2	T44.3X3	T44.3X4	T44.3X5	T44.3X6
Ethosuximide	T42.2X1	T42.2X2	T42.2X3	T42.2X4	T42.2X5	T42.2X6
Ethotoin	T42.0X1	T42.0X2	T42.0X3	T42.0X4	T42.0X5	T42.0X6
Ethoxazene	T37.91	T37.92	T37.93	T37.94	T37.95	T37.96
Ethoxazorutoside	T46.991	T46.992	T46.993	T46.994	T46.995	T46.996
2-Ethoxyethanol	T52.3X1	T52.3X2	T52.3X3	T52.3X4	—	—
Ethoxzolamide	T50.2X1	T50.2X2	T50.2X3	T50.2X4	T50.2X5	T50.2X6
Ethyl						
acetate	T52.8X1	T52.8X2	T52.8X3	T52.8X4		
alcohol	T51.0X1	T51.0X2	T51.0X3	T51.0X4	—	—
beverage	T51.0X1	T51.0X2	T51.0X3	T51.0X4	—	—
aldehyde (vapor)	T59.891	T59.892	T59.893	T59.894		
liquid	T52.8X1	T52.8X2	T52.8X3	T52.8X4	—	—
aminobenzoate	T41.3X1	T41.3X2	T41.3X3	T41.3X4	T41.3X5	T41.3X6
aminophenothiazine	T43.3X1	T43.3X2	T43.3X3	T43.3X4	T43.3X5	T43.3X6
benzoate	T52.8X1	T52.8X2	T52.8X3	T52.8X4	—	—
biscoumacetate	T45.511	T45.512	T45.513	T45.514	T45.515	T45.516
bromide (anesthetic)	T41.0X1	T41.0X2	T41.0X3	T41.0X4	T41.0X5	T41.0X6
carbamate	T45.1X1	T45.1X2	T45.1X3	T45.1X4	T45.1X5	T45.1X6
carbinol	T51.3X1	T51.3X2	T51.3X3	T51.3X4	—	—
carbonate	T52.8X1	T52.8X2	T52.8X3	T52.8X4	—	—
chaulmoograte	T37.1X1	T37.1X2	T37.1X3	T37.1X4	T37.1X5	T37.1X6
chloride (anesthetic)	T41.0X1	T41.0X2	T41.0X3	T41.0X4	T41.0X5	T41.0X6
anesthetic (local)	T41.3X1	T41.3X2	T41.3X3	T41.3X4	T41.3X5	T41.3X6
inhaled	T41.0X1	T41.0X2	T41.0X3	T41.0X4	T41.0X5	T41.0X6
local	T49.4X1	T49.4X2	T49.4X3	T49.4X4	T49.4X5	T49.4X6
solvent	T53.6X1	T53.6X2	T53.6X3	T53.6X4	—	—
dibunate	T48.3X1	T48.3X2	T48.3X3	T48.3X4	T48.3X5	T48.3X6
dichloroarsine (vapor)	T57.0X1	T57.0X2	T57.0X3	T57.0X4	—	—
estranol	T38.7X1	T38.7X2	T38.7X3	T38.7X4	T38.7X5	T38.7X6
ether — see also ether	T52.8X1	T52.8X2	T52.8X3	T52.8X4	—	—
formate NEC (solvent)	T52.0X1	T52.0X2	T52.0X3	T52.0X4	—	—
fumarate	T49.4X1	T49.4X2	T49.4X3	T49.4X4	T49.4X5	T49.4X6
hydroxyisobutyrate NEC (solvent)	T52.8X1	T52.8X2	T52.8X3	T52.8X4	—	—
iodoacetate	T59.3X1	T59.3X2	T59.3X3	T59.3X4	—	—
lactate NEC (solvent)	T52.8X1	T52.8X2	T52.8X3	T52.8X4	—	—
loflazepate	T42.4X1	T42.4X2	T42.4X3	T42.4X4	T42.4X5	T42.4X6

Substance	Poisoning, Accidental (Unintentional)	Poisoning, Intentional Self-Harm	Poisoning, Assault	Poisoning, Undetermined	Adverse Effect	Underdosing
Ethyl (Continued)						
mercuric chloride	T56.1X1	T56.1X2	T56.1X3	T56.1X4	—	—
methylcarbinol	T51.8X1	T51.8X2	T51.8X3	T51.8X4	—	—
morphine	T40.2X1	T40.2X2	T40.2X3	T40.2X4	T40.2X5	T40.2X6
noradrenaline	T48.6X1	T48.6X2	T48.6X3	T48.6X4	T48.6X5	T48.6X6
oxybutyrate NEC (solvent)	T52.8X1	T52.8X2	T52.8X3	T52.8X4		
Ethylene (gas)	T59.891	T59.892	T59.893	T59.894	—	—
anesthetic (general)	T41.0X1	T41.0X2	T41.0X3	T41.0X4	T41.0X5	T41.0X6
chlorohydrin	T52.8X1	T52.8X2	T52.8X3	T52.8X4		
vapor	T53.6X1	T53.6X2	T53.6X3	T53.6X4		
dichloride	T52.8X1	T52.8X2	T52.8X3	T52.8X4		
vapor	T53.6X1	T53.6X2	T53.6X3	T53.6X4		
dinitrate	T52.3X1	T52.3X2	T52.3X3	T52.3X4		
glycol(s)	T52.8X1	T52.8X2	T52.8X3	T52.8X4		
dinitrate	T52.3X1	T52.3X2	T52.3X3	T52.3X4		
monobutyl ether	T52.3X1	T52.3X2	T52.3X3	T52.3X4		
imine	T54.1X1	T54.1X2	T54.1X3	T54.1X4		
oxide (fumigant) (nonmedicinal)	T59.891	T59.892	T59.893	T59.894	—	—
medicinal	T49.0X1	T49.0X2	T49.0X3	T49.0X4	T49.0X5	T49.0X6
Ethylenediamine theophylline	T48.6X1	T48.6X2	T48.6X3	T48.6X4	T48.6X5	T48.6X6
Ethylenediaminetetra-acetic acid	T50.6X1	T50.6X2	T50.6X3	T50.6X4	T50.6X5	T50.6X6
Ethylenedinitrilotetra-acetate	T50.6X1	T50.6X2	T50.6X3	T50.6X4	T50.6X5	T50.6X6
Ethylestrenol	T38.7X1	T38.7X2	T38.7X3	T38.7X4	T38.7X5	T38.7X6
Ethylhydroxycellulose	T47.4X1	T47.4X2	T47.4X3	T47.4X4	T47.4X5	T47.4X6
Ethylidene						
chloride NEC	T53.6X1	T53.6X2	T53.6X3	T53.6X4	—	—
diacetate	T60.3X1	T60.3X2	T60.3X3	T60.3X4	—	—
dicoumarin	T45.511	T45.512	T45.513	T45.514	T45.515	T45.516
dicoumarol	T45.511	T45.512	T45.513	T45.514	T45.515	T45.516
diethyl ether	T52.0X1	T52.0X2	T52.0X3	T52.0X4	—	—
Ethylmorphine	T40.2X1	T40.2X2	T40.2X3	T40.2X4	T40.2X5	T40.2X6
Ethylnorepinephrine	T48.6X1	T48.6X2	T48.6X3	T48.6X4	T48.6X5	T48.6X6
Ethylparachlorophen-oxyisobutyrate	T46.6X1	T46.6X2	T46.6X3	T46.6X4	T46.6X5	T46.6X6
Ethynodiol	T38.4X1	T38.4X2	T38.4X3	T38.4X4	T38.4X5	T38.4X6
with mestranol diacetate	T38.4X1	T38.4X2	T38.4X3	T38.4X4	T38.4X5	T38.4X6
Etidocaine	T41.3X1	T41.3X2	T41.3X3	T41.3X4	T41.3X5	T41.3X6
infiltration (subcutaneous)	T41.3X1	T41.3X2	T41.3X3	T41.3X4	T41.3X5	T41.3X6
nerve (peripheral) (plexus)	T41.3X1	T41.3X2	T41.3X3	T41.3X4	T41.3X5	T41.3X6
Etidronate	T50.991	T50.992	T50.993	T50.994	T50.995	T50.996
Etidronic acid (disodium salt)	T50.991	T50.992	T50.993	T50.994	T50.995	T50.996
Etifoxine	T42.6X1	T42.6X2	T42.6X3	T42.6X4	T42.6X5	T42.6X6

◀ New ◀ Revised ~~deleted~~ Deleted

Substance	Poisoning, Accidental (Unintentional)	Poisoning, Intentional Self-Harm	Poisoning, Assault	Poisoning, Undetermined	Adverse Effect	Underdosing
	External Cause (T-Code)					
Etilefrine	T44.4X1	T44.4X2	T44.4X3	T44.4X4	T44.4X5	T44.4X6
Etilfen	T42.3X1	T42.3X2	T42.3X3	T42.3X4	T42.3X5	T42.3X6
Etinodiol	T38.4X1	T38.4X2	T38.4X3	T38.4X4	T38.4X5	T38.4X6
Etiroxate	T46.6X1	T46.6X2	T46.6X3	T46.6X4	T46.6X5	T46.6X6
Etizolam	T42.4X1	T42.4X2	T42.4X3	T42.4X4	T42.4X5	T42.4X6
Etodolac	T39.391	T39.392	T39.393	T39.394	T39.395	T39.396
Etofamide	T37.3X1	T37.3X2	T37.3X3	T37.3X4	T37.3X5	T37.3X6
Etofibrate	T46.6X1	T46.6X2	T46.6X3	T46.6X4	T46.6X5	T46.6X6
Etofylline	T46.7X1	T46.7X2	T46.7X3	T46.7X4	T46.7X5	T46.7X6
clofibrate	T46.6X1	T46.6X2	T46.6X3	T46.6X4	T46.6X5	T46.6X6
Etoglucid	T45.1X1	T45.1X2	T45.1X3	T45.1X4	T45.1X5	T45.1X6
Etomidate	T41.1X1	T41.1X2	T41.1X3	T41.1X4	T41.1X5	T41.1X6
Etomide	T39.8X1	T39.8X2	T39.8X3	T39.8X4	T39.8X5	T39.8X6
Etomidoline	T44.3X1	T44.3X2	T44.3X3	T44.3X4	T44.3X5	T44.3X6
Etoposide	T45.1X1	T45.1X2	T45.1X3	T45.1X4	T45.1X5	T45.1X6
Etorphine	T40.2X1	T40.2X2	T40.2X3	T40.2X4	T40.2X5	T40.2X6
Etoval	T42.3X1	T42.3X2	T42.3X3	T42.3X4	T42.3X5	T42.3X6
Etozolin	T50.1X1	T50.1X2	T50.1X3	T50.1X4	T50.1X5	T50.1X6
Etretinate	T50.991	T50.992	T50.993	T50.994	T50.995	T50.996
Etryptamine	T43.691	T43.692	T43.693	T43.694	T43.695	T43.696
Etybenzatropine	T44.3X1	T44.3X2	T44.3X3	T44.3X4	T44.3X5	T44.3X6
Etynodiol	T38.4X1	T38.4X2	T38.4X3	T38.4X4	T38.4X5	T38.4X6
Eucaine	T41.3X1	T41.3X2	T41.3X3	T41.3X4	T41.3X5	T41.3X6
Eucalyptus oil	T49.7X1	T49.7X2	T49.7X3	T49.7X4	T49.7X5	T49.7X6
Eucatropine	T49.5X1	T49.5X2	T49.5X3	T49.5X4	T49.5X5	T49.5X6
Eucodal	T40.2X1	T40.2X2	T40.2X3	T40.2X4	T40.2X5	T40.2X6
Euneryl	T42.3X1	T42.3X2	T42.3X3	T42.3X4	T42.3X5	T42.3X6
Euphthalmine	T44.3X1	T44.3X2	T44.3X3	T44.3X4	T44.3X5	T44.3X6
Eurax	T49.0X1	T49.0X2	T49.0X3	T49.0X4	T49.0X5	T49.0X6
Euresol	T49.4X1	T49.4X2	T49.4X3	T49.4X4	T49.4X5	T49.4X6
Euthroid	T38.1X1	T38.1X2	T38.1X3	T38.1X4	T38.1X5	T38.1X6
Evans blue	T50.8X1	T50.8X2	T50.8X3	T50.8X4	T50.8X5	T50.8X6
Evipal	T42.3X1	T42.3X2	T42.3X3	T42.3X4	T42.3X5	T42.3X6
sodium	T41.1X1	T41.1X2	T41.1X3	T41.1X4	T41.1X5	T41.1X6
Evipan	T42.3X1	T42.3X2	T42.3X3	T42.3X4	T42.3X5	T42.3X6
sodium	T41.1X1	T41.1X2	T41.1X3	T41.1X4	T41.1X5	T41.1X6
Exalamide	T49.0X1	T49.0X2	T49.0X3	T49.0X4	T49.0X5	T49.0X6
Exalgin	T39.1X1	T39.1X2	T39.1X3	T39.1X4	T39.1X5	T39.1X6
Excipients, pharmaceutical	T50.901	T50.902	T50.903	T50.904	T50.905	T50.906
Exhaust gas (engine) (motor vehicle)	T58.01	T58.02	T58.03	T58.04	—	—
Ex-Lax (phenolphthalein)	T47.2X1	T47.2X2	T47.2X3	T47.2X4	T47.2X5	T47.2X6
Expectorant NEC	T48.4X1	T48.4X2	T48.4X3	T48.4X4	T48.4X5	T48.4X6

Substance	Poisoning, Accidental (Unintentional)	Poisoning, Intentional Self-Harm	Poisoning, Assault	Poisoning, Undetermined	Adverse Effect	Underdosing
	External Cause (T-Code)					
Extended insulin zinc suspension	T38.3X1	T38.3X2	T38.3X3	T38.3X4	T38.3X5	T38.3X6
External medications (skin) (mucous membrane)	T49.91	T49.92	T49.93	T49.94	T49.95	T49.96
dental agent	T49.7X1	T49.7X2	T49.7X3	T49.7X4	T49.7X5	T49.7X6
ENT agent	T49.6X1	T49.6X2	T49.6X3	T49.6X4	T49.6X5	T49.6X6
ophthalmic preparation	T49.5X1	T49.5X2	T49.5X3	T49.5X4	T49.5X5	T49.5X6
specified NEC	T49.8X1	T49.8X2	T49.8X3	T49.8X4	T49.8X5	T49.8X6
Extrapyramidal antagonist NEC	T44.3X1	T44.3X2	T44.3X3	T44.3X4	T44.3X5	T44.3X6
Eye agents (anti-infective)	T49.5X1	T49.5X2	T49.5X3	T49.5X4	T49.5X5	T49.5X6
Eye drug NEC	T49.5X1	T49.5X2	T49.5X3	T49.5X4	T49.5X5	T49.5X6
F						
FAC (fluorouracil + doxorubicin + cyclophosphamide)	T45.1X1	T45.1X2	T45.1X3	T45.1X4	T45.1X5	T45.1X6
Factor						
I (fibrinogen)	T45.8X1	T45.8X2	T45.8X3	T45.8X4	T45.8X5	T45.8X6
III (thromboplastin)	T45.8X1	T45.8X2	T45.8X3	T45.8X4	T45.8X5	T45.8X6
VIII (antihemophilic Factor) (Concentrate)	T45.8X1	T45.8X2	T45.8X3	T45.8X4	T45.8X5	T45.8X6
IX complex	T45.7X1	T45.7X2	T45.7X3	T45.7X4	T45.7X5	T45.7X6
human	T45.8X1	T45.8X2	T45.8X3	T45.8X4	T45.8X5	T45.8X6
Famotidine	T47.0X1	T47.0X2	T47.0X3	T47.0X4	T47.0X5	T47.0X6
Fat suspension, intravenous	T50.991	T50.992	T50.993	T50.994	T50.995	T50.996
Fazadinium bromide	T48.1X1	T48.1X2	T48.1X3	T48.1X4	T48.1X5	T48.1X6
Febarbamate	T42.3X1	T42.3X2	T42.3X3	T42.3X4	T42.3X5	T42.3X6
Fecal softener	T47.4X1	T47.4X2	T47.4X3	T47.4X4	T47.4X5	T47.4X6
Fedrilate	T48.3X1	T48.3X2	T48.3X3	T48.3X4	T48.3X5	T48.3X6
Felodipine	T46.1X1	T46.1X2	T46.1X3	T46.1X4	T46.1X5	T46.1X6
Felypressin	T38.891	T38.892	T38.893	T38.894	T38.895	T38.896
Femoxetine	T43.221	T43.222	T43.223	T43.224	T43.225	T43.226
Fenalcomine	T46.3X1	T46.3X2	T46.3X3	T46.3X4	T46.3X5	T46.3X6
Fenamisal	T37.1X1	T37.1X2	T37.1X3	T37.1X4	T37.1X5	T37.1X6
Fenazone	T39.2X1	T39.2X2	T39.2X3	T39.2X4	T39.2X5	T39.2X6
Fenbendazole	T37.4X1	T37.4X2	T37.4X3	T37.4X4	T37.4X5	T37.4X6
Fenbutrazate	T50.5X1	T50.5X2	T50.5X3	T50.5X4	T50.5X5	T50.5X6
Fencamfamine	T43.691	T43.692	T43.693	T43.694	T43.695	T43.696
Fendiline	T46.1X1	T46.1X2	T46.1X3	T46.1X4	T46.1X5	T46.1X6
Fenetylline	T43.691	T43.692	T43.693	T43.694	T43.695	T43.696
Fenflumizole	T39.391	T39.392	T39.393	T39.394	T39.395	T39.396
Fenfluramine	T50.5X1	T50.5X2	T50.5X3	T50.5X4	T50.5X5	T50.5X6
Fenobarbital	T42.3X1	T42.3X2	T42.3X3	T42.3X4	T42.3X5	T42.3X6
Fenofibrate	T46.6X1	T46.6X2	T46.6X3	T46.6X4	T46.6X5	T46.6X6
Fenoprofen	T39.311	T39.312	T39.313	T39.314	T39.315	T39.316
Fenoterol	T48.6X1	T48.6X2	T48.6X3	T48.6X4	T48.6X5	T48.6X6

◀ New   ◀| Revised   deleted Deleted

TABLE OF DRUGS AND CHEMICALS

TABLE OF DRUGS AND CHEMICALS

Substance	External Cause (T-Code)					
	Poisoning, Accidental (Unintentional)	Poisoning, Intentional Self-Harm	Poisoning, Assault	Poisoning, Undetermined	Adverse Effect	Underdosing
Fenoverine	T44.3X1	T44.3X2	T44.3X3	T44.3X4	T44.3X5	T44.3X6
Fenoxazoline	T48.5X1	T48.5X2	T48.5X3	T48.5X4	T48.5X5	T48.5X6
Fenproporex	T50.5X1	T50.5X2	T50.5X3	T50.5X4	T50.5X5	T50.5X6
Fenquizone	T50.2X1	T50.2X2	T50.2X3	T50.2X4	T50.2X5	T50.2X6
Fentanyl	T40.4X1	T40.4X2	T40.4X3	T40.4X4	T40.4X5	T40.4X6
Fentazin	T43.3X1	T43.3X2	T43.3X3	T43.3X4	T43.3X5	T43.3X6
Fenthion	T60.0X1	T60.0X2	T60.0X3	T60.0X4	—	—
Fenticlor	T49.0X1	T49.0X2	T49.0X3	T49.0X4	T49.0X5	T49.0X6
Fenylbutazone	T39.2X1	T39.2X2	T39.2X3	T39.2X4	T39.2X5	T39.2X6
Feprazone	T39.2X1	T39.2X2	T39.2X3	T39.2X4	T39.2X5	T39.2X6
Fer de lance (bite) (venom)	T63.061	T63.062	T63.063	T63.064	—	—
Ferric — see also Iron						
chloride	T45.4X1	T45.4X2	T45.4X3	T45.4X4	T45.4X5	T45.4X6
citrate	T45.4X1	T45.4X2	T45.4X3	T45.4X4	T45.4X5	T45.4X6
hydroxide						
colloidal	T45.4X1	T45.4X2	T45.4X3	T45.4X4	T45.4X5	T45.4X6
polymaltose	T45.4X1	T45.4X2	T45.4X3	T45.4X4	T45.4X5	T45.4X6
pyrophosphate	T45.4X1	T45.4X2	T45.4X3	T45.4X4	T45.4X5	T45.4X6
Ferritin	T45.4X1	T45.4X2	T45.4X3	T45.4X4	T45.4X5	T45.4X6
Ferrocholinate	T45.4X1	T45.4X2	T45.4X3	T45.4X4	T45.4X5	T45.4X6
Ferrodextrane	T45.4X1	T45.4X2	T45.4X3	T45.4X4	T45.4X5	T45.4X6
Ferropolimaler	T45.4X1	T45.4X2	T45.4X3	T45.4X4	T45.4X5	T45.4X6
Ferrous — see also Iron						
phosphate	T45.4X1	T45.4X2	T45.4X3	T45.4X4	T45.4X5	T45.4X6
salt	T45.4X1	T45.4X2	T45.4X3	T45.4X4	T45.4X5	T45.4X6
with folic acid	T45.4X1	T45.4X2	T45.4X3	T45.4X4	T45.4X5	T45.4X6
Ferrous fumarate, gluconate, lactate, salt NEC, sulfate (medicinal)	T45.4X1	T45.4X2	T45.4X3	T45.4X4	T45.4X5	T45.4X6
Ferrovanadium (fumes)	T59.891	T59.892	T59.893	T59.894	—	—
Ferrum — see Iron						
Fertilizers NEC	T65.891	T65.892	T65.893	T65.894	—	—
with herbicide mixture	T60.3X1	T60.3X2	T60.3X3	T60.3X4	—	—
Fetoxilate	T47.6X1	T47.6X2	T47.6X3	T47.6X4	T47.6X5	T47.6X6
Fiber, dietary	T47.4X1	T47.4X2	T47.4X3	T47.4X4	T47.4X5	T47.4X6
Fibrinogen (human)	T45.8X1	T45.8X2	T45.8X3	T45.8X4	T45.8X5	T45.8X6
Fibrinolysin (human)	T45.691	T45.692	T45.693	T45.694	T45.695	T45.696
Fibrinolysis						
affecting drug	T45.601	T45.602	T45.603	T45.604	T45.605	T45.606
inhibitor NEC	T45.621	T45.622	T45.623	T45.624	T45.625	T45.626
Fibrinolytic drug	T45.611	T45.612	T45.613	T45.614	T45.615	T45.616
Filix mas	T37.4X1	T37.4X2	T37.4X3	T37.4X4	T37.4X5	T37.4X6
Filtering cream	T49.3X1	T49.3X2	T49.3X3	T49.3X4	T49.3X5	T49.3X6

Substance	External Cause (T-Code)					
	Poisoning, Accidental (Unintentional)	Poisoning, Intentional Self-Harm	Poisoning, Assault	Poisoning, Undetermined	Adverse Effect	Underdosing
Fiorinal	T39.011	T39.012	T39.013	T39.014	T39.015	T39.016
Firedamp	T59.891	T59.892	T59.893	T59.894	—	—
Fish, noxious, nonbacterial	T61.91	T61.92	T61.93	T61.94	—	—
ciguatera	T61.01	T61.02	T61.03	T61.04	—	—
scombroid	T61.11	T61.12	T61.13	T61.14	—	—
shell	T61.781	T61.782	T61.783	T61.784	—	—
specified NEC	T61.771	T61.772	T61.773	T61.774	—	—
Flagyl	T37.3X1	T37.3X2	T37.3X3	T37.3X4	T37.3X5	T37.3X6
Flavine adenine dinucleotide	T45.2X1	T45.2X2	T45.2X3	T45.2X4	T45.2X5	T45.2X6
Flavodic acid	T46.991	T46.992	T46.993	T46.994	T46.995	T46.996
Flavoxate	T44.3X1	T44.3X2	T44.3X3	T44.3X4	T44.3X5	T44.3X6
Flaxedil	T48.1X1	T48.1X2	T48.1X3	T48.1X4	T48.1X5	T48.1X6
Flaxseed (medicinal)	T49.3X1	T49.3X2	T49.3X3	T49.3X4	T49.3X5	T49.3X6
Flecainide	T46.2X1	T46.2X2	T46.2X3	T46.2X4	T46.2X5	T46.2X6
Fleroxacin	T36.8X1	T36.8X2	T36.8X3	T36.8X4	T36.8X5	T36.8X6
Floctafenine	T39.8X1	T39.8X2	T39.8X3	T39.8X4	T39.8X5	T39.8X6
Flomax	T44.6X1	T44.6X2	T44.6X3	T44.6X4	T44.6X5	T44.6X6
Flomoxef	T36.1X1	T36.1X2	T36.1X3	T36.1X4	T36.1X5	T36.1X6
Flopropione	T44.3X1	T44.3X2	T44.3X3	T44.3X4	T44.3X5	T44.3X6
Florantyrone	T47.5X1	T47.5X2	T47.5X3	T47.5X4	T47.5X5	T47.5X6
Floraquin	T37.8X1	T37.8X2	T37.8X3	T37.8X4	T37.8X5	T37.8X6
Florinef	T38.0X1	T38.0X2	T38.0X3	T38.0X4	T38.0X5	T38.0X6
ENT agent	T49.6X1	T49.6X2	T49.6X3	T49.6X4	T49.6X5	T49.6X6
ophthalmic preparation	T49.5X1	T49.5X2	T49.5X3	T49.5X4	T49.5X5	T49.5X6
topical NEC	T49.0X1	T49.0X2	T49.0X3	T49.0X4	T49.0X5	T49.0X6
Flowers of sulfur	T49.4X1	T49.4X2	T49.4X3	T49.4X4	T49.4X5	T49.4X6
Floxuridine	T45.1X1	T45.1X2	T45.1X3	T45.1X4	T45.1X5	T45.1X6
Fluanisone	T43.4X1	T43.4X2	T43.4X3	T43.4X4	T43.4X5	T43.4X6
Flubendazole	T37.4X1	T37.4X2	T37.4X3	T37.4X4	T37.4X5	T37.4X6
Fluclorolone acetonide	T49.0X1	T49.0X2	T49.0X3	T49.0X4	T49.0X5	T49.0X6
Flucloxacillin	T36.0X1	T36.0X2	T36.0X3	T36.0X4	T36.0X5	T36.0X6
Fluconazole	T37.8X1	T37.8X2	T37.8X3	T37.8X4	T37.8X5	T37.8X6
Flucytosine	T37.8X1	T37.8X2	T37.8X3	T37.8X4	T37.8X5	T37.8X6
Fludeoxyglucose (18F)	T50.8X1	T50.8X2	T50.8X3	T50.8X4	T50.8X5	T50.8X6
Fludiazepam	T42.4X1	T42.4X2	T42.4X3	T42.4X4	T42.4X5	T42.4X6
Fludrocortisone	T50.0X1	T50.0X2	T50.0X3	T50.0X4	T50.0X5	T50.0X6
ENT agent	T49.6X1	T49.6X2	T49.6X3	T49.6X4	T49.6X5	T49.6X6
ophthalmic preparation	T49.5X1	T49.5X2	T49.5X3	T49.5X4	T49.5X5	T49.5X6
topical NEC	T49.0X1	T49.0X2	T49.0X3	T49.0X4	T49.0X5	T49.0X6
Fludroxycortide	T49.0X1	T49.0X2	T49.0X3	T49.0X4	T49.0X5	T49.0X6
Flufenamic acid	T39.391	T39.392	T39.393	T39.394	T39.395	T39.396
Fluindione	T45.511	T45.512	T45.513	T45.514	T45.515	T45.516

◀ New ◀ Revised ~~deleted~~ Deleted

Substance	Poisoning, Accidental (Unintentional)	Poisoning, Intentional Self-Harm	Poisoning, Assault	Poisoning, Undetermined	Adverse Effect	Underdosing
Flumequine	T37.8X1	T37.8X2	T37.8X3	T37.8X4	T37.8X5	T37.8X6
Flumethasone	T49.0X1	T49.0X2	T49.0X3	T49.0X4	T49.0X5	T49.0X6
Flumethiazide	T50.2X1	T50.2X2	T50.2X3	T50.2X4	T50.2X5	T50.2X6
Flumidin	T37.5X1	T37.5X2	T37.5X3	T37.5X4	T37.5X5	T37.5X6
Flunarizine	T46.7X1	T46.7X2	T46.7X3	T46.7X4	T46.7X5	T46.7X6
Flunidazole	T37.8X1	T37.8X2	T37.8X3	T37.8X4	T37.8X5	T37.8X6
Flunisolide	T48.6X1	T48.6X2	T48.6X3	T48.6X4	T48.6X5	T48.6X6
Flunitrazepam	T42.4X1	T42.4X2	T42.4X3	T42.4X4	T42.4X5	T42.4X6
Fluocinolone (acetonide)	T49.0X1	T49.0X2	T49.0X3	T49.0X4	T49.0X5	T49.0X6
Fluocinonide	T49.0X1	T49.0X2	T49.0X3	T49.0X4	T49.0X5	T49.0X6
Fluocortin (butyl)	T49.0X1	T49.0X2	T49.0X3	T49.0X4	T49.0X5	T49.0X6
Fluocortolone	T49.0X1	T49.0X2	T49.0X3	T49.0X4	T49.0X5	T49.0X6
Fluohydrocortisone	T38.0X1	T38.0X2	T38.0X3	T38.0X4	T38.0X5	T38.0X6
ENT agent	T49.6X1	T49.6X2	T49.6X3	T49.6X4	T49.6X5	T49.6X6
ophthalmic preparation	T49.5X1	T49.5X2	T49.5X3	T49.5X4	T49.5X5	T49.5X6
topical NEC	T49.0X1	T49.0X2	T49.0X3	T49.0X4	T49.0X5	T49.0X6
Fluonid	T49.0X1	T49.0X2	T49.0X3	T49.0X4	T49.0X5	T49.0X6
Fluopromazine	T43.3X1	T43.3X2	T43.3X3	T43.3X4	T43.3X5	T43.3X6
Fluoroacetate	T60.8X1	T60.8X2	T60.8X3	T60.8X4	—	—
Fluorescein	T50.8X1	T50.8X2	T50.8X3	T50.8X4	T50.8X5	T50.8X6
Fluorhydrocortisone	T50.0X1	T50.0X2	T50.0X3	T50.0X4	T50.0X5	T50.0X6
Fluoride (nonmedicinal) (pesticide) (sodium) NEC	T60.8X1	T60.8X2	T60.8X3	T60.8X4	—	—
hydrogen — see Hydrofluoric acid						
medicinal NEC	T50.991	T50.992	T50.993	T50.994	T50.995	T50.996
dental use	T49.7X1	T49.7X2	T49.7X3	T49.7X4	T49.7X5	T49.7X6
not pesticide NEC	T54.91	T54.92	T54.93	T54.94	—	—
stannous	T49.7X1	T49.7X2	T49.7X3	T49.7X4	T49.7X5	T49.7X6
Fluorinated corticosteroids	T38.0X1	T38.0X2	T38.0X3	T38.0X4	T38.0X5	T38.0X6
Fluorine (gas)	T59.5X1	T59.5X2	T59.5X3	T59.5X4	—	—
salt — see Fluoride(s)						
Fluoristan	T49.7X1	T49.7X2	T49.7X3	T49.7X4	T49.7X5	T49.7X6
Fluormetholone	T49.0X1	T49.0X2	T49.0X3	T49.0X4	T49.0X5	T49.0X6
Fluoroacetate	T60.8X1	T60.8X2	T60.8X3	T60.8X4	—	—
Fluorocarbon monomer	T53.6X1	T53.6X2	T53.6X3	T53.6X4	—	—
Fluorocytosine	T37.8X1	T37.8X2	T37.8X3	T37.8X4	T37.8X5	T37.8X6
Fluorodeoxyuridine	T45.1X1	T45.1X2	T45.1X3	T45.1X4	T45.1X5	T45.1X6
Fluorometholone	T49.0X1	T49.0X2	T49.0X3	T49.0X4	T49.0X5	T49.0X6
ophthalmic preparation	T49.5X1	T49.5X2	T49.5X3	T49.5X4	T49.5X5	T49.5X6
Fluorophosphate insecticide	T60.0X1	T60.0X2	T60.0X3	T60.0X4	—	—
Fluorosol	T46.3X1	T46.3X2	T46.3X3	T46.3X4	T46.3X5	T46.3X6
Fluorouracil	T45.1X1	T45.1X2	T45.1X3	T45.1X4	T45.1X5	T45.1X6

Substance	Poisoning, Accidental (Unintentional)	Poisoning, Intentional Self-Harm	Poisoning, Assault	Poisoning, Undetermined	Adverse Effect	Underdosing
Fluorphenylalanine	T49.5X1	T49.5X2	T49.5X3	T49.5X4	T49.5X5	T49.5X6
Fluothane	T41.0X1	T41.0X2	T41.0X3	T41.0X4	T41.0X5	T41.0X6
Fluoxetine	T43.221	T43.222	T43.223	T43.224	T43.225	T43.226
Fluoxymesterone	T38.7X1	T38.7X2	T38.7X3	T38.7X4	T38.7X5	T38.7X6
Flupenthixol	T43.4X1	T43.4X2	T43.4X3	T43.4X4	T43.4X5	T43.4X6
Flupentixol	T43.4X1	T43.4X2	T43.4X3	T43.4X4	T43.4X5	T43.4X6
Fluphenazine	T43.3X1	T43.3X2	T43.3X3	T43.3X4	T43.3X5	T43.3X6
Fluprednidene	T49.0X1	T49.0X2	T49.0X3	T49.0X4	T49.0X5	T49.0X6
Fluprednisolone	T38.0X1	T38.0X2	T38.0X3	T38.0X4	T38.0X5	T38.0X6
Fluradoline	T39.8X1	T39.8X2	T39.8X3	T39.8X4	T39.8X5	T39.8X6
Flurandrenolide	T49.0X1	T49.0X2	T49.0X3	T49.0X4	T49.0X5	T49.0X6
Flurandrenolone	T49.0X1	T49.0X2	T49.0X3	T49.0X4	T49.0X5	T49.0X6
Flurazepam	T42.4X1	T42.4X2	T42.4X3	T42.4X4	T42.4X5	T42.4X6
Flurbiprofen	T39.311	T39.312	T39.313	T39.314	T39.315	T39.316
Flurobate	T49.0X1	T49.0X2	T49.0X3	T49.0X4	T49.0X5	T49.0X6
Flurotyl	T43.291	T43.292	T43.293	T43.294	T43.295	T43.296
Fluroxene	T41.0X1	T41.0X2	T41.0X3	T41.0X4	T41.0X5	T41.0X6
Fluspirilene	T43.591	T43.592	T43.593	T43.594	T43.595	T43.596
Flutamide	T38.6X1	T38.6X2	T38.6X3	T38.6X4	T38.6X5	T38.6X6
Flutazolam	T42.4X1	T42.4X2	T42.4X3	T42.4X4	T42.4X5	T42.4X6
Fluticasone propionate	T38.0X1	T38.0X2	T38.0X3	T38.0X4	T38.0X5	T38.0X6
Flutoprazepam	T42.4X1	T42.4X2	T42.4X3	T42.4X4	T42.4X5	T42.4X6
Flutropium bromide	T48.6X1	T48.6X2	T48.6X3	T48.6X4	T48.6X5	T48.6X6
Fluvoxamine	T43.221	T43.222	T43.223	T43.224	T43.225	T43.226
Folacin	T45.8X1	T45.8X2	T45.8X3	T45.8X4	T45.8X5	T45.8X6
Folic acid	T45.8X1	T45.8X2	T45.8X3	T45.8X4	T45.8X5	T45.8X6
with ferrous salt	T45.2X1	T45.2X2	T45.2X3	T45.2X4	T45.2X5	T45.2X6
antagonist	T45.1X1	T45.1X2	T45.1X3	T45.1X4	T45.1X5	T45.1X6
Folinic acid	T45.8X1	T45.8X2	T45.8X3	T45.8X4	T45.8X5	T45.8X6
Folium stramoniae	T48.6X1	T48.6X2	T48.6X3	T48.6X4	T48.6X5	T48.6X6
Follicle-stimulating hormone, human	T38.811	T38.812	T38.813	T38.814	T38.815	T38.816
Folpet	T60.3X1	T60.3X2	T60.3X3	T60.3X4	—	—
Fominoben	T48.3X1	T48.3X2	T48.3X3	T48.3X4	T48.3X5	T48.3X6
Food, foodstuffs, noxious, nonbacterial, NEC	T62.91	T62.92	T62.93	T62.94	—	—
berries	T62.1X1	T62.1X2	T62.1X3	T62.1X4	—	—
fish — see also Fish	T61.91	T61.92	T61.93	T61.94	—	—
mushrooms	T62.0X1	T62.0X2	T62.0X3	T62.0X4	—	—
plants	T62.2X1	T62.2X2	T62.2X3	T62.2X4	—	—
seafood	T61.91	T61.92	T61.93	T61.94	—	—
specified NEC	T61.8X1	T61.8X2	T61.8X3	T61.8X4	—	—
seeds	T62.2X1	T62.2X2	T62.2X3	T62.2X4	—	—

◀ New ◀|| Revised ~~deleted~~ Deleted

TABLE OF DRUGS AND CHEMICALS

Substance	Poisoning, Accidental (Unintentional)	Poisoning, Intentional Self-Harm	Poisoning, Assault	Poisoning, Undetermined	Adverse Effect	Underdosing
Food, foodstuffs, noxious, nonbacterial, NEC *(Continued)*						
shellfish	T61.781	T61.782	T61.783	T61.784	—	—
specified NEC	T62.8X1	T62.8X2	T62.8X3	T62.8X4	—	—
Fool's parsley	T62.2X1	T62.2X2	T62.2X3	T62.2X4	—	—
Formaldehyde (solution), gas or vapor	T59.2X1	T59.2X2	T59.2X3	T59.2X4	—	—
fungicide	T60.3X1	T60.3X2	T60.3X3	T60.3X4	—	—
Formalin	T59.2X1	T59.2X2	T59.2X3	T59.2X4	—	—
fungicide	T60.3X1	T60.3X2	T60.3X3	T60.3X4	—	—
vapor	T59.2X1	T59.2X2	T59.2X3	T59.2X4	—	—
Formic acid	T54.2X1	T54.2X2	T54.2X3	T54.2X4	—	—
vapor	T59.891	T59.892	T59.893	T59.894	—	—
Foscarnet sodium	T37.5X1	T37.5X2	T37.5X3	T37.5X4	T37.5X5	T37.5X6
Fosfestrol	T38.5X1	T38.5X2	T38.5X3	T38.5X4	T38.5X5	T38.5X6
Fosfomycin	T36.8X1	T36.8X2	T36.8X3	T36.8X4	T36.8X5	T36.8X6
Fosfonet sodium	T37.5X1	T37.5X2	T37.5X3	T37.5X4	T37.5X5	T37.5X6
Fosinopril	T46.4X1	T46.4X2	T46.4X3	T46.4X4	T46.4X5	T46.4X6
sodium	T46.4X1	T46.4X2	T46.4X3	T46.4X4	T46.4X5	T46.4X6
Fowler's solution	T57.0X1	T57.0X2	T57.0X3	T57.0X4	—	—
Foxglove	T62.2X1	T62.2X2	T62.2X3	T62.2X4	—	—
Framycetin	T36.5X1	T36.5X2	T36.5X3	T36.5X4	T36.5X5	T36.5X6
Frangula	T47.2X1	T47.2X2	T47.2X3	T47.2X4	T47.2X5	T47.2X6
extract	T47.2X1	T47.2X2	T47.2X3	T47.2X4	T47.2X5	T47.2X6
Frei antigen	T50.8X1	T50.8X2	T50.8X3	T50.8X4	T50.8X5	T50.8X6
Freon	T53.5X1	T53.5X2	T53.5X3	T53.5X4	—	—
Fructose	T50.3X1	T50.3X2	T50.3X3	T50.3X4	T50.3X5	T50.3X6
Frusemide	T50.1X1	T50.1X2	T50.1X3	T50.1X4	T50.1X5	T50.1X6
FSH	T38.811	T38.812	T38.813	T38.814	T38.815	T38.816
Ftorafur	T45.1X1	T45.1X2	T45.1X3	T45.1X4	T45.1X5	T45.1X6
Fuel						
automobile	T52.0X1	T52.0X2	T52.0X3	T52.0X4	—	—
exhaust gas, not in transit	T58.01	T58.02	T58.03	T58.04	—	—
vapor NEC	T52.0X1	T52.0X2	T52.0X3	T52.0X4	—	—
gas (domestic use) — *see also Carbon, monoxide, fuel, utility*	T59.891	T59.892	T59.893	T59.894	—	—
utility	T59.891	T59.892	T59.893	T59.894	—	—
in mobile container	T59.891	T59.892	T59.893	T59.894	—	—
incomplete combustion of — *see Carbon, monoxide, fuel, utility*						
piped (natural)	T59.891	T59.892	T59.893	T59.894	—	—
industrial, incomplete combustion	T58.8X1	T58.8X2	T58.8X3	T58.8X4	—	—

Substance	Poisoning, Accidental (Unintentional)	Poisoning, Intentional Self-Harm	Poisoning, Assault	Poisoning, Undetermined	Adverse Effect	Underdosing
Fugillin	T36.8X1	T36.8X2	T36.8X3	T36.8X4	T36.8X5	T36.8X6
Fulminate of mercury	T56.1X1	T56.1X2	T56.1X3	T56.1X4	—	—
Fulvicin	T36.7X1	T36.7X2	T36.7X3	T36.7X4	T36.7X5	T36.7X6
Fumadil	T36.8X1	T36.8X2	T36.8X3	T36.8X4	T36.8X5	T36.8X6
Fumagillin	T36.8X1	T36.8X2	T36.8X3	T36.8X4	T36.8X5	T36.8X6
Fumaric acid	T49.4X1	T49.4X2	T49.4X3	T49.4X4	T49.4X5	T49.4X6
Fumes (from)	T59.91	T59.92	T59.93	T59.94	—	—
carbon monoxide — *see Carbon, monoxide*						
charcoal (domestic use) — *see Charcoal, fumes*						
chloroform — *see Chloroform*						
coke (in domestic stoves, fireplaces) — *see Coke, fumes*						
corrosive NEC	T54.91	T54.92	T54.93	T54.94	—	—
ether — *see ether*						
freons	T53.5X1	T53.5X2	T53.5X3	T53.5X4	—	—
hydrocarbons	T59.891	T59.892	T59.893	T59.894	—	—
petroleum (liquefied)	T59.891	T59.892	T59.893	T59.894	—	—
distributed through pipes (pure or mixed with air)	T59.891	T59.892	T59.893	T59.894	—	—
lead — *see lead*						
metal — *see Metals, or the specified metal*						
nitrogen dioxide	T59.0X1	T59.0X2	T59.0X3	T59.0X4	—	—
pesticides — *see Pesticides*						
petroleum (liquefied)	T59.891	T59.892	T59.893	T59.894	—	—
distributed through pipes (pure or mixed with air)	T59.891	T59.892	T59.893	T59.894	—	—
polyester	T59.891	T59.892	T59.893	T59.894	—	—
specified source NEC — *see also substance specified*	T59.891	T59.892	T59.893	T59.894	—	—
sulfur dioxide	T59.1X1	T59.1X2	T59.1X3	T59.1X4	—	—
Fumigant NEC	T60.91	T60.92	T60.93	T60.94	—	—
Fungi, noxious, used as food	T62.0X1	T62.0X2	T62.0X3	T62.0X4	—	—
Fungicide NEC (nonmedicinal)	T60.3X1	T60.3X2	T60.3X3	T60.3X4	—	—
Fungizone	T36.7X1	T36.7X2	T36.7X3	T36.7X4	T36.7X5	T36.7X6
topical	T49.0X1	T49.0X2	T49.0X3	T49.0X4	T49.0X5	T49.0X6
Furacin	T49.0X1	T49.0X2	T49.0X3	T49.0X4	T49.0X5	T49.0X6
Furadantin	T37.91	T37.92	T37.93	T37.94	T37.95	T37.96
Furazolidone	T37.8X1	T37.8X2	T37.8X3	T37.8X4	T37.8X5	T37.8X6
Furazolium chloride	T49.0X1	T49.0X2	T49.0X3	T49.0X4	T49.0X5	T49.0X6
Furfural	T52.8X1	T52.8X2	T52.8X3	T52.8X4	—	—

◀ New   ◀ Revised   ~~deleted~~ Deleted

Substance	Poisoning, Accidental (Unintentional)	Poisoning, Intentional Self-Harm	Poisoning, Assault	Poisoning, Undetermined	Adverse Effect	Underdosing
Furnace (coal burning) (domestic), gas from industrial	T58.2X1	T58.2X2	T58.2X3	T58.2X4	—	—
industrial	T58.8X1	T58.8X2	T58.8X3	T58.8X4	—	—
Furniture polish	T65.891	T65.892	T65.893	T65.894	—	—
Furosemide	T50.1X1	T50.1X2	T50.1X3	T50.1X4	T50.1X5	T50.1X6
Furoxone	T37.91	T37.92	T37.93	T37.94	T37.95	T37.96
Fursultiamine	T45.2X1	T45.2X2	T45.2X3	T45.2X4	T45.2X5	T45.2X6
Fusafungine	T36.8X1	T36.8X2	T36.8X3	T36.8X4	T36.8X5	T36.8X6
Fusel oil (any) (amyl) (butyl) (propyl), vapor	T51.3X1	T51.3X2	T51.3X3	T51.3X4	—	—
Fusidate (ethanolamine) (sodium)	T36.8X1	T36.8X2	T36.8X3	T36.8X4	T36.8X5	T36.8X6
Fusidic acid	T36.8X1	T36.8X2	T36.8X3	T36.8X4	T36.8X5	T36.8X6
Fytic acid, nonasodium	T50.6X1	T50.6X2	T50.6X3	T50.6X4	T50.6X5	T50.6X6

G

Substance	Poisoning, Accidental (Unintentional)	Poisoning, Intentional Self-Harm	Poisoning, Assault	Poisoning, Undetermined	Adverse Effect	Underdosing
GABA	T43.8X1	T43.8X2	T43.8X3	T43.8X4	T43.8X5	T43.8X6
Gadopentetic acid	T50.8X1	T50.8X2	T50.8X3	T50.8X4	T50.8X5	T50.8X6
Galactose	T50.3X1	T50.3X2	T50.3X3	T50.3X4	T50.3X5	T50.3X6
b-Galactosidase	T47.5X1	T47.5X2	T47.5X3	T47.5X4	T47.5X5	T47.5X6
Galantamine	T44.0X1	T44.0X2	T44.0X3	T44.0X4	T44.0X5	T44.0X6
Gallamine (triethiodide)	T48.1X1	T48.1X2	T48.1X3	T48.1X4	T48.1X5	T48.1X6
Gallium citrate	T50.991	T50.992	T50.993	T50.994	T50.995	T50.996
Gallopamil	T46.1X1	T46.1X2	T46.1X3	T46.1X4	T46.1X5	T46.1X6
Gamboge	T47.2X1	T47.2X2	T47.2X3	T47.2X4	T47.2X5	T47.2X6
Gamimune	T50.Z11	T50.Z12	T50.Z13	T50.Z14	T50.Z15	T50.Z16
Gamma-aminobutyric acid	T43.8X1	T43.8X2	T43.8X3	T43.8X4	T43.8X5	T43.8X6
Gamma-benzene hexachloride (medicinal)	T49.0X1	T49.0X2	T49.0X3	T49.0X4	T49.0X5	T49.0X6
nonmedicinal, vapor	T53.6X1	T53.6X2	T53.6X3	T53.6X4	—	—
Gamma-BHC (medicinal) — see also Gamma-benzene hexachloride	T49.0X1	T49.0X2	T49.0X3	T49.0X4	T49.0X5	T49.0X6
Gamma globulin	T50.Z11	T50.Z12	T50.Z13	T50.Z14	T50.Z15	T50.Z16
Gamulin	T50.Z11	T50.Z12	T50.Z13	T50.Z14	T50.Z15	T50.Z16
Ganciclovir (sodium)	T37.5X1	T37.5X2	T37.5X3	T37.5X4	T37.5X5	T37.5X6
Ganglionic blocking drug NEC	T44.2X1	T44.2X2	T44.2X3	T44.2X4	T44.2X5	T44.2X6
specified NEC	T44.2X1	T44.2X2	T44.2X3	T44.2X4	T44.2X5	T44.2X6
Ganja	T40.7X1	T40.7X2	T40.7X3	T40.7X4	T40.7X5	T40.7X6
Garamycin	T36.5X1	T36.5X2	T36.5X3	T36.5X4	T36.5X5	T36.5X6
ophthalmic preparation	T49.5X1	T49.5X2	T49.5X3	T49.5X4	T49.5X5	T49.5X6
topical NEC	T49.0X1	T49.0X2	T49.0X3	T49.0X4	T49.0X5	T49.0X6
Gardenal	T42.3X1	T42.3X2	T42.3X3	T42.3X4	T42.3X5	T42.3X6
Gardepanyl	T42.3X1	T42.3X2	T42.3X3	T42.3X4	T42.3X5	T42.3X6

Substance	Poisoning, Accidental (Unintentional)	Poisoning, Intentional Self-Harm	Poisoning, Assault	Poisoning, Undetermined	Adverse Effect	Underdosing
Gas	T59.91	T59.92	T59.93	T59.94	—	—
acetylene	T59.891	T59.892	T59.893	T59.894	—	—
incomplete combustion of	T58.11	T58.12	T58.13	T58.14	—	—
air contaminants, source or type not specified	T59.91	T59.92	T59.93	T59.94	—	—
anesthetic	T41.0X1	T41.0X2	T41.0X3	T41.0X4	T41.0X5	T41.0X6
blast furnace	T58.8X1	T58.8X2	T58.8X3	T58.8X4	—	—
butane — see butane						
carbon monoxide — see Carbon, monoxide						
chlorine	T59.4X1	T59.4X2	T59.4X3	T59.4X4	—	—
coal	T58.2X1	T58.2X2	T58.2X3	T58.2X4	—	—
cyanide	T57.3X1	T57.3X2	T57.3X3	T57.3X4	—	—
dicyanogen	T65.0X1	T65.0X2	T65.0X3	T65.0X4	—	—
domestic — see Domestic gas	T57.91	T57.92	T57.93	T57.94		
exhaust	T57.91	T57.92	T57.93	T57.94	—	—
from utility (for cooking, heating, or lighting) (after combustion) — see Carbon, monoxide, fuel, utility						
prior to combustion	T59.891	T59.892	T59.893	T59.894	—	—
from wood or coal-burning stove or fireplace	T57.91	T57.92	T57.93	T57.94	—	—
fuel (domestic use) (after combustion) — see also Carbon, monoxide, fuel	T57.91	T57.92	T57.93	T57.94	—	—
industrial use	T58.8X1	T58.8X2	T58.8X3	T58.8X4	—	—
prior to combustion	T59.891	T59.892	T59.893	T59.894	—	—
utility	T59.891	T59.892	T59.893	T59.894	—	—
in mobile container	T59.891	T59.892	T59.893	T59.894	—	—
incomplete combustion of — see Carbon, monoxide, fuel, utility						
piped (natural)	T59.891	T59.892	T59.893	T59.894	—	—
garage	T58.01	T58.02	T58.03	T58.04	—	—
hydrocarbon NEC	T59.891	T59.892	T59.893	T59.894	—	—
incomplete combustion of — see Carbon, monoxide, fuel, utility						
liquefied — see butane						
piped	T59.891	T59.892	T59.893	T59.894	—	—
hydrocyanic acid	T65.0X1	T65.0X2	T65.0X3	T65.0X4	—	—

◀ New ◀ Revised deleted Deleted

TABLE OF DRUGS AND CHEMICALS

Substance	Poisoning, Accidental (Unintentional)	Poisoning, Intentional Self-Harm	Poisoning, Assault	Poisoning, Undetermined	Adverse Effect	Underdosing
Gas (Continued)						
illuminating (after combustion)	T58.11	T58.12	T58.13	T58.14	—	—
prior to combustion	T59.891	T59.892	T59.893	T59.894	—	—
incomplete combustion, any — see Carbon, monoxide						
kiln	T58.8X1	T58.8X2	T58.8X3	T58.8X4	—	—
lacrimogenic	T59.3X1	T59.3X2	T59.3X3	T59.3X4	—	—
liquefied petroleum — see butane						
marsh	T59.891	T59.892	T59.893	T59.894	—	—
motor exhaust, not in transit	T58.01	T58.02	T58.03	T58.04	—	—
mustard, not in war	T59.891	T59.892	T59.893	T59.894	—	—
natural	T59.891	T59.892	T59.893	T59.894	—	—
nerve, not in war	T59.91	T59.92	T59.93	T59.94	—	—
oil	T52.0X1	T52.0X2	T52.0X3	T52.0X4	—	—
petroleum (liquefied) (distributed in mobile containers)	T59.891	T59.892	T59.893	T59.894	—	—
piped (pure or mixed with air)	T59.891	T59.892	T59.893	T59.894	—	—
piped (manufactured) (natural) NEC	T59.891	T59.892	T59.893	T59.894	—	—
producer	T58.8X1	T58.8X2	T58.8X3	T58.8X4	—	—
propane — see propane						
refrigerant (chlorofluorocarbon)	T53.5X1	T53.5X2	T53.5X3	T53.5X4	—	—
not chlorofluoro-carbon	T59.891	T59.892	T59.893	T59.894	—	—
sewer	T59.91	T59.92	T59.93	T59.94	—	—
specified source NEC	T59.91	T59.92	T59.93	T59.94	—	—
stove (after combustion)	T58.11	T58.12	T58.13	T58.14	—	—
tear	T59.3X1	T59.3X2	T59.3X3	T59.3X4	—	—
therapeutic	T41.5X1	T41.5X2	T41.5X3	T41.5X4	T41.5X5	T41.5X6
utility (for cooking, heating, or lighting) (piped) NEC	T59.891	T59.892	T59.893	T59.894	—	—
in mobile container	T59.891	T59.892	T59.893	T59.894	—	—
incomplete combustion of — see Carbon, monoxide, fuel, utility						
piped (natural)	T59.891	T59.892	T59.893	T59.894	—	—
water	T58.11	T58.12	T58.13	T58.14	—	—
incomplete combustion of — see Carbon, monoxide, fuel, utility						

Substance	Poisoning, Accidental (Unintentional)	Poisoning, Intentional Self-Harm	Poisoning, Assault	Poisoning, Undetermined	Adverse Effect	Underdosing
Gas NEC	T59.91	T59.92	T59.93	T59.94	—	—
acetylene	T59.891	T59.892	T59.893	T59.894	—	—
incomplete combustion of	T58.11	T58.12	T58.13	T58.14	—	—
air contaminants, source or type not specified	T59.91	T59.92	T59.93	T59.94	—	—
anesthetic	T41.0X1	T41.0X2	T41.0X3	T41.0X4	T41.0X5	T41.0X6
blast furnace	T58.8X1	T58.8X2	T58.8X3	T58.8X4	—	—
butane — see butane						
carbon monoxide — see Carbon, monoxide						
chlorine	T59.4X1	T59.4X2	T59.4X3	T59.4X4	—	—
coal	T58.2X1	T58.2X2	T58.2X3	T58.2X4	—	—
cyanide	T57.3X1	T57.3X2	T57.3X3	T57.3X4	—	—
dicyanogen	T65.0X1	T65.0X2	T65.0X3	T65.0X4	—	—
domestic — see Domestic gas	T57.91	T57.92	T57.93	T57.94	—	—
exhaust	T57.91	T57.92	T57.93	T57.94	—	—
from utility (for cooking, heating, or lighting) (after combustion) — see Carbon, monoxide, fuel, utility						
prior to combustion	T59.891	T59.892	T59.893	T59.894	—	—
from wood or coal-burning stove or fireplace	T57.91	T57.92	T57.93	T57.94	—	—
fuel (domestic use) (after combustion) — see also Carbon, monoxide, fuel	T57.91	T57.92	T57.93	T57.94	—	—
industrial use	T58.8X1	T58.8X2	T58.8X3	T58.8X4	—	—
prior to combustion	T59.891	T59.892	T59.893	T59.894	—	—
utility	T59.891	T59.892	T59.893	T59.894	—	—
in mobile container	T59.891	T59.892	T59.893	T59.894	—	—
incomplete combustion of — see Carbon, monoxide, fuel, utility						
piped (natural)	T59.891	T59.892	T59.893	T59.894	—	—
garage	T58.01	T58.02	T58.03	T58.04	—	—
hydrocarbon NEC	T59.891	T59.892	T59.893	T59.894	—	—
incomplete combustion of — see Carbon, monoxide, fuel, utility						
liquefied — see butane						
piped	T59.891	T59.892	T59.893	T59.894	—	—
hydrocyanic acid	T65.0X1	T65.0X2	T65.0X3	T65.0X4	—	—

◄ New ◄◄ Revised deleted Deleted

Substance	External Cause (T-Code)					
	Poisoning, Accidental (Unintentional)	Poisoning, Intentional Self-Harm	Poisoning, Assault	Poisoning, Undetermined	Adverse Effect	Underdosing
Gas (Continued)						
illuminating (after combustion)	T58.11	T58.12	T58.13	T58.14	—	—
prior to combustion	T59.891	T59.892	T59.893	T59.894	—	—
incomplete combustion, any — see Carbon, monoxide						
kiln	T58.8X1	T58.8X2	T58.8X3	T58.8X4	—	—
lacrimogenic	T59.3X1	T59.3X2	T59.3X3	T59.3X4	—	—
liquefied petroleum — see butane						
marsh	T59.891	T59.892	T59.893	T59.894	—	—
motor exhaust, not in transit	T58.01	T58.02	T58.03	T58.04	—	—
mustard, not in war	T59.891	T59.892	T59.893	T59.894	—	—
natural	T59.891	T59.892	T59.893	T59.894	—	—
nerve, not in war	T59.91	T59.92	T59.93	T59.94	—	—
oil	T52.0X1	T52.0X2	T52.0X3	T52.0X4	—	—
petroleum (liquefied) (distributed in mobile containers)	T59.891	T59.892	T59.893	T59.894	—	—
piped (pure or mixed with air)	T59.891	T59.892	T59.893	T59.894	—	—
piped (manufactured) (natural) NEC	T59.891	T59.892	T59.893	T59.894	—	—
producer	T58.8X1	T58.8X2	T58.8X3	T58.8X4	—	—
propane — see propane						
refrigerant (chlorofluoro-carbon)	T53.5X1	T53.5X2	T53.5X3	T53.5X4	—	—
not chlorofluoro-carbon	T59.891	T59.892	T59.893	T59.894	—	—
sewer	T59.91	T59.92	T59.93	T59.94	—	—
specified source NEC	T59.91	T59.92	T59.93	T59.94	—	—
stove (after combustion)	T58.11	T58.12	T58.13	T58.14	—	—
tear	T59.3X1	T59.3X2	T59.3X3	T59.3X4	—	—
therapeutic	T41.5X1	T41.5X2	T41.5X3	T41.5X4	T41.5X5	T41.5X6
utility (for cooking, heating, or lighting) (piped) NEC	T59.891	T59.892	T59.893	T59.894	—	—
in mobile container	T59.891	T59.892	T59.893	T59.894	—	—
incomplete combustion of — see Carbon, monoxide, fuel, utility						
piped (natural)	T59.891	T59.892	T59.893	T59.894	—	—
water	T58.11	T58.12	T58.13	T58.14	—	—
incomplete combustion of — see Carbon, monoxide, fuel, utility						

Substance	External Cause (T-Code)					
	Poisoning, Accidental (Unintentional)	Poisoning, Intentional Self-Harm	Poisoning, Assault	Poisoning, Undetermined	Adverse Effect	Underdosing
Gaseous substance — see Gas						
Gasoline	T52.0X1	T52.0X2	T52.0X3	T52.0X4	—	—
vapor	T52.0X1	T52.0X2	T52.0X3	T52.0X4	—	—
Gastric enzymes	T47.5X1	T47.5X2	T47.5X3	T47.5X4	T47.5X5	T47.5X6
Gastrografin	T50.8X1	T50.8X2	T50.8X3	T50.8X4	T50.8X5	T50.8X6
Gastrointestinal drug	T47.91	T47.92	T47.93	T47.94	T47.95	T47.96
biological	T47.8X1	T47.8X2	T47.8X3	T47.8X4	T47.8X5	T47.8X6
specified NEC	T47.8X1	T47.8X2	T47.8X3	T47.8X4	T47.8X5	T47.8X6
Gaultheria procumbens	T62.2X1	T62.2X2	T62.2X3	T62.2X4	—	—
Gelatin (intravenous)	T45.8X1	T45.8X2	T45.8X3	T45.8X4	T45.8X5	T45.8X6
absorbable (sponge)	T45.7X1	T45.7X2	T45.7X3	T45.7X4	T45.7X5	T45.7X6
Gefarnate	T44.3X1	T44.3X2	T44.3X3	T44.3X4	T44.3X5	T44.3X6
Gelfilm	T49.8X1	T49.8X2	T49.8X3	T49.8X4	T49.8X5	T49.8X6
Gelfoam	T45.7X1	T45.7X2	T45.7X3	T45.7X4	T45.7X5	T45.7X6
Gelsemine	T50.991	T50.992	T50.993	T50.994	T50.995	T50.996
Gelsemium (sempervirens)	T62.2X1	T62.2X2	T62.2X3	T62.2X4	—	—
Gemeprost	T48.0X1	T48.0X2	T48.0X3	T48.0X4	T48.0X5	T48.0X6
Gemfibrozil	T46.6X1	T46.6X2	T46.6X3	T46.6X4	T46.6X5	T46.6X6
Gemonil	T42.3X1	T42.3X2	T42.3X3	T42.3X4	T42.3X5	T42.3X6
Gentamicin	T36.5X1	T36.5X2	T36.5X3	T36.5X4	T36.5X5	T36.5X6
ophthalmic preparation	T49.5X1	T49.5X2	T49.5X3	T49.5X4	T49.5X5	T49.5X6
topical NEC	T49.0X1	T49.0X2	T49.0X3	T49.0X4	T49.0X5	T49.0X6
Gentian	T47.5X1	T47.5X2	T47.5X3	T47.5X4	T47.5X5	T47.5X6
violet	T49.0X1	T49.0X2	T49.0X3	T49.0X4	T49.0X5	T49.0X6
Gepefrine	T44.4X1	T44.4X2	T44.4X3	T44.4X4	T44.4X5	T44.4X6
Gestonorone caproate	T38.5X1	T38.5X2	T38.5X3	T38.5X4	T38.5X5	T38.5X6
Gexane	T49.0X1	T49.0X2	T49.0X3	T49.0X4	T49.0X5	T49.0X6
Gila monster (venom)	T63.111	T63.112	T63.113	T63.114	—	—
Ginger	T47.5X1	T47.5X2	T47.5X3	T47.5X4	T47.5X5	T47.5X6
Jamaica — see Jamaica, ginger						
Gitalin	T46.0X1	T46.0X2	T46.0X3	T46.0X4	T46.0X5	T46.0X6
amorphous	T46.0X1	T46.0X2	T46.0X3	T46.0X4	T46.0X5	T46.0X6
Gitaloxin	T46.0X1	T46.0X2	T46.0X3	T46.0X4	T46.0X5	T46.0X6
Gitoxin	T46.0X1	T46.0X2	T46.0X3	T46.0X4	T46.0X5	T46.0X6
Glafenine	T39.8X1	T39.8X2	T39.8X3	T39.8X4	T39.8X5	T39.8X6
Glandular extract (medicinal) NEC	T50.Z91	T50.Z92	T50.Z93	T50.Z94	T50.Z95	T50.Z96
Glaucarubin	T37.3X1	T37.3X2	T37.3X3	T37.3X4	T37.3X5	T37.3X6
Glibenclamide	T38.3X1	T38.3X2	T38.3X3	T38.3X4	T38.3X5	T38.3X6
Glibornuride	T38.3X1	T38.3X2	T38.3X3	T38.3X4	T38.3X5	T38.3X6
Gliclazide	T38.3X1	T38.3X2	T38.3X3	T38.3X4	T38.3X5	T38.3X6
Glimidine	T38.3X1	T38.3X2	T38.3X3	T38.3X4	T38.3X5	T38.3X6

◀ New ◀▮ Revised ~~deleted~~ Deleted

Substance	External Cause (T-Code)					
	Poisoning, Accidental (Unintentional)	Poisoning, Intentional Self-Harm	Poisoning, Assault	Poisoning, Undetermined	Adverse Effect	Underdosing
Glipizide	T38.3X1	T38.3X2	T38.3X3	T38.3X4	T38.3X5	T38.3X6
Gliquidone	T38.3X1	T38.3X2	T38.3X3	T38.3X4	T38.3X5	T38.3X6
Glisolamide	T38.3X1	T38.3X2	T38.3X3	T38.3X4	T38.3X5	T38.3X6
Glisoxepide	T38.3X1	T38.3X2	T38.3X3	T38.3X4	T38.3X5	T38.3X6
Globin zinc insulin	T38.3X1	T38.3X2	T38.3X3	T38.3X4	T38.3X5	T38.3X6
Globulin						
antilymphocytic	T50.Z11	T50.Z12	T50.Z13	T50.Z14	T50.Z15	T50.Z16
antirhesus	T50.Z11	T50.Z12	T50.Z13	T50.Z14	T50.Z15	T50.Z16
antivenin	T50.Z11	T50.Z12	T50.Z13	T50.Z14	T50.Z15	T50.Z16
antiviral	T50.Z11	T50.Z12	T50.Z13	T50.Z14	T50.Z15	T50.Z16
Glucagon	T38.3X1	T38.3X2	T38.3X3	T38.3X4	T38.3X5	T38.3X6
Glucocorticoids	T38.0X1	T38.0X2	T38.0X3	T38.0X4	T38.0X5	T38.0X6
Glucocorticosteroid	T38.0X1	T38.0X2	T38.0X3	T38.0X4	T38.0X5	T38.0X6
Gluconic acid	T50.991	T50.992	T50.993	T50.994	T50.995	T50.996
Glucosamine sulfate	T39.4X1	T39.4X2	T39.4X3	T39.4X4	T39.4X5	T39.4X6
Glucose	T50.3X1	T50.3X2	T50.3X3	T50.3X4	T50.3X5	T50.3X6
with sodium chloride	T50.3X1	T50.3X2	T50.3X3	T50.3X4	T50.3X5	T50.3X6
Glucosulfone sodium	T37.1X1	T37.1X2	T37.1X3	T37.1X4	T37.1X5	T37.1X6
Glucurolactone	T47.8X1	T47.8X2	T47.8X3	T47.8X4	T47.8X5	T47.8X6
Glue NEC	T52.8X1	T52.8X2	T52.8X3	T52.8X4	—	—
Glutamic acid	T47.5X1	T47.5X2	T47.5X3	T47.5X4	T47.5X5	T47.5X6
Glutaral (medicinal)	T49.0X1	T49.0X2	T49.0X3	T49.0X4	T49.0X5	T49.0X6
nonmedicinal	T65.891	T65.892	T65.893	T65.894	—	—
Glutaraldehyde (nonmedicinal)	T65.891	T65.892	T65.893	T65.894	—	—
medicinal	T49.0X1	T49.0X2	T49.0X3	T49.0X4	T49.0X5	T49.0X6
Glutathione	T50.6X1	T50.6X2	T50.6X3	T50.6X4	T50.6X5	T50.6X6
Glutethimide	T42.6X1	T42.6X2	T42.6X3	T42.6X4	T42.6X5	T42.6X6
Glyburide	T38.3X1	T38.3X2	T38.3X3	T38.3X4	T38.3X5	T38.3X6
Glycerin	T47.4X1	T47.4X2	T47.4X3	T47.4X4	T47.4X5	T47.4X6
Glycerol	T47.4X1	T47.4X2	T47.4X3	T47.4X4	T47.4X5	T47.4X6
borax	T49.6X1	T49.6X2	T49.6X3	T49.6X4	T49.6X5	T49.6X6
intravenous	T50.3X1	T50.3X2	T50.3X3	T50.3X4	T50.3X5	T50.3X6
iodinated	T48.4X1	T48.4X2	T48.4X3	T48.4X4	T48.4X5	T48.4X6
Glycerophosphate	T50.991	T50.992	T50.993	T50.994	T50.995	T50.996
Glyceryl						
gualacolate	T48.4X1	T48.4X2	T48.4X3	T48.4X4	T48.4X5	T48.4X6
nitrate	T46.3X1	T46.3X2	T46.3X3	T46.3X4	T46.3X5	T46.3X6
triacetate (topical)	T49.0X1	T49.0X2	T49.0X3	T49.0X4	T49.0X5	T49.0X6
trinitrate	T46.3X1	T46.3X2	T46.3X3	T46.3X4	T46.3X5	T46.3X6
Glycine	T50.3X1	T50.3X2	T50.3X3	T50.3X4	T50.3X5	T50.3X6
Glyclopyramide	T38.3X1	T38.3X2	T38.3X3	T38.3X4	T38.3X5	T38.3X6
Glycobiarsol	T37.3X1	T37.3X2	T37.3X3	T37.3X4	T37.3X5	T37.3X6
Glycols (ether)	T52.3X1	T52.3X2	T52.3X3	T52.3X4	—	—
Glyconiazide	T37.1X1	T37.1X2	T37.1X3	T37.1X4	T37.1X5	T37.1X6
Glycopyrrolate	T44.3X1	T44.3X2	T44.3X3	T44.3X4	T44.3X5	T44.3X6
Glycopyrronium	T44.3X1	T44.3X2	T44.3X3	T44.3X4	T44.3X5	T44.3X6
bromide	T44.3X1	T44.3X2	T44.3X3	T44.3X4	T44.3X5	T44.3X6
Glycoside, cardiac (stimulant)	T46.0X1	T46.0X2	T46.0X3	T46.0X4	T46.0X5	T46.0X6
Glycyclamide	T38.3X1	T38.3X2	T38.3X3	T38.3X4	T38.3X5	T38.3X6
Glycyrrhiza extract	T48.4X1	T48.4X2	T48.4X3	T48.4X4	T48.4X5	T48.4X6
Glycyrrhizic acid	T48.4X1	T48.4X2	T48.4X3	T48.4X4	T48.4X5	T48.4X6
Glycyrrhizinate potassium	T48.4X1	T48.4X2	T48.4X3	T48.4X4	T48.4X5	T48.4X6
Glymidine sodium	T38.3X1	T38.3X2	T38.3X3	T38.3X4	T38.3X5	T38.3X6
Glyphosate	T60.3X1	T60.3X2	T60.3X3	T60.3X4	—	—
Glyphylline	T48.6X1	T48.6X2	T48.6X3	T48.6X4	T48.6X5	T48.6X6
Gold						
colloidal (198Au)	T45.1X1	T45.1X2	T45.1X3	T45.1X4	T45.1X5	T45.1X6
salts	T39.4X1	T39.4X2	T39.4X3	T39.4X4	T39.4X5	T39.4X6
Golden sulfide of antimony	T56.891	T56.892	T56.893	T56.894	—	—
Goldylocks	T62.2X1	T62.2X2	T62.2X3	T62.2X4	—	—
Gonadal tissue extract	T38.901	T38.902	T38.903	T38.904	T38.905	T38.906
female	T38.5X1	T38.5X2	T38.5X3	T38.5X4	T38.5X5	T38.5X6
male	T38.7X1	T38.7X2	T38.7X3	T38.7X4	T38.7X5	T38.7X6
Gonadorelin	T38.891	T38.892	T38.893	T38.894	T38.895	T38.896
Gonadotropin	T38.891	T38.892	T38.893	T38.894	T38.895	T38.896
chorionic	T38.891	T38.892	T38.893	T38.894	T38.895	T38.896
pituitary	T38.811	T38.812	T38.813	T38.814	T38.815	T38.816
Goserelin	T45.1X1	T45.1X2	T45.1X3	T45.1X4	T45.1X5	T45.1X6
Grain alcohol	T51.0X1	T51.0X2	T51.0X3	T51.0X4	—	—
Gramicidin	T49.0X1	T49.0X2	T49.0X3	T49.0X4	T49.0X5	T49.0X6
Granisetron	T45.0X1	T45.0X2	T45.0X3	T45.0X4	T45.0X5	T45.0X6
Gratiola officinalis	T62.2X1	T62.2X2	T62.2X3	T62.2X4	—	—
Grease	T65.891	T65.892	T65.893	T65.894	—	—
Green hellebore	T62.2X1	T62.2X2	T62.2X3	T62.2X4	—	—
Green soap	T49.2X1	T49.2X2	T49.2X3	T49.2X4	T49.2X5	T49.2X6
Grifulvin	T36.7X1	T36.7X2	T36.7X3	T36.7X4	T36.7X5	T36.7X6
Griseofulvin	T36.7X1	T36.7X2	T36.7X3	T36.7X4	T36.7X5	T36.7X6
Growth hormone	T38.811	T38.812	T38.813	T38.814	T38.815	T38.816
Guaiacol derivatives	T48.4X1	T48.4X2	T48.4X3	T48.4X4	T48.4X5	T48.4X6
Guaiac reagent	T50.991	T50.992	T50.993	T50.994	T50.995	T50.996
Guaifenesin	T48.4X1	T48.4X2	T48.4X3	T48.4X4	T48.4X5	T48.4X6
Guaimesal	T48.4X1	T48.4X2	T48.4X3	T48.4X4	T48.4X5	T48.4X6
Guaiphenesin	T48.4X1	T48.4X2	T48.4X3	T48.4X4	T48.4X5	T48.4X6
Guamecycline	T36.4X1	T36.4X2	T36.4X3	T36.4X4	T36.4X5	T36.4X6

◄ New ◄ Revised ~~deleted~~ Deleted

Substance	Poisoning, Accidental (Unintentional)	Poisoning, Intentional Self-Harm	Poisoning, Assault	Poisoning, Undetermined	Adverse Effect	Underdosing
Guanabenz	T46.5X1	T46.5X2	T46.5X3	T46.5X4	T46.5X5	T46.5X6
Guanacline	T46.5X1	T46.5X2	T46.5X3	T46.5X4	T46.5X5	T46.5X6
Guanadrel	T46.5X1	T46.5X2	T46.5X3	T46.5X4	T46.5X5	T46.5X6
Guanatol	T37.2X1	T37.2X2	T37.2X3	T37.2X4	T37.2X5	T37.2X6
Guanethidine	T46.5X1	T46.5X2	T46.5X3	T46.5X4	T46.5X5	T46.5X6
Guanfacine	T46.5X1	T46.5X2	T46.5X3	T46.5X4	T46.5X5	T46.5X6
Guano	T65.891	T65.892	T65.893	T65.894	—	—
Guanochlor	T46.5X1	T46.5X2	T46.5X3	T46.5X4	T46.5X5	T46.5X6
Guanoclor	T46.5X1	T46.5X2	T46.5X3	T46.5X4	T46.5X5	T46.5X6
Guanoctine	T46.5X1	T46.5X2	T46.5X3	T46.5X4	T46.5X5	T46.5X6
Guanoxabenz	T46.5X1	T46.5X2	T46.5X3	T46.5X4	T46.5X5	T46.5X6
Guanoxan	T46.5X1	T46.5X2	T46.5X3	T46.5X4	T46.5X5	T46.5X6
Guar gum (medicinal)	T46.6X1	T46.6X2	T46.6X3	T46.6X4	T46.6X5	T46.6X6
H						
Hachimycin	T36.7X1	T36.7X2	T36.7X3	T36.7X4	T36.7X5	T36.7X6
Hair						
dye	T49.4X1	T49.4X2	T49.4X3	T49.4X4	T49.4X5	T49.4X6
preparation NEC	T49.4X1	T49.4X2	T49.4X3	T49.4X4	T49.4X5	T49.4X6
Halazepam	T42.4X1	T42.4X2	T42.4X3	T42.4X4	T42.4X5	T42.4X6
Halcinolone	T49.0X1	T49.0X2	T49.0X3	T49.0X4	T49.0X5	T49.0X6
Halcinonide	T49.0X1	T49.0X2	T49.0X3	T49.0X4	T49.0X5	T49.0X6
Halethazole	T49.0X1	T49.0X2	T49.0X3	T49.0X4	T49.0X5	T49.0X6
Hallucinogen NEC	T40.901	T40.902	T40.903	T40.904	T40.905	T40.906
Halofantrine	T37.2X1	T37.2X2	T37.2X2	T37.2X4	T37.2X5	T37.2X6
Halofenate	T46.6X1	T46.6X2	T46.6X3	T46.6X4	T46.6X5	T46.6X6
Halometasone	T49.0X1	T49.0X2	T49.0X3	T49.0X4	T49.0X5	T49.0X6
Haloperidol	T43.4X1	T43.4X2	T43.4X3	T43.4X4	T43.4X5	T43.4X6
Haloprogin	T49.0X1	T49.0X2	T49.0X3	T49.0X4	T49.0X5	T49.0X6
Halotex	T49.0X1	T49.0X2	T49.0X3	T49.0X4	T49.0X5	T49.0X6
Halothane	T41.0X1	T41.0X2	T41.0X3	T41.0X4	T41.0X5	T41.0X6
Haloxazolam	T42.4X1	T42.4X2	T42.4X3	T42.4X4	T42.4X5	T42.4X6
Halquinols	T49.0X1	T49.0X2	T49.0X3	T49.0X4	T49.0X5	T49.0X6
Hamamelis	T49.2X1	T49.2X2	T49.2X3	T49.2X4	T49.2X5	T49.2X6
Haptendextran	T45.8X1	T45.8X2	T45.8X3	T45.8X4	T45.8X5	T45.8X6
Harmonyl	T46.5X1	T46.5X2	T46.5X3	T46.5X4	T46.5X5	T46.5X6
Hartmann's solution	T50.3X1	T50.3X2	T50.3X3	T50.3X4	T50.3X5	T50.3X6
Hashish	T40.7X1	T40.7X2	T40.7X3	T40.7X4	T40.7X5	T40.7X6
Hawaiian Woodrose seeds	T40.991	T40.992	T40.993	T40.994	—	—
HCB	T60.3X1	T60.3X2	T60.3X3	T60.3X4	—	—
HCH	T53.6X1	T53.6X2	T53.6X3	T53.6X4	—	—
medicinal	T49.0X1	T49.0X2	T49.0X3	T49.0X4	T49.0X5	T49.0X6

Substance	Poisoning, Accidental (Unintentional)	Poisoning, Intentional Self-Harm	Poisoning, Assault	Poisoning, Undetermined	Adverse Effect	Underdosing
HCN	T57.3X1	T57.3X2	T57.3X3	T57.3X4	—	—
Headache cures, drugs, powders NEC	T50.901	T50.902	T50.903	T50.904	T50.905	T50.906
Heavenly Blue (morning glory)	T40.991	T40.992	T40.993	T40.994	—	—
Heavy metal antidote	T45.8X1	T45.8X2	T45.8X3	T45.8X4	T45.8X5	T45.8X6
Hedaquinium	T49.0X1	T49.0X2	T49.0X3	T49.0X4	T49.0X5	T49.0X6
Hedge hyssop	T62.2X1	T62.2X2	T62.2X3	T62.2X4	—	—
Heet	T49.8X1	T49.8X2	T49.8X3	T49.8X4	T49.8X5	T49.8X6
Helium	T48.991	T48.992	T48.993	T48.994	T48.995	T48.996
Helenin	T37.4X1	T37.4X2	T37.4X3	T37.4X4	T37.4X5	T37.4X6
Hellebore (black) (green) (white)	T62.2X1	T62.2X2	T62.2X3	T62.2X4	—	—
Helium (nonmedicinal) NEC	T59.891	T59.892	T59.893	T59.894	—	—
medicinal	T48.991	T48.992	T48.993	T48.994	T48.995	T48.996
Hematin	T45.8X1	T45.8X2	T45.8X3	T45.8X4	T45.8X5	T45.8X6
Hematinic preparation	T45.8X1	T45.8X2	T45.8X3	T45.8X4	T45.8X5	T45.8X6
Hemlock	T62.2X1	T62.2X2	T62.2X3	T62.2X4	—	—
Hemostatic	T45.621	T45.622	T45.623	T45.624	T45.625	T45.626
drug, systemic	T45.621	T45.622	T45.623	T45.624	T45.625	T45.626
Hemostyptic	T49.4X1	T49.4X2	T49.4X3	T49.4X4	T49.4X5	T49.4X6
Henbane	T62.2X1	T62.2X2	T62.2X3	T62.2X4	—	—
Heparin (sodium)	T45.511	T45.512	T45.513	T45.514	T45.515	T45.516
action reverser	T45.7X1	T45.7X2	T45.7X3	T45.7X4	T45.7X5	T45.7X6
Heparin-fraction	T45.511	T45.512	T45.513	T45.514	T45.515	T45.516
Heparinoid (systemic)	T45.511	T45.512	T45.513	T45.514	T45.515	T45.516
Hepatic secretion stimulant	T47.8X1	T47.8X2	T47.8X3	T47.8X4	T47.8X5	T47.8X6
Hepatitis B						
immune globulin	T50.Z11	T50.Z12	T50.Z13	T50.Z14	T50.Z15	T50.Z16
vaccine	T50.B91	T50.B92	T50.B93	T50.B94	T50.B95	T50.B96
Hepronicate	T46.7X1	T46.7X2	T46.7X3	T46.7X4	T46.7X5	T46.7X6
Heptabarb	T42.3X1	T42.3X2	T42.3X3	T42.3X4	T42.3X5	T42.3X6
Heptabarbitone	T42.3X1	T42.3X2	T42.3X3	T42.3X4	T42.3X5	T42.3X6
Heptabarbital	T42.3X1	T42.3X2	T42.3X3	T42.3X4	T42.3X5	T42.3X6
Heptachlor	T60.1X1	T60.1X2	T60.1X3	T60.1X4	—	—
Heptalgin	T40.2X1	T40.2X2	T40.2X3	T40.2X4	T40.2X5	T40.2X6
Heptaminol	T46.3X1	T46.3X2	T46.3X3	T46.3X4	T46.3X5	T46.3X6
Herbicide NEC	T60.3X1	T60.3X2	T60.3X3	T60.3X4	—	—
Heroin	T40.1X1	T40.1X2	T40.1X3	T40.1X4	—	—
Herplex	T49.5X1	T49.5X2	T49.5X3	T49.5X4	T49.5X5	T49.5X6
HES	T45.8X1	T45.8X2	T45.8X3	T45.8X4	T45.8X5	T45.8X6
Hesperidin	T46.991	T46.992	T46.993	T46.994	T46.995	T46.996
Hetacillin	T36.0X1	T36.0X2	T36.0X3	T36.0X4	T36.0X5	T36.0X6

TABLE OF DRUGS AND CHEMICALS

TABLE OF DRUGS AND CHEMICALS

Substance	External Cause (T-Code)					
	Poisoning, Accidental (Unintentional)	Poisoning, Intentional Self-Harm	Poisoning, Assault	Poisoning, Undetermined	Adverse Effect	Underdosing
Hetastarch	T45.8X1	T45.8X2	T45.8X3	T45.8X4	T45.8X5	T45.8X6
HETP	T60.0X1	T60.0X2	T60.0X3	T60.0X4	—	—
Hexachlorobenzene (vapor)	T60.3X1	T60.3X2	T60.3X3	T60.3X4	—	—
Hexachlorocyclohexane	T53.6X1	T53.6X2	T53.6X3	T53.6X4	—	—
Hexachlorophene	T49.0X1	T49.0X2	T49.0X3	T49.0X4	T49.0X5	T49.0X6
Hexadiline	T46.3X1	T46.3X2	T46.3X3	T46.3X4	T46.3X5	T46.3X6
Hexadimethrine (bromide)	T45.7X1	T45.7X2	T45.7X3	T45.7X4	T45.7X5	T45.7X6
Hexadylamine	T46.3X1	T46.3X2	T46.3X3	T46.3X4	T46.3X5	T46.3X6
Hexaethyl tetraphosphate	T60.0X1	T60.0X2	T60.0X3	T60.0X4	—	—
Hexafluorenium bromide	T48.1X1	T48.1X2	T48.1X3	T48.1X4	T48.1X5	T48.1X6
Hexafluorodiethyl ether	T43.291	T43.292	T43.293	T43.294	T43.295	T43.296
Hexafluronium (bromide)	T48.1X1	T48.1X2	T48.1X3	T48.1X4	T48.1X5	T48.1X6
Hexahydrobenzol	T52.8X1	T52.8X2	T52.8X3	T52.8X4	—	—
Hexahydrocresol(s)	T51.8X1	T51.8X2	T51.8X3	T51.8X4	—	—
arsenide	T57.0X1	T57.0X2	T57.0X3	T57.0X4	—	—
arseniurated	T57.0X1	T57.0X2	T57.0X3	T57.0X4	—	—
cyanide	T57.3X1	T57.3X2	T57.3X3	T57.3X4	—	—
gas	T59.891	T59.892	T59.893	T59.894	—	—
Fluoride (liquid)	T57.8X1	T57.8X2	T57.8X3	T57.8X4	—	—
vapor	T59.891	T59.892	T59.893	T59.894	—	—
phophorated	T60.0X1	T60.0X2	T60.0X3	T60.0X4	—	—
sulfate	T57.8X1	T57.8X2	T57.8X3	T57.8X4	—	—
sulfide (gas)	T59.6X1	T59.6X2	T59.6X3	T59.6X4	—	—
arseniurated	T57.0X1	T57.0X2	T57.0X3	T57.0X4	—	—
sulfurated	T57.8X1	T57.8X2	T57.8X3	T57.8X4	—	—
Hexahydrophenol	T51.8X1	T51.8X2	T51.8X3	T51.8X4	—	—
Hexa-germ	T49.2X1	T49.2X2	T49.2X3	T49.2X4	T49.2X5	T49.2X6
Hexalen	T51.8X1	T51.8X2	T51.8X3	T51.8X4	—	—
Hexamethonium bromide	T44.2X1	T44.2X2	T44.2X3	T44.2X4	T44.2X5	T44.2X6
Hexamethylene	T52.8X1	T52.8X2	T52.8X3	T52.8X4	—	—
Hexamethylmelamine	T45.1X1	T45.1X2	T45.1X3	T45.1X4	T45.1X5	T45.1X6
Hexamidine	T49.0X1	T49.0X2	T49.0X3	T49.0X4	T49.0X5	T49.0X6
Hexamine (mandelate)	T37.8X1	T37.8X2	T37.8X3	T37.8X4	T37.8X5	T37.8X6
Hexanone, 2-hexanone	T52.4X1	T52.4X2	T52.4X3	T52.4X4	—	—
Hexanuorenium	T48.1X1	T48.1X2	T48.1X3	T48.1X4	T48.1X5	T48.1X6
Hexapropymate	T42.6X1	T42.6X2	T42.6X3	T42.6X4	T42.6X5	T42.6X6
Hexasonium iodide	T44.3X1	T44.3X2	T44.3X3	T44.3X4	T44.3X5	T44.3X6
Hexcarbacholine bromide	T48.1X1	T48.1X2	T48.1X3	T48.1X4	T48.1X5	T48.1X6
Hexemal	T42.3X1	T42.3X2	T42.3X3	T42.3X4	T42.3X5	T42.3X6
Hexestrol	T38.5X1	T38.5X2	T38.5X3	T38.5X4	T38.5X5	T38.5X6
Hexethal (sodium)	T42.3X1	T42.3X2	T42.3X3	T42.3X4	T42.3X5	T42.3X6
Hexetidine	T37.8X1	T37.8X2	T37.8X3	T37.8X4	T37.8X5	T37.8X6

Substance	External Cause (T-Code)					
	Poisoning, Accidental (Unintentional)	Poisoning, Intentional Self-Harm	Poisoning, Assault	Poisoning, Undetermined	Adverse Effect	Underdosing
Hexobarbital	T42.3X1	T42.3X2	T42.3X3	T42.3X4	T42.3X5	T42.3X6
rectal	T41.291	T41.292	T41.293	T41.294	T41.295	T41.296
sodium	T41.1X1	T41.1X2	T41.1X3	T41.1X4	T41.1X5	T41.1X6
Hexobendine	T46.3X1	T46.3X2	T46.3X3	T46.3X4	T46.3X5	T46.3X6
Hexocyclium	T44.3X1	T44.3X2	T44.3X3	T44.3X4	T44.3X5	T44.3X6
metilsulfate	T44.3X1	T44.3X2	T44.3X3	T44.3X4	T44.3X5	T44.3X6
Hexoestrol	T38.5X1	T38.5X2	T38.5X3	T38.5X4	T38.5X5	T38.5X6
Hexone	T52.4X1	T52.4X2	T52.4X3	T52.4X4	—	—
Hexoprenaline	T48.6X1	T48.6X2	T48.6X3	T48.6X4	T48.6X5	T48.6X6
Hexylcaine	T41.3X1	T41.3X2	T41.3X3	T41.3X4	T41.3X5	T41.3X6
Hexylresorcinol	T52.2X1	T52.2X2	T52.2X3	T52.2X4	—	—
HGH (human growth hormone)	T38.811	T38.812	T38.813	T38.814	T38.815	T38.816
Hinkle's pills	T47.2X1	T47.2X2	T47.2X3	T47.2X4	T47.2X5	T47.2X6
Histalog	T50.8X1	T50.8X2	T50.8X3	T50.8X4	T50.8X5	T50.8X6
Histamine (phosphate)	T50.8X1	T50.8X2	T50.8X3	T50.8X4	T50.8X5	T50.8X6
Histoplasmin	T50.8X1	T50.8X2	T50.8X3	T50.8X4	T50.8X5	T50.8X6
Holly berries	T62.2X1	T62.2X2	T62.2X3	T62.2X4	—	—
Homatropine	T44.3X1	T44.3X2	T44.3X3	T44.3X4	T44.3X5	T44.3X6
methylbromide	T44.3X1	T44.3X2	T44.3X3	T44.3X4	T44.3X5	T44.3X6
Homochlorcyclizine	T45.0X1	T45.0X2	T45.0X3	T45.0X4	T45.0X5	T45.0X6
Homosalate	T49.3X1	T49.3X2	T49.3X3	T49.3X4	T49.3X5	T49.3X6
Homo-tet	T50.Z11	T50.Z12	T50.Z13	T50.Z14	T50.Z15	T50.Z16
Hormone	T38.801	T38.802	T38.803	T38.804	T38.805	T38.806
adrenal cortical steroids	T38.0X1	T38.0X2	T38.0X3	T38.0X4	T38.0X5	T38.0X6
androgenic	T38.7X1	T38.7X2	T38.7X3	T38.7X4	T38.7X5	T38.7X6
anterior pituitary NEC	T38.811	T38.812	T38.813	T38.814	T38.815	T38.816
antidiabetic agents	T38.3X1	T38.3X2	T38.3X3	T38.3X4	T38.3X5	T38.3X6
antidiuretic	T38.891	T38.892	T38.893	T38.894	T38.895	T38.896
cancer therapy	T45.1X1	T45.1X2	T45.1X3	T45.1X4	T45.1X5	T45.1X6
follicle stimulating	T38.811	T38.812	T38.813	T38.814	T38.815	T38.816
gonadotropic	T38.891	T38.892	T38.893	T38.894	T38.895	T38.896
pituitary	T38.811	T38.812	T38.813	T38.814	T38.815	T38.816
growth	T38.811	T38.812	T38.813	T38.814	T38.815	T38.816
luteinizing	T38.811	T38.812	T38.813	T38.814	T38.815	T38.816
ovarian	T38.5X1	T38.5X2	T38.5X3	T38.5X4	T38.5X5	T38.5X6
oxytocic	T48.0X1	T48.0X2	T48.0X3	T48.0X4	T48.0X5	T48.0X6
parathyroid (derivatives)	T50.991	T50.992	T50.993	T50.994	T50.995	T50.996
pituitary (posterior) NEC	T38.891	T38.892	T38.893	T38.894	T38.895	T38.896
anterior	T38.811	T38.812	T38.813	T38.814	T38.815	T38.816
specified, NEC	T38.891	T38.892	T38.893	T38.894	T38.895	T38.896
thyroid	T38.1X1	T38.1X2	T38.1X3	T38.1X4	T38.1X5	T38.1X6
Hornet (sting)	T63.451	T63.452	T63.453	T63.454	—	—

◀ New ◀ Revised ~~deleted~~ Deleted

Substance	Poisoning, Accidental (Unintentional)	Poisoning, Intentional Self-Harm	Poisoning, Assault	Poisoning, Undetermined	Adverse Effect	Underdosing
Horse anti-human lymphocytic serum	T50.Z11	T50.Z12	T50.Z13	T50.Z14	T50.Z15	T50.Z16
Horticulture agent NEC	T65.91	T65.92	T65.93	T65.94	—	—
with pesticide	T60.91	T60.92	T60.93	T60.94	—	—
Human						
albumin	T45.8X1	T45.8X2	T45.8X3	T45.8X4	T45.8X5	T45.8X6
growth hormone (HGH)	T38.811	T38.812	T38.813	T38.814	T38.815	T38.816
immune serum	T50.Z11	T50.Z12	T50.Z13	T50.Z14	T50.Z15	T50.Z16
Hyaluronidase	T45.3X1	T45.3X2	T45.3X3	T45.3X4	T45.3X5	T45.3X6
Hyazyme	T45.3X1	T45.3X2	T45.3X3	T45.3X4	T45.3X5	T45.3X6
Hycodan	T40.2X1	T40.2X2	T40.2X3	T40.2X4	T40.2X5	T40.2X6
Hydantoin derivative NEC	T42.0X1	T42.0X2	T42.0X3	T42.0X4	T42.0X5	T42.0X6
Hydeltra	T38.0X1	T38.0X2	T38.0X3	T38.0X4	T38.0X5	T38.0X6
Hydergine	T44.6X1	T44.6X2	T44.6X3	T44.6X4	T44.6X5	T44.6X6
Hydrabamine penicillin	T36.0X1	T36.0X2	T36.0X3	T36.0X4	T36.0X5	T36.0X6
Hydralazine	T46.5X1	T46.5X2	T46.5X3	T46.5X4	T46.5X5	T46.5X6
Hydrargaphen	T49.0X1	T49.0X2	T49.0X3	T49.0X4	T49.0X5	T49.0X6
Hydrargyri amino-chloridum	T49.0X1	T49.0X2	T49.0X3	T49.0X4	T49.0X5	T49.0X6
Hydrastine	T48.291	T48.292	T48.293	T48.294	T48.295	T48.296
Hydrazine	T54.1X1	T54.1X2	T54.1X3	T54.1X4	—	—
monoamine oxidase inhibitors	T43.1X1	T43.1X2	T43.1X3	T43.1X4	T43.1X5	T43.1X6
Hydrazoic acid, azides	T54.2X1	T54.2X2	T54.2X3	T54.2X4	—	—
Hydriodic acid	T48.4X1	T48.4X2	T48.4X3	T48.4X4	T48.4X5	T48.4X6
Hydrocarbon gas	T59.891	T59.892	T59.893	T59.894	—	—
incomplete combustion of — see Carbon, monoxide, fuel, utility						
liquefied (mobile container)	T59.891	T59.892	T59.893	T59.894	—	—
piped (natural)	T59.891	T59.892	T59.893	T59.894	—	—
Hydrochloric acid (liquid)	T54.2X1	T54.2X2	T54.2X3	T54.2X4	—	—
medicinal (digestant)	T47.5X1	T47.5X2	T47.5X3	T47.5X4	T47.5X5	T47.5X6
vapor	T59.891	T59.892	T59.893	T59.894	—	—
Hydrochlorothiazide	T50.2X1	T50.2X2	T50.2X3	T50.2X4	T50.2X5	T50.2X6
Hydrocodone	T40.2X1	T40.2X2	T40.2X3	T40.2X4	T40.2X5	T40.2X6
Hydrocortisone (derivatives)	T38.0X1	T38.0X2	T38.0X3	T38.0X4	T38.0X5	T38.0X6
aceponate	T49.0X1	T49.0X2	T49.0X3	T49.0X4	T49.0X5	T49.0X6
ENT agent	T49.6X1	T49.6X2	T49.6X3	T49.6X4	T49.6X5	T49.6X6
ophthalmic preparation	T49.5X1	T49.5X2	T49.5X3	T49.5X4	T49.5X5	T49.5X6
topical NEC	T49.0X1	T49.0X2	T49.0X3	T49.0X4	T49.0X5	T49.0X6
Hydrocortone	T38.0X1	T38.0X2	T38.0X3	T38.0X4	T38.0X5	T38.0X6
ENT agent	T49.6X1	T49.6X2	T49.6X3	T49.6X4	T49.6X5	T49.6X6
ophthalmic preparation	T49.5X1	T49.5X2	T49.5X3	T49.5X4	T49.5X5	T49.5X6
topical NEC	T49.0X1	T49.0X2	T49.0X3	T49.0X4	T49.0X5	T49.0X6

Substance	Poisoning, Accidental (Unintentional)	Poisoning, Intentional Self-Harm	Poisoning, Assault	Poisoning, Undetermined	Adverse Effect	Underdosing
Hydrocyanic acid (liquid)	T57.3X1	T57.3X2	T57.3X3	T57.3X4	—	—
gas	T65.0X1	T65.0X2	T65.0X3	T65.0X4	—	—
Hydroflumethiazide	T50.2X1	T50.2X2	T50.2X3	T50.2X4	T50.2X5	T50.2X6
Hydrofluoric acid (liquid)	T54.2X1	T54.2X2	T54.2X3	T54.2X4	—	—
vapor	T59.891	T59.892	T59.893	T59.894	—	—
Hydrogen	T59.891	T59.892	T59.893	T59.894	—	—
arsenide	T57.0X1	T57.0X2	T57.0X3	T57.0X4	—	—
arseniureted	T57.0X1	T57.0X2	T57.0X3	T57.0X4	—	—
chloride	T57.8X1	T57.8X2	T57.8X3	T57.8X4	—	—
cyanide (salts)	T57.3X1	T57.3X2	T57.3X3	T57.3X4	—	—
gas	T57.3X1	T57.3X2	T57.3X3	T57.3X4	—	—
Fluoride	T59.5X1	T59.5X2	T59.5X3	T59.5X4	—	—
vapor	T59.5X1	T59.5X2	T59.5X3	T59.5X4	—	—
peroxide	T49.0X1	T49.0X2	T49.0X3	T49.0X4	T49.0X5	T49.0X6
phosphureted	T57.1X1	T57.1X2	T57.1X3	T57.1X4	—	—
sulfide	T59.6X1	T59.6X2	T59.6X3	T59.6X4	—	—
arseniureted	T57.0X1	T57.0X2	T57.0X3	T57.0X4	—	—
sulfureted	T59.6X1	T59.6X2	T59.6X3	T59.6X4	—	—
Hydromethylpyridine	T46.7X1	T46.7X2	T46.7X3	T46.7X4	T46.7X5	T46.7X6
Hydromorphinol	T40.2X1	T40.2X2	T40.2X3	T40.2X4	—	—
Hydromorphinone	T40.2X1	T40.2X2	T40.2X3	T40.2X4	T40.2X5	T40.2X6
Hydromorphone	T40.2X1	T40.2X2	T40.2X3	T40.2X4	T40.2X5	T40.2X6
Hydromox	T50.2X1	T50.2X2	T50.2X3	T50.2X4	T50.2X5	T50.2X6
Hydrophilic lotion	T49.3X1	T49.3X2	T49.3X3	T49.3X4	T49.3X5	T49.3X6
Hydroquinidine	T46.2X1	T46.2X2	T46.2X3	T46.2X4	T46.2X5	T46.2X6
Hydroquinone	T52.2X1	T52.2X2	T52.2X3	T52.2X4	—	—
vapor	T59.891	T59.892	T59.893	T59.894	—	—
Hydrosulfuric acid (gas)	T59.6X1	T59.6X2	T59.6X3	T59.6X4	—	—
Hydrotalcite	T47.1X1	T47.1X2	T47.1X3	T47.1X4	T47.1X5	T47.1X6
Hydrous wool fat	T49.3X1	T49.3X2	T49.3X3	T49.3X4	T49.3X5	T49.3X6
Hydroxide, caustic	T54.3X1	T54.3X2	T54.3X3	T54.3X4	—	—
Hydroxocobalamin	T45.8X1	T45.8X2	T45.8X3	T45.8X4	T45.8X5	T45.8X6
Hydroxyamphetamine	T49.5X1	T49.5X2	T49.5X3	T49.5X4	T49.5X5	T49.5X6
Hydroxycarbamide	T45.1X1	T45.1X2	T45.1X3	T45.1X4	T45.1X5	T45.1X6
Hydroxychloroquine	T37.8X1	T37.8X2	T37.8X3	T37.8X4	T37.8X5	T37.8X6
Hydroxydihydrocodeinone	T40.2X1	T40.2X2	T40.2X3	T40.2X4	T40.2X5	T40.2X6
Hydroxyestrone	T38.5X1	T38.5X2	T38.5X3	T38.5X4	T38.5X5	T38.5X6
Hydroxyethyl starch	T45.8X1	T45.8X2	T45.8X3	T45.8X4	T45.8X5	T45.8X6
Hydroxymethylpentanone	T52.4X1	T52.4X2	T52.4X3	T52.4X4	—	—
Hydroxyphenamate	T43.591	T43.592	T43.593	T43.594	T43.595	T43.596
Hydroxyphenylbutazone	T39.2X1	T39.2X2	T39.2X3	T39.2X4	T39.2X5	T39.2X6

TABLE OF DRUGS AND CHEMICALS

TABLE OF DRUGS AND CHEMICALS

Substance	Poisoning, Accidental (Unintentional)	Poisoning, Intentional Self-Harm	Poisoning, Assault	Poisoning, Undetermined	Adverse Effect	Underdosing
Hydroxyprogesterone	T38.5X1	T38.5X2	T38.5X3	T38.5X4	T38.5X5	T38.5X6
caproate	T38.5X1	T38.5X2	T38.5X3	T38.5X4	T38.5X5	T38.5X6
Hydroxyquinoline (derivatives) NEC	T37.8X1	T37.8X2	T37.8X3	T37.8X4	T37.8X5	T37.8X6
Hydroxystilbamidine	T37.3X1	T37.3X2	T37.3X3	T37.3X4	T37.3X5	T37.3X6
Hydroxytoluene (nonmedicinal)	T54.0X1	T54.0X2	T54.0X3	T54.0X4	—	—
medicinal	T49.0X1	T49.0X2	T49.0X3	T49.0X4	T49.0X5	T49.0X6
Hydroxyurea	T45.1X1	T45.1X2	T45.1X3	T45.1X4	T45.1X5	T45.1X6
Hydroxyzine	T43.591	T43.592	T43.593	T43.594	T43.595	T43.596
Hyoscine	T44.3X1	T44.3X2	T44.3X3	T44.3X4	T44.3X5	T44.3X6
Hyoscyamine	T44.3X1	T44.3X2	T44.3X3	T44.3X4	T44.3X5	T44.3X6
Hyoscyamus	T44.3X1	T44.3X2	T44.3X3	T44.3X4	T44.3X5	T44.3X6
dry extract	T44.3X1	T44.3X2	T44.3X3	T44.3X4	T44.3X5	T44.3X6
Hypaque	T50.8X1	T50.8X2	T50.8X3	T50.8X4	T50.8X5	T50.8X6
Hypertussis	T50.Z11	T50.Z12	T50.Z13	T50.Z14	T50.Z15	T50.Z16
Hypnotic	T42.71	T42.72	T42.73	T42.74	T42.75	T42.76
anticonvulsant	T42.71	T42.72	T42.73	T42.74	T42.75	T42.76
specified NEC	T42.6X1	T42.6X2	T42.6X3	T42.6X4	T42.6X5	T42.6X6
Hypochlorite	T49.0X1	T49.0X2	T49.0X3	T49.0X4	T49.0X5	T49.0X6
Hypophysis, posterior	T38.891	T38.892	T38.893	T38.894	T38.895	T38.896
Hypotensive NEC	T46.5X1	T46.5X2	T46.5X3	T46.5X4	T46.5X5	T46.5X6
Hypromellose	T49.5X1	T49.5X2	T49.5X3	T49.5X4	T49.5X5	T49.5X6

I

Substance	Poisoning, Accidental (Unintentional)	Poisoning, Intentional Self-Harm	Poisoning, Assault	Poisoning, Undetermined	Adverse Effect	Underdosing
Ibacitabine	T37.5X1	T37.5X2	T37.5X3	T37.5X4	T37.5X5	T37.5X6
Ibopamine	T44.991	T44.992	T44.993	T44.994	T44.995	T44.996
Ibufenac	T39.311	T39.312	T39.313	T39.314	T39.315	T39.316
Ibuprofen	T39.311	T39.312	T39.313	T39.314	T39.315	T39.316
Ibuproxam	T39.311	T39.312	T39.313	T39.314	T39.315	T39.316
Ibuterol	T48.6X1	T48.6X2	T48.6X3	T48.6X4	T48.6X5	T48.6X6
Ichthammol	T49.0X1	T49.0X2	T49.0X3	T49.0X4	T49.0X5	T49.0X6
Ichthyol	T49.4X1	T49.4X2	T49.4X3	T49.4X4	T49.4X5	T49.4X6
Idarubicin	T45.1X1	T45.1X2	T45.1X3	T45.1X4	T45.1X5	T45.1X6
Idrocilamide	T42.8X1	T42.8X2	T42.8X3	T42.8X4	T42.8X5	T42.8X6
Ifenprodil	T46.7X1	T46.7X2	T46.7X3	T46.7X4	T46.7X5	T46.7X6
Ifosfamide	T45.1X1	T45.1X2	T45.1X3	T45.1X4	T45.1X5	T45.1X6
Iletin	T38.3X1	T38.3X2	T38.3X3	T38.3X4	T38.3X5	T38.3X6
Ilex	T62.2X1	T62.2X2	T62.2X3	T62.2X4	—	—
Illuminating gas (after combustion)	T58.11	T58.12	T58.13	T58.14	—	—
prior to combustion	T59.891	T59.892	T59.893	T59.894	—	—
Ilopan	T45.2X1	T45.2X2	T45.2X3	T45.2X4	T45.2X5	T45.2X6
Iloprost	T46.7X1	T46.7X2	T46.7X3	T46.7X4	T46.7X5	T46.7X6

Substance	Poisoning, Accidental (Unintentional)	Poisoning, Intentional Self-Harm	Poisoning, Assault	Poisoning, Undetermined	Adverse Effect	Underdosing
Ilotycin	T36.3X1	T36.3X2	T36.3X3	T36.3X4	T36.3X5	T36.3X6
ophthalmic preparation	T49.5X1	T49.5X2	T49.5X3	T49.5X4	T49.5X5	T49.5X6
topical NEC	T49.0X1	T49.0X2	T49.0X3	T49.0X4	T49.0X5	T49.0X6
Imidazole-4-carboxamide	T45.1X1	T45.1X2	T45.1X3	T45.1X4	T45.1X5	T45.1X6
Imipenem	T36.0X1	T36.0X2	T36.0X3	T36.0X4	T36.0X5	T36.0X6
Imipramine	T43.011	T43.012	T43.013	T43.014	T43.015	T43.016
Iminostilbene	T42.1X1	T42.1X2	T42.1X3	T42.1X4	T42.1X5	T42.1X6
Immu-G	T50.Z11	T50.Z12	T50.Z13	T50.Z14	T50.Z15	T50.Z16
Immuglobin	T50.Z11	T50.Z12	T50.Z13	T50.Z14	T50.Z15	T50.Z16
Immune						
globulin	T50.Z11	T50.Z12	T50.Z13	T50.Z14	T50.Z15	T50.Z16
serum globulin	T50.Z11	T50.Z12	T50.Z13	T50.Z14	T50.Z15	T50.Z16
Immunoglobin human (intravenous) (normal)	T50.Z11	T50.Z12	T50.Z13	T50.Z14	T50.Z15	T50.Z16
unmodified	T50.Z11	T50.Z12	T50.Z13	T50.Z14	T50.Z15	T50.Z16
Immunosuppressive drug	T45.1X1	T45.1X2	T45.1X3	T45.1X4	T45.1X5	T45.1X6
Immu-tetanus	T50.Z11	T50.Z12	T50.Z13	T50.Z14	T50.Z15	T50.Z16
Indalpine	T43.221	T43.222	T43.223	T43.224	T43.225	T43.226
Indanazoline	T48.5X1	T48.5X2	T48.5X3	T48.5X4	T48.5X5	T48.5X6
Indandione (derivatives)	T45.511	T45.512	T45.513	T45.514	T45.515	T45.516
Indapamide	T46.5X1	T46.5X2	T46.5X3	T46.5X4	T46.5X5	T46.5X6
Indendione (derivatives)	T45.511	T45.512	T45.513	T45.514	T45.515	T45.516
Indenolol	T44.7X1	T44.7X2	T44.7X3	T44.7X4	T44.7X5	T44.7X6
Inderal	T44.7X1	T44.7X2	T44.7X3	T44.7X4	T44.7X5	T44.7X6
Indian						
hemp	T40.7X1	T40.7X2	T40.7X3	T40.7X4	T40.7X5	T40.7X6
tobacco	T62.2X1	T62.2X2	T62.2X3	T62.2X4	—	—
Indigo carmine	T50.8X1	T50.8X2	T50.8X3	T50.8X4	T50.8X5	T50.8X6
Indobufen	T45.521	T45.522	T45.523	T45.524	T45.525	T45.526
Indocin	T39.2X1	T39.2X2	T39.2X3	T39.2X4	T39.2X5	T39.2X6
Indocyanine green	T50.8X1	T50.8X2	T50.8X3	T50.8X4	T50.8X5	T50.8X6
Indometacin	T39.391	T39.392	T39.393	T39.394	T39.395	T39.396
Indomethacin	T39.391	T39.392	T39.393	T39.394	T39.395	T39.396
farnesil	T39.4X1	T39.4X2	T39.4X3	T39.4X4	T39.4X5	T39.4X6
Indoramin	T44.6X1	T44.6X2	T44.6X3	T44.6X4	T44.6X5	T44.6X6
Industrial						
alcohol	T51.0X1	T51.0X2	T51.0X3	T51.0X4	—	—
fumes	T59.891	T59.892	T59.893	T59.894	—	—
solvents (fumes) (vapors)	T52.91	T52.92	T52.93	T52.94	—	—
Influenza vaccine	T50.B91	T50.B92	T50.B93	T50.B94	T50.B95	T50.B96
Ingested substance NEC	T65.91	T65.92	T65.93	T65.94	—	—
INH	T37.1X1	T37.1X2	T37.1X3	T37.1X4	T37.1X5	T37.1X6

◀ New   ◀ Revised   ~~deleted~~ Deleted

Substance	Poisoning, Accidental (Unintentional)	Poisoning, Intentional Self-Harm	Poisoning, Assault	Poisoning, Undetermined	Adverse Effect	Underdosing
Inhalation, gas (noxious) — see Gas						
Inhibitor						
angiotensin-converting enzyme	T46.4X1	T46.4X2	T46.4X3	T46.4X4	T46.4X5	T46.4X6
carbonic anhydrase	T50.2X1	T50.2X2	T50.2X3	T50.2X4	T50.2X5	T50.2X6
fibrinolysis	T45.621	T45.622	T45.623	T45.624	T45.625	T45.626
monoamine oxidase NEC	T43.1X1	T43.1X2	T43.1X3	T43.1X4	T43.1X5	T43.1X6
hydrazine	T43.1X1	T43.1X2	T43.1X3	T43.1X4	T43.1X5	T43.1X6
postsynaptic	T43.8X1	T43.8X2	T43.8X3	T43.8X4	T43.8X5	T43.8X6
prothrombin synthesis	T45.511	T45.512	T45.513	T45.514	T45.515	T45.516
Ink	T65.891	T65.892	T65.893	T65.894	—	—
Inorganic substance NEC	T57.91	T57.92	T57.93	T57.94	—	—
Inosine pranobex	T37.5X1	T37.5X2	T37.5X3	T37.5X4	T37.5X5	T37.5X6
Inositol	T50.991	T50.992	T50.993	T50.994	T50.995	T50.996
nicotinate	T46.7X1	T46.7X2	T46.7X3	T46.7X4	T46.7X5	T46.7X6
Inproquone	T45.1X1	T45.1X2	T45.1X3	T45.1X4	T45.1X5	T45.1X6
Insect (sting), venomous	T63.481	T63.482	T63.483	T63.484	—	—
ant	T63.421	T63.422	T63.423	T63.424	—	—
bee	T63.441	T63.442	T63.443	T63.444	—	—
caterpillar	T63.431	T63.432	T63.433	T63.434	—	—
hornet	T63.451	T63.452	T63.453	T63.454	—	—
wasp	T63.461	T63.462	T63.463	T63.464	—	—
Insecticide NEC	T60.91	T60.92	T60.93	T60.94	—	—
carbamate	T60.0X1	T60.0X2	T60.0X3	T60.0X4	—	—
chlorinated	T60.1X1	T60.1X2	T60.1X3	T60.1X4	—	—
mixed	T60.91	T60.92	T60.93	T60.94	—	—
organochlorine	T60.1X1	T60.1X2	T60.1X3	T60.1X4	—	—
organophosphorus	T60.0X1	T60.0X2	T60.0X3	T60.0X4	—	—
Insular tissue extract	T38.3X1	T38.3X2	T38.3X3	T38.3X4	T38.3X5	T38.3X6
Insulin (amorphous) (globin) (isophane) (Lente) (NPH) (Semilente) (Ultralente)	T38.3X1	T38.3X2	T38.3X3	T38.3X4	T38.3X5	T38.3X6
defalan	T38.3X1	T38.3X2	T38.3X3	T38.3X4	T38.3X5	T38.3X6
human	T38.3X1	T38.3X2	T38.3X3	T38.3X4	T38.3X5	T38.3X6
injection, soluble	T38.3X1	T38.3X2	T38.3X3	T38.3X4	T38.3X5	T38.3X6
biphasic	T38.3X1	T38.3X2	T38.3X3	T38.3X4	T38.3X5	T38.3X6
intermediate acting	T38.3X1	T38.3X2	T38.3X3	T38.3X4	T38.3X5	T38.3X6
protamine zinc	T38.3X1	T38.3X2	T38.3X3	T38.3X4	T38.3X5	T38.3X6
slow acting	T38.3X1	T38.3X2	T38.3X3	T38.3X4	T38.3X5	T38.3X6
zinc						
protamine injection	T38.3X1	T38.3X2	T38.3X3	T38.3X4	T38.3X5	T38.3X6
suspension (amorphous) (crystalline)	T38.3X1	T38.3X2	T38.3X3	T38.3X4	T38.3X5	T38.3X6

Substance	Poisoning, Accidental (Unintentional)	Poisoning, Intentional Self-Harm	Poisoning, Assault	Poisoning, Undetermined	Adverse Effect	Underdosing
Interferon (alpha) (beta) (gamma)	T37.5X1	T37.5X2	T37.5X3	T37.5X4	T37.5X5	T37.5X6
Intestinal motility control drug	T47.6X1	T47.6X2	T47.6X3	T47.6X4	T47.6X5	T47.6X6
biological	T47.8X1	T47.8X2	T47.8X3	T47.8X4	T47.8X5	T47.8X6
Intranarcon	T41.1X1	T41.1X2	T41.1X3	T41.1X4	T41.1X5	T41.1X6
Intravenous						
amino acids	T50.991	T50.992	T50.993	T50.994	T50.995	T50.996
fat suspension	T50.991	T50.992	T50.993	T50.994	T50.995	T50.996
Inulin	T50.8X1	T50.8X2	T50.8X3	T50.8X4	T50.8X5	T50.8X6
Invert sugar	T50.3X1	T50.3X2	T50.3X3	T50.3X4	T50.3X5	T50.3X6
Inza — see Naproxen						
Iobenzamic acid	T50.8X1	T50.8X2	T50.8X3	T50.8X4	T50.8X5	T50.8X6
Iocarmic acid	T50.8X1	T50.8X2	T50.8X3	T50.8X4	T50.8X5	T50.8X6
Iocetamic acid	T50.8X1	T50.8X2	T50.8X3	T50.8X4	T50.8X5	T50.8X6
Iodamide	T50.8X1	T50.8X2	T50.8X3	T50.8X4	T50.8X5	T50.8X6
Iodide NEC — see also Iodine	T49.0X1	T49.0X2	T49.0X3	T49.0X4	T49.0X5	T49.0X6
mercury (ointment)	T49.0X1	T49.0X2	T49.0X3	T49.0X4	T49.0X5	T49.0X6
methylate	T49.0X1	T49.0X2	T49.0X3	T49.0X4	T49.0X5	T49.0X6
potassium (expectorant) NEC	T48.4X1	T48.4X2	T48.4X3	T48.4X4	T48.4X5	T48.4X6
Iodinated						
contrast medium	T50.8X1	T50.8X2	T50.8X3	T50.8X4	T50.8X5	T50.8X6
glycerol	T48.4X1	T48.4X2	T48.4X3	T48.4X4	T48.4X5	T48.4X6
human serum albumin (131I)	T50.8X1	T50.8X2	T50.8X3	T50.8X4	T50.8X5	T50.8X6
Iodine (antiseptic, external) (tincture) NEC	T49.0X1	T49.0X2	T49.0X3	T49.0X4	T49.0X5	T49.0X6
125 — see also Radiation sickness, and Exposure to radioactivce isotopes	T50.8X1	T50.8X2	T50.8X3	T50.8X4	T50.8X5	T50.8X6
therapeutic	T50.991	T50.992	T50.993	T50.994	T50.995	T50.996
131 — see also Radiation sickness, and Exposure to radioactivce isotopes	T50.8X1	T50.8X2	T50.8X3	T50.8X4	T50.8X5	T50.8X6
therapeutic	T38.2X1	T38.2X2	T38.2X3	T38.2X4	T38.2X5	T38.2X6
diagnostic	T50.8X1	T50.8X2	T50.8X3	T50.8X4	T50.8X5	T50.8X6
for thyroid conditions (antithyroid)	T38.2X1	T38.2X2	T38.2X3	T38.2X4	T38.2X5	T38.2X6
solution	T49.0X1	T49.0X2	T49.0X3	T49.0X4	T49.0X5	T49.0X6
vapor	T59.891	T59.892	T59.893	T59.894	—	—
Iodipamide	T50.8X1	T50.8X2	T50.8X3	T50.8X4	T50.8X5	T50.8X6
Iodized (poppy seed) oil	T50.8X1	T50.8X2	T50.8X3	T50.8X4	T50.8X5	T50.8X6
Iodobismitol	T37.8X1	T37.8X2	T37.8X3	T37.8X4	T37.8X5	T37.8X6
Iodochlorhydroxyquin	T37.8X1	T37.8X2	T37.8X3	T37.8X4	T37.8X5	T37.8X6
topical	T49.0X1	T49.0X2	T49.0X3	T49.0X4	T49.0X5	T49.0X6
Iodochlorhydroxyquino-line	T37.8X1	T37.8X2	T37.8X3	T37.8X4	T37.8X5	T37.8X6
Iodocholesterol (131I)	T50.8X1	T50.8X2	T50.8X3	T50.8X4	T50.8X5	T50.8X6

Substance	External Cause (T-Code)					
	Poisoning, Accidental (Unintentional)	Poisoning, Intentional Self-Harm	Poisoning, Assault	Poisoning, Undetermined	Adverse Effect	Underdosing
Iodoform	T49.0X1	T49.0X2	T49.0X3	T49.0X4	T49.0X5	T49.0X6
Iodohippuric acid	T50.8X1	T50.8X2	T50.8X3	T50.8X4	T50.8X5	T50.8X6
Iodopanoic acid	T50.8X1	T50.8X2	T50.8X3	T50.8X4	T50.8X5	T50.8X6
Iodophthalein (sodium)	T50.8X1	T50.8X2	T50.8X3	T50.8X4	T50.8X5	T50.8X6
Iodopyracet	T50.8X1	T50.8X2	T50.8X3	T50.8X4	T50.8X5	T50.8X6
Iodoquinol	T37.8X1	T37.8X2	T37.8X3	T37.8X4	T37.8X5	T37.8X6
Iodoxamic acid	T50.8X1	T50.8X2	T50.8X3	T50.8X4	T50.8X5	T50.8X6
Iofendylate	T50.8X1	T50.8X2	T50.8X3	T50.8X4	T50.8X5	T50.8X6
Ioglycamic acid	T50.8X1	T50.8X2	T50.8X3	T50.8X4	T50.8X5	T50.8X6
Iohexol	T50.8X1	T50.8X2	T50.8X3	T50.8X4	T50.8X5	T50.8X6
Ion exchange resin						
anion	T47.8X1	T47.8X2	T47.8X3	T47.8X4	T47.8X5	T47.8X6
cation	T50.3X1	T50.3X2	T50.3X3	T50.3X4	T50.3X5	T50.3X6
cholestyramine	T46.6X1	T46.6X2	T46.6X3	T46.6X4	T46.6X5	T46.6X6
intestinal	T47.8X1	T47.8X2	T47.8X3	T47.8X4	T47.8X5	T47.8X6
Iopamidol	T50.8X1	T50.8X2	T50.8X3	T50.8X4	T50.8X5	T50.8X6
Iopanoic acid	T50.8X1	T50.8X2	T50.8X3	T50.8X4	T50.8X5	T50.8X6
Iophenoic acid	T50.8X1	T50.8X2	T50.8X3	T50.8X4	T50.8X5	T50.8X6
Iopodate, sodium	T50.8X1	T50.8X2	T50.8X3	T50.8X4	T50.8X5	T50.8X6
Iopodic acid	T50.8X1	T50.8X2	T50.8X3	T50.8X4	T50.8X5	T50.8X6
Iopromide	T50.8X1	T50.8X2	T50.8X3	T50.8X4	T50.8X5	T50.8X6
Iopydol	T50.8X1	T50.8X2	T50.8X3	T50.8X4	T50.8X5	T50.8X6
Iotalamic acid	T50.8X1	T50.8X2	T50.8X3	T50.8X4	T50.8X5	T50.8X6
Iothalamate	T50.8X1	T50.8X2	T50.8X3	T50.8X4	T50.8X5	T50.8X6
Iothiouracil	T38.2X1	T38.2X2	T38.2X3	T38.2X4	T38.2X5	T38.2X6
Iotrol	T50.8X1	T50.8X2	T50.8X3	T50.8X4	T50.8X5	T50.8X6
Iotrolan	T50.8X1	T50.8X2	T50.8X3	T50.8X4	T50.8X5	T50.8X6
Iotroxate	T50.8X1	T50.8X2	T50.8X3	T50.8X4	T50.8X5	T50.8X6
Iotroxic acid	T50.8X1	T50.8X2	T50.8X3	T50.8X4	T50.8X5	T50.8X6
Ioversol	T50.8X1	T50.8X2	T50.8X3	T50.8X4	T50.8X5	T50.8X6
Ioxaglate	T50.8X1	T50.8X2	T50.8X3	T50.8X4	T50.8X5	T50.8X6
Ioxaglic acid	T50.8X1	T50.8X2	T50.8X3	T50.8X4	T50.8X5	T50.8X6
Ioxitalamic acid	T50.8X1	T50.8X2	T50.8X3	T50.8X4	T50.8X5	T50.8X6
Ipecac	T47.7X1	T47.7X2	T47.7X3	T47.7X4	T47.7X5	T47.7X6
Ipecacuanha	T48.4X1	T48.4X2	T48.4X3	T48.4X4	T48.4X5	T48.4X6
Ipodate, calcium	T50.8X1	T50.8X2	T50.8X3	T50.8X4	T50.8X5	T50.8X6
Ipral	T42.3X1	T42.3X2	T42.3X3	T42.3X4	T42.3X5	T42.3X6
Ipratropium (bromide)	T48.6X1	T48.6X2	T48.6X3	T48.6X4	T48.6X5	T48.6X6
Ipriflavone	T46.3X1	T46.3X2	T46.3X3	T46.3X4	T46.3X5	T46.3X6
Iprindole	T43.011	T43.012	T43.013	T43.014	T43.015	T43.016
Iproclozide	T43.1X1	T43.1X2	T43.1X3	T43.1X4	T43.1X5	T43.1X6
Iprofenin	T50.8X1	T50.8X2	T50.8X3	T50.8X4	T50.8X5	T50.8X6

Substance	External Cause (T-Code)					
	Poisoning, Accidental (Unintentional)	Poisoning, Intentional Self-Harm	Poisoning, Assault	Poisoning, Undetermined	Adverse Effect	Underdosing
Iproheptine	T49.2X1	T49.2X2	T49.2X3	T49.2X4	T49.2X5	T49.2X6
Iproniazid	T43.1X1	T43.1X2	T43.1X3	T43.1X4	T43.1X5	T43.1X6
Iproplatin	T45.1X1	T45.1X2	T45.1X3	T45.1X4	T45.1X5	T45.1X6
Iproveratril	T46.1X1	T46.1X2	T46.1X3	T46.1X4	T46.1X5	T46.1X6
Iron (compounds) (medicinal) NEC	T45.4X1	T45.4X2	T45.4X3	T45.4X4	T45.4X5	T45.4X6
ammonium	T45.4X1	T45.4X2	T45.4X3	T45.4X4	T45.4X5	T45.4X6
dextran injection	T45.4X1	T45.4X2	T45.4X3	T45.4X4	T45.4X5	T45.4X6
nonmedicinal	T56.891	T56.892	T56.893	T56.894	—	—
salts	T45.4X1	T45.4X2	T45.4X3	T45.4X4	T45.4X5	T45.4X6
sorbitex	T45.4X1	T45.4X2	T45.4X3	T45.4X4	T45.4X5	T45.4X6
sorbitol citric acid complex	T45.4X1	T45.4X2	T45.4X3	T45.4X4	T45.4X5	T45.4X6
Irrigating fluid (vaginal)	T49.8X1	T49.8X2	T49.8X3	T49.8X4	T49.8X5	T49.8X6
eye	T49.5X1	T49.5X2	T49.5X3	T49.5X4	T49.5X5	T49.5X6
Isepamicin	T36.5X1	T36.5X2	T36.5X3	T36.5X4	T36.5X5	T36.5X6
Isoaminile (citrate)	T48.3X1	T48.3X2	T48.3X3	T48.3X4	T48.3X5	T48.3X6
Isoamyl nitrite	T46.3X1	T46.3X2	T46.3X3	T46.3X4	T46.3X5	T46.3X6
Isobenzan	T60.1X1	T60.1X2	T60.1X3	T60.1X4	—	—
Isobutyl acetate	T52.8X1	T52.8X2	T52.8X3	T52.8X4	—	—
Isocarboxazid	T43.1X1	T43.1X2	T43.1X3	T43.1X4	T43.1X5	T43.1X6
Isoconazole	T49.0X1	T49.0X2	T49.0X3	T49.0X4	T49.0X5	T49.0X6
Isocyanate	T65.0X1	T65.0X2	T65.0X3	T65.0X4	—	—
Isoephedrine	T44.991	T44.992	T44.993	T44.994	T44.995	T44.996
Isoetarine	T48.6X1	T48.6X2	T48.6X3	T48.6X4	T48.6X5	T48.6X6
Isoethadione	T42.2X1	T42.2X2	T42.2X3	T42.2X4	T42.2X5	T42.2X6
Isoetharine	T44.5X1	T44.5X2	T44.5X3	T44.5X4	T44.5X5	T44.5X6
Isoflurane	T41.0X1	T41.0X2	T41.0X3	T41.0X4	T41.0X5	T41.0X6
Isoflurophate	T44.0X1	T44.0X2	T44.0X3	T44.0X4	T44.0X5	T44.0X6
Isomaltose, ferric complex	T45.4X1	T45.4X2	T45.4X3	T45.4X4	T45.4X5	T45.4X6
Isometheptene	T44.3X1	T44.3X2	T44.3X3	T44.3X4	T44.3X5	T44.3X6
Isoniazid	T37.1X1	T37.1X2	T37.1X3	T37.1X4	T37.1X5	T37.1X6
with						
rifampicin	T36.6X1	T36.6X2	T36.6X3	T36.6X4	T36.6X5	T36.6X6
thioacetazone	T37.1X1	T37.1X2	T37.1X3	T37.1X4	T37.1X5	T37.1X6
Isonicotinic acid hydrazide	T37.1X1	T37.1X2	T37.1X3	T37.1X4	T37.1X5	T37.1X6
Isonipecaine	T40.4X1	T40.4X2	T40.4X3	T40.4X4	T40.4X5	T40.4X6
Isopentaquine	T37.2X1	T37.2X2	T37.2X3	T37.2X4	T37.2X5	T37.2X6
Isophane insulin	T38.3X1	T38.3X2	T38.3X3	T38.3X4	T38.3X5	T38.3X6
Isophorone	T65.891	T65.892	T65.893	T65.894	—	—
Isophosphamide	T45.1X1	T45.1X2	T45.1X3	T45.1X4	T45.1X5	T45.1X6
Isopregnenone	T38.5X1	T38.5X2	T38.5X3	T38.5X4	T38.5X5	T38.5X6
Isoprenaline	T48.6X1	T48.6X2	T48.6X3	T48.6X4	T48.6X5	T48.6X6
Isopromethazine	T43.3X1	T43.3X2	T43.3X3	T43.3X4	T43.3X5	T43.3X6

◀ New   ◀ Revised   deleted Deleted

Substance	Poisoning, Accidental (Unintentional)	Poisoning, Intentional Self-Harm	Poisoning, Assault	Poisoning, Undetermined	Adverse Effect	Underdosing
Isopropamide	T44.3X1	T44.3X2	T44.3X3	T44.3X4	T44.3X5	T44.3X6
iodide	T44.3X1	T44.3X2	T44.3X3	T44.3X4	T44.3X5	T44.3X6
Isopropanol	T51.2X1	T51.2X2	T51.2X3	T51.2X4	—	—
Isopropyl						
acetate	T52.8X1	T52.8X2	T52.8X3	T52.8X4	—	—
alcohol	T51.2X1	T51.2X2	T51.2X3	T51.2X4	—	—
medicinal	T49.4X1	T49.4X2	T49.4X3	T49.4X4	T49.4X5	T49.4X6
ether	T52.8X1	T52.8X2	T52.8X3	T52.8X4	—	—
Isopropylaminophena-zone	T39.2X1	T39.2X2	T39.2X3	T39.2X4	T39.2X5	T39.2X6
Isoproterenol	T48.6X1	T48.6X2	T48.6X3	T48.6X4	T48.6X5	T48.6X6
Isosorbide dinitrate	T46.3X1	T46.3X2	T46.3X3	T46.3X4	T46.3X5	T46.3X6
Isothipendyl	T45.0X1	T45.0X2	T45.0X3	T45.0X4	T45.0X5	T45.0X6
Isotretinoin	T50.991	T50.992	T50.993	T50.994	T50.995	T50.996
Isoxazolyl penicillin	T36.0X1	T36.0X2	T36.0X3	T36.0X4	T36.0X5	T36.0X6
Isoxicam	T39.391	T39.392	T39.393	T39.394	T39.395	T39.396
Isoxsuprine	T46.7X1	T46.7X2	T46.7X3	T46.7X4	T46.7X5	T46.7X6
Ispagula	T47.4X1	T47.4X2	T47.4X3	T47.4X4	T47.4X5	T47.4X6
husk	T47.4X1	T47.4X2	T47.4X3	T47.4X4	T47.4X5	T47.4X6
Isradipine	T46.1X1	T46.1X2	T46.1X3	T46.1X4	T46.1X5	T46.1X6
l-thyroxine sodium	T38.1X1	T38.1X2	T38.1X3	T38.1X4	T38.1X5	T38.1X6
Itraconazole	T37.8X1	T37.8X2	T37.8X3	T37.8X4	T37.8X5	T37.8X6
Itramin tosilate	T46.3X1	T46.3X2	T46.3X3	T46.3X4	T46.3X5	T46.3X6
Ivermectin	T37.4X1	T37.4X2	T37.4X3	T37.4X4	T37.4X5	T37.4X6
Izoniazid	T37.1X1	T37.1X2	T37.1X3	T37.1X4	T37.1X5	T37.1X6
with thioacetazone	T37.1X1	T37.1X2	T37.1X3	T37.1X4	T37.1X5	T37.1X6
J						
Jalap	T47.2X1	T47.2X2	T47.2X3	T47.2X4	T47.2X5	T47.2X6
Jamaica						
dogwood (bark)	T39.8X1	T39.8X2	T39.8X3	T39.8X4	T39.8X5	T39.8X6
ginger	T65.891	T65.892	T65.893	T65.894	—	—
root	T62.2X1	T62.2X2	T62.2X3	T62.2X4	—	—
Jatropha	T62.2X1	T62.2X2	T62.2X3	T62.2X4	—	—
curcas	T62.2X1	T62.2X2	T62.2X3	T62.2X4	—	—
Jectofer	T45.4X1	T45.4X2	T45.4X3	T45.4X4	T45.4X5	T45.4X6
Jellyfish (sting)	T63.621	T63.622	T63.623	T63.624		
Jequirity (bean)	T62.2X1	T62.2X2	T62.2X3	T62.2X4		
Jimson weed (stramonium)	T62.2X1	T62.2X2	T62.2X3	T62.2X4	—	—
seeds	T62.2X1	T62.2X2	T62.2X3	T62.2X4	—	—
Josamycin	T36.3X1	T36.3X2	T36.3X3	T36.3X4	T36.3X5	T36.3X6
Juniper tar	T49.1X1	T49.1X2	T49.1X3	T49.1X4	T49.1X5	T49.1X6

Substance	Poisoning, Accidental (Unintentional)	Poisoning, Intentional Self-Harm	Poisoning, Assault	Poisoning, Undetermined	Adverse Effect	Underdosing
K						
Kallidinogenase	T46.7X1	T46.7X2	T46.7X3	T46.7X4	T46.7X5	T46.7X6
Kallikrein	T46.7X1	T46.7X2	T46.7X3	T46.7X4	T46.7X5	T46.7X6
Kanamycin	T36.5X1	T36.5X2	T36.5X3	T36.5X4	T36.5X5	T36.5X6
Kantrex	T36.5X1	T36.5X2	T36.5X3	T36.5X4	T36.5X5	T36.5X6
Kaolin	T47.6X1	T47.6X2	T47.6X3	T47.6X4	T47.6X5	T47.6X6
light	T47.6X1	T47.6X2	T47.6X3	T47.6X4	T47.6X5	T47.6X6
Karaya (gum)	T47.4X1	T47.4X2	T47.4X3	T47.4X4	T47.4X5	T47.4X6
Kebuzone	T39.2X1	T39.2X2	T39.2X3	T39.2X4	T39.2X5	T39.2X6
Kelevan	T60.1X1	T60.1X2	T60.1X3	T60.1X4	—	—
Kemithal	T41.1X1	T41.1X2	T41.1X3	T41.1X4	T41.1X5	T41.1X6
Kenacort	T38.0X1	T38.0X2	T38.0X3	T38.0X4	T38.0X5	T38.0X6
Keratolytic drug NEC	T49.4X1	T49.4X2	T49.4X3	T49.4X4	T49.4X5	T49.4X6
anthracene	T49.4X1	T49.4X2	T49.4X3	T49.4X4	T49.4X5	T49.4X6
Keratoplastic NEC	T49.4X1	T49.4X2	T49.4X3	T49.4X4	T49.4X5	T49.4X6
Kerosene, kerosine (fuel) (solvent) NEC	T52.0X1	T52.0X2	T52.0X3	T52.0X4	—	—
insecticide	T52.0X1	T52.0X2	T52.0X3	T52.0X4	—	—
vapor	T52.0X1	T52.0X2	T52.0X3	T52.0X4	—	—
Ketamine	T41.291	T41.292	T41.293	T41.294	T41.295	T41.296
Ketazolam	T42.4X1	T42.4X2	T42.4X3	T42.4X4	T42.4X5	T42.4X6
Ketazon	T39.2X1	T39.2X2	T39.2X3	T39.2X4	T39.2X5	T39.2X6
Ketobemidone	T40.4X1	T40.4X2	T40.4X3	T40.4X4	—	—
Ketoconazole	T49.0X1	T49.0X2	T49.0X3	T49.0X4	T49.0X5	T49.0X6
Ketols	T52.4X1	T52.4X2	T52.4X3	T52.4X4	—	—
Ketone oils	T52.4X1	T52.4X2	T52.4X3	T52.4X4	—	—
Ketoprofen	T39.311	T39.312	T39.313	T39.314	T39.315	T39.316
Ketorolac	T39.8X1	T39.8X2	T39.8X3	T39.8X4	T39.8X5	T39.8X6
Ketotifen	T45.0X1	T45.0X2	T45.0X3	T45.0X4	T45.0X5	T45.0X6
Khat	T43.691	T43.692	T43.693	T43.694	—	—
Khellin	T46.3X1	T46.3X2	T46.3X3	T46.3X4	T46.3X5	T46.3X6
Khelloside	T46.3X1	T46.3X2	T46.3X3	T46.3X4	T46.3X5	T46.3X6
Kiln gas or vapor (carbon monoxide)	T58.8X1	T58.8X2	T58.8X3	T58.8X4	—	—
Kitasamycin	T36.3X1	T36.3X2	T36.3X3	T36.3X4	T36.3X5	T36.3X6
Konsyl	T47.4X1	T47.4X2	T47.4X3	T47.4X4	T47.4X5	T47.4X6
Kosam seed	T62.2X1	T62.2X2	T62.2X3	T62.2X4	—	—
Krait (venom)	T63.091	T63.092	T63.093	T63.094	—	—
Kwell (insecticide)	T60.1X1	T60.1X2	T60.1X3	T60.1X4	—	—
anti-infective (topical)	T49.0X1	T49.0X2	T49.0X3	T49.0X4	T49.0X5	T49.0X6

◀ New   ◀ Revised   ~~deleted~~ Deleted

Substance	Poisoning, Accidental (Unintentional)	Poisoning, Intentional Self-Harm	Poisoning, Assault	Poisoning, Undetermined	Adverse Effect	Underdosing
L						
Labetalol	T44.8X1	T44.8X2	T44.8X3	T44.8X4	T44.8X5	T44.8X6
Laburnum (seeds)	T62.2X1	T62.2X2	T62.2X3	T62.2X4	—	—
leaves	T62.2X1	T62.2X2	T62.2X3	T62.2X4	—	—
Lachesine	T49.5X1	T49.5X2	T49.5X3	T49.5X4	T49.5X5	T49.5X6
Lacidipine	T46.5X1	T46.5X2	T46.5X3	T46.5X4	T46.5X5	T46.5X6
Lacquer	T65.6X1	T65.6X2	T65.6X3	T65.6X4	—	—
Lacrimogenic gas	T59.3X1	T59.3X2	T59.3X3	T59.3X4	—	—
Lactated potassic saline	T50.3X1	T50.3X2	T50.3X3	T50.3X4	T50.3X5	T50.3X6
Lactic acid	T49.8X1	T49.8X2	T49.8X3	T49.8X4	T49.8X5	T49.8X6
Lactobacillus						
acidophilus	T47.6X1	T47.6X2	T47.6X3	T47.6X4	T47.6X5	T47.6X6
compound	T47.6X1	T47.6X2	T47.6X3	T47.6X4	T47.6X5	T47.6X6
bifidus, lyophilized	T47.6X1	T47.6X2	T47.6X3	T47.6X4	T47.6X5	T47.6X6
bulgaricus	T47.6X1	T47.6X2	T47.6X3	T47.6X4	T47.6X5	T47.6X6
sporogenes	T47.6X1	T47.6X2	T47.6X3	T47.6X4	T47.6X5	T47.6X6
Lactoflavin	T45.2X1	T45.2X2	T45.2X3	T45.2X4	T45.2X5	T45.2X6
Lactose (as excipient)	T50.901	T50.902	T50.903	T50.904	T50.905	T50.906
Lactuca (virosa) (extract)	T42.6X1	T42.6X2	T42.6X3	T42.6X4	T42.6X5	T42.6X6
Lactucarium	T42.6X1	T42.6X2	T42.6X3	T42.6X4	T42.6X5	T42.6X6
Lactulose	T47.3X1	T47.3X2	T47.3X3	T47.3X4	T47.3X5	T47.3X6
Laevo — *see Levo-*						
Lanatosides	T46.0X1	T46.0X2	T46.0X3	T46.0X4	T46.0X5	T46.0X6
Lanolin	T49.3X1	T49.3X2	T49.3X3	T49.3X4	T49.3X5	T49.3X6
Largactil	T43.3X1	T43.3X2	T43.3X3	T43.3X4	T43.3X5	T43.3X6
Larkspur	T62.2X1	T62.2X2	T62.2X3	T62.2X4	—	—
Laroxyl	T43.011	T43.012	T43.013	T43.014	T43.015	T43.016
Lassar's paste	T49.4X1	T49.4X2	T49.4X3	T49.4X4	T49.4X5	T49.4X6
Lasix	T50.1X1	T50.1X2	T50.1X3	T50.1X4	T50.1X5	T50.1X6
Latamoxef	T36.1X1	T36.1X2	T36.1X3	T36.1X4	T36.1X5	T36.1X6
Latex	T65.811	T65.812	T65.813	T65.814	—	—
Lathyrus (seed)	T62.2X1	T62.2X2	T62.2X3	T62.2X4	—	—
Laudanum	T40.0X1	T40.0X2	T40.0X3	T40.0X4	T40.0X5	T40.0X6
Laudexium	T48.1X1	T48.1X2	T48.1X3	T48.1X4	T48.1X5	T48.1X6
Laughing gas	T41.0X1	T41.0X2	T41.0X3	T41.0X4	T41.0X5	T41.0X6
Laurel, black or cherry	T62.2X1	T62.2X2	T62.2X3	T62.2X4	—	—
Laurolinium	T49.0X1	T49.0X2	T49.0X3	T49.0X4	T49.0X5	T49.0X6
Lauryl sulfoacetate	T49.2X1	T49.2X2	T49.2X3	T49.2X4	T49.2X5	T49.2X6

Substance	Poisoning, Accidental (Unintentional)	Poisoning, Intentional Self-Harm	Poisoning, Assault	Poisoning, Undetermined	Adverse Effect	Underdosing
Laxative NEC	T47.4X1	T47.4X2	T47.4X3	T47.4X4	T47.4X5	T47.4X6
osmotic	T47.3X1	T47.3X2	T47.3X3	T47.3X4	T47.3X5	T47.3X6
saline	T47.3X1	T47.3X2	T47.3X3	T47.3X4	T47.3X5	T47.3X6
stimulant	T47.2X1	T47.2X2	T47.2X3	T47.2X4	T47.2X5	T47.2X6
L-dopa	T42.8X1	T42.8X2	T42.8X3	T42.8X4	T42.8X5	T42.8X6
Lead (dust) (fumes) (vapor) NEC	T56.0X1	T56.0X2	T56.0X3	T56.0X4	—	—
acetate	T49.2X1	T49.2X2	T49.2X3	T49.2X4	T49.2X5	T49.2X6
alkyl (fuel additive)	T56.0X1	T56.0X2	T56.0X3	T56.0X4	—	—
anti-infectives	T37.8X1	T37.8X2	T37.8X3	T37.8X4	T37.8X5	T37.8X6
antiknock compound (tetraethyl)	T56.0X1	T56.0X2	T56.0X3	T56.0X4	—	—
arsenate, arsenite (dust) (herbicide) (insecticide) (vapor)	T57.0X1	T57.0X2	T57.0X3	T57.0X4	—	—
carbonate	T56.0X1	T56.0X2	T56.0X3	T56.0X4	—	—
paint	T56.0X1	T56.0X2	T56.0X3	T56.0X4	—	—
chromate	T56.0X1	T56.0X2	T56.0X3	T56.0X4	—	—
paint	T56.0X1	T56.0X2	T56.0X3	T56.0X4	—	—
dioxide	T56.0X1	T56.0X2	T56.0X3	T56.0X4	—	—
inorganic	T56.0X1	T56.0X2	T56.0X3	T56.0X4	—	—
iodide	T56.0X1	T56.0X2	T56.0X3	T56.0X4	—	—
pigment (paint)	T56.0X1	T56.0X2	T56.0X3	T56.0X4	—	—
monoxide (dust)	T56.0X1	T56.0X2	T56.0X3	T56.0X4	—	—
paint	T56.0X1	T56.0X2	T56.0X3	T56.0X4	—	—
organic	T56.0X1	T56.0X2	T56.0X3	T56.0X4	—	—
oxide	T56.0X1	T56.0X2	T56.0X3	T56.0X4	—	—
paint	T56.0X1	T56.0X2	T56.0X3	T56.0X4	—	—
paint	T56.0X1	T56.0X2	T56.0X3	T56.0X4	—	—
salts	T56.0X1	T56.0X2	T56.0X3	T56.0X4	—	—
specified compound NEC	T56.0X1	T56.0X2	T56.0X3	T56.0X4	—	—
tetra-ethyl	T56.0X1	T56.0X2	T56.0X3	T56.0X4	—	—
Lebanese red	T40.7X1	T40.7X2	T40.7X3	T40.7X4	T40.7X5	T40.7X6
Lefetamine	T39.8X1	T39.8X2	T39.8X3	T39.8X4	T39.8X5	T39.8X6
Lenperone	T43.4X1	T43.4X2	T43.4X3	T43.4X4	T43.4X5	T43.4X6
Lente lietin (insulin)	T38.3X1	T38.3X2	T38.3X3	T38.3X4	T38.3X5	T38.3X6
Leptazol	T50.7X1	T50.7X2	T50.7X3	T50.7X4	T50.7X5	T50.7X6
Leptophos	T60.0X1	T60.0X2	T60.0X3	T60.0X4	—	—
Leritine	T40.2X1	T40.2X2	T40.2X3	T40.2X4	T40.2X5	T40.2X6
Letosteine	T48.4X1	T48.4X2	T48.4X3	T48.4X4	T48.4X5	T48.4X6
Letter	T38.1X1	T38.1X2	T38.1X3	T38.1X4	T38.1X5	T38.1X6
Lettuce opium	T42.6X1	T42.6X2	T42.6X3	T42.6X4	T42.6X5	T42.6X6
Leucinocaine	T41.3X1	T41.3X2	T41.3X3	T41.3X4	T41.3X5	T41.3X6

◀ New ◀ Revised ~~deleted~~ Deleted

Substance	Poisoning, Accidental (Unintentional)	Poisoning, Intentional Self-Harm	Poisoning, Assault	Poisoning, Undetermined	Adverse Effect	Underdosing
Leucocianidol	T46.991	T46.992	T46.993	T46.994	T46.995	T46.996
Leucovorin (factor)	T45.8X1	T45.8X2	T45.8X3	T45.8X4	T45.8X5	T45.8X6
Leukeran	T45.1X1	T45.1X2	T45.1X3	T45.1X4	T45.1X5	T45.1X6
Leuprolide	T38.891	T38.892	T38.893	T38.894	T38.895	T38.896
Levalbuterol	T48.6X1	T48.6X2	T48.6X3	T48.6X4	T48.6X5	T48.6X6
Levallorphan	T50.7X1	T50.7X2	T50.7X3	T50.7X4	T50.7X5	T50.7X6
Levamisole	T37.4X1	T37.4X2	T37.4X3	T37.4X4	T37.4X5	T37.4X6
Levanil	T42.6X1	T42.6X2	T42.6X3	T42.6X4	T42.6X5	T42.6X6
Levarterenol	T44.4X1	T44.4X2	T44.4X3	T44.4X4	T44.4X5	T44.4X6
Levdropropizine	T48.3X1	T48.3X2	T48.3X3	T48.3X4	T48.3X5	T48.3X6
Levobunolol	T49.5X1	T49.5X2	T49.5X3	T49.5X4	T49.5X5	T49.5X6
Levocabastine (hydrochloride)	T45.0X1	T45.0X2	T45.0X3	T45.0X4	T45.0X5	T45.0X6
Levocarnitine	T50.991	T50.992	T50.993	T50.994	T50.995	T50.996
Levodopa	T42.8X1	T42.8X2	T42.8X3	T42.8X4	T42.8X5	T42.8X6
with carbidopa	T42.8X1	T42.8X2	T42.8X3	T42.8X4	T42.8X5	T42.8X6
Levo-dromoran	T40.2X1	T40.2X2	T40.2X3	T40.2X4	T40.2X5	T40.2X6
Levoglutamide	T50.991	T50.992	T50.993	T50.994	T50.995	T50.996
Levoid	T38.1X1	T38.1X2	T38.1X3	T38.1X4	T38.1X5	T38.1X6
Levo-iso-methadone	T40.3X1	T40.3X2	T40.3X3	T40.3X4	T40.3X5	T40.3X6
Levomepromazine	T43.3X1	T43.3X2	T43.3X3	T43.3X4	T43.3X5	T43.3X6
Levonordefrin	T49.6X1	T49.6X2	T49.6X3	T49.6X4	T49.6X5	T49.6X6
Levonorgestrel	T38.4X1	T38.4X2	T38.4X3	T38.4X4	T38.4X5	T38.4X6
with ethinylestradiol	T38.5X1	T38.5X2	T38.5X3	T38.5X4	T38.5X5	T38.5X6
Levopromazine	T43.3X1	T43.3X2	T43.3X3	T43.3X4	T43.3X5	T43.3X6
Levoprome	T42.6X1	T42.6X2	T42.6X3	T42.6X4	T42.6X5	T42.6X6
Levopropoxyphene	T40.4X1	T40.4X2	T40.4X3	T40.4X4	T40.4X5	T40.4X6
Levopropylhexedrine	T50.5X1	T50.5X2	T50.5X3	T50.5X4	T50.5X5	T50.5X6
Levoproxyphylline	T48.6X1	T48.6X2	T48.6X3	T48.6X4	T48.6X5	T48.6X6
Levorphanol	T40.4X1	T40.4X2	T40.4X3	T40.4X4	T40.4X5	T40.4X6
Levothyroxine	T38.1X1	T38.1X2	T38.1X3	T38.1X4	T38.1X5	T38.1X6
sodium	T38.1X1	T38.1X2	T38.1X3	T38.1X4	T38.1X5	T38.1X6
Levsin	T44.3X1	T44.3X2	T44.3X3	T44.3X4	T44.3X5	T44.3X6
Levulose	T50.3X1	T50.3X2	T50.3X3	T50.3X4	T50.3X5	T50.3X6
Lewisite (gas), not in war	T57.0X1	T57.0X2	T57.0X3	T57.0X4	—	—
Librium	T42.4X1	T42.4X2	T42.4X3	T42.4X4	T42.4X5	T42.4X6
Lidex	T49.0X1	T49.0X2	T49.0X3	T49.0X4	T49.0X5	T49.0X6
Lidocaine	T41.3X1	T41.3X2	T41.3X3	T41.3X4	T41.3X5	T41.3X6
regional	T41.3X1	T41.3X2	T41.3X3	T41.3X4	T41.3X5	T41.3X6
spinal	T41.3X1	T41.3X2	T41.3X3	T41.3X4	T41.3X5	T41.3X6
Lidofenin	T50.8X1	T50.8X2	T50.8X3	T50.8X4	T50.8X5	T50.8X6
Lidoflazine	T46.1X1	T46.1X2	T46.1X3	T46.1X4	T46.1X5	T46.1X6
Lighter fluid	T52.0X1	T52.0X2	T52.0X3	T52.0X4	—	—

Substance	Poisoning, Accidental (Unintentional)	Poisoning, Intentional Self-Harm	Poisoning, Assault	Poisoning, Undetermined	Adverse Effect	Underdosing
Lignin hemicellulose	T47.6X1	T47.6X2	T47.6X3	T47.6X4	T47.6X5	T47.6X6
Lignocaine	T41.3X1	T41.3X2	T41.3X3	T41.3X4	T41.3X5	T41.3X6
regional	T41.3X1	T41.3X2	T41.3X3	T41.3X4	T41.3X5	T41.3X6
spinal	T41.3X1	T41.3X2	T41.3X3	T41.3X4	T41.3X5	T41.3X6
Ligroin(e) (solvent)	T52.0X1	T52.0X2	T52.0X3	T52.0X4	—	—
vapor	T59.891	T59.892	T59.893	T59.894		
Ligustrum vulgare	T62.2X1	T62.2X2	T62.2X3	T62.2X4	—	—
Lily of the valley	T62.2X1	T62.2X2	T62.2X3	T62.2X4	—	—
Lime (chloride)	T54.3X1	T54.3X2	T54.3X3	T54.3X4		
Limonene	T52.8X1	T52.8X2	T52.8X3	T52.8X4		
Lincomycin	T36.8X1	T36.8X2	T36.8X3	T36.8X4	T36.8X5	T36.8X6
Lindane (insecticide) (nonmedicinal) (vapor)	T53.6X1	T53.6X2	T53.6X3	T53.6X4	—	—
medicinal	T49.0X1	T49.0X2	T49.0X3	T49.0X4	T49.0X5	T49.0X6
Liniments NEC	T49.91	T49.92	T49.93	T49.94	T49.95	T49.96
Linoleic acid	T46.6X1	T46.6X2	T46.6X3	T46.6X4	T46.6X5	T46.6X6
Linolenic acid	T46.6X1	T46.6X2	T46.6X3	T46.6X4	T46.6X5	T46.6X6
Linseed	T47.4X1	T47.4X2	T47.4X3	T47.4X4	T47.4X5	T47.4X6
Liothyronine	T38.1X1	T38.1X2	T38.1X3	T38.1X4	T38.1X5	T38.1X6
Liotrix	T38.1X1	T38.1X2	T38.1X3	T38.1X4	T38.1X5	T38.1X6
Lipancreatin	T47.5X1	T47.5X2	T47.5X3	T47.5X4	T47.5X5	T47.5X6
Lipo-alprostadil	T46.7X1	T46.7X2	T46.7X3	T46.7X4	T46.7X5	T46.7X6
Lipo-Lutin	T38.5X1	T38.5X2	T38.5X3	T38.5X4	T38.5X5	T38.5X6
Lipotropic drug NEC	T50.901	T50.902	T50.903	T50.904	T50.905	T50.906
Liquefied petroleum gases	T59.891	T59.892	T59.893	T59.894	—	—
piped (pure or mixed with air)	T59.891	T59.892	T59.893	T59.894	—	—
Liquid						
paraffin	T47.4X1	T47.4X2	T47.4X3	T47.4X4	T47.4X5	T47.4X6
petrolatum	T47.4X1	T47.4X2	T47.4X3	T47.4X4	T47.4X5	T47.4X6
topical	T49.3X1	T49.3X2	T49.3X3	T49.3X4	T49.3X5	T49.3X6
specified NEC	T65.891	T65.892	T65.893	T65.894	—	—
substance	T65.91	T65.92	T65.93	T65.94	—	—
Liquor creosolis compositus	T65.891	T65.892	T65.893	T65.894	—	—
Liquorice	T48.4X1	T48.4X2	T48.4X3	T48.4X4	T48.4X5	T48.4X6
extract	T47.8X1	T47.8X2	T47.8X3	T47.8X4	T47.8X5	T47.8X6
Lirugen	T50.991	T50.992	T50.993	T50.994	T50.995	T50.996
Lisinopril	T46.4X1	T46.4X2	T46.4X3	T46.4X4	T46.4X5	T46.4X6
Lisuride	T42.8X1	T42.8X2	T42.8X3	T42.8X4	T42.8X5	T42.8X6
Lithane	T43.8X1	T43.8X2	T43.8X3	T43.8X4	T43.8X5	T43.8X6
Lithium	T56.891	T56.892	T56.893	T56.894	—	—
gluconate	T43.591	T43.592	T43.593	T43.594	T43.595	T43.596
salts (carbonate)	T43.591	T43.592	T43.593	T43.594	T43.595	T43.596

◀ New ◀ Revised ~~deleted~~ Deleted

Substance	Poisoning, Accidental (Unintentional)	Poisoning, Intentional Self-Harm	Poisoning, Assault	Poisoning, Undetermined	Adverse Effect	Underdosing
Lithonate	T43.8X1	T43.8X2	T43.8X3	T43.8X4	T43.8X5	T43.8X6
Liver						
extract	T45.8X1	T45.8X2	T45.8X3	T45.8X4	T45.8X5	T45.8X6
for parenteral use	T45.8X1	T45.8X2	T45.8X3	T45.8X4	T45.8X5	T45.8X6
fraction 1	T45.8X1	T45.8X2	T45.8X3	T45.8X4	T45.8X5	T45.8X6
hydrolysate	T45.8X1	T45.8X2	T45.8X3	T45.8X4	T45.8X5	T45.8X6
Lizard (bite) (venom)	T63.121	T63.122	T63.123	T63.124	—	—
LMD	T45.8X1	T45.8X2	T45.8X3	T45.8X4	T45.8X5	T45.8X6
Lobelia	T62.2X1	T62.2X2	T62.2X3	T62.2X4	—	—
Lobeline	T50.7X1	T50.7X2	T50.7X3	T50.7X4	T50.7X5	T50.7X6
Local action drug NEC	T49.8X1	T49.8X2	T49.8X3	T49.8X4	T49.8X5	T49.8X6
Locorten	T49.0X1	T49.0X2	T49.0X3	T49.0X4	T49.0X5	T49.0X6
Lofepramine	T43.011	T43.012	T43.013	T43.014	T43.015	T43.016
Lolium temulentum	T62.2X1	T62.2X2	T62.2X3	T62.2X4	—	—
Lomotil	T47.6X1	T47.6X2	T47.6X3	T47.6X4	T47.6X5	T47.6X6
Lomustine	T45.1X1	T45.1X2	T45.1X3	T45.1X4	T45.1X5	T45.1X6
Lonidamine	T45.1X1	T45.1X2	T45.1X3	T45.1X4	T45.1X5	T45.1X6
Loperamide	T47.6X1	T47.6X2	T47.6X3	T47.6X4	T47.6X5	T47.6X6
Loprazolam	T42.4X1	T42.4X2	T42.4X3	T42.4X4	T42.4X5	T42.4X6
Lorajmine	T46.2X1	T46.2X2	T46.2X3	T46.2X4	T46.2X5	T46.2X6
Loratidine	T45.0X1	T45.0X2	T45.0X3	T45.0X4	T45.0X5	T45.0X6
Lorazepam	T42.4X1	T42.4X2	T42.4X3	T42.4X4	T42.4X5	T42.4X6
Lorcainide	T46.2X1	T46.2X2	T46.2X3	T46.2X4	T46.2X5	T46.2X6
Lormetazepam	T42.4X1	T42.4X2	T42.4X3	T42.4X4	T42.4X5	T42.4X6
Lotions NEC	T49.91	T49.92	T49.93	T49.94	T49.95	T49.96
Lotusate	T42.3X1	T42.3X2	T42.3X3	T42.3X4	T42.3X5	T42.3X6
Lovastatin	T46.6X1	T46.6X2	T46.6X3	T46.6X4	T46.6X5	T46.6X6
Loxapine	T43.591	T43.592	T43.593	T43.594	T43.595	T43.596
Lowila	T49.2X1	T49.2X2	T49.2X3	T49.2X4	T49.2X5	T49.2X6
Lozenges (throat)	T49.6X1	T49.6X2	T49.6X3	T49.6X4	T49.6X5	T49.6X6
LSD	T40.8X1	T40.8X2	T40.8X3	T40.8X4	—	—
L-Tryptophan — see amino acid						
Lubricant, eye	T49.5X1	T49.5X2	T49.5X3	T49.5X4	T49.5X5	T49.5X6
Lubricating oil NEC	T52.0X1	T52.0X2	T52.0X3	T52.0X4	—	—
Lucanthone	T37.4X1	T37.4X2	T37.4X3	T37.4X4	T37.4X5	T37.4X6
Luminal	T42.3X1	T42.3X2	T42.3X3	T42.3X4	T42.3X5	T42.3X6
Lung irritant (gas) NEC	T59.91	T59.92	T59.93	T59.94	—	—
Luteinizing hormone	T38.811	T38.812	T38.813	T38.814	T38.815	T38.816
Lutocylol	T38.5X1	T38.5X2	T38.5X3	T38.5X4	T38.5X5	T38.5X6
Lutromone	T38.5X1	T38.5X2	T38.5X3	T38.5X4	T38.5X5	T38.5X6
Lututrin	T48.291	T48.292	T48.293	T48.294	T48.295	T48.296
Lye (Concentrated)	T54.3X1	T54.3X2	T54.3X3	T54.3X4	—	—

Substance	Poisoning, Accidental (Unintentional)	Poisoning, Intentional Self-Harm	Poisoning, Assault	Poisoning, Undetermined	Adverse Effect	Underdosing
Lygranum (skin test)	T50.8X1	T50.8X2	T50.8X3	T50.8X4	T50.8X5	T50.8X6
Lymecycline	T36.4X1	T36.4X2	T36.4X3	T36.4X4	T36.4X5	T36.4X6
Lymphogranuloma venereum antigen	T50.8X1	T50.8X2	T50.8X3	T50.8X4	T50.8X5	T50.8X6
Lynestrenol	T38.4X1	T38.4X2	T38.4X3	T38.4X4	T38.4X5	T38.4X6
Lypressin	T38.891	T38.892	T38.893	T38.894	T38.895	T38.896
Lyovac Sodium Edecrin	T50.1X1	T50.1X2	T50.1X3	T50.1X4	T50.1X5	T50.1X6
Lysergic acid diethylamide	T40.8X1	T40.8X2	T40.8X3	T40.8X4	—	—
Lysergide	T40.8X1	T40.8X2	T40.8X3	T40.8X4	—	—
Lysine vasopressin	T38.891	T38.892	T38.893	T38.894	T38.895	T38.896
Lysol	T54.1X1	T54.1X2	T54.1X3	T54.1X4	—	—
Lysozyme	T49.0X1	T49.0X2	T49.0X3	T49.0X4	T49.0X5	T49.0X6
Lytta (vitatta)	T49.8X1	T49.8X2	T49.8X3	T49.8X4	T49.8X5	T49.8X6
M						
Mace	T59.3X1	T59.3X2	T59.3X3	T59.3X4	—	—
Macrogol	T50.991	T50.992	T50.993	T50.994	T50.995	T50.996
Macrolide						
anabolic drug	T38.7X1	T38.7X2	T38.7X3	T38.7X4	T38.7X5	T38.7X6
antibiotic	T36.3X1	T36.3X2	T36.3X3	T36.3X4	T36.3X5	T36.3X6
Mafenide	T49.0X1	T49.0X2	T49.0X3	T49.0X4	T49.0X5	T49.0X6
Magaldrate	T47.1X1	T47.1X2	T47.1X3	T47.1X4	T47.1X5	T47.1X6
Magic mushroom	T40.991	T40.992	T40.993	T40.994	—	—
Magnamycin	T36.8X1	T36.8X2	T36.8X3	T36.8X4	T36.8X5	T36.8X6
Magnesia magma	T47.1X1	T47.1X2	T47.1X3	T47.1X4	T47.1X5	T47.1X6
Magnesium NEC	T56.891	T56.892	T56.893	T56.894	—	—
carbonate	T47.1X1	T47.1X2	T47.1X3	T47.1X4	T47.1X5	T47.1X6
citrate	T47.4X1	T47.4X2	T47.4X3	T47.4X4	T47.4X5	T47.4X6
hydroxide	T47.1X1	T47.1X2	T47.1X3	T47.1X4	T47.1X5	T47.1X6
oxide	T47.1X1	T47.1X2	T47.1X3	T47.1X4	T47.1X5	T47.1X6
peroxide	T49.0X1	T49.0X2	T49.0X3	T49.0X4	T49.0X5	T49.0X6
salicylate	T39.091	T39.092	T39.093	T39.094	T39.095	T39.096
silicofluoride	T50.3X1	T50.3X2	T50.3X3	T50.3X4	T50.3X5	T50.3X6
sulfate	T47.4X1	T47.4X2	T47.4X3	T47.4X4	T47.4X5	T47.4X6
thiosulfate	T45.0X1	T45.0X2	T45.0X3	T45.0X4	T45.0X5	T45.0X6
trisilicate	T47.1X1	T47.1X2	T47.1X3	T47.1X4	T47.1X5	T47.1X6
Malathion (medicinal)	T49.0X1	T49.0X2	T49.0X3	T49.0X4	T49.0X5	T49.0X6
insecticide	T60.0X1	T60.0X2	T60.0X3	T60.0X4	—	—
Male fern extract	T37.4X1	T37.4X2	T37.4X3	T37.4X4	T37.4X5	T37.4X6
M-AMSA	T45.1X1	T45.1X2	T45.1X3	T45.1X4	T45.1X5	T45.1X6
Mandelic acid	T37.8X1	T37.8X2	T37.8X3	T37.8X4	T37.8X5	T37.8X6
Manganese (dioxide) (salts)	T57.2X1	T57.2X2	T57.2X3	T57.2X4	—	—
medicinal	T50.991	T50.992	T50.993	T50.994	T50.995	T50.996

◀ New ◀ Revised ~~deleted~~ Deleted

Substance	Poisoning, Accidental (Unintentional)	Poisoning, Intentional Self-Harm	Poisoning, Assault	Poisoning, Undetermined	Adverse Effect	Underdosing
Mannitol	T47.3X1	T47.3X2	T47.3X3	T47.3X4	T47.3X5	T47.3X6
hexanitrate	T46.3X1	T46.3X2	T46.3X3	T46.3X4	T46.3X5	T46.3X6
Mannomustine	T45.1X1	T45.1X2	T45.1X3	T45.1X4	T45.1X5	T45.1X6
MAO inhibitors	T43.1X1	T43.1X2	T43.1X3	T43.1X4	T43.1X5	T43.1X6
Mapharsen	T37.8X1	T37.8X2	T37.8X3	T37.8X4	T37.8X5	T37.8X6
Maphenide	T49.0X1	T49.0X2	T49.0X3	T49.0X4	T49.0X5	T49.0X6
Maprotiline	T43.021	T43.022	T43.023	T43.024	T43.025	T43.026
Marcaine	T41.3X1	T41.3X2	T41.3X3	T41.3X4	T41.3X5	T41.3X6
infiltration (subcutaneous)	T41.3X1	T41.3X2	T41.3X3	T41.3X4	T41.3X5	T41.3X6
nerve block (peripheral) (plexus)	T41.3X1	T41.3X2	T41.3X3	T41.3X4	T41.3X5	T41.3X6
Marezine	T45.0X1	T45.0X2	T45.0X3	T45.0X4	T45.0X5	T45.0X6
Marihuana	T40.7X1	T40.7X2	T40.7X3	T40.7X4	T40.7X5	T40.7X6
Marijuana	T40.7X1	T40.7X2	T40.7X3	T40.7X4	T40.7X5	T40.7X6
Marine (sting)	T63.691	T63.692	T63.693	T63.694	—	—
animals (sting)	T63.691	T63.692	T63.693	T63.694	—	—
plants (sting)	T63.711	T63.712	T63.713	T63.714	—	—
Marplan	T43.1X1	T43.1X2	T43.1X3	T43.1X4	T43.1X5	T43.1X6
Marsh gas	T59.891	T59.892	T59.893	T59.894	—	—
Marsilid	T43.1X1	T43.1X2	T43.1X3	T43.1X4	T43.1X5	T43.1X6
Matulane	T45.1X1	T45.1X2	T45.1X3	T45.1X4	T45.1X5	T45.1X6
Mazindol	T50.5X1	T50.5X2	T50.5X3	T50.5X4	T50.5X5	T50.5X6
MCPA	T60.3X1	T60.3X2	T60.3X3	T60.3X4	—	—
MDMA	T43.621	T43.622	T43.623	T43.624	T43.625	T43.626
Meadow saffron	T62.2X1	T62.2X2	T62.2X3	T62.2X4	—	—
Measles virus vaccine (attenuated)	T50.B91	T50.B92	T50.B93	T50.B94	T50.B95	T50.B96
Meat, noxious	T62.8X1	T62.8X2	T62.8X3	T62.8X4	—	—
Meballymal	T42.3X1	T42.3X2	T42.3X3	T42.3X4	T42.3X5	T42.3X6
Mebanazine	T43.1X1	T43.1X2	T43.1X3	T43.1X4	T43.1X5	T43.1X6
Mebaral	T42.3X1	T42.3X2	T42.3X3	T42.3X4	T42.3X5	T42.3X6
Mebendazole	T37.4X1	T37.4X2	T37.4X3	T37.4X4	T37.4X5	T37.4X6
Mebeverine	T44.3X1	T44.3X2	T44.3X3	T44.3X4	T44.3X5	T44.3X6
Mebhydrolin	T45.0X1	T45.0X2	T45.0X3	T45.0X4	T45.0X5	T45.0X6
Mebumal	T42.3X1	T42.3X2	T42.3X3	T42.3X4	T42.3X5	T42.3X6
Mebutamate	T43.591	T43.592	T43.593	T43.594	T43.595	T43.596
Mecamylamine	T44.2X1	T44.2X2	T44.2X3	T44.2X4	T44.2X5	T44.2X6
Mechlorethamine	T45.1X1	T45.1X2	T45.1X3	T45.1X4	T45.1X5	T45.1X6
Mecillinam	T36.0X1	T36.0X2	T36.0X3	T36.0X4	T36.0X5	T36.0X6
Meclizine (hydrochloride)	T45.0X1	T45.0X2	T45.0X3	T45.0X4	T45.0X5	T45.0X6
Meclocycline	T36.4X1	T36.4X2	T36.4X3	T36.4X4	T36.4X5	T36.4X6
Meclofenamate	T39.391	T39.392	T39.393	T39.394	T39.395	T39.396
Meclofenamic acid	T39.391	T39.392	T39.393	T39.394	T39.395	T39.396

Substance	Poisoning, Accidental (Unintentional)	Poisoning, Intentional Self-Harm	Poisoning, Assault	Poisoning, Undetermined	Adverse Effect	Underdosing
Meclofenoxate	T43.691	T43.692	T43.693	T43.694	T43.695	T43.696
Meclozine	T45.0X1	T45.0X2	T45.0X3	T45.0X4	T45.0X5	T45.0X6
Mecobalamin	T45.8X1	T45.8X2	T45.8X3	T45.8X4	T45.8X5	T45.8X6
Mecoprop	T60.3X1	T60.3X2	T60.3X3	T60.3X4	—	—
Mecrilate	T49.3X1	T49.3X2	T49.3X3	T49.3X4	T49.3X5	T49.3X6
Mecysteine	T48.4X1	T48.4X2	T48.4X3	T48.4X4	T48.4X5	T48.4X6
Medazepam	T42.4X1	T42.4X2	T42.4X3	T42.4X4	T42.4X5	T42.4X6
Medicament NEC	T50.901	T50.902	T50.903	T50.904	T50.905	T50.906
Medinal	T42.3X1	T42.3X2	T42.3X3	T42.3X4	T42.3X5	T42.3X6
Medomin	T42.3X1	T42.3X2	T42.3X3	T42.3X4	T42.3X5	T42.3X6
Medrogestone	T38.5X1	T38.5X2	T38.5X3	T38.5X4	T38.5X5	T38.5X6
Medroxalol	T44.8X1	T44.8X2	T44.8X3	T44.8X4	T44.8X5	T44.8X6
Medroxyprogesterone acetate (depot)	T38.5X1	T38.5X2	T38.5X3	T38.5X4	T38.5X5	T38.5X6
Medrysone	T49.0X1	T49.0X2	T49.0X3	T49.0X4	T49.0X5	T49.0X6
Mefenamic acid	T39.391	T39.392	T39.393	T39.394	T39.395	T39.396
Mefenorex	T50.5X1	T50.5X2	T50.5X3	T50.5X4	T50.5X5	T50.5X6
Mefloquine	T37.2X1	T37.2X2	T37.2X3	T37.2X4	T37.2X5	T37.2X6
Mefruside	T50.2X1	T50.2X2	T50.2X3	T50.2X4	T50.2X5	T50.2X6
Megahallucinogen	T40.901	T40.902	T40.903	T40.904	T40.905	T40.906
Megestrol	T38.5X1	T38.5X2	T38.5X3	T38.5X4	T38.5X5	T38.5X6
Meglumine						
antimoniate	T37.8X1	T37.8X2	T37.8X3	T37.8X4	T37.8X5	T37.8X6
diatrizoate	T50.8X1	T50.8X2	T50.8X3	T50.8X4	T50.8X5	T50.8X6
iodipamide	T50.8X1	T50.8X2	T50.8X3	T50.8X4	T50.8X5	T50.8X6
iotroxate	T50.8X1	T50.8X2	T50.8X3	T50.8X4	T50.8X5	T50.8X6
MEK (methyl ethyl ketone)	T52.4X1	T52.4X2	T52.4X3	T52.4X4	—	—
Meladrazine	T44.3X1	T44.3X2	T44.3X3	T44.3X4	T44.3X5	T44.3X6
Meladinin	T49.3X1	T49.3X2	T49.3X3	T49.3X4	T49.3X5	T49.3X6
Melaleuca alternifolia oil	T49.0X1	T49.0X2	T49.0X3	T49.0X4	T49.0X5	T49.0X6
Melanizing agents	T49.3X1	T49.3X2	T49.3X3	T49.3X4	T49.3X5	T49.3X6
Melanocyte-stimulating hormone	T38.891	T38.892	T38.893	T38.894	T38.895	T38.896
Melarsonyl potassium	T37.3X1	T37.3X2	T37.3X3	T37.3X4	T37.3X5	T37.3X6
Melarsoprol	T37.3X1	T37.3X2	T37.3X3	T37.3X4	T37.3X5	T37.3X6
Melia azedarach	T62.2X1	T62.2X2	T62.2X3	T62.2X4	—	—
Melitracen	T43.011	T43.012	T43.013	T43.014	T43.015	T43.016
Mellaril	T43.3X1	T43.3X2	T43.3X3	T43.3X4	T43.3X5	T43.3X6
Meloxine	T49.3X1	T49.3X2	T49.3X3	T49.3X4	T49.3X5	T49.3X6
Melperone	T43.4X1	T43.4X2	T43.4X3	T43.4X4	T43.4X5	T43.4X6
Melphalan	T45.1X1	T45.1X2	T45.1X3	T45.1X4	T45.1X5	T45.1X6
Memantine	T43.8X1	T43.8X2	T43.8X3	T43.8X4	T43.8X5	T43.8X6

TABLE OF DRUGS AND CHEMICALS

Substance	Poisoning, Accidental (Unintentional)	Poisoning, Intentional Self-Harm	Poisoning, Assault	Poisoning, Undetermined	Adverse Effect	Underdosing
Menadiol	T45.7X1	T45.7X2	T45.7X3	T45.7X4	T45.7X5	T45.7X6
sodium sulfate	T45.7X1	T45.7X2	T45.7X3	T45.7X4	T45.7X5	T45.7X6
Menadione	T45.7X1	T45.7X2	T45.7X3	T45.7X4	T45.7X5	T45.7X6
sodium bisulfite	T45.7X1	T45.7X2	T45.7X3	T45.7X4	T45.7X5	T45.7X6
Menaphthone	T45.7X1	T45.7X2	T45.7X3	T45.7X4	T45.7X5	T45.7X6
Menaquinone	T45.7X1	T45.7X2	T45.7X3	T45.7X4	T45.7X5	T45.7X6
Menatetrenone	T45.7X1	T45.7X2	T45.7X3	T45.7X4	T45.7X5	T45.7X6
Meningococcal vaccine	T50.A91	T50.A92	T50.A93	T50.A94	T50.A95	T50.A96
Menningovax (-AC) (-C)	T50.A91	T50.A92	T50.A93	T50.A94	T50.A95	T50.A96
Menotropins	T38.811	T38.812	T38.813	T38.814	T38.815	T38.816
Menthol	T48.5X1	T48.5X2	T48.5X3	T48.5X4	T48.5X5	T48.5X6
Mepacrine	T37.2X1	T37.2X2	T37.2X3	T37.2X4	T37.2X5	T37.2X6
Meparfynol	T42.6X1	T42.6X2	T42.6X3	T42.6X4	T42.6X5	T42.6X6
Mepartricin	T36.7X1	T36.7X2	T36.7X3	T36.7X4	T36.7X5	T36.7X6
Mepazine	T43.3X1	T43.3X2	T43.3X3	T43.3X4	T43.3X5	T43.3X6
Mepenzolate	T44.3X1	T44.3X2	T44.3X3	T44.3X4	T44.3X5	T44.3X6
bromide	T44.3X1	T44.3X2	T44.3X3	T44.3X4	T44.3X5	T44.3X6
Meperidine	T40.4X1	T40.4X2	T40.4X3	T40.4X4	T40.4X5	T40.4X6
Mephebarbital	T42.3X1	T42.3X2	T42.3X3	T42.3X4	T42.3X5	T42.3X6
Mephenamin(e)	T42.8X1	T42.8X2	T42.8X3	T42.8X4	T42.8X5	T42.8X6
Mephenesin	T42.8X1	T42.8X2	T42.8X3	T42.8X4	T42.8X5	T42.8X6
Mephenhydramine	T45.0X1	T45.0X2	T45.0X3	T45.0X4	T45.0X5	T45.0X6
Mephenoxalone	T42.8X1	T42.8X2	T42.8X3	T42.8X4	T42.8X5	T42.8X6
Mephentermine	T44.991	T44.992	T44.993	T44.994	T44.995	T44.996
Mephenytoin	T42.0X1	T42.0X2	T42.0X3	T42.0X4	T42.0X5	T42.0X6
with phenobarbital	T42.3X1	T42.3X2	T42.3X3	T42.3X4	T42.3X5	T42.3X6
Mephobarbital	T42.3X1	T42.3X2	T42.3X3	T42.3X4	T42.3X5	T42.3X6
Mephosfolan	T60.0X1	T60.0X2	T60.0X3	T60.0X4	—	—
Mepindolol	T44.7X1	T44.7X2	T44.7X3	T44.7X4	T44.7X5	T44.7X6
Mepiperphenidol	T44.3X1	T44.3X2	T44.3X3	T44.3X4	T44.3X5	T44.3X6
Mepitiostane	T38.7X1	T38.7X2	T38.7X3	T38.7X4	T38.7X5	T38.7X6
Mepivacaine	T41.3X1	T41.3X2	T41.3X3	T41.3X4	T41.3X5	T41.3X6
epidural	T41.3X1	T41.3X2	T41.3X3	T41.3X4	T41.3X5	T41.3X6
Meprednisone	T38.0X1	T38.0X2	T38.0X3	T38.0X4	T38.0X5	T38.0X6
Meprobam	T43.591	T43.592	T43.593	T43.594	T43.595	T43.596
Meprobamate	T43.591	T43.592	T43.593	T43.594	T43.595	T43.596
Meproscillarin	T46.0X1	T46.0X2	T46.0X3	T46.0X4	T46.0X5	T46.0X6
Meprylcaine	T41.3X1	T41.3X2	T41.3X3	T41.3X4	T41.3X5	T41.3X6
Meptazinol	T39.8X1	T39.8X2	T39.8X3	T39.8X4	T39.8X5	T39.8X6
Mepyramine	T45.0X1	T45.0X2	T45.0X3	T45.0X4	T45.0X5	T45.0X6
Mequitazine	T43.3X1	T43.3X2	T43.3X3	T43.3X4	T43.3X5	T43.3X6
Meralluride	T50.2X1	T50.2X2	T50.2X3	T50.2X4	T50.2X5	T50.2X6

Substance	Poisoning, Accidental (Unintentional)	Poisoning, Intentional Self-Harm	Poisoning, Assault	Poisoning, Undetermined	Adverse Effect	Underdosing
Merbaphen	T50.2X1	T50.2X2	T50.2X3	T50.2X4	T50.2X5	T50.2X6
Merbromin	T49.0X1	T49.0X2	T49.0X3	T49.0X4	T49.0X5	T49.0X6
Mercaptobenzothiazole salts	T49.0X1	T49.0X2	T49.0X3	T49.0X4	T49.0X5	T49.0X6
Mercaptomerin	T50.2X1	T50.2X2	T50.2X3	T50.2X4	T50.2X5	T50.2X6
Mercaptopurine	T45.1X1	T45.1X2	T45.1X3	T45.1X4	T45.1X5	T45.1X6
Mercumatilin	T50.2X1	T50.2X2	T50.2X3	T50.2X4	T50.2X5	T50.2X6
Mercuramide	T50.2X1	T50.2X2	T50.2X3	T50.2X4	T50.2X5	T50.2X6
Mercurochrome	T49.0X1	T49.0X2	T49.0X3	T49.0X4	T49.0X5	T49.0X6
Mercurophylline	T50.2X1	T50.2X2	T50.2X3	T50.2X4	T50.2X5	T50.2X6
Mercury, mercurial, mercuric, mercurous (compounds) (cyanide) (fumes) (nonmedicinal) (vapor) NEC	T56.1X1	T56.1X2	T56.1X3	T56.1X4	—	—
ammoniated	T49.0X1	T49.0X2	T49.0X3	T49.0X4	T49.0X5	T49.0X6
anti-infective						
local	T49.0X1	T49.0X2	T49.0X3	T49.0X4	T49.0X5	T49.0X6
systemic	T37.8X1	T37.8X2	T37.8X3	T37.8X4	T37.8X5	T37.8X6
topical	T49.0X1	T49.0X2	T49.0X3	T49.0X4	T49.0X5	T49.0X6
chloride (ammoniated)	T49.0X1	T49.0X2	T49.0X3	T49.0X4	T49.0X5	T49.0X6
fungicide	T56.1X1	T56.1X2	T56.1X3	T56.1X4	—	—
diuretic NEC	T50.2X1	T50.2X2	T50.2X3	T50.2X4	T50.2X5	T50.2X6
fungicide	T56.1X1	T56.1X2	T56.1X3	T56.1X4	—	—
organic (fungicide)	T56.1X1	T56.1X2	T56.1X3	T56.1X4	—	—
oxide, yellow	T49.0X1	T49.0X2	T49.0X3	T49.0X4	T49.0X5	T49.0X6
Mersalyl	T50.2X1	T50.2X2	T50.2X3	T50.2X4	T50.2X5	T50.2X6
Merthiolate	T49.0X1	T49.0X2	T49.0X3	T49.0X4	T49.0X5	T49.0X6
ophthalmic preparation	T49.5X1	T49.5X2	T49.5X3	T49.5X4	T49.5X5	T49.5X6
Meruvax	T50.B91	T50.B92	T50.B93	T50.B94	T50.B95	T50.B96
Mesalazine	T47.8X1	T47.8X2	T47.8X3	T47.8X4	T47.8X5	T47.8X6
Mescal buttons	T40.991	T40.992	T40.993	T40.994	—	—
Mescaline	T40.991	T40.992	T40.993	T40.994	—	—
Mesna	T48.4X1	T48.4X2	T48.4X3	T48.4X4	T48.4X5	T48.4X6
Mesoglycan	T46.6X1	T46.6X2	T46.6X3	T46.6X4	T46.6X5	T46.6X6
Mesoridazine	T43.3X1	T43.3X2	T43.3X3	T43.3X4	T43.3X5	T43.3X6
Mestanolone	T38.7X1	T38.7X2	T38.7X3	T38.7X4	T38.7X5	T38.7X6
Mesterolone	T38.7X1	T38.7X2	T38.7X3	T38.7X4	T38.7X5	T38.7X6
Mestranol	T38.5X1	T38.5X2	T38.5X3	T38.5X4	T38.5X5	T38.5X6
Mesulergine	T42.8X1	T42.8X2	T42.8X3	T42.8X4	T42.8X5	T42.8X6
Mesulfen	T49.0X1	T49.0X2	T49.0X3	T49.0X4	T49.0X5	T49.0X6
Mesuximide	T42.2X1	T42.2X2	T42.2X3	T42.2X4	T42.2X5	T42.2X6
Metabutethamine	T41.3X1	T41.3X2	T41.3X3	T41.3X4	T41.3X5	T41.3X6
Metactesylacetate	T49.0X1	T49.0X2	T49.0X3	T49.0X4	T49.0X5	T49.0X6

◀ New ◀ Revised ~~deleted~~ Deleted

Substance	Poisoning, Accidental (Unintentional)	Poisoning, Intentional Self-Harm	Poisoning, Assault	Poisoning, Undetermined	Adverse Effect	Underdosing
Metacycline	T36.4X1	T36.4X2	T36.4X3	T36.4X4	T36.4X5	T36.4X6
Metaldehyde (snail killer) NEC	T60.8X1	T60.8X2	T60.8X3	T60.8X4	—	—
Metals (heavy) (nonmedicinal)	T56.91	T56.92	T56.93	T56.94	—	—
dust, fumes, or vapor NEC	T56.91	T56.92	T56.93	T56.94	—	—
light NEC	T56.91	T56.92	T56.93	T56.94	—	—
dust, fumes, or vapor NEC	T56.91	T56.92	T56.93	T56.94	—	—
specified NEC	T56.891	T56.892	T56.893	T56.894	—	—
thallium	T56.811	T56.812	T56.813	T56.814	—	—
Metamfetamine	T43.621	T43.622	T43.623	T43.624	T43.625	T43.626
Metamizole sodium	T39.2X1	T39.2X2	T39.2X3	T39.2X4	T39.2X5	T39.2X6
Metampicillin	T36.0X1	T36.0X2	T36.0X3	T36.0X4	T36.0X5	T36.0X6
Metamucil	T47.4X1	T47.4X2	T47.4X3	T47.4X4	T47.4X5	T47.4X6
Metaphen	T49.0X1	T49.0X2	T49.0X3	T49.0X4	T49.0X5	T49.0X6
Metandienone	T38.7X1	T38.7X2	T38.7X3	T38.7X4	T38.7X5	T38.7X6
Metandrostenolone	T38.7X1	T38.7X2	T38.7X3	T38.7X4	T38.7X5	T38.7X6
Metaphos	T60.0X1	T60.0X2	T60.0X3	T60.0X4	—	—
Metapramine	T43.011	T43.012	T43.013	T43.014	T43.015	T43.016
Metaproterenol	T48.291	T48.292	T48.293	T48.294	T48.295	T48.296
Metaraminol	T44.4X1	T44.4X2	T44.4X3	T44.4X4	T44.4X5	T44.4X6
Metaxalone	T42.8X1	T42.8X2	T42.8X3	T42.8X4	T42.8X5	T42.8X6
Metenolone	T38.7X1	T38.7X2	T38.7X3	T38.7X4	T38.7X5	T38.7X6
Metergoline	T42.8X1	T42.8X2	T42.8X3	T42.8X4	T42.8X5	T42.8X6
Metescufylline	T46.991	T46.992	T46.993	T46.994	T46.995	T46.996
Metetoin	T42.0X1	T42.0X2	T42.0X3	T42.0X4	T42.0X5	T42.0X6
Metformin	T38.3X1	T38.3X2	T38.3X3	T38.3X4	T38.3X5	T38.3X6
Methacholine	T44.1X1	T44.1X2	T44.1X3	T44.1X4	T44.1X5	T44.1X6
Methacycline	T36.4X1	T36.4X2	T36.4X3	T36.4X4	T36.4X5	T36.4X6
Methadone	T40.3X1	T40.3X2	T40.3X3	T40.3X4	T40.3X5	T40.3X6
Methallenestril	T38.5X1	T38.5X2	T38.5X3	T38.5X4	T38.5X5	T38.5X6
Methallenoestril	T38.5X1	T38.5X2	T38.5X3	T38.5X4	T38.5X5	T38.5X6
Methamphetamine	T43.621	T43.622	T43.623	T43.624	T43.625	T43.626
Methampyrone	T39.2X1	T39.2X2	T39.2X3	T39.2X4	T39.2X5	T39.2X6
Methandienone	T38.7X1	T38.7X2	T38.7X3	T38.7X4	T38.7X5	T38.7X6
Methandriol	T38.7X1	T38.7X2	T38.7X3	T38.7X4	T38.7X5	T38.7X6
Methandrostenolone	T38.7X1	T38.7X2	T38.7X3	T38.7X4	T38.7X5	T38.7X6
Methane	T59.891	T59.892	T59.893	T59.894	—	—
Methanethiol	T59.891	T59.892	T59.893	T59.894	—	—
Methaniazide	T37.1X1	T37.1X2	T37.1X3	T37.1X4	T37.1X5	T37.1X6
Methanol (vapor)	T51.1X1	T51.1X2	T51.1X3	T51.1X4	—	—
Methantheline	T44.3X1	T44.3X2	T44.3X3	T44.3X4	T44.3X5	T44.3X6
Methanthelinium bromide	T44.3X1	T44.3X2	T44.3X3	T44.3X4	T44.3X5	T44.3X6
Methaphenilene	T45.0X1	T45.0X2	T45.0X3	T45.0X4	T45.0X5	T45.0X6

Substance	Poisoning, Accidental (Unintentional)	Poisoning, Intentional Self-Harm	Poisoning, Assault	Poisoning, Undetermined	Adverse Effect	Underdosing
Methapyrilene	T45.0X1	T45.0X2	T45.0X3	T45.0X4	T45.0X5	T45.0X6
Methaqualone (compound)	T42.6X1	T42.6X2	T42.6X3	T42.6X4	T42.6X5	T42.6X6
Metharbital	T42.3X1	T42.3X2	T42.3X3	T42.3X4	T42.3X5	T42.3X6
Methazolamide	T50.2X1	T50.2X2	T50.2X3	T50.2X4	T50.2X5	T50.2X6
Methdilazine	T43.3X1	T43.3X2	T43.3X3	T43.3X4	T43.3X5	T43.3X6
Methedrine	T43.621	T43.622	T43.623	T43.624	T43.625	T43.626
Methenamine (mandelate)	T37.8X1	T37.8X2	T37.8X3	T37.8X4	T37.8X5	T37.8X6
Methenolone	T38.7X1	T38.7X2	T38.7X3	T38.7X4	T38.7X5	T38.7X6
Methergine	T48.0X1	T48.0X2	T48.0X3	T48.0X4	T48.0X5	T48.0X6
Methetoin	T42.0X1	T42.0X2	T42.0X3	T42.0X4	T42.0X5	T42.0X6
Methiacil	T38.2X1	T38.2X2	T38.2X3	T38.2X4	T38.2X5	T38.2X6
Methicillin	T36.0X1	T36.0X2	T36.0X3	T36.0X4	T36.0X5	T36.0X6
Methimazole	T38.2X1	T38.2X2	T38.2X3	T38.2X4	T38.2X5	T38.2X6
Methiodal sodium	T50.8X1	T50.8X2	T50.8X3	T50.8X4	T50.8X5	T50.8X6
Methionine	T50.991	T50.992	T50.993	T50.994	T50.995	T50.996
Methisazone	T37.5X1	T37.5X2	T37.5X3	T37.5X4	T37.5X5	T37.5X6
Methisoprinol	T37.5X1	T37.5X2	T37.5X3	T37.5X4	T37.5X5	T37.5X6
Methitural	T42.3X1	T42.3X2	T42.3X3	T42.3X4	T42.3X5	T42.3X6
Methixene	T44.3X1	T44.3X2	T44.3X3	T44.3X4	T44.3X5	T44.3X6
Methobarbital, methobarbitone	T42.3X1	T42.3X2	T42.3X3	T42.3X4	T42.3X5	T42.3X6
Methocarbamol	T42.8X1	T42.8X2	T42.8X3	T42.8X4	T42.8X5	T42.8X6
skeletal muscle relaxant	T48.1X1	T48.1X2	T48.1X3	T48.1X4	T48.1X5	T48.1X6
Methohexital	T41.1X1	T41.1X2	T41.1X3	T41.1X4	T41.1X5	T41.1X6
Methohexitone	T41.1X1	T41.1X2	T41.1X3	T41.1X4	T41.1X5	T41.1X6
Methoin	T42.0X1	T42.0X2	T42.0X3	T42.0X4	T42.0X5	T42.0X6
Methopholine	T39.8X1	T39.8X2	T39.8X3	T39.8X4	T39.8X5	T39.8X6
Methopromazine	T43.3X1	T43.3X2	T43.3X3	T43.3X4	T43.3X5	T43.3X6
Methorate	T48.3X1	T48.3X2	T48.3X3	T48.3X4	T48.3X5	T48.3X6
Methoserpidine	T46.5X1	T46.5X2	T46.5X3	T46.5X4	T46.5X5	T46.5X6
Methotrexate	T45.1X1	T45.1X2	T45.1X3	T45.1X4	T45.1X5	T45.1X6
Methotrimeprazine	T43.3X1	T43.3X2	T43.3X3	T43.3X4	T43.3X5	T43.3X6
Methoxa-Dome	T49.3X1	T49.3X2	T49.3X3	T49.3X4	T49.3X5	T49.3X6
Methoxamine	T44.4X1	T44.4X2	T44.4X3	T44.4X4	T44.4X5	T44.4X6
Methoxsalen	T50.991	T50.992	T50.993	T50.994	T50.995	T50.996
Methoxyaniline	T65.3X1	T65.3X2	T65.3X3	T65.3X4	—	—
Methoxybenzyl penicillin	T36.0X1	T36.0X2	T36.0X3	T36.0X4	T36.0X5	T36.0X6
Methoxychlor	T53.7X1	T53.7X2	T53.7X3	T53.7X4	—	—
Methoxy-DDT	T53.7X1	T53.7X2	T53.7X3	T53.7X4	—	—
2-Methoxyethanol	T52.3X1	T52.3X2	T52.3X3	T52.3X4	—	—
Methoxyflurane	T41.0X1	T41.0X2	T41.0X3	T41.0X4	T41.0X5	T41.0X6
Methoxyphenamine	T48.6X1	T48.6X2	T48.6X3	T48.6X4	T48.6X5	T48.6X6
Methoxypromazine	T43.3X1	T43.3X2	T43.3X3	T43.3X4	T43.3X5	T43.3X6

◀ New ◀ Revised ~~deleted~~ Deleted

TABLE OF DRUGS AND CHEMICALS

Substance	Poisoning, Accidental (Unintentional)	Poisoning, Intentional Self-Harm	Poisoning, Assault	Poisoning, Undetermined	Adverse Effect	Underdosing
5-Methoxypsoralen (5-MOP)	T50.991	T50.992	T50.993	T50.994	T50.995	T50.996
8-Methoxypsoralen (8-MOP)	T50.991	T50.992	T50.993	T50.994	T50.995	T50.996
Methscopolamine bromide	T44.3X1	T44.3X2	T44.3X3	T44.3X4	T44.3X5	T44.3X6
Methsuximide	T42.2X1	T42.2X2	T42.2X3	T42.2X4	T42.2X5	T42.2X6
Methyclothiazide	T50.2X1	T50.2X2	T50.2X3	T50.2X4	T50.2X5	T50.2X6
Methyl						
acetate	T52.4X1	T52.4X2	T52.4X3	T52.4X4	—	—
acetone	T52.4X1	T52.4X2	T52.4X3	T52.4X4	—	—
acrylate	T65.891	T65.892	T65.893	T65.894	—	—
alcohol	T51.1X1	T51.1X2	T51.1X3	T51.1X4	—	—
aminophenol	T65.3X1	T65.3X2	T65.3X3	T65.3X4	—	—
amphetamine	T43.621	T43.622	T43.623	T43.624	T43.625	T43.626
androstanolone	T38.7X1	T38.7X2	T38.7X3	T38.7X4	T38.7X5	T38.7X6
atropine	T44.3X1	T44.3X2	T44.3X3	T44.3X4	T44.3X5	T44.3X6
benzene	T52.2X1	T52.2X2	T52.2X3	T52.2X4	—	—
benzoate	T52.8X1	T52.8X2	T52.8X3	T52.8X4	—	—
benzol	T52.2X1	T52.2X2	T52.2X3	T52.2X4	—	—
bromide (gas)	T59.891	T59.892	T59.893	T59.894	—	—
fumigant	T60.8X1	T60.8X2	T60.8X3	T60.8X4	—	—
butanol	T51.3X1	T51.3X2	T51.3X3	T51.3X4	—	—
carbinol	T51.1X1	T51.1X2	T51.1X3	T51.1X4	—	—
carbonate	T52.8X1	T52.8X2	T52.8X3	T52.8X4	—	—
CCNU	T45.1X1	T45.1X2	T45.1X3	T45.1X4	T45.1X5	T45.1X6
cellosolve	T52.91	T52.92	T52.93	T52.94	—	—
cellulose	T47.4X1	T47.4X2	T47.4X3	T47.4X4	T47.4X5	T47.4X6
chloride (gas)	T59.891	T59.892	T59.893	T59.894	—	—
chloroformate	T59.3X1	T59.3X2	T59.3X3	T59.3X4	—	—
cyclohexane	T52.8X1	T52.8X2	T52.8X3	T52.8X4	—	—
cyclohexanol	T51.8X1	T51.8X2	T51.8X3	T51.8X4	—	—
cyclohexanone	T52.8X1	T52.8X2	T52.8X3	T52.8X4	—	—
cyclohexyl acetate	T52.8X1	T52.8X2	T52.8X3	T52.8X4	—	—
demeton	T60.0X1	T60.0X2	T60.0X3	T60.0X4	—	—
dihydromorphinone	T40.2X1	T40.2X2	T40.2X3	T40.2X4	T40.2X5	T40.2X6
ergometrine	T48.0X1	T48.0X2	T48.0X3	T48.0X4	T48.0X5	T48.0X6
ergonovine	T48.0X1	T48.0X2	T48.0X3	T48.0X4	T48.0X5	T48.0X6
ethyl ketone	T52.4X1	T52.4X2	T52.4X3	T52.4X4	—	—
glucamine antimonate	T37.8X1	T37.8X2	T37.8X3	T37.8X4	T37.8X5	T37.8X6
hydrazine	T65.891	T65.892	T65.893	T65.894	—	—
iodide	T65.891	T65.892	T65.893	T65.894	—	—
isobutyl ketone	T52.4X1	T52.4X2	T52.4X3	T52.4X4	—	—
isothiocyanate	T60.3X1	T60.3X2	T60.3X3	T60.3X4	—	—
mercaptan	T59.891	T59.892	T59.893	T59.894	—	—

Substance	Poisoning, Accidental (Unintentional)	Poisoning, Intentional Self-Harm	Poisoning, Assault	Poisoning, Undetermined	Adverse Effect	Underdosing
Methyl (Continued)						
morphine NEC	T40.2X1	T40.2X2	T40.2X3	T40.2X4	T40.2X5	T40.2X6
nicotinate	T49.4X1	T49.4X2	T49.4X3	T49.4X4	T49.4X5	T49.4X6
paraben	T49.0X1	T49.0X2	T49.0X3	T49.0X4	T49.0X5	T49.0X6
parafynol	T42.6X1	T42.6X2	T42.6X3	T42.6X4	T42.6X5	T42.6X6
parathion	T60.0X1	T60.0X2	T60.0X3	T60.0X4	—	—
peridol	T43.4X1	T43.4X2	T43.4X3	T43.4X4	T43.4X5	T43.4X6
phenidate	T43.631	T43.632	T43.633	T43.634	T43.635	T43.636
prednisolone	T38.0X1	T38.0X2	T38.0X3	T38.0X4	T38.0X5	T38.0X6
ENT agent	T49.6X1	T49.6X2	T49.6X3	T49.6X4	T49.6X5	T49.6X6
ophthalmic preparation	T49.5X1	T49.5X2	T49.5X3	T49.5X4	T49.5X5	T49.5X6
topical NEC	T49.0X1	T49.0X2	T49.0X3	T49.0X4	T49.0X5	T49.0X6
propylcarbinol	T51.3X1	T51.3X2	T51.3X3	T51.3X4	—	—
rosaniline NEC	T49.0X1	T49.0X2	T49.0X3	T49.0X4	T49.0X5	T49.0X6
salicylate	T49.2X1	T49.2X2	T49.2X3	T49.2X4	T49.2X5	T49.2X6
sulfate (fumes)	T59.891	T59.892	T59.893	T59.894	—	—
liquid	T52.8X1	T52.8X2	T52.8X3	T52.8X4	—	—
sulfonal	T42.6X1	T42.6X2	T42.6X3	T42.6X4	T42.6X5	T42.6X6
testosterone	T38.7X1	T38.7X2	T38.7X3	T38.7X4	T38.7X5	T38.7X6
thiouracil	T38.2X1	T38.2X2	T38.2X3	T38.2X4	T38.2X5	T38.2X6
Methylamphetamine	T43.621	T43.622	T43.623	T43.624	T43.625	T43.626
Methylated spirit	T51.1X1	T51.1X2	T51.1X3	T51.1X4	—	—
Methylatropine nitrate	T44.3X1	T44.3X2	T44.3X3	T44.3X4	T44.3X5	T44.3X6
Methylbenactyzium bromide	T44.3X1	T44.3X2	T44.3X3	T44.3X4	T44.3X5	T44.3X6
Methylbenzethonium chloride	T49.0X1	T49.0X2	T49.0X3	T49.0X4	T49.0X5	T49.0X6
Methylcellulose	T47.4X1	T47.4X2	T47.4X3	T47.4X4	T47.4X5	T47.4X6
laxative	T47.4X1	T47.4X2	T47.4X3	T47.4X4	T47.4X5	T47.4X6
Methylchlorophenoxy-acetic acid	T60.3X1	T60.3X2	T60.3X3	T60.3X4	—	—
Methyldopa	T46.5X1	T46.5X2	T46.5X3	T46.5X4	T46.5X5	T46.5X6
Methyldopate	T46.5X1	T46.5X2	T46.5X3	T46.5X4	T46.5X5	T46.5X6
Methylene						
blue	T50.6X1	T50.6X2	T50.6X3	T50.6X4	T50.6X5	T50.6X6
chloride or dichloride (solvent) NEC	T53.4X1	T53.4X2	T53.4X3	T53.4X4	—	—
Methylenedioxyamphet-amine	T43.621	T43.622	T43.623	T43.624	T43.625	T43.626
Methylenedioxymethamphetamine	T43.621	T43.622	T43.623	T43.624	T43.625	T43.626
Methylergometrine	T48.0X1	T48.0X2	T48.0X3	T48.0X4	T48.0X5	T48.0X6
Methylergonovine	T48.0X1	T48.0X2	T48.0X3	T48.0X4	T48.0X5	T48.0X6
Methylestrenolone	T38.5X1	T38.5X2	T38.5X3	T38.5X4	T38.5X5	T38.5X6
Methylethyl cellulose	T50.991	T50.992	T50.993	T50.994	T50.995	T50.996
Methylhexabital	T42.3X1	T42.3X2	T42.3X3	T42.3X4	T42.3X5	T42.3X6
Methylmorphine	T40.2X1	T40.2X2	T40.2X3	T40.2X4	T40.2X5	T40.2X6

◀ New ◀ Revised deleted Deleted

	External Cause (T-Code)					
Substance	Poisoning, Accidental (Unintentional)	Poisoning, Intentional Self-Harm	Poisoning, Assault	Poisoning, Undetermined	Adverse Effect	Underdosing
Methylparaben (ophthalmic)	T49.5X1	T49.5X2	T49.5X3	T49.5X4	T49.5X5	T49.5X6
Methylparafynol	T42.6X1	T42.6X2	T42.6X3	T42.6X4	T42.6X5	T42.6X6
Methylpentynol, methylpenthynol	T42.6X1	T42.6X2	T42.6X3	T42.6X4	T42.6X5	T42.6X6
Methylphenidate	T43.631	T43.632	T43.633	T43.634	T43.635	T43.636
Methylphenobarbital	T42.3X1	T42.3X2	T42.3X3	T42.3X4	T42.3X5	T42.3X6
Methylpolysiloxane	T47.1X1	T47.1X2	T47.1X3	T47.1X4	T47.1X5	T47.1X6
Methylprednisolone — *see Methyl, prednisolone*						
Methylrosaniline	T49.0X1	T49.0X2	T49.0X3	T49.0X4	T49.0X5	T49.0X6
Methylrosanilinium chloride	T49.0X1	T49.0X2	T49.0X3	T49.0X4	T49.0X5	T49.0X6
Methyltestosterone	T38.7X1	T38.7X2	T38.7X3	T38.7X4	T38.7X5	T38.7X6
Methylthionine chloride	T50.6X1	T50.6X2	T50.6X3	T50.6X4	T50.6X5	T50.6X6
Methylthioninium chloride	T50.6X1	T50.6X2	T50.6X3	T50.6X4	T50.6X5	T50.6X6
Methylthiouracil	T38.2X1	T38.2X2	T38.2X3	T38.2X4	T38.2X5	T38.2X6
Methyprylon	T42.6X1	T42.6X2	T42.6X3	T42.6X4	T42.6X5	T42.6X6
Methysergide	T46.5X1	T46.5X2	T46.5X3	T46.5X4	T46.5X5	T46.5X6
Metiamide	T47.1X1	T47.1X2	T47.1X3	T47.1X4	T47.1X5	T47.1X6
Meticillin	T36.0X1	T36.0X2	T36.0X3	T36.0X4	T36.0X5	T36.0X6
Meticrane	T50.2X1	T50.2X2	T50.2X3	T50.2X4	T50.2X5	T50.2X6
Metildigoxin	T46.0X1	T46.0X2	T46.0X3	T46.0X4	T46.0X5	T46.0X6
Metipranolol	T49.5X1	T49.5X2	T49.5X3	T49.5X4	T49.5X5	T49.5X6
Metirosine	T46.5X1	T46.5X2	T46.5X3	T46.5X4	T46.5X5	T46.5X6
Metisazone	T37.5X1	T37.5X2	T37.5X3	T37.5X4	T37.5X5	T37.5X6
Metixene	T44.3X1	T44.3X2	T44.3X3	T44.3X4	T44.3X5	T44.3X6
Metizoline	T48.5X1	T48.5X2	T48.5X3	T48.5X4	T48.5X5	T48.5X6
Metoclopramide	T45.0X1	T45.0X2	T45.0X3	T45.0X4	T45.0X5	T45.0X6
Metofenazate	T43.3X1	T43.3X2	T43.3X3	T43.3X4	T43.3X5	T43.3X6
Metofoline	T39.8X1	T39.8X2	T39.8X3	T39.8X4	T39.8X5	T39.8X6
Metolazone	T50.2X1	T50.2X2	T50.2X3	T50.2X4	T50.2X5	T50.2X6
Metopon	T40.2X1	T40.2X2	T40.2X3	T40.2X4	T40.2X5	T40.2X6
Metoprine	T45.1X1	T45.1X2	T45.1X3	T45.1X4	T45.1X5	T45.1X6
Metoprolol	T44.7X1	T44.7X2	T44.7X3	T44.7X4	T44.7X5	T44.7X6
Metrifonate	T60.0X1	T60.0X2	T60.0X3	T60.0X4	—	—
Metrizamide	T50.8X1	T50.8X2	T50.8X3	T50.8X4	T50.8X5	T50.8X6
Metrizoic acid	T50.8X1	T50.8X2	T50.8X3	T50.8X4	T50.8X5	T50.8X6
Metronidazole	T37.8X1	T37.8X2	T37.8X3	T37.8X4	T37.8X5	T37.8X6
Metycaine	T41.3X1	T41.3X2	T41.3X3	T41.3X4	T41.3X5	T41.3X6
infiltration (subcutaneous)	T41.3X1	T41.3X2	T41.3X3	T41.3X4	T41.3X5	T41.3X6
nerve block (peripheral) (plexus)	T41.3X1	T41.3X2	T41.3X3	T41.3X4	T41.3X5	T41.3X6
topical (surface)	T41.3X1	T41.3X2	T41.3X3	T41.3X4	T41.3X5	T41.3X6
Metyrapone	T50.8X1	T50.8X2	T50.8X3	T50.8X4	T50.8X5	T50.8X6
Mevinphos	T60.0X1	T60.0X2	T60.0X3	T60.0X4	—	—

	External Cause (T-Code)					
Substance	Poisoning, Accidental (Unintentional)	Poisoning, Intentional Self-Harm	Poisoning, Assault	Poisoning, Undetermined	Adverse Effect	Underdosing
Mexazolam	T42.4X1	T42.4X2	T42.4X3	T42.4X4	T42.4X5	T42.4X6
Mexenone	T49.3X1	T49.3X2	T49.3X3	T49.3X4	T49.3X5	T49.3X6
Mexiletine	T46.2X1	T46.2X2	T46.2X3	T46.2X4	T46.2X5	T46.2X6
Mezereon	T62.2X1	T62.2X2	T62.2X3	T62.2X4	—	—
berries	T62.1X1	T62.1X2	T62.1X3	T62.1X4	—	—
Mezlocillin	T36.0X1	T36.0X2	T36.0X3	T36.0X4	T36.0X5	T36.0X6
Mianserin	T43.021	T43.022	T43.023	T43.024	T43.025	T43.026
Micatin	T49.0X1	T49.0X2	T49.0X3	T49.0X4	T49.0X5	T49.0X6
Miconazole	T49.0X1	T49.0X2	T49.0X3	T49.0X4	T49.0X5	T49.0X6
Micronomicin	T36.5X1	T36.5X2	T36.5X3	T36.5X4	T36.5X5	T36.5X6
Midazolam	T42.4X1	T42.4X2	T42.4X3	T42.4X4	T42.4X5	T42.4X6
Midecamycin	T36.3X1	T36.3X2	T36.3X3	T36.3X4	T36.3X5	T36.3X6
Mifepristone	T38.6X1	T38.6X2	T38.6X3	T38.6X4	T38.6X5	T38.6X6
Milk of magnesia	T47.1X1	T47.1X2	T47.1X3	T47.1X4	T47.1X5	T47.1X6
Millipede (tropical) (venomous)	T63.411	T63.412	T63.413	T63.414	—	—
Miltown	T43.591	T43.592	T43.593	T43.594	T43.595	T43.596
Milverine	T44.3X1	T44.3X2	T44.3X3	T44.3X4	T44.3X5	T44.3X6
Minaprine	T43.291	T43.292	T43.293	T43.294	T43.295	T43.296
Minaxolone	T41.291	T41.292	T41.293	T41.294	T41.295	T41.296
Mineral						
acids	T54.2X1	T54.2X2	T54.2X3	T54.2X4	—	—
oil (laxative) (medicinal)	T47.4X1	T47.4X2	T47.4X3	T47.4X4	T47.4X5	T47.4X6
emulsion	T47.2X1	T47.2X2	T47.2X3	T47.2X4	T47.2X5	T47.2X6
nonmedicinal	T52.0X1	T52.0X2	T52.0X3	T52.0X4	—	—
topical	T49.3X1	T49.3X2	T49.3X3	T49.3X4	T49.3X5	T49.3X6
salt NEC	T50.3X1	T50.3X2	T50.3X3	T50.3X4	T50.3X5	T50.3X6
spirits	T52.0X1	T52.0X2	T52.0X3	T52.0X4	—	—
Mineralocorticosteroid	T50.0X1	T50.0X2	T50.0X3	T50.0X4	T50.0X5	T50.0X6
Minocycline	T36.4X1	T36.4X2	T36.4X3	T36.4X4	T36.4X5	T36.4X6
Minoxidil	T46.7X1	T46.7X2	T46.7X3	T46.7X4	T46.7X5	T46.7X6
Miokamycin	T36.3X1	T36.3X2	T36.3X3	T36.3X4	T36.3X5	T36.3X6
Miotic drug	T49.5X1	T49.5X2	T49.5X3	T49.5X4	T49.5X5	T49.5X6
Mipafox	T60.0X1	T60.0X2	T60.0X3	T60.0X4	—	—
Mirex	T60.1X1	T60.1X2	T60.1X3	T60.1X4	—	—
Mirtazapine	T43.021	T43.022	T43.023	T43.024	T43.025	T43.026
Misonidazole	T37.3X1	T37.3X2	T37.3X3	T37.3X4	T37.3X5	T37.3X6
Misoprostol	T47.1X1	T47.1X2	T47.1X3	T47.1X4	T47.1X5	T47.1X6
Mithramycin	T45.1X1	T45.1X2	T45.1X3	T45.1X4	T45.1X5	T45.1X6
Mitobronitol	T45.1X1	T45.1X2	T45.1X3	T45.1X4	T45.1X5	T45.1X6
Mitoguazone	T45.1X1	T45.1X2	T45.1X3	T45.1X4	T45.1X5	T45.1X6
Mitolactol	T45.1X1	T45.1X2	T45.1X3	T45.1X4	T45.1X5	T45.1X6
Mitomycin	T45.1X1	T45.1X2	T45.1X3	T45.1X4	T45.1X5	T45.1X6

◀ New　◀ Revised　~~deleted~~ Deleted

TABLE OF DRUGS AND CHEMICALS

Substance	External Cause (T-Code)					
	Poisoning, Accidental (Unintentional)	Poisoning, Intentional Self-Harm	Poisoning, Assault	Poisoning, Undetermined	Adverse Effect	Underdosing
Mitopodozide	T45.1X1	T45.1X2	T45.1X3	T45.1X4	T45.1X5	T45.1X6
Mitotane	T45.1X1	T45.1X2	T45.1X3	T45.1X4	T45.1X5	T45.1X6
Mitoxantrone	T45.1X1	T45.1X2	T45.1X3	T45.1X4	T45.1X5	T45.1X6
Mivacurium chloride	T48.1X1	T48.1X2	T48.1X3	T48.1X4	T48.1X5	T48.1X6
Miyari bacteria	T47.6X1	T47.6X2	T47.6X3	T47.6X4	T47.6X5	T47.6X6
Moclobemide	T43.1X1	T43.1X2	T43.1X3	T43.1X4	T43.1X5	T43.1X6
Moderil	T46.5X1	T46.5X2	T46.5X3	T46.5X4	T46.5X5	T46.5X6
Mofebutazone	T39.2X1	T39.2X2	T39.2X3	T39.2X4	T39.2X5	T39.2X6
Mogadon—see Nitrazepam						
Molindone	T43.591	T43.592	T43.593	T43.594	T43.595	T43.596
Molsidomine	T46.3X1	T46.3X2	T46.3X3	T46.3X4	T46.3X5	T46.3X6
Mometasone	T49.0X1	T49.0X2	T49.0X3	T49.0X4	T49.0X5	T49.0X6
Monistat	T49.0X1	T49.0X2	T49.0X3	T49.0X4	T49.0X5	T49.0X6
Monkshood	T62.2X1	T62.2X2	T62.2X3	T62.2X4	—	—
Monoamine oxidase inhibitor NEC	T43.1X1	T43.1X2	T43.1X3	T43.1X4	T43.1X5	T43.1X6
hydrazine	T43.1X1	T43.1X2	T43.1X3	T43.1X4	T43.1X5	T43.1X6
Monobenzone	T49.4X1	T49.4X2	T49.4X3	T49.4X4	T49.4X5	T49.4X6
Monochloroacetic acid	T60.3X1	T60.3X2	T60.3X3	T60.3X4	—	—
Monochlorobenzene	T53.7X1	T53.7X2	T53.7X3	T53.7X4	—	—
Monoethanolamine	T46.8X1	T46.8X2	T46.8X3	T46.8X4	T46.8X5	T46.8X6
oleate	T46.8X1	T46.8X2	T46.8X3	T46.8X4	T46.8X5	T46.8X6
Monooctanoin	T50.991	T50.992	T50.993	T50.994	T50.995	T50.996
Monophenylbutazone	T39.2X1	T39.2X2	T39.2X3	T39.2X4	T39.2X5	T39.2X6
Monosodium glutamate	T65.891	T65.892	T65.893	T65.894	—	—
Monosulfiram	T49.0X1	T49.0X2	T49.0X3	T49.0X4	T49.0X5	T49.0X6
Monoxide, carbon—see Carbon, monoxide	T57.91	T57.92	T57.93	T57.94	—	—
Monoxidine hydrochloride	T46.1X1	T46.1X2	T46.1X3	T46.1X4	T46.1X5	T46.1X6
Monuron	T60.3X1	T60.3X2	T60.3X3	T60.3X4	—	—
Moperone	T43.4X1	T43.4X2	T43.4X3	T43.4X4	T43.4X5	T43.4X6
Mopidamol	T45.1X1	T45.1X2	T45.1X3	T45.1X4	T45.1X5	T45.1X6
MOPP (mechlorethamine + vincristine + prednisone + procarbazine)	T45.1X1	T45.1X2	T45.1X3	T45.1X4	T45.1X5	T45.1X6
Morfin	T40.2X1	T40.2X2	T40.2X3	T40.2X4	T40.2X5	T40.2X6
Morinamide	T37.1X1	T37.1X2	T37.1X3	T37.1X4	T37.1X5	T37.1X6
Morning glory seeds	T40.991	T40.992	T40.993	T40.994	—	—
Moroxydine	T37.5X1	T37.5X2	T37.5X3	T37.5X4	T37.5X5	T37.5X6
Morphazinamide	T37.1X1	T37.1X2	T37.1X3	T37.1X4	T37.1X5	T37.1X6
Morphine	T40.2X1	T40.2X2	T40.2X3	T40.2X4	T40.2X5	T40.2X6
antagonist	T50.7X1	T50.7X2	T50.7X3	T50.7X4	T50.7X5	T50.7X6
Morpholinylethylmorphine	T40.2X1	T40.2X2	T40.2X3	T40.2X4	—	—
Morsuximide	T42.2X1	T42.2X2	T42.2X3	T42.2X4	T42.2X5	T42.2X6

Substance	External Cause (T-Code)					
	Poisoning, Accidental (Unintentional)	Poisoning, Intentional Self-Harm	Poisoning, Assault	Poisoning, Undetermined	Adverse Effect	Underdosing
Mosapramine	T43.591	T43.592	T43.593	T43.594	T43.595	T43.596
Moth balls—see also Pesticides	T60.2X1	T60.2X2	T60.2X3	T60.2X4	—	—
naphthalene	T60.2X1	T60.2X2	T60.2X3	T60.2X4	—	—
paradichlorobenzene	T60.1X1	T60.1X2	T60.1X3	T60.1X4	—	—
Motor exhaust gas	T58.01	T58.02	T58.03	T58.04	—	—
Mouthwash (antiseptic) (zinc chloride)	T49.6X1	T49.6X2	T49.6X3	T49.6X4	T49.6X5	T49.6X6
Moxastine	T45.0X1	T45.0X2	T45.0X3	T45.0X4	T45.0X5	T45.0X6
Moxaverine	T44.3X1	T44.3X2	T44.3X3	T44.3X4	T44.3X5	T44.3X6
Moxifensine	T43.291	T43.292	T43.293	T43.294	T43.295	T43.296
Moxisylyte	T46.7X1	T46.7X2	T46.7X3	T46.7X4	T46.7X5	T46.7X6
Mucilage, plant	T47.4X1	T47.4X2	T47.4X3	T47.4X4	T47.4X5	T47.4X6
Mucolytic drug	T48.4X1	T48.4X2	T48.4X3	T48.4X4	T48.4X5	T48.4X6
Mucomyst	T48.4X1	T48.4X2	T48.4X3	T48.4X4	T48.4X5	T48.4X6
Mucous membrane agents (external)	T49.91	T49.92	T49.93	T49.94	T49.95	T49.96
specified NEC	T49.8X1	T49.8X2	T49.8X3	T49.8X4	T49.8X5	T49.8X6
Mumps						
immune globulin (human)	T50.Z11	T50.Z12	T50.Z13	T50.Z14	T50.Z15	T50.Z16
skin test antigen	T50.8X1	T50.8X2	T50.8X3	T50.8X4	T50.8X5	T50.8X6
vaccine	T50.B91	T50.B92	T50.B93	T50.B94	T50.B95	T50.B96
Mumpsvax	T50.B91	T50.B92	T50.B93	T50.B94	T50.B95	T50.B96
Mupirocin	T49.0X1	T49.0X2	T49.0X3	T49.0X4	T49.0X5	T49.0X6
Muriatic acid—see Hydrochloric acid						
Muromonab-CD3	T45.1X1	T45.1X2	T45.1X3	T45.1X4	T45.1X5	T45.1X6
Muscle relaxant—see Relaxant, muscle						
Muscle-action drug NEC	T48.201	T48.202	T48.203	T48.204	T48.205	T48.206
Muscle affecting agents NEC	T48.201	T48.202	T48.203	T48.204	T48.205	T48.206
oxytocic	T48.0X1	T48.0X2	T48.0X3	T48.0X4	T48.0X5	T48.0X6
relaxants	T48.201	T48.202	T48.203	T48.204	T48.205	T48.206
central nervous system	T42.8X1	T42.8X2	T42.8X3	T42.8X4	T42.8X5	T42.8X6
skeletal	T48.1X1	T48.1X2	T48.1X3	T48.1X4	T48.1X5	T48.1X6
smooth	T44.3X1	T44.3X2	T44.3X3	T44.3X4	T44.3X5	T44.3X6
Muscle-tone depressant, central NEC	T42.8X1	T42.8X2	T42.8X3	T42.8X4	T42.8X5	T42.8X6
specified NEC	T42.8X1	T42.8X2	T42.8X3	T42.8X4	T42.8X5	T42.8X6
Mushroom, noxious	T62.0X1	T62.0X2	T62.0X3	T62.0X4	—	—
Mussel, noxious	T61.781	T61.782	T61.783	T61.784	—	—
Mustard (emetic)	T47.7X1	T47.7X2	T47.7X3	T47.7X4	T47.7X5	T47.7X6
black	T47.7X1	T47.7X2	T47.7X3	T47.7X4	T47.7X5	T47.7X6
gas, not in war	T59.91	T59.92	T59.93	T59.94	—	—
nitrogen	T45.1X1	T45.1X2	T45.1X3	T45.1X4	T45.1X5	T45.1X6

◀ New   ◀ Revised   ~~deleted~~ Deleted

Substance	Poisoning, Accidental (Unintentional)	Poisoning, Intentional Self-Harm	Poisoning, Assault	Poisoning, Undetermined	Adverse Effect	Underdosing
Mustine	T45.1X1	T45.1X2	T45.1X3	T45.1X4	T45.1X5	T45.1X6
M-vac	T45.1X1	T45.1X2	T45.1X3	T45.1X4	T45.1X5	T45.1X6
Mycifradin	T36.5X1	T36.5X2	T36.5X3	T36.5X4	T36.5X5	T36.5X6
topical	T49.0X1	T49.0X2	T49.0X3	T49.0X4	T49.0X5	T49.0X6
Mycitracin	T36.8X1	T36.8X2	T36.8X3	T36.8X4	T36.8X5	T36.8X6
ophthalmic preparation	T49.5X1	T49.5X2	T49.5X3	T49.5X4	T49.5X5	T49.5X6
Mycostatin	T36.7X1	T36.7X2	T36.7X3	T36.7X4	T36.7X5	T36.7X6
topical	T49.0X1	T49.0X2	T49.0X3	T49.0X4	T49.0X5	T49.0X6
Mycotoxins	T64.81	T64.82	T64.83	T64.84	—	—
aflatoxin	T64.01	T64.02	T64.03	T64.04	—	—
specified NEC	T64.81	T64.82	T64.83	T64.84	—	—
Mydriacyl	T44.3X1	T44.3X2	T44.3X3	T44.3X4	T44.3X5	T44.3X6
Mydriatic drug	T49.5X1	T49.5X2	T49.5X3	T49.5X4	T49.5X5	T49.5X6
Myelobromal	T45.1X1	T45.1X2	T45.1X3	T45.1X4	T45.1X5	T45.1X6
Myleran	T45.1X1	T45.1X2	T45.1X3	T45.1X4	T45.1X5	T45.1X6
Myochrysin(e)	T39.2X1	T39.2X2	T39.2X3	T39.2X4	T39.2X5	T39.2X6
Myoneural blocking agents	T48.1X1	T48.1X2	T48.1X3	T48.1X4	T48.1X5	T48.1X6
Myralact	T49.0X1	T49.0X2	T49.0X3	T49.0X4	T49.0X5	T49.0X6
Myristica fragrans	T62.2X1	T62.2X2	T62.2X3	T62.2X4	—	—
Myristicin	T65.891	T65.892	T65.893	T65.894	—	—
Mysoline	T42.3X1	T42.3X2	T42.3X3	T42.3X4	T42.3X5	T42.3X6
N						
Nabilone	T40.7X1	T40.7X2	T40.7X3	T40.7X4	T40.7X5	T40.7X6
Nabumetone	T39.391	T39.392	T39.393	T39.394	T39.395	T39.396
Nadolol	T44.7X1	T44.7X2	T44.7X3	T44.7X4	T44.7X5	T44.7X6
Nafcillin	T36.0X1	T36.0X2	T36.0X3	T36.0X4	T36.0X5	T36.0X6
Nafoxidine	T38.6X1	T38.6X2	T38.6X3	T38.6X4	T38.6X5	T38.6X6
Naftazone	T46.991	T46.992	T46.993	T46.994	T46.995	T46.996
Naftidrofuryl (oxalate)	T46.7X1	T46.7X2	T46.7X3	T46.7X4	T46.7X5	T46.7X6
Naftifine	T49.0X1	T49.0X2	T49.0X3	T49.0X4	T49.0X5	T49.0X6
Nail polish remover	T52.91	T52.92	T52.93	T52.94	—	—
Nalbuphine	T40.4X1	T40.4X2	T40.4X3	T40.4X4	T40.4X5	T40.4X6
Naled	T60.0X1	T60.0X2	T60.0X3	T60.0X4	—	—
Nalidixic acid	T37.8X1	T37.8X2	T37.8X3	T37.8X4	T37.8X5	T37.8X6
Nalorphine	T50.7X1	T50.7X2	T50.7X3	T50.7X4	T50.7X5	T50.7X6
Naloxone	T50.7X1	T50.7X2	T50.7X3	T50.7X4	T50.7X5	T50.7X6
Naltrexone	T50.7X1	T50.7X2	T50.7X3	T50.7X4	T50.7X5	T50.7X6
Namenda	T43.8X1	T43.8X2	T43.8X3	T43.8X4	T43.8X5	T43.8X6
Nandrolone	T38.7X1	T38.7X2	T38.7X3	T38.7X4	T38.7X5	T38.7X6
Naphazoline	T48.5X1	T48.5X2	T48.5X3	T48.5X4	T48.5X5	T48.5X6
Naphtha (painters') (petroleum)	T52.0X1	T52.0X2	T52.0X3	T52.0X4	—	—
solvent	T52.0X1	T52.0X2	T52.0X3	T52.0X4	—	—
vapor	T52.0X1	T52.0X2	T52.0X3	T52.0X4	—	—
Naphthalene (non-chlorinated)	T60.2X1	T60.2X2	T60.2X3	T60.2X4	—	—
chlorinated	T60.1X1	T60.1X2	T60.1X3	T60.1X4	—	—
vapor	T60.1X1	T60.1X2	T60.1X3	T60.1X4	—	—
insecticide or moth repellent	T60.2X1	T60.2X2	T60.2X3	T60.2X4	—	—
chlorinated	T60.1X1	T60.1X2	T60.1X3	T60.1X4	—	—
vapor	T60.2X1	T60.2X2	T60.2X3	T60.2X4	—	—
chlorinated	T60.1X1	T60.1X2	T60.1X3	T60.1X4	—	—
Naphthol	T65.891	T65.892	T65.893	T65.894	—	—
Naphthylamine	T65.891	T65.892	T65.893	T65.894	—	—
Naphthylthiourea (ANTU)	T60.4X1	T60.4X2	T60.4X3	T60.4X4	—	—
Naprosyn — see Naproxen						
Naproxen	T39.311	T39.312	T39.313	T39.314	T39.315	T39.316
Narcotic (drug)	T40.601	T40.602	T40.603	T40.604	T40.605	T40.606
analgesic NEC	T40.601	T40.602	T40.603	T40.604	T40.605	T40.606
antagonist	T50.7X1	T50.7X2	T50.7X3	T50.7X4	T50.7X5	T50.7X6
specified NEC	T40.691	T40.692	T40.693	T40.694	T40.695	T40.696
synthetic	T40.4X1	T40.4X2	T40.4X3	T40.4X4	T40.4X5	T40.4X6
Narcotine	T48.3X1	T48.3X2	T48.3X3	T48.3X4	T48.3X5	T48.3X6
Nardil	T43.1X1	T43.1X2	T43.1X3	T43.1X4	T43.1X5	T43.1X6
Nasal drug NEC	T49.6X1	T49.6X2	T49.6X3	T49.6X4	T49.6X5	T49.6X6
Natamycin	T49.0X1	T49.0X2	T49.0X3	T49.0X4	T49.0X5	T49.0X6
Natrium cyanide — see Cyanide(s)						
Natural gas	T59.891	T59.892	T59.893	T59.894	—	—
incomplete combustion	T57.91	T57.92	T57.93	T57.94	—	—
Natural						
blood (product)	T45.8X1	T45.8X2	T45.8X3	T45.8X4	T45.8X5	T45.8X6
gas (piped)	T59.891	T59.892	T59.893	T59.894	—	—
incomplete combustion	T58.11	T58.12	T58.13	T58.14	—	—
Nealbarbital	T42.3X1	T42.3X2	T42.3X3	T42.3X4	T42.3X5	T42.3X6
Nectadon	T48.3X1	T48.3X2	T48.3X3	T48.3X4	T48.3X5	T48.3X6
Nedocromil	T48.6X1	T48.6X2	T48.6X3	T48.6X4	T48.6X5	T48.6X6
Nefopam	T39.8X1	T39.8X2	T39.8X3	T39.8X4	T39.8X5	T39.8X6
Nematocyst (sting)	T63.691	T63.692	T63.693	T63.694	—	—
Nembutal	T42.3X1	T42.3X2	T42.3X3	T42.3X4	T42.3X5	T42.3X6
Nemonapride	T43.591	T43.592	T43.593	T43.594	T43.595	T43.596
Neoarsphenamine	T37.8X1	T37.8X2	T37.8X3	T37.8X4	T37.8X5	T37.8X6

TABLE OF DRUGS AND CHEMICALS

Substance	Poisoning, Accidental (Unintentional)	Poisoning, Intentional Self-Harm	Poisoning, Assault	Poisoning, Undetermined	Adverse Effect	Underdosing
Neocinchophen	T50.4X1	T50.4X2	T50.4X3	T50.4X4	T50.4X5	T50.4X6
Neomycin (derivatives)	T36.5X1	T36.5X2	T36.5X3	T36.5X4	T36.5X5	T36.5X6
with						
bacitracin	T49.0X1	T49.0X2	T49.0X3	T49.0X4	T49.0X5	T49.0X6
neostigmine	T44.0X1	T44.0X2	T44.0X3	T44.0X4	T44.0X5	T44.0X6
ENT agent	T49.6X1	T49.6X2	T49.6X3	T49.6X4	T49.6X5	T49.6X6
ophthalmic preparation	T49.5X1	T49.5X2	T49.5X3	T49.5X4	T49.5X5	T49.5X6
topical NEC	T49.0X1	T49.0X2	T49.0X3	T49.0X4	T49.0X5	T49.0X6
Neonal	T42.3X1	T42.3X2	T42.3X3	T42.3X4	T42.3X5	T42.3X6
Neoprontosil	T37.0X1	T37.0X2	T37.0X3	T37.0X4	T37.0X5	T37.0X6
Neosalvarsan	T37.8X1	T37.8X2	T37.8X3	T37.8X4	T37.8X5	T37.8X6
Neosilversalvarsan	T37.8X1	T37.8X2	T37.8X3	T37.8X4	T37.8X5	T37.8X6
Neosporin	T36.8X1	T36.8X2	T36.8X3	T36.8X4	T36.8X5	T36.8X6
ENT agent	T49.6X1	T49.6X2	T49.6X3	T49.6X4	T49.6X5	T49.6X6
opthalmic preparation	T49.5X1	T49.5X2	T49.5X3	T49.5X4	T49.5X5	T49.5X6
topical NEC	T49.0X1	T49.0X2	T49.0X3	T49.0X4	T49.0X5	T49.0X6
Neostigmine bromide	T44.0X1	T44.0X2	T44.0X3	T44.0X4	T44.0X5	T44.0X6
Neraval	T42.3X1	T42.3X2	T42.3X3	T42.3X4	T42.3X5	T42.3X6
Neravan	T42.3X1	T42.3X2	T42.3X3	T42.3X4	T42.3X5	T42.3X6
Nerium oleander	T62.2X1	T62.2X2	T62.2X3	T62.2X4	—	—
Nerve gas, not in war	T59.91	T59.92	T59.93	T59.94	—	—
Nesacaine	T41.3X1	T41.3X2	T41.3X3	T41.3X4	T41.3X5	T41.3X6
infiltration (subcutaneous)	T41.3X1	T41.3X2	T41.3X3	T41.3X4	T41.3X5	T41.3X6
nerve block (peripheral) (plexus)	T41.3X1	T41.3X2	T41.3X3	T41.3X4	T41.3X5	T41.3X6
Netilmicin	T36.5X1	T36.5X2	T36.5X3	T36.5X4	T36.5X5	T36.5X6
Neurobarb	T42.3X1	T42.3X2	T42.3X3	T42.3X4	T42.3X5	T42.3X6
Neuroleptic drug NEC	T43.501	T43.502	T43.503	T43.504	T43.505	T43.506
Neuromuscular blocking drug	T48.1X1	T48.1X2	T48.1X3	T48.1X4	T48.1X5	T48.1X6
Neutral insulin injection	T38.3X1	T38.3X2	T38.3X3	T38.3X4	T38.3X5	T38.3X6
Neutral spirits	T51.0X1	T51.0X2	T51.0X3	T51.0X4	—	—
beverage	T51.0X1	T51.0X2	T51.0X3	T51.0X4	—	—
Niacin	T46.7X1	T46.7X2	T46.7X3	T46.7X4	T46.7X5	T46.7X6
Niacinamide	T45.2X1	T45.2X2	T45.2X3	T45.2X4	T45.2X5	T45.2X6
Nialamide	T43.1X1	T43.1X2	T43.1X3	T43.1X4	T43.1X5	T43.1X6
Niaprazine	T42.6X1	T42.6X2	T42.6X3	T42.6X4	T42.6X5	T42.6X6
Nicametate	T46.7X1	T46.7X2	T46.7X3	T46.7X4	T46.7X5	T46.7X6
Nicardipine	T46.1X1	T46.1X2	T46.1X3	T46.1X4	T46.1X5	T46.1X6
Nicergoline	T46.7X1	T46.7X2	T46.7X3	T46.7X4	T46.7X5	T46.7X6
Nickel (carbonyl) (tetra-carbonyl) (fumes) (vapor)	T56.891	T56.892	T56.893	T56.894	—	—

Substance	Poisoning, Accidental (Unintentional)	Poisoning, Intentional Self-Harm	Poisoning, Assault	Poisoning, Undetermined	Adverse Effect	Underdosing
Nickelocene	T56.891	T56.892	T56.893	T56.894	—	—
Niclosamide	T37.4X1	T37.4X2	T37.4X3	T37.4X4	T37.4X5	T37.4X6
Nicofuranose	T46.7X1	T46.7X2	T46.7X3	T46.7X4	T46.7X5	T46.7X6
Nicomorphine	T40.2X1	T40.2X2	T40.2X3	T40.2X4	—	—
Nicorandil	T46.3X1	T46.3X2	T46.3X3	T46.3X4	T46.3X5	T46.3X6
Nicotiana (plant)	T62.2X1	T62.2X2	T62.2X3	T62.2X4	—	—
Nicotinamide	T45.2X1	T45.2X2	T45.2X3	T45.2X4	T45.2X5	T45.2X6
Nicotine (insecticide) (spray) (sulfate) NEC	T60.2X1	T60.2X2	T60.2X3	T60.2X4	—	—
from tobacco	T65.291	T65.292	T65.293	T65.294	—	—
cigarettes	T65.221	T65.222	T65.223	T65.224	—	—
not insecticide	T65.291	T65.292	T65.293	T65.294	—	—
Nicotinic acid	T46.7X1	T46.7X2	T46.7X3	T46.7X4	T46.7X5	T46.7X6
Nicotinyl alcohol	T46.7X1	T46.7X2	T46.7X3	T46.7X4	T46.7X5	T46.7X6
Nicoumalone	T45.511	T45.512	T45.513	T45.514	T45.515	T45.516
Nifedipine	T46.1X1	T46.1X2	T46.1X3	T46.1X4	T46.1X5	T46.1X6
Nifenazone	T39.2X1	T39.2X2	T39.2X3	T39.2X4	T39.2X5	T39.2X6
Nifuraldezone	T37.91	T37.92	T37.93	T37.94	T37.95	T37.96
Nifuratel	T37.8X1	T37.8X2	T37.8X3	T37.8X4	T37.8X5	T37.8X6
Nifurtimox	T37.3X1	T37.3X2	T37.3X3	T37.3X4	T37.3X5	T37.3X6
Nifurtoinol	T37.8X1	T37.8X2	T37.8X3	T37.8X4	T37.8X5	T37.8X6
Nightshade, deadly (solanum) — see also Belladonna	T62.2X1	T62.2X2	T62.2X3	T62.2X4	—	—
berry	T62.1X1	T62.1X2	T62.1X3	T62.1X4	—	—
Nikethamide	T50.7X1	T50.7X2	T50.7X3	T50.7X4	T50.7X5	T50.7X6
Nilstat	T36.7X1	T36.7X2	T36.7X3	T36.7X4	T36.7X5	T36.7X6
topical	T49.0X1	T49.0X2	T49.0X3	T49.0X4	T49.0X5	T49.0X6
Nilutamide	T38.6X1	T38.6X2	T38.6X3	T38.6X4	T38.6X5	T38.6X6
Nimesulide	T39.391	T39.392	T39.393	T39.394	T39.395	T39.396
Nimetazepam	T42.4X1	T42.4X2	T42.4X3	T42.4X4	T42.4X5	T42.4X6
Nimodipine	T46.1X1	T46.1X2	T46.1X3	T46.1X4	T46.1X5	T46.1X6
Nimorazole	T37.3X1	T37.3X2	T37.3X3	T37.3X4	T37.3X5	T37.3X6
Nimustine	T45.1X1	T45.1X2	T45.1X3	T45.1X4	T45.1X5	T45.1X6
Niridazole	T37.4X1	T37.4X2	T37.4X3	T37.4X4	T37.4X5	T37.4X6
Nisentil	T40.2X1	T40.2X2	T40.2X3	T40.2X4	T40.2X5	T40.2X6
Nisoldipine	T46.1X1	T46.1X2	T46.1X3	T46.1X4	T46.1X5	T46.1X6
Nitramine	T65.3X1	T65.3X2	T65.3X3	T65.3X4	—	—
Nitrate, organic	T46.3X1	T46.3X2	T46.3X3	T46.3X4	T46.3X5	T46.3X6
Nitrazepam	T42.4X1	T42.4X2	T42.4X3	T42.4X4	T42.4X5	T42.4X6
Nitrefazole	T50.6X1	T50.6X2	T50.6X3	T50.6X4	T50.6X5	T50.6X6
Nitrendipine	T46.1X1	T46.1X2	T46.1X3	T46.1X4	T46.1X5	T46.1X6

◀ New ◀ Revised ~~deleted~~ Deleted

TABLE OF DRUGS AND CHEMICALS

	External Cause (T-Code)					
Substance	Poisoning, Accidental (Unintentional)	Poisoning, Intentional Self-Harm	Poisoning, Assault	Poisoning, Undetermined	Adverse Effect	Underdosing
Nitric						
acid (liquid)	T54.2X1	T54.2X2	T54.2X3	T54.2X4	—	—
vapor	T59.891	T59.892	T59.893	T59.894	—	—
oxide (gas)	T59.0X1	T59.0X2	T59.0X3	T59.0X4	—	—
Nitrimidazine	T37.3X1	T37.3X2	T37.3X3	T37.3X4	T37.3X5	T37.3X6
Nitrite, amyl (medicinal) (vapor)	T46.3X1	T46.3X2	T46.3X3	T46.3X4	T46.3X5	T46.3X6
Nitroaniline	T65.3X1	T65.3X2	T65.3X3	T65.3X4		
vapor	T59.891	T59.892	T59.893	T59.894		
Nitrobenzene, nitrobenzol	T65.3X1	T65.3X2	T65.3X3	T65.3X4		
vapor	T65.3X1	T65.3X2	T65.3X3	T65.3X4		
Nitrocellulose	T65.891	T65.892	T65.893	T65.894	—	—
lacquer	T65.891	T65.892	T65.893	T65.894	—	—
Nitrodiphenyl	T65.3X1	T65.3X2	T65.3X3	T65.3X4		
Nitrofural	T49.0X1	T49.0X2	T49.0X3	T49.0X4	T49.0X5	T49.0X6
Nitrofurantoin	T37.8X1	T37.8X2	T37.8X3	T37.8X4	T37.8X5	T37.8X6
Nitrofurazone	T49.0X1	T49.0X2	T49.0X3	T49.0X4	T49.0X5	T49.0X6
Nitrogen	T59.0X1	T59.0X2	T59.0X3	T59.0X4	—	—
mustard	T45.1X1	T45.1X2	T45.1X3	T45.1X4	T45.1X5	T45.1X6
Nitroglycerin, nitro-glycerol (medicinal)	T46.3X1	T46.3X2	T46.3X3	T46.3X4	T46.3X5	T46.3X6
nonmedicinal	T65.5X1	T65.5X2	T65.5X3	T65.5X4	—	—
fumes	T65.5X1	T65.5X2	T65.5X3	T65.5X4	—	—
Nitroglycol	T52.3X1	T52.3X2	T52.3X3	T52.3X4		
Nitrohydrochloric acid	T54.2X1	T54.2X2	T54.2X3	T54.2X4		
Nitromersol	T49.0X1	T49.0X2	T49.0X3	T49.0X4	T49.0X5	T49.0X6
Nitronaphthalene	T65.891	T65.892	T65.893	T65.894		
Nitrophenol	T54.0X1	T54.0X2	T54.0X3	T54.0X4	—	—
Nitropropane	T52.8X1	T52.8X2	T52.8X3	T52.8X4	—	—
Nitroprusside	T46.5X1	T46.5X2	T46.5X3	T46.5X4	T46.5X5	T46.5X6
Nitrosodimethylamine	T65.3X1	T65.3X2	T65.3X3	T65.3X4	—	—
Nitrothiazol	T37.4X1	T37.4X2	T37.4X3	T37.4X4	T37.4X5	T37.4X6
Nitrotoluene, nitrotoluol	T65.3X1	T65.3X2	T65.3X3	T65.3X4		
vapor	T65.3X1	T65.3X2	T65.3X3	T65.3X4	—	—
Nitrous						
acid (liquid)	T54.2X1	T54.2X2	T54.2X3	T54.2X4	—	—
fumes	T59.891	T59.892	T59.893	T59.894	—	—
ether spirit	T46.3X1	T46.3X2	T46.3X3	T46.3X4	T46.3X5	T46.3X6
oxide	T41.0X1	T41.0X2	T41.0X3	T41.0X4	T41.0X5	T41.0X6
Nitroxoline	T37.8X1	T37.8X2	T37.8X3	T37.8X4	T37.8X5	T37.8X6
Nitrozone	T49.0X1	T49.0X2	T49.0X3	T49.0X4	T49.0X5	T49.0X6
Nizatidine	T47.0X1	T47.0X2	T47.0X3	T47.0X4	T47.0X5	T47.0X6

	External Cause (T-Code)					
Substance	Poisoning, Accidental (Unintentional)	Poisoning, Intentional Self-Harm	Poisoning, Assault	Poisoning, Undetermined	Adverse Effect	Underdosing
Nizofenone	T43.8X1	T43.8X2	T43.8X3	T43.8X4	T43.8X5	T43.8X6
Noctec	T42.6X1	T42.6X2	T42.6X3	T42.6X4	T42.6X5	T42.6X6
Noludar	T42.6X1	T42.6X2	T42.6X3	T42.6X4	T42.6X5	T42.6X6
Noptil	T42.3X1	T42.3X2	T42.3X3	T42.3X4	T42.3X5	T42.3X6
Nomegestrol	T38.5X1	T38.5X2	T38.5X3	T38.5X4	T38.5X5	T38.5X6
Nomifensine	T43.291	T43.292	T43.293	T43.294	T43.295	T43.296
Nonoxinol	T49.8X1	T49.8X2	T49.8X3	T49.8X4	T49.8X5	T49.8X6
Nonylphenoxy (polyethoxy-ethanol)	T49.8X1	T49.8X2	T49.8X3	T49.8X4	T49.8X5	T49.8X6
Noptil	T42.3X1	T42.3X2	T42.3X3	T42.3X4	T42.3X5	T42.3X6
Noradrenaline	T44.4X1	T44.4X2	T44.4X3	T44.4X4	T44.4X5	T44.4X6
Noramidopyrine	T39.2X1	T39.2X2	T39.2X3	T39.2X4	T39.2X5	T39.2X6
methanesulfonate sodium	T39.2X1	T39.2X2	T39.2X3	T39.2X4	T39.2X5	T39.2X6
Norbormide	T60.4X1	T60.4X2	T60.4X3	T60.4X4	—	—
Nordazepam	T42.4X1	T42.4X2	T42.4X3	T42.4X4	T42.4X5	T42.4X6
Norepinephrine	T44.4X1	T44.4X2	T44.4X3	T44.4X4	T44.4X5	T44.4X6
Norethandrolone	T38.7X1	T38.7X2	T38.7X3	T38.7X4	T38.7X5	T38.7X6
Norethindrone	T38.4X1	T38.4X2	T38.4X3	T38.4X4	T38.4X5	T38.4X6
Norethisterone (acetate) (enantate)	T38.4X1	T38.4X2	T38.4X3	T38.4X4	T38.4X5	T38.4X6
with ethinylestradiol	T38.5X1	T38.5X2	T38.5X3	T38.5X4	T38.5X5	T38.5X6
Noretynodrel	T38.5X1	T38.5X2	T38.5X3	T38.5X4	T38.5X5	T38.5X6
Norfenefrine	T44.4X1	T44.4X2	T44.4X3	T44.4X4	T44.4X5	T44.4X6
Norfloxacin	T36.8X1	T36.8X2	T36.8X3	T36.8X4	T36.8X5	T36.8X6
Norgestrel	T38.4X1	T38.4X2	T38.4X3	T38.4X4	T38.4X5	T38.4X6
Norgestrienone	T38.4X1	T38.4X2	T38.4X3	T38.4X4	T38.4X5	T38.4X6
Norlestrin	T38.4X1	T38.4X2	T38.4X3	T38.4X4	T38.4X5	T38.4X6
Norlutin	T38.4X1	T38.4X2	T38.4X3	T38.4X4	T38.4X5	T38.4X6
Normal serum albumin (human), salt-poor	T45.8X1	T45.8X2	T45.8X3	T45.8X4	T45.8X5	T45.8X6
Normethandrone	T38.5X1	T38.5X2	T38.5X3	T38.5X4	T38.5X5	T38.5X6
Normison — see Benzodiazepines						
Normorphine	T40.2X1	T40.2X2	T40.2X3	T40.2X4	—	—
Norpseudoephedrine	T50.5X1	T50.5X2	T50.5X3	T50.5X4	T50.5X5	T50.5X6
Nortestosterone (furanpropionate)	T38.7X1	T38.7X2	T38.7X3	T38.7X4	T38.7X5	T38.7X6
Nortriptyline	T43.011	T43.012	T43.013	T43.014	T43.015	T43.016
Noscapine	T48.3X1	T48.3X2	T48.3X3	T48.3X4	T48.3X5	T48.3X6
Nose preparations	T49.6X1	T49.6X2	T49.6X3	T49.6X4	T49.6X5	T49.6X6
Novobiocin	T36.5X1	T36.5X2	T36.5X3	T36.5X4	T36.5X5	T36.5X6
Novocain (infiltration) (topical)	T41.3X1	T41.3X2	T41.3X3	T41.3X4	T41.3X5	T41.3X6
nerve block (peripheral) (plexus)	T41.3X1	T41.3X2	T41.3X3	T41.3X4	T41.3X5	T41.3X6
spinal	T41.3X1	T41.3X2	T41.3X3	T41.3X4	T41.3X5	T41.3X6

◀ New ◀‖ Revised ~~deleted~~ Deleted

TABLE OF DRUGS AND CHEMICALS

Substance	Poisoning, Accidental (Unintentional)	Poisoning, Intentional Self-Harm	Poisoning, Assault	Poisoning, Undetermined	Adverse Effect	Underdosing
Noxious foodstuff	T62.91	T62.92	T62.93	T62.94	—	—
specified NEC	T62.8X1	T62.8X2	T62.8X3	T62.8X4	—	—
Noxiptiline	T43.011	T43.012	T43.013	T43.014	T43.015	T43.016
Noxytiolin	T49.0X1	T49.0X2	T49.0X3	T49.0X4	T49.0X5	T49.0X6
NPH Iletin (insulin)	T38.3X1	T38.3X2	T38.3X3	T38.3X4	T38.3X5	T38.3X6
Numorphan	T40.2X1	T40.2X2	T40.2X3	T40.2X4	T40.2X5	T40.2X6
Nunol	T42.3X1	T42.3X2	T42.3X3	T42.3X4	T42.3X5	T42.3X6
Nupercaine (spinal anesthetic)	T41.3X1	T41.3X2	T41.3X3	T41.3X4	T41.3X5	T41.3X6
topical (surface)	T41.3X1	T41.3X2	T41.3X3	T41.3X4	T41.3X5	T41.3X6
Nutmeg oil (liniment)	T49.3X1	T49.3X2	T49.3X3	T49.3X4	T49.3X5	T49.3X6
Nutritional supplement	T50.901	T50.902	T50.903	T50.904	T50.905	T50.906
Nux vomica	T65.1X1	T65.1X2	T65.1X3	T65.1X4	—	—
Nydrazid	T37.1X1	T37.1X2	T37.1X3	T37.1X4	T37.1X5	T37.1X6
Nylidrin	T46.7X1	T46.7X2	T46.7X3	T46.7X4	T46.7X5	T46.7X6
Nystatin	T36.7X1	T36.7X2	T36.7X3	T36.7X4	T36.7X5	T36.7X6
topical	T49.0X1	T49.0X2	T49.0X3	T49.0X4	T49.0X5	T49.0X6
Nytol	T45.0X1	T45.0X2	T45.0X3	T45.0X4	T45.0X5	T45.0X6
O						
Obidoxime chloride	T50.6X1	T50.6X2	T50.6X3	T50.6X4	T50.6X5	T50.6X6
Octafonium (chloride)	T49.3X1	T49.3X2	T49.3X3	T49.3X4	T49.3X5	T49.3X6
Octamethyl pyrophosphoramide	T60.0X1	T60.0X2	T60.0X3	T60.0X4	—	—
Octanoin	T50.991	T50.992	T50.993	T50.994	T50.995	T50.996
Octatropine methylbromide	T44.3X1	T44.3X2	T44.3X3	T44.3X4	T44.3X5	T44.3X6
Octotiamine	T45.2X1	T45.2X2	T45.2X3	T45.2X4	T45.2X5	T45.2X6
Octoxinol (9)	T49.8X1	T49.8X2	T49.8X3	T49.8X4	T49.8X5	T49.8X6
Octreotide	T38.991	T38.992	T38.993	T38.994	T38.995	T38.996
Octyl nitrite	T46.3X1	T46.3X2	T46.3X3	T46.3X4	T46.3X5	T46.3X6
Oestradiol	T38.5X1	T38.5X2	T38.5X3	T38.5X4	T38.5X5	T38.5X6
Oestriol	T38.5X1	T38.5X2	T38.5X3	T38.5X4	T38.5X5	T38.5X6
Oestrogen	T38.5X1	T38.5X2	T38.5X3	T38.5X4	T38.5X5	T38.5X6
Oestrone	T38.5X1	T38.5X2	T38.5X3	T38.5X4	T38.5X5	T38.5X6
Ofloxacin	T36.8X1	T36.8X2	T36.8X3	T36.8X4	T36.8X5	T36.8X6
Oil (of)	T65.891	T65.892	T65.893	T65.894	—	—
bitter almond	T62.8X1	T62.8X2	T62.8X3	T62.8X4	—	—
cloves	T49.7X1	T49.7X2	T49.7X3	T49.7X4	T49.7X5	T49.7X6
colors	T65.6X1	T65.6X2	T65.6X3	T65.6X4	—	—
fumes	T59.891	T59.892	T59.893	T59.894	—	—
lubricating	T52.0X1	T52.0X2	T52.0X3	T52.0X4	—	—
Niobe	T52.8X1	T52.8X2	T52.8X3	T52.8X4	—	—
Oil (of) (Continued)						
vitriol (liquid)	T54.2X1	T54.2X2	T54.2X3	T54.2X4	—	—
fumes	T54.2X1	T54.2X2	T54.2X3	T54.2X4	—	—
wintergreen (bitter) NEC	T49.3X1	T49.3X2	T49.3X3	T49.3X4	T49.3X5	T49.3X6
Oily preparation (for skin)	T49.3X1	T49.3X2	T49.3X3	T49.3X4	T49.3X5	T49.3X6
Ointment NEC	T49.3X1	T49.3X2	T49.3X3	T49.3X4	T49.3X5	T49.3X6
Olanzapine	T43.591	T43.592	T43.593	T43.594	T43.595	T43.596
Oleander	T62.2X1	T62.2X2	T62.2X3	T62.2X4	—	—
Oleandomycin	T36.3X1	T36.3X2	T36.3X3	T36.3X4	T36.3X5	T36.3X6
Oleandrin	T46.0X1	T46.0X2	T46.0X3	T46.0X4	T46.0X5	T46.0X6
Oleic acid	T46.6X1	T46.6X2	T46.6X3	T46.6X4	T46.6X5	T46.6X6
Oleovitamin A	T45.2X1	T45.2X2	T45.2X3	T45.2X4	T45.2X5	T45.2X6
Oleum ricini	T47.2X1	T47.2X2	T47.2X3	T47.2X4	T47.2X5	T47.2X6
Olive oil (medicinal) NEC	T47.4X1	T47.4X2	T47.4X3	T47.4X4	T47.4X5	T47.4X6
Olivomycin	T45.1X1	T45.1X2	T45.1X3	T45.1X4	T45.1X5	T45.1X6
Olsalazine	T47.8X1	T47.8X2	T47.8X3	T47.8X4	T47.8X5	T47.8X6
Omeprazole	T47.1X1	T47.1X2	T47.1X3	T47.1X4	T47.1X5	T47.1X6
OMPA	T60.0X1	T60.0X2	T60.0X3	T60.0X4	—	—
Ondansetron	T45.0X1	T45.0X2	T45.0X3	T45.0X4	T45.0X5	T45.0X6
Oncovin	T45.1X1	T45.1X2	T45.1X3	T45.1X4	T45.1X5	T45.1X6
Ophthaine	T41.3X1	T41.3X2	T41.3X3	T41.3X4	T41.3X5	T41.3X6
Ophthetic	T41.3X1	T41.3X2	T41.3X3	T41.3X4	T41.3X5	T41.3X6
Opiate NEC	T40.601	T40.602	T40.603	T40.604	T40.605	T40.606
antagonists	T50.7X1	T50.7X2	T50.7X3	T50.7X4	T50.7X5	T50.7X6
Opioid NEC	T40.2X1	T40.2X2	T40.2X3	T40.2X4	T40.2X5	T40.2X6
Opipramol	T43.011	T43.012	T43.013	T43.014	T43.015	T43.016
Opium alkaloids (total)	T40.0X1	T40.0X2	T40.0X3	T40.0X4	T40.0X5	T40.0X6
standardized powdered	T40.0X1	T40.0X2	T40.0X3	T40.0X4	T40.0X5	T40.0X6
tincture (camphorated)	T40.0X1	T40.0X2	T40.0X3	T40.0X4	T40.0X5	T40.0X6
Oracon	T38.4X1	T38.4X2	T38.4X3	T38.4X4	T38.4X5	T38.4X6
Oragrafin	T50.8X1	T50.8X2	T50.8X3	T50.8X4	T50.8X5	T50.8X6
Oral contraceptives	T38.4X1	T38.4X2	T38.4X3	T38.4X4	T38.4X5	T38.4X6
Oral rehydration salts	T50.3X1	T50.3X2	T50.3X3	T50.3X4	T50.3X5	T50.3X6
Orazamide	T50.991	T50.992	T50.993	T50.994	T50.995	T50.996
Orciprenaline	T48.291	T48.292	T48.293	T48.294	T48.295	T48.296
Organidin	T48.4X1	T48.4X2	T48.4X3	T48.4X4	T48.4X5	T48.4X6
Organonitrate NEC	T46.3X1	T46.3X2	T46.3X3	T46.3X4	T46.3X5	T46.3X6
Organophosphates	T60.0X1	T60.0X2	T60.0X3	T60.0X4	—	—
Orimune	T50.B91	T50.B92	T50.B93	T50.B94	T50.B95	T50.B96
Orinase	T38.3X1	T38.3X2	T38.3X3	T38.3X4	T38.3X5	T38.3X6
Ormeloxifene	T38.6X1	T38.6X2	T38.6X3	T38.6X4	T38.6X5	T38.6X6

◄ New ◄ Revised ~~deleted~~ Deleted

Substance	External Cause (T-Code) Poisoning, Accidental (Unintentional)	Poisoning, Intentional Self-Harm	Poisoning, Assault	Poisoning, Undetermined	Adverse Effect	Underdosing
Ornidazole	T37.3X1	T37.3X2	T37.3X3	T37.3X4	T37.3X5	T37.3X6
Ornithine aspartate	T50.991	T50.992	T50.993	T50.994	T50.995	T50.996
Ornoprostil	T47.1X1	T47.1X2	T47.1X3	T47.1X4	T47.1X5	T47.1X6
Orphenadrine (hydrochloride)	T42.8X1	T42.8X2	T42.8X3	T42.8X4	T42.8X5	T42.8X6
Ortal (sodium)	T42.3X1	T42.3X2	T42.3X3	T42.3X4	T42.3X5	T42.3X6
Orthoboric acid	T49.0X1	T49.0X2	T49.0X3	T49.0X4	T49.0X5	T49.0X6
ENT agent	T49.6X1	T49.6X2	T49.6X3	T49.6X4	T49.6X5	T49.6X6
ophthalmic preparation	T49.5X1	T49.5X2	T49.5X3	T49.5X4	T49.5X5	T49.5X6
Orthocaine	T41.3X1	T41.3X2	T41.3X3	T41.3X4	T41.3X5	T41.3X6
Orthodichlorobenzene	T53.7X1	T53.7X2	T53.7X3	T53.7X4	—	—
Ortho-Novum	T38.4X1	T38.4X2	T38.4X3	T38.4X4	T38.4X5	T38.4X6
Orthotolidine (reagent)	T54.2X1	T54.2X2	T54.2X3	T54.2X4	—	—
Osmic acid (liquid)	T54.2X1	T54.2X2	T54.2X3	T54.2X4	—	—
fumes	T54.2X1	T54.2X2	T54.2X3	T54.2X4	—	—
Osmotic diuretics	T50.2X1	T50.2X2	T50.2X3	T50.2X4	T50.2X5	T50.2X6
Otilonium bromide	T44.3X1	T44.3X2	T44.3X3	T44.3X4	T44.3X5	T44.3X6
Otorhinolaryngological drug NEC	T49.6X1	T49.6X2	T49.6X3	T49.6X4	T49.6X5	T49.6X6
Ouabain(e)	T46.0X1	T46.0X2	T46.0X3	T46.0X4	T46.0X5	T46.0X6
Ovarian						
hormone	T38.5X1	T38.5X2	T38.5X3	T38.5X4	T38.5X5	T38.5X6
stimulant	T38.5X1	T38.5X2	T38.5X3	T38.5X4	T38.5X5	T38.5X6
Ovral	T38.4X1	T38.4X2	T38.4X3	T38.4X4	T38.4X5	T38.4X6
Ovulen	T38.4X1	T38.4X2	T38.4X3	T38.4X4	T38.4X5	T38.4X6
Oxacillin	T36.0X1	T36.0X2	T36.0X3	T36.0X4	T36.0X5	T36.0X6
Oxalic acid	T54.2X1	T54.2X2	T54.2X3	T54.2X4	—	—
ammonium salt	T50.991	T50.992	T50.993	T50.994	T50.995	T50.996
Oxamniquine	T37.4X1	T37.4X2	T37.4X3	T37.4X4	T37.4X5	T37.4X6
Oxanamide	T43.591	T43.592	T43.593	T43.594	T43.595	T43.596
Oxandrolone	T38.7X1	T38.7X2	T38.7X3	T38.7X4	T38.7X5	T38.7X6
Oxantel	T37.4X1	T37.4X2	T37.4X3	T37.4X4	T37.4X5	T37.4X6
Oxapium iodide	T44.3X1	T44.3X2	T44.3X3	T44.3X4	T44.3X5	T44.3X6
Oxaprotiline	T43.021	T43.022	T43.023	T43.024	T43.025	T43.026
Oxaprozin	T39.311	T39.312	T39.313	T39.314	T39.315	T39.316
Oxatomide	T45.0X1	T45.0X2	T45.0X3	T45.0X4	T45.0X5	T45.0X6
Oxazepam	T42.4X1	T42.4X2	T42.4X3	T42.4X4	T42.4X5	T42.4X6
Oxazimedrine	T50.5X1	T50.5X2	T50.5X3	T50.5X4	T50.5X5	T50.5X6
Oxazolam	T42.4X1	T42.4X2	T42.4X3	T42.4X4	T42.4X5	T42.4X6
Oxazolidine derivatives	T42.2X1	T42.2X2	T42.2X3	T42.2X4	T42.2X5	T42.2X6
Oxazolidinedione (derivative)	T42.2X1	T42.2X2	T42.2X3	T42.2X4	T42.2X5	T42.2X6
Ox bile extract	T47.5X1	T47.5X2	T47.5X3	T47.5X4	T47.5X5	T47.5X6
Oxcarbazepine	T42.1X1	T42.1X2	T42.1X3	T42.1X4	T42.1X5	T42.1X6
Oxedrine	T44.4X1	T44.4X2	T44.4X3	T44.4X4	T44.4X5	T44.4X6

Substance	External Cause (T-Code) Poisoning, Accidental (Unintentional)	Poisoning, Intentional Self-Harm	Poisoning, Assault	Poisoning, Undetermined	Adverse Effect	Underdosing
Oxeladin (citrate)	T48.3X1	T48.3X2	T48.3X3	T48.3X4	T48.3X5	T48.3X6
Oxendolone	T38.5X1	T38.5X2	T38.5X3	T38.5X4	T38.5X5	T38.5X6
Oxetacaine	T41.3X1	T41.3X2	T41.3X3	T41.3X4	T41.3X5	T41.3X6
Oxethazine	T41.3X1	T41.3X2	T41.3X3	T41.3X4	T41.3X5	T41.3X6
Oxetorone	T39.8X1	T39.8X2	T39.8X3	T39.8X4	T39.8X5	T39.8X6
Oxiconazole	T49.0X1	T49.0X2	T49.0X3	T49.0X4	T49.0X5	T49.0X6
Oxidizing agent NEC	T54.91	T54.92	T54.93	T54.94	—	—
Oxipurinol	T50.4X1	T50.4X2	T50.4X3	T50.4X4	T50.4X5	T50.4X6
Oxitriptan	T43.291	T43.292	T43.293	T43.294	T43.295	T43.296
Oxitropium bromide	T48.6X1	T48.6X2	T48.6X3	T48.6X4	T48.6X5	T48.6X6
Oxodipine	T46.1X1	T46.1X2	T46.1X3	T46.1X4	T46.1X5	T46.1X6
Oxolamine	T48.3X1	T48.3X2	T48.3X3	T48.3X4	T48.3X5	T48.3X6
Oxolinic acid	T37.8X1	T37.8X2	T37.8X3	T37.8X4	T37.8X5	T37.8X6
Oxomemazine	T43.3X1	T43.3X2	T43.3X3	T43.3X4	T43.3X5	T43.3X6
Oxophenarsine	T37.3X1	T37.3X2	T37.3X3	T37.3X4	T37.3X5	T37.3X6
Oxprenolol	T44.7X1	T44.7X2	T44.7X3	T44.7X4	T44.7X5	T44.7X6
Oxsoralen	T49.3X1	T49.3X2	T49.3X3	T49.3X4	T49.3X5	T49.3X6
Oxtriphylline	T48.6X1	T48.6X2	T48.6X3	T48.6X4	T48.6X5	T48.6X6
Oxybate sodium	T41.291	T41.292	T41.293	T41.294	T41.295	T41.296
Oxybuprocaine	T41.3X1	T41.3X2	T41.3X3	T41.3X4	T41.3X5	T41.3X6
Oxybutynin	T44.3X1	T44.3X2	T44.3X3	T44.3X4	T44.3X5	T44.3X6
Oxychlorosene	T49.0X1	T49.0X2	T49.0X3	T49.0X4	T49.0X5	T49.0X6
Oxycodone	T40.2X1	T40.2X2	T40.2X3	T40.2X4	T40.2X5	T40.2X6
Oxyfedrine	T46.3X1	T46.3X2	T46.3X3	T46.3X4	T46.3X5	T46.3X6
Oxygen	T41.5X1	T41.5X2	T41.5X3	T41.5X4	T41.5X5	T41.5X6
Oxylone	T49.0X1	T49.0X2	T49.0X3	T49.0X4	T49.0X5	T49.0X6
ophthalmic preparation	T49.5X1	T49.5X2	T49.5X3	T49.5X4	T49.5X5	T49.5X6
Oxymesterone	T38.7X1	T38.7X2	T38.7X3	T38.7X4	T38.7X5	T38.7X6
Oxymetazoline	T48.5X1	T48.5X2	T48.5X3	T48.5X4	T48.5X5	T48.5X6
Oxymetholone	T38.7X1	T38.7X2	T38.7X3	T38.7X4	T38.7X5	T38.7X6
Oxymorphone	T40.2X1	T40.2X2	T40.2X3	T40.2X4	T40.2X5	T40.2X6
Oxypertine	T43.591	T43.592	T43.593	T43.594	T43.595	T43.596
Oxyphenbutazone	T39.2X1	T39.2X2	T39.2X3	T39.2X4	T39.2X5	T39.2X6
Oxyphencyclimine	T44.3X1	T44.3X2	T44.3X3	T44.3X4	T44.3X5	T44.3X6
Oxyphenisatine	T47.2X1	T47.2X2	T47.2X3	T47.2X4	T47.2X5	T47.2X6
Oxyphenonium bromide	T44.3X1	T44.3X2	T44.3X3	T44.3X4	T44.3X5	T44.3X6
Oxypolygelatin	T45.8X1	T45.8X2	T45.8X3	T45.8X4	T45.8X5	T45.8X6
Oxyquinoline (derivatives)	T37.8X1	T37.8X2	T37.8X3	T37.8X4	T37.8X5	T37.8X6
Oxytetracycline	T36.4X1	T36.4X2	T36.4X3	T36.4X4	T36.4X5	T36.4X6
Oxytocic drug NEC	T48.0X1	T48.0X2	T48.0X3	T48.0X4	T48.0X5	T48.0X6
Oxytocin (synthetic)	T48.0X1	T48.0X2	T48.0X3	T48.0X4	T48.0X5	T48.0X6
Ozone	T59.891	T59.892	T59.893	T59.894	—	—

◀ New   ◀ Revised   ~~deleted~~ Deleted

Substance	External Cause (T-Code)					
	Poisoning, Accidental (Unintentional)	Poisoning, Intentional Self-Harm	Poisoning, Assault	Poisoning, Undetermined	Adverse Effect	Underdosing
P						
PABA	T49.3X1	T49.3X2	T49.3X3	T49.3X4	T49.3X5	T49.3X6
Packed red cells	T45.8X1	T45.8X2	T45.8X3	T45.8X4	T45.8X5	T45.8X6
Padimate	T49.3X1	T49.3X2	T49.3X3	T49.3X4	T49.3X5	T49.3X6
Paint NEC	T65.6X1	T65.6X2	T65.6X3	T65.6X4	—	—
cleaner	T52.91	T52.92	T52.93	T52.94		
fumes NEC	T59.891	T59.892	T59.893	T59.894	—	—
lead (fumes)	T56.0X1	T56.0X2	T56.0X3	T56.0X4		
solvent NEC	T52.8X1	T52.8X2	T52.8X3	T52.8X4	—	—
stripper	T52.8X1	T52.8X2	T52.8X3	T52.8X4	—	—
Palfium	T40.2X1	T40.2X2	T40.2X3	T40.2X4	—	—
Palm kernel oil	T50.991	T50.992	T50.993	T50.994	T50.995	T50.996
Paludrine	T37.2X1	T37.2X2	T37.2X3	T37.2X4	T37.2X5	T37.2X6
PAM (pralidoxime)	T50.6X1	T50.6X2	T50.6X3	T50.6X4	T50.6X5	T50.6X6
Pamaquine (naphthoute)	T37.2X1	T37.2X2	T37.2X3	T37.2X4	T37.2X5	T37.2X6
Panadol	T39.1X1	T39.1X2	T39.1X3	T39.1X4	T39.1X5	T39.1X6
Pancreatic						
digestive secretion stimulant	T47.8X1	T47.8X2	T47.8X3	T47.8X4	T47.8X5	T47.8X6
dornase	T45.3X1	T45.3X2	T45.3X3	T45.3X4	T45.3X5	T45.3X6
Pancreatin	T47.5X1	T47.5X2	T47.5X3	T47.5X4	T47.5X5	T47.5X6
Pancrelipase	T47.5X1	T47.5X2	T47.5X3	T47.5X4	T47.5X5	T47.5X6
Pancuronium (bromide)	T48.1X1	T48.1X2	T48.1X3	T48.1X4	T48.1X5	T48.1X6
Pangamic acid	T45.2X1	T45.2X2	T45.2X3	T45.2X4	T45.2X5	T45.2X6
Panthenol	T45.2X1	T45.2X2	T45.2X3	T45.2X4	T45.2X5	T45.2X6
topical	T49.8X1	T49.8X2	T49.8X3	T49.8X4	T49.8X5	T49.8X6
Pantopon	T40.0X1	T40.0X2	T40.0X3	T40.0X4	T40.0X5	T40.0X6
Pantothenic acid	T45.2X1	T45.2X2	T45.2X3	T45.2X4	T45.2X5	T45.2X6
Panwarfin	T45.511	T45.512	T45.513	T45.514	T45.515	T45.516
Papain	T47.5X1	T47.5X2	T47.5X3	T47.5X4	T47.5X5	T47.5X6
digestant	T47.5X1	T47.5X2	T47.5X3	T47.5X4	T47.5X5	T47.5X6
Papaveretum	T40.0X1	T40.0X2	T40.0X3	T40.0X4	T40.0X5	T40.0X6
Papaverine	T44.3X1	T44.3X2	T44.3X3	T44.3X4	T44.3X5	T44.3X6
Para-acetamidophenol	T39.1X1	T39.1X2	T39.1X3	T39.1X4	T39.1X5	T39.1X6
Para-aminobenzoic acid	T49.3X1	T49.3X2	T49.3X3	T49.3X4	T49.3X5	T49.3X6
Para-aminophenol derivatives	T39.1X1	T39.1X2	T39.1X3	T39.1X4	T39.1X5	T39.1X6
Para-aminosalicylic acid	T37.1X1	T37.1X2	T37.1X3	T37.1X4	T37.1X5	T37.1X6
Paracetaldehyde	T42.6X1	T42.6X2	T42.6X3	T42.6X4	T42.6X5	T42.6X6
Paracetamol	T39.1X1	T39.1X2	T39.1X3	T39.1X4	T39.1X5	T39.1X6
Parachlorophenol (camphorated)	T49.0X1	T49.0X2	T49.0X3	T49.0X4	T49.0X5	T49.0X6
Paracodin	T40.2X1	T40.2X2	T40.2X3	T40.2X4	T40.2X5	T40.2X6
Paradione	T42.2X1	T42.2X2	T42.2X3	T42.2X4	T42.2X5	T42.2X6

Substance	External Cause (T-Code)					
	Poisoning, Accidental (Unintentional)	Poisoning, Intentional Self-Harm	Poisoning, Assault	Poisoning, Undetermined	Adverse Effect	Underdosing
Paraffin(s) (wax)	T52.0X1	T52.0X2	T52.0X3	T52.0X4	—	—
liquid (medicinal)	T47.4X1	T47.4X2	T47.4X3	T47.4X4	T47.4X5	T47.4X6
nonmedicinal	T52.0X1	T52.0X2	T52.0X3	T52.0X4	—	—
Paraformaldehyde	T60.3X1	T60.3X2	T60.3X3	T60.3X4	—	—
Paraldehyde	T42.6X1	T42.6X2	T42.6X3	T42.6X4	T42.6X5	T42.6X6
Paramethadione	T42.2X1	T42.2X2	T42.2X3	T42.2X4	T42.2X5	T42.2X6
Paramethasone	T38.0X1	T38.0X2	T38.0X3	T38.0X4	T38.0X5	T38.0X6
acetate	T49.0X1	T49.0X2	T49.0X3	T49.0X4	T49.0X5	T49.0X6
Paraoxon	T60.0X1	T60.0X2	T60.0X3	T60.0X4		
Paraquat	T60.3X1	T60.3X2	T60.3X3	T60.3X4	—	—
Parasympatholytic NEC	T44.3X1	T44.3X2	T44.3X3	T44.3X4	T44.3X5	T44.3X6
Parasympathomimetic drug NEC	T44.1X1	T44.1X2	T44.1X3	T44.1X4	T44.1X5	T44.1X6
Parathion	T60.0X1	T60.0X2	T60.0X3	T60.0X4	—	—
Parathormone	T50.991	T50.992	T50.993	T50.994	T50.995	T50.996
Parathyroid extract	T50.991	T50.992	T50.993	T50.994	T50.995	T50.996
Paratyphoid vaccine	T50.A91	T50.A92	T50.A93	T50.A94	T50.A95	T50.A96
Paredrine	T44.4X1	T44.4X2	T44.4X3	T44.4X4	T44.4X5	T44.4X6
Paregoric	T40.0X1	T40.0X2	T40.0X3	T40.0X4	T40.0X5	T40.0X6
Pargyline	T46.5X1	T46.5X2	T46.5X3	T46.5X4	T46.5X5	T46.5X6
Paris green	T57.0X1	T57.0X2	T57.0X3	T57.0X4	—	—
insecticide	T57.0X1	T57.0X2	T57.0X3	T57.0X4	—	—
Parnate	T43.1X1	T43.1X2	T43.1X3	T43.1X4	T43.1X5	T43.1X6
Paromomycin	T36.5X1	T36.5X2	T36.5X3	T36.5X4	T36.5X5	T36.5X6
Paroxypropione	T45.1X1	T45.1X2	T45.1X3	T45.1X4	T45.1X5	T45.1X6
Parzone	T40.2X1	T40.2X2	T40.2X3	T40.2X4	T40.2X5	T40.2X6
PAS	T37.1X1	T37.1X2	T37.1X3	T37.1X4	T37.1X5	T37.1X6
Pasiniazid	T37.1X1	T37.1X2	T37.1X3	T37.1X4	T37.1X5	T37.1X6
PBB (polybrominated biphenyls)	T65.891	T65.892	T65.893	T65.894	—	—
PCB	T65.891	T65.892	T65.893	T65.894	—	—
PCP						
meaning pentachlorophenol	T60.1X1	T60.1X2	T60.1X3	T60.1X4	—	—
fungicide	T60.3X1	T60.3X2	T60.3X3	T60.3X4	—	—
herbicide	T60.3X1	T60.3X2	T60.3X3	T60.3X4	—	—
insecticide	T60.1X1	T60.1X2	T60.1X3	T60.1X4	—	—
meaning phencyclidine	T40.991	T40.992	T40.993	T40.994	—	—
Peach kernel oil (emulsion)	T47.4X1	T47.4X2	T47.4X3	T47.4X4	T47.4X5	T47.4X6
Peanut oil (emulsion) NEC	T47.4X1	T47.4X2	T47.4X3	T47.4X4	T47.4X5	T47.4X6
topical	T49.3X1	T49.3X2	T49.3X3	T49.3X4	T49.3X5	T49.3X6
Pearly Gates (morning glory seeds)	T40.991	T40.992	T40.993	T40.994	—	—
Pecazine	T43.3X1	T43.3X2	T43.3X3	T43.3X4	T43.3X5	T43.3X6
Pectin	T47.6X1	T47.6X2	T47.6X3	T47.6X4	T47.6X5	T47.6X6

◀ New   ◀ Revised   ~~deleted~~ Deleted

Substance	External Cause (T-Code)					
	Poisoning, Accidental (Unintentional)	Poisoning, Intentional Self-Harm	Poisoning, Assault	Poisoning, Undetermined	Adverse Effect	Underdosing
Pefloxacin	T37.8X1	T37.8X2	T37.8X3	T37.8X4	T37.8X5	T37.8X6
Pegademase, bovine	T50.Z91	T50.Z92	T50.Z93	T50.Z94	T50.Z95	T50.Z96
Pelletierine tannate	T37.4X1	T37.4X2	T37.4X3	T37.4X4	T37.4X5	T37.4X6
Pemirolast (potassium)	T48.6X1	T48.6X2	T48.6X3	T48.6X4	T48.6X5	T48.6X6
Pemoline	T50.7X1	T50.7X2	T50.7X3	T50.7X4	T50.7X5	T50.7X6
Pempidine	T44.2X1	T44.2X2	T44.2X3	T44.2X4	T44.2X5	T44.2X6
Penamecillin	T36.0X1	T36.0X2	T36.0X3	T36.0X4	T36.0X5	T36.0X6
Penbutolol	T44.7X1	T44.7X2	T44.7X3	T44.7X4	T44.7X5	T44.7X6
Penethamate	T36.0X1	T36.0X2	T36.0X3	T36.0X4	T36.0X5	T36.0X6
Penfluridol	T43.591	T43.592	T43.593	T43.594	T43.595	T43.596
Penflutizide	T50.2X1	T50.2X2	T50.2X3	T50.2X4	T50.2X5	T50.2X6
Pengitoxin	T46.0X1	T46.0X2	T46.0X3	T46.0X4	T46.0X5	T46.0X6
Penicillamine	T50.6X1	T50.6X2	T50.6X3	T50.6X4	T50.6X5	T50.6X6
Penicillin (any)	T36.0X1	T36.0X2	T36.0X3	T36.0X4	T36.0X5	T36.0X6
Penicillinase	T45.3X1	T45.3X2	T45.3X3	T45.3X4	T45.3X5	T45.3X6
Penicilloyl polylysine	T50.8X1	T50.8X2	T50.8X3	T50.8X4	T50.8X5	T50.8X6
Penimepicycline	T36.4X1	T36.4X2	T36.4X3	T36.4X4	T36.4X5	T36.4X6
Pentachloroethane	T53.6X1	T53.6X2	T53.6X3	T53.6X4	—	—
Pentachloronaphthalene	T53.7X1	T53.7X2	T53.7X3	T53.7X4	—	—
Pentachlorophenol (pesticide)	T60.1X1	T60.1X2	T60.1X3	T60.1X4	—	—
fungicide	T60.3X1	T60.3X2	T60.3X3	T60.3X4	—	—
herbicide	T60.3X1	T60.3X2	T60.3X3	T60.3X4	—	—
insecticide	T60.1X1	T60.1X2	T60.1X3	T60.1X4	—	—
Pentaerythritol tetranitrate	T46.3X1	T46.3X2	T46.3X3	T46.3X4	T46.3X5	T46.3X6
Pentaerythritol	T46.3X1	T46.3X2	T46.3X3	T46.3X4	T46.3X5	T46.3X6
chloral	T42.6X1	T42.6X2	T42.6X3	T42.6X4	T42.6X5	T42.6X6
tetranitrate NEC	T46.3X1	T46.3X2	T46.3X3	T46.3X4	T46.3X5	T46.3X6
Pentagastrin	T50.8X1	T50.8X2	T50.8X3	T50.8X4	T50.8X5	T50.8X6
Pentalin	T53.6X1	T53.6X2	T53.6X3	T53.6X4	—	—
Pentamethonium bromide	T44.2X1	T44.2X2	T44.2X3	T44.2X4	T44.2X5	T44.2X6
Pentamidine	T37.3X1	T37.3X2	T37.3X3	T37.3X4	T37.3X5	T37.3X6
Pentanol	T51.3X1	T51.3X2	T51.3X3	T51.3X4	—	—
Pentapyrrolinium (bitartrate)	T44.2X1	T44.2X2	T44.2X3	T44.2X4	T44.2X5	T44.2X6
Pentaquine	T37.2X1	T37.2X2	T37.2X3	T37.2X4	T37.2X5	T37.2X6
Pentazocine	T40.4X1	T40.4X2	T40.4X3	T40.4X4	T40.4X5	T40.4X6
Pentetrazole	T50.7X1	T50.7X2	T50.7X3	T50.7X4	T50.7X5	T50.7X6
Penthienate bromide	T44.3X1	T44.3X2	T44.3X3	T44.3X4	T44.3X5	T44.3X6
Pentifylline	T46.7X1	T46.7X2	T46.7X3	T46.7X4	T46.7X5	T46.7X6
Pentobarbital	T42.3X1	T42.3X2	T42.3X3	T42.3X4	T42.3X5	T42.3X6
sodium	T42.3X1	T42.3X2	T42.3X3	T42.3X4	T42.3X5	T42.3X6
Pentobarbitone	T42.3X1	T42.3X2	T42.3X3	T42.3X4	T42.3X5	T42.3X6
Pentolonium tartrate	T44.2X1	T44.2X2	T44.2X3	T44.2X4	T44.2X5	T44.2X6

Substance	External Cause (T-Code)					
	Poisoning, Accidental (Unintentional)	Poisoning, Intentional Self-Harm	Poisoning, Assault	Poisoning, Undetermined	Adverse Effect	Underdosing
Pentosan polysulfate (sodium)	T39.8X1	T39.8X2	T39.8X3	T39.8X4	T39.8X5	T39.8X6
Pentostatin	T45.1X1	T45.1X2	T45.1X3	T45.1X4	T45.1X5	T45.1X6
Pentothal	T41.1X1	T41.1X2	T41.1X3	T41.1X4	T41.1X5	T41.1X6
Pentoxifylline	T46.7X1	T46.7X2	T46.7X3	T46.7X4	T46.7X5	T46.7X6
Pentoxyverine	T48.3X1	T48.3X2	T48.3X3	T48.3X4	T48.3X5	T48.3X6
Pentrinat	T46.3X1	T46.3X2	T46.3X3	T46.3X4	T46.3X5	T46.3X6
Pentylenetetrazole	T50.7X1	T50.7X2	T50.7X3	T50.7X4	T50.7X5	T50.7X6
Pentylsalicylamide	T37.1X1	T37.1X2	T37.1X3	T37.1X4	T37.1X5	T37.1X6
Pentymal	T42.3X1	T42.3X2	T42.3X3	T42.3X4	T42.3X5	T42.3X6
Peplomycin	T45.1X1	T45.1X2	T45.1X3	T45.1X4	T45.1X5	T45.1X6
Peppermint (oil)	T47.5X1	T47.5X2	T47.5X3	T47.5X4	T47.5X5	T47.5X6
Pepsin	T47.5X1	T47.5X2	T47.5X3	T47.5X4	T47.5X5	T47.5X6
digestant	T47.5X1	T47.5X2	T47.5X3	T47.5X4	T47.5X5	T47.5X6
Pepstatin	T47.1X1	T47.1X2	T47.1X3	T47.1X4	T47.1X5	T47.1X6
Peptavlon	T50.8X1	T50.8X2	T50.8X3	T50.8X4	T50.8X5	T50.8X6
Perazine	T43.3X1	T43.3X2	T43.3X3	T43.3X4	T43.3X5	T43.3X6
Percaine (spinal)	T41.3X1	T41.3X2	T41.3X3	T41.3X4	T41.3X5	T41.3X6
topical (surface)	T41.3X1	T41.3X2	T41.3X3	T41.3X4	T41.3X5	T41.3X6
Perchloroethylene	T53.3X1	T53.3X2	T53.3X3	T53.3X4	—	—
medicinal	T37.4X1	T37.4X2	T37.4X3	T37.4X4	T37.4X5	T37.4X6
vapor	T53.3X1	T53.3X2	T53.3X3	T53.3X4	—	—
Percodan	T40.2X1	T40.2X2	T40.2X3	T40.2X4	T40.2X5	T40.2X6
Percogesic — see also acetaminophen	T45.0X1	T45.0X2	T45.0X3	T45.0X4	T45.0X5	T45.0X6
Percorten	T38.0X1	T38.0X2	T38.0X3	T38.0X4	T38.0X5	T38.0X6
Pergolide	T42.8X1	T42.8X2	T42.8X3	T42.8X4	T42.8X5	T42.8X6
Pergonal	T38.811	T38.812	T38.813	T38.814	T38.815	T38.816
Perhexilene	T46.3X1	T46.3X2	T46.3X3	T46.3X4	T46.3X5	T46.3X6
Perhexiline (maleate)	T46.3X1	T46.3X2	T46.3X3	T46.3X4	T46.3X5	T46.3X6
Periactin	T45.0X1	T45.0X2	T45.0X3	T45.0X4	T45.0X5	T45.0X6
Periciazine	T43.3X1	T43.3X2	T43.3X3	T43.3X4	T43.3X5	T43.3X6
Periclor	T42.6X1	T42.6X2	T42.6X3	T42.6X4	T42.6X5	T42.6X6
Perindopril	T46.4X1	T46.4X2	T46.4X3	T46.4X4	T46.4X5	T46.4X6
Perisoxal	T39.8X1	T39.8X2	T39.8X3	T39.8X4	T39.8X5	T39.8X6
Peritrate	T46.3X1	T46.3X2	T46.3X3	T46.3X4	T46.3X5	T46.3X6
Peritoneal dialysis solution	T50.3X1	T50.3X2	T50.3X3	T50.3X4	T50.3X5	T50.3X6
Perlapine	T42.4X1	T42.4X2	T42.4X3	T42.4X4	T42.4X5	T42.4X6
Permanganate	T65.891	T65.892	T65.893	T65.894	—	—
Permethrin	T60.1X1	T60.1X2	T60.1X3	T60.1X4	—	—
Pernocton	T42.3X1	T42.3X2	T42.3X3	T42.3X4	T42.3X5	T42.3X6
Pernoston	T42.3X1	T42.3X2	T42.3X3	T42.3X4	T42.3X5	T42.3X6
Peronine	T40.2X1	T40.2X2	T40.2X3	T40.2X4	—	—
Perphenazine	T43.3X1	T43.3X2	T43.3X3	T43.3X4	T43.3X5	T43.3X6

◀ New   ◀ Revised   ~~deleted~~ Deleted

Substance	Poisoning, Accidental (Unintentional)	Poisoning, Intentional Self-Harm	Poisoning, Assault	Poisoning, Undetermined	Adverse Effect	Underdosing
Pertofrane	T43.011	T43.012	T43.013	T43.014	T43.015	T43.016
Pertussis						
immune serum (human)	T50.Z11	T50.Z12	T50.Z13	T50.Z14	T50.Z15	T50.Z16
vaccine (with diphtheria toxoid) (with tetanus toxoid)	T50.A11	T50.A12	T50.A13	T50.A14	T50.A15	T50.A16
Peruvian balsam	T49.0X1	T49.0X2	T49.0X3	T49.0X4	T49.0X5	T49.0X6
Peruvoside	T46.0X1	T46.0X2	T46.0X3	T46.0X4	T46.0X5	T46.0X6
Pesticide (dust) (fumes) (vapor) NEC	T60.91	T60.92	T60.93	T60.94	—	—
arsenic	T57.0X1	T57.0X2	T57.0X3	T57.0X4	—	—
chlorinated	T60.1X1	T60.1X2	T60.1X3	T60.1X4	—	—
cyanide	T65.0X1	T65.0X2	T65.0X3	T65.0X4	—	—
kerosene	T52.0X1	T52.0X2	T52.0X3	T52.0X4	—	—
mixture (of compounds)	T60.91	T60.92	T60.93	T60.94	—	—
naphthalene	T60.2X1	T60.2X2	T60.2X3	T60.2X4	—	—
organochlorine (compounds)	T60.1X1	T60.1X2	T60.1X3	T60.1X4	—	—
petroleum (distillate) (products) NEC	T60.8X1	T60.8X2	T60.8X3	T60.8X4	—	—
specified ingredient NEC	T60.8X1	T60.8X2	T60.8X3	T60.8X4	—	—
strychnine	T65.1X1	T65.1X2	T65.1X3	T65.1X4	—	—
thallium	T60.4X1	T60.4X2	T60.4X3	T60.4X4	—	—
Pethidine	T40.4X1	T40.4X2	T40.4X3	T40.4X4	T40.4X5	T40.4X6
Petrichloral	T42.6X1	T42.6X2	T42.6X3	T42.6X4	T42.6X5	T42.6X6
Petrol	T52.0X1	T52.0X2	T52.0X3	T52.0X4	—	—
vapor	T52.0X1	T52.0X2	T52.0X3	T52.0X4	—	—
Petrolatum	T49.3X1	T49.3X2	T49.3X3	T49.3X4	T49.3X5	T49.3X6
hydrophilic	T49.3X1	T49.3X2	T49.3X3	T49.3X4	T49.3X5	T49.3X6
liquid	T47.4X1	T47.4X2	T47.4X3	T47.4X4	T47.4X5	T47.4X6
topical	T49.3X1	T49.3X2	T49.3X3	T49.3X4	T49.3X5	T49.3X6
nonmedicinal	T52.0X1	T52.0X2	T52.0X3	T52.0X4	—	—
red veterinary	T49.3X1	T49.3X2	T49.3X3	T49.3X4	T49.3X5	T49.3X6
white	T49.3X1	T49.3X2	T49.3X3	T49.3X4	T49.3X5	T49.3X6
Petroleum (products) NEC	T52.0X1	T52.0X2	T52.0X3	T52.0X4	—	—
benzine(s) — see Ligroin						
ether — see Ligroin						
jelly — see Petrolatum						
naphtha — see Ligroin						
pesticide	T60.8X1	T60.8X2	T60.8X3	T60.8X4	—	—
solids	T52.0X1	T52.0X2	T52.0X3	T52.0X4	—	—
solvents	T52.0X1	T52.0X2	T52.0X3	T52.0X4	—	—
vapor	T52.0X1	T52.0X2	T52.0X3	T52.0X4	—	—
Peyote	T40.991	T40.992	T40.993	T40.994	—	—
Phanodorm, phanodorn	T42.3X1	T42.3X2	T42.3X3	T42.3X4	T42.3X5	T42.3X6

Substance	Poisoning, Accidental (Unintentional)	Poisoning, Intentional Self-Harm	Poisoning, Assault	Poisoning, Undetermined	Adverse Effect	Underdosing
Phanquinone	T37.3X1	T37.3X2	T37.3X3	T37.3X4	T37.3X5	T37.3X6
Phanquone	T37.3X1	T37.3X2	T37.3X3	T37.3X4	T37.3X5	T37.3X6
Pharmaceutical						
adjunct NEC	T50.901	T50.902	T50.903	T50.904	T50.905	T50.906
excipient NEC	T50.901	T50.902	T50.903	T50.904	T50.905	T50.906
sweetener	T50.901	T50.902	T50.903	T50.904	T50.905	T50.906
viscous agent	T50.901	T50.902	T50.903	T50.904	T50.905	T50.906
Phemitone	T42.3X1	T42.3X2	T42.3X3	T42.3X4	T42.3X5	T42.3X6
Phenacaine	T41.3X1	T41.3X2	T41.3X3	T41.3X4	T41.3X5	T41.3X6
Phenacemide	T42.6X1	T42.6X2	T42.6X3	T42.6X4	T42.6X5	T42.6X6
Phenacetin	T39.1X1	T39.1X2	T39.1X3	T39.1X4	T39.1X5	T39.1X6
Phenadoxone	T40.2X1	T40.2X2	T40.2X3	T40.2X4	—	—
Phenaglycodol	T43.591	T43.592	T43.593	T43.594	T43.595	T43.596
Phenantoin	T42.0X1	T42.0X2	T42.0X3	T42.0X4	T42.0X5	T42.0X6
Phenaphthazine reagent	T50.991	T50.992	T50.993	T50.994	T50.995	T50.996
Phenazocine	T40.4X1	T40.4X2	T40.4X3	T40.4X4	T40.4X5	T40.4X6
Phenazone	T39.2X1	T39.2X2	T39.2X3	T39.2X4	T39.2X5	T39.2X6
Phenazopyridine	T39.8X1	T39.8X2	T39.8X3	T39.8X4	T39.8X5	T39.8X6
Phenbenicillin	T36.0X1	T36.0X2	T36.0X3	T36.0X4	T36.0X5	T36.0X6
Phenbutrazate	T50.5X1	T50.5X2	T50.5X3	T50.5X4	T50.5X5	T50.5X6
Phencyclidine	T40.991	T40.992	T40.993	T40.994	T40.995	T40.996
Phendimetrazine	T50.5X1	T50.5X2	T50.5X3	T50.5X4	T50.5X5	T50.5X6
Phenelzine	T43.1X1	T43.1X2	T43.1X3	T43.1X4	T43.1X5	T43.1X6
Phenemal	T42.3X1	T42.3X2	T42.3X3	T42.3X4	T42.3X5	T42.3X6
Phenergan	T42.6X1	T42.6X2	T42.6X3	T42.6X4	T42.6X5	T42.6X6
Pheneticillin	T36.0X1	T36.0X2	T36.0X3	T36.0X4	T36.0X5	T36.0X6
Pheneturide	T42.6X1	T42.6X2	T42.6X3	T42.6X4	T42.6X5	T42.6X6
Phenformin	T38.3X1	T38.3X2	T38.3X3	T38.3X4	T38.3X5	T38.3X6
Phenglutarimide	T44.3X1	T44.3X2	T44.3X3	T44.3X4	T44.3X5	T44.3X6
Phenicarbazide	T39.8X1	T39.8X2	T39.8X3	T39.8X4	T39.8X5	T39.8X6
Phenindamine	T45.0X1	T45.0X2	T45.0X3	T45.0X4	T45.0X5	T45.0X6
Phenindione	T45.511	T45.512	T45.513	T45.514	T45.515	T45.516
Pheniprazine	T43.1X1	T43.1X2	T43.1X3	T43.1X4	T43.1X5	T43.1X6
Pheniramine	T45.0X1	T45.0X2	T45.0X3	T45.0X4	T45.0X5	T45.0X6
Phenisatin	T47.2X1	T47.2X2	T47.2X3	T47.2X4	T47.2X5	T47.2X6
Phenmetrazine	T50.5X1	T50.5X2	T50.5X3	T50.5X4	T50.5X5	T50.5X6
Phenobal	T42.3X1	T42.3X2	T42.3X3	T42.3X4	T42.3X5	T42.3X6
Phenobarbital	T42.3X1	T42.3X2	T42.3X3	T42.3X4	T42.3X5	T42.3X6
with						
mephenytoin	T42.3X1	T42.3X2	T42.3X3	T42.3X4	T42.3X5	T42.3X6
phenytoin	T42.3X1	T42.3X2	T42.3X3	T42.3X4	T42.3X5	T42.3X6
sodium	T42.3X1	T42.3X2	T42.3X3	T42.3X4	T42.3X5	T42.3X6

◀ New   ◀ Revised   ~~deleted~~ Deleted

	External Cause (T-Code)					
Substance	Poisoning, Accidental (Unintentional)	Poisoning, Intentional Self-Harm	Poisoning, Assault	Poisoning, Undetermined	Adverse Effect	Underdosing
Phenobarbitone	T42.3X1	T42.3X2	T42.3X3	T42.3X4	T42.3X5	T42.3X6
Phenobutiodil	T50.8X1	T50.8X2	T50.8X3	T50.8X4	T50.8X5	T50.8X6
Phenoctide	T49.0X1	T49.0X2	T49.0X3	T49.0X4	T49.0X5	T49.0X6
Phenol	T49.0X1	T49.0X2	T49.0X3	T49.0X4	T49.0X5	T49.0X6
disinfectant	T54.0X1	T54.0X2	T54.0X3	T54.0X4	—	—
in oil injection	T46.8X1	T46.8X2	T46.8X3	T46.8X4	T46.8X5	T46.8X6
medicinal	T49.1X1	T49.1X2	T49.1X3	T49.1X4	T49.1X5	T49.1X6
nonmedicinal NEC	T54.0X1	T54.0X2	T54.0X3	T54.0X4	—	—
pesticide	T60.8X1	T60.8X2	T60.8X3	T60.8X4	—	—
red	T50.8X1	T50.8X2	T50.8X3	T50.8X4	T50.8X5	T50.8X6
Phenolic preparation	T49.1X1	T49.1X2	T49.1X3	T49.1X4	T49.1X5	T49.1X6
Phenolphthalein	T47.2X1	T47.2X2	T47.2X3	T47.2X4	T47.2X5	T47.2X6
Phenolsulfonphthalein	T50.8X1	T50.8X2	T50.8X3	T50.8X4	T50.8X5	T50.8X6
Phenomorphan	T40.2X1	T40.2X2	T40.2X3	T40.2X4	—	—
Phenonyl	T42.3X1	T42.3X2	T42.3X3	T42.3X4	T42.3X5	T42.3X6
Phenoperidine	T40.4X1	T40.4X2	T40.4X3	T40.4X4	—	—
Phenopyrazone	T46.991	T46.992	T46.993	T46.994	T46.995	T46.996
Phenoquin	T50.4X1	T50.4X2	T50.4X3	T50.4X4	T50.4X5	T50.4X6
Phenothiazine (psychotropic) NEC	T43.3X1	T43.3X2	T43.3X3	T43.3X4	T43.3X5	T43.3X6
insecticide	T60.2X1	T60.2X2	T60.2X3	T60.2X4	—	—
Phenothrin	T49.0X1	T49.0X2	T49.0X3	T49.0X4	T49.0X5	T49.0X6
Phenoxybenzamine	T46.7X1	T46.7X2	T46.7X3	T46.7X4	T46.7X5	T46.7X6
Phenoxyethanol	T49.0X1	T49.0X2	T49.0X3	T49.0X4	T49.0X5	T49.0X6
Phenoxymethyl penicillin	T36.0X1	T36.0X2	T36.0X3	T36.0X4	T36.0X5	T36.0X6
Phenprobamate	T42.8X1	T42.8X2	T42.8X3	T42.8X4	T42.8X5	T42.8X6
Phenprocoumon	T45.511	T45.512	T45.513	T45.514	T45.515	T45.516
Phensuximide	T42.2X1	T42.2X2	T42.2X3	T42.2X4	T42.2X5	T42.2X6
Phentermine	T50.5X1	T50.5X2	T50.5X3	T50.5X4	T50.5X5	T50.5X6
Phenthicillin	T36.0X1	T36.0X2	T36.0X3	T36.0X4	T36.0X5	T36.0X6
Phentolamine	T46.7X1	T46.7X2	T46.7X3	T46.7X4	T46.7X5	T46.7X6
Phenyl						
butazone	T39.2X1	T39.2X2	T39.2X3	T39.2X4	T39.2X5	T39.2X6
enediamine	T65.3X1	T65.3X2	T65.3X3	T65.3X4	—	—
hydrazine	T65.3X1	T65.3X2	T65.3X3	T65.3X4	—	—
antineoplastic	T45.1X1	T45.1X2	T45.1X3	T45.1X4	T45.1X5	T45.1X6
mercuric compounds — see Mercury						
salicylate	T49.3X1	T49.3X2	T49.3X3	T49.3X4	T49.3X5	T49.3X6
Phenylalanine mustard	T45.1X1	T45.1X2	T45.1X3	T45.1X4	T45.1X5	T45.1X6
Phenylbutazone	T39.2X1	T39.2X2	T39.2X3	T39.2X4	T39.2X5	T39.2X6
Phenylenediamine	T65.3X1	T65.3X2	T65.3X3	T65.3X4	—	—
Phenylephrine	T44.4X1	T44.4X2	T44.4X3	T44.4X4	T44.4X5	T44.4X6

	External Cause (T-Code)					
Substance	Poisoning, Accidental (Unintentional)	Poisoning, Intentional Self-Harm	Poisoning, Assault	Poisoning, Undetermined	Adverse Effect	Underdosing
Phenylethylbiguanide	T38.3X1	T38.3X2	T38.3X3	T38.3X4	T38.3X5	T38.3X6
Phenylmercuric						
acetate	T49.0X1	T49.0X2	T49.0X3	T49.0X4	T49.0X5	T49.0X6
borate	T49.0X1	T49.0X2	T49.0X3	T49.0X4	T49.0X5	T49.0X6
nitrate	T49.0X1	T49.0X2	T49.0X3	T49.0X4	T49.0X5	T49.0X6
Phenylmethylbarbitone	T42.3X1	T42.3X2	T42.3X3	T42.3X4	T42.3X5	T42.3X6
Phenylpropanol	T47.5X1	T47.5X2	T47.5X3	T47.5X4	T47.5X5	T47.5X6
Phenylpropanolamine	T44.991	T44.992	T44.993	T44.994	T44.995	T44.996
Phenylsulfthion	T60.0X1	T60.0X2	T60.0X3	T60.0X4	—	—
Phenyltoloxamine	T45.0X1	T45.0X2	T45.0X3	T45.0X4	T45.0X5	T45.0X6
Phenyramidol, phenyramidon	T39.8X1	T39.8X2	T39.8X3	T39.8X4	T39.8X5	T39.8X6
Phenytoin	T42.0X1	T42.0X2	T42.0X3	T42.0X4	T42.0X5	T42.0X6
with Phenobarbital	T42.3X1	T42.3X2	T42.3X3	T42.3X4	T42.3X5	T42.3X6
pHisoHex	T49.2X1	T49.2X2	T49.2X3	T49.2X4	T49.2X5	T49.2X6
Pholcodine	T48.3X1	T48.3X2	T48.3X3	T48.3X4	T48.3X5	T48.3X6
Pholedrine	T46.991	T46.992	T46.993	T46.994	T46.995	T46.996
Phorate	T60.0X1	T60.0X2	T60.0X3	T60.0X4	—	—
Phosdrin	T60.0X1	T60.0X2	T60.0X3	T60.0X4	—	—
Phosfolan	T60.0X1	T60.0X2	T60.0X3	T60.0X4	—	—
Phosgene (gas)	T59.891	T59.892	T59.893	T59.894	—	—
Phosphamidon	T60.0X1	T60.0X2	T60.0X3	T60.0X4	—	—
Phosphate	T65.891	T65.892	T65.893	T65.894	—	—
laxative	T47.4X1	T47.4X2	T47.4X3	T47.4X4	T47.4X5	T47.4X6
organic	T60.0X1	T60.0X2	T60.0X3	T60.0X4	—	—
solvent	T52.91	T52.92	T52.93	T52.94	—	—
tricresyl	T65.891	T65.892	T65.893	T65.894	—	—
Phosphine	T57.1X1	T57.1X2	T57.1X3	T57.1X4	—	—
fumigant	T57.1X1	T57.1X2	T57.1X3	T57.1X4	—	—
Phospholine	T49.5X1	T49.5X2	T49.5X3	T49.5X4	T49.5X5	T49.5X6
Phosphoric acid	T54.2X1	T54.2X2	T54.2X3	T54.2X4	—	—
Phosphorus (compound) NEC	T57.1X1	T57.1X2	T57.1X3	T57.1X4	—	—
pesticide	T60.0X1	T60.0X2	T60.0X3	T60.0X4	—	—
Phthalates	T65.891	T65.892	T65.893	T65.894	—	—
Phthalic anhydride	T65.891	T65.892	T65.893	T65.894	—	—
Phthalimidoglutarimide	T42.6X1	T42.6X2	T42.6X3	T42.6X4	T42.6X5	T42.6X6
Phthalylsulfathiazole	T37.0X1	T37.0X2	T37.0X3	T37.0X4	T37.0X5	T37.0X6
Phylloquinone	T45.7X1	T45.7X2	T45.7X3	T45.7X4	T45.7X5	T45.7X6
Physeptone	T40.3X1	T40.3X2	T40.3X3	T40.3X4	T40.3X5	T40.3X6
Physostigma venenosum	T62.2X1	T62.2X2	T62.2X3	T62.2X4	—	—
Physostigmine	T49.5X1	T49.5X2	T49.5X3	T49.5X4	T49.5X5	T49.5X6
Phytolacca decandra	T62.2X1	T62.2X2	T62.2X3	T62.2X4	—	—
berries	T62.1X1	T62.1X2	T62.1X3	T62.1X4	—	—

TABLE OF DRUGS AND CHEMICALS

Substance	Poisoning, Accidental (Unintentional)	Poisoning, Intentional Self-Harm	Poisoning, Assault	Poisoning, Undetermined	Adverse Effect	Underdosing
Phytomenadione	T45.7X1	T45.7X2	T45.7X3	T45.7X4	T45.7X5	T45.7X6
Phytonadione	T45.7X1	T45.7X2	T45.7X3	T45.7X4	T45.7X5	T45.7X6
Picoperine	T48.3X1	T48.3X2	T48.3X3	T48.3X4	T48.3X5	T48.3X6
Picosulfate (sodium)	T47.2X1	T47.2X2	T47.2X3	T47.2X4	T47.2X5	T47.2X6
Picric (acid)	T54.2X1	T54.2X2	T54.2X3	T54.2X4	—	—
Picrotoxin	T50.7X1	T50.7X2	T50.7X3	T50.7X4	T50.7X5	T50.7X6
Piketoprofen	T49.0X1	T49.0X2	T49.0X3	T49.0X4	T49.0X5	T49.0X6
Pilocarpine	T44.1X1	T44.1X2	T44.1X3	T44.1X4	T44.1X5	T44.1X6
Pilocarpus (jaborandi) extract	T44.1X1	T44.1X2	T44.1X3	T44.1X4	T44.1X5	T44.1X6
Pilsicainide (hydrochloride)	T46.2X1	T46.2X2	T46.2X3	T46.2X4	T46.2X5	T46.2X6
Pimaricin	T36.7X1	T36.7X2	T36.7X3	T36.7X4	T36.7X5	T36.7X6
Pimeclone	T50.7X1	T50.7X2	T50.7X3	T50.7X4	T50.7X5	T50.7X6
Pimelic ketone	T52.8X1	T52.8X2	T52.8X3	T52.8X4	—	—
Pimethixene	T45.0X1	T45.0X2	T45.0X3	T45.0X4	T45.0X5	T45.0X6
Piminodine	T40.2X1	T40.2X2	T40.2X3	T40.2X4	T40.2X5	T40.2X6
Pimozide	T43.591	T43.592	T43.593	T43.594	T43.595	T43.596
Pinacidil	T46.5X1	T46.5X2	T46.5X3	T46.5X4	T46.5X5	T46.5X6
Pinaverium bromide	T44.3X1	T44.3X2	T44.3X3	T44.3X4	T44.3X5	T44.3X6
Pinazepam	T42.4X1	T42.4X2	T42.4X3	T42.4X4	T42.4X5	T42.4X6
Pindolol	T44.7X1	T44.7X2	T44.7X3	T44.7X4	T44.7X5	T44.7X6
Pindone	T60.4X1	T60.4X2	T60.4X3	T60.4X4	—	—
Pine oil (disinfectant)	T65.891	T65.892	T65.893	T65.894	—	—
Pinkroot	T37.4X1	T37.4X2	T37.4X3	T37.4X4	T37.4X5	T37.4X6
Pipadone	T40.2X1	T40.2X2	T40.2X3	T40.2X4	—	—
Pipamazine	T45.0X1	T45.0X2	T45.0X3	T45.0X4	T45.0X5	T45.0X6
Pipamperone	T43.4X1	T43.4X2	T43.4X3	T43.4X4	T43.4X5	T43.4X6
Pipazetate	T48.3X1	T48.3X2	T48.3X3	T48.3X4	T48.3X5	T48.3X6
Pipemidic acid	T37.8X1	T37.8X2	T37.8X3	T37.8X4	T37.8X5	T37.8X6
Pipenzolate bromide	T44.3X1	T44.3X2	T44.3X3	T44.3X4	T44.3X5	T44.3X6
Piperacetazine	T43.3X1	T43.3X2	T43.3X3	T43.3X4	T43.3X5	T43.3X6
Piperacillin	T36.0X1	T36.0X2	T36.0X3	T36.0X4	T36.0X5	T36.0X6
Piperazine	T37.4X1	T37.4X2	T37.4X3	T37.4X4	T37.4X5	T37.4X6
estrone sulfate	T38.5X1	T38.5X2	T38.5X3	T38.5X4	T38.5X5	T38.5X6
Piper cubeba	T62.2X1	T62.2X2	T62.2X3	T62.2X4	—	—
Piperidione	T48.3X1	T48.3X2	T48.3X3	T48.3X4	—	—
Piperidolate	T44.3X1	T44.3X2	T44.3X3	T44.3X4	T44.3X5	T44.3X6
Piperocaine	T41.3X1	T41.3X2	T41.3X3	T41.3X4	T41.3X5	T41.3X6
infiltration (subcutaneous)	T41.3X1	T41.3X2	T41.3X3	T41.3X4	T41.3X5	T41.3X6
nerve block (peripheral) (plexus)	T41.3X1	T41.3X2	T41.3X3	T41.3X4	T41.3X5	T41.3X6
topical (surface)	T41.3X1	T41.3X2	T41.3X3	T41.3X4	T41.3X5	T41.3X6
Piperonyl butoxide	T60.8X1	T60.8X2	T60.8X3	T60.8X4	—	—
Pipethanate	T44.3X1	T44.3X2	T44.3X3	T44.3X4	T44.3X5	T44.3X6

Substance	Poisoning, Accidental (Unintentional)	Poisoning, Intentional Self-Harm	Poisoning, Assault	Poisoning, Undetermined	Adverse Effect	Underdosing
Pipobroman	T45.1X1	T45.1X2	T45.1X3	T45.1X4	T45.1X5	T45.1X6
Pipofezine	T43.0X1	T43.0X2	T43.0X3	T43.0X4	T43.0X5	T43.0X6
Pipotiazine	T43.3X1	T43.3X2	T43.3X3	T43.3X4	T43.3X5	T43.3X6
Pipoxizine	T45.0X1	T45.0X2	T45.0X3	T45.0X4	T45.0X5	T45.0X6
Pipradrol	T43.691	T43.692	T43.693	T43.694	T43.695	T43.696
Piprinhydrinate	T45.0X1	T45.0X2	T45.0X3	T45.0X4	T45.0X5	T45.0X6
Pirarubicin	T45.1X1	T45.1X2	T45.1X3	T45.1X4	T45.1X5	T45.1X6
Pirazinamide	T37.1X1	T37.1X2	T37.1X3	T37.1X4	T37.1X5	T37.1X6
Pirbuterol	T48.6X1	T48.6X2	T48.6X3	T48.6X4	T48.6X5	T48.6X6
Pirenzepine	T47.1X1	T47.1X2	T47.1X3	T47.1X4	T47.1X5	T47.1X6
Piretanide	T50.1X1	T50.1X2	T50.1X3	T50.1X4	T50.1X5	T50.1X6
Piribedil	T42.8X1	T42.8X2	T42.8X3	T42.8X4	T42.8X5	T42.8X6
Piridoxilate	T46.3X1	T46.3X2	T46.3X3	T46.3X4	T46.3X5	T46.3X6
Piritramide	T40.4X1	T40.4X2	T40.4X3	T40.4X4	—	—
Pirlindole	T43.0X1	T43.0X2	T43.0X3	T43.0X4	T43.0X5	T43.0X6
Piromidic acid	T37.8X1	T37.8X2	T37.8X3	T37.8X4	T37.8X5	T37.8X6
Piroxicam	T39.391	T39.392	T39.393	T39.394	T39.395	T39.396
beta-cyclodextrin complex	T39.8X1	T39.8X2	T39.8X3	T39.8X4	T39.8X5	T39.8X6
Pirozadil	T46.6X1	T46.6X2	T46.6X3	T46.6X4	T46.6X5	T46.6X6
Piscidia (bark) (erythrina)	T39.8X1	T39.8X2	T39.8X3	T39.8X4	T39.8X5	T39.8X6
Pitch	T65.891	T65.892	T65.893	T65.894	—	—
Pitkin's solution	T41.3X1	T41.3X2	T41.3X3	T41.3X4	T41.3X5	T41.3X6
Pitocin	T48.0X1	T48.0X2	T48.0X3	T48.0X4	T48.0X5	T48.0X6
Pitressin (tannate)	T38.891	T38.892	T38.893	T38.894	T38.895	T38.896
Pituitary extracts (posterior)	T38.891	T38.892	T38.893	T38.894	T38.895	T38.896
anterior	T38.811	T38.812	T38.813	T38.814	T38.815	T38.816
Pituitrin	T38.891	T38.892	T38.893	T38.894	T38.895	T38.896
Pivampicillin	T36.0X1	T36.0X2	T36.0X3	T36.0X4	T36.0X5	T36.0X6
Pivmecillinam	T36.0X1	T36.0X2	T36.0X3	T36.0X4	T36.0X5	T36.0X6
Placental hormone	T38.891	T38.892	T38.893	T38.894	T38.895	T38.896
Placidyl	T42.6X1	T42.6X2	T42.6X3	T42.6X4	T42.6X5	T42.6X6
Plague vaccine	T50.A91	T50.A92	T50.A93	T50.A94	T50.A95	T50.A96
Plant						
food or fertilizer NEC	T65.891	T65.892	T65.893	T65.894	—	—
containing herbicide	T60.3X1	T60.3X2	T60.3X3	T60.3X4	—	—
noxious, used as food	T62.2X1	T62.2X2	T62.2X3	T62.2X4	—	—
berries	T62.1X1	T62.1X2	T62.1X3	T62.1X4	—	—
seeds	T62.2X1	T62.2X2	T62.2X3	T62.2X4	—	—
specified type NEC	T62.2X1	T62.2X2	T62.2X3	T62.2X4	—	—
Plasma	T45.8X1	T45.8X2	T45.8X3	T45.8X4	T45.8X5	T45.8X6
expander NEC	T45.8X1	T45.8X2	T45.8X3	T45.8X4	T45.8X5	T45.8X6
protein fraction (human)	T45.8X1	T45.8X2	T45.8X3	T45.8X4	T45.8X5	T45.8X6

◀ New ◀ Revised ~~deleted~~ Deleted

Substance	External Cause (T-Code)					
	Poisoning, Accidental (Unintentional)	Poisoning, Intentional Self-Harm	Poisoning, Assault	Poisoning, Undetermined	Adverse Effect	Underdosing
Plasmanate	T45.8X1	T45.8X2	T45.8X3	T45.8X4	T45.8X5	T45.8X6
Plasminogen (tissue) activator	T45.611	T45.612	T45.613	T45.614	T45.615	T45.616
Plaster dressing	T49.3X1	T49.3X2	T49.3X3	T49.3X4	T49.3X5	T49.3X6
Plastic dressing	T49.3X1	T49.3X2	T49.3X3	T49.3X4	T49.3X5	T49.3X6
Plegicil	T43.3X1	T43.3X2	T43.3X3	T43.3X4	T43.3X5	T43.3X6
Plicamycin	T45.1X1	T45.1X2	T45.1X3	T45.1X4	T45.1X5	T45.1X6
Podophyllotoxin	T49.8X1	T49.8X2	T49.8X3	T49.8X4	T49.8X5	T49.8X6
Podophyllum (resin)	T49.4X1	T49.4X2	T49.4X3	T49.4X4	T49.4X5	T49.4X6
Poison NEC	T65.91	T65.92	T65.93	T65.94	—	—
Poisonous berries	T62.1X1	T62.1X2	T62.1X3	T62.1X4	—	—
Pokeweed (any part)	T62.2X1	T62.2X2	T62.2X3	T62.2X4	—	—
Poldine metilsulfate	T44.3X1	T44.3X2	T44.3X3	T44.3X4	T44.3X5	T44.3X6
Polidexide (sulfate)	T46.6X1	T46.6X2	T46.6X3	T46.6X4	T46.6X5	T46.6X6
Polidocanol	T46.8X1	T46.8X2	T46.8X3	T46.8X4	T46.8X5	T46.8X6
Poliomyelitis vaccine	T50.B91	T50.B92	T50.B93	T50.B94	T50.B95	T50.B96
Polish (car) (floor) (furniture) (metal) (porcelain) (silver)	T65.891	T65.892	T65.893	T65.894	—	—
abrasive	T65.891	T65.892	T65.893	T65.894	—	—
porcelain	T65.891	T65.892	T65.893	T65.894	—	—
Poloxalkol	T47.4X1	T47.4X2	T47.4X3	T47.4X4	T47.4X5	T47.4X6
Poloxamer	T47.4X1	T47.4X2	T47.4X3	T47.4X4	T47.4X5	T47.4X6
Polyaminostyrene resins	T50.3X1	T50.3X2	T50.3X3	T50.3X4	T50.3X5	T50.3X6
Polycarbophil	T47.4X1	T47.4X2	T47.4X3	T47.4X4	T47.4X5	T47.4X6
Polychlorinated biphenyl	T65.891	T65.892	T65.893	T65.894	—	—
Polycycline	T36.4X1	T36.4X2	T36.4X3	T36.4X4	T36.4X5	T36.4X6
Polyester fumes	T59.891	T59.892	T59.893	T59.894	—	—
Polyester resin hardener	T52.91	T52.92	T52.93	T52.94	—	—
fumes	T59.891	T59.892	T59.893	T59.894	—	—
Polyestradiol phosphate	T38.5X1	T38.5X2	T38.5X3	T38.5X4	T38.5X5	T38.5X6
Polyethanolamine alkyl sulfate	T49.2X1	T49.2X2	T49.2X3	T49.2X4	T49.2X5	T49.2X6
Polyethylene adhesive	T49.3X1	T49.3X2	T49.3X3	T49.3X4	T49.3X5	T49.3X6
Polyferose	T45.4X1	T45.4X2	T45.4X3	T45.4X4	T45.4X5	T45.4X6
Polygeline	T45.8X1	T45.8X2	T45.8X3	T45.8X4	T45.8X5	T45.8X6
Polymyxin	T36.8X1	T36.8X2	T36.8X3	T36.8X4	T36.8X5	T36.8X6
B	T36.8X1	T36.8X2	T36.8X3	T36.8X4	T36.8X5	T36.8X6
ENT agent	T49.6X1	T49.6X2	T49.6X3	T49.6X4	T49.6X5	T49.6X6
ophthalmic preparation	T49.5X1	T49.5X2	T49.5X3	T49.5X4	T49.5X5	T49.5X6
topical NEC	T49.0X1	T49.0X2	T49.0X3	T49.0X4	T49.0X5	T49.0X6
E sulfate (eye preparation)	T49.5X1	T49.5X2	T49.5X3	T49.5X4	T49.5X5	T49.5X6
Polynoxylin	T49.0X1	T49.0X2	T49.0X3	T49.0X4	T49.0X5	T49.0X6
Polyoestradiol phosphate	T38.5X1	T38.5X2	T38.5X3	T38.5X4	T38.5X5	T38.5X6
Polyoxymethyleneurea	T49.0X1	T49.0X2	T49.0X3	T49.0X4	T49.0X5	T49.0X6

Substance	External Cause (T-Code)					
	Poisoning, Accidental (Unintentional)	Poisoning, Intentional Self-Harm	Poisoning, Assault	Poisoning, Undetermined	Adverse Effect	Underdosing
Polysilane	T47.8X1	T47.8X2	T47.8X3	T47.8X4	T47.8X5	T47.8X6
Polytetrafluoroethylene (inhaled)	T59.891	T59.892	T59.893	T59.894	—	—
Polythiazide	T50.2X1	T50.2X2	T50.2X3	T50.2X4	T50.2X5	T50.2X6
Polyvidone	T45.8X1	T45.8X2	T45.8X3	T45.8X4	T45.8X5	T45.8X6
Polyvinylpyrrolidone	T45.8X1	T45.8X2	T45.8X3	T45.8X4	T45.8X5	T45.8X6
Pontocaine (hydrochloride) (infiltration) (topical)	T41.3X1	T41.3X2	T41.3X3	T41.3X4	T41.3X5	T41.3X6
nerve block (peripheral) (plexus)	T41.3X1	T41.3X2	T41.3X3	T41.3X4	T41.3X5	T41.3X6
spinal	T41.3X1	T41.3X2	T41.3X3	T41.3X4	T41.3X5	T41.3X6
Porfiromycin	T45.1X1	T45.1X2	T45.1X3	T45.1X4	T45.1X5	T45.1X6
Posterior pituitary hormone NEC	T38.891	T38.892	T38.893	T38.894	T38.895	T38.896
Pot	T40.7X1	T40.7X2	T40.7X3	T40.7X4	T40.7X5	T40.7X6
Potash (caustic)	T54.3X1	T54.3X2	T54.3X3	T54.3X4	—	—
Potassic saline injection (lactated)	T50.3X1	T50.3X2	T50.3X3	T50.3X4	T50.3X5	T50.3X6
Potassium (salts) NEC	T50.3X1	T50.3X2	T50.3X3	T50.3X4	T50.3X5	T50.3X6
aminobenzoate	T45.8X1	T45.8X2	T45.8X3	T45.8X4	T45.8X5	T45.8X6
aminosalicylate	T37.1X1	T37.1X2	T37.1X3	T37.1X4	T37.1X5	T37.1X6
antimony 'tartrate'	T37.8X1	T37.8X2	T37.8X3	T37.8X4	T37.8X5	T37.8X6
arsenite (solution)	T57.0X1	T57.0X2	T57.0X3	T57.0X4	—	—
bichromate	T56.2X1	T56.2X2	T56.2X3	T56.2X4	—	—
bisulfate	T47.3X1	T47.3X2	T47.3X3	T47.3X4	T47.3X5	T47.3X6
bromide	T42.6X1	T42.6X2	T42.6X3	T42.6X4	T42.6X5	T42.6X6
canrenoate	T50.0X1	T50.0X2	T50.0X3	T50.0X4	T50.0X5	T50.0X6
carbonate	T54.3X1	T54.3X2	T54.3X3	T54.3X4	—	—
chlorate NEC	T65.891	T65.892	T65.893	T65.894	—	—
chloride	T50.3X1	T50.3X2	T50.3X3	T50.3X4	T50.3X5	T50.3X6
citrate	T50.991	T50.992	T50.993	T50.994	T50.995	T50.996
cyanide	T65.0X1	T65.0X2	T65.0X3	T65.0X4	—	—
ferric hexacyanoferrate (medicinal)	T50.6X1	T50.6X2	T50.6X3	T50.6X4	T50.6X5	T50.6X6
nonmedicinal	T65.891	T65.892	T65.893	T65.894	—	—
Fluoride	T57.8X1	T57.8X2	T57.8X3	T57.8X4	—	—
glucaldrate	T47.1X1	T47.1X2	T47.1X3	T47.1X4	T47.1X5	T47.1X6
hydroxide	T54.3X1	T54.3X2	T54.3X3	T54.3X4	—	—
iodate	T49.0X1	T49.0X2	T49.0X3	T49.0X4	T49.0X5	T49.0X6
iodide	T48.4X1	T48.4X2	T48.4X3	T48.4X4	T48.4X5	T48.4X6
nitrate	T57.8X1	T57.8X2	T57.8X3	T57.8X4	—	—
oxalate	T65.891	T65.892	T65.893	T65.894	—	—
perchlorate (nonmedicinal) NEC	T65.891	T65.892	T65.893	T65.894	—	—
antithyroid	T38.2X1	T38.2X2	T38.2X3	T38.2X4	T38.2X5	T38.2X6
medicinal	T38.2X1	T38.2X2	T38.2X3	T38.2X4	T38.2X5	T38.2X6

◀ New ◀ Revised ~~deleted~~ Deleted

TABLE OF DRUGS AND CHEMICALS

Substance	Poisoning, Accidental (Unintentional)	Poisoning, Intentional Self-Harm	Poisoning, Assault	Poisoning, Undetermined	Adverse Effect	Underdosing
Permanganate (nonmedicinal)	T65.891	T65.892	T65.893	T65.894	—	—
medicinal	T49.0X1	T49.0X2	T49.0X3	T49.0X4	T49.0X5	T49.0X6
sulfate	T47.2X1	T47.2X2	T47.2X3	T47.2X4	T47.2X5	T47.2X6
Potassium-removing resin	T50.3X1	T50.3X2	T50.3X3	T50.3X4	T50.3X5	T50.3X6
Potassium-retaining drug	T50.3X1	T50.3X2	T50.3X3	T50.3X4	T50.3X5	T50.3X6
Povidone	T45.8X1	T45.8X2	T45.8X3	T45.8X4	T45.8X5	T45.8X6
iodine	T49.0X1	T49.0X2	T49.0X3	T49.0X4	T49.0X5	T49.0X6
Practolol	T44.7X1	T44.7X2	T44.7X3	T44.7X4	T44.7X5	T44.7X6
Prajmalium bitartrate	T46.2X1	T46.2X2	T46.2X3	T46.2X4	T46.2X5	T46.2X6
Pralidoxime (iodide)	T50.6X1	T50.6X2	T50.6X3	T50.6X4	T50.6X5	T50.6X6
chloride	T50.6X1	T50.6X2	T50.6X3	T50.6X4	T50.6X5	T50.6X6
Pramiverine	T44.3X1	T44.3X2	T44.3X3	T44.3X4	T44.3X5	T44.3X6
Pramocaine	T49.1X1	T49.1X2	T49.1X3	T49.1X4	T49.1X5	T49.1X6
Pramoxine	T49.1X1	T49.1X2	T49.1X3	T49.1X4	T49.1X5	T49.1X6
Prasterone	T38.7X1	T38.7X2	T38.7X3	T38.7X4	T38.7X5	T38.7X6
Pravastatin	T46.6X1	T46.6X2	T46.6X3	T46.6X4	T46.6X5	T46.6X6
Prazepam	T42.4X1	T42.4X2	T42.4X3	T42.4X4	T42.4X5	T42.4X6
Praziquantel	T37.4X1	T37.4X2	T37.4X3	T37.4X4	T37.4X5	T37.4X6
Prazitone	T43.291	T43.292	T43.293	T43.294	T43.295	T43.296
Prazosin	T44.6X1	T44.6X2	T44.6X3	T44.6X4	T44.6X5	T44.6X6
Prednicarbate	T49.0X1	T49.0X2	T49.0X3	T49.0X4	T49.0X5	T49.0X6
Prednimustine	T45.1X1	T45.1X2	T45.1X3	T45.1X4	T45.1X5	T45.1X6
Prednisolone	T38.0X1	T38.0X2	T38.0X3	T38.0X4	T38.0X5	T38.0X6
ENT agent	T49.6X1	T49.6X2	T49.6X3	T49.6X4	T49.6X5	T49.6X6
ophthalmic preparation	T49.5X1	T49.5X2	T49.5X3	T49.5X4	T49.5X5	T49.5X6
steaglate	T49.0X1	T49.0X2	T49.0X3	T49.0X4	T49.0X5	T49.0X6
topical NEC	T49.0X1	T49.0X2	T49.0X3	T49.0X4	T49.0X5	T49.0X6
Prednisone	T38.0X1	T38.0X2	T38.0X3	T38.0X4	T38.0X5	T38.0X6
Prednylidene	T38.0X1	T38.0X2	T38.0X3	T38.0X4	T38.0X5	T38.0X6
Pregnandiol	T38.5X1	T38.5X2	T38.5X3	T38.5X4	T38.5X5	T38.5X6
Pregneninolone	T38.5X1	T38.5X2	T38.5X3	T38.5X4	T38.5X5	T38.5X6
Preludin	T43.691	T43.692	T43.693	T43.694	T43.695	T43.696
Premarin	T38.5X1	T38.5X2	T38.5X3	T38.5X4	T38.5X5	T38.5X6
Premedication anesthetic	T41.201	T41.202	T41.203	T41.204	T41.205	T41.206
Prenalterol	T44.5X1	T44.5X2	T44.5X3	T44.5X4	T44.5X5	T44.5X6
Prenoxdiazine	T48.3X1	T48.3X2	T48.3X3	T48.3X4	T48.3X5	T48.3X6
Prenylamine	T46.3X1	T46.3X2	T46.3X3	T46.3X4	T46.3X5	T46.3X6
Preparation, local	T49.4X1	T49.4X2	T49.4X3	T49.4X4	T49.4X5	T49.4X6
Preparation H	T49.8X1	T49.8X2	T49.8X3	T49.8X4	T49.8X5	T49.8X6
Preservative (nonmedicinal)	T65.891	T65.892	T65.893	T65.894	—	—
medicinal	T50.901	T50.902	T50.903	T50.904	T50.905	T50.906
wood	T60.91	T60.92	T60.93	T60.94	—	—

Substance	Poisoning, Accidental (Unintentional)	Poisoning, Intentional Self-Harm	Poisoning, Assault	Poisoning, Undetermined	Adverse Effect	Underdosing
Prethcamide	T50.7X1	T50.7X2	T50.7X3	T50.7X4	T50.7X5	T50.7X6
Pride of China	T62.2X1	T62.2X2	T62.2X3	T62.2X4	—	—
Pridinol	T44.3X1	T44.3X2	T44.3X3	T44.3X4	T44.3X5	T44.3X6
Prifinium bromide	T44.3X1	T44.3X2	T44.3X3	T44.3X4	T44.3X5	T44.3X6
Prilocaine	T41.3X1	T41.3X2	T41.3X3	T41.3X4	T41.3X5	T41.3X6
infiltration (subcutaneous)	T41.3X1	T41.3X2	T41.3X3	T41.3X4	T41.3X5	T41.3X6
nerve block (peripheral) (plexus)	T41.3X1	T41.3X2	T41.3X3	T41.3X4	T41.3X5	T41.3X6
regional	T41.3X1	T41.3X2	T41.3X3	T41.3X4	T41.3X5	T41.3X6
Primaquine	T37.2X1	T37.2X2	T37.2X3	T37.2X4	T37.2X5	T37.2X6
Primidone	T42.6X1	T42.6X2	T42.6X3	T42.6X4	T42.6X5	T42.6X6
Primula (veris)	T62.2X1	T62.2X2	T62.2X3	T62.2X4	—	—
Prinadol	T40.2X1	T40.2X2	T40.2X3	T40.2X4	T40.2X5	T40.2X6
Priscol, Priscoline	T44.6X1	T44.6X2	T44.6X3	T44.6X4	T44.6X5	T44.6X6
Pristinamycin	T36.3X1	T36.3X2	T36.3X3	T36.3X4	T36.3X5	T36.3X6
Privet	T62.2X1	T62.2X2	T62.2X3	T62.2X4	—	—
berries	T62.1X1	T62.1X2	T62.1X3	T62.1X4	—	—
Privine	T44.4X1	T44.4X2	T44.4X3	T44.4X4	T44.4X5	T44.4X6
Pro-Banthine	T44.3X1	T44.3X2	T44.3X3	T44.3X4	T44.3X5	T44.3X6
Probarbital	T42.3X1	T42.3X2	T42.3X3	T42.3X4	T42.3X5	T42.3X6
Probenecid	T50.4X1	T50.4X2	T50.4X3	T50.4X4	T50.4X5	T50.4X6
Probucol	T46.6X1	T46.6X2	T46.6X3	T46.6X4	T46.6X5	T46.6X6
Procainamide	T46.2X1	T46.2X2	T46.2X3	T46.2X4	T46.2X5	T46.2X6
Procaine	T41.3X1	T41.3X2	T41.3X3	T41.3X4	T41.3X5	T41.3X6
benzylpenicillin	T36.0X1	T36.0X2	T36.0X3	T36.0X4	T36.0X5	T36.0X6
nerve block (peripheral) (plexus)	T41.3X1	T41.3X2	T41.3X3	T41.3X4	T41.3X5	T41.3X6
penicillin G	T36.0X1	T36.0X2	T36.0X3	T36.0X4	T36.0X5	T36.0X6
regional	T41.3X1	T41.3X2	T41.3X3	T41.3X4	T41.3X5	T41.3X6
spinal	T41.3X1	T41.3X2	T41.3X3	T41.3X4	T41.3X5	T41.3X6
Procalmidol	T43.591	T43.592	T43.593	T43.594	T43.595	T43.596
Procarbazine	T45.1X1	T45.1X2	T45.1X3	T45.1X4	T45.1X5	T45.1X6
Procaterol	T44.5X1	T44.5X2	T44.5X3	T44.5X4	T44.5X5	T44.5X6
Prochlorperazine	T43.3X1	T43.3X2	T43.3X3	T43.3X4	T43.3X5	T43.3X6
Procyclidine	T44.3X1	T44.3X2	T44.3X3	T44.3X4	T44.3X5	T44.3X6
Producer gas	T58.8X1	T58.8X2	T58.8X3	T58.8X4	—	—
Profadol	T40.4X1	T40.4X2	T40.4X3	T40.4X4	T40.4X5	T40.4X6
Profenamine	T44.3X1	T44.3X2	T44.3X3	T44.3X4	T44.3X5	T44.3X6
Profenil	T44.3X1	T44.3X2	T44.3X3	T44.3X4	T44.3X5	T44.3X6
Proflavine	T49.0X1	T49.0X2	T49.0X3	T49.0X4	T49.0X5	T49.0X6
Progabide	T42.6X1	T42.6X2	T42.6X3	T42.6X4	T42.6X5	T42.6X6
Progestin	T38.5X1	T38.5X2	T38.5X3	T38.5X4	T38.5X5	T38.5X6
oral contraceptive	T38.4X1	T38.4X2	T38.4X3	T38.4X4	T38.4X5	T38.4X6

◀ New ◀ Revised ~~deleted~~ Deleted

Substance	External Cause (T-Code)					
	Poisoning, Accidental (Unintentional)	Poisoning, Intentional Self-Harm	Poisoning, Assault	Poisoning, Undetermined	Adverse Effect	Underdosing
Progesterone	T38.5X1	T38.5X2	T38.5X3	T38.5X4	T38.5X5	T38.5X6
Progestogen NEC	T38.5X1	T38.5X2	T38.5X3	T38.5X4	T38.5X5	T38.5X6
Progestone	T38.5X1	T38.5X2	T38.5X3	T38.5X4	T38.5X5	T38.5X6
Proglumide	T47.1X1	T47.1X2	T47.1X3	T47.1X4	T47.1X5	T47.1X6
Proguanil	T37.2X1	T37.2X2	T37.2X3	T37.2X4	T37.2X5	T37.2X6
Prolactin	T38.811	T38.812	T38.813	T38.814	T38.815	T38.816
Prolintane	T43.691	T43.692	T43.693	T43.694	T43.695	T43.696
Proloid	T38.1X1	T38.1X2	T38.1X3	T38.1X4	T38.1X5	T38.1X6
Proluton	T38.5X1	T38.5X2	T38.5X3	T38.5X4	T38.5X5	T38.5X6
Promacetin	T37.1X1	T37.1X2	T37.1X3	T37.1X4	T37.1X5	T37.1X6
Promazine	T43.3X1	T43.3X2	T43.3X3	T43.3X4	T43.3X5	T43.3X6
Promedol	T40.2X1	T40.2X2	T40.2X3	T40.2X4	—	—
Promegestone	T38.5X1	T38.5X2	T38.5X3	T38.5X4	T38.5X5	T38.5X6
Promethazine (teoclate)	T43.3X1	T43.3X2	T43.3X3	T43.3X4	T43.3X5	T43.3X6
Promin	T37.1X1	T37.1X2	T37.1X3	T37.1X4	T37.1X5	T37.1X6
Pronase	T45.3X1	T45.3X2	T45.3X3	T45.3X4	T45.3X5	T45.3X6
Pronestyl (hydrochloride)	T46.2X1	T46.2X2	T46.2X3	T46.2X4	T46.2X5	T46.2X6
Pronetalol	T44.7X1	T44.7X2	T44.7X3	T44.7X4	T44.7X5	T44.7X6
Prontosil	T37.0X1	T37.0X2	T37.0X3	T37.0X4	T37.0X5	T37.0X6
Propachlor	T60.3X1	T60.3X2	T60.3X3	T60.3X4	—	—
Propafenone	T46.2X1	T46.2X2	T46.2X3	T46.2X4	T46.2X5	T46.2X6
Propallylonal	T42.3X1	T42.3X2	T42.3X3	T42.3X4	T42.3X5	T42.3X6
Propamidine	T49.0X1	T49.0X2	T49.0X3	T49.0X4	T49.0X5	T49.0X6
Propane (distributed in mobile container)	T59.891	T59.892	T59.893	T59.894	—	—
distributed through pipes	T59.891	T59.892	T59.893	T59.894	—	—
incomplete combustion	T57.11	T57.12	T57.13	T57.14	—	—
Propanidid	T41.291	T41.292	T41.293	T41.294	T41.295	T41.296
Propanil	T60.3X1	T60.3X2	T60.3X3	T60.3X4	—	—
1-Propanol	T51.3X1	T51.3X2	T51.3X3	T51.3X4	—	—
2-Propanol	T51.2X1	T51.2X2	T51.2X3	T51.2X4	—	—
Propantheline	T44.3X1	T44.3X2	T44.3X3	T44.3X4	T44.3X5	T44.3X6
bromide	T44.3X1	T44.3X2	T44.3X3	T44.3X4	T44.3X5	T44.3X6
Proparacaine	T41.3X1	T41.3X2	T41.3X3	T41.3X4	T41.3X5	T41.3X6
Propatylnitrate	T46.3X1	T46.3X2	T46.3X3	T46.3X4	T46.3X5	T46.3X6
Propicillin	T36.0X1	T36.0X2	T36.0X3	T36.0X4	T36.0X5	T36.0X6
Propiolactone	T49.0X1	T49.0X2	T49.0X3	T49.0X4	T49.0X5	T49.0X6
Propiomazine	T45.0X1	T45.0X2	T45.0X3	T45.0X4	T45.0X5	T45.0X6
Propionaldehyde (medicinal)	T42.6X1	T42.6X2	T42.6X3	T42.6X4	T42.6X5	T42.6X6
Propionate (calcium) (sodium)	T49.0X1	T49.0X2	T49.0X3	T49.0X4	T49.0X5	T49.0X6
Propion gel	T49.0X1	T49.0X2	T49.0X3	T49.0X4	T49.0X5	T49.0X6

Substance	External Cause (T-Code)					
	Poisoning, Accidental (Unintentional)	Poisoning, Intentional Self-Harm	Poisoning, Assault	Poisoning, Undetermined	Adverse Effect	Underdosing
Propitocaine	T41.3X1	T41.3X2	T41.3X3	T41.3X4	T41.3X5	T41.3X6
infiltration (subcutaneous)	T41.3X1	T41.3X2	T41.3X3	T41.3X4	T41.3X5	T41.3X6
nerve block (peripheral) (plexus)	T41.3X1	T41.3X2	T41.3X3	T41.3X4	T41.3X5	T41.3X6
Propofol	T41.291	T41.292	T41.293	T41.294	T41.295	T41.296
Propoxur	T60.0X1	T60.0X2	T60.0X3	T60.0X4	—	—
Propoxycaine	T41.3X1	T41.3X2	T41.3X3	T41.3X4	T41.3X5	T41.3X6
infiltration (subcutaneous)	T41.3X1	T41.3X2	T41.3X3	T41.3X4	T41.3X5	T41.3X6
nerve block (peripheral) (plexus)	T41.3X1	T41.3X2	T41.3X3	T41.3X4	T41.3X5	T41.3X6
topical (surface)	T41.3X1	T41.3X2	T41.3X3	T41.3X4	T41.3X5	T41.3X6
Propoxyphene	T40.4X1	T40.4X2	T40.4X3	T40.4X4	T40.4X5	T40.4X6
Propranolol	T44.7X1	T44.7X2	T44.7X3	T44.7X4	T44.7X5	T44.7X6
Propyl						
alcohol	T51.3X1	T51.3X2	T51.3X3	T51.3X4	—	—
carbinol	T51.3X1	T51.3X2	T51.3X3	T51.3X4	—	—
hexadrine	T44.4X1	T44.4X2	T44.4X3	T44.4X4	T44.4X5	T44.4X6
iodone	T50.8X1	T50.8X2	T50.8X3	T50.8X4	T50.8X5	T50.8X6
thiouracil	T38.2X1	T38.2X2	T38.2X3	T38.2X4	T38.2X5	T38.2X6
Propylaminophenothiazine	T43.3X1	T43.3X2	T43.3X3	T43.3X4	T43.3X5	T43.3X6
Propylene	T59.891	T59.892	T59.893	T59.894	—	—
Propylhexedrine	T48.5X1	T48.5X2	T48.5X3	T48.5X4	T48.5X5	T48.5X6
Propyliodone	T50.8X1	T50.8X2	T50.8X3	T50.8X4	T50.8X5	T50.8X6
Propylthiouracil	T38.2X1	T38.2X2	T38.2X3	T38.2X4	T38.2X5	T38.2X6
Propylparaben (ophthalmic)	T49.5X1	T49.5X2	T49.5X3	T49.5X4	T49.5X5	T49.5X6
Propyphenazone	T39.2X1	T39.2X2	T39.2X3	T39.2X4	T39.2X5	T39.2X6
Proquazone	T39.391	T39.392	T39.393	T39.394	T39.395	T39.396
Proscillaridin	T46.0X1	T46.0X2	T46.0X3	T46.0X4	T46.0X5	T46.0X6
Prostacyclin	T45.521	T45.522	T45.523	T45.524	T45.525	T45.526
Prostaglandin (I2)	T45.521	T45.522	T45.523	T45.524	T45.525	T45.526
E1	T46.7X1	T46.7X2	T46.7X3	T46.7X4	T46.7X5	T46.7X6
E2	T48.0X1	T48.0X2	T48.0X3	T48.0X4	T48.0X5	T48.0X6
F2 alpha	T48.0X1	T48.0X2	T48.0X3	T48.0X4	T48.0X5	T48.0X6
Prostigmin	T44.0X1	T44.0X2	T44.0X3	T44.0X4	T44.0X5	T44.0X6
Prosultiamine	T45.2X1	T45.2X2	T45.2X3	T45.2X4	T45.2X5	T45.2X6
Protamine sulfate	T45.7X1	T45.7X2	T45.7X3	T45.7X4	T45.7X5	T45.7X6
zinc insulin	T38.3X1	T38.3X2	T38.3X3	T38.3X4	T38.3X5	T38.3X6
Protease	T47.5X1	T47.5X2	T47.5X3	T47.5X4	T47.5X5	T47.5X6
Protectant, skin NEC	T49.3X1	T49.3X2	T49.3X3	T49.3X4	T49.3X5	T49.3X6
Protein hydrolysate	T50.991	T50.992	T50.993	T50.994	T50.995	T50.996
Prothiaden — see Dothiepin hydrochloride						
Prothionamide	T37.1X1	T37.1X2	T37.1X3	T37.1X4	T37.1X5	T37.1X6

◄ New ◄| Revised ~~deleted~~ Deleted

Substance	Poisoning, Accidental (Unintentional)	Poisoning, Intentional Self-Harm	Poisoning, Assault	Poisoning, Undetermined	Adverse Effect	Underdosing
Prothipendyl	T43.591	T43.592	T43.593	T43.594	T43.595	T43.596
Prothoate	T60.0X1	T60.0X2	T60.0X3	T60.0X4	—	—
Prothrombin						
activator	T45.7X1	T45.7X2	T45.7X3	T45.7X4	T45.7X5	T45.7X6
synthesis inhibitor	T45.511	T45.512	T45.513	T45.514	T45.515	T45.516
Protionamide	T37.1X1	T37.1X2	T37.1X3	T37.1X4	T37.1X5	T37.1X6
Protirelin	T38.891	T38.892	T38.893	T38.894	T38.895	T38.896
Protokylol	T48.6X1	T48.6X2	T48.6X3	T48.6X4	T48.6X5	T48.6X6
Protopam	T50.6X1	T50.6X2	T50.6X3	T50.6X4	T50.6X5	T50.6X6
Protoveratrine(s) (A) (B)	T46.5X1	T46.5X2	T46.5X3	T46.5X4	T46.5X5	T46.5X6
Protriptyline	T43.011	T43.012	T43.013	T43.014	T43.015	T43.016
Provera	T38.5X1	T38.5X2	T38.5X4	T38.5X4	T38.5X5	T38.5X6
Provitamin A	T45.2X1	T45.2X2	T45.2X3	T45.2X4	T45.2X5	T45.2X6
Proxibarbal	T42.3X1	T42.3X2	T42.3X3	T42.3X4	T42.3X5	T42.3X6
Proxymetacaine	T41.3X1	T41.3X2	T41.3X3	T41.3X4	T41.3X5	T41.3X6
Proxyphylline	T48.6X1	T48.6X2	T48.6X3	T48.6X4	T48.6X5	T48.6X6
Prozac — see Fluoxetine hydrochloride						
Prunus						
laurocerasus	T62.2X1	T62.2X2	T62.2X3	T62.2X4	—	—
virginiana	T62.2X1	T62.2X2	T62.2X3	T62.2X4	—	—
Prussian blue						
commercial	T65.891	T65.892	T65.893	T65.894	—	—
therapeutic	T50.6X1	T50.6X2	T50.6X3	T50.6X4	T50.6X5	T50.6X6
Prussic acid	T65.0X1	T65.0X2	T65.0X3	T65.0X4	—	—
vapor	T57.3X1	T57.3X2	T57.3X3	T57.3X4	—	—
Pseudoephedrine	T44.991	T44.992	T44.993	T44.994	T44.995	T44.996
Psilocin	T40.991	T40.992	T40.993	T40.994	—	—
Psilocybin	T40.991	T40.992	T40.993	T40.994	—	—
Psilocybine	T40.991	T40.992	T40.993	T40.994	—	—
Psoralene (nonmedicinal)	T65.891	T65.892	T65.893	T65.894	—	—
Psoralens (medicinal)	T50.991	T50.992	T50.993	T50.994	T50.995	T50.996
PSP (phenolsulfonphthalein)	T50.8X1	T50.8X2	T50.8X3	T50.8X4	T50.8X5	T50.8X6
Psychodysleptic drug NEC	T40.901	T40.902	T40.903	T40.904	T40.905	T40.906
Psychostimulant	T43.601	T43.602	T43.603	T43.604	T43.605	T43.606
amphetamine	T43.621	T43.622	T43.623	T43.624	T43.625	T43.626
caffeine	T43.611	T43.612	T43.613	T43.614	T43.615	T43.616
methylphenidate	T43.631	T43.632	T43.633	T43.634	T43.635	T43.636
specified NEC	T43.691	T43.692	T43.693	T43.694	T43.695	T43.696
Psychotherapeutic drug NEC	T43.91	T43.92	T43.93	T43.94	T43.95	T43.96
antidepressants — see also Antidepressant	T43.201	T43.202	T43.203	T43.204	T43.205	T43.206

Substance	Poisoning, Accidental (Unintentional)	Poisoning, Intentional Self-Harm	Poisoning, Assault	Poisoning, Undetermined	Adverse Effect	Underdosing
Psychotherapeutic drug NEC (Continued)						
specified NEC	T43.8X1	T43.8X2	T43.8X3	T43.8X4	T43.8X5	T43.8X6
tranquilizers NEC	T43.501	T43.502	T43.503	T43.504	T43.505	T43.506
Psychotomimetic agents	T40.901	T40.902	T40.903	T40.904	T40.905	T40.906
Psychotropic drug NEC	T43.91	T43.92	T43.93	T43.94	T43.95	T43.96
specified NEC	T43.8X1	T43.8X2	T43.8X3	T43.8X4	T43.8X5	T43.8X6
Psyllium hydrophilic mucilloid	T47.4X1	T47.4X2	T47.4X3	T47.4X4	T47.4X5	T47.4X6
Pteroylglutamic acid	T45.8X1	T45.8X2	T45.8X3	T45.8X4	T45.8X5	T45.8X6
Pteroyltriglutamate	T45.1X1	T45.1X2	T45.1X3	T45.1X4	T45.1X5	T45.1X6
PTFE — see Polytetrafluoroethylene						
Pulp						
devitalizing paste	T49.7X1	T49.7X2	T49.7X3	T49.7X4	T49.7X5	T49.7X6
dressing	T49.7X1	T49.7X2	T49.7X3	T49.7X4	T49.7X5	T49.7X6
Pulsatilla	T62.2X1	T62.2X2	T62.2X3	T62.2X4	—	—
Pumpkin seed extract	T37.4X1	T37.4X2	T37.4X3	T37.4X4	T37.4X5	T37.4X6
Purex (bleach)	T54.91	T54.92	T54.93	T54.94		
Purgative NEC — see also Cathartic	T47.4X1	T47.4X2	T47.4X3	T47.4X4	T47.4X5	T47.4X6
Purine analogue (antineoplastic)	T45.1X1	T45.1X2	T45.1X3	T45.1X4	T45.1X5	T45.1X6
Purine diuretics	T50.2X1	T50.2X2	T50.2X3	T50.2X4	T50.2X5	T50.2X6
Purinethol	T45.1X1	T45.1X2	T45.1X3	T45.1X4	T45.1X5	T45.1X6
PVP	T45.8X1	T45.8X2	T45.8X3	T45.8X4	T45.8X5	T45.8X6
Pyrabital	T39.8X1	T39.8X2	T39.8X3	T39.8X4	T39.8X5	T39.8X6
Pyramidon	T39.2X1	T39.2X2	T39.2X3	T39.2X4	T39.2X5	T39.2X6
Pyrantel	T37.4X1	T37.4X2	T37.4X3	T37.4X4	T37.4X5	T37.4X6
Pyrathiazine	T45.0X1	T45.0X2	T45.0X3	T45.0X4	T45.0X5	T45.0X6
Pyrazinamide	T37.1X1	T37.1X2	T37.1X3	T37.1X4	T37.1X5	T37.1X6
Pyrazinoic acid (amide)	T37.1X1	T37.1X2	T37.1X3	T37.1X4	T37.1X5	T37.1X6
Pyrazole (derivatives)	T39.2X1	T39.2X2	T39.2X3	T39.2X4	T39.2X5	T39.2X6
Pyrazolone analgesic NEC	T39.2X1	T39.2X2	T39.2X3	T39.2X4	T39.2X5	T39.2X6
Pyrethrin, pyrethrum (nonmedicinal)	T60.2X1	T60.2X2	T60.2X3	T60.2X4	—	—
Pyrethrum extract	T49.0X1	T49.0X2	T49.0X3	T49.0X4	T49.0X5	T49.0X6
Pyribenzamine	T45.0X1	T45.0X2	T45.0X3	T45.0X4	T45.0X5	T45.0X6
Pyridine	T52.8X1	T52.8X2	T52.8X3	T52.8X4	—	—
aldoxime methiodide	T50.6X1	T50.6X2	T50.6X3	T50.6X4	T50.6X5	T50.6X6
aldoxime methyl chloride	T50.6X1	T50.6X2	T50.6X3	T50.6X4	T50.6X5	T50.6X6
vapor	T59.891	T59.892	T59.893	T59.894	—	—
Pyridium	T39.8X1	T39.8X2	T39.8X3	T39.8X4	T39.8X5	T39.8X6
Pyridostigmine bromide	T44.0X1	T44.0X2	T44.0X3	T44.0X4	T44.0X5	T44.0X6
Pyridoxal phosphate	T45.2X1	T45.2X2	T45.2X3	T45.2X4	T45.2X5	T45.2X6

◀ New　◀ Revised　~~deleted~~ Deleted

Substance	Poisoning, Accidental (Unintentional)	Poisoning, Intentional Self-Harm	Poisoning, Assault	Poisoning, Undetermined	Adverse Effect	Underdosing
Pyridoxine	T45.2X1	T45.2X2	T45.2X3	T45.2X4	T45.2X5	T45.2X6
Pyrilamine	T45.0X1	T45.0X2	T45.0X3	T45.0X4	T45.0X5	T45.0X6
Pyrimethamine	T37.2X1	T37.2X2	T37.2X3	T37.2X4	T37.2X5	T37.2X6
with sulfadoxine	T37.2X1	T37.2X2	T37.2X3	T37.2X4	T37.2X5	T37.2X6
Pyrimidine antagonist	T45.1X1	T45.1X2	T45.1X3	T45.1X4	T45.1X5	T45.1X6
Pyriminil	T60.4X1	T60.4X2	T60.4X3	T60.4X4	—	—
Pyrithione zinc	T49.4X1	T49.4X2	T49.4X3	T49.4X4	T49.4X5	T49.4X6
Pyrithyldione	T42.6X1	T42.6X2	T42.6X3	T42.6X4	T42.6X5	T42.6X6
Pyrogallic acid	T49.0X1	T49.0X2	T49.0X3	T49.0X4	T49.0X5	T49.0X6
Pyrogallol	T49.0X1	T49.0X2	T49.0X3	T49.0X4	T49.0X5	T49.0X6
Pyroxylin	T49.3X1	T49.3X2	T49.3X3	T49.3X4	T49.3X5	T49.3X6
Pyrrobutamine	T45.0X1	T45.0X2	T45.0X3	T45.0X4	T45.0X5	T45.0X6
Pyrrolizidine alkaloids	T62.8X1	T62.8X2	T62.8X3	T62.8X4	—	—
Pyrvinium chloride	T37.4X1	T37.4X2	T37.4X3	T37.4X4	T37.4X5	T37.4X6
PZI	T38.3X1	T38.3X2	T38.3X3	T38.3X4	T38.3X5	T38.3X6
Q						
Quaalude	T42.6X1	T42.6X2	T42.6X3	T42.6X4	T42.6X5	T42.6X6
Quarternary ammonium						
anti-infective	T49.0X1	T49.0X2	T49.0X3	T49.0X4	T49.0X5	T49.0X6
ganglion blocking	T44.2X1	T44.2X2	T44.2X3	T44.2X4	T44.2X5	T44.2X6
parasympatholytic	T44.3X1	T44.3X2	T44.3X3	T44.3X4	T44.3X5	T44.3X6
Quazepam	T42.4X1	T42.4X2	T42.4X3	T42.4X4	T42.4X5	T42.4X6
Quicklime	T54.3X1	T54.3X2	T54.3X3	T54.3X4	—	—
Quillaja extract	T48.4X1	T48.4X2	T48.4X3	T48.4X4	T48.4X5	T48.4X6
Quinacrine	T37.2X1	T37.2X2	T37.2X3	T37.2X4	T37.2X5	T37.2X6
Quinaglute	T46.2X1	T46.2X2	T46.2X3	T46.2X4	T46.2X5	T46.2X6
Quinalbarbital	T42.3X1	T42.3X2	T42.3X3	T42.3X4	T42.3X5	T42.3X6
Quinalbarbitone sodium	T42.3X1	T42.3X2	T42.3X3	T42.3X4	T42.3X5	T42.3X6
Quinalphos	T60.0X1	T60.0X2	T60.0X3	T60.0X4	—	—
Quinapril	T46.4X1	T46.4X2	T46.4X3	T46.4X4	T46.4X5	T46.4X6
Quinestradiol	T38.5X1	T38.5X2	T38.5X3	T38.5X4	T38.5X5	T38.5X6
Quinestradol	T38.5X1	T38.5X2	T38.5X3	T38.5X4	T38.5X5	T38.5X6
Quinestrol	T38.5X1	T38.5X2	T38.5X3	T38.5X4	T38.5X5	T38.5X6
Quinethazone	T50.2X1	T50.2X2	T50.2X3	T50.2X4	T50.2X5	T50.2X6
Quingestanol	T38.4X1	T38.4X2	T38.4X3	T38.4X4	T38.4X5	T38.4X6
Quinidine	T46.2X1	T46.2X2	T46.2X3	T46.2X4	T46.2X5	T46.2X6
Quinine	T37.2X1	T37.2X2	T37.2X3	T37.2X4	T37.2X5	T37.2X6
Quiniobine	T37.8X1	T37.8X2	T37.8X3	T37.8X4	T37.8X5	T37.8X6
Quinisocaine	T49.1X1	T49.1X2	T49.1X3	T49.1X4	T49.1X5	T49.1X6
Quinocide	T37.2X1	T37.2X2	T37.2X3	T37.2X4	T37.2X5	T37.2X6
Quinoline (derivatives) NEC	T37.8X1	T37.8X2	T37.8X3	T37.8X4	T37.8X5	T37.8X6

Substance	Poisoning, Accidental (Unintentional)	Poisoning, Intentional Self-Harm	Poisoning, Assault	Poisoning, Undetermined	Adverse Effect	Underdosing
Quinupramine	T43.011	T43.012	T43.013	T43.014	T43.015	T43.016
Quotane	T41.3X1	T41.3X2	T41.3X3	T41.3X4	T41.3X5	T41.3X6
R						
Rabies						
immune globulin (human)	T50.Z11	T50.Z12	T50.Z13	T50.Z14	T50.Z15	T50.Z16
vaccine	T50.B91	T50.B92	T50.B93	T50.B94	T50.B95	T50.B96
Racemoramide	T40.2X1	T40.2X2	T40.2X3	T40.2X4	—	—
Racemorphan	T40.2X1	T40.2X2	T40.2X3	T40.2X4	T40.2X5	T40.2X6
Racepinefrin	T44.5X1	T44.5X2	T44.5X3	T44.5X4	T44.5X5	T44.5X6
Raclopride	T43.591	T43.592	T43.593	T43.594	T43.595	T43.596
Radiator alcohol	T51.1X1	T51.1X2	T51.1X3	T51.1X4	—	—
Radioactive drug NEC	T50.8X1	T50.8X2	T50.8X3	T50.8X4	T50.8X5	T50.8X6
Radio-opaque (drugs) (materials)	T50.8X1	T50.8X2	T50.8X3	T50.8X4	T50.8X5	T50.8X6
Ramifenazone	T39.2X1	T39.2X2	T39.2X3	T39.2X4	T39.2X5	T39.2X6
Ramipril	T46.4X1	T46.4X2	T46.4X3	T46.4X4	T46.4X5	T46.4X6
Ranitidine	T47.0X1	T47.0X2	T47.0X3	T47.0X4	T47.0X5	T47.0X6
Ranunculus	T62.2X1	T62.2X2	T62.2X3	T62.2X4	—	—
Rat poison NEC	T60.4X1	T60.4X2	T60.4X3	T60.4X4	—	—
Rattlesnake (venom)	T63.011	T63.012	T63.013	T63.014		
Raubasine	T46.7X1	T46.7X2	T46.7X3	T46.7X4	T46.7X5	T46.7X6
Raudixin	T46.5X1	T46.5X2	T46.5X3	T46.5X4	T46.5X5	T46.5X6
Rautensin	T46.5X1	T46.5X2	T46.5X3	T46.5X4	T46.5X5	T46.5X6
Rautina	T46.5X1	T46.5X2	T46.5X3	T46.5X4	T46.5X5	T46.5X6
Rautotal	T46.5X1	T46.5X2	T46.5X3	T46.5X4	T46.5X5	T46.5X6
Rauwiloid	T46.5X1	T46.5X2	T46.5X3	T46.5X4	T46.5X5	T46.5X6
Rauwoldin	T46.5X1	T46.5X2	T46.5X3	T46.5X4	T46.5X5	T46.5X6
Rauwolfia (alkaloids)	T46.5X1	T46.5X2	T46.5X3	T46.5X4	T46.5X5	T46.5X6
Razoxane	T45.1X1	T45.1X2	T45.1X3	T45.1X4	T45.1X5	T45.1X6
Realgar	T57.0X1	T57.0X2	T57.0X3	T57.0X4	—	—
Recombinant (R) — *see specific protein*						
Red blood cells, packed	T45.8X1	T45.8X2	T45.8X3	T45.8X4	T45.8X5	T45.8X6
Red squill (scilliroside)	T60.4X1	T60.4X2	T60.4X3	T60.4X4	—	—
Reducing agent, industrial NEC	T65.891	T65.892	T65.893	T65.894	—	—
Refrigerant gas (chlorofluoro-carbon)	T53.5X1	T53.5X2	T53.5X3	T53.5X4	—	—
not chlorofluoro-carbon	T59.891	T59.892	T59.893	T59.894	—	—
Regroton	T50.2X1	T50.2X2	T50.2X3	T50.2X4	T50.2X5	T50.2X6
Rehydration salts (oral)	T50.3X1	T50.3X2	T50.3X3	T50.3X4	T50.3X5	T50.3X6
Rela	T42.8X1	T42.8X2	T42.8X3	T42.8X4	T42.8X5	T42.8X6

◀ New   ◀ Revised   ~~deleted~~ Deleted

TABLE OF DRUGS AND CHEMICALS

Substance	Poisoning, Accidental (Unintentional)	Poisoning, Intentional Self-Harm	Poisoning, Assault	Poisoning, Undetermined	Adverse Effect	Underdosing
Relaxant, muscle						
anesthetic	T48.1X1	T48.1X2	T48.1X3	T48.1X4	T48.1X5	T48.1X6
central nervous system	T42.8X1	T42.8X2	T42.8X3	T42.8X4	T42.8X5	T42.8X6
skeletal NEC	T48.1X1	T48.1X2	T48.1X3	T48.1X4	T48.1X5	T48.1X6
smooth NEC	T44.3X1	T44.3X2	T44.3X3	T44.3X4	T44.3X5	T44.3X6
Remoxipride	T43.591	T43.592	T43.593	T43.594	T43.595	T43.596
Renese	T50.2X1	T50.2X2	T50.2X3	T50.2X4	T50.2X5	T50.2X6
Renografin	T50.8X1	T50.8X2	T50.8X3	T50.8X4	T50.8X5	T50.8X6
Replacement solution	T50.3X1	T50.3X2	T50.3X3	T50.3X4	T50.3X5	T50.3X6
Reproterol	T48.6X1	T48.6X2	T48.6X3	T48.6X4	T48.6X5	T48.6X6
Rescinnamine	T46.5X1	T46.5X2	T46.5X3	T46.5X4	T46.5X5	T46.5X6
Reserpin(e)	T46.5X1	T46.5X2	T46.5X3	T46.5X4	T46.5X5	T46.5X6
Resorcin, resorcinol (nonmedicinal)	T65.891	T65.892	T65.893	T65.894	—	—
medicinal	T49.4X1	T49.4X2	T49.4X3	T49.4X4	T49.4X5	T49.4X6
Respaire	T48.4X1	T48.4X2	T48.4X3	T48.4X4	T48.4X5	T48.4X6
Respiratory drug NEC	T48.901	T48.902	T48.903	T48.904	T48.905	T48.906
antiasthmatic NEC	T48.6X1	T48.6X2	T48.6X3	T48.6X4	T48.6X5	T48.6X6
anti-common-cold NEC	T48.5X1	T48.5X2	T48.5X3	T48.5X4	T48.5X5	T48.5X6
expectorant NEC	T48.4X1	T48.4X2	T48.4X3	T48.4X4	T48.4X5	T48.4X6
stimulant	T48.901	T48.902	T48.903	T48.904	T48.905	T48.906
Retinoic acid	T49.0X1	T49.0X2	T49.0X3	T49.0X4	T49.0X5	T49.0X6
Retinol	T45.2X1	T45.2X2	T45.2X3	T45.2X4	T45.2X5	T45.2X6
Rh (D) immune globulin (human)	T50.Z11	T50.Z12	T50.Z13	T50.Z14	T50.Z15	T50.Z16
Rhodine	T39.011	T39.012	T39.013	T39.014	T39.015	T39.016
RhoGAM	T50.Z11	T50.Z12	T50.Z13	T50.Z14	T50.Z15	T50.Z16
Rhubarb						
dry extract	T47.2X1	T47.2X2	T47.2X3	T47.2X4	T47.2X5	T47.2X6
tincture, compound	T47.2X1	T47.2X2	T47.2X3	T47.2X4	T47.2X5	T47.2X6
Ribavirin	T37.5X1	T37.5X2	T37.5X3	T37.5X4	T37.5X5	T37.5X6
Riboflavin	T45.2X1	T45.2X2	T45.2X3	T45.2X4	T45.2X5	T45.2X6
Ribostamycin	T36.5X1	T36.5X2	T36.5X3	T36.5X4	T36.5X5	T36.5X6
Ricin	T62.2X1	T62.2X2	T62.2X3	T62.2X4	—	—
Ricinus communis	T62.2X1	T62.2X2	T62.2X3	T62.2X4	—	—
Rickettsial vaccine NEC	T50.A91	T50.A92	T50.A93	T50.A94	T50.A95	T50.A96
Rifabutin	T36.6X1	T36.6X2	T36.6X3	T36.6X4	T36.6X5	T36.6X6
Rifamide	T36.6X1	T36.6X2	T36.6X3	T36.6X4	T36.6X5	T36.6X6
Rifampicin	T36.6X1	T36.6X2	T36.6X3	T36.6X4	T36.6X5	T36.6X6
with isoniazid	T37.1X1	T37.1X2	T37.1X3	T37.1X4	T37.1X5	T37.1X6
Rifampin	T36.6X1	T36.6X2	T36.6X3	T36.6X4	T36.6X5	T36.6X6
Rifamycin	T36.6X1	T36.6X2	T36.6X3	T36.6X4	T36.6X5	T36.6X6
Rifaximin	T36.6X1	T36.6X2	T36.6X3	T36.6X4	T36.6X5	T36.6X6

Substance	Poisoning, Accidental (Unintentional)	Poisoning, Intentional Self-Harm	Poisoning, Assault	Poisoning, Undetermined	Adverse Effect	Underdosing
Rimantadine	T37.5X1	T37.5X2	T37.5X3	T37.5X4	T37.5X5	T37.5X6
Rimazolium metilsulfate	T39.8X1	T39.8X2	T39.8X3	T39.8X4	T39.8X5	T39.8X6
Rimifon	T37.1X1	T37.1X2	T37.1X3	T37.1X4	T37.1X5	T37.1X6
Rimiterol	T48.6X1	T48.6X2	T48.6X3	T48.6X4	T48.6X5	T48.6X6
Ringer (lactate) solution	T50.3X1	T50.3X2	T50.3X3	T50.3X4	T50.3X5	T50.3X6
Ristocetin	T36.8X1	T36.8X2	T36.8X3	T36.8X4	T36.8X5	T36.8X6
Ritalin	T43.631	T43.632	T43.633	T43.634	T43.635	T43.636
Ritodrine	T44.5X1	T44.5X2	T44.5X3	T44.5X4	T44.5X5	T44.5X6
Roach killer — *see Insecticide*						
Rociverine	T44.3X1	T44.3X2	T44.3X3	T44.3X4	T44.3X5	T44.3X6
Rocky Mountain spotted fever vaccine	T50.A91	T50.A92	T50.A93	T50.A94	T50.A95	T50.A96
Rodenticide NEC	T60.4X1	T60.4X2	T60.4X3	T60.4X4	—	—
Rohypnol	T42.4X1	T42.4X2	T42.4X3	T42.4X4	T42.4X5	T42.4X6
Rokitamycin	T36.3X1	T36.3X2	T36.3X3	T36.3X4	T36.3X5	T36.3X6
Rolaids	T47.1X1	T47.1X2	T47.1X3	T47.1X4	T47.1X5	T47.1X6
Rolitetracycline	T36.4X1	T36.4X2	T36.4X3	T36.4X4	T36.4X5	T36.4X6
Romilar	T48.3X1	T48.3X2	T48.3X3	T48.3X4	T48.3X5	T48.3X6
Ronifibrate	T46.6X1	T46.6X2	T46.6X3	T46.6X4	T46.6X5	T46.6X6
Rosaprostol	T47.1X1	T47.1X2	T47.1X3	T47.1X4	T47.1X5	T47.1X6
Rose bengal sodium (131I)	T50.8X1	T50.8X2	T50.8X3	T50.8X4	T50.8X5	T50.8X6
Rose water ointment	T49.3X1	T49.3X2	T49.3X3	T49.3X4	T49.3X5	T49.3X6
Rosoxacin	T37.8X1	T37.8X2	T37.8X3	T37.8X4	T37.8X5	T37.8X6
Rotenone	T60.2X1	T60.2X2	T60.2X3	T60.2X4	—	—
Rotoxamine	T45.0X1	T45.0X2	T45.0X3	T45.0X4	T45.0X5	T45.0X6
Rough-on-rats	T60.4X1	T60.4X2	T60.4X3	T60.4X4	—	—
Roxatidine	T47.0X1	T47.0X2	T47.0X3	T47.0X4	T47.0X5	T47.0X6
Roxithromycin	T36.3X1	T36.3X2	T36.3X3	T36.3X4	T36.3X5	T36.3X6
Rt-PA	T45.611	T45.612	T45.613	T45.614	T45.615	T45.616
Rubbing alcohol	T51.2X1	T51.2X2	T51.2X3	T51.2X4	—	—
Rubefacient	T49.4X1	T49.4X2	T49.4X3	T49.4X4	T49.4X5	T49.4X6
Rubella vaccine	T50.B91	T50.B92	T50.B93	T50.B94	T50.B95	T50.B96
Rubelogen	T50.B91	T50.B92	T50.B93	T50.B94	T50.B95	T50.B96
Rubeovax	T50.991	T50.992	T50.993	T50.994	T50.995	T50.996
Rubidium chloride Rb82	T50.8X1	T50.8X2	T50.8X3	T50.8X4	T50.8X5	T50.8X6
Rubidomycin	T45.1X1	T45.1X2	T45.1X3	T45.1X4	T45.1X5	T45.1X6
Rue	T62.2X1	T62.2X2	T62.2X3	T62.2X4	—	—
Rufocromomycin	T45.1X1	T45.1X2	T45.1X3	T45.1X4	T45.1X5	T45.1X6
Russel's viper venin	T45.7X1	T45.7X2	T45.7X3	T45.7X4	T45.7X5	T45.7X6
Ruta (graveolens)	T62.2X1	T62.2X2	T62.2X3	T62.2X4	—	—
Rutinum	T46.991	T46.992	T46.993	T46.994	T46.995	T46.996
Rutoside	T46.991	T46.992	T46.993	T46.994	T46.995	T46.996

◀ New   ◀ Revised   ~~deleted~~ Deleted

Substance	Poisoning, Accidental (Unintentional)	Poisoning, Intentional Self-Harm	Poisoning, Assault	Poisoning, Undetermined	Adverse Effect	Underdosing
S						
Sabadilla (plant)	T62.2X1	T62.2X2	T62.2X3	T62.2X4	—	—
pesticide	T60.2X1	T60.2X2	T60.2X3	T60.2X4	—	—
Saccharated iron oxide	T45.8X1	T45.8X2	T45.8X3	T45.8X4	T45.8X5	T45.8X6
Saccharin	T50.901	T50.902	T50.903	T50.904	T50.905	T50.906
Saccharomyces boulardii	T47.6X1	T47.6X2	T47.6X3	T47.6X4	T47.6X5	T47.6X6
Safflower oil	T46.6X1	T46.6X2	T46.6X3	T46.6X4	T46.6X5	T46.6X6
Safrazine	T43.1X1	T43.1X2	T43.1X3	T43.1X4	T43.1X5	T43.1X6
Salazosulfapyridine	T37.0X1	T37.0X2	T37.0X3	T37.0X4	T37.0X5	T37.0X6
Salbutamol	T48.6X1	T48.6X2	T48.6X3	T48.6X4	T48.6X5	T48.6X6
Salicylamide	T39.091	T39.092	T39.093	T39.094	T39.095	T39.096
Salicylate NEC	T39.091	T39.092	T39.093	T39.094	T39.095	T39.096
methyl	T49.3X1	T49.3X2	T49.3X3	T49.3X4	T49.3X5	T49.3X6
theobromine calcium	T50.2X1	T50.2X2	T50.2X3	T50.2X4	T50.2X5	T50.2X6
Salicylazosulfapyridine	T37.0X1	T37.0X2	T37.0X3	T37.0X4	T37.0X5	T37.0X6
Salicylhydroxamic acid	T49.0X1	T49.0X2	T49.0X3	T49.0X4	T49.0X5	T49.0X6
Salicylic acid	T49.4X1	T49.4X2	T49.4X3	T49.4X4	T49.4X5	T49.4X6
with benzoic acid	T49.4X1	T49.4X2	T49.4X3	T49.4X4	T49.4X5	T49.4X6
congeners	T39.091	T39.092	T39.093	T39.094	T39.095	T39.096
derivative	T39.091	T39.092	T39.093	T39.094	T39.095	T39.096
salts	T39.091	T39.092	T39.093	T39.094	T39.095	T39.096
Salinazid	T37.1X1	T37.1X2	T37.1X3	T37.1X4	T37.1X5	T37.1X6
Salmeterol	T48.6X1	T48.6X2	T48.6X3	T48.6X4	T48.6X5	T48.6X6
Salol	T49.3X1	T49.3X2	T49.3X3	T49.3X4	T49.3X5	T49.3X6
Salsalate	T39.091	T39.092	T39.093	T39.094	T39.095	T39.096
Salt substitute	T50.901	T50.902	T50.903	T50.904	T50.905	T50.906
Salt-replacing drug	T50.901	T50.902	T50.903	T50.904	T50.905	T50.906
Salt-retaining mineralocorticoid	T50.0X1	T50.0X2	T50.0X3	T50.0X4	T50.0X5	T50.0X6
Saluretic NEC	T50.2X1	T50.2X2	T50.2X3	T50.2X4	T50.2X5	T50.2X6
Saluron	T50.2X1	T50.2X2	T50.2X3	T50.2X4	T50.2X5	T50.2X6
Salvarsan 606 (neosilver) (silver)	T37.8X1	T37.8X2	T37.8X3	T37.8X4	T37.8X5	T37.8X6
Sambucus canadensis	T62.2X1	T62.2X2	T62.2X3	T62.2X4	—	—
berry	T62.1X1	T62.1X2	T62.1X3	T62.1X4	—	—
Sandril	T46.5X1	T46.5X2	T46.5X3	T46.5X4	T46.5X5	T46.5X6
Sanguinaria canadensis	T62.2X1	T62.2X2	T62.2X3	T62.2X4	—	—
Saniflush (cleaner)	T54.2X1	T54.2X2	T54.2X3	T54.2X4	—	—
Santonin	T37.4X1	T37.4X2	T37.4X3	T37.4X4	T37.4X5	T37.4X6
Santyl	T49.8X1	T49.8X2	T49.8X3	T49.8X4	T49.8X5	T49.8X6
Saralasin	T46.5X1	T46.5X2	T46.5X3	T46.5X4	T46.5X5	T46.5X6
Sarcolysin	T45.1X1	T45.1X2	T45.1X3	T45.1X4	T45.1X5	T45.1X6
Sarkomycin	T45.1X1	T45.1X2	T45.1X3	T45.1X4	T45.1X5	T45.1X6
Saroten	T43.011	T43.012	T43.013	T43.014	T43.015	T43.016

Substance	Poisoning, Accidental (Unintentional)	Poisoning, Intentional Self-Harm	Poisoning, Assault	Poisoning, Undetermined	Adverse Effect	Underdosing
Saturnine — *see Lead*						
Savin (oil)	T49.4X1	T49.4X2	T49.4X3	T49.4X4	T49.4X5	T49.4X6
Scammony	T47.2X1	T47.2X2	T47.2X3	T47.2X4	T47.2X5	T47.2X6
Scarlet red	T49.8X1	T49.8X2	T49.8X3	T49.8X4	T49.8X5	T49.8X6
Scheele's green	T57.0X1	T57.0X2	T57.0X3	T57.0X4	—	—
insecticide	T57.0X1	T57.0X2	T57.0X3	T57.0X4	—	—
Schizontozide (blood) (tissue)	T37.2X1	T37.2X2	T37.2X3	T37.2X4	T37.2X5	T37.2X6
Schradan	T60.0X1	T60.0X2	T60.0X3	T60.0X4	—	—
Schweinfurth green	T57.0X1	T57.0X2	T57.0X3	T57.0X4	—	—
insecticide	T57.0X1	T57.0X2	T57.0X3	T57.0X4	—	—
Scilla, rat poison	T60.4X1	T60.4X2	T60.4X3	T60.4X4	—	—
Scillaren	T60.4X1	T60.4X2	T60.4X3	T60.4X4	—	—
Sclerosing agent	T46.8X1	T46.8X2	T46.8X3	T46.8X4	T46.8X5	T46.8X6
Scombrotoxin	T61.11	T61.12	T61.13	T61.14	—	—
Scopolamine	T44.3X1	T44.3X2	T44.3X3	T44.3X4	T44.3X5	T44.3X6
Scopolia extract	T44.3X1	T44.3X2	T44.3X3	T44.3X4	T44.3X5	T44.3X6
Scouring powder	T65.891	T65.892	T65.893	T65.894	—	—
Sea						
anemone (sting)	T63.631	T63.632	T63.633	T63.634	—	—
cucumber (sting)	T63.691	T63.692	T63.693	T63.694	—	—
snake (bite) (venom)	T63.091	T63.092	T63.093	T63.094	—	—
urchin spine (puncture)	T63.691	T63.692	T63.693	T63.694	—	—
Seafood	T61.91	T61.92	T61.93	T61.94	—	—
specified NEC	T61.8X1	T61.8X2	T61.8X3	T61.8X4	—	—
Secbutabarbital	T42.3X1	T42.3X2	T42.3X3	T42.3X4	T42.3X5	T42.3X6
Secbutabarbitone	T42.3X1	T42.3X2	T42.3X3	T42.3X4	T42.3X5	T42.3X6
Secnidazole	T37.3X1	T37.3X2	T37.3X3	T37.3X4	T37.3X5	T37.3X6
Secobarbital	T42.3X1	T42.3X2	T42.3X3	T42.3X4	T42.3X5	T42.3X6
Seconal	T42.3X1	T42.3X2	T42.3X3	T42.3X4	T42.3X5	T42.3X6
Secretin	T50.8X1	T50.8X2	T50.8X3	T50.8X4	T50.8X5	T50.8X6
Sedative NEC	T42.71	T42.72	T42.73	T42.74	T42.75	T42.76
mixed NEC	T42.6X1	T42.6X2	T42.6X3	T42.6X4	T42.6X5	T42.6X6
Sedormid	T42.6X1	T42.6X2	T42.6X3	T42.6X4	T42.6X5	T42.6X6
Seed disinfectant or dressing	T60.8X1	T60.8X2	T60.8X3	T60.8X4	—	—
Seeds (poisonous)	T62.2X1	T62.2X2	T62.2X3	T62.2X4	—	—
Selegiline	T42.8X1	T42.8X2	T42.8X3	T42.8X4	T42.8X5	T42.8X6
Selenium NEC	T56.891	T56.892	T56.893	T56.894	—	—
disulfide or sulfide	T49.4X1	T49.4X2	T49.4X3	T49.4X4	T49.4X5	T49.4X6
fumes	T59.891	T59.892	T59.893	T59.894	—	—
sulfide	T49.4X1	T49.4X2	T49.4X3	T49.4X4	T49.4X5	T49.4X6
Selenomethionine (75Se)	T50.8X1	T50.8X2	T50.8X3	T50.8X4	T50.8X5	T50.8X6
Selsun	T49.4X1	T49.4X2	T49.4X3	T49.4X4	T49.4X5	T49.4X6

TABLE OF DRUGS AND CHEMICALS

	External Cause (T-Code)					
Substance	Poisoning, Accidental (Unintentional)	Poisoning, Intentional Self-Harm	Poisoning, Assault	Poisoning, Undetermined	Adverse Effect	Underdosing
Semustine	T45.1X1	T45.1X2	T45.1X3	T45.1X4	T45.1X5	T45.1X6
Senega syrup	T48.4X1	T48.4X2	T48.4X3	T48.4X4	T48.4X5	T48.4X6
Senna	T47.2X1	T47.2X2	T47.2X3	T47.2X4	T47.2X5	T47.2X6
Sennoside A+B	T47.2X1	T47.2X2	T47.2X3	T47.2X4	T47.2X5	T47.2X6
Septisol	T49.2X1	T49.2X2	T49.2X3	T49.2X4	T49.2X5	T49.2X6
Seractide	T38.811	T38.812	T38.813	T38.814	T38.815	T38.816
Serax	T42.4X1	T42.4X2	T42.4X3	T42.4X4	T42.4X5	T42.4X6
Serenesil	T42.6X1	T42.6X2	T42.6X3	T42.6X4	T42.6X5	T42.6X6
Serenium (hydrochloride)	T37.91	T37.92	T37.93	T37.94	T37.95	T37.96
Serepax — see Oxazepam						
Sermorelin	T38.891	T38.892	T38.893	T38.894	T38.895	T38.896
Sernyl	T41.1X1	T41.1X2	T41.1X3	T41.1X4	T41.1X5	T41.1X6
Serotonin	T50.991	T50.992	T50.993	T50.994	T50.995	T50.996
Serpasil	T46.5X1	T46.5X2	T46.5X3	T46.5X4	T46.5X5	T46.5X6
Serrapeptase	T45.3X1	T45.3X2	T45.3X3	T45.3X4	T45.3X5	T45.3X6
Serum						
antibotulinus	T50.Z11	T50.Z12	T50.Z13	T50.Z14	T50.Z15	T50.Z16
anticytotoxic	T50.Z11	T50.Z12	T50.Z13	T50.Z14	T50.Z15	T50.Z16
antidiphtheria	T50.Z11	T50.Z12	T50.Z13	T50.Z14	T50.Z15	T50.Z16
antimeningococcus	T50.Z11	T50.Z12	T50.Z13	T50.Z14	T50.Z15	T50.Z16
anti-Rh	T50.Z11	T50.Z12	T50.Z13	T50.Z14	T50.Z15	T50.Z16
anti-snake-bite	T50.Z11	T50.Z12	T50.Z13	T50.Z14	T50.Z15	T50.Z16
antitetanic	T50.Z11	T50.Z12	T50.Z13	T50.Z14	T50.Z15	T50.Z16
antitoxic	T50.Z11	T50.Z12	T50.Z13	T50.Z14	T50.Z15	T50.Z16
complement (inhibitor)	T45.8X1	T45.8X2	T45.8X3	T45.8X4	T45.8X5	T45.8X6
convalescent	T50.Z11	T50.Z12	T50.Z13	T50.Z14	T50.Z15	T50.Z16
hemolytic complement	T45.8X1	T45.8X2	T45.8X3	T45.8X4	T45.8X5	T45.8X6
immune (human)	T50.Z11	T50.Z12	T50.Z13	T50.Z14	T50.Z15	T50.Z16
protective NEC	T50.Z11	T50.Z12	T50.Z13	T50.Z14	T50.Z15	T50.Z16
Setastine	T45.0X1	T45.0X2	T45.0X3	T45.0X4	T45.0X5	T45.0X6
Setoperone	T43.591	T43.592	T43.593	T43.594	T43.595	T43.596
Sewer gas	T59.91	T59.92	T59.93	T59.94	—	—
Shampoo	T55.0X1	T55.0X2	T55.0X3	T55.0X4	—	—
Shellfish, noxious, nonbacterial	T61.781	T61.782	T61.783	T61.784	—	—
Sildenafil	T46.7X1	T46.7X2	T46.7X3	T46.7X4	T46.7X5	T46.7X6
Silibinin	T50.991	T50.992	T50.993	T50.994	T50.995	T50.996
Silicone NEC	T65.891	T65.892	T65.893	T65.894	—	—
medicinal	T49.3X1	T49.3X2	T49.3X3	T49.3X4	T49.3X5	T49.3X6
Silvadene	T49.0X1	T49.0X2	T49.0X3	T49.0X4	T49.0X5	T49.0X6
Silver	T49.0X1	T49.0X2	T49.0X3	T49.0X4	T49.0X5	T49.0X6
anti-infectives	T49.0X1	T49.0X2	T49.0X3	T49.0X4	T49.0X5	T49.0X6
arsphenamine	T37.8X1	T37.8X2	T37.8X3	T37.8X4	T37.8X5	T37.8X6

	External Cause (T-Code)					
Substance	Poisoning, Accidental (Unintentional)	Poisoning, Intentional Self-Harm	Poisoning, Assault	Poisoning, Undetermined	Adverse Effect	Underdosing
Silver (Continued)						
colloidal	T49.0X1	T49.0X2	T49.0X3	T49.0X4	T49.0X5	T49.0X6
nitrate	T49.0X1	T49.0X2	T49.0X3	T49.0X4	T49.0X5	T49.0X6
ophthalmic preparation	T49.5X1	T49.5X2	T49.5X3	T49.5X4	T49.5X5	T49.5X6
toughened (keratolytic)	T49.4X1	T49.4X2	T49.4X3	T49.4X4	T49.4X5	T49.4X6
nonmedicinal (dust)	T56.891	T56.892	T56.893	T56.894	—	—
protein	T49.5X1	T49.5X2	T49.5X3	T49.5X4	T49.5X5	T49.5X6
salvarsan	T37.8X1	T37.8X2	T37.8X3	T37.8X4	T37.8X5	T37.8X6
sulfadiazine	T49.4X1	T49.4X2	T49.4X3	T49.4X4	T49.4X5	T49.4X6
Silymarin	T50.991	T50.992	T50.993	T50.994	T50.995	T50.996
Simaldrate	T47.1X1	T47.1X2	T47.1X3	T47.1X4	T47.1X5	T47.1X6
Simazine	T60.3X1	T60.3X2	T60.3X3	T60.3X4	—	—
Simethicone	T47.1X1	T47.1X2	T47.1X3	T47.1X4	T47.1X5	T47.1X6
Simfibrate	T46.6X1	T46.6X2	T46.6X3	T46.6X4	T46.6X5	T46.6X6
Simvastatin	T46.6X1	T46.6X2	T46.6X3	T46.6X4	T46.6X5	T46.6X6
Sincalide	T50.8X1	T50.8X2	T50.8X3	T50.8X4	T50.8X5	T50.8X6
Sinequan	T43.011	T43.012	T43.013	T43.014	T43.015	T43.016
Singoserp	T46.5X1	T46.5X2	T46.5X3	T46.5X4	T46.5X5	T46.5X6
Sintrom	T45.511	T45.512	T45.513	T45.514	T45.515	T45.516
Sisomicin	T36.5X1	T36.5X2	T36.5X3	T36.5X4	T36.5X5	T36.5X6
Sitosterols	T46.6X1	T46.6X2	T46.6X3	T46.6X4	T46.6X5	T46.6X6
Skeletal muscle relaxants	T48.1X1	T48.1X2	T48.1X3	T48.1X4	T48.1X5	T48.1X6
Skin						
agents (external)	T49.91	T49.92	T49.93	T49.94	T49.95	T49.96
specified NEC	T49.8X1	T49.8X2	T49.8X3	T49.8X4	T49.8X5	T49.8X6
test antigen	T50.8X1	T50.8X2	T50.8X3	T50.8X4	T50.8X5	T50.8X6
Sleep-eze	T45.0X1	T45.0X2	T45.0X3	T45.0X4	T45.0X5	T45.0X6
Sleeping draught, pill	T42.71	T42.72	T42.73	T42.74	T42.75	T42.76
Smallpox vaccine	T50.B11	T50.B12	T50.B13	T50.B14	T50.B15	T50.B16
Smelter fumes NEC	T56.91	T56.92	T56.93	T56.94	—	—
Smog	T59.1X1	T59.1X2	T59.1X3	T59.1X4	—	—
Smoke NEC	T59.811	T59.812	T59.813	T59.814	—	—
Smooth muscle relaxant	T44.3X1	T44.3X2	T44.3X3	T44.3X4	T44.3X5	T44.3X6
Snail killer NEC	T60.8X1	T60.8X2	T60.8X3	T60.8X4	—	—
Snake venom or bite	T63.001	T63.002	T63.003	T63.004	—	—
hemocoagulase	T45.7X1	T45.7X2	T45.7X3	T45.7X4	T45.7X5	T45.7X6
Snuff	T65.211	T65.212	T65.213	T65.214	—	—
Soap (powder) (product)	T55.0X1	T55.0X2	T55.0X3	T55.0X4	—	—
enema	T47.4X1	T47.4X2	T47.4X3	T47.4X4	T47.4X5	T47.4X6
medicinal, soft	T49.2X1	T49.2X2	T49.2X3	T49.2X4	T49.2X5	T49.2X6
superfatted	T49.2X1	T49.2X2	T49.2X3	T49.2X4	T49.2X5	T49.2X6
Sobrerol	T48.4X1	T48.4X2	T48.4X3	T48.4X4	T48.4X5	T48.4X6

◀ New   ◀ Revised   ~~deleted~~ Deleted

Substance	Poisoning, Accidental (Unintentional)	Poisoning, Intentional Self-Harm	Poisoning, Assault	Poisoning, Undetermined	Adverse Effect	Underdosing
Soda (caustic)	T54.3X1	T54.3X2	T54.3X3	T54.3X4	—	—
bicarb	T47.1X1	T47.1X2	T47.1X3	T47.1X4	T47.1X5	T47.1X6
chlorinated — see Sodium, hypochlorite						
Sodium						
acetosulfone	T37.1X1	T37.1X2	T37.1X3	T37.1X4	T37.1X5	T37.1X6
acetrizoate	T50.8X1	T50.8X2	T50.8X3	T50.8X4	T50.8X5	T50.8X6
acid phosphate	T50.3X1	T50.3X2	T50.3X3	T50.3X4	T50.3X5	T50.3X6
alginate	T47.8X1	T47.8X2	T47.8X3	T47.8X4	T47.8X5	T47.8X6
amidotrizoate	T50.8X1	T50.8X2	T50.8X3	T50.8X4	T50.8X5	T50.8X6
aminopterin	T45.1X1	T45.1X2	T45.1X3	T45.1X4	T45.1X5	T45.1X6
amylosulfate	T47.8X1	T47.8X2	T47.8X3	T47.8X4	T47.8X5	T47.8X6
amytal	T42.3X1	T42.3X2	T42.3X3	T42.3X4	T42.3X5	T42.3X6
antimony gluconate	T37.3X1	T37.3X2	T37.3X3	T37.3X4	T37.3X5	T37.3X6
arsenate	T57.0X1	T57.0X2	T57.0X3	T57.0X4	—	—
aurothiomalate	T39.4X1	T39.4X2	T39.4X3	T39.4X4	T39.4X5	T39.4X6
aurothiosulfate	T39.4X1	T39.4X2	T39.4X3	T39.4X4	T39.4X5	T39.4X6
barbiturate	T42.3X1	T42.3X2	T42.3X3	T42.3X4	T42.3X5	T42.3X6
basic phosphate	T47.4X1	T47.4X2	T47.4X3	T47.4X4	T47.4X5	T47.4X6
bicarbonate	T47.1X1	T47.1X2	T47.1X3	T47.1X4	T47.1X5	T47.1X6
bichromate	T57.8X1	T57.8X2	T57.8X3	T57.8X4	—	—
biphosphate	T50.3X1	T50.3X2	T50.3X3	T50.3X4	T50.3X5	T50.3X6
bisulfate	T65.891	T65.892	T65.893	T65.894	—	—
borate						
cleanser	T57.8X1	T57.8X2	T57.8X3	T57.8X4	—	—
eye	T49.5X1	T49.5X2	T49.5X3	T49.5X4	T49.5X5	T49.5X6
therapeutic	T49.8X1	T49.8X2	T49.8X3	T49.8X4	T49.8X5	T49.8X6
bromide	T42.6X1	T42.6X2	T42.6X3	T42.6X4	T42.6X5	T42.6X6
cacodylate (nonmedicinal) NEC	T50.8X1	T50.8X2	T50.8X3	T50.8X4	T50.8X5	T50.8X6
anti-infective	T37.8X1	T37.8X2	T37.8X3	T37.8X4	T37.8X5	T37.8X6
herbicide	T60.3X1	T60.3X2	T60.3X3	T60.3X4	—	—
calcium edetate	T45.8X1	T45.8X2	T45.8X3	T45.8X4	T45.8X5	T45.8X6
carbonate NEC	T54.3X1	T54.3X2	T54.3X3	T54.3X4	—	—
chlorate NEC	T65.891	T65.892	T65.893	T65.894	—	—
herbicide	T54.91	T54.92	T54.93	T54.94	—	—
chloride	T50.3X1	T50.3X2	T50.3X3	T50.3X4	T50.3X5	T50.3X6
with glucose	T50.3X1	T50.3X2	T50.3X3	T50.3X4	T50.3X5	T50.3X6
chromate	T65.891	T65.892	T65.893	T65.894	—	—
citrate	T50.991	T50.992	T50.993	T50.994	T50.995	T50.996
cromoglicate	T48.6X1	T48.6X2	T48.6X3	T48.6X4	T48.6X5	T48.6X6
cyanide	T65.0X1	T65.0X2	T65.0X3	T65.0X4	—	—
cyclamate	T50.3X1	T50.3X2	T50.3X3	T50.3X4	T50.3X5	T50.3X6
Sodium (Continued)						
dehydrocholate	T45.8X1	T45.8X2	T45.8X3	T45.8X4	T45.8X5	T45.8X6
diatrizoate	T50.8X1	T50.8X2	T50.8X3	T50.8X4	T50.8X5	T50.8X6
dibunate	T48.4X1	T48.4X2	T48.4X3	T48.4X4	T48.4X5	T48.4X6
dioctyl sulfosuccinate	T47.4X1	T47.4X2	T47.4X3	T47.4X4	T47.4X5	T47.4X6
dipantoyl ferrate	T45.8X1	T45.8X2	T45.8X3	T45.8X4	T45.8X5	T45.8X6
edetate	T45.8X1	T45.8X2	T45.8X3	T45.8X4	T45.8X5	T45.8X6
ethacrynate	T50.1X1	T50.1X2	T50.1X3	T50.1X4	T50.1X5	T50.1X6
feredetate	T45.8X1	T45.8X2	T45.8X3	T45.8X4	T45.8X5	T45.8X6
Fluoride — see Fluoride						
fluoroacetate (dust) (pesticide)	T60.4X1	T60.4X2	T60.4X3	T60.4X4	—	—
free salt	T50.3X1	T50.3X2	T50.3X3	T50.3X4	T50.3X5	T50.3X6
fusidate	T36.8X1	T36.8X2	T36.8X3	T36.8X4	T36.8X5	T36.8X6
glucaldrate	T47.1X1	T47.1X2	T47.1X3	T47.1X4	T47.1X5	T47.1X6
glucosulfone	T37.1X1	T37.1X2	T37.1X3	T37.1X4	T37.1X5	T37.1X6
glutamate	T45.8X1	T45.8X2	T45.8X3	T45.8X4	T45.8X5	T45.8X6
hydrogen carbonate	T50.3X1	T50.3X2	T50.3X3	T50.3X4	T50.3X5	T50.3X6
hydroxide	T54.3X1	T54.3X2	T54.3X3	T54.3X4	—	—
hypochlorite (bleach) NEC	T54.3X1	T54.3X2	T54.3X3	T54.3X4	—	—
disinfectant	T54.3X1	T54.3X2	T54.3X3	T54.3X4	—	—
medicinal (anti-infective) (external)	T49.0X1	T49.0X2	T49.0X3	T49.0X4	T49.0X5	T49.0X6
vapor	T54.3X1	T54.3X2	T54.3X3	T54.3X4	—	—
hyposulfite	T49.0X1	T49.0X2	T49.0X3	T49.0X4	T49.0X5	T49.0X6
indigotin disulfonate	T50.8X1	T50.8X2	T50.8X3	T50.8X4	T50.8X5	T50.8X6
iodide	T50.991	T50.992	T50.993	T50.994	T50.995	T50.996
I-131	T50.8X1	T50.8X2	T50.8X3	T50.8X4	T50.8X5	T50.8X6
therapeutic	T38.2X1	T38.2X2	T38.2X3	T38.2X4	T38.2X5	T38.2X6
iodohippurate (131I)	T50.8X1	T50.8X2	T50.8X3	T50.8X4	T50.8X5	T50.8X6
iopodate	T50.8X1	T50.8X2	T50.8X3	T50.8X4	T50.8X5	T50.8X6
iothalamate	T50.8X1	T50.8X2	T50.8X3	T50.8X4	T50.8X5	T50.8X6
iron edetate	T45.4X1	T45.4X2	T45.4X3	T45.4X4	T45.4X5	T45.4X6
lactate (compound solution)	T45.8X1	T45.8X2	T45.8X3	T45.8X4	T45.8X5	T45.8X6
lauryl (sulfate)	T49.2X1	T49.2X2	T49.2X3	T49.2X4	T49.2X5	T49.2X6
(L)-triiodothyronine	T38.1X1	T38.1X2	T38.1X3	T38.1X4	T38.1X5	T38.1X6
magnesium citrate	T50.991	T50.992	T50.993	T50.994	T50.995	T50.996
mersalate	T50.2X1	T50.2X2	T50.2X3	T50.2X4	T50.2X5	T50.2X6
metasilicate	T65.891	T65.892	T65.893	T65.894	—	—
metrizoate	T50.8X1	T50.8X2	T50.8X3	T50.8X4	T50.8X5	T50.8X6
monofluoroacetate (pesticide)	T60.1X1	T60.1X2	T60.1X3	T60.1X4	—	—
morrhuate	T46.8X1	T46.8X2	T46.8X3	T46.8X4	T46.8X5	T46.8X6
nafcillin	T36.0X1	T36.0X2	T36.0X3	T36.0X4	T36.0X5	T36.0X6

◀ New ◀ Revised ~~deleted~~ Deleted

Substance	External Cause (T-Code)					
	Poisoning, Accidental (Unintentional)	Poisoning, Intentional Self-Harm	Poisoning, Assault	Poisoning, Undetermined	Adverse Effect	Underdosing
Sodium (Continued)						
nitrate (oxidizing agent)	T65.891	T65.892	T65.893	T65.894	—	—
nitrite	T50.6X1	T50.6X2	T50.6X3	T50.6X4	T50.6X5	T50.6X6
nitroferricyanide	T46.5X1	T46.5X2	T46.5X3	T46.5X4	T46.5X5	T46.5X6
nitroprusside	T46.5X1	T46.5X2	T46.5X3	T46.5X4	T46.5X5	T46.5X6
oxalate	T65.891	T65.892	T65.893	T65.894	—	—
oxide/peroxide	T65.891	T65.892	T65.893	T65.894	—	—
oxybate	T41.291	T41.292	T41.293	T41.294	T41.295	T41.296
para-aminohippurate	T50.8X1	T50.8X2	T50.8X3	T50.8X4	T50.8X5	T50.8X6
perborate (nonmedicinal) NEC	T65.891	T65.892	T65.893	T65.894	—	—
medicinal	T49.0X1	T49.0X2	T49.0X3	T49.0X4	T49.0X5	T49.0X6
soap	T55.0X1	T55.0X2	T55.0X3	T55.0X4	—	—
percarbonate — see Sodium, perborate						
pertechnetate Tc99m	T50.8X1	T50.8X2	T50.8X3	T50.8X4	T50.8X5	T50.8X6
phosphate						
cellulose	T45.8X1	T45.8X2	T45.8X3	T45.8X4	T45.8X5	T45.8X6
dibasic	T47.2X1	T47.2X2	T47.2X3	T47.2X4	T47.2X5	T47.2X6
monobasic	T47.2X1	T47.2X2	T47.2X3	T47.2X4	T47.2X5	T47.2X6
phytate	T50.6X1	T50.6X2	T50.6X3	T50.6X4	T50.6X5	T50.6X6
picosulfate	T47.2X1	T47.2X2	T47.2X3	T47.2X4	T47.2X5	T47.2X6
polyhydroxyaluminium monocarbonate	T47.1X1	T47.1X2	T47.1X3	T47.1X4	T47.1X5	T47.1X6
polystyrene sulfonate	T50.3X1	T50.3X2	T50.3X3	T50.3X4	T50.3X5	T50.3X6
propionate	T49.0X1	T49.0X2	T49.0X3	T49.0X4	T49.0X5	T49.0X6
propyl hydroxybenzoate	T50.991	T50.992	T50.993	T50.994	T50.995	T50.996
psylliate	T46.8X1	T46.8X2	T46.8X3	T46.8X4	T46.8X5	T46.8X6
removing resins	T50.3X1	T50.3X2	T50.3X3	T50.3X4	T50.3X5	T50.3X6
salicylate	T39.091	T39.092	T39.093	T39.094	T39.095	T39.096
salt NEC	T50.3X1	T50.3X2	T50.3X3	T50.3X4	T50.3X5	T50.3X6
selenate	T60.2X1	T60.2X2	T60.2X3	T60.2X4	—	—
stibogluconate	T37.3X1	T37.3X2	T37.3X3	T37.3X4	T37.3X5	T37.3X6
sulfate	T47.4X1	T47.4X2	T47.4X3	T47.4X4	T47.4X5	T47.4X6
sulfoxone	T37.1X1	T37.1X2	T37.1X3	T37.1X4	T37.1X5	T37.1X6
tetradecyl sulfate	T46.8X1	T46.8X2	T46.8X3	T46.8X4	T46.8X5	T46.8X6
thiopental	T41.1X1	T41.1X2	T41.1X3	T41.1X4	T41.1X5	T41.1X6
thiosalicylate	T39.091	T39.092	T39.093	T39.094	T39.095	T39.096
thiosulfate	T50.6X1	T50.6X2	T50.6X3	T50.6X4	T50.6X5	T50.6X6
tolbutamide	T38.3X1	T38.3X2	T38.3X3	T38.3X4	T38.3X5	T38.3X6
l-triiodothyronine	T38.1X1	T38.1X2	T38.1X3	T38.1X4	T38.1X5	T38.1X6
tyropanoate	T50.8X1	T50.8X2	T50.8X3	T50.8X4	T50.8X5	T50.8X6
valproate	T42.6X1	T42.6X2	T42.6X3	T42.6X4	T42.6X5	T42.6X6
versenate	T50.6X1	T50.6X2	T50.6X3	T50.6X4	T50.6X5	T50.6X6

Substance	External Cause (T-Code)					
	Poisoning, Accidental (Unintentional)	Poisoning, Intentional Self-Harm	Poisoning, Assault	Poisoning, Undetermined	Adverse Effect	Underdosing
Sodium-free salt	T50.901	T50.902	T50.903	T50.904	T50.905	T50.906
Sodium-removing resin	T50.3X1	T50.3X2	T50.3X3	T50.3X4	T50.3X5	T50.3X6
Soft soap	T55.0X1	T55.0X2	T55.0X3	T55.0X4	—	—
Solanine	T62.2X1	T62.2X2	T62.2X3	T62.2X4	—	—
berries	T62.1X1	T62.1X2	T62.1X3	T62.1X4	—	—
Solanum dulcamara	T62.2X1	T62.2X2	T62.2X3	T62.2X4	—	—
berries	T62.1X1	T62.1X2	T62.1X3	T62.1X4	—	—
Solapsone	T37.1X1	T37.1X2	T37.1X3	T37.1X4	T37.1X5	T37.1X6
Solar lotion	T49.3X1	T49.3X2	T49.3X3	T49.3X4	T49.3X5	T49.3X6
Solasulfone	T37.1X1	T37.1X2	T37.1X3	T37.1X4	T37.1X5	T37.1X6
Soldering fluid	T65.891	T65.892	T65.893	T65.894	—	—
Solid substance	T65.91	T65.92	T65.93	T65.94		
specified NEC	T65.891	T65.892	T65.893	T65.894	—	—
Solvent, industrial NEC	T52.91	T52.92	T52.93	T52.94		
naphtha	T52.0X1	T52.0X2	T52.0X3	T52.0X4	—	—
petroleum	T52.0X1	T52.0X2	T52.0X3	T52.0X4	—	—
specified NEC	T52.8X1	T52.8X2	T52.8X3	T52.8X4		
Soma	T42.8X1	T42.8X2	T42.8X3	T42.8X4	T42.8X5	T42.8X6
Somatorelin	T38.891	T38.892	T38.893	T38.894	T38.895	T38.896
Somatostatin	T38.991	T38.992	T38.993	T38.994	T38.995	T38.996
Somatotropin	T38.811	T38.812	T38.813	T38.814	T38.815	T38.816
Somatrem	T38.811	T38.812	T38.813	T38.814	T38.815	T38.816
Somatropin	T38.811	T38.812	T38.813	T38.814	T38.815	T38.816
Sominex	T45.0X1	T45.0X2	T45.0X3	T45.0X4	T45.0X5	T45.0X6
Somnos	T42.6X1	T42.6X2	T42.6X3	T42.6X4	T42.6X5	T42.6X6
Somonal	T42.3X1	T42.3X2	T42.3X3	T42.3X4	T42.3X5	T42.3X6
Soneryl	T42.3X1	T42.3X2	T42.3X3	T42.3X4	T42.3X5	T42.3X6
Soothing syrup	T50.901	T50.902	T50.903	T50.904	T50.905	T50.906
Sopor	T42.6X1	T42.6X2	T42.6X3	T42.6X4	T42.6X5	T42.6X6
Soporific	T42.71	T42.72	T42.73	T42.74	T42.75	T42.76
Soporific drug	T42.71	T42.72	T42.73	T42.74	T42.75	T42.76
specified type NEC	T42.6X1	T42.6X2	T42.6X3	T42.6X4	T42.6X5	T42.6X6
Sorbide nitrate	T46.3X1	T46.3X2	T46.3X3	T46.3X4	T46.3X5	T46.3X6
Sorbitol	T47.4X1	T47.4X2	T47.4X3	T47.4X4	T47.4X5	T47.4X6
Sotalol	T44.7X1	T44.7X2	T44.7X3	T44.7X4	T44.7X5	T44.7X6
Sotradecol	T46.8X1	T46.8X2	T46.8X3	T46.8X4	T46.8X5	T46.8X6
Soysterol	T46.6X1	T46.6X2	T46.6X3	T46.6X4	T46.6X5	T46.6X6
Spacoline	T44.3X1	T44.3X2	T44.3X3	T44.3X4	T44.3X5	T44.3X6
Spanish fly	T49.8X1	T49.8X2	T49.8X3	T49.8X4	T49.8X5	T49.8X6
Sparine	T43.3X1	T43.3X2	T43.3X3	T43.3X4	T43.3X5	T43.3X6
Sparteine	T48.0X1	T48.0X2	T48.0X3	T48.0X4	T48.0X5	T48.0X6

◀ New ◀ Revised ~~deleted~~ Deleted

Substance	Poisoning, Accidental (Unintentional)	Poisoning, Intentional Self-Harm	Poisoning, Assault	Poisoning, Undetermined	Adverse Effect	Underdosing
Spasmolytic						
anticholinergics	T44.3X1	T44.3X2	T44.3X3	T44.3X4	T44.3X5	T44.3X6
autonomic	T44.3X1	T44.3X2	T44.3X3	T44.3X4	T44.3X5	T44.3X6
bronchial NEC	T48.6X1	T48.6X2	T48.6X3	T48.6X4	T48.6X5	T48.6X6
quaternary ammonium	T44.3X1	T44.3X2	T44.3X3	T44.3X4	T44.3X5	T44.3X6
skeletal muscle NEC	T48.1X1	T48.1X2	T48.1X3	T48.1X4	T48.1X5	T48.1X6
Spectinomycin	T36.5X1	T36.5X2	T36.5X3	T36.5X4	T36.5X5	T36.5X6
Speed	T43.621	T43.622	T43.623	T43.624	T43.625	T43.626
Spermicide	T49.8X1	T49.8X2	T49.8X3	T49.8X4	T49.8X5	T49.8X6
Spider (bite) (venom)	T63.391	T63.392	T63.393	T63.394	—	—
antivenin	T50.Z11	T50.Z12	T50.Z13	T50.Z14	T50.Z15	T50.Z16
Spigelia (root)	T37.4X1	T37.4X2	T37.4X3	T37.4X4	T37.4X5	T37.4X6
Spindle inactivator	T50.4X1	T50.4X2	T50.4X3	T50.4X4	T50.4X5	T50.4X6
Spiperone	T43.4X1	T43.4X2	T43.4X3	T43.4X4	T43.4X5	T43.4X6
Spiramycin	T36.3X1	T36.3X2	T36.3X3	T36.3X4	T36.3X5	T36.3X6
Spirapril	T46.4X1	T46.4X2	T46.4X3	T46.4X4	T46.4X5	T46.4X6
Spirilene	T43.591	T43.592	T43.593	T43.594	T43.595	T43.596
Spirit(s) (neutral) NEC	T51.0X1	T51.0X2	T51.0X3	T51.0X4	—	—
beverage	T51.0X1	T51.0X2	T51.0X3	T51.0X4	—	—
industrial	T51.0X1	T51.0X2	T51.0X3	T51.0X4		
mineral	T52.0X1	T52.0X2	T52.0X3	T52.0X4		
of salt — see Hydrochloric acid						
surgical	T51.0X1	T51.0X2	T51.0X3	T51.0X4	—	—
Spironolactone	T50.0X1	T50.0X2	T50.0X3	T50.0X4	T50.0X5	T50.0X6
Spiroperidol	T43.4X1	T43.4X2	T43.4X3	T43.4X4	T43.4X5	T43.4X6
Sponge, absorbable (gelatin)	T45.7X1	T45.7X2	T45.7X3	T45.7X4	T45.7X5	T45.7X6
Sporostacin	T49.0X1	T49.0X2	T49.0X3	T49.0X4	T49.0X5	T49.0X6
Spray (aerosol)	T65.91	T65.92	T65.93	T65.94	—	—
cosmetic	T65.891	T65.892	T65.893	T65.894	—	—
medicinal NEC	T50.901	T50.902	T50.903	T50.904	T50.905	T50.906
pesticides — see Pesticides						
specified content — see specific substance						
Spurge flax	T62.2X1	T62.2X2	T62.2X3	T62.2X4	—	—
Spurges	T62.2X1	T62.2X2	T62.2X3	T62.2X4	—	—
Sputum viscosity-lowering drug	T48.4X1	T48.4X2	T48.4X3	T48.4X4	T48.4X5	T48.4X6
Squill	T46.0X1	T46.0X2	T46.0X3	T46.0X4	T46.0X5	T46.0X6
rat poison	T60.4X1	T60.4X2	T60.4X3	T60.4X4	—	—
Squirting cucumber (cathartic)	T47.2X1	T47.2X2	T47.2X3	T47.2X4	T47.2X5	T47.2X6
Stains	T65.6X1	T65.6X2	T65.6X3	T65.6X4	—	—
Stannous fluoride	T49.7X1	T49.7X2	T49.7X3	T49.7X4	T49.7X5	T49.7X6
Stanolone	T38.7X1	T38.7X2	T38.7X3	T38.7X4	T38.7X5	T38.7X6

Substance	Poisoning, Accidental (Unintentional)	Poisoning, Intentional Self-Harm	Poisoning, Assault	Poisoning, Undetermined	Adverse Effect	Underdosing
Stanozolol	T38.7X1	T38.7X2	T38.7X3	T38.7X4	T38.7X5	T38.7X6
Staphisagria or stavesacre (pediculicide)	T49.0X1	T49.0X2	T49.0X3	T49.0X4	T49.0X5	T49.0X6
Starch	T50.901	T50.902	T50.903	T50.904	T50.905	T50.906
Stelazine	T43.3X1	T43.3X2	T43.3X3	T43.3X4	T43.3X5	T43.3X6
Stemetil	T43.3X1	T43.3X2	T43.3X3	T43.3X4	T43.3X5	T43.3X6
Stepronin	T48.4X1	T48.4X2	T48.4X3	T48.4X4	T48.4X5	T48.4X6
Sterculia	T47.4X1	T47.4X2	T47.4X3	T47.4X4	T47.4X5	T47.4X6
Sternutator gas	T59.891	T59.892	T59.893	T59.894	—	—
Steroid	T38.0X1	T38.0X2	T38.0X3	T38.0X4	T38.0X5	T38.0X6
anabolic	T38.7X1	T38.7X2	T38.7X3	T38.7X4	T38.7X5	T38.7X6
androgenic	T38.7X1	T38.7X2	T38.7X3	T38.7X4	T38.7X5	T38.7X6
antineoplastic, hormone	T38.7X1	T38.7X2	T38.7X3	T38.7X4	T38.7X5	T38.7X6
estrogen	T38.5X1	T38.5X2	T38.5X3	T38.5X4	T38.5X5	T38.5X6
ENT agent	T49.6X1	T49.6X2	T49.6X3	T49.6X4	T49.6X5	T49.6X6
ophthalmic preparation	T49.5X1	T49.5X2	T49.5X3	T49.5X4	T49.5X5	T49.5X6
topical NEC	T49.0X1	T49.0X2	T49.0X3	T49.0X4	T49.0X5	T49.0X6
Stibine	T56.891	T56.892	T56.893	T56.894	—	—
Stibogluconate	T37.3X1	T37.3X2	T37.3X3	T37.3X4	T37.3X5	T37.3X6
Stibophen	T37.4X1	T37.4X2	T37.4X3	T37.4X4	T37.4X5	T37.4X6
Stilbamidine (isetionate)	T37.3X1	T37.3X2	T37.3X3	T37.3X4	T37.3X5	T37.3X6
Stilbestrol	T38.5X1	T38.5X2	T38.5X3	T38.5X4	T38.5X5	T38.5X6
Stilboestrol	T38.5X1	T38.5X2	T38.5X3	T38.5X4	T38.5X5	T38.5X6
Stimulant						
central nervous system — see also Psychostimulant	T43.601	T43.602	T43.603	T43.604	T43.605	T43.606
analeptics	T50.7X1	T50.7X2	T50.7X3	T50.7X4	T50.7X5	T50.7X6
opiate antagonist	T50.7X1	T50.7X2	T50.7X3	T50.7X4	T50.7X5	T50.7X6
psychotherapeutic NEC — see also Psychotherapeutic drug	T43.601	T43.602	T43.603	T43.604	T43.605	T43.606
specified NEC	T43.691	T43.692	T43.693	T43.694	T43.695	T43.696
respiratory	T48.901	T48.902	T48.903	T48.904	T48.905	T48.906
Stone-dissolving drug	T50.901	T50.902	T50.903	T50.904	T50.905	T50.906
Storage battery (cells) (acid)	T54.2X1	T54.2X2	T54.2X3	T54.2X4	—	—
Stovaine	T41.3X1	T41.3X2	T41.3X3	T41.3X4	T41.3X5	T41.3X6
infiltration (subcutaneous)	T41.3X1	T41.3X2	T41.3X3	T41.3X4	T41.3X5	T41.3X6
nerve block (peripheral) (plexus)	T41.3X1	T41.3X2	T41.3X3	T41.3X4	T41.3X5	T41.3X6
spinal	T41.3X1	T41.3X2	T41.3X3	T41.3X4	T41.3X5	T41.3X6
topical (surface)	T41.3X1	T41.3X2	T41.3X3	T41.3X4	T41.3X5	T41.3X6
Stovarsal	T37.8X1	T37.8X2	T37.8X3	T37.8X4	T37.8X5	T37.8X6
Stove gas — see Gas, stove	T57.91	T57.92	T57.93	T57.94	—	—

TABLE OF DRUGS AND CHEMICALS

Substance	Poisoning, Accidental (Unintentional)	Poisoning, Intentional Self-Harm	Poisoning, Assault	Poisoning, Undetermined	Adverse Effect	Underdosing
Stoxil	T49.5X1	T49.5X2	T49.5X3	T49.5X4	T49.5X5	T49.5X6
Stramonium	T48.6X1	T48.6X2	T48.6X3	T48.6X4	T48.6X5	T48.6X6
natural state	T62.2X1	T62.2X2	T62.2X3	T62.2X4	—	—
Streptodornase	T45.3X1	T45.3X2	T45.3X3	T45.3X4	T45.3X5	T45.3X6
Streptoduocin	T36.5X1	T36.5X2	T36.5X3	T36.5X4	T36.5X5	T36.5X6
Streptokinase	T45.611	T45.612	T45.613	T45.614	T45.615	T45.616
Streptomycin (derivative)	T36.5X1	T36.5X2	T36.5X3	T36.5X4	T36.5X5	T36.5X6
Streptonivicin	T36.5X1	T36.5X2	T36.5X3	T36.5X4	T36.5X5	T36.5X6
Streptovarycin	T36.5X1	T36.5X2	T36.5X3	T36.5X4	T36.5X5	T36.5X6
Streptozocin	T45.1X1	T45.1X2	T45.1X3	T45.1X4	T45.1X5	T45.1X6
Streptozotocin	T45.1X1	T45.1X2	T45.1X3	T45.1X4	T45.1X5	T45.1X6
Stripper (paint) (solvent)	T52.8X1	T52.8X2	T52.8X3	T52.8X4	—	—
Strobane	T60.1X1	T60.1X2	T60.1X3	T60.1X4	—	—
Strofantina	T46.0X1	T46.0X2	T46.0X3	T46.0X4	T46.0X5	T46.0X6
Strophanthin (g) (k)	T46.0X1	T46.0X2	T46.0X3	T46.0X4	T46.0X5	T46.0X6
Strophanthus	T46.0X1	T46.0X2	T46.0X3	T46.0X4	T46.0X5	T46.0X6
Strophantin	T46.0X1	T46.0X2	T46.0X3	T46.0X4	T46.0X5	T46.0X6
Strophantin-g	T46.0X1	T46.0X2	T46.0X3	T46.0X4	T46.0X5	T46.0X6
Strychnine (nonmedicinal) (pesticide) (salts)	T65.1X1	T65.1X2	T65.1X3	T65.1X4	—	—
medicinal	T48.291	T48.292	T48.293	T48.294	T48.295	T48.296
Strychnos (ignatii) — see Strychnine						
Styramate	T42.8X1	T42.8X2	T42.8X3	T42.8X4	T42.8X5	T42.8X6
Styrene	T65.891	T65.892	T65.893	T65.894	—	—
Succinimide, antiepileptic or anticonvulsant	T42.2X1	T42.2X2	T42.2X3	T42.2X4	T42.2X5	T42.2X6
mercuric — see Mercury						
Succinylcholine	T48.1X1	T48.1X2	T48.1X3	T48.1X4	T48.1X5	T48.1X6
Succinylsulfathiazole	T37.0X1	T37.0X2	T37.0X3	T37.0X4	T37.0X5	T37.0X6
Sucralfate	T47.1X1	T47.1X2	T47.1X3	T47.1X4	T47.1X5	T47.1X6
Sucrose	T50.3X1	T50.3X2	T50.3X3	T50.3X4	T50.3X5	T50.3X6
Sufentanil	T40.4X1	T40.4X2	T40.4X3	T40.4X4	T40.4X5	T40.4X6
Sulbactam	T36.0X1	T36.0X2	T36.0X3	T36.0X4	T36.0X5	T36.0X6
Sulbenicillin	T36.0X1	T36.0X2	T36.0X3	T36.0X4	T36.0X5	T36.0X6
Sulbentine	T49.0X1	T49.0X2	T49.0X3	T49.0X4	T49.0X5	T49.0X6
Sulfacetamide	T49.0X1	T49.0X2	T49.0X3	T49.0X4	T49.0X5	T49.0X6
ophthalmic preparation	T49.5X1	T49.5X2	T49.5X3	T49.5X4	T49.5X5	T49.5X6
Sulfachlorpyridazine	T37.0X1	T37.0X2	T37.0X3	T37.0X4	T37.0X5	T37.0X6
Sulfacitine	T37.0X1	T37.0X2	T37.0X3	T37.0X4	T37.0X5	T37.0X6
Sulfadiasulfone sodium	T37.0X1	T37.0X2	T37.0X3	T37.0X4	T37.0X5	T37.0X6
Sulfadiazine	T37.0X1	T37.0X2	T37.0X3	T37.0X4	T37.0X5	T37.0X6
silver (topical)	T49.0X1	T49.0X2	T49.0X3	T49.0X4	T49.0X5	T49.0X6
Sulfadimethoxine	T37.0X1	T37.0X2	T37.0X3	T37.0X4	T37.0X5	T37.0X6
Sulfadimidine	T37.0X1	T37.0X2	T37.0X3	T37.0X4	T37.0X5	T37.0X6
Sulfadoxine	T37.0X1	T37.0X2	T37.0X3	T37.0X4	T37.0X5	T37.0X6
with pyrimethamine	T37.2X1	T37.2X2	T37.2X3	T37.2X4	T37.2X5	T37.2X6
Sulfaethidole	T37.0X1	T37.0X2	T37.0X3	T37.0X4	T37.0X5	T37.0X6
Sulfafurazole	T37.0X1	T37.0X2	T37.0X3	T37.0X4	T37.0X5	T37.0X6
Sulfaguanidine	T37.0X1	T37.0X2	T37.0X3	T37.0X4	T37.0X5	T37.0X6
Sulfalene	T37.0X1	T37.0X2	T37.0X3	T37.0X4	T37.0X5	T37.0X6
Sulfaloxate	T37.0X1	T37.0X2	T37.0X3	T37.0X4	T37.0X5	T37.0X6
Sulfaloxic acid	T37.0X1	T37.0X2	T37.0X3	T37.0X4	T37.0X5	T37.0X6
Sulfamazone	T39.2X1	T39.2X2	T39.2X3	T39.2X4	T39.2X5	T39.2X6
Sulfamerazine	T37.0X1	T37.0X2	T37.0X3	T37.0X4	T37.0X5	T37.0X6
Sulfameter	T37.0X1	T37.0X2	T37.0X3	T37.0X4	T37.0X5	T37.0X6
Sulfamethazine	T37.0X1	T37.0X2	T37.0X3	T37.0X4	T37.0X5	T37.0X6
Sulfamethizole	T37.0X1	T37.0X2	T37.0X3	T37.0X4	T37.0X5	T37.0X6
Sulfamethoxazole	T37.0X1	T37.0X2	T37.0X3	T37.0X4	T37.0X5	T37.0X6
with trimethoprim	T36.8X1	T36.8X2	T36.8X3	T36.8X4	T36.8X5	T36.8X6
Sulfamethoxydiazine	T37.0X1	T37.0X2	T37.0X3	T37.0X4	T37.0X5	T37.0X6
Sulfamethoxypyridazine	T37.0X1	T37.0X2	T37.0X3	T37.0X4	T37.0X5	T37.0X6
Sulfamethylthiazole	T37.0X1	T37.0X2	T37.0X3	T37.0X4	T37.0X5	T37.0X6
Sulfametoxydiazine	T37.0X1	T37.0X2	T37.0X3	T37.0X4	T37.0X5	T37.0X6
Sulfamidopyrine	T39.2X1	T39.2X2	T39.2X3	T39.2X4	T39.2X5	T39.2X6
Sulfamonomethoxine	T37.0X1	T37.0X2	T37.0X3	T37.0X4	T37.0X5	T37.0X6
Sulfamoxole	T37.0X1	T37.0X2	T37.0X3	T37.0X4	T37.0X5	T37.0X6
Sulfamylon	T49.0X1	T49.0X2	T49.0X3	T49.0X4	T49.0X5	T49.0X6
Sulfan blue (diagnostic dye)	T50.8X1	T50.8X2	T50.8X3	T50.8X4	T50.8X5	T50.8X6
Sulfanilamide	T37.0X1	T37.0X2	T37.0X3	T37.0X4	T37.0X5	T37.0X6
Sulfanilylguanidine	T37.0X1	T37.0X2	T37.0X3	T37.0X4	T37.0X5	T37.0X6
Sulfaperin	T37.0X1	T37.0X2	T37.0X3	T37.0X4	T37.0X5	T37.0X6
Sulfaphenazole	T37.0X1	T37.0X2	T37.0X3	T37.0X4	T37.0X5	T37.0X6
Sulfaphenylthiazole	T37.0X1	T37.0X2	T37.0X3	T37.0X4	T37.0X5	T37.0X6
Sulfaproxyline	T37.0X1	T37.0X2	T37.0X3	T37.0X4	T37.0X5	T37.0X6
Sulfapyridine	T37.0X1	T37.0X2	T37.0X3	T37.0X4	T37.0X5	T37.0X6
Sulfapyrimidine	T37.0X1	T37.0X2	T37.0X3	T37.0X4	T37.0X5	T37.0X6
Sulfarsphenamine	T37.8X1	T37.8X2	T37.8X3	T37.8X4	T37.8X5	T37.8X6
Sulfasalazine	T37.0X1	T37.0X2	T37.0X3	T37.0X4	T37.0X5	T37.0X6
Sulfasuxidine	T37.0X1	T37.0X2	T37.0X3	T37.0X4	T37.0X5	T37.0X6
Sulfasymazine	T37.0X1	T37.0X2	T37.0X3	T37.0X4	T37.0X5	T37.0X6
Sulfated amylopectin	T47.8X1	T47.8X2	T47.8X3	T47.8X4	T47.8X5	T47.8X6
Sulfathiazole	T37.0X1	T37.0X2	T37.0X3	T37.0X4	T37.0X5	T37.0X6
Sulfatostearate	T49.2X1	T49.2X2	T49.2X3	T49.2X4	T49.2X5	T49.2X6
Sulfinpyrazone	T50.4X1	T50.4X2	T50.4X3	T50.4X4	T50.4X5	T50.4X6

◄ New ◄ Revised ~~deleted~~ Deleted

Substance	Poisoning, Accidental (Unintentional)	Poisoning, Intentional Self-Harm	Poisoning, Assault	Poisoning, Undetermined	Adverse Effect	Underdosing
Sulfiram	T49.0X1	T49.0X2	T49.0X3	T49.0X4	T49.0X5	T49.0X6
Sulfisomidine	T37.0X1	T37.0X2	T37.0X3	T37.0X4	T37.0X5	T37.0X6
Sulfisoxazole	T37.0X1	T37.0X2	T37.0X3	T37.0X4	T37.0X5	T37.0X6
ophthalmic preparation	T49.5X1	T49.5X2	T49.5X3	T49.5X4	T49.5X5	T49.5X6
Sulfobromophthalein (sodium)	T50.8X1	T50.8X2	T50.8X3	T50.8X4	T50.8X5	T50.8X6
Sulfobromphthalein	T50.8X1	T50.8X2	T50.8X3	T50.8X4	T50.8X5	T50.8X6
Sulfogaiacol	T48.4X1	T48.4X2	T48.4X3	T48.4X4	T48.4X5	T48.4X6
Sulfomyxin	T36.8X1	T36.8X2	T36.8X3	T36.8X4	T36.8X5	T36.8X6
Sulfonal	T42.6X1	T42.6X2	T42.6X3	T42.6X4	T42.6X5	T42.6X6
Sulfonamide NEC	T37.0X1	T37.0X2	T37.0X3	T37.0X4	T37.0X5	T37.0X6
eye	T49.5X1	T49.5X2	T49.5X3	T49.5X4	T49.5X5	T49.5X6
Sulfonazide	T37.1X1	T37.1X2	T37.1X3	T37.1X4	T37.1X5	T37.1X6
Sulfones	T37.1X1	T37.1X2	T37.1X3	T37.1X4	T37.1X5	T37.1X6
Sulfonethylmethane	T42.6X1	T42.6X2	T42.6X3	T42.6X4	T42.6X5	T42.6X6
Sulfonmethane	T42.6X1	T42.6X2	T42.6X3	T42.6X4	T42.6X5	T42.6X6
Sulfonphthal, sulfonphthol	T50.8X1	T50.8X2	T50.8X3	T50.8X4	T50.8X5	T50.8X6
Sulfonylurea derivatives, oral	T38.3X1	T38.3X2	T38.3X3	T38.3X4	T38.3X5	T38.3X6
Sulforidazine	T43.3X1	T43.3X2	T43.3X3	T43.3X4	T43.3X5	T43.3X6
Sulfoxone	T37.1X1	T37.1X2	T37.1X3	T37.1X4	T37.1X5	T37.1X6
Sulfur, sulfurated, sulfuric, sulfurous, sulfuryl (compounds NEC) (medicinal)	T49.4X1	T49.4X2	T49.4X3	T49.4X4	T49.4X5	T49.4X6
acid	T54.2X1	T54.2X2	T54.2X3	T54.2X4	—	—
dioxide (gas)	T59.1X1	T59.1X2	T59.1X3	T59.1X4	—	—
ether — see Ether(s)						
hydrogen	T59.6X1	T59.6X2	T59.6X3	T59.6X4	—	—
medicinal (keratolytic) (ointment) NEC	T49.4X1	T49.4X2	T49.4X3	T49.4X4	T49.4X5	T49.4X6
ointment	T49.0X1	T49.0X2	T49.0X3	T49.0X4	T49.0X5	T49.0X6
pesticide (vapor)	T60.91	T60.92	T60.93	T60.94	—	—
vapor NEC	T59.891	T59.892	T59.893	T59.894	—	—
Sulfuric acid	T54.2X1	T54.2X2	T54.2X3	T54.2X4	—	—
Sulglicotide	T47.1X1	T47.1X2	T47.1X3	T47.1X4	T47.1X5	T47.1X6
Sulindac	T39.391	T39.392	T39.393	T39.394	T39.395	T39.396
Sulisatin	T47.2X1	T47.2X2	T47.2X3	T47.2X4	T47.2X5	T47.2X6
Sulisobenzone	T49.3X1	T49.3X2	T49.3X3	T49.3X4	T49.3X5	T49.3X6
Sulkowitch's reagent	T50.8X1	T50.8X2	T50.8X3	T50.8X4	T50.8X5	T50.8X6
Sulmetozine	T44.3X1	T44.3X2	T44.3X3	T44.3X4	T44.3X5	T44.3X6
Suloctidil	T46.7X1	T46.7X2	T46.7X3	T46.7X4	T46.7X5	T46.7X6
Sulph — see also Sulf-						
Sulphadiazine	T37.0X1	T37.0X2	T37.0X3	T37.0X4	T37.0X5	T37.0X6

Substance	Poisoning, Accidental (Unintentional)	Poisoning, Intentional Self-Harm	Poisoning, Assault	Poisoning, Undetermined	Adverse Effect	Underdosing
Sulphadimethoxine	T37.0X1	T37.0X2	T37.0X3	T37.0X4	T37.0X5	T37.0X6
Sulphadimidine	T37.0X1	T37.0X2	T37.0X3	T37.0X4	T37.0X5	T37.0X6
Sulphadione	T37.1X1	T37.1X2	T37.1X3	T37.1X4	T37.1X5	T37.1X6
Sulphafurazole	T37.0X1	T37.0X2	T37.0X3	T37.0X4	T37.0X5	T37.0X6
Sulphamethizole	T37.0X1	T37.0X2	T37.0X3	T37.0X4	T37.0X5	T37.0X6
Sulphamethoxazole	T37.0X1	T37.0X2	T37.0X3	T37.0X4	T37.0X5	T37.0X6
Sulphan blue	T50.8X1	T50.8X2	T50.8X3	T50.8X4	T50.8X5	T50.8X6
Sulphaphenazole	T37.0X1	T37.0X2	T37.0X3	T37.0X4	T37.0X5	T37.0X6
Sulphapyridine	T37.0X1	T37.0X2	T37.0X3	T37.0X4	T37.0X5	T37.0X6
Sulphasalazine	T37.0X1	T37.0X2	T37.0X3	T37.0X4	T37.0X5	T37.0X6
Sulphinpyrazone	T50.4X1	T50.4X2	T50.4X3	T50.4X4	T50.4X5	T50.4X6
Sulpiride	T43.591	T43.592	T43.593	T43.594	T43.595	T43.596
Sulprostone	T48.0X1	T48.0X2	T48.0X3	T48.0X4	T48.0X5	T48.0X6
Sulpyrine	T39.2X1	T39.2X2	T39.2X3	T39.2X4	T39.2X5	T39.2X6
Sultamicillin	T36.0X1	T36.0X2	T36.0X3	T36.0X4	T36.0X5	T36.0X6
Sulthiame	T42.6X1	T42.6X2	T42.6X3	T42.6X4	T42.6X5	T42.6X6
Sultiame	T42.6X1	T42.6X2	T42.6X3	T42.6X4	T42.6X5	T42.6X6
Sultopride	T43.591	T43.592	T43.593	T43.594	T43.595	T43.596
Sumatriptan	T39.8X1	T39.8X2	T39.8X3	T39.8X4	T39.8X5	T39.8X6
Sunflower seed oil	T46.6X1	T46.6X2	T46.6X3	T46.6X4	T46.6X5	T46.6X6
Superinone	T48.4X1	T48.4X2	T48.4X3	T48.4X4	T48.4X5	T48.4X6
Suprofen	T39.311	T39.312	T39.313	T39.314	T39.315	T39.316
Suramin (sodium)	T37.4X1	T37.4X2	T37.4X3	T37.4X4	T37.4X5	T37.4X6
Surfacaine	T41.3X1	T41.3X2	T41.3X3	T41.3X4	T41.3X5	T41.3X6
Surital	T41.1X1	T41.1X2	T41.1X3	T41.1X4	T41.1X5	T41.1X6
Sutilains	T45.3X1	T45.3X2	T45.3X3	T45.3X4	T45.3X5	T45.3X6
Suxamethonium (chloride)	T48.1X1	T48.1X2	T48.1X3	T48.1X4	T48.1X5	T48.1X6
Suxethonium (chloride)	T48.1X1	T48.1X2	T48.1X3	T48.1X4	T48.1X5	T48.1X6
Suxibuzone	T39.2X1	T39.2X2	T39.2X3	T39.2X4	T39.2X5	T39.2X6
Sweet oil (birch)	T49.3X1	T49.3X2	T49.3X3	T49.3X4	T49.3X5	T49.3X6
Sweet niter spirit	T46.3X1	T46.3X2	T46.3X3	T46.3X4	T46.3X5	T46.3X6
Sweetener	T50.901	T50.902	T50.903	T50.904	T50.905	T50.906
Sym-dichloroethyl ether	T53.6X1	T53.6X2	T53.6X3	T53.6X4	—	—
Sympatholytic NEC	T44.8X1	T44.8X2	T44.8X3	T44.8X4	T44.8X5	T44.8X6
haloalkylamine	T44.8X1	T44.8X2	T44.8X3	T44.8X4	T44.8X5	T44.8X6
Sympathomimetic NEC	T44.901	T44.902	T44.903	T44.904	T44.905	T44.906
anti-common-cold	T48.5X1	T48.5X2	T48.5X3	T48.5X4	T48.5X5	T48.5X6
bronchodilator	T48.6X1	T48.6X2	T48.6X3	T48.6X4	T48.6X5	T48.6X6
specified NEC	T44.991	T44.992	T44.993	T44.994	T44.995	T44.996
Synagis	T50.B91	T50.B92	T50.B93	T50.B94	T50.B95	T50.B96
Synalar	T49.0X1	T49.0X2	T49.0X3	T49.0X4	T49.0X5	T49.0X6
Synthroid	T38.1X1	T38.1X2	T38.1X3	T38.1X4	T38.1X5	T38.1X6

◀ New   ◀ Revised   ~~deleted~~ Deleted

Substance	External Cause (T-Code)					
	Poisoning, Accidental (Unintentional)	Poisoning, Intentional Self-Harm	Poisoning, Assault	Poisoning, Undetermined	Adverse Effect	Underdosing
Syntocinon	T48.0X1	T48.0X2	T48.0X3	T48.0X4	T48.0X5	T48.0X6
Syrosingopine	T46.5X1	T46.5X2	T46.5X3	T46.5X4	T46.5X5	T46.5X6
Systemic drug	T45.91	T45.92	T45.93	T45.94	T45.95	T45.96
specified NEC	T45.8X1	T45.8X2	T45.8X3	T45.8X4	T45.8X5	T45.8X6
2,4,5-T	T60.3X1	T60.3X2	T60.3X3	T60.3X4	—	—
T						
Tablets — see also specified substance	T50.901	T50.902	T50.903	T50.904	T50.905	T50.906
Tace	T38.5X1	T38.5X2	T38.5X3	T38.5X4	T38.5X5	T38.5X6
Tacrine	T44.0X1	T44.0X2	T44.0X3	T44.0X4	T44.0X5	T44.0X6
Tadalafil	T46.7X1	T46.7X2	T46.7X3	T46.7X4	T46.7X5	T46.7X6
Talampicillin	T36.0X1	T36.0X2	T36.0X3	T36.0X4	T36.0X5	T36.0X6
Talbutal	T42.3X1	T42.3X2	T42.3X3	T42.3X4	T42.3X5	T42.3X6
Talc powder	T49.3X1	T49.3X2	T49.3X3	T49.3X4	T49.3X5	T49.3X6
Talcum	T49.3X1	T49.3X2	T49.3X3	T49.3X4	T49.3X5	T49.3X6
Taleranol	T38.6X1	T38.6X2	T38.6X3	T38.6X4	T38.6X5	T38.6X6
Tamoxifen	T38.6X1	T38.6X2	T38.6X3	T38.6X4	T38.6X5	T38.6X6
Tamsulosin	T44.6X1	T44.6X2	T44.6X3	T44.6X4	T44.6X5	T44.6X6
Tandearil, tanderil	T39.2X1	T39.2X2	T39.2X3	T39.2X4	T39.2X5	T39.2X6
Tannic acid	T49.2X1	T49.2X2	T49.2X3	T49.2X4	T49.2X5	T49.2X6
medicinal (astringent)	T49.2X1	T49.2X2	T49.2X3	T49.2X4	T49.2X5	T49.2X6
Tannin — see Tannic acid						
Tansy	T62.2X1	T62.2X2	T62.2X3	T62.2X4	—	—
TAO	T36.3X1	T36.3X2	T36.3X3	T36.3X4	T36.3X5	T36.3X6
Tapazole	T38.2X1	T38.2X2	T38.2X3	T38.2X4	T38.2X5	T38.2X6
Tar NEC	T52.0X1	T52.0X2	T52.0X3	T52.0X4	—	—
camphor	T60.1X1	T60.1X2	T60.1X3	T60.1X4	—	—
distillate	T49.1X1	T49.1X2	T49.1X3	T49.1X4	T49.1X5	T49.1X6
fumes	T59.891	T59.892	T59.893	T59.894	—	—
medicinal	T49.1X1	T49.1X2	T49.1X3	T49.1X4	T49.1X5	T49.1X6
ointment	T49.1X1	T49.1X2	T49.1X3	T49.1X4	T49.1X5	T49.1X6
Taractan	T43.591	T43.592	T43.593	T43.594	T43.595	T43.596
Tarantula (venomous)	T63.321	T63.322	T63.323	T63.324	—	—
Tartar emetic	T37.8X1	T37.8X2	T37.8X3	T37.8X4	T37.8X5	T37.8X6
Tartaric acid	T65.891	T65.892	T65.893	T65.894	—	—
Tartrated antimony (anti-infective)	T37.8X1	T37.8X2	T37.8X3	T37.8X4	T37.8X5	T37.8X6
Tartrate, laxative	T47.4X1	T47.4X2	T47.4X3	T47.4X4	T47.4X5	T47.4X6
Tauromustine	T45.1X1	T45.1X2	T45.1X3	T45.1X4	T45.1X5	T45.1X6
TCA — see Trichloroacetic acid						
TCDD	T53.7X1	T53.7X2	T53.7X3	T53.7X4	—	—
TDI (vapor)	T65.0X1	T65.0X2	T65.0X3	T65.0X4	—	—

Substance	External Cause (T-Code)					
	Poisoning, Accidental (Unintentional)	Poisoning, Intentional Self-Harm	Poisoning, Assault	Poisoning, Undetermined	Adverse Effect	Underdosing
Tear						
gas	T59.3X1	T59.3X2	T59.3X3	T59.3X4	—	—
solution	T49.5X1	T49.5X2	T49.5X3	T49.5X4	T49.5X5	T49.5X6
Teclothiazide	T50.2X1	T50.2X2	T50.2X3	T50.2X4	T50.2X5	T50.2X6
Teclozan	T37.3X1	T37.3X2	T37.3X3	T37.3X4	T37.3X5	T37.3X6
Tegafur	T45.1X1	T45.1X2	T45.1X3	T45.1X4	T45.1X5	T45.1X6
Tegretol	T42.1X1	T42.1X2	T42.1X3	T42.1X4	T42.1X5	T42.1X6
Teicoplanin	T36.8X1	T36.8X2	T36.8X3	T36.8X4	T36.8X5	T36.8X6
Telepaque	T50.8X1	T50.8X2	T50.8X3	T50.8X4	T50.8X5	T50.8X6
Tellurium	T56.891	T56.892	T56.893	T56.894	—	—
fumes	T56.891	T56.892	T56.893	T56.894	—	—
TEM	T45.1X1	T45.1X2	T45.1X3	T45.1X4	T45.1X5	T45.1X6
Temazepam	T42.4X1	T42.4X2	T42.4X3	T42.4X4	T42.4X5	T42.4X6
Temocillin	T36.0X1	T36.0X2	T36.0X3	T36.0X4	T36.0X5	T36.0X6
Tenamfetamine	T43.621	T43.622	T43.623	T43.624	T43.625	T43.626
Teniposide	T45.1X1	T45.1X2	T45.1X3	T45.1X4	T45.1X5	T45.1X6
Tenitramine	T46.3X1	T46.3X2	T46.3X3	T46.3X4	T46.3X5	T46.3X6
Tenoglicin	T48.4X1	T48.4X2	T48.4X3	T48.4X4	T48.4X5	T48.4X6
Tenonitrozole	T37.3X1	T37.3X2	T37.3X3	T37.3X4	T37.3X5	T37.3X6
Tenoxicam	T39.391	T39.392	T39.393	T39.394	T39.395	T39.396
TEPA	T45.1X1	T45.1X2	T45.1X3	T45.1X4	T45.1X5	T45.1X6
TEPP	T60.0X1	T60.0X2	T60.0X3	T60.0X4	—	—
Teprotide	T46.5X1	T46.5X2	T46.5X3	T46.5X4	T46.5X5	T46.5X6
Terazosin	T44.6X1	T44.6X2	T44.6X3	T44.6X4	T44.6X5	T44.6X6
Terbufos	T60.0X1	T60.0X2	T60.0X3	T60.0X4	—	—
Terbutaline	T48.6X1	T48.6X2	T48.6X3	T48.6X4	T48.6X5	T48.6X6
Terconazole	T49.0X1	T49.0X2	T49.0X3	T49.0X4	T49.0X5	T49.0X6
Terfenadine	T45.0X1	T45.0X2	T45.0X3	T45.0X4	T45.0X5	T45.0X6
Teriparatide (acetate)	T50.991	T50.992	T50.993	T50.994	T50.995	T50.996
Terizidone	T37.1X1	T37.1X2	T37.1X3	T37.1X4	T37.1X5	T37.1X6
Terlipressin	T38.891	T38.892	T38.893	T38.894	T38.895	T38.896
Terodiline	T46.3X1	T46.3X2	T46.3X3	T46.3X4	T46.3X5	T46.3X6
Teroxalene	T37.4X1	T37.4X2	T37.4X3	T37.4X4	T37.4X5	T37.4X6
Terpin(cis) hydrate	T48.4X1	T48.4X2	T48.4X3	T48.4X4	T48.4X5	T48.4X6
Terramycin	T36.4X1	T36.4X2	T36.4X3	T36.4X4	T36.4X5	T36.4X6
Tertatolol	T44.7X1	T44.7X2	T44.7X3	T44.7X4	T44.7X5	T44.7X6
Tessalon	T48.3X1	T48.3X2	T48.3X3	T48.3X4	T48.3X5	T48.3X6
Testolactone	T38.7X1	T38.7X2	T38.7X3	T38.7X4	T38.7X5	T38.7X6
Testosterone	T38.7X1	T38.7X2	T38.7X3	T38.7X4	T38.7X5	T38.7X6
Tetanus toxoid or vaccine	T50.A91	T50.A92	T50.A93	T50.A94	T50.A95	T50.A96
antitoxin	T50.Z11	T50.Z12	T50.Z13	T50.Z14	T50.Z15	T50.Z16
immune globulin (human)	T50.Z11	T50.Z12	T50.Z13	T50.Z14	T50.Z15	T50.Z16

◀ New ◀ Revised ~~deleted~~ Deleted

Substance	Poisoning, Accidental (Unintentional)	Poisoning, Intentional Self-Harm	Poisoning, Assault	Poisoning, Undetermined	Adverse Effect	Underdosing
Tetanus toxoid or vaccine *(Continued)*						
toxoid	T50.A91	T50.A92	T50.A93	T50.A94	T50.A95	T50.A96
with diphtheria toxoid	T50.A21	T50.A22	T50.A23	T50.A24	T50.A25	T50.A26
with pertussis	T50.A11	T50.A12	T50.A13	T50.A14	T50.A15	T50.A16
Tetrabenazine	T43.591	T43.592	T43.593	T43.594	T43.595	T43.596
Tetracaine	T41.3X1	T41.3X2	T41.3X3	T41.3X4	T41.3X5	T41.3X6
nerve block (peripheral) (plexus)	T41.3X1	T41.3X2	T41.3X3	T41.3X4	T41.3X5	T41.3X6
regional	T41.3X1	T41.3X2	T41.3X3	T41.3X4	T41.3X5	T41.3X6
spinal	T41.3X1	T41.3X2	T41.3X3	T41.3X4	T41.3X5	T41.3X6
Tetrachlorethylene — *see Tetrachloroethylene*						
Tetrachlormethiazide	T50.2X1	T50.2X2	T50.2X3	T50.2X4	T50.2X5	T50.2X6
2,3,7,8-Tetrachlorodibenzo-p-dioxin	T53.7X1	T53.7X2	T53.7X3	T53.7X4	—	—
Tetrachloroethane	T53.6X1	T53.6X2	T53.6X3	T53.6X4	—	—
vapor	T53.6X1	T53.6X2	T53.6X3	T53.6X4	—	—
paint or varnish	T53.6X1	T53.6X2	T53.6X3	T53.6X4	—	—
Tetrachloroethylene (liquid)	T53.3X1	T53.3X2	T53.3X3	T53.3X4	—	—
medicinal	T37.4X1	T37.4X2	T37.4X3	T37.4X4	T37.4X5	T37.4X6
vapor	T53.3X1	T53.3X2	T53.3X3	T53.3X4	—	—
Tetrachloromethane — *see Carbon tetrachloride*						
Tetracosactide	T38.811	T38.812	T38.813	T38.814	T38.815	T38.816
Tetracosactrin	T38.811	T38.812	T38.813	T38.814	T38.815	T38.816
Tetracycline	T36.4X1	T36.4X2	T36.4X3	T36.4X4	T36.4X5	T36.4X6
ophthalmic preparation	T49.5X1	T49.5X2	T49.5X3	T49.5X4	T49.5X5	T49.5X6
topical NEC	T49.0X1	T49.0X2	T49.0X3	T49.0X4	T49.0X5	T49.0X6
Tetradifon	T60.8X1	T60.8X2	T60.8X3	T60.8X4	—	—
Tetradotoxin	T61.771	T61.772	T61.773	T61.774	—	—
Tetraethyl						
lead	T56.0X1	T56.0X2	T56.0X3	T56.0X4	—	—
pyrophosphate	T60.0X1	T60.0X2	T60.0X3	T60.0X4	—	—
Tetraethylammonium chloride	T44.2X1	T44.2X2	T44.2X3	T44.2X4	T44.2X5	T44.2X6
Tetraethylthiuram disulfide	T50.6X1	T50.6X2	T50.6X3	T50.6X4	T50.6X5	T50.6X6
Tetrahydroaminoacridine	T44.0X1	T44.0X2	T44.0X3	T44.0X4	T44.0X5	T44.0X6
Tetrahydrocannabinol	T40.7X1	T40.7X2	T40.7X3	T40.7X4	T40.7X5	T40.7X6
Tetrahydrofuran	T52.8X1	T52.8X2	T52.8X3	T52.8X4	—	—
Tetrahydronaphthalene	T52.8X1	T52.8X2	T52.8X3	T52.8X4	—	—
Tetrahydrozoline	T49.5X1	T49.5X2	T49.5X3	T49.5X4	T49.5X5	T49.5X6
Tetralin	T52.8X1	T52.8X2	T52.8X3	T52.8X4	—	—
Tetramethrin	T60.2X1	T60.2X2	T60.2X3	T60.2X4	—	—

Substance	Poisoning, Accidental (Unintentional)	Poisoning, Intentional Self-Harm	Poisoning, Assault	Poisoning, Undetermined	Adverse Effect	Underdosing
Tetramethylthiuram (disulfide) NEC	T60.3X1	T60.3X2	T60.3X3	T60.3X4	—	—
medicinal	T49.0X1	T49.0X2	T49.0X3	T49.0X4	T49.0X5	T49.0X6
Tetramisole	T37.4X1	T37.4X2	T37.4X3	T37.4X4	T37.4X5	T37.4X6
Tetranicotinoyl fructose	T46.7X1	T46.7X2	T46.7X3	T46.7X4	T46.7X5	T46.7X6
Tetronal	T42.6X1	T42.6X2	T42.6X3	T42.6X4	T42.6X5	T42.6X6
Tetrazepam	T42.4X1	T42.4X2	T42.4X3	T42.4X4	T42.4X5	T42.4X6
Tetryl	T65.3X1	T65.3X2	T65.3X3	T65.3X4	—	—
Tetrylammonium chloride	T44.2X1	T44.2X2	T44.2X3	T44.2X4	T44.2X5	T44.2X6
Tetryzoline	T49.5X1	T49.5X2	T49.5X3	T49.5X4	T49.5X5	T49.5X6
Thalidomide	T45.1X1	T45.1X2	T45.1X3	T45.1X4	T45.1X5	T45.1X6
Thallium (compounds) (dust) NEC	T56.811	T56.812	T56.813	T56.814	—	—
pesticide	T60.4X1	T60.4X2	T60.4X3	T60.4X4	—	—
THC	T40.7X1	T40.7X2	T40.7X3	T40.7X4	T40.7X5	T40.7X6
Thebacon	T48.3X1	T48.3X2	T48.3X3	T48.3X4	T48.3X5	T48.3X6
Thebaine	T40.2X1	T40.2X2	T40.2X3	T40.2X4	T40.2X5	T40.2X6
Thenoic acid	T49.6X1	T49.6X2	T49.6X3	T49.6X4	T49.6X5	T49.6X6
Thenyldiamine	T45.0X1	T45.0X2	T45.0X3	T45.0X4	T45.0X5	T45.0X6
Theobromine (calcium salicylate)	T48.6X1	T48.6X2	T48.6X3	T48.6X4	T48.6X5	T48.6X6
sodium salicylate	T48.6X1	T48.6X2	T48.6X3	T48.6X4	T48.6X5	T48.6X6
Theophyllamine	T48.6X1	T48.6X2	T48.6X3	T48.6X4	T48.6X5	T48.6X6
Theophylline	T48.6X1	T48.6X2	T48.6X3	T48.6X4	T48.6X5	T48.6X6
aminobenzoic acid	T48.6X1	T48.6X2	T48.6X3	T48.6X4	T48.6X5	T48.6X6
ethylenediamine	T48.6X1	T48.6X2	T48.6X3	T48.6X4	T48.6X5	T48.6X6
piperazine p-amino-benzoate	T48.6X1	T48.6X2	T48.6X3	T48.6X4	T48.6X5	T48.6X6
Thiabendazole	T37.4X1	T37.4X2	T37.4X3	T37.4X4	T37.4X5	T37.4X6
Thialbarbital	T41.1X1	T41.1X2	T41.1X3	T41.1X4	T41.1X5	T41.1X6
Thiamazole	T38.2X1	T38.2X2	T38.2X3	T38.2X4	T38.2X5	T38.2X6
Thiambutosine	T37.1X1	T37.1X2	T37.1X3	T37.1X4	T37.1X5	T37.1X6
Thiamine	T45.2X1	T45.2X2	T45.2X3	T45.2X4	T45.2X5	T45.2X6
Thiamphenicol	T36.2X1	T36.2X2	T36.2X3	T36.2X4	T36.2X5	T36.2X6
Thiamylal	T41.1X1	T41.1X2	T41.1X3	T41.1X4	T41.1X5	T41.1X6
sodium	T41.1X1	T41.1X2	T41.1X3	T41.1X4	T41.1X5	T41.1X6
Thiazesim	T43.291	T43.292	T43.293	T43.294	T43.295	T43.296
Thiazides (diuretics)	T50.2X1	T50.2X2	T50.2X3	T50.2X4	T50.2X5	T50.2X6
Thiazinamium metilsulfate	T43.3X1	T43.3X2	T43.3X3	T43.3X4	T43.3X5	T43.3X6
Thiethylperazine	T43.3X1	T43.3X2	T43.3X3	T43.3X4	T43.3X5	T43.3X6
Thimerosal	T49.0X1	T49.0X2	T49.0X3	T49.0X4	T49.0X5	T49.0X6
ophthalmic preparation	T49.5X1	T49.5X2	T49.5X3	T49.5X4	T49.5X5	T49.5X6
Thioacetazone	T37.1X1	T37.1X2	T37.1X3	T37.1X4	T37.1X5	T37.1X6
with isoniazid	T37.1X1	T37.1X2	T37.1X3	T37.1X4	T37.1X5	T37.1X6
Thiobarbital sodium	T41.1X1	T41.1X2	T41.1X3	T41.1X4	T41.1X5	T41.1X6

◀ New ◀ Revised ~~deleted~~ Deleted

TABLE OF DRUGS AND CHEMICALS

Substance	Poisoning, Accidental (Unintentional)	Poisoning, Intentional Self-Harm	Poisoning, Assault	Poisoning, Undetermined	Adverse Effect	Underdosing
Thiobarbiturate anesthetic	T41.1X1	T41.1X2	T41.1X3	T41.1X4	T41.1X5	T41.1X6
Thiobismol	T37.8X1	T37.8X2	T37.8X3	T37.8X4	T37.8X5	T37.8X6
Thiobutabarbital sodium	T41.1X1	T41.1X2	T41.1X3	T41.1X4	T41.1X5	T41.1X6
Thiocarbamate (insecticide)	T60.0X1	T60.0X2	T60.0X3	T60.0X4	—	—
Thiocarbamide	T38.2X1	T38.2X2	T38.2X3	T38.2X4	T38.2X5	T38.2X6
Thiocarbarsone	T37.8X1	T37.8X2	T37.8X3	T37.8X4	T37.8X5	T37.8X6
Thiocarlide	T37.1X1	T37.1X2	T37.1X3	T37.1X4	T37.1X5	T37.1X6
Thioctamide	T50.991	T50.992	T50.993	T50.994	T50.995	T50.996
Thioctic acid	T50.991	T50.992	T50.993	T50.994	T50.995	T50.996
Thiofos	T60.0X1	T60.0X2	T60.0X3	T60.0X4	—	—
Thioglycolate	T49.4X1	T49.4X2	T49.4X3	T49.4X4	T49.4X5	T49.4X6
Thioglycolic acid	T65.891	T65.892	T65.893	T65.894		
Thioguanine	T45.1X1	T45.1X2	T45.1X3	T45.1X4	T45.1X5	T45.1X6
Thiomercaptomerin	T50.2X1	T50.2X2	T50.2X3	T50.2X4	T50.2X5	T50.2X6
Thiomerin	T50.2X1	T50.2X2	T50.2X3	T50.2X4	T50.2X5	T50.2X6
Thiomersal	T49.0X1	T49.0X2	T49.0X3	T49.0X4	T49.0X5	T49.0X6
Thionazin	T60.0X1	T60.0X2	T60.0X3	T60.0X4	—	—
Thiopental (sodium)	T41.1X1	T41.1X2	T41.1X3	T41.1X4	T41.1X5	T41.1X6
Thiopentone (sodium)	T41.1X1	T41.1X2	T41.1X3	T41.1X4	T41.1X5	T41.1X6
Thiopropazate	T43.3X1	T43.3X2	T43.3X3	T43.3X4	T43.3X5	T43.3X6
Thioproperazine	T43.3X1	T43.3X2	T43.3X3	T43.3X4	T43.3X5	T43.3X6
Thioridazine	T43.3X1	T43.3X2	T43.3X3	T43.3X4	T43.3X5	T43.3X6
Thiosinamine	T49.3X1	T49.3X2	T49.3X3	T49.3X4	T49.3X5	T49.3X6
Thiotepa	T45.1X1	T45.1X2	T45.1X3	T45.1X4	T45.1X5	T45.1X6
Thiothixene	T43.4X1	T43.4X2	T43.4X3	T43.4X4	T43.4X5	T43.4X6
Thiouracil (benzyl) (methyl) (propyl)	T38.2X1	T38.2X2	T38.2X3	T38.2X4	T38.2X5	T38.2X6
Thiourea	T38.2X1	T38.2X2	T38.2X3	T38.2X4	T38.2X5	T38.2X6
Thiphenamil	T44.3X1	T44.3X2	T44.3X3	T44.3X4	T44.3X5	T44.3X6
Thiram	T60.3X1	T60.3X2	T60.3X3	T60.3X4	—	—
medicinal	T49.2X1	T49.2X2	T49.2X3	T49.2X4	T49.2X5	T49.2X6
Thonzylamine (systemic)	T45.0X1	T45.0X2	T45.0X3	T45.0X4	T45.0X5	T45.0X6
mucosal decongestant	T48.5X1	T48.5X2	T48.5X3	T48.5X4	T48.5X5	T48.5X6
Thorazine	T43.3X1	T43.3X2	T43.3X3	T43.3X4	T43.3X5	T43.3X6
Thorium dioxide suspension	T50.8X1	T50.8X2	T50.8X3	T50.8X4	T50.8X5	T50.8X6
Thornapple	T62.2X1	T62.2X2	T62.2X3	T62.2X4	—	—
Throat drug NEC	T49.6X1	T49.6X2	T49.6X3	T49.6X4	T49.6X5	T49.6X6
Thrombin	T45.7X1	T45.7X2	T45.7X3	T45.7X4	T45.7X5	T45.7X6
Thrombolysin	T45.611	T45.612	T45.613	T45.614	T45.615	T45.616
Thromboplastin	T45.7X1	T45.7X2	T45.7X3	T45.7X4	T45.7X5	T45.7X6
Thurfyl nicotinate	T46.7X1	T46.7X2	T46.7X3	T46.7X4	T46.7X5	T46.7X6
Thymol	T49.0X1	T49.0X2	T49.0X3	T49.0X4	T49.0X5	T49.0X6

Substance	Poisoning, Accidental (Unintentional)	Poisoning, Intentional Self-Harm	Poisoning, Assault	Poisoning, Undetermined	Adverse Effect	Underdosing
Thymopentin	T37.5X1	T37.5X2	T37.5X3	T37.5X4	T37.5X5	T37.5X6
Thymoxamine	T46.7X1	T46.7X2	T46.7X3	T46.7X4	T46.7X5	T46.7X6
Thymus extract	T38.891	T38.892	T38.893	T38.894	T38.895	T38.896
Thyreotrophic hormone	T38.811	T38.812	T38.813	T38.814	T38.815	T38.816
Thyroglobulin	T38.1X1	T38.1X2	T38.1X3	T38.1X4	T38.1X5	T38.1X6
Thyroid (hormone)	T38.1X1	T38.1X2	T38.1X3	T38.1X4	T38.1X5	T38.1X6
Thyrolar	T38.1X1	T38.1X2	T38.1X3	T38.1X4	T38.1X5	T38.1X6
Thyrotrophin	T38.811	T38.812	T38.813	T38.814	T38.815	T38.816
Thyrotropic hormone	T38.811	T38.812	T38.813	T38.814	T38.815	T38.816
Thyroxine	T38.1X1	T38.1X2	T38.1X3	T38.1X4	T38.1X5	T38.1X6
Tiabendazole	T37.4X1	T37.4X2	T37.4X3	T37.4X4	T37.4X5	T37.4X6
Tiamizide	T50.2X1	T50.2X2	T50.2X3	T50.2X4	T50.2X5	T50.2X6
Tianeptine	T43.291	T43.292	T43.293	T43.294	T43.295	T43.296
Tiapamil	T46.1X1	T46.1X2	T46.1X3	T46.1X4	T46.1X5	T46.1X6
Tiapride	T43.591	T43.592	T43.593	T43.594	T43.595	T43.596
Tiaprofenic acid	T39.311	T39.312	T39.313	T39.314	T39.315	T39.316
Tiaramide	T39.8X1	T39.8X2	T39.8X3	T39.8X4	T39.8X5	T39.8X6
Ticarcillin	T36.0X1	T36.0X2	T36.0X3	T36.0X4	T36.0X5	T36.0X6
Ticlatone	T49.0X1	T49.0X2	T49.0X3	T49.0X4	T49.0X5	T49.0X6
Ticlopidine	T45.521	T45.522	T45.523	T45.524	T45.525	T45.526
Ticrynafen	T50.1X1	T50.1X2	T50.1X3	T50.1X4	T50.1X5	T50.1X6
Tidiacic	T50.991	T50.992	T50.993	T50.994	T50.995	T50.996
Tiemonium	T44.3X1	T44.3X2	T44.3X3	T44.3X4	T44.3X5	T44.3X6
iodide	T44.3X1	T44.3X2	T44.3X3	T44.3X4	T44.3X5	T44.3X6
Tienilic acid	T50.1X1	T50.1X2	T50.1X3	T50.1X4	T50.1X5	T50.1X6
Tifenamil	T44.3X1	T44.3X2	T44.3X3	T44.3X4	T44.3X5	T44.3X6
Tigan	T45.0X1	T45.0X2	T45.0X3	T45.0X4	T45.0X5	T45.0X6
Tigloidine	T44.3X1	T44.3X2	T44.3X3	T44.3X4	T44.3X5	T44.3X6
Tilactase	T47.5X1	T47.5X2	T47.5X3	T47.5X4	T47.5X5	T47.5X6
Tiletamine	T41.291	T41.292	T41.293	T41.294	T41.295	T41.296
Tilidine	T40.4X1	T40.4X2	T40.4X3	T40.4X4	—	—
Timepidium bromide	T44.3X1	T44.3X2	T44.3X3	T44.3X4	T44.3X5	T44.3X6
Timiperone	T43.4X1	T43.4X2	T43.4X3	T43.4X4	T43.4X5	T43.4X6
Timolol	T44.7X1	T44.7X2	T44.7X3	T44.7X4	T44.7X5	T44.7X6
Tin (chloride) (dust) (oxide) NEC	T56.6X1	T56.6X2	T56.6X3	T56.6X4	—	—
anti-infectives	T37.8X1	T37.8X2	T37.8X3	T37.8X4	T37.8X5	T37.8X6
Tincture, iodine — see Iodine						
Tindal	T43.3X1	T43.3X2	T43.3X3	T43.3X4	T43.3X5	T43.3X6
Tinidazole	T37.3X1	T37.3X2	T37.3X3	T37.3X4	T37.3X5	T37.3X6
Tinoridine	T39.8X1	T39.8X2	T39.8X3	T39.8X4	T39.8X5	T39.8X6
Tiocarlide	T37.1X1	T37.1X2	T37.1X3	T37.1X4	T37.1X5	T37.1X6
Tioclomarol	T45.511	T45.512	T45.513	T45.514	T45.515	T45.516

◀ New ◀ Revised ~~deleted~~ Deleted

Substance	Poisoning, Accidental (Unintentional)	Poisoning, Intentional Self-Harm	Poisoning, Assault	Poisoning, Undetermined	Adverse Effect	Underdosing
Tioconazole	T49.0X1	T49.0X2	T49.0X3	T49.0X4	T49.0X5	T49.0X6
Tioguanine	T45.1X1	T45.1X2	T45.1X3	T45.1X4	T45.1X5	T45.1X6
Tiopronin	T50.991	T50.992	T50.993	T50.994	T50.995	T50.996
Tiotixene	T43.4X1	T43.4X2	T43.4X3	T43.4X4	T43.4X5	T43.4X6
Tioxolone	T49.4X1	T49.4X2	T49.4X3	T49.4X4	T49.4X5	T49.4X6
Tipepidine	T48.3X1	T48.3X2	T48.3X3	T48.3X4	T48.3X5	T48.3X6
Tiquizium bromide	T44.3X1	T44.3X2	T44.3X3	T44.3X4	T44.3X5	T44.3X6
Tiratricol	T38.1X1	T38.1X2	T38.1X3	T38.1X4	T38.1X5	T38.1X6
Tisopurine	T50.4X1	T50.4X2	T50.4X3	T50.4X4	T50.4X5	T50.4X6
Titanium (compounds) (vapor)	T56.891	T56.892	T56.893	T56.894	—	—
dioxide	T49.3X1	T49.3X2	T49.3X3	T49.3X4	T49.3X5	T49.3X6
ointment	T49.3X1	T49.3X2	T49.3X3	T49.3X4	T49.3X5	T49.3X6
oxide	T49.3X1	T49.3X2	T49.3X3	T49.3X4	T49.3X5	T49.3X6
tetrachloride	T56.891	T56.892	T56.893	T56.894	—	—
Titanocene	T56.891	T56.892	T56.893	T56.894	—	—
Titroid	T38.1X1	T38.1X2	T38.1X3	T38.1X4	T38.1X5	T38.1X6
Tizanidine	T42.8X1	T42.8X2	T42.8X3	T42.8X4	T42.8X5	T42.8X6
TMTD	T60.3X1	T60.3X2	T60.3X3	T60.3X4		
TNT (fumes)	T65.3X1	T65.3X2	T65.3X3	T65.3X4	—	—
Toadstool	T62.0X1	T62.0X2	T62.0X3	T62.0X4		
Tobacco NEC	T65.291	T65.292	T65.293	T65.294		
cigarettes	T65.221	T65.222	T65.223	T65.224	—	—
Indian	T62.2X1	T62.2X2	T62.2X3	T62.2X4	—	—
smoke, second-hand	T65.221	T65.222	T65.223	T65.224	—	—
Tobramycin	T36.5X1	T36.5X2	T36.5X3	T36.5X4	T36.5X5	T36.5X6
Tocainide	T46.2X1	T46.2X2	T46.2X3	T46.2X4	T46.2X5	T46.2X6
Tocoferol	T45.2X1	T45.2X2	T45.2X3	T45.2X4	T45.2X5	T45.2X6
Tocopherol	T45.2X1	T45.2X2	T45.2X3	T45.2X4	T45.2X5	T45.2X6
acetate	T45.2X1	T45.2X2	T45.2X3	T45.2X4	T45.2X5	T45.2X6
Tocosamine	T48.0X1	T48.0X2	T48.0X3	T48.0X4	T48.0X5	T48.0X6
Todralazine	T46.5X1	T46.5X2	T46.5X3	T46.5X4	T46.5X5	T46.5X6
Tofisopam	T42.4X1	T42.4X2	T42.4X3	T42.4X4	T42.4X5	T42.4X6
Tofranil	T43.011	T43.012	T43.013	T43.014	T43.015	T43.016
Toilet deodorizer	T65.891	T65.892	T65.893	T65.894	—	—
Tolamolol	T44.7X1	T44.7X2	T44.7X3	T44.7X4	T44.7X5	T44.7X6
Tolazamide	T38.3X1	T38.3X2	T38.3X3	T38.3X4	T38.3X5	T38.3X6
Tolazoline	T46.7X1	T46.7X2	T46.7X3	T46.7X4	T46.7X5	T46.7X6
Tolbutamide (sodium)	T38.3X1	T38.3X2	T38.3X3	T38.3X4	T38.3X5	T38.3X6
Tolciclate	T49.0X1	T49.0X2	T49.0X3	T49.0X4	T49.0X5	T49.0X6
Tolmetin	T39.391	T39.392	T39.393	T39.394	T39.395	T39.396
Tolnaftate	T49.0X1	T49.0X2	T49.0X3	T49.0X4	T49.0X5	T49.0X6
Tolonidine	T46.5X1	T46.5X2	T46.5X3	T46.5X4	T46.5X5	T46.5X6

Substance	Poisoning, Accidental (Unintentional)	Poisoning, Intentional Self-Harm	Poisoning, Assault	Poisoning, Undetermined	Adverse Effect	Underdosing
Toloxatone	T42.6X1	T42.6X2	T42.6X3	T42.6X4	T42.6X5	T42.6X6
Tolperisone	T44.3X1	T44.3X2	T44.3X3	T44.3X4	T44.3X5	T44.3X6
Tolserol	T42.8X1	T42.8X2	T42.8X3	T42.8X4	T42.8X5	T42.8X6
Toluene (liquid)	T52.2X1	T52.2X2	T52.2X3	T52.2X4		
diisocyanate	T65.0X1	T65.0X2	T65.0X3	T65.0X4	—	—
Toluidine	T65.891	T65.892	T65.893	T65.894		
vapor	T59.891	T59.892	T59.893	T59.894		
Toluol (liquid)	T52.2X1	T52.2X2	T52.2X3	T52.2X4	—	—
vapor	T52.2X1	T52.2X2	T52.2X3	T52.2X4		
Toluylenediamine	T65.3X1	T65.3X2	T65.3X3	T65.3X4		
Tolylene-2,4-diisocyanate	T65.0X1	T65.0X2	T65.0X3	T65.0X4	—	—
Tonic NEC	T50.901	T50.902	T50.903	T50.904	T50.905	T50.906
Topical action drug NEC	T49.91	T49.92	T49.93	T49.94	T49.95	T49.96
ear, nose or throat	T49.6X1	T49.6X2	T49.6X3	T49.6X4	T49.6X5	T49.6X6
eye	T49.5X1	T49.5X2	T49.5X3	T49.5X4	T49.5X5	T49.5X6
skin	T49.91	T49.92	T49.93	T49.94	T49.95	T49.96
specified NEC	T49.8X1	T49.8X2	T49.8X3	T49.8X4	T49.8X5	T49.8X6
Toquizine	T44.3X1	T44.3X2	T44.3X3	T44.3X4	T44.3X5	T44.3X6
Toremifene	T38.6X1	T38.6X2	T38.6X3	T38.6X4	T38.6X5	T38.6X6
Tosylchloramide sodium	T49.8X1	T49.8X2	T49.8X3	T49.8X4	T49.8X5	T49.8X6
Toxaphene (dust) (spray)	T60.1X1	T60.1X2	T60.1X3	T60.1X4	—	—
Toxin, diphtheria (Schick Test)	T50.8X1	T50.8X2	T50.8X3	T50.8X4	T50.8X5	T50.8X6
Toxoid						
combined	T50.A21	T50.A22	T50.A23	T50.A24	T50.A25	T50.A26
diphtheria	T50.A91	T50.A92	T50.A93	T50.A94	T50.A95	T50.A96
tetanus	T50.A91	T50.A92	T50.A93	T50.A94	T50.A95	T50.A96
Trace element NEC	T45.8X1	T45.8X2	T45.8X3	T45.8X4	T45.8X5	T45.8X6
Tractor fuel NEC	T52.0X1	T52.0X2	T52.0X3	T52.0X4	—	—
Tragacanth	T50.991	T50.992	T50.993	T50.994	T50.995	T50.996
Tramadol	T40.4X1	T40.4X2	T40.4X3	T40.4X4	T40.4X5	T40.4X6
Tramazoline	T48.5X1	T48.5X2	T48.5X3	T48.5X4	T48.5X5	T48.5X6
Tranexamic acid	T45.621	T45.622	T45.623	T45.624	T45.625	T45.626
Tranilast	T45.0X1	T45.0X2	T45.0X3	T45.0X4	T45.0X5	T45.0X6
Tranquilizer NEC	T43.501	T43.502	T43.503	T43.504	T43.505	T43.506
with hypnotic or sedative	T42.6X1	T42.6X2	T42.6X3	T42.6X4	T42.6X5	T42.6X6
benzodiazepine NEC	T42.4X1	T42.4X2	T42.4X3	T42.4X4	T42.4X5	T42.4X6
butyrophenone NEC	T43.4X1	T43.4X2	T43.4X3	T43.4X4	T43.4X5	T43.4X6
carbamate	T43.591	T43.592	T43.593	T43.594	T43.595	T43.596
dimethylamine	T43.3X1	T43.3X2	T43.3X3	T43.3X4	T43.3X5	T43.3X6
ethylamine	T43.3X1	T43.3X2	T43.3X3	T43.3X4	T43.3X5	T43.3X6
hydroxyzine	T43.591	T43.592	T43.593	T43.594	T43.595	T43.596
major NEC	T43.501	T43.502	T43.503	T43.504	T43.505	T43.506

◀ New ◀ Revised ~~deleted~~ Deleted

TABLE OF DRUGS AND CHEMICALS

	External Cause (T-Code)					
Substance	Poisoning, Accidental (Unintentional)	Poisoning, Intentional Self-Harm	Poisoning, Assault	Poisoning, Undetermined	Adverse Effect	Underdosing
Tranquilizer NEC *(Continued)*						
penothiazine NEC	T43.3X1	T43.3X2	T43.3X3	T43.3X4	T43.3X5	T43.3X6
phenothiazine-based	T43.3X1	T43.3X2	T43.3X3	T43.3X4	T43.3X5	T43.3X6
piperazine NEC	T43.3X1	T43.3X2	T43.3X3	T43.3X4	T43.3X5	T43.3X6
piperidine	T43.3X1	T43.3X2	T43.3X3	T43.3X4	T43.3X5	T43.3X6
propylamine	T43.3X1	T43.3X2	T43.3X3	T43.3X4	T43.3X5	T43.3X6
specified NEC	T43.591	T43.592	T43.593	T43.594	T43.595	T43.596
thioxanthene NEC	T43.591	T43.592	T43.593	T43.594	T43.595	T43.596
Tranxene	T42.4X1	T42.4X2	T42.4X3	T42.4X4	T42.4X5	T42.4X6
Tranylcypromine	T43.1X1	T43.1X2	T43.1X3	T43.1X4	T43.1X5	T43.1X6
Trapidil	T46.3X1	T46.3X2	T46.3X3	T46.3X4	T46.3X5	T46.3X6
Trasentine	T44.3X1	T44.3X2	T44.3X3	T44.3X4	T44.3X5	T44.3X6
Travert	T50.3X1	T50.3X2	T50.3X3	T50.3X4	T50.3X5	T50.3X6
Trazodone	T43.211	T43.212	T43.213	T43.214	T43.215	T43.216
Trecator	T37.1X1	T37.1X2	T37.1X3	T37.1X4	T37.1X5	T37.1X6
Treosulfan	T45.1X1	T45.1X2	T45.1X3	T45.1X4	T45.1X5	T45.1X6
Tretamine	T45.1X1	T45.1X2	T45.1X3	T45.1X4	T45.1X5	T45.1X6
Tretinoin	T49.0X1	T49.0X2	T49.0X3	T49.0X4	T49.0X5	T49.0X6
Tretoquinol	T48.6X1	T48.6X2	T48.6X3	T48.6X4	T48.6X5	T48.6X6
Triacetin	T49.0X1	T49.0X2	T49.0X3	T49.0X4	T49.0X5	T49.0X6
Triacetoxyanthracene	T49.4X1	T49.4X2	T49.4X3	T49.4X4	T49.4X5	T49.4X6
Triacetyloleandomycin	T36.3X1	T36.3X2	T36.3X3	T36.3X4	T36.3X5	T36.3X6
Triamcinolone	T38.0X1	T38.0X2	T38.0X3	T38.0X4	T38.0X5	T38.0X6
ENT agent	T49.6X1	T49.6X2	T49.6X3	T49.6X4	T49.6X5	T49.6X6
hexacetonide	T49.0X1	T49.0X2	T49.0X3	T49.0X4	T49.0X5	T49.0X6
ophthalmic preparation	T49.5X1	T49.5X2	T49.5X3	T49.5X4	T49.5X5	T49.5X6
topical NEC	T49.0X1	T49.0X2	T49.0X3	T49.0X4	T49.0X5	T49.0X6
Triampyzine	T44.3X1	T44.3X2	T44.3X3	T44.3X4	T44.3X5	T44.3X6
Triamterene	T50.2X1	T50.2X2	T50.2X3	T50.2X4	T50.2X5	T50.2X6
Triazine (herbicide)	T60.3X1	T60.3X2	T60.3X3	T60.3X4	—	—
Triaziquone	T45.1X1	T45.1X2	T45.1X3	T45.1X4	T45.1X5	T45.1X6
Triazolam	T42.4X1	T42.4X2	T42.4X3	T42.4X4	T42.4X5	T42.4X6
Triazole (herbicide)	T60.3X1	T60.3X2	T60.3X3	T60.3X4	—	—
Tribenoside	T46.991	T46.992	T46.993	T46.994	T46.995	T46.996
Tribromacetaldehyde	T42.6X1	T42.6X2	T42.6X3	T42.6X4	T42.6X5	T42.6X6
Tribromoethanol, rectal	T41.291	T41.292	T41.293	T41.294	T41.295	T41.296
Tribromomethane	T42.6X1	T42.6X2	T42.6X3	T42.6X4	T42.6X5	T42.6X6
Trichlorethane	T53.2X1	T53.2X2	T53.2X3	T53.2X4	—	—
Trichlorethylene	T53.2X1	T53.2X2	T53.2X3	T53.2X4	—	—
Trichlorfon	T60.0X1	T60.0X2	T60.0X3	T60.0X4	—	—
Trichlormethiazide	T50.2X1	T50.2X2	T50.2X3	T50.2X4	T50.2X5	T50.2X6
Trichlormethine	T45.1X1	T45.1X2	T45.1X3	T45.1X4	T45.1X5	T45.1X6

	External Cause (T-Code)					
Substance	Poisoning, Accidental (Unintentional)	Poisoning, Intentional Self-Harm	Poisoning, Assault	Poisoning, Undetermined	Adverse Effect	Underdosing
Trichloroacetic acid, Trichloracetic acid	T54.2X1	T54.2X2	T54.2X3	T54.2X4	—	—
medicinal	T49.4X1	T49.4X2	T49.4X3	T49.4X4	T49.4X5	T49.4X6
Trichloroethane	T53.2X1	T53.2X2	T53.2X3	T53.2X4	—	—
Trichloroethanol	T42.6X1	T42.6X2	T42.6X3	T42.6X4	T42.6X5	T42.6X6
Trichloroethylene (liquid) (vapor)	T53.2X1	T53.2X2	T53.2X3	T53.2X4	—	—
anesthetic (gas)	T41.0X1	T41.0X2	T41.0X3	T41.0X4	T41.0X5	T41.0X6
vapor NEC	T53.2X1	T53.2X2	T53.2X3	T53.2X4	—	—
Trichloroethyl phosphate	T42.6X1	T42.6X2	T42.6X3	T42.6X4	T42.6X5	T42.6X6
Trichlorofluoromethane NEC	T53.5X1	T53.5X2	T53.5X3	T53.5X4	—	—
Trichloronate	T60.0X1	T60.0X2	T60.0X3	T60.0X4	—	—
2,4,5-Trichlorophen-oxyacetic acid	T60.3X1	T60.3X2	T60.3X3	T60.3X4	—	—
Trichloropropane	T53.6X1	T53.6X2	T53.6X3	T53.6X4	—	—
Trichlorotriethylamine	T45.1X1	T45.1X2	T45.1X3	T45.1X4	T45.1X5	T45.1X6
Trichomonacides NEC	T37.3X1	T37.3X2	T37.3X3	T37.3X4	T37.3X5	T37.3X6
Trichomycin	T36.7X1	T36.7X2	T36.7X3	T36.7X4	T36.7X5	T36.7X6
Triclobisonium chloride	T49.0X1	T49.0X2	T49.0X3	T49.0X4	T49.0X5	T49.0X6
Triclocarban	T49.0X1	T49.0X2	T49.0X3	T49.0X4	T49.0X5	T49.0X6
Triclofos	T42.6X1	T42.6X2	T42.6X3	T42.6X4	T42.6X5	T42.6X6
Triclosan	T49.0X1	T49.0X2	T49.0X3	T49.0X4	T49.0X5	T49.0X6
Tricresyl phosphate	T65.891	T65.892	T65.893	T65.894	—	—
solvent	T52.91	T52.92	T52.93	T52.94	—	—
Tricyclamol chloride	T44.3X1	T44.3X2	T44.3X3	T44.3X4	T44.3X5	T44.3X6
Tridesilon	T49.0X1	T49.0X2	T49.0X3	T49.0X4	T49.0X5	T49.0X6
Tridihexethyl iodide	T44.3X1	T44.3X2	T44.3X3	T44.3X4	T44.3X5	T44.3X6
Tridione	T42.2X1	T42.2X2	T42.2X3	T42.2X4	T42.2X5	T42.2X6
Trientine	T45.8X1	T45.8X2	T45.8X3	T45.8X4	T45.8X5	T45.8X6
Triethanolamine NEC	T54.3X1	T54.3X2	T54.3X3	T54.3X4	—	—
detergent	T54.3X1	T54.3X2	T54.3X3	T54.3X4	—	—
trinitrate (biphosphate)	T46.3X1	T46.3X2	T46.3X3	T46.3X4	T46.3X5	T46.3X6
Triethanomelamine	T45.1X1	T45.1X2	T45.1X3	T45.1X4	T45.1X5	T45.1X6
Triethylenemelamine	T45.1X1	T45.1X2	T45.1X3	T45.1X4	T45.1X5	T45.1X6
Triethylenephosphoramide	T45.1X1	T45.1X2	T45.1X3	T45.1X4	T45.1X5	T45.1X6
Triethylenethiophosphoramide	T45.1X1	T45.1X2	T45.1X3	T45.1X4	T45.1X5	T45.1X6
Trifluoperazine	T43.3X1	T43.3X2	T43.3X3	T43.3X4	T43.3X5	T43.3X6
Trifluoroethyl vinyl ether	T41.0X1	T41.0X2	T41.0X3	T41.0X4	T41.0X5	T41.0X6
Trifluperidol	T43.4X1	T43.4X2	T43.4X3	T43.4X4	T43.4X5	T43.4X6
Triflupromazine	T43.3X1	T43.3X2	T43.3X3	T43.3X4	T43.3X5	T43.3X6
Trifluridine	T37.5X1	T37.5X2	T37.5X3	T37.5X4	T37.5X5	T37.5X6
Triflusal	T45.521	T45.522	T45.523	T45.524	T45.525	T45.526
Trihexyphenidyl	T44.3X1	T44.3X2	T44.3X3	T44.3X4	T44.3X5	T44.3X6
Triiodothyronine	T38.1X1	T38.1X2	T38.1X3	T38.1X4	T38.1X5	T38.1X6

◀ New ◀|| Revised ~~deleted~~ Deleted

Substance	Poisoning, Accidental (Unintentional)	Poisoning, Intentional Self-Harm	Poisoning, Assault	Poisoning, Undetermined	Adverse Effect	Underdosing
Trilene	T41.0X1	T41.0X2	T41.0X3	T41.0X4	T41.0X5	T41.0X6
Trilostane	T38.991	T38.992	T38.993	T38.994	T38.995	T38.996
Trimebutine	T44.3X1	T44.3X2	T44.3X3	T44.3X4	T44.3X5	T44.3X6
Trimecaine	T41.3X1	T41.3X2	T41.3X3	T41.3X4	T41.3X5	T41.3X6
Trimeprazine (tartrate)	T44.3X1	T44.3X2	T44.3X3	T44.3X4	T44.3X5	T44.3X6
Trimetaphan camsilate	T44.2X1	T44.2X2	T44.2X3	T44.2X4	T44.2X5	T44.2X6
Trimetazidine	T46.7X1	T46.7X2	T46.7X3	T46.7X4	T46.7X5	T46.7X6
Trimethadione	T42.2X1	T42.2X2	T42.2X3	T42.2X4	T42.2X5	T42.2X6
Trimethaphan	T44.2X1	T44.2X2	T44.2X3	T44.2X4	T44.2X5	T44.2X6
Trimethidinium	T44.2X1	T44.2X2	T44.2X3	T44.2X4	T44.2X5	T44.2X6
Trimethobenzamide	T45.0X1	T45.0X2	T45.0X3	T45.0X4	T45.0X5	T45.0X6
Trimethoprim	T37.8X1	T37.8X2	T37.8X3	T37.8X4	T37.8X5	T37.8X6
with sulfamethoxazole	T36.8X1	T36.8X2	T36.8X3	T36.8X4	T36.8X5	T36.8X6
Trimethylcarbinol	T51.3X1	T51.3X2	T51.3X3	T51.3X4	—	—
Trimethylpsoralen	T49.3X1	T49.3X2	T49.3X3	T49.3X4	T49.3X5	T49.3X6
Trimeton	T45.0X1	T45.0X2	T45.0X3	T45.0X4	T45.0X5	T45.0X6
Trimetrexate	T45.1X1	T45.1X2	T45.1X3	T45.1X4	T45.1X5	T45.1X6
Trimipramine	T43.011	T43.012	T43.013	T43.014	T43.015	T43.016
Trimustine	T45.1X1	T45.1X2	T45.1X3	T45.1X4	T45.1X5	T45.1X6
Trinitrine	T46.3X1	T46.3X2	T46.3X3	T46.3X4	T46.3X5	T46.3X6
Trinitrobenzol	T65.3X1	T65.3X2	T65.3X3	T65.3X4	—	—
Trinitrophenol	T65.3X1	T65.3X2	T65.3X3	T65.3X4	—	—
Trinitrotoluene (fumes)	T65.3X1	T65.3X2	T65.3X3	T65.3X4	—	—
Trional	T42.6X1	T42.6X2	T42.6X3	T42.6X4	T42.6X5	T42.6X6
Triorthocresyl phosphate	T65.891	T65.892	T65.893	T65.894	—	—
Trioxide of arsenic	T57.0X1	T57.0X2	T57.0X3	T57.0X4	—	—
Trioxysalen	T49.4X1	T49.4X2	T49.4X3	T49.4X4	T49.4X5	T49.4X6
Tripamide	T50.2X1	T50.2X2	T50.2X3	T50.2X4	T50.2X5	T50.2X6
Triparanol	T46.6X1	T46.6X2	T46.6X3	T46.6X4	T46.6X5	T46.6X6
Tripelennamine	T45.0X1	T45.0X2	T45.0X3	T45.0X4	T45.0X5	T45.0X6
Triperiden	T44.3X1	T44.3X2	T44.3X3	T44.3X4	T44.3X5	T44.3X6
Triperidol	T43.4X1	T43.4X2	T43.4X3	T43.4X4	T43.4X5	T43.4X6
Triphenylphosphate	T65.891	T65.892	T65.893	T65.894	—	—
Triple						
bromides	T42.6X1	T42.6X2	T42.6X3	T42.6X4	T42.6X5	T42.6X6
carbonate	T47.1X1	T47.1X2	T47.1X3	T47.1X4	T47.1X5	T47.1X6
vaccine						
DPT	T50.A11	T50.A12	T50.A13	T50.A14	T50.A15	T50.A16
including pertussis	T50.A11	T50.A12	T50.A13	T50.A14	T50.A15	T50.A16
MMR	T50.B91	T50.B92	—	—	—	—
Triprolidine	T45.0X1	T45.0X2	T45.0X3	T45.0X4	T45.0X5	T45.0X6
Trisodium hydrogen edetate	T50.6X1	T50.6X2	T50.6X3	T50.6X4	T50.6X5	T50.6X6

Substance	Poisoning, Accidental (Unintentional)	Poisoning, Intentional Self-Harm	Poisoning, Assault	Poisoning, Undetermined	Adverse Effect	Underdosing
Trisoralen	T49.3X1	T49.3X2	T49.3X3	T49.3X4	T49.3X5	T49.3X6
Trisulfapyrimidines	T37.0X1	T37.0X2	T37.0X3	T37.0X4	T37.0X5	T37.0X6
Trithiozine	T44.3X1	T44.3X2	T44.3X3	T44.3X4	T44.3X5	T44.3X6
Tritiozine	T44.3X1	T44.3X2	T44.3X3	T44.3X4	T44.3X5	T44.3X6
Tritoqualine	T45.0X1	T45.0X2	T45.0X3	T45.0X4	T45.0X5	T45.0X6
Trofosfamide	T45.1X1	T45.1X2	T45.1X3	T45.1X4	T45.1X5	T45.1X6
Troleandomycin	T36.3X1	T36.3X2	T36.3X3	T36.3X4	T36.3X5	T36.3X6
Trolnitrate (phosphate)	T46.3X1	T46.3X2	T46.3X3	T46.3X4	T46.3X5	T46.3X6
Tromantadine	T37.5X1	T37.5X2	T37.5X3	T37.5X4	T37.5X5	T37.5X6
Trometamol	T50.2X1	T50.2X2	T50.2X3	T50.2X4	T50.2X5	T50.2X6
Tromethamine	T50.2X1	T50.2X2	T50.2X3	T50.2X4	T50.2X5	T50.2X6
Tronothane	T41.3X1	T41.3X2	T41.3X3	T41.3X4	T41.3X5	T41.3X6
Tropacine	T44.3X1	T44.3X2	T44.3X3	T44.3X4	T44.3X5	T44.3X6
Tropatepine	T44.3X1	T44.3X2	T44.3X3	T44.3X4	T44.3X5	T44.3X6
Tropicamide	T44.3X1	T44.3X2	T44.3X3	T44.3X4	T44.3X5	T44.3X6
Trospium chloride	T44.3X1	T44.3X2	T44.3X3	T44.3X4	T44.3X5	T44.3X6
Troxerutin	T46.991	T46.992	T46.993	T46.994	T46.995	T46.996
Troxidone	T42.2X1	T42.2X2	T42.2X3	T42.2X4	T42.2X5	T42.2X6
Tryparsamide	T37.3X1	T37.3X2	T37.3X3	T37.3X4	T37.3X5	T37.3X6
Trypsin	T45.3X1	T45.3X2	T45.3X3	T45.3X4	T45.3X5	T45.3X6
Tryptizol	T43.011	T43.012	T43.013	T43.014	T43.015	T43.016
TSH	T38.811	T38.812	T38.813	T38.814	T38.815	T38.816
Tuaminoheptane	T48.5X1	T48.5X2	T48.5X3	T48.5X4	T48.5X5	T48.5X6
Tuberculin, purified protein derivative (PPD)	T50.8X1	T50.8X2	T50.8X3	T50.8X4	T50.8X5	T50.8X6
Tubocurare	T48.1X1	T48.1X2	T48.1X3	T48.1X4	T48.1X5	T48.1X6
Tubocurarine (chloride)	T48.1X1	T48.1X2	T48.1X3	T48.1X4	T48.1X5	T48.1X6
Tulobuterol	T48.6X1	T48.6X2	T48.6X3	T48.6X4	T48.6X5	T48.6X6
Turpentine (spirits of)	T52.8X1	T52.8X2	T52.8X3	T52.8X4	—	—
vapor	T52.8X1	T52.8X2	T52.8X3	T52.8X4	—	—
Tybamate	T43.591	T43.592	T43.593	T43.594	T43.595	T43.596
Tyloxapol	T48.4X1	T48.4X2	T48.4X3	T48.4X4	T48.4X5	T48.4X6
Tymazoline	T48.5X1	T48.5X2	T48.5X3	T48.5X4	T48.5X5	T48.5X6
Typhoid-paratyphoid vaccine	T50.A91	T50.A92	T50.A93	T50.A94	T50.A95	T50.A96
Typhus vaccine	T50.A91	T50.A92	T50.A93	T50.A94	T50.A95	T50.A96
Tyropanoate	T50.8X1	T50.8X2	T50.8X3	T50.8X4	T50.8X5	T50.8X6
Tyrothricin	T49.6X1	T49.6X2	T49.6X3	T49.6X4	T49.6X5	T49.6X6
ENT agent	T49.6X1	T49.6X2	T49.6X3	T49.6X4	T49.6X5	T49.6X6
ophthalmic preparation	T49.5X1	T49.5X2	T49.5X3	T49.5X4	T49.5X5	T49.5X6
U						
Ufenamate	T39.391	T39.392	T39.393	T39.394	T39.395	T39.396
Ultraviolet light protectant	T49.3X1	T49.3X2	T49.3X3	T49.3X4	T49.3X5	T49.3X6

◀ New ◀ Revised ~~deleted~~ Deleted

Substance	Poisoning, Accidental (Unintentional)	Poisoning, Intentional Self-Harm	Poisoning, Assault	Poisoning, Undetermined	Adverse Effect	Underdosing
Undecenoic acid	T49.0X1	T49.0X2	T49.0X3	T49.0X4	T49.0X5	T49.0X6
Undecoylium	T49.0X1	T49.0X2	T49.0X3	T49.0X4	T49.0X5	T49.0X6
Undecylenic acid (derivatives)	T49.0X1	T49.0X2	T49.0X3	T49.0X4	T49.0X5	T49.0X6
Unna's boot	T49.3X1	T49.3X2	T49.3X3	T49.3X4	T49.3X5	T49.3X6
Unsaturated fatty acid	T46.6X1	T46.6X2	T46.6X3	T46.6X4	T46.6X5	T46.6X6
Uracil mustard	T45.1X1	T45.1X2	T45.1X3	T45.1X4	T45.1X5	T45.1X6
Uramustine	T45.1X1	T45.1X2	T45.1X3	T45.1X4	T45.1X5	T45.1X6
Urapidil	T46.5X1	T46.5X2	T46.5X3	T46.5X4	T46.5X5	T46.5X6
Urari	T48.1X1	T48.1X2	T48.1X3	T48.1X4	T48.1X5	T48.1X6
Urate oxidase	T50.4X1	T50.4X2	T50.4X3	T50.4X4	T50.4X5	T50.4X6
Urea	T47.3X1	T47.3X2	T47.3X3	T47.3X4	T47.3X5	T47.3X6
peroxide	T49.0X1	T49.0X2	T49.0X3	T49.0X4	T49.0X5	T49.0X6
stibamine	T37.4X1	T37.4X2	T37.4X3	T37.4X4	T37.4X5	T37.4X6
topical	T49.8X1	T49.8X2	T49.8X3	T49.8X4	T49.8X5	T49.8X6
Urethane	T45.1X1	T45.1X2	T45.1X3	T45.1X4	T45.1X5	T45.1X6
Urginea (maritima) (scilla) — see Squill						
Uric acid metabolism drug NEC	T50.4X1	T50.4X2	T50.4X3	T50.4X4	T50.4X5	T50.4X6
Uricosuric agent	T50.4X1	T50.4X2	T50.4X3	T50.4X4	T50.4X5	T50.4X6
Urinary anti-infective	T37.8X1	T37.8X2	T37.8X3	T37.8X4	T37.8X5	T37.8X6
Urofollitropin	T38.811	T38.812	T38.813	T38.814	T38.815	T38.816
Urokinase	T45.611	T45.612	T45.613	T45.614	T45.615	T45.616
Urokon	T50.8X1	T50.8X2	T50.8X3	T50.8X4	T50.8X5	T50.8X6
Ursodeoxycholic acid	T50.991	T50.992	T50.993	T50.994	T50.995	T50.996
Ursodiol	T50.991	T50.992	T50.993	T50.994	T50.995	T50.996
Urtica	T62.2X1	T62.2X2	T62.2X3	T62.2X4	—	—
Utility gas — see Gas, utility						
V						
Vaccine NEC	T50.Z91	T50.Z92	T50.Z93	T50.Z94	T50.Z95	T50.Z96
antineoplastic	T50.Z91	T50.Z92	T50.Z93	T50.Z94	T50.Z95	T50.Z96
bacterial NEC	T50.A91	T50.A92	T50.A93	T50.A94	T50.A95	T50.A96
with						
other bacterial component	T50.A91	T50.A92	T50.A93	T50.A94	T50.A95	T50.A96
pertussis component	T50.A91	T50.A92	T50.A93	T50.A94	T50.A95	T50.A96
viral-rickettsial component	T50.A91	T50.A92	T50.A93	T50.A94	T50.A95	T50.A96
mixed NEC	T50.A91	T50.A92	T50.A93	T50.A94	T50.A95	T50.A96
BCG	T50.A91	T50.A92	T50.A93	T50.A94	T50.A95	T50.A96
cholera	T50.A91	T50.A92	T50.A93	T50.A94	T50.A95	T50.A96
diphtheria	T50.A91	T50.A92	T50.A93	T50.A94	T50.A95	T50.A96
with tetanus	T50.A21	T50.A22	T50.A23	T50.A24	T50.A25	T50.A26
and pertussis	T50.A11	T50.A12	T50.A13	T50.A14	T50.A15	T50.A16

Substance	Poisoning, Accidental (Unintentional)	Poisoning, Intentional Self-Harm	Poisoning, Assault	Poisoning, Undetermined	Adverse Effect	Underdosing
Vaccine NEC *(Continued)*						
influenza	T50.B91	T50.B92	T50.B93	T50.B94	T50.B95	T50.B96
measles	T50.B91	T50.B92	T50.B93	T50.B94	T50.B95	T50.B96
with mumps and rubella	T50.B91	T50.B92	T50.B93	T50.B94	T50.B95	T50.B96
meningococcal	T50.A91	T50.A92	T50.A93	T50.A94	T50.A95	T50.A96
mumps	T50.B91	T50.B92	T50.B93	T50.B94	T50.B95	T50.B96
paratyphoid	T50.A91	T50.A92	T50.A93	T50.A94	T50.A95	T50.A96
pertussis	T50.A11	T50.A12	T50.A13	T50.A14	T50.A15	T50.A16
with diphtheria	T50.A11	T50.A12	T50.A13	T50.A14	T50.A15	T50.A16
and tetanus	T50.A11	T50.A12	T50.A13	T50.A14	T50.A15	T50.A16
plague	T50.A91	T50.A92	T50.A93	T50.A94	T50.A95	T50.A96
poliomyelitis	T50.B91	T50.B92	T50.B93	T50.B94	T50.B95	T50.B96
poliovirus	T50.B91	T50.B92	T50.B93	T50.B94	T50.B95	T50.B96
rabies	T50.B91	T50.B92	T50.B93	T50.B94	T50.B95	T50.B96
respiratory syncytial virus	T50.B91	T50.B92	T50.B93	T50.B94	T50.B95	T50.B96
rickettsial NEC	T50.A91	T50.A92	T50.A93	T50.A94	T50.A95	T50.A96
with						
bacterial component	T50.A21	T50.A22	T50.A23	T50.A24	T50.A25	T50.A26
Rocky Mountain spotted fever	T50.A91	T50.A92	T50.A93	T50.A94	T50.A95	T50.A96
rubella	T50.B91	T50.B92	T50.B93	T50.B94	T50.B95	T50.B96
sabin oral	T50.B91	T50.B92	T50.B93	T50.B94	T50.B95	T50.B96
smallpox	T50.B11	T50.B12	T50.B13	T50.B14	T50.B15	T50.B16
TAB	T50.A91	T50.A92	T50.A93	T50.A94	T50.A95	T50.A96
tetanus	T50.A91	T50.A92	T50.A93	T50.A94	T50.A95	T50.A96
typhoid	T50.A91	T50.A92	T50.A93	T50.A94	T50.A95	T50.A96
typhus	T50.A91	T50.A92	T50.A93	T50.A94	T50.A95	T50.A96
viral NEC	T50.B91	T50.B92	T50.B93	T50.B94	T50.B95	T50.B96
yellow fever	T50.B91	T50.B92	T50.B93	T50.B94	T50.B95	T50.B96
Vaccinia immune globulin	T50.Z11	T50.Z12	T50.Z13	T50.Z14	T50.Z15	T50.Z16
Vaginal contraceptives	T49.8X1	T49.8X2	T49.8X3	T49.8X4	T49.8X5	T49.8X6
Valerian						
root	T42.6X1	T42.6X2	T42.6X3	T42.6X4	T42.6X5	T42.6X6
tincture	T42.6X1	T42.6X2	T42.6X3	T42.6X4	T42.6X5	T42.6X6
Valethamate bromide	T44.3X1	T44.3X2	T44.3X3	T44.3X4	T44.3X5	T44.3X6
Valisone	T49.0X1	T49.0X2	T49.0X3	T49.0X4	T49.0X5	T49.0X6
Valium	T42.4X1	T42.4X2	T42.4X3	T42.4X4	T42.4X5	T42.4X6
Valmid	T42.6X1	T42.6X2	T42.6X3	T42.6X4	T42.6X5	T42.6X6
Valnoctamide	T42.6X1	T42.6X2	T42.6X3	T42.6X4	T42.6X5	T42.6X6
Valproate (sodium)	T42.6X1	T42.6X2	T42.6X3	T42.6X4	T42.6X5	T42.6X6
Valproic acid	T42.6X1	T42.6X2	T42.6X3	T42.6X4	T42.6X5	T42.6X6
Valpromide	T42.6X1	T42.6X2	T42.6X3	T42.6X4	T42.6X5	T42.6X6
Vanadium	T56.891	T56.892	T56.893	T56.894	—	—

◀ New ◀ Revised ~~deleted~~ Deleted

	External Cause (T-Code)					
Substance	Poisoning, Accidental (Unintentional)	Poisoning, Intentional Self-Harm	Poisoning, Assault	Poisoning, Undetermined	Adverse Effect	Underdosing
Vancomycin	T36.8X1	T36.8X2	T36.8X3	T36.8X4	T36.8X5	T36.8X6
Vapor — *see also Gas*	T59.91	T59.92	T59.93	T59.94	—	—
kiln (carbon monoxide)	T58.8X1	T58.8X2	T58.8X3	T58.8X4	—	—
lead — *see lead*						
specified source NEC	T59.891	T59.892	T59.893	T59.894	—	—
Vardenafil	T46.7X1	T46.7X2	T46.7X3	T46.7X4	T46.7X5	T46.7X6
Varicose reduction drug	T46.8X1	T46.8X2	T46.8X3	T46.8X4	T46.8X5	T46.8X6
Varnish	T65.4X1	T65.4X2	T65.4X3	T65.4X4	—	—
cleaner	T52.91	T52.92	T52.93	T52.94	—	—
Vaseline	T49.3X1	T49.3X2	T49.3X3	T49.3X4	T49.3X5	T49.3X6
Vasodilan	T46.7X1	T46.7X2	T46.7X3	T46.7X4	T46.7X5	T46.7X6
Vasodilator						
coronary NEC	T46.3X1	T46.3X2	T46.3X3	T46.3X4	T46.3X5	T46.3X6
peripheral NEC	T46.7X1	T46.7X2	T46.7X3	T46.7X4	T46.7X5	T46.7X6
Vasopressin	T38.891	T38.892	T38.893	T38.894	T38.895	T38.896
Vasopressor drugs	T38.891	T38.892	T38.893	T38.894	T38.895	T38.896
Vecuronium bromide	T48.1X1	T48.1X2	T48.1X3	T48.1X4	T48.1X5	T48.1X6
Vegetable extract, astringent	T49.2X1	T49.2X2	T49.2X3	T49.2X4	T49.2X5	T49.2X6
Venlafaxine	T43.211	T43.212	T43.213	T43.214	T43.215	T43.216
Venom, venomous (bite) (sting)	T63.91	T63.92	T63.93	T63.94	—	—
amphibian NEC	T63.831	T63.832	T63.833	T63.834	—	—
animal NEC	T63.891	T63.892	T63.893	T63.894	—	—
ant	T63.421	T63.422	T63.423	T63.424	—	—
arthropod NEC	T63.481	T63.482	T63.483	T63.484	—	—
bee	T63.441	T63.442	T63.443	T63.444	—	—
centipede	T63.411	T63.412	T63.413	T63.414	—	—
fish	T63.591	T63.592	T63.593	T63.594	—	—
frog	T63.811	T63.812	T63.813	T63.814	—	—
hornet	T63.451	T63.452	T63.453	T63.454	—	—
insect NEC	T63.481	T63.482	T63.483	T63.484	—	—
lizard	T63.121	T63.122	T63.123	T63.124	—	—
marine						
animals	T63.691	T63.692	T63.693	T63.694	—	—
bluebottle	T63.611	T63.612	T63.613	T63.614	—	—
jellyfish NEC	T63.621	T63.622	T63.623	T63.624	—	—
Portugese Man-o-war	T63.611	T63.612	T63.613	T63.614	—	—
sea anemone	T63.631	T63.632	T63.633	T63.634	—	—
specified NEC	T63.691	T63.692	T63.693	T63.694	—	—
fish	T63.591	T63.592	T63.593	T63.594	—	—
plants	T63.711	T63.712	T63.713	T63.714	—	—
sting ray	T63.511	T63.512	T63.513	T63.514	—	—

	External Cause (T-Code)					
Substance	Poisoning, Accidental (Unintentional)	Poisoning, Intentional Self-Harm	Poisoning, Assault	Poisoning, Undetermined	Adverse Effect	Underdosing
Venom, venomous *(Continued)*						
millipede (tropical)	T63.411	T63.412	T63.413	T63.414	—	—
plant NEC	T63.791	T63.792	T63.793	T63.794	—	—
marine	T63.711	T63.712	T63.713	T63.714	—	—
reptile	T63.191	T63.192	T63.193	T63.194	—	—
gila monster	T63.111	T63.112	T63.113	T63.114	—	—
lizard NEC	T63.121	T63.122	T63.123	T63.124	—	—
scorpion	T63.2X1	T63.2X2	T63.2X3	T63.2X4	—	—
snake	T63.001	T63.002	T63.003	T63.004	—	—
African NEC	T63.081	T63.082	T63.083	T63.084	—	—
American (North) (South) NEC	T63.061	T63.062	T63.063	T63.064	—	—
Asian	T63.081	T63.082	T63.083	T63.084	—	—
Australian	T63.071	T63.072	T63.073	T63.074	—	—
cobra	T63.041	T63.042	T63.043	T63.044	—	—
coral snake	T63.021	T63.022	T63.023	T63.024	—	—
rattlesnake	T63.011	T63.012	T63.013	T63.014	—	—
specified NEC	T63.091	T63.092	T63.093	T63.094	—	—
taipan	T63.031	T63.032	T63.033	T63.034	—	—
specified NEC	T63.891	T63.892	T63.893	T63.894	—	—
spider	T63.301	T63.302	T63.303	T63.304	—	—
black widow	T63.311	T63.312	T63.313	T63.314	—	—
brown recluse	T63.331	T63.332	T63.333	T63.334	—	—
specified NEC	T63.391	T63.392	T63.393	T63.394	—	—
tarantula	T63.321	T63.322	T63.323	T63.324	—	—
sting ray	T63.511	T63.512	T63.513	T63.514	—	—
toad	T63.821	T63.822	T63.823	T63.824	—	—
wasp	T63.461	T63.462	T63.463	T63.464	—	—
Venous sclerosing drug NEC	T46.8X1	T46.8X2	T46.8X3	T46.8X4	T46.8X5	T46.8X6
Ventolin — *see Albuterol*						
Verapamil	T46.1X1	T46.1X2	T46.1X3	T46.1X4	T46.1X5	T46.1X6
Veramon	T42.3X1	T42.3X2	T42.3X3	T42.3X4	T42.3X5	T42.3X6
Veratrine	T46.5X1	T46.5X2	T46.5X3	T46.5X4	T46.5X5	T46.5X6
Veratrum						
album	T62.2X1	T62.2X2	T62.2X3	T62.2X4	—	—
alkaloids	T46.5X1	T46.5X2	T46.5X3	T46.5X4	T46.5X5	T46.5X6
viride	T62.2X1	T62.2X2	T62.2X3	T62.2X4	—	—
Verdigris	T60.3X1	T60.3X2	T60.3X3	T60.3X4	—	—
Veronal	T42.3X1	T42.3X2	T42.3X3	T42.3X4	T42.3X5	T42.3X6
Veroxil	T37.4X1	T37.4X2	T37.4X3	T37.4X4	T37.4X5	T37.4X6
Versenate	T50.6X1	T50.6X2	T50.6X3	T50.6X4	T50.6X5	T50.6X6

TABLE OF DRUGS AND CHEMICALS

TABLE OF DRUGS AND CHEMICALS

Substance	Poisoning, Accidental (Unintentional)	Poisoning, Intentional Self-Harm	Poisoning, Assault	Poisoning, Undetermined	Adverse Effect	Underdosing
Versidyne	T39.8X1	T39.8X2	T39.8X3	T39.8X4	T39.8X5	T39.8X6
Vetrabutine	T48.0X1	T48.0X2	T48.0X3	T48.0X4	T48.0X5	T48.0X6
Vidarabine	T37.5X1	T37.5X2	T37.5X3	T37.5X4	T37.5X5	T37.5X6
Vienna						
green	T57.0X1	T57.0X2	T57.0X3	T57.0X4	—	—
insecticide	T60.2X1	T60.2X2	T60.2X3	T60.2X4	—	—
red	T57.0X1	T57.0X2	T57.0X3	T57.0X4	—	—
pharmaceutical dye	T50.991	T50.992	T50.993	T50.994	T50.995	T50.996
Vigabatrin	T42.6X1	T42.6X2	T42.6X3	T42.6X4	T42.6X5	T42.6X6
Viloxazine	T43.291	T43.292	T43.293	T43.294	T43.295	T43.296
Viminol	T39.8X1	T39.8X2	T39.8X3	T39.8X4	T39.8X5	T39.8X6
Vinbarbital, vinbarbitone	T42.3X1	T42.3X2	T42.3X3	T42.3X4	T42.3X5	T42.3X6
Vinblastine	T45.1X1	T45.1X2	T45.1X3	T45.1X4	T45.1X5	T45.1X6
Vinburnine	T46.7X1	T46.7X2	T46.7X3	T46.7X4	T46.7X5	T46.7X6
Vincamine	T45.1X1	T45.1X2	T45.1X3	T45.1X4	T45.1X5	T45.1X6
Vincristine	T45.1X1	T45.1X2	T45.1X3	T45.1X4	T45.1X5	T45.1X6
Vindesine	T45.1X1	T45.1X2	T45.1X3	T45.1X4	T45.1X5	T45.1X6
Vinesthene, vinethene	T41.0X1	T41.0X2	T41.0X3	T41.0X4	T41.0X5	T41.0X6
Vinorelbine tartrate	T45.1X1	T45.1X2	T45.1X3	T45.1X4	T45.1X5	T45.1X6
Vinpocetine	T46.7X1	T46.7X2	T46.7X3	T46.7X4	T46.7X5	T46.7X6
Vinyl						
acetate	T65.891	T65.892	T65.893	T65.894	—	—
bital	T42.3X1	T42.3X2	T42.3X3	T42.3X4	T42.3X5	T42.3X6
bromide	T65.891	T65.892	T65.893	T65.894	—	—
chloride	T59.891	T59.892	T59.893	T59.894	—	—
ether	T41.0X1	T41.0X2	T41.0X3	T41.0X4	T41.0X5	T41.0X6
Vinylbital	T42.3X1	T42.3X2	T42.3X3	T42.3X4	T42.3X5	T42.3X6
Vinylidene chloride	T65.891	T65.892	T65.893	T65.894	—	—
Vioform	T37.8X1	T37.8X2	T37.8X3	T37.8X4	T37.8X5	T37.8X6
topical	T49.0X1	T49.0X2	T49.0X3	T49.0X4	T49.0X5	T49.0X6
Viomycin	T36.8X1	T36.8X2	T36.8X3	T36.8X4	T36.8X5	T36.8X6
Viosterol	T45.2X1	T45.2X2	T45.2X3	T45.2X4	T45.2X5	T45.2X6
Viper (venom)	T63.091	T63.092	T63.093	T63.094	—	—
Viprynium	T37.4X1	T37.4X2	T37.4X3	T37.4X4	T37.4X5	T37.4X6
Viquidil	T46.7X1	T46.7X2	T46.7X3	T46.7X4	T46.7X5	T46.7X6
Viral vaccine NEC	T50.B91	T50.B92	T50.B93	T50.B94	T50.B95	T50.B96
Virginiamycin	T36.8X1	T36.8X2	T36.8X3	T36.8X4	T36.8X5	T36.8X6
Virugon	T37.5X1	T37.5X2	T37.5X3	T37.5X4	T37.5X5	T37.5X6
Viscous agent	T50.901	T50.902	T50.903	T50.904	T50.905	T50.906
Visine	T49.5X1	T49.5X2	T49.5X3	T49.5X4	T49.5X5	T49.5X6
Visnadine	T46.3X1	T46.3X2	T46.3X3	T46.3X4	T46.3X5	T46.3X6

Substance	Poisoning, Accidental (Unintentional)	Poisoning, Intentional Self-Harm	Poisoning, Assault	Poisoning, Undetermined	Adverse Effect	Underdosing
Vitamin NEC	T45.2X1	T45.2X2	T45.2X3	T45.2X4	T45.2X5	T45.2X6
A	T45.2X1	T45.2X2	T45.2X3	T45.2X4	T45.2X5	T45.2X6
B NEC	T45.2X1	T45.2X2	T45.2X3	T45.2X4	T45.2X5	T45.2X6
nicotinic acid	T46.7X1	T46.7X2	T46.7X3	T46.7X4	T46.7X5	T46.7X6
B1	T45.2X1	T45.2X2	T45.2X3	T45.2X4	T45.2X5	T45.2X6
B2	T45.2X1	T45.2X2	T45.2X3	T45.2X4	T45.2X5	T45.2X6
B6	T45.2X1	T45.2X2	T45.2X3	T45.2X4	T45.2X5	T45.2X6
B12	T45.2X1	T45.2X2	T45.2X3	T45.2X4	T45.2X5	T45.2X6
B15	T45.2X1	T45.2X2	T45.2X3	T45.2X4	T45.2X5	T45.2X6
C	T45.2X1	T45.2X2	T45.2X3	T45.2X4	T45.2X5	T45.2X6
D	T45.2X1	T45.2X2	T45.2X3	T45.2X4	T45.2X5	T45.2X6
D2	T45.2X1	T45.2X2	T45.2X3	T45.2X4	T45.2X5	T45.2X6
D3	T45.2X1	T45.2X2	T45.2X3	T45.2X4	T45.2X5	T45.2X6
E	T45.2X1	T45.2X2	T45.2X3	T45.2X4	T45.2X5	T45.2X6
E acetate	T45.2X1	T45.2X2	T45.2X3	T45.2X4	T45.2X5	T45.2X6
hematopoietic	T45.8X1	T45.8X2	T45.8X3	T45.8X4	T45.8X5	T45.8X6
K NEC	T45.7X1	T45.7X2	T45.7X3	T45.7X4	T45.7X5	T45.7X6
K1	T45.7X1	T45.7X2	T45.7X3	T45.7X4	T45.7X5	T45.7X6
K2	T45.7X1	T45.7X2	T45.7X3	T45.7X4	T45.7X5	T45.7X6
PP	T45.2X1	T45.2X2	T45.2X3	T45.2X4	T45.2X5	T45.2X6
ulceroprotectant	T47.1X1	T47.1X2	T47.1X3	T47.1X4	T47.1X5	T47.1X6
Vleminckx's solution	T49.4X1	T49.4X2	T49.4X3	T49.4X4	T49.4X5	T49.4X6
Voltaren — *see Diclofenac sodium*						
W						
Warfarin	T45.511	T45.512	T45.513	T45.514	T45.515	T45.516
rodenticide	T60.4X1	T60.4X2	T60.4X3	T60.4X4	—	—
sodium	T45.511	T45.512	T45.513	T45.514	T45.515	T45.516
Wasp (sting)	T63.461	T63.462	T63.463	T63.464	—	—
Water						
balance drug	T50.3X1	T50.3X2	T50.3X3	T50.3X4	T50.3X5	T50.3X6
distilled	T50.3X1	T50.3X2	T50.3X3	T50.3X4	T50.3X5	T50.3X6
gas — *see Gas, water*						
incomplete combustion of — *see Carbon, monoxide, fuel, utility*						
hemlock	T62.2X1	T62.2X2	T62.2X3	T62.2X4	—	—
moccasin (venom)	T63.061	T63.062	T63.063	T63.064	—	—
purified	T50.3X1	T50.3X2	T50.3X3	T50.3X4	T50.3X5	T50.3X6
Wax (paraffin) (petroleum)	T52.0X1	T52.0X2	T52.0X3	T52.0X4	—	—
automobile	T65.891	T65.892	T65.893	T65.894	—	—
floor	T52.0X1	T52.0X2	T52.0X3	T52.0X4	—	—

◀ New   ◀ Revised   ~~deleted~~ Deleted

Substance	Poisoning, Accidental (Unintentional)	Poisoning, Intentional Self-Harm	Poisoning, Assault	Poisoning, Undetermined	Adverse Effect	Underdosing
Weed killers NEC	T60.3X1	T60.3X2	T60.3X3	T60.3X4	—	—
Welldorm	T42.6X1	T42.6X2	T42.6X3	T42.6X4	T42.6X5	T42.6X6
White						
arsenic	T57.0X1	T57.0X2	T57.0X3	T57.0X4	—	—
hellebore	T62.2X1	T62.2X2	T62.2X3	T62.2X4	—	—
lotion (keratolytic)	T49.4X1	T49.4X2	T49.4X3	T49.4X4	T49.4X5	T49.4X6
spirit	T52.0X1	T52.0X2	T52.0X3	T52.0X4	—	—
Whitewash	T65.891	T65.892	T65.893	T65.894	—	—
Whole blood (human)	T45.8X1	T45.8X2	T45.8X3	T45.8X4	T45.8X5	T45.8X6
Wild						
black cherry	T62.2X1	T62.2X2	T62.2X3	T62.2X4	—	—
poisonous plants NEC	T62.2X1	T62.2X2	T62.2X3	T62.2X4	—	—
Window cleaning fluid	T65.891	T65.892	T65.893	T65.894	—	—
Wintergreen (oil)	T49.3X1	T49.3X2	T49.3X3	T49.3X4	T49.3X5	T49.3X6
Wisterine	T62.2X1	T62.2X2	T62.2X3	T62.2X4	—	—
Witch hazel	T49.2X1	T49.2X2	T49.2X3	T49.2X4	T49.2X5	T49.2X6
Wood alcohol or spirit	T51.1X1	T51.1X2	T51.1X3	T51.1X4	—	—
Wool fat (hydrous)	T49.3X1	T49.3X2	T49.3X3	T49.3X4	T49.3X5	T49.3X6
Woorali	T48.1X1	T48.1X2	T48.1X3	T48.1X4	T48.1X5	T48.1X6
Wormseed, American	T37.4X1	T37.4X2	T37.4X3	T37.4X4	T37.4X5	T37.4X6
X						
Xamoterol	T44.5X1	T44.5X2	T44.5X3	T44.5X4	T44.5X5	T44.5X6
Xanthine diuretics	T50.2X1	T50.2X2	T50.2X3	T50.2X4	T50.2X5	T50.2X6
Xanthinol nicotinate	T46.7X1	T46.7X2	T46.7X3	T46.7X4	T46.7X5	T46.7X6
Xanthotoxin	T49.3X1	T49.3X2	T49.3X3	T49.3X4	T49.3X5	T49.3X6
Xantinol nicotinate	T46.7X1	T46.7X2	T46.7X3	T46.7X4	T46.7X5	T46.7X6
Xantocillin	T36.0X1	T36.0X2	T36.0X3	T36.0X4	T36.0X5	T36.0X6
Xenon (127Xe) (133Xe)	T50.8X1	T50.8X2	T50.8X3	T50.8X4	T50.8X5	T50.8X6
Xenysalate	T49.4X1	T49.4X2	T49.4X3	T49.4X4	T49.4X5	T49.4X6
Xibornol	T37.8X1	T37.8X2	T37.8X3	T37.8X4	T37.8X5	T37.8X6
Xigris	T45.511	T45.512	T45.513	T45.514	T45.515	T45.516
Xipamide	T50.2X1	T50.2X2	T50.2X3	T50.2X4	T50.2X5	T50.2X6
Xylene (vapor)	T52.2X1	T52.2X2	T52.2X3	T52.2X4	—	—
Xylocaine (infiltration) (topical)	T41.3X1	T41.3X2	T41.3X3	T41.3X4	T41.3X5	T41.3X6
nerve block (peripheral) (plexus)	T41.3X1	T41.3X2	T41.3X3	T41.3X4	T41.3X5	T41.3X6
spinal	T41.3X1	T41.3X2	T41.3X3	T41.3X4	T41.3X5	T41.3X6
Xylol (vapor)	T52.2X1	T52.2X2	T52.2X3	T52.2X4	—	—
Xylometazoline	T48.5X1	T48.5X2	T48.5X3	T48.5X4	T48.5X5	T48.5X6

Substance	Poisoning, Accidental (Unintentional)	Poisoning, Intentional Self-Harm	Poisoning, Assault	Poisoning, Undetermined	Adverse Effect	Underdosing
Y						
Yeast	T45.2X1	T45.2X2	T45.2X3	T45.2X4	T45.2X5	T45.2X6
dried	T45.2X1	T45.2X2	T45.2X3	T45.2X4	T45.2X5	T45.2X6
Yellow						
fever vaccine	T50.B91	T50.B92	T50.B93	T50.B94	T50.B95	T50.B96
jasmine	T62.2X1	T62.2X2	T62.2X3	T62.2X4	—	—
phenolphthalein	T47.2X1	T47.2X2	T47.2X3	T47.2X4	T47.2X5	T47.2X6
Yew	T62.2X1	T62.2X2	T62.2X3	T62.2X4	—	—
Yohimbic acid	T40.991	T40.992	T40.993	T40.994	T40.995	T40.996
Z						
Zactane	T39.8X1	T39.8X2	T39.8X3	T39.8X4	T39.8X5	T39.8X6
Zalcitabine	T37.5X1	T37.5X2	T37.5X3	T37.5X4	T37.5X5	T37.5X6
Zaroxolyn	T50.2X1	T50.2X2	T50.2X3	T50.2X4	T50.2X5	T50.2X6
Zephiran (topical)	T49.0X1	T49.0X2	T49.0X3	T49.0X4	T49.0X5	T49.0X6
ophthalmic preparation	T49.5X1	T49.5X2	T49.5X3	T49.5X4	T49.5X5	T49.5X6
Zeranol	T38.7X1	T38.7X2	T38.7X3	T38.7X4	T38.7X5	T38.7X6
Zerone	T51.1X1	T51.1X2	T51.1X3	T51.1X4	—	—
Zidovudine	T37.5X1	T37.5X2	T37.5X3	T37.5X4	T37.5X5	T37.5X6
Zimeldine	T43.221	T43.222	T43.223	T43.224	T43.225	T43.226
Zinc (compounds) (fumes) (vapor) NEC	T56.5X1	T56.5X2	T56.5X3	T56.5X4	—	—
anti-infectives	T49.0X1	T49.0X2	T49.0X3	T49.0X4	T49.0X5	T49.0X6
antivaricose	T46.8X1	T46.8X2	T46.8X3	T46.8X4	T46.8X5	T46.8X6
bacitracin	T49.0X1	T49.0X2	T49.0X3	T49.0X4	T49.0X5	T49.0X6
chloride (mouthwash)	T49.6X1	T49.6X2	T49.6X3	T49.6X4	T49.6X5	T49.6X6
chromate	T56.5X1	T56.5X2	T56.5X3	T56.5X4	—	—
gelatin	T49.3X1	T49.3X2	T49.3X3	T49.3X4	T49.3X5	T49.3X6
oxide	T49.3X1	T49.3X2	T49.3X3	T49.3X4	T49.3X5	T49.3X6
plaster	T49.3X1	T49.3X2	T49.3X3	T49.3X4	T49.3X5	T49.3X6
peroxide	T49.0X1	T49.0X2	T49.0X3	T49.0X4	T49.0X5	T49.0X6
pesticides	T56.5X1	T56.5X2	T56.5X3	T56.5X4	—	—
phosphide	T60.4X1	T60.4X2	T60.4X3	T60.4X4	—	—
pyrithionate	T49.4X1	T49.4X2	T49.4X3	T49.4X4	T49.4X5	T49.4X6
stearate	T49.3X1	T49.3X2	T49.3X3	T49.3X4	T49.3X5	T49.3X6
sulfate	T49.5X1	T49.5X2	T49.5X3	T49.5X4	T49.5X5	T49.5X6
ENT agent	T49.6X1	T49.6X2	T49.6X3	T49.6X4	T49.6X5	T49.6X6
ophthalmic solution	T49.5X1	T49.5X2	T49.5X3	T49.5X4	T49.5X5	T49.5X6
topical NEC	T49.0X1	T49.0X2	T49.0X3	T49.0X4	T49.0X5	T49.0X6
undecylenate	T49.0X1	T49.0X2	T49.0X3	T49.0X4	T49.0X5	T49.0X6

◀ New   ◀ Revised   ~~deleted~~ Deleted

	External Cause (T-Code)					
Substance	Poisoning, Accidental (Unintentional)	Poisoning, Intentional Self-Harm	Poisoning, Assault	Poisoning, Undetermined	Adverse Effect	Underdosing
Zineb	T60.0X1	T60.0X2	T60.0X3	T60.0X4	—	—
Zinostatin	T45.1X1	T45.1X2	T45.1X3	T45.1X4	T45.1X5	T45.1X6
Zipeprol	T48.3X1	T48.3X2	T48.3X3	T48.3X4	T48.3X5	T48.3X6
Zofenopril	T46.4X1	T46.4X2	T46.4X3	T46.4X4	T46.4X5	T46.4X6
Zolpidem	T42.6X1	T42.6X2	T42.6X3	T42.6X4	T42.6X5	T42.6X6
Zomepirac	T39.391	T39.392	T39.393	T39.394	T39.395	T39.396
Zopiclone	T42.6X1	T42.6X2	T42.6X3	T42.6X4	T42.6X5	T42.6X6

	External Cause (T-Code)					
Substance	Poisoning, Accidental (Unintentional)	Poisoning, Intentional Self-Harm	Poisoning, Assault	Poisoning, Undetermined	Adverse Effect	Underdosing
Zorubicin	T45.1X1	T45.1X2	T45.1X3	T45.1X4	T45.1X5	T45.1X6
Zotepine	T43.591	T43.592	T43.593	T43.594	T43.595	T43.596
Zovant	T45.511	T45.512	T45.513	T45.514	T45.515	T45.516
Zoxazolamine	T42.8X1	T42.8X2	T42.8X3	T42.8X4	T42.8X5	T42.8X6
Zuclopenthixol	T43.4X1	T43.4X2	T43.4X3	T43.4X4	T43.4X5	T43.4X6
Zygadenus (venenosus)	T62.2X1	T62.2X2	T62.2X3	T62.2X4	—	—
Zyprexa	T43.591	T43.592	T43.593	T43.594	T43.595	T43.596

◀ New   ◀ Revised   deleted Deleted

External Cause
of Injuries Index

A

Abandonment (causing exposure to weather conditions) (with intent to injure or kill) NEC X58

Abuse (adult) (child) (mental) (physical) (sexual) X58

Accident (to) X58
aircraft (in transit) (powered) —see also Accident, transport, aircraft
due to, caused by cataclysm —see Forces of nature, by type
animal-drawn vehicle —see Accident, transport, animal-drawn vehicle occupant
animal-rider —see Accident, transport, animal-rider
automobile —see Accident, transport, car occupant
bare foot water skiier V94.4
boat, boating —see also Accident, watercraft
striking swimmer
powered V94.11
unpowered V94.12
bus —see Accident, transport, bus occupant
cable car, not on rails V98.0
on rails —see Accident, transport, streetcar occupant
car —see Accident, transport, car occupant
caused by, due to
animal NEC W64
chain hoist W24.0
cold (excessive) —see Exposure, cold
corrosive liquid, substance —see Table of Drugs and Chemicals
cutting or piercing instrument —see Contact, with, by type of instrument
drive belt W24.0
electric
current —see Exposure, electric current
motor —see also Contact, with, by type of machine W31.3
current (of) W86.8
environmental factor NEC X58
explosive material —see Explosion
fire, flames —see Exposure, fire
firearm missile —see Discharge, firearm by type
heat (excessive) —see Heat
hot —see Contact, with, hot
ignition —see Ignition
lifting device W24.0
lightning —see subcategory T75.0
causing fire —see Exposure, fire
machine, machinery —see Contact, with, by type of machine
natural factor NEC X58
pulley (block) W24.0
radiation —see Radiation
steam X13.1
inhalation X13.0
pipe X16
thunderbolt —see subcategory T75.0
causing fire —see Exposure, fire
transmission device W24.1
coach —see Accident, transport, bus occupant
coal car —see Accident, transport, industrial vehicle occupant
diving —see also Fall, into, water
with
drowning or submersion —see Drowning
forklift —see Accident, transport, industrial vehicle occupant
heavy transport vehicle NOS —see Accident, transport, truck occupant
ice yacht V98.2

Accident (Continued)
in
medical, surgical procedure
as, or due to misadventure —see Misadventure
causing an abnormal reaction or later complication without mention of misadventure —see also Complication of or following, by type of procedure Y84.9
land yacht V98.1
late effect of —see W00-X58 with 7th character S
logging car —see Accident, transport, industrial vehicle occupant
machine, machinery —see also Contact, with, by type of machine
on board watercraft V93.69
explosion —see Explosion, in, watercraft
fire —see Burn, on board watercraft
powered craft V93.63
ferry boat V93.61
fishing boat V93.62
jetskis V93.63
liner V93.61
merchant ship V93.60
passenger ship V93.61
sailboat V93.64
mine tram —see Accident, transport, industrial vehicle occupant
mobility scooter (motorized) —see Accident, transport, pedestrian, conveyance, specified type NEC
motor scooter —see Accident, transport, motorcyclist
motor vehicle NOS (traffic) —see also Accident, transport V89.2
nontraffic V89.0
three-wheeled NOS —see Accident, transport, three-wheeled motor vehicle occupant
motorcycle NOS —see Accident, transport, motorcyclist
nonmotor vehicle NOS (nontraffic) —see also Accident, transport V89.1
traffic NOS V89.3
nontraffic (victim's mode of transport NOS) V88.9
collision (between) V88.7
bus and truck V88.5
car and:
bus V88.3
pickup V88.2
three-wheeled motor vehicle V88.0
train V88.6
truck V88.4
two-wheeled motor vehicle V88.0
van V88.2
specified vehicle NEC and:
three-wheeled motor vehicle V88.1
two-wheeled motor vehicle V88.1
known mode of transport —see Accident, transport, by type of vehicle
noncollision V88.8
on board watercraft V93.89
powered craft V93.83
ferry boat V93.81
fishing boat V93.82
jetskis V93.83
liner V93.81
merchant ship V93.80
passenger ship V93.81
unpowered craft V93.88
canoe V93.85
inflatable V93.86
in tow
recreational V94.31
specified NEC V94.32
kayak V93.85

Accident (Continued)
on board watercraft (Continued)
unpowered craft (Continued)
sailboat V93.84
surf-board V93.88
water skis V93.87
windsurfer V93.88
parachutist V97.29
entangled in object V97.21
injured on landing V97.22
pedal cycle —see Accident, transport, pedal cyclist
pedestrian (on foot)
with
another pedestrian W51
with fall W03
due to ice or snow W00.0
on pedestrian conveyance NEC V00.09
roller skater (in-line) V00.01
skate boarder V00.02
transport vehicle —see Accident, transport
on pedestrian conveyance —see Accident, transport, pedestrian, conveyance
pick-up truck or van —see Accident, transport, pickup truck occupant
quarry truck —see Accident, transport, industrial vehicle occupant
railway vehicle (any) (in motion) —see Accident, transport, railway vehicle occupant
due to cataclysm —see Forces of nature, by type
scooter (non-motorized) —see Accident, transport, pedestrian, conveyance, scooter
sequelae of —see W00-X58 with 7th character S
skateboard —see Accident, transport, pedestrian, conveyance, skateboard
ski (ing) —see Accident, transport, pedestrian, conveyance
lift V98.3
specified cause NEC X58
streetcar —see Accident, transport, streetcar occupant
traffic (victim's mode of transport NOS) V87.9
collision (between) V87.7
bus and truck V87.5
car and:
bus V87.3
pickup V87.2
three-wheeled motor vehicle V87.0
train V87.6
truck V87.4
two-wheeled motor vehicle V87.0
van V87.2
specified vehicle NEC and:
three-wheeled motor vehicle V87.1
two-wheeled motor vehicle V87.1
known mode of transport —see Accident, transport, by type of vehicle
noncollision V87.8
transport (involving injury to) V99
18 wheeler —see Accident, transport, truck occupant
agricultural vehicle occupant (nontraffic) V84.9
driver V84.5
hanger-on V84.7
passenger V84.6
traffic V84.3
driver V84.0
hanger-on V84.2
passenger V84.1
while boarding or alighting V84.4

▶ New   ⇒ Revised   ~~deleted~~ Deleted   ● Use Additional Character(s)

Accident *(Continued)*
 transport *(Continued)*
  aircraft NEC V97.89
   military NEC V97.818
    with civilian aircraft V97.810
    civilian injured by V97.811
   occupant injured (in)
    nonpowered craft accident
     V96.9
     balloon V96.00
      collision V96.03
      crash V96.01
      explosion V96.05
      fire V96.04
      forced landing V96.02
      specified type NEC V96.09
     glider V96.20
      collision V96.23
      crash V96.21
      explosion V96.25
      fire V96.24
      forced landing V96.22
      specified type NEC V96.29
     hang glider V96.10
      collision V96.13
      crash V96.11
      explosion V96.15
      fire V96.14
      forced landing V96.12
      specified type NEC V96.19
     specified craft NEC V96.8
    powered craft accident V95.9
     fixed wing NEC
      commercial V95.30
       collision V95.33
       crash V95.31
       explosion V95.35
       fire V95.34
       forced landing V95.32
       specified type NEC
        V95.39
      private V95.20
       collision V95.23
       crash V95.21
       explosion V95.25
       fire V95.24
       forced landing V95.22
       specified type NEC
        V95.29
     glider V95.10
      collision V95.13
      crash V95.11
      explosion V95.15
      fire V95.14
      forced landing V95.12
      specified type NEC V95.19
     helicopter V95.00
      collision V95.03
      crash V95.01
      explosion V95.05
      fire V95.04
      forced landing V95.02
      specified type NEC V95.09
     spacecraft V95.40
      collision V95.43
      crash V95.41
      explosion V95.45
      fire V95.44
      forced landing V95.42
      specified type NEC V95.49
     specified craft NEC V95.8
     ultralight V95.10
      collision V95.13
      crash V95.11
      explosion V95.15
      fire V95.14
      forced landing V95.12
      specified type NEC V95.19
   specified accident NEC V97.0
   while boarding or alighting
    V97.1

Accident *(Continued)*
 transport *(Continued)*
  aircraft NEC *(Continued)*
   person (injured by)
    falling from, in or on aircraft V97.0
    machinery on aircraft V97.89
    on ground with aircraft involvement
     V97.39
    rotating propeller V97.32
    struck by object falling from aircraft
     V97.31
    sucked into aircraft jet V97.33
    while boarding or alighting aircraft
     V97.1
  airport (battery-powered) passenger
   vehicle —*see* Accident, transport,
   industrial vehicle occupant
  all-terrain vehicle occupant (nontraffic)
   V86.95
   driver V86.55
   dune buggy —*see* Accident, transport,
    dune buggy occupant
   hanger-on V86.75
   passenger V86.65
   snowmobile —*see* Accident, transport,
    snowmobile occupant
   specified type NEC V86.99
   traffic V86.35
    driver V86.05
    hanger-on V86.25
    passenger V86.15
   while boarding or alighting V86.45
  ambulance occupant (traffic) V86.31
   driver V86.01
   hanger-on V86.21
   nontraffic V86.91
    driver V86.51
    hanger-on V86.71
    passenger V86.61
   passenger V86.11
   while boarding or alighting V86.41
  animal-drawn vehicle occupant (in)
   V80.929
   collision (with)
    animal V80.12
     being ridden V80.711
    animal-drawn vehicle V80.721
    bus V80.42
    car V80.42
    fixed or stationary object V80.82
    military vehicle V80.920
    nonmotor vehicle V80.791
    pedal cycle V80.22
    pedestrian V80.12
    pickup V80.42
    railway train or vehicle V80.62
    specified motor vehicle NEC V80.52
    streetcar V80.731
    truck V80.42
    two-or three-wheeled motor vehicle
     V80.32
    van V80.42
   noncollision V80.02
   specified circumstance NEC V80.928
  animal-rider V80.919
   collision (with)
    animal V80.11
     being ridden V80.710
    animal-drawn vehicle V80.720
    bus V80.41
    car V80.41
    fixed or stationary object V80.81
    military vehicle V80.910
    nonmotor vehicle V80.790
    pedal cycle V80.21
    pedestrian V80.11
    pickup V80.41
    railway train or vehicle V80.61
    specified motor vehicle NEC V80.51
    streetcar V80.730
    truck V80.41

Accident *(Continued)*
 transport *(Continued)*
  animal-rider *(Continued)*
   collision *(Continued)*
    two- or three-wheeled motor vehicle
     V80.31
    van V80.41
   noncollision V80.018
    specified as horse rider V80.010
   specified circumstance NEC V80.918
  armored car —*see* Accident, transport,
   truck occupant
  battery-powered truck (baggage) (mail) —
   see Accident, transport, industrial
   vehicle occupant
  bus occupant V79.9
   collision (with)
    animal (traffic) V70.9
     being ridden (traffic) V76.9
      nontraffic V76.3
       while boarding or alighting V76.4
      nontraffic V70.3
       while boarding or alighting V70.4
    animal-drawn vehicle (traffic) V76.9
     nontraffic V76.3
      while boarding or alighting V76.4
    bus (traffic) V74.9
     nontraffic V74.3
      while boarding or alighting V74.4
    car (traffic) V73.9
     nontraffic V73.3
      while boarding or alighting V73.4
    motor vehicle NOS (traffic) V79.60
     nontraffic V79.20
     specified type NEC (traffic) V79.69
      nontraffic V79.29
    pedal cycle (traffic) V71.9
     nontraffic V71.3
      while boarding or alighting V71.4
    pickup truck (traffic) V73.9
     nontraffic V73.3
      while boarding or alighting V73.4
    railway vehicle (traffic) V75.9
     nontraffic V75.3
      while boarding or alighting V75.4
    specified vehicle NEC (traffic) V76.9
     nontraffic V76.3
      while boarding or alighting V76.4
    stationary object (traffic) V77.9
     nontraffic V77.3
      while boarding or alighting V77.4
    streetcar (traffic) V76.9
     nontraffic V76.3
      while boarding or alighting V76.4
    three wheeled motor vehicle (traffic)
     V72.9
     nontraffic V72.3
      while boarding or alighting V72.4
    truck (traffic) V74.9
     nontraffic V74.3
      while boarding or alighting V74.4
    two wheeled motor vehicle (traffic)
     V72.9
     nontraffic V72.3
      while boarding or alighting V72.4
    van (traffic) V73.9
     nontraffic V73.3
      while boarding or alighting V73.4
   driver
    collision (with)
     animal (traffic) V70.5
      being ridden (traffic) V76.5
       nontraffic V76.0
      nontraffic V70.0
     animal-drawn vehicle (traffic)
      V76.5
       nontraffic V76.0
     bus (traffic) V74.5
      nontraffic V74.0
     car (traffic) V73.5
      nontraffic V73.0

Accident (Continued)
  transport (Continued)
    bus occupant (Continued)
      driver (Continued)
        collision (Continued)
          motor vehicle NOS (traffic) V79.40
            nontraffic V79.00
            specified type NEC (traffic)
              V79.49
              nontraffic V79.09
          pedal cycle (traffic) V71.5
            nontraffic V71.0
          pickup truck (traffic) V73.5
            nontraffic V73.0
          railway vehicle (traffic) V75.5
            nontraffic V75.0
          specified vehicle NEC (traffic)
            V76.5
            nontraffic V76.0
          stationary object (traffic) V77.5
            nontraffic V77.0
          streetcar (traffic) V76.5
            nontraffic V76.0
          three wheeled motor vehicle
            (traffic) V72.5
            nontraffic V72.0
          truck (traffic) V74.5
            nontraffic V74.0
          two wheeled motor vehicle (traffic)
            V72.5
            nontraffic V72.0
          van (traffic) V73.5
            nontraffic V73.0
        noncollision accident (traffic) V78.5
          nontraffic V78.0
      hanger-on
        collision (with)
          animal (traffic) V70.7
            being ridden (traffic) V76.7
              nontraffic V76.2
            nontraffic V70.2
          animal-drawn vehicle (traffic) V76.7
            nontraffic V76.2
          bus (traffic) V74.7
            nontraffic V74.2
          car (traffic) V73.7
            nontraffic V73.2
          pedal cycle (traffic) V71.7
            nontraffic V71.2
          pickup truck (traffic) V73.7
            nontraffic V73.2
          railway vehicle (traffic) V75.7
            nontraffic V75.2
          specified vehicle NEC (traffic) V76.7
            nontraffic V76.2
          stationary object (traffic) V77.7
            nontraffic V77.2
          streetcar (traffic) V76.7
            nontraffic V76.2
          three wheeled motor vehicle
            (traffic) V72.7
            nontraffic V72.2
          truck (traffic) V74.7
            nontraffic V74.2
          two wheeled motor vehicle (traffic)
            V72.7
            nontraffic V72.2
          van (traffic) V73.7
            nontraffic V73.2
        noncollision accident (traffic) V78.7
          nontraffic V78.2
      noncollision accident (traffic) V78.9
        nontraffic V78.3
        while boarding or alighting V78.4
      nontraffic V79.3
      passenger
        collision (with)
          animal (traffic) V70.6
            being ridden (traffic) V76.6
              nontraffic V76.1
            nontraffic V70.1

Accident (Continued)
  transport (Continued)
    bus occupant (Continued)
      passenger (Continued)
        collision (Continued)
          animal-drawn vehicle (traffic) V76.6
            nontraffic V76.1
          bus (traffic) V74.6
            nontraffic V74.1
          car (traffic) V73.6
            nontraffic V73.1
          motor vehicle NOS (traffic) V79.50
            nontraffic V79.10
            specified type NEC (traffic)
              V79.59
              nontraffic V79.19
          pedal cycle (traffic) V71.6
            nontraffic V71.1
          pickup truck (traffic) V73.6
            nontraffic V73.1
          railway vehicle (traffic) V75.6
            nontraffic V75.1
          specified vehicle NEC (traffic) V76.6
            nontraffic V76.1
          stationary object (traffic) V77.6
            nontraffic V77.1
          streetcar (traffic) V76.6
            nontraffic V76.1
          three wheeled motor vehicle
            (traffic) V72.6
            nontraffic V72.1
          truck (traffic) V74.6
            nontraffic V74.1
          two wheeled motor vehicle (traffic)
            V72.6
            nontraffic V72.1
          van (traffic) V73.6
            nontraffic V73.1
        noncollision accident (traffic) V78.6
          nontraffic V78.1
      specified type NEC V79.88
      military vehicle V79.81
    cable car, not on rails V98.0
      on rails —see Accident, transport,
        streetcar occupant
    car occupant V49.9
      ambulance occupant —see Accident,
        transport, ambulance occupant
      collision (with)
        animal (traffic) V40.9
          being ridden (traffic) V46.9
            nontraffic V46.3
            while boarding or alighting
              V46.4
          nontraffic V40.3
          while boarding or alighting V40.4
        animal-drawn vehicle (traffic) V46.9
          nontraffic V46.3
          while boarding or alighting V46.4
        bus (traffic) V44.9
          nontraffic V44.3
          while boarding or alighting V44.4
        car (traffic) V43.92
          nontraffic V43.32
          while boarding or alighting V43.42
        motor vehicle NOS (traffic) V49.60
          nontraffic V49.20
          specified type NEC (traffic) V49.69
            nontraffic V49.29
        pedal cycle (traffic) V41.9
          nontraffic V41.3
          while boarding or alighting V41.4
        pickup truck (traffic) V43.93
          nontraffic V43.33
          while boarding or alighting V43.43
        railway vehicle (traffic) V45.9
          nontraffic V45.3
          while boarding or alighting V45.4
        specified vehicle NEC (traffic) V46.9
          nontraffic V46.3
          while boarding or alighting V46.4

Accident (Continued)
  transport (Continued)
    car occupant (Continued)
      collision (Continued)
        sport utility vehicle (traffic) V43.91
          nontraffic V43.31
          while boarding or alighting V43.41
      ➡stationary object (traffic) V47.9
        ➡nontraffic V47.3
          while boarding or alighting V47.4
        streetcar (traffic) V46.9
          nontraffic V46.3
          while boarding or alighting V46.4
        three wheeled motor vehicle (traffic)
          V42.9
          nontraffic V42.3
          while boarding or alighting V42.4
        truck (traffic) V44.9
          nontraffic V44.3
          while boarding or alighting V44.4
        two wheeled motor vehicle (traffic)
          V42.9
          nontraffic V42.3
          while boarding or alighting V42.4
        van (traffic) V43.94
          nontraffic V43.34
          while boarding or alighting V43.44
      driver
        collision (with)
          animal (traffic) V40.5
            being ridden (traffic) V46.5
              nontraffic V46.0
            nontraffic V40.0
          animal-drawn vehicle (traffic) V46.5
            nontraffic V46.0
          bus (traffic) V44.5
            nontraffic V44.0
          car (traffic) V43.52
            nontraffic V43.02
          motor vehicle NOS (traffic) V49.40
            nontraffic V49.00
            specified type NEC (traffic)
              V49.49
              nontraffic V49.09
          pedal cycle (traffic) V41.5
            nontraffic V41.0
          pickup truck (traffic) V43.53
            nontraffic V43.03
          railway vehicle (traffic) V45.5
            nontraffic V45.0
          specified vehicle NEC (traffic) V46.5
            nontraffic V46.0
          sport utility vehicle (traffic) V43.51
            nontraffic V43.01
        ➡stationary object (traffic) V47.5
          ➡nontraffic V47.0
          streetcar (traffic) V46.5
            nontraffic V46.0
          three wheeled motor vehicle
            (traffic) V42.5
            nontraffic V42.0
          truck (traffic) V44.5
            nontraffic V44.0
          two wheeled motor vehicle (traffic)
            V42.5
            nontraffic V42.0
          van (traffic) V43.54
            nontraffic V43.04
        noncollision accident (traffic) V48.5
          nontraffic V48.0
      hanger-on
        collision (with)
          animal (traffic) V40.7
            being ridden (traffic) V46.7
              nontraffic V46.2
            nontraffic V40.2
          animal-drawn vehicle (traffic)
            V46.7
            nontraffic V46.2
          bus (traffic) V44.7
            nontraffic V44.2

▶ New   ⇒ Revised   ~~deleted~~ Deleted   ● Use Additional Character(s)

Accident *(Continued)*
  transport *(Continued)*
    car occupant *(Continued)*
      hanger-on *(Continued)*
        collision *(Continued)*
          car (traffic) V43.72
            nontraffic V43.22
          pedal cycle (traffic) V41.7
            nontraffic V41.2
          pickup truck (traffic) V43.73
            nontraffic V43.23
          railway vehicle (traffic) V45.7
            nontraffic V45.2
          specified vehicle NEC (traffic) V46.7
            nontraffic V46.2
          sport utility vehicle (traffic) V43.71
            nontraffic V43.21
          stationary object (traffic) V47.7
            nontraffic V47.2
          streetcar (traffic) V46.7
            nontraffic V46.2
          three wheeled motor vehicle
            (traffic) V42.7
            nontraffic V42.2
          truck (traffic) V44.7
            nontraffic V44.2
          two wheeled motor vehicle (traffic)
            V42.7
            nontraffic V42.2
          van (traffic) V43.74
            nontraffic V43.24
        noncollision accident (traffic) V48.7
         nontraffic V48.2
      noncollision accident (traffic) V48.9
        nontraffic V48.3
        while boarding or alighting V48.4
      nontraffic V49.3
      passenger
        collision (with)
          animal (traffic) V40.6
            being ridden (traffic) V46.6
              nontraffic V46.1
            nontraffic V40.1
          animal-drawn vehicle (traffic) V46.6
            nontraffic V46.1
          bus (traffic) V44.6
            nontraffic V44.1
          car (traffic) V43.62
            nontraffic V43.12
          motor vehicle NOS (traffic) V49.50
            nontraffic V49.10
            specified type NEC (traffic) V49.59
              nontraffic V49.19
          pedal cycle (traffic) V41.6
            nontraffic V41.1
          pickup truck (traffic) V43.63
            nontraffic V43.13
          railway vehicle (traffic) V45.6
            nontraffic V45.1
          specified vehicle NEC (traffic) V46.6
            nontraffic V46.1
          sport utility vehicle (traffic) V43.61
            nontraffic V43.11
          ➡stationary object (traffic) V47.6
           ➡nontraffic V47.1
          streetcar (traffic) V46.6
            nontraffic V46.1
          three wheeled motor vehicle
            (traffic) V42.6
            nontraffic V42.1
          truck (traffic) V44.6
            nontraffic V44.1
          two wheeled motor vehicle (traffic)
            V42.6
            nontraffic V42.1
          van (traffic) V43.64
            nontraffic V43.14
        noncollision accident (traffic) V48.6
         nontraffic V48.1
      specified type NEC V49.88
      military vehicle V49.81

Accident *(Continued)*
  transport *(Continued)*
    coal car —*see* Accident, transport,
      industrial vehicle occupant
    construction vehicle occupant (nontraffic)
      V85.9
      driver V85.5
      hanger-on V85.7
      passenger V85.6
      traffic V85.3
        driver V85.0
        hanger-on V85.2
        passenger V85.1
      while boarding or alighting V85.4
    ➡dirt bike rider (nontraffic) V86.96
      ▶driver V86.56
      ▶hanger-on V86.76
      ▶passenger V86.66
      ▶traffic V86.36
        ▶driver V86.06
        ▶hanger-on V86.26
        ▶passenger V86.16
      ▶while boarding or alighting V86.46
    due to cataclysm —*see* Forces of nature,
      by type
    dune buggy occupant (nontraffic) V86.93
      driver V86.53
      hanger-on V86.73
      passenger V86.63
      traffic V86.33
        driver V86.03
        hanger-on V86.23
        passenger V86.13
      while boarding or alighting V86.43
    forklift —*see* Accident, transport,
      industrial vehicle occupant
    go cart —*see* Accident, transport, all-terrain
      vehicle occupant
    golf cart —*see* Accident, transport,
      all-terrain vehicle occupant
    heavy transport vehicle occupant —
      see Accident, transport, truck occupant
    ice yacht V98.2
    industrial vehicle occupant (nontraffic)
      V83.9
      driver V83.5
      hanger-on V83.7
      passenger V83.6
      traffic V83.3
        driver V83.0
        hanger-on V83.2
        passenger V83.1
      while boarding or alighting V83.4
    interurban electric car —*see* Accident,
      transport, streetcar
    land yacht V98.1
    logging car —*see* Accident, transport,
      industrial vehicle occupant
    military vehicle occupant (traffic) V86.34
      driver V86.04
      hanger-on V86.24
      nontraffic V86.94
        driver V86.54
        hanger-on V86.74
        passenger V86.64
      passenger V86.14
      while boarding or alighting V86.44
    mine tram —*see* Accident, transport,
      industrial vehicle occupant
    motor vehicle NEC occupant (traffic) V89.2
    motorcoach —*see* Accident, transport,
      bus occupant
    ▶motor/cross bike rider —*see also* Accident,
      transport, dirt bike rider V86.96
    motorcyclist V29.9
      collision (with)
        animal (traffic) V20.9
          being ridden (traffic) V26.9
            nontraffic V26.2
            while boarding or alighting V26.3
          nontraffic V20.2
          while boarding or alighting V20.3

Accident *(Continued)*
  transport *(Continued)*
    motorcyclist *(Continued)*
      collision *(Continued)*
        animal-drawn vehicle (traffic) V26.9
          nontraffic V26.2
          while boarding or alighting V26.3
        bus (traffic) V24.9
          nontraffic V24.2
          while boarding or alighting V24.3
        car (traffic) V23.9
          nontraffic V23.2
          while boarding or alighting V23.3
        motor vehicle NOS (traffic) V29.60
          nontraffic V29.20
          specified type NEC (traffic) V29.69
            nontraffic V29.29
        pedal cycle (traffic) V21.9
          nontraffic V21.2
          while boarding or alighting V21.3
        pickup truck (traffic) V23.9
          nontraffic V23.2
          while boarding or alighting V23.3
        railway vehicle (traffic) V25.9
          nontraffic V25.2
          while boarding or alighting V25.3
        specified vehicle NEC (traffic) V26.9
          nontraffic V26.2
          while boarding or alighting V26.3
        stationary object (traffic) V27.9
          nontraffic V27.2
          while boarding or alighting V27.3
        streetcar (traffic) V26.9
          nontraffic V26.2
          while boarding or alighting V26.3
        three wheeled motor vehicle (traffic)
          V22.9
          nontraffic V22.2
          while boarding or alighting V22.3
        truck (traffic) V24.9
          nontraffic V24.2
          while boarding or alighting V24.3
        two wheeled motor vehicle (traffic)
          V22.9
          nontraffic V22.2
          while boarding or alighting V22.3
        van (traffic) V23.9
          nontraffic V23.2
          while boarding or alighting V23.3
      driver
        collision (with)
          animal (traffic) V20.4
            being ridden (traffic) V26.4
              nontraffic V26.0
            nontraffic V20.0
          animal-drawn vehicle (traffic) V26.4
            nontraffic V26.0
          bus (traffic) V24.4
            nontraffic V24.0
          car (traffic) V23.4
            nontraffic V23.0
          motor vehicle NOS (traffic) V29.40
            nontraffic V29.00
            specified type NEC (traffic)
              V29.49
              nontraffic V29.09
          pedal cycle (traffic) V21.4
            nontraffic V21.0
          pickup truck (traffic) V23.4
            nontraffic V23.0
          railway vehicle (traffic) V25.4
            nontraffic V25.0
          specified vehicle NEC (traffic) V26.4
            nontraffic V26.0
          stationary object (traffic) V27.4
            nontraffic V27.0
          streetcar (traffic) V26.4
            nontraffic V26.0
          three wheeled motor vehicle
            (traffic) V22.4
            nontraffic V22.0

Accident *(Continued)*
  transport *(Continued)*
    motorcyclist *(Continued)*
      driver *(Continued)*
        collision *(Continued)*
          truck (traffic) V24.4
            nontraffic V24.0
          two wheeled motor vehicle (traffic) V22.4
            nontraffic V22.0
          van (traffic) V23.4
            nontraffic V23.0
        noncollision accident (traffic) V28.4
          nontraffic V28.0
      noncollision accident (traffic) V28.9
        nontraffic V28.2
        while boarding or alighting V28.3
      nontraffic V29.3
      passenger
        collision (with)
          animal (traffic) V20.5
            being ridden (traffic) V26.5
              nontraffic V26.1
            nontraffic V20.1
          animal-drawn vehicle (traffic) V26.5
            nontraffic V26.1
          bus (traffic) V24.5
            nontraffic V24.1
          car (traffic) V23.5
            nontraffic V23.1
          motor vehicle NOS (traffic) V29.50
            nontraffic V29.10
            specified type NEC (traffic) V29.59
              nontraffic V29.19
          pedal cycle (traffic) V21.5
            nontraffic V21.1
          pickup truck (traffic) V23.5
            nontraffic V23.1
          railway vehicle (traffic) V25.5
            nontraffic V25.1
          specified vehicle NEC (traffic) V26.5
            nontraffic V26.1
          stationary object (traffic) V27.5
            nontraffic V27.1
          streetcar (traffic) V26.5
            nontraffic V26.1
          three wheeled motor vehicle (traffic) V22.5
            nontraffic V22.1
          truck (traffic) V24.5
            nontraffic V24.1
          two wheeled motor vehicle (traffic) V22.5
            nontraffic V22.1
          van (traffic) V23.5
            nontraffic V23.1
        noncollision accident (traffic) V28.5
          nontraffic V28.1
      specified type NEC V29.88
      military vehicle V29.81
    occupant (of)
      aircraft (powered) V95.9
        fixed wing
          commercial —*see* Accident, transport, aircraft, occupant, powered, fixed wing, commercial
          private —*see* Accident, transport, aircraft, occupant, powered, fixed wing, private
        nonpowered V96.9
        specified NEC V95.8
      airport battery-powered vehicle —*see* Accident, transport, industrial vehicle occupant
      all-terrain vehicle (ATV) —*see* Accident, transport, all-terrain vehicle occupant
      animal-drawn vehicle —*see* Accident, transport, animal-drawn vehicle occupant

Accident *(Continued)*
  transport *(Continued)*
    occupant *(Continued)*
      automobile —*see* Accident, transport, car occupant
      balloon V96.00
      battery-powered vehicle —*see* Accident, transport, industrial vehicle occupant
      bicycle —*see* Accident, transport, pedal cyclist
        motorized —*see* Accident, transport, motorcycle rider
      boat NEC —*see* Accident, watercraft
      bulldozer —*see* Accident, transport, construction vehicle occupant
      bus —*see* Accident, transport, bus occupant
      cable car (on rails) —*see also* Accident, transport, streetcar occupant
        not on rails V98.0
      car —*see also* Accident, transport, car occupant
        cable (on rails) —*see also* Accident, transport, streetcar occupant
        not on rails V98.0
      coach —*see* Accident, transport, bus occupant
      coal-car —*see* Accident, transport, industrial vehicle occupant
      digger —*see* Accident, transport, construction vehicle occupant
      dump truck —*see* Accident, transport, construction vehicle occupant
      earth-leveler —*see* Accident, transport, construction vehicle occupant
      farm machinery (self-propelled) —*see* Accident, transport, agricultural vehicle occupant
      forklift —*see* Accident, transport, industrial vehicle occupant
      glider (unpowered) V96.20
        hang V96.10
        powered (microlight) (ultralight) —*see* Accident, transport, aircraft, occupant, powered, glider
      glider (unpowered) NEC V96.20
      hang-glider V96.10
      harvester —*see* Accident, transport, agricultural vehicle occupant
      heavy (transport) vehicle —*see* Accident, transport, truck occupant
      helicopter —*see* Accident, transport, aircraft, occupant, helicopter
      ice-yacht V98.2
      kite (carrying person) V96.8
      land-yacht V98.1
      logging car —*see* Accident, transport, industrial vehicle occupant
      mechanical shovel —*see* Accident, transport, construction vehicle occupant
      microlight —*see* Accident, transport, aircraft, occupant, powered, glider
      minibus —*see* Accident, transport, pickup truck occupant
      minivan —*see* Accident, transport, pickup truck occupant
      moped —*see* Accident, transport, motorcycle
      motor scooter —*see* Accident, transport, motorcycle
      motorcycle (with sidecar) —*see* Accident, transport, motorcycle
      ▶off-road motor-vehicle —*see also* Accident, transport, all-terrain vehicle occupant V86.99
      pedal cycle —*see also* Accident, transport, pedal cyclist
      pick-up (truck) —*see* Accident, transport, pickup truck occupant

Accident *(Continued)*
  transport *(Continued)*
    occupant *(Continued)*
      railway (train) (vehicle) (subterranean) (elevated) —*see* Accident, transport, railway vehicle occupant
      rickshaw —*see* Accident, transport, pedal cycle
        pedal driven —*see* Accident, transport, pedal cyclist
      road-roller —*see* Accident, transport, construction vehicle occupant
      ship NOS V94.9
      ski-lift (chair) (gondola) V98.3
      snowmobile —*see* Accident, transport, snowmobile occupant
      spacecraft, spaceship —*see* Accident, transport, aircraft, occupant, spacecraft
      sport utility vehicle —*see* Accident, transport, pickup truck occupant
      streetcar (interurban) (operating on public street or highway) —*see* Accident, transport, streetcar occupant
      SUV —*see* Accident, transport, pickup truck occupant
      téléférique V98.0
      three-wheeled vehicle (motorized) —*see also* Accident, transport, three-wheeled motor vehicle occupant
        nonmotorized —*see* Accident, transport, pedal cycle
      tractor (farm) (and trailer) —*see* Accident, transport, agricultural vehicle occupant
      train —*see* Accident, transport, railway vehicle occupant
      tram —*see* Accident, transport, streetcar occupant
        in mine or quarry —*see* Accident, transport, industrial vehicle occupant
      tricycle —*see* Accident, transport, pedal cycle
        motorized —*see* Accident, transport, three-wheeled motor vehicle
      trolley —*see* Accident, transport, streetcar occupant
        in mine or quarry —*see* Accident, transport, industrial vehicle occupant
      tub, in mine or quarry —*see* Accident, transport, industrial vehicle occupant
      ultralight —*see* Accident, transport, aircraft, occupant, powered, glider
      van —*see* Accident, transport, van occupant
      vehicle NEC V89.9
        heavy transport —*see* Accident, transport, truck occupant
        motor (traffic) NEC V89.2
          nontraffic NEC V89.0
      watercraft NOS V94.9
        causing drowning —*see* Drowning, resulting from accident to boat
    ▶off-road motor-vehicle —*see also* Accident, transport, all-terrain vehicle occupant V86.99
    parachutist V97.29
      after accident to aircraft —*see* Accident, transport, aircraft
      entangled in object V97.21
      injured on landing V97.22
    pedal cyclist V19.9
      collision (with)
        animal (traffic) V10.9
          being ridden (traffic) V16.9
            nontraffic V16.2
            while boarding or alighting V16.3

▶ New   ⇒ Revised   ~~deleted~~ Deleted   ● Use Additional Character(s)

Accident *(Continued)*
  transport *(Continued)*
    pedal cyclist *(Continued)*
      collision *(Continued)*
        animal (traffic) V10.9 *(Continued)*
          nontraffic V10.2
            while boarding or alighting V10.3
        animal-drawn vehicle (traffic) V16.9
          nontraffic V16.2
            while boarding or alighting V16.3
        bus (traffic) V14.9
          nontraffic V14.2
            while boarding or alighting V14.3
        car (traffic) V13.9
          nontraffic V13.2
            while boarding or alighting V13.3
        motor vehicle NOS (traffic) V19.60
          nontraffic V19.20
          specified type NEC (traffic) V19.69
            nontraffic V19.29
        pedal cycle (traffic) V11.9
          nontraffic V11.2
            while boarding or alighting V11.3
        pickup truck (traffic) V13.9
          nontraffic V13.2
            while boarding or alighting V13.3
        railway vehicle (traffic) V15.9
          nontraffic V15.2
            while boarding or alighting V15.3
        specified vehicle NEC (traffic) V16.9
          nontraffic V16.2
            while boarding or alighting V16.3
        stationary object (traffic) V17.9
          nontraffic V17.2
            while boarding or alighting V17.3
        streetcar (traffic) V16.9
          nontraffic V16.2
            while boarding or alighting V16.3
        three wheeled motor vehicle (traffic) V12.9
          nontraffic V12.2
            while boarding or alighting V12.3
        truck (traffic) V14.9
          nontraffic V14.2
            while boarding or alighting V14.3
        two wheeled motor vehicle (traffic) V12.9
          nontraffic V12.2
            while boarding or alighting V12.3
        van (traffic) V13.9
          nontraffic V13.2
            while boarding or alighting V13.3
      driver
        collision (with)
          animal (traffic) V10.4
            being ridden (traffic) V16.4
              nontraffic V16.0
            nontraffic V10.0
          animal-drawn vehicle (traffic) V16.4
            nontraffic V16.0
          bus (traffic) V14.4
            nontraffic V14.0
          car (traffic) V13.4
            nontraffic V13.0
          motor vehicle NOS (traffic) V19.40
            nontraffic V19.00
            specified type NEC (traffic) V19.49
              nontraffic V19.09
          pedal cycle (traffic) V11.4
            nontraffic V11.0
          pickup truck (traffic) V13.4
            nontraffic V13.0
          railway vehicle (traffic) V15.4
            nontraffic V15.0
          specified vehicle NEC (traffic) V16.4
            nontraffic V16.0
          stationary object (traffic) V17.4
            nontraffic V17.0
          streetcar (traffic) V16.4
            nontraffic V16.0
          three wheeled motor vehicle (traffic) V12.4
            nontraffic V12.0

Accident *(Continued)*
  transport *(Continued)*
    pedal cyclist *(Continued)*
      driver *(Continued)*
        collision *(Continued)*
          truck (traffic) V14.4
            nontraffic V14.0
          two wheeled motor vehicle (traffic) V12.4
            nontraffic V12.0
          van (traffic) V13.4
            nontraffic V13.0
        noncollision accident (traffic) V18.4
          nontraffic V18.0
      noncollision accident (traffic) V18.9
        nontraffic V18.2
        while boarding or alighting V18.3
      nontraffic V19.3
      passenger
        collision (with)
          animal (traffic) V10.5
            being ridden (traffic) V16.5
              nontraffic V16.1
            nontraffic V10.1
          animal-drawn vehicle (traffic) V16.5
            nontraffic V16.1
          bus (traffic) V14.5
            nontraffic V14.1
          car (traffic) V13.5
            nontraffic V13.1
          motor vehicle NOS (traffic) V19.50
            nontraffic V19.10
            specified type NEC (traffic) V19.59
              nontraffic V19.19
          pedal cycle (traffic) V11.5
            nontraffic V11.1
          pickup truck (traffic) V13.5
            nontraffic V13.1
          railway vehicle (traffic) V15.5
            nontraffic V15.1
          specified vehicle NEC (traffic) V16.5
            nontraffic V16.1
          stationary object (traffic) V17.5
            nontraffic V17.1
          streetcar (traffic) V16.5
            nontraffic V16.1
          three wheeled motor vehicle (traffic) V12.5
            nontraffic V12.1
          truck (traffic) V14.5
            nontraffic V14.1
          two wheeled motor vehicle (traffic) V12.5
            nontraffic V12.1
          van (traffic) V13.5
            nontraffic V13.1
        noncollision accident (traffic) V18.5
          nontraffic V18.1
      specified type NEC V19.88
      military vehicle V19.81
    pedestrian
      conveyance (occupant) V09.9
        babystroller V00.828
          collision (with) V09.9
            animal being ridden or animal drawn vehicle V06.99
              nontraffic V06.09
              traffic V06.19
            bus or heavy transport V04.99
              nontraffic V04.09
              traffic V04.19
            car V03.99
              nontraffic V03.09
              traffic V03.19
            pedal cycle V01.99
              nontraffic V01.09
              traffic V01.19
            pick-up truck or van V03.99
              nontraffic V03.09
              traffic V03.19

Accident *(Continued)*
  transport *(Continued)*
    pedestrian *(Continued)*
      conveyance *(Continued)*
        babystroller *(Continued)*
          collision *(Continued)*
            railway (train) (vehicle) V05.99
              nontraffic V05.09
              traffic V05.19
            stationary object V00.822
            streetcar V06.99
              nontraffic V06.09
              traffic V06.19
            two- or three-wheeled motor vehicle V02.99
              nontraffic V02.09
              traffic V02.19
            vehicle V09.9
              animal-drawn V06.99
                nontraffic V06.09
                traffic V06.19
              motor
                nontraffic V09.00
                traffic V09.20
        fall V00.821
        nontraffic V09.1
          involving motor vehicle NEC V09.00
        traffic V09.3
          involving motor vehicle NEC V09.20
        flat-bottomed NEC V00.388
          collision (with) V09.9
            animal being ridden or animal drawn vehicle V06.99
              nontraffic V06.09
              traffic V06.19
            bus or heavy transport V04.99
              nontraffic V04.09
              traffic V04.19
            car V03.99
              nontraffic V03.09
              traffic V03.19
            pedal cycle V01.99
              nontraffic V01.09
              traffic V01.19
            pick-up truck or van V03.99
              nontraffic V03.09
              traffic V03.19
            railway (train) (vehicle) V05.99
              nontraffic V05.09
              traffic V05.19
            stationary object V00.382
            streetcar V06.99
              nontraffic V06.09
              traffic V06.19
            two-or three-wheeled motor vehicle V02.99
              nontraffic V02.09
              traffic V02.19
            vehicle V09.9
              animal-drawn V06.99
                nontraffic V06.09
                traffic V06.19
              motor
                nontraffic V09.00
                traffic V09.20
        fall V00.381
        nontraffic V09.1
          involving motor vehicle NEC V09.00
        snow
          board —*see* Accident, transport, pedestrian, conveyance, snow board
          ski —*see* Accident, transport, pedestrian, conveyance, skis (snow)
        traffic V09.3
          involving motor vehicle NEC V09.20

Accident (Continued)
  transport (Continued)
    pedestrian (Continued)
      conveyance (Continued)
        gliding type NEC V00.288
          collision (with) V09.9
            animal being ridden or animal
              drawn vehicle V06.99
              nontraffic V06.09
              traffic V06.19
            bus or heavy transport
              V04.99
              nontraffic V04.09
              traffic V04.19
            car V03.99
              nontraffic V03.09
              traffic V03.19
            pedal cycle V01.99
              nontraffic V01.09
              traffic V01.19
            pick-up truck or van V03.99
              nontraffic V03.09
              traffic V03.19
            railway (train) (vehicle) V05.99
              nontraffic V05.09
              traffic V05.19
            stationary object V00.282
            streetcar V06.99
              nontraffic V06.09
              traffic V06.19
            two- or three-wheeled motor
              vehicle V02.99
              nontraffic V02.09
              traffic V02.19
            vehicle V09.9
              animal-drawn V06.99
                nontraffic V06.09
                traffic V06.19
              motor
                nontraffic V09.00
                traffic V09.20
          fall V00.281
        heelies —see Accident, transport,
          pedestrian, conveyance,
          heelies
        ice skate —see Accident, transport,
          pedestrian, conveyance, ice
          skate
        nontraffic V09.1
          involving motor vehicle NEC
            V09.00
        sled —see Accident, transport,
          pedestrian, conveyance, sled
        traffic V09.3
          involving motor vehicle NEC
            V09.20
          wheelies —see Accident,
            transport, pedestrian,
            conveyance, heelies
       heelies V00.158
        colliding with stationary object
          V00.152
        fall V00.151
       ice skates V00.218
        collision (with) V09.9
          animal being ridden or animal
            drawn vehicle V06.99
            nontraffic V06.09
            traffic V06.19
          bus or heavy transport V04.99
            nontraffic V04.09
            traffic V04.19
          car V03.99
            nontraffic V03.09
            traffic V03.19
          pedal cycle V01.99
            nontraffic V01.09
            traffic V01.19
          pick-up truck or van V03.99
            nontraffic V03.09
            traffic V03.19

Accident (Continued)
  transport (Continued)
    pedestrian (Continued)
      conveyance (Continued)
        ice skates (Continued)
          collision (Continued)
            railway (train) (vehicle)
              V05.99
              nontraffic V05.09
              traffic V05.19
            stationary object V00.212
            streetcar V06.99
              nontraffic V06.09
              traffic V06.19
            two- or three-wheeled motor
              vehicle V02.99
              nontraffic V02.09
              traffic V02.19
            vehicle V09.9
              animal-drawn V06.99
                nontraffic V06.09
                traffic V06.19
              motor
                nontraffic V09.00
                traffic V09.20
          fall V00.211
          nontraffic V09.1
            involving motor vehicle NEC
              V09.00
          traffic V09.3
            involving motor vehicle NEC
              V09.20
        motorized mobility scooter
          V00.838
          collision with stationary object
            V00.832
          fall from V00.831
        nontraffic V09.1
          involving motor vehicle
            V09.00
            military V09.01
            specified type NEC V09.09
        roller skates (non in-line) V00.128
          collision (with) V09.9
            animal being ridden or animal
              drawn vehicle V06.91
              nontraffic V06.01
              traffic V06.11
            bus or heavy transport
              V04.91
              nontraffic V04.01
              traffic V04.11
            car V03.91
              nontraffic V03.01
              traffic V03.11
            pedal cycle V01.91
              nontraffic V01.01
              traffic V01.11
            pick-up truck or van V03.91
              nontraffic V03.01
              traffic V03.11
            railway (train) (vehicle)
              V05.91
              nontraffic V05.01
              traffic V05.11
            stationary object V00.122
            streetcar V06.91
              nontraffic V06.01
              traffic V06.11
            two- or three-wheeled motor
              vehicle V02.91
              nontraffic V02.01
              traffic V02.11
            vehicle V09.9
              animal-drawn V06.91
                nontraffic V06.01
                traffic V06.11
              motor
                nontraffic V09.00
                traffic V09.20
          fall V00.121

Accident (Continued)
  transport (Continued)
    pedestrian (Continued)
      conveyance (Continued)
        roller skates (Continued)
          in-line V00.118
            collision —see also Accident,
              transport, pedestrian,
              conveyance occupant, roller
              skates, collision
              with stationary object
                V00.112
            fall V00.111
            nontraffic V09.1
              involving motor vehicle NEC
                V09.00
            traffic V09.3
              involving motor vehicle NEC
                V09.20
        rolling shoes V00.158
          colliding with stationary object
            V00.152
          fall V00.151
        rolling type NEC V00.188
          collision (with) V09.9
            animal being ridden or animal
              drawn vehicle V06.99
              nontraffic V06.09
              traffic V06.19
            bus or heavy transport V04.99
              nontraffic V04.09
              traffic V04.19
            car V03.99
              nontraffic V03.09
              traffic V03.19
            pedal cycle V01.99
              nontraffic V01.09
              traffic V01.19
            pick-up truck or van V03.99
              nontraffic V03.09
              traffic V03.19
            railway (train) (vehicle)
              V05.99
              nontraffic V05.09
              traffic V05.19
            stationary object V00.182
            streetcar V06.99
              nontraffic V06.09
              traffic V06.19
            two- or three-wheeled motor
              vehicle V02.99
              nontraffic V02.09
              traffic V02.19
            vehicle V09.9
              animal-drawn V06.99
                nontraffic V06.09
                traffic V06.19
              motor
                nontraffic V09.00
                traffic V09.20
          fall V00.181
        in-line roller skate —see Accident,
          transport, pedestrian,
          conveyance, roller skate,
          in-line
        nontraffic V09.1
          involving motor vehicle NEC
            V09.00
        roller skate —see Accident,
          transport, pedestrian,
          conveyance, roller skate
        scooter (non-motorized) —
          see Accident, transport,
          pedestrian, conveyance,
          scooter
        skateboard —see Accident,
          transport, pedestrian,
          conveyance, skateboard
        traffic V09.3
          involving motor vehicle NEC
            V09.20

▶ New   ➡ Revised   ~~deleted~~ Deleted   ● Use Additional Character(s)

Accident (Continued)
  transport (Continued)
    pedestrian (Continued)
      conveyance (Continued)
        scooter (non-motorized) V00.148
          collision (with) V09.9
            animal being ridden or animal
              drawn vehicle V06.99
              nontraffic V06.09
              traffic V06.19
            bus or heavy transport
              V04.99
              nontraffic V04.09
              traffic V04.19
            car V03.99
              nontraffic V03.09
              traffic V03.19
            pedal cycle V01.99
              nontraffic V01.09
              traffic V01.19
            pick-up truck or van V03.99
              nontraffic V03.09
              traffic V03.19
            railway (train) (vehicle)
              V05.99
              nontraffic V05.09
              traffic V05.19
            stationary object V00.142
            streetcar V06.99
              nontraffic V06.09
              traffic V06.19
            two- or three-wheeled motor
              vehicle V02.99
              nontraffic V02.09
              traffic V02.19
            vehicle V09.9
              animal-drawn V06.99
                nontraffic V06.09
                traffic V06.19
              motor
                nontraffic V09.00
                traffic V09.20
          fall V00.141
          nontraffic V09.1
            involving motor vehicle NEC
              V09.00
          traffic V09.3
            involving motor vehicle NEC
              V09.20
        skate board V00.138
          collision (with) V09.9
            animal being ridden or
              animal drawn vehicle
              V06.92
              nontraffic V06.02
              traffic V06.12
            bus or heavy transport
              V04.92
              nontraffic V04.02
              traffic V04.12
            car V03.92
              nontraffic V03.02
              traffic V03.12
            pedal cycle V01.92
              nontraffic V01.02
              traffic V01.12
            pick-up truck or van V03.92
              nontraffic V03.02
              traffic V03.12
            railway (train) (vehicle)
              V05.92
              nontraffic V05.02
              traffic V05.12
            stationary object V00.132
            streetcar V06.92
              nontraffic V06.02
              traffic V06.12
            two- or three-wheeled motor
              vehicle V02.92
              nontraffic V02.02
              traffic V02.12

Accident (Continued)
  transport (Continued)
    pedestrian (Continued)
      conveyance (Continued)
        skate board (Continued)
          collision (Continued)
            vehicle V09.9
              animal-drawn V06.92
                nontraffic V06.02
                traffic V06.12
              motor
                nontraffic V09.00
                traffic V09.20
          fall V00.131
          nontraffic V09.1
            involving motor vehicle NEC
              V09.00
          traffic V09.3
            involving motor vehicle NEC
              V09.20
        skis (snow) V00.328
          collision (with) V09.9
            animal being ridden or animal
              drawn vehicle V06.99
              nontraffic V06.09
              traffic V06.19
            bus or heavy transport V04.99
              nontraffic V04.09
              traffic V04.19
            car V03.99
              nontraffic V03.09
              traffic V03.19
            pedal cycle V01.99
              nontraffic V01.09
              traffic V01.19
            pick-up truck or van V03.99
              nontraffic V03.09
              traffic V03.19
            railway (train) (vehicle) V05.99
              nontraffic V05.09
              traffic V05.19
            stationary object V00.322
            streetcar V06.99
              nontraffic V06.09
              traffic V06.19
            two- or three-wheeled motor
              vehicle V02.99
              nontraffic V02.09
              traffic V02.19
            vehicle V09.9
              animal-drawn V06.99
                nontraffic V06.09
                traffic V06.19
              motor
                nontraffic V09.00
                traffic V09.20
          fall V00.321
          nontraffic V09.1
            involving motor vehicle NEC
              V09.00
          traffic V09.3
            involving motor vehicle NEC
              V09.20
        sled V00.228
          collision (with) V09.9
            animal being ridden or animal
              drawn vehicle V06.99
              nontraffic V06.09
              traffic V06.19
            bus or heavy transport V04.99
              nontraffic V04.09
              traffic V04.19
            car V03.99
              nontraffic V03.09
              traffic V03.19
            pedal cycle V01.99
              nontraffic V01.09
              traffic V01.19
            pick-up truck or van V03.99
              nontraffic V03.09
              traffic V03.19

Accident (Continued)
  transport (Continued)
    pedestrian (Continued)
      conveyance (Continued)
        sled (Continued)
          collision (Continued)
            railway (train) (vehicle)
              V05.99
              nontraffic V05.09
              traffic V05.19
            stationary object V00.222
            streetcar V06.99
              nontraffic V06.09
              traffic V06.19
            two- or three-wheeled motor
              vehicle V02.99
              nontraffic V02.09
              traffic V02.19
            vehicle V09.9
              animal-drawn V06.99
                nontraffic V06.09
                traffic V06.19
              motor
                nontraffic V09.00
                traffic V09.20
          fall V00.221
          nontraffic V09.1
            involving motor vehicle NEC
              V09.00
          traffic V09.3
            involving motor vehicle NEC
              V09.20
        snow board V00.318
          collision (with) V09.9
            animal being ridden or animal
              drawn vehicle V06.99
              nontraffic V06.09
              traffic V06.19
            bus or heavy transport V04.99
              nontraffic V04.09
              traffic V04.19
            car V03.99
              nontraffic V03.09
              traffic V03.19
            pedal cycle V01.99
              nontraffic V01.09
              traffic V01.19
            pick-up truck or van V03.99
              nontraffic V03.09
              traffic V03.19
            railway (train) (vehicle) V05.99
              nontraffic V05.09
              traffic V05.19
            stationary object V00.312
            streetcar V06.99
              nontraffic V06.09
              traffic V06.19
            two- or three-wheeled motor
              vehicle V02.99
              nontraffic V02.09
              traffic V02.19
            vehicle V09.9
              animal-drawn V06.99
                nontraffic V06.09
                traffic V06.19
              motor
                nontraffic V09.00
                traffic V09.20
          fall V00.311
          nontraffic V09.1
            involving motor vehicle NEC
              V09.00
          traffic V09.3
            involving motor vehicle NEC
              V09.20
        specified type NEC V00.898
          collision (with) V09.9
            animal being ridden or animal
              drawn vehicle V06.99
              nontraffic V06.09
              traffic V06.19

Accident *(Continued)*
  transport *(Continued)*
    pedestrian *(Continued)*
      conveyance *(Continued)*
        specified type NEC *(Continued)*
          collision *(Continued)*
            bus or heavy transport V04.99
              nontraffic V04.09
              traffic V04.19
            car V03.99
              nontraffic V03.09
              traffic V03.19
            pedal cycle V01.99
              nontraffic V01.09
              traffic V01.19
            pick-up truck or van V03.99
              nontraffic V03.09
              traffic V03.19
            railway (train) (vehicle) V05.99
              nontraffic V05.09
              traffic V05.19
            stationary object V00.892
            streetcar V06.99
              nontraffic V06.09
              traffic V06.19
            two- or three-wheeled motor vehicle V02.99
              nontraffic V02.09
              traffic V02.19
            vehicle V09.9
              animal-drawn V06.99
                nontraffic V06.09
                traffic V06.19
              motor
                nontraffic V09.00
                traffic V09.20
          fall V00.891
          nontraffic V09.1
            involving motor vehicle NEC V09.00
          traffic V09.3
            involving motor vehicle NEC V09.20
        traffic V09.3
          involving motor vehicle V09.20
            military V09.21
            specified type NEC V09.29
        wheelchair (powered) V00.818
          collision (with) V09.9
            animal being ridden or animal drawn vehicle V06.99
              nontraffic V06.09
              traffic V06.19
            bus or heavy transport V04.99
              nontraffic V04.09
              traffic V04.19
            car V03.99
              nontraffic V03.09
              traffic V03.19
            pedal cycle V01.99
              nontraffic V01.09
              traffic V01.19
            pick-up truck or van V03.99
              nontraffic V03.09
              traffic V03.19
            railway (train) (vehicle) V05.99
              nontraffic V05.09
              traffic V05.19
            stationary object V00.812
            streetcar V06.99
              nontraffic V06.09
              traffic V06.19
            two- or three-wheeled motor vehicle V02.99
              nontraffic V02.09
              traffic V02.19

Accident *(Continued)*
  transport *(Continued)*
    pedestrian *(Continued)*
      conveyance *(Continued)*
        wheelchair *(Continued)*
          collision *(Continued)*
            vehicle V09.9
              animal-drawn V06.99
                nontraffic V06.09
                traffic V06.19
              motor
                nontraffic V09.00
                traffic V09.20
          fall V00.811
          nontraffic V09.1
            involving motor vehicle NEC V09.00
          traffic V09.3
            involving motor vehicle NEC V09.20
        wheeled shoe V00.158
          colliding with stationary object V00.152
          fall V00.151
      on foot *—see also* Accident, pedestrian
        collision (with)
          animal being ridden or animal drawn vehicle V06.90
            nontraffic V06.00
            traffic V06.10
          bus or heavy transport V04.90
            nontraffic V04.00
            traffic V04.10
          car V03.90
            nontraffic V03.00
            traffic V03.10
          pedal cycle V01.90
            nontraffic V01.00
            traffic V01.10
          pick-up truck or van V03.90
            nontraffic V03.00
            traffic V03.10
          railway (train) (vehicle) V05.90
            nontraffic V05.00
            traffic V05.10
          streetcar V06.90
            nontraffic V06.00
            traffic V06.10
          two- or three-wheeled motor vehicle V02.90
            nontraffic V02.00
            traffic V02.10
          vehicle V09.9
            animal-drawn V06.90
              nontraffic V06.00
              traffic V06.10
            motor
              nontraffic V09.00
              traffic V09.20
         nontraffic V09.1
          involving motor vehicle V09.00
            military V09.01
            specified type NEC V09.09
        traffic V09.3
          involving motor vehicle V09.20
            military V09.21
            specified type NEC V09.29
      person NEC (unknown way or transportation) V99
      collision (between)
        bus (with)
          heavy transport vehicle (traffic) V87.5
            nontraffic V88.5
        car (with)
          nontraffic V88.5
          bus (traffic) V87.3
            nontraffic V88.3
          heavy transport vehicle (traffic) V87.4
            nontraffic V88.4

Accident *(Continued)*
  transport *(Continued)*
    person NEC *(Continued)*
      collision *(Continued)*
        car *(Continued)*
          pick-up truck or van (traffic) V87.2
            nontraffic V88.2
          train or railway vehicle (traffic) V87.6
            nontraffic V88.6
          two- or three-wheeled motor vehicle (traffic) V87.0
            nontraffic V88.0
          motor vehicle (traffic) NEC V87.7
            nontraffic V88.7
          two- or three-wheeled vehicle (with) (traffic)
            motor vehicle NEC V87.1
            nontraffic V88.1
         nonmotor vehicle (collision) (noncollision) (traffic) V87.9
          nontraffic V88.9
    pickup truck occupant V59.9
      collision (with)
        animal (traffic) V50.9
          being ridden (traffic) V56.9
            nontraffic V56.3
            while boarding or alighting V56.4
          nontraffic V50.3
            while boarding or alighting V50.4
        animal-drawn vehicle (traffic) V56.9
          nontraffic V56.3
          while boarding or alighting V56.4
        bus (traffic) V54.9
          nontraffic V54.3
          while boarding or alighting V54.4
        car (traffic) V53.9
          nontraffic V53.3
          while boarding or alighting V53.4
        motor vehicle NOS (traffic) V59.60
          nontraffic V59.20
          specified type NEC (traffic) V59.69
            nontraffic V59.29
        pedal cycle (traffic) V51.9
          nontraffic V51.3
          while boarding or alighting V51.4
        pickup truck (traffic) V53.9
          nontraffic V53.3
          while boarding or alighting V53.4
        railway vehicle (traffic) V55.9
          nontraffic V55.3
          while boarding or alighting V55.4
        specified vehicle NEC (traffic) V56.9
          nontraffic V56.3
          while boarding or alighting V56.4
        stationary object (traffic) V57.9
          nontraffic V57.3
          while boarding or alighting V57.4
        streetcar (traffic) V56.9
          nontraffic V56.3
          while boarding or alighting V56.4
        three wheeled motor vehicle (traffic) V52.9
          nontraffic V52.3
          while boarding or alighting V52.4
        truck (traffic) V54.9
          nontraffic V54.3
          while boarding or alighting V54.4
        two wheeled motor vehicle (traffic) V52.9
          nontraffic V52.3
          while boarding or alighting V52.4
        van (traffic) V53.9
          nontraffic V53.3
          while boarding or alighting V53.4
    driver
      collision (with)
        animal (traffic) V50.5
          being ridden (traffic) V56.5
            nontraffic V56.0
          nontraffic V50.0

▶ New   ⇒ Revised   ~~deleted~~ Deleted   ● Use Additional Character(s)

Accident *(Continued)*
  transport *(Continued)*
    pickup truck occupant *(Continued)*
      driver *(Continued)*
        collision *(Continued)*
          animal-drawn vehicle (traffic)
            V56.5
            nontraffic V56.0
          bus (traffic) V54.5
            nontraffic V54.0
          car (traffic) V53.5
            nontraffic V53.0
          motor vehicle NOS (traffic) V59.40
            nontraffic V59.00
            specified type NEC (traffic)
              V59.49
            nontraffic V59.09
          pedal cycle (traffic) V51.5
            nontraffic V51.0
          pickup truck (traffic) V53.5
            nontraffic V53.0
          railway vehicle (traffic) V55.5
            nontraffic V55.0
          specified vehicle NEC (traffic) V56.5
            nontraffic V56.0
          stationary object (traffic) V57.5
            nontraffic V57.0
          streetcar (traffic) V56.5
            nontraffic V56.0
          three wheeled motor vehicle
            (traffic) V52.5
            nontraffic V52.0
          truck (traffic) V54.5
            nontraffic V54.0
          two wheeled motor vehicle (traffic)
            V52.5
            nontraffic V52.0
          van (traffic) V53.5
            nontraffic V53.0
        noncollision accident (traffic) V58.5
          nontraffic V58.0
      hanger-on
        collision (with)
          animal (traffic) V50.7
            being ridden (traffic) V56.7
              nontraffic V56.2
            nontraffic V50.2
          animal-drawn vehicle (traffic) V56.7
            nontraffic V56.2
          bus (traffic) V54.7
            nontraffic V54.2
          car (traffic) V53.7
            nontraffic V53.2
          pedal cycle (traffic) V51.7
            nontraffic V51.2
          pickup truck (traffic) V53.7
            nontraffic V53.2
          railway vehicle (traffic) V55.7
            nontraffic V55.2
          specified vehicle NEC (traffic) V56.7
            nontraffic V56.2
          stationary object (traffic) V57.7
            nontraffic V57.2
          streetcar (traffic) V56.7
            nontraffic V56.2
          three wheeled motor vehicle
            (traffic) V52.7
            nontraffic V52.2
          truck (traffic) V54.7
            nontraffic V54.2
          two wheeled motor vehicle (traffic)
            V52.7
            nontraffic V52.2
          van (traffic) V53.7
            nontraffic V53.2
        noncollision accident (traffic) V58.7
          nontraffic V58.2
      noncollision accident (traffic) V58.9
        nontraffic V58.3
        while boarding or alighting V58.4
      nontraffic V59.3

Accident *(Continued)*
  transport *(Continued)*
    pickup truck occupant *(Continued)*
      passenger
        collision (with)
          animal (traffic) V50.6
            being ridden (traffic) V56.6
              nontraffic V56.1
            nontraffic V50.1
          animal-drawn vehicle (traffic)
            V56.6
            nontraffic V56.1
          bus (traffic) V54.6
            nontraffic V54.1
          car (traffic) V53.6
            nontraffic V53.1
          motor vehicle NOS (traffic) V59.50
            nontraffic V59.10
            specified type NEC (traffic)
              V59.59
            nontraffic V59.19
          pedal cycle (traffic) V51.6
            nontraffic V51.1
          pickup truck (traffic) V53.6
            nontraffic V53.1
          railway vehicle (traffic) V55.6
            nontraffic V55.1
          specified vehicle NEC (traffic) V56.6
            nontraffic V56.1
          stationary object (traffic) V57.6
            nontraffic V57.1
          streetcar (traffic) V56.6
            nontraffic V56.1
          three wheeled motor vehicle
            (traffic) V52.6
            nontraffic V52.1
          truck (traffic) V54.6
            nontraffic V54.1
          two wheeled motor vehicle (traffic)
            V52.6
            nontraffic V52.1
          van (traffic) V53.6
            nontraffic V53.1
        noncollision accident (traffic) V58.6
          nontraffic V58.1
      specified type NEC V59.88
        military vehicle V59.81
    quarry truck —*see* Accident, transport,
        industrial vehicle occupant
    race car —*see* Accident, transport, motor
        vehicle NEC occupant
    railway vehicle occupant V81.9
      collision (with) V81.3
        motor vehicle (non-military) (traffic)
          V81.1
        military V81.83
        nontraffic V81.0
        rolling stock V81.2
        specified object NEC V81.3
      during derailment V81.7
        with antecedent collision —*see*
            Accident, transport, railway
            vehicle occupant, collision
      explosion V81.81
      fall (in railway vehicle) V81.5
        during derailment V81.7
          with antecedent collision —*see*
              Accident, transport, railway
              vehicle occupant, collision
        from railway vehicle V81.6
          during derailment V81.7
            with antecedent collision —*see*
                Accident, transport,
                railway vehicle occupant,
                collision
        while boarding or alighting V81.4
      fire V81.81
      object falling onto train V81.82
      specified type NEC V81.89
      while boarding or alighting V81.4
    ski lift V98.3

Accident *(Continued)*
  transport *(Continued)*
    snowmobile occupant (nontraffic)
        V86.92
      driver V86.52
      hanger-on V86.72
      passenger V86.62
      traffic V86.32
        driver V86.02
        hanger-on V86.22
        passenger V86.12
      while boarding or alighting V86.42
      specified NEC V98.8
    sport utility vehicle occupant —*see also*
        Accident, transport, pickup truck
        occupant
    streetcar occupant V82.9
      collision (with) V82.3
        motor vehicle (traffic) V82.1
          nontraffic V82.0
        rolling stock V82.2
      during derailment V82.7
        with antecedent collision —*see*
            Accident, transport, streetcar
            occupant, collision
      fall (in streetcar) V82.5
        during derailment V82.7
          with antecedent collision —*see*
              Accident, transport, streetcar
              occupant, collision
        from streetcar V82.6
          during derailment V82.7
            with antecedent collision —*see*
                Accident, transport, streetcar
                occupant, collision
          while boarding or alighting
            V82.4
        while boarding or alighting V82.4
      specified type NEC V82.8
      while boarding or alighting V82.4
    three-wheeled motor vehicle occupant
        V39.9
      collision (with)
        animal (traffic) V30.9
          being ridden (traffic) V36.9
            nontraffic V36.3
            while boarding or alighting
              V36.4
          nontraffic V30.3
          while boarding or alighting
            V30.4
        animal-drawn vehicle (traffic)
          V36.9
          nontraffic V36.3
          while boarding or alighting
            V36.4
        bus (traffic) V34.9
          nontraffic V34.3
          while boarding or alighting
            V34.4
        car (traffic) V33.9
          nontraffic V33.3
          while boarding or alighting
            V33.4
        motor vehicle NOS (traffic) V39.60
          nontraffic V39.20
          specified type NEC (traffic)
            V39.69
          nontraffic V39.29
        pedal cycle (traffic) V31.9
          nontraffic V31.3
          while boarding or alighting
            V31.4
        pickup truck (traffic) V33.9
          nontraffic V33.3
          while boarding or alighting
            V33.4
        railway vehicle (traffic) V35.9
          nontraffic V35.3
          while boarding or alighting
            V35.4

A

Accident *(Continued)*
  transport *(Continued)*
    three-wheeled motor vehicle occupant
      (Continued)
      collision *(Continued)*
        specified vehicle NEC (traffic) V36.9
          nontraffic V36.3
          while boarding or alighting V36.4
        stationary object (traffic) V37.9
          nontraffic V37.3
          while boarding or alighting V37.4
        streetcar (traffic) V36.9
          nontraffic V36.3
          while boarding or alighting V36.4
        three wheeled motor vehicle (traffic)
          V32.9
          nontraffic V32.3
          while boarding or alighting V32.4
        truck (traffic) V34.9
          nontraffic V34.3
          while boarding or alighting V34.4
        two wheeled motor vehicle (traffic)
          V32.9
          nontraffic V32.3
          while boarding or alighting V32.4
        van (traffic) V33.9
          nontraffic V33.3
          while boarding or alighting V33.4
      driver
        collision (with)
          animal (traffic) V30.5
            being ridden (traffic) V36.5
              nontraffic V36.0
            nontraffic V30.0
          animal-drawn vehicle (traffic) V36.5
            nontraffic V36.0
          bus (traffic) V34.5
            nontraffic V34.0
          car (traffic) V33.5
            nontraffic V33.0
          motor vehicle NOS (traffic) V39.40
            nontraffic V39.00
            specified type NEC (traffic)
              V39.49
              nontraffic V39.09
          pedal cycle (traffic) V31.5
            nontraffic V31.0
          pickup truck (traffic) V33.5
            nontraffic V33.0
          railway vehicle (traffic) V35.5
            nontraffic V35.0
          specified vehicle NEC (traffic) V36.5
            nontraffic V36.0
          stationary object (traffic) V37.5
            nontraffic V37.0
          streetcar (traffic) V36.5
            nontraffic V36.0
          three wheeled motor vehicle
            (traffic) V32.5
            nontraffic V32.0
          truck (traffic) V34.5
            nontraffic V34.0
          two wheeled motor vehicle (traffic)
            V32.5
            nontraffic V32.0
          van (traffic) V33.5
            nontraffic V33.0
        noncollision accident (traffic) V38.5
          nontraffic V38.0
      hanger-on
        collision (with)
          animal (traffic) V30.7
            being ridden (traffic) V36.7
              nontraffic V36.2
            nontraffic V30.2
          animal-drawn vehicle (traffic) V36.7
            nontraffic V36.2
          bus (traffic) V34.7
            nontraffic V34.2
          car (traffic) V33.7
            nontraffic V33.2

Accident *(Continued)*
  transport *(Continued)*
    three-wheeled motor vehicle occupant
      (Continued)
      hanger-on *(Continued)*
        collision *(Continued)*
          pedal cycle (traffic) V31.7
            nontraffic V31.2
          pickup truck (traffic) V33.7
            nontraffic V33.2
          railway vehicle (traffic) V35.7
            nontraffic V35.2
          specified vehicle NEC (traffic) V36.7
            nontraffic V36.2
          stationary object (traffic) V37.7
            nontraffic V37.2
          streetcar (traffic) V36.7
            nontraffic V36.2
          three wheeled motor vehicle
            (traffic) V32.7
            nontraffic V32.2
          truck (traffic) V34.7
            nontraffic V34.2
          two wheeled motor vehicle (traffic)
            V32.7
            nontraffic V32.2
          van (traffic) V33.7
            nontraffic V33.2
        noncollision accident (traffic) V38.7
          nontraffic V38.2
      noncollision accident (traffic) V38.9
        nontraffic V38.3
        while boarding or alighting V38.4
      nontraffic V39.3
      passenger
        collision (with)
          animal (traffic) V30.6
            being ridden (traffic) V36.6
              nontraffic V36.1
            nontraffic V30.1
          animal-drawn vehicle (traffic) V36.6
            nontraffic V36.1
          bus (traffic) V34.6
            nontraffic V34.1
          car (traffic) V33.6
            nontraffic V33.1
          motor vehicle NOS (traffic) V39.50
            nontraffic V39.10
            specified type NEC (traffic)
              V39.59
              nontraffic V39.19
          pedal cycle (traffic) V31.6
            nontraffic V31.1
          pickup truck (traffic) V33.6
            nontraffic V33.1
          railway vehicle (traffic) V35.6
            nontraffic V35.1
          specified vehicle NEC (traffic)
            V36.6
            nontraffic V36.1
          stationary object (traffic) V37.6
            nontraffic V37.1
          streetcar (traffic) V36.6
            nontraffic V36.1
          three wheeled motor vehicle
            (traffic) V32.6
            nontraffic V32.1
          truck (traffic) V34.6
            nontraffic V34.1
          two wheeled motor vehicle (traffic)
            V32.6
            nontraffic V32.1
          van (traffic) V33.6
            nontraffic V33.1
        noncollision accident (traffic) V38.6
          nontraffic V38.1
      specified type NEC V39.89
        military vehicle V39.81
      tractor (farm) (and trailer) —*see* Accident,
        transport, agricultural vehicle
        occupant

Accident *(Continued)*
  transport *(Continued)*
    tram —*see* Accident, transport, streetcar
      in mine or quarry —*see* Accident,
        transport, industrial vehicle
        occupant
    trolley —*see* Accident, transport, streetcar
      in mine or quarry —*see* Accident,
        transport, industrial vehicle
        occupant
    truck (heavy) occupant V69.9
      collision (with)
        animal (traffic) V60.9
          being ridden (traffic) V66.9
            nontraffic V66.3
              while boarding or alighting V66.4
          nontraffic V60.3
          while boarding or alighting V60.4
        animal-drawn vehicle (traffic) V66.9
          nontraffic V66.3
          while boarding or alighting V66.4
        bus (traffic) V64.9
          nontraffic V64.3
          while boarding or alighting V64.4
        car (traffic) V63.9
          nontraffic V63.3
          while boarding or alighting V63.4
        motor vehicle NOS (traffic) V69.60
          nontraffic V69.20
          specified type NEC (traffic) V69.69
            nontraffic V69.29
        pedal cycle (traffic) V61.9
          nontraffic V61.3
          while boarding or alighting V61.4
        pickup truck (traffic) V63.9
          nontraffic V63.3
          while boarding or alighting V63.4
        railway vehicle (traffic) V65.9
          nontraffic V65.3
          while boarding or alighting V65.4
        specified vehicle NEC (traffic) V66.9
          nontraffic V66.3
          while boarding or alighting V66.4
        stationary object (traffic) V67.9
          nontraffic V67.3
          while boarding or alighting V67.4
        streetcar (traffic) V66.9
          nontraffic V66.3
          while boarding or alighting V66.4
        three wheeled motor vehicle (traffic)
          V62.9
          nontraffic V62.3
          while boarding or alighting V62.4
        truck (traffic) V64.9
          nontraffic V64.3
          while boarding or alighting V64.4
        two wheeled motor vehicle (traffic)
          V62.9
          nontraffic V62.3
          while boarding or alighting V62.4
        van (traffic) V63.9
          nontraffic V63.3
          while boarding or alighting V63.4
      driver
        collision (with)
          animal (traffic) V60.5
            being ridden (traffic) V66.5
              nontraffic V66.0
            nontraffic V60.0
          animal-drawn vehicle (traffic)
            V66.5
            nontraffic V66.0
          bus (traffic) V64.5
            nontraffic V64.0
          car (traffic) V63.5
            nontraffic V63.0
          motor vehicle NOS (traffic) V69.40
            nontraffic V69.00
            specified type NEC (traffic)
              V69.49
              nontraffic V69.09

▶ New   ⇒ Revised   ~~deleted~~ Deleted   ● Use Additional Character(s)

Accident *(Continued)*
  transport *(Continued)*
    truck occupant *(Continued)*
      driver *(Continued)*
        collision *(Continued)*
          pedal cycle (traffic) V61.5
            nontraffic V61.0
          pickup truck (traffic) V63.5
            nontraffic V63.0
          railway vehicle (traffic) V65.5
            nontraffic V65.0
          specified vehicle NEC (traffic) V66.5
            nontraffic V66.0
          stationary object (traffic) V67.5
            nontraffic V67.0
          streetcar (traffic) V66.5
            nontraffic V66.0
          three wheeled motor vehicle
            (traffic) V62.5
            nontraffic V62.0
          truck (traffic) V64.5
            nontraffic V64.0
          two wheeled motor vehicle (traffic)
            V62.5
            nontraffic V62.0
          van (traffic) V63.5
            nontraffic V63.0
        noncollision accident (traffic) V68.5
          nontraffic V68.0
      dump —*see* Accident, transport,
        construction vehicle occupant
      hanger-on
        collision (with)
          animal (traffic) V60.7
            being ridden (traffic) V66.7
              nontraffic V66.2
            nontraffic V60.2
          animal-drawn vehicle (traffic) V66.7
            nontraffic V66.2
          bus (traffic) V64.7
            nontraffic V64.2
          car (traffic) V63.7
            nontraffic V63.2
          pedal cycle (traffic) V61.7
            nontraffic V61.2
          pickup truck (traffic) V63.7
            nontraffic V63.2
          railway vehicle (traffic) V65.7
            nontraffic V65.2
          specified vehicle NEC (traffic) V66.7
            nontraffic V66.2
          stationary object (traffic) V67.7
            nontraffic V67.2
          streetcar (traffic) V66.7
            nontraffic V66.2
          three wheeled motor vehicle
            (traffic) V62.7
            nontraffic V62.2
          truck (traffic) V64.7
            nontraffic V64.2
          two wheeled motor vehicle (traffic)
            V62.7
            nontraffic V62.2
          van (traffic) V63.7
            nontraffic V63.2
        noncollision accident (traffic) V68.7
          nontraffic V68.2
      noncollision accident (traffic) V68.9
        nontraffic V68.3
        while boarding or alighting V68.4
      nontraffic V69.3
      passenger
        collision (with)
          animal (traffic) V60.6
            being ridden (traffic) V66.6
              nontraffic V66.1
            nontraffic V60.1
          animal-drawn vehicle (traffic) V66.6
            nontraffic V66.1
          bus (traffic) V64.6
            nontraffic V64.1

Accident *(Continued)*
  transport *(Continued)*
    truck occupant *(Continued)*
      passenger *(Continued)*
        collision *(Continued)*
          car (traffic) V63.6
            nontraffic V63.1
          motor vehicle NOS (traffic) V69.50
            nontraffic V69.10
            specified type NEC (traffic)
              V69.59
              nontraffic V69.19
          pedal cycle (traffic) V61.6
            nontraffic V61.1
          pickup truck (traffic) V63.6
            nontraffic V63.1
          railway vehicle (traffic) V65.6
            nontraffic V65.1
          specified vehicle NEC (traffic)
            V66.6
            nontraffic V66.1
          stationary object (traffic) V67.6
            nontraffic V67.1
          streetcar (traffic) V66.6
            nontraffic V66.1
          three wheeled motor vehicle
            (traffic) V62.6
            nontraffic V62.1
          truck (traffic) V64.6
            nontraffic V64.1
          two wheeled motor vehicle (traffic)
            V62.6
            nontraffic V62.1
          van (traffic) V63.6
            nontraffic V63.1
        noncollision accident (traffic) V68.6
          nontraffic V68.1
      pickup —*see* Accident, transport, pickup
        truck occupant
      specified type NEC V69.88
      military vehicle V69.81
    van occupant V59.9
      collision (with)
        animal (traffic) V50.9
          being ridden (traffic) V56.9
            nontraffic V56.3
            while boarding or alighting
              V56.4
          nontraffic V50.3
          while boarding or alighting V50.4
        animal-drawn vehicle (traffic) V56.9
          nontraffic V56.3
          while boarding or alighting V56.4
        bus (traffic) V54.9
          nontraffic V54.3
          while boarding or alighting V54.4
        car (traffic) V53.9
          nontraffic V53.3
          while boarding or alighting V53.4
        motor vehicle NOS (traffic) V59.60
          nontraffic V59.20
          specified type NEC (traffic) V59.69
            nontraffic V59.29
        pedal cycle (traffic) V51.9
          nontraffic V51.3
          while boarding or alighting V51.4
        pickup truck (traffic) V53.9
          nontraffic V53.3
          while boarding or alighting V53.4
        railway vehicle (traffic) V55.9
          nontraffic V55.3
          while boarding or alighting V55.4
        specified vehicle NEC (traffic) V56.9
          nontraffic V56.3
          while boarding or alighting V56.4
        stationary object (traffic) V57.9
          nontraffic V57.3
          while boarding or alighting V57.4
        streetcar (traffic) V56.9
          nontraffic V56.3
          while boarding or alighting V56.4

Accident *(Continued)*
  transport *(Continued)*
    van occupant *(Continued)*
      collision *(Continued)*
        three wheeled motor vehicle (traffic)
          V52.9
          nontraffic V52.3
          while boarding or alighting V52.4
        truck (traffic) V54.9
          nontraffic V54.3
          while boarding or alighting V54.4
        two wheeled motor vehicle (traffic)
          V52.9
          nontraffic V52.3
          while boarding or alighting V52.4
        van (traffic) V53.9
          nontraffic V53.3
          while boarding or alighting V53.4
      driver
        collision (with)
          animal (traffic) V50.5
            being ridden (traffic) V56.5
              nontraffic V56.0
            nontraffic V50.0
          animal-drawn vehicle (traffic) V56.5
            nontraffic V56.0
          bus (traffic) V54.5
            nontraffic V54.0
          car (traffic) V53.5
            nontraffic V53.0
          motor vehicle NOS (traffic) V59.40
            nontraffic V59.00
            specified type NEC (traffic)
              V59.49
              nontraffic V59.09
          pedal cycle (traffic) V51.5
            nontraffic V51.0
          pickup truck (traffic) V53.5
            nontraffic V53.0
          railway vehicle (traffic) V55.5
            nontraffic V55.0
          specified vehicle NEC (traffic) V56.5
            nontraffic V56.0
          stationary object (traffic) V57.5
            nontraffic V57.0
          streetcar (traffic) V56.5
            nontraffic V56.0
          three wheeled motor vehicle
            (traffic) V52.5
            nontraffic V52.0
          truck (traffic) V54.5
            nontraffic V54.0
          two wheeled motor vehicle (traffic)
            V52.5
            nontraffic V52.0
          van (traffic) V53.5
            nontraffic V53.0
        noncollision accident (traffic) V58.5
          nontraffic V58.0
      hanger-on
        collision (with)
          animal (traffic) V50.7
            being ridden (traffic) V56.7
              nontraffic V56.2
            nontraffic V50.2
          animal-drawn vehicle (traffic) V56.7
            nontraffic V56.2
          bus (traffic) V54.7
            nontraffic V54.2
          car (traffic) V53.7
            nontraffic V53.2
          pedal cycle (traffic) V51.7
            nontraffic V51.2
          pickup truck (traffic) V53.7
            nontraffic V53.2
          railway vehicle (traffic) V55.7
            nontraffic V55.2
          specified vehicle NEC (traffic) V56.7
            nontraffic V56.2
          stationary object (traffic) V57.7
            nontraffic V57.2

A

Accident (Continued)
  transport (Continued)
    van occupant (Continued)
      hanger-on (Continued)
        collision (Continued)
          streetcar (traffic) V56.7
            nontraffic V56.2
          three wheeled motor vehicle
              (traffic) V52.7
            nontraffic V52.2
          truck (traffic) V54.7
            nontraffic V54.2
          two wheeled motor vehicle (traffic)
              V52.7
            nontraffic V52.2
          van (traffic) V53.7
            nontraffic V53.2
        noncollision accident (traffic) V58.7
          nontraffic V58.2
      noncollision accident (traffic) V58.9
        nontraffic V58.3
        while boarding or alighting V58.4
      nontraffic V59.3
      passenger
        collision (with)
          animal (traffic) V50.6
            being ridden (traffic) V56.6
              nontraffic V56.1
            nontraffic V50.1
          animal-drawn vehicle (traffic) V56.6
            nontraffic V56.1
          bus (traffic) V54.6
            nontraffic V54.1
          car (traffic) V53.6
            nontraffic V53.1
          motor vehicle NOS (traffic) V59.50
            nontraffic V59.10
            specified type NEC (traffic) V59.59
              nontraffic V59.19
          pedal cycle (traffic) V51.6
            nontraffic V51.1
          pickup truck (traffic) V53.6
            nontraffic V53.1
          railway vehicle (traffic) V55.6
            nontraffic V55.1
          specified vehicle NEC (traffic) V56.6
            nontraffic V56.1
          stationary object (traffic) V57.6
            nontraffic V57.1
          streetcar (traffic) V56.6
            nontraffic V56.1
          three wheeled motor vehicle
              (traffic) V52.6
            nontraffic V52.1
          truck (traffic) V54.6
            nontraffic V54.1
          two wheeled motor vehicle (traffic)
              V52.6
            nontraffic V52.1
          van (traffic) V53.6
            nontraffic V53.1
        noncollision accident (traffic) V58.6
          nontraffic V58.1
      specified type NEC V59.88
      military vehicle V59.81
    watercraft occupant —see Accident,
        watercraft
  vehicle NEC V89.9
    animal-drawn NEC —see Accident,
        transport, animal-drawn vehicle
        occupant
    special
      agricultural —see Accident, transport,
          agricultural vehicle occupant
      construction —see Accident, transport,
          construction vehicle occupant
      industrial —see Accident, transport,
          industrial vehicle occupant
      three-wheeled NEC (motorized) —see
          Accident, transport, three-wheeled
          motor vehicle occupant

Accident (Continued)
  watercraft V94.9
    causing
      drowning —see Drowning, due to,
          accident to, watercraft
      injury NEC V91.89
        crushed between craft and object
            V91.19
          powered craft V91.13
            ferry boat V91.11
            fishing boat V91.12
            jetskis V91.13
            liner V91.11
            merchant ship V91.10
            passenger ship V91.11
          unpowered craft V91.18
            canoe V91.15
            inflatable V91.16
            kayak V91.15
            sailboat V91.14
            surf-board V91.18
            windsurfer V91.18
        fall on board V91.29
          powered craft V91.23
            ferry boat V91.21
            fishing boat V91.22
            jetskis V91.23
            liner V91.21
            merchant ship V91.20
            passenger ship V91.21
          unpowered craft
            canoe V91.25
            inflatable V91.26
            kayak V91.25
            sailboat V91.24
        fire on board causing burn V91.09
          powered craft V91.03
            ferry boat V91.01
            fishing boat V91.02
            jetskis V91.03
            liner V91.01
            merchant ship V91.00
            passenger ship V91.01
          unpowered craft V91.08
            canoe V91.05
            inflatable V91.06
            kayak V91.05
            sailboat V91.04
            surf-board V91.08
            water skis V91.07
            windsurfer V91.08
        hit by falling object V91.39
          powered craft V91.33
            ferry boat V91.31
            fishing boat V91.32
            jetskis V91.33
            liner V91.31
            merchant ship V91.30
            passenger ship V91.31
          unpowered craft V91.38
            canoe V91.35
            inflatable V91.36
            kayak V91.35
            sailboat V91.34
            surf-board V91.38
            water skis V91.37
            windsurfer V91.38
        specified type NEC V91.89
          powered craft V91.83
            ferry boat V91.81
            fishing boat V91.82
            jetskis V91.83
            liner V91.81
            merchant ship V91.80
            passenger ship V91.81
          unpowered craft V91.88
            canoe V91.85
            inflatable V91.86
            kayak V91.85
            sailboat V91.84
            surf-board V91.88

Accident (Continued)
  watercraft (Continued)
    causing (Continued)
      injury NEC (Continued)
        specified type NEC (Continued)
          unpowered craft (Continued)
            water skis V91.87
            windsurfer V91.88
    due to, caused by cataclysm —see Forces of
        nature, by type
    military NEC V94.818
      with civilian watercraft V94.810
      civilian in water injured by V94.811
    nonpowered, struck by
        nonpowered vessel V94.22
        powered vessel V94.21
    specified type NEC V94.89
    striking swimmer
      powered V94.11
      unpowered V94.12
Acid throwing (assault) Y08.89
Activity (involving) (of victim at time of event)
    Y93.9
  aerobic and step exercise (class) Y93.A3
  alpine skiing Y93.23
  animal care NEC Y93.K9
  arts and handcrafts NEC Y93.D9
  athletics NEC Y93.79
  athletics played as a team or group NEC
      Y93.69
  athletics played individually NEC Y93.59
  baking Y93.G3
  ballet Y93.41
  barbells Y93.B3
  BASE (Building, Antenna, Span, Earth)
      jumping Y93.33
  baseball Y93.64
  basketball Y93.67
  bathing (personal) Y93.E1
  beach volleyball Y93.68
  bike riding Y93.55
  blackout game Y93.85
  boogie boarding Y93.18
  bowling Y93.54
  boxing Y93.71
  brass instrument playing Y93.J4
  building construction Y93.H3
  bungee jumping Y93.34
  calisthenics Y93.A2
  canoeing (in calm and turbulent water) Y93.16
  capture the flag Y93.6A
  cardiorespiratory exercise NEC Y93.A9
  caregiving (providing) NEC Y93.F9
    bathing Y93.F1
    lifting Y93.F2
  cellular
    communication device Y93.C2
    telephone Y93.C2
  challenge course Y93.A5
  cheerleading Y93.45
  choking game Y93.85
  circuit training Y93.A4
  cleaning
    floor Y93.E5
  climbing NEC Y93.39
    mountain Y93.31
    rock Y93.31
    wall Y93.31
  clothing care and maintenance NEC Y93.E9
  combatives Y93.75
  computer
    keyboarding Y93.C1
    technology NEC Y93.C9
  confidence course Y93.A5
  construction (building) Y93.H3
  cooking and baking Y93.G3
  cool down exercises Y93.A2
  cricket Y93.69
  crocheting Y93.D1
  cross country skiing Y93.24
  dancing (all types) Y93.41

▶ New   ➡ Revised   ~~deleted~~ Deleted   ● Use Additional Character(s)

Activity (Continued)

digging
  dirt Y93.H1
dirt digging Y93.H1
dishwashing Y93.G1
diving (platform) (springboard) Y93.12
  underwater Y93.15
dodge ball Y93.6A
downhill skiing Y93.23
drum playing Y93.J2
dumbbells Y93.B3
electronic
  devices NEC Y93.C9
    hand held interactive Y93.C2
  game playing (using) (with)
    interactive device Y93.C2
    keyboard or other stationary device
      Y93.C1
elliptical machine Y93.A1
exercise(s)
  machines ((primarily) for)
    cardiorespiratory conditioning Y93.A1
    muscle strengthening Y93.B1
  muscle strengthening (non-machine) NEC
    Y93.B9
external motion NEC Y93.I9
  rollercoaster Y93.I1
fainting game Y93.85
field hockey Y93.65
figure skating (pairs) (singles) Y93.21
flag football Y93.62
floor mopping and cleaning Y93.E5
food preparation and clean up Y93.G1
football (American) NOS Y93.61
  flag Y93.62
  tackle Y93.61
  touch Y93.62
four square Y93.6A
free weights Y93.B3
frisbee (ultimate) Y93.74
furniture
  building Y93.D3
  finishing Y93.D3
  repair Y93.D3
game playing (electronic)
  using interactive device Y93.C2
  using keyboard or other stationary device
    Y93.C1
gardening Y93.H2
golf Y93.53
grass drills Y93.A6
grilling and smoking food Y93.G2
grooming and shearing an animal Y93.K3
guerilla drills Y93.A6
gymnastics (rhythmic) Y93.43
hand held interactive electronic device Y93.C2
handball Y93.73
handcrafts NEC Y93.D9
hang gliding Y93.35
hiking (on level or elevated terrain) Y93.01
hockey (ice) Y93.22
  field Y93.65
horseback riding Y93.52
household (interior) maintenance NEC Y93.
  E9
ice NEC Y93.29
  dancing Y93.21
  hockey Y93.22
  skating Y93.21
inline roller skating Y93.51
ironing Y93.E4
judo Y93.75
jumping (off) NEC Y93.39
  BASE (Building, Antenna, Span, Earth)
    Y93.33
  bungee Y93.34
  jacks Y93.A2
  rope Y93.56
jumping jacks Y93.A2
jumping rope Y93.56
karate Y93.75

kayaking (in calm and turbulent water) Y93.16
keyboarding (computer) Y93.C1
kickball Y93.6A
knitting Y93.D1
lacrosse Y93.65
land maintenance NEC Y93.H9
landscaping Y93.H2
laundry Y93.E2
machines (exercise)
  primarily for cardiorespiratory
    conditioning Y93.A1
  primarily for muscle strengthening Y93.B1
maintenance
  exterior building NEC Y93.H9
  household (interior) NEC Y93.E9
  land Y93.H9
  property Y93.H9
marching (on level or elevated terrain) Y93.01
martial arts Y93.75
microwave oven Y93.G3
milking an animal Y93.K2
mopping (floor) Y93.E5
mountain climbing Y93.31
muscle strengthening
  exercises (non-machine) NEC Y93.B9
  machines Y93.B1
musical keyboard (electronic) playing Y93.J1
nordic skiing Y93.24
obstacle course Y93.A5
oven (microwave) Y93.G3
packing up and unpacking in moving to a
  new residence Y93.E6
parasailing Y93.19
pass out game Y93.85
percussion instrument playing NEC Y93.J2
personal
  bathing and showering Y93.E1
  hygiene NEC Y93.E8
  showering Y93.E1
physical games generally associated with
  school recess, summer camp and
  children Y93.6A
physical training NEC Y93.A9
piano playing Y93.J1
pilates Y93.B4
platform diving Y93.12
playing musical instrument
  brass instrument Y93.J4
  drum Y93.J2
  musical keyboard (electronic) Y93.J1
  percussion instrument NEC Y93.J2
  piano Y93.J1
  string instrument Y93.J3
  winds instrument Y93.J4
property maintenance
  exterior NEC Y93.H9
  interior NEC Y93.E9
pruning (garden and lawn) Y93.H2
pull-ups Y93.B2
push-ups Y93.B2
racquetball Y93.73
rafting (in calm and turbulent water) Y93.16
raking (leaves) Y93.H1
rappelling Y93.32
refereeing a sports activity Y93.81
residential relocation Y93.E6
rhythmic gymnastics Y93.43
rhythmic movement NEC Y93.49
riding
  horseback Y93.52
  rollercoaster Y93.I1
rock climbing Y93.31
roller skating (inline) Y93.51
rollercoaster riding Y93.I1
rough housing and horseplay Y93.83
rowing (in calm and turbulent water)
  Y93.16
rugby Y93.63
SCUBA diving Y93.15
sewing Y93.D2

shoveling Y93.H1
  dirt Y93.H1
  snow Y93.H1
showering (personal) Y93.E1
sit-ups Y93.B2
skateboarding Y93.51
skating (ice) Y93.21
  roller Y93.51
skiing (alpine) (downhill) Y93.23
  cross country Y93.24
  nordic Y93.24
  water Y93.17
sledding (snow) Y93.23
sleeping (sleep) Y93.84
smoking and grilling food Y93.G2
snorkeling Y93.15
snow NEC Y93.29
  boarding Y93.23
  shoveling Y93.H1
  sledding Y93.23
  tubing Y93.23
soccer Y93.66
softball Y93.64
specified NEC Y93.89
spectator at an event Y93.82
sports NEC Y93.79
  sports played as a team or group NEC
    Y93.69
  sports played individually NEC Y93.59
springboard diving Y93.12
squash Y93.73
stationary bike Y93.A1
step (stepping) exercise (class) Y93.A3
stepper machine Y93.A1
stove Y93.G3
string instrument playing Y93.J3
surfing Y93.18
  wind Y93.18
swimming Y93.11
tackle football Y93.61
tap dancing Y93.41
tennis Y93.73
tobogganing Y93.23
touch football Y93.62
track and field events (non-running) Y93.57
  running Y93.02
trampoline Y93.44
treadmill Y93.A1
trimming shrubs Y93.H2
tubing (in calm and turbulent water) Y93.16
  snow Y93.23
ultimate frisbee Y93.74
underwater diving Y93.15
unpacking in moving to a new residence
  Y93.E6
use of stove, oven and microwave oven Y93.
  G3
vacuuming Y93.E3
volleyball (beach) (court) Y93.68
wake boarding Y93.17
walking (on level or elevated terrain) Y93.01
  an animal Y93.K1
walking an animal Y93.K1
wall climbing Y93.31
warm up and cool down exercises Y93.A2
water NEC Y93.19
  aerobics Y93.14
  craft NEC Y93.19
  exercise Y93.14
  polo Y93.13
  skiing Y93.17
  sliding Y93.18
  survival training and testing Y93.19
weeding (garden and lawn) Y93.H2
wind instrument playing Y93.J4
windsurfing Y93.18
wrestling Y93.72
yoga Y93.42
Adverse effect of drugs —see Table of Drugs
  and Chemicals

A

Aerosinusitis —*see* Air, pressure
After-effect, late —*see* Sequelae
Air
  blast in war operations —*see* War operations, air blast
  pressure
    change, rapid
      during
        ascent W94.29
          while (in) (surfacing from)
            aircraft W94.23
            deep water diving W94.21
            underground W94.22
        descent W94.39
          in
            aircraft W94.31
            water W94.32
      high, prolonged W94.0
      low, prolonged W94.12
      due to residence or long visit at high altitude W94.11
Alpine sickness W94.11
Altitude sickness W94.11
Anaphylactic shock, anaphylaxis —*see* Table of Drugs and Chemicals
Andes disease W94.11
Arachnidism, arachnoidism X58
Arson (with intent to injure or kill) X97
Asphyxia, asphyxiation
  by
    food (bone) (seed) —*see* categories T17 and T18
    gas —*see also* Table of Drugs and Chemicals
      legal
        execution —*see* Legal, intervention, gas
        intervention —*see* Legal, intervention, gas
  from
    fire —*see also* Exposure, fire
      in war operations —*see* War operations, fire
    ignition —*see* Ignition
    vomitus T17.81
  in war operations —*see* War operations, restriction of airway
Aspiration
  food (any type) (into respiratory tract) (with asphyxia, obstruction respiratory tract, suffocation) —*see* categories T17 and T18
  foreign body —*see* Foreign body, aspiration
  vomitus (with asphyxia, obstruction respiratory tract, suffocation) T17.81
Assassination (attempt) —*see* Assault
Assault (homicidal) (by) (in) Y09
  arson X97
  bite (of human being) Y04.1
  bodily force Y04.8
    bite Y04.1
    bumping into Y04.2
    sexual —*see* subcategories T74.0, T76.0
    unarmed fight Y04.0

Assault *(Continued)*
  bomb X96.9
    antipersonnel X96.0
    fertilizer X96.3
    gasoline X96.1
    letter X96.2
    petrol X96.1
    pipe X96.3
    specified NEC X96.8
  brawl (hand) (fists) (foot) (unarmed) Y04.0
  burning, burns (by fire) NEC X97
    acid Y08.89
    caustic, corrosive substance Y08.89
    chemical from swallowing caustic, corrosive substance —*see* Table of Drugs and Chemicals
    cigarette(s) X97
    hot object X98.9
      fluid NEC X98.2
      household appliance X98.3
      specified NEC X98.8
      steam X98.0
      tap water X98.1
      vapors X98.0
    scalding —*see* Assault, burning
    steam X98.0
    vitriol Y08.89
  caustic, corrosive substance (gas) Y08.89
  crashing of
    aircraft Y08.81
    motor vehicle Y03.8
      pushed in front of Y02.0
      run over Y03.0
      specified NEC Y03.8
  cutting or piercing instrument X99.9
    dagger X99.2
    glass X99.0
    knife X99.1
    specified NEC X99.8
    sword X99.2
  dagger X99.2
  drowning (in) X92.9
    bathtub X92.0
    natural water X92.3
    specified NEC X92.8
    swimming pool X92.1
      following fall X92.2
  dynamite X96.8
  explosive(s) (material) X96.9
  fight (hand) (fists) (foot) (unarmed) Y04.0
    with weapon —*see* Assault, by type of weapon
  fire X97
  firearm X95.9
    airgun X95.01
    handgun X93
    hunting rifle X94.1
    larger X94.9
      specified NEC X94.8
    machine gun X94.2
    shotgun X94.0
    specified NEC X95.8

Assault *(Continued)*
  from high place Y01
  gunshot (wound) NEC —*see* Assault, firearm, by type
  incendiary device X97
  injury Y09
    to child due to criminal abortion attempt NEC Y08.89
  knife X99.1
  late effect of —*see* X92-Y08 with 7th character S
  placing before moving object NEC Y02.8
    motor vehicle Y02.0
  poisoning —*see* categories T36-T65 with 7th character S
  puncture, any part of body —*see* Assault, cutting or piercing instrument
  pushing
    before moving object NEC Y02.8
      motor vehicle Y02.0
      subway train Y02.1
      train Y02.1
  rape T74.2-●
  scalding —*see* Assault, burning
  sequelae of —*see* X92-Y08 with 7th character S
  sexual (by bodily force) T74.2-●
  shooting —*see* Assault, firearm
  specified means NEC Y08.89
  stab, any part of body —*see* Assault, cutting or piercing instrument
  steam X98.0
  striking against
    other person Y04.2
    sports equipment Y08.09
      baseball bat Y08.02
      hockey stick Y08.01
  struck by
    sports equipment Y08.09
      baseball bat Y08.02
      hockey stick Y08.01
  submersion —*see* Assault, drowning
  violence Y09
  weapon Y09
    blunt Y00
    cutting or piercing —*see* Assault, cutting or piercing instrument
    firearm —*see* Assault, firearm
  wound Y09
    cutting —*see* Assault, cutting or piercing instrument
    gunshot —*see* Assault, firearm
    knife X99.1
    piercing —*see* Assault, cutting or piercing instrument
    puncture —*see* Assault, cutting or piercing instrument
    stab —*see* Assault, cutting or piercing instrument
Attack by mammals NEC W55.89
Avalanche —*see* Landslide
Aviator's disease —*see* Air, pressure

▶ New   ⇒ Revised   ~~deleted~~ Deleted   ● Use Additional Character(s)

B

Barotitis, barodontalgia, barosinusitis,
  barotrauma (otitic) (sinus) —*see* Air,
  pressure
Battered (baby) (child) (person) (syndrome)
  X58
Bayonet wound W26.1
  in
    legal intervention —*see* Legal,
      intervention, sharp object,
      bayonet
    war operations —*see* War operations,
      combat
  stated as undetermined whether accidental or
    intentional Y28.8
  suicide (attempt) X78.2
Bean in nose —*see* categories T17 and T18
Bed set on fire NEC —*see* Exposure, fire,
  uncontrolled, building, bed
Beheading (by guillotine)
  homicide X99.9
  legal execution —*see* Legal, intervention
Bending, injury in (prolonged) (static) X50.1
Bends —*see* Air, pressure, change
Bite, bitten by
  alligator W58.01
  arthropod (nonvenomous) NEC W57
  bull W55.21
  cat W55.01
  cow W55.21
  crocodile W58.11
  dog W54.0
  goat W55.31
  hoof stock NEC W55.31
  horse W55.11
  human being (accidentally) W50.3
    with intent to injure or kill Y04.1
    as, or caused by, a crowd or human
      stampede (with fall) W52
    assault Y04.1
    homicide (attempt) Y04.1
    in
      fight Y04.1
  insect (nonvenomous) W57
  lizard (nonvenomous) W59.01
  mammal NEC W55.81
    marine W56.31
  marine animal (nonvenomous) W56.81
  millipede W57
  moray eel W56.51
  mouse W53.01
  person(s) (accidentally) W50.3
    with intent to injure or kill Y04.1
    as, or caused by, a crowd or human
      stampede (with fall) W52
    assault Y04.1
    homicide (attempt) Y04.1
    in
      fight Y04.1
  pig W55.41
  raccoon W55.51
  rat W53.11
  reptile W59.81
    lizard W59.01
    snake W59.11
    turtle W59.21
    terrestrial W59.81
  rodent W53.81
    mouse W53.01
    rat W53.11
    specified NEC W53.81
    squirrel W53.21
  shark W56.41
  sheep W55.31
  snake (nonvenomous) W59.11
  spider (nonvenomous) W57
  squirrel W53.21
Blast (air) in war operations —*see* War
  operations, blast
Blizzard X37.2

Blood alcohol level Y90.9
  20-39mg/100ml Y90.1
  40-59mg/100ml Y90.2
  60-79mg/100ml Y90.3
  80-99mg/100ml Y90.4
  100-119mg/100ml Y90.5
  120-199mg/100ml Y90.6
  200-239mg/100ml Y90.7
  less than 20mg/100ml Y90.0
  presence in blood, level not specified
    Y90.9
Blow X58
  by law-enforcing agent, police (on duty) —*see*
    Legal, intervention, manhandling
  blunt object —*see* Legal, intervention, blunt
    object
Blowing up —*see* Explosion
Brawl (hand) (fists) (foot) Y04.0
Breakage (accidental) (part of)
  ladder (causing fall) W11
  scaffolding (causing fall) W12
Broken
  glass, contact with —*see* Contact, with, glass
  power line (causing electric shock) W85
Bumping against, into (accidentally)
  object NEC W22.8
    with fall —*see* Fall, due to, bumping
      against, object
    caused by crowd or human stampede
      (with fall) W52
    sports equipment W21.9
  person(s) W51
    with fall W03
      due to ice or snow W00.0
    assault Y04.2
    caused by, a crowd or human stampede
      (with fall) W52
    homicide (attempt) Y04.2
  sports equipment W21.9
Burn, burned, burning (accidental) (by) (from)
  (on)
  acid NEC —*see* Table of Drugs and
    Chemicals
  bed linen —*see* Exposure, fire, uncontrolled,
    in building, bed
  blowtorch X08.8
    with ignition of clothing NEC X06.2
      nightwear X05
  bonfire, campfire (controlled) —*see also*
    Exposure, fire, controlled, not in
    building
    uncontrolled —*see* Exposure, fire,
      uncontrolled, not in building
  candle X08.8
    with ignition of clothing NEC X06.2
      nightwear X05
  caustic liquid, substance (external) (internal)
    NEC —*see* Table of Drugs and
    Chemicals
  chemical (external) (internal) —*see also* Table
    of Drugs and Chemicals
    in war operations —*see* War operations, fire
  cigar(s) or cigarette(s) X08.8
    with ignition of clothing NEC X06.2
      nightwear X05
  clothes, clothing NEC (from controlled fire)
    X06.2
    with conflagration —*see* Exposure, fire,
      uncontrolled, building
      not in building or structure —*see*
        Exposure, fire, uncontrolled, not in
        building
  cooker (hot) X15.8
    stated as undetermined whether accidental
      or intentional Y27.3
    suicide (attempt) X77.3
  electric blanket X16
  engine (hot) X17
  fire, flames —*see* Exposure, fire
  flare, Very pistol —*see* Discharge, firearm
    NEC

Burn, burned, burning (Continued)
  heat
    from appliance (electrical) (household)
      X15.8
      cooker X15.8
      hotplate X15.2
      kettle X15.8
      light bulb X15.8
      saucepan X15.3
      skillet X15.3
      stated as undetermined whether
        accidental or intentional Y27.3
      stove X15.0
      suicide (attempt) X77.3
      toaster X15.1
    in local application or packing during
      medical or surgical procedure
      Y63.5
  heating
    appliance, radiator or pipe X16
  homicide (attempt) —*see* Assault, burning
  hot
    air X14.1
    cooker X15.8
    drink X10.0
    engine X17
    fat X10.2
    fluid NEC X12
    food X10.1
    gases X14.1
    heating appliance X16
    household appliance NEC X15.8
    kettle X15.8
    liquid NEC X12
    machinery X17
    metal (molten) (liquid) NEC X18
    object (not producing fire or flames) NEC
      X19
    oil (cooking) X10.2
    pipe(s) X16
    radiator X16
    saucepan (glass) (metal) X15.3
    stove (kitchen) X15.0
    substance NEC X19
      caustic or corrosive NEC —*see* Table of
        Drugs and Chemicals
    toaster X15.1
    tool X17
    vapor X13.1
    water (tap) —*see* Contact, with, hot, tap
      water
  hotplate X15.2
    suicide (attempt) X77.3
  ignition —*see* Ignition
  in war operations —*see* War operations, fire
  inflicted by other person X97
    by hot objects, hot vapor, and steam —*see*
      Assault, burning, hot object
  internal, from swallowed caustic, corrosive
    liquid, substance —*see* Table of Drugs
    and Chemicals
  iron (hot) X15.8
    stated as undetermined whether accidental
      or intentional Y27.3
    suicide (attempt) X77.3
  kettle (hot) X15.8
    stated as undetermined whether accidental
      or intentional Y27.3
    suicide (attempt) X77.3
  lamp (flame) X08.8
    with ignition of clothing NEC X06.2
      nightwear X05
  lighter (cigar) (cigarette) X08.8
    with ignition of clothing NEC X06.2
      nightwear X05
  lightning —*see* subcategory T75.0
    causing fire —*see* Exposure, fire
  liquid (boiling) (hot) NEC X12
    stated as undetermined whether accidental
      or intentional Y27.2
    suicide (attempt) X77.2

Burn, burned, burning *(Continued)*
  local application of externally applied
      substance in medical or surgical care
      Y63.5
  machinery (hot) X17
  matches X08.8
    with ignition of clothing NEC X06.2
      nightwear X05
  mattress —*see* Exposure, fire, uncontrolled,
      building, bed
  medicament, externally applied Y63.5
  metal (hot) (liquid) (molten) NEC X18
  nightwear (nightclothes, nightdress, gown,
      pajamas, robe) X05
  object (hot) NEC X19
  on board watercraft
    due to
        accident to watercraft V91.09
          powered craft V91.03
            ferry boat V91.01
            fishing boat V91.02
            jetskis V91.03
            liner V91.01
            merchant ship V91.00
            passenger ship V91.01
          unpowered craft V91.08
            canoe V91.05
            inflatable V91.06
            kayak V91.05
            sailboat V91.04
            surf-board V91.08
            water skis V91.07
            windsurfer V91.08
        fire on board V93.09
          ferry boat V93.01
          fishing boat V93.02
          jetskis V93.03
          liner V93.01
          merchant ship V93.00
          passenger ship V93.01
          powered craft NEC V93.03
          sailboat V93.04

Burn, burned, burning *(Continued)*
  on board watercraft *(Continued)*
    due to *(Continued)*
        specified heat source NEC on board
            V93.19
          ferry boat V93.11
          fishing boat V93.12
          jetskis V93.13
          liner V93.11
          merchant ship V93.10
          passenger ship V93.11
          powered craft NEC V93.13
          sailboat V93.14
  pipe (hot) X16
    smoking X08.8
      with ignition of clothing NEC X06.2
        nightwear X05
  powder —*see* Powder burn
  radiator (hot) X16
  saucepan (hot) (glass) (metal) X15.3
    stated as undetermined whether
        accidental or intentional
        Y27.3
    suicide (attempt) X77.3
  self-inflicted X76
    stated as undetermined whether
        accidental or intentional
        Y26
  stated as undetermined whether
      accidental or intentional Y27.0
  steam X13.1
    pipe X16
      stated as undetermined whether
          accidental or intentional
          Y27.8
    stated as undetermined whether
        accidental or intentional Y27.0
    suicide (attempt) X77.0
  stove (hot) (kitchen) X15.0
    stated as undetermined whether
        accidental or intentional Y27.3
    suicide (attempt) X77.3

Burn, burned, burning *(Continued)*
  substance (hot) NEC X19
    boiling X12
      stated as undetermined whether
          accidental or intentional Y27.2
      suicide (attempt) X77.2
    molten (metal) X18
  suicide (attempt) NEC X76
    hot
      household appliance X77.3
      object X77.9
    stated as undetermined whether accidental or
        intentional Y27.0
  therapeutic misadventure
    heat in local application or packing during
        medical or surgical procedure Y63.5
    overdose of radiation Y63.2
  toaster (hot) X15.1
    stated as undetermined whether accidental
        or intentional Y27.3
    suicide (attempt) X77.3
  tool (hot) X17
  torch, welding X08.8
    with ignition of clothing NEC X06.2
      nightwear X05
  trash fire (controlled) —*see* Exposure, fire,
      controlled, not in building
    uncontrolled —*see* Exposure, fire,
        uncontrolled, not in building
  vapor (hot) X13.1
    stated as undetermined whether accidental
        or intentional Y27.0
    suicide (attempt) X77.0
  Very pistol —*see* Discharge, firearm NEC
Butted by animal W55.82
  bull W55.22
  cow W55.22
  goat W55.32
  horse W55.12
  pig W55.42
  sheep W55.32

▶ New   ➡ Revised   ~~deleted~~ Deleted   ● Use Additional Character(s)

C

Caisson disease —*see* Air, pressure, change
Campfire (exposure to) (controlled) —*see also* Exposure, fire, controlled, not in building
  uncontrolled —*see* Exposure, fire, uncontrolled, not in building
Capital punishment (any means) —*see* Legal, intervention
Car sickness T75.3
Casualty (not due to war) NEC X58
  war —*see* War operations
Cat
  bite W55.01
  scratch W55.03
Cataclysm, cataclysmic (any injury) NEC —*see* Forces of nature
Catching fire —*see* Exposure, fire
Caught
  between
    folding object W23.0
    objects (moving) (stationary and moving) W23.0
      and machinery —*see* Contact, with, by type of machine
      stationary W23.1
    sliding door and door frame W23.0
  by, in
    machinery (moving parts of) —*see* Contact, with, by type of machine
    washing-machine wringer W23.0
  under packing crate (due to losing grip) W23.1
Cave-in caused by cataclysmic earth surface movement or eruption —*see* Landslide
Change(s) in air pressure —*see* Air, pressure, change
Choked, choking (on) (any object except food or vomitus)
  food (bone) (seed) —*see* categories T17 and T18
  vomitus T17.81-•
Civil insurrection —*see* War operations
Cloudburst (any injury) X37.8
Cold, exposure to (accidental) (excessive) (extreme) (natural) (place) NEC —*see* Exposure, cold
Collapse
  building W20.1
    burning (uncontrolled fire) X00.2
  dam or man-made structure (causing earth movement) X36.0
  machinery —*see* Contact, with, by type of machine
  structure W20.1
    burning (uncontrolled fire) X00.2
Collision (accidental) NEC —*see also* Accident, transport V89.9
  pedestrian W51
    with fall W03
      due to ice or snow W00.0
      involving pedestrian conveyance —*see* Accident, transport, pedestrian, conveyance
    and
      crowd or human stampede (with fall) W52
      object W22.8
        with fall —*see* Fall, due to, bumping against, object
  person(s) —*see* Collision, pedestrian
  transport vehicle NEC V89.9
    and
      avalanche, fallen or not moving —*see* Accident, transport
        falling or moving —*see* Landslide
      landslide, fallen or not moving —*see* Accident, transport
        falling or moving —*see* Landslide

Collision NEC *(Continued)*
  transport vehicle NEC *(Continued)*
    due to cataclysm —*see* Forces of nature, by type
    intentional, purposeful suicide (attempt) —*see* Suicide, collision
Combustion, spontaneous —*see* Ignition
Complication (delayed) of or following (medical or surgical procedure) Y84.9
  with misadventure —*see* Misadventure
  amputation of limb(s) Y83.5
  anastomosis (arteriovenous) (blood vessel) (gastrojejunal) (tendon) (natural or artificial material) Y83.2
  aspiration (of fluid) Y84.4
    tissue Y84.8
  biopsy Y84.8
  blood
    sampling Y84.7
    transfusion
      procedure Y84.8
  bypass Y83.2
  catheterization (urinary) Y84.6
    cardiac Y84.0
  colostomy Y83.3
  cystostomy Y83.3
  dialysis (kidney) Y84.1
  drug —*see* Table of Drugs and Chemicals
  due to misadventure —*see* Misadventure
  duodenostomy Y83.3
  electroshock therapy Y84.3
  external stoma, creation of Y83.3
  formation of external stoma Y83.3
  gastrostomy Y83.3
  graft Y83.2
  hypothermia (medically-induced) Y84.8
  implant, implantation (of)
    artificial
      internal device (cardiac pacemaker) (electrodes in brain) (heart valve prosthesis) (orthopedic) Y83.1
      material or tissue (for anastomosis or bypass) Y83.2
        with creation of external stoma Y83.3
    natural tissues (for anastomosis or bypass) Y83.2
      with creation of external stoma Y83.3
  infusion
    procedure Y84.8
  injection —*see* Table of Drugs and Chemicals
    procedure Y84.8
  insertion of gastric or duodenal sound Y84.5
  insulin-shock therapy Y84.3
  paracentesis (abdominal) (thoracic) (aspirative) Y84.4
  procedures other than surgical operation —*see* Complication of or following, by type of procedure
  radiological procedure or therapy Y84.2
  removal of organ (partial) (total) NEC Y83.6
  sampling
    blood Y84.7
    fluid NEC Y84.4
    tissue Y84.8
  shock therapy Y84.3
  surgical operation NEC —*see also* Complication of or following, by type of operation Y83.9
    reconstructive NEC Y83.4
      with
        anastomosis, bypass or graft Y83.2
        formation of external stoma Y83.3
    specified NEC Y83.8
  transfusion —*see also* Table of Drugs and Chemicals
    procedure Y84.8
  transplant, transplantation (heart) (kidney) (liver) (whole organ, any) Y83.0
    partial organ Y83.4
  ureterostomy Y83.3

Complication of or following *(Continued)*
  vaccination —*see also* Table of Drugs and Chemicals
    procedure Y84.8
Compression
  divers' squeeze —*see* Air, pressure, change
  trachea by
    food (lodged in esophagus) —*see* categories T17 and T18
    vomitus (lodged in esophagus) T17.81-•
Conflagration —*see* Exposure, fire, uncontrolled
Constriction (external)
  hair W49.01
  jewelry W49.04
  ring W49.04
  rubber band W49.03
  specified item NEC W49.09
  string W49.02
  thread W49.02
Contact (accidental)
  with
    abrasive wheel (metalworking) W31.1
    alligator W58.09
      bite W58.01
      crushing W58.03
      strike W58.02
    amphibian W62.9
      frog W62.0
      toad W62.1
    animal (nonvenomous) NEC W64
      marine W56.89
        bite W56.81
        dolphin —*see* Contact, with, dolphin
        fish NEC —*see* Contact, with, fish
        mammal —*see* Contact, with, mammal, marine
        orca —*see* Contact, with, orca
        sea lion —*see* Contact, with, sea lion
        shark —*see* Contact, with, shark
        strike W56.82
    animate mechanical force NEC W64
    arrow W21.89
      not thrown, projected or falling W45.8
    arthropods (nonvenomous) W57
    axe W27.0
    band-saw (industrial) W31.2
    bayonet —*see* Bayonet wound
    bee(s) X58
    bench-saw (industrial) W31.2
    bird W61.99
      bite W61.91
      chicken —*see* Contact, with, chicken
      duck —*see* Contact, with, duck
      goose —*see* Contact, with, goose
      macaw —*see* Contact, with, macaw
      parrot —*see* Contact, with, parrot
      psittacine —*see* Contact, with, psittacine
      strike W61.92
      turkey —*see* Contact, with, turkey
    blender W29.0
    boiling water X12
      stated as undetermined whether accidental or intentional Y27.2
      suicide (attempt) X77.2
    bore, earth-drilling or mining (land) (seabed) W31.0
    buffalo —*see* Contact, with, hoof stock NEC
    bull W55.29
      bite W55.21
      gored W55.22
      strike W55.22
    bumper cars W31.81
    camel —*see* Contact, with, hoof stock NEC
    can
      lid W26.8
      opener W27.4
        powered W29.0
    cat W55.09
      bite W55.01
      scratch W55.03
    caterpillar (venomous) X58

Contact *(Continued)*
  with *(Continued)*
    centipede (venomous) X58
    chain
      hoist W24.0
        agricultural operations W30.89
      saw W29.3
    chicken W61.39
      peck W61.33
      strike W61.32
    chisel W27.0
    circular saw W31.2
    cobra X58
    combine (harvester) W30.0
    conveyer belt W24.1
    cooker (hot) X15.8
      stated as undetermined whether
        accidental or intentional Y27.3
      suicide (attempt) X77.3
    coral X58
    cotton gin W31.82
    cow W55.29
      bite W55.21
      strike W55.22
    crane W24.0
      agricultural operations W30.89
    crocodile W58.19
      bite W58.11
      crushing W58.13
      strike W58.12
    dagger W26.1
      stated as undetermined whether
        accidental or intentional Y28.2
      suicide (attempt) X78.2
    dairy equipment W31.82
    dart W21.89
      not thrown, projected or falling W45.8
    deer —*see* Contact, with, hoof stock
      NEC
    derrick W24.0
      agricultural operations W30.89
      hay W30.2
    dog W54.8
      bite W54.0
      strike W54.1
    dolphin W56.09
      bite W56.01
      strike W56.02
    donkey —*see* Contact, with, hoof stock
      NEC
    drill (powered) W29.8
      earth (land) (seabed) W31.0
      nonpowered W27.8
    drive belt W24.0
      agricultural operations W30.89
    dry ice —*see* Exposure, cold, man-made
    dryer (clothes) (powered) (spin) W29.2
    duck W61.69
      bite W61.61
      strike W61.62
    earth(-)
      drilling machine (industrial) W31.0
      scraping machine in stationary use
        W31.83
    edge of stiff paper W26.2
    electric
      beater W29.0
      blanket X16
      fan W29.2
        commercial W31.82
      knife W29.1
      mixer W29.0
    elevator (building) W24.0
      agricultural operations W30.89
      grain W30.3
    engine(s), hot NEC X17
    excavating machine W31.0
    farm machine W30.9
    feces —*see* Contact, with, by type of
      animal
    fer de lance X58

Contact *(Continued)*
  with *(Continued)*
    fish W56.59
      bite W56.51
      shark —*see* Contact, with, shark
      strike W56.52
    flying horses W31.81
    forging (metalworking) machine
      W31.1
    fork W27.4
    forklift (truck) W24.0
      agricultural operations W30.89
    frog W62.0
    garden
      cultivator (powered) W29.3
        riding W30.89
      fork W27.1
    gas turbine W31.3
    Gila monster X58
    giraffe —*see* Contact, with, hoof stock
      NEC
    glass (sharp) (broken) W25
      with subsequent fall W18.02
      assault X99.0
      due to fall —*see* Fall, by type
      stated as undetermined whether
        accidental or intentional Y28. 0
      suicide (attempt) X78.0
    goat W55.39
      bite W55.31
      strike W55.32
    goose W61.59
      bite W61.51
      strike W61.52
    hand
      saw W27.0
      tool (not powered) NEC W27.8
        powered W29.8
    harvester W30.0
    hay-derrick W30.2
    heat NEC X19
      from appliance (electrical)
        (household) —*see* Contact, with,
        hot, household appliance
      heating appliance X16
    heating
      appliance (hot) X16
      pad (electric) X16
    hedge-trimmer (powered) W29.3
    hoe W27.1
    hoist (chain) (shaft) NEC W24.0
      agricultural W30.89
    hoof stock NEC W55.39
      bite W55.31
      strike W55.32
    hornet(s) X58
    horse W55.19
      bite W55.11
      strike W55.12
    hot
      air X14.1
        inhalation X14.0
      cooker X15.8
      drinks X10.0
      engine X17
      fats X10.2
      fluids NEC X12
        assault X98.2
        suicide (attempt) X77.2
        undetermined whether accidental or
          intentional Y27.2
      food X10.1
      gases X14.1
        inhalation X14.0
      heating appliance X16
      household appliance X15.8
        assault X98.3
        cooker X15.8
        hotplate X15.2
        kettle X15.8
        light bulb X15.8

Contact *(Continued)*
  with *(Continued)*
    hot *(Continued)*
      household appliance *(Continued)*
        object NEC X19
          assault X98.8
          stated as undetermined whether
            accidental or intentional Y27.9
          suicide (attempt) X77.8
        saucepan X15.3
        skillet X15.3
        stated as undetermined whether
          accidental or intentional Y27.3
        stove X15.0
        suicide (attempt) X77.3
        toaster X15.1
      kettle X15.8
      light bulb X15.8
      liquid NEC —*see also* Burn X12
        drinks X10.0
        stated as undetermined whether
          accidental or intentional Y27.2
        suicide (attempt) X77.2
        tap water X11.8
          stated as undetermined whether
            accidental or intentional Y27.1
          suicide (attempt) X77.1
      machinery X17
      metal (molten) (liquid) NEC X18
      object (not producing fire or flames)
        NEC X19
      oil (cooking) X10.2
      pipe X16
      plate X15.2
      radiator X16
      saucepan (glass) (metal) X15.3
      skillet X15.3
      stove (kitchen) X15.0
      substance NEC X19
      tap-water X11.8
        assault X98.1
        heated on stove X12
          stated as undetermined whether
            accidental or intentional Y27.2
          suicide (attempt) X77.2
        in bathtub X11.0
        running X11.1
        stated as undetermined whether
          accidental or intentional Y27.1
        suicide (attempt) X77.1
      toaster X15.1
      tool X17
      vapors X13.1
        inhalation X13.0
      water (tap) X11.8
        boiling X12
          stated as undetermined whether
            accidental or intentional Y27.2
          suicide (attempt) X77.2
        heated on stove X12
          stated as undetermined whether
            accidental or intentional Y27.2
          suicide (attempt) X77.2
        in bathtub X11.0
        running X11.1
        stated as undetermined whether
          accidental or intentional Y27.1
        suicide (attempt) X77.1
    hotplate X15.2
    ice-pick W27.4
    insect (nonvenomous) NEC W57
    kettle (hot) X15.8
    knife W26.0
      assault X99.1
      electric W29.1
      stated as undetermined whether
        accidental or intentional Y28.1
      suicide (attempt) X78.1
    lathe (metalworking) W31.1
      turnings W45.8
      woodworking W31.2

▶ New   ⟹ Revised   ~~deleted~~ Deleted   ● Use Additional Character(s)

Contact *(Continued)*
  with *(Continued)*
    lawnmower (powered) (ridden) W28
      causing electrocution W86.8
        suicide (attempt) X83.1
      unpowered W27.1
    lift, lifting (devices) W24.0
      agricultural operations W30.89
      shaft W24.0
    liquefied gas —*see* Exposure, cold,
      man-made
    liquid air, hydrogen, nitrogen —*see*
      Exposure, cold, man-made
    lizard (nonvenomous) W59.09
      bite W59.01
      strike W59.02
    llama —*see* Contact, with, hoof stock NEC
    macaw W61.19
      bite W61.11
      strike W61.12
    machine, machinery W31.9
      abrasive wheel W31.1
      agricultural including animal-powered
        W30.9
        combine harvester W30.0
        grain storage elevator W30.3
        hay derrick W30.2
        power take-off device W30.1
        reaper W30.0
        specified NEC W30.89
        thresher W30.0
        transport vehicle, stationary W30.81
      band saw W31.2
      bench saw W31.2
      circular saw W31.2
      commercial NEC W31.82
      drilling, metal (industrial) W31.1
      earth-drilling W31.0
      earthmoving or scraping W31.89
      excavating W31.89
      forging machine W31.1
      gas turbine W31.3
      hot X17
      internal combustion engine W31.3
      land drill W31.0
      lathe W31.1
      lifting (devices) W24.0
      metal drill W31.1
      metalworking (industrial) W31.1
      milling, metal W31.1
      mining W31.0
      molding W31.2
      overhead plane W31.2
      power press, metal W31.1
      prime mover W31.3
      printing W31.89
      radial saw W31.2
      recreational W31.81
      roller-coaster W31.81
      rolling mill, metal W31.1
      sander W31.2
      seabed drill W31.0
      shaft
        hoist W31.0
        lift W31.0
      specified NEC W31.89
      spinning W31.89
      steam engine W31.3
      transmission W24.1
      undercutter W31.0
      water driven turbine W31.3
      weaving W31.89
      woodworking or forming (industrial)
        W31.2
    mammal (feces) (urine) W55.89
      bull —*see* Contact, with, bull
      cat —*see* Contact, with, cat
      cow —*see* Contact, with, cow
      goat —*see* Contact, with, goat
      hoof stock —*see* Contact, with, hoof
        stock

Contact *(Continued)*
  with *(Continued)*
    mammal *(Continued)*
      horse —*see* Contact, with, horse
      marine W56.39
        dolphin —*see* Contact, with, dolphin
        orca —*see* Contact, with, orca
        sea lion —*see* Contact, with, sea lion
        specified NEC W56.39
          bite W56.31
          strike W56.32
      pig —*see* Contact, with, pig
      raccoon —*see* Contact, with, raccoon
      rodent —*see* Contact, with, rodent
      sheep —*see* Contact, with, sheep
      specified NEC W55.89
        bite W55.81
        strike W55.82
    marine
      animal W56.89
        bite W56.81
        dolphin —*see* Contact, with, dolphin
        fish NEC —*see* Contact, with, fish
        mammal —*see* Contact, with,
          mammal, marine
        orca —*see* Contact, with, orca
        sea lion —*see* Contact, with, sea lion
        shark —*see* Contact, with, shark
        strike W56.82
    meat
      grinder (domestic) W29.0
        industrial W31.82
        nonpowered W27.4
      slicer (domestic) W29.0
        industrial W31.82
    merry go round W31.81
    metal, (hot) (liquid) (molten) NEC X18
    millipede W57
    nail W45.0
      gun W29.4
    needle (sewing) W27.3
      hypodermic W46.0
        contaminated W46.1
    object (blunt) NEC
      hot NEC X19
      legal intervention —*see* Legal,
        intervention, blunt object
      sharp NEC W45.8
        inflicted by other person NEC W45.8
          stated as
            intentional homicide (attempt) —
              see Assault, cutting or
              piercing instrument
        legal intervention —*see* Legal,
          intervention, sharp object
        self-inflicted X78.9
    orca W56.29
      bite W56.21
      strike W56.22
    overhead plane W31.2
    paper (as sharp object) W26.2
    paper-cutter W27.5
    parrot W61.09
      bite W61.01
      strike W61.02
    pig W55.49
      bite W55.41
      strike W55.42
    pipe, hot X16
    pitchfork W27.1
    plane (metal) (wood) W27.0
      overhead W31.2
    plant thorns, spines, sharp leaves or other
      mechanisms W60
    powered
      garden cultivator W29.3
      household appliance, implement, or
        machine W29.8
      saw (industrial) W31.2
        hand W29.8
    printing machine W31.89

Contact *(Continued)*
  with *(Continued)*
    psittacine bird W61.29
      bite W61.21
      macaw —*see* Contact, with, macaw
      parrot —*see* Contact, with, parrot
      strike W61.22
    pulley (block) (transmission) W24.0
      agricultural operations W30.89
    raccoon W55.59
      bite W55.51
      strike W55.52
    radial-saw (industrial) W31.2
    radiator (hot) X16
    rake W27.1
    rattlesnake X58
    reaper W30.0
    reptile W59.89
      lizard —*see* Contact, with, lizard
      snake —*see* Contact, with, snake
      specified NEC W59.89
        bite W59.81
        crushing W59.83
        strike W59.82
      turtle —*see* Contact, with, turtle
    rivet gun (powered) W29.4
    road scraper —*see* Accident, transport,
      construction vehicle
    rodent (feces) (urine) W53.89
      bite W53.81
      mouse W53.09
        bite W53.01
      rat W53.19
        bite W53.11
      specified NEC W53.89
        bite W53.81
      squirrel W53.29
        bite W53.21
    roller coaster W31.81
    rope NEC W24.0
      agricultural operations W30.89
    saliva —*see* Contact, with, by type of
      animal
    sander W29.8
      industrial W31.2
    saucepan (hot) (glass) (metal) X15.3
    saw W27.0
      band (industrial) W31.2
      bench (industrial) W31.2
      chain W29.3
      hand W27.0
    sawing machine, metal W31.1
    scissors W27.2
    scorpion X58
    screwdriver W27.0
      powered W29.8
    sea
      anemone, cucumber or urchin (spine)
        X58
      lion W56.19
        bite W56.11
        strike W56.12
    serpent —*see* Contact, with, snake, by type
    sewing-machine (electric) (powered) W29.2
      not powered W27.8
    shaft (hoist) (lift) (transmission) NEC W24.0
      agricultural W30.89
    shark W56.49
      bite W56.41
      strike W56.42
    sharp object(s) W26.9
      specified NEC W26.8
    shears (hand) W27.2
      powered (industrial) W31.1
        domestic W29.2
    sheep W55.39
      bite W55.31
      strike W55.32
    shovel W27.8
      steam —*see* Accident, transport,
        construction vehicle

▶ New   ⇒ Revised   ~~deleted~~ Deleted   ● Use Additional Character(s)

Contact *(Continued)*
  with *(Continued)*
    snake (nonvenomous) W59.19
      bite W59.11
      crushing W59.13
      strike W59.12
    spade W27.1
    spider (venomous) X58
    spin-drier W29.2
    spinning machine W31.89
    splinter W45.8
    sports equipment W21.9
    staple gun (powered) W29.8
    steam X13.1
      engine W31.3
      inhalation X13.0
      pipe X16
      shovel W31.89
    stove (hot) (kitchen) X15.0
    substance, hot NEC X19
      molten (metal) X18
    sword W26.1
      assault X99.2
      stated as undetermined whether
          accidental or intentional
          Y28.2
      suicide (attempt) X78.2
    tarantula X58
    thresher W30.0
    tin can lid W26.8
    toad W62.1
    toaster (hot) X15.1
    tool W27.8
      hand (not powered) W27.8
        auger W27.0
        axe W27.0
        can opener W27.4
        chisel W27.0
        fork W27.4
        garden W27.1
        handsaw W27.0
        hoe W27.1
        ice-pick W27.4
        kitchen utensil W27.4
        manual
          lawn mower W27.1
          sewing machine W27.8
        meat grinder W27.4
        needle (sewing) W27.3
          hypodermic W46.0
            contaminated W46.1
        paper cutter W27.5
        pitchfork W27.1
        rake W27.1
        scissors W27.2
        screwdriver W27.0
        specified NEC W27.8
        workbench W27.0
      hot X17
      powered W29.8
        blender W29.0
          commercial W31.82
        can opener W29.0
          commercial W31.82
        chainsaw W29.3
        clothes dryer W29.2
          commercial W31.82
        dishwasher W29.2
          commercial W31.82
        edger W29.3
        electric fan W29.2
          commercial W31.82
        electric knife W29.1
        food processor W29.0
          commercial W31.82
        garbage disposal W29.0
          commercial W31.82

Contact *(Continued)*
  with *(Continued)*
    tool *(Continued)*
      powered *(Continued)*
        garden tool W29.3
        hedge trimmer W29.3
        ice maker W29.0
          commercial W31.82
        kitchen appliance W29.0
          commercial W31.82
        lawn mower W28
        meat grinder W29.0
          commercial W31.82
        mixer W29.0
          commercial W31.82
        rototiller W29.3
        sewing machine W29.2
          commercial W31.82
        washing machine W29.2
          commercial W31.82
    transmission device (belt, cable, chain,
        gear, pinion, shaft) W24.1
      agricultural operations W30.89
    turbine (gas) (water-driven) W31.3
    turkey W61.49
      peck W61.43
      strike W61.42
    turtle (nonvenomous) W59.29
      bite W59.21
      strike W59.22
      terrestrial W59.89
        bite W59.81
        crushing W59.83
        strike W59.82
    under-cutter W31.0
    urine —*see* Contact, with, by type of animal
  vehicle
    agricultural use (transport) —*see*
        Accident, transport, agricultural
        vehicle
      not on public highway W30.81
    industrial use (transport) —*see*
        Accident, transport, industrial
        vehicle
      not on public highway W31.83
    off-road use (transport) —*see* Accident,
        transport, all-terrain or off-road
        vehicle
      not on public highway W31.83
    special construction use (transport) —*see*
        Accident, transport, construction
        vehicle
      not on public highway W31.83
  venomous
    animal X58
    arthropods X58
    lizard X58
    marine animal NEC X58
    marine plant NEC X58
    millipedes (tropical) X58
    plant(s) X58
    snake X58
    spider X58
  viper X58
  washing-machine (powered) W29.2
  wasp X58
  weaving-machine W31.89
  winch W24.0
    agricultural operations W30.89
  wire NEC W24.0
    agricultural operations W30.89
  wood slivers W45.8
  yellow jacket X58
  zebra —*see* Contact, with, hoof stock NEC
pressure X50.9
stress X50.9
Coup de soleil X32

Crash
  aircraft (in transit) (powered) V95.9
    balloon V96.01
    fixed wing NEC (private) V95.21
      commercial V95.31
    glider V96.21
      hang V96.11
      powered V95.11
    helicopter V95.01
    in war operations —*see* War operations,
        destruction of aircraft
    microlight V95.11
    nonpowered V96.9
      specified NEC V96.8
    powered NEC V95.8
    stated as
      homicide (attempt) Y08.81
      suicide (attempt) X83.0
    ultralight V95.11
  spacecraft V95.41
  transport vehicle NEC —*see also* Accident,
      transport V89.9
    homicide (attempt) Y03.8
    motor NEC (traffic) V89.2
      homicide (attempt) Y03.8
      suicide (attempt) —*see* Suicide, collision
Cruelty (mental) (physical) (sexual) X58
Crushed (accidentally) X58
  between objects (moving) (stationary and
      moving) W23.0
    stationary W23.1
  by
    alligator W58.03
    avalanche NEC —*see* Landslide
    cave-in W20.0
      caused by cataclysmic earth surface
          movement —*see* Landslide
    crocodile W58.13
    crowd or human stampede W52
    falling
      aircraft V97.39
        in war operations —*see* War
            operations, destruction of aircraft
      earth, material W20.0
        caused by cataclysmic earth surface
            movement —*see* Landslide
      object NEC W20.8
    landslide NEC —*see* Landslide
    lizard (nonvenomous) W59.09
    machinery —*see* Contact, with, by type of
        machine
    reptile NEC W59.89
    snake (nonvenomous) W59.13
  in
    machinery —*see* Contact, with, by type of
        machine
Cut, cutting (any part of body) (accidental) —
    see also Contact, with, by object or machine
  during medical or surgical treatment as
      misadventure —*see* Index to Diseases
      and Injuries, Complications
  homicide (attempt) —*see* Assault, cutting or
      piercing instrument
  inflicted by other person —*see* Assault,
      cutting or piercing instrument
  legal
    execution —*see* Legal, intervention
    intervention —*see* Legal, intervention,
        sharp object
  machine NEC —*see also* Contact, with, by
      type of machine W31.9
  self-inflicted —*see* Suicide, cutting or piercing
      instrument
  suicide (attempt) —*see* Suicide, cutting or
      piercing instrument
Cyclone (any injury) X37.1

▶ New   ⇒ Revised   ~~deleted~~ Deleted   • Use Additional Character(s)

D

Decapitation (accidental circumstances)
  NEC X58
  homicide X99.9
  legal execution —*see* Legal, intervention
Dehydration from lack of water X58
Deprivation X58
Derailment (accidental)
  railway (rolling stock) (train) (vehicle)
    (without antecedent collision) V81.7
    with antecedent collision —*see* Accident,
      transport, railway vehicle occupant
  streetcar (without antecedent collision)
    V82.7
    with antecedent collision —*see* Accident,
      transport, streetcar occupant
Descent
  parachute (voluntary) (without accident to
    aircraft) V97.29
    due to accident to aircraft —*see* Accident,
      transport, aircraft
Desertion X58
Destitution X58
Disability, late effect or sequela of injury —*see*
  Sequelae
Discharge (accidental)
  airgun W34.010
    assault X95.01
    homicide (attempt) X95.01
    stated as undetermined whether accidental
      or intentional Y24.0
    suicide (attempt) X74.01
  BB gun —*see* Discharge, airgun
  firearm (accidental) W34.00
    assault X95.9
    handgun (pistol) (revolver) W32.0
      assault X93
      homicide (attempt) X93
      legal intervention —*see* Legal,
        intervention, firearm, handgun
      stated as undetermined whether
        accidental or intentional Y22
      suicide (attempt) X72
    homicide (attempt) X95.9
    hunting rifle W33.02
      assault X94.1
      homicide (attempt) X94.1
      legal intervention
        injuring
          bystander Y35.032
          law enforcement personnel
            Y35.031
          suspect Y35.033
      stated as undetermined whether
        accidental or intentional Y23.1
      suicide (attempt) X73.1
    larger W33.00
      assault X94.9
      homicide (attempt) X94.9
      hunting rifle —*see* Discharge, firearm,
        hunting rifle
      legal intervention —*see* Legal,
        intervention, firearm by type of
        firearm
      machine gun —*see* Discharge, firearm,
        machine gun
      shotgun —*see* Discharge, firearm,
        shotgun
      specified NEC W33.09
        assault X94.8
        homicide (attempt) X94.8
        legal intervention
          injuring
            bystander Y35.092
            law enforcement personnel
              Y35.091
            suspect Y35.093
        stated as undetermined whether
          accidental or intentional Y23.8
        suicide (attempt) X73.8

Discharge *(Continued)*
  firearm *(Continued)*
    larger *(Continued)*
      stated as undetermined whether
        accidental or intentional Y23.9
      suicide (attempt) X73.9
    legal intervention
      injuring
        bystander Y35.002
        law enforcement personnel Y35.001
        suspect Y35.03
      using rubber bullet
        injuring
          bystander Y35.042
          law enforcement personnel
            Y35.041
          suspect Y35.043
    machine gun W33.03
      assault X94.2
      homicide (attempt) X94.2
      legal intervention —*see* Legal,
        intervention, firearm, machine gun
      stated as undetermined whether
        accidental or intentional Y23.3
      suicide (attempt) X73.2
    pellet gun —*see* Discharge, airgun
    shotgun W33.01
      assault X94.0
      homicide (attempt) X94.0
      legal intervention —*see* Legal,
        intervention, firearm, specified NEC
      stated as undetermined whether
        accidental or intentional Y23.0
      suicide (attempt) X73.0
    specified NEC W34.09
      assault X95.8
      homicide (attempt) X95.8
      legal intervention —*see* Legal,
        intervention, firearm, specified NEC
      stated as undetermined whether
        accidental or intentional Y24.8
      suicide (attempt) X74.8
    stated as undetermined whether accidental
      or intentional Y24.9
    suicide (attempt) X74.9
    Very pistol W34.09
      assault X95.8
      homicide (attempt) X95.8
      stated as undetermined whether
        accidental or intentional Y24.8
      suicide (attempt) X74.8
  firework(s) W39
    stated as undetermined whether accidental
      or intentional Y25
  gas-operated gun NEC W34.018
    airgun —*see* Discharge, airgun
    assault X95.09
    homicide (attempt) X95.09
    paintball gun —*see* Discharge, paintball
      gun
    stated as undetermined whether accidental
      or intentional Y24.8
    suicide (attempt) X74.09
  gun NEC —*see also* Discharge, firearm NEC
    air —*see* Discharge, airgun
    BB —*see* Discharge, airgun
    for single hand use —*see* Discharge,
      firearm, handgun
    hand —*see* Discharge, firearm, handgun
    machine —*see* Discharge, firearm, machine
      gun
    other specified —*see* Discharge, firearm
      NEC
    paintball —*see* Discharge, paintball gun
    pellet —*see* Discharge, airgun
  handgun —*see* Discharge, firearm, handgun
  machine gun —*see* Discharge, firearm,
    machine gun
  paintball gun W34.011
    assault X95.02
    homicide (attempt) X95.02

Discharge *(Continued)*
  paintball gun *(Continued)*
    stated as undetermined whether accidental
      or intentional Y24.8
    suicide (attempt) X74.02
  pistol —*see* Discharge, firearm, handgun
    flare —*see* Discharge, firearm, Very pistol
    pellet —*see* Discharge, airgun
    Very —*see* Discharge, firearm, Very pistol
  revolver —*see* Discharge, firearm, handgun
  rifle (hunting) —*see* Discharge, firearm,
    hunting rifle
  shotgun —*see* Discharge, firearm, shotgun
  spring-operated gun NEC W34.018
    assault X95.09
    homicide (attempt) X95.09
    stated as undetermined whether accidental
      or intentional Y24.8
    suicide (attempt) X74.09
Disease
  Andes W94.11
  aviator's —*see* Air, pressure
  range W94.11
Diver's disease, palsy, paralysis, squeeze —*see*
  Air, pressure
Diving (into water) —*see* Accident, diving
Dog bite W54.0
Dragged by transport vehicle NEC —*see also*
  Accident, transport V09.9
Drinking poison (accidental) —*see* Table of
  Drugs and Chemicals
Dropped (accidentally) while being carried or
  supported by other person W04
Drowning (accidental) W74
  assault X92.9
  due to
    accident (to)
      machinery —*see* Contact, with, by type
        of machine
      watercraft V90.89
        burning V90.29
          powered V90.23
            fishing boat V90.22
            jetskis V90.23
            merchant ship V90.20
            passenger ship V90.21
          unpowered V90.28
            canoe V90.25
            inflatable V90.26
            kayak V90.25
            sailboat V90.24
            water skis V90.27
        crushed V90.39
          powered V90.33
            fishing boat V90.32
            jetskis V90.33
            merchant ship V90.30
            passenger ship V90.31
          unpowered V90.38
            canoe V90.35
            inflatable V90.36
            kayak V90.35
            sailboat V90.34
            water skis V90.37
        overturning V90.09
          powered V90.03
            fishing boat V90.02
            jetskis V90.03
            merchant ship V90.00
            passenger ship V90.01
          unpowered V90.08
            canoe V90.05
            inflatable V90.06
            kayak V90.05
            sailboat V90.04
        sinking V90.19
          powered V90.13
            fishing boat V90.12
            jetskis V90.13
            merchant ship V90.10
            passenger ship V90.11

Drowning (Continued)
  due to (Continued)
    accident (Continued)
      watercraft (Continued)
        sinking (Continued)
          unpowered V90.18
            canoe V90.15
            inflatable V90.16
            kayak V90.15
            sailboat V90.14
          specified type NEC V90.89
            powered V90.83
              fishing boat V90.82
              jetskis V90.83
              merchant ship V90.80
              passenger ship V90.81
            unpowered V90.88
              canoe V90.85
              inflatable V90.86
              kayak V90.85
              sailboat V90.84
              water skis V90.87
    avalanche —see Landslide
    cataclysmic
      earth surface movement NEC —see
        Forces of nature, earth movement
      storm —see Forces of nature, cataclysmic
        storm
    cloudburst X37.8
    cyclone X37.1
    fall overboard (from) V92.09
      powered craft V92.03
        ferry boat V92.01
        fishing boat V92.02
        jetskis V92.03
        liner V92.01
        merchant ship V92.00
        passenger ship V92.01
      resulting from
        accident to watercraft —see Drowning,
          due to, accident to, watercraft
        being washed overboard (from)
          V92.29
          powered craft V92.23
            ferry boat V92.21
            fishing boat V92.22
            jetskis V92.23
            liner V92.21
            merchant ship V92.20
            passenger ship V92.21
          unpowered craft V92.28
            canoe V92.25
            inflatable V92.26
            kayak V92.25
            sailboat V92.24
            surf-board V92.28
            water skis V92.27
            windsurfer V92.28
        motion of watercraft V92.19
          powered craft V92.13
            ferry boat V92.11
            fishing boat V92.12
            jetskis V92.13
            liner V92.11
            merchant ship V92.10
            passenger ship V92.11
          unpowered craft
            canoe V92.15
            inflatable V92.16
            kayak V92.15
            sailboat V92.14
      unpowered craft V92.08
        canoe V92.05
        inflatable V92.06
        kayak V92.05

Drowning (Continued)
  due to (Continued)
    fall overboard (Continued)
      unpowered craft (Continued)
        sailboat V92.04
        surf-board V92.08
        water skis V92.07
        windsurfer V92.08
    hurricane X37.0
    jumping into water from watercraft
      (involved in accident) —see also
      Drowning, due to, accident to,
      watercraft
      without accident to or on watercraft
        W16.711
    tidal wave NEC —see Forces of nature,
      tidal wave
    torrential rain X37.8
  following
    fall
      into
        bathtub W16.211
        bucket W16.221
        fountain —see Drowning, following,
          fall, into, water, specified NEC
        quarry —see Drowning, following,
          fall, into, water, specified NEC
        reservoir —see Drowning, following,
          fall, into, water, specified NEC
        swimming-pool W16.011
          stated as undetermined whether
            accidental or intentional
            Y21.3
          striking
            bottom W16.021
            wall W16.031
          suicide (attempt) X71.2
        water NOS W16.41
          natural (lake) (open sea) (river)
            (stream) (pond) W16.111
          striking
            bottom W16.121
            side W16.131
          specified NEC W16.311
          striking
            bottom W16.321
            wall W16.331
      overboard NEC —see Drowning, due to,
        fall overboard
    jump or dive
      from boat W16.711
        striking bottom W16.721
      into
        fountain —see Drowning, following,
          jump or dive, into, water,
          specified NEC
        quarry —see Drowning, following,
          jump or dive, into, water,
          specified NEC
        reservoir —see Drowning, following,
          jump or dive, into, water,
          specified NEC
        swimming-pool W16.511
          striking
            bottom W16.521
            wall W16.531
          suicide (attempt) X71.2
        water NOS W16.91
          natural (lake) (open sea) (river)
            (stream) (pond) W16.611
          specified NEC W16.811
          striking
            bottom W16.821
            wall W16.831
          striking bottom W16.621

Drowning (Continued)
  homicide (attempt) X92.9
  in
    bathtub (accidental) W65
      assault X92.0
      following fall W16.211
        stated as undetermined whether
          accidental or intentional
          Y21.1
      stated as undetermined whether
        accidental or intentional Y21.0
      suicide (attempt) X71.0
    lake —see Drowning, in, natural water
    natural water (lake) (open sea) (river)
      (stream) (pond) W69
      assault X92.3
      following
        dive or jump W16.611
          striking bottom W16.621
        fall W16.111
          striking
            bottom W16.121
            side W16.131
      stated as undetermined whether
        accidental or intentional Y21.4
      suicide (attempt) X71.3
    quarry —see Drowning, in, specified place
      NEC
    quenching tank —see Drowning, in,
      specified place NEC
    reservoir —see Drowning, in, specified
      place NEC
    river —see Drowning, in, natural water
    sea —see Drowning, in, natural water
    specified place NEC W73
      assault X92.8
      following
        dive or jump W16.811
          striking
            bottom W16.821
            wall W16.831
        fall W16.311
          striking
            bottom W16.321
            wall W16.331
      stated as undetermined whether
        accidental or intentional Y21.8
      suicide (attempt) X71.8
    stream —see Drowning, in, natural water
    swimming-pool W67
      assault X92.1
        following fall X92.2
      following
        dive or jump W16.511
          striking
            bottom W16.521
            wall W16.531
        fall W16.011
          striking
            bottom W16.021
            wall W16.031
      stated as undetermined whether
        accidental or intentional Y21.2
        following fall Y21.3
      suicide (attempt) X71.1
        following fall X71.2
    war operations —see War operations,
      restriction of airway
  resulting from accident to watercraft —see
    Drowning, due to, accident, watercraft
  self-inflicted X71.9
  stated as undetermined whether accidental or
    intentional Y21.9
  suicide (attempt) X71.9

▶ New   ⇒ Revised   ~~deleted~~ Deleted   ● Use Additional Character(s)

E

Earth (surface) movement NEC —see Forces of nature, earth movement
Earth falling (on) W20.0
  caused by cataclysmic earth surface movement or eruption —see Landslide
Earthquake (any injury) X34
Effect(s) (adverse) of
  air pressure (any) —see Air, pressure
  cold, excessive (exposure to) —see Exposure, cold
  heat (excessive) —see Heat
  hot place (weather) —see Heat
  insolation X30
  late —see Sequelae
  motion —see Motion
  nuclear explosion or weapon in war operations —see War operations, nuclear weapon
  radiation —see Radiation
  travel —see Travel
Electric shock (accidental) (by) (in) —see Exposure, electric current
Electrocution (accidental) —see Exposure, electric current
Endotracheal tube wrongly placed during anesthetic procedure Y65.3
Entanglement
  in
    bed linen, causing suffocation —see category T71
    wheel of pedal cycle V19.88
Entry of foreign body or material —see Foreign body
Environmental pollution related condition —see Z57
Execution, legal (any method) —see Legal, intervention
Exhaustion
  cold —see Exposure, cold
  due to excessive exertion —see also Overexertion X50.9
  heat —see Heat
Explosion (accidental) (of) (with secondary fire) W40.9
  acetylene W40.1
  aerosol can W36.1
  air tank (compressed) (in machinery) W36.2
  aircraft (in transit) (powered) NEC V95.9
    balloon V96.05
    fixed wing NEC (private) V95.25
      commercial V95.35
    glider V96.25
      hang V96.15
      powered V95.15
    helicopter V95.05
    in war operations —see War operations, destruction of aircraft
    microlight V95.15
    nonpowered V96.9
      specified NEC V96.8
    powered NEC V95.8
    stated as
      homicide (attempt) Y03.8
      suicide (attempt) X83.0
    ultralight V95.15
  anesthetic gas in operating room W40.1
  antipersonnel bomb W40.8
    assault X96.0
    homicide (attempt) X96.0
    suicide (attempt) X75
  assault X96.9
  bicycle tire W37.0
  blasting (cap) (materials) W40.0
  boiler (machinery), not on transport vehicle W35
    on watercraft —see Explosion, in, watercraft
  butane W40.1
  caused by other person X96.9
  coal gas W40.1

Explosion (Continued)
  detonator W40.0
  dump (munitions) W40.8
  dynamite W40.0
    in
      assault X96.8
      homicide (attempt) X96.8
      legal intervention
        injuring
          bystander Y35.112
          law enforcement personnel Y35.111
          suspect Y35.113
      suicide (attempt) X75
  explosive (material) W40.9
    gas W40.1
    in blasting operation W40.0
    specified NEC W40.8
      in
        assault X96.8
        homicide (attempt) X96.8
        legal intervention
          injuring
            bystander Y35.192
            law enforcement personnel Y35.191
            suspect Y35.193
        suicide (attempt) X75
  factory (munitions) W40.8
  fertilizer bomb W40.8
    assault X96.3
    homicide (attempt) X96.3
    suicide (attempt) X75
  fire-damp W40.1
  firearm (parts) NEC W34.19
    airgun W34.110
    BB gun W34.110
    gas, air or spring-operated gun NEC W34.118
    handgun W32.1
    hunting rifle W33.12
    larger firearm W33.10
      specified NEC W33.19
    machine gun W33.13
    paintball gun W34.111
    pellet gun W34.110
    shotgun W33.11
    Very pistol [flare] W34.19
  fireworks W39
  gas (coal) (explosive) W40.1
    cylinder W36.9
      aerosol can W36.1
      air tank W36.2
      pressurized W36.3
      specified NEC W36.8
  gasoline (fumes) (tank) not in moving motor vehicle W40.1
    bomb W40.8
      assault X96.1
      homicide (attempt) X96.1
      suicide (attempt) X75
    in motor vehicle —see Accident, transport, by type of vehicle
  grain store W40.8
  grenade W40.8
    in
      assault X96.8
      homicide (attempt) X96.8
      legal intervention
        injuring
          bystander Y35.192
          law enforcement personnel Y35.191
          suspect Y35.193
      suicide (attempt) X75
  handgun (parts) —see Explosion, firearm, handgun (parts)
  homicide (attempt) X96.9
    antipersonnel bomb —see Explosion, antipersonnel bomb
    fertilizer bomb —see Explosion, fertilizer bomb

Explosion (Continued)
  homicide (Continued)
    gasoline bomb —see Explosion, gasoline bomb
    letter bomb —see Explosion, letter bomb
    pipe bomb —see Explosion, pipe bomb
    specified NEC X96.8
  hose, pressurized W37.8
  hot water heater, tank (in machinery) W35
    on watercraft —see Explosion, in, watercraft
  in, on
    dump W40.8
    factory W40.8
    mine (of explosive gases) NEC W40.1
    watercraft V93.59
      powered craft V93.53
        ferry boat V93.51
        fishing boat V93.52
        jetskis V93.53
        liner V93.51
        merchant ship V93.50
        passenger ship V93.51
        sailboat V93.54
  letter bomb W40.8
    assault X96.2
    homicide (attempt) X96.2
    suicide (attempt) X75
  machinery —see also Contact, with, by type of machine
    on board watercraft —see Explosion, in, watercraft
    pressure vessel —see Explosion, by type of vessel
  methane W40.1
  mine W40.1
  missile NEC W40.8
  mortar bomb W40.8
    in
      assault X96.8
      homicide (attempt) X96.8
      legal intervention
        injuring
          bystander Y35.192
          law enforcement personnel Y35.191
          suspect Y35.193
      suicide (attempt) X75
  munitions (dump) (factory) W40.8
  pipe, pressurized W37.8
    bomb W40.8
      assault X96.4
      homicide (attempt) X96.4
      suicide (attempt) X75
  pressure, pressurized
    cooker W38
    gas tank (in machinery) W36.3
    hose W37.8
    pipe W37.8
    specified device NEC W38
    tire W37.8
      bicycle W37.0
    vessel (in machinery) W38
  propane W40.1
  self-inflicted X75
  shell (artillery) NEC W40.8
    during war operations —see War operations, explosion
    in
      legal intervention
        injuring
          bystander Y35.122
          law enforcement personnel Y35.121
          suspect Y35.123
    war —see War operations, explosion
  spacecraft V95.45
  stated as undetermined whether accidental or intentional Y25
  steam or water lines (in machinery) W37.8
  stove W40.9
  suicide (attempt) X75

▶ New   ⟹ Revised   ~~deleted~~ Deleted   ● Use Additional Character(s)

▶ New   ⇒ Revised   ~~deleted~~ Deleted   ● Use Additional Character(s)

Exposure *(Continued)*
    prolonged in deep-freeze unit or refrigerator
        W93.2
    radiation —*see* Radiation
    smoke —*see also* Exposure, fire
        tobacco, second hand Z77.22
    specified factors NEC X58
    sunlight X32
        man-made (sun lamp) W89.8
            tanning bed W89.1
    supersonic waves W42.0
    transmission line(s), electric W85
    vibration W49.9

Exposure *(Continued)*
    waves
        infrasound W49.9
        sound W42.9
        supersonic W42.0
    weather NEC —*see* Forces of nature
External cause status Y99.9
    child assisting in compensated work for
        family Y99.8
    civilian activity done for financial or other
        compensation Y99.0
    civilian activity done for income or pay
        Y99.0

External cause status *(Continued)*
    family member assisting in compensated
        work for other family member Y99.8
    hobby not done for income Y99.8
    leisure activity Y99.8
    military activity Y99.1
    off-duty activity of military personnel Y99.8
    recreation or sport not for income or while a
        student Y99.8
    specified NEC Y99.8
    student activity Y99.8
    volunteer activity Y99.2

F

Factors, supplemental
  alcohol
    blood level
      less than 20mg/100ml Y90.0
      presence in blood, level not specified
        Y90.9
      20-39mg/100ml Y90.1
      40-59mg/100ml Y90.2
      60-79mg/100ml Y90.3
      80-99mg/100ml Y90.4
      100-119mg/100ml Y90.5
      120-199mg/100ml Y90.6
      200-239mg/100ml Y90.7
      240mg/100ml or more Y90.8
    presence in blood, but level not specified
      Y90.9
  environmental-pollution-related condition —
    see Z57
  nosocomial condition Y95
  work-related condition Y99.0
Failure
  in suture or ligature during surgical
    procedure Y65.2
  mechanical, of instrument or apparatus
    (any) (during any medical or surgical
    procedure) Y65.8
  sterile precautions (during medical and
    surgical care) —see Misadventure,
    failure, sterile precautions, by type of
    procedure
  to
    introduce tube or instrument Y65.4
      endotracheal tube during anesthesia Y65.3
    make curve (transport vehicle) NEC —see
      Accident, transport
    remove tube or instrument Y65.4
Fall, falling (accidental) W19
  building W20.1
    burning (uncontrolled fire) X00.3
  down
    embankment W17.81
    escalator W10.0
    hill W17.81
    ladder W11
    ramp W10.2
    stairs, steps W10.9
  due to
    bumping against
      object W18.00
        sharp glass W18.02
        specified NEC W18.09
        sports equipment W18.01
      person W03
        due to ice or snow W00.0
        on pedestrian conveyance —see
          Accident, transport, pedestrian,
          conveyance
    collision with another person W03
      due to ice or snow W00.0
      involving pedestrian conveyance —see
        Accident, transport, pedestrian,
        conveyance
    grocery cart tipping over W17.82
    ice or snow W00.9
      from one level to another W00.2
      on stairs or steps W00.1
      involving pedestrian conveyance —see
        Accident, transport, pedestrian,
        conveyance
      on same level W00.0
    slipping (on moving sidewalk) W01.0
      with subsequent striking against object
        W01.10
        furniture W01.190
        sharp object W01.119
          glass W01.110
          power tool or machine W01.111
          specified NEC W01.118
        specified NEC W01.198

Fall, falling (Continued)
  due to (Continued)
    striking against
      object W18.00
        sharp glass W18.02
        specified NEC W18.09
        sports equipment W18.01
      person W03
        due to ice or snow W00.0
        on pedestrian conveyance —see
          Accident, transport, pedestrian,
          conveyance
  earth (with asphyxia or suffocation (by
    pressure)) —see Earth, falling
  from, off, out of
    aircraft NEC (with accident to aircraft
      NEC) V97.0
      while boarding or alighting V97.1
    balcony W13.0
    bed W06
    boat, ship, watercraft NEC (with
      drowning or submersion) —
      see Drowning, due to, fall
      overboard
      with hitting bottom or object V94.0
    bridge W13.1
    building W13.9
      burning (uncontrolled fire) X00.3
    cavity W17.2
    chair W07
    cherry picker W17.89
    cliff W15
    dock W17.4
    embankment W17.81
    escalator W10.0
    flagpole W13.8
    furniture NEC W08
    grocery cart W17.82
    haystack W17.89
    high place NEC W17.89
      stated as undetermined whether
        accidental or intentional Y30
    hole W17.2
    incline W10.2
    ladder W11
    lifting device W17.89
    machine, machinery —see also Contact,
      with, by type of machine
      not in operation W17.89
    manhole W17.1
    mobile elevated work platform [MEWP]
      W17.89
    motorized mobility scooter W05.2
    one level to another NEC W17.89
      intentional, purposeful, suicide
        (attempt) X80
      stated as undetermined whether
        accidental or intentional Y30
    pit W17.2
    playground equipment W09.8
      jungle gym W09.2
      slide W09.0
      swing W09.1
    quarry W17.89
    railing W13.9
    ramp W10.2
    roof W13.2
    scaffolding W12
    scooter (nonmotorized) W05.1
      motorized mobility W05.2
    sky lift W17.89
    stairs, steps W10.9
      curb W10.1
      due to ice or snow W00.1
      escalator W10.0
      incline W10.2
      ramp W10.2
      sidewalk curb W10.1
      specified NEC W10.8
    stepladder W11
    storm drain W17.1

Fall, falling (Continued)
  from, off, out of (Continued)
    streetcar NEC V82.6
      with antecedent collision —see
        Accident, transport, streetcar
        occupant
      while boarding or alighting V82.4
    structure NEC W13.8
      burning (uncontrolled fire) X00.3
    table W08
    toilet W18.11
      with subsequent striking against object
        W18.12
    train NEC V81.6
      during derailment (without antecedent
        collision) V81.7
      with antecedent collision —see
        Accident, transport, railway
        vehicle occupant
      while boarding or alighting V81.4
    transport vehicle after collision —see
      Accident, transport, by type of
      vehicle, collision
    tree W14
    vehicle (in motion) NEC —see also
      Accident, transport V89.9
      motor NEC —see also Accident,
        transport, occupant, by type of
        vehicle V87.8
      stationary W17.89
        while boarding or alighting —see
          Accident, transport, by type of
          vehicle, while boarding or
          alighting
    viaduct W13.8
    wall W13.8
    watercraft —see also Drowning, due to, fall
      overboard
      with hitting bottom or object V94.0
    well W17.0
    wheelchair, non-moving W05.0
      powered —see Accident, transport,
        pedestrian, conveyance occupant,
        specified type NEC
    window W13.4
  in, on
    aircraft NEC V97.0
      with accident to aircraft V97.0
      while boarding or alighting
        V97.1
    bathtub (empty) W18.2
      filled W16.212
        causing drowning W16.211
    escalator W10.0
    incline W10.2
    ladder W11
    machine, machinery —see Contact, with,
      by type of machine
    object, edged, pointed or sharp (with
      cut) —see Fall, by type
    playground equipment W09.8
      jungle gym W09.2
      slide W09.0
      swing W09.1
    ramp W10.2
    scaffolding W12
    shower W18.2
      causing drowning W16.211
    staircase, stairs, steps W10.9
      curb W10.1
      due to ice or snow W00.1
      escalator W10.0
      incline W10.2
      specified NEC W10.8
    streetcar (without antecedent collision)
      V82.5
      with antecedent collision —see
        Accident, transport, streetcar
        occupant
      while boarding or alighting
        V82.4

▶ New   ➡ Revised   ~~deleted~~ Deleted   ● Use Additional Character(s)

▶ New   ⇒ Revised   ~~deleted~~ Deleted   ● Use Additional Character(s)

F, G, & H

Forces of nature *(Continued)*
    radiation (natural) X39.08
        radon X39.01
    radon X39.01
    specified force NEC X39.8
    storm surge X37.0
    structure collapse causing
        earth movement
            X36.0
    sunlight X32
    tidal wave X37.41
        due to
            earthquake X37.41
            landslide X37.43
            storm X37.42
            volcanic eruption X37.41
    tornado X37.1

Forces of nature *(Continued)*
    tsunami X37.41
    twister X37.1
    typhoon X37.0
    volcanic eruption X35
Foreign body
    aspiration —*see* Index to Diseases and
        Injuries, Foreign body, respitory
        tract
    embedded in skin W45
    entering through skin W45.8
        can lid W26.2
        nail W45.0
        paper W26.2
        specified NEC 45.8
        splinter W45.8

Forest fire (exposure to) —*see* Exposure, fire,
    uncontrolled, not in building
Found injured X58
    from exposure (to) —*see* Exposure
    on
        highway, road(way), street V89.9
        railway right of way V81.9
Fracture (circumstances unknown or
    unspecified) X58
    due to specified cause NEC X58
Freezing —*see* Exposure, cold
Frostbite X31
    due to man-made conditions —*see* Exposure,
        cold, man-made
Frozen —*see* Exposure, cold

G

Gored by bull W55.22
Gunshot wound W34.00

H

Hailstones, injured by X39.8
Hanged herself or himself —*see* Hanging,
    self-inflicted
Hanging (accidental) —*see also* category T71
    legal execution —*see* Legal, intervention,
        specified means NEC
Heat (effects of) (excessive) X30
    due to
        man-made conditions W92
            on board watercraft V93.29
                fishing boat V93.22
                merchant ship V93.20
                passenger ship V93.21
                sailboat V93.24
                specified powered craft NEC V93.23
        weather (conditions) X30

Heat *(Continued)*
    from
        electric heating apparatus causing
            burning X16
        nuclear explosion in war operations —
            see War operations, nuclear
            weapons
        inappropriate in local application or
            packing in medical or surgical
            procedure Y63.5
Hemorrhage
    delayed following medical or surgical
        treatment without mention of
        misadventure —*see* Index to Diseases
        and Injuries, Complication(s)
    during medical or surgical treatment as
        misadventure —*see* Index to Diseases
        and Injuries, Complication(s)

High
    altitude (effects) —*see* Air, pressure, low
    level of radioactivity, effects —*see* Radiation
    pressure (effects) —*see* Air, pressure, high
    temperature, effects —*see* Heat
Hit, hitting (accidental) by —*see* Struck by
Hitting against —*see* Striking against
Homicide (attempt) (justifiable) —*see* Assault
Hot
    place, effects —*see also* Heat
    weather, effects X30
House fire (uncontrolled) —*see* Exposure, fire,
    uncontrolled, building
Humidity, causing problem X39.8
Hunger X58
Hurricane (any injury) X37.0
Hypobarism, hypobaropathy —*see* Air,
    pressure, low

▶ New   ⇒ Revised   ~~deleted~~ Deleted   ● Use Additional Character(s)

I

Ictus
caloris —*see also* Heat
solaris X3Ø
Ignition (accidental) —*see also* Exposure, fire
X08.8
anesthetic gas in operating room W4Ø.1
apparel X06.2
from highly flammable material X04
nightwear X05
bed linen (sheets) (spreads) (pillows)
(mattress) —*see* Exposure, fire,
uncontrolled, building, bed
benzine X04
clothes, clothing NEC (from controlled fire)
X06.2
from
highly flammable material X04
ether X04
in operating room W4Ø.1
explosive material —*see* Explosion
gasoline X04
jewelry (plastic) (any) X06.Ø
kerosene X04
material
explosive —*see* Explosion
highly flammable with secondary
explosion X04
nightwear X05
paraffin X04
petrol X04
Immersion (accidental) —*see also* Drowning
hand or foot due to cold (excessive) X31
Implantation of quills of porcupine
W55.89
Inanition (from) (hunger) X58
thirst X58.8
Inappropriate operation performed
correct operation on wrong side or body
part (wrong side) (wrong site)
Y65.53
operation intended for another patient done
on wrong patient Y65.52
wrong operation performed on correct
patient Y65.51
Inattention after, at birth (homicidal intent)
(infanticidal intent) X58
Incident, adverse
device
anesthesiology Y70.8
accessory Y70.2
diagnostic Y70.0
miscellaneous Y70.8
monitoring Y70.0
prosthetic Y70.2
rehabilitative Y70.1
surgical Y70.3
therapeutic Y70.1
cardiovascular Y71.8
accessory Y71.2
diagnostic Y71.0
miscellaneous Y71.8
monitoring Y71.0
prosthetic Y71.2
rehabilitative Y71.1
surgical Y71.3
therapeutic Y71.1
gastroenterology Y73.8
accessory Y73.2
diagnostic Y73.0
miscellaneous Y73.8
monitoring Y73.0
prosthetic Y73.2
rehabilitative Y73.1
surgical Y73.3
therapeutic Y73.1
general
hospital Y74.8
accessory Y74.2
diagnostic Y74.0

Incident, adverse *(Continued)*
device *(Continued)*
general *(Continued)*
hospital *(Continued)*
miscellaneous Y74.8
monitoring Y74.0
prosthetic Y74.2
rehabilitative Y74.1
surgical Y74.3
therapeutic Y74.1
surgical Y81.8
accessory Y81.2
diagnostic Y81.0
miscellaneous Y81.8
monitoring Y81.0
prosthetic Y81.2
rehabilitative Y81.1
surgical Y81.3
therapeutic Y81.1
gynecological Y76.8
accessory Y76.2
diagnostic Y76.0
miscellaneous Y76.8
monitoring Y76.0
prosthetic Y76.2
rehabilitative Y76.1
surgical Y76.3
therapeutic Y76.1
medical Y82.9
specified type NEC Y82.8
neurological Y75.8
accessory Y75.2
diagnostic Y75.0
miscellaneous Y75.8
monitoring Y75.0
prosthetic Y75.2
rehabilitative Y75.1
surgical Y75.3
therapeutic Y75.1
obstetrical Y76.8
accessory Y76.2
diagnostic Y76.0
miscellaneous Y76.8
monitoring Y76.0
prosthetic Y76.2
rehabilitative Y76.1
surgical Y76.3
therapeutic Y76.1
ophthalmic Y77.8
accessory Y77.2
diagnostic Y77.0
miscellaneous Y77.8
monitoring Y77.0
prosthetic Y77.2
rehabilitative Y77.1
surgical Y77.3
therapeutic Y77.1
orthopedic Y79.8
accessory Y79.2
diagnostic Y79.0
miscellaneous Y79.8
monitoring Y79.0
prosthetic Y79.2
rehabilitative Y79.1
surgical Y79.3
therapeutic Y79.1
otorhinolaryngological Y72.8
accessory Y72.2
diagnostic Y72.0
miscellaneous Y72.8
monitoring Y72.0
prosthetic Y72.2
rehabilitative Y72.1
surgical Y72.3
therapeutic Y72.1
personal use Y74.8
accessory Y74.2
diagnostic Y74.0
miscellaneous Y74.8
monitoring Y74.0
prosthetic Y74.2

Incident, adverse *(Continued)*
device *(Continued)*
personal use *(Continued)*
rehabilitative Y74.1
surgical Y74.3
therapeutic Y74.1
physical medicine Y80.8
accessory Y80.2
diagnostic Y80.0
miscellaneous Y80.8
monitoring Y80.0
prosthetic Y80.2
rehabilitative Y80.1
surgical Y80.3
therapeutic Y80.1
plastic surgical Y81.8
accessory Y81.2
diagnostic Y81.0
miscellaneous Y81.8
monitoring Y81.0
prosthetic Y81.2
rehabilitative Y81.1
surgical Y81.3
therapeutic Y81.1
radiological Y78.8
accessory Y78.2
diagnostic Y78.0
miscellaneous Y78.8
monitoring Y78.0
prosthetic Y78.2
rehabilitative Y78.1
surgical Y78.3
therapeutic Y78.1
urology Y73.8
accessory Y73.2
diagnostic Y73.0
miscellaneous Y73.8
monitoring Y73.0
prosthetic Y73.2
rehabilitative Y73.1
surgical Y73.3
therapeutic Y73.1
Incineration (accidental) —*see* Exposure, fire
Infanticide —*see* Assault
Infrasound waves (causing injury) W49.9
Ingestion
foreign body (causing injury) (with
obstruction) —*see* Foreign body,
alimentary canal
poisonous
plant(s) X58
substance NEC —*see* Table of Drugs and
Chemicals
Inhalation
excessively cold substance, man-made —*see*
Exposure, cold, man-made
food (any type) (into respiratory tract) (with
asphyxia, obstruction respiratory tract,
suffocation) —*see* categories T17 and T18
foreign body —*see* Foreign body, aspiration
gastric contents (with asphyxia, obstruction
respiratory passage, suffocation) T17.81-●
hot air or gases X14.0
liquid air, hydrogen, nitrogen W93.12
suicide (attempt) X83.2
steam X13.0
assault X98.0
stated as undetermined whether accidental
or intentional Y27.0
suicide (attempt) X77.0
toxic gas —*see* Table of Drugs and
Chemicals
vomitus (with asphyxia, obstruction
respiratory passage, suffocation) T17.81-●
Injury, injured (accidental(ly)) NOS X58
by, caused by, from
assault —*see* Assault
law-enforcing agent, police, in course
of legal intervention —*see* Legal
intervention
suicide (attempt) X83.8

I, J, & K

Injury, injured NOS (Continued)
  due to, in
    civil insurrection —see War
        operations
    fight —see also Assault, fight
        Y04.0
    war operations —see War
        operations
  homicide —see also Assault Y09
  inflicted (by)
    in course of arrest (attempted), suppression
        of disturbance, maintenance of order,
        by law-enforcing agents —see Legal
        intervention

Injury, injured NOS (Continued)
  inflicted (Continued)
    other person
      stated as
        accidental X58
        intentional, homicide (attempt) —see
            Assault
        undetermined whether accidental or
            intentional Y33
    purposely (inflicted) by other person(s) —see
        Assault
    self-inflicted X83.8
      stated as accidental X58
    specified cause NEC X58

Injury, injured NOS (Continued)
    undetermined whether accidental or
        intentional Y33
  Insolation, effects X30
  Insufficient nourishment X58
  Interruption of respiration (by)
    food (lodged in esophagus) —see categories
        T17 and T18
    vomitus (lodged in esophagus) T17.81-●
  Intervention, legal —see Legal intervention
  Intoxication
    drug —see Table of Drugs and Chemicals
    poison —see Table of Drugs and
        Chemicals

J

Jammed (accidentally)
  between objects (moving) (stationary and
      moving) W23.0
    stationary W23.1
Jumped, jumping
  before moving object NEC X81.8
    motor vehicle X81.0
    subway train X81.1
    train X81.1
    undetermined whether accidental or
        intentional Y31
  from
    boat (into water) voluntarily,
        without accident (to or on boat)
        W16.712
      with
        accident to or on boat —see Accident,
            watercraft
        drowning or submersion W16.711
          suicide (attempt) X71.3

Jumped, jumping (Continued)
  from (Continued)
    boat voluntarily, without accident
        (Continued)
      striking bottom W16.722
        causing drowning W16.721
    building —see also Jumped, from,
        high place W13.9
      burning (uncontrolled fire)
          X00.5
    high place NEC W17.89
      suicide (attempt) X80
      undetermined whether accidental or
          intentional Y30
    structure —see also Jumped, from, high
        place W13.9
      burning (uncontrolled fire)
          X00.5
  into water W16.92
    causing drowning W16.91
    from, off watercraft —see Jumped, from,
        boat

Jumped, jumping (Continued)
  into water (Continued)
    in
      natural body W16.612
        causing drowning W16.611
        striking bottom W16.622
          causing drowning W16.621
      specified place NEC W16.812
        causing drowning W16.811
        striking
          bottom W16.822
            causing drowning W16.821
          wall W16.832
            causing drowning W16.831
      swimming pool W16.512
        causing drowning W16.511
        striking
          bottom W16.522
            causing drowning W16.521
          wall W16.532
            causing drowning W16.531
    suicide (attempt) X71.3

K

Kicked by
  animal NEC W55.82
  person(s) (accidentally) W50.1
    with intent to injure or kill Y04.0
    as, or caused by, a crowd or human
        stampede (with fall) W52
    assault Y04.0
    homicide (attempt) Y04.0
    in
      fight Y04.0
      legal intervention
        injuring
          bystander Y35.812
          law enforcement personnel
              Y35.811
          suspect Y35.813

Kicking
  against
    object W22.8
      sports equipment W21.9
      stationary W22.09
        sports equipment W21.89
    person —see Striking against, person
    sports equipment W21.9
  carpet stretcher with knee X50.3
Killed, killing (accidentally) NOS —see also
    Injury X58
  in
    action —see War operations
    brawl, fight (hand) (fists) (foot) Y04.0
      by weapon —see also Assault
        cutting, piercing —see Assault, cutting
            or piercing instrument
        firearm —see Discharge, firearm, by
            type, homicide

Killed, killing NOS (Continued)
  self
    stated as
      accident NOS X58
      suicide —see Suicide
      undetermined whether accidental or
          intentional Y33
Kneeling (prolonged) (static) X50.1
Knocked down (accidentally) (by) NOS X58
  animal (not being ridden) NEC —see also
      Struck by, by type of animal
  crowd or human stampede W52
  person W51
    in brawl, fight Y04.0
  transport vehicle NEC —see also Accident,
      transport V09.9

▶ New   ⇒ Revised   ~~deleted~~ Deleted   ● Use Additional Character(s)

L

Laceration NEC —*see* Injury
Lack of
care (helpless person) (infant) (newborn) X58
food except as result of abandonment or
neglect X58
due to abandonment or neglect X58
water except as result of transport accident X58
due to transport accident —*see* Accident,
transport, by type
helpless person, infant, newborn X58
Landslide (falling on transport vehicle) X36.1
caused by collapse of man-made structure
X36.0
Late effect —*see* Sequelae
Legal
execution (any method) —*see* Legal,
intervention
intervention (by)
baton —*see* Legal, intervention, blunt
object, baton
bayonet —*see* Legal, intervention, sharp
object, bayonet
blow —*see* Legal, intervention,
manhandling
blunt object
baton
injuring
bystander Y35.312
law enforcement personnel Y35.311
suspect Y35.313
injuring
bystander Y35.302
law enforcement personnel Y35.301
suspect Y35.303
specified NEC
injuring
bystander Y35.392
law enforcement personnel Y35.391
suspect Y35.393
stave
injuring
bystander Y35.392
law enforcement personnel Y35.391
suspect Y35.393
bomb —*see* Legal, intervention, explosive
cutting or piercing instrument —*see* Legal,
intervention, sharp object
dynamite —*see* Legal, intervention,
explosive, dynamite
explosive(s)
dynamite
injuring
bystander Y35.112
law enforcement personnel Y35.111
suspect Y35.113
grenade
injuring
bystander Y35.192
law enforcement personnel Y35.191
suspect Y35.193
injuring
bystander Y35.102
law enforcement personnel Y35.101
suspect Y35.103

Legal (*Continued*)
intervention (*Continued*)
explosive (*Continued*)
mortar bomb
injuring
bystander Y35.192
law enforcement personnel
Y35.191
suspect Y35.193
shell
injuring
bystander Y35.122
law enforcement personnel Y35.121
suspect Y35.123
specified NEC
injuring
bystander Y35.192
law enforcement personnel Y35.191
suspect Y35.193
firearm(s) (discharge)
handgun
injuring
bystander Y35.022
law enforcement personnel Y35.021
suspect Y35.023
injuring
bystander Y35.002
law enforcement personnel Y35.001
suspect Y35.003
machine gun
injuring
bystander Y35.012
law enforcement personnel Y35.011
suspect Y35.013
rifle pellet
injuring
bystander Y35.032
law enforcement personnel Y35.031
suspect Y35.033
rubber bullet
injuring
bystander Y35.042
law enforcement personnel Y35.041
suspect Y35.043
shotgun —*see* Legal, intervention,
firearm, specified NEC
specified NEC
injuring
bystander Y35.092
law enforcement personnel Y35.091
suspect Y35.093
gas (asphyxiation) (poisoning)
injuring
bystander Y35.202
law enforcement personnel Y35.201
suspect Y35.203
specified NEC
injuring
bystander Y35.292
law enforcement personnel Y35.291
suspect Y35.293
tear gas
injuring
bystander Y35.212
law enforcement personnel Y35.211
suspect Y35.213

Legal (*Continued*)
intervention (*Continued*)
grenade —*see* Legal, intervention,
explosive, grenade
injuring
bystander Y35.92
law enforcement personnel Y35.91
suspect Y35.93
late effect (of) —*see* with 7th character S
Y35
manhandling
injuring
bystander Y35.812
law enforcement personnel Y35.811
suspect Y35.813
sequelae (of) —*see* with 7th character S
Y35
sharp objects
bayonet
injuring
bystander Y35.412
law enforcement personnel
Y35.411
suspect Y35.413
injuring
bystander Y35.402
law enforcement personnel Y35.401
suspect Y35.403
specified NEC
injuring
bystander Y35.492
law enforcement personnel Y35.491
suspect Y35.493
specified means NEC
injuring
bystander Y35.892
law enforcement personnel Y35.891
suspect Y35.893
stabbing —*see* Legal, intervention, sharp
object
stave —*see* Legal, intervention, blunt
object, stave
tear gas —*see* Legal, intervention, gas, tear
gas
truncheon —*see* Legal, intervention, blunt
object, stave
Lifting —*see also* Overexertion
heavy objects X50.0
weights X50.0
Lightning (shock) (stroke) (struck by) —*see*
subcategory T75.0
causing fire —*see* Exposure, fire
Loss of control (transport vehicle) NEC —*see*
Accident, transport
Lost at sea NOS —*see* Drowning, due to, fall
overboard
Low
pressure (effects) —*see* Air, pressure, low
temperature (effects) —*see* Exposure, cold
Lying before train, vehicle or other moving
object X81.8
subway train X81.1
train X81.1
undetermined whether accidental or
intentional Y31
Lynching —*see* Assault

M

Malfunction (mechanism or component) (of)
  firearm
    airgun W34.10
    BB gun W34.110
    gas, air or spring-operated gun NEC
      W34.118
    handgun W32.1
    hunting rifle W33.12
    larger firearm W33.10
      specified NEC W33.19
    machine gun W33.13
    paintball gun W34.111
    pellet gun W34.110
    shotgun W33.11
    specified NEC W34.19
    Very pistol [flare] W34.19
  handgun —*see* Malfunction, firearm,
    handgun
Maltreatment —*see* Perpetrator
Mangled (accidentally) NOS X58
Manhandling (in brawl, fight) Y04.0
  legal intervention —*see* Legal, intervention,
    manhandling
Manslaughter (nonaccidental) —*see* Assault
Mauled by animal NEC W55.89
Medical procedure, complication of
  (delayed or as an abnormal reaction
    without mention of misadventure) —*see*
    Complication of or following, by specified
    type of procedure
  due to or as a result of misadventure —*see*
    Misadventure
Melting (due to fire) —*see also* Exposure, fire
  apparel NEC X06.3
  clothes, clothing NEC X06.3
    nightwear X05
  fittings or furniture (burning building)
    (uncontrolled fire) X00.8
  nightwear X05
  plastic jewelry X06.1
Mental cruelty X58
Military operations (injuries to military and
    civilians occuring during peacetime on
    military property and during routine
    military exercises and operations) (by)
    (from) (involving) Y37.90-•
  air blast Y37.20-•
  aircraft
    destruction —*see* Military operations,
      destruction of aircraft
    airway restriction —*see* Military operations,
      restriction of airways
    asphyxiation —*see* Military operations,
      restriction of airways
  biological weapons Y37.6X-•
  blast Y37.20-•
  blast fragments Y37.20-•
  blast wave Y37.20-•
  blast wind Y37.20-•
  bomb Y37.20-•
    dirty Y37.50-•
    gasoline Y37.31-•
    incendiary Y37.31-•
    petrol Y37.31-•
  bullet Y37.43-•
    incendiary Y37.32-•
    rubber Y37.41-•
  chemical weapons Y37.7X-•
  combat
    hand to hand (unarmed) combat
      Y37.44-•
    using blunt or piercing object Y37.45-•
  conflagration —*see* Military operations, fire
  conventional warfare NEC Y37.49-•
  depth-charge Y37.01-•
  destruction of aircraft Y37.10-•
    due to
      air to air missile Y37.11-•
      collision with other aircraft Y37.12-•

Military operations (*Continued*)
  destruction of aircraft (*Continued*)
    due to (*Continued*)
      detonation (accidental) of onboard
        munitions and explosives Y37.14-•
      enemy fire or explosives Y37.11-•
      explosive placed on aircraft Y37.11-•
      onboard fire Y37.13-•
      rocket propelled grenade [RPG] Y37.11-•
      small arms fire Y37.11-•
      surface to air missile Y37.11-•
      specified NEC Y37.19-•
  detonation (accidental) of
    onboard marine weapons Y37.05-•
    own munitions or munitions launch device
      Y37.24-•
  dirty bomb Y37.50-•
  explosion (of) Y37.20-•
    aerial bomb Y37.21-•
    bomb NOS —*see also* Military operations,
      bomb(s) Y37.20-•
    fragments Y37.20-•
    grenade Y37.29-•
    guided missile Y37.22-•
    improvised explosive device [IED]
      (person-borne) (roadside) (vehicle-
      borne) Y37.23-•
    land mine Y37.29-•
    marine mine (at sea) (in harbor) Y37.02-•
    marine weapon Y37.00-•
      specified NEC Y37.09-•
    own munitions or munitions launch device
      (accidental) Y37.24-•
    sea-based artillery shell Y37.03-•
    specified NEC Y37.29-•
    torpedo Y37.04-•
  fire Y37.30-•
    specified NEC Y37.39-•
  firearms
    discharge Y37.43-•
    pellets Y37.42-•
  flamethrower Y37.33-•
  fragments (from) (of)
    improvised explosive device [IED]
      (person-borne) (roadside) (vehicle-
      borne) Y37.26-•
    munitions Y37.25-•
    specified NEC Y37.29-•
    weapons Y37.27-•
  friendly fire Y37.92-•
  hand to hand (unarmed) combat Y37.44-•
  hot substances —*see* Military operations, fire
  incendiary bullet Y37.32-•
  nuclear weapon (effects of) Y37.50-•
    acute radiation exposure Y37.54-•
    blast pressure Y37.51-•
    direct blast Y37.51-•
    direct heat Y37.53-•
    fallout exposure Y37.54-•
    fireball Y37.53-•
    indirect blast (struck or crushed by blast
      debris) (being thrown by blast)
      Y37.52-•
    ionizing radiation (immediate exposure)
      Y37.54-•
    nuclear radiation Y37.54-•
    radiation
      ionizing (immediate exposure) Y37.54-•
      nuclear Y37.54-•
      thermal Y37.53-•
    secondary effects Y37.54-•
    specified NEC Y37.59-•
    thermal radiation Y37.53-•
  restriction of air (airway)
    intentional Y37.46-•
    unintentional Y37.47-•
  rubber bullets Y37.41-•
  shrapnel NOS Y37.29-•
  suffocation —*see* Military operations,
    restriction of airways
  unconventional warfare NEC Y37.7X-•

Military operations (*Continued*)
  underwater blast NOS Y37.00-•
  warfare
    conventional NEC Y37.49-•
    unconventional NEC Y37.7X-•
  weapon of mass destruction [WMD]
    Y37.91-•
  weapons
    biological weapons Y37.6X-•
    chemical Y37.7X-•
    nuclear (effects of) Y37.50-•
      acute radiation exposure Y37.54-•
      blast pressure Y37.51-•
      direct blast Y37.51-•
      direct heat Y37.53-•
      fallout exposure Y37.54-•
      fireball Y37.53-•
      radiation
        ionizing (immediate exposure)
          Y37.54-•
        nuclear Y37.54-•
        thermal Y37.53-•
      secondary effects Y37.54-•
      specified NEC Y37.59-•
    of mass destruction [WMD] Y37.91-•
Misadventure(s) to patient(s) during surgical
** or medical care** Y69
  contaminated medical or biological substance
    (blood, drug, fluid) Y64.9
    administered (by) NEC Y64.9
      immunization Y64.1
      infusion Y64.0
      injection Y64.1
      specified means NEC Y64.8
      transfusion Y64.0
      vaccination Y64.1
  excessive amount of blood or other fluid
    during transfusion or infusion Y63.0
  failure
    in dosage Y63.9
      electroshock therapy Y63.4
      inappropriate temperature (too hot or
        too cold) in local application and
        packing Y63.5
      infusion
        excessive amount of fluid Y63.0
        incorrect dilution of fluid Y63.1
      insulin-shock therapy Y63.4
      nonadministration of necessary drug or
        biological substance Y63.6
      overdose —*see* Table of Drugs and
        Chemicals
      radiation, in therapy Y63.2
    radiation
      overdose Y63.2
    specified procedure NEC Y63.8
    transfusion
      excessive amount of blood Y63.0
  mechanical, of instrument or apparatus
    (any) (during any procedure) Y65.8
  sterile precautions (during procedure)
    Y62.9
    aspiration of fluid or tissue (by puncture
      or catheterization, except heart)
      Y62.6
    biopsy (except needle aspiration)
      Y62.8
      needle (aspirating) Y62.6
    blood sampling Y62.6
    catheterization Y62.6
      heart Y62.5
    dialysis (kidney) Y62.2
    endoscopic examination Y62.4
    enema Y62.8
    immunization Y62.3
    infusion Y62.1
    injection Y62.3
    needle biopsy Y62.6
    paracentesis (abdominal) (thoracic)
      Y62.6
    perfusion Y62.2

▶ New   ⇒ Revised   ~~deleted~~ Deleted   • Use Additional Character(s)

Misadventure(s) to patient(s) during surgical
   or medical care *(Continued)*
   failure *(Continued)*
      sterile precautions *(Continued)*
         puncture (lumbar) Y62.6
         removal of catheter or packing
            Y62.8
         specified procedure NEC Y62.8
         surgical operation Y62.0
         transfusion Y62.1
         vaccination Y62.3
      suture or ligature during surgical
         procedure Y65.2
      to introduce or to remove tube or
         instrument —*see* Failure, to
   hemorrhage —*see* Index to Diseases and
      Injuries, Complication(s)
   inadvertent exposure of patient to radiation
      Y63.3
   inappropriate
      operation performed —*see*
         Inappropriate operation
         performed
      temperature (too hot or too cold) in
         local application or packing
         Y63.5

Misadventure(s) to patient(s) during surgical
   or medical care *(Continued)*
   infusion —*see also* Misadventure, by type,
      infusion Y69
      excessive amount of fluid Y63.0
      incorrect dilution of fluid Y63.1
      wrong fluid Y65.1
   mismatched blood in transfusion Y65.0
   nonadministration of necessary drug or
      biological substance Y63.6
   overdose —*see* Table of Drugs and
      Chemicals
   radiation (in therapy) Y63.2
   perforation —*see* Index to Diseases and
      Injuries, Complication(s)
   performance of inappropriate operation —*see*
      Inappropriate operation performed
   puncture —*see* Index to Diseases and Injuries,
      Complication(s)
   specified type NEC Y65.8
      failure
         suture or ligature during surgical
            operation Y65.2
         to introduce or to remove tube or
            instrument —*see* Failure, to
      infusion of wrong fluid Y65.1

Misadventure(s) to patient(s) during surgical
   or medical care *(Continued)*
   specified type NEC *(Continued)*
      performance of inappropriate operation —
         see Inappropriate operation performed
      transfusion of mismatched blood Y65.0
      wrong
         fluid in infusion Y65.1
         placement of endotracheal tube during
            anesthetic procedure Y65.3
   transfusion —*see* Misadventure, by type,
      transfusion
      excessive amount of blood Y63.0
      mismatched blood Y65.0
   wrong
      drug given in error —*see* Table of Drugs
         and Chemicals
      fluid in infusion Y65.1
      placement of endotracheal tube during
         anesthetic procedure Y65.3
Mismatched blood in transfusion Y65.0
Motion sickness T75.3
Mountain sickness W94.11
Mudslide (of cataclysmic nature) —*see*
   Landslide
Murder (attempt) —*see* Assault

N

Nail
   contact with W45.0
      gun W29.4
   embedded in skin W45.0
Neglect (criminal) (homicidal intent) X58

Noise (causing injury) (pollution) W42.9
   supersonic W42.0
Nonadministration (of)
   drug or biological substance (necessary)
      Y63.6
   surgical and medical care Y66
Nosocomial condition Y95

O

Object
   falling
      from, in, on, hitting
         machinery —*see* Contact, with, by type
            of machine
   set in motion by
      accidental explosion or rupture of pressure
         vessel W38
      firearm —*see* Discharge, firearm, by type
      machine (ry) —*see* Contact, with, by type
         of machine
Overdose (drug) —*see* Table of Drugs and
   Chemicals
   radiation Y63.2

Overexertion X50.9
   from
      prolonged static or awkward postures
         X50.1
      repetitive movements X50.3
      specified strenuous movements or postures
         NEC X50.9
      strenuous movement or load X50.0
Overexposure (accidental) (to)
   cold —*see also* Exposure, cold X31
      due to man-made conditions —*see*
         Exposure, cold, man-made
   heat —*see also* Heat X30
   radiation —*see* Radiation
   radioactivity W88.0
   sun (sunburn) X32

Overexposure *(Continued)*
   weather NEC —*see* Forces of nature
   wind NEC —*see* Forces of nature
Overheated —*see* Heat
Overturning (accidental)
   machinery —*see* Contact, with, by type of
      machine
   transport vehicle NEC —*see also* Accident,
      transport V89.9
   watercraft (causing drowning,
      submersion) —*see also* Drowning, due to,
      accident to, watercraft, overturning
   causing injury except drowning or
      submersion —*see* Accident, watercraft,
         causing, injury NEC

P

Parachute descent (voluntary) (without accident to aircraft) V97.29
  due to accident to aircraft —*see* Accident, transport, aircraft
Pecked by bird W61.99
Perforation during medical or surgical treatment as misadventure —*see* Index to Diseases and Injuries, Complication(s)
Perpetrator, perpetration, of assault, maltreatment and neglect (by) Y07.9
  boyfriend Y07.03
  brother Y07.410
    stepbrother Y07.435
  coach Y07.53
  cousin
    female Y07.491
    male Y07.490
  daycare provider Y07.519
    at-home
      adult care Y07.512
      childcare Y07.510
    care center
      adult care Y07.513
      childcare Y07.511
  family member NEC Y07.499
  father Y07.11
    adoptive Y07.13
    foster Y07.420
    stepfather Y07.430
  foster father Y07.420
  foster mother Y07.421
  girl friend Y07.04
  healthcare provider Y07.529
    mental health Y07.521
    specified NEC Y07.528
  husband Y07.01
  instructor Y07.53
  mother Y07.12
    adoptive Y07.14
    foster Y07.421
    stepmother Y07.433
  nonfamily member Y07.50
    specified NEC Y07.59
  nurse Y07.528
  occupational therapist Y07.528
  partner of parent
    female Y07.434
    male Y07.432
  physical therapist Y07.528
  sister Y07.411
  speech therapist Y07.528
  stepbrother Y07.435
  stepfather Y07.430
  stepmother Y07.433
  stepsister Y07.436
  teacher Y07.53
  wife Y07.02
Piercing —*see* Contact, with, by type of object or machine
Pinched
  between objects (moving) (stationary and moving) W23.0
    stationary W23.1
Pinned under machine (ry) —*see* Contact, with, by type of machine
Place of occurrence Y92.9
  abandoned house Y92.89
  airplane Y92.813
  airport Y92.520
  ambulatory health services establishment NEC Y92.538
  ambulatory surgery center Y92.530
  amusement park Y92.831
  apartment (co-op) —*see* Place of occurrence, residence, apartment
  assembly hall Y92.29
  bank Y92.510
  barn Y92.71
  baseball field Y92.320

Place of occurrence *(Continued)*
  basketball court Y92.310
  beach Y92.832
  boarding house —*see* Place of occurrence, residence, boarding house
  boat Y92.814
  bowling alley Y92.39
  bridge Y92.89
  building under construction Y92.61
  bus Y92.811
    station Y92.521
  cafe Y92.511
  campsite Y92.833
  campus —*see* Place of occurrence, school
  canal Y92.89
  car Y92.810
  casino Y92.59
  children's home —*see* Place of occurrence, residence, institutional, orphanage
  church Y92.22
  cinema Y92.26
  clubhouse Y92.29
  coal pit Y92.64
  college (community) Y92.214
  condominium —*see* Place of occurrence, residence, apartment
  construction area —*see* Place of occurrence, industrial and construction area
  convalescent home —*see* Place of occurrence, residence, institutional, nursing home
  court-house Y92.240
  cricket ground Y92.328
  cultural building Y92.258
    art gallery Y92.250
    museum Y92.251
    music hall Y92.252
    opera house Y92.253
    specified NEC Y92.258
    theater Y92.254
  dancehall Y92.252
  day nursery Y92.210
  dentist office Y92.531
  derelict house Y92.89
  desert Y92.820
  dock NOS Y92.89
  dockyard Y92.62
  doctor's office Y92.531
  dormitory —*see* Place of occurrence, residence, institutional, school dormitory
  dry dock Y92.62
  factory (building) (premises) Y92.63
  farm (land under cultivation) (outbuildings) Y92.79
    barn Y92.71
    chicken coop Y92.72
    field Y92.73
    hen house Y92.72
    house —*see* Place of occurrence, residence, house
    orchard Y92.74
    specified NEC Y92.79
  football field Y92.321
  forest Y92.821
  freeway Y92.411
  gallery Y92.250
  garage (commercial) Y92.59
    boarding house Y92.044
    military base Y92.135
    mobile home Y92.025
    nursing home Y92.124
    orphanage Y92.114
    private house Y92.015
    reform school Y92.155
  gas station Y92.524
  gasworks Y92.69
  golf course Y92.39
  gravel pit Y92.64
  grocery Y92.512
  gymnasium Y92.39
  handball court Y92.318
  harbor Y92.89

Place of occurrence *(Continued)*
  harness racing course Y92.39
  healthcare provider office Y92.531
  highway (interstate) Y92.411
  hill Y92.828
  hockey rink Y92.330
  home —*see* Place of occurrence, residence
  hospice —*see* Place of occurrence, residence, institutional, nursing home
  hospital Y92.239
    cafeteria Y92.233
    corridor Y92.232
    operating room Y92.234
    patient
      bathroom Y92.231
      room Y92.230
    specified NEC Y92.238
  hotel Y92.59
  house —*see also* Place of occurrence, residence
    abandoned Y92.89
    under construction Y92.61
  industrial and construction area (yard) Y92.69
    building under construction Y92.61
    dock Y92.62
    dry dock Y92.62
    factory Y92.63
    gasworks Y92.69
    mine Y92.64
    oil rig Y92.65
    pit Y92.64
    power station Y92.69
    shipyard Y92.62
    specified NEC Y92.69
    tunnel under construction Y92.69
    workshop Y92.69
  kindergarten Y92.211
  lacrosse field Y92.328
  lake Y92.828
  library Y92.241
  mall Y92.59
  market Y92.512
  marsh Y92.828
  military
    base —*see* Place of occurrence, residence, institutional, military base
    training ground Y92.84
  mine Y92.64
  mosque Y92.22
  motel Y92.59
  motorway (interstate) Y92.411
  mountain Y92.828
  movie-house Y92.26
  museum Y92.251
  music-hall Y92.252
  not applicable Y92.9
  nuclear power station Y92.69
  nursing home —*see* Place of occurrence, residence, institutional, nursing home
  office building Y92.59
  offshore installation Y92.65
  oil rig Y92.65
  old people's home —*see* Place of occurrence, residence, institutional, specified NEC
  opera-house Y92.253
  orphanage —*see* Place of occurrence, residence, institutional, orphanage
  outpatient surgery center Y92.530
  park (public) Y92.830
    amusement Y92.831
  parking garage Y92.89
    lot Y92.481
  pavement Y92.480
  physician office Y92.531
  polo field Y92.328
  pond Y92.828
  post office Y92.242
  power station Y92.69
  prairie Y92.828
  prison —*see* Place of occurrence, residence, institutional, prison

▶ New   ⇒ Revised   ~~deleted~~ Deleted   ● Use Additional Character(s)

Place of occurrence (Continued)
  public
    administration building Y92.248
      city hall Y92.243
      courthouse Y92.240
      library Y92.241
      post office Y92.242
      specified NEC Y92.248
    building NEC Y92.29
    hall Y92.29
    place NOS Y92.89
  race course Y92.39
  radio station Y92.59
  railway line (bridge) Y92.85
  ranch (outbuildings) —see Place of
      occurrence, farm
  recreation area Y92.838
    amusement park Y92.831
    beach Y92.832
    campsite Y92.833
    park (public) Y92.830
    seashore Y92.832
    specified NEC Y92.838
  reform school —see Place of occurrence,
      residence, institutional, reform school
  religious institution Y92.22
  residence (non-institutional) (private) Y92.009
    apartment Y92.039
      bathroom Y92.031
      bedroom Y92.032
      kitchen Y92.030
      specified NEC Y92.038
    bathroom Y92.002
    bedroom Y92.003
    boarding house Y92.049
      bathroom Y92.041
      bedroom Y92.042
      driveway Y92.043
      garage Y92.044
      garden Y92.046
      kitchen Y92.040
      specified NEC Y92.048
      swimming pool Y92.045
      yard Y92.046
    dining room Y92.001
    garden Y92.007
    home Y92.009
    house, single family Y92.019
      bathroom Y92.012
      bedroom Y92.013
      dining room Y92.011
      driveway Y92.014
      garage Y92.015
      garden Y92.017
      kitchen Y92.010
      specified NEC Y92.018
      swimming pool Y92.016
      yard Y92.017
    institutional Y92.10
      children's home —see Place of
          occurrence, residence, institutional,
          orphanage
      hospice —see Place of occurrence,
          residence, institutional, nursing
          home
      military base Y92.139
        barracks Y92.133
        garage Y92.135
        garden Y92.137
        kitchen Y92.130
        mess hall Y92.131
        specified NEC Y92.138
        swimming pool Y92.136
        yard Y92.137
      nursing home Y92.129
        bathroom Y92.121
        bedroom Y92.122
        driveway Y92.123
        garage Y92.124
        garden Y92.126
        kitchen Y92.120

Place of occurrence (Continued)
  residence (Continued)
    institutional (Continued)
      nursing home (Continued)
        specified NEC Y92.128
        swimming pool Y92.125
        yard Y92.126
      orphanage Y92.119
        bathroom Y92.111
        bedroom Y92.112
        driveway Y92.113
        garage Y92.114
        garden Y92.116
        kitchen Y92.110
        specified NEC Y92.118
        swimming pool Y92.115
        yard Y92.116
      prison Y92.149
        bathroom Y92.142
        cell Y92.143
        courtyard Y92.147
        dining room Y92.141
        kitchen Y92.140
        specified NEC Y92.148
        swimming pool Y92.146
      reform school Y92.159
        bathroom Y92.152
        bedroom Y92.153
        dining room Y92.151
        driveway Y92.154
        garage Y92.155
        garden Y92.157
        kitchen Y92.150
        specified NEC Y92.158
        swimming pool Y92.156
        yard Y92.157
      school dormitory Y92.169
        bathroom Y92.162
        bedroom Y92.163
        dining room Y92.161
        kitchen Y92.160
        specified NEC Y92.168
      specified NEC Y92.199
        bathroom Y92.192
        bedroom Y92.193
        dining room Y92.191
        driveway Y92.194
        garage Y92.195
        garden Y92.197
        kitchen Y92.190
        specified NEC Y92.198
        swimming pool Y92.196
        yard Y92.197
    kitchen Y92.000
    mobile home Y92.029
      bathroom Y92.022
      bedroom Y92.023
      dining room Y92.021
      driveway Y92.024
      garage Y92.025
      garden Y92.027
      kitchen Y92.020
      specified NEC Y92.028
      swimming pool Y92.026
      yard Y92.027
    specified place in residence NEC Y92.008
    specified residence type NEC Y92.099
      bathroom Y92.091
      bedroom Y92.092
      driveway Y92.093
      garage Y92.094
      garden Y92.096
      kitchen Y92.090
      specified NEC Y92.098
      swimming pool Y92.095
      yard Y92.096
  restaurant Y92.511
  riding school Y92.39
  river Y92.828
  road Y92.488
  rodeo ring Y92.39

Place of occurrence (Continued)
  rugby field Y92.328
  same day surgery center Y92.530
  sand pit Y92.64
  school (private) (public) (state) Y92.219
    college Y92.214
    daycare center Y92.210
    elementary school Y92.211
    high school Y92.213
    kindergarten Y92.211
    middle school Y92.212
    specified NEC Y92.218
    trace school Y92.215
    university Y92.214
    vocational school Y92.215
  sea (shore) Y92.832
  senior citizen center Y92.29
  service area
    airport Y92.520
    bus station Y92.521
    gas station Y92.524
    highway rest stop Y92.523
    railway station Y92.522
  shipyard Y92.62
  shop (commercial) Y92.513
  sidewalk Y92.480
  silo Y92.79
  skating rink (roller) Y92.331
    ice Y92.330
  slaughter house Y92.86
  soccer field Y92.322
  specified place NEC Y92.89
  sports area Y92.39
    athletic
      court Y92.318
        basketball Y92.310
        specified NEC Y92.318
        squash Y92.311
        tennis Y92.312
      field Y92.328
        baseball Y92.320
        cricket ground Y92.328
        football Y92.321
        hockey Y92.328
        soccer Y92.322
        specified NEC Y92.328
    golf course Y92.39
    gymnasium Y92.39
    riding school Y92.39
    skating rink (roller) Y92.331
      ice Y92.330
    stadium Y92.39
    swimming pool Y92.34
  squash court Y92.311
  stadium Y92.39
  steeplechasing course Y92.39
  store Y92.512
  stream Y92.828
  street and highway Y92.410
    bike path Y92.482
    freeway Y92.411
    highway ramp Y92.415
    interstate highway Y92.411
    local residential or business street
        Y92.414
    motorway Y92.411
    parking lot Y92.481
    parkway Y92.412
    sidewalk Y92.480
    specified NEC Y92.488
    state road Y92.413
  subway car Y92.816
  supermarket Y92.512
  swamp Y92.828
  swimming pool (public) Y92.34
    private (at) Y92.095
      boarding house Y92.045
      military base Y92.136
      mobile home Y92.026
      nursing home Y92.125
      orphanage Y92.115

Place of occurrence *(Continued)*
  swimming pool *(Continued)*
    private *(Continued)*
      prison Y92.146
      reform school Y92.156
      single family residence
        Y92.016
  synagogue Y92.22
  television station Y92.59
  tennis court Y92.312
  theater Y92.254
  trade area Y92.59
    bank Y92.510
    cafe Y92.511
    casino Y92.59
    garage Y92.59
    hotel Y92.59
    market Y92.512
    office building Y92.59
    radio station Y92.59
    restaurant Y92.511
    shop Y92.513
    shopping mall Y92.59
    store Y92.512
    supermarket Y92.512
    television station Y92.59
    warehouse Y92.59
  trailer park, residential —*see* Place of
    occurrence, residence, mobile
    home
  trailer site NOS Y92.89
  train Y92.815
    station Y92.522
  truck Y92.812
  tunnel under construction Y92. 69
  university Y92.214
  urgent (health) care center Y92.532
  vehicle (transport) Y92.818
    airplane Y92.813
    boat Y92.814
    bus Y92.811
    car Y92.810
    specified NEC Y92.818
    subway car Y92.816
    train Y92.815
    truck Y92.812
  warehouse Y92.59
  water reservoir Y92.89
  wilderness area Y92.828
    desert Y92.820
    forest Y92.821
    marsh Y92.828
    mountain Y92.828
    prairie Y92.828
    specified NEC Y92.828
    swamp Y92.828
  workshop Y92.69
  yard, private Y92.096
    boarding house Y92.046
    mobile home Y92.027
    single family house Y92.017

Place of occurrence *(Continued)*
  youth center Y92.29
  zoo (zoological garden) Y92.834
Plumbism —*see* Table of Drugs and Chemicals,
  lead
Poisoning (accidental) (by) —*see also* Table of
  Drugs and Chemicals
  by plant, thorns, spines, sharp leaves or other
    mechanisms NEC X58
  carbon monoxide
    generated by
      motor vehicle —*see* Accident, transport
      watercraft (in transit) (not in transit)
        V93.89
        ferry boat V93.81
        fishing boat V93.82
        jet skis V93.83
        liner V93.81
        merchant ship V93.80
        passenger ship V93.81
        powered craft NEC V93.83
  caused by injection of poisons into skin by
    plant thorns, spines, sharp leaves X58
    marine or sea plants (venomous) X58
  exhaust gas
    generated by
      motor vehicle —*see* Accident, transport
      watercraft (in transit) (not in transit)
        V93.89
        ferry boat V93.81
        fishing boat V93.82
        jet skis V93.83
        liner V93.81
        merchant ship V93.80
        passenger ship V93.81
        powered craft NEC V93.83
  fumes or smoke due to
    explosion —*see also* Explosion W40.9
    fire —*see* Exposure, fire
    ignition —*see* Ignition
  gas
    in legal intervention —*see* Legal,
      intervention, gas
    legal execution —*see* Legal, intervention,
      gas
  in war operations —*see* War operations
  legal
  execution —*see* Legal, intervention, gas
  intervention
      by gas —*see* Legal, intervention, gas
      other specified means —*see* Legal,
        intervention, specified means
        NEC
Powder burn (by) (from)
  airgun W34.110
  BB gun W34.110
  firearm NEC W34.19
  gas, air or spring-operated gun NEC
    W34.118
  handgun W32.1
  hunting rifle W33.12

Powder burn *(Continued)*
  larger firearm W33.10
    specified NEC W33.19
  machine gun W33.13
  paintball gun W34.111
  pellet gun W34.110
  shotgun W33.11
  Very pistol [flare] W34.19
Premature cessation (of) surgical and medical
  care Y66
Privation (food) (water) X58
Procedure (operation)
  correct, on wrong side or body part (wrong
    side) (wrong site) Y65.53
  intended for another patient done on wrong
    patient Y65.52
  performed on patient not scheduled for
    surgery Y65.52
  performed on wrong patient Y65.52
  wrong, performed on correct patient Y65.51
Prolonged
  sitting in transport vehicle —*see* Travel, by
    type of vehicle
  stay in
    high altitude as cause of anoxia,
      barodontalgia, barotitis or hypoxia
      W94.11
    weightless environment X52
Pulling, excessive —*see also* Overexertion
  X50.9
Puncture, puncturing —*see also* Contact, with,
  by type of object or machine
  by
    plant thorns, spines, sharp leaves or other
      mechanisms NEC W60
  during medical or surgical treatment as
    misadventure —*see* Index to Diseases
    and Injuries, Complication(s)
Pushed, pushing (accidental) (injury in)
  by other person(s) (accidental) W51
    with fall W03
      due to ice or snow W00.0
    as, or caused by, a crowd or human
      stampede (with fall) W52
    before moving object NEC Y02.8
      motor vehicle Y02.0
      subway train Y02.1
      train Y02.1
    from
      high place NEC
        in accidental circumstances W17.89
        stated as
          intentional, homicide (attempt) Y01
          undetermined whether accidental
            or intentional Y30
      transport vehicle NEC —*see also*
        Accident, transport V89.9
        stated as
          intentional, homicide (attempt)
            Y08.89
    overexertion X50.9

▶ New   ⇒ Revised   ~~deleted~~ Deleted   ● Use Additional Character(s)

R

Radiation (exposure to)
arc lamps W89.Ø
atomic power plant (malfunction) NEC
      W88.1
complication of or abnormal reaction to
      medical radiotherapy Y84.2
electromagnetic, ionizing W88.Ø
gamma rays W88.1
in
   war operations (from or following
         nuclear explosion) —see also War
         operations
   inadvertent exposure of patient (receiving
         test or therapy) Y63.3
infrared (heaters and lamps) W90.1
   excessive heat from W92
ionized, ionizing (particles, artificially
      accelerated)
   radioisotopes W88.1
   specified NEC W88.8
   x-rays W88.Ø
isotopes, radioactive —see Radiation,
      radioactive isotopes
laser(s) W90.2
   in war operations —see War operations
   misadventure in medical care Y63.2
light sources (man-made visible and
      ultraviolet) W89.9
   natural X32
   specified NEC W89.8
   tanning bed W89.1
   welding light W89.Ø
man-made visible light W89.9
   specified NEC W89.8
   tanning bed W89.1
   welding light W89.Ø
microwave W90.8
misadventure in medical or surgical
      procedure Y63.2

Radiation (Continued)
natural NEC X39.Ø8
   radon X39.Ø1
overdose (in medical or surgical procedure)
      Y63.2
radar W90.Ø
radioactive isotopes (any) W88.1
   atomic power plant malfunction W88.1
   misadventure in medical or surgical
         treatment Y63.2
radiofrequency W90.Ø
radium NEC W88.1
sun X32
ultraviolet (light) (man-made) W89.9
   natural X32
   specified NEC W89.8
   tanning bed W89.1
   welding light W89.Ø
welding arc, torch, or light W89.Ø
   excessive heat from W92
x-rays (hard) (soft) W88.Ø
Range disease W94.11
Rape (attempted) T74.2- ●
Rat bite W53.11
Reaching (prolonged) (static) X50.1
Reaction, abnormal to medical procedure —see
      also Complication of or following, by type
      of procedure Y84.9
with misadventure —see Misadventure
biologicals —see Table of Drugs and
      Chemicals
drugs —see Table of Drugs and Chemicals
vaccine —see Table of Drugs and
      Chemicals
Recoil
airgun W34.11Ø
BB gun W34.11Ø
firearm NEC W34.19
gas, air or spring-operated gun NEC W34.118

Recoil (Continued)
handgun W32.1
hunting rifle W33.12
larger firearm W33.1Ø
   specified NEC W33.19
machine gun W33.13
paintball gun W34.111
pellet W34.11Ø
shotgun W33.11
Very pistol [flare] W34.19
Reduction in
atmospheric pressure —see Air, pressure,
      change
Rock falling on or hitting (accidentally)
      (person) W20.8
in cave-in W20.Ø
Run over (accidentally) (by)
animal (not being ridden) NEC W55.89
machinery —see Contact, with, by specified
      type of machine
transport vehicle NEC —see also Accident,
      transport V09.9
   intentional homicide (attempt) Y03.0
   motor NEC V09.20
      intentional homicide (attempt) Y03.0
Running
before moving object X81.8
   motor vehicle X81.0
Running off, away
animal (being ridden) —see also Accident,
      transport V80.918
   not being ridden W55.89
animal-drawn vehicle NEC —see also
      Accident, transport V80.928
highway, road(way), street
   transport vehicle NEC —see also Accident,
      transport V89.9
Rupture pressurized devices —see Explosion,
      by type of device

S

Saturnism —see Table of Drugs and Chemicals, lead
Scald, scalding (accidental) (by) (from) (in) X19
  air (hot) X14.1
  gases (hot) X14.1
  homicide (attempt) —see Assault, burning, hot object
  inflicted by other person
    stated as intentional, homicide (attempt) — see Assault, burning, hot object
  liquid (boiling) (hot) NEC X12
    stated as undetermined whether accidental or intentional Y27.2
    suicide (attempt) X77.2
  local application of externally applied substance in medical or surgical care Y63.5
  metal (molten) (liquid) (hot) NEC X18
  self-inflicted X77.9
  stated as undetermined whether accidental or intentional Y27.8
  steam X13.1
    assault X98.0
    stated as undetermined whether accidental or intentional Y27.0
    suicide (attempt) X77.0
  suicide (attempt) X77.9
  vapor (hot) X13.1
    assault X98.0
    stated as undetermined whether accidental or intentional Y27.0
    suicide (attempt) X77.0
Scratched by
  cat W55.03
  person(s) (accidentally) W50.4
    with intent to injure or kill Y04.0
    as, or caused by, a crowd or human stampede (with fall) W52
    assault Y04.0
    homicide (attempt) Y04.0
    in
      fight Y04.0
      legal intervention
        injuring
          bystander Y35.892
          law enforcement personnel Y35.891
          suspect Y35.893
Seasickness T75.3
Self-harm NEC —see also External cause by type, undetermined whether accidental or intentional
  intentional —see Suicide
  poisoning NEC —see Table of drugs and biologicals, accident
Self-inflicted (injury) NEC —see also External cause by type, undetermined whether accidental or intentional
  intentional —see Suicide
  poisoning NEC —see Table of drugs and biologicals, accident
Sequelae (of)
  accident NEC —see W00-X58 with 7th character S
  assault (homicidal) (any means) —see X92-Y08 with 7th character S
  homicide, attempt (any means) —see X92-Y08 with 7th character S
  injury undetermined whether accidentally or purposely inflicted —see Y21-Y33 with 7th character S
  intentional self-harm (classifiable to X71-X83) —see X71-X83 with 7th character S
  legal intervention (see with 7th character S Y35)
  motor vehicle accident —see V00-V99 with 7th character S
  suicide, attempt (any means) —see X71-X83 with 7th character S

Sequelae (Continued)
  transport accident —see V00-V99 with 7th character S
  war operations —see War operations
Shock
  electric —see Exposure, electric current
  from electric appliance (any) (faulty) W86.8
    domestic W86.0
    suicide (attempt) X83.1
Shooting, shot (accidental (ly)) —see also Discharge, firearm, by type
  herself or himself —see Discharge, firearm by type, self-inflicted
  homicide (attempt) —see Discharge, firearm by type, homicide
  in war operations —see War operations
  inflicted by other person —see Discharge, firearm by type, homicide
    accidental —see Discharge, firearm, by type of firearm
  legal
    execution —see Legal, intervention, firearm
    intervention —see Legal, intervention, firearm
  self-inflicted —see Discharge, firearm by type, suicide
    accidental —see Discharge, firearm, by type of firearm
  suicide (attempt) —see Discharge, firearm by type, suicide
Shoving (accidentally) by other person —see Pushed, by other person
Sickness
  alpine W94.11
  motion —see Motion
  mountain W94.11
Sinking (accidental)
  watercraft (causing drowning, submersion) —see also Drowning, due to, accident to, watercraft, sinking
    causing injury except drowning or submersion —see Accident, watercraft, causing, injury NEC
Siriasis X32
Sitting (prolonged) (static) X50.1
Slashed wrists —see Cut, self-inflicted
Slipping (accidental) (on same level) (with fall) W01.0
  without fall W18.40
    due to
      specified NEC W18.49
      stepping from one level to another W18.43
      stepping into hole or opening W18.42
      stepping on object W18.41
  on
    ice W00.0
      with skates —see Accident, transport, pedestrian, conveyance
    mud W01.0
    oil W01.0
    snow W00.0
      with skis —see Accident, transport, pedestrian, conveyance
    surface (slippery) (wet) NEC W01.0
Sliver, wood, contact with W45.8
Smoldering (due to fire) —see Exposure, fire
Sodomy (attempted) by force T74.2-●
Sound waves (causing injury) W42.9
  supersonic W42.0
Splinter, contact with W45.8
Stab, stabbing —see Cut
Standing (prolonged) (static) X50.1
Starvation X58
Status of external cause Y99.9
  child assisting in compensated work for family Y99.8
  civilian activity done for financial or other compensation Y99.0
  civilian activity done for income or pay Y99.0

Status of external cause (Continued)
  family member assisting in compensated work for other family member Y99.8
  hobby not done for income Y99.8
  leisure activity Y99.8
  military activity Y99.1
  off-duty activity of military personnel Y99.8
  recreation or sport not for income or while a student Y99.8
  specified NEC Y99.8
  student activity Y99.8
  volunteer activity Y99.2
Stepped on
  by
    animal (not being ridden) NEC W55.89
    crowd or human stampede W52
    person W50.0
Stepping on
  object W22.8
    with fall W18.31
    sports equipment W21.9
    stationary W22.09
      sports equipment W21.89
  person W51
    by crowd or human stampede W52
  sports equipment W21.9
Sting
  arthropod, nonvenomous W57
  insect, nonvenomous W57
Storm (cataclysmic) —see Forces of nature, cataclysmic storm
Straining, excessive —see also Overexertion X50.9
Strangling —see Strangulation
Strangulation (accidental) —see category T71
Strenuous movements —see also Overexertion X50.9
Striking against
  airbag (automobile) W22.10
    driver side W22.11
    front passenger side W22.12
    specified NEC W22.19
  bottom when
    diving or jumping into water (in) W16.822
      causing drowning W16.821
      from boat W16.722
        causing drowning W16.721
      natural body W16.622
        causing drowning W16.821
      swimming pool W16.522
        causing drowning W16.521
    falling into water (in) W16.322
      causing drowning W16.321
      fountain —see Striking against, bottom when, falling into water, specified NEC
      natural body W16.122
        causing drowning W16.121
      reservoir —see Striking against, bottom when, falling into water, specified NEC
      specified NEC W16.322
        causing drowning W16.321
      swimming pool W16.022
        causing drowning W16.021
  diving board (swimming-pool) W21.4
  object W22.8
    with
      drowning or submersion —see Drowning
      fall —see Fall, due to, bumping against, object
    caused by crowd or human stampede (with fall) W52
    furniture W22.03
    lamppost W22.02
    sports equipment W21.9
    stationary W22.09
      sports equipment W21.89
    wall W22.01

▶ New   ⇒ Revised   ~~deleted~~ Deleted   ● Use Additional Character(s)

Striking against (*Continued*)
  person(s) W51
    with fall W03
      due to ice or snow W00.0
    as, or caused by, a crowd or human
        stampede (with fall) W52
    assault Y04.2
    homicide (attempt) Y04.2
  sports equipment W21.9
  wall (when) W22.01
    diving or jumping into water (in) W16.832
      causing drowning W16.831
      swimming pool W16.532
        causing drowning W16.531
    falling into water (in) W16.332
      causing drowning W16.331
      fountain —*see* Striking against, wall
        when, falling into water, specified
        NEC
      natural body W16.132
        causing drowning W16.131
      reservoir —*see* Striking against, wall
        when, falling into water, specified
        NEC
      specified NEC W16.332
        causing drowning W16.331
      swimming pool W16.032
        causing drowning W16.031
    swimming pool (when) W22.042
      causing drowning W22.041
      diving or jumping into water W16.532
        causing drowning W16.531
      falling into water W16.032
        causing drowning W16.031
Struck (accidentally) by
  airbag (automobile) W22.10
    driver side W22.11
    front passenger side W22.12
    specified NEC W22.19
  alligator W58.02
  animal (not being ridden) NEC W55.89
  avalanche —*see* Landslide
  ball (hit) (thrown) W21.00
    assault Y08.09
    baseball W21.03
    basketball W21.05
    football W21.01
    golf ball W21.04
    football W21.01
    soccer W21.02
    softball W21.07
    specified NEC W21.09
    volleyball W21.06
  bat or racquet
    baseball bat W21.11
      assault Y08.02
    golf club W21.13
      assault Y08.09
    specified NEC W21.19
      assault Y08.09
    tennis racquet W21.12
      assault Y08.09
  bullet —*see also* Discharge, firearm by type
    in war operations —*see* War operations
  crocodile W58.12
  dog W54.1
  flare, Very pistol —*see* Discharge, firearm
    NEC
  hailstones X39.8
  hockey (ice)
    field
      puck W21.221
      stick W21.211
    puck W21.220
    stick W21.210
      assault Y08.01
  landslide —*see* Landslide
  law-enforcement agent (on duty) —*see* Legal,
    intervention, manhandling
    with blunt object —*see* Legal, intervention,
      blunt object

Struck by (*Continued*)
  lightning —*see* subcategory T75.0
    causing fire —*see* Exposure, fire
  machine —*see* Contact, with, by type of
    machine
  mammal NEC W55.89
    marine W56.32
  marine animal W56.82
  missile
    firearm —*see* Discharge, firearm by type
    in war operations —*see* War operations,
      missile
  object W22.8
    blunt W22.8
      assault Y00
      suicide (attempt) X79
      undetermined whether accidental or
        intentional Y29
    falling W20.8
      from, in, on
        building W20.1
          burning (uncontrolled fire) X00.4
        cataclysmic
          earth surface movement NEC —*see*
            Landslide
          storm —*see* Forces of nature,
            cataclysmic storm
        cave-in W20.0
        earthquake X34
        machine (in operation) —*see* Contact,
          with, by type of machine
        structure W20.1
          burning X00.4
        transport vehicle (in motion) —*see*
          Accident, transport, by type of
          vehicle
        watercraft V93.49
          due to
            accident to craft V91.39
              powered craft V91.33
                ferry boat V91.31
                fishing boat V91.32
                jetskis V91.33
                liner V91.31
                merchant ship V91.30
                passenger ship V91.31
             unpowered craft V91.38
                canoe V91.35
                inflatable V91.36
                kayak V91.35
                sailboat V91.34
                surf-board V91.38
                windsurfer V91.38
            powered craft V93.43
              ferry boat V93.41
              fishing boat V93.42
              jetskis V93.43
              liner V93.41
              merchant ship V93.40
              passenger ship V93.41
            unpowered craft V93.48
              sailboat V93.44
              surf-board V93.48
              windsurfer V93.48
    moving NEC W20.8
    projected W20.8
      assault Y00
      in sports W21.9
        assault Y08.09
        ball W21.00
          baseball W21.03
          basketball W21.05
          football W21.01
          golf ball W21.04
          soccer W21.02
          softball W21.07
          specified NEC W21.09
          volleyball W21.06
        bat or racquet
          baseball bat W21.11
            assault Y08.02

Struck by (*Continued*)
  object (*Continued*)
    projected (*Continued*)
      in sports (*Continued*)
        bat or racquet (*Continued*)
          golf club W21.13
            assault Y08.09-•
          specified NEC W21.19
            assault Y08.09
          tennis racquet W21.12
            assault Y08.09
        hockey (ice)
          field
            puck W21.221
            stick W21.211
          puck W21.220
          stick W21.210
            assault Y08.01
        specified NEC W21.89
    set in motion by explosion —*see* Explosion
    thrown W20.8
      assault Y00
      in sports W21.9
        assault Y08.09
        ball W21.00
          baseball W21.03
          basketball W21.05
          football W21.01
          golf ball W21.04
          soccer W21.02
          soft ball W21.07
          specified NEC W21.09
          volleyball W21.06
        bat or racquet
          baseball bat W21.11
            assault Y08.02
          golf club W21.13
            assault Y08.09
          specified NEC W21.19
            assault Y08.09
          tennis racquet W21.12
            assault Y08.09
        hockey (ice)
          field
            puck W21.221
            stick W21.211
          puck W21.220
          stick W21.210
            assault Y08.01
        specified NEC W21.89
  other person(s) W50.0
    with
      blunt object W22.8
        intentional, homicide (attempt) Y00
        sports equipment W21.9
        undetermined whether accidental or
          intentional Y29
      fall W03
        due to ice or snow W00.0
      as, or caused by, a crowd or human
        stampede (with fall) W52
    assault Y04.2
    homicide (attempt) Y04.2
    in legal intervention
      injuring
        bystander Y35.812
        law enforcement personnel Y35.811
        suspect Y35.813
    sports equipment W21.9
  police (on duty) —*see* Legal, intervention,
    manhandling
    with blunt object —*see* Legal, intervention,
      blunt object
  sports equipment W21.9
    assault Y08.09
    ball W21.00
      baseball W21.03
      basketball W21.05
      football W21.01
      golf ball W21.04
      soccer W21.02

Struck by (Continued)
  sports equipment (Continued)
    ball (Continued)
      soft ball W21.07
      specified NEC W21.09
      volleyball W21.06
    bat or racquet
      baseball bat W21.11
        assault Y08.02
      golf club W21.13
        assault Y08.09
      specified NEC W21.19
      tennis racquet W21.12
        assault Y08.09
    cleats (shoe) W21.31
    foot wear NEC W21.39
    football helmet W21.81
    hockey (ice)
      field
        puck W21.221
        stick W21.211
      puck W21.220
      stick W21.210
        assault Y08.01
    skate blades W21.32
    specified NEC W21.89
      assault Y08.09
  thunderbolt —*see* subcategory
    T75.0
  causing fire —*see* Exposure, fire
  transport vehicle NEC —*see also* Accident,
    transport V09.9
    intentional, homicide (attempt) Y03.0
    motor NEC —*see also* Accident, transport
      V09.20
      homicide Y03.0
  vehicle (transport) NEC —*see* Accident,
    transport, by type of vehicle
  stationary (falling from jack,
    hydraulic lift, ramp)
    W20.8
Stumbling
  without fall W18.40
    due to
      specified NEC W18.49
      stepping from one level to another
        W18.43
      stepping into hole or opening W18.42
      stepping on object W18.41
  over
    animal NEC W01.0
      with fall W18.09
    carpet, rug or (small) object W22.8
      with fall W18.09
    person W51
      with fall W03
        due to ice or snow W00.0

Submersion (accidental) —*see* Drowning
Suffocation (accidental) (by external means)
  (by pressure) (mechanical) —*see also*
    category T71
  due to, by
    avalanche —*see* Landslide
    explosion —*see* Explosion
    fire —*see* Exposure, fire
    food, any type (aspiration) (ingestion)
      (inhalation) —*see* categories T17 and
      T18
    ignition —*see* Ignition
    landslide —*see* Landslide
    machine (ry) —*see* Contact, with, by type
      of machine
    vomitus (aspiration) (inhalation)
      T17.81-●
  in
    burning building X00.8
Suicide, suicidal (attempted) (by) X83.8
  blunt object X79
  burning, burns X76
    hot object X77.9
      fluid NEC X77.2
      household appliance X77.3
      specified NEC X77.8
      steam X77.0
      tap water X77.1
      vapors X77.0
  caustic substance —*see* Table of Drugs and
    Chemicals
  cold, extreme X83.2
  collision of motor vehicle with
    motor vehicle X82.0
    specified NEC X82.8
    train X82.1
    tree X82.2
  crashing of aircraft X83.0
  cut (any part of body) X78.9
  cutting or piercing instrument X78.9
    dagger X78.2
    glass X78.0
    knife X78.1
    specified NEC X78.8
    sword X78.2
  drowning (in) X71.9
    bathtub X71.0
    natural water X71.3
    specified NEC X71.8
    swimming pool X71.1
      following fall X71.2
  electrocution X83.1
  explosive(s) (material) X75
  fire, flames X76
  firearm X74.9
    airgun X74.01
    handgun X72

Suicide, suicidal (Continued)
  firearm (Continued)
    hunting rifle X73.1
    larger X73.9
      specified NEC X73.8
    machine gun X73.2
    shotgun X73.0
    specified NEC X74.8
  hanging X83.8
  hot object —*see* Suicide, burning, hot object
  jumping
    before moving object X81.8
      motor vehicle X81.0
      subway train X81.1
      train X81.1
    from high place X80
  late effect of attempt —*see* X71-X83 with 7th
    character S
  lying before moving object, train, vehicle X81.8
  poisoning —*see* Table of Drugs and
    Chemicals
  puncture (any part of body) —*see* Suicide,
    cutting or piercing instrument
  scald —*see* Suicide, burning, hot object
  sequelae of attempt —*see* X71-X83 with 7th
    character S
  sharp object (any) —*see* Suicide, cutting or
    piercing instrument
  shooting —*see* Suicide, firearm
  specified means NEC X83.8
  stab (any part of body) —*see* Suicide, cutting
    or piercing instrument
  steam, hot vapors X77.0
  strangulation X83.8
  submersion —*see* Suicide, drowning
  suffocation X83.8
  wound NEC X83.8
Sunstroke X32
Supersonic waves (causing injury) W42.0
Surgical procedure, complication of (delayed
  or as an abnormal reaction without
  mention of misadventure) —*see also*
  Complication of or following, by type of
  procedure
  due to or as a result of misadventure —*see*
    Misadventure
Swallowed, swallowing
  foreign body —*see* Foreign body, alimentary
    canal
  poison —*see* Table of Drugs and Chemicals
  substance
    caustic or corrosive —*see* Table of Drugs
      and Chemicals
      poisonous —*see* Table of Drugs and
        Chemicals

▶ New   ⮕ Revised   ~~deleted~~ Deleted   ● Use Additional Character(s)

T

Tackle in sport W03
Terrorism (involving) Y38.8Ø
  biological weapons Y38.6X-●
  chemical weapons Y38.7X-●
  conflagration Y38.3X-●
  drowning and submersion Y38.89-●
  explosion Y38.2X-●
    destruction of aircraft Y38.1X-●
    marine weapons Y38.ØX-●
  fire Y38.3X-●
  firearms Y38.4X-●
  hot substances Y38.3X-●
  lasers Y38.89-●
  nuclear weapons Y38.5X-●
  piercing or stabbing instruments
    Y38.89-●
  secondary effects Y38.9X-●
  specified method NEC Y38.89-●
  suicide bomber Y38.81-●
Thirst X58
Threat to breathing
  aspiration —see Aspiration
  due to cave-in, falling earth or substance
    NEC —see category T71
Thrown (accidentally)
  against part (any) of or object in transport
    vehicle (in motion) NEC —see also
    Accident, transport

Thrown (Continued)
  from
    high place, homicide (attempt) YØ1
    machinery —see Contact, with, by type of
      machine
    transport vehicle NEC —see also Accident,
      transport V89.9
  off —see Thrown, from
Thunderbolt —see subcategory T75.Ø
  causing fire —see Exposure, fire
Tidal wave (any injury) NEC —see Forces of
  nature, tidal wave
Took
  overdose (drug) —see Table of Drugs and
    Chemicals
  poison —see Table of Drugs and
    Chemicals
Tornado (any injury) X37.1
Torrential rain (any injury) X37.8
Torture X58
Trampled by animal NEC W55.89
Trapped (accidentally)
  between objects (moving) (stationary and
    moving) —see Caught
  by part (any) of
    motorcycle V29.88
    pedal cycle V19.88
    transport vehicle NEC —see also Accident,
      transport V89.9
Travel (effects) (sickness) T75.3

Tree falling on or hitting (accidentally)
  (person) W20.8
Tripping
  without fall W18.4Ø
    due to
      specified NEC W18.49
      stepping from one level to another
        W18.43
      stepping into hole or opening
        W18.42
      stepping on object W18.41
  over
    animal WØ1.Ø
      with fall WØ1.Ø
    carpet, rug or (small) object W22.8
      with fall W18.09
    person W51
      with fall WØ3
        due to ice or snow WØØ.Ø
Twisted by person(s) (accidentally) W5Ø.2
  with intent to injure or kill YØ4.Ø
  as, or caused by, a crowd or human stampede
    (with fall) W52
  assault YØ4.Ø
  homicide (attempt) YØ4.Ø
  in
    fight YØ4.Ø
    legal intervention —see Legal, intervention,
      manhandling
Twisting (prolonged) (static) X5Ø.1

U

Underdosing of necessary drugs, medicaments
  or biological substances Y63.6
Undetermined intent (contact)
  (exposure)
  automobile collision Y32
  blunt object Y29
  drowning (submersion) (in) Y21.9
    bathtub Y21.Ø
      after fall Y21.1
    natural water (lake) (ocean) (pond) (river)
      (stream) Y21.4
    specified place NEC Y21.8
    swimming pool Y21.2
      after fall Y21.3
  explosive material Y25
  fall, jump or push from high place Y3Ø
  falling, lying or running before moving object
    Y31
  fire Y26

Undetermined intent (Continued)
  firearm discharge Y24.9
    airgun (BB) (pellet) Y24.Ø
    handgun (pistol) (revolver)
      Y22
    hunting rifle Y23.1
    larger Y23.9
      hunting rifle Y23.1
      machine gun Y23.3
      military Y23.2
      shotgun Y23.Ø
      specified type NEC Y23.8
    machine gun Y23.3
    military Y23.2
    shotgun Y23.Ø
    specified type NEC Y24.8
    Very pistol Y24.8
  hot object Y27.9
    fluid NEC Y27.2
    household appliance Y27.3
    specified object NEC Y27.8

Undetermined intent (Continued)
  hot object (Continued)
    steam Y27.Ø
    tap water Y27.1
    vapor Y27.Ø
  jump, fall or push from high place Y3Ø
  lying, falling or running before moving object
    Y31
  motor vehicle crash Y32
  push, fall or jump from high place Y3Ø
  running, falling or lying before moving object
    Y31
  sharp object Y28.9
    dagger Y28.2
    glass Y28.Ø
    knife Y28.1
    specified object NEC Y28.8
    sword Y28.2
  smoke Y26
  specified event NEC Y33
Use of hand as hammer X5Ø.3

V

Vibration (causing injury) W49.9
Victim (of)
  avalanche —see Landslide
  earth movements NEC —see Forces of nature,
    earth movement
  earthquake X34

Victim (Continued)
  flood —see Flood
  landslide —see Landslide
  lightning —see subcategory T75.Ø
    causing fire —see Exposure, fire
  storm (cataclysmic) NEC —see Forces of
    nature, cataclysmic storm
  volcanic eruption X35

Volcanic eruption (any injury) X35
Vomitus, gastric contents in air passages (with
  asphyxia, obstruction or
  suffocation) T17.81-●

▶ New   ➡ Revised   ~~deleted~~ Deleted   ● Use Additional Character(s)

T, U, & V

W

Walked into stationary object (any) W22.09
  furniture W22.03
  lamppost W22.02
  wall W22.01
War operations (injuries to military personnel
    and civilians during war, civil insurrection
    and peacekeeping missions) (by) (from)
    (involving) Y36.90-●
  after cessation of hostilities Y36.89-●
    explosion (of)
      bomb placed during war operations
        Y36.82-●
      mine placed during war operations
        Y36.81-●
    specified NEC Y36.88-●
  air blast Y36.20-●
  aircraft
    destruction —see War operations,
      destruction of aircraft
    airway restriction —see War operations,
      restriction of airways
  asphyxiation —see War operations, restriction
    of airways
  biological weapons Y36.6X-●
  blast Y36.20-●
  blast fragments Y36.20-●
  blast wave Y36.20-●
  blast wind Y36.20-●
  bomb Y36.20-●
    dirty Y36.50-●
    gasoline Y36.31-●
    incendiary Y36.31-●
    petrol Y36.31-●
  bullet Y36.43-●
    incendiary Y36.32-●
    rubber Y36.41-●
  chemical weapons Y36.7X-●
  combat
    hand to hand (unarmed) combat Y36.44-●
    using blunt or piercing object Y36.45-●
  conflagration —see War operations, fire
  conventional warfare NEC Y36.49-●
  depth-charge Y36.01-●
  destruction of aircraft Y36.10-●
    due to
      air to air missile Y36.11-●
      collision with other aircraft Y36.12-●
      detonation (accidental) of onboard
        munitions and explosives Y36.14-●
      enemy fire or explosives Y36.11-●
      explosive placed on aircraft Y36.11-●
      onboard fire Y36.13-●
      rocket propelled grenade [RPG] Y36.11-●
      small arms fire Y36.11-●
      surface to air missile Y36.11-●
    specified NEC Y36.19-●
  detonation (accidental) of
    onboard marine weapons Y36.05-●
    own munitions or munitions launch device
      Y36.24-●

War operations (Continued)
  dirty bomb Y36.50-●
  explosion (of) Y36.20-●
    aerial bomb Y36.21-●
    after cessation of hostilities
      bomb placed during war operations
        Y36.82-●
      mine placed during war operations
        Y36.81-●
    bomb NOS —see also War operations,
      bomb(s) Y36.20-●
    fragments Y36.20-●
    grenade Y36.29-●
    guided missile Y36.22-●
    improvised explosive device [IED]
      (person-borne) (roadside)
      (vehicle-borne) Y36.23-●
    land mine Y36.29-●
    marine mine (at sea) (in harbor)
      Y36.02-●
    marine weapon Y36.00-●
      specified NEC Y36.09-●
    own munitions or munitions launch
      device (accidental) of Y36.24-●
    sea-based artillery shell Y36.03-●
    specified NEC Y36.29-●
    torpedo Y36.04-●
  fire Y36.30-●
    specified NEC Y36.39-●
  firearms
    discharge Y36.43-●
    pellets Y36.42-●
  flamethrower Y36.33-●
  fragments (from) (of)
    improvised explosive device [IED]
      (person-borne) (roadside)
      (vehicle-borne) Y36.26-●
    munitions Y36.25-●
    specified NEC Y36.29-●
    weapons Y36.27-●
  friendly fire Y36.92
  hand to hand (unarmed) combat
    Y36.44-●
  hot substances —see War operations,
    fire
  incendiary bullet Y36.32-●
  nuclear weapon (effects of) Y36.50-●
    acute radiation exposure Y36.54-●
    blast pressure Y36.51-●
    direct blast Y36.51-●
    direct heat Y36.53-●
    fallout exposure Y36.54-●
    fireball Y36.53-●
    indirect blast (struck or crushed by blast
      debris) (being thrown by blast)
      Y36.52-●
    ionizing radiation (immediate exposure)
      Y36.54-●
    nuclear radiation Y36.54-●
    radiation
      ionizing (immediate exposure)
        Y36.54-●

War operations (Continued)
  nuclear weapon (Continued)
    radiation (Continued)
      nuclear Y36.54-●
      thermal Y36.53-●
    secondary effects Y36.54-●
    specified NEC Y36.59-●
    thermal radiation Y36.53-●
  restriction of air (airway)
    intentional Y36.46-●
    unintentional Y36.47-●
  rubber bullets Y36.41-●
  shrapnel NOS Y36.29-●
  suffocation —see War operations, restriction
    of airways
  unconventional warfare NEC Y36.7X-●
  underwater blast NOS Y36.00-●
  warfare
    conventional NEC Y36.49-●
    unconventional NEC Y36.7X-●
  weapon of mass destruction [WMD] Y36.91
  weapons
    biological weapons Y36.6X-●
    chemical Y36.7X-●
    nuclear (effects of) Y36.50-●
      acute radiation exposure Y36.54-●
      blast pressure Y36.51-●
      direct blast Y36.51-●
      direct heat Y36.53-●
      fallout exposure Y36.54-●
      fireball Y36.53-●
      radiation
        ionizing (immediate exposure)
          Y36.54-●
        nuclear Y36.54-●
        thermal Y36.53-●
      secondary effects Y36.54-●
      specified NEC Y36.59-●
    of mass destruction [WMD] Y36.91-●
Washed
  away by flood —see Flood
  off road by storm (transport vehicle) —see
    Forces of nature, cataclysmic storm
Weather exposure NEC —see Forces of nature
Weightlessness (causing injury) (effects of) (in
    spacecraft, real or simulated) X52
Work related condition Y99.0
Wound (accidental) NEC —see also Injury X58
  battle —see also War operations Y36.90
  gunshot —see Discharge, firearm by type
Wreck transport vehicle NEC —see also
    Accident, transport V89.9
Wrong
  device implanted into correct surgical site
    Y65.51
  fluid in infusion Y65.1
  patient, procedure performed on Y65.52
  procedure (operation) on correct patient
    Y65.51

▶ New   ➡ Revised   ~~deleted~~ Deleted   ● Use Additional Character(s)

PART III

ICD-10-CM Tabular List of Diseases and Injuries

CHAPTER 1

CERTAIN INFECTIOUS AND PARASITIC DISEASES (A00–B99)

OGCR Chapter-Specific Coding Guidelines

1. **Chapter 1: Certain Infectious and Parasitic Diseases (A00-B99)**

   a. **Human Immunodeficiency Virus (HIV) Infections**

      1) **Code only confirmed cases**

      Code only confirmed cases of HIV infection/illness. This is an exception to the hospital inpatient guideline Section II, H.

      In this context, "confirmation" does not require documentation of positive serology or culture for HIV; the provider's diagnostic statement that the patient is HIV positive, or has an HIV-related illness is sufficient.

      2) **Selection and sequencing of HIV codes**

         (a) **Patient admitted for HIV-related condition**

         If a patient is admitted for an HIV-related condition, the principal diagnosis should be B20, Human immunodeficiency virus [HIV] disease followed by additional diagnosis codes for all reported HIV-related conditions.

         (b) **Patient with HIV disease admitted for unrelated condition**

         If a patient with HIV disease is admitted for an unrelated condition (such as a traumatic injury), the code for the unrelated condition (e.g., the nature of injury code) should be the principal diagnosis. Other diagnoses would be B20 followed by additional diagnosis codes for all reported HIV-related conditions.

         (c) **Whether the patient is newly diagnosed**

         Whether the patient is newly diagnosed or has had previous admissions/encounters for HIV conditions is irrelevant to the sequencing decision.

         (d) **Asymptomatic human immunodeficiency virus**

         Z21, Asymptomatic human immunodeficiency virus [HIV] infection status, is to be applied when the patient without any documentation of symptoms is listed as being "HIV positive," "known HIV," "HIV test positive," or similar terminology. Do not use this code if the term "AIDS" is used or if the patient is treated for any HIV-related illness or is described as having any condition(s) resulting from his/her HIV positive status; use B20 in these cases.

         (e) **Patients with inconclusive HIV serology**

         Patients with inconclusive HIV serology, but no definitive diagnosis or manifestations of the illness, may be assigned code R75, Inconclusive laboratory evidence of human immunodeficiency virus [HIV].

         (f) **Previously diagnosed HIV-related illness**

         Patients with any known prior diagnosis of an HIV-related illness should be coded to B20. Once a patient has developed an HIV-related illness, the patient should always be assigned code B20 on every subsequent admission/encounter. Patients previously diagnosed with any HIV illness (B20) should never be assigned to R75 or Z21, Asymptomatic human immunodeficiency virus [HIV] infection status.

         (g) **HIV Infection in Pregnancy, Childbirth and the Puerperium**

         During pregnancy, childbirth or the puerperium, a patient admitted (or presenting for a health care encounter) because of an HIV-related illness should receive a principal diagnosis code of O98.7-, Human immunodeficiency [HIV] disease complicating pregnancy, childbirth and the puerperium, followed by B20 and the code(s) for the HIV-related illness(es). Codes from Chapter 15 always take sequencing priority.

         Patients with asymptomatic HIV infection status admitted (or presenting for a health care encounter) during pregnancy, childbirth, or the puerperium should receive codes of O98.7- and Z21.

         (h) **Encounters for testing for HIV**

         If a patient is being seen to determine his/her HIV status, use code Z11.4, Encounter for screening for human immunodeficiency virus [HIV]. Use additional codes for any associated high risk behavior.

         If a patient with signs or symptoms is being seen for HIV testing, code the signs and symptoms. An additional counseling code Z71.7, Human immunodeficiency virus [HIV] counseling,

may be used if counseling is provided during the encounter for the test.

When a patient returns to be informed of his/her HIV test results and the test result is negative, use code Z71.7, Human immunodeficiency virus [HIV] counseling.

If the results are positive, see previous guidelines and assign codes as appropriate.

   b. **Infectious agents as the cause of diseases classified to other chapters**

   Certain infections are classified in chapters other than Chapter 1 and no organism is identified as part of the infection code. In these instances, it is necessary to use an additional code from Chapter 1 to identify the organism. A code from category B95, Streptococcus, Staphylococcus, and Enterococcus as the cause of diseases classified to other chapters, B96, Other bacterial agents as the cause of diseases classified to other chapters, or B97, Viral agents as the cause of diseases classified to other chapters, is to be used as an additional code to identify the organism. An instructional note will be found at the infection code advising that an additional organism code is required.

   c. **Infections resistant to antibiotics**

   Many bacterial infections are resistant to current antibiotics. It is necessary to identify all infections documented as antibiotic resistant. Assign a code from category Z16, Resistance to antimicrobial drugs, following the infection code only if the infection code does not identify drug resistance.

   d. **Sepsis, Severe Sepsis, and Septic Shock**

      1) **Coding of Sepsis and Severe Sepsis**

         (a) **Sepsis**

         For a diagnosis of sepsis, assign the appropriate code for the underlying systemic infection. If the type of infection or causal organism is not further specified, assign code A41.9, Sepsis, unspecified organism.

         A code from subcategory R65.2, Severe sepsis, should not be assigned unless severe sepsis or an associated acute organ dysfunction is documented.

            (i) Negative or inconclusive blood cultures and sepsis
            Negative or inconclusive blood cultures do not preclude a diagnosis of sepsis in patients with clinical evidence of the condition, however, the provider should be queried.

            (ii) Urosepsis
            The term urosepsis is a nonspecific term. It is not to be considered synonymous with sepsis. It has no default code in the Alphabetic Index. Should a provider use this term, he/she must be queried for clarification.

            (iii) Sepsis with organ dysfunction
            If a patient has sepsis and associated acute organ dysfunction or multiple organ dysfunction (MOD), follow the instructions for coding severe sepsis.

            (iv) Acute organ dysfunction that is not clearly associated with the sepsis
            If a patient has sepsis and an acute organ dysfunction, but the medical record documentation indicates that the acute organ dysfunction is related to a medical condition other than the sepsis, do not assign a code from subcategory R65.2, Severe sepsis. An acute organ dysfunction must be associated with the sepsis in order to assign the severe sepsis code. If the documentation is not clear as to whether an acute organ dysfunction is related to the sepsis or another medical condition, query the provider.

         (b) **Severe sepsis**

         The coding of severe sepsis requires a minimum of 2 codes: first a code for the underlying systemic infection, followed by a code from subcategory R65.2, Severe sepsis. If the causal organism is not documented, assign code A41.9, Sepsis, unspecified organism, for the infection. Additional code(s) for the associated acute organ dysfunction are also required.

         Due to the complex nature of severe sepsis, some cases may require querying the provider prior to assignment of the codes.

2) Septic shock

(a) Septic shock generally refers to circulatory failure associated with severe sepsis, and therefore, it represents a type of acute organ dysfunction.

For all cases of septic shock, the code for the systemic infection should be sequenced first, followed by code R65.21, Severe sepsis with septic shock or code T81.12, Postprocedural septic shock. Any additional codes for the other acute organ dysfunctions should also be assigned. As noted in the sequencing instructions in the Tabular List, the code for septic shock cannot be assigned as a principal diagnosis.

3) Sequencing of severe sepsis

If severe sepsis is present on admission, and meets the definition of principal diagnosis, the underlying systemic infection should be assigned as principal diagnosis followed by the appropriate code from subcategory R65.2 as required by the sequencing rules in the Tabular List. A code from subcategory R65.2 can never be assigned as a principal diagnosis.

When severe sepsis develops during an encounter (it was not present on admission) the underlying systemic infection and the appropriate code from subcategory R65.2 should be assigned as secondary diagnoses.

Severe sepsis may be present on admission but the diagnosis may not be confirmed until sometime after admission. If the documentation is not clear whether severe sepsis was present on admission, the provider should be queried.

4) Sepsis and severe sepsis with a localized infection

If the reason for admission is both sepsis or severe sepsis and a localized infection, such as pneumonia or cellulitis, a code(s) for the underlying systemic infection should be assigned first and the code for the localized infection should be assigned as a secondary diagnosis. If the patient has severe sepsis, a code from subcategory R65.2 should also be assigned as a secondary diagnosis. If the patient is admitted with a localized infection, such as pneumonia, and sepsis/severe sepsis doesn't develop until after admission, the localized infection should be assigned first, followed by the appropriate sepsis/severe sepsis codes.

5) Sepsis due to a postprocedural infection

(a) Documentation of causal relationship

As with all postprocedural complications, code assignment is based on the provider's documentation of the relationship between the infection and the procedure.

(b) Sepsis due to a postprocedural infection

For such cases, the postprocedural infection code, such as, T80.2, Infections following infusion, transfusion, and therapeutic injection, T81.4, Infection following a procedure, T88.0, Infection following immunization, or O86.0, Infection of obstetric surgical wound, should be coded first, followed by the code for the specific infection. If the patient has severe sepsis the appropriate code from subcategory R65.2 should also be assigned with the additional code(s) for any acute organ dysfunction.

(c) Postprocedural infection and postprocedural septic shock

In cases where a postprocedural infection has occurred and has resulted in severe sepsis the code for the precipitating complication such as code T81.4, Infection following a procedure, or O86.0, Infection of obstetrical surgical wound should be coded first followed by code R65.20, Severe sepsis without septic shock. A Code for the systemic infection should also be assigned.

If a postprocedural infection has resulted in postprocedural septic shock, the code for the precipitating complication such as code T81.4, Infection following a procedure, or O86.0, Infection of obstetrical surgical wound should be coded first followed by code T81.12-, Postprocedural septic shock. A code for the systemic infection should also be assigned.

6) Sepsis and severe sepsis associated with a noninfectious process (condition)

In some cases a noninfectious process (condition), such as trauma, may lead to an infection which can result in sepsis or severe sepsis. If sepsis or severe sepsis is documented as associated with a noninfectious condition, such as a burn or serious injury, and this condition meets the definition for principal diagnosis, the code for the noninfectious condition should be sequenced first, followed by the code for the resulting infection. If severe sepsis is present, a code from subcategory R65.2 should also be assigned with any associated organ dysfunction(s) codes. It is not necessary to assign a code from subcategory R65.1, Systemic inflammatory response syndrome (SIRS) of non-infectious origin, for these cases.

If the infection meets the definition of principal diagnosis it should be sequenced before the non-infectious condition. When both the associated non-infectious condition and the infection meet the definition of principal diagnosis either may be assigned as principal diagnosis.

Only one code from category R65, Symptoms and signs specifically associated with systemic inflammation and infection, should be assigned. Therefore, when a non-infectious condition leads to an infection resulting in severe sepsis, assign the appropriate code from subcategory R65.2, Severe sepsis. Do not additionally assign a code from subcategory R65.1, Systemic inflammatory response syndrome (SIRS) of non-infectious origin.

See Section I.C.18. SIRS due to non-infectious process

7) Sepsis and septic shock complicating abortion, pregnancy, childbirth, and the puerperium

See Section I.C.15. Sepsis and septic shock complicating abortion, pregnancy, childbirth and the puerperium

8) Newborn sepsis

See Section I.C.16. f. Bacterial sepsis of Newborn

e. Methicillin Resistant Staphylococcus aureus (MRSA) Conditions

1) Selection and sequencing of MRSA codes

(a) Combination codes for MRSA infection

When a patient is diagnosed with an infection that is due to methicillin resistant *Staphylococcus aureus* (MRSA), and that infection has a combination code that includes the causal organism (e.g., sepsis, pneumonia) assign the appropriate combination code for the condition (e.g., code A41.02, Sepsis due to Methicillin resistant Staphylococcus aureus or code J15.212, Pneumonia due to Methicillin resistant Staphylococcus aureus). Do not assign code B95.62, Methicillin resistant Staphylococcus aureus infection as the cause of diseases classified elsewhere, as an additional code because the combination code includes the type of infection and the MRSA organism. Do not assign a code from subcategory Z16.11, Resistance to penicillins, as an additional diagnosis.

See Section C.1. for instructions on coding and sequencing of sepsis and severe sepsis.

(b) Other codes for MRSA infection

When there is documentation of a current infection (e.g., wound infection, stitch abscess, urinary tract infection) due to MRSA, and that infection does not have a combination code that includes the causal organism, assign the appropriate code to identify the condition along with code B95.62, Methicillin resistant Staphylococcus aureus infection as the cause of diseases classified elsewhere for the MRSA infection. Do not assign a code from subcategory Z16.11, Resistance to penicillins.

(c) Methicillin susceptible Staphylococcus aureus (MSSA) and MRSA colonization

The condition or state of being colonized or carrying MSSA or MRSA is called colonization or carriage, while an individual person is described as being colonized or being a carrier. Colonization means that MSSA or MSRA is present on or in the body without necessarily causing illness. A positive MRSA colonization test might be documented by the provider as "MRSA screen positive" or "MRSA nasal swab positive".

Assign code Z22.322, Carrier or suspected carrier of Methicillin resistant Staphylococcus aureus, for patients documented as having MRSA colonization. Assign code Z22.321, Carrier or suspected carrier of Methicillin susceptible Staphylococcus aureus, for patient documented as having MSSA colonization. Colonization is not necessarily indicative of a disease process or as the cause of a specific condition the patient may have unless documented as such by the provider.

(d) MRSA colonization and infection

If a patient is documented as having both MRSA colonization and infection during a hospital admission, code Z22.322, Carrier or suspected carrier of Methicillin resistant Staphylococcus aureus, and a code for the MRSA infection may both be assigned.

f. Zika virus infections

1) Code only confirmed cases

Code only a confirmed diagnosis of Zika virus (A92.5, Zika virus disease) as documented by the provider. This is an exception to the hospital inpatient guideline Section II, H.

In this context, "confirmation" does not require documentation of the type of test performed; the physician's diagnostic statement that the condition is confirmed is sufficient. This code should be assigned regardless of the stated mode of transmission.

If the provider documents "suspected", "possible" or "probable" Zika, do not assign code A92.5. Assign a code(s) explaining the reason for encounter (such as fever, rash, or joint pain) or Z20.828, Contact with and (suspected) exposure to other viral communicable diseases.

CHAPTER 1 (A00-B99)

CHAPTER 1

CERTAIN INFECTIOUS AND PARASITIC DISEASES (A00-B99)

| Includes | diseases generally recognized as communicable or transmissible |

Use additional code to identify resistance to antimicrobial drugs (Z16.-)

| Excludes1 | certain localized infections - see body system-related chapters |

| Excludes2 | carrier or suspected carrier of infectious disease (Z22.-) |

infectious and parasitic diseases complicating pregnancy, childbirth and the puerperium (O98.-)

infectious and parasitic diseases specific to the perinatal period (P35-P39)

influenza and other acute respiratory infections (J00-J22)

This chapter contains the following blocks:

A00-A09	Intestinal infectious diseases
A15-A19	Tuberculosis
A20-A28	Certain zoonotic bacterial diseases
A30-A49	Other bacterial diseases
A50-A64	Infections with a predominantly sexual mode of transmission
A65-A69	Other spirochetal diseases
A70-A74	Other diseases caused by chlamydiae
A75-A79	Rickettsioses
A80-A89	Viral and prion infections of the central nervous system
A90-A99	Arthropod-borne viral fevers and viral hemorrhagic fevers
B00-B09	Viral infections characterized by skin and mucous membrane lesions
B10	Other human herpesviruses
B15-B19	Viral hepatitis
B20	Human immunodeficiency virus [HIV] disease
B25-B34	Other viral diseases
B35-B49	Mycoses
B50-B64	Protozoal diseases
B65-B83	Helminthiases
B85-B89	Pediculosis, acariasis and other infestations
B90-B94	Sequelae of infectious and parasitic diseases
B95-B97	Bacterial and viral infectious agents
B99	Other infectious diseases

INTESTINAL INFECTIOUS DISEASES (A00-A09)

● **A00 Cholera**
A serious, often deadly, infectious disease of the small intestine
(Ex) **For category A00 CC codes: See PDX Collection 2**

A00.0 Cholera due to Vibrio cholerae 01, biovar cholerae
Classical cholera

A00.1 Cholera due to Vibrio cholerae 01, biovar eltor
Cholera eltor

A00.9 Cholera, unspecified

● **A01 Typhoid and paratyphoid fevers**
Caused by Salmonella typhi and Salmonella paratyphi A, B, and C bacteria
(Ex) **For category A01 CC codes: See PDX Collection 3**

● **A01.0 Typhoid fever**
Infection due to Salmonella typhi

A01.00 Typhoid fever, unspecified

A01.01 Typhoid meningitis

A01.02 Typhoid fever with heart involvement
Typhoid endocarditis
Typhoid myocarditis

A01.03 Typhoid pneumonia
A01.04 Typhoid arthritis
A01.05 Typhoid osteomyelitis
A01.09 Typhoid fever with other complications

A01.1 Paratyphoid fever A
A01.2 Paratyphoid fever B
A01.3 Paratyphoid fever C
A01.4 Paratyphoid fever, unspecified
Infection due to Salmonella paratyphi NOS

● **A02 Other salmonella infections**
| Includes | infection or foodborne intoxication due to any Salmonella species other than S. typhi and S. paratyphi |

A02.0 Salmonella enteritis
Salmonellosis
(Ex) See PDX Collection 4

A02.1 Salmonella sepsis
(Ex) See PDX Collection 5

● **A02.2 Localized salmonella infections**

A02.20 Localized salmonella infection, unspecified
Specified in the documentation as localized, but unspecified as to type

A02.21 Salmonella meningitis
Specified as localized in the meninges
(Ex) See PDX Collection 6

A02.22 Salmonella pneumonia
Specified as localized in the lungs
(Ex) See PDX Collection 7

A02.23 Salmonella arthritis
Specified as localized in the joints
(Ex) See PDX Collection 8

A02.24 Salmonella osteomyelitis
Specified as localized in bone
(Ex) See PDX Collection 9

A02.25 Salmonella pyelonephritis
Salmonella tubulo-interstitial nephropathy
(Ex) See PDX Collection 10

A02.29 Salmonella with other localized infection
Specified as localized (because it is still under localized heading) but does not assign into any of the above codes
(Ex) See PDX Collection 10

A02.8 Other specified salmonella infections
Any specified salmonella infection which does NOT assign into any of the above codes (not specified as localized)
(Ex) See PDX Collection 11

A02.9 Salmonella infection, unspecified
Unspecified in the documentation as to specific type of salmonella
(Ex) See PDX Collection 12

Item 1-1 Salmonella is a bacterium that lives in the intestines of fowl and mammals and can spread to humans through improper food preparation and cooking. Salmonellosis is an infection with the bacterium. Symptoms include diarrhea, fever, and abdominal cramps 12 to 72 hours after infection. The illness usually lasts 4 to 7 days, and most persons recover without treatment. The diarrhea may be so severe that the patient needs to be hospitalized. Patients with immunocompromised systems in chronic, ill health are more likely to have the infection invade their bloodstream with life-threatening results. For example, patients with sickle cell disease are more prone to salmonella osteomyelitis than others.

▶ New   ⇒ Revised   ~~deleted~~ Deleted   Excludes 1   Excludes 2   Includes   Use additional   Code first   Code also   Key words

OGCR Official Guidelines   ● Unacceptable Principal Diagnosis   X Assign placeholder X   ● Use Additional Character(s)   ▶ Manifestation Code   **Coding Clinic**

● **A03   Shigellosis**
An infectious disease caused by bacteria (Shigella)

A03.0   Shigellosis due to Shigella dysenteriae 🏥
Group A shigellosis [Shiga-Kruse dysentery]
Ⓔ See PDX Collection 13

A03.1   Shigellosis due to Shigella flexneri
Group B shigellosis

A03.2   Shigellosis due to Shigella boydii
Group C shigellosis

A03.3   Shigellosis due to Shigella sonnei
Group D shigellosis

A03.8   Other shigellosis

A03.9   Shigellosis, unspecified
Bacillary dysentery NOS

● **A04   Other bacterial intestinal infections**

Excludes1   bacterial foodborne intoxications, NEC (A05.-)
tuberculous enteritis (A18.32)

Ⓔ For category A04 CC codes A04.0-A04.4: See PDX Collection 14
For category A04 CC codes A04.5-A04.8: See PDX Collection 15

A04.0   Enteropathogenic Escherichia coli infection 🏥
Pertaining to or producing intestinal disease

A04.1   Enterotoxigenic Escherichia coli infection 🏥
Producing or containing intestinal toxin

A04.2   Enteroinvasive Escherichia coli infection 🏥
Capable of penetrating and spreading through intestinal mucosal epithelium

A04.3   Enterohemorrhagic Escherichia coli infection 🏥
Causing bloody diarrhea, resulting from microorganisms

A04.4   Other intestinal Escherichia coli infections 🏥
Escherichia coli enteritis NOS

A04.5   Campylobacter enteritis 🏥
Spiral shaped bacterium

A04.6   Enteritis due to Yersinia enterocolitica 🏥
Excludes1   extraintestinal yersiniosis (A28.2)
Transmitted by infected food /water and person-to-person contact, affecting intestinal tract

● **A04.7   Enterocolitis due to Clostridium difficile**
Foodborne intoxication by Clostridium difficile
Pseudomembraneous colitis
Marked by fibrinous deposit (false membrane) with enmeshed necrotic cells

▶ **A04.71   Enterocolitis due to Clostridium difficile, recurrent** 🏥

▶ **A04.72   Enterocolitis due to Clostridium difficile, not specified as recurrent** 🏥

A04.8   Other specified bacterial intestinal infections 🏥

A04.9   Bacterial intestinal infection, unspecified 🏥
Bacterial enteritis NOS
Ⓔ See PDX Collection 16

Figure 1-1 Electron micrograph of escherichia coli (E. coli) expressing P fimbriae. (Getty Image)

Item 1–2   *Escherichia coli [E. coli]* is a gram-negative bacterium found in the intestinal tracts of humans and animals and is usually nonpathogenic. Pathogenic strains can cause diarrhea or pyogenic (pus-producing) infections. Can be a threat to food safety.

● **A05   Other bacterial foodborne intoxications, not elsewhere classified**

⇒ **Excludes1**   Clostridium difficile foodborne intoxication and infection (A04.7-)
Escherichia coli infection (A04.0-A04.4)
listeriosis (A32.-)
salmonella foodborne intoxication and infection (A02.-)
toxic effect of noxious foodstuffs (T61-T62)

Ⓔ For category A05 CC codes unless otherwise indicated: See PDX Collection 17

A05.0   Foodborne staphylococcal intoxication 🏥

A05.1   Botulism food poisoning 🏥
Botulism NOS
Classical foodborne intoxication due to Clostridium botulinum

Excludes1   infant botulism (A48.51)
wound botulism (A48.52)

Ⓔ See PDX Collection 18

A05.2   Foodborne Clostridium perfringens [Clostridium welchii] intoxication 🏥
Type A causes gas gangrene and necrotizing colitis; major cause of food poisoning in humans
Enteritis necroticans
Pig-bel
Ⓔ See PDX Collection 19

A05.3   Foodborne Vibrio parahaemolyticus intoxication 🏥
Organism that survives only in high salt environment (halophilic), major cause of gastroenteritis due to consumption of raw or improperly cooked fish/seafood

A05.4   Foodborne Bacillus cereus intoxication 🏥
Spore-forming species commonly found in soil, causes food poisoning from formation of intestinal toxins in contaminated foods

A05.5   Foodborne Vibrio vulnificus intoxication 🏥
Species that survives in high salt environment (halophilic) with infection by eating raw seafood causes septicemia and cellulitis

A05.8   Other specified bacterial foodborne intoxications 🏥

A05.9   Bacterial foodborne intoxication, unspecified

● **A06   Amebiasis**
An intestinal illness caused by the microscopic parasite Entamoeba histolytica

Includes   infection due to Entamoeba histolytica
Excludes1   other protozoal intestinal diseases (A07.-)
Excludes2   acanthamebiasis (B60.1-)
Naegleriasis (B60.2)

A06.0   Acute amebic dysentery 🏥
Acute amebiasis
Intestinal amebiasis NOS
Ⓔ See PDX Collection 20

A06.1   Chronic intestinal amebiasis 🏥
Ⓔ See PDX Collection 20

A06.2   Amebic nondysenteric colitis 🏥
Pertaining to single cell microorganism
Ⓔ See PDX Collection 21

A06.3   Ameboma of intestine 🏥
Tumorlike mass produced by localized inflammation often in intestine
Ameboma NOS
Ⓔ See PDX Collection 22

A06.4   Amebic liver abscess 🏥
Hepatic amebiasis
Ⓔ See PDX Collection 23

CHAPTER 1 (A00-B99)

N Newborn Age: 0   P Pediatric Age: 0–17   M Maternity DX: 12–55   A Adult Age: 15–124   ♀ Females Only   ♂ Males Only

🏥 Complication\Comorbidity   🏥 Major C\C   Ⓔ CC/MCC Exclusions   🏥 Hospital-Acquired Condition

A06.5   **Amebic lung abscess** 🔎
     Amebic abscess of lung (and liver)
     (Ex) See PDX Collection 24

A06.6   **Amebic brain abscess** 🔎
     Amebic abscess of brain (and liver) (and lung)
     (Ex) See PDX Collection 25

A06.7   **Cutaneous amebiasis**

● **A06.8**   **Amebic infection of other sites**
     (Ex) For category A06.8 CC codes: See PDX Collection 22

     A06.81   **Amebic cystitis** 🔎

     A06.82   **Other amebic genitourinary infections** 🔎
         Amebic balanitis
         Amebic vesiculitis
         Amebic vulvovaginitis

     A06.89   **Other amebic infections** 🔎
         Amebic appendicitis
         Amebic splenic abscess

A06.9   **Amebiasis, unspecified**

● **A07**   **Other protozoal intestinal diseases**
     (Ex) For category A07 CC codes unless otherwise indicated: See PDX Collection 26

     A07.0   **Balantidiasis**
         Balantidial dysentery
         Infection by protozoa that may cause diarrhea and dysentery,
         with ulceration of colonic mucous membranes

     A07.1   **Giardiasis [lambliasis]**
         Common infection in small intestine spread by contaminated
         food, water, or direct person-to-person contact

     A07.2   **Cryptosporidiosis** 🔎
         Human infection with protozoa usually seen as self-limited
         diarrhea in those who work with cattle

     A07.3   **Isosporiasis** 🔎
         Human intestinal disease caused by protozoa
         Infection due to Isospora belli and Isospora hominis
         Intestinal coccidiosis
         Isosporosis

     A07.4   **Cyclosporiasis** 🔎
         Infection by protozoa with most common species infecting
         humans being C cayetanensis
         (Ex) See PDX Collection 27

     A07.8   **Other specified protozoal intestinal diseases** 🔎
         Intestinal microsporidiosis
         Intestinal trichomoniasis
         Sarcocystosis
         Sarcosporidiosis

     A07.9   **Protozoal intestinal disease, unspecified** 🔎
         Flagellate diarrhea
         Protozoal colitis
         Protozoal diarrhea
         Protozoal dysentery

● **A08**   **Viral and other specified intestinal infections**
     Excludes1   influenza with involvement of gastrointestinal
             tract (J09.X3, J10.2, J11.2)
     (Ex) For category A08 CC codes: See PDX Collection 28

     A08.0   **Rotaviral enteritis** 🔎

●   **A08.1**   **Acute gastroenteropathy due to Norwalk agent and**
         other small round viruses

     A08.11   **Acute gastroenteropathy due to Norwalk**
             agent 🔎
         Acute gastroenteropathy due to Norovirus
         Acute gastroenteropathy due to Norwalk-like
         agent

     A08.19   **Acute gastroenteropathy due to other small**
             round viruses 🔎
         Acute gastroenteropathy due to small round
         virus [SRV] NOS

     A08.2   **Adenoviral enteritis** 🔎

● **A08.3**   **Other viral enteritis**

     A08.31   **Calicivirus enteritis** 🔎

     A08.32   **Astrovirus enteritis** 🔎

     A08.39   **Other viral enteritis** 🔎
         Coxsackie virus enteritis
         Echovirus enteritis
         Enterovirus enteritis NEC
         Torovirus enteritis

A08.4   **Viral intestinal infection, unspecified**
     Viral enteritis NOS
     Viral gastroenteritis NOS
     Viral gastroenteropathy NOS
     Coding Clinic: 2016, Q3, P12

A08.8   **Other specified intestinal infections**

A09   **Infectious gastroenteritis and colitis, unspecified** 🔎
     Infectious colitis NOS
     Infectious enteritis NOS
     Infectious gastroenteritis NOS

     Excludes1   colitis NOS (K52.9)
             diarrhea NOS (R19.7)
             enteritis NOS (K52.9)
             gastroenteritis NOS (K52.9)
             noninfective gastroenteritis and colitis,
               unspecified (K52.9)
     (Ex) See PDX Collection 17

TUBERCULOSIS (A15-A19)

Includes   infections due to Mycobacterium tuberculosis
             and Mycobacterium bovis

Excludes1   congenital tuberculosis (P37.0)
             nonspecific reaction to test for tuberculosis
               without active tuberculosis (R76.1-)
             pneumoconiosis associated with tuberculosis, any
               type in A15 (J65)
             positive PPD (R76.11)
             positive tuberculin skin test without active
               tuberculosis (R76.11)
             sequelae of tuberculosis (B90.-)
             silicotuberculosis (J65)

● **A15**   **Respiratory tuberculosis**
     (Ex) For category A15 CC codes unless otherwise indicated: See PDX Collection 29

     A15.0   **Tuberculosis of lung** 🔎
         Tuberculous bronchiectasis
         Chronic dilatation of bronchi
         Tuberculous fibrosis of lung
         Tuberculous pneumonia
         Tuberculous pneumothorax

Figure 1-2   Far advanced bilateral pulmonary tuberculosis before and after 8 months of treatment with streptomycin, PAS, and isoniazid. (Getty Image)

Item 1–3   **Tuberculosis** is a common and deadly infectious disease caused by the *Mycobacterium tuberculosis* organism. The first tuberculosis infection is called the **primary infection** and most commonly attacks the lungs but can affect the central nervous system, lymphatic system, circulatory system, genitourinary system, bones, joints, and even the skin. A **Ghon** lesion is the **initial lesion.** A **secondary lesion** occurs when the tubercle bacilli are carried to other areas.

▶ New   ⟹ Revised   ~~deleted~~ Deleted   Excludes 1   Excludes 2   Includes   Use additional   Code first   Code also   Key words

OGCR Official Guidelines   ● Unacceptable Principal Diagnosis   X Assign placeholder X   ▶ Use Additional Character(s)   ▶ Manifestation Code   **Coding Clinic**

Item 1-4 Although it primarily affects the lungs, the bacteria *Mycobacterium tuberculosis* can travel from the pulmonary circulation to virtually any organ in the body, much as a cancer metastasizes to a secondary site. If the immune system becomes compromised by age or disease, what would otherwise be a self-limiting primary tuberculosis in the lungs will develop in other organs. These are known as extrapulmonary sites.

A15.4   Tuberculosis of intrathoracic lymph nodes
     Tuberculosis of hilar lymph nodes
     Tuberculosis of mediastinal lymph nodes
     Tuberculosis of tracheobronchial lymph nodes
     Excludes1   tuberculosis specified as primary (A15.7)

A15.5   Tuberculosis of larynx, trachea and bronchus
     Tuberculosis of bronchus
     Tuberculosis of glottis
     Tuberculosis of larynx
     Tuberculosis of trachea

A15.6   Tuberculous pleurisy
     Tuberculosis of pleura
     Tuberculous empyema
     Excludes1   primary respiratory tuberculosis (A15.7)

A15.7   Primary respiratory tuberculosis
     (Ex) See PDX Collection 30

A15.8   Other respiratory tuberculosis
     Mediastinal tuberculosis
     Nasopharyngeal tuberculosis
     Tuberculosis of nose
     Tuberculosis of sinus [any nasal]
     (Ex) See PDX Collection 31

A15.9   Respiratory tuberculosis unspecified
     (Ex) See PDX Collection 31

● **A17   Tuberculosis of nervous system**

A17.0   Tuberculous meningitis
     Tuberculosis of meninges (cerebral) (spinal)
     Tuberculous leptomeningitis
     Excludes1   tuberculous meningoencephalitis
                   (A17.82)
     (Ex) See PDX Collection 32

A17.1   Meningeal tuberculoma
     Tuberculoma of meninges (cerebral) (spinal)
     Excludes2   tuberculoma of brain and spinal cord
                   (A17.81)
     (Ex) See PDX Collection 32

● **A17.8   Other tuberculosis of nervous system**

     A17.81   Tuberculoma of brain and spinal cord
         Tuberculous abscess of brain and spinal cord
         (Ex) See PDX Collection 33

     A17.82   Tuberculous meningoencephalitis
         Inflammation of brain and meninges; AKA
         cerebromeningitis and encephalomeningitis
         Tuberculous myelitis
         (Ex) See PDX Collection 33

     A17.83   Tuberculous neuritis
         Tuberculous mononeuropathy
         (Ex) No exclusions

     A17.89   Other tuberculosis of nervous system
         Tuberculous polyneuropathy
         (Ex) See PDX Collection 34

A17.9   Tuberculosis of nervous system, unspecified
     (Ex) See PDX Collection 35

● **A18   Tuberculosis of other organs**

● **A18.0   Tuberculosis of bones and joints**

     A18.01   Tuberculosis of spine
         Pott's disease or curvature of spine
         Tuberculous arthritis
         Tuberculous osteomyelitis of spine
         Tuberculous spondylitis
         (Ex) See PDX Collection 36

     A18.02   Tuberculous arthritis of other joints
         Tuberculosis of hip (joint)
         Tuberculosis of knee (joint)
         (Ex) See PDX Collection 37

     A18.03   Tuberculosis of other bones
         Tuberculous mastoiditis
         Tuberculous osteomyelitis
         (Ex) See PDX Collection 38

     A18.09   Other musculoskeletal tuberculosis
         Tuberculous myositis
         Tuberculous synovitis
         Tuberculous tenosynovitis
         (Ex) See PDX Collection 39

● **A18.1   Tuberculosis of genitourinary system**

     A18.10   Tuberculosis of genitourinary system, unspecified
         (Ex) See PDX Collection 40

     A18.11   Tuberculosis of kidney and ureter
         (Ex) See PDX Collection 41

     A18.12   Tuberculosis of bladder
         (Ex) See PDX Collection 41

     A18.13   Tuberculosis of other urinary organs
         Tuberculous urethritis
         (Ex) See PDX Collection 41

     A18.14   Tuberculosis of prostate ♂
         (Ex) See PDX Collection 42

     A18.15   Tuberculosis of other male genital organs ♂
         (Ex) See PDX Collection 42

     A18.16   Tuberculosis of cervix ♀
         (Ex) See PDX Collection 43

     A18.17   Tuberculous female pelvic inflammatory disease ♀
         Tuberculous endometritis
         Tuberculous oophoritis and salpingitis
         Oophoritis = inflammation of ovary
         Salpingitis = inflammation of fallopian tube
         (Ex) See PDX Collection 43

     A18.18   Tuberculosis of other female genital organs ♀
         Tuberculous ulceration of vulva
         (Ex) See PDX Collection 43

A18.2   Tuberculous peripheral lymphadenopathy
     Tuberculous adenitis
     Excludes2   tuberculosis of bronchial and mediastinal
                 lymph nodes (A15.4)
                 tuberculosis of mesenteric and
                 retroperitoneal lymph nodes
                 (A18.39)
                 tuberculous tracheobronchial adenopathy
                 (A15.4)
     (Ex) See PDX Collection 44

● **A18.3   Tuberculosis of intestines, peritoneum and mesenteric glands**
     (Ex) **For category A18.3 CC codes:** See PDX Collection 45

     A18.31   Tuberculous peritonitis
         Tuberculous ascites

     A18.32   Tuberculous enteritis
         Tuberculosis of anus and rectum
         Tuberculosis of intestine (large) (small)

     A18.39   Retroperitoneal tuberculosis
         Tuberculosis of mesenteric glands
         Tuberculosis of retroperitoneal (lymph glands)

CHAPTER 1 (A00-B99)

A

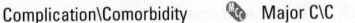

N   Newborn Age: 0   **P**   Pediatric Age: 0-17   **M**   Maternity DX: 12-55   **A**   Adult Age: 15-124   ♀   Females Only   ♂   Males Only

   Complication\Comorbidity   Major C\C   (Ex) CC/MCC Exclusions   Hospital-Acquired Condition

639

A18.4 **Tuberculosis of skin and subcutaneous tissue** 🔑
  Erythema induratum, tuberculous
  Lupus excedens
  Lupus vulgaris NOS
  Lupus vulgaris of eyelid
    *Cutaneous tuberculosis characterized by reddish brown
      plaque on skin surrounded by papules and nodules*
  Scrofuloderma
    *Type of cutaneous tuberculosis, with direct extension of
      tuberculosis into skin from underlying structures;
      AKA tuberculosis colliquativa*
  Tuberculosis of external ear
    Excludes2 lupus erythematosus (L93.-)
        lupus NOS (M32.9)
        systemic (M32.-)
    (Ex:) See PDX Collection 30

● **A18.5** **Tuberculosis of eye**
    Excludes2 lupus vulgaris of eyelid (A18.4)
      (Ex:) For category A18.5 CC codes: See PDX Collection 46
  A18.50 **Tuberculosis of eye, unspecified** 🔑
  A18.51 **Tuberculous episcleritis** 🔑
      Inflammation of episclera and adjacent tissues
  A18.52 **Tuberculous keratitis** 🔑
      Tuberculous interstitial keratitis
      Tuberculous keratoconjunctivitis (interstitial)
        (phlyctenular)
      Inflammation of cornea and conjunctiva
  A18.53 **Tuberculous chorioretinitis** 🔑
      *Inflammation of choroid and retina;
        retinochoroiditis*
  A18.54 **Tuberculous iridocyclitis** 🔑
      Inflammation of iris and ciliary body
  A18.59 **Other tuberculosis of eye** 🔑
      Tuberculous conjunctivitis
  A18.6 **Tuberculosis of (inner) (middle) ear** 🔑
      Tuberculous otitis media
      Excludes2 tuberculosis of external ear (A18.4)
          tuberculous mastoiditis (A18.03)
      (Ex:) See PDX Collection 47
  A18.7 **Tuberculosis of adrenal glands** 🔑
      Tuberculous Addison's disease
      (Ex:) See PDX Collection 48
● **A18.8** **Tuberculosis of other specified organs**
  A18.81 **Tuberculosis of thyroid gland** 🔑
      (Ex:) See PDX Collection 49
  A18.82 **Tuberculosis of other endocrine glands** 🔑
      Tuberculosis of pituitary gland
      Tuberculosis of thymus gland
      (Ex:) See PDX Collection 35
  A18.83 **Tuberculosis of digestive tract organs, not
      elsewhere classified** 🔑
      Excludes1 tuberculosis of intestine (A18.32)
      (Ex:) See PDX Collection 45
  A18.84 **Tuberculosis of heart** 🔑
      Tuberculous cardiomyopathy
      Tuberculous endocarditis
      Tuberculous myocarditis
      Tuberculous pericarditis
      (Ex:) See PDX Collection 35
  A18.85 **Tuberculosis of spleen** 🔑
      (Ex:) See PDX Collection 50
  A18.89 **Tuberculosis of other sites** 🔑
      Tuberculosis of muscle
      Tuberculous cerebral arteritis
      (Ex:) See PDX Collection 35

Item 1–5 **Miliary tuberculosis** can be a life-threatening condition. If a tuberculous lesion enters a blood vessel, immense dissemination of tuberculous organisms can occur if the immune system is weak. High-risk populations— children under 4 years of age, the elderly, or the immunocompromised— are particularly prone to this type of infection. The lesions will have a millet seedlike appearance on chest x-ray. Bronchial washings and biopsy may aid in diagnosis.

● **A19** **Miliary tuberculosis**
    Includes   disseminated tuberculosis
        generalized tuberculosis
        tuberculous polyserositis
      (Ex:) For category A19 CC codes: See PDX Collection 51
  A19.0 **Acute miliary tuberculosis of a single specified site** 🔑
  A19.1 **Acute miliary tuberculosis of multiple sites** 🔑
  A19.2 **Acute miliary tuberculosis, unspecified** 🔑
  A19.8 **Other miliary tuberculosis** 🔑
  A19.9 **Miliary tuberculosis, unspecified** 🔑

CERTAIN ZOONOTIC BACTERIAL DISEASES (A20-A28)

● **A20** **Plague**
    *Infectious disease caused by a Yersinia pestis bacterium, transmitted
      by a rodent flea bite or handling of infected animal*
    Includes   infection due to Yersinia pestis
  A20.0 **Bubonic plague** 🔑
      (Ex:) See PDX Collection 52
  A20.1 **Cellulocutaneous plague** 🔑
      Skin and subcutaneous tissue plague
      (Ex:) See PDX Collection 52
  A20.2 **Pneumonic plague** 🔑
      (Ex:) See PDX Collection 53
  A20.3 **Plague meningitis** 🔑
      (Ex:) See PDX Collection 54
  A20.7 **Septicemic plague** 🔑
      (Ex:) See PDX Collection 55
  A20.8 **Other forms of plague** 🔑
      Abortive plague
      Asymptomatic plague
      Pestis minor
        Systemic bacterial disease
      (Ex:) See PDX Collection 54
  A20.9 **Plague, unspecified** 🔑
      (Ex:) See PDX Collection 56

● **A21** **Tularemia**
    *Caused by Francisella tularensis bacterium found in rodents, rabbits,
      and hares and transmitted to humans by contact with infected
      animal tissues or by ticks, biting flies, or mosquitoes*
    Includes   deer-fly fever
        infection due to Francisella tularensis
        rabbit fever
    Coding Clinic: 2016, Q4, P25
  A21.0 **Ulceroglandular tularemia** 🔑
      *Most common form of tularemia in humans is painful,
        swollen, erythematous papule at point of inoculation
        that ruptures to form shallow ulcer*
      (Ex:) See PDX Collection 57
  A21.1 **Oculoglandular tularemia** 🔑
      *Primary site of entry is conjunctival sac, results in
        granulomatous corneal lesions*
      Ophthalmic tularemia
      (Ex:) See PDX Collection 58
  A21.2 **Pulmonary tularemia** 🔑
      (Ex:) See PDX Collection 59

▶ New   ⮞ Revised   ~~deleted~~ Deleted   Excludes 1   Excludes 2   Includes   Use additional   Code first   Code also   Key words
OGCR Official Guidelines   ● Unacceptable Principal Diagnosis   X Assign placeholder X   ● Use Additional Character(s)   ▐ Manifestation Code   **Coding Clinic**

A21.3   Gastrointestinal tularemia 🦠
    Abdominal tularemia
    (Ex) See PDX Collection 60

A21.7   Generalized tularemia 🦠
    (Ex) See PDX Collection 61

A21.8   Other forms of tularemia 🦠
    (Ex) See PDX Collection 61

A21.9   Tularemia, unspecified 🦠
    (Ex) See PDX Collection 61

● **A22   Anthrax**
An acute infectious disease caused by the spore-forming Bacillus anthracis; occurs in humans exposed to infected animals or tissue from infected animals

    Includes   infection due to Bacillus anthracis

A22.0   Cutaneous anthrax 🦠
    Malignant carbuncle
    Malignant pustule
    (Ex) See PDX Collection 62

A22.1   Pulmonary anthrax 🦠
    Inhalation anthrax
    Ragpicker's disease
    Woolsorter's disease
    (Ex) See PDX Collection 63

A22.2   Gastrointestinal anthrax 🦠
    (Ex) See PDX Collection 64

A22.7   Anthrax sepsis 🦠
    Infectious bacterial disease
    MCC when PDx is its own MCC
    (Ex) See PDX Collection 5

A22.8   Other forms of anthrax 🦠
    Anthrax meningitis
    (Ex) See PDX Collection 65

A22.9   Anthrax, unspecified 🦠
    (Ex) See PDX Collection 66

● **A23   Brucellosis**
    Includes   Malta fever
               Mediterranean fever
               undulant fever

A23.0   Brucellosis due to Brucella melitensis
    Resulting in flu-like symptoms that may lead to chronic symptoms that include recurrent fevers, joint pain, and fatigue

A23.1   Brucellosis due to Brucella abortus
    Most common cause of brucellosis in humans; AKA Bang bacillus

A23.2   Brucellosis due to Brucella suis
    Species found primarily in pigs, rabbits, and reindeer

A23.3   Brucellosis due to Brucella canis
    Species that causes respiratory tract infection in humans

A23.8   Other brucellosis 🦠
    (Ex) See PDX Collection 67

A23.9   Brucellosis, unspecified 🦠
    (Ex) See PDX Collection 67

● **A24   Glanders and melioidosis**
Infection, usually of rodents, which spreads to other animals and humans, caused by Burkholderia pseudomallei through break in skin contaminated with infested soil or water
    (Ex) **For category A24 CC codes unless otherwise indicated:** See PDX Collection 69

A24.0   Glanders 🦠
    Infection due to Pseudomonas mallei
    Malleus
    (Ex) See PDX Collection 68

A24.1   Acute and fulminating melioidosis 🦠
    Melioidosis pneumonia
    Melioidosis sepsis

A24.2   Subacute and chronic melioidosis 🦠

A24.3   Other melioidosis 🦠

A24.9   Melioidosis, unspecified 🦠
    Infection due to Pseudomonas pseudomallei NOS
    Whitmore's disease

● **A25   Rat-bite fevers**
RBF, infectious disease caused by Streptobacillus moniliformis or Spirillum minus.
    (Ex) **For category A25 CC codes:** See PDX Collection 70

A25.0   Spirillosis 🦠
    Any disease condition caused by spirilla
    Sodoku

A25.1   Streptobacillosis 🦠
    Acute, febrile human illness caused by bacteria transmitted by rats in most cases, passed from rodent to human via rodent's urine or mucous secretions; AKA rat fever
    Epidemic arthritic erythema
    Haverhill fever
    Streptobacillary rat-bite fever

A25.9   Rat-bite fever, unspecified 🦠

● **A26   Erysipeloid**
Infection with Erysipelothrix rhusiopathiae, occurring often as occupational disease resulting from handling infected fish, shellfish, meat, or poultry

A26.0   Cutaneous erysipeloid
    Erythema migrans

A26.7   Erysipelothrix sepsis 🦠
    MCC when PDx is its own MCC
    (Ex) See PDX Collection 71

A26.8   Other forms of erysipeloid

A26.9   Erysipeloid, unspecified

● **A27   Leptospirosis**
Occurs most commonly in the tropics
    (Ex) **For category A27 CC codes unless otherwise indicated:** See PDX Collection 72

A27.0   Leptospirosis icterohemorrhagica 🦠
    Leptospiral or spirochetal jaundice (hemorrhagic)
    Weil's disease

● **A27.8   Other forms of leptospirosis**

A27.81   Aseptic meningitis in leptospirosis 🦠
    (Ex) See PDX Collection 73

A27.89   Other forms of leptospirosis 🦠

A27.9   Leptospirosis, unspecified 🦠

● **A28   Other zoonotic bacterial diseases, not elsewhere classified**
    (Ex) **For category A28 CC codes unless otherwise indicated:** See PDX Collection 74

A28.0   Pasteurellosis 🦠
    Infection of humans or other animals by species of Pasteurella

A28.1   Cat-scratch disease 🦠
    Cat-scratch fever
    (Ex) See PDX Collection 75

A28.2   Extraintestinal yersiniosis 🦠
    Infection from Yersinia enterocolitica; AKA enteric yersiniosis, intestinal yersiniosis, Yersinia enteritis
    Excludes1   enteritis due to Yersinia enterocolitica (A04.6)
                plague (A20.-)

A28.8   Other specified zoonotic bacterial diseases, not elsewhere classified

A28.9   Zoonotic bacterial disease, unspecified 🦠

Item 1-6 Brucellosis: An infectious disease caused by the bacterium Brucella. Humans are infected by contact with contaminated animals or animal products. In humans brucellosis symptoms that are similar to the flu include fever, sweats, headaches, back pains, and physical weakness. Severe infections of the central nervous system or lining of the heart may occur. Brucellosis can also cause chronic symptoms that include recurrent fevers, joint pain, and fatigue.

CHAPTER 1 (A00-B99)

OTHER BACTERIAL DISEASES (A30-A49)

● **A30 Leprosy [Hansen's disease]**
Chronic infectious disease attacking the skin, peripheral nerves, and mucous membranes

| **Includes** | infection due to Mycobacterium leprae |
| **Excludes1** | sequelae of leprosy (B92) |

A30.0 Indeterminate leprosy 🖐
I leprosy
Ex: See PDX Collection 76

A30.1 Tuberculoid leprosy 🖐
TT leprosy
Ex: See PDX Collection 77

A30.2 Borderline tuberculoid leprosy 🖐
BT leprosy
Ex: See PDX Collection 78

A30.3 Borderline leprosy 🖐
BB leprosy
Ex: See PDX Collection 78

A30.4 Borderline lepromatous leprosy 🖐
BL leprosy
Ex: See PDX Collection 78

A30.5 Lepromatous leprosy 🖐
LL leprosy
Ex: See PDX Collection 79

A30.8 Other forms of leprosy 🖐
Ex: See PDX Collection 80

A30.9 Leprosy, unspecified 🖐
Ex: See PDX Collection 81

● **A31 Infection due to other mycobacteria**
Excludes2 leprosy (A30.-)
tuberculosis (A15-A19)
Ex: For category A31 CC codes unless otherwise indicated: See PDX Collection 83

A31.0 Pulmonary mycobacterial infection 🖐
Infection due to Mycobacterium avium
Infection due to Mycobacterium intracellulare [Battey bacillus]
Infection due to Mycobacterium kansasii
Ex: See PDX Collection 82

A31.1 Cutaneous mycobacterial infection 🖐
Buruli ulcer
Infection due to Mycobacterium marinum
Infection due to Mycobacterium ulcerans

A31.2 Disseminated mycobacterium avium-intracellulare complex (DMAC) 🖐
MAC sepsis

A31.8 Other mycobacterial infections 🖐

A31.9 Mycobacterial infection, unspecified 🖐
Atypical mycobacterial infection NOS
Mycobacteriosis NOS

● **A32 Listeriosis**
Infection caused by Listeria monocytogenes

| **Includes** | listerial foodborne infection |
| **Excludes1** | neonatal (disseminated) listeriosis (P37.2) |

Ex: For category A32 CC codes unless otherwise indicated: See PDX Collection 74

A32.0 Cutaneous listeriosis 🖐

● **A32.1 Listerial meningitis and meningoencephalitis**
A32.11 Listerial meningitis 🖐
A32.12 Listerial meningoencephalitis 🖐

A32.7 Listerial sepsis 🖐
MCC when PDx is its own MCC
Ex: See PDX Collection 71

Item 1-7 Diptheria: A highly contagious bacterial disease that results in the formation of an adherent membrane in the throat that may lead to suffocation. In its most poisonous form, it attacks the heart and lungs. It is spread by direct physical contact or breathing the aerosolized secretions of infected individuals. The exact location is specified in the codes.

● **A32.8 Other forms of listeriosis**
A32.81 Oculoglandular listeriosis 🖐
Primary infection site is conjunctival sac, which if untreated may result in perforation of cornea and optic atrophy

A32.82 Listerial endocarditis 🖐
Exudative and proliferative inflammatory condition of endocardium caused by listeria bacteria

A32.89 Other forms of listeriosis 🖐
Listerial cerebral arteritis

A32.9 Listeriosis, unspecified 🖐

A33 Tetanus neonatorum 🖐   N
Neonate = newborn
Ex: See PDX Collection 84

A34 Obstetrical tetanus ♀ 🖐   M
Ex: See PDX Collection 85

A35 Other tetanus 🖐
Tetanus NOS
Excludes1 tetanus neonatorum (A33)
obstetrical tetanus (A34)
Ex: See PDX Collection 86

● **A36 Diphtheria**
Ex: For category A36 CC codes unless otherwise indicated: See PDX Collection 87

A36.0 Pharyngeal diphtheria 🖐
Diphtheritic membranous angina
Tonsillar diphtheria

A36.1 Nasopharyngeal diphtheria 🖐

A36.2 Laryngeal diphtheria 🖐
Diphtheritic laryngotracheitis

A36.3 Cutaneous diphtheria 🖐
Excludes2 erythrasma (L08.1)

● **A36.8 Other diphtheria**
A36.81 Diphtheritic cardiomyopathy 🖐
Diphtheritic myocarditis
Ex: See PDX Collection 88

A36.82 Diphtheritic radiculomyelitis 🖐
A36.83 Diphtheritic polyneuritis 🖐
A36.84 Diphtheritic tubulo-interstitial nephropathy 🖐
A36.85 Diphtheritic cystitis 🖐
A36.86 Diphtheritic conjunctivitis 🖐
A36.89 Other diphtheritic complications 🖐
Diphtheritic peritonitis

A36.9 Diphtheria, unspecified 🖐

● **A37 Whooping cough**
Pertussis is a highly contagious disease caused by the bacterium Bordetella pertussis and results in a whooping sounding cough.
Ex: For category A37 CC codes A37.00, A37.10, A37.80, A37.90: See PDX Collection 89
For category A37 CC codes A37.01, A37.11, A37.81, A37.91: See PDX Collection 90

● **A37.0 Whooping cough due to Bordetella pertussis**
A37.00 Whooping cough due to Bordetella pertussis without pneumonia 🖐

A37.01 Whooping cough due to Bordetella pertussis with pneumonia 🖐
MCC when PDx is its own MCC

▶ New   ⇒ Revised   ~~deleted~~ Deleted | Excludes 1 | | Excludes 2 | | Includes | | Use additional | | Code first | | Code also | | Key words |

OGCR Official Guidelines   ● Unacceptable Principal Diagnosis   X Assign placeholder X   ● Use Additional Character(s)   ▶ Manifestation Code   **Coding Clinic**

● **A37.1**   **Whooping cough due to Bordetella parapertussis**

     A37.10   Whooping cough due to Bordetella parapertussis without pneumonia 🦠

     A37.11   Whooping cough due to Bordetella parapertussis with pneumonia 🦠
         MCC when PDx is its own MCC

● **A37.8**   **Whooping cough due to other Bordetella species**

     A37.80   Whooping cough due to other Bordetella species without pneumonia 🦠

     A37.81   Whooping cough due to other Bordetella species with pneumonia 🦠
         MCC when PDx is its own MCC

● **A37.9**   **Whooping cough, unspecified species**

     A37.90   Whooping cough, unspecified species without pneumonia 🦠

     A37.91   Whooping cough, unspecified species with pneumonia 🦠
         MCC when PDx is its own MCC

● **A38**   **Scarlet fever**
     Most commonly caused by the bacteria Streptococcus pneumoniae and Neisseria meningitides

     Includes   scarlatina

     Excludes2   streptococcal sore throat (J02.0)

     (Ex) **For category A38 CC codes:** See PDX Collection 91

     A38.0   Scarlet fever with otitis media 🦠

     A38.1   Scarlet fever with myocarditis 🦠

     A38.8   Scarlet fever with other complications 🦠

     A38.9   Scarlet fever, uncomplicated 🦠
         Scarlet fever, NOS

● **A39**   **Meningococcal infection**
     Most commonly caused by the bacteria Streptococcus pneumoniae and Neisseria meningitides

     A39.0   Meningococcal meningitis 🦠
         (Ex) See PDX Collection 92

     A39.1   Waterhouse-Friderichsen syndrome 🦠
         Fulminating complication of meningococcemia
         Meningococcal hemorrhagic adrenalitis
         Meningococcic adrenal syndrome
         (Ex) See PDX Collection 93

     A39.2   Acute meningococcemia 🦠
         (Ex) See PDX Collection 94

     A39.3   Chronic meningococcemia 🦠
         (Ex) See PDX Collection 94

     A39.4   Meningococcemia, unspecified 🦠
         (Ex) See PDX Collection 94

● **A39.5**   **Meningococcal heart disease**

     A39.50   Meningococcal carditis, unspecified 🦠
         (Ex) See PDX Collection 95

     A39.51   Meningococcal endocarditis 🦠
         (Ex) See PDX Collection 96

     A39.52   Meningococcal myocarditis 🦠
         (Ex) See PDX Collection 97

     A39.53   Meningococcal pericarditis 🦠
         (Ex) See PDX Collection 98

● **A39.8**   **Other meningococcal infections**

     A39.81   Meningococcal encephalitis 🦠
         (Ex) See PDX Collection 99

     A39.82   Meningococcal retrobulbar neuritis 🦠
         Optic neuritis in portion of optic nerve posterior to eyeball; AKA postocular optic neuritis
         (Ex) See PDX Collection 100

     A39.83   Meningococcal arthritis 🦠
         (Ex) See PDX Collection 101

     A39.84   Postmeningococcal arthritis 🦠
         (Ex) See PDX Collection 101

     A39.89   Other meningococcal infections 🦠
         Meningococcal conjunctivitis
         (Ex) See PDX Collection 102

     A39.9   Meningococcal infection, unspecified 🦠
         Meningococcal disease NOS
         (Ex) See PDX Collection 102

● **A40**   **Streptococcal sepsis**
     Code first
         postprocedural streptococcal sepsis (T81.4-)
         streptococcal sepsis during labor (O75.3)
         streptococcal sepsis following abortion or ectopic or molar pregnancy (O03-O07, O08.0)
         streptococcal sepsis following immunization (T88.0)
         streptococcal sepsis following infusion, transfusion or therapeutic injection (T80.2-)

     Excludes1   neonatal (P36.0-P36.1)
         puerperal sepsis (O85)
         sepsis due to Streptococcus, group D (A41.81)

     (Ex) **For category A40 CC codes unless otherwise indicated:** See PDX Collection 71

     A40.0   Sepsis due to streptococcus, group A 🦠

     A40.1   Sepsis due to streptococcus, group B 🦠

     A40.3   Sepsis due to Streptococcus pneumoniae 🦠
         Pneumococcal sepsis
         (Ex) No exclusions

     A40.8   Other streptococcal sepsis 🦠

     A40.9   Streptococcal sepsis, unspecified 🦠

● **A41**   **Other sepsis**
     Code first
         postprocedural sepsis (T81.4-)
         sepsis during labor (O75.3)
         sepsis following abortion, ectopic or molar pregnancy (O03-O07, O08.0)
         sepsis following immunization (T88.0)
         sepsis following infusion, transfusion or therapeutic injection (T80.2-)

     Excludes1   bacteremia NOS (R78.81)
         neonatal (P36.-)
         puerperal sepsis (O85)
         streptococcal sepsis (A40.-)

     Excludes2   sepsis (due to) (in) actinomycotic (A42.7)
         sepsis (due to) (in) anthrax (A22.7)
         sepsis (due to) (in) candidal (B37.7)
         sepsis (due to) (in) Erysipelothrix (A26.7)
         sepsis (due to) (in) extraintestinal yersiniosis (A28.2)
         sepsis (due to) (in) gonococcal (A54.86)
         sepsis (due to) (in) herpesviral (B00.7)
         sepsis (due to) (in) listerial (A32.7)
         sepsis (due to) (in) melioidosis (A24.1)
         sepsis (due to) (in) meningococcal (A39.2-A39.4)
         sepsis (due to) (in) plague (A20.7)
         sepsis (due to) (in) tularemia (A21.7)
         toxic shock syndrome (A48.3)

     (Ex) **For category A41 CC codes:** See PDX Collection 71
     Coding Clinic: 2016, Q1, P39

● **A41.0**   **Sepsis due to Staphylococcus aureus**

     A41.01   Sepsis due to Methicillin susceptible Staphylococcus aureus 🦠
         MSSA sepsis
         Staphylococcus aureus sepsis NOS

     A41.02   Sepsis due to Methicillin resistant Staphylococcus aureus 🦠

     A41.1   Sepsis due to other specified staphylococcus 🦠
         Coagulase negative staphylococcus sepsis

     A41.2   Sepsis due to unspecified staphylococcus 🦠

CHAPTER 1 (A00-B99)

N Newborn Age: 0   **P** Pediatric Age: 0-17   **M** Maternity DX: 12-55   **A** Adult Age: 15-124   ♀ Females Only   ♂ Males Only

🦠 Complication\Comorbidity   🦠 Major C\C   (Ex) CC/MCC Exclusions   🦠 Hospital-Acquired Condition

643

CHAPTER 1 (A00-B99)

A41.3   Sepsis due to Hemophilus influenzae 🔖

A41.4   Sepsis due to anaerobes 🔖
> **Excludes1**   gas gangrene (A48.0)

● A41.5   Sepsis due to other Gram-negative organisms

     A41.50   **Gram-negative sepsis, unspecified** 🔖
         Gram-negative sepsis NOS

     A41.51   Sepsis due to Escherichia coli [E. coli] 🔖

     A41.52   Sepsis due to Pseudomonas 🔖
         Pseudomonas aeroginosa

     A41.53   Sepsis due to Serratia 🔖

     A41.59   Other Gram-negative sepsis 🔖

● A41.8   Other specified sepsis

     A41.81   Sepsis due to Enterococcus 🔖

     A41.89   Other specified sepsis 🔖
         Coding Clinic: 2016, Q3, P8-14

A41.9   Sepsis, unspecified organism 🔖
     Septicemia NOS

● A42   **Actinomycosis**
> **Excludes1**   actinomycetoma (B47.1)

A42.0   Pulmonary actinomycosis 🔖
     (Ex:) See PDX Collection 103

A42.1   Abdominal actinomycosis 🔖
     (Ex:) See PDX Collection 104

A42.2   Cervicofacial actinomycosis 🔖
     (Ex:) See PDX Collection 105

A42.7   Actinomycotic sepsis 🔖
     (Ex:) See PDX Collection 71

● A42.8   Other forms of actinomycosis
     (Ex:) For category A42.8 CC codes: See PDX Collection 106

     A42.81   Actinomycotic meningitis 🔖

     A42.82   Actinomycotic encephalitis 🔖

     A42.89   Other forms of actinomycosis 🔖

A42.9   Actinomycosis, unspecified 🔖
     (Ex:) See PDX Collection 106

● A43   **Nocardiosis**

A43.0   Pulmonary nocardiosis 🔖
     (Ex:) See PDX Collection 103

A43.1   Cutaneous nocardiosis 🔖
     (Ex:) See PDX Collection 107

A43.8   Other forms of nocardiosis 🔖
     (Ex:) See PDX Collection 106

A43.9   Nocardiosis, unspecified 🔖
     (Ex:) See PDX Collection 106

● A44   **Bartonellosis**
     (Ex:) For category A44 CC codes: See PDX Collection 108

A44.0   Systemic bartonellosis 🔖
     Oroya fever

A44.1   Cutaneous and mucocutaneous bartonellosis 🔖
     Verruga peruana

A44.8   Other forms of bartonellosis 🔖

A44.9   Bartonellosis, unspecified 🔖

A46   **Erysipelas**
> **Excludes1**   postpartum or puerperal erysipelas (O86.89)

Item 1-8   **Gas gangrene** is a necrotizing subcutaneous infection that will cause tissue death. Patients with poor circulation (e.g., diabetes, peripheral nephropathy) will have low oxygen content in their tissues (hypoxia), which allows the Clostridium bacteria to flourish. Gas gangrene often occurs at the site of a surgical wound or trauma. Onset is sudden and dramatic. Treatment can include debridement, amputation, and/or hyperbaric oxygen treatments.

● A48   **Other bacterial diseases, not elsewhere classified**
> **Excludes1**   actinomycetoma (B47.1)

A48.0   Gas gangrene 🔖
     Clostridial cellulitis
     Clostridial myonecrosis
     (Ex:) See PDX Collection 109

A48.1   Legionnaires' disease 🔖
     (Ex:) See PDX Collection 110

A48.2   Nonpneumonic Legionnaires' disease [Pontiac fever]

A48.3   Toxic shock syndrome 🔖
     Use additional code to identify the organism (B95, B96)
> **Excludes1**   endotoxic shock NOS (R57.8)
>   sepsis NOS (A41.9)
     (Ex:) See PDX Collection 111

A48.4   Brazilian purpuric fever
     Systemic Hemophilus aegyptius infection

● A48.5   Other specified botulism
     Non-foodborne intoxication due to toxins of
         Clostridium botulinum [C. botulinum]
> **Excludes1**   food poisoning due to toxins of
>   Clostridium botulinum (A05.1)

     A48.51   Infant botulism 🔖   P
         (Ex:) See PDX Collection 18

     A48.52   Wound botulism 🔖
         Non-foodborne botulism NOS
         Use additional code for associated wound
         (Ex:) See PDX Collection 18

A48.8   Other specified bacterial diseases

● A49   **Bacterial infection of unspecified site**
> **Excludes1**   bacterial agents as the cause of diseases classified
>   elsewhere (B95-B96)
>   chlamydial infection NOS (A74.9)
>   meningococcal infection NOS (A39.9)
>   rickettsial infection NOS (A79.9)
>   spirochetal infection NOS (A69.9)

● A49.0   Staphylococcal infection, unspecified site

     A49.01   **Methicillin susceptible Staphylococcus aureus infection, unspecified site**
         Methicillin susceptible Staphylococcus aureus (MSSA) infection
         Staphylococcus aureus infection NOS

     A49.02   **Methicillin resistant Staphylococcus aureus infection, unspecified site**
         Methicillin resistant Staphylococcus aureus (MRSA) infection

A49.1   Streptococcal infection, unspecified site

A49.2   Hemophilus influenzae infection, unspecified site
     Any of seven bacterium of genus Haemophilus

A49.3   Mycoplasma infection, unspecified site
     Bacterium of class Mollicutes, unusual group of bacteria distinguished by absence of cell wall

A49.8   Other bacterial infections of unspecified site

A49.9   Bacterial infection, unspecified
> **Excludes1**   bacteremia NOS (R78.81)

▶ New   ⇒ Revised   ~~deleted~~ Deleted   Excludes 1   Excludes 2   Includes   Use additional   Code first   Code also   Key words

644

OGCR Official Guidelines   ● Unacceptable Principal Diagnosis   X Assign placeholder X   ● Use Additional Character(s)   ▶ Manifestation Code   **Coding Clinic**

Figure 1-3 Chancre of primary syphilis. (From James WD, Berger TG, Elston DM: Andrews' Diseases of the Skin: Clinical Dermatology, Philadelphia, Saunders Elsevier, 2006)

Item 1–9 Syphilis, also known as lues, is the most serious of the venereal diseases caused by *Treponema pallidum*. The **primary** stage is characterized by an ulceration known as **chancre,** which usually appears on the genitals but can also develop on the anus, lips, tonsils, breasts, or fingers. Syphilis is easy to cure in its early stages. A single intramuscular injection of penicillin will usually cure a person who has had syphilis for less than a year.

The **secondary** stage is characterized by a rash that can affect any area of the body. **Latent** syphilis is divided into **early,** which is diagnosed within two years of infection, and **late,** which is diagnosed two years or more after infection. Additional doses of penicillin or another antibiotic are needed to treat someone who has had syphilis for longer than a year. For those allergic to penicillin, there are other antibiotic treatments. **Congenital** syphilis is also labeled **early** or **late** based on the time of diagnosis.

INFECTIONS WITH A PREDOMINANTLY SEXUAL MODE OF TRANSMISSION (A50-A64)

Excludes1 human immunodeficiency virus [HIV] disease (B20)
nonspecific and nongonococcal urethritis (N34.1)
Reiter's disease (M02.3-)

● **A50 Congenital syphilis**
  ● **A50.0 Early congenital syphilis, symptomatic**
      Any congenital syphilitic condition specified as early or manifest less than two years after birth
      (Ex) For category A50.0 CC codes: See PDX Collection 112
      A50.01 Early congenital syphilitic oculopathy 🔖
      A50.02 Early congenital syphilitic osteochondropathy 🔖
      A50.03 Early congenital syphilitic pharyngitis 🔖
          Early congenital syphilitic laryngitis
      A50.04 Early congenital syphilitic pneumonia 🔖
      A50.05 Early congenital syphilitic rhinitis 🔖
      A50.06 Early cutaneous congenital syphilis 🔖
      A50.07 Early mucocutaneous congenital syphilis 🔖
      A50.08 Early visceral congenital syphilis 🔖
      A50.09 Other early congenital syphilis, symptomatic 🔖
    A50.1 Early congenital syphilis, latent
        Congenital syphilis without clinical manifestations, with positive serological reaction and negative spinal fluid test, less than two years after birth
    A50.2 Early congenital syphilis, unspecified 🔖
        Congenital syphilis NOS less than two years after birth
        (Ex) See PDX Collection 113
  ● **A50.3 Late congenital syphilitic oculopathy**
      Excludes1 Hutchinson's triad (A50.53)
      (Ex) For category A50.3 CC codes: See PDX Collection 112
      A50.30 Late congenital syphilitic oculopathy, unspecified 🔖
      A50.31 Late congenital syphilitic interstitial keratitis 🔖
      A50.32 Late congenital syphilitic chorioretinitis 🔖
      A50.39 Other late congenital syphilitic oculopathy 🔖

● **A50.4 Late congenital neurosyphilis [juvenile neurosyphilis]**
    Use additional code to identify any associated mental disorder
    Excludes1 Hutchinson's triad (A50.53)
    (Ex) For category A50.4 CC codes unless otherwise indicated: See PDX Collection 114
    A50.40 Late congenital neurosyphilis, unspecified 🔖
        Juvenile neurosyphilis NOS
    A50.41 Late congenital syphilitic meningitis 🔖
        (Ex) See PDX Collection 115
    A50.42 Late congenital syphilitic encephalitis 🔖
    A50.43 Late congenital syphilitic polyneuropathy 🔖
    A50.44 Late congenital syphilitic optic nerve atrophy 🔖
        (Ex) See PDX Collection 112
    A50.45 Juvenile general paresis 🔖
        Dementia paralytica juvenilis
        Juvenile tabetoparetic neurosyphilis
    A50.49 Other late congenital neurosyphilis 🔖
        Juvenile tabes dorsalis
● **A50.5 Other late congenital syphilis, symptomatic**
    Any congenital syphilitic condition specified as late or manifest two years or more after birth
    (Ex) For category A50.5 CC codes: See PDX Collection 112
    A50.51 Clutton's joints 🔖
    A50.52 Hutchinson's teeth 🔖
    A50.53 Hutchinson's triad 🔖
    A50.54 Late congenital cardiovascular syphilis 🔖
    A50.55 Late congenital syphilitic arthropathy 🔖
    A50.56 Late congenital syphilitic osteochondropathy 🔖
    A50.57 Syphilitic saddle nose 🔖
    A50.59 Other late congenital syphilis, symptomatic 🔖
  A50.6 Late congenital syphilis, latent
      Congenital syphilis without clinical manifestations, with positive serological reaction and negative spinal fluid test, two years or more after birth.
  A50.7 Late congenital syphilis, unspecified
      Congenital syphilis NOS two years or more after birth.
  A50.9 Congenital syphilis, unspecified

● **A51 Early syphilis**
    A51.0 Primary genital syphilis
        Syphilitic chancre NOS
    A51.1 Primary anal syphilis
    A51.2 Primary syphilis of other sites
  ● **A51.3 Secondary syphilis of skin and mucous membranes**
      A51.31 Condyloma latum 🔖
          (Ex) See PDX Collection 112
      A51.32 Syphilitic alopecia 🔖
          (Ex) See PDX Collection 116
      A51.39 Other secondary syphilis of skin 🔖
          Syphilitic leukoderma
          Syphilitic mucous patch
          Excludes1 late syphilitic leukoderma (A52.79)
          (Ex) See PDX Collection 112
  ● **A51.4 Other secondary syphilis**
      A51.41 Secondary syphilitic meningitis 🔖
          (Ex) See PDX Collection 117
      A51.42 Secondary syphilitic female pelvic disease ♀ 🔖
          (Ex) See PDX Collection 113
      A51.43 Secondary syphilitic oculopathy 🔖
          Secondary syphilitic chorioretinitis
          Secondary syphilitic iridocyclitis, iritis
          Secondary syphilitic uveitis
          (Ex) See PDX Collection 112

N Newborn Age: 0   **P** Pediatric Age: 0–17   **M** Maternity DX: 12–55   **A** Adult Age: 15–124   ♀ Females Only   ♂ Males Only
🔖 Complication\Comorbidity   🔖 Major C\C   (Ex) CC/MCC Exclusions   🔖 Hospital-Acquired Condition

645

A51.44   **Secondary syphilitic nephritis** 🔑
    Ⓔ See PDX Collection 113

A51.45   **Secondary syphilitic hepatitis** 🔑
    Ⓔ See PDX Collection 118

A51.46   **Secondary syphilitic osteopathy** 🔑
    Ⓔ See PDX Collection 119

A51.49   **Other secondary syphilitic conditions** 🔑
    Secondary syphilitic lymphadenopathy
    Secondary syphilitic myositis
    Ⓔ No exclusions

A51.5   **Early syphilis, latent**
    Syphilis (acquired) without clinical manifestations, with
    positive serological reaction and negative spinal
    fluid test, less than two years after infection.

A51.9   **Early syphilis, unspecified**

● **A52   Late syphilis**

  ● **A52.0   Cardiovascular and cerebrovascular syphilis**
    Ⓔ For category A52.0 CC codes: See PDX Collection 114

A52.00   **Cardiovascular syphilis, unspecified** 🔑

A52.01   **Syphilitic aneurysm of aorta** 🔑

A52.02   **Syphilitic aortitis** 🔑

A52.03   **Syphilitic endocarditis** 🔑
    Syphilitic aortic valve incompetence or stenosis
    Syphilitic mitral valve stenosis
    Syphilitic pulmonary valve regurgitation

A52.04   **Syphilitic cerebral arteritis** 🔑

A52.05   **Other cerebrovascular syphilis** 🔑
    Syphilitic cerebral aneurysm (ruptured) (non-ruptured)
    Syphilitic cerebral thrombosis

A52.06   **Other syphilitic heart involvement** 🔑
    Syphilitic coronary artery disease
    Syphilitic myocarditis
    Syphilitic pericarditis

A52.09   **Other cardiovascular syphilis** 🔑

  ● **A52.1   Symptomatic neurosyphilis**
    Ⓔ For category A52.1 CC codes unless otherwise indicated: See PDX Collection 114

A52.10   **Symptomatic neurosyphilis, unspecified** 🔑

A52.11   **Tabes dorsalis** 🔑
    Cognitive decline with progressive degeneration of
    posterior columns, roots, and ganglia of spinal
    cord, occur 15-20 years after initial infection
    of syphilis; AKA Duchenne disease
    Locomotor ataxia (progressive)
    Tabetic neurosyphilis

A52.12   **Other cerebrospinal syphilis** 🔑

A52.13   **Late syphilitic meningitis** 🔑
    Ⓔ See PDX Collection 115

A52.14   **Late syphilitic encephalitis** 🔑

A52.15   **Late syphilitic neuropathy** 🔑
    Late syphilitic acoustic neuritis
    Late syphilitic optic (nerve) atrophy
    Late syphilitic polyneuropathy
    Late syphilitic retrobulbar neuritis

A52.16   **Charcôt's arthropathy (tabetic)** 🔑
    Progressive musculoskeletal condition characterized
    by joint dislocation, fractures, and deformities,
    results in progressive destruction of bone and
    soft tissue of weight-bearing joints

A52.17   **General paresis** 🔑
    Chronic meningoencephalitis results in loss of
    cortical function, or progressive dementia
    and generalized paralysis, occurring 10-20
    years after initial infection of syphilis; AKA
    Bayle disease, dementia paralytica, paralytic
    dementiaparetic neurosyphilis, syphilitic
    meningoencephalitis
    Dementia paralytica

A52.19   **Other symptomatic neurosyphilis** 🔑
    Syphilitic parkinsonism

A52.2   **Asymptomatic neurosyphilis** 🔑
    Ⓔ See PDX Collection 114

A52.3   **Neurosyphilis, unspecified** 🔑
    Gumma (syphilitic)
    Destructive lesions of syphilis
    Syphilis (late)
    Syphiloma
    Ⓔ See PDX Collection 114

● **A52.7   Other symptomatic late syphilis**
    Ⓔ For category A52.7 CC codes unless otherwise indicated: See PDX Collection 116

A52.71   **Late syphilitic oculopathy** 🔑
    Late syphilitic chorioretinitis
    Late syphilitic episcleritis
    Ⓔ See PDX Collection 120

A52.72   **Syphilis of lung and bronchus** 🔑

A52.73   **Symptomatic late syphilis of other respiratory organs** 🔑

A52.74   **Syphilis of liver and other viscera** 🔑
    Late syphilitic peritonitis

A52.75   **Syphilis of kidney and ureter** 🔑
    Syphilitic glomerular disease

A52.76   **Other genitourinary symptomatic late syphilis** 🔑
    Late syphilitic female pelvic inflammatory disease

A52.77   **Syphilis of bone and joint** 🔑

A52.78   **Syphilis of other musculoskeletal tissue** 🔑
    Late syphilitic bursitis
    Syphilis [stage unspecified] of bursa
    Syphilis [stage unspecified] of muscle
    Syphilis [stage unspecified] of synovium
    Syphilis [stage unspecified] of tendon

A52.79   **Other symptomatic late syphilis** 🔑
    Late syphilitic leukoderma
    Syphilis of adrenal gland
    Syphilis of pituitary gland
    Syphilis of thyroid gland
    Syphilitic splenomegaly
    Excludes1   syphilitic leukoderma (secondary) (A51.39)

A52.8   **Late syphilis, latent**
    Syphilis (acquired) without clinical manifestations, with
    positive serological reaction and negative spinal
    fluid test, two years or more after infection

A52.9   **Late syphilis, unspecified**

● **A53   Other and unspecified syphilis**

A53.0   **Latent syphilis, unspecified as early or late**
    Latent syphilis NOS
    Positive serological reaction for syphilis

A53.9   **Syphilis, unspecified**
    Infection due to Treponema pallidum NOS
    Syphilis (acquired) NOS
    Excludes1   syphilis NOS under two years of age (A50.2)

● **A54   Gonococcal infection**

  ● **A54.0   Gonococcal infection of lower genitourinary tract without periurethral or accessory gland abscess**
    Excludes1   gonococcal infection with genitourinary gland abscess (A54.1)
        gonococcal infection with periurethral abscess (A54.1)
    Ⓔ For category A54.0 CC codes: See PDX Collection 121

A54.00   **Gonococcal infection of lower genitourinary tract, unspecified** 🔑

A54.01   **Gonococcal cystitis and urethritis, unspecified** 🔑

A54.02   **Gonococcal vulvovaginitis, unspecified** ♀ 🔑

A54.03   **Gonococcal cervicitis, unspecified** ♀ 🔑

A54.09   **Other gonococcal infection of lower genitourinary tract** 🔑

CHAPTER 1 (A00-B99)

Item 1-10 An STD (sexually transmitted disease) caused by **Neisseria gonorrhoeae** that flourishes in the warm, moist areas of the reproductive tract. Untreated gonorrhea spreads to other parts of the body, causing inflammation of the testes or prostate or pelvic inflammatory disease (PID).

A54.1 Gonococcal infection of lower genitourinary tract with periurethral and accessory gland abscess 🔹
    Gonococcal Bartholin's gland abscess

● **A54.2 Gonococcal pelviperitonitis and other gonococcal genitourinary infection**
    (Ex) For category A54.2 CC codes: See PDX Collection 121

  A54.21 Gonococcal infection of kidney and ureter 🔹
  A54.22 Gonococcal prostatitis ♂ 🔹
  A54.23 Gonococcal infection of other male genital organs ♂ 🔹
    Gonococcal epididymitis
    Gonococcal orchitis
  A54.24 Gonococcal female pelvic inflammatory disease ♀ 🔹
    Gonococcal pelviperitonitis
    Excludes1 gonococcal peritonitis (A54.85)
  A54.29 Other gonococcal genitourinary infections 🔹

● **A54.3 Gonococcal infection of eye**
    (Ex) For category A54.3 CC codes: See PDX Collection 116

  A54.30 Gonococcal infection of eye, unspecified 🔹
  A54.31 Gonococcal conjunctivitis 🔹
    Form of bacterial conjunctivitis contracted by newborns during delivery; AKA neonatal conjunctivitis
    Ophthalmia neonatorum due to gonococcus
  A54.32 Gonococcal iridocyclitis 🔹
    Inflammation of iris and of ciliary body due to gonococcal infection
  A54.33 Gonococcal keratitis 🔹
    Inflammation of cornea due to gonococcal infection; AKA keratoconjunctivitis, keratopathy
  A54.39 Other gonococcal eye infection 🔹
    Gonococcal endophthalmia

● **A54.4 Gonococcal infection of musculoskeletal system**
    (Ex) For category A54.4 CC codes: See PDX Collection 122

  A54.40 Gonococcal infection of musculoskeletal system, unspecified 🔹
  A54.41 Gonococcal spondylopathy 🔹
    Disorder of vertebrae due to gonococcal infection; AKA rachiopathy
  A54.42 Gonococcal arthritis 🔹
    Excludes2 gonococcal infection of spine (A54.41)
  A54.43 Gonococcal osteomyelitis 🔹
    Excludes2 gonococcal infection of spine (A54.41)
  A54.49 Gonococcal infection of other musculoskeletal tissue 🔹
    Gonococcal bursitis
    Gonococcal myositis
    Gonococcal synovitis
    Gonococcal tenosynovitis

A54.5 Gonococcal pharyngitis
A54.6 Gonococcal infection of anus and rectum

● **A54.8 Other gonococcal infections**
  A54.81 Gonococcal meningitis 🔹
    (Ex) See PDX Collection 117
  A54.82 Gonococcal brain abscess 🔹
    (Ex) See PDX Collection 123

  A54.83 Gonococcal heart infection 🔹
    Gonococcal endocarditis
    Gonococcal myocarditis
    Gonococcal pericarditis
    (Ex) See PDX Collection 124
  A54.84 Gonococcal pneumonia 🔹
    (Ex) See PDX Collection 123
  A54.85 Gonococcal peritonitis 🔹
    Excludes1 gonococcal pelviperitonitis (A54.24)
    (Ex) See PDX Collection 125
  A54.86 Gonococcal sepsis 🔹
    MCC when PDx is its own MCC
    (Ex) See PDX Collection 71
  A54.89 Other gonococcal infections 🔹
    Gonococcal keratoderma
    Gonococcal lymphadenitis
    (Ex) See PDX Collection 123

A54.9 Gonococcal infection, unspecified 🔹
    (Ex) See PDX Collection 123

A55 Chlamydial lymphogranuloma (venereum)
  Climatic or tropical bubo
  Durand-Nicolas-Favre disease
  Esthiomene
  Lymphogranuloma inguinale

● **A56 Other sexually transmitted chlamydial diseases**
  Includes sexually transmitted diseases due to Chlamydia trachomatis
  Excludes1 neonatal chlamydial conjunctivitis (P39.1)
        neonatal chlamydial pneumonia (P23.1)
  Excludes2 chlamydial lymphogranuloma (A55)
        conditions classified to A74.-

● **A56.0 Chlamydial infection of lower genitourinary tract**
  A56.00 Chlamydial infection of lower genitourinary tract, unspecified
  A56.01 Chlamydial cystitis and urethritis
  A56.02 Chlamydial vulvovaginitis ♀
  A56.09 Other chlamydial infection of lower genitourinary tract
    Chlamydial cervicitis

● **A56.1 Chlamydial infection of pelviperitoneum and other genitourinary organs**
  A56.11 Chlamydial female pelvic inflammatory disease ♀
  A56.19 Other chlamydial genitourinary infection
    Chlamydial epididymitis
    Chlamydial orchitis

A56.2 Chlamydial infection of genitourinary tract, unspecified
A56.3 Chlamydial infection of anus and rectum
A56.4 Chlamydial infection of pharynx
A56.8 Sexually transmitted chlamydial infection of other sites

A57 Chancroid
  Ulcus molle
  Sexually transmitted infection caused by bacteria, Haemophilus ducreyi

A58 Granuloma inguinale
  Chronic, progressive, ulcerative granulomatous disease
  Donovanosis

CHAPTER 1 (A00-B99)

N Newborn Age: 0   P Pediatric Age: 0–17   M Maternity DX: 12–55   A Adult Age: 15–124   ♀ Females Only   ♂ Males Only

🔹 Complication\Comorbidity   🔹 Major C\C   (Ex) CC/MCC Exclusions   🔹 Hospital-Acquired Condition

CHAPTER 1 (A00-B99)

● **A59　Trichomoniasis**

　　Excludes2　intestinal trichomoniasis (A07.8)

　　A common STD caused by a parasite, Trichomonas vaginalis

　● **A59.0　Urogenital trichomoniasis**

　　　A59.00　Urogenital trichomoniasis, unspecified

　　　　　Fluor (vaginalis) due to Trichomonas

　　　　　Leukorrhea (vaginalis) due to Trichomonas

　　　A59.01　Trichomonal vulvovaginitis ♀

　　　A59.02　Trichomonal prostatitis ♂

　　　A59.03　Trichomonal cystitis and urethritis

　　　A59.09　Other urogenital trichomoniasis

　　　　　Common sexually transmitted disease (STD) caused by single-celled protozoan parasite; AKA trich

　　　　　Trichomonas cervicitis

　　A59.8　Trichomoniasis of other sites

　　A59.9　Trichomoniasis, unspecified

● **A60　Anogenital herpesviral [herpes simplex] infections**

　● **A60.0　Herpesviral infection of genitalia and urogenital tract**

　　　A60.00　Herpesviral infection of urogenital system, unspecified

　　　A60.01　Herpesviral infection of penis ♂

　　　A60.02　Herpesviral infection of other male genital organs ♂

　　　A60.03　Herpesviral cervicitis ♀

　　　A60.04　Herpesviral vulvovaginitis ♀

　　　　　Herpesviral [herpes simplex] ulceration

　　　　　Herpesviral [herpes simplex] vaginitis

　　　　　Herpesviral [herpes simplex] vulvitis

　　　A60.09　Herpesviral infection of other urogenital tract

　　A60.1　Herpesviral infection of perianal skin and rectum

　　A60.9　Anogenital herpesviral infection, unspecified

● **A63　Other predominantly sexually transmitted diseases, not elsewhere classified**

　　Excludes2　molluscum contagiosum (B08.1)

　　　　　　　papilloma of cervix (D26.0)

　　A63.0　Anogenital (venereal) warts

　　　　Anogenital warts due to (human) papillomavirus [HPV]

　　　　Condyloma acuminatum

　　A63.8　Other specified predominantly sexually transmitted diseases

● **A64　Unspecified sexually transmitted disease**

OTHER SPIROCHETAL DISEASES (A65-A69)

　　Excludes2　leptospirosis (A27.-)

　　　　　　　syphilis (A50-A53)

A65　Nonvenereal syphilis

　　Bejel

　　Endemic syphilis

　　Njovera

● **A66　Yaws**

　　Endemic, infectious, tropical disease caused by spirochete, spread by direct contact; AKA frambesia, framboesia, frambesia tropica

　　Includes　bouba

　　　　　　frambesia (tropica)

　　　　　　pian

　　A66.0　Initial lesions of yaws

　　　　Chancre of yaws

　　　　Frambesia, initial or primary

　　　　Initial frambesial ulcer

　　　　Mother yaw

　　A66.1　Multiple papillomata and wet crab yaws

　　　　Frambesioma

　　　　Pianoma

　　　　Plantar or palmar papilloma of yaws

　　A66.2　Other early skin lesions of yaws

　　　　Cutaneous yaws, less than five years after infection

　　　　Early yaws (cutaneous)(macular)(maculopapular) (micropapular)(papular)

　　　　Frambeside of early yaws

　　A66.3　Hyperkeratosis of yaws

　　　　Hypertrophy of stratum corneum of skin in which there are small, hard, verrucous scales

　　　　Ghoul hand

　　　　Hyperkeratosis, palmar or plantar (early) (late) due to yaws

　　　　Worm-eaten soles

　　A66.4　Gummata and ulcers of yaws

　　　　Small, rubbery granuloma with necrotic center and inflamed characteristic of advanced stage of syphilis; AKA syphiloma

　　　　Gummatous frambeside

　　　　Nodular late yaws (ulcerated)

　　A66.5　Gangosa

　　　　Manifestation of yaws that develops in the soft palate and spreads eroding bone, cartilage, and soft tissue

　　　　Rhinopharyngitis mutilans

　　A66.6　Bone and joint lesions of yaws

　　　　Yaws ganglion

　　　　Yaws goundou

　　　　Yaws gumma, bone

　　　　Yaws gummatous osteitis or periostitis

　　　　Yaws hydrarthrosis

　　　　Yaws osteitis

　　　　Yaws periostitis (hypertrophic)

　　A66.7　Other manifestations of yaws

　　　　Juxta-articular nodules of yaws

　　　　Mucosal yaws

　　A66.8　Latent yaws

　　　　Yaws without clinical manifestations, with positive serology

　　A66.9　Yaws, unspecified

● **A67　Pinta [carate]**

　　Group of nonvenereal diseases caused by Treponema species

　　A67.0　Primary lesions of pinta

　　　　Chancre (primary) of pinta

　　　　Papule (primary) of pinta

　　A67.1　Intermediate lesions of pinta

　　　　Erythematous plaques of pinta

　　　　Hyperchromic lesions of pinta

　　　　Hyperkeratosis of pinta

　　　　Pintids

　　A67.2　Late lesions of pinta

　　　　Achromic skin lesions of pinta

　　　　Cicatricial skin lesions of pinta

　　　　Dyschromic skin lesions of pinta

　　A67.3　Mixed lesions of pinta

　　　　Achromic with hyperchromic skin lesions of pinta [carate]

　　A67.9　Pinta, unspecified

● **A68　Relapsing fevers**

　　Includes　recurrent fever

　　Excludes2　Lyme disease (A69.2-)

　　(Ex) **For category A68 CC codes:** See PDX Collection 108

　　A68.0　Louse-borne relapsing fever 🗝

　　　　Relapsing fever due to Borrelia recurrentis

　　A68.1　Tick-borne relapsing fever 🗝

　　　　Relapsing fever due to any Borrelia species other than Borrelia recurrentis

　　A68.9　Relapsing fever, unspecified 🗝

▶ New　　⟹ Revised　　~~deleted~~ Deleted　　Excludes 1　　Excludes 2　　Includes　　Use additional　　Code first　　Code also　　Key words

OGCR Official Guidelines　　● Unacceptable Principal Diagnosis　　X Assign placeholder X　　● Use Additional Character(s)　　▶ Manifestation Code　　Coding Clinic

Item 1-11 Cancrum oris, also known as **noma** or **gangrenous stomatitis,** begins as an ulcer of the gingiva and results in a progressive gangrenous process.

● **A69   Other spirochetal infections**

    A69.0   Necrotizing ulcerative stomatitis
        Cancrum oris
        Fusospirochetal gangrene
        Noma
        Stomatitis gangrenosa

    A69.1   Other Vincent's infections 🔲
        Fusospirochetal pharyngitis
        Necrotizing ulcerative (acute) gingivitis
        Necrotizing ulcerative (acute) gingivostomatitis
        Spirochetal stomatitis
        Trench mouth
        Vincent's angina
        Vincent's gingivitis
        (Ex) See PDX Collection 126

● **A69.2   Lyme disease**
        Erythema chronicum migrans due to Borrelia
          burgdorferi
        (Ex) For category A69.2 CC codes: See PDX Collection 108

    A69.20   Lyme disease, unspecified 🔲
    A69.21   Meningitis due to Lyme disease 🔲
    A69.22   Other neurologic disorders in Lyme disease 🔲
        Cranial neuritis
        Meningoencephalitis
        Polyneuropathy
    A69.23   Arthritis due to Lyme disease 🔲
    A69.29   Other conditions associated with Lyme disease 🔲
        Myopericarditis due to Lyme disease
        Coding Clinic: 2016, Q3, P12

    A69.8   Other specified spirochetal infections
    A69.9   Spirochetal infection, unspecified

OTHER DISEASES CAUSED BY CHLAMYDIAE (A70-A74)

    Excludes1 sexually transmitted chlamydial diseases
             (A55-A56)

● **A70   Chlamydia psittaci infections** 🔲
    Ornithosis
    Parrot fever
    Psittacosis
    (Ex) See PDX Collection 127

● **A71   Trachoma**
    Excludes1 sequelae of trachoma (B94.0)

    A71.0   Initial stage of trachoma
        Trachoma dubium

    A71.1   Active stage of trachoma
        Granular conjunctivitis (trachomatous)
        Trachomatous follicular conjunctivitis
        Trachomatous pannus

    A71.9   Trachoma, unspecified

● **A74   Other diseases caused by chlamydiae**
    Excludes1 neonatal chlamydial conjunctivitis (P39.1)
             neonatal chlamydial pneumonia (P23.1)
             Reiter's disease (M02.3-)
             sexually transmitted chlamydial diseases
               (A55-A56)
    Excludes2 chlamydial pneumonia (J16.0)

    A74.0   Chlamydial conjunctivitis
        Paratrachoma

●   **A74.8   Other chlamydial diseases**
    A74.81   Chlamydial peritonitis
    A74.89   Other chlamydial diseases

    A74.9   Chlamydial infection, unspecified
        Chlamydiosis NOS

Item 1-12 Rickettsioses are diseases spread from ticks, lice, fleas, or mites to humans.
    Typhus is spread to humans chiefly by the fleas of rats.
    Endemic identifies a disease as being present in low numbers of humans at all times, whereas **epidemic** identifies a disease as being present in high numbers of humans at a specific time. Morbidity (death) is higher in epidemic diseases.
    Brill's disease, also known as **Brill-Zinsser disease,** is spread from human to human by body lice and also from the lice of flying squirrels. **Scrub typhus** is spread in the same ways as Brill's disease.
    Malaria is spread to humans by mosquitoes.

RICKETTSIOSES (A75-A79)

● **A75   Typhus fever**
    Excludes1 rickettsiosis due to Ehrlichia sennetsu (A79.81)
    (Ex) For category A75 CC codes unless otherwise indicated: See PDX Collection 108

    A75.0   Epidemic louse-borne typhus fever due to Rickettsia prowazekii 🔲
        Organisms transmitted between humans via louse
        Classical typhus (fever)
        Epidemic (louse-borne) typhus

    A75.1   Recrudescent typhus [Brill's disease] 🔲
        Brill-Zinsser disease

    A75.2   Typhus fever due to Rickettsia typhi 🔲
        Murine (flea-borne) typhus

    A75.3   Typhus fever due to Rickettsia tsutsugamushi 🔲
        Scrub (mite-borne) typhus
        Tsutsugamushi fever

    A75.9   Typhus fever, unspecified 🔲
        Typhus (fever) NOS
        (Ex) See PDX Collection 128

● **A77   Spotted fever [tick-borne rickettsioses]**
    (Ex) For category A77 CC codes: See PDX Collection 108

    A77.0   Spotted fever due to Rickettsia rickettsii 🔲
        Rocky Mountain spotted fever
        Sao Paulo fever

    A77.1   Spotted fever due to Rickettsia conorii 🔲
        African tick typhus
        Boutonneuse fever
        India tick typhus
        Kenya tick typhus
        Marseilles fever
        Mediterranean tick fever

    A77.2   Spotted fever due to Rickettsia siberica 🔲
        North Asian tick fever
        Siberian tick typhus

    A77.3   Spotted fever due to Rickettsia australis 🔲
        Queensland tick typhus

●   **A77.4   Ehrlichiosis**
    Type of tick-borne fever caused by bacteria infection
    Excludes1 Rickettsiosis due to Ehrlichia sennetsu
             (A79.81)

    A77.40   Ehrlichiosis, unspecified 🔲
    A77.41   Ehrlichiosis chafeensis [E. chafeensis] 🔲
    A77.49   Other ehrlichiosis 🔲

    A77.8   Other spotted fevers 🔲
    A77.9   Spotted fever, unspecified 🔲
        Tick-borne typhus NOS

● **A78   Q fever** 🔲
    Infection due to Coxiella burnetii
    Nine Mile fever
    Quadrilateral fever
    (Ex) See PDX Collection 108

N Newborn Age: 0   **P** Pediatric Age: 0–17   **M** Maternity DX: 12–55   **A** Adult Age: 15–124   ♀ Females Only   ♂ Males Only

🔲 Complication\Comorbidity   🔲 Major C\C   (Ex) CC/MCC Exclusions   🔲 Hospital-Acquired Condition

649

CHAPTER 1 (A00-B99)

● **A79 Other rickettsioses**
(Ex) For category A79 CC codes unless otherwise indicated: See PDX Collection 129

  A79.0 Trench fever 🔲
    Quintan fever
    Wolhynian fever
    (Ex) See PDX Collection 108

  A79.1 Rickettsialpox due to Rickettsia akari 🔲
    Kew Garden fever
    Vesicular rickettsiosis

● **A79.8 Other specified rickettsioses**
    A79.81 Rickettsiosis due to Ehrlichia sennetsu 🔲
    A79.89 Other specified rickettsioses 🔲

  A79.9 Rickettsiosis, unspecified 🔲
    Rickettsial infection NOS

VIRAL AND PRION INFECTIONS OF THE CENTRAL NERVOUS SYSTEM (A80-A89)

Excludes1 postpolio syndrome (G14)
          sequelae of poliomyelitis (B91)
          sequelae of viral encephalitis (B94.1)

● **A80 Acute poliomyelitis**
(Ex) For category A80 CC codes: See PDX Collection 130

  A80.0 Acute paralytic poliomyelitis, vaccine-associated 🔲
  A80.1 Acute paralytic poliomyelitis, wild virus, imported 🔲
  A80.2 Acute paralytic poliomyelitis, wild virus, indigenous 🔲
● **A80.3 Acute paralytic poliomyelitis, other and unspecified**
    A80.30 Acute paralytic poliomyelitis, unspecified 🔲
    A80.39 Other acute paralytic poliomyelitis 🔲
  A80.4 Acute nonparalytic poliomyelitis
  A80.9 Acute poliomyelitis, unspecified

● **A81 Atypical virus infections of central nervous system**
Includes diseases of the central nervous system caused by prions
Use additional code to identify:
  dementia with behavioral disturbance (F02.81)
  dementia without behavioral disturbance (F02.80)

● **A81.0 Creutzfeldt-Jakob disease**
(Ex) For category A81.0 CC codes: See PDX Collection 131

  A81.00 Creutzfeldt-Jakob disease, unspecified 🔲
    Jakob-Creutzfeldt disease, unspecified

  A81.01 Variant Creutzfeldt-Jakob disease 🔲
    vCJD

  A81.09 Other Creutzfeldt-Jakob disease 🔲
    CJD
    Familial Creutzfeldt-Jakob disease
    Iatrogenic Creutzfeldt-Jakob disease
    Sporadic Creutzfeldt-Jakob disease
    Subacute spongiform encephalopathy (with dementia)

  A81.1 Subacute sclerosing panencephalitis 🔲
    Type of viral encephalitis that causes parenchymatous lesions in gray and white matter of brain
    Dawson's inclusion body encephalitis
    Van Bogaert's sclerosing leukoencephalopathy
    (Ex) See PDX Collection 132

  A81.2 Progressive multifocal leukoencephalopathy 🔲
    Group of diseases affecting white matter of brain
    Multifocal leukoencephalopathy NOS
    (Ex) See PDX Collection 133

● **A81.8 Other atypical virus infections of central nervous system**
(Ex) For category A81.8 CC codes unless otherwise indicated: See PDX Collection 135

  A81.81 Kuru 🔲
    (Ex) See PDX Collection 134
  A81.82 Gerstmann-Sträussler-Scheinker syndrome 🔲
    GSS syndrome
  A81.83 Fatal familial insomnia 🔲
    FFI
  A81.89 Other atypical virus infections of central nervous system 🔲

  A81.9 Atypical virus infection of central nervous system, unspecified 🔲
    Prion diseases of the central nervous system NOS
    (Ex) See PDX Collection 134

● **A82 Rabies**
Viral disease affecting the central nervous system and transmitted from infected mammals to man.
(Ex) For category A82 CC codes: See PDX Collection 136

  A82.0 Sylvatic rabies 🔲
  A82.1 Urban rabies 🔲
  A82.9 Rabies, unspecified 🔲

● **A83 Mosquito-borne viral encephalitis**
Inflammation of the brain caused most commonly by Herpes Simplex virus.
Includes mosquito-borne viral meningoencephalitis
Excludes2 Venezuelan equine encephalitis (A92.2)
          West Nile fever (A92.3-)
          West Nile virus (A92.3-)
(Ex) For category A83 CC codes: See PDX Collection 137

  A83.0 Japanese encephalitis 🔲
  A83.1 Western equine encephalitis 🔲
  A83.2 Eastern equine encephalitis 🔲
  A83.3 St. Louis encephalitis 🔲
  A83.4 Australian encephalitis 🔲
    Kunjin virus disease
  A83.5 California encephalitis 🔲
    California meningoencephalitis
    La Crosse encephalitis
  A83.6 Rocio virus disease 🔲
    Mosquito-borne virus
  A83.8 Other mosquito-borne viral encephalitis 🔲
  A83.9 Mosquito-borne viral encephalitis, unspecified 🔲

● **A84 Tick-borne viral encephalitis**
Includes tick-borne viral meningoencephalitis
(Ex) For category A84 CC codes: See PDX Collection 137

  A84.0 Far Eastern tick-borne encephalitis [Russian spring-summer encephalitis] 🔲
  A84.1 Central European tick-borne encephalitis 🔲
  A84.8 Other tick-borne viral encephalitis 🔲
    Louping ill
    Powassan virus disease
  A84.9 Tick-borne viral encephalitis, unspecified 🔲

Item 1-13 Acute Poliomyelitis: Also called infantile paralysis and is caused by the poliovirus, which enters the body orally and infects the intestinal wall and then enters the blood stream and central nervous system, causing muscle weakness and paralysis. This disease has been nearly eradicated with the polio vaccine.

▶ New   ⇒ Revised   ~~deleted~~ Deleted   Excludes 1   Excludes 2   Includes   Use additional   Code first   Code also   Key words
OGCR Official Guidelines   ● Unacceptable Principal Diagnosis   X Assign placeholder X   ● Use Additional Character(s)   ▶ Manifestation Code   **Coding Clinic**

Item 1-14 Encephalitis is an inflammation of the brain most often caused by a virus but may also be caused by a bacteria and most commonly transmitted by a mosquito. **Myelitis** is an inflammation of the spinal cord that may disrupt CNS function. Untreated myelitis may rapidly lead to permanent damage to the spinal cord. **Encephalomyelitis** is a general term for an inflammation of the brain and spinal cord.

● **A85   Other viral encephalitis, not elsewhere classified**

> **Includes**   specified viral encephalomyelitis NEC
> specified viral meningoencephalitis NEC
>
> **Excludes1**   benign myalgic encephalomyelitis (G93.3)
> encephalitis due to cytomegalovirus (B25.8)
> encephalitis due to herpesvirus NEC (B10.0-)
> encephalitis due to herpesvirus [herpes simplex]
>   (B00.4)
> encephalitis due to measles virus (B05.0)
> encephalitis due to mumps virus (B26.2)
> encephalitis due to poliomyelitis virus (A80.-)
> encephalitis due to zoster (B02.0)
> lymphocytic choriomeningitis (A87.2)

> (Ex) **For category A85 CC codes unless otherwise indicated:** See PDX Collection 138

     A85.0   Enteroviral encephalitis 🔵
         Enteroviral encephalomyelitis

     A85.1   Adenoviral encephalitis 🔵
         Adenoviral meningoencephalitis

     A85.2   Arthropod-borne viral encephalitis, unspecified 🔵

> **Excludes1**   West nile virus with encephalitis (A92.31)
> (Ex) See PDX Collection 137

     A85.8   Other specified viral encephalitis 🔵
         Encephalitis lethargica
         Von Economo-Cruchet disease

● **A86   Unspecified viral encephalitis** 🔵
     Viral encephalomyelitis NOS
     Viral meningoencephalitis NOS
     (Ex) See PDX Collection 139

● **A87   Viral meningitis**

> **Excludes1**   meningitis due to herpesvirus [herpes simplex]
>   (B00.3)
> meningitis due to measles virus (B05.1)
> meningitis due to mumps virus (B26.1)
> meningitis due to poliomyelitis virus (A80.-)
> meningitis due to zoster (B02.1)

> (Ex) **For category A87 CC codes unless otherwise indicated:** See PDX Collection 140

     A87.0   Enteroviral meningitis 🔵
         Group of common viruses responsible for the majority of viral
           meningitis
         Coxsackievirus meningitis
         Echovirus meningitis

     A87.1   Adenoviral meningitis 🔵

     A87.2   Lymphocytic choriomeningitis 🔵
         Lymphocytic meningoencephalitis
         (Ex) See PDX Collection 141

     A87.8   Other viral meningitis 🔵

     A87.9   Viral meningitis, unspecified 🔵

● **A88   Other viral infections of central nervous system, not elsewhere classified**

> **Excludes1**   viral encephalitis NOS (A86)
> viral meningitis NOS (A87.9)

     A88.0   Enteroviral exanthematous fever [Boston exanthem] 🔵
         Infectious skin eruption
         (Ex) See PDX Collection 137

     A88.1   Epidemic vertigo

     A88.8   Other specified viral infections of central nervous system 🔵
         (Ex) See PDX Collection 138

  A89   Unspecified viral infection of central nervous system 🔵
     (Ex) See PDX Collection 139

OGCR   Section I. C.1.f.

Certain Infectious and Parasitic Diseases (A00-B99)

Zika virus infections

Code only confirmed cases

Code only a confirmed diagnosis of Zika virus (A92.5, Zika virus disease) as documented by the provider. This is an exception to the hospital inpatient guideline Section II, H.

In this context, "confirmation" does not require documentation of the type of test performed; the physician's diagnostic statement that the condition is confirmed is sufficient. This code should be assigned regardless of the stated mode of transmission.

If the provider documents "suspected", "possible" or "probable" Zika, do not assign code A92.5. Assign a code(s) explaining the reason for encounter (such as fever, rash, or joint pain) or Z20.828, Contact with and (suspected) exposure to other viral communicable diseases.

ARTHROPOD-BORNE VIRAL FEVERS AND VIRAL HEMORRHAGIC FEVERS (A90-A99)

  A90   Dengue fever [classical dengue] 🔵
     Acute, self-limited disease, characterized by fever, prostration, severe
       muscle pains, headache, rash, lymphadenopathy, and leukopenia,
       caused by dengue virus; AKA breakbone, dandy

> **Excludes1**   dengue hemorrhagic fever (A91)
> (Ex) See PDX Collection 142
> **Coding Clinic: 2016, Q3, P13**

  A91   Dengue hemorrhagic fever 🔵
     Serious follow-up to regular dengue, with symptoms of hemorrhage
     (Ex) See PDX Collection 143

● **A92   Other mosquito-borne viral fevers**

> **Excludes1**   Ross River disease (B33.1)

     A92.0   Chikungunya virus disease 🔵
         Transmitted by mosquitoes
         Chikungunya (hemorrhagic) fever
         (Ex) See PDX Collection 143

     A92.1   O'nyong-nyong fever 🔵
         Acute, nonfatal febrile disease transmitted by mosquitoes,
           which clinically resembles dengue and chikungunya
         (Ex) See PDX Collection 144

     A92.2   Venezuelan equine fever 🔵
         Venezuelan equine encephalitis
         Venezuelan equine encephalomyelitis virus disease
         (Ex) See PDX Collection 144

● **A92.3   West Nile virus infection**
         West Nile fever
         (Ex) **For category A92.3 CC codes:** See PDX Collection 145

       A92.30   West Nile virus infection, unspecified 🔵
           West Nile fever NOS
           West Nile fever without complications
           West Nile virus NOS

       A92.31   West Nile virus infection with encephalitis 🔵
           West Nile encephalitis
           West Nile encephalomyelitis
           Coding Clinic: 2016, Q3, P13

       A92.32   West Nile virus infection with other neurologic manifestation 🔵
           Use additional code to specify the neurologic manifestation

       A92.39   West Nile virus infection with other complications 🔵
           Use additional code to specify the other conditions

     A92.4   Rift Valley fever 🔵
         (Ex) See PDX Collection 144

     A92.5   Zika virus disease 🔵
         Zika virus fever
         Zika virus infection
         Zika NOS
         (Ex) See PDX Collection 144
         Coding Clinic: 2016, Q4, P4-7, 121

     A92.8   Other specified mosquito-borne viral fevers 🔵
         (Ex) See PDX Collection 144

     A92.9   Mosquito-borne viral fever, unspecified 🔵
         (Ex) See PDX Collection 143

CHAPTER 1 (A00-B99)

CHAPTER 1 (A00-B99)

● **A93** Other arthropod-borne viral fevers, not elsewhere classified

    A93.0 Oropouche virus disease 🔖
        Tropical viral infection
        Oropouche fever
        Ⓔⓧ See PDX Collection 144

    A93.1 Sandfly fever 🔖
        Pappataci fever
        Phlebotomus fever
        Ⓔⓧ See PDX Collection 143

    A93.2 Colorado tick fever 🔖
        Ⓔⓧ See PDX Collection 143

    A93.8 Other specified arthropod-borne viral fevers 🔖
        Piry virus disease
        Vesicular stomatitis virus disease [Indiana fever]
        Ⓔⓧ See PDX Collection 143

● **A94** Unspecified arthropod-borne viral fever 🔖
    Arboviral fever NOS
    Arbovirus infection NOS
    Ⓔⓧ See PDX Collection 143

● **A95** Yellow fever
    Acute infectious disease transmitted by mosquitoes
    Ⓔⓧ For category A95 CC codes: See PDX Collection 146

    A95.0 Sylvatic yellow fever 🔖
        Jungle yellow fever

    A95.1 Urban yellow fever 🔖

    A95.9 Yellow fever, unspecified 🔖

● **A96** Arenaviral hemorrhagic fever
    Virus that causes various hemorrhagic fevers
    Ⓔⓧ For category A96 CC codes: See PDX Collection 147

    A96.0 Junin hemorrhagic fever 🔖
        Argentinian hemorrhagic fever

    A96.1 Machupo hemorrhagic fever 🔖
        Transmitted by contact with infected rodents
        Bolivian hemorrhagic fever

    A96.2 Lassa fever
        Acute type of hemorrhagic fever caused by contact with
        disease carrying mouse or person

    A96.8 Other arenaviral hemorrhagic fevers 🔖

    A96.9 Arenaviral hemorrhagic fever, unspecified 🔖

● **A98** Other viral hemorrhagic fevers, not elsewhere classified
    <u>Excludes1</u> chikungunya hemorrhagic fever (A92.0)
                   dengue hemorrhagic fever (A91)
    Ⓔⓧ For category A98 CC codes unless otherwise indicated: See PDX Collection 143

    A98.0 Crimean-Congo hemorrhagic fever 🔖
        Virus transmitted by ticks and contact with blood, secretions,
        or fluids from infected humans or animals
        Central Asian hemorrhagic fever

    A98.1 Omsk hemorrhagic fever 🔖
        Transmitted to humans by bites of infected ticks or contact
        with infected muskrats

    A98.2 Kyasanur Forest disease 🔖
        Transmitted via infected monkeys, voles, ticks

    A98.3 Marburg virus disease
        Rare, acute, often fatal type of hemorrhagic fever

    A98.4 Ebola virus disease

    A98.5 Hemorrhagic fever with renal syndrome 🔖
        Epidemic hemorrhagic fever
        Korean hemorrhagic fever
        Russian hemorrhagic fever
        Hantaan virus disease
        Hantavirus disease with renal manifestations
        Nephropathia epidemica
        Songo fever
        <u>Excludes1</u> hantavirus (cardio)-pulmonary syndrome
                      (B33.4)
        Ⓔⓧ See PDX Collection 148

    A98.8 Other specified viral hemorrhagic fevers 🔖

● **A99** Unspecified viral hemorrhagic fever 🔖
    Ⓔⓧ See PDX Collection 143

Figure 1-4 Primary herpes simplex in and around the mouth. The infection is usually acquired from siblings or parents and is readily transmitted to other direct contacts. (Getty Image)

Item 1–15 **Herpes** is a viral disease for which there is no cure. There are two types of the herpes simplex virus: **Type I** causes **cold sores** or **fever blisters,** and **Type II** causes **genital herpes.** The virus can be spread from a sore on the lips to the genitals or from the genitals to the lips.

VIRAL INFECTIONS CHARACTERIZED BY SKIN AND MUCOUS MEMBRANE LESIONS (B00-B09)

● **B00** Herpesviral [herpes simplex] infections
    <u>Excludes1</u> congenital herpesviral infections (P35.2)
    <u>Excludes2</u> anogenital herpesviral infection (A60.-)
                   gammaherpesviral mononucleosis (B27.0-)
                   herpangina (B08.5)

    B00.0 Eczema herpeticum
        Cutaneous eruption caused by herpes simplex virus (HSV)
        type 1, HSV-2, coxsackievirus A16, or vaccinia virus
        Kaposi's varicelliform eruption

    B00.1 Herpesviral vesicular dermatitis
        Vesicle formation; characteristics include formation of blisters
        and scabs on feet and legs
        Herpes simplex facialis
        Herpes simplex labialis
        Herpes simplex otitis externa
        Vesicular dermatitis of ear
        Vesicular dermatitis of lip

    B00.2 Herpesviral gingivostomatitis and pharyngotonsillitis 🔖
        Inflammation involving both gingivae and oral mucosa
        Herpesviral pharyngitis
        Inflammation of pharynx and tonsils; AKA
        tonsillopharyngitis
        Ⓔⓧ See PDX Collection 149

    B00.3 Herpesviral meningitis 🔖
        Ⓔⓧ See PDX Collection 150

    B00.4 Herpesviral encephalitis 🔖
        Herpesviral meningoencephalitis
        Simian B disease
        <u>Excludes1</u> herpesviral encephalitis due to herpesvirus 6
                     and 7 (B10.01, B10.09)
                     non-simplex herpesviral encephalitis
                     (B10.0-)
        Ⓔⓧ See PDX Collection 151

●   **B00.5** Herpesviral ocular disease
        Ⓔⓧ For category B00.5 CC codes: See PDX Collection 152

        B00.50 Herpesviral ocular disease, unspecified 🔖

        B00.51 Herpesviral iridocyclitis 🔖
             Herpesviral iritis
             Herpesviral uveitis, anterior

        B00.52 Herpesviral keratitis 🔖
             Herpesviral keratoconjunctivitis

        B00.53 Herpesviral conjunctivitis 🔖

        B00.59 Other herpesviral disease of eye 🔖
             Herpesviral dermatitis of eyelid

    B00.7 Disseminated herpesviral disease 🔖
        Herpesviral sepsis
        Ⓔⓧ See PDX Collection 153

▶ New   ⇒ Revised   ~~deleted~~ Deleted   Excludes 1   Excludes 2   Includes   Use additional   Code first   Code also   Key words

OGCR Official Guidelines   ● Unacceptable Principal Diagnosis   X Assign placeholder X   🔖 Use Additional Character(s)   ▌Manifestation Code   **Coding Clinic**

● B00.8 **Other forms of herpesviral infections**

B00.81 **Herpesviral hepatitis**
Ⓔ See PDX Collection 154

B00.82 **Herpes simplex myelitis**
Ⓔ See PDX Collection 155

B00.89 **Other herpesviral infection**
Herpesviral whitlow
Ⓔ See PDX Collection 156

B00.9 **Herpesviral infection, unspecified**
Herpes simplex infection NOS

● B01 **Varicella [chickenpox]**
Very contagious disease caused by the varicella zoster virus that results in an itchy outbreak of skin blisters (varicella). The same virus causes shingles (zoster).

B01.0 **Varicella meningitis**
Ⓔ See PDX Collection 157

● B01.1 **Varicella encephalitis, myelitis and encephalomyelitis**
Postchickenpox encephalitis, myelitis and encephalomyelitis

B01.11 **Varicella encephalitis and encephalomyelitis**
Postchickenpox encephalitis and encephalomyelitis
Ⓔ See PDX Collection 158

B01.12 **Varicella myelitis**
Postchickenpox myelitis
Ⓔ See PDX Collection 159

B01.2 **Varicella pneumonia**
Ⓔ See PDX Collection 160

● B01.8 **Varicella with other complications**
Ⓔ For category B01.8 CC codes: See PDX Collection 157

B01.81 **Varicella keratitis**

B01.89 **Other varicella complications**

B01.9 **Varicella without complication**
Varicella NOS
Ⓔ See PDX Collection 157

● B02 **Zoster [herpes zoster]**

Includes	shingles
	zona

B02.0 **Zoster encephalitis**
Zoster meningoencephalitis
Ⓔ See PDX Collection 161

B02.1 **Zoster meningitis**
Ⓔ See PDX Collection 162

● B02.2 **Zoster with other nervous system involvement**
Ⓔ For category B02.2 CC codes unless otherwise indicated: See PDX Collection 161

B02.21 **Postherpetic geniculate ganglionitis**

B02.22 **Postherpetic trigeminal neuralgia**

B02.23 **Postherpetic polyneuropathy**

B02.24 **Postherpetic myelitis**
Herpes zoster myelitis
Ⓔ See PDX Collection 163

B02.29 **Other postherpetic nervous system involvement**
Postherpetic radiculopathy

Figure 1-5 Photograph of eyelids with marginal blepharitis. (From Hoyt CS, Taylor D: Pediatric Ophthalmology and Strabismus, London, Elsevier Saunders, 2005)

Item 1-17 Blepharitis is a common condition in which the eyelid is swollen and yellow scaling and conjunctivitis develop. Usually the hair on the scalp and brow is involved.

● B02.3 **Zoster ocular disease**
Ⓔ For category B02.3 CC codes: See PDX Collection 164

B02.30 **Zoster ocular disease, unspecified**

B02.31 **Zoster conjunctivitis**

B02.32 **Zoster iridocyclitis**

B02.33 **Zoster keratitis**
Herpes zoster keratoconjunctivitis

B02.34 **Zoster scleritis**

B02.39 **Other herpes zoster eye disease**
Zoster blepharitis

B02.7 **Disseminated zoster**
Ⓔ See PDX Collection 165

B02.8 **Zoster with other complications**
Herpes zoster otitis externa
Ⓔ See PDX Collection 165

B02.9 **Zoster without complications**
Zoster NOS

● B03 **Smallpox**
Note: In 1980 the 33rd World Health Assembly declared that smallpox had been eradicated. The classification is maintained for surveillance purposes.
Ⓔ See PDX Collection 166

● B04 **Monkeypox**
Disease occurring in captive monkeys and other mammals that may be transmitted to humans, clinically similar to smallpox
Ⓔ See PDX Collection 167

● B05 **Measles**

Includes	morbilli
Excludes1	subacute sclerosing panencephalitis (A81.1)

B05.0 **Measles complicated by encephalitis**
Postmeasles encephalitis
Ⓔ See PDX Collection 168

B05.1 **Measles complicated by meningitis**
Postmeasles meningitis
Ⓔ See PDX Collection 169

B05.2 **Measles complicated by pneumonia**
Postmeasles pneumonia
Ⓔ See PDX Collection 170

B05.3 **Measles complicated by otitis media**
Postmeasles otitis media

B05.4 **Measles with intestinal complications**
Ⓔ See PDX Collection 169

● B05.8 **Measles with other complications**

B05.81 **Measles keratitis and keratoconjunctivitis**
Ⓔ See PDX Collection 171

B05.89 **Other measles complications**
Ⓔ See PDX Collection 169

B05.9 **Measles without complication**
Measles NOS

CHAPTER 1 (A00-B99)

Item 1-16 Zoster: Also known as *shingles* and is caused by the same virus as chickenpox. After exposure, the virus lies dormant in nerve tissue and is activated by factors including aging, stress, suppression of the immune system, and certain medication. It begins as a unilateral rash that leads to blisters and sores on the skin. It may involve the nerve pathways of the eye, forehead, nose, and eyelids and may be very painful with long-term systemic effects.

N Newborn Age: 0   P Pediatric Age: 0–17   M Maternity DX: 12–55   A Adult Age: 15–124   ♀ Females Only   ♂ Males Only

Ⓒ Complication\Comorbidity   Ⓜ Major C\C   Ⓔ CC/MCC Exclusions   Ⓗ Hospital-Acquired Condition

● **B06**   **Rubella [German measles]**
    Excludes1   congenital rubella (P35.0)
 ● **B06.0**   **Rubella with neurological complications**
     Ⓔⓧ **For category B06.0 CC codes:** See PDX Collection 172
     B06.00   **Rubella with neurological complication, unspecified** 🔑
     B06.01   **Rubella encephalitis** 🔑
            Rubella meningoencephalitis
     B06.02   **Rubella meningitis** 🔑
     B06.09   **Other neurological complications of rubella** 🔑
 ● **B06.8**   **Rubella with other complications**
     B06.81   **Rubella pneumonia** 🔑
         Ⓔⓧ See PDX Collection 172
     B06.82   **Rubella arthritis** 🔑
         Ⓔⓧ See PDX Collection 173
     B06.89   **Other rubella complications** 🔑
         Ⓔⓧ See PDX Collection 172
   B06.9   **Rubella without complication**
        Rubella NOS

● **B07**   **Viral warts**
    Includes   verruca simplex
              verruca vulgaris
              viral warts due to human papillomavirus
    Excludes2   anogenital (venereal) warts (A63.0)
              papilloma of bladder (D41.4)
              papilloma of cervix (D26.0)
              papilloma larynx (D14.1)
   B07.0   **Plantar wart**
        Verruca plantaris
   B07.8   **Other viral warts**
        Common wart
        Flat wart
        Verruca plana
   B07.9   **Viral wart, unspecified**

● **B08**   **Other viral infections characterized by skin and mucous membrane lesions, not elsewhere classified**
    Excludes1   vesicular stomatitis virus disease (A93.8)
 ● **B08.0**   **Other orthopoxvirus infections**
     Excludes2   monkeypox (B04)
   ● **B08.01**   **Cowpox and vaccinia not from vaccine**
       B08.010   **Cowpox**
       B08.011   **Vaccinia not from vaccine**
         Excludes1   vaccinia (from vaccination) (generalized) (T88.1)
     B08.02   **Orf virus disease**
         Contagious pustular dermatitis
         Ecthyma contagiosum
     B08.03   **Pseudocowpox [milker's node]**
     B08.04   **Paravaccinia, unspecified**
     B08.09   **Other orthopoxvirus infections**
         Orthopoxvirus infection NOS
   B08.1   **Molluscum contagiosum**
        Various skin diseases characterized by soft, rounded, cutaneous lesions
 ● **B08.2**   **Exanthema subitum [sixth disease] Roseola infantum**
        Acute, short-lived high fever in infants and young children followed by a rash mainly on the trunk, caused by human herpesvirus 6
     B08.20   **Exanthema subitum [sixth disease], unspecified Roseola infantum, unspecified**   P
     B08.21   **Exanthema subitum [sixth disease] due to human herpesvirus 6 Roseola infantum due to human herpesvirus 6**   P
         Virus results in sudden rash; infection results in lifelong persistence
     B08.22   **Exanthema subitum [sixth disease] due to human herpesvirus 7 Roseola infantum due to human herpesvirus 7**   P

   B08.3   **Erythema infectiosum [fifth disease]** 🔑
        Moderately contagious, epidemic disease in children caused by B19 virus; onset of rash that begins as redness of cheeks, later there is rash on trunk and limbs; when this fades, there may be central clearing that leaves lacelike pattern
        Ⓔⓧ See PDX Collection 174
   B08.4   **Enteroviral vesicular stomatitis with exanthem**
        Hand, foot and mouth disease
        Check your documentation—this code is HAND, foot, and mouth disease. Code B08.8 is foot and mouth disease.
   B08.5   **Enteroviral vesicular pharyngitis**
        Herpangina
 ● **B08.6**   **Parapoxvirus infections**
     B08.60   **Parapoxvirus infection, unspecified**
     B08.61   **Bovine stomatitis**
     B08.62   **Sealpox**
     B08.69   **Other parapoxvirus infections**
 ● **B08.7**   **Yatapoxvirus infections**
     B08.70   **Yatapoxvirus infection, unspecified**
     B08.71   **Tanapox virus disease** 🔑
         Ⓔⓧ See PDX Collection 167
     B08.72   **Yaba pox virus disease**
         Yaba monkey tumor disease
     B08.79   **Other yatapoxvirus infections**
   B08.8   **Other specified viral infections characterized by skin and mucous membrane lesions**
        Enteroviral lymphonodular pharyngitis
        Foot-and-mouth disease
        Check your documentation. Code B08.4 is for HAND, foot, and mouth disease.
        Poxvirus NEC

● **B09**   **Unspecified viral infection characterized by skin and mucous membrane lesions**
        Viral enanthema NOS
        Viral exanthema NOS

OTHER HUMAN HERPESVIRUSES (B10)

● **B10**   **Other human herpesviruses**
    Excludes2   cytomegalovirus (B25.9)
            Epstein-Barr virus (B27.0-)
            herpes NOS (B00.9)
            herpes simplex (B00.-)
            herpes zoster (B02.-)
            human herpesvirus NOS (B00.-)
            human herpesvirus 1 and 2 (B00.-)
            human herpesvirus 3 (B01.-, B02.-)
            human herpesvirus 4 (B27.0-)
            human herpesvirus 5 (B25.-)
            varicella (B01.-)
            zoster (B02.-)
 ● **B10.0**   **Other human herpesvirus encephalitis**
     Excludes2   herpes encephalitis NOS (B00.4)
            herpes simplex encephalitis (B00.4)
            human herpesvirus encephalitis (B00.4)
            simian B herpes virus encephalitis (B00.4)
     Ⓔⓧ **For category B10.0 CC codes:** See PDX Collection 151
     B10.01   **Human herpesvirus 6 encephalitis** 🔑
         Sudden rash or roseola
     B10.09   **Other human herpesvirus encephalitis** 🔑
         Human herpesvirus 7 encephalitis
         Virus closely related to human herpesvirus 6, but not known to cause any disease

▶ New   ⇒ Revised   ~~deleted~~ Deleted   Excludes 1   Excludes 2   Includes   Use additional   Code first   Code also   Key words
OGCR Official Guidelines   ● Unacceptable Principal Diagnosis   X Assign placeholder X   ● Use Additional Character(s)   ▶ Manifestation Code   **Coding Clinic**

Figure 1-6 Hepatitis B viral infection. **A.** Liver parenchyma showing hepatocytes with diffuse granular cytoplasm, so-called ground glass hepatocytes (H&E). **B.** Immunoperoxidase stains from the same case, showing cytoplasmic inclusions of viral particles. (From Kumar: Robbins and Cotran: Pathologic Basis of Disease, ed 8, Saunders, An Imprint of Elsevier, 2009)

Item 1–18   Hepatitis A (HAV) was formerly called epidemic, infectious, short-incubation, or acute catarrhal jaundice hepatitis. The primary transmission mode is the oral–fecal route. **Hepatitis B (HBV)** was formerly called long-incubation period, serum, or homologous serum hepatitis. Transmission modes are through blood from infected persons and from body fluids of infected mother to neonate. **Hepatitis C (HCV)**, caused by the hepatitis C virus, is primarily transfusion associated. **Hepatitis D (HDV)**, also called delta hepatitis, is caused by the hepatitis D virus in patients formerly or currently infected with hepatitis B. **Hepatitis E (HEV)** is also called enterically transmitted non-A, non-B hepatitis. The primary transmission mode is the oral–fecal route, usually through contaminated water.

- **B10.8   Other human herpesvirus infection**
  - **B10.81   Human herpesvirus 6 infection**
    Causative agent of exanthema subitum that results in sudden rash
  - **B10.82   Human herpesvirus 7 infection**
    Closely related to human herpesvirus 6, but not known cause any disease
  - **B10.89   Other human herpesvirus infection**
    Human herpesvirus 8 infection
    May be the cause of Kaposi sarcoma, a malignant tumor
    Kaposi's sarcoma-associated herpesvirus infection

VIRAL HEPATITIS (B15-B19)

Excludes1	sequelae of viral hepatitis (B94.2)
Excludes2	cytomegaloviral hepatitis (B25.1)
	herpesviral [herpes simplex] hepatitis (B00.81)

- **B15   Acute hepatitis A**
  - (Ex) **For category B15 CC codes:** See PDX Collection 175
  - **B15.0   Hepatitis A with hepatic coma**
  - **B15.9   Hepatitis A without hepatic coma**
    Hepatitis A (acute) (viral) NOS

- **B16   Acute hepatitis B**
  - (Ex) **For category B16 CC codes:** See PDX Collection 175
  - **B16.0   Acute hepatitis B with delta-agent with hepatic coma**
  - **B16.1   Acute hepatitis B with delta-agent without hepatic coma**
  - **B16.2   Acute hepatitis B without delta-agent with hepatic coma**
  - **B16.9   Acute hepatitis B without delta-agent and without hepatic coma**
    Hepatitis B (acute) (viral) NOS
    Coding Clinic: 2016, Q3, P13

Figure 1-7 Kaposi's sarcoma. There are large confluent hyperpigmented patch-stage lesions with lymphedema. (From Kanski, JJ: Clinical Diagnosis in Ophthalmology, London, Elsevier Mosby, 2006)

Item 1–19   AIDS (acquired immune deficiency syndrome) is caused by **HIV** (human immunodeficiency virus). HIV affects certain white blood cells (T-4 lymphocytes) and destroys the ability of the cells to fight infections, making patients susceptible to a host of infectious diseases (e.g., **Pneumocystis carinii pneumonia (PCP), Kaposi's sarcoma,** and **lymphoma). AIDS-related complex (ARC)** is an early stage of AIDS in which tests for HIV are positive but the symptoms are mild.

- **B17   Other acute viral hepatitis**
  - (Ex) **For category B17 CC codes:** See PDX Collection 175
  - **B17.0   Acute delta-(super) infection of hepatitis B carrier**
  - **B17.1   Acute hepatitis C**
    - **B17.10   Acute hepatitis C without hepatic coma**
      Acute hepatitis C NOS
    - **B17.11   Acute hepatitis C with hepatic coma**
  - **B17.2   Acute hepatitis E**
  - **B17.8   Other specified acute viral hepatitis**
    Hepatitis non-A non-B (acute) (viral) NEC
  - **B17.9   Acute viral hepatitis, unspecified**
    Acute hepatitis NOS
    Acute infectious hepatitis NOS

- **B18   Chronic viral hepatitis**
  - **Includes**   Carrier of viral hepatitis
  - (Ex) **For category B18 CC codes:** See PDX Collection 175
  - **B18.0   Chronic viral hepatitis B with delta-agent**
  - **B18.1   Chronic viral hepatitis B without delta-agent**
    Carrier of viral hepatitis B
    Chronic (viral) hepatitis B
  - **B18.2   Chronic viral hepatitis C**
    Carrier of viral hepatitis C
    Coding Clinic: 2017, Q1, P41
  - **B18.8   Other chronic viral hepatitis**
    Carrier of other viral hepatitis
  - **B18.9   Chronic viral hepatitis, unspecified**
    Carrier of unspecified viral hepatitis

- **B19   Unspecified viral hepatitis**
  - (Ex) **For category B19 CC codes:** See PDX Collection 175
  - **B19.0   Unspecified viral hepatitis with hepatic coma**
  - **B19.1   Unspecified viral hepatitis B**
    - **B19.10   Unspecified viral hepatitis B without hepatic coma**
      Unspecified viral hepatitis B NOS
    - **B19.11   Unspecified viral hepatitis B with hepatic coma**
  - **B19.2   Unspecified viral hepatitis C**
    - **B19.20   Unspecified viral hepatitis C without hepatic coma**
      Viral hepatitis C NOS
    - **B19.21   Unspecified viral hepatitis C with hepatic coma**
  - **B19.9   Unspecified viral hepatitis without hepatic coma**
    Viral hepatitis NOS

CHAPTER 1 (A00-B99)

N Newborn Age: 0   **P** Pediatric Age: 0–17   **M** Maternity DX: 12–55   **A** Adult Age: 15–124   ♀ Females Only   ♂ Males Only

🔖 Complication\Comorbidity   🔖 Major C\C   (Ex) CC/MCC Exclusions   🔖 Hospital-Acquired Condition

CHAPTER 1 (A00–B99)

OGCR Section I. C.1.a.

Certain Infectious and Parasitic Diseases (A00–B99)

a. Human Immunodeficiency Virus (HIV) Infections

  1) Code only confirmed cases

    Code only confirmed cases of HIV infection illness. This is an exception to the hospital inpatient guideline Section II, H.

    In this context, "confirmation" does not require documentation of positive serology or culture for HIV; the provider's diagnostic statement that the patient is HIV positive, or has an HIV-related illness is sufficient.

HUMAN IMMUNODEFICIENCY VIRUS [HIV] DISEASE (B20)

B20   **Human immunodeficiency virus [HIV] disease** 🔖

    Includes   acquired immune deficiency syndrome [AIDS]
                     AIDS-related complex [ARC]
                     HIV infection, symptomatic

    Code first Human immunodeficiency virus [HIV] disease complicating pregnancy, childbirth and the puerperium, if applicable (O98.7-)

    Use additional code(s) to identify all manifestations of HIV infection

    Excludes1   asymptomatic human immunodeficiency virus [HIV] infection status (Z21)
                   exposure to HIV virus (Z20.6)
                   inconclusive serologic evidence of HIV (R75)

    Ⓔⓧ See PDX Collection 176

OTHER VIRAL DISEASES (B25–B34)

● **B25**   **Cytomegaloviral disease**
    AKA: HCMV or Human Herpesvirus 5 (HHV-5)

    Excludes1   congenital cytomegalovirus infection (P35.1)
                   cytomegaloviral mononucleosis (B27.1-)

    B25.0   **Cytomegaloviral pneumonitis** 🔖
          MCC when PDx is its own MCC
          Ⓔⓧ See PDX Collection 110

    B25.1   **Cytomegaloviral hepatitis** 🔖
          CC when PDx is its own CC
          Ⓔⓧ No exclusions

    B25.2   **Cytomegaloviral pancreatitis** 🔖
          MCC when PDx is its own MCC
          Ⓔⓧ See PDX Collection 177

    B25.8   **Other cytomegaloviral diseases** 🔖
          Cytomegaloviral encephalitis
          Ⓔⓧ See PDX Collection 178

    B25.9   **Cytomegaloviral disease, unspecified** 🔖
          Ⓔⓧ See PDX Collection 178

● **B26**   **Mumps**

    Includes   epidemic parotitis
                 infectious parotitis
    Acute, contagious, viral disease

    B26.0   **Mumps orchitis** ♂ 🔖
          Ⓔⓧ See PDX Collection 179

    B26.1   **Mumps meningitis** 🔖
          Ⓔⓧ See PDX Collection 180

    B26.2   **Mumps encephalitis** 🔖
          Ⓔⓧ See PDX Collection 181

    B26.3   **Mumps pancreatitis** 🔖
          Ⓔⓧ See PDX Collection 182

● **B26.8**   **Mumps with other complications**
    Ⓔⓧ **For category B26.8 CC codes unless otherwise indicated:** See PDX Collection 184

    B26.81   **Mumps hepatitis** 🔖
          Ⓔⓧ See PDX Collection 183

    B26.82   **Mumps myocarditis** 🔖

    B26.83   **Mumps nephritis** 🔖

    B26.84   **Mumps polyneuropathy** 🔖
          Ⓔⓧ See PDX Collection 185

    B26.85   **Mumps arthritis** 🔖

    B26.89   **Other mumps complications** 🔖

    B26.9   **Mumps without complication**
          Mumps NOS
          Mumps parotitis NOS

● **B27**   **Infectious mononucleosis**

    Includes   glandular fever
                 monocytic angina
                 Pfeiffer's disease

● **B27.0**   **Gammaherpesviral mononucleosis**
    AKA: Pfeiffer's disease, infective mononucleosis
    Mononucleosis due to Epstein-Barr virus

    B27.00   **Gammaherpesviral mononucleosis without complication**
          Infective mononucleosis

    B27.01   **Gammaherpesviral mononucleosis with polyneuropathy**

    B27.02   **Gammaherpesviral mononucleosis with meningitis**

    B27.09   **Gammaherpesviral mononucleosis with other complications**
          Hepatomegaly in gammaherpesviral mononucleosis

● **B27.1**   **Cytomegaloviral mononucleosis**
    Infectious disease resembling infectious mononucleosis

    B27.10   **Cytomegaloviral mononucleosis without complications**

    B27.11   **Cytomegaloviral mononucleosis with polyneuropathy**

    B27.12   **Cytomegaloviral mononucleosis with meningitis**

    B27.19   **Cytomegaloviral mononucleosis with other complication**
          Hepatomegaly in cytomegaloviral mononucleosis

● **B27.8**   **Other infectious mononucleosis**

    B27.80   **Other infectious mononucleosis without complication**

    B27.81   **Other infectious mononucleosis with polyneuropathy**

    B27.82   **Other infectious mononucleosis with meningitis**

    B27.89   **Other infectious mononucleosis with other complication**
          Hepatomegaly in other infectious mononucleosis

● **B27.9**   **Infectious mononucleosis, unspecified**

    B27.90   **Infectious mononucleosis, unspecified without complication**

    B27.91   **Infectious mononucleosis, unspecified with polyneuropathy**

    B27.92   **Infectious mononucleosis, unspecified with meningitis**

    B27.99   **Infectious mononucleosis, unspecified with other complication**
          Hepatomegaly in unspecified infectious mononucleosis

▶ New   ⇨ Revised   ~~deleted~~ Deleted   Excludes 1   Excludes 2   Includes   Use additional   Code first   Code also   Key words

OGCR Official Guidelines   ● Unacceptable Principal Diagnosis   X Assign placeholder X   ● Use Additional Character(s)   ▶ Manifestation Code   Coding Clinic

● **B30   Viral conjunctivitis**

> **Excludes1**   herpesviral [herpes simplex] ocular disease
> (B00.5)
> ocular zoster (B02.3)

B30.0   Keratoconjunctivitis due to adenovirus
Epidemic keratoconjunctivitis
Shipyard eye

B30.1   Conjunctivitis due to adenovirus
Acute adenoviral follicular conjunctivitis
Swimming-pool conjunctivitis

B30.2   Viral pharyngoconjunctivitis

B30.3   Acute epidemic hemorrhagic conjunctivitis (enteroviral)
Conjunctivitis due to coxsackievirus 24
Conjunctivitis due to enterovirus 70
Hemorrhagic conjunctivitis (acute)(epidemic)

B30.8   Other viral conjunctivitis
Newcastle conjunctivitis

B30.9   Viral conjunctivitis, unspecified

● **B33   Other viral diseases, not elsewhere classified**

B33.0   Epidemic myalgia
*Acute infectious disease, caused by group A coxsackie viruses
or other enteroviruses with symptoms that include
sudden pain in chest or upper abdomen with fever*
Bornholm disease

B33.1   Ross River disease 🦠
Epidemic polyarthritis and exanthema
Ross River fever
ⒺⓍ See PDX Collection 144

● **B33.2   Viral carditis**
Coxsackie (virus) carditis

> **B33.20   Viral carditis, unspecified** 🦠
> ⒺⓍ See PDX Collection 186

> **B33.21   Viral endocarditis** 🦠
> ⒺⓍ See PDX Collection 187

> **B33.22   Viral myocarditis** 🦠
> ⒺⓍ See PDX Collection 186

> **B33.23   Viral pericarditis** 🦠
> ⒺⓍ See PDX Collection 188

> **B33.24   Viral cardiomyopathy**

B33.3   Retrovirus infections, not elsewhere classified
Retrovirus infection NOS

B33.4   Hantavirus (cardio)-pulmonary syndrome [HPS] [HCPS] 🦠
Hantavirus disease with pulmonary manifestations
Sin nombre virus disease

> Use additional code to identify any associated acute
> kidney failure (N17.9)

> **Excludes1**   hantavirus disease with renal
> manifestations (A98.5)
> hemorrhagic fever with renal
> manifestations (A98.5)

ⒺⓍ See PDX Collection 189

B33.8   Other specified viral diseases

> **Excludes1**   anogenital human papillomavirus
> infection (A63.0)
> viral warts due to human papillomavirus
> infection (B07)

● **B34   Viral infection of unspecified site**

> **Excludes1**   anogenital human papillomavirus infection
> (A63.0)
> cytomegaloviral disease NOS (B25.9)
> herpesvirus [herpes simplex] infection NOS
> (B00.9)
> retrovirus infection NOS (B33.3)
> viral agents as the cause of diseases classified
> elsewhere (B97.-)
> viral warts due to human papillomavirus
> infection (B07)

B34.0   Adenovirus infection, unspecified

B34.1   Enterovirus infection, unspecified
Intestinal tract infection
Coxsackievirus infection NOS
Echovirus infection NOS

B34.2   Coronavirus infection, unspecified

> **Excludes1**   pneumonia due to SARS-associated
> coronavirus (J12.81)

B34.3   Parvovirus infection, unspecified 🦠
ⒺⓍ See PDX Collection 174

B34.4   Papovavirus infection, unspecified

B34.8   Other viral infections of unspecified site

B34.9   Viral infection, unspecified
Viremia NOS
Coding Clinic: 2016, Q3, P10

MYCOSES (B35-B49)

> **Excludes2**   hypersensitivity pneumonitis due to organic dust
> (J67.-)
> mycosis fungoides (C84.0-)

● **B35   Dermatophytosis**
AKA tinea or ringworm

> **Includes**   favus
> infections due to species of Epidermophyton,
> Micro-sporum and Trichophyton
> tinea, any type except those in B36.-

B35.0   Tinea barbae and tinea capitis
Beard ringworm
Kerion
Scalp ringworm
Sycosis, mycotic

B35.1   Tinea unguium
*White patches or pits on surface or edges of nails, followed by
infection under nail plate*
Dermatophytic onychia
Dermatophytosis of nail
Onychomycosis
Ringworm of nails

B35.2   Tinea manuum
Tinea of hands
Dermatophytosis of hand
Hand ringworm

B35.3   Tinea pedis
Tinea affecting feet
Athlete's foot
Dermatophytosis of foot
Foot ringworm

B35.4   Tinea corporis
Infecting skin areas other than hands
Ringworm of the body

N Newborn Age: 0   **P** Pediatric Age: 0–17   **M** Maternity DX: 12–55   **A** Adult Age: 15–124   ♀ Females Only   ♂ Males Only

🦠 Complication\Comorbidity   🦠 Major C\C   ⒺⓍ CC/MCC Exclusions   🦠 Hospital-Acquired Condition

657

CHAPTER 1 (A00-B99)

CHAPTER 1 (A00-B99)

B35.5 Tinea imbricata
Chronic tropical tinea corporis; AKA Oriental ringworm, tinea inguinalis, tinea cruris
Tokelau

B35.6 Tinea cruris
In groin or perineal area, spreading to adjacent regions; AKA jock itch, eczema marginatum, ringworm of groin, or t inguinalis
Dhobi itch
Groin ringworm
Jock itch

B35.8 Other dermatophytoses
Disseminated dermatophytosis
Granulomatous dermatophytosis

B35.9 Dermatophytosis, unspecified
Ringworm NOS

● **B36 Other superficial mycoses**

B36.0 Pityriasis versicolor
Common, chronic, symptomless disorder that includes macular patches of various sizes and shapes; AKA liver spots
Tinea flava
Tinea versicolor

B36.1 Tinea nigra
Minor fungal infection, with dark lesions, usually on skin of hands
Keratomycosis nigricans palmaris
Microsporosis nigra
Pityriasis nigra

B36.2 White piedra
White to light brown nodules on hair of beard, axilla, or groin; AKA trichosporosis
Tinea blanca

B36.3 Black piedra
Characterized by small black or brown nodules on shafts of scalp hair

B36.8 Other specified superficial mycoses

B36.9 Superficial mycosis, unspecified

● **B37 Candidiasis**

Includes candidosis
moniliasis

Excludes1 neonatal candidiasis (P37.5)

B37.0 Candidal stomatitis 🦠
Oral thrush
(Ex:) See PDX Collection 190

B37.1 Pulmonary candidiasis 🦠
Candidal bronchitis
Candidal pneumonia
(Ex:) See PDX Collection 190

B37.2 Candidiasis of skin and nail
Candidal onychia
Candidal paronychia

Excludes2 diaper dermatitis (L22)

B37.3 Candidiasis of vulva and vagina ♀
Candidal vulvovaginitis
Monilial vulvovaginitis
Vaginal thrush

● **B37.4 Candidiasis of other urogenital sites**
(Ex:) For category B37.4 CC codes: See PDX Collection 191

B37.41 Candidal cystitis and urethritis 🦠 🦠

B37.42 Candidal balanitis ♂
Male condition only

B37.49 Other urogenital candidiasis 🦠 🦠
Candidal pyelonephritis

B37.5 Candidal meningitis 🦠
(Ex:) See PDX Collection 192

B37.6 Candidal endocarditis 🦠
(Ex:) See PDX Collection 190

Figure 1-8 Oral candidiasis (thrush). (From James WD, Berger T, Elston D: Andrews' Diseases of the Skin: Clinical Dermatology, 11e, Saunders, 2011)

Item 1–20 Candidiasis, also called oidiomycosis or moniliasis, is a fungal infection. It most often appears on moist cutaneous areas of the body but can also be responsible for a variety of systemic infections such as endocarditis, meningitis, arthritis, and myositis. Antifungal medications cure most yeast infections.

B37.7 Candidal sepsis 🦠
Disseminated candidiasis systemic candidiasis
MCC when PDx is its own MCC
(Ex:) See PDX Collection 193

● **B37.8 Candidiasis of other sites**
(Ex:) For category B37.8 CC codes unless otherwise indicated: See PDX Collection 190

B37.81 Candidal esophagitis 🦠

B37.82 Candidal enteritis 🦠
Candidal proctitis

B37.83 Candidal cheilitis 🦠
Inflammation affecting lip

B37.84 Candidal otitis externa 🦠
Inflammation of external auditory canal

B37.89 Other sites of candidiasis 🦠
Infection manifested by invasive candidiasis
Candidal osteomyelitis
(Ex:) See PDX Collection 194

B37.9 Candidiasis, unspecified
Thrush NOS

● **B38 Coccidioidomycosis**
Fungal disease; AKA coccidioidosis, coccidioidal granuloma, Posadas, or Posadas-Wernicke disease

B38.0 Acute pulmonary coccidioidomycosis 🦠
(Ex:) See PDX Collection 195

B38.1 Chronic pulmonary coccidioidomycosis 🦠
(Ex:) See PDX Collection 196

B38.2 Pulmonary coccidioidomycosis, unspecified 🦠
(Ex:) See PDX Collection 196

B38.3 Cutaneous coccidioidomycosis 🦠
(Ex:) See PDX Collection 197

B38.4 Coccidioidomycosis meningitis 🦠
(Ex:) See PDX Collection 198

B38.7 Disseminated coccidioidomycosis 🦠
Generalized coccidioidomycosis
(Ex:) See PDX Collection 199

● **B38.8 Other forms of coccidioidomycosis**

B38.81 Prostatic coccidioidomycosis ♂ 🦠
(Ex:) See PDX Collection 197

B38.89 Other forms of coccidioidomycosis 🦠
(Ex:) See PDX Collection 199

B38.9 Coccidioidomycosis, unspecified 🦠
(Ex:) See PDX Collection 199

▶ New   ⇒ Revised   ~~deleted~~ Deleted   Excludes 1   Excludes 2   Includes   Use additional   Code first   Code also   Key words
OGCR Official Guidelines   ● Unacceptable Principal Diagnosis   X Assign placeholder X   ❚ Use Additional Character(s)   ❚ Manifestation Code   **Coding Clinic**

Item 1-21 Bird and bat droppings that fall into the soil give rise to a fungus that can spread airborne spores. When inhaled into the lungs, these spores divide and multiply into lesions. Histoplasmosis capsulatum takes three forms: primary (lodged in the lungs only), chronic (resembles TB), and disseminated (infection has moved to other organs). This is an opportunistic infection in immunosuppressed patients.

● **B39   Histoplasmosis**
    Infection resulting from inhalation or ingestion of spores; AKA Darling disease
    Code first *associated AIDS (B20)*
    Use additional code for any associated manifestations, such as:
      endocarditis (I39)
      meningitis (G02)
      pericarditis (I32)
      retinitits (H32)

   B39.0   Acute pulmonary histoplasmosis capsulati 🦠
      Ⓔⓧ See PDX Collection 200

   B39.1   Chronic pulmonary histoplasmosis capsulati 🦠
      Ⓔⓧ See PDX Collection 200

   B39.2   Pulmonary histoplasmosis capsulati, unspecified 🦠
      Ⓔⓧ See PDX Collection 200

   B39.3   Disseminated histoplasmosis capsulati 🦠
      Generalized histoplasmosis capsulati
      Ⓔⓧ See PDX Collection 201

   B39.4   Histoplasmosis capsulati, unspecified
      American histoplasmosis

   B39.5   Histoplasmosis duboisii
      African histoplasmosis

   B39.9   Histoplasmosis, unspecified

● **B40   Blastomycosis**
    Rare and potentially fatal infection caused by inhaling fungus found in moist soil in temperate climates.
    Excludes1   Brazilian blastomycosis (B41.-)
               keloidal blastomycosis (B48.0)
    Ⓔⓧ **For category B40 CC codes:** See PDX Collection 202

   B40.0   Acute pulmonary blastomycosis 🦠
   B40.1   Chronic pulmonary blastomycosis 🦠
   B40.2   Pulmonary blastomycosis, unspecified 🦠
   B40.3   Cutaneous blastomycosis 🦠
   B40.7   Disseminated blastomycosis 🦠
      Generalized blastomycosis

  ● **B40.8   Other forms of blastomycosis**
      B40.81   Blastomycotic meningoencephalitis 🦠
         Meningomyelitis due to blastomycosis
      B40.89   Other forms of blastomycosis 🦠
   B40.9   Blastomycosis, unspecified 🦠

● **B41   Paracoccidioidomycosis**
    Fungal infection usually chronic that begins in lungs, spreads to mucocutaneous areas which may extend to skin, tonsils, gastrointestinal lymphatics, liver, and spleen; AKA Almeida or Lutz-Splendore-Almeida disease, Brazilian or South American blastomycosis, or paracoccidioidal granuloma
    Includes   Brazilian blastomycosis
           Lutz' disease
    Ⓔⓧ **For category B41 CC codes:** See PDX Collection 203

   B41.0   Pulmonary paracoccidioidomycosis 🦠
   B41.7   Disseminated paracoccidioidomycosis 🦠
      Generalized paracoccidioidomycosis
   B41.8   Other forms of paracoccidioidomycosis 🦠
   B41.9   Paracoccidioidomycosis, unspecified 🦠

● **B42   Sporotrichosis**
    Chronic fungal infection with nodular lesions
   B42.0   Pulmonary sporotrichosis
   B42.1   Lymphocutaneous sporotrichosis
   B42.7   Disseminated sporotrichosis
      Generalized sporotrichosis

  ● **B42.8   Other forms of sporotrichosis**
      B42.81   Cerebral sporotrichosis
         Meningitis due to sporotrichosis
      B42.82   Sporotrichosis arthritis
      B42.89   Other forms of sporotrichosis
   B42.9   Sporotrichosis, unspecified

● **B43   Chromomycosis and pheomycotic abscess**
    Chronic fungal infection of skin, initiated at site of puncture affecting lower limb or foot (mossy foot)
   B43.0   Cutaneous chromomycosis
      Dermatitis verrucosa
   B43.1   Pheomycotic brain abscess
      Cerebral chromomycosis
   B43.2   Subcutaneous pheomycotic abscess and cyst
   B43.8   Other forms of chromomycosis
   B43.9   Chromomycosis, unspecified

● **B44   Aspergillosis**
    Infection marked by inflammatory lesions in skin, ear, orbit, nasal sinuses, lungs, and occasionally bones and meninges
    Includes   aspergilloma
    Ⓔⓧ **For category B44 CC codes unless otherwise indicated:** See PDX Collection 204

   B44.0   Invasive pulmonary aspergillosis 🦠
      MCC when PDx is its own MCC
      Ⓔⓧ See PDX Collection 110
   B44.1   Other pulmonary aspergillosis 🦠
   B44.2   Tonsillar aspergillosis 🦠
   B44.7   Disseminated aspergillosis 🦠
      Generalized aspergillosis

  ● **B44.8   Other forms of aspergillosis**
      B44.81   Allergic bronchopulmonary aspergillosis 🦠
         Ⓔⓧ See PDX Collection 205
      B44.89   Other forms of aspergillosis 🦠
   B44.9   Aspergillosis, unspecified 🦠

● **B45   Cryptococcosis**
    Infection in the immunocompromised and fatal if left untreated; AKA torulosis, Buschke, or Busse-Buschke disease
    Ⓔⓧ **For category B45 CC codes unless otherwise indicated:** See PDX Collection 206

   B45.0   Pulmonary cryptococcosis 🦠
   B45.1   Cerebral cryptococcosis 🦠
      Cryptococcal meningitis
      Cryptococcosis meningocerebralis
      MCC when PDx is its own MCC
      Ⓔⓧ See PDX Collection 207
   B45.2   Cutaneous cryptococcosis 🦠
   B45.3   Osseous cryptococcosis 🦠
   B45.7   Disseminated cryptococcosis 🦠
      Generalized cryptococcosis
   B45.8   Other forms of cryptococcosis 🦠
   B45.9   Cryptococcosis, unspecified 🦠

CHAPTER 1 (A00-B99)

N Newborn Age: 0   **P** Pediatric Age: 0–17   **M** Maternity DX: 12–55   **A** Adult Age: 15–124   ♀ Females Only   ♂ Males Only

🦠 Complication\Comorbidity   🦠 Major C\C   Ⓔⓧ CC/MCC Exclusions   🦠 Hospital-Acquired Condition

659

● B46   Zygomycosis
Fungal infections including subcutaneous lesions and infection of sinuses, brain, or lungs
(Ex) **For category B46 CC codes: See PDX Collection 208**

   B46.0   Pulmonary mucormycosis 🔎
Fungal infection affecting lung

   B46.1   Rhinocerebral mucormycosis 🔎

   B46.2   Gastrointestinal mucormycosis 🔎

   B46.3   Cutaneous mucormycosis 🔎
Subcutaneous mucormycosis

   B46.4   Disseminated mucormycosis 🔎
Generalized mucormycosis

   B46.5   Mucormycosis, unspecified 🔎

   B46.8   Other zygomycoses 🔎
Entomophthoromycosis

   B46.9   Zygomycosis, unspecified 🔎
Phycomycosis NOS

● B47   Mycetoma
Slow progressive, destructive fungal infection of cutaneous and subcutaneous tissues, fascia, and bone, primarily seen in foot (Madura foot) or leg

   B47.0   Eumycetoma 🔎
Madura foot, mycotic Maduromycosis
(Ex) See PDX Collection 209

   B47.1   Actinomycetoma 🔎
(Ex) See PDX Collection 106

   B47.9   Mycetoma, unspecified 🔎
Madura foot NOS
(Ex) See PDX Collection 210

● B48   Other mycoses, not elsewhere classified

   B48.0   Lobomycosis
Infection with symptoms of red, smooth, hard cutaneous nodules resembling keloids
Keloidal blastomycosis
Lobo's disease

   B48.1   Rhinosporidiosis
Chronic, localized granulomatous fungal infection, affecting mucocutaneous tissues, usually of nose characterized by polyps, papillomas, and wartlike lesions

   B48.2   Allescheriasis 🔎
Fungal infection
Infection due to Pseudallescheria boydii
    Excludes1   eumycetoma (B47.0)
(Ex) See PDX Collection 211

   B48.3   Geotrichosis 🔎
Fungal infection usually of bronchi, lungs, mouth, or intestinal tract
Geotrichum stomatitis
(Ex) See PDX Collection 212

   B48.4   Penicillosis 🔎
Fungal infection
(Ex) See PDX Collection 204

   B48.8   Other specified mycoses 🔎
Adiaspiromycosis
Infection of tissue and organs by Alternaria
Infection of tissue and organs by Drechslera
Infection of tissue and organs by Fusarium
Infection of tissue and organs by saprophytic fungi NEC
(Ex) See PDX Collection 213

● B49   Unspecified mycosis 🔎
Fungemia NOS
(Ex) See PDX Collection 212

PROTOZOAL DISEASES (B50-B64)

   Excludes1   amebiasis (A06.-)
           other protozoal intestinal diseases (A07.-)

● B50   Plasmodium falciparum malaria
Severe form of malaria that can be fatal
    Includes   mixed infections of Plasmodium falciparum with any other Plasmodium species
(Ex) **For category B50 CC codes: See PDX Collection 214**

   B50.0   Plasmodium falciparum malaria with cerebral complications 🔎
Cerebral malaria NOS

   B50.8   Other severe and complicated Plasmodium falciparum malaria 🔎
Severe or complicated Plasmodium falciparum malaria NOS

   B50.9   Plasmodium falciparum malaria, unspecified 🔎

● B51   Plasmodium vivax malaria
    Includes   mixed infections of Plasmodium vivax with other Plasmodium species, except Plasmodium falciparum
    Excludes1   plasmodium vivav with Plasmodium falciparum (B50.-)
(Ex) **For category B51 CC codes unless otherwise indicated: See PDX Collection 214**

   B51.0   Plasmodium vivax malaria with rupture of spleen 🔎

   B51.8   Plasmodium vivax malaria with other complications 🔎

   B51.9   Plasmodium vivax malaria without complication 🔎
Plasmodium vivax malaria NOS
(Ex) See PDX Collection 215

● B52   Plasmodium malariae malaria
Causes fever that recurs at approximately three-day intervals (quartan fever), longer than two-day (tertian) intervals of other malarial parasites
    Includes   mixed infections of Plasmodium malariae with other Plasmodium species, except Plasmodium falciparum and Plasmodium vivax
    Excludes1   plasmodium falciparum (B50.-)
            plasmodium vivax (B51.-)
(Ex) **For category B52 CC codes unless otherwise indicated: See PDX Collection 214**

   B52.0   Plasmodium malariae malaria with nephropathy 🔎
CC when PDx is its own CC
(Ex) See PDX Collection 216

   B52.8   Plasmodium malariae malaria with other complications 🔎

   B52.9   Plasmodium malariae malaria without complication 🔎
Plasmodium malariae malaria NOS

● B53   Other specified malaria
(Ex) **For category B53 CC codes unless otherwise indicated: See PDX Collection 214**

   B53.0   Plasmodium ovale malaria 🔎
Least diagnosed type of malaria spread by female mosquitoes of rare species
    Excludes1   plasmodium ovale with Plasmodium falciparum (B50.-)
            plasmodium ovale with Plasmodium malariae (B52.-)
            plasmodium ovale with Plasmodium vivax (B51.-)

   B53.1   Malaria due to simian plasmodia 🔎
Malaria-like disease (parasite infection)
    Excludes1   malaria due to simian plasmodia with Plasmodium falciparum (B50.-)
            malaria due to simian plasmodia with Plasmodium malariae (B52.-)
            malaria due to simian plasmodia with Plasmodium ovale (B53.0)
            malaria due to simian plasmodia with Plasmodium vivax (B51.-)

   B53.8   Other malaria, not elsewhere classified 🔎

▶ New   ⇒ Revised   ~~deleted~~ Deleted   Excludes 1   Excludes 2   Includes   Use additional   Code first   Code also   Key words
OGCR Official Guidelines   ● Unacceptable Principal Diagnosis   X Assign placeholder X   ● Use Additional Character(s)   ▶ Manifestation Code   **Coding Clinic**

B54   **Unspecified malaria** 🔖
    (Ex) See PDX Collection 217

● **B55**   **Leishmaniasis**
    Protozoal infection
    (Ex) **For category B55 CC codes:** See PDX Collection 218

    B55.0   **Visceral leishmaniasis** 🔖
         Kala-azar
         Post-kala-azar dermal leishmaniasis

    B55.1   **Cutaneous leishmaniasis** 🔖
    B55.2   **Mucocutaneous leishmaniasis** 🔖
    B55.9   **Leishmaniasis, unspecified** 🔖

● **B56**   **African trypanosomiasis**
    Human African trypanosomiasis (HAT) is transmitted by fly bites
    (Ex) **For category B56 CC codes:** See PDX Collection 218

    B56.0   **Gambiense trypanosomiasis** 🔖
         Infection due to Trypanosoma brucei gambiense
         West African sleeping sickness

    B56.1   **Rhodesiense trypanosomiasis** 🔖
         East African sleeping sickness
         Infection due to Trypanosoma brucei rhodesiense

    B56.9   **African trypanosomiasis, unspecified** 🔖
         Sleeping sickness NOS

● **B57**   **Chagas' disease**
    Tropical parasitic disease

    | **Includes** | American trypanosomiasis |
                  infection due to Trypanosoma cruzi

    B57.0   **Acute Chagas' disease with heart involvement** 🔖
         Acute Chagas' disease with myocarditis
         (Ex) See PDX Collection 219

    B57.1   **Acute Chagas' disease without heart involvement** 🔖
         Acute Chagas' disease NOS
         (Ex) See PDX Collection 218

    B57.2   **Chagas' disease (chronic) with heart involvement** 🔖
         American trypanosomiasis NOS
         Chagas' disease (chronic) NOS
         Chagas' disease (chronic) with myocarditis
         Trypanosomiasis NOS
         (Ex) See PDX Collection 219

   ● **B57.3**   **Chagas' disease (chronic) with digestive system involvement**
         (Ex) **For category B57.3 CC codes:** See PDX Collection 218

      B57.30   **Chagas' disease with digestive system involvement, unspecified** 🔖
      B57.31   **Megaesophagus in Chagas' disease** 🔖
      B57.32   **Megacolon in Chagas' disease** 🔖
      B57.39   **Other digestive system involvement in Chagas' disease** 🔖

   ● **B57.4**   **Chagas' disease (chronic) with nervous system involvement**
         (Ex) **For category B57.4 CC codes:** See PDX Collection 218

      B57.40   **Chagas' disease with nervous system involvement, unspecified** 🔖
      B57.41   **Meningitis in Chagas' disease** 🔖
      B57.42   **Meningoencephalitis in Chagas' disease** 🔖
      B57.49   **Other nervous system involvement in Chagas' disease** 🔖

    B57.5   **Chagas' disease (chronic) with other organ involvement** 🔖
         (Ex) See PDX Collection 218

Item 1–22   **Toxoplasmosis** is caused by the protozoa **Toxoplasma gondii**, of which the house cat can be a host. Human infection occurs when contact is made with materials containing the pathogen, such as feces, contaminated soil, or ingestion of infected lamb, goat, or pork. Of the infected, very few have symptoms because a healthy person's immune system keeps the parasite from causing illness. When the immune system is compromised, symptoms may occur. Clinical symptoms include flu-like symptoms, but the disease progresses to include the eyes and the brain in babies.

● **B58**   **Toxoplasmosis**
    Infection by protozoon transmitted in cysts in feces of cats

    | **Includes** | infection due to Toxoplasma gondii |
    | **Excludes1** | congenital toxoplasmosis (P37.1) |

   ● **B58.0**   **Toxoplasma oculopathy**

      B58.00   **Toxoplasma oculopathy, unspecified** 🔖
           (Ex) See PDX Collection 220

      B58.01   **Toxoplasma chorioretinitis** 🔖
           (Ex) See PDX Collection 221

      B58.09   **Other toxoplasma oculopathy** 🔖
           Toxoplasma uveitis
           (Ex) See PDX Collection 222

    B58.1   **Toxoplasma hepatitis** 🔖
         (Ex) See PDX Collection 223

    B58.2   **Toxoplasma meningoencephalitis** 🔖
         (Ex) See PDX Collection 224

    B58.3   **Pulmonary toxoplasmosis** 🔖
         (Ex) See PDX Collection 225

   ● **B58.8**   **Toxoplasmosis with other organ involvement**
         (Ex) **For category B58.8 CC codes unless otherwise indicated:** See PDX Collection 220

      B58.81   **Toxoplasma myocarditis** 🔖
           (Ex) See PDX Collection 226

      B58.82   **Toxoplasma myositis** 🔖
      B58.83   **Toxoplasma tubulo-interstitial nephropathy** 🔖
           Toxoplasma pyelonephritis
      B58.89   **Toxoplasmosis with other organ involvement** 🔖

    B58.9   **Toxoplasmosis, unspecified** 🔖
         (Ex) See PDX Collection 227

    B59   **Pneumocystosis** 🔖
         Caused by fungus
         Pneumonia due to Pneumocystis carinii
         Pneumonia due to Pneumocystis jiroveci
         (Ex) See PDX Collection 228

● **B60**   **Other protozoal diseases, not elsewhere classified**

    | **Excludes1** | cryptosporidiosis (A07.2) |
                  intestinal microsporidiosis (A07.8)
                  isosporiasis (A07.3)

    B60.0   **Babesiosis** 🔖
         Tickborne disease caused by microscopic organisms
         Piroplasmosis
         (Ex) See PDX Collection 218

   ● **B60.1**   **Acanthamebiasis**
         (Ex) **For category B60.1 CC codes:** See PDX Collection 229

      B60.10   **Acanthamebiasis, unspecified** 🔖
      B60.11   **Meningoencephalitis due to Acanthamoeba (culbertsoni)**
      B60.12   **Conjunctivitis due to Acanthamoeba**
   ● **B60.13**   **Keratoconjunctivitis due to Acanthamoeba**
      B60.19   **Other acanthamebic disease** 🔖

    B60.2   **Naegleriasis** 🔖
         Infection with microscopic organisms
         Primary amebic meningoencephalitis
         (Ex) See PDX Collection 229

    B60.8   **Other specified protozoal diseases**
         Microsporidiosis

    B64   **Unspecified protozoal disease**

| N | Newborn Age: 0 | P | Pediatric Age: 0–17 | M | Maternity DX: 12–55 | A | Adult Age: 15–124 | ♀ Females Only | ♂ Males Only |
| 🔖 Complication\Comorbidity | | 🔖 Major C\C | | (Ex) CC/MCC Exclusions | | 🔖 Hospital-Acquired Condition | | | |

HELMINTHIASES (B65-B83)

Diseases or infestations caused by parasitic worms

● **B65** **Schistosomiasis [bilharziasis]**
Infection with flukes (flat parasitic worms)

    Includes snail fever

    Ⓔ **For category B65 CC codes:** See PDX Collection 230

    B65.0 **Schistosomiasis due to Schistosoma haematobium [urinary schistosomiasis]** 🔖

    B65.1 **Schistosomiasis due to Schistosoma mansoni [intestinal schistosomiasis]** 🔖

    B65.2 **Schistosomiasis due to Schistosoma japonicum** 🔖
        Asiatic schistosomiasis

    B65.3 **Cercarial dermatitis** 🔖
        Swimmer's itch

    B65.8 **Other schistosomiasis** 🔖
        Infection due to Schistosoma intercalatum
        Infection due to Schistosoma mattheei
        Infection due to Schistosoma mekongi

    B65.9 **Schistosomiasis, unspecified** 🔖

● **B66** **Other fluke infections**
Trematode (parasitic worms)

    Ⓔ **For category B66 CC codes:** See PDX Collection 231

    B66.0 **Opisthorchiasis** 🔖
        Infection due to cat liver fluke
        Infection due to Opisthorchis (felineus)(viverrini)

    B66.1 **Clonorchiasis** 🔖
        Chinese liver fluke disease
        Infection due to Clonorchis sinensis
        Oriental liver fluke disease

    B66.2 **Dicroceliasis** 🔖
        Liver fluke
        Infection due to Dicrocoelium dendriticum
        Lancet fluke infection

    B66.3 **Fascioliasis** 🔖
        Infection due to Fasciola gigantica
        Infection due to Fasciola hepatica
        Infection due to Fasciola indica
        Sheep liver fluke disease

    B66.4 **Paragonimiasis** 🔖
        Infection due to Paragonimus species
        Lung fluke disease
        Pulmonary distomiasis

    B66.5 **Fasciolopsiasis** 🔖
        Largest intestinal fluke in humans
        Infection due to Fasciolopsis buski
        Intestinal distomiasis

    B66.8 **Other specified fluke infections** 🔖
        Echinostomiasis
        Heterophyiasis
        Metagonimiasis
        Nanophyetiasis
        Watsoniasis

    B66.9 **Fluke infection, unspecified**

● **B67** **Echinococcosis**
Larval forms of tapeworms usually of liver or lungs

    Includes hydatidosis

    B67.0 **Echinococcus granulosus infection of liver** 🔖
        Ⓔ See PDX Collection 232

    B67.1 **Echinococcus granulosus infection of lung** 🔖
        Ⓔ See PDX Collection 233

    B67.2 **Echinococcus granulosus infection of bone** 🔖
        Ⓔ See PDX Collection 234

Item 1-23 Echinococcosis: Also known as hydatid disease; is caused by Echinococcus granulosus, E. multilocularis, and E. vogeli tapeworms; and is contracted from infected food. Found in southern South America, the Mediterranean, the Middle East, central Asia, and Africa and uncommon in the United States but has been reported in California, New Mexico, Arizona and Utah. The disease is treated with medication over a long course as it is resistive.

    B67.3 **Echinococcus granulosus infection, other and multiple sites**

        B67.31 **Echinococcus granulosus infection, thyroid gland** 🔖
            Ⓔ See PDX Collection 235

        B67.32 **Echinococcus granulosus infection, multiple sites** 🔖
            Ⓔ See PDX Collection 234

        B67.39 **Echinococcus granulosus infection, other sites** 🔖
            Ⓔ See PDX Collection 234

    B67.4 **Echinococcus granulosus infection, unspecified** 🔖
        Dog tapeworm (infection)
        Ⓔ See PDX Collection 236

    B67.5 **Echinococcus multilocularis infection of liver** 🔖
        Ⓔ See PDX Collection 237

●   **B67.6** **Echinococcus multilocularis infection, other and multiple sites**
        Ⓔ **For category B67.6 CC codes:** See PDX Collection 238

        B67.61 **Echinococcus multilocularis infection, multiple sites** 🔖

        B67.69 **Echinococcus multilocularis infection, other sites** 🔖

    B67.7 **Echinococcus multilocularis infection, unspecified** 🔖
        Ⓔ See PDX Collection 239

    B67.8 **Echinococcosis, unspecified, of liver** 🔖
        Ⓔ See PDX Collection 240

●   **B67.9** **Echinococcosis, other and unspecified**
        Ⓔ **For category B67.9 CC codes:** See PDX Collection 240

        B67.90 **Echinococcosis, unspecified** 🔖
            Echinococcosis NOS

        B67.99 **Other echinococcosis** 🔖

● **B68** **Taeniasis**
Intestinal tapeworm (cestode) infection from raw or undercooked meat of infected animal

    Excludes1 cysticercosis (B69.-)

    B68.0 **Taenia solium taeniasis** 🔖
        Pork tapeworm (infection)
        Ⓔ See PDX Collection 241

    B68.1 **Taenia saginata taeniasis** 🔖
        Beef tapeworm (infection)
        Infection due to adult tapeworm Taenia saginata
        Ⓔ See PDX Collection 242

    B68.9 **Taeniasis, unspecified** 🔖
        Ⓔ See PDX Collection 242

● **B69** **Cysticercosis**
Systemic illness caused by the larvae of pork tapeworm

    Includes cysticerciasis infection due to larval form of Taenia solium

    Ⓔ **For category B69 CC codes:** See PDX Collection 242

    B69.0 **Cysticercosis of central nervous system** 🔖

    B69.1 **Cysticercosis of eye** 🔖

●   **B69.8** **Cysticercosis of other sites**

        B69.81 **Myositis in cysticercosis** 🔖

        B69.89 **Cysticercosis of other sites** 🔖

    B69.9 **Cysticercosis, unspecified** 🔖

▶ New   ➡ Revised   ~~deleted~~ Deleted   Excludes 1   Excludes 2   Includes   Use additional   Code first   Code also   Key words

OGCR Official Guidelines   ● Unacceptable Principal Diagnosis   X Assign placeholder X   🔖 Use Additional Character(s)   ▶ Manifestation Code   Coding Clinic

662

● **B70   Diphyllobothriasis and sparganosis**
Infection with tapeworms seen most often from inadequately cooked fish
Ⓔⓧ *For category B70 CC codes:* See PDX Collection 242

    B70.0   Diphyllobothriasis
        Diphyllobothrium (adult) (latum) (pacificum) infection
        Fish tapeworm (infection)
        Excludes2   larval diphyllobothriasis (B70.1)

    B70.1   Sparganosis 🔖
        Infection with migrating tapeworm larvae, which invade subcutaneous tissues, causing inflammation and fibrosis that resembles cellulitis
        Infection due to Sparganum (mansoni) (proliferum)
        Infection due to Spirometra larva
        Larval diphyllobothriasis
        Spirometrosis

● **B71   Other cestode infections**
Ⓔⓧ *For category B71 CC codes:* See PDX Collection 242

    B71.0   Hymenolepiasis 🔖
        Intestinal infestation with tapeworms
        Dwarf tapeworm infection
        Rat tapeworm (infection)

    B71.1   Dipylidiasis 🔖
        Infection with tapeworm common to dogs and cats and seen in children having close contact with infected pets

    B71.8   Other specified cestode infections 🔖
        Infection by the larval stage of a tapeworm, usually through fruit or vegetables
        Coenurosis

    B71.9   Cestode infection, unspecified
        Tapeworm (infection) NOS

    B72   Dracunculiasis 🔖
        Infection with roundworms
        Includes   guinea worm infection
                  infection due to Dracunculus medinensis
        Ⓔⓧ See PDX Collection 243

● **B73   Onchocerciasis**
Infection with parasitic worm
    Includes   onchocerca volvulus infection
                  onchocercosis
                  river blindness

  ● **B73.0   Onchocerciasis with eye disease**
        Ⓔⓧ *For category B73 CC codes:* See PDX Collection 243

        B73.00   Onchocerciasis with eye involvement, unspecified 🔖

        B73.01   Onchocerciasis with endophthalmitis 🔖

        B73.02   Onchocerciasis with glaucoma 🔖

        B73.09   Onchocerciasis with other eye involvement 🔖
            Infestation of eyelid due to onchocerciasis

    B73.1   Onchocerciasis without eye disease 🔖

● **B74   Filariasis**
Infestation with slender threadlike worms
    Excludes2   onchocerciasis (B73)
               tropical (pulmonary) eosinophilia NOS (J82)
    Ⓔⓧ *For category B74 CC codes:* See PDX Collection 243

    B74.0   Filariasis due to Wuchereria bancrofti 🔖
        Bancroftian elephantiasis
        Bancroftian filariasis

    B74.1   Filariasis due to Brugia malayi 🔖

    B74.2   Filariasis due to Brugia timori 🔖

    B74.3   Loiasis 🔖
        Infection with round worms growing in subcutaneous connective tissue
        Calabar swelling
        Eyeworm disease of Africa
        Loa loa infection

    B74.4   Mansonelliasis 🔖
        Infection with filarial parasite
        Infection due to Mansonella ozzardi
        Infection due to Mansonella perstans
        Infection due to Mansonella streptocerca

    B74.8   Other filariases 🔖
        Dirofilariasis

    B74.9   Filariasis, unspecified 🔖

● **B75   Trichinellosis** 🔖
Infestation with parasitic roundworms ingested in undercooked contaminated meat
    Includes   infection due to Trichinella species trichiniasis
    Ⓔⓧ See PDX Collection 244

● **B76   Hookworm diseases**
Occurs in hot, humid parts of world where larvae are soil borne, enter digestive tract through skin of feet/legs or in contaminated food/ water; AKA ground itch
    Includes   uncinariasis
    Ⓔⓧ *For category B76 CC codes:* See PDX Collection 245

    B76.0   Ancylostomiasis 🔖
        Infection due to Ancylostoma species

    B76.1   Necatoriasis 🔖
        Infection due to Necator americanus

    B76.8   Other hookworm diseases 🔖

    B76.9   Hookworm disease, unspecified 🔖
        Cutaneous larva migrans NOS

● **B77   Ascariasis**
Infection by roundworm in small intestine
    Includes   ascaridiasis
                  roundworm infection

    B77.0   Ascariasis with intestinal complications 🔖
        Ⓔⓧ See PDX Collection 246

  ● **B77.8   Ascariasis with other complications**
        B77.81   Ascariasis pneumonia 🔖
            MCC when PDx is its own MCC
            Ⓔⓧ See PDX Collection 247

        B77.89   Ascariasis with other complications 🔖
            Ⓔⓧ See PDX Collection 246

    B77.9   Ascariasis, unspecified 🔖
        Ⓔⓧ See PDX Collection 246

● **B78   Strongyloidiasis**
Infection with adult female roundworms
    Excludes1   trichostrongyliasis (B81.2)
    Ⓔⓧ *For category B78 CC codes:* See PDX Collection 246

    B78.0   Intestinal strongyloidiasis 🔖

    B78.1   Cutaneous strongyloidiasis 🔖

    B78.7   Disseminated strongyloidiasis 🔖

    B78.9   Strongyloidiasis, unspecified 🔖

    B79   Trichuriasis 🔖
    Intestinal infection with roundworms
    Includes   trichocephaliasis
                  whipworm (disease)(infection)
    Ⓔⓧ See PDX Collection 246

    B80   Enterobiasis 🔖
    Intestinal infection with pinworms
    Includes   oxyuriasis
                  pinworm infection
                  threadworm infection
    Ⓔⓧ See PDX Collection 246

CHAPTER 1 (A00–B99)

N Newborn Age: 0   **P** Pediatric Age: 0–17   **M** Maternity DX: 12–55   **A** Adult Age: 15–124   ♀ Females Only   ♂ Males Only

🔖 Complication\Comorbidity   🔖 Major C\C   Ⓔⓧ CC/MCC Exclusions   🔖 Hospital-Acquired Condition

CHAPTER 1 (A00-B99)

● **B81** **Other intestinal helminthiases, not elsewhere classified**
Diseases or infestations caused by parasitic worms

> **Excludes1** ➡ angiostrongyliasis due to:
> > ▶ Angiostrongylus cantonensis (B83.2)
> > ▶ Parastrongylus cantonensis (B83.2)

(Ex:) For category B81 CC codes B81.0-B81.2: See PDX Collection 246
     For category B81 CC codes B81.3-B81.8: See PDX Collection 248

B81.0 **Anisakiasis** 🔖
Roundworm infection via contaminated undercooked infected fish or marine mammals
Infection due to Anisakis larva

B81.1 **Intestinal capillariasis** 🔖
Infestation with of parasites (nematodes)
Capillariasis NOS
Infection due to Capillaria philippinensis

> **Excludes2** hepatic capillariasis (B83.8)

B81.2 **Trichostrongyliasis** 🔖

B81.3 **Intestinal angiostrongyliasis** 🔖
➡ Angiostrongyliasis due to:
> ▶ Angiostrongylus costaricensis (B83.2)
> ▶ Parastrongylus costaricensis (B83.2)

B81.4 **Mixed intestinal helminthiases** 🔖
Infection due to intestinal helminths classified to more than one of the categories B65.0-B81.3 and B81.8
Mixed helminthiasis NOS

B81.8 **Other specified intestinal helminthiases** 🔖
Infection due to Oesophagostomum species [esophagostomiasis]
Infection due to Ternidens diminutus [ternidensiasis]

● **B82** **Unspecified intestinal parasitism**

B82.0 **Intestinal helminthiasis, unspecified** 🔖
Infected with worms
(Ex:) See PDX Collection 248

B82.9 **Intestinal parasitism, unspecified**

● **B83** **Other helminthiases**
Caused by parasitic worms

> **Excludes1** capillariasis NOS (B81.1)
> **Excludes2** intestinal capillariasis (B81.1)

B83.0 **Visceral larva migrans**
Prolonged migration of nematode larvae
Toxocariasis

B83.1 **Gnathostomiasis**
Infection with nematode occurring from ingested undercooked fish contaminated with larvae; larvae migrate to subcutaneous tissue or deeper tissues, results are abscesses
Wandering swelling

B83.2 **Angiostrongyliasis due to Parastrongylus cantonensis**
Nematode infection caused by eating contaminated raw snails, slugs, or paratenic hosts such as prawns or crabs; larval worms migrate to central nervous system resulting in eosinophilic meningitis
Eosinophilic meningoencephalitis due to Parastrongylus cantonensis

> **Excludes2** intestinal angiostrongyliasis (B81.3)

B83.3 **Syngamiasis**
Infestation with gapeworm from turkey, pheasant, guinea fowl, goose, and wild birds
Syngamosis

B83.4 **Internal hirudiniasis**
Infestation by leeches

> **Excludes2** external hirudiniasis (B88.3)

B83.8 **Other specified helminthiases**
Parasitic worm infestation
Acanthocephaliasis
Gongylonemiasis
Hepatic capillariasis
Metastrongyliasis
Thelaziasis

B83.9 **Helminthiasis, unspecified**
Worms NOS

> **Excludes1** intestinal helminthiasis NOS (B82.0)

PEDICULOSIS, ACARIASIS AND OTHER INFESTATIONS (B85-B89)

● **B85** **Pediculosis and phthiriasis**
Infestation of lice

B85.0 **Pediculosis due to Pediculus humanus capitis**
Head-louse infestation

B85.1 **Pediculosis due to Pediculus humanus corporis**
Body-louse infestation

B85.2 **Pediculosis, unspecified**

B85.3 **Phthiriasis**
Crab or pubic lice
Infestation by crab-louse
Infestation by Phthirus pubis

B85.4 **Mixed pediculosis and phthiriasis**
Infestation classifiable to more than one of the categories B85.0-B85.3

B86 **Scabies**
Contagious dermatitis caused by mites
Sarcoptic itch

● **B87** **Myiasis**
Infestation by fly maggots

> **Includes** infestation by larva of flies

B87.0 **Cutaneous myiasis**
Creeping myiasis

B87.1 **Wound myiasis**
Traumatic myiasis

B87.2 **Ocular myiasis**

B87.3 **Nasopharyngeal myiasis**
Laryngeal myiasis

B87.4 **Aural myiasis**

● **B87.8** **Myiasis of other sites**

B87.81 **Genitourinary myiasis**

B87.82 **Intestinal myiasis**

B87.89 **Myiasis of other sites**

B87.9 **Myiasis, unspecified**

● **B88** **Other infestations**

B88.0 **Other acariasis**
Acarine dermatitis
Dermatitis due to Demodex species
Dermatitis due to Dermanyssus gallinae
Dermatitis due to Liponyssoides sanguineus
Trombiculosis

> **Excludes2** scabies (B86)

B88.1 **Tungiasis [sandflea infestation]**
Inflammatory skin disease caused by infestation of fleas

B88.2 **Other arthropod infestations**
Scarabiasis

B88.3 **External hirudiniasis**
Leech infestation NOS

> **Excludes2** internal hirudiniasis (B83.4)

B88.8 **Other specified infestations**
Infection of topical fresh water fish parasite
Ichthyoparasitism due to Vandellia cirrhosa
Linguatulosis
Porocephaliasis

B88.9 **Infestation, unspecified**
Infestation (skin) NOS
Infestation by mites NOS
Skin parasites NOS

B89 **Unspecified parasitic disease**

▶ New   ➡ Revised   ~~deleted~~ Deleted   Excludes 1   Excludes 2   Includes   Use additional   Code first   Code also   Key words

OGCR Official Guidelines   ● Unacceptable Principal Diagnosis   X Assign placeholder X   ● Use Additional Character(s)   ▶ Manifestation Code   Coding Clinic

SEQUELAE OF INFECTIOUS AND PARASITIC DISEASES (B90-B94)

Note: Categories B90-B94 are to be used to indicate conditions in categories A00-B89 as the cause of sequelae, which are themselves classified elsewhere. The 'sequelae' include conditions specified as such; they also include residuals of diseases classifiable to the above categories if there is evidence that the disease itself is no longer present. Codes from these categories are not to be used for chronic infections. Code chronic current infections to active infectious disease as appropriate.

Code first condition resulting from (sequela) the infectious or parasitic disease

● **B90   Sequelae of tuberculosis**
     Condition resulting from tuberculosis
    B90.0   Sequelae of central nervous system tuberculosis
    B90.1   Sequelae of genitourinary tuberculosis
    B90.2   Sequelae of tuberculosis of bones and joints
    B90.8   Sequelae of tuberculosis of other organs
            Excludes2   sequelae of respiratory tuberculosis (B90.9)
    B90.9   Sequelae of respiratory and unspecified tuberculosis
            Sequelae of tuberculosis NOS

B91   Sequelae of poliomyelitis
        Excludes1   postpolio syndrome (G14)

B92   Sequelae of leprosy

● **B94   Sequelae of other and unspecified infectious and parasitic diseases**
    B94.0   Sequelae of trachoma
    B94.1   Sequelae of viral encephalitis
    B94.2   Sequelae of viral hepatitis
    B94.8   Sequelae of other specified infectious and parasitic diseases
    B94.9   Sequelae of unspecified infectious and parasitic disease
    OGCR Section I.C.1.b.

> Certain infectious and parasitic diseases
>
> Infectious agents as the cause of diseases classified to other chapters
>
> Certain infections are classified in chapters other than Chapter 1 and no organism is identified as part of the infection code. In these instances, it is necessary to use an additional code from Chapter 1 to identify the organism. A code from category B95, Streptococcus, Staphylococcus, and Enterococcus as the cause of diseases classified to other chapters, B96, Other bacterial agents as the cause of diseases classified to other chapters, or B97, Viral agents as the cause of diseases classified to other chapters, is to be used as an additional code to identify the organism. An instructional note will be found at the infection code advising that an additional organism code is required.

BACTERIAL AND VIRAL INFECTIOUS AGENTS (B95-B97)

Note: These categories are provided for use as supplementary or additional codes to identify the infectious agent(s) in diseases classified elsewhere.
    Code the disease first, then the bacterium. Do not report codes from B95-B97 for sepsis.

● **B95   Streptococcus, Staphylococcus, and Enterococcus as the cause of diseases classified elsewhere**
    ● **B95.0   Streptococcus, group A, as the cause of diseases classified elsewhere**
    ● **B95.1   Streptococcus, group B, as the cause of diseases classified elsewhere**
    ● **B95.2   Enterococcus as the cause of diseases classified elsewhere**

● **B95.3   Streptococcus pneumoniae as the cause of diseases classified elsewhere**
● **B95.4   Other streptococcus as the cause of diseases classified elsewhere**
● **B95.5   Unspecified streptococcus as the cause of diseases classified elsewhere**
● **B95.6   Staphylococcus aureus as the cause of diseases classified elsewhere**
    ● **B95.61   Methicillin susceptible Staphylococcus aureus infection as the cause of diseases classified elsewhere**
            Methicillin susceptible Staphylococcus aureus (MSSA) infection as the cause of diseases classified elsewhere
            Staphylococcus aureus infection NOS as the cause of diseases classified elsewhere
    ● **B95.62   Methicillin resistant Staphylococcus aureus infection as the cause of diseases classified elsewhere**
            Methicillin resistant staphylococcus aureus (MRSA) infection as the cause of diseases classified elsewhere
            Coding Clinic: 2016, Q1, P13
● **B95.7   Other staphylococcus as the cause of diseases classified elsewhere**
● **B95.8   Unspecified staphylococcus as the cause of diseases classified elsewhere**

● **B96   Other bacterial agents as the cause of diseases classified elsewhere**
    ● **B96.0   Mycoplasma pneumoniae [M. pneumoniae] as the cause of diseases classified elsewhere**
            Pleuro-pneumonia-like-organism [PPLO]
    ● **B96.1   Klebsiella pneumoniae [K. pneumoniae] as the cause of diseases classified elsewhere**
    ● **B96.2   Escherichia coli [E. coli] as the cause of diseases classified elsewhere**
        ● **B96.20   Unspecified Escherichia coli [E. coli] as the cause of diseases classified elsewhere**
                Escherichia coli [E. coli] NOS
        ● **B96.21   Shiga toxin-producing Escherichia coli [E. coli] (STEC) O157 as the cause of diseases classified elsewhere**
                E. coli O157:H- (nonmotile) with confirmation of Shiga toxin
                E. coli O157 with confirmation of Shiga toxin when H antigen is unknown, or is not H7
                O157:H7 Escherichia coli [E.coli] with or without confirmation of Shiga toxin-production
                Shiga toxin-producing Escherichia coli [E.coli] O157:H7 with or without confirmation of Shiga toxin-production
                STEC O157:H7 with or without confirmation of Shiga toxin-production
        ● **B96.22   Other specified Shiga toxin-producing Escherichia coli [E. coli] (STEC) as the cause of diseases classified elsewhere**
                Non-O157 Shiga toxin-producing Escherichia coli [E.coli]
                Non-O157 Shiga toxin-producing Escherichia coli [E.coli] with known O group
        ● **B96.23   Unspecified Shiga toxin-producing Escherichia coli [E. coli] (STEC) as the cause of diseases classified elsewhere**
                Shiga toxin-producing Escherichia coli [E. coli] with unspecified O group
                STEC NOS
        ● **B96.29   Other Escherichia coli [E. coli] as the cause of diseases classified elsewhere**
                Non-Shiga toxin-producing E. coli

CHAPTER 1 (A00-B99)

- **B96.3** Hemophilus influenzae [H. influenzae] as the cause of diseases classified elsewhere
- **B96.4** Proteus (mirabilis) (morganii) as the cause of diseases classified elsewhere
- **B96.5** Pseudomonas (aeruginosa) (mallei) (pseudomallei) as the cause of diseases classified elsewhere
  Coding Clinic: 2015, Q1, P18
- **B96.6** Bacteroides fragilis [B. fragilis] as the cause of diseases classified elsewhere
- **B96.7** Clostridium perfringens [C. perfringens] as the cause of diseases classified elsewhere
- **B96.8** Other specified bacterial agents as the cause of diseases classified elsewhere
  - **B96.81** Helicobacter pylori [H. pylori] as the cause of diseases classified elsewhere
  - **B96.82** Vibrio vulnificus as the cause of diseases classified elsewhere
  - **B96.89** Other specified bacterial agents as the cause of diseases classified elsewhere

- **B97** Viral agents as the cause of diseases classified elsewhere
  - **B97.0** Adenovirus as the cause of diseases classified elsewhere
  - **B97.1** Enterovirus as the cause of diseases classified elsewhere
    - **B97.10** Unspecified enterovirus as the cause of diseases classified elsewhere
    - **B97.11** Coxsackievirus as the cause of diseases classified elsewhere
    - **B97.12** Echovirus as the cause of diseases classified elsewhere
    - **B97.19** Other enterovirus as the cause of diseases classified elsewhere
  - **B97.2** Coronavirus as the cause of diseases classified elsewhere
    - **B97.21** SARS-associated coronavirus as the cause of diseases classified elsewhere
      Excludes1 pneumonia due to SARS-associated coronavirus (J12.81)
      (Ex) See PDX Collection 249
    - **B97.29** Other coronavirus as the cause of diseases classified elsewhere

Item 1–24 **Retrovirus** develops by copying its RNA, genetic materials, into the DNA, which then produces new virus particles. It is from the Retroviridae virus family. **Human T-cell lymphotropic virus, Type I (HTLV-I)** is also called human T-cell leukemia virus, Type I, and is a retrovirus thought to cause T-cell leukemia/lymphoma. **Human T-cell lymphotropic virus, Type II (HTLV-II),** is also called human T-cell leukemia virus, Type II, and is a retrovirus associated with hematologic disorders.

     HIV-2 is one of the serotypes of HIV and is usually confined to West Africa, whereas HIV-**1** is found worldwide.

- **B97.3** Retrovirus as the cause of diseases classified elsewhere
  Excludes1 human immunodeficiency virus [HIV] disease (B20)
  - **B97.30** Unspecified retrovirus as the cause of diseases classified elsewhere
  - **B97.31** Lentivirus as the cause of diseases classified elsewhere
  - **B97.32** Oncovirus as the cause of diseases classified elsewhere
  - **B97.33** Human T-cell lymphotrophic virus, type I [HTLV-I] as the cause of diseases classified elsewhere
    (Ex) See PDX Collection 250
  - **B97.34** Human T-cell lymphotrophic virus, type II [HTLV-II] as the cause of diseases classified elsewhere
    (Ex) See PDX Collection 251
  - **B97.35** Human immunodeficiency virus, type 2 [HIV 2] as the cause of diseases classified elsewhere
    (Ex) See PDX Collection 252
  - **B97.39** Other retrovirus as the cause of diseases classified elsewhere
- **B97.4** Respiratory syncytial virus as the cause of diseases classified elsewhere
- **B97.5** Reovirus as the cause of diseases classified elsewhere
- **B97.6** Parvovirus as the cause of diseases classified elsewhere
- **B97.7** Papillomavirus as the cause of diseases classified elsewhere
- **B97.8** Other viral agents as the cause of diseases classified elsewhere
  - **B97.81** Human metapneumovirus as the cause of diseases classified elsewhere
  - **B97.89** Other viral agents as the cause of diseases classified elsewhere
    Coding Clinic: 2016, Q3, P8-10, 14

OTHER INFECTIOUS DISEASES (B99)

- **B99** Other and unspecified infectious diseases
  - **B99.8** Other infectious disease
  - **B99.9** Unspecified infectious disease

▶ New   ⇒ Revised   ~~deleted~~ Deleted   Excludes 1   Excludes 2   Includes   Use additional   Code first   Code also   Key words
OGCR Official Guidelines   ● Unacceptable Principal Diagnosis   X Assign placeholder X   ● Use Additional Character(s)   ❱ Manifestation Code   **Coding Clinic**

CHAPTER 2

NEOPLASMS (C00-D49)

OGCR Chapter-Specific Coding Guidelines

2. Chapter 2: Neoplasms (C00-D49)
General guidelines
Chapter 2 of the ICD-10-CM contains the codes for most benign and all malignant neoplasms. Certain benign neoplasms, such as prostatic adenomas, may be found in the specific body system chapters. To properly code a neoplasm it is necessary to determine from the record if the neoplasm is benign, in-situ, malignant, or of uncertain histologic behavior. If malignant, any secondary (metastatic) sites should also be determined.

Primary malignant neoplasms overlapping site boundaries
A primary malignant neoplasm that overlaps two or more contiguous (next to each other) sites should be classified to the subcategory/code .8 ('overlapping lesion'), unless the combination is specifically indexed elsewhere. For multiple neoplasms of the same site that are not contiguous such as tumors in different quadrants of the same breast, codes for each site should be assigned.

Malignant neoplasm of ectopic tissue
Malignant neoplasms of ectopic tissue are to be coded to the site of origin mentioned, e.g., ectopic pancreatic malignant neoplasms involving the stomach are coded to **malignant neoplasm of** pancreas, unspecified (C25.9).

The neoplasm table in the Alphabetic Index should be referenced first. However, if the histological term is documented, that term should be referenced first, rather than going immediately to the Neoplasm Table, in order to determine which column in the Neoplasm Table is appropriate. For example, if the documentation indicates "adenoma," refer to the term in the Alphabetic Index to review the entries under this term and the instructional note to "see also neoplasm, by site, benign." The table provides the proper code based on the type of neoplasm and the site. It is important to select the proper column in the table that corresponds to the type of neoplasm. The Tabular List should then be referenced to verify that the correct code has been selected from the table and that a more specific site code does not exist.

See Section I.C.21. Factors influencing health status and contact with health services, Status, for information regarding Z15.0, codes for genetic susceptibility to cancer.

a. Treatment directed at the malignancy
If the treatment is directed at the malignancy, designate the malignancy as the principal diagnosis.

The only exception to this guideline is if a patient admission/encounter is solely for the administration of chemotherapy, immunotherapy or **external beam** radiation therapy, assign the appropriate Z51.— code as the first-listed or principal diagnosis, and the diagnosis or problem for which the service is being performed as a secondary diagnosis.

b. Treatment of secondary site
When a patient is admitted because of a primary neoplasm with metastasis and treatment is directed toward the secondary site only, the secondary neoplasm is designated as the principal diagnosis even though the primary malignancy is still present.

c. Coding and sequencing of complications
Coding and sequencing of complications associated with the malignancies or with the therapy thereof are subject to the following guidelines:

1) Anemia associated with malignancy
When admission/encounter is for management of an anemia associated with the malignancy, and the treatment is only for anemia, the appropriate code for the malignancy is sequenced as the principal or first-listed diagnosis followed by the appropriate code for the anemia (such as code D63.0, Anemia in neoplastic disease).

2) Anemia associated with chemotherapy, immunotherapy and radiation therapy
When the admission/encounter is for management of an anemia associated with an adverse effect of the administration of chemotherapy or immunotherapy and the only treatment is for the anemia, the anemia code is sequenced first followed by the appropriate codes for the neoplasm and the adverse effect

(T45.1X5, Adverse effect of antineoplastic and immunosuppressive drugs).

When the admission/encounter is for management of an anemia associated with an adverse effect of radiotherapy, the anemia code should be sequenced first, followed by the appropriate neoplasm code and code Y84.2, Radiological procedure and radiotherapy as the cause of abnormal reaction of the patient, or of later complication, without mention of misadventure at the time of the procedure.

3) Management of dehydration due to the malignancy
When the admission/encounter is for management of dehydration due to the malignancy and only the dehydration is being treated (intravenous rehydration), the dehydration is sequenced first, followed by the code(s) for the malignancy.

4) Treatment of a complication resulting from a surgical procedure
When the admission/encounter is for treatment of a complication resulting from a surgical procedure, designate the complication as the principal or first-listed diagnosis if treatment is directed at resolving the complication.

d. Primary malignancy previously excised
When a primary malignancy has been previously excised or eradicated from its site and there is no further treatment directed to that site and there is no evidence of any existing primary malignancy, a code from category Z85, Personal history of malignant neoplasm, should be used to indicate the former site of the malignancy. Any mention of extension, invasion, or metastasis to another site is coded as a secondary malignant neoplasm to that site. The secondary site may be the principal or first-listed with the Z85 code used as a secondary code.

e. Admissions/Encounters involving chemotherapy, immunotherapy and radiation therapy

1) Episode of care involves surgical removal of neoplasm
When an episode of care involves the surgical removal of a neoplasm, primary or secondary site, followed by adjunct chemotherapy or radiation treatment during the same episode of care, the code for the neoplasm should be assigned as principal or first-listed diagnosis.

2) Patient admission/encounter solely for administration of chemotherapy, immunotherapy and radiation therapy
If a patient admission/encounter is solely for the administration of chemotherapy, immunotherapy or **external beam** radiation therapy assign code Z51.0, Encounter for antineoplastic radiation therapy, or Z51.11, Encounter for antineoplastic chemotherapy, or Z51.12, Encounter for antineoplastic immunotherapy as the first-listed or principal diagnosis. If a patient receives more than one of these therapies during the same admission more than one of these codes may be assigned, in any sequence.

The malignancy for which the therapy is being administered should be assigned as a secondary diagnosis.

If a patient admission/encounter is for the insertion or implantation of radioactive elements (e.g., brachytherapy) the appropriate code for the malignancy is sequenced as the principal or first-listed diagnosis. Code Z51.0 should not be assigned.

3) Patient admitted for radiation therapy, chemotherapy or immunotherapy and develops complications
When a patient is admitted for the purpose of **external beam** radiotherapy, immunotherapy or chemotherapy and develops complications such as uncontrolled nausea and vomiting or dehydration, the principal or first-listed diagnosis is Z51.0, Encounter for antineoplastic radiation therapy, or Z51.11, Encounter for antineoplastic chemotherapy, or Z51.12, Encounter for antineoplastic immunotherapy followed by any codes for the complications.

When a patient is admitted for the purpose of insertion or implantation of radioactive elements (e.g., brachytherapy) and develops complications such as uncontrolled nausea and vomiting or dehydration, the principal or first-listed diagnosis is the appropriate code for the malignancy followed by any codes for the complications.

f. Admission/encounter to determine extent of malignancy
When the reason for admission/encounter is to determine the extent of the malignancy, or for a procedure such as paracentesis or thoracentesis, the primary malignancy or appropriate metastatic site is designated as the principal or first-listed

diagnosis, even though chemotherapy or radiotherapy is administered.

g. Symptoms, signs, and abnormal findings listed in Chapter 18 associated with neoplasms

Symptoms, signs, and ill-defined conditions listed in Chapter 18 characteristic of, or associated with, an existing primary or secondary site malignancy cannot be used to replace the malignancy as principal or first-listed diagnosis, regardless of the number of admissions or encounters for treatment and care of the neoplasm.

See section I.C.21. Factors influencing health status and contact with health services, Encounter for prophylactic organ removal.

h. Admission/encounter for pain control/management

See Section I.C.6. for information on coding admission/encounter for pain control/management.

i. Malignancy in two or more noncontiguous sites

A patient may have more than one malignant tumor in the same organ. These tumors may represent different primaries or metastatic disease, depending on the site. Should the documentation be unclear, the provider should be queried as to the status of each tumor so that the correct codes can be assigned.

j. Disseminated malignant neoplasm, unspecified

Code C80.0, Disseminated malignant neoplasm, unspecified, is for use only in those cases where the patient has advanced metastatic disease and no known primary or secondary sites are specified. It should not be used in place of assigning codes for the primary site and all known secondary sites.

k. Malignant neoplasm without specification of site

Code C80.1, Malignant (primary) neoplasm, unspecified, equates to Cancer, unspecified. This code should only be used when no determination can be made as to the primary site of a malignancy. This code should rarely be used in the inpatient setting.

l. Sequencing of neoplasm codes

1) Encounter for treatment of primary malignancy

If the reason for the encounter is for treatment of a primary malignancy, assign the malignancy as the principal/first-listed diagnosis. The primary site is to be sequenced first, followed by any metastatic sites.

2) Encounter for treatment of secondary malignancy

When an encounter is for a primary malignancy with metastasis and treatment is directed toward the metastatic (secondary) site(s) only, the metastatic site(s) is designated as the principal/first-listed diagnosis. The primary malignancy is coded as an additional code.

3) Malignant neoplasm in a pregnant patient

When a pregnant woman has a malignant neoplasm, a code from subcategory O9A.1-, Malignant neoplasm complicating pregnancy, childbirth, and the puerperium, should be sequenced first, followed by the appropriate code from Chapter 2 to indicate the type of neoplasm.

4) Encounter for complication associated with a neoplasm

When an encounter is for management of a complication associated with a neoplasm, such as dehydration, and the treatment is only for the complication, the complication is coded first, followed by the appropriate code(s) for the neoplasm.

The exception to this guideline is anemia. When the admission/encounter is for management of an anemia associated with the malignancy, and the treatment is only for anemia, the appropriate code for the malignancy is sequenced as the principal or first-listed diagnosis followed by code D63.0, Anemia in neoplastic disease.

5) Complication from surgical procedure for treatment of a neoplasm

When an encounter is for treatment of a complication resulting from a surgical procedure performed for the treatment of the neoplasm, designate the complication as the principal/first-listed diagnosis. See guideline regarding the coding of a current malignancy versus personal history to determine if the code for the neoplasm should also be assigned.

6) Pathologic fracture due to a neoplasm

When an encounter is for a pathological fracture due to a neoplasm, and the focus of treatment is the fracture, a code from subcategory M84.5, Pathological fracture in neoplastic disease, should be sequenced first, followed by the code for the neoplasm.

If the focus of treatment is the neoplasm with an associated pathological fracture, the neoplasm code should be sequenced first, followed by a code from M84.5 for the pathological fracture.

m. Current malignancy versus personal history of malignancy

When a primary malignancy has been excised but further treatment, such as an additional surgery for the malignancy, radiation therapy or chemotherapy is directed to that site, the primary malignancy code should be used until treatment is completed.

When a primary malignancy has been previously excised or eradicated from its site, there is no further treatment (of the malignancy) directed to that site, and there is no evidence of any existing primary malignancy, a code from category Z85, Personal history of malignant neoplasm, should be used to indicate the former site of the malignancy.

See Section I.C.21. Factors influencing health status and contact with health services, History (of)

n. Leukemia, Multiple Myeloma, and Malignant Plasma Cell Neoplasms in remission versus personal history

The categories for leukemia, and category C90, Multiple myeloma and malignant plasma cell neoplasms, have codes indicating whether or not the leukemia has achieved remission. There are also codes Z85.6, Personal history of leukemia, and Z85.79, Personal history of other malignant neoplasms of lymphoid, hematopoietic and related tissues. If the documentation is unclear, as to whether the leukemia has achieved remission, the provider should be queried.

See Section I.C.21. Factors influencing health status and contact with health services, History (of)

o. Aftercare following surgery for neoplasm

See Section I.C.21. Factors influencing health status and contact with health services, Aftercare

p. Follow-up care for completed treatment of a malignancy

See Section I.C.21. Factors influencing health status and contact with health services, Follow-up

q. Prophylactic organ removal for prevention of malignancy

See Section I.C. 21, Factors influencing health status and contact with health services, Prophylactic organ removal

r. Malignant neoplasm associated with transplanted organ

A malignant neoplasm of a transplanted organ should be coded as a transplant complication. Assign first the appropriate code from category T86.-, Complications of transplanted organs and tissue, followed by code C80.2, Malignant neoplasm associated with transplanted organ. Use an additional code for the specific malignancy.

Item 2–1 Neoplasm: Neo = new, plasm = growth, development, formation. This new growth (mass, tumor) can be malignant or benign, which is confirmed by the pathology report. Do not assign a code to a neoplasm until you review the pathology report. Certain CPT codes will specify benign or malignant lesion, so be certain the diagnosis code supports the procedure code.

CHAPTER 2

NEOPLASMS (C00-D49)

This chapter contains the following blocks:

C00-C14	Malignant neoplasms of lip, oral cavity and pharynx
C15-C26	Malignant neoplasms of digestive organs
C30-C39	Malignant neoplasms of respiratory and intrathoracic organs
C40-C41	Malignant neoplasms of bone and articular cartilage
C43-C44	Melanoma and other malignant neoplasms of skin
C45-C49	Malignant neoplasms of mesothelial and soft tissue
C50	Malignant neoplasms of breast
C51-C58	Malignant neoplasms of female genital organs
C60-C63	Malignant neoplasms of male genital organs
C64-C68	Malignant neoplasms of urinary tract
C69-C72	Malignant neoplasms of eye, brain and other parts of central nervous system
C73-C75	Malignant neoplasms of thyroid and other endocrine glands
C7A	Malignant neuroendocrine tumors
C7B	Secondary neuroendocrine tumors
C76-C80	Malignant neoplasms of ill-defined, other secondary and unspecified sites
C81-C96	Malignant neoplasms of lymphoid, hematopoietic and related tissue
D00-D09	In situ neoplasms
D10-D36	Benign neoplasms, except benign neuroendocrine tumors
D3A	Benign neuroendocrine tumors
D37-D48	Neoplasms of uncertain behavior, polycythemia vera and myelodysplastic syndromes
D49	Neoplasms of unspecified behavior

Notes: Functional activity

All neoplasms are classified in this chapter, whether they are functionally active or not. An additional code from Chapter 4 may be used, to identify functional activity associated with any neoplasm.

Morphology [Histology]

Chapter 2 classifies neoplasms primarily by site (topography), with broad groupings for behavior, malignant, in situ, benign, etc. The Table of Neoplasms should be used to identify the correct topography code. In a few cases, such as for malignant melanoma and certain neuroendocrine tumors, the morphology (histologic type) is included in the category and codes.

Primary malignant neoplasms overlapping site boundaries

A primary malignant neoplasm that overlaps two or more contiguous (next to each other) sites should be classified to the subcategory/code .8 ('overlapping lesion'), unless the combination is specifically indexed elsewhere. For multiple neoplasms of the same site that are not contiguous, such as tumors in different quadrants of the same breast, codes for each site should be assigned.

Malignant neoplasm of ectopic tissue

Malignant neoplasms of ectopic tissue are to be coded to the site mentioned, e.g., ectopic pancreatic malignant neoplasms are coded to pancreas, unspecified (C25.9).

MALIGNANT NEOPLASMS (C00-C96)

MALIGNANT NEOPLASMS, STATED OR PRESUMED TO BE PRIMARY (OF SPECIFIED SITES), AND CERTAIN SPECIFIED HISTOLOGIES, EXCEPT NEUROENDOCRINE, AND OF LYMPHOID, HEMATOPOIETIC AND RELATED TISSUE (C00-C75)

MALIGNANT NEOPLASMS OF LIP, ORAL CAVITY AND PHARYNX (C00-C14)

● **C00   Malignant neoplasm of lip**

Use additional code to identify:
alcohol abuse and dependence (F10.-)
history of tobacco dependence (Z87.891)
tobacco dependence (F17.-)
tobacco use (Z72.0)

> **Excludes1**   malignant melanoma of lip (C43.0)
> Merkel cell carcinoma of lip (C4A.0)
> other and unspecified malignant neoplasm of skin of lip (C44.0-)

C00.0   Malignant neoplasm of external upper lip
Malignant neoplasm of lipstick area of upper lip
Malignant neoplasm of upper lip NOS
Malignant neoplasm of vermilion border of upper lip

C00.1   Malignant neoplasm of external lower lip
Malignant neoplasm of lower lip NOS
Malignant neoplasm of lipstick area of lower lip
Malignant neoplasm of vermilion border of lower lip

C00.2   Malignant neoplasm of external lip, unspecified
Malignant neoplasm of vermilion border of lip NOS

C00.3   Malignant neoplasm of upper lip, inner aspect
Malignant neoplasm of buccal aspect of upper lip
Malignant neoplasm of frenulum of upper lip
Malignant neoplasm of mucosa of upper lip
Malignant neoplasm of oral aspect of upper lip

C00.4   Malignant neoplasm of lower lip, inner aspect
Malignant neoplasm of buccal aspect of lower lip
Malignant neoplasm of frenulum of lower lip
Malignant neoplasm of mucosa of lower lip
Malignant neoplasm of oral aspect of lower lip

C00.5   Malignant neoplasm of lip, unspecified, inner aspect
Malignant neoplasm of buccal aspect of lip, unspecified
Malignant neoplasm of frenulum of lip, unspecified
Malignant neoplasm of mucosa of lip, unspecified
Malignant neoplasm of oral aspect of lip, unspecified

C00.6   Malignant neoplasm of commissure of lip, unspecified
Commissure: Site of union of corresponding parts

C00.8   Malignant neoplasm of overlapping sites of lip

C00.9   Malignant neoplasm of lip, unspecified

CHAPTER 2 (C00-D49)

N Newborn Age: 0   P Pediatric Age: 0–17   M Maternity DX: 12–55   A Adult Age: 15–124   ♀ Females Only   ♂ Males Only
🔹 Complication\Comorbidity   🔸 Major C\C   (Ex.) CC/MCC Exclusions   🔹 Hospital-Acquired Condition

669

CHAPTER 2 (C00-D49)

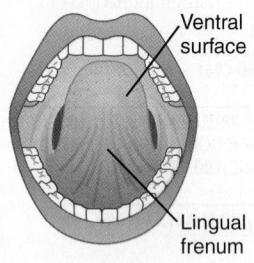

Figure 2-1 Anatomical structures of the mouth and lips. **A.** Transitional or vermilion borders. Lips are connected to the gums by frenulum. **B.** Dorsal surface. **C.** Ventral surface.

C01 Malignant neoplasm of base of tongue
Malignant neoplasm of dorsal surface of base of tongue
Malignant neoplasm of fixed part of tongue NOS
Malignant neoplasm of posterior third of tongue

Use additional code to identify:
alcohol abuse and dependence (F10.-)
history of tobacco dependence (Z87.891)
tobacco dependence (F17.-)
tobacco use (Z72.0)

● **C02 Malignant neoplasm of other and unspecified parts of tongue**
Use additional code to identify:
alcohol abuse and dependence (F10.-)
history of tobacco dependence (Z87.891)
tobacco dependence (F17.-)
tobacco use (Z72.0)

C02.0 Malignant neoplasm of dorsal surface of tongue
Malignant neoplasm of anterior two-thirds of tongue, dorsal surface
> **Excludes2** malignant neoplasm of dorsal surface of base of tongue (C01)

C02.1 Malignant neoplasm of border of tongue
Malignant neoplasm of tip of tongue

C02.2 Malignant neoplasm of ventral surface of tongue
Malignant neoplasm of anterior two-thirds of tongue, ventral surface
Malignant neoplasm of frenulum linguae

C02.3 Malignant neoplasm of anterior two-thirds of tongue, part unspecified
Malignant neoplasm of middle third of tongue NOS
Malignant neoplasm of mobile part of tongue NOS

C02.4 Malignant neoplasm of lingual tonsil
Lingual tonsil: Aggregation of lymph follicles at root of tongue
> **Excludes2** malignant neoplasm of tonsil NOS (C09.9)

C02.8 Malignant neoplasm of overlapping sites of tongue
Malignant neoplasm of two or more contiguous sites of tongue

C02.9 Malignant neoplasm of tongue, unspecified

● **C03 Malignant neoplasm of gum**
> **Includes** malignant neoplasm of alveolar (ridge) mucosa
> malignant neoplasm of gingiva

Use additional code to identify:
alcohol abuse and dependence (F10.-)
history of tobacco dependence (Z87.891)
tobacco dependence (F17.-)
tobacco use (Z72.0)
> **Excludes2** malignant odontogenic neoplasms (C41.0-C41.1)

C03.0 Malignant neoplasm of upper gum
C03.1 Malignant neoplasm of lower gum
C03.9 Malignant neoplasm of gum, unspecified

● **C04 Malignant neoplasm of floor of mouth**
Use additional code to identify:
alcohol abuse and dependence (F10.-)
history of tobacco dependence (Z87.891)
tobacco dependence (F17.-)
tobacco use (Z72.0)

C04.0 Malignant neoplasm of anterior floor of mouth
Malignant neoplasm of anterior to the premolar-canine junction

C04.1 Malignant neoplasm of lateral floor of mouth

C04.8 Malignant neoplasm of overlapping sites of floor of mouth

C04.9 Malignant neoplasm of floor of mouth, unspecified

● **C05 Malignant neoplasm of palate**
Use additional code to identify:
alcohol abuse and dependence (F10.-)
history of tobacco dependence (Z87.891)
tobacco dependence (F17.-)
tobacco use (Z72.0)
> **Excludes1** Kaposi's sarcoma of palate (C46.2)

C05.0 Malignant neoplasm of hard palate
C05.1 Malignant neoplasm of soft palate
> **Excludes2** malignant neoplasm of nasopharyngeal surface of soft palate (C11.3)

C05.2 Malignant neoplasm of uvula
C05.8 Malignant neoplasm of overlapping sites of palate
C05.9 Malignant neoplasm of palate, unspecified
Malignant neoplasm of roof of mouth

● **C06 Malignant neoplasm of other and unspecified parts of mouth**
Use additional code to identify:
alcohol abuse and dependence (F10.-)
history of tobacco dependence (Z87.891)
tobacco dependence (F17.-)
tobacco use (Z72.0)

C06.0 Malignant neoplasm of cheek mucosa
Malignant neoplasm of buccal mucosa NOS
Malignant neoplasm of internal cheek

C06.1 Malignant neoplasm of vestibule of mouth
Malignant neoplasm of buccal sulcus (upper) (lower)
Malignant neoplasm of labial sulcus (upper) (lower)

C06.2 Malignant neoplasm of retromolar area

● **C06.8 Malignant neoplasm of overlapping sites of other and unspecified parts of mouth**

C06.80 Malignant neoplasm of overlapping sites of unspecified parts of mouth

C06.89 Malignant neoplasm of overlapping sites of other parts of mouth
'book leaf' neoplasm [ventral surface of tongue and floor of mouth]

C06.9 Malignant neoplasm of mouth, unspecified
Malignant neoplasm of minor salivary gland, unspecified site
Malignant neoplasm of oral cavity NOS

▶ New   ➠ Revised   ~~deleted~~ Deleted   Excludes 1   Excludes 2   Includes   Use additional   Code first   Code also   Key words

OGCR Official Guidelines   ● Unacceptable Principal Diagnosis   X Assign placeholder X   ● Use Additional Character(s)   ▶ Manifestation Code   **Coding Clinic**

Parotid gland

Sublingual gland

Submandibular gland

Figure 2-2 Major salivary glands.

C07　Malignant neoplasm of parotid gland
　　Use additional code to identify:
　　　alcohol abuse and dependence (F10.-)
　　　exposure to environmental tobacco smoke (Z77.22)
　　　exposure to tobacco smoke in the perinatal period (P96.81)
　　　history of tobacco dependence (Z87.891)
　　　occupational exposure to environmental tobacco smoke
　　　　(Z57.31)
　　　tobacco dependence (F17.-)
　　　tobacco use (Z72.0)

●**C08　Malignant neoplasm of other and unspecified major salivary glands**
　　　Includes　malignant neoplasm of salivary ducts
　　Use additional code to identify:
　　　alcohol abuse and dependence (F10.-)
　　　exposure to environmental tobacco smoke (Z77.22)
　　　exposure to tobacco smoke in the perinatal period (P96.81)
　　　history of tobacco dependence (Z87.891)
　　　occupational exposure to environmental tobacco smoke
　　　　(Z57.31)
　　　tobacco dependence (F17.-)
　　　tobacco use (Z72.0)
　　　Excludes1　malignant neoplasms of specified minor salivary
　　　　　　　　　glands which are classified according to their
　　　　　　　　　anatomical location
　　　Excludes2　malignant neoplasms of minor salivary glands
　　　　　　　　　NOS (C06.9)
　　　　　　　　　malignant neoplasm of parotid gland (C07)
　　C08.0　**Malignant neoplasm of submandibular gland**
　　　　　Malignant neoplasm of submaxillary gland
　　C08.1　**Malignant neoplasm of sublingual gland**
　　C08.9　**Malignant neoplasm of major salivary gland, unspecified**
　　　　　Malignant neoplasm of salivary gland (major) NOS

　　★**(See Plate 61 on page 73.)**

●**C09　Malignant neoplasm of tonsil**
　　Use additional code to identify:
　　　alcohol abuse and dependence (F10.-)
　　　exposure to environmental tobacco smoke (Z77.22)
　　　exposure to tobacco smoke in the perinatal period (P96.81)
　　　history of tobacco dependence (Z87.891)
　　　occupational exposure to environmental tobacco smoke
　　　　(Z57.31)
　　　tobacco dependence (F17.-)
　　　tobacco use (Z72.0)
　　　Excludes2　malignant neoplasm of lingual tonsil (C02.4)
　　　　　　　　　malignant neoplasm of pharyngeal tonsil (C11.1)
　　C09.0　**Malignant neoplasm of tonsillar fossa**
　　　　　*Surface of palatine (two masses of lymphatic tissue on sides of
　　　　　　throat) tonsils*
　　C09.1　**Malignant neoplasm of tonsillar pillar (anterior) (posterior)**
　　　　　*Extension from palatine (two masses of lymphatic tissue on
　　　　　　sides of throat) tonsils*
　　C09.8　**Malignant neoplasm of overlapping sites of tonsil**
　　C09.9　**Malignant neoplasm of tonsil, unspecified**
　　　　　Malignant neoplasm of tonsil NOS
　　　　　Malignant neoplasm of faucial tonsils
　　　　　Malignant neoplasm of palatine tonsils

●**C10　Malignant neoplasm of oropharynx**
　　　Area of throat at back of mouth
　　Use additional code to identify:
　　　alcohol abuse and dependence (F10.-)
　　　exposure to environmental tobacco smoke (Z77.22)
　　　exposure to tobacco smoke in the perinatal period (P96.81)
　　　history of tobacco dependence (Z87.891)
　　　occupational exposure to environmental tobacco smoke
　　　　(Z57.31)
　　　tobacco dependence (F17.-)
　　　tobacco use (Z72.0)
　　　Excludes2　malignant neoplasm of tonsil (C09.-)
　　C10.0　**Malignant neoplasm of vallecula**
　　　　　Vallecula, depression or furrow
　　C10.1　**Malignant neoplasm of anterior surface of epiglottis**
　　　　　Malignant neoplasm of epiglottis, free border [margin]
　　　　　Malignant neoplasm of glossoepiglottic fold(s)
　　　　　Excludes2　malignant neoplasm of epiglottis
　　　　　　　　　　　(suprahyoid portion) NOS (C32.1)
　　C10.2　**Malignant neoplasm of lateral wall of oropharynx**
　　C10.3　**Malignant neoplasm of posterior wall of oropharynx**
　　C10.4　**Malignant neoplasm of branchial cleft**
　　　　　*Congenital slitlike openings formed between branchial arches
　　　　　　pharyngeal groove*
　　　　　Malignant neoplasm of branchial cyst [site of neoplasm]
　　C10.8　**Malignant neoplasm of overlapping sites of oropharynx**
　　　　　Malignant neoplasm of junctional region of oropharynx
　　C10.9　**Malignant neoplasm of oropharynx, unspecified**

●**C11　Malignant neoplasm of nasopharynx**
　　Use additional code to identify:
　　　exposure to environmental tobacco smoke (Z77.22)
　　　exposure to tobacco smoke in the perinatal period (P96.81)
　　　history of tobacco dependence (Z87.891)
　　　occupational exposure to environmental tobacco smoke
　　　　(Z57.31)
　　　tobacco dependence (F17.-)
　　　tobacco use (Z72.0)
　　C11.0　**Malignant neoplasm of superior wall of nasopharynx**
　　　　　Part of pharynx that lies above soft palate
　　　　　Malignant neoplasm of roof of nasopharynx
　　C11.1　**Malignant neoplasm of posterior wall of nasopharynx**
　　　　　Malignant neoplasm of adenoid
　　　　　Malignant neoplasm of pharyngeal tonsil
　　C11.2　**Malignant neoplasm of lateral wall of nasopharynx**
　　　　　Malignant neoplasm of fossa of Rosenmüller
　　　　　Malignant neoplasm of opening of auditory tube
　　　　　Malignant neoplasm of pharyngeal recess
　　C11.3　**Malignant neoplasm of anterior wall of nasopharynx**
　　　　　Malignant neoplasm of floor of nasopharynx
　　　　　Malignant neoplasm of nasopharyngeal (anterior)
　　　　　　(posterior) surface of soft palate
　　　　　Malignant neoplasm of posterior margin of nasal
　　　　　　choana
　　　　　Malignant neoplasm of posterior margin of nasal
　　　　　　septum
　　C11.8　**Malignant neoplasm of overlapping sites of nasopharynx**
　　C11.9　**Malignant neoplasm of nasopharynx, unspecified**
　　　　　Malignant neoplasm of nasopharyngeal wall NOS

C12　Malignant neoplasm of pyriform sinus
　　　Malignant neoplasm of pyriform fossa
　　Use additional code to identify:
　　　exposure to environmental tobacco smoke (Z77.22)
　　　exposure to tobacco smoke in the perinatal period (P96.81)
　　　history of tobacco dependence (Z87.891)
　　　occupational exposure to environmental tobacco smoke
　　　　(Z57.31)
　　　tobacco dependence (F17.-)
　　　tobacco use (Z72.0)

CHAPTER 2 (C00-D49)

N Newborn Age: 0　　**P** Pediatric Age: 0–17　　**M** Maternity DX: 12–55　　**A** Adult Age: 15–124　　♀ Females Only　　♂ Males Only

 Complication\Comorbidity　　 Major C\C　　(Ex) CC/MCC Exclusions　　Hospital-Acquired Condition

671

CHAPTER 2 (C00-D49)

● C13   **Malignant neoplasm of hypopharynx**

Use additional code to identify:
exposure to environmental tobacco smoke (Z77.22)
exposure to tobacco smoke in the perinatal period (P96.81)
history of tobacco dependence (Z87.891)
occupational exposure to environmental tobacco smoke (Z57.31)
tobacco dependence (F17.-)
tobacco use (Z72.0)

Excludes2   malignant neoplasm of pyriform sinus (C12)

C13.0   **Malignant neoplasm of postcricoid region**
Behind the cricoid cartilage of neck

C13.1   **Malignant neoplasm of aryepiglottic fold, hypopharyngeal aspect**
Arytenoepiglottic fold, triangular opening between side of epiglottis and apex of arytenoid cartilage
Malignant neoplasm of aryepiglottic fold, marginal zone
Malignant neoplasm of aryepiglottic fold NOS
Malignant neoplasm of interarytenoid fold, marginal zone
Malignant neoplasm of interarytenoid fold NOS

    Excludes2   malignant neoplasm of aryepiglottic fold or interarytenoid fold, laryngeal aspect (C32.1)

C13.2   **Malignant neoplasm of posterior wall of hypopharynx**

C13.8   **Malignant neoplasm of overlapping sites of hypopharynx**

C13.9   **Malignant neoplasm of hypopharynx, unspecified**
Malignant neoplasm of hypopharyngeal wall NOS

● C14   **Malignant neoplasm of other and ill-defined sites in the lip, oral cavity and pharynx**

Use additional code to identify:
alcohol abuse and dependence (F10.-)
exposure to environmental tobacco smoke (Z77.22)
exposure to tobacco smoke in the perinatal period (P96.81)
history of tobacco dependence (Z87.891)
occupational exposure to environmental tobacco smoke (Z57.31)
tobacco dependence (F17.-)
tobacco use (Z72.0)

Excludes1   malignant neoplasm of oral cavity NOS (C06.9)

C14.0   **Malignant neoplasm of pharynx, unspecified**

C14.2   **Malignant neoplasm of Waldeyer's ring**

C14.8   **Malignant neoplasm of overlapping sites of lip, oral cavity and pharynx**
Primary malignant neoplasm of two or more contiguous sites of lip, oral cavity and pharynx

    Excludes1   'book leaf' neoplasm [ventral surface of tongue and floor of mouth] (C06.89)

MALIGNANT NEOPLASM OF DIGESTIVE ORGANS (C15-C26)

Excludes1   Kaposi's sarcoma of gastrointestinal sites (C46.4)

Excludes2   gastrointestinal stromal tumors (C49.A-)

● C15   **Malignant neoplasms of esophagus**

Use additional code to identify:
alcohol abuse and dependence (F10.-)

(Ex) **For category C15 CC codes:** See PDX Collection 253

C15.3   **Malignant neoplasm of upper third of esophagus** 🔍

C15.4   **Malignant neoplasm of middle third of esophagus** 🔍

C15.5   **Malignant neoplasm of lower third of esophagus** 🔍

    Excludes1   malignant neoplasm of cardio-esophageal junction (C16.0)

C15.8   **Malignant neoplasm of overlapping sites of esophagus** 🔍

C15.9   **Malignant neoplasm of esophagus, unspecified** 🔍

● C16   **Malignant neoplasm of stomach**

Use additional code to identify:
alcohol abuse and dependence (F10.-)

Excludes2   malignant carcinoid tumor of the stomach (C7A.092)

(Ex) **For category C16 CC codes:** See PDX Collection 254

C16.0   **Malignant neoplasm of cardia** 🔍
Malignant neoplasm of cardiac orifice
Malignant neoplasm of cardio-esophageal junction
Malignant neoplasm of esophagus and stomach
Malignant neoplasm of gastro-esophageal junction

C16.1   **Malignant neoplasm of fundus of stomach** 🔍

C16.2   **Malignant neoplasm of body of stomach** 🔍

C16.3   **Malignant neoplasm of pyloric antrum** 🔍
Malignant neoplasm of gastric antrum

C16.4   **Malignant neoplasm of pylorus** 🔍
Malignant neoplasm of prepylorus
Malignant neoplasm of pyloric canal

C16.5   **Malignant neoplasm of lesser curvature of stomach, unspecified** 🔍
Malignant neoplasm of lesser curvature of stomach, not classifiable to C16.1-C16.4

C16.6   **Malignant neoplasm of greater curvature of stomach, unspecified** 🔍
Malignant neoplasm of greater curvature of stomach, not classifiable to C16.0-C16.4

C16.8   **Malignant neoplasm of overlapping sites of stomach** 🔍

C16.9   **Malignant neoplasm of stomach, unspecified** 🔍
Gastric cancer NOS

Figure 2-3 The esophagus is the muscular tube that connects the pharynx and the stomach. The 10 inch (25 cm) long esophagus is divided into three parts: **cervical, thoracic,** and **abdominal.**

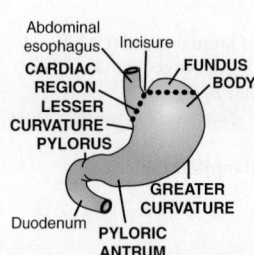

Figure 2-4 Parts of the stomach.

Item 2–2 The esophagus opens into the stomach through the **cardiac orifice,** also called the **cardioesophageal junction.** The **cardia** is adjacent to the cardiac orifice. The stomach widens into the **greater** and **lesser curvatures.** The **pyloric antrum** precedes the **pylorus,** which opens to the duodenum.

▶ New   ➠ Revised   ~~deleted~~ Deleted   Excludes 1   Excludes 2   Includes   Use additional   Code first   Code also   Key words

OGCR Official Guidelines   ● Unacceptable Principal Diagnosis   X Assign placeholder X   ● Use Additional Character(s)   ▌ Manifestation Code   **Coding Clinic**

672

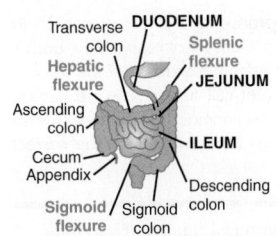

Figure 2-5 Small intestine and colon.

● **C17 Malignant neoplasm of small intestine**
    Excludes1   malignant carcinoid tumor of the small intestine
    (C7A.01)

C17.0 Malignant neoplasm of duodenum 🔖
    First or proximal portion of small intestine, extending from pylorus to jejunum
    Ⓔ See PDX Collection 255

C17.1 Malignant neoplasm of jejunum 🔖
    Second section of small intestine, extending from duodenum to ileum
    Ⓔ See PDX Collection 256

C17.2 Malignant neoplasm of ileum 🔖
    Distal and longest portion of small intestine, extending from jejunum to cecum
        Excludes1   malignant neoplasm of ileocecal valve
        (C18.0)
    Ⓔ See PDX Collection 257

C17.3 Meckel's diverticulum, malignant 🔖
    Appendage of ileum
        Excludes1   Meckel's diverticulum, congenital (Q43.0)
    Ⓔ See PDX Collection 258

C17.8 Malignant neoplasm of overlapping sites of small intestine 🔖
    Ⓔ See PDX Collection 259

C17.9 Malignant neoplasm of small intestine, unspecified 🔖
    Ⓔ See PDX Collection 259

● **C18 Malignant neoplasm of colon**
    Excludes1   malignant carcinoid tumors of the colon (C7A.02)

C18.0 Malignant neoplasm of cecum 🔖
    First section of large intestine
    Malignant neoplasm of ileocecal valve
    Ⓔ See PDX Collection 260

C18.1 Malignant neoplasm of appendix 🔖
    Blind ended tube connected to the cecum; AKA vermiform appendix
    Ⓔ See PDX Collection 261

C18.2 Malignant neoplasm of ascending colon 🔖
    Ascending colon is between cecum and right colic flexure
    Ⓔ See PDX Collection 262

C18.3 Malignant neoplasm of hepatic flexure 🔖
    A flexure is a bending in a structure or organ. Note the three flexures illustrated in Figure 2–5.
    Ⓔ See PDX Collection 263

C18.4 Malignant neoplasm of transverse colon 🔖
    Portion of colon that runs transversely across upper part of abdomen, between right and left colic flexures
    Ⓔ See PDX Collection 264

C18.5 Malignant neoplasm of splenic flexure 🔖
    Bend at junction of transverse and descending colon
    Ⓔ See PDX Collection 265

C18.6 Malignant neoplasm of descending colon 🔖
    Portion between left colic flexure and sigmoid colon at pelvic brim; AKA iliac colon
    Ⓔ See PDX Collection 266

C18.7 Malignant neoplasm of sigmoid colon 🔖
    S-shaped part of colon extending from pelvic brim to third segment of sacrum
    Malignant neoplasm of sigmoid (flexure)
        Excludes1   malignant neoplasm of rectosigmoid
        junction (C19)
    Ⓔ See PDX Collection 267

C18.8 Malignant neoplasm of overlapping sites of colon 🔖
    Ⓔ See PDX Collection 268

C18.9 Malignant neoplasm of colon, unspecified 🔖
    Malignant neoplasm of large intestine NOS
    Ⓔ See PDX Collection 268

C19 Malignant neoplasm of rectosigmoid junction 🔖
    Malignant neoplasm of colon with rectum
    Malignant neoplasm of rectosigmoid (colon)
        Excludes1   malignant carcinoid tumors of the colon
        (C7A.02-)
    Ⓔ See PDX Collection 269

C20 Malignant neoplasm of rectum 🔖
    Malignant neoplasm of rectal ampulla
        Excludes1   malignant carcinoid tumor of the rectum
        (C7A.026)
    Ⓔ See PDX Collection 270

● **C21 Malignant neoplasm of anus and anal canal**
        Excludes2   malignant carcinoid tumors of the colon
        (C7A.02-)
        malignant melanoma of anal margin (C43.51)
        malignant melanoma of anal skin (C43.51)
        malignant melanoma of perianal skin (C43.51)
        other and unspecified malignant neoplasm of
            anal margin (C44.500, C44.510, C44.520,
            C44.590)
        other and unspecified malignant neoplasm
            of anal skin (C44.500, C44.510, C44.520,
            C44.590)
        other and unspecified malignant neoplasm of
            perianal skin (C44.500, C44.510, C44.520,
            C44.590)
    Ⓔ For category C21 CC codes C21.0-C21.1: See PDX Collection 271
       For category C21 CC codes C21.2-C21.8: See PDX Collection 272

C21.0 Malignant neoplasm of anus, unspecified 🔖

C21.1 Malignant neoplasm of anal canal 🔖
    Terminal part of large intestine
    Malignant neoplasm of anal sphincter

C21.2 Malignant neoplasm of cloacogenic zone 🔖

C21.8 Malignant neoplasm of overlapping sites of rectum, anus and anal canal 🔖
    Malignant neoplasm of anorectal junction
    Malignant neoplasm of anorectum
    Primary malignant neoplasm of two or more
        contiguous sites of rectum, anus and anal canal

CHAPTER 2 (C00-D49)

N Newborn Age: 0   **P** Pediatric Age: 0–17   **M** Maternity DX: 12–55   **A** Adult Age: 15–124   ♀ Females Only   ♂ Males Only

🔖 Complication\Comorbidity   🔖 Major C\C   Ⓔ CC/MCC Exclusions   🔖 Hospital-Acquired Condition

673

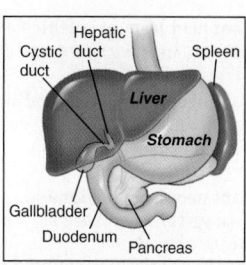

Figure 2-6 Diagram of liver, gallbladder, hepatic duct, pancreas, and spleen. (From Thibodeau and Patton: Anatomy and Physiology, ed 7, Mosby, 2010)

Item 2-3 Islets of Langerhans (endocrine producing cells comprising 1% to 2% of the pancreatic mass) make and secrete hormones that regulate the body's production of insulin, glucagon, and stomach acid. Breakdown of the insulin-producing cells can cause diabetes mellitus. Islet cell tumors can be benign or malignant and include glucagonomas, insulinomas, gastrinomas, and neuroendocrine tumor. The neoplasm table must be consulted for the correct neoplasm code.

Figure 2-7 Paranasal sinuses. (From Buck CJ: Step-by-Step Medical Coding, ed 2016, St. Louis, Elsevier, 2016)

● **C22 Malignant neoplasm of liver and intrahepatic bile ducts**
Intrahepatic: Within liver
Use additional code to identify:
    alcohol abuse and dependence (F10.-)
    hepatitis B (B16.-, B18.0-B18.1) hepatitis C (B17.1-, B18.2)
> **Excludes1**   malignant neoplasm of biliary tract NOS (C24.9)
>   secondary malignant neoplasm of liver and intrahepatic bile duct (C78.7)

Ⓔ **For category C22 CC codes:** See PDX Collection 273

C22.0 Liver cell carcinoma 🔑
Hepatocellular carcinoma
Hepatoma

C22.1 Intrahepatic bile duct carcinoma 🔑
Cholangiocarcinoma
Adenocarcinoma (cancer that originates in glandular tissue) arising from epithelium of intrahepatic bile ducts
> **Excludes1**   malignant neoplasm of hepatic duct (C24.0)

C22.2 Hepatoblastoma 🔑
Malignant intrahepatic tumor

C22.3 Angiosarcoma of liver 🔑
Kupffer cell sarcoma

C22.4 Other sarcomas of liver 🔑

C22.7 Other specified carcinomas of liver 🔑

C22.8 Malignant neoplasm of liver, primary, unspecified as to type 🔑

C22.9 Malignant neoplasm of liver, not specified as primary or secondary 🔑

  C23 Malignant neoplasm of gallbladder 🔑
Ⓔ See PDX Collection 274

● **C24 Malignant neoplasm of other and unspecified parts of biliary tract**
> **Excludes1**   malignant neoplasm of intrahepatic bile duct (C22.1)

C24.0 Malignant neoplasm of extrahepatic bile duct 🔑 .
Extrahepatic = outside the liver
Malignant neoplasm of biliary duct or passage NOS
Malignant neoplasm of common bile duct
Malignant neoplasm of cystic duct
Malignant neoplasm of hepatic duct
Ⓔ See PDX Collection 275

C24.1 Malignant neoplasm of ampulla of Vater 🔑
Union of pancreatic duct and common bile duct
Ⓔ See PDX Collection 276

C24.8 Malignant neoplasm of overlapping sites of biliary tract 🔑
Malignant neoplasm involving both intrahepatic and extrahepatic bile ducts
Primary malignant neoplasm of two or more contiguous sites of biliary tract
Ⓔ See PDX Collection 277

C24.9 Malignant neoplasm of biliary tract, unspecified 🔑
Ⓔ See PDX Collection 277

● **C25 Malignant neoplasm of pancreas**
Check documentation for specific site.
Code also exocrine pancreatic insufficiency (K86.81)
Use additional code to identify:
    alcohol abuse and dependence (F10.-)
Ⓔ **For category C25 CC codes:** See PDX Collection 278

C25.0 Malignant neoplasm of head of pancreas 🔑
C25.1 Malignant neoplasm of body of pancreas 🔑
C25.2 Malignant neoplasm of tail of pancreas 🔑
C25.3 Malignant neoplasm of pancreatic duct 🔑
C25.4 Malignant neoplasm of endocrine pancreas 🔑
Malignant neoplasm of islets of Langerhans
That part of the pancreas that acts as endocrine gland and consists of islets of Langerhans
Use additional code to identify any functional activity.

C25.7 Malignant neoplasm of other parts of pancreas 🔑
Malignant neoplasm of neck of pancreas
C25.8 Malignant neoplasm of overlapping sites of pancreas 🔑
C25.9 Malignant neoplasm of pancreas, unspecified 🔑

● **C26 Malignant neoplasm of other and ill-defined digestive organs**
> **Excludes1**   malignant neoplasm of peritoneum and retroperitoneum (C48.-)

C26.0 Malignant neoplasm of intestinal tract, part unspecified
Malignant neoplasm of intestine NOS
C26.1 Malignant neoplasm of spleen
> **Excludes1**   Hodgkin lymphoma (C81.-)
>   non-Hodgkin lymphoma (C82-C85)

C26.9 Malignant neoplasm of ill-defined sites within the digestive system
Malignant neoplasm of alimentary canal or tract NOS
Malignant neoplasm of gastrointestinal tract NOS
> **Excludes1**   malignant neoplasm of abdominal NOS (C76.2)
>   malignant neoplasm of intra-abdominal NOS (C76.2)

▶ New   ⇒ Revised   ~~deleted~~ Deleted   Excludes 1   Excludes 2   Includes   Use additional   Code first   Code also   Key words
OGCR Official Guidelines   ● Unacceptable Principal Diagnosis   X Assign placeholder X   ● Use Additional Character(s)   ❱ Manifestation Code   **Coding Clinic**

CHAPTER 2 (C00-D49)

MALIGNANT NEOPLASMS OF RESPIRATORY AND INTRATHORACIC ORGANS (C30-C39)

Includes	malignant neoplasm of middle ear	
Excludes1	mesothelioma (C45.-)	

● **C30   Malignant neoplasm of nasal cavity and middle ear**

C30.0   Malignant neoplasm of nasal cavity
Malignant neoplasm of cartilage of nose
Malignant neoplasm of nasal concha
Malignant neoplasm of internal nose
Malignant neoplasm of septum of nose
Malignant neoplasm of vestibule of nose
Anterior part of nasal cavity

Excludes1   malignant neoplasm of nasal bone (C41.0)
malignant neoplasm of nose NOS (C76.0)
malignant neoplasm of olfactory bulb (C72.2-)
malignant neoplasm of posterior margin of nasal septum and choana (C11.3)
malignant melanoma of skin of nose (C43.31)
malignant neoplasm of turbinates (C41.0)
other and unspecified malignant neoplasm of skin of nose C44.301, C44.311, C44.321, C44.391)

C30.1   Malignant neoplasm of middle ear
Malignant neoplasm of antrum tympanicum
Boney cavity or chamber
Malignant neoplasm of auditory tube
Malignant neoplasm of eustachian tube
Malignant neoplasm of inner ear
Malignant neoplasm of mastoid air cells
Malignant neoplasm of tympanic cavity

Excludes1   malignant neoplasm of auricular canal (external) (C43.2-, C44.2-)
malignant neoplasm of bone of ear (meatus) (C41.0)
malignant neoplasm of cartilage of ear (C49.0)
malignant melanoma of skin of (external) ear (C43.2-)
other and unspecified malignant neoplasm of skin of (external) ear (C44.2-)

● **C31   Malignant neoplasm of accessory sinuses**
Paired sinuses in bones of face

C31.0   Malignant neoplasm of maxillary sinus
Malignant neoplasm of antrum (Highmore) (maxillary)

C31.1   Malignant neoplasm of ethmoidal sinus

C31.2   Malignant neoplasm of frontal sinus

C31.3   Malignant neoplasm of sphenoid sinus

C31.8   Malignant neoplasm of overlapping sites of accessory sinuses

C31.9   Malignant neoplasm of accessory sinus, unspecified

● **C32   Malignant neoplasm of larynx**
Use additional code to identify:
alcohol abuse and dependence (F10.-)
exposure to environmental tobacco smoke (Z77.22)
exposure to tobacco smoke in the perinatal period (P96.81)
history of tobacco dependence (Z87.891)
occupational exposure to environmental tobacco smoke (Z57.31)
tobacco dependence (F17.-)
tobacco use (Z72.0)

C32.0   Malignant neoplasm of glottis
Vocal apparatus of larynx, consisting of true vocal cords (plicae vocales) and opening between them (rima glottidis)
Malignant neoplasm of intrinsic larynx
Malignant neoplasm of laryngeal commissure (anterior) (posterior)
Malignant neoplasm of vocal cord (true) NOS
True vocal cords ("lower vocal folds") produce vocalization when air from the lungs passes between them. Check your documentation. Code C32.1 is for malignant neoplasm of the false vocal cords.

C32.1   Malignant neoplasm of supraglottis
Area of pharynx above glottis
Malignant neoplasm of aryepiglottic fold or interarytenoid fold, laryngeal aspect
Malignant neoplasm of epiglottis (suprahyoid portion) NOS
Malignant neoplasm of extrinsic larynx
Malignant neoplasm of false vocal cord
False vocal cords ("upper vocal folds") are not involved in vocalization. Check your documentation. Code C32.0 is for true vocal cords.
Malignant neoplasm of posterior (laryngeal) surface of epiglottis
Malignant neoplasm of ventricular bands

Excludes2   malignant neoplasm of anterior surface of epiglottis (C10.1)
malignant neoplasm of aryepiglottic fold or interarytenoid fold, hypopharyngeal aspect (C13.1)
malignant neoplasm of aryepiglottic fold or interarytenoid fold, marginal zone (C13.1)
malignant neoplasm of aryepiglottic fold or interarytenoid fold NOS (C13.1)

C32.2   Malignant neoplasm of subglottis
Lowest part of larynx from just below vocal cords down to top of trachea

C32.3   Malignant neoplasm of laryngeal cartilage
Cartilages of larynx, including cricoid, thyroid, and epiglottic, and two each of arytenoid, corniculate, and cuneiform

C32.8   Malignant neoplasm of overlapping sites of larynx

C32.9   Malignant neoplasm of larynx, unspecified

● **C33   Malignant neoplasm of trachea** 🦠
Use additional code to identify:
exposure to environmental tobacco smoke (Z77.22)
exposure to tobacco smoke in the perinatal period (P96.81)
history of tobacco dependence (Z87.891)
occupational exposure to environmental tobacco smoke (Z57.31)
tobacco dependence (F17.-)
tobacco use (Z72.0)
(Ex) See PDX Collection 279

CHAPTER 2 (C00-D49)

N Newborn Age: 0   **P** Pediatric Age: 0–17   **M** Maternity DX: 12–55   **A** Adult Age: 15–124   ♀ Females Only   ♂ Males Only

🦠 Complication\Comorbidity   🦠 Major C\C   (Ex) CC/MCC Exclusions   🦠 Hospital-Acquired Condition

675

● **C34**   **Malignant neoplasm of bronchus and lung**
     Use additional code to identify:
       exposure to environmental tobacco smoke (Z77.22)
       exposure to tobacco smoke in the perinatal period (P96.81)
       history of tobacco dependence (Z87.891)
       occupational exposure to environmental tobacco smoke
         (Z57.31)
       tobacco dependence (F17.-)
       tobacco use (Z72.0)

     Excludes1   Kaposi's sarcoma of lung (C46.5-)
                malignant carcinoid tumor of the bronchus and
                  lung (C7A.090)

● **C34.0**   **Malignant neoplasm of main bronchus**
       Malignant neoplasm of carina
         Ridgelike structure
       Malignant neoplasm of hilus (of lung)
         Anatomic depression or pit
       (Ex) **For category C34.0 CC codes:** See PDX Collection 280

     C34.00   **Malignant neoplasm of unspecified main**
               bronchus

     C34.01   **Malignant neoplasm of right main bronchus**

     C34.02   **Malignant neoplasm of left main bronchus**

● **C34.1**   **Malignant neoplasm of upper lobe, bronchus or lung**
       (Ex) **For category C34.1 CC codes:** See PDX Collection 281

     C34.10   **Malignant neoplasm of unspecified bronchus**
               or lung

     C34.11   **Malignant neoplasm of upper lobe, right**
               bronchus or lung

     C34.12   **Malignant neoplasm of upper lobe, left**
               bronchus or lung

   C34.2   **Malignant neoplasm of middle lobe, bronchus or**
      lung
       (Ex) See PDX Collection 282

● **C34.3**   **Malignant neoplasm of lower lobe, bronchus or lung**
       (Ex) **For category C34.4 CC codes:** See PDX Collection 283

     C34.30   **Malignant neoplasm of lower lobe, unspecified**
               bronchus or lung

     C34.31   **Malignant neoplasm of lower lobe, right**
               bronchus or lung

     C34.32   **Malignant neoplasm of lower lobe, left**
               bronchus or lung

● **C34.8**   **Malignant neoplasm of overlapping sites of bronchus**
      and lung
       (Ex) **For category C34.8 CC codes:** See PDX Collection 284

     C34.80   **Malignant neoplasm of overlapping sites**
               of unspecified bronchus and lung

     C34.81   **Malignant neoplasm of overlapping sites of**
               right bronchus and lung

     C34.82   **Malignant neoplasm of overlapping sites of left**
               bronchus and lung

● **C34.9**   **Malignant neoplasm of unspecified part of bronchus or**
      lung
       (Ex) **For category C34.9 CC codes:** See PDX Collection 284

     C34.90   **Malignant neoplasm of unspecified part of**
               unspecified bronchus or lung
               Lung cancer NOS

     C34.91   **Malignant neoplasm of unspecified part of**
               right bronchus or lung

     C34.92   **Malignant neoplasm of unspecified part of left**
               bronchus or lung

● **C37**   **Malignant neoplasm of thymus**
     Excludes1   malignant carcinoid tumor of the thymus
                  (C7A.091)
     (Ex) See PDX Collection 285

● **C38**   **Malignant neoplasm of heart, mediastinum and pleura**
     Excludes1   mesothelioma (C45.-)
     (Ex) **For category C38 CC codes unless otherwise indicated:** See PDX Collection 287

   C38.0   **Malignant neoplasm of heart**
       Malignant neoplasm of pericardium
      Excludes1   malignant neoplasm of great vessels
                   (C49.3)
       (Ex) See PDX Collection 286

   C38.1   **Malignant neoplasm of anterior mediastinum**

   C38.2   **Malignant neoplasm of posterior mediastinum**

   C38.3   **Malignant neoplasm of mediastinum,**
      part unspecified

   C38.4   **Malignant neoplasm of pleura**
       (Ex) See PDX Collection 288

   C38.8   **Malignant neoplasm of overlapping sites of heart,**
      mediastinum and pleura
       Pleura are comprised of serous membrane that lines the
         thoracic cavity (parietal) and covers the lungs (visceral).

● **C39**   **Malignant neoplasm of other and ill-defined sites in the**
     respiratory system and intrathoracic organs
     Intrathoracic: within thorax/chest
     Use additional code to identify:
       exposure to environmental tobacco smoke (Z77.22)
       exposure to tobacco smoke in the perinatal period (P96.81)
       history of tobacco dependence (Z87.891)
       occupational exposure to environmental tobacco smoke
         (Z57.31)
       tobacco dependence (F17.-)
       tobacco use (Z72.0)

     Excludes1   intrathoracic malignant neoplasm NOS (C76.1)
                thoracic malignant neoplasm NOS (C76.1)

   C39.0   **Malignant neoplasm of upper respiratory tract,**
      part unspecified

   C39.9   **Malignant neoplasm of lower respiratory tract,**
      part unspecified
       Malignant neoplasm of respiratory tract NOS

MALIGNANT NEOPLASMS OF BONE AND ARTICULAR CARTILAGE (C40-C41)

     Includes   malignant neoplasm of cartilage (articular) (joint)
                 malignant neoplasm of periosteum
     Excludes1   malignant neoplasm of bone marrow NOS (C96.9)
                 malignant neoplasm of synovia (C49.-)

● **C40**   **Malignant neoplasm of bone and articular cartilage of limbs**
     Use additional code to identify major osseous defect, if
     applicable (M89.7-)

● **C40.0**   **Malignant neoplasm of scapula and long bones of upper**
      limb
       (Ex) **For category C40.0 CC codes:** See PDX Collection 289

     C40.00   **Malignant neoplasm of scapula and long bones**
               of unspecified upper limb

     C40.01   **Malignant neoplasm of scapula and long bones**
               of right upper limb

     C40.02   **Malignant neoplasm of scapula and long bones**
               of left upper limb

● **C40.1**   **Malignant neoplasm of short bones of upper limb**
       (Ex) **For category C40.1 CC codes:** See PDX Collection 290

     C40.10   **Malignant neoplasm of short bones**
               of unspecified upper limb

     C40.11   **Malignant neoplasm of short bones of right**
               upper limb

     C40.12   **Malignant neoplasm of short bones of left**
               upper limb

▶ New   ⇒ Revised   ~~deleted~~ Deleted   Excludes 1   Excludes 2   Includes   Use additional   Code first   Code also   Key words
OGCR Official Guidelines   ● Unacceptable Principal Diagnosis   X Assign placeholder X   ● Use Additional Character(s)   ⟩ Manifestation Code   **Coding Clinic**

Frontal bone
Nasal bone
Zygomatic bone
Orbit
Maxilla
Mandible
Clavicle
Manubrium
Scapula
Costal cartilage
Xiphoid process
Humerus
Radius
Ulna
Carpals
Metacarpals
Phalanges
Femur
Patella
Tibia
Fibula
Tarsals
Metatarsals
Phalanges
Sternum
Ribs
Vertebral column
Coxal (hip) bone
Ilium
Sacrum
Coccyx
Pubis
Ischium
Greater trochanter

Axial skeleton
Appendicular skeleton

Figure 2-8   Diagram of skeleton of trunk and limbs with bones labeled. (From Thibodeau and Patton: Anatomy and Physiology, ed 7, Mosby, 2010)

● **C40.2   Malignant neoplasm of long bones of lower limb**
(Ex) For category C40.2 CC codes: See PDX Collection 291

    C40.20   Malignant neoplasm of long bones of unspecified lower limb 🦠

    C40.21   Malignant neoplasm of long bones of right lower limb 🦠

    C40.22   Malignant neoplasm of long bones of left lower limb 🦠

● **C40.3   Malignant neoplasm of short bones of lower limb**
(Ex) For category C40.3 CC codes: See PDX Collection 292

    C40.30   Malignant neoplasm of short bones of unspecified lower limb 🦠

    C40.31   Malignant neoplasm of short bones of right lower limb 🦠

    C40.32   Malignant neoplasm of short bones of left lower limb 🦠

● **C40.8   Malignant neoplasm of overlapping sites of bone and articular cartilage of limb**
(Ex) For category C40.8 CC codes: See PDX Collection 293

    C40.80   Malignant neoplasm of overlapping sites of bone and articular cartilage of unspecified limb 🦠

    C40.81   Malignant neoplasm of overlapping sites of bone and articular cartilage of right limb 🦠

    C40.82   Malignant neoplasm of overlapping sites of bone and articular cartilage of left limb 🦠

● **C40.9   Malignant neoplasm of unspecified bones and articular cartilage of limb**
(Ex) For category C40.9 CC codes: See PDX Collection 293

    C40.90   Malignant neoplasm of unspecified bones and articular cartilage of unspecified limb 🦠

    C40.91   Malignant neoplasm of unspecified bones and articular cartilage of right limb 🦠

    C40.92   Malignant neoplasm of unspecified bones and articular cartilage of left limb 🦠

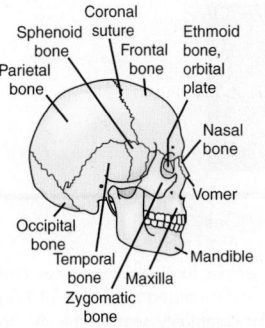

Figure 2-9   Bones of the skull.

Coronal suture
Sphenoid bone
Parietal bone
Frontal bone
Ethmoid bone, orbital plate
Nasal bone
Vomer
Occipital bone
Temporal bone
Zygomatic bone
Maxilla
Mandible

● **C41   Malignant neoplasm of bone and articular cartilage of other and unspecified sites**

    Excludes1   malignant neoplasm of bones of limbs (C40.-)
      malignant neoplasm of cartilage of ear (C49.0)
      malignant neoplasm of cartilage of eyelid (C49.0)
      malignant neoplasm of cartilage of larynx (C32.3)
      malignant neoplasm of cartilage of limbs (C40.-)
      malignant neoplasm of cartilage of nose (C30.0)

    C41.0   Malignant neoplasm of bones of skull and face 🦠
      Malignant neoplasm of maxilla (superior)
      Malignant neoplasm of orbital bone

      Excludes2   carcinoma, any type except intraosseous or odontogenic of:
        maxillary sinus (C31.0)
        upper jaw (C03.0)
      malignant neoplasm of jaw bone (lower) (C41.1)
    (Ex) See PDX Collection 294

    C41.1   Malignant neoplasm of mandible 🦠
      Malignant neoplasm of inferior maxilla
      Malignant neoplasm of lower jaw bone

      Excludes2   carcinoma, any type except intraosseous or odontogenic of:
        jaw NOS (C03.9)
        lower (C03.1)
      malignant neoplasm of upper jaw bone (C41.0)
    (Ex) See PDX Collection 295

    C41.2   Malignant neoplasm of vertebral column 🦠
      Excludes1   malignant neoplasm of sacrum and coccyx (C41.4)
    (Ex) See PDX Collection 296

    C41.3   Malignant neoplasm of ribs, sternum and clavicle 🦠
    (Ex) See PDX Collection 297

    C41.4   Malignant neoplasm of pelvic bones, sacrum and coccyx 🦠
    (Ex) See PDX Collection 298

    C41.9   Malignant neoplasm of bone and articular cartilage, unspecified 🦠
    (Ex) See PDX Collection 293

MELANOMA AND OTHER MALIGNANT NEOPLASMS OF SKIN (C43-C44)

● **C43   Malignant melanoma of skin**
    Excludes1   melanoma in situ (D03.-)
    Excludes2   malignant melanoma of skin of genital organs (C51-C52, C60.-, C63.-)
      Merkel cell carcinoma (C4A.-)
      sites other than skin-code to malignant neoplasm of the site

    C43.0   Malignant melanoma of lip
      Excludes1   malignant neoplasm of vermilion border of lip (C00.0-C00.2)

CHAPTER 2 (C00-D49)

Figure 2-10 Malignant melanoma of skin. (Getty Image)

Item 2–4 Malignant melanoma is a serious form of skin cancer that affects the melanocytes (pigment-forming cells) and is caused by ultraviolet (UV) rays from the sun that damage skin. It is most commonly seen in the 40- to 60-year-olds with fair skin, blue or green eyes, and red or blond hair who sunburn easily.

Melanoma can spread very rapidly and is the most deadly form of skin cancer. It is less common than other types of skin cancer. The rate of melanoma is increasing and currently is the leading cause of death from skin disease.

● **C43.1 Malignant melanoma of eyelid, including canthus**
    Canthus: Either corner of eye where upper and lower eyelids meet
    C43.10 Malignant melanoma of unspecified eyelid, including canthus
    C43.11 Malignant melanoma of right eyelid, including canthus
    C43.12 Malignant melanoma of left eyelid, including canthus
● **C43.2 Malignant melanoma of ear and external auricular canal**
    C43.20 Malignant melanoma of unspecified ear and external auricular canal
    C43.21 Malignant melanoma of right ear and external auricular canal
    C43.22 Malignant melanoma of left ear and external auricular canal
● **C43.3 Malignant melanoma of other and unspecified parts of face**
    C43.30 Malignant melanoma of unspecified part of face
    C43.31 Malignant melanoma of nose
    C43.39 Malignant melanoma of other parts of face
  C43.4 Malignant melanoma of scalp and neck
● **C43.5 Malignant melanoma of trunk**
    Excludes2   malignant neoplasm of anus NOS (C21.0)
                    malignant neoplasm of scrotum (C63.2)
    C43.51 Malignant melanoma of anal skin
        Malignant melanoma of anal margin
        Malignant melanoma of perianal skin
    C43.52 Malignant melanoma of skin of breast
    C43.59 Malignant melanoma of other part of trunk
● **C43.6 Malignant melanoma of upper limb, including shoulder**
    C43.60 Malignant melanoma of upper limb, including shoulder, unspecified side
    C43.61 Malignant melanoma of right upper limb, including shoulder
    C43.62 Malignant melanoma of left upper limb, including shoulder
● **C43.7 Malignant melanoma of lower limb, including hip**
    C43.70 Malignant melanoma of unspecified lower limb, including hip
    C43.71 Malignant melanoma of right lower limb, including hip
    C43.72 Malignant melanoma of left lower limb, including hip
  C43.8 Malignant melanoma of overlapping sites of skin
  C43.9 Malignant melanoma of skin, unspecified
    Malignant melanoma of unspecified site of skin
    Melanoma (malignant) NOS

● **C4A Merkel cell carcinoma**
  C4A.0 Merkel cell carcinoma of lip
    Excludes1   malignant neoplasm of vermilion border of lip (C00.0-C00.2)
● **C4A.1 Merkel cell carcinoma of eyelid, including canthus**
    C4A.10 Merkel cell carcinoma of unspecified eyelid, including canthus
    C4A.11 Merkel cell carcinoma of right eyelid, including canthus
    C4A.12 Merkel cell carcinoma of left eyelid, including canthus
● **C4A.2 Merkel cell carcinoma of ear and external auricular canal**
    C4A.20 Merkel cell carcinoma of unspecified ear and external auricular canal
    C4A.21 Merkel cell carcinoma of right ear and external auricular canal
    C4A.22 Merkel cell carcinoma of left ear and external auricular canal
● **C4A.3 Merkel cell carcinoma of other and unspecified parts of face**
    C4A.30 Merkel cell carcinoma of unspecified part of face
    C4A.31 Merkel cell carcinoma of nose
    C4A.39 Merkel cell carcinoma of other parts of face
  C4A.4 Merkel cell carcinoma of scalp and neck
● **C4A.5 Merkel cell carcinoma of trunk**
    Excludes2   malignant neoplasm of anus NOS (C21.0)
                    malignant neoplasm of scrotum (C63.2)
    C4A.51 Merkel cell carcinoma of anal skin
        Merkel cell carcinoma of anal margin
        Merkel cell carcinoma of perianal skin
    C4A.52 Merkel cell carcinoma of skin of breast
    C4A.59 Merkel cell carcinoma of other part of trunk
● **C4A.6 Merkel cell carcinoma of upper limb, including shoulder**
    C4A.60 Merkel cell carcinoma of unspecified upper limb, including shoulder
    C4A.61 Merkel cell carcinoma of right upper limb, including shoulder
    C4A.62 Merkel cell carcinoma of left upper limb, including shoulder
● **C4A.7 Merkel cell carcinoma of lower limb, including hip**
    C4A.70 Merkel cell carcinoma of unspecified lower limb, including hip
    C4A.71 Merkel cell carcinoma of right lower limb, including hip
    C4A.72 Merkel cell carcinoma of left lower limb, including hip
  C4A.8 Merkel cell carcinoma of overlapping sites
  C4A.9 Merkel cell carcinoma, unspecified
    Merkel cell carcinoma of unspecified site
    Merkel cell carcinoma NOS

● **C44 Other and unspecified malignant neoplasm of skin**
    Includes   malignant neoplasm of sebaceous glands
              malignant neoplasm of sweat glands
    Excludes1   Kaposi's sarcoma of skin (C46.0)
              malignant melanoma of skin (C43.-)
              malignant neoplasm of skin of genital organs (C51-C52, C60.-, C63.2)
              Merkel cell carcinoma (C4A.-)
● **C44.0 Other and unspecified malignant neoplasm of skin of lip**
    Excludes1   malignant neoplasm of lip (C00.-)
    C44.00 Unspecified malignant neoplasm of skin of lip
    C44.01 Basal cell carcinoma of skin of lip
    C44.02 Squamous cell carcinoma of skin of lip
    C44.09 Other specified malignant neoplasm of skin of lip

CHAPTER 2 (C00-D49)

● C44.1   Other and unspecified malignant neoplasm of skin of eyelid, including canthus

   Excludes1   connective tissue of eyelid (C49.Ø)

   ● C44.1Ø   Unspecified malignant neoplasm of skin of eyelid, including canthus

      C44.1Ø1   Unspecified malignant neoplasm of skin of unspecified eyelid, including canthus

      C44.1Ø2   Unspecified malignant neoplasm of skin of right eyelid, including canthus

      C44.1Ø9   Unspecified malignant neoplasm of skin of left eyelid, including canthus

   ● C44.11   Basal cell carcinoma of skin of eyelid, including canthus

      C44.111   Basal cell carcinoma of skin of unspecified eyelid, including canthus

      C44.112   Basal cell carcinoma of skin of right eyelid, including canthus

      C44.119   Basal cell carcinoma of skin of left eyelid, including canthus

   ● C44.12   Squamous cell carcinoma of skin of eyelid, including canthus

      C44.121   Squamous cell carcinoma of skin of unspecified eyelid, including canthus

      C44.122   Squamous cell carcinoma of skin of right eyelid, including canthus

      C44.129   Squamous cell carcinoma of skin of left eyelid, including canthus

   ● C44.19   Other specified malignant neoplasm of skin of eyelid, including canthus

      C44.191   Other specified malignant neoplasm of skin of unspecified eyelid, including canthus

      C44.192   Other specified malignant neoplasm of skin of right eyelid, including canthus

      C44.199   Other specified malignant neoplasm of skin of left eyelid, including canthus

● C44.2   Other and unspecified malignant neoplasm of skin of ear and external auricular canal

   Excludes1   connective tissue of ear (C49.Ø)

   ● C44.2Ø   Unspecified malignant neoplasm of skin of ear and external auricular canal

      C44.2Ø1   Unspecified malignant neoplasm of skin of unspecified ear and external auricular canal

      C44.2Ø2   Unspecified malignant neoplasm of skin of right ear and external auricular canal

      C44.2Ø9   Unspecified malignant neoplasm of skin of left ear and external auricular canal

   ● C44.21   Basal cell carcinoma of skin of ear and external auricular canal

      C44.211   Basal cell carcinoma of skin of unspecified ear and external auricular canal

      C44.212   Basal cell carcinoma of skin of right ear and external auricular canal

      C44.219   Basal cell carcinoma of skin of left ear and external auricular canal

● C44.22   Squamous cell carcinoma of skin of ear and external auricular canal

      C44.221   Squamous cell carcinoma of skin of unspecified ear and external auricular canal

      C44.222   Squamous cell carcinoma of skin of right ear and external auricular canal

      C44.229   Squamous cell carcinoma of skin of left ear and external auricular canal

   ● C44.29   Other specified malignant neoplasm of skin of ear and external auricular canal

      C44.291   Other specified malignant neoplasm of skin of unspecified ear and external auricular canal

      C44.292   Other specified malignant neoplasm of skin of right ear and external auricular canal

      C44.299   Other specified malignant neoplasm of skin of left ear and external auricular canal

● C44.3   Other and unspecified malignant neoplasm of skin of other and unspecified parts of face

   ● C44.3Ø   Unspecified malignant neoplasm of skin of other and unspecified parts of face

      C44.3ØØ   Unspecified malignant neoplasm of skin of unspecified part of face

      C44.3Ø1   Unspecified malignant neoplasm of skin of nose

      C44.3Ø9   Unspecified malignant neoplasm of skin of other parts of face

   ● C44.31   Basal cell carcinoma of skin of other and unspecified parts of face

      C44.31Ø   Basal cell carcinoma of skin of unspecified parts of face

      C44.311   Basal cell carcinoma of skin of nose

      C44.319   Basal cell carcinoma of skin of other parts of face
                Coding Clinic: 2Ø17, Q1, P4

   ● C44.32   Squamous cell carcinoma of skin of other and unspecified parts of face

      C44.32Ø   Squamous cell carcinoma of skin of unspecified parts of face

      C44.321   Squamous cell carcinoma of skin of nose

      C44.329   Squamous cell carcinoma of skin of other parts of face

   ● C44.39   Other specified malignant neoplasm of skin of other and unspecified parts of face

      C44.39Ø   Other specified malignant neoplasm of skin of unspecified parts of face

      C44.391   Other specified malignant neoplasm of skin of nose

      C44.399   Other specified malignant neoplasm of skin of other parts of face

● C44.4   Other and unspecified malignant neoplasm of skin of scalp and neck

      C44.4Ø   Unspecified malignant neoplasm of skin of scalp and neck

      C44.41   Basal cell carcinoma of skin of scalp and neck

      C44.42   Squamous cell carcinoma of skin of scalp and neck

      C44.49   Other specified malignant neoplasm of skin of scalp and neck

● **C44.5**   **Other and unspecified malignant neoplasm of skin of trunk**

> **Excludes1**   anus NOS (C21.0)
> scrotum (C63.2)

  ● **C44.50**   Unspecified malignant neoplasm of skin of trunk

    C44.500   Unspecified malignant neoplasm of anal skin
> Unspecified malignant neoplasm of anal margin
> Unspecified malignant neoplasm of perianal skin

    C44.501   Unspecified malignant neoplasm of skin of breast

    C44.509   Unspecified malignant neoplasm of skin of other part of trunk

  ● **C44.51**   Basal cell carcinoma of skin of trunk

    C44.510   Basal cell carcinoma of anal skin
> Basal cell carcinoma of anal margin
> Basal cell carcinoma of perianal skin

    C44.511   Basal cell carcinoma of skin of breast

    C44.519   Basal cell carcinoma of skin of other part of trunk

  ● **C44.52**   Squamous cell carcinoma of skin of trunk

    C44.520   Squamous cell carcinoma of anal skin
> Squamous cell carcinoma of anal margin
> Squamous cell carcinoma of perianal skin

    C44.521   Squamous cell carcinoma of skin of breast

    C44.529   Squamous cell carcinoma of skin of other part of trunk

  ● **C44.59**   Other specified malignant neoplasm of skin of trunk

    C44.590   Other specified malignant neoplasm of anal skin
> Other specified malignant neoplasm of anal margin
> Other specified malignant neoplasm of perianal skin

    C44.591   Other specified malignant neoplasm of skin of breast

    C44.599   Other specified malignant neoplasm of skin of other part of trunk

● **C44.6**   **Other and unspecified malignant neoplasm of skin of upper limb, including shoulder**

  ● **C44.60**   Unspecified malignant neoplasm of skin of upper limb, including shoulder

    C44.601   Unspecified malignant neoplasm of skin of unspecified upper limb, including shoulder

    C44.602   Unspecified malignant neoplasm of skin of right upper limb, including shoulder

    C44.609   Unspecified malignant neoplasm of skin of left upper limb, including shoulder

  ● **C44.61**   Basal cell carcinoma of skin of upper limb, including shoulder

    C44.611   Basal cell carcinoma of skin of unspecified upper limb, including shoulder

    C44.612   Basal cell carcinoma of skin of right upper limb, including shoulder

    C44.619   Basal cell carcinoma of skin of left upper limb, including shoulder

  ● **C44.62**   Squamous cell carcinoma of skin of upper limb, including shoulder

    C44.621   Squamous cell carcinoma of skin of unspecified upper limb, including shoulder

    C44.622   Squamous cell carcinoma of skin of right upper limb, including shoulder

    C44.629   Squamous cell carcinoma of skin of left upper limb, including shoulder

  ● **C44.69**   Other specified malignant neoplasm of skin of upper limb, including shoulder

    C44.691   Other specified malignant neoplasm of skin of unspecified upper limb, including shoulder

    C44.692   Other specified malignant neoplasm of skin of right upper limb, including shoulder

    C44.699   Other specified malignant neoplasm of skin of left upper limb, including shoulder

● **C44.7**   **Other and unspecified malignant neoplasm of skin of lower limb, including hip**

  ● **C44.70**   Unspecified malignant neoplasm of skin of lower limb, including hip

    C44.701   Unspecified malignant neoplasm of skin of unspecified lower limb, including hip

    C44.702   Unspecified malignant neoplasm of skin of right lower limb, including hip

    C44.709   Unspecified malignant neoplasm of skin of left lower limb, including hip

  ● **C44.71**   Basal cell carcinoma of skin of lower limb, including hip

    C44.711   Basal cell carcinoma of skin of unspecified lower limb, including hip

    C44.712   Basal cell carcinoma of skin of right lower limb, including hip

    C44.719   Basal cell carcinoma of skin of left lower limb, including hip

  ● **C44.72**   Squamous cell carcinoma of skin of lower limb, including hip

    C44.721   Squamous cell carcinoma of skin of unspecified lower limb, including hip

    C44.722   Squamous cell carcinoma of skin of right lower limb, including hip

    C44.729   Squamous cell carcinoma of skin of left lower limb, including hip

  ● **C44.79**   Other specified malignant neoplasm of skin of lower limb, including hip

    C44.791   Other specified malignant neoplasm of skin of unspecified lower limb, including hip

    C44.792   Other specified malignant neoplasm of skin of right lower limb, including hip

    C44.799   Other specified malignant neoplasm of skin of left lower limb, including hip

● **C44.8**   **Other and unspecified malignant neoplasm of overlapping sites of skin**

  C44.80   Unspecified malignant neoplasm of overlapping sites of skin

  C44.81   Basal cell carcinoma of overlapping sites of skin

  C44.82   Squamous cell carcinoma of overlapping sites of skin

  C44.89   Other specified malignant neoplasm of overlapping sites of skin

▶ New   ⇒ Revised   ~~deleted~~ Deleted   Excludes 1   Excludes 2   Includes   Use additional   Code first   Code also   Key words

OGCR Official Guidelines   ● Unacceptable Principal Diagnosis   X Assign placeholder X   ● Use Additional Character(s)   ▌ Manifestation Code   **Coding Clinic**

● **C44.9**   **Other and unspecified malignant neoplasm of skin, unspecified**

    C44.90   **Unspecified malignant neoplasm of skin, unspecified**
        Malignant neoplasm of unspecified site of skin

    C44.91   **Basal cell carcinoma of skin, unspecified**

    C44.92   **Squamous cell carcinoma of skin, unspecified**

    C44.99   **Other specified malignant neoplasm of skin, unspecified**

MALIGNANT NEOPLASMS OF MESOTHELIAL AND SOFT TISSUE (C45-C49)

● **C45**   **Mesothelioma**
    Malignant cells develop in protective lining that covers internal organs (mesothelium) caused by exposure to asbestos

    C45.0   **Mesothelioma of pleura** 🔾
        Excludes1   other malignant neoplasm of pleura (C38.4)
        (Ex) See PDX Collection 288
        Coding Clinic: 2017, Q2, P11

    C45.1   **Mesothelioma of peritoneum** 🔾
        Mesothelioma of cul-de-sac
        Mesothelioma of mesentery
        Mesothelioma of mesocolon
        Mesothelioma of omentum
        Mesothelioma of peritoneum (parietal) (pelvic)
        Excludes1   other malignant neoplasm of soft tissue of peritoneum (C48.-)
        (Ex) See PDX Collection 299

    C45.2   **Mesothelioma of pericardium** 🔾
        Excludes1   other malignant neoplasm of pericardium (C38.0)
        (Ex) See PDX Collection 286

    C45.7   **Mesothelioma of other sites**

    C45.9   **Mesothelioma, unspecified**

● **C46**   **Kaposi's sarcoma**
    Code first any human immunodeficiency virus [HIV] disease (B20)

    C46.0   **Kaposi's sarcoma of skin** 🔾
        (Ex) See PDX Collection 300

    C46.1   **Kaposi's sarcoma of soft tissue** 🔾
        Kaposi's sarcoma of blood vessel
        Kaposi's sarcoma of connective tissue
        Kaposi's sarcoma of fascia
        Kaposi's sarcoma of ligament
        Kaposi's sarcoma of lymphatic(s) NEC
        Kaposi's sarcoma of muscle
        Excludes2   Kaposi's sarcoma of lymph glands and nodes (C46.3)
        (Ex) See PDX Collection 301

    C46.2   **Kaposi's sarcoma of palate** 🔾
        (Ex) See PDX Collection 302

    C46.3   **Kaposi's sarcoma of lymph nodes** 🔾
        (Ex) See PDX Collection 303

    C46.4   **Kaposi's sarcoma of gastrointestinal sites** 🔾
        (Ex) See PDX Collection 304

Figure 2-11   Kaposi's sarcoma. There are large confluent hyperpigmented patch-stage lesions with lymphedema. (From Goldman L, Ausiello D, Arend W, Armitage J, Clemmons D, Drazen J, Griggs R, et al: Cecil Medicine: Expert Consult, 23e, Saunders, 2007)

Item 2-5   **Kaposi's sarcoma** is a cancer that causes patches of abnormal tissue to grow under the skin; in the lining of the mouth, nose, and throat; or in other organs, often beginning and spreading to other organs. Patients who have had organ transplants or patients with AIDS are at high risk for this malignancy.

● **C46.5**   **Kaposi's sarcoma of lung**
    (Ex) For category C46.5 CC codes: See PDX Collection 284

    C46.50   **Kaposi's sarcoma of unspecified lung** 🔾

    C46.51   **Kaposi's sarcoma of right lung** 🔾

    C46.52   **Kaposi's sarcoma of left lung** 🔾

    C46.7   **Kaposi's sarcoma of other sites** 🔾
        (Ex) See PDX Collection 305

    C46.9   **Kaposi's sarcoma, unspecified** 🔾
        Kaposi's sarcoma of unspecified site
        (Ex) See PDX Collection 306

● **C47**   **Malignant neoplasm of peripheral nerves and autonomic nervous system**
    Includes   malignant neoplasm of sympathetic and parasympathetic nerves and ganglia
    Excludes1   Kaposi's sarcoma of soft tissue (C46.1)
    (Ex) For category C47 CC Codes: See PDX Collection 307

    C47.0   **Malignant neoplasm of peripheral nerves of head, face and neck** 🔾
        Excludes1   malignant neoplasm of peripheral nerves of orbit (C69.6-)

● **C47.1**   **Malignant neoplasm of peripheral nerves of upper limb, including shoulder**

    C47.10   **Malignant neoplasm of peripheral nerves of unspecified upper limb, including shoulder** 🔾

    C47.11   **Malignant neoplasm of peripheral nerves of right upper limb, including shoulder** 🔾

    C47.12   **Malignant neoplasm of peripheral nerves of left upper limb, including shoulder** 🔾

● **C47.2**   **Malignant neoplasm of peripheral nerves of lower limb, including hip**

    C47.20   **Malignant neoplasm of peripheral nerves of unspecified lower limb, including hip** 🔾

    C47.21   **Malignant neoplasm of peripheral nerves of right lower limb, including hip** 🔾

    C47.22   **Malignant neoplasm of peripheral nerves of left lower limb, including hip** 🔾

    C47.3   **Malignant neoplasm of peripheral nerves of thorax** 🔾

    C47.4   **Malignant neoplasm of peripheral nerves of abdomen** 🔾

    C47.5   **Malignant neoplasm of peripheral nerves of pelvis** 🔾

    C47.6   **Malignant neoplasm of peripheral nerves of trunk, unspecified** 🔾
        Malignant neoplasm of peripheral nerves of unspecified part of trunk

    C47.8   **Malignant neoplasm of overlapping sites of peripheral nerves and autonomic nervous system** 🔾

    C47.9   **Malignant neoplasm of peripheral nerves and autonomic nervous system, unspecified** 🔾
        Malignant neoplasm of unspecified site of peripheral nerves and autonomic nervous system

● **C48**   **Malignant neoplasm of retroperitoneum and peritoneum**
    Excludes1   Kaposi's sarcoma of connective tissue (C46.1)
        mesothelioma (C45.-)
    (Ex) For category C48 unless otherwise indicated: See PDX Collection 299

    C48.0   **Malignant neoplasm of retroperitoneum** 🔾
        Behind/outside of peritoneum
        (Ex) See PDX Collection 308

    C48.1   **Malignant neoplasm of specified parts of peritoneum** 🔾
        Serous membrane lining abdominopelvic walls and covering viscera
        Malignant neoplasm of cul-de-sac
        Malignant neoplasm of mesentery
        Malignant neoplasm of mesocolon
        Malignant neoplasm of omentum
        Malignant neoplasm of parietal peritoneum
        Malignant neoplasm of pelvic peritoneum

    C48.2   **Malignant neoplasm of peritoneum, unspecified** 🔾

    C48.8   **Malignant neoplasm of overlapping sites of retroperitoneum and peritoneum** 🔾

CHAPTER 2 (C00-D49)

N Newborn Age: 0   **P** Pediatric Age: 0–17   **M** Maternity DX: 12–55   **A** Adult Age: 15–124   ♀ Females Only   ♂ Males Only

🔾 Complication\Comorbidity   🔾 Major C\C   (Ex) CC/MCC Exclusions   🔾 Hospital-Acquired Condition

681

● **C49   Malignant neoplasm of other connective and soft tissue**

Includes   malignant neoplasm of blood vessel
malignant neoplasm of bursa
malignant neoplasm of cartilage
malignant neoplasm of fascia
malignant neoplasm of fat
malignant neoplasm of ligament, except uterine
malignant neoplasm of lymphatic vessel
malignant neoplasm of muscle
malignant neoplasm of synovia
malignant neoplasm of tendon (sheath)

Excludes1   malignant neoplasm of cartilage (of):
articular (C40-C41)
larynx (C32.3)
nose (C30.0)
malignant neoplasm of connective tissue of breast (C50.-)

Excludes2   Kaposi's sarcoma of soft tissue (C46.1)
malignant neoplasm of heart (C38.0)
malignant neoplasm of peripheral nerves and autonomic nervous system (C47.-)
malignant neoplasm of peritoneum (C48.2)
malignant neoplasm of retroperitoneum (C48.0)
malignant neoplasm of uterine ligament (C57.3)
mesothelioma (C45.-)

Ex) **For category C49 unless otherwise indicated:** See PDX Collection 307

C49.0   **Malignant neoplasm of connective and soft tissue of head, face and neck** 🔑
Malignant neoplasm of connective tissue of ear
Malignant neoplasm of connective tissue of eyelid

Excludes1   connective tissue of orbit (C69.6-)

● **C49.1**   **Malignant neoplasm of connective and soft tissue of upper limb, including shoulder**

C49.10   **Malignant neoplasm of connective and soft tissue of unspecified upper limb, including shoulder** 🔑

C49.11   **Malignant neoplasm of connective and soft tissue of right upper limb, including shoulder** 🔑

C49.12   **Malignant neoplasm of connective and soft tissue of left upper limb, including shoulder** 🔑

● **C49.2**   **Malignant neoplasm of connective and soft tissue of lower limb, including hip**

C49.20   **Malignant neoplasm of connective and soft tissue of unspecified lower limb, including hip** 🔑

C49.21   **Malignant neoplasm of connective and soft tissue of right lower limb, including hip** 🔑

C49.22   **Malignant neoplasm of connective and soft tissue of left lower limb, including hip** 🔑

C49.3   **Malignant neoplasm of connective and soft tissue of thorax** 🔑
Malignant neoplasm of axilla
Malignant neoplasm of diaphragm
Malignant neoplasm of great vessels

Excludes1   malignant neoplasm of breast (C50.-)
malignant neoplasm of heart (C38.0)
malignant neoplasm of mediastinum (C38.1-C38.3)
malignant neoplasm of thymus (C37)

Coding Clinic: 2015, Q3, P19

C49.4   **Malignant neoplasm of connective and soft tissue of abdomen** 🔑
Malignant neoplasm of abdominal wall
Malignant neoplasm of hypochondrium

C49.5   **Malignant neoplasm of connective and soft tissue of pelvis** 🔑
Malignant neoplasm of buttock
Malignant neoplasm of groin
Malignant neoplasm of perineum

C49.6   **Malignant neoplasm of connective and soft tissue of trunk, unspecified** 🔑
Malignant neoplasm of back NOS

C49.8   **Malignant neoplasm of overlapping sites of connective and soft tissue** 🔑
Primary malignant neoplasm of two or more contiguous sites of connective and soft tissue

C49.9   **Malignant neoplasm of connective and soft tissue, unspecified** 🔑

● **C49.A**   **Gastrointestinal stromal tumor**
Coding Clinic: 2016, Q4, P8

C49.A0   **Gastrointestinal stromal tumor, unspecified site** 🔑

C49.A1   **Gastrointestinal stromal tumor of esophagus** 🔑

C49.A2   **Gastrointestinal stromal tumor of stomach** 🔑
Ex) See PDX Collection 511

C49.A3   **Gastrointestinal stromal tumor of small intestine** 🔑

C49.A4   **Gastrointestinal stromal tumor of large intestine** 🔑

C49.A5   **Gastrointestinal stromal tumor of rectum** 🔑

C49.A9   **Gastrointestinal stromal tumor of other sites** 🔑

MALIGNANT NEOPLASMS OF BREAST (C50)

● **C50   Malignant neoplasm of breast**

Includes   connective tissue of breast
Paget's disease of breast
Paget's disease of nipple
Intraductal carcinoma of breast characterized by eczema-like inflammatory skin changes

Use additional code to identify estrogen receptor status (Z17.0, Z17.1)

Excludes1   skin of breast (C44.501, C44.511, C44.521, C44.591)

● **C50.0**   **Malignant neoplasm of nipple and areola**

● **C50.01**   **Malignant neoplasm of nipple and areola, female**

C50.011   **Malignant neoplasm of nipple and areola, right female breast** ♀

C50.012   **Malignant neoplasm of nipple and areola, left female breast** ♀

C50.019   **Malignant neoplasm of nipple and areola, unspecified female breast** ♀

● **C50.02**   **Malignant neoplasm of nipple and areola, male**

C50.021   **Malignant neoplasm of nipple and areola, right male breast** ♂

C50.022   **Malignant neoplasm of nipple and areola, left male breast** ♂

C50.029   **Malignant neoplasm of nipple and areola, unspecified male breast** ♂

Figure 2-12   Female breast quadrants and axillary tail.

AXILLARY TAIL
UPPER-INNER
UPPER-OUTER
Nipple and areola
Central portion
LOWER-OUTER
LOWER-INNER

▶ New   ➡ Revised   ~~deleted~~ Deleted   Excludes 1   Excludes 2   Includes   Use additional   Code first   Code also   Key words
OGCR Official Guidelines   ● Unacceptable Principal Diagnosis   X Assign placeholder X   ● Use Additional Character(s)   ▌ Manifestation Code   **Coding Clinic**

● **C50.1   Malignant neoplasm of central portion of breast**
   ● **C50.11   Malignant neoplasm of central portion of breast, female**
      C50.111   Malignant neoplasm of central portion of right female breast ♀
      C50.112   Malignant neoplasm of central portion of left female breast ♀
      C50.119   Malignant neoplasm of central portion of unspecified female breast ♀
   ● **C50.12   Malignant neoplasm of central portion of breast, male**
      C50.121   Malignant neoplasm of central portion of right male breast ♂
      C50.122   Malignant neoplasm of central portion of left male breast ♂
      C50.129   Malignant neoplasm of central portion of unspecified male breast ♂

● **C50.2   Malignant neoplasm of upper-inner quadrant of breast**
   ● **C50.21   Malignant neoplasm of upper-inner quadrant of breast, female**
      C50.211   Malignant neoplasm of upper-inner quadrant of right female breast ♀
      C50.212   Malignant neoplasm of upper-inner quadrant of left female breast ♀
      C50.219   Malignant neoplasm of upper-inner quadrant of unspecified female breast ♀
   ● **C50.22   Malignant neoplasm of upper-inner quadrant of breast, male**
      C50.221   Malignant neoplasm of upper-inner quadrant of right male breast ♂
      C50.222   Malignant neoplasm of upper-inner quadrant of left male breast ♂
      C50.229   Malignant neoplasm of upper-inner quadrant of unspecified male breast ♂

● **C50.3   Malignant neoplasm of lower-inner quadrant of breast**
   ● **C50.31   Malignant neoplasm of lower-inner quadrant of breast, female**
      C50.311   Malignant neoplasm of lower-inner quadrant of right female breast ♀
      C50.312   Malignant neoplasm of lower-inner quadrant of left female breast ♀
      C50.319   Malignant neoplasm of lower-inner quadrant of unspecified female breast ♀
   ● **C50.32   Malignant neoplasm of lower-inner quadrant of breast, male**
      C50.321   Malignant neoplasm of lower-inner quadrant of right male breast ♂
      C50.322   Malignant neoplasm of lower-inner quadrant of left male breast ♂
      C50.329   Malignant neoplasm of lower-inner quadrant of unspecified male breast ♂

● **C50.4   Malignant neoplasm of upper-outer quadrant of breast**
   ● **C50.41   Malignant neoplasm of upper-outer quadrant of breast, female**
      C50.411   Malignant neoplasm of upper-outer quadrant of right female breast ♀
      C50.412   Malignant neoplasm of upper-outer quadrant of left female breast ♀
      C50.419   Malignant neoplasm of upper-outer quadrant of unspecified female breast ♀

● **C50.42   Malignant neoplasm of upper-outer quadrant of breast, male**
      C50.421   Malignant neoplasm of upper-outer quadrant of right male breast ♂
      C50.422   Malignant neoplasm of upper-outer quadrant of left male breast ♂
      C50.429   Malignant neoplasm of upper-outer quadrant of unspecified male breast ♂

● **C50.5   Malignant neoplasm of lower-outer quadrant of breast**
   ● **C50.51   Malignant neoplasm of lower-outer quadrant of breast, female**
      C50.511   Malignant neoplasm of lower-outer quadrant of right female breast ♀
      C50.512   Malignant neoplasm of lower-outer quadrant of left female breast ♀
      C50.519   Malignant neoplasm of lower-outer quadrant of unspecified female breast ♀
   ● **C50.52   Malignant neoplasm of lower-outer quadrant of breast, male**
      C50.521   Malignant neoplasm of lower-outer quadrant of right male breast ♂
      C50.522   Malignant neoplasm of lower-outer quadrant of left male breast ♂
      C50.529   Malignant neoplasm of lower-outer quadrant of unspecified male breast ♂

● **C50.6   Malignant neoplasm of axillary tail of breast**
   ● **C50.61   Malignant neoplasm of axillary tail of breast, female**
      C50.611   Malignant neoplasm of axillary tail of right female breast ♀
      C50.612   Malignant neoplasm of axillary tail of left female breast ♀
      C50.619   Malignant neoplasm of axillary tail of unspecified female breast ♀
   ● **C50.62   Malignant neoplasm of axillary tail of breast, male**
      C50.621   Malignant neoplasm of axillary tail of right male breast ♂
      C50.622   Malignant neoplasm of axillary tail of left male breast ♂
      C50.629   Malignant neoplasm of axillary tail of unspecified male breast ♂

● **C50.8   Malignant neoplasm of overlapping sites of breast**
   ● **C50.81   Malignant neoplasm of overlapping sites of breast, female**
      C50.811   Malignant neoplasm of overlapping sites of right female breast ♀
      C50.812   Malignant neoplasm of overlapping sites of left female breast ♀
      C50.819   Malignant neoplasm of overlapping sites of unspecified female breast ♀
   ● **C50.82   Malignant neoplasm of overlapping sites of breast, male**
      C50.821   Malignant neoplasm of overlapping sites of right male breast ♂
      C50.822   Malignant neoplasm of overlapping sites of left male breast ♂
      C50.829   Malignant neoplasm of overlapping sites of unspecified male breast ♂

● **C50.9   Malignant neoplasm of breast of unspecified site**
   ● **C50.91   Malignant neoplasm of breast of unspecified site, female**
      C50.911   Malignant neoplasm of unspecified site of right female breast ♀
      C50.912   Malignant neoplasm of unspecified site of left female breast ♀
      C50.919   Malignant neoplasm of unspecified site of unspecified female breast ♀

CHAPTER 2 (C00–D49)

N Newborn Age: 0   **P** Pediatric Age: 0–17   **M** Maternity DX: 12–55   **A** Adult Age: 15–124   ♀ Females Only   ♂ Males Only

🔖 Complication\Comorbidity   🔖 Major C\C   Ⓔⓧ CC/MCC Exclusions   🔖 Hospital-Acquired Condition

683

CHAPTER 2 (C00-D49)

● **C50.92** Malignant neoplasm of breast of unspecified site, male
     C50.921 Malignant neoplasm of unspecified site of right male breast ♂
     C50.922 Malignant neoplasm of unspecified site of left male breast ♂
     C50.929 Malignant neoplasm of unspecified site of unspecified male breast ♂

MALIGNANT NEOPLASMS OF FEMALE GENITAL ORGANS (C51-C58)

> **Includes** malignant neoplasm of skin of female genital organs

● **C51** Malignant neoplasm of vulva
> **Excludes1** carcinoma in situ of vulva (D07.1)

   C51.0 Malignant neoplasm of labium majus ♀
     Outer folds of skin external female genitalia
     Malignant neoplasm of Bartholin's [greater vestibular] gland
   C51.1 Malignant neoplasm of labium minus ♀
     Two inner folds surrounding vulva in female genitalia
   C51.2 Malignant neoplasm of clitoris ♀
   C51.8 Malignant neoplasm of overlapping sites of vulva ♀
   C51.9 Malignant neoplasm of vulva, unspecified ♀
     Malignant neoplasm of external female genitalia NOS
     Malignant neoplasm of pudendum

   C52 Malignant neoplasm of vagina ♀
> **Excludes1** carcinoma in situ of vagina (D07.2)

● **C53** Malignant neoplasm of cervix uteri
> **Excludes1** carcinoma in situ of cervix uteri (D06.-)

   C53.0 Malignant neoplasm of endocervix ♀
     Inside the cervix
   C53.1 Malignant neoplasm of exocervix ♀
     Outside the cervix
   C53.8 Malignant neoplasm of overlapping sites of cervix uteri ♀
   C53.9 Malignant neoplasm of cervix uteri, unspecified ♀

● **C54** Malignant neoplasm of corpus uteri
   C54.0 Malignant neoplasm of isthmus uteri ♀
     Constricted part of uterus between cervix and body
     Malignant neoplasm of lower uterine segment
   C54.1 Malignant neoplasm of endometrium ♀
     Lining of uterus
   C54.2 Malignant neoplasm of myometrium ♀
     Middle layer of uterine wall consisting of smooth muscle supporting stromal and vascular tissue
   C54.3 Malignant neoplasm of fundus uteri ♀
     Top rounded portion of uterus
   C54.8 Malignant neoplasm of overlapping sites of corpus uteri ♀
     Main body of uterus
   C54.9 Malignant neoplasm of corpus uteri, unspecified ♀

   C55 Malignant neoplasm of uterus, part unspecified ♀

● **C56** Malignant neoplasm of ovary
> Use additional code to identify any functional activity
> (Ex) For category C56 CC Codes: See PDX Collection 309

   C56.1 Malignant neoplasm of right ovary ♀
   C56.2 Malignant neoplasm of left ovary ♀
   C56.9 Malignant neoplasm of unspecified ovary ♀

● **C57** Malignant neoplasm of other and unspecified female genital organs
 ● **C57.0** Malignant neoplasm of fallopian tube
     Malignant neoplasm of oviduct
     Malignant neoplasm of uterine tube
     C57.00 Malignant neoplasm of unspecified fallopian tube ♀
     C57.01 Malignant neoplasm of right fallopian tube ♀
     C57.02 Malignant neoplasm of left fallopian tube ♀
 ● **C57.1** Malignant neoplasm of broad ligament
     C57.10 Malignant neoplasm of unspecified broad ligament ♀
     C57.11 Malignant neoplasm of right broad ligament ♀
     C57.12 Malignant neoplasm of left broad ligament ♀
 ● **C57.2** Malignant neoplasm of round ligament
     C57.20 Malignant neoplasm of unspecified round ligament ♀
     C57.21 Malignant neoplasm of right round ligament ♀
     C57.22 Malignant neoplasm of left round ligament ♀
   C57.3 Malignant neoplasm of parametrium ♀
     Malignant neoplasm of uterine ligament NOS
   C57.4 Malignant neoplasm of uterine adnexa, unspecified ♀
   C57.7 Malignant neoplasm of other specified female genital organs ♀
     Malignant neoplasm of wolffian body or duct
   C57.8 Malignant neoplasm of overlapping sites of female genital organs ♀
     Primary malignant neoplasm of two or more contiguous sites of the female genital organs whose point of origin cannot be determined
     Primary tubo-ovarian malignant neoplasm whose point of origin cannot be determined
     Primary utero-ovarian malignant neoplasm whose point of origin cannot be determined
   C57.9 Malignant neoplasm of female genital organ, unspecified ♀
     Malignant neoplasm of female genitourinary tract NOS

   C58 Malignant neoplasm of placenta ♀   M
> **Includes** choriocarcinoma NOS
> chorionepithelioma NOS
> **Excludes1** chorioadenoma (destruens) (D39.2)
> hydatidiform mole NOS (O01.9)
> invasive hydatidiform mole (D39.2)
> male choriocarcinoma NOS (C62.9-)
> malignant hydatidiform mole (D39.2)

MALIGNANT NEOPLASMS OF MALE GENITAL ORGANS (C60-C63)

> **Includes** malignant neoplasm of skin of male genital organs

● **C60** Malignant neoplasm of penis
   C60.0 Malignant neoplasm of prepuce ♂
     Malignant neoplasm of foreskin
   C60.1 Malignant neoplasm of glans penis ♂
   C60.2 Malignant neoplasm of body of penis ♂
     Malignant neoplasm of corpus cavernosum
   C60.8 Malignant neoplasm of overlapping sites of penis ♂
   C60.9 Malignant neoplasm of penis, unspecified ♂
     Malignant neoplasm of skin of penis NOS

Figure 2-13 Cervix uteri.

▶ New   ⇒ Revised   ~~deleted~~ Deleted   Excludes 1   Excludes 2   Includes   Use additional   Code first   Code also   Key words
OGCR Official Guidelines   ● Unacceptable Principal Diagnosis   X Assign placeholder X   ● Use Additional Character(s)   ▷ Manifestation Code   **Coding Clinic**

Urinary bladder
Symphysis pubis
Sacrum
Rectum
SPERMATIC CORD,
SEMINAL VESICLE
VAS DEFERENS
Prostate gland
PENIS
Anus
EPIDIDYMIS
Bulbourethral gland
GLANS PENIS
Urethra
TUNICA VAGINALIS
Testis
SCROTUM

Figure 2-14 Penis and other male genital organs.

C61 Malignant neoplasm of prostate ♂
Use additional code to identify:
hormone sensitivity status (Z19.1-Z19.2)
rising PSA following treatment for malignant neoplasm of prostate (R97.21)
Excludes1 malignant neoplasm of seminal vesicle (C63.7)

● **C62 Malignant neoplasm of testis**
Use additional code to identify any functional activity.
● **C62.0 Malignant neoplasm of undescended testis**
Malignant neoplasm of ectopic testis
Malignant neoplasm of retained testis
    C62.00 Malignant neoplasm of unspecified undescended testis ♂
    C62.01 Malignant neoplasm of undescended right testis ♂
    C62.02 Malignant neoplasm of undescended left testis ♂
● **C62.1 Malignant neoplasm of descended testis**
Malignant neoplasm of scrotal testis
    C62.10 Malignant neoplasm of unspecified descended testis, unspecified side ♂
    C62.11 Malignant neoplasm of descended right testis ♂
    C62.12 Malignant neoplasm of descended left testis ♂
● **C62.9 Malignant neoplasm of testis, unspecified whether descended or undescended**
    C62.90 Malignant neoplasm of unspecified testis, unspecified whether descended or undescended ♂
Malignant neoplasm of testis NOS
    C62.91 Malignant neoplasm of right testis, unspecified whether descended or undescended ♂
    C62.92 Malignant neoplasm of left testis, unspecified whether descended or undescended ♂

● **C63 Malignant neoplasm of other and unspecified male genital organs**
● **C63.0 Malignant neoplasm of epididymis**
    C63.00 Malignant neoplasm of unspecified epididymis ♂
    C63.01 Malignant neoplasm of right epididymis ♂
    C63.02 Malignant neoplasm of left epididymis ♂
● **C63.1 Malignant neoplasm of spermatic cord**
    C63.10 Malignant neoplasm of unspecified spermatic cord ♂
    C63.11 Malignant neoplasm of right spermatic cord ♂
    C63.12 Malignant neoplasm of left spermatic cord ♂
 C63.2 Malignant neoplasm of scrotum ♂
Malignant neoplasm of skin of scrotum
 C63.7 Malignant neoplasm of other specified male genital organs ♂
Malignant neoplasm of seminal vesicle
Malignant neoplasm of tunica vaginalis

C63.8 Malignant neoplasm of overlapping sites of male genital organs ♂
Primary malignant neoplasm of two or more contiguous sites of male genital organs whose point of origin cannot be determined
C63.9 Malignant neoplasm of male genital organ, unspecified ♂
Malignant neoplasm of male genitourinary tract NOS

MALIGNANT NEOPLASMS OF URINARY TRACT (C64-C68)

● **C64 Malignant neoplasm of kidney, except renal pelvis**
Excludes1 malignant carcinoid tumor of the kidney (C7A.093)
malignant neoplasm of renal calyces (C65.-)
malignant neoplasm of renal pelvis (C65.-)
(Ex) For category C64 CC Codes: See PDX Collection 310
    C64.1 Malignant neoplasm of right kidney, except renal pelvis 🔖
    C64.2 Malignant neoplasm of left kidney, except renal pelvis 🔖
    C64.9 Malignant neoplasm of unspecified kidney, except renal pelvis 🔖

● **C65 Malignant neoplasm of renal pelvis**
Includes malignant neoplasm of pelviureteric junction
malignant neoplasm of renal calyces
(Ex) For category C65 CC Codes: See PDX Collection 310
    C65.1 Malignant neoplasm of right renal pelvis 🔖
    C65.2 Malignant neoplasm of left renal pelvis 🔖
    C65.9 Malignant neoplasm of unspecified renal pelvis 🔖

● **C66 Malignant neoplasm of ureter**
Excludes1 malignant neoplasm of ureteric orifice of bladder (C67.6)
(Ex) For category C66 CC Codes: See PDX Collection 311
    C66.1 Malignant neoplasm of right ureter 🔖
    C66.2 Malignant neoplasm of left ureter 🔖
    C66.9 Malignant neoplasm of unspecified ureter 🔖

● **C67 Malignant neoplasm of bladder**
C67.0 Malignant neoplasm of trigone of bladder
Triangular area formed by three openings in the floor of urinary bladder
C67.1 Malignant neoplasm of dome of bladder
Vaulted roof
C67.2 Malignant neoplasm of lateral wall of bladder
Side walls
C67.3 Malignant neoplasm of anterior wall of bladder
Front wall
C67.4 Malignant neoplasm of posterior wall of bladder
Back wall
C67.5 Malignant neoplasm of bladder neck
Joining of bladder and urethra
Malignant neoplasm of internal urethral orifice
C67.6 Malignant neoplasm of ureteric orifice
Opening from bladder to ureters
C67.7 Malignant neoplasm of urachus
Embryonic canal that connects the urinary bladder with the structure that forms the umbilical cord (allantois)
C67.8 Malignant neoplasm of overlapping sites of bladder
C67.9 Malignant neoplasm of bladder, unspecified
Coding Clinic: 2017, Q1, P6; 2016, Q1, P19

CHAPTER 2 (C00-D49)

● **C68 Malignant neoplasm of other and unspecified urinary organs**

> **Excludes1** malignant neoplasm of female genitourinary tract NOS (C57.9)
>
> malignant neoplasm of male genitourinary tract NOS (C63.9)

> (Ex) **For category C68 CC codes C68.0-C68.1:** See PDX Collection 312
>
> **For category C68 CC codes C68.8-C68.9:** See PDX Collection 313

C68.0 Malignant neoplasm of urethra 🔖

> **Excludes1** malignant neoplasm of urethral orifice of bladder (C67.5)

C68.1 Malignant neoplasm of paraurethral glands 🔖

> *Group of glands of female urethra drained by paraurethral ducts; AKA Skene glands, female prostate*

C68.8 Malignant neoplasm of overlapping sites of urinary organs 🔖

> Primary malignant neoplasm of two or more contiguous sites of urinary organs whose point of origin cannot be determined

C68.9 Malignant neoplasm of urinary organ, unspecified 🔖

> Malignant neoplasm of urinary system NOS

MALIGNANT NEOPLASMS OF EYE, BRAIN AND OTHER PARTS OF CENTRAL NERVOUS SYSTEM (C69-C72)

● **C69 Malignant neoplasm of eye and adnexa**

> **Excludes1** malignant neoplasm of connective tissue of eyelid (C49.0)
>
> malignant neoplasm of eyelid (skin) (C43.1-, C44.1-)
>
> malignant neoplasm of optic nerve (C72.3-)

● **C69.0 Malignant neoplasm of conjunctiva**

C69.00 Malignant neoplasm of unspecified conjunctiva

C69.01 Malignant neoplasm of right conjunctiva

C69.02 Malignant neoplasm of left conjunctiva

● **C69.1 Malignant neoplasm of cornea**

C69.10 Malignant neoplasm of unspecified cornea

C69.11 Malignant neoplasm of right cornea

C69.12 Malignant neoplasm of left cornea

● **C69.2 Malignant neoplasm of retina**

> **Excludes1** dark area on retina (D49.81)
>
> neoplasm of unspecified behavior of retina and choroid (D49.81)
>
> retinal freckle (D49.81)

C69.20 Malignant neoplasm of unspecified retina

C69.21 Malignant neoplasm of right retina

C69.22 Malignant neoplasm of left retina

● **C69.3 Malignant neoplasm of choroid**

C69.30 Malignant neoplasm of unspecified choroid

C69.31 Malignant neoplasm of right choroid

C69.32 Malignant neoplasm of left choroid

● **C69.4 Malignant neoplasm of ciliary body**

C69.40 Malignant neoplasm of unspecified ciliary body

C69.41 Malignant neoplasm of right ciliary body

C69.42 Malignant neoplasm of left ciliary body

● **C69.5 Malignant neoplasm of lacrimal gland and duct**

> Malignant neoplasm of lacrimal sac
>
> Malignant neoplasm of nasolacrimal duct

C69.50 Malignant neoplasm of unspecified lacrimal gland and duct

C69.51 Malignant neoplasm of right lacrimal gland and duct

C69.52 Malignant neoplasm of left lacrimal gland and duct

● **C69.6 Malignant neoplasm of orbit**

> Malignant neoplasm of connective tissue of orbit
>
> Malignant neoplasm of extraocular muscle
>
> Malignant neoplasm of peripheral nerves of orbit
>
> Malignant neoplasm of retrobulbar tissue
>
> Malignant neoplasm of retro-ocular tissue

> **Excludes1** malignant neoplasm of orbital bone (C41.0)

C69.60 Malignant neoplasm of unspecified orbit

C69.61 Malignant neoplasm of right orbit

C69.62 Malignant neoplasm of left orbit

● **C69.8 Malignant neoplasm of overlapping sites of eye and adnexa**

C69.80 Malignant neoplasm of overlapping sites of unspecified eye and adnexa

C69.81 Malignant neoplasm of overlapping sites of right eye and adnexa

C69.82 Malignant neoplasm of overlapping sites of left eye and adnexa

● **C69.9 Malignant neoplasm of unspecified site of eye**

> Malignant neoplasm of eyeball

C69.90 Malignant neoplasm of unspecified site of unspecified eye

C69.91 Malignant neoplasm of unspecified site of right eye

C69.92 Malignant neoplasm of unspecified site of left eye

● **C70 Malignant neoplasm of meninges**

C70.0 Malignant neoplasm of cerebral meninges 🔖

> (Ex) See PDX Collection 314

C70.1 Malignant neoplasm of spinal meninges 🔖

> (Ex) See PDX Collection 315

C70.9 Malignant neoplasm of meninges, unspecified 🔖

> (Ex) See PDX Collection 314

● **C71 Malignant neoplasm of brain**

> **Excludes1** malignant neoplasm of cranial nerves (C72.2-C72.5)
>
> retrobulbar malignant neoplasm (C69.6-)

> (Ex) **For category C71 CC codes:** See PDX Collection 316

C71.0 Malignant neoplasm of cerebrum, except lobes and ventricles 🔖

> Malignant neoplasm of supratentorial NOS

C71.1 Malignant neoplasm of frontal lobe 🔖

C71.2 Malignant neoplasm of temporal lobe 🔖

C71.3 Malignant neoplasm of parietal lobe 🔖

C71.4 Malignant neoplasm of occipital lobe 🔖

C71.5 Malignant neoplasm of cerebral ventricle 🔖

> **Excludes1** malignant neoplasm of fourth cerebral ventricle (C71.7)

C71.6 Malignant neoplasm of cerebellum 🔖

C71.7 Malignant neoplasm of brain stem 🔖

> Malignant neoplasm of fourth cerebral ventricle
>
> Infratentorial malignant neoplasm NOS

C71.8 Malignant neoplasm of overlapping sites of brain 🔖

C71.9 Malignant neoplasm of brain, unspecified 🔖

Figure 2-15 The brain.

▶ New   ⇒ Revised   ~~deleted~~ Deleted   Excludes 1   Excludes 2   Includes   Use additional   Code first   Code also   Key words

OGCR Official Guidelines   ● Unacceptable Principal Diagnosis   X Assign placeholder X   ● Use Additional Character(s)   ▶ Manifestation Code   **Coding Clinic**

● **C72**   **Malignant neoplasm of spinal cord, cranial nerves and other parts of central nervous system**

> **Excludes1**   malignant neoplasm of meninges (C70.-)
> malignant neoplasm of peripheral nerves and autonomic nervous system (C47.-)
> (Ex) For category C72 unless otherwise indicated: See PDX Collection 318

    C72.0   **Malignant neoplasm of spinal cord** 🦠
> (Ex) See PDX Collection 317

    C72.1   **Malignant neoplasm of cauda equina** 🦠
> *Lower end of spinal column*
> (Ex) See PDX Collection 317

   ● **C72.2**   **Malignant neoplasm of olfactory nerve**
> Malignant neoplasm of olfactory bulb

      C72.20   **Malignant neoplasm of unspecified olfactory nerve** 🦠

      C72.21   **Malignant neoplasm of right olfactory nerve** 🦠
      C72.22   **Malignant neoplasm of left olfactory nerve** 🦠

   ● **C72.3**   **Malignant neoplasm of optic nerve**

      C72.30   **Malignant neoplasm of unspecified optic nerve** 🦠

      C72.31   **Malignant neoplasm of right optic nerve** 🦠
      C72.32   **Malignant neoplasm of left optic nerve** 🦠

   ● **C72.4**   **Malignant neoplasm of acoustic nerve**

      C72.40   **Malignant neoplasm of unspecified acoustic nerve** 🦠

      C72.41   **Malignant neoplasm of right acoustic nerve** 🦠
      C72.42   **Malignant neoplasm of left acoustic nerve** 🦠

   ● **C72.5**   **Malignant neoplasm of other and unspecified cranial nerves**

      C72.50   **Malignant neoplasm of unspecified cranial nerve** 🦠
> Malignant neoplasm of cranial nerve NOS

      C72.59   **Malignant neoplasm of other cranial nerves** 🦠

    C72.9   **Malignant neoplasm of central nervous system, unspecified** 🦠
> Malignant neoplasm of unspecified site of central nervous system
> Malignant neoplasm of nervous system NOS
> (Ex) See PDX Collection 319

MALIGNANT NEOPLASMS OF THYROID AND OTHER ENDOCRINE GLANDS (C73-C75)

    C73   **Malignant neoplasm of thyroid gland**
> Use additional code to identify any functional activity

● **C74**   **Malignant neoplasm of adrenal gland**
> (Ex) For category C74 CC codes: See PDX Collection 320

   ● **C74.0**   **Malignant neoplasm of cortex of adrenal gland**

      C74.00   **Malignant neoplasm of cortex of unspecified adrenal gland** 🦠

      C74.01   **Malignant neoplasm of cortex of right adrenal gland** 🦠

      C74.02   **Malignant neoplasm of cortex of left adrenal gland** 🦠

   ● **C74.1**   **Malignant neoplasm of medulla of adrenal gland**
> *Pair of glands situated on top of or above each kidney ("suprarenal")*

      C74.10   **Malignant neoplasm of medulla of unspecified adrenal gland** 🦠

      C74.11   **Malignant neoplasm of medulla of right adrenal gland** 🦠

      C74.12   **Malignant neoplasm of medulla of left adrenal gland** 🦠

● **C74.9**   **Malignant neoplasm of unspecified part of adrenal gland**

      C74.90   **Malignant neoplasm of unspecified part of unspecified adrenal gland** 🦠

      C74.91   **Malignant neoplasm of unspecified part of right adrenal gland** 🦠

      C74.92   **Malignant neoplasm of unspecified part of left adrenal gland** 🦠

● **C75**   **Malignant neoplasm of other endocrine glands and related structures**

> **Excludes1**   malignant carcinoid tumors (C7A.0-)
> malignant neoplasm of adrenal gland (C74.-)
> malignant neoplasm of endocrine pancreas (C25.4)
> malignant neoplasm of islets of Langerhans (C25.4)
> malignant neoplasm of ovary (C56.-)
> malignant neoplasm of testis (C62.-)
> malignant neoplasm of thymus (C37)
> malignant neoplasm of thyroid gland (C73)
> malignant neuroendocrine tumors (C7A.-)

    C75.0   **Malignant neoplasm of parathyroid gland** 🦠
> (Ex) See PDX Collection 321

    C75.1   **Malignant neoplasm of pituitary gland** 🦠
> (Ex) See PDX Collection 322

    C75.2   **Malignant neoplasm of craniopharyngeal duct** 🦠
> (Ex) See PDX Collection 322

    C75.3   **Malignant neoplasm of pineal gland** 🦠
> (Ex) See PDX Collection 323

    C75.4   **Malignant neoplasm of carotid body** 🦠
> (Ex) See PDX Collection 324

    C75.5   **Malignant neoplasm of aortic body and other paraganglia** 🦠
> (Ex) See PDX Collection 325

    C75.8   **Malignant neoplasm with pluriglandular involvement, unspecified** 🦠
> (Ex) See PDX Collection 326

    C75.9   **Malignant neoplasm of endocrine gland, unspecified** 🦠
> (Ex) See PDX Collection 326

MALIGNANT NEUROENDOCRINE TUMORS (C7A)

● **C7A**   **Malignant neuroendocrine tumors**
> Code also any associated multiple endocrine neoplasia [MEN] syndromes (E31.2-)
> Use additional code to identify any associated endocrine syndrome, such as:
> carcinoid syndrome (E34.0)

> **Excludes2**   malignant pancreatic islet cell tumors (C25.4)
> Merkel cell carcinoma (C4A.-)

   ● **C7A.0**   **Malignant carcinoid tumors**

      C7A.00   **Malignant carcinoid tumor of unspecified site** 🦠
> (Ex) See PDX Collection 346

    ● **C7A.01**   **Malignant carcinoid tumors of the small intestine**

       C7A.010   **Malignant carcinoid tumor of the duodenum** 🦠
> (Ex) See PDX Collection 347

       C7A.011   **Malignant carcinoid tumor of the jejunum** 🦠
> (Ex) See PDX Collection 348

       C7A.012   **Malignant carcinoid tumor of the ileum** 🦠
> (Ex) See PDX Collection 349

       C7A.019   **Malignant carcinoid tumor of the small intestine, unspecified portion** 🦠
> (Ex) See PDX Collection 350

N Newborn Age: 0   **P** Pediatric Age: 0–17   **M** Maternity DX: 12–55   **A** Adult Age: 15–124   ♀ Females Only   ♂ Males Only

🦠 Complication\Comorbidity   🦠 Major C\C   (Ex) CC/MCC Exclusions   🦠 Hospital-Acquired Condition

687

CHAPTER 2 (C00-D49)

C7A.02 Malignant carcinoid tumors of the appendix, large intestine, and rectum

C7A.020 Malignant carcinoid tumor of the appendix
Ex: See PDX Collection 351

C7A.021 Malignant carcinoid tumor of the cecum
Ex: See PDX Collection 352

C7A.022 Malignant carcinoid tumor of the ascending colon
Ex: See PDX Collection 353

C7A.023 Malignant carcinoid tumor of the transverse colon
Ex: See PDX Collection 354

C7A.024 Malignant carcinoid tumor of the descending colon
Ex: See PDX Collection 355

C7A.025 Malignant carcinoid tumor of the sigmoid colon
Ex: See PDX Collection 356

C7A.026 Malignant carcinoid tumor of the rectum
Ex: See PDX Collection 357

C7A.029 Malignant carcinoid tumor of the large intestine, unspecified portion
Malignant carcinoid tumor of the colon NOS
Ex: See PDX Collection 358

C7A.09 Malignant carcinoid tumors of other sites
Ex: For category C7A.09 CC codes unless otherwise indicated: See PDX Collection 361

C7A.090 Malignant carcinoid tumor of the bronchus and lung
Ex: See PDX Collection 359

C7A.091 Malignant carcinoid tumor of the thymus
Ex: See PDX Collection 360

C7A.092 Malignant carcinoid tumor of the stomach

C7A.093 Malignant carcinoid tumor of the kidney
Ex: See PDX Collection 362

C7A.094 Malignant carcinoid tumor of the foregut, unspecified

C7A.095 Malignant carcinoid tumor of the midgut, unspecified

C7A.096 Malignant carcinoid tumor of the hindgut, unspecified

C7A.098 Malignant carcinoid tumors of other sites
Ex: See PDX Collection 346

C7A.1 Malignant poorly differentiated neuroendocrine tumors
Malignant poorly differentiated neuroendocrine tumor NOS
Malignant poorly differentiated neuroendocrine carcinoma, any site
High grade neuroendocrine carcinoma, any site
Ex: See PDX Collection 346

C7A.8 Other malignant neuroendocrine tumors
Secondary neuroendocrine tumors (C7B)
Ex: See PDX Collection 346

SECONDARY NEUROENDOCRINE TUMORS (C7B)

C7B Secondary neuroendocrine tumors
Use additional code to identify any functional activity

C7B.0 Secondary carcinoid tumors

C7B.00 Secondary carcinoid tumors, unspecified site

C7B.01 Secondary carcinoid tumors of distant lymph nodes
Ex: See PDX Collection 363

C7B.02 Secondary carcinoid tumors of liver
Ex: See PDX Collection 364

C7B.03 Secondary carcinoid tumors of bone
Ex: See PDX Collection 365

C7B.04 Secondary carcinoid tumors of peritoneum
Mesentary metastasis of carcinoid tumor
Ex: See PDX Collection 366

C7B.09 Secondary carcinoid tumors of other sites
Ex: See PDX Collection 367

C7B.1 Secondary Merkel cell carcinoma
Merkel cell carcinoma nodal presentation
Merkel cell carcinoma visceral metastatic presentation

C7B.8 Other secondary neuroendocrine tumors
Ex: See PDX Collection 367

MALIGNANT NEOPLASMS OF ILL-DEFINED, OTHER SECONDARY AND UNSPECIFIED SITES (C76-C80)

C76 Malignant neoplasm of other and ill-defined sites
Excludes1 malignant neoplasm of female genitourinary tract NOS (C57.9)
malignant neoplasm of male genitourinary tract NOS (C63.9)
malignant neoplasm of lymphoid, hematopoietic and related tissue (C81-C96)
malignant neoplasm of skin (C44.-)
malignant neoplasm of unspecified site NOS (C80.1)

C76.0 Malignant neoplasm of head, face and neck
Malignant neoplasm of cheek NOS
Malignant neoplasm of nose NOS

C76.1 Malignant neoplasm of thorax
Intrathoracic malignant neoplasm NOS
Malignant neoplasm of axilla NOS
Thoracic malignant neoplasm NOS

C76.2 Malignant neoplasm of abdomen

C76.3 Malignant neoplasm of pelvis
Malignant neoplasm of groin NOS
Malignant neoplasm of sites overlapping systems within the pelvis
Rectovaginal (septum) malignant neoplasm
Between rectum and vagina
Rectovesical (septum) malignant neoplasm
Between rectum and urinary bladder; AKA vesicorectal

C76.4 Malignant neoplasm of upper limb
C76.40 Malignant neoplasm of unspecified upper limb
C76.41 Malignant neoplasm of right upper limb
C76.42 Malignant neoplasm of left upper limb

C76.5 Malignant neoplasm of lower limb
C76.50 Malignant neoplasm of unspecified lower limb
C76.51 Malignant neoplasm of right lower limb
C76.52 Malignant neoplasm of left lower limb

C76.8 Malignant neoplasm of other specified ill-defined sites
Malignant neoplasm of overlapping ill-defined sites

● **C77**   **Secondary and unspecified malignant neoplasm of lymph nodes**

> **Excludes1**   malignant neoplasm of lymph nodes, specified as primary (C81-C86, C88, C96.-)
> mesentary metastasis of carcinoid tumor (C7B.04)
> secondary carcinoid tumors of distant lymph nodes (C7B.01)

> (Ex) **For category C77 CC codes:** See PDX Collection 303

     C77.0   **Secondary and unspecified malignant neoplasm of lymph nodes of head, face and neck** 🔖
> Secondary and unspecified malignant neoplasm of supraclavicular lymph nodes

     C77.1   **Secondary and unspecified malignant neoplasm of intrathoracic lymph nodes** 🔖

     C77.2   **Secondary and unspecified malignant neoplasm of intra-abdominal lymph nodes** 🔖

     C77.3   **Secondary and unspecified malignant neoplasm of axilla and upper limb lymph nodes** 🔖
> Secondary and unspecified malignant neoplasm of pectoral lymph nodes

     C77.4   **Secondary and unspecified malignant neoplasm of inguinal and lower limb lymph nodes** 🔖

     C77.5   **Secondary and unspecified malignant neoplasm of intrapelvic lymph nodes** 🔖

     C77.8   **Secondary and unspecified malignant neoplasm of lymph nodes of multiple regions** 🔖

     C77.9   **Secondary and unspecified malignant neoplasm of lymph node, unspecified** 🔖

● **C78**   **Secondary malignant neoplasm of respiratory and digestive organs**

> **Excludes1**   secondary carcinoid tumors of liver (C7B.02)
> secondary carcinoid tumors of peritoneum (C7B.04)

> **Excludes2**   lymph node metastases (C77.0)

    ● **C78.0**   **Secondary malignant neoplasm of lung**
> (Ex) **For category C78.0 CC Codes:** See PDX Collection 327

     C78.00   **Secondary malignant neoplasm of unspecified lung** 🔖

     C78.01   **Secondary malignant neoplasm of right lung** 🔖

     C78.02   **Secondary malignant neoplasm of left lung** 🔖

     C78.1   **Secondary malignant neoplasm of mediastinum** 🔖
> *Thoracic cavity between pleural cavities*
> (Ex) See PDX Collection 328

     C78.2   **Secondary malignant neoplasm of pleura** 🔖
> *Serous membrane covering lungs and lining thoracic cavity*
> (Ex) See PDX Collection 329

    ● **C78.3**   **Secondary malignant neoplasm of other and unspecified respiratory organs**
> (Ex) **For category C78.3 CC Codes:** See PDX Collection 330

     C78.30   **Secondary malignant neoplasm of unspecified respiratory organ** 🔖

     C78.39   **Secondary malignant neoplasm of other respiratory organs** 🔖

     C78.4   **Secondary malignant neoplasm of small intestine** 🔖
> (Ex) See PDX Collection 331

     C78.5   **Secondary malignant neoplasm of large intestine and rectum** 🔖
> (Ex) See PDX Collection 332

     C78.6   **Secondary malignant neoplasm of retroperitoneum and peritoneum** 🔖
> (Ex) See PDX Collection 333
> **Coding Clinic: 2017, Q2, P12**

     C78.7   **Secondary malignant neoplasm of liver and intrahepatic bile duct** 🔖
> (Ex) See PDX Collection 334

Item 2–6   The adrenal glands are a pair of glands situated on top of or above each kidney ("suprarenal") and chiefly responsible for regulating the stress response through the synthesis of corticosteroids and catecholamines, including cortisol and adrenaline.

    ● **C78.8**   **Secondary malignant neoplasm of other and unspecified digestive organs**
> (Ex) **For category C78.8 CC Codes:** See PDX Collection 335

     C78.80   **Secondary malignant neoplasm of unspecified digestive organ** 🔖

     C78.89   **Secondary malignant neoplasm of other digestive organs** 🔖
> Code also exocrine pancreatic insufficiency (K86.81)

● **C79**   **Secondary malignant neoplasm of other and unspecified sites**

> **Excludes1**   secondary carcinoid tumors (C7B.-)
> secondary neuroendocrine tumors (C7B.-)
> ~~lymph node metastases (C77.0)~~

    ● **C79.0**   **Secondary malignant neoplasm of kidney and renal pelvis**
> (Ex) **For category C79.0 CC Codes:** See PDX Collection 336

     C79.00   **Secondary malignant neoplasm of unspecified kidney and renal pelvis** 🔖

     C79.01   **Secondary malignant neoplasm of right kidney and renal pelvis** 🔖

     C79.02   **Secondary malignant neoplasm of left kidney and renal pelvis** 🔖

    ● **C79.1**   **Secondary malignant neoplasm of bladder and other and unspecified urinary organs**
> (Ex) **For category C79.1 CC Codes:** See PDX Collection 336

     C79.10   **Secondary malignant neoplasm of unspecified urinary organs** 🔖

     C79.11   **Secondary malignant neoplasm of bladder** 🔖
> ▶ **Excludes2**   lymph node metastases (C77.0)

     C79.19   **Secondary malignant neoplasm of other urinary organs** 🔖

     C79.2   **Secondary malignant neoplasm of skin** 🔖
> **Excludes1**   secondary Merkel cell carcinoma (C7B.1)
> (Ex) See PDX Collection 337

    ● **C79.3**   **Secondary malignant neoplasm of brain and cerebral meninges**

     C79.31   **Secondary malignant neoplasm of brain** 🔖
> (Ex) See PDX Collection 338

     C79.32   **Secondary malignant neoplasm of cerebral meninges** 🔖
> (Ex) See PDX Collection 339

    ● **C79.4**   **Secondary malignant neoplasm of other and unspecified parts of nervous system**
> (Ex) **For category C79.4 CC codes:** See PDX Collection 339

     C79.40   **Secondary malignant neoplasm of unspecified part of nervous system** 🔖

     C79.49   **Secondary malignant neoplasm of other parts of nervous system** 🔖

    ● **C79.5**   **Secondary malignant neoplasm of bone and bone marrow**
> **Excludes1**   secondary carcinoid tumors of bone (C7B.03)
> (Ex) **For category C79.5 CC codes:** See PDX Collection 340

     C79.51   **Secondary malignant neoplasm of bone** 🔖

     C79.52   **Secondary malignant neoplasm of bone marrow** 🔖

    ● **C79.6**   **Secondary malignant neoplasm of ovary**
> (Ex) **For category C79.6 CC codes:** See PDX Collection 341

     C79.60   **Secondary malignant neoplasm of unspecified ovary** ♀ 🔖

     C79.61   **Secondary malignant neoplasm of right ovary** ♀ 🔖

     C79.62   **Secondary malignant neoplasm of left ovary** ♀ 🔖

CHAPTER 2 (C00-D49)

N Newborn Age: 0   **P** Pediatric Age: 0–17   **M** Maternity DX: 12–55   **A** Adult Age: 15–124   ♀ Females Only   ♂ Males Only

🔖 Complication\Comorbidity   🔖 Major C\C   (Ex) CC/MCC Exclusions   🔖 Hospital-Acquired Condition

● **C79.7** Secondary malignant neoplasm of adrenal gland
  (Ex) *For category C79.7 CC codes: See PDX Collection 342*

   C79.70 Secondary malignant neoplasm of unspecified adrenal gland 🔖

   C79.71 Secondary malignant neoplasm of right adrenal gland 🔖

   C79.72 Secondary malignant neoplasm of left adrenal gland 🔖

● **C79.8** Secondary malignant neoplasm of other specified sites

   C79.81 Secondary malignant neoplasm of breast 🔖
     (Ex) See PDX Collection 343

   C79.82 Secondary malignant neoplasm of genital organs 🔖
     (Ex) See PDX Collection 344

   C79.89 Secondary malignant neoplasm of other specified sites 🔖
     (Ex) See PDX Collection 345
     Coding Clinic: 2017, Q2, P11

C79.9 Secondary malignant neoplasm of unspecified site 🔖
   Metastatic cancer NOS
   Metastatic disease NOS
   Excludes1 carcinomatosis NOS (C80.0)
              generalized cancer NOS (C80.0)
              malignant (primary) neoplasm of unspecified site (C80.1)
   (Ex) See PDX Collection 345

OGCR Section I.C.2.j and k

> Disseminated malignant neoplasm, unspecified
>
> j. Code C80.0, Disseminated malignant neoplasm, unspecified, is for use only in those cases where the patient has advanced metastatic disease and no known primary or secondary sites are specified. It should not be used in place of assigning codes for the primary site and all known secondary sites.
>
> Malignant neoplasm without specification of site
>
> k. Code C80.1, Malignant (primary) neoplasm, unspecified, equates to Cancer, unspecified. This code should only be used when no determination can be made as to the primary site of a malignancy. This code should rarely be used in the inpatient setting.

● **C80** Malignant neoplasm without specification of site
   Excludes1 malignant carcinoid tumor of unspecified site (C7A.00)
              malignant neoplasm of specified multiple sites-code to each site

   C80.0 Disseminated malignant neoplasm, unspecified 🔖
     Carcinomatosis NOS
     Generalized cancer, unspecified site (primary) (secondary)
     Generalized malignancy, unspecified site (primary) (secondary)
     (Ex) See PDX Collection 345

   C80.1 Malignant (primary) neoplasm, unspecified
     Cancer NOS
     Cancer unspecified site (primary)
     Carcinoma unspecified site (primary)
     Malignancy unspecified site (primary)
     Excludes1 secondary malignant neoplasm of unspecified site (C79.9)

● **C80.2** Malignant neoplasm associated with transplanted organ 🔖
     Code first complication of transplanted organ (T86.-)
     Use additional code to identify the specific malignancy
     (Ex) See PDX Collection 345

★ **(See Plate 315 on page 49.)**

MALIGNANT NEOPLASMS OF LYMPHOID, HEMATOPOIETIC AND RELATED TISSUE (C81-C96)

Excludes2 Kaposi's sarcoma of lymph nodes (C46.3)
           secondary and unspecified neoplasm of lymph nodes (C77.-)
           secondary neoplasm of bone marrow (C79.52)
           secondary neoplasm of spleen (C78.89)

● **C81** Hodgkin lymphoma
   Form of malignant lymphoma with four types, nodular sclerosis, mixed cellularity, lymphocyte depleted, and lymphocyte predominant
   Excludes1 personal history of Hodgkin lymphoma (Z85.71)

● **C81.0** Nodular lymphocyte predominant Hodgkin lymphoma
   Least aggressive, least common, typically no symptoms
   Lymphocytic-histiocytic predominance Hodgkin's disease

   C81.00 Nodular lymphocyte predominant Hodgkin lymphoma, unspecified site 🔖
     (Ex) See PDX Collection 368

   C81.01 Nodular lymphocyte predominant Hodgkin lymphoma, lymph nodes of head, face, and neck 🔖
     (Ex) See PDX Collection 369

   C81.02 Nodular lymphocyte predominant Hodgkin lymphoma, intrathoracic lymph nodes 🔖
     (Ex) See PDX Collection 370

   C81.03 Nodular lymphocyte predominant Hodgkin lymphoma, intra-abdominal lymph nodes 🔖
     (Ex) See PDX Collection 371

   C81.04 Nodular lymphocyte predominant Hodgkin lymphoma, lymph nodes of axilla and upper limb 🔖
     (Ex) See PDX Collection 372

   C81.05 Nodular lymphocyte predominant Hodgkin lymphoma, lymph nodes of inguinal region and lower limb 🔖
     (Ex) See PDX Collection 373

   C81.06 Nodular lymphocyte predominant Hodgkin lymphoma, intrapelvic lymph nodes 🔖
     (Ex) See PDX Collection 374

   C81.07 Nodular lymphocyte predominant Hodgkin lymphoma, spleen 🔖
     (Ex) See PDX Collection 375

   C81.08 Nodular lymphocyte predominant Hodgkin lymphoma, lymph nodes of multiple sites 🔖
     (Ex) See PDX Collection 368

   C81.09 Nodular lymphocyte predominant Hodgkin lymphoma, extranodal and solid organ sites 🔖
     (Ex) See PDX Collection 368

● **C81.1** Nodular sclerosis Hodgkin lymphoma
   Nodular sclerosis classical Hodgkin lymphoma
   Moderately aggressive; most common in young adults

   C81.10 Nodular sclerosis Hodgkin lymphoma, unspecified site 🔖
     (Ex) See PDX Collection 376

   C81.11 Nodular sclerosis Hodgkin lymphoma, lymph nodes of head, face, and neck 🔖
     (Ex) See PDX Collection 377

   C81.12 Nodular sclerosis Hodgkin lymphoma, intrathoracic lymph nodes 🔖
     (Ex) See PDX Collection 378

   C81.13 Nodular sclerosis Hodgkin lymphoma, intra-abdominal lymph nodes 🔖
     (Ex) See PDX Collection 379

   C81.14 Nodular sclerosis Hodgkin lymphoma, lymph nodes of axilla and upper limb 🔖
     (Ex) See PDX Collection 380

   C81.15 Nodular sclerosis Hodgkin lymphoma, lymph nodes of inguinal region and lower limb 🔖
     (Ex) See PDX Collection 381

▶ New   ⇒ Revised   ~~deleted~~ Deleted   Excludes 1   Excludes 2   Includes   Use additional   Code first   Code also   Key words
OGCR Official Guidelines   ● Unacceptable Principal Diagnosis   X Assign placeholder X   ● Use Additional Character(s)   ▸ Manifestation Code   **Coding Clinic**

C81.16   Nodular sclerosis Hodgkin lymphoma, intrapelvic lymph nodes
         (Ex) See PDX Collection 382

C81.17   Nodular sclerosis Hodgkin lymphoma, spleen
         (Ex) See PDX Collection 383

C81.18   Nodular sclerosis Hodgkin lymphoma, lymph nodes of multiple sites
         (Ex) See PDX Collection 376

C81.19   Nodular sclerosis Hodgkin lymphoma, extranodal and solid organ sites
         (Ex) See PDX Collection 376

● C81.2   **Mixed cellularity Hodgkin lymphoma**
          Mixed cellularity classical Hodgkin lymphoma
          A type of Hodgkin's that is moderately aggressive with mixed cell types

C81.20   Mixed cellularity Hodgkin lymphoma, unspecified site
         (Ex) See PDX Collection 384

C81.21   Mixed cellularity Hodgkin lymphoma, lymph nodes of head, face, and neck
         (Ex) See PDX Collection 385

C81.22   Mixed cellularity Hodgkin lymphoma, intrathoracic lymph nodes
         (Ex) See PDX Collection 386

C81.23   Mixed cellularity Hodgkin lymphoma, intra-abdominal lymph nodes
         (Ex) See PDX Collection 387

C81.24   Mixed cellularity Hodgkin lymphoma, lymph nodes of axilla and upper limb
         (Ex) See PDX Collection 388

C81.25   Mixed cellularity Hodgkin lymphoma, lymph nodes of inguinal region and lower limb
         (Ex) See PDX Collection 389

C81.26   Mixed cellularity Hodgkin lymphoma, intrapelvic lymph nodes
         (Ex) See PDX Collection 390

C81.27   Mixed cellularity Hodgkin lymphoma, spleen
         (Ex) See PDX Collection 391

C81.28   Mixed cellularity Hodgkin lymphoma, lymph nodes of multiple sites
         (Ex) See PDX Collection 384

C81.29   Mixed cellularity Hodgkin lymphoma, extranodal and solid organ sites
         (Ex) See PDX Collection 384

● C81.3   **Lymphocyte depleted Hodgkin lymphoma**
          Lymphocyte depleted classical Hodgkin lymphoma
          Most aggressive type with poor prognosis

C81.30   Lymphocyte depleted Hodgkin lymphoma, unspecified site
         (Ex) See PDX Collection 392

C81.31   Lymphocyte depleted Hodgkin lymphoma, lymph nodes of head, face, and neck
         (Ex) See PDX Collection 393

C81.32   Lymphocyte depleted Hodgkin lymphoma, intrathoracic lymph nodes
         (Ex) See PDX Collection 394

C81.33   Lymphocyte depleted Hodgkin lymphoma, intra-abdominal lymph nodes
         (Ex) See PDX Collection 395

C81.34   Lymphocyte depleted Hodgkin lymphoma, lymph nodes of axilla and upper limb
         (Ex) See PDX Collection 396

C81.35   Lymphocyte depleted Hodgkin lymphoma, lymph nodes of inguinal region and lower limb
         (Ex) See PDX Collection 397

C81.36   Lymphocyte depleted Hodgkin lymphoma, intrapelvic lymph nodes
         (Ex) See PDX Collection 398

C81.37   Lymphocyte depleted Hodgkin lymphoma, spleen
         (Ex) See PDX Collection 399

C81.38   Lymphocyte depleted Hodgkin lymphoma, lymph nodes of multiple sites
         (Ex) See PDX Collection 400

C81.39   Lymphocyte depleted Hodgkin lymphoma, extranodal and solid organ sites
         (Ex) See PDX Collection 392

● C81.4   **Lymphocyte-rich Hodgkin lymphoma**
          Lymphocyte-rich classical Hodgkin lymphoma
          Excludes1   nodular lymphocyte predominant Hodgkin lymphoma (C81.0-)

C81.40   Lymphocyte-rich Hodgkin lymphoma, unspecified site
         (Ex) See PDX Collection 368

C81.41   Lymphocyte-rich Hodgkin lymphoma, lymph nodes of head, face, and neck
         (Ex) See PDX Collection 369

C81.42   Lymphocyte-rich Hodgkin lymphoma, intrathoracic lymph nodes
         (Ex) See PDX Collection 370

C81.43   Lymphocyte-rich Hodgkin lymphoma, intra-abdominal lymph nodes
         (Ex) See PDX Collection 371

C81.44   Lymphocyte-rich Hodgkin lymphoma, lymph nodes of axilla and upper limb
         (Ex) See PDX Collection 372

C81.45   Lymphocyte-rich Hodgkin lymphoma, lymph nodes of inguinal region and lower limb
         (Ex) See PDX Collection 373

C81.46   Lymphocyte-rich Hodgkin lymphoma, intrapelvic lymph nodes
         (Ex) See PDX Collection 374

C81.47   Lymphocyte-rich Hodgkin lymphoma, spleen
         (Ex) See PDX Collection 375

C81.48   Lymphocyte-rich Hodgkin lymphoma, lymph nodes of multiple sites
         (Ex) See PDX Collection 368

C81.49   Lymphocyte-rich Hodgkin lymphoma, extranodal and solid organ sites
         (Ex) See PDX Collection 368

● C81.7   **Other Hodgkin lymphoma**
          Classical Hodgkin lymphoma NOS
          Other classical Hodgkin lymphoma

C81.70   Other Hodgkin lymphoma, unspecified site
         (Ex) See PDX Collection 401

C81.71   Other Hodgkin lymphoma, lymph nodes of head, face, and neck
         (Ex) See PDX Collection 402

C81.72   Other Hodgkin lymphoma, intrathoracic lymph nodes
         (Ex) See PDX Collection 403

C81.73   Other Hodgkin lymphoma, intra-abdominal lymph nodes
         (Ex) See PDX Collection 404

C81.74   Other Hodgkin lymphoma, lymph nodes of axilla and upper limb
         (Ex) See PDX Collection 405

C81.75   Other Hodgkin lymphoma, lymph nodes of inguinal region and lower limb
         (Ex) See PDX Collection 406

C81.76   Other Hodgkin lymphoma, intrapelvic lymph nodes
         (Ex) See PDX Collection 407

C81.77   Other Hodgkin lymphoma, spleen
         (Ex) See PDX Collection 408

C81.78   Other Hodgkin lymphoma, lymph nodes of multiple sites
         (Ex) See PDX Collection 401

C81.79   Other Hodgkin lymphoma, extranodal and solid organ sites
         (Ex) See PDX Collection 401

CHAPTER 2 (C00–D49)

● C81.9 Hodgkin lymphoma, unspecified

C81.90 Hodgkin lymphoma, unspecified, unspecified site 🔖
Ex: See PDX Collection 409

C81.91 Hodgkin lymphoma, unspecified, lymph nodes of head, face, and neck 🔖
Ex: See PDX Collection 410

C81.92 Hodgkin lymphoma, unspecified, intrathoracic lymph nodes 🔖
Ex: See PDX Collection 411

C81.93 Hodgkin lymphoma, unspecified, intra-abdominal lymph nodes 🔖
Ex: See PDX Collection 412

C81.94 Hodgkin lymphoma, unspecified, lymph nodes of axilla and upper limb 🔖
Ex: See PDX Collection 413

C81.95 Hodgkin lymphoma, unspecified, lymph nodes of inguinal region and lower limb 🔖
Ex: See PDX Collection 414

C81.96 Hodgkin lymphoma, unspecified, intrapelvic lymph nodes 🔖
Ex: See PDX Collection 415

C81.97 Hodgkin lymphoma, unspecified, spleen 🔖
Ex: See PDX Collection 416

C81.98 Hodgkin lymphoma, unspecified, lymph nodes of multiple sites 🔖
Ex: See PDX Collection 409

C81.99 Hodgkin lymphoma, unspecified, extranodal and solid organ sites 🔖
Ex: No exclusions

● C82 Follicular lymphoma
Group of malignant lymphomas

Includes   follicular lymphoma with or without diffuse areas

Excludes1 mature T/NK-cell lymphomas (C84.-)
personal history of non-Hodgkin lymphoma (Z85.72)

● C82.0 Follicular lymphoma grade I

C82.00 Follicular lymphoma grade I, unspecified site 🔖
Ex: See PDX Collection 417

C82.01 Follicular lymphoma grade I, lymph nodes of head, face, and neck 🔖
Ex: See PDX Collection 418

C82.02 Follicular lymphoma grade I, intrathoracic lymph nodes 🔖
Ex: See PDX Collection 419

C82.03 Follicular lymphoma grade I, intra-abdominal lymph nodes 🔖
Ex: See PDX Collection 420

C82.04 Follicular lymphoma grade I, lymph nodes of axilla and upper limb 🔖
Ex: See PDX Collection 421

C82.05 Follicular lymphoma grade I, lymph nodes of inguinal region and lower limb 🔖
Ex: See PDX Collection 422

C82.06 Follicular lymphoma grade I, intrapelvic lymph nodes 🔖
Ex: See PDX Collection 423

C82.07 Follicular lymphoma grade I, spleen 🔖
Ex: See PDX Collection 424

C82.08 Follicular lymphoma grade I, lymph nodes of multiple sites 🔖
Ex: See PDX Collection 425

C82.09 Follicular lymphoma grade I, extranodal and solid organ sites 🔖
Ex: See PDX Collection 417

● C82.1 Follicular lymphoma grade II

C82.10 Follicular lymphoma grade II, unspecified site 🔖
Ex: See PDX Collection 417

C82.11 Follicular lymphoma grade II, lymph nodes of head, face, and neck 🔖
Ex: See PDX Collection 418

C82.12 Follicular lymphoma grade II, intrathoracic lymph nodes 🔖
Ex: See PDX Collection 419

C82.13 Follicular lymphoma grade II, intra-abdominal lymph nodes 🔖
Ex: See PDX Collection 420

C82.14 Follicular lymphoma grade II, lymph nodes of axilla and upper limb 🔖
Ex: See PDX Collection 421

C82.15 Follicular lymphoma grade II, lymph nodes of inguinal region and lower limb 🔖
Ex: See PDX Collection 422

C82.16 Follicular lymphoma grade II, intrapelvic lymph nodes 🔖
Ex: See PDX Collection 423

C82.17 Follicular lymphoma grade II, spleen 🔖
Ex: See PDX Collection 424

C82.18 Follicular lymphoma grade II, lymph nodes of multiple sites 🔖
Ex: See PDX Collection 425

C82.19 Follicular lymphoma grade II, extranodal and solid organ sites 🔖
Ex: See PDX Collection 417

● C82.2 Follicular lymphoma grade III, unspecified

C82.20 Follicular lymphoma grade III, unspecified, unspecified site 🔖
Ex: See PDX Collection 417

C82.21 Follicular lymphoma grade III, unspecified, lymph nodes of head, face, and neck 🔖
Ex: See PDX Collection 418

C82.22 Follicular lymphoma grade III, unspecified, intrathoracic lymph nodes 🔖
Ex: See PDX Collection 419

C82.23 Follicular lymphoma grade III, unspecified, intra-abdominal lymph nodes 🔖
Ex: See PDX Collection 420

C82.24 Follicular lymphoma grade III, unspecified, lymph nodes of axilla and upper limb 🔖
Ex: See PDX Collection 421

C82.25 Follicular lymphoma grade III, unspecified, lymph nodes of inguinal region and lower limb 🔖
Ex: See PDX Collection 422

C82.26 Follicular lymphoma grade III, unspecified, intrapelvic lymph nodes 🔖
Ex: See PDX Collection 423

C82.27 Follicular lymphoma grade III, unspecified, spleen 🔖
Ex: See PDX Collection 424

C82.28 Follicular lymphoma grade III, unspecified, lymph nodes of multiple sites 🔖
Ex: See PDX Collection 425

C82.29 Follicular lymphoma grade III, unspecified, extranodal and solid organ sites 🔖
Ex: See PDX Collection 417

● **C82.3　Follicular lymphoma grade IIIa**

    C82.30　Follicular lymphoma grade IIIa, unspecified site 🔗
        Ex: See PDX Collection 417

    C82.31　Follicular lymphoma grade IIIa, lymph nodes of head, face, and neck 🔗
        Ex: See PDX Collection 418

    C82.32　Follicular lymphoma grade IIIa, intrathoracic lymph nodes 🔗
        Ex: See PDX Collection 419

    C82.33　Follicular lymphoma grade IIIa, intra-abdominal lymph nodes 🔗
        Ex: See PDX Collection 420

    C82.34　Follicular lymphoma grade IIIa, lymph nodes of axilla and upper limb 🔗
        Ex: See PDX Collection 421

    C82.35　Follicular lymphoma grade IIIa, lymph nodes of inguinal region and lower limb 🔗
        Ex: See PDX Collection 422

    C82.36　Follicular lymphoma grade IIIa, intrapelvic lymph nodes 🔗
        Ex: See PDX Collection 423

    C82.37　Follicular lymphoma grade IIIa, spleen 🔗
        Ex: See PDX Collection 424

    C82.38　Follicular lymphoma grade IIIa, lymph nodes of multiple sites 🔗
        Ex: See PDX Collection 425

    C82.39　Follicular lymphoma grade IIIa, extranodal and solid organ sites 🔗
        Ex: See PDX Collection 417

● **C82.4　Follicular lymphoma grade IIIb**

    C82.40　Follicular lymphoma grade IIIb, unspecified site 🔗
        Ex: See PDX Collection 417

    C82.41　Follicular lymphoma grade IIIb, lymph nodes of head, face, and neck 🔗
        Ex: See PDX Collection 418

    C82.42　Follicular lymphoma grade IIIb, intrathoracic lymph nodes 🔗
        Ex: See PDX Collection 419

    C82.43　Follicular lymphoma grade IIIb, intra-abdominal lymph nodes 🔗
        Ex: See PDX Collection 420

    C82.44　Follicular lymphoma grade IIIb, lymph nodes of axilla and upper limb 🔗
        Ex: See PDX Collection 421

    C82.45　Follicular lymphoma grade IIIb, lymph nodes of inguinal region and lower limb 🔗
        Ex: See PDX Collection 422

    C82.46　Follicular lymphoma grade IIIb, intrapelvic lymph nodes 🔗
        Ex: See PDX Collection 423

    C82.47　Follicular lymphoma grade IIIb, spleen 🔗
        Ex: See PDX Collection 424

    C82.48　Follicular lymphoma grade IIIb, lymph nodes of multiple sites 🔗
        Ex: See PDX Collection 425

    C82.49　Follicular lymphoma grade IIIb, extranodal and solid organ sites 🔗
        Ex: See PDX Collection 417

● **C82.5　Diffuse follicle center lymphoma**

    C82.50　Diffuse follicle center lymphoma, unspecified site 🔗
        Ex: See PDX Collection 426

    C82.51　Diffuse follicle center lymphoma, lymph nodes of head, face, and neck 🔗
        Ex: See PDX Collection 427

    C82.52　Diffuse follicle center lymphoma, intrathoracic lymph nodes 🔗
        Ex: See PDX Collection 428

    C82.53　Diffuse follicle center lymphoma, intra-abdominal lymph nodes 🔗
        Ex: See PDX Collection 429

    C82.54　Diffuse follicle center lymphoma, lymph nodes of axilla and upper limb 🔗
        Ex: See PDX Collection 430

    C82.55　Diffuse follicle center lymphoma, lymph nodes of inguinal region and lower limb 🔗
        Ex: See PDX Collection 431

    C82.56　Diffuse follicle center lymphoma, intrapelvic lymph nodes 🔗
        Ex: See PDX Collection 432

    C82.57　Diffuse follicle center lymphoma, spleen 🔗
        Ex: See PDX Collection 433

    C82.58　Diffuse follicle center lymphoma, lymph nodes of multiple sites 🔗
        Ex: See PDX Collection 434

    C82.59　Diffuse follicle center lymphoma, extranodal and solid organ sites 🔗
        Ex: See PDX Collection 426

● **C82.6　Cutaneous follicle center lymphoma**

    C82.60　Cutaneous follicle center lymphoma, unspecified site 🔗
        Ex: See PDX Collection 417

    C82.61　Cutaneous follicle center lymphoma, lymph nodes of head, face, and neck 🔗
        Ex: See PDX Collection 418

    C82.62　Cutaneous follicle center lymphoma, intrathoracic lymph nodes 🔗
        Ex: See PDX Collection 419

    C82.63　Cutaneous follicle center lymphoma, intra-abdominal lymph nodes 🔗
        Ex: See PDX Collection 420

    C82.64　Cutaneous follicle center lymphoma, lymph nodes of axilla and upper limb 🔗
        Ex: See PDX Collection 421

    C82.65　Cutaneous follicle center lymphoma, lymph nodes of inguinal region and lower limb 🔗
        Ex: See PDX Collection 422

    C82.66　Cutaneous follicle center lymphoma, intrapelvic lymph nodes 🔗
        Ex: See PDX Collection 423

    C82.67　Cutaneous follicle center lymphoma, spleen 🔗
        Ex: See PDX Collection 424

    C82.68　Cutaneous follicle center lymphoma, lymph nodes of multiple sites 🔗
        Ex: See PDX Collection 425

    C82.69　Cutaneous follicle center lymphoma, extranodal and solid organ sites 🔗
        Ex: See PDX Collection 417

CHAPTER 2 (C00–D49)

N Newborn Age: 0　　**P** Pediatric Age: 0–17　　**M** Maternity DX: 12–55　　**A** Adult Age: 15–124　　♀ Females Only　　♂ Males Only

🔗 Complication\Comorbidity　　🔗 Major C\C　　Ex: CC/MCC Exclusions　　🔗 Hospital-Acquired Condition

693

CHAPTER 2 (C00-D49)

● **C82.8** **Other types of follicular lymphoma**

    C82.80 Other types of follicular lymphoma, unspecified site 🔗
        Ex: See PDX Collection 417

    C82.81 Other types of follicular lymphoma, lymph nodes of head, face, and neck 🔗
        Ex: See PDX Collection 418

    C82.82 Other types of follicular lymphoma, intrathoracic lymph nodes 🔗
        Ex: See PDX Collection 419

    C82.83 Other types of follicular lymphoma, intra-abdominal lymph nodes 🔗
        Ex: See PDX Collection 420

    C82.84 Other types of follicular lymphoma, lymph nodes of axilla and upper limb 🔗
        Ex: See PDX Collection 421

    C82.85 Other types of follicular lymphoma, lymph nodes of inguinal region and lower limb 🔗
        Ex: See PDX Collection 422

    C82.86 Other types of follicular lymphoma, intrapelvic lymph nodes 🔗
        Ex: See PDX Collection 423

    C82.87 Other types of follicular lymphoma, spleen 🔗
        Ex: See PDX Collection 424

    C82.88 Other types of follicular lymphoma, lymph nodes of multiple sites 🔗
        Ex: See PDX Collection 425

    C82.89 Other types of follicular lymphoma, extranodal and solid organ sites 🔗
        Ex: See PDX Collection 417

● **C82.9** **Follicular lymphoma, unspecified**

    C82.90 Follicular lymphoma, unspecified, unspecified site 🔗
        Ex: See PDX Collection 417

    C82.91 Follicular lymphoma, unspecified, lymph nodes of head, face, and neck 🔗
        Ex: See PDX Collection 418

    C82.92 Follicular lymphoma, unspecified, intrathoracic lymph nodes 🔗
        Ex: See PDX Collection 419

    C82.93 Follicular lymphoma, unspecified, intra-abdominal lymph nodes 🔗
        Ex: See PDX Collection 420

    C82.94 Follicular lymphoma, unspecified, lymph nodes of axilla and upper limb 🔗
        Ex: See PDX Collection 421

    C82.95 Follicular lymphoma, unspecified, lymph nodes of inguinal region and lower limb 🔗
        Ex: See PDX Collection 422

    C82.96 Follicular lymphoma, unspecified, intrapelvic lymph nodes 🔗
        Ex: See PDX Collection 423

    C82.97 Follicular lymphoma, unspecified, spleen 🔗
        Ex: See PDX Collection 424

    C82.98 Follicular lymphoma, unspecified, lymph nodes of multiple sites 🔗
        Ex: See PDX Collection 425

    C82.99 Follicular lymphoma, unspecified, extranodal and solid organ sites 🔗
        Ex: See PDX Collection 417

● **C83** **Non-follicular lymphoma**

    Excludes1 personal history of non-Hodgkin lymphoma (Z85.72)

● **C83.0** **Small cell B-cell lymphoma**
    Lymphoplasmacytic lymphoma
    Nodal marginal zone lymphoma
    Non-leukemic variant of B-CLL
    Splenic marginal zone lymphoma

    Excludes1 chronic lymphocytic leukemia (C91.1)
        mature T/NK-cell lymphomas (C84.-)
        Waldenström macroglobulinemia (C88.0)

    C83.00 Small cell B-cell lymphoma, unspecified site 🔗
        Ex: See PDX Collection 435

    C83.01 Small cell B-cell lymphoma, lymph nodes of head, face, and neck 🔗
        Ex: See PDX Collection 436

    C83.02 Small cell B-cell lymphoma, intrathoracic lymph nodes 🔗
        Ex: See PDX Collection 437

    C83.03 Small cell B-cell lymphoma, intra-abdominal lymph nodes 🔗
        Ex: See PDX Collection 438

    C83.04 Small cell B-cell lymphoma, lymph nodes of axilla and upper limb 🔗
        Ex: See PDX Collection 439

    C83.05 Small cell B-cell lymphoma, lymph nodes of inguinal region and lower limb 🔗
        Ex: See PDX Collection 440

    C83.06 Small cell B-cell lymphoma, intrapelvic lymph nodes 🔗
        Ex: See PDX Collection 441

    C83.07 Small cell B-cell lymphoma, spleen 🔗
        Ex: See PDX Collection 442

    C83.08 Small cell B-cell lymphoma, lymph nodes of multiple sites 🔗
        Ex: See PDX Collection 435

    C83.09 Small cell B-cell lymphoma, extranodal and solid organ sites 🔗
        Ex: See PDX Collection 435

● **C83.1** **Mantle cell lymphoma**
    Centrocytic lymphoma
    Malignant lymphomatous polyposis

    C83.10 Mantle cell lymphoma, unspecified site 🔗
        Ex: See PDX Collection 426

    C83.11 Mantle cell lymphoma, lymph nodes of head, face, and neck 🔗
        Ex: See PDX Collection 427

    C83.12 Mantle cell lymphoma, intrathoracic lymph nodes 🔗
        Ex: See PDX Collection 428

    C83.13 Mantle cell lymphoma, intra-abdominal lymph nodes 🔗
        Ex: See PDX Collection 429

    C83.14 Mantle cell lymphoma, lymph nodes of axilla and upper limb 🔗
        Ex: See PDX Collection 430

    C83.15 Mantle cell lymphoma, lymph nodes of inguinal region and lower limb 🔗
        Ex: See PDX Collection 431

    C83.16 Mantle cell lymphoma, intrapelvic lymph nodes 🔗
        Ex: See PDX Collection 432

▶ New   ⇒ Revised   deleted Deleted   Excludes 1   Excludes 2   Includes   Use additional   Code first   Code also   Key words

OGCR Official Guidelines   ● Unacceptable Principal Diagnosis   X Assign placeholder X   ● Use Additional Character(s)   ▶ Manifestation Code   **Coding Clinic**

C83.17   Mantle cell lymphoma, spleen
          Ex: See PDX Collection 433

C83.18   Mantle cell lymphoma, lymph nodes of
          multiple sites
          Ex: See PDX Collection 434

C83.19   Mantle cell lymphoma, extranodal and solid
          organ sites
          Ex: See PDX Collection 426

● C83.3   Diffuse large B-cell lymphoma
          Anaplastic diffuse large B-cell lymphoma
          CD30-positive diffuse large B-cell lymphoma
          Centroblastic diffuse large B-cell lymphoma
          Diffuse large B-cell lymphoma, subtype not specified
          Immunoblastic diffuse large B-cell lymphoma
          Plasmablastic diffuse large B-cell lymphoma
          Diffuse large B-cell lymphoma, subtype not specified
          T-cell rich diffuse large B-cell lymphoma
          Excludes1   mediastinal (thymic) large B-cell
                      lymphoma (C85.2-)
                      mature T/NK-cell lymphomas (C84.-)

C83.30   Diffuse large B-cell lymphoma, unspecified
          site
          Ex: See PDX Collection 443

C83.31   Diffuse large B-cell lymphoma, lymph nodes of
          head, face, and neck
          Ex: See PDX Collection 444

C83.32   Diffuse large B-cell lymphoma, intrathoracic
          lymph nodes
          Ex: See PDX Collection 445

C83.33   Diffuse large B-cell lymphoma, intra-
          abdominal lymph nodes
          Ex: See PDX Collection 446

C83.34   Diffuse large B-cell lymphoma, lymph nodes of
          axilla and upper limb
          Ex: See PDX Collection 447

C83.35   Diffuse large B-cell lymphoma, lymph nodes of
          inguinal region and lower limb
          Ex: See PDX Collection 448

C83.36   Diffuse large B-cell lymphoma, intrapelvic
          lymph nodes
          Ex: See PDX Collection 449

C83.37   Diffuse large B-cell lymphoma, spleen
          Ex: See PDX Collection 450

C83.38   Diffuse large B-cell lymphoma, lymph nodes of
          multiple sites
          Ex: See PDX Collection 443

C83.39   Diffuse large B-cell lymphoma, extranodal and
          solid organ sites
          Ex: See PDX Collection 443

● C83.5   Lymphoblastic (diffuse) lymphoma
          Highly malignant type of non-Hodgkin lymphoma with
              diffuse infiltration
          B-precursor lymphoma
          Lymphoblastic B-cell lymphoma
          Lymphoblastic lymphoma NOS
          Lymphoblastic T-cell lymphoma
          T-precursor lymphoma

C83.50   Lymphoblastic (diffuse) lymphoma, unspecified
          site
          Ex: See PDX Collection 451

C83.51   Lymphoblastic (diffuse) lymphoma, lymph
          nodes of head, face, and neck
          Ex: See PDX Collection 452

C83.52   Lymphoblastic (diffuse) lymphoma,
          intrathoracic lymph nodes
          Ex: See PDX Collection 453

C83.53   Lymphoblastic (diffuse) lymphoma, intra-
          abdominal lymph nodes
          Ex: See PDX Collection 454

C83.54   Lymphoblastic (diffuse) lymphoma, lymph
          nodes of axilla and upper limb
          Ex: See PDX Collection 455

C83.55   Lymphoblastic (diffuse) lymphoma, lymph
          nodes of inguinal region and lower limb
          Ex: See PDX Collection 456

C83.56   Lymphoblastic (diffuse) lymphoma, intrapelvic
          lymph nodes
          Ex: See PDX Collection 457

C83.57   Lymphoblastic (diffuse) lymphoma, spleen
          Ex: See PDX Collection 458

C83.58   Lymphoblastic (diffuse) lymphoma, lymph
          nodes of multiple sites
          Ex: See PDX Collection 451

C83.59   Lymphoblastic (diffuse) lymphoma, extranodal
          and solid organ sites
          Ex: See PDX Collection 451

● C83.7   Burkitt lymphoma
          Form of small cell lymphoma
          Atypical Burkitt lymphoma
          Burkitt-like lymphoma
          Excludes1   mature B-cell leukemia Burkitt type
                      (C91.A-)

C83.70   Burkitt lymphoma, unspecified site
          Ex: See PDX Collection 459

C83.71   Burkitt lymphoma, lymph nodes of head, face,
          and neck
          Ex: See PDX Collection 460

C83.72   Burkitt lymphoma, intrathoracic lymph
          nodes
          Ex: See PDX Collection 461

C83.73   Burkitt lymphoma, intra-abdominal lymph
          nodes
          Ex: See PDX Collection 462

C83.74   Burkitt lymphoma, lymph nodes of axilla and
          upper limb
          Ex: See PDX Collection 463

C83.75   Burkitt lymphoma, lymph nodes of inguinal
          region and lower limb
          Ex: See PDX Collection 464

C83.76   Burkitt lymphoma, intrapelvic lymph nodes
          Ex: See PDX Collection 465

C83.77   Burkitt lymphoma, spleen
          Ex: See PDX Collection 466

C83.78   Burkitt lymphoma, lymph nodes of multiple
          sites
          Ex: See PDX Collection 459

C83.79   Burkitt lymphoma, extranodal and solid organ
          sites
          Ex: See PDX Collection 459

CHAPTER 2 (C00-D49)

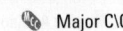

● **C83.8**   **Other non-follicular lymphoma**
Intravascular large B-cell lymphoma
Lymphoid granulomatosis
Primary effusion B-cell lymphoma

> **Excludes1**   mediastinal (thymic) large B-cell lymphoma (C85.2-)
> T-cell rich B-cell lymphoma (C83.3-)

    C83.80   Other non-follicular lymphoma, unspecified site 🔊
> (Ex:) See PDX Collection 435

    C83.81   Other non-follicular lymphoma, lymph nodes of head, face, and neck 🔊
> (Ex:) See PDX Collection 436

    C83.82   Other non-follicular lymphoma, intrathoracic lymph nodes 🔊
> (Ex:) See PDX Collection 437

    C83.83   Other non-follicular lymphoma, intra-abdominal lymph nodes 🔊
> (Ex:) See PDX Collection 438

    C83.84   Other non-follicular lymphoma, lymph nodes of axilla and upper limb 🔊
> (Ex:) See PDX Collection 439

    C83.85   Other non-follicular lymphoma, lymph nodes of inguinal region and lower limb 🔊
> (Ex:) See PDX Collection 440

    C83.86   Other non-follicular lymphoma, intrapelvic lymph nodes 🔊
> (Ex:) See PDX Collection 441

    C83.87   Other non-follicular lymphoma, spleen 🔊
> (Ex:) See PDX Collection 442

    C83.88   Other non-follicular lymphoma, lymph nodes of multiple sites 🔊
> (Ex:) See PDX Collection 435

    C83.89   Other non-follicular lymphoma, extranodal and solid organ sites 🔊
> (Ex:) See PDX Collection 435

● **C83.9**   **Non-follicular (diffuse) lymphoma, unspecified**

    C83.90   Non-follicular (diffuse) lymphoma, unspecified, unspecified site 🔊
> (Ex:) See PDX Collection 435

    C83.91   Non-follicular (diffuse) lymphoma, unspecified, lymph nodes of head, face, and neck 🔊
> (Ex:) See PDX Collection 436

    C83.92   Non-follicular (diffuse) lymphoma, unspecified, intrathoracic lymph nodes 🔊
> (Ex:) See PDX Collection 437

    C83.93   Non-follicular (diffuse) lymphoma, unspecified, intra-abdominal lymph nodes 🔊
> (Ex:) See PDX Collection 438

    C83.94   Non-follicular (diffuse) lymphoma, unspecified, lymph nodes of axilla and upper limb 🔊
> (Ex:) See PDX Collection 439

    C83.95   Non-follicular (diffuse) lymphoma, unspecified, lymph nodes of inguinal region and lower limb 🔊
> (Ex:) See PDX Collection 440

    C83.96   Non-follicular (diffuse) lymphoma, unspecified, intrapelvic lymph nodes 🔊
> (Ex:) See PDX Collection 441

    C83.97   Non-follicular (diffuse) lymphoma, unspecified, spleen 🔊
> (Ex:) See PDX Collection 442

    C83.98   Non-follicular (diffuse) lymphoma, unspecified, lymph nodes of multiple sites 🔊
> (Ex:) See PDX Collection 435

    C83.99   Non-follicular (diffuse) lymphoma, unspecified, extranodal and solid organ sites 🔊
> (Ex:) See PDX Collection 435

● **C84**   **Mature T/NK-cell lymphomas**

> **Excludes1**   personal history of non-Hodgkin lymphoma (Z85.72)

● **C84.0**   **Mycosis fungoides**
Chronic or rapidly progressive form of cutaneous T-cell lymphoma; AKA granuloma fungoides

> **Excludes1**   peripheral T-cell lymphoma, not classified (C84.4-)

    C84.00   Mycosis fungoides, unspecified site 🔊
> (Ex:) See PDX Collection 467

    C84.01   Mycosis fungoides, lymph nodes of head, face, and neck 🔊
> (Ex:) See PDX Collection 468

    C84.02   Mycosis fungoides, intrathoracic lymph nodes 🔊
> (Ex:) See PDX Collection 469

    C84.03   Mycosis fungoides, intra-abdominal lymph nodes 🔊
> (Ex:) See PDX Collection 470

    C84.04   Mycosis fungoides, lymph nodes of axilla and upper limb 🔊
> (Ex:) See PDX Collection 471

    C84.05   Mycosis fungoides, lymph nodes of inguinal region and lower limb 🔊
> (Ex:) See PDX Collection 472

    C84.06   Mycosis fungoides, intrapelvic lymph nodes 🔊
> (Ex:) See PDX Collection 473

    C84.07   Mycosis fungoides, spleen 🔊
> (Ex:) See PDX Collection 474

    C84.08   Mycosis fungoides, lymph nodes of multiple sites 🔊
> (Ex:) See PDX Collection 475

    C84.09   Mycosis fungoides, extranodal and solid organ sites 🔊
> (Ex:) See PDX Collection 467

● **C84.1**   **Sézary disease**
Type of cutaneous lymphoma affecting T-cells

    C84.10   Sézary disease, unspecified site 🔊
> (Ex:) See PDX Collection 476

    C84.11   Sézary disease, lymph nodes of head, face, and neck 🔊
> (Ex:) See PDX Collection 477

    C84.12   Sézary disease, intrathoracic lymph nodes 🔊
> (Ex:) See PDX Collection 478

    C84.13   Sézary disease, intra-abdominal lymph nodes 🔊
> (Ex:) See PDX Collection 479

    C84.14   Sézary disease, lymph nodes of axilla and upper limb 🔊
> (Ex:) See PDX Collection 480

    C84.15   Sézary disease, lymph nodes of inguinal region and lower limb 🔊
> (Ex:) See PDX Collection 481

    C84.16   Sézary disease, intrapelvic lymph nodes 🔊
> (Ex:) See PDX Collection 482

    C84.17   Sézary disease, spleen 🔊
> (Ex:) See PDX Collection 483

    C84.18   Sézary disease, lymph nodes of multiple sites 🔊
> (Ex:) See PDX Collection 484

    C84.19   Sézary disease, extranodal and solid organ sites 🔊
> (Ex:) See PDX Collection 476

● **C84.4**   **Peripheral T-cell lymphoma, not classified**
Diverse group of blood carcinomas originating from T-cells, requiring aggressive chemotherapy
Lennert's lymphoma
Lymphoepithelioid lymphoma
Mature T-cell lymphoma, not elsewhere classified

     C84.40   Peripheral T-cell lymphoma, not classified, unspecified site 🖱
       (Ex) See PDX Collection 426

     C84.41   Peripheral T-cell lymphoma, not classified, lymph nodes of head, face, and neck 🖱
       (Ex) See PDX Collection 427

     C84.42   Peripheral T-cell lymphoma, not classified, intrathoracic lymph nodes 🖱
       (Ex) See PDX Collection 428

     C84.43   Peripheral T-cell lymphoma, not classified, intra-abdominal lymph nodes 🖱
       (Ex) See PDX Collection 429

     C84.44   Peripheral T-cell lymphoma, not classified, lymph nodes of axilla and upper limb 🖱
       (Ex) See PDX Collection 430

     C84.45   Peripheral T-cell lymphoma, not classified, lymph nodes of inguinal region and lower limb 🖱
       (Ex) See PDX Collection 431

     C84.46   Peripheral T-cell lymphoma, not classified, intrapelvic lymph nodes 🖱
       (Ex) See PDX Collection 432

     C84.47   Peripheral T-cell lymphoma, not classified, spleen 🖱
       (Ex) See PDX Collection 433

     C84.48   Peripheral T-cell lymphoma, not classified, lymph nodes of multiple sites 🖱
       (Ex) See PDX Collection 434

     C84.49   Peripheral T-cell lymphoma, not classified, extranodal and solid organ sites 🖱
       (Ex) See PDX Collection 426

● **C84.6**   **Anaplastic large cell lymphoma, ALK-positive**
Anaplastic large cell lymphoma, CD30-positive

     C84.60   Anaplastic large cell lymphoma, ALK-positive, unspecified site 🖱
       (Ex) See PDX Collection 426

     C84.61   Anaplastic large cell lymphoma, ALK-positive, lymph nodes of head, face, and neck 🖱
       (Ex) See PDX Collection 427

     C84.62   Anaplastic large cell lymphoma, ALK-positive, intrathoracic lymph nodes 🖱
       (Ex) See PDX Collection 428

     C84.63   Anaplastic large cell lymphoma, ALK-positive, intra-abdominal lymph nodes 🖱
       (Ex) See PDX Collection 429

     C84.64   Anaplastic large cell lymphoma, ALK-positive, lymph nodes of axilla and upper limb 🖱
       (Ex) See PDX Collection 430

     C84.65   Anaplastic large cell lymphoma, ALK-positive, lymph nodes of inguinal region and lower limb 🖱
       (Ex) See PDX Collection 431

     C84.66   Anaplastic large cell lymphoma, ALK-positive, intrapelvic lymph nodes 🖱
       (Ex) See PDX Collection 432

     C84.67   Anaplastic large cell lymphoma, ALK-positive, spleen 🖱
       (Ex) See PDX Collection 433

     C84.68   Anaplastic large cell lymphoma, ALK-positive, lymph nodes of multiple sites 🖱
       (Ex) See PDX Collection 434

     C84.69   Anaplastic large cell lymphoma, ALK-positive, extranodal and solid organ sites 🖱
       (Ex) See PDX Collection 426

Item 2–7 Lymphosarcoma, also known as malignant lymphoma, is a cancer of the lymph system exhibiting abnormal cells encompassing an entire lymph node creating a diffuse pattern without any definite organization. Diffuse pattern lymphoma has a more unfavorable survival outlook than those with a follicular or nodular pattern. Reticulosarcoma is the most common aggressive form of non-Hodgkin's lymphoma.

● **C84.7**   **Anaplastic large cell lymphoma, ALK-negative**
     Excludes1   primary cutaneous CD30-positive T-cell proliferations (C86.6-)

     C84.70   Anaplastic large cell lymphoma, ALK-negative, unspecified site 🖱
       (Ex) See PDX Collection 426

     C84.71   Anaplastic large cell lymphoma, ALK-negative, lymph nodes of head, face, and neck 🖱
       (Ex) See PDX Collection 427

     C84.72   Anaplastic large cell lymphoma, ALK-negative, intrathoracic lymph nodes 🖱
       (Ex) See PDX Collection 428

     C84.73   Anaplastic large cell lymphoma, ALK-negative, intra-abdominal lymph nodes 🖱
       (Ex) See PDX Collection 429

     C84.74   Anaplastic large cell lymphoma, ALK-negative, lymph nodes of axilla and upper limb 🖱
       (Ex) See PDX Collection 430

     C84.75   Anaplastic large cell lymphoma, ALK-negative, lymph nodes of inguinal region and lower limb 🖱
       (Ex) See PDX Collection 431

     C84.76   Anaplastic large cell lymphoma, ALK-negative, intrapelvic lymph nodes 🖱
       (Ex) See PDX Collection 432

     C84.77   Anaplastic large cell lymphoma, ALK-negative, spleen 🖱
       (Ex) See PDX Collection 433

     C84.78   Anaplastic large cell lymphoma, ALK-negative, lymph nodes of multiple sites 🖱
       (Ex) See PDX Collection 434

     C84.79   Anaplastic large cell lymphoma, ALK-negative, extranodal and solid organ sites 🖱
       (Ex) See PDX Collection 426

● **C84.A**   **Cutaneous T-cell lymphoma, unspecified**

     C84.A0   Cutaneous T-cell lymphoma, unspecified, unspecified site 🖱
       (Ex) See PDX Collection 426

     C84.A1   Cutaneous T-cell lymphoma, unspecified lymph nodes of head, face, and neck 🖱
       (Ex) See PDX Collection 427

     C84.A2   Cutaneous T-cell lymphoma, unspecified, intrathoracic lymph nodes 🖱
       (Ex) See PDX Collection 428

     C84.A3   Cutaneous T-cell lymphoma, unspecified, intra-abdominal lymph nodes 🖱
       (Ex) See PDX Collection 429

     C84.A4   Cutaneous T-cell lymphoma, unspecified, lymph nodes of axilla and upper limb 🖱
       (Ex) See PDX Collection 430

     C84.A5   Cutaneous T-cell lymphoma, unspecified, lymph nodes of inguinal region and lower limb 🖱
       (Ex) See PDX Collection 431

     C84.A6   Cutaneous T-cell lymphoma, unspecified, intrapelvic lymph nodes 🖱
       (Ex) See PDX Collection 432

     C84.A7   Cutaneous T-cell lymphoma, unspecified, spleen 🖱
       (Ex) See PDX Collection 433

     C84.A8   Cutaneous T-cell lymphoma, unspecified, lymph nodes of multiple sites 🖱
       (Ex) See PDX Collection 434

     C84.A9   Cutaneous T-cell lymphoma, unspecified, extranodal and solid organ sites 🖱
       (Ex) See PDX Collection 426

CHAPTER 2 (C00-D49)

N Newborn Age: 0   **P** Pediatric Age: 0–17   **M** Maternity DX: 12–55   **A** Adult Age: 15–124   ♀ Females Only   ♂ Males Only

🖱 Complication\Comorbidity   🖱 Major C\C   (Ex) CC/MCC Exclusions   🖱 Hospital-Acquired Condition   **697**

- **C84.Z** **Other mature T/NK-cell lymphomas**

  Note: If T-cell lineage or involvement is mentioned in conjunction with a specific lymphoma, code to the more specific description.

  Excludes1   angioimmunoblastic T-cell lymphoma (C86.5)
  blastic NK-cell lymphoma (C86.4)
  enteropathy-type T-cell lymphoma (C86.2)
  extranodal NK-cell lymphoma, nasal type (C86.0)
  hepatosplenic T-cell lymphoma (C86.1)
  primary cutaneous CD30-positive T-cell proliferations (C86.6)
  subcutaneous panniculitis-like T-cell lymphoma (C86.3)
  T-cell leukemia (C91.1-)

  C84.Z0 **Other mature T/NK-cell lymphomas, unspecified site** 🖐
  Ex See PDX Collection 426

  C84.Z1 **Other mature T/NK-cell lymphomas, lymph nodes of head, face, and neck** 🖐
  Ex See PDX Collection 427

  C84.Z2 **Other mature T/NK-cell lymphomas, intrathoracic lymph nodes** 🖐
  Ex See PDX Collection 428

  C84.Z3 **Other mature T/NK-cell lymphomas, intra-abdominal lymph nodes** 🖐
  Ex See PDX Collection 429

  C84.Z4 **Other mature T/NK-cell lymphomas, lymph nodes of axilla and upper limb** 🖐
  Ex See PDX Collection 430

  C84.Z5 **Other mature T/NK-cell lymphomas, lymph nodes of inguinal region and lower limb** 🖐
  Ex See PDX Collection 431

  C84.Z6 **Other mature T/NK-cell lymphomas, intrapelvic lymph nodes** 🖐
  Ex See PDX Collection 432

  C84.Z7 **Other mature T/NK-cell lymphomas, spleen** 🖐
  Ex See PDX Collection 433

  C84.Z8 **Other mature T/NK-cell lymphomas, lymph nodes of multiple sites** 🖐
  Ex See PDX Collection 434

  C84.Z9 **Other mature T/NK-cell lymphomas, extranodal and solid organ sites** 🖐
  Ex See PDX Collection 426

- **C84.9** **Mature T/NK-cell lymphomas, unspecified**
  NK/T cell lymphoma NOS

  Excludes1   mature T-cell lymphoma, not elsewhere classified (C84.4-)

  C84.90 **Mature T/NK-cell lymphomas, unspecified, unspecified site** 🖐
  Ex See PDX Collection 426

  C84.91 **Mature T/NK-cell lymphomas, unspecified, lymph nodes of head, face, and neck** 🖐
  Ex See PDX Collection 427

  C84.92 **Mature T/NK-cell lymphomas, unspecified, intrathoracic lymph nodes** 🖐
  Ex See PDX Collection 428

  C84.93 **Mature T/NK-cell lymphomas, unspecified, intra-abdominal lymph nodes** 🖐
  Ex See PDX Collection 429

  C84.94 **Mature T/NK-cell lymphomas, unspecified, lymph nodes of axilla and upper limb** 🖐
  Ex See PDX Collection 430

  C84.95 **Mature T/NK-cell lymphomas, unspecified, lymph nodes of inguinal region and lower limb** 🖐
  Ex See PDX Collection 431

  C84.96 **Mature T/NK-cell lymphomas, unspecified, intrapelvic lymph nodes** 🖐
  Ex See PDX Collection 432

  C84.97 **Mature T/NK-cell lymphomas, unspecified, spleen** 🖐
  Ex See PDX Collection 433

  C84.98 **Mature T/NK-cell lymphomas, unspecified, lymph nodes of multiple sites** 🖐
  Ex See PDX Collection 434

  C84.99 **Mature T/NK-cell lymphomas, unspecified, extranodal and solid organ sites** 🖐
  Ex See PDX Collection 426

- **C85** **Other specified and unspecified types of non-Hodgkin lymphoma**

  Excludes1   other specified types of T/NK-cell lymphoma (C86.-)
  personal history of non-Hodgkin lymphoma (Z85.72)

- **C85.1** **Unspecified B-cell lymphoma**

  Note: If B-cell lineage or involvement is mentioned in conjunction with a specific lymphoma, code to the more specific description.

  C85.10 **Unspecified B-cell lymphoma, unspecified site** 🖐
  Ex See PDX Collection 426

  C85.11 **Unspecified B-cell lymphoma, lymph nodes of head, face, and neck** 🖐
  Ex See PDX Collection 427

  C85.12 **Unspecified B-cell lymphoma, intrathoracic lymph nodes** 🖐
  Ex See PDX Collection 428

  C85.13 **Unspecified B-cell lymphoma, intra-abdominal lymph nodes** 🖐
  Ex See PDX Collection 429

  C85.14 **Unspecified B-cell lymphoma, lymph nodes of axilla and upper limb** 🖐
  Ex See PDX Collection 430

  C85.15 **Unspecified B-cell lymphoma, lymph nodes of inguinal region and lower limb** 🖐
  Ex See PDX Collection 431

  C85.16 **Unspecified B-cell lymphoma, intrapelvic lymph nodes** 🖐
  Ex See PDX Collection 432

  C85.17 **Unspecified B-cell lymphoma, spleen** 🖐
  Ex See PDX Collection 433

  C85.18 **Unspecified B-cell lymphoma, lymph nodes of multiple sites** 🖐
  Ex See PDX Collection 434

  C85.19 **Unspecified B-cell lymphoma, extranodal and solid organ sites** 🖐
  Ex See PDX Collection 426

- **C85.2** **Mediastinal (thymic) large B-cell lymphoma**

  C85.20 **Mediastinal (thymic) large B-cell lymphoma, unspecified site** 🖐
  Ex See PDX Collection 426

  C85.21 **Mediastinal (thymic) large B-cell lymphoma, lymph nodes of head, face, and neck** 🖐
  Ex See PDX Collection 427

  C85.22 **Mediastinal (thymic) large B-cell lymphoma, intrathoracic lymph nodes** 🖐
  Ex See PDX Collection 428

  C85.23 **Mediastinal (thymic) large B-cell lymphoma, intra-abdominal lymph nodes** 🖐
  Ex See PDX Collection 429

  C85.24 **Mediastinal (thymic) large B-cell lymphoma, lymph nodes of axilla and upper limb** 🖐
  Ex See PDX Collection 430

  C85.25 **Mediastinal (thymic) large B-cell lymphoma, lymph nodes of inguinal region and lower limb** 🖐
  Ex See PDX Collection 431

  C85.26 **Mediastinal (thymic) large B-cell lymphoma, intrapelvic lymph nodes** 🖐
  Ex See PDX Collection 432

▶ New   ⟶ Revised   ~~deleted~~ Deleted   Excludes 1   Excludes 2   Includes   Use additional   Code first   Code also   Key words
OGCR Official Guidelines   ● Unacceptable Principal Diagnosis   X Assign placeholder X   ● Use Additional Character(s)   ▶ Manifestation Code   **Coding Clinic**

C85.27   **Mediastinal (thymic) large B-cell lymphoma, spleen** 🔹
(Ex) See PDX Collection 433

C85.28   **Mediastinal (thymic) large B-cell lymphoma, lymph nodes of multiple sites** 🔹
(Ex) See PDX Collection 434

C85.29   **Mediastinal (thymic) large B-cell lymphoma, extranodal and solid organ sites** 🔹
(Ex) See PDX Collection 426

● **C85.8**   **Other specified types of non-Hodgkin lymphoma**

C85.80   **Other specified types of non-Hodgkin lymphoma, unspecified site** 🔹
(Ex) See PDX Collection 426

C85.81   **Other specified types of non-Hodgkin lymphoma, lymph nodes of head, face, and neck** 🔹
(Ex) See PDX Collection 427

C85.82   **Other specified types of non-Hodgkin lymphoma, intrathoracic lymph nodes** 🔹
(Ex) See PDX Collection 428

C85.83   **Other specified types of non-Hodgkin lymphoma, intra-abdominal lymph nodes** 🔹
(Ex) See PDX Collection 429

C85.84   **Other specified types of non-Hodgkin lymphoma, lymph nodes of axilla and upper limb** 🔹
(Ex) See PDX Collection 430

C85.85   **Other specified types of non-Hodgkin lymphoma, lymph nodes of inguinal region and lower limb** 🔹
(Ex) See PDX Collection 431

C85.86   **Other specified types of non-Hodgkin lymphoma, intrapelvic lymph nodes** 🔹
(Ex) See PDX Collection 432

C85.87   **Other specified types of non-Hodgkin lymphoma, spleen** 🔹
(Ex) See PDX Collection 433

C85.88   **Other specified types of non-Hodgkin lymphoma, lymph nodes of multiple sites** 🔹
(Ex) See PDX Collection 434

C85.89   **Other specified types of non-Hodgkin lymphoma, extranodal and solid organ sites** 🔹
(Ex) See PDX Collection 426

● **C85.9**   **Non-Hodgkin lymphoma, unspecified**
Lymphoma NOS
Malignant lymphoma NOS
Non-Hodgkin lymphoma NOS

C85.90   **Non-Hodgkin lymphoma, unspecified, unspecified site** 🔹
(Ex) See PDX Collection 426

C85.91   **Non-Hodgkin lymphoma, unspecified, lymph nodes of head, face, and neck** 🔹
(Ex) See PDX Collection 427

C85.92   **Non-Hodgkin lymphoma, unspecified, intrathoracic lymph nodes** 🔹
(Ex) See PDX Collection 428

C85.93   **Non-Hodgkin lymphoma, unspecified, intra-abdominal lymph nodes** 🔹
(Ex) See PDX Collection 429

C85.94   **Non-Hodgkin lymphoma, unspecified, lymph nodes of axilla and upper limb** 🔹
(Ex) See PDX Collection 430

C85.95   **Non-Hodgkin lymphoma, unspecified, lymph nodes of inguinal region and lower limb** 🔹
(Ex) See PDX Collection 431

C85.96   **Non-Hodgkin lymphoma, unspecified, intrapelvic lymph nodes** 🔹
(Ex) See PDX Collection 432

C85.97   **Non-Hodgkin lymphoma, unspecified, spleen** 🔹
(Ex) See PDX Collection 433

C85.98   **Non-Hodgkin lymphoma, unspecified, lymph nodes of multiple sites** 🔹
(Ex) See PDX Collection 434

C85.99   **Non-Hodgkin lymphoma, unspecified, extranodal and solid organ sites** 🔹
(Ex) See PDX Collection 426

● **C86**   **Other specified types of T/NK-cell lymphoma**

Excludes1   anaplastic large cell lymphoma, ALK negative (C84.7-)
anaplastic large cell lymphoma, ALK positive (C84.6-)
mature T/NK-cell lymphomas (C84.-)
other specified types of non-Hodgkin lymphoma (C85.8-)

C86.0   **Extranodal NK/T-cell lymphoma, nasal type** 🔹
(Ex) See PDX Collection 427

C86.1   **Hepatosplenic T-cell lymphoma** 🔹
Alpha-beta and gamma delta types
(Ex) See PDX Collection 433

C86.2   **Enteropathy-type (intestinal) T-cell lymphoma** 🔹
Enteropathy associated T-cell lymphoma
(Ex) See PDX Collection 429

C86.3   **Subcutaneous panniculitis-like T-cell lymphoma** 🔹
(Ex) See PDX Collection 429

C86.4   **Blastic NK-cell lymphoma** 🔹
▶Blastic plasmacytoid dendritic cell neoplasm (BPDCN)
(Ex) See PDX Collection 426

C86.5   **Angioimmunoblastic T-cell lymphoma** 🔹
Angioimmunoblastic lymphadenopathy with dysproteinemia (AILD)
(Ex) See PDX Collection 435

C86.6   **Primary cutaneous CD30-positive T-cell proliferations** 🔹
Lymphomatoid papulosis
Primary cutaneous anaplastic large cell lymphoma
Primary cutaneous CD30-positive large T-cell lymphoma
(Ex) See PDX Collection 435

● **C88**   **Malignant immunoproliferative diseases and certain other B-cell lymphomas**
Diseases involving immune system

Excludes1   B-cell lymphoma, unspecified (C85.1-)
personal history of other malignant neoplasms of lymphoid, hematopoietic and related tissues (Z85.79)

C88.0   **Waldenström's macroglobulinemia**
Lymphoplasmacytic lymphoma with IgM-production
Macroglobulinemia (idiopathic) (primary)

Excludes1   small cell B-cell lymphoma (C83.0)

C88.2   **Heavy chain disease** 🔹
Franklin disease
Gamma heavy chain disease
Mu heavy chain disease
(Ex) See PDX Collection 485

C88.3   **Immunoproliferative small intestinal disease** 🔹
Alpha heavy chain disease
Mediterranean lymphoma
(Ex) See PDX Collection 485

C88.4   **Extranodal marginal zone B-cell lymphoma of mucosa-associated lymphoid tissue [MALT-lymphoma]** 🔹
Lymphoma of skin-associated lymphoid tissue [SALT-lymphoma]
Lymphoma of bronchial-associated lymphoid tissue [BALT-lymphoma]

Excludes1   high malignant (diffuse large B-cell) lymphoma (C83.3-)
(Ex) See PDX Collection 426

C88.8   **Other malignant immunoproliferative diseases** 🔹
(Ex) See PDX Collection 486

C88.9   **Malignant immunoproliferative disease, unspecified** 🔹
Immunoproliferative disease NOS
(Ex) See PDX Collection 485

N Newborn Age: 0   **P** Pediatric Age: 0–17   **M** Maternity DX: 12–55   **A** Adult Age: 15–124   ♀ Females Only   ♂ Males Only
🔹 Complication\Comorbidity   🔹 Major C\C   (Ex) CC/MCC Exclusions   🔹 Hospital-Acquired Condition

699

Item 2–8 **Multiple myeloma** is a cancer of a plasma cell (a type of white blood cell) and is an incurable but treatable disease. Immunoproliferative neoplasm is a term for diseases (mostly cancers) in which the immune system cells proliferate.

● **C90**   **Multiple myeloma and malignant plasma cell neoplasms**

      Excludes1   personal history of other malignant neoplasms of lymphoid, hematopoietic and related tissues (Z85.79)

      (Ex) **For category C90 CC codes:** See PDX Collection 485

   ● **C90.0**   **Multiple myeloma**
         Kahler's disease
         Medullary plasmacytoma
         Myelomatosis
         Plasma cell myeloma

        Excludes1   solitary myeloma (C90.3-)
                      solitary plasmacytoma (C90.3-)

      C90.00   **Multiple myeloma not having achieved remission** 🔊
           Multiple myeloma with failed remission
           Multiple myeloma NOS

      C90.01   **Multiple myeloma in remission** 🔊
      C90.02   **Multiple myeloma in relapse** 🔊

   ● **C90.1**   **Plasma cell leukemia**
        Rare type of acute leukemia
        Plasmacytic leukemia

      C90.10   **Plasma cell leukemia not having achieved remission** 🔊
           Plasma cell leukemia with failed remission
           Plasma cell leukemia NOS

      C90.11   **Plasma cell leukemia in remission** 🔊
      C90.12   **Plasma cell leukemia in relapse** 🔊

   ● **C90.2**   **Extramedullary plasmacytoma**
        Malignant monoclonal plasma cell tumor growing in soft tissue; AKA plasma cell dyscrasias

      C90.20   **Extramedullary plasmacytoma not having achieved remission** 🔊
           Extramedullary plasmacytoma with failed remission
           Extramedullary plasmacytoma NOS

      C90.21   **Extramedullary plasmacytoma in remission** 🔊
      C90.22   **Extramedullary plasmacytoma in relapse** 🔊

   ● **C90.3**   **Solitary plasmacytoma**
        Localized malignant plasma cell tumor NOS
        Plasmacytoma NOS
        Solitary myeloma

      C90.30   **Solitary plasmacytoma not having achieved remission** 🔊
           Solitary plasmacytoma with failed remission
           Solitary plasmacytoma NOS

      C90.31   **Solitary plasmacytoma in remission** 🔊
      C90.32   **Solitary plasmacytoma in relapse** 🔊

● **C91**   **Lymphoid leukemia**
      Type of leukemia affecting circulating cells of lymphoid origin

      Excludes1   personal history of leukemia (Z85.6)

      (Ex) **For category C91 CC codes unless otherwise indicated:** See PDX Collection 485

   ● **C91.0**   **Acute lymphoblastic leukemia [ALL]**
        Note: Code C91.0 should only be used for T-cell and B-cell precursor leukemia

      C91.00   **Acute lymphoblastic leukemia not having achieved remission** 🔊
           Acute lymphoblastic leukemia with failed remission
           Acute lymphoblastic leukemia NOS

      C91.01   **Acute lymphoblastic leukemia, in remission** 🔊
      C91.02   **Acute lymphoblastic leukemia, in relapse** 🔊

Item 2–9 Leukemia is a cancer (acute or chronic) of the blood-forming tissues of the bone marrow. Blood cells all start out as stem cells. They mature and become red cells, white cells, or platelets. There are three main types of leukocytes (white cells that fight infection): monocytes, lymphocytes, and granulocytes. **Acute monocytic leukemia** (AML) affects monocytes. **Acute lymphoid leukemia** (ALL) affects lymphocytes, and **acute myeloid leukemia** (AML) affects cells that typically develop into white blood cells (not lymphocytes), though it may develop in other blood cells.

   ● **C91.1**   **Chronic lymphocytic leukemia of B-cell type**
        Lymphoplasmacytic leukemia
        Richter syndrome

      Excludes1   lymphoplasmacytic lymphoma (C83.0-)

      C91.10   **Chronic lymphocytic leukemia of B-cell type not having achieved remission** 🔊
           Chronic lymphocytic leukemia of B-cell type with failed remission
           Chronic lymphocytic leukemia of B-cell type NOS

      C91.11   **Chronic lymphocytic leukemia of B-cell type in remission** 🔊
      C91.12   **Chronic lymphocytic leukemia of B-cell type in relapse** 🔊

   ● **C91.3**   **Prolymphocytic leukemia of B-cell type**
        Chronic leukemia with symptoms of large number of circulating lymphocytes

      C91.30   **Prolymphocytic leukemia of B-cell type not having achieved remission** 🔊
           Prolymphocytic leukemia of B-cell type with failed remission
           Prolymphocytic leukemia of B-cell type NOS

      C91.31   **Prolymphocytic leukemia of B-cell type, in remission** 🔊
      C91.32   **Prolymphocytic leukemia of B-cell type, in relapse** 🔊

   ● **C91.4**   **Hairy cell leukemia**
        Chronic leukemia with splenomegaly and excessive number of abnormal large mononuclear cells covered by hairlike villi
        Leukemic reticuloendotheliosis

      (Ex) **For category C91.4 CC codes:** See PDX Collection 487

      C91.40   **Hairy cell leukemia not having achieved remission** 🔊
           Hairy cell leukemia with failed remission
           Hairy cell leukemia NOS

      C91.41   **Hairy cell leukemia, in remission** 🔊
      C91.42   **Hairy cell leukemia, in relapse** 🔊

   ● **C91.5**   **Adult T-cell lymphoma/leukemia (HTLV-1-associated)**
        Acute variant of adult T-cell lymphoma/leukemia (HTLV-1-associated)
        Chronic variant of adult T-cell lymphoma/leukemia (HTLV-1-associated)
        Lymphomatoid variant of adult T-cell lymphoma/leukemia (HTLV-1-associated)
        Smouldering variant of adult T-cell lymphoma/leukemia (HTLV-1-associated)

      C91.50   **Adult T-cell lymphoma/leukemia (HTLV-1-associated) not having achieved remission** 🔊 A
           Adult T-cell lymphoma/leukemia (HTLV-1-associated) with failed remission
           Adult T-cell lymphoma/leukemia (HTLV-1-associated) NOS

      C91.51   **Adult T-cell lymphoma/leukemia (HTLV-1-associated), in remission** 🔊 A
      C91.52   **Adult T-cell lymphoma/leukemia (HTLV-1-associated), in relapse** 🔊 A

▶ New   ⇒ Revised   ~~deleted~~ Deleted   Excludes 1   Excludes 2   Includes   Use additional   Code first   Code also   Key words
OGCR Official Guidelines   ● Unacceptable Principal Diagnosis   X Assign placeholder X   ● Use Additional Character(s)   🔊 Manifestation Code   **Coding Clinic**

● **C91.6   Prolymphocytic leukemia of T-cell type**
     C91.60   Prolymphocytic leukemia of T-cell type not having achieved remission 🔒
         Prolymphocytic leukemia of T-cell type with failed remission
         Prolymphocytic leukemia of T-cell type NOS
     C91.61   Prolymphocytic leukemia of T-cell type, in remission 🔒
     C91.62   Prolymphocytic leukemia of T-cell type, in relapse 🔒

● **C91.A   Mature B-cell leukemia Burkitt-type**
     Excludes1   Burkitt lymphoma (C83.7-)
     C91.A0   Mature B-cell leukemia Burkitt-type not having achieved remission 🔒
         Mature B-cell leukemia Burkitt-type with failed remission
         Mature B-cell leukemia Burkitt-type NOS
     C91.A1   Mature B-cell leukemia Burkitt-type, in remission 🔒
     C91.A2   Mature B-cell leukemia Burkitt-type, in relapse 🔒

● **C91.Z   Other lymphoid leukemia**
     T-cell large granular lymphocytic leukemia (associated with rheumatoid arthritis)
     C91.Z0   Other lymphoid leukemia not having achieved remission 🔒
         Other lymphoid leukemia with failed remission
         Other lymphoid leukemia NOS
     C91.Z1   Other lymphoid leukemia, in remission 🔒
     C91.Z2   Other lymphoid leukemia, in relapse 🔒

● **C91.9   Lymphoid leukemia, unspecified**
     C91.90   Lymphoid leukemia, unspecified not having achieved remission 🔒
         Lymphoid leukemia with failed remission
         Lymphoid leukemia NOS
     C91.91   Lymphoid leukemia, unspecified, in remission 🔒
     C91.92   Lymphoid leukemia, unspecified, in relapse 🔒

● **C92   Myeloid leukemia**
     Includes   granulocytic leukemia
                 myelogenous leukemia
     Excludes1   personal history of leukemia (Z85.6)
     (Ex) **For category C92 CC codes: See PDX Collection 485**

● **C92.0   Acute myeloblastic leukemia**
     Acute myeloblastic leukemia, minimal differentiation
     Acute myeloblastic leukemia (with maturation)
     Acute myeloblastic leukemia 1/ETO
     Acute myeloblastic leukemia M0
     Acute myeloblastic leukemia M1
     Acute myeloblastic leukemia M2
     Acute myeloblastic leukemia with t(8;21)
     Acute myeloblastic leukemia (without a FAB classification) NOS
     Refractory anemia with excess blasts in transformation [RAEB T]
     Excludes1   acute exacerbation of chronic myeloid leukemia (C92.10)
                 refractory anemia with excess of blasts not in transformation (D46.2-)
     C92.00   Acute myeloblastic leukemia, not having achieved remission 🔒
         Acute myeloblastic leukemia with failed remission
         Acute myeloblastic leukemia NOS
     C92.01   Acute myeloblastic leukemia, in remission 🔒
     C92.02   Acute myeloblastic leukemia, in relapse 🔒

● **C92.1   Chronic myeloid leukemia, BCR/ABL-positive**
     Chronic myelogenous leukemia, Philadelphia chromosome (Ph1) positive
     Chronic myelogenous leukemia, t(9;22) (q34;q11)
     Chronic myelogenous leukemia with crisis of blast cells
     Excludes1   atypical chronic myeloid leukemia BCR/ABL-negative (C92.2-)
                 chronic myelomonocytic leukemia (C93.1-)
                 chronic myeloproliferative disease (D47.1)
     C92.10   Chronic myeloid leukemia, BCR/ABL-positive, not having achieved remission 🔒
         Chronic myeloid leukemia, BCR/ABL-positive with failed remission
         Chronic myeloid leukemia, BCR/ABL-positive NOS
         Coding Clinic: 2017, Q1, P7
     C92.11   Chronic myeloid leukemia, BCR/ABL-positive, in remission 🔒
     C92.12   Chronic myeloid leukemia, BCR/ABL-positive, in relapse 🔒

● **C92.2   Atypical chronic myeloid leukemia, BCR/ABL-negative**
     C92.20   Atypical chronic myeloid leukemia, BCR/ABL-negative, not having achieved remission 🔒
         Atypical chronic myeloid leukemia, BCR/ABL-negative with failed remission
         Atypical chronic myeloid leukemia, BCR/ABL-negative NOS
     C92.21   Atypical chronic myeloid leukemia, BCR/ABL-negative, in remission 🔒
     C92.22   Atypical chronic myeloid leukemia, BCR/ABL-negative, in relapse 🔒

● **C92.3   Myeloid sarcoma**
     A malignant tumor of immature myeloid cells
     Chloroma
     Granulocytic sarcoma
     C92.30   Myeloid sarcoma, not having achieved remission 🔒
         Myeloid sarcoma with failed remission
         Myeloid sarcoma NOS
     C92.31   Myeloid sarcoma, in remission 🔒
     C92.32   Myeloid sarcoma, in relapse 🔒

● **C92.4   Acute promyelocytic leukemia**
     AML M3
     AML Me with t(15;17) and variants
     C92.40   Acute promyelocytic leukemia, not having achieved remission 🔒
         Acute promyelocytic leukemia with failed remission
         Acute promyelocytic leukemia NOS
     C92.41   Acute promyelocytic leukemia, in remission 🔒
     C92.42   Acute promyelocytic leukemia, in relapse 🔒

● **C92.5   Acute myelomonocytic leukemia**
     AML M4
     AML M4 Eo with inv(16) or t(16;16)
     C92.50   Acute myelomonocytic leukemia, not having achieved remission 🔒
         Acute myelomonocytic leukemia with failed remission
         Acute myelomonocytic leukemia NOS
     C92.51   Acute myelomonocytic leukemia, in remission 🔒
     C92.52   Acute myelomonocytic leukemia, in relapse 🔒

N Newborn Age: 0   **P** Pediatric Age: 0–17   **M** Maternity DX: 12–55   **A** Adult Age: 15–124   ♀ Females Only   ♂ Males Only

🔒 Complication\Comorbidity   ◆ Major C\C   (Ex) CC/MCC Exclusions   🔒 Hospital-Acquired Condition

701

CHAPTER 2 (C00–D49)

● **C92.6**   Acute myeloid leukemia with 11q23-abnormality
     Acute myeloid leukemia with variation of MLL-gene

    C92.60   Acute myeloid leukemia with 11q23-abnormality not having achieved remission 🔒
       Acute myeloid leukemia with 11q23-abnormality with failed remission
       Acute myeloid leukemia with 11q23-abnormality NOS

    C92.61   Acute myeloid leukemia with 11q23-abnormality in remission 🔒

    C92.62   Acute myeloid leukemia with 11q23-abnormality in relapse 🔒

● **C92.A**   Acute myeloid leukemia with multilineage dysplasia
     Acute myeloid leukemia with dysplasia of remaining hematopoesis and/or myelodysplastic disease in its history

    C92.A0   Acute myeloid leukemia with multilineage dysplasia, not having achieved remission 🔒
       Acute myeloid leukemia with multilineage dysplasia with failed remission
       Acute myeloid leukemia with multilineage dysplasia NOS

    C92.A1   Acute myeloid leukemia with multilineage dysplasia, in remission 🔒

    C92.A2   Acute myeloid leukemia with multilineage dysplasia, in relapse 🔒

● **C92.Z**   Other myeloid leukemia

    C92.Z0   Other myeloid leukemia not having achieved remission 🔒
       Myeloid leukemia NEC with failed remission
       Myeloid leukemia NEC

    C92.Z1   Other myeloid leukemia, in remission 🔒

    C92.Z2   Other myeloid leukemia, in relapse 🔒

● **C92.9**   Myeloid leukemia, unspecified

    C92.90   Myeloid leukemia, unspecified, not having achieved remission 🔒
       Myeloid leukemia, unspecified with failed remission
       Myeloid leukemia, unspecified NOS

    C92.91   Myeloid leukemia, unspecified in remission 🔒

    C92.92   Myeloid leukemia, unspecified in relapse 🔒

●● **C93**   Monocytic leukemia

   | **Includes** | monocytoid leukemia |
   | **Excludes1** | personal history of leukemia (Z85.6) |

   Ⓔ **For category C93 CC codes:** See PDX Collection 485

● **C93.0**   Acute monoblastic/monocytic leukemia
     AML M5
     AML M5a
     AML M5b

    C93.00   Acute monoblastic/monocytic leukemia, not having achieved remission 🔒
       Acute monoblastic/monocytic leukemia with failed remission
       Acute monoblastic/monocytic leukemia NOS

    C93.01   Acute monoblastic/monocytic leukemia, in remission 🔒

    C93.02   Acute monoblastic/monocytic leukemia, in relapse 🔒

● **C93.1**   Chronic myelomonocytic leukemia
     Chronic monocytic leukemia
     CMML-1
     CMML-2
     CMML with eosinophilia

    C93.10   Chronic myelomonocytic leukemia not having achieved remission 🔒
       Chronic myelomonocytic leukemia with failed remission
       Chronic myelomonocytic leukemia NOS

    C93.11   Chronic myelomonocytic leukemia, in remission 🔒

    C93.12   Chronic myelomonocytic leukemia, in relapse 🔒

● **C93.3**   Juvenile myelomonocytic leukemia

    C93.30   Juvenile myelomonocytic leukemia, not having achieved remission 🔒   P
       Juvenile myelomonocytic leukemia with failed remission
       Juvenile myelomonocytic leukemia NOS

    C93.31   Juvenile myelomonocytic leukemia, in remission 🔒   P

    C93.32   Juvenile myelomonocytic leukemia, in relapse 🔒   P

● **C93.Z**   Other monocytic leukemia

    C93.Z0   Other monocytic leukemia, not having achieved remission 🔒
       Other monocytic leukemia NOS

    C93.Z1   Other monocytic leukemia, in remission 🔒

    C93.Z2   Other monocytic leukemia, in relapse 🔒

● **C93.9**   Monocytic leukemia, unspecified

    C93.90   Monocytic leukemia, unspecified, not having achieved remission 🔒
       Monocytic leukemia, unspecified with failed remission
       Monocytic leukemia, unspecified NOS

    C93.91   Monocytic leukemia, unspecified in remission 🔒

    C93.92   Monocytic leukemia, unspecified in relapse 🔒

● **C94**   Other leukemias of specified cell type

Excludes1	leukemic reticuloendotheliosis (C91.4-)
	myelodysplastic syndromes (D46.-)
	personal history of leukemia (Z85.6)
	plasma cell leukemia (C90.1-)

   Ⓔ **For category C94 CC codes unless otherwise indicated:** See PDX Collection 485

● **C94.0**   Acute erythroid leukemia
     Acute myeloid leukemia M6(a)(b)
     Erythroleukemia

    C94.00   Acute erythroid leukemia, not having achieved remission 🔒
       Acute erythroid leukemia with failed remission
       Acute erythroid leukemia NOS

    C94.01   Acute erythroid leukemia, in remission 🔒

    C94.02   Acute erythroid leukemia, in relapse 🔒

● **C94.2**   Acute megakaryoblastic leukemia
     Acute myeloid leukemia M7
     Acute megakaryocytic leukemia

    C94.20   Acute megakaryoblastic leukemia not having achieved remission 🔒
       Acute megakaryoblastic leukemia with failed remission
       Acute megakaryoblastic leukemia NOS

    C94.21   Acute megakaryoblastic leukemia, in remission 🔒

    C94.22   Acute megakaryoblastic leukemia, in relapse 🔒

CHAPTER 2 (C00-D49)

▶ New   ⇒ Revised   ~~deleted~~ Deleted   Excludes 1   Excludes 2   Includes   Use additional   Code first   Code also   Key words
OGCR Official Guidelines   ● Unacceptable Principal Diagnosis   X Assign placeholder X   🔒 Use Additional Character(s)   ▸ Manifestation Code   **Coding Clinic**

● **C94.3   Mast cell leukemia**

    C94.30   Mast cell leukemia not having achieved remission 🔖
       Mast cell leukemia with failed remission
       Mast cell leukemia NOS

    C94.31   Mast cell leukemia, in remission 🔖

    C94.32   Mast cell leukemia, in relapse 🔖

● **C94.4   Acute panmyelosis with myelofibrosis**
    Acute myelofibrosis

     Excludes1   myelofibrosis NOS (D75.81)
                 secondary myelofibrosis NOS (D75.81)

     (Ex) **For category C94.4 CC codes:** See PDX Collection 488

    C94.40   Acute panmyelosis with myelofibrosis not having achieved remission 🔖
       Acute myelofibrosis NOS
       Acute panmyelosis with myelofibrosis with failed remission
       Acute panmyelosis NOS

    C94.41   Acute panmyelosis with myelofibrosis, in remission 🔖

    C94.42   Acute panmyelosis with myelofibrosis, in relapse 🔖

   C94.6   Myelodysplastic disease, not classified 🔖
     Myeloproliferative disease, not classified
     (Ex) See PDX Collection 488

● **C94.8   Other specified leukemias**
    Aggressive NK-cell leukemia
    Acute basophilic leukemia

    C94.80   Other specified leukemias not having achieved remission 🔖
       Other specified leukemia with failed remission
       Other specified leukemias NOS

    C94.81   Other specified leukemias, in remission 🔖

    C94.82   Other specified leukemias, in relapse 🔖

● **C95   Leukemia of unspecified cell type**

     Excludes1   personal history of leukemia (Z85.6)
     (Ex) **For category C95 CC codes:** See PDX Collection 485

   ● **C95.0   Acute leukemia of unspecified cell type**
     Acute bilineal leukemia
     Acute mixed lineage leukemia
     Biphenotypic acute leukemia
     Stem cell leukemia of unclear lineage

      Excludes1   acute exacerbation of unspecified chronic leukemia (C95.10)

    C95.00   Acute leukemia of unspecified cell type not having achieved remission 🔖
       Acute leukemia of unspecified cell type with failed remission
       Acute leukemia NOS

    C95.01   Acute leukemia of unspecified cell type, in remission 🔖

    C95.02   Acute leukemia of unspecified cell type, in relapse 🔖

   ● **C95.1   Chronic leukemia of unspecified cell type**

    C95.10   Chronic leukemia of unspecified cell type not having achieved remission 🔖
       Chronic leukemia of unspecified cell type with failed remission
       Chronic leukemia NOS

    C95.11   Chronic leukemia of unspecified cell type, in remission 🔖

    C95.12   Chronic leukemia of unspecified cell type, in relapse 🔖

● **C95.9   Leukemia, unspecified**

    C95.90   Leukemia, unspecified not having achieved remission 🔖
       Leukemia, unspecified with failed remission
       Leukemia NOS

    C95.91   Leukemia, unspecified, in remission 🔖

    C95.92   Leukemia, unspecified, in relapse 🔖

● **C96   Other and unspecified malignant neoplasms of lymphoid, hematopoietic and related tissue**

     Excludes1   personal history of other malignant neoplasms of lymphoid, hematopoietic and related tissues (Z85.79)

   C96.0   Multifocal and multisystemic (disseminated) Langerhans-cell histiocytosis 🔖
     Histiocytosis X, multisystemic
     Letterer-Siwe disease

     Excludes1   adult pulmonary Langerhans cell histiocytosis (J84.82)
                 multifocal and unisystemic Langerhans-cell histiocytosis (C96.5)
                 unifocal Langerhans-cell histiocytosis (C96.6)

     (Ex) See PDX Collection 489

▶ ● **C96.2   Malignant mast cell neoplasm**
     ~~Aggressive systemic mastocytosis~~
     ~~Mast cell sarcoma~~

     Excludes1 ▶ indolent mastocytosis (D47.02)
                 mast cell leukemia (C94.30)
                 mastocytosis (congenital) (cutaneous) (Q82.2)
     (Ex) **For category C96.2 CC codes:** See PDX Collection 490

    ▶ **C96.20   Malignant mast cell neoplasm, unspecified** 🔖

    ▶ **C96.21   Aggressive systemic mastocytosis** 🔖

    ▶ **C96.22   Mast cell sarcoma** 🔖

    ▶ **C96.29   Other malignant mast cell neoplasm** 🔖

   C96.4   Sarcoma of dendritic cells (accessory cells) 🔖
     Follicular dendritic cell sarcoma
     Interdigitating dendritic cell sarcoma
     Langerhans cell sarcoma
     (Ex) See PDX Collection 491

   C96.5   Multifocal and unisystemic Langerhans-cell histiocytosis 🔖
     Hand-Schüller-Christian disease
     Histiocytosis X, multifocal

     Excludes1   multifocal and multisystemic (disseminated) Langerhans-cell histiocytosis (C96.0)
                 unifocal Langerhans-cell histiocytosis (C96.6)

     (Ex) See PDX Collection 492

   C96.6   Unifocal Langerhans-cell histiocytosis 🔖
     Eosinophilic granuloma
     Histiocytosis X, unifocal
     Histiocytosis X NOS
     Langerhans-cell histiocytosis NOS

     Excludes1   multifocal and multisysemic (disseminated) Langerhans-cell histiocytosis (C96.0)
                 multifocal and unisystemic Langerhans-cell histiocytosis (C96.5)

     (Ex) See PDX Collection 492

   C96.A   Histiocytic sarcoma 🔖
     Malignant histiocytosis
     (Ex) See PDX Collection 493

   C96.Z   Other specified malignant neoplasms of lymphoid, hematopoietic and related tissue 🔖
     (Ex) See PDX Collection 491

   C96.9   Malignant neoplasm of lymphoid, hematopoietic and related tissue, unspecified 🔖
     (Ex) See PDX Collection 491

N Newborn Age: 0   **P** Pediatric Age: 0–17   **M** Maternity DX: 12–55   **A** Adult Age: 15–124   ♀ Females Only   ♂ Males Only

🔖 Complication\Comorbidity   🔖 Major C\C   (Ex) CC/MCC Exclusions   🔖 Hospital-Acquired Condition

703

CHAPTER 2 (C00-D49)

IN SITU NEOPLASMS (D00-D09)

In situ is carcinoma involving cells in localized tissues that has not spread to nearby tissues

Includes   Bowen's disease
           erythroplasia
           grade III intraepithelial neoplasia
           Queyrat's erythroplasia

● **D00   Carcinoma in situ of oral cavity, esophagus and stomach**
     Excludes1   melanoma in situ (D03.-)

   ● **D00.0   Carcinoma in situ of lip, oral cavity and pharynx**
         Use additional code to identify:
         exposure to environmental tobacco smoke (Z77.22)
         exposure to tobacco smoke in the perinatal period (P96.81)
         history of tobacco dependence (Z87.891)
         occupational exposure to environmental tobacco smoke (Z57.31)
         tobacco dependence (F17.-)
         tobacco use (Z72.0)
         Excludes1   carcinoma in situ of aryepiglottic fold or interarytenoid fold, laryngeal aspect (D02.0)
                    carcinoma in situ of epiglottis NOS (D02.0)
                    carcinoma in situ of epiglottis suprahyoid portion (D02.0)
                    carcinoma in situ of skin of lip (D03.0, D04.0)

      D00.00   Carcinoma in situ of oral cavity, unspecified site
      D00.01   Carcinoma in situ of labial mucosa and vermilion border
      D00.02   Carcinoma in situ of buccal mucosa
      D00.03   Carcinoma in situ of gingiva and edentulous alveolar ridge
      D00.04   Carcinoma in situ of soft palate
      D00.05   Carcinoma in situ of hard palate
      D00.06   Carcinoma in situ of floor of mouth
      D00.07   Carcinoma in situ of tongue
      D00.08   Carcinoma in situ of pharynx
         Carcinoma in situ of aryepiglottic fold NOS
         Carcinoma in situ of hypopharyngeal aspect of aryepiglottic fold
         Carcinoma in situ of marginal zone of aryepiglottic fold

   D00.1   Carcinoma in situ of esophagus
   D00.2   Carcinoma in situ of stomach

● **D01   Carcinoma in situ of other and unspecified digestive organs**
     Excludes1   melanoma in situ (D03.-)

   D01.0   Carcinoma in situ of colon
         Excludes1   carcinoma in situ of rectosigmoid junction (D01.1)

   D01.1   Carcinoma in situ of rectosigmoid junction
   D01.2   Carcinoma in situ of rectum
   D01.3   Carcinoma in situ of anus and anal canal
         Anal intraepithelial neoplasia III [AIN III]
         Severe dysplasia of anus
         Excludes1   anal intraepithelial neoplasia I and II [AIN I and AIN II] (K62.82)
                    carcinoma in situ of anal margin (D04.5)
                    carcinoma in situ of anal skin (D04.5)
                    carcinoma in situ of perianal skin (D04.5)

   ● **D01.4   Carcinoma in situ of other and unspecified parts of intestine**
         Excludes1   carcinoma in situ of ampulla of Vater (D01.5)

      D01.40   Carcinoma in situ of unspecified part of intestine
      D01.49   Carcinoma in situ of other parts of intestine

   D01.5   Carcinoma in situ of liver, gallbladder and bile ducts
         Carcinoma in situ of ampulla of Vater
   D01.7   Carcinoma in situ of other specified digestive organs
         Carcinoma in situ of pancreas
   D01.9   Carcinoma in situ of digestive organ, unspecified

● **D02   Carcinoma in situ of middle ear and respiratory system**
     Use additional code to identify:
     exposure to environmental tobacco smoke (Z77.22)
     exposure to tobacco smoke in the perinatal period (P96.81)
     history of tobacco dependence (Z87.891)
     occupational exposure to environmental tobacco smoke (Z57.31)
     tobacco dependence (F17.-)
     tobacco use (Z72.0)
     Excludes1   melanoma in situ (D03.-)

   D02.0   Carcinoma in situ of larynx
         Carcinoma in situ of aryepiglottic fold or interarytenoid fold, laryngeal aspect
         Carcinoma in situ of epiglottis (suprahyoid portion)
         Excludes1   carcinoma in situ of aryepiglottic fold or interarytenoid fold NOS (D00.08)
                    carcinoma in situ of hypopharyngeal aspect (D00.08)
                    carcinoma in situ of marginal zone (D00.08)

   D02.1   Carcinoma in situ of trachea
   ● **D02.2   Carcinoma in situ of bronchus and lung**
      D02.20   Carcinoma in situ of unspecified bronchus and lung
      D02.21   Carcinoma in situ of right bronchus and lung
      D02.22   Carcinoma in situ of left bronchus and lung

   D02.3   Carcinoma in situ of other parts of respiratory system
         Carcinoma in situ of accessory sinuses
         Carcinoma in situ of middle ear
         Carcinoma in situ of nasal cavities
         Excludes1   carcinoma in situ of ear (external) (skin) (D04.2-)
                    carcinoma in situ of nose NOS (D09.8)
                    carcinoma in situ of skin of nose (D04.3)

   D02.4   Carcinoma in situ of respiratory system, unspecified

● **D03   Melanoma in situ**
   D03.0   Melanoma in situ of lip
   ● **D03.1   Melanoma in situ of eyelid, including canthus**
      D03.10   Melanoma in situ of unspecified eyelid, including canthus
      D03.11   Melanoma in situ of right eyelid, including canthus
      D03.12   Melanoma in situ of left eyelid, including canthus

   ● **D03.2   Melanoma in situ of ear and external auricular canal**
      D03.20   Melanoma in situ of unspecified ear and external auricular canal
      D03.21   Melanoma in situ of right ear and external auricular canal
      D03.22   Melanoma in situ of left ear and external auricular canal

● **D03.3 Melanoma in situ of other and unspecified parts of face**
    D03.30 Melanoma in situ of unspecified part of face
    D03.39 Melanoma in situ of other parts of face
  D03.4 Melanoma in situ of scalp and neck
● **D03.5** Melanoma in situ of trunk
    D03.51 Melanoma in situ of anal skin
        Melanoma in situ of anal margin
        Melanoma in situ of perianal skin
    D03.52 Melanoma in situ of breast (skin) (soft tissue)
    D03.59 Melanoma in situ of other part of trunk
● **D03.6** Melanoma in situ of upper limb, including shoulder
    D03.60 Melanoma in situ of unspecified upper limb, including shoulder
    D03.61 Melanoma in situ of right upper limb, including shoulder
    D03.62 Melanoma in situ of left upper limb, including shoulder
● **D03.7** Melanoma in situ of lower limb, including hip
    D03.70 Melanoma in situ of unspecified lower limb, including hip
    D03.71 Melanoma in situ of right lower limb, including hip
    D03.72 Melanoma in situ of left lower limb, including hip
  D03.8 Melanoma in situ of other sites
    Melanoma in situ of scrotum
    Excludes1 carcinoma in situ of scrotum (D07.61)
  D03.9 Melanoma in situ, unspecified

● **D04 Carcinoma in situ of skin**
    Excludes1 erythroplasia of Queyrat (penis) NOS (D07.4)
        melanoma in situ (D03.-)
  D04.0 Carcinoma in situ of skin of lip
    Excludes1 carcinoma in situ of vermilion border of lip (D00.01)
● **D04.1** Carcinoma in situ of skin of eyelid, including canthus
    D04.10 Carcinoma in situ of skin of unspecified eyelid, including canthus
    D04.11 Carcinoma in situ of skin of right eyelid, including canthus
    D04.12 Carcinoma in situ of skin of left eyelid, including canthus
● **D04.2** Carcinoma in situ of skin of ear and external auricular canal
    D04.20 Carcinoma in situ of skin of unspecified ear and external auricular canal
    D04.21 Carcinoma in situ of skin of right ear and external auricular canal
    D04.22 Carcinoma in situ of skin of left ear and external auricular canal
● **D04.3** Carcinoma in situ of skin of other and unspecified parts of face
    D04.30 Carcinoma in situ of skin of unspecified part of face
    D04.39 Carcinoma in situ of skin of other parts of face
  D04.4 Carcinoma in situ of skin of scalp and neck
  D04.5 Carcinoma in situ of skin of trunk
    Carcinoma in situ of anal margin
    Carcinoma in situ of anal skin
    Carcinoma in situ of perianal skin
    Carcinoma in situ of skin of breast
    Excludes1 carcinoma in situ of anus NOS (D01.3)
        carcinoma in situ of scrotum (D07.61)
        carcinoma in situ of skin of genital organs (D07.-)

● **D04.6** Carcinoma in situ of skin of upper limb, including shoulder
    D04.60 Carcinoma in situ of skin of unspecified upper limb, including shoulder
    D04.61 Carcinoma in situ of skin of right upper limb, including shoulder
    D04.62 Carcinoma in situ of skin of left upper limb, including shoulder
● **D04.7** Carcinoma in situ of skin of lower limb, including hip
    D04.70 Carcinoma in situ of skin of unspecified lower limb, including hip
    D04.71 Carcinoma in situ of skin of right lower limb, including hip
    D04.72 Carcinoma in situ of skin of left lower limb, including hip
  D04.8 Carcinoma in situ of skin of other sites
  D04.9 Carcinoma in situ of skin, unspecified

● **D05 Carcinoma in situ of breast**
    Excludes1 carcinoma in situ of skin of breast (D04.5)
        melanoma in situ of breast (skin) (D03.5)
        Paget's disease of breast or nipple (C50.-)
● **D05.0** Lobular carcinoma in situ of breast
    D05.00 Lobular carcinoma in situ of unspecified breast
    D05.01 Lobular carcinoma in situ of right breast
    D05.02 Lobular carcinoma in situ of left breast
● **D05.1** Intraductal carcinoma in situ of breast
    D05.10 Intraductal carcinoma in situ of unspecified breast
    D05.11 Intraductal carcinoma in situ of right breast
    D05.12 Intraductal carcinoma in situ of left breast
● **D05.8** Other specified type of carcinoma in situ of breast
    D05.80 Other specified type of carcinoma in situ of unspecified breast
    D05.81 Other specified type of carcinoma in situ of right breast
    D05.82 Other specified type of carcinoma in situ of left breast
● **D05.9** Unspecified type of carcinoma in situ of breast
    D05.90 Unspecified type of carcinoma in situ of unspecified breast
    D05.91 Unspecified type of carcinoma in situ of right breast
    D05.92 Unspecified type of carcinoma in situ of left breast

● **D06 Carcinoma in situ of cervix uteri**
    Includes cervical adenocarcinoma in situ
        cervical intraepithelial glandular neoplasia
        cervical intraepithelial neoplasia III [CIN III]
        severe dysplasia of cervix uteri
    Excludes1 cervical intraepithelial neoplasia II [CIN II] (N87.1)
        cytologic evidence of malignancy of cervix without histologic confirmation (R87.614)
        high grade squamous intraepithelial lesion (HGSIL) of cervix (R87.613)
        melanoma in situ of cervix (D03.5)
        moderate cervical dysplasia (N87.1)
  D06.0 Carcinoma in situ of endocervix ♀
  D06.1 Carcinoma in situ of exocervix ♀
  D06.7 Carcinoma in situ of other parts of cervix ♀
  D06.9 Carcinoma in situ of cervix, unspecified ♀

CHAPTER 2 (C00-D49)

N Newborn Age: 0   **P** Pediatric Age: 0–17   **M** Maternity DX: 12–55   **A** Adult Age: 15–124   ♀ Females Only   ♂ Males Only

🅒 Complication\Comorbidity   🅜 Major C\C   (Ex) CC/MCC Exclusions   🅗 Hospital-Acquired Condition

705

CHAPTER 2 (C00-D49)

● **D07**   **Carcinoma in situ of other and unspecified genital organs**
     Excludes1   melanoma in situ of trunk (D03.5)

D07.0   Carcinoma in situ of endometrium ♀

D07.1   Carcinoma in situ of vulva ♀
     Severe dysplasia of vulva
     Vulvar intraepithelial neoplasia III [VIN III]
     Excludes1   moderate dysplasia of vulva (N90.1)
                 vulvar intraepithelial neoplasia II [VIN II] (N90.1)

D07.2   Carcinoma in situ of vagina ♀
     Severe dysplasia of vagina
     Vaginal intraepithelial neoplasia III [VIN III]
     Excludes1   moderate dysplasia of vagina (N89.1)
                 vaginal intraepithelial neoplasia II [VIN II] (N89.1)

● **D07.3**   Carcinoma in situ of other and unspecified female genital organs
     D07.30   Carcinoma in situ of unspecified female genital organs ♀
     D07.39   Carcinoma in situ of other female genital organs ♀

D07.4   Carcinoma in situ of penis ♂
     Erythroplasia of Queyrat NOS

D07.5   Carcinoma in situ of prostate ♂
     Prostatic intraepithelial neoplasia III (PIN III)
     Severe dysplasia of prostate
     Excludes1   dysplasia (mild) (moderate) of prostate (N42.3-)
                 prostatic intraepithelial neoplasia II [PIN II] (N42.3-)

● **D07.6**   Carcinoma in situ of other and unspecified male genital organs
     D07.60   Carcinoma in situ of unspecified male genital organs ♂
     D07.61   Carcinoma in situ of scrotum ♂
     D07.69   Carcinoma in situ of other male genital organs ♂

● **D09**   **Carcinoma in situ of other and unspecified sites**
     Excludes1   melanoma in situ (D03.-)

D09.0   Carcinoma in situ of bladder

● **D09.1**   Carcinoma in situ of other and unspecified urinary organs
     D09.10   Carcinoma in situ of unspecified urinary organ
     D09.19   Carcinoma in situ of other urinary organs

● **D09.2**   Carcinoma in situ of eye
     Excludes1   carcinoma in situ of skin of eyelid (D04.1-)
     D09.20   Carcinoma in situ of unspecified eye
     D09.21   Carcinoma in situ of right eye
     D09.22   Carcinoma in situ of left eye

D09.3   Carcinoma in situ of thyroid and other endocrine glands
     Excludes1   carcinoma in situ of endocrine pancreas (D01.7)
                 carcinoma in situ of ovary (D07.39)
                 carcinoma in situ of testis (D07.69)

D09.8   Carcinoma in situ of other specified sites

D09.9   Carcinoma in situ, unspecified

Figure 2-16   The esophagus is the muscular tube that connects the pharynx and the stomach. The 10 inch (25 cm) long esophagus is divided into three parts: **cervical, thoracic,** and **abdominal.**

BENIGN NEOPLASMS, EXCEPT BENIGN NEUROENDOCRINE TUMORS (D10-D36)

● **D10**   **Benign neoplasm of mouth and pharynx**
     D10.0   Benign neoplasm of lip
         Benign neoplasm of lip (frenulum) (inner aspect) (mucosa) (vermilion border)
         Excludes1   benign neoplasm of skin of lip (D22.0, D23.0)

     D10.1   Benign neoplasm of tongue
         Benign neoplasm of lingual tonsil

     D10.2   Benign neoplasm of floor of mouth

●   **D10.3**   Benign neoplasm of other and unspecified parts of mouth
     D10.30   Benign neoplasm of unspecified part of mouth
     D10.39   Benign neoplasm of other parts of mouth
         Benign neoplasm of minor salivary gland NOS
         Excludes1   benign odontogenic neoplasms (D16.4-D16.5)
                 benign neoplasm of mucosa of lip (D10.0)
                 benign neoplasm of nasopharyngeal surface of soft palate (D10.6)

     D10.4   Benign neoplasm of tonsil
         Benign neoplasm of tonsil (faucial) (palatine)
         Excludes1   benign neoplasm of lingual tonsil (D10.1)
                 benign neoplasm of pharyngeal tonsil (D10.6)
                 benign neoplasm of tonsillar fossa (D10.5)
                 benign neoplasm of tonsillar pillars (D10.5)

     D10.5   Benign neoplasm of other parts of oropharynx
         Division of pharynx lying between soft palate and upper edge of epiglottis
         Benign neoplasm of epiglottis, anterior aspect
         Benign neoplasm of tonsillar fossa
         Benign neoplasm of tonsillar pillars
         Benign neoplasm of vallecula
         Excludes1   benign neoplasm of epiglottis NOS (D14.1)
                 benign neoplasm of epiglottis, suprahyoid portion (D14.1)

▶ New   ⇒ Revised   ~~deleted~~ Deleted   Excludes 1   Excludes 2   Includes   Use additional   Code first   Code also   Key words
OGCR Official Guidelines   ● Unacceptable Principal Diagnosis   X Assign placeholder X   ● Use Additional Character(s)   ▶ Manifestation Code   **Coding Clinic**

D10.6 **Benign neoplasm of nasopharynx**
Segment of pharynx that lies above soft palate
Benign neoplasm of pharyngeal tonsil
Benign neoplasm of posterior margin of septum and choanae

D10.7 **Benign neoplasm of hypopharynx**
Segment of pharynx that lies below upper edge of epiglottis and opens into larynx and esophagus

D10.9 **Benign neoplasm of pharynx, unspecified**

● **D11 Benign neoplasm of major salivary glands**

Excludes1   benign neoplasms of specified minor salivary glands which are classified according to their anatomical location
benign neoplasms of minor salivary glands NOS (D10.39)

D11.0 **Benign neoplasm of parotid gland**

D11.7 **Benign neoplasm of other major salivary glands**
Benign neoplasm of sublingual salivary gland
Benign neoplasm of submandibular salivary gland

D11.9 **Benign neoplasm of major salivary gland, unspecified**

● **D12 Benign neoplasm of colon, rectum, anus and anal canal**

Excludes1   benign carcinoid tumors of the large intestine, and rectum (D3A.02-)
Coding Clinic: 2017, Q1, P15; 2015, Q2, P14

D12.0 **Benign neoplasm of cecum**
Benign neoplasm of ileocecal valve

D12.1 **Benign neoplasm of appendix**

Excludes1   benign carcinoid tumor of the appendix (D3A.020)

D12.2 **Benign neoplasm of ascending colon**
Coding Clinic: 2017, Q1, P15

D12.3 **Benign neoplasm of transverse colon**
Benign neoplasm of hepatic flexure
Benign neoplasm of splenic flexure
Flexure is a bending in a structure or organ. Note the three flexures illustrated in Figure 2–17. Hepatic = liver, sigmoid = colon, splenic = spleen.
Coding Clinic: 2017, Q1, P16

D12.4 **Benign neoplasm of descending colon**
Coding Clinic: 2015, Q2, P14

D12.5 **Benign neoplasm of sigmoid colon**

D12.6 **Benign neoplasm of colon, unspecified**
Adenomatosis of colon
Benign neoplasm of large intestine NOS
Polyposis (hereditary) of colon
Excludes1   inflammatory polyp of colon (K51.4-)
polyp of colon NOS (K63.5)
Coding Clinic: 2017, Q1, P8-9

D12.7 **Benign neoplasm of rectosigmoid junction**
Angle where sigmoid colon becomes rectum

D12.8 **Benign neoplasm of rectum**
Excludes1   benign carcinoid tumor of the rectum (D3A.026)

D12.9 **Benign neoplasm of anus and anal canal**
Benign neoplasm of anus NOS
Excludes1   benign neoplasm of anal margin (D22.5, D23.5)
benign neoplasm of anal skin (D22.5, D23.5)
benign neoplasm of perianal skin (D22.5, D23.5)

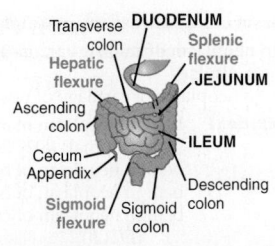

Figure 2-17 Small intestine and colon.

● **D13 Benign neoplasm of other and ill-defined parts of digestive system**

Excludes1   benign stromal tumors of digestive system (D21.4)

D13.0 **Benign neoplasm of esophagus**

D13.1 **Benign neoplasm of stomach**
Excludes1   benign carcinoid tumor of the stomach (D3A.092)

D13.2 **Benign neoplasm of duodenum**
Excludes1   benign carcinoid tumor of the duodenum (D3A.010)

● D13.3 **Benign neoplasm of other and unspecified parts of small intestine**
Excludes1   benign carcinoid tumors of the small intestine (D3A.01-)
benign neoplasm of ileocecal valve (D12.0)

D13.30 **Benign neoplasm of unspecified part of small intestine**

D13.39 **Benign neoplasm of other parts of small intestine**

D13.4 **Benign neoplasm of liver**
Benign neoplasm of intrahepatic bile ducts

D13.5 **Benign neoplasm of extrahepatic bile ducts**
Extensions of common hepatic bile duct (tube that collects bile from liver)

D13.6 **Benign neoplasm of pancreas**
Excludes1   benign neoplasm of endocrine pancreas (D13.7)

D13.7 **Benign neoplasm of endocrine pancreas**
Pancreatic islets: Cells scattered throughout pancreas
Islet cell tumor
Benign neoplasm of islets of Langerhans
Use additional code to identify any functional activity.

D13.9 **Benign neoplasm of ill-defined sites within the digestive system**
Benign neoplasm of digestive system NOS
Benign neoplasm of intestine NOS
Benign neoplasm of spleen

CHAPTER 2 (C00-D49)

CHAPTER 2 (C00-D49)

● **D14** Benign neoplasm of middle ear and respiratory system

    D14.0 Benign neoplasm of middle ear, nasal cavity and accessory sinuses

        Benign neoplasm of cartilage of nose

        Excludes1   benign neoplasm of auricular canal (external) (D22.2-, D23.2-)

            benign neoplasm of bone of ear (D16.4)

            benign neoplasm of bone of nose (D16.4)

            benign neoplasm of cartilage of ear (D21.0)

            benign neoplasm of ear (external) (skin) (D22.2-, D23.2-)

            benign neoplasm of nose NOS (D36.7)

            benign neoplasm of skin of nose (D22.39, D23.39)

            benign neoplasm of olfactory bulb (D33.3)

            benign neoplasm of posterior margin of septum and choanae (D10.6)

            polyp of accessory sinus (J33.8)

            polyp of ear (middle) (H74.4)

            polyp of nasal (cavity) (J33.-)

    D14.1 Benign neoplasm of larynx

        Adenomatous polyp of larynx

        Benign neoplasm of epiglottis (suprahyoid portion)

        Horseshoe shaped bone in anterior midline of neck between chin and thyroid cartilage

        Excludes1   benign neoplasm of epiglottis, anterior aspect (D10.5)

            polyp (nonadenomatous) of vocal cord or larynx (J38.1)

    D14.2 Benign neoplasm of trachea

●   **D14.3** Benign neoplasm of bronchus and lung

        Excludes1   benign carcinoid tumor of the bronchus and lung (D3A.090)

        D14.30 Benign neoplasm of unspecified bronchus and lung

        D14.31 Benign neoplasm of right bronchus and lung

        D14.32 Benign neoplasm of left bronchus and lung

    D14.4 Benign neoplasm of respiratory system, unspecified

● **D15** Benign neoplasm of other and unspecified intrathoracic organs

    Excludes1   benign neoplasm of mesothelial tissue (D19.-)

    D15.0 Benign neoplasm of thymus

        Excludes1   benign carcinoid tumor of the thymus (D3A.091)

    D15.1 Benign neoplasm of heart

        Excludes1   benign neoplasm of great vessels (D21.3)

    D15.2 Benign neoplasm of mediastinum

    D15.7 Benign neoplasm of other specified intrathoracic organs

    D15.9 Benign neoplasm of intrathoracic organ, unspecified

● **D16** Benign neoplasm of bone and articular cartilage

    Excludes1   benign neoplasm of connective tissue of ear (D21.0)

            benign neoplasm of connective tissue of eyelid (D21.0)

            benign neoplasm of connective tissue of larynx (D14.1)

            benign neoplasm of connective tissue of nose (D14.0)

            benign neoplasm of synovia (D21.-)

●   **D16.0** Benign neoplasm of scapula and long bones of upper limb

        D16.00 Benign neoplasm of scapula and long bones of unspecified upper limb

        D16.01 Benign neoplasm of scapula and long bones of right upper limb

        D16.02 Benign neoplasm of scapula and long bones of left upper limb

● **D16.1** Benign neoplasm of short bones of upper limb

    D16.10 Benign neoplasm of short bones of unspecified upper limb

    D16.11 Benign neoplasm of short bones of right upper limb

    D16.12 Benign neoplasm of short bones of left upper limb

● **D16.2** Benign neoplasm of long bones of lower limb

    D16.20 Benign neoplasm of long bones of unspecified lower limb

    D16.21 Benign neoplasm of long bones of right lower limb

    D16.22 Benign neoplasm of long bones of left lower limb

● **D16.3** Benign neoplasm of short bones of lower limb

    D16.30 Benign neoplasm of short bones of unspecified lower limb

    D16.31 Benign neoplasm of short bones of right lower limb

    D16.32 Benign neoplasm of short bones of left lower limb

    D16.4 Benign neoplasm of bones of skull and face

        Benign neoplasm of maxilla (superior)

        Benign neoplasm of orbital bone

        Cavity or socket of skull in which eye and its appendages are located

        Keratocyst of maxilla

        Keratocystic odontogenic tumor of maxilla

        Excludes2   benign neoplasm of lower jaw bone (D16.5)

    D16.5 Benign neoplasm of lower jaw bone

        Keratocyst of mandible

        Keratocystic odontogenic tumor of mandible

    D16.6 Benign neoplasm of vertebral column

        Excludes1   benign neoplasm of sacrum and coccyx (D16.8)

    D16.7 Benign neoplasm of ribs, sternum and clavicle

    D16.8 Benign neoplasm of pelvic bones, sacrum and coccyx

    D16.9 Benign neoplasm of bone and articular cartilage, unspecified

● **D17** Benign lipomatous neoplasm

    Slow-growing benign tumors (rubbery masses) of mature fat cells enclosed in a thin fibrous capsule

    D17.0 Benign lipomatous neoplasm of skin and subcutaneous tissue of head, face and neck

    D17.1 Benign lipomatous neoplasm of skin and subcutaneous tissue of trunk

●   **D17.2** Benign lipomatous neoplasm of skin and subcutaneous tissue of limb

        D17.20 Benign lipomatous neoplasm of skin and subcutaneous tissue of unspecified limb

        D17.21 Benign lipomatous neoplasm of skin and subcutaneous tissue of right arm

        D17.22 Benign lipomatous neoplasm of skin and subcutaneous tissue of left arm

        D17.23 Benign lipomatous neoplasm of skin and subcutaneous tissue of right leg

        D17.24 Benign lipomatous neoplasm of skin and subcutaneous tissue of left leg

●   **D17.3** Benign lipomatous neoplasm of skin and subcutaneous tissue of other and unspecified sites

        D17.30 Benign lipomatous neoplasm of skin and subcutaneous tissue of unspecified sites

        D17.39 Benign lipomatous neoplasm of skin and subcutaneous tissue of other sites

    D17.4 Benign lipomatous neoplasm of intrathoracic organs

▶ New   ⇒ Revised   deleted Deleted   Excludes 1   Excludes 2   Includes   Use additional   Code first   Code also   Key words

OGCR Official Guidelines   ● Unacceptable Principal Diagnosis   X Assign placeholder X   ● Use Additional Character(s)   ▶ Manifestation Code   **Coding Clinic**

Figure 2-18 Hemangioma of skin and subcutaneous tissue. (Getty Image)

Item 2–10 Hemangiomas are abnormally dense collections of dilated capillaries that occur on the skin or in internal organs. Hemangiomas are both deep and superficial and undergo a rapid growth phase when the size increases rapidly, followed by a rest phase, in which the tumor changes very little, followed by an involutional phase in which the tumor begins to and can disappear altogether. **Lymphangiomas** or cystic hygroma are benign collections of overgrown lymph vessels and, although rare, may occur anywhere but most commonly on the head and neck of children and infants. Visceral organs, lungs, and gastrointestinal tract may also be involved.

D17.5 Benign lipomatous neoplasm of intra-abdominal organs

> Excludes1 benign lipomatous neoplasm of peritoneum and retroperitoneum (D17.79)

D17.6 Benign lipomatous neoplasm of spermatic cord ♂

● D17.7 Benign lipomatous neoplasm of other sites

> **D17.71 Benign lipomatous neoplasm of kidney**
>
> **D17.72 Benign lipomatous neoplasm of other genitourinary organ**
>
> **D17.79 Benign lipomatous neoplasm of other sites**
>> Benign lipomatous neoplasm of peritoneum
>> Benign lipomatous neoplasm of retroperitoneum

D17.9 Benign lipomatous neoplasm, unspecified
> Lipoma NOS

● D18 Hemangioma and lymphangioma, any site

> Excludes1 benign neoplasm of glomus jugulare (D35.6)
> blue or pigmented nevus (D22.-)
> nevus NOS (D22.-)
> vascular nevus (Q82.5)

● D18.0 Hemangioma
> *Common type of vascular malformation*
> Angioma NOS
> Cavernous nevus

> **D18.00 Hemangioma unspecified site**
>
> **D18.01 Hemangioma of skin and subcutaneous tissue**
>
> **D18.02 Hemangioma of intracranial structures**
>
> **D18.03 Hemangioma of intra-abdominal structures**
>
> **D18.09 Hemangioma of other sites**

D18.1 Lymphangioma, any site

● D19 Benign neoplasm of mesothelial tissue
> *Mesothelial tissue is the membrane lining several body cavities*

D19.0 Benign neoplasm of mesothelial tissue of pleura

D19.1 Benign neoplasm of mesothelial tissue of peritoneum

D19.7 Benign neoplasm of mesothelial tissue of other sites

D19.9 Benign neoplasm of mesothelial tissue, unspecified
> Benign mesothelioma NOS

● D20 Benign neoplasm of soft tissue of retroperitoneum and peritoneum

> Excludes1 benign lipomatous neoplasm of peritoneum and retroperitoneum (D17.79)
> benign neoplasm of mesothelial tissue (D19.-)

D20.0 Benign neoplasm of soft tissue of retroperitoneum

D20.1 Benign neoplasm of soft tissue of peritoneum

● D21 Other benign neoplasms of connective and other soft tissue

> Includes benign neoplasm of blood vessel
> benign neoplasm of bursa
> benign neoplasm of cartilage
> benign neoplasm of fascia
> benign neoplasm of fat
> benign neoplasm of ligament, except uterine
> benign neoplasm of lymphatic channel
> benign neoplasm of muscle
> benign neoplasm of synovia
> benign neoplasm of tendon (sheath)
> benign stromal tumors

> Excludes1 benign neoplasm of articular cartilage (D16.-)
> benign neoplasm of cartilage of larynx (D14.1)
> benign neoplasm of cartilage of nose (D14.0)
> benign neoplasm of connective tissue of breast (D24.-)
> benign neoplasm of peripheral nerves and autonomic nervous system (D36.1-)
> benign neoplasm of peritoneum (D20.1)
> benign neoplasm of retroperitoneum (D20.0)
> benign neoplasm of uterine ligament, any (D28.2)
> benign neoplasm of vascular tissue (D18.-)
> hemangioma (D18.0-)
> lipomatous neoplasm (D17.-)
> lymphangioma (D18.1)
> uterine leiomyoma (D25.-)

D21.0 Benign neoplasm of connective and other soft tissue of head, face and neck
> Benign neoplasm of connective tissue of ear
> Benign neoplasm of connective tissue of eyelid

> Excludes1 benign neoplasm of connective tissue of orbit (D31.6-)

● D21.1 Benign neoplasm of connective and other soft tissue of upper limb, including shoulder

> **D21.10 Benign neoplasm of connective and other soft tissue of unspecified upper limb, including shoulder**
>
> **D21.11 Benign neoplasm of connective and other soft tissue of right upper limb, including shoulder**
>
> **D21.12 Benign neoplasm of connective and other soft tissue of left upper limb, including shoulder**

● D21.2 Benign neoplasm of connective and other soft tissue of lower limb, including hip

> **D21.20 Benign neoplasm of connective and other soft tissue of unspecified lower limb, including hip**
>
> **D21.21 Benign neoplasm of connective and other soft tissue of right lower limb, including hip**
>
> **D21.22 Benign neoplasm of connective and other soft tissue of left lower limb, including hip**

D21.3 Benign neoplasm of connective and other soft tissue of thorax
> Benign neoplasm of axilla
> Benign neoplasm of diaphragm
> Benign neoplasm of great vessels

> Excludes1 benign neoplasm of heart (D15.1)
> benign neoplasm of mediastinum (D15.2)
> benign neoplasm of thymus (D15.0)

D21.4 Benign neoplasm of connective and other soft tissue of abdomen
> Benign stromal tumors of abdomen

D21.5 Benign neoplasm of connective and other soft tissue of pelvis

> Excludes1 benign neoplasm of any uterine ligament (D28.2)
> uterine leiomyoma (D25.-)

D21.6 Benign neoplasm of connective and other soft tissue of trunk, unspecified
> Benign neoplasm of back NOS

D21.9 Benign neoplasm of connective and other soft tissue, unspecified

CHAPTER 2 (C00-D49)

N Newborn Age: 0   **P** Pediatric Age: 0–17   **M** Maternity DX: 12–55   **A** Adult Age: 15–124   ♀ Females Only   ♂ Males Only

Complication\Comorbidity   Major C\C   (Ex) CC/MCC Exclusions   Hospital-Acquired Condition

● **D22   Melanocytic nevi**

    Includes   atypical nevus
                   blue hairy pigmented nevus
                   nevus NOS

    D22.0   Melanocytic nevi of lip
        Skin lesions composed of nests of nevus cells with macules/
        papules

●   **D22.1   Melanocytic nevi of eyelid, including canthus**
        D22.10   Melanocytic nevi of unspecified eyelid, including canthus
        D22.11   Melanocytic nevi of right eyelid, including canthus
        D22.12   Melanocytic nevi of left eyelid, including canthus

●   **D22.2   Melanocytic nevi of ear and external auricular canal**
        D22.20   Melanocytic nevi of unspecified ear and external auricular canal
        D22.21   Melanocytic nevi of right ear and external auricular canal
        D22.22   Melanocytic nevi of left ear and external auricular canal

●   **D22.3   Melanocytic nevi of other and unspecified parts of face**
        D22.30   Melanocytic nevi of unspecified part of face
        D22.39   Melanocytic nevi of other parts of face

    D22.4   Melanocytic nevi of scalp and neck

    D22.5   Melanocytic nevi of trunk
        Melanocytic nevi of anal margin
        Melanocytic nevi of anal skin
        Melanocytic nevi of perianal skin
        Melanocytic nevi of skin of breast

●   **D22.6   Melanocytic nevi of upper limb, including shoulder**
        D22.60   Melanocytic nevi of unspecified upper limb, including shoulder
        D22.61   Melanocytic nevi of right upper limb, including shoulder
        D22.62   Melanocytic nevi of left upper limb, including shoulder

●   **D22.7   Melanocytic nevi of lower limb, including hip**
        D22.70   Melanocytic nevi of unspecified lower limb, including hip
        D22.71   Melanocytic nevi of right lower limb, including hip
        D22.72   Melanocytic nevi of left lower limb, including hip

    D22.9   Melanocytic nevi, unspecified

● **D23   Other benign neoplasms of skin**

    Includes   benign neoplasm of hair follicles
                   benign neoplasm of sebaceous glands
                   benign neoplasm of sweat glands

    Excludes1   benign lipomatous neoplasms of skin (D17.0-D17.3)
                     melanocytic nevi (D22.-)

    D23.0   Other benign neoplasm of skin of lip
        Excludes1   benign neoplasm of vermilion border of lip (D10.0)

●   **D23.1   Other benign neoplasm of skin of eyelid, including canthus**
        D23.10   Other benign neoplasm of skin unspecified of eyelid, including canthus
        D23.11   Other benign neoplasm of skin of right eyelid, including canthus
        D23.12   Other benign neoplasm of skin of left eyelid, including canthus

●   **D23.2   Other benign neoplasm of skin of ear and external auricular canal**
        D23.20   Other benign neoplasm of skin of unspecified ear and external auricular canal
        D23.21   Other benign neoplasm of skin of right ear and external auricular canal
        D23.22   Other benign neoplasm of skin of left ear and external auricular canal

●   **D23.3   Other benign neoplasm of skin of other and unspecified parts of face**
        D23.30   Other benign neoplasm of skin of unspecified part of face
        D23.39   Other benign neoplasm of skin of other parts of face

    D23.4   Other benign neoplasm of skin of scalp and neck

    D23.5   Other benign neoplasm of skin of trunk
        Other benign neoplasm of anal margin
        Other benign neoplasm of anal skin
        Other benign neoplasm of perianal skin
        Other benign neoplasm of skin of breast
        Excludes1   benign neoplasm of anus NOS (D12.9)

●   **D23.6   Other benign neoplasm of skin of upper limb, including shoulder**
        D23.60   Other benign neoplasm of skin of unspecified upper limb, including shoulder
        D23.61   Other benign neoplasm of skin of right upper limb, including shoulder
        D23.62   Other benign neoplasm of skin of left upper limb, including shoulder

●   **D23.7   Other benign neoplasm of skin of lower limb, including hip**
        D23.70   Other benign neoplasm of skin of unspecified lower limb, including hip
        D23.71   Other benign neoplasm of skin of right lower limb, including hip
        D23.72   Other benign neoplasm of skin of left lower limb, including hip

    D23.9   Other benign neoplasm of skin, unspecified

● **D24   Benign neoplasm of breast**

    Includes   benign neoplasm of connective tissue of breast
                   benign neoplasm of soft parts of breast
                   fibroadenoma of breast

    Excludes2   adenofibrosis of breast (N60.2)
                   benign cyst of breast (N60.-)
                   benign mammary dysplasia (N60.-)
                   benign neoplasm of skin of breast (D22.5, D23.5)
                   fibrocystic disease of breast (N60.-)

    D24.1   Benign neoplasm of right breast
        Coding Clinic: 2017, Q1, P5

    D24.2   Benign neoplasm of left breast

    D24.9   Benign neoplasm of unspecified breast

● **D25   Leiomyoma of uterus**
    Benign tumors or nodules of the uterine wall

    Includes   uterine fibroid
                   uterine fibromyoma
                   uterine myoma

    D25.0   Submucous leiomyoma of uterus ♀

    D25.1   Intramural leiomyoma of uterus ♀
        Interstitial leiomyoma of uterus

    D25.2   Subserosal leiomyoma of uterus ♀
        Subperitoneal leiomyoma of uterus

    D25.9   Leiomyoma of uterus, unspecified ♀

▶ New   ⮕ Revised   ~~deleted~~ Deleted   Excludes 1   Excludes 2   Includes   Use additional   Code first   Code also   Key words
OGCR Official Guidelines   ● Unacceptable Principal Diagnosis   X Assign placeholder X   ● Use Additional Character(s)   ▶ Manifestation Code   **Coding Clinic**

● **D26   Other benign neoplasms of uterus**
    D26.0   Other benign neoplasm of cervix uteri ♀
    D26.1   Other benign neoplasm of corpus uteri ♀
    D26.7   Other benign neoplasm of other parts of uteri ♀
    D26.9   Other benign neoplasm of uterus, unspecified ♀

Item 2–11   Teratoma: terat = monster, oma = mass, tumor. Alternate terms: dermoid cyst of the ovary, ovarian teratoma. Teratomas are neoplasms and arise from germ cells (ovaries in female and testes in male) and can be benign or malignant. Teratomas have been known to contain hair, nails, and teeth, giving them a bizarre ("monster") appearance.

● **D27   Benign neoplasm of ovary**
    Use additional code to identify any functional activity.
    Excludes2   corpus albicans cyst (N83.2-)
                corpus luteum cyst (N83.1-)
                endometrial cyst (N80.1)
                follicular (atretic) cyst (N83.0-)
                graafian follicle cyst (N83.0-)
                ovarian cyst NEC (N83.2-)
                ovarian retention cyst (N83.2-)
    D27.0   Benign neoplasm of right ovary ♀
    D27.1   Benign neoplasm of left ovary ♀
    D27.9   Benign neoplasm of unspecified ovary ♀
               Ovarian teratoma

● **D28   Benign neoplasm of other and unspecified female genital organs**
    Includes   adenomatous polyp
             benign neoplasm of skin of female genital organs
             benign teratoma
    Excludes1   epoophoron cyst (Q50.5)
               fimbrial cyst (Q50.4)
               Gartner's duct cyst (Q52.4)
               parovarian cyst (Q50.5)
    D28.0   Benign neoplasm of vulva ♀
    D28.1   Benign neoplasm of vagina ♀
    D28.2   Benign neoplasm of uterine tubes and ligaments ♀
               Benign neoplasm of fallopian tube
               Benign neoplasm of uterine ligament (broad) (round)
    D28.7   Benign neoplasm of other specified female genital organs ♀
    D28.9   Benign neoplasm of female genital organ, unspecified ♀

● **D29   Benign neoplasm of male genital organs**
    Includes   benign neoplasm of skin of male genital organs
    D29.0   Benign neoplasm of penis ♂
    D29.1   Benign neoplasm of prostate ♂
          Excludes1   enlarged prostate (N40.-)
   ● **D29.2**   Benign neoplasm of testis
          Use additional code to identify any functional activity.
          D29.20   Benign neoplasm of unspecified testis ♂
          D29.21   Benign neoplasm of right testis ♂
          D29.22   Benign neoplasm of left testis ♂
   ● **D29.3**   Benign neoplasm of epididymis
          D29.30   Benign neoplasm of unspecified epididymis ♂
          D29.31   Benign neoplasm of right epididymis ♂
          D29.32   Benign neoplasm of left epididymis ♂
    D29.4   Benign neoplasm of scrotum ♂
          Benign neoplasm of skin of scrotum
    D29.8   Benign neoplasm of other specified male genital organs ♂
          Benign neoplasm of seminal vesicle
          Benign neoplasm of spermatic cord
          Benign neoplasm of tunica vaginalis
    D29.9   Benign neoplasm of male genital organ, unspecified ♂

● **D30   Benign neoplasm of urinary organs**
   ● **D30.0**   Benign neoplasm of kidney
          Excludes1   benign carcinoid tumor of the kidney (D3A.093)
               benign neoplasm of renal calyces (D30.1-)
               benign neoplasm of renal pelvis (D30.1-)
          D30.00   Benign neoplasm of unspecified kidney
          D30.01   Benign neoplasm of right kidney
          D30.02   Benign neoplasm of left kidney
   ● **D30.1**   Benign neoplasm of renal pelvis
          D30.10   Benign neoplasm of unspecified renal pelvis
          D30.11   Benign neoplasm of right renal pelvis
          D30.12   Benign neoplasm of left renal pelvis
   ● **D30.2**   Benign neoplasm of ureter
          Excludes1   benign neoplasm of ureteric orifice of bladder (D30.3)
          D30.20   Benign neoplasm of unspecified ureter
          D30.21   Benign neoplasm of right ureter
          D30.22   Benign neoplasm of left ureter
    D30.3   Benign neoplasm of bladder
          Benign neoplasm of ureteric orifice of bladder
          Benign neoplasm of urethral orifice of bladder
    D30.4   Benign neoplasm of urethra
          Excludes1   benign neoplasm of urethral orifice of bladder (D30.3)
    D30.8   Benign neoplasm of other specified urinary organs
          Benign neoplasm of paraurethral glands
    D30.9   Benign neoplasm of urinary organ, unspecified
          Benign neoplasm of urinary system NOS

● **D31   Benign neoplasm of eye and adnexa**
    Excludes1   benign neoplasm of connective tissue of eyelid (D21.0)
               benign neoplasm of optic nerve (D33.3)
               benign neoplasm of skin of eyelid (D22.1-, D23.1-)
   ● **D31.0**   Benign neoplasm of conjunctiva
          D31.00   Benign neoplasm of unspecified conjunctiva
          D31.01   Benign neoplasm of right conjunctiva
          D31.02   Benign neoplasm of left conjunctiva
   ● **D31.1**   Benign neoplasm of cornea
          D31.10   Benign neoplasm of unspecified cornea
          D31.11   Benign neoplasm of right cornea
          D31.12   Benign neoplasm of left cornea
   ● **D31.2**   Benign neoplasm of retina
          Excludes1   dark area on retina (D49.81)
               hemangioma of retina (D49.81)
               neoplasm of unspecified behavior of retina and choroid (D49.81)
               retinal freckle (D49.81)
          D31.20   Benign neoplasm of unspecified retina
          D31.21   Benign neoplasm of right retina
          D31.22   Benign neoplasm of left retina
   ● **D31.3**   Benign neoplasm of choroid
          D31.30   Benign neoplasm of unspecified choroid
          D31.31   Benign neoplasm of right choroid
          D31.32   Benign neoplasm of left choroid
   ● **D31.4**   Benign neoplasm of ciliary body
          D31.40   Benign neoplasm of unspecified ciliary body
          D31.41   Benign neoplasm of right ciliary body
          D31.42   Benign neoplasm of left ciliary body

● **D31.5 Benign neoplasm of lacrimal gland and duct**
Benign neoplasm of lacrimal sac
Benign neoplasm of nasolacrimal duct

    D31.50 Benign neoplasm of unspecified lacrimal gland and duct

    D31.51 Benign neoplasm of right lacrimal gland and duct

    D31.52 Benign neoplasm of left lacrimal gland and duct

● **D31.6 Benign neoplasm of unspecified site of orbit**
Benign neoplasm of connective tissue of orbit
Benign neoplasm of extraocular muscle
Benign neoplasm of peripheral nerves of orbit
Benign neoplasm of retrobulbar tissue
Benign neoplasm of retro-ocular tissue

    Excludes1   benign neoplasm of orbital bone (D16.4)

    D31.60 Benign neoplasm of unspecified site of unspecified orbit

    D31.61 Benign neoplasm of unspecified site of right orbit

    D31.62 Benign neoplasm of unspecified site of left orbit

● **D31.9 Benign neoplasm of unspecified part of eye**
Benign neoplasm of eyeball

    D31.90 Benign neoplasm of unspecified part of unspecified eye

    D31.91 Benign neoplasm of unspecified part of right eye

    D31.92 Benign neoplasm of unspecified part of left eye

● **D32 Benign neoplasm of meninges**

    D32.0 Benign neoplasm of cerebral meninges

    D32.1 Benign neoplasm of spinal meninges

    D32.9 Benign neoplasm of meninges, unspecified
       Meningioma NOS

● **D33 Benign neoplasm of brain and other parts of central nervous system**

    Excludes1   angioma (D18.0-)
             benign neoplasm of meninges (D32.-)
             benign neoplasm of peripheral nerves and
                autonomic nervous system (D36.1-)
             hemangioma (D18.0-)
             neurofibromatosis (Q85.0-)
             retro-ocular benign neoplasm (D31.6-)

    D33.0 Benign neoplasm of brain, supratentorial
Benign neoplasm of cerebral ventricle
Benign neoplasm of cerebrum
Benign neoplasm of frontal lobe
Benign neoplasm of occipital lobe
Benign neoplasm of parietal lobe
Benign neoplasm of temporal lobe

    Excludes1   benign neoplasm of fourth ventricle (D33.1)

    D33.1 Benign neoplasm of brain, infratentorial
Benign neoplasm of brain stem
Benign neoplasm of cerebellum
Benign neoplasm of fourth ventricle

    D33.2 Benign neoplasm of brain, unspecified

    D33.3 Benign neoplasm of cranial nerves
Benign neoplasm of olfactory bulb

    D33.4 Benign neoplasm of spinal cord

    D33.7 Benign neoplasm of other specified parts of central nervous system

    D33.9 Benign neoplasm of central nervous system, unspecified
Benign neoplasm of nervous system (central) NOS

D34 Benign neoplasm of thyroid gland
Use additional code to identify any functional activity.

● **D35 Benign neoplasm of other and unspecified endocrine glands**
Use additional code to identify any functional activity.

    Excludes1   benign neoplasm of endocrine pancreas (D13.7)
             benign neoplasm of ovary (D27.-)
             benign neoplasm of testis (D29.2.-)
             benign neoplasm of thymus (D15.0)

● **D35.0 Benign neoplasm of adrenal gland**

    D35.00 Benign neoplasm of unspecified adrenal gland

    D35.01 Benign neoplasm of right adrenal gland

    D35.02 Benign neoplasm of left adrenal gland

    D35.1 Benign neoplasm of parathyroid gland

    D35.2 Benign neoplasm of pituitary gland

    D35.3 Benign neoplasm of craniopharyngeal duct

    D35.4 Benign neoplasm of pineal gland

    D35.5 Benign neoplasm of carotid body

    D35.6 Benign neoplasm of aortic body and other paraganglia
Benign tumor of glomus jugulare

    D35.7 Benign neoplasm of other specified endocrine glands

    D35.9 Benign neoplasm of endocrine gland, unspecified
Benign neoplasm of unspecified endocrine gland

● **D36 Benign neoplasm of other and unspecified sites**

    D36.0 Benign neoplasm of lymph nodes

    Excludes1   lymphangioma (D18.1)

● **D36.1 Benign neoplasm of peripheral nerves and autonomic nervous system**

    Excludes1   benign neoplasm of peripheral nerves of
               orbit (D31.6-)
             neurofibromatosis (Q85.0-)

    D36.10 Benign neoplasm of peripheral nerves and autonomic nervous system, unspecified

    D36.11 Benign neoplasm of peripheral nerves and autonomic nervous system of face, head, and neck

    D36.12 Benign neoplasm of peripheral nerves and autonomic nervous system, upper limb, including shoulder

    D36.13 Benign neoplasm of peripheral nerves and autonomic nervous system of lower limb, including hip

    D36.14 Benign neoplasm of peripheral nerves and autonomic nervous system of thorax

    D36.15 Benign neoplasm of peripheral nerves and autonomic nervous system of abdomen

    D36.16 Benign neoplasm of peripheral nerves and autonomic nervous system of pelvis

    D36.17 Benign neoplasm of peripheral nerves and autonomic nervous system of trunk, unspecified

    D36.7 Benign neoplasm of other specified sites
Benign neoplasm of nose NOS

    D36.9 Benign neoplasm, unspecified site

▶ New   ⇒ Revised   ~~deleted~~ Deleted   Excludes 1   Excludes 2   Includes   Use additional   Code first   Code also   Key words

OGCR Official Guidelines   ● Unacceptable Principal Diagnosis   X Assign placeholder X   ● Use Additional Character(s)   ▶ Manifestation Code   **Coding Clinic**

BENIGN NEUROENDOCRINE TUMORS (D3A)

- **D3A** **Benign neuroendocrine tumors**

  Code also any associated multiple endocrine neoplasia [MEN] syndromes (E31.2-)

  Use additional code to identify any associated endocrine syndrome, such as:
  carcinoid syndrome (E34.0)

  Excludes2   benign pancreatic islet cell tumors (D13.7)

  - **D3A.0** **Benign carcinoid tumors**

    D3A.00 **Benign carcinoid tumor of unspecified site**
    Carcinoid tumor NOS

    - **D3A.01** **Benign carcinoid tumors of the small intestine**

      D3A.010 **Benign carcinoid tumor of the duodenum**

      D3A.011 **Benign carcinoid tumor of the jejunum**

      D3A.012 **Benign carcinoid tumor of the ileum**

      D3A.019 **Benign carcinoid tumor of the small intestine, unspecified portion**

    - **D3A.02** **Benign carcinoid tumors of the appendix, large intestine, and rectum**

      D3A.020 **Benign carcinoid tumor of the appendix**

      D3A.021 **Benign carcinoid tumor of the cecum**

      D3A.022 **Benign carcinoid tumor of the ascending colon**

      D3A.023 **Benign carcinoid tumor of the transverse colon**

      D3A.024 **Benign carcinoid tumor of the descending colon**

      D3A.025 **Benign carcinoid tumor of the sigmoid colon**

      D3A.026 **Benign carcinoid tumor of the rectum**

      D3A.029 **Benign carcinoid tumor of the large intestine, unspecified portion**
      Benign carcinoid tumor of the colon NOS

    - **D3A.09** **Benign carcinoid tumors of other sites**

      D3A.090 **Benign carcinoid tumor of the bronchus and lung**

      D3A.091 **Benign carcinoid tumor of the thymus**

      D3A.092 **Benign carcinoid tumor of the stomach**

      D3A.093 **Benign carcinoid tumor of the kidney**

      D3A.094 **Benign carcinoid tumor of the foregut, unspecified**

      D3A.095 **Benign carcinoid tumor of the midgut, unspecified**

      D3A.096 **Benign carcinoid tumor of the hindgut, unspecified**

      D3A.098 **Benign carcinoid tumors of other sites**

  - **D3A.8** **Other benign neuroendocrine tumors**
    Neuroendocrine tumor NOS

Figure 2-19 Major salivary glands.

Parotid gland

Sublingual gland

Submandibular gland

NEOPLASMS OF UNCERTAIN BEHAVIOR, POLYCYTHEMIA VERA AND MYELODYSPLASTIC SYNDROMES (D37-D48)

Note: Categories D37-D44, and D48 classify by site neoplasms of uncertain behavior, i.e., histologic confirmation whether the neoplasm is malignant or benign cannot be made.

Excludes1   neoplasms of unspecified behavior (D49.-)

- **D37** **Neoplasm of uncertain behavior of oral cavity and digestive organs**

  Excludes1   stromal tumors of uncertain behavior of digestive system (D48.1)

  - **D37.0** **Neoplasm of uncertain behavior of lip, oral cavity and pharynx**

    Excludes1   neoplasm of uncertain behavior of aryepiglottic fold or interarytenoid fold, laryngeal aspect (D38.0)
    neoplasm of uncertain behavior of epiglottis NOS (D38.0)
    neoplasm of uncertain behavior of skin of lip (D48.5)
    neoplasm of uncertain behavior of suprahyoid portion of epiglottis (D38.0)

    D37.01 **Neoplasm of uncertain behavior of lip**
    Neoplasm of uncertain behavior of vermilion border of lip

    D37.02 **Neoplasm of uncertain behavior of tongue**

    - **D37.03** **Neoplasm of uncertain behavior of the major salivary glands**

      D37.030 **Neoplasm of uncertain behavior of the parotid salivary glands**

      D37.031 **Neoplasm of uncertain behavior of the sublingual salivary glands**

      D37.032 **Neoplasm of uncertain behavior of the submandibular salivary glands**

      D37.039 **Neoplasm of uncertain behavior of the major salivary glands, unspecified**

    D37.04 **Neoplasm of uncertain behavior of the minor salivary glands**
    Neoplasm of uncertain behavior of submucosal salivary glands of lip
    Neoplasm of uncertain behavior of submucosal salivary glands of cheek
    Neoplasm of uncertain behavior of submucosal salivary glands of hard palate
    Neoplasm of uncertain behavior of submucosal salivary glands of soft palate

    D37.05 **Neoplasm of uncertain behavior of pharynx**
    Neoplasm of uncertain behavior of aryepiglottic fold of pharynx NOS
    Neoplasm of uncertain behavior of hypopharyngeal aspect of aryepiglottic fold of pharynx
    Neoplasm of uncertain behavior of marginal zone of aryepiglottic fold of pharynx

    D37.09 **Neoplasm of uncertain behavior of other specified sites of the oral cavity**

CHAPTER 2 (C00-D49)

N   Newborn Age: 0   **P**   Pediatric Age: 0–17   **M**   Maternity DX: 12–55   **A**   Adult Age: 15–124   ♀   Females Only   ♂   Males Only

🄒 Complication\Comorbidity   🅜 Major C\C   ⓔ CC/MCC Exclusions   🄗 Hospital-Acquired Condition

713

D37.1   Neoplasm of uncertain behavior of **stomach**

D37.2   Neoplasm of uncertain behavior of **small intestine**

D37.3   Neoplasm of uncertain behavior of **appendix**

D37.4   Neoplasm of uncertain behavior of **colon**

D37.5   Neoplasm of uncertain behavior of **rectum**
Neoplasm of uncertain behavior of rectosigmoid junction
Rectosigmoid junction: Angle where sigmoid colon becomes rectum

D37.6   Neoplasm of uncertain behavior of **liver, gallbladder and bile ducts**
Neoplasm of uncertain behavior of ampulla of Vater
Ampulla of Vater: Enlarged segment of ducts from liver and pancreas at entry point to small intestine

D37.8   Neoplasm of uncertain behavior of other **specified digestive organs**
Neoplasm of uncertain behavior of anal canal
Neoplasm of uncertain behavior of anal sphincter
Neoplasm of uncertain behavior of anus NOS
Neoplasm of uncertain behavior of esophagus
Neoplasm of uncertain behavior of intestine NOS
Neoplasm of uncertain behavior of pancreas

> **Excludes1**   neoplasm of uncertain behavior of anal margin (D48.5)
> neoplasm of uncertain behavior of anal skin (D48.5)
> neoplasm of uncertain behavior of perianal skin (D48.5)

D37.9   Neoplasm of uncertain behavior of digestive organ, **unspecified**

● **D38**   Neoplasm of uncertain behavior of **middle ear and respiratory and intrathoracic organs**

> **Excludes1**   neoplasm of uncertain behavior of heart (D48.7)

D38.0   Neoplasm of uncertain behavior of **larynx**
Neoplasm of uncertain behavior of aryepiglottic fold or interarytenoid fold, laryngeal aspect
Neoplasm of uncertain behavior of epiglottis (suprahyoid portion)

> **Excludes1**   neoplasm of uncertain behavior of aryepiglottic fold or interarytenoid fold NOS (D37.05)
> neoplasm of uncertain behavior of hypopharyngeal aspect of aryepiglottic fold (D37.05)
> neoplasm of uncertain behavior of marginal zone of aryepiglottic fold (D37.05)

D38.1   Neoplasm of uncertain behavior of **trachea, bronchus and lung**

D38.2   Neoplasm of uncertain behavior of **pleura**

D38.3   Neoplasm of uncertain behavior of **mediastinum**

D38.4   Neoplasm of uncertain behavior of **thymus**

D38.5   Neoplasm of uncertain behavior of other **respiratory organs**
Neoplasm of uncertain behavior of accessory sinuses
Neoplasm of uncertain behavior of cartilage of nose
Neoplasm of uncertain behavior of middle ear
Neoplasm of uncertain behavior of nasal cavities

> **Excludes1**   neoplasm of uncertain behavior of ear (external) (skin) (D48.5)
> neoplasm of uncertain behavior of nose NOS (D48.7)
> neoplasm of uncertain behavior of skin of nose (D48.5)

D38.6   Neoplasm of uncertain behavior of respiratory organ, **unspecified**

● **D39**   Neoplasm of uncertain behavior of **female genital organs**

D39.0   Neoplasm of uncertain behavior of **uterus** ♀

● **D39.1**   Neoplasm of uncertain behavior of **ovary**
Use additional code to identify any functional activity.

D39.10   Neoplasm of uncertain behavior of **unspecified** ovary ♀

D39.11   Neoplasm of uncertain behavior of **right** ovary ♀

D39.12   Neoplasm of uncertain behavior of **left ovary** ♀

D39.2   Neoplasm of uncertain behavior of **placenta** ♀   M
Chorioadenoma destruens
Invasive hydatidiform mole
Malignant hydatidiform mole

> **Excludes1**   hydatidiform mole NOS (O01.9)

D39.8   Neoplasm of uncertain behavior of other **specified female genital organs** ♀
Neoplasm of uncertain behavior of skin of female genital organs

D39.9   Neoplasm of uncertain behavior of female genital organ, **unspecified** ♀

● **D40**   Neoplasm of uncertain behavior of **male genital organs**

D40.0   Neoplasm of uncertain behavior of **prostate** ♂

● **D40.1**   Neoplasm of uncertain behavior of **testis**

D40.10   Neoplasm of uncertain behavior of **unspecified** testis ♂

D40.11   Neoplasm of uncertain behavior of **right** testis ♂

D40.12   Neoplasm of uncertain behavior of **left testis** ♂

D40.8   Neoplasm of uncertain behavior of other **specified male genital organs** ♂
Neoplasm of uncertain behavior of skin of male genital organs

D40.9   Neoplasm of uncertain behavior of male genital organ, **unspecified** ♂

● **D41**   Neoplasm of uncertain behavior of **urinary organs**

● **D41.0**   Neoplasm of uncertain behavior of **kidney**

> **Excludes1**   neoplasm of uncertain behavior of renal pelvis (D41.1-)

D41.00   Neoplasm of uncertain behavior of **unspecified** kidney

D41.01   Neoplasm of uncertain behavior of **right kidney**

D41.02   Neoplasm of uncertain behavior of **left kidney**

● **D41.1**   Neoplasm of uncertain behavior of **renal pelvis**

D41.10   Neoplasm of uncertain behavior of **unspecified** renal pelvis

D41.11   Neoplasm of uncertain behavior of **right renal** pelvis

D41.12   Neoplasm of uncertain behavior of **left renal** pelvis

● **D41.2**   Neoplasm of uncertain behavior of **ureter**

D41.20   Neoplasm of uncertain behavior of **unspecified** ureter

D41.21   Neoplasm of uncertain behavior of **right ureter**

D41.22   Neoplasm of uncertain behavior of **left ureter**

D41.3   Neoplasm of uncertain behavior of **urethra**

D41.4   Neoplasm of uncertain behavior of **bladder**

D41.8   Neoplasm of uncertain behavior of other **specified urinary organs**

D41.9   Neoplasm of uncertain behavior of **unspecified urinary organ**

● **D42 Neoplasm of uncertain behavior of meninges**

  D42.0 **Neoplasm of uncertain behavior of cerebral meninges**

  D42.1 **Neoplasm of uncertain behavior of spinal meninges**

  D42.9 **Neoplasm of uncertain behavior of meninges, unspecified**

● **D43 Neoplasm of uncertain behavior of brain and central nervous system**

  Excludes1 neoplasm of uncertain behavior of peripheral nerves and autonomic nervous system (D48.2)

  D43.0 **Neoplasm of uncertain behavior of brain, supratentorial**
  Superior to tentorium of cerebellum
  Neoplasm of uncertain behavior of cerebral ventricle
  Neoplasm of uncertain behavior of cerebrum
  Neoplasm of uncertain behavior of frontal lobe
  Neoplasm of uncertain behavior of occipital lobe
  Neoplasm of uncertain behavior of parietal lobe
  Neoplasm of uncertain behavior of temporal lobe

  Excludes1 neoplasm of uncertain behavior of fourth ventricle (D43.1)

  D43.1 **Neoplasm of uncertain behavior of brain, infratentorial**
  Beneath the tentorium of cerebellum
  Neoplasm of uncertain behavior of brain stem
  Neoplasm of uncertain behavior of cerebellum
  Neoplasm of uncertain behavior of fourth ventricle

  D43.2 **Neoplasm of uncertain behavior of brain, unspecified**

  D43.3 **Neoplasm of uncertain behavior of cranial nerves**

  D43.4 **Neoplasm of uncertain behavior of spinal cord**

  D43.8 **Neoplasm of uncertain behavior of other specified parts of central nervous system**

  D43.9 **Neoplasm of uncertain behavior of central nervous system, unspecified**
  Neoplasm of uncertain behavior of nervous system (central) NOS

● **D44 Neoplasm of uncertain behavior of endocrine glands**

  Excludes1 multiple endocrine adenomatosis (E31.2-)
  multiple endocrine neoplasia (E31.2-)
  neoplasm of uncertain behavior of endocrine pancreas (D37.8)
  neoplasm of uncertain behavior of ovary (D39.1-)
  neoplasm of uncertain behavior of testis (D40.1-)
  neoplasm of uncertain behavior of thymus (D38.4)

  D44.0 **Neoplasm of uncertain behavior of thyroid gland**

  ● D44.1 **Neoplasm of uncertain behavior of adrenal gland**
  Use additional code to identify any functional activity.

    D44.10 **Neoplasm of uncertain behavior of unspecified adrenal gland**

    D44.11 **Neoplasm of uncertain behavior of right adrenal gland**

    D44.12 **Neoplasm of uncertain behavior of left adrenal gland**

  D44.2 **Neoplasm of uncertain behavior of parathyroid gland**

  D44.3 **Neoplasm of uncertain behavior of pituitary gland**
  Use additional code to identify any functional activity.

  D44.4 **Neoplasm of uncertain behavior of craniopharyngeal duct**

  D44.5 **Neoplasm of uncertain behavior of pineal gland**

  D44.6 **Neoplasm of uncertain behavior of carotid body**

  D44.7 **Neoplasm of uncertain behavior of aortic body and other paraganglia**
  Coding Clinic: 2016, Q4, P26

  D44.9 **Neoplasm of uncertain behavior of unspecified endocrine gland**

D45 **Polycythemia vera**

  Excludes1 familial polycythemia (D75.0)
  secondary polycythemia (D75.1)

  Primary polycythemia. Secondary polycythemia is D75.1. Check your documentation. Polycythemia is caused by too many red blood cells, which increase the thickness of blood (viscosity). This can cause engorgement of the spleen (splenomegaly) with extra RBCs and potential clot formation.

● **D46 Myelodysplastic syndromes**
  Use additional code for adverse effect, if applicable, to identify drug (T36-T50 with fifth or sixth character 5)

  Excludes2 drug-induced aplastic anemia (D61.1)

  D46.0 **Refractory anemia without ring sideroblasts, so stated**
  Refractory anemia without sideroblasts, without excess of blasts

  D46.1 **Refractory anemia with ring sideroblasts RARS**

  ● D46.2 **Refractory anemia with excess of blasts [RAEB]**
  Form of myelodysplasia with increased immature white blood cells (blasts) in bone marrow

    D46.20 **Refractory anemia with excess of blasts, unspecified RAEB NOS**

    D46.21 **Refractory anemia with excess of blasts 1 RAEB 1**
    Bone marrow disease which results in insufficient RBCs (anemia) in which level of blasts is less than 10%

    D46.22 **Refractory anemia with excess of blasts 2 RAEB 2** 🐾
    Bone marrow disease manifested by insufficient numbers of RBCs (anemia) with level of blasts 10-20%
    (Ex) See PDX Collection 488

  D46.A **Refractory cytopenia with multilineage dysplasia**

  D46.B **Refractory cytopenia with multilineage dysplasia and ring sideroblasts**
  RCMD RS

  D46.C **Myelodysplastic syndrome with isolated del(5q) chromosomal abnormality** 🐾
  Myelodysplastic syndrome with 5q deletion
  5q minus syndrome NOS
  (Ex) See PDX Collection 488

  D46.4 **Refractory anemia, unspecified**

  D46.Z **Other myelodysplastic syndromes**
  Excludes1 chronic myelomonocytic leukemia (C93.1-)

  D46.9 **Myelodysplastic syndrome, unspecified**
  Myelodysplasia NOS

● **D47 Other neoplasms of uncertain behavior of lymphoid, hematopoietic and related tissue**

  ➡● D47.0 **Mast cell neoplasms of uncertain behavior**
  ~~Indolent systemic mastocytosis~~
  ~~Mast cell tumor NOS~~
  ~~Mastocytoma NOS~~

    Excludes1 ~~malignant mast cell tumor (C96.2)~~
    ~~mastocytosis (congenital) (cutaneous) (Q82.2)~~
    ▸congenital cutaneous mastocytosis (Q82.2-)
    ▸histiocytic neoplasms of uncertain behavior (D47.Z9)
    ▸malignant mast cell neoplasm (C96.2-)
    (Ex) **For category D47.0 CC codes:** See PDX Collection 494

  ▸ D47.01 **Cutaneous mastocytosis** 🐾
    ▸Diffuse cutaneous mastocytosis
    ▸Maculopapular cutaneous mastocytosis
    ▸Solitary mastocytoma
    ▸Telangiectasia macularis eruptiva perstans
    ▸Urticaria pigmentosa
    ▸ **Excludes1** congenital (diffuse) (maculopapular) cutaneous mastocytosis (Q82.2)
    ▸congenital urticaria pigmentosa (Q82.2)
    ▸extracutaneous mastocytoma (D47.09)

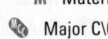

N Newborn Age: 0   **P** Pediatric Age: 0–17   **M** Maternity DX: 12–55   **A** Adult Age: 15–124   ♀ Females Only   ♂ Males Only

🐾 Complication\Comorbidity   🐾 Major C\C   (Ex) CC/MCC Exclusions   🐾 Hospital-Acquired Condition

715

CHAPTER 2 (C00-D49)

► **D47.02 Systemic mastocytosis**
► Indolent systemic mastocytosis
► Isolated bone marrow mastocytosis
► Smoldering systemic mastocytosis
► Systemic mastocytosis, with an associated hematological non-mast cell lineage disease (SM-AHNMD)
► Code also if applicable, any associated hematological non-mast cell lineage disease, such as:
► acute myeloid leukemia (C92.6-, C92.A-)
► chronic myelomonocytic leukemia (C93.1-)
► essential thrombocytosis (D47.3)
► hypereosinophilic syndrome (D72.1)
► myelodysplastic syndrome (D46.9)
► myeloproliferative syndrome (D47.1)
► non-Hodgkin lymphoma (C82-C85)
► plasma cell myeloma (C90.0-)
► polycythemia vera (D45)
► **Excludes1** aggressive systemic mastocytosis (C96.21)
► mast cell leukemia (C94.3-)
► **D47.09 Other mast cell neoplasms of uncertain behavior**
► Extracutaneous mastocytoma
► Mast cell tumor NOS
► Mastocytoma NOS
► Mastocytosis NOS

D47.1 Chronic myeloproliferative disease
Chronic neutrophilic leukemia
Myeloproliferative disease, unspecified
Excludes1 atypical chronic myeloid leukemia BCR/ABL-negative (C92.2-)
chronic myeloid leukemia BCR/ABL-positive (C92.1-)
myelofibrosis NOS (D75.81)
myelophthisic anemia (D61.82)
myelophthisis (D61.82)
secondary myelofibrosis NOS (D75.81)
(Ex) See PDX Collection 488

D47.2 Monoclonal gammopathy
Monoclonal gammopathy of undetermined significance [MGUS]

D47.3 Essential (hemorrhagic) thrombocythemia
Essential thrombocytosis
Idiopathic hemorrhagic thrombocythemia

D47.4 Osteomyelofibrosis
Chronic idiopathic myelofibrosis
Myelofibrosis (idiopathic) (with myeloid metaplasia)
Myelosclerosis (megakaryocytic) with myeloid metaplasia
Secondary myelofibrosis in myeloproliferative disease
Excludes1 acute myelofibrosis (C94.4-)

● **D47.Z Other specified neoplasms of uncertain behavior of lymphoid, hematopoietic and related tissue**
● **D47.Z1 Post-transplant lymphoproliferative disorder (PTLD)**
Code first complications of transplanted organs and tissue (T86.-)
(Ex) See PDX Collection 495
D47.Z2 Castleman disease
Code also if applicable human herpesvirus 8 infection (B10.89)
Excludes2 Kaposi's sarcoma (C46-)
(Ex) See PDX Collection 488
Coding Clinic: 2016, Q4, P8
D47.Z9 Other specified neoplasms of uncertain behavior of lymphoid, hematopoietic and related tissue
Histiocytic tumors of uncertain behavior
(Ex) See PDX Collection 488

D47.9 Neoplasm of uncertain behavior of lymphoid, hematopoietic and related tissue, unspecified
Lymphoproliferative disease NOS
(Ex) See PDX Collection 488

● **D48 Neoplasm of uncertain behavior of other and unspecified sites**
Excludes1 neurofibromatosis (nonmalignant) (Q85.0-)
D48.0 Neoplasm of uncertain behavior of bone and articular cartilage
Excludes1 neoplasm of uncertain behavior of cartilage of ear (D48.1)
neoplasm of uncertain behavior of cartilage of larynx (D38.0)
neoplasm of uncertain behavior of cartilage of nose (D38.5)
neoplasm of uncertain behavior of connective tissue of eyelid (D48.1)
neoplasm of uncertain behavior of synovia (D48.1)
D48.1 Neoplasm of uncertain behavior of connective and other soft tissue
Neoplasm of uncertain behavior of connective tissue of ear
Neoplasm of uncertain behavior of connective tissue of eyelid
Stromal tumors of uncertain behavior of digestive system
Excludes1 neoplasm of uncertain behavior of articular cartilage (D48.0)
neoplasm of uncertain behavior of cartilage of larynx (D38.0)
neoplasm of uncertain behavior of cartilage of nose (D38.5)
neoplasm of uncertain behavior of connective tissue of breast (D48.6-)
D48.2 Neoplasm of uncertain behavior of peripheral nerves and autonomic nervous system
Excludes1 neoplasm of uncertain behavior of peripheral nerves of orbit (D48.7)
D48.3 Neoplasm of uncertain behavior of retroperitoneum
D48.4 Neoplasm of uncertain behavior of peritoneum
D48.5 Neoplasm of uncertain behavior of skin
Neoplasm of uncertain behavior of anal margin
Neoplasm of uncertain behavior of anal skin
Neoplasm of uncertain behavior of perianal skin
Neoplasm of uncertain behavior of skin of breast
Excludes1 neoplasm of uncertain behavior of anus NOS (D37.8)
neoplasm of uncertain behavior of skin of genital organs (D39.8, D40.8)
neoplasm of uncertain behavior of vermilion border of lip (D37.0)
● **D48.6 Neoplasm of uncertain behavior of breast**
Neoplasm of uncertain behavior of connective tissue of breast
Cystosarcoma phyllodes
Excludes1 neoplasm of uncertain behavior of skin of breast (D48.5)
D48.60 Neoplasm of uncertain behavior of unspecified breast
D48.61 Neoplasm of uncertain behavior of right breast
D48.62 Neoplasm of uncertain behavior of left breast
D48.7 Neoplasm of uncertain behavior of other specified sites
Neoplasm of uncertain behavior of eye
Neoplasm of uncertain behavior of heart
Neoplasm of uncertain behavior of peripheral nerves of orbit
Excludes1 neoplasm of uncertain behavior of connective tissue (D48.1)
neoplasm of uncertain behavior of skin of eyelid (D48.5)
D48.9 Neoplasm of uncertain behavior, unspecified

► New ⇒ Revised ~~deleted~~ Deleted Excludes 1 Excludes 2 Includes Use additional Code first Code also Key words
OGCR Official Guidelines ● Unacceptable Principal Diagnosis X Assign placeholder X ● Use Additional Character(s) ▶ Manifestation Code **Coding Clinic**

CHAPTER 2 (C00-D49)

● **D49 Neoplasms of unspecified behavior**

> **Note:** Category D49 classifies by site neoplasms of unspecified morphology and behavior. The term 'mass,' unless otherwise stated, is not to be regarded as a neoplastic growth.

> **Includes**   'growth' NOS
> neoplasm NOS
> new growth NOS
> tumor NOS

> **Excludes1**   neoplasms of uncertain behavior (D37-D44, D48)

D49.0 Neoplasm of unspecified behavior of digestive system

> **Excludes1**   neoplasm of unspecified behavior of margin of anus (D49.2)
> neoplasm of unspecified behavior of perianal skin (D49.2)
> neoplasm of unspecified behavior of skin of anus (D49.2)

D49.1 Neoplasm of unspecified behavior of respiratory system

D49.2 Neoplasm of unspecified behavior of bone, soft tissue, and skin

> **Excludes1**   neoplasm of unspecified behavior of anal canal (D49.0)
> neoplasm of unspecified behavior of anus NOS (D49.0)
> neoplasm of unspecified behavior of bone marrow (D49.89)
> neoplasm of unspecified behavior of cartilage of larynx (D49.1)
> neoplasm of unspecified behavior of cartilage of nose (D49.1)
> neoplasm of unspecified behavior of connective tissue of breast (D49.3)
> neoplasm of unspecified behavior of skin of genital organs (D49.59)
> neoplasm of unspecified behavior of vermilion border of lip (D49.0)

D49.3 Neoplasm of unspecified behavior of breast

> **Excludes1**   neoplasm of unspecified behavior of skin of breast (D49.2)

D49.4 Neoplasm of unspecified behavior of bladder

● **D49.5 Neoplasm of unspecified behavior of other genitourinary organs**

● **D49.51 Neoplasm of unspecified behavior of kidney**

> **D49.511 Neoplasm of unspecified behavior of right kidney**
> Coding Clinic: 2016, Q4, P9

> **D49.512 Neoplasm of unspecified behavior of left kidney**
> Coding Clinic: 2016, Q4, P9

> **D49.519 Neoplasm of unspecified behavior of unspecified kidney**
> Coding Clinic: 2016, Q4, P9

> **D49.59 Neoplasm of unspecified behavior of other genitourinary organ**
> Coding Clinic: 2016, Q4, P9

D49.6 Neoplasm of unspecified behavior of brain

> **Excludes1**   neoplasm of unspecified behavior of cerebral meninges (D49.7)
> neoplasm of unspecified behavior of cranial nerves (D49.7)

D49.7 Neoplasm of unspecified behavior of endocrine glands and other parts of nervous system

> **Excludes1**   neoplasm of unspecified behavior of peripheral, sympathetic, and parasympathetic nerves and ganglia (D49.2)

● **D49.8 Neoplasm of unspecified behavior of other specified sites**

> **Excludes1**   neoplasm of unspecified behavior of eyelid (skin) (D49.2)
> neoplasm of unspecified behavior of eyelid cartilage (D49.2)
> neoplasm of unspecified behavior of great vessels (D49.2)
> neoplasm of unspecified behavior of optic nerve (D49.7)

> **D49.81 Neoplasm of unspecified behavior of retina and choroid**
> Dark area on retina
> Retinal freckle

> **D49.89 Neoplasm of unspecified behavior of other specified sites**

D49.9 Neoplasm of unspecified behavior of unspecified site

CHAPTER 2 (C00-D49)

OGCR Chapter-Specific Coding Guidelines

    3.   **Chapter 3: Disease of the blood and blood-forming organs and certain disorders involving the immune mechanism (D50-D89)**
        Reserved for future guideline expansion

CHAPTER 3

DISEASES OF THE BLOOD AND BLOOD-FORMING ORGANS AND CERTAIN DISORDERS INVOLVING THE IMMUNE MECHANISM (D50-D89)

    Excludes2   autoimmune disease (systemic) NOS (M35.9)
        certain conditions originating in the perinatal period (P00-P96)
        complications of pregnancy, childbirth and the puerperium (O00-O9A)
        congenital malformations, deformations and chromosomal abnormalities (Q00-Q99)
        endocrine, nutritional and metabolic diseases (E00-E88)
        human immunodeficiency virus [HIV] disease (B20)
        injury, poisoning and certain other consequences of external causes (S00-T88)
        neoplasms (C00-D49)
        symptoms, signs and abnormal clinical and laboratory findings, not elsewhere classified (R00-R94)

    This chapter contains the following blocks:

D50-D53	Nutritional anemias
D55-D59	Hemolytic anemias
D60-D64	Aplastic and other anemias and other bone marrow failure syndromes
D65-D69	Coagulation defects, purpura and other hemorrhagic conditions
D70-D77	Other disorders of blood and blood-forming organs
D78	Intraoperative and postprocedural complications of the spleen
D80-D89	Certain disorders involving the immune mechanism

NUTRITIONAL ANEMIAS (D50-D53)

● **D50**   **Iron deficiency anemia**
    A disease characterized by a decrease in the number of red cells (hemoglobin) in the blood.

    Includes   asiderotic anemia
                hypochromic anemia

    D50.0   **Iron deficiency anemia secondary to blood loss (chronic)**
        Posthemorrhagic anemia (chronic)

        Excludes1   acute posthemorrhagic anemia (D62)
                    congenital anemia from fetal blood loss (P61.3)

    D50.1   **Sideropenic dysphagia**
        Web-like growth of membranes in throat that makes swallowing difficult
        Kelly-Paterson syndrome
        Plummer-Vinson syndrome

    D50.8   **Other iron deficiency anemias**
        Iron deficiency anemia due to inadequate dietary iron intake

    D50.9   **Iron deficiency anemia, unspecified**

● **D51**   **Vitamin B12 deficiency anemia**

    Excludes1   vitamin B12 deficiency (E53.8)

    D51.0   **Vitamin B12 deficiency anemia due to intrinsic factor deficiency**
        Addison anemia
        Biermer anemia
        Pernicious (congenital) anemia
        Congenital intrinsic factor deficiency

    D51.1   **Vitamin B12 deficiency anemia due to selective vitamin B12 malabsorption with proteinuria**
        Imerslund (Gräsbeck) syndrome
        Megaloblastic hereditary anemia

    D51.2   **Transcobalamin II deficiency**

    D51.3   **Other dietary vitamin B12 deficiency anemia**
        Vegan anemia

    D51.8   **Other vitamin B12 deficiency anemias**

    D51.9   **Vitamin B12 deficiency anemia, unspecified**

● **D52**   **Folate deficiency anemia**

    Excludes1   folate deficiency without anemia (E53.8)

    D52.0   **Dietary folate deficiency anemia**
        Nutritional megaloblastic anemia

    D52.1   **Drug-induced folate deficiency anemia**
        Use additional code for adverse effect, if applicable, to identify drug (T36-T50 with fifth or sixth character 5)

    D52.8   **Other folate deficiency anemias**

    D52.9   **Folate deficiency anemia, unspecified**
        Folic acid deficiency anemia NOS

● **D53**   **Other nutritional anemias**

    Includes   megaloblastic anemia unresponsive to vitamin B12 or folate therapy

    D53.0   **Protein deficiency anemia**
        Amino-acid deficiency anemia
        Orotaciduric anemia

        Excludes1   Lesch-Nyhan syndrome (E79.1)

    D53.1   **Other megaloblastic anemias, not elsewhere classified**
        Megaloblastic anemia NOS

        Excludes1   Di Guglielmo's disease (C94.0)

    D53.2   **Scorbutic anemia**
        Anemia resulting from deficiency of ascorbic acid (vitamin C)

        Excludes1   scurvy (E54)

    D53.8   **Other specified nutritional anemias**
        Anemia associated with deficiency of copper
        Anemia associated with deficiency of molybdenum
        Anemia associated with deficiency of zinc

        Excludes1   nutritional deficiencies without anemia, such as:
                copper deficiency NOS (E61.0)
                molybdenum deficiency NOS (E61.5)
                zinc deficiency NOS (E60)

    D53.9   **Nutritional anemia, unspecified**
        Simple chronic anemia

        Excludes1   anemia NOS (D64.9)

HEMOLYTIC ANEMIAS (D55-D59)

● **D55**   **Anemia due to enzyme disorders**

    Excludes1   drug-induced enzyme deficiency anemia (D59.2)

    D55.0   **Anemia due to glucose-6-phosphate dehydrogenase [G6PD] deficiency**
        Favism
        G6PD deficiency anemia

    D55.1   **Anemia due to other disorders of glutathione metabolism**
        Anemia (due to) enzyme deficiencies, except G6PD, related to the hexose monophosphate [HMP] shunt pathway
        Anemia (due to) hemolytic nonspherocytic (hereditary), type I

▶ New   ⇒ Revised   ~~deleted~~ Deleted   Excludes 1   Excludes 2   Includes   Use additional   Code first   Code also   Key words
OGCR Official Guidelines   ● Unacceptable Principal Diagnosis   X Assign placeholder X   ● Use Additional Character(s)   ▮ Manifestation Code   **Coding Clinic**

D55.2   **Anemia due to disorders of glycolytic enzymes**
  Hemolytic nonspherocytic (hereditary) anemia, type II
  Hexokinase deficiency anemia
  Pyruvate kinase [PK] deficiency anemia
  Triose-phosphate isomerase deficiency anemia
  Excludes1 disorders of glycolysis not associated
      with anemia (E74.8)

D55.3   **Anemia due to disorders of nucleotide metabolism**

D55.8   **Other anemias due to enzyme disorders**

D55.9   **Anemia due to enzyme disorder, unspecified**

● **D56**   **Thalassemia**
*Hereditary disorders characterized by low production of hemoglobin
or excessive destruction of red blood cells*
  Excludes1 sickle-cell thalassemia (D57.4-)

D56.0   **Alpha thalassemia**
  Alpha thalassemia major
  Hemoglobin H Constant Spring
  Hemoglobin H disease
  Hydrops fetalis due to alpha thalassemia
  Severe alpha thalassemia
  Triple gene defect alpha thalassemia
  Use additional code, if applicable, for hydrops fetalis
    due to alpha thalassemia (P56.99)
  Excludes1 alpha thalassemia trait or minor (D56.3)
      asymptomatic alpha thalassemia (D56.3)
      hydrops fetalis due to isoimmunization
       (P56.0)
      hydrops fetalis not due to immune
       hemolysis (P83.2)

D56.1   **Beta thalassemia**
  Beta thalassemia major
  Cooley's anemia
  Homozygous beta thalassemia
  Severe beta thalassemia
  Thalassemia intermedia
  Thalassemia major
  Excludes1 beta thalassemia minor (D56.3)
      beta thalassemia trait (D56.3)
      delta-beta thalassemia (D56.2)
      hemoglobin E-beta thalassemia (D56.5)
      sickle-cell beta thalassemia (D57.4-)

D56.2   **Delta-beta thalassemia**
  Homozygous delta-beta thalassemia
  Excludes1 delta-beta thalassemia minor (D56.3)
      delta-beta thalassemia trait (D56.3)

D56.3   **Thalassemia minor**
*Genetic disorders that have in common defective production
of hemoglobin*
  Alpha thalassemia minor
  Alpha thalassemia silent carrier
  Alpha thalassemia trait
  Beta thalassemia minor
  Beta thalassemia trait
  Delta-beta thalassemia minor
  Delta-beta thalassemia trait
  Thalassemia trait NOS
  Excludes1 alpha thalassemia (D56.0)
      beta thalassemia (D56.1)
      delta-beta thalassemia (D56.2)
      hemoglobin E-beta thalassemia (D56.5)
      sickle-cell trait (D57.3)

D56.4   **Hereditary persistence of fetal hemoglobin [HPFH]**
Persistent production of hemoglobin

D56.5   **Hemoglobin E-beta thalassemia**
  Excludes1 beta thalassemia (D56.1)
      beta thalassemia minor (D56.3)
      beta thalassemia trait (D56.3)
      delta-beta thalassemia (D56.2)
      delta-beta thalassemia trait (D56.3)
      hemoglobin E disease (D58.2)
      other hemoglobinopathies (D58.2)
      sickle-cell beta thalassemia (D57.4-)

D56.8   **Other thalassemias**
  Dominant thalassemia
  Hemoglobin C thalassemia
  Mixed thalassemia
  Thalassemia with other hemoglobinopathy
  Excludes1 hemoglobin C disease (D58.2)
      hemoglobin E disease (D58.2)
      other hemoglobinopathies (D58.2)
      sickle cell anemia (D57.-)
      sickle-cell thalassemia (D57.4)

D56.9   **Thalassemia, unspecified**
  Mediterranean anemia (with other hemoglobinopathy)

● **D57**   **Sickle-cell disorders**
*Inherited disease in which red blood cells, normally disc-shaped,
become crescent shaped*
  Use additional code for any associated fever (R50.81)
  Excludes1 other hemoglobinopathies (D58.-)
  (Ex) **For category D57 CC codes: See PDX Collection 496**

● **D57.0**   **Hb-SS disease with crisis**
  Sickle-cell disease NOS with crisis
  Hb-SS disease with vasoocclusive pain
  D57.00 Hb-SS disease with crisis, unspecified 🔹
  D57.01 Hb-SS disease with acute chest syndrome 🔹
  D57.02 Hb-SS disease with splenic sequestration 🔹

D57.1   **Sickle-cell disease without crisis Hb-SS disease without
crisis**
  Sickle-cell anemia NOS
  Sickle-cell disease NOS
  Sickle-cell disorder NOS

● **D57.2**   **Sickle-cell/Hb-C disease**
  Hb-SC disease
  Hb-S/Hb-C disease
  D57.20 Sickle-cell/Hb-C disease without crisis
 ● D57.21 Sickle-cell/Hb-C disease with crisis
    D57.211 Sickle-cell/Hb-C disease with acute
      chest syndrome 🔹 🔹
      CC when PDX is its own CC
    D57.212 Sickle-cell/Hb-C disease with splenic
      sequestration 🔹
    D57.219 Sickle-cell/Hb-C disease with
      crisis, unspecified 🔹
      Sickle-cell/Hb-C disease with crisis
      NOS

D57.3   **Sickle-cell trait**
  Hb-S trait
  Heterozygous hemoglobin S

● **D57.4**   **Sickle-cell thalassemia**
  Sickle-cell beta thalassemia
  Thalassemia Hb-S disease
  D57.40 Sickle-cell thalassemia without crisis
    Microdrepanocytosis
    Sickle-cell thalassemia NOS
 ● D57.41 Sickle-cell thalassemia with crisis
    *Sickle-cell "crisis" is precipitated when abnormally
    crescent-shaped red blood cells form clots and
    interrupt blood flow to major organs, causing
    severe pain and organ damage.*
    Sickle-cell thalassemia with vasoocclusive pain
    D57.411 Sickle-cell thalassemia with acute
      chest syndrome 🔹 🔹
      CC when PDX is its own CC
    D57.412 Sickle-cell thalassemia with splenic
      sequestration 🔹
    D57.419 Sickle-cell thalassemia with
      crisis, unspecified 🔹
      Sickle-cell thalassemia with crisis
      NOS

CHAPTER 3 (D50-D89)

N Newborn Age: 0 P Pediatric Age: 0–17 M Maternity DX: 12–55 A Adult Age: 15–124 ♀ Females Only ♂ Males Only

 Complication\Comorbidity 🔹 Major C\C (Ex) CC/MCC Exclusions 🔹 Hospital-Acquired Condition

719

CHAPTER 3 (D50-D89)

● **D57.8   Other sickle-cell disorders**
Hb-SD disease
Hb-SE disease

     D57.80   Other sickle-cell disorders without crisis

     ● **D57.81   Other sickle-cell disorders with crisis**

         D57.811   Other sickle-cell disorders with acute chest syndrome 🗨

         D57.812   Other sickle-cell disorders with splenic sequestration 🗨

         D57.819   Other sickle-cell disorders with crisis, unspecified 🗨
Other sickle-cell disorders with crisis NOS

● **D58   Other hereditary hemolytic anemias**
Genetic condition in which bone marrow is unable to compensate for premature destruction of red blood cells

     Excludes1   hemolytic anemia of the newborn (P55.-)

     D58.0   Hereditary spherocytosis
Presence of spherocytes (spherically shaped red blood cells)
Acholuric (familial) jaundice
Congenital (spherocytic) hemolytic icterus
Minkowski-Chauffard syndrome

     D58.1   Hereditary elliptocytosis
Presence of large numbers of elliptocytes in blood
Elliptocytosis (congenital)
Ovalocytosis (congenital) (hereditary)

     D58.2   Other hemoglobinopathies
Abnormal hemoglobin NOS
Congenital Heinz body anemia
Hb-C disease
Hb-D disease
Hb-E disease
Hemoglobinopathy NOS
Unstable hemoglobin hemolytic disease

         Excludes1   familial polycythemia (D75.0)
Hb-M disease (D74.0)
hemoglobin E-beta thalassemia (D56.5)
hereditary persistence of fetal hemoglobin [HPFH] (D56.4)
high-altitude polycythemia (D75.1)
methemoglobinemia (D74.-)
other hemoglobinopathies with thalassemia (D56.8)

     D58.8   Other specified hereditary hemolytic anemias 🗨
Stomatocytosis
Ⓔⓧ See PDX Collection 497

     D58.9   Hereditary hemolytic anemia, unspecified 🗨
Ⓔⓧ See PDX Collection 497

● **D59   Acquired hemolytic anemia**
Ⓔⓧ For category D59 CC codes: See PDX Collection 496

     D59.0   Drug-induced autoimmune hemolytic anemia 🗨
Use additional code for adverse effect, if applicable, to identify drug (T36-T50 with fifth or sixth character 5)

     D59.1   Other autoimmune hemolytic anemias 🗨
Autoimmune hemolytic disease (cold type) (warm type)
Chronic cold hemagglutinin disease
Cold agglutinin disease
Cold agglutinin hemoglobinuria
Cold type (secondary) (symptomatic) hemolytic anemia
Warm type (secondary) (symptomatic) hemolytic anemia

         Excludes1   Evans syndrome (D69.41)
hemolytic disease of newborn (P55.-)
paroxysmal cold hemoglobinuria (D59.6)

     D59.2   Drug-induced nonautoimmune hemolytic anemia 🗨
Drug-induced enzyme deficiency anemia
Use additional code for adverse effect, if applicable, to identify drug (T36-T50 with fifth or sixth character 5)

     D59.3   Hemolytic-uremic syndrome 🗨
Use additional code to identify associated:
E. coli infection (B96.2-)
Pneumococcal pneumonia (J13)
Shigella dysenteriae (A03.9)

     D59.4   Other nonautoimmune hemolytic anemias 🗨
Mechanical hemolytic anemia
Microangiopathic hemolytic anemia
Toxic hemolytic anemia

     D59.5   Paroxysmal nocturnal hemoglobinuria [Marchiafava-Micheli]

         Excludes1   hemoglobinuria NOS (R82.3)

     D59.6   Hemoglobinuria due to hemolysis from other external causes
Hemoglobinuria from exertion
March hemoglobinuria
Paroxysmal cold hemoglobinuria
Use additional code (Chapter 20) to identify external cause

         Excludes1   hemoglobinuria NOS (R82.3)

     D59.8   Other acquired hemolytic anemias

     D59.9   Acquired hemolytic anemia, unspecified 🗨
Idiopathic hemolytic anemia, chronic

APLASTIC AND OTHER ANEMIAS AND OTHER BONE MARROW FAILURE SYNDROMES (D60-D64)

● **D60   Acquired pure red cell aplasia [erythroblastopenia]**
Deficiency of erythroblasts

     Includes   red cell aplasia (acquired) (adult) (with thymoma)
     Excludes1   congenital red cell aplasia (D61.01)
Ⓔⓧ For category D60 CC codes: See PDX Collection 496

     D60.0   Chronic acquired pure red cell aplasia 🗨
Lack of development of blood cell

     D60.1   Transient acquired pure red cell aplasia 🗨

     D60.8   Other acquired pure red cell aplasias 🗨

     D60.9   Acquired pure red cell aplasia, unspecified 🗨

● **D61   Other aplastic anemias and other bone marrow failure syndromes**

     Excludes1   neutropenia (D70.-)

     ● **D61.0   Constitutional aplastic anemia**
Condition where bone marrow is unable to produce blood cells

         D61.01   Constitutional (pure) red blood cell aplasia 🗨
Blackfan-Diamond syndrome
Congenital (pure) red cell aplasia
Familial hypoplastic anemia
Primary (pure) red cell aplasia
Red cell (pure) aplasia of infants

             Excludes1   acquired red cell aplasia (D60.9)
Ⓔⓧ See PDX Collection 498

         D61.09   Other constitutional aplastic anemia 🗨
Fanconi's anemia
Pancytopenia with malformations
Ⓔⓧ See PDX Collection 499

     D61.1   Drug-induced aplastic anemia 🗨
Use additional code for adverse effect, if applicable, to identify drug (T36-T50 with fifth or sixth character 5)
Ⓔⓧ See PDX Collection 496

     D61.2   Aplastic anemia due to other external agents 🗨
Code first, if applicable, toxic effects of substances chiefly nonmedicinal as to source (T51-T65)
Ⓔⓧ See PDX Collection 496

     D61.3   Idiopathic aplastic anemia 🗨
Ⓔⓧ See PDX Collection 496

▶ New   ⮕ Revised   ~~deleted~~ Deleted   Excludes 1   Excludes 2   Includes   Use additional   Code first   Code also   Key words

OGCR Official Guidelines   ● Unacceptable Principal Diagnosis   X Assign placeholder X   ● Use Additional Character(s)   ▶ Manifestation Code   **Coding Clinic**

● **D61.8　Other specified aplastic anemias and other bone marrow failure syndromes**
　　(Ex:) **For category D61.8 CC codes unless otherwise indicated:** See PDX Collection 500

　● **D61.81　Pancytopenia**
　　　　　Marked deficiency of all the blood elements: Red blood cells (erythrocytes), white blood cells (leukocytes), and platelets (thrombocytes). Check laboratory results.

　　　　　Excludes1　pancytopenia (due to) (with) aplastic anemia (D61.9)
　　　　　　　　　pancytopenia (due to) (with) bone marrow infiltration (D61.82)
　　　　　　　　　pancytopenia (due to) (with) congenital (pure) red cell aplasia (D61.01)
　　　　　　　　　pancytopenia (due to) (with) hairy cell leukemia (C91.4-)
　　　　　　　　　pancytopenia (due to) (with) human immunodeficiency virus disease (B20.-)
　　　　　　　　　pancytopenia (due to) (with) leukoerythroblastic anemia (D61.82)
　　　　　　　　　pancytopenia (due to) (with) myeloproliferative disease (D47.1)

　　　　　Excludes2　pancytopenia (due to) (with) myelodysplastic syndromes (D46.-)

　　　　D61.810　Antineoplastic chemotherapy induced pancytopenia 🍷
　　　　　　Excludes2　aplastic anemia due to antineoplastic chemotherapy (D61.1)

　　　　D61.811　Other drug-induced pancytopenia 🍷
　　　　　　Excludes2　aplastic anemia due to drugs (D61.1)

　　　　D61.818　Other pancytopenia 🍷

　　D61.82　Myelophthisis 🍷
　　　　　Leukoerythroblastic anemia
　　　　　Myelophthisic anemia
　　　　　Panmyelophthisis
　　　　　Code also the underlying disorder, such as:
　　　　　　malignant neoplasm of breast (C50.-)
　　　　　　tuberculosis (A15.-)

　　　　　Excludes1　idiopathic myelofibrosis (D47.1)
　　　　　　　　　myelofibrosis NOS (D75.81)
　　　　　　　　　myelofibrosis with myeloid metaplasia (D47.4)
　　　　　　　　　primary myelofibrosis (D47.1)
　　　　　　　　　secondary myelofibrosis (D75.81)

　　D61.89　Other specified aplastic anemias and other bone marrow failure syndromes 🍷
　　　　　(Ex:) See PDX Collection 496

D61.9　Aplastic anemia, unspecified 🍷
　　　Hypoplastic anemia NOS
　　　Medullary hypoplasia
　　　(Ex:) See PDX Collection 496

D62　Acute posthemorrhagic anemia 🍷
　　Excludes1　anemia due to chronic blood loss (D50.0)
　　　　　blood loss anemia NOS (D50.0)
　　　　　congenital anemia from fetal blood loss (P61.3)
　　(Ex:) See PDX Collection 501

● **D63　Anemia in chronic diseases classified elsewhere**
　▶ *D63.0　Anemia in neoplastic disease*
　　　　Code first neoplasm (C00-D49)

　　　　Excludes1　~~anemia due to antineoplastic chemotherapy (D64.81)~~
　　　　　　　aplastic anemia due to antineoplastic chemotherapy (D61.1)

　　▶ **Excludes2**　anemia due to antineoplastic chemotherapy (D64.81)

　　OGCR Section I.C.2.e.2.

　　　2) Anemia associated with chemotherapy, immunotherapy and radiation therapy
　　　When the admission/encounter is for management of an anemia associated with an adverse effect of the administration of chemotherapy or immunotherapy and the only treatment is for the anemia, the anemia code is sequenced first followed by the appropriate codes for the neoplasm and the adverse effect (T45.1X5, Adverse effect of antineoplastic and immunosuppressive drugs).

　▶ *D63.1　Anemia in chronic kidney disease*
　　　　Erythropoietin resistant anemia (EPO resistant anemia)
　　　　Code first underlying chronic kidney disease (CKD) (N18.-)

　▶ *D63.8　Anemia in other chronic diseases classified elsewhere*
　　　　Code first underlying disease, such as:
　　　　　diphyllobothriasis (B70.0)
　　　　　hookworm disease (B76.0-B76.9)
　　　　　hypothyroidism (E00.0-E03.9)
　　　　　malaria (B50.0-B54)
　　　　　symptomatic late syphilis (A52.79)
　　　　　tuberculosis (A18.89)

● **D64　Other anemias**
　　Excludes1　refractory anemia (D46.-)
　　　　　refractory anemia with excess blasts in transformation [RAEB T] (C92.0-)

　　D64.0　Hereditary sideroblastic anemia
　　　　Abnormal production RBCs (erythrocytes)
　　　　Sex-linked hypochromic sideroblastic anemia

　▶ **D64.1　*Secondary sideroblastic anemia due to disease***
　　　　Code first underlying disease

　　D64.2　Secondary sideroblastic anemia due to drugs and toxins
　　　　Code first poisoning due to drug or toxin, if applicable (T36-T65 with fifth or sixth character 1-4 or 6)
　　　　Use additional code for adverse effect, if applicable, to identify drug (T36-T50 with fifth or sixth character 5)

　　D64.3　Other sideroblastic anemias
　　　　Sideroblastic anemia NOS
　　　　Pyridoxine-responsive sideroblastic anemia NEC

　　D64.4　Congenital dyserythropoietic anemia
　　　　Any of several rare hereditary anemias, mostly types of macrocytic anemia
　　　　Dyshematopoietic anemia (congenital)

　　　　Excludes1　Blackfan-Diamond syndrome (D61.01)
　　　　　　　Di Guglielmo's disease (C94.0)

● **D64.8　Other specified anemias**
　　D64.81　Anemia due to antineoplastic chemotherapy
　　　　　Antineoplastic chemotherapy induced anemia

　　　　　Excludes1　aplastic anemia due to antineoplastic chemotherapy (D61.1)

　　　　　Excludes2　anemia in neoplastic disease (D63.0)

　　D64.89　Other specified anemias
　　　　　Infantile pseudoleukemia

　　D64.9　Anemia, unspecified
　　　　　Coding Clinic: 2017, Q1, P7

CHAPTER 3 (D50-D89)

N　Newborn Age: 0　　P　Pediatric Age: 0–17　　M　Maternity DX: 12–55　　A　Adult Age: 15–124　　♀　Females Only　　♂　Males Only
🍷 Complication\Comorbidity　　🍷 Major C\C　　(Ex:) CC/MCC Exclusions　　🍷 Hospital-Acquired Condition

COAGULATION DEFECTS, PURPURA AND OTHER HEMORRHAGIC CONDITIONS (D65-D69)

D65   **Disseminated intravascular coagulation [defibrination syndrome]** 🔖

Blood clots form and consume all coagulation proteins and platelets and disrupt normal coagulation, resulting in abnormal bleeding

Afibrinogenemia, acquired
Consumption coagulopathy
Diffuse or disseminated intravascular coagulation [DIC]
Fibrinolytic hemorrhage, acquired
Fibrinolytic purpura
Purpura fulminans

> **Excludes1**   disseminated intravascular coagulation (complicating):
> abortion or ectopic or molar pregnancy (O00-O07, O08.1)
> in newborn (P60)
> pregnancy, childbirth and the puerperium (O45.0, O46.0, O67.0, O72.3)

Ⓔ See PDX Collection 502

D66   **Hereditary factor VIII deficiency** 🔖

Inherited coagulation disorder carried by females but most often affecting males

Classical hemophilia
Deficiency factor VIII (with functional defect)
Hemophilia NOS
Hemophilia A

> **Excludes1**   factor VIII deficiency with vascular defect (D68.0)

Ⓔ See PDX Collection 502

D67   **Hereditary factor IX deficiency** 🔖

Christmas disease
Factor IX deficiency (with functional defect)
Hemophilia B
Plasma thromboplastin component [PTC] deficiency

Ⓔ See PDX Collection 502

● **D68**   **Other coagulation defects**

> **Excludes1**   abnormal coagulation profile (R79.1)
> coagulation defects complicating abortion or ectopic or molar pregnancy (O00-O07, O08.1)
> coagulation defects complicating pregnancy, childbirth and the puerperium (O45.0, O46.0, O67.0, O72.3)

Coding Clinic: 2016, Q1, P14

D68.0   **Von Willebrand's disease** 🔖

Congenital bleeding disorder
Angiohemophilia
Factor VIII deficiency with vascular defect
Vascular hemophilia

> **Excludes1**   capillary fragility (hereditary) (D69.8)
> factor VIII deficiency NOS (D66)
> factor VIII deficiency with functional defect (D66)

Ⓔ See PDX Collection 502

D68.1   **Hereditary factor XI deficiency** 🔖

Deficiency of blood coagulation resulting in systemic blood-clotting defect
Hemophilia C
Plasma thromboplastin antecedent [PTA] deficiency
Rosenthal's disease

Ⓔ See PDX Collection 502

D68.2   **Hereditary deficiency of other clotting factors** 🔖

Blood clotting disorders caused by hereditary deficiencies of one or more clotting factors
AC globulin deficiency
Congenital afibrinogenemia
Deficiency of factor I [fibrinogen]
Deficiency of factor II [prothrombin]
Deficiency of factor V [labile]
Deficiency of factor VII [stable]
Deficiency of factor X [Stuart-Prower]
Deficiency of factor XII [Hageman]
Deficiency of factor XIII [fibrin stabilizing]
Dysfibrinogenemia (congenital)
Hypoproconvertinemia
Owren's disease
Proaccelerin deficiency

Ⓔ See PDX Collection 502

● **D68.3**   **Hemorrhagic disorder due to circulating anticoagulants**

Blood clotting disorders caused by anticoagulants (warfarin and heparin)

● **D68.31**   **Hemorrhagic disorder due to intrinsic circulating anticoagulants, antibodies, or inhibitors**

D68.311   **Acquired hemophilia** 🔖

Autoimmune hemophilia
Autoimmune inhibitors to clotting factors
Secondary hemophilia

Ⓔ See PDX Collection 503

D68.312   **Antiphospholipid antibody with hemorrhagic disorder** 🔖

Lupus anticoagulant (LAC) with hemorrhagic disorder
Systemic lupus erythematosus [SLE] inhibitor with hemorrhagic disorder

> **Excludes1**   antiphospholipid antibody, finding without diagnosis (R76.0)
> antiphospholipid antibody syndrome (D68.61)
> antiphospholipid antibody with hypercoagulable state (D68.61)
> lupus anticoagulant (LAC) finding without diagnosis (R76.0)
> lupus anticoagulant (LAC) with hypercoagulable state (D68.62)
> systemic lupus erythematosus [SLE] inhibitor finding without diagnosis (R76.0)
> systemic lupus erythematosus [SLE] inhibitor with hypercoagulable state (D68.62)

Ⓔ See PDX Collection 504

D68.318   **Other hemorrhagic disorder due to intrinsic circulating anticoagulants, antibodies, or inhibitors**

Antithromboplastinemia
Antithromboplastinogenemia
Hemorrhagic disorder due to intrinsic increase in antithrombin
Hemorrhagic disorder due to intrinsic increase in anti-VIIIa
Hemorrhagic disorder due to intrinsic increase in anti-IXa
Hemorrhagic disorder due to intrinsic increase in anti-XIa

Ⓔ See PDX Collection 503

▶ New   ⟹ Revised   ~~deleted~~ Deleted   Excludes 1   Excludes 2   Includes   Use additional   Code first   Code also   Key words

OGCR Official Guidelines   ● Unacceptable Principal Diagnosis   X Assign placeholder X   ● Use Additional Character(s)   ▌ Manifestation Code   **Coding Clinic**

D68.32 **Hemorrhagic disorder due to extrinsic circulating anticoagulants** 🔹
     Drug-induced hemorrhagic disorder
     Hemorrhagic disorder due to increase in anti-IIa
     Hemorrhagic disorder due to increase in anti-Xa
     Hyperheparinemia
     Use additional code for adverse effect, if applicable, to identify drug (T45.515, T45.525)
     (Ex:) See PDX Collection 502
     Coding Clinic: 2016, Q1, P14-15

D68.4 **Acquired coagulation factor deficiency** 🔹
     Deficiency of coagulation factor due to liver disease
     Deficiency of coagulation factor due to vitamin K deficiency
     Excludes1   vitamin K deficiency of newborn (P53)
     (Ex:) See PDX Collection 502

●**D68.5** **Primary thrombophilia**
     AKA idiopathic thrombocytopenia, may be acquired or congenital and is a common cause of coagulation disorders.
     Primary hypercoagulable states
     Excludes1   antiphospholipid syndrome (D68.61)
       lupus anticoagulant (D68.62)
       secondary activated protein C resistance (D68.69)
       secondary antiphospholipid antibody syndrome (D68.69)
       secondary lupus anticoagulant with hypercoagulable state (D68.69)
       secondary systemic lupus erythematosus [SLE] inhibitor with hypercoagulable state (D68.69)
       systemic lupus erythematosus [SLE] inhibitor finding without diagnosis (R76.0)
       systemic lupus erythematosus [SLE] inhibitor with hemorrhagic disorder (D68.312)
       thrombotic thrombocytopenic purpura (M31.1)
     (Ex:) For category D68.5 CC codes: See PDX Collection 505

D68.51 **Activated protein C resistance** 🔹
     Factor V Leiden mutation

D68.52 **Prothrombin gene mutation** 🔹

D68.59 **Other primary thrombophilia** 🔹
     Antithrombin III deficiency
     Hypercoagulable state NOS
     Primary hypercoagulable state NEC
     Primary thrombophilia NEC
     Protein C deficiency
     Protein S deficiency
     Thrombophilia NOS

●**D68.6** **Other thrombophilia**
     Other hypercoagulable states
     Excludes1   diffuse or disseminated intravascular coagulation [DIC] (D65)
       heparin induced thrombocytopenia (HIT) (D75.82)
       hyperhomocysteinemia (E72.11)
     (Ex:) For category D68.6 CC codes: See PDX Collection 505

D68.61 **Antiphospholipid syndrome** 🔹
     Anticardiolipin syndrome
     Antiphospholipid antibody syndrome
     Excludes1   anti-phospholipid antibody, finding without diagnosis (R76.0)
       anti-phospholipid antibody with hemorrhagic disorder (D68.312)
       lupus anticoagulant syndrome (D68.62)

D68.62 **Lupus anticoagulant syndrome** 🔹
     Lupus anticoagulant
     Presence of systemic lupus erythematosus [SLE] inhibitor
     Excludes1   anticardiolipin syndrome (D68.61)
       antiphospholipid syndrome (D68.61)
       lupus anticoagulant (LAC) finding without diagnosis (R76.0)
       lupus anticoagulant (LAC) with hemorrhagic disorder (D68.312)

D68.69 **Other thrombophilia** 🔹
     Hypercoagulable states NEC
     Secondary hypercoagulable state NOS

D68.8 **Other specified coagulation defects** 🔹
     Excludes1   hemorrhagic disease of newborn (P53)
     (Ex:) See PDX Collection 502

D68.9 **Coagulation defect, unspecified** 🔹
     (Ex:) See PDX Collection 502

●**D69** **Purpura and other hemorrhagic conditions**
     Group of conditions characterized by small hemorrhages in skin, mucous membranes, or serosal surfaces
     Excludes1   benign hypergammaglobulinemic purpura (D89.0)
       cryoglobulinemic purpura (D89.1)
       essential (hemorrhagic) thrombocythemia (D47.3)
       hemorrhagic thrombocythemia (D47.3)
       purpura fulminans (D65)
       thrombotic thrombocytopenic purpura (M31.1)
       Waldenström hypergammaglobulinemic purpura (D89.0)

D69.0 **Allergic purpura** 🔹
     Allergic vasculitis
     Nonthrombocytopenic hemorrhagic purpura
     Nonthrombocytopenic idiopathic purpura
     Purpura anaphylactoid
     Purpura Henoch(-Schönlein)
     Purpura rheumatica
     Vascular purpura
     Excludes1   thrombocytopenic hemorrhagic purpura (D69.3)
     (Ex:) See PDX Collection 502

CHAPTER 3 (D50-D89)

D69.1 **Qualitative platelet defects**
Bernard-Soulier [giant platelet] syndrome
Glanzmann's disease
Grey platelet syndrome
Thromboasthenia (hemorrhagic) (hereditary)
Thrombocytopathy
Excludes1 von Willebrand's disease (D68.0)

D69.2 **Other nonthrombocytopenic purpura**
Purpura NOS
Purpura simplex
Senile purpura

D69.3 **Immune thrombocytopenic purpura**
Hemorrhagic (thrombocytopenic) purpura
Idiopathic thrombocytopenic purpura
Tidal platelet dysgenesis
(Ex) See PDX Collection 502

● D69.4 **Other primary thrombocytopenia**
Excludes1 transient neonatal thrombocytopenia (P61.0)
Wiskott-Aldrich syndrome (D82.0)

D69.41 **Evans syndrome**
Acquired hemolytic anemia and thrombocytopenia
(Ex) See PDX Collection 502

D69.42 **Congenital and hereditary thrombocytopenia purpura**
Congenital thrombocytopenia
Hereditary thrombocytopenia
Code first congenital or hereditary disorder, such as:
thrombocytopenia with absent radius (TAR syndrome) (Q87.2)
(Ex) See PDX Collection 502

D69.49 **Other primary thrombocytopenia**
Megakaryocytic hypoplasia
Primary thrombocytopenia NOS

● D69.5 **Secondary thrombocytopenia**
Acquired reduction of number of platelets required for blood clotting
Excludes1 heparin induced thrombocytopenia (HIT) (D75.82)
transient thrombocytopenia of newborn (P61.0)

D69.51 **Posttransfusion purpura**
Posttransfusion purpura from whole blood (fresh) or blood products PTP

D69.59 **Other secondary thrombocytopenia**

D69.6 **Thrombocytopenia, unspecified**

D69.8 **Other specified hemorrhagic conditions**
Capillary fragility (hereditary)
Vascular pseudohemophilia

D69.9 **Hemorrhagic condition, unspecified**

OTHER DISORDERS OF BLOOD AND BLOOD-FORMING ORGANS (D70-D77)

● D70 **Neutropenia**
Decrease in number of neutrophils (type of white blood cell)
Includes agranulocytosis
decreased absolute neurophile count (ANC)
Use additional code for any associated:
fever (R50.81)
mucositis (J34.81, K12.3-, K92.81, N76.81)
Excludes1 neutropenic splenomegaly (D73.81)
transient neonatal neutropenia (P61.5)

D70.0 **Congenital agranulocytosis**
Reduced numbers of neutrophils (type of white blood cell)
Congenital neutropenia
Infantile genetic agranulocytosis
Kostmann's disease

D70.1 **Agranulocytosis secondary to cancer chemotherapy**
Decreased numbers of granulocytes (type of white blood cell)
Code also *underlying neoplasm*
Use additional code for adverse effect, if applicable, to identify drug (T45.1X5)

D70.2 **Other drug-induced agranulocytosis**
Use additional code for adverse effect, if applicable, to identify drug (T36-T50 with fifth or sixth character 5)

D70.3 **Neutropenia due to infection**

D70.4 **Cyclic neutropenia**
Chronic neutropenia (low number of type of white blood cell)
Cyclic hematopoiesis
Periodic neutropenia

D70.8 **Other neutropenia**

D70.9 **Neutropenia, unspecified**

D71 **Functional disorders of polymorphonuclear neutrophils**
Polymorphonuclear: varying shapes of nucleus; AKA PMNs
Cell membrane receptor complex [CR3] defect
Chronic (childhood) granulomatous disease
Congenital dysphagocytosis
Progressive septic granulomatosis

● D72 **Other disorders of white blood cells**
Excludes1 basophilia (D72.824)
immunity disorders (D80-D89)
neutropenia (D70)
preleukemia (syndrome) (D46.9)

D72.0 **Genetic anomalies of leukocytes**
Alder (granulation) (granulocyte) anomaly
Alder syndrome
Hereditary leukocytic hypersegmentation
Hereditary leukocytic hyposegmentation
Hereditary leukomelanopathy
May-Hegglin (granulation) (granulocyte) anomaly
May-Hegglin syndrome
Pelger-Huët (granulation) (granulocyte) anomaly
Pelger-Huët syndrome
Excludes1 Chédiak (-Steinbrinck)-Higashi syndrome (E70.330)

D72.1 **Eosinophilia**
Formation and accumulation of high number of white cells in blood/tissue
Allergic eosinophilia
Hereditary eosinophilia
Excludes1 Löffler's syndrome (J82)
pulmonary eosinophilia (J82)

● D72.8 **Other specified disorders of white blood cells**
Excludes1 leukemia (C91-C95)

● D72.81 **Decreased white blood cell count**
Excludes1 neutropenia (D70.-)

D72.810 **Lymphocytopenia**
Decreased lymphocytes
Reduction in number of lympho cytes in blood

D72.818 **Other decreased white blood cell count**
Basophilic leukopenia
Eosinophilic leukopenia
Monocytopenia
Other decreased leukocytes
Plasmacytopenia

D72.819 **Decreased white blood cell count, unspecified**
Decreased leukocytes, unspecified
Leukocytopenia, unspecified
Leukopenia
Excludes1 malignant leukopenia (D70.9)

● **D72.82   Elevated white blood cell count**
    Excludes1   eosinophilia (D72.1)

D72.820   Lymphocytosis (symptomatic)
    Elevated lymphocytes
    Excess of normal lymphocytes

D72.821   Monocytosis (symptomatic)
    Excludes1   infectious
                   mononucleosis
                   (B27.-)

D72.822   Plasmacytosis
    Presence of excess plasma cells

D72.823   Leukemoid reaction
    Basophilic leukemoid reaction
    Leukemoid reaction NOS
    Lymphocytic leukemoid reaction
    Monocytic leukemoid reaction
    Myelocytic leukemoid reaction
    Neutrophilic leukemoid reaction

D72.824   Basophilia
    Increase of basophils in blood

D72.825   Bandemia
    Bandemia without diagnosis of
       specific infection
    Excess number of band cells (immature
       white blood cells) released by bone
       marrow
    Excludes1   confirmed infection
                   -code to infection
                   leukemia (C91.-,
                   C92.-, C93.-,
                   C94.-, C95.-)

D72.828   Other elevated white blood cell count

**D72.829   Elevated white blood cell
count, unspecified**
    Elevated leukocytes, unspecified
    Leukocytosis, unspecified

D72.89   Other specified disorders of white blood cells
    Abnormality of white blood cells NEC

D72.9   Disorder of white blood cells, unspecified
    Abnormal leukocyte differential NOS

● **D73   Diseases of spleen**

D73.0   Hyposplenism
    Diminished functioning of spleen
    Atrophy of spleen
    Excludes1   asplenia (congenital) (Q89.01)
                   postsurgical absence of spleen (Z90.81)

D73.1   Hypersplenism
    Accelerated function of spleen
    Excludes1   neutropenic splenomegaly (D73.81)
                   primary splenic neutropenia (D73.81)
                   splenitis, splenomegaly in late syphilis
                    (A52.79)
                   splenitis, splenomegaly in tuberculosis
                    (A18.85)
                   splenomegaly NOS (R16.1)
                   splenomegaly congenital (Q89.0)

D73.2   Chronic congestive splenomegaly
    Enlargement of spleen

D73.3   Abscess of spleen

D73.4   Cyst of spleen

D73.5   Infarction of spleen
    Splenic rupture, nontraumatic
    Torsion of spleen
    Excludes1   rupture of spleen due to Plasmodium
                    vivax malaria (B51.0)
                   traumatic rupture of spleen (S36.03-)

● **D73.8   Other diseases of spleen**

D73.81   Neutropenic splenomegaly
    Werner-Schultz disease
    Enlarged spleen responding to inadequate number
       of neutrophils

D73.89   Other diseases of spleen
    Fibrosis of spleen NOS
    Perisplenitis
    Splenitis NOS

D73.9   Disease of spleen, unspecified

● **D74   Methemoglobinemia**
    Excessive methemoglobin (form of hemoglobin)
    (Ex) **For category D74 CC codes:** See PDX Collection 506

D74.0   Congenital methemoglobinemia 🔖
    Congenital NADH-methemoglobin reductase
       deficiency
    Hemoglobin-M [Hb-M] disease
    Methemoglobinemia, hereditary

D74.8   Other methemoglobinemias 🔖
    Acquired methemoglobinemia (with
       sulfhemoglobinemia)
    Toxic methemoglobinemia

D74.9   Methemoglobinemia, unspecified 🔖

● **D75   Other and unspecified diseases of blood and blood-forming
organs**
    Excludes2   acute lymphadenitis (L04.-)
                   chronic lymphadenitis (I88.1)
                   enlarged lymph nodes (R59.-)
                   hypergammaglobulinemia NOS (D89.2)
                   lymphadenitis NOS (I88.9)
                   mesenteric lymphadenitis (acute) (chronic) (I88.0)

D75.0   Familial erythrocytosis
    Genetic mutation of gene that results in increased circulating
       RBCs
    Benign polycythemia
    Familial polycythemia
    Excludes1   hereditary ovalocytosis (D58.1)

D75.1   Secondary polycythemia
    Increase in total red cell mass
    Acquired polycythemia
    Emotional polycythemia
    Erythrocytosis NOS
    Hypoxemic polycythemia
    Nephrogenous polycythemia
    Polycythemia due to erythropoietin
    Polycythemia due to fall in plasma volume
    Polycythemia due to high altitude
    Polycythemia due to stress
    Polycythemia NOS
    Relative polycythemia
    Excludes1   polycythemia neonatorum (P61.1)
                   polycythemia vera (D45)

CHAPTER 3 (D50-D89)

N Newborn Age: 0   **P** Pediatric Age: 0–17   **M** Maternity DX: 12–55   **A** Adult Age: 15–124   ♀ Females Only   ♂ Males Only

🔖 Complication\Comorbidity   🔖 Major C\C   (Ex) CC/MCC Exclusions   🔖 Hospital-Acquired Condition

725

● **D75.8** **Other specified diseases of blood and blood-forming organs**

▷ **D75.81** *Myelofibrosis* 🔖
    Replacing bone marrow by fibrous tissue
    Myelofibrosis NOS
    Secondary myelofibrosis NOS

    Code first the underlying disorder, such as:
      malignant neoplasm of breast (C50.-)

    Use additional code, if applicable, for associated therapy-related myelodysplastic syndrome (D46.-)

    Use additional code for adverse effect, if applicable, to identify drug (T45.1X5)

    Excludes1 acute myelofibrosis (C94.4-)
                idiopathic myelofibrosis (D47.1)
                leukoerythroblastic anemia (D61.82)
                myelofibrosis with myeloid metaplasia (D47.4)
                myelophthisic anemia (D61.82)
                myelophthisis (D61.82)
                primary myelofibrosis (D47.1)

    Ⓔˣ See PDX Collection 488

D75.82 Heparin induced thrombocytopenia (HIT)

D75.89 Other specified diseases of blood and blood-forming organs

D75.9 Disease of blood and blood-forming organs, unspecified

● **D76** **Other specified diseases with participation of lymphoreticular and reticulohistiocytic tissue**

Excludes1 (Abt-) Letterer-Siwe disease (C96.0)
            eosinophilic granuloma (C96.6)
            Hand-Schüller-Christian disease (C96.5)
            histiocytic medullary reticulosis (C96.9)
            histiocytic sarcoma (C96.A)
            histiocytosis X, multifocal (C96.5)
            histiocytosis X, unifocal (C96.6)
            Langerhans-cell histiocytosis, multifocal (C96.5)
            Langerhans-cell histiocytosis NOS (C96.6)
            Langerhans-cell histiocytosis, unifocal (C96.6)
            leukemic reticuloendotheliosis (C91.4-)
            lipomelanotic reticulosis (I89.8)
            malignant histiocytosis (C96.A)
            malignant reticulosis (C86.0)
            nonlipid reticuloendotheliosis (C96.0)

Ⓔˣ For category D76 CC codes: See PDX Collection 507

D76.1 **Hemophagocytic lymphohistiocytosis** 🔖
    Familial hemophagocytic reticulosis
    Histiocytoses of mononuclear phagocytes

D76.2 **Hemophagocytic syndrome, infection-associated** 🔖
    Use additional code to identify infectious agent or disease.

D76.3 **Other histiocytosis syndromes** 🔖
    Reticulohistiocytoma (giant-cell)
    Sinus histiocytosis with massive lymphadenopathy
    Xanthogranuloma

▷ **D77** *Other disorders of blood and blood-forming organs in diseases classified elsewhere*

    Code first underlying disease, such as:
      amyloidosis (E85.-)
      congenital early syphilis (A50.0)
      echinococcosis (B67.0-B67.9)
      malaria (B50.0-B54)
      schistosomiasis [bilharziasis] (B65.0-B65.9)
      vitamin C deficiency (E54)

    Excludes1 rupture of spleen due to Plasmodium vivax malaria (B51.0)
                splenitis, splenomegaly in late syphilis (A52.79)
                splenitis, splenomegaly in tuberculosis (A18.85)

INTRAOPERATIVE AND POSTPROCEDURAL COMPLICATIONS OF THE SPLEEN (D78)

● **D78** **Intraoperative and postprocedural complications of the spleen**
    Coding Clinic: 2016, Q4, P9

● **D78.0** **Intraoperative hemorrhage and hematoma of the spleen complicating a procedure**

    Excludes1 intraoperative hemorrhage and hematoma of the spleen due to accidental puncture or laceration during a procedure (D78.1-)

    Ⓔˣ For category D78.0 CC codes: See PDX Collection 508

D78.01 Intraoperative hemorrhage and hematoma of the spleen complicating a procedure on the spleen 🔖

D78.02 Intraoperative hemorrhage and hematoma of the spleen complicating other procedure 🔖

● **D78.1** **Accidental puncture and laceration of the spleen during a procedure**

    Ⓔˣ For category D78.1 CC codes: See PDX Collection 509

D78.11 Accidental puncture and laceration of the spleen during a procedure on the spleen 🔖

D78.12 Accidental puncture and laceration of the spleen during other procedure 🔖

● **D78.2** **Postprocedural hemorrhage of the spleen following a procedure**

    Ⓔˣ For category D78.2 CC codes: See PDX Collection 508

D78.21 Postprocedural hemorrhage of the spleen following a procedure on the spleen 🔖

D78.22 Postprocedural hemorrhage of the spleen following other procedure 🔖

● **D78.3** **Postprocedural hematoma and seroma of the spleen following a procedure**

    Ⓔˣ For category D78.3 CC codes: See PDX Collection 508

D78.31 Postprocedural hematoma of the spleen following a procedure on the spleen 🔖

D78.32 Postprocedural hematoma of the spleen following other procedure 🔖

D78.33 Postprocedural seroma of the spleen following a procedure on the spleen 🔖

D78.34 Postprocedural seroma of the spleen following other procedure 🔖

● **D78.8** **Other intraoperative and postprocedural complications of the spleen**

    Use additional code, if applicable, to further specify disorder

    Ⓔˣ For category D78.8 CC codes: See PDX Collection 510

D78.81 Other intraoperative complications of the spleen 🔖

D78.89 Other postprocedural complications of the spleen 🔖

▶ New   ⇛ Revised   ~~deleted~~ Deleted   Excludes 1   Excludes 2   Includes   Use additional   Code first   Code also   Key words
OGCR Official Guidelines   ● Unacceptable Principal Diagnosis   X Assign placeholder X   ● Use Additional Character(s)   ▷ Manifestation Code   Coding Clinic

CERTAIN DISORDERS INVOLVING THE IMMUNE MECHANISM (D80-D89)

Includes   defects in the complement system
immunodeficiency disorders, except human
immunodeficiency virus [HIV] disease
sarcoidosis

Excludes1   autoimmune disease (systemic) NOS (M35.9)
functional disorders of polymorphonuclear
neutrophils (D71)
human immunodeficiency virus [HIV] disease
(B20)

● **D80   Immunodeficiency with predominantly antibody defects**
(Ex) For category D80 CC codes unless otherwise indicated: See PDX Collection 511

D80.0   Hereditary hypogammaglobulinemia 🔾
Autosomal recessive agammaglobulinemia (Swiss type)
X-linked agammaglobulinemia [Bruton] (with growth
hormone deficiency)

D80.1   Nonfamilial hypogammaglobulinemia 🔾
Abnormally low levels of all classes of immunoglobulins
Agammaglobulinemia with immunoglobulin-bearing
B-lymphocytes
Common variable agammaglobulinemia [CVAgamma]
Hypogammaglobulinemia NOS
(Ex) See PDX Collection 512

D80.2   Selective deficiency of immunoglobulin A [IgA] 🔾
(Ex) See PDX Collection 512

D80.3   Selective deficiency of immunoglobulin G [IgG] subclasses 🔾

D80.4   Selective deficiency of immunoglobulin M [IgM] 🔾

D80.5   Immunodeficiency with increased immunoglobulin M [IgM] 🔾

D80.6   Antibody deficiency with near-normal immunoglobulins or with hyperimmunoglobulinemia 🔾
Abnormally high levels of immunoglobulins in serum

D80.7   Transient hypogammaglobulinemia of infancy 🔾

D80.8   Other immunodeficiencies with predominantly antibody defects 🔾
Kappa light chain deficiency

D80.9   Immunodeficiency with predominantly antibody defects, unspecified 🔾

● **D81   Combined immunodeficiencies**
Excludes1   autosomal recessive agammaglobulinemia (Swiss type) (D80.0)
(Ex) For category D81 CC codes unless otherwise indicated: See PDX Collection 511

D81.0   Severe combined immunodeficiency [SCID] with reticular dysgenesis 🔾

D81.1   Severe combined immunodeficiency [SCID] with low T- and B-cell numbers 🔾

D81.2   Severe combined immunodeficiency [SCID] with low or normal B-cell numbers 🔾

D81.3   Adenosine deaminase [ADA] deficiency 🔾
(Ex) See PDX Collection 513

D81.4   Nezelof's syndrome 🔾

D81.5   Purine nucleoside phosphorylase [PNP] deficiency 🔾
(Ex) See PDX Collection 513

D81.6   Major histocompatibility complex class I deficiency 🔾
Bare lymphocyte syndrome

D81.7   Major histocompatibility complex class II deficiency 🔾

● **D81.8   Other combined immunodeficiencies**

● **D81.81   Biotin-dependent carboxylase deficiency**
Multiple carboxylase deficiency

Excludes1   biotin-dependent carboxylase
deficiency due to dietary
deficiency of biotin (E53.8)

D81.810   Biotinidase deficiency

D81.818   Other biotin-dependent carboxylase deficiency
Holocarboxylase synthetase
deficiency
Other multiple carboxylase
deficiency

D81.819   Biotin-dependent carboxylase deficiency, unspecified
Multiple carboxylase deficiency,
unspecified

D81.89   Other combined immunodeficiencies 🔾

D81.9   Combined immunodeficiency, unspecified 🔾
Severe combined immunodeficiency disorder [SCID]
NOS

● **D82   Immunodeficiency associated with other major defects**
Excludes1   ataxia telangiectasia [Louis-Bar] (G11.3)

D82.0   Wiskott-Aldrich syndrome 🔾
X-linked immunodeficiency
Immunodeficiency with thrombocytopenia and eczema
(Ex) See PDX Collection 511

D82.1   Di George's syndrome 🔾
*Congenital disorder with defective development of third and
fourth pharyngeal pouches*
Pharyngeal pouch syndrome
Thymic alymphoplasia
Thymic aplasia or hypoplasia with immunodeficiency
(Ex) See PDX Collection 511

D82.2   Immunodeficiency with short-limbed stature

D82.3   Immunodeficiency following hereditary defective response to Epstein-Barr virus
X-linked lymphoproliferative disease

D82.4   Hyperimmunoglobulin E [IgE] syndrome
*Suspected genetic defect that produces high levels of antibody
immunoglobulin (IgE) that causes skin and lung
infections and eczema*

D82.8   Immunodeficiency associated with other specified major defects

D82.9   Immunodeficiency associated with major defect, unspecified

● **D83   Common variable immunodeficiency**
(Ex) For category D83 CC codes: See PDX Collection 511

D83.0   Common variable immunodeficiency with predominant abnormalities of B-cell numbers and function 🔾

D83.1   Common variable immunodeficiency with predominant immunoregulatory T-cell disorders 🔾

D83.2   Common variable immunodeficiency with autoantibodies to B- or T-cells 🔾

D83.8   Other common variable immunodeficiencies 🔾

D83.9   Common variable immunodeficiency, unspecified 🔾

CHAPTER 3 (D50-D89)

Item 3-1 Sarcoidosis: A symptom of an inflammation producing tiny lumps of cells (granulomas) in various organs, most commonly the lungs and lymph nodes, that affect organ function. Cause is unknown occurring primarily in 20- to 40-year-olds, African-American, especially women, and those of Asian, German, Irish, Scandinavian, and Puerto Rican heritage.

● **D84   Other immunodeficiencies**

D84.0   Lymphocyte function antigen-1 [LFA-1] defect

D84.1   Defects in the complement system
C1 esterase inhibitor [C1-INH] deficiency

D84.8   Other specified immunodeficiencies 🔖
(Ex:) See PDX Collection 511

D84.9   Immunodeficiency, unspecified 🔖
(Ex:) See PDX Collection 511

● **D86   Sarcoidosis**

D86.0   Sarcoidosis of lung

D86.1   Sarcoidosis of lymph nodes

D86.2   Sarcoidosis of lung with sarcoidosis of lymph nodes

D86.3   Sarcoidosis of skin

● **D86.8   Sarcoidosis of other sites**

D86.81   Sarcoid meningitis

D86.82   Multiple cranial nerve palsies in sarcoidosis

D86.83   Sarcoid iridocyclitis
Rare large tumor with irregular surface of iris

D86.84   Sarcoid pyelonephritis
Systemic disease of unknown etiology characterized by chronic granulomatous inflammation with tissue destruction of pelvis kidney
Tubulo-interstitial nephropathy in sarcoidosis

D86.85   Sarcoid myocarditis

D86.86   Sarcoid arthropathy
Polyarthritis in sarcoidosis

D86.87   Sarcoid myositis
Granumloma of muscle

D86.89   Sarcoidosis of other sites
Hepatic granuloma
Uveoparotid fever [Heerfordt]

D86.9   Sarcoidosis, unspecified

● **D89   Other disorders involving the immune mechanism, not elsewhere classified**

Excludes1   hyperglobulinemia NOS (R77.1)
monoclonal gammopathy (of undetermined significance) (D47.2)

Excludes2   transplant failure and rejection (T86.-)

D89.0   Polyclonal hypergammaglobulinemia
Benign hypergammaglobulinemic purpura
Polyclonal gammopathy NOS

D89.1   Cryoglobulinemia
Cryoglobulin (proteins) in blood that precipitate temperatures below 98.6° F; usually symptomatic of underlying disease
Cryoglobulinemic purpura
Cryoglobulinemic vasculitis
Essential cryoglobulinemia
Idiopathic cryoglobulinemia
Mixed cryoglobulinemia
Primary cryoglobulinemia
Secondary cryoglobulinemia

D89.2   Hypergammaglobulinemia, unspecified

D89.3   Immune reconstitution syndrome
Immune reconstitution inflammatory syndrome [IRIS]
Use additional code for adverse effect, if applicable, to identify drug (T36-T50 with fifth or sixth character 5)

● **D89.4   Mast cell activation syndrome and related disorders**

➡ **Excludes1**   aggressive systemic mastocytosis (C96.21)
➡ congenital cutaneous mastocytosis (Q82.2)
~~indolent systemic mastocytosis (D47.0)~~
~~malignant mastocytoma (C96.2)~~
▶ (non-congenital) cutaneous mastocytosis (D47.01)
▶ (indolent) systemic mastocytosis (D47.02)
▶ malignant mast cell neoplasm (C96.2-)
▶ malignant mastocytoma (C96.29)
mast cell leukemia (C94.3-)
~~mastocytoma (D47.0)~~
~~systemic mastocytosis associated with a clonal hematologic non-mast cell lineage disease (SM-AHNMD) (D47.0)~~
▶ mast cell sarcoma (C96.22)
▶ mastocytoma NOS (D47.09)
▶ other mast cell neoplasms of uncertain behavior (D47.09)
▶ systemic mastocytosis associated with a clonal hematologic non-mast cell lineage disease (SM-AHNMD) (D47.02)

Coding Clinic: 2016, Q4, P11

D89.40   Mast cell activation, unspecified
Mast cell activation disorder, unspecified
Mast cell activation syndrome, NOS

D89.41   Monoclonal mast cell activation syndrome
Coding Clinic: 2016, Q4, P11

D89.42   Idiopathic mast cell activation syndrome
Coding Clinic: 2016, Q4, P11

D89.43   Secondary mast cell activation
Secondary mast cell activation syndrome
Code also underlying etiology, if known
Coding Clinic: 2016, Q4, P11

D89.49   Other mast cell activation disorder
Other mast cell activation syndrome
Coding Clinic: 2016, Q4, P11

● **D89.8   Other specified disorders involving the immune mechanism, not elsewhere classified**

● **D89.81   Graft-versus-host disease**
Code first underlying cause, such as:
complications of transplanted organs and tissue (T86.-)
complications of blood transfusion (T80.89)
Use additional code to identify associated manifestations, such as:
desquamative dermatitis (L30.8)
diarrhea (R19.7)
elevated bilirubin (R17)
hair loss (L65.9)
(Ex:) For category D89.81 CC codes: See PDX Collection 514

● **D89.810   Acute graft-versus-host disease** 🔖

● **D89.811   Chronic graft-versus-host disease** 🔖

● **D89.812   Acute on chronic graft-versus-host disease** 🔖

● **D89.813   Graft-versus-host disease, unspecified** 🔖

D89.82   Autoimmune lymphoproliferative syndrome [ALPS]

D89.89   Other specified disorders involving the immune mechanism, not elsewhere classified
Excludes1   human immunodeficiency virus disease (B20)

D89.9   Disorder involving the immune mechanism, unspecified
Immune disease NOS
Coding Clinic: 2015, Q3, P22

▶ New   ⇒ Revised   ~~deleted~~ Deleted   Excludes 1   Excludes 2   Includes   Use additional   Code first   Code also   Key words

OGCR Official Guidelines   ● Unacceptable Principal Diagnosis   X Assign placeholder X   ● Use Additional Character(s)   ▶ Manifestation Code   **Coding Clinic**

CHAPTER 4

ENDOCRINE, NUTRITIONAL AND METABOLIC DISEASES (E00-E89)

OGCR Chapter-Specific Coding Guidelines

4. **Chapter 4: Endocrine, Nutritional, and Metabolic Diseases (E00-E89)**

a. **Diabetes mellitus**

The diabetes mellitus codes are combination codes that include the type of diabetes mellitus, the body system affected, and the complications affecting that body system. As many codes within a particular category as are necessary to describe all of the complications of the disease may be used. They should be sequenced based on the reason for a particular encounter. Assign as many codes from categories E08 – E13 as needed to identify all of the associated conditions that the patient has.

1) **Type of diabetes**

The age of a patient is not the sole determining factor, though most type 1 diabetics develop the condition before reaching puberty. For this reason type 1 diabetes mellitus is also referred to as juvenile diabetes.

2) **Type of diabetes mellitus not documented**

If the type of diabetes mellitus is not documented in the medical record the default is E11.-, Type 2 diabetes mellitus.

3) **Diabetes mellitus and the use of insulin oral hypoglycemics**

If the documentation in a medical record does not indicate the type of diabetes but does indicate that the patient uses insulin, code E11, Type 2 diabetes mellitus, should be assigned. **An additional code should be assigned from category Z79 to identify the long-term (current) use of insulin or oral hypoglycemic drugs. If the patient is treated with both oral medications and insulin, only the code for long-term (current) use of insulin should be assigned. Code Z79.4 should not be assigned if insulin is given temporarily to bring a type 2 patient's blood sugar under control during an encounter.**

4) **Diabetes mellitus in pregnancy and gestational diabetes**

See Section I.C.15. Diabetes mellitus in pregnancy.
See Section I.C.15. Gestational (pregnancy induced) diabetes

5) **Complications due to insulin pump malfunction**

(a) **Underdose of insulin due to insulin pump failure**

An underdose of insulin due to an insulin pump failure should be assigned to a code from subcategory T85.6, Mechanical complication of other specified internal and external prosthetic devices, implants and grafts, that specifies the type of pump malfunction, as the principal or first-listed code, followed by code T38.3X6-, Underdosing of insulin and oral hypoglycemic

[antidiabetic] drugs. Additional codes for the type of diabetes mellitus and any associated complications due to the underdosing should also be assigned.

(b) **Overdose of insulin due to insulin pump failure**

The principal or first-listed code for an encounter due to an insulin pump malfunction resulting in an overdose of insulin, should also be T85.6-, Mechanical complication of other specified internal and external prosthetic devices, implants and grafts, followed by code T38.3X1-, Poisoning by insulin and oral hypoglycemic [antidiabetic] drugs, accidental (unintentional).

6) **Secondary diabetes mellitus**

Codes under categories E08, Diabetes mellitus due to underlying condition, E09, Drug or chemical induced diabetes mellitus and E13, Other specified diabetes mellitus, identify complications/ manifestations associated with secondary diabetes mellitus. Secondary diabetes is always caused by another condition or event (e.g., cystic fibrosis, malignant neoplasm of pancreas, pancreatectomy, adverse effect of drug, or poisoning).

(a) **Secondary diabetes mellitus and the use of insulin or hypoglycemic drugs**

For patients with secondary diabetes mellitus who routinely use insulin or oral hypoglycemic drugs, an additional code from category Z79 should be assigned to identify the long-term (current) use of insulin or oral hypoglycemic drugs. If the patient is treated with both oral medications and insulin, only the code for long-term (current) use of insulin should be assigned. Code Z79.4 should not be assigned if insulin is given temporarily to bring a type 2 patient's blood sugar under control during an encounter.

(b) **Assigning and sequencing secondary diabetes codes and its causes**

The sequencing of the secondary diabetes codes in relationship to codes for the cause of the diabetes is based on the Tabular List instructions for categories E08, E09 and E13.

(i) **Secondary diabetes mellitus due to pancreatectomy** For postpancreatectomy diabetes mellitus (lack of insulin due to the surgical removal of all or part of the pancreas), assign code E89.1, Postprocedural hypoinsulinemia. Assign a code from category E13 and a code from subcategory Z90.41-, Acquired absence of pancreas, as additional codes.

(ii) **Secondary diabetes due to drugs** Secondary diabetes may be caused by an adverse effect of correctly administered medications, poisoning or sequela of poisoning.

See section I.C.19.e for coding of adverse effects and poisoning, and section I.C.20 for external cause code reporting.

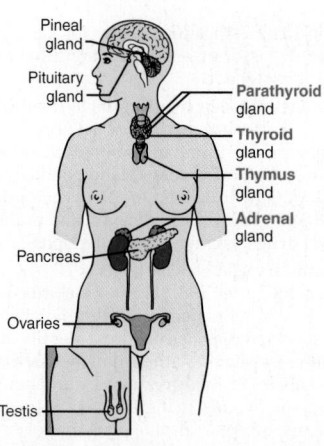

Figure 4-1 The endocrine system. (From Buck CJ: Step-by-Step Medical Coding, ed 2016, St. Louis, Elsevier, 2016)

CHAPTER 4

ENDOCRINE, NUTRITIONAL AND METABOLIC DISEASES (E00-E89)

All neoplasms, whether functionally active or not, are classified in Chapter 2. Appropriate codes in this chapter (i.e., E05.8, E07.0, E16-E31, E34.-) may be used as additional codes to indicate either functional activity by neoplasms and ectopic endocrine tissue or hyperfunction and hypofunction of endocrine glands associated with neoplasms and other conditions classified elsewhere.

Excludes1 transitory endocrine and metabolic disorders specific to newborn (P70-P74)

This chapter contains the following blocks:

E00-E07	Disorders of thyroid gland
E08-E13	Diabetes mellitus
E15-E16	Other disorders of glucose regulation and pancreatic internal secretion
E20-E35	Disorders of other endocrine glands
E36	Intraoperative complications of endocrine system
E40-E46	Malnutrition
E50-E64	Other nutritional deficiencies
E65-E68	Overweight, obesity and other hyperalimentation
E70-E88	Metabolic disorders
E89	Postprocedural endocrine and metabolic complications and disorders, not elsewhere classified

DISORDERS OF THYROID GLAND (E00-E07)

● **E00** **Congenital iodine-deficiency syndrome**

Use additional code (F70-F79) to identify associated intellectual disabilities.

Excludes1 subclinical iodine-deficiency hypothyroidism (E02)

E00.0 **Congenital iodine-deficiency syndrome, neurological type**
Endemic cretinism, neurological type

E00.1 **Congenital iodine-deficiency syndrome, myxedematous type**
Dry, waxy type of swelling (nonpitting edema) with abnormal deposits of mucin in skin (mucinosis) and other tissues
Endemic hypothyroid cretinism
Endemic cretinism, myxedematous type

E00.2 **Congenital iodine-deficiency syndrome, mixed type**
Endemic cretinism, mixed type

E00.9 **Congenital iodine-deficiency syndrome, unspecified**
Congenital iodine-deficiency hypothyroidism NOS
Endemic cretinism NOS

Figure 4-2 Goiter is an enlargement of the thyroid gland.

Item 4–1 Simple goiter indicates no nodules are present. The most common type of goiter is a **diffuse colloidal,** also called a **nontoxic** or **endemic** goiter.

● **E01** **Iodine-deficiency related thyroid disorders and allied conditions**

Excludes1 congenital iodine-deficiency syndrome (E00.-)
subclinical iodine-deficiency hypothyroidism (E02)

E01.0 **Iodine-deficiency related diffuse (endemic) goiter**
Thyroid gland is enlarged

E01.1 **Iodine-deficiency related multinodular (endemic) goiter**
Iodine-deficiency related nodular goiter

E01.2 **Iodine-deficiency related (endemic) goiter, unspecified**
Endemic goiter NOS

E01.8 **Other iodine-deficiency related thyroid disorders and allied conditions**
Acquired iodine-deficiency hypothyroidism NOS

E02 **Subclinical iodine-deficiency hypothyroidism**

● **E03** **Other hypothyroidism**

Excludes1 iodine-deficiency related hypothyroidism (E00-E02)
postprocedural hypothyroidism (E89.0)

E03.0 **Congenital hypothyroidism with diffuse goiter**
Congenital parenchymatous goiter (nontoxic)
Congenital goiter (nontoxic) NOS

Excludes1 transitory congenital goiter with normal function (P72.0)

E03.1 **Congenital hypothyroidism without goiter**
Aplasia of thyroid (with myxedema)
Congenital atrophy of thyroid
Congenital hypothyroidism NOS

E03.2 **Hypothyroidism due to medicaments and other exogenous substances**
Code first poisoning due to drug or toxin, if applicable (T36-T65 with fifth or sixth character 1-4 or 6)

Use additional code for adverse effect, if applicable, to identify drug (T36-T50 with fifth or sixth character 5)

E03.3 **Postinfectious hypothyroidism**

E03.4 **Atrophy of thyroid (acquired)**

Excludes1 congenital atrophy of thyroid (E03.1)

E03.5 **Myxedema coma** 🔖
Often fatal complication of long-term hypothyroidism
Ⓔⓧ See PDX Collection 515

E03.8 **Other specified hypothyroidism**

E03.9 **Hypothyroidism, unspecified**
Myxedema NOS

Item 4–2 Hypothyroidism is a condition in which there are insufficient levels of thyroxine. **Cretinism** is congenital hypothyroidism, which can result in mental and physical retardation.

- **E04   Other nontoxic goiter**
  > **Excludes1**   congenital goiter (NOS) (diffuse) (parenchymatous) (E03.0)
  > iodine-deficiency related goiter (E00-E02)

  - **E04.0   Nontoxic diffuse goiter**
    Thyroid gland is enlarged
    Diffuse (colloid) nontoxic goiter
    Simple nontoxic goiter

  - **E04.1   Nontoxic single thyroid nodule**
    Colloid nodule (cystic) (thyroid)
    Nontoxic uninodular goiter
    Thyroid (cystic) nodule NOS

  - **E04.2   Nontoxic multinodular goiter**
    Enlarged thyroid gland with multiple nodules
    Cystic goiter NOS
    Multinodular (cystic) goiter NOS

  - **E04.8   Other specified nontoxic goiter**

  - **E04.9   Nontoxic goiter, unspecified**
    Goiter NOS
    Nodular goiter (nontoxic) NOS

- **E05   Thyrotoxicosis [hyperthyroidism]**
  Enlarged thyroid gland with multiple nodules
  > **Excludes1**   chronic thyroiditis with transient thyrotoxicosis (E06.2)
  > neonatal thyrotoxicosis (P72.1)
  > (Ex) **For category E05 CC codes:** See PDX Collection 516

  - **E05.0   Thyrotoxicosis with diffuse goiter**
    Exophthalmic or toxic goiter NOS
    Graves' disease
    Toxic diffuse goiter

    - **E05.00   Thyrotoxicosis with diffuse goiter without thyrotoxic crisis or storm**
    - **E05.01   Thyrotoxicosis with diffuse goiter with thyrotoxic crisis or storm** 🔖

  - **E05.1   Thyrotoxicosis with toxic single thyroid nodule**
    Thyrotoxicosis with toxic uninodular goiter

    - **E05.10   Thyrotoxicosis with toxic single thyroid nodule without thyrotoxic crisis or storm**
    - **E05.11   Thyrotoxicosis with toxic single thyroid nodule with thyrotoxic crisis or storm** 🔖

  - **E05.2   Thyrotoxicosis with toxic multinodular goiter**
    Toxic nodular goiter NOS

    - **E05.20   Thyrotoxicosis with toxic multinodular goiter without thyrotoxic crisis or storm**
    - **E05.21   Thyrotoxicosis with toxic multinodular goiter with thyrotoxic crisis or storm** 🔖

  - **E05.3   Thyrotoxicosis from ectopic thyroid tissue**
    - **E05.30   Thyrotoxicosis from ectopic thyroid tissue without thyrotoxic crisis or storm**
    - **E05.31   Thyrotoxicosis from ectopic thyroid tissue with thyrotoxic crisis or storm** 🔖

- **E05.4   Thyrotoxicosis factitia**
  - **E05.40   Thyrotoxicosis factitia without thyrotoxic crisis or storm**
  - **E05.41   Thyrotoxicosis factitia with thyrotoxic crisis or storm** 🔖

- **E05.8   Other thyrotoxicosis**
  Overproduction of thyroid-stimulating hormone
  - **E05.80   Other thyrotoxicosis without thyrotoxic crisis or storm**
  - **E05.81   Other thyrotoxicosis with thyrotoxic crisis or storm** 🔖

- **E05.9   Thyrotoxicosis, unspecified**
  Hyperthyroidism NOS
  - **E05.90   Thyrotoxicosis, unspecified without thyrotoxic crisis or storm**
  - **E05.91   Thyrotoxicosis, unspecified with thyrotoxic crisis or storm** 🔖

- **E06   Thyroiditis**
  An inflammation of the thyroid gland which results in an inability to convert iodine into thyroid hormone
  > **Excludes1**   postpartum thyroiditis (O90.5)

  - **E06.0   Acute thyroiditis** 🔖
    Abscess of thyroid
    Pyogenic thyroiditis
    Suppurative thyroiditis
    Use additional code (B95-B97) to identify infectious agent.
    (Ex) See PDX Collection 517

  - **E06.1   Subacute thyroiditis**
    Inflammation of thyroid gland following viral upper respiratory infection
    de Quervain thyroiditis
    Giant-cell thyroiditis
    Granulomatous thyroiditis
    Nonsuppurative thyroiditis
    Viral thyroiditis
    > **Excludes1**   autoimmune thyroiditis (E06.3)

  - **E06.2   Chronic thyroiditis with transient thyrotoxicosis**
    Chronic inflammation of thyroid gland with intermittent overproduction of thyroid hormone
    > **Excludes1**   autoimmune thyroiditis (E06.3)

  - **E06.3   Autoimmune thyroiditis**
    Hashimoto's thyroiditis
    Hashitoxicosis (transient)
    Lymphadenoid goiter
    Lymphocytic thyroiditis
    Struma lymphomatosa

  - **E06.4   Drug-induced thyroiditis**
    Use additional code for adverse effect, if applicable, to identify drug (T36-T50 with fifth or sixth character 5)

  - **E06.5   Other chronic thyroiditis**
    Chronic fibrous thyroiditis
    Chronic thyroiditis NOS
    Ligneous thyroiditis
    Riedel thyroiditis

  - **E06.9   Thyroiditis, unspecified**

Figure 4-3   Graves' disease. In Graves' disease, exophthalmos often looks more pronounced than it actually is because of the extreme lid retraction that may occur. This patient, for instance, had minimal proptosis of the left eye but marked lid retraction. (From Lissauer T, Clayden G, and Craft A: Illustrated Textbook of Paediatrics, Edinburgh, Mosby, 2015)

Item 4–3   Thyrotoxicosis is a condition caused by excessive amounts of the thyroid hormone thyroxine production or hyperthyroidism. **Graves' disease is associated with hyperthyroidism** (known as **Basedow's disease** in Europe).

CHAPTER 4 (E00-E90)

N   Newborn Age: 0   P   Pediatric Age: 0–17   M   Maternity DX: 12–55   A   Adult Age: 15–124   ♀   Females Only   ♂   Males Only

🔖 Complication\Comorbidity   🔖 Major C\C   (Ex) CC/MCC Exclusions   🔖 Hospital-Acquired Condition

● **E07 Other disorders of thyroid**

E07.0 Hypersecretion of calcitonin
C-cell hyperplasia of thyroid
Hypersecretion of thyrocalcitonin

E07.1 Dyshormogenetic goiter
Group of several types of goiter resulting from enzyme defects in hormone synthesis
Familial dyshormogenetic goiter
Pendred's syndrome

Excludes1 transitory congenital goiter with normal function (P72.0)

● **E07.8 Other specified disorders of thyroid**

E07.81 Sick-euthyroid syndrome
Euthyroid sick-syndrome

E07.89 Other specified disorders of thyroid
Abnormality of thyroid-binding globulin
Hemorrhage of thyroid
Infarction of thyroid

E07.9 Disorder of thyroid, unspecified

OGCR Section I.C.4.a.

Diabetes mellitus

The diabetes mellitus codes are combination codes that include the type of diabetes mellitus, body system affected, and the complications affecting that body system. As many codes within a particular category as are necessary to describe all of the complications of the disease may be used. They should be sequenced based on the reason for a particular visit. Assign as many codes from categories E08–E13 as needed to identify all of the associated conditions that the patient has.

DIABETES MELLITUS (E08-E13)
A metabolic disease that results in persistent hyperglycemia.
Coding Clinic: 2016, Q4, P142

● **E08 Diabetes mellitus due to underlying condition**

Code first the underlying condition, such as:
congenital rubella (P35.0)
Cushing's syndrome (E24.-)
cystic fibrosis (E84.-)
malignant neoplasm (C00-C96)
malnutrition (E40-E46)
pancreatitis and other diseases of the pancreas (K85-K86.-)

Use additional code to identify control using:
insulin (Z79.4)
oral antidiabetic drugs (Z79.84)
oral hypoglycemic drugs (Z79.84)

Excludes1 drug or chemical induced diabetes mellitus (E09.-)
gestational diabetes (O24.4-)
neonatal diabetes mellitus (P70.2)
postpancreatectomy diabetes mellitus (E13.-)
postprocedural diabetes mellitus (E13.-)
secondary diabetes mellitus NEC (E13.-)
type 1 diabetes mellitus (E10.-)
type 2 diabetes mellitus (E11.-)

● **E08.0 Diabetes mellitus due to underlying condition with hyperosmolarity**
Ⓔⓧ For category E08.0 CC codes: See PDX Collection 518

E08.00 *Diabetes mellitus due to underlying condition with hyperosmolarity without nonketotic hyperglycemic-hyperosmolar coma (NKHHC)*

E08.01 *Diabetes mellitus due to underlying condition with hyperosmolarity with coma*

● **E08.1 Diabetes mellitus due to underlying condition with ketoacidosis**
Ⓔⓧ For category E08.1 CC codes: See PDX Collection 518

E08.10 *Diabetes mellitus due to underlying condition with ketoacidosis without coma*

E08.11 *Diabetes mellitus due to underlying condition with ketoacidosis with coma*

● **E08.2 Diabetes mellitus due to underlying condition with kidney complications**

E08.21 *Diabetes mellitus due to underlying condition with diabetic nephropathy*
Diabetes mellitus due to underlying condition with intercapillary glomerulosclerosis
Diabetes mellitus due to underlying condition with intracapillary glomerulonephrosis
Diabetes mellitus due to underlying condition with Kimmelstiel-Wilson disease

E08.22 *Diabetes mellitus due to underlying condition with diabetic chronic kidney disease*
Use additional code to identify stage of chronic kidney disease (N18.1-N18.6)

E08.29 *Diabetes mellitus due to underlying condition with other diabetic kidney complication*
Renal tubular degeneration in diabetes mellitus due to underlying condition

● **E08.3 Diabetes mellitus due to underlying condition with ophthalmic complications**
Changes in blood vessels of retina in which blood vessels swell and leak fluid into retinal surface.
Coding Clinic: 2016, Q4, P11

● **E08.31 Diabetes mellitus due to underlying condition with unspecified diabetic retinopathy**

E08.311 *Diabetes mellitus due to underlying condition with unspecified diabetic retinopathy with macular edema*

E08.319 *Diabetes mellitus due to underlying condition with unspecified diabetic retinopathy without macular edema*

● **E08.32 Diabetes mellitus due to underlying condition with mild nonproliferative diabetic retinopathy**
Diabetes mellitus due to underlying condition with nonproliferative diabetic retinopathy NOS

One of the following 7th characters is to be assigned to codes in subcategory E08.32 to designate laterality of the disease:

1	right eye
2	left eye
3	bilateral
9	unspecified eye

● **E08.321** *Diabetes mellitus due to underlying condition with mild nonproliferative diabetic retinopathy with macular edema*

● **E08.329** *Diabetes mellitus due to underlying condition with mild nonproliferative diabetic retinopathy without macular edema*

● **E08.33 Diabetes mellitus due to underlying condition with moderate nonproliferative diabetic retinopathy**

One of the following 7th characters is to be assigned to codes in subcategory E08.33 to designate laterality of the disease:

1	right eye
2	left eye
3	bilateral
9	unspecified eye

● **E08.331** *Diabetes mellitus due to underlying condition with moderate nonproliferative diabetic retinopathy with macular edema*

● **E08.339** *Diabetes mellitus due to underlying condition with moderate nonproliferative diabetic retinopathy without macular edema*

▶ New   ⇒ Revised   ~~deleted~~ Deleted   Excludes 1   Excludes 2   Includes   Use additional   Code first   Code also   Key words

732   OGCR Official Guidelines   ● Unacceptable Principal Diagnosis   X Assign placeholder X   ● Use Additional Character(s)   ▶ Manifestation Code   Coding Clinic

● **E08.34** **Diabetes mellitus due to underlying condition with severe nonproliferative diabetic retinopathy**

One of the following 7th characters is to be assigned to codes in subcategory E08.34 to designate laterality of the disease:

1	right eye
2	left eye
3	bilateral
9	unspecified eye

● ▶ *E08.341*   *Diabetes mellitus due to underlying condition with severe nonproliferative diabetic retinopathy with macular edema*

● ▶ *E08.349*   *Diabetes mellitus due to underlying condition with severe nonproliferative diabetic retinopathy without macular edema*

● **E08.35** **Diabetes mellitus due to underlying condition with proliferative diabetic retinopathy**

One of the following 7th characters is to be assigned to codes in subcategory E08.35 to designate laterality of the disease:

1	right eye
2	left eye
3	bilateral
9	unspecified eye

● ▶ *E08.351*   *Diabetes mellitus due to underlying condition with proliferative diabetic retinopathy with macular edema*

● ▶ *E08.352*   *Diabetes mellitus due to underlying condition with proliferative diabetic retinopathy with traction retinal detachment involving the macula*

● ▶ *E08.353*   *Diabetes mellitus due to underlying condition with proliferative diabetic retinopathy with traction retinal detachment not involving the macula*

● ▶ *E08.354*   *Diabetes mellitus due to underlying condition with proliferative diabetic retinopathy with combined traction retinal detachment and rhegmatogenous retinal detachment*

● ▶ *E08.355*   *Diabetes mellitus due to underlying condition with stable proliferative diabetic retinopathy*

● ▶ *E08.359*   *Diabetes mellitus due to underlying condition with proliferative diabetic retinopathy without macular edema*

▶ *E08.36*   *Diabetes mellitus due to underlying condition with diabetic cataract*

X ● ▶ *E08.37*   *Diabetes mellitus due to underlying condition with diabetic macular edema, resolved following treatment*

One of the following 7th characters is to be assigned to code E08.37 to designate laterality of the disease:

1	right eye
2	left eye
3	bilateral
9	unspecified eye

▶ *E08.39*   *Diabetes mellitus due to underlying condition with other diabetic ophthalmic complication*

Use additional code to identify manifestation, such as:
diabetic glaucoma (H40-H42)

● **E08.4** **Diabetes mellitus due to underlying condition with neurological complications**

▶ *E08.40*   *Diabetes mellitus due to underlying condition with diabetic neuropathy, unspecified*

▶ *E08.41*   *Diabetes mellitus due to underlying condition with diabetic mononeuropathy*

▶ *E08.42*   *Diabetes mellitus due to underlying condition with diabetic polyneuropathy*

Diabetes mellitus due to underlying condition with diabetic neuralgia

▶ *E08.43*   *Diabetes mellitus due to underlying condition with diabetic autonomic (poly)neuropathy*

Diabetes mellitus due to underlying condition with diabetic gastroparesis

▶ *E08.44*   *Diabetes mellitus due to underlying condition with diabetic amyotrophy*

▶ *E08.49*   *Diabetes mellitus due to underlying condition with other diabetic neurological complication*

● **E08.5** **Diabetes mellitus due to underlying condition with circulatory complications**

▶ *E08.51*   *Diabetes mellitus due to underlying condition with diabetic peripheral angiopathy without gangrene*

▶ *E08.52*   *Diabetes mellitus due to underlying condition with diabetic peripheral angiopathy with gangrene* 🔖

Diabetes mellitus due to underlying condition with diabetic gangrene

CC when PDx is its own CC

Ex: See PDX Collection 519

▶ *E08.59*   *Diabetes mellitus due to underlying condition with other circulatory complications*

● **E08.6** **Diabetes mellitus due to underlying condition with other specified complications**

● **E08.61** **Diabetes mellitus due to underlying condition with diabetic arthropathy**

▶ *E08.610*   *Diabetes mellitus due to underlying condition with diabetic neuropathic arthropathy*

Diabetes mellitus due to underlying condition with Charcôt's joints

▶ *E08.618*   *Diabetes mellitus due to underlying condition with other diabetic arthropathy*

● **E08.62** **Diabetes mellitus due to underlying condition with skin complications**

▶ *E08.620*   *Diabetes mellitus due to underlying condition with diabetic dermatitis*

Diabetes mellitus due to underlying condition with diabetic necrobiosis lipoidica

▶ *E08.621*   *Diabetes mellitus due to underlying condition with foot ulcer*

Use additional code to identify site of ulcer (L97.4-, L97.5-)

▶ *E08.622*   *Diabetes mellitus due to underlying condition with other skin ulcer*

Use additional code to identify site of ulcer (L97.1-L97.9, L98.41-L98.49)

▶ *E08.628*   *Diabetes mellitus due to underlying condition with other skin complications*

● **E08.63** **Diabetes mellitus due to underlying condition with oral complications**

▶ *E08.630*   *Diabetes mellitus due to underlying condition with periodontal disease*

▶ *E08.638*   *Diabetes mellitus due to underlying condition with other oral complications*

CHAPTER 4 (E00-E90)

- **E08.64 Diabetes mellitus due to underlying condition with hypoglycemia**
  - ▸ *E08.641 Diabetes mellitus due to underlying condition with hypoglycemia with coma* 🔖
    - (Ex) See PDX Collection 518
  - ▸ *E08.649 Diabetes mellitus due to underlying condition with hypoglycemia without coma*
  - ▸ *E08.65 Diabetes mellitus due to underlying condition with hyperglycemia*
  - ▸ *E08.69 Diabetes mellitus due to underlying condition with other specified complication*
    - Use additional code to identify complication
- ▸ *E08.8 Diabetes mellitus due to underlying condition with unspecified complications*
- ▸ *E08.9 Diabetes mellitus due to underlying condition without complications*

- **E09 Drug or chemical induced diabetes mellitus**
  - *Code first poisoning due to drug or toxin, if applicable (T36-T65 with fifth or sixth character 1-4 or 6)*
  - Use additional code for adverse effect, if applicable, to identify drug (T36-T50 with fifth or sixth character 5)
  - Use additional code to identify control using:
    - insulin (Z79.4)
    - oral antidiabetic drugs (Z79.84)
    - oral hypoglycemic drugs (Z79.84)
  - **Excludes1** diabetes mellitus due to underlying condition (E08.-)
    - gestational diabetes (O24.4-)
    - neonatal diabetes mellitus (P70.2)
    - postpancreatectomy diabetes mellitus (E13.-)
    - postprocedural diabetes mellitus (E13.-)
    - secondary diabetes mellitus NEC (E13.-)
    - type 1 diabetes mellitus (E10.-)
    - type 2 diabetes mellitus (E11.-)
  - **E09.0 Drug or chemical induced diabetes mellitus with hyperosmolarity**
    - (Ex) For category E09.0 CC codes: See PDX Collection 518
    - **E09.00 Drug or chemical induced diabetes mellitus with hyperosmolarity without nonketotic hyperglycemic-hyperosmolar coma (NKHHC)** 🔖🔖
    - **E09.01 Drug or chemical induced diabetes mellitus with hyperosmolarity with coma** 🔖🔖
  - **E09.1 Drug or chemical induced diabetes mellitus with ketoacidosis**
    - (Ex) For category E09.1 CC codes: See PDX Collection 518
    - **E09.10 Drug or chemical induced diabetes mellitus with ketoacidosis without coma** 🔖🔖
    - **E09.11 Drug or chemical induced diabetes mellitus with ketoacidosis with coma** 🔖
  - **E09.2 Drug or chemical induced diabetes mellitus with kidney complications**
    - **E09.21 Drug or chemical induced diabetes mellitus with diabetic nephropathy**
      - Drug or chemical induced diabetes mellitus with intercapillary glomerulosclerosis
      - Drug or chemical induced diabetes mellitus with intracapillary glomerulonephrosis
      - Drug or chemical induced diabetes mellitus with Kimmelstiel-Wilson disease
    - **E09.22 Drug or chemical induced diabetes mellitus with diabetic chronic kidney disease**
      - Use additional code to identify stage of chronic kidney disease (N18.1-N18.6)
    - **E09.29 Drug or chemical induced diabetes mellitus with other diabetic kidney complication**
      - Drug or chemical induced diabetes mellitus with renal tubular degeneration

- **E09.3 Drug or chemical induced diabetes mellitus with ophthalmic complications**
  - Coding Clinic: 2016, Q4, P11
  - **E09.31 Drug or chemical induced diabetes mellitus with unspecified diabetic retinopathy**
    - **E09.311 Drug or chemical induced diabetes mellitus with unspecified diabetic retinopathy with macular edema**
    - **E09.319 Drug or chemical induced diabetes mellitus with unspecified diabetic retinopathy without macular edema**
  - **E09.32 Drug or chemical induced diabetes mellitus with mild nonproliferative diabetic retinopathy**
    - Drug or chemical induced diabetes mellitus with nonproliferative diabetic retinopathy NOS
    - One of the following 7th characters is to be assigned to codes in subcategory E09.32 to designate laterality of the disease:

1	right eye
2	left eye
3	bilateral
9	unspecified eye

    - **E09.321 Drug or chemical induced diabetes mellitus with mild nonproliferative diabetic retinopathy with macular edema**
    - **E09.329 Drug or chemical induced diabetes mellitus with mild nonproliferative diabetic retinopathy without macular edema**
  - **E09.33 Drug or chemical induced diabetes mellitus with moderate nonproliferative diabetic retinopathy**
    - One of the following 7th characters is to be assigned to codes in subcategory E09.33 to designate laterality of the disease:

1	right eye
2	left eye
3	bilateral
9	unspecified eye

    - **E09.331 Drug or chemical induced diabetes mellitus with moderate nonproliferative diabetic retinopathy with macular edema**
    - **E09.339 Drug or chemical induced diabetes mellitus with moderate nonproliferative diabetic retinopathy without macular edema**
  - **E09.34 Drug or chemical induced diabetes mellitus with severe nonproliferative diabetic retinopathy**
    - One of the following 7th characters is to be assigned to codes in subcategory E09.34 to designate laterality of the disease:

1	right eye
2	left eye
3	bilateral
9	unspecified eye

    - **E09.341 Drug or chemical induced diabetes mellitus with severe nonproliferative diabetic retinopathy with macular edema**
    - **E09.349 Drug or chemical induced diabetes mellitus with severe nonproliferative diabetic retinopathy without macular edema**

734

▶ New ⇒ Revised ~~deleted~~ Deleted | Excludes 1 | Excludes 2 | Includes | Use additional | Code first | Code also | Key words

OGCR Official Guidelines ● Unacceptable Principal Diagnosis X Assign placeholder X ● Use Additional Character(s) ▸ Manifestation Code **Coding Clinic**

● **E09.35**   **Drug or chemical induced diabetes mellitus with proliferative diabetic retinopathy**

> One of the following 7th characters is to be assigned to codes in subcategory E09.35 to designate laterality of the disease:

1	right eye
2	left eye
3	bilateral
9	unspecified eye

  ● **E09.351**   Drug or chemical induced diabetes mellitus with proliferative diabetic retinopathy with macular edema

  ● **E09.352**   Drug or chemical induced diabetes mellitus with proliferative diabetic retinopathy with traction retinal detachment involving the macula

  ● **E09.353**   Drug or chemical induced diabetes mellitus with proliferative diabetic retinopathy with traction retinal detachment not involving the macula

  ● **E09.354**   Drug or chemical induced diabetes mellitus with proliferative diabetic retinopathy with combined traction retinal detachment and rhegmatogenous retinal detachment

  ● **E09.355**   Drug or chemical induced diabetes mellitus with stable proliferative diabetic retinopathy

  ● **E09.359**   Drug or chemical induced diabetes mellitus with proliferative diabetic retinopathy without macular edema

E09.36   Drug or chemical induced diabetes mellitus with diabetic cataract

X ● **E09.37**   Drug or chemical induced diabetes mellitus with diabetic macular edema, resolved following treatment

> One of the following 7th characters is to be assigned to code E09.37 to designate laterality of the disease:

1	right eye
2	left eye
3	bilateral
9	unspecified eye

E09.39   Drug or chemical induced diabetes mellitus with other diabetic ophthalmic complication

> Use additional code to identify manifestation, such as:
> diabetic glaucoma (H40-H42)

● **E09.4**   **Drug or chemical induced diabetes mellitus with neurological complications**

E09.40   Drug or chemical induced diabetes mellitus with neurological complications with diabetic neuropathy, unspecified

E09.41   Drug or chemical induced diabetes mellitus with neurological complications with diabetic mononeuropathy

E09.42   Drug or chemical induced diabetes mellitus with neurological complications with diabetic polyneuropathy
> Drug or chemical induced diabetes mellitus with diabetic neuralgia

E09.43   Drug or chemical induced diabetes mellitus with neurological complications with diabetic autonomic (poly)neuropathy
> Drug or chemical induced diabetes mellitus with diabetic gastroparesis

E09.44   Drug or chemical induced diabetes mellitus with neurological complications with diabetic amyotrophy

E09.49   Drug or chemical induced diabetes mellitus with neurological complications with other diabetic neurological complication

● **E09.5**   **Drug or chemical induced diabetes mellitus with circulatory complications**

E09.51   Drug or chemical induced diabetes mellitus with diabetic peripheral angiopathy without gangrene

E09.52   Drug or chemical induced diabetes mellitus with diabetic peripheral angiopathy with gangrene 🔖
> Drug or chemical induced diabetes mellitus with diabetic gangrene
> CC when PDx is its own CC
> (Ex) See PDX Collection 519

E09.59   Drug or chemical induced diabetes mellitus with other circulatory complications

● **E09.6**   **Drug or chemical induced diabetes mellitus with other specified complications**

  ● **E09.61**   Drug or chemical induced diabetes mellitus with diabetic arthropathy

    E09.610   Drug or chemical induced diabetes mellitus with diabetic neuropathic arthropathy
> Drug or chemical induced diabetes mellitus with Charcôt's joints
> *Progressive degeneration of weight-bearing joint*

    E09.618   Drug or chemical induced diabetes mellitus with other diabetic arthropathy

  ● **E09.62**   Drug or chemical induced diabetes mellitus with skin complications

    E09.620   Drug or chemical induced diabetes mellitus with diabetic dermatitis
> Drug or chemical induced diabetes mellitus with diabetic necrobiosis lipoidica
> *Necrotizing skin condition*

    E09.621   Drug or chemical induced diabetes mellitus with foot ulcer
> Use additional code to identify site of ulcer (L97.4-, L97.5-)

    E09.622   Drug or chemical induced diabetes mellitus with other skin ulcer
> Use additional code to identify site of ulcer (L97.1-L97.9, L98.41-L98.49)

    E09.628   Drug or chemical induced diabetes mellitus with other skin complications

  ● **E09.63**   Drug or chemical induced diabetes mellitus with oral complications

    E09.630   Drug or chemical induced diabetes mellitus with periodontal disease

    E09.638   Drug or chemical induced diabetes mellitus with other oral complications

  ● **E09.64**   Drug or chemical induced diabetes mellitus with hypoglycemia

    E09.641   Drug or chemical induced diabetes mellitus with hypoglycemia with coma 🔖
> (Ex) See PDX Collection 518

    E09.649   Drug or chemical induced diabetes mellitus with hypoglycemia without coma

    E09.65   Drug or chemical induced diabetes mellitus with hyperglycemia

    E09.69   Drug or chemical induced diabetes mellitus with other specified complication
> Use additional code to identify complication

E09.8   Drug or chemical induced diabetes mellitus with unspecified complications

E09.9   Drug or chemical induced diabetes mellitus without complications

● E10   Type 1 diabetes mellitus

Includes   brittle diabetes (mellitus)
diabetes (mellitus) due to autoimmune process
diabetes (mellitus) due to immune mediated
    pancreatic islet beta-cell destruction
idiopathic diabetes (mellitus)
juvenile onset diabetes (mellitus)
ketosis-prone diabetes (mellitus)

Excludes 1   diabetes mellitus due to underlying condition
    (E08.-)
drug or chemical induced diabetes mellitus (E09.-)
gestational diabetes (O24.4-)
hyperglycemia NOS (R73.9)
neonatal diabetes mellitus (P70.2)
postpancreatectomy diabetes mellitus (E13.-)
postprocedural diabetes mellitus (E13.-)
secondary diabetes mellitus NEC (E13.-)
type 2 diabetes mellitus (E11.-)

● E10.1   Type 1 diabetes mellitus with ketoacidosis
*Acidosis accompanied by accumulation of ketone bodies
(ketosis) in body tissues and fluids*
Ⓔⓧ **For category E.10.1 CC codes: See PDX Collection 520**

    **E10.10   Type 1 diabetes mellitus with ketoacidosis
without coma** 🔖 🔖
Coding Clinic: 2013, Q3, P20

    **E10.11   Type 1 diabetes mellitus with ketoacidosis with
coma** 🔖

● E10.2   Type 1 diabetes mellitus with kidney complications
    **E10.21   Type 1 diabetes mellitus with diabetic
nephropathy**
Type 1 diabetes mellitus with intercapillary
    glomerulosclerosis
Type 1 diabetes mellitus with intracapillary
    glomerulonephrosis
Type 1 diabetes mellitus with Kimmelstiel-
    Wilson disease

    **E10.22   Type 1 diabetes mellitus with diabetic chronic
kidney disease**
Use additional code to identify stage of chronic
    kidney disease (N18.1-N18.6)

    **E10.29   Type 1 diabetes mellitus with other diabetic
kidney complication**
Type 1 diabetes mellitus with renal tubular
    degeneration
Coding Clinic: 2016, Q1, P13

● E10.3   Type 1 diabetes mellitus with ophthalmic complications
Coding Clinic: 2016, Q4, P11

    **● E10.31   Type 1 diabetes mellitus with unspecified
diabetic retinopathy**
        **E10.311   Type 1 diabetes mellitus
with unspecified diabetic retinopathy
with macular edema**

        **E10.319   Type 1 diabetes mellitus
with unspecified diabetic retinopathy
without macular edema**

    **● E10.32   Type 1 diabetes mellitus with mild
nonproliferative diabetic retinopathy**
Type 1 diabetes mellitus with nonproliferative
    diabetic retinopathy NOS

One of the following 7th characters is to be
assigned to codes in subcategory E10.32 to
designate laterality of the disease:

1	right eye
2	left eye
3	bilateral
9	unspecified eye

        **● E10.321   Type 1 diabetes mellitus with mild
nonproliferative diabetic retinopathy
with macular edema**

        **● E10.329   Type 1 diabetes mellitus with mild
nonproliferative diabetic retinopathy
without macular edema**

**● E10.33   Type 1 diabetes mellitus with moderate
nonproliferative diabetic retinopathy**
One of the following 7th characters is to be
assigned to codes in subcategory E10.33 to
designate laterality of the disease:

1	right eye
2	left eye
3	bilateral
9	unspecified eye

    **● E10.331   Type 1 diabetes mellitus with
moderate nonproliferative diabetic
retinopathy with macular edema**

    **● E10.339   Type 1 diabetes mellitus with
moderate nonproliferative diabetic
retinopathy without macular edema**

**● E10.34   Type 1 diabetes mellitus with severe
nonproliferative diabetic retinopathy**
One of the following 7th characters is to be
assigned to codes in subcategory E10.34 to
designate laterality of the disease:

1	right eye
2	left eye
3	bilateral
9	unspecified eye

    **● E10.341   Type 1 diabetes mellitus with severe
nonproliferative diabetic retinopathy
with macular edema**

    **● E10.349   Type 1 diabetes mellitus with severe
nonproliferative diabetic retinopathy
without macular edema**

**● E10.35   Type 1 diabetes mellitus with proliferative
diabetic retinopathy**
One of the following 7th characters is to be
assigned to codes in subcategory E10.35 to
designate laterality of the disease:

1	right eye
2	left eye
3	bilateral
9	unspecified eye

    **● E10.351   Type 1 diabetes mellitus with
proliferative diabetic retinopathy
with macular edema**

    **● E10.352   Type 1 diabetes mellitus with
proliferative diabetic retinopathy
with traction retinal detachment
involving the macula**

    **● E10.353   Type 1 diabetes mellitus with
proliferative diabetic retinopathy
with traction retinal detachment not
involving the macula**

    **● E10.354   Type 1 diabetes mellitus with
proliferative diabetic retinopathy
with combined traction retinal
detachment and rhegmatogenous
retinal detachment**

    **● E10.355   Type 1 diabetes mellitus with stable
proliferative diabetic retinopathy**

    **● E10.359   Type 1 diabetes mellitus with
proliferative diabetic retinopathy
without macular edema**

    E10.36   Type 1 diabetes mellitus with diabetic cataract

X ● **E10.37** **Type 1 diabetes mellitus with diabetic macular edema, resolved following treatment**

> One of the following 7th characters is to be assigned to code E10.37 to designate laterality of the disease:

> | | |
> |---|---|
> | 1 | right eye |
> | 2 | left eye |
> | 3 | bilateral |
> | 9 | unspecified eye |

E10.39 **Type 1 diabetes mellitus with other diabetic ophthalmic complication**

> Use additional code to identify manifestation, such as:
> diabetic glaucoma (H40-H42)

● **E10.4** **Type 1 diabetes mellitus with neurological complications**

E10.40 **Type 1 diabetes mellitus with diabetic neuropathy, unspecified**

E10.41 **Type 1 diabetes mellitus with diabetic mononeuropathy**

E10.42 **Type 1 diabetes mellitus with diabetic polyneuropathy**

> Type 1 diabetes mellitus with diabetic neuralgia

E10.43 **Type 1 diabetes mellitus with diabetic autonomic (poly)neuropathy**

> Type 1 diabetes mellitus with diabetic gastroparesis

E10.44 **Type 1 diabetes mellitus with diabetic amyotrophy**

E10.49 **Type 1 diabetes mellitus with other diabetic neurological complication**

● **E10.5** **Type 1 diabetes mellitus with circulatory complications**

E10.51 **Type 1 diabetes mellitus with diabetic peripheral angiopathy without gangrene**

E10.52 **Type 1 diabetes mellitus with diabetic peripheral angiopathy with gangrene**

> Type 1 diabetes mellitus with diabetic gangrene 🔖
> CC when PDx is its own CC
> (Ex:) See PDX Collection 519

E10.59 **Type 1 diabetes mellitus with other circulatory complications**

● **E10.6** **Type 1 diabetes mellitus with other specified complications**

● **E10.61** **Type 1 diabetes mellitus with diabetic arthropathy**

E10.610 **Type 1 diabetes mellitus with diabetic neuropathic arthropathy**

> Type 1 diabetes mellitus with Charcôt's joints

E10.618 **Type 1 diabetes mellitus with other diabetic arthropathy**

● **E10.62** **Type 1 diabetes mellitus with skin complications**

E10.620 **Type 1 diabetes mellitus with diabetic dermatitis**

> Type 1 diabetes mellitus with diabetic necrobiosis lipoidica

E10.621 **Type 1 diabetes mellitus with foot ulcer**

> Use additional code to identify site of ulcer (L97.4-, L97.5-)

E10.622 **Type 1 diabetes mellitus with other skin ulcer**

> Use additional code to identify site of ulcer (L97.1-L97.9, L98.41-L98.49)

E10.628 **Type 1 diabetes mellitus with other skin complications**

● **E10.63** **Type 1 diabetes mellitus with oral complications**

E10.630 **Type 1 diabetes mellitus with periodontal disease**

E10.638 **Type 1 diabetes mellitus with other oral complications**

● **E10.64** **Type 1 diabetes mellitus with hypoglycemia**

E10.641 **Type 1 diabetes mellitus with hypoglycemia with coma** 🔖
> (Ex:) See PDX Collection 520

E10.649 **Type 1 diabetes mellitus with hypoglycemia without coma**
> Coding Clinic: 2016, Q1, P13

E10.65 **Type 1 diabetes mellitus with hyperglycemia**
> Coding Clinic: 2013, Q3, P20

E10.69 **Type 1 diabetes mellitus with other specified complication**

> Use additional code to identify complication

E10.8 **Type 1 diabetes mellitus with unspecified complications**

E10.9 **Type 1 diabetes mellitus without complications**

● **E11** **Type 2 diabetes mellitus**

Includes diabetes (mellitus) due to insulin secretory defect
diabetes NOS
insulin resistant diabetes (mellitus)

Use additional code to identify control using:
insulin (Z79.4)
oral antidiabetic drugs (Z79.84)
oral hypoglycemic drugs (Z79.84)

Excludes1 diabetes mellitus due to underlying condition (E08.-)
drug or chemical induced diabetes mellitus (E09.-)
gestational diabetes (O24.4-)
neonatal diabetes mellitus (P70.2)
postpancreatectomy diabetes mellitus (E13.-)
postprocedural diabetes mellitus (E13.-)
secondary diabetes mellitus NEC (E13.-)
type 1 diabetes mellitus (E10.-)
> Coding Clinic: 2016, Q4, P121, Q2, P10

● **E11.0** **Type 2 diabetes mellitus with hyperosmolarity**
> (Ex:) For category E11.0 CC codes: See PDX Collection 518

E11.00 **Type 2 diabetes mellitus with hyperosmolarity without nonketotic hyperglycemic-hyperosmolar coma (NKHHC)** 🔖 🔖

E11.01 **Type 2 diabetes mellitus with hyperosmolarity with coma** 🔖 🔖

▶ ● **E11.1** **Type 2 diabetes mellitus with ketoacidosis**
> (Ex:) For category E11.1 CC codes: See PDX Collection 518

▶ **E11.10** **Type 2 diabetes mellitus with ketoacidosis without coma** 🔖

▶ **E11.11** **Type 2 diabetes mellitus with ketoacidosis with coma** 🔖

● **E11.2** **Type 2 diabetes mellitus with kidney complications**

E11.21 **Type 2 diabetes mellitus with diabetic nephropathy**

> Type 2 diabetes mellitus with intercapillary glomerulosclerosis
> Type 2 diabetes mellitus with intracapillary glomerulonephrosis
> Type 2 diabetes mellitus with Kimmelstiel-Wilson disease

E11.22 **Type 2 diabetes mellitus with diabetic chronic kidney disease**

> Use additional code to identify stage of chronic kidney disease (N18.1-N18.6)
> Coding Clinic: 2016, Q2, P36, Q1, P13

E11.29 **Type 2 diabetes mellitus with other diabetic kidney complication**

> Type 2 diabetes mellitus with renal tubular degeneration

CHAPTER 4 (E00-E90)

CHAPTER 4 (E00-E90)

- **E11.3**   **Type 2 diabetes mellitus with ophthalmic complications**
  Coding Clinic: 2016, Q4, P11

  - **E11.31**   Type 2 diabetes mellitus with unspecified diabetic retinopathy

    - **E11.311**   Type 2 diabetes mellitus with unspecified diabetic retinopathy with macular edema

    - **E11.319**   Type 2 diabetes mellitus with unspecified diabetic retinopathy without macular edema
      Coding Clinic: 2013, Q3, P20

  - **E11.32**   Type 2 diabetes mellitus with mild nonproliferative diabetic retinopathy

    Type 2 diabetes mellitus with nonproliferative diabetic retinopathy NOS

    One of the following 7th characters is to be assigned to codes in subcategory E11.32 to designate laterality of the disease:

1	right eye
2	left eye
3	bilateral
9	unspecified eye

    - **E11.321**   Type 2 diabetes mellitus with mild nonproliferative diabetic retinopathy with macular edema

    - **E11.329**   Type 2 diabetes mellitus with mild nonproliferative diabetic retinopathy without macular edema

  - **E11.33**   Type 2 diabetes mellitus with moderate nonproliferative diabetic retinopathy

    One of the following 7th characters is to be assigned to codes in subcategory E11.33 to designate laterality of the disease:

1	right eye
2	left eye
3	bilateral
9	unspecified eye

    - **E11.331**   Type 2 diabetes mellitus with moderate nonproliferative diabetic retinopathy with macular edema

    - **E11.339**   Type 2 diabetes mellitus with moderate nonproliferative diabetic retinopathy without macular edema

  - **E11.34**   Type 2 diabetes mellitus with severe nonproliferative diabetic retinopathy

    One of the following 7th characters is to be assigned to codes in subcategory E11.34 to designate laterality of the disease:

1	right eye
2	left eye
3	bilateral
9	unspecified eye

    - **E11.341**   Type 2 diabetes mellitus with severe nonproliferative diabetic retinopathy with macular edema

    - **E11.349**   Type 2 diabetes mellitus with severe nonproliferative diabetic retinopathy without macular edema

  - **E11.35**   Type 2 diabetes mellitus with proliferative diabetic retinopathy

    One of the following 7th characters is to be assigned to codes in subcategory E11.35 to designate laterality of the disease:

1	right eye
2	left eye
3	bilateral
9	unspecified eye

    - **E11.351**   Type 2 diabetes mellitus with proliferative diabetic retinopathy with macular edema

    - **E11.352**   Type 2 diabetes mellitus with proliferative diabetic retinopathy with traction retinal detachment involving the macula

    - **E11.353**   Type 2 diabetes mellitus with proliferative diabetic retinopathy with traction retinal detachment not involving the macula

    - **E11.354**   Type 2 diabetes mellitus with proliferative diabetic retinopathy with combined traction retinal detachment and rhegmatogenous retinal detachment

    - **E11.355**   Type 2 diabetes mellitus with stable proliferative diabetic retinopathy

    - **E11.359**   Type 2 diabetes mellitus with proliferative diabetic retinopathy without macular edema

  - **E11.36**   Type 2 diabetes mellitus with diabetic cataract
    Coding Clinic: 2016, Q2, P36

  - X **E11.37**   Type 2 diabetes mellitus with diabetic macular edema, resolved following treatment

    One of the following 7th characters is to be assigned to code E11.37 to designate laterality of the disease:

1	right eye
2	left eye
3	bilateral
9	unspecified eye

  - **E11.39**   Type 2 diabetes mellitus with other diabetic ophthalmic complication

    Use additional code to identify manifestation, such as:
    diabetic glaucoma (H40-H42)

- **E11.4**   **Type 2 diabetes mellitus with neurological complications**

  - **E11.40**   Type 2 diabetes mellitus with diabetic neuropathy, unspecified

  - **E11.41**   Type 2 diabetes mellitus with diabetic mononeuropathy

  - **E11.42**   Type 2 diabetes mellitus with diabetic polyneuropathy

    Type 2 diabetes mellitus with diabetic neuralgia
    Coding Clinic: 2016, Q1, P13

  - **E11.43**   Type 2 diabetes mellitus with diabetic autonomic (poly)neuropathy

    Type 2 diabetes mellitus with diabetic gastroparesis
    Coding Clinic: 2016, Q2, P36

  - **E11.44**   Type 2 diabetes mellitus with diabetic amyotrophy
    Coding Clinic: 2016, Q2, P36

  - **E11.49**   Type 2 diabetes mellitus with other diabetic neurological complication

▶ New   ⇒ Revised   ~~deleted~~ Deleted   Excludes 1   Excludes 2   Includes   Use additional   Code first   Code also   Key words
OGCR Official Guidelines   ● Unacceptable Principal Diagnosis   X Assign placeholder X   ● Use Additional Character(s)   ▶ Manifestation Code   Coding Clinic

● **E11.5**   **Type 2 diabetes mellitus with circulatory complications**

    E11.51   **Type 2 diabetes mellitus with diabetic peripheral angiopathy without gangrene**

    E11.52   **Type 2 diabetes mellitus with diabetic peripheral angiopathy with gangrene**

        Type 2 diabetes mellitus with diabetic gangrene 🔖

        CC when PDx is its own CC

        (Ex) See PDX Collection 519

    E11.59   **Type 2 diabetes mellitus with other circulatory complications**

● **E11.6**   **Type 2 diabetes mellitus with other specified complications**

   ● **E11.61**   **Type 2 diabetes mellitus with diabetic arthropathy**

      E11.610   **Type 2 diabetes mellitus with diabetic neuropathic arthropathy**

        Type 2 diabetes mellitus with Charcôt's joints

        Coding Clinic: 2016, Q2, P36

      E11.618   **Type 2 diabetes mellitus with other diabetic arthropathy**

        Coding Clinic: 2016, Q2, P36

   ● **E11.62**   **Type 2 diabetes mellitus with skin complications**

      E11.620   **Type 2 diabetes mellitus with diabetic dermatitis**

        Type 2 diabetes mellitus with diabetic necrobiosis lipoidica

      E11.621   **Type 2 diabetes mellitus with foot ulcer**

        Use additional code to identify site of ulcer (L97.4-, L97.5-)

        Coding Clinic: 2016, Q1, P12

      E11.622   **Type 2 diabetes mellitus with other skin ulcer**

        Use additional code to identify site of ulcer (L97.1-L97.9, L98.41-L98.49)

      E11.628   **Type 2 diabetes mellitus with other skin complications**

   ● **E11.63**   **Type 2 diabetes mellitus with oral complications**

      E11.630   **Type 2 diabetes mellitus with periodontal disease**

      E11.638   **Type 2 diabetes mellitus with other oral complications**

   ● **E11.64**   **Type 2 diabetes mellitus with hypoglycemia**

      E11.641   **Type 2 diabetes mellitus with hypoglycemia with coma** 🔖

        (Ex) See PDX Collection 518

      E11.649   **Type 2 diabetes mellitus with hypoglycemia without coma**

        Coding Clinic: 2016, Q3, P42; 2015, Q3, P21

    E11.65   **Type 2 diabetes mellitus with hyperglycemia**

        Coding Clinic: 2013, Q3, P20

    E11.69   **Type 2 diabetes mellitus with other specified complication**

        Use additional code to identify complication

        Use this code with E11.65 to report DKA in a Type 2 patient

        Coding Clinic: 2016, Q4, P142

   E11.8   **Type 2 diabetes mellitus with unspecified complications**

   E11.9   **Type 2 diabetes mellitus without complications**

        MCE: Questionable admission when principal dx

        Coding Clinic: 2016, Q4, P142, Q2, P36

● **E13**   **Other specified diabetes mellitus**

   Includes   diabetes mellitus due to genetic defects of beta-cell function

        diabetes mellitus due to genetic defects in insulin action

        postpancreatectomy diabetes mellitus

        postprocedural diabetes mellitus

        secondary diabetes mellitus NEC

Use additional code to identify control using:
   insulin (Z79.4)
   oral antidiabetic drugs (Z79.84)
   oral hypoglycemic drugs (Z79.84)

   Excludes1   diabetes (mellitus) due to autoimmune process (E10.-)

        diabetes (mellitus) due to immune mediated pancreatic islet beta-cell destruction (E10.-)

        diabetes mellitus due to underlying condition (E08.-)

        drug or chemical induced diabetes mellitus (E09.-)

        gestational diabetes (O24.4-)

        neonatal diabetes mellitus (P70.2)

        type 1 diabetes mellitus (E10.-)

        ~~type 2 diabetes mellitus (E11.-)~~

● **E13.0**   **Other specified diabetes mellitus with hyperosmolarity**

        (Ex) For category E13.0 CC codes: See PDX Collection 518

    E13.00   **Other specified diabetes mellitus with hyperosmolarity without nonketotic hyperglycemic-hyperosmolar coma (NKHHC)** 🔖 🔖

       ▶ **Excludes2**   type 2 diabetes mellitus (E11.-)

    E13.01   **Other specified diabetes mellitus with hyperosmolarity with coma** 🔖 🔖

● **E13.1**   **Other specified diabetes mellitus with ketoacidosis**

        (Ex) For category E13.1 CC codes: See PDX Collection 518

    E13.10   **Other specified diabetes mellitus with ketoacidosis without coma** 🔖 🔖

        Coding Clinic: 2016, Q2, P10; 2013, Q1, P26

    E13.11   **Other specified diabetes mellitus with ketoacidosis with coma** 🔖

● **E13.2**   **Other specified diabetes mellitus with kidney complications**

    E13.21   **Other specified diabetes mellitus with diabetic nephropathy**

        Other specified diabetes mellitus with intercapillary glomerulosclerosis

        Other specified diabetes mellitus with intracapillary glomerulonephrosis

        Other specified diabetes mellitus with Kimmelstiel-Wilson disease

    E13.22   **Other specified diabetes mellitus with diabetic chronic kidney disease**

        Use additional code to identify stage of chronic kidney disease (N18.1-N18.6)

    E13.29   **Other specified diabetes mellitus with other diabetic kidney complication**

        Other specified diabetes mellitus with renal tubular degeneration

● **E13.3**   **Other specified diabetes mellitus with ophthalmic complications**

        Coding Clinic: 2016, Q4, P11

   ● **E13.31**   **Other specified diabetes mellitus with unspecified diabetic retinopathy**

      E13.311   **Other specified diabetes mellitus with unspecified diabetic retinopathy with macular edema**

      E13.319   **Other specified diabetes mellitus with unspecified diabetic retinopathy without macular edema**

CHAPTER 4 (E00-E90)

N Newborn Age: 0   **P** Pediatric Age: 0–17   **M** Maternity DX: 12–55   **A** Adult Age: 15–124   ♀ Females Only   ♂ Males Only

🔖 Complication\Comorbidity   🔖 Major C\C   (Ex) CC/MCC Exclusions   🔖 Hospital-Acquired Condition

739

● **E13.32** **Other specified diabetes mellitus with mild nonproliferative diabetic retinopathy**

Other specified diabetes mellitus with nonproliferative diabetic retinopathy NOS

One of the following 7th characters is to be assigned to codes in subcategory E13.32 to designate laterality of the disease:

1	right eye
2	left eye
3	bilateral
9	unspecified eye

● **E13.321** **Other specified diabetes mellitus with mild nonproliferative diabetic retinopathy with macular edema**

● **E13.329** **Other specified diabetes mellitus with mild nonproliferative diabetic retinopathy without macular edema**

● **E13.33** **Other specified diabetes mellitus with moderate nonproliferative diabetic retinopathy**

One of the following 7th characters is to be assigned to codes in subcategory E13.33 to designate laterality of the disease:

1	right eye
2	left eye
3	bilateral
9	unspecified eye

● **E13.331** **Other specified diabetes mellitus with moderate nonproliferative diabetic retinopathy with macular edema**

● **E13.339** **Other specified diabetes mellitus with moderate nonproliferative diabetic retinopathy without macular edema**

● **E13.34** **Other specified diabetes mellitus with severe nonproliferative diabetic retinopathy**

One of the following 7th characters is to be assigned to codes in subcategory E13.34 to designate laterality of the disease:

1	right eye
2	left eye
3	bilateral
9	unspecified eye

● **E13.341** **Other specified diabetes mellitus with severe nonproliferative diabetic retinopathy with macular edema**

● **E13.349** **Other specified diabetes mellitus with severe nonproliferative diabetic retinopathy without macular edema**

● **E13.35** **Other specified diabetes mellitus with proliferative diabetic retinopathy**

One of the following 7th characters is to be assigned to codes in subcategory E13.35 to designate laterality of the disease:

1	right eye
2	left eye
3	bilateral
9	unspecified eye

● **E13.351** **Other specified diabetes mellitus with proliferative diabetic retinopathy with macular edema**

● **E13.352** **Other specified diabetes mellitus with proliferative diabetic retinopathy with traction retinal detachment involving the macula**

● **E13.353** **Other specified diabetes mellitus with proliferative diabetic retinopathy with traction retinal detachment not involving the macula**

● **E13.354** **Other specified diabetes mellitus with proliferative diabetic retinopathy with combined traction retinal detachment and rhegmatogenous retinal detachment**

● **E13.355** **Other specified diabetes mellitus with stable proliferative diabetic retinopathy**

● **E13.359** **Other specified diabetes mellitus with proliferative diabetic retinopathy without macular edema**

E13.36 **Other specified diabetes mellitus with diabetic cataract**

X ● **E13.37** **Other specified diabetes mellitus with diabetic macular edema, resolved following treatment**

One of the following 7th characters is to be assigned to code E13.37 to designate laterality of the disease:

1	right eye
2	left eye
3	bilateral
9	unspecified eye

E13.39 **Other specified diabetes mellitus with other diabetic ophthalmic complication**

Use additional code to identify manifestation, such as:
diabetic glaucoma (H40-H42)

● **E13.4** **Other specified diabetes mellitus with neurological complications**

E13.40 **Other specified diabetes mellitus with diabetic neuropathy, unspecified**

E13.41 **Other specified diabetes mellitus with diabetic mononeuropathy**

E13.42 **Other specified diabetes mellitus with diabetic polyneuropathy**

Other specified diabetes mellitus with diabetic neuralgia

E13.43 **Other specified diabetes mellitus with diabetic autonomic (poly)neuropathy**

Other specified diabetes mellitus with diabetic gastroparesis

E13.44 **Other specified diabetes mellitus with diabetic amyotrophy**

E13.49 **Other specified diabetes mellitus with other diabetic neurological complication**

● **E13.5** **Other specified diabetes mellitus with circulatory complications**

E13.51 **Other specified diabetes mellitus with diabetic peripheral angiopathy without gangrene**

E13.52 **Other specified diabetes mellitus with diabetic peripheral angiopathy with gangrene**

Other specified diabetes mellitus with diabetic gangrene ⊙
CC when PDx is its own CC
Ⓔⓧ See PDX Collection 519

E13.59 **Other specified diabetes mellitus with other circulatory complications**

● **E13.6** **Other specified diabetes mellitus with other specified complications**

● **E13.61** **Other specified diabetes mellitus with diabetic arthropathy**

E13.610 **Other specified diabetes mellitus with diabetic neuropathic arthropathy**

Other specified diabetes mellitus with Charcôt's joints

E13.618 **Other specified diabetes mellitus with other diabetic arthropathy**

▶ New   ⟹ Revised   d̶e̶l̶e̶t̶e̶d̶ Deleted   Excludes 1   Excludes 2   Includes   Use additional   Code first   Code also   Key words

OGCR Official Guidelines   ● Unacceptable Principal Diagnosis   X Assign placeholder X   ● Use Additional Character(s)   ▶ Manifestation Code   **Coding Clinic**

● **E13.62** **Other specified diabetes mellitus with skin complications**

    E13.620 **Other specified diabetes mellitus with diabetic dermatitis**
        Other specified diabetes mellitus with diabetic necrobiosis lipoidica

    E13.621 **Other specified diabetes mellitus with foot ulcer**
        Use additional code to identify site of ulcer (L97.4-, L97.5-)

    E13.622 **Other specified diabetes mellitus with other skin ulcer**
        Use additional code to identify site of ulcer (L97.1-L97.9, L98.41-L98.49)

    E13.628 **Other specified diabetes mellitus with other skin complications**

● **E13.63** **Other specified diabetes mellitus with oral complications**

    E13.630 **Other specified diabetes mellitus with periodontal disease**

    E13.638 **Other specified diabetes mellitus with other oral complications**

● **E13.64** **Other specified diabetes mellitus with hypoglycemia**

    E13.641 **Other specified diabetes mellitus with hypoglycemia with coma**
        (Ex:) See PDX Collection 518

    E13.649 **Other specified diabetes mellitus with hypoglycemia without coma**

    E13.65 **Other specified diabetes mellitus with hyperglycemia**

    E13.69 **Other specified diabetes mellitus with other specified complication**
        Use additional code to identify complication

E13.8 **Other specified diabetes mellitus with unspecified complications**

E13.9 **Other specified diabetes mellitus without complications**
    MCE: Questionable admission when principal dx

OTHER DISORDERS OF GLUCOSE REGULATION AND PANCREATIC INTERNAL SECRETION (E15-E16)

E15 **Nondiabetic hypoglycemic coma**
    Includes drug-induced insulin coma in nondiabetic hyperinsulinism with hypoglycemic coma hypoglycemic coma NOS
    (Ex:) See PDX Collection 520

● **E16** **Other disorders of pancreatic internal secretion**

    E16.0 **Drug-induced hypoglycemia without coma**
        ➡ **Excludes1** diabetes with hypoglycemia without coma (E09.649)
        Use additional code for adverse effect, if applicable, to identify drug (T36-T50 with fifth or sixth character 5)

    E16.1 **Other hypoglycemia**
        Functional hyperinsulinism
        Functional nonhyperinsulinemic hypoglycemia
        Hyperinsulinism NOS
        Hyperplasia of pancreatic islet beta cells NOS
        Excludes1 diabetes with hypoglycemia (E08.649, E10.649, E11.649, E13.649)
        hypoglycemia in infant of diabetic mother (P70.1)
        neonatal hypoglycemia (P70.4)

E16.2 **Hypoglycemia, unspecified**
    Excludes1 diabetes with hypoglycemia (E08.649, E10.649, E11.649, E13.649)
    Coding Clinic: 2016, Q3, P42

E16.3 **Increased secretion of glucagon**
    Hyperplasia of pancreatic endocrine cells with glucagon excess

E16.4 **Increased secretion of gastrin**
    Hypergastrinemia
    Hyperplasia of pancreatic endocrine cells with gastrin excess
    Zollinger-Ellison syndrome

E16.8 **Other specified disorders of pancreatic internal secretion**
    Increased secretion from endocrine pancreas of growth hormone-releasing hormone
    Increased secretion from endocrine pancreas of pancreatic polypeptide
    Increased secretion from endocrine pancreas of somatostatin
    Increased secretion from endocrine pancreas of vasoactive-intestinal polypeptide

E16.9 **Disorder of pancreatic internal secretion, unspecified**
    Islet-cell hyperplasia NOS
    Pancreatic endocrine cell hyperplasia NOS

DISORDERS OF OTHER ENDOCRINE GLANDS (E20-E35)

Excludes1 galactorrhea (N64.3)
    gynecomastia (N62)

● **E20** **Hypoparathyroidism**
  Greatly reduced function of parathyroid glands; AKA parathyroid insufficiency
    Excludes1 Di George's syndrome (D82.1)
    postprocedural hypoparathyroidism (E89.2)
    tetany NOS (R29.0)
    transitory neonatal hypoparathyroidism (P71.4)

E20.0 **Idiopathic hypoparathyroidism**
  Rare condition, unknown cause; short dwarf-like with round face

E20.1 **Pseudohypoparathyroidism**
  Hereditary condition resembling hypoparathyroidism, but caused by inability to respond to parathyroid hormone

E20.8 **Other hypoparathyroidism**

E20.9 **Hypoparathyroidism, unspecified**
    Parathyroid tetany

● **E21** **Hyperparathyroidism and other disorders of parathyroid gland**
    Excludes1 adult osteomalacia (M83.-)
    ectopic hyperparathyroidism (E34.2)
    familial hypocalciuric hypercalcemia (E83.52)
    hungry bone syndrome (E83.81)
    infantile and juvenile osteomalacia (E55.0)

E21.0 **Primary hyperparathyroidism**
    Hyperplasia of parathyroid
    Osteitis fibrosa cystica generalisata [von Recklinghausen's disease of bone]

E21.1 **Secondary hyperparathyroidism, not elsewhere classified**
    Excludes1 secondary hyperparathyroidism of renal origin (N25.81)

Item 4-4 Hyperparathyroidism is an overactive parathyroid gland that secretes excessive parathormone, causing increased levels of circulating calcium. This results in a loss of calcium in the bone (osteoporosis).

Hypoparathyroidism is an underactive parathyroid gland that results in decreased levels of circulating calcium. The primary manifestation is **tetany**, a continuous muscle spasm.

Figure 4-4 Tetany caused by hypoparathyroidism.

CHAPTER 4 (E00-E90)

Item 4–5 **Hyperadrenalism** is overactivity of the adrenal cortex, which secretes corticosteroid hormones. Excessive glucocorticoid hormone results in hyperglycemia **(Cushing's syndrome),** and excessive aldosterone results in **Conn's syndrome. Adrenogenital syndrome** is the result of excessive secretion of androgens, male hormones, which stimulates premature sexual development. **Hypoadrenalism, Addison's disease,** is a condition in which the adrenal glands atrophy.

Figure 4-5 Centripetal and generalized obesity and dorsal kyphosis in a woman with Cushing's disease. (From Salvo SG: Mosby's Pathology for Massage Therapists, St. Louis, MO: Mosby/Elsevier, 2009)

E21.2 **Other hyperparathyroidism**
　　　　　Tertiary hyperparathyroidism
　　　　　Excludes1　familial hypocalciuric hypercalcemia
　　　　　　　　　　　　(E83.52)

E21.3 **Hyperparathyroidism, unspecified**

E21.4 **Other specified disorders of parathyroid gland**

E21.5 **Disorder of parathyroid gland, unspecified**

● **E22** **Hyperfunction of pituitary gland**
　　　Excludes1　Cushing's syndrome (E24.-)
　　　　　　　　　Nelson's syndrome (E24.1)
　　　　　　　　　overproduction of ACTH not associated with
　　　　　　　　　　　Cushing's disease (E27.0)
　　　　　　　　　overproduction of pituitary ACTH (E24.0)
　　　　　　　　　overproduction of thyroid-stimulating hormone
　　　　　　　　　　　(E05.8-)
　　　(Ex) **For category E22 CC codes unless otherwise indicated:** See PDX Collection 521

E22.0 **Acromegaly and pituitary gigantism**
　　　　　Chronic disease caused by hypersecretion of growth hormone
　　　　　Overproduction of growth hormone
　　　　　Excludes1　constitutional gigantism (E34.4)
　　　　　　　　　　　constitutional tall stature (E34.4)
　　　　　　　　　　　increased secretion from endocrine
　　　　　　　　　　　　pancreas of growth hormone-
　　　　　　　　　　　　releasing hormone (E16.8)

E22.1 **Hyperprolactinemia** 🔖
　　　　　Increased levels of prolactin
　　　　　Use additional code for adverse effect, if applicable,
　　　　　　to identify drug (T36-T50 with fifth or sixth
　　　　　　character 5)

E22.2 **Syndrome of inappropriate secretion of antidiuretic
　　　　　hormone** 🔖
　　　　　(Ex) See PDX Collection 522

E22.8 **Other hyperfunction of pituitary gland** 🔖
　　　　　Central precocious puberty

E22.9 **Hyperfunction of pituitary gland, unspecified** 🔖

● **E23** **Hypofunction and other disorders of the pituitary gland**
　　　Includes　the listed conditions whether the disorder is in
　　　　　　　　　the pituitary or the hypothalamus
　　　Excludes1　postprocedural hypopituitarism (E89.3)

E23.0 **Hypopituitarism** 🔖
　　　　　Fertile eunuch syndrome
　　　　　Hypogonadotropic hypogonadism
　　　　　Idiopathic growth hormone deficiency
　　　　　Isolated deficiency of gonadotropin
　　　　　Isolated deficiency of growth hormone
　　　　　Isolated deficiency of pituitary hormone
　　　　　Kallmann's syndrome
　　　　　Lorain-Levi short stature
　　　　　Necrosis of pituitary gland (postpartum)
　　　　　Panhypopituitarism
　　　　　Pituitary cachexia
　　　　　Pituitary insufficiency NOS
　　　　　Pituitary short stature
　　　　　Sheehan's syndrome
　　　　　Simmonds' disease
　　　　　(Ex) See PDX Collection 523

E23.1 **Drug-induced hypopituitarism**
　　　　　Use additional code for adverse effect, if applicable,
　　　　　　to identify drug (T36-T50 with fifth or sixth
　　　　　　character 5)

E23.2 **Diabetes insipidus** 🔖
　　　　　Excludes1　nephrogenic diabetes insipidus (N25.1)
　　　　　(Ex) See PDX Collection 524

E23.3 **Hypothalamic dysfunction, not elsewhere classified**
　　　　　Excludes1　Prader-Willi syndrome (Q87.1)
　　　　　　　　　　　Russell-Silver syndrome (Q87.1)

E23.6 **Other disorders of pituitary gland**
　　　　　Abscess of pituitary
　　　　　Adiposogenital dystrophy

E23.7 **Disorder of pituitary gland, unspecified**

● **E24** **Cushing's syndrome**
　　　Excludes1　congenital adrenal hyperplasia (E25.0)
　　　(Ex) **For category E24 CC codes:** See PDX Collection 525

E24.0 **Pituitary-dependent Cushing's disease** 🔖
　　　　　Overproduction of pituitary ACTH
　　　　　Pituitary-dependent hypercorticalism

E24.1 **Nelson's syndrome**

E24.2 **Drug-induced Cushing's syndrome** 🔖
　　　　　Use additional code for adverse effect, if applicable,
　　　　　　to identify drug (T36-T50 with fifth or sixth
　　　　　　character 5)

E24.3 **Ectopic ACTH syndrome** 🔖

E24.4 **Alcohol-induced pseudo-Cushing's syndrome** 🔖

E24.8 **Other Cushing's syndrome** 🔖

E24.9 **Cushing's syndrome, unspecified** 🔖

● **E25** **Adrenogenital disorders**
　　　Disorder of production of steroid hormone in adrenal gland
　　　Includes　adrenogenital syndromes, virilizing or
　　　　　　　　　feminizing, whether acquired or due to
　　　　　　　　　adrenal hyperplasia consequent on inborn
　　　　　　　　　enzyme defects in hormone synthesis
　　　　　　　　　female adrenal pseudohermaphroditism
　　　　　　　　　female heterosexual precocious pseudopuberty
　　　　　　　　　male isosexual precocious pseudopuberty
　　　　　　　　　male macrogenitosomia praecox
　　　　　　　　　male sexual precocity with adrenal hyperplasia
　　　　　　　　　male virilization (female)
　　　Excludes1　indeterminate sex and pseudohermaphroditism
　　　　　　　　　(Q56)
　　　　　　　　　chromosomal abnormalities (Q90-Q99)

E25.0 **Congenital adrenogenital disorders associated with
　　　　　enzyme deficiency**
　　　　　Congenital adrenal hyperplasia
　　　　　21-Hydroxylase deficiency
　　　　　Salt-losing congenital adrenal hyperplasia

E25.8 **Other adrenogenital disorders**
　　　　　Idiopathic adrenogenital disorder
　　　　　Use additional code for adverse effect, if applicable,
　　　　　　to identify drug (T36-T50 with fifth or sixth
　　　　　　character 5)

E25.9 **Adrenogenital disorder, unspecified**
　　　　　Adrenogenital syndrome NOS

▶ New　⇒ Revised　~~deleted~~ Deleted　Excludes 1　Excludes 2　Includes　Use additional　Code first　Code also　Key words

OGCR Official Guidelines　● Unacceptable Principal Diagnosis　X Assign placeholder X　◐ Use Additional Character(s)　▸ Manifestation Code　**Coding Clinic**

● **E26   Hyperaldosteronism**
Abnormality of electrolyte metabolism caused by excessive secretion of aldosterone

   ● **E26.0   Primary hyperaldosteronism**

      E26.01   Conn's syndrome
        Code also adrenal adenoma (D35.0-)

      E26.02   Glucocorticoid-remediable aldosteronism
        Familial aldosteronism type I

      E26.09   Other primary hyperaldosteronism
        Primary aldosteronism due to adrenal hyperplasia (bilateral)

   E26.1   Secondary hyperaldosteronism

   ● **E26.8   Other hyperaldosteronism**

      E26.81   Bartter's syndrome

      E26.89   Other hyperaldosteronism

   E26.9   Hyperaldosteronism, unspecified
      Aldosteronism NOS
      Hyperaldosteronism NOS

● **E27   Other disorders of adrenal gland**
   (Ex) For category E27 CC codes: See PDX Collection 526

   E27.0   Other adrenocortical overactivity 🔹
      Overproduction of ACTH, not associated with Cushing's disease
      Premature adrenarche
      Excludes1   Cushing's syndrome (E24.-)

   E27.1   Primary adrenocortical insufficiency 🔹
      Addison's disease
      Autoimmune adrenalitis
      Excludes1   Addison only phenotype adrenoleukodystrophy (E71.528)
         amyloidosis (E85.-)
         tuberculous Addison's disease (A18.7)
         Waterhouse-Friderichsen syndrome (A39.1)

   E27.2   Addisonian crisis 🔹
      Acute onset of adrenocortical insufficiency
      Adrenal crisis
      Adrenocortical crisis

   E27.3   Drug-induced adrenocortical insufficiency 🔹
      Use additional code for adverse effect, if applicable, to identify drug (T36-T50 with fifth or sixth character 5)

   ● **E27.4   Other and unspecified adrenocortical insufficiency**
      Excludes1   adrenoleukodystrophy [Addison-Schilder] (E71.528)
         Waterhouse-Friderichsen syndrome (A39.1)

      E27.40   Unspecified adrenocortical insufficiency 🔹
        Adrenocortical insufficiency NOS
        Hypoaldosteronism

      E27.49   Other adrenocortical insufficiency 🔹
        Adrenal hemorrhage
        Adrenal infarction

   E27.5   Adrenomedullary hyperfunction 🔹
      Adrenomedullary hyperplasia
      Catecholamine hypersecretion

   E27.8   Other specified disorders of adrenal gland
      Abnormality of cortisol-binding globulin

   E27.9   Disorder of adrenal gland, unspecified

● **E28   Ovarian dysfunction**
   Excludes1   isolated gonadotropin deficiency (E23.0)
       postprocedural ovarian failure (E89.4-)

   E28.0   Estrogen excess ♀
      Use additional code for adverse effect, if applicable, to identify drug (T36-T50 with fifth or sixth character 5)

   E28.1   Androgen excess ♀
      Hypersecretion of ovarian androgens
      Use additional code for adverse effect, if applicable, to identify drug (T36-T50 with fifth or sixth character 5)

   E28.2   Polycystic ovarian syndrome ♀
      Sclerocystic ovary syndrome
      Stein-Leventhal syndrome

   ● **E28.3   Primary ovarian failure**
      Excludes1   pure gonadal dysgenesis (Q99.1)
        Turner's syndrome (Q96.-)

     ● **E28.31   Premature menopause**

       E28.310   Symptomatic premature menopause ♀   A
         Symptoms such as flushing, sleeplessness, headache, lack of concentration, associated with premature menopause

       E28.319   Asymptomatic premature menopause ♀   A
         Premature menopause NOS

      E28.39   Other primary ovarian failure ♀
        Decreased estrogen
        Resistant ovary syndrome

   E28.8   Other ovarian dysfunction ♀
      Ovarian hyperfunction NOS
      Excludes1   postprocedural ovarian failure (E89.4-)

   E28.9   Ovarian dysfunction, unspecified ♀

● **E29   Testicular dysfunction**
   Excludes1   androgen insensitivity syndrome (E34.5-)
       azoospermia or oligospermia NOS (N46.0-N46.1)
       isolated gonadotropin deficiency (E23.0)
       Klinefelter's syndrome (Q98.0-Q98.1, Q98.4)

   E29.0   Testicular hyperfunction ♂
      Hypersecretion of testicular hormones

   E29.1   Testicular hypofunction ♂
      Defective biosynthesis of testicular androgen NOS
      5-delta-Reductase deficiency (with male pseudohermaphroditism)
      Testicular hypogonadism NOS
      Use additional code for adverse effect, if applicable, to identify drug (T36-T50 with fifth or sixth character 5)
      Excludes1   postprocedural testicular hypofunction (E89.5)

   E29.8   Other testicular dysfunction ♂

   E29.9   Testicular dysfunction, unspecified ♂

● **E30   Disorders of puberty, not elsewhere classified**

   E30.0   Delayed puberty
      Constitutional delay of puberty
      Delayed sexual development

   E30.1   Precocious puberty   P
      Sexual maturation at earlier age than normal, or before age 8 in girls and 9 in boys, usually hormonal; AKA sexual precocity or pubertas praecox
      Precocious menstruation
      Excludes1   Albright (-McCune) (-Sternberg) syndrome (Q78.1)
        central precocious puberty (E22.8)
        congenital adrenal hyperplasia (E25.0)
        female heterosexual precocious pseudopuberty (E25.-)
        male isosexual precocious pseudopuberty (E25.-)

   E30.8   Other disorders of puberty   P
      Premature thelarche

   E30.9   Disorder of puberty, unspecified

N Newborn Age: 0   **P** Pediatric Age: 0–17   **M** Maternity DX: 12–55   **A** Adult Age: 15–124   ♀ Females Only   ♂ Males Only

 Complication\Comorbidity   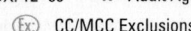 Major C\C   (Ex) CC/MCC Exclusions   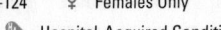 Hospital-Acquired Condition

743

CHAPTER 4 (E00-E90)

● **E31   Polyglandular dysfunction**

     Excludes1   ataxia telangiectasia [Louis-Bar] (G11.3)
                       dystrophia myotonica [Steinert] (G71.11)
                       pseudohypoparathyroidism (E20.1)

   E31.0   Autoimmune polyglandular failure
           Schmidt's syndrome

   E31.1   Polyglandular hyperfunction

       Excludes1   multiple endocrine adenomatosis (E31.2-)
                       multiple endocrine neoplasia (E31.2-)

 ● **E31.2   Multiple endocrine neoplasia [MEN] syndromes**
         Adenomatous hyperplasia and malignant tumors in
            endocrine glands
         Multiple endocrine adenomatosis

         Code also any associated malignancies and other
            conditions associated with the syndromes

      E31.20   Multiple endocrine neoplasia [MEN]
              syndrome, unspecified
               Multiple endocrine adenomatosis NOS
               Multiple endocrine neoplasia [MEN]
                  syndrome NOS

      E31.21   Multiple endocrine neoplasia [MEN] type I
              Wermer's syndrome

      E31.22   Multiple endocrine neoplasia [MEN] type IIA
              Sipple's syndrome

      E31.23   Multiple endocrine neoplasia [MEN] type IIB

   E31.8   Other polyglandular dysfunction

   E31.9   Polyglandular dysfunction, unspecified

● **E32   Diseases of thymus**

     Excludes1   aplasia or hypoplasia of thymus with
                     immunodeficiency (D82.1)
                   myasthenia gravis (G70.0)

   E32.0   Persistent hyperplasia of thymus
           Hypertrophy of thymus

   E32.1   Abscess of thymus 🔖
          Ⓔⓧ See PDX Collection 527

   E32.8   Other diseases of thymus

       Excludes1   aplasia or hypoplasia with
                     immunodeficiency (D82.1)
                   thymoma (D15.0)

   E32.9   Disease of thymus, unspecified

● **E34   Other endocrine disorders**

     Excludes1   pseudohypoparathyroidism (E20.1)

   E34.0   Carcinoid syndrome 🔖

       Note: May be used as an additional code to identify
            functional activity associated with a carcinoid
            tumor.
         Ⓔⓧ See PDX Collection 528

   E34.1   Other hypersecretion of intestinal hormones

   E34.2   Ectopic hormone secretion, not elsewhere classified

       Excludes1   ectopic ACTH syndrome (E24.3)

   E34.3   Short stature due to endocrine disorder
           Constitutional short stature
           Laron-type short stature

       Excludes1   achondroplastic short stature (Q77.4)
                     hypochondroplastic short stature (Q77.4)
                   nutritional short stature (E45)
                   pituitary short stature (E23.0)
                   progeria (E34.8)
                   renal short stature (N25.0)
                   Russell-Silver syndrome (Q87.1)
                   short-limbed stature with
                      immunodeficiency (D82.2)
                   short stature in specific dysmorphic
                      syndromes - code to syndrome - see
                      Alphabetical Index
                   short stature NOS (R62.52)

   E34.4   Constitutional tall stature
           Constitutional gigantism

 ● **E34.5   Androgen insensitivity syndrome**

      E34.50   Androgen insensitivity syndrome, unspecified
              Androgen insensitivity NOS

      E34.51   Complete androgen insensitivity syndrome
              Complete androgen insensitivity
              de Quervain syndrome
              Goldberg-Maxwell syndrome

      E34.52   Partial androgen insensitivity syndrome
              Partial androgen insensitivity
              Reifenstein syndrome

   E34.8   Other specified endocrine disorders
           Pineal gland dysfunction
           Progeria

       Excludes2   pseudohypoparathyroidism (E20.1)

   E34.9   Endocrine disorder, unspecified
           Endocrine disturbance NOS
           Hormone disturbance NOS

▸ **E35   *Disorders of endocrine glands in diseases classified elsewhere***

     Code first underlying disease, such as:
       late congenital syphilis of thymus gland [Dubois disease]
         (A50.5)
     Use additional code, if applicable, to identify:
       sequelae of tuberculosis of other organs (B90.8)

     Excludes1   Echinococcus granulosus infection of thyroid
                     gland (B67.3)
                   meningococcal hemorrhagic adrenalitis (A39.1)
                   syphilis of endocrine gland (A52.79)
                   tuberculosis of adrenal gland, except calcification
                     (A18.7)
                   tuberculosis of endocrine gland NEC (A18.82)
                   tuberculosis of thyroid gland (A18.81)
                   Waterhouse-Friderichsen syndrome (A39.1)

INTRAOPERATIVE COMPLICATIONS OF ENDOCRINE SYSTEM (E36)

● **E36   Intraoperative complications of endocrine system**

     Excludes2   postprocedural endocrine and metabolic
                     complications and disorders, not elsewhere
                   classified (E89.-)

 ● **E36.0   Intraoperative hemorrhage and hematoma of an**
         endocrine system organ or structure complicating a
         procedure

       Excludes1   intraoperative hemorrhage and
                     hematoma of an endocrine system
                   organ or structure due to accidental
                   puncture or laceration during a
                   procedure (E36.1-)
         Ⓔⓧ For category E36.0 CC codes: See PDX Collection 529

      E36.01   Intraoperative hemorrhage and hematoma of an
              endocrine system organ or structure
              complicating an endocrine system procedure 🔖

      E36.02   Intraoperative hemorrhage and hematoma of an
              endocrine system organ or structure
              complicating other procedure 🔖

 ● **E36.1   Accidental puncture and laceration of an endocrine**
         system organ or structure during a procedure
         Ⓔⓧ For category E36.1 CC codes: See PDX Collection 509

      E36.11   Accidental puncture and laceration of an
              endocrine system organ or structure during an
              endocrine system procedure 🔖

      E36.12   Accidental puncture and laceration of an
              endocrine system organ or structure during
              other procedure 🔖

   E36.8   Other intraoperative complications of endocrine system
           Use additional code, if applicable, to further specify
           disorder

▶ New   ⟿ Revised   ~~deleted~~ Deleted   Excludes 1   Excludes 2   Includes   Use additional   Code first   Code also   Key words

OGCR Official Guidelines   ● Unacceptable Principal Diagnosis   X Assign placeholder X   ● Use Additional Character(s)   ▸ Manifestation Code   **Coding Clinic**

MALNUTRITION (E40-E46)

Excludes1   intestinal malabsorption (K90.-)
         sequelae of protein-calorie malnutrition (E64.0)

Excludes2   nutritional anemias (D50-D53)
         starvation (T73.0)

E40   Kwashiorkor 🔖
Malnutrition produced by severe protein deficiency
Severe malnutrition with nutritional edema with
   dyspigmentation of skin and hair
   Excludes1   marasmic kwashiorkor (E42)
   (Ex) See PDX Collection 530

E41   Nutritional marasmus 🔖
Severe malnutrition with marasmus
   Excludes1   marasmic kwashiorkor (E42)
   (Ex) See PDX Collection 530

E42   Marasmic kwashiorkor 🔖
Severe protein malnutrition
Intermediate form severe protein-calorie malnutrition
Severe protein-calorie malnutrition with signs of both
   kwashiorkor and marasmus
   (Ex) See PDX Collection 530

E43   Unspecified severe protein-calorie malnutrition 🔖
Starvation edema
   (Ex) See PDX Collection 530

● E44   Protein-calorie malnutrition of moderate and mild degree
   (Ex) **For category E44 CC codes:** See PDX Collection 530

   E44.0   Moderate protein-calorie malnutrition 🔖

   E44.1   Mild protein-calorie malnutrition 🔖

**E45   Retarded development following protein-calorie
malnutrition** 🔖
Nutritional short stature
Nutritional stunting
Physical retardation due to malnutrition
   (Ex) See PDX Collection 530

E46   Unspecified protein-calorie malnutrition 🔖
Malnutrition NOS
Protein-calorie imbalance NOS
   Excludes1   nutritional deficiency NOS (E63.9)
   (Ex) See PDX Collection 530

OTHER NUTRITIONAL DEFICIENCIES (E50-E64)

Excludes2   nutritional anemias (D50-D53)

● E50   Vitamin A deficiency
   Excludes1   sequelae of vitamin A deficiency (E64.1)

   E50.0   Vitamin A deficiency with conjunctival xerosis

   **E50.1   Vitamin A deficiency with Bitot's spot and conjunctival
       xerosis**
       Bitot's spot in the young child

   E50.2   Vitamin A deficiency with corneal xerosis

   E50.3   Vitamin A deficiency with corneal ulceration and xerosis

   E50.4   Vitamin A deficiency with keratomalacia
       *Eye disorder that results in dry cornea caused by vitamin A
       deficiency*

   E50.5   Vitamin A deficiency with night blindness

   E50.6   Vitamin A deficiency with xerophthalmic scars of cornea
       *Abnormal dryness and thickening of conjunctiva and cornea
       due to vitamin A deficiency*

   E50.7   Other ocular manifestations of vitamin A deficiency
       Xerophthalmia NOS

Item 4–6   Bitot's spots are the result of a buildup of keratin debris found on the superficial surface the conjunctiva; oval, triangular, or irregular in shape; and a sign of vitamin A deficiency and associated with night blindness. The disease may progress to **keratomalacia,** which can result in eventual prolapse of the iris and loss of the lens.

Figure 4-6   Bitot's spot on the conjunctiva.

   E50.8   Other manifestations of vitamin A deficiency
       Follicular keratosis
       Xeroderma

   E50.9   Vitamin A deficiency, unspecified
       Hypovitaminosis A NOS

● E51   Thiamine deficiency
   Excludes1   sequelae of thiamine deficiency (E64.8)

   ● E51.1   Beriberi
     (Ex) **For category E51.1 CC codes:** See PDX Collection 531

     E51.11   Dry beriberi 🔖
         *Thiamine deficiency with nervous system
         manifestation most often caused by excessive
         alcohol consumption*
         Beriberi NOS
         Beriberi with polyneuropathy

     E51.12   Wet beriberi 🔖
         *Thiamine deficiency with cardiovascular
         manifestation most often caused by excessive
         alcohol consumption*
         Beriberi with cardiovascular manifestations
         Cardiovascular beriberi
         Shoshin disease

   E51.2   Wernicke's encephalopathy 🔖
       *Acute disease of brain due to thiamine deficiency most often
       associated with excessive alcohol consumption*
       (Ex) See PDX Collection 531

   E51.8   Other manifestations of thiamine deficiency 🔖
       (Ex) See PDX Collection 531

   E51.9   Thiamine deficiency, unspecified 🔖
       (Ex) See PDX Collection 531

E52   Niacin deficiency [pellagra]
Niacin (-tryptophan) deficiency
Nicotinamide deficiency
Pellagra (alcoholic)
   Excludes1   sequelae of niacin deficiency (E64.8)

Figure 4-7   The sharply demarcated, characteristic scaling dermatitis of pellagra. (From James WD, Berger TG, Elston DM: Andrews' Diseases of the Skin: Clinical Dermatology, Philadelphia, Saunders Elsevier, 2006)

Item 4–7   Pellagra is associated with a deficiency of niacin and its precursor, **tryptophan.** Characteristics of the condition include diarrhea, dermatitis on exposed skin surfaces, dementia, and death. It is prevalent in developing countries where nutrition is inadequate. **Beriberi** is associated with thiamine deficiency.

CHAPTER 4 (E00-E90)

N   Newborn Age: 0   P   Pediatric Age: 0–17   M   Maternity DX: 12–55   A   Adult Age: 15–124   ♀   Females Only   ♂   Males Only

🔖   Complication\Comorbidity   🔖   Major C\C   (Ex)   CC/MCC Exclusions   🔖   Hospital-Acquired Condition

CHAPTER 4 (E00-E90)

● **E53** **Deficiency of other B group vitamins**
    Excludes1 sequelae of vitamin B deficiency (E64.8)

    E53.0 **Riboflavin deficiency** 🔗
        Ariboflavinosis
        Vitamin B2 deficiency
        (Ex) See PDX Collection 531

    E53.1 **Pyridoxine deficiency**
        Vitamin B6 deficiency
        Excludes1 pyridoxine-responsive sideroblastic anemia (D64.3)

    E53.8 **Deficiency of other specified B group vitamins**
        Biotin deficiency
        Cyanocobalamin deficiency
        Folate deficiency
        Folic acid deficiency
        Pantothenic acid deficiency
        Vitamin B12 deficiency
        Excludes1 folate deficiency anemia (D52.-)
                     vitamin B12 deficiency anemia (D51.-)

    E53.9 **Vitamin B deficiency, unspecified**

● **E54** **Ascorbic acid deficiency**
    Deficiency of vitamin C
    Scurvy
    Excludes1 scorbutic anemia (D53.2)
                sequelae of vitamin C deficiency (E64.2)

● **E55** **Vitamin D deficiency**
    Excludes1 adult osteomalacia (M83.-)
               osteoporosis (M80.-)
               sequelae of rickets (E64.3)

    E55.0 **Rickets, active** 🔗
        Infantile osteomalacia
        Juvenile osteomalacia
        Softening of bone
        Excludes1 celiac rickets (K90.0)
                 Crohn's rickets (K50.-)
                 hereditary vitamin D-dependent rickets (E83.32)
                 inactive rickets (E64.3)
                 renal rickets (N25.0)
                 sequelae of rickets (E64.3)
                 vitamin D-resistant rickets (E83.31)
        (Ex) See PDX Collection 532

    E55.9 **Vitamin D deficiency, unspecified**
        Avitaminosis D

● **E56** **Other vitamin deficiencies**
    Excludes1 sequelae of other vitamin deficiencies (E64.8)

    E56.0 **Deficiency of vitamin E**

    E56.1 **Deficiency of vitamin K**
        Excludes1 deficiency of coagulation factor due to vitamin K deficiency (D68.4)
                 vitamin K deficiency of newborn (P53)

    E56.8 **Deficiency of other vitamins**

    E56.9 **Vitamin deficiency, unspecified**

● **E58** **Dietary calcium deficiency**
    Excludes1 disorders of calcium metabolism (E83.5-)
                sequelae of calcium deficiency (E64.8)

● **E59** **Dietary selenium deficiency**
    Keshan disease
    Excludes1 sequelae of selenium deficiency (E64.8)

● **E60** **Dietary zinc deficiency**

● **E61** **Deficiency of other nutrient elements**
    Use additional code for adverse effect, if applicable, to identify drug (T36-T50 with fifth or sixth character 5)
    Excludes1 disorders of mineral metabolism (E83.-)
                iodine deficiency related thyroid disorders (E00-E02)
                sequelae of malnutrition and other nutritional deficiencies (E64.-)

    E61.0 **Copper deficiency**

    E61.1 **Iron deficiency**
        Excludes1 iron deficiency anemia (D50.-)

    E61.2 **Magnesium deficiency**

    E61.3 **Manganese deficiency**

    E61.4 **Chromium deficiency**

    E61.5 **Molybdenum deficiency**

    E61.6 **Vanadium deficiency**

    E61.7 **Deficiency of multiple nutrient elements**

    E61.8 **Deficiency of other specified nutrient elements**

    E61.9 **Deficiency of nutrient element, unspecified**

● **E63** **Other nutritional deficiencies**
    Excludes1 dehydration (E86.0)
                failure to thrive, adult (R62.7)
                failure to thrive, child (R62.51)
                feeding problems in newborn (P92.-)
                sequelae of malnutrition and other nutritional deficiencies (E64.-)

    E63.0 **Essential fatty acid [EFA] deficiency**

    E63.1 **Imbalance of constituents of food intake**

    E63.8 **Other specified nutritional deficiencies**

    E63.9 **Nutritional deficiency, unspecified**

● **E64** **Sequelae of malnutrition and other nutritional deficiencies**
    Pathological condition resulting from disease, injury, or other trauma
    Note: This category is to be used to indicate conditions in categories E43, E44, E46, E50-E63 as the cause of sequelae, which are themselves classified elsewhere. The 'sequelae' include conditions specified as such; they also include the late effects of diseases classifiable to the above categories if the disease itself is no longer present
    Code first condition resulting from (sequela) of malnutrition and other nutritional deficiencies

    E64.0 **Sequelae of protein-calorie malnutrition** 🔗
        Excludes2 retarded development following protein-calorie malnutrition (E45)
        (Ex) See PDX Collection 530

    E64.1 **Sequelae of vitamin A deficiency**

    E64.2 **Sequelae of vitamin C deficiency**

    E64.3 **Sequelae of rickets**

    E64.8 **Sequelae of other nutritional deficiencies**

    E64.9 **Sequelae of unspecified nutritional deficiency**

▶ New   ⇒ Revised   ~~deleted~~ Deleted   Excludes 1   Excludes 2   Includes   Use additional   Code first   Code also   Key words
OGCR Official Guidelines   ● Unacceptable Principal Diagnosis   X Assign placeholder X   ● Use Additional Character(s)   ▶ Manifestation Code   **Coding Clinic**

OVERWEIGHT, OBESITY AND OTHER HYPERALIMENTATION (E65-E68)

E65   Localized adiposity
     Fat pad

● E66   Overweight and obesity

     Code first obesity complicating pregnancy, childbirth and the puerperium, if applicable (O99.21-)

     Use additional code to identify body mass index (BMI), if known (Z68.-)

     Excludes1   adiposogenital dystrophy (E23.6)
                          lipomatosis NOS (E88.2)
                          lipomatosis dolorosa [Dercum] (E88.2)
                          Prader-Willi syndrome (Q87.1)

   ● E66.0   Obesity due to excess calories

       E66.01   Morbid (severe) obesity due to excess calories 🔹

            Excludes1   morbid (severe) obesity with alveolar hypoventilation (E66.2)

       E66.09   Other obesity due to excess calories
              MCE: Questionable admission when principal dx

   E66.1   Drug-induced obesity
        MCE: Questionable admission when principal dx
        Use additional code for adverse effect, if applicable, to identify drug (T36-T50 with fifth or sixth character 5)

   E66.2   Morbid (severe) obesity with alveolar hypoventilation 🔹
        Uncommon condition of unknown cause leading to inadequate ventilation in lungs, even though lungs and airways are normal
        Obesity hypoventilation syndrome (OHS)
        Pickwickian syndrome
        (Ex) See PDX Collection 533

   E66.3   Overweight

   E66.8   Other obesity
        MCE: Questionable admission when principal dx

   E66.9   Obesity, unspecified
        Obesity NOS
        MCE: Questionable admission when principal dx

● E67   Other hyperalimentation
     Ingestion of more than optimal amount of nutrients

     Excludes1   hyperalimentation NOS (R63.2)
                          sequelae of hyperalimentation (E68)

   E67.0   Hypervitaminosis A

   E67.1   Hypercarotinemia

   E67.2   Megavitamin-B6 syndrome

   E67.3   Hypervitaminosis D

   E67.8   Other specified hyperalimentation

E68   Sequelae of hyperalimentation
     Code first condition resulting from (sequela) of hyperalimentation

METABOLIC DISORDERS (E70-E88)

     Excludes1   androgen insensitivity syndrome (E34.5-)
                          congenital adrenal hyperplasia (E25.0)
                          Ehlers-Danlos syndrome (Q79.6)
                          hemolytic anemias attributable to enzyme disorders (D55.-)
                          Marfan's syndrome (Q87.4)
                          5-alpha-reductase deficiency (E29.1)

● E70   Disorders of aromatic amino-acid metabolism
     (Ex) **For category E70 CC codes:** See PDX Collection 534

   E70.0   Classical phenylketonuria 🔹
        Inherited disorder that increases to harmful levels amino acid phenylalanine

   E70.1   Other hyperphenylalaninemias 🔹

● E70.2   Disorders of tyrosine metabolism
     Excludes1   transitory tyrosinemia of newborn (P74.5)

   E70.20   Disorder of tyrosine metabolism, unspecified 🔹
        Tyrosine: Nonessential amino acid occurring in most proteins

   E70.21   Tyrosinemia 🔹
        Congenital amino acid metabolism
        Hypertyrosinemia

   E70.29   Other disorders of tyrosine metabolism 🔹
        Alkaptonuria
        Ochronosis

● E70.3   Albinism
     Congenital condition of reduced or absent pigment in eyes, skin, and hair

   E70.30   Albinism, unspecified 🔹

   ● E70.31   Ocular albinism
       E70.310   X-linked ocular albinism 🔹
       E70.311   Autosomal recessive ocular albinism 🔹
       E70.318   Other ocular albinism 🔹
       E70.319   Ocular albinism, unspecified 🔹

   ● E70.32   Oculocutaneous albinism
       Partial or total lack of melanin pigment in eyes

       Excludes1   Chediak-Higashi syndrome (E70.330)
                          Hermansky-Pudlak syndrome (E70.331)

       E70.320   Tyrosinase negative oculocutaneous albinism 🔹
            Albinism I
            Oculocutaneous albinism ty-neg

       E70.321   Tyrosinase positive oculocutaneous albinism 🔹
            Albinism II
            Oculocutaneous albinism ty-pos

       E70.328   Other oculocutaneous albinism 🔹
            Cross syndrome

       E70.329   Oculocutaneous albinism, unspecified 🔹

   ● E70.33   Albinism with hematologic abnormality
       E70.330   Chediak-Higashi syndrome 🔹
       E70.331   Hermansky-Pudlak syndrome 🔹
       E70.338   Other albinism with hematologic abnormality 🔹
       E70.339   Albinism with hematologic abnormality, unspecified 🔹

   E70.39   Other specified albinism 🔹
        Piebaldism

● E70.4   Disorders of histidine metabolism
   E70.40   Disorders of histidine metabolism, unspecified 🔹
   E70.41   Histidinemia 🔹
   E70.49   Other disorders of histidine metabolism 🔹

E70.5   Disorders of tryptophan metabolism 🔹

E70.8   Other disorders of aromatic amino-acid metabolism 🔹

E70.9   Disorder of aromatic amino-acid metabolism, unspecified 🔹

N Newborn Age: 0   **P** Pediatric Age: 0–17   **M** Maternity DX: 12–55   **A** Adult Age: 15–124   ♀ Females Only   ♂ Males Only

🔹 Complication\Comorbidity   🔹 Major C\C   (Ex) CC/MCC Exclusions   🔹 Hospital-Acquired Condition

747

CHAPTER 4 (E00-E90)

● E71   **Disorders of branched-chain amino-acid metabolism and fatty-acid metabolism**

    E71.0   **Maple-syrup-urine disease** 🔑
        Due to defect in amino acid catabolism, causing severe ketoacidosis with smell of maple syrup in urine and on body
        Ⓔ See PDX Collection 534

●   **E71.1**   **Other disorders of branched-chain amino-acid metabolism**
        Ⓔ **For category E71.1 CC codes:** See PDX Collection 534

●   **E71.11**   **Branched-chain organic acidurias**
        E71.110   **Isovaleric acidemia** 🔑
        E71.111   **3-methylglutaconic aciduria** 🔑
        E71.118   **Other branched-chain organic acidurias** 🔑

●   **E71.12**   **Disorders of propionate metabolism**
        E71.120   **Methylmalonic acidemia** 🔑
        E71.121   **Propionic acidemia** 🔑
        E71.128   **Other disorders of propionate metabolism** 🔑

      E71.19   **Other disorders of branched-chain amino-acid metabolism** 🔑
        Hyperleucine-isoleucinemia
        Hypervalinemia

    E71.2   **Disorder of branched-chain amino-acid metabolism, unspecified** 🔑
        Ⓔ See PDX Collection 534

●   **E71.3**   **Disorders of fatty-acid metabolism**
      Excludes1   peroxisomal disorders (E71.5)
                Refsum's disease (G60.1)
                Schilder's disease (G37.0)
      Excludes2   carnitine deficiency due to inborn error of metabolism (E71.42)

      E71.30   **Disorder of fatty-acid metabolism, unspecified**
●   **E71.31**   **Disorders of fatty-acid oxidation**
        Ⓔ **For category E71.31 CC codes:** See PDX Collection 535

        E71.310   **Long chain/very long chain acyl CoA dehydrogenase deficiency** 🔑
            LCAD
            VLCAD

        E71.311   **Medium chain acyl CoA dehydrogenase deficiency** 🔑
            MCAD

        E71.312   **Short chain acyl CoA dehydrogenase deficiency** 🔑
            SCAD

        E71.313   **Glutaric aciduria type II** 🔑
            Glutaric aciduria type II A
            Glutaric aciduria type II B
            Glutaric aciduria type II C
            Excludes1   glutaric aciduria (type 1) NOS (E72.3)

        E71.314   **Muscle carnitine palmitoyltransferase deficiency** 🔑
        E71.318   **Other disorders of fatty-acid oxidation** 🔑

      E71.32   **Disorders of ketone metabolism** 🔑
        Ⓔ See PDX Collection 535

      E71.39   **Other disorders of fatty-acid metabolism** 🔑
        Ⓔ See PDX Collection 492

●   **E71.4**   **Disorders of carnitine metabolism**
      Excludes1   muscle carnitine palmitoyltransferase deficiency (E71.314)

      E71.40   **Disorder of carnitine metabolism, unspecified**
      E71.41   **Primary carnitine deficiency**
      E71.42   **Carnitine deficiency due to inborn errors of metabolism**
        Code also associated inborn error or metabolism

      E71.43   **Iatrogenic carnitine deficiency**
        Iatrogenic: Outcomes from activity of physicians
        Carnitine deficiency due to hemodialysis
        Carnitine deficiency due to Valproic acid therapy

●   **E71.44**   **Other secondary carnitine deficiency**
        E71.440   **Ruvalcaba-Myhre-Smith syndrome**
        E71.448   **Other secondary carnitine deficiency**

●   **E71.5**   **Peroxisomal disorders**
      Class of conditions which lead to disorders of lipid metabolism
      Excludes1   Schilder's disease (G37.0)
      Ⓔ **For category E71.5 CC codes:** See PDX Collection 536

      E71.50   **Peroxisomal disorder, unspecified** 🔑
●   **E71.51**   **Disorders of peroxisome biogenesis**
        Group 1 peroxisomal disorders
        Excludes1   Refsum's disease (G60.1)

        E71.510   **Zellweger syndrome** 🔑
        E71.511   **Neonatal adrenoleukodystrophy** 🔑
            Excludes1   X-linked adrenoleuko-dystrophy (E71.42-)

        E71.518   **Other disorders of peroxisome biogenesis** 🔑

●   **E71.52**   **X-linked adrenoleukodystrophy**
        E71.520   **Childhood cerebral X-linked adrenoleukodystrophy** 🔑
        E71.521   **Adolescent X-linked adrenoleukodystrophy** 🔑
        E71.522   **Adrenomyeloneuropathy** 🔑
        E71.528   **Other X-linked adrenoleukodystrophy** 🔑
            Addison only phenotype adrenoleukodystrophy
            Addison-Schilder adrenoleukodystrophy

        E71.529   **X-linked adrenoleukodystrophy, unspecified type** 🔑

      E71.53   **Other group 2 peroxisomal disorders** 🔑
●   **E71.54**   **Other peroxisomal disorders**
        E71.540   **Rhizomelic chondrodysplasia punctata** 🔑
            Rare, severe, inherited disorder with limb shortening, bone and cartilage abnormalities, abnormal facial appearance, severe mental retardation, psychomotor retardation, and cataracts
            Excludes1   chondrodysplasia punctata NOS (Q77.3)

        E71.541   **Zellweger-like syndrome** 🔑
        E71.542   **Other group 3 peroxisomal disorders** 🔑
        E71.548   **Other peroxisomal disorders** 🔑

▶ New   ⇒ Revised   ~~deleted~~ Deleted   Excludes 1   Excludes 2   Includes   Use additional   Code first   Code also   Key words

OGCR Official Guidelines   ● Unacceptable Principal Diagnosis   X Assign placeholder X   ● Use Additional Character(s)   ▸ Manifestation Code   **Coding Clinic**

● **E72   Other disorders of amino-acid metabolism**

     Excludes1   disorders of:
         aromatic amino-acid metabolism (E70.-)
         branched-chain amino-acid metabolism
           (E71.0-E71.2)
         fatty-acid metabolism (E71.3)
         purine and pyrimidine metabolism (E79.-)
         gout (M1A.-, M10.-)

     (Ex) **For category E72 CC codes unless otherwise noted:** See PDX Collection 534

● **E72.0   Disorders of amino-acid transport**

     Excludes1   disorders of tryptophan metabolism
          (E70.5)

   **E72.00   Disorders of amino-acid
          transport, unspecified**

   E72.01   Cystinuria
         *Hereditary aminoaciduria due to impairment of
         renal transport with predominant symptom of
         urinary cystine calculi*

   E72.02   Hartnup's disease
         Inborn error of metabolism

   E72.03   Lowe's syndrome
         *X-linked disorder with rickets, hydrophthalmia,
         congenital glaucoma, cataracts, mental
         retardation, and renal tubule dysfunction*

         Use additional code for associated glaucoma
          (H42)
         (Ex) No exclusion

   E72.04   Cystinosis
         *Genetic disease with excessive depostits of amino
         acid cystine in cells*
         Fanconi (-de Toni) (-Debré) syndrome with
          cystinosis

       Excludes1   Fanconi (-de Toni) (-Debré)
            syndrome without
            cystinosis (E72.09)

   E72.09   Other disorders of amino-acid transport
         Fanconi (-de Toni) (-Debré) syndrome,
          unspecified

● **E72.1   Disorders of sulfur-bearing amino-acid metabolism**

     Excludes1   cystinosis (E72.04)
          cystinuria (E72.01)
          transcobalamin II deficiency (D51.2)

   **E72.10   Disorders of sulfur-bearing amino-acid
          metabolism, unspecified**

   E72.11   Homocystinuria
         Cystathionine synthase deficiency

   **E72.12   Methylenetetrahydrofolate reductase
          deficiency**

   **E72.19   Other disorders of sulfur-bearing amino-acid
          metabolism**
         Cystathioninuria
         Methioninemia
         Sulfite oxidase deficiency

● **E72.2   Disorders of urea cycle metabolism**

     Excludes1   disorders of ornithine metabolism (E72.4)

   **E72.20   Disorder of urea cycle
          metabolism, unspecified**
         Hyperammonemia
         Elevated levels of ammonia

       Excludes1   hyperammonemia-
            hyperornithinemia-
            homocitrullinemia
            syndrome E72.4
            transient hyperammonemia of
            newborn (P74.6)

   E72.21   Argininemia
         *Disorder in which deficiency of enzyme arginase
         causes build up of arginine and ammonia in
         blood*

   E72.22   Arginosuccinic aciduria
         *Gene disorder of urea cycle resulting accumulation
         of ammonia*

   E72.23   Citrullinemia
         *Urea cycle disorder that causes ammonia and other
         toxic substances to accumulate in blood*

   E72.29   Other disorders of urea cycle metabolism

● **E72.3   Disorders of lysine and hydroxylysine metabolism**
       Glutaric aciduria NOS
       Glutaric aciduria (type I)
       Hydroxylysinemia
       Hyperlysinemia

     Excludes1   glutaric aciduria type II (E71.313)
          Refsum's disease (G60.1)
          Zellweger syndrome (E71.510)

● **E72.4   Disorders of ornithine metabolism**
       Hyperammonemia-Hyperornithinemia-
         Homocitrullinemia syndrome
       Ornithinemia (types I, II)
       Ornithine transcarbamylase deficiency

     Excludes1   hereditary choroidal dystrophy (H31.2-)

● **E72.5   Disorders of glycine metabolism**

   E72.50   Disorder of glycine metabolism, unspecified

   E72.51   Non-ketotic hyperglycinemia

   E72.52   Trimethylaminuria

   E72.53   Hyperoxaluria
         Oxalosis
         Oxaluria

   E72.59   Other disorders of glycine metabolism
         D-glycericacidemia
         Hyperhydroxyprolinemia
         Hyperprolinemia (types I, II)
         Sarcosinemia

   E72.8   Other specified disorders of amino-acid metabolism
       Disorders of beta-amino-acid metabolism
       Disorders of gamma-glutamyl cycle

   E72.9   Disorder of amino-acid metabolism, unspecified

● **E73   Lactose intolerance**
     *Intolerance for lactose, due to inherited deficiency of lactase activity in
     intestinal mucosa*

   E73.0   Congenital lactase deficiency

   E73.1   Secondary lactase deficiency

   E73.8   Other lactose intolerance

   E73.9   Lactose intolerance, unspecified

● **E74   Other disorders of carbohydrate metabolism**

     Excludes1   diabetes mellitus (E08-E13)
          hypoglycemia NOS (E16.2)
          increased secretion of glucagon (E16.3)
          mucopolysaccharidosis (E76.0-E76.3)

     (Ex) **For category E74 CC codes:** See PDX Collection 534

● **E74.0   Glycogen storage disease**

   E74.00   Glycogen storage disease, unspecified

   E74.01   von Gierke's disease
         Type I glycogen storage disease

   E74.02   Pompe disease
         Cardiac glycogenosis
         Type II glycogen storage disease

   E74.03   Cori disease
         Forbes' disease
         Type III glycogen storage disease

   E74.04   McArdle disease
         Type V glycogen storage disease

   E74.09   Other glycogen storage disease
         Andersen disease
         Hers disease
         Tauri disease
         Glycogen storage disease, types 0, IV, VI-XI
         Liver phosphorylase deficiency
         Muscle phosphofructokinase deficiency

CHAPTER 4 (E00-E90)

CHAPTER 4 (E00-E90)

● E74.1 **Disorders of fructose metabolism**
   Excludes1   muscle phosphofructokinase deficiency (E74.09)

   E74.10 **Disorder of fructose metabolism, unspecified**

   E74.11 **Essential fructosuria**
      Fructokinase deficiency

   E74.12 **Hereditary fructose intolerance**
      Fructosemia

   E74.19 **Other disorders of fructose metabolism**
      Fructose-1, 6-diphosphatase deficiency

● E74.2 **Disorders of galactose metabolism**

   E74.20 **Disorders of galactose metabolism, unspecified**

   E74.21 **Galactosemia**
      Genetic disorders resulting from defective simple sugar (galactose) metabolism

   E74.29 **Other disorders of galactose metabolism**
      Galactokinase deficiency

● E74.3 **Other disorders of intestinal carbohydrate absorption**
   Excludes2 lactose intolerance (E73.-)

   E74.31 **Sucrase-isomaltase deficiency**
      Deficiency in metabolism in intestinal mucosa results in malabsorption of sucrose and starch

   E74.39 **Other disorders of intestinal carbohydrate absorption**
      Disorder of intestinal carbohydrate absorption NOS
      Glucose-galactose malabsorption
      Sucrase deficiency

● E74.4 **Disorders of pyruvate metabolism and gluconeogenesis**
     Deficiency of phosphoenolpyruvate carboxykinase
     Deficiency of pyruvate carboxylase
     Deficiency of pyruvate dehydrogenase
   Excludes1 disorders of pyruvate metabolism and gluconeogenesis with anemia (D55.-)
             Leigh's syndrome (G31.82)

  E74.8 **Other specified disorders of carbohydrate metabolism**
     Essential pentosuria
     Renal glycosuria

  E74.9 **Disorder of carbohydrate metabolism, unspecified**

● E75 **Disorders of sphingolipid metabolism and other lipid storage disorders**
   Excludes1 mucolipidosis, types I-III (E77.0-E77.1)
            Refsum's disease (G60.1)

● E75.0 **GM2 gangliosidosis**
   Rare metabolic disorder that causes destruction of nerve cells of brain and spinal cord
   (Ex:) **For category E75.0 CC codes: See PDX Collection 537**

   E75.00 **GM2 gangliosidosis, unspecified**

   E75.01 **Sandhoff disease**

   E75.02 **Tay-Sachs disease**

   E75.09 **Other GM2 gangliosidosis**
      Adult GM2 gangliosidosis
      Juvenile GM2 gangliosidosis

● E75.1 **Other and unspecified gangliosidosis**
   (Ex:) **For category E75.1 CC codes: See PDX Collection 537**

   E75.10 **Unspecified gangliosidosis**
      Gangliosidosis NOS

   E75.11 **Mucolipidosis IV**
      Disorder with symptoms of psychomotor retardation and severe visual impairment

   E75.19 **Other gangliosidosis**
      GM1 gangliosidosis
      GM3 gangliosidosis

Item 4–8 **Leukodystrophy** is characterized by degeneration and/or failure of the myelin formation of the central nervous system and sometimes of the peripheral nervous system. The disease is inherited and progressive.

● E75.2 **Other sphingolipidosis**
   Lysosomal (a particle in a cytoplasm cell that contains digestive enzymes) storage diseases with symptoms of abnormal storage of amino acids
   Excludes1 adrenoleukodystrophy [Addison-Schilder] (E71.528)

   E75.21 **Fabry (-Anderson) disease**

   E75.22 **Gaucher disease**

   E75.23 **Krabbe disease**
      (Ex:) See PDX Collection 538

  ● E75.24 **Niemann-Pick disease**

     E75.240 **Niemann-Pick disease type A**
     E75.241 **Niemann-Pick disease type B**
     E75.242 **Niemann-Pick disease type C**
     E75.243 **Niemann-Pick disease type D**
     E75.248 **Other Niemann-Pick disease**
     E75.249 **Niemann-Pick disease, unspecified**

   E75.25 **Metachromatic leukodystrophy**
      (Ex:) See PDX Collection 538

   E75.29 **Other sphingolipidosis**
      Farber's syndrome
      Sulfatase deficiency
      Sulfatide lipidosis
      (Ex:) See PDX Collection 538

  E75.3 **Sphingolipidosis, unspecified**

  E75.4 **Neuronal ceroid lipofuscinosis**
     Batten disease
     Bielschowsky-Jansky disease
     Kufs disease
     Spielmeyer-Vogt disease
     (Ex:) See PDX Collection 537

  E75.5 **Other lipid storage disorders**
     Cerebrotendinous cholesterosis [van Bogaert-Scherer-Epstein]
     Wolman's disease

  E75.6 **Lipid storage disorder, unspecified**

● E76 **Disorders of glycosaminoglycan metabolism**
   (Ex:) For category E76 CC codes: See PDX Collection 539

  ● E76.0 **Mucopolysaccharidosis, type I**
   Inborn metabolic disorder of enzymes that break down carbohydrates

   E76.01 **Hurler's syndrome**
   E76.02 **Hurler-Scheie syndrome**
   E76.03 **Scheie's syndrome**

  E76.1 **Mucopolysaccharidosis, type II**
   Inborn metabolic disorder of enzymes that break down carbohydrates occurs in 2-4 year old males
   Hunter's syndrome

  ● E76.2 **Other mucopolysaccharidoses**

  ● E76.21 **Morquio mucopolysaccharidoses**

     E76.210 **Morquio A mucopolysaccharidoses**
       Classic Morquio syndrome
       Morquio syndrome A
       Mucopolysaccharidosis, type IVA

     E76.211 **Morquio B mucopolysaccharidoses**
       Morquio-like mucopolysaccharidoses
       Morquio-like syndrome
       Morquio syndrome B
       Mucopolysaccharidosis, type IVB

     E76.219 **Morquio mucopolysaccharidoses, unspecified**
       Morquio syndrome
       Mucopolysaccharidosis, type IV

▶ New   ⇒ Revised   ~~deleted~~ Deleted   Excludes 1   Excludes 2   Includes   Use additional   Code first   Code also   Key words
OGCR Official Guidelines   ● Unacceptable Principal Diagnosis   X Assign placeholder X   ● Use Additional Character(s)   ▶ Manifestation Code   **Coding Clinic**

E76.22   **Sanfilippo mucopolysaccharidoses** 🔖
  Mucopolysaccharidosis, type III (A) (B) (C) (D)
  Sanfilippo A syndrome
  Sanfilippo B syndrome
  Sanfilippo C syndrome
  Sanfilippo D syndrome

E76.29   **Other mucopolysaccharidoses** 🔖
  beta-Glucuronidase deficiency
  Maroteaux-Lamy (mild) (severe) syndrome
  Mucopolysaccharidosis, types VI, VII

E76.3   **Mucopolysaccharidosis, unspecified** 🔖

E76.8   **Other disorders of glucosaminoglycan metabolism** 🔖

E76.9   **Glucosaminoglycan metabolism disorder, unspecified** 🔖

● **E77   Disorders of glycoprotein metabolism**

E77.0   **Defects in post-translational modification of lysosomal enzymes**
  Mucolipidosis II [I-cell disease]
  Mucolipidosis III [pseudo-Hurler polydystrophy]

E77.1   **Defects in glycoprotein degradation**
  Aspartylglucosaminuria
  Fucosidosis
  Mannosidosis
  Sialidosis [mucolipidosis I]

E77.8   **Other disorders of glycoprotein metabolism**

E77.9   **Disorder of glycoprotein metabolism, unspecified**

● **E78   Disorders of lipoprotein metabolism and other lipidemias**
  Excludes1   sphingolipidosis (E75.0-E75.3)

● E78.0   **Pure hypercholesterolemia**
  Coding Clinic: 2016, Q4, P13

E78.00   **Pure hypercholesterolemia, unspecified**
  Fredrickson's hyperlipoproteinemia, type IIa
  Hyperbetalipoproteinemia
  Low-density-lipoprotein-type [LDL] hyperlipoproteinemia
  ▶ (Pure) hypercholesterolemia NOS
  Coding Clinic: 2016, Q4, P13

E78.01   **Familial hypercholesterolemia**
  Coding Clinic: 2016, Q4, P13

E78.1   **Pure hyperglyceridemia**
  Elevated fasting triglycerides
  Endogenous hyperglyceridemia
  Fredrickson's hyperlipoproteinemia, type IV
  Hyperlipidemia, group B
  Hyperprebetalipoproteinemia
  Very-low-density-lipoprotein-type [VLDL] hyperlipoproteinemia

E78.2   **Mixed hyperlipidemia**
  Broad- or floating-betalipoproteinemia
  Combined hyperlipidemia NOS
  Elevated cholesterol with elevated triglycerides NEC
  Fredrickson's hyperlipoproteinemia, type IIb or III
  Hyperbetalipoproteinemia with prebetalipoproteinemia
  Hypercholesteremia with endogenous hyperglyceridemia
  Hyperlipidemia, group C
  Tubo-eruptive xanthoma
  Xanthoma tuberosum
  Excludes1   cerebrotendinous cholesterosis [van Bogaert-Scherer-Epstein] (E75.5)
  familial combined hyperlipidemia (E78.4)

E78.3   **Hyperchylomicronemia**
  Chylomicron retention disease
  Fredrickson's hyperlipoproteinemia, type I or V
  Hyperlipidemia, group D
  Mixed hyperglyceridemia

E78.4   **Other hyperlipidemia**
  Familial combined hyperlipidemia

E78.5   **Hyperlipidemia, unspecified**

E78.6   **Lipoprotein deficiency**
  Abetalipoproteinemia
  Depressed HDL cholesterol
  High-density lipoprotein deficiency
  Hypoalphalipoproteinemia
  Hypobetalipoproteinemia (familial)
  Lecithin cholesterol acyltransferase deficiency
  Tangier disease

● E78.7   **Disorders of bile acid and cholesterol metabolism**
  Excludes1   Niemann-Pick disease type C (E75.242)
  🔖 For category E78.7 CC codes: See PDX Collection 540

E78.70   **Disorder of bile acid and cholesterol metabolism, unspecified**

E78.71   **Barth syndrome** 🔖

E78.72   **Smith-Lemli-Opitz syndrome** 🔖

E78.79   **Other disorders of bile acid and cholesterol metabolism**

● E78.8   **Other disorders of lipoprotein metabolism**

E78.81   **Lipoid dermatoarthritis**

E78.89   **Other lipoprotein metabolism disorders**

E78.9   **Disorder of lipoprotein metabolism, unspecified**

● **E79   Disorders of purine and pyrimidine metabolism**
  Purines, along with pyrimidines, signal RNA and DNA production
  Excludes1   Ataxia-telangiectasia (Q87.1)
  Bloom's syndrome (Q82.8)
  Cockayne's syndrome (Q87.1)
  calculus of kidney (N20.0)
  combined immunodeficiency disorders (D81.-)
  Fanconi's anemia (D61.09)
  gout (M1A.-, M10.-)
  orotaciduric anemia (D53.0)
  progeria (E34.8)
  Werner's syndrome (E34.8)
  xeroderma pigmentosum (Q82.1)
  🔖 For category E79 CC codes: See PDX Collection 513

E79.0   **Hyperuricemia without signs of inflammatory arthritis and tophaceous disease**
  Asymptomatic hyperuricemia

E79.1   **Lesch-Nyhan syndrome** 🔖
  HGPRT deficiency

E79.2   **Myoadenylate deaminase deficiency** 🔖

E79.8   **Other disorders of purine and pyrimidine metabolism** 🔖
  Hereditary xanthinuria

E79.9   **Disorder of purine and pyrimidine metabolism, unspecified** 🔖

● **E80   Disorders of porphyrin and bilirubin metabolism**
  Group of chemical compounds in RBC's that combine with iron to form heme
  Includes   defects of catalase and peroxidase
  🔖 For category E80 CC codes unless otherwise indicated: See PDX Collection 513

E80.0   **Hereditary erythropoietic porphyria** 🔖
  Congenital erythropoietic porphyria
  Erythropoietic protoporphyria

E80.1   **Porphyria cutanea tarda** 🔖

● E80.2   **Other and unspecified porphyria**

E80.20   **Unspecified porphyria** 🔖
  Porphyria NOS

E80.21   **Acute intermittent (hepatic) porphyria** 🔖

E80.29   **Other porphyria** 🔖
  Hereditary coproporphyria

E80.3   **Defects of catalase and peroxidase** 🔖
  Acatalasia [Takahara]
  🔖 See PDX Collection 492

E80.4   **Gilbert syndrome**

E80.5   **Crigler-Najjar syndrome**

E80.6   **Other disorders of bilirubin metabolism**
  Dubin-Johnson syndrome
  Rotor's syndrome

E80.7   **Disorder of bilirubin metabolism, unspecified**

CHAPTER 4 (E00-E90)

● **E83**   **Disorders of mineral metabolism**
    Excludes1   dietary mineral deficiency (E58-E61)
           parathyroid disorders (E20-E21)
           vitamin D deficiency (E55.-)

● **E83.0**   **Disorders of copper metabolism**
    E83.00   **Disorder of copper metabolism, unspecified**
    E83.01   **Wilson's disease**
        Code also associated Kayser Fleischer ring
        (H18.04-)
    E83.09   **Other disorders of copper metabolism**
        Menkes' (kinky hair) (steely hair) disease

● **E83.1**   **Disorders of iron metabolism**
    Excludes1   iron deficiency anemia (D50.-)
           sideroblastic anemia (D64.0-D64.3)
    E83.10   **Disorder of iron metabolism, unspecified**
  ● **E83.11**   **Hemochromatosis**
      ▶ **Excludes1**   GALD (P78.84)
          ▶Gestational alloimmune liver
            disease (P78.84)
          ▶Neonatal hemochromatosis
            (P78.84)
      E83.110   **Hereditary hemochromatosis**
          Bronzed diabetes
          Pigmentary cirrhosis (of liver)
          Primary (hereditary)
            hemochromatosis
      E83.111   **Hemochromatosis due to repeated red blood cell transfusions**
          Iron overload due to repeated red
            blood cell transfusions
          Transfusion (red blood cell)
            associated hemochromatosis
      E83.118   **Other hemochromatosis**
      E83.119   **Hemochromatosis, unspecified**
    E83.19   **Other disorders of iron metabolism**
        Use additional code, if applicable, for
        idiopathic pulmonary hemosiderosis
        (J84.03)

   E83.2   **Disorders of zinc metabolism**
        Acrodermatitis enteropathica

● **E83.3**   **Disorders of phosphorus metabolism and phosphatases**
    Excludes1   adult osteomalacia (M83.-)
           osteoporosis (M80.-)
    E83.30   **Disorder of phosphorus metabolism, unspecified**
    E83.31   **Familial hypophosphatemia**
        Vitamin D-resistant osteomalacia
        Vitamin D-resistant rickets
      Excludes1   vitamin D-deficiency rickets
            (E55.0)
    E83.32   **Hereditary vitamin D-dependent rickets (type 1) (type 2)**
        25-hydroxyvitamin D 1-alpha-hydroxylase
          deficiency
        Pseudovitamin D deficiency
        Vitamin D receptor defect
    E83.39   **Other disorders of phosphorus metabolism**
        Acid phosphatase deficiency
        Hypophosphatasia

● **E83.4**   **Disorders of magnesium metabolism**
    E83.40   **Disorders of magnesium metabolism, unspecified**
    E83.41   **Hypermagnesemia**
        Coding Clinic: 2016, Q4, P55
    E83.42   **Hypomagnesemia**
    E83.49   **Other disorders of magnesium metabolism**

● **E83.5**   **Disorders of calcium metabolism**
    Excludes1   chondrocalcinosis (M11.1-M11.2)
           hungry bone syndrome (E83.81)
           hyperparathyroidism (E21.0-E21.3)
    E83.50   **Unspecified disorder of calcium metabolism**
    E83.51   **Hypocalcemia**
    E83.52   **Hypercalcemia**
        Familial hypocalciuric hypercalcemia
    E83.59   **Other disorders of calcium metabolism**
        Idiopathic hypercalciuria

● **E83.8**   **Other disorders of mineral metabolism**
    E83.81   **Hungry bone syndrome**
    E83.89   **Other disorders of mineral metabolism**

   E83.9   **Disorder of mineral metabolism, unspecified**

● **E84**   **Cystic fibrosis**
    Includes   mucoviscidosis
        Code also exocrine pancreatic insufficiency (K86.81)
        (Ex) **For category E84 CC codes: See PDX Collection 541**

   E84.0   **Cystic fibrosis with pulmonary manifestations** 🔗
        Use additional code to identify any infectious organism
        present, such as:
        Pseudomonas (B96.5)

● **E84.1**   **Cystic fibrosis with intestinal manifestations**
    E84.11   **Meconium ileus in cystic fibrosis** 🔗   N
      Excludes1   meconium ileus not due to cystic
            fibrosis (P76.0)
    E84.19   **Cystic fibrosis with other intestinal manifestations** 🔗
        Distal intestinal obstruction syndrome

   E84.8   **Cystic fibrosis with other manifestations** 🔗
   E84.9   **Cystic fibrosis, unspecified** 🔗

● **E85**   **Amyloidosis**
    A disorder resulting from the abnormal deposition of a particular
    protein (amyloid) into tissues of the body
    ~~Excludes1 Alzheimer's disease (G30.0-)~~
    ▶ **Excludes2**   Alzheimer's disease (G30.0-)
    (Ex) **For category E85CC codes: See PDX Collection 542**

   E85.0   **Non-neuropathic heredofamilial amyloidosis** 🔗
        Hereditary amyloid nephropathy
    ▶Code also associated disorders, such as:
      ▶autoinflammatory syndromes (M04.-)
    ▶ **Excludes2**   Transthyretin-related (ATTR) familial
            amyloid cardiomyopathy (E85.4)

   E85.1   **Neuropathic heredofamilial amyloidosis** 🔗
        Amyloid polyneuropathy (Portuguese)
    ▶Transthyretin-related (ATTR) familial amyloid
        polyneuropathy
    Coding Clinic: 2012, Q4, P100

   E85.2   **Heredofamilial amyloidosis, unspecified** 🔗
   E85.3   **Secondary systemic amyloidosis** 🔗
        Hemodialysis-associated amyloidosis

   E85.4   **Organ-limited amyloidosis** 🔗
        Localized amyloidosis
    ▶Transthyretin-related (ATTR) familial amyloid
        cardiomyopathy

● **E85.8**   **Other amyloidosis**
   ▶ **E85.81**   **Light chain (AL) amyloidosis** 🔗
   ▶ **E85.82**   **Wild-type transthyretin-related (ATTR) amyloidosis** 🔗
        ▶Senile systemic amyloidosis (SSA)
   ▶ **E85.89**   **Other amyloidosis** 🔗

   E85.9   **Amyloidosis, unspecified** 🔗

▶ New   ⟹ Revised   ~~deleted~~ Deleted   Excludes 1   Excludes 2   Includes   Use additional   Code first   Code also   Key words

OGCR Official Guidelines   ● Unacceptable Principal Diagnosis   X Assign placeholder X   ● Use Additional Character(s)   ▶ Manifestation Code   **Coding Clinic**

● **E86**   **Volume depletion**

    Excludes1   dehydration of newborn (P74.1)
                   hypovolemic shock NOS (R57.1)
                   postprocedural hypovolemic shock (T81.19)
                   traumatic hypovolemic shock (T79.4)

    Use additional code(s) for any associated disorders of electrolyte and acid-base balance (E87.-)

    E86.0   **Dehydration**
           Excessive loss of body water

    E86.1   **Hypovolemia**
           Diminished volume of circulating blood
           Depletion of volume of plasma

    E86.9   **Volume depletion, unspecified**

● **E87**   **Other disorders of fluid, electrolyte and acid-base balance**

    Excludes1   diabetes insipidus (E23.2)
                   electrolyte imbalance associated with hyperemesis gravidarum (O21.1)
                   electrolyte imbalance following ectopic or molar pregnancy (O08.5)
                   familial periodic paralysis (G72.3)

    (Ex) For category E87 CC codes: See PDX Collection 543

    E87.0   **Hyperosmolality and hypernatremia** 🔖
           Sodium [Na] excess
           Sodium [Na] overload

    E87.1   **Hypo-osmolality and hyponatremia** 🔖
           Sodium [Na] deficiency
           Excludes1   syndrome of inappropriate secretion of antidiuretic hormone (E22.2)

    E87.2   **Acidosis** 🔖
           Acidosis NOS
           Lactic acidosis
           Metabolic acidosis
           Respiratory acidosis
           Excludes1   diabetic acidosis - see categories E08-E10, E13 with ketoacidosis

    E87.3   **Alkalosis** 🔖
           Alkalosis NOS
           Metabolic alkalosis
           Respiratory alkalosis

    E87.4   **Mixed disorder of acid-base balance** 🔖

    E87.5   **Hyperkalemia**
           Potassium [K] excess
           Potassium [K] overload

    E87.6   **Hypokalemia**
           Potassium [K] deficiency

●   **E87.7**   **Fluid overload**
           Excludes1   edema NOS (R60.9)
                      fluid retention (R60.9)

        E87.70   **Fluid overload, unspecified**

        E87.71   **Transfusion associated circulatory overload**
                  Fluid overload due to transfusion (blood) (blood components) TACO

        E87.79   **Other fluid overload**

    E87.8   **Other disorders of electrolyte and fluid balance, not elsewhere classified**
           Electrolyte imbalance NOS
           Hyperchloremia
           Hypochloremia

● **E88**   **Other and unspecified metabolic disorders**

    Use additional codes for associated conditions

    Excludes1   histiocytosis X (chronic) (C96.6)

●   **E88.0**   **Disorders of plasma-protein metabolism, not elsewhere classified**

        Excludes1   disorder of lipoprotein metabolism (E78.-)
                      monoclonal gammopathy (of undetermined significance) (D47.2)
                      polyclonal hypergammaglobulinemia (D89.0)
                      Waldenström macroglobulinemia (C88.0)

        E88.01   **Alpha-1-antitrypsin deficiency AAT deficiency**

        E88.09   **Other disorders of plasma-protein metabolism, not elsewhere classified**
                Bisalbuminemia

    E88.1   **Lipodystrophy, not elsewhere classified**
           Defective fat metabolism resulting in absence of subcutaneous fat
           Lipodystrophy NOS
           Excludes1   Whipple's disease (K90.81)

    E88.2   **Lipomatosis, not elsewhere classified**
           Abnormal tumorlike accumulations of fat in tissue
           Lipomatosis NOS
           Lipomatosis (Check) dolorosa [Dercum]

    E88.3   **Tumor lysis syndrome** 🔖
           Tumor lysis syndrome (spontaneous)
           Tumor lysis syndrome following antineoplastic drug chemotherapy
           Use additional code for adverse effect, if applicable, to identify drug (T45.1X5)
           (Ex) See PDX Collection 544

●   **E88.4**   **Mitochondrial metabolism disorders**
           Congenital disorder of metabolism
        Excludes1   disorders of pyruvate metabolism (E74.4)
                      Kearns-Sayre syndrome (H49.81)
                      Leber's disease (H47.22)
                      Leigh's encephalopathy (G31.82)
                      Mitochondrial myopathy, NEC (G71.3)
                      Reye's syndrome (G93.7)
           (Ex) For category E88.4 CC codes: See PDX Collection 545

        E88.40   **Mitochondrial metabolism disorder, unspecified** 🔖

        E88.41   **MELAS syndrome** 🔖
                Mitochondrial myopathy, encephalopathy, lactic acidosis and stroke-like episodes

        E88.42   **MERRF syndrome** 🔖
                Myoclonic epilepsy associated with ragged-red fibers
                Code also progressive myoclonic epilepsy (G40.3-)

        E88.49   **Other mitochondrial metabolism disorders** 🔖

●   **E88.8**   **Other specified metabolic disorders**

        E88.81   **Metabolic syndrome**
                Dysmetabolic syndrome X
                Use additional codes for associated manifestations, such as:
                obesity (E66.-)

        E88.89   **Other specified metabolic disorders**
                Launois-Bensaude adenolipomatosis
                Excludes1   adult pulmonary Langerhans cell histiocytosis (J84.82)

    E88.9   **Metabolic disorder, unspecified**

Item 4-9   Circulating fluid volume is regulated by the amount of water and sodium ingested, excreted by the kidneys into the urine, and lost through the gastrointestinal tract, lungs, and skin. To maintain blood volume within a normal range, the kidneys regulate the amount of water and sodium lost into the urine. Too much (**fluid overload**) or too little fluid volume (**volume depletion**) will affect blood pressure. Severe cases of vomiting, diarrhea, bleeding, and burns (fluid loss through exposed burn surface area) can contribute to fluid loss. Internal body environment must maintain a precise balance (homeostasis) between too much fluid and too little fluid. This complex balancing mechanism is critical to good health.

N   Newborn Age: 0   P   Pediatric Age: 0–17   M   Maternity DX: 12–55   A   Adult Age: 15–124   ♀   Females Only   ♂   Males Only

🔖   Complication\Comorbidity   🔖   Major C\C   (Ex)   CC/MCC Exclusions   🔖   Hospital-Acquired Condition

CHAPTER 4 (E00-E90)

CHAPTER 4 (E00-E90)

POSTPROCEDURAL ENDOCRINE AND METABOLIC COMPLICATIONS AND DISORDERS, NOT ELSEWHERE CLASSIFIED (E89)

● E89   **Postprocedural endocrine and metabolic complications and disorders, not elsewhere classified**

     Excludes2   intraoperative complications of endocrine system organ or structure (E36.0-, E36.1-, E36.8)

   E89.0   **Postprocedural hypothyroidism**
       Postirradiation hypothyroidism
       Postsurgical hypothyroidism

   E89.1   **Postprocedural hypoinsulinemia** 🗝
       Postpancreatectomy hyperglycemia
       Postsurgical hypoinsulinemia

       Use additional code, if applicable, to identify:
         acquired absence of pancreas (Z90.41-)
         diabetes mellitus (postpancreatectomy)
           (postprocedural) (E13.-)
         insulin use (Z79.4)

       Excludes1   transient postprocedural hyperglycemia (R73.9)
               transient postprocedural hypoglycemia (E16.2)

       (Ex:) See PDX Collection 520

   E89.2   **Postprocedural hypoparathyroidism**
       Parathyroprival tetany

   E89.3   **Postprocedural hypopituitarism**
       Postirradiation hypopituitarism

● E89.4   **Postprocedural ovarian failure**

     E89.40   **Asymptomatic postprocedural ovarian failure** ♀
         Postprocedural ovarian failure NOS

     E89.41   **Symptomatic postprocedural ovarian failure** ♀
         Symptoms such as flushing, sleeplessness, headache, lack of concentration, associated with postprocedural menopause

   E89.5   **Postprocedural testicular hypofunction** ♂

   E89.6   **Postprocedural adrenocortical (-medullary) hypofunction** 🗝
       (Ex:) See PDX Collection 526

● E89.8   **Other postprocedural endocrine and metabolic complications and disorders**
       (Ex:) For category E89.8 CC codes: See PDX Collection 546
       Coding Clinic: 2016, Q4, P9

   ● E89.81   **Postprocedural hemorrhage of an endocrine system organ or structure following a procedure**

     E89.810   **Postprocedural hemorrhage of an endocrine system organ or structure following an endocrine system procedure** 🗝

     E89.811   **Postprocedural hemorrhage of an endocrine system organ or structure following other procedure** 🗝

   ● E89.82   **Postprocedural hematoma and seroma of an endocrine system organ or structure**

     E89.820   **Postprocedural hematoma of an endocrine system organ or structure following an endocrine system procedure** 🗝

     E89.821   **Postprocedural hematoma of an endocrine system organ or structure following other procedure** 🗝

     E89.822   **Postprocedural seroma of an endocrine system organ or structure following an endocrine system procedure** 🗝

     E89.823   **Postprocedural seroma of an endocrine system organ or structure following other procedure** 🗝

     E89.89   **Other postprocedural endocrine and metabolic complications and disorders** 🗝

       Use additional code, if applicable, to further specify disorder

▶ New   ⫴ Revised   ~~deleted~~ Deleted   Excludes 1   Excludes 2   Includes   Use additional   Code first   Code also   Key words
OGCR Official Guidelines   ● Unacceptable Principal Diagnosis   X Assign placeholder X   ● Use Additional Character(s)   ▌ Manifestation Code   **Coding Clinic**

CHAPTER 5

MENTAL, BEHAVIORAL AND NEURODEVELOPMENTAL DISORDERS (F01-F99)

OGCR Chapter-Specific Coding Guidelines

5. Chapter 5: Mental, Behavioral and Neurodevelopmental disorders (F01 – F99)

a. Pain disorders related to psychological factors

Assign code F45.41, for pain that is exclusively related to psychological disorders. As indicated by the Excludes 1 note under category G89, a code from category G89 should not be assigned with code F45.41

Code F45.42, Pain disorders with related psychological factors, should be used with a code from category G89, Pain, not elsewhere classified, if there is documentation of a psychological component for a patient with acute or chronic pain.

See Section I.C.6. Pain

c. Mental and behavioral disorders due to psychoactive substance use

1) In Remission

Selection of codes for "in remission" for categories F10-F19, Mental and behavioral disorders due to psychoactive substance use (categories F10-F19 with -11, -.21) requires the provider's clinical judgment. The appropriate codes for "in remission" are assigned only on the basis of provider documentation (as defined in the Official Guidelines for Coding and Reporting), unless otherwise instructed by the classification.

Mild substance use disorders in early or sustained remission are classified to the appropriate codes for substance abuse in remission, and moderate or severe substance use disorders in early or sustained remission are classified to the appropriate codes for substance dependence in remission.

2) Psychoactive Substance Use, Abuse and Dependence

When the provider documentation refers to use, abuse and dependence of the same substance (e.g. alcohol, opioid, cannabis, etc.), only one code should be assigned to identify the pattern of use based on the following hierarchy:

- If both use and abuse are documented, assign only the code for abuse
- If both abuse and dependence are documented, assign only the code for dependence
- If use, abuse and dependence are all documented, assign only the code for dependence
- If both use and dependence are documented, assign only the code for dependence

3) Psychoactive Substance Use *Disorders*

As with all other diagnoses, the codes for psychoactive substance use **disorders** (F10.9-, F11.9-, F12.9-, F13.9-, F14.9-, F15.9-, F16.9-) should only be assigned based on provider documentation and when they meet the definition of a reportable diagnosis (see Section III, Reporting Additional Diagnoses). The codes are to be used only when the psychoactive substance use is associated with a **physical,** mental or behavioral disorder, and such a relationship is documented by the provider.

CHAPTER 5

MENTAL, BEHAVIORAL AND NEURODEVELOPMENTAL DISORDERS (F01-F99)

Includes	disorders of psychological development
Excludes2	symptoms, signs and abnormal clinical laboratory findings, not elsewhere classified (R00-R99)

This chapter contains the following blocks:

F01-F09	Mental disorders due to known physiological conditions
F10-F19	Mental and behavioral disorders due to psychoactive substance use
F20-F29	Schizophrenia, schizotypal, delusional, and other non-mood psychotic disorders
F30-F39	Mood [affective] disorders
F40-F48	Anxiety, dissociative, stress-related, somatoform and other nonpsychotic mental disorders
F50-F59	Behavioral syndromes associated with physiological disturbances and physical factors
F60-F69	Disorders of adult personality and behavior
F70-F79	Intellectual disabilities
F80-F89	Pervasive and specific developmental disorders
F90-F98	Behavioral and emotional disorders with onset usually occurring in childhood and adolescence
F99	Unspecified mental disorder

MENTAL DISORDERS DUE TO KNOWN PHYSIOLOGICAL CONDITIONS (F01-F09)

This block comprises a range of mental disorders grouped together on the basis of their having in common a demonstrable etiology in cerebral disease, brain injury, or other insult leading to cerebral dysfunction. The dysfunction may be primary, as in diseases, injuries, and insults that affect the brain directly and selectively; or secondary, as in systemic diseases and disorders that attack the brain only as one of the multiple organs or systems of the body that are involved.

● **F01**   **Vascular dementia**

Vascular dementia as a result of infarction of the brain due to vascular disease, including hypertensive cerebrovascular disease.

   Includes   arteriosclerotic dementia

Code first the underlying physiological condition or sequelae of cerebrovascular disease.

● **F01.5**   **Vascular dementia**

   ● **F01.50**   **Vascular dementia without behavioral disturbance**   A

       Major neurocognitive disorder without behavioral disturbance

   ● **F01.51**   **Vascular dementia with behavioral disturbance** 🔖   A

       Major neurocognitive disorder due to vascular disease, with behavioral disturbance

       Major neurocognitive disorder with aggressive behavior

       Major neurocognitive disorder with combative behavior

       Major neurocognitive disorder with violent behavior

       Vascular dementia with aggressive behavior

       Vascular dementia with combative behavior

       Vascular dementia with violent behavior

       Use additional code, if applicable, to identify wandering in vascular dementia (Z91.83)

       (Ex:) See PDX Collection 547

N   Newborn Age: 0   **P**   Pediatric Age: 0–17   **M**   Maternity DX: 12–55   **A**   Adult Age: 15–124   ♀   Females Only   ♂   Males Only

🔖   Complication\Comorbidity   🔖   Major C\C   (Ex:)   CC/MCC Exclusions   🔖   Hospital-Acquired Condition   755

CHAPTER 5 (F01-F99)

● **F02**   **Dementia in other diseases classified elsewhere**

Code first the underlying physiological condition, such as:

Alzheimer's (G30.-)
cerebral lipidosis (E75.4)
Creutzfeldt-Jakob disease (A81.0-)
dementia with Lewy bodies (G31.83)
dementia with Parkinsonism (G31.83)
epilepsy and recurrent seizures (G40.-)
frontotemporal dementia (G31.09)
hepatolenticular degeneration (E83.0)
human immunodeficiency virus [HIV] disease (B20)
Huntington's disease (G10)
hypercalcemia (E83.52)
hypothyroidism, acquired (E00-E03.-)
intoxications (T36-T65)
Jakob-Creutzfeldt disease (A81.0-)
multiple sclerosis (G35)
neurosyphilis (A52.17)
niacin deficiency [pellagra] (E52)
Parkinson's disease (G20)
Pick's disease (G31.01)
polyarteritis nodosa (M30.0)
prion disease (A81.9)
systemic lupus erythematosus (M32.-)
traumatic brain injury (S06.-)
trypanosomiasis (B56.-, B57.-)
vitamin B deficiency (E53.8)

Includes   Major neurocognitive disorder in other diseases
classified elsewhere

Excludes2   dementia in alcohol and psychoactive substance
disorders (F10-F19, with .17, .27, .97)
vascular dementia (F01.5-)

Coding Clinic: 2016, Q4, P141

● **F02.8**   **Dementia in other diseases classified elsewhere**

▷ **F02.80**   *Dementia in other diseases classified elsewhere
without behavioral disturbance*
Dementia in other diseases classified elsewhere
NOS
Major neurocognitive disorder in other
diseases classified elsewhere
Coding Clinic: 2017, Q1, P43; 2016, Q2, P6

▷ **F02.81**   *Dementia in other diseases classified elsewhere
with behavioral disturbance* 🔗
Dementia in other diseases classified elsewhere
with aggressive behavior
Dementia in other diseases classified elsewhere
with combative behavior
Dementia in other diseases classified elsewhere
with violent behavior
Major neurocognitive disorder in other
diseases classified elsewhere with
aggressive behavior
Major neurocognitive disorder in other
diseases classified elsewhere with
combative behavior
Major neurocognitive disorder in other
diseases classified elsewhere with violent
behavior
Use additional code, if applicable, to identify
wandering in dementia in conditions
classified elsewhere (Z91.83)
(Ex) See PDX Collection 548
Coding Clinic: 2017, Q2, P8, Q1, P43

Item 5-1 Psychosis was a term formerly applied to any mental disorder
but is now restricted to disturbances of a great magnitude in which there is a
personality disintegration and loss of contact with reality.

● **F03**   **Unspecified dementia**
Presenile dementia NOS
Presenile psychosis NOS
Primary degenerative dementia NOS
Senile dementia NOS
Senile dementia depressed or paranoid type
Senile psychosis NOS

Excludes1   senility NOS (R41.81)

Excludes2   mild memory disturbance due to known
physiological condition (F06.8)
senile dementia with delirium or acute
confusional state (F05)

● **F03.9**   **Unspecified dementia**

F03.90   **Unspecified dementia without behavioral
disturbance**   A
Dementia NOS
Coding Clinic: 2012, Q4, P92

F03.91   **Unspecified dementia with behavioral
disturbance** 🔗   A
Unspecified dementia with aggressive behavior
Unspecified dementia with combative behavior
Unspecified dementia with violent behavior
Use additional code, if applicable, to identify
wandering in unspecified dementia
(Z91.83)
(Ex) See PDX Collection 548

● **F04**   **Amnestic disorder due to known physiological condition**
Korsakov's psychosis or syndrome, nonalcoholic
Code first the underlying physiological condition

Excludes1   amnesia NOS (R41.3)
anterograde amnesia (R41.1)
dissociative amnesia (F44.0)
retrograde amnesia (R41.2)

Excludes2   alcohol-induced or unspecified Korsakov's
syndrome (F10.26, F10.96)
Korsakov's syndrome induced by other
psychoactive substances (F13.26, F13.96,
F19.16, F19.26, F19.96)

● **F05**   **Delirium due to known physiological condition** 🔗
Acute or subacute brain syndrome
Acute or subacute confusional state (nonalcoholic)
Acute or subacute infective psychosis
Acute or subacute organic reaction
Acute or subacute psycho-organic syndrome
Delirium of mixed etiology
Delirium superimposed on dementia
Sundowning
Code first the underlying physiological condition

Excludes1   delirium NOS (R41.0)

Excludes2   delirium tremens alcohol-induced or unspecified
(F10.231, F10.921)
(Ex) See PDX Collection 549

● **F06**   **Other mental disorders due to known physiological condition**

Includes   mental disorders due to endocrine disorder
mental disorders due to exogenous hormone
mental disorders due to exogenous toxic
substance
mental disorders due to primary cerebral disease
mental disorders due to somatic illness
mental disorders due to systemic disease
affecting the brain

Code first the underlying physiological condition

Excludes1   unspecified dementia (F03)

Excludes2   delirium due to known physiological condition
(F05)
dementia as classified in F01-F02
other mental disorders associated with alcohol
and other psychoactive substances (F10-F19)
(Ex) For category F06 CC codes: See PDX Collection 550

▶ New   ⇒ Revised   deleted Deleted   Excludes 1   Excludes 2   Includes   Use additional   Code first   Code also   Key words

OGCR Official Guidelines   ● Unacceptable Principal Diagnosis   X Assign placeholder X   ● Use Additional Character(s)   ▷ Manifestation Code   **Coding Clinic**

● **F06.0**   **Psychotic disorder with hallucinations** due to known physiological condition
Organic hallucinatory state (nonalcoholic)

> **Excludes2**   hallucinations and perceptual disturbance induced by alcohol and other psychoactive substances (F10-F19 with .151, .251, .951)
> schizophrenia (F20.-)

● **F06.1**   **Catatonic disorder** due to known physiological condition
Catatonia associated with another mental disorder
Catatonia NOS

> **Excludes1**   catatonic stupor (R40.1)
> stupor NOS (R40.1)

> **Excludes2**   catatonic schizophrenia (F20.2)
> dissociative stupor (F44.2)

● **F06.2**   **Psychotic disorder with delusions** due to known physiological condition
Paranoid and paranoid-hallucinatory organic states
Schizophrenia-like psychosis in epilepsy

> **Excludes2**   alcohol and drug-induced psychotic disorder (F10-F19 with .150, .250, .950)
> brief psychotic disorder (F23)
> delusional disorder (F22)
> schizophrenia (F20.-)

● **F06.3**   **Mood disorder** due to known physiological condition

> **Excludes2**   mood disorders due to alcohol and other psychoactive substances (F10-F19 with .14, .24, .94)
> mood disorders, not due to known physiological condition or unspecified (F30-F39)

  ● **F06.30**   **Mood disorder due to known physiological condition, unspecified**

  ● **F06.31**   **Mood disorder due to known physiological condition with depressive features**
  ▶ Depressive disorder due to known physiological condition, with depressive features

  ● **F06.32**   **Mood disorder due to known physiological condition with major depressive-like episode**
  ▶ Depressive disorder due to known physiological condition, with major depressive-like episode

  ● **F06.33**   **Mood disorder due to known physiological condition with manic features**
  ▶ Bipolar and related disorder due to a known physiological condition, with manic features
  ▶ Bipolar and related disorder due to known physiological condition, with manic- or hypomanic-like episodes

  ● **F06.34**   **Mood disorder due to known physiological condition with mixed features**
  ▶ Bipolar and related disorder due to known physiological condition, with mixed features
  ▶ Depressive disorder due to known physiological condition, with mixed features

● **F06.4**   **Anxiety disorder** due to known physiological condition

> **Excludes2**   anxiety disorders due to alcohol and other psychoactive substances (F10-F19 with .180, .280, .980)
> anxiety disorders, not due to known physiological condition or unspecified (F40.-, F41.-)

● **F06.8**   **Other specified mental disorders** due to known physiological condition
Epileptic psychosis NOS
▶ Obsessive-compulsive and related disorder due to a known physiological condition
Organic dissociative disorder
Organic emotionally labile [asthenic] disorder

● **F07**   **Personality and behavioral disorders** due to known physiological condition
Code first the underlying physiological condition

● **F07.0**   **Personality change** due to known physiological condition
Frontal lobe syndrome
Limbic epilepsy personality syndrome
Lobotomy syndrome
Organic personality disorder
Organic pseudopsychopathic personality
Organic pseudoretarded personality
Postleucotomy syndrome

Code first underlying physiological condition

> **Excludes1**   mild cognitive impairment (G31.84)
> postconcussional syndrome (F07.81)
> postencephalitic syndrome (F07.89)
> signs and symptoms involving emotional state (R45.-)

> **Excludes2**   specific personality disorder (F60.-)

● **F07.8**   **Other personality and behavioral disorders** due to known physiological condition

  ● **F07.81**   **Postconcussional syndrome**
  Postcontusional syndrome (encephalopathy)
  Post-traumatic brain syndrome, nonpsychotic

  Use additional code to identify associated post-traumatic headache, if applicable (G44.3-)

  > **Excludes1**   current concussion (brain) (S06.0-)
  > postencephalitic syndrome (F07.89)

  ● **F07.89**   **Other personality and behavioral disorders due to known physiological condition**
  Postencephalitic syndrome
  Damage to temporal brain lobes with memory loss and abnormal behavior
  Right hemispheric organic affective disorder

● **F07.9**   **Unspecified personality and behavioral disorder** due to known physiological condition
Organic psychosyndrome
Due to exposure to organic solvents

● **F09**   **Unspecified mental disorder** due to known physiological condition
Mental disorder NOS due to known physiological condition
Organic brain syndrome NOS
Organic mental disorder NOS
Organic psychosis NOS
Symptomatic psychosis NOS

Code first the underlying physiological condition

> **Excludes1**   psychosis NOS (F29)

MENTAL AND BEHAVIORAL DISORDERS DUE TO PSYCHOACTIVE SUBSTANCE USE (F10-F19)

● **F10**   **Alcohol related disorders**
Use additional code for blood alcohol level, if applicable (Y90.-)
(Ex) **For category F10 CC codes:** See PDX Collection 550

● **F10.1**   **Alcohol abuse**

> **Excludes1**   alcohol dependence (F10.2-)
> alcohol use, unspecified (F10.9-)

  F10.10   **Alcohol abuse, uncomplicated**
  Alcohol use disorder, mild

  ▶ **F10.11**   **Alcohol abuse, in remission**
  ▶ Alcohol use disorder, mild, in early remission
  ▶ Alcohol use disorder, mild, in sustained remission

  ● **F10.12**   **Alcohol abuse with intoxication**

    F10.120   **Alcohol abuse with intoxication, uncomplicated**

    F10.121   **Alcohol abuse with intoxication, delirium**

    F10.129   **Alcohol abuse with intoxication, unspecified**

N   Newborn Age: 0   P   Pediatric Age: 0–17   M   Maternity DX: 12–55   A   Adult Age: 15–124   ♀   Females Only   ♂   Males Only

Complication\Comorbidity   Major C\C   (Ex) CC/MCC Exclusions   Hospital-Acquired Condition

CHAPTER 5 (F01-F99)

F10.14   **Alcohol abuse with alcohol-induced mood disorder** 🔖
Alcohol use disorder, mild, with alcohol-induced bipolar or related disorder
Alcohol use disorder, mild, with alcohol-induced depressive disorder

● **F10.15**   **Alcohol abuse with alcohol-induced psychotic disorder**
F10.150   Alcohol abuse with alcohol-induced psychotic disorder with delusions
F10.151   Alcohol abuse with alcohol-induced psychotic disorder with hallucinations 🔖
F10.159   Alcohol abuse with alcohol-induced psychotic disorder, unspecified 🔖

● **F10.18**   **Alcohol abuse with other alcohol-induced disorders**
F10.180   Alcohol abuse with alcohol-induced anxiety disorder 🔖
F10.181   Alcohol abuse with alcohol-induced sexual dysfunction 🔖
F10.182   Alcohol abuse with alcohol-induced sleep disorder
F10.188   Alcohol abuse with other alcohol-induced disorder 🔖

F10.19   **Alcohol abuse with unspecified alcohol-induced disorder** 🔖

● **F10.2**   **Alcohol dependence**
> **Excludes1**   alcohol abuse (F10.1-)
> alcohol use, unspecified (F10.9-)
> **Excludes2**   toxic effect of alcohol (T51.0-)

F10.20   **Alcohol dependence, uncomplicated**
Alcohol use disorder, moderate
Alcohol use disorder, severe

F10.21   **Alcohol dependence, in remission**
▶Alcohol use disorder, moderate, in early remission
▶Alcohol use disorder, moderate, in sustained remission
▶Alcohol use disorder, severe, in early remission
▶Alcohol use disorder, severe, in sustained remission

● **F10.22**   **Alcohol dependence with intoxication**
Acute drunkenness (in alcoholism)
> **Excludes2**   alcohol dependence with withdrawal (F10.23-)

F10.220   Alcohol dependence with intoxication, uncomplicated
F10.221   Alcohol dependence with intoxication delirium 🔖
F10.229   Alcohol dependence with intoxication, unspecified

● **F10.23**   **Alcohol dependence with withdrawal**
> **Excludes2**   alcohol dependence with intoxication (F10.22-)

F10.230   Alcohol dependence with withdrawal, uncomplicated 🔖
F10.231   Alcohol dependence with withdrawal delirium 🔖
F10.232   Alcohol dependence with withdrawal with perceptual disturbance 🔖
F10.239   Alcohol dependence with withdrawal, unspecified 🔖
Coding Clinic: 2015, Q2, P15

F10.24   **Alcohol dependence with alcohol-induced mood disorder** 🔖
Alcohol use disorder, moderate, with alcohol-induced bipolar or related disorder
Alcohol use disorder, moderate, with alcohol-induced depressive disorder
Alcohol use disorder, severe, with alcohol-induced bipolar or related disorder
Alcohol use disorder, severe, with alcohol-induced depressive disorder

● **F10.25**   **Alcohol dependence with alcohol-induced psychotic disorder**
F10.250   Alcohol dependence with alcohol-induced psychotic disorder with delusions
F10.251   Alcohol dependence with alcohol-induced psychotic disorder with hallucinations 🔖
F10.259   Alcohol dependence with alcohol-induced psychotic disorder, unspecified 🔖

F10.26   **Alcohol dependence with alcohol-induced persisting amnestic disorder**
Alcohol use disorder, moderate, with alcohol-induced major neurocognitive disorder, amnestic-confabulatory type
Alcohol use disorder, severe, with alcohol-induced major neurocognitive disorder, amnestic-confabulatory type

F10.27   **Alcohol dependence with alcohol-induced persisting dementia** 🔖
Alcohol use disorder, moderate, with alcohol-induced major neurocognitive disorder, nonamnestic-confabulatory type
Alcohol use disorder, severe, with alcohol-induced major neurocognitive disorder, nonamnestic-confabulatory type

● **F10.28**   **Alcohol dependence with other alcohol-induced disorders**
F10.280   Alcohol dependence with alcohol-induced anxiety disorder 🔖
F10.281   Alcohol dependence with alcohol-induced sexual dysfunction 🔖
F10.282   Alcohol dependence with alcohol-induced sleep disorder
F10.288   Alcohol dependence with other alcohol-induced disorder 🔖
Alcohol use disorder, moderate, with alcohol-induced mild neurocognitive disorder
Alcohol use disorder, severe, with alcohol-induced mild neurocognitive disorder

F10.29   **Alcohol dependence with unspecified alcohol-induced disorder** 🔖

● **F10.9**   **Alcohol use, unspecified**
> **Excludes1**   alcohol abuse (F10.1-)
> alcohol dependence (F10.2-)

● **F10.92**   **Alcohol use, unspecified with intoxication**
F10.920   Alcohol use, unspecified with intoxication, uncomplicated
F10.921   Alcohol use, unspecified with intoxication delirium 🔖
F10.929   Alcohol use, unspecified with intoxication, unspecified

F10.94   **Alcohol use, unspecified with alcohol-induced mood disorder** 🔖
Alcohol-induced bipolar or related disorder, without use disorder
Alcohol-induced depressive disorder, without use disorder

▶ New   ⇒ Revised   ~~deleted~~ Deleted   Excludes 1   Excludes 2   Includes   Use additional   Code first   Code also   Key words
OGCR Official Guidelines   ● Unacceptable Principal Diagnosis   X Assign placeholder X   ● Use Additional Character(s)   ▶ Manifestation Code   **Coding Clinic**

● **F10.95**　Alcohol use, unspecified with alcohol-induced psychotic disorder

　　F10.950　Alcohol use, unspecified with alcohol-induced psychotic disorder with delusions

　　F10.951　Alcohol use, unspecified with alcohol-induced psychotic disorder with hallucinations 🔖

　　F10.959　Alcohol use, unspecified with alcohol-induced psychotic disorder, unspecified 🔖
　　　　　　Alcohol-induced psychotic disorder without use disorder

F10.96　Alcohol use, unspecified with alcohol-induced persisting amnestic disorder
　　　　Alcohol-induced major neurocognitive disorder, amnestic-confabulatory type, without use disorder

F10.97　Alcohol use, unspecified with alcohol-induced persisting dementia
　　　　Alcohol-induced major neurocognitive disorder, nonamnestic-confabulatory type, without use disorder

● **F10.98**　Alcohol use, unspecified with other alcohol-induced disorders

　　F10.980　Alcohol use, unspecified with alcohol-induced anxiety disorder 🔖
　　　　　　Alcohol-induced anxiety disorder, without use disorder

　　F10.981　Alcohol use, unspecified with alcohol-induced sexual dysfunction 🔖
　　　　　　Alcohol-induced sexual dysfunction, without use disorder

　　F10.982　Alcohol use, unspecified with alcohol-induced sleep disorder
　　　　　　Alcohol-induced sleep disorder, without use disorder

　　F10.988　Alcohol use, unspecified with other alcohol-induced disorder 🔖
　　　　　　Alcohol-induced mild neurocognitive disorder, without use disorder

F10.99　Alcohol use, unspecified with unspecified alcohol-induced disorder 🔖

● **F11**　**Opioid related disorders**
　　(Ex) For category F11 CC codes unless otherwise indicated: See PDX Collection 550

● **F11.1**　Opioid abuse

　　Excludes1　opioid dependence (F11.2-)
　　　　　　　opioid use, unspecified (F11.9-)

　　F11.10　Opioid abuse, uncomplicated
　　　　　　Opioid use disorder, mild

▶ **F11.11**　Opioid abuse, in remission
　　　　　▶Opioid use disorder, mild, in early remission
　　　　　▶Opioid use disorder, mild, in sustained remission

● **F11.12**　Opioid abuse with intoxication

　　F11.120　Opioid abuse with intoxication, uncomplicated

　　F11.121　Opioid abuse with intoxication delirium 🔖

　　F11.122　Opioid abuse with intoxication with perceptual disturbance

　　F11.129　Opioid abuse with intoxication, unspecified

　　F11.14　Opioid abuse with opioid-induced mood disorder
　　　　　　Opioid use disorder, mild, with opioid-induced depressive disorder

● **F11.15**　Opioid abuse with opioid-induced psychotic disorder

　　F11.150　Opioid abuse with opioid-induced psychotic disorder with delusions 🔖

　　F11.151　Opioid abuse with opioid-induced psychotic disorder with hallucinations 🔖

　　F11.159　Opioid abuse with opioid-induced psychotic disorder, unspecified

● **F11.18**　Opioid abuse with other opioid-induced disorder

　　F11.181　Opioid abuse with opioid-induced sexual dysfunction

　　F11.182　Opioid abuse with opioid-induced sleep disorder

　　F11.188　Opioid abuse with other opioid-induced disorder

F11.19　Opioid abuse with unspecified opioid-induced disorder

● **F11.2**　Opioid dependence

　　Excludes1　opioid abuse (F11.1-)
　　　　　　　opioid use, unspecified (F11.9-)

　　Excludes2　opioid poisoning (T40.0--T40.2-)

　　F11.20　Opioid dependence, uncomplicated 🔖
　　　　　　Opioid use disorder, moderate
　　　　　　Opioid use disorder, severe
　　　　　　(Ex) No exclusions

　　F11.21　Opioid dependence, in remission
　　　　　▶Opioid use disorder, moderate, in early remission
　　　　　▶Opioid use disorder, moderate, in sustained remission
　　　　　▶Opioid use disorder, severe, in early remission
　　　　　▶Opioid use disorder, severe, in sustained remission

● **F11.22**　Opioid dependence with intoxication

　　Excludes1　opioid dependence with withdrawal (F11.23)

　　F11.220　Opioid dependence with intoxication, uncomplicated

　　F11.221　Opioid dependence with intoxication delirium 🔖

　　F11.222　Opioid dependence with intoxication with perceptual disturbance 🔖
　　　　　　(Ex) No exclusions

　　F11.229　Opioid dependence with intoxication, unspecified

　　F11.23　Opioid dependence with withdrawal 🔖

　　Excludes1　opioid dependence with intoxication (F11.22-)

　　F11.24　Opioid dependence with opioid-induced mood disorder
　　　　　　Opioid use disorder, moderate, with opioid-induced depressive disorder

● **F11.25**　Opioid dependence with opioid-induced psychotic disorder

　　F11.250　Opioid dependence with opioid-induced psychotic disorder with delusions 🔖

　　F11.251　Opioid dependence with opioid-induced psychotic disorder with hallucinations 🔖

　　F11.259　Opioid dependence with opioid-induced psychotic disorder, unspecified 🔖
　　　　　　(Ex) No exclusions

● **F11.28**　Opioid dependence with other opioid-induced disorder
　　(Ex) For category F11.28 CC codes: No exclusions

　　F11.281　Opioid dependence with opioid-induced sexual dysfunction 🔖

　　F11.282　Opioid dependence with opioid-induced sleep disorder 🔖

　　F11.288　Opioid dependence with other opioid-induced disorder 🔖

F11.29　Opioid dependence with unspecified opioid-induced disorder

N Newborn Age: 0　　**P** Pediatric Age: 0–17　　**M** Maternity DX: 12–55　　**A** Adult Age: 15–124　　♀ Females Only　　♂ Males Only

🔖 Complication\Comorbidity　　🔖 Major C\C　　(Ex) CC/MCC Exclusions　　🔖 Hospital-Acquired Condition

759

● **F11.9**   **Opioid use, unspecified**
    Excludes1   opioid abuse (F11.1-)
              opioid dependence (F11.2-)
   F11.90   Opioid use, unspecified, uncomplicated
● **F11.92**   Opioid use, unspecified with intoxication
      Excludes1   opioid use, unspecified with
                  withdrawal (F11.93)
     F11.920   Opioid use, unspecified with
            intoxication, uncomplicated
     F11.921   Opioid use, unspecified with
            intoxication delirium
            Opioid-induced delirium
     F11.922   Opioid use, unspecified with
            intoxication with perceptual
            disturbance
     F11.929   Opioid use, unspecified with
            intoxication, unspecified
   F11.93   Opioid use, unspecified with withdrawal
      Excludes1   opioid use, unspecified with
                  intoxication (F11.92-)
   F11.94   Opioid use, unspecified with opioid-induced
        mood disorder
        Opioid-induced depressive disorder, without
            use disorder
● **F11.95**   Opioid use, unspecified with opioid-induced
        psychotic disorder
     F11.950   Opioid use, unspecified with
            opioid-induced psychotic disorder
            with delusions
     F11.951   Opioid use, unspecified with
            opioid-induced psychotic disorder
            with hallucinations
     F11.959   Opioid use, unspecified with
            opioid-induced psychotic disorder,
            unspecified
● **F11.98**   Opioid use, unspecified with other specified
        opioid-induced disorder
     F11.981   Opioid use, unspecified with opioid-
            induced sexual dysfunction
            Opioid-induced sexual dysfunction,
               without use disorder
     F11.982   Opioid use, unspecified with opioid-
            induced sleep disorder
            Opioid-induced sleep disorder,
               without use disorder
     F11.988   Opioid use, unspecified with other
            opioid-induced disorder
            Opioid-induced anxiety disorder,
               without use disorder
   F11.99   Opioid use, unspecified with unspecified
        opioid-induced disorder

● **F12**   **Cannabis related disorders**
     Includes   marijuana
     (Ex) For category F12 CC codes: See PDX Collection 550
 ● **F12.1**   **Cannabis abuse**
      Excludes1   cannabis dependence (F12.2-)
              cannabis use, unspecified (F12.9-)
   F12.10   Cannabis abuse, uncomplicated
        Cannabis use disorder, mild
▶ **F12.11**   Cannabis abuse, in remission
       ▶Cannabis use disorder, mild, in early remission
       ▶Cannabis use disorder, mild, in sustained
          remission
● **F12.12**   Cannabis abuse with intoxication
     F12.120   Cannabis abuse with intoxication,
            uncomplicated
     F12.121   Cannabis abuse with intoxication
            delirium
     F12.122   Cannabis abuse with intoxication
            with perceptual disturbance
     F12.129   Cannabis abuse with
            intoxication, unspecified

● **F12.15**   Cannabis abuse with psychotic disorder
     F12.150   Cannabis abuse with psychotic
            disorder with delusions
     F12.151   Cannabis abuse with psychotic
            disorder with hallucinations
     F12.159   Cannabis abuse with psychotic
            disorder, unspecified
● **F12.18**   Cannabis abuse with other cannabis-induced
        disorder
     F12.180   Cannabis abuse with cannabis-
            induced anxiety disorder
     F12.188   Cannabis abuse with other cannabis-
            induced disorder
            Cannabis use disorder, mild,
               with cannabis-induced sleep
               disorder
   F12.19   Cannabis abuse with unspecified cannabis-
        induced disorder
● **F12.2**   **Cannabis dependence**
     Excludes1   cannabis abuse (F12.1-)
              cannabis use, unspecified (F12.9-)
     Excludes2   cannabis poisoning (T40.7-)
   F12.20   Cannabis dependence, uncomplicated
        Cannabis use disorder, moderate
        Cannabis use disorder, severe
   F12.21   Cannabis dependence, in remission
       ▶Cannabis use disorder, moderate, in early
          remission
       ▶Cannabis use disorder, moderate, in sustained
          remission
       ▶Cannabis use disorder, severe, in early
          remission
       ▶Cannabis use disorder, severe, in sustained
          remission
● **F12.22**   Cannabis dependence with intoxication
     F12.220   Cannabis dependence with
            intoxication, uncomplicated
     F12.221   Cannabis dependence with
            intoxication delirium
     F12.222   Cannabis dependence with
            intoxication with perceptual
            disturbance
     F12.229   Cannabis dependence with
            intoxication, unspecified
● **F12.25**   Cannabis dependence with psychotic disorder
     F12.250   Cannabis dependence with psychotic
            disorder with delusions
     F12.251   Cannabis dependence with psychotic
            disorder with hallucinations
     F12.259   Cannabis dependence with psychotic
            disorder, unspecified
● **F12.28**   Cannabis dependence with other cannabis-
        induced disorder
     F12.280   Cannabis dependence with cannabis-
            induced anxiety disorder
     F12.288   Cannabis dependence with other
            cannabis-induced disorder
            Cannabis use disorder, moderate,
              with cannabis-induced sleep
              disorder
            Cannabis use disorder, severe, with
              cannabis-induced sleep
              disorder
            Cannabis withdrawal
   F12.29   Cannabis dependence with unspecified
        cannabis-induced disorder

▶ New   ⇒ Revised   ~~deleted~~ Deleted   Excludes 1   Excludes 2   Includes   Use additional   Code first   Code also   Key words
OGCR Official Guidelines   ● Unacceptable Principal Diagnosis   X Assign placeholder X   ● Use Additional Character(s)   ▶ Manifestation Code   **Coding Clinic**

● **F12.9   Cannabis use, unspecified**

> **Excludes1**   cannabis abuse (F12.1-)
> cannabis dependence (F12.2-)

F12.90   Cannabis use, unspecified, uncomplicated

● **F12.92   Cannabis use, unspecified with intoxication**

F12.920   Cannabis use, unspecified with intoxication, uncomplicated

F12.921   Cannabis use, unspecified with intoxication delirium 🔴

F12.922   Cannabis use, unspecified with intoxication with perceptual disturbance

F12.929   Cannabis use, unspecified with intoxication, unspecified

● **F12.95   Cannabis use, unspecified with psychotic disorder**

F12.950   Cannabis use, unspecified with psychotic disorder with delusions 🔴

F12.951   Cannabis use, unspecified with psychotic disorder with hallucinations 🔴

F12.959   Cannabis use, unspecified with psychotic disorder, unspecified
> Cannabis-induced psychotic disorder, without use disorder

● **F12.98   Cannabis use, unspecified with other cannabis-induced disorder**

F12.980   Cannabis use, unspecified with anxiety disorder
> Cannabis-induced anxiety disorder, without use disorder

F12.988   Cannabis use, unspecified with other cannabis-induced disorder
> Cannabis-induced sleep disorder, without use disorder

F12.99   Cannabis use, unspecified with unspecified cannabis-induced disorder

● **F13   Sedative, hypnotic, or anxiolytic related disorders**
> (Ex) For category F13 CC codes unless otherwise indicated: See PDX Collection 550

● **F13.1   Sedative, hypnotic or anxiolytic-related abuse**

> **Excludes1**   sedative, hypnotic or anxiolytic-related dependence (F13.2-)
> sedative, hypnotic, or anxiolytic use, unspecified (F13.9-)

F13.10   Sedative, hypnotic or anxiolytic abuse, uncomplicated
> Sedative, hypnotic, or anxiolytic use disorder, mild

▶ **F13.11   Sedative, hypnotic or anxiolytic abuse, in remission**
> ▶Sedative, hypnotic or anxiolytic use disorder, mild, in early remission
> ▶Sedative, hypnotic or anxiolytic use disorder, mild, in sustained remission

● **F13.12   Sedative, hypnotic or anxiolytic abuse with intoxication**

F13.120   Sedative, hypnotic or anxiolytic abuse with intoxication, uncomplicated

F13.121   Sedative, hypnotic or anxiolytic abuse with intoxication delirium 🔴

F13.129   Sedative, hypnotic or anxiolytic abuse with intoxication, unspecified

F13.14   Sedative, hypnotic or anxiolytic abuse with sedative, hypnotic or anxiolytic-induced mood disorder
> ⇒Sedative, hypnotic, or anxiolytic use disorder, mild, with sedative, hypnotic, or anxiolytic-induced bipolar or related disorder
> ⇒Sedative, hypnotic, or anxiolytic use disorder, mild, with sedative, hypnotic, or anxiolytic-induced depressive disorder

● **F13.15   Sedative, hypnotic or anxiolytic abuse with sedative, hypnotic or anxiolytic-induced psychotic disorder**

F13.150   Sedative, hypnotic or anxiolytic abuse with sedative, hypnotic or anxiolytic-induced psychotic disorder with delusions 🔴

F13.151   Sedative, hypnotic or anxiolytic abuse with sedative, hypnotic or anxiolytic-induced psychotic disorder with hallucinations 🔴

F13.159   Sedative, hypnotic or anxiolytic abuse with sedative, hypnotic or anxiolytic-induced psychotic disorder, unspecified

● **F13.18   Sedative, hypnotic or anxiolytic abuse with other sedative, hypnotic or anxiolytic-induced disorders**

F13.180   Sedative, hypnotic or anxiolytic abuse with sedative, hypnotic or anxiolytic-induced anxiety disorder

F13.181   Sedative, hypnotic or anxiolytic abuse with sedative, hypnotic or anxiolytic-induced sexual dysfunction

F13.182   Sedative, hypnotic or anxiolytic abuse with sedative, hypnotic or anxiolytic-induced sleep disorder

F13.188   Sedative, hypnotic or anxiolytic abuse with other sedative, hypnotic or anxiolytic-induced disorder

F13.19   Sedative, hypnotic or anxiolytic abuse with unspecified sedative, hypnotic or anxiolytic-induced disorder

● **F13.2   Sedative, hypnotic or anxiolytic-related dependence**

> **Excludes1**   sedative, hypnotic or anxiolytic-related abuse (F13.1-)
> sedative, hypnotic, or anxiolytic use, unspecified (F13.9-)

> **Excludes2**   sedative, hypnotic, or anxiolytic poisoning (T42.-)

F13.20   Sedative, hypnotic or anxiolytic dependence, uncomplicated 🔴
> (Ex) No exclusions

F13.21   Sedative, hypnotic or anxiolytic dependence, in remission
> ▶Sedative, hypnotic or anxiolytic use disorder, moderate, in early remission
> ▶Sedative, hypnotic or anxiolytic use disorder, moderate, in sustained remission
> ▶Sedative, hypnotic or anxiolytic use disorder, severe, in early remission
> ▶Sedative, hypnotic or anxiolytic use disorder, severe, in sustained remission

● **F13.22   Sedative, hypnotic or anxiolytic dependence with intoxication**

> **Excludes1**   sedative, hypnotic or anxiolytic dependence with withdrawal (F13.23-)

F13.220   Sedative, hypnotic or anxiolytic dependence with intoxication, uncomplicated

F13.221   Sedative, hypnotic or anxiolytic dependence with intoxication delirium 🔴

F13.229   Sedative, hypnotic or anxiolytic dependence with intoxication, unspecified

CHAPTER 5 (F01-F99)

N Newborn Age: 0   P Pediatric Age: 0–17   M Maternity DX: 12–55   A Adult Age: 15–124   ♀ Females Only   ♂ Males Only

🔴 Complication\Comorbidity   🔴 Major C\C   (Ex:) CC/MCC Exclusions   🔴 Hospital-Acquired Condition

● **F13.23** **Sedative, hypnotic or anxiolytic dependence with withdrawal**
Sedative, hypnotic, or anxiolytic use disorder, moderate
Sedative, hypnotic, or anxiolytic use disorder, severe

> **Excludes1**   sedative, hypnotic or anxiolytic dependence with intoxication (F13.22-)

    F13.230 **Sedative, hypnotic or anxiolytic dependence with withdrawal, uncomplicated**

    F13.231 **Sedative, hypnotic or anxiolytic dependence with withdrawal delirium**

    F13.232 **Sedative, hypnotic or anxiolytic dependence with withdrawal with perceptual disturbance**
Sedative, hypnotic, or anxiolytic withdrawal with perceptual disturbances

    F13.239 **Sedative, hypnotic or anxiolytic dependence with withdrawal, unspecified**
Sedative, hypnotic, or anxiolytic withdrawal without perceptual disturbances

  F13.24 **Sedative, hypnotic or anxiolytic dependence with sedative, hypnotic or anxiolytic-induced mood disorder**
➡ Sedative, hypnotic, or anxiolytic use disorder, moderate, with sedative, hypnotic, or anxiolytic-induced bipolar or related disorder
➡ Sedative, hypnotic, or anxiolytic use disorder, moderate, with sedative, hypnotic, or anxiolytic-induced depressive disorder
Sedative, hypnotic, or anxiolytic use disorder, severe, with sedative, hypnotic, or anxiolytic-induced bipolar or related disorder
➡ Sedative, hypnotic, or anxiolytic use disorder, severe, with sedative, hypnotic, or anxiolytic-induced depressive disorder

● **F13.25** **Sedative, hypnotic or anxiolytic dependence with sedative, hypnotic or anxiolytic-induced psychotic disorder**

    F13.250 **Sedative, hypnotic or anxiolytic dependence with sedative, hypnotic or anxiolytic-induced psychotic disorder with delusions**

    F13.251 **Sedative, hypnotic or anxiolytic dependence with sedative, hypnotic or anxiolytic-induced psychotic disorder with hallucinations**

    F13.259 **Sedative, hypnotic or anxiolytic dependence with sedative, hypnotic or anxiolytic-induced psychotic disorder, unspecified**
(Ex:) No exclusions

  F13.26 **Sedative, hypnotic or anxiolytic dependence with sedative, hypnotic or anxiolytic-induced persisting amnestic disorder**
(Ex:) No exclusions

  F13.27 **Sedative, hypnotic or anxiolytic dependence with sedative, hypnotic or anxiolytic-induced persisting dementia**
➡ Sedative, hypnotic, or anxiolytic use disorder, moderate, with sedative, hypnotic, or anxiolytic-induced major neurocognitive disorder
Sedative, hypnotic, or anxiolytic use disorder, severe, with sedative, hypnotic, or anxiolytic-induced major neurocognitive disorder

● **F13.28** **Sedative, hypnotic or anxiolytic dependence with other sedative, hypnotic or anxiolytic-induced disorders**
(Ex:) **For category F13.28 CC codes:** No exclusions

    F13.280 **Sedative, hypnotic or anxiolytic dependence with sedative, hypnotic or anxiolytic-induced anxiety disorder**

    F13.281 **Sedative, hypnotic or anxiolytic dependence with sedative, hypnotic or anxiolytic-induced sexual dysfunction**

    F13.282 **Sedative, hypnotic or anxiolytic dependence with sedative, hypnotic or anxiolytic-induced sleep disorder**

    F13.288 **Sedative, hypnotic or anxiolytic dependence with other sedative, hypnotic or anxiolytic-induced disorder**
➡ Sedative, hypnotic, or anxiolytic use disorder, moderate, with sedative, hypnotic, or anxiolytic-induced mild neurocognitive disorder
➡ Sedative, hypnotic, or anxiolytic use disorder, severe, with sedative, hypnotic, or anxiolytic-induced mild neurocognitive disorder

  F13.29 **Sedative, hypnotic or anxiolytic dependence with unspecified sedative, hypnotic or anxiolytic-induced disorder**

● **F13.9** **Sedative, hypnotic or anxiolytic-related use, unspecified**

> **Excludes1**   sedative, hypnotic or anxiolytic-related abuse (F13.1-)
> sedative, hypnotic or anxiolytic-related dependence (F13.2-)

  F13.90 **Sedative, hypnotic, or anxiolytic use, unspecified, uncomplicated**

● **F13.92** **Sedative, hypnotic or anxiolytic use, unspecified with intoxication**

> **Excludes1**   sedative, hypnotic or anxiolytic use, unspecified with withdrawal (F13.93-)

    F13.920 **Sedative, hypnotic or anxiolytic use, unspecified with intoxication, uncomplicated**

    F13.921 **Sedative, hypnotic or anxiolytic use, unspecified with intoxication delirium**
Sedative, hypnotic, or anxiolytic-induced delirium

    F13.929 **Sedative, hypnotic or anxiolytic use, unspecified with intoxication, unspecified**

● **F13.93** **Sedative, hypnotic or anxiolytic use, unspecified with withdrawal**

> **Excludes1**   sedative, hypnotic or anxiolytic use, unspecified with intoxication (F13.92-)

    F13.930 **Sedative, hypnotic or anxiolytic use, unspecified with withdrawal, uncomplicated**

    F13.931 **Sedative, hypnotic or anxiolytic use, unspecified with withdrawal delirium**

    F13.932 **Sedative, hypnotic or anxiolytic use, unspecified with withdrawal with perceptual disturbances**

    F13.939 **Sedative, hypnotic or anxiolytic use, unspecified with withdrawal, unspecified**

▶ New   ➡ Revised   ~~deleted~~ Deleted   Excludes 1   Excludes 2   Includes   Use additional   Code first   Code also   Key words
OGCR Official Guidelines   ● Unacceptable Principal Diagnosis   X Assign placeholder X   ▶ Use Additional Character(s)   ▶ Manifestation Code   **Coding Clinic**

F13.94 Sedative, hypnotic or anxiolytic use, unspecified with sedative, hypnotic or anxiolytic-induced mood disorder
Sedative, hypnotic, or anxiolytic-induced bipolar or related disorder, without use disorder
Sedative, hypnotic, or anxiolytic-induced depressive disorder, without use disorder

● **F13.95 Sedative, hypnotic or anxiolytic use, unspecified with sedative, hypnotic or anxiolytic-induced psychotic disorder**

　　F13.950 Sedative, hypnotic or anxiolytic use, unspecified with sedative, hypnotic or anxiolytic-induced psychotic disorder with delusions 🅒

　　F13.951 Sedative, hypnotic or anxiolytic use, unspecified with sedative, hypnotic or anxiolytic-induced psychotic disorder with hallucinations 🅒

　　F13.959 Sedative, hypnotic or anxiolytic use, unspecified with sedative, hypnotic or anxiolytic-induced psychotic disorder, unspecified
　　　➡ Sedative, hypnotic, or anxiolytic-induced psychotic disorder, without use disorder

F13.96 Sedative, hypnotic or anxiolytic use, unspecified with sedative, hypnotic or anxiolytic-induced persisting amnestic disorder

F13.97 Sedative, hypnotic or anxiolytic use, unspecified with sedative, hypnotic or anxiolytic-induced persisting dementia 🅒
➡ Sedative, hypnotic, or anxiolytic-induced major neurocognitive disorder, without use disorder

● **F13.98 Sedative, hypnotic or anxiolytic use, unspecified with other sedative, hypnotic or anxiolytic-induced disorders**

　　F13.980 Sedative, hypnotic or anxiolytic use, unspecified with sedative, hypnotic or anxiolytic-induced anxiety disorder
　　　➡ Sedative, hypnotic, or anxiolytic-induced anxiety disorder, without use disorder

　　F13.981 Sedative, hypnotic or anxiolytic use, unspecified with sedative, hypnotic or anxiolytic-induced sexual dysfunction
　　　➡ Sedative, hypnotic, or anxiolytic-induced sexual dysfunction disorder, without use disorder

　　F13.982 Sedative, hypnotic or anxiolytic use, unspecified with sedative, hypnotic or anxiolytic-induced sleep disorder
　　　➡ Sedative, hypnotic, or anxiolytic-induced sleep disorder, without use disorder

　　F13.988 Sedative, hypnotic or anxiolytic use, unspecified with other sedative, hypnotic or anxiolytic-induced disorder
　　　➡ Sedative, hypnotic, or anxiolytic-induced mild neurocognitive disorder

F13.99 Sedative, hypnotic or anxiolytic use, unspecified with unspecified sedative, hypnotic or anxiolytic-induced disorder

● **F14 Cocaine related disorders**
　Excludes2 other stimulant-related disorders (F15.-)
　🅔🅧 For category F14 CC codes unless otherwise indicated: See PDX Collection 550

● **F14.1 Cocaine abuse**
　Excludes1 cocaine dependence (F14.2-)
　　　　　　cocaine use, unspecified (F14.9-)

　　F14.10 Cocaine abuse, uncomplicated
　　　Cocaine use disorder, mild

▶ **F14.11 Cocaine abuse, in remission**
　　▶ Cocaine use disorder, mild, in early remission
　　▶ Cocaine use disorder, mild, in sustained remission

● **F14.12 Cocaine abuse with intoxication**

　　F14.120 Cocaine abuse with intoxication, uncomplicated

　　F14.121 Cocaine abuse with intoxication with delirium 🅒

　　F14.122 Cocaine abuse with intoxication with perceptual disturbance

　　F14.129 Cocaine abuse with intoxication, unspecified

　F14.14 Cocaine abuse with cocaine-induced mood disorder
　　Cocaine use disorder, mild, with cocaine-induced bipolar or related disorder
　　Cocaine use disorder, mild, with cocaine-induced depressive disorder

● **F14.15 Cocaine abuse with cocaine-induced psychotic disorder**

　　F14.150 Cocaine abuse with cocaine-induced psychotic disorder with delusions 🅒

　　F14.151 Cocaine abuse with cocaine-induced psychotic disorder with hallucinations 🅒

　　F14.159 Cocaine abuse with cocaine-induced psychotic disorder, unspecified

● **F14.18 Cocaine abuse with other cocaine-induced disorder**

　　F14.180 Cocaine abuse with cocaine-induced anxiety disorder

　　F14.181 Cocaine abuse with cocaine-induced sexual dysfunction

　　F14.182 Cocaine abuse with cocaine-induced sleep disorder

　　F14.188 Cocaine abuse with other cocaine-induced disorder
　　　Cocaine use disorder, mild, with cocaine-induced obsessive-compulsive or related disorder

　F14.19 Cocaine abuse with unspecified cocaine-induced disorder

● **F14.2 Cocaine dependence**
　Excludes1 cocaine abuse (F14.1-)
　　　　　　cocaine use, unspecified (F14.9-)
　Excludes2 cocaine poisoning (T40.5-)

　　F14.20 Cocaine dependence, uncomplicated 🅒
　　　Cocaine use disorder, moderate
　　　Cocaine use disorder, severe
　　　🅔🅧 No exclusions

　　F14.21 Cocaine dependence, in remission
　　▶ Cocaine use disorder, moderate, in early remission
　　▶ Cocaine use disorder, moderate, in sustained remission
　　▶ Cocaine use disorder, severe, in early remission
　　▶ Cocaine use disorder, severe, in sustained remission
　　Coding Clinic: 2017, Q2, P27

CHAPTER 5 (F01-F99)

N Newborn Age: 0   P Pediatric Age: 0–17   M Maternity DX: 12–55   A Adult Age: 15–124   ♀ Females Only   ♂ Males Only
🅒 Complication\Comorbidity   🅜 Major C\C   🅔🅧 CC/MCC Exclusions   🅗 Hospital-Acquired Condition

763

● **F14.22**   Cocaine dependence with intoxication
　　　Excludes1　cocaine dependence with withdrawal (F14.23)

　　F14.220　Cocaine dependence with intoxication, uncomplicated

　　F14.221　Cocaine dependence with intoxication delirium 🔊

　　F14.222　Cocaine dependence with intoxication with perceptual disturbance 🔊
　　　　(Ex) No exclusions

　　F14.229　Cocaine dependence with intoxication, unspecified 🔊
　　　　(Ex) No exclusions

F14.23　Cocaine dependence with withdrawal 🔊
　　Excludes1　cocaine dependence with intoxication (F14.22-)

F14.24　Cocaine dependence with cocaine-induced mood disorder
　　Cocaine use disorder, moderate, with cocaine-induced bipolar or related disorder
　　Cocaine use disorder, moderate, with cocaine-induced depressive disorder
　　Cocaine use disorder, severe, with cocaine-induced bipolar or related disorder
　　Cocaine use disorder, severe, with cocaine-induced depressive disorder

● **F14.25**　Cocaine dependence with cocaine-induced psychotic disorder

　　F14.250　Cocaine dependence with cocaine-induced psychotic disorder with delusions 🔊

　　F14.251　Cocaine dependence with cocaine-induced psychotic disorder with hallucinations 🔊

　　F14.259　Cocaine dependence with cocaine-induced psychotic disorder, unspecified 🔊
　　　　(Ex) No exclusions

● **F14.28**　Cocaine dependence with other cocaine-induced disorder
　　(Ex) For category F14.28 CC codes: No exclusions

　　F14.280　Cocaine dependence with cocaine-induced anxiety disorder 🔊

　　F14.281　Cocaine dependence with cocaine-induced sexual dysfunction 🔊

　　F14.282　Cocaine dependence with cocaine-induced sleep disorder 🔊

　　F14.288　Cocaine dependence with other cocaine-induced disorder 🔊
　　　　Cocaine use disorder, moderate, with cocaine-induced obsessive-compulsive or related disorder
　　　　Cocaine use disorder, severe, with cocaine-induced obsessive-compulsive or related disorder

F14.29　Cocaine dependence with unspecified cocaine-induced disorder

● **F14.9**　Cocaine use, unspecified
　　Excludes1　cocaine abuse (F14.1-)
　　　　　　　cocaine dependence (F14.2-)

　　F14.90　Cocaine use, unspecified, uncomplicated

● **F14.92**　Cocaine use, unspecified with intoxication

　　F14.920　Cocaine use, unspecified with intoxication, uncomplicated

　　F14.921　Cocaine use, unspecified with intoxication delirium 🔊

　　F14.922　Cocaine use, unspecified with intoxication with perceptual disturbance

　　F14.929　Cocaine use, unspecified with intoxication, unspecified

F14.94　Cocaine use, unspecified with cocaine-induced mood disorder
　　Cocaine-induced bipolar or related disorder, without use disorder
　　Cocaine-induced depressive disorder, without use disorder

● **F14.95**　Cocaine use, unspecified with cocaine-induced psychotic disorder

　　F14.950　Cocaine use, unspecified with cocaine-induced psychotic disorder with delusions 🔊

　　F14.951　Cocaine use, unspecified with cocaine-induced psychotic disorder with hallucinations 🔊

　　F14.959　Cocaine use, unspecified with cocaine-induced psychotic disorder, unspecified
　　　　Cocaine-induced psychotic disorder, without use disorder

● **F14.98**　Cocaine use, unspecified with other specified cocaine-induced disorder

　　F14.980　Cocaine use, unspecified with cocaine-induced anxiety disorder
　　　　Cocaine-induced anxiety disorder, without use disorder

　　F14.981　Cocaine use, unspecified with cocaine-induced sexual dysfunction
　　　　Cocaine-induced sexual dysfunction, without use disorder

　　F14.982　Cocaine use, unspecified with cocaine-induced sleep disorder
　　　　Cocaine-induced sleep disorder, without use disorder

　　F14.988　Cocaine use, unspecified with other cocaine-induced disorder
　　　　Cocaine-induced obsessive-compulsive or related disorder

F14.99　Cocaine use, unspecified with unspecified cocaine-induced disorder

● **F15**　**Other stimulant related disorders**
　　Includes　amphetamine-related disorders
　　　　　　　caffeine
　　Excludes2　cocaine-related disorders (F14.-)
　　(Ex) For category F15 CC codes unless otherwise indicated: See PDX Collection 550

● **F15.1**　Other stimulant abuse
　　Excludes1　other stimulant dependence (F15.2-)
　　　　　　　other stimulant use, unspecified (F15.9-)

　　F15.10　Other stimulant abuse, uncomplicated
　　　　Amphetamine type substance use disorder, mild
　　　　Other or unspecified stimulant use disorder, mild

▶ **F15.11**　Other stimulant abuse, in remission
　　▶Amphetamine type substance use disorder, mild, in early remission
　　▶Amphetamine type substance use disorder, mild, in sustained remission
　　▶Other or unspecified stimulant use disorder, mild, in early remission
　　▶Other or unspecified stimulant use disorder, mild, in sustained remission

● **F15.12**　Other stimulant abuse with intoxication

　　F15.120　Other stimulant abuse with intoxication, uncomplicated

　　F15.121　Other stimulant abuse with intoxication delirium 🔊

F15.122   **Other stimulant abuse with intoxication with perceptual disturbance**
     Amphetamine or other stimulant use disorder, mild, with amphetamine or other stimulant intoxication, with perceptual disturbances

F15.129   **Other stimulant abuse with intoxication, unspecified**
     Amphetamine or other stimulant use disorder, mild, with amphetamine or other stimulant intoxication, without perceptual disturbances

F15.14   **Other stimulant abuse with stimulant-induced mood disorder**
     Amphetamine or other stimulant use disorder, mild, with amphetamine or other stimulant-induced bipolar or related disorder
     Amphetamine or other stimulant use disorder, mild, with amphetamine or other stimulant-induced depressive disorder

● **F15.15**   **Other stimulant abuse with stimulant-induced psychotic disorder**

F15.150   **Other stimulant abuse with stimulant-induced psychotic disorder with delusions** 🕭

F15.151   **Other stimulant abuse with stimulant-induced psychotic disorder with hallucinations** 🕭

F15.159   **Other stimulant abuse with stimulant-induced psychotic disorder, unspecified**

● **F15.18**   **Other stimulant abuse with other stimulant-induced disorder**

F15.180   **Other stimulant abuse with stimulant-induced anxiety disorder**

F15.181   **Other stimulant abuse with stimulant-induced sexual dysfunction**

F15.182   **Other stimulant abuse with stimulant-induced sleep disorder**

F15.188   **Other stimulant abuse with other stimulant-induced disorder**
     Amphetamine or other stimulant use disorder, mild, with amphetamine or other stimulant-induced obsessive-compulsive or related disorder

F15.19   **Other stimulant abuse with unspecified stimulant-induced disorder**

● **F15.2**   **Other stimulant dependence**
     Excludes1   other stimulant abuse (F15.1-)
                 other stimulant use, unspecified (F15.9-)

F15.20   **Other stimulant dependence, uncomplicated** 🕭
     Amphetamine type substance use disorder, moderate
     Amphetamine type substance use disorder, severe
     Other or unspecified stimulant use disorder, moderate
     Other or unspecified stimulant use disorder, severe
     (Ex) No exclusions

F15.21   **Other stimulant dependence, in remission**
     ▶Amphetamine type substance use disorder, moderate, in early remission
     ▶Amphetamine type substance use disorder, moderate, in sustained remission
     ▶Amphetamine type substance use disorder, severe, in early remission
     ▶Amphetamine type substance use disorder, severe, in sustained remission
     ▶Other or unspecified stimulant use disorder, moderate, in early remission
     ▶Other or unspecified stimulant use disorder, moderate, in sustained remission
     ▶Other or unspecified stimulant use disorder, severe, in early remission
     ▶Other or unspecified stimulant use disorder, severe, in sustained remission

● **F15.22**   **Other stimulant dependence with intoxication**
     Excludes1   other stimulant dependence with withdrawal (F15.23)

F15.220   **Other stimulant dependence with intoxication, uncomplicated**

F15.221   **Other stimulant dependence with intoxication delirium** 🕭

F15.222   **Other stimulant dependence with intoxication with perceptual disturbance** 🕭
     Amphetamine or other stimulant use disorder, moderate, with amphetamine or other stimulant intoxication, with perceptual disturbances
     Amphetamine or other stimulant use disorder, severe, with amphetamine or other stimulant intoxication, with perceptual disturbances
     (Ex) No exclusions

F15.229   **Other stimulant dependence with intoxication, unspecified**
     Amphetamine or other stimulant use disorder, moderate, with amphetamine or other stimulant intoxication, without perceptual disturbances
     Amphetamine or other stimulant use disorder, severe, with amphetamine or other stimulant intoxication, without perceptual disturbances

F15.23   **Other stimulant dependence with withdrawal** 🕭
     Amphetamine or other stimulant withdrawal
     Excludes1   other stimulant dependence with intoxication (F15.22-)

F15.24   **Other stimulant dependence with stimulant-induced mood disorder**
     Amphetamine or other stimulant use disorder, moderate, with amphetamine or other stimulant-induced bipolar or related disorder
     Amphetamine or other stimulant use disorder, moderate, with amphetamine or other stimulant-induced depressive disorder
     Amphetamine or other stimulant use disorder, severe, with amphetamine or other stimulant-induced bipolar or related disorder
     Amphetamine or other stimulant use disorder, severe, with amphetamine or other stimulant-induced depressive disorder

● F15.25   Other stimulant dependence with stimulant-
           induced psychotic disorder
  F15.250 Other stimulant dependence with
           stimulant-induced psychotic disorder
           with delusions 🔖
  F15.251 Other stimulant dependence with
           stimulant-induced psychotic disorder
           with hallucinations 🔖
  F15.259 Other stimulant dependence with
           stimulant-induced psychotic
           disorder, unspecified 🔖
           ⓔ No exclusions

● F15.28   Other stimulant dependence with other
           stimulant-induced disorder
           ⓔ For category F15.28 CC codes: No exclusions
  F15.280 Other stimulant dependence with
           stimulant-induced anxiety disorder 🔖
  F15.281 Other stimulant dependence with
           stimulant-induced sexual
           dysfunction 🔖
  F15.282 Other stimulant dependence with
           stimulant-induced sleep disorder 🔖
  F15.288 Other stimulant dependence with
           other stimulant-induced disorder 🔖
           ⟹ Amphetamine or other stimulant
               use disorder, moderate, with
               amphetamine or other
               stimulant-induced obsessive-
               compulsive or related
               disorder
           ⟹ Amphetamine or other stimulant
               use disorder, severe, with
               amphetamine or other stimulant-
               induced obsessive-compulsive
               or related disorder

  F15.29   Other stimulant dependence with unspecified
           stimulant-induced disorder

● F15.9   Other stimulant use, unspecified
          Excludes1   other stimulant abuse (F15.1-)
                      other stimulant dependence (F15.2-)
  F15.90   Other stimulant use, unspecified, uncomplicated
● F15.92   Other stimulant use, unspecified with
           intoxication
          Excludes1   other stimulant use, unspecified
                      with withdrawal (F15.93)
  F15.920 Other stimulant use, unspecified with
           intoxication, uncomplicated
  F15.921 Other stimulant use, unspecified with
           intoxication delirium 🔖
           Amphetamine or other stimulant-
               induced delirium
  F15.922 Other stimulant use, unspecified
           with intoxication with perceptual
           disturbance
  F15.929 Other stimulant use, unspecified with
           intoxication, unspecified
           Caffeine intoxication
  F15.93   Other stimulant use, unspecified with
           withdrawal 🔖
           Caffeine withdrawal
          Excludes1   other stimulant use, unspecified
                      with intoxication (F15.92-)
  F15.94   Other stimulant use, unspecified with
           stimulant-induced mood disorder
           Amphetamine or other stimulant-induced
               bipolar or related disorder, without use
               disorder
           Amphetamine or other stimulant-induced
               depressive disorder, without use
               disorder

● F15.95   Other stimulant use, unspecified with
           stimulant-induced psychotic disorder
  F15.950 Other stimulant use, unspecified with
           stimulant-induced psychotic disorder
           with delusions 🔖
  F15.951 Other stimulant use, unspecified with
           stimulant-induced psychotic disorder
           with hallucinations 🔖
  F15.959 Other stimulant use, unspecified with
           stimulant-induced psychotic disorder,
           unspecified
           ⟹ Amphetamine or other stimulant-
               induced psychotic disorder,
               without use disorder

● F15.98   Other stimulant use, unspecified with other
           stimulant-induced disorder
  F15.980 Other stimulant use, unspecified with
           stimulant-induced anxiety disorder
           Amphetamine or other stimulant-
               induced anxiety disorder,
               without use disorder
           Caffeine-induced anxiety disorder,
               without use disorder
  F15.981 Other stimulant use, unspecified with
           stimulant-induced sexual dysfunction
           Amphetamine or other stimulant-
               induced sexual dysfunction,
               without use disorder
  F15.982 Other stimulant use, unspecified with
           stimulant-induced sleep disorder
           Amphetamine or other stimulant-
               induced sleep disorder, without
               use disorder
           Caffeine-induced sleep disorder,
               without use disorder
  F15.988 Other stimulant use, unspecified with
           other stimulant-induced disorder
           Amphetamine or other stimulant-
               induced obsessive-compulsive
               or related disorder, without use
               disorder
  F15.99   Other stimulant use, unspecified with
           unspecified stimulant-induced disorder

● F16   Hallucinogen related disorders
        Includes   ecstasy
                   PCP
                   phencyclidine
        ⓔ For category F16 CC codes unless otherwise indicated: See PDX Collection 550
● F16.1   Hallucinogen abuse
        Excludes1   hallucinogen dependence (F16.2-)
                    hallucinogen use, unspecified (F16.9-)
  F16.10   Hallucinogen abuse, uncomplicated
           Other hallucinogen use disorder, mild
           Phencyclidine use disorder, mild
▶ F16.11   Hallucinogen abuse, in remission
           ▶ Other hallucinogen use disorder, mild, in early
               remission
           ▶ Other hallucinogen use disorder, mild, in
               sustained remission
           ▶ Phencyclidine use disorder, mild, in early
               remission
           ▶ Phencyclidine use disorder, mild, in sustained
               remission
● F16.12   Hallucinogen abuse with intoxication
  F16.120 Hallucinogen abuse with intoxication,
           uncomplicated
  F16.121 Hallucinogen abuse with intoxication
           with delirium 🔖
  F16.122 Hallucinogen abuse with intoxication
           with perceptual disturbance
  F16.129 Hallucinogen abuse with
           intoxication, unspecified

▶ New   ⟹ Revised   ~~deleted~~ Deleted   Excludes 1   Excludes 2   Includes   Use additional   Code first   Code also   Key words
OGCR Official Guidelines   ● Unacceptable Principal Diagnosis   X Assign placeholder X   ● Use Additional Character(s)   ▶ Manifestation Code   Coding Clinic

F16.14   Hallucinogen abuse with hallucinogen-induced mood disorder
> Other hallucinogen use disorder, mild, with other hallucinogen-induced bipolar or related disorder
> Other hallucinogen use disorder, mild, with other hallucinogen-induced depressive disorder
> Phencyclidine use disorder, mild, with phencyclidine-induced bipolar or related disorder
> Phencyclidine use disorder, mild, with phencyclidine-induced depressive disorder

● **F16.15**   Hallucinogen abuse with hallucinogen-induced psychotic disorder

     F16.150   Hallucinogen abuse with hallucinogen-induced psychotic disorder with delusions

     F16.151   Hallucinogen abuse with hallucinogen-induced psychotic disorder with hallucinations

     F16.159   Hallucinogen abuse with hallucinogen-induced psychotic disorder, unspecified

● **F16.18**   Hallucinogen abuse with other hallucinogen-induced disorder

     F16.180   Hallucinogen abuse with hallucinogen-induced anxiety disorder

     F16.183   Hallucinogen abuse with hallucinogen persisting perception disorder (flashbacks)

     F16.188   Hallucinogen abuse with other hallucinogen-induced disorder

   F16.19   Hallucinogen abuse with unspecified hallucinogen-induced disorder

● **F16.2**   Hallucinogen dependence

> **Excludes1**   hallucinogen abuse (F16.1-)
> hallucinogen use, unspecified (F16.9-)

   F16.20   Hallucinogen dependence, uncomplicated
> Other hallucinogen use disorder, moderate
> Other hallucinogen use disorder, severe
> Phencyclidine use disorder, moderate
> Phencyclidine use disorder, severe
> (Ex) No exclusions

   F16.21   Hallucinogen dependence, in remission
> ▶Other hallucinogen use disorder, moderate, in early remission
> ▶Other hallucinogen use disorder, moderate, in sustained remission
> ▶Other hallucinogen use disorder, severe, in early remission
> ▶Other hallucinogen use disorder, severe, in sustained remission
> ▶Phencyclidine use disorder, moderate, in early remission
> ▶Phencyclidine use disorder, moderate, in sustained remission
> ▶Phencyclidine use disorder, severe, in early remission
> ▶Phencyclidine use disorder, severe, in sustained remission

● **F16.22**   Hallucinogen dependence with intoxication

     F16.220   Hallucinogen dependence with intoxication, uncomplicated

     F16.221   Hallucinogen dependence with intoxication with delirium

     F16.229   Hallucinogen dependence with intoxication, unspecified

F16.24   Hallucinogen dependence with hallucinogen-induced mood disorder
> Other hallucinogen use disorder, moderate, with other hallucinogen-induced bipolar or related disorder
> Other hallucinogen use disorder, moderate, with other hallucinogen-induced depressive disorder
> Other hallucinogen use disorder, severe, with other hallucinogen-induced bipolar or related disorder
> Other hallucinogen use disorder, severe, with other hallucinogen-induced depressive disorder
> Phencyclidine use disorder, moderate, with phencyclidine-induced bipolar or related disorder
> Phencyclidine use disorder, moderate, with phencyclidine-induced depressive disorder
> Phencyclidine use disorder, severe, with phencyclidine-induced bipolar or related disorder
> Phencyclidine use disorder, severe, with phencyclidine-induced depressive disorder

● **F16.25**   Hallucinogen dependence with hallucinogen-induced psychotic disorder

     F16.250   Hallucinogen dependence with hallucinogen-induced psychotic disorder with delusions

     F16.251   Hallucinogen dependence with hallucinogen-induced psychotic disorder with hallucinations

     F16.259   Hallucinogen dependence with hallucinogen-induced psychotic disorder, unspecified
> (Ex) No exclusions

● **F16.28**   Hallucinogen dependence with other hallucinogen-induced disorder
> (Ex) For category F16.28 CC codes: No exclusions

     F16.280   Hallucinogen dependence with hallucinogen-induced anxiety disorder

     F16.283   Hallucinogen dependence with hallucinogen persisting perception disorder (flashbacks)

     F16.288   Hallucinogen dependence with other hallucinogen-induced disorder

   F16.29   Hallucinogen dependence with unspecified hallucinogen-induced disorder

● **F16.9**   Hallucinogen use, unspecified

> **Excludes1**   hallucinogen abuse (F16.1-)
> hallucinogen dependence (F16.2-)

   F16.90   Hallucinogen use, unspecified, uncomplicated

● **F16.92**   Hallucinogen use, unspecified with intoxication

     F16.920   Hallucinogen use, unspecified with intoxication, uncomplicated

     F16.921   Hallucinogen use, unspecified with intoxication with delirium
> Other hallucinogen intoxication delirium

     F16.929   Hallucinogen use, unspecified with intoxication, unspecified

   F16.94   Hallucinogen use, unspecified with hallucinogen-induced mood disorder
> Other hallucinogen-induced bipolar or related disorder, without use disorder
> Other hallucinogen-induced depressive disorder, without use disorder
> Phencyclidine-induced bipolar or related disorder, without use disorder
> Phencyclidine-induced depressive disorder, without use disorder

CHAPTER 5 (F01-F99)

CHAPTER 5 (F01-F99)

● **F16.95** Hallucinogen use, unspecified with hallucinogen-induced psychotic disorder

  F16.950 Hallucinogen use, unspecified with hallucinogen-induced psychotic disorder with delusions ☜

  F16.951 Hallucinogen use, unspecified with hallucinogen-induced psychotic disorder with hallucinations ☜

  F16.959 Hallucinogen use, unspecified with hallucinogen-induced psychotic disorder, unspecified
    Other hallucinogen-induced psychotic disorder, without use disorder
    Phencyclidine-induced psychotic disorder, without use disorder

● **F16.98** Hallucinogen use, unspecified with other specified hallucinogen-induced disorder

  F16.980 Hallucinogen use, unspecified with hallucinogen-induced anxiety disorder
    Other hallucinogen-induced anxiety disorder, without use disorder
    Phencyclidine-induced anxiety disorder, without use disorder

  F16.983 Hallucinogen use, unspecified with hallucinogen persisting perception disorder (flashbacks)

  F16.988 Hallucinogen use, unspecified with other hallucinogen-induced disorder

  F16.99 Hallucinogen use, unspecified with unspecified hallucinogen-induced disorder

● **F17**   **Nicotine dependence**

  Excludes1   history of tobacco dependence (Z87.891)
      tobacco use NOS (Z72.0)

  Excludes2   tobacco use (smoking) during pregnancy, childbirth and the puerperium (O99.33-)
      toxic effect of nicotine (T65.2-)

  Ⓔ **For category F17 CC codes:** See PDX Collection 550

● **F17.2**   **Nicotine dependence**

  ● **F17.20** Nicotine dependence, unspecified

    ● **F17.200** Nicotine dependence, unspecified, uncomplicated
      Tobacco use disorder, mild
      Tobacco use disorder, moderate
      Tobacco use disorder, severe
      Coding Clinic: 2016, Q1, P37

    ● **F17.201** Nicotine dependence, unspecified, in remission
      ▶ Tobacco use disorder, mild, in early remission
      ▶ Tobacco use disorder, mild, in sustained remission
      ▶ Tobacco use disorder, moderate, in early remission
      ▶ Tobacco use disorder, moderate, in sustained remission
      ▶ Tobacco use disorder, severe, in early remission
      ▶ Tobacco use disorder, severe, in sustained remission

    F17.203 Nicotine dependence unspecified, with withdrawal ☜
      Tobacco withdrawal

    F17.208 Nicotine dependence, unspecified, with other nicotine-induced disorders

    F17.209 Nicotine dependence, unspecified, with unspecified nicotine-induced disorders

  ● **F17.21** Nicotine dependence, cigarettes

    ● **F17.210** Nicotine dependence, cigarettes, uncomplicated
      Coding Clinic: 2017, Q2, P28-29

    ● **F17.211** Nicotine dependence, cigarettes, in remission
      ▶ Tobacco use disorder, cigarettes, mild, in early remission
      ▶ Tobacco use disorder, cigarettes, mild, in sustained remission
      ▶ Tobacco use disorder, cigarettes, moderate, in early remission
      ▶ Tobacco use disorder, cigarettes, moderate, in sustained remission
      ▶ Tobacco use disorder, cigarettes, severe, in early remission
      ▶ Tobacco use disorder, cigarettes, severe, in sustained remission

    F17.213 Nicotine dependence, cigarettes, with withdrawal ☜

    F17.218 Nicotine dependence, cigarettes, with other nicotine-induced disorders

    F17.219 Nicotine dependence, cigarettes, with unspecified nicotine-induced disorders

  ● **F17.22** Nicotine dependence, chewing tobacco

    ● **F17.220** Nicotine dependence, chewing tobacco, uncomplicated

    ● **F17.221** Nicotine dependence, chewing tobacco, in remission
      ▶ Tobacco use disorder, chewing tobacco, mild, in early remission
      ▶ Tobacco use disorder, chewing tobacco, mild, in sustained remission
      ▶ Tobacco use disorder, chewing tobacco, moderate, in early remission
      ▶ Tobacco use disorder, chewing tobacco, moderate, in sustained remission
      ▶ Tobacco use disorder, chewing tobacco, severe, in early remission
      ▶ Tobacco use disorder, chewing tobacco, severe, in sustained remission

    F17.223 Nicotine dependence, chewing tobacco, with withdrawal ☜

    F17.228 Nicotine dependence, chewing tobacco, with other nicotine-induced disorders

    F17.229 Nicotine dependence, chewing tobacco, with unspecified nicotine-induced disorders

  ● **F17.29** Nicotine dependence, other tobacco product

    ● **F17.290** Nicotine dependence, other tobacco product, uncomplicated
      Coding Clinic: 2017, Q2, P28-29

    ● **F17.291** Nicotine dependence, other tobacco product, in remission
      ▶ Tobacco use disorder, other tobacco product, mild, in early remission
      ▶ Tobacco use disorder, other tobacco product, mild, in sustained remission
      ▶ Tobacco use disorder, other tobacco product, moderate, in early remission
      ▶ Tobacco use disorder, other tobacco product, moderate, in sustained remission
      ▶ Tobacco use disorder, other tobacco product, severe, in early remission
      ▶ Tobacco use disorder, other tobacco product, severe, in sustained remission

▶ New   ⇒ Revised   ~~deleted~~ Deleted   Excludes 1   Excludes 2   Includes   Use additional   Code first   Code also   Key words
OGCR Official Guidelines   ● Unacceptable Principal Diagnosis   X Assign placeholder X   ● Use Additional Character(s)   ▌ Manifestation Code   **Coding Clinic**

F17.293   Nicotine dependence, other tobacco product, with withdrawal

F17.298   Nicotine dependence, other tobacco product, with other nicotine-induced disorders

F17.299   Nicotine dependence, other tobacco product, with unspecified nicotine-induced disorders

● **F18**   **Inhalant related disorders**

Includes   volatile solvents

(Ex) For category F18 CC codes unless otherwise indicated: See PDX Collection 550

● **F18.1**   **Inhalant abuse**

Excludes1   inhalant dependence (F18.2-)
inhalant use, unspecified (F18.9-)

F18.10   **Inhalant abuse, uncomplicated**
Inhalant use disorder, mild

▶ F18.11   **Inhalant abuse, in remission**
▶ Inhalant use disorder, mild, in early remission
▶ Inhalant use disorder, mild, in sustained remission

● F18.12   **Inhalant abuse with intoxication**

F18.120   **Inhalant abuse with intoxication, uncomplicated**

F18.121   **Inhalant abuse with intoxication delirium**

F18.129   **Inhalant abuse with intoxication, unspecified**

F18.14   **Inhalant abuse with inhalant-induced mood disorder**
Inhalant use disorder, mild, with inhalant-induced depressive disorder

● F18.15   **Inhalant abuse with inhalant-induced psychotic disorder**

F18.150   **Inhalant abuse with inhalant-induced psychotic disorder with delusions**

F18.151   **Inhalant abuse with inhalant-induced psychotic disorder with hallucinations**

F18.159   **Inhalant abuse with inhalant-induced psychotic disorder, unspecified**

F18.17   **Inhalant abuse with inhalant-induced dementia**
Inhalant use disorder, mild, with inhalant-induced major neurocognitive disorder

● F18.18   **Inhalant abuse with other inhalant-induced disorders**

F18.180   **Inhalant abuse with inhalant-induced anxiety disorder**

F18.188   **Inhalant abuse with other inhalant-induced disorder**
Inhalant use disorder, mild, with inhalant-induced mild neurocognitive disorder

F18.19   **Inhalant abuse with unspecified inhalant-induced disorder**

● **F18.2**   **Inhalant dependence**

Excludes1   inhalant abuse (F18.1-)
inhalant use, unspecified (F18.9-)

F18.20   **Inhalant dependence, uncomplicated**
Inhalant use disorder, moderate
Inhalant use disorder, severe
(Ex) No exclusions

F18.21   **Inhalant dependence, in remission**
▶ Inhalant use disorder, moderate, in early remission
▶ Inhalant use disorder, moderate, in sustained remission
▶ Inhalant use disorder, severe, in early remission
▶ Inhalant use disorder, severe, in sustained remission

● F18.22   **Inhalant dependence with intoxication**

F18.220   **Inhalant dependence with intoxication, uncomplicated**

F18.221   **Inhalant dependence with intoxication delirium**

F18.229   **Inhalant dependence with intoxication, unspecified**

F18.24   **Inhalant dependence with inhalant-induced mood disorder**
Inhalant use disorder, moderate, with inhalant-induced depressive disorder
Inhalant use disorder, severe, with inhalant-induced depressive disorder

● F18.25   **Inhalant dependence with inhalant-induced psychotic disorder**

F18.250   **Inhalant dependence with inhalant-induced psychotic disorder with delusions**

F18.251   **Inhalant dependence with inhalant-induced psychotic disorder with hallucinations**

F18.259   **Inhalant dependence with inhalant-induced psychotic disorder, unspecified**
(Ex) No exclusions

F18.27   **Inhalant dependence with inhalant-induced dementia**
Inhalant use disorder, moderate, with inhalant-induced major neurocognitive disorder
Inhalant use disorder, severe, with inhalant-induced major neurocognitive disorder

● F18.28   **Inhalant dependence with other inhalant-induced disorders**
(Ex) For category F18.28 CC codes: No exclusions

F18.280   **Inhalant dependence with inhalant-induced anxiety disorder**

F18.288   **Inhalant dependence with other inhalant-induced disorder**
Inhalant use disorder, moderate, with inhalant-induced mild neurocognitive disorder
Inhalant use disorder, severe, with inhalant-induced mild neurocognitive disorder

F18.29   **Inhalant dependence with unspecified inhalant-induced disorder**

● **F18.9**   **Inhalant use, unspecified**

Excludes1   inhalant abuse (F18.1-)
inhalant dependence (F18.2-)

F18.90   **Inhalant use, unspecified, uncomplicated**

● F18.92   **Inhalant use, unspecified with intoxication**

F18.920   **Inhalant use, unspecified with intoxication, uncomplicated**

F18.921   **Inhalant use, unspecified with intoxication with delirium**

F18.929   **Inhalant use, unspecified with intoxication, unspecified**

F18.94   **Inhalant use, unspecified with inhalant-induced mood disorder**
Inhalant-induced depressive disorder

● F18.95   **Inhalant use, unspecified with inhalant-induced psychotic disorder**

F18.950   **Inhalant use, unspecified with inhalant-induced psychotic disorder with delusions**

F18.951   **Inhalant use, unspecified with inhalant-induced psychotic disorder with hallucinations**

F18.959   **Inhalant use, unspecified with inhalant-induced psychotic disorder, unspecified**

F18.97 Inhalant use, unspecified with inhalant-induced persisting dementia
Inhalant-induced major neurocognitive disorder

● **F18.98** Inhalant use, unspecified with other inhalant-induced disorders

    F18.980 Inhalant use, unspecified with inhalant-induced anxiety disorder

    F18.988 Inhalant use, unspecified with other inhalant-induced disorder
         Inhalant-induced mild neurocognitive disorder

F18.99 Inhalant use, unspecified with unspecified inhalant-induced disorder

● **F19** Other psychoactive substance related disorders

    Includes   polysubstance drug use (indiscriminate drug use)

    (Ex) For category F19 CC codes unless otherwise indicated: See PDX Collection 550

● **F19.1** Other psychoactive substance abuse

    Excludes1   other psychoactive substance dependence (F19.2-)
             other psychoactive substance use, unspecified (F19.9-)

    F19.10 Other psychoactive substance abuse, uncomplicated
         Other (or unknown) substance use disorder, mild

▶ **F19.11** Other psychoactive substance abuse, in remission
        ▶Other (or unknown) substance use disorder, mild, in early remission
        ▶Other (or unknown) substance use disorder, mild, in sustained remission

● **F19.12** Other psychoactive substance abuse with intoxication

    F19.120 Other psychoactive substance abuse with intoxication, uncomplicated

    F19.121 Other psychoactive substance abuse with intoxication delirium

    F19.122 Other psychoactive substance abuse with intoxication with perceptual disturbances

    F19.129 Other psychoactive substance abuse with intoxication, unspecified

    F19.14 Other psychoactive substance abuse with psychoactive substance-induced mood disorder
         Other (or unknown) substance use disorder, mild, with other (or unknown) substance-induced bipolar or related disorder
         Other (or unknown) substance use disorder, mild, with other (or unknown) substance-induced depressive disorder

● **F19.15** Other psychoactive substance abuse with psychoactive substance-induced psychotic disorder

    F19.150 Other psychoactive substance abuse with psychoactive substance-induced psychotic disorder with delusions

    F19.151 Other psychoactive substance abuse with psychoactive substance-induced psychotic disorder with hallucinations

    F19.159 Other psychoactive substance abuse with psychoactive substance-induced psychotic disorder, unspecified

    F19.16 Other psychoactive substance abuse with psychoactive substance-induced persisting amnestic disorder

    F19.17 Other psychoactive substance abuse with psychoactive substance-induced persisting dementia
         Other (or unknown) substance use disorder, mild, with other (or unknown) substance-induced major neurocognitive disorder

● **F19.18** Other psychoactive substance abuse with other psychoactive substance-induced disorders

    F19.180 Other psychoactive substance abuse with psychoactive substance-induced anxiety disorder

    F19.181 Other psychoactive substance abuse with psychoactive substance-induced sexual dysfunction

    F19.182 Other psychoactive substance abuse with psychoactive substance-induced sleep disorder

    F19.188 Other psychoactive substance abuse with other psychoactive substance-induced disorder
         Other (or unknown) substance use disorder, mild, with other (or unknown) substance-induced mild neurocognitive disorder
         Other (or unknown) substance use disorder, mild, with other (or unknown) substance-induced obsessive-compulsive or related disorder

    F19.19 Other psychoactive substance abuse with unspecified psychoactive substance-induced disorder

● **F19.2** Other psychoactive substance dependence

    Excludes1   other psychoactive substance abuse (F19.1-)
             other psychoactive substance use, unspecified (F19.9-)

    F19.20 Other psychoactive substance dependence, uncomplicated
         Other (or unknown) substance use disorder, moderate
         Other (or unknown) substance use disorder, severe
         (Ex) No exclusions

    F19.21 Other psychoactive substance dependence, in remission
        ▶Other (or unknown) substance use disorder, moderate, in early remission
        ▶Other (or unknown) substance use disorder, moderate, in sustained remission
        ▶Other (or unknown) substance use disorder, severe, in early remission
        ▶Other (or unknown) substance use, severe, in sustained remission

● **F19.22** Other psychoactive substance dependence with intoxication

    Excludes1   other psychoactive substance dependence with withdrawal (F19.23-)

    F19.220 Other psychoactive substance dependence with intoxication, uncomplicated

    F19.221 Other psychoactive substance dependence with intoxication delirium

    F19.222 Other psychoactive substance dependence with intoxication with perceptual disturbance
         (Ex) No exclusions

    F19.229 Other psychoactive substance dependence with intoxication, unspecified

▶ New   ⇒ Revised   ~~deleted~~ Deleted   Excludes 1   Excludes 2   Includes   Use additional   Code first   Code also   Key words
OGCR Official Guidelines   ● Unacceptable Principal Diagnosis   X Assign placeholder X   ● Use Additional Character(s)   ▶ Manifestation Code   **Coding Clinic**

- **F19.23 Other psychoactive substance dependence with withdrawal**
  - **Excludes1** other psychoactive substance dependence with intoxication (F19.22-)
  - **F19.230 Other psychoactive substance dependence with withdrawal, uncomplicated** 🔹
  - **F19.231 Other psychoactive substance dependence with withdrawal delirium** 🔹
  - **F19.232 Other psychoactive substance dependence with withdrawal with perceptual disturbance** 🔹
  - **F19.239 Other psychoactive substance dependence with withdrawal, unspecified** 🔹
- **F19.24 Other psychoactive substance dependence with psychoactive substance-induced mood disorder**
  - Other (or unknown) substance use disorder, moderate, with other (or unknown) substance-induced bipolar or related disorder
  - Other (or unknown) substance use disorder, moderate, with other (or unknown) substance-induced depressive disorder
  - Other (or unknown) substance use disorder, severe, with other (or unknown) substance-induced bipolar or related disorder
  - Other (or unknown) substance use disorder, severe, with other (or unknown) substance-induced depressive disorder
- **F19.25 Other psychoactive substance dependence with psychoactive substance-induced psychotic disorder**
  - **F19.250 Other psychoactive substance dependence with psychoactive substance-induced psychotic disorder with delusions** 🔹
  - **F19.251 Other psychoactive substance dependence with psychoactive substance-induced psychotic disorder with hallucinations** 🔹
  - **F19.259 Other psychoactive substance dependence with psychoactive substance-induced psychotic disorder, unspecified** 🔹
    - (Ex) No exclusions
- **F19.26 Other psychoactive substance dependence with psychoactive substance-induced persisting amnestic disorder** 🔹
    - (Ex) No exclusions
- **F19.27 Other psychoactive substance dependence with psychoactive substance-induced persisting dementia** 🔹
  - Other (or unknown) substance use disorder, moderate, with other (or unknown) substance-induced major neurocognitive disorder
  - Other (or unknown) substance use disorder, severe, with other (or unknown) substance-induced major neurocognitive disorder
- **F19.28 Other psychoactive substance dependence with other psychoactive substance-induced disorders**
    - (Ex) For category F19.28 CC codes: No exclusions
  - **F19.280 Other psychoactive substance dependence with psychoactive substance-induced anxiety disorder** 🔹
  - **F19.281 Other psychoactive substance dependence with psychoactive substance-induced sexual dysfunction** 🔹
  - **F19.282 Other psychoactive substance dependence with psychoactive substance-induced sleep disorder** 🔹
  - **F19.288 Other psychoactive substance dependence with other psychoactive substance-induced disorder** 🔹
    - Other (or unknown) substance use disorder, moderate, with other (or unknown) substance-induced mild neurocognitive disorder
    - Other (or unknown) substance use disorder, severe, with other (or unknown) substance-induced mild neurocognitive disorder
    - Other (or unknown) substance use disorder, moderate, with other (or unknown) substance-induced obsessive-compulsive or related disorder
    - Other (or unknown) substance use disorder, severe, with other (or unknown) substance-induced obsessive-compulsive or related disorder
- **F19.29 Other psychoactive substance dependence with unspecified psychoactive substance-induced disorder**
- **F19.9 Other psychoactive substance use, unspecified**
  - **Excludes1** other psychoactive substance abuse (F19.1-)
    - other psychoactive substance dependence (F19.2-)
  - **F19.90 Other psychoactive substance use, unspecified, uncomplicated**
  - **F19.92 Other psychoactive substance use, unspecified with intoxication**
    - **Excludes1** other psychoactive substance use, unspecified with withdrawal (F19.93)
    - **F19.920 Other psychoactive substance use, unspecified with intoxication, uncomplicated**
    - **F19.921 Other psychoactive substance use, unspecified with intoxication with delirium** 🔹
      - Other (or unknown) substance-induced delirium
    - **F19.922 Other psychoactive substance use, unspecified with intoxication with perceptual disturbance**
    - **F19.929 Other psychoactive substance use, unspecified with intoxication, unspecified**
- **F19.93 Other psychoactive substance use, unspecified with withdrawal**
  - **Excludes1** other psychoactive substance use, unspecified with intoxication (F19.92-)
  - **F19.930 Other psychoactive substance use, unspecified with withdrawal, uncomplicated** 🔹
  - **F19.931 Other psychoactive substance use, unspecified with withdrawal delirium** 🔹
  - **F19.932 Other psychoactive substance use, unspecified with withdrawal with perceptual disturbance** 🔹
  - **F19.939 Other psychoactive substance use, unspecified with withdrawal, unspecified** 🔹

F19.94   **Other psychoactive substance use, unspecified with psychoactive substance-induced mood disorder**
Other (or unknown) substance-induced bipolar or related disorder, without use disorder
Other (or unknown) substance-induced depressive disorder, without use disorder

● **F19.95**   **Other psychoactive substance use, unspecified with psychoactive substance-induced psychotic disorder**

     F19.950   **Other psychoactive substance use, unspecified with psychoactive substance-induced psychotic disorder with delusions** 🔗

     F19.951   **Other psychoactive substance use, unspecified with psychoactive substance-induced psychotic disorder with hallucinations** 🔗

     F19.959   **Other psychoactive substance use, unspecified with psychoactive substance-induced psychotic disorder, unspecified**
         Other or unknown substance-induced psychotic disorder, without use disorder

   F19.96   **Other psychoactive substance use, unspecified with psychoactive substance-induced persisting amnestic disorder**

   F19.97   **Other psychoactive substance use, unspecified with psychoactive substance-induced persisting dementia** 🔗
      Other (or unknown) substance-induced major neurocognitive disorder, without use disorder

● **F19.98**   **Other psychoactive substance use, unspecified with other psychoactive substance-induced disorders**

     F19.980   **Other psychoactive substance use, unspecified with psychoactive substance-induced anxiety disorder**
         Other (or unknown) substance-induced anxiety disorder, without use disorder

     F19.981   **Other psychoactive substance use, unspecified with psychoactive substance-induced sexual dysfunction**
         Other (or unknown) substance-induced sexual dysfunction, without use disorder

     F19.982   **Other psychoactive substance use, unspecified with psychoactive substance-induced sleep disorder**
         Other (or unknown) substance-induced sleep disorder, without use disorder

     F19.988   **Other psychoactive substance use, unspecified with other psychoactive substance-induced disorder**
         Other (or unknown) substance-induced mild neurocognitive disorder, without use disorder
         Other (or unknown) substance-induced obsessive-compulsive or related disorder, without use disorder

   F19.99   **Other psychoactive substance use, unspecified with unspecified psychoactive substance-induced disorder**

SCHIZOPHRENIA, SCHIZOTYPAL, DELUSIONAL, AND OTHER NON-MOOD PSYCHOTIC DISORDERS (F20-F29)

● **F20**   **Schizophrenia**
Personality disorders characterized by multiple mental and behavioral irregularities (may exhibit disorganized thinking, delusions, and auditory hallucinations)

   Excludes1   brief psychotic disorder (F23)
             cyclic schizophrenia (F25.0)
             mood [affective] disorders with psychotic symptoms (F30.2, F31.2, F31.5, F31.64, F32.3, F33.3)
             schizoaffective disorder (F25.-)
             schizophrenic reaction NOS (F23)

   Excludes2   schizophrenic reaction in:
             alcoholism (F10.15-, F10.25-, F10.95-)
             brain disease (F06.2)
             epilepsy (F06.2)
             psychoactive drug use (F11-F19 with .15, .25, .95)
             schizotypal disorder (F21)

   (Ex:) **For category F20 CC codes:** See PDX Collection 551

   F20.0   **Paranoid schizophrenia** 🔗
      Paraphrenic schizophrenia

     Excludes1   involutional paranoid state (F22)
             paranoia (F22)

   F20.1   **Disorganized schizophrenia** 🔗
      Hebephrenic schizophrenia
      Hebephrenia

   F20.2   **Catatonic schizophrenia** 🔗
      Schizophrenic catalepsy
      Schizophrenic catatonia
      Schizophrenic flexibilitas cerea

     Excludes1   catatonic stupor (R40.1)

   F20.3   **Undifferentiated schizophrenia**
      Atypical schizophrenia

     Excludes1   acute schizophrenia-like psychotic disorder (F23)

     Excludes2   post-schizophrenic depression (F32.89)

   F20.5   **Residual schizophrenia** 🔗
      Restzustand (schizophrenic)
      Schizophrenic residual state

● **F20.8**   **Other schizophrenia**

     F20.81   **Schizophreniform disorder** 🔗
         Schizophreniform psychosis NOS

     F20.89   **Other schizophrenia** 🔗
         Cenesthopathic schizophrenia
         Simple schizophrenia

   F20.9   **Schizophrenia, unspecified**

   F21   **Schizotypal disorder**
Personality disorder characterized by need for social isolation, odd behavior and thinking, and often unconventional beliefs
      Borderline schizophrenia
      Latent schizophrenia
      Latent schizophrenic reaction
      Prepsychotic schizophrenia
      Prodromal schizophrenia
      Pseudoneurotic schizophrenia
      Pseudopsychopathic schizophrenia
      Schizotypal personality disorder

     Excludes2   Asperger's syndrome (F84.5)
             schizoid personality disorder (F60.1)

▶ New   ⇛ Revised   ~~deleted~~ Deleted   Excludes 1   Excludes 2   Includes   Use additional   Code first   Code also   Key words
OGCR Official Guidelines   ● Unacceptable Principal Diagnosis   X Assign placeholder X   ▶ Use Additional Character(s)   ▷ Manifestation Code   **Coding Clinic**

F22   **Delusional disorders**
Delusional dysmorphophobia
Involutional paranoid state
Paranoia
Paranoia querulans
Paranoid psychosis
Paranoid state
Paraphrenia (late)
Sensitiver Beziehungswahn

> **Excludes1**   mood [affective] disorders with psychotic symptoms (F30.2, F31.2, F31.5, F31.64, F32.3, F33.3)
> paranoid schizophrenia (F20.0)

> **Excludes2**   paranoid personality disorder (F60.0)
> paranoid psychosis, psychogenic (F23)
> paranoid reaction (F23)

F23   **Brief psychotic disorder**
Paranoid reaction
Psychogenic paranoid psychosis

> **Excludes2**   mood [affective] disorders with psychotic symptoms (F30.2, F31.2, F31.5, F31.64, F32.3, F33.3)

> (Ex) No exclusions

F24   **Shared psychotic disorder**
Folie à deux
Induced paranoid disorder
Induced psychotic disorder

● **F25**   **Schizoaffective disorders**
Mental disorder exhibiting major depressive episode, manic episode, or mixed episode occurs with symptoms of schizophrenia, and mood disorder

> **Excludes1**   mood [affective] disorders with psychotic symptoms (F30.2, F31.2, F31.5, F31.64, F32.3, F33.3)
> schizophrenia (F20.-)

F25.0   **Schizoaffective disorder, bipolar type**
Cyclic schizophrenia
Schizoaffective disorder, manic type
Schizoaffective disorder, mixed type
Schizoaffective psychosis, bipolar type
~~Schizophreniform psychosis, manic type~~

F25.1   **Schizoaffective disorder, depressive type**
Schizoaffective psychosis, depressive type
~~Schizophreniform psychosis, depressive type~~

F25.8   **Other schizoaffective disorders**

F25.9   **Schizoaffective disorder, unspecified**
Schizoaffective psychosis NOS

F28   **Other psychotic disorder not due to a substance or known physiological condition**
Chronic hallucinatory psychosis
▶Other specified schizophrenia spectrum and other psychotic disorder

F29   **Unspecified psychosis not due to a substance or known physiological condition**
Psychosis NOS
▶Unspecified schizophrenia spectrum and other psychotic disorder

> **Excludes1**   mental disorder NOS (F99)
> unspecified mental disorder due to known physiological condition (F09)

MOOD [AFFECTIVE] DISORDERS (F30-F39)

● **F30**   **Manic episode**
Elevated, expansive, or irritable mood

> **Includes**   bipolar disorder, single manic episode
> mixed affective episode

> **Excludes1**   bipolar disorder (F31.-)
> major depressive disorder, single episode (F32.-)
> major depressive disorder, recurrent (F33.-)

> (Ex) **For category F30 CC codes unless otherwise indicated:** See PDX Collection 551

● **F30.1**   **Manic episode without psychotic symptoms**

F30.10   **Manic episode without psychotic symptoms, unspecified**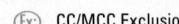

F30.11   **Manic episode without psychotic symptoms, mild**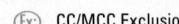

F30.12   **Manic episode without psychotic symptoms, moderate**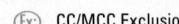

F30.13   **Manic episode, severe, without psychotic symptoms**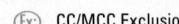
> (Ex) See PDX Collection 552

F30.2   **Manic episode, severe with psychotic symptoms**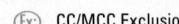
Manic stupor
Mania with mood-congruent psychotic symptoms
Mania with mood-incongruent psychotic symptoms

F30.3   **Manic episode in partial remission**

F30.4   **Manic episode in full remission**

F30.8   **Other manic episodes**
Abnormality of mood resembling mania but less intense
Hypomania

F30.9   **Manic episode, unspecified**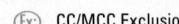
Mania NOS

● **F31**   **Bipolar disorder**
Mood disorders with history of manic, mixed, or hypomanic episodes

> **Includes**   ▶bipolar I disorder
> ▶bipolar type I disorder
> manic-depressive illness
> manic-depressive psychosis
> manic-depressive reaction

> **Excludes1**   bipolar disorder, single manic episode (F30.-)
> major depressive disorder, single episode (F32.-)
> major depressive disorder, recurrent (F33.-)

> **Excludes2**   cyclothymia (F34.0)

> (Ex) **For category F31 CC codes unless otherwise indicated:** See PDX Collection 551

F31.0   **Bipolar disorder, current episode hypomanic**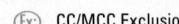

● **F31.1**   **Bipolar disorder, current episode manic without psychotic features**

F31.10   **Bipolar disorder, current episode manic without psychotic features, unspecified**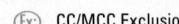

F31.11   **Bipolar disorder, current episode manic without psychotic features, mild**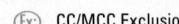

F31.12   **Bipolar disorder, current episode manic without psychotic features, moderate**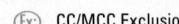

F31.13   **Bipolar disorder, current episode manic without psychotic features, severe**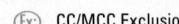
> (Ex) See PDX Collection 553

F31.2   **Bipolar disorder, current episode manic severe with psychotic features**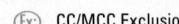
Bipolar disorder, current episode manic with mood-congruent psychotic symptoms
Bipolar disorder, current episode manic with mood-incongruent psychotic symptoms
▶Bipolar I disorder, current or most recent episode manic with psychotic features

● **F31.3**   **Bipolar disorder, current episode depressed, mild or moderate severity**

F31.30   **Bipolar disorder, current episode depressed, mild or moderate severity, unspecified**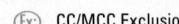

F31.31   **Bipolar disorder, current episode depressed, mild**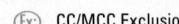

F31.32   **Bipolar disorder, current episode depressed, moderate**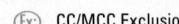

F31.4   **Bipolar disorder, current episode depressed, severe, without psychotic features**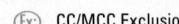
> (Ex) See PDX Collection 554

F31.5   **Bipolar disorder, current episode depressed, severe, with psychotic features**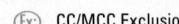
Bipolar disorder, current episode depressed with mood-incongruent psychotic symptoms
Bipolar disorder, current episode depressed with mood-congruent psychotic symptoms
▶Bipolar I disorder, current or most recent episode depressed, with psychotic features

N Newborn Age: 0   **P** Pediatric Age: 0–17   **M** Maternity DX: 12–55   **A** Adult Age: 15–124   ♀ Females Only   ♂ Males Only

 Complication\Comorbidity   Major C\C   (Ex) CC/MCC Exclusions   Hospital-Acquired Condition

773

CHAPTER 5 (F01-F99)

● F31.6   **Bipolar disorder, current episode mixed**

    F31.60   **Bipolar disorder, current episode mixed, unspecified** 🗨

    F31.61   **Bipolar disorder, current episode mixed, mild** 🗨

    F31.62   **Bipolar disorder, current episode mixed, moderate** 🗨

    F31.63   **Bipolar disorder, current episode mixed, severe, without psychotic features** 🗨
        (Ex) See PDX Collection 554

    F31.64   **Bipolar disorder, current episode mixed, severe, with psychotic features** 🗨
        Bipolar disorder, current episode mixed with mood-congruent psychotic symptoms
        Bipolar disorder, current episode mixed with mood-incongruent psychotic symptoms

● F31.7   **Bipolar disorder, currently in remission**

    F31.70   **Bipolar disorder, currently in remission, most recent episode unspecified**

    F31.71   **Bipolar disorder, in partial remission, most recent episode hypomanic**

    F31.72   **Bipolar disorder, in full remission, most recent episode hypomanic**

    F31.73   **Bipolar disorder, in partial remission, most recent episode manic**

    F31.74   **Bipolar disorder, in full remission, most recent episode manic**

    F31.75   **Bipolar disorder, in partial remission, most recent episode depressed**

    F31.76   **Bipolar disorder, in full remission, most recent episode depressed**

    F31.77   **Bipolar disorder, in partial remission, most recent episode mixed**

    F31.78   **Bipolar disorder, in full remission, most recent episode mixed**

● F31.8   **Other bipolar disorders**

    F31.81   **Bipolar II disorder** 🗨
        ▶ Bipolar disorder, type 2

    F31.89   **Other bipolar disorder** 🗨
        Recurrent manic episodes NOS

    F31.9   **Bipolar disorder, unspecified**
        ▶ Manic depression

● F32   **Major depressive disorder, single episode**

    Includes   single episode of agitated depression
        single episode of depressive reaction
        single episode of major depression
        single episode of psychogenic depression
        single episode of reactive depression
        single episode of vital depression

    Excludes1   bipolar disorder (F31.-)
        manic episode (F30.-)
        recurrent depressive disorder (F33.-)

    Excludes2   adjustment disorder (F43.2)

    F32.0   **Major depressive disorder, single episode, mild** 🗨
        (Ex) See PDX Collection 555

    F32.1   **Major depressive disorder, single episode, moderate** 🗨
        (Ex) See PDX Collection 555

    F32.2   **Major depressive disorder, single episode, severe without psychotic features** 🗨
        (Ex) See PDX Collection 555

    F32.3   **Major depressive disorder, single episode, severe with psychotic features** 🗨
        Single episode of major depression with mood-congruent psychotic symptoms
        Single episode of major depression with mood-incongruent psychotic symptoms
        Single episode of major depression with psychotic symptoms
        Single episode of psychogenic depressive psychosis
        Single episode of psychotic depression
        Single episode of reactive depressive psychosis
        (Ex) See PDX Collection 555

    F32.4   **Major depressive disorder, single episode, in partial remission**

    F32.5   **Major depressive disorder, single episode, in full remission**

● F32.8   **Other depressive episodes**

    F32.81   **Premenstrual dysphoric disorder** ♀
        Excludes1   premenstrual tension syndrome (N94.3)
        Coding Clinic: 2016, Q4, P14

    F32.89   **Other specified depressive episodes**
        Atypical depression
        Post-schizophrenic depression
        Single episode of 'masked' depression NOS
        Coding Clinic: 2016, Q4, P14

    F32.9   **Major depressive disorder, single episode, unspecified**
        Depression NOS
        Depressive disorder NOS
        Major depression NOS

● F33   **Major depressive disorder, recurrent**

    Includes   recurrent episodes of depressive reaction
        recurrent episodes of endogenous depression
        recurrent episodes of major depression
        recurrent episodes of psychogenic depression
        recurrent episodes of reactive depression
        recurrent episodes of seasonal depressive disorder
        recurrent episodes of vital depression

    Excludes1   bipolar disorder (F31.-)
        manic episode (F30.-)

    (Ex) For category F33 CC codes unless otherwise indicated: See PDX Collection 555

    F33.0   **Major depressive disorder, recurrent, mild** 🗨

    F33.1   **Major depressive disorder, recurrent, moderate** 🗨

    F33.2   **Major depressive disorder, recurrent severe without psychotic features** 🗨

    F33.3   **Major depressive disorder, recurrent, severe with psychotic symptoms** 🗨
        Endogenous depression with psychotic symptoms
        ▶ Major depressive disorder, recurrent, with psychotic features
        Recurrent severe episodes of major depression with mood-congruent psychotic symptoms
        Recurrent severe episodes of major depression with mood-incongruent psychotic symptoms
        Recurrent severe episodes of major depression with psychotic symptoms
        Recurrent severe episodes of psychogenic depressive psychosis
        Recurrent severe episodes of psychotic depression
        Recurrent severe episodes of reactive depressive psychosis
        (Ex) See PDX Collection 551

● F33.4   **Major depressive disorder, recurrent, in remission**

    F33.40   **Major depressive disorder, recurrent, in remission, unspecified** 🗨

    F33.41   **Major depressive disorder, recurrent, in partial remission**

    F33.42   **Major depressive disorder, recurrent, in full remission**

    F33.8   **Other recurrent depressive disorders** 🗨
        Recurrent brief depressive episodes
        (Ex) See PDX Collection 551

    F33.9   **Major depressive disorder, recurrent, unspecified** 🗨
        Monopolar depression NOS

▶ New   ⇒ Revised   ~~deleted~~ Deleted   Excludes 1   Excludes 2   Includes   Use additional   Code first   Code also   Key words
OGCR Official Guidelines   ● Unacceptable Principal Diagnosis   X Assign placeholder X   ● Use Additional Character(s)   ▎ Manifestation Code   **Coding Clinic**

Figure 5-1 PET scan of depressed individual's brain before and after recovery. (From Fortinash KM: Psychiatric Mental Health Nursing, ed 4, St. Louis, Mosby, 2008)

● **F34**   **Persistent mood [affective] disorders**

  F34.0   **Cyclothymic disorder**
    Affective personality disorder
    Cycloid personality
    Cyclothymia
    Cyclothymic personality

  F34.1   **Dysthymic disorder**
    Depressive neurosis
    Depressive personality disorder
    Dysthymia
    Neurotic depression
    Persistent anxiety depression
    Persistent depressive disorder
    Excludes2   anxiety depression (mild or not persistent) (F41.8)

 ● **F34.8**   **Other persistent mood [affective] disorders**
    (Ex) For category F34.8 CC codes: See PDX Collection 551

    F34.81   **Disruptive mood dysregulation disorder**
      Coding Clinic: 2016, Q4, P14

    F34.89   **Other specified persistent mood disorders**
      Coding Clinic: 2016, Q4, P14

  F34.9   **Persistent mood [affective] disorder, unspecified**
    (Ex) See PDX Collection 551

  F39   **Unspecified mood [affective] disorder**
    Affective psychosis NOS

ANXIETY, DISSOCIATIVE, STRESS-RELATED, SOMATOFORM AND OTHER NONPSYCHOTIC MENTAL DISORDERS (F40-F48)

● **F40**   **Phobic anxiety disorders**
    Irrational fear with avoidance of the feared subject, activity, or situation even though the individual knows that the reaction is excessive

 ● **F40.0**   **Agoraphobia**
    Intense, irrational fear of open spaces
    F40.00   **Agoraphobia, unspecified**
    F40.01   **Agoraphobia with panic disorder**
      Panic disorder with agoraphobia
      Excludes1   panic disorder without agoraphobia (F41.0)
    F40.02   **Agoraphobia without panic disorder**

 ● **F40.1**   **Social phobias**
    Anthropophobia
    ▶Social anxiety disorder
    Social anxiety disorder of childhood
    Social neurosis
    F40.10   **Social phobia, unspecified**
    F40.11   **Social phobia, generalized**

 ● **F40.2**   **Specific (isolated) phobias**
    Excludes2   dysmorphophobia (nondelusional) (F45.22)
      nosophobia (F45.22)
  ● **F40.21**   **Animal type phobia**
    F40.210   **Arachnophobia**
      Fear of spiders
    F40.218   **Other animal type phobia**
  ● **F40.22**   **Natural environment type phobia**
    F40.220   **Fear of thunderstorms**
    F40.228   **Other natural environment type phobia**
  ● **F40.23**   **Blood, injection, injury type phobia**
    F40.230   **Fear of blood**
    F40.231   **Fear of injections and transfusions**
    F40.232   **Fear of other medical care**
    F40.233   **Fear of injury**
  ● **F40.24**   **Situational type phobia**
    F40.240   **Claustrophobia**
      Fear of closed spaces
    F40.241   **Acrophobia**
      Fear of heights
    F40.242   **Fear of bridges**
    F40.243   **Fear of flying**
    F40.248   **Other situational type phobia**
  ● **F40.29**   **Other specified phobia**
    F40.290   **Androphobia**
      Fear of men
    F40.291   **Gynephobia**
      Fear of women
    F40.298   **Other specified phobia**

  F40.8   **Other phobic anxiety disorders**
    Phobic anxiety disorder of childhood

  F40.9   **Phobic anxiety disorder, unspecified**
    Phobia NOS
    Phobic state NOS

● **F41**   **Other anxiety disorders**
    Excludes2   anxiety in:
      acute stress reaction (F43.0)
      transient adjustment reaction (F43.2)
      neurasthenia (F48.8)
      psychophysiologic disorders (F45.-)
      separation anxiety (F93.0)

 ➡ **F41.0**   **Panic disorder [episodic paroxysmal anxiety]**
    Panic attack
    Panic state
    Excludes1   panic disorder with agoraphobia (F40.01)

  F41.1   **Generalized anxiety disorder**
    Anxiety neurosis
    Anxiety reaction
    Anxiety state
    Overanxious disorder
    Excludes2   neurasthenia (F48.8)

  F41.3   **Other mixed anxiety disorders**
  F41.8   **Other specified anxiety disorders**
    Anxiety depression (mild or not persistent)
    Anxiety hysteria
    Mixed anxiety and depressive disorder
  F41.9   **Anxiety disorder, unspecified**
    Anxiety NOS

● **F42**   **Obsessive-compulsive disorder**
    Anxiety disorder with recurrent obsessions or compulsions
    Excludes2   obsessive-compulsive personality (disorder) (F60.5)
      obsessive-compulsive symptoms occurring in depression (F32-F33)
      obsessive-compulsive symptoms occurring in schizophrenia (F20.-)

CHAPTER 5 (F01-F99)

N Newborn Age: 0   P Pediatric Age: 0–17   M Maternity DX: 12–55   A Adult Age: 15–124   ♀ Females Only   ♂ Males Only
  Complication\Comorbidity   Major C\C   (Ex) CC/MCC Exclusions   Hospital-Acquired Condition
775

CHAPTER 5 (F01-F99)

F42.2   **Mixed obsessional thoughts and acts**
             Coding Clinic: 2016, Q4, P15

F42.3   **Hoarding disorder**
             Coding Clinic: 2016, Q4, P14-15

F42.4   **Excoriation (skin-picking) disorder**
             Excludes1   factitial dermatitis (L98.1)
                              other specified behavioral and emotional
                                 disorders with onset usually
                                 occurring in early childhood and
                                 adolescence (F98.8)
             Coding Clinic: 2016, Q4, P14-15

F42.8   **Other obsessive-compulsive disorder**
             Anancastic neurosis
             Obsessive-compulsive neurosis
             Coding Clinic: 2016, Q4, P15

F42.9   **Obsessive-compulsive disorder, unspecified**
             Coding Clinic: 2016, Q4, P15

● **F43**   **Reaction to severe stress and adjustment disorders**

F43.0   **Acute stress reaction**
             Acute crisis reaction
             Acute reaction to stress
             Combat and operational stress reaction
             Combat fatigue
             Crisis state
             Psychic shock

● **F43.1** **Post-traumatic stress disorder (PTSD)**
             Traumatic neurosis

       F43.10   **Post-traumatic stress disorder, unspecified**

       F43.11   **Post-traumatic stress disorder, acute**

       F43.12   **Post-traumatic stress disorder, chronic**

● **F43.2** **Adjustment disorders**
             Culture shock
             Grief reaction
             Hospitalism in children
             Excludes2   separation anxiety disorder of childhood
                              (F93.0)

       F43.20   **Adjustment disorder, unspecified**

       F43.21   **Adjustment disorder with depressed mood**

       F43.22   **Adjustment disorder with anxiety**

       F43.23   **Adjustment disorder with mixed anxiety and
                    depressed mood**

       F43.24   **Adjustment disorder with disturbance of
                    conduct**

       F43.25   **Adjustment disorder with mixed disturbance of
                    emotions and conduct**

       F43.29   **Adjustment disorder with other symptoms**

F43.8   **Other reactions to severe stress**
             Other specified trauma and stressor-related disorder

F43.9   **Reaction to severe stress, unspecified**
             Trauma and stressor-related disorder, NOS

● **F44**   **Dissociative and conversion disorders**
             Includes   conversion hysteria
                             conversion reaction
                             hysteria
                             hysterical psychosis
             Excludes2   malingering [conscious simulation] (Z76.5)

F44.0   **Dissociative amnesia**
             Sudden loss of memory for personal information
             Excludes1   amnesia NOS (R41.3)
                              anterograde amnesia (R41.1)
                              dissociative amnesia with dissociative
                                 fugue (F44.1)
                              retrograde amnesia (R41.2)
             Excludes2   alcohol-or other psychoactive substance-
                                 induced amnestic disorder (F10, F13,
                                 F19 with .26, .96)
                              amnestic disorder due to known
                                 physiological condition (F04)
                              postictal amnesia in epilepsy (G40.-)

F44.1   **Dissociative fugue**
             *Characterized by episode of sudden, unexpected travel with
                amnesia for past and partial to total confusion about
                identity or assumption of new identity*
             Dissociative amnesia with dissociative fugue
             Excludes2   postictal fugue in epilepsy (G40.-)

F44.2   **Dissociative stupor**
             *Profound diminution or absence of voluntary movement and
                responsiveness to external stimuli*
             Excludes1   catatonic stupor (R40.1)
                              stupor NOS (R40.1)
             Excludes2   catatonic disorder due to known
                                 physiological condition (F06.1)
                              depressive stupor (F32, F33)
                              manic stupor (F30, F31)

F44.4   **Conversion disorder with motor symptom or deficit**
             ▶Conversion disorder with abnormal movement
             ▶Conversion disorder with speech symptoms
             ▶Conversion disorder with swallowing symptoms
             ▶Conversion disorder with weakness/paralysis
             Dissociative motor disorders
             Psychogenic aphonia
             Psychogenic dysphonia

F44.5   **Conversion disorder with seizures or convulsions**
             ▶Conversion disorder with attacks or seizures
             Dissociative convulsions

F44.6   **Conversion disorder with sensory symptom or deficit**
             ▶Conversion disorder with anesthesia or sensory loss
             ▶Conversion disorder with special sensory symptoms
             Dissociative anesthesia and sensory loss
             Psychogenic deafness

F44.7   **Conversion disorder with mixed symptom presentation**

● **F44.8** **Other dissociative and conversion disorders**

       F44.81   **Dissociative identity disorder**
                    Multiple personality disorder

       F44.89   **Other dissociative and conversion disorders**
                    Ganser's syndrome
                    Psychogenic confusion
                    Psychogenic twilight state
                    Trance and possession disorders

F44.9   **Dissociative and conversion disorder, unspecified**
             Dissociative disorder NOS

OGCR Section I.C.5.a.

Pain disorders related to psychological factors

Assign code F45.41, for pain that is exclusively related to psychological
disorders. As indicated by the Excludes 1 note under category G89,
a code from category G89 should not be assigned with code F45.41
Code F45.42, Pain disorders with related psychological factors, should
be used with a code from category G89, Pain, not elsewhere classified,
if there is documentation of a psychological component for a patient
with acute or chronic pain.

See Section I.C.6. Pain

● **F45**   **Somatoform disorders**
             *Mental disorders characterized by symptoms suggesting general
                medical condition*
             Excludes2   dissociative and conversion disorders (F44.-)
                              factitious disorders (F68.1-)
                              hair-plucking (F63.3)
                              lalling (F80.0)
                              lisping (F80.0)
                              malingering [conscious simulation] (Z76.5)
                              nail-biting (F98.8)
                              psychological or behavioral factors associated
                                 with disorders or diseases classified
                                 elsewhere (F54)
                              sexual dysfunction, not due to a substance or
                                 known physiological condition (F52.-)
                              thumb-sucking (F98.8)
                              tic disorders (in childhood and adolescence) (F95.-)
                              Tourette's syndrome (F95.2)
                              trichotillomania (F63.3)

F45.0   **Somatization disorder**
             Briquet's disorder
             Multiple psychosomatic disorder

▶ New   ▬▶ Revised   ~~deleted~~ Deleted   Excludes 1   Excludes 2   Includes   Use additional   Code first   Code also   Key words
OGCR Official Guidelines   ● Unacceptable Principal Diagnosis   X Assign placeholder X   ● Use Additional Character(s)   ▶ Manifestation Code   Coding Clinic

F45.1   Undifferentiated somatoform disorder
Somatic symptom disorder
Undifferentiated psychosomatic disorder

● **F45.2   Hypochondriacal disorders**
Persistent, unrealistic preoccupation with possibility of having serious disease

Excludes2   delusional dysmorphophobia (F22)
fixed delusions about bodily functions or shape (F22)

F45.20   Hypochondriacal disorder, unspecified

F45.21   Hypochondriasis
Hypochondriacal neurosis
Illness anxiety disorder

F45.22   Body dysmorphic disorder
Dysmorphophobia (nondelusional)
Nosophobia

F45.29   Other hypochondriacal disorders

● **F45.4   Pain disorders related to psychological factors**

Excludes1   pain NOS (R52)

F45.41   Pain disorder exclusively related to psychological factors
Somatoform pain disorder (persistent)

F45.42   Pain disorder with related psychological factors
Code also associated acute or chronic pain (G89.-)

F45.8   Other somatoform disorders
Psychogenic dysmenorrhea
Psychogenic dysphagia, including 'globus hystericus'
Psychogenic pruritus
Psychogenic torticollis
Somatoform autonomic dysfunction
Teeth grinding

Excludes1   sleep related teeth grinding (G47.63)
Coding Clinic: 2016, Q4, P118

F45.9   Somatoform disorder, unspecified
Psychosomatic disorder NOS

● **F48   Other nonpsychotic mental disorders**

F48.1   Depersonalization-derealization syndrome

F48.2   Pseudobulbar affect
Involuntary emotional expression disorder
Code first underlying cause, if known, such as:
amyotrophic lateral sclerosis (G12.21)
multiple sclerosis (G35)
sequelae of cerebrovascular disease (I69.-)
sequelae of traumatic intracranial injury (S06.-)

F48.8   Other specified nonpsychotic mental disorders
Dhat syndrome
Neurasthenia
Occupational neurosis, including writer's cramp
Psychasthenia
Psychasthenic neurosis
Psychogenic syncope

F48.9   Nonpsychotic mental disorder, unspecified
Neurosis NOS

BEHAVIORAL SYNDROMES ASSOCIATED WITH PHYSIOLOGICAL DISTURBANCES AND PHYSICAL FACTORS (F50-F59)

● **F50   Eating disorders**

Excludes1   anorexia NOS (R63.0)
feeding difficulties (R63.3)
▶feeding problems of newborn (P92.-)
polyphagia (R63.2)

Excludes2   feeding disorder in infancy or childhood (F98.2-)

● **F50.0   Anorexia nervosa**

Excludes1   loss of appetite (R63.0)
psychogenic loss of appetite (F50.89)

(Ex) **For category F50.0 CC codes: See PDX Collection 556**

F50.00   Anorexia nervosa, unspecified 🔹

F50.01   Anorexia nervosa, restricting type 🔹

F50.02   Anorexia nervosa, binge eating/purging type 🔹

Excludes1   bulimia nervosa (F50.2)

F50.2   Bulimia nervosa 🔹
Bulimia NOS
Hyperorexia nervosa

Excludes1   anorexia nervosa, binge eating/purging type (F50.02)

(Ex) See PDX Collection 557

● **F50.8   Other eating disorders**

Excludes2   pica of infancy and childhood (F98.3)

F50.81   Binge eating disorder
Coding Clinic: 2016, Q4, P15

▶ **F50.82   Avoidant/restrictive food intake disorder**

F50.89   Other specified eating disorder
Pica in adults
Psychogenic loss of appetite
Coding Clinic: 2016, Q4, P16

F50.9   Eating disorder, unspecified
Atypical anorexia nervosa
Atypical bulimia nervosa
▶Feeding or eating disorder, unspecified
▶Other specified feeding disorder

● **F51   Sleep disorders not due to a substance or known physiological condition**

Excludes2   organic sleep disorders (G47.-)

● **F51.0   Insomnia not due to a substance or known physiological condition**

Excludes2   alcohol related insomnia (F10.182, F10.282, F10.982)
drug-related insomnia (F11.182, F11.282, F11.982, F13.182, F13.282, F13.982, F14.182, F14.282, F14.982, F15.182, F15.282, F15.982, F19.182, F19.282, F19.982)
insomnia NOS (G47.0-)
insomnia due to known physiological condition (G47.0-)
organic insomnia (G47.0-)
sleep deprivation (Z72.820)

F51.01   Primary insomnia
Idiopathic insomnia

F51.02   Adjustment insomnia

F51.03   Paradoxical insomnia

F51.04   Psychophysiologic insomnia

F51.05   Insomnia due to other mental disorder
Code also associated mental disorder

F51.09   Other insomnia not due to a substance or known physiological condition

● **F51.1   Hypersomnia not due to a substance or known physiological condition**
Hypersomnia: Excessive sleeping/sleepiness

Excludes2   alcohol related hypersomnia (F10.182, F10.282, F10.982)
drug-related hypersomnia (F11.182, F11.282, F11.982, F13.182, F13.282, F13.982, F14.182, F14.282, F14.982, F15.182, F15.282, F15.982, F19.182, F19.282, F19.982)
hypersomnia NOS (G47.10)
hypersomnia due to known physiological condition (G47.10)
idiopathic hypersomnia (G47.11, G47.12)
narcolepsy (G47.4-)

F51.11   Primary hypersomnia

F51.12   Insufficient sleep syndrome

Excludes1   sleep deprivation (Z72.820)

F51.13   Hypersomnia due to other mental disorder
Code also associated mental disorder

F51.19   Other hypersomnia not due to a substance or known physiological condition

F51.3   Sleepwalking [somnambulism]
▶Non-rapid eye movement sleep arousal disorders, sleepwalking type

---

N Newborn Age: 0   P Pediatric Age: 0–17   M Maternity DX: 12–55   A Adult Age: 15–124   ♀ Females Only   ♂ Males Only

 Complication\Comorbidity   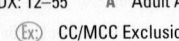 Major C\C   (Ex) CC/MCC Exclusions   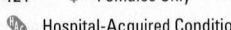 Hospital-Acquired Condition

F51.4 **Sleep terrors [night terrors]**
▶Non-rapid eye movement sleep arousal disorders, sleep
terror type

F51.5 **Nightmare disorder**
Dream anxiety disorder

F51.8 **Other sleep disorders not due to a substance or known
physiological condition**

F51.9 **Sleep disorder not due to a substance or known
physiological condition, unspecified**
Emotional sleep disorder NOS

● **F52** **Sexual dysfunction not due to a substance or known
physiological condition**
Excludes2 Dhat syndrome (F48.8)

F52.0 **Hypoactive sexual desire disorder**
Total loss of feeling of sexual pleasure
Lack or loss of sexual desire
▶Male hypoactive sexual desire disorder
Sexual anhedonia
Excludes1 decreased libido (R68.82)

F52.1 **Sexual aversion disorder**
Sexual aversion and lack of sexual enjoyment

● **F52.2** **Sexual arousal disorders**
Failure of genital response

F52.21 **Male erectile disorder** ♂
▶Erectile disorder
Psychogenic impotence
Excludes1 impotence of organic origin
(N52.-)
impotence NOS (N52.-)

F52.22 **Female sexual arousal disorder** ♀
▶Female sexual interest/arousal disorder

● **F52.3** **Orgasmic disorder**
Inhibited orgasm
Psychogenic anorgasmy

F52.31 **Female orgasmic disorder** ♀

F52.32 **Male orgasmic disorder** ♂
Delayed ejaculation

F52.4 **Premature ejaculation** ♂

F52.5 **Vaginismus not due to a substance or known
physiological condition** ♀
Psychogenic vaginismus
Excludes2 vaginismus (due to a known
physiological condition) (N94.2)

F52.6 **Dyspareunia not due to a substance or known
physiological condition**
Dyspareunia: Difficult or painful sexual intercourse
Genito-pelvic pain penetration disorder
Psychogenic dyspareunia
Excludes2 dyspareunia (due to a known
physiological condition) (N94.1-)

F52.8 **Other sexual dysfunction not due to a substance or
known physiological condition**
Excessive sexual drive
Nymphomania
Satyriasis

● **F52.9** **Unspecified sexual dysfunction not due to a substance or
known physiological condition**
Sexual dysfunction NOS

F53 **Puerperal psychosis** ♀   M
Postpartum depression
*Acute mental illness with sudden onset following childbirth with
symptoms of affective psychosis, disorientation, and confusion
are prevalent*
Excludes1 mood disorders with psychotic features (F30.2,
F31.2, F31.5, F31.64, F32.3, F33.3)
postpartum dysphoria (O90.6)
psychosis in schizophrenia, schizotypal,
delusional, and other psychotic disorders
(F20-F29)

▶ **F54** *Psychological and behavioral factors associated with disorders
or diseases classified elsewhere*
Psychological factors affecting physical conditions
Code first the associated physical disorder, such as:
asthma (J45.-)
dermatitis (L23-L25)
gastric ulcer (K25.-)
mucous colitis (K58.-)
ulcerative colitis (K51.-)
urticaria (L50.-)
Excludes2 tension-type headache (G44.2)

● **F55** **Abuse of non-psychoactive substances**
Excludes2 abuse of psychoactive substances (F10-F19)
F55.0 **Abuse of antacids**
F55.1 **Abuse of herbal or folk remedies**
F55.2 **Abuse of laxatives**
F55.3 **Abuse of steroids or hormones**
F55.4 **Abuse of vitamins**
F55.8 **Abuse of other non-psychoactive substances**

F59 **Unspecified behavioral syndromes associated with
physiological disturbances and physical factors**
Psychogenic physiological dysfunction NOS

DISORDERS OF ADULT PERSONALITY AND BEHAVIOR (F60-F69)

● **F60** **Specific personality disorders**
*Long-term patterns of thoughts and behaviors causing serious
problems with relationships and work.*

F60.0 **Paranoid personality disorder**
Hostile, devious, and combative response to disappointments
Expansive paranoid personality (disorder)
Fanatic personality (disorder)
Querulant personality (disorder)
Paranoid personality (disorder)
Sensitive paranoid personality (disorder)
Excludes2 paranoia (F22)
paranoia querulans (F22)
paranoid psychosis (F22)
paranoid schizophrenia (F20.0)
paranoid state (F22)

F60.1 **Schizoid personality disorder**
*Detachment from social relationships with minimal emotional
experiences and expressions*
Excludes2 Asperger's syndrome (F84.5)
delusional disorder (F22)
schizoid disorder of childhood (F84.5)
schizophrenia (F20.-)
schizotypal disorder (F21)

F60.2   Antisocial personality disorder
Continuous and chronic antisocial behavior
Amoral personality (disorder)
Asocial personality (disorder)
Dissocial personality disorder
Psychopathic personality (disorder)
Sociopathic personality (disorder)

Excludes1   conduct disorders (F91.-)

Excludes2   borderline personality disorder (F60.3)

F60.3   Borderline personality disorder
*Instability of mood, self-image or sense of self, and
    interpersonal relationships*
Aggressive personality (disorder)
Emotionally unstable personality disorder
Explosive personality (disorder)

Excludes2   antisocial personality disorder (F60.2)

F60.4   Histrionic personality disorder
*Personality disorder with excessive emotional and attention-
    seeking behavior*
Hysterical personality (disorder)
Psychoinfantile personality (disorder)

F60.5   Obsessive-compulsive personality disorder
Anankastic personality (disorder)
Compulsive personality (disorder)
Obsessional personality (disorder)

Excludes2   obsessive-compulsive disorder (F42-)

F60.6   Avoidant personality disorder
Anxious personality disorder

F60.7   Dependent personality disorder
Asthenic personality (disorder)
Inadequate personality (disorder)
Passive personality (disorder)

● **F60.8   Other specific personality disorders**

F60.81   Narcissistic personality disorder
*Vanity, conceit, egotism or indifference to plight
    of others*

F60.89   Other specific personality disorders
Eccentric personality disorder
'Haltlose' type personality disorder
Immature personality disorder
Passive-aggressive personality disorder
Psychoneurotic personality disorder
Self-defeating personality disorder

F60.9   Personality disorder, unspecified
Character disorder NOS
Character neurosis NOS
Pathological personality NOS

● **F63   Impulse disorders**

Excludes2   habitual excessive use of alcohol or psychoactive
            substances (F10-F19)
            impulse disorders involving sexual behavior (F65.-)

F63.0   Pathological gambling
Compulsive gambling
▶Gambling disorder

Excludes1   gambling and betting NOS (Z72.6)
Excludes2   excessive gambling by manic patients
            (F30, F31)
            gambling in antisocial personality
            disorder (F60.2)

F63.1   Pyromania
Pathological fire-setting

Excludes2   fire-setting (by) (in):
            adult with antisocial personality
            disorder (F60.2)
            alcohol or psychoactive substance
            intoxication (F10-F19)
            conduct disorders (F91.-)
            mental disorders due to known
            physiological condition (F01-F09)
            schizophrenia (F20.-)

F63.2   Kleptomania
Pathological stealing

Excludes1   shoplifting as the reason for observation
            for suspected mental disorder
            (Z03.8)

Excludes2   depressive disorder with stealing
            (F31-F33)
            stealing due to underlying mental
            condition-code to mental condition
            stealing in mental disorders due to known
            physiological condition (F01-F09)

F63.3   Trichotillomania
Hair plucking

Excludes2   other stereotyped movement disorder
            (F98.4)

● **F63.8   Other impulse disorders**

F63.81   Intermittent explosive disorder

F63.89   Other impulse disorders

F63.9   Impulse disorder, unspecified
Impulse control disorder NOS

● **F64   Gender identity disorders**

F64.0   Transsexualism
Gender identity disorder in adolescence and
    adulthood
Gender dysphoria in adolescents and adults
Coding Clinic: 2016, Q4, P16

F64.1   Dual role transvestism
Use additional code to identify sex reassignment status
    (Z87.890)

Excludes1   gender identity disorder in childhood
            (F64.2)

Excludes2   fetishistic transvestism (F65.1)
Coding Clinic: 2016, Q4, P16

F64.2   Gender identity disorder of childhood   P
Gender dysphoria in children

Excludes1   gender identity disorder in adolescence
            and adulthood (F64.0)

Excludes2   sexual maturation disorder (F66)

F64.8   Other gender identity disorders
▶Other specified gender dysphoria

F64.9   Gender identity disorder, unspecified
▶Gender dysphoria, unspecified
Gender-role disorder NOS

● **F65   Paraphilias**

F65.0   Fetishism
*Intense sexual urges and arousing fantasies using inanimate
    objects*
▶Fetishistic disorder

F65.1   Transvestic fetishism
*Intense sexual urges, arousal, or orgasm associated with
    fantasized/actual cross-dressing*
Fetishistic transvestism
▶Transvestic disorder

F65.2   Exhibitionism
▶Exhibitionistic disorder

F65.3   Voyeurism
*Sexual urges or arousal involving real or fantasized
    observation of unsuspecting people who are naked,
    disrobing, or engaging in sexual activity*
▶Voyeuristic disorder

F65.4   Pedophilia
▶Pedophilic disorder

N Newborn Age: 0   **P** Pediatric Age: 0–17   **M** Maternity DX: 12–55   **A** Adult Age: 15–124   ♀ Females Only   ♂ Males Only

🔵 Complication\Comorbidity   🔵 Major C\C   (Ex) CC/MCC Exclusions   🔵 Hospital-Acquired Condition   779

● **F65.5**   **Sadomasochism**

     F65.50   **Sadomasochism, unspecified**

     F65.51   **Sexual masochism**
         ▶Sexual masochism disorder

     F65.52   **Sexual sadism**
         ▶Sexual sadism disorder

● **F65.8**   **Other paraphilias**

     F65.81   **Frotteurism**
         Sexual arousal or orgasm is achieved by rubbing up against another person (or fantasies of), in crowded place with unsuspecting victim
         ▶Frotteuristic disorder

     F65.89   **Other paraphilias**
         Necrophilia
         ▶Other specified paraphilic disorder

     F65.9   **Paraphilia, unspecified**
         ▶Paraphilic disorder, unspecified
         Sexual deviation NOS

F66   **Other sexual disorders**
     Sexual maturation disorder
     Sexual relationship disorder

● **F68**   **Other disorders of adult personality and behavior**

● **F68.1**   **Factitious disorder**
     Compensation neurosis
     Elaboration of physical symptoms for psychological reasons
     Hospital hopper syndrome
     Münchhausen's syndrome
     Peregrinating patient

     Excludes2   factitial dermatitis (L98.1)
         person feigning illness (with obvious motivation) (Z76.5)

     (Ex:) **For category F68.1 CC codes:** See PDX Collection 551

     F68.10   **Factitious disorder, unspecified** 🗞

     F68.11   **Factitious disorder with predominantly psychological signs and symptoms**

     F68.12   **Factitious disorder with predominantly physical signs and symptoms** 🗞

     F68.13   **Factitious disorder with combined psychological and physical signs and symptoms**

     F68.8   **Other specified disorders of adult personality and behavior**

F69   **Unspecified disorder of adult personality and behavior**   A

INTELLECTUAL DISABILITIES (F70-F79)

Code first any associated physical or developmental disorders

     Excludes1   borderline intellectual functioning, IQ above 70 to 84 (R41.83)

F70   **Mild intellectual disabilities**
     IQ level 50-55 to approximately 70
     Mild mental subnormality

F71   **Moderate intellectual disabilities**
     IQ level 35-40 to 50-55
     Moderate mental subnormality

F72   **Severe intellectual disabilities** 🗞
     IQ 20-25 to 35-40
     Severe mental subnormality
     (Ex:) See PDX Collection 558

F73   **Profound intellectual disabilities** 🗞
     IQ level below 20-25
     Profound mental subnormality
     (Ex:) See PDX Collection 558

F78   **Other intellectual disabilities**

F79   **Unspecified intellectual disabilities**
     Mental deficiency NOS
     Mental subnormality NOS

PERVASIVE AND SPECIFIC DEVELOPMENTAL DISORDERS (F80-F89)

● **F80**   **Specific developmental disorders of speech and language**

     F80.0   **Phonological disorder**
         Communication disorder of unknown cause, characterized by failure to use age-appropriate sounds
         Dyslalia
         Functional speech articulation disorder
         Lalling
         Lisping
         Phonological developmental disorder
         Speech articulation developmental disorder
         Speech-sound disorder

         Excludes1   speech articulation impairment due to aphasia NOS (R47.01)
            speech articulation impairment due to apraxia (R48.2)

         Excludes2   speech articulation impairment due to hearing loss (F80.4)
            speech articulation impairment due to intellectual disabilities (F70-F79)
            speech articulation impairment with expressive language developmental disorder (F80.1)
            speech articulation impairment with mixed receptive expressive language developmental disorder (F80.2)

     F80.1   **Expressive language disorder**
         Developmental dysphasia or aphasia, expressive type

         Excludes1   mixed receptive-expressive language disorder (F80.2)
            dysphasia and aphasia NOS (R47.-)

         Excludes2   acquired aphasia with epilepsy [Landau-Kleffner] (G40.80-)
            intellectual disabilities (F70-F79)
            pervasive developmental disorders (F84.-)
            selective mutism (F94.0)

     F80.2   **Mixed receptive-expressive language disorder**
         Developmental dysphasia or aphasia, receptive type
         Developmental Wernicke's aphasia

         Excludes1   central auditory processing disorder (H93.25)
            dysphasia or aphasia NOS (R47.-)
            expressive language disorder (F80.1)
            expressive type dysphasia or aphasia (F80.1)
            word deafness (H93.25)

         Excludes2   acquired aphasia with epilepsy [Landau-Kleffner] (G40.80-)
            intellectual disabilities (F70-F79)
            pervasive developmental disorders (F84.-)
            selective mutism (F94.0)

     F80.4   **Speech and language development delay due to hearing loss**

         Code also type of hearing loss (H90.-, H91.-)

● **F80.8**   **Other developmental disorders of speech or language**

     F80.81   **Childhood onset fluency disorder**
         Cluttering NOS
         Stuttering NOS

         Excludes1   adult onset fluency disorder (F98.5)
            fluency disorder in conditions classified elsewhere (R47.82)
            fluency disorder (stuttering) following cerebrovascular disease (I69. with final characters -23)

▶ New   ⇒ Revised   ~~deleted~~ Deleted   Excludes 1   Excludes 2   Includes   Use additional   Code first   Code also   Key words

OGCR Official Guidelines   ● Unacceptable Principal Diagnosis   X Assign placeholder X   ● Use Additional Character(s)   ▶ Manifestation Code   **Coding Clinic**

F80.82   Social pragmatic communication disorder
> **Excludes1**   Asperger's syndrome (F84.5)
>   autistic disorder (F84.0)
> Coding Clinic: 2016, Q4, P16

F80.89   Other developmental disorders of speech and language
> Coding Clinic: 2017, Q1, P27

F80.9   Developmental disorder of speech and language, unspecified
Communication disorder NOS
Language disorder NOS

● **F81   Specific developmental disorders of scholastic skills**

F81.0   Specific reading disorder
'Backward reading'
Developmental dyslexia
▶ Specific learning disorder, with impairment in reading
Specific reading retardation
> **Excludes1**   alexia NOS (R48.0)
>   dyslexia NOS (R48.0)

F81.2   Mathematics disorder
Developmental acalculia
Developmental arithmetical disorder
Developmental Gerstmann's syndrome
▶ Specific learning disorder, with impairment in mathematics
> **Excludes1**   acalculia NOS (R48.8)
> **Excludes2**   arithmetical difficulties associated with a reading disorder (F81.0)
>   arithmetical difficulties associated with a spelling disorder (F81.81)
>   arithmetical difficulties due to inadequate teaching (Z55.8)

● **F81.8   Other developmental disorders of scholastic skills**

F81.81   Disorder of written expression
▶ Specific learning disorder, with impairment in written expression
Specific spelling disorder

F81.89   Other developmental disorders of scholastic skills

● **F81.9   Developmental disorder of scholastic skills, unspecified**
Knowledge acquisition disability NOS
Learning disability NOS
Learning disorder NOS

● **F82   Specific developmental disorder of motor function**
Clumsy child syndrome
Developmental coordination disorder
Developmental dyspraxia
> **Excludes1**   abnormalities of gait and mobility (R26.-)
>   lack of coordination (R27.-)
> **Excludes2**   lack of coordination secondary to intellectual disabilities (F70-F79)

● **F84   Pervasive developmental disorders**
Use additional code to identify any associated medical condition and intellectual disabilities.
(Ex) For category F84 CC codes unless otherwise indicated: See PDX Collection 551

F84.0   Autistic disorder 🐾
Autism spectrum disorder
Infantile autism
Infantile psychosis
Kanner's syndrome
> **Excludes1**   Asperger's syndrome (F84.5)
> Coding Clinic: 2017, Q1, P27

F84.2   Rett's syndrome 🐾
Neurodevelopmental disorder
> **Excludes1**   Asperger's syndrome (F84.5)
>   Autistic disorder (F84.0)
>   other childhood disintegrative disorder (F84.3)
(Ex) See PDX Collection 537

F84.3   Other childhood disintegrative disorder 🐾   P
Dementia infantilis
At least two years of normal development followed by significant loss of language abilities, social skills, bowel/bladder control, motor skills
Disintegrative psychosis
Heller's syndrome
At least two years of normal development followed by significant loss of language abilities, social skills, bowel/bladder control, motor skills
Symbiotic psychosis
Abnormal relationship to mothering figure, characterized by intense separation anxiety, severe regression, giving up of useful speech, and autism
Use additional code to identify any associated neurological condition.
> **Excludes1**   Asperger's syndrome (F84.5)
>   Autistic disorder (F84.0)
>   Rett's syndrome (F84.2)

F84.5   Asperger's syndrome 🐾
Developmental disorder
Asperger's disorder
Autistic psychopathy
Schizoid disorder of childhood

F84.8   Other pervasive developmental disorders 🐾
Overactive disorder associated with intellectual disabilities and stereotyped movements

F84.9   Pervasive developmental disorder, unspecified 🐾
Atypical autism

F88   Other disorders of psychological development
Developmental agnosia
Global developmental delay
Other specified neurodevelopmental disorder

F89   Unspecified disorder of psychological development
Developmental disorder NOS
Neurodevelopmental disorder NOS

BEHAVIORAL AND EMOTIONAL DISORDERS WITH ONSET USUALLY OCCURRING IN CHILDHOOD AND ADOLESCENCE (F90-F98)

Note: Codes within categories F90-F98 may be used regardless of the age of a patient. These disorders generally have onset within the childhood or adolescent years, but may continue throughout life or not be diagnosed until adulthood.

● **F90   Attention-deficit hyperactivity disorders**
Attention deficit disorder with hyperactivity=ADHD
> **Includes**   attention deficit disorder with hyperactivity
>   attention deficit syndrome with hyperactivity
> **Excludes2**   anxiety disorders (F40.-, F41.-)
>   mood [affective] disorders (F30-F39)
>   pervasive developmental disorders (F84.-)
>   schizophrenia (F20.-)

F90.0   Attention-deficit hyperactivity disorder, predominantly inattentive type
▶ Attention-deficit/hyperactivity disorder, predominantly inattentive presentation

F90.1   Attention-deficit hyperactivity disorder, predominantly hyperactive type
▶ Attention-deficit/hyperactivity disorder, predominantly hyperactive impulsive presentation

F90.2   Attention-deficit hyperactivity disorder, combined type
▶ Attention-deficit/hyperactivity disorder, combined presentation

F90.8   Attention-deficit hyperactivity disorder, other type

F90.9   Attention-deficit hyperactivity disorder, unspecified type
Attention-deficit hyperactivity disorder of childhood or adolescence NOS
Attention-deficit hyperactivity disorder NOS

CHAPTER 5 (F01-F99)

● **F91**   **Conduct disorders**
Childhood/adolescence disruptive behavior disorder

    Excludes1   antisocial behavior (Z72.81-)
                    antisocial personality disorder (F60.2)

    Excludes2   conduct problems associated with attention-deficit hyperactivity disorder (F90.-)
                    mood [affective] disorders (F30-F39)
                    pervasive developmental disorders (F84.-)
                    schizophrenia (F20.-)

   F91.0   **Conduct disorder confined to family context**

   F91.1   **Conduct disorder, childhood-onset type**
           Unsocialized conduct disorder
           Conduct disorder, solitary aggressive type
           Unsocialized aggressive disorder

   F91.2   **Conduct disorder, adolescent-onset type**
           Socialized conduct disorder
           Conduct disorder, group type

   F91.3   **Oppositional defiant disorder**

   F91.8   **Other conduct disorders**
           Other specified conduct disorder
           Other specified disruptive disorder

   F91.9   **Conduct disorder, unspecified**
           Behavioral disorder NOS
           Conduct disorder NOS
           Disruptive behavior disorder NOS
           Disruptive disorder NOS

● **F93**   **Emotional disorders with onset specific to childhood**

   F93.0   **Separation anxiety disorder of childhood**

    Excludes2   mood [affective] disorders (F30-F39)
                    nonpsychotic mental disorders (F40-F48)
                    phobic anxiety disorder of childhood (F40.8)
                    social phobia (F40.1)

   F93.8   **Other childhood emotional disorders**
           Identity disorder

    Excludes2   gender identity disorder of childhood (F64.2)

   F93.9   **Childhood emotional disorder, unspecified**

● **F94**   **Disorders of social functioning with onset specific to childhood and adolescence**

   F94.0   **Selective mutism**
           Elective mutism

    Excludes2   pervasive developmental disorders (F84.-)
                    schizophrenia (F20.-)
                    specific developmental disorders of speech and language (F80.-)
                    transient mutism as part of separation anxiety in young children (F93.0)

   F94.1   **Reactive attachment disorder of childhood**
           Use additional code to identify any associated failure to thrive or growth retardation

    Excludes1   disinhibited attachment disorder of childhood (F94.2)
                    normal variation in pattern of selective attachment

    Excludes2   Asperger's syndrome (F84.5)
                    maltreatment syndromes (T74.-)
                    sexual or physical abuse in childhood, resulting in psychosocial problems (Z62.81-)

   F94.2   **Disinhibited attachment disorder of childhood**
           Affectionless psychopathy
           Institutional syndrome

    Excludes1   reactive attachment disorder of childhood (F94.1)

    Excludes2   Asperger's syndrome (F84.5)
                    attention-deficit hyperactivity disorders (F90.-)
                    hospitalism in children (F43.2-)

   F94.8   **Other childhood disorders of social functioning**

   F94.9   **Childhood disorder of social functioning, unspecified**

● **F95**   **Tic disorder**
Involuntary twitch

   F95.0   **Transient tic disorder**
           Provisional tic disorder

   F95.1   **Chronic motor or vocal tic disorder**

   F95.2   **Tourette's disorder**
           Combined vocal and multiple motor tic disorder [de la Tourette]
           Tourette's syndrome

   F95.8   **Other tic disorders**

   F95.9   **Tic disorder, unspecified**
           Tic NOS

● **F98**   **Other behavioral and emotional disorders with onset usually occurring in childhood and adolescence**

    Excludes2   breath-holding spells (R06.89)
                    gender identity disorder of childhood (F64.2)
                    Kleine-Levin syndrome (G47.13)
                    obsessive-compulsive disorder (F42-)
                    sleep disorders not due to a substance or known physiological condition (F51.-)

   F98.0   **Enuresis not due to a substance or known physiological condition**
           Enuresis: Urinary incontinence
           Enuresis (primary) (secondary) of nonorganic origin
           Functional enuresis
           Psychogenic enuresis
           Urinary incontinence of nonorganic origin

    Excludes1   enuresis NOS (R32)

   F98.1   **Encopresis not due to a substance or known physiological condition**
           Encopresis: Fecal incontinence
           Functional encopresis
           Incontinence of feces of nonorganic origin
           Psychogenic encopresis

           Use additional code to identify the cause of any coexisting constipation.

    Excludes1   encopresis NOS (R15.-)

● **F98.2**   **Other feeding disorders of infancy and childhood**

    Excludes1   feeding difficulties (R63.3)

    Excludes2   anorexia nervosa and other eating disorders (F50.-)
                    feeding problems of newborn (P92.-)
                    pica of infancy or childhood (F98.3)

   F98.21   **Rumination disorder of infancy**

   F98.29   **Other feeding disorders of infancy and early childhood**

   F98.3   **Pica of infancy and childhood**
           Craving and eating substances such as paint, clay, or dirt to replace a nutritional deficit in the body.

Item 5–2 Enuresis: Bed wetting by children at night. Causes can be either psychological or medical (diabetes, urinary tract infections, or abnormalities). **Encopresis:** Overflow incontinence of bowels sometimes resulting from chronic constipation or fecal impaction. Check the documentation for additional diagnoses.

▶ New   ⇒ Revised   ~~deleted~~ Deleted   Excludes 1   Excludes 2   Includes   Use additional   Code first   Code also   Key words

OGCR Official Guidelines   ● Unacceptable Principal Diagnosis   X Assign placeholder X   ● Use Additional Character(s)   ▶ Manifestation Code   **Coding Clinic**

F98.4   Stereotyped movement disorders
    Stereotype/habit disorder
    Excludes1   abnormal involuntary movements (R25.-)
    Excludes2   compulsions in obsessive-compulsive
                        disorder (F42-)
                    hair plucking (F63.3)
                    movement disorders of organic origin
                        (G20-G25)
                    nail-biting (F98.8)
                    nose-picking (F98.8)
                    stereotypies that are part of a broader
                        psychiatric condition (F01-F95)
                    thumb-sucking (F98.8)
                    tic disorders (F95.-)
                    trichotillomania (F63.3)

F98.5   Adult onset fluency disorder
    Excludes1   childhood onset fluency disorder (F80.81)
                    dysphasia (R47.02)
                    fluency disorder in conditions classified
                        elsewhere (R47.82)
                    fluency disorder (stuttering) following
                        cerebrovascular disease (I69. with
                        final characters -23)
                    tic disorders (F95.-)

**F98.8   Other specified behavioral and emotional disorders with
          onset usually occurring in childhood and adolescence**
    Excessive masturbation
    Nail-biting
    Nose-picking
    Thumb-sucking

**F98.9   Unspecified behavioral and emotional disorders with
          onset usually occurring in childhood and adolescence**

UNSPECIFIED MENTAL DISORDER (F99)

F99   Mental disorder, not otherwise specified
    Mental illness NOS
    Excludes1   unspecified mental disorder due to known
                        physiological condition (F09)

CHAPTER 6

DISEASES OF THE NERVOUS SYSTEM
(G00-G99)

OGCR Chapter-Specific Coding Guidelines

6. Chapter 6: Diseases of the Nervous System (G00-G99)

a. Dominant/nondominant side

Codes from category G81, Hemiplegia and hemiparesis, and subcategories, G83.1, Monoplegia of lower limb, G83.2, Monoplegia of upper limb, and G83.3, Monoplegia, unspecified, identify whether the dominant or nondominant side is affected. Should the affected side be documented, but not specified as dominant or nondominant, and the classification system does not indicate a default, code selection is as follows:

- For ambidextrous patients, the default should be dominant.
- If the left side is affected, the default is non-dominant.
- If the right side is affected, the default is dominant.

b. Pain - Category G89

1) General coding information

Codes in category G89, Pain, not elsewhere classified, may be used in conjunction with codes from other categories and chapters to provide more detail about acute or chronic pain and neoplasm-related pain, unless otherwise indicated below.

If the pain is not specified as acute or chronic, post-thoracotomy, postprocedural, or neoplasm-related, do not assign codes from category G89.

A code from category G89 should not be assigned if the underlying (definitive) diagnosis is known, unless the reason for the encounter is pain control/management and not management of the underlying condition.

When an admission or encounter is for a procedure aimed at treating the underlying condition (e.g., spinal fusion, kyphoplasty), a code for the underlying condition (e.g., vertebral fracture, spinal stenosis) should be assigned as the principal diagnosis. No code from category G89 should be assigned.

(a) Category G89 Codes as Principal or First-Listed Diagnosis

Category G89 codes are acceptable as principal diagnosis or the first-listed code:

- When pain control or pain management is the reason for the admission/encounter (e.g., a patient with displaced intervertebral disc, nerve impingement and severe back pain presents for injection of steroid into the spinal canal). The underlying cause of the pain should be reported as an additional diagnosis, if known.
- When a patient is admitted for the insertion of a neurostimulator for pain control, assign the appropriate pain code as the principal or first-listed diagnosis. When an admission or encounter is for a procedure aimed at treating the underlying condition and a neurostimulator is inserted for pain control during the same admission/encounter, a code for the underlying condition should be assigned as the principal diagnosis and the appropriate pain code should be assigned as a secondary diagnosis.

(b) Use of Category G89 Codes in Conjunction with Site Specific Pain Codes

(i) Assigning Category G89 and Site-Specific Pain Codes

Codes from category G89 may be used in conjunction with codes that identify the site of pain (including codes from chapter 18) if the category G89 code provides additional information. For example, if the code describes the site of the pain, but does not fully describe whether the pain is acute or chronic, then both codes should be assigned.

(ii) Sequencing of Category G89 Codes with Site-Specific Pain Codes

The sequencing of category G89 codes with site-specific pain codes (including chapter 18 codes), is dependent on the circumstances of the encounter/admission as follows:

- If the encounter is for pain control or pain management, assign the code from category G89 followed by the code identifying the specific site of pain (e.g., encounter for pain management for acute neck pain from trauma is assigned code G89.11, Acute pain due to trauma, followed by code M54.2, Cervicalgia, to identify the site of pain).
- If the encounter is for any other reason except pain control or pain management, and a related definitive diagnosis has not been established (confirmed) by the provider, assign the code for the specific site of pain first, followed by the appropriate code from category G89.

2) Pain due to devices, implants and grafts
See Section I.C.19. Pain due to medical devices

3) Postoperative Pain

The provider's documentation should be used to guide the coding of postoperative pain, as well as Section III. Reporting Additional Diagnoses and Section IV. Diagnostic Coding and Reporting in the Outpatient Setting.

The default for post-thoracotomy and other postoperative pain not specified as acute or chronic is the code for the acute form.

Routine or expected postoperative pain immediately after surgery should not be coded.

(a) Postoperative pain not associated with specific postoperative complication

Postoperative pain not associated with a specific postoperative complication is assigned to the appropriate postoperative pain code in category G89.

(b) Postoperative pain associated with specific postoperative complication

Postoperative pain associated with a specific postoperative complication (such as painful wire sutures) is assigned to the appropriate code(s) found in Chapter 19, Injury, poisoning, and certain other consequences of external causes. If appropriate, use additional code(s) from category G89 to identify acute or chronic pain (G89.18 or G89.28).

4) Chronic pain

Chronic pain is classified to subcategory G89.2. There is no time frame defining when pain becomes chronic pain. The provider's documentation should be used to guide use of these codes.

5) Neoplasm Related Pain

Code G89.3 is assigned to pain documented as being related, associated or due to cancer, primary or secondary malignancy, or tumor. This code is assigned regardless of whether the pain is acute or chronic.

This code may be assigned as the principal or first-listed code when the stated reason for the admission/encounter is documented as pain control/pain management. The underlying neoplasm should be reported as an additional diagnosis.

When the reason for the admission/encounter is management of the neoplasm and the pain associated with the neoplasm is also documented, code G89.3 may be assigned as an additional diagnosis. It is not necessary to assign an additional code for the site of the pain.

See Section I.C.2 for instructions on the sequencing of neoplasms for all other stated reasons for the admission/encounter (except for pain control/pain management).

6) Chronic pain syndrome

Central pain syndrome (G89.0) and chronic pain syndrome (G89.4) are different than the term "chronic pain," and therefore codes should only be used when the provider has specifically documented this condition.

See Section I.C.5. Pain disorders related to psychological factors

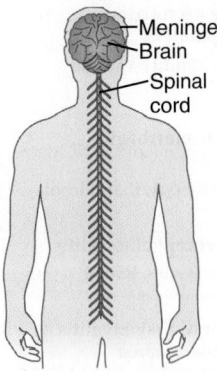
— Meninges
— Brain
— Spinal cord

Figure 6-1 The brain and spinal cord make up the central nervous system.

Item 6-1 The two major classifications of the nervous system are the peripheral nervous system and the central nervous system (CNS). The central nervous system is comprised of the brain and the spinal cord. The peripheral nervous system is comprised of the parasympathetic and sympathetic systems. **Encephalitis** is the swelling of the brain. **Meningitis** is swelling of the covering of the brain, the meninges. Types and causes of brain infections are:

Type	Cause
purulent	bacterial
aseptic/abacterial	viral
chronic meningitis	mycobacterial and fungal

CHAPTER 6

DISEASES OF THE NERVOUS SYSTEM (G00-G99)

> **Excludes2** certain conditions originating in the perinatal period (P04-P96)
> certain infectious and parasitic diseases (A00-B99)
> complications of pregnancy, childbirth and the puerperium (O00-O9A)
> congenital malformations, deformations, and chromosomal abnormalities (Q00-Q99)
> endocrine, nutritional and metabolic diseases (E00-E88)
> injury, poisoning and certain other consequences of external causes (S00-T88)
> neoplasms (C00-D49)
> symptoms, signs and abnormal clinical and laboratory findings, not elsewhere classified (R00-R94)

This chapter contains the following blocks:

G00-G09	Inflammatory diseases of the central nervous system
G10-G14	Systemic atrophies primarily affecting the central nervous system
G20-G26	Extrapyramidal and movement disorders
G30-G32	Other degenerative diseases of the nervous system
G35-G37	Demyelinating diseases of the central nervous system
G40-G47	Episodic and paroxysmal disorders
G50-G59	Nerve, nerve root and plexus disorders
G60-G65	Polyneuropathies and other disorders of the peripheral nervous system
G70-G73	Diseases of myoneural junction and muscle
G80-G83	Cerebral palsy and other paralytic syndromes
G89-G99	Other disorders of the nervous system

INFLAMMATORY DISEASES OF THE CENTRAL NERVOUS SYSTEM (G00-G09)

● **G00 Bacterial meningitis, not elsewhere classified**
An infection of the cerebrospinal fluid surrounding the spinal cord and brain.

> **Includes** bacterial arachnoiditis
> bacterial leptomeningitis
> bacterial meningitis
> bacterial pachymeningitis

➡ **Excludes1** bacterial meningoencephalitis (G04.2)
➡ bacterial meningomyelitis (G04.2)
~~meningomyelitis (G04.2)~~

(Ex:) **For category G00 CC codes:** See PDX Collection 207

G00.0 Hemophilus meningitis 🦠
Meningitis due to Hemophilus influenzae

G00.1 Pneumococcal meningitis 🦠
Meningitis due to Streptococcal pneumoniae

G00.2 Streptococcal meningitis 🦠
Use additional code to further identify organism (B95.0-B95.5)

G00.3 Staphylococcal meningitis 🦠
Use additional code to further identify organism (B95.61-B95.8)

G00.8 Other bacterial meningitis 🦠
Meningitis due to Escherichia coli
Meningitis due to Friedländer bacillus
Meningitis due to Klebsiella
Use additional code to further identify organism (B96.-)

G00.9 Bacterial meningitis, unspecified 🦠
Meningitis due to gram-negative bacteria, unspecified
Purulent meningitis NOS
Pyogenic meningitis NOS
Suppurative meningitis NOS

▶ **G01 Meningitis in bacterial diseases classified elsewhere** 🦠
Code first underlying disease

> **Excludes1** meningitis (in):
> gonococcal (A54.81)
> leptospirosis (A27.81)
> listeriosis (A32.11)
> Lyme disease (A69.21)
> meningococcal (A39.0)
> neurosyphilis (A52.13)
> tuberculosis (A17.0)
> meningoencephalitis and meningomyelitis in bacterial diseases classified elsewhere (G05)

(Ex:) See PDX Collection 207

▶ **G02 Meningitis in other infectious and parasitic diseases classified elsewhere** 🦠

> *Code first underlying disease, such as:*
> African trypanosomiasis (B56.-)
> poliovirus infection (A80.-)

> **Excludes1** candidal meningitis (B37.5)
> coccidioidomycosis meningitis (B38.4)
> cryptococcal meningitis (B45.1)
> herpesviral [herpes simplex] meningitis (B00.3)
> infectious mononucleosis complicated by meningitis (B27.- with fourth character 2)
> measles complicated by meningitis (B05.1)
> meningoencephalitis and meningomyelitis in other infectious and parasitic diseases classified elsewhere (G05)
> mumps meningitis (B26.1)
> rubella meningitis (B06.02)
> varicella [chickenpox] meningitis (B01.0)
> zoster meningitis (B02.1)

(Ex:) See PDX Collection 559

N Newborn Age: 0   P Pediatric Age: 0-17   M Maternity DX: 12-55   A Adult Age: 15-124   ♀ Females Only   ♂ Males Only

🦠 Complication\Comorbidity   🦠 Major C\C   (Ex:) CC/MCC Exclusions   🦠 Hospital-Acquired Condition

● **G03**   **Meningitis due to other and unspecified causes**

> **Includes**   arachnoiditis NOS
> leptomeningitis NOS
> meningitis NOS
> pachymeningitis NOS

> **Excludes1**   meningoencephalitis (G04.-)
> meningomyelitis (G04.-)

> (Ex:) **For category G03 CC codes unless otherwise indicated:** See PDX Collection 207

> **G03.0**   **Nonpyogenic meningitis** 🔎
> Aseptic meningitis
> Nonbacterial meningitis

> **G03.1**   **Chronic meningitis** 🔎

> **G03.2**   **Benign recurrent meningitis [Mollaret]** 🔎
> (Ex:) See PDX Collection 140

> **G03.8**   **Meningitis due to other specified causes** 🔎

> **G03.9**   **Meningitis, unspecified** 🔎
> Arachnoiditis (spinal) NOS

● **G04**   **Encephalitis, myelitis and encephalomyelitis**

> **Includes**   acute ascending myelitis
> meningoencephalitis
> meningomyelitis

> **Excludes1**   encephalopathy NOS (G93.40)
> other noninfectious acute disseminated
> encephalomyelitis (noninfectious ADEM)
> (G04.81)

> **Excludes2**   acute transverse myelitis (G37.3-)
> alcoholic encephalopathy (G31.2)
> benign myalgic encephalomyelitis (G93.3)
> multiple sclerosis (G35)
> subacute necrotizing myelitis (G37.4)
> toxic encephalitis (G92)
> toxic encephalopathy (G92)

● **G04.0**   **Acute disseminated encephalitis and encephalomyelitis (ADEM)**

> **Excludes1**   acute necrotizing hemorrhagic
> encephalopathy (G04.3-)

> (Ex:) **For category G04.0 CC codes unless otherwise indicated:** See PDX Collection 560

> **G04.00**   **Acute disseminated encephalitis and encephalomyelitis, unspecified** 🔎

> ▶ **G04.01**   *Postinfectious acute disseminated encephalitis and encephalomyelitis (postinfectious ADEM)* 🔎

> > **Excludes1**   post chickenpox encephalitis (B01.1)
> > post measles encephalitis (B05.0)
> > post measles myelitis (B05.1)

> **G04.02**   **Postimmunization acute disseminated encephalitis, myelitis and encephalomyelitis** 🔎
> Encephalitis, post immunization
> Encephalomyelitis, post immunization
> Use additional code to identify the vaccine
> (T50.A-, T50.B-, T50.Z-)
> (Ex:) No exclusions

> **G04.1**   **Tropical spastic paraplegia** 🔎
> (Ex:) See PDX Collection 561

> **G04.2**   **Bacterial meningoencephalitis and meningomyelitis, not elsewhere classified** 🔎
> (Ex:) See PDX Collection 207

● **G04.3**   **Acute necrotizing hemorrhagic encephalopathy**
> *Sudden and severe CNS disease with pathology of hemorrhages and necrosis of white matter*

> > **Excludes1**   acute disseminated encephalitis and encephalomyelitis (G04.0-)

> **G04.30**   **Acute necrotizing hemorrhagic encephalopathy, unspecified** 🔎
> (Ex:) No exclusions

> **G04.31**   **Postinfectious acute necrotizing hemorrhagic encephalopathy** 🔎
> (Ex:) See PDX Collection 560

> **G04.32**   **Postimmunization acute necrotizing hemorrhagic encephalopathy** 🔎
> Use additional code to identify vaccine
> (T50.A-, T50.B-, T50.Z-)
> (Ex:) No exclusions

> **G04.39**   **Other acute necrotizing hemorrhagic encephalopathy** 🔎
> Code also underlying etiology, if applicable
> (Ex:) No exclusions

● **G04.8**   **Other encephalitis, myelitis and encephalomyelitis**
> Code also any associated seizure (G40.-, R56.9)
> (Ex:) **For category G04.8 CC codes:** See PDX Collection 560

> **G04.81**   **Other encephalitis and encephalomyelitis** 🔎
> Noninfectious acute disseminated encephalomyelitis (noninfectious ADEM)

> **G04.89**   **Other myelitis** 🔎

● **G04.9**   **Encephalitis, myelitis and encephalomyelitis, unspecified**
> (Ex:) **For category G04.9 CC codes:** See PDX Collection 562

> **G04.90**   **Encephalitis and encephalomyelitis, unspecified** 🔎
> Ventriculitis (cerebral) NOS

> **G04.91**   **Myelitis, unspecified** 🔎

● **G05**   **Encephalitis, myelitis and encephalomyelitis in diseases classified elsewhere**

> *Code first underlying disease, such as:*
> human immunodeficiency virus [HIV] disease (B20)
> poliovirus (A80.-)
> suppurative otitis media (H66.01-H66.4)
> trichinellosis (B75)

> **Excludes1**   adenoviral encephalitis, myelitis and encephalomyelitis (A85.1)
> congenital toxoplasmosis encephalitis, myelitis and encephalomyelitis (P37.1)
> cytomegaloviral encephalitis, myelitis and encephalomyelitis (B25.8)
> encephalitis, myelitis and encephalomyelitis (in) measles (B05.0)
> encephalitis, myelitis and encephalomyelitis (in) systemic lupus erythematosus (M32.19)
> enteroviral encephalitis, myelitis and encephalomyelitis (A85.0)
> eosinophilic meningoencephalitis (B83.2)
> herpesviral [herpes simplex] encephalitis, myelitis and encephalomyelitis (B00.4)
> listerial encephalitis, myelitis and encephalomyelitis (A32.12)
> meningococcal encephalitis, myelitis and encephalomyelitis (A39.81)
> mumps encephalitis, myelitis and encephalomyelitis (B26.2)
> postchickenpox encephalitis, myelitis and encephalomyelitis (B01.1-)
> rubella encephalitis, myelitis and encephalomyelitis (B06.01)
> toxoplasmosis encephalitis, myelitis and encephalomyelitis (B58.2)
> zoster encephalitis, myelitis and encephalomyelitis (B02.0)

> (Ex:) **For category G05 CC codes:** See PDX Collection 560

> ▶ **G05.3**   *Encephalitis and encephalomyelitis in diseases classified elsewhere* 🔎
> Meningoencephalitis in diseases classified elsewhere

> ▶ **G05.4**   *Myelitis in diseases classified elsewhere* 🔎
> Meningomyelitis in diseases classified elsewhere

▶ New   ⇒ Revised   ~~deleted~~ Deleted   Excludes 1   Excludes 2   Includes   Use additional   Code first   Code also   Key words

OGCR Official Guidelines   ● Unacceptable Principal Diagnosis   X Assign placeholder X   ● Use Additional Character(s)   ▶ Manifestation Code   **Coding Clinic**

● **G06   Intracranial and intraspinal abscess and granuloma**
    An accumulation of pus in either the brain or spinal cord
    Use additional code (B95-B97) to identify infectious agent.

     G06.0   Intracranial abscess and granuloma 🔖
         Brain [any part] abscess (embolic)
         Cerebellar abscess (embolic)
         Cerebral abscess (embolic)
         Intracranial epidural abscess or granuloma
         Intracranial extradural abscess or granuloma
         Intracranial subdural abscess or granuloma
         Otogenic abscess (embolic)
         Excludes1   tuberculous intracranial abscess and
                          granuloma (A17.81)
         (Ex) See PDX Collection 563

     G06.1   Intraspinal abscess and granuloma 🔖
         Abscess (embolic) of spinal cord [any part]
         Intraspinal epidural abscess or granuloma
         Intraspinal extradural abscess or granuloma
         Intraspinal subdural abscess or granuloma
         Excludes1   tuberculous intraspinal abscess and
                          granuloma (A17.81)
         (Ex) See PDX Collection 564

     G06.2   Extradural and subdural abscess, unspecified 🔖
         (Ex) See PDX Collection 565

▹ *G07   Intracranial and intraspinal abscess and granuloma in diseases classified elsewhere* 🔖
    Code first underlying disease, such as:
         schistosomiasis granuloma of brain (B65.-)
     Excludes1   abscess of brain:
                   amebic (A06.6)
                   chromomycotic (B43.1)
                   gonococcal (A54.82)
                   tuberculous (A17.81)
                   tuberculoma of meninges (A17.1)
     (Ex) See PDX Collection 565

● **G08   Intracranial and intraspinal phlebitis and thrombophlebitis** 🔖
     Septic embolism of intracranial or intraspinal venous sinuses
         and veins
     Septic endophlebitis of intracranial or intraspinal venous
         sinuses and veins
     Septic phlebitis of intracranial or intraspinal venous sinuses
         and veins
     Septic thrombophlebitis of intracranial or intraspinal venous
         sinuses and veins
     Septic thrombosis of intracranial or intraspinal venous sinuses
         and veins
     Excludes1   intracranial phlebitis and thrombophlebitis
                   complicating:
                   abortion, ectopic or molar pregnancy
                       (O00-O07, O08.7)
                   pregnancy, childbirth and the puerperium
                       (O22.5, O87.3)
                   nonpyogenic intracranial phlebitis and
                       thrombophlebitis (I67.6)
     Excludes2   intracranial phlebitis and thrombophlebitis
                   complicating nonpyogenic intraspinal
                   phlebitis and thrombophlebitis (G95.1)
     (Ex) See PDX Collection 565

G09   Sequelae of inflammatory diseases of central nervous system
     Note: Category G09 is to be used to indicate conditions
         whose primary classification is to G00-G08 as the cause of
         sequelae, themselves classifiable elsewhere. The 'sequelae'
         include conditions specified as residuals.
     Code first condition resulting from (sequela) of inflammatory diseases
         of central nervous system

Item 6-2 Huntington's chorea is an inherited degenerative disorder of the central nervous system and is characterized by ceaseless, jerky movements and progressive cognitive and behavioral deterioration.

SYSTEMIC ATROPHIES PRIMARILY AFFECTING THE CENTRAL NERVOUS SYSTEM (G10-G14)

G10   Huntington's disease 🔖
    Genetic disease with degeneration of cells of the nervous system,
        including brain
     Huntington's chorea
     Huntington's dementia
  ▸Code also dementia in other diseases classified elsewhere
         without behavioral disturbance (F02.80)
     (Ex) See PDX Collection 566

● **G11   Hereditary ataxia**
    Genetic neurological disorder affecting coordination
     Excludes2   cerebral palsy (G80.-)
                   hereditary and idiopathic neuropathy (G60.-)
                   metabolic disorders (E70-E88)
     (Ex) For category G11 CC codes unless otherwise indicated: See PDX Collection 567

     G11.0   Congenital nonprogressive ataxia 🔖
     G11.1   Early-onset cerebellar ataxia 🔖
         Early-onset cerebellar ataxia with essential tremor
         Early-onset cerebellar ataxia with myoclonus [Hunt's
             ataxia]
         Early-onset cerebellar ataxia with retained tendon reflexes
         Friedreich's ataxia (autosomal recessive)
         X-linked recessive spinocerebellar ataxia
     G11.2   Late-onset cerebellar ataxia 🔖   A
     G11.3   Cerebellar ataxia with defective DNA repair 🔖
         Ataxia telangiectasia [Louis-Bar]
         Excludes2   Cockayne's syndrome (Q87.1)
                   other disorders of purine and pyrimidine
                       metabolism (E79.-)
                   xeroderma pigmentosum (Q82.1)
     G11.4   Hereditary spastic paraplegia 🔖
         (Ex) See PDX Collection 568
     G11.8   Other hereditary ataxias 🔖
     G11.9   Hereditary ataxia, unspecified 🔖
         Hereditary cerebellar ataxia NOS
         Hereditary cerebellar degeneration
         Hereditary cerebellar disease
         Hereditary cerebellar syndrome
         (Ex) See PDX Collection 569

● **G12   Spinal muscular atrophy and related syndromes**
     (Ex) For category G12 CC codes: See PDX Collection 570
     **G12.0   Infantile spinal muscular atrophy, type I
            [Werdnig-Hoffman]** 🔖
     G12.1   Other inherited spinal muscular atrophy 🔖
         Adult form spinal muscular atrophy
         Childhood form, type II spinal muscular atrophy
         Distal spinal muscular atrophy
         Juvenile form, type III spinal muscular atrophy
             [Kugelberg-Welander]
         Progressive bulbar palsy of childhood [Fazio-Londe]
         Scapuloperoneal form spinal muscular atrophy
● **G12.2   Motor neuron disease**
         Progressive disease of motor neurons that carry impulses to
             muscles to move
         G12.20   Motor neuron disease, unspecified 🔖
         G12.21   Amyotrophic lateral sclerosis 🔖   A
            Lou Gehrig's disease (ALS)
            ~~Progressive spinal muscle atrophy~~
         G12.22   Progressive bulbar palsy 🔖
         ▸ **G12.23   Primary lateral sclerosis** 🔖
         ▸ **G12.24   Familial motor neuron disease** 🔖
         ▸ **G12.25   Progressive spinal muscle atrophy** 🔖
         G12.29   Other motor neuron disease 🔖
            ~~Familial motor neuron disease~~
            ~~Primary lateral sclerosis~~

N Newborn Age: 0   **P** Pediatric Age: 0-17   **M** Maternity DX: 12-55   **A** Adult Age: 15-124   ♀ Females Only   ♂ Males Only

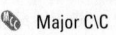 Complication\Comorbidity   🔖 Major C\C   (Ex) CC/MCC Exclusions   🔖 Hospital-Acquired Condition   787

G12.8　Other spinal muscular atrophies and related syndromes 🔖

G12.9　Spinal muscular atrophy, **unspecified** 🔖

● **G13**　Systemic atrophies primarily affecting central nervous system in diseases classified elsewhere

▸ *G13.0　Paraneoplastic neuromyopathy and neuropathy*
Carcinomatous neuromyopathy
Sensorial paraneoplastic neuropathy [Denny Brown]
Code first underlying neoplasm (C00-D49)

▸ *G13.1　Other systemic atrophy primarily affecting central nervous system in neoplastic disease*
Paraneoplastic limbic encephalopathy
Code first underlying neoplasm (C00-D49)

▸ *G13.2　Systemic atrophy primarily affecting the central nervous system in myxedema*
Code first underlying disease, such as:
hypothyroidism (E03.-)
myxedematous congenital iodine deficiency (E00.1)

▸ *G13.8　Systemic atrophy primarily affecting central nervous system in other diseases classified elsewhere*
Code first underlying disease

G14　Postpolio syndrome
Includes　Postpolio myelitic syndrome
Excludes1　sequelae of poliomyelitis (B91)

EXTRAPYRAMIDAL AND MOVEMENT DISORDERS (G20-G26)

G20　Parkinson's disease
Progressive disease of the nervous system that affects muscle coordination
Hemiparkinsonism
Idiopathic Parkinsonism or Parkinson's disease
Paralysis agitans
Parkinsonism or Parkinson's disease NOS
Primary Parkinsonism or Parkinson's disease
Excludes1　dementia with Parkinsonism (G31.83)
Coding Clinic: 2017, Q2, P7-8; 2016, Q2, P7

● **G21**　Secondary parkinsonism
Symptoms of Parkinson's caused by medicines, illness, or other nervous system disorder
Excludes1　dementia with Parkinsonism (G31.83)
Huntington's disease (G10)
Shy-Drager syndrome (G90.3)
syphilitic Parkinsonism (A52.19)

G21.0　Malignant neuroleptic syndrome 🔖
Use additional code for adverse effect, if applicable, to identify drug (T43.3X5, T43.4X5, T43.505, T43.595)
Excludes1　neuroleptic induced parkinsonism (G21.11)
Ⓔ See PDX Collection 571

● G21.1　Other drug-induced secondary parkinsonism
Ⓔ For category G21.1 CC codes: See PDX Collection 572

G21.11　Neuroleptic induced parkinsonism 🔖
Use additional code for adverse effect, if applicable, to identify drug (T43.3X5, T43.4X5, T43.505, T43.595)
Excludes1　malignant neuroleptic syndrome (G21.0)

G21.19　Other drug induced secondary parkinsonism 🔖
▸Other medication-induced parkinsonism
Use additional code for adverse effect, if applicable, to identify drug (T36-T50 with fifth or sixth character 5)

G21.2　Secondary parkinsonism due to other external agents 🔖
Code first (T51-T65) to identify external agent

G21.3　Postencephalitic parkinsonism 🔖

G21.4　Vascular parkinsonism 🔖

G21.8　Other secondary parkinsonism 🔖

G21.9　Secondary parkinsonism, unspecified 🔖

● **G23**　Other degenerative diseases of basal ganglia
Excludes2　multi-system degeneration of the autonomic nervous system (G90.3)
Ⓔ For category G23 CC codes: See PDX Collection 573

G23.0　Hallervorden-Spatz disease 🔖
Pigmentary pallidal degeneration

G23.1　Progressive supranuclear ophthalmoplegia [Steele-Richardson-Olszewski] 🔖
Progressive supranuclear palsy

G23.2　Striatonigral degeneration 🔖

G23.8　Other specified degenerative diseases of basal ganglia 🔖
Calcification of basal ganglia

G23.9　Degenerative disease of basal ganglia, **unspecified** 🔖

● **G24**　Dystonia
Involuntary movements
Includes　dyskinesia
Excludes2　athetoid cerebral palsy (G80.3)

● G24.0　Drug induced dystonia
Use additional code for adverse effect, if applicable, to identify drug (T36-T50 with fifth or sixth character 5)

G24.01　Drug induced **subacute** dyskinesia
Drug induced blepharospasm
Drug induced orofacial dyskinesia
Neuroleptic induced tardive dyskinesia
Tardive dyskinesia

G24.02　Drug induced **acute** dystonia 🔖
Acute dystonic reaction to drugs
Neuroleptic induced acute dystonia
Ⓔ See PDX Collection 574

G24.09　Other drug induced dystonia 🔖
Ⓔ See PDX Collection 574

G24.1　Genetic torsion dystonia
Dystonia deformans progressiva
Dystonia musculorum deformans
Familial torsion dystonia
Idiopathic familial dystonia
Idiopathic (torsion) dystonia NOS
(Schwalbe-) Ziehen-Oppenheim disease

G24.2　Idiopathic nonfamilial dystonia 🔖
Ⓔ See PDX Collection 574

G24.3　Spasmodic torticollis
Head tilts toward one side and chin is elevated and turned toward opposite side (wry neck)
Excludes1　congenital torticollis (Q68.0)
hysterical torticollis (F44.4)
ocular torticollis (R29.891)
psychogenic torticollis (F45.8)
torticollis NOS (M43.6)
traumatic recurrent torticollis (S13.4)

G24.4　Idiopathic orofacial dystonia
Orofacial dyskinesia
Excludes1　drug induced orofacial dyskinesia (G24.01)

G24.5　Blepharospasm
Tonic spasm of orbicularis oculi muscle, producing closure of eyelids
Excludes1　drug induced blepharospasm (G24.01)

G24.8　Other dystonia 🔖
Acquired torsion dystonia NOS
Ⓔ See PDX Collection 574

G24.9　Dystonia, **unspecified**
Dyskinesia NOS

- **G25 Other extrapyramidal and movement disorders**
  Extrapyramidal: Other than pyramidal tracts
       Excludes2   sleep related movement disorders (G47.6-)
  - **G25.0 Essential tremor**
    Familial tremor
         Excludes1   tremor NOS (R25.1)
  - **G25.1 Drug-induced tremor**
    Use additional code for adverse effect, if applicable, to identify drug (T36-T50 with fifth or sixth character 5)
  - **G25.2 Other specified forms of tremor**
    Intention tremor
  - **G25.3 Myoclonus**
    Shocklike contractions muscle(s)
    Drug-induced myoclonus
    Palatal myoclonus
    Use additional code for adverse effect, if applicable, to identify drug (T36-T50 with fifth or sixth character 5)
         Excludes1   facial myokymia (G51.4)
                           myoclonic epilepsy (G40.-)
  - **G25.4 Drug-induced chorea**
    Use additional code for adverse effect, if applicable, to identify drug (T36-T50 with fifth or sixth character 5)
  - **G25.5 Other chorea**
    Continual, involuntary, jerky, movements
    Chorea NOS
         Excludes1   chorea NOS with heart involvement (I02.0)
                           Huntington's chorea (G10)
                           rheumatic chorea (I02.-)
                           Sydenham's chorea (I02.-)
  - **G25.6 Drug induced tics and other tics of organic origin**
    - **G25.61 Drug induced tics**
      Use additional code for adverse effect, if applicable, to identify drug (T36-T50 with fifth or sixth character 5)
    - **G25.69 Other tics of organic origin**
           Excludes1   habit spasm (F95.9)
                             tic NOS (F95.9)
                             Tourette's syndrome (F95.2)
  - **G25.7 Other and unspecified drug induced movement disorders**
    Use additional code for adverse effect, if applicable, to identify drug (T36-T50 with fifth or sixth character 5)
    - **G25.70 Drug induced movement disorder, unspecified**
    - **G25.71 Drug induced akathisia**
      Drug induced acathisia
      Neuroleptic induced acute akathisia
      ▶Tardive akathisia
    - **G25.79 Other drug induced movement disorders**
  - **G25.8 Other specified extrapyramidal and movement disorders**
    - **G25.81 Restless legs syndrome**
    - **G25.82 Stiff-man syndrome** 🖝
      (Ex:) See PDX Collection 575
    - **G25.83 Benign shuddering attacks**
    - **G25.89 Other specified extrapyramidal and movement disorders**
  - **G25.9 Extrapyramidal and movement disorder, unspecified** 🖝
    (Ex:) See PDX Collection 575

- **G26 *Extrapyramidal and movement disorders in diseases classified elsewhere***
  Code first underlying disease

OTHER DEGENERATIVE DISEASES OF THE NERVOUS SYSTEM (G30-G32)

- **G30 Alzheimer's disease**
  Progressive central neurodegenerative disorder
       Includes   Alzheimer's dementia senile and presenile forms
  Use additional code to identify:
    delirium, if applicable (F05)
    dementia with behavioral disturbance (F02.81)
    dementia without behavioral disturbance (F02.80)
       Excludes1   senile degeneration of brain NEC (G31.1)
                         senile dementia NOS (F03)
                         senility NOS (R41.81)
  - **G30.0 Alzheimer's disease with early onset**
  - **G30.1 Alzheimer's disease with late onset**   A
  - **G30.8 Other Alzheimer's disease**
  - **G30.9 Alzheimer's disease, unspecified**
    Coding Clinic: 2017, Q1, P43; 2016, Q2, P6; 2012, Q4, P95

- **G31 Other degenerative diseases of nervous system, not elsewhere classified**
  Use additional code to identify:
    dementia with behavioral disturbance (F02.81)
    dementia without behavioral disturbance (F02.80)
       Excludes2   Reye's syndrome (G93.7)
  - **G31.0 Frontotemporal dementia**
    - **G31.01 Pick's disease**
      Primary progressive aphasia
      Progressive isolated aphasia
    - **G31.09 Other frontotemporal dementia**
      Frontal dementia
  - **G31.1 Senile degeneration of brain, not elsewhere classified**
         Excludes1   Alzheimer's disease (G30.-)
                           senility NOS (R41.81)
  - **G31.2 Degeneration of nervous system due to alcohol**
    Alcoholic cerebellar ataxia
    Alcoholic cerebellar degeneration
    Alcoholic cerebral degeneration
    Alcoholic encephalopathy
    Dysfunction of the autonomic nervous system due to alcohol
    Code also associated alcoholism (F10.-)
  - **G31.8 Other specified degenerative diseases of nervous system**
    - **G31.81 Alpers' disease** 🖝
      Rare neuronal degeneration of cerebral cortex disease of young children
      Grey-matter degeneration
      (Ex:) See PDX Collection 537
      Coding Clinic: 2017, Q2, P7
    - **G31.82 Leigh's disease** 🖝
      Rare neurometabolic disorder that affects central nervous system
      Subacute necrotizing encephalopathy
      (Ex:) See PDX Collection 537
    - **G31.83 Dementia with Lewy bodies**
      Closely allied to Parkinson's Disease
      Dementia with Parkinsonism
      Lewy body dementia
      Lewy body disease
      Coding Clinic: 2017, Q2, P7; 2016, Q4, P141

N Newborn Age: 0   **P** Pediatric Age: 0–17   **M** Maternity DX: 12–55   **A** Adult Age: 15–124   ♀ Females Only   ♂ Males Only

🖝 Complication\Comorbidity   🖝 Major C\C   (Ex:) CC/MCC Exclusions   🖝 Hospital-Acquired Condition

789

CHAPTER 6 (G00-G99)

G31.84   **Mild cognitive impairment, so stated**
▶Mild neurocognitive disorder

Excludes1   age related cognitive decline (R41.81)
altered mental status (R41.82)
cerebral degeneration (G31.9)
change in mental status (R41.82)
cognitive deficits following (sequelae of) cerebral hemorrhage or infarction (I69.01-, I69.11-, I69.21-, I69.31-, I69.81-, I69.91-)
cognitive impairment due to intracranial or head injury (S06.-)
dementia (F01.-, F02.-, F03)
mild memory disturbance (F06.8)
neurologic neglect syndrome (R41.4)
personality change, nonpsychotic (F68.8)

G31.85   **Corticobasal degeneration**

G31.89   **Other specified degenerative diseases of nervous system**

G31.9   **Degenerative disease of nervous system, unspecified**

● **G32**   **Other degenerative disorders of nervous system in diseases classified elsewhere**

▶ *G32.0*   *Subacute combined degeneration of spinal cord in diseases classified elsewhere*
Dana-Putnam syndrome
Sclerosis of spinal cord (combined) (dorsolateral) (posterolateral)

Code first underlying disease, such as:
anemia (D51.9)
dietary (D51.3)
pernicious (D51.0)
vitamin B12 deficiency (E53.8)

Excludes1   syphilitic combined degeneration of spinal cord (A52.11)
(Ex:) See PDX Collection 576

● **G32.8**   **Other specified degenerative disorders of nervous system in diseases classified elsewhere**

Code first underlying disease, such as:
amyloidosis cerebral degeneration (E85.-)
cerebral degeneration (due to) hypothyroidism (E00.0-E03.9)
cerebral degeneration (due to) neoplasm (C00-D49)
cerebral degeneration (due to) vitamin B deficiency, except thiamine (E52-E53.-)

Excludes1   superior hemorrhagic polioencephalitis [Wernicke's encephalopathy] (E51.2)

▶ *G32.81*   *Cerebellar ataxia in diseases classified elsewhere*

Code first underlying disease, such as:
celiac disease (with gluten ataxia) (K90.0)
cerebellar ataxia (in) neoplastic disease (paraneoplastic cerebellar degeneration) (C00-D49)
non-celiac gluten ataxia (M35.9)

Excludes1   systemic atrophy primarily affecting the central nervous system in alcoholic cerebellar ataxia (G31.2)
systemic atrophy primarily affecting the central nervous system in myxedema (G13.2)
(Ex:) See PDX Collection 567

▶ *G32.89*   *Other specified degenerative disorders of nervous system in diseases classified elsewhere*
Degenerative encephalopathy in diseases classified elsewhere

Item 6–3   Multiple sclerosis (MS) is a nervous system disease affecting the brain and spinal cord by damaging the myelin sheath surrounding and protecting nerve cells. The damage slows down/blocks messages between the brain and body. Symptoms are: visual disturbances, muscle weakness, coordination and balance issues, numbness, prickling, thinking and memory problems. The cause is unknown, though it is thought that it may be an autoimmune disease. It affects women more than men, between 20 and 40 years of age. MS can be mild, but it may cause the loss of ability to write, walk, and speak. There is no cure, but medication may slow or control symptoms.

DEMYELINATING DISEASES OF THE CENTRAL NERVOUS SYSTEM (G35-G37)

G35   **Multiple sclerosis**
Destruction of central nervous system; four types: relapsing remitting, secondary progressive, primary progressive, and progressive relapsing
Disseminated multiple sclerosis
Generalized multiple sclerosis
Multiple sclerosis NOS
Multiple sclerosis of brain stem
Multiple sclerosis of cord

● **G36**   **Other acute disseminated demyelination**
Excludes1   postinfectious encephalitis and encephalomyelitis NOS (G04.01)
(Ex:) For category G36 CC codes unless otherwise indicated: See PDX Collection 578

G36.0   **Neuromyelitis optica [Devic]**
Inflammatory disorder in which immune system attacks optic nerves and spinal cord producing inflammation of optic nerve (optic neuritis) and spinal cord (myelitis)
Demyelination in optic neuritis
Excludes1   optic neuritis NOS (H46)
(Ex:) See PDX Collection 577

G36.1   **Acute and subacute hemorrhagic leukoencephalitis [Hurst]**

G36.8   **Other specified acute disseminated demyelination**

G36.9   **Acute disseminated demyelination, unspecified**

● **G37**   **Other demyelinating diseases of central nervous system**
Destruction of central nervous system

G37.0   **Diffuse sclerosis of central nervous system**
Periaxial encephalitis
Schilder's disease
Excludes1   X linked adrenoleukodystrophy (E71.52-)
(Ex:) See PDX Collection 579

G37.1   **Central demyelination of corpus callosum**
(Ex:) See PDX Collection 578

G37.2   **Central pontine myelinolysis**
(Ex:) See PDX Collection 578

G37.3   **Acute transverse myelitis in demyelinating disease of central nervous system**
Acute transverse myelitis NOS
Acute transverse myelopathy
Excludes1   multiple sclerosis (G35)
neuromyelitis optica [Devic] (G36.0)
(Ex:) See PDX Collection 580

G37.4   **Subacute necrotizing myelitis of central nervous system**
(Ex:) See PDX Collection 562

G37.5   **Concentric sclerosis [Baló] of central nervous system**
(Ex:) See PDX Collection 579

G37.8   **Other specified demyelinating diseases of central nervous system**
(Ex:) See PDX Collection 578

G37.9   **Demyelinating disease of central nervous system, unspecified**
(Ex:) See PDX Collection 578

▶ New   ⇒ Revised   deleted Deleted   Excludes 1   Excludes 2   Includes   Use additional   Code first   Code also   Key words
OGCR Official Guidelines   ● Unacceptable Principal Diagnosis   X Assign placeholder X   ● Use Additional Character(s)   ▶ Manifestation Code   **Coding Clinic**

EPISODIC AND PAROXYSMAL DISORDERS (G40-G47)

● **G40 Epilepsy and recurrent seizures**

Note: The following terms are to be considered equivalent to intractable: pharmacoresistant (pharmacologically resistant), treatment resistant, refractory (medically) and poorly controlled

Excludes1 conversion disorder with seizures (F44.5)
convulsions NOS (R56.9)
post traumatic seizures (R56.1)
seizure (convulsive) NOS (R56.9)
seizure of newborn (P90)

Excludes2 hippocampal sclerosis (G93.81)
mesial temporal sclerosis (G93.81)
temporal sclerosis (G93.81)
Todd's paralysis (G83.84)

● **G40.0 Localization-related (focal) (partial) idiopathic epilepsy and epileptic syndromes with seizures of localized onset**
Benign childhood epilepsy with centrotemporal EEG spikes
Childhood epilepsy with occipital EEG paroxysms

Excludes1 adult onset localization-related epilepsy (G40.1-, G40.2-)

● **G40.00 Localization-related (focal) (partial) idiopathic epilepsy and epileptic syndromes with seizures of localized onset, not intractable**
Localization-related (focal) (partial) idiopathic epilepsy and epileptic syndromes with seizures of localized onset without intractability

G40.001 Localization-related (focal) (partial) idiopathic epilepsy and epileptic syndromes with seizures of localized onset, not intractable, with status epilepticus 🦠
⓮ See PDX Collection 581

G40.009 Localization-related (focal) (partial) idiopathic epilepsy and epileptic syndromes with seizures of localized onset, not intractable, without status epilepticus 🦠
Localization-related (focal) (partial) idiopathic epilepsy and epileptic syndromes with seizures of localized onset NOS
⓮ See PDX Collection 581

● **G40.01 Localization-related (focal) (partial) idiopathic epilepsy and epileptic syndromes with seizures of localized onset, intractable**

G40.011 Localization-related (focal) (partial) idiopathic epilepsy and epileptic syndromes with seizures of localized onset, intractable, with status epilepticus 🦠
⓮ See PDX Collection 582

G40.019 Localization-related (focal) (partial) idiopathic epilepsy and epileptic syndromes with seizures of localized onset, intractable, without status epilepticus 🦠
⓮ See PDX Collection 582

● **G40.1 Localization-related (focal) (partial) symptomatic epilepsy and epileptic syndromes with simple partial seizures**
Attacks without alteration of consciousness
Epilepsia partialis continua [Kozhevnikof]
Simple partial seizures developing into secondarily generalized seizures

● **G40.10 Localization-related (focal) (partial) symptomatic epilepsy and epileptic syndromes with simple partial seizures, not intractable**
Localization-related (focal) (partial) symptomatic epilepsy and epileptic syndromes with simple partial seizures without intractability

G40.101 Localization-related (focal) (partial) symptomatic epilepsy and epileptic syndromes with simple partial seizures, not intractable, with status epilepticus 🦠
⓮ See PDX Collection 581

G40.109 Localization-related (focal) (partial) symptomatic epilepsy and epileptic syndromes with simple partial seizures, not intractable, without status epilepticus 🦠
Localization-related (focal) (partial) symptomatic epilepsy and epileptic syndromes with simple partial seizures NOS
⓮ See PDX Collection 581

● **G40.11 Localization-related (focal) (partial) symptomatic epilepsy and epileptic syndromes with simple partial seizures, intractable**

G40.111 Localization-related (focal) (partial) symptomatic epilepsy and epileptic syndromes with simple partial seizures, intractable, with status epilepticus 🦠
⓮ See PDX Collection 582

G40.119 Localization-related (focal) (partial) symptomatic epilepsy and epileptic syndromes with simple partial seizures, intractable, without status epilepticus 🦠
⓮ See PDX Collection 582

● **G40.2 Localization-related (focal) (partial) symptomatic epilepsy and epileptic syndromes with complex partial seizures**
Attacks with alteration of consciousness, often with automatisms
Complex partial seizures developing into secondarily generalized seizures

● **G40.20 Localization-related (focal) (partial) symptomatic epilepsy and epileptic syndromes with complex partial seizures, not intractable**
Localization-related (focal) (partial) symptomatic epilepsy and epileptic syndromes with complex partial seizures without intractability

G40.201 Localization-related (focal) (partial) symptomatic epilepsy and epileptic syndromes with complex partial seizures, not intractable, with status epilepticus 🦠
⓮ See PDX Collection 581

G40.209 Localization-related (focal) (partial) symptomatic epilepsy and epileptic syndromes with complex partial seizures, not intractable, without status epilepticus 🦠
Localization-related (focal) (partial) symptomatic epilepsy and epileptic syndromes with complex partial seizures NOS
⓮ See PDX Collection 581

CHAPTER 6 (G00-G99)

CHAPTER 6 (G00-G99)

● **G40.21** Localization-related (focal) (partial) symptomatic epilepsy and epileptic syndromes with complex partial seizures, **intractable**

    G40.211 Localization-related (focal) (partial) symptomatic epilepsy and epileptic syndromes with complex partial seizures, intractable, **with status epilepticus**
      Ex: See PDX Collection 582

    G40.219 Localization-related (focal) (partial) symptomatic epilepsy and epileptic syndromes with complex partial seizures, intractable, **without status epilepticus**
      Ex: See PDX Collection 582

● **G40.3** Generalized idiopathic epilepsy and epileptic syndromes

    Code also MERRF syndrome, if applicable (E88.42)

 ● **G40.30** Generalized idiopathic epilepsy and epileptic syndromes, **not intractable**
    Generalized idiopathic epilepsy and epileptic syndromes without intractability

    G40.301 Generalized idiopathic epilepsy and epileptic syndromes, not intractable, **with status epilepticus**
      Ex: See PDX Collection 583

    G40.309 Generalized idiopathic epilepsy and epileptic syndromes, not intractable, **without status epilepticus**
      Generalized idiopathic epilepsy and epileptic syndromes NOS

 ● **G40.31** Generalized idiopathic epilepsy and epileptic syndromes, **intractable**

    G40.311 Generalized idiopathic epilepsy and epileptic syndromes, intractable, **with status epilepticus**
      Ex: See PDX Collection 583

    G40.319 Generalized idiopathic epilepsy and epileptic syndromes, intractable, **without status epilepticus**
      Ex: See PDX Collection 583

● **G40.A** Absence epileptic syndrome
    Childhood absence epilepsy [pyknolepsy]
    Juvenile absence epilepsy
    Absence epileptic syndrome, NOS

 ● **G40.A0** Absence epileptic syndrome, **not intractable**

    G40.A01 Absence epileptic syndrome, not intractable, **with status epilepticus**

    G40.A09 Absence epileptic syndrome, not intractable, **without status epilepticus**

 ● **G40.A1** Absence epileptic syndrome, **intractable**

    G40.A11 Absence epileptic syndrome, intractable, **with status epilepticus**
      Ex: See PDX Collection 582

    G40.A19 Absence epileptic syndrome, intractable, **without status epilepticus**
      Ex: See PDX Collection 582

● **G40.B** Juvenile myoclonic epilepsy [impulsive petit mal]
    Ex: For category G40.B CC codes: See PDX Collection 582

 ● **G40.B0** Juvenile myoclonic epilepsy, **not intractable**

    G40.B01 Juvenile myoclonic epilepsy, not intractable, **with status epilepticus**

    G40.B09 Juvenile myoclonic epilepsy, not intractable, **without status epilepticus**

 ● **G40.B1** Juvenile myoclonic epilepsy, **intractable**

    G40.B11 Juvenile myoclonic epilepsy, intractable, **with status epilepticus**

    G40.B19 Juvenile myoclonic epilepsy, intractable, **without status epilepticus**

● **G40.4** Other generalized epilepsy and epileptic syndromes
    Epilepsy with grand mal seizures on awakening
    Epilepsy with myoclonic absences
    Epilepsy with myoclonic-astatic seizures
    Grand mal seizure NOS
    Nonspecific atonic epileptic seizures
    Nonspecific clonic epileptic seizures
    Nonspecific myoclonic epileptic seizures
    Nonspecific tonic epileptic seizures
    Nonspecific tonic-clonic epileptic seizures
    Symptomatic early myoclonic encephalopathy

 ● **G40.40** Other generalized epilepsy and epileptic syndromes, **not intractable**
    Other generalized epilepsy and epileptic syndromes without intractability
    Other generalized epilepsy and epileptic syndromes NOS

    G40.401 Other generalized epilepsy and epileptic syndromes, not intractable, **with status epilepticus**

    G40.409 Other generalized epilepsy and epileptic syndromes, not intractable, **without status epilepticus**

 ● **G40.41** Other generalized epilepsy and epileptic syndromes, **intractable**

    G40.411 Other generalized epilepsy and epileptic syndromes, intractable, **with status epilepticus**
      Ex: See PDX Collection 582

    G40.419 Other generalized epilepsy and epileptic syndromes, intractable, **without status epilepticus**
      Ex: See PDX Collection 582

● **G40.5** Epileptic seizures related to **external causes**
    Epileptic seizures related to alcohol
    Epileptic seizures related to drugs
    Epileptic seizures related to hormonal changes
    Epileptic seizures related to sleep deprivation
    Epileptic seizures related to stress

    Code also, if applicable, associated epilepsy and recurrent seizures (G40.-)

    Use additional code for adverse effect, if applicable, to identify drug (T36-T50 with fifth or sixth character 5)
    Ex: For category G40.5 CC codes: See PDX Collection 582

 ● **G40.50** Epileptic seizures related to external causes, **not intractable**

    G40.501 Epileptic seizures related to external causes, not intractable, **with status epilepticus**

    G40.509 Epileptic seizures related to external causes, not intractable, **without status epilepticus**
      Epileptic seizures related to external causes, NOS

● **G40.8   Other epilepsy and recurrent seizures**
     Epilepsies and epileptic syndromes undetermined as to
          whether they are focal or generalized
     Landau-Kleffner syndrome
     (Ex) **For category G40.8 CC codes unless otherwise indicated:** See PDX
          Collection 582

   ● **G40.80   Other epilepsy**
        G40.801   Other epilepsy, not intractable, with
                   status epilepticus 🔗
                   Other epilepsy without intractability
                        with status epilepticus

        G40.802   Other epilepsy, not intractable,
                   without status epilepticus 🔗
                   Other epilepsy NOS
                   Other epilepsy without intractability
                        without status epilepticus

        G40.803   Other epilepsy, intractable, with
                   status epilepticus 🔗

        G40.804   Other epilepsy, intractable, without
                   status epilepticus 🔗

   ● **G40.81   Lennox-Gastaut syndrome**
        G40.811   Lennox-Gastaut syndrome, not
                   intractable, with status epilepticus 🔗

        G40.812   Lennox-Gastaut syndrome, not
                   intractable, without status
                   epilepticus 🔗

        G40.813   Lennox-Gastaut syndrome,
                   intractable, with status epilepticus 🔗

        G40.814   Lennox-Gastaut syndrome, intractable,
                   without status epilepticus 🔗

   ● **G40.82   Epileptic spasms**
        Infantile spasms
        Salaam attacks
        West's syndrome
        G40.821   Epileptic spasms, not intractable, with
                   status epilepticus 🔗
                   (Ex) See PDX Collection 581

        G40.822   Epileptic spasms, not intractable,
                   without status epilepticus 🔗
                   (Ex) See PDX Collection 581

        G40.823   Epileptic spasms, intractable, with
                   status epilepticus 🔗

        G40.824   Epileptic spasms, intractable,
                   without status epilepticus 🔗

   ○ **G40.89   Other seizures** 🔗
        Excludes1   post traumatic seizures (R56.1)
                        recurrent seizures NOS (G40.909)
                        seizure NOS (R56.9)

● **G40.9   Epilepsy, unspecified**
   ● **G40.90   Epilepsy, unspecified, not intractable**
        Epilepsy, unspecified, without intractability
        G40.901   Epilepsy, unspecified, not intractable,
                   with status epilepticus

        G40.909   Epilepsy, unspecified, not intractable,
                   without status epilepticus
                   Epilepsy NOS
                   Epileptic convulsions NOS
                   Epileptic fits NOS
                   Epileptic seizures NOS
                   Recurrent seizures NOS
                   Seizure disorder NOS

   ● **G40.91   Epilepsy, unspecified, intractable**
        Intractable seizure disorder NOS
        (Ex) **For category G40.91 CC codes:** See PDX Collection 582
        G40.911   Epilepsy, unspecified, intractable,
                   with status epilepticus 🔗

        G40.919   Epilepsy, unspecified, intractable,
                   without status epilepticus 🔗

Item 6–4   Migraine headache is described as an intense pulsing or throbbing
pain in one area of the head. It can be accompanied by extreme sensitivity to
light (photophobic) and sound and is three times more common in women than
in men. Symptoms include nausea and vomiting. Research indicates migraine
headaches are caused by inherited abnormalities in genes that control the
activities of certain cell populations in the brain.

● **G43   Migraine**
     Note: The following terms are to be considered equivalent
          to intractable: pharmacoresistant (pharmacologically
          resistant), treatment resistant, refractory (medically) and
          poorly controlled
     Use additional code for adverse effect, if applicable, to identify
          drug (T36-T50 with fifth or sixth character 5)
     Excludes1   headache NOS (R51)
                     lower half migraine (G44.00)
     Excludes2   headache syndromes (G44.-)

   ● **G43.0   Migraine without aura**
        *Neurological disorder, generally recurring headaches without
             early symptom (aura)*
        Common migraine
        Excludes1   chronic migraine without aura (G43.7-)

      ● **G43.00   Migraine without aura, not intractable**
             *Neurological disorder, generally recurring
                  headaches without early symptom (aura);
                  resistant to cure, relief, or control*
             Migraine without aura without mention of
                  refractory migraine
             G43.001   Migraine without aura, not
                        intractable, with status migrainosus

             G43.009   Migraine without aura, not
                        intractable, without status
                        migrainosus
                        Migraine without aura NOS

      ● **G43.01   Migraine without aura, intractable**
             *Intractable migraine: Not easily cured or managed;
                  relentless pain from a migraine*
             Migraine without aura with refractory
                  migraine
             G43.011   Migraine without aura, intractable,
                        with status migrainosus

             G43.019   Migraine without aura, intractable,
                        without status migrainosus

   ● **G43.1   Migraine with aura**
        Basilar migraine
        Classical migraine
        Migraine equivalents
        Migraine preceded or accompanied by transient focal
             neurological phenomena
        Migraine triggered seizures
        Migraine with acute-onset aura
        Migraine with aura without headache (migraine
             equivalents)
        Migraine with prolonged aura
        Migraine with typical aura
        Retinal migraine
        Code also any associated seizure (G40.-, R56.9)
        Excludes1   persistent migraine aura (G43.5-, G43.6-)

      ● **G43.10   Migraine with aura, not intractable**
             Migraine with aura without mention of
                  refractory migraine
             G43.101   Migraine with aura, not intractable,
                        with status migrainosus

             G43.109   Migraine with aura, not intractable,
                        without status migrainosus
                        Migraine with aura NOS

      ● **G43.11   Migraine with aura, intractable**
             Migraine with aura with refractory migraine
             G43.111   Migraine with aura, intractable, with
                        status migrainosus

             G43.119   Migraine with aura, intractable,
                        without status migrainosus

CHAPTER 6 (G00-G99)

G43.4 Hemiplegic migraine
Inherited migraine disorder causing temporary paralysis of one side of body followed by severe headache and nausea
Familial migraine
Sporadic migraine

- **G43.40 Hemiplegic migraine, not intractable**
  Hemiplegic migraine without refractory migraine
  - **G43.401 Hemiplegic migraine, not intractable, with status migrainosus**
  - **G43.409 Hemiplegic migraine, not intractable, without status migrainosus**
    Hemiplegic migraine NOS
- **G43.41 Hemiplegic migraine, intractable**
  Hemiplegic migraine with refractory migraine
  - **G43.411 Hemiplegic migraine, intractable, with status migrainosus**
  - **G43.419 Hemiplegic migraine, intractable, without status migrainosus**

G43.5 Persistent migraine aura without cerebral infarction

- **G43.50 Persistent migraine aura without cerebral infarction, not intractable**
  Persistent migraine aura without cerebral infarction, without refractory migraine
  - **G43.501 Persistent migraine aura without cerebral infarction, not intractable, with status migrainosus**
  - **G43.509 Persistent migraine aura without cerebral infarction, not intractable, without status migrainosus**
    Persistent migraine aura NOS
- **G43.51 Persistent migraine aura without cerebral infarction, intractable**
  Persistent migraine aura without cerebral infarction, with refractory migraine
  - **G43.511 Persistent migraine aura without cerebral infarction, intractable, with status migrainosus**
  - **G43.519 Persistent migraine aura without cerebral infarction, intractable, without status migrainosus**

G43.6 Persistent migraine aura with cerebral infarction
Visual, motor, or psychic disturbances, paresthesias, and related neurologic abnormalities accompanying migraine
Code also the type of cerebral infarction (I63.-)

- **G43.60 Persistent migraine aura with cerebral infarction, not intractable**
  Persistent migraine aura with cerebral infarction, without refractory migraine
  Ex: For category G43.6 CC codes unless otherwise indicated: See PDX Collection 584
  - **G43.601 Persistent migraine aura with cerebral infarction, not intractable, with status migrainosus**
  - **G43.609 Persistent migraine aura with cerebral infarction, not intractable, without status migrainosus**
    Ex: See PDX Collection 585

- **G43.61 Persistent migraine aura with cerebral infarction, intractable**
  Persistent migraine aura with cerebral infarction, with refractory migraine
  - **G43.611 Persistent migraine aura with cerebral infarction, intractable, with status migrainosus**
  - **G43.619 Persistent migraine aura with cerebral infarction, intractable, without status migrainosus**

G43.7 Chronic migraine without aura
Transformed migraine
Excludes1 migraine without aura (G43.0-)

- **G43.70 Chronic migraine without aura, not intractable**
  Chronic migraine without aura, without refractory migraine
  - **G43.701 Chronic migraine without aura, not intractable, with status migrainosus**
  - **G43.709 Chronic migraine without aura, not intractable, without status migrainosus**
    Chronic migraine without aura NOS
- **G43.71 Chronic migraine without aura, intractable**
  Chronic migraine without aura, with refractory migraine
  - **G43.711 Chronic migraine without aura, intractable, with status migrainosus**
  - **G43.719 Chronic migraine without aura, intractable, without status migrainosus**

G43.A Cyclical vomiting

- **G43.A0 Cyclical vomiting, not intractable**
  Cyclical vomiting, without refractory migraine
- **G43.A1 Cyclical vomiting, intractable**
  Cyclical vomiting, with refractory migraine

G43.B Ophthalmoplegic migraine

- **G43.B0 Ophthalmoplegic migraine, not intractable**
  Ophthalmoplegic migraine, without refractory migraine
- **G43.B1 Ophthalmoplegic migraine, intractable**
  Ophthalmoplegic migraine, with refractory migraine

G43.C Periodic headache syndromes in child or adult

- **G43.C0 Periodic headache syndromes in child or adult, not intractable**
  Periodic headache syndromes in child or adult, without refractory migraine
- **G43.C1 Periodic headache syndromes in child or adult, intractable**
  Periodic headache syndromes in child or adult, with refractory migraine

G43.D Abdominal migraine

- **G43.D0 Abdominal migraine, not intractable**
  Abdominal migraine, without refractory migraine
- **G43.D1 Abdominal migraine, intractable**
  Abdominal migraine, with refractory migraine

G43.8 Other migraine

- **G43.80 Other migraine, not intractable**
  Other migraine, without refractory migraine
  - **G43.801 Other migraine, not intractable, with status migrainosus**
  - **G43.809 Other migraine, not intractable, without status migrainosus**
- **G43.81 Other migraine, intractable**
  Other migraine, with refractory migraine
  - **G43.811 Other migraine, intractable, with status migrainosus**
  - **G43.819 Other migraine, intractable, without status migrainosus**

▶ New ⟹ Revised ~~deleted~~ Deleted Excludes 1 Excludes 2 Includes Use additional Code first Code also Key words
OGCR Official Guidelines ● Unacceptable Principal Diagnosis X Assign placeholder X ● Use Additional Character(s) ▸ Manifestation Code **Coding Clinic**

● **G43.82 Menstrual migraine, not intractable**
    Menstrual headache, not intractable
    Menstrual migraine, without refractory
      migraine
    Menstrually related migraine, not intractable
    Pre-menstrual headache, not intractable
    Pre-menstrual migraine, not intractable
    Pure menstrual migraine, not intractable
    Code also associated premenstrual tension
      syndrome (N94.3)

      G43.821 Menstrual migraine, not intractable, with status migrainosus ♀

      G43.829 Menstrual migraine, not intractable, without status migrainosus ♀
          Menstrual migraine NOS

● **G43.83 Menstrual migraine, intractable**
    Menstrual headache, intractable
    Menstrual migraine, with refractory migraine
    Menstrually related migraine, intractable
    Pre-menstrual headache, intractable
    Pre-menstrual migraine, intractable
    Pure menstrual migraine, intractable
    Code also associated premenstrual tension
      syndrome (N94.3)

      G43.831 Menstrual migraine, intractable, with status migrainosus ♀

      G43.839 Menstrual migraine, intractable, without status migrainosus ♀

● **G43.9 Migraine, unspecified**

  ● **G43.90 Migraine, unspecified, not intractable**
    Migraine, unspecified, without refractory
      migraine

      G43.901 Migraine, unspecified, not intractable, with status migrainosus
          Status migrainosus NOS

      G43.909 Migraine, unspecified, not intractable, without status migrainosus
          Migraine NOS

  ● **G43.91 Migraine, unspecified, intractable**
    Migraine, unspecified, with refractory
      migraine

      G43.911 Migraine, unspecified, intractable, with status migrainosus

      G43.919 Migraine, unspecified, intractable, without status migrainosus

● **G44 Other headache syndromes**
  Excludes1   headache NOS (R51)
  Excludes2   atypical facial pain (G50.1)
          headache due to lumbar puncture (G97.1)
          migraines (G43.-)
          trigeminal neuralgia (G50.0)

  ● **G44.0 Cluster headaches and other trigeminal autonomic cephalgias (TAC)**

    ● **G44.00 Cluster headache syndrome, unspecified**
      Ciliary neuralgia
      Cluster headache NOS
      Histamine cephalgia
      Lower half migraine
      Migrainous neuralgia

      G44.001 Cluster headache syndrome, unspecified, intractable

      G44.009 Cluster headache syndrome, unspecified, not intractable
          Cluster headache syndrome NOS

    ● **G44.01 Episodic cluster headache**
      G44.011 Episodic cluster headache, intractable

      G44.019 Episodic cluster headache, not intractable
          Episodic cluster headache NOS

● **G44.02 Chronic cluster headache**
    G44.021 Chronic cluster headache, intractable

    G44.029 Chronic cluster headache, not intractable
        Chronic cluster headache NOS

● **G44.03 Episodic paroxysmal hemicrania**
    Paroxysmal hemicrania NOS

    G44.031 Episodic paroxysmal hemicrania, intractable

    G44.039 Episodic paroxysmal hemicrania, not intractable
        Episodic paroxysmal hemicrania NOS

● **G44.04 Chronic paroxysmal hemicrania**
  Unilateral headache

    G44.041 Chronic paroxysmal hemicrania, intractable

    G44.049 Chronic paroxysmal hemicrania, not intractable
        Chronic paroxysmal hemicrania NOS

● **G44.05 Short lasting unilateral neuralgiform headache with conjunctival injection and tearing (SUNCT)**

    G44.051 Short lasting unilateral neuralgiform headache with conjunctival injection and tearing (SUNCT), intractable

    G44.059 Short lasting unilateral neuralgiform headache with conjunctival injection and tearing (SUNCT), not intractable
        Short lasting unilateral neuralgiform headache with conjunctival injection and tearing (SUNCT) NOS

● **G44.09 Other trigeminal autonomic cephalgias (TAC)**
  Cluster headaches

    G44.091 Other trigeminal autonomic cephalgias (TAC), intractable

    G44.099 Other trigeminal autonomic cephalgias (TAC), not intractable

G44.1 Vascular headache, not elsewhere classified
  Excludes2   cluster headache (G44.0)
          complicated headache syndromes (G44.5-)
          drug-induced headache (G44.4-)
          migraine (G43.-)
          other specified headache syndromes (G44.8-)
          post-traumatic headache (G44.3-)
          tension-type headache (G44.2-)

● **G44.2 Tension-type headache**

  ● **G44.20 Tension-type headache, unspecified**
      G44.201 Tension-type headache, unspecified, intractable

      G44.209 Tension-type headache, unspecified, not intractable
          Tension headache NOS

  ● **G44.21 Episodic tension-type headache**
      G44.211 Episodic tension-type headache, intractable

      G44.219 Episodic tension-type headache, not intractable
          Episodic tension-type headache NOS

  ● **G44.22 Chronic tension-type headache**
      G44.221 Chronic tension-type headache, intractable

      G44.229 Chronic tension-type headache, not intractable
          Chronic tension-type headache NOS

CHAPTER 6 (G00-G99)

N Newborn Age: 0   **P** Pediatric Age: 0–17   **M** Maternity DX: 12–55   **A** Adult Age: 15–124   ♀ Females Only   ♂ Males Only

   Complication\Comorbidity   Major C\C   (Ex) CC/MCC Exclusions   Hospital-Acquired Condition

795

● **G44.3   Post-traumatic headache**

  ● **G44.30   Post-traumatic headache, unspecified**

    G44.301   Post-traumatic headache, unspecified, intractable

    G44.309   Post-traumatic headache, unspecified, not intractable
        Post-traumatic headache NOS

  ● **G44.31   Acute post-traumatic headache**

    G44.311   Acute post-traumatic headache, intractable

    G44.319   Acute post-traumatic headache, not intractable
        Acute post-traumatic headache NOS

  ● **G44.32   Chronic post-traumatic headache**

    G44.321   Chronic post-traumatic headache, intractable

    G44.329   Chronic post-traumatic headache, not intractable
        Chronic post-traumatic headache NOS

● **G44.4   Drug-induced headache, not elsewhere classified**
    Medication overuse headache

    Use additional code for adverse effect, if applicable, to identify drug (T36-T50 with fifth or sixth character 5)

    G44.40   Drug-induced headache, not elsewhere classified, not intractable

    G44.41   Drug-induced headache, not elsewhere classified, intractable

● **G44.5   Complicated headache syndromes**

    G44.51   Hemicrania continua
        Persistent unilateral headache

    G44.52   New daily persistent headache (NDPH)

    G44.53   Primary thunderclap headache

    G44.59   Other complicated headache syndrome

● **G44.8   Other specified headache syndromes**

    G44.81   Hypnic headache
        Benign primary headaches

    G44.82   Headache associated with sexual activity
        Orgasmic headache
        Preorgasmic headache

    G44.83   Primary cough headache

    G44.84   Primary exertional headache

    G44.85   Primary stabbing headache

    G44.89   Other headache syndrome

● **G45   Transient cerebral ischemic attacks and related syndromes**

    Excludes1   neonatal cerebral ischemia (P91.0)
        transient retinal artery occlusion (H34.0-)

    (Ex:) **For category G45 CC codes unless otherwise indicated:** See PDX Collection 586

    G45.0   Vertebro-basilar artery syndrome 🔊

    G45.1   Carotid artery syndrome (hemispheric) 🔊

    G45.2   Multiple and bilateral precerebral artery syndromes 🔊

    G45.3   Amaurosis fugax 🔊
        Transient visual loss in one eye
        (Ex:) See PDX Collection 587

    G45.4   Transient global amnesia
        Episode of short-term memory loss, nonrecurrent, lasting few hours

        Excludes1   amnesia NOS (R41.3)

    G45.8   Other transient cerebral ischemic attacks and related syndromes 🔊

    G45.9   Transient cerebral ischemic attack, unspecified 🔊
        Spasm of cerebral artery
        TIA
        Transient cerebral ischemia NOS

● **G46   Vascular syndromes of brain in cerebrovascular diseases**
    Code first underlying cerebrovascular disease (I60-I69)

    G46.0   Middle cerebral artery syndrome 🔊
        (Ex:) See PDX Collection 586

    G46.1   Anterior cerebral artery syndrome 🔊
        (Ex:) See PDX Collection 586

    G46.2   Posterior cerebral artery syndrome 🔊
        (Ex:) See PDX Collection 586

    G46.3   Brain stem stroke syndrome
        Benedikt syndrome
        Claude syndrome
        Foville syndrome
        Millard-Gubler syndrome
        Wallenberg syndrome
        Weber syndrome

    G46.4   Cerebellar stroke syndrome

    G46.5   Pure motor lacunar syndrome
        Occlusion of single deep penetrating artery

    G46.6   Pure sensory lacunar syndrome

    G46.7   Other lacunar syndromes

    G46.8   Other vascular syndromes of brain in cerebrovascular diseases

● **G47   Sleep disorders**

    Excludes2   nightmares (F51.5)
        nonorganic sleep disorders (F51.-)
        sleep terrors (F51.4)
        sleepwalking (F51.3)

  ● **G47.0   Insomnia**

    Excludes2   alcohol related insomnia (F10.182, F10.282, F10.982)
        drug-related insomnia (F11.182, F11.282, F11.982, F13.182, F13.282, F13.982, F14.182, F14.282, F14.982, F15.182, F15.282, F15.982, F19.182, F19.282, F19.982)
        idiopathic insomnia (F51.01)
        insomnia due to a mental disorder (F51.05)
        insomnia not due to a substance or known physiological condition (F51.0-)
        nonorganic insomnia (F51.0-)
        primary insomnia (F51.01)
        sleep apnea (G47.3-)

    G47.00   Insomnia, unspecified
        Insomnia NOS

    G47.01   Insomnia due to medical condition
        Code also associated medical condition

    G47.09   Other insomnia

  ● **G47.1   Hypersomnia**

    Excludes2   alcohol-related hypersomnia (F10.182, F10.282, F10.982)
        drug-related hypersomnia (F11.182, F11.282, F11.982, F13.182, F13.282, F13.982, F14.182, F14.282, F14.982, F15.182, F15.282, F15.982, F19.182, F19.282, F19.982)
        hypersomnia due to a mental disorder (F51.13)
        hypersomnia not due to a substance or known physiological condition (F51.1-)
        primary hypersomnia (F51.11)
        sleep apnea (G47.3-)

    G47.10   Hypersomnia, unspecified
        Hypersomnia NOS

    G47.11   Idiopathic hypersomnia with long sleep time
        Idiopathic hypersomnia NOS

    G47.12   Idiopathic hypersomnia without long sleep time

    G47.13   Recurrent hypersomnia
        Kleine-Levin syndrome
        Menstrual related hypersomnia

▶ New   ⇒ Revised   ~~deleted~~ Deleted   Excludes 1   Excludes 2   Includes   Use additional   Code first   Code also   Key words

796   OGCR Official Guidelines   ● Unacceptable Principal Diagnosis   X Assign placeholder X   ● Use Additional Character(s)   ▷ Manifestation Code   **Coding Clinic**

G47.14   **Hypersomnia due to medical condition**
> Code also associated medical condition

G47.19   **Other hypersomnia**

● G47.2   **Circadian rhythm sleep disorders**
> Disorders of the sleep wake schedule
> Inversion of nyctohemeral rhythm
> Inversion of sleep rhythm

G47.20   **Circadian rhythm sleep disorder, unspecified type**
> Sleep wake schedule disorder NOS

G47.21   **Circadian rhythm sleep disorder, delayed sleep phase type**
> Delayed sleep phase syndrome

G47.22   **Circadian rhythm sleep disorder, advanced sleep phase type**

G47.23   **Circadian rhythm sleep disorder, irregular sleep wake type**
> Irregular sleep-wake pattern

G47.24   **Circadian rhythm sleep disorder, free running type**
> ▶Circadian rhythm sleep disorder, non-24-hour sleep-wake type

G47.25   **Circadian rhythm sleep disorder, jet lag type**

G47.26   **Circadian rhythm sleep disorder, shift work type**

▷ *G47.27*   *Circadian rhythm sleep disorder in conditions classified elsewhere*
> *Code first underlying condition*

G47.29   **Other circadian rhythm sleep disorder**

● G47.3   **Sleep apnea**
> *Characterized by episodes in which breathing stops during sleep*
> Code also any associated underlying condition
> **Excludes1**   apnea NOS (R06.81)
>   Cheyne-Stokes breathing (R06.3)
>   pickwickian syndrome (E66.2)
>   sleep apnea of newborn (P28.3)

G47.30   **Sleep apnea, unspecified**
> Sleep apnea NOS

G47.31   **Primary central sleep apnea**
> ▶Idiopathic central sleep apnea

G47.32   **High altitude periodic breathing**

G47.33   **Obstructive sleep apnea (adult) (pediatric)**
> ▶Obstructive sleep apnea hypopnea
>> **Excludes1**   obstructive sleep apnea of newborn (P28.3)

G47.34   **Idiopathic sleep related nonobstructive alveolar hypoventilation**
> Sleep related hypoxia

G47.35   **Congenital central alveolar hypoventilation syndrome**

▷ *G47.36*   *Sleep related hypoventilation in conditions classified elsewhere*
> Sleep related hypoxemia in conditions classified elsewhere
> *Code first underlying condition*

▷ *G47.37*   *Central sleep apnea in conditions classified elsewhere*
> *Code first underlying condition*

G47.39   **Other sleep apnea**

● G47.4   **Narcolepsy and cataplexy**
> *Cataplexy is a disorder evidenced by seizures including minor slacking of the facial muscles to complete collapse and often affects people who have* **narcolepsy***, a disorder in which there is great difficulty remaining awake during the daytime.*

● G47.41   **Narcolepsy**
> G47.411   **Narcolepsy with cataplexy**
> G47.419   **Narcolepsy without cataplexy**
>> Narcolepsy NOS

● G47.42   **Narcolepsy in conditions classified elsewhere**
> *Code first underlying condition*
> ▷ *G47.421*   *Narcolepsy in conditions classified elsewhere with cataplexy*
> ▷ *G47.429*   *Narcolepsy in conditions classified elsewhere without cataplexy*

● G47.5   **Parasomnia**
> **Excludes1**   alcohol induced parasomnia (F10.182, F10.282, F10.982)
>   drug induced parasomnia (F11.182, F11.282, F11.982, F13.182, F13.282, F13.982, F14.182, F14.282, F14.982, F15.182, F15.282, F15.982, F19.182, F19.282, F19.982)
>   parasomnia not due to a substance or known physiological condition (F51.8)

G47.50   **Parasomnia, unspecified**
> Parasomnia NOS

G47.51   **Confusional arousals**

G47.52   **REM sleep behavior disorder**

G47.53   **Recurrent isolated sleep paralysis**

▷ *G47.54*   *Parasomnia in conditions classified elsewhere*
> *Code first underlying condition*

G47.59   **Other parasomnia**

● G47.6   **Sleep related movement disorders**
> **Excludes2**   restless legs syndrome (G25.81)

G47.61   **Periodic limb movement disorder**
> ~~Periodic limb movement disorder~~

G47.62   **Sleep related leg cramps**

G47.63   **Sleep related bruxism**
> **Excludes1**   psychogenic bruxism (F45.8)
> **Coding Clinic: 2016, Q4, P118**

G47.69   **Other sleep related movement disorders**

● G47.8   **Other sleep disorders**
> ▶Other specified sleep-wake disorder

G47.9   **Sleep disorder, unspecified**
> Sleep disorder NOS
> ▶Unspecified sleep-wake disorder

★ **(See Plate 118 on page 54.)**

NERVE, NERVE ROOT AND PLEXUS DISORDERS (G50-G59)

> **Excludes1**   current traumatic nerve, nerve root and plexus disorders - see Injury, nerve by body region
>   neuralgia NOS (M79.2)
>   neuritis NOS (M79.2)
>   peripheral neuritis in pregnancy (O26.82-)
>   radiculitis NOS (M54.1-)

● G50   **Disorders of trigeminal nerve**
> **Includes**   disorders of 5th cranial nerve

G50.0   **Trigeminal neuralgia**
> Syndrome of paroxysmal facial pain
> Tic douloureux

G50.1   **Atypical facial pain**

G50.8   **Other disorders of trigeminal nerve**

G50.9   **Disorder of trigeminal nerve, unspecified**

Item 6–5   Trigeminal neuralgia, tic douloureux, is a pain syndrome diagnosed from the patient's history alone. The condition is characterized by pain and a brief facial spasm or tic. Pain is unilateral and follows the sensory distribution of cranial nerve V, typically radiating to the maxillary (V2) or mandibular (V3) area.

CHAPTER 6 (G00-G99)

N Newborn Age: 0   **P** Pediatric Age: 0–17   **M** Maternity DX: 12–55   **A** Adult Age: 15–124   ♀ Females Only   ♂ Males Only

Complication\Comorbidity   Major C\C   (Ex) CC/MCC Exclusions   Hospital-Acquired Condition

797

Item 6-6 The most common facial nerve disorder is **Bell's Palsy,** which occurs suddenly and results in facial drooping unilaterally. This disorder is the result of a reaction to a virus that causes the facial nerve in the ear to swell resulting in pressure in the bony canal.

● **G51**   **Facial nerve disorders**

     Includes   disorders of 7th cranial nerve

     G51.0   **Bell's palsy**
           Facial palsy

     G51.1   **Geniculate ganglionitis**
           Rare disorder with symptoms of severe pain deep in ear,
              spreading to ear canal, outer ear, mastoid or eye regions

           Excludes1   postherpetic geniculate ganglionitis
                          (B02.21)

     G51.2   **Melkersson's syndrome**
           Melkersson-Rosenthal syndrome

     G51.3   **Clonic hemifacial spasm**

     G51.4   **Facial myokymia**
           Involuntary facial muscle movement

     G51.8   **Other disorders of facial nerve**

     G51.9   **Disorder of facial nerve, unspecified**

● **G52**   **Disorders of other cranial nerves**

     Excludes2   disorders of acoustic [8th] nerve (H93.3)
                  disorders of optic [2nd] nerve (H46, H47.0)
                  paralytic strabismus due to nerve palsy
                     (H49.0-H49.2)

     G52.0   **Disorders of olfactory nerve**
           Disorders of 1st cranial nerve

     G52.1   **Disorders of glossopharyngeal nerve**
           Disorder of 9th cranial nerve
           Glossopharyngeal neuralgia

     G52.2   **Disorders of vagus nerve**
           Disorders of pneumogastric [10th] nerve

     G52.3   **Disorders of hypoglossal nerve**
           Disorders of 12th cranial nerve

     G52.7   **Disorders of multiple cranial nerves**
           Polyneuritis cranialis

     G52.8   **Disorders of other specified cranial nerves**

     G52.9   **Cranial nerve disorder, unspecified**

▶ *G53*   *Cranial nerve disorders in diseases classified elsewhere*

     Code first underlying disease, such as:
          neoplasm (C00-D49)

     Excludes1   multiple cranial nerve palsy in sarcoidosis
                   (D86.82)
                  multiple cranial nerve palsy in syphilis (A52.15)
                  postherpetic geniculate ganglionitis (B02.21)
                  postherpetic trigeminal neuralgia (B02.22)

● **G54**   **Nerve root and plexus disorders**

     Raiculopathy (nerve root disorder) caused by pressure on nerve root,
        most common cause is herniation of intervertebral disk. Plexus
        disorders (plexopathies) are due to compression or injury.

     Excludes1   current traumatic nerve root and plexus disorders
                   - see nerve injury by body region
                  intervertebral disc disorders (M50-M51)
                  neuralgia or neuritis NOS (M79.2)
                  neuritis or radiculitis brachial NOS (M54.13)
                  neuritis or radiculitis lumbar NOS (M54.16)
                  neuritis or radiculitis lumbosacral NOS (M54.17)
                  neuritis or radiculitis thoracic NOS (M54.14)
                  radiculitis NOS (M54.10)
                  radiculopathy NOS (M54.10)
                  spondylosis (M47.-)

     G54.0   **Brachial plexus disorders**
           Thoracic outlet syndrome

     G54.1   **Lumbosacral plexus disorders**

     G54.2   **Cervical root disorders, not elsewhere classified**

● **G54.3**   **Thoracic root disorders, not elsewhere classified**

     G54.4   **Lumbosacral root disorders, not elsewhere classified**

     G54.5   **Neuralgic amyotrophy**
           Parsonage-Aldren-Turner syndrome
           Shoulder-girdle neuritis

           Excludes1   neuralgic amyotrophy in diabetes
                          mellitus (E08-E13 with .44)

     G54.6   **Phantom limb syndrome with pain**
           Sensations (cramping, itching) in a limb that no longer
              exists

     G54.7   **Phantom limb syndrome without pain**
           Phantom limb syndrome NOS

     G54.8   **Other nerve root and plexus disorders**

     G54.9   **Nerve root and plexus disorder, unspecified**

▶ *G55*   *Nerve root and plexus compressions in diseases classified elsewhere*

     Code first underlying disease, such as:
          neoplasm (C00-D49)

     Excludes1   nerve root compression (due to) (in) ankylosing
                   spondylitis (M45.-)
                  nerve root compression (due to) (in)dorsopathies
                  (M53.-, M54.-)
                  nerve root compression (due to) (in)intervertebral
                  disc disorders (M50.1.-, M51.1.-)
                  nerve root compression (due to) (in)
                  spondylopathies (M46.-, M48.-)

★ **(See Plates 472 and 473 on pages 56 and 57.)**

● **G56**   **Mononeuropathies of upper limb**

     Excludes1   current traumatic nerve disorder - see nerve
                   injury by body region

   ● **G56.0**   **Carpal tunnel syndrome**

         G56.00   **Carpal tunnel syndrome, unspecified upper**
                  limb

         G56.01   **Carpal tunnel syndrome, right upper limb**

         G56.02   **Carpal tunnel syndrome, left upper limb**

         G56.03   **Carpal tunnel syndrome, bilateral upper**
                  limbs
                  Coding Clinic: 2016, Q4, P17

   ● **G56.1**   **Other lesions of median nerve**

         G56.10   **Other lesions of median nerve, unspecified side**

         G56.11   **Other lesions of median nerve, right upper limb**

         G56.12   **Other lesions of median nerve, left upper limb**

         G56.13   **Other lesions of median nerve, bilateral upper**
                  limbs
                  Coding Clinic: 2016, Q4, P17

   ● **G56.2**   **Lesion of ulnar nerve**
              Tardy ulnar nerve palsy

         G56.20   **Lesion of ulnar nerve, unspecified upper limb**

         G56.21   **Lesion of ulnar nerve, right upper limb**

         G56.22   **Lesion of ulnar nerve, left upper limb**

         G56.23   **Lesion of ulnar nerve, bilateral upper limbs**
                  Coding Clinic: 2016, Q4, P17

   ● **G56.3**   **Lesion of radial nerve**

         G56.30   **Lesion of radial nerve, unspecified upper limb**

         G56.31   **Lesion of radial nerve, right upper limb**

         G56.32   **Lesion of radial nerve, left upper limb**

         G56.33   **Lesion of radial nerve, bilateral upper limbs**
                  Coding Clinic: 2016, Q4, P17

▶ New   ⇒ Revised   ~~deleted~~ Deleted   Excludes 1   Excludes 2   Includes   Use additional   Code first   Code also   Key words

OGCR Official Guidelines   ● Unacceptable Principal Diagnosis   X Assign placeholder X   ● Use Additional Character(s)   ▶ Manifestation Code   **Coding Clinic**

G56.4 Causalgia of upper limb
　　　　Intense burning pain and sensitivity to slight touch
　　　　Complex regional pain syndrome II of upper limb
　　　　　Excludes1　complex regional pain syndrome I of
　　　　　　　　　　　lower limb (G90.52-)
　　　　　　　　　　complex regional pain syndrome I of
　　　　　　　　　　　upper limb (G90.51-)
　　　　　　　　　　complex regional pain syndrome II of
　　　　　　　　　　　lower limb (G57.7-)
　　　　　　　　　　reflex sympathetic dystrophy of lower
　　　　　　　　　　　limb (G90.52-)
　　　　　　　　　　reflex sympathetic dystrophy (G90.51-)
　　　G56.40　Causalgia of unspecified upper limb
　　　G56.41　Causalgia of right upper limb
　　　G56.42　Causalgia of left upper limb
　　　G56.43　Causalgia of bilateral upper limbs
　　　　　　　Coding Clinic: 2016, Q4, P17

G56.8 Other specified mononeuropathies of upper limb
　　　　Disease of a single nerve
　　　　Interdigital neuroma of upper limb
　　　G56.80　Other specified mononeuropathies
　　　　　　　of unspecified upper limb
　　　G56.81　Other specified mononeuropathies of right
　　　　　　　upper limb
　　　G56.82　Other specified mononeuropathies of left upper
　　　　　　　limb
　　　G56.83　Other specified mononeuropathies of bilateral
　　　　　　　upper limbs
　　　　　　　Coding Clinic: 2016, Q4, P17

G56.9 Unspecified mononeuropathy of upper limb
　　　　Disease of a single nerve
　　　G56.90　Unspecified mononeuropathy of unspecified
　　　　　　　upper limb
　　　G56.91　Unspecified mononeuropathy of right upper
　　　　　　　limb
　　　G56.92　Unspecified mononeuropathy of left upper limb
　　　G56.93　Unspecified mononeuropathy of bilateral upper
　　　　　　　limbs
　　　　　　　Coding Clinic: 2016, Q4, P17

G57 Mononeuropathies of lower limb
　　　　　Excludes1　current traumatic nerve disorder - see nerve
　　　　　　　　　　injury by body region

★**(See Plates 544 and 545 on pages 58 and 59.)**

G57.0 Lesion of sciatic nerve
　　　　　Excludes1　sciatica NOS (M54.3-)
　　　　　Excludes2　sciatica attributed to intervertebral disc
　　　　　　　　　　disorder (M51.1.-)
　　　G57.00　Lesion of sciatic nerve, unspecified lower limb
　　　G57.01　Lesion of sciatic nerve, right lower limb
　　　G57.02　Lesion of sciatic nerve, left lower limb
　　　G57.03　Lesion of sciatic nerve, bilateral lower limbs
　　　　　　　Coding Clinic: 2016, Q4, P1

G57.1 Meralgia paresthetica
　　　　Numbness or pain in outer thigh caused by injury to nerve
　　　　Lateral cutaneous nerve of thigh syndrome
　　　G57.10　Meralgia paresthetica, unspecified lower limb
　　　G57.11　Meralgia paresthetica, right lower limb
　　　G57.12　Meralgia paresthetica, left lower limb
　　　G57.13　Meralgia paresthetica, bilateral lower limbs
　　　　　　　Coding Clinic: 2016, Q4, P1

G57.2 Lesion of femoral nerve
　　　G57.20　Lesion of femoral nerve, unspecified lower limb
　　　G57.21　Lesion of femoral nerve, right lower limb
　　　G57.22　Lesion of femoral nerve, left lower limb
　　　G57.23　Lesion of femoral nerve, bilateral lower limbs
　　　　　　　Coding Clinic: 2016, Q4, P1

G57.3 Lesion of lateral popliteal nerve
　　　　Peroneal nerve palsy
　　　G57.30　Lesion of lateral popliteal nerve, unspecified
　　　　　　　lower limb
　　　G57.31　Lesion of lateral popliteal nerve, right lower limb
　　　G57.32　Lesion of lateral popliteal nerve, left lower limb
　　　G57.33　Lesion of lateral popliteal nerve, bilateral lower
　　　　　　　limbs
　　　　　　　Coding Clinic: 2016, Q4, P1

G57.4 Lesion of medial popliteal nerve
　　　G57.40　Lesion of medial popliteal nerve, unspecified
　　　　　　　lower limb
　　　G57.41　Lesion of medial popliteal nerve, right lower
　　　　　　　limb
　　　G57.42　Lesion of medial popliteal nerve, left lower limb
　　　G57.43　Lesion of medial popliteal nerve, bilateral
　　　　　　　lower limbs
　　　　　　　Coding Clinic: 2016, Q4, P1

G57.5 Tarsal tunnel syndrome
　　　G57.50　Tarsal tunnel syndrome, unspecified lower limb
　　　G57.51　Tarsal tunnel syndrome, right lower limb
　　　G57.52　Tarsal tunnel syndrome, left lower limb
　　　G57.53　Tarsal tunnel syndrome, bilateral lower limbs
　　　　　　　Coding Clinic: 2016, Q4, P1

G57.6 Lesion of plantar nerve
　　　　Morton's metatarsalgia
　　　G57.60　Lesion of plantar nerve, unspecified lower limb
　　　G57.61　Lesion of plantar nerve, right lower limb
　　　G57.62　Lesion of plantar nerve, left lower limb
　　　G57.63　Lesion of plantar nerve, bilateral lower limbs
　　　　　　　Coding Clinic: 2016, Q4, P1

G57.7 Causalgia of lower limb
　　　　Complex regional pain syndrome II of lower limb
　　　　　Excludes1　complex regional pain syndrome I of
　　　　　　　　　　lower limb (G90.52-)
　　　　　　　　　　complex regional pain syndrome I of
　　　　　　　　　　　upper limb (G90.51-)
　　　　　　　　　　complex regional pain syndrome II of
　　　　　　　　　　　upper limb (G56.4-)
　　　　　　　　　　reflex sympathetic dystrophy of lower
　　　　　　　　　　　limb (G90.52-)
　　　　　　　　　　reflex sympathetic dystrophy of upper
　　　　　　　　　　　limb (G90.51-)
　　　G57.70　Causalgia of unspecified lower limb
　　　G57.71　Causalgia of right lower limb
　　　G57.72　Causalgia of left lower limb
　　　G57.73　Causalgia of bilateral lower limbs
　　　　　　　Coding Clinic: 2016, Q4, P1

G57.8 Other specified mononeuropathies of lower limb
　　　　Interdigital neuroma of lower limb
　　　G57.80　Other specified mononeuropathies
　　　　　　　of unspecified lower limb
　　　G57.81　Other specified mononeuropathies of right
　　　　　　　lower limb
　　　G57.82　Other specified mononeuropathies of left lower
　　　　　　　limb
　　　G57.83　Other specified mononeuropathies of bilateral
　　　　　　　lower limbs
　　　　　　　Coding Clinic: 2016, Q4, P17

G57.9 Unspecified mononeuropathy of lower limb
　　　G57.90　Unspecified mononeuropathy of unspecified
　　　　　　　lower limb
　　　G57.91　Unspecified mononeuropathy of right lower limb
　　　G57.92　Unspecified mononeuropathy of left lower limb
　　　G57.93　Unspecified mononeuropathy of bilateral lower
　　　　　　　limbs
　　　　　　　Coding Clinic: 2016, Q4, P17

CHAPTER 6 (G00-G99)

CHAPTER 6 (GØØ-G99)

● **G58   Other mononeuropathies**
     G58.0   Intercostal neuropathy
     G58.7   Mononeuritis multiplex
     G58.8   Other specified mononeuropathies
     G58.9   Mononeuropathy, unspecified

▌ **G59   Mononeuropathy in diseases classified elsewhere**
     Code first underlying disease
     Excludes1   diabetic mononeuropathy (E08-E13 with .41)
                    syphilitic nerve paralysis (A52.19)
                    syphilitic neuritis (A52.15)
                    tuberculous mononeuropathy (A17.83)

**POLYNEUROPATHIES AND OTHER DISORDERS OF
THE PERIPHERAL NERVOUS SYSTEM (G60-G65)**

     Excludes1   neuralgia NOS (M79.2)
                    neuritis NOS (M79.2)
                    peripheral neuritis in pregnancy (O26.82-)
                    radiculitis NOS (M54.10)

● **G60   Hereditary and idiopathic neuropathy**
     G60.0   Hereditary motor and sensory neuropathy
          Charcot-Marie-Tooth disease
          Déjerine-Sottas disease
          Hereditary motor and sensory neuropathy, types I-IV
          Hypertrophic neuropathy of infancy
          Peroneal muscular atrophy (axonal type) (hypertrophic
             type)
          Roussy-Lévy syndrome
     G60.1   Refsum's disease 🔖
          Genetic disorder affecting fatty acid metabolism
          Infantile Refsum disease
          (Ex.) See PDX Collection 588
     G60.2   Neuropathy in association with hereditary ataxia
     G60.3   Idiopathic progressive neuropathy
     G60.8   Other hereditary and idiopathic neuropathies
          Dominantly inherited sensory neuropathy
          Morvan's disease
          Nelaton's syndrome
          Recessively inherited sensory neuropathy
     G60.9   Hereditary and idiopathic neuropathy, unspecified

Item 6-7 The **peripheral nervous system** consists of 31 pairs of spinal nerves, 12 pairs of cranial nerves, and the autonomic nerves, which are divided into the parasympathetic and sympathetic nerves. The cranial nerves are: olfactory (I), optic (II), oculomotor (III), trochlear (IV), trigeminal (V), abducens (VI), facial (VII), vestibulocochlear (VIII), glossopharyngeal (IX), vagus (X), accessory (XI), and hypoglossal (XII).

● **G61   Inflammatory polyneuropathy**
     G61.0   Guillain-Barré syndrome 🔖
          Autoimmune disease affecting peripheral nervous system
          Acute (post-)infective polyneuritis
          Miller Fisher Syndrome
          (Ex.) See PDX Collection 92
     G61.1   Serum neuropathy
          Use additional code for adverse effect, if applicable, to
             identify serum (T50.-)
● **G61.8   Other inflammatory polyneuropathies**
          **G61.81   Chronic inflammatory demyelinating
                      polyneuritis** 🔖
                 (Ex.) See PDX Collection 589
          G61.82   Multifocal motor neuropathy
                 MMN
          G61.89   Other inflammatory polyneuropathies
     G61.9   Inflammatory polyneuropathy, unspecified

● **G62   Other and unspecified polyneuropathies**
     G62.0   Drug-induced polyneuropathy
          Use additional code for adverse effect, if applicable,
             to identify drug (T36-T50 with fifth or sixth
             character 5)
     G62.1   Alcoholic polyneuropathy
          Malfunction of many peripheral nerves throughout the body
     G62.2   Polyneuropathy due to other toxic agents
          Code first (T51-T65) to identify toxic agent

Figure 6-2 Actions of parasympathetic and sympathetic nerves. (From Chabner: The Language of Medicine, ed 9, St. Louis, Saunders, 2011)

▶ New   ⇒ Revised   d̶e̶l̶e̶t̶e̶d̶ Deleted   Excludes 1   Excludes 2   Includes   Use additional   Code first   Code also   Key words
OGCR Official Guidelines   ● Unacceptable Principal Diagnosis   X Assign placeholder X   ● Use Additional Character(s)   ▌ Manifestation Code   **Coding Clinic**

● **G62.8 Other specified polyneuropathies**

  G62.81 Critical illness polyneuropathy 🔹
     Acute motor neuropathy
     (Ex) See PDX Collection 590

  G62.82 Radiation-induced polyneuropathy
     Use additional external cause code (W88-W90, X39.0-) to identify cause
     Coding Clinic: 2016, Q4, P18

  G62.89 Other specified polyneuropathies
     Coding Clinic: 2016, Q2, P11

G62.9 Polyneuropathy, unspecified
  Neuropathy NOS

▸ *G63* *Polyneuropathy in diseases classified elsewhere*

  Code first underlying disease, such as:
    amyloidosis (E85.-)
    endocrine disease, except diabetes (E00-E07, E15-E16, E20-E34)
    metabolic diseases (E70-E88)
    neoplasm (C00-D49)
    nutritional deficiency (E40-E64)

  Excludes1 polyneuropathy (in):
      diabetes mellitus (E08-E13 with .42)
      diphtheria (A36.83)
      infectious mononucleosis (B27.0-B27.9 with 1)
      Lyme disease (A69.22)
      mumps (B26.84)
      postherpetic (B02.23)
      rheumatoid arthritis (M05.33)
      scleroderma (M34.83)
      systemic lupus erythematosus (M32.19)
  Coding Clinic: 2012, Q4, P100

G64 Other disorders of peripheral nervous system
  Disorder of peripheral nervous system NOS

● **G65 Sequelae of inflammatory and toxic polyneuropathies**

  Code first condition resulting from (sequela) of inflammatory and toxic polyneuropathies

  G65.0 Sequelae of Guillain-Barré syndrome

  G65.1 Sequelae of other inflammatory polyneuropathy

  G65.2 Sequelae of toxic polyneuropathy

DISEASES OF MYONEURAL JUNCTION AND MUSCLE (G70-G73)

● **G70 Myasthenia gravis and other myoneural disorders**
  Excludes1 botulism (A05.1, A48.51-A48.52)
      transient neonatal myasthenia gravis (P94.0)

● **G70.0 Myasthenia gravis**
  Acquired and results in fatigable muscle weakness exacerbated by activity and improved with rest

  G70.00 Myasthenia gravis without (acute) exacerbation
     Myasthenia gravis NOS

  G70.01 Myasthenia gravis with (acute) exacerbation 🔹
     Myasthenia gravis in crisis
     (Ex) See PDX Collection 591

G70.1 Toxic myoneural disorders
  Dysfunction at junction of muscle and motor nerve (myoneural junction)
  Code first (T51-T65) to identify toxic agent

G70.2 Congenital and developmental myasthenia

● **G70.8 Other specified myoneural disorders**

  G70.80 Lambert-Eaton syndrome, unspecified 🔹
     Lambert-Eaton syndrome NOS
     (Ex) See PDX Collection 591

▸ *G70.81* *Lambert-Eaton syndrome in disease classified elsewhere* 🔹

    Code first underlying disease
    Excludes1 Lambert-Eaton syndrome in neoplastic disease (G73.1)
    (Ex) See PDX Collection 591

  G70.89 Other specified myoneural disorders

G70.9 Myoneural disorder, unspecified

● **G71 Primary disorders of muscles**
  Excludes2 arthrogryposis multiplex congenita (Q74.3)
      metabolic disorders (E70-E88)
      myositis (M60.-)

G71.0 Muscular dystrophy 🔹
  Autosomal recessive, childhood type, muscular dystrophy resembling Duchenne or Becker muscular dystrophy
  Benign [Becker] muscular dystrophy
  Benign scapuloperoneal muscular dystrophy with early contractures [Emery-Dreifuss]
  Congenital muscular dystrophy NOS
  Congenital muscular dystrophy with specific morphological abnormalities of the muscle fiber
  Distal muscular dystrophy
  Facioscapulohumeral muscular dystrophy
  Limb-girdle muscular dystrophy
  Ocular muscular dystrophy
  Oculopharyngeal muscular dystrophy
  Scapuloperoneal muscular dystrophy
  Severe [Duchenne] muscular dystrophy
  (Ex) See PDX Collection 592

● **G71.1 Myotonic disorders**
  Inherited disorder that affects muscles tone

  G71.11 Myotonic muscular dystrophy
     Dystrophia myotonica [Steinert]
     Myotonia atrophica
     Myotonic dystrophy
     Proximal myotonic myopathy (PROMM)
     Steinert disease

  G71.12 Myotonia congenita
     Acetazolamide responsive myotonia congenita
     Dominant myotonia congenita [Thomsen disease]
     Myotonia levior
     Recessive myotonia congenita [Becker disease]

  G71.13 Myotonic chondrodystrophy
     Chondrodystrophic myotonia
     Congenital myotonic chondrodystrophy
     Schwartz-Jampel disease

  G71.14 Drug induced myotonia
     Use additional code for adverse effect, if applicable, to identify drug (T36-T50 with fifth or sixth character 5)

  G71.19 Other specified myotonic disorders
     Myotonia fluctuans
     Myotonia permanens
     Neuromyotonia [Isaacs]
     Paramyotonia congenita (of von Eulenburg)
     Pseudomyotonia
     Symptomatic myotonia

G71.2 Congenital myopathies 🔹
  Central core disease
  Fiber-type disproportion
  Minicore disease
  Multicore disease
  Myotubular (centronuclear) myopathy
  Nemaline myopathy

  Excludes1 arthrogryposis multiplex congenita (Q74.3)
  (Ex) See PDX Collection 592

Item 6-8 Muscular dystrophies (MD) are a group of rare inherited muscle diseases. Voluntary muscles become progressively weaker. In the late stages of MD, fat and connective tissue replace muscle fibers. In some types of muscular dystrophy, heart muscles, other involuntary muscles, and other organs are affected. **Myopathies** is a general term for neuromuscular diseases in which the muscle fibers dysfunction for any one of many reasons, resulting in muscular weakness.

N Newborn Age: 0   **P** Pediatric Age: 0–17   **M** Maternity DX: 12–55   **A** Adult Age: 15–124   ♀ Females Only   ♂ Males Only

🔹 Complication\Comorbidity   🔹 Major C\C   (Ex) CC/MCC Exclusions   🔹 Hospital-Acquired Condition

G71.3 Mitochondrial myopathy, not elsewhere classified
Myopathies associated with increased number of enlarged, often abnormal, mitochondria in muscle fibers

> **Excludes1** Kearns-Sayre syndrome (H49.81)
> Leber's disease (H47.21)
> Leigh's encephalopathy (G31.82)
> mitochondrial metabolism disorders
> (E88.4.-)
> Reye's syndrome (G93.7)

G71.8 Other primary disorders of muscles

G71.9 Primary disorder of muscle, unspecified
Hereditary myopathy NOS

● **G72 Other and unspecified myopathies**

> **Excludes1** arthrogryposis multiplex congenita (Q74.3)
> dermatopolymyositis (M33.-)
> ischemic infarction of muscle (M62.2-)
> myositis (M60.-)
> polymyositis (M33.2.-)

G72.0 Drug-induced myopathy 🔖

Use additional code for adverse effect, if applicable, to identify drug (T36-T50 with fifth or sixth character 5)
(Ex:) See PDX Collection 593

G72.1 Alcoholic myopathy 🔖

Use additional code to identify alcoholism (F10.-)
(Ex:) See PDX Collection 593

G72.2 Myopathy due to other toxic agents 🔖

Code first (T51-T65) *to identify toxic agent*
(Ex:) See PDX Collection 593

G72.3 Periodic paralysis
Familial periodic paralysis
Hyperkalemic periodic paralysis (familial)
Hypokalemic periodic paralysis (familial)
Myotonic periodic paralysis (familial)
Normokalemic paralysis (familial)
Potassium sensitive periodic paralysis

> **Excludes1** paramyotonia congenita (of von
> Eulenburg) (G71.19)

● **G72.4 Inflammatory and immune myopathies, not elsewhere classified**

G72.41 Inclusion body myositis [IBM]

G72.49 Other inflammatory and immune myopathies, not elsewhere classified
Inflammatory myopathy NOS

● **G72.8 Other specified myopathies**

G72.81 Critical illness myopathy 🔖
Acute necrotizing myopathy
Acute quadriplegic myopathy
Intensive care (ICU) myopathy
Myopathy of critical illness
(Ex:) See PDX Collection 594

G72.89 Other specified myopathies

G72.9 Myopathy, unspecified

● **G73 Disorders of myoneural junction and muscle in diseases classified elsewhere**
(Ex:) For category G73 CC codes: See PDX Collection 591

●▸ **G73.1 Lambert-Eaton syndrome in neoplastic disease** 🔖
Rare autoimmune disorder affecting calcium channels of nerve-muscle (neuromuscular) junction

Code first underlying neoplasm (C00-D49)

> **Excludes1** Lambert-Eaton syndrome not associated
> with neoplasm (G70.80-G70.81)

▸ **G73.3 Myasthenic syndromes in other diseases classified elsewhere** 🔖

Code first underlying disease, such as:
neoplasm (C00-D49)
thyrotoxicosis (E05.-)

▸ **G73.7 Myopathy in diseases classified elsewhere**

Code first underlying disease, such as:
hyperparathyroidism (E21.0, E21.3)
hypoparathyroidism (E20.-)
glycogen storage disease (E74.0)
lipid storage disorders (E75.-)

> **Excludes1** myopathy in:
> rheumatoid arthritis (M05.32)
> sarcoidosis (D86.87)
> scleroderma (M34.82)
> sicca syndrome [Sjögren] (M35.03)
> systemic lupus erythematosus (M32.19)

CEREBRAL PALSY AND OTHER PARALYTIC SYNDROMES (G80-G83)

● **G80 Cerebral palsy**

> **Excludes1** hereditary spastic paraplegia (G11.4)

G80.0 Spastic quadriplegic cerebral palsy 🔖
Congenital spastic paralysis (cerebral)
(Ex:) See PDX Collection 595

G80.1 Spastic diplegic cerebral palsy 🔖
Spastic cerebral palsy NOS
(Ex:) See PDX Collection 596

G80.2 Spastic hemiplegic cerebral palsy 🔖
(Ex:) See PDX Collection 597

G80.3 Athetoid cerebral palsy 🔖
Result of damage to cerebellum or basal ganglia responsible for processing neuromuscular signals
Double athetosis (syndrome)
Dyskinetic cerebral palsy
Dystonic cerebral palsy
Vogt disease
(Ex:) See PDX Collection 598

G80.4 Ataxic cerebral palsy
Poor muscle tone and coordination

G80.8 Other cerebral palsy
Mixed cerebral palsy syndromes

G80.9 Cerebral palsy, unspecified
Cerebral palsy NOS

OGCR Section I.C.6.a.

Dominant/nondominant side

Codes from category G81, Hemiplegia and hemiparesis, and subcategories, G83.1, Monoplegia of lower limb, G83.2, Monoplegia of upper limb, and G83.3, Monoplegia, unspecified, identify whether the dominant and nondominant side is affected. Should the affected side be documented, but not specified as dominant or nondominant, and the classification system does not indicate a default, code selection is as follows:

- For ambidextrous patients, the default should be dominant.
- If the left side is affected, the default is non-dominant.
- If the right side is affected, the default is dominant.

● **G81 Hemiplegia and hemiparesis**

Note: This category is to be used only when hemiplegia (complete)(incomplete) is reported without further specification, or is stated to be old or longstanding but of unspecified cause. The category is also for use in multiple coding to identify these types of hemiplegia resulting from any cause.

> **Excludes1** congenital cerebral palsy (G80.-)
> hemiplegia and hemiparesis due to sequela of
> cerebrovascular disease (I69.05-, I69.15-,
> I69.25-, I69.35-, I69.85-, I69.95-)

(Ex:) For category G81 CC codes: See PDX Collection 561
Coding Clinic: 2012, Q4, P106

● **G81.0 Flaccid hemiplegia**
Paralysis of half of body with loss of tone of muscles of paralyzed part and absence of tendon reflexes

G81.00 Flaccid hemiplegia affecting unspecified side 🔖

G81.01 Flaccid hemiplegia affecting right dominant side 🔖

Item 6–9 Hemiplegia is complete paralysis of one side of the body—arm, leg, and trunk. **Hemiparesis** is a generalized weakness or incomplete paralysis of one side of the body. If most activities (eating, writing) are performed with the right hand, the right is the dominant side, and the left is the nondominant side. **Quadriplegia,** also called tetraplegia, is the complete paralysis of all four limbs. **Quadriparesis** is the incomplete paralysis of all four limbs. Nerve damage in C1–C4 is associated with lower limb paralysis, and C5–C7 damage is associated with upper limb paralysis. **Diplegia** is the paralysis of the upper limbs. **Monoplegia** is the complete paralysis of one limb.

G81.02	**Flaccid hemiplegia affecting left dominant side** 🔖
G81.03	**Flaccid hemiplegia affecting right nondominant side** 🔖
G81.04	**Flaccid hemiplegia affecting left nondominant side** 🔖

● **G81.1 Spastic hemiplegia**
Paralysis of half of body with spasticity of muscles of paralyzed part and increased tendon reflexes

G81.10	**Spastic hemiplegia affecting unspecified side** 🔖
G81.11	**Spastic hemiplegia affecting right dominant side** 🔖
G81.12	**Spastic hemiplegia affecting left dominant side** 🔖
G81.13	**Spastic hemiplegia affecting right nondominant side** 🔖
G81.14	**Spastic hemiplegia affecting left nondominant side** 🔖

● **G81.9 Hemiplegia, unspecified**

G81.90	**Hemiplegia, unspecified affecting unspecified side** 🔖
G81.91	**Hemiplegia, unspecified affecting right dominant side** 🔖
G81.92	**Hemiplegia, unspecified affecting left dominant side** 🔖
G81.93	**Hemiplegia, unspecified affecting right nondominant side** 🔖
G81.94	**Hemiplegia, unspecified affecting left nondominant side** 🔖

Coding Clinic: 2015, Q1, P26

● **G82 Paraplegia (paraparesis) and quadriplegia (quadriparesis)**
Note: This category is to be used only when the listed conditions are reported without further specification, or are stated to be old or longstanding but of unspecified cause. The category is also for use in multiple coding to identify these conditions resulting from any cause.

> **Excludes1** congenital cerebral palsy (G80.-)
> functional quadriplegia (R53.2)
> hysterical paralysis (F44.4)

● **G82.2 Paraplegia**
Paralysis of both lower limbs NOS
Paraparesis (lower) NOS
Paraplegia (lower) NOS
(Ex) **For category G82.2 CC codes:** See PDX Collection 561

G82.20	**Paraplegia, unspecified** 🔖
G82.21	**Paraplegia, complete** 🔖
G82.22	**Paraplegia, incomplete** 🔖

● **G82.5 Quadriplegia**
Paralysis of all limbs; AKA tetraplegia
(Ex) **For category G82.5 CC codes:** See PDX Collection 595

G82.50	**Quadriplegia, unspecified** 🔖
G82.51	**Quadriplegia, C1-C4 complete** 🔖
G82.52	**Quadriplegia, C1-C4 incomplete** 🔖
G82.53	**Quadriplegia, C5-C7 complete** 🔖
G82.54	**Quadriplegia, C5-C7 incomplete** 🔖

● **G83 Other paralytic syndromes**
Note: This category is to be used only when the listed conditions are reported without further specification, or are stated to be old or longstanding but of unspecified cause. The category is also for use in multiple coding to identify these conditions resulting from any cause.

> **Includes** paralysis (complete) (incomplete), except as in G80-G82

● **G83.0 Diplegia of upper limbs** 🔖
Paralysis affecting limbs on both sides; AKA bilateral paralysis
Diplegia (upper)
Paralysis of both upper limbs
(Ex) See PDX Collection 599

● **G83.1 Monoplegia of lower limb**
Paralysis of limb on one side
Paralysis of lower limb

> **Excludes1** monoplegia of lower limbs due to sequela of cerebrovascular disease (I69.04-, I69.14-, I69.24-, I69.34-, I69.84-, I69.94-)

Coding Clinic: 2012, Q4, P106

G83.10	**Monoplegia of lower limb affecting unspecified side**
G83.11	**Monoplegia of lower limb affecting right dominant side**
G83.12	**Monoplegia of lower limb affecting left dominant side**
G83.13	**Monoplegia of lower limb affecting right nondominant side**
G83.14	**Monoplegia of lower limb affecting left nondominant side**

● **G83.2 Monoplegia of upper limb**
Paralysis of upper limb

> **Excludes1** monoplegia of upper limbs due to sequela of cerebrovascular disease (I69.03-, I69.13-, I69.23-, I69.33-, I69.83-, I69.93-)

Coding Clinic: 2012, Q4, P106

G83.20	**Monoplegia of upper limb affecting unspecified side**
G83.21	**Monoplegia of upper limb affecting right dominant side**
G83.22	**Monoplegia of upper limb affecting left dominant side**
G83.23	**Monoplegia of upper limb affecting right nondominant side**
G83.24	**Monoplegia of upper limb affecting left nondominant side**

● **G83.3 Monoplegia, unspecified**
Coding Clinic: 2012, Q4, P106

G83.30	**Monoplegia, unspecified affecting unspecified side**
G83.31	**Monoplegia, unspecified affecting right dominant side**
G83.32	**Monoplegia, unspecified affecting left dominant side**
G83.33	**Monoplegia, unspecified affecting right nondominant side**
G83.34	**Monoplegia, unspecified affecting left nondominant side**

● **G83.4 Cauda equina syndrome** 🔖
Aching pain due to compression of spinal nerve roots
Neurogenic bladder due to cauda equina syndrome

> **Excludes1** cord bladder NOS (G95.89)
> neurogenic bladder NOS (N31.9)
> (Ex) See PDX Collection 600

● **G83.5 Locked-in state** 🔖
(Ex) See PDX Collection 601

CHAPTER 6 (G00-G99)

N Newborn Age: 0   P Pediatric Age: 0–17   M Maternity DX: 12–55   A Adult Age: 15–124   ♀ Females Only   ♂ Males Only
🔖 Complication\Comorbidity   🔖 Major C\C   (Ex) CC/MCC Exclusions   🔖 Hospital-Acquired Condition

803

CHAPTER 6 (G00-G99)

● **G83.8   Other specified paralytic syndromes**

    Excludes1   paralytic syndromes due to current spinal
                    cord injury-code to spinal cord
                    injury (S14, S24, S34)

      G83.81   Brown-Séquard syndrome

      G83.82   Anterior cord syndrome

      G83.83   Posterior cord syndrome

      G83.84   Todd's paralysis (postepileptic)

      G83.89   Other specified paralytic syndromes

    G83.9   Paralytic syndrome, unspecified

OTHER DISORDERS OF THE NERVOUS SYSTEM (G89-G99)

● **G89   Pain, not elsewhere classified**

    Code also related psychological factors associated with pain
        (F45.42)

    Excludes1   generalized pain NOS (R52)
                    pain disorders exclusively related to
                        psychological factors (F45.41)
                    pain NOS (R52)

    Excludes2   atypical face pain (G50.1)
                    headache syndromes (G44.-)
                    localized pain, unspecified type - code to pain by
                        site, such as:
                        abdomen pain (R10.-)
                        back pain (M54.9)
                        breast pain (N64.4)
                        chest pain (R07.1-R07.9)
                        ear pain (H92.0-)
                        eye pain (H57.1)
                        headache (R51)
                        joint pain (M25.5-)
                        limb pain (M79.6-)
                        lumbar region pain (M54.5)
                        painful urination (R30.9)
                        pelvic and perineal pain (R10.2)
                        shoulder pain (M25.51-)
                        spine pain (M54.-)
                        throat pain (R07.0)
                        tongue pain (K14.6)
                        tooth pain (K08.8)
                    renal colic (N23)
                    migraines (G43.-)
                    myalgia (M79.1)
                    pain from prosthetic devices, implants, and grafts
                        (T82.84, T83.84, T84.84, T85.84-)
                    phantom limb syndrome with pain (G54.6)
                    vulvar vestibulitis (N94.810)
                    vulvodynia (N94.81-)

    G89.0   Central pain syndrome
            *Neurological condition causing intractable pain resulting
                from damage to CNS*
            Déjérine-Roussy syndrome
            Myelopathic pain syndrome
            Thalamic pain syndrome (hyperesthetic)

● **G89.1   Acute pain, not elsewhere classified**

      G89.11   Acute pain due to trauma

      G89.12   Acute post-thoracotomy pain
                Post-thoracotomy pain NOS

      G89.18   Other acute postprocedural pain
                Postoperative pain NOS
                Postprocedural pain NOS

● **G89.2   Chronic pain, not elsewhere classified**

    Excludes1   causalgia, lower limb (G57.7-)
                    causalgia, upper limb (G56.4-)
                    central pain syndrome (G89.0)
                    chronic pain syndrome (G89.4)
                    complex regional pain syndrome II, lower
                        limb (G57.7-)
                    complex regional pain syndrome II,
                        upper limb (G56.4-)
                    neoplasm related chronic pain (G89.3)
                    reflex sympathetic dystrophy (G90.5-)

      G89.21   Chronic pain due to trauma

      G89.22   Chronic post-thoracotomy pain

      G89.28   Other chronic postprocedural pain
                Other chronic postoperative pain

      G89.29   Other chronic pain

    G89.3   Neoplasm related pain (acute) (chronic)
            Cancer associated pain
            Pain due to malignancy (primary) (secondary)
            Tumor associated pain

    G89.4   Chronic pain syndrome
            Chronic pain associated with significant psychosocial
                dysfunction

● **G90   Disorders of autonomic nervous system**

    Excludes1   dysfunction of the autonomic nervous system
                    due to alcohol (G31.2)

● **G90.0   Idiopathic peripheral autonomic neuropathy**

      G90.01   Carotid sinus syncope
                Carotid sinus syndrome

      **G90.09   Other idiopathic peripheral autonomic
                neuropathy**
                Idiopathic peripheral autonomic neuropathy
                    NOS

    G90.1   Familial dysautonomia [Riley-Day]
            Inherited disorder that affects nerve function

    G90.2   Horner's syndrome
            Due to damage of the sympathetic nervous system
            Bernard(-Horner) syndrome
            Cervical sympathetic dystrophy or paralysis

    **G90.3   Multi-system degeneration of the autonomic nervous
            system** 🔑
            Neurogenic orthostatic hypotension [Shy-Drager]
            Excludes1   orthostatic hypotension NOS (I95.1)
            (Ex.) See PDX Collection 573

    G90.4   Autonomic dysreflexia
            Syndrome resulting from lesions of spinal cord
            Use additional code to identify the cause, such as:
                fecal impaction (K56.41)
                pressure ulcer (pressure area) (L89.-)
                urinary tract infection (N39.0)

● **G90.5   Complex regional pain syndrome I (CRPS I)**
            Reflex sympathetic dystrophy
            Excludes1   causalgia of lower limb (G57.7-)
                            causalgia of upper limb (G56.4-)
                            complex regional pain syndrome II of
                                lower limb (G57.7-)
                            complex regional pain syndrome II of
                                upper limb (G56.4-)
            (Ex.) For category G90.5 CC codes unless otherwise indicated: See PDX
            Collection 603

      **G90.50   Complex regional pain syndrome I,
                unspecified** 🔑
                (Ex.) See PDX Collection 602

● **G90.51   Complex regional pain syndrome I of upper
            limb**

      **G90.511   Complex regional pain syndrome I of
                right upper limb** 🔑

      **G90.512   Complex regional pain syndrome I of
                left upper limb** 🔑

      **G90.513   Complex regional pain syndrome I of
                upper limb, bilateral** 🔑

      **G90.519   Complex regional pain syndrome I
                of unspecified upper limb** 🔑

● **G90.52   Complex regional pain syndrome I of lower
            limb**

      **G90.521   Complex regional pain syndrome I of
                right lower limb** 🔑

      **G90.522   Complex regional pain syndrome I of
                left lower limb** 🔑

      **G90.523   Complex regional pain syndrome I of
                lower limb, bilateral** 🔑

      **G90.529   Complex regional pain syndrome I
                of unspecified lower limb** 🔑

      **G90.59   Complex regional pain syndrome I of other
                specified site** 🔑

▶ New   ⇒ Revised   ~~deleted~~ Deleted   Excludes 1   Excludes 2   Includes   Use additional   Code first   Code also   Key words

OGCR Official Guidelines   ● Unacceptable Principal Diagnosis   X Assign placeholder X   ● Use Additional Character(s)   ▶ Manifestation Code   **Coding Clinic**

G90.8   Other disorders of autonomic nervous system

G90.9   Disorder of the autonomic nervous system, unspecified

● **G91   Hydrocephalus**

Dilatation of cerebral ventricles, accompanied by accumulation of cerebrospinal fluid

> **Includes**   acquired hydrocephalus

> **Excludes1**   Arnold-Chiari syndrome with hydrocephalus (Q07.-)
> congenital hydrocephalus (Q03.-)
> spina bifida with hydrocephalus (Q05.-)

Ⓔ For category G91 CC codes unless otherwise indicated: See PDX Collection 605

G91.0   Communicating hydrocephalus 🔖

Secondary normal pressure hydrocephalus

Ⓔ See PDX Collection 604

G91.1   Obstructive hydrocephalus 🔖

G91.2   (Idiopathic) normal pressure hydrocephalus 🔖

Normal pressure hydrocephalus NOS

Ⓔ See PDX Collection 604

G91.3   Post-traumatic hydrocephalus, unspecified 🔖

▸ **G91.4   Hydrocephalus in diseases classified elsewhere**

Code first underlying condition, such as:
congenital syphilis (A50.4-)
neoplasm (C00-D49)

> **Excludes1**   hydrocephalus due to congenital toxoplasmosis (P37.1)

G91.8   Other hydrocephalus 🔖

G91.9   Hydrocephalus, unspecified 🔖

● **G92   Toxic encephalopathy** 🔖

Disorder or disease of brain caused by chemicals
Toxic encephalitis
Toxic metabolic encephalopathy

▸ *Code first if applicable, drug induced (T36-T50) (T51-T65) to identify toxic agent*

Ⓔ See PDX Collection 606

Coding Clinic: 2017, Q1, P39-40

● **G93   Other disorders of brain**

G93.0   Cerebral cysts

Arachnoid cyst
Porencephalic cyst, acquired

> **Excludes1**   acquired periventricular cysts of newborn (P91.1)
> congenital cerebral cysts (Q04.6)

G93.1   Anoxic brain damage, not elsewhere classified 🔖

Permanent brain damage by lack of oxygen perfusion through brain tissues.

> **Excludes1**   cerebral anoxia due to anesthesia during labor and delivery (O74.3)
> cerebral anoxia due to anesthesia during the puerperium (O89.2)
> neonatal anoxia (P84)

Ⓔ See PDX Collection 607

G93.2   Benign intracranial hypertension

> **Excludes1**   hypertensive encephalopathy (I67.4)

G93.3   Postviral fatigue syndrome

Benign myalgic encephalomyelitis

> **Excludes1**   chronic fatigue syndrome NOS (R53.82)

● **G93.4   Other and unspecified encephalopathy**

> **Excludes1**   alcoholic encephalopathy (G31.2)
> encephalopathy in diseases classified elsewhere (G94)
> hypertensive encephalopathy (I67.4)
> toxic (metabolic) encephalopathy (G92)

Coding Clinic: 2017, Q2, P9

G93.40   Encephalopathy, unspecified 🔖

Ⓔ See PDX Collection 608

G93.41   Metabolic encephalopathy 🔖

Septic encephalopathy

Ⓔ See PDX Collection 609

Coding Clinic: 2017, Q2, P8; 2016, Q3, P42; 2015, Q3, P21

G93.49   Other encephalopathy 🔖

Encephalopathy NEC

Ⓔ See PDX Collection 610

Coding Clinic: 2017, Q2, P9

G93.5   Compression of brain 🔖

Arnold-Chiari type 1 compression of brain
Compression of brain (stem)
Herniation of brain (stem)

> **Excludes1**   diffuse traumatic compression of brain (S06.2-)
> focal traumatic compression of brain (S06.3-)

Ⓔ See PDX Collection 611

G93.6   Cerebral edema 🔖

> **Excludes1**   cerebral edema due to birth injury (P11.0)
> traumatic cerebral edema (S06.1-)

Ⓔ See PDX Collection 612

G93.7   Reye's syndrome 🔖   P

Life-threatening neurological condition, usually follows viral illness

▸ *Code first (poisoning due to salicylates, if applicable (T39.0-, with sixth character 1-4)*
~~(T39.0-), if salicylates-induced~~

▸ Use additional code for adverse effect due to salicylates, if applicable (T39.0-, with sixth character 5)

Ⓔ See PDX Collection 613

● **G93.8   Other specified disorders of brain**

G93.81   Temporal sclerosis

Hippocampal sclerosis
Mesial temporal sclerosis

G93.82   Brain death 🔖

Ⓔ See PDX Collection 515

G93.89   Other specified disorders of brain

Postradiation encephalopathy

Coding Clinic: 2016, Q4, P7

G93.9   Disorder of brain, unspecified

▸ **G94   Other disorders of brain in diseases classified elsewhere**

Code first underlying disease

> **Excludes1**   encephalopathy in congenital syphilis (A50.49)
> encephalopathy in influenza (J09.X9, J10.81, J11.81)
> encephalopathy in syphilis (A52.19)
> hydrocephalus in diseases classified elsewhere (G91.4)

Coding Clinic: 2017, Q2, P8

● **G95   Other and unspecified diseases of spinal cord**

> **Excludes2**   myelitis (G04.-)

G95.0   Syringomyelia and syringobulbia 🔖

Ⓔ See PDX Collection 614

● **G95.1   Vascular myelopathies**

> **Excludes2**   intraspinal phlebitis and thrombophlebitis, except non-pyogenic (G08)

Ⓔ For category G95.1 CC codes: See PDX Collection 603

G95.11   Acute infarction of spinal cord (embolic) (nonembolic)

Anoxia of spinal cord
Arterial thrombosis of spinal cord

G95.19   Other vascular myelopathies 🔖

Edema of spinal cord
Hematomyelia
Nonpyogenic intraspinal phlebitis and thrombophlebitis
Subacute necrotic myelopathy

● **G95.2   Other and unspecified cord compression**

Ⓔ For category G95.2 CC codes: See PDX Collection 615

G95.20   Unspecified cord compression 🔖

G95.29   Other cord compression 🔖

N   Newborn Age: 0   **P**   Pediatric Age: 0–17   **M**   Maternity DX: 12–55   **A**   Adult Age: 15–124   ♀   Females Only   ♂   Males Only

 Complication\Comorbidity   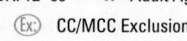 Major C\C   Ⓔ CC/MCC Exclusions   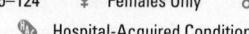 Hospital-Acquired Condition

805

CHAPTER 6 (G00-G99)

● **G95.8 Other specified diseases of spinal cord**

> **Excludes1**   neurogenic bladder NOS (N31.9)
> neurogenic bladder due to cauda equina syndrome (G83.4)
> neuromuscular dysfunction of bladder without spinal cord lesion (N31.-)

(Ex:) **For category G95.8 CC codes:** See PDX Collection 603

G95.81 Conus medullaris syndrome 🔧
Damage to gray matter and/or nerve roots in lower end of spinal cord

G95.89 Other specified diseases of spinal cord 🔧
Cord bladder NOS
Drug-induced myelopathy
Radiation-induced myelopathy

> **Excludes1**   myelopathy NOS (G95.9)

G95.9 Disease of spinal cord, unspecified 🔧
Myelopathy NOS
(Ex:) See PDX Collection 615

● **G96 Other disorders of central nervous system**

G96.0 Cerebrospinal fluid leak 🔧

> **Excludes1**   cerebrospinal fluid leak from spinal puncture (G97.0)

(Ex:) See PDX Collection 616

● **G96.1 Disorders of meninges, not elsewhere classified**

G96.11 Dural tear 🔧

> **Excludes1**   accidental puncture or laceration of dura during a procedure (G97.41)

(Ex:) See PDX Collection 509

G96.12 Meningeal adhesions (cerebral) (spinal)

G96.19 Other disorders of meninges, not elsewhere classified

G96.8 Other specified disorders of central nervous system

G96.9 Disorder of central nervous system, unspecified

● **G97 Intraoperative and postprocedural complications and disorders of nervous system, not elsewhere classified**

> **Excludes2**   intraoperative and postprocedural cerebrovascular infarction (I97.81-, I97.82-)

Coding Clinic: 2016, Q4, P9

G97.0 Cerebrospinal fluid leak from spinal puncture 🔧
(Ex:) See PDX Collection 617

G97.1 Other reaction to spinal and lumbar puncture
Headache due to lumbar puncture

G97.2 Intracranial hypotension following ventricular shunting 🔧
(Ex:) See PDX Collection 617

G97.3 Intraoperative hemorrhage and hematoma of a nervous system organ or structure complicating a procedure

> **Excludes1**   intraoperative hemorrhage and hematoma of a nervous system organ or structure due to accidental puncture and laceration during a procedure (G97.4-)

(Ex:) **For category G97.3 CC codes:** See PDX Collection 618

G97.31 Intraoperative hemorrhage and hematoma of a nervous system organ or structure complicating a nervous system procedure 🔧

G97.32 Intraoperative hemorrhage and hematoma of a nervous system organ or structure complicating other procedure 🔧

● **G97.4 Accidental puncture and laceration of a nervous system organ or structure during a procedure**
(Ex:) **For category G97.4 CC codes:** See PDX Collection 509

G97.41 Accidental puncture or laceration of dura during a procedure 🔧
Incidental (inadvertent) durotomy

G97.48 Accidental puncture and laceration of other nervous system organ or structure during a nervous system procedure 🔧

G97.49 Accidental puncture and laceration of other nervous system organ or structure during other procedure 🔧

● **G97.5 Postprocedural hemorrhage of a nervous system organ or structure following a procedure**
(Ex:) **For category G97.5 CC codes:** See PDX Collection 619

G97.51 Postprocedural hemorrhage of a nervous system organ or structure following a nervous system procedure 🔧

G97.52 Postprocedural hemorrhage of a nervous system organ or structure following other procedure 🔧

● **G97.6 Postprocedural hematoma and seroma of a nervous system organ or structure following a procedure**
(Ex:) **For category G97.6 CC codes:** See PDX Collection 619

G97.61 Postprocedural hematoma of a nervous system organ or structure following a nervous system procedure 🔧

G97.62 Postprocedural hematoma of a nervous system organ or structure following other procedure 🔧

G97.63 Postprocedural seroma of a nervous system organ or structure following a nervous system procedure 🔧

G97.64 Postprocedural seroma of a nervous system organ or structure following other procedure 🔧

● **G97.8 Other intraoperative and postprocedural complications and disorders of nervous system**
Use additional code to further specify disorder
(Ex:) **For category G97.8 CC codes:** See PDX Collection 617

G97.81 Other intraoperative complications of nervous system 🔧

G97.82 Other postprocedural complications and disorders of nervous system 🔧

● **G98 Other disorders of nervous system not elsewhere classified**

> **Includes**   nervous system disorder NOS

G98.0 Neurogenic arthritis, not elsewhere classified
Nonsyphilitic neurogenic arthropathy NEC
Nonsyphilitic neurogenic spondylopathy NEC

> **Excludes1**   spondylopathy (in):
> syringomyelia and syringobulbia (G95.0)
> tabes dorsalis (A52.11)

G98.8 Other disorders of nervous system
Nervous system disorder NOS

● **G99 Other disorders of nervous system in diseases classified elsewhere**

▷ *G99.0 Autonomic neuropathy in diseases classified elsewhere* 🔧
Code first underlying disease, such as:
amyloidosis (E85.-)
gout (M1A.-, M10.-)
hyperthyroidism (E05.-)

> **Excludes1**   diabetic autonomic neuropathy (E08-E13 with .43)

(Ex:) See PDX Collection 620

▷ *G99.2 Myelopathy in diseases classified elsewhere* 🔧
Code first underlying disease, such as:
neoplasm (C00-D49)

> **Excludes1**   myelopathy in:
> intervertebral disease (M50.0-, M51.0-)
> spondylosis (M47.0-, M47.1-)

(Ex:) See PDX Collection 603

▷ *G99.8 Other specified disorders of nervous system in diseases classified elsewhere*
Code first underlying disorder, such as:
amyloidosis (E85.-)
avitaminosis (E56.9)

> **Excludes1**   nervous system involvement in:
> cysticercosis (B69.0)
> rubella (B06.0-)
> syphilis (A52.1-)

▶ New   ⇒ Revised   ~~deleted~~ Deleted   Excludes 1   Excludes 2   Includes   Use additional   Code first   Code also   Key words

OGCR Official Guidelines   ● Unacceptable Principal Diagnosis   X Assign placeholder X   🔧 Use Additional Character(s)   ▷ Manifestation Code   **Coding Clinic**

CHAPTER 7

DISEASES OF THE EYE AND ADNEXA (H00-H59)

OGCR Chapter-Specific Coding Guidelines

7. Chapter 7: Diseases of the Eye and Adnexa (H00-H59)

a. Glaucoma

1) **Assigning Glaucoma Codes**

Assign as many codes from category H40, Glaucoma, as needed to identify the type of glaucoma, the affected eye, and the glaucoma stage.

2) **Bilateral glaucoma with same type and stage**

When a patient has bilateral glaucoma and both eyes are documented as being the same type and stage, and there is a code for bilateral glaucoma, report only the code for the type of glaucoma, bilateral, with the seventh character for the stage.

When a patient has bilateral glaucoma and both eyes are documented as being the same type and stage, and the classification does not provide a code for bilateral glaucoma (i.e. subcategories H40.10, H40.11 and H40.20) report only one code for the type of glaucoma with the appropriate seventh character for the stage.

3) **Bilateral glaucoma stage with different types or stages**

When a patient has bilateral glaucoma and each eye is documented as having a different type or stage, and the classification distinguishes laterality, assign the appropriate code for each eye rather than the code for bilateral glaucoma.

When a patient has bilateral glaucoma and each eye is documented as having a different type, and the classification does not distinguish laterality (i.e. subcategories H40.10, H40.11 and H40.20), assign one code for each type of glaucoma with the appropriate seventh character for the stage.

When a patient has bilateral glaucoma and each eye is documented as having the same type, but different stage, and the classification does not distinguish laterality (i.e. subcategories H40.10, H40.11 and H40.20), assign a code for the type of glaucoma for each eye with the seventh character for the specific glaucoma stage documented for each eye.

4) **Patient admitted with glaucoma and stage evolves during the admission**

If a patient is admitted with glaucoma and the stage progresses during the admission, assign the code for highest stage documented.

5) **Indeterminate stage glaucoma**

Assignment of the seventh character "4" for "indeterminate stage" should be based on the clinical documentation. The seventh character "4" is used for glaucomas whose stage cannot be clinically determined. This seventh character should not be confused with the seventh character "0", unspecified, which should be assigned when there is no documentation regarding the stage of the glaucoma.

b. Blindness

If "blindness" or "low vision" of both eyes is documented but the visual impairment category is not documented, assign code H54.3, Unqualified visual loss, both eyes. If "blindness" or "low vision" in one eye is documented but the visual impairment category is not documented, assign a code from H54.6-, Unqualified visual loss, one eye. If "blindness" or "visual loss" is documented without any information about whether one or both eyes are affected, assign code H54.7, Unspecified visual loss.

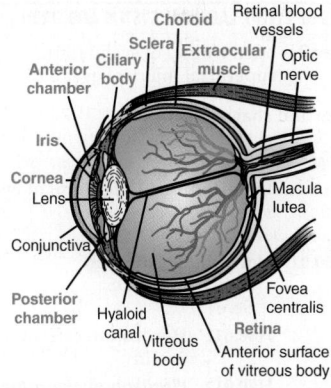

Figure 7-1 Eye and ocular adnexa. (From Buck CJ: Step-by-Step Medical Coding, ed 2016, St. Louis, Elsevier, 2016)

★ **(See Plate 87 on page 63.)**

CHAPTER 7

DISEASES OF THE EYE AND ADNEXA (H00-H59)

Note: Use an external cause code following the code for the eye condition, if applicable, to identify the cause of the eye condition

Excludes2   certain conditions originating in the perinatal period (P04-P96)
certain infectious and parasitic diseases (A00-B99)
complications of pregnancy, childbirth and the puerperium (O00-O9A)
congenital malformations, deformations, and chromosomal abnormalities (Q00-Q99)
diabetes mellitus related eye conditions (E09.3-, E10.3-, E11.3-, E13.3-)
endocrine, nutritional and metabolic diseases (E00-E88)
injury (trauma) of eye and orbit (S05.-)
injury, poisoning and certain other consequences of external causes (S00-T88)
neoplasms (C00-D49)
symptoms, signs and abnormal clinical and laboratory findings, not elsewhere classified (R00-R94)
syphilis related eye disorders (A50.01, A50.3-, A51.43, A52.71)

This chapter contains the following blocks:

H00-H05	Disorders of eyelid, lacrimal system and orbit
H10-H11	Disorders of conjunctiva
H15-H22	Disorders of sclera, cornea, iris and ciliary body
H25-H28	Disorders of lens
H30-H36	Disorders of choroid and retina
H40-H42	Glaucoma
H43-H44	Disorders of vitreous body and globe
H46-H47	Disorders of optic nerve and visual pathways
H49-H52	Disorders of ocular muscles, binocular movement, accommodation and refraction
H53-H54	Visual disturbances and blindness
H55-H57	Other disorders of eye and adnexa
H59	Intraoperative and postprocedural complications and disorders of eye and adnexa, not elsewhere classified

DISORDERS OF EYELID, LACRIMAL SYSTEM AND ORBIT (H00-H05)

Excludes2   open wound of eyelid (S01.1-)
                superficial injury of eyelid (S00.1-, S00.2-)

● **H00**   **Hordeolum and chalazion**
Hordeolum: inflammatory staphylococcal infection of sebaceous glands of eyelids; AKA stye. Chalazion: eyelid mass

● **H00.0**   **Hordeolum (externum) (internum) of eyelid**
Bacterial infection (staphylococcus) of the sebaceous gland of the eyelid (stye)

● **H00.01**   **Hordeolum externum**
Hordeolum NOS
Stye

H00.011   Hordeolum externum right upper eyelid

H00.012   Hordeolum externum right lower eyelid

H00.013   Hordeolum externum right eye, unspecified eyelid

H00.014   Hordeolum externum left upper eyelid

H00.015   Hordeolum externum left lower eyelid

H00.016   Hordeolum externum left eye, unspecified eyelid

H00.019   Hordeolum externum unspecified eye, unspecified eyelid

● **H00.02**   **Hordeolum internum**
Infection of meibomian gland

H00.021   Hordeolum internum right upper eyelid

H00.022   Hordeolum internum right lower eyelid

H00.023   Hordeolum internum right eye, unspecified eyelid

H00.024   Hordeolum internum left upper eyelid

H00.025   Hordeolum internum left lower eyelid

H00.026   Hordeolum internum left eye, unspecified eyelid

H00.029   Hordeolum internum unspecified eye, unspecified eyelid

● **H00.03**   **Abscess of eyelid**
Furuncle of eyelid

H00.031   Abscess of right upper eyelid

H00.032   Abscess of right lower eyelid

H00.033   Abscess of eyelid right eye, unspecified eyelid

H00.034   Abscess of left upper eyelid

H00.035   Abscess of left lower eyelid

H00.036   Abscess of eyelid left eye, unspecified eyelid

H00.039   Abscess of eyelid unspecified eye, unspecified eyelid

● **H00.1**   **Chalazion**
Often caused by accumulation of meibomian gland secretions resulting from a blockage of duct.
Meibomian (gland) cyst

Excludes2   infected meibomian gland (H00.02-)

H00.11   Chalazion right upper eyelid

H00.12   Chalazion right lower eyelid

H00.13   Chalazion right eye, unspecified eyelid

H00.14   Chalazion left upper eyelid

H00.15   Chalazion left lower eyelid

H00.16   Chalazion left eye, unspecified eyelid

H00.19   Chalazion unspecified eye, unspecified eyelid

● **H01**   **Other inflammation of eyelid**

● **H01.0**   **Blepharitis**
Inflammation of eyelids

Excludes1   blepharoconjunctivitis (H10.5-)

● **H01.00**   **Unspecified blepharitis**

H01.001   Unspecified blepharitis right upper eyelid

H01.002   Unspecified blepharitis right lower eyelid

H01.003   Unspecified blepharitis right eye, unspecified eyelid

H01.004   Unspecified blepharitis left upper eyelid

H01.005   Unspecified blepharitis left lower eyelid

H01.006   Unspecified blepharitis left eye, unspecified eyelid

H01.009   Unspecified blepharitis unspecified eye, unspecified eyelid

● **H01.01**   **Ulcerative blepharitis**

H01.011   Ulcerative blepharitis right upper eyelid

H01.012   Ulcerative blepharitis right lower eyelid

H01.013   Ulcerative blepharitis right eye, unspecified eyelid

H01.014   Ulcerative blepharitis left upper eyelid

H01.015   Ulcerative blepharitis left lower eyelid

H01.016   Ulcerative blepharitis left eye, unspecified eyelid

H01.019   Ulcerative blepharitis unspecified eye, unspecified eyelid

● **H01.02**   **Squamous blepharitis**

H01.021   Squamous blepharitis right upper eyelid

H01.022   Squamous blepharitis right lower eyelid

H01.023   Squamous blepharitis right eye, unspecified eyelid

H01.024   Squamous blepharitis left upper eyelid

H01.025   Squamous blepharitis left lower eyelid

H01.026   Squamous blepharitis left eye, unspecified eyelid

H01.029   Squamous blepharitis unspecified eye, unspecified eyelid

● **H01.1**   **Noninfectious dermatoses of eyelid**

● **H01.11**   **Allergic dermatitis of eyelid**
Contact dermatitis of eyelid

H01.111   Allergic dermatitis of right upper eyelid

H01.112   Allergic dermatitis of right lower eyelid

H01.113   Allergic dermatitis of right eye, unspecified eyelid

H01.114   Allergic dermatitis of left upper eyelid

H01.115   Allergic dermatitis of left lower eyelid

H01.116   Allergic dermatitis of left eye, unspecified eyelid

H01.119   Allergic dermatitis of unspecified eye, unspecified eyelid

▶ New   ⇒ Revised   deleted Deleted   Excludes 1   Excludes 2   Includes   Use additional   Code first   Code also   Key words
OGCR Official Guidelines   ● Unacceptable Principal Diagnosis   X Assign placeholder X   ● Use Additional Character(s)   ▶ Manifestation Code   **Coding Clinic**

● **H01.12**   Discoid lupus erythematosus of eyelid

     H01.121   Discoid lupus erythematosus of right upper eyelid

     H01.122   Discoid lupus erythematosus of right lower eyelid

     H01.123   Discoid lupus erythematosus of right eye, unspecified eyelid

     H01.124   Discoid lupus erythematosus of left upper eyelid

     H01.125   Discoid lupus erythematosus of left lower eyelid

     H01.126   Discoid lupus erythematosus of left eye, unspecified eyelid

     H01.129   Discoid lupus erythematosus of unspecified eye, unspecified eyelid

● **H01.13**   Eczematous dermatitis of eyelid

     H01.131   Eczematous dermatitis of right upper eyelid

     H01.132   Eczematous dermatitis of right lower eyelid

     H01.133   Eczematous dermatitis of right eye, unspecified eyelid

     H01.134   Eczematous dermatitis of left upper eyelid

     H01.135   Eczematous dermatitis of left lower eyelid

     H01.136   Eczematous dermatitis of left eye, unspecified eyelid

     H01.139   Eczematous dermatitis of unspecified eye, unspecified eyelid

● **H01.14**   Xeroderma of eyelid

     Abnormally dry

     H01.141   Xeroderma of right upper eyelid

     H01.142   Xeroderma of right lower eyelid

     H01.143   Xeroderma of right eye, unspecified eyelid

     H01.144   Xeroderma of left upper eyelid

     H01.145   Xeroderma of left lower eyelid

     H01.146   Xeroderma of left eye, unspecified eyelid

     H01.149   Xeroderma of unspecified eye, unspecified eyelid

  H01.8   Other specified inflammations of eyelid

  H01.9   Unspecified inflammation of eyelid

     Inflammation of eyelid NOS

● **H02**   Other disorders of eyelid

     Turning inward (inversion) of eyelid margin and ingrowing eyelashes

     Excludes1   congenital malformations of eyelid (Q10.0-Q10.3)

● **H02.0**   Entropion and trichiasis of eyelid

● **H02.00**   Unspecified entropion of eyelid

     H02.001   Unspecified entropion of right upper eyelid

     H02.002   Unspecified entropion of right lower eyelid

     H02.003   Unspecified entropion of right eye, unspecified eyelid

     H02.004   Unspecified entropion of left upper eyelid

Figure 7-2   Right lower eyelid entropion. Note the inward rotation of the tarsal plate about the horizontal axis and the resultant contact between the mucocutaneous junction and ocular surface. (From Glynn M, Drake WM, Hutchison R: Hutchison's Clinical Methods: An Integrated Approach to Clinical Practice, Edinburgh, Saunders/Elsevier, 2012)

     H02.005   Unspecified entropion of left lower eyelid

     H02.006   Unspecified entropion of left eye, unspecified eyelid

     H02.009   Unspecified entropion of unspecified eye, unspecified eyelid

● **H02.01**   Cicatricial entropion of eyelid

     Scar

     H02.011   Cicatricial entropion of right upper eyelid

     H02.012   Cicatricial entropion of right lower eyelid

     H02.013   Cicatricial entropion of right eye, unspecified eyelid

     H02.014   Cicatricial entropion of left upper eyelid

     H02.015   Cicatricial entropion of left lower eyelid

     H02.016   Cicatricial entropion of left eye, unspecified eyelid

     H02.019   Cicatricial entropion of unspecified eye, unspecified eyelid

● **H02.02**   Mechanical entropion of eyelid

     Turning inward (inversion) of eyelid margin due to lack of support

     H02.021   Mechanical entropion of right upper eyelid

     H02.022   Mechanical entropion of right lower eyelid

     H02.023   Mechanical entropion of right eye, unspecified eyelid

     H02.024   Mechanical entropion of left upper eyelid

     H02.025   Mechanical entropion of left lower eyelid

     H02.026   Mechanical entropion of left eye, unspecified eyelid

     H02.029   Mechanical entropion of unspecified eye, unspecified eyelid

● **H02.03**   Senile entropion of eyelid

     Turning inward (inversion) of eyelid margin due to aging

     H02.031   Senile entropion of right upper eyelid   A

     H02.032   Senile entropion of right lower eyelid   A

     H02.033   Senile entropion of right eye, unspecified eyelid   A

     H02.034   Senile entropion of left upper eyelid   A

     H02.035   Senile entropion of left lower eyelid   A

     H02.036   Senile entropion of left eye, unspecified eyelid   A

     H02.039   Senile entropion of unspecified eye, unspecified eyelid   A

● **H02.04**   Spastic entropion of eyelid

     Turning inward (inversion) of eyelid margin caused by spasm of muscle

     H02.041   Spastic entropion of right upper eyelid

     H02.042   Spastic entropion of right lower eyelid

     H02.043   Spastic entropion of right eye, unspecified eyelid

     H02.044   Spastic entropion of left upper eyelid

     H02.045   Spastic entropion of left lower eyelid

     H02.046   Spastic entropion of left eye, unspecified eyelid

     H02.049   Spastic entropion of unspecified eye, unspecified eyelid

CHAPTER 7 (H00-H59)

▶● **H02.05** **Trichiasis without entropion**
Ingrowing hairs of eyelashes

➠ **H02.051** Trichiasis without entropion **right upper** eyelid

➠ **H02.052** Trichiasis without entropion **right lower** eyelid

➠ **H02.053** Trichiasis without entropion **right eye, unspecified** eyelid

➠ **H02.054** Trichiasis without entropion **left upper** eyelid

➠ **H02.055** Trichiasis without entropion **left lower** eyelid

➠ **H02.056** Trichiasis without entropion **left eye, unspecified** eyelid

➠ **H02.059** Trichiasis without entropion **unspecified** eye, **unspecified** eyelid

● **H02.1** **Ectropion of eyelid**
Eversion (pulling away) of eyelid

● **H02.10** **Unspecified ectropion of eyelid**

H02.101 Unspecified ectropion of **right upper** eyelid

H02.102 Unspecified ectropion of **right lower** eyelid

H02.103 Unspecified ectropion of **right eye, unspecified** eyelid

H02.104 Unspecified ectropion of **left upper** eyelid

H02.105 Unspecified ectropion of **left lower** eyelid

H02.106 Unspecified ectropion of **left eye, unspecified** eyelid

H02.109 Unspecified ectropion of **unspecified eye, unspecified** eyelid

● **H02.11** **Cicatricial ectropion of eyelid**
Pulling of eyelid down and away from eye due to scar or tightening

H02.111 Cicatricial ectropion of **right upper** eyelid

H02.112 Cicatricial ectropion of **right lower** eyelid

H02.113 Cicatricial ectropion of **right eye, unspecified** eyelid

H02.114 Cicatricial ectropion of **left upper** eyelid

H02.115 Cicatricial ectropion of **left lower** eyelid

H02.116 Cicatricial ectropion of **left eye, unspecified** eyelid

H02.119 Cicatricial ectropion of **unspecified eye, unspecified** eyelid

● **H02.12** **Mechanical ectropion of eyelid**
Eversion (pulling away) of eyelid due to lack of support

H02.121 Mechanical ectropion of **right upper** eyelid

H02.122 Mechanical ectropion of **right lower** eyelid

H02.123 Mechanical ectropion of **right eye, unspecified** eyelid

H02.124 Mechanical ectropion of **left upper** eyelid

H02.125 Mechanical ectropion of **left lower** eyelid

H02.126 Mechanical ectropion of **left eye, unspecified** eyelid

H02.129 Mechanical ectropion of **unspecified eye, unspecified** eyelid

● **H02.13** **Senile ectropion of eyelid**
Eversion (pulling away) of eyelid due to age

H02.131 Senile ectropion of **right upper** eyelid A

H02.132 Senile ectropion of **right lower** eyelid A

H02.133 Senile ectropion of **right eye, unspecified** eyelid A

H02.134 Senile ectropion of **left upper** eyelid A

H02.135 Senile ectropion of **left lower** eyelid A

H02.136 Senile ectropion of **left eye, unspecified** eyelid A

H02.139 Senile ectropion of **unspecified eye, unspecified** eyelid A

● **H02.14** **Spastic ectropion of eyelid**
Eversion (pulling away) of eyelid due to tonic muscle spasm

H02.141 Spastic ectropion of **right upper** eyelid

H02.142 Spastic ectropion of **right lower** eyelid

H02.143 Spastic ectropion of **right eye, unspecified** eyelid

H02.144 Spastic ectropion of **left upper** eyelid

H02.145 Spastic ectropion of **left lower** eyelid

H02.146 Spastic ectropion of **left eye, unspecified** eyelid

H02.149 Spastic ectropion of **unspecified eye, unspecified** eyelid

● **H02.2** **Lagophthalmos**
Condition in which eye cannot completely close

● **H02.20** **Unspecified lagophthalmos**

H02.201 Unspecified lagophthalmos **right upper** eyelid

H02.202 Unspecified lagophthalmos **right lower** eyelid

H02.203 Unspecified lagophthalmos **right eye, unspecified** eyelid

H02.204 Unspecified lagophthalmos **left upper** eyelid

H02.205 Unspecified lagophthalmos **left lower** eyelid

H02.206 Unspecified lagophthalmos **left eye, unspecified** eyelid

H02.209 Unspecified lagophthalmos **unspecified eye, unspecified** eyelid

● **H02.21** **Cicatricial lagophthalmos**
Upper or lower eyelid does not close due to scar or tightening

H02.211 Cicatricial lagophthalmos **right upper** eyelid

H02.212 Cicatricial lagophthalmos **right lower** eyelid

H02.213 Cicatricial lagophthalmos **right eye, unspecified** eyelid

H02.214 Cicatricial lagophthalmos **left upper** eyelid

H02.215 Cicatricial lagophthalmos **left lower** eyelid

H02.216 Cicatricial lagophthalmos **left eye, unspecified** eyelid

H02.219 Cicatricial lagophthalmos **unspecified eye, unspecified** eyelid

▶ New   ➠ Revised   ~~deleted~~ Deleted   Excludes 1   Excludes 2   Includes   Use additional   Code first   Code also   Key words
OGCR Official Guidelines   ● Unacceptable Principal Diagnosis   X Assign placeholder X   ● Use Additional Character(s)   ❚ Manifestation Code   **Coding Clinic**

● **H02.22 Mechanical lagophthalmos**
Inability to close lids due to structural disorder
  H02.221 Mechanical lagophthalmos right upper eyelid
  H02.222 Mechanical lagophthalmos right lower eyelid
  H02.223 Mechanical lagophthalmos right eye, unspecified eyelid
  H02.224 Mechanical lagophthalmos left upper eyelid
  H02.225 Mechanical lagophthalmos left lower eyelid
  H02.226 Mechanical lagophthalmos left eye, unspecified eyelid
  H02.229 Mechanical lagophthalmos unspecified eye, unspecified eyelid

● **H02.23 Paralytic lagophthalmos**
Eyelids do not close due to paralysis
  H02.231 Paralytic lagophthalmos right upper eyelid
  H02.232 Paralytic lagophthalmos right lower eyelid
  H02.233 Paralytic lagophthalmos right eye, unspecified eyelid
  H02.234 Paralytic lagophthalmos left upper eyelid
  H02.235 Paralytic lagophthalmos left lower eyelid
  H02.236 Paralytic lagophthalmos left eye, unspecified eyelid
  H02.239 Paralytic lagophthalmos unspecified eye, unspecified eyelid

★**(See Plate 81, middle, on page 65.)**

● **H02.3 Blepharochalasis**
Relaxation of skin of eyelid, due to atrophy of intercellular tissue
Pseudoptosis
  H02.30 Blepharochalasis unspecified eye, unspecified eyelid
  H02.31 Blepharochalasis right upper eyelid
  H02.32 Blepharochalasis right lower eyelid
  H02.33 Blepharochalasis right eye, unspecified eyelid
  H02.34 Blepharochalasis left upper eyelid
  H02.35 Blepharochalasis left lower eyelid
  H02.36 Blepharochalasis left eye, unspecified eyelid

● **H02.4 Ptosis of eyelid**
Falling forward, drooping, sagging of eyelid
  ● **H02.40 Unspecified ptosis of eyelid**
    H02.401 Unspecified ptosis of right eyelid
    H02.402 Unspecified ptosis of left eyelid
    H02.403 Unspecified ptosis of bilateral eyelids
    H02.409 Unspecified ptosis of unspecified eyelid
  ● **H02.41 Mechanical ptosis of eyelid**
    H02.411 Mechanical ptosis of right eyelid
    H02.412 Mechanical ptosis of left eyelid
    H02.413 Mechanical ptosis of bilateral eyelids
    H02.419 Mechanical ptosis of unspecified eyelid

Item 7–1 Ptosis of eyelid is drooping of the upper eyelid over the pupil when the eyes are fully opened resulting from nerve or muscle damage, which may require surgical correction.

● **H02.42 Myogenic ptosis of eyelid**
  H02.421 Myogenic ptosis of right eyelid
  H02.422 Myogenic ptosis of left eyelid
  H02.423 Myogenic ptosis of bilateral eyelids
  H02.429 Myogenic ptosis of unspecified eyelid
● **H02.43 Paralytic ptosis of eyelid**
Neurogenic ptosis of eyelid
  H02.431 Paralytic ptosis of right eyelid
  H02.432 Paralytic ptosis of left eyelid
  H02.433 Paralytic ptosis of bilateral eyelids
  H02.439 Paralytic ptosis unspecified eyelid
● **H02.5 Other disorders affecting eyelid function**
  Excludes2 blepharospasm (G24.5)
    organic tic (G25.69)
    psychogenic tic (F95.-)
● **H02.51 Abnormal innervation syndrome**
  H02.511 Abnormal innervation syndrome right upper eyelid
  H02.512 Abnormal innervation syndrome right lower eyelid
  H02.513 Abnormal innervation syndrome right eye, unspecified eyelid
  H02.514 Abnormal innervation syndrome left upper eyelid
  H02.515 Abnormal innervation syndrome left lower eyelid
  H02.516 Abnormal innervation syndrome left eye, unspecified eyelid
  H02.519 Abnormal innervation syndrome unspecified eye, unspecified eyelid
● **H02.52 Blepharophimosis**
Drooping of eyelid with reduced lid size
Ankyloblepharon
  H02.521 Blepharophimosis right upper eyelid
  H02.522 Blepharophimosis right lower eyelid
  H02.523 Blepharophimosis right eye, unspecified eyelid
  H02.524 Blepharophimosis left upper eyelid
  H02.525 Blepharophimosis left lower eyelid
  H02.526 Blepharophimosis left eye, unspecified eyelid
  H02.529 Blepharophimosis unspecified eye, unspecified lid
● **H02.53 Eyelid retraction**
Eyelid lag
  H02.531 Eyelid retraction right upper eyelid
  H02.532 Eyelid retraction right lower eyelid
  H02.533 Eyelid retraction right eye, unspecified eyelid
  H02.534 Eyelid retraction left upper eyelid
  H02.535 Eyelid retraction left lower eyelid
  H02.536 Eyelid retraction left eye, unspecified eyelid
  H02.539 Eyelid retraction unspecified eye, unspecified lid
  H02.59 Other disorders affecting eyelid function
Deficient blink reflex
Sensory disorders

Figure 7-3 Ptosis of eyelid. (From Kanski JJ: Clinical Diagnosis in Ophthalmology, London, Elsevier Mosby, 2006)

CHAPTER 7 (H00-H59)

● **H02.6**   **Xanthelasma of eyelid**
Yellow-to-orange patches or pimples clustered together on eyelid

     H02.60   Xanthelasma of unspecified eye, unspecified eyelid

     H02.61   Xanthelasma of right upper eyelid

     H02.62   Xanthelasma of right lower eyelid

     H02.63   Xanthelasma of right eye, unspecified eyelid

     H02.64   Xanthelasma of left upper eyelid

     H02.65   Xanthelasma of left lower eyelid

     H02.66   Xanthelasma of left eye, unspecified eyelid

● **H02.7**   **Other and unspecified degenerative disorders of eyelid and periocular area**

     H02.70   Unspecified degenerative disorders of eyelid and periocular area

   ● H02.71   **Chloasma of eyelid and periocular area**
Dyspigmentation of eyelid
Hyperpigmentation of eyelid

       H02.711   Chloasma of right upper eyelid and periocular area

       H02.712   Chloasma of right lower eyelid and periocular area

       H02.713   Chloasma of right eye, unspecified eyelid and periocular area

       H02.714   Chloasma of left upper eyelid and periocular area

       H02.715   Chloasma of left lower eyelid and periocular area

       H02.716   Chloasma of left eye, unspecified eyelid and periocular area

       H02.719   Chloasma of unspecified eye, unspecified eyelid and periocular area

   ● H02.72   **Madarosis of eyelid and periocular area**
Loss of eyelashes and/or eyebrows
Hypotrichosis of eyelid

       H02.721   Madarosis of right upper eyelid and periocular area

       H02.722   Madarosis of right lower eyelid and periocular area

       H02.723   Madarosis of right eye, unspecified eyelid and periocular area

       H02.724   Madarosis of left upper eyelid and periocular area

       H02.725   Madarosis of left lower eyelid and periocular area

       H02.726   Madarosis of left eye, unspecified eyelid and periocular area

       H02.729   Madarosis of unspecified eye, unspecified eyelid and periocular area

   ● H02.73   **Vitiligo of eyelid and periocular area**
Skin pigmentation disease characterized by white patches
Hypopigmentation of eyelid

       H02.731   Vitiligo of right upper eyelid and periocular area

       H02.732   Vitiligo of right lower eyelid and periocular area

       H02.733   Vitiligo of right eye, unspecified eyelid and periocular area

       H02.734   Vitiligo of left upper eyelid and periocular area

       H02.735   Vitiligo of left lower eyelid and periocular area

       H02.736   Vitiligo of left eye, unspecified eyelid and periocular area

       H02.739   Vitiligo of unspecified eye, unspecified eyelid and periocular area

     H02.79   Other degenerative disorders of eyelid and periocular area

● **H02.8**   **Other specified disorders of eyelid**

   ● H02.81   **Retained foreign body in eyelid**
Use additional code to identify the type of retained foreign body (Z18.-)

       Excludes1   laceration of eyelid with foreign body (S01.12-)
retained intraocular foreign body (H44.6-, H44.7-)
superficial foreign body of eyelid and periocular area (S00.25-)

       H02.811   Retained foreign body in right upper eyelid

       H02.812   Retained foreign body in right lower eyelid

       H02.813   Retained foreign body in right eye, unspecified eyelid

       H02.814   Retained foreign body in left upper eyelid

       H02.815   Retained foreign body in left lower eyelid

       H02.816   Retained foreign body in left eye, unspecified eyelid

       H02.819   Retained foreign body in unspecified eye, unspecified eyelid

   ● H02.82   **Cysts of eyelid**
Sebaceous cyst of eyelid

       H02.821   Cysts of right upper eyelid

       H02.822   Cysts of right lower eyelid

       H02.823   Cysts of right eye, unspecified eyelid

       H02.824   Cysts of left upper eyelid

       H02.825   Cysts of left lower eyelid

       H02.826   Cysts of left eye, unspecified eyelid

       H02.829   Cysts of unspecified eye, unspecified eyelid

   ● H02.83   **Dermatochalasis of eyelid**
Skin is inelastic and hangs loosely in folds

       H02.831   Dermatochalasis of right upper eyelid

       H02.832   Dermatochalasis of right lower eyelid

       H02.833   Dermatochalasis of right eye, unspecified eyelid

       H02.834   Dermatochalasis of left upper eyelid

       H02.835   Dermatochalasis of left lower eyelid

       H02.836   Dermatochalasis of left eye, unspecified eyelid

       H02.839   Dermatochalasis of unspecified eye, unspecified eyelid

   ● H02.84   **Edema of eyelid**
Hyperemia of eyelid

       H02.841   Edema of right upper eyelid

       H02.842   Edema of right lower eyelid

       H02.843   Edema of right eye, unspecified eyelid

       H02.844   Edema of left upper eyelid

       H02.845   Edema of left lower eyelid

       H02.846   Edema of left eye, unspecified eyelid

       H02.849   Edema of unspecified eye, unspecified eyelid

   ● H02.85   **Elephantiasis of eyelid**
Massive secondary lymphedema with hypertrophy of skin and subcutaneous tissues (pachyderma)

       H02.851   Elephantiasis of right upper eyelid

       H02.852   Elephantiasis of right lower eyelid

       H02.853   Elephantiasis of right eye, unspecified eyelid

       H02.854   Elephantiasis of left upper eyelid

       H02.855   Elephantiasis of left lower eyelid

▶ New   ⇛ Revised   ~~deleted~~ Deleted   Excludes 1   Excludes 2   Includes   Use additional   Code first   Code also   Key words

OGCR Official Guidelines   ● Unacceptable Principal Diagnosis   X Assign placeholder X   ● Use Additional Character(s)   ▶ Manifestation Code   **Coding Clinic**

H02.856   Elephantiasis of left eye, unspecified eyelid

H02.859   Elephantiasis of unspecified eye, unspecified eyelid

● H02.86   **Hypertrichosis of eyelid**
Excessive growth of hair

H02.861   Hypertrichosis of right upper eyelid

H02.862   Hypertrichosis of right lower eyelid

H02.863   Hypertrichosis of right eye, unspecified eyelid

H02.864   Hypertrichosis of left upper eyelid

H02.865   Hypertrichosis of left lower eyelid

H02.866   Hypertrichosis of left eye, unspecified eyelid

H02.869   Hypertrichosis of unspecified eye, unspecified eyelid

● H02.87   **Vascular anomalies of eyelid**

H02.871   Vascular anomalies of right upper eyelid

H02.872   Vascular anomalies of right lower eyelid

H02.873   Vascular anomalies of right eye, unspecified eyelid

H02.874   Vascular anomalies of left upper eyelid

H02.875   Vascular anomalies of left lower eyelid

H02.876   Vascular anomalies of left eye, unspecified eyelid

H02.879   Vascular anomalies of unspecified eye, unspecified eyelid

H02.89   Other specified disorders of eyelid
Hemorrhage of eyelid

H02.9   **Unspecified disorder of eyelid**
Disorder of eyelid NOS

● **H04   Disorders of lacrimal system**

    Excludes1   congenital malformations of lacrimal system (Q10.4-Q10.6)

● H04.0   **Dacryoadenitis**
Inflammation of lacrimal gland

    ● H04.00   Unspecified dacryoadenitis

H04.001   Unspecified dacryoadenitis, right lacrimal gland

H04.002   Unspecified dacryoadenitis, left lacrimal gland

H04.003   Unspecified dacryoadenitis, bilateral lacrimal glands

H04.009   Unspecified dacryoadenitis, unspecified lacrimal gland

    ● H04.01   Acute dacryoadenitis

H04.011   Acute dacryoadenitis, right lacrimal gland

H04.012   Acute dacryoadenitis, left lacrimal gland

H04.013   Acute dacryoadenitis, bilateral lacrimal glands

H04.019   Acute dacryoadenitis, unspecified lacrimal gland

★ **(See Plate 82 on page 67.)**

    ● H04.02   Chronic dacryoadenitis

H04.021   Chronic dacryoadenitis, right lacrimal gland

H04.022   Chronic dacryoadenitis, left lacrimal gland

H04.023   Chronic dacryoadenitis, bilateral lacrimal gland

H04.029   Chronic dacryoadenitis, unspecified lacrimal gland

    ● H04.03   Chronic enlargement of lacrimal gland

H04.031   Chronic enlargement of right lacrimal gland

H04.032   Chronic enlargement of left lacrimal gland

H04.033   Chronic enlargement of bilateral lacrimal glands

H04.039   Chronic enlargement of unspecified lacrimal gland

● H04.1   **Other disorders of lacrimal gland**

    ● H04.11   Dacryops
Watery eye or distention of lacrimal duct due to fluid

H04.111   Dacryops of right lacrimal gland

H04.112   Dacryops of left lacrimal gland

H04.113   Dacryops of bilateral lacrimal glands

H04.119   Dacryops of unspecified lacrimal gland

    ● H04.12   Dry eye syndrome
Tear film insufficiency, NOS

H04.121   Dry eye syndrome of right lacrimal gland

H04.122   Dry eye syndrome of left lacrimal gland

H04.123   Dry eye syndrome of bilateral lacrimal glands

H04.129   Dry eye syndrome of unspecified lacrimal gland

    ● H04.13   Lacrimal cyst
Lacrimal cystic degeneration

H04.131   Lacrimal cyst right lacrimal gland

H04.132   Lacrimal cyst left lacrimal gland

H04.133   Lacrimal cyst bilateral lacrimal glands

H04.139   Lacrimal cyst unspecified lacrimal gland

    ● H04.14   Primary lacrimal gland atrophy

H04.141   Primary lacrimal gland atrophy, right lacrimal gland

H04.142   Primary lacrimal gland atrophy, left lacrimal gland

H04.143   Primary lacrimal gland atrophy, bilateral lacrimal glands

H04.149   Primary lacrimal gland atrophy, unspecified lacrimal gland

    ● H04.15   Secondary lacrimal gland atrophy

H04.151   Secondary lacrimal gland atrophy, right lacrimal gland

H04.152   Secondary lacrimal gland atrophy, left lacrimal gland

H04.153   Secondary lacrimal gland atrophy, bilateral lacrimal glands

H04.159   Secondary lacrimal gland atrophy, unspecified lacrimal gland

    ● H04.16   Lacrimal gland dislocation

H04.161   Lacrimal gland dislocation, right lacrimal gland

H04.162   Lacrimal gland dislocation, left lacrimal gland

Figure 7-4   Lacrimal apparatus. (From Buck CJ: Step-by-Step Medical Coding, 2016, St. Louis, Elsevier, 2016)

CHAPTER 7 (H00-H59)

H04.163   Lacrimal gland dislocation, bilateral lacrimal glands

H04.169   Lacrimal gland dislocation, unspecified lacrimal gland

H04.19   Other specified disorders of lacrimal gland

● H04.2   Epiphora
Overflow of tears due to stricture of lacrimal passages; AKA lacrimation

● H04.20   Unspecified epiphora

H04.201   Unspecified epiphora, right lacrimal gland

H04.202   Unspecified epiphora, left lacrimal gland

H04.203   Unspecified epiphora, bilateral lacrimal glands

H04.209   Unspecified epiphora, unspecified lacrimal gland

● H04.21   Epiphora due to excess lacrimation

H04.211   Epiphora due to excess lacrimation, right lacrimal gland

H04.212   Epiphora due to excess lacrimation, left lacrimal gland

H04.213   Epiphora due to excess lacrimation, bilateral lacrimal glands

H04.219   Epiphora due to excess lacrimation, unspecified lacrimal gland

● H04.22   Epiphora due to insufficient drainage

H04.221   Epiphora due to insufficient drainage, right lacrimal gland

H04.222   Epiphora due to insufficient drainage, left lacrimal gland

H04.223   Epiphora due to insufficient drainage, bilateral lacrimal glands

H04.229   Epiphora due to insufficient drainage, unspecified lacrimal gland

● H04.3   Acute and unspecified inflammation of lacrimal passages

Excludes1   neonatal dacryocystitis (P39.1)

● H04.30   Unspecified dacryocystitis

H04.301   Unspecified dacryocystitis of right lacrimal passage

H04.302   Unspecified dacryocystitis of left lacrimal passage

H04.303   Unspecified dacryocystitis of bilateral lacrimal passages

H04.309   Unspecified dacryocystitis of unspecified lacrimal passage

● H04.31   Phlegmonous dacryocystitis
Cellulitis of lacrimal sac

H04.311   Phlegmonous dacryocystitis of right lacrimal passage

H04.312   Phlegmonous dacryocystitis of left lacrimal passage

H04.313   Phlegmonous dacryocystitis of bilateral lacrimal passages

H04.319   Phlegmonous dacryocystitis of unspecified lacrimal passage

● H04.32   Acute dacryocystitis
Acute dacryopericystitis

H04.321   Acute dacryocystitis of right lacrimal passage

H04.322   Acute dacryocystitis of left lacrimal passage

H04.323   Acute dacryocystitis of bilateral lacrimal passages

H04.329   Acute dacryocystitis of unspecified lacrimal passage

● H04.33   Acute lacrimal canaliculitis

H04.331   Acute lacrimal canaliculitis of right lacrimal passage

H04.332   Acute lacrimal canaliculitis of left lacrimal passage

H04.333   Acute lacrimal canaliculitis of bilateral lacrimal passages

H04.339   Acute lacrimal canaliculitis of unspecified lacrimal passage

● H04.4   Chronic inflammation of lacrimal passages

● H04.41   Chronic dacryocystitis
Inflammation of lacrimal sac

H04.411   Chronic dacryocystitis of right lacrimal passage

H04.412   Chronic dacryocystitis of left lacrimal passage

H04.413   Chronic dacryocystitis of bilateral lacrimal passages

H04.419   Chronic dacryocystitis of unspecified lacrimal passage

● H04.42   Chronic lacrimal canaliculitis
Inflammation of lacrimal ducts

H04.421   Chronic lacrimal canaliculitis of right lacrimal passage

H04.422   Chronic lacrimal canaliculitis of left lacrimal passage

H04.423   Chronic lacrimal canaliculitis of bilateral lacrimal passages

H04.429   Chronic lacrimal canaliculitis of unspecified lacrimal passage

● H04.43   Chronic lacrimal mucocele
Accumulation of mucous secretion

H04.431   Chronic lacrimal mucocele of right lacrimal passage

H04.432   Chronic lacrimal mucocele of left lacrimal passage

H04.433   Chronic lacrimal mucocele of bilateral lacrimal passages

H04.439   Chronic lacrimal mucocele of unspecified lacrimal passage

● H04.5   Stenosis and insufficiency of lacrimal passages

● H04.51   Dacryolith
Concretion in lacrimal sac/duct; AKA lacrimal calculus

H04.511   Dacryolith of right lacrimal passage

H04.512   Dacryolith of left lacrimal passage

H04.513   Dacryolith of bilateral lacrimal passages

H04.519   Dacryolith of unspecified lacrimal passage

● H04.52   Eversion of lacrimal punctum
Turning out of lacrimal drainage opening

H04.521   Eversion of right lacrimal punctum

H04.522   Eversion of left lacrimal punctum

H04.523   Eversion of bilateral lacrimal punctum

H04.529   Eversion of unspecified lacrimal punctum

● H04.53   Neonatal obstruction of nasolacrimal duct

Excludes1   congenital stenosis and stricture of lacrimal duct (Q10.5)

H04.531   Neonatal obstruction of right nasolacrimal duct   N

H04.532   Neonatal obstruction of left nasolacrimal duct   N

H04.533   Neonatal obstruction of bilateral nasolacrimal duct   N

H04.539   Neonatal obstruction of unspecified nasolacrimal duct   N

▶ New   ⇒ Revised   ~~deleted~~ Deleted   Excludes 1   Excludes 2   Includes   Use additional   Code first   Code also   Key words
OGCR Official Guidelines   ● Unacceptable Principal Diagnosis   X Assign placeholder X   ● Use Additional Character(s)   ▷ Manifestation Code   **Coding Clinic**

● H04.54 Stenosis of lacrimal canaliculi
   H04.541 Stenosis of right lacrimal canaliculi
   H04.542 Stenosis of left lacrimal canaliculi
   H04.543 Stenosis of bilateral lacrimal canaliculi
   H04.549 Stenosis of unspecified lacrimal canaliculi
● H04.55 Acquired stenosis of nasolacrimal duct
   H04.551 Acquired stenosis of right nasolacrimal duct
   H04.552 Acquired stenosis of left nasolacrimal duct
   H04.553 Acquired stenosis of bilateral nasolacrimal duct
   H04.559 Acquired stenosis of unspecified nasolacrimal duct
● H04.56 Stenosis of lacrimal punctum
   H04.561 Stenosis of right lacrimal punctum
   H04.562 Stenosis of left lacrimal punctum
   H04.563 Stenosis of bilateral lacrimal punctum
   H04.569 Stenosis of unspecified lacrimal punctum
● H04.57 Stenosis of lacrimal sac
   H04.571 Stenosis of right lacrimal sac
   H04.572 Stenosis of left lacrimal sac
   H04.573 Stenosis of bilateral lacrimal sac
   H04.579 Stenosis of unspecified lacrimal sac
● H04.6 Other changes of lacrimal passages
  ● H04.61 Lacrimal fistula
    H04.611 Lacrimal fistula right lacrimal passage
    H04.612 Lacrimal fistula left lacrimal passage
    H04.613 Lacrimal fistula bilateral lacrimal passages
    H04.619 Lacrimal fistula unspecified lacrimal passage
  H04.69 Other changes of lacrimal passages
● H04.8 Other disorders of lacrimal system
  ● H04.81 Granuloma of lacrimal passages
    Inflammatory response due to infectious or noninfectious agents
    H04.811 Granuloma of right lacrimal passage
    H04.812 Granuloma of left lacrimal passage
    H04.813 Granuloma of bilateral lacrimal passages
    H04.819 Granuloma of unspecified lacrimal passage
  H04.89 Other disorders of lacrimal system
  H04.9 Disorder of lacrimal system, unspecified

● H05 **Disorders of orbit**
  Excludes1 congenital malformation of orbit (Q10.7)
● H05.0 Acute inflammation of orbit
  H05.00 Unspecified acute inflammation of orbit
  ● H05.01 Cellulitis of orbit
    Infection of soft tissue of orbit
    Abscess of orbit
    (Ex) **For category H05.01 CC codes:** See PDX Collection 621
    H05.011 Cellulitis of right orbit 🔖
    H05.012 Cellulitis of left orbit 🔖
    H05.013 Cellulitis of bilateral orbits 🔖
    H05.019 Cellulitis of unspecified orbit 🔖

● H05.02 Osteomyelitis of orbit
    Infection of boney orbit of eye
    (Ex) **For category H05.02 CC codes:** See PDX Collection 622
    H05.021 Osteomyelitis of right orbit 🔖
    H05.022 Osteomyelitis of left orbit 🔖
    H05.023 Osteomyelitis of bilateral orbits 🔖
    H05.029 Osteomyelitis of unspecified orbit 🔖
● H05.03 Periostitis of orbit
    Inflammation of periosteum (membrane covering bone surface)
    (Ex) **For category H05.03 CC codes:** See PDX Collection 623
    H05.031 Periostitis of right orbit 🔖
    H05.032 Periostitis of left orbit 🔖
    H05.033 Periostitis of bilateral orbits 🔖
    H05.039 Periostitis of unspecified orbit 🔖
● H05.04 Tenonitis of orbit
    Inflammation of tenon capsule (space enclosing fascia of Tenon between eyeball and fat of orbit)
    H05.041 Tenonitis of right orbit
    H05.042 Tenonitis of left orbit
    H05.043 Tenonitis of bilateral orbits
    H05.049 Tenonitis of unspecified orbit
● H05.1 Chronic inflammatory disorders of orbit
  H05.10 Unspecified chronic inflammatory disorders of orbit
  ● H05.11 Granuloma of orbit
    Pseudotumor (inflammatory) of orbit
    H05.111 Granuloma of right orbit
    H05.112 Granuloma of left orbit
    H05.113 Granuloma of bilateral orbits
    H05.119 Granuloma of unspecified orbit
  ● H05.12 Orbital myositis
    Inflammation of extraocular muscles of orbit
    H05.121 Orbital myositis, right orbit
    H05.122 Orbital myositis, left orbit
    H05.123 Orbital myositis, bilateral
    H05.129 Orbital myositis, unspecified orbit
● H05.2 Exophthalmic conditions
    Bulging eyes
  H05.20 Unspecified exophthalmos
  ● H05.21 Displacement (lateral) of globe
    H05.211 Displacement (lateral) of globe, right eye
    H05.212 Displacement (lateral) of globe, left eye
    H05.213 Displacement (lateral) of globe, bilateral
    H05.219 Displacement (lateral) of globe, unspecified eye
  ● H05.22 Edema of orbit
    Orbital congestion
    H05.221 Edema of right orbit
    H05.222 Edema of left orbit
    H05.223 Edema of bilateral orbit
    H05.229 Edema of unspecified orbit
  ● H05.23 Hemorrhage of orbit
    H05.231 Hemorrhage of right orbit
    H05.232 Hemorrhage of left orbit
    H05.233 Hemorrhage of bilateral orbit
    H05.239 Hemorrhage of unspecified orbit

CHAPTER 7 (H00–H59)

N Newborn Age: 0   P Pediatric Age: 0–17   M Maternity DX: 12–55   A Adult Age: 15–124   ♀ Females Only   ♂ Males Only
🔖 Complication\Comorbidity   🔖 Major C\C   (Ex) CC/MCC Exclusions   🔖 Hospital-Acquired Condition
815

Figure 7-5   Exophthalmos. (From Black JM, Hokanson JH: Medical-Surgical Nursing: Clinical Management for Positive Outcomes, St. Louis, Saunders Elsevier, 2009)

● **H05.24**   **Constant exophthalmos**
     Constant bulging eyes, often symptom of Graves disease
     H05.241   Constant exophthalmos, **right** eye
     H05.242   Constant exophthalmos, **left** eye
     H05.243   Constant exophthalmos, **bilateral**
     H05.249   Constant exophthalmos, **unspecified** eye

● **H05.25**   **Intermittent exophthalmos**
     Intermittent bulging eye occurring with bending forward or sharp turning of head
     H05.251   Intermittent exophthalmos, **right** eye
     H05.252   Intermittent exophthalmos, **left** eye
     H05.253   Intermittent exophthalmos, **bilateral**
     H05.259   Intermittent exophthalmos, **unspecified** eye

● **H05.26**   **Pulsating exophthalmos**
     Bulging eyes with pulsation and bruit, often due to aneurysm pushing eye forward
     H05.261   Pulsating exophthalmos, **right** eye
     H05.262   Pulsating exophthalmos, **left** eye
     H05.263   Pulsating exophthalmos, **bilateral**
     H05.269   Pulsating exophthalmos, **unspecified** eye

● **H05.3**   **Deformity of orbit**
     Excludes1   congenital deformity of orbit (Q10.7)
                hypertelorism (Q75.2)
     H05.30   **Unspecified deformity of orbit**
●   H05.31   **Atrophy of orbit**
     H05.311   Atrophy of **right** orbit
     H05.312   Atrophy of **left** orbit
     H05.313   Atrophy of **bilateral** orbit
     H05.319   Atrophy of **unspecified** orbit
●   H05.32   **Deformity of orbit due to bone disease**
     Code also associated bone disease
     H05.321   Deformity of **right** orbit due to bone disease
     H05.322   Deformity of **left** orbit due to bone disease
     H05.323   Deformity of **bilateral** orbits due to bone disease
     H05.329   Deformity of **unspecified** orbit due to bone disease
●   H05.33   **Deformity of orbit due to trauma or surgery**
     H05.331   Deformity of **right** orbit due to trauma or surgery
     H05.332   Deformity of **left** orbit due to trauma or surgery
     H05.333   Deformity of **bilateral** orbits due to trauma or surgery
     H05.339   Deformity of **unspecified** orbit due to trauma or surgery
●   H05.34   **Enlargement of orbit**
     H05.341   Enlargement of **right** orbit
     H05.342   Enlargement of **left** orbit
     H05.343   Enlargement of **bilateral** orbits
     H05.349   Enlargement of **unspecified** orbit
●   H05.35   **Exostosis of orbit**
     H05.351   Exostosis of **right** orbit
     H05.352   Exostosis of **left** orbit
     H05.353   Exostosis of **bilateral** orbits
     H05.359   Exostosis of **unspecified** orbit

● **H05.4**   **Enophthalmos**
     Recessed eyeball into orbit
●   H05.40   **Unspecified enophthalmos**
     H05.401   Unspecified enophthalmos, **right** eye
     H05.402   Unspecified enophthalmos, **left** eye
     H05.403   Unspecified enophthalmos, **bilateral**
     H05.409   Unspecified enophthalmos, **unspecified** eye
●   H05.41   **Enophthalmos due to atrophy of orbital tissue**
     H05.411   Enophthalmos due to atrophy of orbital tissue, **right** eye
     H05.412   Enophthalmos due to atrophy of orbital tissue, **left** eye
     H05.413   Enophthalmos due to atrophy of orbital tissue, **bilateral**
     H05.419   Enophthalmos due to atrophy of orbital tissue, **unspecified** eye
●   H05.42   **Enophthalmos due to trauma or surgery**
     H05.421   Enophthalmos due to trauma or surgery, **right** eye
     H05.422   Enophthalmos due to trauma or surgery, **left** eye
     H05.423   Enophthalmos due to trauma or surgery, **bilateral**
     H05.429   Enophthalmos due to trauma or surgery, **unspecified** eye

● **H05.5**   **Retained (old) foreign body following penetrating wound of orbit**
     Retrobulbar foreign body
     Use additional code to identify the type of retained foreign body (Z18.-)
     Excludes1   current penetrating wound of orbit (S05.4-)
     Excludes2   retained foreign body of eyelid (H02.81-)
                retained intraocular foreign body (H44.6-, H44.7-)
     H05.50   Retained (old) foreign body following penetrating wound of **unspecified** orbit
     H05.51   Retained (old) foreign body following penetrating wound of **right** orbit
     H05.52   Retained (old) foreign body following penetrating wound of **left** orbit
     H05.53   Retained (old) foreign body following penetrating wound of **bilateral** orbits

● **H05.8**   **Other disorders of orbit**
●   H05.81   **Cyst of orbit**
     Encephalocele of orbit
     H05.811   Cyst of **right** orbit
     H05.812   Cyst of **left** orbit
     H05.813   Cyst of **bilateral** orbits
     H05.819   Cyst of **unspecified** orbit

▶ New   ⇒ Revised   ~~deleted~~ Deleted   Excludes 1   Excludes 2   Includes   Use additional   Code first   Code also   Key words

816

OGCR Official Guidelines   ● Unacceptable Principal Diagnosis   X Assign placeholder X   ● Use Additional Character(s)   ▌ Manifestation Code   **Coding Clinic**

● **H05.82   Myopathy of extraocular muscles**
Weakness of muscles of eye

   H05.821   **Myopathy of extraocular muscles, right orbit**

   H05.822   **Myopathy of extraocular muscles, left orbit**

   H05.823   **Myopathy of extraocular muscles, bilateral**

   H05.829   **Myopathy of extraocular muscles, unspecified orbit**

H05.89   **Other disorders of orbit**

H05.9   **Unspecified disorder of orbit**

DISORDERS OF CONJUNCTIVA (H10-H11)

★ **(See Plate 81, upper, on page 66.)**

● **H10   Conjunctivitis**
Inflammation of membrane of the inside of the eyelid or on surface of eye (conjunctiva)

   Excludes1   keratoconjunctivitis (H16.2-)

● **H10.0   Mucopurulent conjunctivitis**

   ● **H10.01   Acute follicular conjunctivitis**

      H10.011   **Acute follicular conjunctivitis, right eye**

      H10.012   **Acute follicular conjunctivitis, left eye**

      H10.013   **Acute follicular conjunctivitis, bilateral**

      H10.019   **Acute follicular conjunctivitis, unspecified eye**

   ● **H10.02   Other mucopurulent conjunctivitis**

      H10.021   **Other mucopurulent conjunctivitis, right eye**

      H10.022   **Other mucopurulent conjunctivitis, left eye**

      H10.023   **Other mucopurulent conjunctivitis, bilateral**

      H10.029   **Other mucopurulent conjunctivitis, unspecified eye**

● **H10.1   Acute atopic conjunctivitis**
Acute papillary conjunctivitis

   H10.10   **Acute atopic conjunctivitis, unspecified eye**

   H10.11   **Acute atopic conjunctivitis, right eye**

   H10.12   **Acute atopic conjunctivitis, left eye**

   H10.13   **Acute atopic conjunctivitis, bilateral**

● **H10.2   Other acute conjunctivitis**

   ● **H10.21   Acute toxic conjunctivitis**
   Acute chemical conjunctivitis
   Code first (T51-T65) to identify chemical and intent

      Excludes1   burn and corrosion of eye and adnexa (T26.-)

      H10.211   **Acute toxic conjunctivitis, right eye**

      H10.212   **Acute toxic conjunctivitis, left eye**

      H10.213   **Acute toxic conjunctivitis, bilateral**

      H10.219   **Acute toxic conjunctivitis, unspecified eye**

   ● **H10.22   Pseudomembranous conjunctivitis**

      H10.221   **Pseudomembranous conjunctivitis, right eye**

      H10.222   **Pseudomembranous conjunctivitis, left eye**

      H10.223   **Pseudomembranous conjunctivitis, bilateral**

      H10.229   **Pseudomembranous conjunctivitis, unspecified eye**

● **H10.23   Serous conjunctivitis, except viral**

   Excludes1   viral conjunctivitis (B30.-)

      H10.231   **Serous conjunctivitis, except viral, right eye**

      H10.232   **Serous conjunctivitis, except viral, left eye**

      H10.233   **Serous conjunctivitis, except viral, bilateral**

      H10.239   **Serous conjunctivitis, except viral, unspecified eye**

● **H10.3   Unspecified acute conjunctivitis**

   Excludes1   ophthalmia neonatorum NOS (P39.1)

   H10.30   **Unspecified acute conjunctivitis, unspecified eye**

   H10.31   **Unspecified acute conjunctivitis, right eye**

   H10.32   **Unspecified acute conjunctivitis, left eye**

   H10.33   **Unspecified acute conjunctivitis, bilateral**

● **H10.4   Chronic conjunctivitis**

   ● **H10.40   Unspecified chronic conjunctivitis**

      H10.401   **Unspecified chronic conjunctivitis, right eye**

      H10.402   **Unspecified chronic conjunctivitis, left eye**

      H10.403   **Unspecified chronic conjunctivitis, bilateral**

      H10.409   **Unspecified chronic conjunctivitis, unspecified eye**

   ● **H10.41   Chronic giant papillary conjunctivitis**
   Inflammation of membrane of the inside of the eyelid or on surface of eye often associated with contact lens wear

      H10.411   **Chronic giant papillary conjunctivitis, right eye**

      H10.412   **Chronic giant papillary conjunctivitis, left eye**

      H10.413   **Chronic giant papillary conjunctivitis, bilateral**

      H10.419   **Chronic giant papillary conjunctivitis, unspecified eye**

   ● **H10.42   Simple chronic conjunctivitis**

      H10.421   **Simple chronic conjunctivitis, right eye**

      H10.422   **Simple chronic conjunctivitis, left eye**

      H10.423   **Simple chronic conjunctivitis, bilateral**

      H10.429   **Simple chronic conjunctivitis, unspecified eye**

   ● **H10.43   Chronic follicular conjunctivitis**
   Inflammation of membrane of the inside of the eyelid or on surface of eye due to topical medications or infection

      H10.431   **Chronic follicular conjunctivitis, right eye**

      H10.432   **Chronic follicular conjunctivitis, left eye**

      H10.433   **Chronic follicular conjunctivitis, bilateral**

      H10.439   **Chronic follicular conjunctivitis, unspecified eye**

   ● **H10.44   Vernal conjunctivitis**
   Affecting children, especially boys in which there are flattened papules with thick, gelatinous exudate on conjunctivae on inside of upper lid

      Excludes1   vernal keratoconjunctivitis with limbar and corneal involvement (H16.26-)

   H10.45   **Other chronic allergic conjunctivitis**

CHAPTER 7 (H00-H59)

● **H10.5   Blepharoconjunctivitis**
   Inflammation of eyelids and conjunctiva
   ● **H10.50   Unspecified blepharoconjunctivitis**
      H10.501   Unspecified blepharoconjunctivitis, right eye
      H10.502   Unspecified blepharoconjunctivitis, left eye
      H10.503   Unspecified blepharoconjunctivitis, bilateral
      H10.509   Unspecified blepharoconjunctivitis, unspecified eye
   ● **H10.51   Ligneous conjunctivitis**
      H10.511   Ligneous conjunctivitis, right eye
      H10.512   Ligneous conjunctivitis, left eye
      H10.513   Ligneous conjunctivitis, bilateral
      H10.519   Ligneous conjunctivitis, unspecified eye
   ● **H10.52   Angular blepharoconjunctivitis**
      H10.521   Angular blepharoconjunctivitis, right eye
      H10.522   Angular blepharoconjunctivitis, left eye
      H10.523   Angular blepharoconjunctivitis, bilateral
      H10.529   Angular blepharoconjunctivitis, unspecified eye
   ● **H10.53   Contact blepharoconjunctivitis**
      H10.531   Contact blepharoconjunctivitis, right eye
      H10.532   Contact blepharoconjunctivitis, left eye
      H10.533   Contact blepharoconjunctivitis, bilateral
      H10.539   Contact blepharoconjunctivitis, unspecified eye
● **H10.8   Other conjunctivitis**
   ● **H10.81   Pingueculitis**
      Inflammation of a yellow, raised thickening on the white of the eye associated with chronic dry eyes
         Excludes1   pinguecula (H11.15-)
      H10.811   Pingueculitis, right eye
      H10.812   Pingueculitis, left eye
      H10.813   Pingueculitis, bilateral
      H10.819   Pingueculitis, unspecified eye
   H10.89   Other conjunctivitis
   H10.9   Unspecified conjunctivitis
● **H11   Other disorders of conjunctiva**
      Excludes1   keratoconjunctivitis (H16.2-)
   ● **H11.0   Pterygium of eye**
         Excludes1   pseudopterygium (H11.81-)
      ● **H11.00   Unspecified pterygium of eye**
         H11.001   Unspecified pterygium of right eye
         H11.002   Unspecified pterygium of left eye
         H11.003   Unspecified pterygium of eye, bilateral
         H11.009   Unspecified pterygium of unspecified eye
      ● **H11.01   Amyloid pterygium**
         H11.011   Amyloid pterygium of right eye
         H11.012   Amyloid pterygium of left eye
         H11.013   Amyloid pterygium of eye, bilateral
         H11.019   Amyloid pterygium of unspecified eye

Figure 7-6   Double pterygium. Note both nasal and temporal pterygia in a 57-year-old farmer. (From Brightbill FS, McDonnell PJ: Corneal Surgery: Theory, Technique and Tissue, S.l., Mosby Elsevier, 2009)

Item 7-2   Pterygium is Greek for batlike. The condition is characterized by a membrane that extends from the limbus to the center of the cornea and resembles a wing.

● **H11.02   Central pterygium of eye**
   H11.021   Central pterygium of right eye
   H11.022   Central pterygium of left eye
   H11.023   Central pterygium of eye, bilateral
   H11.029   Central pterygium of unspecified eye
● **H11.03   Double pterygium of eye**
   H11.031   Double pterygium of right eye
   H11.032   Double pterygium of left eye
   H11.033   Double pterygium of eye, bilateral
   H11.039   Double pterygium of unspecified eye
● **H11.04   Peripheral pterygium of eye, stationary**
   H11.041   Peripheral pterygium, stationary, right eye
   H11.042   Peripheral pterygium, stationary, left eye
   H11.043   Peripheral pterygium, stationary, bilateral
   H11.049   Peripheral pterygium, stationary, unspecified eye
● **H11.05   Peripheral pterygium of eye, progressive**
   H11.051   Peripheral pterygium, progressive, right eye
   H11.052   Peripheral pterygium, progressive, left eye
   H11.053   Peripheral pterygium, progressive, bilateral
   H11.059   Peripheral pterygium, progressive, unspecified eye
● **H11.06   Recurrent pterygium of eye**
   H11.061   Recurrent pterygium of right eye
   H11.062   Recurrent pterygium of left eye
   H11.063   Recurrent pterygium of eye, bilateral
   H11.069   Recurrent pterygium of unspecified eye
● **H11.1   Conjunctival degenerations and deposits**
      Excludes2   pseudopterygium (H11.81)
   H11.10   Unspecified conjunctival degenerations
   ● **H11.11   Conjunctival deposits**
      H11.111   Conjunctival deposits, right eye
      H11.112   Conjunctival deposits, left eye
      H11.113   Conjunctival deposits, bilateral
      H11.119   Conjunctival deposits, unspecified eye
   ● **H11.12   Conjunctival concretions**
      White to yellow nodules within or beneath conjunctiva
      H11.121   Conjunctival concretions, right eye
      H11.122   Conjunctival concretions, left eye
      H11.123   Conjunctival concretions, bilateral
      H11.129   Conjunctival concretions, unspecified eye
   ● **H11.13   Conjunctival pigmentations**
      Conjunctival argyrosis [argyria]
      H11.131   Conjunctival pigmentations, right eye
      H11.132   Conjunctival pigmentations, left eye
      H11.133   Conjunctival pigmentations, bilateral
      H11.139   Conjunctival pigmentations, unspecified eye

▶ New   ⇒ Revised   ~~deleted~~ Deleted   Excludes 1   Excludes 2   Includes   Use additional   Code first   Code also   Key words

818   OGCR Official Guidelines   ● Unacceptable Principal Diagnosis   X Assign placeholder X   ● Use Additional Character(s)   ▶ Manifestation Code   Coding Clinic

● **H11.14 Conjunctival xerosis, unspecified**
> **Excludes1**   xerosis of conjunctiva due to vitamin A deficiency (E50.0, E50.1)

    H11.141   Conjunctival xerosis, unspecified, **right eye**

    H11.142   Conjunctival xerosis, unspecified, **left eye**

    H11.143   Conjunctival xerosis, unspecified, **bilateral**

    H11.149   Conjunctival xerosis, unspecified, **unspecified eye**

● **H11.15 Pinguecula**
> *Yellowish spot near sclerocorneal junction, usually on nasal side; associated with aging*
> **Excludes1**   pingueculitis (H10.81-)

    H11.151   Pinguecula, **right eye**

    H11.152   Pinguecula, **left eye**

    H11.153   Pinguecula, **bilateral**

    H11.159   Pinguecula, **unspecified eye**

● **H11.2 Conjunctival scars**

    ● **H11.21 Conjunctival adhesions and strands (localized)**

       H11.211   Conjunctival adhesions and strands (localized), **right eye**

       H11.212   Conjunctival adhesions and strands (localized), **left eye**

       H11.213   Conjunctival adhesions and strands (localized), **bilateral**

       H11.219   Conjunctival adhesions and strands (localized), **unspecified eye**

    ● **H11.22 Conjunctival granuloma**

       H11.221   Conjunctival granuloma, **right eye**

       H11.222   Conjunctival granuloma, **left eye**

       H11.223   Conjunctival granuloma, **bilateral**

       H11.229   Conjunctival granuloma, **unspecified**

    ● **H11.23 Symblepharon**
> *Adhesion between tarsal conjunctiva and bulbar conjunctiva*

       H11.231   Symblepharon, **right eye**

       H11.232   Symblepharon, **left eye**

       H11.233   Symblepharon, **bilateral**

       H11.239   Symblepharon, **unspecified eye**

    ● **H11.24 Scarring of conjunctiva**

       H11.241   Scarring of conjunctiva, **right eye**

       H11.242   Scarring of conjunctiva, **left eye**

       H11.243   Scarring of conjunctiva, **bilateral**

       H11.249   Scarring of conjunctiva, **unspecified eye**

● **H11.3 Conjunctival hemorrhage**
> Subconjunctival hemorrhage

    H11.30   Conjunctival hemorrhage, **unspecified eye**

    H11.31   Conjunctival hemorrhage, **right eye**

    H11.32   Conjunctival hemorrhage, **left eye**

    H11.33   Conjunctival hemorrhage, **bilateral**

● **H11.4 Other conjunctival vascular disorders and cysts**

    ● **H11.41 Vascular abnormalities of conjunctiva**
> Conjunctival aneurysm

       H11.411   Vascular abnormalities of conjunctiva, **right eye**

       H11.412   Vascular abnormalities of conjunctiva, **left eye**

       H11.413   Vascular abnormalities of conjunctiva, **bilateral**

       H11.419   Vascular abnormalities of conjunctiva, **unspecified eye**

● **H11.42 Conjunctival edema**

    H11.421   Conjunctival edema, **right eye**

    H11.422   Conjunctival edema, **left eye**

    H11.423   Conjunctival edema, **bilateral**

    H11.429   Conjunctival edema, **unspecified eye**

● **H11.43 Conjunctival hyperemia**

    H11.431   Conjunctival hyperemia, **right eye**

    H11.432   Conjunctival hyperemia, **left eye**

    H11.433   Conjunctival hyperemia, **bilateral**

    H11.439   Conjunctival hyperemia, **unspecified eye**

● **H11.44 Conjunctival cysts**

    H11.441   Conjunctival cysts, **right eye**

    H11.442   Conjunctival cysts, **left eye**

    H11.443   Conjunctival cysts, **bilateral**

    H11.449   Conjunctival cysts, **unspecified eye**

● **H11.8 Other specified disorders of conjunctiva**

    ● **H11.81 Pseudopterygium of conjunctiva**
> *Conjunctival scar attached to cornea*

       H11.811   Pseudopterygium of conjunctiva, **right eye**

       H11.812   Pseudopterygium of conjunctiva, **left eye**

       H11.813   Pseudopterygium of conjunctiva, **bilateral**

       H11.819   Pseudopterygium of conjunctiva, **unspecified eye**

    ● **H11.82 Conjunctivochalasis**
> *Conjunctiva bulges over eyelid margin or covers lower punctum*

       H11.821   Conjunctivochalasis, **right eye**

       H11.822   Conjunctivochalasis, **left eye**

       H11.823   Conjunctivochalasis, **bilateral**

       H11.829   Conjunctivochalasis, **unspecified eye**

    H11.89   **Other specified disorders of conjunctiva**

    H11.9   **Unspecified disorder of conjunctiva**

DISORDERS OF SCLERA, CORNEA, IRIS AND CILIARY BODY (H15-H22)

● **H15 Disorders of sclera**

    ● **H15.0 Scleritis**
> *Inflammation of the white (sclera and episclera) of the eye.*

       ● **H15.00 Unspecified scleritis**

          H15.001   Unspecified scleritis, **right eye**

          H15.002   Unspecified scleritis, **left eye**

          H15.003   Unspecified scleritis, **bilateral**

          H15.009   Unspecified scleritis, **unspecified eye**

       ● **H15.01 Anterior scleritis**

          H15.011   Anterior scleritis, **right eye**

          H15.012   Anterior scleritis, **left eye**

          H15.013   Anterior scleritis, **bilateral**

          H15.019   Anterior scleritis, **unspecified eye**

       ● **H15.02 Brawny scleritis**
> *Swelling around the cornea that is gelantinous in appearance*

          H15.021   Brawny scleritis, **right eye**

          H15.022   Brawny scleritis, **left eye**

          H15.023   Brawny scleritis, **bilateral**

          H15.029   Brawny scleritis, **unspecified eye**

       ● **H15.03 Posterior scleritis**
> Sclerotenonitis

          H15.031   Posterior scleritis, **right eye**

          H15.032   Posterior scleritis, **left eye**

          H15.033   Posterior scleritis, **bilateral**

          H15.039   Posterior scleritis, **unspecified eye**

N Newborn Age: 0   **P** Pediatric Age: 0–17   **M** Maternity DX: 12–55   **A** Adult Age: 15–124   ♀ Females Only   ♂ Males Only

Complication\Comorbidity   Major C\C   (Ex) CC/MCC Exclusions   Hospital-Acquired Condition

CHAPTER 7 (H00-H59)

819

● H15.04   Scleritis with corneal involvement
    H15.041   Scleritis with corneal involvement, right eye
    H15.042   Scleritis with corneal involvement, left eye
    H15.043   Scleritis with corneal involvement, bilateral
    H15.049   Scleritis with corneal involvement, unspecified eye

● H15.05   Scleromalacia perforans
    Necrotic without inflammation; usually associated with rheumatoid arthritis
    H15.051   Scleromalacia perforans, right eye
    H15.052   Scleromalacia perforans, left eye
    H15.053   Scleromalacia perforans, bilateral
    H15.059   Scleromalacia perforans, unspecified eye

● H15.09   Other scleritis
    Scleral abscess
    H15.091   Other scleritis, right eye
    H15.092   Other scleritis, left eye
    H15.093   Other scleritis, bilateral
    H15.099   Other scleritis, unspecified eye

● H15.1   Episcleritis
    Inflammation of the white (sclera and episclera) of the eye.

● H15.10   Unspecified episcleritis
    H15.101   Unspecified episcleritis, right eye
    H15.102   Unspecified episcleritis, left eye
    H15.103   Unspecified episcleritis, bilateral
    H15.109   Unspecified episcleritis, unspecified eye

● H15.11   Episcleritis periodica fugax
    Transient, recurrent inflammation of portion of episclera (connective tissue on the surface of the sclera)
    H15.111   Episcleritis periodica fugax, right eye
    H15.112   Episcleritis periodica fugax, left eye
    H15.113   Episcleritis periodica fugax, bilateral
    H15.119   Episcleritis periodica fugax, unspecified eye

● H15.12   Nodular episcleritis
    Characterized by tender, localized, moveable nodule within inflamed area
    H15.121   Nodular episcleritis, right eye
    H15.122   Nodular episcleritis, left eye
    H15.123   Nodular episcleritis, bilateral
    H15.129   Nodular episcleritis, unspecified eye

● H15.8   Other disorders of sclera
    Excludes2   blue sclera (Q13.5)
                degenerative myopia (H44.2-)

● H15.81   Equatorial staphyloma
    H15.811   Equatorial staphyloma, right eye
    H15.812   Equatorial staphyloma, left eye
    H15.813   Equatorial staphyloma, bilateral
    H15.819   Equatorial staphyloma, unspecified eye

● H15.82   Localized anterior staphyloma
    H15.821   Localized anterior staphyloma, right eye
    H15.822   Localized anterior staphyloma, left eye
    H15.823   Localized anterior staphyloma, bilateral
    H15.829   Localized anterior staphyloma, unspecified eye

● H15.83   Staphyloma posticum
    H15.831   Staphyloma posticum, right eye
    H15.832   Staphyloma posticum, left eye
    H15.833   Staphyloma posticum, bilateral
    H15.839   Staphyloma posticum, unspecified eye

● H15.84   Scleral ectasia
    H15.841   Scleral ectasia, right eye
    H15.842   Scleral ectasia, left eye
    H15.843   Scleral ectasia, bilateral
    H15.849   Scleral ectasia, unspecified eye

● H15.85   Ring staphyloma
    H15.851   Ring staphyloma, right eye
    H15.852   Ring staphyloma, left eye
    H15.853   Ring staphyloma, bilateral
    H15.859   Ring staphyloma, unspecified eye

  H15.89   Other disorders of sclera
  H15.9   Unspecified disorder of sclera

● H16   Keratitis
● H16.0   Corneal ulcer

● H16.00   Unspecified corneal ulcer
    H16.001   Unspecified corneal ulcer, right eye
    H16.002   Unspecified corneal ulcer, left eye
    H16.003   Unspecified corneal ulcer, bilateral
    H16.009   Unspecified corneal ulcer, unspecified eye

● H16.01   Central corneal ulcer
    H16.011   Central corneal ulcer, right eye
    H16.012   Central corneal ulcer, left eye
    H16.013   Central corneal ulcer, bilateral
    H16.019   Central corneal ulcer, unspecified eye

● H16.02   Ring corneal ulcer
    H16.021   Ring corneal ulcer, right eye
    H16.022   Ring corneal ulcer, left eye
    H16.023   Ring corneal ulcer, bilateral
    H16.029   Ring corneal ulcer, unspecified eye

● H16.03   Corneal ulcer with hypopyon
    H16.031   Corneal ulcer with hypopyon, right eye
    H16.032   Corneal ulcer with hypopyon, left eye
    H16.033   Corneal ulcer with hypopyon, bilateral
    H16.039   Corneal ulcer with hypopyon, unspecified eye

Marginal   Ring   Central   Rosacea   Mooren's
(catarrhal) ulcer   ulcer   corneal ulcer   ulcer   (rodent) ulcer

Figure 7-7   Corneal ulcers: marginal, ring, central corneal, rosacea, and Mooren's.

Item 7-3   An infected ulcer is usually called a **serpiginous** or **hypopyon** ulcer which is a pus sac in the anterior chamber of the eye. **Marginal** ulcers are usually asymptomatic, not primary, and are often superficial and simple. More severe marginal ulcers spread to form a ring ulcer. **Ring** ulcers can extend around the entire corneal periphery. **Central corneal** ulcers develop when there is an abrasion to the epithelium and an infection develops in the eroded area. The **pyocyaneal** ulcer is the most serious corneal infection, which, if left untreated, can lead to loss of the eye.

▶ New   ➡ Revised   ~~deleted~~ Deleted   Excludes 1   Excludes 2   Includes   Use additional   Code first   Code also   Key words
OGCR Official Guidelines   ● Unacceptable Principal Diagnosis   X Assign placeholder X   ● Use Additional Character(s)   ▶ Manifestation Code   **Coding Clinic**

● **H16.04   Marginal corneal ulcer**
     H16.041   Marginal corneal ulcer, right eye
     H16.042   Marginal corneal ulcer, left eye
     H16.043   Marginal corneal ulcer, bilateral
     H16.049   Marginal corneal ulcer, unspecified eye

● **H16.05   Mooren's corneal ulcer**
     H16.051   Mooren's corneal ulcer, right eye
     H16.052   Mooren's corneal ulcer, left eye
     H16.053   Mooren's corneal ulcer, bilateral
     H16.059   Mooren's corneal ulcer, unspecified eye

● **H16.06   Mycotic corneal ulcer**
     H16.061   Mycotic corneal ulcer, right eye
     H16.062   Mycotic corneal ulcer, left eye
     H16.063   Mycotic corneal ulcer, bilateral
     H16.069   Mycotic corneal ulcer, unspecified eye

● **H16.07   Perforated corneal ulcer**
     H16.071   Perforated corneal ulcer, right eye
     H16.072   Perforated corneal ulcer, left eye
     H16.073   Perforated corneal ulcer, bilateral
     H16.079   Perforated corneal ulcer, unspecified eye

● **H16.1   Other and unspecified superficial keratitis without conjunctivitis**

● **H16.10   Unspecified superficial keratitis**
     H16.101   Unspecified superficial keratitis, right eye
     H16.102   Unspecified superficial keratitis, left eye
     H16.103   Unspecified superficial keratitis, bilateral
     H16.109   Unspecified superficial keratitis, unspecified eye

● **H16.11   Macular keratitis**
     Areolar keratitis
     Nummular keratitis
     Stellate keratitis
     Striate keratitis
     H16.111   Macular keratitis, right eye
     H16.112   Macular keratitis, left eye
     H16.113   Macular keratitis, bilateral
     H16.119   Macular keratitis, unspecified eye

● **H16.12   Filamentary keratitis**
     H16.121   Filamentary keratitis, right eye
     H16.122   Filamentary keratitis, left eye
     H16.123   Filamentary keratitis, bilateral
     H16.129   Filamentary keratitis, unspecified eye

● **H16.13   Photokeratitis**
     Snow blindness
     Welders' keratitis
     H16.131   Photokeratitis, right eye
     H16.132   Photokeratitis, left eye
     H16.133   Photokeratitis, bilateral
     H16.139   Photokeratitis, unspecified eye

● **H16.14   Punctate keratitis**
     H16.141   Punctate keratitis, right eye
     H16.142   Punctate keratitis, left eye
     H16.143   Punctate keratitis, bilateral
     H16.149   Punctate keratitis, unspecified eye

● **H16.2   Keratoconjunctivitis**

● **H16.20   Unspecified keratoconjunctivitis**
     Superficial keratitis with conjunctivitis NOS
     H16.201   Unspecified keratoconjunctivitis, right eye
     H16.202   Unspecified keratoconjunctivitis, left eye
     H16.203   Unspecified keratoconjunctivitis, bilateral
     H16.209   Unspecified keratoconjunctivitis, unspecified eye

● **H16.21   Exposure keratoconjunctivitis**
     H16.211   Exposure keratoconjunctivitis, right eye
     H16.212   Exposure keratoconjunctivitis, left eye
     H16.213   Exposure keratoconjunctivitis, bilateral
     H16.219   Exposure keratoconjunctivitis, unspecified eye

● **H16.22   Keratoconjunctivitis sicca, not specified as Sjögren's**
     Excludes1   Sjogren's syndrome (M35.01)
     H16.221   Keratoconjunctivitis sicca, not specified as Sjögren's, right eye
     H16.222   Keratoconjunctivitis sicca, not specified as Sjögren's, left eye
     H16.223   Keratoconjunctivitis sicca, not specified as Sjögren's, bilateral
     H16.229   Keratoconjunctivitis sicca, not specified as Sjögren's, unspecified eye

● **H16.23   Neurotrophic keratoconjunctivitis**
     H16.231   Neurotrophic keratoconjunctivitis, right eye
     H16.232   Neurotrophic keratoconjunctivitis, left eye
     H16.233   Neurotrophic keratoconjunctivitis, bilateral
     H16.239   Neurotrophic keratoconjunctivitis, unspecified eye

● **H16.24   Ophthalmia nodosa**
     H16.241   Ophthalmia nodosa, right eye
     H16.242   Ophthalmia nodosa, left eye
     H16.243   Ophthalmia nodosa, bilateral
     H16.249   Ophthalmia nodosa, unspecified eye

● **H16.25   Phlyctenular keratoconjunctivitis**
     H16.251   Phlyctenular keratoconjunctivitis, right eye
     H16.252   Phlyctenular keratoconjunctivitis, left eye
     H16.253   Phlyctenular keratoconjunctivitis, bilateral
     H16.259   Phlyctenular keratoconjunctivitis, unspecified eye

● **H16.26   Vernal keratoconjunctivitis, with limbar and corneal involvement**
     Excludes1   vernal conjunctivitis without limbar and corneal involvement (H10.44)
     H16.261   Vernal keratoconjunctivitis, with limbar and corneal involvement, right eye
     H16.262   Vernal keratoconjunctivitis, with limbar and corneal involvement, left eye

CHAPTER 7 (H00–H59)

N   Newborn Age: 0   P   Pediatric Age: 0–17   M   Maternity DX: 12–55   A   Adult Age: 15–124   ♀   Females Only   ♂   Males Only
🦠 Complication\Comorbidity   🦠 Major C\C   (Ex)   CC/MCC Exclusions   🦠 Hospital-Acquired Condition

H16.263   Vernal keratoconjunctivitis, with limbar and corneal involvement, bilateral

H16.269   Vernal keratoconjunctivitis, with limbar and corneal involvement, unspecified eye

● H16.29 Other keratoconjunctivitis

H16.291   Other keratoconjunctivitis, right eye

H16.292   Other keratoconjunctivitis, left eye

H16.293   Other keratoconjunctivitis, bilateral

H16.299   Other keratoconjunctivitis, unspecified eye

● H16.3 Interstitial and deep keratitis

● H16.30 Unspecified interstitial keratitis

H16.301   Unspecified interstitial keratitis, right eye

H16.302   Unspecified interstitial keratitis, left eye

H16.303   Unspecified interstitial keratitis, bilateral

H16.309   Unspecified interstitial keratitis, unspecified eye

● H16.31 Corneal abscess

H16.311   Corneal abscess, right eye

H16.312   Corneal abscess, left eye

H16.313   Corneal abscess, bilateral

H16.319   Corneal abscess, unspecified eye

● H16.32 Diffuse interstitial keratitis
      Cogan's syndrome

H16.321   Diffuse interstitial keratitis, right eye

H16.322   Diffuse interstitial keratitis, left eye

H16.323   Diffuse interstitial keratitis, bilateral

H16.329   Diffuse interstitial keratitis, unspecified eye

● H16.33 Sclerosing keratitis

H16.331   Sclerosing keratitis, right eye

H16.332   Sclerosing keratitis, left eye

H16.333   Sclerosing keratitis, bilateral

H16.339   Sclerosing keratitis, unspecified eye

● H16.39 Other interstitial and deep keratitis

H16.391   Other interstitial and deep keratitis, right eye

H16.392   Other interstitial and deep keratitis, left eye

H16.393   Other interstitial and deep keratitis, bilateral

H16.399   Other interstitial and deep keratitis, unspecified eye

● H16.4 Corneal neovascularization

● H16.40 Unspecified corneal neovascularization

H16.401   Unspecified corneal neovascularization, right eye

H16.402   Unspecified corneal neovascularization, left eye

H16.403   Unspecified corneal neovascularization, bilateral

H16.409   Unspecified corneal neovascularization, unspecified eye

● H16.41 Ghost vessels (corneal)

H16.411   Ghost vessels (corneal), right eye

H16.412   Ghost vessels (corneal), left eye

H16.413   Ghost vessels (corneal), bilateral

H16.419   Ghost vessels (corneal), unspecified eye

● H16.42 Pannus (corneal)

H16.421   Pannus (corneal), right eye

H16.422   Pannus (corneal), left eye

H16.423   Pannus (corneal), bilateral

H16.429   Pannus (corneal), unspecified eye

● H16.43 Localized vascularization of cornea

H16.431   Localized vascularization of cornea, right eye

H16.432   Localized vascularization of cornea, left eye

H16.433   Localized vascularization of cornea, bilateral

H16.439   Localized vascularization of cornea, unspecified eye

● H16.44 Deep vascularization of cornea

H16.441   Deep vascularization of cornea, right eye

H16.442   Deep vascularization of cornea, left eye

H16.443   Deep vascularization of cornea, bilateral

H16.449   Deep vascularization of cornea, unspecified eye

● H16.8 Other keratitis

H16.9 Unspecified keratitis

● H17 Corneal scars and opacities

● H17.0 Adherent leukoma

H17.00   Adherent leukoma, unspecified eye

H17.01   Adherent leukoma, right eye

H17.02   Adherent leukoma, left eye

H17.03   Adherent leukoma, bilateral

● H17.1 Central corneal opacity

H17.10   Central corneal opacity, unspecified eye

H17.11   Central corneal opacity, right eye

H17.12   Central corneal opacity, left eye

H17.13   Central corneal opacity, bilateral

● H17.8 Other corneal scars and opacities

● H17.81 Minor opacity of cornea
      Corneal nebula

H17.811   Minor opacity of cornea, right eye

H17.812   Minor opacity of cornea, left eye

H17.813   Minor opacity of cornea, bilateral

H17.819   Minor opacity of cornea, unspecified eye

● H17.82 Peripheral opacity of cornea

H17.821   Peripheral opacity of cornea, right eye

H17.822   Peripheral opacity of cornea, left eye

H17.823   Peripheral opacity of cornea, bilateral

H17.829   Peripheral opacity of cornea, unspecified eye

H17.89   Other corneal scars and opacities

H17.9 Unspecified corneal scar and opacity

● H18 Other disorders of cornea

● H18.0 Corneal pigmentations and deposits

● H18.00 Unspecified corneal deposit

H18.001   Unspecified corneal deposit, right eye

H18.002   Unspecified corneal deposit, left eye

H18.003   Unspecified corneal deposit, bilateral

H18.009   Unspecified corneal deposit, unspecified eye

● H18.01 Anterior corneal pigmentations
      Staehli's line

H18.011   Anterior corneal pigmentations, right eye

H18.012   Anterior corneal pigmentations, left eye

▶ New   ⇒ Revised   deleted Deleted   Excludes 1   Excludes 2   Includes   Use additional   Code first   Code also   Key words

OGCR Official Guidelines   ● Unacceptable Principal Diagnosis   X Assign placeholder X   ● Use Additional Character(s)   ▷ Manifestation Code   Coding Clinic

H18.013   **Anterior corneal pigmentations, bilateral**

H18.019   **Anterior corneal pigmentations, unspecified eye**

● H18.02   Argentous corneal deposits

    H18.021   Argentous corneal deposits, right eye

    H18.022   Argentous corneal deposits, left eye

    H18.023   Argentous corneal deposits, bilateral

    H18.029   Argentous corneal deposits, unspecified eye

● H18.03   Corneal deposits in metabolic disorders

    Code also associated metabolic disorder

    H18.031   Corneal deposits in metabolic disorders, right eye

    H18.032   Corneal deposits in metabolic disorders, left eye

    H18.033   Corneal deposits in metabolic disorders, bilateral

    H18.039   Corneal deposits in metabolic disorders, unspecified eye

● H18.04   Kayser-Fleischer ring

    Code also associated Wilson's disease (E83.01)

    H18.041   Kayser-Fleischer ring, right eye

    H18.042   Kayser-Fleischer ring, left eye

    H18.043   Kayser-Fleischer ring, bilateral

    H18.049   Kayser-Fleischer ring, unspecified eye

● H18.05   Posterior corneal pigmentations

    Krukenberg's spindle

    H18.051   Posterior corneal pigmentations, right eye

    H18.052   Posterior corneal pigmentations, left eye

    H18.053   Posterior corneal pigmentations, bilateral

    H18.059   Posterior corneal pigmentations, unspecified eye

● H18.06   Stromal corneal pigmentations

    Hematocornea

    H18.061   Stromal corneal pigmentations, right eye

    H18.062   Stromal corneal pigmentations, left eye

    H18.063   Stromal corneal pigmentations, bilateral

    H18.069   Stromal corneal pigmentations, unspecified eye

● H18.1   Bullous keratopathy

    H18.10   Bullous keratopathy, unspecified eye

    H18.11   Bullous keratopathy, right eye

    H18.12   Bullous keratopathy, left eye

    H18.13   Bullous keratopathy, bilateral

● H18.2   Other and unspecified corneal edema

    H18.20   Unspecified corneal edema

   ● H18.21   Corneal edema secondary to contact lens

     Excludes2   other corneal disorders due to contact lens (H18.82-)

    H18.211   Corneal edema secondary to contact lens, right eye

    H18.212   Corneal edema secondary to contact lens, left eye

    H18.213   Corneal edema secondary to contact lens, bilateral

    H18.219   Corneal edema secondary to contact lens, unspecified eye

● H18.22   Idiopathic corneal edema

    H18.221   Idiopathic corneal edema, right eye

    H18.222   Idiopathic corneal edema, left eye

    H18.223   Idiopathic corneal edema, bilateral

    H18.229   Idiopathic corneal edema, unspecified eye

● H18.23   Secondary corneal edema

    H18.231   Secondary corneal edema, right eye

    H18.232   Secondary corneal edema, left eye

    H18.233   Secondary corneal edema, bilateral

    H18.239   Secondary corneal edema, unspecified eye

● H18.3   Changes of corneal membranes

    H18.30   Unspecified corneal membrane change

   ● H18.31   Folds and rupture in Bowman's membrane

    H18.311   Folds and rupture in Bowman's membrane, right eye

    H18.312   Folds and rupture in Bowman's membrane, left eye

    H18.313   Folds and rupture in Bowman's membrane, bilateral

    H18.319   Folds and rupture in Bowman's membrane, unspecified eye

   ● H18.32   Folds in Descemet's membrane

    H18.321   Folds in Descemet's membrane, right eye

    H18.322   Folds in Descemet's membrane, left eye

    H18.323   Folds in Descemet's membrane, bilateral

    H18.329   Folds in Descemet's membrane, unspecified eye

   ● H18.33   Rupture in Descemet's membrane

    H18.331   Rupture in Descemet's membrane, right eye

    H18.332   Rupture in Descemet's membrane, left eye

    H18.333   Rupture in Descemet's membrane, bilateral

    H18.339   Rupture in Descemet's membrane, unspecified eye

● H18.4   Corneal degeneration

    Excludes1   Mooren's ulcer (H16.0-)

              recurrent erosion of cornea (H18.83-)

    H18.40   Unspecified corneal degeneration

   ● H18.41   Arcus senilis

    Senile corneal changes

    H18.411   Arcus senilis, right eye

    H18.412   Arcus senilis, left eye

    H18.413   Arcus senilis, bilateral

    H18.419   Arcus senilis, unspecified eye

   ● H18.42   Band keratopathy

    H18.421   Band keratopathy, right eye

    H18.422   Band keratopathy, left eye

    H18.423   Band keratopathy, bilateral

    H18.429   Band keratopathy, unspecified eye

    H18.43   Other calcerous corneal degeneration

   ● H18.44   Keratomalacia

    Excludes1   keratomalacia due to vitamin A deficiency (E50.4)

    H18.441   Keratomalacia, right eye

    H18.442   Keratomalacia, left eye

    H18.443   Keratomalacia, bilateral

    H18.449   Keratomalacia, unspecified eye

CHAPTER 7 (H00-H59)

● H18.45   Nodular corneal degeneration
    H18.451   Nodular corneal degeneration, right eye
    H18.452   Nodular corneal degeneration, left eye
    H18.453   Nodular corneal degeneration, bilateral
    H18.459   Nodular corneal degeneration, unspecified eye

● H18.46   Peripheral corneal degeneration
    H18.461   Peripheral corneal degeneration, right eye
    H18.462   Peripheral corneal degeneration, left eye
    H18.463   Peripheral corneal degeneration, bilateral
    H18.469   Peripheral corneal degeneration, unspecified eye

    H18.49   Other corneal degeneration

● H18.5   Hereditary corneal dystrophies
    H18.50   Unspecified hereditary corneal dystrophies
    H18.51   Endothelial corneal dystrophy
       Fuchs' dystrophy
    H18.52   Epithelial (juvenile) corneal dystrophy
    H18.53   Granular corneal dystrophy
    H18.54   Lattice corneal dystrophy
    H18.55   Macular corneal dystrophy
    H18.59   Other hereditary corneal dystrophies

● H18.6   Keratoconus
 ● H18.60   Keratoconus, unspecified
    H18.601   Keratoconus, unspecified, right eye
    H18.602   Keratoconus, unspecified, left eye
    H18.603   Keratoconus, unspecified, bilateral
    H18.609   Keratoconus, unspecified, unspecified eye

 ● H18.61   Keratoconus, stable
    H18.611   Keratoconus, stable, right eye
    H18.612   Keratoconus, stable, left eye
    H18.613   Keratoconus, stable, bilateral
    H18.619   Keratoconus, stable, unspecified eye

 ● H18.62   Keratoconus, unstable
       Acute hydrops
    H18.621   Keratoconus, unstable, right eye
    H18.622   Keratoconus, unstable, left eye
    H18.623   Keratoconus, unstable, bilateral
    H18.629   Keratoconus, unstable, unspecified eye

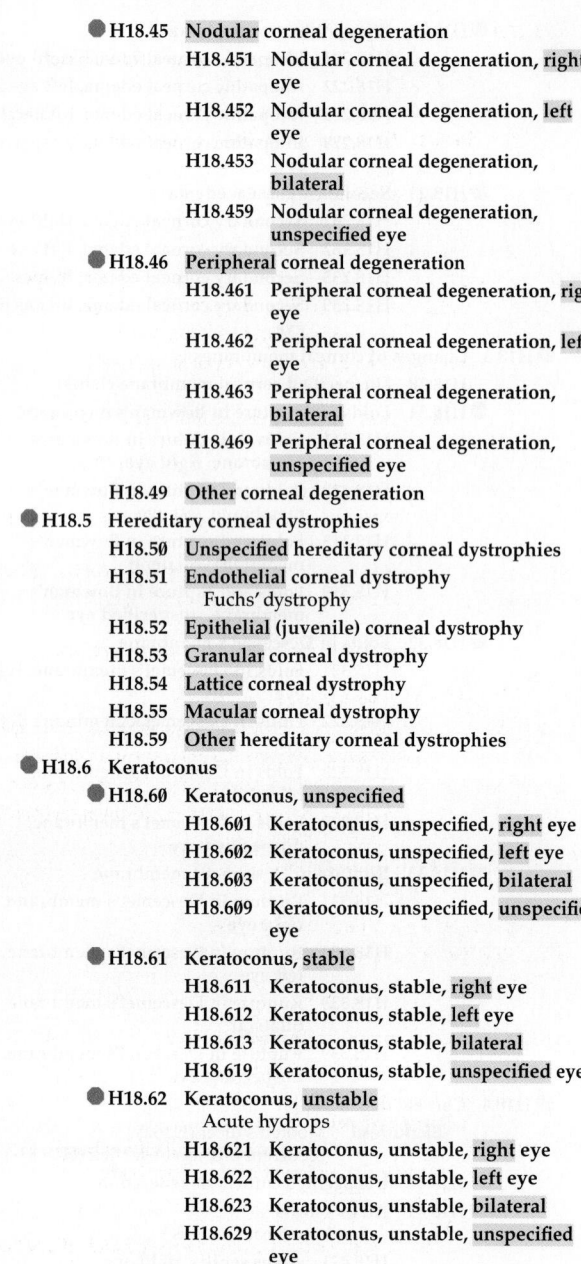

Figure 7-8 Lateral view of the displacement of the cone apex in keratoconus. (From Yanoff: Ophthalmology, ed 3, Mosby, Inc., 2008)

Item 7–4 Keratoconus results in corneal degeneration that begins in childhood, gradually changes the cornea from a round to cone shape, decreasing visual acuity. Treatment includes contact lenses. In severe cases the need for corneal transplant may be the treatment of choice; however, newer technologies may use high frequency radio energy to shrink the edges of the cornea, pulling the central area back to a more normal shape. It can help delay or avoid the need for a corneal transplantation.

● H18.7   Other and unspecified corneal deformities
   Excludes1   congenital malformations of cornea (Q13.3-Q13.4)
    H18.70   Unspecified corneal deformity

● H18.71   Corneal ectasia
    H18.711   Corneal ectasia, right eye
    H18.712   Corneal ectasia, left eye
    H18.713   Corneal ectasia, bilateral
    H18.719   Corneal ectasia, unspecified eye

● H18.72   Corneal staphyloma
    H18.721   Corneal staphyloma, right eye
    H18.722   Corneal staphyloma, left eye
    H18.723   Corneal staphyloma, bilateral
    H18.729   Corneal staphyloma, unspecified eye

● H18.73   Descemetocele
    H18.731   Descemetocele, right eye
    H18.732   Descemetocele, left eye
    H18.733   Descemetocele, bilateral
    H18.739   Descemetocele, unspecified eye

● H18.79   Other corneal deformities
    H18.791   Other corneal deformities, right eye
    H18.792   Other corneal deformities, left eye
    H18.793   Other corneal deformities, bilateral
    H18.799   Other corneal deformities, unspecified eye

● H18.8   Other specified disorders of cornea
 ● H18.81   Anesthesia and hypoesthesia of cornea
    H18.811   Anesthesia and hypoesthesia of cornea, right eye
    H18.812   Anesthesia and hypoesthesia of cornea, left eye
    H18.813   Anesthesia and hypoesthesia of cornea, bilateral
    H18.819   Anesthesia and hypoesthesia of cornea, unspecified eye

 ● H18.82   Corneal disorder due to contact lens
   Excludes2   corneal edema due to contact lens (H18.21-)
    H18.821   Corneal disorder due to contact lens, right eye
    H18.822   Corneal disorder due to contact lens, left eye
    H18.823   Corneal disorder due to contact lens, bilateral
    H18.829   Corneal disorder due to contact lens, unspecified eye

 ● H18.83   Recurrent erosion of cornea
    H18.831   Recurrent erosion of cornea, right eye
    H18.832   Recurrent erosion of cornea, left eye
    H18.833   Recurrent erosion of cornea, bilateral
    H18.839   Recurrent erosion of cornea, unspecified eye

 ● H18.89   Other specified disorders of cornea
    H18.891   Other specified disorders of cornea, right eye
    H18.892   Other specified disorders of cornea, left eye
    H18.893   Other specified disorders of cornea, bilateral
    H18.899   Other specified disorders of cornea, unspecified eye

H18.9   Unspecified disorder of cornea

▶ New   ⟼ Revised   ~~deleted~~ Deleted   Excludes 1   Excludes 2   Includes   Use additional   Code first   Code also   Key words

OGCR Official Guidelines   ● Unacceptable Principal Diagnosis   X Assign placeholder X   ● Use Additional Character(s)   ▶ Manifestation Code   **Coding Clinic**

● **H20   Iridocyclitis**
  ● **H20.0   Acute and subacute iridocyclitis**
     Acute anterior uveitis
     Acute cyclitis
     Acute iritis
     Subacute anterior uveitis
     Subacute cyclitis
     Subacute iritis
     Excludes1   iridocyclitis, iritis, uveitis (due to) (in)
         diabetes mellitus (E08-E13 with .39)
       iridocyclitis, iritis, uveitis (due to) (in)
         diphtheria (A36.89)
       iridocyclitis, iritis, uveitis (due to) (in)
         gonococcal (A54.32)
       iridocyclitis, iritis, uveitis (due to) (in)
         herpes (simplex) (B00.51)
       iridocyclitis, iritis, uveitis (due to) (in)
         herpes zoster (B02.32)
       iridocyclitis, iritis, uveitis (due to) (in)
         late congenital syphilis (A50.39)
       iridocyclitis, iritis, uveitis (due to) (in)
         late syphilis (A52.71)
       iridocyclitis, iritis, uveitis (due to) (in)
         sarcoidosis (D86.83)
       iridocyclitis, iritis, uveitis (due to) (in)
         syphilis (A51.43)
       iridocyclitis, iritis, uveitis (due to) (in)
         toxoplasmosis (B58.09)
       iridocyclitis, iritis, uveitis (due to) (in)
         tuberculosis (A18.54)
    Ⓔⓧ **For category H20 CC codes:** See PDX Collection 624
    H20.00   Unspecified acute and subacute iridocyclitis 🅒
  ● **H20.01   Primary iridocyclitis**
    H20.011   Primary iridocyclitis, right eye 🅒
    H20.012   Primary iridocyclitis, left eye 🅒
    H20.013   Primary iridocyclitis, bilateral 🅒
    H20.019   Primary iridocyclitis, unspecified eye 🅒
  ● **H20.02   Recurrent acute iridocyclitis**
    H20.021   Recurrent acute iridocyclitis, right eye 🅒
    H20.022   Recurrent acute iridocyclitis, left eye 🅒
    H20.023   Recurrent acute iridocyclitis, bilateral 🅒
    H20.029   Recurrent acute iridocyclitis, unspecified eye 🅒
  ● **H20.03   Secondary infectious iridocyclitis**
    H20.031   Secondary infectious iridocyclitis, right eye 🅒
    H20.032   Secondary infectious iridocyclitis, left eye 🅒
    H20.033   Secondary infectious iridocyclitis, bilateral 🅒
    H20.039   Secondary infectious iridocyclitis, unspecified eye 🅒
  ● **H20.04   Secondary noninfectious iridocyclitis**
    H20.041   Secondary noninfectious iridocyclitis, right eye
    H20.042   Secondary noninfectious iridocyclitis, left eye
    H20.043   Secondary noninfectious iridocyclitis, bilateral
    H20.049   Secondary noninfectious iridocyclitis, unspecified eye
  ● **H20.05   Hypopyon**
    H20.051   Hypopyon, right eye
    H20.052   Hypopyon, left eye
    H20.053   Hypopyon, bilateral
    H20.059   Hypopyon, unspecified eye

● **H20.1   Chronic iridocyclitis**
    Use additional code for any associated cataract
    (H26.21-)
    Excludes2   posterior cyclitis (H30.2-)
    H20.10   Chronic iridocyclitis, unspecified eye
    H20.11   Chronic iridocyclitis, right eye
    H20.12   Chronic iridocyclitis, left eye
    H20.13   Chronic iridocyclitis, bilateral
● **H20.2   Lens-induced iridocyclitis**
    H20.20   Lens-induced iridocyclitis, unspecified eye
    H20.21   Lens-induced iridocyclitis, right eye
    H20.22   Lens-induced iridocyclitis, left eye
    H20.23   Lens-induced iridocyclitis, bilateral
● **H20.8   Other iridocyclitis**
    Excludes2   glaucomatocyclitis crises (H40.4-)
       posterior cyclitis (H30.2-)
       sympathetic uveitis (H44.13-)
  ● **H20.81   Fuchs' heterochromic cyclitis**
    H20.811   Fuchs' heterochromic cyclitis, right eye
    H20.812   Fuchs' heterochromic cyclitis, left eye
    H20.813   Fuchs' heterochromic cyclitis, bilateral
    H20.819   Fuchs' heterochromic cyclitis, unspecified eye
  ● **H20.82   Vogt-Koyanagi syndrome**
    H20.821   Vogt-Koyanagi syndrome, right eye
    H20.822   Vogt-Koyanagi syndrome, left eye
    H20.823   Vogt-Koyanagi syndrome, bilateral
    H20.829   Vogt-Koyanagi syndrome, unspecified eye
  H20.9   Unspecified iridocyclitis 🅒
    Uveitis NOS

● **H21   Other disorders of iris and ciliary body**
    Excludes2   sympathetic uveitis (H44.1-)
  ● **H21.0   Hyphema**
    Excludes1   traumatic hyphema (S05.1-)
    H21.00   Hyphema, unspecified eye
    H21.01   Hyphema, right eye
    H21.02   Hyphema, left eye
    H21.03   Hyphema, bilateral
  ● **H21.1   Other vascular disorders of iris and ciliary body**
    Neovascularization of iris or ciliary body
    Rubeosis iridis
    Rubeosis of iris
  ● **H21.1X   Other vascular disorders of iris and ciliary body**
    H21.1X1   Other vascular disorders of iris and ciliary body, right eye
    H21.1X2   Other vascular disorders of iris and ciliary body, left eye
    H21.1X3   Other vascular disorders of iris and ciliary body, bilateral
    H21.1X9   Other vascular disorders of iris and ciliary body, unspecified eye
  ● **H21.2   Degeneration of iris and ciliary body**
  ● **H21.21   Degeneration of chamber angle**
    H21.211   Degeneration of chamber angle, right eye
    H21.212   Degeneration of chamber angle, left eye
    H21.213   Degeneration of chamber angle, bilateral
    H21.219   Degeneration of chamber angle, unspecified eye

CHAPTER 7 (H00-H59)

N Newborn Age: 0   P Pediatric Age: 0–17   M Maternity DX: 12–55   A Adult Age: 15–124   ♀ Females Only   ♂ Males Only
🅒 Complication\Comorbidity   🅜 Major C\C   Ⓔⓧ CC/MCC Exclusions   🅗 Hospital-Acquired Condition

825

● **H21.22**   Degeneration of ciliary body
     H21.221   Degeneration of ciliary body, right eye
     H21.222   Degeneration of ciliary body, left eye
     H21.223   Degeneration of ciliary body, bilateral
     H21.229   Degeneration of ciliary body, unspecified eye

● **H21.23**   Degeneration of iris (pigmentary)
     Translucency of iris
     H21.231   Degeneration of iris (pigmentary), right eye
     H21.232   Degeneration of iris (pigmentary), left eye
     H21.233   Degeneration of iris (pigmentary), bilateral
     H21.239   Degeneration of iris (pigmentary), unspecified eye

● **H21.24**   Degeneration of pupillary margin
     H21.241   Degeneration of pupillary margin, right eye
     H21.242   Degeneration of pupillary margin, left eye
     H21.243   Degeneration of pupillary margin, bilateral
     H21.249   Degeneration of pupillary margin, unspecified eye

● **H21.25**   Iridoschisis
     H21.251   Iridoschisis, right eye
     H21.252   Iridoschisis, left eye
     H21.253   Iridoschisis, bilateral
     H21.259   Iridoschisis, unspecified eye

● **H21.26**   Iris atrophy (essential) (progressive)
     H21.261   Iris atrophy (essential) (progressive), right eye
     H21.262   Iris atrophy (essential) (progressive), left eye
     H21.263   Iris atrophy (essential) (progressive), bilateral
     H21.269   Iris atrophy (essential) (progressive), unspecified eye

● **H21.27**   Miotic pupillary cyst
     H21.271   Miotic pupillary cyst, right eye
     H21.272   Miotic pupillary cyst, left eye
     H21.273   Miotic pupillary cyst, bilateral
     H21.279   Miotic pupillary cyst, unspecified eye

     H21.29   Other iris atrophy

● **H21.3**   Cyst of iris, ciliary body and anterior chamber
     Excludes2   miotic pupillary cyst (H21.27-)

● **H21.30**   Idiopathic cysts of iris, ciliary body or anterior chamber
     Cyst of iris, ciliary body or anterior chamber NOS
     H21.301   Idiopathic cysts of iris, ciliary body or anterior chamber, right eye
     H21.302   Idiopathic cysts of iris, ciliary body or anterior chamber, left eye
     H21.303   Idiopathic cysts of iris, ciliary body or anterior chamber, bilateral
     H21.309   Idiopathic cysts of iris, ciliary body or anterior chamber, unspecified eye

● **H21.31**   Exudative cysts of iris or anterior chamber
     H21.311   Exudative cysts of iris or anterior chamber, right eye
     H21.312   Exudative cysts of iris or anterior chamber, left eye
     H21.313   Exudative cysts of iris or anterior chamber, bilateral
     H21.319   Exudative cysts of iris or anterior chamber, unspecified eye

● **H21.32**   Implantation cysts of iris, ciliary body or anterior chamber
     H21.321   Implantation cysts of iris, ciliary body or anterior chamber, right eye
     H21.322   Implantation cysts of iris, ciliary body or anterior chamber, left eye
     H21.323   Implantation cysts of iris, ciliary body or anterior chamber, bilateral
     H21.329   Implantation cysts of iris, ciliary body or anterior chamber, unspecified eye

● **H21.33**   Parasitic cyst of iris, ciliary body or anterior chamber
     (Ex) **For category H21.33 CC codes:** See PDX Collection 625
     H21.331   Parasitic cyst of iris, ciliary body or anterior chamber, right eye
     H21.332   Parasitic cyst of iris, ciliary body or anterior chamber, left eye
     H21.333   Parasitic cyst of iris, ciliary body or anterior chamber, bilateral
     H21.339   Parasitic cyst of iris, ciliary body or anterior chamber, unspecified eye

● **H21.34**   Primary cyst of pars plana
     H21.341   Primary cyst of pars plana, right eye
     H21.342   Primary cyst of pars plana, left eye
     H21.343   Primary cyst of pars plana, bilateral
     H21.349   Primary cyst of pars plana, unspecified eye

● **H21.35**   Exudative cyst of pars plana
     H21.351   Exudative cyst of pars plana, right eye
     H21.352   Exudative cyst of pars plana, left eye
     H21.353   Exudative cyst of pars plana, bilateral
     H21.359   Exudative cyst of pars plana, unspecified eye

● **H21.4**   Pupillary membranes
     Iris bombé
     Pupillary occlusion
     Pupillary seclusion
     Excludes1   congenital pupillary membranes (Q13.8)
     H21.40   Pupillary membranes, unspecified eye
     H21.41   Pupillary membranes, right eye
     H21.42   Pupillary membranes, left eye
     H21.43   Pupillary membranes, bilateral

● **H21.5**   Other and unspecified adhesions and disruptions of iris and ciliary body
     Excludes1   corectopia (Q13.2)

● **H21.50**   Unspecified adhesions of iris
     Synechia (iris) NOS
     H21.501   Unspecified adhesions of iris, right eye
     H21.502   Unspecified adhesions of iris, left eye
     H21.503   Unspecified adhesions of iris, bilateral
     H21.509   Unspecified adhesions of iris and ciliary body, unspecified eye

● **H21.51**   Anterior synechiae (iris)
     H21.511   Anterior synechiae (iris), right eye
     H21.512   Anterior synechiae (iris), left eye
     H21.513   Anterior synechiae (iris), bilateral
     H21.519   Anterior synechiae (iris), unspecified eye

● **H21.52**   Goniosynechiae
     H21.521   Goniosynechiae, right eye
     H21.522   Goniosynechiae, left eye
     H21.523   Goniosynechiae, bilateral
     H21.529   Goniosynechiae, unspecified eye

● **H21.53   Iridodialysis**
     H21.531   Iridodialysis, **right eye**
     H21.532   Iridodialysis, **left eye**
     H21.533   Iridodialysis, **bilateral**
     H21.539   Iridodialysis, **unspecified** eye

● **H21.54   Posterior synechiae (iris)**
     H21.541   Posterior synechiae (iris), **right eye**
     H21.542   Posterior synechiae (iris), **left eye**
     H21.543   Posterior synechiae (iris), **bilateral**
     H21.549   Posterior synechiae (iris), **unspecified** eye

● **H21.55   Recession of chamber angle**
     H21.551   Recession of chamber angle, **right eye**
     H21.552   Recession of chamber angle, **left eye**
     H21.553   Recession of chamber angle, **bilateral**
     H21.559   Recession of chamber angle, **unspecified** eye

● **H21.56   Pupillary abnormalities**
     Deformed pupil
     Ectopic pupil
     Rupture of sphincter, pupil
     Excludes1   congenital deformity of pupil (Q13.2-)
     H21.561   Pupillary abnormality, **right eye**
     H21.562   Pupillary abnormality, **left eye**
     H21.563   Pupillary abnormality, **bilateral**
     H21.569   Pupillary abnormality, **unspecified** eye

● **H21.8   Other specified disorders of iris and ciliary body**
     H21.81   Floppy iris syndrome
         Intraoperative floppy iris syndrome (IFIS)
         Use additional code for adverse effect, if applicable, to identify drug (T36-T50 with fifth or sixth character 5)
     H21.82   Plateau iris syndrome (post-iridectomy) (postprocedural)
     H21.89   Other specified disorders of iris and ciliary body

H21.9   Unspecified disorder of iris and ciliary body

▸ *H22   Disorders of iris and ciliary body in diseases classified elsewhere*
     Code first underlying disease, such as:
     gout (M1A.-, M10.-)
     leprosy (A30.-)
     parasitic disease (B89)

DISORDERS OF LENS (H25-H28)

● **H25   Age-related cataract**
     Senile cataract
     Excludes2   capsular glaucoma with pseudoexfoliation of lens (H40.1-)

● **H25.0   Age-related incipient cataract**
    ● H25.01   Cortical age-related cataract
     H25.011   Cortical age-related cataract, **right** eye   A
     H25.012   Cortical age-related cataract, **left** eye   A
     H25.013   Cortical age-related cataract, **bilateral**   A
     H25.019   Cortical age-related cataract, **unspecified** eye   A
    ● H25.03   Anterior subcapsular polar age-related cataract
     H25.031   Anterior subcapsular polar age-related cataract, **right** eye   A
     H25.032   Anterior subcapsular polar age-related cataract, **left** eye   A
     H25.033   Anterior subcapsular polar age-related cataract, **bilateral**   A
     H25.039   Anterior subcapsular polar age-related cataract, **unspecified** eye   A

Figure 7-9   Age-related cataract. Nuclear sclerosis and cortical lens opacities are present. (From Ignatavicius DD, Workman ML: Medical-Surgical Nursing: Patient-Centered Collaborative Care, St. Louis, MO, Saunders/Elsevier, 2010)

Item 7-5 Senile cataracts are linked to the aging process. The most common area for the formation of a cataract is the cortical area of the lens. **Polar cataracts** can be either anterior or posterior. **Anterior polar cataracts** are more common and are small, white, capsular cataracts located on the anterior portion of the lens. **Total cataracts,** also called **complete** or **mature,** cause an opacity of all fibers of the lens. **Hypermature** describes a mature cataract with a swollen, milky cortex that covers the entire lens. **Immature,** also called **incipient,** cataracts have a clear cortex and are only slightly opaque. Treatment for all cataracts is the removal of the lens.

● **H25.04   Posterior subcapsular polar age-related cataract**
     H25.041   Posterior subcapsular polar age-related cataract, **right eye**   A
     H25.042   Posterior subcapsular polar age-related cataract, **left eye**   A
     H25.043   Posterior subcapsular polar age-related cataract, **bilateral**   A
     H25.049   Posterior subcapsular polar age-related cataract, **unspecified** eye   A
    ● H25.09   Other age-related incipient cataract
     Coronary age-related cataract
     Punctate age-related cataract
     Water clefts
     H25.091   Other age-related incipient cataract, **right eye**   A
     H25.092   Other age-related incipient cataract, **left eye**   A
     H25.093   Other age-related incipient cataract, **bilateral**   A
     H25.099   Other age-related incipient cataract, **unspecified** eye   A

● **H25.1   Age-related nuclear cataract**
     Cataracta brunescens
     Nuclear sclerosis cataract
     H25.10   Age-related nuclear cataract, **unspecified** eye   A
     H25.11   Age-related nuclear cataract, **right eye**   A
     H25.12   Age-related nuclear cataract, **left eye**   A
         Coding Clinic: 2016, Q1, P33
     H25.13   Age-related nuclear cataract, **bilateral**   A
         Coding Clinic: 2016, Q1, P32

● **H25.2   Age-related cataract, morgagnian type**
     Age-related hypermature cataract
     H25.20   Age-related cataract, morgagnian type, **unspecified** eye   A
     H25.21   Age-related cataract, morgagnian type, **right** eye   A
     H25.22   Age-related cataract, morgagnian type, **left eye**   A
     H25.23   Age-related cataract, morgagnian type, **bilateral**   A

● **H25.8   Other age-related cataract**
    ● H25.81   Combined forms of age-related cataract
     H25.811   Combined forms of age-related cataract, **right eye**   A
     H25.812   Combined forms of age-related cataract, **left eye**   A
     H25.813   Combined forms of age-related cataract, **bilateral**   A
     H25.819   Combined forms of age-related cataract, **unspecified** eye   A
     H25.89   Other age-related cataract

H25.9   Unspecified age-related cataract   A

CHAPTER 7 (H00-H59)

● **H26 Other cataract**

    Excludes1   congenital cataract (Q12.0)

  ● **H26.0 Infantile and juvenile cataract**

    ● **H26.00 Unspecified infantile and juvenile cataract**

      H26.001   Unspecified infantile and juvenile cataract, right eye   P

      H26.002   Unspecified infantile and juvenile cataract, left eye   P

      H26.003   Unspecified infantile and juvenile cataract, bilateral   P

      H26.009   Unspecified infantile and juvenile cataract, unspecified eye   P

    ● **H26.01 Infantile and juvenile cortical, lamellar, or zonular cataract**

      H26.011   Infantile and juvenile cortical, lamellar, or zonular cataract, right eye   P

      H26.012   Infantile and juvenile cortical, lamellar, or zonular cataract, left eye   P

      H26.013   Infantile and juvenile cortical, lamellar, or zonular cataract, bilateral   P

      H26.019   Infantile and juvenile cortical, lamellar, or zonular cataract, unspecified eye   P

    ● **H26.03 Infantile and juvenile nuclear cataract**

      H26.031   Infantile and juvenile nuclear cataract, right eye   P

      H26.032   Infantile and juvenile nuclear cataract, left eye   P

      H26.033   Infantile and juvenile nuclear cataract, bilateral   P

      H26.039   Infantile and juvenile nuclear cataract, unspecified eye   P

    ● **H26.04 Anterior subcapsular polar infantile and juvenile cataract**

      H26.041   Anterior subcapsular polar infantile and juvenile cataract, right eye   P

      H26.042   Anterior subcapsular polar infantile and juvenile cataract, left eye   P

      H26.043   Anterior subcapsular polar infantile and juvenile cataract, bilateral   P

      H26.049   Anterior subcapsular polar infantile and juvenile cataract, unspecified eye   P

    ● **H26.05 Posterior subcapsular polar infantile and juvenile cataract**

      H26.051   Posterior subcapsular polar infantile and juvenile cataract, right eye   P

      H26.052   Posterior subcapsular polar infantile and juvenile cataract, left eye   P

      H26.053   Posterior subcapsular polar infantile and juvenile cataract, bilateral   P

      H26.059   Posterior subcapsular polar infantile and juvenile cataract, unspecified eye   P

    ● **H26.06 Combined forms of infantile and juvenile cataract**

      H26.061   Combined forms of infantile and juvenile cataract, right eye   P

      H26.062   Combined forms of infantile and juvenile cataract, left eye   P

      H26.063   Combined forms of infantile and juvenile cataract bilateral   P

      H26.069   Combined forms of infantile and juvenile cataract, unspecified eye   P

    H26.09   Other infantile and juvenile cataract   P

  ● **H26.1 Traumatic cataract**

    Use additional code (Chapter 20) to identify external cause

    ● **H26.10 Unspecified traumatic cataract**

      H26.101   Unspecified traumatic cataract, right eye

      H26.102   Unspecified traumatic cataract, left eye

      H26.103   Unspecified traumatic cataract, bilateral

      H26.109   Unspecified traumatic cataract, unspecified eye

    ● **H26.11 Localized traumatic opacities**

      H26.111   Localized traumatic opacities, right eye

      H26.112   Localized traumatic opacities, left eye

      H26.113   Localized traumatic opacities, bilateral

      H26.119   Localized traumatic opacities, unspecified eye

    ● **H26.12 Partially resolved traumatic cataract**

      H26.121   Partially resolved traumatic cataract, right eye

      H26.122   Partially resolved traumatic cataract, left eye

      H26.123   Partially resolved traumatic cataract, bilateral

      H26.129   Partially resolved traumatic cataract, unspecified eye

    ● **H26.13 Total traumatic cataract**

      H26.131   Total traumatic cataract, right eye

      H26.132   Total traumatic cataract, left eye

      H26.133   Total traumatic cataract, bilateral

      H26.139   Total traumatic cataract, unspecified eye

  ● **H26.2 Complicated cataract**

    H26.20   Unspecified complicated cataract

      Cataracta complicata NOS

    ● **H26.21 Cataract with neovascularization**

      Code also associated condition, such as: chronic iridocyclitis (H20.1-)

      H26.211   Cataract with neovascularization, right eye

      H26.212   Cataract with neovascularization, left eye

      H26.213   Cataract with neovascularization, bilateral

      H26.219   Cataract with neovascularization, unspecified eye

    ● **H26.22 Cataract secondary to ocular disorders (degenerative) (inflammatory)**

      Code also associated ocular disorder

      H26.221   Cataract secondary to ocular disorders (degenerative) (inflammatory), right eye

      H26.222   Cataract secondary to ocular disorders (degenerative) (inflammatory), left eye

      H26.223   Cataract secondary to ocular disorders (degenerative) (inflammatory), bilateral

      H26.229   Cataract secondary to ocular disorders (degenerative) (inflammatory), unspecified eye

    ● **H26.23 Glaucomatous flecks (subcapsular)**

      Code first underlying glaucoma (H40-H42)

      H26.231   Glaucomatous flecks (subcapsular), right eye

      H26.232   Glaucomatous flecks (subcapsular), left eye

▶ New   ⮞ Revised   ~~deleted~~ Deleted   Excludes 1   Excludes 2   Includes   Use additional   Code first   Code also   Key words

OGCR Official Guidelines   ● Unacceptable Principal Diagnosis   X Assign placeholder X   ● Use Additional Character(s)   ▶ Manifestation Code   Coding Clinic

H26.233   Glaucomatous flecks (subcapsular), bilateral

H26.239   Glaucomatous flecks (subcapsular), unspecified eye

● H26.3   **Drug-induced cataract**
Toxic cataract

Use additional code for adverse effect, if applicable, to identify drug (T36-T50 with fifth or sixth character 5)

H26.30   Drug-induced cataract, unspecified eye

H26.31   Drug-induced cataract, right eye

H26.32   Drug-induced cataract, left eye

H26.33   Drug-induced cataract, bilateral

● H26.4   **Secondary cataract**

H26.40   Unspecified secondary cataract

● H26.41   **Soemmering's ring**

H26.411   Soemmering's ring, right eye

H26.412   Soemmering's ring, left eye

H26.413   Soemmering's ring, bilateral

H26.419   Soemmering's ring, unspecified eye

● H26.49   **Other secondary cataract**

H26.491   Other secondary cataract, right eye

H26.492   Other secondary cataract, left eye

H26.493   Other secondary cataract, bilateral

H26.499   Other secondary cataract, unspecified eye

H26.8   **Other specified cataract**

H26.9   **Unspecified cataract**

● H27   **Other disorders of lens**

Excludes1   congenital lens malformations (Q12.-)
mechanical complications of intraocular lens implant (T85.2)
pseudophakia (Z96.1)

● H27.0   **Aphakia**
Acquired absence of lens
Acquired aphakia
Aphakia due to trauma

Excludes1   cataract extraction status (Z98.4-)
congenital absence of lens (Q12.3)
congenital aphakia (Q12.3)

H27.00   Aphakia, unspecified eye

H27.01   Aphakia, right eye

H27.02   Aphakia, left eye

H27.03   Aphakia, bilateral

● H27.1   **Dislocation of lens**

H27.10   Unspecified dislocation of lens

● H27.11   **Subluxation of lens**

H27.111   Subluxation of lens, right eye

H27.112   Subluxation of lens, left eye

H27.113   Subluxation of lens, bilateral

H27.119   Subluxation of lens, unspecified eye

● H27.12   **Anterior dislocation of lens**

H27.121   Anterior dislocation of lens, right eye

H27.122   Anterior dislocation of lens, left eye

H27.123   Anterior dislocation of lens, bilateral

H27.129   Anterior dislocation of lens, unspecified eye

● H27.13   **Posterior dislocation of lens**

H27.131   Posterior dislocation of lens, right eye

H27.132   Posterior dislocation of lens, left eye

H27.133   Posterior dislocation of lens, bilateral

H27.139   Posterior dislocation of lens, unspecified eye

H27.8   **Other specified disorders of lens**

H27.9   **Unspecified disorder of lens**

◗ H28   *Cataract in diseases classified elsewhere*
Code first underlying disease, such as:
hypoparathyroidism (E20.-)
myotonia (G71.1-)
myxedema (E03.-)
protein-calorie malnutrition (E40-E46)

Excludes1   cataract in diabetes mellitus (E08.36, E09.36, E10.36, E11.36, E13.36)

DISORDERS OF CHOROID AND RETINA (H30-H36)

★ **(See Plate 90 on page 64.)**

● H30   **Chorioretinal inflammation**

● H30.0   **Focal chorioretinal inflammation**
Focal chorioretinitis
Focal choroiditis
Focal retinitis
Focal retinochoroiditis

● H30.00   **Unspecified focal chorioretinal inflammation**
Focal chorioretinitis NOS
Focal choroiditis NOS
Focal retinitis NOS
Focal retinochoroiditis NOS

H30.001   Unspecified focal chorioretinal inflammation, right eye

H30.002   Unspecified focal chorioretinal inflammation, left eye

H30.003   Unspecified focal chorioretinal inflammation, bilateral

H30.009   Unspecified focal chorioretinal inflammation, unspecified eye

● H30.01   **Focal chorioretinal inflammation, juxtapapillary**

H30.011   Focal chorioretinal inflammation, juxtapapillary, right eye

H30.012   Focal chorioretinal inflammation, juxtapapillary, left eye

H30.013   Focal chorioretinal inflammation, juxtapapillary, bilateral

H30.019   Focal chorioretinal inflammation, juxtapapillary, unspecified eye

● H30.02   **Focal chorioretinal inflammation of posterior pole**

H30.021   Focal chorioretinal inflammation of posterior pole, right eye

H30.022   Focal chorioretinal inflammation of posterior pole, left eye

H30.023   Focal chorioretinal inflammation of posterior pole, bilateral

H30.029   Focal chorioretinal inflammation of posterior pole, unspecified eye

● H30.03   **Focal chorioretinal inflammation, peripheral**

H30.031   Focal chorioretinal inflammation, peripheral, right eye

H30.032   Focal chorioretinal inflammation, peripheral, left eye

H30.033   Focal chorioretinal inflammation, peripheral, bilateral

H30.039   Focal chorioretinal inflammation, peripheral, unspecified eye

● H30.04   **Focal chorioretinal inflammation, macular or paramacular**

H30.041   Focal chorioretinal inflammation, macular or paramacular, right eye

H30.042   Focal chorioretinal inflammation, macular or paramacular, left eye

H30.043   Focal chorioretinal inflammation, macular or paramacular, bilateral

H30.049   Focal chorioretinal inflammation, macular or paramacular, unspecified eye

CHAPTER 7 (H00-H59)

N Newborn Age: 0   **P** Pediatric Age: 0–17   **M** Maternity DX: 12–55   **A** Adult Age: 15–124   ♀ Females Only   ♂ Males Only

🔖 Complication\Comorbidity   🔖 Major C\C   ⓔⓍ CC/MCC Exclusions   🔖 Hospital-Acquired Condition

829

CHAPTER 7 (H00–H59)

● **H30.1 Disseminated chorioretinal inflammation**
Disseminated chorioretinitis
Disseminated choroiditis
Disseminated retinitis
Disseminated retinochoroiditis

Excludes2 exudative retinopathy (H35.02-)

(Ex) For category H30.1 CC codes: See PDX Collection 626

● **H30.10 Unspecified disseminated chorioretinal inflammation**
Disseminated chorioretinitis NOS
Disseminated choroiditis NOS
Disseminated retinitis NOS
Disseminated retinochoroiditis NOS

H30.101 Unspecified disseminated chorioretinal inflammation, right eye

H30.102 Unspecified disseminated chorioretinal inflammation, left eye

H30.103 Unspecified disseminated chorioretinal inflammation, bilateral

H30.109 Unspecified disseminated chorioretinal inflammation, unspecified eye

● **H30.11 Disseminated chorioretinal inflammation of posterior pole**
H30.111 Disseminated chorioretinal inflammation of posterior pole, right eye

H30.112 Disseminated chorioretinal inflammation of posterior pole, left eye

H30.113 Disseminated chorioretinal inflammation of posterior pole, bilateral

H30.119 Disseminated chorioretinal inflammation of posterior pole, unspecified eye

● **H30.12 Disseminated chorioretinal inflammation, peripheral**
H30.121 Disseminated chorioretinal inflammation, peripheral right eye

H30.122 Disseminated chorioretinal inflammation, peripheral, left eye

H30.123 Disseminated chorioretinal inflammation, peripheral, bilateral

H30.129 Disseminated chorioretinal inflammation, peripheral, unspecified eye

● **H30.13 Disseminated chorioretinal inflammation, generalized**
H30.131 Disseminated chorioretinal inflammation, generalized, right eye

H30.132 Disseminated chorioretinal inflammation, generalized, left eye

H30.133 Disseminated chorioretinal inflammation, generalized, bilateral

H30.139 Disseminated chorioretinal inflammation, generalized, unspecified eye

● **H30.14 Acute posterior multifocal placoid pigment epitheliopathy**
H30.141 Acute posterior multifocal placoid pigment epitheliopathy, right eye

H30.142 Acute posterior multifocal placoid pigment epitheliopathy, left eye

H30.143 Acute posterior multifocal placoid pigment epitheliopathy, bilateral

H30.149 Acute posterior multifocal placoid pigment epitheliopathy, unspecified eye

● **H30.2 Posterior cyclitis**
Pars planitis

H30.20 Posterior cyclitis, unspecified eye

H30.21 Posterior cyclitis, right eye

H30.22 Posterior cyclitis, left eye

H30.23 Posterior cyclitis, bilateral

● **H30.8 Other chorioretinal inflammations**
● **H30.81 Harada's disease**
H30.811 Harada's disease, right eye

H30.812 Harada's disease, left eye

H30.813 Harada's disease, bilateral

H30.819 Harada's disease, unspecified eye

● **H30.89 Other chorioretinal inflammations**
(Ex) For category H30.89 CC codes: See PDX Collection 626

H30.891 Other chorioretinal inflammations, right eye

H30.892 Other chorioretinal inflammations, left eye

H30.893 Other chorioretinal inflammations, bilateral

H30.899 Other chorioretinal inflammations, unspecified eye

● **H30.9 Unspecified chorioretinal inflammation**
Chorioretinitis NOS
Choroiditis NOS
Neuroretinitis NOS
Retinitis NOS
Retinochoroiditis NOS

(Ex) For category H30.9 CC codes: See PDX Collection 626

H30.90 Unspecified chorioretinal inflammation, unspecified eye

H30.91 Unspecified chorioretinal inflammation, right eye

H30.92 Unspecified chorioretinal inflammation, left eye

H30.93 Unspecified chorioretinal inflammation, bilateral

● **H31 Other disorders of choroid**
● **H31.0 Chorioretinal scars**

Excludes2 postsurgical chorioretinal scars (H59.81-)

● **H31.00 Unspecified chorioretinal scars**
H31.001 Unspecified chorioretinal scars, right eye

H31.002 Unspecified chorioretinal scars, left eye

H31.003 Unspecified chorioretinal scars, bilateral

H31.009 Unspecified chorioretinal scars, unspecified eye

● **H31.01 Macula scars of posterior pole (postinflammatory) (post-traumatic)**

Excludes1 postprocedural chorioretinal scar (H59.81-)

H31.011 Macula scars of posterior pole (postinflammatory) (post-traumatic), right eye

H31.012 Macula scars of posterior pole (postinflammatory) (post-traumatic), left eye

▶ New   ⇒ Revised   ~~deleted~~ Deleted   Excludes 1   Excludes 2   Includes   Use additional   Code first   Code also   Key words

OGCR Official Guidelines   ● Unacceptable Principal Diagnosis   X Assign placeholder X   ▶ Use Additional Character(s)   ▶ Manifestation Code   **Coding Clinic**

H31.013   Macula scars of posterior pole (postinflammatory) (post-traumatic), bilateral

H31.019   Macula scars of posterior pole (postinflammatory) (post-traumatic), unspecified eye

● H31.02   Solar retinopathy

H31.021   Solar retinopathy, right eye

H31.022   Solar retinopathy, left eye

H31.023   Solar retinopathy, bilateral

H31.029   Solar retinopathy, unspecified eye

● H31.09   Other chorioretinal scars

H31.091   Other chorioretinal scars, right eye

H31.092   Other chorioretinal scars, left eye

H31.093   Other chorioretinal scars, bilateral

H31.099   Other chorioretinal scars, unspecified eye

● H31.1   Choroidal degeneration

Excludes2   angioid streaks of macula (H35.33)

● H31.10   Unspecified choroidal degeneration
Choroidal sclerosis NOS

H31.101   Choroidal degeneration, unspecified, right eye

H31.102   Choroidal degeneration, unspecified, left eye

H31.103   Choroidal degeneration, unspecified, bilateral

H31.109   Choroidal degeneration, unspecified, unspecified eye

● H31.11   Age-related choroidal atrophy

H31.111   Age-related choroidal atrophy, right eye   A

H31.112   Age-related choroidal atrophy, left eye   A

H31.113   Age-related choroidal atrophy, bilateral   A

H31.119   Age-related choroidal atrophy, unspecified eye   A

● H31.12   Diffuse secondary atrophy of choroid

H31.121   Diffuse secondary atrophy of choroid, right eye

H31.122   Diffuse secondary atrophy of choroid, left eye

H31.123   Diffuse secondary atrophy of choroid, bilateral

H31.129   Diffuse secondary atrophy of choroid, unspecified eye

● H31.2   Hereditary choroidal dystrophy

Excludes2   hyperornithinemia (E72.4)
ornithinemia (E72.4)

H31.20   Hereditary choroidal dystrophy, unspecified

H31.21   Choroideremia

H31.22   Choroidal dystrophy (central areolar) (generalized) (peripapillary)

H31.23   Gyrate atrophy, choroid

H31.29   Other hereditary choroidal dystrophy

● H31.3   Choroidal hemorrhage and rupture

● H31.30   Unspecified choroidal hemorrhage

H31.301   Unspecified choroidal hemorrhage, right eye

H31.302   Unspecified choroidal hemorrhage, left eye

H31.303   Unspecified choroidal hemorrhage, bilateral

H31.309   Unspecified choroidal hemorrhage, unspecified eye

● H31.31   Expulsive choroidal hemorrhage

H31.311   Expulsive choroidal hemorrhage, right eye

H31.312   Expulsive choroidal hemorrhage, left eye

H31.313   Expulsive choroidal hemorrhage, bilateral

H31.319   Expulsive choroidal hemorrhage, unspecified eye

● H31.32   Choroidal rupture
Ex: For category H31.32 CC codes: See PDX Collection 627

H31.321   Choroidal rupture, right eye 🐾

H31.322   Choroidal rupture, left eye 🐾

H31.323   Choroidal rupture, bilateral 🐾

H31.329   Choroidal rupture, unspecified eye 🐾

● H31.4   Choroidal detachment
Ex: For category H31.4 CC codes: See PDX Collection 627

● H31.40   Unspecified choroidal detachment

H31.401   Unspecified choroidal detachment, right eye 🐾

H31.402   Unspecified choroidal detachment, left eye 🐾

H31.403   Unspecified choroidal detachment, bilateral 🐾

H31.409   Unspecified choroidal detachment, unspecified eye 🐾

● H31.41   Hemorrhagic choroidal detachment

H31.411   Hemorrhagic choroidal detachment, right eye 🐾

H31.412   Hemorrhagic choroidal detachment, left eye 🐾

H31.413   Hemorrhagic choroidal detachment, bilateral 🐾

H31.419   Hemorrhagic choroidal detachment, unspecified eye 🐾

● H31.42   Serous choroidal detachment

H31.421   Serous choroidal detachment, right eye 🐾

H31.422   Serous choroidal detachment, left eye 🐾

H31.423   Serous choroidal detachment, bilateral 🐾

H31.429   Serous choroidal detachment, unspecified eye 🐾

H31.8   Other specified disorders of choroid

H31.9   Unspecified disorder of choroid

▷ H32   *Chorioretinal disorders in diseases classified elsewhere*

Code first underlying disease, such as:
congenital toxoplasmosis (P37.1)
histoplasmosis (B39.-)
leprosy (A30.-)

Excludes1   chorioretinitis (in):
toxoplasmosis (acquired) (B58.01)
tuberculosis (A18.53)

● H33   Retinal detachments and breaks

Excludes1   detachment of retinal pigment epithelium (H35.72-, H35.73-)

● H33.0   Retinal detachment with retinal break
Rhegmatogenous retinal detachment

Excludes1   serous retinal detachment (without retinal break) (H33.2-)

● H33.00   Unspecified retinal detachment with retinal break

H33.001   Unspecified retinal detachment with retinal break, right eye

H33.002   Unspecified retinal detachment with retinal break, left eye

N Newborn Age: 0   **P** Pediatric Age: 0–17   **M** Maternity DX: 12–55   **A** Adult Age: 15–124   ♀ Females Only   ♂ Males Only

🐾 Complication\Comorbidity   🐾 Major C\C   Ex: CC/MCC Exclusions   🐾 Hospital-Acquired Condition

831

CHAPTER 7 (H00–H59)

NON-RHEGMATOGENOUS
RETINAL DETACHMENT

VITREOUS DETACHMENT

RHEGMATOGENOUS
RETINAL
DETACHMENT

Figure 7-10 Retinal detachment. (From Kumar: Robbins and Cotran: Pathologic Basis of Disease, ed 7, Saunders, 2005)

Item 7-6 Retinal detachments and defects are conditions of the eye in which the retina separates from the underlying tissue. Initial detachment may be localized, requiring rapid treatment (medical emergency) to avoid the entire retina from detaching which leads to vision loss and blindness.

H33.003   Unspecified retinal detachment with retinal break, bilateral
H33.009   Unspecified retinal detachment with retinal break, unspecified eye

● H33.01   Retinal detachment with single break
H33.011   Retinal detachment with single break, right eye
H33.012   Retinal detachment with single break, left eye
H33.013   Retinal detachment with single break, bilateral
H33.019   Retinal detachment with single break, unspecified eye

● H33.02   Retinal detachment with multiple breaks
H33.021   Retinal detachment with multiple breaks, right eye
H33.022   Retinal detachment with multiple breaks, left eye
H33.023   Retinal detachment with multiple breaks, bilateral
H33.029   Retinal detachment with multiple breaks, unspecified eye

● H33.03   Retinal detachment with giant retinal tear
H33.031   Retinal detachment with giant retinal tear, right eye
H33.032   Retinal detachment with giant retinal tear, left eye
H33.033   Retinal detachment with giant retinal tear, bilateral
H33.039   Retinal detachment with giant retinal tear, unspecified eye

● H33.04   Retinal detachment with retinal dialysis
H33.041   Retinal detachment with retinal dialysis, right eye
H33.042   Retinal detachment with retinal dialysis, left eye
H33.043   Retinal detachment with retinal dialysis, bilateral
H33.049   Retinal detachment with retinal dialysis, unspecified eye

● H33.05   Total retinal detachment
H33.051   Total retinal detachment, right eye
H33.052   Total retinal detachment, left eye
H33.053   Total retinal detachment, bilateral
H33.059   Total retinal detachment, unspecified eye

● H33.1   Retinoschisis and retinal cysts
Excludes1   congenital retinoschisis (Q14.1) microcystoid degeneration of retina (H35.42-)

● H33.10   Unspecified retinoschisis
H33.101   Unspecified retinoschisis, right eye
H33.102   Unspecified retinoschisis, left eye
H33.103   Unspecified retinoschisis, bilateral
H33.109   Unspecified retinoschisis, unspecified eye

● H33.11   Cyst of ora serrata
H33.111   Cyst of ora serrata, right eye
H33.112   Cyst of ora serrata, left eye
H33.113   Cyst of ora serrata, bilateral
H33.119   Cyst of ora serrata, unspecified eye

● H33.12   Parasitic cyst of retina
(Ex) For category H33.12 CC codes: See PDX Collection 625
H33.121   Parasitic cyst of retina, right eye 🔧
H33.122   Parasitic cyst of retina, left eye 🔧
H33.123   Parasitic cyst of retina, bilateral 🔧
H33.129   Parasitic cyst of retina, unspecified eye 🔧

● H33.19   Other retinoschisis and retinal cysts
Pseudocyst of retina
H33.191   Other retinoschisis and retinal cysts, right eye
H33.192   Other retinoschisis and retinal cysts, left eye
H33.193   Other retinoschisis and retinal cysts, bilateral
H33.199   Other retinoschisis and retinal cysts, unspecified eye

● H33.2   Serous retinal detachment
Retinal detachment NOS
Retinal detachment without retinal break
Excludes1   central serous chorioretinopathy (H35.71-)
(Ex) For category H33.2 CC codes: See PDX Collection 628
H33.20   Serous retinal detachment, unspecified eye 🔧
H33.21   Serous retinal detachment, right eye 🔧
H33.22   Serous retinal detachment, left eye 🔧
H33.23   Serous retinal detachment, bilateral 🔧

▶ New   ⟹ Revised   ~~deleted~~ Deleted   Excludes 1   Excludes 2   Includes   Use additional   Code first   Code also   Key words
OGCR Official Guidelines   ● Unacceptable Principal Diagnosis   X Assign placeholder X   🔧 Use Additional Character(s)   ▷ Manifestation Code   Coding Clinic

● **H33.3**   **Retinal breaks without detachment**

     Excludes1   chorioretinal scars after surgery for detachment (H59.81-)

                     peripheral retinal degeneration without break (H35.4-)

   ● **H33.30**   Unspecified retinal break

       H33.301   Unspecified retinal break, right eye

       H33.302   Unspecified retinal break, left eye

       H33.303   Unspecified retinal break, bilateral

       H33.309   Unspecified retinal break, unspecified eye

   ● **H33.31**   Horseshoe tear of retina without detachment

       Operculum of retina without detachment

       H33.311   Horseshoe tear of retina without detachment, right eye

       H33.312   Horseshoe tear of retina without detachment, left eye

       H33.313   Horseshoe tear of retina without detachment, bilateral

       H33.319   Horseshoe tear of retina without detachment, unspecified eye

   ● **H33.32**   Round hole of retina without detachment

       H33.321   Round hole, right eye

       H33.322   Round hole, left eye

       H33.323   Round hole, bilateral

       H33.329   Round hole, unspecified eye

   ● **H33.33**   Multiple defects of retina without detachment

       H33.331   Multiple defects of retina without detachment, right eye

       H33.332   Multiple defects of retina without detachment, left eye

       H33.333   Multiple defects of retina without detachment, bilateral

       H33.339   Multiple defects of retina without detachment, unspecified eye

● **H33.4**   **Traction detachment of retina**

     Proliferative vitreo-retinopathy with retinal detachment

     (Ex) **For category H33.4 CC codes:** See PDX Collection 628

       H33.40   Traction detachment of retina, unspecified eye 🔒

       H33.41   Traction detachment of retina, right eye 🔒

       H33.42   Traction detachment of retina, left eye 🔒

       H33.43   Traction detachment of retina, bilateral 🔒

   H33.8   Other retinal detachments 🔒

     (Ex) See PDX Collection 628

● **H34**   **Retinal vascular occlusions**

     Blockage in vessel of the retina

     Excludes1   amaurosis fugax (G45.3)

     (Ex) **For category H34 CC codes:** See PDX Collection 587

   ● **H34.0**   Transient retinal artery occlusion

       H34.00   Transient retinal artery occlusion, unspecified eye 🔒

       H34.01   Transient retinal artery occlusion, right eye 🔒

       H34.02   Transient retinal artery occlusion, left eye 🔒

       H34.03   Transient retinal artery occlusion, bilateral 🔒

   ● **H34.1**   Central retinal artery occlusion

       H34.10   Central retinal artery occlusion, unspecified eye 🔒

       H34.11   Central retinal artery occlusion, right eye 🔒

       H34.12   Central retinal artery occlusion, left eye 🔒

       H34.13   Central retinal artery occlusion, bilateral 🔒

   ● **H34.2**   Other retinal artery occlusions

     ● **H34.21**   Partial retinal artery occlusion

       Hollenhorst's plaque

       Retinal microembolism

       H34.211   Partial retinal artery occlusion, right eye 🔒

       H34.212   Partial retinal artery occlusion, left eye 🔒

       H34.213   Partial retinal artery occlusion, bilateral 🔒

       H34.219   Partial retinal artery occlusion, unspecified eye 🔒

     ● **H34.23**   Retinal artery branch occlusion

       H34.231   Retinal artery branch occlusion, right eye 🔒

       H34.232   Retinal artery branch occlusion, left eye 🔒

       H34.233   Retinal artery branch occlusion, bilateral 🔒

       H34.239   Retinal artery branch occlusion, unspecified eye 🔒

   ● **H34.8**   Other retinal vascular occlusions

     Coding Clinic: 2016, Q4, P19

     ● **H34.81**   Central retinal vein occlusion

       One of the following 7th characters is to be assigned to codes in subcategory H34.81 to designate the severity of the occlusion:

0	with macular edema
1	with retinal neovascularization
2	stable
	Old central retinal vein occlusion

       ● H34.811   Central retinal vein occlusion, right eye 🔒

       ● H34.812   Central retinal vein occlusion, left eye 🔒

       ● H34.813   Central retinal vein occlusion, bilateral 🔒

       ● H34.819   Central retinal vein occlusion, unspecified eye 🔒

     ● **H34.82**   Venous engorgement

       Incipient retinal vein occlusion

       Partial retinal vein occlusion

       H34.821   Venous engorgement, right eye

       H34.822   Venous engorgement, left eye

       H34.823   Venous engorgement, bilateral

       H34.829   Venous engorgement, unspecified eye

     ● **H34.83**   Tributary (branch) retinal vein occlusion

       One of the following 7th characters is to be assigned to codes in subcategory H34.83 to designate the severity of the occlusion:

0	with macular edema
1	with retinal neovascularization
2	stable
	Old tributary (branch) retinal vein occlusion

       ● H34.831   Tributary (branch) retinal vein occlusion, right eye

       ● H34.832   Tributary (branch) retinal vein occlusion, left eye

       ● H34.833   Tributary (branch) retinal vein occlusion, bilateral

       ● H34.839   Tributary (branch) retinal vein occlusion, unspecified eye

   H34.9   Unspecified retinal vascular occlusion 🔒

N   Newborn Age: 0   P   Pediatric Age: 0–17   M   Maternity DX: 12–55   A   Adult Age: 15–124   ♀ Females Only   ♂ Males Only

🔒 Complication\Comorbidity   🔒 Major C\C   (Ex) CC/MCC Exclusions   🔒 Hospital-Acquired Condition

● **H35 Other retinal disorders**

Excludes2 diabetic retinal disorders (E08.311-E08.359,
E09.311-E09.359, E10.311-E10.359,
E11.311-E11.359, E13.311-E13.359)

● **H35.0 Background retinopathy and retinal vascular changes**
Code also any associated hypertension (I10.-)

OGCR Section I. C.9.a.5.

Hypertensive Retinopathy

Subcategory H35.0, Background retinopathy and
retinal vascular changes, should be used with a
code from category I10–I15, Hypertensive disease to
include the systemic hypertension. The sequencing is
based on the reason for the encounter.

H35.00 Unspecified background retinopathy
● **H35.01 Changes in retinal vascular appearance**
Retinal vascular sheathing

H35.011 Changes in retinal vascular
appearance, right eye

H35.012 Changes in retinal vascular
appearance, left eye

H35.013 Changes in retinal vascular
appearance, bilateral

H35.019 Changes in retinal vascular
appearance, unspecified eye

● **H35.02 Exudative retinopathy**
Coats retinopathy

H35.021 Exudative retinopathy, right eye

H35.022 Exudative retinopathy, left eye

H35.023 Exudative retinopathy, bilateral

H35.029 Exudative retinopathy, unspecified
eye

● **H35.03 Hypertensive retinopathy**

H35.031 Hypertensive retinopathy, right eye

H35.032 Hypertensive retinopathy, left eye

H35.033 Hypertensive retinopathy, bilateral

H35.039 Hypertensive retinopathy, unspecified
eye

● **H35.04 Retinal micro-aneurysms, unspecified**

H35.041 Retinal micro-aneurysms,
unspecified, right eye

H35.042 Retinal micro-aneurysms,
unspecified, left eye

H35.043 Retinal micro-aneurysms,
unspecified, bilateral

H35.049 Retinal micro-aneurysms,
unspecified, unspecified eye

● **H35.05 Retinal neovascularization, unspecified**

H35.051 Retinal neovascularization,
unspecified, right eye

H35.052 Retinal neovascularization,
unspecified, left eye

H35.053 Retinal neovascularization,
unspecified, bilateral

H35.059 Retinal neovascularization,
unspecified, unspecified eye

● **H35.06 Retinal vasculitis**
Eales disease
Retinal perivasculitis

H35.061 Retinal vasculitis, right eye

H35.062 Retinal vasculitis, left eye

H35.063 Retinal vasculitis, bilateral

H35.069 Retinal vasculitis, unspecified eye

● **H35.07 Retinal telangiectasis**

H35.071 Retinal telangiectasis, right eye

H35.072 Retinal telangiectasis, left eye

H35.073 Retinal telangiectasis, bilateral

H35.079 Retinal telangiectasis, unspecified eye

H35.09 Other intraretinal microvascular abnormalities
Retinal varices

● **H35.1 Retinopathy of prematurity**

● **H35.10 Retinopathy of prematurity, unspecified**
Retinopathy of prematurity NOS

H35.101 Retinopathy of prematurity,
unspecified, right eye

H35.102 Retinopathy of prematurity,
unspecified, left eye

H35.103 Retinopathy of prematurity,
unspecified, bilateral

H35.109 Retinopathy of prematurity,
unspecified, unspecified eye

● **H35.11 Retinopathy of prematurity, stage 0**

H35.111 Retinopathy of prematurity, stage 0,
right eye

H35.112 Retinopathy of prematurity, stage 0,
left eye

H35.113 Retinopathy of prematurity, stage 0,
bilateral

H35.119 Retinopathy of prematurity, stage 0,
unspecified eye

● **H35.12 Retinopathy of prematurity, stage 1**

H35.121 Retinopathy of prematurity, stage 1,
right eye

H35.122 Retinopathy of prematurity, stage 1,
left eye

H35.123 Retinopathy of prematurity, stage 1,
bilateral

H35.129 Retinopathy of prematurity, stage 1,
unspecified eye

● **H35.13 Retinopathy of prematurity, stage 2**

H35.131 Retinopathy of prematurity, stage 2,
right eye

H35.132 Retinopathy of prematurity, stage 2,
left eye

H35.133 Retinopathy of prematurity, stage 2,
bilateral

H35.139 Retinopathy of prematurity, stage 2,
unspecified eye

● **H35.14 Retinopathy of prematurity, stage 3**

H35.141 Retinopathy of prematurity, stage 3,
right eye

H35.142 Retinopathy of prematurity, stage 3,
left eye

H35.143 Retinopathy of prematurity, stage 3,
bilateral

H35.149 Retinopathy of prematurity, stage 3,
unspecified eye

● **H35.15 Retinopathy of prematurity, stage 4**

H35.151 Retinopathy of prematurity, stage 4,
right eye

H35.152 Retinopathy of prematurity, stage 4,
left eye

H35.153 Retinopathy of prematurity, stage 4,
bilateral

H35.159 Retinopathy of prematurity, stage 4,
unspecified eye

834

▶ New ⇒ Revised ~~deleted~~ Deleted Excludes 1 Excludes 2 Includes Use additional Code first Code also Key words
OGCR Official Guidelines ● Unacceptable Principal Diagnosis X Assign placeholder X ● Use Additional Character(s) ▶ Manifestation Code **Coding Clinic**

● H35.16   Retinopathy of prematurity, stage 5
     H35.161   Retinopathy of prematurity, stage 5, right eye
     H35.162   Retinopathy of prematurity, stage 5, left eye
     H35.163   Retinopathy of prematurity, stage 5, bilateral
     H35.169   Retinopathy of prematurity, stage 5, unspecified eye

● H35.17   Retrolental fibroplasia
     H35.171   Retrolental fibroplasia, right eye
     H35.172   Retrolental fibroplasia, left eye
     H35.173   Retrolental fibroplasia, bilateral
     H35.179   Retrolental fibroplasia, unspecified eye

● H35.2   Other non-diabetic proliferative retinopathy
     Proliferative vitreo-retinopathy

> **Excludes1**   proliferative vitreo-retinopathy with retinal detachment (H33.4-)

     H35.20   Other non-diabetic proliferative retinopathy, unspecified eye
     H35.21   Other non-diabetic proliferative retinopathy, right eye
     H35.22   Other non-diabetic proliferative retinopathy, left eye
     H35.23   Other non-diabetic proliferative retinopathy, bilateral

● H35.3   Degeneration of macula and posterior pole
     H35.30   Unspecified macular degeneration   A
        Age-related macular degeneration

● H35.31   Nonexudative age-related macular degeneration
        Atrophic age-related macular degeneration
        Dry age-related macular degeneration

One of the following 7th characters is to be assigned to codes in subcategory H35.31 to designate the stage of the disease:

Ø	stage unspecified
1	early dry stage
2	intermediate dry stage
3	advanced atrophic without subfoveal involvement
	advanced dry stage
4	advanced atrophic with subfoveal involvement

     ● H35.311   Nonexudative age-related macular degeneration, right eye   A
           Coding Clinic: 2016, Q4, P20-21
     ● H35.312   Nonexudative age-related macular degeneration, left eye   A
           Coding Clinic: 2016, Q4, P20-21
     ● H35.313   Nonexudative age-related macular degeneration, bilateral   A
           Coding Clinic: 2016, Q4, P20
     ● H35.319   Nonexudative age-related macular degeneration, unspecified eye   A
           Coding Clinic: 2016, Q4, P20

● H35.32   Exudative age-related macular degeneration
        Wet age-related macular degeneration

One of the following 7th characters is to be assigned to codes in subcategory H35.32 to designate the stage of the disease:

Ø	stage unspecified
1	with active choroidal neovascularization
2	with inactive choroidal neovascularization
	with involuted or regressed neovascularization
3	with inactive scar

Coding Clinic: 2016, Q4, P20

     ● H35.321   Exudative age-related macular degeneration, right eye   A
     ● H35.322   Exudative age-related macular degeneration, left eye   A
     ● H35.323   Exudative age-related macular degeneration, bilateral   A
     ● H35.329   Exudative age-related macular degeneration, unspecified eye   A

     H35.33   Angioid streaks of macula

● H35.34   Macular cyst, hole, or pseudohole
     H35.341   Macular cyst, hole, or pseudohole, right eye
     H35.342   Macular cyst, hole, or pseudohole, left eye
     H35.343   Macular cyst, hole, or pseudohole, bilateral
     H35.349   Macular cyst, hole, or pseudohole, unspecified eye

● H35.35   Cystoid macular degeneration

> **Excludes1**   cystoid macular edema following cataract surgery (H59.03-)

     H35.351   Cystoid macular degeneration, right eye
     H35.352   Cystoid macular degeneration, left eye
     H35.353   Cystoid macular degeneration, bilateral
     H35.359   Cystoid macular degeneration, unspecified eye

● H35.36   Drusen (degenerative) of macula
     H35.361   Drusen (degenerative) of macula, right eye
           Coding Clinic: 2016, Q4, P21
     H35.362   Drusen (degenerative) of macula, left eye
           Coding Clinic: 2016, Q4, P21
     H35.363   Drusen (degenerative) of macula, bilateral
           Coding Clinic: 2017, Q1, P51
     H35.369   Drusen (degenerative) of macula, unspecified eye

● H35.37   Puckering of macula
     H35.371   Puckering of macula, right eye
     H35.372   Puckering of macula, left eye
     H35.373   Puckering of macula, bilateral
     H35.379   Puckering of macula, unspecified eye

CHAPTER 7 (HØØ-H59)

Item 7-7 Macular degeneration is typically age-related, chronic, and is evidenced by deterioration of the macula (the part of the retina that provides for central field vision), resulting in blurred vision or a blind spot in the center of visual field while not affecting peripheral vision.

N Newborn Age: Ø   **P** Pediatric Age: Ø–17   **M** Maternity DX: 12–55   **A** Adult Age: 15–124   ♀ Females Only   ♂ Males Only

Complication\Comorbidity   Major C\C   (Ex) CC/MCC Exclusions   Hospital-Acquired Condition

835

● **H35.38**   **Toxic maculopathy**
> *Code first poisoning due to drug or toxin, if applicable (T36-T65 with fifth or sixth character 1-4 or 6)*

> Use additional code for adverse effect, if applicable, to identify drug (T36-T50 with fifth or sixth character 5)

     H35.381   Toxic maculopathy, right eye
     H35.382   Toxic maculopathy, left eye
     H35.383   Toxic maculopathy, bilateral
     H35.389   Toxic maculopathy, unspecified eye

● **H35.4**   **Peripheral retinal degeneration**
> **Excludes1**   hereditary retinal degeneration (dystrophy) (H35.5-)
> peripheral retinal degeneration with retinal break (H33.3-)

     H35.40   Unspecified peripheral retinal degeneration

● **H35.41**   **Lattice degeneration of retina**
> Palisade degeneration of retina

     H35.411   Lattice degeneration of retina, right eye
     H35.412   Lattice degeneration of retina, left eye
     H35.413   Lattice degeneration of retina, bilateral
     H35.419   Lattice degeneration of retina, unspecified eye

● **H35.42**   **Microcystoid degeneration of retina**
     H35.421   Microcystoid degeneration of retina, right eye
     H35.422   Microcystoid degeneration of retina, left eye
     H35.423   Microcystoid degeneration of retina, bilateral
     H35.429   Microcystoid degeneration of retina, unspecified eye

● **H35.43**   **Paving stone degeneration of retina**
     H35.431   Paving stone degeneration of retina, right eye
     H35.432   Paving stone degeneration of retina, left eye
     H35.433   Paving stone degeneration of retina, bilateral
     H35.439   Paving stone degeneration of retina, unspecified eye

● **H35.44**   **Age-related reticular degeneration of retina**
     H35.441   Age-related reticular degeneration of retina, right eye   A
     H35.442   Age-related reticular degeneration of retina, left eye   A
     H35.443   Age-related reticular degeneration of retina, bilateral   A
     H35.449   Age-related reticular degeneration of retina, unspecified eye   A

● **H35.45**   **Secondary pigmentary degeneration**
     H35.451   Secondary pigmentary degeneration, right eye
     H35.452   Secondary pigmentary degeneration, left eye
     H35.453   Secondary pigmentary degeneration, bilateral
     H35.459   Secondary pigmentary degeneration, unspecified eye

● **H35.46**   **Secondary vitreoretinal degeneration**
     H35.461   Secondary vitreoretinal degeneration, right eye
     H35.462   Secondary vitreoretinal degeneration, left eye
     H35.463   Secondary vitreoretinal degeneration, bilateral
     H35.469   Secondary vitreoretinal degeneration, unspecified eye

● **H35.5**   **Hereditary retinal dystrophy**
> **Excludes1**   dystrophies primarily involving Bruch's membrane (H31.1-)

     H35.50   Unspecified hereditary retinal dystrophy
     H35.51   Vitreoretinal dystrophy
     H35.52   Pigmentary retinal dystrophy
> Albipunctate retinal dystrophy
> Retinitis pigmentosa
> Tapetoretinal dystrophy

     H35.53   Other dystrophies primarily involving the sensory retina
> Stargardt's disease

     H35.54   Dystrophies primarily involving the retinal pigment epithelium
> Vitelliform retinal dystrophy

● **H35.6**   **Retinal hemorrhage**
     H35.60   Retinal hemorrhage, unspecified eye
     H35.61   Retinal hemorrhage, right eye
     H35.62   Retinal hemorrhage, left eye
     H35.63   Retinal hemorrhage, bilateral

● **H35.7**   **Separation of retinal layers**
> **Excludes1**   retinal detachment (serous) (H33.2-)
> rhegmatogenous retinal detachment (H33.0-)

> (Ex) **For category H35.7 CC codes:** See PDX Collection 628

     H35.70   Unspecified separation of retinal layers 🔘

● **H35.71**   **Central serous chorioretinopathy**
     H35.711   Central serous chorioretinopathy, right eye
     H35.712   Central serous chorioretinopathy, left eye
     H35.713   Central serous chorioretinopathy, bilateral
     H35.719   Central serous chorioretinopathy, unspecified eye

● **H35.72**   **Serous detachment of retinal pigment epithelium**
     H35.721   Serous detachment of retinal pigment epithelium, right eye 🔘
     H35.722   Serous detachment of retinal pigment epithelium, left eye 🔘
     H35.723   Serous detachment of retinal pigment epithelium, bilateral 🔘
     H35.729   Serous detachment of retinal pigment epithelium, unspecified eye 🔘

● **H35.73**   **Hemorrhagic detachment of retinal pigment epithelium**
     H35.731   Hemorrhagic detachment of retinal pigment epithelium, right eye 🔘
     H35.732   Hemorrhagic detachment of retinal pigment epithelium, left eye 🔘
     H35.733   Hemorrhagic detachment of retinal pigment epithelium, bilateral 🔘
     H35.739   Hemorrhagic detachment of retinal pigment epithelium, unspecified eye 🔘

▶ New   ⇒ Revised   ~~deleted~~ Deleted   Excludes 1   Excludes 2   Includes   Use additional   Code first   Code also   Key words

OGCR Official Guidelines   ● Unacceptable Principal Diagnosis   X Assign placeholder X   ● Use Additional Character(s)   ▶ Manifestation Code   **Coding Clinic**

H35.8   Other specified retinal disorders
>   **Excludes2**   retinal hemorrhage (H35.6-)
> H35.81   Retinal edema
>   Retinal cotton wool spots
> H35.82   Retinal ischemia 🔖
>   (Ex) See PDX Collection 629
> H35.89   Other specified retinal disorders
H35.9   Unspecified retinal disorder

▶ **H36   Retinal disorders in diseases classified elsewhere**
>   Code first underlying disease, such as:
>   lipid storage disorders (E75.-)
>   sickle-cell disorders (D57.-)
>   **Excludes1**   arteriosclerotic retinopathy (H35.0-)
>   diabetic retinopathy (E08.3-, E09.3-, E10.3-,
>   E11.3-, E13.3-)

GLAUCOMA (H40-H42)

● H40   **Glaucoma**
>   *Intraocular pressure (IOP) that is too high results from too much
>   aqueous humor and because of excess production or inadequate
>   drainage, optic nerve damage and vision loss may occur.*
>   **Excludes1**   absolute glaucoma (H44.51-)
>   congenital glaucoma (Q15.0)
>   traumatic glaucoma due to birth injury (P15.3)
> ● H40.0   Glaucoma suspect
>   ● H40.00   Preglaucoma, unspecified
>   H40.001   Preglaucoma, unspecified, right eye
>   H40.002   Preglaucoma, unspecified, left eye
>   H40.003   Preglaucoma, unspecified, bilateral
>   H40.009   Preglaucoma, unspecified, unspecified
>   eye
>   ● H40.01   Open angle with borderline findings, low risk
>   Open angle, low risk
>   H40.011   Open angle with borderline findings,
>   low risk, right eye
>   H40.012   Open angle with borderline findings,
>   low risk, left eye
>   H40.013   Open angle with borderline findings,
>   low risk, bilateral
>   H40.019   Open angle with borderline findings,
>   low risk, unspecified eye
>   ● H40.02   Open angle with borderline findings, high risk
>   Open angle, high risk
>   H40.021   Open angle with borderline findings,
>   high risk, right eye
>   H40.022   Open angle with borderline findings,
>   high risk, left eye
>   H40.023   Open angle with borderline findings,
>   high risk, bilateral
>   H40.029   Open angle with borderline findings,
>   high risk, unspecified eye
>   ● H40.03   Anatomical narrow angle
>   Primary angle closure suspect
>   H40.031   Anatomical narrow angle, right eye
>   H40.032   Anatomical narrow angle, left eye
>   H40.033   Anatomical narrow angle, bilateral
>   H40.039   Anatomical narrow angle, unspecified
>   eye
>   ● H40.04   Steroid responder
>   H40.041   Steroid responder, right eye
>   H40.042   Steroid responder, left eye
>   H40.043   Steroid responder, bilateral
>   H40.049   Steroid responder, unspecified eye

● H40.05   Ocular hypertension
> H40.051   Ocular hypertension, right eye
> H40.052   Ocular hypertension, left eye
> H40.053   Ocular hypertension, bilateral
> H40.059   Ocular hypertension, unspecified eye
● H40.06   Primary angle closure without glaucoma
>   damage
> H40.061   Primary angle closure without
>   glaucoma damage, right eye
> H40.062   Primary angle closure without
>   glaucoma damage, left eye
> H40.063   Primary angle closure without
>   glaucoma damage, bilateral
> H40.069   Primary angle closure without
>   glaucoma damage, unspecified eye
● H40.1   Open-angle glaucoma
> X ● H40.10   Unspecified open-angle glaucoma
>   One of the following 7th characters is to be
>   assigned to code H40.10 to designate the
>   stage of glaucoma

0	stage unspecified
1	mild stage
2	moderate stage
3	severe stage
4	indeterminate stage

> ● H40.11   Primary open-angle glaucoma
>   Chronic simple glaucoma
>   One of the following 7th characters is to be
>   assigned to each code in subcategory
>   H40.11 to designate the stage of
>   glaucoma

0	stage unspecified
1	mild stage
2	moderate stage
3	severe stage
4	indeterminate stage

>   **Coding Clinic: 2016, Q4, P22**
> ● H40.111   Primary open-angle glaucoma, right
>   eye
> ● H40.112   Primary open-angle glaucoma, left
>   eye
> ● H40.113   Primary open-angle glaucoma,
>   bilateral
> ● H40.119   Primary open-angle glaucoma,
>   unspecified eye
> ● H40.12   Low-tension glaucoma
>   One of the following 7th characters is to be
>   assigned to each code in subcategory
>   H40.12 to designate the stage of
>   glaucoma

0	stage unspecified
1	mild stage
2	moderate stage
3	severe stage
4	indeterminate stage

> ●● H40.121   Low-tension glaucoma, right eye
> ●● H40.122   Low-tension glaucoma, left eye
> ●● H40.123   Low-tension glaucoma, bilateral
> ●● H40.129   Low-tension glaucoma, unspecified
>   eye

CHAPTER 7 (H00-H59)

N   Newborn Age: 0   P   Pediatric Age: 0–17   M   Maternity DX: 12–55   A   Adult Age: 15–124   ♀   Females Only   ♂   Males Only

🔖 Complication\Comorbidity   🔖 Major C\C   (Ex) CC/MCC Exclusions   🔖 Hospital-Acquired Condition

CHAPTER 7 (H00-H59)

● H40.13   Pigmentary glaucoma

One of the following 7th characters is to be assigned to each code in subcategory H40.13 to designate the stage of glaucoma

0	stage unspecified
1	mild stage
2	moderate stage
3	severe stage
4	indeterminate stage

●● H40.131   Pigmentary glaucoma, right eye

●● H40.132   Pigmentary glaucoma, left eye

●● H40.133   Pigmentary glaucoma, bilateral

●● H40.139   Pigmentary glaucoma, unspecified eye

● H40.14   Capsular glaucoma with pseudoexfoliation of lens

One of the following 7th characters is to be assigned to each code in subcategory H40.14 to designate the stage of glaucoma

0	stage unspecified
1	mild stage
2	moderate stage
3	severe stage
4	indeterminate stage

● H40.141   Capsular glaucoma with pseudoexfoliation of lens, right eye

● H40.142   Capsular glaucoma with pseudoexfoliation of lens, left eye

● H40.143   Capsular glaucoma with pseudoexfoliation of lens, bilateral

● H40.149   Capsular glaucoma with pseudoexfoliation of lens, unspecified eye

● H40.15   Residual stage of open-angle glaucoma

● H40.151   Residual stage of open-angle glaucoma, right eye

● H40.152   Residual stage of open-angle glaucoma, left eye

● H40.153   Residual stage of open-angle glaucoma, bilateral

● H40.159   Residual stage of open-angle glaucoma, unspecified eye

● H40.2   Primary angle-closure glaucoma

Excludes1   aqueous misdirection (H40.83-)
malignant glaucoma (H40.83-)

X ● H40.20   Unspecified primary angle-closure glaucoma

One of the following 7th characters is to be assigned to code H40.20 to designate the stage of glaucoma

0	stage unspecified
1	mild stage
2	moderate stage
3	severe stage
4	indeterminate stage

● H40.21   Acute angle-closure glaucoma

Acute angle-closure glaucoma attack
Acute angle-closure glaucoma crisis
(Ex) **For category H40.21 CC codes: See PDX Collection 630**

H40.211   Acute angle-closure glaucoma, right eye 🌀

H40.212   Acute angle-closure glaucoma, left eye 🌀

H40.213   Acute angle-closure glaucoma, bilateral 🌀

H40.219   Acute angle-closure glaucoma, unspecified eye 🌀

● H40.22   Chronic angle-closure glaucoma

Chronic primary angle closure glaucoma

One of the following 7th characters is to be assigned to each code in subcategory H40.22 to designate the stage of glaucoma

0	stage unspecified
1	mild stage
2	moderate stage
3	severe stage
4	indeterminate stage

● H40.221   Chronic angle-closure glaucoma, right eye

● H40.222   Chronic angle-closure glaucoma, left eye

● H40.223   Chronic angle-closure glaucoma, bilateral

● H40.229   Chronic angle-closure glaucoma, unspecified eye

● H40.23   Intermittent angle-closure glaucoma

H40.231   Intermittent angle-closure glaucoma, right eye

H40.232   Intermittent angle-closure glaucoma, left eye

H40.233   Intermittent angle-closure glaucoma, bilateral

H40.239   Intermittent angle-closure glaucoma, unspecified eye

● H40.24   Residual stage of angle-closure glaucoma

H40.241   Residual stage of angle-closure glaucoma, right eye

H40.242   Residual stage of angle-closure glaucoma, left eye

H40.243   Residual stage of angle-closure glaucoma, bilateral

H40.249   Residual stage of angle-closure glaucoma, unspecified eye

● H40.3   Glaucoma secondary to eye trauma

Code also underlying condition

One of the following 7th characters is to be assigned to each code in subcategory H40.3 to designate the stage of glaucoma

0	stage unspecified
1	mild stage
2	moderate stage
3	severe stage
4	indeterminate stage

X ● H40.30   Glaucoma secondary to eye trauma, unspecified eye

X ● H40.31   Glaucoma secondary to eye trauma, right eye

X ● H40.32   Glaucoma secondary to eye trauma, left eye

X ● H40.33   Glaucoma secondary to eye trauma, bilateral

▶ New   ⇒ Revised   ~~deleted~~ Deleted   Excludes 1   Excludes 2   Includes   Use additional   Code first   Code also   Key words

OGCR Official Guidelines   ● Unacceptable Principal Diagnosis   X Assign placeholder X   ● Use Additional Character(s)   ▶ Manifestation Code   **Coding Clinic**

● H40.4 **Glaucoma secondary to eye inflammation**
Code also underlying condition
One of the following 7th characters is to be assigned to each code in subcategory H40.4 to designate the stage of glaucoma

Ø	stage unspecified
1	mild stage
2	moderate stage
3	severe stage
4	indeterminate stage

X● H40.40 Glaucoma secondary to eye inflammation, unspecified eye

X● H40.41 Glaucoma secondary to eye inflammation, right eye

X● H40.42 Glaucoma secondary to eye inflammation, left eye

X● H40.43 Glaucoma secondary to eye inflammation, bilateral

● H40.5 **Glaucoma secondary to other eye disorders**
Code also underlying eye disorder
One of the following 7th characters is to be assigned to each code in subcategory H40.5 to designate the stage of glaucoma

Ø	stage unspecified
1	mild stage
2	moderate stage
3	severe stage
4	indeterminate stage

X● H40.50 Glaucoma secondary to other eye disorders, unspecified eye

X● H40.51 Glaucoma secondary to other eye disorders, right eye

X● H40.52 Glaucoma secondary to other eye disorders, left eye

X● H40.53 Glaucoma secondary to other eye disorders, bilateral

● H40.6 **Glaucoma secondary to drugs**
Use additional code for adverse effect, if applicable, to identify drug (T36-T50 with fifth or sixth character 5)
One of the following 7th characters is to be assigned to each code in subcategory H40.6 to designate the stage of glaucoma

Ø	stage unspecified
1	mild stage
2	moderate stage
3	severe stage
4	indeterminate stage

X● H40.60 Glaucoma secondary to drugs, unspecified eye
X● H40.61 Glaucoma secondary to drugs, right eye
X● H40.62 Glaucoma secondary to drugs, left eye
X● H40.63 Glaucoma secondary to drugs, bilateral

● H40.8 **Other glaucoma**
● H40.81 **Glaucoma with increased episcleral venous pressure**
H40.811 Glaucoma with increased episcleral venous pressure, right eye
H40.812 Glaucoma with increased episcleral venous pressure, left eye
H40.813 Glaucoma with increased episcleral venous pressure, bilateral
H40.819 Glaucoma with increased episcleral venous pressure, unspecified eye

● H40.82 **Hypersecretion glaucoma**
H40.821 Hypersecretion glaucoma, right eye
H40.822 Hypersecretion glaucoma, left eye
H40.823 Hypersecretion glaucoma, bilateral
H40.829 Hypersecretion glaucoma, unspecified eye

● H40.83 **Aqueous misdirection**
Malignant glaucoma
H40.831 Aqueous misdirection, right eye
H40.832 Aqueous misdirection, left eye
H40.833 Aqueous misdirection, bilateral
H40.839 Aqueous misdirection, unspecified eye

H40.89 **Other specified glaucoma**

H40.9 **Unspecified glaucoma**

▌ H42 *Glaucoma in diseases classified elsewhere*
Code first underlying condition, such as:
amyloidosis (E85.-)
aniridia (Q13.1)
▶ glaucoma (in) diabetes mellitus (E08.39, E09.39, E10.39, E11.39, E13.39)
Lowe's syndrome (E72.03)
Reiger's anomaly (Q13.81)
specified metabolic disorder (E70-E88)

Excludes1 glaucoma (in) onchocerciasis (B73.02)
glaucoma (in) syphilis (A52.71)
glaucoma (in) tuberculous (A18.59)
~~glaucoma (in) diabetes mellitus (E08.39, E09.39, E10.39, E11.39, E13.39)~~

DISORDERS OF VITREOUS BODY AND GLOBE (H43-H44)

● H43 **Disorders of vitreous body**
● H43.0 **Vitreous prolapse**
Excludes1 vitreous syndrome following cataract surgery (H59.0-)
traumatic vitreous prolapse (S05.2-)
H43.00 Vitreous prolapse, unspecified eye
H43.01 Vitreous prolapse, right eye
H43.02 Vitreous prolapse, left eye
H43.03 Vitreous prolapse, bilateral

● H43.1 **Vitreous hemorrhage**
H43.10 Vitreous hemorrhage, unspecified eye
H43.11 Vitreous hemorrhage, right eye
H43.12 Vitreous hemorrhage, left eye
H43.13 Vitreous hemorrhage, bilateral

● H43.2 **Crystalline deposits in vitreous body**
H43.20 Crystalline deposits in vitreous body, unspecified eye
H43.21 Crystalline deposits in vitreous body, right eye
H43.22 Crystalline deposits in vitreous body, left eye
H43.23 Crystalline deposits in vitreous body, bilateral

● H43.3 **Other vitreous opacities**
● H43.31 **Vitreous membranes and strands**
H43.311 Vitreous membranes and strands, right eye
H43.312 Vitreous membranes and strands, left eye
H43.313 Vitreous membranes and strands, bilateral
H43.319 Vitreous membranes and strands, unspecified eye

● **H43.39 Other vitreous opacities**
Vitreous floaters
Small clumps of cells that float in the vitreous of the eye, appearing as black specks or dots in the field of vision and common in the aging eye.

H43.391   Other vitreous opacities, **right eye**

H43.392   Other vitreous opacities, **left eye**

H43.393   Other vitreous opacities, **bilateral**

H43.399   Other vitreous opacities, **unspecified eye**

● **H43.8 Other disorders of vitreous body**
Excludes1   proliferative vitreo-retinopathy with retinal detachment (H33.4)
Excludes2   vitreous abscess (H44.02-)

● **H43.81 Vitreous degeneration**
Vitreous detachment

H43.811   Vitreous degeneration, **right eye**

H43.812   Vitreous degeneration, **left eye**

H43.813   Vitreous degeneration, **bilateral**

H43.819   Vitreous degeneration, **unspecified eye**

● **H43.82 Vitreomacular adhesion**
Vitreomacular traction

H43.821   Vitreomacular adhesion, **right eye**   A

H43.822   Vitreomacular adhesion, **left eye**   A

H43.823   Vitreomacular adhesion, **bilateral**   A

H43.829   Vitreomacular adhesion, **unspecified eye**   A

H43.89   Other disorders of vitreous body

H43.9   Unspecified disorder of vitreous body

● **H44 Disorders of globe**
Includes   disorders affecting multiple structures of eye

● **H44.0 Purulent endophthalmitis**
Use additional code to identify organism
Excludes1   bleb associated endophthalmitis (H59.4-)

● **H44.00 Unspecified purulent endophthalmitis**
(Ex:) For category H44.00 CC codes: See PDX Collection 625

H44.001   Unspecified purulent endophthalmitis, **right eye**

H44.002   Unspecified purulent endophthalmitis, **left eye**

H44.003   Unspecified purulent endophthalmitis, **bilateral**

H44.009   Unspecified purulent endophthalmitis, **unspecified eye**

● **H44.01 Panophthalmitis (acute)**
(Ex:) For category H44.01 CC codes: See PDX Collection 625

H44.011   Panophthalmitis (acute), **right eye**

H44.012   Panophthalmitis (acute), **left eye**

H44.013   Panophthalmitis (acute), **bilateral**

H44.019   Panophthalmitis (acute), **unspecified eye**

● **H44.02 Vitreous abscess (chronic)**
(Ex:) For category H44.02 CC codes: See PDX Collection 631

H44.021   Vitreous abscess (chronic), **right eye**

H44.022   Vitreous abscess (chronic), **left eye**

H44.023   Vitreous abscess (chronic), **bilateral**

H44.029   Vitreous abscess (chronic), **unspecified eye**

● **H44.1 Other endophthalmitis**
Excludes1   bleb associated endophthalmitis (H59.4-)
Excludes2   ophthalmia nodosa (H16.2-)

● **H44.11 Panuveitis**
(Ex:) For category H44.11 CC codes: See PDX Collection 632

H44.111   Panuveitis, **right eye**

H44.112   Panuveitis, **left eye**

H44.113   Panuveitis, **bilateral**

H44.119   Panuveitis, **unspecified eye**

● **H44.12 Parasitic endophthalmitis, unspecified**
(Ex:) For category H44.12 CC codes: See PDX Collection 625

H44.121   Parasitic endophthalmitis, unspecified, **right eye**

H44.122   Parasitic endophthalmitis, unspecified, **left eye**

H44.123   Parasitic endophthalmitis, unspecified, **bilateral**

H44.129   Parasitic endophthalmitis, unspecified, **unspecified eye**

● **H44.13 Sympathetic uveitis**
(Ex:) For category H44.13 CC codes: See PDX Collection 632

H44.131   Sympathetic uveitis, **right eye**

H44.132   Sympathetic uveitis, **left eye**

H44.133   Sympathetic uveitis, **bilateral**

H44.139   Sympathetic uveitis, **unspecified eye**

H44.19   **Other endophthalmitis**
(Ex:) See PDX Collection 625

● **H44.2 Degenerative myopia**
Malignant myopia

H44.20   Degenerative myopia, **unspecified eye**

H44.21   Degenerative myopia, **right eye**

H44.22   Degenerative myopia, **left eye**

H44.23   Degenerative myopia, **bilateral**

▶● **H44.2A Degenerative myopia with choroidal neovascularization**
▶ Use Additional code for any associated choroid disorders (H31.-)

▶ H44.2A1   Degenerative myopia with choroidal neovascularization, **right eye**

▶ H44.2A2   Degenerative myopia with choroidal neovascularization, **left eye**

▶ H44.2A3   Degenerative myopia with choroidal neovascularization, **bilateral eye**

▶ H44.2A9   Degenerative myopia with choroidal neovascularization, **unspecified eye**

▶● **H44.2B Degenerative myopia with macular hole**

▶ H44.2B1   Degenerative myopia with macular hole, **right eye**

▶ H44.2B2   Degenerative myopia with macular hole, **left eye**

▶ H44.2B3   Degenerative myopia with macular hole, **bilateral eye**

▶ H44.2B9   Degenerative myopia with macular hole, **unspecified eye**

▶● **H44.2C Degenerative myopia with retinal detachment**
▶ Use Additional code to identify the retinal detachment (H33.-)

▶ H44.2C1   Degenerative myopia with retinal detachment, **right eye**

▶ H44.2C2   Degenerative myopia with retinal detachment, **left eye**

▶ H44.2C3   Degenerative myopia with retinal detachment, **bilateral eye**

▶ H44.2C9   Degenerative myopia with retinal detachment, **unspecified eye**

▶ New   ⇒ Revised   ~~deleted~~ Deleted   Excludes 1   Excludes 2   Includes   Use additional   Code first   Code also   Key words
OGCR Official Guidelines   ● Unacceptable Principal Diagnosis   X Assign placeholder X   ● Use Additional Character(s)   ▌ Manifestation Code   **Coding Clinic**

▶● **H44.2D** Degenerative myopia with foveoschisis
   ▶ H44.2D1 Degenerative myopia with foveoschisis, right eye
   ▶ H44.2D2 Degenerative myopia with foveoschisis, left eye
   ▶ H44.2D3 Degenerative myopia with foveoschisis, bilateral eye
   ▶ H44.2D9 Degenerative myopia with foveoschisis, unspecified eye
▶● **H44.2E** Degenerative myopia with other maculopathy
   ▶ H44.2E1 Degenerative myopia with other maculopathy, right eye
   ▶ H44.2E2 Degenerative myopia with other maculopathy, left eye
   ▶ H44.2E3 Degenerative myopia with other maculopathy, bilateral eye
   ▶ H44.2E9 Degenerative myopia with other maculopathy, unspecified eye
● **H44.3** Other and unspecified degenerative disorders of globe
  H44.30 Unspecified degenerative disorder of globe
  ● H44.31 Chalcosis
    H44.311 Chalcosis, right eye
    H44.312 Chalcosis, left eye
    H44.313 Chalcosis, bilateral
    H44.319 Chalcosis, unspecified eye
  ● H44.32 Siderosis of eye
    H44.321 Siderosis of eye, right eye
    H44.322 Siderosis of eye, left eye
    H44.323 Siderosis of eye, bilateral
    H44.329 Siderosis of eye, unspecified eye
  ● H44.39 Other degenerative disorders of globe
    H44.391 Other degenerative disorders of globe, right eye
    H44.392 Other degenerative disorders of globe, left eye
    H44.393 Other degenerative disorders of globe, bilateral
    H44.399 Other degenerative disorders of globe, unspecified eye
● **H44.4** Hypotony of eye
  H44.40 Unspecified hypotony of eye
  ● H44.41 Flat anterior chamber hypotony of eye
    H44.411 Flat anterior chamber hypotony of right eye
    H44.412 Flat anterior chamber hypotony of left eye
    H44.413 Flat anterior chamber hypotony of eye, bilateral
    H44.419 Flat anterior chamber hypotony of unspecified eye
  ● H44.42 Hypotony of eye due to ocular fistula
    H44.421 Hypotony of right eye due to ocular fistula
    H44.422 Hypotony of left eye due to ocular fistula
    H44.423 Hypotony of eye due to ocular fistula, bilateral
    H44.429 Hypotony of unspecified eye due to ocular fistula

● H44.43 Hypotony of eye due to other ocular disorders
    H44.431 Hypotony of eye due to other ocular disorders, right eye
    H44.432 Hypotony of eye due to other ocular disorders, left eye
    H44.433 Hypotony of eye due to other ocular disorders, bilateral
    H44.439 Hypotony of eye due to other ocular disorders, unspecified eye
● H44.44 Primary hypotony of eye
    H44.441 Primary hypotony of right eye
    H44.442 Primary hypotony of left eye
    H44.443 Primary hypotony of eye, bilateral
    H44.449 Primary hypotony of unspecified eye
● **H44.5** Degenerated conditions of globe
  H44.50 Unspecified degenerated conditions of globe
  ● H44.51 Absolute glaucoma
    H44.511 Absolute glaucoma, right eye
    H44.512 Absolute glaucoma, left eye
    H44.513 Absolute glaucoma, bilateral
    H44.519 Absolute glaucoma, unspecified eye
  ● H44.52 Atrophy of globe
    Phthisis bulbi
    H44.521 Atrophy of globe, right eye
    H44.522 Atrophy of globe, left eye
    H44.523 Atrophy of globe, bilateral
    H44.529 Atrophy of globe, unspecified eye
  ● H44.53 Leucocoria
    H44.531 Leucocoria, right eye
    H44.532 Leucocoria, left eye
    H44.533 Leucocoria, bilateral
    H44.539 Leucocoria, unspecified eye
● H44.6 Retained (old) intraocular foreign body, magnetic
  Use additional code to identify magnetic foreign body (Z18.11)
  Excludes1 current intraocular foreign body (S05.-)
  Excludes2 retained foreign body in eyelid (H02.81-)
    retained (old) foreign body following penetrating wound of orbit (H05.5-)
    retained (old) intraocular foreign body, nonmagnetic (H44.7-)
  ● H44.60 Unspecified retained (old) intraocular foreign body, magnetic
    H44.601 Unspecified retained (old) intraocular foreign body, magnetic, right eye
    H44.602 Unspecified retained (old) intraocular foreign body, magnetic, left eye
    H44.603 Unspecified retained (old) intraocular foreign body, magnetic, bilateral
    H44.609 Unspecified retained (old) intraocular foreign body, magnetic, unspecified eye
  ● H44.61 Retained (old) magnetic foreign body in anterior chamber
    H44.611 Retained (old) magnetic foreign body in anterior chamber, right eye
    H44.612 Retained (old) magnetic foreign body in anterior chamber, left eye
    H44.613 Retained (old) magnetic foreign body in anterior chamber, bilateral
    H44.619 Retained (old) magnetic foreign body in anterior chamber, unspecified eye

N Newborn Age: 0   P Pediatric Age: 0–17   M Maternity DX: 12–55   A Adult Age: 15–124   ♀ Females Only   ♂ Males Only
Complication\Comorbidity   Major C\C   (Ex) CC/MCC Exclusions   Hospital-Acquired Condition
841

CHAPTER 7 (H00-H59)

CHAPTER 7 (H00-H59)

● H44.62   Retained (old) magnetic foreign body in iris or ciliary body

    H44.621   Retained (old) magnetic foreign body in iris or ciliary body, right eye

    H44.622   Retained (old) magnetic foreign body in iris or ciliary body, left eye

    H44.623   Retained (old) magnetic foreign body in iris or ciliary body, bilateral

    H44.629   Retained (old) magnetic foreign body in iris or ciliary body, unspecified eye

● H44.63   Retained (old) magnetic foreign body in lens

    H44.631   Retained (old) magnetic foreign body in lens, right eye

    H44.632   Retained (old) magnetic foreign body in lens, left eye

    H44.633   Retained (old) magnetic foreign body in lens, bilateral

    H44.639   Retained (old) magnetic foreign body in lens, unspecified eye

● H44.64   Retained (old) magnetic foreign body in posterior wall of globe

    H44.641   Retained (old) magnetic foreign body in posterior wall of globe, right eye

    H44.642   Retained (old) magnetic foreign body in posterior wall of globe, left eye

    H44.643   Retained (old) magnetic foreign body in posterior wall of globe, bilateral

    H44.649   Retained (old) magnetic foreign body in posterior wall of globe, unspecified eye

● H44.65   Retained (old) magnetic foreign body in vitreous body

    H44.651   Retained (old) magnetic foreign body in vitreous body, right eye

    H44.652   Retained (old) magnetic foreign body in vitreous body, left eye

    H44.653   Retained (old) magnetic foreign body in vitreous body, bilateral

    H44.659   Retained (old) magnetic foreign body in vitreous body, unspecified eye

● H44.69   Retained (old) intraocular foreign body, magnetic, in other or multiple sites

    H44.691   Retained (old) intraocular foreign body, magnetic, in other or multiple sites, right eye

    H44.692   Retained (old) intraocular foreign body, magnetic, in other or multiple sites, left eye

    H44.693   Retained (old) intraocular foreign body, magnetic, in other or multiple sites, bilateral

    H44.699   Retained (old) intraocular foreign body, magnetic, in other or multiple sites, unspecified eye

● H44.7   Retained (old) intraocular foreign body, nonmagnetic

    Use additional code to identify nonmagnetic foreign body (Z18.01-Z18.10, Z18.12, Z18.2-Z18.9)

    Excludes1   current intraocular foreign body (S05.-)

    Excludes2   retained foreign body in eyelid (H02.81-)
                retained (old) foreign body following penetrating wound of orbit (H05.5-)
                retained (old) intraocular foreign body, magnetic (H44.6-)

● H44.70   Unspecified retained (old) intraocular foreign body, nonmagnetic

    H44.701   Unspecified retained (old) intraocular foreign body, nonmagnetic, right eye

    H44.702   Unspecified retained (old) intraocular foreign body, nonmagnetic, left eye

    H44.703   Unspecified retained (old) intraocular foreign body, nonmagnetic, bilateral

    H44.709   Unspecified retained (old) intraocular foreign body, nonmagnetic, unspecified eye
            Retained (old) intraocular foreign body NOS

● H44.71   Retained (nonmagnetic) (old) foreign body in anterior chamber

    H44.711   Retained (nonmagnetic) (old) foreign body in anterior chamber, right eye

    H44.712   Retained (nonmagnetic) (old) foreign body in anterior chamber, left eye

    H44.713   Retained (nonmagnetic) (old) foreign body in anterior chamber, bilateral

    H44.719   Retained (nonmagnetic) (old) foreign body in anterior chamber, unspecified eye

● H44.72   Retained (nonmagnetic) (old) foreign body in iris or ciliary body

    H44.721   Retained (nonmagnetic) (old) foreign body in iris or ciliary body, right eye

    H44.722   Retained (nonmagnetic) (old) foreign body in iris or ciliary body, left eye

    H44.723   Retained (nonmagnetic) (old) foreign body in iris or ciliary body, bilateral

    H44.729   Retained (nonmagnetic) (old) foreign body in iris or ciliary body, unspecified eye

● H44.73   Retained (nonmagnetic) (old) foreign body in lens

    H44.731   Retained (nonmagnetic) (old) foreign body in lens, right eye

    H44.732   Retained (nonmagnetic) (old) foreign body in lens, left eye

    H44.733   Retained (nonmagnetic) (old) foreign body in lens, bilateral

    H44.739   Retained (nonmagnetic) (old) foreign body in lens, unspecified eye

● H44.74   Retained (nonmagnetic) (old) foreign body in posterior wall of globe

    H44.741   Retained (nonmagnetic) (old) foreign body in posterior wall of globe, right eye

    H44.742   Retained (nonmagnetic) (old) foreign body in posterior wall of globe, left eye

    H44.743   Retained (nonmagnetic) (old) foreign body in posterior wall of globe, bilateral

    H44.749   Retained (nonmagnetic) (old) foreign body in posterior wall of globe, unspecified eye

● H44.75   Retained (nonmagnetic) (old) foreign body in vitreous body

    H44.751   Retained (nonmagnetic) (old) foreign body in vitreous body, right eye

    H44.752   Retained (nonmagnetic) (old) foreign body in vitreous body, left eye

    H44.753   Retained (nonmagnetic) (old) foreign body in vitreous body, bilateral

    H44.759   Retained (nonmagnetic) (old) foreign body in vitreous body, unspecified eye

● H44.79 Retained (old) intraocular foreign body, nonmagnetic, in other or multiple sites

   H44.791 Retained (old) intraocular foreign body, nonmagnetic, in other or multiple sites, right eye

   H44.792 Retained (old) intraocular foreign body, nonmagnetic, in other or multiple sites, left eye

   H44.793 Retained (old) intraocular foreign body, nonmagnetic, in other or multiple sites, bilateral

   H44.799 Retained (old) intraocular foreign body, nonmagnetic, in other or multiple sites, unspecified eye

● H44.8 Other disorders of globe

   ● H44.81 Hemophthalmos

      H44.811 Hemophthalmos, right eye

      H44.812 Hemophthalmos, left eye

      H44.813 Hemophthalmos, bilateral

      H44.819 Hemophthalmos, unspecified eye

   ● H44.82 Luxation of globe

      H44.821 Luxation of globe, right eye

      H44.822 Luxation of globe, left eye

      H44.823 Luxation of globe, bilateral

      H44.829 Luxation of globe, unspecified eye

   H44.89 Other disorders of globe

H44.9 Unspecified disorder of globe

★ **(See Plate 86 on page 55.)**

DISORDERS OF OPTIC NERVE AND VISUAL PATHWAYS (H46-H47)

● H46 Optic neuritis

   Excludes2 ischemic optic neuropathy (H47.01-)
   neuromyelitis optica [Devic] (G36.0)

   Ex: For category H46 CC codes: See PDX Collection 633

   ● H46.0 Optic papillitis

      H46.00 Optic papillitis, unspecified eye

      H46.01 Optic papillitis, right eye

      H46.02 Optic papillitis, left eye

      H46.03 Optic papillitis, bilateral

   ● H46.1 Retrobulbar neuritis
      Retrobulbar neuritis NOS

      Excludes1 syphilitic retrobulbar neuritis (A52.15)

      H46.10 Retrobulbar neuritis, unspecified eye

      H46.11 Retrobulbar neuritis, right eye

      H46.12 Retrobulbar neuritis, left eye

      H46.13 Retrobulbar neuritis, bilateral

   H46.2 Nutritional optic neuropathy

   H46.3 Toxic optic neuropathy
      Code first (T51-T65) *to identify cause*

   H46.8 Other optic neuritis

   H46.9 Unspecified optic neuritis

● H47 Other disorders of optic [2nd] nerve and visual pathways

   ● H47.0 Disorders of optic nerve, not elsewhere classified

      ● H47.01 Ischemic optic neuropathy

         H47.011 Ischemic optic neuropathy, right eye

         H47.012 Ischemic optic neuropathy, left eye

         H47.013 Ischemic optic neuropathy, bilateral

         H47.019 Ischemic optic neuropathy, unspecified eye

   ● H47.02 Hemorrhage in optic nerve sheath

      H47.021 Hemorrhage in optic nerve sheath, right eye

      H47.022 Hemorrhage in optic nerve sheath, left eye

      H47.023 Hemorrhage in optic nerve sheath, bilateral

      H47.029 Hemorrhage in optic nerve sheath, unspecified eye

   ● H47.03 Optic nerve hypoplasia

      H47.031 Optic nerve hypoplasia, right eye

      H47.032 Optic nerve hypoplasia, left eye

      H47.033 Optic nerve hypoplasia, bilateral

      H47.039 Optic nerve hypoplasia, unspecified eye

   ● H47.09 Other disorders of optic nerve, not elsewhere classified
      Compression of optic nerve

      H47.091 Other disorders of optic nerve, not elsewhere classified, right eye

      H47.092 Other disorders of optic nerve, not elsewhere classified, left eye

      H47.093 Other disorders of optic nerve, not elsewhere classified, bilateral

      H47.099 Other disorders of optic nerve, not elsewhere classified, unspecified eye

● H47.1 Papilledema

   H47.10 Unspecified papilledema
      Ex: See PDX Collection 634

   H47.11 Papilledema associated with increased intracranial pressure
      Ex: See PDX Collection 634

   H47.12 Papilledema associated with decreased ocular pressure

   H47.13 Papilledema associated with retinal disorder

   ● H47.14 Foster-Kennedy syndrome

      H47.141 Foster-Kennedy syndrome, right eye

      H47.142 Foster-Kennedy syndrome, left eye

      H47.143 Foster-Kennedy syndrome, bilateral

      H47.149 Foster-Kennedy syndrome, unspecified eye

Figure 7-11 *Stages of papilledema according to the Frisén grading scale.* **A,** Very eary papilledema (Frisén stage 1). **B,** Early papilledema (Frisén stage 2). **C,** Moderate papilledema (Frisén stage 3). **D,** Marked papilledema (Frisén stage 4). **E,** Severe papilledema. (From Youmans JR, Winn HR: Youmans Neurological Surgery, Philadelphia, PA, Elsevier/Saunders, 2011)

Item 7-8 Papilledema is swelling of the optic disc caused by increased intracranial pressure. It is most often bilateral and occurs quickly (hours) or over weeks of time. It is a common symptom of a brain tumor. The term should not be used to describe optic disc swelling with underlying infectious, infiltrative, or inflammatory etiologies.

CHAPTER 7 (H00-H59)

● **H47.2**   **Optic atrophy**

    H47.20   Unspecified optic atrophy

●   **H47.21**   Primary optic atrophy

       H47.211   Primary optic atrophy, right eye

       H47.212   Primary optic atrophy, left eye

       H47.213   Primary optic atrophy, bilateral

       H47.219   Primary optic atrophy, unspecified eye

    H47.22   Hereditary optic atrophy

       Leber's optic atrophy

●   **H47.23**   Glaucomatous optic atrophy

       H47.231   Glaucomatous optic atrophy, right eye

       H47.232   Glaucomatous optic atrophy, left eye

       H47.233   Glaucomatous optic atrophy, bilateral

       H47.239   Glaucomatous optic atrophy, unspecified eye

●   **H47.29**   Other optic atrophy

       Temporal pallor of optic disc

       H47.291   Other optic atrophy, right eye

       H47.292   Other optic atrophy, left eye

       H47.293   Other optic atrophy, bilateral

       H47.299   Other optic atrophy, unspecified eye

● **H47.3**   **Other disorders of optic disc**

●   **H47.31**   Coloboma of optic disc

       H47.311   Coloboma of optic disc, right eye

       H47.312   Coloboma of optic disc, left eye

       H47.313   Coloboma of optic disc, bilateral

       H47.319   Coloboma of optic disc, unspecified eye

●   **H47.32**   Drusen of optic disc

       H47.321   Drusen of optic disc, right eye

       H47.322   Drusen of optic disc, left eye

       H47.323   Drusen of optic disc, bilateral

       H47.329   Drusen of optic disc, unspecified eye

●   **H47.33**   Pseudopapilledema of optic disc

       H47.331   Pseudopapilledema of optic disc, right eye

       H47.332   Pseudopapilledema of optic disc, left eye

       H47.333   Pseudopapilledema of optic disc, bilateral

       H47.339   Pseudopapilledema of optic disc, unspecified eye

●   **H47.39**   Other disorders of optic disc

       H47.391   Other disorders of optic disc, right eye

       H47.392   Other disorders of optic disc, left eye

       H47.393   Other disorders of optic disc, bilateral

       H47.399   Other disorders of optic disc, unspecified eye

● **H47.4**   **Disorders of optic chiasm**

      Code also underlying condition

      (Ex) **For category H47.4 CC codes:** See PDX Collection 635

    H47.41   Disorders of optic chiasm in (due to) inflammatory disorders

    H47.42   Disorders of optic chiasm in (due to) neoplasm

    H47.43   Disorders of optic chiasm in (due to) vascular disorders

    H47.49   Disorders of optic chiasm in (due to) other disorders

● **H47.5**   **Disorders of other visual pathways**

      Disorders of optic tracts, geniculate nuclei and optic radiations

      Code also underlying condition

      (Ex) **For category H47.5 CC codes:** See PDX Collection 635

●   **H47.51**   Disorders of visual pathways in (due to) inflammatory disorders

       H47.511   Disorders of visual pathways in (due to) inflammatory disorders, right side

       H47.512   Disorders of visual pathways in (due to) inflammatory disorders, left side

       H47.519   Disorders of visual pathways in (due to) inflammatory disorders, unspecified side

●   **H47.52**   Disorders of visual pathways in (due to) neoplasm

       H47.521   Disorders of visual pathways in (due to) neoplasm, right side

       H47.522   Disorders of visual pathways in (due to) neoplasm, left side

       H47.529   Disorders of visual pathways in (due to) neoplasm, unspecified side

●   **H47.53**   Disorders of visual pathways in (due to) vascular disorders

       H47.531   Disorders of visual pathways in (due to) vascular disorders, right side

       H47.532   Disorders of visual pathways in (due to) vascular disorders, left side

       H47.539   Disorders of visual pathways in (due to) vascular disorders, unspecified side

● **H47.6**   **Disorders of visual cortex**

      Code also underlying condition

      Excludes1   injury to visual cortex S04.04

      (Ex) **For category H47.6 CC codes:** See PDX Collection 636

●   **H47.61**   Cortical blindness

       H47.611   Cortical blindness, right side of brain

       H47.612   Cortical blindness, left side of brain

       H47.619   Cortical blindness, unspecified side of brain

●   **H47.62**   Disorders of visual cortex in (due to) inflammatory disorders

       H47.621   Disorders of visual cortex in (due to) inflammatory disorders, right side of brain

       H47.622   Disorders of visual cortex in (due to) inflammatory disorders, left side of brain

       H47.629   Disorders of visual cortex in (due to) inflammatory disorders, unspecified side of brain

●   **H47.63**   Disorders of visual cortex in (due to) neoplasm

       H47.631   Disorders of visual cortex in (due to) neoplasm, right side of brain

       H47.632   Disorders of visual cortex in (due to) neoplasm, left side of brain

       H47.639   Disorders of visual cortex in (due to) neoplasm, unspecified side of brain

▶ New   ⇒ Revised   ~~deleted~~ Deleted   Excludes 1   Excludes 2   Includes   Use additional   Code first   Code also   Key words

OGCR Official Guidelines   ● Unacceptable Principal Diagnosis   X Assign placeholder X   ● Use Additional Character(s)   ▶ Manifestation Code   **Coding Clinic**

● H47.64   Disorders of visual cortex in (due to) vascular
           disorders
    H47.641   Disorders of visual cortex in (due to)
              vascular disorders, right side of
              brain 🔖
    H47.642   Disorders of visual cortex in (due to)
              vascular disorders, left side of
              brain 🔖
    H47.649   Disorders of visual cortex in (due to)
              vascular disorders, unspecified side of
              brain 🔖

H47.9   Unspecified disorder of visual pathways

DISORDERS OF OCULAR MUSCLES, BINOCULAR MOVEMENT, ACCOMMODATION AND REFRACTION (H49-H52)

Excludes2   nystagmus and other irregular eye movements
                (H55)

● H49   Paralytic strabismus
        Excludes2   internal ophthalmoplegia (H52.51-)
                        internuclear ophthalmoplegia (H51.2-)
                        progressive supranuclear ophthalmoplegia
                        (G23.1)

● H49.0   Third [oculomotor] nerve palsy
    H49.00   Third [oculomotor] nerve palsy, unspecified eye
    H49.01   Third [oculomotor] nerve palsy, right eye
    H49.02   Third [oculomotor] nerve palsy, left eye
    H49.03   Third [oculomotor] nerve palsy, bilateral
● H49.1   Fourth [trochlear] nerve palsy
    H49.10   Fourth [trochlear] nerve palsy, unspecified eye
    H49.11   Fourth [trochlear] nerve palsy, right eye
    H49.12   Fourth [trochlear] nerve palsy, left eye
    H49.13   Fourth [trochlear] nerve palsy, bilateral
● H49.2   Sixth [abducent] nerve palsy
    H49.20   Sixth [abducent] nerve palsy, unspecified eye
    H49.21   Sixth [abducent] nerve palsy, right eye
    H49.22   Sixth [abducent] nerve palsy, left eye
    H49.23   Sixth [abducent] nerve palsy, bilateral
● H49.3   Total (external) ophthalmoplegia
    H49.30   Total (external) ophthalmoplegia, unspecified
             eye
    H49.31   Total (external) ophthalmoplegia, right eye
    H49.32   Total (external) ophthalmoplegia, left eye
    H49.33   Total (external) ophthalmoplegia, bilateral
● H49.4   Progressive external ophthalmoplegia
          Excludes1   Kearns-Sayre syndrome (H49.81-)
    H49.40   Progressive external ophthalmoplegia,
             unspecified eye
    H49.41   Progressive external ophthalmoplegia, right eye
    H49.42   Progressive external ophthalmoplegia, left eye
    H49.43   Progressive external ophthalmoplegia, bilateral

Item 7–9   Strabismus or esotropia (crossed eyes) is a condition of the
extraocular eye muscles, resulting in an inability of the eyes to focus and also
affects depth perception.

Figure 7-12   **A.** Image of strabismus. **B.** Exotropia. (**A** from Yanoff:
Ophthalmology, ed 3, Mosby, Inc., 2008. **B** from Zitelli BJ, Davis HW,
Pediatric Physical Diagnosis: Atlas of Pediatric Physical Diagnosis,
Philadelphia, Elsevier Saunders, 2012)

● H49.8   Other paralytic strabismus
    ● H49.81   Kearns-Sayre syndrome
               Progressive external ophthalmoplegia with
               pigmentary retinopathy
               Use additional code for other manifestation,
               such as:
               heart block (I45.9)
               Ⓔ **For category H49.81 CC codes:** See PDX Collection 545
        H49.811   Kearns-Sayre syndrome, right eye 🔖
        H49.812   Kearns-Sayre syndrome, left eye 🔖
        H49.813   Kearns-Sayre syndrome, bilateral 🔖
        H49.819   Kearns-Sayre syndrome, unspecified
                  eye 🔖
    ● H49.88   Other paralytic strabismus
               External ophthalmoplegia NOS
        H49.881   Other paralytic strabismus, right eye
        H49.882   Other paralytic strabismus, left eye
        H49.883   Other paralytic strabismus, bilateral
        H49.889   Other paralytic strabismus,
                  unspecified eye
    H49.9   Unspecified paralytic strabismus

● H50   Other strabismus
    ● H50.0   Esotropia
              Convergent concomitant strabismus
              Excludes1   intermittent esotropia (H50.31-, H50.32)
        H50.00   Unspecified esotropia
        ● H50.01   Monocular esotropia
            H50.011   Monocular esotropia, right eye
            H50.012   Monocular esotropia, left eye
        ● H50.02   Monocular esotropia with A pattern
            H50.021   Monocular esotropia with A pattern,
                      right eye
            H50.022   Monocular esotropia with A pattern,
                      left eye
        ● H50.03   Monocular esotropia with V pattern
            H50.031   Monocular esotropia with V pattern,
                      right eye
            H50.032   Monocular esotropia with V pattern,
                      left eye

CHAPTER 7 (H00-H59)

- ● H50.04   Monocular esotropia with other noncomitancies
  - H50.041   Monocular esotropia with other noncomitancies, right eye
  - H50.042   Monocular esotropia with other noncomitancies, left eye
- H50.05   Alternating esotropia
- H50.06   Alternating esotropia with A pattern
- H50.07   Alternating esotropia with V pattern
- H50.08   Alternating esotropia with other noncomitancies
- ● H50.1   Exotropia

  Misalignment in which one eye deviates outward (away from nose) while the other fixates normally

  Divergent concomitant strabismus

  Excludes1   intermittent exotropia (H50.33-, H50.34)
  - H50.10   Unspecified exotropia
  - ● H50.11   Monocular exotropia
    - H50.111   Monocular exotropia, right eye
    - H50.112   Monocular exotropia, left eye
  - ● H50.12   Monocular exotropia with A pattern
    - H50.121   Monocular exotropia with A pattern, right eye
    - H50.122   Monocular exotropia with A pattern, left eye
  - ● H50.13   Monocular exotropia with V pattern
    - H50.131   Monocular exotropia with V pattern, right eye
    - H50.132   Monocular exotropia with V pattern, left eye
  - ● H50.14   Monocular exotropia with other noncomitancies
    - H50.141   Monocular exotropia with other noncomitancies, right eye
    - H50.142   Monocular exotropia with other noncomitancies, left eye
  - H50.15   Alternating exotropia
  - H50.16   Alternating exotropia with A pattern
  - H50.17   Alternating exotropia with V pattern
  - H50.18   Alternating exotropia with other noncomitancies
- ● H50.2   Vertical strabismus

  Hypertropia
  - H50.21   Vertical strabismus, right eye
  - H50.22   Vertical strabismus, left eye
- ● H50.3   Intermittent heterotropia

  Displacement of an organ or part of an organ from its normal position
  - H50.30   Unspecified intermittent heterotropia
  - ● H50.31   Intermittent monocular esotropia
    - H50.311   Intermittent monocular esotropia, right eye
    - H50.312   Intermittent monocular esotropia, left eye
  - H50.32   Intermittent alternating esotropia
  - ● H50.33   Intermittent monocular exotropia
    - H50.331   Intermittent monocular exotropia, right eye
    - H50.332   Intermittent monocular exotropia, left eye
  - H50.34   Intermittent alternating exotropia

- ● H50.4   Other and unspecified heterotropia
  - H50.40   Unspecified heterotropia
  - ● H50.41   Cyclotropia
    - H50.411   Cyclotropia, right eye
    - H50.412   Cyclotropia, left eye
  - H50.42   Monofixation syndrome
  - H50.43   Accommodative component in esotropia
- ● H50.5   Heterophoria

  One or both eyes wander away from the position where both eyes are looking together in the same direction
  - H50.50   Unspecified heterophoria
  - H50.51   Esophoria

    Eye deviates inward (toward the nose)
  - H50.52   Exophoria

    Eye deviates outward (toward the ear)
  - H50.53   Vertical heterophoria
  - H50.54   Cyclophoria
  - H50.55   Alternating heterophoria
- ● H50.6   Mechanical strabismus
  - H50.60   Mechanical strabismus, unspecified
  - ● H50.61   Brown's sheath syndrome
    - H50.611   Brown's sheath syndrome, right eye
    - H50.612   Brown's sheath syndrome, left eye
  - H50.69   Other mechanical strabismus

    Strabismus due to adhesions

    Traumatic limitation of duction of eye muscle
- ● H50.8   Other specified strabismus
  - ● H50.81   Duane's syndrome
    - H50.811   Duane's syndrome, right eye
    - H50.812   Duane's syndrome, left eye
  - H50.89   Other specified strabismus
- H50.9   Unspecified strabismus

- ● H51   Other disorders of binocular movement
  - H51.0   Palsy (spasm) of conjugate gaze
  - ● H51.1   Convergence insufficiency and excess
    - H51.11   Convergence insufficiency
    - H51.12   Convergence excess
  - ● H51.2   Internuclear ophthalmoplegia
    - H51.20   Internuclear ophthalmoplegia, unspecified eye
    - H51.21   Internuclear ophthalmoplegia, right eye
    - H51.22   Internuclear ophthalmoplegia, left eye
    - H51.23   Internuclear ophthalmoplegia, bilateral
  - H51.8   Other specified disorders of binocular movement
  - H51.9   Unspecified disorder of binocular movement
- ● H52   Disorders of refraction and accommodation
  - ● H52.0   Hypermetropia
    - H52.00   Hypermetropia, unspecified eye
    - H52.01   Hypermetropia, right eye
    - H52.02   Hypermetropia, left eye
    - H52.03   Hypermetropia, bilateral
  - ● H52.1   Myopia

    Excludes1   degenerative myopia (H44.2-)
    - H52.10   Myopia, unspecified eye
    - H52.11   Myopia, right eye
    - H52.12   Myopia, left eye
    - H52.13   Myopia, bilateral

▶ New   ⇒ Revised   ~~deleted~~ Deleted   Excludes 1   Excludes 2   Includes   Use additional   Code first   Code also   Key words

OGCR Official Guidelines   ● Unacceptable Principal Diagnosis   X Assign placeholder X   ● Use Additional Character(s)   ▷ Manifestation Code   **Coding Clinic**

Item 7–10 Disorders of refraction: **Hypermetropia,** or farsightedness, means focus at a distance is adequate but not on close objects. **Myopia** is near-sightedness or short-sightedness and means the focus on nearby objects is clear but distant objects appear blurred. **Astigmatism** is warping of the curvature of the cornea so light rays entering do not meet a single focal point, resulting in a distorted image. **Anisometropia** is unequal refractive power in which one eye may be myopic (near-sighted) and the other hyperopic (far-sighted). **Presbyopia** is the loss of focus on near objects, which occurs with age because the lens loses elasticity.

- H52.2   Astigmatism
  - H52.20   Unspecified astigmatism
    - H52.201   Unspecified astigmatism, right eye
    - H52.202   Unspecified astigmatism, left eye
    - H52.203   Unspecified astigmatism, bilateral
    - H52.209   Unspecified astigmatism, unspecified eye
  - H52.21   Irregular astigmatism
    - H52.211   Irregular astigmatism, right eye
    - H52.212   Irregular astigmatism, left eye
    - H52.213   Irregular astigmatism, bilateral
    - H52.219   Irregular astigmatism, unspecified eye
  - H52.22   Regular astigmatism
    - H52.221   Regular astigmatism, right eye
    - H52.222   Regular astigmatism, left eye
    - H52.223   Regular astigmatism, bilateral
    - H52.229   Regular astigmatism, unspecified eye
- H52.3   Anisometropia and aniseikonia
  - H52.31   Anisometropia
  - H52.32   Aniseikonia
- H52.4   Presbyopia
- H52.5   Disorders of accommodation
  - H52.51   Internal ophthalmoplegia (complete) (total)
    - H52.511   Internal ophthalmoplegia (complete) (total), right eye
    - H52.512   Internal ophthalmoplegia (complete) (total), left eye
    - H52.513   Internal ophthalmoplegia (complete) (total), bilateral
    - H52.519   Internal ophthalmoplegia (complete) (total), unspecified eye
  - H52.52   Paresis of accommodation
    - H52.521   Paresis of accommodation, right eye
    - H52.522   Paresis of accommodation, left eye
    - H52.523   Paresis of accommodation, bilateral
    - H52.529   Paresis of accommodation, unspecified eye
  - H52.53   Spasm of accommodation
    - H52.531   Spasm of accommodation, right eye
    - H52.532   Spasm of accommodation, left eye
    - H52.533   Spasm of accommodation, bilateral
    - H52.539   Spasm of accommodation, unspecified eye
- H52.6   Other disorders of refraction
- H52.7   Unspecified disorder of refraction

VISUAL DISTURBANCES AND BLINDNESS (H53-H54)

- H53   Visual disturbances
  - H53.0   Amblyopia ex anopsia
    - **Excludes1**   amblyopia due to vitamin A deficiency (E50.5)
    - H53.00   Unspecified amblyopia
      - H53.001   Unspecified amblyopia, right eye
      - H53.002   Unspecified amblyopia, left eye
      - H53.003   Unspecified amblyopia, bilateral
      - H53.009   Unspecified amblyopia, unspecified eye
    - H53.01   Deprivation amblyopia
      - H53.011   Deprivation amblyopia, right eye
      - H53.012   Deprivation amblyopia, left eye
      - H53.013   Deprivation amblyopia, bilateral
      - H53.019   Deprivation amblyopia, unspecified eye
    - H53.02   Refractive amblyopia
      - H53.021   Refractive amblyopia, right eye
      - H53.022   Refractive amblyopia, left eye
      - H53.023   Refractive amblyopia, bilateral
      - H53.029   Refractive amblyopia, unspecified eye
    - H53.03   Strabismic amblyopia
      - **Excludes1**   strabismus (H50.-)
      - H53.031   Strabismic amblyopia, right eye
      - H53.032   Strabismic amblyopia, left eye
      - H53.033   Strabismic amblyopia, bilateral
      - H53.039   Strabismic amblyopia, unspecified eye
    - H53.04   Amblyopia suspect
      - **Coding Clinic: 2016, Q4, P22**
      - H53.041   Amblyopia suspect, right eye
      - H53.042   Amblyopia suspect, left eye
      - H53.043   Amblyopia suspect, bilateral
      - H53.049   Amblyopia suspect, unspecified eye
  - H53.1   Subjective visual disturbances
    - **Excludes1**   subjective visual disturbances due to vitamin A deficiency (E50.5)
      - visual hallucinations (R44.1)
    - H53.10   Unspecified subjective visual disturbances
    - H53.11   Day blindness
      - Hemeralopia
    - H53.12   Transient visual loss
      - Scintillating scotoma
      - **Excludes1**   amaurosis fugax (G45.3-)
        - transient retinal artery occlusion (H34.0-)
      - (Ex) **For category H53.12 CC codes:** See PDX Collection 637
      - H53.121   Transient visual loss, right eye 🦠
      - H53.122   Transient visual loss, left eye 🦠
      - H53.123   Transient visual loss, bilateral 🦠
      - H53.129   Transient visual loss, unspecified eye 🦠
    - H53.13   Sudden visual loss
      - (Ex) **For category H53.13 CC codes:** See PDX Collection 637
      - H53.131   Sudden visual loss, right eye 🦠
      - H53.132   Sudden visual loss, left eye 🦠
      - H53.133   Sudden visual loss, bilateral 🦠
      - H53.139   Sudden visual loss, unspecified eye 🦠

CHAPTER 7 (H00-H59)

N Newborn Age: 0   **P** Pediatric Age: 0–17   **M** Maternity DX: 12–55   **A** Adult Age: 15–124   ♀ Females Only   ♂ Males Only

🦠 Complication\Comorbidity   🦠 Major C\C   (Ex) CC/MCC Exclusions   🦠 Hospital-Acquired Condition

847

● **H53.14**   **Visual discomfort**
Asthenopia
Photophobia

    H53.141   **Visual discomfort, right eye**

    H53.142   **Visual discomfort, left eye**

    H53.143   **Visual discomfort, bilateral**

    H53.149   **Visual discomfort, unspecified**

H53.15   **Visual distortions of shape and size**
Metamorphopsia

H53.16   **Psychophysical visual disturbances**

H53.19   **Other subjective visual disturbances**
Visual halos

H53.2   **Diplopia**
Double vision

● **H53.3**   **Other and unspecified disorders of binocular vision**

    H53.30   **Unspecified disorder of binocular vision**

    H53.31   **Abnormal retinal correspondence**

    H53.32   **Fusion with defective stereopsis**

    H53.33   **Simultaneous visual perception without fusion**

    H53.34   **Suppression of binocular vision**

● **H53.4**   **Visual field defects**

    H53.40   **Unspecified visual field defects**

    ● **H53.41**   **Scotoma involving central area**
Central scotoma

       H53.411   **Scotoma involving central area, right eye**

       H53.412   **Scotoma involving central area, left eye**

       H53.413   **Scotoma involving central area, bilateral**

       H53.419   **Scotoma involving central area, unspecified eye**

    ● **H53.42**   **Scotoma of blind spot area**
Enlarged blind spot

       H53.421   **Scotoma of blind spot area, right eye**

       H53.422   **Scotoma of blind spot area, left eye**

       H53.423   **Scotoma of blind spot area, bilateral**

       H53.429   **Scotoma of blind spot area, unspecified eye**

    ● **H53.43**   **Sector or arcuate defects**
Arcuate scotoma
Bjerrum scotoma

       H53.431   **Sector or arcuate defects, right eye**

       H53.432   **Sector or arcuate defects, left eye**

       H53.433   **Sector or arcuate defects, bilateral**

       H53.439   **Sector or arcuate defects, unspecified eye**

    ● **H53.45**   **Other localized visual field defect**
Peripheral visual field defect
Ring scotoma NOS
Scotoma NOS

       H53.451   **Other localized visual field defect, right eye**

       H53.452   **Other localized visual field defect, left eye**

       H53.453   **Other localized visual field defect, bilateral**

       H53.459   **Other localized visual field defect, unspecified eye**

● **H53.46**   **Homonymous bilateral field defects**
Homonymous hemianopia
Homonymous hemianopsia
Quadrant anopia
Quadrant anopsia

    H53.461   **Homonymous bilateral field defects, right side**

    H53.462   **Homonymous bilateral field defects, left side**

    H53.469   **Homonymous bilateral field defects, unspecified side**
Homonymous bilateral field defects NOS

H53.47   **Heteronymous bilateral field defects**
Heteronymous hemianop(s)ia

● **H53.48**   **Generalized contraction of visual field**

    H53.481   **Generalized contraction of visual field, right eye**

    H53.482   **Generalized contraction of visual field, left eye**

    H53.483   **Generalized contraction of visual field, bilateral**

    H53.489   **Generalized contraction of visual field, unspecified eye**

● **H53.5**   **Color vision deficiencies**
Color blindness

    Excludes2   day blindness (H53.11)

    H53.50   **Unspecified color vision deficiencies**
Color blindness NOS

    H53.51   **Achromatopsia**

    H53.52   **Acquired color vision deficiency**

    H53.53   **Deuteranomaly**
Deuteranopia

    H53.54   **Protanomaly**
Protanopia

    H53.55   **Tritanomaly**
Tritanopia

    H53.59   **Other color vision deficiencies**

● **H53.6**   **Night blindness**

    Excludes1   night blindness due to vitamin A deficiency (E50.5)

    H53.60   **Unspecified night blindness**

    H53.61   **Abnormal dark adaptation curve**

    H53.62   **Acquired night blindness**

    H53.63   **Congenital night blindness**

    H53.69   **Other night blindness**

● **H53.7**   **Vision sensitivity deficiencies**

    H53.71   **Glare sensitivity**

    H53.72   **Impaired contrast sensitivity**

H53.8   **Other visual disturbances**

H53.9   **Unspecified visual disturbance**

▶ New   ⇒ Revised   ~~deleted~~ Deleted   Excludes 1   Excludes 2   Includes   Use additional   Code first   Code also   Key words

OGCR Official Guidelines   ● Unacceptable Principal Diagnosis   X Assign placeholder X   ● Use Additional Character(s)   ▌ Manifestation Code   Coding Clinic

● **H54** **Blindness and low vision**

> **Note:** For definition of visual impairment categories see table below.
>
> *Code first any associated underlying cause of the blindness*
>
> **Excludes1** amaurosis fugax (G45.3)

● **H54.0** **Blindness, both eyes**

> Visual impairment categories 3, 4, 5 in both eyes.

▶● **H54.0X** **Blindness, both eyes, different category levels**

▶ **H54.0X3** **Blindness right eye, category 3**

▶ **H54.0X33** Blindness right eye category 3, blindness left eye category 3

▶ **H54.0X34** Blindness right eye category 3, blindness left eye category 4

▶ **H54.0X35** Blindness right eye category 3, blindness left eye category 5

▶● **H54.0X4** **Blindness right eye, category 4**

▶ **H54.0X43** Blindness right eye category 4, blindness left eye category 3

▶ **H54.0X44** Blindness right eye category 4, blindness left eye category 4

▶ **H54.0X45** Blindness right eye category 4, blindness left eye category 5

▶● **H54.0X5** **Blindness right eye, category 5**

▶ **H54.0X53** Blindness right eye category 5, blindness left eye category 3

▶ **H54.0X54** Blindness right eye category 5, blindness left eye category 4

▶ **H54.0X55** Blindness right eye category 5, blindness left eye category 5

● **H54.1** **Blindness, one eye, low vision other eye**

> Visual impairment categories 3, 4, 5 in one eye, with categories 1 or 2 in the other eye.

H54.10 Blindness, one eye, low vision other eye, unspecified eyes

● **H54.11** **Blindness, right eye, low vision left eye**

▶● **H54.113** **Blindness right eye category 3, low vision left eye**

▶ **H54.1131** Blindness right eye category 3, low vision left eye category 1

▶ **H54.1132** Blindness right eye category 3, low vision left eye category 2

▶● **H54.114** **Blindness right eye category 4, low vision left eye**

▶ **H54.1141** Blindness right eye category 4, low vision left eye category 1

▶ **H54.1142** Blindness right eye category 4, low vision left eye category 2

▶● **H54.115** **Blindness right eye category 5, low vision left eye**

▶ **H54.1151** Blindness right eye category 5, low vision left eye category 1

▶ **H54.1152** Blindness right eye category 5, low vision left eye category 2

● **H54.12** **Blindness, left eye, low vision right eye**

▶● **H54.121** **Low vision right eye category 1, blindness left eye**

▶ **H54.1213** Low vision right eye category 1, blindness left eye category 3

▶ **H54.1214** Low vision right eye category 1, blindness left eye category 4

▶ **H54.1215** Low vision right eye category 1, blindness left eye category 5

▶● **H54.122** **Low vision right eye category 2, blindness left eye**

▶ **H54.1223** Low vision right eye category 2, blindness left eye category 3

▶ **H54.1224** Low vision right eye category 2, blindness left eye category 4

▶ **H54.1225** Low vision right eye category 2, blindness left eye category 5

● **H54.2** **Low vision, both eyes**

> Visual impairment categories 1 or 2 in both eyes.

▶● **H54.2X** **Low vision, both eyes, different category levels**

▶● **H54.2X1** **Low vision, right eye, category 1**

▶ **H54.2X11** Low vision right eye category 1, low vision left eye category 1

▶ **H54.2X12** Low vision right eye category 1, low vision left eye category 2

▶● **H54.2X2** **Low vision, right eye, category 2**

▶ **H54.2X21** Low vision right eye category 2, low vision left eye category 1

▶ **H54.2X22** Low vision right eye category 2, low vision left eye category 2

H54.3 **Unqualified visual loss, both eyes**

> Visual impairment category 9 in both eyes.

N Newborn Age: 0   **P** Pediatric Age: 0–17   **M** Maternity DX: 12–55   **A** Adult Age: 15–124   ♀ Females Only   ♂ Males Only

🅒 Complication\Comorbidity   🅜 Major C\C   (Ex) CC/MCC Exclusions   🅗 Hospital-Acquired Condition

849

CHAPTER 7 (H00-H59)

CHAPTER 7 (H00–H59)

● **H54.4**   **Blindness, one eye**
     Visual impairment categories 3, 4, 5 in one eye [normal vision in other eye]

     H54.40   Blindness, one eye, unspecified eye

● **H54.41**   Blindness, right eye, normal vision left eye

▶● **H54.413**   Blindness, right eye, category 3

     ▶ **H54.413A**   Blindness right eye category 3, normal vision left eye

▶● **H54.414**   Blindness, right eye, category 4

     ▶ **H54.414A**   Blindness right eye category 4, normal vision left eye

▶● **H54.415**   Blindness, right eye, category 5

     ▶ **H54.415A**   Blindness right eye category 5, normal vision left eye

● **H54.42**   Blindness, left eye, normal vision right eye

▶● **H54.42A**   Blindness, left eye, category 3-5

     ▶ **H54.42A3**   Blindness left eye category 3, normal vision right eye

     ▶ **H54.42A4**   Blindness left eye category 4, normal vision right eye

     ▶ **H54.42A5**   Blindness left eye category 5, normal vision right eye

● **H54.5**   **Low vision, one eye**
     Visual impairment categories 1 or 2 in one eye [normal vision in other eye].

     H54.50   Low vision, one eye, unspecified eye

● **H54.51**   Low vision, right eye, normal vision left eye

▶● **H54.511**   Low vision, right eye, category 1-2

     ▶ **H54.511A**   Low vision right eye category 1, normal vision left eye

     ▶ **H54.512A**   Low vision right eye category 2, normal vision left eye

● **H54.52**   Low vision, left eye, normal vision right eye

▶● **H54.52A**   Low vision, left eye, category 1-2

     ▶ **H54.52A1**   Low vision left eye category 1, normal vision right eye

     ▶ **H54.52A2**   Low vision left eye category 2, normal vision right eye

● **H54.6**   **Unqualified visual loss, one eye**
     Visual impairment category 9 in one eye [normal vision in other eye].

     H54.60   Unqualified visual loss, one eye, unspecified

     H54.61   Unqualified visual loss, right eye, normal vision left eye

     H54.62   Unqualified visual loss, left eye, normal vision right eye

● **H54.7**   **Unspecified visual loss**
     Visual impairment category 9 NOS

H54.8   **Legal blindness, as defined in USA**
     Blindness NOS according to USA definition

     Excludes1   legal blindness with specification of impairment level (H54.0-H54.7)

Note: The table below gives a classification of severity of visual impairment recommended by a WHO Study Group on the Prevention of Blindness, Geneva, 6-10 November 1972.

The term 'low vision' in category H54 comprises categories 1 and 2 of the table, the term 'blindness' categories 3, 4 and 5, and the term 'unqualified visual loss' category 9.

If the extent of the visual field is taken into account, patients with a field no greater than 10 but greater than 5 around central fixation should be placed in category 3 and patients with a field no greater than 5 around central fixation should be placed in category 4, even if the central acuity is not impaired.

(Document 508 compliance requires all cells in the following table to be filled.)

Category of visual impairment	Visual acuity with best possible correction	
	Maximum less than:	Minimum equal to or better than:
—	6/18	6/60
3/10 (0.3)	1/10 (0.1)	—
20/70	20/200	—
—	6/60	3/60
1/10 (0.1)	1/20 (0.05)	—
20/200	20/400	—
—	3/60	1/60 (finger counting at one meter)
1/20 (0.05)	1/50 (0.02)	—
20/400	5/300 (20/1200)	—
—	1/60 (finger counting at one meter)	Light perception
1/50 (0.02)	—	—
5/300	—	—
—	No light perception	
—	Undetermined or unspecified	—

OGCR Section I.C.7.b.

Blindness
If "blindness" or "low vision" of both eyes is documented but the visual impairment category is not documented, assign code H54.3, Unqualified visual loss, both eyes. If "blindness" or "low vision" in one eye is documented but the visual impairment category is not documented, assign a code from H54.6-, Unqualified visual loss, one eye. If "blindness" or "visual loss" is documented without any information about whether one or both eyes are affected, assign code H54.7, Unspecified visual loss.

▶ New   ⇒ Revised   ~~deleted~~ Deleted   Excludes 1   Excludes 2   Includes   Use additional   Code first   Code also   Key words

OGCR Official Guidelines   ● Unacceptable Principal Diagnosis   X Assign placeholder X   ● Use Additional Character(s)   ▌ Manifestation Code   **Coding Clinic**

OTHER DISORDERS OF EYE AND ADNEXA (H55-H57)

● H55　Nystagmus and other irregular eye movements
  ● H55.0　Nystagmus
     Rapid, involuntary movements of the eyes in the horizontal or vertical direction
    H55.00　Unspecified nystagmus
    H55.01　Congenital nystagmus
    H55.02　Latent nystagmus
    H55.03　Visual deprivation nystagmus
    H55.04　Dissociated nystagmus
    H55.09　Other forms of nystagmus
  ● H55.8　Other irregular eye movements
    H55.81　Saccadic eye movements
    H55.89　Other irregular eye movements

● H57　Other disorders of eye and adnexa
  ● H57.0　Anomalies of pupillary function
    H57.00　Unspecified anomaly of pupillary function
    H57.01　Argyll Robertson pupil, atypical
      Excludes1　syphilitic Argyll Robertson pupil (A52.19)
    H57.02　Anisocoria
    H57.03　Miosis
    H57.04　Mydriasis
    ● H57.05　Tonic pupil
      H57.051　Tonic pupil, right eye
      H57.052　Tonic pupil, left eye
      H57.053　Tonic pupil, bilateral
      H57.059　Tonic pupil, unspecified eye
    H57.09　Other anomalies of pupillary function
  ● H57.1　Ocular pain
    H57.10　Ocular pain, unspecified eye
    H57.11　Ocular pain, right eye
    H57.12　Ocular pain, left eye
    H57.13　Ocular pain, bilateral
  H57.8　Other specified disorders of eye and adnexa
  ● H57.9　Unspecified disorder of eye and adnexa

INTRAOPERATIVE AND POSTPROCEDURAL COMPLICATIONS AND DISORDERS OF EYE AND ADNEXA, NOT ELSEWHERE CLASSIFIED (H59)

● H59　Intraoperative and postprocedural complications and disorders of eye and adnexa, not elsewhere classified
  Excludes1　mechanical complication of intraocular lens (T85.2)
    mechanical complication of other ocular prosthetic devices, implants and grafts (T85.3)
    pseudophakia (Z96.1)
    secondary cataracts (H26.4-)
  ● H59.0　Disorders of the eye following cataract surgery
    (Ex) *For category H59.0 CC codes: See PDX Collection 638*
    ● H59.01　Keratopathy (bullous aphakic) following cataract surgery
      Vitreal corneal syndrome
      Vitreous (touch) syndrome
      H59.011　Keratopathy (bullous aphakic) following cataract surgery, right eye
      H59.012　Keratopathy (bullous aphakic) following cataract surgery, left eye
      H59.013　Keratopathy (bullous aphakic) following cataract surgery, bilateral
      H59.019　Keratopathy (bullous aphakic) following cataract surgery, unspecified eye

  ● H59.02　Cataract (lens) fragments in eye following cataract surgery
    H59.021　Cataract (lens) fragments in eye following cataract surgery, right eye
    H59.022　Cataract (lens) fragments in eye following cataract surgery, left eye
    H59.023　Cataract (lens) fragments in eye following cataract surgery, bilateral
    H59.029　Cataract (lens) fragments in eye following cataract surgery, unspecified eye
  ● H59.03　Cystoid macular edema following cataract surgery
    H59.031　Cystoid macular edema following cataract surgery, right eye
    H59.032　Cystoid macular edema following cataract surgery, left eye
    H59.033　Cystoid macular edema following cataract surgery, bilateral
    H59.039　Cystoid macular edema following cataract surgery, unspecified eye
  ● H59.09　Other disorders of the eye following cataract surgery
    H59.091　Other disorders of the right eye following cataract surgery
    H59.092　Other disorders of the left eye following cataract surgery
    H59.093　Other disorders of the eye following cataract surgery, bilateral
    H59.099　Other disorders of unspecified eye following cataract surgery
  ● H59.1　Intraoperative hemorrhage and hematoma of eye and adnexa complicating a procedure
    Excludes1　intraoperative hemorrhage and hematoma of eye and adnexa due to accidental puncture or laceration during a procedure (H59.2-)
    (Ex) *For category H59.1 CC codes: See PDX Collection 639*
  ● H59.11　Intraoperative hemorrhage and hematoma of eye and adnexa complicating an ophthalmic procedure
    H59.111　Intraoperative hemorrhage and hematoma of right eye and adnexa complicating an ophthalmic procedure
    H59.112　Intraoperative hemorrhage and hematoma of left eye and adnexa complicating an ophthalmic procedure
    H59.113　Intraoperative hemorrhage and hematoma of eye and adnexa complicating an ophthalmic procedure, bilateral
    H59.119　Intraoperative hemorrhage and hematoma of unspecified eye and adnexa complicating an ophthalmic procedure

N Newborn Age: 0　　**P** Pediatric Age: 0–17　　**M** Maternity DX: 12–55　　**A** Adult Age: 15–124　　♀ Females Only　　♂ Males Only
🌑 Complication\Comorbidity　　🌑 Major C\C　　(Ex) CC/MCC Exclusions　　🌑 Hospital-Acquired Condition

851

CHAPTER 7 (H00-H59)

● H59.12   Intraoperative hemorrhage and hematoma of eye and adnexa complicating other procedure

     H59.121   Intraoperative hemorrhage and hematoma of right eye and adnexa complicating other procedure 🔖

     H59.122   Intraoperative hemorrhage and hematoma of left eye and adnexa complicating other procedure 🔖

     H59.123   Intraoperative hemorrhage and hematoma of eye and adnexa complicating other procedure, bilateral 🔖

     H59.129   Intraoperative hemorrhage and hematoma of unspecified eye and adnexa complicating other procedure 🔖

● H59.2   Accidental puncture and laceration of eye and adnexa during a procedure

     (Ex:) For category H59.2 CC codes: See PDX Collection 509

   ● H59.21   Accidental puncture and laceration of eye and adnexa during an ophthalmic procedure

     H59.211   Accidental puncture and laceration of right eye and adnexa during an ophthalmic procedure 🔖

     H59.212   Accidental puncture and laceration of left eye and adnexa during an ophthalmic procedure 🔖

     H59.213   Accidental puncture and laceration of eye and adnexa during an ophthalmic procedure, bilateral 🔖

     H59.219   Accidental puncture and laceration of unspecified eye and adnexa during an ophthalmic procedure 🔖

   ● H59.22   Accidental puncture and laceration of eye and adnexa during other procedure

     H59.221   Accidental puncture and laceration of right eye and adnexa during other procedure 🔖

     H59.222   Accidental puncture and laceration of left eye and adnexa during other procedure 🔖

     H59.223   Accidental puncture and laceration of eye and adnexa during other procedure, bilateral 🔖

     H59.229   Accidental puncture and laceration of unspecified eye and adnexa during other procedure 🔖

● H59.3   Postprocedural hemorrhage, hematoma, and seroma of eye and adnexa following other procedure

     (Ex:) For category H59.3 CC codes: See PDX Collection 639

     Coding Clinic: 2016, Q4, P10

   ● H59.31   Postprocedural hemorrhage of eye and adnexa following an ophthalmic procedure

     H59.311   Postprocedural hemorrhage of right eye and adnexa following an ophthalmic procedure 🔖

     H59.312   Postprocedural hemorrhage of left eye and adnexa following an ophthalmic procedure 🔖

     H59.313   Postprocedural hemorrhage of eye and adnexa following an ophthalmic procedure, bilateral 🔖

     H59.319   Postprocedural hemorrhage of unspecified eye and adnexa following an ophthalmic procedure 🔖

● H59.32   Postprocedural hemorrhage of eye and adnexa following other procedure

     H59.321   Postprocedural hemorrhage of right eye and adnexa following other procedure 🔖

     H59.322   Postprocedural hemorrhage of left eye and adnexa following other procedure 🔖

     H59.323   Postprocedural hemorrhage of eye and adnexa following other procedure, bilateral 🔖

     H59.329   Postprocedural hemorrhage of unspecified eye and adnexa following other procedure 🔖

● H59.33   Postprocedural hematoma of eye and adnexa following an ophthalmic procedure

     H59.331   Postprocedural hematoma of right eye and adnexa following an ophthalmic procedure 🔖

     H59.332   Postprocedural hematoma of left eye and adnexa following an ophthalmic procedure 🔖

     H59.333   Postprocedural hematoma of eye and adnexa following an ophthalmic procedure, bilateral 🔖

     H59.339   Postprocedural hematoma of unspecified eye and adnexa following an ophthalmic procedure 🔖

● H59.34   Postprocedural hematoma of eye and adnexa following other procedure

     H59.341   Postprocedural hematoma of right eye and adnexa following other procedure 🔖

     H59.342   Postprocedural hematoma of left eye and adnexa following other procedure 🔖

     H59.343   Postprocedural hematoma of eye and adnexa following other procedure, bilateral 🔖

     H59.349   Postprocedural hematoma of unspecified eye and adnexa following other procedure 🔖

● H59.35   Postprocedural seroma of eye and adnexa following an ophthalmic procedure

     H59.351   Postprocedural seroma of right eye and adnexa following an ophthalmic procedure 🔖

     H59.352   Postprocedural seroma of left eye and adnexa following an ophthalmic procedure 🔖

     H59.353   Postprocedural seroma of eye and adnexa following an ophthalmic procedure, bilateral 🔖

     H59.359   Postprocedural seroma of unspecified eye and adnexa following an ophthalmic procedure 🔖

● H59.36   Postprocedural seroma of eye and adnexa following other procedure

     H59.361   Postprocedural seroma of right eye and adnexa following other procedure 🔖

     H59.362   Postprocedural seroma of left eye and adnexa following other procedure 🔖

     H59.363   Postprocedural seroma of eye and adnexa following other procedure, bilateral 🔖

     H59.369   Postprocedural seroma of unspecified eye and adnexa following other procedure 🔖

▶ New   ⇒ Revised   ~~deleted~~ Deleted   Excludes 1   Excludes 2   Includes   Use additional   Code first   Code also   Key words

OGCR Official Guidelines   ● Unacceptable Principal Diagnosis   X Assign placeholder X   ● Use Additional Character(s)   ▸ Manifestation Code   **Coding Clinic**

● **H59.4** **Inflammation (infection) of postprocedural bleb**
Postprocedural blebitis

> **Excludes1**   filtering (vitreous) bleb after glaucoma
> surgery status (Z98.83)

H59.40   Inflammation (infection) of postprocedural
bleb, unspecified

H59.41   Inflammation (infection) of postprocedural
bleb, stage 1

H59.42   Inflammation (infection) of postprocedural
bleb, stage 2

H59.43   Inflammation (infection) of postprocedural
bleb, stage 3
Bleb endophthalmitis

● **H59.8** **Other intraoperative and postprocedural complications
and disorders of eye and adnexa, not elsewhere
classified**
(Ex) **For category H59.8 CC codes:** See PDX Collection 638

● **H59.81**   **Chorioretinal scars after surgery for detachment**

H59.811   Chorioretinal scars after surgery for
detachment, right eye 🖉

H59.812   Chorioretinal scars after surgery for
detachment, left eye 🖉

H59.813   Chorioretinal scars after surgery for
detachment, bilateral 🖉

H59.819   Chorioretinal scars after surgery for
detachment, unspecified eye 🖉

H59.88   Other intraoperative complications of eye and
adnexa, not elsewhere classified 🖉

H59.89   Other postprocedural complications and
disorders of eye and adnexa, not elsewhere
classified 🖉

N Newborn Age: 0   **P** Pediatric Age: 0–17   **M** Maternity DX: 12–55   **A** Adult Age: 15–124   ♀ Females Only   ♂ Males Only

🖉 Complication\Comorbidity   🖉 Major C\C   (Ex) CC/MCC Exclusions   🖉 Hospital-Acquired Condition

853

CHAPTER 8

DISEASES OF THE EAR AND MASTOID PROCESS (H60-H95)

OGCR Chapter-Specific Coding Guidelines

> 8. Chapter 8: Diseases of the Ear and Mastoid Process (H60-H95)
> Reserved for future guideline expansion

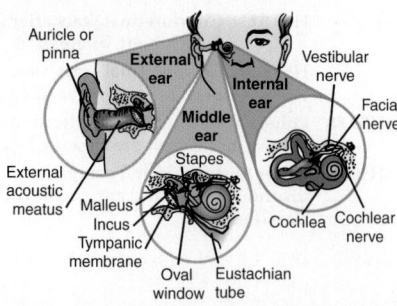

Figure 8-1 Auditory system. (From Buck CJ: Step-by-Step Medical Coding, ed 2016, St. Louis, Elsevier, 2016)

★**(See Plate 92 on page 68.)**

CHAPTER 8

DISEASES OF THE EAR AND MASTOID PROCESS (H60-H95)

Note: Use an external cause code following the code for the ear condition, if applicable, to identify the cause of the ear condition

> **Excludes2**   certain conditions originating in the perinatal period (P04-P96)
> certain infectious and parasitic diseases (A00-B99)
> complications of pregnancy, childbirth and the puerperium (O00-O9A)
> congenital malformations, deformations and chromosomal abnormalities (Q00-Q99)
> endocrine, nutritional and metabolic diseases (E00-E88)
> injury, poisoning and certain other consequences of external causes (S00-T88)
> neoplasms (C00-D49)
> symptoms, signs and abnormal clinical and laboratory findings, not elsewhere classified (R00-R94)

This chapter contains the following blocks:

H60-H62	Diseases of external ear
H65-H75	Diseases of middle ear and mastoid
H80-H83	Diseases of inner ear
H90-H94	Other disorders of ear
H95	Intraoperative and postprocedural complications and disorders of ear and mastoid process, not elsewhere classified

DISEASES OF EXTERNAL EAR (H60-H62)

● **H60   Otitis externa**

  ● **H60.0   Abscess of external ear**
      Boil of external ear
      Carbuncle of auricle or external auditory canal
      Furuncle of external ear

      H60.00   Abscess of external ear, unspecified ear
      H60.01   Abscess of right external ear
      H60.02   Abscess of left external ear
      H60.03   Abscess of external ear, bilateral

● **H60.1   Cellulitis of external ear**
    Cellulitis of auricle
    Cellulitis of external auditory canal

  H60.10   Cellulitis of external ear, unspecified ear
  H60.11   Cellulitis of right external ear
  H60.12   Cellulitis of left external ear
  H60.13   Cellulitis of external ear, bilateral

● **H60.2   Malignant otitis externa**
    Ex: For category H60.2 CC codes: See PDX Collection 640

  H60.20   Malignant otitis externa, unspecified ear 🔖
  H60.21   Malignant otitis externa, right ear 🔖
  H60.22   Malignant otitis externa, left ear 🔖
  H60.23   Malignant otitis externa, bilateral 🔖

● **H60.3   Other infective otitis externa**

  ● H60.31   Diffuse otitis externa
      H60.311   Diffuse otitis externa, right ear
      H60.312   Diffuse otitis externa, left ear
      H60.313   Diffuse otitis externa, bilateral
      H60.319   Diffuse otitis externa, unspecified ear

  ● H60.32   Hemorrhagic otitis externa
      H60.321   Hemorrhagic otitis externa, right ear
      H60.322   Hemorrhagic otitis externa, left ear
      H60.323   Hemorrhagic otitis externa, bilateral
      H60.329   Hemorrhagic otitis externa, unspecified ear

  ● H60.33   Swimmer's ear
      H60.331   Swimmer's ear, right ear
      H60.332   Swimmer's ear, left ear
      H60.333   Swimmer's ear, bilateral
      H60.339   Swimmer's ear, unspecified ear

  ● H60.39   Other infective otitis externa
      H60.391   Other infective otitis externa, right ear
      H60.392   Other infective otitis externa, left ear
      H60.393   Other infective otitis externa, bilateral
      H60.399   Other infective otitis externa, unspecified ear

● **H60.4   Cholesteatoma of external ear**
    Keratosis obturans of external ear (canal)

    Excludes2   cholesteatoma of middle ear (H71.-)
        recurrent cholesteatoma of postmastoidectomy cavity (H95.0-)

  H60.40   Cholesteatoma of external ear, unspecified ear
  H60.41   Cholesteatoma of right external ear
  H60.42   Cholesteatoma of left external ear
  H60.43   Cholesteatoma of external ear, bilateral

● **H60.5   Acute noninfective otitis externa**

  ● H60.50   Unspecified acute noninfective otitis externa
      Acute otitis externa NOS
      H60.501   Unspecified acute noninfective otitis externa, right ear
      H60.502   Unspecified acute noninfective otitis externa, left ear
      H60.503   Unspecified acute noninfective otitis externa, bilateral
      H60.509   Unspecified acute noninfective otitis externa, unspecified ear

  ● H60.51   Acute actinic otitis externa
      H60.511   Acute actinic otitis externa, right ear
      H60.512   Acute actinic otitis externa, left ear
      H60.513   Acute actinic otitis externa, bilateral
      H60.519   Acute actinic otitis externa, unspecified ear

●H60.52 Acute chemical otitis externa
    H60.521 Acute chemical otitis externa, right ear
    H60.522 Acute chemical otitis externa, left ear
    H60.523 Acute chemical otitis externa, bilateral
    H60.529 Acute chemical otitis externa, unspecified ear

●H60.53 Acute contact otitis externa
    H60.531 Acute contact otitis externa, right ear
    H60.532 Acute contact otitis externa, left ear
    H60.533 Acute contact otitis externa, bilateral
    H60.539 Acute contact otitis externa, unspecified ear

●H60.54 Acute eczematoid otitis externa
    H60.541 Acute eczematoid otitis externa, right ear
    H60.542 Acute eczematoid otitis externa, left ear
    H60.543 Acute eczematoid otitis externa, bilateral
    H60.549 Acute eczematoid otitis externa, unspecified ear

●H60.55 Acute reactive otitis externa
    H60.551 Acute reactive otitis externa, right ear
    H60.552 Acute reactive otitis externa, left ear
    H60.553 Acute reactive otitis externa, bilateral
    H60.559 Acute reactive otitis externa, unspecified ear

●H60.59 Other noninfective acute otitis externa
    H60.591 Other noninfective acute otitis externa, right ear
    H60.592 Other noninfective acute otitis externa, left ear
    H60.593 Other noninfective acute otitis externa, bilateral
    H60.599 Other noninfective acute otitis externa, unspecified ear

●H60.6 Unspecified chronic otitis externa
    H60.60 Unspecified chronic otitis externa, unspecified ear
    H60.61 Unspecified chronic otitis externa, right ear
    H60.62 Unspecified chronic otitis externa, left ear
    H60.63 Unspecified chronic otitis externa, bilateral

●H60.8 Other otitis externa
    ●H60.8X Other otitis externa
        H60.8X1 Other otitis externa, right ear
        H60.8X2 Other otitis externa, left ear
        H60.8X3 Other otitis externa, bilateral
        H60.8X9 Other otitis externa, unspecified ear

●H60.9 Unspecified otitis externa
    H60.90 Unspecified otitis externa, unspecified ear
    H60.91 Unspecified otitis externa, right ear
    H60.92 Unspecified otitis externa, left ear
    H60.93 Unspecified otitis externa, bilateral

●H61 Other disorders of external ear
  ●H61.0 Chondritis and perichondritis of external ear
    Chondrodermatitis nodularis chronica helicis
    Perichondritis of auricle
    Perichondritis of pinna
    ●H61.00 Unspecified perichondritis of external ear
        H61.001 Unspecified perichondritis of right external ear
        H61.002 Unspecified perichondritis of left external ear
        H61.003 Unspecified perichondritis of external ear, bilateral
        H61.009 Unspecified perichondritis of external ear, unspecified ear

●H61.01 Acute perichondritis of external ear
    H61.011 Acute perichondritis of right external ear
    H61.012 Acute perichondritis of left external ear
    H61.013 Acute perichondritis of external ear, bilateral
    H61.019 Acute perichondritis of external ear, unspecified ear

●H61.02 Chronic perichondritis of external ear
    H61.021 Chronic perichondritis of right external ear
    H61.022 Chronic perichondritis of left external ear
    H61.023 Chronic perichondritis of external ear, bilateral
    H61.029 Chronic perichondritis of external ear, unspecified ear

●H61.03 Chondritis of external ear
    Chondritis of auricle
    Chondritis of pinna
    H61.031 Chondritis of right external ear
    H61.032 Chondritis of left external ear
        Coding Clinic: 2015, Q1, P18
    H61.033 Chondritis of external ear, bilateral
    H61.039 Chondritis of external ear, unspecified ear

●H61.1 Noninfective disorders of pinna
    Excludes2 cauliflower ear (M95.1-)
                 gouty tophi of ear (M1A.-)
  ●H61.10 Unspecified noninfective disorders of pinna
    Disorder of pinna NOS
    H61.101 Unspecified noninfective disorders of pinna, right ear
    H61.102 Unspecified noninfective disorders of pinna, left ear
    H61.103 Unspecified noninfective disorders of pinna, bilateral
    H61.109 Unspecified noninfective disorders of pinna, unspecified ear

●H61.11 Acquired deformity of pinna
    Acquired deformity of auricle
    Excludes2 cauliflower ear (M95.1-)
    H61.111 Acquired deformity of pinna, right ear
    H61.112 Acquired deformity of pinna, left ear
    H61.113 Acquired deformity of pinna, bilateral
    H61.119 Acquired deformity of pinna, unspecified ear

●H61.12 Hematoma of pinna
    Hematoma of auricle
    H61.121 Hematoma of pinna, right ear
    H61.122 Hematoma of pinna, left ear
    H61.123 Hematoma of pinna, bilateral
    H61.129 Hematoma of pinna, unspecified ear

●H61.19 Other noninfective disorders of pinna
    H61.191 Noninfective disorders of pinna, right ear
    H61.192 Noninfective disorders of pinna, left ear
    H61.193 Noninfective disorders of pinna, bilateral
    H61.199 Noninfective disorders of pinna, unspecified ear

CHAPTER 8 (H60–H95)

● **H61.2 Impacted cerumen**
Wax in ear

   H61.20 Impacted cerumen, unspecified ear
   MCE: Questionable admission when principal dx

   H61.21 Impacted cerumen, right ear
   MCE: Questionable admission when principal dx

   H61.22 Impacted cerumen, left ear
   MCE: Questionable admission when principal dx

   H61.23 Impacted cerumen, bilateral
   MCE: Questionable admission when principal dx

● **H61.3 Acquired stenosis of external ear canal**
Collapse of external ear canal

   Excludes1 postprocedural stenosis of external ear
   canal (H95.81-)

   ● **H61.30 Acquired stenosis of external ear canal,
   unspecified**

      **H61.301 Acquired stenosis of right external ear
      canal, unspecified**

      **H61.302 Acquired stenosis of left external ear
      canal, unspecified**

      **H61.303 Acquired stenosis of external ear
      canal, unspecified, bilateral**

      **H61.309 Acquired stenosis of external ear
      canal, unspecified, unspecified ear**

   ● **H61.31 Acquired stenosis of external ear canal
   secondary to trauma**

      **H61.311 Acquired stenosis of right external ear
      canal secondary to trauma**

      **H61.312 Acquired stenosis of left external ear
      canal secondary to trauma**

      **H61.313 Acquired stenosis of external ear
      canal secondary to trauma, bilateral**

      **H61.319 Acquired stenosis of external
      ear canal secondary to trauma,
      unspecified ear**

   ● **H61.32 Acquired stenosis of external ear canal
   secondary to inflammation and infection**

      **H61.321 Acquired stenosis of right external ear
      canal secondary to inflammation and
      infection**

      **H61.322 Acquired stenosis of left external ear
      canal secondary to inflammation and
      infection**

      **H61.323 Acquired stenosis of external ear
      canal secondary to inflammation and
      infection, bilateral**

      **H61.329 Acquired stenosis of external ear
      canal secondary to inflammation and
      infection, unspecified ear**

   ● **H61.39 Other acquired stenosis of external ear canal**

      **H61.391 Other acquired stenosis of right
      external ear canal**

      **H61.392 Other acquired stenosis of left
      external ear canal**

      **H61.393 Other acquired stenosis of external
      ear canal, bilateral**

      **H61.399 Other acquired stenosis of external
      ear canal, unspecified ear**

● **H61.8 Other specified disorders of external ear**

   ● **H61.81 Exostosis of external canal**

      H61.811 Exostosis of right external canal

      H61.812 Exostosis of left external canal

      H61.813 Exostosis of external canal, bilateral

      **H61.819 Exostosis of external canal,
      unspecified ear**

   ● **H61.89 Other specified disorders of external ear**

      **H61.891 Other specified disorders of right
      external ear**

      **H61.892 Other specified disorders of left
      external ear**

      **H61.893 Other specified disorders of external
      ear, bilateral**

      **H61.899 Other specified disorders of external
      ear, unspecified ear**

● **H61.9 Disorder of external ear, unspecified**

   **H61.90 Disorder of external ear, unspecified,
   unspecified ear**

   H61.91 Disorder of right external ear, unspecified

   H61.92 Disorder of left external ear, unspecified

   H61.93 Disorder of external ear, unspecified, bilateral

● **H62 Disorders of external ear in diseases classified elsewhere**

   ● **H62.4 Otitis externa in other diseases classified elsewhere**

   Code first underlying disease, such as:
   erysipelas (A46)
   impetigo (L01.0)

   Excludes1 otitis externa (in):
   candidiasis (B37.84)
   herpes viral [herpes simplex] (B00.1)
   herpes zoster (B02.8)

   ▌ *H62.40 Otitis externa in other diseases classified
   elsewhere, unspecified ear*

   ▌ *H62.41 Otitis externa in other diseases classified
   elsewhere, right ear*

   ▌ *H62.42 Otitis externa in other diseases classified
   elsewhere, left ear*

   ▌ *H62.43 Otitis externa in other diseases classified
   elsewhere, bilateral*

   ● **H62.8 Other disorders of external ear in diseases classified
   elsewhere**

   Code first underlying disease, such as:
   gout (M1A.-, M10.-)

   ● **H62.8X Other disorders of external ear in diseases
   classified elsewhere**

      ▌ *H62.8X1 Other disorders of right external ear in
      diseases classified elsewhere*

      ▌ *H62.8X2 Other disorders of left external ear in
      diseases classified elsewhere*

      ▌ *H62.8X3 Other disorders of external ear in
      diseases classified elsewhere, bilateral*

      ▌ *H62.8X9 Other disorders of external ear
      in diseases classified elsewhere,
      unspecified ear*

DISEASES OF MIDDLE EAR AND MASTOID (H65-H75)

★ **(See Plate 94 on page 69.)**

● **H65 Nonsuppurative otitis media**
*Bacterial or viral infection or inflammation of the middle ear; may result
in fluid accumulation with pain and temporary hearing loss.*

   Includes nonsuppurative otitis media with myringitis

   Use additional code for any associated perforated tympanic
   membrane (H72.-)

   Use additional code to identify:
   exposure to environmental tobacco smoke (Z77.22)
   exposure to tobacco smoke in the perinatal period (P96.81)
   history of tobacco dependence (Z87.891)
   occupational exposure to environmental tobacco smoke
   (Z57.31)
   tobacco dependence (F17.-)
   tobacco use (Z72.0)

   ● **H65.0 Acute serous otitis media**
   Acute and subacute secretory otitis

      H65.00 Acute serous otitis media, unspecified ear

      H65.01 Acute serous otitis media, right ear

      H65.02 Acute serous otitis media, left ear

      H65.03 Acute serous otitis media, bilateral

      H65.04 Acute serous otitis media, recurrent, right ear

      H65.05 Acute serous otitis media, recurrent, left ear

      H65.06 Acute serous otitis media, recurrent, bilateral

      **H65.07 Acute serous otitis media, recurrent,
      unspecified ear**

▶ New   ⇒ Revised   ~~deleted~~ Deleted   Excludes 1   Excludes 2   Includes   Use additional   Code first   Code also   Key words

OGCR Official Guidelines   ● Unacceptable Principal Diagnosis   X Assign placeholder X   ● Use Additional Character(s)   ▌ Manifestation Code   **Coding Clinic**

● H65.1   Other acute nonsuppurative otitis media
    Excludes1   otitic barotrauma (T70.0)
                otitis media (acute) NOS (H66.9)

  ● H65.11   Acute and subacute allergic otitis media
      (mucoid) (sanguinous) (serous)

    H65.111   Acute and subacute allergic otitis
        media (mucoid) (sanguinous)
        (serous), right ear

    H65.112   Acute and subacute allergic otitis
        media (mucoid) (sanguinous)
        (serous), left ear

    H65.113   Acute and subacute allergic otitis
        media (mucoid) (sanguinous)
        (serous), bilateral

    H65.114   Acute and subacute allergic otitis
        media (mucoid) (sanguinous)
        (serous), recurrent, right ear

    H65.115   Acute and subacute allergic otitis
        media (mucoid) (sanguinous)
        (serous), recurrent, left ear

    H65.116   Acute and subacute allergic otitis
        media (mucoid) (sanguinous)
        (serous), recurrent, bilateral

    H65.117   Acute and subacute allergic otitis
        media (mucoid) (sanguinous)
        (serous), recurrent, unspecified ear

    H65.119   Acute and subacute allergic otitis
        media (mucoid) (sanguinous)
        (serous), unspecified ear

  ● H65.19   Other acute nonsuppurative otitis media
      Acute and subacute mucoid otitis media
      Acute and subacute nonsuppurative otitis
        media NOS
      Acute and subacute sanguinous otitis media
      Acute and subacute seromucinous otitis media

    H65.191   Other acute nonsuppurative otitis
        media, right ear

    H65.192   Other acute nonsuppurative otitis
        media, left ear

    H65.193   Other acute nonsuppurative otitis
        media, bilateral

    H65.194   Other acute nonsuppurative otitis
        media, recurrent, right ear

    H65.195   Other acute nonsuppurative otitis
        media, recurrent, left ear

    H65.196   Other acute nonsuppurative otitis
        media, recurrent, bilateral

    H65.197   Other acute nonsuppurative otitis
        media recurrent, unspecified ear

    H65.199   Other acute nonsuppurative otitis
        media, unspecified ear

● H65.2   Chronic serous otitis media
    Chronic tubotympanal catarrh

  H65.20   Chronic serous otitis media, unspecified ear
  H65.21   Chronic serous otitis media, right ear
  H65.22   Chronic serous otitis media, left ear
  H65.23   Chronic serous otitis media, bilateral

● H65.3   Chronic mucoid otitis media
    Chronic mucinous otitis media
    Chronic secretory otitis media
    Chronic transudative otitis media
    Glue ear

    Excludes1   adhesive middle ear disease (H74.1)

  H65.30   Chronic mucoid otitis media, unspecified ear
  H65.31   Chronic mucoid otitis media, right ear
  H65.32   Chronic mucoid otitis media, left ear
  H65.33   Chronic mucoid otitis media, bilateral

● H65.4   Other chronic nonsuppurative otitis media

  ● H65.41   Chronic allergic otitis media
    H65.411   Chronic allergic otitis media, right ear
    H65.412   Chronic allergic otitis media, left ear

    H65.413   Chronic allergic otitis media, bilateral
    H65.419   Chronic allergic otitis media,
        unspecified ear

  ● H65.49   Other chronic nonsuppurative otitis media
      Chronic exudative otitis media
      Chronic nonsuppurative otitis media NOS
      Chronic otitis media with effusion (nonpurulent)
      Chronic seromucinous otitis media

    H65.491   Other chronic nonsuppurative otitis
        media, right ear

    H65.492   Other chronic nonsuppurative otitis
        media, left ear

    H65.493   Other chronic nonsuppurative otitis
        media, bilateral

    H65.499   Other chronic nonsuppurative otitis
        media, unspecified ear

● H65.9   Unspecified nonsuppurative otitis media
    Allergic otitis media NOS
    Catarrhal otitis media NOS
    Exudative otitis media NOS
    Mucoid otitis media NOS
    Otitis media with effusion (nonpurulent) NOS
    Secretory otitis media NOS
    Seromucinous otitis media NOS
    Serous otitis media NOS
    Transudative otitis media NOS

  H65.90   Unspecified nonsuppurative otitis media,
      unspecified ear

  H65.91   Unspecified nonsuppurative otitis media, right
      ear

  H65.92   Unspecified nonsuppurative otitis media, left ear

  H65.93   Unspecified nonsuppurative otitis media,
      bilateral

● H66   Suppurative and unspecified otitis media
    Suppurative: Discharging pus

    Includes   suppurative and unspecified otitis media with
                myringitis

    Use additional code to identify:
      exposure to environmental tobacco smoke (Z77.22)
      exposure to tobacco smoke in the perinatal period (P96.81)
      history of tobacco dependence (Z87.891)
      occupational exposure to environmental tobacco smoke (Z57.31)
      tobacco dependence (F17.-)
      tobacco use (Z72.0)

  ● H66.0   Acute suppurative otitis media

    ● H66.00   Acute suppurative otitis media without
        spontaneous rupture of ear drum

      H66.001   Acute suppurative otitis media
          without spontaneous rupture of ear
          drum, right ear
          Coding Clinic: 2016, Q1, P34

      H66.002   Acute suppurative otitis media
          without spontaneous rupture of ear
          drum, left ear

      H66.003   Acute suppurative otitis media
          without spontaneous rupture of ear
          drum, bilateral

      H66.004   Acute suppurative otitis media
          without spontaneous rupture of ear
          drum, recurrent, right ear

      H66.005   Acute suppurative otitis media
          without spontaneous rupture of ear
          drum, recurrent, left ear

      H66.006   Acute suppurative otitis media
          without spontaneous rupture of ear
          drum, recurrent, bilateral

      H66.007   Acute suppurative otitis media
          without spontaneous rupture of ear
          drum, recurrent, unspecified ear

      H66.009   Acute suppurative otitis media
          without spontaneous rupture of ear
          drum, unspecified ear

● **H66.01** **Acute suppurative otitis media with spontaneous rupture of ear drum**

H66.011 Acute suppurative otitis media with spontaneous rupture of ear drum, right ear

H66.012 Acute suppurative otitis media with spontaneous rupture of ear drum, left ear

H66.013 Acute suppurative otitis media with spontaneous rupture of ear drum, bilateral

H66.014 Acute suppurative otitis media with spontaneous rupture of ear drum, recurrent, right ear

H66.015 Acute suppurative otitis media with spontaneous rupture of ear drum, recurrent, left ear

H66.016 Acute suppurative otitis media with spontaneous rupture of ear drum, recurrent, bilateral

H66.017 Acute suppurative otitis media with spontaneous rupture of ear drum, recurrent, unspecified ear

H66.019 Acute suppurative otitis media with spontaneous rupture of ear drum, unspecified ear

● **H66.1** **Chronic tubotympanic suppurative otitis media**
Benign chronic suppurative otitis media
Chronic tubotympanic disease
Use additional code for any associated perforated tympanic membrane (H72.-)

H66.10 Chronic tubotympanic suppurative otitis media, unspecified

H66.11 Chronic tubotympanic suppurative otitis media, right ear

H66.12 Chronic tubotympanic suppurative otitis media, left ear

H66.13 Chronic tubotympanic suppurative otitis media, bilateral

● **H66.2** **Chronic atticoantral suppurative otitis media**
Chronic atticoantral disease
Use additional code for any associated perforated tympanic membrane (H72.-)

H66.20 Chronic atticoantral suppurative otitis media, unspecified ear

H66.21 Chronic atticoantral suppurative otitis media, right ear

H66.22 Chronic atticoantral suppurative otitis media, left ear

H66.23 Chronic atticoantral suppurative otitis media, bilateral

● **H66.3** **Other chronic suppurative otitis media**
Chronic suppurative otitis media NOS
Use additional code for any associated perforated tympanic membrane (H72.-)

Excludes1 tuberculous otitis media (A18.6)

● **H66.3X** **Other chronic suppurative otitis media**

H66.3X1 Other chronic suppurative otitis media, right ear

H66.3X2 Other chronic suppurative otitis media, left ear

H66.3X3 Other chronic suppurative otitis media, bilateral

H66.3X9 Other chronic suppurative otitis media, unspecified ear

● **H66.4** **Suppurative otitis media, unspecified**
Purulent otitis media NOS
Use additional code for any associated perforated tympanic membrane (H72.-)

H66.40 Suppurative otitis media, unspecified, unspecified ear

H66.41 Suppurative otitis media, unspecified, right ear

H66.42 Suppurative otitis media, unspecified, left ear

H66.43 Suppurative otitis media, unspecified, bilateral

● **H66.9** **Otitis media, unspecified**
Otitis media NOS
Acute otitis media NOS
Chronic otitis media NOS
Use additional code for any associated perforated tympanic membrane (H72.-)

H66.90 Otitis media, unspecified, unspecified ear

H66.91 Otitis media, unspecified, right ear

H66.92 Otitis media, unspecified, left ear

H66.93 Otitis media, unspecified, bilateral

● **H67** **Otitis media in diseases classified elsewhere**
Code first underlying disease, such as:
viral disease NEC (B00-B34)
Use additional code for any associated perforated tympanic membrane (H72.-)

Excludes1 otitis media in:
influenza (J09.X9, J10.83, J11.83)
measles (B05.3)
scarlet fever (A38.0)
tuberculosis (A18.6)

▷ *H67.1* *Otitis media in diseases classified elsewhere, right ear*

▷ *H67.2* *Otitis media in diseases classified elsewhere, left ear*

▷ *H67.3* *Otitis media in diseases classified elsewhere, bilateral*

▷ *H67.9* *Otitis media in diseases classified elsewhere, unspecified ear*

● **H68** **Eustachian salpingitis and obstruction**

● **H68.0** **Eustachian salpingitis**

● **H68.00** **Unspecified Eustachian salpingitis**

H68.001 Unspecified Eustachian salpingitis, right ear

H68.002 Unspecified Eustachian salpingitis, left ear

H68.003 Unspecified Eustachian salpingitis, bilateral

H68.009 Unspecified Eustachian salpingitis, unspecified ear

● **H68.01** **Acute Eustachian salpingitis**

H68.011 Acute Eustachian salpingitis, right ear

H68.012 Acute Eustachian salpingitis, left ear

H68.013 Acute Eustachian salpingitis, bilateral

H68.019 Acute Eustachian salpingitis, unspecified ear

● **H68.02** **Chronic Eustachian salpingitis**

H68.021 Chronic Eustachian salpingitis, right ear

H68.022 Chronic Eustachian salpingitis, left ear

H68.023 Chronic Eustachian salpingitis, bilateral

H68.029 Chronic Eustachian salpingitis, unspecified ear

- H68.1 **Obstruction of Eustachian tube**
    Stenosis of Eustachian tube
    Stricture of Eustachian tube
    - H68.10 **Unspecified obstruction of Eustachian tube**
        - H68.101 Unspecified obstruction of Eustachian tube, right ear
        - H68.102 Unspecified obstruction of Eustachian tube, left ear
        - H68.103 Unspecified obstruction of Eustachian tube, bilateral
        - H68.109 Unspecified obstruction of Eustachian tube, unspecified ear
    - H68.11 **Osseous obstruction of Eustachian tube**
        - H68.111 Osseous obstruction of Eustachian tube, right ear
        - H68.112 Osseous obstruction of Eustachian tube, left ear
        - H68.113 Osseous obstruction of Eustachian tube, bilateral
        - H68.119 Osseous obstruction of Eustachian tube, unspecified ear
    - H68.12 **Intrinsic cartilagenous obstruction of Eustachian tube**
        - H68.121 Intrinsic cartilagenous obstruction of Eustachian tube, right ear
        - H68.122 Intrinsic cartilagenous obstruction of Eustachian tube, left ear
        - H68.123 Intrinsic cartilagenous obstruction of Eustachian tube, bilateral
        - H68.129 Intrinsic cartilagenous obstruction of Eustachian tube, unspecified ear
    - H68.13 **Extrinsic cartilagenous obstruction of Eustachian tube**
        Compression of Eustachian tube
        - H68.131 Extrinsic cartilagenous obstruction of Eustachian tube, right ear
        - H68.132 Extrinsic cartilagenous obstruction of Eustachian tube, left ear
        - H68.133 Extrinsic cartilagenous obstruction of Eustachian tube, bilateral
        - H68.139 Extrinsic cartilagenous obstruction of Eustachian tube, unspecified ear
- H69 **Other and unspecified disorders of Eustachian tube**
    - H69.0 **Patulous Eustachian tube**
        - H69.00 Patulous Eustachian tube, unspecified ear
        - H69.01 Patulous Eustachian tube, right ear
        - H69.02 Patulous Eustachian tube, left ear
        - H69.03 Patulous Eustachian tube, bilateral
    - H69.8 **Other specified disorders of Eustachian tube**
        - H69.80 Other specified disorders of Eustachian tube, unspecified ear
        - H69.81 Other specified disorders of Eustachian tube, right ear
        - H69.82 Other specified disorders of Eustachian tube, left ear
        - H69.83 Other specified disorders of Eustachian tube, bilateral
    - H69.9 **Unspecified Eustachian tube disorder**
        - H69.90 Unspecified Eustachian tube disorder, unspecified ear
        - H69.91 Unspecified Eustachian tube disorder, right ear
        - H69.92 Unspecified Eustachian tube disorder, left ear
        - H69.93 Unspecified Eustachian tube disorder, bilateral

- H70 **Mastoiditis and related conditions**
    - H70.0 **Acute mastoiditis**
        Abscess of mastoid
        Empyema of mastoid
        (Ex) For category H70.0 CC codes: See PDX Collection 641
        - H70.00 **Acute mastoiditis without complications**
            - H70.001 Acute mastoiditis without complications, right ear
            - H70.002 Acute mastoiditis without complications, left ear
            - H70.003 Acute mastoiditis without complications, bilateral
            - H70.009 Acute mastoiditis without complications, unspecified ear
        - H70.01 **Subperiosteal abscess of mastoid**
            - H70.011 Subperiosteal abscess of mastoid, right ear
            - H70.012 Subperiosteal abscess of mastoid, left ear
            - H70.013 Subperiosteal abscess of mastoid, bilateral
            - H70.019 Subperiosteal abscess of mastoid, unspecified ear
        - H70.09 **Acute mastoiditis with other complications**
            - H70.091 Acute mastoiditis with other complications, right ear
            - H70.092 Acute mastoiditis with other complications, left ear
            - H70.093 Acute mastoiditis with other complications, bilateral
            - H70.099 Acute mastoiditis with other complications, unspecified ear
    - H70.1 **Chronic mastoiditis**
        Caries of mastoid
        Fistula of mastoid
        Excludes1 tuberculous mastoiditis (A18.03)
        - H70.10 Chronic mastoiditis, unspecified ear
        - H70.11 Chronic mastoiditis, right ear
        - H70.12 Chronic mastoiditis, left ear
        - H70.13 Chronic mastoiditis, bilateral
    - H70.2 **Petrositis**
        Inflammation of petrous bone
        - H70.20 **Unspecified petrositis**
            - H70.201 Unspecified petrositis, right ear
            - H70.202 Unspecified petrositis, left ear
            - H70.203 Unspecified petrositis, bilateral
            - H70.209 Unspecified petrositis, unspecified ear
        - H70.21 **Acute petrositis**
            - H70.211 Acute petrositis, right ear
            - H70.212 Acute petrositis, left ear
            - H70.213 Acute petrositis, bilateral
            - H70.219 Acute petrositis, unspecified ear
        - H70.22 **Chronic petrositis**
            - H70.221 Chronic petrositis, right ear
            - H70.222 Chronic petrositis, left ear
            - H70.223 Chronic petrositis, bilateral
            - H70.229 Chronic petrositis, unspecified ear

Item 8-1 Mastoiditis is an infection of the portion of the temporal bone of the skull that is behind the ear (mastoid process) caused by an untreated otitis media, leading to an infection of the surrounding structures which may include the brain.

CHAPTER 8 (H60-H95)

● **H70.8**   **Other mastoiditis and related conditions**
      Excludes1   preauricular sinus and cyst (Q18.1)
                       sinus, fistula, and cyst of branchial cleft
                       (Q18.0)
    ● **H70.81**   **Postauricular fistula**
       H70.811   Postauricular fistula, **right ear**
       H70.812   Postauricular fistula, **left ear**
       H70.813   Postauricular fistula, **bilateral**
       H70.819   Postauricular fistula, **unspecified ear**
    ● **H70.89**   **Other mastoiditis and related conditions**
       H70.891   Other mastoiditis and related conditions, **right ear**
       H70.892   Other mastoiditis and related conditions, **left ear**
       H70.893   Other mastoiditis and related conditions, **bilateral**
       H70.899   Other mastoiditis and related conditions, **unspecified ear**
● **H70.9**   **Unspecified mastoiditis**
      H70.90   Unspecified mastoiditis, **unspecified ear**
      H70.91   Unspecified mastoiditis, **right ear**
      H70.92   Unspecified mastoiditis, **left ear**
      H70.93   Unspecified mastoiditis, **bilateral**

● **H71**   **Cholesteatoma of middle ear**
      Excludes2   cholesteatoma of external ear (H60.4-)
                       recurrent cholesteatoma of postmastoidectomy
                       cavity (H95.0-)
    ● **H71.0**   **Cholesteatoma of attic**
       H71.00   Cholesteatoma of attic, **unspecified ear**
       H71.01   Cholesteatoma of attic, **right ear**
       H71.02   Cholesteatoma of attic, **left ear**
       H71.03   Cholesteatoma of attic, **bilateral**
    ● **H71.1**   **Cholesteatoma of tympanum**
       H71.10   Cholesteatoma of tympanum, **unspecified ear**
       H71.11   Cholesteatoma of tympanum, **right ear**
       H71.12   Cholesteatoma of tympanum, **left ear**
       H71.13   Cholesteatoma of tympanum, **bilateral**
    ● **H71.2**   **Cholesteatoma of mastoid**
       H71.20   Cholesteatoma of mastoid, **unspecified ear**
       H71.21   Cholesteatoma of mastoid, **right ear**
       H71.22   Cholesteatoma of mastoid, **left ear**
       H71.23   Cholesteatoma of mastoid, **bilateral**
    ● **H71.3**   **Diffuse cholesteatosis**
       H71.30   Diffuse cholesteatosis, **unspecified ear**
       H71.31   Diffuse cholesteatosis, **right ear**
       H71.32   Diffuse cholesteatosis, **left ear**
       H71.33   Diffuse cholesteatosis, **bilateral**
    ● **H71.9**   **Unspecified cholesteatoma**
       H71.90   Unspecified cholesteatoma, **unspecified ear**
       H71.91   Unspecified cholesteatoma, **right ear**
       H71.92   Unspecified cholesteatoma, **left ear**
       H71.93   Unspecified cholesteatoma, **bilateral**

★ **(See Plate 93 on page 69.)**

● **H72**   **Perforation of tympanic membrane**
      Hole or rupture in ear drum
      Includes   persistent post-traumatic perforation of ear drum
                       postinflammatory perforation of ear drum
      Code first any associated otitis media (H65.-, H66.1-, H66.2-,
         H66.3-, H66.4-, H66.9-, H67.-)
      Excludes1   acute suppurative otitis media with rupture of
                       the tympanic membrane (H66.01-)
                       traumatic rupture of ear drum (S09.2-)
    ● **H72.0**   **Central perforation of tympanic membrane**
       H72.00   Central perforation of tympanic membrane, **unspecified ear**
       H72.01   Central perforation of tympanic membrane, **right ear**
       H72.02   Central perforation of tympanic membrane, **left ear**
       H72.03   Central perforation of tympanic membrane, **bilateral**
    ● **H72.1**   **Attic perforation of tympanic membrane**
      Perforation of pars flaccida
       H72.10   Attic perforation of tympanic membrane, **unspecified ear**
       H72.11   Attic perforation of tympanic membrane, **right ear**
       H72.12   Attic perforation of tympanic membrane, **left ear**
       H72.13   Attic perforation of tympanic membrane, **bilateral**
    ● **H72.2**   **Other marginal perforations of tympanic membrane**
      ● **H72.2X**   **Other marginal perforations of tympanic membrane**
         H72.2X1   Other marginal perforations of tympanic membrane, **right ear**
         H72.2X2   Other marginal perforations of tympanic membrane, **left ear**
         H72.2X3   Other marginal perforations of tympanic membrane, **bilateral**
         H72.2X9   Other marginal perforations of tympanic membrane, **unspecified ear**
    ● **H72.8**   **Other perforations of tympanic membrane**
      ● **H72.81**   **Multiple perforations of tympanic membrane**
         H72.811   Multiple perforations of tympanic membrane, **right ear**
         H72.812   Multiple perforations of tympanic membrane, **left ear**
         H72.813   Multiple perforations of tympanic membrane, **bilateral**
         H72.819   Multiple perforations of tympanic membrane, **unspecified ear**
      ● **H72.82**   **Total perforations of tympanic membrane**
         H72.821   Total perforations of tympanic membrane, **right ear**
         H72.822   Total perforations of tympanic membrane, **left ear**
         H72.823   Total perforations of tympanic membrane, **bilateral**
         H72.829   Total perforations of tympanic membrane, **unspecified ear**
    ● **H72.9**   **Unspecified perforation of tympanic membrane**
       H72.90   Unspecified perforation of tympanic membrane, **unspecified ear**
       H72.91   Unspecified perforation of tympanic membrane, **right ear**
       H72.92   Unspecified perforation of tympanic membrane, **left ear**
       H72.93   Unspecified perforation of tympanic membrane, **bilateral**

▶ New   ⇒ Revised   ~~deleted~~ Deleted   Excludes 1   Excludes 2   Includes   Use additional   Code first   Code also   Key words
OGCR Official Guidelines   ● Unacceptable Principal Diagnosis   X Assign placeholder X   ● Use Additional Character(s)   ▶ Manifestation Code   **Coding Clinic**

- H73　Other disorders of tympanic membrane
  - H73.0　Acute myringitis
    - Excludes1　acute myringitis with otitis media (H65, H66)
    - H73.00　Unspecified acute myringitis
      Acute tympanitis NOS
      - H73.001　Acute myringitis, right ear
      - H73.002　Acute myringitis, left ear
      - H73.003　Acute myringitis, bilateral
      - H73.009　Acute myringitis, unspecified ear
    - H73.01　Bullous myringitis
      - H73.011　Bullous myringitis, right ear
      - H73.012　Bullous myringitis, left ear
      - H73.013　Bullous myringitis, bilateral
      - H73.019　Bullous myringitis, unspecified ear
    - H73.09　Other acute myringitis
      - H73.091　Other acute myringitis, right ear
      - H73.092　Other acute myringitis, left ear
      - H73.093　Other acute myringitis, bilateral
      - H73.099　Other acute myringitis, unspecified ear
  - H73.1　Chronic myringitis
    Chronic tympanitis
    - Excludes1　chronic myringitis with otitis media (H65, H66)
    - H73.10　Chronic myringitis, unspecified ear
    - H73.11　Chronic myringitis, right ear
    - H73.12　Chronic myringitis, left ear
    - H73.13　Chronic myringitis, bilateral
  - H73.2　Unspecified myringitis
    - H73.20　Unspecified myringitis, unspecified ear
    - H73.21　Unspecified myringitis, right ear
    - H73.22　Unspecified myringitis, left ear
    - H73.23　Unspecified myringitis, bilateral
  - H73.8　Other specified disorders of tympanic membrane
    - H73.81　Atrophic flaccid tympanic membrane
      - H73.811　Atrophic flaccid tympanic membrane, right ear
      - H73.812　Atrophic flaccid tympanic membrane, left ear
      - H73.813　Atrophic flaccid tympanic membrane, bilateral
      - H73.819　Atrophic flaccid tympanic membrane, unspecified ear
    - H73.82　Atrophic nonflaccid tympanic membrane
      - H73.821　Atrophic nonflaccid tympanic membrane, right ear
      - H73.822　Atrophic nonflaccid tympanic membrane, left ear
      - H73.823　Atrophic nonflaccid tympanic membrane, bilateral
      - H73.829　Atrophic nonflaccid tympanic membrane, unspecified ear
    - H73.89　Other specified disorders of tympanic membrane
      - H73.891　Other specified disorders of tympanic membrane, right ear
      - H73.892　Other specified disorders of tympanic membrane, left ear
      - H73.893　Other specified disorders of tympanic membrane, bilateral
      - H73.899　Other specified disorders of tympanic membrane, unspecified ear

- H73.9　Unspecified disorder of tympanic membrane
  - H73.90　Unspecified disorder of tympanic membrane, unspecified ear
  - H73.91　Unspecified disorder of tympanic membrane, right ear
  - H73.92　Unspecified disorder of tympanic membrane, left ear
  - H73.93　Unspecified disorder of tympanic membrane, bilateral
- H74　Other disorders of middle ear mastoid
  - Excludes2　mastoiditis (H70.-)
  - H74.0　Tympanosclerosis
    - H74.01　Tympanosclerosis, right ear
    - H74.02　Tympanosclerosis, left ear
    - H74.03　Tympanosclerosis, bilateral
    - H74.09　Tympanosclerosis, unspecified ear
  - H74.1　Adhesive middle ear disease
    Adhesive otitis
    - Excludes1　glue ear (H65.3-)
    - H74.11　Adhesive right middle ear disease
    - H74.12　Adhesive left middle ear disease
    - H74.13　Adhesive middle ear disease, bilateral
    - H74.19　Adhesive middle ear disease, unspecified ear
  - H74.2　Discontinuity and dislocation of ear ossicles
    - H74.20　Discontinuity and dislocation of ear ossicles, unspecified ear
    - H74.21　Discontinuity and dislocation of right ear ossicles
    - H74.22　Discontinuity and dislocation of left ear ossicles
    - H74.23　Discontinuity and dislocation of ear ossicles, bilateral
  - H74.3　Other acquired abnormalities of ear ossicles
    - H74.31　Ankylosis of ear ossicles
      - H74.311　Ankylosis of ear ossicles, right ear
      - H74.312　Ankylosis of ear ossicles, left ear
      - H74.313　Ankylosis of ear ossicles, bilateral
      - H74.319　Ankylosis of ear ossicles, unspecified ear
    - H74.32　Partial loss of ear ossicles
      - H74.321　Partial loss of ear ossicles, right ear
      - H74.322　Partial loss of ear ossicles, left ear
      - H74.323　Partial loss of ear ossicles, bilateral
      - H74.329　Partial loss of ear ossicles, unspecified ear
    - H74.39　Other acquired abnormalities of ear ossicles
      - H74.391　Other acquired abnormalities of right ear ossicles
      - H74.392　Other acquired abnormalities of left ear ossicles
      - H74.393　Other acquired abnormalities of ear ossicles, bilateral
      - H74.399　Other acquired abnormalities of ear ossicles, unspecified ear
  - H74.4　Polyp of middle ear
    - H74.40　Polyp of middle ear, unspecified ear
    - H74.41　Polyp of right middle ear
    - H74.42　Polyp of left middle ear
    - H74.43　Polyp of middle ear, bilateral

CHAPTER 8 (H60–H95)

CHAPTER 8 (H60-H95)

● H74.8 Other specified disorders of middle ear and mastoid
 ● H74.8X Other specified disorders of middle ear and mastoid
  H74.8X1 Other specified disorders of right middle ear and mastoid
  H74.8X2 Other specified disorders of left middle ear and mastoid
  H74.8X3 Other specified disorders of middle ear and mastoid, bilateral
  H74.8X9 Other specified disorders of middle ear and mastoid, unspecified ear
● H74.9 Unspecified disorder of middle ear and mastoid
  H74.90 Unspecified disorder of middle ear and mastoid, unspecified ear
  H74.91 Unspecified disorder of right middle ear and mastoid
  H74.92 Unspecified disorder of left middle ear and mastoid
  H74.93 Unspecified disorder of middle ear and mastoid, bilateral

● H75 Other disorders of middle ear and mastoid in diseases classified elsewhere
 Code first underlying disease
 ● H75.0 Mastoiditis in infectious and parasitic diseases classified elsewhere
  Excludes1 mastoiditis (in):
   syphilis (A52.77)
   tuberculosis (A18.03)
  ▶ *H75.00 Mastoiditis in infectious and parasitic diseases classified elsewhere, unspecified ear*
  ▶ *H75.01 Mastoiditis in infectious and parasitic diseases classified elsewhere, right ear*
  ▶ *H75.02 Mastoiditis in infectious and parasitic diseases classified elsewhere, left ear*
  ▶ *H75.03 Mastoiditis in infectious and parasitic diseases classified elsewhere, bilateral*
 ● H75.8 Other specified disorders of middle ear and mastoid in diseases classified elsewhere
  ▶ *H75.80 Other specified disorders of middle ear and mastoid in diseases classified elsewhere, unspecified ear*
  ▶ *H75.81 Other specified disorders of right middle ear and mastoid in diseases classified elsewhere*
  ▶ *H75.82 Other specified disorders of left middle ear and mastoid in diseases classified elsewhere*
  ▶ *H75.83 Other specified disorders of middle ear and mastoid in diseases classified elsewhere, bilateral*

DISEASES OF INNER EAR (H80-H83)

★ **(See Plate 95 on page 69.)**

● H80 Otosclerosis
 Inherited middle ear spongelike bone growth causing hearing loss
 Includes Otospongiosis
 ● H80.0 Otosclerosis involving oval window, nonobliterative
  H80.00 Otosclerosis involving oval window, nonobliterative, unspecified ear
  H80.01 Otosclerosis involving oval window, nonobliterative, right ear
  H80.02 Otosclerosis involving oval window, nonobliterative, left ear
  H80.03 Otosclerosis involving oval window, nonobliterative, bilateral
 ● H80.1 Otosclerosis involving oval window, obliterative
  H80.10 Otosclerosis involving oval window, obliterative, unspecified ear
  H80.11 Otosclerosis involving oval window, obliterative, right ear

H80.12 Otosclerosis involving oval window, obliterative, left ear
H80.13 Otosclerosis involving oval window, obliterative, bilateral
● H80.2 Cochlear otosclerosis
 Otosclerosis involving otic capsule
 Otosclerosis involving round window
 H80.20 Cochlear otosclerosis, unspecified ear
 H80.21 Cochlear otosclerosis, right ear
 H80.22 Cochlear otosclerosis, left ear
 H80.23 Cochlear otosclerosis, bilateral
● H80.8 Other otosclerosis
 H80.80 Other otosclerosis, unspecified ear
 H80.81 Other otosclerosis, right ear
 H80.82 Other otosclerosis, left ear
 H80.83 Other otosclerosis, bilateral
● H80.9 Unspecified otosclerosis
 H80.90 Unspecified otosclerosis, unspecified ear
 H80.91 Unspecified otosclerosis, right ear
 H80.92 Unspecified otosclerosis, left ear
 H80.93 Unspecified otosclerosis, bilateral

● H81 Disorders of vestibular function
 Excludes1 epidemic vertigo (A88.1)
  vertigo NOS (R42)
 ● H81.0 Ménière's disease
  Vestibular disorder that produces recurring symptoms including severe and intermittent hearing loss including the feeling of ear pressure or pain
  Labyrinthine hydrops
  Ménière's syndrome or vertigo
  H81.01 Ménière's disease, right ear
  H81.02 Ménière's disease, left ear
  H81.03 Ménière's disease, bilateral
  H81.09 Ménière's disease, unspecified ear
 ● H81.1 Benign paroxysmal vertigo
  H81.10 Benign paroxysmal vertigo, unspecified ear
  H81.11 Benign paroxysmal vertigo, right ear
  H81.12 Benign paroxysmal vertigo, left ear
  H81.13 Benign paroxysmal vertigo, bilateral
 ● H81.2 Vestibular neuronitis
  H81.20 Vestibular neuronitis, unspecified ear
  H81.21 Vestibular neuronitis, right ear
  H81.22 Vestibular neuronitis, left ear
  H81.23 Vestibular neuronitis, bilateral
 ● H81.3 Other peripheral vertigo
  ● H81.31 Aural vertigo
   H81.311 Aural vertigo, right ear
   H81.312 Aural vertigo, left ear
   H81.313 Aural vertigo, bilateral
   H81.319 Aural vertigo, unspecified ear
  ● H81.39 Other peripheral vertigo
   Lermoyez' syndrome
   Otogenic vertigo
   Peripheral vertigo NOS
   H81.391 Other peripheral vertigo, right ear
   H81.392 Other peripheral vertigo, left ear
   H81.393 Other peripheral vertigo, bilateral
   H81.399 Other peripheral vertigo, unspecified ear
 ● H81.4 Vertigo of central origin
  Central positional nystagmus
  H81.41 Vertigo of central origin, right ear
  H81.42 Vertigo of central origin, left ear
  H81.43 Vertigo of central origin, bilateral
  H81.49 Vertigo of central origin, unspecified ear

▶ New   ⟹ Revised   ~~deleted~~ Deleted   Excludes 1   Excludes 2   Includes   Use additional   Code first   Code also   Key words
OGCR Official Guidelines   ● Unacceptable Principal Diagnosis   X Assign placeholder X   ● Use Additional Character(s)   ▶ Manifestation Code   **Coding Clinic**
862

H81.8   Other disorders of vestibular function

   H81.8X   Other disorders of vestibular function

     H81.8X1   Other disorders of vestibular function, right ear

     H81.8X2   Other disorders of vestibular function, left ear

     H81.8X3   Other disorders of vestibular function, bilateral

     H81.8X9   Other disorders of vestibular function, unspecified ear

H81.9   Unspecified disorder of vestibular function
> Vertiginous syndrome NOS

   H81.90   Unspecified disorder of vestibular function, unspecified ear

   H81.91   Unspecified disorder of vestibular function, right ear

   H81.92   Unspecified disorder of vestibular function, left ear

   H81.93   Unspecified disorder of vestibular function, bilateral

H82   Vertiginous syndromes in diseases classified elsewhere
> *Code first underlying disease*

   Excludes1   epidemic vertigo (A88.1)

   H82.1   *Vertiginous syndromes in diseases classified elsewhere, right ear*

   H82.2   *Vertiginous syndromes in diseases classified elsewhere, left ear*

   H82.3   *Vertiginous syndromes in diseases classified elsewhere, bilateral*

   H82.9   *Vertiginous syndromes in diseases classified elsewhere, unspecified ear*

H83   Other diseases of inner ear

   H83.0   Labyrinthitis
> *Balance disorder that follows URI or head injury*

     H83.01   Labyrinthitis, right ear

     H83.02   Labyrinthitis, left ear

     H83.03   Labyrinthitis, bilateral

     H83.09   Labyrinthitis, unspecified ear

   H83.1   Labyrinthine fistula

     H83.11   Labyrinthine fistula, right ear

     H83.12   Labyrinthine fistula, left ear

     H83.13   Labyrinthine fistula, bilateral

     H83.19   Labyrinthine fistula, unspecified ear

   H83.2   Labyrinthine dysfunction
> Labyrinthine hypersensitivity
> Labyrinthine hypofunction
> Labyrinthine loss of function

     H83.2X   Labyrinthine dysfunction

       H83.2X1   Labyrinthine dysfunction, right ear

       H83.2X2   Labyrinthine dysfunction, left ear

       H83.2X3   Labyrinthine dysfunction, bilateral

       H83.2X9   Labyrinthine dysfunction, unspecified ear

   H83.3   Noise effects on inner ear
> Acoustic trauma of inner ear
> Noise-induced hearing loss of inner ear

     H83.3X   Noise effects on inner ear

       H83.3X1   Noise effects on right inner ear

       H83.3X2   Noise effects on left inner ear

       H83.3X3   Noise effects on inner ear, bilateral

       H83.3X9   Noise effects on inner ear, unspecified ear

H83.8   Other specified diseases of inner ear

   H83.8X   Other specified diseases of inner ear

     H83.8X1   Other specified diseases of right inner ear

     H83.8X2   Other specified diseases of left inner ear

     H83.8X3   Other specified diseases of inner ear, bilateral

     H83.8X9   Other specified diseases of inner ear, unspecified ear

H83.9   Unspecified disease of inner ear

   H83.90   Unspecified disease of inner ear, unspecified ear

   H83.91   Unspecified disease of right inner ear

   H83.92   Unspecified disease of left inner ear

   H83.93   Unspecified disease of inner ear, bilateral

OTHER DISORDERS OF EAR (H90-H94)

H90   Conductive and sensorineural hearing loss

   Excludes1   deaf nonspeaking NEC (H91.3)
> deafness NOS (H91.9-)
> hearing loss NOS (H91.9-)
> noise-induced hearing loss (H83.3-)
> ototoxic hearing loss (H91.0-)
> sudden (idiopathic) hearing loss (H91.2-)

   H90.0   Conductive hearing loss, bilateral

   H90.1   Conductive hearing loss, unilateral with unrestricted hearing on the contralateral side

     H90.11   Conductive hearing loss, unilateral, right ear, with unrestricted hearing on the contralateral side

     H90.12   Conductive hearing loss, unilateral, left ear, with unrestricted hearing on the contralateral side

   H90.2   Conductive hearing loss, unspecified
> Conductive deafness NOS

   H90.3   Sensorineural hearing loss, bilateral

   H90.4   Sensorineural hearing loss, unilateral with unrestricted hearing on the contralateral side

     H90.41   Sensorineural hearing loss, unilateral, right ear, with unrestricted hearing on the contralateral side

     H90.42   Sensorineural hearing loss, unilateral, left ear, with unrestricted hearing on the contralateral side

   H90.5   Unspecified sensorineural hearing loss
> Central hearing loss NOS
> Congenital deafness NOS
> Neural hearing loss NOS
> Perceptive hearing loss NOS
> Sensorineural deafness NOS
> Sensory hearing loss NOS

     Excludes1   abnormal auditory perception (H93.2-)
> psychogenic deafness (F44.6)

   H90.6   Mixed conductive and sensorineural hearing loss, bilateral
> **Coding Clinic: 2015, Q2, P7**

   H90.7   Mixed conductive and sensorineural hearing loss, unilateral with unrestricted hearing on the contralateral side

     H90.71   Mixed conductive and sensorineural hearing loss, unilateral, right ear, with unrestricted hearing on the contralateral side

     H90.72   Mixed conductive and sensorineural hearing loss, unilateral, left ear, with unrestricted hearing on the contralateral side

   H90.8   Mixed conductive and sensorineural hearing loss, unspecified

- ● **H90.A** **Conductive and sensorineural hearing loss with restricted hearing on the contralateral side**
  Coding Clinic: 2016, Q4, P23-24
  - ● **H90.A1** Conductive hearing loss, unilateral, with restricted hearing on the contralateral side
    - **H90.A11** Conductive hearing loss, unilateral, right ear with restricted hearing on the contralateral side
    - **H90.A12** Conductive hearing loss, unilateral, left ear with restricted hearing on the contralateral side
      Coding Clinic: 2016, Q4, P25
  - ● **H90.A2** Sensorineural hearing loss, unilateral, with restricted hearing on the contralateral side
    - **H90.A21** Sensorineural hearing loss, unilateral, right ear, with restricted hearing on the contralateral side
    - **H90.A22** Sensorineural hearing loss, unilateral, left ear, with restricted hearing on the contralateral side
  - ● **H90.A3** Mixed conductive and sensorineural hearing loss, unilateral with restricted hearing on the contralateral side
    - **H90.A31** Mixed conductive and sensorineural hearing loss, unilateral, right ear with restricted hearing on the contralateral side
    - **H90.A32** Mixed conductive and sensorineural hearing loss, unilateral, left ear with restricted hearing on the contralateral side

- ● **H91** **Other and unspecified hearing loss**
  Excludes1   abnormal auditory perception (H93.2-)
  hearing loss as classified in H90.-
  impacted cerumen (H61.2-)
  noise-induced hearing loss (H83.3-)
  psychogenic deafness (F44.6)
  transient ischemic deafness (H93.01-)
  - ● **H91.0** Ototoxic hearing loss
    Code first poisoning due to drug or toxin, if applicable (T36-T65 with fifth or sixth character 1-4 or 6)
    Use additional code for adverse effect, if applicable, to identify drug (T36-T50 with fifth or sixth character 5)
    - **H91.01** Ototoxic hearing loss, right ear
    - **H91.02** Ototoxic hearing loss, left ear
    - **H91.03** Ototoxic hearing loss, bilateral
    - **H91.09** Ototoxic hearing loss, unspecified ear
  - ● **H91.1** Presbycusis
    Presbyacusia
    - **H91.10** Presbycusis, unspecified ear
    - **H91.11** Presbycusis, right ear
    - **H91.12** Presbycusis, left ear
    - **H91.13** Presbycusis, bilateral
  - ● **H91.2** Sudden idiopathic hearing loss
    Sudden hearing loss NOS
    - **H91.20** Sudden idiopathic hearing loss, unspecified ear
    - **H91.21** Sudden idiopathic hearing loss, right ear
    - **H91.22** Sudden idiopathic hearing loss, left ear
    - **H91.23** Sudden idiopathic hearing loss, bilateral
  - **H91.3** Deaf nonspeaking, not elsewhere classified
  - ● **H91.8** Other specified hearing loss
    - ● **H91.8X** Other specified hearing loss
      - **H91.8X1** Other specified hearing loss, right ear
      - **H91.8X2** Other specified hearing loss, left ear
      - **H91.8X3** Other specified hearing loss, bilateral
      - **H91.8X9** Other specified hearing loss, unspecified ear

- ● **H91.9** Unspecified hearing loss
  Deafness NOS
  High frequency deafness
  Low frequency deafness
  - **H91.90** Unspecified hearing loss, unspecified ear
  - **H91.91** Unspecified hearing loss, right ear
  - **H91.92** Unspecified hearing loss, left ear
  - **H91.93** Unspecified hearing loss, bilateral

- ● **H92** **Otalgia and effusion of ear**
  - ● **H92.0** Otalgia
    - **H92.01** Otalgia, right ear
    - **H92.02** Otalgia, left ear
    - **H92.03** Otalgia, bilateral
    - **H92.09** Otalgia, unspecified ear
  - ● **H92.1** Otorrhea
    Excludes1   leakage of cerebrospinal fluid through ear (G96.0)
    - **H92.10** Otorrhea, unspecified ear
    - **H92.11** Otorrhea, right ear
    - **H92.12** Otorrhea, left ear
    - **H92.13** Otorrhea, bilateral
  - ● **H92.2** Otorrhagia
    Excludes1   traumatic otorrhagia - code to injury
    - **H92.20** Otorrhagia, unspecified ear
    - **H92.21** Otorrhagia, right ear
    - **H92.22** Otorrhagia, left ear
    - **H92.23** Otorrhagia, bilateral

- ● **H93** **Other disorders of ear, not elsewhere classified**
  - ● **H93.0** Degenerative and vascular disorders of ear
    Excludes1   presbycusis (H91.1)
    - ● **H93.01** Transient ischemic deafness
      - **H93.011** Transient ischemic deafness, right ear
      - **H93.012** Transient ischemic deafness, left ear
      - **H93.013** Transient ischemic deafness, bilateral
      - **H93.019** Transient ischemic deafness, unspecified ear
    - ● **H93.09** Unspecified degenerative and vascular disorders of ear
      - **H93.091** Unspecified degenerative and vascular disorders of right ear
      - **H93.092** Unspecified degenerative and vascular disorders of left ear
      - **H93.093** Unspecified degenerative and vascular disorders of ear, bilateral
      - **H93.099** Unspecified degenerative and vascular disorders of unspecified ear
  - ● **H93.1** Tinnitus
    Perception of sound (ringing, buzzing, humming, whistling tunes, or singing)
    - **H93.11** Tinnitus, right ear
    - **H93.12** Tinnitus, left ear
    - **H93.13** Tinnitus, bilateral
    - **H93.19** Tinnitus, unspecified ear
  - ● **H93.A** Pulsatile tinnitus
    Coding Clinic: 2016, Q4, P25
    - **H93.A1** Pulsatile tinnitus, right ear
      Coding Clinic: 2016, Q4, P26
    - **H93.A2** Pulsatile tinnitus, left ear
    - **H93.A3** Pulsatile tinnitus, bilateral
    - **H93.A9** Pulsatile tinnitus, unspecified ear

▶ New   ⇒ Revised   ~~deleted~~ Deleted   Excludes 1   Excludes 2   Includes   Use additional   Code first   Code also   Key words
OGCR Official Guidelines   ● Unacceptable Principal Diagnosis   X Assign placeholder X   ● Use Additional Character(s)   ▌Manifestation Code   Coding Clinic

- **H93.2 Other abnormal auditory perceptions**
  - **Excludes2** auditory hallucinations (R44.0)
  - **H93.21 Auditory recruitment**
    - H93.211 Auditory recruitment, right ear
    - H93.212 Auditory recruitment, left ear
    - H93.213 Auditory recruitment, bilateral
    - H93.219 Auditory recruitment, unspecified ear
  - **H93.22 Diplacusis**
    - H93.221 Diplacusis, right ear
    - H93.222 Diplacusis, left ear
    - H93.223 Diplacusis, bilateral
    - H93.229 Diplacusis, unspecified ear
  - **H93.23 Hyperacusis**
    - H93.231 Hyperacusis, right ear
    - H93.232 Hyperacusis, left ear
    - H93.233 Hyperacusis, bilateral
    - H93.239 Hyperacusis, unspecified ear
  - **H93.24 Temporary auditory threshold shift**
    - H93.241 Temporary auditory threshold shift, right ear
    - H93.242 Temporary auditory threshold shift, left ear
    - H93.243 Temporary auditory threshold shift, bilateral
    - H93.249 Temporary auditory threshold shift, unspecified ear
  - **H93.25 Central auditory processing disorder**
    - Congenital auditory imperception
    - Word deafness
    - **Excludes1** mixed receptive-expressive language disorder (F80.2)
  - **H93.29 Other abnormal auditory perceptions**
    - H93.291 Other abnormal auditory perceptions, right ear
    - H93.292 Other abnormal auditory perceptions, left ear
    - H93.293 Other abnormal auditory perceptions, bilateral
    - H93.299 Other abnormal auditory perceptions, unspecified ear
- **H93.3 Disorders of acoustic nerve**
  - Disorder of 8th cranial nerve
  - **Excludes1** acoustic neuroma (D33.3)
    - syphilitic acoustic neuritis (A52.15)
  - **H93.3X Disorders of acoustic nerve**
    - H93.3X1 Disorders of right acoustic nerve
    - H93.3X2 Disorders of left acoustic nerve
    - H93.3X3 Disorders of bilateral acoustic nerves
    - H93.3X9 Disorders of unspecified acoustic nerve
- **H93.8 Other specified disorders of ear**
  - **H93.8X Other specified disorders of ear**
    - H93.8X1 Other specified disorders of right ear
    - H93.8X2 Other specified disorders of left ear
    - H93.8X3 Other specified disorders of ear, bilateral
    - H93.8X9 Other specified disorders of ear, unspecified ear
- **H93.9 Unspecified disorder of ear**
  - **H93.90 Unspecified disorder of ear, unspecified ear**
  - **H93.91 Unspecified disorder of right ear**
  - **H93.92 Unspecified disorder of left ear**
  - **H93.93 Unspecified disorder of ear, bilateral**

- **H94 Other disorders of ear in diseases classified elsewhere**
  - **H94.0 Acoustic neuritis in infectious and parasitic diseases classified elsewhere**
    - *Code first underlying disease, such as:*
      - parasitic disease (B65-B89)
    - **Excludes1** acoustic neuritis (in):
      - herpes zoster (B02.29)
      - syphilis (A52.15)
    - *H94.00 Acoustic neuritis in infectious and parasitic diseases classified elsewhere, unspecified ear*
    - *H94.01 Acoustic neuritis in infectious and parasitic diseases classified elsewhere, right ear*
    - *H94.02 Acoustic neuritis in infectious and parasitic diseases classified elsewhere, left ear*
    - *H94.03 Acoustic neuritis in infectious and parasitic diseases classified elsewhere, bilateral*
  - **H94.8 Other specified disorders of ear in diseases classified elsewhere**
    - *Code first underlying disease, such as:*
      - congenital syphilis (A50.0)
    - **Excludes1** aural myiasis (B87.4)
      - syphilitic labyrinthitis (A52.79)
    - *H94.80 Other specified disorders of ear in diseases classified elsewhere, unspecified ear*
    - *H94.81 Other specified disorders of right ear in diseases classified elsewhere*
    - *H94.82 Other specified disorders of left ear in diseases classified elsewhere*
    - *H94.83 Other specified disorders of ear in diseases classified elsewhere, bilateral*
- **H95 Intraoperative and postprocedural complications and disorders of ear and mastoid process, not elsewhere classified**
  - Coding Clinic: 2016, Q4, P10
  - **H95.0 Recurrent cholesteatoma of postmastoidectomy cavity**
    - **H95.00 Recurrent cholesteatoma of postmastoidectomy cavity, unspecified ear**
    - **H95.01 Recurrent cholesteatoma of postmastoidectomy cavity, right ear**
    - **H95.02 Recurrent cholesteatoma of postmastoidectomy cavity, left ear**
    - **H95.03 Recurrent cholesteatoma of postmastoidectomy cavity, bilateral ears**
  - **H95.1 Other disorders of ear and mastoid process following mastoidectomy**
    - **H95.11 Chronic inflammation of postmastoidectomy cavity**
      - H95.111 Chronic inflammation of postmastoidectomy cavity, right ear
      - H95.112 Chronic inflammation of postmastoidectomy cavity, left ear
      - H95.113 Chronic inflammation of postmastoidectomy cavity, bilateral ears
      - H95.119 Chronic inflammation of postmastoidectomy cavity, unspecified ear
    - **H95.12 Granulation of postmastoidectomy cavity**
      - H95.121 Granulation of postmastoidectomy cavity, right ear
      - H95.122 Granulation of postmastoidectomy cavity, left ear
      - H95.123 Granulation of postmastoidectomy cavity, bilateral ears
      - H95.129 Granulation of postmastoidectomy cavity, unspecified ear

CHAPTER 8 (H60-H95)

N Newborn Age: 0   P Pediatric Age: 0–17   M Maternity DX: 12–55   A Adult Age: 15–124   ♀ Females Only   ♂ Males Only
🅒 Complication\Comorbidity   🅒 Major C\C   (Ex) CC/MCC Exclusions   🅗 Hospital-Acquired Condition
865

● H95.13   Mucosal cyst of postmastoidectomy cavity

    H95.131   Mucosal cyst of postmastoidectomy cavity, right ear

    H95.132   Mucosal cyst of postmastoidectomy cavity, left ear

    H95.133   Mucosal cyst of postmastoidectomy cavity, bilateral ears

    H95.139   Mucosal cyst of postmastoidectomy cavity, unspecified ear

● H95.19   Other disorders following mastoidectomy

    H95.191   Other disorders following mastoidectomy, right ear

    H95.192   Other disorders following mastoidectomy, left ear

    H95.193   Other disorders following mastoidectomy, bilateral ears

    H95.199   Other disorders following mastoidectomy, unspecified ear

● H95.2   Intraoperative hemorrhage and hematoma of ear and mastoid process complicating a procedure

    Excludes1   intraoperative hemorrhage and hematoma of ear and mastoid process due to accidental puncture or laceration during a procedure (H95.3-)

    (Ex) **For category H95.2 CC codes:** See PDX Collection 642

    H95.21   Intraoperative hemorrhage and hematoma of ear and mastoid process complicating a procedure on the ear and mastoid process

    H95.22   Intraoperative hemorrhage and hematoma of ear and mastoid process complicating other procedure

● H95.3   Accidental puncture and laceration of ear and mastoid process during a procedure

    (Ex) **For category H95.3 CC codes:** See PDX Collection 509

    H95.31   Accidental puncture and laceration of the ear and mastoid process during a procedure on the ear and mastoid process

    H95.32   Accidental puncture and laceration of the ear and mastoid process during other procedure

● H95.4   Postprocedural hemorrhage of ear and mastoid process following a procedure

    (Ex) **For category H95.4 CC codes:** See PDX Collection 642

    H95.41   Postprocedural hemorrhage of ear and mastoid process following a procedure on the ear and mastoid process

    H95.42   Postprocedural hemorrhage of ear and mastoid process following other procedure

● H95.5   Postprocedural hematoma and seroma of ear and mastoid process following a procedure

    (Ex) **For category H95.5 CC codes:** See PDX Collection 642

    H95.51   Postprocedural hematoma of ear and mastoid process following a procedure on the ear and mastoid process

    H95.52   Postprocedural hematoma of ear and mastoid process following other procedure

    H95.53   Postprocedural seroma of ear and mastoid process following a procedure on the ear and mastoid process

    H95.54   Postprocedural seroma of ear and mastoid process following other procedure

● H95.8   Other intraoperative and postprocedural complications and disorders of the ear and mastoid process, not elsewhere classified

    Excludes2   postprocedural complications and disorders following mastoidectomy (H95.0-, H95.1-)

    (Ex) **For category H95.8 CC codes:** See PDX Collection 643

    ● H95.81   Postprocedural stenosis of external ear canal

        H95.811   Postprocedural stenosis of right external ear canal

        H95.812   Postprocedural stenosis of left external ear canal

        H95.813   Postprocedural stenosis of external ear canal, bilateral

        H95.819   Postprocedural stenosis of unspecified external ear canal

    H95.88   Other intraoperative complications and disorders of the ear and mastoid process, not elsewhere classified

        Use additional code, if applicable, to further specify disorder

    H95.89   Other postprocedural complications and disorders of the ear and mastoid process, not elsewhere classified

        Use additional code, if applicable, to further specify disorder

CHAPTER 9

DISEASES OF THE CIRCULATORY SYSTEM (I00-I99)

OGCR Chapter-Specific Coding Guidelines

9. **Chapter 9: Diseases of the Circulatory System (I00-I99)**

   a. **Hypertension**

   The classification presumes a causal relationship between hypertension and heart involvement and between hypertension and kidney involvement, as the two conditions are linked by the term "with" in the Alphabetic Index. These conditions should be coded as related even in the absence of provider documentation explicitly linking them, unless the documentation clearly states the conditions are unrelated.

   For hypertension and conditions not specifically linked by relational terms such as "with," "associated with" or "due to" in the classification, provider documentation must link the conditions in order to code them as related.

   1) **Hypertension with Heart Disease**

   Hypertension with heart conditions classified to I50.- or I51.4-I51.9, are assigned to, a code from category I11, Hypertensive heart disease. Use additional code(s) from category I50, Heart failure, to identify the type(s) of heart failure in those patients with heart failure.

   The same heart conditions (I50.-, I51.4-I51.9) with hypertension, are coded separately if the provider has specifically documented a different cause. Sequence according to the circumstances of the admission/encounter.

   2) **Hypertensive Chronic Kidney Disease**

   Assign codes from category I12, Hypertensive chronic kidney disease, when both hypertension and a condition classifiable to category N18, Chronic kidney disease (CKD), are present. CKD should not be coded as hypertensive if the physician has specifically documented a different cause.

   The appropriate code from category N18 should be used as a secondary code with a code from category I12 to identify the stage of chronic kidney disease.

   See Section I.C.14. Chronic kidney disease.

   If a patient has hypertensive chronic kidney disease and acute renal failure, an additional code for the acute renal failure is required.

   3) **Hypertensive Heart and Chronic Kidney Disease**

   Assign codes from combination category I13, Hypertensive heart and chronic kidney disease, when there is hypertension with both heart and kidney involvement. If heart failure is present, assign an additional code from category I50 to identify the type of heart failure.

   The appropriate code from category N18, Chronic kidney disease, should be used as a secondary code with a code from category I13 to identify the stage of chronic kidney disease.

   See Section I.C.14. Chronic kidney disease.

   The codes in category I13, Hypertensive heart and chronic kidney disease, are combination codes that include hypertension, heart disease and chronic kidney disease. The Includes note at I13 specifies that the conditions included at I11 and I12 are included together in I13. If a patient has hypertension, heart disease and chronic kidney disease then a code from I13 should be used, not individual codes for hypertension, heart disease and chronic kidney disease, or codes from I11 or I12.

   For patients with both acute renal failure and chronic kidney disease an additional code for acute renal failure is required.

   4) **Hypertensive Cerebrovascular Disease**

   For hypertensive cerebrovascular disease, first assign the appropriate code from categories I60-I69, followed by the appropriate hypertension code.

   5) **Hypertensive Retinopathy**

   Subcategory H35.0, Background retinopathy and retinal vascular changes, should be used with a code from category I10 – I15, Hypertensive disease to include the systemic hypertension. The sequencing is based on the reason for the encounter.

   6) **Hypertension, Secondary**

   Secondary hypertension is due to an underlying condition. Two codes are required: one to identify the underlying etiology and one from category I15 to identify the hypertension. Sequencing of codes is determined by the reason for admission/encounter.

   7) **Hypertension, Transient**

   Assign code R03.0, Elevated blood pressure reading without diagnosis of hypertension, unless patient has an established diagnosis of hypertension. Assign code O13.-, Gestational [pregnancy-induced] hypertension without significant proteinuria, or O14.-, Pre-eclampsia, for transient hypertension of pregnancy.

   8) **Hypertension, Controlled**

   This diagnostic statement usually refers to an existing state of hypertension under control by therapy. Assign the appropriate code from categories I10-I15, Hypertensive diseases.

   9) **Hypertension, Uncontrolled**

   Uncontrolled hypertension may refer to untreated hypertension or hypertension not responding to current therapeutic regimen. In either case, assign the appropriate code from categories I10-I15, Hypertensive diseases.

   10) **Hypertensive Crisis**

   Assign a code from category I16, Hypertensive crisis, for documented hypertensive urgency, hypertensive emergency or unspecified hypertensive crisis. Code also any identified hypertensive disease (I10-I15). The sequencing is based on the reason for the encounter.

   10) **Pulmonary Hypertension**

   Pulmonary hypertension is classified to category I27, Other pulmonary heart diseases. For secondary pulmonary hypertension (I27.1, I27.2-), code also any associated conditions or adverse effects of drugs or toxins. The sequencing is based on the reason for the encounter.

   b. **Atherosclerotic Coronary Artery Disease and Angina**

   ICD-10-CM has combination codes for atherosclerotic heart disease with angina pectoris. The subcategories for these codes are I25.11, Atherosclerotic heart disease of native coronary artery with angina pectoris and I25.7, Atherosclerosis of coronary artery bypass graft(s) and coronary artery of transplanted heart with angina pectoris.

   When using one of these combination codes it is not necessary to use an additional code for angina pectoris. A causal relationship can be assumed in a patient with both atherosclerosis and angina pectoris, unless the documentation indicates the angina is due to something other than the atherosclerosis.

   If a patient with coronary artery disease is admitted due to an acute myocardial infarction (AMI), the AMI should be sequenced before the coronary artery disease.

   See Section I.C.9. Acute myocardial infarction (AMI)

   c. **Intraoperative and Postprocedural Cerebrovascular Accident**

   Medical record documentation should clearly specify the cause-and-effect relationship between the medical intervention and the cerebrovascular accident in order to assign a code for intraoperative or postprocedural cerebrovascular accident.

   Proper code assignment depends on whether it was an infarction or hemorrhage and whether it occurred intraoperatively or postoperatively. If it was a cerebral hemorrhage, code assignment depends on the type of procedure performed.

   d. **Sequelae of Cerebrovascular Disease**

   1) **Category I69, Sequelae of Cerebrovascular disease**

   Category I69 is used to indicate conditions classifiable to categories I60-I67 as the causes of sequela (neurologic deficits), themselves classified elsewhere. These "late effects" include neurologic deficits that persist after initial onset of conditions classifiable to categories I60-I67. The neurologic deficits caused by cerebrovascular disease may be present from the onset or may arise at any time after the onset of the condition classifiable to categories I60-I67.

   Codes from category I69, Sequelae of cerebrovascular disease, that specify hemiplegia, hemiparesis and monoplegia identify whether the dominant or nondominant side is affected. Should the affected side be documented, but not specified as dominant or nondominant, and the classification system does not indicate a default, code selection is as follows:

   - For ambidextrous patients, the default should be dominant.
   - If the left side is affected, the default is non-dominant.
   - If the right side is affected, the default is dominant.

   2) **Codes from category I69 with codes from I60-I67**

   Codes from category I69 may be assigned on a health care record with codes from I60-I67, if the patient has a current cerebrovascular disease and deficits from an old cerebrovascular disease.

3) Codes from category I69 and Personal history of transient ischemic attack (TIA) and cerebral infarction (Z86.73)

Codes from category I69 should not be assigned if the patient does not have neurologic deficits.

See Section I.C.21. 4. History (of) for use of personal history codes

e. **Acute myocardial infarction (AMI)**

1) **Type 1 ST elevation myocardial infarction (STEMI) and non ST elevation myocardial infarction (NSTEMI)**

The ICD-10-CM codes for acute **type 1** myocardial infarction (AMI) identify the site, such as anterolateral wall or true posterior wall. Subcategories I21.0-I21.2 and code I21.3 are used for **type 1** ST elevation myocardial infarction (STEMI). Code I21.4, Non-ST elevation (NSTEMI) myocardial infarction, is used for **type 1** non ST elevation myocardial infarction (NSTEMI) and nontransmural MIs.

If **a type 1** NSTEMI evolves to STEMI, assign the STEMI code. If **a type 1** STEMI converts to NSTEMI due to thrombolytic therapy, it is still coded as STEMI.

For encounters occurring while the myocardial infarction is equal to, or less than, four weeks old, including transfers to another acute setting or a postacute setting, and the myocardial infarction meets the definition for "other diagnoses" (see Section III, Reporting Additional Diagnoses), codes from category I21 may continue to be reported. For encounters after the 4 week time frame and the patient is still receiving care related to the myocardial infarction, the appropriate aftercare code should be assigned, rather than a code from category I21. For old or healed myocardial infarctions not requiring further care, code I25.2, Old myocardial infarction, may be assigned.

2) **Acute myocardial infarction, unspecified**

Code **I21.9, Acute myocardial infarction, unspecified,** is the default for unspecified acute myocardial infarction **or unspecified type.** If only type 1 STEMI or transmural MI without the site is documented, assign code I21.3, **ST elevation (STEMI) myocardial infarction of unspecified site.**

3) **AMI documented as nontransmural or subendocardial but site provided**

If an AMI is documented as nontransmural or subendocardial, but the site is provided, it is still coded as a subendocardial AMI.

See Section I.C.21.3 for information on coding status post administration of tPA in a different facility within the last 24 hours.

4) **Subsequent acute myocardial infarction**

A code from category I22, Subsequent ST elevation (STEMI) and non ST elevation (NSTEMI) myocardial infarction, is to be used when a patient who has suffered **a type 1 or unspecified** AMI has a new AMI within the 4 week time frame of the initial AMI. A code from category I22 must be used in conjunction with a code from category I21. The sequencing of the I22 and I21 codes depends on the circumstances of the encounter.

Do not assign code I22 for subsequent myocardial infarctions other than type 1 or unspecified. For subsequent type 2 AMI assign only code I21.A1. For subsequent type 4 or type 5 AMI, assign only code I21.A9.

5) Other Types of Myocardial Infarction

The ICD-10-CM provides codes for different types of myocardial infarction. Type 1 myocardial infarctions are assigned to codes I21.0-I21.4.

Type 2 myocardial infarction, and myocardial infarction due to demand ischemia or secondary to ischemic balance, is assigned to code I21.A1, Myocardial infarction type 2 with a code for the underlying cause. Do not assign code I24.8, Other forms of acute ischemic heart disease for the demand ischemia. Sequencing of type 2 AMI or the underlying cause is dependent on the circumstances of admission. When a type 2 AMI code is described as NSTEMI or STEMI, only assign code I21.A1. Codes I21.01-I21.4 should only be assigned for type 1 AMIs.

Acute myocardial infarctions type 3, 4a, 4b, 4c and 5 are assigned to code I21.A9, Other myocardial infarction type.

The "Code also" and "Code first" notes should be followed related to complications, and for coding of postprocedural myocardial infarctions during or following cardiac surgery.

Figure 9-1 Cardiovascular valves.

Item 9–1 Rheumatic fever is the inflammation of the valve(s) of the heart, usually the mitral or aortic, which leads to valve damage. Rheumatic heart inflammations are usually **pericarditis** (sac surrounding heart), **endocarditis** (heart cavity), or **myocarditis** (heart muscle).

CHAPTER 9

DISEASES OF THE CIRCULATORY SYSTEM (I00-I99)

Excludes2   certain conditions originating in the perinatal period (P04-P96)
certain infectious and parasitic diseases (A00-B99)
complications of pregnancy, childbirth and the puerperium (O00-O9A)
congenital malformations, deformations, and chromosomal abnormalities (Q00-Q99)
endocrine, nutritional and metabolic diseases (E00-E88)
injury, poisoning and certain other consequences of external causes (S00-T88)
neoplasms (C00-D49)
symptoms, signs and abnormal clinical and laboratory findings, not elsewhere classified (R00-R94)
systemic connective tissue disorders (M30-M36)
transient cerebral ischemic attacks and related syndromes (G45.-)

This chapter contains the following blocks:

I00-I02	Acute rheumatic fever
I05-I09	Chronic rheumatic heart diseases
I10-I16	Hypertensive diseases
I20-I25	Ischemic heart diseases
I26-I28	Pulmonary heart disease and diseases of pulmonary circulation
I30-I52	Other forms of heart disease
I60-I69	Cerebrovascular diseases
I70-I79	Diseases of arteries, arterioles and capillaries
I80-I89	Diseases of veins, lymphatic vessels and lymph nodes, not elsewhere classified
I95-I99	Other and unspecified disorders of the circulatory system

ACUTE RHEUMATIC FEVER (I00-I02)

I00   **Rheumatic fever without heart involvement**

     Includes   arthritis, rheumatic, acute or subacute
     Excludes1   rheumatic fever with heart involvement (I01.0-I01.9)

● **I01**   **Rheumatic fever with heart involvement**

     Excludes1   chronic diseases of rheumatic origin (I05-I09) unless rheumatic fever is also present or there is evidence of reactivation or activity of the rheumatic process.

   I01.0   **Acute rheumatic pericarditis** 🔹
       Any condition in I00 with pericarditis
       Rheumatic pericarditis (acute)

       Excludes1   acute pericarditis not specified as rheumatic (I30.-)

       (Ex) See PDX Collection 188

   I01.1   **Acute rheumatic endocarditis** 🔹
       Any condition in I00 with endocarditis or valvulitis
       Acute rheumatic valvulitis
       (Ex) See PDX Collection 644

▶ New   ⇒ Revised   ~~deleted~~ Deleted   Excludes 1   Excludes 2   Includes   Use additional   Code first   Code also   Key words

OGCR Official Guidelines   ● Unacceptable Principal Diagnosis   X Assign placeholder X   ● Use Additional Character(s)   ▌ Manifestation Code   **Coding Clinic**

Item 9–2 Rheumatic chorea, also called Sydenham's, juvenile, minor, simple, or St. Vitus' dance, is a major symptom of rheumatic fever and is characterized by ceaseless, involuntary, jerky, purposeless movements.

I01.2   **Acute rheumatic myocarditis** 🔾
      Any condition in I00 with myocarditis
      Ⓔⓧ See PDX Collection 186

I01.8   **Other acute rheumatic heart disease** 🔾
      Any condition in I00 with other or multiple types of heart involvement
      Acute rheumatic pancarditis
      Ⓔⓧ See PDX Collection 645

I01.9   **Acute rheumatic heart disease, unspecified** 🔾
      Any condition in I00 with unspecified type of heart involvement
      Rheumatic carditis, acute
      Rheumatic heart disease, active or acute
      Ⓔⓧ See PDX Collection 646

● **I02**   **Rheumatic chorea**
    Includes   Sydenham's chorea
    Excludes1   chorea NOS (G25.5)
                 Huntington's chorea (G10)

I02.0   **Rheumatic chorea with heart involvement** 🔾
      Chorea NOS with heart involvement
      Rheumatic chorea with heart involvement of any type classifiable under I01.-
      Ⓔⓧ See PDX Collection 645

I02.9   **Rheumatic chorea without heart involvement** 🔾
      Rheumatic chorea NOS
      Ⓔⓧ See PDX Collection 646

CHRONIC RHEUMATIC HEART DISEASES (I05-I09)

● **I05**   **Rheumatic mitral valve diseases**
    Includes   conditions classifiable to both I05.0 and I05.2-I05.9, whether specified as rheumatic or not
    Excludes1   mitral valve disease specified as nonrheumatic (I34.-)
                 mitral valve disease with aortic and/or tricuspid valve involvement (I08.-)

I05.0   **Rheumatic mitral stenosis**
      Mitral (valve) obstruction (rheumatic)

I05.1   **Rheumatic mitral insufficiency**
      Rheumatic mitral incompetence
      Rheumatic mitral regurgitation
      Excludes1   mitral insufficiency not specified as rheumatic (I34.0)

I05.2   **Rheumatic mitral stenosis with insufficiency**
      Rheumatic mitral stenosis with incompetence or regurgitation

I05.8   **Other rheumatic mitral valve diseases**
      Rheumatic mitral (valve) failure

I05.9   **Rheumatic mitral valve disease, unspecified**
      Rheumatic mitral (valve) disorder (chronic) NOS

● **I06**   **Rheumatic aortic valve diseases**
    Excludes1   aortic valve disease not specified as rheumatic (I35.-)
                 aortic valve disease with mitral and/or tricuspid valve involvement (I08.-)

I06.0   **Rheumatic aortic stenosis**
      Rheumatic aortic (valve) obstruction

I06.1   **Rheumatic aortic insufficiency**
      Rheumatic aortic incompetence
      Rheumatic aortic regurgitation

★ **(See Plate 244 on page 78.)**

Item 9–3 Mitral stenosis is the narrowing of the mitral valve separating the left atrium from the left ventricle. **Mitral insufficiency** is the improper closure of the mitral valve which may lead to enlargement (hypertrophy) of the left atrium.

Item 9–4 Aortic stenosis is the narrowing of the aortic valve located between the left ventricle and the aorta. **Aortic insufficiency** is the improper closure of the aortic valve which may lead to enlargement (hypertrophy) of the left ventricle.

I06.2   **Rheumatic aortic stenosis with insufficiency**
      Rheumatic aortic stenosis with incompetence or regurgitation

I06.8   **Other rheumatic aortic valve diseases**

I06.9   **Rheumatic aortic valve disease, unspecified**
      Rheumatic aortic (valve) disease NOS

● **I07**   **Rheumatic tricuspid valve diseases**
    Includes   rheumatic tricuspid valve diseases specified as rheumatic or unspecified
    Excludes1   tricuspid valve disease specified as nonrheumatic (I36.-)
                 tricuspid valve disease with aortic and/or mitral valve involvement (I08.-)

I07.0   **Rheumatic tricuspid stenosis**
      Tricuspid (valve) stenosis (rheumatic)

I07.1   **Rheumatic tricuspid insufficiency**
      Tricuspid (valve) insufficiency (rheumatic)

I07.2   **Rheumatic tricuspid stenosis and insufficiency**

I07.8   **Other rheumatic tricuspid valve diseases**

I07.9   **Rheumatic tricuspid valve disease, unspecified**
      Rheumatic tricuspid valve disorder NOS

● **I08**   **Multiple valve diseases**
    Includes   multiple valve diseases specified as rheumatic or unspecified
    Excludes1   endocarditis, valve unspecified (I38)
                 multiple valve disease specified a nonrheumatic (I34.-, I35.-, I36.-, I37.-, I38.-, Q22.-, Q23.-, Q24.8-)
                 rheumatic valve disease NOS (I09.1)

I08.0   **Rheumatic disorders of both mitral and aortic valves**
      Involvement of both mitral and aortic valves specified as rheumatic or unspecified

I08.1   **Rheumatic disorders of both mitral and tricuspid valves**

I08.2   **Rheumatic disorders of both aortic and tricuspid valves**

I08.3   **Combined rheumatic disorders of mitral, aortic and tricuspid valves**

I08.8   **Other rheumatic multiple valve diseases**

I08.9   **Rheumatic multiple valve disease, unspecified**

● **I09**   **Other rheumatic heart diseases**
I09.0   **Rheumatic myocarditis** 🔾
      Excludes1   myocarditis not specified as rheumatic (I51.4)
      Ⓔⓧ See PDX Collection 647

I09.1   **Rheumatic diseases of endocardium, valve unspecified**
      Rheumatic endocarditis (chronic)
      Rheumatic valvulitis (chronic)
      Excludes1   endocarditis, valve unspecified (I38)

I09.2   **Chronic rheumatic pericarditis** 🔾
      Adherent pericardium, rheumatic
      Chronic rheumatic mediastinopericarditis
      Chronic rheumatic myopericarditis
      Excludes1   chronic pericarditis not specified as rheumatic (I31.-)
      Ⓔⓧ See PDX Collection 188

● **I09.8**   **Other specified rheumatic heart diseases**
    I09.81   **Rheumatic heart failure** 🔾
        Use additional code to identify type of heart failure (I50.-)
        Ⓔⓧ See PDX Collection 648

    I09.89   **Other specified rheumatic heart diseases**
        Rheumatic disease of pulmonary valve

I09.9   **Rheumatic heart disease, unspecified**
      Rheumatic carditis
      Excludes1   rheumatoid carditis (M05.31)

N Newborn Age: 0   P Pediatric Age: 0–17   M Maternity DX: 12–55   A Adult Age: 15–124   ♀ Females Only   ♂ Males Only

🔾 Complication\Comorbidity   🔾 Major C\C   Ⓔⓧ CC/MCC Exclusions   🔾 Hospital-Acquired Condition

CHAPTER 9 (I00-I99)

Item 9–5 Hypertension is caused by high arterial blood pressure in the arteries. **Essential, primary,** or **idiopathic** hypertension occurs without identifiable organic cause. **Secondary** hypertension is that which has an organic cause. **Malignant** hypertension is severely elevated blood pressure. **Benign** hypertension is mildly elevated blood pressure.

HYPERTENSIVE DISEASES (I10-I16)

Use additional code to identify:
exposure to environmental tobacco smoke (Z77.22)
history of tobacco dependence (Z87.891)
occupational exposure to environmental tobacco smoke (Z57.31)
tobacco dependence (F17.-)
tobacco use (Z72.0)

Excludes1   neonatal hypertension (P29.2)
primary pulmonary hypertension (I27.0)

Excludes2   hypertensive disease complicating pregnancy, childbirth and the puerperium (O10-O11, O13-O16)

I10   **Essential (primary) hypertension**
     Includes   high blood pressure
hypertension (arterial) (benign) (essential) (malignant) (primary) (systemic)

     Excludes1   hypertensive disease complicating pregnancy, childbirth and the puerperium (O10-O11, O13-O16)

     Excludes2   essential (primary) hypertension involving vessels of brain (I60-I69)
essential (primary) hypertension involving vessels of eye (H35.0-)

     MCE: Questionable admission when principal dx

● **I11**   **Hypertensive heart disease**
➡   **Includes**   any condition in I50.-, I51.4-I51.9 due to hypertension

   I11.0   **Hypertensive heart disease with heart failure**
Hypertensive heart failure
Use additional code to identify type of heart failure (I50.-)
Coding Clinic: 2017, Q1, P47

   I11.9   **Hypertensive heart disease without heart failure**
Hypertensive heart disease NOS

OGCR   Section I.C.9.a.2.

Hypertensive Chronic Kidney Disease

Assign codes from category I12, Hypertensive chronic kidney disease, when both hypertension and a condition classifiable to category N18, Chronic kidney disease (CKD), are present. **CKD should not be coded as hypertensive if the physician has specifically documented a different cause.**

The appropriate code from category N18 should be used as a secondary code with a code from category I12 to identify the stage of chronic kidney disease.
See Section I.C.14. Chronic kidney disease.

If a patient has hypertensive chronic kidney disease and acute renal failure, an additional code for the acute renal failure is required.

● **I12**   **Hypertensive chronic kidney disease**
     Includes   any condition in N18 and N26 - due to hypertension
arteriosclerosis of kidney
arteriosclerotic nephritis (chronic) (interstitial)
hypertensive nephropathy
nephrosclerosis

     Excludes1   hypertension due to kidney disease (I15.0, I15.1)
renovascular hypertension (I15.0)
secondary hypertension (I15.-)

     Excludes2   acute kidney failure (N17.-)
Coding Clinic: 2016, Q4, P123

   I12.0   **Hypertensive chronic kidney disease with stage 5 chronic kidney disease or end stage renal disease** 🔒
Use additional code to identify the stage of chronic kidney disease (N18.5, N18.6)
(Ex) See PDX Collection 649
Coding Clinic: 2016, Q3, P23

   I12.9   **Hypertensive chronic kidney disease with stage 1 through stage 4 chronic kidney disease, or unspecified chronic kidney disease**
Hypertensive chronic kidney disease NOS
Hypertensive renal disease NOS
Use additional code to identify the stage of chronic kidney disease (N18.1-N18.4, N18.9)

OGCR   Section I.c.9.a.3.

Hypertensive Heart and Chronic Kidney Disease

Assign codes from combination category I13, Hypertensive heart and chronic kidney disease, when **there is hypertension with both heart and kidney involvement.** If heart failure is present, assign an additional code from category I50 to identify the type of heart failure.

The appropriate code from category N18, Chronic kidney disease, should be used as a secondary code with a code from category I13 to identify the stage of chronic kidney disease.
See Section I.C.14. Chronic kidney disease.

The codes in category I13, Hypertensive heart and chronic kidney disease, are combination codes that include hypertension, heart disease and chronic kidney disease. The Includes note at I13 specifies that the conditions included at I11 and I12 are included together in I13. If a patient has hypertension, heart disease and chronic kidney disease then a code from I13 should be used, not individual codes for hypertension, heart disease and chronic kidney disease, or codes from I11 or I12.

For patients with both acute renal failure and chronic kidney disease an additional code for acute renal failure is required.

● **I13**   **Hypertensive heart and chronic kidney disease**
     Includes   any condition in I11.- with any condition in I12.-
cardiorenal disease
cardiovascular renal disease
(Ex) For category I13 CC codes: See PDX Collection 650
Coding Clinic: 2016, Q4, P123

   I13.0   **Hypertensive heart and chronic kidney disease with heart failure and stage 1 through stage 4 chronic kidney disease, or unspecified chronic kidney disease** 🔒
Use additional code to identify type of heart failure (I50.-)
Use additional code to identify stage of chronic kidney disease (N18.1-N18.4, N18.9)

● **I13.1**   **Hypertensive heart and chronic kidney disease without heart failure**
     I13.10   **Hypertensive heart and chronic kidney disease without heart failure, with stage 1 through stage 4 chronic kidney disease, or unspecified chronic kidney disease**
Hypertensive heart disease and hypertensive chronic kidney disease NOS
Use additional code to identify the stage of chronic kidney disease (N18.1-N18.4, N18.9)

     I13.11   **Hypertensive heart and chronic kidney disease without heart failure, with stage 5 chronic kidney disease, or end stage renal disease** 🔒
Use additional code to identify the stage of chronic kidney disease (N18.5, N18.6)

   I13.2   **Hypertensive heart and chronic kidney disease with heart failure and with stage 5 chronic kidney disease, or end stage renal disease** 🔒
Use additional code to identify type of heart failure (I50.-)
Use additional code to identify the stage of chronic kidney disease (N18.5, N18.6)

▶ New   ⟹ Revised   ~~deleted~~ Deleted   Excludes 1   Excludes 2   Includes   Use additional   Code first   Code also   Key words
OGCR Official Guidelines   ● Unacceptable Principal Diagnosis   X Assign placeholder X   ● Use Additional Character(s)   ▷ Manifestation Code   **Coding Clinic**

● **I15   Secondary hypertension**
    Code also underlying condition
    Excludes1   postprocedural hypertension (I97.3)
    Excludes2   secondary hypertension involving vessels of
                        brain (I60-I69)
                    secondary hypertension involving vessels of eye
                        (H35.0-)
    I15.0   Renovascular hypertension
    I15.1   Hypertension secondary to other renal disorders
                Coding Clinic: 2016, Q3, P23
    I15.2   Hypertension secondary to endocrine disorders
    I15.8   Other secondary hypertension
    I15.9   Secondary hypertension, unspecified

● **I16   Hypertensive crisis**
    Code also any identified hypertensive disease (I10-I15)
    Coding Clinic: 2016, Q4, P26-27, 123
    I16.0   Hypertensive urgency 🗟
                (Ex) No exclusions
    I16.1   Hypertensive emergency
    I16.9   Hypertensive crisis, unspecified 🗟
                (Ex) No exclusions

ISCHEMIC HEART DISEASES (I20-I25)

Use additional code to identify presence of hypertension
(I10-I16)

● **I20   Angina pectoris**
    Chest pain/discomfort due to lack of oxygen to the heart muscle.
    Principal symptom of myocardial infarction.
    Use additional code to identify:
        exposure to environmental tobacco smoke (Z77.22)
        history of tobacco dependence (Z87.891)
        occupational exposure to environmental tobacco smoke
            (Z57.31)
        tobacco dependence (F17.-)
        tobacco use (Z72.0)
    Excludes1   angina pectoris with atherosclerotic heart disease
                        of native coronary arteries (I25.1-)
                    atherosclerosis of coronary artery bypass graft(s)
                        and coronary artery of transplanted heart
                        with angina pectoris (I25.7-)
                    postinfarction angina (I23.7)
    I20.0   Unstable angina 🗟
                Accelerated angina
                Crescendo angina
                De novo effort angina
                Intermediate coronary syndrome
                Preinfarction syndrome
                Worsening effort angina
                (Ex) See PDX Collection 651
    I20.1   Angina pectoris with documented spasm 🗟
                Angiospastic angina
                Prinzmetal angina
                Spasm-induced angina
                Variant angina
                (Ex) See PDX Collection 652

I20.8   Other forms of angina pectoris
            Angina equivalent
            Angina of effort
            Coronary slow flow syndrome
            Stable angina
            Stenocardia
            Use additional code(s) for symptoms associated with
                angina equivalent
I20.9   Angina pectoris, unspecified
            Angina NOS
            Anginal syndrome
            Cardiac angina
            Ischemic chest pain

➡ **I21   Acute myocardial infarction**
    Includes   cardiac infarction
                    coronary (artery) embolism
                    coronary (artery) occlusion
                    coronary (artery) rupture
                    coronary (artery) thrombosis
                    infarction of heart, myocardium, or ventricle
                    myocardial infarction specified as acute or with a
                        stated duration of 4 weeks (28 days) or less
                        from onset
    Use additional code, if applicable, to identify:
        exposure to environmental tobacco smoke (Z77.22)
        history of tobacco dependence (Z87.891)
        occupational exposure to environmental tobacco smoke
            (Z57.31)
        status post administration of tPA (rtPA) in a different facility
            within the last 24 hours prior to admission to current
            facility (Z92.82)
        tobacco dependence (F17.-)
        tobacco use (Z72.0)
    Excludes2   old myocardial infarction (I25.2)
                    postmyocardial infarction syndrome (I24.1)
                ➡subsequent type 1 myocardial infarction (I22.-)
    (Ex) For category I21 CC codes: See PDX Collection 653
    Coding Clinic: 2016, Q4, P140; 2013, Q1, P25-26; 2012, Q4, P103
    ● **I21.0   ST elevation (STEMI) myocardial infarction of anterior**
                wall
                ▶Type 1 ST elevation myocardial infarction of anterior
                    wall
                    Coding Clinic: 2013, Q1, P26
                I21.01   ST elevation (STEMI) myocardial infarction
                            involving left main coronary artery 🗟
                I21.02   ST elevation (STEMI) myocardial infarction
                            involving left anterior descending coronary
                            artery 🗟
                            ST elevation (STEMI) myocardial infarction
                                involving diagonal coronary artery
                            Coding Clinic: 2013, Q1, P26
                I21.09   ST elevation (STEMI) myocardial infarction
                            involving other coronary artery of anterior
                            wall 🗟
                            Acute transmural myocardial infarction of
                                anterior wall
                            Anteroapical transmural (Q wave) infarction
                                (acute)
                            Anterolateral transmural (Q wave) infarction
                                (acute)
                            Anteroseptal transmural (Q wave) infarction
                                (acute)
                            Transmural (Q wave) infarction (acute) (of)
                                anterior (wall) NOS
                            Coding Clinic: 2012, Q4, P102, 104

N Newborn Age: 0   **P** Pediatric Age: 0–17   **M** Maternity DX: 12–55   **A** Adult Age: 15–124   ♀ Females Only   ♂ Males Only

🗟 Complication\Comorbidity   🗟 Major C\C   (Ex) CC/MCC Exclusions   🗟 Hospital-Acquired Condition

871

● **I21.1** **ST elevation (STEMI) myocardial infarction of inferior wall**
▶Type 1 ST elevation myocardial infarction of inferior wall
Coding Clinic: 2013, Q1, P26

I21.11 **ST elevation (STEMI) myocardial infarction involving right coronary artery** 🔖
Inferoposterior transmural (Q wave) infarction (acute)

I21.19 **ST elevation (STEMI) myocardial infarction involving other coronary artery of inferior wall** 🔖
Acute transmural myocardial infarction of inferior wall
Inferolateral transmural (Q wave) infarction (acute)
Transmural (Q wave) infarction (acute) (of) diaphragmatic wall
Transmural (Q wave) infarction (acute) (of) inferior (wall) NOS

Excludes2   ST elevation (STEMI) myocardial infarction involving left circumflex coronary artery (I21.21)

Coding Clinic: 2012, Q4, P97

● **I21.2** **ST elevation (STEMI) myocardial infarction of other sites**
▶Type 1 ST elevation myocardial infarction of other sites
Coding Clinic: 2013, Q1, P26

I21.21 **ST elevation (STEMI) myocardial infarction involving left circumflex coronary artery** 🔖
ST elevation (STEMI) myocardial infarction involving oblique marginal coronary artery

I21.29 **ST elevation (STEMI) myocardial infarction involving other sites** 🔖
Acute transmural myocardial infarction of other sites
Apical-lateral transmural (Q wave) infarction (acute)
Basal-lateral transmural (Q wave) infarction (acute)
High lateral transmural (Q wave) infarction (acute)
Lateral (wall) NOS transmural (Q wave) infarction (acute)
Posterior (true) transmural (Q wave) infarction (acute)
Posterobasal transmural (Q wave) infarction (acute)
Posterolateral transmural (Q wave) infarction (acute)
Posteroseptal transmural (Q wave) infarction (acute)
Septal transmural (Q wave) infarction (acute) NOS

OGCR Section I.c.9.e.2.

Acute myocardial infarction, unspecified

Code **I21.9, Acute myocardial infarction, unspecified,** is the default for unspecified acute myocardial infarction **or unspecified type.** If only type 1 STEMI or transmural MI without the site is documented, assign I21.3, **ST elevation (STEMI) myocardial infarction of unspecified site.**

I21.3 **ST elevation (STEMI) myocardial infarction of unspecified site** 🔖
Acute transmural myocardial infarction of unspecified site
~~Myocardial infarction (acute) NOS~~
Transmural (Q wave) myocardial infarction NOS
▶Type 1 ST elevation myocardial infarction of unspecified site
Coding Clinic: 2013, Q1, P26

I21.4 **Non-ST elevation (NSTEMI) myocardial infarction** 🔖
Acute subendocardial myocardial infarction
Non-Q wave myocardial infarction NOS
Nontransmural myocardial infarction NOS
▶Type 1 non-ST elevation myocardial infarction
Coding Clinic: 2017, Q1, P44; 2015, Q2, P16; 2013, Q1, P26

▶ **I21.9** **Acute myocardial infarction, unspecified** 🔖
▶Myocardial infarction (acute) NOS

▶● **I21.A** **Other type of myocardial infarction**

▶ **I21.A1** **Myocardial infarction type 2** 🔖
▶Myocardial infarction due to demand ischemia
▶Myocardial infarction secondary to ischemic imbalance
▶ Code also the underlying cause, if known and applicable, such as:
▶anemia (D50.0-D64.9)
▶chronic obstructive pulmonary disease (J44.-)
▶heart failure (I50.-)
▶paroxysmal tachycardia (I47.0-I47.9)
▶renal failure (N17.0-N19)
▶shock (R57.0-R57.9)

▶ **I21.A9** **Other myocardial infarction type** 🔖
▶Myocardial infarction associated with revascularization procedure
▶Myocardial infarction type 3
▶Myocardial infarction type 4a
▶Myocardial infarction type 4b
▶Myocardial infarction type 4c
▶Myocardial infarction type 5
▶ *Code first, if applicable, postprocedural myocardial infarction following cardiac surgery (I97.190), or postprocedural myocardial infarction during cardiac surgery (I97.790)*
▶ Code also complication, if known and applicable, such as:
▶(acute) stent occlusion (T82.897-)
▶(acute) stent stenosis (T82.857-)
▶(acute) stent thrombosis (T82.867-)
▶cardiac arrest due to underlying cardiac condition (I46.2)
▶complication of percutaneous coronary intervention (PCI) (I97.89)
▶occlusion of coronary artery bypass graft (T82.218-)

● **I22** **Subsequent ST elevation (STEMI) and non-ST elevation (NSTEMI) myocardial infarction**

Includes   acute myocardial infarction occurring within four weeks (28 days) of a previous acute myocardial infarction, regardless of site
cardiac infarction
coronary (artery) embolism
coronary (artery) occlusion
coronary (artery) rupture
coronary (artery) thrombosis
infarction of heart, myocardium, or ventricle
recurrent myocardial infarction
reinfarction of myocardium
rupture of heart, myocardium, or ventricle
▶subsequent type 1 myocardial infarction

▶ **Excludes1**   subsequent myocardial infarction, type 2 (I21.A1)
▶subsequent myocardial infarction of other type (type 3) (type 4) (type 5) (I21.A9)

Use additional code, if applicable, to identify:
exposure to environmental tobacco smoke (Z77.22)
history of tobacco dependence (Z87.891)
occupational exposure to environmental tobacco smoke (Z57.31)
status post administration of tPA (rtPA) in a different facility within the last 24 hours prior to admission to current facility (Z92.82)
tobacco dependence (F17.-)
tobacco use (Z72.0)
Ⓔⓧ **For category I22 CC codes:** See PDX Collection 653
Coding Clinic: 2013, Q1, P25; 2012, Q4, P103

▶ New   ⇒ Revised   ~~deleted~~ Deleted   Excludes 1   Excludes 2   Includes   Use additional   Code first   Code also   Key words
OGCR Official Guidelines   ● Unacceptable Principal Diagnosis   X Assign placeholder X   ● Use Additional Character(s)   ▶ Manifestation Code   **Coding Clinic**

I22.0   **Subsequent ST elevation (STEMI) myocardial infarction of anterior wall** 🔖

     Subsequent acute transmural myocardial infarction of anterior wall

     Subsequent transmural (Q wave) infarction (acute)(of) anterior (wall) NOS

     Subsequent anteroapical transmural (Q wave) infarction (acute)

     Subsequent anterolateral transmural (Q wave) infarction (acute)

     Subsequent anteroseptal transmural (Q wave) infarction (acute)

I22.1   **Subsequent ST elevation (STEMI) myocardial infarction of inferior wall** 🔖

     Subsequent acute transmural myocardial infarction of inferior wall

     Subsequent transmural (Q wave) infarction (acute)(of) diaphragmatic wall

     Subsequent transmural (Q wave) infarction (acute)(of) inferior (wall) NOS

     Subsequent inferolateral transmural (Q wave) infarction (acute)

     Subsequent inferoposterior transmural (Q wave) infarction (acute)

     Coding Clinic: 2012, Q4, P97, 102, 104

I22.2   **Subsequent non-ST elevation (NSTEMI) myocardial infarction** 🔖

     Subsequent acute subendocardial myocardial infarction

     Subsequent non-Q wave myocardial infarction NOS

     Subsequent nontransmural myocardial infarction NOS

I22.8   **Subsequent ST elevation (STEMI) myocardial infarction of other sites** 🔖

     Subsequent acute transmural myocardial infarction of other sites

     Subsequent apical-lateral transmural (Q wave) myocardial infarction (acute)

     Subsequent basal-lateral transmural (Q wave) myocardial infarction (acute)

     Subsequent high lateral transmural (Q wave) myocardial infarction (acute)

     Subsequent transmural (Q wave) myocardial infarction (acute)(of) lateral (wall) NOS

     Subsequent posterior (true) transmural (Q wave) myocardial infarction (acute)

     Subsequent posterobasal transmural (Q wave) myocardial infarction (acute)

     Subsequent posterolateral transmural (Q wave) myocardial infarction (acute)

     Subsequent posteroseptal transmural (Q wave) myocardial infarction (acute)

     Subsequent septal NOS transmural (Q wave) myocardial infarction (acute)

I22.9   **Subsequent ST elevation (STEMI) myocardial infarction of unspecified site** 🔖

     Subsequent acute myocardial infarction of unspecified site

     Subsequent myocardial infarction (acute) NOS

● **I23**   **Certain current complications following ST elevation (STEMI) and non-ST elevation (NSTEMI) myocardial infarction (within the 28 day period)**

     (Ex:) **For category I23 CC codes unless otherwise indicated:** See PDX Collection 654

     Coding Clinic: 2017, Q2, P11

I23.0   **Hemopericardium as current complication following acute myocardial infarction** 🔖   A

     Excludes1   hemopericardium not specified as current complication following acute myocardial infarction (I31.2)

I23.1   **Atrial septal defect as current complication following acute myocardial infarction** 🔖   A

     Excludes1   acquired atrial septal defect not specified as current complication following acute myocardial infarction (I51.0)

I23.2   **Ventricular septal defect as current complication following acute myocardial infarction** 🔖   A

     Excludes1   acquired ventricular septal defect not specified as current complication following acute myocardial infarction (I51.0)

I23.3   **Rupture of cardiac wall without hemopericardium as current complication following acute myocardial infarction** 🔖   A

     Coding Clinic: 2017, Q2, P11

I23.4   **Rupture of chordae tendineae as current complication following acute myocardial infarction** 🔖

     Excludes1   rupture of chordae tendineae not specified as current complication following acute myocardial infarction (I51.1)

     (Ex:) See PDX Collection 655

I23.5   **Rupture of papillary muscle as current complication following acute myocardial infarction** 🔖

     Excludes1   rupture of papillary muscle not specified as current complication following acute myocardial infarction (I51.2)

     (Ex:) See PDX Collection 656

I23.6   **Thrombosis of atrium, auricular appendage, and ventricle as current complications following acute myocardial infarction** 🔖   A

     Excludes1   thrombosis of atrium, auricular appendage, and ventricle not specified as current complication following acute myocardial infarction (I51.3)

I23.7   **Postinfarction angina** 🔖   A

     Coding Clinic: 2015, Q2, P16-17

I23.8   **Other current complications following acute myocardial infarction** 🔖   A

● **I24**   **Other acute ischemic heart diseases**

     Excludes1   angina pectoris (I20.-)

                 transient myocardial ischemia in newborn (P29.4)

     (Ex:) **For category I24 CC codes unless otherwise indicated:** See PDX Collection 657

I24.0   **Acute coronary thrombosis not resulting in myocardial infarction** 🔖

     Acute coronary (artery) (vein) embolism not resulting in myocardial infarction

     Acute coronary (artery) (vein) occlusion not resulting in myocardial infarction

     Acute coronary (artery) (vein) thromboembolism not resulting in myocardial infarction

     Excludes1   atherosclerotic heart disease (I25.1-)

     Coding Clinic: 2013, Q1, P24

I24.1   **Dressler's syndrome** 🔖

     Postmyocardial infarction syndrome

     Excludes1   postinfarction angina (I23.7)

     (Ex:) See PDX Collection 658

I24.8   **Other forms of acute ischemic heart disease** 🔖

     ▶ **Excludes1**   myocardial infarction due to demand ischemia (I21.A1)

I24.9   **Acute ischemic heart disease, unspecified** 🔖

     Excludes1   ischemic heart disease (chronic) NOS (I25.9)

● **I25**   **Chronic ischemic heart disease**

     Use additional code to identify:

     chronic total occlusion of coronary artery (I25.82)

     exposure to environmental tobacco smoke (Z77.22)

     history of tobacco dependence (Z87.891)

     occupational exposure to environmental tobacco smoke (Z57.31)

     tobacco dependence (F17.-)

     tobacco use (Z72.0)

N Newborn Age: 0   **P** Pediatric Age: 0–17   **M** Maternity DX: 12–55   **A** Adult Age: 15–124   ♀ Females Only   ♂ Males Only

🔖 Complication\Comorbidity   🔖 Major C\C   (Ex:) CC/MCC Exclusions   🔖 Hospital-Acquired Condition

873

Item 9–6 Classification is based on the location of the atherosclerosis. **"Of native coronary artery"** indicates the atherosclerosis is within an original heart artery. **"Of autologous vein bypass graft"** indicates that the atherosclerosis is within a vein graft that was taken from within the patient. **"Of nonautologous biological bypass graft"** indicates the atherosclerosis is within a vessel grafted from other than the patient. **"Of artery bypass graft"** indicates the atherosclerosis is within an artery that was grafted from within the patient.

★ **(See Plates 218 and 219 on pages 74 and 75.)**

● **I25.1 Atherosclerotic heart disease of native coronary artery**
Disease in which fatty deposits form on the walls of arteries
Atherosclerotic cardiovascular disease
Coronary (artery) atheroma
Coronary (artery) atherosclerosis
Coronary (artery) disease
Coronary (artery) sclerosis

Use additional code, if applicable, to identify:
coronary atherosclerosis due to calcified coronary lesion (I25.84)
coronary atherosclerosis due to lipid rich plaque (I25.83)

Excludes2 atheroembolism (I75.-)
atherosclerosis of coronary artery bypass graft(s) and transplanted heart (I25.7-)

I25.10 Atherosclerotic heart disease of native coronary artery without angina pectoris   A
Atherosclerotic heart disease NOS
Coding Clinic: 2015, Q2, P17; 2012, Q4, P92

OGCR See Section I.9.b.

Atherosclerotic Coronary Artery Disease and Angina

ICD-10-CM has combination codes for atherosclerotic heart disease with angina pectoris. The subcategories for these codes are I25.11, Atherosclerotic heart disease of native coronary artery with angina pectoris and I25.7, Atherosclerosis of coronary artery bypass graft(s) and coronary artery of transplanted heart with angina pectoris.

When using one of these combination codes it is not necessary to use an additional code for angina pectoris. A causal relationship can be assumed in a patient with both atherosclerosis and angina pectoris, unless the documentation indicates the angina is due to something other than the atherosclerosis.

If a patient with coronary artery disease is admitted due to an acute myocardial infarction (AMI), the AMI should be sequenced before the coronary artery disease.

See Section I.C.9. Acute myocardial infarction (AMI)

● **I25.11 Atherosclerotic heart disease of native coronary artery with angina pectoris**

I25.110 Atherosclerotic heart disease of native coronary artery with unstable angina pectoris 🔖   A
Excludes1 unstable angina without atherosclerotic heart disease (I20.0)
CC when PDx is its own CC
(Ex) See PDX Collection 651

Figure 9-2 Atherosclerotic plaque.

Atherosclerotic plaque (atheromas)

I25.111 Atherosclerotic heart disease of native coronary artery with angina pectoris with documented spasm   A
Excludes1 angina pectoris with documented spasm without atherosclerotic heart disease (I20.1)

I25.118 Atherosclerotic heart disease of native coronary artery with other forms of angina pectoris   A
Excludes1 other forms of angina pectoris without atherosclerotic heart disease (I20.8)
Coding Clinic: 2015, Q2, P16-17

I25.119 Atherosclerotic heart disease of native coronary artery with unspecified angina pectoris   A
Atherosclerotic heart disease with angina NOS
Atherosclerotic heart disease with ischemic chest pain
Excludes1 unspecified angina pectoris without atherosclerotic heart disease (I20.9)

I25.2 Old myocardial infarction
Healed myocardial infarction
Past myocardial infarction diagnosed by ECG or other investigation, but currently presenting no symptoms

I25.3 Aneurysm of heart 🔖
Mural aneurysm
Ventricular aneurysm
(Ex) See PDX Collection 659

● **I25.4 Coronary artery aneurysm and dissection**
I25.41 Coronary artery aneurysm
Coronary arteriovenous fistula, acquired
Excludes1 congenital coronary (artery) aneurysm (Q24.5)
I25.42 Coronary artery dissection 🔖
(Ex) See PDX Collection 660

I25.5 Ischemic cardiomyopathy
Excludes2 coronary atherosclerosis (I25.1-, I25.7-)

I25.6 Silent myocardial ischemia

● **I25.7 Atherosclerosis of coronary artery bypass graft(s) and coronary artery of transplanted heart with angina pectoris**
Use additional code, if applicable, to identify:
coronary atherosclerosis due to calcified coronary lesion (I25.84)
coronary atherosclerosis due to lipid rich plaque (I25.83)
Excludes1 atherosclerosis of bypass graft(s) of transplanted heart without angina pectoris (I25.812)
atherosclerosis of coronary artery bypass graft(s) without angina pectoris (I25.810)
atherosclerosis of native coronary artery of transplanted heart without angina pectoris (I25.811)
~~embolism or thrombus of coronary artery bypass graft(s) (T82.8-)~~

▶ New   ⇒ Revised   ~~deleted~~ Deleted   Excludes 1   Excludes 2   Includes   Use additional   Code first   Code also   Key words
OGCR Official Guidelines   ● Unacceptable Principal Diagnosis   X Assign placeholder X   ● Use Additional Character(s)   ▶ Manifestation Code   **Coding Clinic**

● **I25.70** **Atherosclerosis of coronary artery bypass graft(s), unspecified, with angina pectoris**

    I25.700 **Atherosclerosis of coronary artery bypass graft(s), unspecified, with unstable angina pectoris**   A

       Excludes1   unstable angina pectoris without atherosclerosis of coronary artery bypass graft (I20.0)

       CC when PDx is its own CC
       (Ex:) See PDX Collection 651

    I25.701 **Atherosclerosis of coronary artery bypass graft(s), unspecified, with angina pectoris with documented spasm**   A

       Excludes1   angina pectoris with documented spasm without atherosclerosis of coronary artery bypass graft (I20.1)

    I25.708 **Atherosclerosis of coronary artery bypass graft(s), unspecified, with other forms of angina pectoris**   A

       Excludes1   other forms of angina pectoris without atherosclerosis of coronary artery bypass graft (I20.8)

    I25.709 **Atherosclerosis of coronary artery bypass graft(s), unspecified, with unspecified angina pectoris**   A

       Excludes1   unspecified angina pectoris without atherosclerosis of coronary artery bypass graft (I20.9)

● **I25.71** **Atherosclerosis of autologous vein coronary artery bypass graft(s) with angina pectoris**

    (Ex:) **For category I25.71 CC codes unless otherwise indicated:** See PDX Collection 662

    I25.710 **Atherosclerosis of autologous vein coronary artery bypass graft(s) with unstable angina pectoris**   A

       Excludes1   unstable angina without atherosclerosis of autologous vein coronary artery bypass graft(s) (I20.0)

       ▶ **Excludes2**   embolism or thrombus of coronary artery bypass graft(s) (T82.8-)

       CC when PDx is its own CC
       (Ex:) See PDX Collection 661

    I25.711 **Atherosclerosis of autologous vein coronary artery bypass graft(s) with angina pectoris with documented spasm**   A

       Excludes1   angina pectoris with documented spasm without atherosclerosis of autologous vein coronary artery bypass graft(s) (I20.1)

    I25.718 **Atherosclerosis of autologous vein coronary artery bypass graft(s) with other forms of angina pectoris**   A

       Excludes1   other forms of angina pectoris without atherosclerosis of autologous vein coronary artery bypass graft(s) (I20.8)

    I25.719 **Atherosclerosis of autologous vein coronary artery bypass graft(s) with unspecified angina pectoris**   A

       Excludes1   unspecified angina pectoris without atherosclerosis of autologous vein coronary artery bypass graft(s) (I20.9)

● **I25.72** **Atherosclerosis of autologous artery coronary artery bypass graft(s) with angina pectoris**

    Atherosclerosis of internal mammary artery graft with angina pectoris

    (Ex:) **For category I25.72 CC codes unless otherwise indicated:** See PDX Collection 662

    I25.720 **Atherosclerosis of autologous artery coronary artery bypass graft(s) with unstable angina pectoris**   A

       Excludes1   unstable angina without atherosclerosis of autologous artery coronary artery bypass graft(s) (I20.0)

       CC when PDx is its own CC
       (Ex:) See PDX Collection 661

    I25.721 **Atherosclerosis of autologous artery coronary artery bypass graft(s) with angina pectoris with documented spasm**   A

       Excludes1   angina pectoris with documented spasm without atherosclerosis of autologous artery coronary artery bypass graft(s) (I20.1)

    I25.728 **Atherosclerosis of autologous artery coronary artery bypass graft(s) with other forms of angina pectoris**   A

       Excludes1   other forms of angina pectoris without atherosclerosis of autologous artery coronary artery bypass graft(s) (I20.8)

    I25.729 **Atherosclerosis of autologous artery coronary artery bypass graft(s) with unspecified angina pectoris**   A

       Excludes1   unspecified angina pectoris without atherosclerosis of autologous artery coronary artery bypass graft(s) (I20.9)

● **I25.73**   **Atherosclerosis of nonautologous biological coronary artery bypass graft(s) with angina pectoris**
> Ⓔⓧ **For category I25.73 CC codes unless otherwise indicated:** See PDX Collection 662

     I25.730   Atherosclerosis of nonautologous biological coronary artery bypass graft(s) with **unstable** angina **pectoris** 🔖   A
> **Excludes1**   unstable angina without atherosclerosis of nonautologous biological coronary artery bypass graft(s) (I20.0)
> CC when PDx is its own CC
> Ⓔⓧ See PDX Collection 661

     I25.731   Atherosclerosis of nonautologous biological coronary artery bypass graft(s) with angina pectoris with **documented spasm** 🔖   A
> **Excludes1**   angina pectoris with documented spasm without atherosclerosis of nonautologous biological coronary artery bypass graft(s) (I20.1)

     I25.738   Atherosclerosis of nonautologous biological coronary artery bypass graft(s) with **other forms of angina pectoris** 🔖   A
> **Excludes1**   other forms of angina pectoris without atherosclerosis of nonautologous biological coronary artery bypass graft(s) (I20.8)

     I25.739   Atherosclerosis of nonautologous biological coronary artery bypass graft(s) with **unspecified angina pectoris** 🔖   A
> **Excludes1**   unspecified angina pectoris without atherosclerosis of nonautologous biological coronary artery bypass graft(s) (I20.9)

● **I25.75**   **Atherosclerosis of native coronary artery of transplanted heart with angina pectoris**
> **Excludes1**   atherosclerosis of native coronary artery of transplanted heart without angina pectoris (I25.811)
> Ⓔⓧ **For category I25.75 CC codes unless otherwise indicated:** See PDX Collection 664

     I25.750   Atherosclerosis of native coronary artery of transplanted heart with **unstable angina** 🔖
> CC when PDx is its own CC
> Ⓔⓧ See PDX Collection 663

     I25.751   Atherosclerosis of native coronary artery of transplanted heart with **angina pectoris with documented spasm** 🔖

     I25.758   Atherosclerosis of native coronary artery of transplanted heart with **other forms of angina pectoris** 🔖

     I25.759   Atherosclerosis of native coronary artery of transplanted heart with **unspecified angina pectoris** 🔖

● **I25.76**   **Atherosclerosis of bypass graft of coronary artery of transplanted heart with angina pectoris**
> **Excludes1**   atherosclerosis of bypass graft of coronary artery of transplanted heart without angina pectoris (I25.812)
> Ⓔⓧ **For category I25.76 CC codes unless otherwise indicated:** See PDX Collection 666

     I25.760   Atherosclerosis of bypass graft of coronary artery of transplanted heart **with unstable angina** 🔖   A
> CC when PDx is its own CC
> Ⓔⓧ See PDX Collection 665

     I25.761   Atherosclerosis of bypass graft of coronary artery of transplanted heart with angina pectoris with **documented spasm** 🔖   A

     I25.768   Atherosclerosis of bypass graft of coronary artery of transplanted heart with **other forms of angina pectoris** 🔖   A

     I25.769   Atherosclerosis of bypass graft of coronary artery of transplanted heart with **unspecified angina pectoris** 🔖   A

● **I25.79**   **Atherosclerosis of other coronary artery bypass graft(s) with angina pectoris**   A
> Ⓔⓧ **For category I25.79 CC codes unless otherwise indicated:** No exclusions

     I25.790   Atherosclerosis of other coronary artery bypass graft(s) with **unstable angina pectoris** 🔖
> **Excludes1**   unstable angina without atherosclerosis of other coronary artery bypass graft(s) (I20.0)
> CC when PDx is its own CC
> Ⓔⓧ See PDX Collection 651

     I25.791   Atherosclerosis of other coronary artery bypass graft(s) with angina pectoris with **documented spasm** 🔖   A
> **Excludes1**   angina pectoris with documented spasm without atherosclerosis of other coronary artery bypass graft(s) (I20.1)

     I25.798   Atherosclerosis of other coronary artery bypass graft(s) with **other forms of angina pectoris** 🔖   A
> **Excludes1**   other forms of angina pectoris without atherosclerosis of other coronary artery bypass graft(s) (I20.8)

     I25.799   Atherosclerosis of other coronary artery bypass graft(s) with **unspecified angina pectoris** 🔖   A
> **Excludes1**   unspecified angina pectoris without atherosclerosis of other coronary artery bypass graft(s) (I20.9)

▶ New   ⟹ Revised   d̶e̶l̶e̶t̶e̶d̶ Deleted   Excludes 1   Excludes 2   Includes   Use additional   Code first   Code also   Key words
OGCR Official Guidelines   ● Unacceptable Principal Diagnosis   X Assign placeholder X   ● Use Additional Character(s)   ▸ Manifestation Code   **Coding Clinic**

● **I25.8**   **Other forms of chronic ischemic heart disease**

   ● **I25.81**   **Atherosclerosis of other coronary vessels without angina pectoris**

       Use additional code, if applicable, to identify:
coronary atherosclerosis due to calcified coronary lesion (I25.84)
coronary atherosclerosis due to lipid rich plaque (I25.83)

       Excludes1   atherosclerotic heart disease of native coronary artery without angina pectoris (I25.10)

       I25.810   **Atherosclerosis of coronary artery bypass graft(s) without angina pectoris** 🅱   A

          Atherosclerosis of coronary artery bypass graft NOS

          Excludes1   atherosclerosis of coronary bypass graft(s) with angina pectoris (I25.70- -I25.73-, I25.79-)

          (Ex) No exclusions

          Coding Clinic: 2016, Q4, P86

       I25.811   **Atherosclerosis of native coronary artery of transplanted heart without angina pectoris** 🅱

          Atherosclerosis of native coronary artery of transplanted heart NOS

          Excludes1   atherosclerosis of native coronary artery of transplanted heart with angina pectoris (I25.75-)

          (Ex) See PDX Collection 664

       I25.812   **Atherosclerosis of bypass graft of coronary artery of transplanted heart without angina pectoris** 🅱   A

          Atherosclerosis of bypass graft of transplanted heart NOS

          Excludes1   atherosclerosis of bypass graft of transplanted heart with angina pectoris (I25.76)

   ● **I25.82**   **Chronic total occlusion of coronary artery**

       Complete occlusion of coronary artery
Total occlusion of coronary artery

       Code first coronary atherosclerosis (I25.1-, I25.7-, I25.81-)

       Excludes1 ➡ acute coronary occlusion with myocardial infarction (I21.0-I21.9, I22.-)
➡ acute coronary occlusion without myocardial infarction (I24.0)

       (Ex) See PDX Collection 666

   ● **I25.83**   **Coronary atherosclerosis due to lipid rich plaque**   A

       Code first coronary atherosclerosis (I25.1-, I25.7-, I25.81-)

   ● **I25.84**   **Coronary atherosclerosis due to calcified coronary lesion**

       Coronary atherosclerosis due to severely calcified coronary lesion

       Code first coronary atherosclerosis (I25.1-, I25.7-, I25.81-)

    I25.89   **Other forms of chronic ischemic heart disease**

● **I25.9**   **Chronic ischemic heart disease, unspecified**

    Ischemic heart disease (chronic) NOS

PULMONARY HEART DISEASE AND DISEASES OF PULMONARY CIRCULATION (I26-I28)

● **I26**   **Pulmonary embolism**

    Includes   pulmonary (acute)(artery)(vein) infarction
pulmonary (acute)(artery)(vein) thromboembolism
pulmonary (acute)(artery)(vein) thrombosis

    Excludes2   chronic pulmonary embolism (I27.82)
personal history of pulmonary embolism (Z86.711)
pulmonary embolism due to trauma (T79.0, T79.1)
pulmonary embolism due to complications of surgical and medical care (T80.0, T81.7-, T82.8-)
pulmonary embolism complicating abortion, ectopic or molar pregnancy (O00-O07, O08.2)
pulmonary embolism complicating pregnancy, childbirth and the puerperium (O88.-)
septic (non-pulmonary) arterial embolism (I76)

  ● **I26.0**   **Pulmonary embolism with acute cor pulmonale**

      (Ex) For category I26.0 CC codes: See PDX Collection 667

   ● **I26.01**   **Septic pulmonary embolism with acute cor pulmonale** 🅱

       Code first underlying infection
MCC when PDx is its own MCC

      I26.02   **Saddle embolus of pulmonary artery with acute cor pulmonale** 🅱 🅱
MCC when PDx is its own MCC

      I26.09   **Other pulmonary embolism with acute cor pulmonale** 🅱 🅱
Acute cor pulmonale NOS
MCC when PDx is its own MCC

  ● **I26.9**   **Pulmonary embolism without acute cor pulmonale**

   ● **I26.90**   **Septic pulmonary embolism without acute cor pulmonale** 🅱

       Code first underlying infection

       (Ex) See PDX Collection 668

      I26.92   **Saddle embolus of pulmonary artery without acute cor pulmonale** 🅱 🅱

       (Ex) See PDX Collection 669

      I26.99   **Other pulmonary embolism without acute cor pulmonale** 🅱 🅱
Acute pulmonary embolism NOS
Pulmonary embolism NOS

       (Ex) See PDX Collection 670

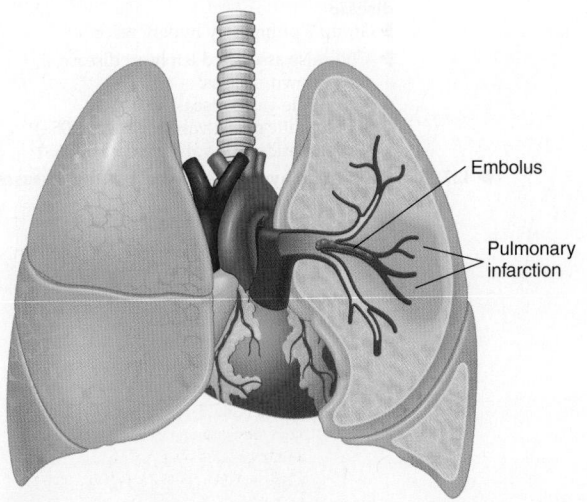

Embolus

Pulmonary infarction

Figure 9-3   Pulmonary Embolism. (From Chabner: The Language of Medicine, ed 8, St. Louis, Saunders, 2007)

CHAPTER 9 (I00-I99)

Item 9–7 Pulmonary heart disease or **cor pulmonale** is right ventricle hypertrophy or RVH as a result of a respiratory disorder increasing back flow pressure to the right ventricle. Left untreated, cor pulmonale leads to right-heart failure and death.

● **I27   Other pulmonary heart diseases**

I27.0   Primary pulmonary hypertension 🔖
▶Heritable pulmonary arterial hypertension
▶Idiopathic pulmonary arterial hypertension
▶Primary group 1 pulmonary hypertension
▶Primary pulmonary arterial hypertension

> **Excludes1**   ~~pulmonary hypertension NOS (I27.2)~~
> ~~secondary pulmonary hypertension (I27.2)~~
> ▶persistent pulmonary hypertension of newborn (P29.30)
> ▶pulmonary hypertension NOS (I27.20)
> ▶secondary pulmonary arterial hypertension (I27.21)
> ▶secondary pulmonary hypertension (I27.29)

(Ex:) See PDX Collection 671

I27.1   Kyphoscoliotic heart disease 🔖
(Ex:) See PDX Collection 533

● **I27.2   Other secondary pulmonary hypertension**
~~Pulmonary hypertension NOS~~

Code also associated underlying condition

> **Excludes1**   Eisenmenger's syndrome (I27.83)
Coding Clinic: 2016, Q2, P8

▶ **I27.20   Pulmonary hypertension, unspecified**
▶Pulmonary hypertension NOS

▶ **I27.21   Secondary pulmonary arterial hypertension**
▶(Associated) (drug-induced) (toxin-induced) pulmonary arterial hypertension NOS
▶(Associated) (drug-induced) (toxin-induced) (secondary) group 1 pulmonary hypertension
> Code also associated conditions if applicable, or adverse effects of drugs or toxins, such as:
> ▶adverse effect of appetite depressants (T50.5X5)
> ▶congenital heart disease (Q20-Q28)
> ▶human immunodeficiency virus [HIV] disease (B20)
> ▶polymyositis (M33.2-)
> ▶portal hypertension (K76.6)
> ▶rheumatoid arthritis (M05.-)
> ▶schistosomiasis (B65.-)
> ▶Sjögren syndrome (M35.0-)
> ▶systemic sclerosis (M34.-)

▶ **I27.22   Pulmonary hypertension due to left heart disease**
▶Group 2 pulmonary hypertension
> Code also associated left heart disease, if known, such as:
> ▶multiple valve disease (I08.-)
> ▶rheumatic mitral valve diseases (I05.-)
> ▶rheumatic aortic valve diseases (I06.-)

▶ **I27.23   Pulmonary hypertension due to lung diseases and hypoxia**
▶Group 3 pulmonary hypertension
> Code also associated lung disease, if known, such as:
> ▶bronchiectasis (J47.-)
> ▶cystic fibrosis with pulmonary manifestations (E84.0)
> ▶interstitial lung disease (J84.-)
> ▶pleural effusion (J90)
> ▶sleep apnea (G47.3-)

▶ **I27.24   Chronic thromboembolic pulmonary hypertension**
▶Group 4 pulmonary hypertension
> ▶ Code also associated pulmonary embolism, if applicable (I26.-, I27.82)

▶ **I27.29   Other secondary pulmonary hypertension**
▶Group 5 pulmonary hypertension
▶Pulmonary hypertension with unclear multifactorial mechanisms
▶Pulmonary hypertension due to hematologic disorders
▶Pulmonary hypertension due to metabolic disorders
▶Pulmonary hypertension due to other systemic disorders
> ▶ Code also other associated disorders, if known, such as:
> ▶chronic myeloid leukemia (C92.10- C92.22)
> ▶essential thrombocythemia (D47.3)
> ▶Gaucher disease (E75.22)
> ▶hypertensive chronic kidney disease with end stage renal disease (I12.0, I12.11, I13.2)
> ▶hyperthyroidism (E05.-)
> ▶hypothyroidism (E00-E03)
> ▶polycythemia vera (D45)
> ▶sarcoidosis (D86.-)

● **I27.8   Other specified pulmonary heart diseases**

I27.81   Cor pulmonale (chronic)
Cor pulmonale NOS
> **Excludes1**   acute cor pulmonale (I26.0-)

I27.82   Chronic pulmonary embolism 🔖
Use additional code, if applicable, for associated long-term (current) use of anticoagulants (Z79.01)
> **Excludes1**   personal history of pulmonary embolism (Z86.711)
(Ex:) See PDX Collection 669

▶ **I27.83   Eisenmenger's syndrome**
▶Eisenmenger's complex
▶(Irreversible) Eisenmenger's disease
▶Pulmonary hypertension with right to left shunt related to congenital heart disease
> ▶ Code also underlying heart defect, if known, such as:
> ▶atrial septal defect (Q21.1)
> ▶Eisenmenger's defect (Q21.8)
> ▶patent ductus arteriosus (Q25.0)
> ▶ventricular septal defect (Q21.0)

I27.89   Other specified pulmonary heart diseases
~~Eisenmenger's complex~~
~~Eisenmenger's syndrome~~
~~**Excludes1**   Eisenmenger's defect (Q21.8)~~

I27.9   Pulmonary heart disease, unspecified
Chronic cardiopulmonary disease

● **I28   Other diseases of pulmonary vessels**
(Ex:) For category I28 CC codes: See PDX Collection 672

I28.0   Arteriovenous fistula of pulmonary vessels 🔖
> **Excludes1**   congenital arteriovenous fistula (Q25.72)

I28.1   Aneurysm of pulmonary artery 🔖
> **Excludes1**   congenital aneurysm (Q25.79)
> congenital arteriovenous aneurysm (Q25.72)

I28.8   Other diseases of pulmonary vessels
Pulmonary arteritis
Pulmonary endarteritis
Rupture of pulmonary vessels
Stenosis of pulmonary vessels
Stricture of pulmonary vessels

I28.9   Disease of pulmonary vessels, unspecified

▶ New   ⇒ Revised   ~~deleted~~ Deleted   Excludes 1   Excludes 2   Includes   Use additional   Code first   Code also   Key words
OGCR Official Guidelines   ● Unacceptable Principal Diagnosis   X Assign placeholder X   ● Use Additional Character(s)   ▌ Manifestation Code   **Coding Clinic**

CHAPTER 9 (I00-I99)

OTHER FORMS OF HEART DISEASE (I30-I52)

● **I30   Acute pericarditis**
Inflammation of pericardium (sac surrounding the heart) caused by an infection

Includes   acute mediastinopericarditis
acute myopericarditis
acute pericardial effusion
acute pleuropericarditis
acute pneumopericarditis

Excludes1   Dressler's syndrome (I24.1)
rheumatic pericarditis (acute) (I01.0)
▶viral pericarditis due to Coxsakie virus (B33.23)

(Ex:) For category I30 CC codes: See PDX Collection 673

I30.0   Acute nonspecific idiopathic pericarditis ◐

I30.1   Infective pericarditis ◐
Pneumococcal pericarditis
Pneumopyopericardium
Purulent pericarditis
Pyopericarditis
Pyopericardium
Pyopneumopericardium
Staphylococcal pericarditis
Streptococcal pericarditis
Suppurative pericarditis
Viral pericarditis

Use additional code (B95-B97) to identify infectious agent

I30.8   Other forms of acute pericarditis ◐

I30.9   Acute pericarditis, unspecified ◐

● **I31   Other diseases of pericardium**

Excludes1   diseases of pericardium specified as rheumatic (I09.2)
postcardiotomy syndrome (I97.0)
traumatic injury to pericardium (S26.-)

(Ex:) For category I31 CC codes unless otherwise indicated: See PDX Collection 188

I31.0   Chronic adhesive pericarditis ◐
Accretio cordis
Adherent pericardium
Adhesive mediastinopericarditis
(Ex:) See PDX Collection 674

I31.1   Chronic constrictive pericarditis ◐
Concretio cordis
Pericardial calcification
(Ex:) See PDX Collection 674

I31.2   Hemopericardium, not elsewhere classified ◐

Excludes1   hemopericardium as current complication following acute myocardial infarction (I23.0)
(Ex:) See PDX Collection 674

I31.3   Pericardial effusion (noninflammatory) ◐
Chylopericardium

Excludes1   acute pericardial effusion (I30.9)

● **I31.4   Cardiac tamponade** ◐
Code first underlying cause

I31.8   Other specified diseases of pericardium ◐
Epicardial plaques
Focal pericardial adhesions

I31.9   Disease of pericardium, unspecified ◐
Pericarditis (chronic) NOS

▶ **I32   Pericarditis in diseases classified elsewhere** ◐
Code first underlying disease

Excludes1   pericarditis (in):
coxsackie (virus) (B33.23)
gonococcal (A54.83)
meningococcal (A39.53)
rheumatoid (arthritis) (M05.31)
syphilitic (A52.06)
systemic lupus erythematosus (M32.12)
tuberculosis (A18.84)
(Ex:) See PDX Collection 673

● **I33   Acute and subacute endocarditis**
Inflammation/infection of lining of heart, affecting heart valves including replacement valves and is usually caused by a bacterial infection

Excludes1   acute rheumatic endocarditis (I01.1)
endocarditis NOS (I38)

(Ex:) For category I33 CC codes: See PDX Collection 675

I33.0   Acute and subacute infective endocarditis ◐
Bacterial endocarditis (acute) (subacute)
Infective endocarditis (acute) (subacute) NOS
Endocarditis lenta (acute) (subacute)
Malignant endocarditis (acute) (subacute)
Purulent endocarditis (acute) (subacute)
Septic endocarditis (acute) (subacute)
Ulcerative endocarditis (acute) (subacute)
Vegetative endocarditis (acute) (subacute)

Use additional code (B95-B97) to identify infectious agent

I33.9   Acute and subacute endocarditis, unspecified ◐
Acute endocarditis NOS
Acute myoendocarditis NOS
Acute periendocarditis NOS
Subacute endocarditis NOS
Subacute myoendocarditis NOS
Subacute periendocarditis NOS

● **I34   Nonrheumatic mitral valve disorders**

Excludes1   mitral valve disease (I05.9)
mitral valve failure (I05.8)
mitral valve stenosis (I05.0)
mitral valve disorder of unspecified cause with diseases of aortic and/or tricuspid valve(s) (I08.-)
mitral valve disorder of unspecified cause with mitral stenosis or obstruction (I05.0)
◀mitral valve disorder specified as congenital (Q23.2, Q23.9)
mitral valve disorder specified as rheumatic (I05.-)

I34.0   Nonrheumatic mitral (valve) insufficiency
Nonrheumatic mitral (valve) incompetence NOS
Nonrheumatic mitral (valve) regurgitation NOS

I34.1   Nonrheumatic mitral (valve) prolapse
Floppy nonrheumatic mitral valve syndrome

Excludes1   Marfan's syndrome (Q87.4-)

I34.2   Nonrheumatic mitral (valve) stenosis

I34.8   Other nonrheumatic mitral valve disorders

I34.9   Nonrheumatic mitral valve disorder, unspecified

● **I35   Nonrheumatic aortic valve disorders**

Excludes1   aortic valve disorder of unspecified cause but with diseases of mitral and/or tricuspid valve(s) (I08.-)
aortic valve disorder specified as congenital (Q23.0, Q23.1)
aortic valve disorder specified as rheumatic (I06.-)
hypertrophic subaortic stenosis (I42.1)

I35.0   Nonrheumatic aortic (valve) stenosis

I35.1   Nonrheumatic aortic (valve) insufficiency
Nonrheumatic aortic (valve) incompetence NOS
Nonrheumatic aortic (valve) regurgitation NOS

I35.2   Nonrheumatic aortic (valve) stenosis with insufficiency

I35.8   Other nonrheumatic aortic valve disorders

I35.9   Nonrheumatic aortic valve disorder, unspecified

CHAPTER 9 (I00-I99)

● **I36**   **Nonrheumatic tricuspid valve disorders**

     Excludes1   tricuspid valve disorders of unspecified cause (I07.-)

              tricuspid valve disorders specified as congenital (Q22.4, Q22.8, Q22.9)

              tricuspid valve disorders specified as rheumatic (I07.-)

              tricuspid valve disorders with aortic and/or mitral valve involvement (I08.-)

   I36.0   **Nonrheumatic tricuspid (valve) stenosis**

   I36.1   **Nonrheumatic tricuspid (valve) insufficiency**
         Nonrheumatic tricuspid (valve) incompetence
         Nonrheumatic tricuspid (valve) regurgitation

   I36.2   **Nonrheumatic tricuspid (valve) stenosis with insufficiency**

   I36.8   **Other nonrheumatic tricuspid valve disorders**

   I36.9   **Nonrheumatic tricuspid valve disorder, unspecified**

● **I37**   **Nonrheumatic pulmonary valve disorders**

     Excludes1   pulmonary valve disorder specified as congenital (Q22.1, Q22.2, Q22.3)

              pulmonary valve disorder specified as rheumatic (I09.89)

   I37.0   **Nonrheumatic pulmonary valve stenosis**

   I37.1   **Nonrheumatic pulmonary valve insufficiency**
         Nonrheumatic pulmonary valve incompetence
         Nonrheumatic pulmonary valve regurgitation

   I37.2   **Nonrheumatic pulmonary valve stenosis with insufficiency**

   I37.8   **Other nonrheumatic pulmonary valve disorders**

   I37.9   **Nonrheumatic pulmonary valve disorder, unspecified**

   I38   **Endocarditis, valve unspecified** 🔍

     Includes   endocarditis (chronic) NOS
              valvular incompetence NOS
              valvular insufficiency NOS
              valvular regurgitation NOS
              valvular stenosis NOS
              valvulitis (chronic) NOS

     Excludes1   congenital insufficiency of cardiac valve NOS (Q24.8)

              congenital stenosis of cardiac valve NOS (Q24.8)

              endocardial fibroelastosis (I42.4)

              endocarditis specified as rheumatic (I09.1)

     (Ex:) See PDX Collection 676

▷ **I39**   *Endocarditis and heart valve disorders in diseases classified elsewhere* 🔍

     Code first underlying disease, such as:
       Q fever (A78)

     Excludes1   endocardial involvement in:
              candidiasis (B37.6)
              gonococcal infection (A54.83)
              Libman-Sacks disease (M32.11)
              listerosis (A32.82)
              meningococcal infection (A39.51)
              rheumatoid arthritis (M05.31)
              syphilis (A52.03)
              tuberculosis (A18.84)
              typhoid fever (A01.02)

     (Ex:) See PDX Collection 676

● **I40**   **Acute myocarditis**
     Inflammation of heart muscle due to infection (viral/bacterial)

     Includes   subacute myocarditis

     Excludes1   acute rheumatic myocarditis (I01.2)

     (Ex:) **For category I40 CC codes:** See PDX Collection 677

   I40.0   **Infective myocarditis** 🔍
         Septic myocarditis

         Use additional code (B95-B97) to identify infectious agent

   I40.1   **Isolated myocarditis** 🔍
         Fiedler's myocarditis
         Giant cell myocarditis
         Idiopathic myocarditis

   I40.8   **Other acute myocarditis** 🔍

   I40.9   **Acute myocarditis, unspecified** 🔍

▷ **I41**   *Myocarditis in diseases classified elsewhere* 🔍

     Code first underlying disease, such as:
       typhus (A75.0-A75.9)

     Excludes1   myocarditis (in):
              Chagas' disease (chronic) (B57.2)
              acute (B57.0)
              coxsackie (virus) infection (B33.22)
              diphtheritic (A36.81)
              gonococcal (A54.83)
              influenzal (J09.X9, J10.82, J11.82)
              meningococcal (A39.52)
              mumps (B26.82)
              rheumatoid arthritis (M05.31)
              sarcoid (D86.85)
              syphilis (A52.06)
              toxoplasmosis (B58.81)
              tuberculous (A18.84)

     (Ex:) See PDX Collection 677

● **I42**   **Cardiomyopathy**
     Disease of the heart muscle resulting in an abnormally enlarged, weakened, thickened, and/or stiffened muscles

     Includes   myocardiopathy

     Code first pre-existing cardiomyopathy complicating pregnancy and puerperium (O99.4)

     Excludes2   ischemic cardiomyopathy (I25.5)
              peripartum cardiomyopathy (O90.3)
              ventricular hypertrophy (I51.7)

     (Ex:) **For category I42 CC codes:** See PDX Collection 678

   I42.0   **Dilated cardiomyopathy** 🔍
         Congestive cardiomyopathy

   I42.1   **Obstructive hypertrophic cardiomyopathy** 🔍
         Hypertrophic subaortic stenosis (idiopathic)

   I42.2   **Other hypertrophic cardiomyopathy** 🔍
         Nonobstructive hypertrophic cardiomyopathy

   I42.3   **Endomyocardial (eosinophilic) disease** 🔍
         Endomyocardial (tropical) fibrosis
         Löffler's endocarditis

   I42.4   **Endocardial fibroelastosis** 🔍
         Congenital cardiomyopathy
         Elastomyofibrosis

   I42.5   **Other restrictive cardiomyopathy** 🔍
         Constrictive cardiomyopathy NOS

   I42.6   **Alcoholic cardiomyopathy** 🔍

         Code also presence of alcoholism (F10.-)

   I42.7   **Cardiomyopathy due to drug and external agent** 🔍

         Code first poisoning due to drug or toxin, if applicable (T36-T65 with fifth or sixth character 1-4 or 6)

         Use additional code for adverse effect, if applicable, to identify drug (T36-T50 with fifth or sixth character 5)

   I42.8   **Other cardiomyopathies** 🔍

   I42.9   **Cardiomyopathy, unspecified** 🔍
         Cardiomyopathy (primary) (secondary) NOS

▶ New   ⇒ Revised   ~~deleted~~ Deleted   Excludes 1   Excludes 2   Includes   Use additional   Code first   Code also   Key words

OGCR Official Guidelines   ● Unacceptable Principal Diagnosis   X Assign placeholder X   🔍 Use Additional Character(s)   ▷ Manifestation Code   **Coding Clinic**

▶ **I43**   *Cardiomyopathy in diseases classified elsewhere* 🅒
> *Code first underlying disease, such as:*
> amyloidosis (E85.-)
> glycogen storage disease (E74.0)
> gout (M10.0-)
> thyrotoxicosis (E05.0-E05.9-)

> **Excludes1**   cardiomyopathy (in):
> coxsackie (virus) (B33.24)
> diphtheria (A36.81)
> sarcoidosis (D86.85)
> tuberculosis (A18.84)

> (Ex) See PDX Collection 678

● **I44**   **Atrioventricular and left bundle-branch block**
> *Conduction problem resulting in arrhythmias/dysrhythmias due to a*
> *lack of electrical impulses being transmitted normally through*
> *the heart*

I44.0   **Atrioventricular block, first degree**

I44.1   **Atrioventricular block, second degree**
> Atrioventricular block, type I and II
> Möbitz block, type I and II
> Second degree block, type I and II
> Wenckebach's block

I44.2   **Atrioventricular block, complete** 🅒
> Complete heart block NOS
> Third degree block
> (Ex) See PDX Collection 679

● **I44.3**   **Other and unspecified atrioventricular block**
> Atrioventricular block NOS

> **I44.30**   **Unspecified atrioventricular block**

> **I44.39**   **Other atrioventricular block**

I44.4   **Left anterior fascicular block**
> MCE: Questionable admission when principal dx

I44.5   **Left posterior fascicular block**
> MCE: Questionable admission when principal dx

● **I44.6**   **Other and unspecified fascicular block**

> **I44.60**   **Unspecified fascicular block**
> Left bundle-branch hemiblock NOS
> MCE: Questionable admission when principal dx

> **I44.69**   **Other fascicular block**
> MCE: Questionable admission when principal dx

I44.7   **Left bundle-branch block, unspecified**
> MCE: Questionable admission when principal dx

● **I45**   **Other conduction disorders**

I45.0   **Right fascicular block**
> MCE: Questionable admission when principal dx

● **I45.1**   **Other and unspecified right bundle-branch block**

> **I45.10**   **Unspecified right bundle-branch block**
> Right bundle-branch block NOS
> MCE: Questionable admission when principal dx

> **I45.19**   **Other right bundle-branch block**
> MCE: Questionable admission when principal dx

I45.2   **Bifascicular block** 🅒
> (Ex) See PDX Collection 679

I45.3   **Trifascicular block** 🅒
> (Ex) See PDX Collection 679

I45.4   **Nonspecific intraventricular block**
> Bundle-branch block NOS

I45.5   **Other specified heart block**
> Sinoatrial block
> Sinoauricular block

> **Excludes1**   heart block NOS (I45.9)

I45.6   **Pre-excitation syndrome**
> Accelerated atrioventricular conduction
> Accessory atrioventricular conduction
> Anomalous atrioventricular excitation
> Lown-Ganong-Levine syndrome
> Pre-excitation atrioventricular conduction
> Wolff-Parkinson-White syndrome

● **I45.8**   **Other specified conduction disorders**

I45.81   **Long QT syndrome**

I45.89   **Other specified conduction disorders** 🅒
> Atrioventricular [AV] dissociation
> Interference dissociation
> Isorhythmic dissociation
> Nonparoxysmal AV nodal tachycardia
> (Ex) See PDX Collection 679
> **Coding Clinic: 2013, Q2, P32**

I45.9   **Conduction disorder, unspecified**
> Heart block NOS
> Stokes-Adams syndrome

● **I46**   **Cardiac arrest**

> **Excludes1**   cardiogenic shock (R57.0)
> (Ex) For category I46 CC codes: See PDX Collection 680

I46.2   **Cardiac arrest due to underlying cardiac condition** 🅜
> *Code first underlying cardiac condition*
> MCC: If patient discharged alive

I46.8   **Cardiac arrest due to other underlying condition** 🅜
> *Code first underlying condition*
> MCC: If patient discharged alive

I46.9   **Cardiac arrest, cause unspecified** 🅜
> MCC: If patient discharged alive

● **I47**   **Paroxysmal tachycardia**
> *Code first tachycardia complicating:*
> abortion or ectopic or molar pregnancy (O00-O07, O08.8)
> obstetric surgery and procedures (O75.4)

> **Excludes1**   tachycardia NOS (R00.0)
> sinoauricular tachycardia NOS (R00.0)
> sinus [sinusal] tachycardia NOS (R00.0)
> (Ex) For category I47 CC codes: See PDX Collection 679

I47.0   **Re-entry ventricular arrhythmia** 🅒

I47.1   **Supraventricular tachycardia** 🅒
> Atrial (paroxysmal) tachycardia
> Atrioventricular [AV] (paroxysmal) tachycardia
> Atrioventricular re-entrant (nodal) tachycardia
> [AVNRT] [AVRT]
> Junctional (paroxysmal) tachycardia
> Nodal (paroxysmal) tachycardia

I47.2   **Ventricular tachycardia** 🅒
> **Coding Clinic: 2013, Q3, P23**

I47.9   **Paroxysmal tachycardia, unspecified**
> Bouveret (-Hoffman) syndrome

● **I48**   **Atrial fibrillation and flutter**
> *Most common abnormal heart rhythm (arrhythmia) presenting*
> *as irregular, rapid beating (tachycardia) of the heart's upper*
> *chamber.*
> (Ex) For category I48 CC codes: See PDX Collection 679

I48.0   **Paroxysmal atrial fibrillation**

I48.1   **Persistent atrial fibrillation** 🅒
> *Rapid contractions of the upper heart chamber*

I48.2   **Chronic atrial fibrillation**
> Permanent atrial fibrillation

I48.3   **Typical atrial flutter** 🅒
> Type I atrial flutter

I48.4   **Atypical atrial flutter** 🅒
> Type II atrial flutter

● **I48.9**   **Unspecified atrial fibrillation and atrial flutter**

I48.91   **Unspecified atrial fibrillation**

I48.92   **Unspecified atrial flutter** 🅒

CHAPTER 9 (I00–I99)

● **I49   Other cardiac arrhythmias**

Code first cardiac arrhythmia complicating:
   abortion or ectopic or molar pregnancy (O00-O07, O08.8)
   obstetric surgery and procedures (O75.4)

Excludes1   ~~bradycardia NOS (R00.1)~~
           neonatal dysrhythmia (P29.1-)
           sinoatrial bradycardia (R00.1)
           sinus bradycardia (R00.1)
           vagal bradycardia (R00.1)

▶ **Excludes2**   bradycardia NOS (R00.1)

● **I49.0   Ventricular fibrillation and flutter**
   (Ex) **For category I49.0 CC codes:** See PDX Collection 679

   I49.01   Ventricular fibrillation 🔍
         MCC: If patient discharged alive

   I49.02   Ventricular flutter 🔍

I49.1   Atrial premature depolarization
       Atrial premature beats

I49.2   Junctional premature depolarization 🔍
       (Ex) See PDX Collection 679

I49.3   Ventricular premature depolarization

● **I49.4   Other and unspecified premature depolarization**

   I49.40   Unspecified premature depolarization
         Premature beats NOS

   I49.49   Other premature depolarization
         Ectopic beats
         Extrasystoles
         Extrasystolic arrhythmias
         Premature contractions

I49.5   Sick sinus syndrome
       Tachycardia-bradycardia syndrome

I49.8   Other specified cardiac arrhythmias
       ▶Brugada syndrome
       Coronary sinus rhythm disorder
       Ectopic rhythm disorder
       Nodal rhythm disorder

I49.9   Cardiac arrhythmia, unspecified
       Arrhythmia (cardiac) NOS

● **I50   Heart failure**

Code first heart failure complicating abortion or ectopic or molar pregnancy (O00-O07, O08.8)
   heart failure due to hypertension (I11.0)
   heart failure due to hypertension with chronic kidney disease (I13.-)
   heart failure following surgery (I97.13-)
   obstetric surgery and procedures (O75.4)
   rheumatic heart failure (I09.81)

Excludes1   neonatal cardiac failure (P29.0)

Excludes2   cardiac arrest (I46.-)

Coding Clinic: 2017, Q1, P47; 2016, Q4, P122-123, Q1, P38; 2015, Q2, P15

⇥ **I50.1   Left ventricular failure, unspecified** 🔍
       Cardiac asthma
       Edema of lung with heart disease NOS
       Edema of lung with heart failure
       Left heart failure
       Pulmonary edema with heart disease NOS
       Pulmonary edema with heart failure

   Excludes1   edema of lung without heart disease or
               heart failure (J81.-)
               pulmonary edema without heart disease
               or failure (J81.-)

       (Ex) See PDX Collection 681

● **I50.2   Systolic (congestive) heart failure**
   ▶Heart failure with reduced ejection fraction [HFrEF]
   ▶Systolic left ventricular heart failure
   ▶ Code also end stage heart failure, if applicable (I50.84)

   Excludes1   combined systolic (congestive) and
               diastolic (congestive) heart failure
               (I50.4-)
   (Ex) **For category I50.2 CC codes:** See PDX Collection 682

   **I50.20   Unspecified systolic (congestive) heart
           failure** 🔍

   I50.21   Acute systolic (congestive) heart failure 🔍
         Presenting a short and relatively severe episode

   I50.22   Chronic systolic (congestive) heart failure 🔍
         Long-lasting, presenting over time

   **I50.23   Acute on chronic systolic (congestive) heart
           failure** 🔍
         *Combination code. What was a chronic condition
          now has an acute exacerbation (to make more
          severe).*
         Coding Clinic: 2013, Q2, P33

● **I50.3   Diastolic (congestive) heart failure**
   ▶Diastolic left ventricular heart failure
   ▶Heart failure with normal ejection fraction
   ▶Heart failure with preserved ejection fraction [HFpEF]
   ▶ Code also end stage heart failure, if applicable (I50.84)

   Excludes1   combined systolic (congestive) and
               diastolic (congestive) heart failure
               (I50.4-)
   (Ex) **For category I50.3 CC codes:** See PDX Collection 682

   **I50.30   Unspecified diastolic (congestive) heart
           failure** 🔍

   I50.31   Acute diastolic (congestive) heart failure 🔍
         Coding Clinic: 2017, Q1, P46

   I50.32   Chronic diastolic (congestive) heart failure 🔍

   **I50.33   Acute on chronic diastolic (congestive) heart
           failure** 🔍

● **I50.4   Combined systolic (congestive) and diastolic
       (congestive) heart failure**
   ▶Combined systolic and diastolic left ventricular heart
     failure
   ▶Heart failure with reduced ejection fraction and
     diastolic dysfunction
   ▶ Code also end stage heart failure, if applicable (I50.84)
   (Ex) **For category I50.4 CC codes:** See PDX Collection 682

   **I50.40   Unspecified combined systolic (congestive) and
           diastolic (congestive) heart failure** 🔍

   **I50.41   Acute combined systolic (congestive) and
           diastolic (congestive) heart failure** 🔍

   **I50.42   Chronic combined systolic (congestive) and
           diastolic (congestive) heart failure** 🔍

   **I50.43   Acute on chronic combined systolic
           (congestive) and diastolic (congestive) heart
           failure** 🔍

▶● **I50.8   Other heart failure**
   ▶● **I50.81   Right heart failure**
           ▶Right ventricular failure

       ▶ **I50.810   Right heart failure, unspecified**
               ▶Right heart failure without mention
                 of left heart failure
               ▶Right ventricular failure NOS

       ▶ **I50.811   Acute right heart failure**
               ▶Acute isolated right heart failure
               ▶Acute (isolated) right ventricular
                 failure

       ▶ **I50.812   Chronic right heart failure**
               ▶Chronic isolated right heart failure
               ▶Chronic (isolated) right ventricular
                 failure

Item 9-8 Congestive heart failure (CHF) is a condition in which the left ventricle of the heart cannot pump enough blood to the body. The blood flow from the heart slows or returns to the heart from the venous system (back flow) resulting in congestion (fluid accumulation) particularly in the abdomen. Most commonly, fluid collects in the lungs and results in shortness of breath, especially when in a reclining position.

▶ New   ⇥ Revised   ~~deleted~~ Deleted   Excludes 1   Excludes 2   Includes   Use additional   Code first   Code also   Key words
OGCR Official Guidelines   ● Unacceptable Principal Diagnosis   X Assign placeholder X   ▶ Use Additional Character(s)   ▶ Manifestation Code   **Coding Clinic**

▶ **I50.813**   **Acute on chronic right heart failure**
- ▶ Acute on chronic isolated right heart failure
- ▶ Acute on chronic (isolated) right ventricular failure
- ▶ Acute decompensation of chronic (isolated) right ventricular failure
- ▶ Acute exacerbation of chronic (isolated) right ventricular failure

▶ **I50.814**   **Right heart failure due to left heart failure**
- ▶ Right ventricular failure secondary to left ventricular failure
- ▶ Code also the type of left ventricular failure, if known (I50.2-I50.43)
- ▶ **Excludes1**   Right heart failure with but not due to left heart failure (I50.82)

▶ **I50.82**   **Biventricular heart failure**
- ▶ Code also the type of left ventricular failure as systolic, diastolic, or combined, if known **(I50.2-I50.43)**

▶ **I50.83**   **High output heart failure**

▶ **I50.84**   **End stage heart failure**
- ▶ Stage D heart failure
- ▶ Code also the type of heart failure as systolic, diastolic, or combined, if known (I50.2-I50.43)

▶ **I50.89**   **Other heart failure**

I50.9   **Heart failure, unspecified**
- Biventricular (heart) failure NOS
- Cardiac, heart or myocardial failure NOS
- Congestive heart disease
- Congestive heart failure NOS
- Right ventricular failure (secondary to left heart failure)

Excludes2   fluid overload (E87.70)

Coding Clinic: 2017, Q1, P45-46; 2015, Q2, P15; 2012, Q4, P92

● **I51**   **Complications and ill-defined descriptions of heart disease**

Excludes1   any condition in I51.4-I51.9 due to hypertension (I11.-)
any condition in I51.4-I51.9 due to hypertension and chronic kidney disease (I13.-)
heart disease specified as rheumatic (I00-I09)

I51.0   **Cardiac septal defect, acquired**   A
- Acquired septal atrial defect (old)
- Acquired septal auricular defect (old)
- Acquired septal ventricular defect (old)

Excludes1   cardiac septal defect as current complication following acute myocardial infarction (I23.1, I23.2)

Ex: See PDX Collection 654

I51.1   **Rupture of chordae tendineae, not elsewhere classified**

Excludes1   rupture of chordae tendineae as current complication following acute myocardial infarction (I23.4)

Ex: See PDX Collection 655

I51.2   **Rupture of papillary muscle, not elsewhere classified**

Excludes1   rupture of papillary muscle as current complication following acute myocardial infarction (I23.5)

Ex: See PDX Collection 656

I51.3   **Intracardiac thrombosis, not elsewhere classified**
- Apical thrombosis (old)
- Atrial thrombosis (old)
- Auricular thrombosis (old)
- Mural thrombosis (old)
- Ventricular thrombosis (old)

Excludes1   intracardiac thrombosis as current complication following acute myocardial infarction (I23.6)

Coding Clinic: 2013, Q1, P24

I51.4   **Myocarditis, unspecified**
- Chronic (interstitial) myocarditis
- Myocardial fibrosis
- Myocarditis NOS

Excludes1   acute or subacute myocarditis (I40.-)

Coding Clinic: 2016, Q4, P122

I51.5   **Myocardial degeneration**
- Fatty degeneration of heart or myocardium
- Myocardial disease
- Senile degeneration of heart or myocardium

Coding Clinic: 2016, Q4, P122

I51.7   **Cardiomegaly**
- Cardiac dilatation
- Cardiac hypertrophy
- Ventricular dilatation

Coding Clinic: 2016, Q4, P122

● **I51.8**   **Other ill-defined heart diseases**

Coding Clinic: 2016, Q4, P122

     I51.81   **Takotsubo syndrome**
- Reversible left ventricular dysfunction following sudden emotional stress
- Stress induced cardiomyopathy
- Takotsubo cardiomyopathy
- Transient left ventricular apical ballooning syndrome

Ex: See PDX Collection 683

     I51.89   **Other ill-defined heart diseases**
- Carditis (acute)(chronic)
- Pancarditis (acute)(chronic)

I51.9   **Heart disease, unspecified**

Coding Clinic: 2016, Q4, P122

▶ **I52**   *Other heart disorders in diseases classified elsewhere*

Code first underlying disease, such as:
- congenital syphilis (A50.5)
- mucopolysaccharidosis (E76.3)
- schistosomiasis (B65.0-B65.9)

Excludes1   heart disease (in):
- gonococcal infection (A54.83)
- meningococcal infection (A39.50)
- rheumatoid arthritis (M05.31)
- syphilis (A52.06)

CEREBROVASCULAR DISEASES (I60-I69)

Use additional code to identify presence of:
- alcohol abuse and dependence (F10.-)
- exposure to environmental tobacco smoke (Z77.22)
- history of tobacco dependence (Z87.891)
- hypertension (I10-I15)
- occupational exposure to environmental tobacco smoke (Z57.31)
- tobacco dependence (F17.-)
- tobacco use (Z72.0)

Excludes1   transient cerebral ischemic attacks and related syndromes (G45.-)
traumatic intracranial hemorrhage (S06.-)

Coding Clinic: 2015, Q4, P40

N Newborn Age: 0   **P** Pediatric Age: 0–17   **M** Maternity DX: 12–55   **A** Adult Age: 15–124   ♀ Females Only   ♂ Males Only

Complication\Comorbidity   Major C\C   Ex: CC/MCC Exclusions   Hospital-Acquired Condition   883

CHAPTER 9 (I00-I99)

● **I60**   **Nontraumatic subarachnoid hemorrhage**

    ~~Includes~~   ~~ruptured cerebral aneurysm~~

    Excludes1   syphilitic ruptured cerebral aneurysm (A52.05)

    Excludes2   sequelae of subarachnoid hemorrhage (I69.0-)

    (Ex:) For category I60 CC codes: See PDX Collection 684

    ● **I60.0**   **Nontraumatic subarachnoid hemorrhage from carotid siphon and bifurcation**

       I60.00   Nontraumatic subarachnoid hemorrhage from unspecified carotid siphon and bifurcation 🔍

       I60.01   Nontraumatic subarachnoid hemorrhage from right carotid siphon and bifurcation 🔍

       I60.02   Nontraumatic subarachnoid hemorrhage from left carotid siphon and bifurcation 🔍

    ● **I60.1**   **Nontraumatic subarachnoid hemorrhage from middle cerebral artery**

       I60.10   Nontraumatic subarachnoid hemorrhage from unspecified middle cerebral artery 🔍

       I60.11   Nontraumatic subarachnoid hemorrhage from right middle cerebral artery 🔍

       I60.12   Nontraumatic subarachnoid hemorrhage from left middle cerebral artery 🔍

      I60.2   **Nontraumatic subarachnoid hemorrhage from anterior communicating artery** 🔍

    ● **I60.3**   **Nontraumatic subarachnoid hemorrhage from posterior communicating artery**

       I60.30   Nontraumatic subarachnoid hemorrhage from unspecified posterior communicating artery 🔍

       I60.31   Nontraumatic subarachnoid hemorrhage from right posterior communicating artery 🔍

       I60.32   Nontraumatic subarachnoid hemorrhage from left posterior communicating artery 🔍

      I60.4   **Nontraumatic subarachnoid hemorrhage from basilar artery** 🔍

    ● **I60.5**   **Nontraumatic subarachnoid hemorrhage from vertebral artery**

       I60.50   Nontraumatic subarachnoid hemorrhage from unspecified vertebral artery 🔍

       I60.51   Nontraumatic subarachnoid hemorrhage from right vertebral artery 🔍

       I60.52   Nontraumatic subarachnoid hemorrhage from left vertebral artery 🔍

      I60.6   **Nontraumatic subarachnoid hemorrhage from other intracranial arteries** 🔍

      I60.7   **Nontraumatic subarachnoid hemorrhage from unspecified intracranial artery** 🔍
       Ruptured (congenital) berry aneurysm
       Ruptured (congenital) cerebral aneurysm
       Subarachnoid hemorrhage (nontraumatic) from cerebral artery NOS
       Subarachnoid hemorrhage (nontraumatic) from communicating artery NOS

       Excludes1   berry aneurysm, nonruptured (I67.1)

      I60.8   **Other nontraumatic subarachnoid hemorrhage** 🔍
       Meningeal hemorrhage
       Rupture of cerebral arteriovenous malformation

      I60.9   **Nontraumatic subarachnoid hemorrhage, unspecified** 🔍

● **I61**   **Nontraumatic intracerebral hemorrhage**

    Excludes2   sequelae of intracerebral hemorrhage (I69.1-)

    (Ex:) For category I61 CC codes: See PDX Collection 684
    Coding Clinic: 2017, Q2, P10

      I61.0   **Nontraumatic intracerebral hemorrhage in hemisphere, subcortical** 🔍
       Deep intracerebral hemorrhage (nontraumatic)
       Coding Clinic: 2016, Q4, P27

      I61.1   **Nontraumatic intracerebral hemorrhage in hemisphere, cortical** 🔍
       Cerebral lobe hemorrhage (nontraumatic)
       Superficial intracerebral hemorrhage (nontraumatic)
       Coding Clinic: 2016, Q4, P28

      I61.2   **Nontraumatic intracerebral hemorrhage in hemisphere, unspecified** 🔍

      I61.3   **Nontraumatic intracerebral hemorrhage in brain stem** 🔍

      I61.4   **Nontraumatic intracerebral hemorrhage in cerebellum** 🔍

      I61.5   **Nontraumatic intracerebral hemorrhage, intraventricular** 🔍

      I61.6   **Nontraumatic intracerebral hemorrhage, multiple localized** 🔍

      I61.8   **Other nontraumatic intracerebral hemorrhage** 🔍

      I61.9   **Nontraumatic intracerebral hemorrhage, unspecified** 🔍

● **I62**   **Other and unspecified nontraumatic intracranial hemorrhage**

    Excludes2   sequelae of intracranial hemorrhage (I69.2)

    (Ex:) For category I62 CC codes: See PDX Collection 684

    ● **I62.0**   **Nontraumatic subdural hemorrhage**

       I62.00   Nontraumatic subdural hemorrhage, unspecified 🔍

       I62.01   Nontraumatic acute subdural hemorrhage 🔍

       I62.02   Nontraumatic subacute subdural hemorrhage 🔍

       I62.03   Nontraumatic chronic subdural hemorrhage 🔍

      I62.1   **Nontraumatic extradural hemorrhage** 🔍
       Nontraumatic epidural hemorrhage

      I62.9   **Nontraumatic intracranial hemorrhage, unspecified** 🔍

★ **(See Plate 141 on page 76.)**

● **I63**   **Cerebral infarction**

    Includes   occlusion and stenosis of cerebral and precerebral arteries, resulting in cerebral infarction

    Use additional code, if applicable, to identify status post administration of tPA (rtPA) in a different facility within the last 24 hours prior to admission to current facility (Z92.82)

    Use additional code, if known, to indicate National Institutes of Health Stroke Scale (NIHSS) score (R29.7-)

    Excludes2   sequelae of cerebral infarction (I69.3-)

    Coding Clinic: 2016, Q4, P28, 61, 127

    ● **I63.0**   **Cerebral infarction due to thrombosis of precerebral arteries**

       I63.00   Cerebral infarction due to thrombosis of unspecified precerebral artery 🔍

       (Ex:) See PDX Collection 685

Cerebral embolus

Cerebral hemorrhage

Cerebral thrombosis

Figure 9-4   Events causing a stroke. (From Shiland: Mastering Healthcare Terminology, ed 1, St. Louis, Mosby, 2003)

▶ New   ⇒ Revised   ~~deleted~~ Deleted   Excludes 1   Excludes 2   Includes   Use additional   Code first   Code also   Key words
OGCR Official Guidelines   ● Unacceptable Principal Diagnosis   X Assign placeholder X   ● Use Additional Character(s)   ▶ Manifestation Code   **Coding Clinic**

● **I63.01 Cerebral infarction due to thrombosis of vertebral artery**
Ⓔ **For category I63.01 CC codes:** See PDX Collection 686

    I63.011 Cerebral infarction due to thrombosis of right vertebral artery 🔖

    I63.012 Cerebral infarction due to thrombosis of left vertebral artery 🔖

    I63.013 Cerebral infarction due to thrombosis of bilateral vertebral arteries 🔖

    I63.019 Cerebral infarction due to thrombosis of unspecified vertebral artery 🔖

I63.02 Cerebral infarction due to thrombosis of basilar artery 🔖
Ⓔ See PDX Collection 685

● **I63.03 Cerebral infarction due to thrombosis of carotid artery**
Ⓔ **For category I63.03 CC codes:** See PDX Collection 687

    I63.031 Cerebral infarction due to thrombosis of right carotid artery 🔖

    I63.032 Cerebral infarction due to thrombosis of left carotid artery 🔖

    I63.033 Cerebral infarction due to thrombosis of bilateral carotid arteries 🔖

    I63.039 Cerebral infarction due to thrombosis of unspecified carotid artery 🔖

I63.09 Cerebral infarction due to thrombosis of other precerebral artery 🔖
Ⓔ See PDX Collection 685

● **I63.1 Cerebral infarction due to embolism of precerebral arteries**

I63.10 Cerebral infarction due to embolism of unspecified precerebral artery 🔖
Ⓔ See PDX Collection 685

● **I63.11 Cerebral infarction due to embolism of vertebral artery**
Ⓔ **For category I63.11 CC codes:** See PDX Collection 686

    I63.111 Cerebral infarction due to embolism of right vertebral artery 🔖

    I63.112 Cerebral infarction due to embolism of left vertebral artery 🔖

    I63.113 Cerebral infarction due to embolism of bilateral vertebral arteries 🔖

    I63.119 Cerebral infarction due to embolism of unspecified vertebral artery 🔖

I63.12 Cerebral infarction due to embolism of basilar artery 🔖
Ⓔ See PDX Collection 685

● **I63.13 Cerebral infarction due to embolism of carotid artery**
Ⓔ **For category I63.13 CC codes:** See PDX Collection 687

    I63.131 Cerebral infarction due to embolism of right carotid artery 🔖

    I63.132 Cerebral infarction due to embolism of left carotid artery 🔖

    I63.133 Cerebral infarction due to embolism of bilateral carotid arteries 🔖

    I63.139 Cerebral infarction due to embolism of unspecified carotid artery 🔖

I63.19 Cerebral infarction due to embolism of other precerebral artery 🔖
Ⓔ See PDX Collection 685

● **I63.2 Cerebral infarction due to unspecified occlusion or stenosis of precerebral arteries**

I63.20 Cerebral infarction due to unspecified occlusion or stenosis of unspecified precerebral arteries 🔖
Ⓔ See PDX Collection 685

● **I63.21 Cerebral infarction due to unspecified occlusion or stenosis of vertebral arteries**
Ⓔ **For category I63.21 CC codes:** See PDX Collection 686

➡ I63.211 Cerebral infarction due to unspecified occlusion or stenosis of right vertebral artery 🔖

➡ I63.212 Cerebral infarction due to unspecified occlusion or stenosis of left vertebral artery 🔖

    I63.213 Cerebral infarction due to unspecified occlusion or stenosis of bilateral vertebral arteries 🔖

    I63.219 Cerebral infarction due to unspecified occlusion or stenosis of unspecified vertebral arteries 🔖

➡ **I63.22 Cerebral infarction due to unspecified occlusion or stenosis of basilar artery** 🔖
Ⓔ See PDX Collection 685

● **I63.23 Cerebral infarction due to unspecified occlusion or stenosis of carotid arteries**
Ⓔ **For category I63.23 CC codes:** See PDX Collection 687

    I63.231 Cerebral infarction due to unspecified occlusion or stenosis of right carotid arteries 🔖

    I63.232 Cerebral infarction due to unspecified occlusion or stenosis of left carotid arteries 🔖

    I63.233 Cerebral infarction due to unspecified occlusion or stenosis of bilateral carotid arteries 🔖

    I63.239 Cerebral infarction due to unspecified occlusion or stenosis of unspecified carotid arteries 🔖

I63.29 Cerebral infarction due to unspecified occlusion or stenosis of other precerebral arteries 🔖
Ⓔ See PDX Collection 685

● **I63.3 Cerebral infarction due to thrombosis of cerebral arteries**
Ⓔ **For category I63.3 CC codes:** See PDX Collection 688

I63.30 Cerebral infarction due to thrombosis of unspecified cerebral artery 🔖

● **I63.31 Cerebral infarction due to thrombosis of middle cerebral artery**

    I63.311 Cerebral infarction due to thrombosis of right middle cerebral artery 🔖

    I63.312 Cerebral infarction due to thrombosis of left middle cerebral artery 🔖

    I63.313 Cerebral infarction due to thrombosis of bilateral middle cerebral arteries 🔖

    I63.319 Cerebral infarction due to thrombosis of unspecified middle cerebral artery 🔖

● **I63.32 Cerebral infarction due to thrombosis of anterior cerebral artery**

    I63.321 Cerebral infarction due to thrombosis of right anterior cerebral artery 🔖

    I63.322 Cerebral infarction due to thrombosis of left anterior cerebral artery 🔖

➡ I63.323 Cerebral infarction due to thrombosis of bilateral anterior cerebral arteries 🔖

    I63.329 Cerebral infarction due to thrombosis of unspecified anterior cerebral artery 🔖

 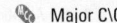
CHAPTER 9 (I00-I99)

● **I63.33** Cerebral infarction due to thrombosis of posterior cerebral artery

   I63.331 Cerebral infarction due to thrombosis of right posterior cerebral artery 🔖

   I63.332 Cerebral infarction due to thrombosis of left posterior cerebral artery 🔖

➡ I63.333 Cerebral infarction to thrombosis of bilateral posterior cerebral arteries 🔖

   I63.339 Cerebral infarction due to thrombosis of unspecified posterior cerebral artery 🔖

● **I63.34** Cerebral infarction due to thrombosis of cerebellar artery

   I63.341 Cerebral infarction due to thrombosis of right cerebellar artery 🔖

   I63.342 Cerebral infarction due to thrombosis of left cerebellar artery 🔖

   I63.343 Cerebral infarction to thrombosis of bilateral cerebellar arteries 🔖

   I63.349 Cerebral infarction due to thrombosis of unspecified cerebellar artery 🔖

   I63.39 Cerebral infarction due to thrombosis of other cerebral artery 🔖

● **I63.4** Cerebral infarction due to embolism of cerebral arteries

   Ⓔⓧ For category I63.4 CC codes: See PDX Collection 688

   I63.40 Cerebral infarction due to embolism of unspecified cerebral artery 🔖

● **I63.41** Cerebral infarction due to embolism of middle cerebral artery

   I63.411 Cerebral infarction due to embolism of right middle cerebral artery 🔖

   I63.412 Cerebral infarction due to embolism of left middle cerebral artery 🔖

   I63.413 Cerebral infarction due to embolism of bilateral middle cerebral arteries 🔖

   I63.419 Cerebral infarction due to embolism of unspecified middle cerebral artery 🔖

● **I63.42** Cerebral infarction due to embolism of anterior cerebral artery

   I63.421 Cerebral infarction due to embolism of right anterior cerebral artery 🔖

   I63.422 Cerebral infarction due to embolism of left anterior cerebral artery 🔖

   I63.423 Cerebral infarction due to embolism of bilateral anterior cerebral arteries 🔖

   I63.429 Cerebral infarction due to embolism of unspecified anterior cerebral artery 🔖

● **I63.43** Cerebral infarction due to embolism of posterior cerebral artery

   I63.431 Cerebral infarction due to embolism of right posterior cerebral artery 🔖

   I63.432 Cerebral infarction due to embolism of left posterior cerebral artery 🔖

   I63.433 Cerebral infarction due to embolism of bilateral posterior cerebral arteries 🔖

   I63.439 Cerebral infarction due to embolism of unspecified posterior cerebral artery 🔖

● **I63.44** Cerebral infarction due to embolism of cerebellar artery

   I63.441 Cerebral infarction due to embolism of right cerebellar artery 🔖

   I63.442 Cerebral infarction due to embolism of left cerebellar artery 🔖

   I63.443 Cerebral infarction due to embolism of bilateral cerebellar arteries 🔖

   I63.449 Cerebral infarction due to embolism of unspecified cerebellar artery 🔖

   I63.49 Cerebral infarction due to embolism of other cerebral artery 🔖

● **I63.5** Cerebral infarction due to unspecified occlusion or stenosis of cerebral arteries

   Ⓔⓧ For category I63.5 CC codes: See PDX Collection 688

   I63.50 Cerebral infarction due to unspecified occlusion or stenosis of unspecified cerebral artery 🔖

● **I63.51** Cerebral infarction due to unspecified occlusion or stenosis of middle cerebral artery

   I63.511 Cerebral infarction due to unspecified occlusion or stenosis of right middle cerebral artery 🔖

   I63.512 Cerebral infarction due to unspecified occlusion or stenosis of left middle cerebral artery 🔖

➡ I63.513 Cerebral infarction due to unspecified occlusion or stenosis of bilateral middle cerebral arteries 🔖

   I63.519 Cerebral infarction due to unspecified occlusion or stenosis of unspecified middle cerebral artery 🔖

● **I63.52** Cerebral infarction due to unspecified occlusion or stenosis of anterior cerebral artery

   I63.521 Cerebral infarction due to unspecified occlusion or stenosis of right anterior cerebral artery 🔖

   I63.522 Cerebral infarction due to unspecified occlusion or stenosis of left anterior cerebral artery 🔖

➡ I63.523 Cerebral infarction due to unspecified occlusion or stenosis of bilateral anterior cerebral arteries 🔖

   I63.529 Cerebral infarction due to unspecified occlusion or stenosis of unspecified anterior cerebral artery 🔖

● **I63.53** Cerebral infarction due to unspecified occlusion or stenosis of posterior cerebral artery

   I63.531 Cerebral infarction due to unspecified occlusion or stenosis of right posterior cerebral artery 🔖

   I63.532 Cerebral infarction due to unspecified occlusion or stenosis of left posterior cerebral artery 🔖

        Coding Clinic: 2017, Q2, P10

➡ I63.533 Cerebral infarction due to unspecified occlusion or stenosis of bilateral posterior cerebral arteries 🔖

   I63.539 Cerebral infarction due to unspecified occlusion or stenosis of unspecified posterior cerebral artery 🔖

● **I63.54**   Cerebral infarction due to unspecified occlusion or stenosis of cerebellar artery

    I63.541   Cerebral infarction due to unspecified occlusion or stenosis of right cerebellar artery 🏥

    I63.542   Cerebral infarction due to unspecified occlusion or stenosis of left cerebellar artery 🏥

    I63.543   Cerebral infarction due to unspecified occlusion or stenosis of bilateral cerebellar arteries 🏥

    I63.549   Cerebral infarction due to unspecified occlusion or stenosis of unspecified cerebellar artery 🏥

  I63.59   Cerebral infarction due to unspecified occlusion or stenosis of other cerebral artery 🏥

I63.6   Cerebral infarction due to cerebral venous thrombosis, nonpyogenic 🏥
   Ⓔ See PDX Collection 688

I63.8   Other cerebral infarction 🏥
   Ⓔ See PDX Collection 688
   Coding Clinic: 2017, Q2, P9

I63.9   Cerebral infarction, unspecified 🏥
   Stroke NOS

   ▶ **Excludes2**   transient cerebral ischemic attacks and related syndromes (G45.-)
   Ⓔ See PDX Collection 688
   Coding Clinic: 2016, Q4, P62; 2015, Q1, P26

● **I65**   Occlusion and stenosis of precerebral arteries, not resulting in cerebral infarction

   Includes   embolism of precerebral artery
      narrowing of precerebral artery
      obstruction (complete) (partial) of precerebral artery
      thrombosis of precerebral artery

   Excludes1   insufficiency, NOS, of precerebral artery (G45.-)
      insufficiency of precerebral arteries causing cerebral infarction (I63.0-I63.2)

● **I65.0**   Occlusion and stenosis of vertebral artery

  I65.01   Occlusion and stenosis of right vertebral artery

  I65.02   Occlusion and stenosis of left vertebral artery

  I65.03   Occlusion and stenosis of bilateral vertebral arteries

  I65.09   Occlusion and stenosis of unspecified vertebral artery

I65.1   Occlusion and stenosis of basilar artery

● **I65.2**   Occlusion and stenosis of carotid artery

  I65.21   Occlusion and stenosis of right carotid artery

  I65.22   Occlusion and stenosis of left carotid artery

  I65.23   Occlusion and stenosis of bilateral carotid arteries

  I65.29   Occlusion and stenosis of unspecified carotid artery

I65.8   Occlusion and stenosis of other precerebral arteries

I65.9   Occlusion and stenosis of unspecified precerebral artery
   Occlusion and stenosis of precerebral artery NOS

● **I66**   Occlusion and stenosis of cerebral arteries, not resulting in cerebral infarction

   Includes   embolism of cerebral artery
      narrowing of cerebral artery
      obstruction (complete) (partial) of cerebral artery
      thrombosis of cerebral artery

   Excludes1   occlusion and stenosis of cerebral artery causing cerebral infarction (I63.3-I63.5)

● **I66.0**   Occlusion and stenosis of middle cerebral artery

  I66.01   Occlusion and stenosis of right middle cerebral artery

  I66.02   Occlusion and stenosis of left middle cerebral artery

  I66.03   Occlusion and stenosis of bilateral middle cerebral arteries

  I66.09   Occlusion and stenosis of unspecified middle cerebral artery

● **I66.1**   Occlusion and stenosis of anterior cerebral artery

  I66.11   Occlusion and stenosis of right anterior cerebral artery

  I66.12   Occlusion and stenosis of left anterior cerebral artery

  I66.13   Occlusion and stenosis of bilateral anterior cerebral arteries

  I66.19   Occlusion and stenosis of unspecified anterior cerebral artery

● **I66.2**   Occlusion and stenosis of posterior cerebral artery

  I66.21   Occlusion and stenosis of right posterior cerebral artery

  I66.22   Occlusion and stenosis of left posterior cerebral artery

  I66.23   Occlusion and stenosis of bilateral posterior cerebral arteries

  I66.29   Occlusion and stenosis of unspecified posterior cerebral artery

I66.3   Occlusion and stenosis of cerebellar arteries

I66.8   Occlusion and stenosis of other cerebral arteries
   Occlusion and stenosis of perforating arteries

I66.9   Occlusion and stenosis of unspecified cerebral artery

● **I67**   Other cerebrovascular diseases

   Excludes2   sequelae of the listed conditions (I69.8)

I67.0   Dissection of cerebral arteries, nonruptured 🏥

   Excludes1   ruptured cerebral arteries (I60.7)
   Ⓔ See PDX Collection 689

I67.1   Cerebral aneurysm, nonruptured
   Cerebral aneurysm NOS
   Cerebral arteriovenous fistula, acquired
   Internal carotid artery aneurysm, intracranial portion
   Internal carotid artery aneurysm, NOS

   Excludes1   congenital cerebral aneurysm, nonruptured (Q28.-)
      ruptured cerebral aneurysm (I60.7)

I67.2   Cerebral atherosclerosis   A
   Atheroma of cerebral and precerebral arteries

I67.3   Progressive vascular leukoencephalopathy 🏥
   Binswanger's disease
   Ⓔ See PDX Collection 133

I67.4   Hypertensive encephalopathy 🏥

   ▶ **Excludes2**   insufficiency, NOS, of precerebral arteries (G45.2)
   Ⓔ See PDX Collection 690

I67.5   Moyamoya disease 🏥
   Ⓔ See PDX Collection 691

I67.6   Nonpyogenic thrombosis of intracranial venous system 🏥
   Nonpyogenic thrombosis of cerebral vein
   Nonpyogenic thrombosis of intracranial venous sinus

   Excludes1   nonpyogenic thrombosis of intracranial venous system causing infarction (I63.6)
   Ⓔ See PDX Collection 692

I67.7   Cerebral arteritis, not elsewhere classified 🏥
   Granulomatous angiitis of the nervous system

   Excludes1   allergic granulomatous angiitis (M30.1)
   Ⓔ See PDX Collection 693

N Newborn Age: 0   **P** Pediatric Age: 0–17   **M** Maternity DX: 12–55   **A** Adult Age: 15–124   ♀ Females Only   ♂ Males Only

🏥 Complication\Comorbidity   🏥 Major C\C   Ⓔ CC/MCC Exclusions   🏥 Hospital-Acquired Condition

887

● **I67.8**   **Other specified cerebrovascular diseases**

     I67.81   **Acute cerebrovascular insufficiency** 🔌
         Acute cerebrovascular insufficiency
           unspecified as to location or reversibility
         (Ex) See PDX Collection 694

     I67.82   **Cerebral ischemia** 🔌
         Chronic cerebral ischemia
         (Ex) See PDX Collection 694

     I67.83   **Posterior reversible encephalopathy syndrome** 🔌
         PRES
         (Ex) See PDX Collection 610

     ● **I67.84**   **Cerebral vasospasm and vasoconstriction**
         (Ex) For category I67.84 CC codes: See PDX Collection 586

         I67.841   **Reversible cerebrovascular vasoconstriction syndrome** 🔌
            Call-Fleming syndrome
            Code first underlying condition, if applicable, such as eclampsia (O15.00-O15.9)

         I67.848   **Other cerebrovascular vasospasm and vasoconstriction** 🔌

     I67.89   **Other cerebrovascular disease** 🔌
         (Ex) See PDX Collection 694

   I67.9   **Cerebrovascular disease, unspecified**

● **I68**   **Cerebrovascular disorders in diseases classified elsewhere**

   ▷ **I68.0**   *Cerebral amyloid angiopathy*
         Code first underlying amyloidosis (E85.-)

   ▷ **I68.2**   *Cerebral arteritis in other diseases classified elsewhere* 🔌
         Code first underlying disease
         Excludes1   cerebral arteritis (in):
              listerosis (A32.89)
              systemic lupus erythematosus (M32.19)
              syphilis (A52.04)
              tuberculosis (A18.89)
         (Ex) See PDX Collection 693

   ▷ **I68.8**   *Other cerebrovascular disorders in diseases classified elsewhere*
         Code first underlying disease
         Excludes1   syphilitic cerebral aneurysm (A52.05)

OGCR   Section I.c.9.d.

> Sequelae of Cerebrovascular Disease
>
> 1) Category I69, Sequelae of Cerebrovascular disease
>
> Category I69 is used to indicate conditions classifiable to categories I60-I67 as the causes of sequela (neurologic deficits), themselves classified elsewhere. These "late effects" include neurologic deficits that persist after initial onset of conditions classifiable to categories I60-I67. The neurologic deficits caused by cerebrovascular disease may be present from the onset of may arise at any time after the onset of the condition classifiable to categories I60-I67.
>
> Codes from category I69, Sequelae of cerebrovascular disease, that specify hemiplegia, hemiparesis and monoplegia identify whether the dominant or nondominant side is affected. Should the affected side be documented, but not specified as dominant or nondominant, and the classification system does not indicate a default, code selection is as follows:
>
> For ambidextrous patients, the default should be dominant.
>
> If the left side is affected, the default is non-dominant.
>
> If the right side is affected, the default is dominant.
>
> 2) Codes from category I69 with codes from I60-I67
>
> Codes from category I69 may be assigned on a health care record with codes from I60-I67, if the patient has a current cerebrovascular disease and deficits from an old cerebrovascular disease.

● **I69**   **Sequelae of cerebrovascular disease**

   Note: Category I69 is to be used to indicate conditions in I60-I67 as the cause of sequelae. The 'sequelae' include conditions specified as such or as residuals which may occur at any time after the onset of the causal condition.

   Excludes1   personal history of cerebral infarction without residual deficit (Z86.73)
         personal history of prolonged reversible ischemic neurologic deficit (PRIND) (Z86.73)
         personal history of reversible ischemic neurologcial deficit (RIND) (Z86.73)
         sequelae of traumatic intracranial injury (S06.-)
         ~~transient ischemic attack (TIA) (G45.9)~~

   Coding Clinic: 2016, Q4, P28; 2015, Q4, P40; 2012, Q4, P107

● **I69.0**   **Sequelae of nontraumatic subarachnoid hemorrhage**

     I69.00   **Unspecified sequelae of nontraumatic subarachnoid hemorrhage**

     ● **I69.01**   **Cognitive deficits following nontraumatic subarachnoid hemorrhage**

         I69.010   **Attention and concentration deficit following nontraumatic subarachnoid hemorrhage**

         I69.011   **Memory deficit following nontraumatic subarachnoid hemorrhage**

         I69.012   **Visuospatial deficit and spatial neglect following nontraumatic subarachnoid hemorrhage**

         I69.013   **Psychomotor deficit following nontraumatic subarachnoid hemorrhage**

         I69.014   **Frontal lobe and executive function deficit following nontraumatic subarachnoid hemorrhage**

         I69.015   **Cognitive social or emotional deficit following nontraumatic subarachnoid hemorrhage**

         I69.018   **Other symptoms and signs involving cognitive functions following nontraumatic subarachnoid hemorrhage**

         I69.019   **Unspecified symptoms and signs involving cognitive functions following nontraumatic subarachnoid hemorrhage**

     ● **I69.02**   **Speech and language deficits following nontraumatic subarachnoid hemorrhage**

         I69.020   **Aphasia following nontraumatic subarachnoid hemorrhage**

         I69.021   **Dysphasia following nontraumatic subarachnoid hemorrhage**

         I69.022   **Dysarthria following nontraumatic subarachnoid hemorrhage**

         I69.023   **Fluency disorder following nontraumatic subarachnoid hemorrhage**
            Stuttering following nontraumatic subarachnoid hemorrhage

         I69.028   **Other speech and language deficits following nontraumatic subarachnoid hemorrhage**

▶ New   ⇒ Revised   ~~deleted~~ Deleted   Excludes 1   Excludes 2   Includes   Use additional   Code first   Code also   Key words

OGCR Official Guidelines   ● Unacceptable Principal Diagnosis   X Assign placeholder X   ● Use Additional Character(s)   ▷ Manifestation Code   **Coding Clinic**

● **I69.03   Monoplegia of upper limb following nontraumatic subarachnoid hemorrhage**

  I69.031   Monoplegia of upper limb following nontraumatic subarachnoid hemorrhage affecting right dominant side

  I69.032   Monoplegia of upper limb following nontraumatic subarachnoid hemorrhage affecting left dominant side

  I69.033   Monoplegia of upper limb following nontraumatic subarachnoid hemorrhage affecting right non-dominant side

  I69.034   Monoplegia of upper limb following nontraumatic subarachnoid hemorrhage affecting left non-dominant side

  I69.039   Monoplegia of upper limb following nontraumatic subarachnoid hemorrhage affecting unspecified side

● **I69.04   Monoplegia of lower limb following nontraumatic subarachnoid hemorrhage**

  I69.041   Monoplegia of lower limb following nontraumatic subarachnoid hemorrhage affecting right dominant side

  I69.042   Monoplegia of lower limb following nontraumatic subarachnoid hemorrhage affecting left dominant side

  I69.043   Monoplegia of lower limb following nontraumatic subarachnoid hemorrhage affecting right non-dominant side

  I69.044   Monoplegia of lower limb following nontraumatic subarachnoid hemorrhage affecting left non-dominant side

  I69.049   Monoplegia of lower limb following nontraumatic subarachnoid hemorrhage affecting unspecified side

● **I69.05   Hemiplegia and hemiparesis following nontraumatic subarachnoid hemorrhage**

  I69.051   Hemiplegia and hemiparesis following nontraumatic subarachnoid hemorrhage affecting right dominant side 🔧
        (Ex) See PDX Collection 695

  I69.052   Hemiplegia and hemiparesis following nontraumatic subarachnoid hemorrhage affecting left dominant side 🔧
        (Ex) See PDX Collection 695

  I69.053   Hemiplegia and hemiparesis following nontraumatic subarachnoid hemorrhage affecting right non-dominant side 🔧
        (Ex) See PDX Collection 696

  I69.054   Hemiplegia and hemiparesis following nontraumatic subarachnoid hemorrhage affecting left non-dominant side 🔧
        (Ex) See PDX Collection 696

  I69.059   Hemiplegia and hemiparesis following nontraumatic subarachnoid hemorrhage affecting unspecified side 🔧
        (Ex) See PDX Collection 697

● **I69.06   Other paralytic syndrome following nontraumatic subarachnoid hemorrhage**

  Use additional code to identify type of paralytic syndrome, such as:
    locked-in state (G83.5)
    quadriplegia (G82.5-)

  Excludes1   hemiplegia/hemiparesis following nontraumatic subarachnoid hemorrhage (I69.05-)
        monoplegia of lower limb following nontraumatic subarachnoid hemorrhage (I69.04-)
        monoplegia of upper limb following nontraumatic subarachnoid hemorrhage (I69.03-)

  I69.061   Other paralytic syndrome following nontraumatic subarachnoid hemorrhage affecting right dominant side

  I69.062   Other paralytic syndrome following nontraumatic subarachnoid hemorrhage affecting left dominant side

  I69.063   Other paralytic syndrome following nontraumatic subarachnoid hemorrhage affecting right non-dominant side

  I69.064   Other paralytic syndrome following nontraumatic subarachnoid hemorrhage affecting left non-dominant side

  I69.065   Other paralytic syndrome following nontraumatic subarachnoid hemorrhage, bilateral

  I69.069   Other paralytic syndrome following nontraumatic subarachnoid hemorrhage affecting unspecified side

● **I69.09   Other sequelae of nontraumatic subarachnoid hemorrhage**

  I69.090   Apraxia following nontraumatic subarachnoid hemorrhage

  I69.091   Dysphagia following nontraumatic subarachnoid hemorrhage

    Use additional code to identify the type of dysphagia, if known (R13.1-)

  I69.092   Facial weakness following nontraumatic subarachnoid hemorrhage

    Facial droop following nontraumatic subarachnoid hemorrhage

  I69.093   Ataxia following nontraumatic subarachnoid hemorrhage

  I69.098   Other sequelae following nontraumatic subarachnoid hemorrhage

    Alterations of sensation following nontraumatic subarachnoid hemorrhage
    Disturbance of vision following nontraumatic subarachnoid hemorrhage

    Use additional code to identify the sequelae

N Newborn Age: 0   **P** Pediatric Age: 0–17   **M** Maternity DX: 12–55   **A** Adult Age: 15–124   ♀ Females Only   ♂ Males Only

🔧 Complication\Comorbidity   🔧 Major C\C   (Ex) CC/MCC Exclusions   🔧 Hospital-Acquired Condition

889

● **I69.1**   **Sequelae of nontraumatic intracerebral hemorrhage**

I69.10   Unspecified sequelae of nontraumatic intracerebral hemorrhage

● **I69.11**   Cognitive deficits following nontraumatic intracerebral hemorrhage

    I69.110   Attention and concentration deficit following nontraumatic intracerebral hemorrhage

    I69.111   Memory deficit following nontraumatic intracerebral hemorrhage

    I69.112   Visuospatial deficit and spatial neglect following nontraumatic intracerebral hemorrhage

    I69.113   Psychomotor deficit following nontraumatic intracerebral hemorrhage

    I69.114   Frontal lobe and executive function deficit following nontraumatic intracerebral hemorrhage

    I69.115   Cognitive social or emotional deficit following nontraumatic intracerebral hemorrhage

    I69.118   Other symptoms and signs involving cognitive functions following nontraumatic intracerebral hemorrhage

    I69.119   Unspecified symptoms and signs involving cognitive functions following nontraumatic intracerebral hemorrhage

● **I69.12**   Speech and language deficits following nontraumatic intracerebral hemorrhage

    I69.120   Aphasia following nontraumatic intracerebral hemorrhage

    I69.121   Dysphasia following nontraumatic intracerebral hemorrhage

    I69.122   Dysarthria following nontraumatic intracerebral hemorrhage

    I69.123   Fluency disorder following nontraumatic intracerebral hemorrhage
        Stuttering following nontraumatic intracerebral hemorrhage

    I69.128   Other speech and language deficits following nontraumatic intracerebral hemorrhage

● **I69.13**   Monoplegia of upper limb following nontraumatic intracerebral hemorrhage

    I69.131   Monoplegia of upper limb following nontraumatic intracerebral hemorrhage affecting right dominant side

    I69.132   Monoplegia of upper limb following nontraumatic intracerebral hemorrhage affecting left dominant side

    I69.133   Monoplegia of upper limb following nontraumatic intracerebral hemorrhage affecting right non-dominant side

    I69.134   Monoplegia of upper limb following nontraumatic intracerebral hemorrhage affecting left non-dominant side

    I69.139   Monoplegia of upper limb following nontraumatic intracerebral hemorrhage affecting unspecified side

● **I69.14**   Monoplegia of lower limb following nontraumatic intracerebral hemorrhage

    I69.141   Monoplegia of lower limb following nontraumatic intracerebral hemorrhage affecting right dominant side

    I69.142   Monoplegia of lower limb following nontraumatic intracerebral hemorrhage affecting left dominant side

    I69.143   Monoplegia of lower limb following nontraumatic intracerebral hemorrhage affecting right non-dominant side

    I69.144   Monoplegia of lower limb following nontraumatic intracerebral hemorrhage affecting left non-dominant side

    I69.149   Monoplegia of lower limb following nontraumatic intracerebral hemorrhage affecting unspecified side

● **I69.15**   Hemiplegia and hemiparesis following nontraumatic intracerebral hemorrhage

    I69.151   Hemiplegia and hemiparesis following nontraumatic intracerebral hemorrhage affecting right dominant side
        Ex: See PDX Collection 695

    I69.152   Hemiplegia and hemiparesis following nontraumatic intracerebral hemorrhage affecting left dominant side
        Ex: See PDX Collection 695

    I69.153   Hemiplegia and hemiparesis following nontraumatic intracerebral hemorrhage affecting right non-dominant side
        Ex: See PDX Collection 696

    I69.154   Hemiplegia and hemiparesis following nontraumatic intracerebral hemorrhage affecting left non-dominant side
        Ex: See PDX Collection 696

    I69.159   Hemiplegia and hemiparesis following nontraumatic intracerebral hemorrhage affecting unspecified side
        Ex: See PDX Collection 697

● **I69.16**   Other paralytic syndrome following nontraumatic intracerebral hemorrhage
    Use additional code to identify type of paralytic syndrome, such as:
    locked-in state (G83.5)
    quadriplegia (G82.5-)

    Excludes1   hemiplegia/hemiparesis following nontraumatic intracerebral hemorrhage (I69.15-)
        monoplegia of lower limb following nontraumatic intracerebral hemorrhage (I69.14-)
        monoplegia of upper limb following nontraumatic intracerebral hemorrhage (I69.13-)

    I69.161   Other paralytic syndrome following nontraumatic intracerebral hemorrhage affecting right dominant side

I69.162   Other paralytic syndrome following nontraumatic intracerebral hemorrhage affecting left dominant side

I69.163   Other paralytic syndrome following nontraumatic intracerebral hemorrhage affecting right non-dominant side

I69.164   Other paralytic syndrome following nontraumatic intracerebral hemorrhage affecting left non-dominant side

I69.165   Other paralytic syndrome following nontraumatic intracerebral hemorrhage, bilateral

I69.169   Other paralytic syndrome following nontraumatic intracerebral hemorrhage affecting unspecified side

● **I69.19**   **Other sequelae of nontraumatic intracerebral hemorrhage**

     I69.190   **Apraxia following nontraumatic intracerebral hemorrhage**

     I69.191   **Dysphagia following nontraumatic intracerebral hemorrhage**

         Use additional code to identify the type of dysphagia, if known (R13.1-)

     I69.192   **Facial weakness following nontraumatic intracerebral hemorrhage**

         Facial droop following nontraumatic intracerebral hemorrhage

     I69.193   **Ataxia following nontraumatic intracerebral hemorrhage**

     I69.198   **Other sequelae of nontraumatic intracerebral hemorrhage**

         Alteration of sensations following nontraumatic intracerebral hemorrhage

         Disturbance of vision following nontraumatic intracerebral hemorrhage

         Use additional code to identify the sequelae

● **I69.2**   **Sequelae of other nontraumatic intracranial hemorrhage**

     I69.20   **Unspecified sequelae of other nontraumatic intracranial hemorrhage**

    ● I69.21   **Cognitive deficits following other nontraumatic intracranial hemorrhage**

     I69.210   **Attention and concentration deficit following other nontraumatic intracranial hemorrhage**

     I69.211   **Memory deficit following other nontraumatic intracranial hemorrhage**

     I69.212   **Visuospatial deficit and spatial neglect following other nontraumatic intracranial hemorrhage**

     I69.213   **Psychomotor deficit following other nontraumatic intracranial hemorrhage**

     I69.214   **Frontal lobe and executive function deficit following other nontraumatic intracranial hemorrhage**

     I69.215   **Cognitive social or emotional deficit following other nontraumatic intracranial hemorrhage**

I69.218   Other symptoms and signs involving cognitive functions following other nontraumatic intracranial hemorrhage

I69.219   Unspecified symptoms and signs involving cognitive functions following other nontraumatic intracranial hemorrhage

● **I69.22**   **Speech and language deficits following other nontraumatic intracranial hemorrhage**

     I69.220   **Aphasia following other nontraumatic intracranial hemorrhage**

     I69.221   **Dysphasia following other nontraumatic intracranial hemorrhage**

     I69.222   **Dysarthria following other nontraumatic intracranial hemorrhage**

     I69.223   **Fluency disorder following other nontraumatic intracranial hemorrhage**

         Stuttering following other nontraumatic intracranial hemorrhage

     I69.228   **Other speech and language deficits following other nontraumatic intracranial hemorrhage**

● **I69.23**   **Monoplegia of upper limb following other nontraumatic intracranial hemorrhage**

     I69.231   **Monoplegia of upper limb following other nontraumatic intracranial hemorrhage affecting right dominant side**

     I69.232   **Monoplegia of upper limb following other nontraumatic intracranial hemorrhage affecting left dominant side**

     I69.233   **Monoplegia of upper limb following other nontraumatic intracranial hemorrhage affecting right non-dominant side**

     I69.234   **Monoplegia of upper limb following other nontraumatic intracranial hemorrhage affecting left non-dominant side**

     I69.239   **Monoplegia of upper limb following other nontraumatic intracranial hemorrhage affecting unspecified side**

● **I69.24**   **Monoplegia of lower limb following other nontraumatic intracranial hemorrhage**

     I69.241   **Monoplegia of lower limb following other nontraumatic intracranial hemorrhage affecting right dominant side**

     I69.242   **Monoplegia of lower limb following other nontraumatic intracranial hemorrhage affecting left dominant side**

     I69.243   **Monoplegia of lower limb following other nontraumatic intracranial hemorrhage affecting right non-dominant side**

     I69.244   **Monoplegia of lower limb following other nontraumatic intracranial hemorrhage affecting left non-dominant side**

     I69.249   **Monoplegia of lower limb following other nontraumatic intracranial hemorrhage affecting unspecified side**

CHAPTER 9 (I00-I99)

N   Newborn Age: 0   **P**   Pediatric Age: 0–17   **M**   Maternity DX: 12–55   **A**   Adult Age: 15–124   ♀   Females Only   ♂   Males Only

     Ⓒ   Complication\Comorbidity   ⓒ   Major C\C   (Ex)   CC/MCC Exclusions   Ⓗ   Hospital-Acquired Condition

891

● **I69.25**   **Hemiplegia and hemiparesis** following other nontraumatic intracranial hemorrhage

   I69.251   **Hemiplegia and hemiparesis following other nontraumatic intracranial hemorrhage affecting right dominant side** 🖐
     Ⓔ See PDX Collection 695

   I69.252   **Hemiplegia and hemiparesis following other nontraumatic intracranial hemorrhage affecting left dominant side** 🖐
     Ⓔ See PDX Collection 695

   I69.253   **Hemiplegia and hemiparesis following other nontraumatic intracranial hemorrhage affecting right non-dominant side** 🖐
     Ⓔ See PDX Collection 696

   I69.254   **Hemiplegia and hemiparesis following other nontraumatic intracranial hemorrhage affecting left non-dominant side** 🖐
     Ⓔ See PDX Collection 696

   I69.259   **Hemiplegia and hemiparesis following other nontraumatic intracranial hemorrhage affecting unspecified side** 🖐
     Ⓔ See PDX Collection 697

● **I69.26**   **Other paralytic syndrome** following other nontraumatic intracranial hemorrhage

   Use additional code to identify type of paralytic syndrome, such as:
     locked-in state (G83.5)
     quadriplegia (G82.5-)

   Excludes1   hemiplegia/hemiparesis following other nontraumatic intracranial hemorrhage (I69.25-)
     monoplegia of lower limb following other nontraumatic intracranial hemorrhage (I69.24-)
     monoplegia of upper limb following other nontraumatic intracranial hemorrhage (I69.23-)

   I69.261   **Other paralytic syndrome following other nontraumatic intracranial hemorrhage affecting right dominant side**

   I69.262   **Other paralytic syndrome following other nontraumatic intracranial hemorrhage affecting left dominant side**

   I69.263   **Other paralytic syndrome following other nontraumatic intracranial hemorrhage affecting right non-dominant side**

   I69.264   **Other paralytic syndrome following other nontraumatic intracranial hemorrhage affecting left non-dominant side**

   I69.265   **Other paralytic syndrome following other nontraumatic intracranial hemorrhage, bilateral**

   I69.269   **Other paralytic syndrome following other nontraumatic intracranial hemorrhage affecting unspecified side**

● **I69.29**   **Other sequelae** of other nontraumatic intracranial hemorrhage

   I69.290   **Apraxia following other nontraumatic intracranial hemorrhage**

   I69.291   **Dysphagia following other nontraumatic intracranial hemorrhage**
     Use additional code to identify the type of dysphagia, if known (R13.1-)

   I69.292   **Facial weakness following other nontraumatic intracranial hemorrhage**
     Facial droop following other nontraumatic intracranial hemorrhage

   I69.293   **Ataxia following other nontraumatic intracranial hemorrhage**

   I69.298   **Other sequelae of other nontraumatic intracranial hemorrhage**
     Alteration of sensation following other nontraumatic intracranial hemorrhage
     Disturbance of vision following other nontraumatic intracranial hemorrhage
     Use additional code to identify the sequelae

● **I69.3**   **Sequelae of cerebral infarction**
   Sequelae of stroke NOS
   Coding Clinic: 2012, Q4, P92, 95

   I69.30   **Unspecified sequelae of cerebral infarction**

● **I69.31**   **Cognitive deficits** following cerebral infarction

   I69.310   **Attention and concentration deficit following cerebral infarction**

   I69.311   **Memory deficit following cerebral infarction**

   I69.312   **Visuospatial deficit and spatial neglect following cerebral infarction**

   I69.313   **Psychomotor deficit following cerebral infarction**

   I69.314   **Frontal lobe and executive function deficit following cerebral infarction**

   I69.315   **Cognitive social or emotional deficit following cerebral infarction**

   I69.318   **Other symptoms and signs involving cognitive functions following cerebral infarction**

   I69.319   **Unspecified symptoms and signs involving cognitive functions following cerebral infarction**

● **I69.32**   **Speech and language deficits** following cerebral infarction

   I69.320   **Aphasia following cerebral infarction**

   I69.321   **Dysphasia following cerebral infarction**
     Coding Clinic: 2012, Q4, P91

   I69.322   **Dysarthria following cerebral infarction**
     ▶ **Excludes2**   transient ischemic attack (TIA) (G45.9)

   I69.323   **Fluency disorder following cerebral infarction**
     Stuttering following cerebral infarction

   I69.328   **Other speech and language deficits following cerebral infarction**

CHAPTER 9 (I00-I99)

● **I69.33** **Monoplegia of upper limb** following cerebral infarction
Coding Clinic: 2017, Q1, P47

     I69.331   Monoplegia of upper limb following cerebral infarction affecting **right dominant side**

     I69.332   Monoplegia of upper limb following cerebral infarction affecting **left dominant side**

     I69.333   Monoplegia of upper limb following cerebral infarction affecting **right non-dominant side**

     I69.334   Monoplegia of upper limb following cerebral infarction affecting **left non-dominant side**

     I69.339   Monoplegia of upper limb following cerebral infarction affecting **unspecified side**

● **I69.34** **Monoplegia of lower limb** following cerebral infarction
Coding Clinic: 2017, Q1, P47

     I69.341   Monoplegia of lower limb following cerebral infarction affecting **right dominant side**

     I69.342   Monoplegia of lower limb following cerebral infarction affecting **left dominant side**

     I69.343   Monoplegia of lower limb following cerebral infarction affecting **right non-dominant side**

     I69.344   Monoplegia of lower limb following cerebral infarction affecting **left non-dominant side**

     I69.349   Monoplegia of lower limb following cerebral infarction affecting **unspecified side**

● **I69.35** **Hemiplegia and hemiparesis** following cerebral infarction

     I69.351   Hemiplegia and hemiparesis following cerebral infarction affecting **right dominant side** 🦠

         ▶ **Excludes2**   transient ischemic attack (TIA) (G45.9)
         (Ex:) See PDX Collection 695
         Coding Clinic: 2015, Q1, P25

     I69.352   Hemiplegia and hemiparesis following cerebral infarction affecting **left dominant side** 🦠
         (Ex:) See PDX Collection 695

     I69.353   Hemiplegia and hemiparesis following cerebral infarction affecting **right non-dominant side** 🦠
         (Ex:) See PDX Collection 696

     I69.354   Hemiplegia and hemiparesis following cerebral infarction affecting **left non-dominant side** 🦠
         (Ex:) See PDX Collection 696
         Coding Clinic: 2012, Q4, P91

     I69.359   Hemiplegia and hemiparesis following cerebral infarction affecting **unspecified side** 🦠
         (Ex:) See PDX Collection 697

● **I69.36** **Other paralytic syndrome** following cerebral infarction
Use additional code to identify type of paralytic syndrome, such as:
locked-in state (G83.5)
quadriplegia (G82.5-)

     Excludes1   hemiplegia/hemiparesis following cerebral infarction (I69.35-)
         monoplegia of lower limb following cerebral infarction (I69.34-)
         monoplegia of upper limb following cerebral infarction (I69.33-)

     I69.361   Other paralytic syndrome following cerebral infarction affecting **right dominant side**

     I69.362   Other paralytic syndrome following cerebral infarction affecting **left dominant side**

     I69.363   Other paralytic syndrome following cerebral infarction affecting **right non-dominant side**

     I69.364   Other paralytic syndrome following cerebral infarction affecting **left non-dominant side**

     I69.365   Other paralytic syndrome following cerebral infarction, **bilateral**

     I69.369   Other paralytic syndrome following cerebral infarction affecting **unspecified side**

● **I69.39** **Other sequelae** of cerebral infarction

     I69.390   **Apraxia** following cerebral infarction

     I69.391   **Dysphagia** following cerebral infarction
         Use additional code to identify the type of dysphagia, if known (R13.1-)

     I69.392   **Facial weakness** following cerebral infarction
         Facial droop following cerebral infarction

     I69.393   **Ataxia** following cerebral infarction

     I69.398   **Other sequelae** of cerebral infarction
         Alteration of sensation following cerebral infarction
         Disturbance of vision following cerebral infarction
         Use additional code to identify the sequelae

● **I69.8** **Sequelae of other cerebrovascular diseases**
     Excludes1   sequelae of traumatic intracranial injury (S06.-)

     I69.80   **Unspecified sequelae** of other cerebrovascular disease

● **I69.81** **Cognitive deficits** following other cerebrovascular disease

     I69.810   **Attention and concentration** deficit following other cerebrovascular disease

     I69.811   **Memory** deficit following other cerebrovascular disease

     I69.812   **Visuospatial** deficit and spatial neglect following other cerebrovascular disease

CHAPTER 9 (I00-I99)

	I69.813	Psychomotor deficit following other cerebrovascular disease
	I69.814	Frontal lobe and executive function deficit following other cerebrovascular disease
	I69.815	Cognitive social or emotional deficit following other cerebrovascular disease
	I69.818	Other symptoms and signs involving cognitive functions following other cerebrovascular disease
	I69.819	Unspecified symptoms and signs involving cognitive functions following other cerebrovascular disease

● I69.82   **Speech and language** deficits following other cerebrovascular disease

	I69.820	Aphasia following other cerebrovascular disease
	I69.821	Dysphasia following other cerebrovascular disease
	I69.822	Dysarthria following other cerebrovascular disease
	I69.823	Fluency disorder following other cerebrovascular disease Stuttering following other cerebrovascular disease
	I69.828	Other speech and language deficits following other cerebrovascular disease

● I69.83   **Monoplegia of upper limb** following other cerebrovascular disease

	I69.831	Monoplegia of upper limb following other cerebrovascular disease affecting **right dominant side**
	I69.832	Monoplegia of upper limb following other cerebrovascular disease affecting **left dominant side**
	I69.833	Monoplegia of upper limb following other cerebrovascular disease affecting **right non-dominant side**
	I69.834	Monoplegia of upper limb following other cerebrovascular disease affecting **left non-dominant side**
	I69.839	Monoplegia of upper limb following other cerebrovascular disease affecting **unspecified** side

● I69.84   **Monoplegia of lower limb** following other cerebrovascular disease

	I69.841	Monoplegia of lower limb following other cerebrovascular disease affecting **right dominant side**
	I69.842	Monoplegia of lower limb following other cerebrovascular disease affecting **left dominant side**
	I69.843	Monoplegia of lower limb following other cerebrovascular disease affecting **right non-dominant side**
	I69.844	Monoplegia of lower limb following other cerebrovascular disease affecting **left non-dominant side**
	I69.849	Monoplegia of lower limb following other cerebrovascular disease affecting **unspecified** side

● I69.85   **Hemiplegia and hemiparesis** following other cerebrovascular disease

	I69.851	Hemiplegia and hemiparesis following other cerebrovascular disease affecting **right dominant side** Ex: See PDX Collection 695
	I69.852	Hemiplegia and hemiparesis following other cerebrovascular disease affecting **left dominant side** Ex: See PDX Collection 695
	I69.853	Hemiplegia and hemiparesis following other cerebrovascular disease affecting **right non-dominant side** Ex: See PDX Collection 696
	I69.854	Hemiplegia and hemiparesis following other cerebrovascular disease affecting **left non-dominant side** Ex: See PDX Collection 696
	I69.859	Hemiplegia and hemiparesis following other cerebrovascular disease affecting **unspecified side** Ex: See PDX Collection 697

● I69.86   **Other paralytic syndrome** following other cerebrovascular disease

Use additional code to identify type of paralytic syndrome, such as:
locked-in state (G83.5)
quadriplegia (G82.5-)

Excludes1   hemiplegia/hemiparesis following other cerebrovascular disease (I69.85-)
monoplegia of lower limb following other cerebrovascular disease (I69.84-)
monoplegia of upper limb following other cerebrovascular disease (I69.83-)

	I69.861	Other paralytic syndrome following other cerebrovascular disease affecting **right dominant side**
	I69.862	Other paralytic syndrome following other cerebrovascular disease affecting **left dominant side**
	I69.863	Other paralytic syndrome following other cerebrovascular disease affecting **right non-dominant side**
	I69.864	Other paralytic syndrome following other cerebrovascular disease affecting **left non-dominant side**
	I69.865	Other paralytic syndrome following other cerebrovascular disease, **bilateral**
	I69.869	Other paralytic syndrome following other cerebrovascular disease affecting **unspecified** side

▶ New   ⟫ Revised   ~~deleted~~ Deleted   Excludes 1   Excludes 2   Includes   Use additional   Code first   Code also   Key words
OGCR Official Guidelines   ● Unacceptable Principal Diagnosis   X Assign placeholder X   ● Use Additional Character(s)   ▌ Manifestation Code   **Coding Clinic**

● I69.89 Other sequelae of other cerebrovascular disease
 I69.890 Apraxia following other cerebrovascular disease
 I69.891 Dysphagia following other cerebrovascular disease
  Use additional code to identify the type of dysphagia, if known (R13.1-)
 I69.892 Facial weakness following other cerebrovascular disease
  Facial droop following other cerebrovascular disease
 I69.893 Ataxia following other cerebrovascular disease
 I69.898 Other sequelae of other cerebrovascular disease
  Alteration of sensation following other cerebrovascular disease
  Disturbance of vision following other cerebrovascular disease
  Use additional code to identify the sequelae

● I69.9 Sequelae of unspecified cerebrovascular diseases
 Excludes1 sequelae of stroke (I69.3)
  sequelae of traumatic intracranial injury (S06.-)
 I69.90 Unspecified sequelae of unspecified cerebrovascular disease
● I69.91 Cognitive deficits following unspecified cerebrovascular disease
 I69.910 Attention and concentration deficit following unspecified cerebrovascular disease
 I69.911 Memory deficit following unspecified cerebrovascular disease
 I69.912 Visuospatial deficit and spatial neglect following unspecified cerebrovascular disease
 I69.913 Psychomotor deficit following unspecified cerebrovascular disease
 I69.914 Frontal lobe and executive function deficit following unspecified cerebrovascular disease
 I69.915 Cognitive social or emotional deficit following unspecified cerebrovascular disease
 I69.918 Other symptoms and signs involving cognitive functions following unspecified cerebrovascular disease
 I69.919 Unspecified symptoms and signs involving cognitive functions following unspecified cerebrovascular disease
● I69.92 Speech and language deficits following unspecified cerebrovascular disease
 I69.920 Aphasia following unspecified cerebrovascular disease
 I69.921 Dysphasia following unspecified cerebrovascular disease
 I69.922 Dysarthria following unspecified cerebrovascular disease
 I69.923 Fluency disorder following unspecified cerebrovascular disease
  Stuttering following unspecified cerebrovascular disease
 I69.928 Other speech and language deficits following unspecified cerebrovascular disease

● I69.93 Monoplegia of upper limb following unspecified cerebrovascular disease
 I69.931 Monoplegia of upper limb following unspecified cerebrovascular disease affecting right dominant side
 I69.932 Monoplegia of upper limb following unspecified cerebrovascular disease affecting left dominant side
 I69.933 Monoplegia of upper limb following unspecified cerebrovascular disease affecting right non-dominant side
 I69.934 Monoplegia of upper limb following unspecified cerebrovascular disease affecting left non-dominant side
 I69.939 Monoplegia of upper limb following unspecified cerebrovascular disease affecting unspecified side
● I69.94 Monoplegia of lower limb following unspecified cerebrovascular disease
 I69.941 Monoplegia of lower limb following unspecified cerebrovascular disease affecting right dominant side
 I69.942 Monoplegia of lower limb following unspecified cerebrovascular disease affecting left dominant side
 I69.943 Monoplegia of lower limb following unspecified cerebrovascular disease affecting right non-dominant side
 I69.944 Monoplegia of lower limb following unspecified cerebrovascular disease affecting left non-dominant side
 I69.949 Monoplegia of lower limb following unspecified cerebrovascular disease affecting unspecified side
● I69.95 Hemiplegia and hemiparesis following unspecified cerebrovascular disease
 I69.951 Hemiplegia and hemiparesis following unspecified cerebrovascular disease affecting right dominant side
  (Ex) See PDX Collection 695
 I69.952 Hemiplegia and hemiparesis following unspecified cerebrovascular disease affecting left dominant side
  (Ex) See PDX Collection 695
 I69.953 Hemiplegia and hemiparesis following unspecified cerebrovascular disease affecting right non-dominant side
  (Ex) See PDX Collection 696
 I69.954 Hemiplegia and hemiparesis following unspecified cerebrovascular disease affecting left non-dominant side
  (Ex) See PDX Collection 696
 I69.959 Hemiplegia and hemiparesis following unspecified cerebrovascular disease affecting unspecified side
  (Ex) See PDX Collection 697

CHAPTER 9 (I00-I99)

CHAPTER 9 (I00-I99)

● **I69.96** **Other paralytic syndrome following unspecified cerebrovascular disease**

Use additional code to identify type of paralytic syndrome, such as:
locked-in state (G83.5)
quadriplegia (G82.5-)

Excludes1 hemiplegia/hemiparesis following unspecified cerebrovascular disease (I69.95-)
monoplegia of lower limb following unspecified cerebrovascular disease (I69.94-)
monoplegia of upper limb following unspecified cerebrovascular disease (I69.93-)

I69.961 Other paralytic syndrome following unspecified cerebrovascular disease affecting right dominant side

I69.962 Other paralytic syndrome following unspecified cerebrovascular disease affecting left dominant side

I69.963 Other paralytic syndrome following unspecified cerebrovascular disease affecting right non-dominant side

I69.964 Other paralytic syndrome following unspecified cerebrovascular disease affecting left non-dominant side

I69.965 Other paralytic syndrome following unspecified cerebrovascular disease, bilateral

I69.969 Other paralytic syndrome following unspecified cerebrovascular disease affecting unspecified side

● **I69.99** **Other sequelae of unspecified cerebrovascular disease**

I69.990 Apraxia following unspecified cerebrovascular disease

I69.991 Dysphagia following unspecified cerebrovascular disease

Use additional code to identify the type of dysphagia, if known (R13.1-)

I69.992 Facial weakness following unspecified cerebrovascular disease
Facial droop following unspecified cerebrovascular disease

I69.993 Ataxia following unspecified cerebrovascular disease

I69.998 Other sequelae following unspecified cerebrovascular disease
Alteration in sensation following unspecified cerebrovascular disease
Disturbance of vision following unspecified cerebrovascular disease
Use additional code to identify the sequelae

DISEASES OF ARTERIES, ARTERIOLES AND CAPILLARIES (I70-I79)

● **I70** **Atherosclerosis**

Includes arteriolosclerosis
arterial degeneration
arteriosclerosis
arteriosclerotic vascular disease
arteriovascular degeneration
atheroma
endarteritis deformans or obliterans
senile arteritis
senile endarteritis
vascular degeneration

Use additional code to identify:
exposure to environmental tobacco smoke (Z77.22)
history of tobacco dependence (Z87.891)
occupational exposure to environmental tobacco smoke (Z57.31)
tobacco dependence (F17.-)
tobacco use (Z72.0)

Excludes2 arteriosclerotic cardiovascular disease (I25.1-)
arteriosclerotic heart disease (I25.1-)
atheroembolism (I75.-)
cerebral atherosclerosis (I67.2)
coronary atherosclerosis (I25.1-)
mesenteric atherosclerosis (K55.1)
precerebral atherosclerosis (I67.2)
primary pulmonary atherosclerosis (I27.0)

I70.0 **Atherosclerosis of aorta** A

I70.1 **Atherosclerosis of renal artery** A
Goldblatt's kidney

Excludes2 atherosclerosis of renal arterioles (I12.-)

★ **(See Plates 500, 501, and 502 on pages 60 – 62.)**

● **I70.2** **Atherosclerosis of native arteries of the extremities**
Mönckeberg's (medial) sclerosis

Use additional code, if applicable, to identify chronic total occlusion of artery of extremity (I70.92)

Excludes2 atherosclerosis of bypass graft of extremities (I70.30-I70.79)

● **I70.20** **Unspecified atherosclerosis of native arteries of extremities**

I70.201 Unspecified atherosclerosis of native arteries of extremities, right leg A

I70.202 Unspecified atherosclerosis of native arteries of extremities, left leg A

I70.203 Unspecified atherosclerosis of native arteries of extremities, bilateral legs A

I70.208 Unspecified atherosclerosis of native arteries of extremities, other extremity A

I70.209 Unspecified atherosclerosis of native arteries of extremities, unspecified extremity A

● **I70.21** **Atherosclerosis of native arteries of extremities with intermittent claudication**

I70.211 Atherosclerosis of native arteries of extremities with intermittent claudication, right leg A

I70.212 Atherosclerosis of native arteries of extremities with intermittent claudication, left leg A

I70.213 Atherosclerosis of native arteries of extremities with intermittent claudication, bilateral legs A

I70.218 Atherosclerosis of native arteries of extremities with intermittent claudication, other extremity A

I70.219 Atherosclerosis of native arteries of extremities with intermittent claudication, unspecified extremity A

▶ New   ⇒ Revised   ~~deleted~~ Deleted   Excludes 1   Excludes 2   Includes   Use additional   Code first   Code also   Key words

OGCR Official Guidelines   ● Unacceptable Principal Diagnosis   X Assign placeholder X   ● Use Additional Character(s)   ▶ Manifestation Code   **Coding Clinic**

● **I70.22**   **Atherosclerosis of native arteries of extremities with rest pain**
> **Includes**   any condition classifiable to I70.21-

   I70.221   **Atherosclerosis of native arteries of extremities with rest pain, right leg**   A

   I70.222   **Atherosclerosis of native arteries of extremities with rest pain, left leg**   A

   I70.223   **Atherosclerosis of native arteries of extremities with rest pain, bilateral legs**   A

   I70.228   **Atherosclerosis of native arteries of extremities with rest pain, other extremity**   A

   I70.229   **Atherosclerosis of native arteries of extremities with rest pain, unspecified extremity**   A

● **I70.23**   **Atherosclerosis of native arteries of right leg with ulceration**
> **Includes**   any condition classifiable to I70.211 and I70.221

Use additional code to identify severity of ulcer (L97.-)

   I70.231   **Atherosclerosis of native arteries of right leg with ulceration of thigh**   A

   I70.232   **Atherosclerosis of native arteries of right leg with ulceration of calf**   A

   I70.233   **Atherosclerosis of native arteries of right leg with ulceration of ankle**   A

   I70.234   **Atherosclerosis of native arteries of right leg with ulceration of heel and midfoot**   A
> Atherosclerosis of native arteries of right leg with ulceration of plantar surface of midfoot

   I70.235   **Atherosclerosis of native arteries of right leg with ulceration of other part of foot**   A
> Atherosclerosis of native arteries of right leg extremities with ulceration of toe

   I70.238   **Atherosclerosis of native arteries of right leg with ulceration of other part of lower right leg**   A

   I70.239   **Atherosclerosis of native arteries of right leg with ulceration of unspecified site**   A

● **I70.24**   **Atherosclerosis of native arteries of left leg with ulceration**
> **Includes**   any condition classifiable to I70.212 and I70.222

Use additional code to identify severity of ulcer (L97.-)

   I70.241   **Atherosclerosis of native arteries of left leg with ulceration of thigh**   A

   I70.242   **Atherosclerosis of native arteries of left leg with ulceration of calf**   A

   I70.243   **Atherosclerosis of native arteries of left leg with ulceration of ankle**   A

   I70.244   **Atherosclerosis of native arteries of left leg with ulceration of heel and midfoot**   A
> Atherosclerosis of native arteries of left leg with ulceration of plantar surface of midfoot

   I70.245   **Atherosclerosis of native arteries of left leg with ulceration of other part of foot**   A
> Atherosclerosis of native arteries of left leg extremities with ulceration of toe

   I70.248   **Atherosclerosis of native arteries of left leg with ulceration of other part of lower left leg**   A

   I70.249   **Atherosclerosis of native arteries of left leg with ulceration of unspecified site**   A

  I70.25   **Atherosclerosis of native arteries of other extremities with ulceration**   A
> **Includes**   any condition classifiable to I70.218 and I70.228

Use additional code to identify the severity of the ulcer (L98.49-)

● **I70.26**   **Atherosclerosis of native arteries of extremities with gangrene**
> **Includes**   any condition classifiable to I70.21-, I70.22-, I70.23-, I70.24-, and I70.25-

Use additional code to identify the severity of any ulcer (L97.-, L98.49-), if applicable

(Ex) For category I70.26 CC codes: See PDX Collection 519

   I70.261   **Atherosclerosis of native arteries of extremities with gangrene, right leg** 🔗   A

   I70.262   **Atherosclerosis of native arteries of extremities with gangrene, left leg** 🔗 A

   I70.263   **Atherosclerosis of native arteries of extremities with gangrene, bilateral legs** 🔗   A

   I70.268   **Atherosclerosis of native arteries of extremities with gangrene, other extremity** 🔗   A

   I70.269   **Atherosclerosis of native arteries of extremities with gangrene, unspecified extremity** 🔗   A

● **I70.29**   **Other atherosclerosis of native arteries of extremities**

   I70.291   **Other atherosclerosis of native arteries of extremities, right leg**

   I70.292   **Other atherosclerosis of native arteries of extremities, left leg**

   I70.293   **Other atherosclerosis of native arteries of extremities, bilateral legs**   A

   I70.298   **Other atherosclerosis of native arteries of extremities, other extremity**   A

   I70.299   **Other atherosclerosis of native arteries of extremities, unspecified extremity**

● **I70.3**   **Atherosclerosis of unspecified type of bypass graft(s) of the extremities**

> Use additional code, if applicable, to identify chronic total occlusion of artery of extremity (I70.92)

> **Excludes1**   embolism or thrombus of bypass graft(s) of extremities (T82.8-)

● **I70.30**   **Unspecified atherosclerosis of unspecified type of bypass graft(s) of the extremities**

   70.301   **Unspecified atherosclerosis of unspecified type of bypass graft(s) of the extremities, right leg**   A

   I70.302   **Unspecified atherosclerosis of unspecified type of bypass graft(s) of the extremities, left leg**   A

I70.303   Unspecified atherosclerosis of unspecified type of bypass graft(s) of the extremities, bilateral legs   A

I70.308   Unspecified atherosclerosis of unspecified type of bypass graft(s) of the extremities, other extremity   A

I70.309   Unspecified atherosclerosis of unspecified type of bypass graft(s) of the extremities, unspecified extremity   A

● I70.31   Atherosclerosis of unspecified type of bypass graft(s) of the extremities with intermittent claudication

I70.311   Atherosclerosis of unspecified type of bypass graft(s) of the extremities with intermittent claudication, right leg   A

I70.312   Atherosclerosis of unspecified type of bypass graft(s) of the extremities with intermittent claudication, left leg   A

I70.313   Atherosclerosis of unspecified type of bypass graft(s) of the extremities with intermittent claudication, bilateral legs   A

I70.318   Atherosclerosis of unspecified type of bypass graft(s) of the extremities with intermittent claudication, other extremity   A

I70.319   Atherosclerosis of unspecified type of bypass graft(s) of the extremities with intermittent claudication, unspecified extremity   A

● I70.32   Atherosclerosis of unspecified type of bypass graft(s) of the extremities with rest pain

Includes   any condition classifiable to I70.31-

I70.321   Atherosclerosis of unspecified type of bypass graft(s) of the extremities with rest pain, right leg   A

I70.322   Atherosclerosis of unspecified type of bypass graft(s) of the extremities with rest pain, left leg   A

I70.323   Atherosclerosis of unspecified type of bypass graft(s) of the extremities with rest pain, bilateral legs   A

I70.328   Atherosclerosis of unspecified type of bypass graft(s) of the extremities with rest pain, other extremity   A

I70.329   Atherosclerosis of unspecified type of bypass graft(s) of the extremities with rest pain, unspecified extremity   A

● I70.33   Atherosclerosis of unspecified type of bypass graft(s) of the right leg with ulceration

Includes   any condition classifiable to I70.311 and I70.321

Use additional code to identify severity of ulcer (L97.-)

Ex) For category I70.33 CC codes: See PDX Collection 698

I70.331   Atherosclerosis of unspecified type of bypass graft(s) of the right leg with ulceration of thigh   A
CC when PDx is its own CC

I70.332   Atherosclerosis of unspecified type of bypass graft(s) of the right leg with ulceration of calf   A
CC when PDx is its own CC

I70.333   Atherosclerosis of unspecified type of bypass graft(s) of the right leg with ulceration of ankle   A
CC when PDx is its own CC

I70.334   Atherosclerosis of unspecified type of bypass graft(s) of the right leg with ulceration of heel and midfoot   A
Atherosclerosis of unspecified type of bypass graft(s) of right leg with ulceration of plantar surface of midfoot
CC when PDx is its own CC

I70.335   Atherosclerosis of unspecified type of bypass graft(s) of the right leg with ulceration of other part of foot   A
Atherosclerosis of unspecified type of bypass graft(s) of the right leg with ulceration of toe

I70.338   Atherosclerosis of unspecified type of bypass graft(s) of the right leg with ulceration of other part of lower leg   A
CC when PDx is its own CC

I70.339   Atherosclerosis of unspecified type of bypass graft(s) of the right leg with ulceration of unspecified site   A
CC when PDx is its own CC

● I70.34   Atherosclerosis of unspecified type of bypass graft(s) of the left leg with ulceration

Includes   any condition classifiable to I70.312 and I70.322

Use additional code to identify severity of ulcer (L97.-)

Ex) For category I70.34 CC codes: See PDX Collection 698

I70.341   Atherosclerosis of unspecified type of bypass graft(s) of the left leg with ulceration of thigh   A
CC when PDx is its own CC

I70.342   Atherosclerosis of unspecified type of bypass graft(s) of the left leg with ulceration of calf   A
CC when PDx is its own CC

I70.343   Atherosclerosis of unspecified type of bypass graft(s) of the left leg with ulceration of ankle   A
CC when PDx is its own CC

I70.344   Atherosclerosis of unspecified type of bypass graft(s) of the left leg with ulceration of heel and midfoot   A
Atherosclerosis of unspecified type of bypass graft(s) of left leg with ulceration of plantar surface of midfoot
CC when PDx is its own CC

I70.345   Atherosclerosis of unspecified type of bypass graft(s) of the left leg with ulceration of other part of foot
Atherosclerosis of unspecified type of bypass graft(s) of the left leg with ulceration of toe

I70.348   Atherosclerosis of unspecified type of bypass graft(s) of the left leg with ulceration of other part of lower leg   A
CC when PDx is its own CC

I70.349   Atherosclerosis of unspecified type of bypass graft(s) of the left leg with ulceration of unspecified site   A
CC when PDx is its own CC

I70.35   Atherosclerosis of unspecified type of bypass graft(s) of other extremity with ulceration   A

Includes   any condition classifiable to I70.318 and I70.328

Use additional code to identify severity of ulcer (L98.49-)

● **I70.36** **Atherosclerosis of unspecified type of bypass graft(s) of the extremities with gangrene**

  Includes any condition classifiable to I70.31-, I70.32-, I70.33-, I70.34-, I70.35

  Use additional code to identify the severity of any ulcer (L97.-, L98.49-), if applicable

  Ex: For category I70.36 CC codes: See PDX Collection 519

  I70.361 Atherosclerosis of unspecified type of bypass graft(s) of the extremities with gangrene, right leg 🔵　　A
    CC when PDx is its own CC

  I70.362 Atherosclerosis of unspecified type of bypass graft(s) of the extremities with gangrene, left leg 🔵　　A
    CC when PDx is its own CC

  I70.363 Atherosclerosis of unspecified type of bypass graft(s) of the extremities with gangrene, bilateral legs 🔵　　A
    CC when PDx is its own CC

  I70.368 Atherosclerosis of unspecified type of bypass graft(s) of the extremities with gangrene, other extremity 🔵　　A
    CC when PDx is its own CC

  I70.369 Atherosclerosis of unspecified type of bypass graft(s) of the extremities with gangrene, unspecified extremity 🔵　　A
    CC when PDx is its own CC

● **I70.39** **Other atherosclerosis of unspecified type of bypass graft(s) of the extremities**

  I70.391 Other atherosclerosis of unspecified type of bypass graft(s) of the extremities, right leg　　A

  I70.392 Other atherosclerosis of unspecified type of bypass graft(s) of the extremities, left leg　　A

  I70.393 Other atherosclerosis of unspecified type of bypass graft(s) of the extremities, bilateral legs　　A

  I70.398 Other atherosclerosis of unspecified type of bypass graft(s) of the extremities, other extremity　　A

  I70.399 Other atherosclerosis of unspecified type of bypass graft(s) of the extremities, unspecified extremity　　A

● **I70.4** **Atherosclerosis of autologous vein bypass graft(s) of the extremities**

  Use additional code, if applicable, to identify chronic total occlusion of artery of extremity (I70.92)

● **I70.40** **Unspecified atherosclerosis of autologous vein bypass graft(s) of the extremities**

  I70.401 Unspecified atherosclerosis of autologous vein bypass graft(s) of the extremities, right leg　　A

  I70.402 Unspecified atherosclerosis of autologous vein bypass graft(s) of the extremities, left leg　　A

  I70.403 Unspecified atherosclerosis of autologous vein bypass graft(s) of the extremities, bilateral legs　　A

  I70.408 Unspecified atherosclerosis of autologous vein bypass graft(s) of the extremities, other extremity　　A

  I70.409 Unspecified atherosclerosis of autologous vein bypass graft(s) of the extremities, unspecified extremity　　A

● **I70.41** **Atherosclerosis of autologous vein bypass graft(s) of the extremities with intermittent claudication**

  I70.411 Atherosclerosis of autologous vein bypass graft(s) of the extremities with intermittent claudication, right leg　　A

  I70.412 Atherosclerosis of autologous vein bypass graft(s) of the extremities with intermittent claudication, left leg　　A

  I70.413 Atherosclerosis of autologous vein bypass graft(s) of the extremities with intermittent claudication, bilateral legs　　A

  I70.418 Atherosclerosis of autologous vein bypass graft(s) of the extremities with intermittent claudication, other extremity　　A

  I70.419 Atherosclerosis of autologous vein bypass graft(s) of the extremities with intermittent claudication, unspecified extremity　　A

● **I70.42** **Atherosclerosis of autologous vein bypass graft(s) of the extremities with rest pain**

  Includes any condition classifiable to I70.41-

  I70.421 Atherosclerosis of autologous vein bypass graft(s) of the extremities with rest pain, right leg　　A

  I70.422 Atherosclerosis of autologous vein bypass graft(s) of the extremities with rest pain, left leg　　A

  I70.423 Atherosclerosis of autologous vein bypass graft(s) of the extremities with rest pain, bilateral legs　　A

  I70.428 Atherosclerosis of autologous vein bypass graft(s) of the extremities with rest pain, other extremity　　A

  I70.429 Atherosclerosis of autologous vein bypass graft(s) of the extremities with rest pain, unspecified extremity　　A

● **I70.43** **Atherosclerosis of autologous vein bypass graft(s) of the right leg with ulceration**

  Includes any condition classifiable to I70.411 and I70.421

  Use additional code to identify severity of ulcer (L97.-)

  Ex: For category I70.43 CC codes: See PDX Collection 698

  I70.431 Atherosclerosis of autologous vein bypass graft(s) of the right leg with ulceration of thigh 🔵　　A
    CC when PDx is its own CC

  I70.432 Atherosclerosis of autologous vein bypass graft(s) of the right leg with ulceration of calf 🔵　　A
    CC when PDx is its own CC

  I70.433 Atherosclerosis of autologous vein bypass graft(s) of the right leg with ulceration of ankle 🔵　　A
    CC when PDx is its own CC

  I70.434 Atherosclerosis of autologous vein bypass graft(s) of the right leg with ulceration of heel and midfoot 🔵　　A
    Atherosclerosis of autologous vein bypass graft(s) of right leg with ulceration of plantar surface of midfoot
    CC when PDx is its own CC

CHAPTER 9 (I00-I99)

N Newborn Age: 0　　**P** Pediatric Age: 0–17　　**M** Maternity DX: 12–55　　**A** Adult Age: 15–124　　♀ Females Only　　♂ Males Only

🔵 Complication\Comorbidity　　🔵 Major C\C　　Ex: CC/MCC Exclusions　　🔵 Hospital-Acquired Condition

899

I70.435   Atherosclerosis of autologous vein bypass graft(s) of the right leg with ulceration of other part of foot   A
> Atherosclerosis of autologous vein bypass graft(s) of right leg with ulceration of toe

I70.438   Atherosclerosis of autologous vein bypass graft(s) of the right leg with ulceration of other part of lower leg 🔗   A
> CC when PDx is its own CC

I70.439   Atherosclerosis of autologous vein bypass graft(s) of the right leg with ulceration of unspecified site 🔗   A
> CC when PDx is its own CC

● **I70.44**   Atherosclerosis of autologous vein bypass graft(s) of the left leg with ulceration
> **Includes**   any condition classifiable to I70.412 and I70.422
>
> Use additional code to identify severity of ulcer (L97.-)
>
> Ⓔ⑂ For category I70.44 CC codes: See PDX Collection 698

I70.441   Atherosclerosis of autologous vein bypass graft(s) of the left leg with ulceration of thigh 🔗   A
> CC when PDx is its own CC

I70.442   Atherosclerosis of autologous vein bypass graft(s) of the left leg with ulceration of calf 🔗   A
> CC when PDx is its own CC

I70.443   Atherosclerosis of autologous vein bypass graft(s) of the left leg with ulceration of ankle 🔗   A
> CC when PDx is its own CC

I70.444   Atherosclerosis of autologous vein bypass graft(s) of the left leg with ulceration of heel and midfoot 🔗   A
> Atherosclerosis of autologous vein bypass graft(s) of left leg with ulceration of plantar surface of midfoot
> CC when PDx is its own CC

I70.445   Atherosclerosis of autologous vein bypass graft(s) of the left leg with ulceration of other part of foot   A
> Atherosclerosis of autologous vein bypass graft(s) of left leg with ulceration of toe

I70.448   Atherosclerosis of autologous vein bypass graft(s) of the left leg with ulceration of other part of lower leg 🔗   A
> CC when PDx is its own CC

I70.449   Atherosclerosis of autologous vein bypass graft(s) of the left leg with ulceration of unspecified site 🔗   A
> CC when PDx is its own CC

I70.45   Atherosclerosis of autologous vein bypass graft(s) of other extremity with ulceration   A
> **Includes**   any condition classifiable to I70.418, I70.428, and I70.438
>
> Use additional code to identify severity of ulcer (L98.49-)

● **I70.46**   Atherosclerosis of autologous vein bypass graft(s) of the extremities with gangrene
> **Includes**   any condition classifiable to I70.41-, I70.42-, and I70.43-, I70.44-, I70.45
>
> Use additional code to identify the severity of any ulcer (L97.-, L98.49-), if applicable
>
> Ⓔ⑂ For category I70.46 CC codes: See PDX Collection 519

I70.461   Atherosclerosis of autologous vein bypass graft(s) of the extremities with gangrene, right leg 🔗   A
> CC when PDx is its own CC

I70.462   Atherosclerosis of autologous vein bypass graft(s) of the extremities with gangrene, left leg 🔗   A
> CC when PDx is its own CC

I70.463   Atherosclerosis of autologous vein bypass graft(s) of the extremities with gangrene, bilateral legs 🔗   A
> CC when PDx is its own CC

I70.468   Atherosclerosis of autologous vein bypass graft(s) of the extremities with gangrene, other extremity 🔗   A
> CC when PDx is its own CC

I70.469   Atherosclerosis of autologous vein bypass graft(s) of the extremities with gangrene, unspecified extremity 🔗   A
> CC when PDx is its own CC

● **I70.49**   Other atherosclerosis of autologous vein bypass graft(s) of the extremities

I70.491   Other atherosclerosis of autologous vein bypass graft(s) of the extremities, right leg   A

I70.492   Other atherosclerosis of autologous vein bypass graft(s) of the extremities, left leg   A

I70.493   Other atherosclerosis of autologous vein bypass graft(s) of the extremities, bilateral legs   A

I70.498   Other atherosclerosis of autologous vein bypass graft(s) of the extremities, other extremity   A

I70.499   Other atherosclerosis of autologous vein bypass graft(s) of the extremities, unspecified extremity   A

● **I70.5**   Atherosclerosis of nonautologous biological bypass graft(s) of the extremities
> Use additional code, if applicable, to identify chronic total occlusion of artery of extremity (I70.92)

● **I70.50**   Unspecified atherosclerosis of nonautologous biological bypass graft(s) of the extremities

I70.501   Unspecified atherosclerosis of nonautologous biological bypass graft(s) of the extremities, right leg   A

I70.502   Unspecified atherosclerosis of nonautologous biological bypass graft(s) of the extremities, left leg   A

I70.503   Unspecified atherosclerosis of nonautologous biological bypass graft(s) of the extremities, bilateral legs   A

I70.508   Unspecified atherosclerosis of nonautologous biological bypass graft(s) of the extremities, other extremity   A

I70.509   Unspecified atherosclerosis of nonautologous biological bypass graft(s) of the extremities, unspecified extremity   A

▶ New   ⇒ Revised   ~~deleted~~ Deleted   Excludes 1   Excludes 2   Includes   Use additional   Code first   Code also   Key words
OGCR Official Guidelines   ● Unacceptable Principal Diagnosis   X Assign placeholder X   ● Use Additional Character(s)   ▌ Manifestation Code   **Coding Clinic**

● I70.51 Atherosclerosis of nonautologous biological bypass graft(s) of the extremities intermittent claudication

   I70.511 Atherosclerosis of nonautologous biological bypass graft(s) of the extremities with intermittent claudication, right leg   A

   I70.512 Atherosclerosis of nonautologous biological bypass graft(s) of the extremities with intermittent claudication, left leg   A

   I70.513 Atherosclerosis of nonautologous biological bypass graft(s) of the extremities with intermittent claudication, bilateral legs   A

   I70.518 Atherosclerosis of nonautologous biological bypass graft(s) of the extremities with intermittent claudication, other extremity   A

   I70.519 Atherosclerosis of nonautologous biological bypass graft(s) of the extremities with intermittent claudication, unspecified extremity   A

● I70.52 Atherosclerosis of nonautologous biological bypass graft(s) of the extremities with rest pain

Includes any condition classifiable to I70.51-

   I70.521 Atherosclerosis of nonautologous biological bypass graft(s) of the extremities with rest pain, right leg   A

   I70.522 Atherosclerosis of nonautologous biological bypass graft(s) of the extremities with rest pain, left leg   A

   I70.523 Atherosclerosis of nonautologous biological bypass graft(s) of the extremities with rest pain, bilateral legs   A

   I70.528 Atherosclerosis of nonautologous biological bypass graft(s) of the extremities with rest pain, other extremity   A

   I70.529 Atherosclerosis of nonautologous biological bypass graft(s) of the extremities with rest pain, unspecified extremity   A

● I70.53 Atherosclerosis of nonautologous biological bypass graft(s) of the right leg with ulceration

Includes any condition classifiable to I70.511 and I70.521

Use additional code to identify severity of ulcer (L97.-)

(Ex) For category I70.53 CC codes: See PDX Collection 698

   I70.531 Atherosclerosis of nonautologous biological bypass graft(s) of the right leg with ulceration of thigh   A
CC when PDx is its own CC

   I70.532 Atherosclerosis of nonautologous biological bypass graft(s) of the right leg with ulceration of calf   A
CC when PDx is its own CC

   I70.533 Atherosclerosis of nonautologous biological bypass graft(s) of the right leg with ulceration of ankle   A
CC when PDx is its own CC

   I70.534 Atherosclerosis of nonautologous biological bypass graft(s) of the right leg with ulceration of heel and midfoot   A
Atherosclerosis of nonautologous biological bypass graft(s) of right leg with ulceration of plantar surface of midfoot
CC when PDx is its own CC

   I70.535 Atherosclerosis of nonautologous biological bypass graft(s) of the right leg with ulceration of other part of foot
Atherosclerosis of nonautologous biological bypass graft(s) of the right leg with ulceration of toe

   I70.538 Atherosclerosis of nonautologous biological bypass graft(s) of the right leg with ulceration of other part of lower leg
CC when PDx is its own CC

   I70.539 Atherosclerosis of nonautologous biological bypass graft(s) of the right leg with ulceration of unspecified site   A
CC when PDx is its own CC

● I70.54 Atherosclerosis of nonautologous biological bypass graft(s) of the left leg with ulceration

Includes any condition classifiable to I70.512 and I70.522

Use additional code to identify severity of ulcer (L97.-)

(Ex) For category I70.54 CC codes: See PDX Collection 698

   I70.541 Atherosclerosis of nonautologous biological bypass graft(s) of the left leg with ulceration of thigh   A
CC when PDx is its own CC

   I70.542 Atherosclerosis of nonautologous biological bypass graft(s) of the left leg with ulceration of calf   A
CC when PDx is its own CC

   I70.543 Atherosclerosis of nonautologous biological bypass graft(s) of the left leg with ulceration of ankle   A
CC when PDx is its own CC

   I70.544 Atherosclerosis of nonautologous biological bypass graft(s) of the left leg with ulceration of heel and midfoot   A
Atherosclerosis of nonautologous biological bypass graft(s) of left leg with ulceration of plantar surface of midfoot
CC when PDx is its own CC

   I70.545 Atherosclerosis of nonautologous biological bypass graft(s) of the left leg with ulceration of other part of foot   A
Atherosclerosis of nonautologous biological bypass graft(s) of the left leg with ulceration of toe

   I70.548 Atherosclerosis of nonautologous biological bypass graft(s) of the left leg with ulceration of other part of lower leg   A
CC when PDx is its own CC

   I70.549 Atherosclerosis of nonautologous biological bypass graft(s) of the left leg with ulceration of unspecified site   A
CC when PDx is its own CC

I70.55 Atherosclerosis of nonautologous biological bypass graft(s) of other extremity with ulceration   A

Includes any condition classifiable to I70.518, I70.528, and I70.538

Use additional code to identify severity of ulcer (L98.49)

CHAPTER 9 (I00-I99)

N Newborn Age: 0   P Pediatric Age: 0–17   M Maternity DX: 12–55   A Adult Age: 15–124   ♀ Females Only   ♂ Males Only
 Complication\Comorbidity   Major C\C   (Ex) CC/MCC Exclusions   Hospital-Acquired Condition
901

● **I70.56 Atherosclerosis of nonautologous biological bypass graft(s) of the extremities with gangrene**

> **Includes** any condition classifiable to I70.51-, I70.52-, and I70.53-, I70.54-, I70.55
>
> Use additional code to identify the severity of any ulcer (L97.-, L98.49-), if applicable
> Ⓔⓧ **For category I70.56 CC codes:** See PDX Collection 519

I70.561 Atherosclerosis of nonautologous biological bypass graft(s) of the extremities with gangrene, right leg 🔗　A
> CC when PDx is its own CC

I70.562 Atherosclerosis of nonautologous biological bypass graft(s) of the extremities with gangrene, left leg 🔗 A
> CC when PDx is its own CC

I70.563 Atherosclerosis of nonautologous biological bypass graft(s) of the extremities with gangrene, bilateral legs 🔗　A
> CC when PDx is its own CC

I70.568 Atherosclerosis of nonautologous biological bypass graft(s) of the extremities with gangrene, other extremity 🔗　A
> CC when PDx is its own CC

I70.569 Atherosclerosis of nonautologous biological bypass graft(s) of the extremities with gangrene, unspecified extremity 🔗　A
> CC when PDx is its own CC

● **I70.59 Other atherosclerosis of nonautologous biological bypass graft(s) of the extremities**

I70.591 Other atherosclerosis of nonautologous biological bypass graft(s) of the extremities, right leg　A

I70.592 Other atherosclerosis of nonautologous biological bypass graft(s) of the extremities, left leg　A

I70.593 Other atherosclerosis of nonautologous biological bypass graft(s) of the extremities, bilateral legs　A

I70.598 Other atherosclerosis of nonautologous biological bypass graft(s) of the extremities, other extremity　A

I70.599 Other atherosclerosis of nonautologous biological bypass graft(s) of the extremities, unspecified extremity　A

● **I70.6 Atherosclerosis of nonbiological bypass graft(s) of the extremities**

> Use additional code, if applicable, to identify chronic total occlusion of artery of extremity (I70.92)

● **I70.60 Unspecified atherosclerosis of nonbiological bypass graft(s) of the extremities**

I70.601 Unspecified atherosclerosis of nonbiological bypass graft(s) of the extremities, right leg　A

I70.602 Unspecified atherosclerosis of nonbiological bypass graft(s) of the extremities, left leg　A

I70.603 Unspecified atherosclerosis of nonbiological bypass graft(s) of the extremities, bilateral legs　A

I70.608 Unspecified atherosclerosis of nonbiological bypass graft(s) of the extremities, other extremity　A

I70.609 Unspecified atherosclerosis of nonbiological bypass graft(s) of the extremities, unspecified extremity　A

● **I70.61 Atherosclerosis of nonbiological bypass graft(s) of the extremities with intermittent claudication**

I70.611 Atherosclerosis of nonbiological bypass graft(s) of the extremities with intermittent claudication, right leg　A

I70.612 Atherosclerosis of nonbiological bypass graft(s) of the extremities with intermittent claudication, left leg　A

I70.613 Atherosclerosis of nonbiological bypass graft(s) of the extremities with intermittent claudication, bilateral legs　A

I70.618 Atherosclerosis of nonbiological bypass graft(s) of the extremities with intermittent claudication, other extremity　A

I70.619 Atherosclerosis of nonbiological bypass graft(s) of the extremities with intermittent claudication, unspecified extremity　A

● **I70.62 Atherosclerosis of nonbiological bypass graft(s) of the extremities with rest pain**

> **Includes** any condition classifiable to I70.61-

I70.621 Atherosclerosis of nonbiological bypass graft(s) of the extremities with rest pain, right leg　A

I70.622 Atherosclerosis of nonbiological bypass graft(s) of the extremities with rest pain, left leg　A

I70.623 Atherosclerosis of nonbiological bypass graft(s) of the extremities with rest pain, bilateral legs　A

I70.628 Atherosclerosis of nonbiological bypass graft(s) of the extremities with rest pain, other extremity　A

I70.629 Atherosclerosis of nonbiological bypass graft(s) of the extremities with rest pain, unspecified extremity　A

● **I70.63 Atherosclerosis of nonbiological bypass graft(s) of the right leg with ulceration**

> **Includes** any condition classifiable to I70.611 and I70.621
>
> Use additional code to identify severity of ulcer (L97.-)
> Ⓔⓧ **For category I70.63 CC codes:** See PDX Collection 698

I70.631 Atherosclerosis of nonbiological bypass graft(s) of the right leg with ulceration of thigh 🔗　A
> CC when PDx is its own CC

I70.632 Atherosclerosis of nonbiological bypass graft(s) of the right leg with ulceration of calf 🔗　A
> CC when PDx is its own CC

I70.633 Atherosclerosis of nonbiological bypass graft(s) of the right leg with ulceration of ankle 🔗　A
> CC when PDx is its own CC

I70.634 Atherosclerosis of nonbiological bypass graft(s) of the right leg with ulceration of heel and midfoot 🔗 A
> Atherosclerosis of nonbiological bypass graft(s) of right leg with ulceration of plantar surface of midfoot
> CC when PDx is its own CC

I70.635 Atherosclerosis of nonbiological bypass graft(s) of the right leg with ulceration of other part of foot　A
> Atherosclerosis of nonbiological bypass graft(s) of the right leg with ulceration of toe

I70.638 Atherosclerosis of nonbiological bypass graft(s) of the right leg with ulceration of other part of lower leg 🦠 A
    CC when PDx is its own CC

I70.639 Atherosclerosis of nonbiological bypass graft(s) of the right leg with ulceration of unspecified site 🦠 A
    CC when PDx is its own CC

● **I70.64** Atherosclerosis of nonbiological bypass graft(s) of the left leg with ulceration
    Includes any condition classifiable to I70.612 and I70.622
    Use additional code to identify severity of ulcer (L97.-)
    (Ex) For category I70.64 CC codes: See PDX Collection 698

I70.641 Atherosclerosis of nonbiological bypass graft(s) of the left leg with ulceration of thigh 🦠 A
    CC when PDx is its own CC

I70.642 Atherosclerosis of nonbiological bypass graft(s) of the left leg with ulceration of calf 🦠 A
    CC when PDx is its own CC

I70.643 Atherosclerosis of nonbiological bypass graft(s) of the left leg with ulceration of ankle 🦠 A
    CC when PDx is its own CC

I70.644 Atherosclerosis of nonbiological bypass graft(s) of the left leg with ulceration of heel and midfoot 🦠 A
    Atherosclerosis of nonbiological bypass graft(s) of left leg with ulceration of plantar surface of midfoot
    CC when PDx is its own CC

I70.645 Atherosclerosis of nonbiological bypass graft(s) of the left leg with ulceration of other part of foot A
    Atherosclerosis of nonbiological bypass graft(s) of the left leg with ulceration of toe

I70.648 Atherosclerosis of nonbiological bypass graft(s) of the left leg with ulceration of other part of lower leg 🦠 A
    CC when PDx is its own CC

I70.649 Atherosclerosis of nonbiological bypass graft(s) of the left leg with ulceration of unspecified site 🦠 A
    CC when PDx is its own CC

I70.65 Atherosclerosis of nonbiological bypass graft(s) of other extremity with ulceration A
    Includes any condition classifiable to I70.618 and I70.628
    Use additional code to identify severity of ulcer (L98.49-)

● **I70.66** Atherosclerosis of nonbiological bypass graft(s) of the extremities with gangrene
    Includes any condition classifiable to I70.61-, I70.62-, I70.63-, I70.64-, I70.65
    Use additional code to identify the severity of any ulcer (L97.-, L98.49-), if applicable
    (Ex) For category I70.66 CC codes: See PDX Collection 519

I70.661 Atherosclerosis of nonbiological bypass graft(s) of the extremities with gangrene, right leg 🦠 A
    CC when PDx is its own CC

I70.662 Atherosclerosis of nonbiological bypass graft(s) of the extremities with gangrene, left leg 🦠 A
    CC when PDx is its own CC

I70.663 Atherosclerosis of nonbiological bypass graft(s) of the extremities with gangrene, bilateral legs 🦠 A
    CC when PDx is its own CC

I70.668 Atherosclerosis of nonbiological bypass graft(s) of the extremities with gangrene, other extremity 🦠 A
    CC when PDx is its own CC

I70.669 Atherosclerosis of nonbiological bypass graft(s) of the extremities with gangrene, unspecified extremity 🦠 A
    CC when PDx is its own CC

● **I70.69** Other atherosclerosis of nonbiological bypass graft(s) of the extremities

I70.691 Other atherosclerosis of nonbiological bypass graft(s) of the extremities, right leg A

I70.692 Other atherosclerosis of nonbiological bypass graft(s) of the extremities, left leg A

I70.693 Other atherosclerosis of nonbiological bypass graft(s) of the extremities, bilateral legs A

I70.698 Other atherosclerosis of nonbiological bypass graft(s) of the extremities, other extremity A

I70.699 Other atherosclerosis of nonbiological bypass graft(s) of the extremities, unspecified extremity A

● **I70.7** Atherosclerosis of other type of bypass graft(s) of the extremities
    Use additional code, if applicable, to identify chronic total occlusion of artery of extremity (I70.92)

● **I70.70** Unspecified atherosclerosis of other type of bypass graft(s) of the extremities

I70.701 Unspecified atherosclerosis of other type of bypass graft(s) of the extremities, right leg A

I70.702 Unspecified atherosclerosis of other type of bypass graft(s) of the extremities, left leg A

I70.703 Unspecified atherosclerosis of other type of bypass graft(s) of the extremities, bilateral legs A

I70.708 Unspecified atherosclerosis of other type of bypass graft(s) of the extremities, other extremity A

I70.709 Unspecified atherosclerosis of other type of bypass graft(s) of the extremities, unspecified extremity A

● **I70.71** Atherosclerosis of other type of bypass graft(s) of the extremities with intermittent claudication

I70.711 Atherosclerosis of other type of bypass graft(s) of the extremities with intermittent claudication, right leg A

I70.712 Atherosclerosis of other type of bypass graft(s) of the extremities with intermittent claudication, left leg A

I70.713 Atherosclerosis of other type of bypass graft(s) of the extremities with intermittent claudication, bilateral legs A

I70.718 Atherosclerosis of other type of bypass graft(s) of the extremities with intermittent claudication, other extremity A

I70.719 Atherosclerosis of other type of bypass graft(s) of the extremities with intermittent claudication, unspecified extremity A

CHAPTER 9 (I00-I99)

●I70.72 Atherosclerosis of other type of bypass graft(s) of the extremities with rest pain

> **Includes** any condition classifiable to I70.71-

I70.721 Atherosclerosis of other type of bypass graft(s) of the extremities with rest pain, right leg A

I70.722 Atherosclerosis of other type of bypass graft(s) of the extremities with rest pain, left leg A

I70.723 Atherosclerosis of other type of bypass graft(s) of the extremities with rest pain, bilateral legs A

I70.728 Atherosclerosis of other type of bypass graft(s) of the extremities with rest pain, other extremity A

I70.729 Atherosclerosis of other type of bypass graft(s) of the extremities with rest pain, unspecified extremity A

●I70.73 Atherosclerosis of other type of bypass graft(s) of the right leg with ulceration

> **Includes** any condition classifiable to I70.711 and I70.721

Use additional code to identify severity of ulcer (L97.-)

Ex) For category I70.73 CC codes: See PDX Collection 698

I70.731 Atherosclerosis of other type of bypass graft(s) of the right leg with ulceration of thigh A
  CC when PDx is its own CC

I70.732 Atherosclerosis of other type of bypass graft(s) of the right leg with ulceration of calf A
  CC when PDx is its own CC

I70.733 Atherosclerosis of other type of bypass graft(s) of the right leg with ulceration of ankle A
  CC when PDx is its own CC

I70.734 Atherosclerosis of other type of bypass graft(s) of the right leg with ulceration of heel and midfoot A
  Atherosclerosis of other type of bypass graft(s) of right leg with ulceration of plantar surface of midfoot
  CC when PDx is its own CC

I70.735 Atherosclerosis of other type of bypass graft(s) of the right leg with ulceration of other part of foot A
  Atherosclerosis of other type of bypass graft(s) of right leg with ulceration of toe

I70.738 Atherosclerosis of other type of bypass graft(s) of the right leg with ulceration of other part of lower leg A
  CC when PDx is its own CC

I70.739 Atherosclerosis of other type of bypass graft(s) of the right leg with ulceration of unspecified site A
  CC when PDx is its own CC

●I70.74 Atherosclerosis of other type of bypass graft(s) of the left leg with ulceration

> **Includes** any condition classifiable to I70.712 and I70.722

Use additional code to identify severity of ulcer (L97.-)

Ex) For category I70.74 CC codes: See PDX Collection 698

I70.741 Atherosclerosis of other type of bypass graft(s) of the left leg with ulceration of thigh A
  CC when PDx is its own CC

I70.742 Atherosclerosis of other type of bypass graft(s) of the left leg with ulceration of calf A
  CC when PDx is its own CC

I70.743 Atherosclerosis of other type of bypass graft(s) of the left leg with ulceration of ankle A
  CC when PDx is its own CC

I70.744 Atherosclerosis of other type of bypass graft(s) of the left leg with ulceration of heel and midfoot A
  Atherosclerosis of other type of bypass graft(s) of left leg with ulceration of plantar surface of midfoot
  CC when PDx is its own CC

I70.745 Atherosclerosis of other type of bypass graft(s) of the left leg with ulceration of other part of foot A
  Atherosclerosis of other type of bypass graft(s) of left leg with ulceration of toe

I70.748 Atherosclerosis of other type of bypass graft(s) of the left leg with ulceration of other part of lower leg A
  CC when PDx is its own CC

I70.749 Atherosclerosis of other type of bypass graft(s) of the left leg with ulceration of unspecified site A
  CC when PDx is its own CC

I70.75 Atherosclerosis of other type of bypass graft(s) of other extremity with ulceration A

> **Includes** any condition classifiable to I70.718 and I70.728

Use additional code to identify severity of ulcer (L98.49)

●I70.76 Atherosclerosis of other type of bypass graft(s) of the extremities with gangrene

> **Includes** any condition classifiable to I70.71-, I70.72-, I70.73-, I70.74-, I70.75

Use additional code to identify the severity of any ulcer (L97.-, L98.49-), if applicable

Ex) For category I70.76 CC codes: See PDX Collection 519

I70.761 Atherosclerosis of other type of bypass graft(s) of the extremities with gangrene, right leg A
  CC when PDx is its own CC

I70.762 Atherosclerosis of other type of bypass graft(s) of the extremities with gangrene, left leg A
  CC when PDx is its own CC

I70.763 Atherosclerosis of other type of bypass graft(s) of the extremities with gangrene, bilateral legs A
  CC when PDx is its own CC

I70.768 Atherosclerosis of other type of bypass graft(s) of the extremities with gangrene, other extremity A
  CC when PDx is its own CC

I70.769 Atherosclerosis of other type of bypass graft(s) of the extremities with gangrene, unspecified extremity A
  CC when PDx is its own CC

● **I70.79**   **Other atherosclerosis of other type of bypass graft(s) of the extremities**

    I70.791   Other atherosclerosis of other type of bypass graft(s) of the extremities, right leg   A

    I70.792   Other atherosclerosis of other type of bypass graft(s) of the extremities, left leg   A

    I70.793   Other atherosclerosis of other type of bypass graft(s) of the extremities, bilateral legs   A

    I70.798   Other atherosclerosis of other type of bypass graft(s) of the extremities, other extremity   A

    I70.799   Other atherosclerosis of other type of bypass graft(s) of the extremities, unspecified extremity   A

I70.8   **Atherosclerosis of other arteries**   A

● **I70.9**   **Other and unspecified atherosclerosis**

   I70.90   **Unspecified atherosclerosis**   A

   I70.91   **Generalized atherosclerosis**   A

   ● **I70.92**   **Chronic total occlusion of artery of the extremities** 🔒   A

     Complete occlusion of artery of the extremities
     Total occlusion of artery of the extremities

     Code first atherosclerosis of arteries of the extremities (I70.2-, I70.3-, I70.4-, I70.5-, I70.6-, I70.7-)

     (Ex) See PDX Collection 699

● **I71**   **Aortic aneurysm and dissection**

   Excludes1   aortic ectasia (I77.81-)
            syphilitic aortic aneurysm (A52.01)
            traumatic aortic aneurysm (S25.09, S35.09)

   (Ex) For category I71 CC codes: See PDX Collection 700

   ● **I71.0**   **Dissection of aorta**

     I71.00   **Dissection of unspecified site of aorta** 🔒

     I71.01   **Dissection of thoracic aorta** 🔒

     I71.02   **Dissection of abdominal aorta** 🔒

     I71.03   **Dissection of thoracoabdominal aorta** 🔒

   I71.1   **Thoracic aortic aneurysm, ruptured** 🔒

   I71.2   **Thoracic aortic aneurysm, without rupture**

   I71.3   **Abdominal aortic aneurysm, ruptured** 🔒

   I71.4   **Abdominal aortic aneurysm, without rupture**

   I71.5   **Thoracoabdominal aortic aneurysm, ruptured** 🔒

   I71.6   **Thoracoabdominal aortic aneurysm, without rupture**

   I71.8   **Aortic aneurysm of unspecified site, ruptured** 🔒

     Rupture of aorta NOS

   I71.9   **Aortic aneurysm of unspecified site, without rupture**

     Aneurysm of aorta
     Dilatation of aorta
     Hyaline necrosis of aorta

● **I72**   **Other aneurysm**

   Includes   aneurysm (cirsoid) (false) (ruptured)

   Excludes2   acquired aneurysm (I77.0)
            aneurysm (of) aorta (I71.-)
            aneurysm (of) arteriovenous NOS (Q27.3-)
            carotid artery dissection (I77.71)
            cerebral (nonruptured) aneurysm (I67.1)
            coronary aneurysm (I25.4)
            coronary artery dissection (I25.42)
            dissection of artery NEC (I77.79)
            dissection of precerebral artery, congenital (nonruptured) (Q28.1)
            heart aneurysm (I25.3)
            iliac artery dissection (I77.72)
      ▶ precerebral artery, congential (nonruptured) (Q28.1)
            pulmonary artery aneurysm (I28.1)
            renal artery dissection (I77.73)
            retinal aneurysm (H35.0)
            ruptured cerebral aneurysm (I60.7)
            varicose aneurysm (I77.0)
            vertebral artery dissection (I77.74)

I72.0   **Aneurysm of carotid artery**

     Aneurysm of common carotid artery
     Aneurysm of external carotid artery
     Aneurysm of internal carotid artery, extracranial portion

     Excludes1   aneurysm of internal carotid artery, intracranial portion (I67.1)
                aneurysm of internal carotid artery NOS (I67.1)

I72.1   **Aneurysm of artery of upper extremity**

I72.2   **Aneurysm of renal artery**

I72.3   **Aneurysm of iliac artery**

I72.4   **Aneurysm of artery of lower extremity**

I72.5   **Aneurysm of other precerebral arteries**

     Aneurysm of basilar artery (trunk)

     Excludes2   aneurysm of carotid artery (I72.0)
                aneurysm of vertebral artery (I72.6)
                dissection of carotid artery (I77.71)
                dissection of other precerebral arteries (I77.75)
                dissection of vertebral artery (I77.74)

   Coding Clinic 2016, Q4, P28

I72.6   **Aneurysm of vertebral artery**

     Excludes2   dissection of vertebral artery (I77.74)
   Coding Clinic 2016, Q4, P28

I72.8   **Aneurysm of other specified arteries**

I72.9   **Aneurysm of unspecified site**

● **I73**   **Other peripheral vascular diseases**

   Excludes2   chilblains (T69.1)
            frostbite (T33-T34)
            immersion hand or foot (T69.0-)
            spasm of cerebral artery (G45.9)

● **I73.0**   **Raynaud's syndrome**

     Diminishing oxygen supply to fingers, toes, nose, and ears when exposed to temperature changes or stress
     Raynaud's disease
     Raynaud's phenomenon (secondary)

   I73.00   **Raynaud's syndrome without gangrene**

   I73.01   **Raynaud's syndrome with gangrene** 🔒
     CC when PDx is its own CC
     (Ex) See PDX Collection 519

I73.1   **Thromboangiitis obliterans [Buerger's disease]**

     Inflammatory occlusive disease resulting in poor circulation to the legs, feet, and sometimes the hands due to progressive inflammatory narrowing and eventually obliteration of the small arteries

Figure 9-5   Raynaud's syndrome. (From Hallett: Comprehensive Vascular and Endovascular Surgery, ed 2, Philadelphia, Mosby Ltd., 2010)

CHAPTER 9 (I00-I99)

● I73.8 **Other specified peripheral vascular diseases**
  Excludes1 diabetic (peripheral) angiopathy
                 (E08-E13 with .51-.52)

  I73.81 **Erythromelalgia**

  I73.89 **Other specified peripheral vascular diseases**
         Acrocyanosis
         Erythrocyanosis
         Simple acroparesthesia [Schultze's type]
         Vasomotor acroparesthesia [Nothnagel's type]

I73.9 **Peripheral vascular disease, unspecified**
      Intermittent claudication
      Peripheral angiopathy NOS
      Spasm of artery
      Excludes1 atherosclerosis of the extremities
                     (I70.2--I70.7-)

● I74 **Arterial embolism and thrombosis**
  Includes embolic infarction
               embolic occlusion
               thrombotic infarction
               thrombotic occlusion

  Code first embolism and thrombosis complicating abortion or
               ectopic or molar pregnancy (O00-O07, O08.2)
               embolism and thrombosis complicating pregnancy, childbirth
               and the puerperium (O88.-)

  Excludes2 atheroembolism (I75.-)
               basilar embolism and thrombosis (I63.0-I63.2,
                 I65.1)
               carotid embolism and thrombosis (I63.0-I63.2,
                 I65.2)
               cerebral embolism and thrombosis (I63.3-I63.5,
                 I66.-)
               coronary embolism and thrombosis (I21-I25)
               mesenteric embolism and thrombosis (K55.0-)
               ophthalmic embolism and thrombosis (H34.-)
               precerebral embolism and thrombosis NOS
                 (I63.0-I63.2, I65.9)
               pulmonary embolism and thrombosis (I26.-)
               renal embolism and thrombosis (N28.0)
               retinal embolism and thrombosis (H34.-)
               septic embolism and thrombosis (I76)
               vertebral embolism and thrombosis (I63.0-I63.2,
                 I65.0)

● I74.0 **Embolism and thrombosis of abdominal aorta**
       (Ex) For category I74.0 CC codes: See PDX Collection 669

       I74.01 **Saddle embolus of abdominal aorta** 🖉

       I74.09 **Other arterial embolism and thrombosis of
               abdominal aorta** 🖉
               Aortic bifurcation syndrome
               Aortoiliac obstruction
               Leriche's syndrome

● I74.1 **Embolism and thrombosis of other and unspecified parts
       of aorta**
       (Ex) For category I74.1 CC codes unless otherwise indicated: See PDX
       Collection 669

       I74.10 **Embolism and thrombosis of unspecified parts
               of aorta** 🖉

       I74.11 **Embolism and thrombosis of thoracic aorta** 🖉
               (Ex) See PDX Collection 701

       I74.19 **Embolism and thrombosis of other parts of
               aorta** 🖉

Item 9-9 An **embolus** is a mass of undissolved matter present in the blood
that is transported by the blood current. A **thrombus** is a blood clot that occludes
or shuts off a vessel. When a thrombus is dislodged, it becomes an embolus.

Embolus

Figure 9-6 An arterial embolus.

I74.2 **Embolism and thrombosis of arteries of the upper
      extremities** 🖉
      (Ex) See PDX Collection 702

I74.3 **Embolism and thrombosis of arteries of the lower
      extremities** 🖉
      (Ex) See PDX Collection 703

I74.4 **Embolism and thrombosis of arteries of extremities,
      unspecified** 🖉
      Peripheral arterial embolism NOS
      (Ex) See PDX Collection 703

I74.5 **Embolism and thrombosis of iliac artery** 🖉
      (Ex) See PDX Collection 704

I74.8 **Embolism and thrombosis of other arteries** 🖉
      (Ex) See PDX Collection 705

I74.9 **Embolism and thrombosis of unspecified artery** 🖉
      (Ex) See PDX Collection 705

● I75 **Atheroembolism**
  Includes atherothrombotic microembolism
               cholesterol embolism

  ● I75.0 **Atheroembolism of extremities**
      ● I75.01 **Atheroembolism of upper extremity**
               (Ex) For category I75.01 CC codes: See PDX Collection 706

               I75.011 **Atheroembolism of right upper
                        extremity** 🖉

               I75.012 **Atheroembolism of left upper
                        extremity** 🖉

               I75.013 **Atheroembolism of bilateral upper
                        extremities** 🖉

               I75.019 **Atheroembolism of unspecified upper
                        extremity** 🖉

      ● I75.02 **Atheroembolism of lower extremity**
               (Ex) For category I75.02 CC codes: See PDX Collection 707

               I75.021 **Atheroembolism of right lower
                        extremity** 🖉

               I75.022 **Atheroembolism of left lower
                        extremity** 🖉

               I75.023 **Atheroembolism of bilateral lower
                        extremities** 🖉

               I75.029 **Atheroembolism of unspecified lower
                        extremity** 🖉

  ● I75.8 **Atheroembolism of other sites**
          I75.81 **Atheroembolism of kidney** 🖉
                  Use additional code for any associated acute
                  kidney failure and chronic kidney disease
                  (N17.-, N18.-)
                  (Ex) See PDX Collection 708

          I75.89 **Atheroembolism of other site** 🖉
                  (Ex) See PDX Collection 709

● I76 **Septic arterial embolism** 🖉
  Code first underlying infection, such as:
     infective endocarditis (I33.0)
     lung abscess (J85.-)
  Use additional code to identify the site of the embolism (I74.-)
  Excludes2 septic pulmonary embolism (I26.01, I26.90)
  (Ex) See PDX Collection 705

● I77 **Other disorders of arteries and arterioles**
  Excludes2 collagen (vascular) diseases (M30-M36)
               hypersensitivity angiitis (M31.0)
               pulmonary artery (I28.-)

  I77.0 **Arteriovenous fistula, acquired**
        Aneurysmal varix
        Arteriovenous aneurysm, acquired
        Excludes1 arteriovenous aneurysm NOS (Q27.3-)
                       presence of arteriovenous shunt (fistula)
                         for dialysis (Z99.2)
                       traumatic - see injury of blood vessel by
                         body region
        Excludes2 cerebral (I67.1)
                       coronary (I25.4)

▶ New   ⇒ Revised   ~~deleted~~ Deleted   Excludes 1   Excludes 2   Includes   Use additional   Code first   Code also   Key words
OGCR Official Guidelines   ● Unacceptable Principal Diagnosis   X Assign placeholder X   ● Use Additional Character(s)   ▶ Manifestation Code   **Coding Clinic**

I77.1   **Stricture of artery**
       Narrowing of artery

I77.2   **Rupture of artery** 🏥
       Erosion of artery
       Fistula of artery
       Ulcer of artery

       Excludes1   traumatic rupture of artery - see injury of
                          blood vessel by body region

       (Ex) See PDX Collection 710

I77.3   **Arterial fibromuscular dysplasia**
       Fibromuscular hyperplasia (of) carotid artery
       Fibromuscular hyperplasia (of) renal artery

I77.4   **Celiac artery compression syndrome** 🏥
       (Ex) See PDX Collection 711

I77.5   **Necrosis of artery** 🏥
       (Ex) See PDX Collection 712

I77.6   **Arteritis, unspecified**
       Aortitis NOS
       Endarteritis NOS

       Excludes1   arteritis or endarteritis:
                        aortic arch (M31.4)
                        cerebral NEC (I67.7)
                        coronary (I25.89)
                        deformans (I70.-)
                        giant cell (M31.5., M31.6)
                        obliterans (I70.-)
                        senile (I70.-)

● I77.7   **Other arterial dissection**

       Excludes2   dissection of aorta (I71.0-)
                        dissection of coronary artery (I25.42)

       (Ex) For category I77.7 CC codes: See PDX Collection 689

     I77.70   **Dissection of unspecified artery** 🏥
             Coding Clinic 2016, Q4, P28

     I77.71   **Dissection of carotid artery** 🏥

     I77.72   **Dissection of iliac artery** 🏥

     I77.73   **Dissection of renal artery** 🏥

     I77.74   **Dissection of vertebral artery** 🏥

         Excludes2   aneurysm of vertebral artery
                          (I72.6)

     I77.75   **Dissection of other precerebral arteries** 🏥
             Dissection of basilar artery (trunk)

         Excludes2   aneurysm of carotid artery
                          (I72.0)
                        aneurysm of other precerebral
                        arteries (I72.5)
                        aneurysm of vertebral artery
                        (I72.6)
                        dissection of carotid artery
                        (I77.71)
                        dissection of vertebral artery
                        (I77.74)

             Coding Clinic 2016, Q4, P28

     I77.76   **Dissection of artery of upper extremity** 🏥
             Coding Clinic 2016, Q4, P28

     I77.77   **Dissection of artery of lower extremity** 🏥
             Coding Clinic 2016, Q4, P28

     I77.79   **Dissection of other specified artery** 🏥
             Coding Clinic 2016, Q4, P28

● I77.8   **Other specified disorders of arteries and arterioles**

     I77.81   **Aortic ectasia**
             Ectasis aorta

         Excludes1   aortic aneurysm and dissection
                          (I71.0-)

         I77.810   **Thoracic aortic ectasia**

         I77.811   **Abdominal aortic ectasia**

         I77.812   **Thoracoabdominal aortic ectasia**

         I77.819   **Aortic ectasia, unspecified site**

     I77.89   **Other specified disorders of arteries and arterioles**

I77.9   **Disorder of arteries and arterioles, unspecified**

● I78   **Diseases of capillaries**

   I78.0   **Hereditary hemorrhagic telangiectasia**
           Rendu-Osler-Weber disease

   I78.1   **Nevus, non-neoplastic**

           Araneus nevus   Spider nevus
           Senile nevus   Stellar nevus

         Excludes1   nevus NOS (D22.-)
                          vascular NOS (Q82.5)

         Excludes2   blue nevus (D22.-)
                          flammeus nevus (Q82.5)
                        hairy nevus (D22.-)
                        melanocytic nevus (D22.-)
                        pigmented nevus (D22.-)
                        portwine nevus (Q82.5)
                        sanguineous nevus (Q82.5)
                        strawberry nevus (Q82.5)
                        verrucous nevus (Q82.5)

   I78.8   **Other diseases of capillaries**

   I78.9   **Disease of capillaries, unspecified**

● I79   **Disorders of arteries, arterioles and capillaries in diseases classified elsewhere**

 ▸ *I79.0*   *Aneurysm of aorta in diseases classified elsewhere*
           Code first underlying disease

         Excludes1   syphilitic aneurysm (A52.01)

 ▸ *I79.1*   *Aortitis in diseases classified elsewhere*
           Code first underlying disease

         Excludes1   syphilitic aortitis (A52.02)

 ▸ *I79.8*   *Other disorders of arteries, arterioles and capillaries in diseases classified elsewhere*
           Code first underlying disease, such as:
              amyloidosis (E85.-)

         Excludes1   diabetic (peripheral) angiopathy
                          (E08-E13 with .51-.52)
                        syphilitic endarteritis (A52.09)
                        tuberculous endarteritis (A18.89)

DISEASES OF VEINS, LYMPHATIC VESSELS AND LYMPH NODES, NOT ELSEWHERE CLASSIFIED (I80-I89)

● I80   **Phlebitis and thrombophlebitis**
       Inflammation of a vein with infiltration of walls (phlebitis).

       Includes   endophlebitis
                    inflammation, vein
                    periphlebitis
                    suppurative phlebitis

       Code first phlebitis and thrombophlebitis complicating
           abortion, ectopic or molar pregnancy (O00-O07, O08.7)
           phlebitis and thrombophlebitis complicating pregnancy,
           childbirth and the puerperium (O22.-, O87.-)

       Excludes1   venous embolism and thrombosis of lower
                          extremities (I82.4-, I82.5-, I82.81-)

● I80.0   **Phlebitis and thrombophlebitis of superficial vessels of lower extremities**
           Phlebitis and thrombophlebitis of femoropopliteal vein

     I80.00   **Phlebitis and thrombophlebitis of superficial vessels of unspecified lower extremity**

     I80.01   **Phlebitis and thrombophlebitis of superficial vessels of right lower extremity**

     I80.02   **Phlebitis and thrombophlebitis of superficial vessels of left lower extremity**

     I80.03   **Phlebitis and thrombophlebitis of superficial vessels of lower extremities, bilateral**

N   Newborn Age: 0   **P**   Pediatric Age: 0–17   **M**   Maternity DX: 12–55   **A**   Adult Age: 15–124   ♀   Females Only   ♂   Males Only

🏥   Complication\Comorbidity   🏥   Major C\C   (Ex)   CC/MCC Exclusions   🏥   Hospital-Acquired Condition

907

CHAPTER 9 (I00-I99)

● **I80.1**   **Phlebitis and thrombophlebitis of femoral vein**
   Ex For category I80.1 CC codes: See PDX Collection 713

    I80.10   Phlebitis and thrombophlebitis of unspecified femoral vein

    I80.11   Phlebitis and thrombophlebitis of right femoral vein

    I80.12   Phlebitis and thrombophlebitis of left femoral vein

    I80.13   Phlebitis and thrombophlebitis of femoral vein, bilateral

● **I80.2**   **Phlebitis and thrombophlebitis of other and unspecified deep vessels of lower extremities**
   Ex For category I80.2 CC codes: See PDX Collection 713

   ● **I80.20**   Phlebitis and thrombophlebitis of unspecified deep vessels of lower extremities

     I80.201   Phlebitis and thrombophlebitis of unspecified deep vessels of right lower extremity

     I80.202   Phlebitis and thrombophlebitis of unspecified deep vessels of left lower extremity

     I80.203   Phlebitis and thrombophlebitis of unspecified deep vessels of lower extremities, bilateral

     I80.209   Phlebitis and thrombophlebitis of unspecified deep vessels of unspecified lower extremity

   ● **I80.21**   Phlebitis and thrombophlebitis of iliac vein

     I80.211   Phlebitis and thrombophlebitis of right iliac vein

     I80.212   Phlebitis and thrombophlebitis of left iliac vein

     I80.213   Phlebitis and thrombophlebitis of iliac vein, bilateral

     I80.219   Phlebitis and thrombophlebitis of unspecified iliac vein

   ● **I80.22**   Phlebitis and thrombophlebitis of popliteal vein

     I80.221   Phlebitis and thrombophlebitis of right popliteal vein

     I80.222   Phlebitis and thrombophlebitis of left popliteal vein

     I80.223   Phlebitis and thrombophlebitis of popliteal vein, bilateral

     I80.229   Phlebitis and thrombophlebitis of unspecified popliteal vein

   ● **I80.23**   Phlebitis and thrombophlebitis of tibial vein

     I80.231   Phlebitis and thrombophlebitis of right tibial vein

     I80.232   Phlebitis and thrombophlebitis of left tibial vein

     I80.233   Phlebitis and thrombophlebitis of tibial vein, bilateral

     I80.239   Phlebitis and thrombophlebitis of unspecified tibial vein

   ● **I80.29**   Phlebitis and thrombophlebitis of other deep vessels of lower extremities

     I80.291   Phlebitis and thrombophlebitis of other deep vessels of right lower extremity

     I80.292   Phlebitis and thrombophlebitis of other deep vessels of left lower extremity

     I80.293   Phlebitis and thrombophlebitis of other deep vessels of lower extremity, bilateral

     I80.299   Phlebitis and thrombophlebitis of other deep vessels of unspecified lower extremity

   I80.3   Phlebitis and thrombophlebitis of lower extremities, unspecified

   I80.8   Phlebitis and thrombophlebitis of other sites

   I80.9   Phlebitis and thrombophlebitis of unspecified site

I81   **Portal vein thrombosis**
   Portal (vein) obstruction
   Excludes2   hepatic vein thrombosis (I82.0)
       phlebitis of portal vein (K75.1)
   Ex See PDX Collection 714

● **I82**   **Other venous embolism and thrombosis**
   Code first venous embolism and thrombosis complicating:
    abortion, ectopic or molar pregnancy (O00-O07, O08.7)
    pregnancy, childbirth and the puerperium (O22.-, O87.-)
   Excludes2   venous embolism and thrombosis (of):
       cerebral (I63.6, I67.6)
       coronary (I21-I25)
       intracranial and intraspinal, septic or NOS (G08)
       intracranial, nonpyogenic (I67.6)
       intraspinal, nonpyogenic (G95.1)
       mesenteric (K55.0-)
       portal (I81)
       pulmonary (I26.-)

   I82.0   **Budd-Chiari syndrome**
    Hepatic vein thrombosis
    Ex See PDX Collection 715

   I82.1   **Thrombophlebitis migrans**
    "White leg" is the other term to describe a migrating thrombus.
    Ex See PDX Collection 716

   ● **I82.2**   **Embolism and thrombosis of vena cava and other thoracic veins**
    Ex For category I82.2 CC codes unless otherwise indicated: See PDX Collection 717

    ● **I82.21**   Embolism and thrombosis of superior vena cava

     I82.210   Acute embolism and thrombosis of superior vena cava
       Embolism and thrombosis of superior vena cava NOS

     I82.211   Chronic embolism and thrombosis of superior vena cava

    ● **I82.22**   Embolism and thrombosis of inferior vena cava
     Ex For category I82.22 CC codes: See PDX Collection 718

     I82.220   Acute embolism and thrombosis of inferior vena cava
       Embolism and thrombosis of inferior vena cava NOS

     I82.221   Chronic embolism and thrombosis of inferior vena cava

    ● **I82.29**   Embolism and thrombosis of other thoracic veins
     Embolism and thrombosis of brachiocephalic (innominate) vein

     I82.290   Acute embolism and thrombosis of other thoracic veins

     I82.291   Chronic embolism and thrombosis of other thoracic veins

   I82.3   Embolism and thrombosis of renal vein
    Ex See PDX Collection 719

▶ New   ⇒ Revised   ~~deleted~~ Deleted   Excludes 1   Excludes 2   Includes   Use additional   Code first   Code also   Key words
OGCR Official Guidelines   ● Unacceptable Principal Diagnosis   X Assign placeholder X   ● Use Additional Character(s)   ▶ Manifestation Code   **Coding Clinic**

● **I82.4** **Acute embolism and thrombosis of deep veins of lower extremity**

      Ⓔ **For category I82.4 CC codes:** See PDX Collection 717

     I82.40 **Acute embolism and thrombosis of unspecified deep veins of lower extremity**

        Deep vein thrombosis NOS

        DVT NOS

        Excludes1   acute embolism and thrombosis of unspecified deep veins of distal lower extremity (I82.4Z-)

                     acute embolism and thrombosis of unspecified deep veins of proximal lower extremity (I82.4Y-)

        I82.401 **Acute embolism and thrombosis of unspecified deep veins of right lower extremity** 🗗 🗗

        I82.402 **Acute embolism and thrombosis of unspecified deep veins of left lower extremity** 🗗 🗗

        I82.403 **Acute embolism and thrombosis of unspecified deep veins of lower extremity, bilateral** 🗗 🗗

        I82.409 **Acute embolism and thrombosis of unspecified deep veins of unspecified lower extremity** 🗗 🗗

    ● **I82.41** **Acute embolism and thrombosis of femoral vein**

        I82.411 **Acute embolism and thrombosis of right femoral vein** 🗗 🗗

        I82.412 **Acute embolism and thrombosis of left femoral vein** 🗗 🗗

        I82.413 **Acute embolism and thrombosis of femoral vein, bilateral** 🗗 🗗

        I82.419 **Acute embolism and thrombosis of unspecified femoral vein** 🗗 🗗

    ● **I82.42** **Acute embolism and thrombosis of iliac vein**

        I82.421 **Acute embolism and thrombosis of right iliac vein** 🗗 🗗

        I82.422 **Acute embolism and thrombosis of left iliac vein** 🗗 🗗

        I82.423 **Acute embolism and thrombosis of iliac vein, bilateral** 🗗 🗗

        I82.429 **Acute embolism and thrombosis of unspecified iliac vein** 🗗 🗗

    ● **I82.43** **Acute embolism and thrombosis of popliteal vein**

        I82.431 **Acute embolism and thrombosis of right popliteal vein** 🗗 🗗

        I82.432 **Acute embolism and thrombosis of left popliteal vein** 🗗 🗗

        I82.433 **Acute embolism and thrombosis of popliteal vein, bilateral** 🗗 🗗

        I82.439 **Acute embolism and thrombosis of unspecified popliteal vein** 🗗 🗗

● **I82.44** **Acute embolism and thrombosis of tibial vein**

        I82.441 **Acute embolism and thrombosis of right tibial vein** 🗗 🗗

        I82.442 **Acute embolism and thrombosis of left tibial vein** 🗗 🗗

        I82.443 **Acute embolism and thrombosis of tibial vein, bilateral** 🗗 🗗

        I82.449 **Acute embolism and thrombosis of unspecified tibial vein** 🗗 🗗

● **I82.49** **Acute embolism and thrombosis of other specified deep vein of lower extremity**

        I82.491 **Acute embolism and thrombosis of other specified deep vein of right lower extremity** 🗗 🗗

        I82.492 **Acute embolism and thrombosis of other specified deep vein of left lower extremity** 🗗 🗗

        I82.493 **Acute embolism and thrombosis of other specified deep vein of lower extremity, bilateral** 🗗 🗗

        I82.499 **Acute embolism and thrombosis of other specified deep vein of unspecified lower extremity** 🗗 🗗

● **I82.4Y** **Acute embolism and thrombosis of unspecified deep veins of proximal lower extremity**

        Acute embolism and thrombosis of deep vein of thigh NOS

        Acute embolism and thrombosis of deep vein of upper leg NOS

        I82.4Y1 **Acute embolism and thrombosis of unspecified deep veins of right proximal lower extremity** 🗗 🗗

        I82.4Y2 **Acute embolism and thrombosis of unspecified deep veins of left proximal lower extremity** 🗗 🗗

        I82.4Y3 **Acute embolism and thrombosis of unspecified deep veins of proximal lower extremity, bilateral** 🗗 🗗

        I82.4Y9 **Acute embolism and thrombosis of unspecified deep veins of unspecified proximal lower extremity** 🗗 🗗

● **I82.4Z** **Acute embolism and thrombosis of unspecified deep veins of distal lower extremity**

        Acute embolism and thrombosis of deep vein of calf NOS

        Acute embolism and thrombosis of deep vein of lower leg NOS

        I82.4Z1 **Acute embolism and thrombosis of unspecified deep veins of right distal lower extremity** 🗗 🗗

        I82.4Z2 **Acute embolism and thrombosis of unspecified deep veins of left distal lower extremity** 🗗 🗗

        I82.4Z3 **Acute embolism and thrombosis of unspecified deep veins of distal lower extremity, bilateral** 🗗 🗗

        I82.4Z9 **Acute embolism and thrombosis of unspecified deep veins of unspecified distal lower extremity** 🗗 🗗

CHAPTER 9 (I00-I99)

CHAPTER 9 (I00–I99)

● **I82.5** **Chronic embolism and thrombosis of deep veins of lower extremity**

Use additional code, if applicable, for associated long-term (current) use of anticoagulants (Z79.01)

Excludes1 personal history of venous embolism and thrombosis (Z86.718)

(Ex:) For category I82.5 CC codes: See PDX Collection 717

● **I82.50** **Chronic embolism and thrombosis of unspecified deep veins of lower extremity**

Excludes1 chronic embolism and thrombosis of unspecified deep veins of distal lower extremity (I82.5Z-)
chronic embolism and thrombosis of unspecified deep veins of proximal lower extremity (I82.5Y-)

I82.501 Chronic embolism and thrombosis of unspecified deep veins of right lower extremity 🔍

I82.502 Chronic embolism and thrombosis of unspecified deep veins of left lower extremity 🔍

I82.503 Chronic embolism and thrombosis of unspecified deep veins of lower extremity, bilateral 🔍

I82.509 Chronic embolism and thrombosis of unspecified deep veins of unspecified lower extremity 🔍

● **I82.51** **Chronic embolism and thrombosis of femoral vein**

I82.511 Chronic embolism and thrombosis of right femoral vein 🔍

I82.512 Chronic embolism and thrombosis of left femoral vein 🔍

I82.513 Chronic embolism and thrombosis of femoral vein, bilateral 🔍

I82.519 Chronic embolism and thrombosis of unspecified femoral vein 🔍

● **I82.52** **Chronic embolism and thrombosis of iliac vein**

I82.521 Chronic embolism and thrombosis of right iliac vein 🔍

I82.522 Chronic embolism and thrombosis of left iliac vein 🔍

I82.523 Chronic embolism and thrombosis of iliac vein, bilateral 🔍

I82.529 Chronic embolism and thrombosis of unspecified iliac vein 🔍

● **I82.53** **Chronic embolism and thrombosis of popliteal vein**

I82.531 Chronic embolism and thrombosis of right popliteal vein 🔍

I82.532 Chronic embolism and thrombosis of left popliteal vein 🔍

I82.533 Chronic embolism and thrombosis of popliteal vein, bilateral 🔍

I82.539 Chronic embolism and thrombosis of unspecified popliteal vein 🔍

● **I82.54** **Chronic embolism and thrombosis of tibial vein**

I82.541 Chronic embolism and thrombosis of right tibial vein 🔍

I82.542 Chronic embolism and thrombosis of left tibial vein 🔍

I82.543 Chronic embolism and thrombosis of tibial vein, bilateral 🔍

I82.549 Chronic embolism and thrombosis of unspecified tibial vein 🔍

● **I82.59** **Chronic embolism and thrombosis of other specified deep vein of lower extremity**

I82.591 Chronic embolism and thrombosis of other specified deep vein of right lower extremity 🔍

I82.592 Chronic embolism and thrombosis of other specified deep vein of left lower extremity 🔍

I82.593 Chronic embolism and thrombosis of other specified deep vein of lower extremity, bilateral 🔍

I82.599 Chronic embolism and thrombosis of other specified deep vein of unspecified lower extremity 🔍

● **I82.5Y** **Chronic embolism and thrombosis of unspecified deep veins of proximal lower extremity**

Chronic embolism and thrombosis of deep veins of thigh NOS
Chronic embolism and thrombosis of deep veins of upper leg NOS

I82.5Y1 Chronic embolism and thrombosis of unspecified deep veins of right proximal lower extremity 🔍

I82.5Y2 Chronic embolism and thrombosis of unspecified deep veins of left proximal lower extremity 🔍

I82.5Y3 Chronic embolism and thrombosis of unspecified deep veins of proximal lower extremity, bilateral 🔍

I82.5Y9 Chronic embolism and thrombosis of unspecified deep veins of unspecified proximal lower extremity 🔍

● **I82.5Z** **Chronic embolism and thrombosis of unspecified deep veins of distal lower extremity**

Chronic embolism and thrombosis of deep veins of calf NOS
Chronic embolism and thrombosis of deep veins of lower leg NOS

I82.5Z1 Chronic embolism and thrombosis of unspecified deep veins of right distal lower extremity 🔍

I82.5Z2 Chronic embolism and thrombosis of unspecified deep veins of left distal lower extremity 🔍

I82.5Z3 Chronic embolism and thrombosis of unspecified deep veins of distal lower extremity, bilateral 🔍

I82.5Z9 Chronic embolism and thrombosis of unspecified deep veins of unspecified distal lower extremity 🔍

Item 9–10 Varicose/Varicosities (varix = singular, varices = plural): Enlarged, engorged, tortuous, twisted vascular vessels (veins, arteries, lymphatics). As such, the condition can present in various parts of the body, although the most familiar locations are the lower extremities. A common complication of varices is thrombophlebitis. Varicosities of the anus and rectum are called hemorrhoids.

Figure 9-7 Varicose veins of the legs. (Getty Image)

▶ New   ⟹ Revised   ~~deleted~~ Deleted   Excludes 1   Excludes 2   Includes   Use additional   Code first   Code also   Key words

OGCR Official Guidelines   ● Unacceptable Principal Diagnosis   X Assign placeholder X   ◗ Use Additional Character(s)   ◗ Manifestation Code   **Coding Clinic**

● **I82.6**   **Acute embolism and thrombosis of veins of upper extremity**
     (Ex) For category I82.6 CC codes: See PDX Collection 717

  ● **I82.60**   **Acute embolism and thrombosis of unspecified veins of upper extremity**

     I82.601   Acute embolism and thrombosis of unspecified veins of right upper extremity 🔾

     I82.602   Acute embolism and thrombosis of unspecified veins of left upper extremity 🔾

     I82.603   Acute embolism and thrombosis of unspecified veins of upper extremity, bilateral 🔾

     I82.609   Acute embolism and thrombosis of unspecified veins of unspecified upper extremity 🔾

  ● **I82.61**   **Acute embolism and thrombosis of superficial veins of upper extremity**
       Acute embolism and thrombosis of antecubital vein
       Acute embolism and thrombosis of basilic vein
       Acute embolism and thrombosis of cephalic vein

     I82.611   Acute embolism and thrombosis of superficial veins of right upper extremity 🔾

     I82.612   Acute embolism and thrombosis of superficial veins of left upper extremity 🔾

     I82.613   Acute embolism and thrombosis of superficial veins of upper extremity, bilateral 🔾

     I82.619   Acute embolism and thrombosis of superficial veins of unspecified upper extremity 🔾

  ● **I82.62**   **Acute embolism and thrombosis of deep veins of upper extremity**
       Acute embolism and thrombosis of brachial vein
       Acute embolism and thrombosis of radial vein
       Acute embolism and thrombosis of ulnar vein

     I82.621   Acute embolism and thrombosis of deep veins of right upper extremity 🔾

     I82.622   Acute embolism and thrombosis of deep veins of left upper extremity 🔾

     I82.623   Acute embolism and thrombosis of deep veins of upper extremity, bilateral 🔾

     I82.629   Acute embolism and thrombosis of deep veins of unspecified upper extremity 🔾

● **I82.7**   **Chronic embolism and thrombosis of veins of upper extremity**
       Use additional code, if applicable, for associated long-term (current) use of anticoagulants (Z79.01)
     Excludes1   personal history of venous embolism and thrombosis (Z86.718)
     (Ex) For category I82.7 CC codes: See PDX Collection 717

  ● **I82.70**   **Chronic embolism and thrombosis of unspecified veins of upper extremity**

     I82.701   Chronic embolism and thrombosis of unspecified veins of right upper extremity 🔾

     I82.702   Chronic embolism and thrombosis of unspecified veins of left upper extremity 🔾

     I82.703   Chronic embolism and thrombosis of unspecified veins of upper extremity, bilateral 🔾

     I82.709   Chronic embolism and thrombosis of unspecified veins of unspecified upper extremity 🔾

  ● **I82.71**   **Chronic embolism and thrombosis of superficial veins of upper extremity**
       Chronic embolism and thrombosis of antecubital vein
       Chronic embolism and thrombosis of basilic vein
       Chronic embolism and thrombosis of cephalic vein

     I82.711   Chronic embolism and thrombosis of superficial veins of right upper extremity 🔾

     I82.712   Chronic embolism and thrombosis of superficial veins of left upper extremity 🔾

     I82.713   Chronic embolism and thrombosis of superficial veins of upper extremity, bilateral 🔾

     I82.719   Chronic embolism and thrombosis of superficial veins of unspecified upper extremity 🔾

  ● **I82.72**   **Chronic embolism and thrombosis of deep veins of upper extremity**
       Chronic embolism and thrombosis of brachial vein
       Chronic embolism and thrombosis of radial vein
       Chronic embolism and thrombosis of ulnar vein

     I82.721   Chronic embolism and thrombosis of deep veins of right upper extremity 🔾

     I82.722   Chronic embolism and thrombosis of deep veins of left upper extremity 🔾

     I82.723   Chronic embolism and thrombosis of deep veins of upper extremity, bilateral 🔾

     I82.729   Chronic embolism and thrombosis of deep veins of unspecified upper extremity 🔾

● **I82.A**   **Embolism and thrombosis of axillary vein**
     (Ex) For category I82.A CC codes: See PDX Collection 717

  ● **I82.A1**   **Acute embolism and thrombosis of axillary vein**

     I82.A11   Acute embolism and thrombosis of right axillary vein 🔾

     I82.A12   Acute embolism and thrombosis of left axillary vein 🔾

     I82.A13   Acute embolism and thrombosis of axillary vein, bilateral 🔾

     I82.A19   Acute embolism and thrombosis of unspecified axillary vein 🔾

  ● **I82.A2**   **Chronic embolism and thrombosis of axillary vein**

     I82.A21   Chronic embolism and thrombosis of right axillary vein 🔾

     I82.A22   Chronic embolism and thrombosis of left axillary vein 🔾

     I82.A23   Chronic embolism and thrombosis of axillary vein, bilateral 🔾

     I82.A29   Chronic embolism and thrombosis of unspecified axillary vein 🔾

N Newborn Age: 0   **P** Pediatric Age: 0–17   **M** Maternity DX: 12–55   **A** Adult Age: 15–124   ♀ Females Only   ♂ Males Only

🔾 Complication\Comorbidity   🔾 Major C\C   (Ex) CC/MCC Exclusions   🔾 Hospital-Acquired Condition

CHAPTER 9 (IØØ-I99)

● **I82.B**   **Embolism and thrombosis of subclavian vein**
  Ex) For category I82.B CC codes: See PDX Collection 717

  ● **I82.B1**   Acute embolism and thrombosis of subclavian vein

    I82.B11   Acute embolism and thrombosis of right subclavian vein 🔍

    I82.B12   Acute embolism and thrombosis of left subclavian vein 🔍

    I82.B13   Acute embolism and thrombosis of subclavian vein, bilateral 🔍

    I82.B19   Acute embolism and thrombosis of unspecified subclavian vein 🔍

  ● **I82.B2**   Chronic embolism and thrombosis of subclavian vein

    I82.B21   Chronic embolism and thrombosis of right subclavian vein 🔍

    I82.B22   Chronic embolism and thrombosis of left subclavian vein 🔍

    I82.B23   Chronic embolism and thrombosis of subclavian vein, bilateral 🔍

    I82.B29   Chronic embolism and thrombosis of unspecified subclavian vein 🔍

● **I82.C**   **Embolism and thrombosis of internal jugular vein**
  Ex) For category I82.C CC codes: See PDX Collection 717

  ● **I82.C1**   Acute embolism and thrombosis of internal jugular vein

    I82.C11   Acute embolism and thrombosis of right internal jugular vein 🔍

    I82.C12   Acute embolism and thrombosis of left internal jugular vein 🔍

    I82.C13   Acute embolism and thrombosis of internal jugular vein, bilateral 🔍

    I82.C19   Acute embolism and thrombosis of unspecified internal jugular vein 🔍

  ● **I82.C2**   Chronic embolism and thrombosis of internal jugular vein

    I82.C21   Chronic embolism and thrombosis of right internal jugular vein 🔍

    I82.C22   Chronic embolism and thrombosis of left internal jugular vein 🔍

    I82.C23   Chronic embolism and thrombosis of internal jugular vein, bilateral 🔍

    I82.C29   Chronic embolism and thrombosis of unspecified internal jugular vein 🔍

● **I82.8**   **Embolism and thrombosis of other specified veins**
  Use additional code, if applicable, for associated long-term (current) use of anticoagulants (Z79.Ø1)
  Ex) For category I82.8 CC codes: See PDX Collection 717

  ● **I82.81**   Embolism and thrombosis of superficial veins of lower extremities
  Embolism and thrombosis of saphenous vein (greater) (lesser)

   ⇒ **I82.811**   Embolism and thrombosis of superficial veins of right lower extremity 🔍

   ⇒ **I82.812**   Embolism and thrombosis of superficial veins of left lower extremity 🔍

    I82.813   Embolism and thrombosis of superficial veins of lower extremities, bilateral 🔍

   ⇒ **I82.819**   Embolism and thrombosis of superficial veins of unspecified lower extremity 🔍

● **I82.89**   **Embolism and thrombosis of other specified veins**

    I82.890   Acute embolism and thrombosis of other specified veins 🔍

    I82.891   Chronic embolism and thrombosis of other specified veins 🔍

● **I82.9**   **Embolism and thrombosis of unspecified vein**
  Ex) For category I82.9 CC codes: See PDX Collection 717

  I82.90   Acute embolism and thrombosis of unspecified vein 🔍
  Embolism of vein NOS
  Thrombosis (vein) NOS

  I82.91   Chronic embolism and thrombosis of unspecified vein 🔍

● **I83**   **Varicose veins of lower extremities**
  Excludes1   varicose veins complicating pregnancy (O22.Ø-)
  varicose veins complicating the puerperium (O87.4)

● **I83.Ø**   **Varicose veins of lower extremities with ulcer**
  Use additional code to identify severity of ulcer (L97.-)

  ● **I83.ØØ**   Varicose veins of unspecified lower extremity with ulcer

    I83.ØØ1   Varicose veins of unspecified lower extremity with ulcer of thigh   A

    I83.ØØ2   Varicose veins of unspecified lower extremity with ulcer of calf   A

    I83.ØØ3   Varicose veins of unspecified lower extremity with ulcer of ankle   A

    I83.ØØ4   Varicose veins of unspecified lower extremity with ulcer of heel and midfoot   A
  Varicose veins of unspecified lower extremity with ulcer of plantar surface of midfoot

    I83.ØØ5   Varicose veins of unspecified lower extremity with ulcer other part of foot   A
  Varicose veins of unspecified lower extremity with ulcer of toe

    I83.ØØ8   Varicose veins of unspecified lower extremity with ulcer other part of lower leg   A

    I83.ØØ9   Varicose veins of unspecified lower extremity with ulcer of unspecified site   A

  ● **I83.Ø1**   Varicose veins of right lower extremity with ulcer

    I83.Ø11   Varicose veins of right lower extremity with ulcer of thigh   A

    I83.Ø12   Varicose veins of right lower extremity with ulcer of calf   A

    I83.Ø13   Varicose veins of right lower extremity with ulcer of ankle   A

    I83.Ø14   Varicose veins of right lower extremity with ulcer of heel and midfoot   A
  Varicose veins of right lower extremity with ulcer of plantar surface of midfoot

    I83.Ø15   Varicose veins of right lower extremity with ulcer other part of foot   A
  Varicose veins of right lower extremity with ulcer of toe

    I83.Ø18   Varicose veins of right lower extremity with ulcer other part of lower leg   A

    I83.Ø19   Varicose veins of right lower extremity with ulcer of unspecified site   A

▶ New   ⇒ Revised   ~~deleted~~ Deleted   Excludes 1   Excludes 2   Includes   Use additional   Code first   Code also   Key words
OGCR Official Guidelines   ● Unacceptable Principal Diagnosis   X Assign placeholder X   ● Use Additional Character(s)   ▶ Manifestation Code   Coding Clinic

● **I83.02**   Varicose veins of left lower extremity with ulcer

I83.021   Varicose veins of left lower extremity with ulcer of thigh   A

I83.022   Varicose veins of left lower extremity with ulcer of calf   A

I83.023   Varicose veins of left lower extremity with ulcer of ankle   A

I83.024   Varicose veins of left lower extremity with ulcer of heel and midfoot   A
     Varicose veins of left lower extremity with ulcer of plantar surface of midfoot

I83.025   Varicose veins of left lower extremity with ulcer other part of foot   A
     Varicose veins of left lower extremity with ulcer of toe

I83.028   Varicose veins of left lower extremity with ulcer other part of lower leg   A

I83.029   Varicose veins of left lower extremity with ulcer of unspecified site   A

● **I83.1**   Varicose veins of lower extremities with inflammation

I83.10   Varicose veins of unspecified lower extremity with inflammation   A

I83.11   Varicose veins of right lower extremity with inflammation   A

I83.12   Varicose veins of left lower extremity with inflammation   A

● **I83.2**   Varicose veins of lower extremities with both ulcer and inflammation

Use additional code to identify severity of ulcer (L97.-)

(Ex) For category I83.2 CC codes: See PDX Collection 720

● **I83.20**   Varicose veins of unspecified lower extremity with both ulcer and inflammation

I83.201   Varicose veins of unspecified lower extremity with both ulcer of thigh and inflammation   A

I83.202   Varicose veins of unspecified lower extremity with both ulcer of calf and inflammation   A

I83.203   Varicose veins of unspecified lower extremity with both ulcer of ankle and inflammation   A

I83.204   Varicose veins of unspecified lower extremity with both ulcer of heel and midfoot and inflammation   A
     Varicose veins of unspecified lower extremity with both ulcer of plantar surface of midfoot and inflammation

I83.205   Varicose veins of unspecified lower extremity with both ulcer other part of foot and inflammation   A
     Varicose veins of unspecified lower extremity with both ulcer of toe and inflammation

I83.208   Varicose veins of unspecified lower extremity with both ulcer of other part of lower extremity and inflammation   A

I83.209   Varicose veins of unspecified lower extremity with both ulcer of unspecified site and inflammation   A

● **I83.21**   Varicose veins of right lower extremity with both ulcer and inflammation

I83.211   Varicose veins of right lower extremity with both ulcer of thigh and inflammation   A

I83.212   Varicose veins of right lower extremity with both ulcer of calf and inflammation   A

I83.213   Varicose veins of right lower extremity with both ulcer of ankle and inflammation   A

I83.214   Varicose veins of right lower extremity with both ulcer of heel and midfoot and inflammation   A
     Varicose veins of right lower extremity with both ulcer of plantar surface of midfoot and inflammation

I83.215   Varicose veins of right lower extremity with both ulcer other part of foot and inflammation   A
     Varicose veins of right lower extremity with both ulcer of toe and inflammation

I83.218   Varicose veins of right lower extremity with both ulcer of other part of lower extremity and inflammation   A

I83.219   Varicose veins of right lower extremity with both ulcer of unspecified site and inflammation   A

● **I83.22**   Varicose veins of left lower extremity with both ulcer and inflammation

I83.221   Varicose veins of left lower extremity with both ulcer of thigh and inflammation   A

I83.222   Varicose veins of left lower extremity with both ulcer of calf and inflammation   A

I83.223   Varicose veins of left lower extremity with both ulcer of ankle and inflammation   A

I83.224   Varicose veins of left lower extremity with both ulcer of heel and midfoot and inflammation   A
     Varicose veins of left lower extremity with both ulcer of plantar surface of midfoot and inflammation

I83.225   Varicose veins of left lower extremity with both ulcer other part of foot and inflammation   A
     Varicose veins of left lower extremity with both ulcer of toe and inflammation

I83.228   Varicose veins of left lower extremity with both ulcer of other part of lower extremity and inflammation   A

I83.229   Varicose veins of left lower extremity with both ulcer of unspecified site and inflammation   A

CHAPTER 9 (I00-I99)

- I83.8   **Varicose veins of lower extremities with other complications**
  - I83.81   **Varicose veins of lower extremities with pain**
    - ⇒ I83.811   Varicose veins of right lower extremity with pain   A
    - ⇒ I83.812   Varicose veins of left lower extremity with pain   A
    - I83.813   Varicose veins of bilateral lower extremities with pain   A
    - ⇒ I83.819   Varicose veins of unspecified lower extremity with pain   A
  - I83.89   **Varicose veins of lower extremities with other complications**
    Varicose veins of lower extremities with edema
    Varicose veins of lower extremities with swelling
    - ⇒ I83.891   Varicose veins of right lower extremity with other complications   A
    - ⇒ I83.892   Varicose veins of left lower extremity with other complications   A
    - I83.893   Varicose veins of bilateral lower extremities with other complications   A
    - ⇒ I83.899   Varicose veins of unspecified lower extremity with other complications   A
- I83.9   **Asymptomatic varicose veins of lower extremities**
  Phlebectasia of lower extremities
  Varicose veins of lower extremities
  Varix of lower extremities
  - I83.90   **Asymptomatic varicose veins of unspecified lower extremity**   A
    Varicose veins NOS
  - I83.91   **Asymptomatic varicose veins of right lower extremity**   A
  - I83.92   **Asymptomatic varicose veins of left lower extremity**   A
  - I83.93   **Asymptomatic varicose veins of bilateral lower extremities**   A

- I85   **Esophageal varices**
  Use additional code to identify:
  alcohol abuse and dependence (F10.-)
  - I85.0   **Esophageal varices**
    Idiopathic esophageal varices
    Primary esophageal varices
    - I85.00   **Esophageal varices without bleeding** 🔗
      Esophageal varices NOS
      (Ex:) See PDX Collection 721
    - I85.01   **Esophageal varices with bleeding** 🔗
      (Ex:) See PDX Collection 722
  - I85.1   **Secondary esophageal varices**
    Esophageal varices secondary to alcoholic liver disease
    Esophageal varices secondary to cirrhosis of liver
    Esophageal varices secondary to schistosomiasis
    Esophageal varices secondary to toxic liver disease
    Code first underlying disease
    - I85.10   **Secondary esophageal varices without bleeding** 🔗
      (Ex:) See PDX Collection 723
    - I85.11   **Secondary esophageal varices with bleeding** 🔗
      (Ex:) See PDX Collection 724

- I86   **Varicose veins of other sites**
  Excludes1   varicose veins of unspecified site (I83.9-)
  Excludes2   retinal varices (H35.0-)
  - I86.0   **Sublingual varices**
  - I86.1   **Scrotal varices** ♂
    Varicocele
  - I86.2   **Pelvic varices**
  - I86.3   **Vulval varices** ♀
    Excludes1   vulval varices complicating childbirth and the puerperium (O87.8)
    vulval varices complicating pregnancy (O22.1-)
  - I86.4   **Gastric varices**
  - I86.8   **Varicose veins of other specified sites**   A
    Varicose ulcer of nasal septum

- I87   **Other disorders of veins**
  - I87.0   **Postthrombotic syndrome**
    Chronic venous hypertension due to deep vein thrombosis
    Postphlebitic syndrome
    Excludes1   chronic venous hypertension without deep vein thrombosis (I87.3-)
    - I87.00   **Postthrombotic syndrome without complications**
      Asymptomatic Postthrombotic syndrome
      - I87.001   Postthrombotic syndrome without complications of right lower extremity
      - I87.002   Postthrombotic syndrome without complications of left lower extremity
      - I87.003   Postthrombotic syndrome without complications of bilateral lower extremity
      - I87.009   Postthrombotic syndrome without complications of unspecified extremity
        Postthrombotic syndrome NOS
    - I87.01   **Postthrombotic syndrome with ulcer**
      Use additional code to specify site and severity of ulcer (L97.-)
      (Ex:) For category I87.01 CC codes: See PDX Collection 725
      - I87.011   Postthrombotic syndrome with ulcer of right lower extremity 🔗
      - I87.012   Postthrombotic syndrome with ulcer of left lower extremity 🔗
      - I87.013   Postthrombotic syndrome with ulcer of bilateral lower extremity 🔗
      - I87.019   Postthrombotic syndrome with ulcer of unspecified lower extremity 🔗
    - I87.02   **Postthrombotic syndrome with inflammation**
      - I87.021   Postthrombotic syndrome with inflammation of right lower extremity
      - I87.022   Postthrombotic syndrome with inflammation of left lower extremity
      - I87.023   Postthrombotic syndrome with inflammation of bilateral lower extremity
      - I87.029   Postthrombotic syndrome with inflammation of unspecified lower extremity

▶ New   ⇒ Revised   ~~deleted~~ Deleted   Excludes 1   Excludes 2   Includes   Use additional   Code first   Code also   Key words
OGCR Official Guidelines   ● Unacceptable Principal Diagnosis   X Assign placeholder X   ● Use Additional Character(s)   ▶ Manifestation Code   **Coding Clinic**

● **I87.03**   **Postthrombotic syndrome with ulcer and inflammation**

> Use additional code to specify site and severity of ulcer (L97.-)
>
> (Ex) **For category I87.03 CC codes:** See PDX Collection 725

     I87.031   **Postthrombotic syndrome with ulcer and inflammation of right lower extremity** 🔖

     I87.032   **Postthrombotic syndrome with ulcer and inflammation of left lower extremity** 🔖

     I87.033   **Postthrombotic syndrome with ulcer and inflammation of bilateral lower extremity** 🔖

     I87.039   **Postthrombotic syndrome with ulcer and inflammation of unspecified lower extremity** 🔖

● **I87.09**   **Postthrombotic syndrome with other complications**

     I87.091   **Postthrombotic syndrome with other complications of right lower extremity**

     I87.092   **Postthrombotic syndrome with other complications of left lower extremity**

     I87.093   **Postthrombotic syndrome with other complications of bilateral lower extremity**

     I87.099   **Postthrombotic syndrome with other complications of unspecified lower extremity**

I87.1   **Compression of vein** 🔖
> Stricture of vein
> Vena cava syndrome (inferior) (superior)
>
> **Excludes2**   compression of pulmonary vein (I28.8)
>
> (Ex) See PDX Collection 726

I87.2   **Venous insufficiency (chronic) (peripheral)**
> Stasis dermatitis
>
> **Excludes1**   stasis dermatitis with varicose veins of lower extremities (I83.1-, I83.2-)

● **I87.3**   **Chronic venous hypertension (idiopathic)**
> Stasis edema
>
> **Excludes1**   chronic venous hypertension due to deep vein thrombosis (I87.0-)
>   varicose veins of lower extremities (I83.-)

   ● **I87.30**   **Chronic venous hypertension (idiopathic) without complications**

> Asymptomatic chronic venous hypertension (idiopathic)

     I87.301   **Chronic venous hypertension (idiopathic) without complications of right lower extremity**

     I87.302   **Chronic venous hypertension (idiopathic) without complications of left lower extremity**

     I87.303   **Chronic venous hypertension (idiopathic) without complications of bilateral lower extremity**

     I87.309   **Chronic venous hypertension (idiopathic) without complications of unspecified lower extremity**
> Chronic venous hypertension NOS

● **I87.31**   **Chronic venous hypertension (idiopathic) with ulcer**

> Use additional code to specify site and severity of ulcer (L97.-)
>
> (Ex) **For category I87.31 CC codes:** See PDX Collection 727

     I87.311   **Chronic venous hypertension (idiopathic) with ulcer of right lower extremity** 🔖

     I87.312   **Chronic venous hypertension (idiopathic) with ulcer of left lower extremity** 🔖

     I87.313   **Chronic venous hypertension (idiopathic) with ulcer of bilateral lower extremity** 🔖

     I87.319   **Chronic venous hypertension (idiopathic) with ulcer of unspecified lower extremity** 🔖

● **I87.32**   **Chronic venous hypertension (idiopathic) with inflammation**

     I87.321   **Chronic venous hypertension (idiopathic) with inflammation of right lower extremity**

     I87.322   **Chronic venous hypertension (idiopathic) with inflammation of left lower extremity**

     I87.323   **Chronic venous hypertension (idiopathic) with inflammation of bilateral lower extremity**

     I87.329   **Chronic venous hypertension (idiopathic) with inflammation of unspecified lower extremity**

● **I87.33**   **Chronic venous hypertension (idiopathic) with ulcer and inflammation**

> Use additional code to specify site and severity of ulcer (L97.-)
>
> (Ex) **For category I87.33 CC codes:** See PDX Collection 727

     I87.331   **Chronic venous hypertension (idiopathic) with ulcer and inflammation of right lower extremity** 🔖

     I87.332   **Chronic venous hypertension (idiopathic) with ulcer and inflammation of left lower extremity** 🔖

     I87.333   **Chronic venous hypertension (idiopathic) with ulcer and inflammation of bilateral lower extremity** 🔖

     I87.339   **Chronic venous hypertension (idiopathic) with ulcer and inflammation of unspecified lower extremity** 🔖

● **I87.39**   **Chronic venous hypertension (idiopathic) with other complications**

     I87.391   **Chronic venous hypertension (idiopathic) with other complications of right lower extremity**

     I87.392   **Chronic venous hypertension (idiopathic) with other complications of left lower extremity**

     I87.393   **Chronic venous hypertension (idiopathic) with other complications of bilateral lower extremity**

     I87.399   **Chronic venous hypertension (idiopathic) with other complications of unspecified lower extremity**

I87.8   **Other specified disorders of veins**
> Phlebosclerosis
> Venofibrosis

I87.9   **Disorder of vein, unspecified**

N   Newborn Age: 0   P   Pediatric Age: 0–17   M   Maternity DX: 12–55   A   Adult Age: 15–124   ♀   Females Only   ♂   Males Only

🔖   Complication\Comorbidity   🔖   Major C\C   (Ex)   CC/MCC Exclusions   🔖   Hospital-Acquired Condition

● **I88**   **Nonspecific lymphadenitis**

> **Excludes1**   acute lymphadenitis, except mesenteric (L04.-)
> enlarged lymph nodes NOS (R59.-)
> human immunodeficiency virus [HIV] disease resulting in generalized lymphadenopathy (B20)

   I88.0   **Nonspecific mesenteric lymphadenitis**
     Mesenteric lymphadenitis (acute)(chronic)

   I88.1   **Chronic lymphadenitis, except mesenteric**
     Adenitis
     Lymphadenitis

   I88.8   **Other nonspecific lymphadenitis**

   I88.9   **Nonspecific lymphadenitis, unspecified**
     Lymphadenitis NOS

● **I89**   **Other noninfective disorders of lymphatic vessels and lymph nodes**

> **Excludes1**   chylocele, tunica vaginalis (nonfilarial) NOS (N50.89)
> enlarged lymph nodes NOS (R59.-)
> filarial chylocele (B74.-)
> hereditary lymphedema (Q82.0)

   I89.0   **Lymphedema, not elsewhere classified**
     Elephantiasis (nonfilarial) NOS
     Lymphangiectasis
     Obliteration, lymphatic vessel
     Praecox lymphedema
     Secondary lymphedema

> **Excludes1**   postmastectomy lymphedema (I97.2)

   I89.1   **Lymphangitis**
     Chronic lymphangitis
     Lymphangitis NOS
     Subacute lymphangitis

> **Excludes1**   acute lymphangitis (L03.-)

   I89.8   **Other specified noninfective disorders of lymphatic vessels and lymph nodes**
     Chylocele (nonfilarial)
     Chylous ascites
     Chylous cyst
     Lipomelanotic reticulosis
     Lymph node or vessel fistula
     Lymph node or vessel infarction
     Lymph node or vessel rupture

   I89.9   **Noninfective disorder of lymphatic vessels and lymph nodes, unspecified**
     Disease of lymphatic vessels NOS

OTHER AND UNSPECIFIED DISORDERS OF THE CIRCULATORY SYSTEM (I95-I99)

● **I95**   **Hypotension**
     Subnormal arterial blood pressure

> **Excludes1**   cardiovascular collapse (R57.9)
> maternal hypotension syndrome (O26.5-)
> nonspecific low blood pressure reading NOS (R03.1)

   I95.0   **Idiopathic hypotension**

   I95.1   **Orthostatic hypotension**
     Hypotension, postural

> *Moving from a sitting or reclining position to a standing position precipitates a sudden drop in blood pressure (hypotension).*

> **Excludes1**   neurogenic orthostatic hypotension [Shy-Drager] (G90.3)
> orthostatic hypotension due to drugs (I95.2)

   I95.2   **Hypotension due to drugs**
     Orthostatic hypotension due to drugs

     Use additional code for adverse effect, if applicable, to identify drug (T36-T50 with fifth or sixth character 5)

   I95.3   **Hypotension of hemodialysis**
     Intra-dialytic hypotension

● **I95.8**   **Other hypotension**

   I95.81   **Postprocedural hypotension**

   I95.89   **Other hypotension**
     Chronic hypotension

   I95.9   **Hypotension, unspecified**

I96   **Gangrene, not elsewhere classified** 🔑
     Gangrenous cellulitis

> **Excludes1**   gangrene in atherosclerosis of native arteries of the extremities (I70.26)
> gangrene of certain specified sites - *see* Alphabetical Index
> ~~gangrene in diabetes mellitus (E08-E13 with .52)~~
> gangrene in hernia (K40.1, K40.4, K41.1, K41.4, K42.1, K43.1-, K44.1, K45.1, K46.1)
> gangrene in other peripheral vascular diseases (I73.-)
> gas gangrene (A48.0)
> pyoderma gangrenosum (L88)

▶ **Excludes2**   gangrene in diabetes mellitus (E08-E13 with .52)

   (Ex:) See PDX Collection 519
   Coding Clinic: 2013, Q2, P35

● **I97**   **Intraoperative and postprocedural complications and disorders of circulatory system, not elsewhere classified**

> **Excludes2**   postprocedural shock (T81.1-)

   I97.0   **Postcardiotomy syndrome**

● **I97.1**   **Other postprocedural cardiac functional disturbances**

> **Excludes2**   acute pulmonary insufficiency following thoracic surgery (J95.1)
> intraoperative cardiac functional disturbances (I97.7-)

   (Ex:) For category I97.1 CC codes: See PDX Collection 728

● **I97.11**   **Postprocedural cardiac insufficiency**

   I97.110   **Postprocedural cardiac insufficiency following cardiac surgery** 🔑

   I97.111   **Postprocedural cardiac insufficiency following other surgery** 🔑

● **I97.12**   **Postprocedural cardiac arrest**

   I97.120   **Postprocedural cardiac arrest following cardiac surgery** 🔑

   I97.121   **Postprocedural cardiac arrest following other surgery** 🔑

● **I97.13**   **Postprocedural heart failure**
     Use additional code to identify the heart failure (I50.-)

   I97.130   **Postprocedural heart failure following cardiac surgery** 🔑

   I97.131   **Postprocedural heart failure following other surgery** 🔑

● **I97.19**   **Other postprocedural cardiac functional disturbances**
     Use additional code, if applicable, to further specify disorder

   I97.190   **Other postprocedural cardiac functional disturbances following cardiac surgery** 🔑

> ▶ Use Additional code, if applicable, for type 4 or type 5 myocardial infarction, to further specify disorder

   I97.191   **Other postprocedural cardiac functional disturbances following other surgery** 🔑

▶ New   ➡ Revised   ~~deleted~~ Deleted   Excludes 1   Excludes 2   Includes   Use additional   Code first   Code also   Key words
OGCR Official Guidelines   ● Unacceptable Principal Diagnosis   X Assign placeholder X   ● Use Additional Character(s)   ▶ Manifestation Code   **Coding Clinic**

I97.2   **Postmastectomy lymphedema syndrome**   A
    Elephantiasis due to mastectomy
    Obliteration of lymphatic vessels

I97.3   **Postprocedural hypertension**

● **I97.4**   **Intraoperative hemorrhage and hematoma of a circulatory system organ or structure complicating a procedure**

    Excludes1   intraoperative hemorrhage and hematoma of a circulatory system organ or structure due to accidental puncture and laceration during a procedure (I97.5-)

    Excludes2   intraoperative cerebrovascular hemorrhage complicating a procedure (G97.3-)

    (Ex) For category I97.4 CC codes: See PDX Collection 729

● **I97.41**   **Intraoperative hemorrhage and hematoma of a circulatory system organ or structure complicating a circulatory system procedure**

    I97.410   Intraoperative hemorrhage and hematoma of a circulatory system organ or structure complicating a cardiac catheterization

    I97.411   Intraoperative hemorrhage and hematoma of a circulatory system organ or structure complicating a cardiac bypass

    I97.418   Intraoperative hemorrhage and hematoma of a circulatory system organ or structure complicating other circulatory system procedure

I97.42   **Intraoperative hemorrhage and hematoma of a circulatory system organ or structure complicating other procedure**
    Coding Clinic: 2016, Q4, P100

● **I97.5**   **Accidental puncture and laceration of a circulatory system organ or structure during a procedure**

    Excludes2   accidental puncture and laceration of brain during a procedure (G97.4-)

    (Ex) For category I97.5 CC codes: See PDX Collection 509

I97.51   **Accidental puncture and laceration of a circulatory system organ or structure during a circulatory system procedure**

I97.52   **Accidental puncture and laceration of a circulatory system organ or structure during other procedure**

● **I97.6**   **Postprocedural hemorrhage, hematoma and seroma of a circulatory system organ or structure following a procedure**

    Excludes2   postprocedural cerebrovascular hemorrhage complicating a procedure (G97.5-)

    (Ex) For category I97.6 CC codes: See PDX Collection 729
    Coding Clinic: 2016, Q4, P10

● **I97.61**   **Postprocedural hemorrhage of a circulatory system organ or structure following a circulatory system procedure**

    I97.610   Postprocedural hemorrhage of a circulatory system organ or structure following a cardiac catheterization

    I97.611   Postprocedural hemorrhage of a circulatory system organ or structure following cardiac bypass

    I97.618   Postprocedural hemorrhage of a circulatory system organ or structure following other circulatory system procedure

● **I97.62**   **Postprocedural hemorrhage, hematoma and seroma of a circulatory system organ or structure following other procedure**

    I97.620   Postprocedural hemorrhage of a circulatory system organ or structure following other procedure

    I97.621   Postprocedural hematoma of a circulatory system organ or structure following other procedure

    I97.622   Postprocedural seroma of a circulatory system organ or structure following other procedure

● **I97.63**   **Postprocedural hematoma of a circulatory system organ or structure following a circulatory system procedure**

    I97.630   Postprocedural hematoma of a circulatory system organ or structure following a cardiac catheterization

    I97.631   Postprocedural hematoma of a circulatory system organ or structure following cardiac bypass

    I97.638   Postprocedural hematoma of a circulatory system organ or structure following other circulatory system procedure

● **I97.64**   **Postprocedural seroma of a circulatory system organ or structure following a circulatory system procedure**

    I97.640   Postprocedural seroma of a circulatory system organ or structure following a cardiac catheterization

    I97.641   Postprocedural seroma of a circulatory system organ or structure following cardiac bypass

    I97.648   Postprocedural seroma of a circulatory system organ or structure following other circulatory system procedure

● **I97.7**   **Intraoperative cardiac functional disturbances**

    Excludes2   acute pulmonary insufficiency following thoracic surgery (J95.1)
      postprocedural cardiac functional disturbances (I97.1-)

    (Ex) For category I97.7 CC codes: See PDX Collection 728

● **I97.71**   **Intraoperative cardiac arrest**

    I97.710   Intraoperative cardiac arrest during cardiac surgery

    I97.711   Intraoperative cardiac arrest during other surgery

● **I97.79**   **Other intraoperative cardiac functional disturbances**

    Use additional code, if applicable, to further specify disorder

    I97.790   Other intraoperative cardiac functional disturbances during cardiac surgery

    I97.791   Other intraoperative cardiac functional disturbances during other surgery

CHAPTER 9 (I00-I99)

● **I97.8**   **Other intraoperative and postprocedural complications and disorders of the circulatory system, not elsewhere classified**

> Use additional code, if applicable, to further specify disorder
>
> Ⓔⓧ **For category I97.8 CC codes unless otherwise indicated:** See PDX Collection 617

  ● **I97.81**   **Intraoperative** cerebrovascular infarction

      I97.810   Intraoperative cerebrovascular infarction during **cardiac surgery** 🔗

      I97.811   Intraoperative cerebrovascular infarction during **other surgery** 🔗

  ● **I97.82**   **Postprocedural** cerebrovascular infarction

      I97.820   Postprocedural cerebrovascular infarction following **cardiac surgery** 🔗

      I97.821   Postprocedural cerebrovascular infarction following **other surgery** 🔗

      I97.88   **Other intraoperative complications of the circulatory system, not elsewhere classified** 🔗

        Ⓔⓧ See PDX Collection 728

      I97.89   **Other postprocedural complications and disorders of the circulatory system, not elsewhere classified** 🔗

        Ⓔⓧ See PDX Collection 728

● **I99**   **Other and unspecified disorders of circulatory system**

   I99.8   **Other disorder of circulatory system**

   I99.9   **Unspecified disorder of circulatory system**

CHAPTER 10

DISEASES OF THE RESPIRATORY SYSTEM (J00-J99)

OGCR Chapter-Specific Coding Guidelines

10. **Chapter 10: Diseases of the Respiratory System (J00-J99)**

a. **Chronic Obstructive Pulmonary Disease [COPD] and Asthma**

1) **Acute exacerbation of chronic obstructive bronchitis and asthma**

The codes in categories J44 and J45 distinguish between uncomplicated cases and those in acute exacerbation. An acute exacerbation is a worsening or a decompensation of a chronic condition. An acute exacerbation is not equivalent to an infection superimposed on a chronic condition, though an exacerbation may be triggered by an infection.

b. **Acute Respiratory Failure**

1) **Acute respiratory failure as principal diagnosis**

A code from subcategory J96.0, Acute respiratory failure, or subcategory J96.2, Acute and chronic respiratory failure, may be assigned as a principal diagnosis when it is the condition established after study to be chiefly responsible for occasioning the admission to the hospital, and the selection is supported by the Alphabetic Index and Tabular List. However, chapter-specific coding guidelines (such as obstetrics, poisoning, HIV, newborn) that provide sequencing direction take precedence.

2) **Acute respiratory failure as secondary diagnosis**

Respiratory failure may be listed as a secondary diagnosis if it occurs after admission, or if it is present on admission, but does not meet the definition of principal diagnosis.

3) **Sequencing of acute respiratory failure and another acute condition**

When a patient is admitted with respiratory failure and another acute condition, (e.g., myocardial infarction, cerebrovascular accident, aspiration pneumonia), the principal diagnosis will not be the same in every situation. This applies whether the other acute condition is a respiratory or nonrespiratory condition. Selection of the principal diagnosis will be dependent on the circumstances of admission. If both the respiratory failure and the other acute condition are equally responsible for occasioning the admission to the hospital, and there are no chapter-specific sequencing rules, the guideline regarding two or more diagnoses that equally meet the definition for principal diagnosis (Section II, C.) may be applied in these situations.

If the documentation is not clear as to whether acute respiratory failure and another condition are equally responsible for occasioning the admission, query the provider for clarification.

c. **Influenza due to certain identified influenza viruses**

Code only confirmed cases of influenza due to certain identified influenza viruses (category J09), and due to other identified influenza virus (category J10). This is an exception to the hospital inpatient guideline Section II, H. (Uncertain Diagnosis).

In this context, "confirmation" does not require documentation of positive laboratory testing specific for avian or other novel influenza A or other identified influenza virus. However, coding should be based on the provider's diagnostic statement that the patient has avian influenza, or other novel influenza A, for category J09, or has another particular identified strain of influenza, such as H1N1 or H3N2, but not identified as novel or variant, for category J10.

If the provider records "suspected" or "possible" or "probable" avian influenza, or novel influenza, or other identified influenza, then the appropriate influenza code from category J11, Influenza due to unidentified influenza virus, should be assigned. A code from category J09, Influenza due to certain identified influenza viruses, should not be assigned nor should a code from category J10, Influenza due to other identified influenza virus.

d. **Ventilator associated Pneumonia**

1) **Documentation of Ventilator associated Pneumonia**

As with all procedural or postprocedural complications, code assignment is based on the provider's documentation of the relationship between the condition and the procedure.

Code J95.851, Ventilator associated pneumonia, should be assigned only when the provider has documented ventilator associated pneumonia (VAP). An additional code to identify the organism (e.g., Pseudomonas aeruginosa, code B96.5) should also be assigned. Do not assign an additional code from categories J12-J18 to identify the type of pneumonia.

Code J95.851 should not be assigned for cases where the patient has pneumonia and is on a mechanical ventilator and the provider has not specifically stated that the pneumonia is ventilator-associated pneumonia. If the documentation is unclear as to whether the patient has a pneumonia that is a complication attributable to the mechanical ventilator, query the provider.

2) **Ventilator associated Pneumonia Develops after Admission**

A patient may be admitted with one type of pneumonia (e.g., code J13, Pneumonia due to Streptococcus pneumonia) and subsequently develop VAP. In this instance, the principal diagnosis would be the appropriate code from categories J12-J18 for the pneumonia diagnosed at the time of admission. Code J95.851, Ventilator associated pneumonia, would be assigned as an additional diagnosis when the provider has also documented the presence of ventilator associated pneumonia.

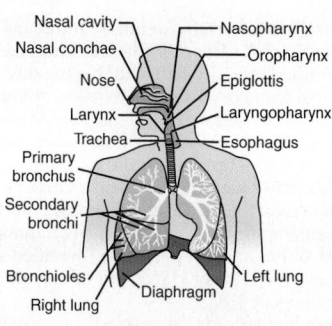

Figure 10-1 Respiratory system. (From Buck CJ: Step-by-Step Medical Coding, ed 2016, St. Louis, Elsevier, 2016)

Figure 10-2 Paranasal sinuses. (From Buck CJ: Step-by-Step Medical Coding, ed 2016, St. Louis, Elsevier, 2016)

Item 10–1 Pharyngitis is painful inflammation of the pharynx (sore throat). Ninety percent of the infections are caused by a virus with the remaining being bacterial and rarely a fungus (candidiasis). Other irritants such as pollutants, chemicals, or smoke may cause similar symptoms.

CHAPTER 10

DISEASES OF THE RESPIRATORY SYSTEM (J00-J99)

Note: When a respiratory condition is described as occurring in more than one site and is not specifically indexed, it should be classified to the lower anatomic site (e.g., tracheobronchitis to bronchitis in J40).

Use additional code, where applicable, to identify:
  exposure to environmental tobacco smoke (Z77.22)
  exposure to tobacco smoke in the perinatal period (P96.81)
  history of tobacco dependence (Z87.891)
  occupational exposure to environmental tobacco smoke (Z57.31)
  tobacco dependence (F17.-)
  tobacco use (Z72.0)

Excludes2 certain conditions originating in the perinatal period (P04-P96)
  certain infectious and parasitic diseases (A00-B99)
  complications of pregnancy, childbirth and the puerperium (O00-O99A)
  congenital malformations, deformations and chromosomal abnormalities (Q00-Q99)
  endocrine, nutritional and metabolic diseases (E00-E88)
  injury, poisoning and certain other consequences of external causes (S00-T88)
  neoplasms (C00-D49)
  smoke inhalation (T59.81-)
  symptoms, signs and abnormal clinical and laboratory findings, not elsewhere classified (R00-R94)

This chapter contains the following blocks:

J00-J06	Acute upper respiratory infections
J09-J18	Influenza and pneumonia
J20-J22	Other acute lower respiratory infections
J30-J39	Other diseases of upper respiratory tract
J40-J47	Chronic lower respiratory diseases
J60-J70	Lung diseases due to external agents
J80-J84	Other respiratory diseases principally affecting the interstitium
J85-J86	Suppurative and necrotic conditions of the lower respiratory tract
J90-J94	Other diseases of the pleura
J95	Intraoperative and postprocedural complications and disorders of respiratory system, not elsewhere classified
J96-J99	Other diseases of the respiratory system

ACUTE UPPER RESPIRATORY INFECTIONS (J00-J06)

Excludes1 chronic obstructive pulmonary disease with acute lower respiratory infection (J44.0)
  influenza virus with other respiratory manifestations (J09.X2, J10.1, J11.1)

J00   Acute nasopharyngitis [common cold]
  Acute rhinitis
  Coryza (acute)
  Infective nasopharyngitis NOS
  Infective rhinitis
  Nasal catarrh, acute
  Nasopharyngitis NOS

  Excludes1 acute pharyngitis (J02.-)
    acute sore throat NOS (J02.9)
    pharyngitis NOS (J02.9)
    rhinitis NOS (J31.0)
    sore throat NOS (J02.9)

  Excludes2 allergic rhinitis (J30.1-J30.9)
    chronic pharyngitis (J31.2)
    chronic rhinitis (J31.0)
    chronic sore throat (J31.2)
    nasopharyngitis, chronic (J31.1)
    vasomotor rhinitis (J30.0)

★ **(See Plate 49 on page 72.)**

● **J01   Acute sinusitis**
  Includes acute abscess of sinus
    acute empyema of sinus
    acute infection of sinus
    acute inflammation of sinus
    acute suppuration of sinus

  Use additional code (B95-B97) to identify infectious agent.
  Excludes1 sinusitis NOS (J32.9)
  Excludes2 chronic sinusitis (J32.0-J32.8)

● **J01.0   Acute maxillary sinusitis**
    Acute antritis

    J01.00   Acute maxillary sinusitis, unspecified
    J01.01   Acute recurrent maxillary sinusitis

● **J01.1   Acute frontal sinusitis**

    J01.10   Acute frontal sinusitis, unspecified
    J01.11   Acute recurrent frontal sinusitis

● **J01.2   Acute ethmoidal sinusitis**

    J01.20   Acute ethmoidal sinusitis, unspecified
    J01.21   Acute recurrent ethmoidal sinusitis

● **J01.3   Acute sphenoidal sinusitis**

    J01.30   Acute sphenoidal sinusitis, unspecified
    J01.31   Acute recurrent sphenoidal sinusitis

● **J01.4   Acute pansinusitis**

    J01.40   Acute pansinusitis, unspecified
    J01.41   Acute recurrent pansinusitis

▶ New   ⇒ Revised   ~~deleted~~ Deleted   Excludes 1   Excludes 2   Includes   Use additional   Code first   Code also   Key words
OGCR Official Guidelines   ● Unacceptable Principal Diagnosis   X Assign placeholder X   ● Use Additional Character(s)   ▶ Manifestation Code   **Coding Clinic**

● **J01.8**   **Other acute sinusitis**

     J01.80   **Other acute sinusitis**
         Acute sinusitis involving more than one sinus but not pansinusitis

     J01.81   **Other acute recurrent sinusitis**
         Acute recurrent sinusitis involving more than one sinus but not pansinusitis

● **J01.9**   **Acute sinusitis, unspecified**

     J01.90   **Acute sinusitis, unspecified**

     J01.91   **Acute recurrent sinusitis, unspecified**

● **J02**   **Acute pharyngitis**

     Includes   acute sore throat

     Excludes1   acute laryngopharyngitis (J06.0)
         peritonsillar abscess (J36)
         pharyngeal abscess (J39.1)
         retropharyngeal abscess (J39.0)

     Excludes2   chronic pharyngitis (J31.2)

     J02.0   **Streptococcal pharyngitis**
         Septic pharyngitis
         Streptococcal sore throat

         Excludes2   scarlet fever (A38.-)

     J02.8   **Acute pharyngitis due to other specified organisms**
         Use additional code (B95-B97) to identify infectious agent

         Excludes1   pharyngitis due to coxsackie virus (B08.5)
         pharyngitis due to gonococcus (A54.5)
         acute pharyngitis due to herpes [simplex] virus (B00.2)
         acute pharyngitis due to infectious mononucleosis (B27.-)
         enteroviral vesicular pharyngitis (B08.5)

     J02.9   **Acute pharyngitis, unspecified**
         Gangrenous pharyngitis (acute)
         Infective pharyngitis (acute) NOS
         Pharyngitis (acute) NOS
         Sore throat (acute) NOS
         Suppurative pharyngitis (acute)
         Ulcerative pharyngitis (acute)

● **J03**   **Acute tonsillitis**

     Inflammation of pharyngeal tonsils caused by virus or bacteria

     Excludes1   acute sore throat (J02.-)
         hypertrophy of tonsils (J35.1)
         peritonsillar abscess (J36)
         sore throat NOS (J02.9)
         streptococcal sore throat (J02.0)

     Excludes2   chronic tonsillitis (J35.0)

● **J03.0**   **Streptococcal tonsillitis**

     J03.00   **Acute streptococcal tonsillitis, unspecified**

     J03.01   **Acute recurrent streptococcal tonsillitis**

● **J03.8**   **Acute tonsillitis due to other specified organisms**
     Use additional code (B95-B97) to identify infectious agent.

     Excludes1   diphtheritic tonsillitis (A36.0)
         herpesviral pharyngotonsillitis (B00.2)
         streptococcal tonsillitis (J03.0)
         tuberculous tonsillitis (A15.8)
         Vincent's tonsillitis (A69.1)

     J03.80   **Acute tonsillitis due to other specified organisms**

     J03.81   **Acute recurrent tonsillitis due to other specified organisms**

● **J03.9**   **Acute tonsillitis, unspecified**
     Follicular tonsillitis (acute)
     Gangrenous tonsillitis (acute)
     Infective tonsillitis (acute)
     Tonsillitis (acute) NOS
     Ulcerative tonsillitis (acute)

     J03.90   **Acute tonsillitis, unspecified**

     J03.91   **Acute recurrent tonsillitis, unspecified**

Item 10–2   **Laryngitis** is an inflammation of the larynx (voice box) resulting in hoarse voice or the complete loss of the voice. **Tracheitis** is an inflammation of the trachea (often following a URI) commonly caused by *staphylococcus aureus* resulting in inspiratory stridor (crowing sound on inspiration) and a croup like cough.

● **J04**   **Acute laryngitis and tracheitis**
     Use additional code (B95-B97) to identify infectious agent.

     Excludes1   acute obstructive laryngitis [croup] and epiglottitis (J05.-)

     Excludes2   laryngismus (stridulus) (J38.5)

     J04.0   **Acute laryngitis**
         Edematous laryngitis (acute)
         Laryngitis (acute) NOS
         Subglottic laryngitis (acute)
         Suppurative laryngitis (acute)
         Ulcerative laryngitis (acute)

         Excludes1   acute obstructive laryngitis (J05.0)
         Excludes2   chronic laryngitis (J37.0)

     ● **J04.1**   **Acute tracheitis**
         Acute viral tracheitis
         Catarrhal tracheitis (acute)
         Tracheitis (acute) NOS

         Excludes2   chronic tracheitis (J42)

     J04.10   **Acute tracheitis without obstruction**

     J04.11   **Acute tracheitis with obstruction**
         Ⓔⓧ See PDX Collection 730

     J04.2   **Acute laryngotracheitis**
         Laryngotracheitis NOS
         Tracheitis (acute) with laryngitis (acute)

         Excludes1   acute obstructive laryngotracheitis (J05.0)
         Excludes2   chronic laryngotracheitis (J37.1)

     ● **J04.3**   **Supraglottitis, unspecified**

     J04.30   **Supraglottitis, unspecified, without obstruction**

     J04.31   **Supraglottitis, unspecified, with obstruction**
         Ⓔⓧ See PDX Collection 731

● **J05**   **Acute obstructive laryngitis [croup] and epiglottitis**
     Use additional code (B95-B97) to identify infectious agent.

     J05.0   **Acute obstructive laryngitis [croup]**
         Obstructive laryngitis (acute) NOS
         Obstructive laryngotracheitis NOS

     ● **J05.1**   **Acute epiglottitis**

         Excludes2   epiglottitis, chronic (J37.0)

     J05.10   **Acute epiglottitis without obstruction**
         Epiglottitis NOS
         Ⓔⓧ See PDX Collection 732

     J05.11   **Acute epiglottitis with obstruction**
         Ⓔⓧ See PDX Collection 730

● **J06**   **Acute upper respiratory infections of multiple and unspecified sites**

     Excludes1   acute respiratory infection NOS (J22)
         streptococcal pharyngitis (J02.0)

     J06.0   **Acute laryngopharyngitis**

     J06.9   **Acute upper respiratory infection, unspecified**
         Upper respiratory disease, acute
         Upper respiratory infection NOS

CHAPTER 10 (J00-J99)

N Newborn Age: 0   **P** Pediatric Age: 0–17   **M** Maternity DX: 12–55   **A** Adult Age: 15–124   ♀ Females Only   ♂ Males Only

Ⓒⓒ Complication\Comorbidity   Ⓜ Major C\C   Ⓔⓧ CC/MCC Exclusions   Hospital-Acquired Condition

921

INFLUENZA AND PNEUMONIA (J09-J18)

Excludes2   allergic or eosinophilic pneumonia (J82)
aspiration pneumonia NOS (J69.0)
meconium pneumonia (P24.01)
neonatal aspiration pneumonia (P24.-)
pneumonia due to solids and liquids (J69.-)
congenital pneumonia (P23.9)
lipid pneumonia (J69.1)
rheumatic pneumonia (I00)
ventilator associated pneumonia (J95.851)

● **J09   Influenza due to certain identified influenza viruses**
Excludes1 ▸ influenza A/H1N1 (J10.-)
influenza due to other influenza viruses (J10.-)
influenza due to unidentified influenza virus (J11.-)
seasonal influenza due to other identified influenza virus (J10.-)
seasonal influenza due to unidentified influenza virus (J11.-)

● **J09.X   Influenza due to identified novel influenza A virus**
Avian influenza
Bird influenza
Influenza A/H5N1
Influenza of other animal origin, not bird or swine
Swine influenza virus (viruses that normally cause infections in pigs)
Coding Clinic: 2016, Q3, P11

J09.X1   Influenza due to identified novel influenza A virus with pneumonia 🔊
Code also , if applicable, associated:
lung abscess (J85.1)
other specified type of pneumonia
Ⓔ⌧ See PDX Collection 110

J09.X2   Influenza due to identified novel influenza A virus with other respiratory manifestations
Influenza due to identified novel influenza A virus NOS
Influenza due to identified novel influenza A virus with laryngitis
Influenza due to identified novel influenza A virus with pharyngitis
Influenza due to identified novel influenza A virus with upper respiratory symptoms
Use additional code, if applicable, for associated:
pleural effusion (J91.8)
sinusitis (J01.-)

J09.X3   Influenza due to identified novel influenza A virus with gastrointestinal manifestations
Influenza due to identified novel influenza A virus gastroenteritis
Excludes1   'intestinal flu' [viral gastroenteritis] (A08.-)

J09.X9   Influenza due to identified novel influenza A virus with other manifestations
Influenza due to identified novel influenza A virus with encephalopathy
Influenza due to identified novel influenza A virus with myocarditis
Influenza due to identified novel influenza A virus with otitis media
Use additional code to identify manifestation

● **J10   Influenza due to other identified influenza virus**
Excludes1   influenza due to avian influenza virus (J09.X-)
influenza due to swine flu (J09.X-)
influenza due to unidentified influenza virus (J11.-)

● **J10.0   Influenza due to other identified influenza virus with pneumonia**
Code also associated lung abscess, if applicable (J85.1)

J10.00   Influenza due to other identified influenza virus with unspecified type of pneumonia 🔊
Ⓔ⌧ See PDX Collection 110

J10.01   Influenza due to other identified influenza virus with the same other identified influenza virus pneumonia 🔊
Ⓔ⌧ See PDX Collection 110

J10.08   Influenza due to other identified influenza virus with other specified pneumonia 🔊
Code also other specified type of pneumonia
Ⓔ⌧ See PDX Collection 733

J10.1   Influenza due to other identified influenza virus with other respiratory manifestations
Influenza due to other identified influenza virus NOS
Influenza due to other identified influenza virus with laryngitis
Influenza due to other identified influenza virus with pharyngitis
Influenza due to other identified influenza virus with upper respiratory symptoms
Use additional code for associated pleural effusion, if applicable (J91.8)
Use additional code for associated sinusitis, if applicable (J01.-)
Coding Clinic: 2016, Q3, P11

J10.2   Influenza due to other identified influenza virus with gastrointestinal manifestations
Influenza due to other identified influenza virus gastroenteritis
Excludes1   'intestinal flu' [viral gastroenteritis] (A08.-)

● **J10.8   Influenza due to other identified influenza virus with other manifestations**

J10.81   Influenza due to other identified influenza virus with encephalopathy

J10.82   Influenza due to other identified influenza virus with myocarditis

J10.83   Influenza due to other identified influenza virus with otitis media
Use additional code for any associated perforated tympanic membrane (H72.-)

J10.89   Influenza due to other identified influenza virus with other manifestations
Use additional codes to identify the manifestations

● **J11   Influenza due to unidentified influenza virus**

● **J11.0   Influenza due to unidentified influenza virus with pneumonia**
Code also associated lung abscess, if applicable (J85.1)
Ⓔ⌧ For category J11.0 CC codes: See PDX Collection 110

J11.00   Influenza due to unidentified influenza virus with unspecified type of pneumonia 🔊
Influenza with pneumonia NOS
Coding Clinic: 2016, Q3, P12

J11.08   Influenza due to unidentified influenza virus with specified pneumonia 🔊
Code also other specified type of pneumonia

▶ New   ➡ Revised   d̶e̶l̶e̶t̶e̶d̶ Deleted   Excludes 1   Excludes 2   Includes   Use additional   Code first   Code also   Key words
OGCR Official Guidelines   ● Unacceptable Principal Diagnosis   X Assign placeholder X   ● Use Additional Character(s)   ▸ Manifestation Code   **Coding Clinic**

J11.1   **Influenza due to unidentified influenza virus with other respiratory manifestations**
> Influenza NOS
> Influenzal laryngitis NOS
> Influenzal pharyngitis NOS
> Influenza with upper respiratory symptoms NOS
> Use additional code for associated pleural effusion, if applicable (J91.8)
> Use additional code for associated sinusitis, if applicable (J01.-)

J11.2   **Influenza due to unidentified influenza virus with gastrointestinal manifestations**
> Influenza gastroenteritis NOS
> **Excludes1**   'intestinal flu' [viral gastroenteritis] (A08.-)

● **J11.8**   **Influenza due to unidentified influenza virus with other manifestations**

J11.81   **Influenza due to unidentified influenza virus with encephalopathy**
> Influenzal encephalopathy NOS

J11.82   **Influenza due to unidentified influenza virus with myocarditis**
> Influenzal myocarditis NOS

J11.83   **Influenza due to unidentified influenza virus with otitis media**
> Influenzal otitis media NOS
> Use additional code for any associated perforated tympanic membrane (H72.-)

J11.89   **Influenza due to unidentified influenza virus with other manifestations**
> Use additional codes to identify the manifestations

● **J12**   **Viral pneumonia, not elsewhere classified**
> **Includes**   bronchopneumonia due to viruses other than influenza viruses
> *Code first* associated influenza, if applicable (J09.X1, J10.0-, J11.0-)
> Code also associated abscess, if applicable (J85.1)
> **Excludes1**   aspiration pneumonia due to anesthesia during labor and delivery (O74.0)
> aspiration pneumonia due to anesthesia during pregnancy (O29)
> aspiration pneumonia due to anesthesia during puerperium (O89.0)
> aspiration pneumonia due to solids and liquids (J69.-)
> aspiration pneumonia NOS (J69.0)
> congenital pneumonia (P23.0)
> congenital rubella pneumonitis (P35.0)
> interstitial pneumonia NOS (J84.9)
> lipid pneumonia (J69.1)
> neonatal aspiration pneumonia (P24.-)
> ⒺⓍ For category J12 CC codes unless otherwise indicated: See PDX Collection 734

J12.0   **Adenoviral pneumonia** 🔖

J12.1   **Respiratory syncytial virus pneumonia** 🔖

J12.2   **Parainfluenza virus pneumonia** 🔖

J12.3   **Human metapneumovirus pneumonia** 🔖

● **J12.8**   **Other viral pneumonia**

J12.81   **Pneumonia due to SARS-associated coronavirus** 🔖
> Severe acute respiratory syndrome NOS
> ⒺⓍ See PDX Collection 735

J12.89   **Other viral pneumonia** 🔖

J12.9   **Viral pneumonia, unspecified** 🔖

Item 10–3   Pneumonia is an infection of the lungs, caused by a variety of microorganisms, including viruses, most commonly the Streptococcus pneumoniae (pneumococcus) bacteria, fungi, and parasites. Pneumonia occurs when the immune system is weakened, often by a URI or influenza.

J13   **Pneumonia due to Streptococcus pneumoniae** 🔖
> Bronchopneumonia due to S. pneumoniae
> *Code first* associated influenza, if applicable (J09.X1, J10.0-, J11.0-)
> Code also associated abscess, if applicable (J85.1)
> **Excludes1**   congenital pneumonia due to S. pneumoniae (P23.6)
> lobar pneumonia, unspecified organism (J18.1)
> pneumonia due to other streptococci (J15.3-J15.4)
> ⒺⓍ See PDX Collection 110

J14   **Pneumonia due to Hemophilus influenzae** 🔖
> Bronchopneumonia due to H. influenzae
> *Code first* associated influenza, if applicable (J09.X1, J10.0-, J11.0-)
> Code also associated abscess, if applicable (J85.1)
> **Excludes1**   congenital pneumonia due to H. influenzae (P23.6)
> ⒺⓍ See PDX Collection 110

● **J15**   **Bacterial pneumonia, not elsewhere classified**
> **Includes**   bronchopneumonia due to bacteria other than S. pneumoniae and H. influenzae
> *Code first* associated influenza, if applicable (J09.X1, J10.0-, J11.0-)
> Code also associated abscess, if applicable (J85.1)
> **Excludes1**   chlamydial pneumonia (J16.0)
> congenital pneumonia (P23.-)
> Legionnaires' disease (A48.1)
> spirochetal pneumonia (A69.8)
> ⒺⓍ For category J15 CC codes: See PDX Collection 110

J15.0   **Pneumonia due to Klebsiella pneumoniae** 🔖

J15.1   **Pneumonia due to Pseudomonas** 🔖

● **J15.2**   **Pneumonia due to staphylococcus**

J15.20   **Pneumonia due to staphylococcus, unspecified** 🔖

● **J15.21**   **Pneumonia due to staphylococcus aureus**

J15.211   **Pneumonia due to Methicillin susceptible Staphylococcus aureus** 🔖
> MSSA pneumonia
> Pneumonia due to Staphylococcus aureus NOS

J15.212   **Pneumonia due to Methicillin resistant Staphylococcus aureus** 🔖

J15.29   **Pneumonia due to other staphylococcus** 🔖

J15.3   **Pneumonia due to streptococcus, group B** 🔖

J15.4   **Pneumonia due to other streptococci** 🔖
> **Excludes1**   pneumonia due to streptococcus, group B (J15.3)
> pneumonia due to Streptococcus pneumoniae (J13)

J15.5   **Pneumonia due to Escherichia coli** 🔖

⇒ **J15.6**   **Pneumonia due to other Gram-negative bacteria** 🔖
> ▶Pneumonia due to other aerobic Gram-negative bacteria
> Pneumonia due to Serratia marcescens

J15.7   **Pneumonia due to Mycoplasma pneumoniae** 🔖

J15.8   **Pneumonia due to other specified bacteria** 🔖

J15.9   **Unspecified bacterial pneumonia** 🔖
> Pneumonia due to gram-positive bacteria

CHAPTER 10 (J00–J99)

N Newborn Age: 0   **P** Pediatric Age: 0–17   **M** Maternity DX: 12–55   **A** Adult Age: 15–124   ♀ Females Only   ♂ Males Only
🔖 Complication\Comorbidity   🔖 Major C\C   ⒺⓍ CC/MCC Exclusions   🔖 Hospital-Acquired Condition

923

● **J16**   **Pneumonia due to other infectious organisms, not elsewhere classified**

> *Code first associated influenza, if applicable (J09.X1, J10.0-, J11.0-)*
>
> Code also associated abscess, if applicable (J85.1)
>
> **Excludes1**   congenital pneumonia (P23.-)
> ornithosis (A70)
> pneumocystosis (B59)
> pneumonia NOS (J18.9)
>
> (Ex:) For category J16 CC codes: See PDX Collection 110

J16.0   **Chlamydial pneumonia** 🔖

J16.8   **Pneumonia due to other specified infectious organisms** 🔖

▷ **J17**   *Pneumonia in diseases classified elsewhere* 🔖

> *Code first underlying disease, such as:*
> Q fever (A78)
> rheumatic fever (I00)
> schistosomiasis (B65.0-B65.9)
>
> **Excludes1**   candidial pneumonia (B37.1)
> chlamydial pneumonia (J16.0)
> gonorrheal pneumonia (A54.84)
> histoplasmosis pneumonia (B39.0-B39.2)
> measles pneumonia (B05.2)
> nocardiosis pneumonia (A43.0)
> pneumocystosis (B59)
> pneumonia due to Pneumocystis carinii (B59)
> pneumonia due to Pneumocystis jiroveci (B59)
> pneumonia in actinomycosis (A42.0)
> pneumonia in anthrax (A22.1)
> pneumonia in ascariasis (B77.81)
> pneumonia in aspergillosis (B44.0-B44.1)
> pneumonia in coccidioidomycosis (B38.0-B38.2)
> pneumonia in cytomegalovirus disease (B25.0)
> pneumonia in toxoplasmosis (B58.3)
> rubella pneumonia (B06.81)
> salmonella pneumonia (A02.22)
> spirochetal infection NEC with pneumonia (A69.8)
> tularemia pneumonia (A21.2)
> typhoid fever with pneumonia (A01.03)
> varicella pneumonia (B01.2)
> whooping cough with pneumonia (A37 with fifth-character 1)
>
> (Ex:) See PDX Collection 110

● **J18**   **Pneumonia, unspecified organism**

> *Code first associated influenza, if applicable (J09.X1, J10.0-, J11.0-)*
>
> **Excludes1**   abscess of lung with pneumonia (J85.1)
> aspiration pneumonia due to anesthesia during labor and delivery (O74.0)
> aspiration pneumonia due to anesthesia during pregnancy (O29)
> aspiration pneumonia due to anesthesia during puerperium (O89.0)
> aspiration pneumonia due to solids and liquids (J69.-)
> aspiration pneumonia NOS (J69.0)
> congenital pneumonia (P23.0)
> drug-induced interstitial lung disorder (J70.2-J70.4)
> interstitial pneumonia NOS (J84.9)
> lipid pneumonia (J69.1)
> neonatal aspiration pneumonia (P24.-)
> pneumonitis due to external agents (J67-J70)
> pneumonitis due to fumes and vapors (J68.0)
> usual interstitial pneumonia (J84.17)
>
> (Ex:) For category J18 CC code unless otherwise indicated: See PDX Collection 110

J18.0   **Bronchopneumonia, unspecified organism** 🔖

> **Excludes1**   hypostatic bronchopneumonia (J18.2)
> lipid pneumonia (J69.1)
>
> **Excludes2**   acute bronchiolitis (J21.-)
> chronic bronchiolitis (J44.9)

J18.1   **Lobar pneumonia, unspecified organism** 🔖
> Coding Clinic: 2016, Q3, P15

J18.2   **Hypostatic pneumonia, unspecified organism** 🔖
> Hypostatic bronchopneumonia
> Passive pneumonia
> (Ex:) See PDX Collection 736

J18.8   **Other pneumonia, unspecified organism** 🔖

J18.9   **Pneumonia, unspecified organism** 🔖
> Coding Clinic: 2016, Q3, P15; 2012, Q4, P94

OTHER ACUTE LOWER RESPIRATORY INFECTIONS (J20-J22)

> **Excludes2**   chronic obstructive pulmonary disease with acute lower respiratory infection (J44.0)

● **J20**   **Acute bronchitis**

> *Inflammation/irritation of the bronchial tubes lasting 2-3 weeks, most commonly caused by a virus*
>
> **Includes**   acute and subacute bronchitis (with) bronchospasm
> acute and subacute bronchitis (with) tracheitis
> acute and subacute bronchitis (with) tracheobronchitis, acute
> acute and subacute fibrinous bronchitis
> acute and subacute membranous bronchitis
> acute and subacute purulent bronchitis
> acute and subacute septic bronchitis
>
> **Excludes1**   bronchitis NOS (J40)
> tracheobronchitis NOS (J40)
>
> **Excludes2**   acute bronchitis with bronchiectasis (J47.0)
> acute bronchitis with chronic obstructive asthma (J44.0)
> acute bronchitis with chronic obstructive pulmonary disease (J44.0)
> allergic bronchitis NOS (J45.909-)
> bronchitis due to chemicals, fumes and vapors (J68.0)
> chronic bronchitis NOS (J42)
> chronic mucopurulent bronchitis (J41.1)
> chronic obstructive bronchitis (J44.-)
> chronic obstructive tracheobronchitis (J44.-)
> chronic simple bronchitis (J41.0)
> chronic tracheobronchitis (J42)

J20.0   **Acute bronchitis due to Mycoplasma pneumoniae**

J20.1   **Acute bronchitis due to Hemophilus influenzae**

J20.2   **Acute bronchitis due to streptococcus**

J20.3   **Acute bronchitis due to coxsackievirus**

J20.4   **Acute bronchitis due to parainfluenza virus**

J20.5   **Acute bronchitis due to respiratory syncytial virus**

J20.6   **Acute bronchitis due to rhinovirus**
> Coding Clinic: 2016, Q3, P10

J20.7   **Acute bronchitis due to echovirus**

J20.8   **Acute bronchitis due to other specified organisms**
> Coding Clinic: 2016, Q3, P11

J20.9   **Acute bronchitis, unspecified**
> Coding Clinic: 2016, Q3, P16

● **J21**   **Acute bronchiolitis**

> *Bronchiolitis obliterans with organizing pneumonia (BOOP) inflammation of bronchioles and surrounding tissue in lung*
>
> **Includes**   acute bronchiolitis with bronchospasm
>
> **Excludes2**   respiratory bronchiolitis interstitial lung disease (J84.115)
>
> (Ex:) For category J21 CC codes unless otherwise indicated: See PDX Collection 738

J21.0   **Acute bronchiolitis due to respiratory syncytial virus** 🔖
> (Ex:) See PDX Collection 737

J21.1   **Acute bronchiolitis due to human metapneumovirus** 🔖

J21.8   **Acute bronchiolitis due to other specified organisms** 🔖

J21.9   **Acute bronchiolitis, unspecified** 🔖
> Bronchiolitis (acute)
>
> **Excludes1**   chronic bronchiolitis (J44.-)

J22   **Unspecified acute lower respiratory infection**
> Acute (lower) respiratory (tract) infection NOS
>
> **Excludes1**   upper respiratory infection (acute) (J06.9)

▶ New   ⇒ Revised   ~~deleted~~ Deleted   Excludes 1   Excludes 2   Includes   Use additional   Code first   Code also   Key words

OGCR Official Guidelines   ● Unacceptable Principal Diagnosis   X Assign placeholder X   ● Use Additional Character(s)   ▷ Manifestation Code   **Coding Clinic**

OTHER DISEASES OF UPPER RESPIRATORY TRACT (J30-J39)

● **J30   Vasomotor and allergic rhinitis**

   Includes   spasmodic rhinorrhea

   Excludes1   allergic rhinitis with asthma (bronchial) (J45.909)
                    rhinitis NOS (J31.0)

   J30.0   Vasomotor rhinitis

   J30.1   Allergic rhinitis due to pollen
            Allergy NOS due to pollen
            Hay fever
            Pollinosis

   J30.2   Other seasonal allergic rhinitis

   J30.5   Allergic rhinitis due to food

 ● **J30.8   Other allergic rhinitis**

      **J30.81   Allergic rhinitis due to animal (cat) (dog) hair
                  and dander**

      J30.89   Other allergic rhinitis
                  Perennial allergic rhinitis

   J30.9   Allergic rhinitis, unspecified

● **J31   Chronic rhinitis, nasopharyngitis and pharyngitis**

   Use additional code to identify:
      exposure to environmental tobacco smoke (Z77.22)
      exposure to tobacco smoke in the perinatal period (P96.81)
      history of tobacco dependence (Z87.891)
      occupational exposure to environmental tobacco smoke
         (Z57.31)
      tobacco dependence (F17.-)
      tobacco use (Z72.0)

   J31.0   Chronic rhinitis
            Atrophic rhinitis (chronic)
            Granulomatous rhinitis (chronic)
            Hypertrophic rhinitis (chronic)
            Obstructive rhinitis (chronic)
            Ozena
            Purulent rhinitis (chronic)
            Rhinitis (chronic) NOS
            Ulcerative rhinitis (chronic)

      Excludes1   allergic rhinitis (J30.1-J30.9)
                       vasomotor rhinitis (J30.0)

   J31.1   Chronic nasopharyngitis

      Excludes2   acute nasopharyngitis (J00)

   J31.2   Chronic pharyngitis
            Chronic sore throat
            Atrophic pharyngitis (chronic)
            Granular pharyngitis (chronic)
            Hypertrophic pharyngitis (chronic)

      Excludes2   acute pharyngitis (J02.9)

● **J32   Chronic sinusitis**

   Includes   sinus abscess
                   sinus empyema
                   sinus infection
                   sinus suppuration

   Use additional code to identify:
      exposure to environmental tobacco smoke (Z77.22)
      exposure to tobacco smoke in the perinatal period (P96.81)
      history of tobacco dependence (Z87.891)
      infectious agent (B95-B97)
      occupational exposure to environmental tobacco smoke
         (Z57.31)
      tobacco dependence (F17.-)
      tobacco use (Z72.0)

   Excludes2   acute sinusitis (J01.-)

   J32.0   Chronic maxillary sinusitis
            Antritis (chronic)
            Maxillary sinusitis NOS

   J32.1   Chronic frontal sinusitis
            Frontal sinusitis NOS

Item 10-4   Nasal polyps are an abnormal growth of tissue (tumor) projecting from a mucous membrane and attached to the surface by a narrow elongated stalk (pedunculated). Nasal polyps usually originate in the ethmoid sinus but also may occur in the maxillary sinus. Symptoms are nasal block, sinusitis, anosmia, and secondary infections.

   J32.2   Chronic ethmoidal sinusitis
            Ethmoidal sinusitis NOS

      Excludes1   Woakes' ethmoiditis (J33.1)

   J32.3   Chronic sphenoidal sinusitis
            Sphenoidal sinusitis NOS

   J32.4   Chronic pansinusitis
            Pansinusitis NOS

   J32.8   Other chronic sinusitis
            Sinusitis (chronic) involving more than one sinus but
               not pansinusitis

   J32.9   Chronic sinusitis, unspecified
            Sinusitis (chronic) NOS

● **J33   Nasal polyp**

   Use additional code to identify:
      exposure to environmental tobacco smoke (Z77.22)
      exposure to tobacco smoke in the perinatal period (P96.81)
      history of tobacco dependence (Z87.891)
      occupational exposure to environmental tobacco smoke
         (Z57.31)
      tobacco dependence (F17.-)
      tobacco use (Z72.0)

   Excludes1   adenomatous polyps (D14.0)

   J33.0   Polyp of nasal cavity
            Choanal polyp
            Nasopharyngeal polyp

   J33.1   Polypoid sinus degeneration
            Woakes' syndrome or ethmoiditis

   J33.8   Other polyp of sinus
            Accessory polyp of sinus
            Ethmoidal polyp of sinus
            Maxillary polyp of sinus
            Sphenoidal polyp of sinus

   J33.9   Nasal polyp, unspecified

● **J34   Other and unspecified disorders of nose and nasal sinuses**

   Excludes2   varicose ulcer of nasal septum (I86.8)

   J34.0   Abscess, furuncle and carbuncle of nose
            Cellulitis of nose
            Necrosis of nose
            Ulceration of nose

   J34.1   Cyst and mucocele of nose and nasal sinus

   J34.2   Deviated nasal septum
            Deflection or deviation of septum (nasal) (acquired)

      Excludes1   congenital deviated nasal septum (Q67.4)

   J34.3   Hypertrophy of nasal turbinates

Deviated
septal
cartilage

Figure 10-3   Deviated nasal septum.

Item 10-5   A **deviated nasal septum** is the displacement of the septal cartilage that separates the nares. This displacement causes obstructed air flow through the nasal passages. A child can be born with this displacement (congenital), or the condition may be acquired through trauma, such as a sports injury. Symptoms include nasal block, sinusitis, and related secondary infections. Septoplasty is surgical repair of this condition.

CHAPTER 10 (J00-J99)

N Newborn Age: 0   **P** Pediatric Age: 0–17   **M** Maternity DX: 12–55   **A** Adult Age: 15–124   ♀ Females Only   ♂ Males Only

🅒 Complication\Comorbidity   🅜 Major C\C   (Ex:) CC/MCC Exclusions   🅗 Hospital-Acquired Condition

CHAPTER 10 (J00-J99)

● **J34.8　Other specified disorders of nose and nasal sinuses**

　　J34.81　Nasal mucositis (ulcerative)

　　　　Code also type of associated therapy, such as:
　　　　　　antineoplastic and immunosuppressive
　　　　　　　drugs (T45.1X-)
　　　　　　radiological procedure and radiotherapy
　　　　　　　(Y84.2)

　　　　Excludes2　gastrointestinal mucositis
　　　　　　　　　(ulcerative) (K92.81)
　　　　　　　　　mucositis (ulcerative) of vagina
　　　　　　　　　　and vulva (N76.81)
　　　　　　　　　oral mucositis (ulcerative)
　　　　　　　　　　(K12.3-)

　　**J34.89　Other specified disorders of nose and nasal
　　　　　　sinuses**
　　　　Perforation of nasal septum NOS
　　　　Rhinolith

J34.9　Unspecified disorder of nose and nasal sinuses

● **J35　Chronic diseases of tonsils and adenoids**

　　Use additional code to identify:
　　　exposure to environmental tobacco smoke (Z77.22)
　　　exposure to tobacco smoke in the perinatal period (P96.81)
　　　history of tobacco dependence (Z87.891)
　　　occupational exposure to environmental tobacco smoke
　　　　(Z57.31)
　　　tobacco dependence (F17.-)
　　　tobacco use (Z72.0)

● **J35.0　Chronic tonsillitis and adenoiditis**

　　　Excludes2　acute tonsillitis (J03.-)

　　J35.01　Chronic tonsillitis

　　J35.02　Chronic adenoiditis

　　J35.03　Chronic tonsillitis and adenoiditis

J35.1　Hypertrophy of tonsils
　　Enlargement of tonsils

　　Excludes1　hypertrophy of tonsils with tonsillitis
　　　　　　　　(J35.0-)

J35.2　Hypertrophy of adenoids
　　Enlargement of adenoids

　　Excludes1　hypertrophy of adenoids with adenoiditis
　　　　　　　　(J35.0-)

J35.3　Hypertrophy of tonsils with hypertrophy of adenoids

　　Excludes1　hypertrophy of tonsils and adenoids with
　　　　　　　　tonsillitis and adenoiditis (J35.03)

J35.8　Other chronic diseases of tonsils and adenoids
　　Adenoid vegetations
　　Amygdalolith
　　Calculus, tonsil
　　Cicatrix of tonsil (and adenoid)
　　Tonsillar tag
　　Ulcer of tonsil

J35.9　Chronic disease of tonsils and adenoids, unspecified
　　Disease (chronic) of tonsils and adenoids NOS

J36　Peritonsillar abscess 🔗

　　Includes　abscess of tonsil
　　　　　　　peritonsillar cellulitis
　　　　　　　quinsy

　　Use additional code (B95-B97) to identify infectious agent.

　　Excludes1　acute tonsillitis (J03.-)
　　　　　　　chronic tonsillitis (J35.0)
　　　　　　　retropharyngeal abscess (J39.0)
　　　　　　　tonsillitis NOS (J03.9-)

　　(Ex) See PDX Collection 739

● **J37　Chronic laryngitis and laryngotracheitis**

　　Use additional code to identify:
　　　exposure to environmental tobacco smoke (Z77.22)
　　　exposure to tobacco smoke in the perinatal period (P96.81)
　　　history of tobacco dependence (Z87.891)
　　　infectious agent (B95-B97)
　　　occupational exposure to environmental tobacco smoke
　　　　(Z57.31)
　　　tobacco dependence (F17.-)
　　　tobacco use (Z72.0)

　　J37.0　Chronic laryngitis
　　　Catarrhal laryngitis
　　　Hypertrophic laryngitis
　　　Sicca laryngitis

　　　Excludes2　acute laryngitis (J04.0)
　　　　　　　　obstructive (acute) laryngitis (J05.0)

　　J37.1　Chronic laryngotracheitis
　　　Laryngitis, chronic, with tracheitis (chronic)
　　　Tracheitis, chronic, with laryngitis

　　　Excludes1　chronic tracheitis (J42)

　　　Excludes2　acute laryngotracheitis (J04.2)
　　　　　　　　acute tracheitis (J04.1)

● **J38　Diseases of vocal cords and larynx, not elsewhere classified**

　　Use additional code to identify:
　　　exposure to environmental tobacco smoke (Z77.22)
　　　exposure to tobacco smoke in the perinatal period (P96.81)
　　　history of tobacco dependence (Z87.891)
　　　occupational exposure to environmental tobacco smoke
　　　　(Z57.31)
　　　tobacco dependence (F17.-)
　　　tobacco use (Z72.0)

　　Excludes1　congenital laryngeal stridor (P28.89)
　　　　　　　obstructive laryngitis (acute) (J05.0)
　　　　　　　postprocedural subglottic stenosis (J95.5)
　　　　　　　stridor (R06.1)
　　　　　　　ulcerative laryngitis (J04.0)

● **J38.0　Paralysis of vocal cords and larynx**
　　Laryngoplegia
　　Paralysis of glottis

　　J38.00　Paralysis of vocal cords and larynx, unspecified

　　J38.01　Paralysis of vocal cords and larynx, unilateral

　　J38.02　Paralysis of vocal cords and larynx, bilateral

　　J38.1　Polyp of vocal cord and larynx

　　　Excludes1　adenomatous polyps (D14.1)

　　J38.2　Nodules of vocal cords
　　　Chorditis (fibrinous)(nodosa)(tuberosa)
　　　Singer's nodes
　　　Teacher's nodes

Figure 10-4　Coronal section of the larynx.

Item 10-6　The **larynx** extends from the tongue to the trachea and is
divided into an upper and lower portion separated by folds. The framework
of the larynx is cartilage composed of the single cricoid, thyroid, and epiglottic
cartilages, and the paired arytenoid, cuneiform, and corniculate cartilages.

▶ New　➡ Revised　~~deleted~~ Deleted　Excludes 1　Excludes 2　Includes　Use additional　Code first　Code also　Key words

OGCR Official Guidelines　● Unacceptable Principal Diagnosis　X Assign placeholder X　● Use Additional Character(s)　▶ Manifestation Code　**Coding Clinic**

J38.3 Other diseases of vocal cords
        Abscess of vocal cords
        Cellulitis of vocal cords
        Granuloma of vocal cords
        Leukokeratosis of vocal cords
        Leukoplakia of vocal cords

J38.4 Edema of larynx
        Edema (of) glottis
        Subglottic edema
        Supraglottic edema
        Excludes1 acute obstructive laryngitis [croup] (J05.0)
                       edematous laryngitis (J04.0)

J38.5 Laryngeal spasm
        Laryngismus (stridulus)

J38.6 Stenosis of larynx

J38.7 Other diseases of larynx
        Abscess of larynx
        Cellulitis of larynx
        Disease of larynx NOS
        Necrosis of larynx
        Pachyderma of larynx
        Perichondritis of larynx
        Ulcer of larynx

●**J39 Other diseases of upper respiratory tract**
        Excludes1 acute respiratory infection NOS (J22)
                       acute upper respiratory infection (J06.9)
                       upper respiratory inflammation due to chemicals,
                          gases, fumes or vapors (J68.2)

J39.0 Retropharyngeal and parapharyngeal abscess 🐾
        Peripharyngeal abscess
        Excludes1 peritonsillar abscess (J36)
        (Ex) See PDX Collection 740

J39.1 Other abscess of pharynx 🐾
        Cellulitis of pharynx
        Nasopharyngeal abscess
        (Ex) See PDX Collection 740

J39.2 Other diseases of pharynx
        Cyst of pharynx
        Edema of pharynx
        Excludes2 chronic pharyngitis (J31.2)
                       ulcerative pharyngitis (J02.9)

**J39.3 Upper respiratory tract hypersensitivity reaction, site
         unspecified**
        Excludes1 hypersensitivity reaction of upper
                          respiratory tract, such as:
                          extrinsic allergic alveolitis (J67.9)
                          pneumoconiosis (J60-J67.9)

J39.8 Other specified diseases of upper respiratory tract

J39.9 Disease of upper respiratory tract, unspecified

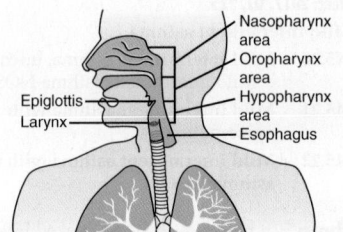

Figure 10-5 The pharynx.

Item 10-7 The **pharynx** is the passage for both food and air between the mouth and the esophagus and is divided into three areas: nasopharynx, oropharynx, and hypopharynx. The hypopharynx branches into the esophagus and the voice box.

Item 10-8 Chronic bronchitis is usually defined as being present in any patient who has persistent cough with sputum production for at least three months in at least two consecutive years. **Simple chronic bronchitis** is marked by a productive cough but no pathological airflow obstruction. **Chronic obstructive pulmonary disease (COPD)** is a group of conditions— bronchitis, emphysema, asthma, bronchiectasis, allergic alveolitis—marked by dyspnea. **Catarrhal** bronchitis is an acute form of bronchitis marked by profuse mucus and pus production (**mucopurulent** discharge). **Croupous** bronchitis, also known as pseudomembranous, fibrinous, plastic, exudative, or membranous, is marked by a violent cough and dyspnea.

CHRONIC LOWER RESPIRATORY DISEASES (J40-J47)
        Excludes1 bronchitis due to chemicals, gases, fumes and
                          vapors (J68.0)
        Excludes2 cystic fibrosis (E84.-)

J40 Bronchitis, not specified as acute or chronic
        Bronchitis NOS
        Catarrhal bronchitis
        Bronchitis with tracheitis NOS
        Tracheobronchitis NOS

        Use additional code to identify:
            exposure to environmental tobacco smoke (Z77.22)
            exposure to tobacco smoke in the perinatal period (P96.81)
            history of tobacco dependence (Z87.891)
            occupational exposure to environmental tobacco smoke
               (Z57.31)
            tobacco dependence (F17.-)
            tobacco use (Z72.0)

        Excludes1 acute bronchitis (J20.-)
                       allergic bronchitis NOS (J45.909-)
                       asthmatic bronchitis NOS (J45.9-)
                       bronchitis due to chemicals, fumes and
                          vapors (J68.0)

●**J41 Simple and mucopurulent chronic bronchitis**
        Use additional code to identify:
            exposure to environmental tobacco smoke (Z77.22)
            exposure to tobacco smoke in the perinatal period (P96.81)
            history of tobacco dependence (Z87.891)
            occupational exposure to environmental tobacco smoke
               (Z57.31)
            tobacco dependence (F17.-)
            tobacco use (Z72.0)

        Excludes1 chronic bronchitis NOS (J42)
                       chronic obstructive bronchitis (J44.-)

J41.0 Simple chronic bronchitis

J41.1 Mucopurulent chronic bronchitis

J41.8 Mixed simple and mucopurulent chronic bronchitis

J42 Unspecified chronic bronchitis
        Chronic bronchitis NOS
        Chronic tracheitis
        Chronic tracheobronchitis

        Use additional code to identify:
            exposure to environmental tobacco smoke (Z77.22)
            exposure to tobacco smoke in the perinatal period (P96.81)
            history of tobacco dependence (Z87.891)
            occupational exposure to environmental tobacco smoke
               (Z57.31)
            tobacco dependence (F17.-)
            tobacco use (Z72.0)

        Excludes1 chronic asthmatic bronchitis (J44.-)
                       chronic bronchitis with airways obstruction (J44.-)
                       chronic emphysematous bronchitis (J44.-)
                       chronic obstructive pulmonary disease NOS
                          (J44.9)
                       simple and mucopurulent chronic bronchitis
                          (J41.-)

CHAPTER 10 (J00-J99)

N Newborn Age: 0   P Pediatric Age: 0-17   M Maternity DX: 12-55   A Adult Age: 15-124   ♀ Females Only   ♂ Males Only

🐾 Complication\Comorbidity   🐾 Major C\C   (Ex) CC/MCC Exclusions   🐾 Hospital-Acquired Condition

● **J43**   **Emphysema**
Use additional code to identify:
exposure to environmental tobacco smoke (Z77.22)
history of tobacco dependence (Z87.891)
occupational exposure to environmental tobacco smoke
(Z57.31)
tobacco dependence (F17.-)
tobacco use (Z72.0)

> **Excludes1**   compensatory emphysema (J98.3)
> emphysema due to inhalation of chemicals, gases,
> fumes or vapors (J68.4)
> emphysema with chronic (obstructive) bronchitis
> (J44.-)
> emphysematous (obstructive) bronchitis (J44.-)
> interstitial emphysema (J98.2)
> mediastinal emphysema (J98.2)
> neonatal interstitial emphysema (P25.0)
> surgical (subcutaneous) emphysema (T81.82)
> traumatic subcutaneous emphysema (T79.7)

J43.0   **Unilateral pulmonary emphysema [MacLeod's
syndrome]**
Swyer-James syndrome
Unilateral emphysema
Unilateral hyperlucent lung
Unilateral pulmonary artery functional hypoplasia
Unilateral transparency of lung

J43.1   **Panlobular emphysema**
Panacinar emphysema

J43.2   **Centrilobular emphysema**

J43.8   **Other emphysema**

J43.9   **Emphysema, unspecified**
Bullous emphysema (lung)(pulmonary)
Emphysema (lung)(pulmonary) NOS
Emphysematous bleb
Vesicular emphysema (lung)(pulmonary)

● **J44**   **Other chronic obstructive pulmonary disease**

> **Includes**   asthma with chronic obstructive pulmonary
> disease
> chronic asthmatic (obstructive) bronchitis
> chronic bronchitis with airways obstruction
> chronic bronchitis with emphysema
> chronic emphysematous bronchitis
> chronic obstructive asthma
> chronic obstructive bronchitis
> chronic obstructive tracheobronchitis

Code also type of asthma, if applicable (J45.-)
Use additional code to identify:
exposure to environmental tobacco smoke (Z77.22)
history of tobacco dependence (Z87.891)
occupational exposure to environmental tobacco smoke
(Z57.31)
tobacco dependence (F17.-)
tobacco use (Z72.0)

> **Excludes1**   bronchiectasis (J47.-)
> chronic bronchitis NOS (J42)
> chronic simple and mucopurulent bronchitis (J41.-)
> chronic tracheitis (J42)
> chronic tracheobronchitis (J42)
> emphysema without chronic bronchitis (J43.-)
> ~~lung diseases due to external agents (J60-J70)~~

Coding Clinic: 2017, Q1, P25; 2016, Q3, P16

J44.0   **Chronic obstructive pulmonary disease with acute lower
respiratory infection** 🔍
~~Use additional code to identify the infection~~
▶ Code also to identify the infection
(Ex:) See PDX Collection 741
Coding Clinic: 2017, Q2, P30, Q1, P24-25; 2016, Q3, P15-16

Figure 10-6   Emphysema. (From Shiland, BJ: Medical Terminology &
Anatomy for ICD-10 Coding, ed 2, Mosby, 2015)

J44.1   **Chronic obstructive pulmonary disease with (acute)
exacerbation** 🔍
Decompensated COPD
Decompensated COPD with (acute) exacerbation

> **Excludes2**   chronic obstructive pulmonary disease
> [COPD] with acute bronchitis (J44.0)
> ▶lung diseases due to external agents
> (J60-J70)

(Ex:) See PDX Collection 741
Coding Clinic: 2017, Q1, P26; 2016, Q3, P15-16, Q1, P36

J44.9   **Chronic obstructive pulmonary disease, unspecified**
Chronic obstructive airway disease NOS
Chronic obstructive lung disease NOS

> ▶ **Excludes2**   lung diseases due to external agents
> (J60-J70)

Coding Clinic: 2017, Q1, P24-25; 2016, Q1, P37

● **J45**   **Asthma**
Allergic (predominantly) asthma
Allergic bronchitis NOS
Allergic rhinitis with asthma
Atopic asthma
Extrinsic allergic asthma
Hay fever with asthma
Idiosyncratic asthma
Intrinsic nonallergic asthma
Nonallergic asthma
Use additional code to identify:
exposure to environmental tobacco smoke (Z77.22)
exposure to tobacco smoke in the perinatal period (P96.81)
history of tobacco dependence (Z87.891)
occupational exposure to environmental tobacco smoke (Z57.31)
tobacco dependence (F17.-)
tobacco use (Z72.0)

> **Excludes1**   detergent asthma (J69.8)
> eosinophilic asthma (J82)
> ~~lung diseases due to external agents (J60-J70)~~
> miner's asthma (J60)
> wheezing NOS (R06.2)
> wood asthma (J67.8)

> **Excludes2**   asthma with chronic obstructive pulmonary
> disease (J44.9)
> chronic asthmatic (obstructive) bronchitis (J44.9)
> chronic obstructive asthma (J44.9)

(Ex:) For category J45 CC codes: See PDX Collection 742
Coding Clinic: 2017, Q1, P25

● **J45.2**   **Mild intermittent asthma**

J45.20   **Mild intermittent asthma, uncomplicated**
Mild intermittent asthma NOS

J45.21   **Mild intermittent asthma with (acute)
exacerbation** 🔍

J45.22   **Mild intermittent asthma with status
asthmaticus** 🔍

Item 10-9   **Asthma** is a bronchial condition marked by airway obstruction,
hyper-responsiveness, and inflammation. **Extrinsic** asthma, also known as allergic
asthma, is characterized by the same symptoms that occur with exposure to allergens
and is divided into the following types: **atopic, occupational, and allergic
bronchopulmonary aspergillosis.** **Intrinsic** asthma occurs in patients
who have no history of allergy or sensitivities to allergens and is divided into the
following types: **nonreaginic and pharmacologic. Status asthmaticus** is
the most severe form of asthma attack and can last for days or weeks.

▶ New   ⮕ Revised   ~~deleted~~ Deleted   Excludes 1   Excludes 2   Includes   Use additional   Code first   Code also   Key words

OGCR Official Guidelines   ● Unacceptable Principal Diagnosis   X Assign placeholder X   🔍 Use Additional Character(s)   ▶ Manifestation Code   **Coding Clinic**

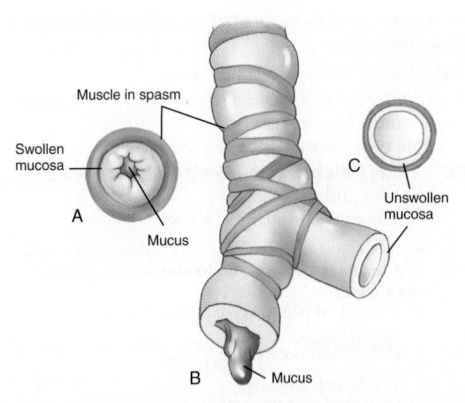

Figure 10-7 Factors causing expiratory obstruction in asthma. **A.** Cross section of a bronchiole occluded by muscle spasm, swollen mucosa, and mucus. **B.** Longitudinal section of an obstructed bronchiole. **C.** Cross-section of a clear bronchiole. (From Shiland: Mastering Healthcare Terminology, ed 1, St. Louis, Mosby, 2003)

● **J45.3 Mild persistent asthma**

    J45.30 Mild persistent asthma, uncomplicated
        Mild persistent asthma NOS

    J45.31 Mild persistent asthma with (acute) exacerbation 🔹
        Coding Clinic: 2016, Q1, P35

    J45.32 Mild persistent asthma with status asthmaticus 🔹

● **J45.4 Moderate persistent asthma**

    J45.40 Moderate persistent asthma, uncomplicated
        Moderate persistent asthma NOS

    J45.41 Moderate persistent asthma with (acute) exacerbation 🔹
        Coding Clinic: 2017, Q1, P26

    J45.42 Moderate persistent asthma with status asthmaticus 🔹

● **J45.5 Severe persistent asthma**

    J45.50 Severe persistent asthma, uncomplicated
        Severe persistent asthma NOS

    J45.51 Severe persistent asthma with (acute) exacerbation 🔹

    J45.52 Severe persistent asthma with status asthmaticus 🔹

● **J45.9 Other and unspecified asthma**

   ● **J45.90 Unspecified asthma**
        Asthmatic bronchitis NOS
        Childhood asthma NOS
        Late onset asthma

      J45.901 Unspecified asthma with (acute) exacerbation 🔹

      J45.902 Unspecified asthma with status asthmaticus 🔹

      J45.909 Unspecified asthma, uncomplicated
        Asthma NOS

        ▶ **Excludes2** lung diseases due to external agents (J60-J70)
        Coding Clinic: 2017, Q1, P25

   ● **J45.99 Other asthma**

      J45.990 Exercise induced bronchospasm

      J45.991 Cough variant asthma

      J45.998 Other asthma

● **J47 Bronchiectasis**

    Includes bronchiolectasis

    Use additional code to identify:
        exposure to environmental tobacco smoke (Z77.22)
        exposure to tobacco smoke in the perinatal period (P96.81)
        history of tobacco dependence (Z87.891)
        occupational exposure to environmental tobacco smoke (Z57.31)
        tobacco dependence (F17.-)
        tobacco use (Z72.0)

    Excludes1 congenital bronchiectasis (Q33.4)
        tuberculous bronchiectasis (current disease) (A15.0)

    (Ex) For category J47 CC codes: See PDX Collection 743

    J47.0 Bronchiectasis with acute lower respiratory infection 🔹
        Bronchiectasis with acute bronchitis
        Use additional code to identify the infection

    J47.1 Bronchiectasis with (acute) exacerbation 🔹

    J47.9 Bronchiectasis, uncomplicated
        Bronchiectasis NOS

LUNG DISEASES DUE TO EXTERNAL AGENTS (J60-J70)

    Excludes2 asthma (J45.-)
        malignant neoplasm of bronchus and lung (C34.-)

● **J60 Coalworker's pneumoconiosis**   A
    Anthracosilicosis
    Anthracosis
    Black lung disease
    Coalworker's lung

    Excludes1 coalworker pneumoconiosis with tuberculosis, any type in A15 (J65)

● **J61 Pneumoconiosis due to asbestos and other mineral fibers**   A
    Asbestosis

    Excludes1 pleural plaque with asbestosis (J92.0)
        pneumoconiosis with tuberculosis, any type in A15 (J65)

● **J62 Pneumoconiosis due to dust containing silica**

    Includes silicotic fibrosis (massive) of lung

    Excludes1 pneumoconiosis with tuberculosis, any type in A15 (J65)

    J62.0 Pneumoconiosis due to talc dust

    J62.8 Pneumoconiosis due to other dust containing silica
        Silicosis NOS

● **J63 Pneumoconiosis due to other inorganic dusts**

    Excludes1 pneumoconiosis with tuberculosis, any type in A15 (J65)

    J63.0 Aluminosis (of lung)

    J63.1 Bauxite fibrosis (of lung)

    J63.2 Berylliosis

    J63.3 Graphite fibrosis (of lung)

    J63.4 Siderosis

    J63.5 Stannosis

    J63.6 Pneumoconiosis due to other specified inorganic dusts

Figure 10-8 Progressive massive fibrosis superimposed on coal workers' pneumoconiosis. The large, blackened scars are located principally in the upper lobe. (From Frazier MS, Drzymkowski JW: Essentials of Human Diseases and Conditions, St. Louis, MO, Saunders, 2004)

Item 10-10 Pneumoconiosis refers to a lung condition resulting from exposure to inorganic or organic airborne particles, such as coal dust or moldy hay, as well as chemical fumes and vapors, such as insecticides. In this condition, the lungs retain the airborne particles.

CHAPTER 10 (J00-J99)

CHAPTER 10 (J00-J99)

J64   Unspecified pneumoconiosis

Excludes1   pneumonoconiosis with tuberculosis, any type in A15 (J65)

J65   Pneumoconiosis associated with tuberculosis
Any condition in J60-J64 with tuberculosis, any type in A15
Silicotuberculosis

● **J66   Airway disease due to specific organic dust**

Excludes2   allergic alveolitis (J67.-)
asbestosis (J61)
bagassosis (J67.1)
farmer's lung (J67.0)
hypersensitivity pneumonitis due to organic dust (J67.-)
reactive airways dysfunction syndrome (J68.3)

J66.0   Byssinosis
Airway disease due to cotton dust

J66.1   Flax-dressers' disease

J66.2   Cannabinosis

J66.8   Airway disease due to other specific organic dusts

● **J67   Hypersensitivity pneumonitis due to organic dust**

Includes   allergic alveolitis and pneumonitis due to inhaled organic dust and particles of fungal, actinomycetic or other origin

Excludes1   pneumonitis due to inhalation of chemicals, gases, fumes or vapors (J68.0)

J67.0   Farmer's lung
Harvester's lung
Haymaker's lung
Moldy hay disease

J67.1   Bagassosis
Bagasse disease
Bagasse pneumonitis

J67.2   Bird fancier's lung
Budgerigar fancier's disease or lung
Pigeon fancier's disease or lung

J67.3   Suberosis
Corkhandler's disease or lung
Corkworker's disease or lung

J67.4   Maltworker's lung
Alveolitis due to Aspergillus clavatus

J67.5   Mushroom-worker's lung

J67.6   Maple-bark-stripper's lung
Alveolitis due to Cryptostroma corticale
Cryptostromosis

J67.7   Air conditioner and humidifier lung 🔖
Allergic alveolitis due to fungal, thermophilic actinomycetes and other organisms growing in ventilation [air conditioning] systems
(Ex.) See PDX Collection 110

J67.8   Hypersensitivity pneumonitis due to other organic dusts 🔖
Cheese-washer's lung
Coffee-worker's lung
Fish-meal worker's lung
Furrier's lung
Sequoiosis
(Ex.) See PDX Collection 110

J67.9   Hypersensitivity pneumonitis due to unspecified organic dust 🔖
Allergic alveolitis (extrinsic) NOS
Hypersensitivity pneumonitis NOS
(Ex.) See PDX Collection 110

● **J68   Respiratory conditions due to inhalation of chemicals, gases, fumes and vapors**

Code first (T51-T65) to identify cause
Use additional code to identify associated respiratory conditions, such as:
acute respiratory failure (J96.0-)

J68.0   Bronchitis and pneumonitis due to chemicals, gases, fumes and vapors 🔖
Chemical bronchitis (acute)
(Ex.) See PDX Collection 110

J68.1   Pulmonary edema due to chemicals, gases, fumes and vapors 🔖
Chemical pulmonary edema (acute) (chronic)

Excludes1   pulmonary edema (acute) (chronic) NOS (J81.-)
(Ex.) See PDX Collection 110

J68.2   Upper respiratory inflammation due to chemicals, gases, fumes and vapors, not elsewhere classified

J68.3   Other acute and subacute respiratory conditions due to chemicals, gases, fumes and vapors
Reactive airways dysfunction syndrome

J68.4   Chronic respiratory conditions due to chemicals, gases, fumes and vapors
Emphysema (diffuse) (chronic) due to inhalation of chemicals, gases, fumes and vapors
Obliterative bronchiolitis (chronic) (subacute) due to inhalation of chemicals, gases, fumes and vapors
Pulmonary fibrosis (chronic) due to inhalation of chemicals, gases, fumes and vapors

Excludes1   chronic pulmonary edema due to chemicals, gases, fumes and vapors (J68.1)

J68.8   Other respiratory conditions due to chemicals, gases, fumes and vapors

J68.9   Unspecified respiratory condition due to chemicals, gases, fumes and vapors

● **J69   Pneumonitis due to solids and liquids**

Excludes1   neonatal aspiration syndromes (P24.-)
postprocedural pneumonitis (J95.4)
(Ex.) **For category J69 CC codes:** See PDX Collection 110

J69.0   Pneumonitis due to inhalation of food and vomit 🔖
Aspiration pneumonia NOS
Aspiration pneumonia (due to) food (regurgitated)
Aspiration pneumonia (due to) gastric secretions
Aspiration pneumonia (due to) milk
Aspiration pneumonia (due to) vomit
Code also any associated foreign body in respiratory tract (T17.-)

Excludes1   chemical pneumonitis due to anesthesia (J95.4)
obstetric aspiration pneumonitis (O74.0)
Coding Clinic: 2017, Q1, P24

J69.1   Pneumonitis due to inhalation of oils and essences 🔖
Exogenous lipoid pneumonia
Lipid pneumonia NOS
Code first (T51-T65) to identify substance

Excludes1   endogenous lipoid pneumonia (J84.89)

J69.8   Pneumonitis due to inhalation of other solids and liquids 🔖
Pneumonitis due to aspiration of blood
Pneumonitis due to aspiration of detergent
Code first (T51-T65) to identify substance

▶ New   ⇒ Revised   deleted Deleted   Excludes 1   Excludes 2   Includes   Use additional   Code first   Code also   Key words
OGCR Official Guidelines   ● Unacceptable Principal Diagnosis   X Assign placeholder X   ● Use Additional Character(s)   ▶ Manifestation Code   Coding Clinic

● **J70**   **Respiratory conditions due to other external agents**

    J70.0   **Acute pulmonary manifestations due to radiation** 🔖
        Radiation pneumonitis
        Use additional code (W88-W90, X39.0-) to identify the
          external cause
        (Ex) See PDX Collection 110

    J70.1   **Chronic and other pulmonary manifestations due to
        radiation** 🔖
        Fibrosis of lung following radiation
        Use additional code (W88-W90, X39.0-) to identify the
          external cause
        (Ex) See PDX Collection 110

    J70.2   **Acute drug-induced interstitial lung disorders**
        Use additional code for adverse effect, if applicable,
          to identify drug (T36-T50 with fifth or sixth
          character 5)
        Excludes1   interstitial pneumonia NOS (J84.9)
                   lymphoid interstitial pneumonia (J84.2)

    J70.3   **Chronic drug-induced interstitial lung disorders**
        Use additional code for adverse effect, if applicable,
          to identify drug (T36-T50 with fifth or sixth
          character 5)
        Excludes1   interstitial pneumonia NOS (J84.9)
                   lymphoid interstitial pneumonia (J84.2)

    J70.4   **Drug-induced interstitial lung disorders, unspecified**
        Use additional code for adverse effect, if applicable,
          to identify drug (T36-T50 with fifth or sixth
          character 5)
        Excludes1   interstitial pneumonia NOS (J84.9)
                   lymphoid interstitial pneumonia (J84.2)

    J70.5   **Respiratory conditions due to smoke inhalation**
        Smoke inhalation NOS
        Excludes1   smoke inhalation due to chemicals, gases,
                   fumes and vapors (J68.9)

    J70.8   **Respiratory conditions due to other specified external
        agents**
        Code first (T51-T65) to identify the external agent

    J70.9   **Respiratory conditions due to unspecified external agent**
        Code first (T51-T65) to identify the external agent

OTHER RESPIRATORY DISEASES PRINCIPALLY AFFECTING THE INTERSTITIUM (J80-J84)

  J80   **Acute respiratory distress syndrome** 🔖
        Acute respiratory distress syndrome in adult or child
        Adult hyaline membrane disease
        Excludes1   respiratory distress syndrome in newborn
                   (perinatal) (P22.0)
        (Ex) See PDX Collection 744
        Coding Clinic: 2017, Q1, P26-27

● **J81**   **Pulmonary edema**
        Use additional code to identify:
          exposure to environmental tobacco smoke (Z77.22)
          history of tobacco dependence (Z87.891)
          occupational exposure to environmental tobacco smoke
            (Z57.31)
          tobacco dependence (F17.-)
          tobacco use (Z72.0)
        Excludes1   chemical (acute) pulmonary edema (J68.1)
                   hypostatic pneumonia (J18.2)
                   passive pneumonia (J18.2)
                   pulmonary edema due to external agents (J60-J70)
                   pulmonary edema with heart disease NOS (I50.1)
                   pulmonary edema with heart failure (I50.1)

    J81.0   **Acute pulmonary edema** 🔖
        Acute edema of lung
        (Ex) See PDX Collection 745
        Coding Clinic: 2017, Q1, P26

    J81.1   **Chronic pulmonary edema** 🔖
        Pulmonary congestion (chronic) (passive)
        Pulmonary edema NOS
        (Ex) See PDX Collection 736

Figure 10-9   Bullous emphysema with large subpleural bullae *(upper left)*. (From Kumar: Robbins and Cotran: Pathologic Basis of Disease, ed 8, Saunders, An Imprint of Elsevier, 2009)

J82   **Pulmonary eosinophilia, not elsewhere classified** 🔖
        Allergic pneumonia
        Eosinophilic asthma
        Eosinophilic pneumonia
        Löffler's pneumonia
        Tropical (pulmonary) eosinophilia NOS
        Excludes1   pulmonary eosinophilia due to aspergillosis
                   (B44.-)
                   pulmonary eosinophilia due to drugs (J70.2-J70.4)
                   pulmonary eosinophilia due to specified parasitic
                     infection (B50-B83)
                   pulmonary eosinophilia due to systemic
                     connective tissue disorders (M30-M36)
                   pulmonary infiltrate NOS (R91.8)
        (Ex) See PDX Collection 746

● **J84**   **Other interstitial pulmonary diseases**
        Excludes1   drug-induced interstitial lung disorders
                   (J70.2-J70.4)
                   interstitial emphysema (J98.2)
                   ~~lung diseases due to external agents (J60-J70)~~
        ▶ **Excludes2**   lung diseases due to external agents (J60-J70)
        (Ex) For category J84 CC codes unless otherwise indicated: See PDX Collection 747

   ● **J84.0**   **Alveolar and parieto-alveolar conditions**
        J84.01   **Alveolar proteinosis** 🔖
        J84.02   **Pulmonary alveolar microlithiasis** 🔖
        ▶ **J84.03**   *Idiopathic pulmonary hemosiderosis* 🔖
            Essential brown induration of lung
            Code first underlying disease, such as:
              disorders of iron metabolism (E83.1-)
            Excludes1   acute idiopathic pulmonary
                       hemorrhage in infants
                       [AIPHI] (R04.81)
        J84.09   **Other alveolar and parieto-alveolar
            conditions** 🔖

   ● **J84.1**   **Other interstitial pulmonary diseases with fibrosis**
        Excludes1   pulmonary fibrosis (chronic) due to
                   inhalation of chemicals, gases, fumes
                   or vapors (J68.4)
                   pulmonary fibrosis (chronic) following
                   radiation (J70.1)

        J84.10   **Pulmonary fibrosis, unspecified**
            Capillary fibrosis of lung
            Cirrhosis of lung (chronic) NOS
            Fibrosis of lung (atrophic) (chronic) (confluent)
               (massive) (perialveolar) (peribronchial)
               NOS
            Induration of lung (chronic) NOS
            Postinflammatory pulmonary fibrosis

N   Newborn Age: 0   **P**   Pediatric Age: 0-17   **M**   Maternity DX: 12-55   **A**   Adult Age: 15-124   ♀   Females Only   ♂   Males Only

🔖 Complication\Comorbidity   🔖 Major C\C   (Ex) CC/MCC Exclusions   🔖 Hospital-Acquired Condition   **931**

CHAPTER 10 (J00-J99)

CHAPTER 10 (JØØ-J99)

● **J84.11   Idiopathic interstitial pneumonia**

     Excludes1   lymphoid interstitial pneumonia (J84.2)

                 pneumocystis pneumonia (B59)

     J84.111   Idiopathic interstitial pneumonia, not otherwise specified

     J84.112   Idiopathic pulmonary fibrosis

           Cryptogenic fibrosing alveolitis

           Idiopathic fibrosing alveolitis

     J84.113   Idiopathic non-specific interstitial pneumonitis

         Excludes1   non-specific interstitial pneumonia NOS, or due to known underlying cause (J84.89)

     J84.114   Acute interstitial pneumonitis 🔖

           Hamman-Rich syndrome

         Excludes1   pneumocystis pneumonia (B59)

     J84.115   Respiratory bronchiolitis interstitial lung disease

     J84.116   Cryptogenic organizing pneumonia 🔖

         Excludes1   organizing pneumonia NOS, or due to known underlying cause (J84.89)

     J84.117   Desquamative interstitial pneumonia 🔖

▸ **J84.17   Other interstitial pulmonary diseases with fibrosis in diseases classified elsewhere**

       Interstitial pneumonia (nonspecific) (usual) due to collagen vascular disease

       Interstitial pneumonia (nonspecific) (usual) in diseases classified elsewhere

       Organizing pneumonia due to collagen vascular disease

       Organizing pneumonia in diseases classified elsewhere

       Code first underlying disease, such as:

          progressive systemic sclerosis (M34.Ø)

          rheumatoid arthritis (MØ5.ØØ-MØ6.9)

          systemic lupus erythematosis (M32.Ø-M32.9)

J84.2   Lymphoid interstitial pneumonia 🔖

     Lymphoid interstitial pneumonitis

● **J84.8   Other specified interstitial pulmonary diseases**

     Excludes1   exogenous lipoid pneumonia (J69.1)

                 unspecified lipoid pneumonia (J69.1)

     J84.81   Lymphangioleiomyomatosis 🔖

           Lymphangiomyomatosis

     J84.82   Adult pulmonary Langerhans cell histiocytosis 🔖   A

           Adult PLCH

     J84.83   Surfactant mutations of the lung 🔖

           Ⓔⓧ See PDX Collection 748

●   **J84.84   Other interstitial lung diseases of childhood**

         Ⓔⓧ For category J84.84 CC codes: See PDX Collection 748

     J84.841   Neuroendocrine cell hyperplasia of infancy 🔖

     J84.842   Pulmonary interstitial glycogenosis 🔖

     J84.843   Alveolar capillary dysplasia with vein misalignment 🔖

     J84.848   Other interstitial lung diseases of childhood 🔖

     J84.89   Other specified interstitial pulmonary diseases

           Endogenous lipoid pneumonia

           Interstitial pneumonitis

           Non-specific interstitial pneumonitis NOS

           Organizing pneumonia NOS

           Code first, if applicable:

             poisoning due to drug or toxin (T51-T65 with fifth or sixth character to indicate intent), for toxic pneumonopathy

             underlying cause of pneumonopathy, if known

           Use additional code, for adverse effect, to identify drug (T36-T5Ø with fifth or sixth character 5), if drug-induced

         Excludes1   cryptogenic organizing pneumonia (J84.116)

                 idiopathic non-specific interstitial pneumonitis (J84.113)

                 lipoid pneumonia, exogenous or unspecified (J69.1)

                 lymphoid interstitial pneumonia (J84.2)

J84.9   Interstitial pulmonary disease, unspecified 🔖

     Interstitial pneumonia NOS

SUPPURATIVE AND NECROTIC CONDITIONS OF THE LOWER RESPIRATORY TRACT (J85-J86)

● **J85   Abscess of lung and mediastinum**

     Use additional code (B95-B97) to identify infectious agent.

     Ⓔⓧ For category J85 CC codes unless otherwise indicated: See PDX Collection 749

     J85.Ø   Gangrene and necrosis of lung 🔖

     J85.1   Abscess of lung with pneumonia 🔖

           Code also the type of pneumonia

     J85.2   Abscess of lung without pneumonia 🔖

           Abscess of lung NOS

     J85.3   Abscess of mediastinum 🔖

           Ⓔⓧ See PDX Collection 75Ø

Item 10–11   Empyema is a condition in which pus accumulates in a body cavity. Empyema **with fistula** occurs when the pus passes from one cavity to another organ or structure.

● **J86   Pyothorax**

     Use additional code (B95-B97) to identify infectious agent.

     Excludes1   abscess of lung (J85.-)

                 pyothorax due to tuberculosis (A15.6)

     Ⓔⓧ For category J86 CC codes: See PDX Collection 751

     J86.Ø   Pyothorax with fistula 🔖

           Bronchocutaneous fistula

           Bronchopleural fistula

           Hepatopleural fistula

           Mediastinal fistula

           Pleural fistula

           Thoracic fistula

           Any condition classifiable to J86.9 with fistula

     J86.9   Pyothorax without fistula 🔖

           Abscess of pleura

           Abscess of thorax

           Empyema (chest) (lung) (pleura)

           Fibrinopurulent pleurisy

           Purulent pleurisy

           Pyopneumothorax

           Septic pleurisy

           Seropurulent pleurisy

           Suppurative pleurisy

▶ New   ⇒ Revised   ~~deleted~~ Deleted   Excludes 1   Excludes 2   Includes   Use additional   Code first   Code also   Key words

OGCR Official Guidelines   ● Unacceptable Principal Diagnosis   X Assign placeholder X   ● Use Additional Character(s)   ▸ Manifestation Code   **Coding Clinic**

OTHER DISEASES OF THE PLEURA (J90-J94)

J90   **Pleural effusion, not elsewhere classified** 🕲
     Encysted pleurisy
     Pleural effusion NOS
     Pleurisy with effusion (exudative) (serous)
       Excludes1   chylous (pleural) effusion (J94.0)
                     malignant pleural effusion (J91.0))
                     pleurisy NOS (R09.1)
                     tuberculous pleural effusion (A15.6)
       (Ex) See PDX Collection 752
       Coding Clinic: 2015, Q2, P16

J91   **Pleural effusion in conditions classified elsewhere**
       Excludes2   pleural effusion in heart failure (I50.-)
                     pleural effusion in systemic lupus erythematosus
                         (M32.13)

     J91.0   *Malignant pleural effusion* 🕲
         Code first underlying neoplasm
         (Ex) See PDX Collection 753

     J91.8   *Pleural effusion in other conditions classified elsewhere* 🕲
         Code first underlying disease, such as:
           filariasis (B74.0-B74.9)
           influenza (J09.X2, J10.1, J11.1)
         (Ex) See PDX Collection 752
         Coding Clinic: 2015, Q2, P16

J92   **Pleural plaque**
       Includes   pleural thickening
     J92.0   **Pleural plaque with presence of asbestos**
     J92.9   **Pleural plaque without asbestos**
         Pleural plaque NOS

J93   **Pneumothorax and air leak**
     Collapsed lung
       Excludes1   congenital or perinatal pneumothorax (P25.1)
                     postprocedural air leak (J95.812)
                     postprocedural pneumothorax (J95.811)
                     traumatic pneumothorax (S27.0)
                     tuberculous (current disease) pneumothorax
                       (A15.-)
                     pyopneumothorax (J86.-)
       (Ex) For category J93 CC codes: See PDX Collection 754

     J93.0   **Spontaneous tension pneumothorax** 🕲
         Tension pneumothorax (most serious type) occurs when air
         (positive pressure) collects in the pleural space

     J93.1   **Other spontaneous pneumothorax**
         J93.11   **Primary spontaneous pneumothorax** 🕲
         J93.12   **Secondary spontaneous pneumothorax** 🕲
              Code first underlying condition, such as:
                catamenial pneumothorax due to
                   endometriosis (N80.8)
                cystic fibrosis (E84.-)
                eosinophilic pneumonia (J82)
                lymphangioleiomyomatosis (J84.81)
                malignant neoplasm of bronchus and lung
                   (C34.-)
                Marfan's syndrome (Q87.4)
                pneumonia due to Pneumocystis carinii
                   (B59)
                secondary malignant neoplasm of lung
                   (C78.0-)
                spontaneous rupture of the esophagus
                   (K22.3)

     J93.8   **Other pneumothorax and air leak**
         J93.81   **Chronic pneumothorax** 🕲
         J93.82   **Other air leak** 🕲
              Persistent air leak
         J93.83   **Other pneumothorax** 🕲
              Acute pneumothorax
              Spontaneous pneumothorax NOS
     J93.9   **Pneumothorax, unspecified** 🕲
         Pneumothorax NOS

J94   **Other pleural conditions**
       Excludes1   pleurisy NOS (R09.1) .
                     traumatic hemopneumothorax (S27.2)
                     traumatic hemothorax (S27.1)
                     tuberculous pleural conditions (current disease)
                       (A15.-)
       (Ex) For category J94 CC codes unless otherwise indicated: See PDX Collection 752

     J94.0   **Chylous effusion** 🕲
         Chyliform effusion
     J94.1   **Fibrothorax**
     J94.2   **Hemothorax** 🕲
         Hemopneumothorax
     J94.8   **Other specified pleural conditions** 🕲
         Hydropneumothorax
         Hydrothorax
         (Ex) No exclusions
     J94.9   **Pleural condition, unspecified**

INTRAOPERATIVE AND POSTPROCEDURAL COMPLICATIONS AND DISORDERS OF RESPIRATORY SYSTEM, NOT ELSEWHERE CLASSIFIED (J95)

J95   **Intraoperative and postprocedural complications and disorders of respiratory system, not elsewhere classified**
       Excludes2   aspiration pneumonia (J69.-)
                     emphysema (subcutaneous) resulting from a
                       procedure (T81.82)
                     hypostatic pneumonia (J18.2)
                     pulmonary manifestations due to radiation
                       (J70.0- J70.1)

     J95.0   **Tracheostomy complications**
         (Ex) For category J95.0 CC codes: See PDX Collection 755
         J95.00   **Unspecified tracheostomy complication** 🕲
         J95.01   **Hemorrhage from tracheostomy stoma** 🕲
         J95.02   **Infection of tracheostomy stoma** 🕲
              Use additional code to identify type of
                   infection, such as:
                  ➧cellulitis of neck (L03.221)
                   sepsis (A40, A41.-)
         J95.03   **Malfunction of tracheostomy stoma** 🕲
              Mechanical complication of tracheostomy
                   stoma
              Obstruction of tracheostomy airway
              Tracheal stenosis due to tracheostomy
         J95.04   **Tracheo-esophageal fistula following tracheostomy** 🕲
         J95.09   **Other tracheostomy complication** 🕲

     J95.1   **Acute pulmonary insufficiency following thoracic surgery** 🕲
         Excludes2   functional disturbances following cardiac
                       surgery (I97.0, I97.1-)
         (Ex) See PDX Collection 756

     J95.2   **Acute pulmonary insufficiency following nonthoracic surgery** 🕲
         Excludes2   functional disturbances following cardiac
                       surgery (I97.0, I97.1-)
         (Ex) See PDX Collection 756

CHAPTER 10 (J00-J99)

N Newborn Age: 0   **P** Pediatric Age: 0-17   **M** Maternity DX: 12-55   **A** Adult Age: 15-124   ♀ Females Only   ♂ Males Only

🕲 Complication\Comorbidity   🕲 Major C\C   (Ex) CC/MCC Exclusions   🕲 Hospital-Acquired Condition

933

CHAPTER 10 (J00-J99)

J95.3 **Chronic pulmonary insufficiency following surgery**
Excludes2 functional disturbances following cardiac surgery (I97.0, I97.1-)
(Ex) See PDX Collection 756

J95.4 **Chemical pneumonitis due to anesthesia**
Mendelson's syndrome
Postprocedural aspiration pneumonia
Use additional code for adverse effect, if applicable, to identify drug (T41.- with fifth or sixth character 5)
Excludes1 aspiration pneumonitis due to anesthesia complicating labor and delivery (O74.0)
aspiration pneumonitis due to anesthesia complicating pregnancy (O29)
aspiration pneumonitis due to anesthesia complicating the puerperium (O89.01)
(Ex) See PDX Collection 757

J95.5 **Postprocedural subglottic stenosis**
(Ex) See PDX Collection 757

J95.6 **Intraoperative hemorrhage and hematoma of a respiratory system organ or structure complicating a procedure**
Excludes1 intraoperative hemorrhage and hematoma of a respiratory system organ or structure due to accidental puncture and laceration during procedure (J95.7-)
(Ex) For category J95.6 CC codes: See PDX Collection 758

J95.61 Intraoperative hemorrhage and hematoma of a respiratory system organ or structure complicating a respiratory system procedure

J95.62 Intraoperative hemorrhage and hematoma of a respiratory system organ or structure complicating other procedure

J95.7 **Accidental puncture and laceration of a respiratory system organ or structure during a procedure**
Excludes2 postprocedural pneumothorax (J95.811)
(Ex) For category J95.7 CC codes: See PDX Collection 509

J95.71 Accidental puncture and laceration of a respiratory system organ or structure during a respiratory system procedure

J95.72 Accidental puncture and laceration of a respiratory system organ or structure during other procedure

J95.8 **Other intraoperative and postprocedural complications and disorders of respiratory system, not elsewhere classified**
Coding Clinic: 2016, Q4, P10

J95.81 Postprocedural pneumothorax and air leak
(Ex) For category J95.81 CC codes: See PDX Collection 754

J95.811 Postprocedural pneumothorax
J95.812 Postprocedural air leak

J95.82 Postprocedural respiratory failure
Excludes1 Respiratory failure in other conditions (J96.-)
(Ex) For category J95.82 CC codes: See PDX Collection 756

J95.821 Acute postprocedural respiratory failure
Postprocedural respiratory failure NOS

J95.822 Acute and chronic postprocedural respiratory failure

J95.83 **Postprocedural hemorrhage of a respiratory system organ or structure following a procedure**
(Ex) For category J95.83 CC codes: See PDX Collection 758

J95.830 Postprocedural hemorrhage of a respiratory system organ or structure following a respiratory system procedure

J95.831 Postprocedural hemorrhage of a respiratory system organ or structure following other procedure

J95.84 **Transfusion-related acute lung injury (TRALI)**
(Ex) See PDX Collection 757

J95.85 **Complication of respirator [ventilator]**
J95.850 Mechanical complication of respirator
Excludes1 encounter for respirator [ventilator] dependence during power failure (Z99.12)
(Ex) See PDX Collection 759

J95.851 Ventilator associated pneumonia
Ventilator associated pneumonitis
Use additional code to identify the organism, if known (B95.-, B96.-, B97.-)
Excludes1 ventilator lung in newborn (P27.8)
(Ex) See PDX Collection 757
Coding Clinic: 2017, Q1, P25

J95.859 Other complication of respirator [ventilator]
(Ex) See PDX Collection 757

J95.86 **Postprocedural hematoma and seroma of a respiratory system organ or structure following a procedure**
(Ex) For category J95.86 CC codes: See PDX Collection 758

J95.860 Postprocedural hematoma of a respiratory system organ or structure following a respiratory system procedure

J95.861 Postprocedural hematoma of a respiratory system organ or structure following other procedure

J95.862 Postprocedural seroma of a respiratory system organ or structure following a respiratory system procedure

J95.863 Postprocedural seroma of a respiratory system organ or structure following other procedure

J95.88 **Other intraoperative complications of respiratory system, not elsewhere classified**
(Ex) See PDX Collection 757

J95.89 **Other postprocedural complications and disorders of respiratory system, not elsewhere classified**
Use additional code to identify disorder, such as:
aspiration pneumonia (J69.-)
bacterial or viral pneumonia (J12-J18)
Excludes2 acute pulmonary insufficiency following thoracic surgery (J95.1)
postprocedural subglottic stenosis (J95.5)
(Ex) See PDX Collection 757

▶ New   ⇒ Revised   ~~deleted~~ Deleted   Excludes 1   Excludes 2   Includes   Use additional   Code first   Code also   Key words
OGCR Official Guidelines   ● Unacceptable Principal Diagnosis   X Assign placeholder X   ● Use Additional Character(s)   ▶ Manifestation Code   **Coding Clinic**

OTHER DISEASES OF THE RESPIRATORY SYSTEM (J96-J99)

J96   Respiratory failure, not elsewhere classified
> **Excludes1** acute respiratory distress syndrome (J80)
> cardiorespiratory failure (R09.2)
> newborn respiratory distress syndrome (P22.0)
> postprocedural respiratory failure (J95.82-)
> respiratory arrest (R09.2)
> respiratory arrest of newborn (P28.81)
> respiratory failure of newborn (P28.5)
>
> (Ex) For category J96 CC codes: See PDX Collection 744

J96.0   Acute respiratory failure
- **J96.00   Acute respiratory failure, unspecified whether with hypoxia or hypercapnia**
  Coding Clinic: 2016, Q3, P14
- **J96.01   Acute respiratory failure with hypoxia**
- **J96.02   Acute respiratory failure with hypercapnia**

J96.1   Chronic respiratory failure
- **J96.10   Chronic respiratory failure, unspecified whether with hypoxia or hypercapnia**
  Coding Clinic: 2016, Q1, P38; 2015, Q1, P21
- **J96.11   Chronic respiratory failure with hypoxia**
- **J96.12   Chronic respiratory failure with hypercapnia**

J96.2   Acute and chronic respiratory failure
  Acute on chronic respiratory failure
- **J96.20   Acute and chronic respiratory failure, unspecified whether with hypoxia or hypercapnia**
- **J96.21   Acute and chronic respiratory failure with hypoxia**
- **J96.22   Acute and chronic respiratory failure with hypercapnia**

J96.9   Respiratory failure, unspecified
- **J96.90   Respiratory failure, unspecified, unspecified whether with hypoxia or hypercapnia**
- **J96.91   Respiratory failure, unspecified with hypoxia**
- **J96.92   Respiratory failure, unspecified with hypercapnia**

J98   Other respiratory disorders
> Use additional code to identify:
> exposure to environmental tobacco smoke (Z77.22)
> exposure to tobacco smoke in the perinatal period (P96.81)
> history of tobacco dependence (Z87.891)
> occupational exposure to environmental tobacco smoke (Z57.31)
> tobacco dependence (F17.-)
> tobacco use (Z72.0)
>
> **Excludes1** newborn apnea (P28.4)
> newborn sleep apnea (P28.3)
>
> **Excludes2** apnea NOS (R06.81)
> sleep apnea (G47.3-)

J98.0   Diseases of bronchus, not elsewhere classified
- **J98.01   Acute bronchospasm**
  > **Excludes1** acute bronchiolitis with bronchospasm (J21.-)
  > acute bronchitis with bronchospasm (J20.-)
  > asthma (J45.-)
  > exercise induced bronchospasm (J45.990)
- **J98.09   Other diseases of bronchus, not elsewhere classified**
  Broncholithiasis
  Calcification of bronchus
  Stenosis of bronchus
  Tracheobronchial collapse
  Tracheobronchial dyskinesia
  Ulcer of bronchus

J98.1   Pulmonary collapse
> **Excludes1** therapeutic collapse of lung status (Z98.3)
>
> (Ex) For category J98.1 CC codes: See PDX Collection 760
- **J98.11   Atelectasis**
  > **Excludes1** newborn atelectasis
  > tuberculous atelectasis (current disease) (A15)
- **J98.19   Other pulmonary collapse**

J98.2   Interstitial emphysema
  Mediastinal emphysema
  > **Excludes1** emphysema NOS (J43.9)
  > emphysema in newborn (P25.0)
  > surgical emphysema (subcutaneous) (T81.82)
  > traumatic subcutaneous emphysema (T79.7)

J98.3   Compensatory emphysema

J98.4   Other disorders of lung
  Calcification of lung
  Cystic lung disease (acquired)
  Lung disease NOS
  Pulmolithiasis
  > **Excludes1** acute interstitial pneumonitis (J84.114)
  > pulmonary insufficiency following surgery (J95.1-J95.2)

J98.5   Diseases of mediastinum, not elsewhere classified
> **Excludes2** abscess of mediastinum (J85.3)
> Coding Clinic: 2016, Q4, P29
- **J98.51   Mediastinitis**
  > *Code first underlying condition, if applicable, such as postoperative mediastinitis (T81.-)*
  > (Ex) No Exclusions
- **J98.59   Other diseases of mediastinum, not elsewhere classified**
  Fibrosis of mediastinum
  Hernia of mediastinum
  Retraction of mediastinum
  (Ex) No Exclusions

J98.6   Disorders of diaphragm
  Diaphragmatitis
  Paralysis of diaphragm
  Relaxation of diaphragm
  > **Excludes1** congenital malformation of diaphragm NEC (Q79.1)
  > congenital diaphragmatic hernia (Q79.0)
  > **Excludes2** diaphragmatic hernia (K44.-)

J98.8   Other specified respiratory disorders

J98.9   Respiratory disorder, unspecified
  Respiratory disease (chronic) NOS

J99   Respiratory disorders in diseases classified elsewhere
> *Code first underlying disease, such as:*
> amyloidosis (E85.-)
> ankylosing spondylitis (M45)
> congenital syphilis (A50.5)
> cryoglobulinemia (D89.1)
> early congenital syphilis (A50.0)
> schistosomiasis (B65.0-B65.9)
>
> **Excludes1** respiratory disorders in:
> amebiasis (A06.5)
> blastomycosis (B40.0-B40.2)
> candidiasis (B37.1)
> coccidioidomycosis (B38.0-B38.2)
> cystic fibrosis with pulmonary manifestations (E84.0)
> dermatomyositis (M33.01, M33.11)
> histoplasmosis (B39.0-B39.2)
> late syphilis (A52.72, A52.73)
> polymyositis (M33.21)
> sicca syndrome (M35.02)
> systemic lupus erythematosus (M32.13)
> systemic sclerosis (M34.81)
> Wegener's granulomatosis (M31.30-M31.31)

CHAPTER 10 (J00-J99)

 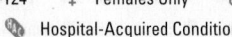

CHAPTER 11

DISEASES OF THE DIGESTIVE SYSTEM (K00-K95)

OGCR Chapter-Specific Coding Guidelines

    11. Chapter 11: Diseases of the Digestive System (K00-K95)
        Reserved for future guideline expansion

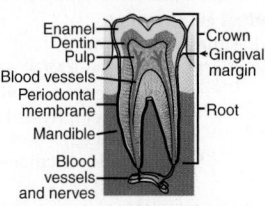

Figure 11-1 Anatomy of a tooth.

Item 11-1 **Anodontia** is the congenital absence of teeth. **Hypodontia** is partial anodontia. **Oligodontia** is the congenital absence of some teeth, whereas **supernumerary** is having more teeth than the normal number. **Mesiodens** are small extra teeth that often appear in pairs, although single small teeth are not uncommon.

CHAPTER 11

DISEASES OF THE DIGESTIVE SYSTEM (K00-K95)

    Excludes2   certain conditions originating in the perinatal period (P04-P96)
          certain infectious and parasitic diseases (A00-B99)
          complications of pregnancy, childbirth and the puerperium (O00-O9A)
          congenital malformations, deformations and chromosomal abnormalities (Q00-Q99)
          endocrine, nutritional and metabolic diseases (E00-E88)
          injury, poisoning and certain other consequences of external causes (S00-T88)
          neoplasms (C00-D49)
          symptoms, signs and abnormal clinical and laboratory findings, not elsewhere classified (R00-R94)

This chapter contains the following blocks:

K00-K14	Diseases of oral cavity and salivary glands
K20-K31	Diseases of esophagus, stomach and duodenum
K35-K38	Diseases of appendix
K40-K46	Hernia
K50-K52	Noninfective enteritis and colitis
K55-K64	Other diseases of intestines
K65-K68	Diseases of peritoneum and retroperitoneum
K70-K77	Diseases of liver
K80-K87	Disorders of gallbladder, biliary tract and pancreas
K90-K95	Other diseases of the digestive system

DISEASES OF ORAL CAVITY AND SALIVARY GLANDS (K00-K14)

● **K00**   **Disorders of tooth development and eruption**
    Excludes2   embedded and impacted teeth (K01.-)

    K00.0   **Anodontia**
          Hypodontia
          Oligodontia
        Excludes1   acquired absence of teeth (K08.1-)

    K00.1   **Supernumerary teeth**
          Distomolar
          Fourth molar
          Mesiodens
          Paramolar
          Supplementary teeth
        Excludes2   supernumerary roots (K00.2)

    K00.2   **Abnormalities of size and form of teeth**
          Concrescence of teeth
          Fusion of teeth
          Gemination of teeth
          Dens evaginatus
          Dens in dente
          Dens invaginatus
          Enamel pearls
          Macrodontia
          Microdontia
          Peg-shaped [conical] teeth
          Supernumerary roots
          Taurodontism
          Tuberculum paramolare
        Excludes1   abnormalities of teeth due to congenital syphilis (A50.5)
                      tuberculum Carabelli, which is regarded as a normal variation and should not be coded

    K00.3   **Mottled teeth**
          Dental fluorosis
          Mottling of enamel
          Nonfluoride enamel opacities
         Excludes2   deposits [accretions] on teeth (K03.6)

    K00.4   **Disturbances in tooth formation**
          Aplasia and hypoplasia of cementum
          Dilaceration of tooth
          Enamel hypoplasia (neonatal) (postnatal) (prenatal)
          Regional odontodysplasia
          Turner's tooth
        Excludes1   Hutchinson's teeth and mulberry molars in congenital syphilis (A50.5)
        Excludes2   mottled teeth (K00.3)

    K00.5   **Hereditary disturbances in tooth structure, not elsewhere classified**
          Amelogenesis imperfecta
          Dentinogenesis imperfecta
          Odontogenesis imperfecta
          Dentinal dysplasia
          Shell teeth

    K00.6   **Disturbances in tooth eruption**
          Dentia praecox
          Natal tooth
          Neonatal tooth
          Premature eruption of tooth
          Premature shedding of primary [deciduous] tooth
          Prenatal teeth
          Retained [persistent] primary tooth
         Excludes2   embedded and impacted teeth (K01.-)

    K00.7   **Teething syndrome**

    K00.8   **Other disorders of tooth development**
          Color changes during tooth formation
          Intrinsic staining of teeth NOS
         Excludes2   posteruptive color changes (K03.7)

    K00.9   **Disorder of tooth development, unspecified**
          Disorder of odontogenesis NOS

● **K01**   **Embedded and impacted teeth**
    Excludes1   abnormal position of fully erupted teeth (M26.3-)

    K01.0   **Embedded teeth**

    K01.1   **Impacted teeth**

▶ New   ⇒ Revised   ~~deleted~~ Deleted   Excludes 1   Excludes 2   Includes   Use additional   Code first   Code also   Key words
OGCR Official Guidelines   ● Unacceptable Principal Diagnosis   X Assign placeholder X   ● Use Additional Character(s)   ▶ Manifestation Code   **Coding Clinic**

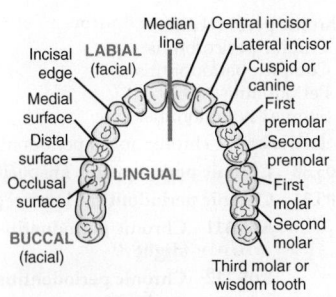

Figure 11-2 The permanent teeth within the dental arch.

Item 11–2 Each dental arch (jaw) normally contains 16 teeth. Tooth decay or **dental caries** is a disease of the enamel, dentin, and cementum of the tooth and can result in a cavity.

● **K02 Dental caries**

    Includes   caries of dentine
                     dental cavities
                     early childhood caries
                     pre-eruptive caries
                     recurrent caries (dentino enamel junction) (enamel) (to the pulp)
                     tooth decay

    K02.3 Arrested dental caries
        Arrested coronal and root caries

●   **K02.5 Dental caries on pit and fissure surface**
        Dental caries on chewing surface of tooth

        K02.51 Dental caries on pit and fissure surface limited to enamel
            White spot lesions [initial caries] on pit and fissure surface of tooth

        K02.52 Dental caries on pit and fissure surface penetrating into dentin
            Primary dental caries, cervical origin

        K02.53 Dental caries on pit and fissure surface penetrating into pulp

●   **K02.6 Dental caries on smooth surface**

        K02.61 Dental caries on smooth surface limited to enamel
            White spot lesions [initial caries] on smooth surface of tooth

        K02.62 Dental caries on smooth surface penetrating into dentin

        K02.63 Dental caries on smooth surface penetrating into pulp

    K02.7 Dental root caries

    K02.9 Dental caries, unspecified

● **K03 Other diseases of hard tissues of teeth**

    Excludes2 bruxism (F45.8)
                   dental caries (K02.-)
                   teeth-grinding NOS (F45.8)

    K03.0 Excessive attrition of teeth
        Approximal wear of teeth
        Occlusal wear of teeth

    K03.1 Abrasion of teeth
        Dentifrice abrasion of teeth
        Habitual abrasion of teeth
        Occupational abrasion of teeth
        Ritual abrasion of teeth
        Traditional abrasion of teeth
        Wedge defect NOS

    K03.2 Erosion of teeth
        Erosion of teeth due to diet
        Erosion of teeth due to drugs and medicaments
        Erosion of teeth due to persistent vomiting
        Erosion of teeth NOS
        Idiopathic erosion of teeth
        Occupational erosion of teeth

    K03.3 Pathological resorption of teeth
        Internal granuloma of pulp
        Resorption of teeth (external)

    K03.4 Hypercementosis
        Cementation hyperplasia

    K03.5 Ankylosis of teeth

    K03.6 Deposits [accretions] on teeth
        Betel deposits [accretions] on teeth
        Black deposits [accretions] on teeth
        Extrinsic staining of teeth NOS
        Green deposits [accretions] on teeth
        Materia alba deposits [accretions] on teeth
        Orange deposits [accretions] on teeth
        Staining of teeth NOS
        Subgingival dental calculus
        Supragingival dental calculus
        Tobacco deposits [accretions] on teeth

    K03.7 Posteruptive color changes of dental hard tissues
        Excludes2 deposits [accretions] on teeth (K03.6)

●   **K03.8 Other specified diseases of hard tissues of teeth**

        K03.81 Cracked tooth
            Excludes1 asymptomatic craze lines in enamel - omit code
                             broken or fractured tooth due to trauma (S02.5)

        K03.89 Other specified diseases of hard tissues of teeth

    K03.9 Disease of hard tissues of teeth, unspecified

K04 Diseases of pulp and periapical tissues
    Coding Clinic: 2016, Q4, P29

●   **K04.0 Pulpitis**
        Acute pulpitis
        Chronic (hyperplastic) (ulcerative) pulpitis
        Ⓔⓧ **For category K04.0 CC codes: See PDX Collection 761**

        K04.01 Reversible pulpitis 🔖

        K04.02 Irreversible pulpitis 🔖

    K04.1 Necrosis of pulp
        Pulpal gangrene

    K04.2 Pulp degeneration
        Denticles
        Pulpal calcifications
        Pulpal stones

    K04.3 Abnormal hard tissue formation in pulp
        Secondary or irregular dentine

    K04.4 Acute apical periodontitis of pulpal origin 🔖
        Acute apical periodontitis NOS
        Excludes1 acute periodontitis (K05.2-)
        Ⓔⓧ See PDX Collection 761

    K04.5 Chronic apical periodontitis
        Apical or periapical granuloma
        Apical periodontitis NOS
        Excludes1 chronic periodontitis (K05.3-)

    K04.6 Periapical abscess with sinus
        Dental abscess with sinus
        Dentoalveolar abscess with sinus

    K04.7 Periapical abscess without sinus
        Dental abscess without sinus
        Dentoalveolar abscess without sinus
        ~~Periapical abscess without sinus~~

    K04.8 Radicular cyst
        Apical (periodontal) cyst
        Periapical cyst
        Residual radicular cyst
        Excludes2 lateral periodontal cyst (K09.0)

●   **K04.9 Other and unspecified diseases of pulp and periapical tissues**

        K04.90 Unspecified diseases of pulp and periapical tissues

        K04.99 Other diseases of pulp and periapical tissues

CHAPTER 11 (K00-K95)

Item 11–3 Acute gingivitis, also known as orilitis or ulitis, is the short-term, severe inflammation of the gums (gingiva) caused by bacteria. **Chronic gingivitis** is persistent inflammation of the gums. When the gingivitis moves into the periodontium it is called periodontitis, also known as paradentitis.

● **K05 Gingivitis and periodontal diseases**
    Use additional code to identify:
        alcohol abuse and dependence (F10.-)
        exposure to environmental tobacco smoke (Z77.22)
        exposure to tobacco smoke in the perinatal period (P96.81)
        history of tobacco dependence (Z87.891)
        occupational exposure to environmental tobacco smoke (Z57.31)
        tobacco dependence (F17.-)
        tobacco use (Z72.0)
    Coding Clinic: 2016, Q4, P29

● **K05.0 Acute gingivitis**
    Excludes1 acute necrotizing ulcerative gingivitis (A69.1)
        herpesviral [herpes simplex] gingivostomatitis (B00.2)
    K05.00 Acute gingivitis, plaque induced
        Acute gingivitis NOS
        Plaque induced gingival disease
    K05.01 Acute gingivitis, non-plaque induced

● **K05.1 Chronic gingivitis**
    Desquamative gingivitis (chronic)
    Gingivitis (chronic) NOS
    Hyperplastic gingivitis (chronic)
    Pregnancy associated gingivitis
    Simple marginal gingivitis (chronic)
    Ulcerative gingivitis (chronic)
    Code first, if applicable, diseases of the digestive system complicating pregnancy (O99.61-)
    K05.10 Chronic gingivitis, plaque induced
        Chronic gingivitis NOS
        Gingivitis NOS
    K05.11 Chronic gingivitis, non-plaque induced

● **K05.2 Aggressive periodontitis**
    Acute pericoronitis
    Excludes1 acute apical periodontitis (K04.4)
        periapical abscess (K04.7)
        periapical abscess with sinus (K04.6)
    K05.20 Aggressive periodontitis, unspecified
●   **K05.21 Aggressive periodontitis, localized**
        Periodontal abscess
        K05.211 Aggressive periodontitis, localized, slight
        K05.212 Aggressive periodontitis, localized, moderate
        K05.213 Aggressive periodontitis, localized, severe
        K05.219 Aggressive periodontitis, localized, unspecified severity
●   **K05.22 Aggressive periodontitis, generalized**
        K05.221 Aggressive periodontitis, generalized, slight
        K05.222 Aggressive periodontitis, generalized, moderate
        K05.223 Aggressive periodontitis, generalized, severe
        K05.229 Aggressive periodontitis, generalized, unspecified severity

● **K05.3 Chronic periodontitis**
    Chronic pericoronitis
    Complex periodontitis
    Periodontitis NOS
    Simplex periodontitis
    Excludes1 chronic apical periodontitis (K04.5)
    K05.30 Chronic periodontitis, unspecified
●   **K05.31 Chronic periodontitis, localized**
        K05.311 Chronic periodontitis, localized, slight
        K05.312 Chronic periodontitis, localized, moderate
        K05.313 Chronic periodontitis, localized, severe
        K05.319 Chronic periodontitis, localized, unspecified severity
●   **K05.32 Chronic periodontitis, generalized**
        K05.321 Chronic periodontitis, generalized, slight
        K05.322 Chronic periodontitis, generalized, moderate
        K05.323 Chronic periodontitis, generalized, severe
        K05.329 Chronic periodontitis, generalized, unspecified severity

K05.4 Periodontosis
    Juvenile periodontosis

K05.5 Other periodontal diseases
    Combined periodontic-endodontic lesion
    Narrow gingival width (of periodontal soft tissue)
    Excludes2 leukoplakia of gingiva (K13.21)

K05.6 Periodontal disease, unspecified

● **K06 Other disorders of gingiva and edentulous alveolar ridge**
    Excludes2 acute gingivitis (K05.0)
        atrophy of edentulous alveolar ridge (K08.2)
        chronic gingivitis (K05.1)
        gingivitis NOS (K05.1)
    Coding Clinic: 2016, Q4, P29
● **K06.0 Gingival recession**
    Gingival recession (postinfective) (postprocedural)
▶●   **K06.01 Gingival recession, localized**
    ▶ **K06.010 Localized gingival recession, unspecified**
        Localized gingival recession, NOS
    ▶ **K06.011 Localized gingival recession, minimal**
    ▶ **K06.012 Localized gingival recession, moderate**
    ▶ **K06.013 Localized gingival recession, severe**
▶●   **K06.02 Gingival recession, generalized**
    ▶ **K06.020 Generalized gingival recession, unspecified**
        Generalized gingival recession, NOS
    ▶ **K06.021 Generalized gingival recession, minimal**
    ▶ **K06.022 Generalized gingival recession, moderate**
    ▶ **K06.023 Generalized gingival recession, severe**

K06.1 Gingival enlargement
    Gingival fibromatosis

K06.2 Gingival and edentulous alveolar ridge lesions associated with trauma
    Irritative hyperplasia of edentulous ridge [denture hyperplasia]
    Use additional code (Chapter 20) to identify external cause or denture status (Z97.2)

▶ New   ⏩ Revised   ~~deleted~~ Deleted   Excludes 1   Excludes 2   Includes   Use additional   Code first   Code also   Key words
OGCR Official Guidelines   ● Unacceptable Principal Diagnosis   X Assign placeholder X   ● Use Additional Character(s)   ▶ Manifestation Code   **Coding Clinic**

K06.3   **Horizontal alveolar bone loss**

K06.8   **Other specified disorders of gingiva and edentulous alveolar ridge**
  Fibrous epulis
  Flabby alveolar ridge
  Giant cell epulis
  Peripheral giant cell granuloma of gingiva
  Pyogenic granuloma of gingiva
  Vertical ridge deficiency
    Excludes2   gingival cyst (K09.0)

K06.9   **Disorder of gingiva and edentulous alveolar ridge, unspecified**

● **K08   Other disorders of teeth and supporting structures**
    Excludes2   dentofacial anomalies [including malocclusion] (M26.-)
                     disorders of jaw (M27.-)
    Coding Clinic: 2016, Q4, P29

K08.0   **Exfoliation of teeth due to systemic causes**
    Code also underlying systemic condition

● K08.1   **Complete loss of teeth**
    Acquired loss of teeth, complete
      Excludes1   congenital absence of teeth (K00.0)
                       exfoliation of teeth due to systemic causes (K08.0)
                       partial loss of teeth (K08.4-)

  ● K08.10   **Complete loss of teeth, unspecified cause**
      K08.101   **Complete loss of teeth, unspecified cause, class I**
      K08.102   **Complete loss of teeth, unspecified cause, class II**
      K08.103   **Complete loss of teeth, unspecified cause, class III**
      K08.104   **Complete loss of teeth, unspecified cause, class IV**
      K08.109   **Complete loss of teeth, unspecified cause, unspecified class**
                 Edentulism NOS

  ● K08.11   **Complete loss of teeth due to trauma**
      K08.111   **Complete loss of teeth due to trauma, class I**
      K08.112   **Complete loss of teeth due to trauma, class II**
      K08.113   **Complete loss of teeth due to trauma, class III**
      K08.114   **Complete loss of teeth due to trauma, class IV**
      K08.119   **Complete loss of teeth due to trauma, unspecified class**

  ● K08.12   **Complete loss of teeth due to periodontal diseases**
      K08.121   **Complete loss of teeth due to periodontal diseases, class I**
      K08.122   **Complete loss of teeth due to periodontal diseases, class II**
      K08.123   **Complete loss of teeth due to periodontal diseases, class III**
      K08.124   **Complete loss of teeth due to periodontal diseases, class IV**
      K08.129   **Complete loss of teeth due to periodontal diseases, unspecified class**

  ● K08.13   **Complete loss of teeth due to caries**
      K08.131   **Complete loss of teeth due to caries, class I**
      K08.132   **Complete loss of teeth due to caries, class II**
      K08.133   **Complete loss of teeth due to caries, class III**
      K08.134   **Complete loss of teeth due to caries, class IV**
      K08.139   **Complete loss of teeth due to caries, unspecified class**

● K08.19   **Complete loss of teeth due to other specified cause**
    K08.191   **Complete loss of teeth due to other specified cause, class I**
    K08.192   **Complete loss of teeth due to other specified cause, class II**
    K08.193   **Complete loss of teeth due to other specified cause, class III**
    K08.194   **Complete loss of teeth due to other specified cause, class IV**
    K08.199   **Complete loss of teeth due to other specified cause, unspecified class**

● K08.2   **Atrophy of edentulous alveolar ridge**
  K08.20   **Unspecified atrophy of edentulous alveolar ridge**
             Atrophy of the mandible NOS
             Atrophy of the maxilla NOS

  K08.21   **Minimal atrophy of the mandible**
             Minimal atrophy of the edentulous mandible

  K08.22   **Moderate atrophy of the mandible**
             Moderate atrophy of the edentulous mandible

  K08.23   **Severe atrophy of the mandible**
             Severe atrophy of the edentulous mandible

  K08.24   **Minimal atrophy of maxilla**
             Minimal atrophy of the edentulous maxilla

  K08.25   **Moderate atrophy of the maxilla**
             Moderate atrophy of the edentulous maxilla

  K08.26   **Severe atrophy of the maxilla**
             Severe atrophy of the edentulous maxilla

K08.3   **Retained dental root**

● K08.4   **Partial loss of teeth**
    Acquired loss of teeth, partial
      Excludes1   complete loss of teeth (K08.1-)
                       congenital absence of teeth (K00.0)
      Excludes2   exfoliation of teeth due to systemic causes (K08.0)

  ● K08.40   **Partial loss of teeth, unspecified cause**
      K08.401   **Partial loss of teeth, unspecified cause, class I**
      K08.402   **Partial loss of teeth, unspecified cause, class II**
      K08.403   **Partial loss of teeth, unspecified cause, class III**
      K08.404   **Partial loss of teeth, unspecified cause, class IV**
      K08.409   **Partial loss of teeth, unspecified cause, unspecified class**
                 Tooth extraction status NOS

  ● K08.41   **Partial loss of teeth due to trauma**
      K08.411   **Partial loss of teeth due to trauma, class I**
      K08.412   **Partial loss of teeth due to trauma, class II**
      K08.413   **Partial loss of teeth due to trauma, class III**
      K08.414   **Partial loss of teeth due to trauma, class IV**
      K08.419   **Partial loss of teeth due to trauma, unspecified class**

  ● K08.42   **Partial loss of teeth due to periodontal diseases**
      K08.421   **Partial loss of teeth due to periodontal diseases, class I**
      K08.422   **Partial loss of teeth due to periodontal diseases, class II**
      K08.423   **Partial loss of teeth due to periodontal diseases, class III**
      K08.424   **Partial loss of teeth due to periodontal diseases, class IV**
      K08.429   **Partial loss of teeth due to periodontal diseases, unspecified class**

● **K08.43** **Partial loss of teeth due to caries**

    K08.431 **Partial loss of teeth due to caries, class I**

    K08.432 **Partial loss of teeth due to caries, class II**

    K08.433 **Partial loss of teeth due to caries, class III**

    K08.434 **Partial loss of teeth due to caries, class IV**

    K08.439 **Partial loss of teeth due to caries, unspecified class**

● **K08.49** **Partial loss of teeth due to other specified cause**

    K08.491 **Partial loss of teeth due to other specified cause, class I**

    K08.492 **Partial loss of teeth due to other specified cause, class II**

    K08.493 **Partial loss of teeth due to other specified cause, class III**

    K08.494 **Partial loss of teeth due to other specified cause, class IV**

    K08.499 **Partial loss of teeth due to other specified cause, unspecified class**

● **K08.5** **Unsatisfactory restoration of tooth**
    Defective bridge, crown, filling
    Defective dental restoration

    Excludes1   dental restoration status (Z98.811)

    Excludes2   endosseous dental implant failure (M27.6-)
                       unsatisfactory endodontic treatment (M27.5-)

    K08.50 **Unsatisfactory restoration of tooth, unspecified**
        Defective dental restoration NOS

    K08.51 **Open restoration margins of tooth**
        Dental restoration failure of marginal integrity
        Open margin on tooth restoration
        Poor gingival margin to tooth restoration

    K08.52 **Unrepairable overhanging of dental restorative materials**
        Overhanging of tooth restoration

● **K08.53** **Fractured dental restorative material**

    Excludes1   cracked tooth (K03.81)
                       traumatic fracture of tooth (S02.5)

    K08.530 **Fractured dental restorative material without loss of material**

    K08.531 **Fractured dental restorative material with loss of material**

    K08.539 **Fractured dental restorative material, unspecified**

    K08.54 **Contour of existing restoration of tooth biologically incompatible with oral health**
        Dental restoration failure of periodontal anatomical integrity
        Unacceptable contours of existing restoration of tooth
        Unacceptable morphology of existing restoration of tooth

    K08.55 **Allergy to existing dental restorative material**
        Use additional code to identify the specific type of allergy

    K08.56 **Poor aesthetic of existing restoration of tooth**
        Dental restoration aesthetically inadequate or displeasing

    K08.59 **Other unsatisfactory restoration of tooth**
        Other defective dental restoration

● **K08.8** **Other specified disorders of teeth and supporting structures**

    K08.81 **Primary occlusal trauma**

    K08.82 **Secondary occlusal trauma**

    K08.89 **Other specified disorders of teeth and supporting structures**
        Enlargement of alveolar ridge NOS
        Insufficient anatomic crown height
        Insufficient clinical crown length
        Irregular alveolar process
        Toothache NOS

    K08.9 **Disorder of teeth and supporting structures, unspecified**

● **K09** **Cysts of oral region, not elsewhere classified**

    Includes   lesions showing histological features both of aneurysmal cyst and of another fibro-osseous lesion

    Excludes2   cysts of jaw (M27.0-, M27.4-)
                       radicular cyst (K04.8)

    K09.0 **Developmental odontogenic cysts**
        Dentigerous cyst
        Eruption cyst
        Follicular cyst
        Gingival cyst
        Lateral periodontal cyst
        Primordial cyst

        Excludes2   keratocysts (D16.4, D16.5)
                            odontogenic keratocystic tumors (D16.4, D16.5)

    K09.1 **Developmental (nonodontogenic) cysts of oral region**
        Cyst (of) incisive canal
        Cyst (of) palatine of papilla
        Globulomaxillary cyst
        Median palatal cyst
        Nasoalveolar cyst
        Nasolabial cyst
        Nasopalatine duct cyst

    K09.8 **Other cysts of oral region, not elsewhere classified**
        Dermoid cyst
        Epidermoid cyst
        Lymphoepithelial cyst
        Epstein's pearl

    K09.9 **Cyst of oral region, unspecified**

★ **(See Plate 61 on page 73.)**

● **K11** **Diseases of salivary glands**
    Use additional code to identify:
        alcohol abuse and dependence (F10.-)
        exposure to environmental tobacco smoke (Z77.22)
        exposure to tobacco smoke in the perinatal period (P96.81)
        history of tobacco dependence (Z87.891)
        occupational exposure to environmental tobacco smoke (Z57.31)
        tobacco dependence (F17.-)
        tobacco use (Z72.0)

    K11.0 **Atrophy of salivary gland**

    K11.1 **Hypertrophy of salivary gland**

Item 11–4 Atrophy is wasting away of a tissue or organ, whereas **hypertrophy** is overdevelopment or enlargement of a tissue or organ. **Sialoadenitis** is salivary gland inflammation. **Parotitis** is the inflammation of the parotid gland. In the epidemic form, parotitis is also known as mumps. **Sialolithiasis** is the formation of calculus within a salivary gland. **Mucocele** is a polyp composed of mucus.

Figure 11-3 Major salivary glands.

Parotid gland
Sublingual gland
Submandibular gland

▶ New   ⟹ Revised   ~~deleted~~ Deleted   Excludes 1   Excludes 2   Includes   Use additional   Code first   Code also   Key words

OGCR Official Guidelines   ● Unacceptable Principal Diagnosis   X Assign placeholder X   ● Use Additional Character(s)   ▌ Manifestation Code   **Coding Clinic**

● **K11.2   Sialoadenitis**
Parotitis
> **Excludes1**   epidemic parotitis (B26.-)
> mumps (B26.-)
> uveoparotid fever [Heerfordt] (D86.89)

K11.20   Sialoadenitis, unspecified

K11.21   Acute sialoadenitis
> **Excludes1**   acute recurrent sialoadenitis (K11.22)

K11.22   Acute recurrent sialoadenitis

K11.23   Chronic sialoadenitis

K11.3   Abscess of salivary gland
Ⓔⓧ See PDX Collection 762

K11.4   Fistula of salivary gland
> **Excludes1**   congenital fistula of salivary gland (Q38.4)
Ⓔⓧ See PDX Collection 762

K11.5   Sialolithiasis
Calculus of salivary gland or duct
Stone of salivary gland or duct

K11.6   Mucocele of salivary gland
Mucous extravasation cyst of salivary gland
Mucous retention cyst of salivary gland
Ranula

K11.7   Disturbances of salivary secretion
Hypoptyalism
Ptyalism
Xerostomia
> **Excludes2**   dry mouth NOS (R68.2)

K11.8   Other diseases of salivary glands
Benign lymphoepithelial lesion of salivary gland
Mikulicz' disease
Necrotizing sialometaplasia
Sialectasia
Stenosis of salivary duct
Stricture of salivary duct
> **Excludes1**   sicca syndrome [Sjögren] (M35.0-)

K11.9   Disease of salivary gland, unspecified
Sialoadenopathy NOS

● **K12   Stomatitis and related lesions**
Use additional code to identify:
alcohol abuse and dependence (F10.-)
exposure to environmental tobacco smoke (Z77.22)
exposure to tobacco smoke in the perinatal period (P96.81)
history of tobacco dependence (Z87.891)
occupational exposure to environmental tobacco smoke (Z57.31)
tobacco dependence (F17.-)
tobacco use (Z72.0)
> **Excludes1**   cancrum oris (A69.0)
> cheilitis (K13.0)
> gangrenous stomatitis (A69.0)
> herpesviral [herpes simplex] gingivostomatitis (B00.2)
> noma (A69.0)

K12.0   Recurrent oral aphthae
Aphthous stomatitis (major) (minor)
Bednar's aphthae
Periadenitis mucosa necrotica recurrens
Recurrent aphthous ulcer
Stomatitis herpetiformis

K12.1   Other forms of stomatitis
Stomatitis NOS
Denture stomatitis
Ulcerative stomatitis
Vesicular stomatitis
> **Excludes1**   acute necrotizing ulcerative stomatitis (A69.1)
> Vincent's stomatitis (A69.1)

K12.2   Cellulitis and abscess of mouth
Cellulitis of mouth (floor)
Submandibular abscess
> **Excludes2**   abscess of salivary gland (K11.3)
> abscess of tongue (K14.0)
> periapical abscess (K04.6-K04.7)
> periodontal abscess (K05.21)
> peritonsillar abscess (J36)
Ⓔⓧ See PDX Collection 763

● **K12.3   Oral mucositis (ulcerative)**
Mucositis (oral) (oropharyneal)
> **Excludes2**   gastrointestinal mucositis (ulcerative) (K92.81)
> mucositis (ulcerative) of vagina and vulva (N76.81)
> nasal mucositis (ulcerative) (J34.81)

K12.30   Oral mucositis (ulcerative), unspecified

K12.31   Oral mucositis (ulcerative) due to antineoplastic therapy
Use additional code for adverse effect, if applicable, to identify antineoplastic and immunosuppressive drugs (T45.1X5)
Use additional code for other antineoplastic therapy, such as:
radiological procedure and radiotherapy (Y84.2)

K12.32   Oral mucositis (ulcerative) due to other drugs
Use additional code for adverse effect, if applicable, to identify drug (T36-T50 with fifth or sixth character 5)

K12.33   Oral mucositis (ulcerative) due to radiation
Use additional external cause code (W88-W90, X39.0-) to identify cause

K12.39   Other oral mucositis (ulcerative)
Viral oral mucositis (ulcerative)

● **K13   Other diseases of lip and oral mucosa**
> **Includes**   epithelial disturbances of tongue
Use additional code to identify:
alcohol abuse and dependence (F10.-)
exposure to environmental tobacco smoke (Z77.22)
exposure to tobacco smoke in the perinatal period (P96.81)
history of tobacco dependence (Z87.891)
occupational exposure to environmental tobacco smoke (Z57.31)
tobacco dependence (F17.-)
tobacco use (Z72.0)
> **Excludes2**   certain disorders of gingiva and edentulous alveolar ridge (K05-K06)
> cysts of oral region (K09.-)
> diseases of tongue (K14.-)
> stomatitis and related lesions (K12.-)

K13.0   Diseases of lips

Abscess of lips	Exfoliative cheilitis
Angular cheilitis	Fistula of lips
Cellulitis of lips	Glandular cheilitis
Cheilitis NOS	Hypertrophy of lips
Cheilodynia	Perlèche NEC
Cheilosis	

> **Excludes1**   ariboflavinosis (E53.0)
> cheilitis due to radiation-related disorders (L55-L59)
> congenital fistula of lips (Q38.0)
> congenital hypertrophy of lips (Q18.6)
> Perlèche due to candidiasis (B37.83)
> Perlèche due to riboflavin deficiency (E53.0)

K13.1   Cheek and lip biting

Item 11–5   Stomatitis is the inflammation of the oral mucosa. **Mucositis** is the inflammation of the mucous membranes lining the digestive tract from the mouth to the anus. It is a common side effect of chemotherapy and of radiotherapy that involves any part of the digestive tract.

CHAPTER 11 (K00-K95)

Figure 11-4 Oral leukoplakia and associated. (From Swartz MH: Textbook of Physical Diagnosis: History and Examination, Philadelphia, PA, Saunders/Elsevier, 2010)

● **K13.2 Leukoplakia and other disturbances of oral epithelium, including tongue**

> Excludes1   carcinoma in situ of oral epithelium (D00.0-)
> hairy leukoplakia (K13.3)

K13.21 Leukoplakia of oral mucosa, including tongue
Considered precancerous and evidenced by thickened white patches of epithelium on mucous membranes
Leukokeratosis of oral mucosa
Leukoplakia of gingiva, lips, tongue

> Excludes1   hairy leukoplakia (K13.3)
> leukokeratosis nicotina palati (K13.24)

K13.22 Minimal keratinized residual ridge mucosa
Minimal keratinization of alveolar ridge mucosa

K13.23 Excessive keratinized residual ridge mucosa
Excessive keratinization of alveolar ridge mucosa

K13.24 Leukokeratosis nicotina palati
Smoker's palate

K13.29 Other disturbances of oral epithelium, including tongue
Erythroplakia of mouth or tongue
Focal epithelial hyperplasia of mouth or tongue
Leukoedema of mouth or tongue
Other oral epithelium disturbances

K13.3 Hairy leukoplakia

K13.4 Granuloma and granuloma-like lesions of oral mucosa
Eosinophilic granuloma
Granuloma pyogenicum
Verrucous xanthoma

K13.5 Oral submucous fibrosis
Submucous fibrosis of tongue

K13.6 Irritative hyperplasia of oral mucosa

> Excludes2   irritative hyperplasia of edentulous ridge [denture hyperplasia] (K06.2)

● **K13.7 Other and unspecified lesions of oral mucosa**

K13.70 Unspecified lesions of oral mucosa

K13.79 Other lesions of oral mucosa
Focal oral mucinosis

★ **(See Plate 58 on page 71.)**

● **K14 Diseases of tongue**
Use additional code to identify:
alcohol abuse and dependence (F10.-)
exposure to environmental tobacco smoke (Z77.22)
history of tobacco dependence (Z87.891)
occupational exposure to environmental tobacco smoke (Z57.31)
tobacco dependence (F17.-)
tobacco use (Z72.0)

> Excludes2   erythroplakia (K13.29)
> focal epithelial hyperplasia (K13.29)
> leukedema of tongue (K13.29)
> leukoplakia of tongue (K13.21)
> hairy leukoplakia (K13.3)
> macroglossia (congenital) (Q38.2)
> submucous fibrosis of tongue (K13.5)

K14.0 Glossitis
Abscess of tongue
Ulceration (traumatic) of tongue

> Excludes1   atrophic glossitis (K14.4)

Figure 11-5   Structure of the tongue.

K14.1 Geographic tongue
Benign migratory glossitis
Glossitis areata exfoliativa

K14.2 Median rhomboid glossitis

K14.3 Hypertrophy of tongue papillae
Black hairy tongue
Coated tongue
Hypertrophy of foliate papillae
Lingua villosa nigra

K14.4 Atrophy of tongue papillae
Atrophic glossitis

K14.5 Plicated tongue
Fissured tongue   Scrotal tongue
Furrowed tongue

> Excludes1   fissured tongue, congenital (Q38.3)

K14.6 Glossodynia
Glossopyrosis   Painful tongue

K14.8 Other diseases of tongue
Atrophy of tongue   Glossocele
Crenated tongue   Glossoptosis
Enlargement of tongue   Hypertrophy of tongue

K14.9 Disease of tongue, unspecified
Glossopathy NOS

DISEASES OF ESOPHAGUS, STOMACH AND DUODENUM (K20-K31)

> Excludes2   hiatus hernia (K44.-)

● **K20 Esophagitis**
Use additional code to identify:
alcohol abuse and dependence (F10.-)

> Excludes1   erosion of esophagus (K22.1-)
> esophagitis with gastro-esophageal reflux disease (K21.0)
> reflux esophagitis (K21.0)
> ulcerative esophagitis (K22.1-)

> Excludes2   eosinophilic gastritis or gastroenteritis (K52.81)

K20.0 Eosinophilic esophagitis

K20.8 Other esophagitis
Abscess of esophagus

K20.9 Esophagitis, unspecified
Esophagitis NOS

● **K21 Gastro-esophageal reflux disease**

> Excludes1   newborn esophageal reflux (P78.83)

K21.0 Gastro-esophageal reflux disease with esophagitis
Reflux esophagitis

K21.9 Gastro-esophageal reflux disease without esophagitis
Esophageal reflux NOS
Coding Clinic: 2016, Q1, P18

● **K22 Other diseases of esophagus**

> Excludes2   esophageal varices (I85.-)

K22.0 Achalasia of cardia
Achalasia NOS
Cardiospasm

> Excludes1   congenital cardiospasm (Q39.5)

▶ New   ⇒ Revised   ~~deleted~~ Deleted   Excludes 1   Excludes 2   Includes   Use additional   Code first   Code also   Key words

942

OGCR Official Guidelines   ● Unacceptable Principal Diagnosis   X Assign placeholder X   ▸ Use Additional Character(s)   ▸ Manifestation Code   **Coding Clinic**

● **K22.1   Ulcer of esophagus**
Barrett's ulcer
Erosion of esophagus
Fungal ulcer of esophagus
Peptic ulcer of esophagus
Ulcer of esophagus due to ingestion of chemicals
Ulcer of esophagus due to ingestion of drugs and
medicaments
Ulcerative esophagitis

*Code first poisoning due to drug or toxin, if applicable
(T36-T65 with fifth or sixth character 1-4 or 6)*

Use additional code for adverse effect, if applicable,
to identify drug (T36-T50 with fifth or sixth
character 5)

Excludes1   Barrett's esophagus (K22.87-)

K22.10   Ulcer of esophagus without bleeding 🖤
Ulcer of esophagus NOS
(Ex:) See PDX Collection 764

K22.11   Ulcer of esophagus with bleeding 🖤
Excludes2   bleeding esophageal varices
(I85.01, I85.11)
(Ex:) See PDX Collection 765

K22.2   Esophageal obstruction
Compression of esophagus
Constriction of esophagus
Stenosis of esophagus
Stricture of esophagus
Excludes1   congenital stenosis or stricture of
esophagus (Q39.3)

K22.3   Perforation of esophagus 🖤
Rupture of esophagus
Excludes1   traumatic perforation of (thoracic)
esophagus (S27.8-)
(Ex:) See PDX Collection 766

K22.4   Dyskinesia of esophagus
Difficulty in moving
Corkscrew esophagus
Diffuse esophageal spasm
Spasm of esophagus
Excludes1   cardiospasm (K22.0)

K22.5   Diverticulum of esophagus, acquired
Esophageal pouch, acquired
Excludes1   diverticulum of esophagus (congenital)
(Q39.6)

K22.6   Gastro-esophageal laceration-hemorrhage syndrome 🖤
Mallory-Weiss syndrome
(Ex:) See PDX Collection 767

Item 11-6   Esophageal reflux is the return flow of the contents of the
stomach to the esophagus and is referred to as GERD and/or "heartburn."
Gastroesophageal reflux is the return flow of the contents of the stomach
and duodenum to the esophagus. **Esophageal leukoplakia** are white
areas on the mucous membrane of the esophagus for which no specific cause
can be identified.

CERVICAL ESOPHAGUS
Left subclavian artery
First rib
Arch of aorta
Diaphragm
THORACIC ESOPHAGUS
ABDOMINAL ESOPHAGUS
Stomach

Figure 11-6   The esophagus is the
muscular tube that connects the pharynx
and the stomach. The 10 inch (25 cm)
long esophagus is divided into three parts:
cervical, thoracic, and **abdominal.**

Item 11-7   Achalasia is a condition in which the smooth muscle
fibers of the esophagus do not relax. Most frequently, this condition
occurs at the esophagogastric sphincter. **Cardiospasm,** also known as
megaesophagus, is achalasia of the thoracic esophagus.

● **K22.7   Barrett's esophagus**
Barrett's disease
Barrett's syndrome
Excludes1   Barrett's ulcer (K22.1)
malignant neoplasm of esophagus
(C15.-)

K22.70   Barrett's esophagus without dysplasia
Barrett's esophagus NOS

● **K22.71   Barrett's esophagus with dysplasia**
**K22.710   Barrett's esophagus with low grade
dysplasia**
**K22.711   Barrett's esophagus with high grade
dysplasia**
**K22.719   Barrett's esophagus with dysplasia,
unspecified**

K22.8   Other specified diseases of esophagus
Hemorrhage of esophagus NOS
Excludes2   esophageal varices (I85.-)
Paterson-Kelly syndrome (D50.1)

K22.9   Disease of esophagus, unspecified

▷ **K23   Disorders of esophagus in diseases classified elsewhere**
Code first underlying disease, such as:
congenital syphilis (A50.5)
Excludes1   late syphilis (A52.79)
megaesophagus due to Chagas' disease (B57.31)
tuberculosis (A18.83)

● **K25   Gastric ulcer**
Includes   erosion (acute) of stomach
pylorus ulcer (peptic)
stomach ulcer (peptic)
Use additional code to identify:
alcohol abuse and dependence (F10.-)
Excludes1   acute gastritis (K29.0-)
peptic ulcer NOS (K27.-)
(Ex:) For category K25 CC codes: See PDX Collection 765

K25.0   Acute gastric ulcer with hemorrhage 🖤
K25.1   Acute gastric ulcer with perforation 🖤
**K25.2   Acute gastric ulcer with both hemorrhage and
perforation** 🖤
K25.3   Acute gastric ulcer without hemorrhage or perforation 🖤
K25.4   Chronic or unspecified gastric ulcer with hemorrhage 🖤
K25.5   Chronic or unspecified gastric ulcer with perforation 🖤
**K25.6   Chronic or unspecified gastric ulcer with both
hemorrhage and perforation** 🖤
K25.7   Chronic gastric ulcer without hemorrhage or perforation
**K25.9   Gastric ulcer, unspecified as acute or chronic, without
hemorrhage or perforation**

A   B   C

Figure 11-7   A. Ulcer. **B.** Perforated ulcer. **C.** Laparoscopic view of a
perforated duodenal ulcer *(arrow)* with fibrinous exudate on the adjacent
peritoneum. (**C** from Feldman: Sleisenger & Fordtran's Gastrointestinal and
Liver Disease, ed 8, Saunders, An Imprint of Elsevier, 2006)

Item 11-8   Gastric ulcers are lesions of the stomach that result in the death
of the tissue and a defect of the surface. **Perforated ulcers** are those in which
the lesion penetrates the gastric wall, leaving a hole. **Peptic ulcers** are lesions
of the stomach or the duodenum. **Peptic** refers to the gastric juice, pepsin.

N Newborn Age: 0   **P** Pediatric Age: 0–17   **M** Maternity DX: 12–55   **A** Adult Age: 15–124   ♀ Females Only   ♂ Males Only

🖤 Complication\Comorbidity   🖤 Major C\C   (Ex:) CC/MCC Exclusions   🖤 Hospital-Acquired Condition

943

● **K26** **Duodenal ulcer**

  Includes erosion (acute) of duodenum
                  duodenum ulcer (peptic)
                  postpyloric ulcer (peptic)

  Use additional code to identify:
    alcohol abuse and dependence (F10.-)

  Excludes1 peptic ulcer NOS (K27.-)

  (Ex) **For category K26 CC codes unless otherwise indicated: See PDX Collection 768**

  K26.0 Acute duodenal ulcer with hemorrhage 🔖

  K26.1 Acute duodenal ulcer with perforation 🔖

  K26.2 Acute duodenal ulcer with both hemorrhage and perforation 🔖

  K26.3 Acute duodenal ulcer without hemorrhage or perforation 🔖
      (Ex) See PDX Collection 769

  K26.4 Chronic or unspecified duodenal ulcer with hemorrhage 🔖
      Coding Clinic: 2016, Q1, P14

  K26.5 Chronic or unspecified duodenal ulcer with perforation 🔖

  K26.6 Chronic or unspecified duodenal ulcer with both hemorrhage and perforation 🔖

  K26.7 Chronic duodenal ulcer without hemorrhage or perforation

  K26.9 Duodenal ulcer, unspecified as acute or chronic, without hemorrhage or perforation

● **K27** **Peptic ulcer, site unspecified**

  Includes gastroduodenal ulcer NOS
                  peptic ulcer NOS

  Use additional code to identify:
    alcohol abuse and dependence (F10.-)

  Excludes1 peptic ulcer of newborn (P78.82)

  (Ex) **For category K27 CC codes: See PDX Collection 768**

  K27.0 Acute peptic ulcer, site unspecified, with hemorrhage 🔖

  K27.1 Acute peptic ulcer, site unspecified, with perforation 🔖

  K27.2 Acute peptic ulcer, site unspecified, with both hemorrhage and perforation 🔖

  K27.3 Acute peptic ulcer, site unspecified, without hemorrhage or perforation 🔖

  K27.4 Chronic or unspecified peptic ulcer, site unspecified, with hemorrhage 🔖

  K27.5 Chronic or unspecified peptic ulcer, site unspecified, with perforation 🔖

  K27.6 Chronic or unspecified peptic ulcer, site unspecified, with both hemorrhage and perforation 🔖

  K27.7 Chronic peptic ulcer, site unspecified, without hemorrhage or perforation 🔖

  K27.9 Peptic ulcer, site unspecified, unspecified as acute or chronic, without hemorrhage or perforation

● **K28** **Gastrojejunal ulcer**

  includes anastomotic ulcer (peptic) or erosion
                gastrocolic ulcer (peptic) or erosion
                gastrointestinal ulcer (peptic) or erosion
                gastrojejunal ulcer (peptic) or erosion
                jejunal ulcer (peptic) or erosion
                marginal ulcer (peptic) or erosion
                stomal ulcer (peptic) or erosion

  Use additional code to identify:
    alcohol abuse and dependence (F10.-)

  Excludes1 primary ulcer of small intestine (K63.3)

  (Ex) **For category K28 CC codes: See PDX Collection 765**

  K28.0 Acute gastrojejunal ulcer with hemorrhage 🔖

  K28.1 Acute gastrojejunal ulcer with perforation 🔖

  K28.2 Acute gastrojejunal ulcer with both hemorrhage and perforation 🔖

  K28.3 Acute gastrojejunal ulcer without hemorrhage or perforation 🔖

  K28.4 Chronic or unspecified gastrojejunal ulcer with hemorrhage 🔖

  K28.5 Chronic or unspecified gastrojejunal ulcer with perforation 🔖

  K28.6 Chronic or unspecified gastrojejunal ulcer with both hemorrhage and perforation 🔖

  K28.7 Chronic gastrojejunal ulcer without hemorrhage or perforation

  K28.9 Gastrojejunal ulcer, unspecified as acute or chronic, without hemorrhage or perforation

● **K29** **Gastritis and duodenitis**

  Excludes1 eosinophilic gastritis or gastroenteritis (K52.81)
                  Zollinger-Ellison syndrome (E16.4)

  (Ex) **For category K29 CC codes: See PDX Collection 770**

● **K29.0** **Acute gastritis**

    Use additional code to identify:
      alcohol abuse and dependence (F10.-)

    Excludes1 erosion (acute) of stomach (K25.-)

    K29.00 Acute gastritis without bleeding

    K29.01 Acute gastritis with bleeding

● **K29.2** **Alcoholic gastritis**

    Use additional code to identify:
      alcohol abuse and dependence (F10.-)

    K29.20 Alcoholic gastritis without bleeding

    K29.21 Alcoholic gastritis with bleeding

● **K29.3** **Chronic superficial gastritis**

    K29.30 Chronic superficial gastritis without bleeding

    K29.31 Chronic superficial gastritis with bleeding 🔖

● **K29.4** **Chronic atrophic gastritis**
    Gastric atrophy

    K29.40 Chronic atrophic gastritis without bleeding

    K29.41 Chronic atrophic gastritis with bleeding 🔖

● **K29.5** **Unspecified chronic gastritis**
    Chronic antral gastritis
    Chronic fundal gastritis

    K29.50 Unspecified chronic gastritis without bleeding

    K29.51 Unspecified chronic gastritis with bleeding 🔖

● **K29.6** **Other gastritis**
    Giant hypertrophic gastritis
    Granulomatous gastritis
    Ménétrier's disease

    K29.60 Other gastritis without bleeding

    K29.61 Other gastritis with bleeding 🔖

● **K29.7** **Gastritis, unspecified**

    K29.70 Gastritis, unspecified, without bleeding

    K29.71 Gastritis, unspecified, with bleeding 🔖

● **K29.8** **Duodenitis**

    K29.80 Duodenitis without bleeding

    K29.81 Duodenitis with bleeding 🔖

● **K29.9** **Gastroduodenitis, unspecified**

    K29.90 Gastroduodenitis, unspecified, without bleeding

    K29.91 Gastroduodenitis, unspecified, with bleeding 🔖

K30 **Functional dyspepsia**
  Indigestion

  Excludes1 dyspepsia NOS (R10.13)
                  heartburn (R12)
                  nervous dyspepsia (F45.8)
                  neurotic dyspepsia (F45.8)
                  psychogenic dyspepsia (F45.8)

Item 11–9 **Gastritis** is a severe inflammation of the stomach. **Atrophic gastritis** is a chronic inflammation of the stomach that results in destruction of the cells of the mucosa of the stomach. Duodenitis is an inflammation of the duodenum, the first section of the small intestine.

▶ New ▥ Revised ~~deleted~~ Deleted Excludes 1 Excludes 2 Includes Use additional Code first Code also Key words
OGCR Official Guidelines ● Unacceptable Principal Diagnosis X Assign placeholder X ● Use Additional Character(s) ▶ Manifestation Code **Coding Clinic**

● **K31**   **Other diseases of stomach and duodenum**
    Includes   functional disorders of stomach
      Excludes2   diabetic gastroparesis (E08.43, E09.43, E10.43,
                   E11.43, E13.43)
                  diverticulum of duodenum (K57.00-K57.13)

    K31.0   **Acute dilatation of stomach** 🔖
        Acute distention of stomach
        (Ex) See PDX Collection 771

    K31.1   **Adult hypertrophic pyloric stenosis** 🔖   A
        Pyloric stenosis NOS
        Excludes1   congenital or infantile pyloric stenosis
                     (Q40.0)
        (Ex) See PDX Collection 772

    K31.2   **Hourglass stricture and stenosis of stomach**
        Excludes1   congenital hourglass stomach (Q40.2)
                     hourglass contraction of stomach (K31.89)

    K31.3   **Pylorospasm, not elsewhere classified**
        Excludes1   congenital or infantile pylorospasm
                     (Q40.0)
                     neurotic pylorospasm (F45.8)
                     psychogenic pylorospasm (F45.8)

    K31.4   **Gastric diverticulum**
        Excludes1   congenital diverticulum of stomach
                     (Q40.2)

    K31.5   **Obstruction of duodenum** 🔖
        Constriction of duodenum
        Duodenal ileus (chronic)
        Stenosis of duodenum
          Narrowing
        Stricture of duodenum
          Narrowing
        Volvulus of duodenum
          Twisting/knotting
        Excludes1   congenital stenosis of duodenum (Q41.0)
        (Ex) See PDX Collection 773

    K31.6   **Fistula of stomach and duodenum** 🔖
        Gastrocolic fistula
        Gastrojejunocolic fistula
        (Ex) See PDX Collection 774

    K31.7   **Polyp of stomach and duodenum**
        Excludes1   adenomatous polyp of stomach (D13.1)

●   **K31.8**   **Other specified diseases of stomach and duodenum**
      ●   **K31.81**   **Angiodysplasia of stomach and duodenum**
           K31.811   **Angiodysplasia of stomach and**
                   duodenum with bleeding 🔖
                   (Ex) See PDX Collection 770
           K31.819   **Angiodysplasia of stomach and**
                   duodenum without bleeding
                   Angiodysplasia of stomach and
                   duodenum NOS

      K31.82   **Dieulafoy lesion (hemorrhagic) of stomach and**
          duodenum 🔖
          Excludes2   Dieulafoy lesion of intestine
                     (K63.81)
          (Ex) See PDX Collection 775

      K31.83   **Achlorhydria**

      K31.84   **Gastroparesis**
          Gastroparalysis
          Code first underlying disease, if known, such as:
            anorexia nervosa (F50.0-)
            diabetes mellitus (E08.43, E09.43, E10.43,
               E11.43, E13.43)
            scleroderma (M34.-)

      K31.89   **Other diseases of stomach and duodenum**
          Coding Clinic: 2017, Q1, P28

    K31.9   **Disease of stomach and duodenum, unspecified**

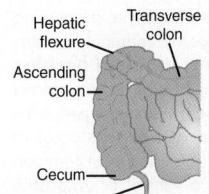

Figure 11-8 Acute appendicitis is the inflammation of the appendix, usually associated with obstruction. Most often this is a disease of adolescents and young adults.

Labels: Hepatic flexure, Transverse colon, Ascending colon, Cecum, Appendix

DISEASES OF APPENDIX (K35-K38)

● **K35**   **Acute appendicitis**
     (Ex) For category K35 CC codes: See PDX Collection 776

    K35.2   **Acute appendicitis with generalized peritonitis** 🔖
        Appendicitis (acute) with generalized (diffuse)
           peritonitis following rupture or perforation of
           appendix
        Perforated appendix NOS
        Ruptured appendix NOS

    K35.3   **Acute appendicitis with localized peritonitis** 🔖
        Acute appendicitis with or without perforation or
           rupture with peritonitis NOS
        Acute appendicitis with or without perforation or
           rupture with localized peritonitis
        Acute appendicitis with peritoneal abscess

●   **K35.8**   **Other and unspecified acute appendicitis**
      K35.80   **Unspecified acute appendicitis** 🔖
          Acute appendicitis NOS
          Acute appendicitis without (localized)
           (generalized) peritonitis

      K35.89   **Other acute appendicitis** 🔖

    K36   **Other appendicitis**
        Chronic appendicitis
        Recurrent appendicitis

    K37   **Unspecified appendicitis**
        Excludes1   -unspecified appendicitis with peritonitis
                   (K35.2-K35.3)

● **K38**   **Other diseases of appendix**
    K38.0   **Hyperplasia of appendix**
    K38.1   **Appendicular concretions**
        Fecalith of appendix
        Stercolith of appendix
    K38.2   **Diverticulum of appendix**
    K38.3   **Fistula of appendix**
    K38.8   **Other specified diseases of appendix**
        Intussusception of appendix
    K38.9   **Disease of appendix, unspecified**

CHAPTER 11 (K00-K95)

Item 11-10 Achlorhydria, also known as gastric anacidity, is the absence of gastric acid.

N   Newborn Age: 0   **P**   Pediatric Age: 0–17   **M**   Maternity DX: 12–55   **A**   Adult Age: 15–124   ♀   Females Only   ♂   Males Only

🔖 Complication\Comorbidity   🔖 Major C\C   (Ex) CC/MCC Exclusions   🔖 Hospital-Acquired Condition

945

Item 11-11 **Hernias** of the groin are the most common type, accounting for 80 percent of all hernias. There are two major types of inguinal hernias: indirect (oblique) affecting men only and direct. **Indirect inguinal hernias** result when the intestines emerge through the abdominal wall in an indirect fashion through the inguinal canal. **Direct inguinal hernias** penetrate through the abdominal wall in a direct fashion. **Femoral hernias** occur at the femoral ring where the femoral vessels enter the thigh and is most common in women. An abdominal wall hernia is also called a ventral or epigastric hernia and occurs in both sexes. Classification is based on location of the hernia and whether there is obstruction or gangrene.

Ventral, epigastric, or incisional hernia occurs on the abdominal surface caused by musculature weakness or a tear at a previous surgical site and is evidenced by a bulge that changes in size, becoming larger with exertion. An **incarcerated** hernia is one in which the intestines become trapped in the hernia. A **strangulated** hernia is one in which the blood supply to the intestines is lost. **Hiatal hernia** occurs when a loop of the stomach protrudes upward through the small opening in the diaphragm through which the esophagus passes, leaving the abdominal cavity and entering the chest. It occurs in both sexes.

Right Lumbar	Umbilical	Left Lumbar
RIGHT INGUINAL OR ILIAC	Hypogastric or pubic	LEFT INGUINAL OR ILIAC

Figure 11-9 Inguinal hernias are those that are located in the inguinal or iliac areas of the abdomen.

HERNIA (K40-K46)

Note: Hernia with both gangrene and obstruction is classified to hernia with gangrene.

Includes   acquired hernia
                 congenital [except diaphragmatic or hiatus] hernia
                 recurrent hernia

● **K40**   **Inguinal hernia**
     Includes   bubonocele
                 direct inguinal hernia
                 double inguinal hernia
                 indirect inguinal hernia
                 inguinal hernia NOS
                 oblique inguinal hernia
                 scrotal hernia
    (Ex) For category K40 CC codes: See PDX Collection 777

  ● **K40.0**   **Bilateral inguinal hernia, with obstruction, without gangrene**
         Inguinal hernia (bilateral) causing obstruction without gangrene
         Incarcerated inguinal hernia (bilateral) without gangrene
         Irreducible inguinal hernia (bilateral) without gangrene
         Strangulated inguinal hernia (bilateral) without gangrene

       K40.00   **Bilateral inguinal hernia, with obstruction, without gangrene, not specified as recurrent**
             Bilateral inguinal hernia, with obstruction, without gangrene NOS

       K40.01   **Bilateral inguinal hernia, with obstruction, without gangrene, recurrent** 🔖

● **K40.1**   **Bilateral inguinal hernia, with gangrene**
       K40.10   **Bilateral inguinal hernia, with gangrene, not specified as recurrent** 🔖
            Bilateral inguinal hernia, with gangrene NOS

       K40.11   **Bilateral inguinal hernia, with gangrene, recurrent** 🔖

● **K40.2**   **Bilateral inguinal hernia, without obstruction or gangrene**
       K40.20   **Bilateral inguinal hernia, without obstruction or gangrene, not specified as recurrent**
            Bilateral inguinal hernia NOS

       K40.21   **Bilateral inguinal hernia, without obstruction or gangrene, recurrent**

● **K40.3**   **Unilateral inguinal hernia, with obstruction, without gangrene**
         Inguinal hernia (unilateral) causing obstruction without gangrene
         Incarcerated inguinal hernia (unilateral) without gangrene
         Irreducible inguinal hernia (unilateral) without gangrene
         Strangulated inguinal hernia (unilateral) without gangrene

       K40.30   **Unilateral inguinal hernia, with obstruction, without gangrene, not specified as recurrent** 🔖
            Inguinal hernia, with obstruction NOS
            Unilateral inguinal hernia, with obstruction, without gangrene NOS

       K40.31   **Unilateral inguinal hernia, with obstruction, without gangrene, recurrent** 🔖

● **K40.4**   **Unilateral inguinal hernia, with gangrene**
       K40.40   **Unilateral inguinal hernia, with gangrene, not specified as recurrent**
            Inguinal hernia with gangrene NOS
            Unilateral inguinal hernia with gangrene NOS

       K40.41   **Unilateral inguinal hernia, with gangrene, recurrent** 🔖

● **K40.9**   **Unilateral inguinal hernia, without obstruction or gangrene**
       K40.90   **Unilateral inguinal hernia, without obstruction or gangrene, not specified as recurrent**
            Inguinal hernia NOS
            Unilateral inguinal hernia NOS

       K40.91   **Unilateral inguinal hernia, without obstruction or gangrene, recurrent**

● **K41**   **Femoral hernia**
  ● **K41.0**   **Bilateral femoral hernia, with obstruction, without gangrene**
         Femoral hernia (bilateral) causing obstruction, without gangrene
         Incarcerated femoral hernia (bilateral), without gangrene
         Irreducible femoral hernia (bilateral), without gangrene
         Strangulated femoral hernia (bilateral), without gangrene
       (Ex) For category K41.0 CC codes: See PDX Collection 778

       K41.00   **Bilateral femoral hernia, with obstruction, without gangrene, not specified as recurrent** 🔖
            Bilateral femoral hernia, with obstruction, without gangrene NOS

       K41.01   **Bilateral femoral hernia, with obstruction, without gangrene, recurrent** 🔖

● **K41.1**   **Bilateral femoral hernia, with gangrene**
       (Ex) For category K41.1 CC codes: See PDX Collection 779

       K41.10   **Bilateral femoral hernia, with gangrene, not specified as recurrent** 🔖
            Bilateral femoral hernia, with gangrene NOS

       K41.11   **Bilateral femoral hernia, with gangrene, recurrent** 🔖

▶ New   ▓ Revised   ~~deleted~~ Deleted   Excludes 1   Excludes 2   Includes   Use additional   Code first   Code also   Key words
OGCR Official Guidelines   ● Unacceptable Principal Diagnosis   X Assign placeholder X   ● Use Additional Character(s)   ▶ Manifestation Code   **Coding Clinic**

● **K41.2** **Bilateral femoral hernia, without obstruction or gangrene**

     K41.20 **Bilateral femoral hernia, without obstruction or gangrene, not specified as recurrent**
         Bilateral femoral hernia NOS

     K41.21 **Bilateral femoral hernia, without obstruction or gangrene, recurrent**

● **K41.3** **Unilateral femoral hernia, with obstruction, without gangrene**
     Femoral hernia (unilateral) causing obstruction, without gangrene
     Incarcerated femoral hernia (unilateral), without gangrene
     Irreducible femoral hernia (unilateral), without gangrene
     Strangulated femoral hernia (unilateral), without gangrene
     (Ex) **For category K41.3 CC codes:** See PDX Collection 778

     K41.30 **Unilateral femoral hernia, with obstruction, without gangrene, not specified as recurrent** 🔹
         Femoral hernia, with obstruction NOS
         Unilateral femoral hernia, with obstruction NOS

     K41.31 **Unilateral femoral hernia, with obstruction, without gangrene, recurrent** 🔹

● **K41.4** **Unilateral femoral hernia, with gangrene**
     (Ex) **For category K41.4 CC codes:** See PDX Collection 779

     K41.40 **Unilateral femoral hernia, with gangrene, not specified as recurrent** 🔹
         Femoral hernia, with gangrene NOS
         Unilateral femoral hernia, with gangrene NOS

     K41.41 **Unilateral femoral hernia, with gangrene, recurrent** 🔹

● **K41.9** **Unilateral femoral hernia, without obstruction or gangrene**

     K41.90 **Unilateral femoral hernia, without obstruction or gangrene, not specified as recurrent**
         Femoral hernia NOS
         Unilateral femoral hernia NOS

     K41.91 **Unilateral femoral hernia, without obstruction or gangrene, recurrent**

● **K42** **Umbilical hernia**

     Includes   paraumbilical hernia

     Excludes1   omphalocele (Q79.2)

     K42.0 **Umbilical hernia with obstruction, without gangrene** 🔹
         Umbilical hernia causing obstruction, without gangrene
         Incarcerated umbilical hernia, without gangrene
         Irreducible umbilical hernia, without gangrene
         Strangulated umbilical hernia, without gangrene
         (Ex) See PDX Collection 780

     K42.1 **Umbilical hernia with gangrene** 🔹
         Gangrenous umbilical hernia
         (Ex) See PDX Collection 781

     K42.9 **Umbilical hernia without obstruction or gangrene**
         Umbilical hernia NOS

● **K43** **Ventral hernia**

     K43.0 **Incisional hernia with obstruction, without gangrene** 🔹
         Incisional hernia causing obstruction, without gangrene
         Incarcerated incisional hernia, without gangrene
         Irreducible incisional hernia, without gangrene
         Strangulated incisional hernia, without gangrene
         (Ex) See PDX Collection 780

     K43.1 **Incisional hernia with gangrene** 🔹
         Gangrenous incisional hernia
         (Ex) See PDX Collection 781

     K43.2 **Incisional hernia without obstruction or gangrene**
         Incisional hernia NOS

     K43.3 **Parastomal hernia with obstruction, without gangrene** 🔹
         Incarcerated parastomal hernia, without gangrene
         Irreducible parastomal hernia, without gangrene
         Parastomal hernia causing obstruction, without gangrene
         Strangulated parastomal hernia, without gangrene
         (Ex) See PDX Collection 780

     K43.4 **Parastomal hernia with gangrene** 🔹
         Gangrenous parastomal hernia
         (Ex) See PDX Collection 781

     K43.5 **Parastomal hernia without obstruction or gangrene**
         Parastomal hernia NOS

     K43.6 **Other and unspecified ventral hernia with obstruction, without gangrene** 🔹
         Epigastric hernia causing obstruction, without gangrene
         Hypogastric hernia causing obstruction, without gangrene
         Incarcerated epigastric hernia without gangrene
         Incarcerated hypogastric hernia without gangrene
         Incarcerated midline hernia without gangrene
         Incarcerated spigelian hernia without gangrene
         Incarcerated subxiphoid hernia without gangrene
         Irreducible epigastric hernia without gangrene
         Irreducible hypogastric hernia without gangrene
         Irreducible midline hernia without gangrene
         Irreducible spigelian hernia without gangrene
         Irreducible subxiphoid hernia without gangrene
         Midline hernia causing obstruction, without gangrene
         Spigelian hernia causing obstruction, without gangrene
         Strangulated epigastric hernia without gangrene
         Strangulated hypogastric hernia without gangrene
         Strangulated midline hernia without gangrene
         Strangulated spigelian hernia without gangrene
         Strangulated subxiphoid hernia without gangrene
         Subxiphoid hernia causing obstruction, without gangrene
         (Ex) See PDX Collection 780

     K43.7 **Other and unspecified ventral hernia with gangrene** 🔹
         Any condition listed under K43.6 specified as gangrenous
         (Ex) See PDX Collection 781

     K43.9 **Ventral hernia without obstruction or gangrene**
         Epigastric hernia
         Ventral hernia NOS

● **K44** **Diaphragmatic hernia**

     Includes   hiatus hernia (esophageal) (sliding) paraesophageal hernia

     Excludes1   congenital diaphragmatic hernia (Q79.0)
                 congenital hiatus hernia (Q40.1)

     (Ex) **For category K44 CC codes:** See PDX Collection 782

     K44.0 **Diaphragmatic hernia with obstruction, without gangrene** 🔹
         Diaphragmatic hernia causing obstruction
         Incarcerated diaphragmatic hernia
         Irreducible diaphragmatic hernia
         Strangulated diaphragmatic hernia

     K44.1 **Diaphragmatic hernia with gangrene** 🔹
         Gangrenous diaphragmatic hernia

     K44.9 **Diaphragmatic hernia without obstruction or gangrene**
         Diaphragmatic hernia NOS
         Coding Clinic: 2017, Q1, P7

CHAPTER 11 (K00-K95)

N Newborn Age: 0   **P** Pediatric Age: 0–17   **M** Maternity DX: 12–55   **A** Adult Age: 15–124   ♀ Females Only   ♂ Males Only

🔹 Complication\Comorbidity   🔹 Major C\C   (Ex) CC/MCC Exclusions   🔹 Hospital-Acquired Condition

947

● **K45　Other abdominal hernia**

　　Includes　abdominal hernia, specified site NEC
　　　　　　　　lumbar hernia
　　　　　　　　obturator hernia
　　　　　　　　pudendal hernia
　　　　　　　　retroperitoneal hernia
　　　　　　　　sciatic hernia

　　K45.0　Other specified abdominal hernia with obstruction, without gangrene 🔖
　　　　　Other specified abdominal hernia causing obstruction
　　　　　Other specified incarcerated abdominal hernia
　　　　　Other specified irreducible abdominal hernia
　　　　　Other specified strangulated abdominal hernia
　　　　　(Ex) See PDX Collection 783

　　K45.1　Other specified abdominal hernia with gangrene 🔖
　　　　　Any condition listed under K45 specified as gangrenous
　　　　　(Ex) See PDX Collection 784

　　K45.8　Other specified abdominal hernia without obstruction or gangrene

● **K46　Unspecified abdominal hernia**

　　Includes　enterocele
　　　　　　　　epiplocele
　　　　　　　　hernia NOS
　　　　　　　　interstitial hernia
　　　　　　　　intestinal hernia
　　　　　　　　intra-abdominal hernia

　　Excludes1　vaginal enterocele (N81.5)

　　K46.0　Unspecified abdominal hernia with obstruction, without gangrene 🔖
　　　　　Unspecified abdominal hernia causing obstruction
　　　　　Unspecified incarcerated abdominal hernia
　　　　　Unspecified irreducible abdominal hernia
　　　　　Unspecified strangulated abdominal hernia
　　　　　(Ex) See PDX Collection 783

　　K46.1　Unspecified abdominal hernia with gangrene 🔖
　　　　　Any condition listed under K46 specified as gangrenous
　　　　　(Ex) See PDX Collection 784

　　K46.9　Unspecified abdominal hernia without obstruction or gangrene
　　　　　Abdominal hernia NOS

★ **(See Plate 284 on page 77.)**

NONINFECTIVE ENTERITIS AND COLITIS (K50-K52)

　　Includes　noninfective inflammatory bowel disease
　　Excludes1　irritable bowel syndrome (K58.-)
　　　　　　　　megacolon (K59.3-)

● **K50　Crohn's disease [regional enteritis]**

　　Includes　granulomatous enteritis

　　Use additional code to identify manifestations, such as:
　　　pyoderma gangrenosum (L88)

　　Excludes1　ulcerative colitis (K51.-)

　　(Ex) **For category K50 CC codes unless otherwise indicated:** See PDX Collection 785

● **K50.0　Crohn's disease of small intestine**
　　　　Crohn's disease [regional enteritis] of duodenum
　　　　Crohn's disease [regional enteritis] of ileum
　　　　Crohn's disease [regional enteritis] of jejunum
　　　　Regional ileitis
　　　　Terminal ileitis

　　Excludes1　Crohn's disease of both small and large intestine (K50.8-)

　　K50.00　Crohn's disease of small intestine without complications 🔖

● **K50.01　Crohn's disease of small intestine with complications**

　　K50.011　Crohn's disease of small intestine with rectal bleeding 🔖

　　K50.012　Crohn's disease of small intestine with intestinal obstruction 🔖
　　　　　CC when PDx is its own CC

　　K50.013　Crohn's disease of small intestine with fistula 🔖
　　　　　CC when PDx is its own CC

　　K50.014　Crohn's disease of small intestine with abscess 🔖
　　　　　CC when PDx is its own CC
　　　　　Coding Clinic: 2012, Q4, P104

　　K50.018　Crohn's disease of small intestine with other complication 🔖

　　K50.019　Crohn's disease of small intestine with unspecified complications 🔖

● **K50.1　Crohn's disease of large intestine**
　　　　Crohn's disease [regional enteritis] of colon
　　　　Crohn's disease [regional enteritis] of large bowel
　　　　Crohn's disease [regional enteritis] of rectum
　　　　Granulomatous colitis
　　　　Regional colitis

　　Excludes1　Crohn's disease of both small and large intestine (K50.8)

　　K50.10　Crohn's disease of large intestine without complications 🔖

● **K50.11　Crohn's disease of large intestine with complications**

　　K50.111　Crohn's disease of large intestine with rectal bleeding 🔖

　　K50.112　Crohn's disease of large intestine with intestinal obstruction 🔖
　　　　　CC when PDx is its own CC

　　K50.113　Crohn's disease of large intestine with fistula 🔖
　　　　　CC when PDx is its own CC

　　K50.114　Crohn's disease of large intestine with abscess 🔖
　　　　　CC when PDx is its own CC
　　　　　Coding Clinic: 2012, Q4, P104

　　K50.118　Crohn's disease of large intestine with other complication 🔖

　　K50.119　Crohn's disease of large intestine with unspecified complications 🔖

● **K50.8　Crohn's disease of both small and large intestine**

　　K50.80　Crohn's disease of both small and large intestine without complications 🔖

● **K50.81　Crohn's disease of both small and large intestine with complications**

　　K50.811　Crohn's disease of both small and large intestine with rectal bleeding 🔖

　　K50.812　Crohn's disease of both small and large intestine with intestinal obstruction 🔖
　　　　　CC when PDx is its own CC

　　K50.813　Crohn's disease of both small and large intestine with fistula 🔖
　　　　　CC when PDx is its own CC

　　K50.814　Crohn's disease of both small and large intestine with abscess 🔖
　　　　　CC when PDx is its own CC
　　　　　Coding Clinic: 2012, Q4, P104

　　K50.818　Crohn's disease of both small and large intestine with other complication 🔖

　　K50.819　Crohn's disease of both small and large intestine with unspecified complications 🔖

Item 11-12　Crohn's disease, also known as **regional enteritis,** is a chronic inflammatory disease of the intestines. Classification is based on location in the small (duodenum, ileum, jejunum) or large (cecum, colon, rectum, anal canal) intestine.

▶ New　⇒ Revised　~~deleted~~ Deleted　Excludes 1　Excludes 2　Includes　Use additional　Code first　Code also　Key words
OGCR Official Guidelines　● Unacceptable Principal Diagnosis　X Assign placeholder X　● Use Additional Character(s)　▌ Manifestation Code　**Coding Clinic**

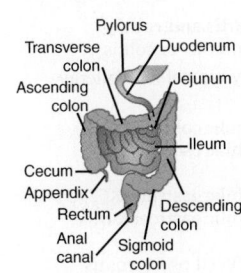

Figure 11-10 Small and large intestines.

Pylorus
Transverse colon
Duodenum
Ascending colon
Jejunum
Ileum
Cecum
Appendix
Rectum
Descending colon
Anal canal
Sigmoid colon

● **K50.9** **Crohn's disease, unspecified**
(Ex) For category K50.9 CC codes: See PDX Collection 786

    K50.90 Crohn's disease, unspecified, without complications 🔹
        Crohn's disease NOS
        Regional enteritis NOS

  ● **K50.91** Crohn's disease, unspecified, with complications
    K50.911 Crohn's disease, unspecified, with rectal bleeding 🔹
    K50.912 Crohn's disease, unspecified, with intestinal obstruction 🔹
        CC when PDx is its own CC
    K50.913 Crohn's disease, unspecified, with fistula 🔹
        CC when PDx is its own CC
    K50.914 Crohn's disease, unspecified, with abscess 🔹
        CC when PDx is its own CC
        Coding Clinic: 2012, Q4, P104
    K50.918 Crohn's disease, unspecified, with other complication 🔹
    K50.919 Crohn's disease, unspecified, with unspecified complications 🔹

● **K51** **Ulcerative colitis**
    Use additional code to identify manifestations, such as: pyoderma gangrenosum (L88)
    Excludes1 Crohn's disease [regional enteritis] (K50.-)
    (Ex) For category K51 CC codes unless otherwise indicated: See PDX Collection 785

  ● **K51.0** **Ulcerative (chronic) pancolitis**
    Backwash ileitis
    K51.00 Ulcerative (chronic) pancolitis without complications 🔹
        Ulcerative (chronic) pancolitis NOS
  ● **K51.01** Ulcerative (chronic) pancolitis with complications
    K51.011 Ulcerative (chronic) pancolitis with rectal bleeding 🔹
    K51.012 Ulcerative (chronic) pancolitis with intestinal obstruction 🔹
        CC when PDx is its own CC
    K51.013 Ulcerative (chronic) pancolitis with fistula 🔹
        CC when PDx is its own CC
    K51.014 Ulcerative (chronic) pancolitis with abscess 🔹
        CC when PDx is its own CC
    K51.018 Ulcerative (chronic) pancolitis with other complication 🔹
    K51.019 Ulcerative (chronic) pancolitis with unspecified complications 🔹

● **K51.2** Ulcerative (chronic) proctitis
    K51.20 Ulcerative (chronic) proctitis without complications 🔹
        Ulcerative (chronic) proctitis NOS
  ● **K51.21** Ulcerative (chronic) proctitis with complications
    K51.211 Ulcerative (chronic) proctitis with rectal bleeding 🔹
    K51.212 Ulcerative (chronic) proctitis with intestinal obstruction 🔹
        CC when PDx is its own CC
    K51.213 Ulcerative (chronic) proctitis with fistula 🔹
        CC when PDx is its own CC
    K51.214 Ulcerative (chronic) proctitis with abscess 🔹
        CC when PDx is its own CC
    K51.218 Ulcerative (chronic) proctitis with other complication 🔹
    K51.219 Ulcerative (chronic) proctitis with unspecified complications 🔹

● **K51.3** Ulcerative (chronic) rectosigmoiditis
    K51.30 Ulcerative (chronic) rectosigmoiditis without complications 🔹
        Ulcerative (chronic) rectosigmoiditis NOS
  ● **K51.31** Ulcerative (chronic) rectosigmoiditis with complications
    K51.311 Ulcerative (chronic) rectosigmoiditis with rectal bleeding 🔹
    K51.312 Ulcerative (chronic) rectosigmoiditis with intestinal obstruction 🔹
        CC when PDx is its own CC
    K51.313 Ulcerative (chronic) rectosigmoiditis with fistula 🔹
        CC when PDx is its own CC
    K51.314 Ulcerative (chronic) rectosigmoiditis with abscess 🔹
        CC when PDx is its own CC
    K51.318 Ulcerative (chronic) rectosigmoiditis with other complication 🔹
    K51.319 Ulcerative (chronic) rectosigmoiditis with unspecified complications 🔹

● **K51.4** Inflammatory polyps of colon
    Excludes1 adenomatous polyp of colon (D12.6)
        polyposis of colon (D12.6)
        polyps of colon NOS (K63.5)
    K51.40 Inflammatory polyps of colon without complications 🔹
        Inflammatory polyps of colon NOS
  ● **K51.41** Inflammatory polyps of colon with complications
    K51.411 Inflammatory polyps of colon with rectal bleeding 🔹
    K51.412 Inflammatory polyps of colon with intestinal obstruction 🔹
        CC when PDx is its own CC
    K51.413 Inflammatory polyps of colon with fistula 🔹
        CC when PDx is its own CC
    K51.414 Inflammatory polyps of colon with abscess 🔹
        CC when PDx is its own CC
    K51.418 Inflammatory polyps of colon with other complication 🔹
    K51.419 Inflammatory polyps of colon with unspecified complications 🔹

Item 11-13 Ulcerative colitis attacks the colonic mucosa and forms abscesses. The disease involves the intestines. Classification is based on the location:
- Enterocolitis: large and small intestine
- Ileocolitis: ileum and colon
- Proctitis: rectum
- Proctosigmoiditis: sigmoid colon and rectum

CHAPTER 11 (K00-K95)

N Newborn Age: 0   P Pediatric Age: 0–17   M Maternity DX: 12–55   A Adult Age: 15–124   ♀ Females Only   ♂ Males Only
🔹 Complication\Comorbidity   Major C\C   (Ex) CC/MCC Exclusions   Hospital-Acquired Condition
949

● **K51.5   Left sided colitis**
　　　Left hemicolitis

　　K51.50   Left sided colitis without complications 🔑
　　　　Left sided colitis NOS

　● **K51.51   Left sided colitis with complications**
　　　　K51.511   Left sided colitis with rectal bleeding 🔑
　　　　K51.512   Left sided colitis with intestinal obstruction 🔑
　　　　　　CC when PDx is its own CC
　　　　K51.513   Left sided colitis with fistula 🔑
　　　　　　CC when PDx is its own CC
　　　　K51.514   Left sided colitis with abscess 🔑
　　　　　　CC when PDx is its own CC
　　　　K51.518   Left sided colitis with other complication 🔑
　　　　K51.519   Left sided colitis with unspecified complications 🔑

● **K51.8   Other ulcerative colitis**
　　K51.80   Other ulcerative colitis without complications 🔑

　● **K51.81   Other ulcerative colitis with complications**
　　　　K51.811   Other ulcerative colitis with rectal bleeding 🔑
　　　　K51.812   Other ulcerative colitis with intestinal obstruction 🔑
　　　　　　CC when PDx is its own CC
　　　　K51.813   Other ulcerative colitis with fistula 🔑
　　　　　　CC when PDx is its own CC
　　　　K51.814   Other ulcerative colitis with abscess 🔑
　　　　　　CC when PDx is its own CC
　　　　K51.818   Other ulcerative colitis with other complication 🔑
　　　　K51.819   Other ulcerative colitis with unspecified complications 🔑

● **K51.9   Ulcerative colitis, unspecified**
　　(Ex) For category K51.9 CC codes: See PDX Collection 787

　　K51.90   Ulcerative colitis, unspecified, without complications 🔑

　● **K51.91   Ulcerative colitis, unspecified, with complications**
　　　　K51.911   Ulcerative colitis, unspecified with rectal bleeding 🔑
　　　　K51.912   Ulcerative colitis, unspecified with intestinal obstruction 🔑
　　　　　　CC when PDx is its own CC
　　　　K51.913   Ulcerative colitis, unspecified with fistula 🔑
　　　　　　CC when PDx is its own CC
　　　　K51.914   Ulcerative colitis, unspecified with abscess 🔑
　　　　　　CC when PDx is its own CC
　　　　K51.918   Ulcerative colitis, unspecified with other complication 🔑
　　　　K51.919   Ulcerative colitis, unspecified with unspecified complications 🔑

● **K52   Other and unspecified noninfective gastroenteritis and colitis**

　　K52.0   Gastroenteritis and colitis due to radiation 🔑
　　　　(Ex) See PDX Collection 788

　　K52.1   Toxic gastroenteritis and colitis 🔑
　　　　Drug-induced gastroenteritis and colitis
　　　　Code first (T51-T65) *to identify toxic agent*
　　　　Use additional code for adverse effect, if applicable, to identify drug (T36-T50 with fifth or sixth character 5)
　　　　(Ex) See PDX Collection 789

● **K52.2   Allergic and dietetic gastroenteritis and colitis**
　　　Food hypersensitivity gastroenteritis or colitis
　　　Use additional code to identify type of food allergy (Z91.01-, Z91.02-)

　　　Excludes2　allergic eosinophilic colitis (K52.82)
　　　　　　　allergic eosinophilic esophagitis (K20.0)
　　　　　　　allergic eosinophilic gastritis (K52.81)
　　　　　　　allergic eosinophilic gastroenteritis (K52.81)
　　　　　　　food protein-induced proctocolitis (K52.82)

　　　Coding Clinic: 2016, Q4, P30-31

　　K52.21   Food protein-induced enterocolitis syndrome
　　　　Use additional code for hypovolemic shock, if present (R57.1)

　　K52.22   Food protein-induced enteropathy

　　K52.29   Other allergic and dietetic gastroenteritis and colitis
　　　　Food hypersensitivity gastroenteritis or colitis
　　　　Immediate gastrointestinal hypersensitivity

　K52.3   Indeterminate colitis
　　　Colonic inflammatory bowel disease unclassified (IBDU)

　　　Excludes1　unspecified colitis (K52.9)

● **K52.8   Other specified noninfective gastroenteritis and colitis**

　　K52.81   Eosinophilic gastritis or gastroenteritis
　　　　Eosinophilic enteritis

　　　Excludes2　eosinophilic esophagitis (K20.0)

　　K52.82   Eosinophilic colitis
　　　　Allergic proctocolitis
　　　　Food-induced eosinophilic proctocolitis
　　　　Food protein-induced proctocolitis
　　　　Milk protein-induced proctocolitis

　● **K52.83   Microscopic colitis**
　　　　Coding Clinic: 2016, Q4, P30-31
　　　　K52.831   Collagenous colitis
　　　　K52.832   Lymphocytic colitis
　　　　K52.838   Other microscopic colitis
　　　　K52.839   Microscopic colitis, unspecified

　　K52.89   Other specified noninfective gastroenteritis and colitis

　K52.9   Noninfective gastroenteritis and colitis, unspecified

Colitis NOS	Ileitis NOS
Enteritis NOS	Jejunitis NOS
Gastroenteritis NOS	Sigmoiditis NOS

　　　Excludes1　diarrhea NOS (R19.7)
　　　　　　　functional diarrhea (K59.1)
　　　　　　　infectious gastroenteritis and colitis NOS (A09)
　　　　　　　neonatal diarrhea (noninfective) (P78.3)
　　　　　　　psychogenic diarrhea (F45.8)

OTHER DISEASES OF INTESTINES (K55-K64)

● **K55   Vascular disorders of intestine**

　　　Excludes1　necrotizing enterocolitis of newborn (P77.-)
　　　(Ex) For category K55 CC codes unless otherwise indicated: See PDX Collection 790

● **K55.0   Acute vascular disorders of intestine**
　　　Infarction of appendices epiploicae
　　　Mesenteric (artery) (vein) embolism
　　　Mesenteric (artery) (vein) infarction
　　　Mesenteric (artery) (vein) thrombosis

　● **K55.01   Acute (reversible) ischemia of small intestine**
　　　　Coding Clinic: 2016, Q4, P32

　　　　K55.011   Focal (segmental) acute (reversible) ischemia of small intestine 🔑
　　　　K55.012   Diffuse acute (reversible) ischemia of small intestine 🔑
　　　　K55.019   Acute (reversible) ischemia of small intestine, extent unspecified 🔑

▶ New　⇒ Revised　~~deleted~~ Deleted　Excludes 1　Excludes 2　Includes　Use additional　Code first　Code also　Key words
OGCR Official Guidelines　● Unacceptable Principal Diagnosis　X Assign placeholder X　● Use Additional Character(s)　▸ Manifestation Code　Coding Clinic

● **K55.02 Acute infarction of small intestine**
Gangrene of small intestine
Necrosis of small intestine
Coding Clinic: 2016, Q4, P32

   K55.021 Focal (segmental) acute infarction of small intestine

   K55.022 Diffuse acute infarction of small intestine

   K55.029 Acute infarction of small intestine, extent unspecified

● **K55.03 Acute (reversible) ischemia of large intestine**
Acute fulminant ischemic colitis
Subacute ischemic colitis
Coding Clinic: 2016, Q4, P32

   K55.031 Focal (segmental) acute (reversible) ischemia of large intestine

   K55.032 Diffuse acute (reversible) ischemia of large intestine

   K55.039 Acute (reversible) ischemia of large intestine, extent unspecified

● **K55.04 Acute infarction of large intestine**
Gangrene of large intestine
Necrosis of large intestine
Coding Clinic: 2016, Q4, P32

   K55.041 Focal (segmental) acute infarction of large intestine

   K55.042 Diffuse acute infarction of large intestine

   K55.049 Acute infarction of large intestine, extent unspecified

● **K55.05 Acute (reversible) ischemia of intestine, part unspecified**

   K55.051 Focal (segmental) acute (reversible) ischemia of intestine, part unspecified

   K55.052 Diffuse acute (reversible) ischemia of intestine, part unspecified

   K55.059 Acute (reversible) ischemia of intestine, part and extent unspecified

● **K55.06 Acute infarction of intestine, part unspecified**
Acute intestinal infarction
Gangrene of intestine
Necrosis of intestine

   K55.061 Focal (segmental) acute infarction of intestine, part unspecified

   K55.062 Diffuse acute infarction of intestine, part unspecified

   K55.069 Acute infarction of intestine, part and extent unspecified

K55.1 Chronic vascular disorders of intestine
Chronic ischemic colitis
Chronic ischemic enteritis
Chronic ischemic enterocolitis
Ischemic stricture of intestine
Mesenteric atherosclerosis
Mesenteric vascular insufficiency
(Ex) See PDX Collection 791

● **K55.2 Angiodysplasia of colon**

   K55.20 Angiodysplasia of colon without hemorrhage

   K55.21 Angiodysplasia of colon with hemorrhage
(Ex) See PDX Collection 770

● **K55.3 Necrotizing enterocolitis**
   Excludes1 necrotizing enterocolitis of newborn (P77.-)
   ⟹ **Excludes2** necrotizing enterocolitis due to Clostridium difficile (A04.7-)

   K55.30 Necrotizing enterocolitis, unspecified
Necrotizing enterocolitis, NOS

   K55.31 Stage 1 necrotizing enterocolitis
Necrotizing enterocolitis without pneumatosis, without perforation
Coding Clinic: 2016, Q4, P32

   K55.32 Stage 2 necrotizing enterocolitis
Necrotizing enterocolitis with pneumatosis, without perforation
Coding Clinic: 2016, Q4, P32

   K55.33 Stage 3 necrotizing enterocolitis
Necrotizing enterocolitis with perforation
Necrotizing enterocolitis with pneumatosis and perforation
Coding Clinic: 2016, Q4, P32

K55.8 Other vascular disorders of intestine
(Ex) See PDX Collection 791

K55.9 Vascular disorder of intestine, unspecified
Ischemic colitis
Ischemic enteritis
Ischemic enterocolitis
(Ex) See PDX Collection 791

● **K56 Paralytic ileus and intestinal obstruction without hernia**
   Excludes1 congenital stricture or stenosis of intestine (Q41-Q42)
      cystic fibrosis with meconium ileus (E84.11)
      ischemic stricture of intestine (K55.1)
      meconium ileus NOS (P76.0)
      neonatal intestinal obstructions classifiable to P76.-
      obstruction of duodenum (K31.5)
   ⟹ postprocedural intestinal obstruction (K91.3-)
      stenosis of anus or rectum (K62.4)
      ~~intestinal obstruction with hernia (K40-K46)~~
   (Ex) For category K56 CC codes: See PDX Collection 792

   K56.0 Paralytic ileus
Paralysis of bowel
Paralysis of colon
Paralysis of intestine
      Excludes1 gallstone ileus (K56.3)
         ileus NOS (K56.7)
      ⟹ obstructive ileus NOS (K56.69-)

   K56.1 Intussusception
Intussusception or invagination of bowel
Intussusception or invagination of colon
Intussusception or invagination of intestine
Intussusception or invagination of rectum
      Excludes2 intussusception of appendix (K38.8)

Figure 11-11 Types of intussusception.

Item 11-14 Intussusception is the prolapse (telescoping) of a part of the intestine into another adjacent part of the intestine. Intussusception may be enteric (ileoileal, jejunoileal, jejunojejunal), colic (colocolic), or intracolic (ileocecal, ileocolic).

N Newborn Age: 0   P Pediatric Age: 0–17   M Maternity DX: 12–55   A Adult Age: 15–124   ♀ Females Only   ♂ Males Only
Complication\Comorbidity   Major C\C   (Ex) CC/MCC Exclusions   Hospital-Acquired Condition

951

CHAPTER 11 (K00-K95)

CHAPTER 11 (K00-K95)

Item 11–15 **Volvulus** is the twisting of a segment of the intestine, resulting in obstruction. Paralytic ileus is paralysis of the intestine. It need not be a complete paralysis, but it must prohibit the passage of food through the intestine and lead to intestinal blockage. It is a common aftermath of some types of surgery.

K56.2   **Volvulus** 🔲
     Strangulation of colon or intestine
     Torsion of colon or intestine
     Twist of colon or intestine
     Excludes2   volvulus of duodenum (K31.5)

K56.3   **Gallstone ileus** 🔲
     Obstruction of intestine by gallstone

● **K56.4**   **Other impaction of intestine**
     K56.41   **Fecal impaction**
           Excludes1   constipation (K59.0-)
                    incomplete defecation (R15.0)

     K56.49   **Other impaction of intestine** 🔲

⇒● **K56.5**   **Intestinal adhesions [bands] with obstruction (postinfection)**
     Abdominal hernia due to adhesions with obstruction
     ⇒ Peritoneal adhesions [bands] with intestinal obstruction (postinfection)
     ▶ **K56.50**   **Intestinal adhesions [bands], unspecified as to partial versus complete obstruction** 🔲
         ▶ Intestinal adhesions with obstruction NOS
     ▶ **K56.51**   **Intestinal adhesions [bands], with partial obstruction** 🔲
         ▶ Intestinal adhesions with incomplete obstruction
     ▶ **K56.52**   **Intestinal adhesions [bands] with complete obstruction** 🔲

● **K56.6**   **Other and unspecified intestinal obstruction**
     ● **K56.60**   **Unspecified intestinal obstruction**
         ~~Intestinal obstruction NOS~~
         Excludes1   intestinal obstruction due to specified condition-code to condition
         Coding Clinic: 2017, Q2, P12
         ▶ **K56.600**   **Partial intestinal obstruction, unspecified as to cause** 🔲
            ▶ Incomplete intestinal obstruction, NOS
         ▶ **K56.601**   **Complete intestinal obstruction, unspecified as to cause** 🔲
         ▶ **K56.609**   **Unspecified intestinal obstruction, unspecified as to partial versus complete obstruction** 🔲
            ▶ Intestinal obstruction NOS

     ● **K56.69**   **Other intestinal obstruction**
         Enterostenosis NOS
         Obstructive ileus NOS
         Occlusion of colon or intestine NOS
         Stenosis of colon or intestine NOS
         Stricture of colon or intestine NOS
         Excludes1   intestinal obstruction due to specified condition-code to condition
         Coding Clinic: 2017, Q2, P12
         ▶ **K56.690**   **Other partial intestinal obstruction** 🔲
            ▶ Other incomplete intestinal obstruction
         ▶ **K56.691**   **Other complete intestinal obstruction** 🔲
         ▶ **K56.699**   **Other intestinal obstruction unspecified as to partial versus complete obstruction** 🔲
            ▶ Other intestinal obstruction, NEC

K56.7   **Ileus, unspecified** 🔲
     ⇒ **Excludes1**   obstructive ileus (K56.69-)
     ▶ **Excludes2**   intestinal obstruction with hernia (K40-K46)
     Coding Clinic: 2017, Q1, P41

● **K57**   **Diverticular disease of intestine**
     Excludes1   congenital diverticulum of intestine (Q43.8)
               Meckel's diverticulum (Q43.0)
     Excludes2   diverticulum of appendix (K38.2)
     (Ex) For category K57 CC codes unless otherwise indicated: See PDX Collection 770

● **K57.0**   **Diverticulitis of small intestine with perforation and abscess**
     Diverticulitis of small intestine with peritonitis
     Excludes1   diverticulitis of both small and large intestine with perforation and abscess (K57.4-)
     K57.00   **Diverticulitis of small intestine with perforation and abscess without bleeding** 🔲
         CC when PDx is its own CC
         (Ex) See PDX Collection 793
     K57.01   **Diverticulitis of small intestine with perforation and abscess with bleeding** 🔲 🔲
         CC when PDx is its own CC

● **K57.1**   **Diverticular disease of small intestine without perforation or abscess**
     Excludes1   diverticular disease of both small and large intestine without perforation or abscess (K57.5-)
     K57.10   **Diverticulosis of small intestine without perforation or abscess without bleeding**
         Diverticular disease of small intestine NOS
     K57.11   **Diverticulosis of small intestine without perforation or abscess with bleeding** 🔲
     K57.12   **Diverticulitis of small intestine without perforation or abscess without bleeding** 🔲
         (Ex) See PDX Collection 793
     K57.13   **Diverticulitis of small intestine without perforation or abscess with bleeding** 🔲

● **K57.2**   **Diverticulitis of large intestine with perforation and abscess**
     Diverticulitis of colon with peritonitis
     Excludes1   diverticulitis of both small and large intestine with perforation and abscess (K57.4-)
     K57.20   **Diverticulitis of large intestine with perforation and abscess without bleeding** 🔲
         CC when PDx is its own CC
         (Ex) See PDX Collection 794
     K57.21   **Diverticulitis of large intestine with perforation and abscess with bleeding** 🔲
         CC when PDx is its own CC

Figure 11-12   Diverticulosis. (From Shiland: Mastering Healthcare Terminology, ed 4, St. Louis, Mosby, 2012)

Item 11–16   **Diverticula** of the intestines are acquired herniations of the mucosa. Diverticulum (singular): Pocket or pouch that bulges outward through a weak spot (herniation) in the colon. Diverticula (plural). **Diverticulosis** is the condition of having diverticula. **Diverticulitis** is inflammation of these pouches or herniations. Classification is based on location (small intestine or colon) and whether it occurs with or without hemorrhage.

▶ New   ⇒ Revised   ~~deleted~~ Deleted   Excludes 1   Excludes 2   Includes   Use additional   Code first   Code also   Key words

952

OGCR Official Guidelines   ● Unacceptable Principal Diagnosis   X Assign placeholder X   ● Use Additional Character(s)   ▌ Manifestation Code   **Coding Clinic**

● **K57.3 Diverticular disease of large intestine without perforation or abscess**
> **Excludes1** diverticular disease of both small and large intestine without perforation or abscess (K57.5-)

K57.30 Diverticulosis of large intestine without perforation or abscess without bleeding
> Diverticular disease of colon NOS

K57.31 Diverticulosis of large intestine without perforation or abscess with bleeding 🦠

K57.32 Diverticulitis of large intestine without perforation or abscess without bleeding 🦠
> (Ex:) See PDX Collection 794

K57.33 Diverticulitis of large intestine without perforation or abscess with bleeding 🦠

● **K57.4 Diverticulitis of both small and large intestine with perforation and abscess**
> Diverticulitis of both small and large intestine with peritonitis

K57.40 Diverticulitis of both small and large intestine with perforation and abscess without bleeding 🦠
> CC when PDx is its own CC
> (Ex:) See PDX Collection 794

K57.41 Diverticulitis of both small and large intestine with perforation and abscess with bleeding 🦠 🦠
> CC when PDx is its own CC

● **K57.5 Diverticular disease of both small and large intestine without perforation or abscess**

K57.50 Diverticulosis of both small and large intestine without perforation or abscess without bleeding
> Diverticular disease of both small and large intestine NOS

K57.51 Diverticulosis of both small and large intestine without perforation or abscess with bleeding 🦠

K57.52 Diverticulitis of both small and large intestine without perforation or abscess without bleeding 🦠
> CC when PDx is its own CC
> (Ex:) See PDX Collection 794

K57.53 Diverticulitis of both small and large intestine without perforation or abscess with bleeding 🦠

● **K57.8 Diverticulitis of intestine, part unspecified, with perforation and abscess**
> Diverticulitis of intestine NOS with peritonitis

K57.80 Diverticulitis of intestine, part unspecified, with perforation and abscess without bleeding 🦠
> CC when PDx is its own CC
> (Ex:) See PDX Collection 794

K57.81 Diverticulitis of intestine, part unspecified, with perforation and abscess with bleeding 🦠 🦠
> CC when PDx is its own CC

● **K57.9 Diverticular disease of intestine, part unspecified, without perforation or abscess**

K57.90 Diverticulosis of intestine, part unspecified, without perforation or abscess without bleeding
> Diverticular disease of intestine NOS

K57.91 Diverticulosis of intestine, part unspecified, without perforation or abscess with bleeding 🦠

K57.92 Diverticulitis of intestine, part unspecified, without perforation or abscess without bleeding 🦠
> (Ex:) See PDX Collection 794

K57.93 Diverticulitis of intestine, part unspecified, without perforation or abscess with bleeding 🦠

● **K58 Irritable bowel syndrome**
> **Includes** irritable colon
> spastic colon

K58.0 Irritable bowel syndrome with diarrhea

K58.1 Irritable bowel syndrome with constipation
> Coding Clinic: 2016, Q4, P32

K58.2 Mixed irritable bowel syndrome
> Coding Clinic: 2016, Q4, P32

K58.8 Other irritable bowel syndrome
> Coding Clinic: 2016, Q4, P32

K58.9 Irritable bowel syndrome without diarrhea
> Irritable bowel syndrome NOS

● **K59 Other functional intestinal disorders**
> **Excludes1** change in bowel habit NOS (R19.4)
> intestinal malabsorption (K90.-)
> psychogenic intestinal disorders (F45.8)
> **Excludes2** functional disorders of stomach (K31.-)

● **K59.0 Constipation**
> Use additional code for adverse effect, if applicable, to identify drug (T36-T50 with fifth or sixth character 5)
> **Excludes1** fecal impaction (K56.41)
> incomplete defecation (R15.0)

K59.00 Constipation, unspecified

K59.01 Slow transit constipation

K59.02 Outlet dysfunction constipation

K59.03 Drug induced constipation
> Use additional code for adverse effect, if applicable, to identify drug (T36-T50 with fifth or sixth character 5)
> Coding Clinic: 2016, Q4, P33

K59.04 Chronic idiopathic constipation
> Functional constipation
> Coding Clinic: 2016, Q4, P33

K59.09 Other constipation
> Chronic constipation

K59.1 Functional diarrhea
> **Excludes1** diarrhea NOS (R19.7)
> irritable bowel syndrome with diarrhea (K58.0)

K59.2 Neurogenic bowel, not elsewhere classified 🦠
> (Ex:) See PDX Collection 795

● **K59.3 Megacolon, not elsewhere classified**
> Dilatation of colon
> *Code first, if applicable (T51-T65) to identify toxic agent*
> **Excludes1** congenital megacolon (aganglionic) (Q43.1)
> megacolon (due to) (in) Chagas' disease (B57.32)
> ▸megacolon (due to) (in) Clostridium difficile (A04.7-)
> megacolon (due to) (in) Hirschsprung's disease (Q43.1)
> (Ex:) For category K59.3 CC codes: See PDX Collection 795
> Coding Clinic: 2016, Q4, P33

K59.31 Toxic megacolon 🦠

K59.39 Other megacolon 🦠
> Megacolon NOS

K59.4 Anal spasm
> Proctalgia fugax

K59.8 Other specified functional intestinal disorders
> Atony of colon Pseudo-obstruction (acute) (chronic) of intestine

K59.9 Functional intestinal disorder, unspecified

CHAPTER 11 (K00-K95)

N Newborn Age: 0   P Pediatric Age: 0–17   M Maternity DX: 12–55   A Adult Age: 15–124   ♀ Females Only   ♂ Males Only
🦠 Complication\Comorbidity   🦠 Major C\C   (Ex:) CC/MCC Exclusions   🦠 Hospital-Acquired Condition

953

Item 11–17 A **fissure** is a groove in the surface, whereas a **fistula** is an abnormal passage. An **abscess** is an accumulation of pus in a tissue cavity resulting from a bacterial or parasitic infection.

● **K60 Fissure and fistula of anal and rectal regions**
> **Excludes1** fissure and fistula of anal and rectal regions with abscess or cellulitis (K61.-)
> **Excludes2** anal sphincter tear (healed) (nontraumatic) (old) (K62.81)

K60.0 Acute anal fissure
K60.1 Chronic anal fissure
K60.2 Anal fissure, unspecified
K60.3 Anal fistula
K60.4 Rectal fistula
> Fistula of rectum to skin
> **Excludes1** rectovaginal fistula (N82.3)
> vesicorectal fistula (N32.1)

K60.5 Anorectal fistula

● **K61 Abscess of anal and rectal regions**
> **Includes** abscess of anal and rectal regions
> cellulitis of anal and rectal regions
> (Ex) For category K61 CC codes: See PDX Collection 796

K61.0 Anal abscess
> Perianal abscess
> **Excludes1** intrasphincteric abscess (K61.4)

K61.1 Rectal abscess
> Perirectal abscess
> **Excludes1** ischiorectal abscess (K61.3)
> Coding Clinic: 2012, Q4, P104

K61.2 Anorectal abscess
K61.3 Ischiorectal abscess
> Abscess of ischiorectal fossa

K61.4 Intrasphincteric abscess

● **K62 Other diseases of anus and rectum**
> **Includes** anal canal
> **Excludes2** colostomy and enterostomy malfunction (K94.0-, K91.4-)
> fecal incontinence (R15.-)
> hemorrhoids (K64.-)

K62.0 Anal polyp
K62.1 Rectal polyp
> **Excludes1** adenomatous polyp (D12.8)

K62.2 Anal prolapse
> Prolapse of anal canal

K62.3 Rectal prolapse
> Prolapse of rectal mucosa

K62.4 Stenosis of anus and rectum
> Stricture of anus (sphincter)

K62.5 Hemorrhage of anus and rectum
> **Excludes1** gastrointestinal bleeding NOS (K92.2)
> melena (K92.1)
> neonatal rectal hemorrhage (P54.2)
> (Ex) See PDX Collection 770

K62.6 Ulcer of anus and rectum
> Solitary ulcer of anus and rectum
> Stercoral ulcer of anus and rectum
> **Excludes1** fissure and fistula of anus and rectum (K60.-)
> ulcerative colitis (K51.-)
> (Ex) See PDX Collection 797

K62.7 Radiation proctitis
> Use additional code to identify the type of radiation (W90.-)

● **K62.8 Other specified diseases of anus and rectum**
> **Excludes2** ulcerative proctitis (K51.2)

K62.81 Anal sphincter tear (healed) (nontraumatic) (old)
> Tear of anus, nontraumatic
> Use additional code for any associated fecal incontinence (R15.-)
> **Excludes2** anal fissure (K60.-)
> anal sphincter tear (healed) (old) complicating delivery (O34.7-)
> traumatic tear of anal sphincter (S31.831)

K62.82 Dysplasia of anus
> Anal intraepithelial neoplasia I and II (AIN I and II) (histologically confirmed)
> Dysplasia of anus NOS
> Mild and moderate dysplasia of anus (histologically confirmed)
> **Excludes1** abnormal results from anal cytologic examination without histologic confirmation (R85.61-)
> anal intraepithelial neoplasia III (D01.3)
> carcinoma in situ of anus (D01.3)
> HGSIL of anus (R85.613)
> severe dysplasia of anus (D01.3)

K62.89 Other specified diseases of anus and rectum
> Proctitis NOS
> Use additional code for any associated fecal incontinence (R15.-)

K62.9 Disease of anus and rectum, unspecified

● **K63 Other diseases of intestine**
K63.0 Abscess of intestine
> **Excludes1** abscess of intestine with Crohn's disease (K50.014, K50.114, K50.814, K50.914)
> abscess of intestine with diverticular disease (K57.0, K57.2, K57.4, K57.8)
> abscess of intestine with ulcerative colitis (K51.014, K51.214, K51.314, K51.414, K51.514, K51.814, K51.914)
> **Excludes2** abscess of anal and rectal regions (K61.-)
> abscess of appendix (K35.3)
> (Ex) See PDX Collection 798

K63.1 Perforation of intestine (nontraumatic)
> Perforation (nontraumatic) of rectum
> **Excludes1** perforation (nontraumatic) of duodenum (K26.-)
> perforation (nontraumatic) of intestine with diverticular disease (K57.0, K57.2, K57.4, K57.8)
> **Excludes2** perforation (nontraumatic) of appendix (K35.2, K35.3)
> (Ex) See PDX Collection 799

K63.2 Fistula of intestine
> **Excludes1** fistula of duodenum (K31.6)
> fistula of intestine with Crohn's disease (K50.013, K50.113, K50.813, K50.913)
> fistula of intestine with ulcerative colitis (K51.013, K51.213, K51.313, K51.413, K51.513, K51.813, K51.913)
> **Excludes2** fistula of anal and rectal regions (K60.-)
> fistula of appendix (K38.3)
> intestinal-genital fistula, female (N82.2-N82.4)
> vesicointestinal fistula (N32.1)
> (Ex) See PDX Collection 800

K63.3   Ulcer of intestine 🔖
Primary ulcer of small intestine

> **Excludes1**   duodenal ulcer (K26.-)
> gastrointestinal ulcer (K28.-)
> gastrojejunal ulcer (K28.-)
> jejunal ulcer (K28.-)
> peptic ulcer, site unspecified (K27.-)
> ulcer of intestine with perforation (K63.1)
> ulcer of anus or rectum (K62.6)
> ulcerative colitis (K51.-)

Ex: See PDX Collection 801

K63.4   Enteroptosis

K63.5   Polyp of colon

> **Excludes1**   adenomatous polyp of colon (D12.6)
> inflammatory polyp of colon (K51.4-)
> polyposis of colon (D12.6)

Coding Clinic: 2017, Q1, P15-16; 2015, Q2, P14

K63.8   Other specified diseases of intestine

K63.81   Dieulafoy lesion of intestine 🔖

> **Excludes2**   Dieulafoy lesion of stomach and duodenum (K31.82)

Ex: See PDX Collection 802

K63.89   Other specified diseases of intestine
Coding Clinic: 2013, Q2, P31

K63.9   Disease of intestine, unspecified

K64   Hemorrhoids and perianal venous thrombosis

> **Includes**   piles
> **Excludes1**   hemorrhoids complicating childbirth and the puerperium (O87.2)
> hemorrhoids complicating pregnancy (O22.4)

K64.0   First degree hemorrhoids
Grade/stage I hemorrhoids
Hemorrhoids (bleeding) without prolapse outside of anal canal

K64.1   Second degree hemorrhoids
Grade/stage II hemorrhoids
Hemorrhoids (bleeding) that prolapse with straining, but retract spontaneously

K64.2   Third degree hemorrhoids
Grade/stage III hemorrhoids
Hemorrhoids (bleeding) that prolapse with straining and require manual replacement back inside anal canal

K64.3   Fourth degree hemorrhoids
Grade/stage IV hemorrhoids
Hemorrhoids (bleeding) with prolapsed tissue that cannot be manually replaced

K64.4   Residual hemorrhoidal skin tags
External hemorrhoids, NOS
Skin tags of anus

K64.5   Perianal venous thrombosis
External hemorrhoids with thrombosis
Perianal hematoma
Thrombosed hemorrhoids NOS

K64.8   Other hemorrhoids
Internal hemorrhoids, without mention of degree
Prolapsed hemorrhoids, degree not specified

K64.9   Unspecified hemorrhoids
Hemorrhoids (bleeding) NOS
Hemorrhoids (bleeding) without mention of degree

DISEASES OF PERITONEUM AND RETROPERITONEUM (K65-K68)

K65   Peritonitis

Use additional code (B95-B97), to identify infectious agent

> **Excludes1**   acute appendicitis with generalized peritonitis (K35.2)
> aseptic peritonitis (T81.6)
> benign paroxysmal peritonitis (E85.0)
> chemical peritonitis (T81.6)
> diverticulitis of both small and large intestine with peritonitis (K57.4-)
> diverticulitis of colon with peritonitis (K57.2-)
> diverticulitis of intestine, NOS, with peritonitis (K57.8-)
> diverticulitis of small intestine with peritonitis (K57.0-)
> gonococcal peritonitis (A54.85)
> neonatal peritonitis (P78.0-P78.1)
> pelvic peritonitis, female (N73.3-N73.5)
> periodic familial peritonitis (E85.0)
> peritonitis due to talc or other foreign substance (T81.6)
> peritonitis in chlamydia (A74.81)
> peritonitis in diphtheria (A36.89)
> peritonitis in syphilis (late) (A52.74)
> peritonitis in tuberculosis (A18.31)
> peritonitis with or following abortion or ectopic or molar pregnancy (O00-O07, O08.0)
> peritonitis with or following appendicitis (K35.-)
> peritonitis with or following diverticular disease of intestine (K57.-)
> puerperal peritonitis (O85)
> retroperitoneal infections (K68.-)

Ex: For category K65 CC codes: See PDX Collection 803

K65.0   Generalized (acute) peritonitis 🔖
Pelvic peritonitis (acute), male
Subphrenic peritonitis (acute)
Suppurative peritonitis (acute)

K65.1   Peritoneal abscess 🔖
Abdominopelvic abscess
Abscess (of) omentum
Abscess (of) peritoneum
Mesenteric abscess
Retrocecal abscess
Subdiaphragmatic abscess
Subhepatic abscess
Subphrenic abscess

K65.2   Spontaneous bacterial peritonitis 🔖

> **Excludes1**   bacterial peritonitis NOS (K65.9)

K65.3   Choleperitonitis 🔖
Peritonitis due to bile

K65.4   Sclerosing mesenteritis 🔖
Fat necrosis of peritoneum
(Idiopathic) sclerosing mesenteric fibrosis
Mesenteric lipodystrophy
Mesenteric panniculitis
Retractile mesenteritis

K65.8   Other peritonitis 🔖
Chronic proliferative peritonitis
Peritonitis due to urine

K65.9   Peritonitis, unspecified 🔖
Bacterial peritonitis NOS
Coding Clinic: 2013, Q2, P31

Item 11-18   Peritonitis is an inflammation of the lining (peritoneum) of the abdominal cavity and surface of the intestines.

Item 11-19   Retroperitoneal infections occur between the posterior parietal peritoneum and posterior abdominal wall where the kidneys, adrenal glands, ureters, duodenum, ascending colon, descending colon, pancreas, and the large vessels and nerves are located.

CHAPTER 11 (K00-K95)

N   Newborn Age: 0   P   Pediatric Age: 0–17   M   Maternity DX: 12–55   A   Adult Age: 15–124   ♀   Females Only   ♂   Males Only

🔖   Complication\Comorbidity   🔖   Major C\C   Ex: CC/MCC Exclusions   🔖   Hospital-Acquired Condition

● **K66** **Other disorders of peritoneum**

　　Excludes2 ascites (R18.-)
　　　　　　　peritoneal effusion (chronic) (R18.8)

　　K66.0 **Peritoneal adhesions (postprocedural) (postinfection)**
　　　　Adhesions (of) abdominal (wall)
　　　　Adhesions (of) diaphragm
　　　　Adhesions (of) intestine
　　　　Adhesions (of) male pelvis
　　　　Adhesions (of) omentum
　　　　Adhesions (of) stomach
　　　　Adhesive bands
　　　　Mesenteric adhesions
　　　　Excludes1 female pelvic adhesions [bands] (N73.6)
　　　　➡ peritoneal adhesions with intestinal obstruction (K56.5-)

　　K66.1 **Hemoperitoneum** 🔖
　　　　Excludes1 traumatic hemoperitoneum (S36.8-)
　　　　Ⓔ⨯ See PDX Collection 804

　　K66.8 **Other specified disorders of peritoneum**
　　K66.9 **Disorder of peritoneum, unspecified**

▷ **K67** *Disorders of peritoneum in infectious diseases classified elsewhere* 🔖
　　Code first underlying disease, such as:
　　　　congenital syphilis (A50.0)
　　　　helminthiasis (B65.0-B83.9)
　　Excludes1 peritonitis in chlamydia (A74.81)
　　　　　　peritonitis in diphtheria (A36.89)
　　　　　　peritonitis in gonococcal (A54.85)
　　　　　　peritonitis in syphilis (late) (A52.74)
　　　　　　peritonitis in tuberculosis (A18.31)
　　Ⓔ⨯ See PDX Collection 803

● **K68** **Disorders of retroperitoneum**
　● **K68.1** **Retroperitoneal abscess**
　　　K68.11 **Postprocedural retroperitoneal abscess** 🔖🔖
　　　　Ⓔ⨯ See PDX Collection 805
　　　K68.12 **Psoas muscle abscess** 🔖
　　　　Ⓔ⨯ See PDX Collection 806
　　　K68.19 **Other retroperitoneal abscess** 🔖
　　　　Ⓔ⨯ See PDX Collection 803
　　K68.9 **Other disorders of retroperitoneum** 🔖
　　　Ⓔ⨯ See PDX Collection 803

DISEASES OF LIVER (K70-K77)

　Excludes1 jaundice NOS (R17)
　Excludes2 hemochromatosis (E83.11-)
　　　　　　Reye's syndrome (G93.7)
　　　　　　viral hepatitis (B15-B19)
　　　　　　Wilson's disease (E83.0)

● **K70** **Alcoholic liver disease**
　　Use additional code to identify:
　　　alcohol abuse and dependence (F10.-)
　　K70.0 **Alcoholic fatty liver**　　　　　　　　　　A
　● **K70.1** **Alcoholic hepatitis**
　　　K70.10 **Alcoholic hepatitis without ascites**　A
　　　K70.11 **Alcoholic hepatitis with ascites**　　A
　　K70.2 **Alcoholic fibrosis and sclerosis of liver**　A
　● **K70.3** **Alcoholic cirrhosis of liver**
　　　Alcoholic cirrhosis NOS
　　　K70.30 **Alcoholic cirrhosis of liver without ascites**　A
　　　K70.31 **Alcoholic cirrhosis of liver with ascites**　A
　● **K70.4** **Alcoholic hepatic failure**
　　　Acute alcoholic hepatic failure
　　　Alcoholic hepatic failure NOS
　　　Chronic alcoholic hepatic failure
　　　Subacute alcoholic hepatic failure
　　　K70.40 **Alcoholic hepatic failure without coma**　A
　　　K70.41 **Alcoholic hepatic failure with coma** 🔖　A
　　　　MCC when PDx is its own MCC
　　　　Ⓔ⨯ See PDX Collection 807
　　K70.9 **Alcoholic liver disease, unspecified**　　A

Item 11-20 Cirrhosis is the progressive fibrosis of the liver resulting in loss of liver function. The main causes of cirrhosis of the liver are alcohol abuse, chronic hepatitis (inflammation of the liver), biliary disease, and excessive amounts of iron. **Alcoholic cirrhosis of the liver** is also called portal, Laënnec's, or fatty nutritional cirrhosis.

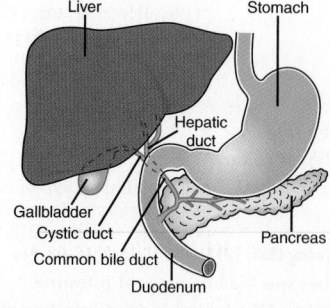

Figure 11-13 Liver and bile ducts.

● **K71** **Toxic liver disease**
　　Includes drug-induced idiosyncratic (unpredictable) liver disease
　　　　　　drug-induced toxic (predictable) liver disease
　　Code first poisoning due to drug or toxin, if applicable (T36-T65 with fifth or sixth character 1-4 or 6)
　　Use additional code for adverse effect, if applicable, to identify drug (T36-T50 with fifth or sixth character 5)
　　Excludes2 alcoholic liver disease (K70.-)
　　　　　　Budd-Chiari syndrome (I82.0)

　　K71.0 **Toxic liver disease with cholestasis**
　　　Cholestasis with hepatocyte injury
　　　'Pure' cholestasis
　● **K71.1** **Toxic liver disease with hepatic necrosis**
　　　Hepatic failure (acute) (chronic) due to drugs
　　　K71.10 **Toxic liver disease with hepatic necrosis, without coma**
　　　K71.11 **Toxic liver disease with hepatic necrosis, with coma** 🔖
　　　　MCC when PDx is its own MCC
　　　　Ⓔ⨯ See PDX Collection 807
　　K71.2 **Toxic liver disease with acute hepatitis**
　　K71.3 **Toxic liver disease with chronic persistent hepatitis**
　　K71.4 **Toxic liver disease with chronic lobular hepatitis**
　● **K71.5** **Toxic liver disease with chronic active hepatitis**
　　　Toxic liver disease with lupoid hepatitis
　　　K71.50 **Toxic liver disease with chronic active hepatitis without ascites**
　　　K71.51 **Toxic liver disease with chronic active hepatitis with ascites**
　　K71.6 **Toxic liver disease with hepatitis, not elsewhere classified**
　　K71.7 **Toxic liver disease with fibrosis and cirrhosis of liver**
　　K71.8 **Toxic liver disease with other disorders of liver**
　　　Toxic liver disease with focal nodular hyperplasia
　　　Toxic liver disease with hepatic granulomas
　　　Toxic liver disease with peliosis hepatis
　　　Toxic liver disease with veno-occlusive disease of liver
　　K71.9 **Toxic liver disease, unspecified**

▶ New　➡ Revised　d̶e̶l̶e̶t̶e̶d̶ Deleted　Excludes 1　Excludes 2　Includes　Use additional　Code first　Code also　Key words

956　OGCR Official Guidelines　● Unacceptable Principal Diagnosis　X Assign placeholder X　● Use Additional Character(s)　▷ Manifestation Code　Coding Clinic

CHAPTER 11 (K00-K95)

● **K72   Hepatic failure, not elsewhere classified**

Includes	fulminant hepatitis NEC, with hepatic failure
	hepatic encephalopathy NOS
	liver (cell) necrosis with hepatic failure
	malignant hepatitis NEC, with hepatic failure
	yellow liver atrophy or dystrophy

Excludes1	alcoholic hepatic failure (K70.4)
	hepatic failure with toxic liver disease (K71.1-)
	icterus of newborn (P55-P59)
	postprocedural hepatic failure (K91.82)

Excludes2	hepatic failure complicating abortion or ectopic or molar pregnancy (O00-O07, O08.8)
	hepatic failure complicating pregnancy, childbirth and the puerperium (O26.6-)
	viral hepatitis with hepatic coma (B15-B19)

● **K72.0   Acute and subacute hepatic failure**
Acute non-viral hepatitis NOS
(Ex) **For category K72.0 CC codes: See PDX Collection 808**
Coding Clinic: 2015, Q2, P17

K72.00   Acute and subacute hepatic failure without coma 🦠
Coding Clinic: 2015, Q2, P17

K72.01   Acute and subacute hepatic failure with coma 🦠
MCC when PDx is its own MCC

● **K72.1   Chronic hepatic failure**

K72.10   Chronic hepatic failure without coma
Coding Clinic: 2017, Q1, P41

K72.11   Chronic hepatic failure with coma 🦠
MCC when PDx is its own MCC
(Ex) See PDX Collection 807

● **K72.9   Hepatic failure, unspecified**

K72.90   Hepatic failure, unspecified without coma

K72.91   Hepatic failure, unspecified with coma 🦠
Hepatic coma NOS
(Ex) See PDX Collection 807
Coding Clinic: 2016, Q2, P35

● **K73   Chronic hepatitis, not elsewhere classified**

Excludes1	alcoholic hepatitis (chronic) (K70.1-)
	drug-induced hepatitis (chronic) (K71.-)
	granulomatous hepatitis (chronic) NEC (K75.3)
	reactive, nonspecific hepatitis (chronic) (K75.2)
	viral hepatitis (chronic) (B15-B19)

K73.0   Chronic persistent hepatitis, not elsewhere classified
K73.1   Chronic lobular hepatitis, not elsewhere classified
K73.2   Chronic active hepatitis, not elsewhere classified
K73.8   Other chronic hepatitis, not elsewhere classified
K73.9   Chronic hepatitis, unspecified

● **K74   Fibrosis and cirrhosis of liver**
Code also, if applicable, viral hepatitis (acute) (chronic) (B15-B19)

Excludes1	alcoholic cirrhosis (of liver) (K70.3)
	alcoholic fibrosis of liver (K70.2)
	cardiac sclerosis of liver (K76.1)
	cirrhosis (of liver) with toxic liver disease (K71.7)
	congenital cirrhosis (of liver) (P78.81)
	pigmentary cirrhosis (of liver) (E83.110)

K74.0   Hepatic fibrosis
K74.1   Hepatic sclerosis
K74.2   Hepatic fibrosis with hepatic sclerosis
K74.3   Primary biliary cirrhosis
Chronic nonsuppurative destructive cholangitis
K74.4   Secondary biliary cirrhosis
K74.5   Biliary cirrhosis, unspecified
● **K74.6   Other and unspecified cirrhosis of liver**

K74.60   Unspecified cirrhosis of liver
Cirrhosis (of liver) NOS

K74.69   Other cirrhosis of liver
Cryptogenic cirrhosis (of liver)
Macronodular cirrhosis (of liver)
Micronodular cirrhosis (of liver)
Mixed type cirrhosis (of liver)
Portal cirrhosis (of liver)
Postnecrotic cirrhosis (of liver)

● **K75   Other inflammatory liver diseases**

Excludes2	toxic liver disease (K71.-)

K75.0   Abscess of liver 🦠
Cholangitic hepatic abscess
Hematogenic hepatic abscess
Hepatic abscess NOS
Lymphogenic hepatic abscess
Pylephlebitic hepatic abscess

Excludes1	amebic liver abscess (A06.4)
	cholangitis without liver abscess (K83.0)
	pylephlebitis without liver abscess (K75.1)

Excludes2	acute or subacute hepatitis NOS (B17.9)
	acute or subacute non-viral hepatitis (K72.0)
	chronic hepatitis NEC (K73.8)

(Ex) See PDX Collection 809

K75.1   Phlebitis of portal vein 🦠
Pylephlebitis

Excludes1	pylephlebitic liver abscess (K75.0)

(Ex) See PDX Collection 809

K75.2   Nonspecific reactive hepatitis

Excludes1	acute or subacute hepatitis (K72.0-)
	chronic hepatitis NEC (K73.-)
	viral hepatitis (B15-B19)

K75.3   Granulomatous hepatitis, not elsewhere classified

Excludes1	acute or subacute hepatitis (K72.0-)
	chronic hepatitis NEC (K73.-)
	viral hepatitis (B15-B19)

K75.4   Autoimmune hepatitis
Lupoid hepatitis NEC

● **K75.8   Other specified inflammatory liver diseases**

K75.81   Nonalcoholic steatohepatitis (NASH)
K75.89   Other specified inflammatory liver diseases

K75.9   Inflammatory liver disease, unspecified
Hepatitis NOS

Excludes1	acute or subacute hepatitis (K72.0-)
	chronic hepatitis NEC (K73.-)
	viral hepatitis (B15-B19)

Coding Clinic: 2015, Q2, P17

● **K76   Other diseases of liver**

Excludes2	alcoholic liver disease (K70.-)
	amyloid degeneration of liver (E85.-)
	cystic disease of liver (congenital) (Q44.6)
	hepatic vein thrombosis (I82.0)
	hepatomegaly NOS (R16.0)
	pigmentary cirrhosis (of liver) (E83.110)
	portal vein thrombosis (I81)
	toxic liver disease (K71.-)

K76.0   Fatty (change of) liver, not elsewhere classified
Nonalcoholic fatty liver disease (NAFLD)

Excludes1	nonalcoholic steatohepatitis (NASH) (K75.81)

K76.1   Chronic passive congestion of liver
Cardiac cirrhosis
Cardiac sclerosis

K76.2   Central hemorrhagic necrosis of liver 🦠

Excludes1	liver necrosis with hepatic failure (K72.-)

(Ex) See PDX Collection 808

K76.3   Infarction of liver 🦠
(Ex) See PDX Collection 808

K76.4   Peliosis hepatis
Hepatic angiomatosis

K76.5   Hepatic veno-occlusive disease

Excludes1	Budd-Chiari syndrome (I82.0)

K76.6   Portal hypertension 🦠
Use additional code for any associated complications, such as:
portal hypertensive gastropathy (K31.89)
(Ex) See PDX Collection 810

CHAPTER 11 (K00-K95)

CHAPTER 11 (K00-K95)

K76.7   **Hepatorenal syndrome** 🔍
         Excludes1   hepatorenal syndrome following labor
                          and delivery (O90.4)
                          postprocedural hepatorenal syndrome
                          (K91.83)
                   (Ex:) See PDX Collection 811

● K76.8   **Other specified diseases of liver**
     ● K76.81   **Hepatopulmonary syndrome**
                 Code first underlying liver disease, such as:
                     alcoholic cirrhosis of liver (K70.3-)
                     cirrhosis of liver without mention of alcohol
                     (K74.6-)
       K76.89   **Other specified diseases of liver**
                     Cyst (simple) of liver
                     Focal nodular hyperplasia of liver
                     Hepatoptosis

     K76.9   **Liver disease, unspecified**

▶ K77   *Liver disorders in diseases classified elsewhere* 🔍
         Code first underlying disease, such as:
             amyloidosis (E85.-)
             congenital syphilis (A50.0, A50.5)
             congenital toxoplasmosis (P37.1)
             schistosomiasis (B65.0-B65.9)
         Excludes1   alcoholic hepatitis (K70.1-)
                          alcoholic liver disease (K70.-)
                          cytomegaloviral hepatitis (B25.1)
                          herpesviral [herpes simplex] hepatitis (B00.81)
                          infectious mononucleosis with liver disease
                          (B27.0-B27.9 with .9)
                          mumps hepatitis (B26.81)
                          sarcoidosis with liver disease (D86.89)
                          secondary syphilis with liver disease (A51.45)
                          syphilis (late) with liver disease (A52.74)
                          toxoplasmosis (acquired) hepatitis (B58.1)
                          tuberculosis with liver disease (A18.83)
                   (Ex:) No exclusions

DISORDERS OF GALLBLADDER, BILIARY TRACT AND PANCREAS (K80–K87)

● K80   **Cholelithiasis**
         Presence or formation of gallstones
         Excludes1   retained cholelithiasis following cholecystectomy
                          (K91.86)

● K80.0   **Calculus of gallbladder with acute cholecystitis**
                     Any condition listed in K80.2 with acute cholecystitis
                     *Check documentation for acute/chronic gallbladder/common
                     bile duct either with or without obstruction.*
       K80.00   **Calculus of gallbladder with acute cholecystitis
                 without obstruction** 🔍
                   (Ex:) See PDX Collection 812
       K80.01   **Calculus of gallbladder with acute cholecystitis
                 with obstruction** 🔍
                   (Ex:) See PDX Collection 813

● K80.1   **Calculus of gallbladder with other cholecystitis**
                   (Ex:) For category K80.1 CC codes unless otherwise indicated: See PDX
                   Collection 813
       K80.10   **Calculus of gallbladder with chronic
                 cholecystitis without obstruction** 🔍
                     Cholelithiasis with cholecystitis NOS
       K80.11   **Calculus of gallbladder with chronic
                 cholecystitis with obstruction** 🔍
       K80.12   **Calculus of gallbladder with acute and chronic
                 cholecystitis without obstruction** 🔍
                   (Ex:) See PDX Collection 812
       K80.13   **Calculus of gallbladder with acute and chronic
                 cholecystitis with obstruction** 🔍
       K80.18   **Calculus of gallbladder with other cholecystitis
                 without obstruction** 🔍
       K80.19   **Calculus of gallbladder with other cholecystitis
                 with obstruction** 🔍

● K80.2   **Calculus of gallbladder without cholecystitis**
                     Cholecystolithiasis without cholecystitis
                     Cholelithiasis (without cholecystitis)
                     Colic (recurrent) of gallbladder (without cholecystitis)
                     Gallstone (impacted) of cystic duct (without
                     cholecystitis)
                     Gallstone (impacted) of gallbladder (without
                     cholecystitis)
       K80.20   **Calculus of gallbladder without cholecystitis
                 without obstruction**
       K80.21   **Calculus of gallbladder without cholecystitis
                 with obstruction** 🔍
                   (Ex:) See PDX Collection 813

● K80.3   **Calculus of bile duct with cholangitis**
                     Any condition listed in K80.5 with cholangitis
       K80.30   **Calculus of bile duct with cholangitis,
                 unspecified, without obstruction** 🔍
                     CC when PDx is its own CC
                   (Ex:) See PDX Collection 814
       K80.31   **Calculus of bile duct with cholangitis,
                 unspecified, with obstruction** 🔍
                     CC when PDx is its own CC
                   (Ex:) See PDX Collection 815
       K80.32   **Calculus of bile duct with acute cholangitis
                 without obstruction** 🔍
                     CC when PDx is its own CC
                   (Ex:) See PDX Collection 814
       K80.33   **Calculus of bile duct with acute cholangitis
                 with obstruction** 🔍
                     CC when PDx is its own CC
                   (Ex:) See PDX Collection 815
       K80.34   **Calculus of bile duct with chronic cholangitis
                 without obstruction** 🔍
                     CC when PDx is its own CC
                   (Ex:) See PDX Collection 814
       K80.35   **Calculus of bile duct with chronic cholangitis
                 with obstruction** 🔍
                     CC when PDx is its own CC
                   (Ex:) See PDX Collection 815
       K80.36   **Calculus of bile duct with acute and chronic
                 cholangitis without obstruction** 🔍
                     CC when PDx is its own CC
                   (Ex:) See PDX Collection 814
       K80.37   **Calculus of bile duct with acute and chronic
                 cholangitis with obstruction** 🔍
                     CC when PDx is its own CC
                   (Ex:) See PDX Collection 815

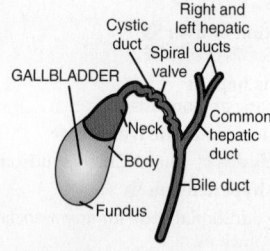

Figure 11-14   Gallbladder and bile ducts.

▶ New   ⟹ Revised   ~~deleted~~ Deleted   Excludes 1   Excludes 2   Includes   Use additional   Code first   Code also   Key words

958   OGCR Official Guidelines   ● Unacceptable Principal Diagnosis   X Assign placeholder X   ▶ Use Additional Character(s)   ▶ Manifestation Code   Coding Clinic

● **K80.4**   **Calculus of bile duct with cholecystitis**
Any condition listed in K80.5 with cholecystitis (with cholangitis)
(Ex) **For category K80.4 CC codes:** See PDX Collection 815

     K80.40   Calculus of bile duct with cholecystitis, unspecified, **without obstruction** 🗇

     K80.41   Calculus of bile duct with cholecystitis, unspecified, **with obstruction** 🗇

     K80.42   Calculus of bile duct with **acute cholecystitis without obstruction** 🗇

     K80.43   Calculus of bile duct with **acute cholecystitis with obstruction** 🗇

     K80.44   Calculus of bile duct with **chronic cholecystitis without obstruction** 🗇

     K80.45   Calculus of bile duct with **chronic cholecystitis with obstruction** 🗇

     K80.46   Calculus of bile duct with **acute and chronic cholecystitis without obstruction** 🗇

     K80.47   Calculus of bile duct with **acute and chronic cholecystitis with obstruction** 🗇

● **K80.5**   **Calculus of bile duct without cholangitis or cholecystitis**
Choledocholithiasis (without cholangitis or cholecystitis)
Gallstone (impacted) of bile duct NOS (without cholangitis or cholecystitis)
Gallstone (impacted) of common duct (without cholangitis or cholecystitis)
Gallstone (impacted) of hepatic duct (without cholangitis or cholecystitis)
Hepatic cholelithiasis (without cholangitis or cholecystitis)
Hepatic colic (recurrent) (without cholangitis or cholecystitis)

     K80.50   Calculus of bile duct without cholangitis or cholecystitis **without obstruction**

     K80.51   Calculus of bile duct without cholangitis or cholecystitis **with obstruction** 🗇
(Ex) See PDX Collection 815

● **K80.6**   **Calculus of gallbladder and bile duct with cholecystitis**

     K80.60   Calculus of gallbladder and bile duct with cholecystitis, unspecified, **without obstruction** 🗇
(Ex) See PDX Collection 815

     K80.61   Calculus of gallbladder and bile duct with cholecystitis, unspecified, **with obstruction** 🗇
(Ex) See PDX Collection 815

     K80.62   Calculus of gallbladder and bile duct with **acute cholecystitis without obstruction** 🗇
(Ex) See PDX Collection 816

     K80.63   Calculus of gallbladder and bile duct with **acute cholecystitis with obstruction** 🗇
(Ex) See PDX Collection 816

     K80.64   Calculus of gallbladder and bile duct with **chronic cholecystitis without obstruction** 🗇
(Ex) See PDX Collection 815

     K80.65   Calculus of gallbladder and bile duct with **chronic cholecystitis with obstruction** 🗇
(Ex) See PDX Collection 815

     K80.66   Calculus of gallbladder and bile duct with **acute and chronic cholecystitis without obstruction** 🗇
(Ex) See PDX Collection 817

     K80.67   Calculus of gallbladder and bile duct with **acute and chronic cholecystitis with obstruction** 🗇
(Ex) See PDX Collection 817

● **K80.7**   **Calculus of gallbladder and bile duct without cholecystitis**

     K80.70   Calculus of gallbladder and bile duct without cholecystitis **without obstruction**

     K80.71   Calculus of gallbladder and bile duct without cholecystitis **with obstruction** 🗇
(Ex) See PDX Collection 815

● **K80.8**   **Other cholelithiasis**

     K80.80   Other cholelithiasis **without obstruction**

     K80.81   Other cholelithiasis **with obstruction** 🗇
(Ex) See PDX Collection 815

● **K81**   **Cholecystitis**
Chronic or acute inflammation of the gallbladder
Excludes1   cholecystitis with cholelithiasis (K80.-)

     K81.0   **Acute cholecystitis** 🗇
Abscess of gallbladder
Angiocholecystitis
Emphysematous (acute) cholecystitis
Empyema of gallbladder
Gangrene of gallbladder
Gangrenous cholecystitis
Suppurative cholecystitis
(Ex) See PDX Collection 818

     K81.1   **Chronic cholecystitis**

     K81.2   **Acute cholecystitis with chronic cholecystitis** 🗇
(Ex) See PDX Collection 819

     K81.9   **Cholecystitis, unspecified**

● **K82**   **Other diseases of gallbladder**
Excludes1   nonvisualization of gallbladder (R93.2)
               postcholecystectomy syndrome (K91.5)
(Ex) **For category K82 CC codes:** See PDX Collection 820

     K82.0   **Obstruction of gallbladder** 🗇
Occlusion of cystic duct or gallbladder without cholelithiasis
Stenosis of cystic duct or gallbladder without cholelithiasis
Stricture of cystic duct or gallbladder without cholelithiasis
Excludes1   obstruction of gallbladder with cholelithiasis (K80.-)

     K82.1   **Hydrops of gallbladder** 🗇
Mucocele of gallbladder

     K82.2   **Perforation of gallbladder** 🗇
Rupture of cystic duct or gallbladder

     K82.3   **Fistula of gallbladder** 🗇
Cholecystocolic fistula
Cholecystoduodenal fistula

     K82.4   **Cholesterolosis of gallbladder**
Strawberry gallbladder
Excludes1   cholesterolosis of gallbladder with cholecystitis (K81.-)
               cholesterolosis of gallbladder with cholelithiasis (K80.-)

     K82.8   **Other specified diseases of gallbladder**
Adhesions of cystic duct or gallbladder
Atrophy of cystic duct or gallbladder
Cyst of cystic duct or gallbladder
Dyskinesia of cystic duct or gallbladder
Hypertrophy of cystic duct or gallbladder
Nonfunctioning of cystic duct or gallbladder
Ulcer of cystic duct or gallbladder

     K82.9   **Disease of gallbladder, unspecified**

CHAPTER 11 (K00-K95)

N   Newborn Age: 0   P   Pediatric Age: 0–17   M   Maternity DX: 12–55   A   Adult Age: 15–124   ♀   Females Only   ♂   Males Only

🗇   Complication\Comorbidity   🗇   Major C\C   (Ex)   CC/MCC Exclusions   🗇   Hospital-Acquired Condition

● **K83**   **Other diseases of biliary tract**
    Excludes1   postcholecystectomy syndrome (K91.5)
    Excludes2   conditions involving the gallbladder (K81-K82)
                 conditions involving the cystic duct (K81-K82)

   K83.0   **Cholangitis** 🔍
      Ascending cholangitis   Sclerosing cholangitis
      Cholangitis NOS   Secondary cholangitis
      Primary cholangitis   Stenosing cholangitis
      Recurrent cholangitis   Suppurative cholangitis
      Excludes1   cholangitic liver abscess (K75.0)
                cholangitis with choledocholithiasis
                    (K80.3-, K80.4-)
                chronic nonsuppurative destructive
                    cholangitis (K74.3)
      (Ex:) See PDX Collection 814

   K83.1   **Obstruction of bile duct** 🔍
      Occlusion of bile duct without cholelithiasis
      Stenosis of bile duct without cholelithiasis
      Stricture of bile duct without cholelithiasis
      Excludes1   congenital obstruction of bile duct (Q44.3)
                obstruction of bile duct with cholelithiasis
                    (K80.-)
      (Ex:) See PDX Collection 821
      Coding Clinic: 2016, Q1, P18

   K83.2   **Perforation of bile duct** 🔍
      Rupture of bile duct
      (Ex:) See PDX Collection 822

   K83.3   **Fistula of bile duct** 🔍
      Choledochoduodenal fistula
      (Ex:) See PDX Collection 822

   K83.4   **Spasm of sphincter of Oddi**

   K83.5   **Biliary cyst**

   K83.8   **Other specified diseases of biliary tract**
      Adhesions of biliary tract
      Atrophy of biliary tract
      Hypertrophy of biliary tract
      Ulcer of biliary tract

   K83.9   **Disease of biliary tract, unspecified**

● **K85**   **Acute pancreatitis**
   Inflammatory process in which pancreatic enzymes autodigest the gland
    Includes   acute (recurrent) pancreatitis
               subacute pancreatitis
   (Ex:) **For category K85 CC codes:** See PDX Collection 177
   Coding Clinic: 2016, Q4, P34

   ● **K85.0**   **Idiopathic acute pancreatitis**
      K85.00   **Idiopathic acute pancreatitis without necrosis or infection** 🔍
      K85.01   **Idiopathic acute pancreatitis with uninfected necrosis** 🔍
      K85.02   **Idiopathic acute pancreatitis with infected necrosis** 🔍

   ● **K85.1**   **Biliary acute pancreatitis**
      Gallstone pancreatitis
      K85.10   **Biliary acute pancreatitis without necrosis or infection** 🔍
      K85.11   **Biliary acute pancreatitis with uninfected necrosis** 🔍
      K85.12   **Biliary acute pancreatitis with infected necrosis** 🔍

Figure 11-15   Pancreatic ductal system.

   ● **K85.2**   **Alcohol induced acute pancreatitis**
      Excludes2   alcohol induced chronic pancreatitis (K86.0)
      K85.20   **Alcohol induced acute pancreatitis without necrosis or infection** 🔍
      K85.21   **Alcohol induced acute pancreatitis with uninfected necrosis** 🔍
      K85.22   **Alcohol induced acute pancreatitis with infected necrosis** 🔍

   ● **K85.3**   **Drug induced acute pancreatitis**
      Use additional code for adverse effect, if applicable, to identify drug (T36-T50 with fifth or sixth character 5)
      Use additional code to identify drug abuse and dependence (F11.-F17.-)
      K85.30   **Drug induced acute pancreatitis without necrosis or infection** 🔍
      K85.31   **Drug induced acute pancreatitis with uninfected necrosis** 🔍
      K85.32   **Drug induced acute pancreatitis with infected necrosis** 🔍

   ● **K85.8**   **Other acute pancreatitis**
      K85.80   **Other acute pancreatitis without necrosis or infection** 🔍
      K85.81   **Other acute pancreatitis with uninfected necrosis** 🔍
      K85.82   **Other acute pancreatitis with infected necrosis** 🔍

   ● **K85.9**   **Acute pancreatitis, unspecified**
      Pancreatitis NOS
      K85.90   **Acute pancreatitis without necrosis or infection, unspecified** 🔍
      K85.91   **Acute pancreatitis with uninfected necrosis, unspecified** 🔍
      K85.92   **Acute pancreatitis with infected necrosis, unspecified** 🔍

● **K86**   **Other diseases of pancreas**
    Excludes2   fibrocystic disease of pancreas (E84.-)
                islet cell tumor (of pancreas) (D13.7)
                pancreatic steatorrhea (K90.3)

   K86.0   **Alcohol-induced chronic pancreatitis** 🔍
      Use additional code to identify:
        alcohol abuse and dependence (F10.-)
      Code also exocrine pancreatic insufficiency (K86.81)
      Excludes2   alcohol induced acute pancreatitis (K85.2-)
      (Ex:) See PDX Collection 823

   K86.1   **Other chronic pancreatitis** 🔍
      Chronic pancreatitis NOS
      Infectious chronic pancreatitis
      Recurrent chronic pancreatitis
      Relapsing chronic pancreatitis
      Code also exocrine pancreatic insufficiency (K86.81)
      (Ex:) See PDX Collection 823

   K86.2   **Cyst of pancreas** 🔍
      (Ex:) See PDX Collection 824

   K86.3   **Pseudocyst of pancreas** 🔍
      (Ex:) See PDX Collection 824

   ● **K86.8**   **Other specified diseases of pancreas**
      Coding Clinic: 2016, Q4, P34
      K86.81   **Exocrine pancreatic insufficiency**
      K86.89   **Other specified diseases of pancreas**
          Aseptic pancreatic necrosis, unrelated to acute pancreatitis
          Atrophy of pancreas
          Calculus of pancreas
          Cirrhosis of pancreas
          Fibrosis of pancreas
          Pancreatic fat necrosis, unrelated to acute pancreatitis
          Pancreatic infantilism
          Pancreatic necrosis NOS, unrelated to acute pancreatitis

   K86.9   **Disease of pancreas, unspecified**

▶ New   ⇒ Revised   ~~deleted~~ Deleted   Excludes 1   Excludes 2   Includes   Use additional   Code first   Code also   Key words
OGCR Official Guidelines   ● Unacceptable Principal Diagnosis   X Assign placeholder X   🔍 Use Additional Character(s)   ▌ Manifestation Code   Coding Clinic

▶ **K87** *Disorders of gallbladder, biliary tract and pancreas in diseases classified elsewhere*

> *Code first underlying disease*
>
> | Excludes1 | cytomegaloviral pancreatitis (B25.2) |
> |---|---|
> | | mumps pancreatitis (B26.3) |
> | | syphilitic gallbladder (A52.74) |
> | | syphilitic pancreas (A52.74) |
> | | tuberculosis of gallbladder (A18.83) |
> | | tuberculosis of pancreas (A18.83) |

OTHER DISEASES OF THE DIGESTIVE SYSTEM (K90-K95)

● **K90 Intestinal malabsorption**

> | Excludes1 | intestinal malabsorption following gastrointestinal surgery (K91.2) |
> |---|---|

Ⓔ **For category K90 cc does unless otherwise indicated:** See PDX Collection 825

K90.0 Celiac disease
Celiac disease with steatorrhea
➠Celiac gluten-sensitive enteropathy
Nontropical sprue
Use additional code for associated disorders including:
dermatitis herpetiformis (L13.0)
gluten ataxia (G32.81)
Code also exocrine pancreatic insufficiency (K86.81)

K90.1 Tropical sprue 🅒
Sprue NOS
Tropical steatorrhea

K90.2 Blind loop syndrome, not elsewhere classified 🅒
Blind loop syndrome NOS

> | Excludes1 | congenital blind loop syndrome (Q43.8) |
> |---|---|
> | | postsurgical blind loop syndrome (K91.2) |

K90.3 Pancreatic steatorrhea 🅒

● **K90.4 Other malabsorption due to intolerance**

> | ➠ Excludes2 | celiac gluten-sensitive enteropathy (K90.0) |
> |---|---|
> | | lactose intolerance (E73.-) |

Coding Clinic: 2016, Q4, P35-36

K90.41 Non-celiac gluten sensitivity 🅒
Gluten sensitivity NOS
Non-celiac gluten sensitive enteropathy

K90.49 Malabsorption due to intolerance, not elsewhere classified 🅒
Malabsorption due to intolerance to carbohydrate
Malabsorption due to intolerance to fat
Malabsorption due to intolerance to protein
Malabsorption due to intolerance to starch

● **K90.8 Other intestinal malabsorption**

K90.81 Whipple's disease 🅒
Ⓔ See PDX Collection 826

K90.89 Other intestinal malabsorption 🅒

K90.9 Intestinal malabsorption, unspecified 🅒

● **K91 Intraoperative and postprocedural complications and disorders of digestive system, not elsewhere classified**

> | Excludes2 | complications of artificial opening of digestive system (K94.-) |
> |---|---|
> | | complications of bariatric procedures (K95.-) |
> | | gastrojejunal ulcer (K28.-) |
> | | postprocedural (radiation) retroperitoneal abscess (K68.11) |
> | | radiation colitis (K52.0) |
> | | radiation gastroenteritis (K52.0) |
> | | radiation proctitis (K62.7) |

Coding Clinic: 2016, Q4, P10

K91.0 Vomiting following gastrointestinal surgery

K91.1 Postgastric surgery syndromes
Dumping syndrome
Postgastrectomy syndrome
Postvagotomy syndrome

K91.2 Postsurgical malabsorption, not elsewhere classified 🅒
Postsurgical blind loop syndrome

> | Excludes1 | malabsorption osteomalacia in adults (M83.2) |
> |---|---|
> | | malabsorption osteoporosis, postsurgical (M80.8-, M81.8) |

Ⓔ See PDX Collection 827

● **K91.3 Postprocedural intestinal obstruction**
Ⓔ **For category K91.3 CC codes:** See PDX Collection 792
Coding Clinic: 2017, Q1, P40-41

▶ **K91.30 Postprocedural intestinal obstruction, unspecified as to partial versus complete** 🅒
▶Postprocedural intestinal obstruction NOS

▶ **K91.31 Postprocedural partial intestinal obstruction** 🅒
▶Postprocedural incomplete intestinal obstruction

▶ **K91.32 Postprocedural complete intestinal obstruction** 🅒

K91.5 Postcholecystectomy syndrome

● **K91.6 Intraoperative hemorrhage and hematoma of a digestive system organ or structure complicating a procedure**

> | Excludes1 | intraoperative hemorrhage and hematoma of a digestive system organ or structure due to accidental puncture and laceration during a procedure (K91.7-) |
> |---|---|

Ⓔ **For category K91.6 CC codes:** See PDX Collection 829

K91.61 Intraoperative hemorrhage and hematoma of a digestive system organ or structure complicating a digestive system procedure 🅒

K91.62 Intraoperative hemorrhage and hematoma of a digestive system organ or structure complicating other procedure 🅒

● **K91.7 Accidental puncture and laceration of a digestive system organ or structure during a procedure**
Ⓔ **For category K91.7 CC codes:** See PDX Collection 509

K91.71 Accidental puncture and laceration of a digestive system organ or structure during a digestive system procedure 🅒

K91.72 Accidental puncture and laceration of a digestive system organ or structure during other procedure 🅒

● **K91.8 Other intraoperative and postprocedural complications and disorders of digestive system**
Ⓔ **For category K91.8 CC codes unless otherwise indicated:** See PDX Collection 828

K91.81 Other intraoperative complications of digestive system 🅒

K91.82 Postprocedural hepatic failure 🅒

K91.83 Postprocedural hepatorenal syndrome 🅒

● **K91.84 Postprocedural hemorrhage of a digestive system organ or structure following a procedure**
Ⓔ **For category K91.84 CC codes:** See PDX Collection 829

K91.840 Postprocedural hemorrhage of a digestive system organ or structure following a digestive system procedure
Coding Clinic: 2016, Q1, P15

K91.841 Postprocedural hemorrhage of a digestive system organ or structure following other procedure 🅒

● **K91.85 Complications of intestinal pouch**

K91.850 Pouchitis 🅒
Inflammation of internal ileoanal pouch

K91.858 Other complications of intestinal pouch 🅒

K91.86 Retained cholelithiasis following cholecystectomy 🅒

● **K91.87** **Postprocedural hematoma and seroma of a digestive system organic or structure following a procedure**
Ex) **For category K97.87 CC codes:** See PDX Collection 829

    K91.870 **Postprocedural hematoma of a digestive system organ or structure following a digestive system procedure** 🔑

    K91.871 **Postprocedural hematoma of a digestive system organ or structure following other procedure** 🔑

    K91.872 **Postprocedural seroma of a digestive system organ or structure following a digestive system procedure** 🔑

    K91.873 **Postprocedural seroma of a digestive system organ or structure following other procedure** 🔑

    K91.89 **Other postprocedural complications and disorders of digestive system** 🔑
      Use additional code, if applicable, to further specify disorder
      Excludes2   postprocedural retroperitoneal abscess (K68.11)
      Ex) See PDX Collection 828
      Coding Clinic: 2017, Q1, P41

● **K92** **Other diseases of digestive system**
    Excludes1   neonatal gastrointestinal hemorrhage (P54.0-P54.3)
    Ex) **For category K92 CC codes unless otherwise indicated:** See PDX Collection 770

    K92.0 **Hematemesis** 🔑
    K92.1 **Melena** 🔑
      Excludes1   occult blood in feces (R19.5)
    K92.2 **Gastrointestinal hemorrhage, unspecified** 🔑
      Gastric hemorrhage NOS
      Intestinal hemorrhage NOS
      Excludes1   acute hemorrhagic gastritis (K29.01)
           hemorrhage of anus and rectum (K62.5)
           angiodysplasia of stomach with hemorrhage (K31.811)
           diverticular disease with hemorrhage (K57.-)
           gastritis and duodenitis with hemorrhage (K29.-)
           peptic ulcer with hemorrhage (K25-K28)

● **K92.8** **Other specified diseases of the digestive system**
    K92.81 **Gastrointestinal mucositis (ulcerative)** 🔑
      Code also type of associated therapy, such as:
        antineoplastic and immunosuppressive drugs (T45.1X-)
        radiological procedure and radiotherapy (Y84.2)
      Excludes2   mucositis (ulcerative) of vagina and vulva (N76.81)
           nasal mucositis (ulcerative) (J34.81)
           oral mucositis (ulcerative) (K12.3-)
      Ex) See PDX Collection 765

    K92.89 **Other specified diseases of the digestive system**
    K92.9 **Disease of digestive system, unspecified**

● **K94** **Complications of artificial openings of the digestive system**
  ● **K94.0** **Colostomy complications**
    Ex) **For category K94.0 CC does unless otherwise indicated:** See PDX Collection 830

    K94.00 **Colostomy complication, unspecified**
    K94.01 **Colostomy hemorrhage** 🔑
    K94.02 **Colostomy infection** 🔑
      Use additional code to specify type of infection, such as:
        cellulitis of abdominal wall (L03.311)
        sepsis (A40.-, A41.-)

    K94.03 **Colostomy malfunction** 🔑
      Mechanical complication of colostomy
      Ex) See PDX Collection 831

    K94.09 **Other complications of colostomy** 🔑

  ● **K94.1** **Enterostomy complications**
    Ex) **For category K94.1 CC does unless otherwise indicated:** See PDX Collection 830

    K94.10 **Enterostomy complication, unspecified**
    K94.11 **Enterostomy hemorrhage** 🔑
    K94.12 **Enterostomy infection** 🔑
      Use additional code to specify type of infection, such as:
        cellulitis of abdominal wall (L03.311)
        sepsis (A40.-, A41.-)

    K94.13 **Enterostomy malfunction** 🔑
      Mechanical complication of enterostomy
      Ex) See PDX Collection 831

    K94.19 **Other complications of enterostomy** 🔑

  ● **K94.2** **Gastrostomy complications**
    K94.20 **Gastrostomy complication, unspecified**
    K94.21 **Gastrostomy hemorrhage** 🔑
    K94.22 **Gastrostomy infection** 🔑
      Use additional code to specify type of infection, such as:
        cellulitis of abdominal wall (L03.311)
        sepsis (A40.-, A41.-)
      Ex) See PDX Collection 828

    K94.23 **Gastrostomy malfunction** 🔑
      Mechanical complication of gastrostomy
      Ex) See PDX Collection 828

    K94.29 **Other complications of gastrostomy** 🔑

  ● **K94.3** **Esophagostomy complications**
    Ex) **For category K94.3 CC codes:** See PDX Collection 828

    K94.30 **Esophagostomy complications, unspecified** 🔑
    K94.31 **Esophagostomy hemorrhage** 🔑
    K94.32 **Esophagostomy infection** 🔑
      Use additional code to identify the infection

    K94.33 **Esophagostomy malfunction** 🔑
      Mechanical complication of esophagostomy

    K94.39 **Other complications of esophagostomy** 🔑

● **K95** **Complications of bariatric procedures**
  Ex) **For category K95 CC codes:** See PDX Collection 828

  ● **K95.0** **Complications of gastric band procedure**
    K95.01 **Infection due to gastric band procedure** 🔑 🔑
      Use additional code to specify type of infection or organism, such as:
        bacterial and viral infectious agents (B95.-, B96.-)
        cellulitis of abdominal wall (L03.311)
        sepsis (A40.-, A41.-)

    K95.09 **Other complications of gastric band procedure** 🔑
      Use additional code, if applicable, to further specify complication

  ● **K95.8** **Complications of other bariatric procedure**
    Excludes1   complications of gastric band surgery (K95.0-)

    K95.81 **Infection due to other bariatric procedure** 🔑 🔑
      Use additional code to specify type of infection or organism, such as:
        bacterial and viral infectious agents (B95.-, B96.-)
        cellulitis of abdominal wall (L03.311)
        sepsis (A40.-, A41.-)

    K95.89 **Other complications of other bariatric procedure** 🔑
      Use additional code, if applicable, to further specify complication

▶ New   ⇒ Revised   ~~deleted~~ Deleted   Excludes 1   Excludes 2   Includes   Use additional   Code first   Code also   Key words
OGCR Official Guidelines   ● Unacceptable Principal Diagnosis   X Assign placeholder X   ● Use Additional Character(s)   ▌ Manifestation Code   **Coding Clinic**

CHAPTER 12

DISEASES OF THE SKIN AND SUBCUTANEOUS TISSUE (L00-L99)

OGCR Chapter-Specific Coding Guidelines

12. **Chapter 12: Diseases of the Skin and Subcutaneous Tissue (L00-L99)**

a. **Pressure ulcer stage codes**

1) **Pressure ulcer stages**

Codes from category L89, Pressure ulcer, identify the site of the pressure ulcer as well as the stage of the ulcer.

The ICD-10-CM classifies pressure ulcer stages based on severity, which is designated by stages 1-4, unspecified stage and unstageable.

Assign as many codes from category L89 as needed to identify all the pressure ulcers the patient has, if applicable.

2) **Unstageable pressure ulcers**

Assignment of the code for unstageable pressure ulcer (L89.--0) should be based on the clinical documentation. These codes are used for pressure ulcers whose stage cannot be clinically determined (e.g., the ulcer is covered by eschar or has been treated with a skin or muscle graft) and pressure ulcers that are documented as deep tissue injury but not documented as due to trauma. This code should not be confused with the codes for unspecified stage (L89.--9). When there is no documentation regarding the stage of the pressure ulcer, assign the appropriate code for unspecified stage (L89.--9).

3) **Documented pressure ulcer stage**

Assignment of the pressure ulcer stage code should be guided by clinical documentation of the stage or documentation of the terms found in the Alphabetic Index. For clinical terms describing the stage that are not found in the Alphabetic Index, and there is no documentation of the stage, the provider should be queried.

4) **Patients admitted with pressure ulcers documented as healed**

No code is assigned if the documentation states that the pressure ulcer is completely healed.

5) **Patients admitted with pressure ulcers documented as healing**

Pressure ulcers described as healing should be assigned the appropriate pressure ulcer stage code based on the documentation in the medical record. If the documentation does not provide information about the stage of the healing pressure ulcer, assign the appropriate code for unspecified stage.

If the documentation is unclear as to whether the patient has a current (new) pressure ulcer or if the patient is being treated for a healing pressure ulcer, query the provider.

For ulcers that were present on admission but healed at the time of discharge, assign the code for the site and stage of the pressure ulcer at the time of admission.

6) **Patient admitted with pressure ulcer evolving into another stage during the admission**

If a patient is admitted to an inpatient hospital with a pressure ulcer at one stage and it progresses to a higher stage, two separate codes should be assigned: one code for the site and stage of the ulcer on admission and a second code for the same ulcer site and the highest stage reported during the stay.

b. **Non-Pressure Chronic Ulcers**

1) **Patients admitted with non-pressure ulcers documented as healed**

No code is assigned if the documentation states that the non-pressure ulcer is completely healed.

2) **Patients admitted with non-pressure ulcers documented as healing**

Non-pressure ulcers described as healing should be assigned the appropriate non-pressure ulcer code based on the documentation in the medical record. If the documentation does not provide information about the severity of the healing non-pressure ulcer, assign the appropriate code for unspecified severity.

If the documentation is unclear as to whether the patient has a current (new) non-pressure ulcer or if the patient is being treated for a healing non-pressure ulcer, query the provider.

For ulcers that were present on admission but healed at the time of discharge, assign the code for the site and severity of the non-pressure ulcer at the time of admission.

3) **Patient admitted with non-pressure ulcer that progresses to another severity level during the admission**

If a patient is admitted to an inpatient hospital with a non-pressure ulcer at one severity level and it progresses to a higher severity level, two separate codes should be assigned: one code for the site and severity level of the ulcer on admission and a second code for the same ulcer site and the highest severity level reported during the stay.

Figure 12-1 Furuncle, also known as a boil, is a staphylococcal infection. The organism enters the body through a hair follicle and so furuncles usually appear in hairy areas of the body. A cluster of furuncles is known as a carbuncle and involves infection into the deep subcutaneous fascia. These usually appear on the back and neck. (**B** from Habif TP, Binnick AN, Meyerson LB: Clinical Dermatology: A Color Guide to Diagnosis and Therapy, S.l., Mosby Elsevier, 2010)

CHAPTER 12

DISEASES OF THE SKIN AND SUBCUTANEOUS TISSUE (L00-L99)

Excludes2   certain conditions originating in the perinatal period (P04-P96)
certain infectious and parasitic diseases (A00-B99)
complications of pregnancy, childbirth and the puerperium (O00-O9A)
congenital malformations, deformations, and chromosomal abnormalities (Q00-Q99)
endocrine, nutritional and metabolic diseases (E00-E88)
lipomelanotic reticulosis (I89.8)
neoplasms (C00-D49)
symptoms, signs and abnormal clinical and laboratory findings, not elsewhere classified (R00-R94)
systemic connective tissue disorders (M30-M36)
viral warts (B07.-)

This chapter contains the following blocks:

L00-L08	Infections of the skin and subcutaneous tissue
L10-L14	Bullous disorders
L20-L30	Dermatitis and eczema
L40-L45	Papulosquamous disorders
L49-L54	Urticaria and erythema
L55-L59	Radiation-related disorders of the skin and subcutaneous tissue
L60-L75	Disorders of skin appendages
L76	Intraoperative and postprocedural complications of skin and subcutaneous tissue
L80-L99	Other disorders of the skin and subcutaneous tissue

CHAPTER 12 (L00-L99)

INFECTIONS OF THE SKIN AND SUBCUTANEOUS TISSUE (L00-L08)

Use additional code (B95-B97) to identify infectious agent.

Excludes2   hordeolum (H00.0)
infective dermatitis (L30.3)
local infections of skin classified in Chapter 1
lupus panniculitis (L93.2)
panniculitis NOS (M79.3)
panniculitis of neck and back (M54.0-)
Perlèche NOS (K13.0)
Perlèche due to candidiasis (B37.0)
Perlèche due to riboflavin deficiency (E53.0)
pyogenic granuloma (L98.0)
relapsing panniculitis [Weber-Christian] (M35.6)
viral warts (B07.-)
zoster (B02.-)

L00   Staphylococcal scalded skin syndrome
Ritter's disease

Use additional code to identify percentage of skin exfoliation (L49.-)

Excludes1   bullous impetigo (L01.03)
pemphigus neonatorum (L01.03)
toxic epidermal necrolysis [Lyell] (L51.2)

● **L01   Impetigo**
Contagious skin infection caused by a streptococcus or staphylococcus aureus, common skin infections among children

Excludes1   impetigo herpetiformis (L40.1)

● **L01.0   Impetigo**
Impetigo contagiosa
Impetigo vulgaris

L01.00   Impetigo, unspecified
Impetigo NOS

L01.01   Non-bullous impetigo

L01.02   Bockhart's impetigo
Impetigo follicularis
Perifolliculitis NOS
Superficial pustular perifolliculitis

L01.03   Bullous impetigo
Impetigo neonatorum
Pemphigus neonatorum
Neonate = newborn

L01.09   Other impetigo
Ulcerative impetigo

L01.1   Impetiginization of other dermatoses

● **L02   Cutaneous abscess, furuncle and carbuncle**
Use additional code to identify organism (B95-B96)

Excludes2   abscess of anus and rectal regions (K61.-)
abscess of female genital organs (external) (N76.4)
abscess of male genital organs (external) (N48.2, N49.-)

● **L02.0   Cutaneous abscess, furuncle and carbuncle of face**

Excludes2   abscess of ear, external (H60.0)
abscess of eyelid (H00.0)
abscess of head [any part, except face] (L02.8)
abscess of lacrimal gland (H04.0)
abscess of lacrimal passages (H04.3)
abscess of mouth (K12.2)
abscess of nose (J34.0)
abscess of orbit (H05.0)
submandibular abscess (K12.2)

L02.01   Cutaneous abscess of face 🔎
(Ex:) No exclusions

L02.02   Furuncle of face
Boil of face
Folliculitis of face

L02.03   Carbuncle of face

● **L02.1   Cutaneous abscess, furuncle and carbuncle of neck**

L02.11   Cutaneous abscess of neck 🔎
(Ex:) See PDX Collection 832

L02.12   Furuncle of neck
Boil of neck
Folliculitis of neck

L02.13   Carbuncle of neck

● **L02.2   Cutaneous abscess, furuncle and carbuncle of trunk**

Excludes1   non-newborn omphalitis (L08.82)
omphalitis of newborn (P38.-)

Excludes2   abscess of breast (N61.1)
abscess of buttocks (L02.3)
abscess of female external genital organs (N76.4)
abscess of male external genital organs (N48.2, N49.-)
abscess of hip (L02.4)

● **L02.21   Cutaneous abscess of trunk**
(Ex:) For category L02.21 CC codes: See PDX Collection 833

L02.211   Cutaneous abscess of abdominal wall 🔎

L02.212   Cutaneous abscess of back [any part, except buttock] 🔎

L02.213   Cutaneous abscess of chest wall 🔎

L02.214   Cutaneous abscess of groin 🔎

L02.215   Cutaneous abscess of perineum 🔎

L02.216   Cutaneous abscess of umbilicus 🔎

L02.219   Cutaneous abscess of trunk, unspecified 🔎

● **L02.22   Furuncle of trunk**
Boil of trunk
Folliculitis of trunk

L02.221   Furuncle of abdominal wall

L02.222   Furuncle of back [any part, except buttock]

L02.223   Furuncle of chest wall

L02.224   Furuncle of groin

L02.225   Furuncle of perineum

L02.226   Furuncle of umbilicus

L02.229   Furuncle of trunk, unspecified

● **L02.23   Carbuncle of trunk**

L02.231   Carbuncle of abdominal wall

L02.232   Carbuncle of back [any part, except buttock]

L02.233   Carbuncle of chest wall

L02.234   Carbuncle of groin

L02.235   Carbuncle of perineum

L02.236   Carbuncle of umbilicus

L02.239   Carbuncle of trunk, unspecified

● **L02.3   Cutaneous abscess, furuncle and carbuncle of buttock**

Excludes1   pilonidal cyst with abscess (L05.01)

L02.31   Cutaneous abscess of buttock 🔎
Cutaneous abscess of gluteal region
(Ex:) See PDX Collection 834

L02.32   Furuncle of buttock
Boil of buttock
Folliculitis of buttock
Furuncle of gluteal region

L02.33   Carbuncle of buttock
Carbuncle of gluteal region

Figure 12-2 Impetigo. A thick, honey-yellow adherent crust covers the entire eroded surface. (From James WD, Elston DM, Berger TG, Andrews GC: Andrews' Diseases of the Skin: Clinical Dermatology, London, Saunders/Elsevier, 2011)

▶ New   ⇒ Revised   ~~deleted~~ Deleted   Excludes 1   Excludes 2   Includes   Use additional   Code first   Code also   Key words

OGCR Official Guidelines   ● Unacceptable Principal Diagnosis   X Assign placeholder X   ▶ Use Additional Character(s)   ▷ Manifestation Code   **Coding Clinic**

L02.4 Cutaneous abscess, furuncle and carbuncle of limb

    Excludes2 Cutaneous abscess, furuncle and carbuncle of groin (L02.214, L02.224, L02.234)

               Cutaneous abscess, furuncle and carbuncle of hand (L02.5-)

               Cutaneous abscess, furuncle and carbuncle of foot (L02.6-)

  L02.41 Cutaneous abscess of limb

    L02.411 Cutaneous abscess of **right axilla**
        Ex: See PDX Collection 835

    L02.412 Cutaneous abscess of **left axilla**
        Ex: See PDX Collection 835

    L02.413 Cutaneous abscess of **right upper limb**
        Ex: See PDX Collection 835

    L02.414 Cutaneous abscess of **left upper limb**
        Ex: See PDX Collection 835

    L02.415 Cutaneous abscess of **right lower limb**
        Ex: See PDX Collection 836

    L02.416 Cutaneous abscess of **left lower limb**
        Ex: See PDX Collection 836

    L02.419 Cutaneous abscess of limb, **unspecified**
        Ex: See PDX Collection 836

  L02.42 Furuncle of limb
    Boil of limb
    Folliculitis of limb

    L02.421 Furuncle of **right axilla**
    L02.422 Furuncle of **left axilla**
    L02.423 Furuncle of **right upper limb**
    L02.424 Furuncle of **left upper limb**
    L02.425 Furuncle of **right lower limb**
    L02.426 Furuncle of **left lower limb**
    L02.429 Furuncle of limb, **unspecified**

  L02.43 Carbuncle of limb
    L02.431 Carbuncle of **right axilla**
    L02.432 Carbuncle of **left axilla**
    L02.433 Carbuncle of **right upper limb**
    L02.434 Carbuncle of **left upper limb**
    L02.435 Carbuncle of **right lower limb**
    L02.436 Carbuncle of **left lower limb**
    L02.439 Carbuncle of limb, **unspecified**

L02.5 Cutaneous abscess, furuncle and carbuncle of hand

  L02.51 Cutaneous abscess of hand
    Ex: For category L02.51 CC codes: See PDX Collection 837

    L02.511 Cutaneous abscess of **right hand**
    L02.512 Cutaneous abscess of **left hand**
    L02.519 Cutaneous abscess of **unspecified hand**

  L02.52 Furuncle hand
    Boil of hand
    Folliculitis of hand

    L02.521 Furuncle **right hand**
    L02.522 Furuncle **left hand**
    L02.529 Furuncle **unspecified hand**

  L02.53 Carbuncle of hand
    L02.531 Carbuncle of **right hand**
    L02.532 Carbuncle of **left hand**
    L02.539 Carbuncle of **unspecified hand**

L02.6 Cutaneous abscess, furuncle and carbuncle of foot

  L02.61 Cutaneous abscess of foot
    Ex: For category L02.61 CC codes: See PDX Collection 838

    L02.611 Cutaneous abscess of **right foot**
    L02.612 Cutaneous abscess of **left foot**
    L02.619 Cutaneous abscess of **unspecified foot**

  L02.62 Furuncle of foot
    Boil of foot
    Folliculitis of foot

    L02.621 Furuncle of **right foot**
    L02.622 Furuncle of **left foot**
    L02.629 Furuncle of **unspecified foot**

  L02.63 Carbuncle of foot
    L02.631 Carbuncle of **right foot**
    L02.632 Carbuncle of **left foot**
    L02.639 Carbuncle of **unspecified foot**

L02.8 Cutaneous abscess, furuncle and carbuncle of other sites

  L02.81 Cutaneous abscess of other sites
    Ex: For category L02.81 CC codes: See PDX Collection 839

    L02.811 Cutaneous abscess of **head [any part, except face]**
    L02.818 Cutaneous abscess of **other sites**

  L02.82 Furuncle of other sites
    Boil of other sites
    Folliculitis of other sites

    L02.821 Furuncle of **head [any part, except face]**
    L02.828 Furuncle of **other sites**

  L02.83 Carbuncle of other sites
    L02.831 Carbuncle of **head [any part, except face]**
    L02.838 Carbuncle of **other sites**

L02.9 Cutaneous abscess, furuncle and carbuncle, unspecified

  L02.91 Cutaneous abscess, **unspecified**
    Ex: See PDX Collection 839

  L02.92 Furuncle, unspecified
    Boil NOS
    Furunculosis NOS

  L02.93 **Carbuncle, unspecified**

L03 Cellulitis and acute lymphangitis

  Excludes2 cellulitis of anal and rectal region (K61.-)
        cellulitis of external auditory canal (H60.1)
        cellulitis of eyelid (H00.0)
        cellulitis of external genital organs (N76.4)
        cellulitis of lacrimal apparatus (H04.3)
        cellulitis of male external genital organs (N48.2, N49.-)
        cellulitis of mouth (K12.2)
        cellulitis of nose (J34.0)
        eosinophilic cellulitis [Wells] (L98.3)
        febrile neutrophilic dermatosis [Sweet] (L98.2)
        lymphangitis (chronic) (subacute) (I89.1)

L03.0 Cellulitis and acute lymphangitis of finger and toe
    Infection of nail
    Onychia
    Paronychia
    Perionychia

  L03.01 Cellulitis of finger
    Felon
    Whitlow

    Excludes1 herpetic whitlow (B00.89)

    L03.011 Cellulitis of **right finger**
    L03.012 Cellulitis of **left finger**
    L03.019 Cellulitis of **unspecified finger**

Item 12-1 Onychia is an inflammation of the tissue surrounding the nail with pus accumulation and loss of the nail, resulting from microscopic pathogens entering through small wounds. **Paronychia** is a nail disease also known as felon or whitlow and is a bacterial or fungal infection.

CHAPTER 12 (L00–L99)

  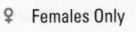

● L03.02   **Acute lymphangitis of finger**
        Hangnail with lymphangitis of finger

L03.021   Acute lymphangitis of **right finger**

L03.022   Acute lymphangitis of **left finger**

L03.029   Acute lymphangitis of **unspecified finger**

● L03.03   **Cellulitis of toe**

L03.031   Cellulitis of **right** toe

L03.032   Cellulitis of **left** toe

L03.039   Cellulitis of **unspecified** toe

● L03.04   **Acute lymphangitis of toe**
        Hangnail with lymphangitis of toe

L03.041   Acute lymphangitis of **right toe**

L03.042   Acute lymphangitis of **left toe**

L03.049   Acute lymphangitis of **unspecified toe**

● L03.1   Cellulitis and acute lymphangitis of **other parts of limb**

● L03.11   **Cellulitis of other parts of limb**

    Excludes2 cellulitis of fingers (L03.01-)
                   cellulitis of toes (L03.03-)
                   groin (L03.314)

L03.111   **Cellulitis of right axilla** 🔖
      (Ex:) See PDX Collection 835

L03.112   **Cellulitis of left axilla** 🔖
      (Ex:) See PDX Collection 835

L03.113   **Cellulitis of right upper limb** 🔖
      (Ex:) See PDX Collection 835

L03.114   **Cellulitis of left upper limb** 🔖
      (Ex:) See PDX Collection 835

L03.115   **Cellulitis of right lower limb** 🔖
      (Ex:) See PDX Collection 836

L03.116   **Cellulitis of left lower limb** 🔖
      (Ex:) See PDX Collection 836

L03.119   **Cellulitis of unspecified part of limb** 🔖
      (Ex:) See PDX Collection 836

● L03.12   **Acute lymphangitis of other parts of limb**

    Excludes2 acute lymphangitis of fingers (L03.2-)
                   acute lymphangitis of toes (L03.04-)
                   acute lymphangitis of groin (L03.324)

L03.121   **Acute lymphangitis of right axilla** 🔖
      (Ex:) See PDX Collection 835

L03.122   **Acute lymphangitis of left axilla** 🔖
      (Ex:) See PDX Collection 835

L03.123   **Acute lymphangitis of right upper limb** 🔖
      (Ex:) See PDX Collection 835

L03.124   **Acute lymphangitis of left upper limb** 🔖
      (Ex:) See PDX Collection 835

L03.125   **Acute lymphangitis of right lower limb** 🔖
      (Ex:) See PDX Collection 836

L03.126   **Acute lymphangitis of left lower limb** 🔖
      (Ex:) See PDX Collection 836

L03.129   **Acute lymphangitis of unspecified part of limb** 🔖
      (Ex:) See PDX Collection 836

Item 12–2   Cellulitis is an acute spreading bacterial infection below the surface of the skin characterized by redness (erythema), warmth, swelling, pain, fever, chills, and enlarged lymph nodes ("swollen glands").

● L03.2   Cellulitis and acute lymphangitis of **face and neck**

● L03.21   Cellulitis and acute lymphangitis of **face**

L03.211   **Cellulitis of face** 🔖

    Excludes2 abscess of orbit (H05.01-)
                   cellulitis of ear (H60.1-)
                   cellulitis of eyelid (H00.0-)
                   cellulitis of head (L03.81)
                   cellulitis of lacrimal apparatus (H04.3)
                   cellulitis of lip (K13.0)
                   cellulitis of mouth (K12.2)
                   cellulitis of nose (internal) (J34.0)
                   cellulitis of orbit (H05.01-)
                   cellulitis of scalp (L03.81)

    (Ex:) See PDX Collection 840

L03.212   **Acute lymphangitis of face** 🔖
      (Ex:) No exclusions

L03.213   **Periorbital cellulitis** 🔖
      Preseptal cellulitis
      (Ex:) See PDX Collection 840
      Coding Clinic: 2016, Q4, P36

● L03.22   Cellulitis and acute lymphangitis of **neck**
    (Ex:) For category L03.22 CC codes: See PDX Collection 832

L03.221   **Cellulitis of neck** 🔖

L03.222   **Acute lymphangitis of neck** 🔖

● L03.3   Cellulitis and acute lymphangitis of **trunk**

● L03.31   **Cellulitis of trunk**

    Excludes2 cellulitis of anal and rectal regions (K61.-)
                   cellulitis of breast NOS (N61.0)
                   cellulitis of female external genital organs (N76.4)
                   cellulitis of male external genital organs (N48.2, N49.-)
                   omphalitis of newborn (P38.-)
                   puerperal cellulitis of breast (O91.2)

    (Ex:) For category L03.31 CC codes unless otherwise indicated: See PDX Collection 833

L03.311   **Cellulitis of abdominal wall** 🔖

    Excludes2 cellulitis of umbilicus (L03.316)
                   cellulitis of groin (L03.314)

L03.312   **Cellulitis of back [any part except buttock]** 🔖

L03.313   **Cellulitis of chest wall** 🔖

L03.314   **Cellulitis of groin** 🔖

L03.315   **Cellulitis of perineum** 🔖

L03.316   **Cellulitis of umbilicus** 🔖

L03.317   **Cellulitis of buttock** 🔖
      (Ex:) See PDX Collection 834

L03.319   **Cellulitis of trunk, unspecified** 🔖

● **L03.32 Acute lymphangitis of trunk**
     (Ex) For category L03.32 CC codes unless otherwise indicated: See PDX Collection 833

     L03.321 Acute lymphangitis of abdominal wall 🔹

     L03.322 Acute lymphangitis of back [any part except buttock] 🔹

     L03.323 Acute lymphangitis of chest wall 🔹

     L03.324 Acute lymphangitis of groin 🔹

     L03.325 Acute lymphangitis of perineum 🔹

     L03.326 Acute lymphangitis of umbilicus 🔹

     L03.327 Acute lymphangitis of buttock 🔹
        (Ex) See PDX Collection 834

     L03.329 Acute lymphangitis of trunk, unspecified 🔹

● **L03.8 Cellulitis and acute lymphangitis of other sites**
     (Ex) For category L03.8 CC codes: See PDX Collection 839

  ● **L03.81 Cellulitis of other sites**

     L03.811 Cellulitis of head [any part, except face] 🔹
        Cellulitis of scalp
        Excludes2 cellulitis of face (L03.211)

     L03.818 Cellulitis of other sites 🔹

  ● **L03.89 Acute lymphangitis of other sites**

     L03.891 Acute lymphangitis of head [any part, except face] 🔹

     L03.898 Acute lymphangitis of other sites 🔹

● **L03.9 Cellulitis and acute lymphangitis, unspecified**
     (Ex) For category L03.9 CC codes: See PDX Collection 839

     L03.90 Cellulitis, unspecified 🔹

     L03.91 Acute lymphangitis, unspecified 🔹
        Excludes1 lymphangitis NOS (I89.1)

● **L04 Acute lymphadenitis**
     Short-term inflammation of lymph nodes which can be regionalized to involve a given area of the lymph system or systemic involving much of the body

     Includes abscess (acute) of lymph nodes, except mesenteric
        acute lymphadenitis, except mesenteric

     Excludes1 chronic or subacute lymphadenitis, except mesenteric (I88.1)
        enlarged lymph nodes (R59.-)
        human immunodeficiency virus [HIV] disease resulting in generalized lymphadenopathy (B20)
        lymphadenitis NOS (I88.9)
        nonspecific mesenteric lymphadenitis (I88.0)

     L04.0 Acute lymphadenitis of face, head and neck

     L04.1 Acute lymphadenitis of trunk

     L04.2 Acute lymphadenitis of upper limb
        Acute lymphadenitis of axilla
        Acute lymphadenitis of shoulder

     L04.3 Acute lymphadenitis of lower limb
        Acute lymphadenitis of hip
        Excludes2 acute lymphadenitis of groin (L04.1)

     L04.8 Acute lymphadenitis of other sites

     L04.9 Acute lymphadenitis, unspecified

Item 12-3 Abscess is a localized collection of pus in tissues or organs and is a sign of infection resulting in swelling and inflammation.

Item 12-4 Pilonidal cyst, also called a coccygeal cyst, is the result of a disorder called pilonidal disease. The cyst usually contains hair and pus.

● **L05 Pilonidal cyst and sinus**

  ● **L05.0 Pilonidal cyst and sinus with abscess**
     (Ex) For category L05.0 CC codes: See PDX Collection 841

     L05.01 Pilonidal cyst with abscess 🔹
        Pilonidal abscess
        Pilonidal dimple with abscess
        Postanal dimple with abscess
        Excludes2 congenital sacral dimple (Q82.6)
           parasacral dimple (Q82.6)

     L05.02 Pilonidal sinus with abscess 🔹
        Coccygeal fistula with abscess
        Coccygeal sinus with abscess
        Pilonidal fistula with abscess

  ● **L05.9 Pilonidal cyst and sinus without abscess**

     L05.91 Pilonidal cyst without abscess
        Pilonidal dimple
        Postanal dimple
        Pilonidal cyst NOS
        Excludes2 congenital sacral dimple (Q82.6)
           parasacral dimple (Q82.6)

     L05.92 Pilonidal sinus without abscess
        Coccygeal fistula
        Coccygeal sinus without abscess
        Pilonidal fistula

● **L08 Other local infections of skin and subcutaneous tissue**

     L08.0 Pyoderma
        Dermatitis gangrenosa
        Purulent dermatitis
        Septic dermatitis
        Suppurative dermatitis
        Excludes1 pyoderma gangrenosum (L88)
           pyoderma vegetans (L08.81)

     L08.1 Erythrasma 🔹
        (Ex) See PDX Collection 107

  ● **L08.8 Other specified local infections of the skin and subcutaneous tissue**

     L08.81 Pyoderma vegetans
        Excludes1 pyoderma gangrenosum (L88)
           pyoderma NOS (L08.0)

     L08.82 Omphalitis not of newborn
        Excludes1 omphalitis of newborn (P38.-)

     L08.89 Other specified local infections of the skin and subcutaneous tissue

     L08.9 Local infection of the skin and subcutaneous tissue, unspecified

---

N   Newborn Age: 0   P   Pediatric Age: 0–17   M   Maternity DX: 12–55   A   Adult Age: 15–124   ♀   Females Only   ♂   Males Only

🔹 Complication\Comorbidity   🔹 Major C\C   (Ex) CC/MCC Exclusions   🔹 Hospital-Acquired Condition

BULLOUS DISORDERS (L10-L14)

Excludes1   benign familial pemphigus [Hailey-Hailey] (Q82.8)
staphylococcal scalded skin syndrome (L00)
toxic epidermal necrolysis [Lyell] (L51.2)

● **L10**   **Pemphigus**

     Excludes1   pemphigus neonatorum (L01.03)

     (Ex) For category L10 CC codes: See PDX Collection 842

     L10.0   **Pemphigus vulgaris** ✎

     L10.1   **Pemphigus vegetans** ✎

     L10.2   **Pemphigus foliaceous** ✎

     L10.3   **Brazilian pemphigus [fogo selvagem]** ✎

     L10.4   **Pemphigus erythematosus** ✎
              Senear-Usher syndrome

     L10.5   **Drug-induced pemphigus** ✎

              Use additional code for adverse effect, if applicable, to identify drug (T36-T50 with fifth or sixth character 5)

     ● **L10.8**   **Other pemphigus**
              L10.81   **Paraneoplastic pemphigus** ✎
              L10.89   **Other pemphigus** ✎

     L10.9   **Pemphigus, unspecified** ✎

● **L11**   **Other acantholytic disorders**

     L11.0   **Acquired keratosis follicularis**

         Excludes1   keratosis follicularis (congenital) [Darier-White] (Q82.8)

     L11.1   **Transient acantholytic dermatosis [Grover]**

     L11.8   **Other specified acantholytic disorders**

     L11.9   **Acantholytic disorder, unspecified**

● **L12**   **Pemphigoid**

     Excludes1   herpes gestationis (O26.4-)
              impetigo herpetiformis (L40.1)

     L12.0   **Bullous pemphigoid** ✎
              (Ex) See PDX Collection 842

     L12.1   **Cicatricial pemphigoid**
              Benign mucous membrane pemphigoid

     L12.2   **Chronic bullous disease of childhood**   P
              Juvenile dermatitis herpetiformis

     ● **L12.3**   **Acquired epidermolysis bullosa**

         Excludes1   epidermolysis bullosa (congenital) (Q81.-)

         (Ex) For category L12.3 CC codes: See PDX Collection 843

         L12.30   **Acquired epidermolysis bullosa, unspecified** ✎

         L12.31   **Epidermolysis bullosa due to drug** ✎

              Use additional code for adverse effect, if applicable, to identify drug (T36-T50 with fifth or sixth character 5)

         L12.35   **Other acquired epidermolysis bullosa** ✎

     L12.8   **Other pemphigoid** ✎
              (Ex) See PDX Collection 842

     L12.9   **Pemphigoid, unspecified** ✎
              (Ex) See PDX Collection 842

Item 12-5   **Dermatitis herpetiformis,** also known as Duhring's disease, is a systemic disease characterized by small blisters (3 to 5 mm) and occasionally large bullae (> 5 mm).

Figure 12-3   Dermatitis herpetiformis. (From Terhorst D: BASICS Dermatologie, München, Elsevier, Urban & Fischer, 2011)

● **L13**   **Other bullous disorders**

     L13.0   **Dermatitis herpetiformis**
              Duhring's disease
              Hydroa herpetiformis

         Excludes1   juvenile dermatitis herpetiformis (L12.2)
                     senile dermatitis herpetiformis (L12.0)

     L13.1   **Subcorneal pustular dermatitis**
              Sneddon-Wilkinson disease

     L13.8   **Other specified bullous disorders**

     L13.9   **Bullous disorder, unspecified**

▷ **L14**   *Bullous disorders in diseases classified elsewhere*
         Code first underlying disease

DERMATITIS AND ECZEMA (L20-L30)

Note: In this block the terms dermatitis and eczema are used synonymously and interchangeably.

     Excludes2   chronic (childhood) granulomatous disease (D71)
                 dermatitis gangrenosa (L08.0)
                 dermatitis herpetiformis (L13.0)
                 dry skin dermatitis (L85.3)
                 factitial dermatitis (L98.1)
                 perioral dermatitis (L71.0)
                 radiation-related disorders of the skin and subcutaneous tissue (L55-L59)
                 stasis dermatitis (I87.2)

● **L20**   **Atopic dermatitis**

     L20.0   **Besnier's prurigo**

     ● **L20.8**   **Other atopic dermatitis**

         Excludes2   circumscribed neurodermatitis (L28.0)

         L20.81   **Atopic neurodermatitis**
              Diffuse neurodermatitis

         L20.82   **Flexural eczema**

         L20.83   **Infantile (acute) (chronic) eczema**   P

         L20.84   **Intrinsic (allergic) eczema**

         L20.89   **Other atopic dermatitis**

     L20.9   **Atopic dermatitis, unspecified**

● **L21**   **Seborrheic dermatitis**

     Excludes2   infective dermatitis (L30.3)
                 seborrheic keratosis (L82.-)

     L21.0   **Seborrhea capitis**
              Cradle cap

     L21.1   **Seborrheic infantile dermatitis**   P

     L21.8   **Other seborrheic dermatitis**

     L21.9   **Seborrheic dermatitis, unspecified**
              Seborrhea NOS

Item 12-6   **Seborrheic dermatitis** is characterized by greasy, scaly, red patches and is associated with oily skin and scalp.

Figure 12-4   Seborrheic dermatitis. (Getty Image)

▶ New   ⟹ Revised   ~~deleted~~ Deleted   Excludes 1   Excludes 2   Includes   Use additional   Code first   Code also   Key words

OGCR Official Guidelines   ● Unacceptable Principal Diagnosis   X Assign placeholder X   ● Use Additional Character(s)   ▷ Manifestation Code   **Coding Clinic**

Item 12–7 Atopic dermatitis, also known as atopic eczema, infantile eczema, disseminated neuro dermatitis, flexural eczema, and *prurigo diathesique* (Besnier), is characterized by intense itching and is often hereditary.

Figure 12-5 Atopic dermatitis. (From Chabner D-E: The Language of Medicine, St. Louis, MO, Saunders/Elsevier, 2007)

L22 Diaper dermatitis
    Diaper erythema
    Diaper rash
    Psoriasiform diaper rash

● **L23 Allergic contact dermatitis**
    Excludes1 allergy NOS (T78.40)
                  contact dermatitis NOS (L25.9)
                  dermatitis NOS (L30.9)

    Excludes2 dermatitis due to substances taken internally
                   (L27.-)
                  dermatitis of eyelid (H01.1-)
                  diaper dermatitis (L22)
                  eczema of external ear (H60.5-)
                  irritant contact dermatitis (L24.-)
                  perioral dermatitis (L71.0)
                  radiation-related disorders of the skin and
                    subcutaneous tissue (L55-L59)

  L23.0 **Allergic contact dermatitis due to metals**
        Allergic contact dermatitis due to chromium
        Allergic contact dermatitis due to nickel

  L23.1 **Allergic contact dermatitis due to adhesives**

  L23.2 **Allergic contact dermatitis due to cosmetics**

  L23.3 **Allergic contact dermatitis due to drugs in contact with skin**
        Use additional code for adverse effect, if applicable,
           to identify drug (T36-T50 with fifth or sixth
           character 5)
      Excludes2 dermatitis due to ingested drugs and
                medicaments (L27.0-L27.1)

  L23.4 **Allergic contact dermatitis due to dyes**

  L23.5 **Allergic contact dermatitis due to other chemical products**
        Allergic contact dermatitis due to cement
        Allergic contact dermatitis due to insecticide
        Allergic contact dermatitis due to plastic
        Allergic contact dermatitis due to rubber

  L23.6 **Allergic contact dermatitis due to food in contact with the skin**
      Excludes2 dermatitis due to ingested food (L27.2)

  L23.7 **Allergic contact dermatitis due to plants, except food**
      Excludes2 allergy NOS due to pollen (J30.1)

  ● **L23.8** **Allergic contact dermatitis due to other agents**
    L23.81 **Allergic contact dermatitis due to animal (cat) (dog) dander**
        Allergic contact dermatitis due to animal (cat) (dog) hair
    L23.89 **Allergic contact dermatitis due to other agents**

  L23.9 **Allergic contact dermatitis, unspecified cause**
        Allergic contact eczema NOS

● **L24 Irritant contact dermatitis**
    Excludes1 allergy NOS (T78.40)
                  contact dermatitis NOS (L25.9)
                  dermatitis NOS (L30.9)

    Excludes2 allergic contact dermatitis (L23.-)
                  dermatitis due to substances taken internally
                   (L27.-)
                  dermatitis of eyelid (H01.1-)
                  diaper dermatitis (L22)
                  eczema of external ear (H60.5-)
                  perioral dermatitis (L71.0)
                  radiation-related disorders of the skin and
                    subcutaneous tissue (L55-L59)

  L24.0 **Irritant contact dermatitis due to detergents**

  L24.1 **Irritant contact dermatitis due to oils and greases**

  L24.2 **Irritant contact dermatitis due to solvents**
        Irritant contact dermatitis due to chlorocompound
        Irritant contact dermatitis due to cyclohexane
        Irritant contact dermatitis due to ester
        Irritant contact dermatitis due to glycol
        Irritant contact dermatitis due to hydrocarbon
        Irritant contact dermatitis due to ketone

  L24.3 **Irritant contact dermatitis due to cosmetics**

  L24.4 **Irritant contact dermatitis due to drugs in contact with skin**
        Use additional code for adverse effect, if applicable,
           to identify drug (T36-T50 with fifth or sixth
           character 5)

  L24.5 **Irritant contact dermatitis due to other chemical products**
        Irritant contact dermatitis due to cement
        Irritant contact dermatitis due to insecticide
        Irritant contact dermatitis due to plastic
        Irritant contact dermatitis due to rubber

  L24.6 **Irritant contact dermatitis due to food in contact with skin**
      Excludes2 dermatitis due to ingested food (L27.2)

  L24.7 **Irritant contact dermatitis due to plants, except food**
      Excludes2 allergy NOS to pollen (J30.1)

  ● **L24.8** **Irritant contact dermatitis due to other agents**
    L24.81 **Irritant contact dermatitis due to metals**
        Irritant contact dermatitis due to chromium
        Irritant contact dermatitis due to nickel
    L24.89 **Irritant contact dermatitis due to other agents**
        Irritant contact dermatitis due to dyes

  L24.9 **Irritant contact dermatitis, unspecified cause**
        Irritant contact eczema NOS

● **L25 Unspecified contact dermatitis**
    Excludes1 allergic contact dermatitis (L23.-)
                  allergy NOS (T78.40)
                  dermatitis NOS (L30.9)
                  irritant contact dermatitis (L24.-)

    Excludes2 dermatitis due to ingested substances (L27.-)
                  dermatitis of eyelid (H01.1-)
                  eczema of external ear (H60.5-)
                  perioral dermatitis (L71.0)
                  radiation-related disorders of the skin and
                    subcutaneous tissue (L55-L59)

  L25.0 **Unspecified contact dermatitis due to cosmetics**

  L25.1 **Unspecified contact dermatitis due to drugs in contact with skin**
        Use additional code for adverse effect, if applicable,
           to identify drug (T36-T50 with fifth or sixth
           character 5)
      Excludes2 dermatitis due to ingested drugs and
                medicaments (L27.0-L27.1)

CHAPTER 12 (L00-L99)

N Newborn Age: 0   **P** Pediatric Age: 0–17   **M** Maternity DX: 12–55   **A** Adult Age: 15–124   ♀ Females Only   ♂ Males Only

    Complication\Comorbidity   Major C\C   Ex CC/MCC Exclusions   Hospital-Acquired Condition   **969**

L25.2 Unspecified contact dermatitis due to dyes

L25.3 Unspecified contact dermatitis due to other chemical products
Unspecified contact dermatitis due to cement
Unspecified contact dermatitis due to insecticide

L25.4 Unspecified contact dermatitis due to food in contact with skin

> **Excludes2** dermatitis due to ingested food (L27.2)

L25.5 Unspecified contact dermatitis due to plants, except food

> **Excludes1** nettle rash (L50.9)

> **Excludes2** allergy NOS due to pollen (J30.1)

L25.8 Unspecified contact dermatitis due to other agents

L25.9 Unspecified contact dermatitis, unspecified cause
Contact dermatitis (occupational) NOS
Contact eczema (occupational) NOS

L26 Exfoliative dermatitis
Hebra's pityriasis

> **Excludes1** Ritter's disease (L00)

● **L27** Dermatitis due to substances taken internally

> **Excludes1** allergy NOS (T78.40)

> **Excludes2** adverse food reaction, except dermatitis (T78.0-T78.1)
> contact dermatitis (L23-L25)
> drug photoallergic response (L56.1)
> drug phototoxic response (L56.0)
> urticaria (L50.-)

L27.0 Generalized skin eruption due to drugs and medicaments taken internally
Use additional code for adverse effect, if applicable, to identify drug (T36-T50 with fifth or sixth character 5)

L27.1 Localized skin eruption due to drugs and medicaments taken internally
Use additional code for adverse effect, if applicable, to identify drug (T36-T50 with fifth or sixth character 5)

L27.2 Dermatitis due to ingested food

> **Excludes2** dermatitis due to food in contact with skin (L23.6, L24.6, L25.4)

L27.8 Dermatitis due to other substances taken internally

L27.9 Dermatitis due to unspecified substance taken internally

● **L28** Lichen simplex chronicus and prurigo

L28.0 Lichen simplex chronicus
Circumscribed neurodermatitis
Lichen NOS

L28.1 Prurigo nodularis

L28.2 Other prurigo
Prurigo NOS   Prurigo mitis
Prurigo Hebra   Urticaria papulosa

● **L29** Pruritus

> **Excludes1** neurotic excoriation (L98.1)
> psychogenic pruritus (F45.8)

L29.0 Pruritus ani

L29.1 Pruritus scroti ♂

L29.2 Pruritus vulvae ♀

L29.3 Anogenital pruritus, unspecified

L29.8 Other pruritus

L29.9 Pruritus, unspecified
Itch NOS

● **L30** Other and unspecified dermatitis

> **Excludes2** contact dermatitis (L23-L25)
> dry skin dermatitis (L85.3)
> small plaque parapsoriasis (L41.3)
> stasis dermatitis (I87.2)

L30.0 Nummular dermatitis

L30.1 Dyshidrosis [pompholyx]

L30.2 Cutaneous autosensitization
Candidid [levurid]   Eczematid
Dermatophytid

L30.3 Infective dermatitis
Infectious eczematoid dermatitis

L30.4 Erythema intertrigo

L30.5 Pityriasis alba

L30.8 Other specified dermatitis

L30.9 Dermatitis, unspecified
Eczema NOS

PAPULOSQUAMOUS DISORDERS (L40-L45)

● **L40** Psoriasis

L40.0 Psoriasis vulgaris
Nummular psoriasis   Plaque psoriasis

L40.1 Generalized pustular psoriasis
Impetigo herpetiformis
Von Zumbusch's disease

L40.2 Acrodermatitis continua

L40.3 Pustulosis palmaris et plantaris

L40.4 Guttate psoriasis

● **L40.5** Arthropathic psoriasis

L40.50 Arthropathic psoriasis, unspecified

L40.51 Distal interphalangeal psoriatic arthropathy

L40.52 Psoriatic arthritis mutilans

L40.53 Psoriatic spondylitis

L40.54 Psoriatic juvenile arthropathy

L40.59 Other psoriatic arthropathy

L40.8 Other psoriasis
Flexural psoriasis

L40.9 Psoriasis, unspecified

● **L41** Parapsoriasis

> **Excludes1** poikiloderma vasculare atrophicans (L94.5)

L41.0 Pityriasis lichenoides et varioliformis acuta
Mucha-Habermann disease

L41.1 Pityriasis lichenoides chronica

L41.3 Small plaque parapsoriasis

L41.4 Large plaque parapsoriasis

L41.5 Retiform parapsoriasis

L41.8 Other parapsoriasis

L41.9 Parapsoriasis, unspecified

L42 Pityriasis rosea

● **L43** Lichen planus

> **Excludes1** lichen planopilaris (L66.1)

L43.0 Hypertrophic lichen planus

L43.1 Bullous lichen planus

L43.2 Lichenoid drug reaction
Use additional code for adverse effect, if applicable, to identify drug (T36-T50 with fifth or sixth character 5)

L43.3 Subacute (active) lichen planus
Lichen planus tropicus

L43.8 Other lichen planus

L43.9 Lichen planus, unspecified

Item 12-8 Psoriasis is a chronic, recurrent inflammatory skin disease characterized by small patches covered with thick silvery scales. **Parapsoriasis** is a treatment-resistant erythroderma. **Pityriasis rosea** is characterized by a herald patch that is a single large lesion and that usually appears on the trunk and is followed by scattered, smaller lesions.

▶ New   ➡ Revised   ~~deleted~~ Deleted   Excludes 1   Excludes 2   Includes   Use additional   Code first   Code also   Key words
OGCR Official Guidelines   ● Unacceptable Principal Diagnosis   X Assign placeholder X   ● Use Additional Character(s)   ▶ Manifestation Code   **Coding Clinic**

L44   Other papulosquamous disorders

　　L44.0   Pityriasis rubra pilaris
　　L44.1   Lichen nitidus
　　L44.2   Lichen striatus
　　L44.3   Lichen ruber moniliformis
　　L44.4   Infantile papular acrodermatitis [Gianotti-Crosti]   P
　　L44.8   Other specified papulosquamous disorders
　　L44.9   Papulosquamous disorder, **unspecified**

L45   Papulosquamous disorders in diseases classified elsewhere
　　Code first underlying disease

URTICARIA AND ERYTHEMA (L49-L54)

　　Excludes1   Lyme disease (A69.2-)
　　　　　　　　　rosacea (L71.-)

L49   Exfoliation due to erythematous conditions according to extent of body surface involved

　　Code first erythematous condition causing exfoliation, such as:
　　　　Ritter's disease (L00)
　　　　(Staphylococcal) scalded skin syndrome (L00)
　　　　Stevens-Johnson syndrome (L51.1)
　　　　Stevens-Johnson syndrome-toxic epidermal necrolysis overlap syndrome (L51.3)
　　　　Toxic epidermal necrolysis (L51.2)

●　L49.0   **Exfoliation due to erythematous condition involving less than 10 percent of body surface**
　　　　　　Exfoliation due to erythematous condition NOS

●　L49.1   **Exfoliation due to erythematous condition involving 10-19 percent of body surface**

●　L49.2   **Exfoliation due to erythematous condition involving 20-29 percent of body surface**

●　L49.3   **Exfoliation due to erythematous condition involving 30-39 percent of body surface** 🔵
　　　　　　ⒺⓍ See PDX Collection 844

●　L49.4   **Exfoliation due to erythematous condition involving 40-49 percent of body surface** 🔵
　　　　　　ⒺⓍ See PDX Collection 845

●　L49.5   **Exfoliation due to erythematous condition involving 50-59 percent of body surface** 🔵
　　　　　　ⒺⓍ See PDX Collection 846

●　L49.6   **Exfoliation due to erythematous condition involving 60-69 percent of body surface** 🔵
　　　　　　ⒺⓍ See PDX Collection 847

●　L49.7   **Exfoliation due to erythematous condition involving 70-79 percent of body surface** 🔵
　　　　　　ⒺⓍ See PDX Collection 848

●　L49.8   **Exfoliation due to erythematous condition involving 80-89 percent of body surface** 🔵
　　　　　　ⒺⓍ See PDX Collection 849

●　L49.9   **Exfoliation due to erythematous condition involving 90 or more percent of body surface** 🔵
　　　　　　ⒺⓍ See PDX Collection 850

Figure 12-6 Erythematous plaques with silvery scales in a patient with psoriasis. (Getty Image)

Figure 12-7 Urticaria (hives). *(Courtesy of David Effron, MD.)* (Getty Image)

Item 12–9 Urticaria is a vascular reaction in which wheals surrounded by a red halo appear and cause severe itching. The causes of urticaria or hives are extensive and varied (e.g., food, heat, cold, drugs, stress, infections).

●L50   Urticaria

　　Excludes1   allergic contact dermatitis (L23.-)
　　　　　　　　　angioneurotic edema (T78.3)
　　　　　　　　　giant urticaria (T78.3)
　　　　　　　　　hereditary angio-edema (D84.1)
　　　　　　　　　Quincke's edema (T78.3)
　　　　　　　　　serum urticaria (T80.6-)
　　　　　　　　　solar urticaria (L56.3)
　　　　　　　　　urticaria neonatorum (P83.8)
　　　　　　　　　urticaria papulosa (L28.2)
　　　　　　　　　urticaria pigmentosa (Q82.2)

　　L50.0   **Allergic urticaria**
　　L50.1   **Idiopathic urticaria**
　　L50.2   **Urticaria due to cold and heat**
　　　　　　Excludes2   familial cold urticaria (M04.2)
　　L50.3   **Dermatographic urticaria**
　　L50.4   **Vibratory urticaria**
　　L50.5   **Cholinergic urticaria**
　　L50.6   **Contact urticaria**
　　L50.8   **Other urticaria**
　　　　　　Chronic urticaria
　　　　　　Recurrent periodic urticaria
　　L50.9   **Urticaria, unspecified**

●L51   Erythema multiforme

　　Use additional code for adverse effect, if applicable, to identify drug (T36-T50 with fifth or sixth character 5)
　　Use additional code to identify associated manifestations, such as:
　　　　arthropathy associated with dermatological disorders (M14.8-)
　　　　conjunctival edema (H11.42)
　　　　conjunctivitis (H10.22-)
　　　　corneal scars and opacities (H17.-)
　　　　corneal ulcer (H16.0-)
　　　　edema of eyelid (H02.84)
　　　　inflammation of eyelid (H01.8)
　　　　keratoconjunctivitis sicca (H16.22-)
　　　　mechanical lagophthalmos (H02.22-)
　　　　stomatitis (K12.-)
　　　　symblepharon (H11.23-)
　　Use additional code to identify percentage of skin exfoliation (L49.-)

　　Excludes1   staphylococcal scalded skin syndrome (L00)
　　　　　　　　　Ritter's disease (L00)
　　ⒺⓍ For category L51 CC codes: See PDX Collection 843

　　L51.0   **Nonbullous erythema multiforme**
　　L51.1   **Stevens-Johnson syndrome** 🔵
　　L51.2   **Toxic epidermal necrolysis [Lyell]** 🔵
　　L51.3   **Stevens-Johnson syndrome-toxic epidermal necrolysis overlap syndrome** 🔵
　　　　　　SJS-TEN overlap syndrome
　　L51.8   **Other erythema multiforme**
　　L51.9   **Erythema multiforme, unspecified**
　　　　　　Erythema iris
　　　　　　Erythema multiforme major NOS
　　　　　　Erythema multiforme minor NOS
　　　　　　Herpes iris

CHAPTER 12 (L00-L99)

N Newborn Age: 0   **P** Pediatric Age: 0–17   **M** Maternity DX: 12–55   **A** Adult Age: 15–124   ♀ Females Only   ♂ Males Only

🔵 Complication\Comorbidity   🔵 Major C\C   ⒺⓍ CC/MCC Exclusions   🔵 Hospital-Acquired Condition

971

L52   Erythema nodosum
     Excludes1   tuberculous erythema nodosum (A18.4)

● **L53   Other erythematous conditions**
     Excludes1   erythema ab igne (L59.0)
               erythema due to external agents in contact with
                   skin (L23-L25)
               erythema intertrigo (L30.4)
     (Ex) **For category L53 CC codes:** See PDX Collection 851

    L53.0 Toxic erythema ⬚
        *Code first poisoning due to drug or toxin, if applicable
        (T36-T65 with fifth or sixth character 1-4 or 6)*
        Use additional code for adverse effect, if applicable,
        to identify drug (T36-T50 with fifth or sixth
        character 5)
        Excludes1 neonatal erythema toxicum (P83.1)

    L53.1 Erythema annulare centrifugum ⬚
    L53.2 Erythema marginatum ⬚
    L53.3 Other chronic figurate erythema ⬚
    L53.8 Other specified erythematous conditions
    L53.9 Erythematous condition, unspecified
        Erythema NOS
        Erythroderma NOS

▶ *L54   Erythema in diseases classified elsewhere*
     Code first underlying disease

RADIATION-RELATED DISORDERS OF THE SKIN AND SUBCUTANEOUS TISSUE (L55-L59)

● **L55   Sunburn**
    L55.0 Sunburn of first degree
    L55.1 Sunburn of second degree
    L55.2 Sunburn of third degree
    L55.9 Sunburn, unspecified

● **L56   Other acute skin changes due to ultraviolet radiation**
    Use additional code to identify the source of the ultraviolet
    radiation (W89, X32)

    L56.0 Drug phototoxic response
        Use additional code for adverse effect, if applicable,
        to identify drug (T36-T50 with fifth or sixth
        character 5)

    L56.1 Drug photoallergic response
        Use additional code for adverse effect, if applicable,
        to identify drug (T36-T50 with fifth or sixth
        character 5)

    L56.2 Photocontact dermatitis [berloque dermatitis]
    L56.3 Solar urticaria
    L56.4 Polymorphous light eruption
    L56.5 Disseminated superficial actinic porokeratosis (DSAP)
    L56.8 Other specified acute skin changes due to ultraviolet
        radiation
    L56.9 Acute skin change due to ultraviolet radiation,
        unspecified

● **L57   Skin changes due to chronic exposure to nonionizing radiation**
   ⟹ Use additional code to identify the source of the ultraviolet
    radiation (W89)

    L57.0 Actinic keratosis
        Keratosis NOS   Solar keratosis
        Senile keratosis
    L57.1 Actinic reticuloid
    L57.2 Cutis rhomboidalis nuchae
    L57.3 Poikiloderma of Civatte
    L57.4 Cutis laxa senilis
        Elastosis senilis
    L57.5 Actinic granuloma

    L57.8 Other skin changes due to chronic exposure to
        nonionizing radiation
        Farmer's skin   Solar dermatitis
        Sailor's skin
    L57.9 Skin changes due to chronic exposure to nonionizing
        radiation, unspecified

● **L58   Radiodermatitis**
    Use additional code to identify the source of the radiation
    (W88, W90)

    L58.0 Acute radiodermatitis
    L58.1 Chronic radiodermatitis
    L58.9 Radiodermatitis, unspecified

● **L59   Other disorders of skin and subcutaneous tissue related to radiation**
    L59.0 Erythema ab igne [dermatitis ab igne]
    L59.8 Other specified disorders of the skin and subcutaneous
        tissue related to radiation
        Coding Clinic: 2017, Q1, P34
    L59.9 Disorder of the skin and subcutaneous tissue related to
        radiation, unspecified

DISORDERS OF SKIN APPENDAGES (L60-L75)

    Excludes1 congenital malformations of integument (Q84.-)

● **L60   Nail disorders**
    Excludes2 clubbing of nails (R68.3)
                 onychia and paronychia (L03.0-)

    L60.0 Ingrowing nail
    L60.1 Onycholysis
    L60.2 Onychogryphosis
    L60.3 Nail dystrophy
    L60.4 Beau's lines
    L60.5 Yellow nail syndrome
    L60.8 Other nail disorders
    L60.9 Nail disorder, unspecified

▶ *L62   Nail disorders in diseases classified elsewhere*
     Code first underlying disease, such as:
      pachydermoperiostosis (M89.4-)

● **L63   Alopecia areata**
    L63.0 Alopecia (capitis) totalis
    L63.1 Alopecia universalis
    L63.2 Ophiasis
    L63.8 Other alopecia areata
    L63.9 Alopecia areata, unspecified

Item 12–10 Alopecia is lack of hair and takes many forms. The most common is male pattern alopecia, also known as **androgenetic alopecia. Telogen effluvium** is early and excessive loss of hair resulting from a trauma to the hair follicle (fever, drugs, surgery, etc.).

Figure 12-8 Male pattern alopecia.

▶ New   ⟹ Revised   ~~deleted~~ Deleted   Excludes 1   Excludes 2   Includes   Use additional   Code first   Code also   Key words

OGCR Official Guidelines   ● Unacceptable Principal Diagnosis   X Assign placeholder X   ● Use Additional Character(s)   ▶ Manifestation Code   Coding Clinic

972

● **L64**   **Androgenic alopecia**
      Includes   male-pattern baldness
      L64.0   **Drug-induced androgenic alopecia**
           Use additional code for adverse effect, if applicable, to identify drug (T36-T50 with fifth or sixth character 5)
      L64.8   **Other androgenic alopecia**
      L64.9   **Androgenic alopecia, unspecified**

● **L65**   **Other nonscarring hair loss**
      Use additional code for adverse effect, if applicable, to identify drug (T36-T50 with fifth or sixth character 5)
      Excludes1   trichotillomania (F63.3)
      L65.0   **Telogen effluvium**
      L65.1   **Anagen effluvium**
      L65.2   **Alopecia mucinosa**
      L65.8   **Other specified nonscarring hair loss**
      L65.9   **Nonscarring hair loss, unspecified**
           Alopecia NOS

● **L66**   **Cicatricial alopecia [scarring hair loss]**
      L66.0   **Pseudopelade**
      L66.1   **Lichen planopilaris**
           Follicular lichen planus
      L66.2   **Folliculitis decalvans**
      L66.3   **Perifolliculitis capitis abscedens**
      L66.4   **Folliculitis ulerythematosa reticulata**
      L66.8   **Other cicatricial alopecia**
           Coding Clinic: 2015, Q1, P19
      L66.9   **Cicatricial alopecia, unspecified**

● **L67**   **Hair color and hair shaft abnormalities**
      Excludes1   monilethrix (Q84.1)
           pili annulati (Q84.1)
           telogen effluvium (L65.0)
      L67.0   **Trichorrhexis nodosa**
      L67.1   **Variations in hair color**
           Canities
           Greyness, hair (premature)
           Heterochromia of hair
           Poliosis circumscripta, acquired
           Poliosis NOS
      L67.8   **Other hair color and hair shaft abnormalities**
           Fragilitas crinium
      L67.9   **Hair color and hair shaft abnormality, unspecified**

● **L68**   **Hypertrichosis**
      Includes   excess hair
      Excludes1   congenital hypertrichosis (Q84.2)
           persistent lanugo (Q84.2)
      L68.0   **Hirsutism**
           Excessive growth of hair
      L68.1   **Acquired hypertrichosis lanuginosa**
      L68.2   **Localized hypertrichosis**
      L68.3   **Polytrichia**
      L68.8   **Other hypertrichosis**
      L68.9   **Hypertrichosis, unspecified**

● **L70**   **Acne**
      Excludes2   acne keloid (L73.0)
      L70.0   **Acne vulgaris**
      L70.1   **Acne conglobata**
      L70.2   **Acne varioliformis**
           Acne necrotica miliaris

      L70.3   **Acne tropica**
      L70.4   **Infantile acne**   P
      L70.5   **Acné excoriée**
           Acné excoriée des jeunes filles
           Picker's acne
      L70.8   **Other acne**
      L70.9   **Acne, unspecified**

● **L71**   **Rosacea**
      Use additional code for adverse effect, if applicable, to identify drug (T36-T50 with fifth or sixth character 5)
      L71.0   **Perioral dermatitis**
      L71.1   **Rhinophyma**
      L71.8   **Other rosacea**
      L71.9   **Rosacea, unspecified**

● **L72**   **Follicular cysts of skin and subcutaneous tissue**
      L72.0   **Epidermal cyst**
   ● **L72.1**   **Pilar and trichodermal cyst**
           L72.11   **Pilar cyst**
           L72.12   **Trichodermal cyst**
               Trichilemmal (proliferating) cyst
      L72.3   **Sebaceous cyst**
           Excludes2   pilar cyst (L72.11)
               trichilemmal (proliferating) cyst (L72.12)
      L72.2   **Steatocystoma multiplex**
      L72.8   **Other follicular cysts of the skin and subcutaneous tissue**
      L72.9   **Follicular cyst of the skin and subcutaneous tissue, unspecified**

● **L73**   **Other follicular disorders**
      L73.0   **Acne keloid**
      L73.1   **Pseudofolliculitis barbae**
      L73.2   **Hidradenitis suppurativa**
      L73.8   **Other specified follicular disorders**
           Sycosis barbae
      L73.9   **Follicular disorder, unspecified**

● **L74**   **Eccrine sweat disorders**
      Excludes2   generalized hyperhidrosis (R61)
      L74.0   **Miliaria rubra**
      L74.1   **Miliaria crystallina**
      L74.2   **Miliaria profunda**
           Miliaria tropicalis
      L74.3   **Miliaria, unspecified**
      L74.4   **Anhidrosis**
           Hypohidrosis
   ● **L74.5**   **Focal hyperhidrosis**
     ● **L74.51**   **Primary focal hyperhidrosis**
           L74.510   **Primary focal hyperhidrosis, axilla**
           L74.511   **Primary focal hyperhidrosis, face**
           L74.512   **Primary focal hyperhidrosis, palms**
           L74.513   **Primary focal hyperhidrosis, soles**
           L74.519   **Primary focal hyperhidrosis, unspecified**
           L74.52   **Secondary focal hyperhidrosis**
               Frey's syndrome
      L74.8   **Other eccrine sweat disorders**
      L74.9   **Eccrine sweat disorder, unspecified**
           Sweat gland disorder NOS

CHAPTER 12 (L00-L99)

● **L75** **Apocrine sweat disorders**

     Excludes1 dyshidrosis (L30.1)
                    hidradenitis suppurativa (L73.2)

     L75.0 **Bromhidrosis**

     L75.1 **Chromhidrosis**

     L75.2 **Apocrine miliaria**
          Fox-Fordyce disease

     L75.8 **Other apocrine sweat disorders**

     L75.9 **Apocrine sweat disorder, unspecified**
          Intraoperative and postprocedural complications of
          skin and subcutaneous tissue (L76)

INTRAOPERATIVE AND POSTPROCEDURAL COMPLICATIONS OF SKIN AND SUBCUTANEOUS TISSUE (L76)

● **L76** **Intraoperative and postprocedural complications of skin and subcutaneous tissue**
     (Ex) For category L76 CC codes unless otherwise indicated: See PDX Collection 852
     Coding Clinic: 2016, Q4, P10

● **L76.0** **Intraoperative hemorrhage and hematoma of skin and subcutaneous tissue complicating a procedure**

     Excludes1 intraoperative hemorrhage and hematoma
                   of skin and subcutaneous tissue due
                   to accidental puncture and laceration
                   during a procedure (L76.1-)

     L76.01 **Intraoperative hemorrhage and hematoma of skin and subcutaneous tissue complicating a dermatologic procedure** 🔲

     L76.02 **Intraoperative hemorrhage and hematoma of skin and subcutaneous tissue complicating other procedure** 🔲

● **L76.1** **Accidental puncture and laceration of skin and subcutaneous tissue during a procedure**
     (Ex) For category L76.1 CC codes: See PDX Collection 509

     L76.11 **Accidental puncture and laceration of skin and subcutaneous tissue during a dermatologic procedure** 🔲

     L76.12 **Accidental puncture and laceration of skin and subcutaneous tissue during other procedure** 🔲

● **L76.2** **Postprocedural hemorrhage of skin and subcutaneous tissue following a procedure**

     L76.21 **Postprocedural hemorrhage of skin and subcutaneous tissue following a dermatologic procedure** 🔲

     L76.22 **Postprocedural hemorrhage of skin and subcutaneous tissue following other procedure** 🔲

● **L76.3** **Postprocedural hematoma and seroma of skin and subcutaneous tissue following a procedure**

     L76.31 **Postprocedural hematoma of skin and subcutaneous tissue following a dermatologic procedure** 🔲

     L76.32 **Postprocedural hematoma of skin and subcutaneous tissue following other procedure** 🔲

     L76.33 **Postprocedural seroma of skin and subcutaneous tissue following a dermatologic procedure** 🔲

     L76.34 **Postprocedural seroma of skin and subcutaneous tissue following other procedure** 🔲

● **L76.8** **Other intraoperative and postprocedural complications of skin and subcutaneous tissue**

     Use additional code, if applicable, to further specify
     disorder

     L76.81 **Other intraoperative complications of skin and subcutaneous tissue**

     L76.82 **Other postprocedural complications of skin and subcutaneous tissue**

OTHER DISORDERS OF THE SKIN AND SUBCUTANEOUS TISSUE (L80-L99)

     L80 **Vitiligo**

         Excludes2 vitiligo of eyelids (H02.73-)
                     vitiligo of vulva (N90.89)

● **L81** **Other disorders of pigmentation**

     Excludes1 birthmark NOS (Q82.5)
                   Peutz-Jeghers syndrome (Q85.8)

     Excludes2 nevus - see Alphabetical Index

     L81.0 **Postinflammatory hyperpigmentation**

     L81.1 **Chloasma**

     L81.2 **Freckles**

     L81.3 **Café au lait spots**

     L81.4 **Other melanin hyperpigmentation**
          Lentigo

     L81.5 **Leukoderma, not elsewhere classified**

     L81.6 **Other disorders of diminished melanin formation**

     L81.7 **Pigmented purpuric dermatosis**
          Angioma serpiginosum

     L81.8 **Other specified disorders of pigmentation**
          Iron pigmentation
          Tattoo pigmentation

     L81.9 **Disorder of pigmentation, unspecified**

● **L82** **Seborrheic keratosis**

     Includes basal cell papilloma
                 dermatosis papulosa nigra
                 Leser-Trélat disease

     Excludes2 seborrheic dermatitis (L21.-)

     L82.0 **Inflamed seborrheic keratosis**

     L82.1 **Other seborrheic keratosis**
          Seborrheic keratosis NOS

     L83 **Acanthosis nigricans**
          Confluent and reticulated papillomatosis

     L84 **Corns and callosities**
          Callus
          Clavus

● **L85** **Other epidermal thickening**

     Excludes2 hypertrophic disorders of the skin (L91.-)

     L85.0 **Acquired ichthyosis**
         Excludes1 congenital ichthyosis (Q80.-)

     L85.1 **Acquired keratosis [keratoderma] palmaris et plantaris**
         Excludes1 inherited keratosis palmaris et plantaris
                       (Q82.8)

     L85.2 **Keratosis punctata (palmaris et plantaris)**

     L85.3 **Xerosis cutis**
         Dry skin dermatitis

     L85.8 **Other specified epidermal thickening**
         Cutaneous horn

     L85.9 **Epidermal thickening, unspecified**

▷ **L86** *Keratoderma in diseases classified elsewhere*
     Firm horny papules that have a cobblestone appearance.

     Code first underlying disease, such as:
         Reiter's disease (M02.3-)

     Excludes1 gonococcal keratoderma (A54.89)
                  gonococcal keratosis (A54.89)
                  keratoderma due to vitamin A deficiency (E50.8)
                  keratosis due to vitamin A deficiency (E50.8)
                  xeroderma due to vitamin A deficiency (E50.8)

▶ New   ⇒ Revised   ~~deleted~~ Deleted   Excludes 1   Excludes 2   Includes   Use additional   Code first   Code also   Key words

OGCR Official Guidelines   ● Unacceptable Principal Diagnosis   X Assign placeholder X   ● Use Additional Character(s)   ▷ Manifestation Code   **Coding Clinic**

● **L87 Transepidermal elimination disorders**
   Excludes1 granuloma annulare (perforating) (L92.0)
   L87.0 Keratosis follicularis et parafollicularis in cutem penetrans
     Kyrle disease
     Hyperkeratosis follicularis penetrans
   L87.1 Reactive perforating collagenosis
   L87.2 Elastosis perforans serpiginosa
   L87.8 Other transepidermal elimination disorders
   L87.9 Transepidermal elimination disorder, unspecified

L88 Pyoderma gangrenosum
   Phagedenic pyoderma
   Excludes1 dermatitis gangrenosa (L08.0)
   (Ex:) See PDX Collection 853
   OGCR Section I.B.14.

General Coding Guidelines

Documentation for BMI, *Depth of* Non-pressure ulcers, Pressure Ulcer Stages, **Coma Scale, and** *NIH Stroke Scale*

For the Body Mass Index (BMI), depth of non-pressure chronic ulcers, pressure ulcer stage, **coma scale, and NIH stroke scale (NIHSS) codes**, code assignment may be based on medical record documentation from clinicians who are not the patient's provider (i.e., physician or other qualified healthcare practitioner legally accountable for establishing the patient's diagnosis), since this information is typically documented by other clinicians involved in the care of the patient (e.g., a dietitian often documents the BMI, a nurse often documents the pressure ulcer stages, **and an emergency medical technician often documents the coma scale**). However, the associated diagnosis (such as overweight, obesity, **acute stroke**, or pressure ulcer) must be documented by the patient's provider. If there is conflicting medical record documentation, either from the same clinician or different clinicians, the patient's attending provider should be queried for clarification.

The BMI, **coma scale, and NHSS** codes should only be reported as secondary diagnoses.

● **L89 Pressure ulcer**
   Includes bed sore   pressure area
          decubitus ulcer   pressure sore
          plaster ulcer
   Code first any associated gangrene (I96)
   Excludes2 decubitus (trophic) ulcer of cervix (uteri) (N86)
     diabetic ulcers (E08.621, E08.622, E09.621, E09.622, E10.621, E10.622, E11.621, E11.622, E13.621, E13.622)
     non-pressure chronic ulcer of skin (L97.-)
     skin infections (L00-L08)
     varicose ulcer (I83.0, I83.2)
   (Ex:) For category L89 CC codes: See PDX Collection 854
   Coding Clinic: 2016, Q4, P124

● **L89.0 Pressure ulcer of elbow**
 ● **L89.00 Pressure ulcer of unspecified elbow**
   L89.000 Pressure ulcer of unspecified elbow, unstageable
   L89.001 Pressure ulcer of unspecified elbow, stage 1
     Healing pressure ulcer of unspecified elbow, stage 1
     Pressure pre-ulcer skin changes limited to persistent focal edema, unspecified elbow
   L89.002 Pressure ulcer of unspecified elbow, stage 2
     Healing pressure ulcer of unspecified elbow, stage 2
     Pressure ulcer with abrasion, blister, partial thickness skin loss involving epidermis and/or dermis, unspecified elbow

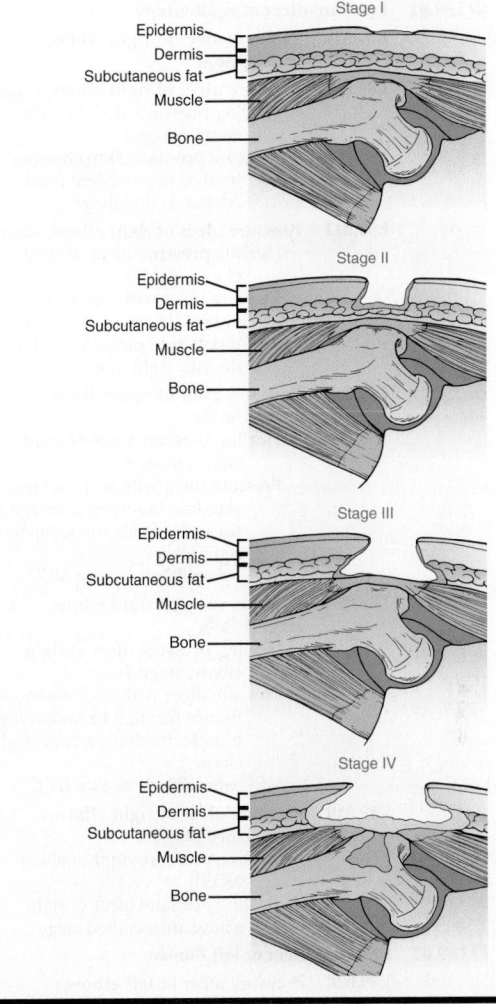

Figure 12-9 Stage I, II, III, and IV of pressure ulcers.

   L89.003 Pressure ulcer of unspecified elbow, stage 3
     Healing pressure ulcer of unspecified elbow, stage 3
     Pressure ulcer with full thickness skin loss involving damage or necrosis of subcutaneous tissue, unspecified elbow
     MCC when PDx is its own MCC
   L89.004 Pressure ulcer of unspecified elbow, stage 4
     Healing pressure ulcer of unspecified elbow, stage 4
     Pressure ulcer with necrosis of soft tissues through to underlying muscle, tendon, or bone, unspecified elbow
     MCC when PDx is its own MCC
   L89.009 Pressure ulcer of unspecified elbow, unspecified stage
     Healing pressure ulcer of elbow NOS
     Healing pressure ulcer of unspecified elbow, unspecified stage

CHAPTER 12 (L00-L99)

CHAPTER 12 (L00-L99)

● **L89.01** **Pressure ulcer of right elbow**

L89.010 **Pressure ulcer of right elbow, unstageable**

L89.011 **Pressure ulcer of right elbow, stage 1**
Healing pressure ulcer of right elbow, stage 1
Pressure pre-ulcer skin changes limited to persistent focal edema, right elbow

L89.012 **Pressure ulcer of right elbow, stage 2**
Healing pressure ulcer of right elbow, stage 2
Pressure ulcer with abrasion, blister, partial thickness skin loss involving epidermis and/or dermis, right elbow

L89.013 **Pressure ulcer of right elbow, stage 3**
Healing pressure ulcer of right elbow, stage 3
Pressure ulcer with full thickness skin loss involving damage or necrosis of subcutaneous tissue, right elbow
MCC when PDx is its own MCC

L89.014 **Pressure ulcer of right elbow, stage 4**
Healing pressure ulcer of right elbow, stage 4
Pressure ulcer with necrosis of soft tissues through to underlying muscle, tendon, or bone, right elbow
MCC when PDx is its own MCC

L89.019 **Pressure ulcer of right elbow, unspecified stage**
Healing pressure right of elbow NOS
➠Healing pressure ulcer of right elbow, unspecified stage

● **L89.02** **Pressure ulcer of left elbow**

L89.020 **Pressure ulcer of left elbow, unstageable**

L89.021 **Pressure ulcer of left elbow, stage 1**
Healing pressure ulcer of left elbow, stage 1
Pressure pre-ulcer skin changes limited to persistent focal edema, left elbow

L89.022 **Pressure ulcer of left elbow, stage 2**
Healing pressure ulcer of left elbow, stage 2
Pressure ulcer with abrasion, blister, partial thickness skin loss involving epidermis and/or dermis, left elbow

L89.023 **Pressure ulcer of left elbow, stage 3**
Healing pressure ulcer of left elbow, stage 3
Pressure ulcer with full thickness skin loss involving damage or necrosis of subcutaneous tissue, left elbow
MCC when PDx is its own MCC

L89.024 **Pressure ulcer of left elbow, stage 4**
Healing pressure ulcer of left elbow, stage 4
Pressure ulcer with necrosis of soft tissues through to underlying muscle, tendon, or bone, left elbow
MCC when PDx is its own MCC

L89.029 **Pressure ulcer of left elbow, unspecified stage**
Healing pressure ulcer of left of elbow NOS
➠Healing pressure ulcer of left elbow, unspecified stage

● **L89.1** **Pressure ulcer of back**

● **L89.10** **Pressure ulcer of unspecified part of back**

L89.100 **Pressure ulcer of unspecified part of back, unstageable**

L89.101 **Pressure ulcer of unspecified part of back, stage 1**
Healing pressure ulcer of unspecified part of back, stage 1
Pressure pre-ulcer skin changes limited to persistent focal edema, unspecified part of back

L89.102 **Pressure ulcer of unspecified part of back, stage 2**
Healing pressure ulcer of unspecified part of back, stage 2
Pressure ulcer with abrasion, blister, partial thickness skin loss involving epidermis and/or dermis, unspecified part of back

L89.103 **Pressure ulcer of unspecified part of back, stage 3**
Healing pressure ulcer of unspecified part of back, stage 3
Pressure ulcer with full thickness skin loss involving damage or necrosis of subcutaneous tissue, unspecified part of back
MCC when PDx is its own MCC

L89.104 **Pressure ulcer of unspecified part of back, stage 4**
Healing pressure ulcer of unspecified part of back, stage 4
Pressure ulcer with necrosis of soft tissues through to underlying muscle, tendon, or bone, unspecified part of back
MCC when PDx is its own MCC

L89.109 **Pressure ulcer of unspecified part of back, unspecified stage**
Healing pressure ulcer of unspecified part of back NOS
Healing pressure ulcer of unspecified part of back, unspecified stage

● **L89.11** **Pressure ulcer of right upper back**
Pressure ulcer of right shoulder blade

L89.110 **Pressure ulcer of right upper back, unstageable**

L89.111 **Pressure ulcer of right upper back, stage 1**
Healing pressure ulcer of right upper back, stage 1
Pressure pre-ulcer skin changes limited to persistent focal edema, right upper back

▶ New   ➠ Revised   ~~deleted~~ Deleted   Excludes 1   Excludes 2   Includes   Use additional   Code first   Code also   Key words
OGCR Official Guidelines   ● Unacceptable Principal Diagnosis   X Assign placeholder X   ● Use Additional Character(s)   ▶ Manifestation Code   Coding Clinic

L89.112   **Pressure ulcer of right upper back, stage 2**
Healing pressure ulcer of right upper back, stage 2
Pressure ulcer with abrasion, blister, partial thickness skin loss involving epidermis and/or dermis, right upper back

L89.113   **Pressure ulcer of right upper back, stage 3** 🕭 🕭
Healing pressure ulcer of right upper back, stage 3
Pressure ulcer with full thickness skin loss involving damage or necrosis of subcutaneous tissue, right upper back
MCC when PDx is its own MCC

L89.114   **Pressure ulcer of right upper back, stage 4** 🕭 🕭
Healing pressure ulcer of right upper back, stage 4
Pressure ulcer with necrosis of soft tissues through to underlying muscle, tendon, or bone, right upper back
MCC when PDx is its own MCC

L89.119   **Pressure ulcer of right upper back, unspecified stage**
Healing pressure ulcer of right upper back NOS
Healing pressure ulcer of right upper back, unspecified stage

● **L89.12**   **Pressure ulcer of left upper back**
Pressure ulcer of left shoulder blade

L89.120   **Pressure ulcer of left upper back, unstageable**

L89.121   **Pressure ulcer of left upper back, stage 1**
Healing pressure ulcer of left upper back, stage 1
Pressure pre-ulcer skin changes limited to persistent focal edema, left upper back

L89.122   **Pressure ulcer of left upper back, stage 2**
Healing pressure ulcer of left upper back, stage 2
Pressure ulcer with abrasion, blister, partial thickness skin loss involving epidermis and/or dermis, left upper back

L89.123   **Pressure ulcer of left upper back, stage 3** 🕭 🕭
Healing pressure ulcer of left upper back, stage 3
Pressure ulcer with full thickness skin loss involving damage or necrosis of subcutaneous tissue, left upper back
MCC when PDx is its own MCC

L89.124   **Pressure ulcer of left upper back, stage 4** 🕭 🕭
Healing pressure ulcer of left upper back, stage 4
Pressure ulcer with necrosis of soft tissues through to underlying muscle, tendon, or bone, left upper back
MCC when PDx is its own MCC

L89.129   **Pressure ulcer of left upper back, unspecified stage**
Healing pressure ulcer of left upper back NOS
Healing pressure ulcer of left upper back, unspecified stage

● **L89.13**   **Pressure ulcer of right lower back**

L89.130   **Pressure ulcer of right lower back, unstageable**

L89.131   **Pressure ulcer of right lower back, stage 1**
Healing pressure ulcer of right lower back, stage 1
Pressure pre-ulcer skin changes limited to persistent focal edema, right lower back

L89.132   **Pressure ulcer of right lower back, stage 2**
Healing pressure ulcer of right lower back, stage 2
Pressure ulcer with abrasion, blister, partial thickness skin loss involving epidermis and/or dermis, right lower back

L89.133   **Pressure ulcer of right lower back, stage 3** 🕭 🕭
Healing pressure ulcer of right lower back, stage 3
Pressure ulcer with full thickness skin loss involving damage or necrosis of subcutaneous tissue, right lower back
MCC when PDx is its own MCC

L89.134   **Pressure ulcer of right lower back, stage 4** 🕭 🕭
Healing pressure ulcer of right lower back, stage 4
Pressure ulcer with necrosis of soft tissues through to underlying muscle, tendon, or bone, right lower back
MCC when PDx is its own MCC

L89.139   **Pressure ulcer of right lower back, unspecified stage**
Healing pressure ulcer of right lower back NOS
Healing pressure ulcer of right lower back, unspecified stage

● **L89.14**   **Pressure ulcer of left lower back**

L89.140   **Pressure ulcer of left lower back, unstageable**

L89.141   **Pressure ulcer of left lower back, stage 1**
Healing pressure ulcer of left lower back, stage 1
Pressure pre-ulcer skin changes limited to persistent focal edema, left lower back

L89.142   **Pressure ulcer of left lower back, stage 2**
Healing pressure ulcer of left lower back, stage 2
Pressure ulcer with abrasion, blister, partial thickness skin loss involving epidermis and/or dermis, left lower back

L89.143   **Pressure ulcer of left lower back, stage 3** 🕭 🕭
Healing pressure ulcer of left lower back, stage 3
Pressure ulcer with full thickness skin loss involving damage or necrosis of subcutaneous tissue, left lower back
MCC when PDx is its own MCC

CHAPTER 12 (L00-L99)

CHAPTER 12 (L00-L99)

L89.144   **Pressure ulcer of left lower back, stage 4** 🔖 🔖
> Healing pressure ulcer of left lower back, stage 4
> Pressure ulcer with necrosis of soft tissues through to underlying muscle, tendon, or bone, left lower back
> MCC when PDx is its own MCC

L89.149   **Pressure ulcer of left lower back, unspecified stage**
> Healing pressure ulcer of left lower back NOS
> Healing pressure ulcer of left lower back, unspecified stage

● **L89.15**   **Pressure ulcer of sacral region**
> Pressure ulcer of coccyx
> Pressure ulcer of tailbone

L89.150   **Pressure ulcer of sacral region, unstageable**

L89.151   **Pressure ulcer of sacral region, stage 1**
> Healing pressure ulcer of sacral region, stage 1
> Pressure pre-ulcer skin changes limited to persistent focal edema, sacral region

L89.152   **Pressure ulcer of sacral region, stage 2**
> Healing pressure ulcer of sacral region, stage 2
> Pressure ulcer with abrasion, blister, partial thickness skin loss involving epidermis and/or dermis, sacral region

L89.153   **Pressure ulcer of sacral region, stage 3** 🔖 🔖
> Healing pressure ulcer of sacral region, stage 3
> Pressure ulcer with full thickness skin loss involving damage or necrosis of subcutaneous tissue, sacral region
> MCC when PDx is its own MCC

L89.154   **Pressure ulcer of sacral region, stage 4** 🔖 🔖
> Healing pressure ulcer of sacral region, stage 4
> Pressure ulcer with necrosis of soft tissues through to underlying muscle, tendon, or bone, sacral region
> MCC when PDx is its own MCC

L89.159   **Pressure ulcer of sacral region, unspecified stage**
> Healing pressure ulcer of sacral region NOS
> Healing pressure ulcer of sacral region, unspecified stage

● **L89.2**   **Pressure ulcer of hip**

● **L89.20**   **Pressure ulcer of unspecified hip**

L89.200   **Pressure ulcer of unspecified hip, unstageable**

L89.201   **Pressure ulcer of unspecified hip, stage 1**
> Healing pressure ulcer of unspecified hip back, stage 1
> Pressure pre-ulcer skin changes limited to persistent focal edema, unspecified hip

L89.202   **Pressure ulcer of unspecified hip, stage 2**
> Healing pressure ulcer of unspecified hip, stage 2
> Pressure ulcer with abrasion, blister, partial thickness skin loss involving epidermis and/or dermis, unspecified hip

L89.203   **Pressure ulcer of unspecified hip, stage 3** 🔖 🔖
> Healing pressure ulcer of unspecified hip, stage 3
> Pressure ulcer with full thickness skin loss involving damage or necrosis of subcutaneous tissue, unspecified hip
> MCC when PDx is its own MCC

L89.204   **Pressure ulcer of unspecified hip, stage 4** 🔖 🔖
> Healing pressure ulcer of unspecified hip, stage 4
> Pressure ulcer with necrosis of soft tissues through to underlying muscle, tendon, or bone, unspecified hip
> MCC when PDx is its own MCC

L89.209   **Pressure ulcer of unspecified hip, unspecified stage**
> Healing pressure ulcer of unspecified hip NOS
> Healing pressure ulcer of unspecified hip, unspecified stage

● **L89.21**   **Pressure ulcer of right hip**

L89.210   **Pressure ulcer of right hip, unstageable**

L89.211   **Pressure ulcer of right hip, stage 1**
> Healing pressure ulcer of right hip back, stage 1
> Pressure pre-ulcer skin changes limited to persistent focal edema, right hip

L89.212   **Pressure ulcer of right hip, stage 2**
> Healing pressure ulcer of right hip, stage 2
> Pressure ulcer with abrasion, blister, partial thickness skin loss involving epidermis and/or dermis, right hip

L89.213   **Pressure ulcer of right hip, stage 3** 🔖 🔖
> Healing pressure ulcer of right hip, stage 3
> Pressure ulcer with full thickness skin loss involving damage or necrosis of subcutaneous tissue, right hip
> MCC when PDx is its own MCC

L89.214   **Pressure ulcer of right hip, stage 4** 🔖 🔖
> Healing pressure ulcer of right hip, stage 4
> Pressure ulcer with necrosis of soft tissues through to underlying muscle, tendon, or bone, right hip
> MCC when PDx is its own MCC

L89.219   **Pressure ulcer of right hip, unspecified stage**
> Healing pressure ulcer of right hip NOS
> Healing pressure ulcer of right hip, unspecified stage

▶ New   ⇒ Revised   ~~deleted~~ Deleted   Excludes 1   Excludes 2   Includes   Use additional   Code first   Code also   Key words

OGCR Official Guidelines   ● Unacceptable Principal Diagnosis   X Assign placeholder X   ● Use Additional Character(s)   ▶ Manifestation Code   **Coding Clinic**

● **L89.22** **Pressure ulcer of left hip**

L89.220 **Pressure ulcer of left hip, unstageable**

L89.221 **Pressure ulcer of left hip, stage 1**
Healing pressure ulcer of left hip back, stage 1
Pressure pre-ulcer skin changes limited to persistent focal edema, left hip

L89.222 **Pressure ulcer of left hip, stage 2**
Healing pressure ulcer of left hip, stage 2
Pressure ulcer with abrasion, blister, partial thickness skin loss involving epidermis and/or dermis, left hip

L89.223 **Pressure ulcer of left hip, stage 3** 🦠 🦠
Healing pressure ulcer of left hip, stage 3
Pressure ulcer with full thickness skin loss involving damage or necrosis of subcutaneous tissue, left hip
MCC when PDx is its own MCC

L89.224 **Pressure ulcer of left hip, stage 4** 🦠 🦠
Healing pressure ulcer of left hip, stage 4
Pressure ulcer with necrosis of soft tissues through to underlying muscle, tendon, or bone, left hip
MCC when PDx is its own MCC

L89.229 **Pressure ulcer of left hip, unspecified stage**
Healing pressure ulcer of left hip NOS
Healing pressure ulcer of left hip, unspecified stage

● **L89.3** **Pressure ulcer of buttock**

● **L89.30** **Pressure ulcer of unspecified buttock**

L89.300 **Pressure ulcer of unspecified buttock, unstageable**

L89.301 **Pressure ulcer of unspecified buttock, stage 1**
Healing pressure ulcer of unspecified buttock, stage 1
Pressure pre-ulcer skin changes limited to persistent focal edema, unspecified buttock

L89.302 **Pressure ulcer of unspecified buttock, stage 2**
Healing pressure ulcer of unspecified buttock, stage 2
Pressure ulcer with abrasion, blister, partial thickness skin loss involving epidermis and/or dermis, unspecified buttock

L89.303 **Pressure ulcer of unspecified buttock, stage 3** 🦠 🦠
Healing pressure ulcer of unspecified buttock, stage 3
Pressure ulcer with full thickness skin loss involving damage or necrosis of subcutaneous tissue, unspecified buttock
MCC when PDx is its own MCC

L89.304 **Pressure ulcer of unspecified buttock, stage 4** 🦠 🦠
Healing pressure ulcer of unspecified buttock, stage 4
Pressure ulcer with necrosis of soft tissues through to underlying muscle, tendon, or bone, unspecified buttock
MCC when PDx is its own MCC

L89.309 **Pressure ulcer of unspecified buttock, unspecified stage**
Healing pressure ulcer of unspecified buttock NOS
Healing pressure ulcer of unspecified buttock, unspecified stage

● **L89.31** **Pressure ulcer of right buttock**

L89.310 **Pressure ulcer of right buttock, unstageable**

L89.311 **Pressure ulcer of right buttock, stage 1**
Healing pressure ulcer of right buttock, stage 1
Pressure pre-ulcer skin changes limited to persistent focal edema, right buttock

L89.312 **Pressure ulcer of right buttock, stage 2**
Healing pressure ulcer of right buttock, stage 2
Pressure ulcer with abrasion, blister, partial thickness skin loss involving epidermis and/or dermis, right buttock

L89.313 **Pressure ulcer of right buttock, stage 3** 🦠 🦠
Healing pressure ulcer of right buttock, stage 3
Pressure ulcer with full thickness skin loss involving damage or necrosis of subcutaneous tissue, right buttock
MCC when PDx is its own MCC

L89.314 **Pressure ulcer of right buttock, stage 4** 🦠 🦠
Healing pressure ulcer of right buttock, stage 4
Pressure ulcer with necrosis of soft tissues through to underlying muscle, tendon, or bone, right buttock
MCC when PDx is its own MCC

L89.319 **Pressure ulcer of right buttock, unspecified stage**
Healing pressure ulcer of right buttock NOS
Healing pressure ulcer of right buttock, unspecified stage

● **L89.32** **Pressure ulcer of left buttock**

L89.320 **Pressure ulcer of left buttock, unstageable**

L89.321 **Pressure ulcer of left buttock, stage 1**
Healing pressure ulcer of left buttock, stage 1
Pressure pre-ulcer skin changes limited to persistent focal edema, left buttock

L89.322 **Pressure ulcer of left buttock, stage 2**
Healing pressure ulcer of left buttock, stage 2
Pressure ulcer with abrasion, blister, partial thickness skin loss involving epidermis and/or dermis, left buttock

N Newborn Age: 0   **P** Pediatric Age: 0–17   **M** Maternity DX: 12–55   **A** Adult Age: 15–124   ♀ Females Only   ♂ Males Only

🦠 Complication\Comorbidity   🦠 Major C\C   (Ex:) CC/MCC Exclusions   🦠 Hospital-Acquired Condition

979

CHAPTER 12 (L00–L99)

CHAPTER 12 (L00-L99)

L89.323   **Pressure ulcer of left buttock, stage 3** 🔖🔖
     Healing pressure ulcer of left buttock, stage 3
     Pressure ulcer with full thickness skin loss involving damage or necrosis of subcutaneous tissue, left buttock
     MCC when PDx is its own MCC

L89.324   **Pressure ulcer of left buttock, stage 4** 🔖🔖
     Healing pressure ulcer of left buttock, stage 4
     Pressure ulcer with necrosis of soft tissues through to underlying muscle, tendon, or bone, left buttock
     MCC when PDx is its own MCC

L89.329   **Pressure ulcer of left buttock, unspecified stage**
     Healing pressure ulcer of left buttock NOS
     Healing pressure ulcer of left buttock, unspecified stage

● **L89.4**   **Pressure ulcer of contiguous site of back, buttock and hip**

L89.40   **Pressure ulcer of contiguous site of back, buttock and hip, unspecified stage**
     Healing pressure ulcer of contiguous site of back, buttock and hip NOS
     Healing pressure ulcer of contiguous site of back, buttock and hip, unspecified stage

L89.41   **Pressure ulcer of contiguous site of back, buttock and hip, stage 1**
     Healing pressure ulcer of contiguous site of back, buttock and hip, stage 1
     Pressure pre-ulcer skin changes limited to persistent focal edema, contiguous site of back, buttock and hip

L89.42   **Pressure ulcer of contiguous site of back, buttock and hip, stage 2**
     Healing pressure ulcer of contiguous site of back, buttock and hip, stage 2
     Pressure ulcer with abrasion, blister, partial thickness skin loss involving epidermis and/or dermis, contiguous site of back, buttock and hip

L89.43   **Pressure ulcer of contiguous site of back, buttock and hip, stage 3** 🔖🔖
     Healing pressure ulcer of contiguous site of back, buttock and hip, stage 3
     Pressure ulcer with full thickness skin loss involving damage or necrosis of subcutaneous tissue, contiguous site of back, buttock and hip
     MCC when PDx is its own MCC

L89.44   **Pressure ulcer of contiguous site of back, buttock and hip, stage 4** 🔖🔖
     Healing pressure ulcer of contiguous site of back, buttock and hip, stage 4
     Pressure ulcer with necrosis of soft tissues through to underlying muscle, tendon, or bone, contiguous site of back, buttock and hip
     MCC when PDx is its own MCC

L89.45   **Pressure ulcer of contiguous site of back, buttock and hip, unstageable**

● **L89.5**   **Pressure ulcer of ankle**

● **L89.50**   **Pressure ulcer of unspecified ankle**

L89.500   **Pressure ulcer of unspecified ankle, unstageable**

L89.501   **Pressure ulcer of unspecified ankle, stage 1**
     Healing pressure ulcer of unspecified ankle, stage 1
     Pressure pre-ulcer skin changes limited to persistent focal edema, unspecified ankle

L89.502   **Pressure ulcer of unspecified ankle, stage 2**
     Healing pressure ulcer of unspecified ankle, stage 2
     Pressure ulcer with abrasion, blister, partial thickness skin loss involving epidermis and/or dermis, unspecified ankle

L89.503   **Pressure ulcer of unspecified ankle, stage 3** 🔖🔖
     Healing pressure ulcer of unspecified ankle, stage 3
     Pressure ulcer with full thickness skin loss involving damage or necrosis of subcutaneous tissue, unspecified ankle
     MCC when PDx is its own MCC

L89.504   **Pressure ulcer of unspecified ankle, stage 4** 🔖🔖
     Healing pressure ulcer of unspecified ankle, stage 4
     Pressure ulcer with necrosis of soft tissues through to underlying muscle, tendon, or bone, unspecified ankle
     MCC when PDx is its own MCC

L89.509   **Pressure ulcer of unspecified ankle, unspecified stage**
     Healing pressure ulcer of unspecified ankle NOS
     Healing pressure ulcer of unspecified ankle, unspecified stage

● **L89.51**   **Pressure ulcer of right ankle**

L89.510   **Pressure ulcer of right ankle, unstageable**

L89.511   **Pressure ulcer of right ankle, stage 1**
     Healing pressure ulcer of right ankle, stage 1
     Pressure pre-ulcer skin changes limited to persistent focal edema, right ankle

L89.512   **Pressure ulcer of right ankle, stage 2**
     Healing pressure ulcer of right ankle, stage 2
     Pressure ulcer with abrasion, blister, partial thickness skin loss involving epidermis and/or dermis, right ankle

L89.513   **Pressure ulcer of right ankle, stage 3** 🔖🔖
     Healing pressure ulcer of right ankle, stage 3
     Pressure ulcer with full thickness skin loss involving damage or necrosis of subcutaneous tissue, right ankle
     MCC when PDx is its own MCC

L89.514   Pressure ulcer of right ankle, stage 4 🔖 🔖
   Healing pressure ulcer of right ankle, stage 4
   Pressure ulcer with necrosis of soft tissues through to underlying muscle, tendon, or bone, right ankle
   MCC when PDx is its own MCC

L89.519   Pressure ulcer of right ankle, unspecified stage
   Healing pressure ulcer of right ankle NOS
   Healing pressure ulcer of right ankle, unspecified stage

● **L89.52   Pressure ulcer of left ankle**

L89.520   Pressure ulcer of left ankle, unstageable

L89.521   Pressure ulcer of left ankle, stage 1
   Healing pressure ulcer of left ankle, stage 1
   Pressure pre-ulcer skin changes limited to persistent focal edema, left ankle

L89.522   Pressure ulcer of left ankle, stage 2
   Healing pressure ulcer of left ankle, stage 2
   Pressure ulcer with abrasion, blister, partial thickness skin loss involving epidermis and/or dermis, left ankle

L89.523   Pressure ulcer of left ankle, stage 3 🔖 🔖
   Healing pressure ulcer of left ankle, stage 3
   Pressure ulcer with full thickness skin loss involving damage or necrosis of subcutaneous tissue, left ankle
   MCC when PDx is its own MCC

L89.524   Pressure ulcer of left ankle, stage 4 🔖 🔖
   Healing pressure ulcer of left ankle, stage 4
   Pressure ulcer with necrosis of soft tissues through to underlying muscle, tendon, or bone, left ankle
   MCC when PDx is its own MCC

L89.529   Pressure ulcer of left ankle, unspecified stage
   Healing pressure ulcer of left ankle NOS
   Healing pressure ulcer of left ankle, unspecified stage

● **L89.6   Pressure ulcer of heel**

● **L89.60   Pressure ulcer of unspecified heel**

L89.600   Pressure ulcer of unspecified heel, unstageable

L89.601   Pressure ulcer of unspecified heel, stage 1
   Healing pressure ulcer of unspecified heel, stage 1
   Pressure pre-ulcer skin changes limited to persistent focal edema, unspecified heel

L89.602   Pressure ulcer of unspecified heel, stage 2
   Healing pressure ulcer of unspecified heel, stage 2
   Pressure ulcer with abrasion, blister, partial thickness skin loss involving epidermis and/or dermis, unspecified heel

L89.603   Pressure ulcer of unspecified heel, stage 3 🔖 🔖
   Healing pressure ulcer of unspecified heel, stage 3
   Pressure ulcer with full thickness skin loss involving damage or necrosis of subcutaneous tissue, unspecified heel
   MCC when PDx is its own MCC

L89.604   Pressure ulcer of unspecified heel, stage 4 🔖 🔖
   Healing pressure ulcer of unspecified heel, stage 4
   Pressure ulcer with necrosis of soft tissues through to underlying muscle, tendon, or bone, unspecified heel
   MCC when PDx is its own MCC

L89.609   Pressure ulcer of unspecified heel, unspecified stage
   Healing pressure ulcer of unspecified heel NOS
   Healing pressure ulcer of unspecified heel, unspecified stage

● **L89.61   Pressure ulcer of right heel**

L89.610   Pressure ulcer of right heel, unstageable

L89.611   Pressure ulcer of right heel, stage 1
   Healing pressure ulcer of right heel, stage 1
   Pressure pre-ulcer skin changes limited to persistent focal edema, right heel

L89.612   Pressure ulcer of right heel, stage 2
   Healing pressure ulcer of right heel, stage 2
   Pressure ulcer with abrasion, blister, partial thickness skin loss involving epidermis and/or dermis, right heel

L89.613   Pressure ulcer of right heel, stage 3 🔖 🔖
   Healing pressure ulcer of right heel, stage 3
   Pressure ulcer with full thickness skin loss involving damage or necrosis of subcutaneous tissue, right heel
   MCC when PDx is its own MCC

L89.614   Pressure ulcer of right heel, stage 4 🔖 🔖
   Healing pressure ulcer of right heel, stage 4
   Pressure ulcer with necrosis of soft tissues through to underlying muscle, tendon, or bone, right heel
   MCC when PDx is its own MCC

L89.619   Pressure ulcer of right heel, unspecified stage
   Healing pressure ulcer of right heel NOS
➥ Healing pressure ulcer of right heel, unspecified stage

● **L89.62 Pressure ulcer of left heel**

L89.620 Pressure ulcer of left heel, unstageable

L89.621 Pressure ulcer of left heel, stage 1
Healing pressure ulcer of left heel, stage 1
Pressure pre-ulcer skin changes limited to persistent focal edema, left heel

L89.622 Pressure ulcer of left heel, stage 2
Healing pressure ulcer of left heel, stage 2
Pressure ulcer with abrasion, blister, partial thickness skin loss involving epidermis and/or dermis, left heel
Coding Clinic: 2016, Q4, P142

L89.623 Pressure ulcer of left heel, stage 3 🐾 🐾
Healing pressure ulcer of left heel, stage 3
Pressure ulcer with full thickness skin loss involving damage or necrosis of subcutaneous tissue, left heel
MCC when PDx is its own MCC
Coding Clinic: 2016, Q4, P142

L89.624 Pressure ulcer of left heel, stage 4 🐾 🐾
Healing pressure ulcer of left heel, stage 4
Pressure ulcer with necrosis of soft tissues through to underlying muscle, tendon, or bone, left heel
MCC when PDx is its own MCC

L89.629 Pressure ulcer of left heel, unspecified stage
Healing pressure ulcer of left heel NOS
Healing pressure ulcer of left heel, unspecified stage

● **L89.8   Pressure ulcer of other site**

● **L89.81 Pressure ulcer of head**
Pressure ulcer of face

L89.810 Pressure ulcer of head, unstageable

L89.811 Pressure ulcer of head, stage 1
Healing pressure ulcer of head, stage 1
Pressure pre-ulcer skin changes limited to persistent focal edema, head

L89.812 Pressure ulcer of head, stage 2
Healing pressure ulcer of head, stage 2
Pressure ulcer with abrasion, blister, partial thickness skin loss involving epidermis and/or dermis, head

L89.813 Pressure ulcer of head, stage 3 🐾 🐾
Healing pressure ulcer of head, stage 3
Pressure ulcer with full thickness skin loss involving damage or necrosis of subcutaneous tissue, head
MCC when PDx is its own MCC

L89.814 Pressure ulcer of head, stage 4 🐾 🐾
Healing pressure ulcer of head, stage 4
Pressure ulcer with necrosis of soft tissues through to underlying muscle, tendon, or bone, head
MCC when PDx is its own MCC

L89.819 Pressure ulcer of head, unspecified stage
Healing pressure ulcer of head NOS
Healing pressure ulcer of head, unspecified stage

● **L89.89 Pressure ulcer of other site**

L89.890 Pressure ulcer of other site, unstageable

L89.891 Pressure ulcer of other site, stage 1
Healing pressure ulcer of other site, stage 1
Pressure pre-ulcer skin changes limited to persistent focal edema, other site

L89.892 Pressure ulcer of other site, stage 2
Healing pressure ulcer of other site, stage 2
Pressure ulcer with abrasion, blister, partial thickness skin loss involving epidermis and/or dermis, other site

L89.893 Pressure ulcer of other site, stage 3 🐾 🐾
Healing pressure ulcer of other site, stage 3
Pressure ulcer with full thickness skin loss involving damage or necrosis of subcutaneous tissue, other site
MCC when PDx is its own MCC

L89.894 Pressure ulcer of other site, stage 4 🐾 🐾
Healing pressure ulcer of other site, stage 4
Pressure ulcer with necrosis of soft tissues through to underlying muscle, tendon, or bone, other site
MCC when PDx is its own MCC

L89.899 Pressure ulcer of other site, unspecified stage
Healing pressure ulcer of other site NOS
Healing pressure ulcer of other site, unspecified stage

● **L89.9   Pressure ulcer of unspecified site**

L89.90 Pressure ulcer of unspecified site, unspecified stage
Healing pressure ulcer of unspecified site NOS
Healing pressure ulcer of unspecified site, unspecified stage

L89.91 Pressure ulcer of unspecified site, stage 1
Healing pressure ulcer of unspecified site, stage 1
Pressure pre-ulcer skin changes limited to persistent focal edema, unspecified site

L89.92 Pressure ulcer of unspecified site, stage 2
Healing pressure ulcer of unspecified site, stage 2
Pressure ulcer with abrasion, blister, partial thickness skin loss involving epidermis and/or dermis, unspecified site

▶ New   ⇒ Revised   ~~deleted~~ Deleted   Excludes 1   Excludes 2   Includes   Use additional   Code first   Code also   Key words
OGCR Official Guidelines   ● Unacceptable Principal Diagnosis   X Assign placeholder X   ● Use Additional Character(s)   ▶ Manifestation Code   **Coding Clinic**

L89.93 Pressure ulcer of unspecified site, stage 3 🔵 🔵
  Healing pressure ulcer of unspecified site,
    stage 3
  Pressure ulcer with full thickness skin
    loss involving damage or necrosis of
    subcutaneous tissue, unspecified site
  MCC when PDx is its own MCC

L89.94 Pressure ulcer of unspecified site, stage 4 🔵 🔵
  Healing pressure ulcer of unspecified site,
    stage 4
  Pressure ulcer with necrosis of soft tissues
    through to underlying muscle, tendon, or
    bone, unspecified site
  MCC when PDx is its own MCC

L89.95 Pressure ulcer of unspecified site, unstageable

🔵 **L90 Atrophic disorders of skin**

L90.0 Lichen sclerosus et atrophicus
  Excludes2 lichen sclerosus of external female genital
      organs (N90.4)
    lichen sclerosus of external male genital
      organs (N48.0)

L90.1 Anetoderma of Schweninger-Buzzi

L90.2 Anetoderma of Jadassohn-Pellizzari

L90.3 Atrophoderma of Pasini and Pierini

L90.4 Acrodermatitis chronica atrophicans

L90.5 Scar conditions and fibrosis of skin
  Adherent scar (skin)
  Cicatrix
  Disfigurement of skin due to scar
  Fibrosis of skin NOS
  Scar NOS
    Excludes2 hypertrophic scar (L91.0)
        keloid scar (L91.0)
    Coding Clinic: 2016, Q2, P5; 2015, Q1, P19

L90.6 Striae atrophicae

L90.8 Other atrophic disorders of skin

L90.9 Atrophic disorder of skin, unspecified

🔵 **L91 Hypertrophic disorders of skin**

L91.0 Keloid scar
  Hypertrophic scar
  Keloid
    Excludes2 acne keloid (L73.0)
        scar NOS (L90.5)

L91.8 Other hypertrophic disorders of the skin

L91.9 Hypertrophic disorder of the skin, unspecified

🔵 **L92 Granulomatous disorders of skin and subcutaneous tissue**
  Excludes2 actinic granuloma (L57.5)

L92.0 Granuloma annulare
  Perforating granuloma annulare

L92.1 Necrobiosis lipoidica, not elsewhere classified
  Excludes1 necrobiosis lipoidica associated with
      diabetes mellitus (E08-E13 with .620)

L92.2 Granuloma faciale [eosinophilic granuloma of skin]

L92.3 Foreign body granuloma of the skin and subcutaneous tissue
  Use additional code to identify the type of retained
    foreign body (Z18.-)

L92.8 Other granulomatous disorders of the skin and subcutaneous tissue

L92.9 Granulomatous disorder of the skin and subcutaneous tissue, unspecified
  ▶ **Excludes2** umbilical granuloma (P83.81)

Item 12-11   Scleroderma means hard skin. It is a group of diseases that causes abnormal growth of connective tissues that support the skin and organs. There are two types: localized scleroderma affecting the skin and systemic scleroderma affecting blood vessels and internal organs and the skin.

🔵 **L93 Lupus erythematosus**
  Use additional code for adverse effect, if applicable, to identify
    drug (T36-T50 with fifth or sixth character 5)
    Excludes1 lupus exedens (A18.4)
        lupus vulgaris (A18.4)
        scleroderma (M34.-)
        systemic lupus erythematosus (M32.-)

L93.0 Discoid lupus erythematosus
  Lupus erythematosus NOS

L93.1 Subacute cutaneous lupus erythematosus

L93.2 Other local lupus erythematosus
  Lupus erythematosus profundus
  Lupus panniculitis

🔵 **L94 Other localized connective tissue disorders**
  Excludes1 systemic connective tissue disorders (M30-M36)

L94.0 Localized scleroderma [morphea]
  Circumscribed scleroderma

L94.1 Linear scleroderma
  En coup de sabre lesion

L94.2 Calcinosis cutis

L94.3 Sclerodactyly

L94.4 Gottron's papules

L94.5 Poikiloderma vasculare atrophicans

L94.6 Ainhum

L94.8 Other specified localized connective tissue disorders

L94.9 Localized connective tissue disorder, unspecified

🔵 **L95 Vasculitis limited to skin, not elsewhere classified**
  Excludes1 angioma serpiginosum (L81.7)
        Henoch(-Schönlein) purpura (D69.0)
        hypersensitivity angiitis (M31.0)
        lupus panniculitis (L93.2)
        panniculitis NOS (M79.3)
        panniculitis of neck and back (M54.0-)
        polyarteritis nodosa (M30.0)
        relapsing panniculitis (M35.6)
        rheumatoid vasculitis (M05.2)
        serum sickness (T80.6-)
        urticaria (L50.-)
        Wegener's granulomatosis (M31.3-)

L95.0 Livedoid vasculitis
  Atrophie blanche (en plaque)

L95.1 Erythema elevatum diutinum

L95.8 Other vasculitis limited to the skin

L95.9 Vasculitis limited to the skin, unspecified

CHAPTER 12 (L00-L99)

● **L97   Non-pressure chronic ulcer of lower limb, not elsewhere classified**

Includes   chronic ulcer of skin of lower limb NOS
non-healing ulcer of skin
non-infected sinus of skin
trophic ulcer NOS
tropical ulcer NOS
ulcer of skin of lower limb NOS

Code first any associated underlying condition, such as:
any associated gangrene (I96)
atherosclerosis of the lower extremities (I70.23-, I70.24-, I70.33-, I70.34-, I70.43-, I70.44-, I70.53-, I70.54-, I70.63-, I70.64-, I70.73-, I70.74-)
chronic venous hypertension (I87.31-, I87.33-)
diabetic ulcers (E08.621, E08.622, E09.621, E09.622, E10.621, E10.622, E11.621, E11.622, E13.621, E13.622)
postphlebitic syndrome (I87.01-, I87.03-)
postthrombotic syndrome (I87.01-, I87.03-)
varicose ulcer (I83.0-, I83.2-)

Excludes2   pressure ulcer (pressure area) (L89.-)
skin infections (L00-L08)
specific infections classified to A00-B99

(Ex:) **For category L97 CC codes:** See PDX Collection 698

● **L97.1   Non-pressure chronic ulcer of thigh**

● **L97.10   Non-pressure chronic ulcer of unspecified thigh**

L97.101   Non-pressure chronic ulcer of unspecified thigh limited to breakdown of skin 🔍

L97.102   Non-pressure chronic ulcer of unspecified thigh with fat layer exposed 🔍

L97.103   Non-pressure chronic ulcer of unspecified thigh with necrosis of muscle 🔍

L97.104   Non-pressure chronic ulcer of unspecified thigh with necrosis of bone 🔍

▶ L97.105   Non-pressure chronic ulcer of unspecified thigh with muscle involvement without evidence of necrosis 🔍

▶ L97.106   Non-pressure chronic ulcer of unspecified thigh with bone involvement without evidence of necrosis 🔍

▶ L97.108   Non-pressure chronic ulcer of unspecified thigh with other specified severity 🔍

L97.109   Non-pressure chronic ulcer of unspecified thigh with unspecified severity 🔍

● **L97.11   Non-pressure chronic ulcer of right thigh**

L97.111   Non-pressure chronic ulcer of right thigh limited to breakdown of skin 🔍

L97.112   Non-pressure chronic ulcer of right thigh with fat layer exposed 🔍

L97.113   Non-pressure chronic ulcer of right thigh with necrosis of muscle 🔍

L97.114   Non-pressure chronic ulcer of right thigh with necrosis of bone 🔍

▶ L97.115   Non-pressure chronic ulcer of right thigh with muscle involvement without evidence of necrosis 🔍

▶ L97.116   Non-pressure chronic ulcer of right thigh with bone involvement without evidence of necrosis 🔍

▶ L97.118   Non-pressure chronic ulcer of right thigh with other specified severity 🔍

L97.119   Non-pressure chronic ulcer of right thigh with unspecified severity 🔍

● **L97.12   Non-pressure chronic ulcer of left thigh**

L97.121   Non-pressure chronic ulcer of left thigh limited to breakdown of skin 🔍

L97.122   Non-pressure chronic ulcer of left thigh with fat layer exposed 🔍

L97.123   Non-pressure chronic ulcer of left thigh with necrosis of muscle 🔍

L97.124   Non-pressure chronic ulcer of left thigh with necrosis of bone 🔍

▶ L97.125   Non-pressure chronic ulcer of left thigh with muscle involvement without evidence of necrosis 🔍

▶ L97.126   Non-pressure chronic ulcer of left thigh with bone involvement without evidence of necrosis 🔍

▶ L97.128   Non-pressure chronic ulcer of left thigh with other specified severity 🔍

L97.129   Non-pressure chronic ulcer of left thigh with unspecified severity 🔍

● **L97.2   Non-pressure chronic ulcer of calf**

● **L97.20   Non-pressure chronic ulcer of unspecified calf**

L97.201   Non-pressure chronic ulcer of unspecified calf limited to breakdown of skin 🔍

L97.202   Non-pressure chronic ulcer of unspecified calf with fat layer exposed 🔍

L97.203   Non-pressure chronic ulcer of unspecified calf with necrosis of muscle 🔍

L97.204   Non-pressure chronic ulcer of unspecified calf with necrosis of bone 🔍

▶ L97.205   Non-pressure chronic ulcer of unspecified calf with muscle involvement without evidence of necrosis 🔍

▶ L97.206   Non-pressure chronic ulcer of unspecified calf with bone involvement without evidence of necrosis 🔍

▶ L97.208   Non-pressure chronic ulcer of unspecified calf with other specified severity 🔍

L97.209   Non-pressure chronic ulcer of unspecified calf with unspecified severity 🔍

● **L97.21   Non-pressure chronic ulcer of right calf**

L97.211   Non-pressure chronic ulcer of right calf limited to breakdown of skin 🔍

L97.212   Non-pressure chronic ulcer of right calf with fat layer exposed 🔍

L97.213   Non-pressure chronic ulcer of right calf with necrosis of muscle 🔍

L97.214   Non-pressure chronic ulcer of right calf with necrosis of bone 🔍

▶ L97.215   Non-pressure chronic ulcer of right calf with muscle involvement without evidence of necrosis 🔍

▶ L97.216   Non-pressure chronic ulcer of right calf with bone involvement without evidence of necrosis 🔍

▶ L97.218   Non-pressure chronic ulcer of right calf with other specified severity 🔍

L97.219   Non-pressure chronic ulcer of right calf with unspecified severity 🔍

▶ New   ⟹ Revised   ~~deleted~~ Deleted   Excludes 1   Excludes 2   Includes   Use additional   Code first   Code also   Key words
OGCR Official Guidelines   ● Unacceptable Principal Diagnosis   X Assign placeholder X   ● Use Additional Character(s)   ▶ Manifestation Code   **Coding Clinic**

● **L97.22 Non-pressure chronic ulcer of left calf**

    L97.221 **Non-pressure chronic ulcer of left calf limited to breakdown of skin** 🦠

    L97.222 **Non-pressure chronic ulcer of left calf with fat layer exposed** 🦠

    L97.223 **Non-pressure chronic ulcer of left calf with necrosis of muscle** 🦠

    L97.224 **Non-pressure chronic ulcer of left calf with necrosis of bone** 🦠

  ▶ L97.225 **Non-pressure chronic ulcer of left calf with muscle involvement without evidence of necrosis** 🦠

  ▶ L97.226 **Non-pressure chronic ulcer of left calf with bone involvement without evidence of necrosis** 🦠

  ▶ L97.228 **Non-pressure chronic ulcer of left calf with other specified severity** 🦠

    L97.229 **Non-pressure chronic ulcer of left calf with unspecified severity** 🦠

● **L97.3 Non-pressure chronic ulcer of ankle**

 ● **L97.30 Non-pressure chronic ulcer of unspecified ankle**

    L97.301 **Non-pressure chronic ulcer of unspecified ankle limited to breakdown of skin** 🦠

    L97.302 **Non-pressure chronic ulcer of unspecified ankle with fat layer exposed** 🦠

    L97.303 **Non-pressure chronic ulcer of unspecified ankle with necrosis of muscle** 🦠

    L97.304 **Non-pressure chronic ulcer of unspecified ankle with necrosis of bone** 🦠

  ▶ L97.305 **Non-pressure chronic ulcer of unspecified ankle with muscle involvement without evidence of necrosis** 🦠

  ▶ L97.306 **Non-pressure chronic ulcer of unspecified ankle with bone involvement without evidence of necrosis** 🦠

  ▶ L97.308 **Non-pressure chronic ulcer of unspecified ankle with other specified severity** 🦠

    L97.309 **Non-pressure chronic ulcer of unspecified ankle with unspecified severity** 🦠

 ● **L97.31 Non-pressure chronic ulcer of right ankle**

    L97.311 **Non-pressure chronic ulcer of right ankle limited to breakdown of skin** 🦠

    L97.312 **Non-pressure chronic ulcer of right ankle with fat layer exposed** 🦠

    L97.313 **Non-pressure chronic ulcer of right ankle with necrosis of muscle** 🦠

    L97.314 **Non-pressure chronic ulcer of right ankle with necrosis of bone** 🦠

  ▶ L97.315 **Non-pressure chronic ulcer of right ankle with muscle involvement without evidence of necrosis** 🦠

  ▶ L97.316 **Non-pressure chronic ulcer of right ankle with bone involvement without evidence of necrosis** 🦠

  ▶ L97.318 **Non-pressure chronic ulcer of right ankle with other specified severity** 🦠

    L97.319 **Non-pressure chronic ulcer of right ankle with unspecified severity** 🦠

● **L97.32 Non-pressure chronic ulcer of left ankle**

    L97.321 **Non-pressure chronic ulcer of left ankle limited to breakdown of skin** 🦠

    L97.322 **Non-pressure chronic ulcer of left ankle with fat layer exposed** 🦠

    L97.323 **Non-pressure chronic ulcer of left ankle with necrosis of muscle** 🦠

    L97.324 **Non-pressure chronic ulcer of left ankle with necrosis of bone** 🦠

  ▶ L97.325 **Non-pressure chronic ulcer of left ankle with muscle involvement without evidence of necrosis** 🦠

  ▶ L97.326 **Non-pressure chronic ulcer of left ankle with bone involvement without evidence of necrosis** 🦠

  ▶ L97.328 **Non-pressure chronic ulcer of left ankle with other specified severity** 🦠

    L97.329 **Non-pressure chronic ulcer of left ankle with unspecified severity** 🦠

● **L97.4 Non-pressure chronic ulcer of heel and midfoot**
    Non-pressure chronic ulcer of plantar surface of midfoot

 ● **L97.40 Non-pressure chronic ulcer of unspecified heel and midfoot**

    L97.401 **Non-pressure chronic ulcer of unspecified heel and midfoot limited to breakdown of skin** 🦠

    L97.402 **Non-pressure chronic ulcer of unspecified heel and midfoot with fat layer exposed** 🦠

    L97.403 **Non-pressure chronic ulcer of unspecified heel and midfoot with necrosis of muscle** 🦠

    L97.404 **Non-pressure chronic ulcer of unspecified heel and midfoot with necrosis of bone** 🦠

  ▶ L97.405 **Non-pressure chronic ulcer of unspecified heel and midfoot with muscle involvement without evidence of necrosis** 🦠

  ▶ L97.406 **Non-pressure chronic ulcer of unspecified heel and midfoot with bone involvement without evidence of necrosis** 🦠

  ▶ L97.408 **Non-pressure chronic ulcer of unspecified heel and midfoot with other specified severity** 🦠

    L97.409 **Non-pressure chronic ulcer of unspecified heel and midfoot with unspecified severity** 🦠

CHAPTER 12 (L00-L99)

● **L97.41**   **Non-pressure chronic ulcer of right heel and midfoot**

     L97.411   Non-pressure chronic ulcer of right heel and midfoot limited to **breakdown of skin** 🔍

     L97.412   Non-pressure chronic ulcer of right heel and midfoot with **fat layer exposed** 🔍

     L97.413   Non-pressure chronic ulcer of right heel and midfoot with **necrosis of muscle** 🔍

     L97.414   Non-pressure chronic ulcer of right heel and midfoot with **necrosis of bone** 🔍

▶   L97.415   Non-pressure chronic ulcer of right heel and midfoot with **muscle involvement** without evidence of **necrosis** 🔍

▶   L97.416   Non-pressure chronic ulcer of right heel and midfoot with **bone involvement** without evidence of **necrosis** 🔍

▶   L97.418   Non-pressure chronic ulcer of right heel and midfoot with **other specified severity** 🔍

     L97.419   Non-pressure chronic ulcer of right heel and midfoot with **unspecified severity** 🔍

● **L97.42**   **Non-pressure chronic ulcer of left heel and midfoot**

     L97.421   Non-pressure chronic ulcer of left heel and midfoot limited to **breakdown of skin** 🔍
               Coding Clinic: 2016, Q1, P13

     L97.422   Non-pressure chronic ulcer of left heel and midfoot with **fat layer exposed** 🔍

     L97.423   Non-pressure chronic ulcer of left heel and midfoot with **necrosis of muscle** 🔍

     L97.424   Non-pressure chronic ulcer of left heel and midfoot with **necrosis of bone** 🔍

▶   L97.425   Non-pressure chronic ulcer of left heel and midfoot with **muscle involvement** without evidence of **necrosis** 🔍

▶   L97.426   Non-pressure chronic ulcer of left heel and midfoot with **bone involvement** without evidence of **necrosis** 🔍

▶   L97.428   Non-pressure chronic ulcer of left heel and midfoot with **other specified severity** 🔍

     L97.429   Non-pressure chronic ulcer of left heel and midfoot with **unspecified severity** 🔍

● **L97.5**   **Non-pressure chronic ulcer of other part of foot**
       Non-pressure chronic ulcer of toe

● **L97.50**   **Non-pressure chronic ulcer of other part of unspecified foot**

     L97.501   Non-pressure chronic ulcer of other part of unspecified foot limited to **breakdown of skin**

     L97.502   Non-pressure chronic ulcer of other part of unspecified foot with **fat layer exposed**

     L97.503   Non-pressure chronic ulcer of other part of unspecified foot with **necrosis of muscle**

     L97.504   Non-pressure chronic ulcer of other part of unspecified foot with **necrosis of bone**

▶   L97.505   Non-pressure chronic ulcer of other part of unspecified foot with **muscle involvement** without evidence of **necrosis** 🔍

▶   L97.506   Non-pressure chronic ulcer of other part of unspecified foot with **bone involvement** without evidence of **necrosis** 🔍

▶   L97.508   Non-pressure chronic ulcer of other part of unspecified foot with **other specified severity** 🔍

     L97.509   Non-pressure chronic ulcer of other part of unspecified foot with **unspecified severity**

● **L97.51**   **Non-pressure chronic ulcer of other part of right foot**

     L97.511   Non-pressure chronic ulcer of other part of right foot limited to **breakdown of skin**

     L97.512   Non-pressure chronic ulcer of other part of right foot with **fat layer exposed**

     L97.513   Non-pressure chronic ulcer of other part of right foot with **necrosis of muscle**

     L97.514   Non-pressure chronic ulcer of other part of right foot with **necrosis of bone**

▶   L97.515   Non-pressure chronic ulcer of other part of right foot with **muscle involvement** without evidence of **necrosis** 🔍

▶   L97.516   Non-pressure chronic ulcer of other part of right foot with **bone involvement** without evidence of **necrosis** 🔍

▶   L97.518   Non-pressure chronic ulcer of other part of right foot with **other specified severity** 🔍

     L97.519   Non-pressure chronic ulcer of other part of right foot with **unspecified severity**

● **L97.52** Non-pressure chronic ulcer of other part of left foot

L97.521 Non-pressure chronic ulcer of other part of left foot limited to breakdown of skin

L97.522 Non-pressure chronic ulcer of other part of left foot with fat layer exposed

L97.523 Non-pressure chronic ulcer of other part of left foot with necrosis of muscle

L97.524 Non-pressure chronic ulcer of other part of left foot with necrosis of bone

▶ **L97.525** Non-pressure chronic ulcer of other part of left foot with muscle involvement without evidence of necrosis 🔗

▶ **L97.526** Non-pressure chronic ulcer of other part of left foot with bone involvement without evidence of necrosis 🔗

▶ **L97.528** Non-pressure chronic ulcer of other part of left foot with other specified severity 🔗

L97.529 Non-pressure chronic ulcer of other part of left foot with unspecified severity

● **L97.8** Non-pressure chronic ulcer of other part of lower leg

● **L97.80** Non-pressure chronic ulcer of other part of unspecified lower leg

L97.801 Non-pressure chronic ulcer of other part of unspecified lower leg limited to breakdown of skin 🔗

L97.802 Non-pressure chronic ulcer of other part of unspecified lower leg with fat layer exposed 🔗

L97.803 Non-pressure chronic ulcer of other part of unspecified lower leg with necrosis of muscle 🔗

L97.804 Non-pressure chronic ulcer of other part of unspecified lower leg with necrosis of bone 🔗

▶ **L97.805** Non-pressure chronic ulcer of other part of unspecified lower leg with muscle involvement without evidence of necrosis 🔗

▶ **L97.806** Non-pressure chronic ulcer of other part of unspecified lower leg with bone involvement without evidence of necrosis 🔗

▶ **L97.808** Non-pressure chronic ulcer of other part of unspecified lower leg with other specified severity 🔗

L97.809 Non-pressure chronic ulcer of other part of unspecified lower leg with unspecified severity 🔗

● **L97.81** Non-pressure chronic ulcer of other part of right lower leg

L97.811 Non-pressure chronic ulcer of other part of right lower leg limited to breakdown of skin 🔗

L97.812 Non-pressure chronic ulcer of other part of right lower leg with fat layer exposed 🔗

L97.813 Non-pressure chronic ulcer of other part of right lower leg with necrosis of muscle 🔗

L97.814 Non-pressure chronic ulcer of other part of right lower leg with necrosis of bone 🔗

▶ **L97.815** Non-pressure chronic ulcer of other part of right lower leg with muscle involvement without evidence of necrosis 🔗

▶ **L97.816** Non-pressure chronic ulcer of other part of right lower leg with bone involvement without evidence of necrosis 🔗

▶ **L97.818** Non-pressure chronic ulcer of other part of right lower leg with other specified severity 🔗

L97.819 Non-pressure chronic ulcer of other part of right lower leg with unspecified severity 🔗

● **L97.82** Non-pressure chronic ulcer of other part of left lower leg

L97.821 Non-pressure chronic ulcer of other part of left lower leg limited to breakdown of skin 🔗

L97.822 Non-pressure chronic ulcer of other part of left lower leg with fat layer exposed 🔗

L97.823 Non-pressure chronic ulcer of other part of left lower leg with necrosis of muscle 🔗

L97.824 Non-pressure chronic ulcer of other part of left lower leg with necrosis of bone 🔗

▶ **L97.825** Non-pressure chronic ulcer of other part of left lower leg with muscle involvement without evidence of necrosis 🔗

▶ **L97.826** Non-pressure chronic ulcer of other part of left lower leg with bone involvement without evidence of necrosis 🔗

▶ **L97.828** Non-pressure chronic ulcer of other part of left lower leg with other specified severity 🔗

L97.829 Non-pressure chronic ulcer of other part of left lower leg with unspecified severity 🔗

● **L97.9**   **Non-pressure chronic ulcer of unspecified part of lower leg**

  ● **L97.90**   Non-pressure chronic ulcer of unspecified part of unspecified lower leg

    L97.901   Non-pressure chronic ulcer of unspecified part of unspecified lower leg limited to breakdown of skin 🔍

    L97.902   Non-pressure chronic ulcer of unspecified part of unspecified lower leg with fat layer exposed 🔍

    L97.903   Non-pressure chronic ulcer of unspecified part of unspecified lower leg with necrosis of muscle 🔍

    L97.904   Non-pressure chronic ulcer of unspecified part of unspecified lower leg with necrosis of bone 🔍

  ▶ **L97.905**   Non-pressure chronic ulcer of unspecified part of unspecified lower leg with muscle involvement without evidence of necrosis 🔍

  ▶ **L97.906**   Non-pressure chronic ulcer of unspecified part of unspecified lower leg with bone involvement without evidence of necrosis 🔍

  ▶ **L97.908**   Non-pressure chronic ulcer of unspecified part of unspecified lower leg with other specified severity 🔍

    L97.909   Non-pressure chronic ulcer of unspecified part of unspecified lower leg with unspecified severity 🔍

  ● **L97.91**   Non-pressure chronic ulcer of unspecified part of right lower leg

    L97.911   Non-pressure chronic ulcer of unspecified part of right lower leg limited to breakdown of skin 🔍

    L97.912   Non-pressure chronic ulcer of unspecified part of right lower leg with fat layer exposed 🔍

    L97.913   Non-pressure chronic ulcer of unspecified part of right lower leg with necrosis of muscle 🔍

    L97.914   Non-pressure chronic ulcer of unspecified part of right lower leg with necrosis of bone 🔍

  ▶ **L97.915**   Non-pressure chronic ulcer of unspecified part of right lower leg with muscle involvement without evidence of necrosis 🔍

  ▶ **L97.916**   Non-pressure chronic ulcer of unspecified part of right lower leg with bone involvement without evidence of necrosis 🔍

  ▶ **L97.918**   Non-pressure chronic ulcer of unspecified part of right lower leg with other specified severity 🔍

    L97.919   Non-pressure chronic ulcer of unspecified part of right lower leg with unspecified severity 🔍

● **L97.92**   Non-pressure chronic ulcer of unspecified part of left lower leg

    L97.921   Non-pressure chronic ulcer of unspecified part of left lower leg limited to breakdown of skin 🔍

    L97.922   Non-pressure chronic ulcer of unspecified part of left lower leg with fat layer exposed 🔍

    L97.923   Non-pressure chronic ulcer of unspecified part of left lower leg with necrosis of muscle 🔍

    L97.924   Non-pressure chronic ulcer of unspecified part of left lower leg with necrosis of bone 🔍

  ▶ **L97.925**   Non-pressure chronic ulcer of unspecified part of left lower leg with muscle involvement without evidence of necrosis 🔍

  ▶ **L97.926**   Non-pressure chronic ulcer of unspecified part of left lower leg with bone involvement without evidence of necrosis 🔍

  ▶ **L97.928**   Non-pressure chronic ulcer of unspecified part of left lower leg with other specified severity 🔍

    L97.929   Non-pressure chronic ulcer of unspecified part of left lower leg with unspecified severity 🔍

● **L98**   **Other disorders of skin and subcutaneous tissue, not elsewhere classified**

  L98.0   **Pyogenic granuloma**

    Excludes2   pyogenic granuloma of gingiva (K06.8)
                  pyogenic granuloma of maxillary alveolar ridge (K04.5)
                  pyogenic granuloma of oral mucosa (K13.4)

  L98.1   **Factitial dermatitis**
    Neurotic excoriation

    Excludes1   Excoriation (skin-picking) disorder (F42.4)

    Coding Clinic: 2016, Q4, P15

  L98.2   **Febrile neutrophilic dermatosis [Sweet]**

  L98.3   **Eosinophilic cellulitis [Wells]** 🔍
    (Ex:) See PDX Collection 839

  ● **L98.4**   **Non-pressure chronic ulcer of skin, not elsewhere classified**
    Chronic ulcer of skin NOS
    Tropical ulcer NOS
    Ulcer of skin NOS

    Excludes2   pressure ulcer (pressure area) (L89.-)
                  gangrene (I96)
                  skin infections (L00-L08)
                  specific infections classified to A00-B99
                  ulcer of lower limb NEC (L97.-)
                  varicose ulcer (I83.0-I82.2)

    ● **L98.41**   Non-pressure chronic ulcer of buttock

      L98.411   Non-pressure chronic ulcer of buttock limited to breakdown of skin

      L98.412   Non-pressure chronic ulcer of buttock with fat layer exposed

▶ New   ▧ Revised   ~~deleted~~ Deleted   Excludes 1   Excludes 2   Includes   Use additional   Code first   Code also   Key words

OGCR Official Guidelines   ● Unacceptable Principal Diagnosis   X Assign placeholder X   ● Use Additional Character(s)   ▶ Manifestation Code   **Coding Clinic**

L98.413   **Non-pressure chronic ulcer of buttock with necrosis of muscle**

L98.414   **Non-pressure chronic ulcer of buttock with necrosis of bone**

▶ L98.415   **Non-pressure chronic ulcer of buttock with muscle involvement without evidence of necrosis** 🔧

▶ L98.416   **Non-pressure chronic ulcer of buttock with bone involvement without evidence of necrosis** 🔧

▶ L98.418   **Non-pressure chronic ulcer of buttock with other specified severity** 🔧

L98.419   **Non-pressure chronic ulcer of buttock with unspecified severity**

● **L98.42   Non-pressure chronic ulcer of back**

L98.421   **Non-pressure chronic ulcer of back limited to breakdown of skin**

L98.422   **Non-pressure chronic ulcer of back with fat layer exposed**

L98.423   **Non-pressure chronic ulcer of back with necrosis of muscle**

L98.424   **Non-pressure chronic ulcer of back with necrosis of bone**

▶ L98.425   **Non-pressure chronic ulcer of back with muscle involvement without evidence of necrosis** 🔧

▶ L98.426   **Non-pressure chronic ulcer of back with bone involvement without evidence of necrosis** 🔧

▶ L98.428   **Non-pressure chronic ulcer of back with other specified severity** 🔧

L98.429   **Non-pressure chronic ulcer of back with unspecified severity**

● **L98.49   Non-pressure chronic ulcer of skin of other sites**

Non-pressure chronic ulcer of skin NOS

L98.491   **Non-pressure chronic ulcer of skin of other sites limited to breakdown of skin**

L98.492   **Non-pressure chronic ulcer of skin of other sites with fat layer exposed**

L98.493   **Non-pressure chronic ulcer of skin of other sites with necrosis of muscle**

L98.494   **Non-pressure chronic ulcer of skin of other sites with necrosis of bone**

▶ L98.495   **Non-pressure chronic ulcer of other sites with muscle involvement without evidence of necrosis** 🔧

▶ L98.496   **Non-pressure chronic ulcer of other sites with bone involvement without evidence of necrosis** 🔧

▶ L98.498   **Non-pressure chronic ulcer of other sites with other specified severity** 🔧

L98.499   **Non-pressure chronic ulcer of skin of other sites with unspecified severity**

L98.5   **Mucinosis of the skin**

Focal mucinosis

Lichen myxedematosus

Reticular erythematous mucinosis

Excludes1   focal oral mucinosis (K13.79)

myxedema (E03.9)

L98.6   **Other infiltrative disorders of the skin and subcutaneous tissue**

Excludes1   hyalinosis cutis et mucosae (E78.89)

L98.7   **Excessive and redundant skin and subcutaneous tissue**

Loose or sagging skin following bariatric surgery weight loss

Loose or sagging skin following dietary weight loss

Loose or sagging skin, NOS

Excludes2   acquired excess or redundant skin of eyelid (H02.3-)

congenital excess or redundant skin of eyelid (Q10.3)

skin changes due to chronic exposure to nonionizing radiation (L57.-)

Coding Clinic: 2016, Q4, P36

L98.8   **Other specified disorders of the skin and subcutaneous tissue**

Coding Clinic: 2013, Q2, P32

L98.9   **Disorder of the skin and subcutaneous tissue, unspecified**

▶ *L99*   *Other disorders of skin and subcutaneous tissue in diseases classified elsewhere*

Code first underlying disease, such as:

amyloidosis (E85.-)

Excludes1   skin disorders in diabetes (E08-E13 with .62)

skin disorders in gonorrhea (A54.89)

skin disorders in syphilis (A51.31, A52.79)

N Newborn Age: 0   **P** Pediatric Age: 0–17   **M** Maternity DX: 12–55   **A** Adult Age: 15–124   ♀ Females Only   ♂ Males Only

🔧 Complication\Comorbidity   🔧 Major C\C   (Ex) CC/MCC Exclusions   🔧 Hospital-Acquired Condition

989

CHAPTER 13

DISEASES OF THE MUSCULOSKELETAL SYSTEM AND CONNECTIVE TISSUE (M00-M99)

OGCR Chapter-Specific Coding Guidelines

13. **Chapter 13: Diseases of the Musculoskeletal System and Connective Tissue (M00-M99)**

    a. Site and laterality

    Most of the codes within Chapter 13 have site and laterality designations. The site represents the bone, joint or the muscle involved. For some conditions where more than one bone, joint or muscle is usually involved, such as osteoarthritis, there is a "multiple sites" code available. For categories where no multiple site code is provided and more than one bone, joint or muscle is involved, multiple codes should be used to indicate the different sites involved.

    1) Bone versus joint

    For certain conditions, the bone may be affected at the upper or lower end, (e.g., avascular necrosis of bone, M87, Osteoporosis, M80, M81). Though the portion of the bone affected may be at the joint, the site designation will be the bone, not the joint.

    b. Acute traumatic versus chronic or recurrent musculoskeletal conditions

    Many musculoskeletal conditions are a result of previous injury or trauma to a site, or are recurrent conditions. Bone, joint or muscle conditions that are the result of a healed injury are usually found in chapter 13. Recurrent bone, joint or muscle conditions are also usually found in chapter 13. Any current, acute injury should be coded to the appropriate injury code from chapter 19. Chronic or recurrent conditions should generally be coded with a code from chapter 13. If it is difficult to determine from the documentation in the record which code is best to describe a condition, query the provider.

    c. Coding of Pathologic Fractures

    7th character A is for use as long as the patient is receiving active treatment for the fracture. While the patient may be seen by a new or different provider over the course of treatment for a pathological fracture, assignment of the 7th character is based on whether the patient is undergoing active treatment and not whether the provider is seeing the patient for the first time.

    7th character, D is to be used for encounters after the patient has completed active treatment **for the fracture and is receiving routine care for the fracture during the healing or recovery phase**. The other 7th characters, listed under each subcategory in the Tabular List, are to be used for subsequent encounters for treatment of problems associated with the healing, such as malunions, nonunions, and sequelae.

    Care for complications of surgical treatment for fracture repairs during the healing or recovery phase should be coded with the appropriate complication codes.

    See Section I.C.19. Coding of traumatic fractures.

    d. Osteoporosis

    Osteoporosis is a systemic condition, meaning that all bones of the musculoskeletal system are affected. Therefore, site is not a component of the codes under category M81, Osteoporosis without current pathological fracture. The site codes under category M80, Osteoporosis with current pathological fracture, identify the site of the fracture, not the osteoporosis.

    1) Osteoporosis without pathological fracture

    Category M81, Osteoporosis without current pathological fracture, is for use for patients with osteoporosis who do not currently have a pathologic fracture due to the osteoporosis, even if they have had a fracture in the past. For patients with a history of osteoporosis fractures, status code Z87.310, Personal history of (healed) osteoporosis fracture, should follow the code from M81.

    2) Osteoporosis with current pathological fracture

    Category M80, Osteoporosis with current pathological fracture, is for patients who have a current pathologic fracture at the time of an encounter. The codes under M80 identify the site of the fracture. A code from category M80, not a traumatic fracture code, should be used for any patient with known osteoporosis who suffers a fracture, even if the patient had a minor fall or trauma, if that fall or trauma would not usually break a normal, healthy bone.

CHAPTER 13

DISEASES OF THE MUSCULOSKELETAL SYSTEM AND CONNECTIVE TISSUE (M00-M99)

Note: Use an external cause code following the code for the musculoskeletal condition, if applicable, to identify the cause of the musculoskeletal condition

Excludes2 arthropathic psoriasis (L40.5-)

certain conditions originating in the perinatal period (P04-P96)

certain infectious and parasitic diseases (A00-B99)

compartment syndrome (traumatic) (T79.A-)

complications of pregnancy, childbirth and the puerperium (O00-O9A)

congenital malformations, deformations, and chromosomal abnormalities (Q00-Q99)

endocrine, nutritional and metabolic diseases (E00-E88)

injury, poisoning and certain other consequences of external causes (S00-T88)

neoplasms (C00-D49)

symptoms, signs and abnormal clinical and laboratory findings, not elsewhere classified (R00-R94)

This chapter contains the following blocks:

M00-M02	Infectious arthropathies
~~M04~~	~~Autoinflammatory syndromes~~
M05-M14	Inflammatory polyarthropathies
M15-M19	Osteoarthritis
M20-M25	Other joint disorders
M26-M27	Dentofacial anomalies [including malocclusion] and other disorders of jaw
M30-M36	Systemic connective tissue disorders
M40-M43	Deforming dorsopathies
M45-M49	Spondylopathies
M50-M54	Other dorsopathies
M60-M63	Disorders of muscles
M65-M67	Disorders of synovium and tendon
M70-M79	Other soft tissue disorders
M80-M85	Disorders of bone density and structure
M86-M90	Other osteopathies
M91-M94	Chondropathies
M95	Other disorders of the musculoskeletal system and connective tissue
M96	Intraoperative and postprocedural complications and disorders of musculoskeletal system, not elsewhere classified
~~M97~~	~~Periprosthetic fracture around internal prosthetic joint~~
M99	Biomechanical lesions, not elsewhere classified

Coding Clinic: 2016, Q4, P124

ARTHROPATHIES (M00-M25)

Includes Disorders affecting predominantly peripheral (limb) joints

INFECTIOUS ARTHROPATHIES (M00-M02)

Note: This block comprises arthropathies due to microbiological agents.

Distinction is made between the following types of etiological relationship:

a) direct infection of joint, where organisms invade synovial tissue and microbial antigen is present in the joint;

b) indirect infection, which may be of two types: a reactive arthropathy, where microbial infection of the body is established but neither organisms nor antigens can be identified in the joint, and a postinfective arthropathy, where microbial antigen is present but recovery of an organism is inconstant and evidence of local multiplication is lacking.

▶ New ⟾ Revised ~~deleted~~ Deleted Excludes 1 Excludes 2 Includes Use additional Code first Code also Key words

OGCR Official Guidelines ● Unacceptable Principal Diagnosis X Assign placeholder X ● Use Additional Character(s) ▶ Manifestation Code **Coding Clinic**

● **M00 Pyogenic arthritis**
  ● **M00.0 Staphylococcal arthritis and polyarthritis**
      Use additional code (B95.61-B95.8) to identify bacterial agent

      Excludes2 infection and inflammatory reaction due to internal joint prosthesis (T84.5-)

    M00.00 Staphylococcal arthritis, unspecified joint 🦠
      Ⓔx See PDX Collection 855
    ● **M00.01 Staphylococcal arthritis, shoulder**
      Ⓔx For category M00.01 CC codes: See PDX Collection 856
      M00.011 Staphylococcal arthritis, right shoulder 🦠
      M00.012 Staphylococcal arthritis, left shoulder 🦠
      M00.019 Staphylococcal arthritis, unspecified shoulder 🦠
    ● **M00.02 Staphylococcal arthritis, elbow**
      Ⓔx For category M00.02 CC codes: See PDX Collection 857
      M00.021 Staphylococcal arthritis, right elbow 🦠
      M00.022 Staphylococcal arthritis, left elbow 🦠
      M00.029 Staphylococcal arthritis, unspecified elbow 🦠
    ● **M00.03 Staphylococcal arthritis, wrist**
      Staphylococcal arthritis of carpal bones
      Ⓔx For category M00.03 CC codes: See PDX Collection 858
      M00.031 Staphylococcal arthritis, right wrist 🦠
      M00.032 Staphylococcal arthritis, left wrist 🦠
      M00.039 Staphylococcal arthritis, unspecified wrist 🦠
    ● **M00.04 Staphylococcal arthritis, hand**
      Staphylococcal arthritis of metacarpus and phalanges
      Ⓔx For category M00.04 CC codes: See PDX Collection 859
      M00.041 Staphylococcal arthritis, right hand 🦠
      M00.042 Staphylococcal arthritis, left hand 🦠
      M00.049 Staphylococcal arthritis, unspecified hand 🦠
    ● **M00.05 Staphylococcal arthritis, hip**
      Ⓔx For category M00.05 CC codes: See PDX Collection 860
      M00.051 Staphylococcal arthritis, right hip 🦠
      M00.052 Staphylococcal arthritis, left hip 🦠
      M00.059 Staphylococcal arthritis, unspecified hip 🦠
    ● **M00.06 Staphylococcal arthritis, knee**
      Ⓔx For category M00.06 CC codes: See PDX Collection 861
      M00.061 Staphylococcal arthritis, right knee 🦠
      M00.062 Staphylococcal arthritis, left knee 🦠
      M00.069 Staphylococcal arthritis, unspecified knee 🦠
    ● **M00.07 Staphylococcal arthritis, ankle and foot**
      Staphylococcal arthritis, tarsus, metatarsus and phalanges
      Ⓔx For category M00.07 CC codes: See PDX Collection 862
      M00.071 Staphylococcal arthritis, right ankle and foot 🦠
      M00.072 Staphylococcal arthritis, left ankle and foot 🦠
      M00.079 Staphylococcal arthritis, unspecified ankle and foot 🦠
    M00.08 Staphylococcal arthritis, vertebrae 🦠
      Ⓔx See PDX Collection 855
    M00.09 Staphylococcal polyarthritis 🦠
      Ⓔx See PDX Collection 855

● **M00.1 Pneumococcal arthritis and polyarthritis**
    M00.10 Pneumococcal arthritis, unspecified joint 🦠
      Ⓔx See PDX Collection 855
    ● **M00.11 Pneumococcal arthritis, shoulder**
      Ⓔx For category M00.11 CC codes: See PDX Collection 856
      M00.111 Pneumococcal arthritis, right shoulder 🦠
      M00.112 Pneumococcal arthritis, left shoulder 🦠
      M00.119 Pneumococcal arthritis, unspecified shoulder 🦠
    ● **M00.12 Pneumococcal arthritis, elbow**
      Ⓔx For category M00.12 CC codes: See PDX Collection 857
      M00.121 Pneumococcal arthritis, right elbow 🦠
      M00.122 Pneumococcal arthritis, left elbow 🦠
      M00.129 Pneumococcal arthritis, unspecified elbow 🦠
    ● **M00.13 Pneumococcal arthritis, wrist**
      Pneumococcal arthritis of carpal bones
      Ⓔx For category M00.13 CC codes: See PDX Collection 858
      M00.131 Pneumococcal arthritis, right wrist 🦠
      M00.132 Pneumococcal arthritis, left wrist 🦠
      M00.139 Pneumococcal arthritis, unspecified wrist 🦠
    ● **M00.14 Pneumococcal arthritis, hand**
      Pneumococcal arthritis of metacarpus and phalanges
      Ⓔx For category M00.14 CC codes: See PDX Collection 859
      M00.141 Pneumococcal arthritis, right hand 🦠
      M00.142 Pneumococcal arthritis, left hand 🦠
      M00.149 Pneumococcal arthritis, unspecified hand 🦠
    ● **M00.15 Pneumococcal arthritis, hip**
      Ⓔx For category M00.15 CC codes: See PDX Collection 860
      M00.151 Pneumococcal arthritis, right hip 🦠
      M00.152 Pneumococcal arthritis, left hip 🦠
      M00.159 Pneumococcal arthritis, unspecified hip 🦠
    ● **M00.16 Pneumococcal arthritis, knee**
      Ⓔx For category M00.16 CC codes: See PDX Collection 861
      M00.161 Pneumococcal arthritis, right knee 🦠
      M00.162 Pneumococcal arthritis, left knee 🦠
      M00.169 Pneumococcal arthritis, unspecified knee 🦠
    ● **M00.17 Pneumococcal arthritis, ankle and foot**
      Pneumococcal arthritis, tarsus, metatarsus and phalanges
      Ⓔx For category M00.17 CC codes: See PDX Collection 862
      M00.171 Pneumococcal arthritis, right ankle and foot 🦠
      M00.172 Pneumococcal arthritis, left ankle and foot 🦠
      M00.179 Pneumococcal arthritis, unspecified ankle and foot 🦠
    M00.18 Pneumococcal arthritis, vertebrae 🦠
      Ⓔx See PDX Collection 855
    M00.19 Pneumococcal polyarthritis 🦠
      Ⓔx See PDX Collection 855

N Newborn Age: 0   P Pediatric Age: 0–17   M Maternity DX: 12–55   A Adult Age: 15–124   ♀ Females Only   ♂ Males Only
🦠 Complication\Comorbidity   🦠 Major C\C   Ⓔx CC/MCC Exclusions   🦠 Hospital-Acquired Condition

CHAPTER 13 (M00-M99)

● **M00.2 Other streptococcal arthritis and polyarthritis**
    Use additional code (B95.0-B95.2, B95.4-B95.5) to
    identify bacterial agent

    **M00.20 Other streptococcal arthritis, unspecified
             joint** 🔍
             Ⓔ See PDX Collection 855

    ● **M00.21 Other streptococcal arthritis, shoulder**
             Ⓔ For category M00.21 CC codes: See PDX Collection 856

        **M00.211 Other streptococcal arthritis, right
                  shoulder** 🔍

        **M00.212 Other streptococcal arthritis, left
                  shoulder** 🔍

        **M00.219 Other streptococcal arthritis,
                  unspecified shoulder** 🔍

    ● **M00.22 Other streptococcal arthritis, elbow**
             Ⓔ For category M00.22 CC codes: See PDX Collection 857

        **M00.221 Other streptococcal arthritis, right
                  elbow** 🔍

        **M00.222 Other streptococcal arthritis, left
                  elbow** 🔍

        **M00.229 Other streptococcal arthritis,
                  unspecified elbow** 🔍

    ● **M00.23 Other streptococcal arthritis, wrist**
             Other streptococcal arthritis of carpal bones
             Ⓔ For category M00.23 CC codes: See PDX Collection 858

        **M00.231 Other streptococcal arthritis, right
                  wrist** 🔍

        **M00.232 Other streptococcal arthritis, left
                  wrist** 🔍

        **M00.239 Other streptococcal arthritis,
                  unspecified wrist** 🔍

    ● **M00.24 Other streptococcal arthritis, hand**
             Other streptococcal arthritis metacarpus and
             phalanges
             Ⓔ For category M00.24 CC codes: See PDX Collection 859

        **M00.241 Other streptococcal arthritis, right
                  hand** 🔍

        **M00.242 Other streptococcal arthritis, left
                  hand** 🔍

        **M00.249 Other streptococcal arthritis,
                  unspecified hand** 🔍

    ● **M00.25 Other streptococcal arthritis, hip**
             Ⓔ For category M00.25 CC codes: See PDX Collection 860

        **M00.251 Other streptococcal arthritis, right
                  hip** 🔍

        **M00.252 Other streptococcal arthritis, left
                  hip** 🔍

        **M00.259 Other streptococcal arthritis,
                  unspecified hip** 🔍

    ● **M00.26 Other streptococcal arthritis, knee**
             Ⓔ For category M00.26 CC codes: See PDX Collection 861

        **M00.261 Other streptococcal arthritis, right
                  knee** 🔍

        **M00.262 Other streptococcal arthritis, left
                  knee** 🔍

        **M00.269 Other streptococcal arthritis,
                  unspecified knee** 🔍

    ● **M00.27 Other streptococcal arthritis, ankle and foot**
             Other streptococcal arthritis, tarsus, metatarsus
             and phalanges
             Ⓔ For category M00.27 CC codes: See PDX Collection 862

        **M00.271 Other streptococcal arthritis, right
                  ankle and foot** 🔍

        **M00.272 Other streptococcal arthritis, left
                  ankle and foot** 🔍

        **M00.279 Other streptococcal arthritis,
                  unspecified ankle and foot** 🔍

    M00.28 Other streptococcal arthritis, vertebrae 🔍
             Ⓔ See PDX Collection 855

    M00.29 Other streptococcal polyarthritis 🔍
             Ⓔ See PDX Collection 855

● **M00.8 Arthritis and polyarthritis due to other bacteria**
    Use additional code (B96) to identify bacteria

    **M00.80 Arthritis due to other bacteria, unspecified
             joint** 🔍
             Ⓔ See PDX Collection 855

    ● **M00.81 Arthritis due to other bacteria, shoulder**
             Ⓔ For category M00.81 CC codes: See PDX Collection 856

        **M00.811 Arthritis due to other bacteria, right
                  shoulder** 🔍

        **M00.812 Arthritis due to other bacteria, left
                  shoulder** 🔍

        **M00.819 Arthritis due to other bacteria,
                  unspecified shoulder** 🔍

    ● **M00.82 Arthritis due to other bacteria, elbow**
             Ⓔ For category M00.82 CC codes: See PDX Collection 857

        **M00.821 Arthritis due to other bacteria, right
                  elbow** 🔍

        **M00.822 Arthritis due to other bacteria, left
                  elbow** 🔍

        **M00.829 Arthritis due to other bacteria,
                  unspecified elbow** 🔍

    ● **M00.83 Arthritis due to other bacteria, wrist**
             Arthritis due to other bacteria, carpal bones
             Ⓔ For category M00.83 CC codes: See PDX Collection 858

        **M00.831 Arthritis due to other bacteria, right
                  wrist** 🔍

        **M00.832 Arthritis due to other bacteria, left
                  wrist** 🔍

        **M00.839 Arthritis due to other bacteria,
                  unspecified wrist** 🔍

    ● **M00.84 Arthritis due to other bacteria, hand**
             Arthritis due to other bacteria, metacarpus and
             phalanges
             Ⓔ For category M00.84 CC codes: See PDX Collection 859

        **M00.841 Arthritis due to other bacteria, right
                  hand** 🔍

        **M00.842 Arthritis due to other bacteria, left
                  hand** 🔍

        **M00.849 Arthritis due to other bacteria,
                  unspecified hand** 🔍

    ● **M00.85 Arthritis due to other bacteria, hip**
             Ⓔ For category M00.85 CC codes: See PDX Collection 860

        **M00.851 Arthritis due to other bacteria, right
                  hip** 🔍

        **M00.852 Arthritis due to other bacteria, left
                  hip** 🔍

        **M00.859 Arthritis due to other bacteria,
                  unspecified hip** 🔍

    ● **M00.86 Arthritis due to other bacteria, knee**
             Ⓔ For category M00.86 CC codes: See PDX Collection 861

        **M00.861 Arthritis due to other bacteria, right
                  knee** 🔍

        **M00.862 Arthritis due to other bacteria, left
                  knee** 🔍

        **M00.869 Arthritis due to other bacteria,
                  unspecified knee** 🔍

    ● **M00.87 Arthritis due to other bacteria, ankle and foot**
             Arthritis due to other bacteria, tarsus,
             metatarsus, and phalanges
             Ⓔ For category M00.87 CC codes: See PDX Collection 862

        **M00.871 Arthritis due to other bacteria, right
                  ankle and foot** 🔍

        **M00.872 Arthritis due to other bacteria, left
                  ankle and foot** 🔍

        **M00.879 Arthritis due to other bacteria,
                  unspecified ankle and foot** 🔍

    M00.88 Arthritis due to other bacteria, vertebrae 🔍
             Ⓔ See PDX Collection 855

    M00.89 Polyarthritis due to other bacteria 🔍
             Ⓔ See PDX Collection 855

M00.9 Pyogenic arthritis, unspecified 🔍
    Infective arthritis NOS
    Ⓔ See PDX Collection 855

▶ New   ⇒ Revised   ~~deleted~~ Deleted   Excludes 1   Excludes 2   Includes   Use additional   Code first   Code also   Key words

OGCR Official Guidelines   ● Unacceptable Principal Diagnosis   X Assign placeholder X   ● Use Additional Character(s)   ▶ Manifestation Code   **Coding Clinic**

● **M01   Direct infections of joint in infectious and parasitic diseases classified elsewhere**

    Code first underlying disease, such as:
      leprosy [Hansen's disease] (A30.-)
      mycoses (B35-B49)
      O'nyong-nyong fever (A92.1)
      paratyphoid fever (A01.1-A01.4)

    Excludes1   arthropathy in Lyme disease (A69.23)
                gonococcal arthritis (A54.42)
                meningococcal arthritis (A39.83)
                mumps arthritis (B26.85)
                postinfective arthropathy (M02.-)
                postmeningococcal arthritis (A39.84)
                reactive arthritis (M02.3)
                rubella arthritis (B06.82)
                sarcoidosis arthritis (D86.86)
                typhoid fever arthritis (A01.04)
                tuberculosis arthritis (A18.01-A18.02)

● **M01.X   Direct infection of joint in infectious and parasitic diseases classified elsewhere**

    (Ex) For category M01.X CC codes unless otherwise indicated: See PDX Collection 863

▸ *M01.X0   Direct infection of unspecified joint in infectious and parasitic diseases classified elsewhere* 🔖

● *M01.X1   Direct infection of shoulder joint in infectious and parasitic diseases classified elsewhere*

    (Ex) For category M01.X1 CC codes: See PDX Collection 864

▸ *M01.X11   Direct infection of right shoulder in infectious and parasitic diseases classified elsewhere* 🔖

▸ *M01.X12   Direct infection of left shoulder in infectious and parasitic diseases classified elsewhere* 🔖

▸ *M01.X19   Direct infection of unspecified shoulder in infectious and parasitic diseases classified elsewhere* 🔖

● *M01.X2   Direct infection of elbow in infectious and parasitic diseases classified elsewhere*

▸ *M01.X21   Direct infection of right elbow in infectious and parasitic diseases classified elsewhere* 🔖

▸ *M01.X22   Direct infection of left elbow in infectious and parasitic diseases classified elsewhere* 🔖

▸ *M01.X29   Direct infection of unspecified elbow in infectious and parasitic diseases classified elsewhere* 🔖

● *M01.X3   Direct infection of wrist in infectious and parasitic diseases classified elsewhere*
     Direct infection of carpal bones in infectious and parasitic diseases classified elsewhere

▸ *M01.X31   Direct infection of right wrist in infectious and parasitic diseases classified elsewhere* 🔖

▸ *M01.X32   Direct infection of left wrist in infectious and parasitic diseases classified elsewhere* 🔖

▸ *M01.X39   Direct infection of unspecified wrist in infectious and parasitic diseases classified elsewhere* 🔖

● *M01.X4   Direct infection of hand in infectious and parasitic diseases classified elsewhere*
     Direct infection of metacarpus and phalanges in infectious and parasitic diseases classified elsewhere

▸ *M01.X41   Direct infection of right hand in infectious and parasitic diseases classified elsewhere* 🔖

▸ *M01.X42   Direct infection of left hand in infectious and parasitic diseases classified elsewhere* 🔖

▸ *M01.X49   Direct infection of unspecified hand in infectious and parasitic diseases classified elsewhere* 🔖

● *M01.X5   Direct infection of hip in infectious and parasitic diseases classified elsewhere*

▸ *M01.X51   Direct infection of right hip in infectious and parasitic diseases classified elsewhere* 🔖

▸ *M01.X52   Direct infection of left hip in infectious and parasitic diseases classified elsewhere* 🔖

▸ *M01.X59   Direct infection of unspecified hip in infectious and parasitic diseases classified elsewhere* 🔖

● *M01.X6   Direct infection of knee in infectious and parasitic diseases classified elsewhere*

▸ *M01.X61   Direct infection of right knee in infectious and parasitic diseases classified elsewhere* 🔖

▸ *M01.X62   Direct infection of left knee in infectious and parasitic diseases classified elsewhere* 🔖

▸ *M01.X69   Direct infection of unspecified knee in infectious and parasitic diseases classified elsewhere* 🔖

● *M01.X7   Direct infection of ankle and foot in infectious and parasitic diseases classified elsewhere*
     Direct infection of tarsus, metatarsus and phalanges in infectious and parasitic diseases classified elsewhere

▸ *M01.X71   Direct infection of right ankle and foot in infectious and parasitic diseases classified elsewhere* 🔖

▸ *M01.X72   Direct infection of left ankle and foot in infectious and parasitic diseases classified elsewhere* 🔖

▸ *M01.X79   Direct infection of unspecified ankle and foot in infectious and parasitic diseases classified elsewhere* 🔖

▸ *M01.X8   Direct infection of vertebrae in infectious and parasitic diseases classified elsewhere* 🔖

▸ *M01.X9   Direct infection of multiple joints in infectious and parasitic diseases classified elsewhere* 🔖

● **M02   Postinfective and reactive arthropathies**

    Code first underlying disease, such as:
      congenital syphilis [Clutton's joints] (A50.5)
      enteritis due to Yersinia enterocolitica (A04.6)
      infective endocarditis (I33.0)
      viral hepatitis (B15-B19)

    Excludes1   Behçet's disease (M35.2)
                direct infections of joint in infectious and parasitic diseases classified elsewhere (M01.-)
                postmeningococcal arthritis (A39.84)
                mumps arthritis (B26.85)
                rubella arthritis (B06.82)
                syphilis arthritis (late) (A52.77)
                rheumatic fever (I00)
                tabetic arthropathy [Charcôt's] (A52.16)

    (Ex) For category M02 CC codes unless otherwise indicated: See PDX Collection 863

● **M02.0   Arthropathy following intestinal bypass**

    M02.00   Arthropathy following intestinal bypass, unspecified site

● **M02.01   Arthropathy following intestinal bypass, shoulder**

    M02.011   Arthropathy following intestinal bypass, right shoulder

    M02.012   Arthropathy following intestinal bypass, left shoulder

    M02.019   Arthropathy following intestinal bypass, unspecified shoulder

● **M02.02** Arthropathy following intestinal bypass, elbow

    M02.021 Arthropathy following intestinal bypass, right elbow

    M02.022 Arthropathy following intestinal bypass, left elbow

    M02.029 Arthropathy following intestinal bypass, unspecified elbow

● **M02.03** Arthropathy following intestinal bypass, wrist
    Arthropathy following intestinal bypass, carpal bones

    M02.031 Arthropathy following intestinal bypass, right wrist

    M02.032 Arthropathy following intestinal bypass, left wrist

    M02.039 Arthropathy following intestinal bypass, unspecified wrist

● **M02.04** Arthropathy following intestinal bypass, hand
    Arthropathy following intestinal bypass, metacarpals and phalanges

    M02.041 Arthropathy following intestinal bypass, right hand

    M02.042 Arthropathy following intestinal bypass, left hand

    M02.049 Arthropathy following intestinal bypass, unspecified hand

● **M02.05** Arthropathy following intestinal bypass, hip

    M02.051 Arthropathy following intestinal bypass, right hip

    M02.052 Arthropathy following intestinal bypass, left hip

    M02.059 Arthropathy following intestinal bypass, unspecified hip

● **M02.06** Arthropathy following intestinal bypass, knee

    M02.061 Arthropathy following intestinal bypass, right knee

    M02.062 Arthropathy following intestinal bypass, left knee

    M02.069 Arthropathy following intestinal bypass, unspecified knee

● **M02.07** Arthropathy following intestinal bypass, ankle and foot
    Arthropathy following intestinal bypass, tarsus, metatarsus and phalanges

    M02.071 Arthropathy following intestinal bypass, right ankle and foot

    M02.072 Arthropathy following intestinal bypass, left ankle and foot

    M02.079 Arthropathy following intestinal bypass, unspecified ankle and foot

    M02.08 Arthropathy following intestinal bypass, vertebrae

    M02.09 Arthropathy following intestinal bypass, multiple sites

● **M02.1** Postdysenteric arthropathy

    M02.10 Postdysenteric arthropathy, unspecified site

● **M02.11** Postdysenteric arthropathy, shoulder

    M02.111 Postdysenteric arthropathy, right shoulder

    M02.112 Postdysenteric arthropathy, left shoulder

    M02.119 Postdysenteric arthropathy, unspecified shoulder

● **M02.12** Postdysenteric arthropathy, elbow

    M02.121 Postdysenteric arthropathy, right elbow

    M02.122 Postdysenteric arthropathy, left elbow

    M02.129 Postdysenteric arthropathy, unspecified elbow

● **M02.13** Postdysenteric arthropathy, wrist
    Postdysenteric arthropathy, carpal bones

    M02.131 Postdysenteric arthropathy, right wrist

    M02.132 Postdysenteric arthropathy, left wrist

    M02.139 Postdysenteric arthropathy, unspecified wrist

● **M02.14** Postdysenteric arthropathy, hand
    Postdysenteric arthropathy, metacarpus and phalanges

    M02.141 Postdysenteric arthropathy, right hand

    M02.142 Postdysenteric arthropathy, left hand

    M02.149 Postdysenteric arthropathy, unspecified hand

● **M02.15** Postdysenteric arthropathy, hip

    M02.151 Postdysenteric arthropathy, right hip

    M02.152 Postdysenteric arthropathy, left hip

    M02.159 Postdysenteric arthropathy, unspecified hip

● **M02.16** Postdysenteric arthropathy, knee
    Ex: For category M02.16 CC codes: See PDX Collection 865

    M02.161 Postdysenteric arthropathy, right knee

    M02.162 Postdysenteric arthropathy, left knee

    M02.169 Postdysenteric arthropathy, unspecified knee

● **M02.17** Postdysenteric arthropathy, ankle and foot
    Postdysenteric arthropathy, tarsus, metatarsus and phalanges

    M02.171 Postdysenteric arthropathy, right ankle and foot

    M02.172 Postdysenteric arthropathy, left ankle and foot

    M02.179 Postdysenteric arthropathy, unspecified ankle and foot

    M02.18 Postdysenteric arthropathy, vertebrae
    Ex: See PDX Collection 866

    M02.19 Postdysenteric arthropathy, multiple sites

● **M02.2** Postimmunization arthropathy

    M02.20 Postimmunization arthropathy, unspecified site

● **M02.21** Postimmunization arthropathy, shoulder

    M02.211 Postimmunization arthropathy, right shoulder

    M02.212 Postimmunization arthropathy, left shoulder

    M02.219 Postimmunization arthropathy, unspecified shoulder

● **M02.22** Postimmunization arthropathy, elbow

    M02.221 Postimmunization arthropathy, right elbow

    M02.222 Postimmunization arthropathy, left elbow

    M02.229 Postimmunization arthropathy, unspecified elbow

● **M02.23** Postimmunization arthropathy, wrist
    Postimmunization arthropathy, carpal bones

    M02.231 Postimmunization arthropathy, right wrist

    M02.232 Postimmunization arthropathy, left wrist

    M02.239 Postimmunization arthropathy, unspecified wrist

▶ New   ⇒ Revised   ~~deleted~~ Deleted   Excludes 1   Excludes 2   Includes   Use additional   Code first   Code also   Key words

OGCR Official Guidelines   ● Unacceptable Principal Diagnosis   X Assign placeholder X   ● Use Additional Character(s)   ▶ Manifestation Code   Coding Clinic

● **M02.24 Postimmunization arthropathy, hand**
Postimmunization arthropathy, metacarpus and phalanges

   M02.241 Postimmunization arthropathy, right hand

   M02.242 Postimmunization arthropathy, left hand

   M02.249 Postimmunization arthropathy, unspecified hand

● **M02.25 Postimmunization arthropathy, hip**

   M02.251 Postimmunization arthropathy, right hip

   M02.252 Postimmunization arthropathy, left hip

   M02.259 Postimmunization arthropathy, unspecified hip

● **M02.26 Postimmunization arthropathy, knee**

   M02.261 Postimmunization arthropathy, right knee

   M02.262 Postimmunization arthropathy, left knee

   M02.269 Postimmunization arthropathy, unspecified knee

● **M02.27 Postimmunization arthropathy, ankle and foot**
Postimmunization arthropathy, tarsus, metatarsus and phalanges

   M02.271 Postimmunization arthropathy, right ankle and foot

   M02.272 Postimmunization arthropathy, left ankle and foot

   M02.279 Postimmunization arthropathy, unspecified ankle and foot

   M02.28 Postimmunization arthropathy, vertebrae

   M02.29 Postimmunization arthropathy, multiple sites

● **M02.3 Reiter's disease**
Reactive arthritis

   M02.30 Reiter's disease, unspecified site ✿
   CC when PDx is its own CC

● **M02.31 Reiter's disease, shoulder**

   M02.311 Reiter's disease, right shoulder ✿
   CC when PDx is its own CC

   M02.312 Reiter's disease, left shoulder ✿
   CC when PDx is its own CC

   M02.319 Reiter's disease, unspecified shoulder ✿
   CC when PDx is its own CC

● **M02.32 Reiter's disease, elbow**

   M02.321 Reiter's disease, right elbow ✿
   CC when PDx is its own CC

   M02.322 Reiter's disease, left elbow ✿
   CC when PDx is its own CC

   M02.329 Reiter's disease, unspecified elbow ✿
   CC when PDx is its own CC

● **M02.33 Reiter's disease, wrist**
Reiter's disease, carpal bones

   M02.331 Reiter's disease, right wrist ✿
   CC when PDx is its own CC

   M02.332 Reiter's disease, left wrist ✿
   CC when PDx is its own CC

   M02.339 Reiter's disease, unspecified wrist ✿
   CC when PDx is its own CC

● **M02.34 Reiter's disease, hand**
Reiter's disease, metacarpus and phalanges

   M02.341 Reiter's disease, right hand ✿
   CC when PDx is its own CC

   M02.342 Reiter's disease, left hand ✿
   CC when PDx is its own CC

   M02.349 Reiter's disease, unspecified hand ✿
   CC when PDx is its own CC

● **M02.35 Reiter's disease, hip**

   M02.351 Reiter's disease, right hip ✿
   CC when PDx is its own CC

   M02.352 Reiter's disease, left hip ✿
   CC when PDx is its own CC

   M02.359 Reiter's disease, unspecified hip ✿
   CC when PDx is its own CC

● **M02.36 Reiter's disease, knee**

   M02.361 Reiter's disease, right knee ✿
   CC when PDx is its own CC

   M02.362 Reiter's disease, left knee ✿
   CC when PDx is its own CC

   M02.369 Reiter's disease, unspecified knee ✿
   CC when PDx is its own CC

● **M02.37 Reiter's disease, ankle and foot**
Reiter's disease, tarsus, metatarsus and phalanges

   M02.371 Reiter's disease, right ankle and foot ✿
   CC when PDx is its own CC

   M02.372 Reiter's disease, left ankle and foot ✿
   CC when PDx is its own CC

   M02.379 Reiter's disease, unspecified ankle and foot ✿
   CC when PDx is its own CC

   M02.38 Reiter's disease, vertebrae ✿
   CC when PDx is its own CC

   M02.39 Reiter's disease, multiple sites ✿
   CC when PDx is its own CC

● **M02.8 Other reactive arthropathies**

   ▶ *M02.80 Other reactive arthropathies, unspecified site* ✿

● **M02.81 Other reactive arthropathies, shoulder**
   (Ex) For category M02.81 CC codes: See PDX Collection 864

   ▶ *M02.811 Other reactive arthropathies, right shoulder* ✿

   ▶ *M02.812 Other reactive arthropathies, left shoulder* ✿

   ▶ *M02.819 Other reactive arthropathies, unspecified shoulder* ✿

● **M02.82 Other reactive arthropathies, elbow**

   ▶ *M02.821 Other reactive arthropathies, right elbow* ✿

   ▶ *M02.822 Other reactive arthropathies, left elbow* ✿

   ▶ *M02.829 Other reactive arthropathies, unspecified elbow* ✿

● **M02.83 Other reactive arthropathies, wrist**
Other reactive arthropathies, carpal bones

   ▶ *M02.831 Other reactive arthropathies, right wrist* ✿

   ▶ *M02.832 Other reactive arthropathies, left wrist* ✿

   ▶ *M02.839 Other reactive arthropathies, unspecified wrist* ✿

● **M02.84 Other reactive arthropathies, hand**
Other reactive arthropathies, metacarpus and phalanges

   ▶ *M02.841 Other reactive arthropathies, right hand* ✿

   ▶ *M02.842 Other reactive arthropathies, left hand* ✿

   ▶ *M02.849 Other reactive arthropathies, unspecified hand* ✿

● **M02.85 Other reactive arthropathies, hip**

   ▶ *M02.851 Other reactive arthropathies, right hip* ✿

   ▶ *M02.852 Other reactive arthropathies, left hip* ✿

   ▶ *M02.859 Other reactive arthropathies, unspecified hip* ✿

CHAPTER 13 (M00–M99)

- **M02.86** Other reactive arthropathies, knee
  - M02.861 *Other reactive arthropathies, right knee*
  - M02.862 *Other reactive arthropathies, left knee*
  - M02.869 *Other reactive arthropathies, unspecified knee*
- **M02.87** Other reactive arthropathies, ankle and foot
  Other reactive arthropathies, tarsus, metatarsus and phalanges
  - M02.871 *Other reactive arthropathies, right ankle and foot*
  - M02.872 *Other reactive arthropathies, left ankle and foot*
  - M02.879 *Other reactive arthropathies, unspecified ankle and foot*
  - M02.88 *Other reactive arthropathies, vertebrae*
  - M02.89 *Other reactive arthropathies, multiple sites*
- M02.9 *Reactive arthropathy, unspecified*

AUTOINFLAMMATORY SYNDROMES (M04)

- **M04** Autoinflammatory syndromes
  Excludes2 Crohn's disease (K50.-)
  Coding Clinic: 2016, Q4, P37
  - **M04.1** Periodic fever syndromes
    Familial Mediterranean fever
    Hyperimmunoglobin D syndrome
    Mevalonate kinase deficiency
    Tumor necrosis factor receptor associated periodic syndrome [TRAPS]
  - **M04.2** Cryopyrin-associated periodic syndromes
    Chronic infantile neurological, cutaneous and articular syndrome [CINCA]
    Familial cold autoinflammatory syndrome
    Familial cold urticaria
    Muckle-Wells syndrome
    Neonatal onset multisystemic inflammatory disorder [NOMID]
  - **M04.8** Other autoinflammatory syndromes
    Blau syndrome
    Deficiency of interleukin 1 receptor antagonist [DIRA]
    Majeed syndrome
    Periodic fever, aphthous stomatitis, pharyngitis, and adenopathy syndrome [PFAPA]
    Pyogenic arthritis, pyoderma gangrenosum, and acne syndrome [PAPA]
  - **M04.9** Autoinflammatory syndrome, unspecified

INFLAMMATORY POLYARTHROPATHIES (M05-M14)

- **M05** Rheumatoid arthritis with rheumatoid factor
  Excludes1 rheumatic fever (I00)
  juvenile rheumatoid arthritis (M08.-)
  rheumatoid arthritis of spine (M45.-)
  - **M05.0** Felty's syndrome
    Rheumatoid arthritis with splenoadenomegaly and leukopenia
    - **M05.00** Felty's syndrome, unspecified site
    - **M05.01** Felty's syndrome, shoulder
      - M05.011 Felty's syndrome, right shoulder
      - M05.012 Felty's syndrome, left shoulder
      - M05.019 Felty's syndrome, unspecified shoulder
    - **M05.02** Felty's syndrome, elbow
      - M05.021 Felty's syndrome, right elbow
      - M05.022 Felty's syndrome, left elbow
      - M05.029 Felty's syndrome, unspecified elbow

Item 13-1   **Rheumatoid arthritis** (RA) is a chronic systemic inflammatory autoimmune disease of undetermined etiology involving primarily the synovial membranes and articular structures of multiple joints. It can also affect other organs, including the eyes, blood vessels, heart, and lungs. The disease is often progressive. In late stages, deformity, ankylosis, and other **inflammatory polyarthropathies** develop.

- **M05.03** Felty's syndrome, wrist
  Felty's syndrome, carpal bones
  - M05.031 Felty's syndrome, right wrist
  - M05.032 Felty's syndrome, left wrist
  - M05.039 Felty's syndrome, unspecified wrist
- **M05.04** Felty's syndrome, hand
  Felty's syndrome, metacarpus and phalanges
  - M05.041 Felty's syndrome, right hand
  - M05.042 Felty's syndrome, left hand
  - M05.049 Felty's syndrome, unspecified hand
- **M05.05** Felty's syndrome, hip
  - M05.051 Felty's syndrome, right hip
  - M05.052 Felty's syndrome, left hip
  - M05.059 Felty's syndrome, unspecified hip
- **M05.06** Felty's syndrome, knee
  - M05.061 Felty's syndrome, right knee
  - M05.062 Felty's syndrome, left knee
  - M05.069 Felty's syndrome, unspecified knee
- **M05.07** Felty's syndrome, ankle and foot
  Felty's syndrome, tarsus, metatarsus and phalanges
  - M05.071 Felty's syndrome, right ankle and foot
  - M05.072 Felty's syndrome, left ankle and foot
  - M05.079 Felty's syndrome, unspecified ankle and foot
  - **M05.09** Felty's syndrome, multiple sites
- **M05.1** Rheumatoid lung disease with rheumatoid arthritis
  - **M05.10** Rheumatoid lung disease with rheumatoid arthritis of unspecified site
  - **M05.11** Rheumatoid lung disease with rheumatoid arthritis of shoulder
    - M05.111 Rheumatoid lung disease with rheumatoid arthritis of right shoulder
    - M05.112 Rheumatoid lung disease with rheumatoid arthritis of left shoulder
    - M05.119 Rheumatoid lung disease with rheumatoid arthritis of unspecified shoulder
  - **M05.12** Rheumatoid lung disease with rheumatoid arthritis of elbow
    - M05.121 Rheumatoid lung disease with rheumatoid arthritis of right elbow
    - M05.122 Rheumatoid lung disease with rheumatoid arthritis of left elbow
    - M05.129 Rheumatoid lung disease with rheumatoid arthritis of unspecified elbow
  - **M05.13** Rheumatoid lung disease with rheumatoid arthritis of wrist
    Rheumatoid lung disease with rheumatoid arthritis, carpal bones
    - M05.131 Rheumatoid lung disease with rheumatoid arthritis of right wrist
    - M05.132 Rheumatoid lung disease with rheumatoid arthritis of left wrist
    - M05.139 Rheumatoid lung disease with rheumatoid arthritis of unspecified wrist

● M05.14 Rheumatoid lung disease with rheumatoid arthritis of hand
    Rheumatoid lung disease with rheumatoid arthritis, metacarpus and phalanges

  M05.141 Rheumatoid lung disease with rheumatoid arthritis of right hand

  M05.142 Rheumatoid lung disease with rheumatoid arthritis of left hand

  M05.149 Rheumatoid lung disease with rheumatoid arthritis of unspecified hand

● M05.15 Rheumatoid lung disease with rheumatoid arthritis of hip

  M05.151 Rheumatoid lung disease with rheumatoid arthritis of right hip

  M05.152 Rheumatoid lung disease with rheumatoid arthritis of left hip

  M05.159 Rheumatoid lung disease with rheumatoid arthritis of unspecified hip

● M05.16 Rheumatoid lung disease with rheumatoid arthritis of knee

  M05.161 Rheumatoid lung disease with rheumatoid arthritis of right knee

  M05.162 Rheumatoid lung disease with rheumatoid arthritis of left knee

  M05.169 Rheumatoid lung disease with rheumatoid arthritis of unspecified knee

● M05.17 Rheumatoid lung disease with rheumatoid arthritis of ankle and foot
    Rheumatoid lung disease with rheumatoid arthritis, tarsus, metatarsus and phalanges

  M05.171 Rheumatoid lung disease with rheumatoid arthritis of right ankle and foot

  M05.172 Rheumatoid lung disease with rheumatoid arthritis of left ankle and foot

  M05.179 Rheumatoid lung disease with rheumatoid arthritis of unspecified ankle and foot

  M05.19 Rheumatoid lung disease with rheumatoid arthritis of multiple sites

● M05.2 Rheumatoid vasculitis with rheumatoid arthritis

  M05.20 Rheumatoid vasculitis with rheumatoid arthritis of unspecified site

● M05.21 Rheumatoid vasculitis with rheumatoid arthritis of shoulder

  M05.211 Rheumatoid vasculitis with rheumatoid arthritis of right shoulder

  M05.212 Rheumatoid vasculitis with rheumatoid arthritis of left shoulder

  M05.219 Rheumatoid vasculitis with rheumatoid arthritis of unspecified shoulder

● M05.22 Rheumatoid vasculitis with rheumatoid arthritis of elbow

  M05.221 Rheumatoid vasculitis with rheumatoid arthritis of right elbow

  M05.222 Rheumatoid vasculitis with rheumatoid arthritis of left elbow

  M05.229 Rheumatoid vasculitis with rheumatoid arthritis of unspecified elbow

● M05.23 Rheumatoid vasculitis with rheumatoid arthritis of wrist
    Rheumatoid vasculitis with rheumatoid arthritis, carpal bones

  M05.231 Rheumatoid vasculitis with rheumatoid arthritis of right wrist

  M05.232 Rheumatoid vasculitis with rheumatoid arthritis of left wrist

  M05.239 Rheumatoid vasculitis with rheumatoid arthritis of unspecified wrist

● M05.24 Rheumatoid vasculitis with rheumatoid arthritis of hand
    Rheumatoid vasculitis with rheumatoid arthritis, metacarpus and phalanges

  M05.241 Rheumatoid vasculitis with rheumatoid arthritis of right hand

  M05.242 Rheumatoid vasculitis with rheumatoid arthritis of left hand

  M05.249 Rheumatoid vasculitis with rheumatoid arthritis of unspecified hand

● M05.25 Rheumatoid vasculitis with rheumatoid arthritis of hip

  M05.251 Rheumatoid vasculitis with rheumatoid arthritis of right hip

  M05.252 Rheumatoid vasculitis with rheumatoid arthritis of left hip

  M05.259 Rheumatoid vasculitis with rheumatoid arthritis of unspecified hip

● M05.26 Rheumatoid vasculitis with rheumatoid arthritis of knee

  M05.261 Rheumatoid vasculitis with rheumatoid arthritis of right knee

  M05.262 Rheumatoid vasculitis with rheumatoid arthritis of left knee

  M05.269 Rheumatoid vasculitis with rheumatoid arthritis of unspecified knee

● M05.27 Rheumatoid vasculitis with rheumatoid arthritis of ankle and foot
    Rheumatoid vasculitis with rheumatoid arthritis, tarsus, metatarsus and phalanges

  M05.271 Rheumatoid vasculitis with rheumatoid arthritis of right ankle and foot

  M05.272 Rheumatoid vasculitis with rheumatoid arthritis of left ankle and foot

  M05.279 Rheumatoid vasculitis with rheumatoid arthritis of unspecified ankle and foot

  M05.29 Rheumatoid vasculitis with rheumatoid arthritis of multiple sites

● M05.3 Rheumatoid heart disease with rheumatoid arthritis
    Rheumatoid carditis
    Rheumatoid endocarditis
    Rheumatoid myocarditis
    Rheumatoid pericarditis

  M05.30 Rheumatoid heart disease with rheumatoid arthritis of unspecified site

● M05.31 Rheumatoid heart disease with rheumatoid arthritis of shoulder

  M05.311 Rheumatoid heart disease with rheumatoid arthritis of right shoulder

  M05.312 Rheumatoid heart disease with rheumatoid arthritis of left shoulder

  M05.319 Rheumatoid heart disease with rheumatoid arthritis of unspecified shoulder

CHAPTER 13 (M00-M99)

● **M05.32** Rheumatoid heart disease with rheumatoid arthritis of **elbow**

    M05.321 Rheumatoid heart disease with rheumatoid arthritis of **right elbow**

    M05.322 Rheumatoid heart disease with rheumatoid arthritis of **left elbow**

    M05.329 Rheumatoid heart disease with rheumatoid arthritis of **unspecified** elbow

● **M05.33** Rheumatoid heart disease with rheumatoid arthritis of **wrist**

    Rheumatoid heart disease with rheumatoid arthritis, carpal bones

    M05.331 Rheumatoid heart disease with rheumatoid arthritis of **right wrist**

    M05.332 Rheumatoid heart disease with rheumatoid arthritis of **left wrist**

    M05.339 Rheumatoid heart disease with rheumatoid arthritis of **unspecified** wrist

● **M05.34** Rheumatoid heart disease with rheumatoid arthritis of **hand**

    Rheumatoid heart disease with rheumatoid arthritis, metacarpus and phalanges

    M05.341 Rheumatoid heart disease with rheumatoid arthritis of **right hand**

    M05.342 Rheumatoid heart disease with rheumatoid arthritis of **left hand**

    M05.349 Rheumatoid heart disease with rheumatoid arthritis of **unspecified** hand

● **M05.35** Rheumatoid heart disease with rheumatoid arthritis of **hip**

    M05.351 Rheumatoid heart disease with rheumatoid arthritis of **right hip**

    M05.352 Rheumatoid heart disease with rheumatoid arthritis of **left hip**

    M05.359 Rheumatoid heart disease with rheumatoid arthritis of **unspecified** hip

● **M05.36** Rheumatoid heart disease with rheumatoid arthritis of **knee**

    M05.361 Rheumatoid heart disease with rheumatoid arthritis of **right knee**

    M05.362 Rheumatoid heart disease with rheumatoid arthritis of **left knee**

    M05.369 Rheumatoid heart disease with rheumatoid arthritis of **unspecified** knee

● **M05.37** Rheumatoid heart disease with rheumatoid arthritis of **ankle and foot**

    Rheumatoid heart disease with rheumatoid arthritis, tarsus, metatarsus and phalanges

    M05.371 Rheumatoid heart disease with rheumatoid arthritis of **right ankle and foot**

    M05.372 Rheumatoid heart disease with rheumatoid arthritis of **left ankle and foot**

    M05.379 Rheumatoid heart disease with rheumatoid arthritis of **unspecified** ankle and foot

M05.39 Rheumatoid heart disease with rheumatoid arthritis of **multiple sites**

● **M05.4** Rheumatoid **myopathy** with rheumatoid arthritis

    (Ex.) For category M05.4 CC codes: See PDX Collection 867

    M05.40 Rheumatoid myopathy with rheumatoid arthritis of **unspecified site** 🔖

        CC when PDx is its own CC

● **M05.41** Rheumatoid myopathy with rheumatoid arthritis of **shoulder**

    M05.411 Rheumatoid myopathy with rheumatoid arthritis of **right shoulder** 🔖

        CC when PDx is its own CC

    M05.412 Rheumatoid myopathy with rheumatoid arthritis of **left shoulder** 🔖

        CC when PDx is its own CC

    M05.419 Rheumatoid myopathy with rheumatoid arthritis of **unspecified shoulder** 🔖

        CC when PDx is its own CC

● **M05.42** Rheumatoid myopathy with rheumatoid arthritis of **elbow**

    M05.421 Rheumatoid myopathy with rheumatoid arthritis of **right elbow** 🔖

        CC when PDx is its own CC

    M05.422 Rheumatoid myopathy with rheumatoid arthritis of **left elbow** 🔖

        CC when PDx is its own CC

    M05.429 Rheumatoid myopathy with rheumatoid arthritis of **unspecified elbow** 🔖

        CC when PDx is its own CC

● **M05.43** Rheumatoid myopathy with rheumatoid arthritis of **wrist**

    Rheumatoid myopathy with rheumatoid arthritis, carpal bones

    M05.431 Rheumatoid myopathy with rheumatoid arthritis of **right wrist** 🔖

        CC when PDx is its own CC

    M05.432 Rheumatoid myopathy with rheumatoid arthritis of **left wrist** 🔖

        CC when PDx is its own CC

    M05.439 Rheumatoid myopathy with rheumatoid arthritis of **unspecified wrist** 🔖

        CC when PDx is its own CC

● **M05.44** Rheumatoid myopathy with rheumatoid arthritis of **hand**

    Rheumatoid myopathy with rheumatoid arthritis, metacarpus and phalanges

    M05.441 Rheumatoid myopathy with rheumatoid arthritis of **right hand** 🔖

        CC when PDx is its own CC

    M05.442 Rheumatoid myopathy with rheumatoid arthritis of **left hand** 🔖

        CC when PDx is its own CC

    M05.449 Rheumatoid myopathy with rheumatoid arthritis of **unspecified hand** 🔖

        CC when PDx is its own CC

● **M05.45** Rheumatoid myopathy with rheumatoid arthritis of **hip**

    M05.451 Rheumatoid myopathy with rheumatoid arthritis of **right hip** 🔖

        CC when PDx is its own CC

    M05.452 Rheumatoid myopathy with rheumatoid arthritis of **left hip** 🔖

    M05.459 Rheumatoid myopathy with rheumatoid arthritis of **unspecified hip** 🔖

        CC when PDx is its own CC

▶ New ⇒ Revised ~~deleted~~ Deleted | Excludes 1 | Excludes 2 | Includes | Use additional | Code first | Code also | Key words

OGCR Official Guidelines ● Unacceptable Principal Diagnosis X Assign placeholder X ● Use Additional Character(s) ▶ Manifestation Code **Coding Clinic**

● **M05.46 Rheumatoid myopathy with rheumatoid arthritis of knee**
    M05.461 Rheumatoid myopathy with rheumatoid arthritis of right knee 🅟
        CC when PDx is its own CC
    M05.462 Rheumatoid myopathy with rheumatoid arthritis of left knee 🅟
        CC when PDx is its own CC
    M05.469 Rheumatoid myopathy with rheumatoid arthritis of unspecified knee 🅟
        CC when PDx is its own CC

● **M05.47 Rheumatoid myopathy with rheumatoid arthritis of ankle and foot**
    Rheumatoid myopathy with rheumatoid arthritis, tarsus, metatarsus and phalanges
    M05.471 Rheumatoid myopathy with rheumatoid arthritis of right ankle and foot 🅟
        CC when PDx is its own CC
    M05.472 Rheumatoid myopathy with rheumatoid arthritis of left ankle and foot 🅟
        CC when PDx is its own CC
    M05.479 Rheumatoid myopathy with rheumatoid arthritis of unspecified ankle and foot 🅟
        CC when PDx is its own CC

    M05.49 Rheumatoid myopathy with rheumatoid arthritis of multiple sites 🅟
        CC when PDx is its own CC

● **M05.5 Rheumatoid polyneuropathy with rheumatoid arthritis**
    M05.50 Rheumatoid polyneuropathy with rheumatoid arthritis of unspecified site

● **M05.51 Rheumatoid polyneuropathy with rheumatoid arthritis of shoulder**
    M05.511 Rheumatoid polyneuropathy with rheumatoid arthritis of right shoulder
    M05.512 Rheumatoid polyneuropathy with rheumatoid arthritis of left shoulder
    M05.519 Rheumatoid polyneuropathy with rheumatoid arthritis of unspecified shoulder

● **M05.52 Rheumatoid polyneuropathy with rheumatoid arthritis of elbow**
    M05.521 Rheumatoid polyneuropathy with rheumatoid arthritis of right elbow
    M05.522 Rheumatoid polyneuropathy with rheumatoid arthritis of left elbow
    M05.529 Rheumatoid polyneuropathy with rheumatoid arthritis of unspecified elbow

● **M05.53 Rheumatoid polyneuropathy with rheumatoid arthritis of wrist**
    Rheumatoid polyneuropathy with rheumatoid arthritis, carpal bones
    M05.531 Rheumatoid polyneuropathy with rheumatoid arthritis of right wrist
    M05.532 Rheumatoid polyneuropathy with rheumatoid arthritis of left wrist
    M05.539 Rheumatoid polyneuropathy with rheumatoid arthritis of unspecified wrist

● **M05.54 Rheumatoid polyneuropathy with rheumatoid arthritis of hand**
    Rheumatoid polyneuropathy with rheumatoid arthritis, metacarpus and phalanges
    M05.541 Rheumatoid polyneuropathy with rheumatoid arthritis of right hand
    M05.542 Rheumatoid polyneuropathy with rheumatoid arthritis of left hand
    M05.549 Rheumatoid polyneuropathy with rheumatoid arthritis of unspecified hand

● **M05.55 Rheumatoid polyneuropathy with rheumatoid arthritis of hip**
    M05.551 Rheumatoid polyneuropathy with rheumatoid arthritis of right hip
    M05.552 Rheumatoid polyneuropathy with rheumatoid arthritis of left hip
    M05.559 Rheumatoid polyneuropathy with rheumatoid arthritis of unspecified hip

● **M05.56 Rheumatoid polyneuropathy with rheumatoid arthritis of knee**
    M05.561 Rheumatoid polyneuropathy with rheumatoid arthritis of right knee
    M05.562 Rheumatoid polyneuropathy with rheumatoid arthritis of left knee
    M05.569 Rheumatoid polyneuropathy with rheumatoid arthritis of unspecified knee

● **M05.57 Rheumatoid polyneuropathy with rheumatoid arthritis of ankle and foot**
    Rheumatoid polyneuropathy with rheumatoid arthritis, tarsus, metatarsus and phalanges
    M05.571 Rheumatoid polyneuropathy with rheumatoid arthritis of right ankle and foot
    M05.572 Rheumatoid polyneuropathy with rheumatoid arthritis of left ankle and foot
    M05.579 Rheumatoid polyneuropathy with rheumatoid arthritis of unspecified ankle and foot

    M05.59 Rheumatoid polyneuropathy with rheumatoid arthritis of multiple sites

● **M05.6 Rheumatoid arthritis with involvement of other organs and systems**
    M05.60 Rheumatoid arthritis of unspecified site with involvement of other organs and systems

● **M05.61 Rheumatoid arthritis of shoulder with involvement of other organs and systems**
    M05.611 Rheumatoid arthritis of right shoulder with involvement of other organs and systems
    M05.612 Rheumatoid arthritis of left shoulder with involvement of other organs and systems
    M05.619 Rheumatoid arthritis of unspecified shoulder with involvement of other organs and systems

● **M05.62 Rheumatoid arthritis of elbow with involvement of other organs and systems**
    M05.621 Rheumatoid arthritis of right elbow with involvement of other organs and systems
    M05.622 Rheumatoid arthritis of left elbow with involvement of other organs and systems
    M05.629 Rheumatoid arthritis of unspecified elbow with involvement of other organs and systems

CHAPTER 13 (M00-M99)

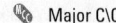

● **M05.63 Rheumatoid arthritis of wrist with involvement of other organs and systems**
Rheumatoid arthritis of carpal bones with involvement of other organs and systems

     M05.631 Rheumatoid arthritis of right wrist with involvement of other organs and systems

     M05.632 Rheumatoid arthritis of left wrist with involvement of other organs and systems

     M05.639 Rheumatoid arthritis of unspecified wrist with involvement of other organs and systems

● **M05.64 Rheumatoid arthritis of hand with involvement of other organs and systems**
Rheumatoid arthritis of metacarpus and phalanges with involvement of other organs and systems

     M05.641 Rheumatoid arthritis of right hand with involvement of other organs and systems

     M05.642 Rheumatoid arthritis of left hand with involvement of other organs and systems

     M05.649 Rheumatoid arthritis of unspecified hand with involvement of other organs and systems

● **M05.65 Rheumatoid arthritis of hip with involvement of other organs and systems**

     M05.651 Rheumatoid arthritis of right hip with involvement of other organs and systems

     M05.652 Rheumatoid arthritis of left hip with involvement of other organs and systems

     M05.659 Rheumatoid arthritis of unspecified hip with involvement of other organs and systems

● **M05.66 Rheumatoid arthritis of knee with involvement of other organs and systems**

     M05.661 Rheumatoid arthritis of right knee with involvement of other organs and systems

     M05.662 Rheumatoid arthritis of left knee with involvement of other organs and systems

     M05.669 Rheumatoid arthritis of unspecified knee with involvement of other organs and systems

● **M05.67 Rheumatoid arthritis of ankle and foot with involvement of other organs and systems**
Rheumatoid arthritis of tarsus, metatarsus and phalanges with involvement of other organs and systems

     M05.671 Rheumatoid arthritis of right ankle and foot with involvement of other organs and systems

     M05.672 Rheumatoid arthritis of left ankle and foot with involvement of other organs and systems

     M05.679 Rheumatoid arthritis of unspecified ankle and foot with involvement of other organs and systems

     M05.69 Rheumatoid arthritis of multiple sites with involvement of other organs and systems

● **M05.7 Rheumatoid arthritis with rheumatoid factor without organ or systems involvement**

     M05.70 Rheumatoid arthritis with rheumatoid factor of unspecified site without organ or systems involvement

● **M05.71 Rheumatoid arthritis with rheumatoid factor of shoulder without organ or systems involvement**

     M05.711 Rheumatoid arthritis with rheumatoid factor of right shoulder without organ or systems involvement

     M05.712 Rheumatoid arthritis with rheumatoid factor of left shoulder without organ or systems involvement

     M05.719 Rheumatoid arthritis with rheumatoid factor of unspecified shoulder without organ or systems involvement

● **M05.72 Rheumatoid arthritis with rheumatoid factor of elbow without organ or systems involvement**

     M05.721 Rheumatoid arthritis with rheumatoid factor of right elbow without organ or systems involvement

     M05.722 Rheumatoid arthritis with rheumatoid factor of left elbow without organ or systems involvement

     M05.729 Rheumatoid arthritis with rheumatoid factor of unspecified elbow without organ or systems involvement

● **M05.73 Rheumatoid arthritis with rheumatoid factor of wrist without organ or systems involvement**

     M05.731 Rheumatoid arthritis with rheumatoid factor of right wrist without organ or systems involvement

     M05.732 Rheumatoid arthritis with rheumatoid factor of left wrist without organ or systems involvement

     M05.739 Rheumatoid arthritis with rheumatoid factor of unspecified wrist without organ or systems involvement

● **M05.74 Rheumatoid arthritis with rheumatoid factor of hand without organ or systems involvement**

     M05.741 Rheumatoid arthritis with rheumatoid factor of right hand without organ or systems involvement

     M05.742 Rheumatoid arthritis with rheumatoid factor of left hand without organ or systems involvement

     M05.749 Rheumatoid arthritis with rheumatoid factor of unspecified hand without organ or systems involvement

● M05.75 Rheumatoid arthritis with rheumatoid factor of hip without organ or systems involvement

    M05.751 Rheumatoid arthritis with rheumatoid factor of right hip without organ or systems involvement

    M05.752 Rheumatoid arthritis with rheumatoid factor of left hip without organ or systems involvement

    M05.759 Rheumatoid arthritis with rheumatoid factor of unspecified hip without organ or systems involvement

● M05.76 Rheumatoid arthritis with rheumatoid factor of knee without organ or systems involvement

    M05.761 Rheumatoid arthritis with rheumatoid factor of right knee without organ or systems involvement

    M05.762 Rheumatoid arthritis with rheumatoid factor of left knee without organ or systems involvement

    M05.769 Rheumatoid arthritis with rheumatoid factor of unspecified knee without organ or systems involvement

● M05.77 Rheumatoid arthritis with rheumatoid factor of ankle and foot without organ or systems involvement

    M05.771 Rheumatoid arthritis with rheumatoid factor of right ankle and foot without organ or systems involvement

    M05.772 Rheumatoid arthritis with rheumatoid factor of left ankle and foot without organ or systems involvement

    M05.779 Rheumatoid arthritis with rheumatoid factor of unspecified ankle and foot without organ or systems involvement

  M05.79 Rheumatoid arthritis with rheumatoid factor of multiple sites without organ or systems involvement

● M05.8 Other rheumatoid arthritis with rheumatoid factor

  M05.80 Other rheumatoid arthritis with rheumatoid factor of unspecified site

● M05.81 Other rheumatoid arthritis with rheumatoid factor of shoulder

    M05.811 Other rheumatoid arthritis with rheumatoid factor of right shoulder

    M05.812 Other rheumatoid arthritis with rheumatoid factor of left shoulder

    M05.819 Other rheumatoid arthritis with rheumatoid factor of unspecified shoulder

● M05.82 Other rheumatoid arthritis with rheumatoid factor of elbow

    M05.821 Other rheumatoid arthritis with rheumatoid factor of right elbow

    M05.822 Other rheumatoid arthritis with rheumatoid factor of left elbow

    M05.829 Other rheumatoid arthritis with rheumatoid factor of unspecified elbow

● M05.83 Other rheumatoid arthritis with rheumatoid factor of wrist

    M05.831 Other rheumatoid arthritis with rheumatoid factor of right wrist

    M05.832 Other rheumatoid arthritis with rheumatoid factor of left wrist

    M05.839 Other rheumatoid arthritis with rheumatoid factor of unspecified wrist

● M05.84 Other rheumatoid arthritis with rheumatoid factor of hand

    M05.841 Other rheumatoid arthritis with rheumatoid factor of right hand

    M05.842 Other rheumatoid arthritis with rheumatoid factor of left hand

    M05.849 Other rheumatoid arthritis with rheumatoid factor of unspecified hand

● M05.85 Other rheumatoid arthritis with rheumatoid factor of hip

    M05.851 Other rheumatoid arthritis with rheumatoid factor of right hip

    M05.852 Other rheumatoid arthritis with rheumatoid factor of left hip

    M05.859 Other rheumatoid arthritis with rheumatoid factor of unspecified hip

● M05.86 Other rheumatoid arthritis with rheumatoid factor of knee

    M05.861 Other rheumatoid arthritis with rheumatoid factor of right knee

    M05.862 Other rheumatoid arthritis with rheumatoid factor of left knee

    M05.869 Other rheumatoid arthritis with rheumatoid factor of unspecified knee

● M05.87 Other rheumatoid arthritis with rheumatoid factor of ankle and foot

    M05.871 Other rheumatoid arthritis with rheumatoid factor of right ankle and foot

    M05.872 Other rheumatoid arthritis with rheumatoid factor of left ankle and foot

    M05.879 Other rheumatoid arthritis with rheumatoid factor of unspecified ankle and foot

  M05.89 Other rheumatoid arthritis with rheumatoid factor of multiple sites

  M05.9 Rheumatoid arthritis with rheumatoid factor, unspecified

● M06 Other rheumatoid arthritis

  ● M06.0 Rheumatoid arthritis without rheumatoid factor

    M06.00 Rheumatoid arthritis without rheumatoid factor, unspecified site

    ● M06.01 Rheumatoid arthritis without rheumatoid factor, shoulder

      M06.011 Rheumatoid arthritis without rheumatoid factor, right shoulder

      M06.012 Rheumatoid arthritis without rheumatoid factor, left shoulder

      M06.019 Rheumatoid arthritis without rheumatoid factor, unspecified shoulder

● **M06.02** Rheumatoid arthritis without rheumatoid
factor, elbow
    M06.021 Rheumatoid arthritis without
rheumatoid factor, right elbow
    M06.022 Rheumatoid arthritis without
rheumatoid factor, left elbow
    M06.029 Rheumatoid arthritis without
rheumatoid factor, unspecified elbow

● **M06.03** Rheumatoid arthritis without rheumatoid
factor, wrist
    M06.031 Rheumatoid arthritis without
rheumatoid factor, right wrist
    M06.032 Rheumatoid arthritis without
rheumatoid factor, left wrist
    M06.039 Rheumatoid arthritis without
rheumatoid factor, unspecified wrist

● **M06.04** Rheumatoid arthritis without rheumatoid
factor, hand
    M06.041 Rheumatoid arthritis without
rheumatoid factor, right hand
    M06.042 Rheumatoid arthritis without
rheumatoid factor, left hand
    M06.049 Rheumatoid arthritis without
rheumatoid factor, unspecified hand

● **M06.05** Rheumatoid arthritis without rheumatoid
factor, hip
    M06.051 Rheumatoid arthritis without
rheumatoid factor, right hip
    M06.052 Rheumatoid arthritis without
rheumatoid factor, left hip
    M06.059 Rheumatoid arthritis without
rheumatoid factor, unspecified hip

● **M06.06** Rheumatoid arthritis without rheumatoid
factor, knee
    M06.061 Rheumatoid arthritis without
rheumatoid factor, right knee
    M06.062 Rheumatoid arthritis without
rheumatoid factor, left knee
    M06.069 Rheumatoid arthritis without
rheumatoid factor, unspecified knee

● **M06.07** Rheumatoid arthritis without rheumatoid
factor, ankle and foot
    M06.071 Rheumatoid arthritis without
rheumatoid factor, right ankle and
foot
    M06.072 Rheumatoid arthritis without
rheumatoid factor, left ankle and foot
    M06.079 Rheumatoid arthritis without
rheumatoid factor, unspecified ankle
and foot

  M06.08 Rheumatoid arthritis without rheumatoid
factor, vertebrae

  M06.09 Rheumatoid arthritis without rheumatoid
factor, multiple sites

M06.1 **Adult-onset Still's disease**   A
    Excludes1 Still's disease NOS (M08.2-)

● **M06.2** **Rheumatoid bursitis**
  M06.20 Rheumatoid bursitis, unspecified site
● M06.21 Rheumatoid bursitis, shoulder
    M06.211 Rheumatoid bursitis, right shoulder
    M06.212 Rheumatoid bursitis, left shoulder
    M06.219 Rheumatoid bursitis, unspecified
shoulder
● M06.22 Rheumatoid bursitis, elbow
    M06.221 Rheumatoid bursitis, right elbow
    M06.222 Rheumatoid bursitis, left elbow
    M06.229 Rheumatoid bursitis, unspecified
elbow
● M06.23 Rheumatoid bursitis, wrist
    M06.231 Rheumatoid bursitis, right wrist
    M06.232 Rheumatoid bursitis, left wrist
    M06.239 Rheumatoid bursitis, unspecified
wrist
● M06.24 Rheumatoid bursitis, hand
    M06.241 Rheumatoid bursitis, right hand
    M06.242 Rheumatoid bursitis, left hand
    M06.249 Rheumatoid bursitis, unspecified
hand
● M06.25 Rheumatoid bursitis, hip
    M06.251 Rheumatoid bursitis, right hip
    M06.252 Rheumatoid bursitis, left hip
    M06.259 Rheumatoid bursitis, unspecified hip
● M06.26 Rheumatoid bursitis, knee
    M06.261 Rheumatoid bursitis, right knee
    M06.262 Rheumatoid bursitis, left knee
    M06.269 Rheumatoid bursitis, unspecified knee
● M06.27 Rheumatoid bursitis, ankle and foot
    M06.271 Rheumatoid bursitis, right ankle and
foot
    M06.272 Rheumatoid bursitis, left ankle and
foot
    M06.279 Rheumatoid bursitis, unspecified
ankle and foot
  M06.28 Rheumatoid bursitis, vertebrae
  M06.29 Rheumatoid bursitis, multiple sites
● **M06.3** **Rheumatoid nodule**
  M06.30 Rheumatoid nodule, unspecified site
● M06.31 Rheumatoid nodule, shoulder
    M06.311 Rheumatoid nodule, right shoulder
    M06.312 Rheumatoid nodule, left shoulder
    M06.319 Rheumatoid nodule, unspecified
shoulder
● M06.32 Rheumatoid nodule, elbow
    M06.321 Rheumatoid nodule, right elbow
    M06.322 Rheumatoid nodule, left elbow
    M06.329 Rheumatoid nodule, unspecified
elbow
● M06.33 Rheumatoid nodule, wrist
    M06.331 Rheumatoid nodule, right wrist
    M06.332 Rheumatoid nodule, left wrist
    M06.339 Rheumatoid nodule, unspecified
wrist

▶ New   ⟹ Revised   ~~deleted~~ Deleted   Excludes 1   Excludes 2   Includes   Use additional   Code first   Code also   Key words
OGCR Official Guidelines   ● Unacceptable Principal Diagnosis   X Assign placeholder X   ● Use Additional Character(s)   ▶ Manifestation Code   **Coding Clinic**

● M06.34　Rheumatoid nodule, hand
　　M06.341　Rheumatoid nodule, right hand
　　M06.342　Rheumatoid nodule, left hand
　　M06.349　Rheumatoid nodule, unspecified hand
● M06.35　Rheumatoid nodule, hip
　　M06.351　Rheumatoid nodule, right hip
　　M06.352　Rheumatoid nodule, left hip
　　M06.359　Rheumatoid nodule, unspecified hip
● M06.36　Rheumatoid nodule, knee
　　M06.361　Rheumatoid nodule, right knee
　　M06.362　Rheumatoid nodule, left knee
　　M06.369　Rheumatoid nodule, unspecified knee
● M06.37　Rheumatoid nodule, ankle and foot
　　M06.371　Rheumatoid nodule, right ankle and foot
　　M06.372　Rheumatoid nodule, left ankle and foot
　　M06.379　Rheumatoid nodule, unspecified ankle and foot
　　M06.38　Rheumatoid nodule, vertebrae
　　M06.39　Rheumatoid nodule, multiple sites
　M06.4　Inflammatory polyarthropathy
　　　Excludes1　polyarthritis NOS (M13.0)
● M06.8　Other specified rheumatoid arthritis
　　M06.80　Other specified rheumatoid arthritis, unspecified site
● M06.81　Other specified rheumatoid arthritis, shoulder
　　M06.811　Other specified rheumatoid arthritis, right shoulder
　　M06.812　Other specified rheumatoid arthritis, left shoulder
　　M06.819　Other specified rheumatoid arthritis, unspecified shoulder
● M06.82　Other specified rheumatoid arthritis, elbow
　　M06.821　Other specified rheumatoid arthritis, right elbow
　　M06.822　Other specified rheumatoid arthritis, left elbow
　　M06.829　Other specified rheumatoid arthritis, unspecified elbow
● M06.83　Other specified rheumatoid arthritis, wrist
　　M06.831　Other specified rheumatoid arthritis, right wrist
　　M06.832　Other specified rheumatoid arthritis, left wrist
　　M06.839　Other specified rheumatoid arthritis, unspecified wrist
● M06.84　Other specified rheumatoid arthritis, hand
　　M06.841　Other specified rheumatoid arthritis, right hand
　　M06.842　Other specified rheumatoid arthritis, left hand
　　M06.849　Other specified rheumatoid arthritis, unspecified hand
● M06.85　Other specified rheumatoid arthritis, hip
　　M06.851　Other specified rheumatoid arthritis, right hip
　　M06.852　Other specified rheumatoid arthritis, left hip
　　M06.859　Other specified rheumatoid arthritis, unspecified hip

● M06.86　Other specified rheumatoid arthritis, knee
　　M06.861　Other specified rheumatoid arthritis, right knee
　　M06.862　Other specified rheumatoid arthritis, left knee
　　M06.869　Other specified rheumatoid arthritis, unspecified knee
● M06.87　Other specified rheumatoid arthritis, ankle and foot
　　M06.871　Other specified rheumatoid arthritis, right ankle and foot
　　M06.872　Other specified rheumatoid arthritis, left ankle and foot
　　M06.879　Other specified rheumatoid arthritis, unspecified ankle and foot
　　M06.88　Other specified rheumatoid arthritis, vertebrae
　　M06.89　Other specified rheumatoid arthritis, multiple sites
　M06.9　Rheumatoid arthritis, unspecified
● M07　Enteropathic arthropathies
　　Code also associated enteropathy, such as:
　　　regional enteritis [Crohn's disease] (K50.-)
　　　ulcerative colitis (K51.-)
　　　Excludes1　psoriatic arthropathies (L40.5-)
● M07.6　Enteropathic arthropathies
　　M07.60　Enteropathic arthropathies, unspecified site
● M07.61　Enteropathic arthropathies, shoulder
　　M07.611　Enteropathic arthropathies, right shoulder
　　M07.612　Enteropathic arthropathies, left shoulder
　　M07.619　Enteropathic arthropathies, unspecified shoulder
● M07.62　Enteropathic arthropathies, elbow
　　M07.621　Enteropathic arthropathies, right elbow
　　M07.622　Enteropathic arthropathies, left elbow
　　M07.629　Enteropathic arthropathies, unspecified elbow
● M07.63　Enteropathic arthropathies, wrist
　　M07.631　Enteropathic arthropathies, right wrist
　　M07.632　Enteropathic arthropathies, left wrist
　　M07.639　Enteropathic arthropathies, unspecified wrist
● M07.64　Enteropathic arthropathies, hand
　　M07.641　Enteropathic arthropathies, right hand
　　M07.642　Enteropathic arthropathies, left hand
　　M07.649　Enteropathic arthropathies, unspecified hand
● M07.65　Enteropathic arthropathies, hip
　　M07.651　Enteropathic arthropathies, right hip
　　M07.652　Enteropathic arthropathies, left hip
　　M07.659　Enteropathic arthropathies, unspecified hip
● M07.66　Enteropathic arthropathies, knee
　　M07.661　Enteropathic arthropathies, right knee
　　M07.662　Enteropathic arthropathies, left knee
　　M07.669　Enteropathic arthropathies, unspecified knee

CHAPTER 13 (M00-M99)

● M07.67 Enteropathic arthropathies, ankle and foot

    M07.671 Enteropathic arthropathies, right ankle and foot

    M07.672 Enteropathic arthropathies, left ankle and foot

    M07.679 Enteropathic arthropathies, unspecified ankle and foot

  M07.68 Enteropathic arthropathies, vertebrae

  M07.69 Enteropathic arthropathies, multiple sites

● M08   Juvenile arthritis

  Code also any associated underlying condition, such as:
    regional enteritis [Crohn's disease] (K50.-)
    ulcerative colitis (K51.-)

  Excludes1   arthropathy in Whipple's disease (M14.8)
              Felty's syndrome (M05.0)
              juvenile dermatomyositis (M33.0-)
              psoriatic juvenile arthropathy (L40.54)

 ● M08.0   Unspecified juvenile rheumatoid arthritis
    Juvenile rheumatoid arthritis with or without rheumatoid factor

    M08.00 Unspecified juvenile rheumatoid arthritis of unspecified site

  ● M08.01 Unspecified juvenile rheumatoid arthritis, shoulder

    M08.011 Unspecified juvenile rheumatoid arthritis, right shoulder

    M08.012 Unspecified juvenile rheumatoid arthritis, left shoulder

    M08.019 Unspecified juvenile rheumatoid arthritis, unspecified shoulder

  ● M08.02 Unspecified juvenile rheumatoid arthritis of elbow

    M08.021 Unspecified juvenile rheumatoid arthritis, right elbow

    M08.022 Unspecified juvenile rheumatoid arthritis, left elbow

    M08.029 Unspecified juvenile rheumatoid arthritis, unspecified elbow

  ● M08.03 Unspecified juvenile rheumatoid arthritis, wrist

    M08.031 Unspecified juvenile rheumatoid arthritis, right wrist

    M08.032 Unspecified juvenile rheumatoid arthritis, left wrist

    M08.039 Unspecified juvenile rheumatoid arthritis, unspecified wrist

  ● M08.04 Unspecified juvenile rheumatoid arthritis, hand

    M08.041 Unspecified juvenile rheumatoid arthritis, right hand

    M08.042 Unspecified juvenile rheumatoid arthritis, left hand

    M08.049 Unspecified juvenile rheumatoid arthritis, unspecified hand

  ● M08.05 Unspecified juvenile rheumatoid arthritis, hip

    M08.051 Unspecified juvenile rheumatoid arthritis, right hip

    M08.052 Unspecified juvenile rheumatoid arthritis, left hip

    M08.059 Unspecified juvenile rheumatoid arthritis, unspecified hip

  ● M08.06 Unspecified juvenile rheumatoid arthritis, knee

    M08.061 Unspecified juvenile rheumatoid arthritis, right knee

    M08.062 Unspecified juvenile rheumatoid arthritis, left knee

    M08.069 Unspecified juvenile rheumatoid arthritis, unspecified knee

 ● M08.07 Unspecified juvenile rheumatoid arthritis, ankle and foot

    M08.071 Unspecified juvenile rheumatoid arthritis, right ankle and foot

    M08.072 Unspecified juvenile rheumatoid arthritis, left ankle and foot

    M08.079 Unspecified juvenile rheumatoid arthritis, unspecified ankle and foot

  M08.08 Unspecified juvenile rheumatoid arthritis, vertebrae

  M08.09 Unspecified juvenile rheumatoid arthritis, multiple sites

 M08.1   Juvenile ankylosing spondylitis

  Excludes1   ankylosing spondylitis in adults (M45.0-)

● M08.2   Juvenile rheumatoid arthritis with systemic onset
  Still's disease NOS

  Excludes1   adult-onset Still's disease (M06.1-)

  M08.20 Juvenile rheumatoid arthritis with systemic onset, unspecified site

 ● M08.21 Juvenile rheumatoid arthritis with systemic onset, shoulder

    M08.211 Juvenile rheumatoid arthritis with systemic onset, right shoulder

    M08.212 Juvenile rheumatoid arthritis with systemic onset, left shoulder

    M08.219 Juvenile rheumatoid arthritis with systemic onset, unspecified shoulder

 ● M08.22 Juvenile rheumatoid arthritis with systemic onset, elbow

    M08.221 Juvenile rheumatoid arthritis with systemic onset, right elbow

    M08.222 Juvenile rheumatoid arthritis with systemic onset, left elbow

    M08.229 Juvenile rheumatoid arthritis with systemic onset, unspecified elbow

 ● M08.23 Juvenile rheumatoid arthritis with systemic onset, wrist

    M08.231 Juvenile rheumatoid arthritis with systemic onset, right wrist

    M08.232 Juvenile rheumatoid arthritis with systemic onset, left wrist

    M08.239 Juvenile rheumatoid arthritis with systemic onset, unspecified wrist

 ● M08.24 Juvenile rheumatoid arthritis with systemic onset, hand

    M08.241 Juvenile rheumatoid arthritis with systemic onset, right hand

    M08.242 Juvenile rheumatoid arthritis with systemic onset, left hand

    M08.249 Juvenile rheumatoid arthritis with systemic onset, unspecified hand

 ● M08.25 Juvenile rheumatoid arthritis with systemic onset, hip

    M08.251 Juvenile rheumatoid arthritis with systemic onset, right hip

    M08.252 Juvenile rheumatoid arthritis with systemic onset, left hip

    M08.259 Juvenile rheumatoid arthritis with systemic onset, unspecified hip

▶ New   ⇒ Revised   ~~deleted~~ Deleted   Excludes 1   Excludes 2   Includes   Use additional   Code first   Code also   Key words

OGCR Official Guidelines   ● Unacceptable Principal Diagnosis   X Assign placeholder X   ● Use Additional Character(s)   ▶ Manifestation Code   Coding Clinic

● M08.26   Juvenile rheumatoid arthritis with systemic onset, knee

    M08.261   Juvenile rheumatoid arthritis with systemic onset, right knee

    M08.262   Juvenile rheumatoid arthritis with systemic onset, left knee

    M08.269   Juvenile rheumatoid arthritis with systemic onset, unspecified knee

● M08.27   Juvenile rheumatoid arthritis with systemic onset, ankle and foot

    M08.271   Juvenile rheumatoid arthritis with systemic onset, right ankle and foot

    M08.272   Juvenile rheumatoid arthritis with systemic onset, left ankle and foot

    M08.279   Juvenile rheumatoid arthritis with systemic onset, unspecified ankle and foot

   M08.28   Juvenile rheumatoid arthritis with systemic onset, vertebrae

   M08.29   Juvenile rheumatoid arthritis with systemic onset, multiple sites

M08.3   Juvenile rheumatoid polyarthritis (seronegative)

● M08.4   Pauciarticular juvenile rheumatoid arthritis

   M08.40   Pauciarticular juvenile rheumatoid arthritis, unspecified site

● M08.41   Pauciarticular juvenile rheumatoid arthritis, shoulder

    M08.411   Pauciarticular juvenile rheumatoid arthritis, right shoulder

    M08.412   Pauciarticular juvenile rheumatoid arthritis, left shoulder

    M08.419   Pauciarticular juvenile rheumatoid arthritis, unspecified shoulder

● M08.42   Pauciarticular juvenile rheumatoid arthritis, elbow

    M08.421   Pauciarticular juvenile rheumatoid arthritis, right elbow

    M08.422   Pauciarticular juvenile rheumatoid arthritis, left elbow

    M08.429   Pauciarticular juvenile rheumatoid arthritis, unspecified elbow

● M08.43   Pauciarticular juvenile rheumatoid arthritis, wrist

    M08.431   Pauciarticular juvenile rheumatoid arthritis, right wrist

    M08.432   Pauciarticular juvenile rheumatoid arthritis, left wrist

    M08.439   Pauciarticular juvenile rheumatoid arthritis, unspecified wrist

● M08.44   Pauciarticular juvenile rheumatoid arthritis, hand

    M08.441   Pauciarticular juvenile rheumatoid arthritis, right hand

    M08.442   Pauciarticular juvenile rheumatoid arthritis, left hand

    M08.449   Pauciarticular juvenile rheumatoid arthritis, unspecified hand

● M08.45   Pauciarticular juvenile rheumatoid arthritis, hip

    M08.451   Pauciarticular juvenile rheumatoid arthritis, right hip

    M08.452   Pauciarticular juvenile rheumatoid arthritis, left hip

    M08.459   Pauciarticular juvenile rheumatoid arthritis, unspecified hip

● M08.46   Pauciarticular juvenile rheumatoid arthritis, knee

    M08.461   Pauciarticular juvenile rheumatoid arthritis, right knee

    M08.462   Pauciarticular juvenile rheumatoid arthritis, left knee

    M08.469   Pauciarticular juvenile rheumatoid arthritis, unspecified knee

● M08.47   Pauciarticular juvenile rheumatoid arthritis, ankle and foot

    M08.471   Pauciarticular juvenile rheumatoid arthritis, right ankle and foot

    M08.472   Pauciarticular juvenile rheumatoid arthritis, left ankle and foot

    M08.479   Pauciarticular juvenile rheumatoid arthritis, unspecified ankle and foot

   M08.48   Pauciarticular juvenile rheumatoid arthritis, vertebrae

● M08.8   Other juvenile arthritis

   M08.80   Other juvenile arthritis, unspecified site

● M08.81   Other juvenile arthritis, shoulder

    M08.811   Other juvenile arthritis, right shoulder

    M08.812   Other juvenile arthritis, left shoulder

    M08.819   Other juvenile arthritis, unspecified shoulder

● M08.82   Other juvenile arthritis, elbow

    M08.821   Other juvenile arthritis, right elbow

    M08.822   Other juvenile arthritis, left elbow

    M08.829   Other juvenile arthritis, unspecified elbow

● M08.83   Other juvenile arthritis, wrist

    M08.831   Other juvenile arthritis, right wrist

    M08.832   Other juvenile arthritis, left wrist

    M08.839   Other juvenile arthritis, unspecified wrist

● M08.84   Other juvenile arthritis, hand

    M08.841   Other juvenile arthritis, right hand

    M08.842   Other juvenile arthritis, left hand

    M08.849   Other juvenile arthritis, unspecified hand

● M08.85   Other juvenile arthritis, hip

    M08.851   Other juvenile arthritis, right hip

    M08.852   Other juvenile arthritis, left hip

    M08.859   Other juvenile arthritis, unspecified hip

● M08.86   Other juvenile arthritis, knee

    M08.861   Other juvenile arthritis, right knee

    M08.862   Other juvenile arthritis, left knee

    M08.869   Other juvenile arthritis, unspecified knee

● M08.87   Other juvenile arthritis, ankle and foot

    M08.871   Other juvenile arthritis, right ankle and foot

    M08.872   Other juvenile arthritis, left ankle and foot

    M08.879   Other juvenile arthritis, unspecified ankle and foot

   M08.88   Other juvenile arthritis, other specified site
       Other juvenile arthritis, vertebrae

   M08.89   Other juvenile arthritis, multiple sites

CHAPTER 13 (M00–M99)

CHAPTER 13 (M00-M99)

● **M08.9 Juvenile arthritis, unspecified**

    Excludes1   juvenile rheumatoid arthritis, unspecified (M08.0-)

    M08.90   Juvenile arthritis, unspecified, unspecified site

● M08.91   Juvenile arthritis, unspecified, shoulder

    M08.911   Juvenile arthritis, unspecified, right shoulder

    M08.912   Juvenile arthritis, unspecified, left shoulder

    M08.919   Juvenile arthritis, unspecified, unspecified shoulder

● M08.92   Juvenile arthritis, unspecified, elbow

    M08.921   Juvenile arthritis, unspecified, right elbow

    M08.922   Juvenile arthritis, unspecified, left elbow

    M08.929   Juvenile arthritis, unspecified, unspecified elbow

● M08.93   Juvenile arthritis, unspecified, wrist

    M08.931   Juvenile arthritis, unspecified, right wrist

    M08.932   Juvenile arthritis, unspecified, left wrist

    M08.939   Juvenile arthritis, unspecified, unspecified wrist

● M08.94   Juvenile arthritis, unspecified, hand

    M08.941   Juvenile arthritis, unspecified, right hand

    M08.942   Juvenile arthritis, unspecified, left hand

    M08.949   Juvenile arthritis, unspecified, unspecified hand

● M08.95   Juvenile arthritis, unspecified, hip

    M08.951   Juvenile arthritis, unspecified, right hip

    M08.952   Juvenile arthritis, unspecified, left hip

    M08.959   Juvenile arthritis, unspecified, unspecified hip

● M08.96   Juvenile arthritis, unspecified, knee

    M08.961   Juvenile arthritis, unspecified, right knee

    M08.962   Juvenile arthritis, unspecified, left knee

    M08.969   Juvenile arthritis, unspecified, unspecified knee

● M08.97   Juvenile arthritis, unspecified, ankle and foot

    M08.971   Juvenile arthritis, unspecified, right ankle and foot

    M08.972   Juvenile arthritis, unspecified, left ankle and foot

    M08.979   Juvenile arthritis, unspecified, unspecified ankle and foot

    M08.98   Juvenile arthritis, unspecified, vertebrae

    M08.99   Juvenile arthritis, unspecified, multiple sites

● **M1A Chronic gout**

    Use additional code to identify:

    Autonomic neuropathy in diseases classified elsewhere (G99.0)

    Calculus of urinary tract in diseases classified elsewhere (N22)

    Cardiomyopathy in diseases classified elsewhere (I43)

    Disorders of external ear in diseases classified elsewhere (H61.1-, H62.8-)

    Disorders of iris and ciliary body in diseases classified elsewhere (H22)

    Glomerular disorders in diseases classified elsewhere (N08)

    Excludes1 gout NOS (M10.-)

    Excludes2 acute gout (M10.-)

    The appropriate 7th character is to be added to each code from category M1A

    | | |
    0   without tophus (tophi)
    1   with tophus (tophi)

● **M1A.0 Idiopathic chronic gout**

    Chronic gouty bursitis

    Primary chronic gout

  X ● M1A.00 Idiopathic chronic gout, unspecified site

  ● M1A.01 Idiopathic chronic gout, shoulder

    ● M1A.011 Idiopathic chronic gout, right shoulder

    ● M1A.012 Idiopathic chronic gout, left shoulder

    ● M1A.019 Idiopathic chronic gout, unspecified shoulder

  ● M1A.02 Idiopathic chronic gout, elbow

    ● M1A.021 Idiopathic chronic gout, right elbow

    ● M1A.022 Idiopathic chronic gout, left elbow

    ● M1A.029 Idiopathic chronic gout, unspecified elbow

  ● M1A.03 Idiopathic chronic gout, wrist

    ● M1A.031 Idiopathic chronic gout, right wrist

    ● M1A.032 Idiopathic chronic gout, left wrist

    ● M1A.039 Idiopathic chronic gout, unspecified wrist

  ● M1A.04 Idiopathic chronic gout, hand

    ● M1A.041 Idiopathic chronic gout, right hand

    ● M1A.042 Idiopathic chronic gout, left hand

    ● M1A.049 Idiopathic chronic gout, unspecified hand

  ● M1A.05 Idiopathic chronic gout, hip

    ● M1A.051 Idiopathic chronic gout, right hip

    ● M1A.052 Idiopathic chronic gout, left hip

    ● M1A.059 Idiopathic chronic gout, unspecified hip

  ● M1A.06 Idiopathic chronic gout, knee

    ● M1A.061 Idiopathic chronic gout, right knee

    ● M1A.062 Idiopathic chronic gout, left knee

    ● M1A.069 Idiopathic chronic gout, unspecified knee

  ● M1A.07 Idiopathic chronic gout, ankle and foot

    ● M1A.071 Idiopathic chronic gout, right ankle and foot

    ● M1A.072 Idiopathic chronic gout, left ankle and foot

    ● M1A.079 Idiopathic chronic gout, unspecified ankle and foot

  X ● M1A.08 Idiopathic chronic gout, vertebrae

  X ● M1A.09 Idiopathic chronic gout, multiple sites

▶ New   ⇒ Revised   ~~deleted~~ Deleted   Excludes 1   Excludes 2   Includes   Use additional   Code first   Code also   Key words

OGCR Official Guidelines   ● Unacceptable Principal Diagnosis   X Assign placeholder X   ● Use Additional Character(s)   ▶ Manifestation Code   **Coding Clinic**

● **M1A.1 Lead-induced** chronic gout
   Code first toxic effects of lead and its compounds (T56.0-)
   X● **M1A.10 Lead-induced** chronic gout, **unspecified site**
   ● **M1A.11 Lead-induced** chronic gout, **shoulder**
      ● **M1A.111 Lead-induced** chronic gout, **right shoulder**
      ● **M1A.112 Lead-induced** chronic gout, **left shoulder**
      ● **M1A.119 Lead-induced** chronic gout, **unspecified shoulder**
   ● **M1A.12 Lead-induced** chronic gout, **elbow**
      ● **M1A.121 Lead-induced** chronic gout, **right elbow**
      ● **M1A.122 Lead-induced** chronic gout, **left elbow**
      ● **M1A.129 Lead-induced** chronic gout, **unspecified elbow**
   ● **M1A.13 Lead-induced** chronic gout, **wrist**
      ● **M1A.131 Lead-induced** chronic gout, **right wrist**
      ● **M1A.132 Lead-induced** chronic gout, **left wrist**
      ● **M1A.139 Lead-induced** chronic gout, **unspecified wrist**
   ● **M1A.14 Lead-induced** chronic gout, **hand**
      ● **M1A.141 Lead-induced** chronic gout, **right hand**
      ● **M1A.142 Lead-induced** chronic gout, **left hand**
      ● **M1A.149 Lead-induced** chronic gout, **unspecified hand**
   ● **M1A.15 Lead-induced** chronic gout, **hip**
      ● **M1A.151 Lead-induced** chronic gout, **right hip**
      ● **M1A.152 Lead-induced** chronic gout, **left hip**
      ● **M1A.159 Lead-induced** chronic gout, **unspecified hip**
   ● **M1A.16 Lead-induced** chronic gout, **knee**
      ● **M1A.161 Lead-induced** chronic gout, **right knee**
      ● **M1A.162 Lead-induced** chronic gout, **left knee**
      ● **M1A.169 Lead-induced** chronic gout, **unspecified knee**
   ● **M1A.17 Lead-induced** chronic gout, **ankle and foot**
      ● **M1A.171 Lead-induced** chronic gout, **right ankle and foot**
      ● **M1A.172 Lead-induced** chronic gout, **left ankle and foot**
      ● **M1A.179 Lead-induced** chronic gout, **unspecified ankle and foot**
   X● **M1A.18 Lead-induced** chronic gout, **vertebrae**
   X● **M1A.19 Lead-induced** chronic gout, **multiple sites**
● **M1A.2 Drug-induced** chronic gout
   Use additional code for adverse effect, if applicable, to identify drug (T36-T50 with fifth or sixth character 5)
   X● **M1A.20 Drug-induced** chronic gout, **unspecified site**
   ● **M1A.21 Drug-induced** chronic gout, **shoulder**
      ● **M1A.211 Drug-induced** chronic gout, **right shoulder**
      ● **M1A.212 Drug-induced** chronic gout, **left shoulder**
      ● **M1A.219 Drug-induced** chronic gout, **unspecified shoulder**
   ● **M1A.22 Drug-induced** chronic gout, **elbow**
      ● **M1A.221 Drug-induced** chronic gout, **right elbow**
      ● **M1A.222 Drug-induced** chronic gout, **left elbow**
      ● **M1A.229 Drug-induced** chronic gout, **unspecified elbow**

● **M1A.23 Drug-induced** chronic gout, **wrist**
   ● **M1A.231 Drug-induced** chronic gout, **right wrist**
   ● **M1A.232 Drug-induced** chronic gout, **left wrist**
   ● **M1A.239 Drug-induced** chronic gout, **unspecified wrist**
● **M1A.24 Drug-induced** chronic gout, **hand**
   ● **M1A.241 Drug-induced** chronic gout, **right hand**
   ● **M1A.242 Drug-induced** chronic gout, **left hand**
   ● **M1A.249 Drug-induced** chronic gout, **unspecified hand**
● **M1A.25 Drug-induced** chronic gout, **hip**
   ● **M1A.251 Drug-induced** chronic gout, **right hip**
   ● **M1A.252 Drug-induced** chronic gout, **left hip**
   ● **M1A.259 Drug-induced** chronic gout, **unspecified hip**
● **M1A.26 Drug-induced** chronic gout, **knee**
   ● **M1A.261 Drug-induced** chronic gout, **right knee**
   ● **M1A.262 Drug-induced** chronic gout, **left knee**
   ● **M1A.269 Drug-induced** chronic gout, **unspecified knee**
● **M1A.27 Drug-induced** chronic gout, **ankle and foot**
   ● **M1A.271 Drug-induced** chronic gout, **right ankle and foot**
   ● **M1A.272 Drug-induced** chronic gout, **left ankle and foot**
   ● **M1A.279 Drug-induced** chronic gout, **unspecified ankle and foot**
X● **M1A.28 Drug-induced** chronic gout, **vertebrae**
X● **M1A.29 Drug-induced** chronic gout, **multiple sites**
● **M1A.3 Chronic gout due to renal impairment**
   Code first associated renal disease
   X● **M1A.30 Chronic gout due to** renal impairment, **unspecified site**
   ● **M1A.31 Chronic gout due to** renal impairment, **shoulder**
      ● **M1A.311 Chronic gout due to** renal impairment, **right shoulder**
      ● **M1A.312 Chronic gout due to** renal impairment, **left shoulder**
      ● **M1A.319 Chronic gout due to** renal impairment, **unspecified shoulder**
   ● **M1A.32 Chronic gout due to** renal impairment, **elbow**
      ● **M1A.321 Chronic gout due to** renal impairment, **right elbow**
      ● **M1A.322 Chronic gout due to** renal impairment, **left elbow**
      ● **M1A.329 Chronic gout due to** renal impairment, **unspecified elbow**
   ● **M1A.33 Chronic gout due to** renal impairment, **wrist**
      ● **M1A.331 Chronic gout due to** renal impairment, **right wrist**
      ● **M1A.332 Chronic gout due to** renal impairment, **left wrist**
      ● **M1A.339 Chronic gout due to** renal impairment, **unspecified wrist**
   ● **M1A.34 Chronic gout due to** renal impairment, **hand**
      ● **M1A.341 Chronic gout due to** renal impairment, **right hand**
      ● **M1A.342 Chronic gout due to** renal impairment, **left hand**
      ● **M1A.349 Chronic gout due to** renal impairment, **unspecified hand**

N Newborn Age: 0   **P** Pediatric Age: 0–17   **M** Maternity DX: 12–55   **A** Adult Age: 15–124   ♀ Females Only   ♂ Males Only

🔖 Complication\Comorbidity   🔖 Major C\C   (Ex) CC/MCC Exclusions   🔖 Hospital-Acquired Condition

1007

CHAPTER 13 (M00–M99)

● M1A.35 Chronic gout due to renal impairment, hip
- ● M1A.351 Chronic gout due to renal impairment, right hip
- ● M1A.352 Chronic gout due to renal impairment, left hip
- ● M1A.359 Chronic gout due to renal impairment, unspecified hip

● M1A.36 Chronic gout due to renal impairment, knee
- ● M1A.361 Chronic gout due to renal impairment, right knee
- ● M1A.362 Chronic gout due to renal impairment, left knee
- ● M1A.369 Chronic gout due to renal impairment, unspecified knee

● M1A.37 Chronic gout due to renal impairment, ankle and foot
- ● M1A.371 Chronic gout due to renal impairment, right ankle and foot
- ● M1A.372 Chronic gout due to renal impairment, left ankle and foot
- ● M1A.379 Chronic gout due to renal impairment, unspecified ankle and foot

X ● M1A.38 Chronic gout due to renal impairment, vertebrae

X ● M1A.39 Chronic gout due to renal impairment, multiple sites

● M1A.4 Other secondary chronic gout
Code first associated condition

X ● M1A.40 Other secondary chronic gout, unspecified site

● M1A.41 Other secondary chronic gout, shoulder
- ● M1A.411 Other secondary chronic gout, right shoulder
- ● M1A.412 Other secondary chronic gout, left shoulder
- ● M1A.419 Other secondary chronic gout, unspecified shoulder

● M1A.42 Other secondary chronic gout, elbow
- ● M1A.421 Other secondary chronic gout, right elbow
- ● M1A.422 Other secondary chronic gout, left elbow
- ● M1A.429 Other secondary chronic gout, unspecified elbow

● M1A.43 Other secondary chronic gout, wrist
- ● M1A.431 Other secondary chronic gout, right wrist
- ● M1A.432 Other secondary chronic gout, left wrist
- ● M1A.439 Other secondary chronic gout, unspecified wrist

● M1A.44 Other secondary chronic gout, hand
- ● M1A.441 Other secondary chronic gout, right hand
- ● M1A.442 Other secondary chronic gout, left hand
- ● M1A.449 Other secondary chronic gout, unspecified hand

● M1A.45 Other secondary chronic gout, hip
- ● M1A.451 Other secondary chronic gout, right hip
- ● M1A.452 Other secondary chronic gout, left hip
- ● M1A.459 Other secondary chronic gout, unspecified hip

● M1A.46 Other secondary chronic gout, knee
- ● M1A.461 Other secondary chronic gout, right knee
- ● M1A.462 Other secondary chronic gout, left knee
- ● M1A.469 Other secondary chronic gout, unspecified knee

● M1A.47 Other secondary chronic gout, ankle and foot
- ● M1A.471 Other secondary chronic gout, right ankle and foot
- ● M1A.472 Other secondary chronic gout, left ankle and foot
- ● M1A.479 Other secondary chronic gout, unspecified ankle and foot

X ● M1A.48 Other secondary chronic gout, vertebrae

X ● M1A.49 Other secondary chronic gout, multiple sites

X ● M1A.9 Chronic gout, unspecified

● M10 Gout
Accumulation of uric acid that results in swollen, red, hot, painful, stiff joints
Acute gout
Gout attack
Gout flare
Podagra
Use additional code to identify:
    Autonomic neuropathy in diseases classified elsewhere (G99.0)
    Calculus of urinary tract in diseases classified elsewhere (N22)
    Cardiomyopathy in diseases classified elsewhere (I43)
    Disorders of external ear in diseases classified elsewhere (H61.1-, H62.8-)
    Disorders of iris and ciliary body in diseases classified elsewhere (H22)
    Glomerular disorders in diseases classified elsewhere (N08)

Excludes2   chronic gout (M1A.-)

● M10.0 Idiopathic gout
Gouty bursitis
Primary gout

  M10.00 Idiopathic gout, unspecified site

● M10.01 Idiopathic gout, shoulder
  M10.011 Idiopathic gout, right shoulder
  M10.012 Idiopathic gout, left shoulder
  M10.019 Idiopathic gout, unspecified shoulder

● M10.02 Idiopathic gout, elbow
  M10.021 Idiopathic gout, right elbow
  M10.022 Idiopathic gout, left elbow
  M10.029 Idiopathic gout, unspecified elbow

● M10.03 Idiopathic gout, wrist
  M10.031 Idiopathic gout, right wrist
  M10.032 Idiopathic gout, left wrist
  M10.039 Idiopathic gout, unspecified wrist

● M10.04 Idiopathic gout, hand
  M10.041 Idiopathic gout, right hand
  M10.042 Idiopathic gout, left hand
  M10.049 Idiopathic gout, unspecified hand

● M10.05 Idiopathic gout, hip
  M10.051 Idiopathic gout, right hip
  M10.052 Idiopathic gout, left hip
  M10.059 Idiopathic gout, unspecified hip

● M10.06 Idiopathic gout, knee
  M10.061 Idiopathic gout, right knee
  M10.062 Idiopathic gout, left knee
  M10.069 Idiopathic gout, unspecified knee

● **M10.07** Idiopathic gout, ankle and foot
  M10.071 Idiopathic gout, right ankle and foot
  M10.072 Idiopathic gout, left ankle and foot
  M10.079 Idiopathic gout, unspecified ankle and foot
  M10.08 Idiopathic gout, vertebrae
  M10.09 Idiopathic gout, multiple sites
● **M10.1** Lead-induced gout
  Code first toxic effects of lead and its compounds (T56.0-)
  M10.10 Lead-induced gout, unspecified site
● **M10.11** Lead-induced gout, shoulder
  M10.111 Lead-induced gout, right shoulder
  M10.112 Lead-induced gout, left shoulder
  M10.119 Lead-induced gout, unspecified shoulder
● **M10.12** Lead-induced gout, elbow
  M10.121 Lead-induced gout, right elbow
  M10.122 Lead-induced gout, left elbow
  M10.129 Lead-induced gout, unspecified elbow
● **M10.13** Lead-induced gout, wrist
  M10.131 Lead-induced gout, right wrist
  M10.132 Lead-induced gout, left wrist
  M10.139 Lead-induced gout, unspecified wrist
● **M10.14** Lead-induced gout, hand
  M10.141 Lead-induced gout, right hand
  M10.142 Lead-induced gout, left hand
  M10.149 Lead-induced gout, unspecified hand
● **M10.15** Lead-induced gout, hip
  M10.151 Lead-induced gout, right hip
  M10.152 Lead-induced gout, left hip
  M10.159 Lead-induced gout, unspecified hip
● **M10.16** Lead-induced gout, knee
  M10.161 Lead-induced gout, right knee
  M10.162 Lead-induced gout, left knee
  M10.169 Lead-induced gout, unspecified knee
● **M10.17** Lead-induced gout, ankle and foot
  M10.171 Lead-induced gout, right ankle and foot
  M10.172 Lead-induced gout, left ankle and foot
  M10.179 Lead-induced gout, unspecified ankle and foot
  M10.18 Lead-induced gout, vertebrae
  M10.19 Lead-induced gout, multiple sites
● **M10.2** Drug-induced gout
  Use additional code for adverse effect, if applicable, to identify drug (T36-T50 with fifth or sixth character 5)
  M10.20 Drug-induced gout, unspecified site
● **M10.21** Drug-induced gout, shoulder
  M10.211 Drug-induced gout, right shoulder
  M10.212 Drug-induced gout, left shoulder
  M10.219 Drug-induced gout, unspecified shoulder
● **M10.22** Drug-induced gout, elbow
  M10.221 Drug-induced gout, right elbow
  M10.222 Drug-induced gout, left elbow
  M10.229 Drug-induced gout, unspecified elbow
● **M10.23** Drug-induced gout, wrist
  M10.231 Drug-induced gout, right wrist
  M10.232 Drug-induced gout, left wrist
  M10.239 Drug-induced gout, unspecified wrist

● **M10.24** Drug-induced gout, hand
  M10.241 Drug-induced gout, right hand
  M10.242 Drug-induced gout, left hand
  M10.249 Drug-induced gout, unspecified hand
● **M10.25** Drug-induced gout, hip
  M10.251 Drug-induced gout, right hip
  M10.252 Drug-induced gout, left hip
  M10.259 Drug-induced gout, unspecified hip
● **M10.26** Drug-induced gout, knee
  M10.261 Drug-induced gout, right knee
  M10.262 Drug-induced gout, left knee
  M10.269 Drug-induced gout, unspecified knee
● **M10.27** Drug-induced gout, ankle and foot
  M10.271 Drug-induced gout, right ankle and foot
  M10.272 Drug-induced gout, left ankle and foot
  M10.279 Drug-induced gout, unspecified ankle and foot
  M10.28 Drug-induced gout, vertebrae
  M10.29 Drug-induced gout, multiple sites
● **M10.3** Gout due to renal impairment
  Code also associated renal disease
  M10.30 Gout due to renal impairment, unspecified site
● **M10.31** Gout due to renal impairment, shoulder
  M10.311 Gout due to renal impairment, right shoulder
  M10.312 Gout due to renal impairment, left shoulder
  M10.319 Gout due to renal impairment, unspecified shoulder
● **M10.32** Gout due to renal impairment, elbow
  M10.321 Gout due to renal impairment, right elbow
  M10.322 Gout due to renal impairment, left elbow
  M10.329 Gout due to renal impairment, unspecified elbow
● **M10.33** Gout due to renal impairment, wrist
  M10.331 Gout due to renal impairment, right wrist
  M10.332 Gout due to renal impairment, left wrist
  M10.339 Gout due to renal impairment, unspecified wrist
● **M10.34** Gout due to renal impairment, hand
  M10.341 Gout due to renal impairment, right hand
  M10.342 Gout due to renal impairment, left hand
  M10.349 Gout due to renal impairment, unspecified hand
● **M10.35** Gout due to renal impairment, hip
  M10.351 Gout due to renal impairment, right hip
  M10.352 Gout due to renal impairment, left hip
  M10.359 Gout due to renal impairment, unspecified hip
● **M10.36** Gout due to renal impairment, knee
  M10.361 Gout due to renal impairment, right knee
  M10.362 Gout due to renal impairment, left knee
  M10.369 Gout due to renal impairment, unspecified knee

CHAPTER 13 (M00-M99)

N Newborn Age: 0   P Pediatric Age: 0-17   M Maternity DX: 12-55   A Adult Age: 15-124   ♀ Females Only   ♂ Males Only
🐾 Complication\Comorbidity   🐾 Major C\C   (Ex) CC/MCC Exclusions   🐾 Hospital-Acquired Condition

1009

CHAPTER 13 (M00-M99)

● M10.37 Gout due to renal impairment, ankle and foot
    M10.371 Gout due to renal impairment, right ankle and foot
    M10.372 Gout due to renal impairment, left ankle and foot
    M10.379 Gout due to renal impairment, unspecified ankle and foot
    M10.38 Gout due to renal impairment, vertebrae
    M10.39 Gout due to renal impairment, multiple sites
● M10.4 Other secondary gout
    Code first associated condition
    M10.40 Other secondary gout, unspecified site
● M10.41 Other secondary gout, shoulder
    M10.411 Other secondary gout, right shoulder
    M10.412 Other secondary gout, left shoulder
    M10.419 Other secondary gout, unspecified shoulder
● M10.42 Other secondary gout, elbow
    M10.421 Other secondary gout, right elbow
    M10.422 Other secondary gout, left elbow
    M10.429 Other secondary gout, unspecified elbow
● M10.43 Other secondary gout, wrist
    M10.431 Other secondary gout, right wrist
    M10.432 Other secondary gout, left wrist
    M10.439 Other secondary gout, unspecified wrist
● M10.44 Other secondary gout, hand
    M10.441 Other secondary gout, right hand
    M10.442 Other secondary gout, left hand
    M10.449 Other secondary gout, unspecified hand
● M10.45 Other secondary gout, hip
    M10.451 Other secondary gout, right hip
    M10.452 Other secondary gout, left hip
    M10.459 Other secondary gout, unspecified hip
● M10.46 Other secondary gout, knee
    M10.461 Other secondary gout, right knee
    M10.462 Other secondary gout, left knee
    M10.469 Other secondary gout, unspecified knee
● M10.47 Other secondary gout, ankle and foot
    M10.471 Other secondary gout, right ankle and foot
    M10.472 Other secondary gout, left ankle and foot
    M10.479 Other secondary gout, unspecified ankle and foot
    M10.48 Other secondary gout, vertebrae
    M10.49 Other secondary gout, multiple sites
  M10.9 Gout, unspecified
    Gout NOS

● M11 Other crystal arthropathies
● M11.0 Hydroxyapatite deposition disease
    M11.00 Hydroxyapatite deposition disease, unspecified site
● M11.01 Hydroxyapatite deposition disease, shoulder
    M11.011 Hydroxyapatite deposition disease, right shoulder
    M11.012 Hydroxyapatite deposition disease, left shoulder
    M11.019 Hydroxyapatite deposition disease, unspecified shoulder

● M11.02 Hydroxyapatite deposition disease, elbow
    M11.021 Hydroxyapatite deposition disease, right elbow
    M11.022 Hydroxyapatite deposition disease, left elbow
    M11.029 Hydroxyapatite deposition disease, unspecified elbow
● M11.03 Hydroxyapatite deposition disease, wrist
    M11.031 Hydroxyapatite deposition disease, right wrist
    M11.032 Hydroxyapatite deposition disease, left wrist
    M11.039 Hydroxyapatite deposition disease, unspecified wrist
● M11.04 Hydroxyapatite deposition disease, hand
    M11.041 Hydroxyapatite deposition disease, right hand
    M11.042 Hydroxyapatite deposition disease, left hand
    M11.049 Hydroxyapatite deposition disease, unspecified hand
● M11.05 Hydroxyapatite deposition disease, hip
    M11.051 Hydroxyapatite deposition disease, right hip
    M11.052 Hydroxyapatite deposition disease, left hip
    M11.059 Hydroxyapatite deposition disease, unspecified hip
● M11.06 Hydroxyapatite deposition disease, knee
    M11.061 Hydroxyapatite deposition disease, right knee
    M11.062 Hydroxyapatite deposition disease, left knee
    M11.069 Hydroxyapatite deposition disease, unspecified knee
● M11.07 Hydroxyapatite deposition disease, ankle and foot
    M11.071 Hydroxyapatite deposition disease, right ankle and foot
    M11.072 Hydroxyapatite deposition disease, left ankle and foot
    M11.079 Hydroxyapatite deposition disease, unspecified ankle and foot
    M11.08 Hydroxyapatite deposition disease, vertebrae
    M11.09 Hydroxyapatite deposition disease, multiple sites
● M11.1 Familial chondrocalcinosis
    M11.10 Familial chondrocalcinosis, unspecified site
● M11.11 Familial chondrocalcinosis, shoulder
    M11.111 Familial chondrocalcinosis, right shoulder
    M11.112 Familial chondrocalcinosis, left shoulder
    M11.119 Familial chondrocalcinosis, unspecified shoulder
● M11.12 Familial chondrocalcinosis, elbow
    M11.121 Familial chondrocalcinosis, right elbow
    M11.122 Familial chondrocalcinosis, left elbow
    M11.129 Familial chondrocalcinosis, unspecified elbow
● M11.13 Familial chondrocalcinosis, wrist
    M11.131 Familial chondrocalcinosis, right wrist
    M11.132 Familial chondrocalcinosis, left wrist
    M11.139 Familial chondrocalcinosis, unspecified wrist

▶ New   ⇒ Revised   ~~deleted~~ Deleted   Excludes 1   Excludes 2   Includes   Use additional   Code first   Code also   Key words
OGCR Official Guidelines   ● Unacceptable Principal Diagnosis   X Assign placeholder X   ● Use Additional Character(s)   》 Manifestation Code   **Coding Clinic**

● M11.14 Familial chondrocalcinosis, hand
    M11.141 Familial chondrocalcinosis, right hand
    M11.142 Familial chondrocalcinosis, left hand
    M11.149 Familial chondrocalcinosis, unspecified hand

● M11.15 Familial chondrocalcinosis, hip
    M11.151 Familial chondrocalcinosis, right hip
    M11.152 Familial chondrocalcinosis, left hip
    M11.159 Familial chondrocalcinosis, unspecified hip

● M11.16 Familial chondrocalcinosis, knee
    M11.161 Familial chondrocalcinosis, right knee
    M11.162 Familial chondrocalcinosis, left knee
    M11.169 Familial chondrocalcinosis, unspecified knee

● M11.17 Familial chondrocalcinosis, ankle and foot
    M11.171 Familial chondrocalcinosis, right ankle and foot
    M11.172 Familial chondrocalcinosis, left ankle and foot
    M11.179 Familial chondrocalcinosis, unspecified ankle and foot

M11.18 Familial chondrocalcinosis, vertebrae
M11.19 Familial chondrocalcinosis, multiple sites

● M11.2 Other chondrocalcinosis
    Chondrocalcinosis NOS
M11.20 Other chondrocalcinosis, unspecified site

● M11.21 Other chondrocalcinosis, shoulder
    M11.211 Other chondrocalcinosis, right shoulder
    M11.212 Other chondrocalcinosis, left shoulder
    M11.219 Other chondrocalcinosis, unspecified shoulder

● M11.22 Other chondrocalcinosis, elbow
    M11.221 Other chondrocalcinosis, right elbow
    M11.222 Other chondrocalcinosis, left elbow
    M11.229 Other chondrocalcinosis, unspecified elbow

● M11.23 Other chondrocalcinosis, wrist
    M11.231 Other chondrocalcinosis, right wrist
    M11.232 Other chondrocalcinosis, left wrist
    M11.239 Other chondrocalcinosis, unspecified wrist

● M11.24 Other chondrocalcinosis, hand
    M11.241 Other chondrocalcinosis, right hand
    M11.242 Other chondrocalcinosis, left hand
    M11.249 Other chondrocalcinosis, unspecified hand

● M11.25 Other chondrocalcinosis, hip
    M11.251 Other chondrocalcinosis, right hip
    M11.252 Other chondrocalcinosis, left hip
    M11.259 Other chondrocalcinosis, unspecified hip

● M11.26 Other chondrocalcinosis, knee
    M11.261 Other chondrocalcinosis, right knee
    M11.262 Other chondrocalcinosis, left knee
    M11.269 Other chondrocalcinosis, unspecified knee

● M11.27 Other chondrocalcinosis, ankle and foot
    M11.271 Other chondrocalcinosis, right ankle and foot
    M11.272 Other chondrocalcinosis, left ankle and foot
    M11.279 Other chondrocalcinosis, unspecified ankle and foot

M11.28 Other chondrocalcinosis, vertebrae
M11.29 Other chondrocalcinosis, multiple sites

● M11.8 Other specified crystal arthropathies
M11.80 Other specified crystal arthropathies, unspecified site

● M11.81 Other specified crystal arthropathies, shoulder
    M11.811 Other specified crystal arthropathies, right shoulder
    M11.812 Other specified crystal arthropathies, left shoulder
    M11.819 Other specified crystal arthropathies, unspecified shoulder

● M11.82 Other specified crystal arthropathies, elbow
    M11.821 Other specified crystal arthropathies, right elbow
    M11.822 Other specified crystal arthropathies, left elbow
    M11.829 Other specified crystal arthropathies, unspecified elbow

● M11.83 Other specified crystal arthropathies, wrist
    M11.831 Other specified crystal arthropathies, right wrist
    M11.832 Other specified crystal arthropathies, left wrist
    M11.839 Other specified crystal arthropathies, unspecified wrist

● M11.84 Other specified crystal arthropathies, hand
    M11.841 Other specified crystal arthropathies, right hand
    M11.842 Other specified crystal arthropathies, left hand
    M11.849 Other specified crystal arthropathies, unspecified hand

● M11.85 Other specified crystal arthropathies, hip
    M11.851 Other specified crystal arthropathies, right hip
    M11.852 Other specified crystal arthropathies, left hip
    M11.859 Other specified crystal arthropathies, unspecified hip

● M11.86 Other specified crystal arthropathies, knee
    M11.861 Other specified crystal arthropathies, right knee
    M11.862 Other specified crystal arthropathies, left knee
    M11.869 Other specified crystal arthropathies, unspecified knee

● M11.87 Other specified crystal arthropathies, ankle and foot
    M11.871 Other specified crystal arthropathies, right ankle and foot
    M11.872 Other specified crystal arthropathies, left ankle and foot
    M11.879 Other specified crystal arthropathies, unspecified ankle and foot

M11.88 Other specified crystal arthropathies, vertebrae
M11.89 Other specified crystal arthropathies, multiple sites

M11.9 Crystal arthropathy, unspecified

CHAPTER 13 (M00-M99)

● **M12** **Other and unspecified arthropathy**

　　Excludes1　arthrosis (M15-M19)
　　　　　　　　cricoarytenoid arthropathy (J38.7)

● **M12.0**　Chronic postrheumatic arthropathy [Jaccoud]

　　M12.00　Chronic postrheumatic arthropathy [Jaccoud], unspecified site

　● M12.01　Chronic postrheumatic arthropathy [Jaccoud], shoulder

　　　M12.011　Chronic postrheumatic arthropathy [Jaccoud], right shoulder

　　　M12.012　Chronic postrheumatic arthropathy [Jaccoud], left shoulder

　　　M12.019　Chronic postrheumatic arthropathy [Jaccoud], unspecified shoulder

　● M12.02　Chronic postrheumatic arthropathy [Jaccoud], elbow

　　　M12.021　Chronic postrheumatic arthropathy [Jaccoud], right elbow

　　　M12.022　Chronic postrheumatic arthropathy [Jaccoud], left elbow

　　　M12.029　Chronic postrheumatic arthropathy [Jaccoud], unspecified elbow

　● M12.03　Chronic postrheumatic arthropathy [Jaccoud], wrist

　　　M12.031　Chronic postrheumatic arthropathy [Jaccoud], right wrist

　　　M12.032　Chronic postrheumatic arthropathy [Jaccoud], left wrist

　　　M12.039　Chronic postrheumatic arthropathy [Jaccoud], unspecified wrist

　● M12.04　Chronic postrheumatic arthropathy [Jaccoud], hand

　　　M12.041　Chronic postrheumatic arthropathy [Jaccoud], right hand

　　　M12.042　Chronic postrheumatic arthropathy [Jaccoud], left hand

　　　M12.049　Chronic postrheumatic arthropathy [Jaccoud], unspecified hand

　● M12.05　Chronic postrheumatic arthropathy [Jaccoud], hip

　　　M12.051　Chronic postrheumatic arthropathy [Jaccoud], right hip

　　　M12.052　Chronic postrheumatic arthropathy [Jaccoud], left hip

　　　M12.059　Chronic postrheumatic arthropathy [Jaccoud], unspecified hip

　● M12.06　Chronic postrheumatic arthropathy [Jaccoud], knee

　　　M12.061　Chronic postrheumatic arthropathy [Jaccoud], right knee

　　　M12.062　Chronic postrheumatic arthropathy [Jaccoud], left knee

　　　M12.069　Chronic postrheumatic arthropathy [Jaccoud], unspecified knee

　● M12.07　Chronic postrheumatic arthropathy [Jaccoud], ankle and foot

　　　M12.071　Chronic postrheumatic arthropathy [Jaccoud], right ankle and foot

　　　M12.072　Chronic postrheumatic arthropathy [Jaccoud], left ankle and foot

　　　M12.079　Chronic postrheumatic arthropathy [Jaccoud], unspecified ankle and foot

　　M12.08　Chronic postrheumatic arthropathy [Jaccoud], other specified site

　　　　　Chronic postrheumatic arthropathy [Jaccoud], vertebrae

　　M12.09　Chronic postrheumatic arthropathy [Jaccoud], multiple sites

● **M12.1**　Kaschin-Beck disease

　　　Osteochondroarthrosis deformans endemica

　　M12.10　Kaschin-Beck disease, unspecified site

　● M12.11　Kaschin-Beck disease, shoulder

　　　M12.111　Kaschin-Beck disease, right shoulder

　　　M12.112　Kaschin-Beck disease, left shoulder

　　　M12.119　Kaschin-Beck disease, unspecified shoulder

　● M12.12　Kaschin-Beck disease, elbow

　　　M12.121　Kaschin-Beck disease, right elbow

　　　M12.122　Kaschin-Beck disease, left elbow

　　　M12.129　Kaschin-Beck disease, unspecified elbow

　● M12.13　Kaschin-Beck disease, wrist

　　　M12.131　Kaschin-Beck disease, right wrist

　　　M12.132　Kaschin-Beck disease, left wrist

　　　M12.139　Kaschin-Beck disease, unspecified wrist

　● M12.14　Kaschin-Beck disease, hand

　　　M12.141　Kaschin-Beck disease, right hand

　　　M12.142　Kaschin-Beck disease, left hand

　　　M12.149　Kaschin-Beck disease, unspecified hand

　● M12.15　Kaschin-Beck disease, hip

　　　M12.151　Kaschin-Beck disease, right hip

　　　M12.152　Kaschin-Beck disease, left hip

　　　M12.159　Kaschin-Beck disease, unspecified hip

　● M12.16　Kaschin-Beck disease, knee

　　　M12.161　Kaschin-Beck disease, right knee

　　　M12.162　Kaschin-Beck disease, left knee

　　　M12.169　Kaschin-Beck disease, unspecified knee

　● M12.17　Kaschin-Beck disease, ankle and foot

　　　M12.171　Kaschin-Beck disease, right ankle and foot

　　　M12.172　Kaschin-Beck disease, left ankle and foot

　　　M12.179　Kaschin-Beck disease, unspecified ankle and foot

　　M12.18　Kaschin-Beck disease, vertebrae

　　M12.19　Kaschin-Beck disease, multiple sites

● **M12.2**　Villonodular synovitis (pigmented)

　　M12.20　Villonodular synovitis (pigmented), unspecified site

　● M12.21　Villonodular synovitis (pigmented), shoulder

　　　M12.211　Villonodular synovitis (pigmented), right shoulder

　　　M12.212　Villonodular synovitis (pigmented), left shoulder

　　　M12.219　Villonodular synovitis (pigmented), unspecified shoulder

　● M12.22　Villonodular synovitis (pigmented), elbow

　　　M12.221　Villonodular synovitis (pigmented), right elbow

　　　M12.222　Villonodular synovitis (pigmented), left elbow

　　　M12.229　Villonodular synovitis (pigmented), unspecified elbow

　● M12.23　Villonodular synovitis (pigmented), wrist

　　　M12.231　Villonodular synovitis (pigmented), right wrist

　　　M12.232　Villonodular synovitis (pigmented), left wrist

　　　M12.239　Villonodular synovitis (pigmented), unspecified wrist

▶ New　⇒ Revised　deleted Deleted　Excludes 1　Excludes 2　Includes　Use additional　Code first　Code also　Key words

OGCR Official Guidelines　● Unacceptable Principal Diagnosis　X Assign placeholder X　▶ Use Additional Character(s)　▌ Manifestation Code　**Coding Clinic**

● M12.24   Villonodular synovitis (pigmented), hand
     M12.241   Villonodular synovitis (pigmented), right hand
     M12.242   Villonodular synovitis (pigmented), left hand
     M12.249   Villonodular synovitis (pigmented), unspecified hand
● M12.25   Villonodular synovitis (pigmented), hip
     M12.251   Villonodular synovitis (pigmented), right hip
     M12.252   Villonodular synovitis (pigmented), left hip
     M12.259   Villonodular synovitis (pigmented), unspecified hip
● M12.26   Villonodular synovitis (pigmented), knee
     M12.261   Villonodular synovitis (pigmented), right knee
     M12.262   Villonodular synovitis (pigmented), left knee
     M12.269   Villonodular synovitis (pigmented), unspecified knee
● M12.27   Villonodular synovitis (pigmented), ankle and foot
     M12.271   Villonodular synovitis (pigmented), right ankle and foot
     M12.272   Villonodular synovitis (pigmented), left ankle and foot
     M12.279   Villonodular synovitis (pigmented), unspecified ankle and foot
     M12.28   Villonodular synovitis (pigmented), other specified site
         Villonodular synovitis (pigmented), vertebrae
     M12.29   Villonodular synovitis (pigmented), multiple sites
● M12.3   Palindromic rheumatism
     M12.30   Palindromic rheumatism, unspecified site
● M12.31   Palindromic rheumatism, shoulder
     M12.311   Palindromic rheumatism, right shoulder
     M12.312   Palindromic rheumatism, left shoulder
     M12.319   Palindromic rheumatism, unspecified shoulder
● M12.32   Palindromic rheumatism, elbow
     M12.321   Palindromic rheumatism, right elbow
     M12.322   Palindromic rheumatism, left elbow
     M12.329   Palindromic rheumatism, unspecified elbow
● M12.33   Palindromic rheumatism, wrist
     M12.331   Palindromic rheumatism, right wrist
     M12.332   Palindromic rheumatism, left wrist
     M12.339   Palindromic rheumatism, unspecified wrist
● M12.34   Palindromic rheumatism, hand
     M12.341   Palindromic rheumatism, right hand
     M12.342   Palindromic rheumatism, left hand
     M12.349   Palindromic rheumatism, unspecified hand
● M12.35   Palindromic rheumatism, hip
     M12.351   Palindromic rheumatism, right hip
     M12.352   Palindromic rheumatism, left hip
     M12.359   Palindromic rheumatism, unspecified hip

● M12.36   Palindromic rheumatism, knee
     M12.361   Palindromic rheumatism, right knee
     M12.362   Palindromic rheumatism, left knee
     M12.369   Palindromic rheumatism, unspecified knee
● M12.37   Palindromic rheumatism, ankle and foot
     M12.371   Palindromic rheumatism, right ankle and foot
     M12.372   Palindromic rheumatism, left ankle and foot
     M12.379   Palindromic rheumatism, unspecified ankle and foot
     M12.38   Palindromic rheumatism, other specified site
         Palindromic rheumatism, vertebrae
     M12.39   Palindromic rheumatism, multiple sites
● M12.4   Intermittent hydrarthrosis
     M12.40   Intermittent hydrarthrosis, unspecified site
● M12.41   Intermittent hydrarthrosis, shoulder
     M12.411   Intermittent hydrarthrosis, right shoulder
     M12.412   Intermittent hydrarthrosis, left shoulder
     M12.419   Intermittent hydrarthrosis, unspecified shoulder
● M12.42   Intermittent hydrarthrosis, elbow
     M12.421   Intermittent hydrarthrosis, right elbow
     M12.422   Intermittent hydrarthrosis, left elbow
     M12.429   Intermittent hydrarthrosis, unspecified elbow
● M12.43   Intermittent hydrarthrosis, wrist
     M12.431   Intermittent hydrarthrosis, right wrist
     M12.432   Intermittent hydrarthrosis, left wrist
     M12.439   Intermittent hydrarthrosis, unspecified wrist
● M12.44   Intermittent hydrarthrosis, hand
     M12.441   Intermittent hydrarthrosis, right hand
     M12.442   Intermittent hydrarthrosis, left hand
     M12.449   Intermittent hydrarthrosis, unspecified hand
● M12.45   Intermittent hydrarthrosis, hip
     M12.451   Intermittent hydrarthrosis, right hip
     M12.452   Intermittent hydrarthrosis, left hip
     M12.459   Intermittent hydrarthrosis, unspecified hip
● M12.46   Intermittent hydrarthrosis, knee
     M12.461   Intermittent hydrarthrosis, right knee
     M12.462   Intermittent hydrarthrosis, left knee
     M12.469   Intermittent hydrarthrosis, unspecified knee
● M12.47   Intermittent hydrarthrosis, ankle and foot
     M12.471   Intermittent hydrarthrosis, right ankle and foot
     M12.472   Intermittent hydrarthrosis, left ankle and foot
     M12.479   Intermittent hydrarthrosis, unspecified ankle and foot
     M12.48   Intermittent hydrarthrosis, other site
     M12.49   Intermittent hydrarthrosis, multiple sites

CHAPTER 13 (M00-M99)

● **M12.5 Traumatic arthropathy**

      Excludes1   current injury-see Alphabetic Index
                  post-traumatic osteoarthritis of first
                     carpometacarpal joint (M18.2-M18.3)
                  post-traumatic osteoarthritis of
                     hip (M16.4-M16.5)
                  post-traumatic osteoarthritis of knee
                     (M17.2-M17.3)
                  post-traumatic osteoarthritis NOS
                     (M19.1-)
                  post-traumatic osteoarthritis of other
                     single joints (M19.1-)

    M12.50 Traumatic arthropathy, unspecified site

● M12.51 Traumatic arthropathy, shoulder

       M12.511 Traumatic arthropathy, right shoulder

       M12.512 Traumatic arthropathy, left shoulder

       M12.519 Traumatic arthropathy, unspecified
                 shoulder

● M12.52 Traumatic arthropathy, elbow

       M12.521 Traumatic arthropathy, right elbow

       M12.522 Traumatic arthropathy, left elbow

       M12.529 Traumatic arthropathy, unspecified
                 elbow

● M12.53 Traumatic arthropathy, wrist

       M12.531 Traumatic arthropathy, right wrist

       M12.532 Traumatic arthropathy, left wrist

       M12.539 Traumatic arthropathy, unspecified
                 wrist

● M12.54 Traumatic arthropathy, hand

       M12.541 Traumatic arthropathy, right hand

       M12.542 Traumatic arthropathy, left hand

       M12.549 Traumatic arthropathy, unspecified
                 hand

● M12.55 Traumatic arthropathy, hip

       M12.551 Traumatic arthropathy, right hip

       M12.552 Traumatic arthropathy, left hip
                 Coding Clinic: 2015, Q1, P17

       M12.559 Traumatic arthropathy, unspecified
                 hip

● M12.56 Traumatic arthropathy, knee

       M12.561 Traumatic arthropathy, right knee

       M12.562 Traumatic arthropathy, left knee

       M12.569 Traumatic arthropathy, unspecified
                 knee

● M12.57 Traumatic arthropathy, ankle and foot

       M12.571 Traumatic arthropathy, right ankle
                 and foot

       M12.572 Traumatic arthropathy, left ankle and
                 foot

       M12.579 Traumatic arthropathy, unspecified
                 ankle and foot

    M12.58 Traumatic arthropathy, other specified site
          Traumatic arthropathy, vertebrae

    M12.59 Traumatic arthropathy, multiple sites

● **M12.8 Other specific arthropathies, not elsewhere classified**
      Transient arthropathy

    M12.80 Other specific arthropathies, not elsewhere
         classified, unspecified site

● M12.81 Other specific arthropathies, not
         classified, shoulder

       M12.811 Other specific arthropathies, not
                 elsewhere classified, right shoulder

       M12.812 Other specific arthropathies, not
                 elsewhere classified, left shoulder

       M12.819 Other specific arthropathies, not
                 elsewhere classified, unspecified
                 shoulder

● M12.82 Other specific arthropathies, not elsewhere
         classified, elbow

       M12.821 Other specific arthropathies, not
                 elsewhere classified, right elbow

       M12.822 Other specific arthropathies, not
                 elsewhere classified, left elbow

       M12.829 Other specific arthropathies, not
                 elsewhere classified, unspecified
                 elbow

● M12.83 Other specific arthropathies, not elsewhere
         classified, wrist

       M12.831 Other specific arthropathies, not
                 elsewhere classified, right wrist

       M12.832 Other specific arthropathies, not
                 elsewhere classified, left wrist

       M12.839 Other specific arthropathies, not
                 elsewhere classified, unspecified wrist

● M12.84 Other specific arthropathies, not elsewhere
         classified, hand

       M12.841 Other specific arthropathies, not
                 elsewhere classified, right hand

       M12.842 Other specific arthropathies, not
                 elsewhere classified, left hand

       M12.849 Other specific arthropathies, not
                 elsewhere classified, unspecified hand

● M12.85 Other specific arthropathies, not elsewhere
         classified, hip

       M12.851 Other specific arthropathies, not
                 elsewhere classified, right hip

       M12.852 Other specific arthropathies, not
                 elsewhere classified, left hip

       M12.859 Other specific arthropathies, not
                 elsewhere classified, unspecified hip

● M12.86 Other specific arthropathies, not elsewhere
         classified, knee

       M12.861 Other specific arthropathies, not
                 elsewhere classified, right knee

       M12.862 Other specific arthropathies, not
                 elsewhere classified, left knee

       M12.869 Other specific arthropathies, not
                 elsewhere classified, unspecified knee

● M12.87 Other specific arthropathies, not elsewhere
         classified, ankle and foot

       M12.871 Other specific arthropathies, not
                 elsewhere classified, right ankle and
                 foot

       M12.872 Other specific arthropathies, not
                 elsewhere classified, left ankle and
                 foot

       M12.879 Other specific arthropathies, not
                 elsewhere classified, unspecified
                 ankle and foot

    M12.88 Other specific arthropathies, not elsewhere
         classified, other specified site
         Other specific arthropathies, not elsewhere
           classified, vertebrae

    M12.89 Other specific arthropathies, not elsewhere
         classified, multiple sites

M12.9 Arthropathy, unspecified

▶ New   ⇛ Revised   ~~deleted~~ Deleted   Excludes 1   Excludes 2   Includes   Use additional   Code first   Code also   Key words

OGCR Official Guidelines   ● Unacceptable Principal Diagnosis   X Assign placeholder X   ● Use Additional Character(s)   ▶ Manifestation Code   **Coding Clinic**

● **M13   Other arthritis**

     Excludes1   arthrosis (M15-M19)
                 osteoarthritis (M15-M19)

   M13.0   Polyarthritis, unspecified

● **M13.1   Monoarthritis, not elsewhere classified**

     M13.10   Monoarthritis, not elsewhere classified, unspecified site

     ● **M13.11   Monoarthritis, not elsewhere classified, shoulder**

       M13.111   Monoarthritis, not elsewhere classified, right shoulder

       M13.112   Monoarthritis, not elsewhere classified, left shoulder

       M13.119   Monoarthritis, not elsewhere classified, unspecified shoulder

     ● **M13.12   Monoarthritis, not elsewhere classified, elbow**

       M13.121   Monoarthritis, not elsewhere classified, right elbow

       M13.122   Monoarthritis, not elsewhere classified, left elbow

       M13.129   Monoarthritis, not elsewhere classified, unspecified elbow

     ● **M13.13   Monoarthritis, not elsewhere classified, wrist**

       M13.131   Monoarthritis, not elsewhere classified, right wrist

       M13.132   Monoarthritis, not elsewhere classified, left wrist

       M13.139   Monoarthritis, not elsewhere classified, unspecified wrist

     ● **M13.14   Monoarthritis, not elsewhere classified, hand**

       M13.141   Monoarthritis, not elsewhere classified, right hand

       M13.142   Monoarthritis, not elsewhere classified, left hand

       M13.149   Monoarthritis, not elsewhere classified, unspecified hand

     ● **M13.15   Monoarthritis, not elsewhere classified, hip**

       M13.151   Monoarthritis, not elsewhere classified, right hip

       M13.152   Monoarthritis, not elsewhere classified, left hip

       M13.159   Monoarthritis, not elsewhere classified, unspecified hip

     ● **M13.16   Monoarthritis, not elsewhere classified, knee**

       M13.161   Monoarthritis, not elsewhere classified, right knee

       M13.162   Monoarthritis, not elsewhere classified, left knee

       M13.169   Monoarthritis, not elsewhere classified, unspecified knee

     ● **M13.17   Monoarthritis, not elsewhere classified, ankle and foot**

       M13.171   Monoarthritis, not elsewhere classified, right ankle and foot

       M13.172   Monoarthritis, not elsewhere classified, left ankle and foot

       M13.179   Monoarthritis, not elsewhere classified, unspecified ankle and foot

● **M13.8   Other specified arthritis**
     Allergic arthritis

     Excludes1   osteoarthritis (M15-M19)

     M13.80   Other specified arthritis, unspecified site

     ● **M13.81   Other specified arthritis, shoulder**

       M13.811   Other specified arthritis, right shoulder

       M13.812   Other specified arthritis, left shoulder

       M13.819   Other specified arthritis, unspecified shoulder

     ● **M13.82   Other specified arthritis, elbow**

       M13.821   Other specified arthritis, right elbow

       M13.822   Other specified arthritis, left elbow

       M13.829   Other specified arthritis, unspecified elbow

     ● **M13.83   Other specified arthritis, wrist**

       M13.831   Other specified arthritis, right wrist

       M13.832   Other specified arthritis, left wrist

       M13.839   Other specified arthritis, unspecified wrist

     ● **M13.84   Other specified arthritis, hand**

       M13.841   Other specified arthritis, right hand

       M13.842   Other specified arthritis, left hand

       M13.849   Other specified arthritis, unspecified hand

     ● **M13.85   Other specified arthritis, hip**

       M13.851   Other specified arthritis, right hip

       M13.852   Other specified arthritis, left hip

       M13.859   Other specified arthritis, unspecified hip

     ● **M13.86   Other specified arthritis, knee**

       M13.861   Other specified arthritis, right knee

       M13.862   Other specified arthritis, left knee

       M13.869   Other specified arthritis, unspecified knee

     ● **M13.87   Other specified arthritis, ankle and foot**

       M13.871   Other specified arthritis, right ankle and foot

       M13.872   Other specified arthritis, left ankle and foot

       M13.879   Other specified arthritis, unspecified ankle and foot

     M13.88   Other specified arthritis, other site

     M13.89   Other specified arthritis, multiple sites

● **M14   Arthropathies in other diseases classified elsewhere**

     Excludes1   arthropathy in:
               diabetes mellitus (E08-E13 with .61-)
               hematological disorders (M36.2-M36.3)
               hypersensitivity reactions (M36.4)
               neoplastic disease (M36.1)
               neurosyphillis (A52.16)
               sarcoidosis (D86.86)
           enteropathic arthropathies (M07.0-)
           juvenile psoriatic arthropathy (L40.54)
           lipoid dermatoarthritis (E78.81)

● **M14.6   Charcôt's joint**
     Neuropathic arthropathy

     Excludes1   Charcôt's joint in diabetes mellitus (E08-E13 with .610)
                 Charcôt's joint in tabes dorsalis (A52.16)

     M14.60   Charcôt's joint, unspecified site

     ● **M14.61   Charcôt's joint, shoulder**

       M14.611   Charcôt's joint, right shoulder

       M14.612   Charcôt's joint, left shoulder

       M14.619   Charcôt's joint, unspecified shoulder

     ● **M14.62   Charcôt's joint, elbow**

       M14.621   Charcôt's joint, right elbow

       M14.622   Charcôt's joint, left elbow

       M14.629   Charcôt's joint, unspecified elbow

     ● **M14.63   Charcôt's joint, wrist**

       M14.631   Charcôt's joint, right wrist

       M14.632   Charcôt's joint, left wrist

       M14.639   Charcôt's joint, unspecified wrist

CHAPTER 13 (M00-M99)

● **M14.64** Charcôt's joint, hand
      M14.641   Charcôt's joint, right hand
      M14.642   Charcôt's joint, left hand
      M14.649   Charcôt's joint, unspecified hand

● **M14.65** Charcôt's joint, hip
      M14.651   Charcôt's joint, right hip
      M14.652   Charcôt's joint, left hip
      M14.659   Charcôt's joint, unspecified hip

● **M14.66** Charcôt's joint, knee
      M14.661   Charcôt's joint, right knee
      M14.662   Charcôt's joint, left knee
      M14.669   Charcôt's joint, unspecified knee

● **M14.67** Charcôt's joint, ankle and foot
      M14.671   Charcôt's joint, right ankle and foot
      M14.672   Charcôt's joint, left ankle and foot
      M14.679   Charcôt's joint, unspecified ankle and foot

   M14.68 Charcôt's joint, vertebrae
   M14.69 Charcôt's joint, multiple sites

● **M14.8** Arthropathies in other specified diseases classified elsewhere
      Code first underlying disease, such as:
        amyloidosis (E85.-)
        erythema multiforme (L51.-)
        erythema nodosum (L52)
        hemochromatosis (E83.11-)
        hyperparathyroidism (E21.-)
        hypothyroidism (E00-E03)
        sickle-cell disorders (D57.-)
        thyrotoxicosis [hyperthyroidism] (E05.-)
        Whipple's disease (K90.81)

  ▷ *M14.80*   *Arthropathies in other specified diseases classified elsewhere, unspecified site*

● **M14.81** Arthropathies in other specified diseases classified elsewhere, shoulder
  ▷ *M14.811*   *Arthropathies in other specified diseases classified elsewhere, right shoulder*
  ▷ *M14.812*   *Arthropathies in other specified diseases classified elsewhere, left shoulder*
  ▷ *M14.819*   *Arthropathies in other specified diseases classified elsewhere, unspecified shoulder*

● **M14.82** Arthropathies in other specified diseases classified elsewhere, elbow
  ▷ *M14.821*   *Arthropathies in other specified diseases classified elsewhere, right elbow*
  ▷ *M14.822*   *Arthropathies in other specified diseases classified elsewhere, left elbow*
  ▷ *M14.829*   *Arthropathies in other specified diseases classified elsewhere, unspecified elbow*

● **M14.83** Arthropathies in other specified diseases classified elsewhere, wrist
  ▷ *M14.831*   *Arthropathies in other specified diseases classified elsewhere, right wrist*
  ▷ *M14.832*   *Arthropathies in other specified diseases classified elsewhere, left wrist*
  ▷ *M14.839*   *Arthropathies in other specified diseases classified elsewhere, unspecified wrist*

● **M14.84** Arthropathies in other specified diseases classified elsewhere, hand
  ▷ *M14.841*   *Arthropathies in other specified diseases classified elsewhere, right hand*
  ▷ *M14.842*   *Arthropathies in other specified diseases classified elsewhere, left hand*
  ▷ *M14.849*   *Arthropathies in other specified diseases classified elsewhere, unspecified hand*

● **M14.85** Arthropathies in other specified diseases classified elsewhere, hip
  ▷ *M14.851*   *Arthropathies in other specified diseases classified elsewhere, right hip*
  ▷ *M14.852*   *Arthropathies in other specified diseases classified elsewhere, left hip*
  ▷ *M14.859*   *Arthropathies in other specified diseases classified elsewhere, unspecified hip*

● **M14.86** Arthropathies in other specified diseases classified elsewhere, knee
  ▷ *M14.861*   *Arthropathies in other specified diseases classified elsewhere, right knee*
  ▷ *M14.862*   *Arthropathies in other specified diseases classified elsewhere, left knee*
  ▷ *M14.869*   *Arthropathies in other specified diseases classified elsewhere, unspecified knee*

● **M14.87** Arthropathies in other specified diseases classified elsewhere, ankle and foot
  ▷ *M14.871*   *Arthropathies in other specified diseases classified elsewhere, right ankle and foot*
  ▷ *M14.872*   *Arthropathies in other specified diseases classified elsewhere, left ankle and foot*
  ▷ *M14.879*   *Arthropathies in other specified diseases classified elsewhere, unspecified ankle and foot*

  ▷ *M14.88*   *Arthropathies in other specified diseases classified elsewhere, vertebrae*
  ▷ *M14.89*   *Arthropathies in other specified diseases classified elsewhere, multiple sites*

OSTEOARTHRITIS (M15-M19)

Osteoarthritis is the most common degenerative joint disease and form of arthritis that breaks down the cartilage causing pain, swelling, and reduced motion in the joints.

   Excludes2   osteoarthritis of spine (M47.-)

● **M15 Polyosteoarthritis**
   Includes   arthritis of multiple sites
   Excludes1   bilateral involvement of single joint (M16-M19)

   M15.0   Primary generalized (osteo)arthritis
   M15.1   Heberden's nodes (with arthropathy)
         Interphalangeal distal osteoarthritis
   M15.2   Bouchard's nodes (with arthropathy)
         Juxtaphalangeal distal osteoarthritis
   M15.3   Secondary multiple arthritis
         Post-traumatic polyosteoarthritis
   M15.4   Erosive (osteo)arthritis
   M15.8   Other polyosteoarthritis
   M15.9   Polyosteoarthritis, unspecified
         Generalized osteoarthritis NOS

● **M16   Osteoarthritis of hip**

     M16.0   Bilateral primary osteoarthritis of hip
         Coding Clinic: 2016, Q4, P146

    ● **M16.1   Unilateral primary osteoarthritis of hip**
         Primary osteoarthritis of hip NOS

         M16.10   Unilateral primary osteoarthritis, unspecified hip

         M16.11   Unilateral primary osteoarthritis, right hip

         M16.12   Unilateral primary osteoarthritis, left hip

     M16.2   Bilateral osteoarthritis resulting from hip dysplasia

    ● **M16.3   Unilateral osteoarthritis resulting from hip dysplasia**
         Dysplastic osteoarthritis of hip NOS

         M16.30   Unilateral osteoarthritis resulting from hip dysplasia, unspecified hip

         M16.31   Unilateral osteoarthritis resulting from hip dysplasia, right hip

         M16.32   Unilateral osteoarthritis resulting from hip dysplasia, left hip

     M16.4   Bilateral post-traumatic osteoarthritis of hip

    ● **M16.5   Unilateral post-traumatic osteoarthritis of hip**
         Post-traumatic osteoarthritis of hip NOS

         M16.50   Unilateral post-traumatic osteoarthritis, unspecified hip

         M16.51   Unilateral post-traumatic osteoarthritis, right hip

         M16.52   Unilateral post-traumatic osteoarthritis, left hip

     M16.6   Other bilateral secondary osteoarthritis of hip

     M16.7   Other unilateral secondary osteoarthritis of hip
         Secondary osteoarthritis of hip NOS

     M16.9   Osteoarthritis of hip, unspecified

● **M17   Osteoarthritis of knee**

     M17.0   Bilateral primary osteoarthritis of knee

    ● **M17.1   Unilateral primary osteoarthritis of knee**
         Primary osteoarthritis of knee NOS

         M17.10   Unilateral primary osteoarthritis, unspecified knee
            Coding Clinic: 2016, Q4, P147

         M17.11   Unilateral primary osteoarthritis, right knee

         M17.12   Unilateral primary osteoarthritis, left knee
            Coding Clinic: 2016, Q4, P146

     M17.2   Bilateral post-traumatic osteoarthritis of knee

    ● **M17.3   Unilateral post-traumatic osteoarthritis of knee**
         Post-traumatic osteoarthritis of knee NOS

         M17.30   Unilateral post-traumatic osteoarthritis, unspecified knee

         M17.31   Unilateral post-traumatic osteoarthritis, right knee

         M17.32   Unilateral post-traumatic osteoarthritis, left knee

     M17.4   Other bilateral secondary osteoarthritis of knee

     M17.5   Other unilateral secondary osteoarthritis of knee
         Secondary osteoarthritis of knee NOS

     M17.9   Osteoarthritis of knee, unspecified
         Coding Clinic: 2016, Q4, P146

● **M18   Osteoarthritis of first carpometacarpal joint**

     M18.0   Bilateral primary osteoarthritis of first carpometacarpal joints

    ● **M18.1   Unilateral primary osteoarthritis of first carpometacarpal joint**
         Primary osteoarthritis of first carpometacarpal joint NOS

         M18.10   Unilateral primary osteoarthritis of first carpometacarpal joint, unspecified hand

         M18.11   Unilateral primary osteoarthritis of first carpometacarpal joint, right hand

         M18.12   Unilateral primary osteoarthritis of first carpometacarpal joint, left hand

     M18.2   Bilateral post-traumatic osteoarthritis of first carpometacarpal joints

    ● **M18.3   Unilateral post-traumatic osteoarthritis of first carpometacarpal joint**
         Post-traumatic osteoarthritis of first carpometacarpal joint NOS

         M18.30   Unilateral post-traumatic osteoarthritis of first carpometacarpal joint, unspecified hand

         M18.31   Unilateral post-traumatic osteoarthritis of first carpometacarpal joint, right hand

         M18.32   Unilateral post-traumatic osteoarthritis of first carpometacarpal joint, left hand

     M18.4   Other bilateral secondary osteoarthritis of first carpometacarpal joints

    ● **M18.5   Other unilateral secondary osteoarthritis of first carpometacarpal joint**
         Secondary osteoarthritis of first carpometacarpal joint NOS

         M18.50   Other unilateral secondary osteoarthritis of first carpometacarpal joint, unspecified hand

         M18.51   Other unilateral secondary osteoarthritis of first carpometacarpal joint, right hand

         M18.52   Other unilateral secondary osteoarthritis of first carpometacarpal joint, left hand

     M18.9   Osteoarthritis of first carpometacarpal joint, unspecified

● **M19   Other and unspecified osteoarthritis**

     Excludes1   polyarthritis (M15.-)
     Excludes2   arthrosis of spine (M47.-)
                 hallux rigidus (M20.2)
                 osteoarthritis of spine (M47.-)

    ● **M19.0   Primary osteoarthritis of other joints**

      ● **M19.01   Primary osteoarthritis, shoulder**

         M19.011   Primary osteoarthritis, right shoulder
            Coding Clinic: 2016, Q4, P145

         M19.012   Primary osteoarthritis, left shoulder

         M19.019   Primary osteoarthritis, unspecified shoulder

      ● **M19.02   Primary osteoarthritis, elbow**

         M19.021   Primary osteoarthritis, right elbow

         M19.022   Primary osteoarthritis, left elbow

         M19.029   Primary osteoarthritis, unspecified elbow

      ● **M19.03   Primary osteoarthritis, wrist**

         M19.031   Primary osteoarthritis, right wrist

         M19.032   Primary osteoarthritis, left wrist

         M19.039   Primary osteoarthritis, unspecified wrist

      ● **M19.04   Primary osteoarthritis, hand**

         Excludes2   primary osteoarthritis of first carpometacarpal joint (M18.0-, M18.1-)

         M19.041   Primary osteoarthritis, right hand

         M19.042   Primary osteoarthritis, left hand

         M19.049   Primary osteoarthritis, unspecified hand

      ● **M19.07   Primary osteoarthritis ankle and foot**

         M19.071   Primary osteoarthritis, right ankle and foot

         M19.072   Primary osteoarthritis, left ankle and foot

         M19.079   Primary osteoarthritis, unspecified ankle and foot

CHAPTER 13 (M00-M99)

- **M19.1   Post-traumatic osteoarthritis of other joints**
  - **M19.11   Post-traumatic osteoarthritis, shoulder**
    - **M19.111   Post-traumatic osteoarthritis, right shoulder**
    - **M19.112   Post-traumatic osteoarthritis, left shoulder**
    - **M19.119   Post-traumatic osteoarthritis, unspecified shoulder**
  - **M19.12   Post-traumatic osteoarthritis, elbow**
    - **M19.121   Post-traumatic osteoarthritis, right elbow**
    - **M19.122   Post-traumatic osteoarthritis, left elbow**
    - **M19.129   Post-traumatic osteoarthritis, unspecified elbow**
  - **M19.13   Post-traumatic osteoarthritis, wrist**
    - **M19.131   Post-traumatic osteoarthritis, right wrist**
    - **M19.132   Post-traumatic osteoarthritis, left wrist**
    - **M19.139   Post-traumatic osteoarthritis, unspecified wrist**
  - **M19.14   Post-traumatic osteoarthritis, hand**
    - **Excludes2**   post-traumatic osteoarthritis of first carpometacarpal joint (M18.2-, M18.3-)
    - **M19.141   Post-traumatic osteoarthritis, right hand**
    - **M19.142   Post-traumatic osteoarthritis, left hand**
    - **M19.149   Post-traumatic osteoarthritis, unspecified hand**
  - **M19.17   Post-traumatic osteoarthritis, ankle and foot**
    - **M19.171   Post-traumatic osteoarthritis, right ankle and foot**
    - **M19.172   Post-traumatic osteoarthritis, left ankle and foot**
    - **M19.179   Post-traumatic osteoarthritis, unspecified ankle and foot**
- **M19.2   Secondary osteoarthritis of other joints**
  - **M19.21   Secondary osteoarthritis, shoulder**
    - **M19.211   Secondary osteoarthritis, right shoulder**
    - **M19.212   Secondary osteoarthritis, left shoulder**
    - **M19.219   Secondary osteoarthritis, unspecified shoulder**
  - **M19.22   Secondary osteoarthritis, elbow**
    - **M19.221   Secondary osteoarthritis, right elbow**
    - **M19.222   Secondary osteoarthritis, left elbow**
    - **M19.229   Secondary osteoarthritis, unspecified elbow**
  - **M19.23   Secondary osteoarthritis, wrist**
    - **M19.231   Secondary osteoarthritis, right wrist**
    - **M19.232   Secondary osteoarthritis, left wrist**
    - **M19.239   Secondary osteoarthritis, unspecified wrist**
  - **M19.24   Secondary osteoarthritis, hand**
    - **M19.241   Secondary osteoarthritis, right hand**
    - **M19.242   Secondary osteoarthritis, left hand**
    - **M19.249   Secondary osteoarthritis, unspecified hand**
  - **M19.27   Secondary osteoarthritis, ankle and foot**
    - **M19.271   Secondary osteoarthritis, right ankle and foot**
    - **M19.272   Secondary osteoarthritis, left ankle and foot**
    - **M19.279   Secondary osteoarthritis, unspecified ankle and foot**

- **M19.9   Osteoarthritis, unspecified site**
  - **M19.90   Unspecified osteoarthritis, unspecified site**
    Arthrosis NOS
    Arthritis NOS
    Osteoarthritis NOS
    Coding Clinic: 2016, Q4, P147
  - **M19.91   Primary osteoarthritis, unspecified site**
    Primary osteoarthritis NOS
  - **M19.92   Post-traumatic osteoarthritis, unspecified site**
    Post-traumatic osteoarthritis NOS
  - **M19.93   Secondary osteoarthritis, unspecified site**
    Secondary osteoarthritis NOS

OTHER JOINT DISORDERS (M20-M25)

Excludes2   joints of the spine (M40-M54)

- **M20   Acquired deformities of fingers and toes**
  - **Excludes1**   acquired absence of fingers and toes (Z89.-)
    congenital absence of fingers and toes (Q71.3-, Q72.3-)
    congenital deformities and malformations of fingers and toes (Q66.-, Q68-Q70, Q74.-)
  - **M20.0   Deformity of finger(s)**
    - **Excludes1**   clubbing of fingers (R68.3)
      palmar fascial fibromatosis [Dupuytren] (M72.0)
      trigger finger (M65.3)
    - **M20.00   Unspecified deformity of finger(s)**
      - **M20.001   Unspecified deformity of right finger(s)**
      - **M20.002   Unspecified deformity of left finger(s)**
      - **M20.009   Unspecified deformity of unspecified finger(s)**
    - **M20.01   Mallet finger**
      - **M20.011   Mallet finger of right finger(s)**
      - **M20.012   Mallet finger of left finger(s)**
      - **M20.019   Mallet finger of unspecified finger(s)**
    - **M20.02   Boutonnière deformity**
      - **M20.021   Boutonnière deformity of right finger(s)**
      - **M20.022   Boutonnière deformity of left finger(s)**
      - **M20.029   Boutonnière deformity of unspecified finger(s)**
    - **M20.03   Swan-neck deformity**
      - **M20.031   Swan-neck deformity of right finger(s)**
      - **M20.032   Swan-neck deformity of left finger(s)**
      - **M20.039   Swan-neck deformity of unspecified finger(s)**
    - **M20.09   Other deformity of finger(s)**
      - **M20.091   Other deformity of right finger(s)**
      - **M20.092   Other deformity of left finger(s)**
      - **M20.099   Other deformity of finger(s), unspecified finger(s)**
  - **M20.1   Hallux valgus (acquired)**
    - **Excludes2**   bunion (M21.6-)
    - **Coding Clinic: 2016, Q4, P38**
    - **M20.10   Hallux valgus (acquired), unspecified foot**
    - **M20.11   Hallux valgus (acquired), right foot**
    - **M20.12   Hallux valgus (acquired), left foot**
  - **M20.2   Hallux rigidus**
    - **M20.20   Hallux rigidus, unspecified foot**
    - **M20.21   Hallux rigidus, right foot**
    - **M20.22   Hallux rigidus, left foot**

▶ New   ⇒ Revised   ~~deleted~~ Deleted   Excludes 1   Excludes 2   Includes   Use additional   Code first   Code also   Key words
OGCR Official Guidelines   ● Unacceptable Principal Diagnosis   X Assign placeholder X   ● Use Additional Character(s)   ▌ Manifestation Code   **Coding Clinic**

Figure 13-1   Hallux valgus.

Item 13-2 Hallux valgus is a sometimes painful structural deformity caused by an inflammation of the bursal sac at the base of the metatarsophalangeal joint (big toe). **Hallux varus** is a deviation of the great toe to the inner side of the foot or away from the next toe.

- ● **M20.3 Hallux varus (acquired)**
  - M20.30   Hallux varus (acquired), unspecified foot
  - M20.31   Hallux varus (acquired), right foot
  - M20.32   Hallux varus (acquired), left foot
- ● **M20.4 Other hammer toe(s) (acquired)**
  - M20.40   Other hammer toe(s) (acquired), unspecified foot
  - M20.41   Other hammer toe(s) (acquired), right foot
  - M20.42   Other hammer toe(s) (acquired), left foot
- ● **M20.5 Other deformities of toe(s) (acquired)**
  - ● **M20.5X Other deformities of toe(s) (acquired)**
    - M20.5X1   Other deformities of toe(s) (acquired), right foot
    - M20.5X2   Other deformities of toe(s) (acquired), left foot
    - M20.5X9   Other deformities of toe(s) (acquired), unspecified foot
- ● **M20.6 Acquired deformities of toe(s), unspecified**
  - M20.60   Acquired deformities of toe(s), unspecified, unspecified foot
  - M20.61   Acquired deformities of toe(s), unspecified, right foot
  - M20.62   Acquired deformities of toe(s), unspecified, left foot
- ● **M21 Other acquired deformities of limbs**
  - **Excludes1**   acquired absence of limb (Z89.-)
    - congenital absence of limbs (Q71-Q73)
    - congenital deformities and malformations of limbs (Q65-Q66, Q68-Q74)
  - **Excludes2**   acquired deformities of fingers or toes (M20.-)
    - coxa plana (M91.2)
- ● **M21.0 Valgus deformity, not elsewhere classified**
  - **Excludes1**   metatarsus valgus (Q66.6)
    - talipes calcaneovalgus (Q66.4)
  - M21.00   Valgus deformity, not elsewhere classified, unspecified site
  - ● **M21.02 Valgus deformity, not elsewhere classified, elbow**
    - Cubitus valgus
    - M21.021   Valgus deformity, not elsewhere classified, right elbow
    - M21.022   Valgus deformity, not elsewhere classified, left elbow
    - M21.029   Valgus deformity, not elsewhere classified, unspecified elbow

Item 13-3 Cubitus valgus is a deformity of the elbow resulting in an increased carrying angle in which the arm extends at the side and the palm faces forward, which results in the forearm and hand extended at a greater than 15 degrees.

Item 13-4 Cubitus varus is a deformity of the elbow resulting in the arm extended at the side and the palm facing forward so that the forearm and hand are held at less than 5 degrees, decreasing the carrying angle.

- ● **M21.05 Valgus deformity, not elsewhere classified, hip**
  - M21.051   Valgus deformity, not elsewhere classified, right hip
  - M21.052   Valgus deformity, not elsewhere classified, left hip
  - M21.059   Valgus deformity, not elsewhere classified, unspecified hip
- ● **M21.06 Valgus deformity, not elsewhere classified, knee**
  - Genu valgum
  - Knock knee
  - M21.061   Valgus deformity, not elsewhere classified, right knee
  - M21.062   Valgus deformity, not elsewhere classified, left knee
  - M21.069   Valgus deformity, not elsewhere classified, unspecified knee
- ● **M21.07 Valgus deformity, not elsewhere classified, ankle**
  - M21.071   Valgus deformity, not elsewhere classified, right ankle
  - M21.072   Valgus deformity, not elsewhere classified, left ankle
  - M21.079   Valgus deformity, not elsewhere classified, unspecified ankle
- ● **M21.1 Varus deformity, not elsewhere classified**
  - **Excludes1**   metatarsus varus (Q66.22)
    - tibia vara (M92.5)
  - M21.10   Varus deformity, not elsewhere classified, unspecified site
  - ● **M21.12 Varus deformity, not elsewhere classified, elbow**
    - Cubitus varus, elbow
    - M21.121   Varus deformity, not elsewhere classified, right elbow
    - M21.122   Varus deformity, not elsewhere classified, left elbow
    - M21.129   Varus deformity, not elsewhere classified, unspecified elbow
  - ● **M21.15 Varus deformity, not elsewhere classified, hip**
    - M21.151   Varus deformity, not elsewhere classified, right hip
    - M21.152   Varus deformity, not elsewhere classified, left hip
    - M21.159   Varus deformity, not elsewhere classified, unspecified
  - ● **M21.16 Varus deformity, not elsewhere classified, knee**
    - Bow leg
    - Genu varum
    - M21.161   Varus deformity, not elsewhere classified, right knee
    - M21.162   Varus deformity, not elsewhere classified, left knee
    - M21.169   Varus deformity, not elsewhere classified, unspecified knee
  - ● **M21.17 Varus deformity, not elsewhere classified, ankle**
    - M21.171   Varus deformity, not elsewhere classified, right ankle
    - M21.172   Varus deformity, not elsewhere classified, left ankle
    - M21.179   Varus deformity, not elsewhere classified, unspecified ankle

CHAPTER 13 (M00-M99)

● **M21.2**   **Flexion** deformity
    M21.20   Flexion deformity, unspecified site
   ● **M21.21**   Flexion deformity, shoulder
       M21.211   Flexion deformity, right shoulder
       M21.212   Flexion deformity, left shoulder
       M21.219   Flexion deformity, unspecified shoulder
   ● **M21.22**   Flexion deformity, elbow
       M21.221   Flexion deformity, right elbow
       M21.222   Flexion deformity, left elbow
       M21.229   Flexion deformity, unspecified elbow
   ● **M21.23**   Flexion deformity, wrist
       M21.231   Flexion deformity, right wrist
       M21.232   Flexion deformity, left wrist
       M21.239   Flexion deformity, unspecified wrist
   ● **M21.24**   Flexion deformity, finger joints
       M21.241   Flexion deformity, right finger joints
       M21.242   Flexion deformity, left finger joints
       M21.249   Flexion deformity, unspecified finger joints
   ● **M21.25**   Flexion deformity, hip
       M21.251   Flexion deformity, right hip
       M21.252   Flexion deformity, left hip
       M21.259   Flexion deformity, unspecified hip
   ● **M21.26**   Flexion deformity, knee
       M21.261   Flexion deformity, right knee
       M21.262   Flexion deformity, left knee
       M21.269   Flexion deformity, unspecified knee
   ● **M21.27**   Flexion deformity, ankle and toes
       M21.271   Flexion deformity, right ankle and toes
       M21.272   Flexion deformity, left ankle and toes
       M21.279   Flexion deformity, unspecified ankle and toes
● **M21.3**   Wrist or foot drop (acquired)
  ● **M21.33**   Wrist drop (acquired)
       M21.331   Wrist drop, right wrist
       M21.332   Wrist drop, left wrist
       M21.339   Wrist drop, unspecified wrist
  ● **M21.37**   Foot drop (acquired)
       M21.371   Foot drop, right foot
       M21.372   Foot drop, left foot
       M21.379   Foot drop, unspecified foot
● **M21.4**   Flat foot [pes planus] (acquired)
    Excludes1   congenital pes planus (Q66.5-)
    M21.40   Flat foot [pes planus] (acquired), unspecified foot
    M21.41   Flat foot [pes planus] (acquired), right foot
    M21.42   Flat foot [pes planus] (acquired), left foot
● **M21.5**   Acquired clawhand, clubhand, clawfoot and clubfoot
    Excludes1   clubfoot, not specified as acquired (Q66.89)
  ● **M21.51**   Acquired clawhand
       M21.511   Acquired clawhand, right hand
       M21.512   Acquired clawhand, left hand
       M21.519   Acquired clawhand, unspecified hand
  ● **M21.52**   Acquired clubhand
       M21.521   Acquired clubhand, right hand
       M21.522   Acquired clubhand, left hand
       M21.529   Acquired clubhand, unspecified hand

  ● **M21.53**   Acquired clawfoot
       M21.531   Acquired clawfoot, right foot
       M21.532   Acquired clawfoot, left foot
       M21.539   Acquired clawfoot, unspecified foot
  ● **M21.54**   Acquired clubfoot
       M21.541   Acquired clubfoot, right foot
       M21.542   Acquired clubfoot, left foot
       M21.549   Acquired clubfoot, unspecified foot
● **M21.6**   Other acquired deformities of foot
    Excludes2   deformities of toe (acquired) (M20.1-M20.6-)
  ● **M21.61**   Bunion
       Coding Clinic: 2016, Q4, P38
       M21.611   Bunion of right foot
       M21.612   Bunion of left foot
       M21.619   Bunion of unspecified foot
  ● **M21.62**   Bunionette
       Coding Clinic: 2016, Q4, P38
       M21.621   Bunionette of right foot
       M21.622   Bunionette of left foot
       M21.629   Bunionette of unspecified foot
  ● **M21.6X**   Other acquired deformities of foot
       M21.6X1   Other acquired deformities of right foot
       M21.6X2   Other acquired deformities of left foot
       M21.6X9   Other acquired deformities of unspecified foot
● **M21.7**   Unequal limb length (acquired)
    Note: The site used should correspond to the shorter limb.
    M21.70   Unequal limb length (acquired), unspecified site
  ● **M21.72**   Unequal limb length (acquired), humerus
       M21.721   Unequal limb length (acquired), right humerus
       M21.722   Unequal limb length (acquired), left humerus
       M21.729   Unequal limb length (acquired), unspecified humerus
  ● **M21.73**   Unequal limb length (acquired), ulna and radius
       M21.731   Unequal limb length (acquired), right ulna
       M21.732   Unequal limb length (acquired), left ulna
       M21.733   Unequal limb length (acquired), right radius
       M21.734   Unequal limb length (acquired), left radius
       M21.739   Unequal limb length (acquired), unspecified ulna and radius
  ● **M21.75**   Unequal limb length (acquired), femur
       M21.751   Unequal limb length (acquired), right femur
       M21.752   Unequal limb length (acquired), left femur
       M21.759   Unequal limb length (acquired), unspecified femur

● M21.76 Unequal limb length (acquired), tibia and fibula

    M21.761 Unequal limb length (acquired), right tibia

    M21.762 Unequal limb length (acquired), left tibia

    M21.763 Unequal limb length (acquired), right fibula

    M21.764 Unequal limb length (acquired), left fibula

    M21.769 Unequal limb length (acquired), unspecified tibia and fibula

● M21.8 Other specified acquired deformities of limbs

    Excludes2 coxa plana (M91.2)

    M21.80 Other specified acquired deformities of unspecified limb

● M21.82 Other specified acquired deformities of upper arm

    M21.821 Other specified acquired deformities of right upper arm

    M21.822 Other specified acquired deformities of left upper arm

    M21.829 Other specified acquired deformities of unspecified upper arm

● M21.83 Other specified acquired deformities of forearm

    M21.831 Other specified acquired deformities of right forearm

    M21.832 Other specified acquired deformities of left forearm

    M21.839 Other specified acquired deformities of unspecified forearm

● M21.85 Other specified acquired deformities of thigh

    M21.851 Other specified acquired deformities of right thigh

    M21.852 Other specified acquired deformities of left thigh

    M21.859 Other specified acquired deformities of unspecified thigh

● M21.86 Other specified acquired deformities of lower leg

    M21.861 Other specified acquired deformities of right lower leg

    M21.862 Other specified acquired deformities of left lower leg

    M21.869 Other specified acquired deformities of unspecified lower leg

● M21.9 Unspecified acquired deformity of limb and hand

    M21.90 Unspecified acquired deformity of unspecified limb

● M21.92 Unspecified acquired deformity of upper arm

    M21.921 Unspecified acquired deformity of right upper arm

    M21.922 Unspecified acquired deformity of left upper arm

    M21.929 Unspecified acquired deformity of unspecified upper arm

● M21.93 Unspecified acquired deformity of forearm

    M21.931 Unspecified acquired deformity of right forearm

    M21.932 Unspecified acquired deformity of left forearm

    M21.939 Unspecified acquired deformity of unspecified forearm

● M21.94 Unspecified acquired deformity of hand

    M21.941 Unspecified acquired deformity of hand, right hand

    M21.942 Unspecified acquired deformity of hand, left hand

    M21.949 Unspecified acquired deformity of hand, unspecified hand

● M21.95 Unspecified acquired deformity of thigh

    M21.951 Unspecified acquired deformity of right thigh

    M21.952 Unspecified acquired deformity of left thigh

    M21.959 Unspecified acquired deformity of unspecified thigh

● M21.96 Unspecified acquired deformity of lower leg

    M21.961 Unspecified acquired deformity of right lower leg

    M21.962 Unspecified acquired deformity of left lower leg

    M21.969 Unspecified acquired deformity of unspecified lower leg

● M22 Disorder of patella

    Excludes1 traumatic dislocation of patella (S83.0-)

● M22.0 Recurrent dislocation of patella

    M22.00 Recurrent dislocation of patella, unspecified knee

    M22.01 Recurrent dislocation of patella, right knee

    M22.02 Recurrent dislocation of patella, left knee

● M22.1 Recurrent subluxation of patella

    Incomplete dislocation of patella

    M22.10 Recurrent subluxation of patella, unspecified knee

    M22.11 Recurrent subluxation of patella, right knee

    M22.12 Recurrent subluxation of patella, left knee

● M22.2 Patellofemoral disorders

    ● M22.2X Patellofemoral disorders

        M22.2X1 Patellofemoral disorders, right knee

        M22.2X2 Patellofemoral disorders, left knee

        M22.2X9 Patellofemoral disorders, unspecified knee

● M22.3 Other derangements of patella

    ● M22.3X Other derangements of patella

        M22.3X1 Other derangements of patella, right knee

        M22.3X2 Other derangements of patella, left knee

        M22.3X9 Other derangements of patella, unspecified knee

● M22.4 Chondromalacia patellae

    M22.40 Chondromalacia patellae, unspecified knee

    M22.41 Chondromalacia patellae, right knee

    M22.42 Chondromalacia patellae, left knee

● M22.8 Other disorders of patella

    ● M22.8X Other disorders of patella

        M22.8X1 Other disorders of patella, right knee

        M22.8X2 Other disorders of patella, left knee

        M22.8X9 Other disorders of patella, unspecified knee

● M22.9 Unspecified disorder of patella

    M22.90 Unspecified disorder of patella, unspecified knee

    M22.91 Unspecified disorder of patella, right knee

    M22.92 Unspecified disorder of patella, left knee

CHAPTER 13 (M00-M99)

● **M23   Internal derangement of knee**

    Excludes1   ankylosis (M24.66)
                 current injury - see injury of knee and lower leg
                     (S80-S89)
                 deformity of knee (M21.-)
                 osteochondritis dissecans (M93.2)
                 recurrent dislocation or subluxation of joints
                     (M24.4)
                 recurrent dislocation or subluxation of patella
                     (M22.0-M22.1)

    ● **M23.0   Cystic meniscus**

       ● **M23.00   Cystic meniscus, unspecified meniscus**
           Cystic meniscus, unspecified lateral meniscus
           Cystic meniscus, unspecified medial meniscus

          M23.000   Cystic meniscus, unspecified lateral meniscus, right knee

          M23.001   Cystic meniscus, unspecified lateral meniscus, left knee

          M23.002   Cystic meniscus, unspecified lateral meniscus, unspecified knee

          M23.003   Cystic meniscus, unspecified medial meniscus, right knee

          M23.004   Cystic meniscus, unspecified medial meniscus, left knee

          M23.005   Cystic meniscus, unspecified medial meniscus, unspecified knee

          M23.006   Cystic meniscus, unspecified meniscus, right knee

          M23.007   Cystic meniscus, unspecified meniscus, left knee

          M23.009   Cystic meniscus, unspecified meniscus, unspecified knee

       ● **M23.01   Cystic meniscus, anterior horn of medial meniscus**

          M23.011   Cystic meniscus, anterior horn of medial meniscus, right knee

          M23.012   Cystic meniscus, anterior horn of medial meniscus, left knee

          M23.019   Cystic meniscus, anterior horn of medial meniscus, unspecified knee

       ● **M23.02   Cystic meniscus, posterior horn of medial meniscus**

          M23.021   Cystic meniscus, posterior horn of medial meniscus, right knee

          M23.022   Cystic meniscus, posterior horn of medial meniscus, left knee

          M23.029   Cystic meniscus, posterior horn of medial meniscus, unspecified knee

       ● **M23.03   Cystic meniscus, other medial meniscus**

          M23.031   Cystic meniscus, other medial meniscus, right knee

          M23.032   Cystic meniscus, other medial meniscus, left knee

          M23.039   Cystic meniscus, other medial meniscus, unspecified knee

       ● **M23.04   Cystic meniscus, anterior horn of lateral meniscus**

          M23.041   Cystic meniscus, anterior horn of lateral meniscus, right knee

          M23.042   Cystic meniscus, anterior horn of lateral meniscus, left knee

          M23.049   Cystic meniscus, anterior horn of lateral meniscus, unspecified knee

       ● **M23.05   Cystic meniscus, posterior horn of lateral meniscus**

          M23.051   Cystic meniscus, posterior horn of lateral meniscus, right knee

          M23.052   Cystic meniscus, posterior horn of lateral meniscus, left knee

          M23.059   Cystic meniscus, posterior horn of lateral meniscus, unspecified knee

---

       ● **M23.06   Cystic meniscus, other lateral meniscus**

          M23.061   Cystic meniscus, other lateral meniscus, right knee

          M23.062   Cystic meniscus, other lateral meniscus, left knee

          M23.069   Cystic meniscus, other lateral meniscus, unspecified knee

★ **(See Plate 509 on page 79.)**

    ● **M23.2   Derangement of meniscus due to old tear or injury**
         Old bucket-handle tear

       ● **M23.20   Derangement of unspecified meniscus due to old tear or injury**
          Derangement of unspecified lateral meniscus due to old tear or injury
          Derangement of unspecified medial meniscus due to old tear or injury

          M23.200   Derangement of unspecified lateral meniscus due to old tear or injury, right knee

          M23.201   Derangement of unspecified lateral meniscus due to old tear or injury, left knee

          M23.202   Derangement of unspecified lateral meniscus due to old tear or injury, unspecified knee

          M23.203   Derangement of unspecified medial meniscus due to old tear or injury, right knee

          M23.204   Derangement of unspecified medial meniscus due to old tear or injury, left knee

          M23.205   Derangement of unspecified medial meniscus due to old tear or injury, unspecified knee

          M23.206   Derangement of unspecified meniscus due to old tear or injury, right knee

          M23.207   Derangement of unspecified meniscus due to old tear or injury, left knee

          M23.209   Derangement of unspecified meniscus due to old tear or injury, unspecified knee

       ● **M23.21   Derangement of anterior horn of medial meniscus due to old tear or injury**

          M23.211   Derangement of anterior horn of medial meniscus due to old tear or injury, right knee

          M23.212   Derangement of anterior horn of medial meniscus due to old tear or injury, left knee

          M23.219   Derangement of anterior horn of medial meniscus due to old tear or injury, unspecified knee

       ● **M23.22   Derangement of posterior horn of medial meniscus due to old tear or injury**

          M23.221   Derangement of posterior horn of medial meniscus due to old tear or injury, right knee

          M23.222   Derangement of posterior horn of medial meniscus due to old tear or injury, left knee

          M23.229   Derangement of posterior horn of medial meniscus due to old tear or injury, unspecified knee

▶ New   ⮕ Revised   ~~deleted~~ Deleted   Excludes 1   Excludes 2   Includes   Use additional   Code first   Code also   Key words
OGCR Official Guidelines   ● Unacceptable Principal Diagnosis   X Assign placeholder X   ▌ Use Additional Character(s)   ▌ Manifestation Code   **Coding Clinic**

● **M23.23** Derangement of other medial meniscus due to old tear or injury

     M23.231 Derangement of other medial meniscus due to old tear or injury, right knee

     M23.232 Derangement of other medial meniscus due to old tear or injury, left knee

     M23.239 Derangement of other medial meniscus due to old tear or injury, unspecified knee

● **M23.24** Derangement of anterior horn of lateral meniscus due to old tear or injury

     M23.241 Derangement of anterior horn of lateral meniscus due to old tear or injury, right knee

     M23.242 Derangement of anterior horn of lateral meniscus due to old tear or injury, left knee

     M23.249 Derangement of anterior horn of lateral meniscus due to old tear or injury, unspecified knee

● **M23.25** Derangement of posterior horn of lateral meniscus due to old tear or injury

     M23.251 Derangement of posterior horn of lateral meniscus due to old tear or injury, right knee

     M23.252 Derangement of posterior horn of lateral meniscus due to old tear or injury, left knee

     M23.259 Derangement of posterior horn of lateral meniscus due to old tear or injury, unspecified knee

● **M23.26** Derangement of other lateral meniscus due to old tear or injury

     M23.261 Derangement of other lateral meniscus due to old tear or injury, right knee

     M23.262 Derangement of other lateral meniscus due to old tear or injury, left knee

     M23.269 Derangement of other lateral meniscus due to old tear or injury, unspecified knee

● **M23.3** Other meniscus derangements

     Degenerate meniscus
     Detached meniscus
     Retained meniscus

● **M23.30** Other meniscus derangements, unspecified meniscus

     Other meniscus derangements, unspecified lateral meniscus
     Other meniscus derangements, unspecified medial meniscus

     M23.300 Other meniscus derangements, unspecified lateral meniscus, right knee

     M23.301 Other meniscus derangements, unspecified lateral meniscus, left knee

     M23.302 Other meniscus derangements, unspecified lateral meniscus, unspecified knee

     M23.303 Other meniscus derangements, unspecified medial meniscus, right knee

     M23.304 Other meniscus derangements, unspecified medial meniscus, left knee

     M23.305 Other meniscus derangements, unspecified medial meniscus, unspecified knee

     M23.306 Other meniscus derangements, unspecified meniscus, right knee

     M23.307 Other meniscus derangements, unspecified meniscus, left knee

     M23.309 Other meniscus derangements, unspecified meniscus, unspecified knee

● **M23.31** Other meniscus derangements, anterior horn of medial meniscus

     M23.311 Other meniscus derangements, anterior horn of medial meniscus, right knee

     M23.312 Other meniscus derangements, anterior horn of medial meniscus, left knee

     M23.319 Other meniscus derangements, anterior horn of medial meniscus, unspecified knee

● **M23.32** Other meniscus derangements, posterior horn of medial meniscus

     M23.321 Other meniscus derangements, posterior horn of medial meniscus, right knee

     M23.322 Other meniscus derangements, posterior horn of medial meniscus, left knee

     M23.329 Other meniscus derangements, posterior horn of medial meniscus, unspecified knee

● **M23.33** Other meniscus derangements, other medial meniscus

     M23.331 Other meniscus derangements, other medial meniscus, right knee

     M23.332 Other meniscus derangements, other medial meniscus, left knee

     M23.339 Other meniscus derangements, other medial meniscus, unspecified knee

● **M23.34** Other meniscus derangements, anterior horn of lateral meniscus

     M23.341 Other meniscus derangements, anterior horn of lateral meniscus, right knee

     M23.342 Other meniscus derangements, anterior horn of lateral meniscus, left knee

     M23.349 Other meniscus derangements, anterior horn of lateral meniscus, unspecified knee

● **M23.35** Other meniscus derangements, posterior horn of lateral meniscus

     M23.351 Other meniscus derangements, posterior horn of lateral meniscus, right knee

     M23.352 Other meniscus derangements, posterior horn of lateral meniscus, left knee

     M23.359 Other meniscus derangements, posterior horn of lateral meniscus, unspecified knee

● **M23.36** Other meniscus derangements, other lateral meniscus

     M23.361 Other meniscus derangements, other lateral meniscus, right knee

     M23.362 Other meniscus derangements, other lateral meniscus, left knee

     M23.369 Other meniscus derangements, other lateral meniscus, unspecified knee

CHAPTER 13 (M00-M99)

N Newborn Age: 0   **P** Pediatric Age: 0–17   **M** Maternity DX: 12–55   **A** Adult Age: 15–124   ♀ Females Only   ♂ Males Only

Complication\Comorbidity   Major C\C   (Ex) CC/MCC Exclusions   Hospital-Acquired Condition

1023

Fibular collateral ligament
Lateral capsular ligament
Fibular
Plate
Tibial collateral ligament
Medial capsular ligament
Tibial

Figure 13-2 Collateral and cruciate ligament of knee. (From DeLee: DeLee and Drez's Orthopaedic Sports Medicine, ed 3, Saunders, 2009)

M23.4 Loose body in knee
  M23.40   Loose body in knee, unspecified knee
  M23.41   Loose body in knee, right knee
  M23.42   Loose body in knee, left knee
M23.5 Chronic instability of knee
  M23.50   Chronic instability of knee, unspecified knee
  M23.51   Chronic instability of knee, right knee
  M23.52   Chronic instability of knee, left knee
M23.6 Other spontaneous disruption of ligament(s) of knee
  M23.60   Other spontaneous disruption of unspecified ligament of knee
    M23.601   Other spontaneous disruption of unspecified ligament of right knee
    M23.602   Other spontaneous disruption of unspecified ligament of left knee
    M23.609   Other spontaneous disruption of unspecified ligament of unspecified knee
  M23.61   Other spontaneous disruption of anterior cruciate ligament of knee
    M23.611   Other spontaneous disruption of anterior cruciate ligament of right knee
    M23.612   Other spontaneous disruption of anterior cruciate ligament of left knee
    M23.619   Other spontaneous disruption of anterior cruciate ligament of unspecified knee
  M23.62   Other spontaneous disruption of posterior cruciate ligament of knee
    M23.621   Other spontaneous disruption of posterior cruciate ligament of right knee
    M23.622   Other spontaneous disruption of posterior cruciate ligament of left knee
    M23.629   Other spontaneous disruption of posterior cruciate ligament of unspecified knee
  M23.63   Other spontaneous disruption of medial collateral ligament of knee
    M23.631   Other spontaneous disruption of medial collateral ligament of right knee
    M23.632   Other spontaneous disruption of medial collateral ligament of left knee
    M23.639   Other spontaneous disruption of medial collateral ligament of unspecified knee
  M23.64   Other spontaneous disruption of lateral collateral ligament of knee
    M23.641   Other spontaneous disruption of lateral collateral ligament of right knee
    M23.642   Other spontaneous disruption of lateral collateral ligament of left knee
    M23.649   Other spontaneous disruption of lateral collateral ligament of unspecified knee

  M23.67   Other spontaneous disruption of capsular ligament of knee
    M23.671   Other spontaneous disruption of capsular ligament of right knee
    M23.672   Other spontaneous disruption of capsular ligament of left knee
    M23.679   Other spontaneous disruption of capsular ligament of unspecified knee
M23.8 Other internal derangements of knee
  Laxity of ligament of knee
  Snapping knee
  M23.8X   Other internal derangements of knee
    M23.8X1   Other internal derangements of right knee
    M23.8X2   Other internal derangements of left knee
    M23.8X9   Other internal derangements of unspecified knee
M23.9 Unspecified internal derangement of knee
  M23.90   Unspecified internal derangement of unspecified knee
  M23.91   Unspecified internal derangement of right knee
  M23.92   Unspecified internal derangement of left knee
M24   Other specific joint derangements
  Excludes1   current injury - see injury of joint by body region
  Excludes2   ganglion (M67.4)
    snapping knee (M23.8-)
    temporomandibular joint disorders (M26.6-)
  M24.0 Loose body in joint
    Excludes2   loose body in knee (M23.4)
    M24.00   Loose body in unspecified joint
    M24.01   Loose body in shoulder
      M24.011   Loose body in right shoulder
      M24.012   Loose body in left shoulder
      M24.019   Loose body in unspecified shoulder
    M24.02   Loose body in elbow
      M24.021   Loose body in right elbow
      M24.022   Loose body in left elbow
      M24.029   Loose body in unspecified elbow
    M24.03   Loose body in wrist
      M24.031   Loose body in right wrist
      M24.032   Loose body in left wrist
      M24.039   Loose body in unspecified wrist
    M24.04   Loose body in finger joints
      M24.041   Loose body in right finger joint(s)
      M24.042   Loose body in left finger joint(s)
      M24.049   Loose body in unspecified finger joint(s)
    M24.05   Loose body in hip
      M24.051   Loose body in right hip
      M24.052   Loose body in left hip
      M24.059   Loose body in unspecified hip
    M24.07   Loose body in ankle and toe joints
      M24.071   Loose body in right ankle
      M24.072   Loose body in left ankle
      M24.073   Loose body in unspecified ankle
      M24.074   Loose body in right toe joint(s)
      M24.075   Loose body in left toe joint(s)
      M24.076   Loose body in unspecified toe joints
    M24.08   Loose body, other site

▶ New   ⮕ Revised   ~~deleted~~ Deleted   Excludes 1   Excludes 2   Includes   Use additional   Code first   Code also   Key words

OGCR Official Guidelines   ● Unacceptable Principal Diagnosis   X Assign placeholder X   ▶ Use Additional Character(s)   ▶ Manifestation Code   **Coding Clinic**

● **M24.1**   **Other articular cartilage disorders**
     Excludes2   chondrocalcinosis (M11.1, M11.2-)
                   internal derangement of knee (M23.-)
                   metastatic calcification (E83.5)
                   ochronosis (E70.2)

    M24.10   Other articular cartilage disorders, unspecified site

● **M24.11**   Other articular cartilage disorders, shoulder
      M24.111   Other articular cartilage disorders, right shoulder
      M24.112   Other articular cartilage disorders, left shoulder
      M24.119   Other articular cartilage disorders, unspecified shoulder

● **M24.12**   Other articular cartilage disorders, elbow
      M24.121   Other articular cartilage disorders, right elbow
      M24.122   Other articular cartilage disorders, left elbow
      M24.129   Other articular cartilage disorders, unspecified elbow

● **M24.13**   Other articular cartilage disorders, wrist
      M24.131   Other articular cartilage disorders, right wrist
      M24.132   Other articular cartilage disorders, left wrist
      M24.139   Other articular cartilage disorders, unspecified wrist

● **M24.14**   Other articular cartilage disorders, hand
      M24.141   Other articular cartilage disorders, right hand
      M24.142   Other articular cartilage disorders, left hand
      M24.149   Other articular cartilage disorders, unspecified hand

● **M24.15**   Other articular cartilage disorders, hip
      M24.151   Other articular cartilage disorders, right hip
      M24.152   Other articular cartilage disorders, left hip
      M24.159   Other articular cartilage disorders, unspecified hip

● **M24.17**   Other articular cartilage disorders, ankle and foot
      M24.171   Other articular cartilage disorders, right ankle
      M24.172   Other articular cartilage disorders, left ankle
      M24.173   Other articular cartilage disorders, unspecified ankle
      M24.174   Other articular cartilage disorders, right foot
      M24.175   Other articular cartilage disorders, left foot
      M24.176   Other articular cartilage disorders, unspecified foot

● **M24.2**   **Disorder of ligament**
     Instability secondary to old ligament injury
     Ligamentous laxity NOS
     Excludes1   familial ligamentous laxity (M35.7)
     Excludes2   internal derangement of knee (M23.5-M23.89)

    M24.20   Disorder of ligament, unspecified site

● **M24.21**   Disorder of ligament, shoulder
      M24.211   Disorder of ligament, right shoulder
      M24.212   Disorder of ligament, left shoulder
      M24.219   Disorder of ligament, unspecified shoulder

● **M24.22**   Disorder of ligament, elbow
      M24.221   Disorder of ligament, right elbow
      M24.222   Disorder of ligament, left elbow
      M24.229   Disorder of ligament, unspecified elbow

● **M24.23**   Disorder of ligament, wrist
      M24.231   Disorder of ligament, right wrist
      M24.232   Disorder of ligament, left wrist
      M24.239   Disorder of ligament, unspecified wrist

● **M24.24**   Disorder of ligament, hand
      M24.241   Disorder of ligament, right hand
      M24.242   Disorder of ligament, left hand
      M24.249   Disorder of ligament, unspecified hand

● **M24.25**   Disorder of ligament, hip
      M24.251   Disorder of ligament, right hip
      M24.252   Disorder of ligament, left hip
      M24.259   Disorder of ligament, unspecified hip

● **M24.27**   Disorder of ligament, ankle and foot
      M24.271   Disorder of ligament, right ankle
      M24.272   Disorder of ligament, left ankle
      M24.273   Disorder of ligament, unspecified ankle
      M24.274   Disorder of ligament, right foot
      M24.275   Disorder of ligament, left foot
      M24.276   Disorder of ligament, unspecified foot

    M24.28   Disorder of ligament, vertebrae

● **M24.3**   **Pathological dislocation of joint, not elsewhere classified**
     Excludes1   congenital dislocation or displacement of joint - see congenital malformations and deformations of the musculoskeletal system (Q65-Q79)
                   current injury - see injury of joints and ligaments by body region
                   recurrent dislocation of joint (M24.4-)

    M24.30   Pathological dislocation of unspecified joint, not elsewhere classified

● **M24.31**   Pathological dislocation of shoulder, not elsewhere classified
      M24.311   Pathological dislocation of right shoulder, not elsewhere classified
      M24.312   Pathological dislocation of left shoulder, not elsewhere classified
      M24.319   Pathological dislocation of unspecified shoulder, not elsewhere classified

● **M24.32**   Pathological dislocation of elbow, not elsewhere classified
      M24.321   Pathological dislocation of right elbow, not elsewhere classified
      M24.322   Pathological dislocation of left elbow, not elsewhere classified
      M24.329   Pathological dislocation of unspecified elbow, not elsewhere classified

● **M24.33**   Pathological dislocation of wrist, not elsewhere classified
      M24.331   Pathological dislocation of right wrist, not elsewhere classified
      M24.332   Pathological dislocation of left wrist, not elsewhere classified
      M24.339   Pathological dislocation of unspecified wrist, not elsewhere classified

CHAPTER 13 (M00-M99)

● **M24.34** Pathological dislocation of hand, not elsewhere classified

     M24.341 Pathological dislocation of right hand, not elsewhere classified

     M24.342 Pathological dislocation of left hand, not elsewhere classified

     M24.349 Pathological dislocation of unspecified hand, not elsewhere classified

● **M24.35** Pathological dislocation of hip, not elsewhere classified

     M24.351 Pathological dislocation of right hip, not elsewhere classified

     M24.352 Pathological dislocation of left hip, not elsewhere classified

     M24.359 Pathological dislocation of unspecified hip, not elsewhere classified

● **M24.36** Pathological dislocation of knee, not elsewhere classified

     M24.361 Pathological dislocation of right knee, not elsewhere classified

     M24.362 Pathological dislocation of left knee, not elsewhere classified

     M24.369 Pathological dislocation of unspecified knee, not elsewhere classified

● **M24.37** Pathological dislocation of ankle and foot, not elsewhere classified

     M24.371 Pathological dislocation of right ankle, not elsewhere classified

     M24.372 Pathological dislocation of left ankle, not elsewhere classified

     M24.373 Pathological dislocation of unspecified ankle, not elsewhere classified

     M24.374 Pathological dislocation of right foot, not elsewhere classified

     M24.375 Pathological dislocation of left foot, not elsewhere classified

     M24.376 Pathological dislocation of unspecified foot, not elsewhere classified

● **M24.4** Recurrent dislocation of joint
     Recurrent subluxation of joint

     Excludes2   recurrent dislocation of patella (M22.Ø-M22.1)
                   recurrent vertebral dislocation (M43.3-, M43.4, M43.5-)

     M24.40 Recurrent dislocation, unspecified joint

● **M24.41** Recurrent dislocation, shoulder

     M24.411 Recurrent dislocation, right shoulder

     M24.412 Recurrent dislocation, left shoulder

     M24.419 Recurrent dislocation, unspecified shoulder

● **M24.42** Recurrent dislocation, elbow

     M24.421 Recurrent dislocation, right elbow

     M24.422 Recurrent dislocation, left elbow

     M24.429 Recurrent dislocation, unspecified elbow

● **M24.43** Recurrent dislocation, wrist

     M24.431 Recurrent dislocation, right wrist

     M24.432 Recurrent dislocation, left wrist

     M24.439 Recurrent dislocation, unspecified wrist

● **M24.44** Recurrent dislocation, hand and finger(s)

     M24.441 Recurrent dislocation, right hand

     M24.442 Recurrent dislocation, left hand

     M24.443 Recurrent dislocation, unspecified hand

     M24.444 Recurrent dislocation, right finger

     M24.445 Recurrent dislocation, left finger

     M24.446 Recurrent dislocation, unspecified finger

● **M24.45** Recurrent dislocation, hip

     M24.451 Recurrent dislocation, right hip

     M24.452 Recurrent dislocation, left hip

     M24.459 Recurrent dislocation, unspecified hip

● **M24.46** Recurrent dislocation, knee

     M24.461 Recurrent dislocation, right knee

     M24.462 Recurrent dislocation, left knee

     M24.469 Recurrent dislocation, unspecified knee

● **M24.47** Recurrent dislocation, ankle, foot and toes

     M24.471 Recurrent dislocation, right ankle

     M24.472 Recurrent dislocation, left ankle

     M24.473 Recurrent dislocation, unspecified ankle

     M24.474 Recurrent dislocation, right foot

     M24.475 Recurrent dislocation, left foot

     M24.476 Recurrent dislocation, unspecified foot

     M24.477 Recurrent dislocation, right toe(s)

     M24.478 Recurrent dislocation, left toe(s)

     M24.479 Recurrent dislocation, unspecified toe(s)

● **M24.5** Contracture of joint

     Excludes1   contracture of muscle without contracture of joint (M62.4-)
                   contracture of tendon (sheath) without contracture of joint (M62.4-)
                   Dupuytren's contracture (M72.Ø)

     Excludes2   acquired deformities of limbs (M2Ø-M21)

     M24.50 Contracture, unspecified joint

● **M24.51** Contracture, shoulder

     M24.511 Contracture, right shoulder

     M24.512 Contracture, left shoulder

     M24.519 Contracture, unspecified shoulder

● **M24.52** Contracture, elbow

     M24.521 Contracture, right elbow

     M24.522 Contracture, left elbow

     M24.529 Contracture, unspecified elbow

● **M24.53** Contracture, wrist

     M24.531 Contracture, right wrist

     M24.532 Contracture, left wrist

     M24.539 Contracture, unspecified wrist

● **M24.54** Contracture, hand

     M24.541 Contracture, right hand

     M24.542 Contracture, left hand

     M24.549 Contracture, unspecified hand

● **M24.55** Contracture, hip

     M24.551 Contracture, right hip
          Coding Clinic: 2016, Q2, P6

     M24.552 Contracture, left hip
          Coding Clinic: 2016, Q2, P6

     M24.559 Contracture, unspecified hip

Item 13–5 **Ankylosis** or arthrokleisis is a consolidation of a joint due to disease, injury, or surgical procedure. Spondylosis is the degeneration of the vertebral processes and formation of osteophytes and commonly occurs with age. **Spondylitis** or ankylosing spondylitis is a type of arthritis that affects the spine or backbone causing back pain and stiffness.

M24.56 Contracture, knee
- M24.561 Contracture, right knee
  - Coding Clinic: 2016, Q2, P6
- M24.562 Contracture, left knee
  - Coding Clinic: 2016, Q2, P6
- M24.569 Contracture, unspecified knee

M24.57 Contracture, ankle and foot
- M24.571 Contracture, right ankle
- M24.572 Contracture, left ankle
- M24.573 Contracture, unspecified ankle
- M24.574 Contracture, right foot
- M24.575 Contracture, left foot
- M24.576 Contracture, unspecified foot

M24.6 Ankylosis of joint
- **Excludes1** stiffness of joint without ankylosis (M25.6-)
- **Excludes2** spine (M43.2-)
- M24.60 Ankylosis, unspecified joint
- M24.61 Ankylosis, shoulder
  - M24.611 Ankylosis, right shoulder
  - M24.612 Ankylosis, left shoulder
  - M24.619 Ankylosis, unspecified shoulder
- M24.62 Ankylosis, elbow
  - M24.621 Ankylosis, right elbow
  - M24.622 Ankylosis, left elbow
  - M24.629 Ankylosis, unspecified elbow
- M24.63 Ankylosis, wrist
  - M24.631 Ankylosis, right wrist
  - M24.632 Ankylosis, left wrist
  - M24.639 Ankylosis, unspecified wrist
- M24.64 Ankylosis, hand
  - M24.641 Ankylosis, right hand
  - M24.642 Ankylosis, left hand
  - M24.649 Ankylosis, unspecified hand
- M24.65 Ankylosis, hip
  - M24.651 Ankylosis, right hip
  - M24.652 Ankylosis, left hip
  - M24.659 Ankylosis, unspecified hip
- M24.66 Ankylosis, knee
  - M24.661 Ankylosis, right knee
  - M24.662 Ankylosis, left knee
  - M24.669 Ankylosis, unspecified knee
- M24.67 Ankylosis, ankle and foot
  - M24.671 Ankylosis, right ankle
  - M24.672 Ankylosis, left ankle
  - M24.673 Ankylosis, unspecified ankle
  - M24.674 Ankylosis, right foot
  - M24.675 Ankylosis, left foot
  - M24.676 Ankylosis, unspecified foot

M24.7 Protrusio acetabuli

M24.8 Other specific joint derangements, not elsewhere classified
- **Excludes2** iliotibial band syndrome (M76.3)
- M24.80 Other specific joint derangements of unspecified joint, not elsewhere classified
- M24.81 Other specific joint derangements of shoulder, not elsewhere classified
  - M24.811 Other specific joint derangements of right shoulder, not elsewhere classified
  - M24.812 Other specific joint derangements of left shoulder, not elsewhere classified
  - M24.819 Other specific joint derangements of unspecified shoulder, not elsewhere classified
- M24.82 Other specific joint derangements of elbow, not elsewhere classified
  - M24.821 Other specific joint derangements of right elbow, not elsewhere classified
  - M24.822 Other specific joint derangements of left elbow, not elsewhere classified
  - M24.829 Other specific joint derangements of unspecified elbow, not elsewhere classified
- M24.83 Other specific joint derangements of wrist, not elsewhere classified
  - M24.831 Other specific joint derangements of right wrist, not elsewhere classified
  - M24.832 Other specific joint derangements of left wrist, not elsewhere classified
  - M24.839 Other specific joint derangements of unspecified wrist, not elsewhere classified
- M24.84 Other specific joint derangements of hand, not elsewhere classified
  - M24.841 Other specific joint derangements of right hand, not elsewhere classified
  - M24.842 Other specific joint derangements of left hand, not elsewhere classified
  - M24.849 Other specific joint derangements of unspecified hand, not elsewhere classified
- M24.85 Other specific joint derangements of hip, not elsewhere classified
  - Irritable hip
  - M24.851 Other specific joint derangements of right hip, not elsewhere classified
  - M24.852 Other specific joint derangements of left hip, not elsewhere classified
  - M24.859 Other specific joint derangements of unspecified hip, not elsewhere classified
- M24.87 Other specific joint derangements of ankle and foot, not elsewhere classified
  - M24.871 Other specific joint derangements of right ankle, not elsewhere classified
  - M24.872 Other specific joint derangements of left ankle, not elsewhere classified
  - M24.873 Other specific joint derangements of unspecified ankle, not elsewhere classified
  - M24.874 Other specific joint derangements of right foot, not elsewhere classified
  - M24.875 Other specific joint derangements left foot, not elsewhere classified
  - M24.876 Other specific joint derangements of unspecified foot, not elsewhere classified

M24.9 Joint derangement, unspecified

CHAPTER 13 (M00-M99)

● **M25 Other joint disorder, not elsewhere classified**

    Excludes2   abnormality of gait and mobility (R26.-)
                acquired deformities of limb (M20-M21)
                calcification of bursa (M71.4-)
                calcification of shoulder (joint) (M75.3)
                calcification of tendon (M65.2-)
                difficulty in walking (R26.2)
                temporomandibular joint disorder (M26.6-)

● **M25.0 Hemarthrosis**

    Excludes1   current injury - see injury of joint by body
                    region
                hemophilic arthropathy (M36.2)

    M25.00 Hemarthrosis, unspecified joint 🔍
        Ⓔ See PDX Collection 868

  ● **M25.01** Hemarthrosis, shoulder
        Ⓔ **For category M25.01 CC codes:** See PDX Collection 869
        M25.011 Hemarthrosis, right shoulder 🔍
        M25.012 Hemarthrosis, left shoulder 🔍
        M25.019 Hemarthrosis, unspecified
                shoulder 🔍

  ● **M25.02** Hemarthrosis, elbow
        Ⓔ **For category M25.02 CC codes:** See PDX Collection 870
        M25.021 Hemarthrosis, right elbow 🔍
        M25.022 Hemarthrosis, left elbow 🔍
        M25.029 Hemarthrosis, unspecified elbow 🔍

  ● **M25.03** Hemarthrosis, wrist
        Ⓔ **For category M25.03 CC codes:** See PDX Collection 871
        M25.031 Hemarthrosis, right wrist 🔍
        M25.032 Hemarthrosis, left wrist 🔍
        M25.039 Hemarthrosis, unspecified wrist 🔍

  ● **M25.04** Hemarthrosis, hand
        Ⓔ **For category M25.04 CC codes:** See PDX Collection 872
        M25.041 Hemarthrosis, right hand 🔍
        M25.042 Hemarthrosis, left hand 🔍
        M25.049 Hemarthrosis, unspecified hand 🔍

  ● **M25.05** Hemarthrosis, hip
        Ⓔ **For category M25.05 CC codes:** See PDX Collection 868
        M25.051 Hemarthrosis, right hip 🔍
        M25.052 Hemarthrosis, left hip 🔍
        M25.059 Hemarthrosis, unspecified hip 🔍

  ● **M25.06** Hemarthrosis, knee
        Ⓔ **For category M25.06 CC codes:** See PDX Collection 873
        M25.061 Hemarthrosis, right knee 🔍
        M25.062 Hemarthrosis, left knee 🔍
        M25.069 Hemarthrosis, unspecified knee 🔍

  ● **M25.07** Hemarthrosis, ankle and foot
        Ⓔ **For category M25.07 CC codes:** See PDX Collection 873
        M25.071 Hemarthrosis, right ankle 🔍
        M25.072 Hemarthrosis, left ankle 🔍
        M25.073 Hemarthrosis, unspecified ankle 🔍
        M25.074 Hemarthrosis, right foot 🔍
        M25.075 Hemarthrosis, left foot 🔍
        M25.076 Hemarthrosis, unspecified foot 🔍

    M25.08 Hemarthrosis, other specified site 🔍
        Hemarthrosis, vertebrae
        Ⓔ See PDX Collection 868

● **M25.1 Fistula of joint**

    M25.10 Fistula, unspecified joint

  ● **M25.11** Fistula, shoulder
        M25.111 Fistula, right shoulder
        M25.112 Fistula, left shoulder
        M25.119 Fistula, unspecified shoulder

  ● **M25.12** Fistula, elbow
        M25.121 Fistula, right elbow
        M25.122 Fistula, left elbow
        M25.129 Fistula, unspecified elbow

  ● **M25.13** Fistula, wrist
        M25.131 Fistula, right wrist
        M25.132 Fistula, left wrist
        M25.139 Fistula, unspecified wrist

  ● **M25.14** Fistula, hand
        M25.141 Fistula, right hand
        M25.142 Fistula, left hand
        M25.149 Fistula, unspecified hand

  ● **M25.15** Fistula, hip
        M25.151 Fistula, right hip
        M25.152 Fistula, left hip
        M25.159 Fistula, unspecified hip

  ● **M25.16** Fistula, knee
        M25.161 Fistula, right knee
        M25.162 Fistula, left knee
        M25.169 Fistula, unspecified knee

  ● **M25.17** Fistula, ankle and foot
        M25.171 Fistula, right ankle
        M25.172 Fistula, left ankle
        M25.173 Fistula, unspecified ankle
        M25.174 Fistula, right foot
        M25.175 Fistula, left foot
        M25.176 Fistula, unspecified foot

    M25.18 Fistula, other specified site
        Fistula, vertebrae

● **M25.2 Flail joint**

    M25.20 Flail joint, unspecified joint

  ● **M25.21** Flail joint, shoulder
        M25.211 Flail joint, right shoulder
        M25.212 Flail joint, left shoulder
        M25.219 Flail joint, unspecified shoulder

  ● **M25.22** Flail joint, elbow
        M25.221 Flail joint, right elbow
        M25.222 Flail joint, left elbow
        M25.229 Flail joint, unspecified elbow

  ● **M25.23** Flail joint, wrist
        M25.231 Flail joint, right wrist
        M25.232 Flail joint, left wrist
        M25.239 Flail joint, unspecified wrist

  ● **M25.24** Flail joint, hand
        M25.241 Flail joint, right hand
        M25.242 Flail joint, left hand
        M25.249 Flail joint, unspecified hand

  ● **M25.25** Flail joint, hip
        M25.251 Flail joint, right hip
        M25.252 Flail joint, left hip
        M25.259 Flail joint, unspecified hip

  ● **M25.26** Flail joint, knee
        M25.261 Flail joint, right knee
        M25.262 Flail joint, left knee
        M25.269 Flail joint, unspecified knee

  ● **M25.27** Flail joint, ankle and foot
        M25.271 Flail joint, right ankle and foot
        M25.272 Flail joint, left ankle and foot
        M25.279 Flail joint, unspecified ankle and foot

    M25.28 Flail joint, other site

● M25.3   **Other instability of joint**
     Excludes1   instability of joint secondary to old ligament injury (M24.2-)
                 instability of joint secondary to removal of joint prosthesis (M96.8-)
     Excludes2   spinal instabilities (M53.2-)
     M25.30   Other instability, unspecified joint
● M25.31   Other instability, shoulder
     M25.311   Other instability, right shoulder
     M25.312   Other instability, left shoulder
     M25.319   Other instability, unspecified shoulder
● M25.32   Other instability, elbow
     M25.321   Other instability, right elbow
     M25.322   Other instability, left elbow
     M25.329   Other instability, unspecified elbow
● M25.33   Other instability, wrist
     M25.331   Other instability, right wrist
     M25.332   Other instability, left wrist
     M25.339   Other instability, unspecified wrist
● M25.34   Other instability, hand
     M25.341   Other instability, right hand
     M25.342   Other instability, left hand
     M25.349   Other instability, unspecified hand
● M25.35   Other instability, hip
     M25.351   Other instability, right hip
     M25.352   Other instability, left hip
     M25.359   Other instability, unspecified hip
● M25.36   Other instability, knee
     M25.361   Other instability, right knee
     M25.362   Other instability, left knee
     M25.369   Other instability, unspecified knee
● M25.37   Other instability, ankle and foot
     M25.371   Other instability, right ankle
     M25.372   Other instability, left ankle
     M25.373   Other instability, unspecified ankle
     M25.374   Other instability, right foot
     M25.375   Other instability, left foot
     M25.376   Other instability, unspecified foot
● M25.4   **Effusion of joint**
     Excludes1   hydrarthrosis in yaws (A66.6)
                 intermittent hydrarthrosis (M12.4-)
                 other infective (teno)synovitis (M65.1-)
     M25.40   Effusion, unspecified joint
● M25.41   Effusion, shoulder
     M25.411   Effusion, right shoulder
     M25.412   Effusion, left shoulder
     M25.419   Effusion, unspecified shoulder
● M25.42   Effusion, elbow
     M25.421   Effusion, right elbow
     M25.422   Effusion, left elbow
     M25.429   Effusion, unspecified elbow
● M25.43   Effusion, wrist
     M25.431   Effusion, right wrist
     M25.432   Effusion, left wrist
     M25.439   Effusion, unspecified wrist
● M25.44   Effusion, hand
     M25.441   Effusion, right hand
     M25.442   Effusion, left hand
     M25.449   Effusion, unspecified hand

● M25.45   Effusion, hip
     M25.451   Effusion, right hip
     M25.452   Effusion, left hip
     M25.459   Effusion, unspecified hip
● M25.46   Effusion, knee
     M25.461   Effusion, right knee
     M25.462   Effusion, left knee
     M25.469   Effusion, unspecified knee
● M25.47   Effusion, ankle and foot
     M25.471   Effusion, right ankle
     M25.472   Effusion, left ankle
     M25.473   Effusion, unspecified ankle
     M25.474   Effusion, right foot
     M25.475   Effusion, left foot
     M25.476   Effusion, unspecified foot
     M25.48   Effusion, other site
● M25.5   **Pain in joint**
     Excludes2   pain in hand (M79.64-)
                 pain in fingers (M79.64-)
                 pain in foot (M79.67-)
                 pain in limb (M79.6-)
                 pain in toes (M79.67-)
     M25.50   Pain in unspecified joint
● M25.51   Pain in shoulder
     M25.511   Pain in right shoulder
     M25.512   Pain in left shoulder
     M25.519   Pain in unspecified shoulder
● M25.52   Pain in elbow
     M25.521   Pain in right elbow
     M25.522   Pain in left elbow
     M25.529   Pain in unspecified elbow
● M25.53   Pain in wrist
     M25.531   Pain in right wrist
     M25.532   Pain in left wrist
     M25.539   Pain in unspecified wrist
● M25.54   Pain in joints of hand
         Coding Clinic: 2016, Q4, P38
     M25.541   Pain in joints of right hand
     M25.542   Pain in joints of left hand
     M25.549   Pain in joints of unspecified hand
                 Pain in joints of hand NOS
● M25.55   Pain in hip
     M25.551   Pain in right hip
     M25.552   Pain in left hip
     M25.559   Pain in unspecified hip
● M25.56   Pain in knee
     M25.561   Pain in right knee
     M25.562   Pain in left knee
     M25.569   Pain in unspecified knee
● M25.57   Pain in ankle and joints of foot
     M25.571   Pain in right ankle and joints of right foot
     M25.572   Pain in left ankle and joints of left foot
     M25.579   Pain in unspecified ankle and joints of unspecified foot

---

N Newborn Age: 0   **P** Pediatric Age: 0–17   **M** Maternity DX: 12–55   **A** Adult Age: 15–124   ♀ Females Only   ♂ Males Only

🝆 Complication\Comorbidity   🝆 Major C\C   (Ex) CC/MCC Exclusions   🝆 Hospital-Acquired Condition

1029

● **M25.6　Stiffness of joint, not elsewhere classified**
　　Excludes1　ankylosis of joint (M24.6-)
　　　　　　　　contracture of joint (M24.5-)
　　M25.60　Stiffness of unspecified joint, not elsewhere classified
● M25.61　Stiffness of shoulder, not elsewhere classified
　　　　M25.611　Stiffness of right shoulder, not elsewhere classified
　　　　M25.612　Stiffness of left shoulder, not elsewhere classified
　　　　M25.619　Stiffness of unspecified shoulder, not elsewhere classified
● M25.62　Stiffness of elbow, not elsewhere classified
　　　　M25.621　Stiffness of right elbow, not elsewhere classified
　　　　M25.622　Stiffness of left elbow, not elsewhere classified
　　　　M25.629　Stiffness of unspecified elbow, not elsewhere classified
● M25.63　Stiffness of wrist, not elsewhere classified
　　　　M25.631　Stiffness of right wrist, not elsewhere classified
　　　　M25.632　Stiffness of left wrist, not elsewhere classified
　　　　M25.639　Stiffness of unspecified wrist, not elsewhere classified
● M25.64　Stiffness of hand, not elsewhere classified
　　　　M25.641　Stiffness of right hand, not elsewhere classified
　　　　M25.642　Stiffness of left hand, not elsewhere classified
　　　　M25.649　Stiffness of unspecified hand, not elsewhere classified
● M25.65　Stiffness of hip, not elsewhere classified
　　　　M25.651　Stiffness of right hip, not elsewhere classified
　　　　M25.652　Stiffness of left hip, not elsewhere classified
　　　　M25.659　Stiffness of unspecified hip, not elsewhere classified
● M25.66　Stiffness of knee, not elsewhere classified
　　　　M25.661　Stiffness of right knee, not elsewhere classified
　　　　M25.662　Stiffness of left knee, not elsewhere classified
　　　　M25.669　Stiffness of unspecified knee, not elsewhere classified
● M25.67　Stiffness of ankle and foot, not elsewhere classified
　　　　M25.671　Stiffness of right ankle, not elsewhere classified
　　　　M25.672　Stiffness of left ankle, not elsewhere classified
　　　　M25.673　Stiffness of unspecified ankle, not elsewhere classified
　　　　M25.674　Stiffness of right foot, not elsewhere classified
　　　　M25.675　Stiffness of left foot, not elsewhere classified
　　　　M25.676　Stiffness of unspecified foot, not elsewhere classified

● M25.7　Osteophyte
　　M25.70　Osteophyte, unspecified joint
● M25.71　Osteophyte, shoulder
　　　　M25.711　Osteophyte, right shoulder
　　　　M25.712　Osteophyte, left shoulder
　　　　M25.719　Osteophyte, unspecified shoulder
● M25.72　Osteophyte, elbow
　　　　M25.721　Osteophyte, right elbow
　　　　M25.722　Osteophyte, left elbow
　　　　M25.729　Osteophyte, unspecified elbow
● M25.73　Osteophyte, wrist
　　　　M25.731　Osteophyte, right wrist
　　　　M25.732　Osteophyte, left wrist
　　　　M25.739　Osteophyte, unspecified wrist
● M25.74　Osteophyte, hand
　　　　M25.741　Osteophyte, right hand
　　　　M25.742　Osteophyte, left hand
　　　　M25.749　Osteophyte, unspecified hand
● M25.75　Osteophyte, hip
　　　　M25.751　Osteophyte, right hip
　　　　M25.752　Osteophyte, left hip
　　　　M25.759　Osteophyte, unspecified hip
● M25.76　Osteophyte, knee
　　　　M25.761　Osteophyte, right knee
　　　　M25.762　Osteophyte, left knee
　　　　M25.769　Osteophyte, unspecified knee
● M25.77　Osteophyte, ankle and foot
　　　　M25.771　Osteophyte, right ankle
　　　　M25.772　Osteophyte, left ankle
　　　　M25.773　Osteophyte, unspecified ankle
　　　　M25.774　Osteophyte, right foot
　　　　M25.775　Osteophyte, left foot
　　　　M25.776　Osteophyte, unspecified foot
　　M25.78　Osteophyte, vertebrae
● M25.8　Other specified joint disorders
　　M25.80　Other specified joint disorders, unspecified joint
● M25.81　Other specified joint disorders, shoulder
　　　　M25.811　Other specified joint disorders, right shoulder
　　　　M25.812　Other specified joint disorders, left shoulder
　　　　M25.819　Other specified joint disorders, unspecified shoulder
● M25.82　Other specified joint disorders, elbow
　　　　M25.821　Other specified joint disorders, right elbow
　　　　M25.822　Other specified joint disorders, left elbow
　　　　M25.829　Other specified joint disorders, unspecified elbow
● M25.83　Other specified joint disorders, wrist
　　　　M25.831　Other specified joint disorders, right wrist
　　　　M25.832　Other specified joint disorders, left wrist
　　　　M25.839　Other specified joint disorders, unspecified wrist

▶ New　⇒ Revised　~~deleted~~ Deleted　Excludes 1　Excludes 2　Includes　Use additional　Code first　Code also　Key words
OGCR Official Guidelines　● Unacceptable Principal Diagnosis　X Assign placeholder X　● Use Additional Character(s)　▶ Manifestation Code　Coding Clinic

● M25.84 Other specified joint disorders, hand
    M25.841 Other specified joint disorders, right hand
    M25.842 Other specified joint disorders, left hand
    M25.849 Other specified joint disorders, unspecified hand

● M25.85 Other specified joint disorders, hip
    M25.851 Other specified joint disorders, right hip
    M25.852 Other specified joint disorders, left hip
    M25.859 Other specified joint disorders, unspecified hip

● M25.86 Other specified joint disorders, knee
    M25.861 Other specified joint disorders, right knee
    M25.862 Other specified joint disorders, left knee
    M25.869 Other specified joint disorders, unspecified knee

● M25.87 Other specified joint disorders, ankle and foot
    M25.871 Other specified joint disorders, right ankle and foot
    M25.872 Other specified joint disorders, left ankle and foot
    M25.879 Other specified joint disorders, unspecified ankle and foot

M25.9 Joint disorder, unspecified

DENTOFACIAL ANOMALIES [INCLUDING MALOCCLUSION] AND OTHER DISORDERS OF JAW (M26-M27)

> **Excludes1** hemifacial atrophy or hypertrophy (Q67.4)
> unilateral condylar hyperplasia or hypoplasia (M27.8)

● **M26 Dentofacial anomalies [including malocclusion]**
  ● M26.0 Major anomalies of jaw size

> **Excludes1** acromegaly (E22.0)
> Robin's syndrome (Q87.0)

    M26.00 Unspecified anomaly of jaw size
    M26.01 Maxillary hyperplasia
    M26.02 Maxillary hypoplasia
    M26.03 Mandibular hyperplasia
    M26.04 Mandibular hypoplasia
    M26.05 Macrogenia
    M26.06 Microgenia
    M26.07 Excessive tuberosity of jaw
        Entire maxillary tuberosity
    M26.09 Other specified anomalies of jaw size

  ● M26.1 Anomalies of jaw-cranial base relationship
    M26.10 Unspecified anomaly of jaw-cranial base relationship
    M26.11 Maxillary asymmetry
    M26.12 Other jaw asymmetry
    M26.19 Other specified anomalies of jaw-cranial base relationship

Figure 13-3 Dentofacial malocclusion.

● M26.2 Anomalies of dental arch relationship
    M26.20 Unspecified anomaly of dental arch relationship
  ● M26.21 Malocclusion, Angle's class
    M26.211 Malocclusion, Angle's class I
        Neutro-occlusion
    M26.212 Malocclusion, Angle's class II
        Disto-occlusion Division I
        Disto-occlusion Division II
    M26.213 Malocclusion, Angle's class III
        Mesio-occlusion
    M26.219 Malocclusion, Angle's class, unspecified

  ● M26.22 Open occlusal relationship
    M26.220 Open anterior occlusal relationship
        Anterior openbite
    M26.221 Open posterior occlusal relationship
        Posterior openbite

    M26.23 Excessive horizontal overlap
        Excessive horizontal overjet
    M26.24 Reverse articulation
        Crossbite (anterior) (posterior)
    M26.25 Anomalies of interarch distance
    M26.29 Other anomalies of dental arch relationship
        Midline deviation of dental arch
        Overbite (excessive) deep
        Overbite (excessive) horizontal
        Overbite (excessive) vertical
        Posterior lingual occlusion of mandibular teeth

● M26.3 Anomalies of tooth position of fully erupted tooth or teeth

> **Excludes2** embedded and impacted teeth (K01.-)

    M26.30 Unspecified anomaly of tooth position of fully erupted tooth or teeth
        Abnormal spacing of fully erupted tooth or teeth NOS
        Displacement of fully erupted tooth or teeth NOS
        Transposition of fully erupted tooth or teeth NOS
    M26.31 Crowding of fully erupted teeth
    M26.32 Excessive spacing of fully erupted teeth
        Diastema of fully erupted tooth or teeth NOS
    M26.33 Horizontal displacement of fully erupted tooth or teeth
        Tipped tooth or teeth
        Tipping of fully erupted tooth
    M26.34 Vertical displacement of fully erupted tooth or teeth
        Extruded tooth
        Infraeruption of tooth or teeth
        Supraeruption of tooth or teeth
    M26.35 Rotation of fully erupted tooth or teeth
    M26.36 Insufficient interocclusal distance of fully erupted teeth (ridge)
        Lack of adequate intermaxillary vertical dimension of fully erupted teeth
    M26.37 Excessive interocclusal distance of fully erupted teeth
        Excessive intermaxillary vertical dimension of fully erupted teeth
        Loss of occlusal vertical dimension of fully erupted teeth
    M26.39 Other anomalies of tooth position of fully erupted tooth or teeth

  M26.4 Malocclusion, unspecified

Item 13–6 Hyperplasia is a condition of overdevelopment, whereas **hypoplasia** is a condition of underdevelopment. **Macrogenia** is overdevelopment of the chin, whereas **microgenia** is underdevelopment of the chin.

N Newborn Age: 0   **P** Pediatric Age: 0–17   **M** Maternity DX: 12–55   **A** Adult Age: 15–124   ♀ Females Only   ♂ Males Only

Ⓒ Complication\Comorbidity   Ⓜ Major C\C   Ⓔ CC/MCC Exclusions   Ⓗ Hospital-Acquired Condition   **1031**

CHAPTER 13 (M00-M99)

● **M26.5   Dentofacial functional abnormalities**

    Excludes1   bruxism (F45.8)
                    teeth-grinding NOS (F45.8)

    M26.50   Dentofacial functional abnormalities, unspecified

    M26.51   Abnormal jaw closure

    M26.52   Limited mandibular range of motion

    M26.53   Deviation in opening and closing of the mandible

    M26.54   Insufficient anterior guidance
            Insufficient anterior occlusal guidance

    M26.55   Centric occlusion maximum intercuspation discrepancy

         Excludes1   centric occlusion NOS (M26.59)

    M26.56   Non-working side interference
            Balancing side interference

    M26.57   Lack of posterior occlusal support

    M26.59   Other dentofacial functional abnormalities
            Centric occlusion (of teeth) NOS
            Malocclusion due to abnormal swallowing
            Malocclusion due to mouth breathing
            Malocclusion due to tongue, lip or finger habits

● **M26.6   Temporomandibular joint disorders**

    Excludes2   current temporomandibular joint dislocation (S03.0)
                      current temporomandibular joint sprain (S03.4)

    Coding Clinic: 2016, Q4, P38-39

   ● M26.60   Temporomandibular joint disorder, unspecified

      M26.601   Right temporomandibular joint disorder, unspecified

      M26.602   Left temporomandibular joint disorder, unspecified

      M26.603   Bilateral temporomandibular joint disorder, unspecified

      M26.609   Unspecified temporomandibular joint disorder, unspecified side
              Temporomandibular joint disorder NOS

   ● M26.61   Adhesions and ankylosis of temporomandibular joint

      M26.611   Adhesions and ankylosis of right temporomandibular joint

      M26.612   Adhesions and ankylosis of left temporomandibular joint

      M26.613   Adhesions and ankylosis of bilateral temporomandibular joint

      M26.619   Adhesions and ankylosis of temporomandibular joint, unspecified side

● M26.62   Arthralgia of temporomandibular joint

    M26.621   Arthralgia of right temporomandibular joint

    M26.622   Arthralgia of left temporomandibular joint

    M26.623   Arthralgia of bilateral temporomandibular joint

    M26.629   Arthralgia of temporomandibular joint, unspecified side

● M26.63   Articular disc disorder of temporomandibular joint

    M26.631   Articular disc disorder of right temporomandibular joint

    M26.632   Articular disc disorder of left temporomandibular joint

    M26.633   Articular disc disorder of bilateral temporomandibular joint

    M26.639   Articular disc disorder of temporomandibular joint, unspecified side

  M26.69   Other specified disorders of temporomandibular joint

● M26.7   Dental alveolar anomalies

  M26.70   Unspecified alveolar anomaly

  M26.71   Alveolar maxillary hyperplasia

  M26.72   Alveolar mandibular hyperplasia

  M26.73   Alveolar maxillary hypoplasia

  M26.74   Alveolar mandibular hypoplasia

  M26.79   Other specified alveolar anomalies

● M26.8   Other dentofacial anomalies

  M26.81   Anterior soft tissue impingement
          Anterior soft tissue impingement on teeth

  M26.82   Posterior soft tissue impingement
          Posterior soft tissue impingement on teeth

  M26.89   Other dentofacial anomalies

  M26.9   Dentofacial anomaly, unspecified

● M27   Other diseases of jaws

  M27.0   Developmental disorders of jaws
         Latent bone cyst of jaw
         Stafne's cyst
         Torus mandibularis
         Torus palatinus

  M27.1   Giant cell granuloma, central
         Giant cell granuloma NOS

     Excludes1   peripheral giant cell granuloma (K06.8)

  M27.2   Inflammatory conditions of jaws
         Osteitis of jaw(s)
         Osteomyelitis (neonatal) jaw(s)
         Osteoradionecrosis jaw(s)
         Periostitis jaw(s)
         Sequestrum of jaw bone

         Use additional code (W88-W90, X39.0) to identify radiation, if radiation-induced

     Excludes2   osteonecrosis of jaw due to drug (M87.180)

  M27.3   Alveolitis of jaws
         Alveolar osteitis
         Dry socket

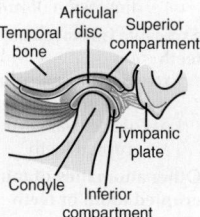

Figure 13-4   Temporomandibular joint.

Item 13–7 Dysfunction of the temporomandibular joint is termed **temporomandibular joint (TMJ) syndrome** and is characterized by pain and tenderness/spasm of the muscles of mastication, joint noise, and in the later stages, limited mandibular movement.

▶ New   ⇛ Revised   ~~deleted~~ Deleted   Excludes 1   Excludes 2   Includes   Use additional   Code first   Code also   Key words

OGCR Official Guidelines   ● Unacceptable Principal Diagnosis   X Assign placeholder X   ● Use Additional Character(s)   ▶ Manifestation Code   **Coding Clinic**

M27.4 Other and unspecified cysts of jaw

> **Excludes1**   cysts of oral region (K09.-)
> latent bone cyst of jaw (M27.0)
> Stafne's cyst (M27.0)

M27.40 Unspecified cyst of jaw
Cyst of jaw NOS

M27.49 Other cysts of jaw
Aneurysmal cyst of jaw
Hemorrhagic cyst of jaw
Traumatic cyst of jaw

M27.5 Periradicular pathology associated with previous endodontic treatment

M27.51 Perforation of root canal space due to endodontic treatment

M27.52 Endodontic overfill

M27.53 Endodontic underfill

M27.59 Other periradicular pathology associated with previous endodontic treatment

M27.6 Endosseous dental implant failure

M27.61 Osseointegration failure of dental implant
Hemorrhagic complications of dental implant placement
Iatrogenic osseointegration failure of dental implant
Osseointegration failure of dental implant due to complications of systemic disease
Osseointegration failure of dental implant due to poor bone quality
Pre-integration failure of dental implant NOS
Pre-osseointegration failure of dental implant

M27.62 Post-osseointegration biological failure of dental implant
Failure of dental implant due to lack of attached gingiva
Failure of dental implant due to occlusal trauma (caused by poor prosthetic design)
Failure of dental implant due to parafunctional habits
Failure of dental implant due to periodontal infection (peri–implantitis)
Failure of dental implant due to poor oral hygiene
Iatrogenic post-osseointegration failure of dental implant
Post-osseointegration failure of dental implant due to complications of systemic disease

M27.63 Post-osseointegration mechanical failure of dental implant
Failure of dental prosthesis causing loss of dental implant
Fracture of dental implant

> **Excludes2**   cracked tooth (K03.81)
> fractured dental restorative material with loss of material (K08.531)
> fractured dental restorative material without loss of material (K08.530)
> fractured tooth (S02.5)

M27.69 Other endosseous dental implant failure
Dental implant failure NOS

M27.8 Other specified diseases of jaws
Cherubism
Exostosis
Fibrous dysplasia
Unilateral condylar hyperplasia
Unilateral condylar hypoplasia

> **Excludes1**   jaw pain (R68.84)

M27.9 Disease of jaws, unspecified

SYSTEMIC CONNECTIVE TISSUE DISORDERS (M30-M36)

> **Includes**   autoimmune disease NOS
> collagen (vascular) disease NOS
> systemic autoimmune disease
> systemic collagen (vascular) disease

> **Excludes1**   autoimmune disease, single organ or single cell-type - code to relevant condition category

M30 Polyarteritis nodosa and related conditions

> **Excludes1**   microscopic polyarteritis (M31.7)

(Ex) For category M30 CC codes unless otherwise indicated: See PDX Collection 874

M30.0 Polyarteritis nodosa 🔖

M30.1 Polyarteritis with lung involvement [Churg-Strauss]🔖
Allergic granulomatous angiitis

M30.2 Juvenile polyarteritis 🔖

M30.3 Mucocutaneous lymph node syndrome [Kawasaki]🔖
(Ex) See PDX Collection 875

M30.8 Other conditions related to polyarteritis nodosa 🔖
Polyangiitis overlap syndrome

M31 Other necrotizing vasculopathies
(Ex) For category M31 CC codes unless otherwise indicated: See PDX Collection 874

M31.0 Hypersensitivity angiitis 🔖
Goodpasture's syndrome

M31.1 Thrombotic microangiopathy 🔖
Thrombotic thrombocytopenic purpura

M31.2 Lethal midline granuloma 🔖

M31.3 Wegener's granulomatosis
Necrotizing respiratory granulomatosis

M31.30 Wegener's granulomatosis without renal involvement 🔖
Wegener's granulomatosis NOS

M31.31 Wegener's granulomatosis with renal involvement 🔖

M31.4 Aortic arch syndrome [Takayasu]🔖

M31.5 Giant cell arteritis with polymyalgia rheumatica

M31.6 Other giant cell arteritis

M31.7 Microscopic polyangiitis 🔖
Microscopic polyarteritis

> **Excludes1**   polyarteritis nodosa (M30.0)

M31.8 Other specified necrotizing vasculopathies 🔖
Hypocomplementemic vasculitis
Septic vasculitis
(Ex) See PDX Collection 712

M31.9 Necrotizing vasculopathy, unspecified 🔖
(Ex) See PDX Collection 712

M32 Systemic lupus erythematosus (SLE)
Autoimmune inflammatory connective tissue disease of unknown cause that occurs most often in women

> **Excludes1**   lupus erythematosus (discoid) (NOS) (L93.0)

M32.0 Drug-induced systemic lupus erythematosus
Use additional code for adverse effect, if applicable, to identify drug (T36-T50 with fifth or sixth character 5)

M32.1 Systemic lupus erythematosus with organ or system involvement

M32.10 Systemic lupus erythematosus, organ or system involvement unspecified

M32.11 Endocarditis in systemic lupus erythematosus 🔖
Libman-Sacks disease
CC when PDx is its own CC
(Ex) See PDX Collection 676

CHAPTER 13 (M00-M99)

CHAPTER 13 (M00-M99)

M32.12 **Pericarditis in systemic lupus erythematosus** 🔒
Lupus pericarditis
CC when PDx is its own CC
(Ex) See PDX Collection 673

M32.13 **Lung involvement in systemic lupus erythematosus**
Pleural effusion due to systemic lupus erythematosus

M32.14 **Glomerular disease in systemic lupus erythematosus**
Lupus renal disease NOS

M32.15 **Tubulo-interstitial nephropathy in systemic lupus erythematosus**

M32.19 **Other organ or system involvement in systemic lupus erythematosus**

M32.8 **Other forms of systemic lupus erythematosus**

M32.9 Systemic lupus erythematosus, **unspecified**
SLE NOS
Systemic lupus erythematosus NOS
Systemic lupus erythematosus without organ involvement

● M33 **Dermatopolymyositis**
(Ex) For category M33 CC codes unless otherwise indicated: See PDX Collection 876

➡● M33.0 **Juvenile dermatomyositis**

➡ M33.00 **Juvenile dermatomyositis, organ involvement unspecified**

➡ M33.01 **Juvenile dermatomyositis with respiratory involvement** 🔒

➡ M33.02 **Juvenile dermatomyositis with myopathy** 🔒
CC when PDx is its own CC
(Ex) See PDX Collection 877

▶ M33.03 **Juvenile dermatomyositis without myopathy** 🔒

➡ M33.09 **Juvenile dermatomyositis with other organ involvement** 🔒

➡● M33.1 **Other dermatomyositis**
▶Adult dermatomyositis

➡ M33.10 **Other dermatomyositis, organ involvement unspecified** 🔒

➡ M33.11 **Other dermatomyositis with respiratory involvement** 🔒

➡ M33.12 **Other dermatomyositis with myopathy** 🔒
CC when PDx is its own CC
(Ex) See PDX Collection 877

▶ M33.13 **Other dermatomyositis without myopathy** 🔒
▶Dermatomyositis NOS

➡ M33.19 **Other dermatomyositis with other organ involvement** 🔒

● M33.2 **Polymyositis**

M33.20 **Polymyositis, organ involvement unspecified** 🔒
(Ex) See PDX Collection 878

M33.21 **Polymyositis with respiratory involvement** 🔒
(Ex) See PDX Collection 878

M33.22 **Polymyositis with myopathy** 🔒
CC when PDx is its own CC
(Ex) See PDX Collection 879

M33.29 **Polymyositis with other organ involvement** 🔒
(Ex) See PDX Collection 878

● M33.9 **Dermatopolymyositis, unspecified**

M33.90 **Dermatopolymyositis, unspecified, organ involvement unspecified** 🔒

M33.91 **Dermatopolymyositis, unspecified with respiratory involvement** 🔒

M33.92 **Dermatopolymyositis, unspecified with myopathy** 🔒
CC when PDx is its own CC
(Ex) See PDX Collection 877

▶ M33.93 **Dermatopolymyositis, unspecified without myopathy** 🔒

M33.99 **Dermatopolymyositis, unspecified with other organ involvement** 🔒

Item 13-8 Polymyalgia rheumatica is a syndrome characterized by aching and morning stiffness and is related to aging and hereditary predisposition.

● M34 **Systemic sclerosis [scleroderma]**
Excludes1 circumscribed scleroderma (L94.0)
neonatal scleroderma (P83.8)

M34.0 **Progressive systemic sclerosis**

M34.1 **CR(E)ST syndrome**
Combination of calcinosis, Raynaud's phenomenon, esophageal dysfunction, sclerodactyly, telangiectasia

M34.2 **Systemic sclerosis induced by drug and chemical**
Code first poisoning due to drug or toxin, if applicable (T36-T65 with fifth or sixth character 1-4 or 6)
Use additional code for adverse effect, if applicable, to identify drug (T36-T50 with fifth or sixth character 5)

● M34.8 **Other forms of systemic sclerosis**

M34.81 **Systemic sclerosis with lung involvement** 🔒
CC when PDx is its own CC
(Ex) No exclusions

M34.82 **Systemic sclerosis with myopathy** 🔒
CC when PDx is its own CC
(Ex) See PDX Collection 867

M34.83 **Systemic sclerosis with polyneuropathy**

M34.89 **Other systemic sclerosis**

M34.9 **Systemic sclerosis, unspecified**

● M35 **Other systemic involvement of connective tissue**
Excludes1 reactive perforating collagenosis (L87.1)

● M35.0 **Sicca syndrome [Sjögren]**

M35.00 **Sicca syndrome, unspecified**

M35.01 **Sicca syndrome with keratoconjunctivitis**

M35.02 **Sicca syndrome with lung involvement**

M35.03 **Sicca syndrome with myopathy** 🔒
CC when PDx is its own CC
(Ex) See PDX Collection 867

M35.04 **Sicca syndrome with tubulo-interstitial nephropathy**
Renal tubular acidosis in sicca syndrome

M35.09 **Sicca syndrome with other organ involvement**

M35.1 **Other overlap syndromes** 🔒
Mixed connective tissue disease
Excludes1 polyangiitis overlap syndrome (M30.8)
(Ex) See PDX Collection 880

M35.2 **Behçet's disease** 🔒
(Ex) See PDX Collection 863

M35.3 **Polymyalgia rheumatica**
Excludes1 polymyalgia rheumatica with giant cell arteritis (M31.5)

M35.4 **Diffuse (eosinophilic) fasciitis**

M35.5 **Multifocal fibrosclerosis** 🔒
(Ex) See PDX Collection 880

M35.6 **Relapsing panniculitis [Weber-Christian]**
Excludes1 lupus panniculitis (L93.2)
panniculitis NOS (M79.3-)

M35.7 **Hypermobility syndrome**
Familial ligamentous laxity
Excludes1 Ehlers-Danlos syndrome (Q79.6)
ligamentous laxity, NOS (M24.2-)

M35.8 **Other specified systemic involvement of connective tissue** 🔒
(Ex) See PDX Collection 880

M35.9 **Systemic involvement of connective tissue, unspecified**
Autoimmune disease (systemic) NOS
Collagen (vascular) disease NOS

▶ New   ➡ Revised   ~~deleted~~ Deleted   Excludes 1   Excludes 2   Includes   Use additional   Code first   Code also   Key words

OGCR Official Guidelines   ● Unacceptable Principal Diagnosis   X Assign placeholder X   🔒 Use Additional Character(s)   ➡ Manifestation Code   **Coding Clinic**

● **M36 Systemic disorders of connective tissue in diseases classified elsewhere**

     Excludes2   arthropathies in diseases classified elsewhere (M14.-)

▷ *M36.0 Dermato(poly)myositis in neoplastic disease* 🔖
     Code first underlying neoplasm (C00-D49)
     (Ex) See PDX Collection 876

▷ *M36.1 Arthropathy in neoplastic disease*
     Code first underlying neoplasm, such as:
         leukemia (C91-C95)
         malignant histiocytosis (C96.A)
         multiple myeloma (C90.0)

▷ *M36.2 Hemophilic arthropathy*
     Hemarthrosis in hemophilic arthropathy
     Code first underlying disease, such as:
         factor VIII deficiency (D66)
         with vascular defect (D68.0)
         factor IX deficiency (D67)
         hemophilia (classical) (D66)
         hemophilia B (D67)
         hemophilia C (D68.1)

▷ *M36.3 Arthropathy in other blood disorders*

▷ *M36.4 Arthropathy in hypersensitivity reactions classified elsewhere*
     Code first underlying disease, such as:
         Henoch (-Schönlein) purpura (D69.0)
         serum sickness (T80.6-)

▷ *M36.8 Systemic disorders of connective tissue in other diseases classified elsewhere*
     Code first underlying disease, such as:
         alkaptonuria (E70.2)
         hypogammaglobulinemia (D80.-)
         ochronosis (E70.2)

DORSOPATHIES (M40-M54)

DEFORMING DORSOPATHIES (M40-M43)

● **M40 Kyphosis and lordosis**
     Excludes1   congenital kyphosis and lordosis (Q76.4)
                 kyphoscoliosis (M41.-)
                 postprocedural kyphosis and lordosis (M96.-)

   ● **M40.0 Postural kyphosis**
     Excludes1   osteochondrosis of spine (M42.-)
     M40.00 Postural kyphosis, site unspecified
     M40.03 Postural kyphosis, cervicothoracic region
     M40.04 Postural kyphosis, thoracic region
     M40.05 Postural kyphosis, thoracolumbar region

Item 13-9   **Kyphosis** is an abnormal curvature of the spine. **Senile kyphosis** is a result of disc degeneration causing ossification (turning to bone). **Adolescent** or **juvenile** kyphosis is also known as **Scheuermann's disease,** a condition in which the discs of the lower thoracic spine herniate, causing the disc space to narrow and the spine to tilt forward. This condition is attributed to poor posture. **Lordosis or swayback** is an abnormal curvature of the spine resulting in an inward curve of the lumbar spine just above the buttocks. **Scoliosis** causes a sideways curve to the spine. The curves are S- or C-shaped, and it is most commonly acquired in late childhood and early teen years, when growth is fast.

   ● **M40.1 Other secondary kyphosis**
     M40.10 Other secondary kyphosis, site unspecified
     M40.12 Other secondary kyphosis, cervical region
     M40.13 Other secondary kyphosis, cervicothoracic region
     M40.14 Other secondary kyphosis, thoracic region
     M40.15 Other secondary kyphosis, thoracolumbar region

   ● **M40.2 Other and unspecified kyphosis**
     ● **M40.20 Unspecified kyphosis**
       M40.202 Unspecified kyphosis, cervical region
       M40.203 Unspecified kyphosis, cervicothoracic region
       M40.204 Unspecified kyphosis, thoracic region
       M40.205 Unspecified kyphosis, thoracolumbar region
       M40.209 Unspecified kyphosis, site unspecified

     ● **M40.29 Other kyphosis**
       M40.292 Other kyphosis, cervical region
       M40.293 Other kyphosis, cervicothoracic region
       M40.294 Other kyphosis, thoracic region
       M40.295 Other kyphosis, thoracolumbar region
       M40.299 Other kyphosis, site unspecified

   ● **M40.3 Flatback syndrome**
     M40.30 Flatback syndrome, site unspecified
     M40.35 Flatback syndrome, thoracolumbar region
     M40.36 Flatback syndrome, lumbar region
     M40.37 Flatback syndrome, lumbosacral region

   ● **M40.4 Postural lordosis**
     Abnormal increase in the normal curvature of the lumbar spine (sway back)
     Acquired lordosis
     M40.40 Postural lordosis, site unspecified
     M40.45 Postural lordosis, thoracolumbar region
     M40.46 Postural lordosis, lumbar region
     M40.47 Postural lordosis, lumbosacral region

   ● **M40.5 Lordosis, unspecified**
     M40.50 Lordosis, unspecified, site unspecified
     M40.55 Lordosis, unspecified, thoracolumbar region
     M40.56 Lordosis, unspecified, lumbar region
     M40.57 Lordosis, unspecified, lumbosacral region

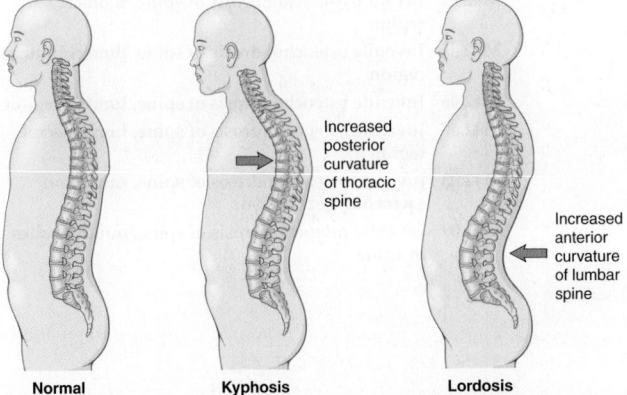

Increased posterior curvature of thoracic spine

Increased anterior curvature of lumbar spine

Normal   **Kyphosis**   **Lordosis**

Figure 13-5   Kyphosis, Lordosis, Scoliosis. (From Chabner: The Language of Medicine, ed 8, St. Louis, Saunders, 2007)

CHAPTER 13 (M00-M99)

N Newborn Age: 0   P Pediatric Age: 0–17   M Maternity DX: 12–55   A Adult Age: 15–124   ♀ Females Only   ♂ Males Only

🔖 Complication\Comorbidity   🔖 Major C\C   (Ex) CC/MCC Exclusions   🔖 Hospital-Acquired Condition

CHAPTER 13 (M00-M99)

● **M41 Scoliosis**

> **Includes**   kyphoscoliosis
> **Excludes1** congenital scoliosis NOS (Q67.5)
> congenital scoliosis due to bony malformation
> (Q76.3)
> postural congenital scoliosis (Q67.5)
> kyphoscoliotic heart disease (I27.1)
> postprocedural scoliosis (M96.-)

● **M41.0 Infantile idiopathic scoliosis**

> **M41.00 Infantile idiopathic scoliosis, site unspecified**
> **M41.02 Infantile idiopathic scoliosis, cervical region**
> **M41.03 Infantile idiopathic scoliosis, cervicothoracic region**
> **M41.04 Infantile idiopathic scoliosis, thoracic region**
> **M41.05 Infantile idiopathic scoliosis, thoracolumbar region**
> **M41.06 Infantile idiopathic scoliosis, lumbar region**
> **M41.07 Infantile idiopathic scoliosis, lumbosacral region**
> **M41.08 Infantile idiopathic scoliosis, sacral and sacrococcygeal region**

● **M41.1 Juvenile and adolescent idiopathic scoliosis**

> ● **M41.11 Juvenile idiopathic scoliosis**
>
>> **M41.112 Juvenile idiopathic scoliosis, cervical region**
>> **M41.113 Juvenile idiopathic scoliosis, cervicothoracic region**
>> **M41.114 Juvenile idiopathic scoliosis, thoracic region**
>> **M41.115 Juvenile idiopathic scoliosis, thoracolumbar region**
>> **M41.116 Juvenile idiopathic scoliosis, lumbar region**
>> **M41.117 Juvenile idiopathic scoliosis, lumbosacral region**
>> **M41.119 Juvenile idiopathic scoliosis, site unspecified**
>
> ● **M41.12 Adolescent scoliosis**
>
>> **M41.122 Adolescent idiopathic scoliosis, cervical region**
>> **M41.123 Adolescent idiopathic scoliosis, cervicothoracic region**
>> **M41.124 Adolescent idiopathic scoliosis, thoracic region**
>> **M41.125 Adolescent idiopathic scoliosis, thoracolumbar region**
>> **M41.126 Adolescent idiopathic scoliosis, lumbar region**
>> **M41.127 Adolescent idiopathic scoliosis, lumbosacral region**
>> **M41.129 Adolescent idiopathic scoliosis, site unspecified**

● **M41.2 Other idiopathic scoliosis**

> **M41.20 Other idiopathic scoliosis, site unspecified**
> **M41.22 Other idiopathic scoliosis, cervical region**
> **M41.23 Other idiopathic scoliosis, cervicothoracic region**
> **M41.24 Other idiopathic scoliosis, thoracic region**
> **M41.25 Other idiopathic scoliosis, thoracolumbar region**
> **M41.26 Other idiopathic scoliosis, lumbar region**
> **M41.27 Other idiopathic scoliosis, lumbosacral region**

● **M41.3 Thoracogenic scoliosis**

> **M41.30 Thoracogenic scoliosis, site unspecified**
> **M41.34 Thoracogenic scoliosis, thoracic region**
> **M41.35 Thoracogenic scoliosis, thoracolumbar region**

● **M41.4 Neuromuscular scoliosis**

> Scoliosis secondary to cerebral palsy, Friedreich's ataxia, poliomyelitis and other neuromuscular disorders
> Code also underlying condition
>
> **M41.40 Neuromuscular scoliosis, site unspecified**
> **M41.41 Neuromuscular scoliosis, occipito-atlanto-axial region**
> **M41.42 Neuromuscular scoliosis, cervical region**
> **M41.43 Neuromuscular scoliosis, cervicothoracic region**
> **M41.44 Neuromuscular scoliosis, thoracic region**
> **M41.45 Neuromuscular scoliosis, thoracolumbar region**
> **M41.46 Neuromuscular scoliosis, lumbar region**
> **M41.47 Neuromuscular scoliosis, lumbosacral region**

● **M41.5 Other secondary scoliosis**

> **M41.50 Other secondary scoliosis, site unspecified**
> **M41.52 Other secondary scoliosis, cervical region**
> **M41.53 Other secondary scoliosis, cervicothoracic region**
> **M41.54 Other secondary scoliosis, thoracic region**
> **M41.55 Other secondary scoliosis, thoracolumbar region**
> **M41.56 Other secondary scoliosis, lumbar region**
> **M41.57 Other secondary scoliosis, lumbosacral region**

● **M41.8 Other forms of scoliosis**

> **M41.80 Other forms of scoliosis, site unspecified**
> **M41.82 Other forms of scoliosis, cervical region**
> **M41.83 Other forms of scoliosis, cervicothoracic region**
> **M41.84 Other forms of scoliosis, thoracic region**
> **M41.85 Other forms of scoliosis, thoracolumbar region**
> **M41.86 Other forms of scoliosis, lumbar region**
> **M41.87 Other forms of scoliosis, lumbosacral region**

> **M41.9 Scoliosis, unspecified**

● **M42 Spinal osteochondrosis**

> ● **M42.0 Juvenile osteochondrosis of spine**
>
> Calvé's disease
> Scheuermann's disease
>
>> **Excludes1** postural kyphosis (M40.0)
>
>> **M42.00 Juvenile osteochondrosis of spine, site unspecified**
>> **M42.01 Juvenile osteochondrosis of spine, occipito-atlanto-axial region**
>> **M42.02 Juvenile osteochondrosis of spine, cervical region**
>> **M42.03 Juvenile osteochondrosis of spine, cervicothoracic region**
>> **M42.04 Juvenile osteochondrosis of spine, thoracic region**
>> **M42.05 Juvenile osteochondrosis of spine, thoracolumbar region**
>> **M42.06 Juvenile osteochondrosis of spine, lumbar region**
>> **M42.07 Juvenile osteochondrosis of spine, lumbosacral region**
>> **M42.08 Juvenile osteochondrosis of spine, sacral and sacrococcygeal region**
>> **M42.09 Juvenile osteochondrosis of spine, multiple sites in spine**

▶ New   ⇒ Revised   ~~deleted~~ Deleted   Excludes 1   Excludes 2   Includes   Use additional   Code first   Code also   Key words

OGCR Official Guidelines   ● Unacceptable Principal Diagnosis   X Assign placeholder X   ● Use Additional Character(s)   ▶ Manifestation Code   Coding Clinic

M42.1   **Adult osteochondrosis of spine**

    M42.10   **Adult osteochondrosis of spine, site unspecified**   A

    M42.11   **Adult osteochondrosis of spine, occipitoatlanto-axial region**   A

    M42.12   **Adult osteochondrosis of spine, cervical region**   A

    M42.13   **Adult osteochondrosis of spine, cervicothoracic region**   A

    M42.14   **Adult osteochondrosis of spine, thoracic region**   A

    M42.15   **Adult osteochondrosis of spine, thoracolumbar region**   A

    M42.16   **Adult osteochondrosis of spine, lumbar region**   A

    M42.17   **Adult osteochondrosis of spine, lumbosacral region**   A

    M42.18   **Adult osteochondrosis of spine, sacral and sacrococcygeal region**   A

    M42.19   **Adult osteochondrosis of spine, multiple sites in spine**   A

M42.9   **Spinal osteochondrosis, unspecified**

M43   **Other deforming dorsopathies**

    Excludes1   congenital spondylolysis and spondylolisthesis (Q76.2)
                hemivertebra (Q76.3-Q76.4)
                Klippel-Feil syndrome (Q76.1)
                lumbarization and sacralization (Q76.4)
                platyspondylisis (Q76.4)
                spina bifida occulta (Q76.0)
                spinal curvature in osteoporosis (M80.-)
                spinal curvature in Paget's disease of bone [osteitis deformans] (M88.-)

M43.0   **Spondylolysis**

    Excludes1   congenital spondylolysis (Q76.2)
                spondylolisthesis (M43.1)

    M43.00   **Spondylolysis, site unspecified**

    M43.01   **Spondylolysis, occipito-atlanto-axial region**

    M43.02   **Spondylolysis, cervical region**

    M43.03   **Spondylolysis, cervicothoracic region**

    M43.04   **Spondylolysis, thoracic region**

    M43.05   **Spondylolysis, thoracolumbar region**

    M43.06   **Spondylolysis, lumbar region**

    M43.07   **Spondylolysis, lumbosacral region**

    M43.08   **Spondylolysis, sacral and sacrococcygeal region**

    M43.09   **Spondylolysis, multiple sites in spine**

M43.1   **Spondylolisthesis**

    Excludes1   acute traumatic of lumbosacral region (S33.1)
                acute traumatic of sites other than lumbosacral - code to Fracture, vertebra, by region
                congenital spondylolisthesis (Q76.2)

    M43.10   **Spondylolisthesis, site unspecified**

    M43.11   **Spondylolisthesis, occipito-atlanto-axial region**

    M43.12   **Spondylolisthesis, cervical region**

    M43.13   **Spondylolisthesis, cervicothoracic region**

    M43.14   **Spondylolisthesis, thoracic region**

    M43.15   **Spondylolisthesis, thoracolumbar region**

    M43.16   **Spondylolisthesis, lumbar region**

    M43.17   **Spondylolisthesis, lumbosacral region**

    M43.18   **Spondylolisthesis, sacral and sacrococcygeal region**

    M43.19   **Spondylolisthesis, multiple sites in spine**

M43.2   **Fusion of spine**
      Ankylosis of spinal joint

    Excludes1   ankylosing spondylitis (M45.0-)
                congenital fusion of spine (Q76.4)

    Excludes2   arthrodesis status (Z98.1)
                pseudoarthrosis after fusion or arthrodesis (M96.0)

    M43.20   **Fusion of spine, site unspecified**

    M43.21   **Fusion of spine, occipito-atlanto-axial region**

    M43.22   **Fusion of spine, cervical region**

    M43.23   **Fusion of spine, cervicothoracic region**

    M43.24   **Fusion of spine, thoracic region**

    M43.25   **Fusion of spine, thoracolumbar region**

    M43.26   **Fusion of spine, lumbar region**

    M43.27   **Fusion of spine, lumbosacral region**

    M43.28   **Fusion of spine, sacral and sacrococcygeal region**

M43.3   **Recurrent atlantoaxial dislocation with myelopathy**

M43.4   **Other recurrent atlantoaxial dislocation**

M43.5   **Other recurrent vertebral dislocation**

    Excludes1   biomechanical lesions NEC (M99.-)

    M43.5X   **Other recurrent vertebral dislocation**

      M43.5X2   **Other recurrent vertebral dislocation, cervical region**

      M43.5X3   **Other recurrent vertebral dislocation, cervicothoracic region**

      M43.5X4   **Other recurrent vertebral dislocation, thoracic region**

      M43.5X5   **Other recurrent vertebral dislocation, thoracolumbar region**

      M43.5X6   **Other recurrent vertebral dislocation, lumbar region**

      M43.5X7   **Other recurrent vertebral dislocation, lumbosacral region**

      M43.5X8   **Other recurrent vertebral dislocation, sacral and sacrococcygeal region**

      M43.5X9   **Other recurrent vertebral dislocation, site unspecified**

M43.6   **Torticollis**

    Excludes1   congenital (sternomastoid) torticollis (Q68.0)
                current injury - see Injury, of spine, by body region ocular torticollis (R29.891)
                psychogenic torticollis (F45.8)
                spasmodic torticollis (G24.3)
                torticollis due to birth injury (P15.2)

M43.8   **Other specified deforming dorsopathies**

    Excludes2   kyphosis and lordosis (M40.-)
                scoliosis (M41.-)

    M43.8X   **Other specified deforming dorsopathies**

      M43.8X1   **Other specified deforming dorsopathies, occipito-atlanto-axial region**

      M43.8X2   **Other specified deforming dorsopathies, cervical region**

      M43.8X3   **Other specified deforming dorsopathies, cervicothoracic region**

      M43.8X4   **Other specified deforming dorsopathies, thoracic region**

      M43.8X5   **Other specified deforming dorsopathies, thoracolumbar region**

      M43.8X6   **Other specified deforming dorsopathies, lumbar region**

      M43.8X7   **Other specified deforming dorsopathies, lumbosacral region**

      M43.8X8   **Other specified deforming dorsopathies, sacral and sacrococcygeal region**

      M43.8X9   **Other specified deforming dorsopathies, site unspecified**

M43.9   **Deforming dorsopathy, unspecified**
      Curvature of spine NOS

CHAPTER 13 (M00-M99)

Item 13-10 Spondylolisthesis is a condition caused by the slipping forward of one disc over another.

SPONDYLOPATHIES (M45-M49)

● **M45 Ankylosing spondylitis**
Rheumatoid arthritis of spine
> **Excludes1**   arthropathy in Reiter's disease (M02.3-)
> juvenile (ankylosing) spondylitis (M08.1)
> **Excludes2**   Behçet's disease (M35.2)

M45.0   Ankylosing spondylitis of multiple sites in spine
M45.1   Ankylosing spondylitis of occipito-atlanto-axial region
M45.2   Ankylosing spondylitis of cervical region
M45.3   Ankylosing spondylitis of cervicothoracic region
M45.4   Ankylosing spondylitis of thoracic region
M45.5   Ankylosing spondylitis of thoracolumbar region
M45.6   Ankylosing spondylitis lumbar region
M45.7   Ankylosing spondylitis of lumbosacral region
M45.8   Ankylosing spondylitis sacral and sacrococcygeal region
M45.9   Ankylosing spondylitis of unspecified sites in spine

● **M46 Other inflammatory spondylopathies**
● **M46.0 Spinal enthesopathy**
Disorder of ligamentous or muscular attachments of spine

M46.00   Spinal enthesopathy, site unspecified
M46.01   Spinal enthesopathy, occipito-atlanto-axial region
M46.02   Spinal enthesopathy, cervical region
M46.03   Spinal enthesopathy, cervicothoracic region
M46.04   Spinal enthesopathy, thoracic region
M46.05   Spinal enthesopathy, thoracolumbar region
M46.06   Spinal enthesopathy, lumbar region
M46.07   Spinal enthesopathy, lumbosacral region
M46.08   Spinal enthesopathy, sacral and sacrococcygeal region
M46.09   Spinal enthesopathy, multiple sites in spine

M46.1   Sacroiliitis, not elsewhere classified

● **M46.2 Osteomyelitis of vertebra**
> (Ex) **For category M46.2 CC codes:** See PDX Collection 881

M46.20   Osteomyelitis of vertebra, site unspecified
M46.21   Osteomyelitis of vertebra, occipito-atlanto-axial region
M46.22   Osteomyelitis of vertebra, cervical region
M46.23   Osteomyelitis of vertebra, cervicothoracic region
M46.24   Osteomyelitis of vertebra, thoracic region
M46.25   Osteomyelitis of vertebra, thoracolumbar region
M46.26   Osteomyelitis of vertebra, lumbar region
M46.27   Osteomyelitis of vertebra, lumbosacral region
M46.28   Osteomyelitis of vertebra, sacral and sacrococcygeal region

● **M46.3 Infection of intervertebral disc (pyogenic)**
Use additional code (B95-B97) to identify infectious agent
> (Ex) **For category M46.3 CC codes:** See PDX Collection 882

M46.30   Infection of intervertebral disc (pyogenic), site unspecified
M46.31   Infection of intervertebral disc (pyogenic), occipito-atlanto-axial region
M46.32   Infection of intervertebral disc (pyogenic), cervical region
M46.33   Infection of intervertebral disc (pyogenic), cervicothoracic region
M46.34   Infection of intervertebral disc (pyogenic), thoracic region

M46.35   Infection of intervertebral disc (pyogenic), thoracolumbar region
M46.36   Infection of intervertebral disc (pyogenic), lumbar region
M46.37   Infection of intervertebral disc (pyogenic), lumbosacral region
M46.38   Infection of intervertebral disc (pyogenic), sacral and sacrococcygeal region
M46.39   Infection of intervertebral disc (pyogenic), multiple sites in spine

● **M46.4 Discitis, unspecified**
M46.40   Discitis, unspecified, site unspecified
M46.41   Discitis, unspecified, occipito-atlanto-axial region
M46.42   Discitis, unspecified, cervical region
M46.43   Discitis, unspecified, cervicothoracic region
M46.44   Discitis, unspecified, thoracic region
M46.45   Discitis, unspecified, thoracolumbar region
M46.46   Discitis, unspecified, lumbar region
M46.47   Discitis, unspecified, lumbosacral region
M46.48   Discitis, unspecified, sacral and sacrococcygeal region
M46.49   Discitis, unspecified, multiple sites in spine

● **M46.5 Other infective spondylopathies**
M46.50   Other infective spondylopathies, site unspecified
M46.51   Other infective spondylopathies, occipitoatlanto-axial region
M46.52   Other infective spondylopathies, cervical region
M46.53   Other infective spondylopathies, cervicothoracic region
M46.54   Other infective spondylopathies, thoracic region
M46.55   Other infective spondylopathies, thoracolumbar region
M46.56   Other infective spondylopathies, lumbar region
M46.57   Other infective spondylopathies, lumbosacral region
M46.58   Other infective spondylopathies, sacral and sacrococcygeal region
M46.59   Other infective spondylopathies, multiple sites in spine

● **M46.8 Other specified inflammatory spondylopathies**
M46.80   Other specified inflammatory spondylopathies, site unspecified
M46.81   Other specified inflammatory spondylopathies, occipito-atlanto-axial region
M46.82   Other specified inflammatory spondylopathies, cervical region
M46.83   Other specified inflammatory spondylopathies, cervicothoracic region
M46.84   Other specified inflammatory spondylopathies, thoracic region
M46.85   Other specified inflammatory spondylopathies, thoracolumbar region
M46.86   Other specified inflammatory spondylopathies, lumbar region
M46.87   Other specified inflammatory spondylopathies, lumbosacral region
M46.88   Other specified inflammatory spondylopathies, sacral and sacrococcygeal region
M46.89   Other specified inflammatory spondylopathies, multiple sites in spine

● M46.9 **Unspecified inflammatory spondylopathy**

    M46.90 **Unspecified inflammatory spondylopathy, site unspecified**

    M46.91 **Unspecified inflammatory spondylopathy, occipito-atlanto-axial region**

    M46.92 **Unspecified inflammatory spondylopathy, cervical region**

    M46.93 **Unspecified inflammatory spondylopathy, cervicothoracic region**

    M46.94 **Unspecified inflammatory spondylopathy, thoracic region**

    M46.95 **Unspecified inflammatory spondylopathy, thoracolumbar region**

    M46.96 **Unspecified inflammatory spondylopathy, lumbar region**

    M46.97 **Unspecified inflammatory spondylopathy, lumbosacral region**

    M46.98 **Unspecified inflammatory spondylopathy, sacral and sacrococcygeal region**

    M46.99 **Unspecified inflammatory spondylopathy, multiple sites in spine**

● **M47 Spondylosis**

    Includes   arthrosis or osteoarthritis of spine
                    degeneration of facet joints

  ● **M47.0 Anterior spinal and vertebral artery compression syndromes**
        Ⓔⓧ For category M47.0 CC codes: See PDX Collection 883

    ● **M47.01 Anterior spinal artery compression syndromes**

       M47.011 **Anterior spinal artery compression syndromes, occipito-atlanto-axial region** 🔾

       M47.012 **Anterior spinal artery compression syndromes, cervical region** 🔾

       M47.013 **Anterior spinal artery compression syndromes, cervicothoracic region** 🔾

       M47.014 **Anterior spinal artery compression syndromes, thoracic region** 🔾

       M47.015 **Anterior spinal artery compression syndromes, thoracolumbar region** 🔾

       M47.016 **Anterior spinal artery compression syndromes, lumbar region** 🔾

       M47.019 **Anterior spinal artery compression syndromes, site unspecified** 🔾

    ● **M47.02 Vertebral artery compression syndromes**

       M47.021 **Vertebral artery compression syndromes, occipito-atlanto-axial region** 🔾

       M47.022 **Vertebral artery compression syndromes, cervical region** 🔾

       M47.029 **Vertebral artery compression syndromes, site unspecified** 🔾

  ● **M47.1 Other spondylosis with myelopathy**
        Spondylogenic compression of spinal cord

        Excludes1   vertebral subluxation (M43.3-M43.59)

    M47.10 **Other spondylosis with myelopathy, site unspecified** 🔾
        Ⓔⓧ See PDX Collection 884

    M47.11 **Other spondylosis with myelopathy, occipito-atlanto-axial region** 🔾
        Ⓔⓧ See PDX Collection 883

    M47.12 **Other spondylosis with myelopathy, cervical region** 🔾
        Ⓔⓧ See PDX Collection 883

    M47.13 **Other spondylosis with myelopathy, cervicothoracic region** 🔾
        Ⓔⓧ See PDX Collection 883

    M47.14 **Other spondylosis with myelopathy, thoracic region** 🔾
        Ⓔⓧ See PDX Collection 885

    M47.15 **Other spondylosis with myelopathy, thoracolumbar region** 🔾
        Ⓔⓧ See PDX Collection 885

    M47.16 **Other spondylosis with myelopathy, lumbar region** 🔾
        Ⓔⓧ See PDX Collection 886

  ● **M47.2 Other spondylosis with radiculopathy**

    M47.20 **Other spondylosis with radiculopathy, site unspecified**

    M47.21 **Other spondylosis with radiculopathy, occipito-atlanto-axial region**

    M47.22 **Other spondylosis with radiculopathy, cervical region**

    M47.23 **Other spondylosis with radiculopathy, cervicothoracic region**

    M47.24 **Other spondylosis with radiculopathy, thoracic region**

    M47.25 **Other spondylosis with radiculopathy, thoracolumbar region**

    M47.26 **Other spondylosis with radiculopathy, lumbar region**

    M47.27 **Other spondylosis with radiculopathy, lumbosacral region**

    M47.28 **Other spondylosis with radiculopathy, sacral and sacrococcygeal region**

  ● **M47.8 Other spondylosis**

    ● **M47.81 Spondylosis without myelopathy or radiculopathy**

       M47.811 **Spondylosis without myelopathy or radiculopathy, occipito-atlanto-axial region**

       M47.812 **Spondylosis without myelopathy or radiculopathy, cervical region**

       M47.813 **Spondylosis without myelopathy or radiculopathy, cervicothoracic region**

       M47.814 **Spondylosis without myelopathy or radiculopathy, thoracic region**

       M47.815 **Spondylosis without myelopathy or radiculopathy, thoracolumbar region**

       M47.816 **Spondylosis without myelopathy or radiculopathy, lumbar region**

       M47.817 **Spondylosis without myelopathy or radiculopathy, lumbosacral region**

       M47.818 **Spondylosis without myelopathy or radiculopathy, sacral and sacrococcygeal region**

       M47.819 **Spondylosis without myelopathy or radiculopathy, site unspecified**

    ● **M47.89 Other spondylosis**

       M47.891 **Other spondylosis, occipito-atlanto-axial region**

       M47.892 **Other spondylosis, cervical region**

       M47.893 **Other spondylosis, cervicothoracic region**

       M47.894 **Other spondylosis, thoracic region**

       M47.895 **Other spondylosis, thoracolumbar region**

       M47.896 **Other spondylosis, lumbar region**

       M47.897 **Other spondylosis, lumbosacral region**

       M47.898 **Other spondylosis, sacral and sacrococcygeal region**

       M47.899 **Other spondylosis, site unspecified**

  M47.9 Spondylosis, unspecified

CHAPTER 13 (M00-M99)

N Newborn Age: 0   **P** Pediatric Age: 0–17   **M** Maternity DX: 12–55   **A** Adult Age: 15–124   ♀ Females Only   ♂ Males Only

🔾 Complication\Comorbidity   🔾 Major C\C   Ⓔⓧ CC/MCC Exclusions   🔾 Hospital-Acquired Condition

1039

CHAPTER 13 (M00–M99)

● M48   **Other spondylopathies**
  ● M48.0   **Spinal stenosis**
    Caudal stenosis
    M48.00   Spinal stenosis, site unspecified
    M48.01   Spinal stenosis, occipito-atlanto-axial region
    M48.02   Spinal stenosis, cervical region
    M48.03   Spinal stenosis, cervicothoracic region
    M48.04   Spinal stenosis, thoracic region
    M48.05   Spinal stenosis, thoracolumbar region
    ● M48.06   Spinal stenosis, lumbar region
      ▶ M48.061   Spinal stenosis, lumbar region without neurogenic claudication
        ▶ Spinal stenosis, lumbar region NOS
      ▶ M48.062   Spinal stenosis, lumbar region with neurogenic claudication
    M48.07   Spinal stenosis, lumbosacral region
    M48.08   Spinal stenosis, sacral and sacrococcygeal region
  ● M48.1   **Ankylosing hyperostosis [Forestier]**
    Diffuse idiopathic skeletal hyperostosis [DISH]
    M48.10   Ankylosing hyperostosis [Forestier], site unspecified
    M48.11   Ankylosing hyperostosis [Forestier], occipito-atlanto-axial region
    M48.12   Ankylosing hyperostosis [Forestier], cervical region
    M48.13   Ankylosing hyperostosis [Forestier], cervicothoracic region
    M48.14   Ankylosing hyperostosis [Forestier], thoracic region
    M48.15   Ankylosing hyperostosis [Forestier], thoracolumbar region
    M48.16   Ankylosing hyperostosis [Forestier], lumbar region
    M48.17   Ankylosing hyperostosis [Forestier], lumbosacral region
    M48.18   Ankylosing hyperostosis [Forestier], sacral and sacrococcygeal region
    M48.19   Ankylosing hyperostosis [Forestier], multiple sites in spine
  ● M48.2   **Kissing spine**
    M48.20   Kissing spine, site unspecified
    M48.21   Kissing spine, occipito-atlanto-axial region
    M48.22   Kissing spine, cervical region
    M48.23   Kissing spine, cervicothoracic region
    M48.24   Kissing spine, thoracic region
    M48.25   Kissing spine, thoracolumbar region
    M48.26   Kissing spine, lumbar region
    M48.27   Kissing spine, lumbosacral region
  ● M48.3   **Traumatic spondylopathy**
    (Ex) For category M48.3 CC codes: See PDX Collection 887
    M48.30   Traumatic spondylopathy, site unspecified 🔍
    M48.31   Traumatic spondylopathy, occipito-atlanto-axial region 🔍
    M48.32   Traumatic spondylopathy, cervical region 🔍
    M48.33   Traumatic spondylopathy, cervicothoracic region 🔍
    M48.34   Traumatic spondylopathy, thoracic region 🔍
    M48.35   Traumatic spondylopathy, thoracolumbar region 🔍
    M48.36   Traumatic spondylopathy, lumbar region 🔍
    M48.37   Traumatic spondylopathy, lumbosacral region 🔍
    M48.38   Traumatic spondylopathy, sacral and sacrococcygeal region 🔍

● M48.4   **Fatigue fracture of vertebra**
  Stress fracture of vertebra
  | **Excludes1** | pathological fracture NOS (M84.4-)
      pathological fracture of vertebra due to neoplasm (M84.58)
      pathological fracture of vertebra due to other diagnosis (M84.68)
      pathological fracture of vertebra due to osteoporosis (M80.-)
      traumatic fracture of vertebrae (S12.0-S12.3-, S22.0-, S32.0-)

  The appropriate 7th character is to be added to each code from subcategory M48.4:

A	initial encounter for fracture
D	subsequent encounter for fracture with routine healing
G	subsequent encounter for fracture with delayed healing
S	sequela of fracture

  X ● M48.40   Fatigue fracture of vertebra, site unspecified
  X ● M48.41   Fatigue fracture of vertebra, occipitoatlanto-axial region
  X ● M48.42   Fatigue fracture of vertebra, cervical region
  X ● M48.43   Fatigue fracture of vertebra, cervicothoracic region
  X ● M48.44   Fatigue fracture of vertebra, thoracic region
  X ● M48.45   Fatigue fracture of vertebra, thoracolumbar region
  X ● M48.46   Fatigue fracture of vertebra, lumbar region
  X ● M48.47   Fatigue fracture of vertebra, lumbosacral region
  X ● M48.48   Fatigue fracture of vertebra, sacral and sacrococcygeal region

● M48.5   **Collapsed vertebra, not elsewhere classified**
  Collapsed vertebra NOS
  Compression fracture of vertebra NOS
  Wedging of vertebra NOS
  | **Excludes1** | current injury - see Injury of spine, by body region
      fatigue fracture of vertebra (M48.4)
      pathological fracture of vertebra due to neoplasm (M84.58)
      pathological fracture of vertebra due to other diagnosis (M84.68)
      pathological fracture of vertebra due to osteoporosis (M80.-)
      pathological fracture NOS (M84.4-)
      stress fracture of vertebra (M48.4-)
      traumatic fracture of vertebra (S12.-, S22.-, S32.-)

  The appropriate 7th character is to be added to each code from subcategory M48.5:

A	initial encounter for fracture
D	subsequent encounter for fracture with routine healing
G	subsequent encounter for fracture with delayed healing
S	sequela of fracture

  (Ex) For category M48.5 CC codes: See PDX Collection 888
  X ● M48.50   Collapsed vertebra, not elsewhere classified, site unspecified A 🔍
  X ● M48.51   Collapsed vertebra, not elsewhere classified, occipito-atlanto-axial region A 🔍

▶ New   ➡ Revised   ~~deleted~~ Deleted | Excludes 1 | | Excludes 2 | | Includes | | Use additional | | Code first | | Code also | | Key words |
OGCR Official Guidelines   ● Unacceptable Principal Diagnosis   X Assign placeholder X   ● Use Additional Character(s)   ▶ Manifestation Code   **Coding Clinic**

X ● M48.52 **Collapsed vertebra, not elsewhere classified, cervical region** A 🔍

X ● M48.53 **Collapsed vertebra, not elsewhere classified, cervicothoracic region** A 🔍

X ● M48.54 **Collapsed vertebra, not elsewhere classified, thoracic region** A 🔍

X ● M48.55 **Collapsed vertebra, not elsewhere classified, thoracolumbar region** A 🔍

X ● M48.56 **Collapsed vertebra, not elsewhere classified, lumbar region** A 🔍

X ● M48.57 **Collapsed vertebra, not elsewhere classified, lumbosacral region** A 🔍

X ● M48.58 **Collapsed vertebra, not elsewhere classified, sacral and sacrococcygeal region** A 🔍

● M48.8 **Other specified spondylopathies**
    Ossification of posterior longitudinal ligament

  ● M48.8X **Other specified spondylopathies**

      M48.8X1 **Other specified spondylopathies, occipito-atlanto-axial region**

      M48.8X2 **Other specified spondylopathies, cervical region**

      M48.8X3 **Other specified spondylopathies, cervicothoracic region**

      M48.8X4 **Other specified spondylopathies, thoracic region**

      M48.8X5 **Other specified spondylopathies, thoracolumbar region**

      M48.8X6 **Other specified spondylopathies, lumbar region**

      M48.8X7 **Other specified spondylopathies, lumbosacral region**

      M48.8X8 **Other specified spondylopathies, sacral and sacrococcygeal region**

      M48.8X9 **Other specified spondylopathies, site unspecified**

  M48.9 **Spondylopathy, unspecified**

● M49 **Spondylopathies in diseases classified elsewhere**

    Includes curvature of spine in diseases classified elsewhere
                  deformity of spine in diseases classified elsewhere
                  kyphosis in diseases classified elsewhere
                  scoliosis in diseases classified elsewhere
                  spondylopathy in diseases classified elsewhere

    Code first underlying disease, such as:
      brucellosis (A23.-)
      Charcot-Marie-Tooth disease (G60.0)
      enterobacterial infections (A01-A04)
      osteitis fibrosa cystica (E21.0)

    Excludes1 curvature of spine in tuberculosis [Pott's] (A18.01)
                   enteropathic arthropathies (M07.-)
                   gonococcal spondylitis (A54.41)
                   neuropathic [tabes dorsalis] spondylitis (A52.11)
                   neuropathic spondylopathy in syringomyelia (G95.0)
                   neuropathic spondylopathy in tabes dorsalis (A52.11)
                   nonsyphilitic neuropathic spondylopathy NEC (G98.0)
                   spondylitis in syphilis (acquired) (A52.77)
                   tuberculous spondylitis (A18.01)
                   typhoid fever spondylitis (A01.05)

● M49.8 **Spondylopathy in diseases classified elsewhere**

  ▸ *M49.80* *Spondylopathy in diseases classified elsewhere, site unspecified*

  ▸ *M49.81* *Spondylopathy in diseases classified elsewhere, occipito-atlanto-axial region*

  ▸ *M49.82* *Spondylopathy in diseases classified elsewhere, cervical region*

  ▸ *M49.83* *Spondylopathy in diseases classified elsewhere, cervicothoracic region*

  ▸ *M49.84* *Spondylopathy in diseases classified elsewhere, thoracic region*

  ▸ *M49.85* *Spondylopathy in diseases classified elsewhere, thoracolumbar region*

  ▸ *M49.86* *Spondylopathy in diseases classified elsewhere, lumbar region*

  ▸ *M49.87* *Spondylopathy in diseases classified elsewhere, lumbosacral region*

  ▸ *M49.88* *Spondylopathy in diseases classified elsewhere, sacral and sacrococcygeal region*

  ▸ *M49.89* *Spondylopathy in diseases classified elsewhere, multiple sites in spine*

OTHER DORSOPATHIES (M50-M54)

  Excludes1 current injury - see injury of spine by body region
                 discitis NOS (M46.4-)

● M50 **Cervical disc disorders**
    Note: Code to the most superior level of disorder.
    Includes cervicothoracic disc disorders with cervicalgia
                  cervicothoracic disc disorders
    Coding Clinic: 2016, Q1, P17

  ● M50.0 **Cervical disc disorder with myelopathy**
      Ⓔ **For category M50.0 CC codes: See PDX Collection 889**

      M50.00 **Cervical disc disorder with myelopathy, unspecified cervical region** 🔍

      M50.01 **Cervical disc disorder with myelopathy, high cervical region** 🔍
              C2-C3 disc disorder with myelopathy
              C3-C4 disc disorder with myelopathy
              Coding Clinic: 2016, Q1, P17

    ● M50.02 **Cervical disc disorder with myelopathy, mid-cervical region**
              Coding Clinic: 2016, Q4, P39-40

        M50.020 **Cervical disc disorder with myelopathy, mid-cervical region, unspecified level** 🔍

        M50.021 **Cervical disc disorder at C4-C5 level with myelopathy** 🔍
                 C4-C5 disc disorder with myelopathy

        M50.022 **Cervical disc disorder at C5-C6 level with myelopathy** 🔍
                 C5-C6 disc disorder with myelopathy

        M50.023 **Cervical disc disorder at C6-C7 level with myelopathy** 🔍
                 C6-C7 disc disorder with myelopathy

      M50.03 **Cervical disc disorder with myelopathy, cervicothoracic region** 🔍
              C7-T1 disc disorder with myelopathy

CHAPTER 13 (M00-M99)

● **M50.1** **Cervical disc disorder with radiculopathy**
    Excludes2 brachial radiculitis NOS (M54.13)

  M50.10 Cervical disc disorder with radiculopathy, unspecified cervical region

  M50.11 Cervical disc disorder with radiculopathy, high cervical region
      C2-C3 disc disorder with radiculopathy
      C3 radiculopathy due to disc disorder
      C3-C4 disc disorder with radiculopathy
      C4 radiculopathy due to disc disorder

● **M50.12** Cervical disc disorder with radiculopathy, mid-cervical region
    Coding Clinic: 2016, Q4, P39-40

    M50.120 Mid-cervical disc disorder, unspecified

    M50.121 Cervical disc disorder at C4-C5 level with radiculopathy
        C4-C5 disc disorder with radiculopathy
        C5 radiculopathy due to disc disorder

    M50.122 Cervical disc disorder at C5-C6 level with radiculopathy
        C5-C6 disc disorder with radiculopathy
        C6 radiculopathy due to disc disorder

    M50.123 Cervical disc disorder at C6-C7 level with radiculopathy
        C6-C7 disc disorder with radiculopathy
        C7 radiculopathy due to disc disorder

  M50.13 Cervical disc disorder with radiculopathy, cervicothoracic region
      C7-T1 disc disorder with radiculopathy
      C8 radiculopathy due to disc disorder

● **M50.2** **Other cervical disc displacement**
  Coding Clinic: 2016, Q4, P40

  M50.20 Other cervical disc displacement, unspecified cervical region

  M50.21 Other cervical disc displacement, high cervical region
      Other C2-C3 cervical disc displacement
      Other C3-C4 cervical disc displacement

● **M50.22** Other cervical disc displacement, mid-cervical region

    M50.220 Other cervical disc displacement, mid-cervical region, unspecified level

    M50.221 Other cervical disc displacement at C4-C5 level
        Other C4-C5 cervical disc displacement

    M50.222 Other cervical disc displacement at C5-C6 level
        Other C5-C6 cervical disc displacement

    M50.223 Other cervical disc displacement at C6-C7 level
        Other C6-C7 cervical disc displacement

  M50.23 Other cervical disc displacement, cervicothoracic region
      Other C7-T1 cervical disc displacement

● **M50.3** **Other cervical disc degeneration**
  Coding Clinic: 2016, Q4, P40

  M50.30 Other cervical disc degeneration, unspecified cervical region

  M50.31 Other cervical disc degeneration, high cervical region
      Other C2-C3 cervical disc degeneration
      Other C3-C4 cervical disc degeneration

● **M50.32** Other cervical disc degeneration, mid-cervical region

    M50.320 Other cervical disc degeneration, mid-cervical region, unspecified level

    M50.321 Other cervical disc degeneration at C4-C5 level
        Other C4-C5 cervical disc degeneration

    M50.322 Other cervical disc degeneration at C5-C6 level
        Other C5-C6 cervical disc degeneration

    M50.323 Other cervical disc degeneration at C6-C7 level
        Other C6-C7 cervical disc degeneration

  M50.33 Other cervical disc degeneration, cervicothoracic region
      Other C7-T1 cervical disc degeneration

● **M50.8** **Other cervical disc disorders**
  Coding Clinic: 2016, Q4, P40

  M50.80 Other cervical disc disorders, unspecified cervical region

  M50.81 Other cervical disc disorders, high cervical region
      Other C2-C3 cervical disc disorders
      Other C3-C4 cervical disc disorders

● **M50.82** Other cervical disc disorders, mid-cervical region

    M50.820 Other cervical disc disorders, mid-cervical region, unspecified level

    M50.821 Other cervical disc disorders at C4-C5 level
        Other C4-C5 cervical disc disorders

    M50.822 Other cervical disc disorders at C5-C6 level
        Other C5-C6 cervical disc disorders

    M50.823 Other cervical disc disorders at C6-C7 level
        Other C6-C7 cervical disc disorders

  M50.83 Other cervical disc disorders, cervicothoracic region
      Other C7-T1 cervical disc disorders

● **M50.9** **Cervical disc disorder, unspecified**
  Coding Clinic: 2016, Q4, P40

  M50.90 Cervical disc disorder, unspecified, unspecified cervical region

  M50.91 Cervical disc disorder, unspecified, high cervical region
      C2-C3 cervical disc disorder, unspecified
      C3-C4 cervical disc disorder, unspecified

CHAPTER 13 (M00-M99)

● M50.92 Cervical disc disorder, unspecified, mid-cervical region
    M50.920 Unspecified cervical disc disorder, mid-cervical region, unspecified level
    M50.921 Unspecified cervical disc disorder at C4-C5 level
        Unspecified C4-C5 cervical disc disorder
    M50.922 Unspecified cervical disc disorder at C5-C6 level
        Unspecified C5-C6 cervical disc disorder
    M50.923 Unspecified cervical disc disorder at C6-C7 level
        Unspecified C6-C7 cervical disc disorder
M50.93 Cervical disc disorder, unspecified, cervicothoracic region
    C7-T1 cervical disc disorder, unspecified

● M51 Thoracic, thoracolumbar, and lumbosacral intervertebral disc disorders
    Excludes2 cervical and cervicothoracic disc disorders (M50.-)
                   sacral and sacrococcygeal disorders (M53.3)

● M51.0 Thoracic, thoracolumbar and lumbosacral intervertebral disc disorders with myelopathy
    (Ex) **For category M51.0 CC codes unless otherwise indicated: See PDX Collection 890**
    M51.04 Intervertebral disc disorders with myelopathy, thoracic region 🔖
    M51.05 Intervertebral disc disorders with myelopathy, thoracolumbar region 🔖
    M51.06 Intervertebral disc disorders with myelopathy, lumbar region 🔖
        (Ex) See PDX Collection 891

● M51.1 Thoracic, thoracolumbar and lumbosacral intervertebral disc disorders with radiculopathy
    Sciatica due to intervertebral disc disorder
    Excludes1 lumbar radiculitis NOS (M54.16)
                   sciatica NOS (M54.3)
    M51.14 Intervertebral disc disorders with radiculopathy, thoracic region
    M51.15 Intervertebral disc disorders with radiculopathy, thoracolumbar region
    M51.16 Intervertebral disc disorders with radiculopathy, lumbar region
    M51.17 Intervertebral disc disorders with radiculopathy, lumbosacral region

● M51.2 Other thoracic, thoracolumbar and lumbosacral intervertebral disc displacement
    Lumbago due to displacement of intervertebral disc
    M51.24 Other intervertebral disc displacement, thoracic region
    M51.25 Other intervertebral disc displacement, thoracolumbar region
    M51.26 Other intervertebral disc displacement, lumbar region
    M51.27 Other intervertebral disc displacement, lumbosacral region

● M51.3 Other thoracic, thoracolumbar and lumbosacral intervertebral disc degeneration
    Coding Clinic: 2013, Q3, P22
    M51.34 Other intervertebral disc degeneration, thoracic region
    M51.35 Other intervertebral disc degeneration, thoracolumbar region

M51.36 Other intervertebral disc degeneration, lumbar region
M51.37 Other intervertebral disc degeneration, lumbosacral region

● M51.4 Schmorl's nodes
    M51.44 Schmorl's nodes, thoracic region
    M51.45 Schmorl's nodes, thoracolumbar region
    M51.46 Schmorl's nodes, lumbar region
    M51.47 Schmorl's nodes, lumbosacral region

● M51.8 Other thoracic, thoracolumbar and lumbosacral intervertebral disc disorders
    M51.84 Other intervertebral disc disorders, thoracic region
    M51.85 Other intervertebral disc disorders, thoracolumbar region
    M51.86 Other intervertebral disc disorders, lumbar region
    M51.87 Other intervertebral disc disorders, lumbosacral region

M51.9 Unspecified thoracic, thoracolumbar and lumbosacral intervertebral disc disorder

● M53 Other and unspecified dorsopathies, not elsewhere classified
    M53.0 Cervicocranial syndrome
        Posterior cervical sympathetic syndrome
    M53.1 Cervicobrachial syndrome
        Excludes2 cervical disc disorder (M50.-)
                       thoracic outlet syndrome (G54.0)

● M53.2 Spinal instabilities
    ● M53.2X Spinal instabilities
        M53.2X1 Spinal instabilities, occipito-atlanto-axial region
        M53.2X2 Spinal instabilities, cervical region
        M53.2X3 Spinal instabilities, cervicothoracic region
        M53.2X4 Spinal instabilities, thoracic region
        M53.2X5 Spinal instabilities, thoracolumbar region
        M53.2X6 Spinal instabilities, lumbar region
        M53.2X7 Spinal instabilities, lumbosacral region
        M53.2X8 Spinal instabilities, sacral and sacrococcygeal region
        M53.2X9 Spinal instabilities, site unspecified

M53.3 Sacrococcygeal disorders, not elsewhere classified
    Coccygodynia

● M53.8 Other specified dorsopathies
    M53.80 Other specified dorsopathies, site unspecified
    M53.81 Other specified dorsopathies, occipito-atlanto-axial region
    M53.82 Other specified dorsopathies, cervical region
    M53.83 Other specified dorsopathies, cervicothoracic region
    M53.84 Other specified dorsopathies, thoracic region
    M53.85 Other specified dorsopathies, thoracolumbar region
    M53.86 Other specified dorsopathies, lumbar region
    M53.87 Other specified dorsopathies, lumbosacral region
    M53.88 Other specified dorsopathies, sacral and sacrococcygeal region

M53.9 Dorsopathy, unspecified

● **M54   Dorsalgia**
   Excludes1   psychogenic dorsalgia (F45.41)
  ● **M54.0   Panniculitis affecting regions of neck and back**
      Excludes1   lupus panniculitis (L93.2)
            panniculitis NOS (M79.3)
            relapsing [Weber-Christian] panniculitis
              (M35.6)
    M54.00   Panniculitis affecting regions of neck and back, site unspecified
    M54.01   Panniculitis affecting regions of neck and back, occipito-atlanto-axial region
    M54.02   Panniculitis affecting regions of neck and back, cervical region
    M54.03   Panniculitis affecting regions of neck and back, cervicothoracic region
    M54.04   Panniculitis affecting regions of neck and back, thoracic region
    M54.05   Panniculitis affecting regions of neck and back, thoracolumbar region
    M54.06   Panniculitis affecting regions of neck and back, lumbar region
    M54.07   Panniculitis affecting regions of neck and back, lumbosacral region
    M54.08   Panniculitis affecting regions of neck and back, sacral and sacrococcygeal region
    M54.09   Panniculitis affecting regions, neck and back, multiple sites in spine
  ● **M54.1   Radiculopathy**
      Brachial neuritis or radiculitis NOS
      Lumbar neuritis or radiculitis NOS
      Lumbosacral neuritis or radiculitis NOS
      Thoracic neuritis or radiculitis NOS
      Radiculitis NOS
      Excludes1   neuralgia and neuritis NOS (M79.2)
            radiculopathy with cervical disc disorder (M50.1)
            radiculopathy with lumbar and other intervertebral disc disorder (M51.1-)
            radiculopathy with spondylosis (M47.2-)
    M54.10   Radiculopathy, site unspecified
    M54.11   Radiculopathy, occipito-atlanto-axial region
    M54.12   Radiculopathy, cervical region
    M54.13   Radiculopathy, cervicothoracic region
    M54.14   Radiculopathy, thoracic region
    M54.15   Radiculopathy, thoracolumbar region
    M54.16   Radiculopathy, lumbar region
    M54.17   Radiculopathy, lumbosacral region
    M54.18   Radiculopathy, sacral and sacrococcygeal region
  M54.2   Cervicalgia
      Excludes1   cervicalgia due to intervertebral cervical disc disorder (M50.-)
  ● **M54.3   Sciatica**
      Excludes1   lesion of sciatic nerve (G57.0)
            sciatica due to intervertebral disc disorder (M51.1-)
            sciatica with lumbago (M54.4-)
    M54.30   Sciatica, unspecified side
    M54.31   Sciatica, right side
    M54.32   Sciatica, left side
  ● **M54.4   Lumbago with sciatica**
      Excludes1   lumbago with sciatica due to intervertebral disc disorder (M51.1-)
    M54.40   Lumbago with sciatica, unspecified side
    M54.41   Lumbago with sciatica, right side
    M54.42   Lumbago with sciatica, left side
      Coding Clinic: 2016, Q2, P7

M54.5   Low back pain
    Loin pain
    Lumbago NOS
    Excludes1   low back strain (S39.012)
          lumbago due to intervertebral disc displacement (M51.2-)
          lumbago with sciatica (M54.4-)
M54.6   Pain in thoracic spine
    Excludes1   pain in thoracic spine due to intervertebral disc disorder (M51.)
● **M54.8   Other dorsalgia**
    Excludes1   dorsalgia in thoracic region (M54.6)
          low back pain (M54.5)
  M54.81   Occipital neuralgia
  M54.89   Other dorsalgia
  M54.9   Dorsalgia, unspecified
    Backache NOS
    Back pain NOS

SOFT TISSUE DISORDERS (M60-M79)

DISORDERS OF MUSCLES (M60-M63)

Excludes1   dermatopolymyositis (M33.-)
      muscular dystrophies and myopathies (G71-G72)
      myopathy in amyloidosis (E85.-)
      myopathy in polyarteritis nodosa (M30.0)
      myopathy in rheumatoid arthritis (M05.32)
      myopathy in scleroderma (M34.-)
      myopathy in Sjögren's syndrome (M35.03)
      myopathy in systemic lupus erythematosus (M32.-)
● **M60   Myositis**
    Excludes2   inclusion body myositis [IBM] (G72.41)
  ● **M60.0   Infective myositis**
      Tropical pyomyositis
      Use additional code (B95-B97) to identify infectious agent
      (Ex) For category M60.0 CC codes: See PDX Collection 806
    ● **M60.00   Infective myositis, unspecified site**
      M60.000   Infective myositis, unspecified right arm 🔗
        Infective myositis, right upper limb NOS
      M60.001   Infective myositis, unspecified left arm 🔗
        Infective myositis, left upper limb NOS
      M60.002   Infective myositis, unspecified arm 🔗
        Infective myositis, upper limb NOS
      M60.003   Infective myositis, unspecified right leg 🔗
        Infective myositis, right lower limb NOS
      M60.004   Infective myositis, unspecified left leg 🔗
        Infective myositis, left lower limb NOS
      M60.005   Infective myositis, unspecified leg 🔗
        Infective myositis, lower limb NOS
      M60.009   Infective myositis, unspecified site 🔗
    ● **M60.01   Infective myositis, shoulder**
      M60.011   Infective myositis, right shoulder 🔗
      M60.012   Infective myositis, left shoulder 🔗
      M60.019   Infective myositis, unspecified shoulder 🔗

▶ New   ⇨ Revised   ~~deleted~~ Deleted   Excludes 1   Excludes 2   Includes   Use additional   Code first   Code also   Key words
OGCR Official Guidelines   ● Unacceptable Principal Diagnosis   X Assign placeholder X   ● Use Additional Character(s)   ▶ Manifestation Code   Coding Clinic

● M60.02 Infective myositis, upper arm
   M60.021 Infective myositis, right upper arm 🔖
   M60.022 Infective myositis, left upper arm 🔖
   M60.029 Infective myositis, unspecified upper arm 🔖
● M60.03 Infective myositis, forearm
   M60.031 Infective myositis, right forearm 🔖
   M60.032 Infective myositis, left forearm 🔖
   M60.039 Infective myositis, unspecified forearm 🔖
● M60.04 Infective myositis, hand and fingers
   M60.041 Infective myositis, right hand 🔖
   M60.042 Infective myositis, left hand 🔖
   M60.043 Infective myositis, unspecified hand 🔖
   M60.044 Infective myositis, right finger(s) 🔖
   M60.045 Infective myositis, left finger(s) 🔖
   M60.046 Infective myositis, unspecified finger(s) 🔖
● M60.05 Infective myositis, thigh
   M60.051 Infective myositis, right thigh 🔖
   M60.052 Infective myositis, left thigh 🔖
   M60.059 Infective myositis, unspecified thigh 🔖
● M60.06 Infective myositis, lower leg
   M60.061 Infective myositis, right lower leg 🔖
   M60.062 Infective myositis, left lower leg 🔖
   M60.069 Infective myositis, unspecified lower leg 🔖
● M60.07 Infective myositis, ankle, foot and toes
   M60.070 Infective myositis, right ankle 🔖
   M60.071 Infective myositis, left ankle 🔖
   M60.072 Infective myositis, unspecified ankle 🔖
   M60.073 Infective myositis, right foot 🔖
   M60.074 Infective myositis, left foot 🔖
   M60.075 Infective myositis, unspecified foot 🔖
   M60.076 Infective myositis, right toe(s) 🔖
   M60.077 Infective myositis, left toe(s) 🔖
   M60.078 Infective myositis, unspecified toe(s) 🔖
   M60.08 Infective myositis, other site 🔖
   M60.09 Infective myositis, multiple sites 🔖
● M60.1 Interstitial myositis
   M60.10 Interstitial myositis of unspecified site
● M60.11 Interstitial myositis, shoulder
   M60.111 Interstitial myositis, right shoulder
   M60.112 Interstitial myositis, left shoulder
   M60.119 Interstitial myositis, unspecified shoulder
● M60.12 Interstitial myositis, upper arm
   M60.121 Interstitial myositis, right upper arm
   M60.122 Interstitial myositis, left upper arm
   M60.129 Interstitial myositis, unspecified upper arm
● M60.13 Interstitial myositis, forearm
   M60.131 Interstitial myositis, right forearm
   M60.132 Interstitial myositis, left forearm
   M60.139 Interstitial myositis, unspecified forearm

● M60.14 Interstitial myositis, hand
   M60.141 Interstitial myositis, right hand
   M60.142 Interstitial myositis, left hand
   M60.149 Interstitial myositis, unspecified hand
● M60.15 Interstitial myositis, thigh
   M60.151 Interstitial myositis, right thigh
   M60.152 Interstitial myositis, left thigh
   M60.159 Interstitial myositis, unspecified thigh
● M60.16 Interstitial myositis, lower leg
   M60.161 Interstitial myositis, right lower leg
   M60.162 Interstitial myositis, left lower leg
   M60.169 Interstitial myositis, unspecified lower leg
● M60.17 Interstitial myositis, ankle and foot
   M60.171 Interstitial myositis, right ankle and foot
   M60.172 Interstitial myositis, left ankle and foot
   M60.179 Interstitial myositis, unspecified ankle and foot
   M60.18 Interstitial myositis, other site
   M60.19 Interstitial myositis, multiple sites
● M60.2 Foreign body granuloma of soft tissue, not elsewhere classified
      Use additional code to identify the type of retained foreign body (Z18.-)
      Excludes1 foreign body granuloma of skin and subcutaneous tissue (L92.3)
   M60.20 Foreign body granuloma of soft tissue, not elsewhere classified, unspecified site
● M60.21 Foreign body granuloma of soft tissue, not elsewhere classified, shoulder
   M60.211 Foreign body granuloma of soft tissue, not elsewhere classified, right shoulder
   M60.212 Foreign body granuloma of soft tissue, not elsewhere classified, left shoulder
   M60.219 Foreign body granuloma of soft tissue, not elsewhere classified, unspecified shoulder
● M60.22 Foreign body granuloma of soft tissue, not elsewhere classified, upper arm
   M60.221 Foreign body granuloma of soft tissue, not elsewhere classified, right upper arm
   M60.222 Foreign body granuloma of soft tissue, not elsewhere classified, left upper arm
   M60.229 Foreign body granuloma of soft tissue, not elsewhere classified, unspecified upper arm
● M60.23 Foreign body granuloma of soft tissue, not elsewhere classified, forearm
   M60.231 Foreign body granuloma of soft tissue, not elsewhere classified, right forearm
   M60.232 Foreign body granuloma of soft tissue, not elsewhere classified, left forearm
   M60.239 Foreign body granuloma of soft tissue, not elsewhere classified, unspecified forearm

CHAPTER 13 (M00-M99)

● M60.24 Foreign body granuloma of soft tissue, not elsewhere classified, **hand**
  M60.241 Foreign body granuloma of soft tissue, not elsewhere classified, **right hand**
  M60.242 Foreign body granuloma of soft tissue, not elsewhere classified, **left hand**
  M60.249 Foreign body granuloma of soft tissue, not elsewhere classified, **unspecified hand**
● M60.25 Foreign body granuloma of soft tissue, not elsewhere classified, **thigh**
  M60.251 Foreign body granuloma of soft tissue, not elsewhere classified, **right thigh**
  M60.252 Foreign body granuloma of soft tissue, not elsewhere classified, **left thigh**
  M60.259 Foreign body granuloma of soft tissue, not elsewhere classified, **unspecified thigh**
● M60.26 Foreign body granuloma of soft tissue, not elsewhere classified, **lower leg**
  M60.261 Foreign body granuloma of soft tissue, not elsewhere classified, **right lower leg**
  M60.262 Foreign body granuloma of soft tissue, not elsewhere classified, **left lower leg**
  M60.269 Foreign body granuloma of soft tissue, not elsewhere classified, **unspecified lower leg**
● M60.27 Foreign body granuloma of soft tissue, not elsewhere classified, **ankle and foot**
  M60.271 Foreign body granuloma of soft tissue, not elsewhere classified, **right ankle and foot**
  M60.272 Foreign body granuloma of soft tissue, not elsewhere classified, **left ankle and foot**
  M60.279 Foreign body granuloma of soft tissue, not elsewhere classified, **unspecified ankle and foot**
  M60.28 Foreign body granuloma of soft tissue, not elsewhere classified, **other site**
● M60.8 Other myositis
  M60.80 Other myositis, **unspecified site**
● M60.81 Other myositis **shoulder**
  M60.811 Other myositis, **right shoulder**
  M60.812 Other myositis, **left shoulder**
  M60.819 Other myositis, **unspecified shoulder**
● M60.82 Other myositis, **upper arm**
  M60.821 Other myositis, **right upper arm**
  M60.822 Other myositis, **left upper arm**
  M60.829 Other myositis, **unspecified upper arm**
● M60.83 Other myositis, **forearm**
  M60.831 Other myositis, **right forearm**
  M60.832 Other myositis, **left forearm**
  M60.839 Other myositis, **unspecified forearm**
● M60.84 Other myositis, **hand**
  M60.841 Other myositis, **right hand**
  M60.842 Other myositis, **left hand**
  M60.849 Other myositis, **unspecified hand**
● M60.85 Other myositis, **thigh**
  M60.851 Other myositis, **right thigh**
  M60.852 Other myositis, **left thigh**
  M60.859 Other myositis, **unspecified thigh**

● M60.86 Other myositis, **lower leg**
  M60.861 Other myositis, **right lower leg**
  M60.862 Other myositis, **left lower leg**
  M60.869 Other myositis, **unspecified lower leg**
● M60.87 Other myositis, **ankle and foot**
  M60.871 Other myositis, **right ankle and foot**
  M60.872 Other myositis, **left ankle and foot**
  M60.879 Other myositis, **unspecified ankle and foot**
  M60.88 Other myositis, **other site**
  M60.89 Other myositis, **multiple sites**
 M60.9 Myositis, **unspecified**

● M61 Calcification and ossification of muscle
 ● M61.0 Myositis ossificans **traumatica**
  M61.00 Myositis ossificans traumatica, **unspecified site**
  ● M61.01 Myositis ossificans traumatica, **shoulder**
   M61.011 Myositis ossificans traumatica, **right shoulder**
   M61.012 Myositis ossificans traumatica, **left shoulder**
   M61.019 Myositis ossificans traumatica, **unspecified shoulder**
  ● M61.02 Myositis ossificans traumatica, **upper arm**
   M61.021 Myositis ossificans traumatica, **right upper arm**
   M61.022 Myositis ossificans traumatica, **left upper arm**
   M61.029 Myositis ossificans traumatica, **unspecified upper arm**
  ● M61.03 Myositis ossificans traumatica, **forearm**
   M61.031 Myositis ossificans traumatica, **right forearm**
   M61.032 Myositis ossificans traumatica, **left forearm**
   M61.039 Myositis ossificans traumatica, **unspecified forearm**
  ● M61.04 Myositis ossificans traumatica, **hand**
   M61.041 Myositis ossificans traumatica, **right hand**
   M61.042 Myositis ossificans traumatica, **left hand**
   M61.049 Myositis ossificans traumatica, **unspecified hand**
  ● M61.05 Myositis ossificans traumatica, **thigh**
   M61.051 Myositis ossificans traumatica, **right thigh**
   M61.052 Myositis ossificans traumatica, **left thigh**
   M61.059 Myositis ossificans traumatica, **unspecified thigh**
  ● M61.06 Myositis ossificans traumatica, **lower leg**
   M61.061 Myositis ossificans traumatica, **right lower leg**
   M61.062 Myositis ossificans traumatica, **left lower leg**
   M61.069 Myositis ossificans traumatica, **unspecified lower leg**
  ● M61.07 Myositis ossificans traumatica, **ankle and foot**
   M61.071 Myositis ossificans traumatica, **right ankle and foot**
   M61.072 Myositis ossificans traumatica, **left ankle and foot**
   M61.079 Myositis ossificans traumatica, **unspecified ankle and foot**
  M61.08 Myositis ossificans traumatica, **other site**
  M61.09 Myositis ossificans traumatica, **multiple sites**

▶ New   ⇒ Revised   deleted Deleted   Excludes 1   Excludes 2   Includes   Use additional   Code first   Code also   Key words
OGCR Official Guidelines   ● Unacceptable Principal Diagnosis   X Assign placeholder X   ● Use Additional Character(s)   ▶ Manifestation Code   **Coding Clinic**

● **M61.1 Myositis ossificans progressiva**
        Fibrodysplasia ossificans progressiva
    M61.10 Myositis ossificans progressiva, unspecified site
● **M61.11** Myositis ossificans progressiva, shoulder
    M61.111 Myositis ossificans progressiva, right shoulder
    M61.112 Myositis ossificans progressiva, left shoulder
    M61.119 Myositis ossificans progressiva, unspecified shoulder
● **M61.12** Myositis ossificans progressiva, upper arm
    M61.121 Myositis ossificans progressiva, right upper arm
    M61.122 Myositis ossificans progressiva, left upper arm
    M61.129 Myositis ossificans progressiva, unspecified arm
● **M61.13** Myositis ossificans progressiva, forearm
    M61.131 Myositis ossificans progressiva, right forearm
    M61.132 Myositis ossificans progressiva, left forearm
    M61.139 Myositis ossificans progressiva, unspecified forearm
● **M61.14** Myositis ossificans progressiva, hand and finger(s)
    M61.141 Myositis ossificans progressiva, right hand
    M61.142 Myositis ossificans progressiva, left hand
    M61.143 Myositis ossificans progressiva, unspecified hand
    M61.144 Myositis ossificans progressiva, right finger(s)
    M61.145 Myositis ossificans progressiva, left finger(s)
    M61.146 Myositis ossificans progressiva, unspecified finger(s)
● **M61.15** Myositis ossificans progressiva, thigh
    M61.151 Myositis ossificans progressiva, right thigh
    M61.152 Myositis ossificans progressiva, left thigh
    M61.159 Myositis ossificans progressiva, unspecified thigh
● **M61.16** Myositis ossificans progressiva, lower leg
    M61.161 Myositis ossificans progressiva, right lower leg
    M61.162 Myositis ossificans progressiva, left lower leg
    M61.169 Myositis ossificans progressiva, unspecified lower leg
● **M61.17** Myositis ossificans progressiva, ankle, foot and toe(s)
    M61.171 Myositis ossificans progressiva, right ankle
    M61.172 Myositis ossificans progressiva, left ankle
    M61.173 Myositis ossificans progressiva, unspecified ankle
    M61.174 Myositis ossificans progressiva, right foot
    M61.175 Myositis ossificans progressiva, left foot

    M61.176 Myositis ossificans progressiva, unspecified foot
    M61.177 Myositis ossificans progressiva, right toe(s)
    M61.178 Myositis ossificans progressiva, left toe(s)
    M61.179 Myositis ossificans progressiva, unspecified toe(s)
    M61.18 Myositis ossificans progressiva, other site
    M61.19 Myositis ossificans progressiva, multiple sites
● **M61.2 Paralytic calcification and ossification of muscle**
        Myositis ossificans associated with quadriplegia or paraplegia
    M61.20 Paralytic calcification and ossification of muscle, unspecified site
● **M61.21** Paralytic calcification and ossification of muscle, shoulder
    M61.211 Paralytic calcification and ossification of muscle, right shoulder
    M61.212 Paralytic calcification and ossification of muscle, left shoulder
    M61.219 Paralytic calcification and ossification of muscle, unspecified shoulder
● **M61.22** Paralytic calcification and ossification of muscle, upper arm
    M61.221 Paralytic calcification and ossification of muscle, right upper arm
    M61.222 Paralytic calcification and ossification of muscle, left upper arm
    M61.229 Paralytic calcification and ossification of muscle, unspecified upper arm
● **M61.23** Paralytic calcification and ossification of muscle, forearm
    M61.231 Paralytic calcification and ossification of muscle, right forearm
    M61.232 Paralytic calcification and ossification of muscle, left forearm
    M61.239 Paralytic calcification and ossification of muscle, unspecified forearm
● **M61.24** Paralytic calcification and ossification of muscle, hand
    M61.241 Paralytic calcification and ossification of muscle, right hand
    M61.242 Paralytic calcification and ossification of muscle, left hand
    M61.249 Paralytic calcification and ossification of muscle, unspecified hand
● **M61.25** Paralytic calcification and ossification of muscle, thigh
    M61.251 Paralytic calcification and ossification of muscle, right thigh
    M61.252 Paralytic calcification and ossification of muscle, left thigh
    M61.259 Paralytic calcification and ossification of muscle, unspecified thigh
● **M61.26** Paralytic calcification and ossification of muscle, lower leg
    M61.261 Paralytic calcification and ossification of muscle, right lower leg
    M61.262 Paralytic calcification and ossification of muscle, left lower leg
    M61.269 Paralytic calcification and ossification of muscle, unspecified lower leg

CHAPTER 13 (M00–M99)

N Newborn Age: 0   **P** Pediatric Age: 0–17   **M** Maternity DX: 12–55   **A** Adult Age: 15–124   ♀ Females Only   ♂ Males Only

🅒 Complication\Comorbidity   🅜 Major C\C   (Ex) CC/MCC Exclusions   🅗 Hospital-Acquired Condition

1047

● **M61.27** Paralytic calcification and ossification of muscle, ankle and foot

     M61.271 Paralytic calcification and ossification of muscle, right ankle and foot

     M61.272 Paralytic calcification and ossification of muscle, left ankle and foot

     M61.279 Paralytic calcification and ossification of muscle, unspecified ankle and foot

   M61.28 Paralytic calcification and ossification of muscle, other site

   M61.29 Paralytic calcification and ossification of muscle, multiple sites

● **M61.3** Calcification and ossification of muscles associated with burns

     Myositis ossificans associated with burns

   M61.30 Calcification and ossification of muscles associated with burns, unspecified site

● **M61.31** Calcification and ossification of muscles associated with burns, shoulder

     M61.311 Calcification and ossification of muscles associated with burns, right shoulder

     M61.312 Calcification and ossification of muscles associated with burns, left shoulder

     M61.319 Calcification and ossification of muscles associated with burns, unspecified shoulder

● **M61.32** Calcification and ossification of muscles associated with burns, upper arm

     M61.321 Calcification and ossification of muscles associated with burns, right upper arm

     M61.322 Calcification and ossification of muscles associated with burns, left upper arm

     M61.329 Calcification and ossification of muscles associated with burns, unspecified upper arm

● **M61.33** Calcification and ossification of muscles associated with burns, forearm

     M61.331 Calcification and ossification of muscles associated with burns, right forearm

     M61.332 Calcification and ossification of muscles associated with burns, left forearm

     M61.339 Calcification and ossification of muscles associated with burns, unspecified forearm

● **M61.34** Calcification and ossification of muscles associated with burns, hand

     M61.341 Calcification and ossification of muscles associated with burns, right hand

     M61.342 Calcification and ossification of muscles associated with burns, left hand

     M61.349 Calcification and ossification of muscles associated with burns, unspecified hand

● **M61.35** Calcification and ossification of muscles associated with burns, thigh

     M61.351 Calcification and ossification of muscles associated with burns, right thigh

     M61.352 Calcification and ossification of muscles associated with burns, left thigh

     M61.359 Calcification and ossification of muscles associated with burns, unspecified thigh

● **M61.36** Calcification and ossification of muscles associated with burns, lower leg

     M61.361 Calcification and ossification of muscles associated with burns, right lower leg

     M61.362 Calcification and ossification of muscles associated with burns, left lower leg

     M61.369 Calcification and ossification of muscles associated with burns, unspecified lower leg

● **M61.37** Calcification and ossification of muscles associated with burns, ankle and foot

     M61.371 Calcification and ossification of muscles associated with burns, right ankle and foot

     M61.372 Calcification and ossification of muscles associated with burns, left ankle and foot

     M61.379 Calcification and ossification of muscles associated with burns, unspecified ankle and foot

   M61.38 Calcification and ossification of muscles associated with burns, other site

   M61.39 Calcification and ossification of muscles associated with burns, multiple sites

● **M61.4** Other calcification of muscle

     Excludes1   calcific tendinitis NOS (M65.2-)

                  calcific tendinitis of shoulder (M75.3)

   M61.40 Other calcification of muscle, unspecified site

● **M61.41** Other calcification of muscle, shoulder

     M61.411 Other calcification of muscle, right shoulder

     M61.412 Other calcification of muscle, left shoulder

     M61.419 Other calcification of muscle, unspecified shoulder

● **M61.42** Other calcification of muscle, upper arm

     M61.421 Other calcification of muscle, right upper arm

     M61.422 Other calcification of muscle, left upper arm

     M61.429 Other calcification of muscle, unspecified upper arm

● **M61.43** Other calcification of muscle, forearm

     M61.431 Other calcification of muscle, right forearm

     M61.432 Other calcification of muscle, left forearm

     M61.439 Other calcification of muscle, unspecified forearm

● **M61.44** Other calcification of muscle, hand

     M61.441 Other calcification of muscle, right hand

     M61.442 Other calcification of muscle, left hand

     M61.449 Other calcification of muscle, unspecified hand

● **M61.45** Other calcification of muscle, thigh

     M61.451 Other calcification of muscle, right thigh

     M61.452 Other calcification of muscle, left thigh

     M61.459 Other calcification of muscle, unspecified thigh

▶ New   ⟹ Revised   ~~deleted~~ Deleted   Excludes 1   Excludes 2   Includes   Use additional   Code first   Code also   Key words

OGCR Official Guidelines   ● Unacceptable Principal Diagnosis   X Assign placeholder X   ● Use Additional Character(s)   ▶ Manifestation Code   Coding Clinic

● M61.46 Other calcification of muscle, lower leg
    M61.461 Other calcification of muscle, right lower leg
    M61.462 Other calcification of muscle, left lower leg
    M61.469 Other calcification of muscle, unspecified lower leg
● M61.47 Other calcification of muscle, ankle and foot
    M61.471 Other calcification of muscle, right ankle and foot
    M61.472 Other calcification of muscle, left ankle and foot
    M61.479 Other calcification of muscle, unspecified ankle and foot
  M61.48 Other calcification of muscle, other site
  M61.49 Other calcification of muscle, multiple sites
● M61.5 Other ossification of muscle
  M61.50 Other ossification of muscle, unspecified site
● M61.51 Other ossification of muscle, shoulder
    M61.511 Other ossification of muscle, right shoulder
    M61.512 Other ossification of muscle, left shoulder
    M61.519 Other ossification of muscle, unspecified shoulder
● M61.52 Other ossification of muscle, upper arm
    M61.521 Other ossification of muscle, right upper arm
    M61.522 Other ossification of muscle, left upper arm
    M61.529 Other ossification of muscle, unspecified upper arm
● M61.53 Other ossification of muscle, forearm
    M61.531 Other ossification of muscle, right forearm
    M61.532 Other ossification of muscle, left forearm
    M61.539 Other ossification of muscle, unspecified forearm
● M61.54 Other ossification of muscle, hand
    M61.541 Other ossification of muscle, right hand
    M61.542 Other ossification of muscle, left hand
    M61.549 Other ossification of muscle, unspecified hand
● M61.55 Other ossification of muscle, thigh
    M61.551 Other ossification of muscle, right thigh
    M61.552 Other ossification of muscle, left thigh
    M61.559 Other ossification of muscle, unspecified thigh
● M61.56 Other ossification of muscle, lower leg
    M61.561 Other ossification of muscle, right lower leg
    M61.562 Other ossification of muscle, left lower leg
    M61.569 Other ossification of muscle, unspecified lower leg
● M61.57 Other ossification of muscle, ankle and foot
    M61.571 Other ossification of muscle, right ankle and foot
    M61.572 Other ossification of muscle, left ankle and foot
    M61.579 Other ossification of muscle, unspecified ankle and foot
  M61.58 Other ossification of muscle, other site
  M61.59 Other ossification of muscle, multiple sites
M61.9 Calcification and ossification of muscle, unspecified

● M62 Other disorders of muscle
  Excludes1 alcoholic myopathy (G72.1)
    cramp and spasm (R25.2)
    drug-induced myopathy (G72.0)
    myalgia (M79.1)
    stiff-man syndrome (G25.82)
  Excludes2 nontraumatic hematoma of muscle (M79.81)
● M62.0 Separation of muscle (nontraumatic)
  Diastasis of muscle
    Excludes1 diastasis recti complicating pregnancy, labor and delivery (O71.8)
      traumatic separation of muscle - see strain of muscle by body region
  M62.00 Separation of muscle (nontraumatic), unspecified site
● M62.01 Separation of muscle (nontraumatic), shoulder
    M62.011 Separation of muscle (nontraumatic), right shoulder
    M62.012 Separation of muscle (nontraumatic), left shoulder
    M62.019 Separation of muscle (nontraumatic), unspecified shoulder
● M62.02 Separation of muscle (nontraumatic), upper arm
    M62.021 Separation of muscle (nontraumatic), right upper arm
    M62.022 Separation of muscle (nontraumatic), left upper arm
    M62.029 Separation of muscle (nontraumatic), unspecified upper arm
● M62.03 Separation of muscle (nontraumatic), forearm
    M62.031 Separation of muscle (nontraumatic), right forearm
    M62.032 Separation of muscle (nontraumatic), left forearm
    M62.039 Separation of muscle (nontraumatic), unspecified forearm
● M62.04 Separation of muscle (nontraumatic), hand
    M62.041 Separation of muscle (nontraumatic), right hand
    M62.042 Separation of muscle (nontraumatic), left hand
    M62.049 Separation of muscle (nontraumatic), unspecified hand
● M62.05 Separation of muscle (nontraumatic), thigh
    M62.051 Separation of muscle (nontraumatic), right thigh
    M62.052 Separation of muscle (nontraumatic), left thigh
    M62.059 Separation of muscle (nontraumatic), unspecified thigh
● M62.06 Separation of muscle (nontraumatic), lower leg
    M62.061 Separation of muscle (nontraumatic), right lower leg
    M62.062 Separation of muscle (nontraumatic), left lower leg
    M62.069 Separation of muscle (nontraumatic), unspecified lower leg
● M62.07 Separation of muscle (nontraumatic), ankle and foot
    M62.071 Separation of muscle (nontraumatic), right ankle and foot
    M62.072 Separation of muscle (nontraumatic), left ankle and foot
    M62.079 Separation of muscle (nontraumatic), unspecified ankle and foot
  M62.08 Separation of muscle (nontraumatic), other site

CHAPTER 13 (M00-M99)

● M62.1   Other rupture of muscle (nontraumatic)
    Excludes1   traumatic rupture of muscle - see strain of muscle by body region
    Excludes2   rupture of tendon (M66.-)
    M62.10   Other rupture of muscle (nontraumatic), unspecified site
● M62.11   Other rupture of muscle (nontraumatic), shoulder
        M62.111   Other rupture of muscle (nontraumatic), right shoulder
        M62.112   Other rupture of muscle (nontraumatic), left shoulder
        M62.119   Other rupture of muscle (nontraumatic), unspecified shoulder
● M62.12   Other rupture of muscle (nontraumatic), upper arm
        M62.121   Other rupture of muscle (nontraumatic), right upper arm
        M62.122   Other rupture of muscle (nontraumatic), left upper arm
        M62.129   Other rupture of muscle (nontraumatic), unspecified upper arm
● M62.13   Other rupture of muscle (nontraumatic), forearm
        M62.131   Other rupture of muscle (nontraumatic), right forearm
        M62.132   Other rupture of muscle (nontraumatic), left forearm
        M62.139   Other rupture of muscle (nontraumatic), unspecified forearm
● M62.14   Other rupture of muscle (nontraumatic), hand
        M62.141   Other rupture of muscle (nontraumatic), right hand
        M62.142   Other rupture of muscle (nontraumatic), left hand
        M62.149   Other rupture of muscle (nontraumatic), unspecified hand
● M62.15   Other rupture of muscle (nontraumatic), thigh
        M62.151   Other rupture of muscle (nontraumatic), right thigh
        M62.152   Other rupture of muscle (nontraumatic), left thigh
        M62.159   Other rupture of muscle (nontraumatic), unspecified thigh
● M62.16   Other rupture of muscle (nontraumatic), lower leg
        M62.161   Other rupture of muscle (nontraumatic), right lower leg
        M62.162   Other rupture of muscle (nontraumatic), left lower leg
        M62.169   Other rupture of muscle (nontraumatic), unspecified lower leg
● M62.17   Other rupture of muscle (nontraumatic), ankle and foot
        M62.171   Other rupture of muscle (nontraumatic), right ankle and foot
        M62.172   Other rupture of muscle (nontraumatic), left ankle and foot
        M62.179   Other rupture of muscle (nontraumatic), unspecified ankle and foot
    M62.18   Other rupture of muscle (nontraumatic), other site

● M62.2   Nontraumatic ischemic infarction of muscle
    Excludes1   compartment syndrome (traumatic) (T79.A-)
                    nontraumatic compartment syndrome (M79.A-)
                    traumatic ischemia of muscle (T79.6)
                    rhabdomyolysis (M62.82)
                    Volkmann's ischemic contracture (T79.6)
    M62.20   Nontraumatic ischemic infarction of muscle, unspecified site
● M62.21   Nontraumatic ischemic infarction of muscle, shoulder
        M62.211   Nontraumatic ischemic infarction of muscle, right shoulder
        M62.212   Nontraumatic ischemic infarction of muscle, left shoulder
        M62.219   Nontraumatic ischemic infarction of muscle, unspecified shoulder
● M62.22   Nontraumatic ischemic infarction of muscle, upper arm
        M62.221   Nontraumatic ischemic infarction of muscle, right upper arm
        M62.222   Nontraumatic ischemic infarction of muscle, left upper arm
        M62.229   Nontraumatic ischemic infarction of muscle, unspecified upper arm
● M62.23   Nontraumatic ischemic infarction of muscle, forearm
        M62.231   Nontraumatic ischemic infarction of muscle, right forearm
        M62.232   Nontraumatic ischemic infarction of muscle, left forearm
        M62.239   Nontraumatic ischemic infarction of muscle, unspecified forearm
● M62.24   Nontraumatic ischemic infarction of muscle, hand
        M62.241   Nontraumatic ischemic infarction of muscle, right hand
        M62.242   Nontraumatic ischemic infarction of muscle, left hand
        M62.249   Nontraumatic ischemic infarction of muscle, unspecified hand
● M62.25   Nontraumatic ischemic infarction of muscle, thigh
        M62.251   Nontraumatic ischemic infarction of muscle, right thigh
        M62.252   Nontraumatic ischemic infarction of muscle, left thigh
        M62.259   Nontraumatic ischemic infarction of muscle, unspecified thigh
● M62.26   Nontraumatic ischemic infarction of muscle, lower leg
        M62.261   Nontraumatic ischemic infarction of muscle, right lower leg
        M62.262   Nontraumatic ischemic infarction of muscle, left lower leg
        M62.269   Nontraumatic ischemic infarction of muscle, unspecified lower leg
● M62.27   Nontraumatic ischemic infarction of muscle, ankle and foot
        M62.271   Nontraumatic ischemic infarction of muscle, right ankle and foot
        M62.272   Nontraumatic ischemic infarction of muscle, left ankle and foot
        M62.279   Nontraumatic ischemic infarction of muscle, unspecified ankle and foot
    M62.28   Nontraumatic ischemic infarction of muscle, other site

▶ New   ⇒ Revised   ~~deleted~~ Deleted   Excludes 1   Excludes 2   Includes   Use additional   Code first   Code also   Key words
OGCR Official Guidelines   ● Unacceptable Principal Diagnosis   X Assign placeholder X   ● Use Additional Character(s)   ▶ Manifestation Code   Coding Clinic

M62.3 Immobility syndrome (paraplegic)
M62.4 Contracture of muscle
         Contracture of tendon (sheath)
         Excludes1   contracture of joint (M24.5-)
    M62.40 Contracture of muscle, unspecified site
 ● M62.41 Contracture of muscle, shoulder
         M62.411 Contracture of muscle, right shoulder
         M62.412 Contracture of muscle, left shoulder
         M62.419 Contracture of muscle, unspecified
                  shoulder
 ● M62.42 Contracture of muscle, upper arm
         M62.421 Contracture of muscle, right upper
                  arm
         M62.422 Contracture of muscle, left upper arm
         M62.429 Contracture of muscle, unspecified
                  upper arm
 ● M62.43 Contracture of muscle, forearm
         M62.431 Contracture of muscle, right forearm
         M62.432 Contracture of muscle, left forearm
         M62.439 Contracture of muscle, unspecified
                  forearm
 ● M62.44 Contracture of muscle, hand
         M62.441 Contracture of muscle, right hand
         M62.442 Contracture of muscle, left hand
         M62.449 Contracture of muscle, unspecified
                  hand
 ● M62.45 Contracture of muscle, thigh
         M62.451 Contracture of muscle, right thigh
         M62.452 Contracture of muscle, left thigh
         M62.459 Contracture of muscle, unspecified
                  thigh
 ● M62.46 Contracture of muscle, lower leg
         M62.461 Contracture of muscle, right lower leg
         M62.462 Contracture of muscle, left lower leg
         M62.469 Contracture of muscle, unspecified
                  lower leg
 ● M62.47 Contracture of muscle, ankle and foot
         M62.471 Contracture of muscle, right ankle
                  and foot
         M62.472 Contracture of muscle, left ankle and
                  foot
         M62.479 Contracture of muscle, unspecified
                  ankle and foot
    M62.48 Contracture of muscle, other site
    M62.49 Contracture of muscle, multiple sites
 ● M62.5 Muscle wasting and atrophy, not elsewhere classified
         Disuse atrophy NEC
         Excludes1   neuralgic amyotrophy (G54.5)
                      ▷progressive muscular atrophy (G12.21)
                        sarcopenia (M62.84)
         Excludes2·   pelvic muscle wasting (N81.84)
    M62.50 Muscle wasting and atrophy, not elsewhere
         classified, unspecified site
 ● M62.51 Muscle wasting and atrophy, not elsewhere
         classified, shoulder
         M62.511 Muscle wasting and atrophy, not
                  elsewhere classified, right shoulder
         M62.512 Muscle wasting and atrophy, not
                  elsewhere classified, left shoulder
         M62.519 Muscle wasting and atrophy, not
                  elsewhere classified, unspecified
                  shoulder

 ● M62.52 Muscle wasting and atrophy, not elsewhere
         classified, upper arm
         M62.521 Muscle wasting and atrophy, not
                  elsewhere classified, right upper arm
         M62.522 Muscle wasting and atrophy, not
                  elsewhere classified, left upper arm
         M62.529 Muscle wasting and atrophy, not
                  elsewhere classified, unspecified
                  upper arm
 ● M62.53 Muscle wasting and atrophy, not elsewhere
         classified, forearm
         M62.531 Muscle wasting and atrophy, not
                  elsewhere classified, right forearm
         M62.532 Muscle wasting and atrophy, not
                  elsewhere classified, left forearm
         M62.539 Muscle wasting and atrophy, not
                  elsewhere classified, unspecified
                  forearm
 ● M62.54 Muscle wasting and atrophy, not elsewhere
         classified, hand
         M62.541 Muscle wasting and atrophy, not
                  elsewhere classified, right hand
         M62.542 Muscle wasting and atrophy, not
                  elsewhere classified, left hand
         M62.549 Muscle wasting and atrophy, not
                  elsewhere classified, unspecified hand
 ● M62.55 Muscle wasting and atrophy, not elsewhere
         classified, thigh
         M62.551 Muscle wasting and atrophy, not
                  elsewhere classified, right thigh
         M62.552 Muscle wasting and atrophy, not
                  elsewhere classified, left thigh
         M62.559 Muscle wasting and atrophy, not
                  elsewhere classified, unspecified
                  thigh
 ● M62.56 Muscle wasting and atrophy, not elsewhere
         classified, lower leg
         M62.561 Muscle wasting and atrophy, not
                  elsewhere classified, right lower leg
         M62.562 Muscle wasting and atrophy, not
                  elsewhere classified, left lower leg
         M62.569 Muscle wasting and atrophy, not
                  elsewhere classified, unspecified
                  lower leg
 ● M62.57 Muscle wasting and atrophy, not elsewhere
         classified, ankle and foot
         M62.571 Muscle wasting and atrophy, not
                  elsewhere classified, right ankle and
                  foot
         M62.572 Muscle wasting and atrophy, not
                  elsewhere classified, left ankle and
                  foot
         M62.579 Muscle wasting and atrophy, not
                  elsewhere classified, unspecified
                  ankle and foot
    M62.58 Muscle wasting and atrophy, not elsewhere
         classified, other site
    M62.59 Muscle wasting and atrophy, not elsewhere
         classified, multiple sites

CHAPTER 13 (M00-M99)

N Newborn Age: 0   **P** Pediatric Age: 0–17   **M** Maternity DX: 12–55   **A** Adult Age: 15–124   ♀ Females Only   ♂ Males Only
      🐾 Complication\Comorbidity   🐾 Major C\C   (Ex) CC/MCC Exclusions   🐾 Hospital-Acquired Condition

1051

● **M62.8 Other specified disorders of muscle**
> **Excludes2**   nontraumatic hematoma of muscle (M79.81)

M62.81 Muscle weakness (generalized)
> **Excludes1**   muscle weakness in sarcopenia (M62.84)

M62.82 Rhabdomyolysis 🔓
> **Excludes1**   traumatic rhabdomyolysis (T79.6)

     (Ex) See PDX Collection 892

● **M62.83 Muscle spasm**
     M62.830 Muscle spasm of back
     M62.831 Muscle spasm of calf
         Charley-horse
     M62.838 Other muscle spasm

M62.84 Sarcopenia
     Age-related sarcopenia
     Code first underlying disease, if applicable, such as:
         disorders of myoneural junction and muscle disease in diseases classified elsewhere (G73.-)
         other and unspecified myopathies (G72.-)
         primary disorders of muscles (G71.-)
     Coding Clinic: 2016, Q4, P41

M62.89 Other specified disorders of muscle
     Muscle (sheath) hernia

M62.9 Disorder of muscle, unspecified

● **M63 Disorders of muscle in diseases classified elsewhere**
> *Code first underlying disease, such as:*
>   leprosy (A30.-)
>   neoplasm (C49.-, C79.89, D21.-, D48.1)
>   schistosomiasis (B65.-)
>   trichinellosis (B75)

> **Excludes1**   myopathy in cysticercosis (B69.81)
>   myopathy in endocrine diseases (G73.7)
>   myopathy in metabolic diseases (G73.7)
>   myopathy in sarcoidosis (D86.87)
>   myopathy in secondary syphilis (A51.49)
>   myopathy in syphilis (late) (A52.78)
>   myopathy in toxoplasmosis (B58.82)
>   myopathy in tuberculosis (A18.09)

● **M63.8 Disorders of muscle in diseases classified elsewhere**
▶ *M63.80 Disorders of muscle in diseases classified elsewhere, unspecified site*

● **M63.81 Disorders of muscle in diseases classified elsewhere, shoulder**
▶ *M63.811 Disorders of muscle in diseases classified elsewhere, right shoulder*
▶ *M63.812 Disorders of muscle in diseases classified elsewhere, left shoulder*
▶ *M63.819 Disorders of muscle in diseases classified elsewhere, unspecified shoulder*

● **M63.82 Disorders of muscle in diseases classified elsewhere, upper arm**
▶ *M63.821 Disorders of muscle in diseases classified elsewhere, right upper arm*
▶ *M63.822 Disorders of muscle in diseases classified elsewhere, left upper arm*
▶ *M63.829 Disorders of muscle in diseases classified elsewhere, unspecified upper arm*

● **M63.83 Disorders of muscle in diseases classified elsewhere, forearm**
▶ *M63.831 Disorders of muscle in diseases classified elsewhere, right forearm*
▶ *M63.832 Disorders of muscle in diseases classified elsewhere, left forearm*
▶ *M63.839 Disorders of muscle in diseases classified elsewhere, unspecified forearm*

● **M63.84 Disorders of muscle in diseases classified elsewhere, hand**
▶ *M63.841 Disorders of muscle in diseases classified elsewhere, right hand*
▶ *M63.842 Disorders of muscle in diseases classified elsewhere, left hand*
▶ *M63.849 Disorders of muscle in diseases classified elsewhere, unspecified hand*

● **M63.85 Disorders of muscle in diseases classified elsewhere, thigh**
▶ *M63.851 Disorders of muscle in diseases classified elsewhere, right thigh*
▶ *M63.852 Disorders of muscle in diseases classified elsewhere, left thigh*
▶ *M63.859 Disorders of muscle in diseases classified elsewhere, unspecified thigh*

● **M63.86 Disorders of muscle in diseases classified elsewhere, lower leg**
▶ *M63.861 Disorders of muscle in diseases classified elsewhere, right lower leg*
▶ *M63.862 Disorders of muscle in diseases classified elsewhere, left lower leg*
▶ *M63.869 Disorders of muscle in diseases classified elsewhere, unspecified lower leg*

● **M63.87 Disorders of muscle in diseases classified elsewhere, ankle and foot**
▶ *M63.871 Disorders of muscle in diseases classified elsewhere, right ankle and foot*
▶ *M63.872 Disorders of muscle in diseases classified elsewhere, left ankle and foot*
▶ *M63.879 Disorders of muscle in diseases classified elsewhere, unspecified ankle and foot*

▶ *M63.88 Disorders of muscle in diseases classified elsewhere, other site*
▶ *M63.89 Disorders of muscle in diseases classified elsewhere, multiple sites*

DISORDERS OF SYNOVIUM AND TENDON (M65-M67)

● **M65 Synovitis and tenosynovitis**
> **Excludes1**   chronic crepitant synovitis of hand and wrist (M70.0-)
>   current injury - see injury of ligament or tendon by body region
>   soft tissue disorders related to use, overuse and pressure (M70.-)

● **M65.0 Abscess of tendon sheath**
> Use additional code (B95-B96) to identify bacterial agent

M65.00 Abscess of tendon sheath, unspecified site

● **M65.01 Abscess of tendon sheath, shoulder**
     M65.011 Abscess of tendon sheath, right shoulder
     M65.012 Abscess of tendon sheath, left shoulder
     M65.019 Abscess of tendon sheath, unspecified shoulder

Item 13-11 Synovitis is an inflammation of a synovial membrane resulting in pain on motion and is characterized by fluctuating swelling due to effusion in a synovial sac. **Tenosynovitis** is an inflammation of a tendon sheath and occurs most commonly in the wrists, hands, and feet. Bursitis is inflammation of a bursa (fluid filled sac) caused by repetitive use, trauma, infection, or systemic inflammatory disease. Bursae act as protectors and facilitate movement between bones and overlapping muscles (deep bursae) or between bones and tendons/skin (superficial bursae).

- M65.02 Abscess of tendon sheath, upper arm
  - M65.021 Abscess of tendon sheath, right upper arm
  - M65.022 Abscess of tendon sheath, left upper arm
  - M65.029 Abscess of tendon sheath, unspecified upper arm
- M65.03 Abscess of tendon sheath, forearm
  - M65.031 Abscess of tendon sheath, right forearm
  - M65.032 Abscess of tendon sheath, left forearm
  - M65.039 Abscess of tendon sheath, unspecified forearm
- M65.04 Abscess of tendon sheath, hand
  - M65.041 Abscess of tendon sheath, right hand
  - M65.042 Abscess of tendon sheath, left hand
  - M65.049 Abscess of tendon sheath, unspecified hand
- M65.05 Abscess of tendon sheath, thigh
  - M65.051 Abscess of tendon sheath, right thigh
  - M65.052 Abscess of tendon sheath, left thigh
  - M65.059 Abscess of tendon sheath, unspecified thigh
- M65.06 Abscess of tendon sheath, lower leg
  - M65.061 Abscess of tendon sheath, right lower leg
  - M65.062 Abscess of tendon sheath, left lower leg
  - M65.069 Abscess of tendon sheath, unspecified lower leg
- M65.07 Abscess of tendon sheath, ankle and foot
  - M65.071 Abscess of tendon sheath, right ankle and foot
  - M65.072 Abscess of tendon sheath, left ankle and foot
  - M65.079 Abscess of tendon sheath, unspecified ankle and foot
  - M65.08 Abscess of tendon sheath, other site
- M65.1 Other infective (teno)synovitis
  - M65.10 Other infective (teno)synovitis, unspecified site
- M65.11 Other infective (teno)synovitis, shoulder
  - M65.111 Other infective (teno)synovitis, right shoulder
  - M65.112 Other infective (teno)synovitis, left shoulder
  - M65.119 Other infective (teno)synovitis, unspecified shoulder
- M65.12 Other infective (teno)synovitis, elbow
  - M65.121 Other infective (teno)synovitis, right elbow
  - M65.122 Other infective (teno)synovitis, left elbow
  - M65.129 Other infective (teno)synovitis, unspecified elbow

- M65.13 Other infective (teno)synovitis, wrist
  - M65.131 Other infective (teno)synovitis, right wrist
  - M65.132 Other infective (teno)synovitis, left wrist
  - M65.139 Other infective (teno)synovitis, unspecified wrist
- M65.14 Other infective (teno)synovitis, hand
  - M65.141 Other infective (teno)synovitis, right hand
  - M65.142 Other infective (teno)synovitis, left hand
  - M65.149 Other infective (teno)synovitis, unspecified hand
- M65.15 Other infective (teno)synovitis, hip
  - M65.151 Other infective (teno)synovitis, right hip
  - M65.152 Other infective (teno)synovitis, left hip
  - M65.159 Other infective (teno)synovitis, unspecified hip
- M65.16 Other infective (teno)synovitis, knee
  - M65.161 Other infective (teno)synovitis, right knee
  - M65.162 Other infective (teno)synovitis, left knee
  - M65.169 Other infective (teno)synovitis, unspecified knee
- M65.17 Other infective (teno)synovitis, ankle and foot
  - M65.171 Other infective (teno)synovitis, right ankle and foot
  - M65.172 Other infective (teno)synovitis, left ankle and foot
  - M65.179 Other infective (teno)synovitis, unspecified ankle and foot
  - M65.18 Other infective (teno)synovitis, other site
  - M65.19 Other infective (teno)synovitis, multiple sites
- M65.2 Calcific tendinitis
  - **Excludes1**   tendinitis as classified in M75-M77
    calcified tendinitis of shoulder (M75.3)
  - M65.20 Calcific tendinitis, unspecified site
- M65.22 Calcific tendinitis, upper arm
  - M65.221 Calcific tendinitis, right upper arm
  - M65.222 Calcific tendinitis, left upper arm
  - M65.229 Calcific tendinitis, unspecified upper arm
- M65.23 Calcific tendinitis, forearm
  - M65.231 Calcific tendinitis, right forearm
  - M65.232 Calcific tendinitis, left forearm
  - M65.239 Calcific tendinitis, unspecified forearm
- M65.24 Calcific tendinitis, hand
  - M65.241 Calcific tendinitis, right hand
  - M65.242 Calcific tendinitis, left hand
  - M65.249 Calcific tendinitis, unspecified hand
- M65.25 Calcific tendinitis, thigh
  - M65.251 Calcific tendinitis, right thigh
  - M65.252 Calcific tendinitis, left thigh
  - M65.259 Calcific tendinitis, unspecified thigh
- M65.26 Calcific tendinitis, lower leg
  - M65.261 Calcific tendinitis, right lower leg
  - M65.262 Calcific tendinitis, left lower leg
  - M65.269 Calcific tendinitis, unspecified lower leg

CHAPTER 13 (M00-M99)

- M65.27 Calcific tendinitis, ankle and foot
  - M65.271 Calcific tendinitis, right ankle and foot
  - M65.272 Calcific tendinitis, left ankle and foot
  - M65.279 Calcific tendinitis, unspecified ankle and foot
  - M65.28 Calcific tendinitis, other site
  - M65.29 Calcific tendinitis, multiple sites
- M65.3 Trigger finger
  Nodular tendinous disease
  - M65.30 Trigger finger, unspecified finger
  - M65.31 Trigger thumb
    - M65.311 Trigger thumb, right thumb
    - M65.312 Trigger thumb, left thumb
    - M65.319 Trigger thumb, unspecified thumb
  - M65.32 Trigger finger, index finger
    - M65.321 Trigger finger, right index finger
    - M65.322 Trigger finger, left index finger
    - M65.329 Trigger finger, unspecified index finger
  - M65.33 Trigger finger, middle finger
    - M65.331 Trigger finger, right middle finger
    - M65.332 Trigger finger, left middle finger
    - M65.339 Trigger finger, unspecified middle finger
  - M65.34 Trigger finger, ring finger
    - M65.341 Trigger finger, right ring finger
    - M65.342 Trigger finger, left ring finger
    - M65.349 Trigger finger, unspecified ring finger
  - M65.35 Trigger finger, little finger
    - M65.351 Trigger finger, right little finger
    - M65.352 Trigger finger, left little finger
    - M65.359 Trigger finger, unspecified little finger
- M65.4 Radial styloid tenosynovitis [de Quervain]
- M65.8 Other synovitis and tenosynovitis
  - M65.80 Other synovitis and tenosynovitis, unspecified site
  - M65.81 Other synovitis and tenosynovitis, shoulder
    - M65.811 Other synovitis and tenosynovitis, right shoulder
    - M65.812 Other synovitis and tenosynovitis, left shoulder
    - M65.819 Other synovitis and tenosynovitis, unspecified shoulder
  - M65.82 Other synovitis and tenosynovitis, upper arm
    - M65.821 Other synovitis and tenosynovitis, right upper arm
    - M65.822 Other synovitis and tenosynovitis, left upper arm
    - M65.829 Other synovitis and tenosynovitis, unspecified upper arm
  - M65.83 Other synovitis and tenosynovitis, forearm
    - M65.831 Other synovitis and tenosynovitis, right forearm
    - M65.832 Other synovitis and tenosynovitis, left forearm
    - M65.839 Other synovitis and tenosynovitis, unspecified forearm
  - M65.84 Other synovitis and tenosynovitis, hand
    - M65.841 Other synovitis and tenosynovitis, right hand
    - M65.842 Other synovitis and tenosynovitis, left hand
    - M65.849 Other synovitis and tenosynovitis, unspecified hand

- M65.85 Other synovitis and tenosynovitis, thigh
  - M65.851 Other synovitis and tenosynovitis, right thigh
  - M65.852 Other synovitis and tenosynovitis, left thigh
  - M65.859 Other synovitis and tenosynovitis, unspecified thigh
- M65.86 Other synovitis and tenosynovitis, lower leg
  - M65.861 Other synovitis and tenosynovitis, right lower leg
  - M65.862 Other synovitis and tenosynovitis, left lower leg
  - M65.869 Other synovitis and tenosynovitis, unspecified lower leg
- M65.87 Other synovitis and tenosynovitis, ankle and foot
  - M65.871 Other synovitis and tenosynovitis, right ankle and foot
  - M65.872 Other synovitis and tenosynovitis, left ankle and foot
  - M65.879 Other synovitis and tenosynovitis, unspecified ankle and foot
  - M65.88 Other synovitis and tenosynovitis, other site
  - M65.89 Other synovitis and tenosynovitis, multiple sites
- M65.9 Synovitis and tenosynovitis, unspecified

- M66 Spontaneous rupture of synovium and tendon
  - **Includes**   rupture that occurs when a normal force is applied to tissues that are inferred to have less than normal strength
  - **Excludes2**   rotator cuff syndrome (M75.1-)
    rupture where an abnormal force is applied to normal tissue - see injury of tendon by body region
  - M66.0 Rupture of popliteal cyst
- M66.1 Rupture of synovium
  Rupture of synovial cyst
  - **Excludes2**   rupture of popliteal cyst (M66.0)
  - M66.10 Rupture of synovium, unspecified joint
  - M66.11 Rupture of synovium, shoulder
    - M66.111 Rupture of synovium, right shoulder
    - M66.112 Rupture of synovium, left shoulder
    - M66.119 Rupture of synovium, unspecified shoulder
  - M66.12 Rupture of synovium, elbow
    - M66.121 Rupture of synovium, right elbow
    - M66.122 Rupture of synovium, left elbow
    - M66.129 Rupture of synovium, unspecified elbow
  - M66.13 Rupture of synovium, wrist
    - M66.131 Rupture of synovium, right wrist
    - M66.132 Rupture of synovium, left wrist
    - M66.139 Rupture of synovium, unspecified wrist
  - M66.14 Rupture of synovium, hand and fingers
    - M66.141 Rupture of synovium, right hand
    - M66.142 Rupture of synovium, left hand
    - M66.143 Rupture of synovium, unspecified hand
    - M66.144 Rupture of synovium, right finger(s)
    - M66.145 Rupture of synovium, left finger(s)
    - M66.146 Rupture of synovium, unspecified finger(s)

● M66.15   Rupture of synovium, hip
     M66.151   Rupture of synovium, right hip
     M66.152   Rupture of synovium, left hip
     M66.159   Rupture of synovium, unspecified hip
● M66.17   Rupture of synovium, ankle, foot and toes
     M66.171   Rupture of synovium, right ankle
     M66.172   Rupture of synovium, left ankle
     M66.173   Rupture of synovium, unspecified ankle
     M66.174   Rupture of synovium, right foot
     M66.175   Rupture of synovium, left foot
     M66.176   Rupture of synovium, unspecified foot
     M66.177   Rupture of synovium, right toe(s)
     M66.178   Rupture of synovium, left toe(s)
     M66.179   Rupture of synovium, unspecified toe(s)
   M66.18   Rupture of synovium, other site
● M66.2   Spontaneous rupture of extensor tendons
   M66.20   Spontaneous rupture of extensor tendons, unspecified site
● M66.21   Spontaneous rupture of extensor tendons, shoulder
     M66.211   Spontaneous rupture of extensor tendons, right shoulder
     M66.212   Spontaneous rupture of extensor tendons, left shoulder
     M66.219   Spontaneous rupture of extensor tendons, unspecified shoulder
● M66.22   Spontaneous rupture of extensor tendons, upper arm
     M66.221   Spontaneous rupture of extensor tendons, right upper arm
     M66.222   Spontaneous rupture of extensor tendons, left upper arm
     M66.229   Spontaneous rupture of extensor tendons, unspecified upper arm
● M66.23   Spontaneous rupture of extensor tendons, forearm
     M66.231   Spontaneous rupture of extensor tendons, right forearm
     M66.232   Spontaneous rupture of extensor tendons, left forearm
     M66.239   Spontaneous rupture of extensor tendons, unspecified forearm
● M66.24   Spontaneous rupture of extensor tendons, hand
     M66.241   Spontaneous rupture of extensor tendons, right hand
     M66.242   Spontaneous rupture of extensor tendons, left hand
     M66.249   Spontaneous rupture of extensor tendons, unspecified hand
● M66.25   Spontaneous rupture of extensor tendons, thigh
     M66.251   Spontaneous rupture of extensor tendons, right thigh
     M66.252   Spontaneous rupture of extensor tendons, left thigh
     M66.259   Spontaneous rupture of extensor tendons, unspecified thigh
● M66.26   Spontaneous rupture of extensor tendons, lower leg
     M66.261   Spontaneous rupture of extensor tendons, right lower leg
     M66.262   Spontaneous rupture of extensor tendons, left lower leg
     M66.269   Spontaneous rupture of extensor tendons, unspecified lower leg

● M66.27   Spontaneous rupture of extensor tendons, ankle and foot
     M66.271   Spontaneous rupture of extensor tendons, right ankle and foot
     M66.272   Spontaneous rupture of extensor tendons, left ankle and foot
     M66.279   Spontaneous rupture of extensor tendons, unspecified ankle and foot
   M66.28   Spontaneous rupture of extensor tendons, other site
   M66.29   Spontaneous rupture of extensor tendons, multiple sites
● M66.3   Spontaneous rupture of flexor tendons
   M66.30   Spontaneous rupture of flexor tendons, unspecified site
● M66.31   Spontaneous rupture of flexor tendons, shoulder
     M66.311   Spontaneous rupture of flexor tendons, right shoulder
     M66.312   Spontaneous rupture of flexor tendons, left shoulder
     M66.319   Spontaneous rupture of flexor tendons, unspecified shoulder
● M66.32   Spontaneous rupture of flexor tendons, upper arm
     M66.321   Spontaneous rupture of flexor tendons, right upper arm
     M66.322   Spontaneous rupture of flexor tendons, left upper arm
     M66.329   Spontaneous rupture of flexor tendons, unspecified upper arm
● M66.33   Spontaneous rupture of flexor tendons, forearm
     M66.331   Spontaneous rupture of flexor tendons, right forearm
     M66.332   Spontaneous rupture of flexor tendons, left forearm
     M66.339   Spontaneous rupture of flexor tendons, unspecified forearm
● M66.34   Spontaneous rupture of flexor tendons, hand
     M66.341   Spontaneous rupture of flexor tendons, right hand
     M66.342   Spontaneous rupture of flexor tendons, left hand
     M66.349   Spontaneous rupture of flexor tendons, unspecified hand
● M66.35   Spontaneous rupture of flexor tendons, thigh
     M66.351   Spontaneous rupture of flexor tendons, right thigh
     M66.352   Spontaneous rupture of flexor tendons, left thigh
     M66.359   Spontaneous rupture of flexor tendons, unspecified thigh
● M66.36   Spontaneous rupture of flexor tendons, lower leg
     M66.361   Spontaneous rupture of flexor tendons, right lower leg
     M66.362   Spontaneous rupture of flexor tendons, left lower leg
     M66.369   Spontaneous rupture of flexor tendons, unspecified lower leg
● M66.37   Spontaneous rupture of flexor tendons, ankle and foot
     M66.371   Spontaneous rupture of flexor tendons, right ankle and foot
     M66.372   Spontaneous rupture of flexor tendons, left ankle and foot
     M66.379   Spontaneous rupture of flexor tendons, unspecified ankle and foot

M66.38   Spontaneous rupture of flexor tendons, other site

M66.39   Spontaneous rupture of flexor tendons, multiple sites

● M66.8   Spontaneous rupture of other tendons

     M66.80   Spontaneous rupture of other tendons, unspecified site

     ● M66.81   Spontaneous rupture of other tendons, shoulder

         M66.811   Spontaneous rupture of other tendons, right shoulder

         M66.812   Spontaneous rupture of other tendons, left shoulder

         M66.819   Spontaneous rupture of other tendons, unspecified shoulder

     ● M66.82   Spontaneous rupture of other tendons, upper arm

         M66.821   Spontaneous rupture of other tendons, right upper arm

         M66.822   Spontaneous rupture of other tendons, left upper arm

         M66.829   Spontaneous rupture of other tendons, unspecified upper arm

     ● M66.83   Spontaneous rupture of other tendons, forearm

         M66.831   Spontaneous rupture of other tendons, right forearm

         M66.832   Spontaneous rupture of other tendons, left forearm

         M66.839   Spontaneous rupture of other tendons, unspecified forearm

     ● M66.84   Spontaneous rupture of other tendons, hand

         M66.841   Spontaneous rupture of other tendons, right hand

         M66.842   Spontaneous rupture of other tendons, left hand

         M66.849   Spontaneous rupture of other tendons, unspecified hand

     ● M66.85   Spontaneous rupture of other tendons, thigh

         M66.851   Spontaneous rupture of other tendons, right thigh

         M66.852   Spontaneous rupture of other tendons, left thigh

         M66.859   Spontaneous rupture of other tendons, unspecified thigh

     ● M66.86   Spontaneous rupture of other tendons, lower leg

         M66.861   Spontaneous rupture of other tendons, right lower leg

         M66.862   Spontaneous rupture of other tendons, left lower leg

         M66.869   Spontaneous rupture of other tendons, unspecified lower leg

     ● M66.87   Spontaneous rupture of other tendons, ankle and foot

         M66.871   Spontaneous rupture of other tendons, right ankle and foot

         M66.872   Spontaneous rupture of other tendons, left ankle and foot

         M66.879   Spontaneous rupture of other tendons, unspecified ankle and foot

     M66.88   Spontaneous rupture of other tendons, other

     M66.89   Spontaneous rupture of other tendons, multiple sites

M66.9   Spontaneous rupture of unspecified tendon

     Rupture at musculotendinous junction, nontraumatic

● M67   Other disorders of synovium and tendon

     Excludes1   palmar fascial fibromatosis [Dupuytren] (M72.0)
                   tendinitis NOS (M77.9-)
                   xanthomatosis localized to tendons (E78.2)

     ● M67.0   Short Achilles tendon (acquired)

         M67.00   Short Achilles tendon (acquired), unspecified ankle

         M67.01   Short Achilles tendon (acquired), right ankle

         M67.02   Short Achilles tendon (acquired), left ankle

     ● M67.2   Synovial hypertrophy, not elsewhere classified

         Excludes1   villonodular synovitis (pigmented) (M12.2-)

         M67.20   Synovial hypertrophy, not elsewhere classified, unspecified site

     ● M67.21   Synovial hypertrophy, not elsewhere classified, shoulder

         M67.211   Synovial hypertrophy, not elsewhere classified, right shoulder

         M67.212   Synovial hypertrophy, not elsewhere classified, left shoulder

         M67.219   Synovial hypertrophy, not elsewhere classified, unspecified shoulder

     ● M67.22   Synovial hypertrophy, not elsewhere classified, upper arm

         M67.221   Synovial hypertrophy, not elsewhere classified, right upper arm

         M67.222   Synovial hypertrophy, not elsewhere classified, left upper arm

         M67.229   Synovial hypertrophy, not elsewhere classified, unspecified upper arm

     ● M67.23   Synovial hypertrophy, not elsewhere classified, forearm

         M67.231   Synovial hypertrophy, not elsewhere classified, right forearm

         M67.232   Synovial hypertrophy, not elsewhere classified, left forearm

         M67.239   Synovial hypertrophy, not elsewhere classified, unspecified forearm

     ● M67.24   Synovial hypertrophy, not elsewhere classified, hand

         M67.241   Synovial hypertrophy, not elsewhere classified, right hand

         M67.242   Synovial hypertrophy, not elsewhere classified, left hand

         M67.249   Synovial hypertrophy, not elsewhere classified, unspecified hand

     ● M67.25   Synovial hypertrophy, not elsewhere classified, thigh

         M67.251   Synovial hypertrophy, not elsewhere classified, right thigh

         M67.252   Synovial hypertrophy, not elsewhere classified, left thigh

         M67.259   Synovial hypertrophy, not elsewhere classified, unspecified thigh

     ● M67.26   Synovial hypertrophy, not elsewhere classified, lower leg

         M67.261   Synovial hypertrophy, not elsewhere classified, right lower leg

         M67.262   Synovial hypertrophy, not elsewhere classified, left lower leg

         M67.269   Synovial hypertrophy, not elsewhere classified, unspecified lower leg

▶ New   ⟹ Revised   ~~deleted~~ Deleted   Excludes 1   Excludes 2   Includes   Use additional   Code first   Code also   Key words

OGCR Official Guidelines   ● Unacceptable Principal Diagnosis   X Assign placeholder X   ● Use Additional Character(s)   ▌ Manifestation Code   Coding Clinic

● M67.27 Synovial hypertrophy, not elsewhere classified, ankle and foot
    M67.271 Synovial hypertrophy, not elsewhere classified, right ankle and foot
    M67.272 Synovial hypertrophy, not elsewhere classified, left ankle and foot
    M67.279 Synovial hypertrophy, not elsewhere classified, unspecified ankle and foot
  M67.28 Synovial hypertrophy, not elsewhere classified, other site
  M67.29 Synovial hypertrophy, not elsewhere classified, multiple sites

● M67.3 **Transient synovitis**
  Toxic synovitis
    Excludes1 palindromic rheumatism (M12.3-)
  M67.30 Transient synovitis, unspecified site
● M67.31 Transient synovitis, shoulder
    M67.311 Transient synovitis, right shoulder
    M67.312 Transient synovitis, left shoulder
    M67.319 Transient synovitis, unspecified shoulder
● M67.32 Transient synovitis, elbow
    M67.321 Transient synovitis, right elbow
    M67.322 Transient synovitis, left elbow
    M67.329 Transient synovitis, unspecified elbow
● M67.33 Transient synovitis, wrist
    M67.331 Transient synovitis, right wrist
    M67.332 Transient synovitis, left wrist
    M67.339 Transient synovitis, unspecified wrist
● M67.34 Transient synovitis, hand
    M67.341 Transient synovitis, right hand
    M67.342 Transient synovitis, left hand
    M67.349 Transient synovitis, unspecified hand
● M67.35 Transient synovitis, hip
    M67.351 Transient synovitis, right hip
    M67.352 Transient synovitis, left hip
    M67.359 Transient synovitis, unspecified hip
● M67.36 Transient synovitis, knee
    M67.361 Transient synovitis, right knee
    M67.362 Transient synovitis, left knee
    M67.369 Transient synovitis, unspecified knee
● M67.37 Transient synovitis, ankle and foot
    M67.371 Transient synovitis, right ankle and foot
    M67.372 Transient synovitis, left ankle and foot
    M67.379 Transient synovitis, unspecified ankle and foot
  M67.38 Transient synovitis, other site
  M67.39 Transient synovitis, multiple sites

● M67.4 **Ganglion**
  Ganglion of joint or tendon (sheath)
    Excludes1 ganglion in yaws (A66.6)
    Excludes2 cyst of bursa (M71.2-M71.3)
            cyst of synovium (M71.2-M71.3)
  M67.40 Ganglion, unspecified site
● M67.41 Ganglion, shoulder
    M67.411 Ganglion, right shoulder
    M67.412 Ganglion, left shoulder
    M67.419 Ganglion, unspecified shoulder

● M67.42 Ganglion, elbow
    M67.421 Ganglion, right elbow
    M67.422 Ganglion, left elbow
    M67.429 Ganglion, unspecified elbow
● M67.43 Ganglion, wrist
    M67.431 Ganglion, right wrist
    M67.432 Ganglion, left wrist
    M67.439 Ganglion, unspecified wrist
● M67.44 Ganglion, hand
    M67.441 Ganglion, right hand
    M67.442 Ganglion, left hand
    M67.449 Ganglion, unspecified hand
● M67.45 Ganglion, hip
    M67.451 Ganglion, right hip
    M67.452 Ganglion, left hip
    M67.459 Ganglion, unspecified hip
● M67.46 Ganglion, knee
    M67.461 Ganglion, right knee
    M67.462 Ganglion, left knee
    M67.469 Ganglion, unspecified knee
● M67.47 Ganglion, ankle and foot
    M67.471 Ganglion, right ankle and foot
    M67.472 Ganglion, left ankle and foot
    M67.479 Ganglion, unspecified ankle and foot
  M67.48 Ganglion, other site
  M67.49 Ganglion, multiple sites

● M67.5 **Plica syndrome**
  Plica knee
  M67.50 Plica syndrome, unspecified knee
  M67.51 Plica syndrome, right knee
  M67.52 Plica syndrome, left knee

● M67.8 **Other specified disorders of synovium and tendon**
  M67.80 Other specified disorders of synovium and tendon, unspecified site
● M67.81 Other specified disorders of synovium and tendon, shoulder
    M67.811 Other specified disorders of synovium, right shoulder
    M67.812 Other specified disorders of synovium, left shoulder
    M67.813 Other specified disorders of tendon, right shoulder
    M67.814 Other specified disorders of tendon, left shoulder
    M67.819 Other specified disorders of synovium and tendon, unspecified shoulder
● M67.82 Other specified disorders of synovium and tendon, elbow
    M67.821 Other specified disorders of synovium, right elbow
    M67.822 Other specified disorders of synovium, left elbow
    M67.823 Other specified disorders of tendon, right elbow
    M67.824 Other specified disorders of tendon, left elbow
    M67.829 Other specified disorders of synovium and tendon, unspecified elbow

CHAPTER 13 (M00-M99)

● M67.83   Other specified disorders of synovium and tendon, wrist
    M67.831   Other specified disorders of synovium, right wrist
    M67.832   Other specified disorders of synovium, left wrist
    M67.833   Other specified disorders of tendon, right wrist
    M67.834   Other specified disorders of tendon, left wrist
    M67.839   Other specified disorders of synovium and tendon, unspecified forearm

● M67.84   Other specified disorders of synovium and tendon, hand
    M67.841   Other specified disorders of synovium, right hand
    M67.842   Other specified disorders of synovium, left hand
    M67.843   Other specified disorders of tendon, right hand
    M67.844   Other specified disorders of tendon, left hand
    M67.849   Other specified disorders of synovium and tendon, unspecified hand

● M67.85   Other specified disorders of synovium and tendon, hip
    M67.851   Other specified disorders of synovium, right hip
    M67.852   Other specified disorders of synovium, left hip
    M67.853   Other specified disorders of tendon, right hip
    M67.854   Other specified disorders of tendon, left hip
    M67.859   Other specified disorders of synovium and tendon, unspecified hip

● M67.86   Other specified disorders of synovium and tendon, knee
    M67.861   Other specified disorders of synovium, right knee
    M67.862   Other specified disorders of synovium, left knee
    M67.863   Other specified disorders of tendon, right knee
    M67.864   Other specified disorders of tendon, left knee
    M67.869   Other specified disorders of synovium and tendon, unspecified knee

● M67.87   Other specified disorders of synovium and tendon, ankle and foot
    M67.871   Other specified disorders of synovium, right ankle and foot
    M67.872   Other specified disorders of synovium, left ankle and foot
    M67.873   Other specified disorders of tendon, right ankle and foot
    M67.874   Other specified disorders of tendon, left ankle and foot
    M67.879   Other specified disorders of synovium and tendon, unspecified ankle and foot

  M67.88   Other specified disorders of synovium and tendon, other site

  M67.89   Other specified disorders of synovium and tendon, multiple sites

● M67.9   Unspecified disorder of synovium and tendon
  M67.90   Unspecified disorder of synovium and tendon, unspecified site
● M67.91   Unspecified disorder of synovium and tendon, shoulder
    M67.911   Unspecified disorder of synovium and tendon, right shoulder
    M67.912   Unspecified disorder of synovium and tendon, left shoulder
    M67.919   Unspecified disorder of synovium and tendon, unspecified shoulder

● M67.92   Unspecified disorder of synovium and tendon, upper arm
    M67.921   Unspecified disorder of synovium and tendon, right upper arm
    M67.922   Unspecified disorder of synovium and tendon, left upper arm
    M67.929   Unspecified disorder of synovium and tendon, unspecified upper arm

● M67.93   Unspecified disorder of synovium and tendon, forearm
    M67.931   Unspecified disorder of synovium and tendon, right forearm
    M67.932   Unspecified disorder of synovium and tendon, left forearm
    M67.939   Unspecified disorder of synovium and tendon, unspecified forearm

● M67.94   Unspecified disorder of synovium and tendon, hand
    M67.941   Unspecified disorder of synovium and tendon, right hand
    M67.942   Unspecified disorder of synovium and tendon, left hand
    M67.949   Unspecified disorder of synovium and tendon, unspecified hand

● M67.95   Unspecified disorder of synovium and tendon, thigh
    M67.951   Unspecified disorder of synovium and tendon, right thigh
    M67.952   Unspecified disorder of synovium and tendon, left thigh
    M67.959   Unspecified disorder of synovium and tendon, unspecified thigh

● M67.96   Unspecified disorder of synovium and tendon, lower leg
    M67.961   Unspecified disorder of synovium and tendon, right lower leg
    M67.962   Unspecified disorder of synovium and tendon, left lower leg
    M67.969   Unspecified disorder of synovium and tendon, unspecified lower leg

● M67.97   Unspecified disorder of synovium and tendon, ankle and foot
    M67.971   Unspecified disorder of synovium and tendon, right ankle and foot
    M67.972   Unspecified disorder of synovium and tendon, left ankle and foot
    M67.979   Unspecified disorder of synovium and tendon, unspecified ankle and foot

  M67.98   Unspecified disorder of synovium and tendon, other site

  M67.99   Unspecified disorder of synovium and tendon, multiple sites

▶ New ⟹ Revised ~~deleted~~ Deleted Excludes 1 Excludes 2 Includes Use additional Code first Code also Key words
OGCR Official Guidelines ● Unacceptable Principal Diagnosis X Assign placeholder X ● Use Additional Character(s) ▶ Manifestation Code Coding Clinic

OTHER SOFT TISSUE DISORDERS (M70-M79)

- **M70   Soft tissue disorders related to use, overuse and pressure**

    Includes   soft tissue disorders of occupational origin

    Use additional external cause code to identify activity causing disorder (Y93.-)

    Excludes1   bursitis NOS (M71.9-)

    Excludes2   bursitis of shoulder (M75.5)
    enthesopathies (M76-M77)
    pressure ulcer (pressure area) (L89.-)

- **M70.0   Crepitant synovitis (acute) (chronic) of hand and wrist**
    - **M70.03   Crepitant synovitis (acute) (chronic), wrist**
        - M70.031   Crepitant synovitis (acute) (chronic), right wrist
        - M70.032   Crepitant synovitis (acute) (chronic), left wrist
        - M70.039   Crepitant synovitis (acute) (chronic), unspecified wrist
    - **M70.04   Crepitant synovitis (acute) (chronic), hand**
        - M70.041   Crepitant synovitis (acute) (chronic), right hand
        - M70.042   Crepitant synovitis (acute) (chronic), left hand
        - M70.049   Crepitant synovitis (acute) (chronic), unspecified hand
- **M70.1   Bursitis of hand**
    - M70.10   Bursitis, unspecified hand
    - M70.11   Bursitis, right hand
    - M70.12   Bursitis, left hand
- **M70.2   Olecranon bursitis**
    - M70.20   Olecranon bursitis, unspecified elbow
    - M70.21   Olecranon bursitis, right elbow
    - M70.22   Olecranon bursitis, left elbow
- **M70.3   Other bursitis of elbow**
    - M70.30   Other bursitis of elbow, unspecified elbow
    - M70.31   Other bursitis of elbow, right elbow
    - M70.32   Other bursitis of elbow, left elbow
- **M70.4   Prepatellar bursitis**
    - M70.40   Prepatellar bursitis, unspecified knee
    - M70.41   Prepatellar bursitis, right knee
    - M70.42   Prepatellar bursitis, left knee
- **M70.5   Other bursitis of knee**
    - M70.50   Other bursitis of knee, unspecified knee
    - M70.51   Other bursitis of knee, right knee
    - M70.52   Other bursitis of knee, left knee
- **M70.6   Trochanteric bursitis**
    Trochanteric tendinitis
    - M70.60   Trochanteric bursitis, unspecified hip
    - M70.61   Trochanteric bursitis, right hip
    - M70.62   Trochanteric bursitis, left hip
- **M70.7   Other bursitis of hip**
    Ischial bursitis
    - M70.70   Other bursitis of hip, unspecified hip
    - M70.71   Other bursitis of hip, right hip
    - M70.72   Other bursitis of hip, left hip

- **M70.8   Other soft tissue disorders related to use, overuse and pressure**
    - M70.80   Other soft tissue disorders related to use, overuse and pressure of unspecified site
    - **M70.81   Other soft tissue disorders related to use, overuse and pressure of shoulder**
        - M70.811   Other soft tissue disorders related to use, overuse and pressure, right shoulder
        - M70.812   Other soft tissue disorders related to use, overuse and pressure, left shoulder
        - M70.819   Other soft tissue disorders related to use, overuse and pressure, unspecified shoulder
    - **M70.82   Other soft tissue disorders related to use, overuse and pressure of upper arm**
        - M70.821   Other soft tissue disorders related to use, overuse and pressure, right upper arm
        - M70.822   Other soft tissue disorders related to use, overuse and pressure, left upper arm
        - M70.829   Other soft tissue disorders related to use, overuse and pressure, unspecified upper arms
    - **M70.83   Other soft tissue disorders related to use, overuse and pressure of forearm**
        - M70.831   Other soft tissue disorders related to use, overuse and pressure, right forearm
        - M70.832   Other soft tissue disorders related to use, overuse and pressure, left forearm
        - M70.839   Other soft tissue disorders related to use, overuse and pressure, unspecified forearm
    - **M70.84   Other soft tissue disorders related to use, overuse and pressure of hand**
        - M70.841   Other soft tissue disorders related to use, overuse and pressure, right hand
        - M70.842   Other soft tissue disorders related to use, overuse and pressure, left hand
        - M70.849   Other soft tissue disorders related to use, overuse and pressure, unspecified hand
    - **M70.85   Other soft tissue disorders related to use, overuse and pressure of thigh**
        - M70.851   Other soft tissue disorders related to use, overuse and pressure, right thigh
        - M70.852   Other soft tissue disorders related to use, overuse and pressure, left thigh
        - M70.859   Other soft tissue disorders related to use, overuse and pressure, unspecified thigh
    - **M70.86   Other soft tissue disorders related to use, overuse and pressure lower leg**
        - M70.861   Other soft tissue disorders related to use, overuse and pressure, right lower leg
        - M70.862   Other soft tissue disorders related to use, overuse and pressure, left lower leg
        - M70.869   Other soft tissue disorders related to use, overuse and pressure, unspecified leg

N   Newborn Age: 0   **P**   Pediatric Age: 0–17   **M**   Maternity DX: 12–55   **A**   Adult Age: 15–124   ♀   Females Only   ♂   Males Only

🔾   Complication\Comorbidity   🔾   Major C\C   (Ex.)   CC/MCC Exclusions   🔾   Hospital-Acquired Condition

1059

CHAPTER 13 (M00-M99)

● **M70.87**   Other soft tissue disorders related to use, overuse and pressure of ankle and foot

     M70.871   Other soft tissue disorders related to use, overuse and pressure, right ankle and foot

     M70.872   Other soft tissue disorders related to use, overuse and pressure, left ankle and foot

     M70.879   Other soft tissue disorders related to use, overuse and pressure, unspecified ankle and foot

   M70.88   Other soft tissue disorders related to use, overuse and pressure other site

   M70.89   Other soft tissue disorders related to use, overuse and pressure multiple sites

● **M70.9**   Unspecified soft tissue disorder related to use, overuse and pressure

   M70.90   Unspecified soft tissue disorder related to use, overuse and pressure of unspecified site

● **M70.91**   Unspecified soft tissue disorder related to use, overuse and pressure of shoulder

     M70.911   Unspecified soft tissue disorder related to use, overuse and pressure, right shoulder

     M70.912   Unspecified soft tissue disorder related to use, overuse and pressure, left shoulder

     M70.919   Unspecified soft tissue disorder related to use, overuse and pressure, unspecified shoulder

● **M70.92**   Unspecified soft tissue disorder related to use, overuse and pressure of upper arm

     M70.921   Unspecified soft tissue disorder related to use, overuse and pressure, right upper arm

     M70.922   Unspecified soft tissue disorder related to use, overuse and pressure, left upper arm

     M70.929   Unspecified soft tissue disorder related to use, overuse and pressure, unspecified upper arm

● **M70.93**   Unspecified soft tissue disorder related to use, overuse and pressure of forearm

     M70.931   Unspecified soft tissue disorder related to use, overuse and pressure, right forearm

     M70.932   Unspecified soft tissue disorder related to use, overuse and pressure, left forearm

     M70.939   Unspecified soft tissue disorder related to use, overuse and pressure, unspecified forearm

● **M70.94**   Unspecified soft tissue disorder related to use, overuse and pressure of hand

     M70.941   Unspecified soft tissue disorder related to use, overuse and pressure, right hand

     M70.942   Unspecified soft tissue disorder related to use, overuse and pressure, left hand

     M70.949   Unspecified soft tissue disorder related to use, overuse and pressure, unspecified hand

● **M70.95**   Unspecified soft tissue disorder related to use, overuse and pressure of thigh

     M70.951   Unspecified soft tissue disorder related to use, overuse and pressure, right thigh

     M70.952   Unspecified soft tissue disorder related to use, overuse and pressure, left thigh

     M70.959   Unspecified soft tissue disorder related to use, overuse and pressure, unspecified thigh

● **M70.96**   Unspecified soft tissue disorder related to use, overuse and pressure lower leg

     M70.961   Unspecified soft tissue disorder related to use, overuse and pressure, right lower leg

     M70.962   Unspecified soft tissue disorder related to use, overuse and pressure, left lower leg

     M70.969   Unspecified soft tissue disorder related to use, overuse and pressure, unspecified lower leg

● **M70.97**   Unspecified soft tissue disorder related to use, overuse and pressure of ankle and foot

     M70.971   Unspecified soft tissue disorder related to use, overuse and pressure, right ankle and foot

     M70.972   Unspecified soft tissue disorder related to use, overuse and pressure, left ankle and foot

     M70.979   Unspecified soft tissue disorder related to use, overuse and pressure, unspecified ankle and foot

   M70.98   Unspecified soft tissue disorder related to use, overuse and pressure other

   M70.99   Unspecified soft tissue disorder related to use, overuse and pressure multiple sites

● **M71**   **Other bursopathies**

   Excludes1   bunion (M20.1)
             bursitis related to use, overuse or pressure (M70.-)
             enthesopathies (M76-M77)

● **M71.0**   **Abscess of bursa**

   Use additional code (B95.-, B96.-) to identify causative organism

   M71.00   Abscess of bursa, unspecified site

● **M71.01**   Abscess of bursa, shoulder

     M71.011   Abscess of bursa, right shoulder

     M71.012   Abscess of bursa, left shoulder

     M71.019   Abscess of bursa, unspecified shoulder

● **M71.02**   Abscess of bursa, elbow

     M71.021   Abscess of bursa, right elbow

     M71.022   Abscess of bursa, left elbow

     M71.029   Abscess of bursa, unspecified elbow

● **M71.03**   Abscess of bursa, wrist

     M71.031   Abscess of bursa, right wrist

     M71.032   Abscess of bursa, left wrist

     M71.039   Abscess of bursa, unspecified wrist

● **M71.04**   Abscess of bursa, hand

     M71.041   Abscess of bursa, right hand

     M71.042   Abscess of bursa, left hand

     M71.049   Abscess of bursa, unspecified hand

▶ New   ➡ Revised   ~~deleted~~ Deleted   Excludes 1   Excludes 2   Includes   Use additional   Code first   Code also   Key words

OGCR Official Guidelines   ● Unacceptable Principal Diagnosis   X Assign placeholder X   ● Use Additional Character(s)   ▶ Manifestation Code   **Coding Clinic**

● M71.05   Abscess of bursa, hip
   M71.051   Abscess of bursa, right hip
   M71.052   Abscess of bursa, left hip
   M71.059   Abscess of bursa, unspecified hip
● M71.06   Abscess of bursa, knee
   M71.061   Abscess of bursa, right knee
   M71.062   Abscess of bursa, left knee
   M71.069   Abscess of bursa, unspecified knee
● M71.07   Abscess of bursa, ankle and foot
   M71.071   Abscess of bursa, right ankle and foot
   M71.072   Abscess of bursa, left ankle and foot
   M71.079   Abscess of bursa, unspecified ankle and foot
  M71.08   Abscess of bursa, other site
  M71.09   Abscess of bursa, multiple sites
● M71.1   Other infective bursitis
   Use additional code (B95.-, B96.-) to identify causative organism
  M71.10   Other infective bursitis, unspecified site
● M71.11   Other infective bursitis, shoulder
   M71.111   Other infective bursitis, right shoulder
   M71.112   Other infective bursitis, left shoulder
   M71.119   Other infective bursitis, unspecified shoulder
● M71.12   Other infective bursitis, elbow
   M71.121   Other infective bursitis, right elbow
   M71.122   Other infective bursitis, left elbow
   M71.129   Other infective bursitis, unspecified elbow
● M71.13   Other infective bursitis, wrist
   M71.131   Other infective bursitis, right wrist
   M71.132   Other infective bursitis, left wrist
   M71.139   Other infective bursitis, unspecified wrist
● M71.14   Other infective bursitis, hand
   M71.141   Other infective bursitis, right hand
   M71.142   Other infective bursitis, left hand
   M71.149   Other infective bursitis, unspecified hand
● M71.15   Other infective bursitis, hip
   M71.151   Other infective bursitis, right hip
   M71.152   Other infective bursitis, left hip
   M71.159   Other infective bursitis, unspecified hip
● M71.16   Other infective bursitis, knee
   M71.161   Other infective bursitis, right knee
   M71.162   Other infective bursitis, left knee
   M71.169   Other infective bursitis, unspecified knee
● M71.17   Other infective bursitis, ankle and foot
   M71.171   Other infective bursitis, right ankle and foot
   M71.172   Other infective bursitis, left ankle and foot
   M71.179   Other infective bursitis, unspecified ankle and foot
  M71.18   Other infective bursitis, other site
  M71.19   Other infective bursitis, multiple sites

● M71.2   Synovial cyst of popliteal space [Baker]
   Popliteal space = popliteal cavity, popliteal fossa. Depression in the posterior aspect of the knee (behind the knee).
   Excludes1   synovial cyst of popliteal space with rupture (M66.0)
  M71.20   Synovial cyst of popliteal space [Baker], unspecified knee
  M71.21   Synovial cyst of popliteal space [Baker], right knee
  M71.22   Synovial cyst of popliteal space [Baker], left knee
● M71.3   Other bursal cyst
   Synovial cyst NOS
   Excludes1   synovial cyst with rupture (M66.1-)
  M71.30   Other bursal cyst, unspecified site
● M71.31   Other bursal cyst, shoulder
   M71.311   Other bursal cyst, right shoulder
   M71.312   Other bursal cyst, left shoulder
   M71.319   Other bursal cyst, unspecified shoulder
● M71.32   Other bursal cyst, elbow
   M71.321   Other bursal cyst, right elbow
   M71.322   Other bursal cyst, left elbow
   M71.329   Other bursal cyst, unspecified elbow
● M71.33   Other bursal cyst, wrist
   M71.331   Other bursal cyst, right wrist
   M71.332   Other bursal cyst, left wrist
   M71.339   Other bursal cyst, unspecified wrist
● M71.34   Other bursal cyst, hand
   M71.341   Other bursal cyst, right hand
   M71.342   Other bursal cyst, left hand
   M71.349   Other bursal cyst, unspecified hand
● M71.35   Other bursal cyst, hip
   M71.351   Other bursal cyst, right hip
   M71.352   Other bursal cyst, left hip
   M71.359   Other bursal cyst, unspecified hip
● M71.37   Other bursal cyst, ankle and foot
   M71.371   Other bursal cyst, right ankle and foot
   M71.372   Other bursal cyst, left ankle and foot
   M71.379   Other bursal cyst, unspecified ankle and foot
  M71.38   Other bursal cyst, other site
  M71.39   Other bursal cyst, multiple sites
● M71.4   Calcium deposit in bursa
   Excludes2   calcium deposit in bursa of shoulder (M75.3)
  M71.40   Calcium deposit in bursa, unspecified site
● M71.42   Calcium deposit in bursa, elbow
   M71.421   Calcium deposit in bursa, right elbow
   M71.422   Calcium deposit in bursa, left elbow
   M71.429   Calcium deposit in bursa, unspecified elbow
● M71.43   Calcium deposit in bursa, wrist
   M71.431   Calcium deposit in bursa, right wrist
   M71.432   Calcium deposit in bursa, left wrist
   M71.439   Calcium deposit in bursa, unspecified wrist
● M71.44   Calcium deposit in bursa, hand
   M71.441   Calcium deposit in bursa, right hand
   M71.442   Calcium deposit in bursa, left hand
   M71.449   Calcium deposit in bursa, unspecified hand

CHAPTER 13 (M00-M99)

CHAPTER 13 (M00-M99)

● M71.45   Calcium deposit in bursa, hip
     M71.451   Calcium deposit in bursa, right hip
     M71.452   Calcium deposit in bursa, left hip
     M71.459   Calcium deposit in bursa, unspecified hip

● M71.46   Calcium deposit in bursa, knee
     M71.461   Calcium deposit in bursa, right knee
     M71.462   Calcium deposit in bursa, left knee
     M71.469   Calcium deposit in bursa, unspecified knee

● M71.47   Calcium deposit in bursa, ankle and foot
     M71.471   Calcium deposit in bursa, right ankle and foot
     M71.472   Calcium deposit in bursa, left ankle and foot
     M71.479   Calcium deposit in bursa, unspecified ankle and foot

   M71.48   Calcium deposit in bursa, other site

   M71.49   Calcium deposit in bursa, multiple sites

● M71.5   Other bursitis, not elsewhere classified
     Excludes1   bursitis NOS (M71.9-)
     Excludes2   bursitis of shoulder (M75.5)
                bursitis of tibial collateral [Pellegrini-Stieda] (M76.4-)

   M71.50   Other bursitis, not elsewhere classified, unspecified site

● M71.52   Other bursitis, not elsewhere classified, elbow
     M71.521   Other bursitis, not elsewhere classified, right elbow
     M71.522   Other bursitis, not elsewhere classified, left elbow
     M71.529   Other bursitis, not elsewhere classified, unspecified elbow

● M71.53   Other bursitis, not elsewhere classified, wrist
     M71.531   Other bursitis, not elsewhere classified, right wrist
     M71.532   Other bursitis, not elsewhere classified, left wrist
     M71.539   Other bursitis, not elsewhere classified, unspecified wrist

● M71.54   Other bursitis, not elsewhere classified, hand
     M71.541   Other bursitis, not elsewhere classified, right hand
     M71.542   Other bursitis, not elsewhere classified, left hand
     M71.549   Other bursitis, not elsewhere classified, unspecified hand

● M71.55   Other bursitis, not elsewhere classified, hip
     M71.551   Other bursitis, not elsewhere classified, right hip
     M71.552   Other bursitis, not elsewhere classified, left hip
     M71.559   Other bursitis, not elsewhere classified, unspecified hip

● M71.56   Other bursitis, not elsewhere classified, knee
     M71.561   Other bursitis, not elsewhere classified, right knee
     M71.562   Other bursitis, not elsewhere classified, left knee
     M71.569   Other bursitis, not elsewhere classified, unspecified knee

● M71.57   Other bursitis, not elsewhere classified, ankle and foot
     M71.571   Other bursitis, not elsewhere classified, right ankle and foot
     M71.572   Other bursitis, not elsewhere classified, left ankle and foot
     M71.579   Other bursitis, not elsewhere classified, unspecified ankle and foot

   M71.58   Other bursitis, not elsewhere classified, other site

● M71.8   Other specified bursopathies
   M71.80   Other specified bursopathies, unspecified site

● M71.81   Other specified bursopathies, shoulder
     M71.811   Other specified bursopathies, right shoulder
     M71.812   Other specified bursopathies, left shoulder
     M71.819   Other specified bursopathies, unspecified shoulder

● M71.82   Other specified bursopathies, elbow
     M71.821   Other specified bursopathies, right elbow
     M71.822   Other specified bursopathies, left elbow
     M71.829   Other specified bursopathies, unspecified elbow

● M71.83   Other specified bursopathies, wrist
     M71.831   Other specified bursopathies, right wrist
     M71.832   Other specified bursopathies, left wrist
     M71.839   Other specified bursopathies, unspecified wrist

● M71.84   Other specified bursopathies, hand
     M71.841   Other specified bursopathies, right hand
     M71.842   Other specified bursopathies, left hand
     M71.849   Other specified bursopathies, unspecified hand

● M71.85   Other specified bursopathies, hip
     M71.851   Other specified bursopathies, right hip
     M71.852   Other specified bursopathies, left hip
     M71.859   Other specified bursopathies, unspecified hip

● M71.86   Other specified bursopathies, knee
     M71.861   Other specified bursopathies, right knee
     M71.862   Other specified bursopathies, left knee
     M71.869   Other specified bursopathies, unspecified knee

● M71.87   Other specified bursopathies, ankle and foot
     M71.871   Other specified bursopathies, right ankle and foot
     M71.872   Other specified bursopathies, left ankle and foot
     M71.879   Other specified bursopathies, unspecified ankle and foot

   M71.88   Other specified bursopathies, other site

   M71.89   Other specified bursopathies, multiple sites

  M71.9   Bursopathy, unspecified
     Bursitis NOS

▶ New   ⇒ Revised   ~~deleted~~ Deleted   Excludes 1   Excludes 2   Includes   Use additional   Code first   Code also   Key words
OGCR Official Guidelines   ● Unacceptable Principal Diagnosis   X Assign placeholder X   ● Use Additional Character(s)   ▌ Manifestation Code   **Coding Clinic**

● **M72 Fibroblastic disorders**

     Excludes2   retroperitoneal fibromatosis (D48.3)

   M72.0 Palmar fascial fibromatosis [Dupuytren]   A

   M72.1 Knuckle pads

   M72.2 Plantar fascial fibromatosis
        Plantar fasciitis

   M72.4 Pseudosarcomatous fibromatosis
        Nodular fasciitis

   M72.6 Necrotizing fasciitis 🦠
        Use additional code (B95.-, B96.-) to identify causative
          organism
        (Ex:) See PDX Collection 806

   M72.8 Other fibroblastic disorders
        Abscess of fascia
        Fasciitis NEC
        Other infective fasciitis
        Use additional code to (B95.-, B96.-) identify causative
          organism

        Excludes1   diffuse (eosinophilic) fasciitis (M35.4)
                    necrotizing fasciitis (M72.6)
                    nodular fasciitis (M72.4)
                    perirenal fasciitis NOS (N13.5)
                    perirenal fasciitis with infection (N13.6)
                    plantar fasciitis (M72.2)

   M72.9 Fibroblastic disorder, unspecified
        Fasciitis NOS
        Fibromatosis NOS

● **M75 Shoulder lesions**

     Excludes2   shoulder-hand syndrome (M89.0-)

  ● **M75.0 Adhesive capsulitis of shoulder**
        Frozen shoulder
        Periarthritis of shoulder

     M75.00 Adhesive capsulitis of unspecified shoulder

     M75.01 Adhesive capsulitis of right shoulder

     M75.02 Adhesive capsulitis of left shoulder
          Coding Clinic: 2015, Q2, P23

  ● **M75.1 Rotator cuff tear or rupture, not specified as traumatic**
        Rotator cuff syndrome
        Supraspinatus syndrome
        Supraspinatus tear or rupture, not specified as
          traumatic

        Excludes1   tear of rotator cuff, traumatic (S46.01-)
        Gradual onset due to repetitive stress to rotator cuff

   ● **M75.10 Unspecified rotator cuff tear or rupture, not specified as traumatic**

      M75.100 Unspecified rotator cuff tear or rupture of unspecified shoulder, not specified as traumatic

      M75.101 Unspecified rotator cuff tear or rupture of right shoulder, not specified as traumatic

      M75.102 Unspecified rotator cuff tear or rupture of left shoulder, not specified as traumatic

   ● **M75.11 Incomplete rotator cuff tear or rupture not specified as traumatic**

      M75.110 Incomplete rotator cuff tear or rupture of unspecified shoulder, not specified as traumatic

      M75.111 Incomplete rotator cuff tear or rupture of right shoulder, not specified as traumatic

      M75.112 Incomplete rotator cuff tear or rupture of left shoulder, not specified as traumatic

  ● **M75.12 Complete rotator cuff tear or rupture not specified as traumatic**

      M75.120 Complete rotator cuff tear or rupture of unspecified shoulder, not specified as traumatic

      M75.121 Complete rotator cuff tear or rupture of right shoulder, not specified as traumatic

      M75.122 Complete rotator cuff tear or rupture of left shoulder, not specified as traumatic

  ● **M75.2 Bicipital tendinitis**

     M75.20 Bicipital tendinitis, unspecified shoulder

     M75.21 Bicipital tendinitis, right shoulder

     M75.22 Bicipital tendinitis, left shoulder

  ● **M75.3 Calcific tendinitis of shoulder**
        Calcified bursa of shoulder

     M75.30 Calcific tendinitis of unspecified shoulder

     M75.31 Calcific tendinitis of right shoulder

     M75.32 Calcific tendinitis of left shoulder

  ● **M75.4 Impingement syndrome of shoulder**

     M75.40 Impingement syndrome of unspecified shoulder

     M75.41 Impingement syndrome of right shoulder

     M75.42 Impingement syndrome of left shoulder

  ● **M75.5 Bursitis of shoulder**

     M75.50 Bursitis of unspecified shoulder

     M75.51 Bursitis of right shoulder

     M75.52 Bursitis of left shoulder

  ● **M75.8 Other shoulder lesions**

     M75.80 Other shoulder lesions, unspecified shoulder

     M75.81 Other shoulder lesions, right shoulder

     M75.82 Other shoulder lesions, left shoulder

  ● **M75.9 Shoulder lesion, unspecified**

     M75.90 Shoulder lesion, unspecified, unspecified shoulder

     M75.91 Shoulder lesion, unspecified, right shoulder

     M75.92 Shoulder lesion, unspecified, left shoulder

● **M76 Enthesopathies, lower limb, excluding foot**

     Excludes2   bursitis due to use, overuse and pressure (M70.-)
                 enthesopathies of ankle and foot (M77.5-)

  ● **M76.0 Gluteal tendinitis**

     M76.00 Gluteal tendinitis, unspecified hip

     M76.01 Gluteal tendinitis, right hip

     M76.02 Gluteal tendinitis, left hip

  ● **M76.1 Psoas tendinitis**

     M76.10 Psoas tendinitis, unspecified hip

     M76.11 Psoas tendinitis, right hip

     M76.12 Psoas tendinitis, left hip

  ● **M76.2 Iliac crest spur**

     M76.20 Iliac crest spur, unspecified hip

     M76.21 Iliac crest spur, right hip

     M76.22 Iliac crest spur, left hip

  ● **M76.3 Iliotibial band syndrome**

     M76.30 Iliotibial band syndrome, unspecified leg

     M76.31 Iliotibial band syndrome, right leg

     M76.32 Iliotibial band syndrome, left leg

  ● **M76.4 Tibial collateral bursitis [Pellegrini-Stieda]**

     M76.40 Tibial collateral bursitis [Pellegrini-Stieda], unspecified leg

     M76.41 Tibial collateral bursitis [Pellegrini-Stieda], right leg

     M76.42 Tibial collateral bursitis [Pellegrini-Stieda], left leg

CHAPTER 13 (M00-M99)

● M76.5 **Patellar tendinitis**
    M76.50 Patellar tendinitis, unspecified knee
    M76.51 Patellar tendinitis, right knee
    M76.52 Patellar tendinitis, left knee

● M76.6 **Achilles tendinitis**
    Achilles bursitis
    M76.60 Achilles tendinitis, unspecified leg
    M76.61 Achilles tendinitis, right leg
    M76.62 Achilles tendinitis, left leg

● M76.7 **Peroneal tendinitis**
    M76.70 Peroneal tendinitis, unspecified leg
    M76.71 Peroneal tendinitis, right leg
    M76.72 Peroneal tendinitis, left leg

● M76.8 **Other specified enthesopathies of lower limb, excluding foot**
    ● M76.81 Anterior tibial syndrome
        M76.811 Anterior tibial syndrome, right leg
        M76.812 Anterior tibial syndrome, left leg
        M76.819 Anterior tibial syndrome, unspecified leg
    ● M76.82 Posterior tibial tendinitis
        M76.821 Posterior tibial tendinitis, right leg
        M76.822 Posterior tibial tendinitis, left leg
        M76.829 Posterior tibial tendinitis, unspecified leg
    ● M76.89 Other specified enthesopathies of lower limb, excluding foot
        M76.891 Other specified enthesopathies of right lower limb, excluding foot
        M76.892 Other specified enthesopathies of left lower limb, excluding foot
        M76.899 Other specified enthesopathies of unspecified lower limb, excluding foot

M76.9 **Unspecified enthesopathy, lower limb, excluding foot**

● M77 **Other enthesopathies**
    Excludes1 bursitis NOS (M71.9-)
    Excludes2 bursitis due to use, overuse and pressure (M70.-)
        osteophyte (M25.7)
        spinal enthesopathy (M46.0-)

● M77.0 **Medial epicondylitis**
    M77.00 Medial epicondylitis, unspecified elbow
    M77.01 Medial epicondylitis, right elbow
    M77.02 Medial epicondylitis, left elbow

● M77.1 **Lateral epicondylitis**
    Tennis elbow
    M77.10 Lateral epicondylitis, unspecified elbow
    M77.11 Lateral epicondylitis, right elbow
    M77.12 Lateral epicondylitis, left elbow

● M77.2 **Periarthritis of wrist**
    M77.20 Periarthritis, unspecified wrist
    M77.21 Periarthritis, right wrist
    M77.22 Periarthritis, left wrist

● M77.3 **Calcaneal spur**
    M77.30 Calcaneal spur, unspecified foot
    M77.31 Calcaneal spur, right foot
    M77.32 Calcaneal spur, left foot

● M77.4 **Metatarsalgia**
    Excludes1 Morton's metatarsalgia (G57.6)
    M77.40 Metatarsalgia, unspecified foot
    M77.41 Metatarsalgia, right foot
    M77.42 Metatarsalgia, left foot

● M77.5 **Other enthesopathy of foot**
    M77.50 Other enthesopathy of unspecified foot
    M77.51 Other enthesopathy of right foot
    M77.52 Other enthesopathy of left foot

M77.8 **Other enthesopathies, not elsewhere classified**

M77.9 **Enthesopathy, unspecified**
    Bone spur NOS
    Capsulitis NOS
    Periarthritis NOS
    Tendinitis NOS

● M79 **Other and unspecified soft tissue disorders, not elsewhere classified**
    Excludes1 psychogenic rheumatism (F45.8)
        soft tissue pain, psychogenic (F45.41)

M79.0 **Rheumatism, unspecified**
    Excludes1 fibromyalgia (M79.7)
        palindromic rheumatism (M12.3-)

M79.1 **Myalgia**
    Myofascial pain syndrome
    Excludes1 fibromyalgia (M79.7)
        myositis (M60.-)

M79.2 **Neuralgia and neuritis, unspecified**
    Excludes1 brachial radiculitis NOS (M54.1)
        lumbosacral radiculitis NOS (M54.1)
        mononeuropathies (G56-G58)
        radiculitis NOS (M54.1)
        sciatica (M54.3-M54.4)

M79.3 **Panniculitis, unspecified**
    Excludes1 lupus panniculitis (L93.2)
        neck and back panniculitis (M54.0-)
        relapsing [Weber-Christian] panniculitis (M35.6)

M79.4 **Hypertrophy of (infrapatellar) fat pad**

M79.5 **Residual foreign body in soft tissue**
    Excludes1 foreign body granuloma of skin and subcutaneous tissue (L92.3)
        foreign body granuloma of soft tissue (M60.2-)

● M79.6 **Pain in limb, hand, foot, fingers and toes**
    Excludes2 pain in joint (M25.5-)
    ● M79.60 Pain in limb, unspecified
        M79.601 Pain in right arm
            Pain in right upper limb NOS
        M79.602 Pain in left arm
            Pain in left upper limb NOS
        M79.603 Pain in arm, unspecified
            Pain in upper limb NOS
        M79.604 Pain in right leg
            Pain in right lower limb NOS
        M79.605 Pain in left leg
            Pain in left lower limb NOS
        M79.606 Pain in leg, unspecified
            Pain in lower limb NOS
        M79.609 Pain in unspecified limb
            Pain in limb NOS
    ● M79.62 Pain in upper arm
        Pain in axillary region
        M79.621 Pain in right upper arm
        M79.622 Pain in left upper arm
        M79.629 Pain in unspecified upper arm
    ● M79.63 Pain in forearm
        M79.631 Pain in right forearm
        M79.632 Pain in left forearm
        M79.639 Pain in unspecified forearm

● **M79.64** Pain in hand and fingers
　　M79.641 Pain in right hand
　　M79.642 Pain in left hand
　　M79.643 Pain in unspecified hand
　　M79.644 Pain in right finger(s)
　　M79.645 Pain in left finger(s)
　　M79.646 Pain in unspecified finger(s)
● **M79.65** Pain in thigh
　　M79.651 Pain in right thigh
　　M79.652 Pain in left thigh
　　M79.659 Pain in unspecified thigh
● **M79.66** Pain in lower leg
　　M79.661 Pain in right lower leg
　　M79.662 Pain in left lower leg
　　M79.669 Pain in unspecified lower leg
● **M79.67** Pain in foot and toes
　　M79.671 Pain in right foot
　　M79.672 Pain in left foot
　　M79.673 Pain in unspecified foot
　　M79.674 Pain in right toe(s)
　　M79.675 Pain in left toe(s)
　　M79.676 Pain in unspecified toe(s)
M79.7 Fibromyalgia
　　Fibromyositis
　　Fibrositis
　　Myofibrositis
● **M79.A** Nontraumatic compartment syndrome
　　Code first, if applicable, associated postprocedural
　　complication
　　Excludes1 compartment syndrome NOS (T79.A-)
　　　　fibromyalgia (M79.7) nontraumatic
　　　　ischemic infarction of muscle
　　　　(M62.2-)
　　　　traumatic compartment syndrome (T79.A-)
● **M79.A1** Nontraumatic compartment syndrome of upper
　　extremity
　　　Nontraumatic compartment syndrome of
　　　shoulder, arm, forearm, wrist, hand, and
　　　fingers
　　　(Ex:) **For category M79.A1 CC codes:** See PDX Collection 893
　　　M79.A11 Nontraumatic compartment syndrome
　　　　of right upper extremity 🖐
　　　M79.A12 Nontraumatic compartment syndrome
　　　　of left upper extremity 🖐
　　　M79.A19 Nontraumatic compartment syndrome
　　　　of unspecified upper extremity 🖐
● **M79.A2** Nontraumatic compartment syndrome of lower
　　extremity
　　　Nontraumatic compartment syndrome of hip,
　　　buttock, thigh, leg, foot, and toes
　　　(Ex:) **For category M79.A2 CC codes:** See PDX Collection 984
　　　M79.A21 Nontraumatic compartment syndrome
　　　　of right lower extremity 🖐
　　　M79.A22 Nontraumatic compartment syndrome
　　　　of left lower extremity 🖐
　　　M79.A29 Nontraumatic compartment syndrome
　　　　of unspecified lower extremity 🖐
　　M79.A3 Nontraumatic compartment syndrome of
　　　abdomen 🖐
　　　(Ex:) See PDX Collection 895
　　M79.A9 Nontraumatic compartment syndrome of other
　　　sites 🖐
　　　(Ex:) See PDX Collection 896
● **M79.8** Other specified soft tissue disorders
　　M79.81 Nontraumatic hematoma of soft tissue
　　　Nontraumatic hematoma of muscle
　　　Nontraumatic seroma of muscle and soft tissue
　　M79.89 Other specified soft tissue disorders
　　　Polyalgia
M79.9 Soft tissue disorder, unspecified

OGCR See Section I.C., Chapter 13.d.

Osteoporosis

Osteoporosis is a systemic condition, meaning that all bones of the musculoskeletal system are affected. Therefore, site is not a component of the codes under category M81, Osteoporosis without current pathological fracture. The site codes under category M80, Osteoporosis with current pathological fracture, identify the site of the fracture, not the osteoporosis.

1) Osteoporosis without pathological fracture

Category M81, Osteoporosis without current pathological fracture, is for use for patients with osteoporosis who do not currently have a pathologic fracture due to the osteoporosis, even if they have had a fracture in the past. For patients with a history of osteoporosis fractures, status code Z87.310, Personal history of (healed) osteoporosis fracture, should follow the code from M81.

2) Osteoporosis with current pathological fracture

Category M80, Osteoporosis with current pathological fracture, is for patients who have a current pathologic fracture at the time of an encounter. The codes under M80 identify the site of the fracture. A code from category M80, not a traumatic fracture code, should be used for any patient with known osteoporosis who suffers a fracture, even if the patient had a minor fall or trauma, if that fall or trauma would not usually break a normal, healthy bone.

OSTEOPATHIES AND CHONDROPATHIES (M80-M94)

DISORDERS OF BONE DENSITY AND STRUCTURE (M80-M85)

M80 Osteoporosis with current pathological fracture
　Excessive skeletal fragility (porous bone) resulting in bone fractures
　　Includes　osteoporosis with current fragility fracture
　　Use additional code to identify major osseous defect, if
　　applicable (M89.7-)
　　Excludes1　collapsed vertebra NOS (M48.5)
　　　　pathological fracture NOS (M84.4)
　　　　wedging of vertebra NOS (M48.5)
　　Excludes2　personal history of (healed) osteoporosis fracture
　　　　(Z87.310)
　　The appropriate 7th character is to be added to each code from
　　category M80:

A	initial encounter for fracture *All encounters involving diagnosis and treatment*
D	subsequent encounter for fracture with routine healing
G	subsequent encounter for fracture with delayed healing *Encounters for attention to casting or fixation devices,* *medication, and follow-up visits during the healing phase*
K	subsequent encounter for fracture with nonunion *Total failure of fracture healing*
P	subsequent encounter for fracture with malunion *Fracture ends do not heal together correctly.*
S	sequela

　　(Ex:) **For category M80[A] CC codes:** See PDX Collection 888
　　　For category M80[K,P] CC codes: See PDX Collection 897
● **M80.0** Age-related osteoporosis with current pathological
　　fracture
　　　Involutional osteoporosis with current pathological
　　　fracture
　　　Osteoporosis NOS with current pathological fracture
　　　Postmenopausal osteoporosis with current pathological
　　　fracture
　　　Senile osteoporosis with current pathological fracture
　　X● **M80.00** Age-related osteoporosis with current
　　　　pathological fracture, unspecified site
　　　　A, K, P 🖐　　　　　　　　　　　　　　A

N Newborn Age: 0　　P Pediatric Age: 0–17　　M Maternity DX: 12–55　　A Adult Age: 15–124　　♀ Females Only　　♂ Males Only

🖐 Complication\Comorbidity　　🖐 Major C\C　　(Ex:) CC/MCC Exclusions　　🖐 Hospital-Acquired Condition

● M80.01 Age-related osteoporosis with current pathological fracture, shoulder
- ● M80.011 Age-related osteoporosis with current pathological fracture, right shoulder A, K, P   A
- ● M80.012 Age-related osteoporosis with current pathological fracture, left shoulder A, K, P   A
- ● M80.019 Age-related osteoporosis with current pathological fracture, unspecified shoulder A, K, P   A

● M80.02 Age-related osteoporosis with current pathological fracture, humerus
- ● M80.021 Age-related osteoporosis with current pathological fracture, right humerus A, K, P   A
- ● M80.022 Age-related osteoporosis with current pathological fracture, left humerus A, K, P   A
- ● M80.029 Age-related osteoporosis with current pathological fracture, unspecified humerus A, K, P   A

● M80.03 Age-related osteoporosis with current pathological fracture, forearm
  Age-related osteoporosis with current pathological fracture of wrist
- ● M80.031 Age-related osteoporosis with current pathological fracture, right forearm A, K, P   A
- ● M80.032 Age-related osteoporosis with current pathological fracture, left forearm A, K, P   A
- ● M80.039 Age-related osteoporosis with current pathological fracture, unspecified forearm A, K, P   A

● M80.04 Age-related osteoporosis with current pathological fracture, hand
- ● M80.041 Age-related osteoporosis with current pathological fracture, right hand A, K, P   A
- ● M80.042 Age-related osteoporosis with current pathological fracture, left hand A, K, P   A
- ● M80.049 Age-related osteoporosis with current pathological fracture, unspecified hand A, K, P   A

● M80.05 Age-related osteoporosis with current pathological fracture, femur
  Age-related osteoporosis with current pathological fracture of hip
- ● M80.051 Age-related osteoporosis with current pathological fracture, right femur A, K, P   A
- ● M80.052 Age-related osteoporosis with current pathological fracture, left femur A, K, P   A
- ● M80.059 Age-related osteoporosis with current pathological fracture, unspecified femur A, K, P   A

● M80.06 Age-related osteoporosis with current pathological fracture, lower leg
- ● M80.061 Age-related osteoporosis with current pathological fracture, right lower leg A, K, P   A
- ● M80.062 Age-related osteoporosis with current pathological fracture, left lower leg A, K, P   A
- ● M80.069 Age-related osteoporosis with current pathological fracture, unspecified lower leg A, K, P   A

● M80.07 Age-related osteoporosis with current pathological fracture, ankle and foot
- ● M80.071 Age-related osteoporosis with current pathological fracture, right ankle and foot A, K, P   A
- ● M80.072 Age-related osteoporosis with current pathological fracture, left ankle and foot A, K, P   A
- ● M80.079 Age-related osteoporosis with current pathological fracture, unspecified ankle and foot A, K, P   A

X ● M80.08 Age-related osteoporosis with current pathological fracture, vertebra(e) A, K, P   A

● M80.8 Other osteoporosis with current pathological fracture
  Drug-induced osteoporosis with current pathological fracture
  Idiopathic osteoporosis with current pathological fracture
  Osteoporosis of disuse with current pathological fracture
  Postoophorectomy osteoporosis with current pathological fracture
  Postsurgical malabsorption osteoporosis with current pathological fracture
  Post-traumatic osteoporosis with current pathological fracture
  Use additional code for adverse effect, if applicable, to identify drug (T36-T50 with fifth or sixth character 5)

X ● M80.80 Other osteoporosis with current pathological fracture, unspecified site A, K, P   A

● M80.81 Other osteoporosis with pathological fracture, shoulder
- ● M80.811 Other osteoporosis with current pathological fracture, right shoulder A, K, P   A
- ● M80.812 Other osteoporosis with current pathological fracture, left shoulder A, K, P   A
- ● M80.819 Other osteoporosis with current pathological fracture, unspecified shoulder A, K, P   A

● M80.82 Other osteoporosis with current pathological fracture, humerus
- ● M80.821 Other osteoporosis with current pathological fracture, right humerus A, K, P   A
- ● M80.822 Other osteoporosis with current pathological fracture, left humerus A, K, P   A
- ● M80.829 Other osteoporosis with current pathological fracture, unspecified humerus A, K, P   A

● M80.83 Other osteoporosis with current pathological fracture, forearm
  Other osteoporosis with current pathological fracture of wrist
- ● M80.831 Other osteoporosis with current pathological fracture, right forearm A, K, P   A
- ● M80.832 Other osteoporosis with current pathological fracture, left forearm A, K, P   A
- ● M80.839 Other osteoporosis with current pathological fracture, unspecified forearm A, K, P   A

● **M80.84** **Other osteoporosis with current pathological fracture, hand**

　● **M80.841** **Other osteoporosis with current pathological fracture, right hand** A, K, P 🦴

　● **M80.842** **Other osteoporosis with current pathological fracture, left hand** A, K, P 🦴

　● **M80.849** **Other osteoporosis with current pathological fracture, unspecified hand** A, K, P 🦴

● **M80.85** **Other osteoporosis with current pathological fracture, femur**
　　Other osteoporosis with current pathological fracture of hip

　● **M80.851** **Other osteoporosis with current pathological fracture, right femur** A, K, P 🦴

　● **M80.852** **Other osteoporosis with current pathological fracture, left femur** A, K, P 🦴

　● **M80.859** **Other osteoporosis with current pathological fracture, unspecified femur** A, K, P 🦴

● **M80.86** **Other osteoporosis with current pathological fracture, lower leg**

　● **M80.861** **Other osteoporosis with current pathological fracture, right lower leg** A, K, P 🦴

　● **M80.862** **Other osteoporosis with current pathological fracture, left lower leg** A, K, P 🦴

　● **M80.869** **Other osteoporosis with current pathological fracture, unspecified lower leg** A, K, P 🦴

● **M80.87** **Other osteoporosis with current pathological fracture, ankle and foot**

　● **M80.871** **Other osteoporosis with current pathological fracture, right ankle and foot** A, K, P 🦴

　● **M80.872** **Other osteoporosis with current pathological fracture, left ankle and foot** A, K, P 🦴

　● **M80.879** **Other osteoporosis with current pathological fracture, unspecified ankle and foot** A, K, P 🦴

X ● **M80.88** **Other osteoporosis with current pathological fracture, vertebra(e)** A, K, P 🦴

● **M81** **Osteoporosis without current pathological fracture**
　　Use additional code to identify:
　　　major osseous defect, if applicable (M89.7-)
　　　personal history of (healed) osteoporosis fracture, if applicable (Z87.310)

　Excludes1　osteoporosis with current pathological fracture (M80.-)
　　　　　　　Sudeck's atrophy (M89.0)

● **M81.0** **Age-related osteoporosis without current pathological fracture** A
　　Involutional osteoporosis without current pathological fracture
　　Osteoporosis NOS
　　Postmenopausal osteoporosis without current pathological fracture
　　Senile osteoporosis without current pathological fracture

● **M81.6** **Localized osteoporosis [Lequesne]**
　　Excludes1　Sudeck's atrophy (M89.0)

● **M81.8** **Other osteoporosis without current pathological fracture**
　　Drug-induced osteoporosis without current pathological fracture
　　Idiopathic osteoporosis without current pathological fracture
　　Osteoporosis of disuse without current pathological fracture
　　Postoophorectomy osteoporosis without current pathological fracture
　　Postsurgical malabsorption osteoporosis without current pathological fracture
　　Post-traumatic osteoporosis without current pathological fracture
　　Use additional code for adverse effect, if applicable, to identify drug (T36-T50 with fifth or sixth character 5)

● **M83** **Adult osteomalacia**
　　Excludes1　infantile and juvenile osteomalacia (E55.0)
　　　　　　　renal osteodystrophy (N25.0)
　　　　　　　rickets (active) (E55.0)
　　　　　　　rickets (active) sequelae (E64.3)
　　　　　　　vitamin D-resistant osteomalacia (E83.3)
　　　　　　　vitamin D-resistant rickets (active) (E83.3)

　M83.0　**Puerperal osteomalacia** ♀　　　　　　　　M

　M83.1　**Senile osteomalacia**　　　　　　　　　　A

　M83.2　**Adult osteomalacia due to malabsorption**　A
　　　　Postsurgical malabsorption osteomalacia in adults

　M83.3　**Adult osteomalacia due to malnutrition**　A

　M83.4　**Aluminum bone disease**

　M83.5　**Other drug-induced osteomalacia in adults**　A
　　　　Use additional code for adverse effect, if applicable, to identify drug (T36-T50 with fifth or sixth character 5)

　M83.8　**Other adult osteomalacia**　　　　　　　A

　M83.9　**Adult osteomalacia, unspecified**　　　　A

● **M84** **Disorder of continuity of bone**
　　Excludes2　traumatic fracture of bone-see fracture, by site

　　(Ex) **For category M84[A] CC codes:** See PDX Collection 888
　　　　For category M84[K,P] CC codes: See PDX Collection 897

● **M84.3** **Stress fracture**
　　Fatigue fracture
　　March fracture
　　Stress fracture NOS
　　Stress reaction
　　Use additional external cause code(s) to identify the cause of the stress fracture

　　Excludes1　pathological fracture NOS (M84.4.-)
　　　　　　　pathological fracture due to osteoporosis (M80.-)
　　　　　　　traumatic fracture (S12.-, S22.-, S32.-, S42.-, S52.-, S62.-, S72.-, S82.-, S92.-)

　　Excludes2　personal history of (healed) stress (fatigue) fracture (Z87.312)
　　　　　　　stress fracture of vertebra (M48.4-)

　　The appropriate 7th character is to be added to each code from subcategory M84.3:

A	initial encounter for fracture
D	subsequent encounter for fracture with routine healing
G	subsequent encounter for fracture with delayed healing
K	subsequent encounter for fracture with nonunion
P	subsequent encounter for fracture with malunion
S	sequela

　　(Ex) **For category M84[A] CC codes:** See PDX Collection 888
　　　　For category M84[K,P] CC codes: See PDX Collection 897

X ● **M84.30** **Stress fracture, unspecified site** K, P 🦴

● **M84.31** **Stress fracture, shoulder**

　● **M84.311** **Stress fracture, right shoulder** K, P 🦴

　● **M84.312** **Stress fracture, left shoulder** K, P 🦴

　● **M84.319** **Stress fracture, unspecified shoulder** K, P 🦴

● M84.32   Stress fracture, humerus
    ● M84.321   Stress fracture, right humerus K, P 🦴
    ● M84.322   Stress fracture, left humerus K, P 🦴
    ● M84.329   Stress fracture, unspecified humerus
                  K, P 🦴

● M84.33   Stress fracture, ulna and radius
    ● M84.331   Stress fracture, right ulna K, P 🦴
    ● M84.332   Stress fracture, left ulna K, P 🦴
    ● M84.333   Stress fracture, right radius K, P 🦴
    ● M84.334   Stress fracture, left radius K, P 🦴
    ● M84.339   Stress fracture, unspecified ulna and
                  radius K, P 🦴

● M84.34   Stress fracture, hand and fingers
    ● M84.341   Stress fracture, right hand K, P 🦴
    ● M84.342   Stress fracture, left hand K, P 🦴
    ● M84.343   Stress fracture, unspecified hand
                  K, P 🦴
    ● M84.344   Stress fracture, right finger(s) K, P 🦴
    ● M84.345   Stress fracture, left finger(s) K, P 🦴
    ● M84.346   Stress fracture, unspecified finger(s)
                  K, P 🦴

● M84.35   Stress fracture, pelvis and femur
        Stress fracture, hip
    ● M84.350   Stress fracture, pelvis K, P 🦴
    ● M84.351   Stress fracture, right femur K, P 🦴
    ● M84.352   Stress fracture, left femur K, P 🦴
    ● M84.353   Stress fracture, unspecified femur
                  K, P 🦴
    ● M84.359   Stress fracture, hip, unspecified
                  K, P 🦴

● M84.36   Stress fracture, tibia and fibula
    ● M84.361   Stress fracture, right tibia K, P 🦴
    ● M84.362   Stress fracture, left tibia K, P 🦴
    ● M84.363   Stress fracture, right fibula K, P 🦴
    ● M84.364   Stress fracture, left fibula K, P 🦴
    ● M84.369   Stress fracture, unspecified tibia and
                  fibula K, P 🦴

● M84.37   Stress fracture, ankle, foot and toes
    ● M84.371   Stress fracture, right ankle K, P 🦴
    ● M84.372   Stress fracture, left ankle K, P 🦴
    ● M84.373   Stress fracture, unspecified ankle
                  K, P 🦴
    ● M84.374   Stress fracture, right foot K, P 🦴
    ● M84.375   Stress fracture, left foot K, P 🦴
    ● M84.376   Stress fracture, unspecified foot
                  K, P 🦴
    ● M84.377   Stress fracture, right toe(s) K, P 🦴
    ● M84.378   Stress fracture, left toe(s) K, P 🦴
    ● M84.379   Stress fracture, unspecified toe(s)
                  K, P 🦴

X ● M84.38   Stress fracture, other site K, P 🦴
       Excludes2   stress fracture of vertebra
                  (M48.4-)

● M84.4   Pathological fracture, not elsewhere classified
      Chronic fracture
      Pathological fracture NOS
    Excludes1   collapsed vertebra NEC (M48.5)
                pathological fracture in neoplastic disease
                  (M84.5-)
                pathological fracture in osteoporosis
                  (M80.-)
                pathological fracture in other disease
                  (M84.6-)
                stress fracture (M84.3-)
                traumatic fracture (S12.-, S22.-, S32.-, S42.-
                , S52.-, S62.-, S72.-, S82.-, S92.-)
    Excludes2   personal history of (healed) pathological
                fracture (Z87.311)
    The appropriate 7th character is to be added to each
       code from subcategory M84.4:

A	initial encounter for fracture
D	subsequent encounter for fracture with routine healing
G	subsequent encounter for fracture with delayed healing
K	subsequent encounter for fracture with nonunion
P	subsequent encounter for fracture with malunion
S	sequela

Ex: For category M80[A] CC codes: See PDX Collection 888
     For category M80[K,P] CC codes: See PDX Collection 897

X ● M84.40   Pathological fracture, unspecified site A, K, P 🦴
● M84.41   Pathological fracture, shoulder
    ● M84.411   Pathological fracture, right shoulder
                  A, K, P 🦴
    ● M84.412   Pathological fracture, left shoulder
                  A, K, P 🦴
    ● M84.419   Pathological fracture, unspecified
                  shoulder A, K, P 🦴
● M84.42   Pathological fracture, humerus
    ● M84.421   Pathological fracture, right humerus
                  A, K, P 🦴
    ● M84.422   Pathological fracture, left humerus
                  A, K, P 🦴
    ● M84.429   Pathological fracture, unspecified
                  humerus A, K, P 🦴
● M84.43   Pathological fracture, ulna and radius
    ● M84.431   Pathological fracture, right ulna
                  A, K, P 🦴
    ● M84.432   Pathological fracture, left ulna
                  A, K, P 🦴
    ● M84.433   Pathological fracture, right radius
                  A, K, P 🦴
    ● M84.434   Pathological fracture, left radius
                  A, K, P 🦴
    ● M84.439   Pathological fracture, unspecified
                  ulna and radius A, K, P 🦴

● **M84.44 Pathological fracture, hand and fingers**
    ● **M84.441 Pathological fracture, right hand**
        A, K, P 🖐
    ● **M84.442 Pathological fracture, left hand**
        A, K, P 🖐
    ● **M84.443 Pathological fracture, unspecified hand** A, K, P 🖐
    ● **M84.444 Pathological fracture, right finger(s)**
        A, K, P 🖐
    ● **M84.445 Pathological fracture, left finger(s)**
        A, K, P 🖐
    ● **M84.446 Pathological fracture, unspecified finger(s)** A, K, P 🖐

● **M84.45 Pathological fracture, femur and pelvis**
    ● **M84.451 Pathological fracture, right femur**
        A, K, P 🖐
    ● **M84.452 Pathological fracture, left femur**
        A, K, P 🖐
    ● **M84.453 Pathological fracture, unspecified femur** A, K, P 🖐
    ● **M84.454 Pathological fracture, pelvis** A, K, P 🖐
        Coding Clinic: 2016, Q4, P43
    ● **M84.459 Pathological fracture, hip, unspecified**
        A, K, P 🖐

● **M84.46 Pathological fracture, tibia and fibula**
    ● **M84.461 Pathological fracture, right tibia**
        A, K, P 🖐
    ● **M84.462 Pathological fracture, left tibia**
        A, K, P 🖐
    ● **M84.463 Pathological fracture, right fibula**
        A, K, P 🖐
    ● **M84.464 Pathological fracture, left fibula**
        A, K, P 🖐
    ● **M84.469 Pathological fracture, unspecified tibia and fibula** A, K, P 🖐

● **M84.47 Pathological fracture, ankle, foot and toes**
    ● **M84.471 Pathological fracture, right ankle**
        A, K, P 🖐
    ● **M84.472 Pathological fracture, left ankle**
        A, K, P 🖐
    ● **M84.473 Pathological fracture, unspecified ankle** A, K, P 🖐
    ● **M84.474 Pathological fracture, right foot**
        A, K, P 🖐
    ● **M84.475 Pathological fracture, left foot**
        A, K, P 🖐
    ● **M84.476 Pathological fracture, unspecified foot**
    ● **M84.477 Pathological fracture, right toe(s)**
        A, K, P 🖐
    ● **M84.478 Pathological fracture, left toe(s)**
        A, K, P 🖐
    ● **M84.479 Pathological fracture, unspecified toe(s)** A, K, P 🖐

X● **M84.48 Pathological fracture, other site** A, K, P 🖐

OGCR Section I.C. 13.C.

Coding of Pathologic Fractures

7th character A is for use as long as the patient is receiving active treatment for the fracture. While the patient may be seen by a new or different provider over the course of treatment for a pathological fracture, assignment of the 7th character is based on whether the patient is undergoing active treatment and not whether the provider is seeing the patient for the first time.

7th character, D is to be used for encounters after the patient has completed active treatment **for the fracture and is receiving routine care for the fracture during the healing or recovery phase**. The other 7th characters, listed under each subcategory in the Tabular List, are to be used for subsequent encounters for treatment of problems associated with the healing, such as malunions, nonunions, and sequelae.

Care for complications of surgical treatment for fracture repairs during the healing or recovery phase should be coded with the appropriate complication codes.

See Section I.C.19. Coding of traumatic fractures.

● **M84.5 Pathological fracture in neoplastic disease**
    Code also underlying neoplasm
    The appropriate 7th character is to be added to each code from subcategory M84.5:

A	initial encounter for fracture
D	subsequent encounter for fracture with routine healing
G	subsequent encounter for fracture with delayed healing
K	subsequent encounter for fracture with nonunion
P	subsequent encounter for fracture with malunion
S	sequela

Ⓔ **For category M8Ø[A] CC codes:** See PDX Collection 888
    For category M8Ø[K,P] CC codes: See PDX Collection 897

X● **M84.5Ø Pathological fracture in neoplastic disease, unspecified site** A, K, P 🖐
● **M84.51 Pathological fracture in neoplastic disease, shoulder**
    ● **M84.511 Pathological fracture in neoplastic disease, right shoulder** A, K, P 🖐
    ● **M84.512 Pathological fracture in neoplastic disease, left shoulder** A, K, P 🖐
    ● **M84.519 Pathological fracture in neoplastic disease, unspecified shoulder** A, K, P 🖐
● **M84.52 Pathological fracture in neoplastic disease, humerus**
    ● **M84.521 Pathological fracture in neoplastic disease, right humerus** A, K, P 🖐
    ● **M84.522 Pathological fracture in neoplastic disease, left humerus** A, K, P 🖐
    ● **M84.529 Pathological fracture in neoplastic disease, unspecified humerus** A, K, P 🖐

CHAPTER 13 (MØØ-M99)

N   Newborn Age: Ø   P   Pediatric Age: Ø–17   M   Maternity DX: 12–55   A   Adult Age: 15–124   ♀   Females Only   ♂   Males Only
🖐 Complication\Comorbidity   🖐 Major C\C   Ⓔ CC/MCC Exclusions   🖐 Hospital-Acquired Condition

1Ø69

- **M84.53** Pathological fracture in neoplastic disease, ulna and radius
  - **M84.531** Pathological fracture in neoplastic disease, right ulna A, K, P
  - **M84.532** Pathological fracture in neoplastic disease, left ulna A, K, P
  - **M84.533** Pathological fracture in neoplastic disease, right radius A, K, P
  - **M84.534** Pathological fracture in neoplastic disease, left radius A, K, P
  - **M84.539** Pathological fracture in neoplastic disease, unspecified ulna and radius A, K, P
- **M84.54** Pathological fracture in neoplastic disease, hand
  - **M84.541** Pathological fracture in neoplastic disease, right hand A, K, P
  - **M84.542** Pathological fracture in neoplastic disease, left hand A, K, P
  - **M84.549** Pathological fracture in neoplastic disease, unspecified hand A, K, P
- **M84.55** Pathological fracture in neoplastic disease, pelvis and femur
  - **M84.550** Pathological fracture in neoplastic disease, pelvis A, K, P
  - **M84.551** Pathological fracture in neoplastic disease, right femur A, K, P
  - **M84.552** Pathological fracture in neoplastic disease, left femur A, K, P
  - **M84.553** Pathological fracture in neoplastic disease, unspecified femur A, K, P
  - **M84.559** Pathological fracture in neoplastic disease, hip, unspecified A, K, P
- **M84.56** Pathological fracture in neoplastic disease, tibia and fibula
  - **M84.561** Pathological fracture in neoplastic disease, right tibia A, K, P
  - **M84.562** Pathological fracture in neoplastic disease, left tibia A, K, P
  - **M84.563** Pathological fracture in neoplastic disease, right fibula A, K, P
  - **M84.564** Pathological fracture in neoplastic disease, left fibula A, K, P
  - **M84.569** Pathological fracture in neoplastic disease, unspecified tibia and fibula A, K, P
- **M84.57** Pathological fracture in neoplastic disease, ankle and foot
  - **M84.571** Pathological fracture in neoplastic disease, right ankle A, K, P
  - **M84.572** Pathological fracture in neoplastic disease, left ankle A, K, P
  - **M84.573** Pathological fracture in neoplastic disease, unspecified ankle A, K, P
  - **M84.574** Pathological fracture in neoplastic disease, right foot A, K, P
  - **M84.575** Pathological fracture in neoplastic disease, left foot A, K, P
  - **M84.576** Pathological fracture in neoplastic disease, unspecified foot A, K, P
- X **M84.58** Pathological fracture in neoplastic disease, other specified site A, K, P
  - Pathological fracture in neoplastic disease, vertebrae

- **M84.6** Pathological fracture in other disease
  - Code also underlying condition
  - **Excludes1** pathological fracture in osteoporosis (M80.-)
  - The appropriate 7th character is to be added to each code from subcategory M84.6:

A	initial encounter for fracture
D	subsequent encounter for fracture with routine healing
G	subsequent encounter for fracture with delayed healing
K	subsequent encounter for fracture with nonunion
P	subsequent encounter for fracture with malunion
S	sequela

  Ex: For category M80[A] CC codes: See PDX Collection 888
  For category M80[K,P] CC codes: See PDX Collection 897

  - X **M84.60** Pathological fracture in other disease, unspecified site A, K, P
  - **M84.61** Pathological fracture in other disease, shoulder
    - **M84.611** Pathological fracture in other disease, right shoulder A, K, P
    - **M84.612** Pathological fracture in other disease, left shoulder A, K, P
    - **M84.619** Pathological fracture in other disease, unspecified shoulder A, K, P
  - **M84.62** Pathological fracture in other disease, humerus
    - **M84.621** Pathological fracture in other disease, right humerus A, K, P
    - **M84.622** Pathological fracture in other disease, left humerus A, K, P
    - **M84.629** Pathological fracture in other disease, unspecified humerus A, K, P
  - **M84.63** Pathological fracture in other disease, ulna and radius
    - **M84.631** Pathological fracture in other disease, right ulna A, K, P
    - **M84.632** Pathological fracture in other disease, left ulna A, K, P
    - **M84.633** Pathological fracture in other disease, right radius A, K, P
    - **M84.634** Pathological fracture in other disease, left radius A, K, P
    - **M84.639** Pathological fracture in other disease, unspecified ulna and radius A, K, P
  - **M84.64** Pathological fracture in other disease, hand
    - **M84.641** Pathological fracture in other disease, right hand A, K, P
    - **M84.642** Pathological fracture in other disease, left hand A, K, P
    - **M84.649** Pathological fracture in other disease, unspecified hand A, K, P
  - **M84.65** Pathological fracture in other disease, pelvis and femur
    - **M84.650** Pathological fracture in other disease, pelvis A, K, P
    - **M84.651** Pathological fracture in other disease, right femur A, K, P
    - **M84.652** Pathological fracture in other disease, left femur A, K, P
    - **M84.653** Pathological fracture in other disease, unspecified femur A, K, P
    - **M84.659** Pathological fracture in other disease, hip, unspecified A, K, P

▶ New   ⟹ Revised   ~~deleted~~ Deleted   Excludes 1   Excludes 2   Includes   Use additional   Code first   Code also   Key words
OGCR Official Guidelines   ● Unacceptable Principal Diagnosis   X Assign placeholder X   ● Use Additional Character(s)   ▶ Manifestation Code   **Coding Clinic**

● **M84.66** Pathological fracture in other disease, tibia and fibula

  ● **M84.661** Pathological fracture in other disease, right tibia A, K, P 🔗

  ● **M84.662** Pathological fracture in other disease, left tibia A, K, P 🔗

  ● **M84.663** Pathological fracture in other disease, right fibula A, K, P 🔗

  ● **M84.664** Pathological fracture in other disease, left fibula A, K, P 🔗

  ● **M84.669** Pathological fracture in other disease, unspecified tibia and fibula A, K, P 🔗

● **M84.67** Pathological fracture in other disease, ankle and foot

  ● **M84.671** Pathological fracture in other disease, right ankle A, K, P 🔗

  ● **M84.672** Pathological fracture in other disease, left ankle A, K, P 🔗

  ● **M84.673** Pathological fracture in other disease, unspecified ankle A, K, P 🔗

  ● **M84.674** Pathological fracture in other disease, right foot A, K, P 🔗

  ● **M84.675** Pathological fracture in other disease, left foot A, K, P 🔗

  ● **M84.676** Pathological fracture in other disease, unspecified foot A, K, P 🔗

X ● **M84.68** Pathological fracture in other disease, other site A, K, P 🔗

● **M84.7** Nontraumatic fracture, not elsewhere classified

  ● **M84.75** Atypical femoral fracture

The appropriate 7th character is to be added to each code from M84.75:

A	initial encounter for fracture
D	subsequent encounter for fracture with routine healing
G	subsequent encounter for fracture with delayed healing
K	subsequent encounter for fracture with nonunion
P	subsequent encounter for fracture with malunion
S	sequela

Ⓔ🅧 **For category M80[A] CC codes:** See PDX Collection 888
For category M80[K,P] CC codes: See PDX Collection 897
Coding Clinic: 2016, Q4, P41

  ● **M84.750** Atypical femoral fracture, unspecified A, K, P 🔗

  ● **M84.751** Incomplete atypical femoral fracture, right leg A, K, P 🔗

  ● **M84.752** Incomplete atypical femoral fracture, left leg A, K, P 🔗

  ● **M84.753** Incomplete atypical femoral fracture, unspecified leg A, K, P 🔗

  ● **M84.754** Complete transverse atypical femoral fracture, right leg A, K, P 🔗

  ● **M84.755** Complete transverse atypical femoral fracture, left leg A, K, P 🔗

  ● **M84.756** Complete transverse atypical femoral fracture, unspecified leg A, K, P 🔗

  ● **M84.757** Complete oblique atypical femoral fracture, right leg A, K, P 🔗

  ● **M84.758** Complete oblique atypical femoral fracture, left leg A, K, P 🔗

  ● **M84.759** Complete oblique atypical femoral fracture, unspecified leg A, K, P 🔗

● **M84.8** Other disorders of continuity of bone

   M84.80 Other disorders of continuity of bone, unspecified site

  ● **M84.81** Other disorders of continuity of bone, shoulder

     M84.811 Other disorders of continuity of bone, right shoulder

     M84.812 Other disorders of continuity of bone, left shoulder

     M84.819 Other disorders of continuity of bone, unspecified shoulder

  ● **M84.82** Other disorders of continuity of bone, humerus

     M84.821 Other disorders of continuity of bone, right humerus

     M84.822 Other disorders of continuity of bone, left humerus

     M84.829 Other disorders of continuity of bone, unspecified humerus

  ● **M84.83** Other disorders of continuity of bone, ulna and radius

     M84.831 Other disorders of continuity of bone, right ulna

     M84.832 Other disorders of continuity of bone, left ulna

     M84.833 Other disorders of continuity of bone, right radius

     M84.834 Other disorders of continuity of bone, left radius

     M84.839 Other disorders of continuity of bone, unspecified ulna and radius

  ● **M84.84** Other disorders of continuity of bone, hand

     M84.841 Other disorders of continuity of bone, right hand

     M84.842 Other disorders of continuity of bone, left hand

     M84.849 Other disorders of continuity of bone, unspecified hand

  ● **M84.85** Other disorders of continuity of bone, pelvic region and thigh

     M84.851 Other disorders of continuity of bone, right pelvic region and thigh

     M84.852 Other disorders of continuity of bone, left pelvic region and thigh

     M84.859 Other disorders of continuity of bone, unspecified pelvic region and thigh

  ● **M84.86** Other disorders of continuity of bone, tibia and fibula

     M84.861 Other disorders of continuity of bone, right tibia

     M84.862 Other disorders of continuity of bone, left tibia

     M84.863 Other disorders of continuity of bone, right fibula

     M84.864 Other disorders of continuity of bone, left fibula

     M84.869 Other disorders of continuity of bone, unspecified tibia and fibula

  ● **M84.87** Other disorders of continuity of bone, ankle and foot

     M84.871 Other disorders of continuity of bone, right ankle and foot

     M84.872 Other disorders of continuity of bone, left ankle and foot

     M84.879 Other disorders of continuity of bone, unspecified ankle and foot

   M84.88 Other disorders of continuity of bone, other site

M84.9 Disorder of continuity of bone, unspecified

CHAPTER 13 (M00-M99)

CHAPTER 13 (M00-M99)

● **M85 Other disorders of bone density and structure**

    Excludes1   osteogenesis imperfecta (Q78.0)
                    osteopetrosis (Q78.2)
                    osteopoikilosis (Q78.8)
                    polyostotic fibrous dysplasia (Q78.1)

  ● **M85.0 Fibrous dysplasia (monostotic)**

      Excludes2   fibrous dysplasia of jaw (M27.8)

    M85.00   Fibrous dysplasia (monostotic), unspecified site

   ● M85.01   Fibrous dysplasia (monostotic), shoulder

       M85.011   Fibrous dysplasia (monostotic), right shoulder

       M85.012   Fibrous dysplasia (monostotic), left shoulder

       M85.019   Fibrous dysplasia (monostotic), unspecified shoulder

   ● M85.02   Fibrous dysplasia (monostotic), upper arm

       M85.021   Fibrous dysplasia (monostotic), right upper arm

       M85.022   Fibrous dysplasia (monostotic), left upper arm

       M85.029   Fibrous dysplasia (monostotic), unspecified upper arm

   ● M85.03   Fibrous dysplasia (monostotic), forearm

       M85.031   Fibrous dysplasia (monostotic), right forearm

       M85.032   Fibrous dysplasia (monostotic), left forearm

       M85.039   Fibrous dysplasia (monostotic), unspecified forearm

   ● M85.04   Fibrous dysplasia (monostotic), hand

       M85.041   Fibrous dysplasia (monostotic), right hand

       M85.042   Fibrous dysplasia (monostotic), left hand

       M85.049   Fibrous dysplasia (monostotic), unspecified hand

   ● M85.05   Fibrous dysplasia (monostotic), thigh

       M85.051   Fibrous dysplasia (monostotic), right thigh

       M85.052   Fibrous dysplasia (monostotic), left thigh

       M85.059   Fibrous dysplasia (monostotic), unspecified thigh

   ● M85.06   Fibrous dysplasia (monostotic), lower leg

       M85.061   Fibrous dysplasia (monostotic), right lower leg

       M85.062   Fibrous dysplasia (monostotic), left lower leg

       M85.069   Fibrous dysplasia (monostotic), unspecified lower leg

   ● M85.07   Fibrous dysplasia (monostotic), ankle and foot

       M85.071   Fibrous dysplasia (monostotic), right ankle and foot

       M85.072   Fibrous dysplasia (monostotic), left ankle and foot

       M85.079   Fibrous dysplasia (monostotic), unspecified ankle and foot

    M85.08   Fibrous dysplasia (monostotic), other site

    M85.09   Fibrous dysplasia (monostotic), multiple sites

● **M85.1 Skeletal fluorosis**

    M85.10   Skeletal fluorosis, unspecified site

   ● M85.11   Skeletal fluorosis, shoulder

       M85.111   Skeletal fluorosis, right shoulder

       M85.112   Skeletal fluorosis, left shoulder

       M85.119   Skeletal fluorosis, unspecified shoulder

   ● M85.12   Skeletal fluorosis, upper arm

       M85.121   Skeletal fluorosis, right upper arm

       M85.122   Skeletal fluorosis, left upper arm

       M85.129   Skeletal fluorosis, unspecified upper arm

   ● M85.13   Skeletal fluorosis, forearm

       M85.131   Skeletal fluorosis, right forearm

       M85.132   Skeletal fluorosis, left forearm

       M85.139   Skeletal fluorosis, unspecified forearm

   ● M85.14   Skeletal fluorosis, hand

       M85.141   Skeletal fluorosis, right hand

       M85.142   Skeletal fluorosis, left hand

       M85.149   Skeletal fluorosis, unspecified hand

   ● M85.15   Skeletal fluorosis, thigh

       M85.151   Skeletal fluorosis, right thigh

       M85.152   Skeletal fluorosis, left thigh

       M85.159   Skeletal fluorosis, unspecified thigh

   ● M85.16   Skeletal fluorosis, lower leg

       M85.161   Skeletal fluorosis, right lower leg

       M85.162   Skeletal fluorosis, left lower leg

       M85.169   Skeletal fluorosis, unspecified lower leg

   ● M85.17   Skeletal fluorosis, ankle and foot

       M85.171   Skeletal fluorosis, right ankle and foot

       M85.172   Skeletal fluorosis, left ankle and foot

       M85.179   Skeletal fluorosis, unspecified ankle and foot

    M85.18   Skeletal fluorosis, other site

    M85.19   Skeletal fluorosis, multiple sites

  M85.2   Hyperostosis of skull

● **M85.3 Osteitis condensans**

    M85.30   Osteitis condensans, unspecified site

   ● M85.31   Osteitis condensans, shoulder

       M85.311   Osteitis condensans, right shoulder

       M85.312   Osteitis condensans, left shoulder

       M85.319   Osteitis condensans, unspecified shoulder

   ● M85.32   Osteitis condensans, upper arm

       M85.321   Osteitis condensans, right upper arm

       M85.322   Osteitis condensans, left upper arm

       M85.329   Osteitis condensans, unspecified upper arm

   ● M85.33   Osteitis condensans, forearm

       M85.331   Osteitis condensans, right forearm

       M85.332   Osteitis condensans, left forearm

       M85.339   Osteitis condensans, unspecified forearm

   ● M85.34   Osteitis condensans, hand

       M85.341   Osteitis condensans, right hand

       M85.342   Osteitis condensans, left hand

       M85.349   Osteitis condensans, unspecified hand

● M85.35 Osteitis condensans, thigh
   M85.351 Osteitis condensans, right thigh
   M85.352 Osteitis condensans, left thigh
   M85.359 Osteitis condensans, unspecified thigh
● M85.36 Osteitis condensans, lower leg
   M85.361 Osteitis condensans, right lower leg
   M85.362 Osteitis condensans, left lower leg
   M85.369 Osteitis condensans, unspecified lower leg
● M85.37 Osteitis condensans, ankle and foot
   M85.371 Osteitis condensans, right ankle and foot
   M85.372 Osteitis condensans, left ankle and foot
   M85.379 Osteitis condensans, unspecified ankle and foot
  M85.38 Osteitis condensans, other site
  M85.39 Osteitis condensans, multiple sites
● M85.4 Solitary bone cyst
   Excludes2 solitary cyst of jaw (M27.4)
  M85.40 Solitary bone cyst, unspecified site
● M85.41 Solitary bone cyst, shoulder
   M85.411 Solitary bone cyst, right shoulder
   M85.412 Solitary bone cyst, left shoulder
   M85.419 Solitary bone cyst, unspecified shoulder
● M85.42 Solitary bone cyst, humerus
   M85.421 Solitary bone cyst, right humerus
   M85.422 Solitary bone cyst, left humerus
   M85.429 Solitary bone cyst, unspecified humerus
● M85.43 Solitary bone cyst, ulna and radius
   M85.431 Solitary bone cyst, right ulna and radius
   M85.432 Solitary bone cyst, left ulna and radius
   M85.439 Solitary bone cyst, unspecified ulna and radius
● M85.44 Solitary bone cyst, hand
   M85.441 Solitary bone cyst, right hand
   M85.442 Solitary bone cyst, left hand
   M85.449 Solitary bone cyst, unspecified hand
● M85.45 Solitary bone cyst, pelvis
   M85.451 Solitary bone cyst, right pelvis
   M85.452 Solitary bone cyst, left pelvis
   M85.459 Solitary bone cyst, unspecified pelvis
● M85.46 Solitary bone cyst, tibia and fibula
   M85.461 Solitary bone cyst, right tibia and fibula
   M85.462 Solitary bone cyst, left tibia and fibula
   M85.469 Solitary bone cyst, unspecified tibia and fibula
● M85.47 Solitary bone cyst, ankle and foot
   M85.471 Solitary bone cyst, right ankle and foot
   M85.472 Solitary bone cyst, left ankle and foot
   M85.479 Solitary bone cyst, unspecified ankle and foot
  M85.48 Solitary bone cyst, other site

● M85.5 Aneurysmal bone cyst
   Excludes2 aneurysmal cyst of jaw (M27.4)
  M85.50 Aneurysmal bone cyst, unspecified site
● M85.51 Aneurysmal bone cyst, shoulder
   M85.511 Aneurysmal bone cyst, right shoulder
   M85.512 Aneurysmal bone cyst, left shoulder
   M85.519 Aneurysmal bone cyst, unspecified shoulder
● M85.52 Aneurysmal bone cyst, upper arm
   M85.521 Aneurysmal bone cyst, right upper arm
   M85.522 Aneurysmal bone cyst, left upper arm
   M85.529 Aneurysmal bone cyst, unspecified upper arm
● M85.53 Aneurysmal bone cyst, forearm
   M85.531 Aneurysmal bone cyst, right forearm
   M85.532 Aneurysmal bone cyst, left forearm
   M85.539 Aneurysmal bone cyst, unspecified forearm
● M85.54 Aneurysmal bone cyst, hand
   M85.541 Aneurysmal bone cyst, right hand
   M85.542 Aneurysmal bone cyst, left hand
   M85.549 Aneurysmal bone cyst, unspecified hand
● M85.55 Aneurysmal bone cyst, thigh
   M85.551 Aneurysmal bone cyst, right thigh
   M85.552 Aneurysmal bone cyst, left thigh
   M85.559 Aneurysmal bone cyst, unspecified thigh
● M85.56 Aneurysmal bone cyst, lower leg
   M85.561 Aneurysmal bone cyst, right lower leg
   M85.562 Aneurysmal bone cyst, left lower leg
   M85.569 Aneurysmal bone cyst, unspecified lower leg
● M85.57 Aneurysmal bone cyst, ankle and foot
   M85.571 Aneurysmal bone cyst, right ankle and foot
   M85.572 Aneurysmal bone cyst, left ankle and foot
   M85.579 Aneurysmal bone cyst, unspecified ankle and foot
  M85.58 Aneurysmal bone cyst, other site
  M85.59 Aneurysmal bone cyst, multiple sites
● M85.6 Other cyst of bone
   Excludes1 cyst of jaw NEC (M27.4)
          osteitis fibrosa cystica generalisata [von Recklinghausen's disease of bone] (E21.0)
  M85.60 Other cyst of bone, unspecified site
● M85.61 Other cyst of bone, shoulder
   M85.611 Other cyst of bone, right shoulder
   M85.612 Other cyst of bone, left shoulder
   M85.619 Other cyst of bone, unspecified shoulder
● M85.62 Other cyst of bone, upper arm
   M85.621 Other cyst of bone, right upper arm
   M85.622 Other cyst of bone, left upper arm
   M85.629 Other cyst of bone, unspecified upper arm
● M85.63 Other cyst of bone, forearm
   M85.631 Other cyst of bone, right forearm
   M85.632 Other cyst of bone, left forearm
   M85.639 Other cyst of bone, unspecified forearm

CHAPTER 13 (M00-M99)

M85.64 Other cyst of bone, hand
  M85.641 Other cyst of bone, right hand
  M85.642 Other cyst of bone, left hand
  M85.649 Other cyst of bone, unspecified hand
M85.65 Other cyst of bone, thigh
  M85.651 Other cyst of bone, right thigh
  M85.652 Other cyst of bone, left thigh
  M85.659 Other cyst of bone, unspecified thigh
M85.66 Other cyst of bone, lower leg
  M85.661 Other cyst of bone, right lower leg
  M85.662 Other cyst of bone, left lower leg
  M85.669 Other cyst of bone, unspecified lower leg
M85.67 Other cyst of bone, ankle and foot
  M85.671 Other cyst of bone, right ankle and foot
  M85.672 Other cyst of bone, left ankle and foot
  M85.679 Other cyst of bone, unspecified ankle and foot
M85.68 Other cyst of bone, other site
M85.69 Other cyst of bone, multiple sites
M85.8 Other specified disorders of bone density and structure
  Hyperostosis of bones, except skull
  Osteosclerosis, acquired

  Excludes1   diffuse idiopathic skeletal hyperostosis [DISH] (M48.1)
              osteosclerosis congenita (Q77.4)
              osteosclerosis fragilitas (generalista) (Q78.2)
              osteosclerosis myelofibrosis (D75.81)

  M85.80 Other specified disorders of bone density and structure, unspecified site
M85.81 Other specified disorders of bone density and structure, shoulder
  M85.811 Other specified disorders of bone density and structure, right shoulder
  M85.812 Other specified disorders of bone density and structure, left shoulder
  M85.819 Other specified disorders of bone density and structure, unspecified shoulder
M85.82 Other specified disorders of bone density and structure, upper arm
  M85.821 Other specified disorders of bone density and structure, right upper arm
  M85.822 Other specified disorders of bone density and structure, left upper arm
  M85.829 Other specified disorders of bone density and structure, unspecified upper arm
M85.83 Other specified disorders of bone density and structure, forearm
  M85.831 Other specified disorders of bone density and structure, right forearm
  M85.832 Other specified disorders of bone density and structure, left forearm
  M85.839 Other specified disorders of bone density and structure, unspecified forearm
M85.84 Other specified disorders of bone density and structure, hand
  M85.841 Other specified disorders of bone density and structure, right hand
  M85.842 Other specified disorders of bone density and structure, left hand
  M85.849 Other specified disorders of bone density and structure, unspecified hand

M85.85 Other specified disorders of bone density and structure, thigh
  M85.851 Other specified disorders of bone density and structure, right thigh
  M85.852 Other specified disorders of bone density and structure, left thigh
  M85.859 Other specified disorders of bone density and structure, unspecified thigh
M85.86 Other specified disorders of bone density and structure, lower leg
  M85.861 Other specified disorders of bone density and structure, right lower leg
  M85.862 Other specified disorders of bone density and structure, left lower leg
  M85.869 Other specified disorders of bone density and structure, unspecified lower leg
M85.87 Other specified disorders of bone density and structure, ankle and foot
  M85.871 Other specified disorders of bone density and structure, right ankle and foot
  M85.872 Other specified disorders of bone density and structure, left ankle and foot
  M85.879 Other specified disorders of bone density and structure, unspecified ankle and foot
  M85.88 Other specified disorders of bone density and structure, other site
  M85.89 Other specified disorders of bone density and structure, multiple sites
M85.9 Disorder of bone density and structure, unspecified

OTHER OSTEOPATHIES (M86-M90)

Excludes1   postprocedural osteopathies (M96.-)

M86 Osteomyelitis
  Use additional code (B95-B97) to identify infectious agent
  Use additional code to identify major osseous defect, if applicable (M89.7-)
  Excludes1   osteomyelitis due to:
              echinococcus (B67.2)
              gonococcus (A54.43)
              salmonella (A02.24)
  Excludes2   ostemyelitis of:
              orbit (H05.0-)
              petrous bone (H70.2-)
              vertebra (M46.2-)
M86.0 Acute hematogenous osteomyelitis
  M86.00 Acute hematogenous osteomyelitis, unspecified site
    (Ex) See PDX Collection 898
  M86.01 Acute hematogenous osteomyelitis, shoulder
    (Ex) For category M86.01 CC codes: See PDX Collection 899
    M86.011 Acute hematogenous osteomyelitis, right shoulder
    M86.012 Acute hematogenous osteomyelitis, left shoulder
    M86.019 Acute hematogenous osteomyelitis, unspecified shoulder
  M86.02 Acute hematogenous osteomyelitis, humerus
    (Ex) For category M86.02 CC codes: See PDX Collection 900
    M86.021 Acute hematogenous osteomyelitis, right humerus
    M86.022 Acute hematogenous osteomyelitis, left humerus
    M86.029 Acute hematogenous osteomyelitis, unspecified humerus

Figure 13-6 Osteomyelitis of the spine. A lateral view of the lower thoracic spine demonstrates destruction of the disk space *(arrow)* as well as destruction of the adjoining vertebral bodies. (From Mettler: Essentials of Radiology, ed 2, Saunders, An Imprint of Elsevier, 2005)

Item 13-12 Osteomyelitis is an inflammation of the bone. **Acute osteomyelitis** is a rapidly destructive, pus-producing infection capable of causing severe bone destruction. **Chronic osteomyelitis** can remain long after the initial acute episode has passed and may lead to a recurrence of the acute phase. **Brodie's abscess** is an encapsulated focal abscess that must be surgically drained. **Periostitis** is an inflammation of the periosteum, a dense membrane composed of fibrous connective tissue that closely wraps all bone, except those with articulating surfaces in joints, which are covered by synovial membranes.

● **M86.03   Acute hematogenous osteomyelitis, radius and ulna**
    (Ex:) For category M86.03 CC codes: See PDX Collection 901

    M86.031   Acute hematogenous osteomyelitis, right radius and ulna

    M86.032   Acute hematogenous osteomyelitis, left radius and ulna

    M86.039   Acute hematogenous osteomyelitis, unspecified radius and ulna

● **M86.04   Acute hematogenous osteomyelitis, hand**
    (Ex:) For category M86.04 CC codes: See PDX Collection 902

    M86.041   Acute hematogenous osteomyelitis, right hand

    M86.042   Acute hematogenous osteomyelitis, left hand

    M86.049   Acute hematogenous osteomyelitis, unspecified hand

● **M86.05   Acute hematogenous osteomyelitis, femur**
    (Ex:) For category M86.05 CC codes: See PDX Collection 903

    M86.051   Acute hematogenous osteomyelitis, right femur

    M86.052   Acute hematogenous osteomyelitis, left femur

    M86.059   Acute hematogenous osteomyelitis, unspecified femur

● **M86.06   Acute hematogenous osteomyelitis, tibia and fibula**
    (Ex:) For category M86.06 CC codes: See PDX Collection 904

    M86.061   Acute hematogenous osteomyelitis, right tibia and fibula

    M86.062   Acute hematogenous osteomyelitis, left tibia and fibula

    M86.069   Acute hematogenous osteomyelitis, unspecified tibia and fibula

● **M86.07   Acute hematogenous osteomyelitis, ankle and foot**
    (Ex:) For category M86.07 CC codes: See PDX Collection 905

    M86.071   Acute hematogenous osteomyelitis, right ankle and foot

    M86.072   Acute hematogenous osteomyelitis, left ankle and foot

    M86.079   Acute hematogenous osteomyelitis, unspecified ankle and foot

    M86.08   Acute hematogenous osteomyelitis, other sites
    (Ex:) See PDX Collection 882

    M86.09   Acute hematogenous osteomyelitis, multiple sites
    (Ex:) See PDX Collection 898

● **M86.1   Other acute osteomyelitis**

    M86.10   Other acute osteomyelitis, unspecified site
    (Ex:) See PDX Collection 898

● **M86.11   Other acute osteomyelitis, shoulder**
    (Ex:) For category M86.11 CC codes: See PDX Collection 899

    M86.111   Other acute osteomyelitis, right shoulder

    M86.112   Other acute osteomyelitis, left shoulder

    M86.119   Other acute osteomyelitis, unspecified shoulder

● **M86.12   Other acute osteomyelitis, humerus**
    (Ex:) For category M86.12 CC codes: See PDX Collection 900

    M86.121   Other acute osteomyelitis, right humerus

    M86.122   Other acute osteomyelitis, left humerus

    M86.129   Other acute osteomyelitis, unspecified humerus

● **M86.13   Other acute osteomyelitis, radius and ulna**
    (Ex:) For category M86.13 CC codes: See PDX Collection 901

    M86.131   Other acute osteomyelitis, right radius and ulna

    M86.132   Other acute osteomyelitis, left radius and ulna

    M86.139   Other acute osteomyelitis, unspecified radius and ulna

● **M86.14   Other acute osteomyelitis, hand**
    (Ex:) For category M86.14 CC codes: See PDX Collection 902

    M86.141   Other acute osteomyelitis, right hand

    M86.142   Other acute osteomyelitis, left hand

    M86.149   Other acute osteomyelitis, unspecified hand

● **M86.15   Other acute osteomyelitis, femur**
    (Ex:) For category M86.15 CC codes: See PDX Collection 903

    M86.151   Other acute osteomyelitis, right femur

    M86.152   Other acute osteomyelitis, left femur

    M86.159   Other acute osteomyelitis, unspecified femur

● **M86.16   Other acute osteomyelitis, tibia and fibula**
    (Ex:) For category M86.16 CC codes: See PDX Collection 904

    M86.161   Other acute osteomyelitis, right tibia and fibula

    M86.162   Other acute osteomyelitis, left tibia and fibula

    M86.169   Other acute osteomyelitis, unspecified tibia and fibula

● **M86.17   Other acute osteomyelitis, ankle and foot**
    (Ex:) For category M86.17 CC codes: See PDX Collection 905

    M86.171   Other acute osteomyelitis, right ankle and foot

    M86.172   Other acute osteomyelitis, left ankle and foot

    M86.179   Other acute osteomyelitis, unspecified ankle and foot

    M86.18   Other acute osteomyelitis, other site
    (Ex:) See PDX Collection 882

    M86.19   Other acute osteomyelitis, multiple sites
    (Ex:) See PDX Collection 898

CHAPTER 13 (M00-M99)

N Newborn Age: 0   P Pediatric Age: 0–17   M Maternity DX: 12–55   A Adult Age: 15–124   ♀ Females Only   ♂ Males Only

  Complication\Comorbidity   Major C\C   (Ex:) CC/MCC Exclusions   Hospital-Acquired Condition

● **M86.2** Subacute osteomyelitis

  M86.20 Subacute osteomyelitis, unspecified site 🔍
    (Ex:) See PDX Collection 898

  ● **M86.21** Subacute osteomyelitis, shoulder
    (Ex:) For category M86.21 CC codes: See PDX Collection 899

    M86.211 Subacute osteomyelitis, right shoulder 🔍
    M86.212 Subacute osteomyelitis, left shoulder 🔍
    M86.219 Subacute osteomyelitis, unspecified shoulder 🔍

  ● **M86.22** Subacute osteomyelitis, humerus
    (Ex:) For category M86.22 CC codes: See PDX Collection 900

    M86.221 Subacute osteomyelitis, right humerus 🔍
    M86.222 Subacute osteomyelitis, left humerus 🔍
    M86.229 Subacute osteomyelitis, unspecified humerus 🔍

  ● **M86.23** Subacute osteomyelitis, radius and ulna
    (Ex:) For category M86.23 CC codes: See PDX Collection 901

    M86.231 Subacute osteomyelitis, right radius and ulna 🔍
    M86.232 Subacute osteomyelitis, left radius and ulna 🔍
    M86.239 Subacute osteomyelitis, unspecified radius and ulna 🔍

  ● **M86.24** Subacute osteomyelitis, hand
    (Ex:) For category M86.24 CC codes: See PDX Collection 902

    M86.241 Subacute osteomyelitis, right hand 🔍
    M86.242 Subacute osteomyelitis, left hand 🔍
    M86.249 Subacute osteomyelitis, unspecified hand 🔍

  ● **M86.25** Subacute osteomyelitis, femur
    (Ex:) For category M86.25 CC codes: See PDX Collection 903

    M86.251 Subacute osteomyelitis, right femur 🔍
    M86.252 Subacute osteomyelitis, left femur 🔍
    M86.259 Subacute osteomyelitis, unspecified femur 🔍

  ● **M86.26** Subacute osteomyelitis, tibia and fibula
    (Ex:) For category M86.26 CC codes: See PDX Collection 904

    M86.261 Subacute osteomyelitis, right tibia and fibula 🔍
    M86.262 Subacute osteomyelitis, left tibia and fibula 🔍
    M86.269 Subacute osteomyelitis, unspecified tibia and fibula 🔍

  ● **M86.27** Subacute osteomyelitis, ankle and foot
    (Ex:) For category M86.27 CC codes: See PDX Collection 905

    M86.271 Subacute osteomyelitis, right ankle and foot 🔍
    M86.272 Subacute osteomyelitis, left ankle and foot 🔍
    M86.279 Subacute osteomyelitis, unspecified ankle and foot 🔍

  M86.28 Subacute osteomyelitis, other site 🔍
    (Ex:) See PDX Collection 882

  M86.29 Subacute osteomyelitis, multiple sites 🔍
    (Ex:) See PDX Collection 898

● **M86.3** Chronic multifocal osteomyelitis
  (Ex:) For category M86.3 CC codes unless otherwise indicated: See PDX Collection 881

  M86.30 Chronic multifocal osteomyelitis, unspecified site 🔍
    (Ex:) See PDX Collection 906

  ● **M86.31** Chronic multifocal osteomyelitis, shoulder

    M86.311 Chronic multifocal osteomyelitis, right shoulder 🔍
    M86.312 Chronic multifocal osteomyelitis, left shoulder 🔍
    M86.319 Chronic multifocal osteomyelitis, unspecified shoulder 🔍

  ● **M86.32** Chronic multifocal osteomyelitis, humerus

    M86.321 Chronic multifocal osteomyelitis, right humerus 🔍
    M86.322 Chronic multifocal osteomyelitis, left humerus 🔍
    M86.329 Chronic multifocal osteomyelitis, unspecified humerus 🔍

  ● **M86.33** Chronic multifocal osteomyelitis, radius and ulna

    M86.331 Chronic multifocal osteomyelitis, right radius and ulna 🔍
    M86.332 Chronic multifocal osteomyelitis, left radius and ulna 🔍
    M86.339 Chronic multifocal osteomyelitis, unspecified radius and ulna 🔍

  ● **M86.34** Chronic multifocal osteomyelitis, hand

    M86.341 Chronic multifocal osteomyelitis, right hand 🔍
    M86.342 Chronic multifocal osteomyelitis, left hand 🔍
    M86.349 Chronic multifocal osteomyelitis, unspecified hand 🔍

  ● **M86.35** Chronic multifocal osteomyelitis, femur

    M86.351 Chronic multifocal osteomyelitis, right femur 🔍
    M86.352 Chronic multifocal osteomyelitis, left femur 🔍
    M86.359 Chronic multifocal osteomyelitis, unspecified femur 🔍

  ● **M86.36** Chronic multifocal osteomyelitis, tibia and fibula

    M86.361 Chronic multifocal osteomyelitis, right tibia and fibula 🔍
    M86.362 Chronic multifocal osteomyelitis, left tibia and fibula 🔍
    M86.369 Chronic multifocal osteomyelitis, unspecified tibia and fibula 🔍

  ● **M86.37** Chronic multifocal osteomyelitis, ankle and foot

    M86.371 Chronic multifocal osteomyelitis, right ankle and foot 🔍
    M86.372 Chronic multifocal osteomyelitis, left ankle and foot 🔍
    M86.379 Chronic multifocal osteomyelitis, unspecified ankle and foot 🔍

  M86.38 Chronic multifocal osteomyelitis, other site 🔍

  M86.39 Chronic multifocal osteomyelitis, multiple sites 🔍

▶ New   ⇒ Revised   ~~deleted~~ Deleted   Excludes 1   Excludes 2   Includes   Use additional   Code first   Code also   Key words
OGCR Official Guidelines   ● Unacceptable Principal Diagnosis   X Assign placeholder X   ● Use Additional Character(s)   ▶ Manifestation Code   **Coding Clinic**

● **M86.4   Chronic osteomyelitis with draining sinus**

    (Ex) **For category M86.4 CC codes unless otherwise indicated:** See PDX Collection 881

    M86.40   Chronic osteomyelitis with draining sinus, unspecified site 🔹

       (Ex) See PDX Collection 906

   ● **M86.41   Chronic osteomyelitis with draining sinus, shoulder**

       M86.411   Chronic osteomyelitis with draining sinus, right shoulder 🔹

       M86.412   Chronic osteomyelitis with draining sinus, left shoulder 🔹

       M86.419   Chronic osteomyelitis with draining sinus, unspecified shoulder 🔹

   ● **M86.42   Chronic osteomyelitis with draining sinus, humerus**

       M86.421   Chronic osteomyelitis with draining sinus, right humerus 🔹

       M86.422   Chronic osteomyelitis with draining sinus, left humerus 🔹

       M86.429   Chronic osteomyelitis with draining sinus, unspecified humerus 🔹

   ● **M86.43   Chronic osteomyelitis with draining sinus, radius and ulna**

       M86.431   Chronic osteomyelitis with draining sinus, right radius and ulna 🔹

       M86.432   Chronic osteomyelitis with draining sinus, left radius and ulna 🔹

       M86.439   Chronic osteomyelitis with draining sinus, unspecified radius and ulna 🔹

   ● **M86.44   Chronic osteomyelitis with draining sinus, hand**

       M86.441   Chronic osteomyelitis with draining sinus, right hand 🔹

       M86.442   Chronic osteomyelitis with draining sinus, left hand 🔹

       M86.449   Chronic osteomyelitis with draining sinus, unspecified hand 🔹

   ● **M86.45   Chronic osteomyelitis with draining sinus, femur**

       M86.451   Chronic osteomyelitis with draining sinus, right femur 🔹

       M86.452   Chronic osteomyelitis with draining sinus, left femur 🔹

       M86.459   Chronic osteomyelitis with draining sinus, unspecified femur 🔹

   ● **M86.46   Chronic osteomyelitis with draining sinus, tibia and fibula**

       M86.461   Chronic osteomyelitis with draining sinus, right tibia and fibula 🔹

       M86.462   Chronic osteomyelitis with draining sinus, left tibia and fibula 🔹

       M86.469   Chronic osteomyelitis with draining sinus, unspecified tibia and fibula 🔹

   ● **M86.47   Chronic osteomyelitis with draining sinus, ankle and foot**

       M86.471   Chronic osteomyelitis with draining sinus, right ankle and foot 🔹

       M86.472   Chronic osteomyelitis with draining sinus, left ankle and foot 🔹

       M86.479   Chronic osteomyelitis with draining sinus, unspecified ankle and foot 🔹

    M86.48   Chronic osteomyelitis with draining sinus, other site 🔹

    M86.49   Chronic osteomyelitis with draining sinus, multiple sites 🔹

● **M86.5   Other chronic hematogenous osteomyelitis**

    (Ex) **For category M86.5 CC codes unless otherwise indicated:** See PDX Collection 881

    M86.50   Other chronic hematogenous osteomyelitis, unspecified site 🔹

       (Ex) See PDX Collection 906

   ● **M86.51   Other chronic hematogenous osteomyelitis, shoulder**

       M86.511   Other chronic hematogenous osteomyelitis, right shoulder 🔹

       M86.512   Other chronic hematogenous osteomyelitis, left shoulder 🔹

       M86.519   Other chronic hematogenous osteomyelitis, unspecified shoulder 🔹

   ● **M86.52   Other chronic hematogenous osteomyelitis, humerus**

       M86.521   Other chronic hematogenous osteomyelitis, right humerus 🔹

       M86.522   Other chronic hematogenous osteomyelitis, left humerus 🔹

       M86.529   Other chronic hematogenous osteomyelitis, unspecified humerus 🔹

   ● **M86.53   Other chronic hematogenous osteomyelitis, radius and ulna**

       M86.531   Other chronic hematogenous osteomyelitis, right radius and ulna 🔹

       M86.532   Other chronic hematogenous osteomyelitis, left radius and ulna 🔹

       M86.539   Other chronic hematogenous osteomyelitis, unspecified radius and ulna 🔹

   ● **M86.54   Other chronic hematogenous osteomyelitis, hand**

       M86.541   Other chronic hematogenous osteomyelitis, right hand 🔹

       M86.542   Other chronic hematogenous osteomyelitis, left hand 🔹

       M86.549   Other chronic hematogenous osteomyelitis, unspecified hand 🔹

   ● **M86.55   Other chronic hematogenous osteomyelitis, femur**

       M86.551   Other chronic hematogenous osteomyelitis, right femur 🔹

       M86.552   Other chronic hematogenous osteomyelitis, left femur 🔹

       M86.559   Other chronic hematogenous osteomyelitis, unspecified femur 🔹

   ● **M86.56   Other chronic hematogenous osteomyelitis, tibia and fibula**

       M86.561   Other chronic hematogenous osteomyelitis, right tibia and fibula 🔹

       M86.562   Other chronic hematogenous osteomyelitis, left tibia and fibula 🔹

       M86.569   Other chronic hematogenous osteomyelitis, unspecified tibia and fibula 🔹

   ● **M86.57   Other chronic hematogenous osteomyelitis, ankle and foot**

       M86.571   Other chronic hematogenous osteomyelitis, right ankle and foot 🔹

       M86.572   Other chronic hematogenous osteomyelitis, left ankle and foot 🔹

       M86.579   Other chronic hematogenous osteomyelitis, unspecified ankle and foot 🔹

    M86.58   Other chronic hematogenous osteomyelitis, other site 🔹

    M86.59   Other chronic hematogenous osteomyelitis, multiple sites 🔹

N   Newborn Age: 0   P   Pediatric Age: 0–17   M   Maternity DX: 12–55   A   Adult Age: 15–124   ♀   Females Only   ♂   Males Only

🔹 Complication\Comorbidity   🔹 Major C\C   (Ex) CC/MCC Exclusions   🔹 Hospital-Acquired Condition

CHAPTER 13 (M00–M99)

● **M86.6 Other chronic osteomyelitis**
  (Ex:) For category M86.6 CC codes unless otherwise indicated: See PDX Collection 881

  M86.60 Other chronic osteomyelitis, unspecified site
    (Ex:) See PDX Collection 906

  ● **M86.61** Other chronic osteomyelitis, shoulder
    M86.611 Other chronic osteomyelitis, right shoulder
    M86.612 Other chronic osteomyelitis, left shoulder
    M86.619 Other chronic osteomyelitis, unspecified shoulder

  ● **M86.62** Other chronic osteomyelitis, humerus
    M86.621 Other chronic osteomyelitis, right humerus
    M86.622 Other chronic osteomyelitis, left humerus
    M86.629 Other chronic osteomyelitis, unspecified humerus

  ● **M86.63** Other chronic osteomyelitis, radius and ulna
    M86.631 Other chronic osteomyelitis, right radius and ulna
    M86.632 Other chronic osteomyelitis, left radius and ulna
    M86.639 Other chronic osteomyelitis, unspecified radius and ulna

  ● **M86.64** Other chronic osteomyelitis, hand
    M86.641 Other chronic osteomyelitis, right hand
    M86.642 Other chronic osteomyelitis, left hand
    M86.649 Other chronic osteomyelitis, unspecified hand

  ● **M86.65** Other chronic osteomyelitis, thigh
    M86.651 Other chronic osteomyelitis, right thigh
    M86.652 Other chronic osteomyelitis, left thigh
    M86.659 Other chronic osteomyelitis, unspecified thigh

  ● **M86.66** Other chronic osteomyelitis, tibia and fibula
    M86.661 Other chronic osteomyelitis, right tibia and fibula
    M86.662 Other chronic osteomyelitis, left tibia and fibula
    M86.669 Other chronic osteomyelitis, unspecified tibia and fibula

  ● **M86.67** Other chronic osteomyelitis, ankle and foot
    M86.671 Other chronic osteomyelitis, right ankle and foot
      Coding Clinic: 2016, Q1, P13
    M86.672 Other chronic osteomyelitis, left ankle and foot
    M86.679 Other chronic osteomyelitis, unspecified ankle and foot

  M86.68 Other chronic osteomyelitis, other site
  M86.69 Other chronic osteomyelitis, multiple sites

● **M86.8 Other osteomyelitis**
  Brodie's abscess
  (Ex:) For category M86.8 CC codes unless otherwise indicated: See PDX Collection 881

  ● **M86.8X** Other osteomyelitis
    M86.8X0 Other osteomyelitis, multiple sites
    M86.8X1 Other osteomyelitis, shoulder

M86.8X2 Other osteomyelitis, upper arm
M86.8X3 Other osteomyelitis, forearm
M86.8X4 Other osteomyelitis, hand
M86.8X5 Other osteomyelitis, thigh
M86.8X6 Other osteomyelitis, lower leg
M86.8X7 Other osteomyelitis, ankle and foot
M86.8X8 Other osteomyelitis, other site
M86.8X9 Other osteomyelitis, unspecified sites
  (Ex:) See PDX Collection 906

M86.9 Osteomyelitis, unspecified
  Infection of bone NOS
  Periostitis without osteomyelitis
  (Ex:) See PDX Collection 906

● **M87 Osteonecrosis**
  Includes avascular necrosis of bone
  Use additional code to identify major osseous defect, if applicable (M89.7-)
  Excludes1 juvenile osteonecrosis (M91-M92)
    osteochondropathies (M90-M93)
  (Ex:) For category M87 CC codes unless otherwise indicated: See PDX Collection 907

  ● **M87.0 Idiopathic aseptic necrosis of bone**
    M87.00 Idiopathic aseptic necrosis of unspecified bone
    ● **M87.01** Idiopathic aseptic necrosis of shoulder
      Idiopathic aseptic necrosis of clavicle and scapula
      (Ex:) For category M87.01 CC codes: See PDX Collection 908
      M87.011 Idiopathic aseptic necrosis of right shoulder
      M87.012 Idiopathic aseptic necrosis of left shoulder
      M87.019 Idiopathic aseptic necrosis of unspecified shoulder

    ● **M87.02** Idiopathic aseptic necrosis of humerus
      (Ex:) For category M87.02 CC codes: See PDX Collection 908
      M87.021 Idiopathic aseptic necrosis of right humerus
      M87.022 Idiopathic aseptic necrosis of left humerus
      M87.029 Idiopathic aseptic necrosis of unspecified humerus

    ● **M87.03** Idiopathic aseptic necrosis of radius, ulna and carpus
      M87.031 Idiopathic aseptic necrosis of right radius
      M87.032 Idiopathic aseptic necrosis of left radius
      M87.033 Idiopathic aseptic necrosis of unspecified radius
      M87.034 Idiopathic aseptic necrosis of right ulna
      M87.035 Idiopathic aseptic necrosis of left ulna
      M87.036 Idiopathic aseptic necrosis of unspecified ulna
      M87.037 Idiopathic aseptic necrosis of right carpus
      M87.038 Idiopathic aseptic necrosis of left carpus
      M87.039 Idiopathic aseptic necrosis of unspecified carpus

● **M87.04** Idiopathic aseptic necrosis of hand and fingers
     Idiopathic aseptic necrosis of metacarpals and
     phalanges of hands

   M87.041 Idiopathic aseptic necrosis of right
            hand 🖐

   M87.042 Idiopathic aseptic necrosis of left
            hand 🖐

   M87.043 Idiopathic aseptic necrosis of
            unspecified hand 🖐

   M87.044 Idiopathic aseptic necrosis of right
            finger(s) 🖐

   M87.045 Idiopathic aseptic necrosis of left
            finger(s) 🖐

   M87.046 Idiopathic aseptic necrosis of
            unspecified finger(s) 🖐

● **M87.05** Idiopathic aseptic necrosis of pelvis and femur

   M87.050 Idiopathic aseptic necrosis of
            pelvis 🖐

   M87.051 Idiopathic aseptic necrosis of right
            femur 🖐
            (Ex:) See PDX Collection 909

   M87.052 Idiopathic aseptic necrosis of left
            femur 🖐
            (Ex:) See PDX Collection 909

   M87.059 Idiopathic aseptic necrosis of
            unspecified femur 🖐
            Idiopathic aseptic necrosis of hip
            NOS
            (Ex:) See PDX Collection 909

● **M87.06** Idiopathic aseptic necrosis of tibia and fibula

   M87.061 Idiopathic aseptic necrosis of right
            tibia 🖐

   M87.062 Idiopathic aseptic necrosis of left
            tibia 🖐

   M87.063 Idiopathic aseptic necrosis of
            unspecified tibia 🖐

   M87.064 Idiopathic aseptic necrosis of right
            fibula 🖐

   M87.065 Idiopathic aseptic necrosis of left
            fibula 🖐

   M87.066 Idiopathic aseptic necrosis of
            unspecified fibula 🖐

● **M87.07** Idiopathic aseptic necrosis of ankle, foot and
          toes
     Idiopathic aseptic necrosis of metatarsus,
     tarsus, and phalanges of toes

   M87.071 Idiopathic aseptic necrosis of right
            ankle 🖐

   M87.072 Idiopathic aseptic necrosis of left
            ankle 🖐

   M87.073 Idiopathic aseptic necrosis of
            unspecified ankle 🖐

   M87.074 Idiopathic aseptic necrosis of right
            foot 🖐
            (Ex:) See PDX Collection 910

   M87.075 Idiopathic aseptic necrosis of left
            foot 🖐
            (Ex:) See PDX Collection 910

   M87.076 Idiopathic aseptic necrosis of
            unspecified foot 🖐
            (Ex:) See PDX Collection 910

   M87.077 Idiopathic aseptic necrosis of right
            toe(s) 🖐

   M87.078 Idiopathic aseptic necrosis of left
            toe(s) 🖐

   M87.079 Idiopathic aseptic necrosis of
            unspecified toe(s) 🖐

M87.08 Idiopathic aseptic necrosis of bone, other site 🖐

M87.09 Idiopathic aseptic necrosis of bone, multiple
         sites 🖐

● **M87.1** Osteonecrosis due to drugs
     Use additional code for adverse effect, if applicable,
     to identify drug (T36-T50 with fifth or sixth
     character 5)
     (Ex:) For category M87 CC codes unless otherwise indicated: See PDX
     Collection 907

   M87.10 Osteonecrosis due to drugs, unspecified bone 🖐

● **M87.11** Osteonecrosis due to drugs, shoulder

   M87.111 Osteonecrosis due to drugs, right
            shoulder 🖐

   M87.112 Osteonecrosis due to drugs, left
            shoulder 🖐

   M87.119 Osteonecrosis due to drugs,
            unspecified shoulder 🖐

● **M87.12** Osteonecrosis due to drugs, humerus
     (Ex:) For category M87.12 CC codes: See PDX Collection 908

   M87.121 Osteonecrosis due to drugs, right
            humerus 🖐

   M87.122 Osteonecrosis due to drugs, left
            humerus 🖐

   M87.129 Osteonecrosis due to drugs,
            unspecified humerus 🖐

● **M87.13** Osteonecrosis due to drugs of radius, ulna and
          carpus

   M87.131 Osteonecrosis due to drugs of right
            radius 🖐

   M87.132 Osteonecrosis due to drugs of left
            radius 🖐

   M87.133 Osteonecrosis due to drugs of
            unspecified radius 🖐

   M87.134 Osteonecrosis due to drugs of right
            ulna 🖐

   M87.135 Osteonecrosis due to drugs of left
            ulna 🖐

   M87.136 Osteonecrosis due to drugs of
            unspecified ulna 🖐

   M87.137 Osteonecrosis due to drugs of right
            carpus 🖐

   M87.138 Osteonecrosis due to drugs of left
            carpus 🖐

   M87.139 Osteonecrosis due to drugs of
            unspecified carpus 🖐

● **M87.14** Osteonecrosis due to drugs, hand and fingers

   M87.141 Osteonecrosis due to drugs, right
            hand 🖐

   M87.142 Osteonecrosis due to drugs, left
            hand 🖐

   M87.143 Osteonecrosis due to drugs,
            unspecified hand 🖐

   M87.144 Osteonecrosis due to drugs, right
            finger(s) 🖐

   M87.145 Osteonecrosis due to drugs, left
            finger(s) 🖐

   M87.146 Osteonecrosis due to drugs,
            unspecified finger(s) 🖐

● **M87.15** Osteonecrosis due to drugs, pelvis and femur
     (Ex:) For category M87.15 CC codes: See PDX Collection 909

   M87.150 Osteonecrosis due to drugs, pelvis 🖐

   M87.151 Osteonecrosis due to drugs, right
            femur 🖐

   M87.152 Osteonecrosis due to drugs, left
            femur 🖐

   M87.159 Osteonecrosis due to drugs,
            unspecified femur 🖐

CHAPTER 13 (M00-M99)

N Newborn Age: 0   P Pediatric Age: 0–17   M Maternity DX: 12–55   A Adult Age: 15–124   ♀ Females Only   ♂ Males Only
          🖐 Complication\Comorbidity   Major C\C   (Ex:) CC/MCC Exclusions   🖐 Hospital-Acquired Condition

● M87.16 Osteonecrosis due to drugs, tibia and fibula
   M87.161 Osteonecrosis due to drugs, right tibia 🐾
   M87.162 Osteonecrosis due to drugs, left tibia 🐾
   M87.163 Osteonecrosis due to drugs, unspecified tibia 🐾
   M87.164 Osteonecrosis due to drugs, right fibula 🐾
   M87.165 Osteonecrosis due to drugs, left fibula 🐾
   M87.166 Osteonecrosis due to drugs, unspecified fibula 🐾

● M87.17 Osteonecrosis due to drugs, ankle, foot and toes
   M87.171 Osteonecrosis due to drugs, right ankle 🐾
   M87.172 Osteonecrosis due to drugs, left ankle 🐾
   M87.173 Osteonecrosis due to drugs, unspecified ankle 🐾
   M87.174 Osteonecrosis due to drugs, right foot 🐾
      Ex: See PDX Collection 910
   M87.175 Osteonecrosis due to drugs, left foot 🐾
      Ex: See PDX Collection 910
   M87.176 Osteonecrosis due to drugs, unspecified foot 🐾
      Ex: See PDX Collection 910
   M87.177 Osteonecrosis due to drugs, right toe(s) 🐾
   M87.178 Osteonecrosis due to drugs, left toe(s) 🐾
   M87.179 Osteonecrosis due to drugs, unspecified toe(s) 🐾

● M87.18 Osteonecrosis due to drugs, other site
   M87.180 Osteonecrosis due to drugs, jaw 🐾
   M87.188 Osteonecrosis due to drugs, other site 🐾

M87.19 Osteonecrosis due to drugs, multiple sites 🐾

● M87.2 Osteonecrosis due to previous trauma
   Ex: For category M87 CC codes unless otherwise indicated: See PDX Collection 907

   M87.20 Osteonecrosis due to previous trauma, unspecified bone 🐾

● M87.21 Osteonecrosis due to previous trauma, shoulder
   M87.211 Osteonecrosis due to previous trauma, right shoulder 🐾
   M87.212 Osteonecrosis due to previous trauma, left shoulder 🐾
   M87.219 Osteonecrosis due to previous trauma, unspecified shoulder 🐾

● M87.22 Osteonecrosis due to previous trauma, humerus
   Ex: For category M87.22 CC codes: See PDX Collection 908
   M87.221 Osteonecrosis due to previous trauma, right humerus 🐾
   M87.222 Osteonecrosis due to previous trauma, left humerus 🐾
   M87.229 Osteonecrosis due to previous trauma, unspecified humerus 🐾

● M87.23 Osteonecrosis due to previous trauma of radius, ulna and carpus
   M87.231 Osteonecrosis due to previous trauma of right radius 🐾
   M87.232 Osteonecrosis due to previous trauma of left radius 🐾
   M87.233 Osteonecrosis due to previous trauma of unspecified radius 🐾
   M87.234 Osteonecrosis due to previous trauma of right ulna 🐾
   M87.235 Osteonecrosis due to previous trauma of left ulna 🐾
   M87.236 Osteonecrosis due to previous trauma of unspecified ulna 🐾
   M87.237 Osteonecrosis due to previous trauma of right carpus 🐾
   M87.238 Osteonecrosis due to previous trauma of left carpus 🐾
   M87.239 Osteonecrosis due to previous trauma of unspecified carpus 🐾

● M87.24 Osteonecrosis due to previous trauma, hand and fingers
   M87.241 Osteonecrosis due to previous trauma, right hand 🐾
   M87.242 Osteonecrosis due to previous trauma, left hand 🐾
   M87.243 Osteonecrosis due to previous trauma, unspecified hand 🐾
   M87.244 Osteonecrosis due to previous trauma, right finger(s) 🐾
   M87.245 Osteonecrosis due to previous trauma, left finger(s) 🐾
   M87.246 Osteonecrosis due to previous trauma, unspecified finger(s) 🐾

● M87.25 Osteonecrosis due to previous trauma, pelvis and femur
   M87.250 Osteonecrosis due to previous trauma, pelvis 🐾
   M87.251 Osteonecrosis due to previous trauma, right femur 🐾
      Ex: See PDX Collection 909
   M87.252 Osteonecrosis due to previous trauma, left femur 🐾
      Ex: See PDX Collection 909
   M87.256 Osteonecrosis due to previous trauma, unspecified femur 🐾
      Ex: See PDX Collection 909

● M87.26 Osteonecrosis due to previous trauma, tibia and fibula
   M87.261 Osteonecrosis due to previous trauma, right tibia 🐾
   M87.262 Osteonecrosis due to previous trauma, left tibia 🐾
   M87.263 Osteonecrosis due to previous trauma, unspecified tibia 🐾
   M87.264 Osteonecrosis due to previous trauma, right fibula 🐾
   M87.265 Osteonecrosis due to previous trauma, left fibula 🐾
   M87.266 Osteonecrosis due to previous trauma, unspecified fibula 🐾

▶ New ⇒ Revised ~~deleted~~ Deleted Excludes 1 Excludes 2 Includes Use additional Code first Code also Key words
OGCR Official Guidelines ● Unacceptable Principal Diagnosis X Assign placeholder X ● Use Additional Character(s) ⟩ Manifestation Code Coding Clinic

● **M87.27 Osteonecrosis due to previous trauma, ankle, foot and toes**

    M87.271 Osteonecrosis due to previous trauma, right ankle 🦴

    M87.272 Osteonecrosis due to previous trauma, left ankle 🦴

    M87.273 Osteonecrosis due to previous trauma, unspecified ankle 🦴

    M87.274 Osteonecrosis due to previous trauma, right foot 🦴
        (Ex) See PDX Collection 910

    M87.275 Osteonecrosis due to previous trauma, left foot 🦴
        (Ex) See PDX Collection 910

    M87.276 Osteonecrosis due to previous trauma, unspecified foot 🦴
        (Ex) See PDX Collection 910

    M87.277 Osteonecrosis due to previous trauma, right toe(s) 🦴

    M87.278 Osteonecrosis due to previous trauma, left toe(s) 🦴

    M87.279 Osteonecrosis due to previous trauma, unspecified toe(s) 🦴

  M87.28 Osteonecrosis due to previous trauma, other site 🦴

  M87.29 Osteonecrosis due to previous trauma, multiple sites 🦴

● **M87.3 Other secondary osteonecrosis**
    (Ex) **For category M87 CC codes unless otherwise indicated:** See PDX Collection 907

  M87.30 Other secondary osteonecrosis, unspecified bone 🦴

● **M87.31 Other secondary osteonecrosis, shoulder**

    M87.311 Other secondary osteonecrosis, right shoulder 🦴

    M87.312 Other secondary osteonecrosis, left shoulder 🦴

    M87.319 Other secondary osteonecrosis, unspecified shoulder 🦴

● **M87.32 Other secondary osteonecrosis, humerus**
    (Ex) **For category M87.32 CC codes:** See PDX Collection 908

    M87.321 Other secondary osteonecrosis, right humerus 🦴

    M87.322 Other secondary osteonecrosis, left humerus 🦴

    M87.329 Other secondary osteonecrosis, unspecified humerus 🦴

● **M87.33 Other secondary osteonecrosis of radius, ulna and carpus**

    M87.331 Other secondary osteonecrosis of right radius 🦴

    M87.332 Other secondary osteonecrosis of left radius 🦴

    M87.333 Other secondary osteonecrosis of unspecified radius 🦴

    M87.334 Other secondary osteonecrosis of right ulna 🦴

    M87.335 Other secondary osteonecrosis of left ulna 🦴

    M87.336 Other secondary osteonecrosis of unspecified ulna 🦴

    M87.337 Other secondary osteonecrosis of right carpus 🦴

    M87.338 Other secondary osteonecrosis of left carpus 🦴

    M87.339 Other secondary osteonecrosis of unspecified carpus 🦴

● **M87.34 Other secondary osteonecrosis, hand and fingers**

    M87.341 Other secondary osteonecrosis, right hand 🦴

    M87.342 Other secondary osteonecrosis, left hand 🦴

    M87.343 Other secondary osteonecrosis, unspecified hand 🦴

    M87.344 Other secondary osteonecrosis, right finger(s) 🦴

    M87.345 Other secondary osteonecrosis, left finger(s) 🦴

    M87.346 Other secondary osteonecrosis, unspecified finger(s) 🦴

● **M87.35 Other secondary osteonecrosis, pelvis and femur**
    (Ex) **For category M87.35 CC codes:** See PDX Collection 909

    M87.350 Other secondary osteonecrosis, pelvis 🦴

    M87.351 Other secondary osteonecrosis, right femur 🦴

    M87.352 Other secondary osteonecrosis, left femur 🦴

    M87.353 Other secondary osteonecrosis, unspecified femur 🦴

● **M87.36 Other secondary osteonecrosis, tibia and fibula**

    M87.361 Other secondary osteonecrosis, right tibia 🦴

    M87.362 Other secondary osteonecrosis, left tibia 🦴

    M87.363 Other secondary osteonecrosis, unspecified tibia 🦴

    M87.364 Other secondary osteonecrosis, right fibula 🦴

    M87.365 Other secondary osteonecrosis, left fibula 🦴

    M87.366 Other secondary osteonecrosis, unspecified fibula 🦴

● **M87.37 Other secondary osteonecrosis, ankle and foot**

    M87.371 Other secondary osteonecrosis, right ankle 🦴

    M87.372 Other secondary osteonecrosis, left ankle 🦴

    M87.373 Other secondary osteonecrosis, unspecified ankle 🦴

    M87.374 Other secondary osteonecrosis, right foot 🦴
        (Ex) See PDX Collection 910

    M87.375 Other secondary osteonecrosis, left foot 🦴
        (Ex) See PDX Collection 910

    M87.376 Other secondary osteonecrosis, unspecified foot 🦴
        (Ex) See PDX Collection 910

    M87.377 Other secondary osteonecrosis, right toe(s) 🦴

    M87.378 Other secondary osteonecrosis, left toe(s) 🦴

    M87.379 Other secondary osteonecrosis, unspecified toe(s) 🦴

  M87.38 Other secondary osteonecrosis, other site 🦴

  M87.39 Other secondary osteonecrosis, multiple sites 🦴

CHAPTER 13 (M00-M99)

CHAPTER 13 (M00-M99)

● **M87.8   Other osteonecrosis**
    Ⓔ For category M87 CC codes unless otherwise indicated: See PDX
    Collection 907

    M87.80   Other osteonecrosis, unspecified bone 🔒

    ● **M87.81   Other osteonecrosis, shoulder**
        M87.811   Other osteonecrosis, right shoulder 🔒
        M87.812   Other osteonecrosis, left shoulder 🔒
        M87.819   Other osteonecrosis, unspecified shoulder 🔒

    ● **M87.82   Other osteonecrosis, humerus**
        Ⓔ For category M87.82 CC codes: See PDX Collection 908
        M87.821   Other osteonecrosis, right humerus 🔒
        M87.822   Other osteonecrosis, left humerus 🔒
        M87.829   Other osteonecrosis, unspecified humerus 🔒

    ● **M87.83   Other osteonecrosis of radius, ulna and carpus**
        M87.831   Other osteonecrosis of right radius 🔒
        M87.832   Other osteonecrosis of left radius 🔒
        M87.833   Other osteonecrosis of unspecified radius 🔒
        M87.834   Other osteonecrosis of right ulna 🔒
        M87.835   Other osteonecrosis of left ulna 🔒
        M87.836   Other osteonecrosis of unspecified ulna 🔒
        M87.837   Other osteonecrosis of right carpus 🔒
        M87.838   Other osteonecrosis of left carpus 🔒
        M87.839   Other osteonecrosis of unspecified carpus 🔒

    ● **M87.84   Other osteonecrosis, hand and fingers**
        M87.841   Other osteonecrosis, right hand 🔒
        M87.842   Other osteonecrosis, left hand 🔒
        M87.843   Other osteonecrosis, unspecified hand 🔒
        M87.844   Other osteonecrosis, right finger(s) 🔒
        M87.845   Other osteonecrosis, left finger(s) 🔒
        M87.849   Other osteonecrosis, unspecified finger(s) 🔒

    ● **M87.85   Other osteonecrosis, pelvis and femur**
        Ⓔ For category M87.85 CC codes: See PDX Collection 909
        M87.850   Other osteonecrosis, pelvis 🔒
        M87.851   Other osteonecrosis, right femur 🔒
        M87.852   Other osteonecrosis, left femur 🔒
        M87.859   Other osteonecrosis, unspecified femur 🔒

    ● **M87.86   Other osteonecrosis, tibia and fibula**
        M87.861   Other osteonecrosis, right tibia 🔒
        M87.862   Other osteonecrosis, left tibia 🔒
        M87.863   Other osteonecrosis, unspecified tibia 🔒
        M87.864   Other osteonecrosis, right fibula 🔒
        M87.865   Other osteonecrosis, left fibula 🔒
        M87.869   Other osteonecrosis, unspecified fibula 🔒

    ● **M87.87   Other osteonecrosis, ankle, foot and toes**
        M87.871   Other osteonecrosis, right ankle 🔒
        M87.872   Other osteonecrosis, left ankle 🔒
        M87.873   Other osteonecrosis, unspecified ankle 🔒
        M87.874   Other osteonecrosis, right foot 🔒
          Ⓔ See PDX Collection 910
        M87.875   Other osteonecrosis, left foot 🔒
          Ⓔ See PDX Collection 910
        M87.876   Other osteonecrosis, unspecified foot 🔒
          Ⓔ See PDX Collection 910

        M87.877   Other osteonecrosis, right toe(s) 🔒
        M87.878   Other osteonecrosis, left toe(s) 🔒
        M87.879   Other osteonecrosis, unspecified toe(s) 🔒

    M87.88   Other osteonecrosis, other site 🔒
    M87.89   Other osteonecrosis, multiple sites 🔒

● **M87.9   Osteonecrosis, unspecified** 🔒
    Necrosis of bone NOS
    Ⓔ For category M87 CC codes unless otherwise indicated: See PDX
    Collection 907

● **M88   Osteitis deformans [Paget's disease of bone]**
    Chronic disorder that results in enlarged and deformed bones. The
    excessive breakdown and formation of bone tissue causes bones
    to weaken and results in bone pain, arthritis, deformities, and
    fractures.

    Excludes1   osteitis deformans in neoplastic disease (M90.6)

    M88.0   Osteitis deformans of skull
    M88.1   Osteitis deformans of vertebrae

● **M88.8   Osteitis deformans of other bones**
    ● **M88.81   Osteitis deformans of shoulder**
        M88.811   Osteitis deformans of right shoulder
        M88.812   Osteitis deformans of left shoulder
        M88.819   Osteitis deformans of unspecified shoulder

    ● **M88.82   Osteitis deformans of upper arm**
        M88.821   Osteitis deformans of right upper arm
        M88.822   Osteitis deformans of left upper arm
        M88.829   Osteitis deformans of unspecified upper arm

    ● **M88.83   Osteitis deformans of forearm**
        M88.831   Osteitis deformans of right forearm
        M88.832   Osteitis deformans of left forearm
        M88.839   Osteitis deformans of unspecified forearm

    ● **M88.84   Osteitis deformans of hand**
        M88.841   Osteitis deformans of right hand
        M88.842   Osteitis deformans of left hand
        M88.849   Osteitis deformans of unspecified hand

    ● **M88.85   Osteitis deformans of thigh**
        M88.851   Osteitis deformans of right thigh
        M88.852   Osteitis deformans of left thigh
        M88.859   Osteitis deformans of unspecified thigh

    ● **M88.86   Osteitis deformans of lower leg**
        M88.861   Osteitis deformans of right lower leg
        M88.862   Osteitis deformans of left lower leg
        M88.869   Osteitis deformans of unspecified lower leg

    ● **M88.87   Osteitis deformans of ankle and foot**
        M88.871   Osteitis deformans of right ankle and foot
        M88.872   Osteitis deformans of left ankle and foot
        M88.879   Osteitis deformans of unspecified ankle and foot

    M88.88   Osteitis deformans of other bones
        Excludes2   osteitis deformans of skull (M88.0)
                   osteitis deformans of vertebrae (M88.1)

    M88.89   Osteitis deformans of multiple sites

    M88.9   Osteitis deformans of unspecified bone

▶ New   ⇒ Revised   ~~deleted~~ Deleted   Excludes 1   Excludes 2   Includes   Use additional   Code first   Code also   Key words

OGCR Official Guidelines   ● Unacceptable Principal Diagnosis   X Assign placeholder X   ● Use Additional Character(s)   ▶ Manifestation Code   **Coding Clinic**

- M89 **Other disorders of bone**
  - M89.0 **Algoneurodystrophy**
    Shoulder-hand syndrome
    Sudeck's atrophy
    Excludes1 causalgia, lower limb (G57.7-)
    causalgia, upper limb (G56.4-)
    complex regional pain syndrome II, lower
    limb (G57.7-)
    complex regional pain syndrome II,
    upper limb (G56.4-)
    reflex sympathetic dystrophy (G90.5-)
    - M89.00 Algoneurodystrophy, unspecified site
    - M89.01 Algoneurodystrophy, shoulder
      - M89.011 Algoneurodystrophy, right shoulder
      - M89.012 Algoneurodystrophy, left shoulder
      - M89.019 Algoneurodystrophy, unspecified
        shoulder
    - M89.02 Algoneurodystrophy, upper arm
      - M89.021 Algoneurodystrophy, right upper arm
      - M89.022 Algoneurodystrophy, left upper arm
      - M89.029 Algoneurodystrophy, unspecified
        upper arm
    - M89.03 Algoneurodystrophy, forearm
      - M89.031 Algoneurodystrophy, right forearm
      - M89.032 Algoneurodystrophy, left forearm
      - M89.039 Algoneurodystrophy, unspecified
        forearm
    - M89.04 Algoneurodystrophy, hand
      - M89.041 Algoneurodystrophy, right hand
      - M89.042 Algoneurodystrophy, left hand
      - M89.049 Algoneurodystrophy, unspecified
        hand
    - M89.05 Algoneurodystrophy, thigh
      - M89.051 Algoneurodystrophy, right thigh
      - M89.052 Algoneurodystrophy, left thigh
      - M89.059 Algoneurodystrophy, unspecified
        thigh
    - M89.06 Algoneurodystrophy, lower leg
      - M89.061 Algoneurodystrophy, right lower leg
      - M89.062 Algoneurodystrophy, left lower leg
      - M89.069 Algoneurodystrophy, unspecified
        lower leg
    - M89.07 Algoneurodystrophy, ankle and foot
      - M89.071 Algoneurodystrophy, right ankle and
        foot
      - M89.072 Algoneurodystrophy, left ankle and
        foot
      - M89.079 Algoneurodystrophy, unspecified
        ankle and foot
    - M89.08 Algoneurodystrophy, other site
    - M89.09 Algoneurodystrophy, multiple sites
  - M89.1 **Physeal arrest**
    Arrest of growth plate
    Epiphyseal arrest
    Growth plate arrest
    - M89.12 Physeal arrest, humerus
      - M89.121 Complete physeal arrest, right
        proximal humerus
      - M89.122 Complete physeal arrest, left proximal
        humerus
      - M89.123 Partial physeal arrest, right proximal
        humerus
      - M89.124 Partial physeal arrest, left proximal
        humerus
      - M89.125 Complete physeal arrest, right distal
        humerus

- M89.126 Complete physeal arrest, left distal
  humerus
- M89.127 Partial physeal arrest, right distal
  humerus
- M89.128 Partial physeal arrest, left distal
  humerus
- M89.129 Physeal arrest, humerus, unspecified
- M89.13 Physeal arrest, forearm
  - M89.131 Complete physeal arrest, right distal
    radius
  - M89.132 Complete physeal arrest, left distal
    radius
  - M89.133 Partial physeal arrest, right distal
    radius
  - M89.134 Partial physeal arrest, left distal
    radius
  - M89.138 Other physeal arrest of forearm
  - M89.139 Physeal arrest, forearm, unspecified
- M89.15 Physeal arrest, femur
  - M89.151 Complete physeal arrest, right
    proximal femur
  - M89.152 Complete physeal arrest, left proximal
    femur
  - M89.153 Partial physeal arrest, right proximal
    femur
  - M89.154 Partial physeal arrest, left proximal
    femur
  - M89.155 Complete physeal arrest, right distal
    femur
  - M89.156 Complete physeal arrest, left distal
    femur
  - M89.157 Partial physeal arrest, right distal
    femur
  - M89.158 Partial physeal arrest, left distal femur
  - M89.159 Physeal arrest, femur, unspecified
- M89.16 Physeal arrest, lower leg
  - M89.160 Complete physeal arrest, right
    proximal tibia
  - M89.161 Complete physeal arrest, left proximal
    tibia
  - M89.162 Partial physeal arrest, right proximal
    tibia
  - M89.163 Partial physeal arrest, left proximal
    tibia
  - M89.164 Complete physeal arrest, right distal
    tibia
  - M89.165 Complete physeal arrest, left distal
    tibia
  - M89.166 Partial physeal arrest, right distal
    tibia
  - M89.167 Partial physeal arrest, left distal tibia
  - M89.168 Other physeal arrest of lower leg
  - M89.169 Physeal arrest, lower leg, unspecified
- M89.18 Physeal arrest, other site
- M89.2 Other disorders of bone development and growth
  - M89.20 Other disorders of bone development and
    growth, unspecified site
  - M89.21 Other disorders of bone development and
    growth, shoulder
    - M89.211 Other disorders of bone development
      and growth, right shoulder
    - M89.212 Other disorders of bone development
      and growth, left shoulder
    - M89.219 Other disorders of bone development
      and growth, unspecified shoulder

CHAPTER 13 (M00-M99)

● M89.22   Other disorders of bone development and growth, humerus

    M89.221   Other disorders of bone development and growth, right humerus

    M89.222   Other disorders of bone development and growth, left humerus

    M89.229   Other disorders of bone development and growth, unspecified humerus

● M89.23   Other disorders of bone development and growth, ulna and radius

    M89.231   Other disorders of bone development and growth, right ulna

    M89.232   Other disorders of bone development and growth, left ulna

    M89.233   Other disorders of bone development and growth, right radius

    M89.234   Other disorders of bone development and growth, left radius

    M89.239   Other disorders of bone development and growth, unspecified ulna and radius

● M89.24   Other disorders of bone development and growth, hand

    M89.241   Other disorders of bone development and growth, right hand

    M89.242   Other disorders of bone development and growth, left hand

    M89.249   Other disorders of bone development and growth, unspecified hand

● M89.25   Other disorders of bone development and growth, femur

    M89.251   Other disorders of bone development and growth, right femur

    M89.252   Other disorders of bone development and growth, left femur

    M89.259   Other disorders of bone development and growth, unspecified femur

● M89.26   Other disorders of bone development and growth, tibia and fibula

    M89.261   Other disorders of bone development and growth, right tibia

    M89.262   Other disorders of bone development and growth, left tibia

    M89.263   Other disorders of bone development and growth, right fibula

    M89.264   Other disorders of bone development and growth, left fibula

    M89.269   Other disorders of bone development and growth, unspecified lower leg

● M89.27   Other disorders of bone development and growth, ankle and foot

    M89.271   Other disorders of bone development and growth, right ankle and foot

    M89.272   Other disorders of bone development and growth, left ankle and foot

    M89.279   Other disorders of bone development and growth, unspecified ankle and foot

  M89.28   Other disorders of bone development and growth, other site

  M89.29   Other disorders of bone development and growth, multiple sites

● M89.3   Hypertrophy of bone

  M89.30   Hypertrophy of bone, unspecified site

● M89.31   Hypertrophy of bone, shoulder

    M89.311   Hypertrophy of bone, right shoulder

    M89.312   Hypertrophy of bone, left shoulder

    M89.319   Hypertrophy of bone, unspecified shoulder

● M89.32   Hypertrophy of bone, humerus

    M89.321   Hypertrophy of bone, right humerus

    M89.322   Hypertrophy of bone, left humerus

    M89.329   Hypertrophy of bone, unspecified humerus

● M89.33   Hypertrophy of bone, ulna and radius

    M89.331   Hypertrophy of bone, right ulna

    M89.332   Hypertrophy of bone, left ulna

    M89.333   Hypertrophy of bone, right radius

    M89.334   Hypertrophy of bone, left radius

    M89.339   Hypertrophy of bone, unspecified ulna and radius

● M89.34   Hypertrophy of bone, hand

    M89.341   Hypertrophy of bone, right hand

    M89.342   Hypertrophy of bone, left hand

    M89.349   Hypertrophy of bone, unspecified hand

● M89.35   Hypertrophy of bone, femur

    M89.351   Hypertrophy of bone, right femur

    M89.352   Hypertrophy of bone, left femur

    M89.359   Hypertrophy of bone, unspecified femur

● M89.36   Hypertrophy of bone, tibia and fibula

    M89.361   Hypertrophy of bone, right tibia

    M89.362   Hypertrophy of bone, left tibia

    M89.363   Hypertrophy of bone, right fibula

    M89.364   Hypertrophy of bone, left fibula

    M89.369   Hypertrophy of bone, unspecified tibia and fibula

● M89.37   Hypertrophy of bone, ankle and foot

    M89.371   Hypertrophy of bone, right ankle and foot

    M89.372   Hypertrophy of bone, left ankle and foot

    M89.379   Hypertrophy of bone, unspecified ankle and foot

  M89.38   Hypertrophy of bone, other site

  M89.39   Hypertrophy of bone, multiple sites

● M89.4   Other hypertrophic osteoarthropathy
    Marie-Bamberger disease
    Pachydermoperiostosis

  M89.40   Other hypertrophic osteoarthropathy, unspecified site

● M89.41   Other hypertrophic osteoarthropathy, shoulder

    M89.411   Other hypertrophic osteoarthropathy, right shoulder

    M89.412   Other hypertrophic osteoarthropathy, left shoulder

    M89.419   Other hypertrophic osteoarthropathy, unspecified shoulder

● M89.42   Other hypertrophic osteoarthropathy, upper arm

    M89.421   Other hypertrophic osteoarthropathy, right upper arm

    M89.422   Other hypertrophic osteoarthropathy, left upper arm

    M89.429   Other hypertrophic osteoarthropathy, unspecified upper arm

● M89.43   Other hypertrophic osteoarthropathy, forearm

    M89.431   Other hypertrophic osteoarthropathy, right forearm

    M89.432   Other hypertrophic osteoarthropathy, left forearm

    M89.439   Other hypertrophic osteoarthropathy, unspecified forearm

▶ New   ⮕ Revised   ~~deleted~~ Deleted   Excludes 1   Excludes 2   Includes   Use additional   Code first   Code also   Key words

OGCR Official Guidelines   ● Unacceptable Principal Diagnosis   X Assign placeholder X   ● Use Additional Character(s)   ▶ Manifestation Code   Coding Clinic

● M89.44   Other hypertrophic osteoarthropathy, hand
     M89.441   Other hypertrophic osteoarthropathy, right hand
     M89.442   Other hypertrophic osteoarthropathy, left hand
     M89.449   Other hypertrophic osteoarthropathy, unspecified hand
● M89.45   Other hypertrophic osteoarthropathy, thigh
     M89.451   Other hypertrophic osteoarthropathy, right thigh
     M89.452   Other hypertrophic osteoarthropathy, left thigh
     M89.459   Other hypertrophic osteoarthropathy, unspecified thigh
● M89.46   Other hypertrophic osteoarthropathy, lower leg
     M89.461   Other hypertrophic osteoarthropathy, right lower leg
     M89.462   Other hypertrophic osteoarthropathy, left lower leg
     M89.469   Other hypertrophic osteoarthropathy, unspecified lower leg
● M89.47   Other hypertrophic osteoarthropathy, ankle and foot
     M89.471   Other hypertrophic osteoarthropathy, right ankle and foot
     M89.472   Other hypertrophic osteoarthropathy, left ankle and foot
     M89.479   Other hypertrophic osteoarthropathy, unspecified ankle and foot
     M89.48   Other hypertrophic osteoarthropathy, other site
     M89.49   Other hypertrophic osteoarthropathy, multiple sites
● M89.5   Osteolysis
     Use additional code to identify major osseous defect, if applicable (M89.7-)
     Excludes2   periprosthetic osteolysis of internal prosthetic joint (T84.05-)
     M89.50   Osteolysis, unspecified site
● M89.51   Osteolysis, shoulder
     M89.511   Osteolysis, right shoulder
     M89.512   Osteolysis, left shoulder
     M89.519   Osteolysis, unspecified shoulder
● M89.52   Osteolysis, upper arm
     M89.521   Osteolysis, right upper arm
     M89.522   Osteolysis, left upper arm
     M89.529   Osteolysis, unspecified upper arm
● M89.53   Osteolysis, forearm
     M89.531   Osteolysis, right forearm
     M89.532   Osteolysis, left forearm
     M89.539   Osteolysis, unspecified forearm
● M89.54   Osteolysis, hand
     M89.541   Osteolysis, right hand
     M89.542   Osteolysis, left hand
     M89.549   Osteolysis, unspecified hand
● M89.55   Osteolysis, thigh
     M89.551   Osteolysis, right thigh
     M89.552   Osteolysis, left thigh
     M89.559   Osteolysis, unspecified thigh
● M89.56   Osteolysis, lower leg
     M89.561   Osteolysis, right lower leg
     M89.562   Osteolysis, left lower leg
     M89.569   Osteolysis, unspecified lower leg

● M89.57   Osteolysis, ankle and foot
     M89.571   Osteolysis, right ankle and foot
     M89.572   Osteolysis, left ankle and foot
     M89.579   Osteolysis, unspecified ankle and foot
     M89.58   Osteolysis, other site
     M89.59   Osteolysis, multiple sites
● M89.6   Osteopathy after poliomyelitis
     Use additional code (B91) to identify previous poliomyelitis
     Excludes1   postpolio syndrome (G14)
     M89.60   Osteopathy after poliomyelitis, unspecified site
● M89.61   Osteopathy after poliomyelitis, shoulder
     M89.611   Osteopathy after poliomyelitis, right shoulder
     M89.612   Osteopathy after poliomyelitis, left shoulder
     M89.619   Osteopathy after poliomyelitis, unspecified shoulder
● M89.62   Osteopathy after poliomyelitis, upper arm
     M89.621   Osteopathy after poliomyelitis, right upper arm
     M89.622   Osteopathy after poliomyelitis, left upper arm
     M89.629   Osteopathy after poliomyelitis, unspecified upper arm
● M89.63   Osteopathy after poliomyelitis, forearm
     M89.631   Osteopathy after poliomyelitis, right forearm
     M89.632   Osteopathy after poliomyelitis, left forearm
     M89.639   Osteopathy after poliomyelitis, unspecified forearm
● M89.64   Osteopathy after poliomyelitis, hand
     M89.641   Osteopathy after poliomyelitis, right hand
     M89.642   Osteopathy after poliomyelitis, left hand
     M89.649   Osteopathy after poliomyelitis, unspecified hand
● M89.65   Osteopathy after poliomyelitis, thigh
     M89.651   Osteopathy after poliomyelitis, right thigh
     M89.652   Osteopathy after poliomyelitis, left thigh
     M89.659   Osteopathy after poliomyelitis, unspecified thigh
● M89.66   Osteopathy after poliomyelitis, lower leg
     M89.661   Osteopathy after poliomyelitis, right lower leg
     M89.662   Osteopathy after poliomyelitis, left lower leg
     M89.669   Osteopathy after poliomyelitis, unspecified lower leg
● M89.67   Osteopathy after poliomyelitis, ankle and foot
     M89.671   Osteopathy after poliomyelitis, right ankle and foot
     M89.672   Osteopathy after poliomyelitis, left ankle and foot
     M89.679   Osteopathy after poliomyelitis, unspecified ankle and foot
     M89.68   Osteopathy after poliomyelitis, other site
     M89.69   Osteopathy after poliomyelitis, multiple sites

CHAPTER 13 (M00-M99)

● **M89.7 Major osseous defect**
Code first underlying disease, if known, such as:
aseptic necrosis of bone (M87.-)
malignant neoplasm of bone (C40.-)
osteolysis (M89.5)
osteomyelitis (M86.-)
osteonecrosis (M87.-)
osteoporosis (M80.-, M81.-)
periprosthetic osteolysis (T84.05-)

M89.70 Major osseous defect, unspecified site

● M89.71 Major osseous defect, shoulder region
Major osseous defect clavicle or scapula
  M89.711 Major osseous defect, right shoulder region
  M89.712 Major osseous defect, left shoulder region
  M89.719 Major osseous defect, unspecified shoulder region

● M89.72 Major osseous defect, humerus
  M89.721 Major osseous defect, right humerus
  M89.722 Major osseous defect, left humerus
  M89.729 Major osseous defect, unspecified humerus

● M89.73 Major osseous defect, forearm
Major osseous defect of radius and ulna
  M89.731 Major osseous defect, right forearm
  M89.732 Major osseous defect, left forearm
  M89.739 Major osseous defect, unspecified forearm

● M89.74 Major osseous defect, hand
Major osseous defect of carpus, fingers, metacarpus
  M89.741 Major osseous defect, right hand
  M89.742 Major osseous defect, left hand
  M89.749 Major osseous defect, unspecified hand

● M89.75 Major osseous defect, pelvic region and thigh
Major osseous defect of femur and pelvis
  M89.751 Major osseous defect, right pelvic region and thigh
  M89.752 Major osseous defect, left pelvic region and thigh
  M89.759 Major osseous defect, unspecified pelvic region and thigh

● M89.76 Major osseous defect, lower leg
Major osseous defect of fibula and tibia
  M89.761 Major osseous defect, right lower leg
  M89.762 Major osseous defect, left lower leg
  M89.769 Major osseous defect, unspecified lower leg

● M89.77 Major osseous defect, ankle and foot
Major osseous defect of metatarsus, tarsus, toes
  M89.771 Major osseous defect, right ankle and foot
  M89.772 Major osseous defect, left ankle and foot
  M89.779 Major osseous defect, unspecified ankle and foot

M89.78 Major osseous defect, other site
M89.79 Major osseous defect, multiple sites

● **M89.8 Other specified disorders of bone**
Infantile cortical hyperostoses
Post-traumatic subperiosteal ossification
● M89.8X Other specified disorders of bone
  M89.8X0 Other specified disorders of bone, multiple sites
  M89.8X1 Other specified disorders of bone, shoulder
  M89.8X2 Other specified disorders of bone, upper arm
  M89.8X3 Other specified disorders of bone, forearm
  M89.8X4 Other specified disorders of bone, hand
  M89.8X5 Other specified disorders of bone, thigh
  M89.8X6 Other specified disorders of bone, lower leg
  M89.8X7 Other specified disorders of bone, ankle and foot
  M89.8X8 Other specified disorders of bone, other site
  M89.8X9 Other specified disorders of bone, unspecified site

M89.9 Disorder of bone, unspecified

● **M90 Osteopathies in diseases classified elsewhere**
Excludes1 osteochondritis, osteomyelitis, and osteopathy (in):
cryptococcosis (B45.3)
diabetes mellitus (E08-E13 with .69-)
gonococcal (A54.43)
neurogenic syphilis (A52.11)
renal osteodystrophy (N25.0)
salmonellosis (A02.24)
secondary syphilis (A51.46)
syphilis (late) (A52.77)

● **M90.5 Osteonecrosis in diseases classified elsewhere**
Code first underlying disease, such as:
caisson disease (T70.3)
hemoglobinopathy (D50-D64)
(Ex) **For category M90.5 CC codes unless otherwise indicated: See PDX Collection 907**

▶ *M90.50 Osteonecrosis in diseases classified elsewhere, unspecified site* 🔍
CC when PDx is its own CC

● M90.51 Osteonecrosis in diseases classified elsewhere, shoulder
(Ex) **For category M90.51 CC codes: See PDX Collection 908**
▶ *M90.511 Osteonecrosis in diseases classified elsewhere, right shoulder* 🔍
CC when PDx is its own CC
▶ *M90.512 Osteonecrosis in diseases classified elsewhere, left shoulder* 🔍
CC when PDx is its own CC
▶ *M90.519 Osteonecrosis in diseases classified elsewhere, unspecified shoulder* 🔍
CC when PDx is its own CC

● M90.52 Osteonecrosis in diseases classified elsewhere, upper arm
▶ *M90.521 Osteonecrosis in diseases classified elsewhere, right upper arm* 🔍
CC when PDx is its own CC
▶ *M90.522 Osteonecrosis in diseases classified elsewhere, left upper arm* 🔍
CC when PDx is its own CC
▶ *M90.529 Osteonecrosis in diseases classified elsewhere, unspecified upper arm* 🔍
CC when PDx is its own CC

▶ New ⇒ Revised ~~deleted~~ Deleted Excludes 1 Excludes 2 Includes Use additional Code first Code also Key words
OGCR Official Guidelines ● Unacceptable Principal Diagnosis X Assign placeholder X ● Use Additional Character(s) ▶ Manifestation Code Coding Clinic

● **M90.53** **Osteonecrosis in diseases classified elsewhere, forearm**

▷ *M90.531*   *Osteonecrosis in diseases classified elsewhere, right forearm* 🔗
     CC when PDx is its own CC

▷ *M90.532*   *Osteonecrosis in diseases classified elsewhere, left forearm* 🔗
     CC when PDx is its own CC

▷ *M90.539*   *Osteonecrosis in diseases classified elsewhere, unspecified forearm* 🔗
     CC when PDx is its own CC

● **M90.54** **Osteonecrosis in diseases classified elsewhere, hand**

▷ *M90.541*   *Osteonecrosis in diseases classified elsewhere, right hand* 🔗
     CC when PDx is its own CC

▷ *M90.542*   *Osteonecrosis in diseases classified elsewhere, left hand* 🔗
     CC when PDx is its own CC

▷ *M90.549*   *Osteonecrosis in diseases classified elsewhere, unspecified hand* 🔗
     CC when PDx is its own CC

● **M90.55** **Osteonecrosis in diseases classified elsewhere, thigh**

     (Ex) For category M90.55 CC codes: See PDX Collection 909

▷ *M90.551*   *Osteonecrosis in diseases classified elsewhere, right thigh* 🔗
     CC when PDx is its own CC

▷ *M90.552*   *Osteonecrosis in diseases classified elsewhere, left thigh* 🔗
     CC when PDx is its own CC

▷ *M90.559*   *Osteonecrosis in diseases classified elsewhere, unspecified thigh* 🔗
     CC when PDx is its own CC

● **M90.56** **Osteonecrosis in diseases classified elsewhere, lower leg**

▷ *M90.561*   *Osteonecrosis in diseases classified elsewhere, right lower leg* 🔗
     CC when PDx is its own CC

▷ *M90.562*   *Osteonecrosis in diseases classified elsewhere, left lower leg* 🔗
     CC when PDx is its own CC

▷ *M90.569*   *Osteonecrosis in diseases classified elsewhere, unspecified lower leg* 🔗
     CC when PDx is its own CC

● **M90.57** **Osteonecrosis in diseases classified elsewhere, ankle and foot**

▷ *M90.571*   *Osteonecrosis in diseases classified elsewhere, right ankle and foot* 🔗
     CC when PDx is its own CC

▷ *M90.572*   *Osteonecrosis in diseases classified elsewhere, left ankle and foot* 🔗
     CC when PDx is its own CC

▷ *M90.579*   *Osteonecrosis in diseases classified elsewhere, unspecified ankle and foot* 🔗
     CC when PDx is its own CC

▷ *M90.58*   *Osteonecrosis in diseases classified elsewhere, other site* 🔗
     CC when PDx is its own CC

▷ *M90.59*   *Osteonecrosis in diseases classified elsewhere, multiple sites* 🔗
     CC when PDx is its own CC

● **M90.6** **Osteitis deformans in neoplastic diseases**
Osteitis deformans in malignant neoplasm of bone
Code first the neoplasm (C40.-, C41.-)

     Excludes1   osteitis deformans [Paget's disease of bone] (M88.-)

▷ *M90.60*   *Osteitis deformans in neoplastic diseases, unspecified site*

● **M90.61** **Osteitis deformans in neoplastic diseases, shoulder**

▷ *M90.611*   *Osteitis deformans in neoplastic diseases, right shoulder*

▷ *M90.612*   *Osteitis deformans in neoplastic diseases, left shoulder*

▷ *M90.619*   *Osteitis deformans in neoplastic diseases, unspecified shoulder*

● **M90.62** **Osteitis deformans in neoplastic diseases, upper arm**

▷ *M90.621*   *Osteitis deformans in neoplastic diseases, right upper arm*

▷ *M90.622*   *Osteitis deformans in neoplastic diseases, left upper arm*

▷ *M90.629*   *Osteitis deformans in neoplastic diseases, unspecified upper arm*

● **M90.63** **Osteitis deformans in neoplastic diseases, forearm**

▷ *M90.631*   *Osteitis deformans in neoplastic diseases, right forearm*

▷ *M90.632*   *Osteitis deformans in neoplastic diseases, left forearm*

▷ *M90.639*   *Osteitis deformans in neoplastic diseases, unspecified forearm*

● **M90.64** **Osteitis deformans in neoplastic diseases, hand**

▷ *M90.641*   *Osteitis deformans in neoplastic diseases, right hand*

▷ *M90.642*   *Osteitis deformans in neoplastic diseases, left hand*

▷ *M90.649*   *Osteitis deformans in neoplastic diseases, unspecified hand*

● **M90.65** **Osteitis deformans in neoplastic diseases, thigh**

▷ *M90.651*   *Osteitis deformans in neoplastic diseases, right thigh*

▷ *M90.652*   *Osteitis deformans in neoplastic diseases, left thigh*

▷ *M90.659*   *Osteitis deformans in neoplastic diseases, unspecified thigh*

● **M90.66** **Osteitis deformans in neoplastic diseases, lower leg**

▷ *M90.661*   *Osteitis deformans in neoplastic diseases, right lower leg*

▷ *M90.662*   *Osteitis deformans in neoplastic diseases, left lower leg*

▷ *M90.669*   *Osteitis deformans in neoplastic diseases, unspecified lower leg*

● **M90.67** **Osteitis deformans in neoplastic diseases, ankle and foot**

▷ *M90.671*   *Osteitis deformans in neoplastic diseases, right ankle and foot*

▷ *M90.672*   *Osteitis deformans in neoplastic diseases, left ankle and foot*

▷ *M90.679*   *Osteitis deformans in neoplastic diseases, unspecified ankle and foot*

▷ *M90.68*   *Osteitis deformans in neoplastic diseases, other site*

▷ *M90.69*   *Osteitis deformans in neoplastic diseases, multiple sites*

CHAPTER 13 (M00-M99)

CHAPTER 13 (M00-M99)

● **M90.8 Osteopathy in diseases classified elsewhere**
   Code first underlying disease, such as:
      rickets (E55.0)
      vitamin-D-resistant rickets (E83.3)
   ◗ *M90.80 Osteopathy in diseases classified elsewhere,*
      unspecified site
● **M90.81 Osteopathy in diseases classified elsewhere,**
   shoulder
      ◗ *M90.811 Osteopathy in diseases classified*
         elsewhere, right shoulder
      ◗ *M90.812 Osteopathy in diseases classified*
         elsewhere, left shoulder
      ◗ *M90.819 Osteopathy in diseases classified*
         elsewhere, unspecified shoulder
● **M90.82 Osteopathy in diseases classified elsewhere,**
   upper arm
      ◗ *M90.821 Osteopathy in diseases classified*
         elsewhere, right upper arm
      ◗ *M90.822 Osteopathy in diseases classified*
         elsewhere, left upper arm
      ◗ *M90.829 Osteopathy in diseases classified*
         elsewhere, unspecified upper arm
● **M90.83 Osteopathy in diseases classified elsewhere,**
   forearm
      ◗ *M90.831 Osteopathy in diseases classified*
         elsewhere, right forearm
      ◗ *M90.832 Osteopathy in diseases classified*
         elsewhere, left forearm
      ◗ *M90.839 Osteopathy in diseases classified*
         elsewhere, unspecified forearm
● **M90.84 Osteopathy in diseases classified elsewhere,**
   hand
      ◗ *M90.841 Osteopathy in diseases classified*
         elsewhere, right hand
      ◗ *M90.842 Osteopathy in diseases classified*
         elsewhere, left hand
      ◗ *M90.849 Osteopathy in diseases classified*
         elsewhere, unspecified hand
● **M90.85 Osteopathy in diseases classified**
   elsewhere, thigh
      ◗ *M90.851 Osteopathy in diseases classified*
         elsewhere, right thigh
      ◗ *M90.852 Osteopathy in diseases classified*
         elsewhere, left thigh
      ◗ *M90.859 Osteopathy in diseases classified*
         elsewhere, unspecified thigh
● **M90.86 Osteopathy in diseases classified elsewhere,**
   lower leg
      ◗ *M90.861 Osteopathy in diseases classified*
         elsewhere, right lower leg
      ◗ *M90.862 Osteopathy in diseases classified*
         elsewhere, left lower leg
      ◗ *M90.869 Osteopathy in diseases classified*
         elsewhere, unspecified lower leg
● **M90.87 Osteopathy in diseases classified elsewhere,**
   ankle and foot
      ◗ *M90.871 Osteopathy in diseases classified*
         elsewhere, right ankle and foot
      ◗ *M90.872 Osteopathy in diseases classified*
         elsewhere, left ankle and foot
      ◗ *M90.879 Osteopathy in diseases classified*
         elsewhere, unspecified ankle and foot
   ◗ *M90.88 Osteopathy in diseases classified elsewhere,*
      other site
   ◗ *M90.89 Osteopathy in diseases classified elsewhere,*
      multiple sites

CHONDROPATHIES (M91-M94)

   Excludes1 postprocedural chondropathies (M96.-)

● **M91 Juvenile osteochondrosis of hip and pelvis**
   Excludes1 slipped upper femoral epiphysis (nontraumatic)
      (M93.0)
   M91.0 Juvenile osteochondrosis of pelvis
      Osteochondrosis (juvenile) of acetabulum
      Osteochondrosis (juvenile) of iliac crest [Buchanan]
      Osteochondrosis (juvenile) of ischiopubic synchondrosis
         [van Neck]
      Osteochondrosis (juvenile) of symphysis pubis [Pierson]
● **M91.1 Juvenile osteochondrosis of head of femur [Legg-Calvé-**
   Perthes]
      M91.10 Juvenile osteochondrosis of head of femur
         [Legg-Calvé-Perthes], unspecified leg
      M91.11 Juvenile osteochondrosis of head of femur
         [Legg-Calvé-Perthes], right leg
      M91.12 Juvenile osteochondrosis of head of femur
         [Legg-Calvé-Perthes], left leg
● **M91.2 Coxa plana**
      Hip deformity due to previous juvenile osteochondrosis
      M91.20 Coxa plana, unspecified hip
      M91.21 Coxa plana, right hip
      M91.22 Coxa plana, left hip
● **M91.3 Pseudocoxalgia**
      M91.30 Pseudocoxalgia, unspecified hip
      M91.31 Pseudocoxalgia, right hip
      M91.32 Pseudocoxalgia, left hip
● **M91.4 Coxa magna**
      M91.40 Coxa magna, unspecified hip
      M91.41 Coxa magna, right hip
      M91.42 Coxa magna, left hip
● **M91.8 Other juvenile osteochondrosis of hip and pelvis**
      Juvenile osteochondrosis after reduction of congenital
         dislocation of hip
      M91.80 Other juvenile osteochondrosis of hip and
         pelvis, unspecified leg
      M91.81 Other juvenile osteochondrosis of hip and
         pelvis, right leg
      M91.82 Other juvenile osteochondrosis of hip and
         pelvis, left leg
● **M91.9 Juvenile osteochondrosis of hip and pelvis, unspecified**
      M91.90 Juvenile osteochondrosis of hip and pelvis,
         unspecified, unspecified leg
      M91.91 Juvenile osteochondrosis of hip and pelvis,
         unspecified, right leg
      M91.92 Juvenile osteochondrosis of hip and pelvis,
         unspecified, left leg
● **M92 Other juvenile osteochondrosis**
● **M92.0 Juvenile osteochondrosis of humerus**
      Osteochondrosis (juvenile) of capitulum of humerus
         [Panner]
      Osteochondrosis (juvenile) of head of humerus [Haas]
      M92.00 Juvenile osteochondrosis of humerus,
         unspecified arm
      M92.01 Juvenile osteochondrosis of humerus, right arm
      M92.02 Juvenile osteochondrosis of humerus, left arm
● **M92.1 Juvenile osteochondrosis of radius and ulna**
      Osteochondrosis (juvenile) of lower ulna [Burns]
      Osteochondrosis (juvenile) of radial head [Brailsford]
      M92.10 Juvenile osteochondrosis of radius and ulna,
         unspecified arm
      M92.11 Juvenile osteochondrosis of radius and ulna,
         right arm
      M92.12 Juvenile osteochondrosis of radius and ulna,
         left arm

▶ New   ⇒ Revised   ~~deleted~~ Deleted   Excludes 1   Excludes 2   Includes   Use additional   Code first   Code also   Key words
OGCR Official Guidelines   ● Unacceptable Principal Diagnosis   X Assign placeholder X   ● Use Additional Character(s)   ◗ Manifestation Code   **Coding Clinic**

● M92.2 Juvenile osteochondrosis, hand
  ● M92.20 Unspecified juvenile osteochondrosis, hand
    M92.201 Unspecified juvenile osteochondrosis, right hand
    M92.202 Unspecified juvenile osteochondrosis, left hand
    M92.209 Unspecified juvenile osteochondrosis, unspecified hand
  ● M92.21 Osteochondrosis (juvenile) of carpal lunate [Kienböck]
    M92.211 Osteochondrosis (juvenile) of carpal lunate [Kienböck], right hand
    M92.212 Osteochondrosis (juvenile) of carpal lunate [Kienböck], left hand
    M92.219 Osteochondrosis (juvenile) of carpal lunate [Kienböck], unspecified hand
  ● M92.22 Osteochondrosis (juvenile) of metacarpal heads [Mauclaire]
    M92.221 Osteochondrosis (juvenile) of metacarpal heads [Mauclaire], right hand
    M92.222 Osteochondrosis (juvenile) of metacarpal heads [Mauclaire], left hand
    M92.229 Osteochondrosis (juvenile) of metacarpal heads [Mauclaire], unspecified hand
  ● M92.29 Other juvenile osteochondrosis, hand
    M92.291 Other juvenile osteochondrosis, right hand
    M92.292 Other juvenile osteochondrosis, left hand
    M92.299 Other juvenile osteochondrosis, unspecified hand
● M92.3 Other juvenile osteochondrosis, upper limb
  M92.30 Other juvenile osteochondrosis, unspecified upper limb
  M92.31 Other juvenile osteochondrosis, right upper limb
  M92.32 Other juvenile osteochondrosis, left upper limb
● M92.4 Juvenile osteochondrosis of patella
  Osteochondrosis (juvenile) of primary patellar center [Köhler]
  Osteochondrosis (juvenile) of secondary patellar center [Sinding Larsen]
  M92.40 Juvenile osteochondrosis of patella, unspecified knee
  M92.41 Juvenile osteochondrosis of patella, right knee
  M92.42 Juvenile osteochondrosis of patella, left knee
● M92.5 Juvenile osteochondrosis of tibia and fibula
  Osteochondrosis (juvenile) of proximal tibia [Blount]
  Osteochondrosis (juvenile) of tibial tubercle [Osgood-Schlatter]
  Tibia vara
  M92.50 Juvenile osteochondrosis of tibia and fibula, unspecified leg
  M92.51 Juvenile osteochondrosis of tibia and fibula, right leg
  M92.52 Juvenile osteochondrosis of tibia and fibula, left leg
● M92.6 Juvenile osteochondrosis of tarsus
  Osteochondrosis (juvenile) of calcaneum [Sever]
  Osteochondrosis (juvenile) of os tibiale externum [Haglund]
  Osteochondrosis (juvenile) of talus [Diaz]
  Osteochondrosis (juvenile) of tarsal navicular [Köhler]
  M92.60 Juvenile osteochondrosis of tarsus, unspecified ankle
  M92.61 Juvenile osteochondrosis of tarsus, right ankle
  M92.62 Juvenile osteochondrosis of tarsus, left ankle

● M92.7 Juvenile osteochondrosis of metatarsus
  Osteochondrosis (juvenile) of fifth metatarsus [Iselin]
  Osteochondrosis (juvenile) of second metatarsus [Freiberg]
  M92.70 Juvenile osteochondrosis of metatarsus, unspecified foot
  M92.71 Juvenile osteochondrosis of metatarsus, right foot
  M92.72 Juvenile osteochondrosis of metatarsus, left foot
M92.8 Other specified juvenile osteochondrosis
  Calcaneal apophysitis
M92.9 Juvenile osteochondrosis, unspecified
  Juvenile apophysitis NOS
  Juvenile epiphysitis NOS
  Juvenile osteochondritis NOS
  Juvenile osteochondrosis NOS
● M93 Other osteochondropathies
  Excludes2 osteochondrosis of spine (M42.-)
● M93.0 Slipped upper femoral epiphysis (nontraumatic)
  Use additional code for associated chondrolysis (M94.3)
  ● M93.00 Unspecified slipped upper femoral epiphysis (nontraumatic)
    M93.001 Unspecified slipped upper femoral epiphysis (nontraumatic), right hip
    M93.002 Unspecified slipped upper femoral epiphysis (nontraumatic), left hip
    M93.003 Unspecified slipped upper femoral epiphysis (nontraumatic), unspecified hip
  ● M93.01 Acute slipped upper femoral epiphysis (nontraumatic)
    M93.011 Acute slipped upper femoral epiphysis (nontraumatic), right hip
    M93.012 Acute slipped upper femoral epiphysis (nontraumatic), left hip
    M93.013 Acute slipped upper femoral epiphysis (nontraumatic), unspecified hip
  ● M93.02 Chronic slipped upper femoral epiphysis (nontraumatic)
    M93.021 Chronic slipped upper femoral epiphysis (nontraumatic), right hip
    M93.022 Chronic slipped upper femoral epiphysis (nontraumatic), left hip
    M93.023 Chronic slipped upper femoral epiphysis (nontraumatic), unspecified hip
  ● M93.03 Acute on chronic slipped upper femoral epiphysis (nontraumatic)
    M93.031 Acute on chronic slipped upper femoral epiphysis (nontraumatic), right hip
    M93.032 Acute on chronic slipped upper femoral epiphysis (nontraumatic), left hip
    M93.033 Acute on chronic slipped upper femoral epiphysis (nontraumatic), unspecified hip
M93.1 Kienböck's disease of adults   A
  Adult osteochondrosis of carpal lunates
● M93.2 Osteochondritis dissecans
  M93.20 Osteochondritis dissecans of unspecified site
  ● M93.21 Osteochondritis dissecans of shoulder
    M93.211 Osteochondritis dissecans, right shoulder
    M93.212 Osteochondritis dissecans, left shoulder
    M93.219 Osteochondritis dissecans, unspecified shoulder

CHAPTER 13 (M00-M99)

● M93.22 Osteochondritis dissecans of elbow
    M93.221 Osteochondritis dissecans, right elbow
    M93.222 Osteochondritis dissecans, left elbow
    M93.229 Osteochondritis dissecans, unspecified elbow

● M93.23 Osteochondritis dissecans of wrist
    M93.231 Osteochondritis dissecans, right wrist
    M93.232 Osteochondritis dissecans, left wrist
    M93.239 Osteochondritis dissecans, unspecified wrist

● M93.24 Osteochondritis dissecans of joints of hand
    M93.241 Osteochondritis dissecans, joints of right hand
    M93.242 Osteochondritis dissecans, joints of left hand
    M93.249 Osteochondritis dissecans, joints of unspecified hand

● M93.25 Osteochondritis dissecans of hip
    M93.251 Osteochondritis dissecans, right hip
    M93.252 Osteochondritis dissecans, left hip
    M93.259 Osteochondritis dissecans, unspecified hip

● M93.26 Osteochondritis dissecans knee
    M93.261 Osteochondritis dissecans, right knee
    M93.262 Osteochondritis dissecans, left knee
    M93.269 Osteochondritis dissecans, unspecified knee

● M93.27 Osteochondritis dissecans of ankle and joints of foot
    M93.271 Osteochondritis dissecans, right ankle and joints of right foot
    M93.272 Osteochondritis dissecans, left ankle and joints of left foot
    M93.279 Osteochondritis dissecans, unspecified ankle and joints of foot

    M93.28 Osteochondritis dissecans other site
    M93.29 Osteochondritis dissecans multiple sites

● M93.8 Other specified osteochondropathies
    M93.80 Other specified osteochondropathies of unspecified site

● M93.81 Other specified osteochondropathies of shoulder
    M93.811 Other specified osteochondropathies, right shoulder
    M93.812 Other specified osteochondropathies, left shoulder
    M93.819 Other specified osteochondropathies, unspecified shoulder

● M93.82 Other specified osteochondropathies of upper arm
    M93.821 Other specified osteochondropathies, right upper arm
    M93.822 Other specified osteochondropathies, left upper arm
    M93.829 Other specified osteochondropathies, unspecified upper arm

● M93.83 Other specified osteochondropathies of forearm
    M93.831 Other specified osteochondropathies, right forearm
    M93.832 Other specified osteochondropathies, left forearm
    M93.839 Other specified osteochondropathies, unspecified forearm

● M93.84 Other specified osteochondropathies of hand
    M93.841 Other specified osteochondropathies, right hand
    M93.842 Other specified osteochondropathies, left hand
    M93.849 Other specified osteochondropathies, unspecified hand

● M93.85 Other specified osteochondropathies of thigh
    M93.851 Other specified osteochondropathies, right thigh
    M93.852 Other specified osteochondropathies, left thigh
    M93.859 Other specified osteochondropathies, unspecified thigh

● M93.86 Other specified osteochondropathies lower leg
    M93.861 Other specified osteochondropathies, right lower leg
    M93.862 Other specified osteochondropathies, left lower leg
    M93.869 Other specified osteochondropathies, unspecified lower leg

● M93.87 Other specified osteochondropathies of ankle and foot
    M93.871 Other specified osteochondropathies, right ankle and foot
    M93.872 Other specified osteochondropathies, left ankle and foot
    M93.879 Other specified osteochondropathies, unspecified ankle and foot

    M93.88 Other specified osteochondropathies other
    M93.89 Other specified osteochondropathies multiple sites

M93.9 Osteochondropathy, unspecified
    Apophysitis NOS
    Epiphysitis NOS
    Osteochondritis NOS
    Osteochondrosis NOS

    M93.90 Osteochondropathy, unspecified of unspecified site

● M93.91 Osteochondropathy, unspecified of shoulder
    M93.911 Osteochondropathy, unspecified, right shoulder
    M93.912 Osteochondropathy, unspecified, left shoulder
    M93.919 Osteochondropathy, unspecified, unspecified shoulder

● M93.92 Osteochondropathy, unspecified of upper arm
    M93.921 Osteochondropathy, unspecified, right upper arm
    M93.922 Osteochondropathy, unspecified, left upper arm
    M93.929 Osteochondropathy, unspecified, unspecified upper arm

● M93.93 Osteochondropathy, unspecified of forearm
    M93.931 Osteochondropathy, unspecified, right forearm
    M93.932 Osteochondropathy, unspecified, left forearm
    M93.939 Osteochondropathy, unspecified, unspecified forearm

● M93.94 Osteochondropathy, unspecified of hand
    M93.941 Osteochondropathy, unspecified, right hand
    M93.942 Osteochondropathy, unspecified, left hand
    M93.949 Osteochondropathy, unspecified, unspecified hand

● M93.95 Osteochondropathy, unspecified of thigh
      M93.951 Osteochondropathy, unspecified, right thigh
      M93.952 Osteochondropathy, unspecified, left thigh
      M93.959 Osteochondropathy, unspecified, unspecified thigh
● M93.96 Osteochondropathy, unspecified lower leg
      M93.961 Osteochondropathy, unspecified, right lower leg
      M93.962 Osteochondropathy, unspecified, left lower leg
      M93.969 Osteochondropathy, unspecified, unspecified lower leg
● M93.97 Osteochondropathy, unspecified of ankle and foot
      M93.971 Osteochondropathy, unspecified, right ankle and foot
      M93.972 Osteochondropathy, unspecified, left ankle and foot
      M93.979 Osteochondropathy, unspecified, unspecified ankle and foot
   M93.98 Osteochondropathy, unspecified other
   M93.99 Osteochondropathy, unspecified multiple sites

● M94 Other disorders of cartilage
   M94.0 Chondrocostal junction syndrome [Tietze]
          Costochondritis
   M94.1 Relapsing polychondritis
● M94.2 Chondromalacia
      Excludes1   chondromalacia patellae (M22.4)
   M94.20 Chondromalacia, unspecified site
● M94.21 Chondromalacia, shoulder
      M94.211 Chondromalacia, right shoulder
      M94.212 Chondromalacia, left shoulder
      M94.219 Chondromalacia, unspecified shoulder
● M94.22 Chondromalacia, elbow
      M94.221 Chondromalacia, right elbow
      M94.222 Chondromalacia, left elbow
      M94.229 Chondromalacia, unspecified elbow
● M94.23 Chondromalacia, wrist
      M94.231 Chondromalacia, right wrist
      M94.232 Chondromalacia, left wrist
      M94.239 Chondromalacia, unspecified wrist
● M94.24 Chondromalacia, joints of hand
      M94.241 Chondromalacia, joints of right hand
      M94.242 Chondromalacia, joints of left hand
      M94.249 Chondromalacia, joints of unspecified hand
● M94.25 Chondromalacia, hip
      M94.251 Chondromalacia, right hip
      M94.252 Chondromalacia, left hip
      M94.259 Chondromalacia, unspecified hip
● M94.26 Chondromalacia, knee
      M94.261 Chondromalacia, right knee
      M94.262 Chondromalacia, left knee
      M94.269 Chondromalacia, unspecified knee
● M94.27 Chondromalacia, ankle and joints of foot
      M94.271 Chondromalacia, right ankle and joints of right foot
      M94.272 Chondromalacia, left ankle and joints of left foot
      M94.279 Chondromalacia, unspecified ankle and joints of foot
   M94.28 Chondromalacia, other site
   M94.29 Chondromalacia, multiple sites

● M94.3 Chondrolysis
      Code first any associated slipped upper femoral epiphysis (nontraumatic) (M93.0-)
● M94.35 Chondrolysis, hip
      M94.351 Chondrolysis, right hip
      M94.352 Chondrolysis, left hip
      M94.359 Chondrolysis, unspecified hip
● M94.8 Other specified disorders of cartilage
● M94.8X Other specified disorders of cartilage
      M94.8X0 Other specified disorders of cartilage, multiple sites
      M94.8X1 Other specified disorders of cartilage, shoulder
      M94.8X2 Other specified disorders of cartilage, upper arm
      M94.8X3 Other specified disorders of cartilage, forearm
      M94.8X4 Other specified disorders of cartilage, hand
      M94.8X5 Other specified disorders of cartilage, thigh
      M94.8X6 Other specified disorders of cartilage, lower leg
      M94.8X7 Other specified disorders of cartilage, ankle and foot
      M94.8X8 Other specified disorders of cartilage, other site
      M94.8X9 Other specified disorders of cartilage, unspecified sites
   M94.9 Disorder of cartilage, unspecified

OTHER DISORDERS OF THE MUSCULOSKELETAL SYSTEM AND CONNECTIVE TISSUE (M95)

● M95 Other acquired deformities of musculoskeletal system and connective tissue
      Excludes2   acquired absence of limbs and organs (Z89-Z90)
                       acquired deformities of limbs (M20-M21)
                       congenital malformations and deformations of the musculoskeletal system (Q65-Q79)
                       deforming dorsopathies (M40-M43)
                       dentofacial anomalies [including malocclusion] (M26.-)
                       postprocedural musculoskeletal disorders (M96.-)
   M95.0 Acquired deformity of nose
      Excludes2   deviated nasal septum (J34.2)
● M95.1 Cauliflower ear
      Excludes2   other acquired deformities of ear (H61.1)
      M95.10 Cauliflower ear, unspecified ear
      M95.11 Cauliflower ear, right ear
      M95.12 Cauliflower ear, left ear
   M95.2 Other acquired deformity of head
   M95.3 Acquired deformity of neck
   M95.4 Acquired deformity of chest and rib
   M95.5 Acquired deformity of pelvis
      Excludes1   maternal care for known or suspected disproportion (O33.-)
   M95.8 Other specified acquired deformities of musculoskeletal system
   M95.9 Acquired deformity of musculoskeletal system, unspecified

N Newborn Age: 0   **P** Pediatric Age: 0–17   **M** Maternity DX: 12–55   **A** Adult Age: 15–124   ♀ Females Only   ♂ Males Only

 Complication\Comorbidity   Major C\C   (Ex) CC/MCC Exclusions   Hospital-Acquired Condition

1091

CHAPTER 13 (M00-M99)

INTRAOPERATIVE AND POSTPROCEDURAL COMPLICATIONS AND DISORDERS OF MUSCULOSKELETAL SYSTEM, NOT ELSEWHERE CLASSIFIED (M96)

M96 **Intraoperative and postprocedural complications and disorders of musculoskeletal system, not elsewhere classified**

    Excludes2   arthropathy following intestinal bypass (M02.0-)
                complications of internal orthopedic prosthetic devices, implants and grafts (T84.-)
                disorders associated with osteoporosis (M80)
                periprosthetic fracture around internal prosthetic joint (M97.-)
                presence of functional implants and other devices (Z96-Z97)

  M96.0 **Pseudarthrosis after fusion or arthrodesis**
        (Ex) No exclusions

  M96.1 **Postlaminectomy syndrome, not elsewhere classified**

  M96.2 **Postradiation kyphosis**

  M96.3 **Postlaminectomy kyphosis**

  M96.4 **Postsurgical lordosis**

  M96.5 **Postradiation scoliosis**

  M96.6 **Fracture of bone following insertion of orthopedic implant, joint prosthesis, or bone plate**
       Intraoperative fracture of bone during insertion of orthopedic implant, joint prosthesis, or bone plate
       Excludes2   complication of internal orthopedic devices, implants or grafts (T84.-)
       (Ex) For category M96.6 CC codes: See PDX Collection 911

    M96.62 **Fracture of humerus following insertion of orthopedic implant, joint prosthesis, or bone plate**
       M96.621 Fracture of humerus following insertion of orthopedic implant, joint prosthesis, or bone plate, right arm
       M96.622 Fracture of humerus following insertion of orthopedic implant, joint prosthesis, or bone plate, left arm
       M96.629 Fracture of humerus following insertion of orthopedic implant, joint prosthesis, or bone plate, unspecified arm

    M96.63 **Fracture of radius or ulna following insertion of orthopedic implant, joint prosthesis, or bone plate**
       M96.631 Fracture of radius or ulna following insertion of orthopedic implant, joint prosthesis, or bone plate, right arm
       M96.632 Fracture of radius or ulna following insertion of orthopedic implant, joint prosthesis, or bone plate, left arm
       M96.639 Fracture of radius or ulna following insertion of orthopedic implant, joint prosthesis, or bone plate, unspecified arm

    M96.65 **Fracture of pelvis following insertion of orthopedic implant, joint prosthesis, or bone plate**

    M96.66 **Fracture of femur following insertion of orthopedic implant, joint prosthesis, or bone plate**
       M96.661 Fracture of femur following insertion of orthopedic implant, joint prosthesis, or bone plate, right leg
       M96.662 Fracture of femur following insertion of orthopedic implant, joint prosthesis, or bone plate, left leg
       M96.669 Fracture of femur following insertion of orthopedic implant, joint prosthesis, or bone plate, unspecified leg

    M96.67 **Fracture of tibia or fibula following insertion of orthopedic implant, joint prosthesis, or bone plate**
       M96.671 Fracture of tibia or fibula following insertion of orthopedic implant, joint prosthesis, or bone plate, right leg
       M96.672 Fracture of tibia or fibula following insertion of orthopedic implant, joint prosthesis, or bone plate, left leg
       M96.679 Fracture of tibia or fibula following insertion of orthopedic implant, joint prosthesis, or bone plate, unspecified leg

    M96.69 **Fracture of other bone following insertion of orthopedic implant, joint prosthesis, or bone plate**

  M96.8 **Other intraoperative and postprocedural complications and disorders of musculoskeletal system, not elsewhere classified**
       Coding Clinic: 2016, Q4, P10

    M96.81 **Intraoperative hemorrhage and hematoma of a musculoskeletal structure complicating a procedure**
       Excludes1   intraoperative hemorrhage and hematoma of a musculoskeletal structure due to accidental puncture and laceration during a procedure (M96.82-)
       (Ex) For category M96.81 CC codes: See PDX Collection 912
       M96.810 Intraoperative hemorrhage and hematoma of a musculoskeletal structure complicating a musculoskeletal system procedure
       M96.811 Intraoperative hemorrhage and hematoma of a musculoskeletal structure complicating other procedure

    M96.82 **Accidental puncture and laceration of a musculoskeletal structure during a procedure**
       (Ex) For category M96.82 CC codes: See PDX Collection 509
       M96.820 Accidental puncture and laceration of a musculoskeletal structure during a musculoskeletal system procedure
       M96.821 Accidental puncture and laceration of a musculoskeletal structure during other procedure

    M96.83 **Postprocedural hemorrhage of a musculoskeletal structure following a procedure**
       (Ex) For category M96.83 CC codes: See PDX Collection 912
       M96.830 Postprocedural hemorrhage of a musculoskeletal structure following a musculoskeletal system procedure
       M96.831 Postprocedural hemorrhage of a musculoskeletal structure following other procedure

    M96.84 **Postprocedural hematoma and seroma of a musculoskeletal structure following a procedure**
       (Ex) For category M96.84 CC codes: See PDX Collection 912
       M96.840 Postprocedural hematoma of a musculoskeletal structure following a musculoskeletal system procedure
       M96.841 Postprocedural hematoma of a musculoskeletal structure following other procedure
          Coding Clinic: 2016, Q4, P10

M96.842 **Postprocedural seroma of a musculoskeletal structure following a musculoskeletal system procedure** 🔹

M96.843 **Postprocedural seroma of a musculoskeletal structure following other procedure** 🔹

M96.89 **Other intraoperative and postprocedural complications and disorders of the musculoskeletal system** 🔹
Instability of joint secondary to removal of joint prosthesis
Use additional code, if applicable, to further specify disorder
(Ex) See PDX Collection 643

PERIPROSTHETIC FRACTURE AROUND INTERNAL PROSTHETIC JOINT (M97)

● M97 **Periprosthetic fracture around internal prosthetic joint**
Excludes2 fracture of bone following insertion of orthopedic implant, joint prosthesis or bone plate (M96.6-)
breakage (fracture) of prosthetic joint (T84.01-)
Coding Clinic: 2016, Q4, P42

The appropriate 7th character is to be added to each code from category M97:

A	initial encounter
D	subsequent encounter
S	sequela

(Ex) For category M97 CC codes: See PDX Collection 911

● M97.0 **Periprosthetic fracture around internal prosthetic hip joint**
X● M97.01 **Periprosthetic fracture around internal prosthetic right hip joint** A 🔹
Coding Clinic: 2016, Q4, P43
X● M97.02 **Periprosthetic fracture around internal prosthetic left hip joint** A 🔹

● M97.1 **Periprosthetic fracture around internal prosthetic knee joint**
X● M97.11 **Periprosthetic fracture around internal prosthetic right knee joint** A 🔹
X● M97.12 **Periprosthetic fracture around internal prosthetic left knee joint** A 🔹

● M97.2 **Periprosthetic fracture around internal prosthetic ankle joint**
X● M97.21 **Periprosthetic fracture around internal prosthetic right ankle joint** A 🔹
X● M97.22 **Periprosthetic fracture around internal prosthetic left ankle joint** A 🔹

● M97.3 **Periprosthetic fracture around internal prosthetic shoulder joint**
X● M97.31 **Periprosthetic fracture around internal prosthetic right shoulder joint** A 🔹
X● M97.32 **Periprosthetic fracture around internal prosthetic left shoulder joint** A 🔹

● M97.4 **Periprosthetic fracture around internal prosthetic elbow joint**
X● M97.41 **Periprosthetic fracture around internal prosthetic right elbow joint** A 🔹
X● M97.42 **Periprosthetic fracture around internal prosthetic left elbow joint** A 🔹

X● M97.8 **Periprosthetic fracture around other internal prosthetic joint** A 🔹
Periprosthetic fracture around internal prosthetic finger joint
Periprosthetic fracture around internal prosthetic spinal joint
Periprosthetic fracture around internal prosthetic toe joint
Periprosthetic fracture around internal prosthetic wrist joint
Use additional code to identify the joint (Z96.6-)
X● M97.9 **Periprosthetic fracture around unspecified internal prosthetic joint** A 🔹

BIOMECHANICAL LESIONS, NOT ELSEWHERE CLASSIFIED (M99)

● M99 **Biomechanical lesions, not elsewhere classified**
Note: This category should not be used if the condition can be classified elsewhere.

● M99.0 **Segmental and somatic dysfunction**
M99.00 **Segmental and somatic dysfunction of head region**
M99.01 **Segmental and somatic dysfunction of cervical region**
M99.02 **Segmental and somatic dysfunction of thoracic region**
M99.03 **Segmental and somatic dysfunction of lumbar region**
M99.04 **Segmental and somatic dysfunction of sacral region**
M99.05 **Segmental and somatic dysfunction of pelvic region**
M99.06 **Segmental and somatic dysfunction of lower extremity**
M99.07 **Segmental and somatic dysfunction of upper extremity**
M99.08 **Segmental and somatic dysfunction of rib cage**
M99.09 **Segmental and somatic dysfunction of abdomen and other regions**

● M99.1 **Subluxation complex (vertebral)**
M99.10 **Subluxation complex (vertebral) of head region** 🔹🔹
(Ex) See PDX Collection 913
M99.11 **Subluxation complex (vertebral) of cervical region** 🔹🔹
(Ex) See PDX Collection 913
M99.12 **Subluxation complex (vertebral) of thoracic region**
M99.13 **Subluxation complex (vertebral) of lumbar region**
M99.14 **Subluxation complex (vertebral) of sacral region**
M99.15 **Subluxation complex (vertebral) of pelvic region**
M99.16 **Subluxation complex (vertebral) of lower extremity**
M99.17 **Subluxation complex (vertebral) of upper extremity**
M99.18 **Subluxation complex (vertebral) of rib cage** 🔹🔹
(Ex) See PDX Collection 914
M99.19 **Subluxation complex (vertebral) of abdomen and other regions**

CHAPTER 13 (M00-M99)

N Newborn Age: 0   **P** Pediatric Age: 0–17   **M** Maternity DX: 12–55   **A** Adult Age: 15–124   ♀ Females Only   ♂ Males Only

🔹 Complication\Comorbidity   🔹 Major C\C   (Ex) CC/MCC Exclusions   🔹 Hospital-Acquired Condition

1093

● **M99.2**   Subluxation stenosis of neural canal

    M99.20   Subluxation stenosis of neural canal of head region

    M99.21   Subluxation stenosis of neural canal of cervical region

    M99.22   Subluxation stenosis of neural canal of thoracic region

    M99.23   Subluxation stenosis of neural canal of lumbar region

    M99.24   Subluxation stenosis of neural canal of sacral region

    M99.25   Subluxation stenosis of neural canal of pelvic region

    M99.26   Subluxation stenosis of neural canal of lower extremity

    M99.27   Subluxation stenosis of neural canal of upper extremity

    M99.28   Subluxation stenosis of neural canal of rib cage

    M99.29   Subluxation stenosis of neural canal of abdomen and other regions

● **M99.3**   Osseous stenosis of neural canal

    M99.30   Osseous stenosis of neural canal of head region

    M99.31   Osseous stenosis of neural canal of cervical region

    M99.32   Osseous stenosis of neural canal of thoracic region

    M99.33   Osseous stenosis of neural canal of lumbar region

    M99.34   Osseous stenosis of neural canal of sacral region

    M99.35   Osseous stenosis of neural canal of pelvic region

    M99.36   Osseous stenosis of neural canal of lower extremity

    M99.37   Osseous stenosis of neural canal of upper extremity

    M99.38   Osseous stenosis of neural canal of rib cage

    M99.39   Osseous stenosis of neural canal of abdomen and other regions

● **M99.4**   Connective tissue stenosis of neural canal

    M99.40   Connective tissue stenosis of neural canal of head region

    M99.41   Connective tissue stenosis of neural canal of cervical region

    M99.42   Connective tissue stenosis of neural canal of thoracic region

    M99.43   Connective tissue stenosis of neural canal of lumbar region

    M99.44   Connective tissue stenosis of neural canal of sacral region

    M99.45   Connective tissue stenosis of neural canal of pelvic region

    M99.46   Connective tissue stenosis of neural canal of lower extremity

    M99.47   Connective tissue stenosis of neural canal of upper extremity

    M99.48   Connective tissue stenosis of neural canal of rib cage

    M99.49   Connective tissue stenosis of neural canal of abdomen and other regions

● **M99.5**   Intervertebral disc stenosis of neural canal

    M99.50   Intervertebral disc stenosis of neural canal of head region

    M99.51   Intervertebral disc stenosis of neural canal of cervical region

    M99.52   Intervertebral disc stenosis of neural canal of thoracic region

    M99.53   Intervertebral disc stenosis of neural canal of lumbar region

    M99.54   Intervertebral disc stenosis of neural canal of sacral region

    M99.55   Intervertebral disc stenosis of neural canal of pelvic region

    M99.56   Intervertebral disc stenosis of neural canal of lower extremity

    M99.57   Intervertebral disc stenosis of neural canal of upper extremity

    M99.58   Intervertebral disc stenosis of neural canal of rib cage

    M99.59   Intervertebral disc stenosis of neural canal of abdomen and other regions

● **M99.6**   Osseous and subluxation stenosis of intervertebral foramina

    M99.60   Osseous and subluxation stenosis of intervertebral foramina of head region

    M99.61   Osseous and subluxation stenosis of intervertebral foramina of cervical region

    M99.62   Osseous and subluxation stenosis of intervertebral foramina of thoracic region

    M99.63   Osseous and subluxation stenosis of intervertebral foramina of lumbar region

    M99.64   Osseous and subluxation stenosis of intervertebral foramina of sacral region

    M99.65   Osseous and subluxation stenosis of intervertebral foramina of pelvic region

    M99.66   Osseous and subluxation stenosis of intervertebral foramina of lower extremity

    M99.67   Osseous and subluxation stenosis of intervertebral foramina of upper extremity

    M99.68   Osseous and subluxation stenosis of intervertebral foramina of rib cage

    M99.69   Osseous and subluxation stenosis of intervertebral foramina of abdomen and other regions

● **M99.7**   Connective tissue and disc stenosis of intervertebral foramina

    M99.70   Connective tissue and disc stenosis of intervertebral foramina of head region

    M99.71   Connective tissue and disc stenosis of intervertebral foramina of cervical region

    M99.72   Connective tissue and disc stenosis of intervertebral foramina of thoracic region

    M99.73   Connective tissue and disc stenosis of intervertebral foramina of lumbar region

    M99.74   Connective tissue and disc stenosis of intervertebral foramina of sacral region

    M99.75   Connective tissue and disc stenosis of intervertebral foramina of pelvic region

    M99.76   Connective tissue and disc stenosis of intervertebral foramina of lower extremity

    M99.77   Connective tissue and disc stenosis of intervertebral foramina of upper extremity

    M99.78   Connective tissue and disc stenosis of intervertebral foramina of rib cage

    M99.79   Connective tissue and disc stenosis of intervertebral foramina of abdomen and other regions

● **M99.8**   Other biomechanical lesions

    M99.80   Other biomechanical lesions of head region

    M99.81   Other biomechanical lesions of cervical region

    M99.82   Other biomechanical lesions of thoracic region

    M99.83   Other biomechanical lesions of lumbar region

    M99.84   Other biomechanical lesions of sacral region

    M99.85   Other biomechanical lesions of pelvic region

    M99.86   Other biomechanical lesions of lower extremity

    M99.87   Other biomechanical lesions of upper extremity

    M99.88   Other biomechanical lesions of rib cage

    M99.89   Other biomechanical lesions of abdomen and other regions

    M99.9   Biomechanical lesion, unspecified

▶ New   ⇒ Revised   ~~deleted~~ Deleted   Excludes 1   Excludes 2   Includes   Use additional   Code first   Code also   Key words

OGCR Official Guidelines   ● Unacceptable Principal Diagnosis   X Assign placeholder X   ● Use Additional Character(s)   ▶ Manifestation Code   **Coding Clinic**

CHAPTER 14

DISEASES OF THE GENITOURINARY SYSTEM (N00-N99)

OGCR Chapter-Specific Coding Guidelines

14. **Chapter 14: Diseases of Genitourinary System (N00-N99)**

a. **Chronic kidney disease**

1) **Stages of chronic kidney disease (CKD)**

The ICD-10-CM classifies CKD based on severity. The severity of CKD is designated by stages 1-5. Stage 2, code N18.2, equates to mild CKD; stage 3, code N18.3, equates to moderate CKD; and stage 4, code N18.4, equates to severe CKD. Code N18.6, End stage renal disease (ESRD), is assigned when the provider has documented end-stage-renal disease (ESRD).

If both a stage of CKD and ESRD are documented, assign code N18.6 only.

2) **Chronic kidney disease and kidney transplant status**

Patients who have undergone kidney transplant may still have some form of chronic kidney disease CKD because the kidney transplant may not fully restore kidney function. Therefore, the presence of CKD alone does not constitute a transplant complication. Assign the appropriate N18 code for the patient's stage of CKD and code Z94.0, Kidney transplant status. If a transplant complication such as failure or rejection or other transplant complication is documented, see section I.C.19.g for information on coding complications of a kidney transplant. If the documentation is unclear as to whether the patient has a complication of the transplant, query the provider.

3) **Chronic kidney disease with other conditions**

Patients with CKD may also suffer from other serious conditions, most commonly diabetes mellitus and hypertension. The sequencing of the CKD code in relationship to codes for other contributing conditions is based on the conventions in the Tabular List.

See I.C.9. Hypertensive chronic kidney disease.
See I.C.19. Chronic kidney disease and kidney transplant complications.

Item 14-1 Nephritis (inflammation) or **nephropathy** (disease) **with lesion of proliferative glomerulonephritis** results from a streptococcal infection.

Nephritis (inflammation) or **nephropathy** (disease) **with lesion of membranous glomerulonephritis** is characterized by deposits along the epithelial side of the basement membrane.

Nephritis (inflammation) or **nephropathy** (disease) **with lesion of membranoproliferative glomerulonephritis** is characterized by alterations in the basement membranes of the kidney and the glomerular cells.

Nephritis (inflammation) or **nephropathy** (disease) **with lesion of rapidly progressive glomerulonephritis** is characterized by rapid and progressive decline in renal function.

Nephritis (inflammation) or **nephropathy** (disease) **with lesion of renal cortical necrosis** is characterized by death of the cortical tissues.

Nephritis (inflammation) or **nephropathy** (disease) **with lesion of renal medullary necrosis** is characterized by death of the tissues that collect urine.

Figure 14-1 Kidneys within the urinary system.

Item 14-2 Glomerulonephritis is nephritis accompanied by inflammation of the glomeruli of the kidney, resulting in the degeneration of the glomeruli and the nephrons.

Acute glomerulonephritis primarily affects children and young adults and is usually a result of a streptococcal infection.

Proliferative glomerulonephritis is the acute form of the disease resulting from a streptococcal infection.

Rapidly progressive glomerulonephritis, also known as **crescentic** or **malignant glomerulonephritis**, is the acute form of the disease, which leads quickly to rapid and progressive decline in renal function.

CHAPTER 14

DISEASES OF THE GENITOURINARY SYSTEM (N00-N99)

Excludes2 certain conditions originating in the perinatal period (P04-P96)
certain infectious and parasitic diseases (A00-B99)
complications of pregnancy, childbirth and the puerperium (O00-O9A)
congenital malformations, deformations and chromosomal abnormalities (Q00-Q99)
endocrine, nutritional and metabolic diseases (E00-E88)
injury, poisoning and certain other consequences of external causes (S00-T88)
neoplasms (C00-D49)
symptoms, signs and abnormal clinical and laboratory findings, not elsewhere classified (R00-R94)

This chapter contains the following blocks:

N00-N08	Glomerular diseases
N10-N16	Renal tubulo-interstitial diseases
N17-N19	Acute kidney failure and chronic kidney disease
N20-N23	Urolithiasis
N25-N29	Other disorders of kidney and ureter
N30-N39	Other diseases of the urinary system
N40-N53	Diseases of male genital organs
N60-N65	Disorders of breast
N70-N77	Inflammatory diseases of female pelvic organs
N80-N98	Noninflammatory disorders of female genital tract
N99	Intraoperative and postprocedural complications and disorders of genitourinary system, not elsewhere classified

GLOMERULAR DISEASES (N00-N08)

Code also any associated kidney failure (N17-N19)

Excludes1 hypertensive chronic kidney disease (I12.-)

● **N00 Acute nephritic syndrome**

Includes acute glomerular disease
acute glomerulonephritis
acute nephritis

Excludes1 acute tubulo-interstitial nephritis (N10)
nephritic syndrome NOS (N05.-)

(Ex) **For category N00 CC codes unless otherwise indicated:** See PDX Collection 915

N00.0 Acute nephritic syndrome with minor glomerular abnormality
Acute nephritic syndrome with minimal change lesion

N00.1 Acute nephritic syndrome with focal and segmental glomerular lesions
Acute nephritic syndrome with focal and segmental hyalinosis
Acute nephritic syndrome with focal and segmental sclerosis
Acute nephritic syndrome with focal glomerulonephritis

CHAPTER 14 (N00-N99)

N00.2 **Acute nephritic syndrome with diffuse membranous glomerulonephritis** 🔖

N00.3 **Acute nephritic syndrome with diffuse mesangial proliferative glomerulonephritis** 🔖

N00.4 **Acute nephritic syndrome with diffuse endocapillary proliferative glomerulonephritis** 🔖

N00.5 **Acute nephritic syndrome with diffuse mesangiocapillary glomerulonephritis** 🔖
    Acute nephritic syndrome with membranoproliferative glomerulonephritis, types 1 and 3, or NOS

N00.6 **Acute nephritic syndrome with dense deposit disease** 🔖
    Acute nephritic syndrome with membranoproliferative glomerulonephritis, type 2

N00.7 **Acute nephritic syndrome with diffuse crescentic glomerulonephritis** 🔖
    Acute nephritic syndrome with extracapillary glomerulonephritis

N00.8 **Acute nephritic syndrome with other morphologic changes** 🔖
    Acute nephritic syndrome with proliferative glomerulonephritis NOS
    ⓔ See PDX Collection 916

N00.9 **Acute nephritic syndrome with unspecified morphologic changes** 🔖

● **N01** **Rapidly progressive nephritic syndrome**

    Includes   rapidly progressive glomerular disease
            rapidly progressive glomerulonephritis
            rapidly progressive nephritis

    Excludes1   nephritic syndrome NOS (N05.-)
    ⓔ For category N01 CC codes: See PDX Collection 915

N01.0 **Rapidly progressive nephritic syndrome with minor glomerular abnormality** 🔖
    Rapidly progressive nephritic syndrome with minimal change lesion

N01.1 **Rapidly progressive nephritic syndrome with focal and segmental glomerular lesions** 🔖
    Rapidly progressive nephritic syndrome with focal and segmental hyalinosis
    Rapidly progressive nephritic syndrome with focal and segmental sclerosis
    Rapidly progressive nephritic syndrome with focal glomerulonephritis

N01.2 **Rapidly progressive nephritic syndrome with diffuse membranous glomerulonephritis** 🔖

N01.3 **Rapidly progressive nephritic syndrome with diffuse mesangial proliferative glomerulonephritis** 🔖

N01.4 **Rapidly progressive nephritic syndrome with diffuse endocapillary proliferative glomerulonephritis** 🔖

N01.5 **Rapidly progressive nephritic syndrome with diffuse mesangiocapillary glomerulonephritis** 🔖
    Rapidly progressive nephritic syndrome with membranoproliferative glomerulonephritis, types 1 and 3, or NOS

N01.6 **Rapidly progressive nephritic syndrome with dense deposit disease** 🔖
    Rapidly progressive nephritic syndrome with membranoproliferative glomerulonephritis, type 2

N01.7 **Rapidly progressive nephritic syndrome with diffuse crescentic glomerulonephritis** 🔖
    Rapidly progressive nephritic syndrome with extracapillary glomerulonephritis

N01.8 **Rapidly progressive nephritic syndrome with other morphologic changes** 🔖
    Rapidly progressive nephritic syndrome with proliferative glomerulonephritis NOS

N01.9 **Rapidly progressive nephritic syndrome with unspecified morphologic changes** 🔖

● **N02** **Recurrent and persistent hematuria**

    Excludes1   acute cystitis with hematuria (N30.01)
            hematuria NOS (R31.9)
            hematuria not associated with specified morphologic lesions (R31.-)
    ⓔ For category N02 CC codes unless otherwise indicated: See PDX Collection 917

N02.0 **Recurrent and persistent hematuria with minor glomerular abnormality** 🔖
    Recurrent and persistent hematuria with minimal change lesion

N02.1 **Recurrent and persistent hematuria with focal and segmental glomerular lesions** 🔖
    Recurrent and persistent hematuria with focal and segmental hyalinosis
    Recurrent and persistent hematuria with focal and segmental sclerosis
    Recurrent and persistent hematuria with focal glomerulonephritis

N02.2 **Recurrent and persistent hematuria with diffuse membranous glomerulonephritis** 🔖

N02.3 **Recurrent and persistent hematuria with diffuse mesangial proliferative glomerulonephritis** 🔖

N02.4 **Recurrent and persistent hematuria with diffuse endocapillary proliferative glomerulonephritis** 🔖

N02.5 **Recurrent and persistent hematuria with diffuse mesangiocapillary glomerulonephritis** 🔖
    Recurrent and persistent hematuria with membranoproliferative glomerulonephritis, types 1 and 3, or NOS

N02.6 **Recurrent and persistent hematuria with dense deposit disease** 🔖
    Recurrent and persistent hematuria with membranoproliferative glomerulonephritis, type 2

N02.7 **Recurrent and persistent hematuria with diffuse crescentic glomerulonephritis** 🔖
    Recurrent and persistent hematuria with extracapillary glomerulonephritis

N02.8 **Recurrent and persistent hematuria with other morphologic changes** 🔖
    Recurrent and persistent hematuria with proliferative glomerulonephritis NOS
    ⓔ See PDX Collection 915

N02.9 **Recurrent and persistent hematuria with unspecified morphologic changes** 🔖
    ⓔ See PDX Collection 915
    Coding Clinic: 2017, Q2, P5

● **N03** **Chronic nephritic syndrome**

    Includes   chronic glomerular disease
            chronic glomerulonephritis
            chronic nephritis

    Excludes1   chronic tubulo-interstitial nephritis (N11.-)
            diffuse sclerosing glomerulonephritis (N05.8-)
            nephritic syndrome NOS (N05.-)
    ⓔ For category N03 CC codes: See PDX Collection 918

N03.0 **Chronic nephritic syndrome with minor glomerular abnormality** 🔖
    Chronic nephritic syndrome with minimal change lesion

N03.1 **Chronic nephritic syndrome with focal and segmental glomerular lesions** 🔖
    Chronic nephritic syndrome with focal and segmental hyalinosis
    Chronic nephritic syndrome with focal and segmental sclerosis
    Chronic nephritic syndrome with focal glomerulonephritis

N03.2 **Chronic nephritic syndrome with diffuse membranous glomerulonephritis** 🔖

N03.3 **Chronic nephritic syndrome with diffuse mesangial proliferative glomerulonephritis** 🔖

N03.4 **Chronic nephritic syndrome with diffuse endocapillary proliferative glomerulonephritis** 🔖

▶ New ⇒ Revised ~~deleted~~ Deleted Excludes 1 Excludes 2 Includes Use additional Code first Code also Key words
OGCR Official Guidelines ● Unacceptable Principal Diagnosis X Assign placeholder X ● Use Additional Character(s) ▸ Manifestation Code Coding Clinic

Item 14–3 Chronic glomerulonephritis (GN) persists over a period of years, with remissions and exacerbation.
    Chronic GN with lesion of proliferative glomerulonephritis results from a streptococcal infection.
    Chronic GN with lesion of membranous glomerulonephritis, also known as membranous nephropathy, is characterized by deposits along the epithelial side of the basement membrane.
    Chronic GN with lesion of membrano-proliferative glomerulonephritis (MPGN) is a group of disorders characterized by alterations in the basement membranes of the kidney and the glomerular cells.
    Chronic GN with lesion of rapidly progressive glomerulonephritis is characterized by necrosis, endothelial proliferation, and mesangial proliferation. The condition is marked by rapid and progressive decline in renal function.

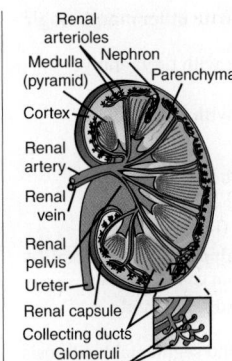

Figure 14-2 Kidney cross section.

N03.5   **Chronic nephritic syndrome with diffuse mesangiocapillary glomerulonephritis** 🔹
     Chronic nephritic syndrome with membranoproliferative glomerulonephritis, types 1 and 3, or NOS

N03.6   **Chronic nephritic syndrome with dense deposit disease** 🔹
     Chronic nephritic syndrome with membranoproliferative glomerulonephritis, type 2

N03.7   **Chronic nephritic syndrome with diffuse crescentic glomerulonephritis** 🔹
     Chronic nephritic syndrome with extracapillary glomerulonephritis

N03.8   **Chronic nephritic syndrome with other morphologic changes** 🔹
     Chronic nephritic syndrome with proliferative glomerulonephritis NOS

N03.9   **Chronic nephritic syndrome with unspecified morphologic changes** 🔹

● N04   **Nephrotic syndrome**
    Includes   congenital nephrotic syndrome
              lipoid nephrosis
    (Ex) **For category N04 CC codes unless otherwise indicated: See PDX Collection 917**

N04.0   **Nephrotic syndrome with minor glomerular abnormality** 🔹
     Nephrotic syndrome with minimal change lesion

N04.1   **Nephrotic syndrome with focal and segmental glomerular lesions** 🔹
     Nephrotic syndrome with focal and segmental hyalinosis
     Nephrotic syndrome with focal and segmental sclerosis
     Nephrotic syndrome with focal glomerulonephritis

N04.2   **Nephrotic syndrome with diffuse membranous glomerulonephritis** 🔹

N04.3   **Nephrotic syndrome with diffuse mesangial proliferative glomerulonephritis** 🔹

N04.4   **Nephrotic syndrome with diffuse endocapillary proliferative glomerulonephritis** 🔹

N04.5   **Nephrotic syndrome with diffuse mesangiocapillary glomerulonephritis** 🔹
     Nephrotic syndrome with membranoproliferative glomerulonephritis, types 1 and 3, or NOS

N04.6   **Nephrotic syndrome with dense deposit disease** 🔹
     Nephrotic syndrome with membranoproliferative glomerulonephritis, type 2

N04.7   **Nephrotic syndrome with diffuse crescentic glomerulonephritis** 🔹
     Nephrotic syndrome with extracapillary glomerulonephritis
     (Ex) See PDX Collection 915

N04.8   **Nephrotic syndrome with other morphologic changes** 🔹
     Nephrotic syndrome with proliferative glomerulonephritis NOS
     (Ex) See PDX Collection 915

N04.9   **Nephrotic syndrome with unspecified morphologic changes** 🔹
     (Ex) See PDX Collection 915

Item 14–4 Nephrotic syndrome (NS) is marked by massive proteinuria (protein in the urine) and water retention. Patients with NS are particularly vulnerable to staphylococcal and pneumococcal infections. NS with lesion of proliferative glomerulonephritis results from a streptococcal infection. NS with lesion of membranous glomerulonephritis results in thickening of the capillary walls. NS with lesion of minimal change glomerulonephritis is usually a benign disorder that occurs mostly in children and requires electron microscopy (biopsy) to verify changes in the glomeruli.

● N05   **Unspecified nephritic syndrome**
    Includes   glomerular disease NOS
              glomerulonephritis NOS
              nephritis NOS
              nephropathy NOS and renal disease NOS with morphological lesion specified in .0-.8
    Excludes1   nephropathy NOS with no stated morphological lesion (N28.9)
              renal disease NOS with no stated morphological lesion (N28.9)
              tubulo-interstitial nephritis NOS (N12)

N05.0   **Unspecified nephritic syndrome with minor glomerular abnormality**
     Unspecified nephritic syndrome with minimal change lesion

N05.1   **Unspecified nephritic syndrome with focal and segmental glomerular lesions**
     Unspecified nephritic syndrome with focal and segmental hyalinosis
     Unspecified nephritic syndrome with focal and segmental sclerosis
     Unspecified nephritic syndrome with focal glomerulonephritis

N05.2   **Unspecified nephritic syndrome with diffuse membranous glomerulonephritis** 🔹
     (Ex) See PDX Collection 918

N05.3   **Unspecified nephritic syndrome with diffuse mesangial proliferative glomerulonephritis** 🔹
     (Ex) See PDX Collection 918

N05.4   **Unspecified nephritic syndrome with diffuse endocapillary proliferative glomerulonephritis** 🔹
     (Ex) See PDX Collection 918

N05.5   **Unspecified nephritic syndrome with diffuse mesangiocapillary glomerulonephritis** 🔹
     Unspecified nephritic syndrome with membranoproliferative glomerulonephritis, types 1 and 3, or NOS
     (Ex) See PDX Collection 918

N05.6   **Unspecified nephritic syndrome with dense deposit disease**
     Unspecified nephritic syndrome with membranoproliferative glomerulonephritis, type 2

N05.7   **Unspecified nephritic syndrome with diffuse crescentic glomerulonephritis**
     Unspecified nephritic syndrome with extracapillary glomerulonephritis

---

N   Newborn Age: Ø   P   Pediatric Age: Ø–17   M   Maternity DX: 12–55   A   Adult Age: 15–124   ♀ Females Only   ♂ Males Only

🔹 Complication\Comorbidity   🔹 Major C\C   (Ex) CC/MCC Exclusions   🔹 Hospital-Acquired Condition

CHAPTER 14 (N00-N99)

N05.8   **Unspecified nephritic syndrome with other morphologic changes**
     Unspecified nephritic syndrome with proliferative glomerulonephritis NOS

N05.9   **Unspecified nephritic syndrome with unspecified morphologic changes**

● **N06**   **Isolated proteinuria with specified morphological lesion**

    Excludes1   proteinuria not associated with specific morphologic lesions (R80.0)

N06.0   **Isolated proteinuria with minor glomerular abnormality**
     Isolated proteinuria with minimal change lesion

N06.1   **Isolated proteinuria with focal and segmental glomerular lesions**
     Isolated proteinuria with focal and segmental hyalinosis
     Isolated proteinuria with focal and segmental sclerosis
     Isolated proteinuria with focal glomerulonephritis

N06.2   **Isolated proteinuria with diffuse membranous glomerulonephritis** 🔗
     Ex: See PDX Collection 918

N06.3   **Isolated proteinuria with diffuse mesangial proliferative glomerulonephritis** 🔗
     Ex: See PDX Collection 918

N06.4   **Isolated proteinuria with diffuse endocapillary proliferative glomerulonephritis** 🔗
     Ex: See PDX Collection 918

N06.5   **Isolated proteinuria with diffuse mesangiocapillary glomerulonephritis** 🔗
     Isolated proteinuria with membranoproliferative glomerulonephritis, types 1 and 3, or NOS
     Ex: See PDX Collection 918

N06.6   **Isolated proteinuria with dense deposit disease**
     Isolated proteinuria with membranoproliferative glomerulonephritis, type 2

N06.7   **Isolated proteinuria with diffuse crescentic glomerulonephritis**
     Isolated proteinuria with extracapillary glomerulonephritis

N06.8   **Isolated proteinuria with other morphologic lesion**
     Isolated proteinuria with proliferative glomerulonephritis NOS

N06.9   **Isolated proteinuria with unspecified morphologic lesion**

● **N07**   **Hereditary nephropathy, not elsewhere classified**

    Excludes2   Alport's syndrome (Q87.81-)
         hereditary amyloid nephropathy (E85.-)
         nail patella syndrome (Q87.2)
         non-neuropathic heredofamilial amyloidosis (E85.-)

N07.0   **Hereditary nephropathy, not elsewhere classified with minor glomerular abnormality**
     Hereditary nephropathy, not elsewhere classified with minimal change lesion

N07.1   **Hereditary nephropathy, not elsewhere classified with focal and segmental glomerular lesions**
     Hereditary nephropathy, not elsewhere classified with focal and segmental hyalinosis
     Hereditary nephropathy, not elsewhere classified with focal and segmental sclerosis
     Hereditary nephropathy, not elsewhere classified with focal glomerulonephritis

N07.2   **Hereditary nephropathy, not elsewhere classified with diffuse membranous glomerulonephritis** 🔗
     Ex: See PDX Collection 918

N07.3   **Hereditary nephropathy, not elsewhere classified with diffuse mesangial proliferative glomerulonephritis** 🔗
     Ex: See PDX Collection 918

N07.4   **Hereditary nephropathy, not elsewhere classified with diffuse endocapillary proliferative glomerulonephritis** 🔗
     Ex: See PDX Collection 918

N07.5   **Hereditary nephropathy, not elsewhere classified with diffuse mesangiocapillary glomerulonephritis** 🔗
     Hereditary nephropathy, not elsewhere classified with membranoproliferative glomerulonephritis, types 1 and 3, or NOS
     Ex: See PDX Collection 918

N07.6   **Hereditary nephropathy, not elsewhere classified with dense deposit disease**
     Hereditary nephropathy, not elsewhere classified with membranoproliferative glomerulonephritis, type 2

N07.7   **Hereditary nephropathy, not elsewhere classified with diffuse crescentic glomerulonephritis**
     Hereditary nephropathy, not elsewhere classified with extracapillary glomerulonephritis

N07.8   **Hereditary nephropathy, not elsewhere classified with other morphologic lesions**
     Hereditary nephropathy, not elsewhere classified with proliferative glomerulonephritis NOS

N07.9   **Hereditary nephropathy, not elsewhere classified with unspecified morphologic lesions**

▶ *N08*   *Glomerular disorders in diseases classified elsewhere*
     Glomerulonephritis
     Nephritis
     Nephropathy

    Code first underlying disease, such as:
     amyloidosis (E85.-)
     congenital syphilis (A50.5)
     cryoglobulinemia (D89.1)
     disseminated intravascular coagulation (D65)
     gout (M1A.-, M10.-)
     microscopic polyangiitis (M31.7)
     multiple myeloma (C90.0-)
     sepsis (A40.0-A41.9)
     sickle-cell disease (D57.0-D57.8)

    Excludes1   glomerulonephritis, nephritis and nephropathy (in):
       antiglomerular basement membrane disease (M31.0)
       diabetes (E08-E13 with .21)
       gonococcal (A54.21)
       Goodpasture's syndrome (M31.0)
       hemolytic-uremic syndrome (D59.3)
       lupus (M32.14)
       mumps (B26.83)
       syphilis (A52.75)
       systemic lupus erythematosus (M32.14)
       Wegener's granulomatosis (M31.31)
     pyelonephritis in diseases classified elsewhere (N16)
     renal tubulo-interstitial disorders classified elsewhere (N16)

▶ New   ⇒ Revised   ~~deleted~~ Deleted   Excludes 1   Excludes 2   Includes   Use additional   Code first   Code also   Key words

OGCR Official Guidelines   ● Unacceptable Principal Diagnosis   X Assign placeholder X   ● Use Additional Character(s)   ▶ Manifestation Code   **Coding Clinic**

Figure 14-3 Acute pyelonephritis. Cortical surface exhibits grayish white areas of inflammation and abscess formation. (From Frazier MS, Drzymkowski JW: Essentials of Human Diseases and Conditions, St. Louis, Saunders/Elsevier, 2009)

Figure 14-4 Hydronephrosis of the kidney, with marked dilatation of pelvis and calyces and thinning of renal parenchyma. (From Kumar: Robbins and Cotran: Pathologic Basis of Disease, ed 8, Saunders, An Imprint of Elsevier, 2009)

Item 14–5 Pyelonephritis is an infection of the kidneys and ureters and may be chronic or acute in one or both kidneys.

RENAL TUBULO-INTERSTITIAL DISEASES (N10-N16)

Includes	pyelonephritis
Excludes1	pyeloureteritis cystica (N28.85)

N10 Acute pyelonephritis 🕮 🕮
Acute infectious interstitial nephritis
Acute pyelitis
Acute tubulo-interstitial nephritis
Hemoglobin nephrosis
Myoglobin nephrosis
Use additional code (B95-B97), to identify infectious agent
(Ex) See PDX Collection 919

● **N11 Chronic tubulo-interstitial nephritis**
Includes   chronic infectious interstitial nephritis
chronic pyelitis
chronic pyelonephritis
Use additional code (B95-B97), to identify infectious agent

N11.0 Nonobstructive reflux-associated chronic pyelonephritis
Pyelonephritis (chronic) associated with (vesicoureteral) reflux
Excludes1   vesicoureteral reflux NOS (N13.70)

N11.1 Chronic obstructive pyelonephritis 🕮
Pyelonephritis (chronic) associated with anomaly of pelviureteric junction
Pyelonephritis (chronic) associated with anomaly of pyeloureteric junction
Pyelonephritis (chronic) associated with crossing of vessel
Pyelonephritis (chronic) associated with kinking of ureter
Pyelonephritis (chronic) associated with obstruction of ureter
Pyelonephritis (chronic) associated with stricture of pelviureteric junction
Pyelonephritis (chronic) associated with stricture of ureter
Excludes1   calculous pyelonephritis (N20.9)
obstructive uropathy (N13.-)
CC when PDx is its own CC
(Ex) See PDX Collection 920

N11.8 Other chronic tubulo-interstitial nephritis 🕮
Nonobstructive chronic pyelonephritis NOS
(Ex) See PDX Collection 921

N11.9 Chronic tubulo-interstitial nephritis, unspecified 🕮 🕮
Chronic interstitial nephritis NOS
Chronic pyelitis NOS
Chronic pyelonephritis NOS
(Ex) See PDX Collection 922

N12 Tubulo-interstitial nephritis, not specified as acute or chronic 🕮 🕮
Interstitial nephritis NOS
Pyelitis NOS
Pyelonephritis NOS
Excludes1   calculous pyelonephritis (N20.9)
(Ex) See PDX Collection 922

● **N13 Obstructive and reflux uropathy**
Excludes2   calculus of kidney and ureter without hydronephrosis (N20.-)
congenital obstructive defects of renal pelvis and ureter (Q62.0-Q62.3)
➡ hydronephrosis with ureteropelvic junction obstruction (Q62.11)
obstructive pyelonephritis (N11.1)
(Ex) **For category N13 CC codes unless otherwise indicated:** See PDX Collection 922

N13.0 Hydronephrosis with ureteropelvic junction obstruction 🕮
Hydronephrosis due to acquired occlusion of ureteropelvic junction
Excludes2   Hydronephrosis with ureteropelvic junction obstruction due to calculus (N13.2)
CC when PDx is its own CC
Coding Clinic: 2016, Q4, P43

N13.1 Hydronephrosis with ureteral stricture, not elsewhere classified 🕮
Excludes1   hydronephrosis with ureteral stricture with infection (N13.6)
CC when PDx is its own CC

N13.2 Hydronephrosis with renal and ureteral calculous obstruction 🕮
Excludes1   hydronephrosis with renal and ureteral calculous obstruction with infection (N13.6)
CC when PDx is its own CC

● **N13.3 Other and unspecified hydronephrosis**
Excludes1   hydronephrosis with infection (N13.6)
N13.30 Unspecified hydronephrosis 🕮
N13.39 Other hydronephrosis 🕮

N13.4 Hydroureter 🕮
Excludes1   congenital hydroureter (Q62.3-)
hydroureter with infection (N13.6)
vesicoureteral-reflux with hydroureter (N13.73-)
(Ex) See PDX Collection 923

N13.5 Crossing vessel and stricture of ureter without hydronephrosis
Kinking and stricture of ureter without hydronephrosis
Excludes1   crossing vessel and stricture of ureter without hydronephrosis with infection (N13.6)
Coding Clinic: 2016, Q4, P43

N13.6 Pyonephrosis 🕮 🕮
Conditions in N13.0-N13.5 with infection
Obstructive uropathy with infection
Use additional code (B95-B97), to identify infectious agent

N Newborn Age: 0   **P** Pediatric Age: 0–17   **M** Maternity DX: 12–55   **A** Adult Age: 15–124   ♀ Females Only   ♂ Males Only

🕮 Complication\Comorbidity   🕮 Major C\C   (Ex) CC/MCC Exclusions   🕮 Hospital-Acquired Condition

1099

CHAPTER 14 (N00-N99)

CHAPTER 14 (N00–N99)

● **N13.7   Vesicoureteral-reflux**

    Excludes1   reflux-associated pyelonephritis (N11.0)

N13.70   Vesicoureteral-reflux, unspecified
Occurs when urine flows from bladder back into ureters
Vesicoureteral-reflux NOS

N13.71   Vesicoureteral-reflux without reflux nephropathy

● **N13.72   Vesicoureteral-reflux with reflux nephropathy without hydroureter**

    N13.721   Vesicoureteral-reflux with reflux nephropathy without hydroureter, unilateral

    N13.722   Vesicoureteral-reflux with reflux nephropathy without hydroureter, bilateral

    N13.729   Vesicoureteral-reflux with reflux nephropathy without hydroureter, unspecified

● **N13.73   Vesicoureteral-reflux with reflux nephropathy with hydroureter**

    N13.731   Vesicoureteral-reflux with reflux nephropathy with hydroureter, unilateral

    N13.732   Vesicoureteral-reflux with reflux nephropathy with hydroureter, bilateral

    N13.739   Vesicoureteral-reflux with reflux nephropathy with hydroureter, unspecified

N13.8   Other obstructive and reflux uropathy 🖰
Urinary tract obstruction due to specified cause
Code first, if applicable, any causal condition first, such as:
enlarged prostate (N40.1)
Ⓔ See PDX Collection 920

N13.9   Obstructive and reflux uropathy, unspecified
Urinary tract obstruction NOS

● **N14   Drug- and heavy-metal-induced tubulo-interstitial and tubular conditions**
Code first poisoning due to drug or toxin, if applicable (T36-T65 with fifth or sixth character 1-4 or 6)
Use additional code for adverse effect, if applicable, to identify drug (T36-T50 with fifth or sixth character 5)

N14.0   Analgesic nephropathy

N14.1   Nephropathy induced by other drugs, medicaments and biological substances

N14.2   Nephropathy induced by unspecified drug, medicament or biological substance

N14.3   Nephropathy induced by heavy metals

N14.4   Toxic nephropathy, not elsewhere classified

● **N15   Other renal tubulo-interstitial diseases**

N15.0   Balkan nephropathy
Balkan endemic nephropathy

N15.1   Renal and perinephric abscess 🖰 🖰
Ⓔ See PDX Collection 919

N15.8   Other specified renal tubulo-interstitial diseases

N15.9   Renal tubulo-interstitial disease, unspecified
Infection of kidney NOS

    Excludes1   urinary tract infection NOS (N39.0)

▷ **N16   *Renal tubulo-interstitial disorders in diseases classified elsewhere***
Pyelonephritis
Tubulo-interstitial nephritis
Code first underlying disease, such as:
brucellosis (A23.0-A23.9)
cryoglobulinemia (D89.1)
glycogen storage disease (E74.0)
leukemia (C91-C95)
lymphoma (C81.0-C85.9, C96.0-C96.9)
multiple myeloma (C90.0-)
sepsis (A40.0-A41.9)
Wilson's disease (E83.0)

    Excludes1   diphtheritic pyelonephritis and tubulo-interstitial nephritis (A36.84)
pyelonephritis and tubulo-interstitial nephritis in candidiasis (B37.49)
pyelonephritis and tubulo-interstitial nephritis in cystinosis (E72.04)
pyelonephritis and tubulo-interstitial nephritis in salmonella infection (A02.25)
pyelonephritis and tubulo-interstitial nephritis in sarcoidosis (D86.84)
pyelonephritis and tubulo-interstitial nephritis in sicca syndrome [Sjogren's] (M35.04)
pyelonephritis and tubulo-interstitial nephritis in systemic lupus erythematosus (M32.15)
pyelonephritis and tubulo-interstitial nephritis in toxoplasmosis (B58.83)
renal tubular degeneration in diabetes (E08-E13 with .29)
syphilitic pyelonephritis and tubulo-interstitial nephritis (A52.75)

ACUTE KIDNEY FAILURE AND CHRONIC KIDNEY DISEASE (N17-N19)

    Excludes2   congenital renal failure (P96.0)
drug- and heavy-metal-induced tubulo-interstitial and tubular conditions (N14.-)
extrarenal uremia (R39.2)
hemolytic-uremic syndrome (D59.3)
hepatorenal syndrome (K76.7)
postpartum hepatorenal syndrome (O90.4)
posttraumatic renal failure (T79.5)
prerenal uremia (R39.2)
renal failure complicating abortion or ectopic or molar pregnancy (O00-O07, O08.4)
renal failure following labor and delivery (O90.4)
renal failure postprocedural (N99.0)

● **N17   Acute kidney failure**
Code also associated underlying condition
    Excludes1   posttraumatic renal failure (T79.5)
Ⓔ **For category N17 CC codes unless otherwise indicated:** See PDX Collection 924

N17.0   Acute kidney failure with tubular necrosis 🖰
Acute tubular necrosis
Renal tubular necrosis
Tubular necrosis NOS

N17.1   Acute kidney failure with acute cortical necrosis 🖰
Acute cortical necrosis
Cortical necrosis NOS
Renal cortical necrosis

N17.2   Acute kidney failure with medullary necrosis 🖰
Medullary [papillary] necrosis NOS
Acute medullary [papillary] necrosis
Renal medullary [papillary] necrosis

N17.8   Other acute kidney failure 🖰
Ⓔ See PDX Collection 925

N17.9   Acute kidney failure, unspecified 🖰
Acute kidney injury (nontraumatic)

    Excludes2   traumatic kidney injury (S37.0-)

▶ New   ⇒ Revised   ~~deleted~~ Deleted   Excludes 1   Excludes 2   Includes   Use additional   Code first   Code also   Key words
OGCR Official Guidelines   ● Unacceptable Principal Diagnosis   X Assign placeholder X   🖰 Use Additional Character(s)   ▷ Manifestation Code   **Coding Clinic**

Item 14–6 Decreased blood flow is the usual cause of **acute renal failure** that offers a good prognosis for recovery.

Chronic renal failure is usually the result of long-standing kidney disease and is a very serious condition that generally results in death.

● **N18 Chronic kidney disease (CKD)**
  Code first any associated:
    diabetic chronic kidney disease (E08.22, E09.22, E10.22, E11.22, E13.22)
    hypertensive chronic kidney disease (I12.-, I13.-)
  Use additional code to identify kidney transplant status, if applicable, (Z94.0)
  Coding Clinic: 2016, Q4, P123

  N18.1 Chronic kidney disease, stage 1
  N18.2 Chronic kidney disease, stage 2 (mild)
  N18.3 Chronic kidney disease, stage 3 (moderate)
  N18.4 Chronic kidney disease, stage 4 (severe) 🔖
      (Ex) See PDX Collection 926
      Coding Clinic: 2013, Q1, P24
  N18.5 Chronic kidney disease, stage 5 🔖
      Excludes1 chronic kidney disease, stage 5 requiring chronic dialysis (N18.6)
      (Ex) See PDX Collection 926
  N18.6 End stage renal disease 🔖
      Chronic kidney disease requiring chronic dialysis
      Use additional code to identify dialysis status (Z99.2)
      (Ex) See PDX Collection 927
      Coding Clinic: 2016, Q3, P23, Q1, P13
  N18.9 Chronic kidney disease, unspecified
      Chronic renal disease
      Chronic renal failure NOS
      Chronic renal insufficiency
      ➡Chronic uremia NOS
      ▶Diffuse sclerosing glomerulonephritis NOS

N19 Unspecified kidney failure
    Uremia NOS
      Excludes1 acute kidney failure (N17.-)
                    chronic kidney disease (N18.-)
                    chronic uremia (N18.9)
                    extrarenal uremia (R39.2)
                    prerenal uremia (R39.2)
                    renal insufficiency (acute) (N28.9)
                    uremia of newborn (P96.0)

UROLITHIASIS (N20-N23)

● **N20 Calculus of kidney and ureter**
    Calculous pyelonephritis
      Excludes1 nephrocalcinosis (E83.5)
                    that with hydronephrosis (N13.2)

  N20.0 Calculus of kidney
      Nephrolithiasis NOS   Staghorn calculus
      Renal calculus   Stone in kidney
      Renal stone
      Coding Clinic: 2017, Q1, P5
  N20.1 Calculus of ureter 🔖
      Ureteric stone
      (Ex) See PDX Collection 928
      Coding Clinic: 2016, Q3, P24
  N20.2 Calculus of kidney with calculus of ureter 🔖
      (Ex) See PDX Collection 928
  N20.9 Urinary calculus, unspecified

Figure 14-5 Multiple urinary calculi.

Multiple calculi

● **N21 Calculus of lower urinary tract**
      Includes   calculus of lower urinary tract with cystitis and urethritis
  N21.0 Calculus in bladder
      Calculus in diverticulum of bladder
      Urinary bladder stone
      Excludes2 staghorn calculus (N20.0)
      Coding Clinic: 2015, Q2, P9
  N21.1 Calculus in urethra
      Excludes2 calculus of prostate (N42.0)
  N21.8 Other lower urinary tract calculus
  N21.9 Calculus of lower urinary tract, unspecified
      Excludes1 calculus of urinary tract NOS (N20.9)

▶ **N22 *Calculus of urinary tract in diseases classified elsewhere***
      Code first underlying disease, such as:
        gout (M1A.-, M10.-)
        schistosomiasis (B65.0-B65.9)

  N23 Unspecified renal colic

OTHER DISORDERS OF KIDNEY AND URETER (N25-N29)
      Excludes2 disorders of kidney and ureter with urolithiasis (N20-N23)

● **N25 Disorders resulting from impaired renal tubular function**
      ~~Excludes1~~ ~~metabolic disorders classifiable to E70-E88~~
  N25.0 Renal osteodystrophy
      Azotemic osteodystrophy
      Phosphate-losing tubular disorders
      Renal rickets
      Renal short stature
      ▶ **Excludes2** metabolic disorders classifiable to E70-E88
  N25.1 Nephrogenic diabetes insipidus 🔖
      Excludes1 diabetes insipidus NOS (E23.2)
      (Ex) See PDX Collection 929
  ● **N25.8 Other disorders resulting from impaired renal tubular function**
      N25.81 Secondary hyperparathyroidism of renal origin 🔖
          Excludes1 secondary hyperparathyroidism, non-renal (E21.1)
          ▶ **Excludes2** metabolic disorders classifiable to E70-E88
          (Ex) See PDX Collection 930
      N25.89 Other disorders resulting from impaired renal tubular function
          Hypokalemic nephropathy
          Lightwood-Albright syndrome
          Renal tubular acidosis NOS
  N25.9 Disorder resulting from impaired renal tubular function, unspecified

● **N26 Unspecified contracted kidney**
      Excludes1 contracted kidney due to hypertension (I12.-)
                    diffuse sclerosing glomerulonephritis (N05.8-)
                    hypertensive nephrosclerosis (arteriolar) (arteriosclerotic) (I12.-)
                    small kidney of unknown cause (N27.-)
  N26.1 Atrophy of kidney (terminal)
  N26.2 Page kidney
  N26.9 Renal sclerosis, unspecified

● **N27 Small kidney of unknown cause**
      Includes   oligonephronia
  N27.0 Small kidney, unilateral
  N27.1 Small kidney, bilateral
  N27.9 Small kidney, unspecified

N Newborn Age: 0   **P** Pediatric Age: 0–17   **M** Maternity DX: 12–55   **A** Adult Age: 15–124   ♀ Females Only   ♂ Males Only

🔖 Complication\Comorbidity   🔖 Major C\C   (Ex) CC/MCC Exclusions   🔖 Hospital-Acquired Condition   1101

● **N28 Other disorders of kidney and ureter, not elsewhere classified**

    N28.0 Ischemia and infarction of kidney 🔍
       Renal artery embolism
       Renal artery obstruction
       Renal artery occlusion
       Renal artery thrombosis
       Renal infarct

        Excludes1 atherosclerosis of renal artery (extrarenal part) (I70.1)
                      congenital stenosis of renal artery (Q27.1)
                      Goldblatt's kidney (I70.1)
        (Ex) See PDX Collection 931

    N28.1 Cyst of kidney, acquired
       ⇒ Cyst (multiple) (solitary) of kidney, (acquired)
        Excludes1 cystic kidney disease (congenital) (Q61.-)

  ● **N28.8 Other specified disorders of kidney and ureter**
        Excludes1 hydroureter (N13.4)
                      ureteric stricture with hydronephrosis (N13.1)
                      ureteric stricture without hydronephrosis (N13.5)

      N28.81 Hypertrophy of kidney
      N28.82 Megaloureter
      N28.83 Nephroptosis
      N28.84 Pyelitis cystica 🔍 🔍
           (Ex) See PDX Collection 922
      N28.85 Pyeloureteritis cystica 🔍 🔍
           (Ex) See PDX Collection 922
      N28.86 Ureteritis cystica 🔍 🔍
           (Ex) See PDX Collection 922
      N28.89 Other specified disorders of kidney and ureter

    N28.9 Disorder of kidney and ureter, unspecified
       Nephropathy NOS
       Renal disease (acute) NOS
       Renal insufficiency (acute)
        Excludes1 chronic renal insufficiency (N18.9)
                      unspecified nephritic syndrome (N05.-)
       Coding Clinic: 2016, Q1, P13

▷ *N29 Other disorders of kidney and ureter in diseases classified elsewhere*
    Code first underlying disease, such as:
       amyloidosis (E85.-)
       nephrocalcinosis (E83.5)
       schistosomiasis (B65.0-B65.9)
        Excludes1 disorders of kidney and ureter in:
                      cystinosis (E72.0)
                      gonorrhea (A54.21)
                      syphilis (A52.75)
                      tuberculosis (A18.11)

OTHER DISEASES OF THE URINARY SYSTEM (N30-N39)

  Excludes1 urinary infection (complicating):
              abortion or ectopic or molar pregnancy (O00-O07, O08.8)
              pregnancy, childbirth and the puerperium (O23.-, O75.3, O86.2-)

● **N30 Cystitis**
  Infection of bladder and irritation in lower urinary tract
  Use additional code to identify infectious agent (B95-B97)
   Excludes1 prostatocystitis (N41.3)

  ● **N30.0 Acute cystitis**
        Excludes1 irradiation cystitis (N30.4-)
                      trigonitis (N30.3-)
        (Ex) **For category N30.0 CC codes:** See PDX Collection 932
      N30.00 Acute cystitis without hematuria 🔍 🔍
      N30.01 Acute cystitis with hematuria 🔍 🔍

  ● **N30.1 Interstitial cystitis (chronic)**
    Ongoing infection of kidney glomeruli and tubules
      N30.10 Interstitial cystitis (chronic) without hematuria
      N30.11 Interstitial cystitis (chronic) with hematuria

  ● **N30.2 Other chronic cystitis**
      N30.20 Other chronic cystitis without hematuria
      N30.21 Other chronic cystitis with hematuria

  ● **N30.3 Trigonitis**
    Inflammation of triangular area of bladder (where the ureters and urethra come together)
    Urethrotrigonitis
      N30.30 Trigonitis without hematuria
      N30.31 Trigonitis with hematuria

  ● **N30.4 Irradiation cystitis**
      (Ex) **For category N30.4 CC codes:** See PDX Collection 932
      N30.40 Irradiation cystitis without hematuria 🔍
      N30.41 Irradiation cystitis with hematuria 🔍

  ● **N30.8 Other cystitis**
    Abscess of bladder
      N30.80 Other cystitis without hematuria
      N30.81 Other cystitis with hematuria

  ● **N30.9 Cystitis, unspecified**
      N30.90 Cystitis, unspecified without hematuria
      N30.91 Cystitis, unspecified with hematuria

● **N31 Neuromuscular dysfunction of bladder, not elsewhere classified**
  Use additional code to identify any associated urinary incontinence (N39.3-N39.4-)
   Excludes1 cord bladder NOS (G95.89)
                 neurogenic bladder due to cauda equina syndrome (G83.4)
                 neuromuscular dysfunction due to spinal cord lesion (G95.89)

  N31.0 Uninhibited neuropathic bladder, not elsewhere classified
  N31.1 Reflex neuropathic bladder, not elsewhere classified
  N31.2 Flaccid neuropathic bladder, not elsewhere classified
    Atonic (motor) (sensory) neuropathic bladder
    Diminished tone of bladder muscle
    Autonomous neuropathic bladder
    Nonreflex neuropathic bladder

  N31.8 Other neuromuscular dysfunction of bladder
  N31.9 Neuromuscular dysfunction of bladder, unspecified
    Neurogenic bladder dysfunction NOS

● **N32 Other disorders of bladder**
   Excludes2 calculus of bladder (N21.0)
                 cystocele (N81.1-)
                 hernia or prolapse of bladder, female (N81.1-)

  N32.0 Bladder-neck obstruction
    Bladder-neck stenosis (acquired)
      Excludes1 congenital bladder-neck obstruction (Q64.3-)

  N32.1 Vesicointestinal fistula 🔍
    Vesicorectal fistula
    (Ex) See PDX Collection 933

  N32.2 Vesical fistula, not elsewhere classified 🔍
      Excludes1 fistula between bladder and female genital tract (N82.0-N82.1)
    (Ex) See PDX Collection 933

  N32.3 Diverticulum of bladder
    Formation of sac from a herniation of wall of bladder
      Excludes1 congenital diverticulum of bladder (Q64.6)
                 diverticulitis of bladder (N30.8-)

● **N32.8　Other specified disorders of bladder**

　N32.81　Overactive bladder
　　　Detrusor muscle hyperactivity
　　　Excludes1　frequent urination due to
　　　　　　　　　specified bladder condition-
　　　　　　　　　code to condition

　N32.89　Other specified disorders of bladder
　　　Bladder hemorrhage
　　　Bladder hypertrophy
　　　Calcified bladder
　　　Contracted bladder

N32.9　Bladder disorder, unspecified

▶ **N33　Bladder disorders in diseases classified elsewhere**
　　Code first underlying disease, such as:
　　　schistosomiasis (B65.0-B65.9)
　　Excludes1　bladder disorder in syphilis (A52.76)
　　　　　　bladder disorder in tuberculosis (A18.12)
　　　　　　candidal cystitis (B37.41)
　　　　　　chlamydial cystitis(A56.01)
　　　　　　cystitis in gonorrhea (A54.01)
　　　　　　cystitis in neurogenic bladder (N31.-)
　　　　　　diphtheritic cystitis (A36.85)
　　　　　　syphilitic cystitis (A52.76)
　　　　　　trichomonal cystitis (A59.03)

● **N34　Urethritis and urethral syndrome**
　　Use additional code (B95-B97), to identify infectious agent
　　Excludes2　Reiter's disease (M02.3-)
　　　　　　urethritis in diseases with a predominantly sexual
　　　　　　　mode of transmission (A50-A64)
　　　　　　urethrotrigonitis (N30.3-)

　N34.0　Urethral abscess 🔵🔵
　　　Abscess (of) Cowper's gland
　　　Abscess (of) Littré's gland
　　　Abscess (of) urethral (gland)
　　　Periurethral abscess
　　　Excludes1　urethral caruncle (N36.2)
　　　(Ex:) See PDX Collection 934

　N34.1　Nonspecific urethritis
　　　Nongonococcal urethritis
　　　Nonvenereal urethritis

　N34.2　Other urethritis
　　　Inflammation of urethra
　　　Meatitis, urethral
　　　Postmenopausal urethritis
　　　Ulcer of urethra (meatus)
　　　Urethritis NOS

　N34.3　Urethral syndrome, unspecified

● **N35　Urethral stricture**
　　Narrowing of lumen of urethra caused by scarring due to infection or injury
　　Excludes1　congenital urethral stricture (Q64.3-)
　　　　　　postprocedural urethral stricture (N99.1-)

　● **N35.0　Post-traumatic urethral stricture**
　　　Urethral stricture due to injury
　　　Excludes1　postprocedural urethral stricture (N99.1-)
　　● **N35.01　Post-traumatic urethral stricture, male**
　　　　N35.010　Post-traumatic urethral stricture, male, meatal ♂
　　　　N35.011　Post-traumatic bulbous urethral stricture ♂
　　　　N35.012　Post-traumatic membranous urethral stricture ♂
　　　　N35.013　Post-traumatic anterior urethral stricture ♂
　　　　N35.014　Post-traumatic urethral stricture, male, unspecified ♂
　　● **N35.02　Post-traumatic urethral stricture, female**
　　　　N35.021　Urethral stricture due to childbirth ♀
　　　　N35.028　Other post-traumatic urethral stricture, female ♀

● **N35.1　Postinfective urethral stricture, not elsewhere classified**
　　Excludes1　urethral stricture associated with
　　　　　　　schistosomiasis (B65.-, N29)
　　　　　　gonococcal urethral stricture (A54.01)
　　　　　　syphilitic urethral stricture (A52.76)
　● **N35.11　Postinfective urethral stricture, not elsewhere classified, male**
　　　N35.111　Postinfective urethral stricture, not elsewhere classified, male, meatal ♂
　⇒ **N35.112　Postinfective bulbous urethral stricture, not elsewhere classified, male** ♂
　⇒ **N35.113　Postinfective membranous urethral stricture, not elsewhere classified, male** ♂
　⇒ **N35.114　Postinfective anterior urethral stricture, not elsewhere classified, male** ♂
　　　N35.119　Postinfective urethral stricture, not elsewhere classified, male, unspecified ♂
　N35.12　Postinfective urethral stricture, not elsewhere classified, female ♀

N35.8　Other urethral stricture
　Excludes1　postprocedural urethral stricture (N99.1-)

N35.9　Urethral stricture, unspecified

● **N36　Other disorders of urethra**
　N36.0　Urethral fistula 🔵
　　　Urethroperineal fistula
　　　Urethrorectal fistula
　　　Urinary fistula NOS
　　　Excludes1　urethroscrotal fistula (N50.89)
　　　　　　urethrovaginal fistula (N82.1)
　　　　　　urethrovesicovaginal fistula (N82.1)
　　　(Ex:) See PDX Collection 935

　N36.1　Urethral diverticulum
　N36.2　Urethral caruncle
　● **N36.4　Urethral functional and muscular disorders**
　　　Use additional code to identify associated urinary stress incontinence (N39.3)
　　N36.41　Hypermobility of urethra
　　N36.42　Intrinsic sphincter deficiency (ISD)
　　N36.43　Combined hypermobility of urethra and intrinsic sphincter deficiency
　　N36.44　Muscular disorders of urethra
　　　　Bladder sphincter dyssynergy

　N36.5　Urethral false passage
　N36.8　Other specified disorders of urethra
　　Excludes1　congenital urethrocele (Q64.7)
　　　　　　female urethrocele (N81.0)
　N36.9　Urethral disorder, unspecified

▶ **N37　Urethral disorders in diseases classified elsewhere**
　　Code first underlying disease
　　Excludes1　urethritis (in):
　　　　　　candidal infection (B37.41)
　　　　　　chlamydial (A56.01)
　　　　　　gonorrhea (A54.01)
　　　　　　syphilis (A52.76)
　　　　　　trichomonal infection (A59.03)
　　　　　　tuberculosis (A18.13)

● **N39**   **Other disorders of urinary system**

     Excludes2   hematuria NOS (R31.-)
           recurrent or persistent hematuria (N02.-)
           recurrent or persistent hematuria with specified
              morphological lesion (N02.-)
           proteinuria NOS (R80.-)

     N39.0   **Urinary tract infection, site not specified** ⊘ ⊘̄

         Use additional code (B95-B97), to identify infectious
           agent

         Excludes1   candidiasis of urinary tract (B37.4-)
              neonatal urinary tract infection (P39.3)
              urinary tract infection of specified site,
                 such as:
                    cystitis (N30.-)
                    urethritis (N34.-)

         (Ex) See PDX Collection 936
         Coding Clinic: 2012, Q4, P94

     N39.3   **Stress incontinence (female) (male)**

         Code also any associated overactive bladder (N32.81)

         Excludes1   mixed incontinence (N39.46)

●   **N39.4**   **Other specified urinary incontinence**

         Code also any associated overactive bladder (N32.81)

         Excludes1   enuresis NOS (R32)
              functional urinary incontinence (R39.81)
              urinary incontinence associated with
                 cognitive impairment (R39.81)
              urinary incontinence NOS (R32)
              urinary incontinence of nonorganic origin
                 (F98.0)

         N39.41   **Urge incontinence**

             Excludes1   mixed incontinence (N39.46)

         N39.42   **Incontinence without sensory awareness**
             Insensible (urinary) incontinence

         N39.43   **Post-void dribbling**

         N39.44   **Nocturnal enuresis**

         N39.45   **Continuous leakage**

         N39.46   **Mixed incontinence**
             Urge and stress incontinence

●   **N39.49**   **Other specified urinary incontinence**

         N39.490   **Overflow incontinence**

         N39.491   **Coital incontinence**
             Coding Clinic: 2016, Q4, P44

         N39.492   **Postural (urinary) incontinence**
             Coding Clinic: 2016, Q4, P44

         N39.498   **Other specified urinary incontinence**
             Reflex incontinence
             Total incontinence

     N39.8   **Other specified disorders of urinary system**

     N39.9   **Disorder of urinary system, unspecified**

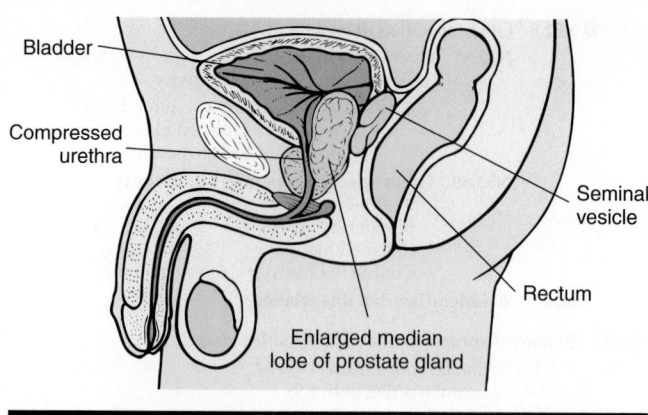

Figure 14-6   Benign prostatic hyperplasia. (From Shiland: Mastering Healthcare Terminology, ed 3, St. Louis, Mosby, 2010)

DISEASES OF MALE GENITAL ORGANS (N40-N53)

★ **(See Plate 387 on page 53.)**

● **N40**   **Benign prostatic hyperplasia**

     Includes   adenofibromatous hypertrophy of prostate
            benign hypertrophy of the prostate
               Enlargement of prostate gland usually occurring
                 with age and causing obstructed urine flow
            benign prostatic hypertrophy
            BPH
            enlarged prostate
            nodular prostate
            polyp of prostate

     Excludes1   benign neoplasms of prostate (adenoma, benign)
              (fibroadenoma) (fibroma) (myoma) (D29.1)
            malignant neoplasm of prostate (C61)

     N40.0   **Benign prostatic hyperplasia without lower urinary tract symptoms** ♂   A
         Enlarged prostate without LUTS
         Enlarged prostate NOS

     N40.1   **Benign prostatic hyperplasia with lower urinary tract symptoms** ♂   A
         Enlarged prostate with LUTS

         Use additional code for associated symptoms, when
           specified:
           incomplete bladder emptying (R39.14)
           nocturia (R35.1)
           straining on urination (R39.16)
           urinary frequency (R35.0)
           urinary hesitancy (R39.11)
           urinary incontinence (N39.4-)
           urinary obstruction (N13.8)
           urinary retention (R33.8)
           urinary urgency (R39.15)
           weak urinary stream (R39.12)

     N40.2   **Nodular prostate without lower urinary tract symptoms** ♂   A
         Nodular prostate without LUTS

     N40.3   **Nodular prostate with lower urinary tract symptoms** ♂   A

         Use additional code for associated symptoms, when
           specified:
           incomplete bladder emptying (R39.14)
           nocturia (R35.1)
           straining on urination (R39.16)
           urinary frequency (R35.0)
           urinary hesitancy (R39.11)
           urinary incontinence (N39.4-)
           urinary obstruction (N13.8)
           urinary retention (R33.8)
           urinary urgency (R39.15)
           weak urinary stream (R39.12)

● **N41   Inflammatory diseases of prostate**
    Use additional code (B95-B97), to identify infectious agent

    N41.0   Acute prostatitis ♂ 🦠   A
       Ⓔ See PDX Collection 937

    N41.1   Chronic prostatitis ♂   A

    N41.2   Abscess of prostate ♂ 🦠   A
       Ⓔ See PDX Collection 937

    N41.3   Prostatocystitis ♂   A

    N41.4   Granulomatous prostatitis ♂   A

    N41.8   Other inflammatory diseases of prostate ♂   A

    N41.9   Inflammatory disease of prostate, unspecified ♂   A
       Prostatitis NOS

● **N42   Other and unspecified disorders of prostate**

    N42.0   Calculus of prostate ♂   A
       Prostatic stone

    N42.1   Congestion and hemorrhage of prostate ♂   A
       Excludes1   enlarged prostate (N40.-)
                 hematuria (R31.-)
                 hyperplasia of prostate (N40.-)
                 inflammatory diseases of prostate (N41.-)

  ● **N42.3   Dysplasia of prostate**
       Coding Clinic: 2016, Q4, P44

    N42.30   Unspecified dysplasia of prostate ♂

    N42.31   Prostatic intraepithelial neoplasia ♂
       PIN
       Prostatic intraepithelial neoplasia I (PIN I)
       Prostatic intraepithelial neoplasia II (PIN II)
       Excludes1   prostatic intraepithelial neoplasia
                 III (PIN III) (D07.5)

    N42.32   Atypical small acinar proliferation of prostate ♂

    N42.39   Other dysplasia of prostate ♂

  ● **N42.8   Other specified disorders of prostate**

    N42.81   Prostatodynia syndrome ♂   A
       Painful prostate syndrome

    N42.82   Prostatosis syndrome ♂   A

    N42.83   Cyst of prostate ♂   A

    N42.89   Other specified disorders of prostate ♂   A

    N42.9   Disorder of prostate, unspecified ♂   A

● **N43   Hydrocele and spermatocele**
       Includes   hydrocele of spermatic cord, testis or tunica vaginalis
       Excludes1   congenital hydrocele (P83.5)

    N43.0   Encysted hydrocele ♂

    N43.1   Infected hydrocele ♂ 🦠
       Use additional code (B95-B97), to identify infectious agent
       Ⓔ See PDX Collection 938

    N43.2   Other hydrocele ♂

    N43.3   Hydrocele, unspecified ♂

  ● **N43.4   Spermatocele of epididymis**
       Spermatic cyst

    N43.40   Spermatocele of epididymis, unspecified ♂

    N43.41   Spermatocele of epididymis, single ♂

    N43.42   Spermatocele of epididymis, multiple ♂

● **N44   Noninflammatory disorders of testis**

  ● **N44.0   Torsion of testis**
       Ⓔ **For category N44.0 CC codes: See PDX Collection 939**

    N44.00   Torsion of testis, unspecified ♂ 🦠

    N44.01   Extravaginal torsion of spermatic cord ♂ 🦠

    N44.02   Intravaginal torsion of spermatic cord ♂ 🦠
       Torsion of spermatic cord NOS

    N44.03   Torsion of appendix testis ♂ 🦠

    N44.04   Torsion of appendix epididymis ♂ 🦠

    N44.1   Cyst of tunica albuginea testis ♂

    N44.2   Benign cyst of testis ♂

    N44.8   Other noninflammatory disorders of the testis ♂

● **N45   Orchitis and epididymitis**
       Orchitis is inflammation of one or both of the testes as a result of mumps or other infection, trauma, or metastasis. Epididymitis is inflammation of the tubular structure that connects the testicle with the vas deferens.
       Use additional code (B95-B97), to identify infectious agent

    N45.1   Epididymitis ♂

    N45.2   Orchitis ♂

    N45.3   Epididymo-orchitis ♂

    N45.4   Abscess of epididymis or testis ♂ 🦠
       Ⓔ See PDX Collection 940

● **N46   Male infertility**
       Excludes1   vasectomy status (Z98.52)

  ● **N46.0   Azoospermia**
       Absolute male infertility
       Male infertility due to germinal (cell) aplasia
       Male infertility due to spermatogenic arrest (complete)

    N46.01   Organic azoospermia ♂   A
       Azoospermia NOS

  ● **N46.02   Azoospermia due to extratesticular causes**
       Code also associated cause

    N46.021   Azoospermia due to drug therapy ♂   A

    N46.022   Azoospermia due to infection ♂   A

    N46.023   Azoospermia due to obstruction of efferent ducts ♂   A

    N46.024   Azoospermia due to radiation ♂   A

    N46.025   Azoospermia due to systemic disease ♂   A

    N46.029   Azoospermia due to other extratesticular causes ♂   A

CHAPTER 14 (N00-N99)

Item 14–7   Hydrocele is a sac of fluid accumulating in the testes membrane.

Blood vessels
Vas deferens
Epididymis
Testis
A   Hydrocele

Figure 14-7   A. Hydrocele. **B.** Newborn with large right hydrocele. (**B** from Nelson WE, Kliegman R: Nelson Textbook of Pediatrics, Philadelphia, Saunders Elsevier, 2011)

Item 14–8 Male infertility is the inability of the female sex partner to conceive after one year of unprotected intercourse.
    Azoospermia is no sperm ejaculated and **oligospermia** is few sperm ejaculated—both resulting in infertility. Extratesticular causes such as injury, infections, radiation, and chemotherapy may also cause male infertility.

N Newborn Age: 0   **P** Pediatric Age: 0–17   **M** Maternity DX: 12–55   **A** Adult Age: 15–124   ♀ Females Only   ♂ Males Only

🦠 Complication\Comorbidity   🦠 Major C\C   Ⓔ CC/MCC Exclusions   🦠 Hospital-Acquired Condition

1105

● **N46.1** **Oligospermia**
    Male infertility due to germinal cell desquamation
    Male infertility due to hypospermatogenesis
    Male infertility due to incomplete spermatogenic arrest

    N46.11 **Organic oligospermia** ♂   A
         Oligospermia NOS

  ● **N46.12** **Oligospermia due to extratesticular causes**
         Code also associated cause

        N46.121 Oligospermia due to drug therapy ♂ A

        N46.122 Oligospermia due to infection ♂   A

        N46.123 Oligospermia due to obstruction of efferent ducts ♂   A

        N46.124 Oligospermia due to radiation ♂   A

        N46.125 Oligospermia due to systemic disease ♂   A

        N46.129 Oligospermia due to other extratesticular causes ♂ A

 N46.8 Other male infertility ♂   A

 N46.9 Male infertility, unspecified ♂   A

● **N47** **Disorders of prepuce**
 N47.0 Adherent prepuce, newborn ♂   N
 N47.1 Phimosis ♂
 N47.2 Paraphimosis ♂
 N47.3 Deficient foreskin ♂
 N47.4 Benign cyst of prepuce ♂
 N47.5 Adhesions of prepuce and glans penis ♂
 N47.6 Balanoposthitis ♂
    Use additional code (B95-B97), to identify infectious agent
    Excludes1 balanitis (N48.1)
 N47.7 Other inflammatory diseases of prepuce ♂
    Use additional code (B95-B97), to identify infectious agent
 N47.8 Other disorders of prepuce ♂

● **N48** **Other disorders of penis**
 N48.0 Leukoplakia of penis ♂
    Balanitis xerotica obliterans
    Kraurosis of penis
    Lichen sclerosus of external male genital organs
    Excludes1 carcinoma in situ of penis (D07.4)
 N48.1 Balanitis ♂
    Use additional code (B95-B97), to identify infectious agent
    Excludes1 amebic balanitis (A06.8)
             balanitis xerotica obliterans (N48.0)
             candidal balanitis (B37.42)
             gonococcal balanitis (A54.23)
             herpesviral [herpes simplex] balanitis (A60.01)

● **N48.2** **Other inflammatory disorders of penis**
    Use additional code (B95-B97), to identify infectious agent
    Excludes1 balanitis (N48.1)
             balanitis xerotica obliterans (N48.0)
             balanoposthitis (N47.6)
    N48.21 Abscess of corpus cavernosum and penis ♂
    N48.22 Cellulitis of corpus cavernosum and penis ♂
    N48.29 Other inflammatory disorders of penis ♂

● **N48.3** **Priapism**
    Painful erection
    Code first underlying cause
    Ⓔ𝔁 **For category N48.3 CC codes:** See PDX Collection 941
    N48.30 Priapism, unspecified ♂ ◐
    N48.31 Priapism due to trauma ♂ ◐
    ▶ *N48.32* *Priapism due to disease classified elsewhere ♂* ◐
    N48.33 Priapism, drug-induced ♂ ◐
    N48.39 Other priapism ♂ ◐
 N48.5 Ulcer of penis ♂
 N48.6 Induration penis plastica ♂
    Peyronie's disease
    Plastic induration of penis
● **N48.8** **Other specified disorders of penis**
    N48.81 Thrombosis of superficial vein of penis ♂
    N48.82 Acquired torsion of penis ♂
         Acquired torsion of penis NOS
         Excludes1 congenital torsion of penis (Q55.63)
    N48.83 Acquired buried penis ♂
         Excludes1 congenital hidden penis (Q55.64)
    N48.89 Other specified disorders of penis ♂
 N48.9 Disorder of penis, unspecified ♂

● **N49** **Inflammatory disorders of male genital organs, not elsewhere classified**
    Use additional code (B95-B97), to identify infectious agent
    Excludes1 inflammation of penis (N48.1, N48.2-)
             orchitis and epididymitis (N45.-)
 N49.0 Inflammatory disorders of seminal vesicle ♂
    Vesiculitis NOS
 N49.1 Inflammatory disorders of spermatic cord, tunica vaginalis and vas deferens ♂
    Vasitis
 N49.2 Inflammatory disorders of scrotum ♂
 N49.3 Fournier gangrene ♂
 N49.8 Inflammatory disorders of other specified male genital organs ♂
    Inflammation of multiple sites in male genital organs
 N49.9 Inflammatory disorder of unspecified male genital organ ♂
    Abscess of unspecified male genital organ
    Boil of unspecified male genital organ
    Carbuncle of unspecified male genital organ
    Cellulitis of unspecified male genital organ

Item 14–9 Seminal vesiculitis is an inflammation of the seminal vesicle. **Spermatocele** is a benign cystic accumulation of sperm arising from the head of the epididymis. **Torsion of the testis** is a medical emergency occurring most commonly in boys 7 to 12 years of age and results from a congenital abnormality of the covering of the testis allowing the testis to twist within its sac and cutting off the blood supply to the testis.

Figure 14-8 **A.** Torsion of testis. **B.** Torsion of the testis. (**B** from Kliegman R, Nelson WE: Nelson Textbook of Pediatrics, Philadelphia, Saunders, 2007)

● **N50   Other and unspecified disorders of male genital organs**

        Excludes2   torsion of testis (N44.0-)

    N50.0   Atrophy of testis ♂

    N50.1   Vascular disorders of male genital organs ♂

        Hematocele, NOS, of male genital organs

        Hemorrhage of male genital organs

        Thrombosis of male genital organs

    N50.3   Cyst of epididymis ♂

●   **N50.8   Other specified disorders of male genital organs**

        Coding Clinic: 2016, Q4, P45

    ● **N50.81   Testicular pain**

        N50.811   Right testicular pain ♂

        N50.812   Left testicular pain ♂

        N50.819   Testicular pain, unspecified ♂

    N50.82   Scrotal pain ♂

    N50.89   Other specified disorders of the male genital organs ♂

        Atrophy of scrotum, seminal vesicle, spermatic cord, tunica vaginalis and vas deferens

        Chylocele, tunica vaginalis (nonfilarial) NOS

        Edema of scrotum, seminal vesicle, spermatic cord, tunica vaginalis and vas deferens

        Hypertrophy of scrotum, seminal vesicle, spermatic cord, tunica vaginalis and vas deferens

        Stricture of spermatic cord, tunica vaginalis, and vas deferens

        Ulcer of scrotum, seminal vesicle, spermatic cord, testis, tunica vaginalis and vas deferens

        Urethroscrotal fistula

    N50.9   Disorder of male genital organs, unspecified ♂

▌ *N51   Disorders of male genital organs in diseases classified elsewhere* ♂

    Code first underlying disease, such as:

      filariasis (B74.0-B74.9)

    Excludes1   amebic balanitis (A06.8)

        candidal balanitis (B37.42)

        gonococcal balanitis (A54.23)

        gonococcal prostatitis (A54.22)

        herpesviral [herpes simplex] balanitis (A60.01)

        trichomonal prostatitis (A59.02)

        tuberculous prostatitis (A18.14)

● **N52   Male erectile dysfunction**

    Excludes1   psychogenic impotence (F52.21)

●   **N52.0   Vasculogenic erectile dysfunction**

    N52.01   Erectile dysfunction due to arterial insufficiency ♂   A

    N52.02   Corporo-venous occlusive erectile dysfunction ♂   A

    N52.03   Combined arterial insufficiency and corporo-venous occlusive erectile dysfunction ♂   A

▌ *N52.1   Erectile dysfunction due to diseases classified elsewhere* ♂   A

    Code first underlying disease

    N52.2   Drug-induced erectile dysfunction ♂   A

●   **N52.3   Postprocedural erectile dysfunction**

    N52.31   Erectile dysfunction following radical prostatectomy ♂   A

    N52.32   Erectile dysfunction following radical cystectomy ♂   A

    N52.33   Erectile dysfunction following urethral surgery ♂   A

    N52.34   Erectile dysfunction following simple prostatectomy ♂   A

    N52.35   Erectile dysfunction following radiation therapy ♂   A

        Coding Clinic: 2016, Q4, P45

    N52.36   Erectile dysfunction following interstitial seed therapy ♂   A

        Coding Clinic: 2016, Q4, P45

    N52.37   Erectile dysfunction following prostate ablative therapy ♂   A

        Erectile dysfunction following cryotherapy

        Erectile dysfunction following other prostate ablative therapies

        Erectile dysfunction following ultrasound ablative therapies

        Coding Clinic: 2016, Q4, P45

    N52.39   Other and unspecified postprocedural erectile dysfunction ♂   A

    N52.8   Other male erectile dysfunction ♂   A

    N52.9   Male erectile dysfunction, unspecified ♂   A

        Impotence NOS

● **N53   Other male sexual dysfunction**

    Excludes1   psychogenic sexual dysfunction (F52.-)

●   **N53.1   Ejaculatory dysfunction**

        Excludes1   premature ejaculation (F52.4)

    N53.11   Retarded ejaculation ♂

    N53.12   Painful ejaculation ♂

    N53.13   Anejaculatory orgasm ♂

    N53.14   Retrograde ejaculation ♂

    N53.19   Other ejaculatory dysfunction ♂

        Ejaculatory dysfunction NOS

    N53.8   Other male sexual dysfunction ♂

    N53.9   Unspecified male sexual dysfunction ♂

DISORDERS OF BREAST (N60-N65)

    Excludes1   disorders of breast associated with childbirth (O91-O92)

● **N60   Benign mammary dysplasia**

    Benign lumpiness of breast

    Includes   fibrocystic mastopathy

●   **N60.0   Solitary cyst of breast**

        Cyst of breast

    N60.01   Solitary cyst of right breast

    N60.02   Solitary cyst of left breast

    N60.09   Solitary cyst of unspecified breast

●   **N60.1   Diffuse cystic mastopathy**

        Cystic breast

        Fibrocystic disease of breast

        Excludes1   diffuse cystic mastopathy with epithelial proliferation (N60.3-)

    N60.11   Diffuse cystic mastopathy of right breast   A

    N60.12   Diffuse cystic mastopathy of left breast   A

    N60.19   Diffuse cystic mastopathy of unspecified breast   A

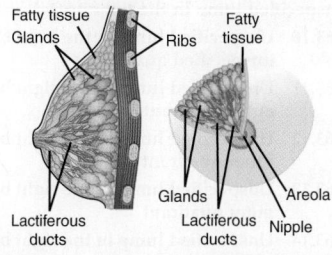

Figure 14-9 Breast.

N Newborn Age: 0   **P** Pediatric Age: 0–17   **M** Maternity DX: 12–55   **A** Adult Age: 15–124   ♀ Females Only   ♂ Males Only

    🔿 Complication\Comorbidity   🔿 Major C\C   (Ex) CC/MCC Exclusions   🔿 Hospital-Acquired Condition   **1107**

CHAPTER 14 (N00-N99)

● N60.2 **Fibroadenosis of breast**
Adenofibrosis of breast
> **Excludes2** fibroadenoma of breast (D24.-)

N60.21 **Fibroadenosis of right breast**
N60.22 **Fibroadenosis of left breast**
N60.29 **Fibroadenosis of unspecified breast**

● N60.3 **Fibrosclerosis of breast**
Cystic mastopathy with epithelial proliferation
N60.31 **Fibrosclerosis of right breast**
N60.32 **Fibrosclerosis of left breast**
N60.39 **Fibrosclerosis of unspecified breast**

● N60.4 **Mammary duct ectasia**
N60.41 **Mammary duct ectasia of right breast**
N60.42 **Mammary duct ectasia of left breast**
N60.49 **Mammary duct ectasia of unspecified breast**

● N60.8 **Other benign mammary dysplasias**
N60.81 **Other benign mammary dysplasias of right breast**
N60.82 **Other benign mammary dysplasias of left breast**
N60.89 **Other benign mammary dysplasias of unspecified breast**

● N60.9 **Unspecified benign mammary dysplasia**
N60.91 **Unspecified benign mammary dysplasia of right breast**
N60.92 **Unspecified benign mammary dysplasia of left breast**
N60.99 **Unspecified benign mammary dysplasia of unspecified breast**

● N61 **Inflammatory disorders of breast**
> **Excludes1** inflammatory carcinoma of breast (C50.9)
> inflammatory disorder of breast associated with childbirth (O91.-)
> neonatal infective mastitis (P39.0)
> thrombophlebitis of breast [Mondor's disease] (I80.8)

N61.0 **Mastitis without abscess**
Infective mastitis (acute) (nonpuerperal) (subacute)
Mastitis (acute) (nonpuerperal) (subacute) NOS
Cellulitis (acute) (nonpuerperal) (subacute) of breast NOS
Cellulitis (acute) (nonpuerperal) (subacute) of nipple NOS

N61.1 **Abscess of the breast and nipple**
Abscess (acute) (chronic) (nonpuerperal) of areola
Abscess (acute) (chronic) (nonpuerperal) of breast
Carbuncle of breast
Mastitis with abscess

N62 **Hypertrophy of breast**
Gynecomastia
Hypertrophy of breast NOS
Massive pubertal hypertrophy of breast
> **Excludes1** breast engorgement of newborn (P83.4)
> disproportion of reconstructed breast (N65.1)

● N63 **Unspecified lump in breast**
Nodule(s) NOS in breast
▶ N63.0 **Unspecified lump in unspecified breast**
▶● N63.1 **Unspecified lump in the right breast**
▶ N63.10 **Unspecified lump in the right breast, unspecified quadrant**
▶ N63.11 **Unspecified lump in the right breast, upper outer quadrant**
▶ N63.12 **Unspecified lump in the right breast, upper inner quadrant**
▶ N63.13 **Unspecified lump in the right breast, lower outer quadrant**
▶ N63.14 **Unspecified lump in the right breast, lower inner quadrant**

▶● N63.2 **Unspecified lump in the left breast**
▶ N63.20 **Unspecified lump in the left breast, unspecified quadrant**
▶ N63.21 **Unspecified lump in the left breast, upper outer quadrant**
▶ N63.22 **Unspecified lump in the left breast, upper inner quadrant**
▶ N63.23 **Unspecified lump in the left breast, lower outer quadrant**
▶ N63.24 **Unspecified lump in the left breast, lower inner quadrant**

▶● N63.3 **Unspecified lump in axillary tail**
▶ N63.31 **Unspecified lump in axillary tail of the right breast**
▶ N63.32 **Unspecified lump in axillary tail of the left breast**

▶● N63.4 **Unspecified lump in breast, subareolar**
▶ N63.41 **Unspecified lump in right breast, subareolar**
▶ N63.42 **Unspecified lump in left breast, subareolar**

● N64 **Other disorders of breast**
> **Excludes2** mechanical complication of breast prosthesis and implant (T85.4-)

N64.0 **Fissure and fistula of nipple**
● N64.1 **Fat necrosis of breast**
Fat necrosis (segmental) of breast
Code first breast necrosis due to breast graft (T85.898)

N64.2 **Atrophy of breast**
N64.3 **Galactorrhea not associated with childbirth**
Excessive or spontaneous flow of milk
N64.4 **Mastodynia**
● N64.5 **Other signs and symptoms in breast**
> **Excludes2** abnormal findings on diagnostic imaging of breast (R92.-)

N64.51 **Induration of breast**
N64.52 **Nipple discharge**
> **Excludes1** abnormal findings in nipple discharge (R89.-)

N64.53 **Retraction of nipple**
N64.59 **Other signs and symptoms in breast**
● N64.8 **Other specified disorders of breast**
N64.81 **Ptosis of breast**   A
> **Excludes1** ptosis of native breast in relation to reconstructed breast (N65.1)

N64.82 **Hypoplasia of breast**   A
Micromastia
> **Excludes1** congenital absence of breast (Q83.0)
> hypoplasia of native breast in relation to reconstructed breast (N65.1)

N64.89 **Other specified disorders of breast**
Galactocele
Subinvolution of breast (postlactational)

N64.9 **Disorder of breast, unspecified**

● N65 **Deformity and disproportion of reconstructed breast**
N65.0 **Deformity of reconstructed breast**   A
Contour irregularity in reconstructed breast
Excess tissue in reconstructed breast
Misshapen reconstructed breast

N65.1 **Disproportion of reconstructed breast**   A
Breast asymmetry between native breast and reconstructed breast
Disproportion between native breast and reconstructed breast

INFLAMMATORY DISEASES OF FEMALE PELVIC ORGANS (N70-N77)

Excludes1   inflammatory diseases of female pelvic organs
complicating:
abortion or ectopic or molar pregnancy
(O00-O07, O08.0)
pregnancy, childbirth and the puerperium
(O23.-, O75.3, O85, O86.-)

★ **(See Plate 360 on page 80.)**

● **N70**   **Salpingitis and oophoritis**
Oophoritis = inflammation of ovary
Salpingitis = inflammation of fallopian tube

     Includes   abscess (of) fallopian tube
abscess (of) ovary
pyosalpinx
salpingo-oophoritis
tubo-ovarian abscess
tubo-ovarian inflammatory disease

     Use additional code (B95-B97), to identify infectious agent

     Excludes1   gonococcal infection (A54.24)
tuberculous infection (A18.17)

   ● **N70.0**   **Acute salpingitis and oophoritis**
Ⓔ **For category N70.0 CC codes:** See PDX Collection 942

     N70.01   Acute salpingitis ♀ 🦠
     N70.02   Acute oophoritis ♀ 🦠
     N70.03   Acute salpingitis and oophoritis ♀ 🦠

   ● **N70.1**   **Chronic salpingitis and oophoritis**
Hydrosalpinx

     N70.11   Chronic salpingitis ♀
     N70.12   Chronic oophoritis ♀
     N70.13   Chronic salpingitis and oophoritis ♀

   ● **N70.9**   **Salpingitis and oophoritis, unspecified**
     N70.91   Salpingitis, unspecified ♀
     N70.92   Oophoritis, unspecified ♀
     N70.93   Salpingitis and oophoritis, unspecified ♀

● **N71**   **Inflammatory disease of uterus, except cervix**

     Includes   endo (myo) metritis
metritis
myometritis
pyometra
uterine abscess

     Use additional code (B95-B97), to identify infectious agent

     Excludes1   hyperplastic endometritis (N85.0-)
infection of uterus following delivery (O85, O86.-)

   N71.0   **Acute inflammatory disease of uterus** ♀ 🦠
Ⓔ See PDX Collection 943

   N71.1   **Chronic inflammatory disease of uterus** ♀

   N71.9   **Inflammatory disease of uterus, unspecified** ♀

Fallopian tube (oviduct)
Corpus uteri
Cervix uteri
Rectum
Vagina
Ovary
Isthmus
Urinary bladder
Symphysis pubis
Clitoris
Urethra
*Mons veneris
*Labium majus
Urethra
*Labium minus
Introitus
Bartholin's glands
Perineum

A   Female Genital System   B   *The three parts of the vulva

Figure 14-10   **A.** Female genital system. **B.** External female genital system. (From Buck CJ: Step-by-Step Medical Coding, ed 2016, St. Louis, Elsevier, 2016)

Item 14-10 Salpingitis is an infection of one or both fallopian tubes. **Oophoritis** is an infection of one or both ovaries.

● **N72**   **Inflammatory disease of cervix uteri** ♀

     Includes   cervicitis (with or without erosion or ectropion)
endocervicitis (with or without erosion or ectropion)
exocervicitis (with or without erosion or ectropion)

     Use additional code (B95-B97), to identify infectious agent

     Excludes1   erosion and ectropion of cervix without cervicitis (N86)

● **N73**   **Other female pelvic inflammatory diseases**

     Use additional code (B95-B97), to identify infectious agent

   N73.0   **Acute parametritis and pelvic cellulitis** ♀ 🦠
Abscess of broad ligament
Abscess of parametrium
Pelvic cellulitis, female
Ⓔ See PDX Collection 942

   N73.1   **Chronic parametritis and pelvic cellulitis** ♀
Any condition in N73.0 specified as chronic

     Excludes1   tuberculous parametritis and pelvic cellutis (A18.17)

   N73.2   **Unspecified parametritis and pelvic cellulitis** ♀
Any condition in N73.0 unspecified whether acute or chronic

   N73.3   **Female acute pelvic peritonitis** ♀ 🦠
Ⓔ See PDX Collection 942

   N73.4   **Female chronic pelvic peritonitis** ♀ 🦠

     Excludes1   tuberculous pelvic (female) peritonitis (A18.17)
Ⓔ See PDX Collection 942

   N73.5   **Female pelvic peritonitis, unspecified** ♀

   N73.6   **Female pelvic peritoneal adhesions (postinfective)** ♀

     Excludes2   postprocedural pelvic peritoneal adhesions (N99.4)

   N73.8   **Other specified female pelvic inflammatory diseases** ♀

   N73.9   **Female pelvic inflammatory disease, unspecified** ♀
Female pelvic infection or inflammation NOS

▌ **N74**   *Female pelvic inflammatory disorders in diseases classified elsewhere* ♀

     Code first underlying disease

     Excludes1   chlamydial cervicitis (A56.02)
chlamydial pelvic inflammatory disease (A56.11)
gonococcal cervicitis (A54.03)
gonococcal pelvic inflammatory disease (A54.24)
herpesviral [herpes simplex] cervicitis (A60.03)
herpesviral [herpes simplex] pelvic inflammatory disease (A60.09)
syphilitic cervicitis (A52.76)
syphilitic pelvic inflammatory disease (A52.76)
trichomonal cervicitis (A59.09)
tuberculous cervicitis (A18.16)
tuberculous pelvic inflammatory disease (A18.17)

● **N75**   **Diseases of Bartholin's gland**

   N75.0   **Cyst of Bartholin's gland** ♀
Cysts filled with liquid or semisolid material

   N75.1   **Abscess of Bartholin's gland** ♀ 🦠
Localized collection of pus
Ⓔ See PDX Collection 944

   N75.8   **Other diseases of Bartholin's gland** ♀
Bartholinitis

   N75.9   **Disease of Bartholin's gland, unspecified** ♀

● **N76**   **Other inflammation of vagina and vulva**

     Use additional code (B95-B97), to identify infectious agent

     Excludes2   senile (atrophic) vaginitis (N95.2)
vulvar vestibulitis (N94.810)

   N76.0   **Acute vaginitis** ♀
Acute vulvovaginitis
Vaginitis NOS
Vulvovaginitis NOS

   N76.1   **Subacute and chronic vaginitis** ♀
Chronic vulvovaginitis
Subacute vulvovaginitis

CHAPTER 14 (N00-N99)

CHAPTER 14 (N00-N99)

N76.2 **Acute vulvitis** ♀
  Vulvitis NOS

N76.3 **Subacute and chronic vulvitis** ♀

N76.4 **Abscess of vulva** ♀ 🔖
  Furuncle of vulva
  Ⓔ See PDX Collection 944

N76.5 **Ulceration of vagina** ♀

N76.6 **Ulceration of vulva** ♀

● N76.8 **Other specified inflammation of vagina and vulva**

  N76.81 **Mucositis (ulcerative) of vagina and vulva** ♀ 🔖

    Code also type of associated therapy, such as:
      antineoplastic and immunosuppressive
        drugs (T45.1X-)
      radiological procedure and radiotherapy
        (Y84.2)

    Excludes2   gastrointestinal mucositis
      (ulcerative) (K92.81)
      nasal mucositis (ulcerative)
        (J34.81)
      oral mucositis (ulcerative) (K12.3-)
    Ⓔ See PDX Collection 945

  N76.89 **Other specified inflammation of vagina and vulva** ♀

● N77 **Vulvovaginal ulceration and inflammation in diseases classified elsewhere**

  ▷ N77.0 *Ulceration of vulva in diseases classified elsewhere* ♀

    Code first underlying disease, such as:
      Behçet's disease (M35.2)

    Excludes1   ulceration of vulva in gonococcal
      infection (A54.02)
      ulceration of vulva in herpesviral [herpes
        simplex] infection (A60.04)
      ulceration of vulva in syphilis (A51.0)
      ulceration of vulva in tuberculosis (A18.18)

  ▷ N77.1 *Vaginitis, vulvitis and vulvovaginitis in diseases classified elsewhere*

    Code first underlying disease, such as:
      pinworm (B80)

    Excludes1   candidial vulvovaginitis (B37.3)
      chlamydial vulvovaginitis (A56.02)
      gonococcal vulvovaginitis (A54.02)
      herpesviral [herpes simplex]
        vulvovaginitis (A60.04)
      trichomonal vulvovaginitis (A59.01)
      tuberculous vulvovaginitis (A18.18)
      vulvovaginitis in early syphilis (A51.0)
      vulvovaginitis in late syphilis (A52.76)

NONINFLAMMATORY DISORDERS OF FEMALE GENITAL TRACT (N80-N98)

● N80 **Endometriosis**

  N80.0 **Endometriosis of uterus** ♀
    Adenomyosis
    Excludes1   stromal endometriosis (D39.0)

  N80.1 **Endometriosis of ovary** ♀

  N80.2 **Endometriosis of fallopian tube** ♀

  N80.3 **Endometriosis of pelvic peritoneum** ♀

  N80.4 **Endometriosis of rectovaginal septum and vagina** ♀

  N80.5 **Endometriosis of intestine** ♀

  N80.6 **Endometriosis in cutaneous scar** ♀

  N80.8 **Other endometriosis** ♀
    ▶ Endometriosis of thorax

  N80.9 **Endometriosis, unspecified** ♀

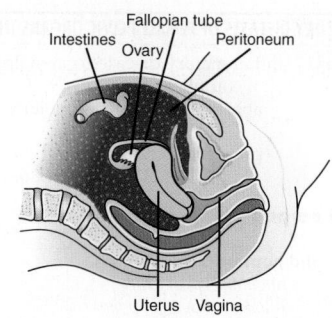

Figure 14-11   Sites of potential endometrial implants.

A   B   C

Figure 14-12   Three stages of uterine prolapse. **A.** Uterus is prolapsed. **B.** Vagina and uterus are prolapsed (incomplete uterovaginal prolapse). **C.** Vagina and uterus are completely prolapsed and are exposed through the external genitalia (complete uterovaginal prolapse).

● N81 **Female genital prolapse**

  Excludes1   genital prolapse complicating pregnancy, labor or
    delivery (O34.5-)
    prolapse and hernia of ovary and fallopian tube
      (N83.4-)
    prolapse of vaginal vault after hysterectomy (N99.3)

  N81.0 **Urethrocele** ♀
    Excludes1   urethrocele with cystocele (N81.1-)
      urethrocele with prolapse of uterus
        (N81.2-N81.4)

● N81.1 **Cystocele**
    Cystocele with urethrocele
    Cystourethrocele
    Excludes1   cystocele with prolapse of uterus
      (N81.2-N81.4)

  N81.10 **Cystocele, unspecified** ♀
    Prolapse of (anterior) vaginal wall NOS

  N81.11 **Cystocele, midline** ♀

  N81.12 **Cystocele, lateral** ♀
    Paravaginal cystocele

  N81.2 **Incomplete uterovaginal prolapse** ♀
    First degree uterine prolapse
    Prolapse of cervix NOS
    Second degree uterine prolapse
    Excludes1   cervical stump prolapse (N81.85)

  N81.3 **Complete uterovaginal prolapse** ♀
    Procidentia (uteri) NOS
    Third degree uterine prolapse

  N81.4 **Uterovaginal prolapse, unspecified** ♀
    Prolapse of uterus NOS

  N81.5 **Vaginal enterocele** ♀
    Excludes1   enterocele with prolapse of uterus
      (N81.2-N81.4)

Item 14–11 Endometriosis is a condition for which no clear cause has been identified. Endometrial tissue is expelled from the uterus into the abdominal cavity and can implant onto a variety of organs. Classification is based on the site of implant of the endometrial tissue.

▶ New   ⇒ Revised   ~~deleted~~ Deleted   Excludes 1   Excludes 2   Includes   Use additional   Code first   Code also   Key words
OGCR Official Guidelines   ● Unacceptable Principal Diagnosis   X Assign placeholder X   ● Use Additional Character(s)   ▷ Manifestation Code   Coding Clinic

N81.6　Rectocele ♀
　　Prolapse of posterior vaginal wall
　　Use additional code for any associated fecal incontinence, if applicable (R15.-)
　　Excludes2　perineocele (N81.81)
　　　　　　　　rectal prolapse (K62.3)
　　　　　　　　rectocele with prolapse of uterus (N81.2-N81.4)

● **N81.8　Other female genital prolapse**
　　N81.81　Perineocele ♀
　　N81.82　Incompetence or weakening of pubocervical tissue ♀
　　N81.83　Incompetence or weakening of rectovaginal tissue ♀
　　N81.84　Pelvic muscle wasting ♀
　　　　Disuse atrophy of pelvic muscles and anal sphincter
　　N81.85　Cervical stump prolapse ♀
　　N81.89　Other female genital prolapse ♀
　　　　Deficient perineum
　　　　Old laceration of muscles of pelvic floor

N81.9　Female genital prolapse, unspecified ♀

● **N82　Fistulae involving female genital tract**
　　Excludes1　vesicointestinal fistulae (N32.1)
　　(Ex) For category N82 CC codes: See PDX Collection 946

　　N82.0　Vesicovaginal fistula ♀ ◐
　　N82.1　Other female urinary-genital tract fistulae ♀ ◐
　　　　Cervicovesical fistula
　　　　Ureterovaginal fistula
　　　　Urethrovaginal fistula
　　　　Uteroureteric fistula
　　　　Uterovesical fistula
　　N82.2　Fistula of vagina to small intestine ♀ ◐
　　N82.3　Fistula of vagina to large intestine ♀ ◐
　　　　Rectovaginal fistula
　　N82.4　Other female intestinal-genital tract fistulae ♀ ◐
　　　　Intestinouterine fistula
　　N82.5　Female genital tract-skin fistulae ♀ ◐
　　　　Uterus to abdominal wall fistula
　　　　Vaginoperineal fistula
　　N82.8　Other female genital tract fistulae ♀ ◐
　　N82.9　Female genital tract fistula, unspecified ♀ ◐

● **N83　Noninflammatory disorders of ovary, fallopian tube and broad ligament**
　　Excludes2　hydrosalpinx (N70.1-)

● **N83.0　Follicular cyst of ovary**
　　　　Cyst of graafian follicle
　　　　Hemorrhagic follicular cyst (of ovary)
　　　　Coding Clinic: 2016, Q4, P46
　　N83.00　Follicular cyst of ovary, unspecified side ♀
　　N83.01　Follicular cyst of right ovary ♀
　　N83.02　Follicular cyst of left ovary ♀

● **N83.1　Corpus luteum cyst**
　　　　Hemorrhagic corpus luteum cyst
　　　　Coding Clinic: 2016, Q4, P46
　　N83.10　Corpus luteum cyst of ovary, unspecified side ♀
　　N83.11　Corpus luteum cyst of right ovary ♀
　　N83.12　Corpus luteum cyst of left ovary ♀

● **N83.2　Other and unspecified ovarian cysts**
　　Excludes1　developmental ovarian cyst (Q50.1)
　　　　　　　　neoplastic ovarian cyst (D27.-)
　　　　　　　　polycystic ovarian syndrome (E28.2)
　　　　　　　　Stein-Leventhal syndrome (E28.2)
　　　　Coding Clinic: 2016, Q4, P46
　● **N83.20　Unspecified ovarian cysts**
　　　　N83.201　Unspecified ovarian cyst, right side ♀

　　　　N83.202　Unspecified ovarian cyst, left side ♀
　　　　N83.209　Unspecified ovarian cyst, unspecified side ♀
　　　　　　Ovarian cyst, NOS
　● **N83.29　Other ovarian cysts**
　　　　Retention cyst of ovary
　　　　Simple cyst of ovary
　　　　N83.291　Other ovarian cyst, right side ♀
　　　　N83.292　Other ovarian cyst, left side ♀
　　　　N83.299　Other ovarian cyst, unspecified side ♀

● **N83.3　Acquired atrophy of ovary and fallopian tube**
　　Coding Clinic: 2016, Q4, P46
　● **N83.31　Acquired atrophy of ovary**
　　　　N83.311　Acquired atrophy of right ovary ♀
　　　　N83.312　Acquired atrophy of left ovary ♀
　　　　N83.319　Acquired atrophy of ovary, unspecified side ♀
　　　　　　Acquired atrophy of ovary, NOS
　● **N83.32　Acquired atrophy of fallopian tube**
　　　　N83.321　Acquired atrophy of right fallopian tube ♀
　　　　N83.322　Acquired atrophy of left fallopian tube ♀
　　　　N83.329　Acquired atrophy of fallopian tube, unspecified side ♀
　　　　　　Acquired atrophy of fallopian tube, NOS
　● **N83.33　Acquired atrophy of ovary and fallopian tube**
　　　　N83.331　Acquired atrophy of right ovary and fallopian tube ♀
　　　　N83.332　Acquired atrophy of left ovary and fallopian tube ♀
　　　　N83.339　Acquired atrophy of ovary and fallopian tube, unspecified side ♀
　　　　　　Acquired atrophy of ovary and fallopian tube, NOS

● **N83.4　Prolapse and hernia of ovary and fallopian tube**
　　Coding Clinic: 2016, Q4, P46
　　N83.40　Prolapse and hernia of ovary and fallopian tube, unspecified side ♀
　　　　Prolapse and hernia of ovary and fallopian tube, NOS
　　N83.41　Prolapse and hernia of right ovary and fallopian tube ♀
　　N83.42　Prolapse and hernia of left ovary and fallopian tube ♀

● **N83.5　Torsion of ovary, ovarian pedicle and fallopian tube**
　　　　Torsion of accessory tube
　　　　(Ex) For category N83.5 CC codes: See PDX Collection 947
　　　　Coding Clinic: 2016, Q4, P46
　● **N83.51　Torsion of ovary and ovarian pedicle**
　　　　N83.511　Torsion of right ovary and ovarian pedicle ♀ ◐
　　　　N83.512　Torsion of left ovary and ovarian pedicle ♀ ◐
　　　　N83.519　Torsion of ovary and ovarian pedicle, unspecified side ♀ ◐
　　　　　　Torsion of ovary and ovarian pedicle, NOS
　● **N83.52　Torsion of fallopian tube**
　　　　Torsion of hydatid of Morgagni
　　　　N83.521　Torsion of right fallopian tube ♀ ◐
　　　　N83.522　Torsion of left fallopian tube ♀ ◐
　　　　N83.529　Torsion of fallopian tube, unspecified side ♀ ◐
　　　　　　Torsion of fallopian tube, NOS
　　N83.53　Torsion of ovary, ovarian pedicle and fallopian tube ♀ ◐

N Newborn Age: 0　　**P** Pediatric Age: 0–17　　**M** Maternity DX: 12–55　　**A** Adult Age: 15–124　　♀ Females Only　　♂ Males Only
　　◐ Complication\Comorbidity　　◐ Major C\C　　(Ex) CC/MCC Exclusions　　◐ Hospital-Acquired Condition

N83.6   Hematosalpinx ♀

> **Excludes1**   hematosalpinx (with) (in):
> > hematocolpos (N89.7)
> > hematometra (N85.7)
> > tubal pregnancy (O00.1-)

N83.7   Hematoma of broad ligament ♀

N83.8   Other noninflammatory disorders of ovary, fallopian tube and broad ligament ♀
> Broad ligament laceration syndrome [Allen-Masters]

N83.9   Noninflammatory disorder of ovary, fallopian tube and broad ligament, unspecified ♀

● **N84   Polyp of female genital tract**

> **Excludes1**   adenomatous polyp (D28.-)
> > placental polyp (O90.89)

N84.0   Polyp of corpus uteri ♀
> Polyp of endometrium
> Polyp of uterus NOS

> > **Excludes1**   polypoid endometrial hyperplasia (N85.0-)

N84.1   Polyp of cervix uteri ♀
> Mucous polyp of cervix

N84.2   Polyp of vagina ♀

N84.3   Polyp of vulva ♀
> Polyp of labia

N84.8   Polyp of other parts of female genital tract ♀

N84.9   Polyp of female genital tract, unspecified ♀

● **N85   Other noninflammatory disorders of uterus, except cervix**

> **Excludes1**   endometriosis (N80.-)
> > inflammatory diseases of uterus (N71.-)
> > noninflammatory disorders of cervix, except malposition (N86-N88)
> > polyp of corpus uteri (N84.0)
> > uterine prolapse (N81.-)

● **N85.0   Endometrial hyperplasia**

N85.00   Endometrial hyperplasia, unspecified ♀
> Hyperplasia (adenomatous) (cystic) (glandular) of endometrium
> Hyperplastic endometritis

N85.01   Benign endometrial hyperplasia ♀
> Endometrial hyperplasia (complex) (simple) without atypia

N85.02   Endometrial intraepithelial neoplasia [EIN] ♀
> Endometrial hyperplasia with atypia

> > **Excludes1**   malignant neoplasm of endometrium (with endometrial intraepithelial neoplasia [EIN]) (C54.1)

N85.2   Hypertrophy of uterus ♀
> Bulky or enlarged uterus

> > **Excludes1**   puerperal hypertrophy of uterus (O90.89)

N85.3   Subinvolution of uterus ♀

> > **Excludes1**   puerperal subinvolution of uterus (O90.89)

N85.4   Malposition of uterus ♀
> Anteversion of uterus
> Retroflexion of uterus
> Retroversion of uterus

> > **Excludes1**   malposition of uterus complicating pregnancy, labor or delivery (O34.5-, O65.5)

N85.5   Inversion of uterus ♀

> > **Excludes1**   current obstetric trauma (O71.2)
> > postpartum inversion of uterus (O71.2)

N85.6   Intrauterine synechiae ♀

N85.7   Hematometra ♀
> Hematosalpinx with hematometra

> > **Excludes1**   hematometra with hematocolpos (N89.7)

N85.8   Other specified noninflammatory disorders of uterus ♀
> Atrophy of uterus, acquired
> Fibrosis of uterus NOS

N85.9   Noninflammatory disorder of uterus, unspecified ♀
> Disorder of uterus NOS

N86   Erosion and ectropion of cervix uteri ♀
> Decubitus (trophic) ulcer of cervix
> Eversion of cervix

> **Excludes1**   erosion and ectropion of cervix with cervicitis (N72)

● **N87   Dysplasia of cervix uteri**

> **Excludes1**   abnormal results from cervical cytologic examination without histologic confirmation (R87.61-)
> > carcinoma in situ of cervix uteri (D06.-)
> > cervical intraepithelial neoplasia III [CIN III] (D06.-)
> > HGSIL of cervix (R87.613)
> > severe dysplasia of cervix uteri (D06.-)

N87.0   Mild cervical dysplasia ♀
> Cervical intraepithelial neoplasia I [CIN I]

N87.1   Moderate cervical dysplasia ♀
> Cervical intraepithelial neoplasia II [CIN II]

N87.9   Dysplasia of cervix uteri, unspecified ♀
> Anaplasia of cervix
> Cervical atypism
> Cervical dysplasia NOS

● **N88   Other noninflammatory disorders of cervix uteri**

> **Excludes2**   inflammatory disease of cervix (N72)
> > polyp of cervix (N84.1)

N88.0   Leukoplakia of cervix uteri ♀

N88.1   Old laceration of cervix uteri ♀
> Adhesions of cervix

> > **Excludes1**   current obstetric trauma (O71.3)

N88.2   Stricture and stenosis of cervix uteri ♀

> > **Excludes1**   stricture and stenosis of cervix uteri complicating labor (O65.5)

N88.3   Incompetence of cervix uteri ♀
> Investigation and management of (suspected) cervical incompetence in a nonpregnant woman

> > **Excludes1**   cervical incompetence complicating pregnancy (O34.3-)

N88.4   Hypertrophic elongation of cervix uteri ♀

N88.8   Other specified noninflammatory disorders of cervix uteri ♀

> > **Excludes1**   current obstetric trauma (O71.3)

N88.9   Noninflammatory disorder of cervix uteri, unspecified ♀

● **N89   Other noninflammatory disorders of vagina**

> **Excludes1**   abnormal results from vaginal cytologic examination without histologic confirmation (R87.62-)
> > carcinoma in situ of vagina (D07.2)
> > HGSIL of vagina (R87.623)
> > inflammation of vagina (N76.-)
> > senile (atrophic) vaginitis (N95.2)
> > severe dysplasia of vagina (D07.2)
> > trichomonal leukorrhea (A59.00)
> > vaginal intraepithelial neoplasia [VAIN], grade III (D07.2)

N89.0   Mild vaginal dysplasia ♀
> Vaginal intraepithelial neoplasia [VAIN], grade I

N89.1   Moderate vaginal dysplasia ♀
> Vaginal intraepithelial neoplasia [VAIN], grade II

N89.3   Dysplasia of vagina, unspecified ♀

N89.4   Leukoplakia of vagina ♀

N89.5   **Stricture and atresia of vagina** ♀
     Vaginal adhesions   Vaginal stenosis
     Excludes1   congenital atresia or stricture (Q52.4)
                postprocedural adhesions of vagina
                    (N99.2)

N89.6   **Tight hymenal ring** ♀
     Rigid hymen   Tight introitus
     Excludes1   imperforate hymen (Q52.3)

N89.7   **Hematocolpos** ♀
     Hematocolpos with hematometra or hematosalpinx
     Coding Clinic: 2016, Q4, P59

N89.8   **Other specified noninflammatory disorders of vagina** ♀
     Leukorrhea NOS
     Old vaginal laceration
     Pessary ulcer of vagina
     Excludes1   current obstetric trauma (O70.-, O71.4,
                O71.7-O71.8)
                old laceration involving muscles of pelvic
                  floor (N81.8)

N89.9   **Noninflammatory disorder of vagina, unspecified** ♀

● **N90**   **Other noninflammatory disorders of vulva and perineum**
     Excludes1   anogenital (venereal) warts (A63.0)
                carcinoma in situ of vulva (D07.1)
                condyloma acuminatum (A63.0)
                current obstetric trauma (O70.-, O71.7-O71.8)
                inflammation of vulva (N76.-)
                severe dysplasia of vulva (D07.1)
                vulvar intraepithelial neoplasm III [VIN III]
                  (D07.1)

N90.0   **Mild vulvar dysplasia** ♀
     Vulvar intraepithelial neoplasia [VIN], grade I

N90.1   **Moderate vulvar dysplasia** ♀
     Vulvar intraepithelial neoplasia [VIN], grade II

N90.3   **Dysplasia of vulva, unspecified** ♀

N90.4   **Leukoplakia of vulva** ♀
     Dystrophy of vulva
     Kraurosis of vulva
     Lichen sclerosus of external female genital organs

N90.5   **Atrophy of vulva** ♀
     Stenosis of vulva

● **N90.6**   **Hypertrophy of vulva**
     Coding Clinic: 2016, Q4, P46

     N90.60   **Unspecified hypertrophy of vulva** ♀
            Unspecified hypertrophy of labia

     N90.61   **Childhood asymmetric labium majus
            enlargement** ♀
            CALME

     N90.69   **Other specified hypertrophy of vulva** ♀
            Other specified hypertrophy of labia

N90.7   **Vulvar cyst** ♀

● **N90.8**   **Other specified noninflammatory disorders of vulva and
perineum**
     ● **N90.81**   **Female genital mutilation status**
            Female genital cutting status

         N90.810   **Female genital mutilation status,
                  unspecified** ♀
                 Female genital cutting status,
                    unspecified
                 Female genital mutilation status NOS

         N90.811   **Female genital mutilation Type I
                  status** ♀
                 Clitorectomy status
                 Female genital cutting Type I status

         N90.812   **Female genital mutilation Type II
                  status** ♀
                 Clitorectomy with excision of labia
                    minora status
                 Female genital cutting Type II status

         N90.813   **Female genital mutilation Type III
                  status** ♀
                 Female genital cutting Type III status
                 Infibulation status

         N90.818   **Other female genital mutilation
                  status** ♀
                 Female genital cutting Type IV status
                 Female genital mutilation Type IV
                    status
                 Other female genital cutting status

     N90.89   **Other specified noninflammatory disorders of
            vulva and perineum** ♀
            Adhesions of vulva
            Hypertrophy of clitoris

N90.9   **Noninflammatory disorder of vulva and perineum,
unspecified** ♀

● **N91**   **Absent, scanty and rare menstruation**
     Excludes1   ovarian dysfunction (E28.-)

N91.0   **Primary amenorrhea** ♀

N91.1   **Secondary amenorrhea** ♀

N91.2   **Amenorrhea, unspecified** ♀

N91.3   **Primary oligomenorrhea** ♀

N91.4   **Secondary oligomenorrhea** ♀

N91.5   **Oligomenorrhea, unspecified** ♀
     Hypomenorrhea NOS

● **N92**   **Excessive, frequent and irregular menstruation**
     Excludes1   postmenopausal bleeding (N95.0)
                precocious puberty (menstruation) (E30.1)

N92.0   **Excessive and frequent menstruation with regular cycle** ♀
     Heavy periods NOS   Polymenorrhea
     Menorrhagia NOS

N92.1   **Excessive and frequent menstruation with irregular
cycle** ♀
     Irregular intermenstrual bleeding
     Irregular, shortened intervals between menstrual bleeding
     Menometrorrhagia
     Metrorrhagia

N92.2   **Excessive menstruation at puberty** ♀   P
     Excessive bleeding associated with onset of menstrual
        periods
     Pubertal menorrhagia
     Puberty bleeding

N92.3   **Ovulation bleeding** ♀
     Regular intermenstrual bleeding

N92.4   **Excessive bleeding in the premenopausal period** ♀
     Climacteric menorrhagia or metrorrhagia
     Menopausal menorrhagia or metrorrhagia
     Preclimacteric menorrhagia or metrorrhagia
     Premenopausal menorrhagia or metrorrhagia

N92.5   **Other specified irregular menstruation** ♀

N92.6   **Irregular menstruation, unspecified** ♀
     Irregular bleeding NOS
     Irregular periods NOS
     Excludes1   irregular menstruation with:
                lengthened intervals or scanty bleeding
                  (N91.3-N91.5)
                shortened intervals or excessive
                  bleeding (N92.1)

● **N93**   **Other abnormal uterine and vaginal bleeding**
     Excludes1   neonatal vaginal hemorrhage (P54.6)
                precocious puberty (menstruation) (E30.1)
                pseudomenses (P54.6)

N93.0   **Postcoital and contact bleeding** ♀

N93.1   **Pre-pubertal vaginal bleeding** ♀
     Coding Clinic: 2016, Q4, P47

N93.8   **Other specified abnormal uterine and vaginal bleeding** ♀
     Dysfunctional or functional uterine or vaginal bleeding
        NOS

N93.9   **Abnormal uterine and vaginal bleeding, unspecified** ♀

CHAPTER 14 (N00-N99)

N   Newborn Age: 0   **P**   Pediatric Age: 0–17   **M**   Maternity DX: 12–55   **A**   Adult Age: 15–124   ♀   Females Only   ♂   Males Only
         ⬤ Complication\Comorbidity   ⬤ Major C\C   (Ex) CC/MCC Exclusions   ⬤ Hospital-Acquired Condition

1113

CHAPTER 14 (N00-N99)

● **N94   Pain and other conditions associated with female genital organs and menstrual cycle**

    N94.0   Mittelschmerz ♀
        Ovulation pain

  ● **N94.1   Dyspareunia**
        Painful intercourse/coitus
        Excludes1   psychogenic dyspareunia (F52.6)
        Coding Clinic: 2016, Q4, P47

        N94.10   Unspecified dyspareunia ♀
        N94.11   Superficial (introital) dyspareunia ♀
        N94.12   Deep dyspareunia ♀
        N94.19   Other specified dyspareunia ♀

    N94.2   Vaginismus ♀
        Vagina tightness
        Excludes1   psychogenic vaginismus (F52.5)

    N94.3   Premenstrual tension syndrome ♀
        AKA: PMS
        ~~Premenstrual dysphoric disorder~~
        Code also associated menstrual migraine (G43.82-, G43.83-)
        Excludes1   Premenstrual dysphoric disorder (F32.81)
        Coding Clinic: 2016, Q4, P14

    N94.4   Primary dysmenorrhea ♀
        Lifelong painful menstruation

    N94.5   Secondary dysmenorrhea ♀
        Later onset of painful menstruation

    N94.6   Dysmenorrhea, unspecified ♀
        Excludes1   psychogenic dysmenorrhea (F45.8)

  ● **N94.8   Other specified conditions associated with female genital organs and menstrual cycle**

     ● **N94.81   Vulvodynia**
        N94.810   Vulvar vestibulitis ♀
        N94.818   Other vulvodynia ♀
        N94.819   Vulvodynia, unspecified ♀
                 Vulvodynia NOS

      N94.89   Other specified conditions associated with female genital organs and menstrual cycle ♀

    N94.9   Unspecified condition associated with female genital organs and menstrual cycle ♀

● **N95   Menopausal and other perimenopausal disorders**
    Menopausal and other perimenopausal disorders due to naturally occurring (age-related) menopause and perimenopause
    Excludes1   excessive bleeding in the premenopausal period (N92.4)
                menopausal and perimenopausal disorders due to artificial or premature menopause (E89.4-, E28.31-)
                premature menopause (E28.31-)
    Excludes2   postmenopausal osteoporosis (M81.0-)
                postmenopausal osteoporosis with current pathological fracture (M80.0-)
                postmenopausal urethritis (N34.2)

    N95.0   Postmenopausal bleeding ♀

    N95.1   Menopausal and female climacteric states ♀
        Symptoms such as flushing, sleeplessness, headache, lack of concentration, associated with natural (age-related) menopause
        Use additional code for associated symptoms
        Excludes1   asymptomatic menopausal state (Z78.0)
                symptoms associated with artificial menopause (E89.41)
                symptoms associated with premature menopause (E28.310)

    N95.2   Postmenopausal atrophic vaginitis ♀
        Senile (atrophic) vaginitis

    N95.8   Other specified menopausal and perimenopausal disorders ♀

    N95.9   Unspecified menopausal and perimenopausal disorder ♀

N96   Recurrent pregnancy loss ♀
    Investigation or care in a nonpregnant woman with history of recurrent pregnancy loss
    Excludes1   recurrent pregnancy loss with current pregnancy (O26.2-)

● **N97   Female infertility**
    Includes   inability to achieve a pregnancy
                sterility, female NOS
    Excludes1   female infertility associated with:
                hypopituitarism (E23.0)
                Stein-Leventhal syndrome (E28.2)
    Excludes2   incompetence of cervix uteri (N88.3)

    N97.0   Female infertility associated with anovulation ♀

    N97.1   Female infertility of tubal origin ♀
        Female infertility associated with congenital anomaly of tube
        Female infertility due to tubal block
        Female infertility due to tubal occlusion
        Female infertility due to tubal stenosis

    N97.2   Female infertility of uterine origin ♀
        Female infertility associated with congenital anomaly of uterus
        Female infertility due to nonimplantation of ovum

    N97.8   Female infertility of other origin ♀

    N97.9   Female infertility, unspecified ♀

● **N98   Complications associated with artificial fertilization**
    (Ex) For category N98 CC codes unless otherwise indicated: See PDX Collection 643

    N98.0   Infection associated with artificial insemination ♀ 🖐
        (Ex) See PDX Collection 948

    N98.1   Hyperstimulation of ovaries ♀ 🖐
        Hyperstimulation of ovaries NOS
        Hyperstimulation of ovaries associated with induced ovulation

    N98.2   Complications of attempted introduction of fertilized ovum following in vitro fertilization ♀ 🖐

    N98.3   Complications of attempted introduction of embryo in embryo transfer ♀ 🖐

    N98.8   Other complications associated with artificial fertilization ♀ 🖐

    N98.9   Complication associated with artificial fertilization, unspecified ♀ 🖐

INTRAOPERATIVE AND POSTPROCEDURAL COMPLICATIONS AND DISORDERS OF GENITOURINARY SYSTEM, NOT ELSEWHERE CLASSIFIED (N99)

● **N99   Intraoperative and postprocedural complications and disorders of genitourinary system, not elsewhere classified**
    Excludes2   irradiation cystitis (N30.4-)
                postoophorectomy osteoporosis with current pathological fracture (M80.8-)
                postoophorectomy osteoporosis without current pathological fracture (M81.8)

    N99.0   Postprocedural (acute) (chronic) kidney failure
        Use additional code to type of kidney disease

  ● **N99.1   Postprocedural urethral stricture**
        Postcatheterization urethral stricture

     ● **N99.11   Postprocedural urethral stricture, male**
        N99.110   Postprocedural urethral stricture, male, meatal ♂
      ➡ **N99.111   Postprocedural bulbous urethral stricture, male ♂**

▶ New   ➡ Revised   ~~deleted~~ Deleted   Excludes 1   Excludes 2   Includes   Use additional   Code first   Code also   Key words

OGCR Official Guidelines   ● Unacceptable Principal Diagnosis   X Assign placeholder X   ● Use Additional Character(s)   ▶ Manifestation Code   Coding Clinic

➡ **N99.112** Postprocedural membranous urethral stricture, male ♂

➡ **N99.113** Postprocedural anterior bulbous urethral stricture, male ♂
  Coding Clinic: 2016, Q4, P48

N99.114 Postprocedural urethral stricture, male, unspecified ♂

N99.115 Postprocedural fossa navicularis urethral stricture ♂
  Coding Clinic: 2016, Q4, P47

N99.12 Postprocedural urethral stricture, female ♀

N99.2 Postprocedural adhesions of vagina ♀

N99.3 Prolapse of vaginal vault after hysterectomy ♀

N99.4 Postprocedural pelvic peritoneal adhesions
  Excludes2   pelvic peritoneal adhesions NOS (N73.6)
  postinfective pelvic peritoneal adhesions (N73.6)

● **N99.5** Complications of stoma of urinary tract
  Excludes2   mechanical complication of urinary catheter (T83.0-)

  ● **N99.51** Complication of cystostomy
  N99.510 Cystostomy hemorrhage
    (Ex) See PDX Collection 949
  N99.511 Cystostomy infection
    (Ex) See PDX Collection 950
  N99.512 Cystostomy malfunction
    (Ex) See PDX Collection 951
  N99.518 Other cystostomy complication
    (Ex) See PDX Collection 949

  ● **N99.52** Complication of incontinent external stoma of urinary tract
  N99.520 Hemorrhage of incontinent external stoma of urinary tract
  N99.521 Infection of incontinent external stoma of urinary tract
    Coding Clinic: 2016, Q4, P48
  N99.522 Malfunction of incontinent external stoma of urinary tract
  N99.523 Herniation of incontinent stoma of urinary tract
    Coding Clinic: 2016, Q4, P48
  N99.524 Stenosis of incontinent stoma of urinary tract
    Coding Clinic: 2016, Q4, P48
  N99.528 Other complication of incontinent external stoma of urinary tract

  ● **N99.53** Complication of continent stoma of urinary tract
  N99.530 Hemorrhage of continent stoma of urinary tract
  N99.531 Infection of continent stoma of urinary tract
  N99.532 Malfunction of continent stoma of urinary tract
  N99.533 Herniation of continent stoma of urinary tract
    Coding Clinic: 2016, Q4, P48
  N99.534 Stenosis of continent stoma of urinary tract
    Coding Clinic: 2016, Q4, P48
  N99.538 Other complication of continent stoma of urinary tract

● **N99.6** Intraoperative hemorrhage and hematoma of a genitourinary system organ or structure complicating a procedure
  Excludes1   intraoperative hemorrhage and hematoma of a genitourinary system organ or structure due to accidental puncture or laceration during a procedure (N99.7-)
  (Ex) For category N99.6 CC codes: See PDX Collection 952

  N99.61 Intraoperative hemorrhage and hematoma of a genitourinary system organ or structure complicating a genitourinary system procedure
  N99.62 Intraoperative hemorrhage and hematoma of a genitourinary system organ or structure complicating other procedure

● **N99.7** Accidental puncture and laceration of a genitourinary system organ or structure during a procedure
  (Ex) For category N99.7 CC codes: See PDX Collection 509

  N99.71 Accidental puncture and laceration of a genitourinary system organ or structure during a genitourinary system procedure
  N99.72 Accidental puncture and laceration of a genitourinary system organ or structure during other procedure

● **N99.8** Other intraoperative and postprocedural complications and disorders of genitourinary system
  Coding Clinic: 2016, Q4, P10
  N99.81 Other intraoperative complications of genitourinary system

  ● **N99.82** Postprocedural hemorrhage of a genitourinary system organ or structure following a procedure
    (Ex) For category N99.82 CC codes: See PDX Collection 952
  N99.820 Postprocedural hemorrhage of a genitourinary system organ or structure following a genitourinary system procedure
  N99.821 Postprocedural hemorrhage of a genitourinary system organ or structure following other procedure

  N99.83 Residual ovary syndrome ♀

  ● **N99.84** Postprocedural hematoma and seroma of a genitourinary system organ or structure following a procedure
    (Ex) For category N99.84 CC codes: See PDX Collection 952
  N99.840 Postprocedural hematoma of a genitourinary system organ or structure following a genitourinary system procedure
  N99.841 Postprocedural hematoma of a genitourinary system organ or structure following other procedure
  N99.842 Postprocedural seroma of a genitourinary system organ or structure following a genitourinary system procedure
  N99.843 Postprocedural seroma of a genitourinary system organ or structure following other procedure

  N99.89 Other postprocedural complications and disorders of genitourinary system

CHAPTER 14 (N00-N99)

CHAPTER 15

PREGNANCY, CHILDBIRTH AND THE PUERPERIUM (O00-O9A)

OGCR Chapter-Specific Coding Guidelines

15. Chapter 15: Pregnancy, Childbirth, and the Puerperium (O00-O9A)

a. General Rules for Obstetric Cases

1) Codes from chapter 15 and sequencing priority

Obstetric cases require codes from chapter 15, codes in the range O00-O9A, Pregnancy, Childbirth, and the Puerperium. Chapter 15 codes have sequencing priority over codes from other chapters. Additional codes from other chapters may be used in conjunction with chapter 15 codes to further specify conditions. Should the provider document that the pregnancy is incidental to the encounter, then code Z33.1, Pregnant state, incidental, should be used in place of any chapter 15 codes. It is the provider's responsibility to state that the condition being treated is not affecting the pregnancy.

2) Chapter 15 codes used only on the maternal record

Chapter 15 codes are to be used only on the maternal record, never on the record of the newborn.

3) Final character for trimester

The majority of codes in Chapter 15 have a final character indicating the trimester of pregnancy. The timeframes for the trimesters are indicated at the beginning of the chapter. If trimester is not a component of a code it is because the condition always occurs in a specific trimester, or the concept of trimester of pregnancy is not applicable. Certain codes have characters for only certain trimesters because the condition does not occur in all trimesters, but it may occur in more than just one.

Assignment of the final character for trimester should be based on the provider's documentation of the trimester (or number of weeks) for the current admission/encounter. This applies to the assignment of trimester for pre-existing conditions as well as those that develop during or are due to the pregnancy. The provider's documentation of the number of weeks may be used to assign the appropriate code identifying the trimester.

Whenever delivery occurs during the current admission, and there is an "in childbirth" option for the obstetric complication being coded, the "in childbirth" code should be assigned.

4) Selection of trimester for inpatient admissions that encompass more than one trimester

In instances when a patient is admitted to a hospital for complications of pregnancy during one trimester and remains in the hospital into a subsequent trimester, the trimester character for the antepartum complication code should be assigned on the basis of the trimester when the complication developed, not the trimester of the discharge. If the condition developed prior to the current admission/encounter or represents a pre-existing condition, the trimester character for the trimester at the time of the admission/encounter should be assigned.

5) Unspecified trimester

Each category that includes codes for trimester has a code for "unspecified trimester." The "unspecified trimester" code should rarely be used, such as when the documentation in the record is insufficient to determine the trimester and it is not possible to obtain clarification.

6) 7th character for Fetus Identification

Where applicable, a 7th character is to be assigned for certain categories (O31, O32, O33.3 - O33.6, O35, O36, O40, O41, O60.1, O60.2, O64, and O69) to identify the fetus for which the complication code applies.

Assign 7th character "0":
- For single gestations
- When the documentation in the record is insufficient to determine the fetus affected and it is not possible to obtain clarification.
- When it is not possible to clinically determine which fetus is affected.

b. Selection of OB Principal or First-listed Diagnosis

1) Routine outpatient prenatal visits

For routine outpatient prenatal visits when no complications are present, a code from category Z34, Encounter for supervision of normal pregnancy, should be used as the first-listed diagnosis. These codes should not be used in conjunction with chapter 15 codes.

2) Supervision of High-Risk Pregnancy

Codes from category O09, Supervision of high-risk pregnancy, are intended for use only during the prenatal period. For complications during the labor or delivery episode as a result of a high-risk pregnancy, assign the applicable complication codes from Chapter 15. If there are no complications during the labor or delivery episode, assign code O80, Encounter for full-term uncomplicated delivery.

For routine prenatal outpatient visits for patients with high-risk pregnancies, a code from category O09, Supervision of high-risk pregnancy, should be used as the first-listed diagnosis. Secondary chapter 15 codes may be used in conjunction with these codes if appropriate.

3) Episodes when no delivery occurs

In episodes when no delivery occurs, the principal diagnosis should correspond to the principal complication of the pregnancy which necessitated the encounter. Should more than one complication exist, all of which are treated or monitored, any of the complications codes may be sequenced first.

4) When a delivery occurs

When an obstetric patient is admitted and delivers during that admission, the condition that prompted the admission should be sequenced as the principal diagnosis. If multiple conditions prompted the admission, sequence the one most related to the delivery as the principal diagnosis. A code for any complication of the delivery should be assigned as an additional diagnosis. In cases of cesarean delivery, if the patient was admitted with a condition that resulted in the performance of a cesarean procedure, that condition should be selected as the principal diagnosis. If the reason for the admission was unrelated to the condition resulting in the cesarean delivery, the condition related to the reason for the admission should be selected as the principal diagnosis.

5) Outcome of delivery

A code from category Z37, Outcome of delivery, should be included on every maternal record when a delivery has occurred. These codes are not to be used on subsequent records or on the newborn record.

c. Pre-existing conditions versus conditions due to the pregnancy

Certain categories in Chapter 15 distinguish between conditions of the mother that existed prior to pregnancy (pre-existing) and those that are a direct result of pregnancy. When assigning codes from Chapter 15, it is important to assess if a condition was pre-existing prior to pregnancy or developed during or due to the pregnancy in order to assign the correct code.

Categories that do not distinguish between pre-existing and pregnancy-related conditions may be used for either. It is acceptable to use codes specifically for the puerperium with codes complicating pregnancy and childbirth if a condition arises postpartum during the delivery encounter.

d. Pre-existing hypertension in pregnancy

Category O10, Pre-existing hypertension complicating pregnancy, childbirth and the puerperium, includes codes for hypertensive heart and hypertensive chronic kidney disease. When assigning one of the O10 codes that includes hypertensive heart disease or hypertensive chronic kidney disease, it is necessary to add a secondary code from the appropriate hypertension category to specify the type of heart failure or chronic kidney disease.

See Section I.C.9. Hypertension.

e. Fetal Conditions Affecting the Management of the Mother

1) Codes from categories O35 and O36

Codes from categories O35, Maternal care for known or suspected fetal abnormality and damage, and O36, Maternal care for other fetal problems, are assigned only when the fetal condition is actually responsible for modifying the management of the mother, i.e., by requiring diagnostic studies, additional observation, special care, or termination of pregnancy. The fact that the fetal condition exists does not justify assigning a code from this series to the mother's record.

2) In utero surgery

In cases when surgery is performed on the fetus, a diagnosis code from category O35, Maternal care for known or suspected fetal abnormality and damage, should be assigned identifying the fetal condition. Assign the appropriate procedure code for the procedure performed.

No code from Chapter 16, the perinatal codes, should be used on the mother's record to identify fetal conditions. Surgery performed in utero on a fetus is still to be coded as an obstetric encounter.

f. HIV Infection in Pregnancy, Childbirth and the Puerperium

During pregnancy, childbirth or the puerperium, a patient admitted because of an HIV-related illness should receive a principal diagnosis from subcategory O98.7-, Human immunodeficiency [HIV] disease complicating pregnancy, childbirth and the puerperium, followed by the code(s) for the HIV-related illness(es).

Patients with asymptomatic HIV infection status admitted during pregnancy, childbirth, or the puerperium should receive codes of O98.7- and Z21, Asymptomatic human immunodeficiency virus [HIV] infection status.

g. Diabetes mellitus in pregnancy

Diabetes mellitus is a significant complicating factor in pregnancy. Pregnant women who are diabetic should be assigned a code from category O24, Diabetes mellitus in pregnancy, childbirth, and the puerperium, first, followed by the appropriate diabetes code(s) (E08-E13) from Chapter 4.

h. **Long term use of insulin and oral hypoglycemics**
See section I.C.4.a.3 for information on the long term use of insulin and oral hypoglycemic.

i. **Gestational (pregnancy induced) diabetes**
Gestational (pregnancy induced) diabetes can occur during the second and third trimester of pregnancy in women who were not diabetic prior to pregnancy. Gestational diabetes can cause complications in the pregnancy similar to those of pre-existing diabetes mellitus. It also puts the woman at greater risk of developing diabetes after the pregnancy. Codes for gestational diabetes are in subcategory O24.4, Gestational diabetes mellitus. No other code from category O24, Diabetes mellitus in pregnancy, childbirth, and the puerperium, should be used with a code from O24.4.

The codes under subcategory O24.4 include diet controlled, insulin controlled, and controlled by oral hypoglycemic drugs. If a patient with gestational diabetes is treated with both diet and insulin, only the code for insulin-controlled is required. If a patient with gestational diabetes is treated with both diet and oral hypoglycemic medications, only the code for "controlled by oral hypoglycemic drugs" is required. Code Z79.4, Long-term (current) use of insulin or code Z79.84, Long-term (current) use of oral hypoglycemic drugs, should not be assigned with codes from subcategory O24.4.

An abnormal glucose tolerance in pregnancy is assigned a code from subcategory O99.81, Abnormal glucose complicating pregnancy, childbirth, and the puerperium.

j. **Sepsis and septic shock complicating abortion, pregnancy, childbirth and the puerperium**
When assigning a chapter 15 code for sepsis complicating abortion, pregnancy, childbirth, and the puerperium, a code for the specific type of infection should be assigned as an additional diagnosis. If severe sepsis is present, a code from subcategory R65.2, Severe sepsis, and code(s) for associated organ dysfunction(s) should also be assigned as additional diagnoses.

k. **Puerperal sepsis**
Code O85, Puerperal sepsis, should be assigned with a secondary code to identify the causal organism (e.g., for a bacterial infection, assign a code from category B95-B96, Bacterial infections in conditions classified elsewhere). A code from category A40, Streptococcal sepsis, or A41, Other sepsis, should not be used for puerperal sepsis. If applicable, use additional codes to identify severe sepsis (R65.2-) and any associated acute organ dysfunction.

l. **Alcohol and tobacco use during pregnancy, childbirth and the puerperium**

1) **Alcohol use during pregnancy, childbirth and the puerperium**
Codes under subcategory O99.31, Alcohol use complicating pregnancy, childbirth, and the puerperium, should be assigned for any pregnancy case when a mother uses alcohol during the pregnancy or postpartum. A secondary code from category F10, Alcohol related disorders, should also be assigned to identify manifestations of the alcohol use.

2) **Tobacco use during pregnancy, childbirth and the puerperium**
Codes under subcategory O99.33, Smoking (tobacco) complicating pregnancy, childbirth, and the puerperium, should be assigned for any pregnancy case when a mother uses any type of tobacco product during the pregnancy or postpartum. A secondary code from category F17, Nicotine dependence, should also be assigned to identify the type of nicotine dependence.

m. **Poisoning, toxic effects, adverse effects and underdosing in a pregnant patient**
A code from subcategory O9A.2, Injury, poisoning and certain other consequences of external causes complicating pregnancy, childbirth, and the puerperium, should be sequenced first, followed by the appropriate injury, poisoning, toxic effect, adverse effect or underdosing code, and then the additional code(s) that specifies the condition caused by the poisoning, toxic effect, adverse effect or underdosing.
See Section I.C.19. Adverse effects, poisoning, underdosing and toxic effects.

n. **Normal Delivery, Code O80**

1) **Encounter for full term uncomplicated delivery**
Code O80 should be assigned when a woman is admitted for a full-term normal delivery and delivers a single, healthy infant without any complications antepartum, during the delivery, or postpartum during the delivery episode. Code O80 is always a principal diagnosis. It is not to be used if any other code from chapter 15 is needed to describe a current complication of the antenatal, delivery, or perinatal period. Additional codes from other chapters may be used with code O80 if they are not related to or are in any way complicating the pregnancy.

2) **Uncomplicated delivery with resolved antepartum complication**
Code O80 may be used if the patient had a complication at some point during the pregnancy, but the complication is not present at the time of the admission for delivery.

3) **Outcome of delivery for O80**
Z37.0, Single live birth, is the only outcome of delivery code appropriate for use with O80.

o. **The Peripartum and Postpartum Periods**

1) **Peripartum and Postpartum periods**
The postpartum period begins immediately after delivery and continues for six weeks following delivery. The peripartum period is defined as the last month of pregnancy to five months postpartum.

2) **Peripartum and postpartum complication**
A postpartum complication is any complication occurring within the six-week period.

3) **Pregnancy-related complications after 6 week period**
Chapter 15 codes may also be used to describe pregnancy-related complications after the peripartum or postpartum period if the provider documents that a condition is pregnancy related.

4) **Admission for routine postpartum care following delivery outside hospital**
When the mother delivers outside the hospital prior to admission and is admitted for routine postpartum care and no complications are noted, code Z39.0, Encounter for care and examination of mother immediately after delivery, should be assigned as the principal diagnosis.

5) **Pregnancy associated cardiomyopathy**
Pregnancy associated cardiomyopathy, code O90.3, is unique in that it may be diagnosed in the third trimester of pregnancy but may continue to progress months after delivery. For this reason, it is referred to as peripartum cardiomyopathy. Code O90.3 is only for use when the cardiomyopathy develops as a result of pregnancy in a woman who did not have pre-existing heart disease.

p. **Code O94, Sequelae of complication of pregnancy, childbirth, and the puerperium**

1) **Code O94**
Code O94, Sequelae of complication of pregnancy, childbirth, and the puerperium, is for use in those cases when an initial complication of a pregnancy develops a sequelae requiring care or treatment at a future date.

2) **After the initial postpartum period**
This code may be used at any time after the initial postpartum period.

3) **Sequencing of Code O94**
This code, like all sequela codes, is to be sequenced following the code describing the sequelae of the complication.

q. **Termination of Pregnancy and Spontaneous abortions**

1) **Abortion with Liveborn Fetus**
When an attempted termination of pregnancy results in a liveborn fetus assign code Z33.2, Encounter for elective termination of pregnancy and a code from category Z37, Outcome of Delivery.

2) **Retained Products of Conception following an abortion**
Subsequent encounters for retained products of conception following a spontaneous abortion or elective termination of pregnancy, **without complications** are assigned O03.4, **Incomplete spontaneous**, abortion **without complication**, or codes O07.4, Failed attempted termination of pregnancy without complication. This advice is appropriate even when the patient was discharged previously with a discharge diagnosis of complete abortion. **If the patient has a specific complication associated with the spontaneous abortion or elective termination of pregnancy in addition to retained products of conception, assign the appropriate complication in category O03 or O07 instead of code O03.4 or O07.4**

3) **Complications leading to abortion**
Codes from Chapter 15 may be used as additional codes to identify any documented complications of the pregnancy in conjunction with codes in categories in O04, O07 and O08.

r. **Abuse in a pregnant patient**
For suspected or confirmed cases of abuse of a pregnant patient, a code(s) from subcategories O9A.3, Physical abuse complicating pregnancy, childbirth, and the puerperium, O9A.4, Sexual abuse complicating pregnancy, childbirth, and the puerperium, and O9A.5, Psychological abuse complicating pregnancy, childbirth, and the puerperium, should be sequenced first, followed by the appropriate codes (if applicable) to identify any associated current injury due to physical abuse, sexual abuse, and the perpetrator of abuse.
See Section I.C.19. Adult and child abuse, neglect and other maltreatment.

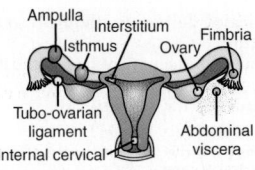

Figure 15-1 Implantation sites of ectopic pregnancy.

Item 15–1 Ectopic pregnancy most often occurs in the fallopian tube. Pregnancy outside the uterus may end in a lifethreatening rupture.

★ **(See Plate 375 on page 52.)**

CHAPTER 15

PREGNANCY, CHILDBIRTH AND THE PUERPERIUM (O00-O9A)

Note: CODES FROM THIS CHAPTER ARE FOR USE ONLY ON MATERNAL RECORDS, NEVER ON NEWBORN RECORDS

Codes from this chapter are for use for conditions related to or aggravated by the pregnancy, childbirth, or by the puerperium (maternal causes or obstetric causes)

Trimesters are counted from the first day of the last menstrual period. They are defined as follows:

1st trimester - less than 14 weeks 0 days

2nd trimester - 14 weeks 0 days to less than 28 weeks 0 days

3rd trimester - 28 weeks 0 days until delivery

Use additional code from category Z3A, Weeks of gestation, to identify the specific week of the pregnancy, if known.

Excludes1 supervision of normal pregnancy (Z34.-)

Excludes2 mental and behavioral disorders associated with the puerperium (F53)
obstetrical tetanus (A34)
postpartum necrosis of pituitary gland (E23.0)
puerperal osteomalacia (M83.0)

This chapter contains the following blocks:

O00-O08	Pregnancy with abortive outcome
O09	Supervision of high risk pregnancy
O10-O16	Edema, proteinuria and hypertensive disorders in pregnancy, childbirth and the puerperium
O20-O29	Other maternal disorders predominantly related to pregnancy
O30-O48	Maternal care related to the fetus and amniotic cavity and possible delivery problems
O60-O77	Complications of labor and delivery
O80, O82	Encounter for delivery
O85-O92	Complications predominantly related to the puerperium
O94-O9A	Other obstetric conditions, not elsewhere classified

PREGNANCY WITH ABORTIVE OUTCOME (O00-O08)

Excludes1 continuing pregnancy in multiple gestation after abortion of one fetus or more (O31.1-, O31.3-)
Coding Clinic: 2016, Q4, P130

● O00 **Ectopic pregnancy**
Includes ruptured ectopic pregnancy
Use additional code from category O08 to identify any associated complication
Ex: For category O00 CC codes: See PDX Collection 953

● O00.0 **Abdominal pregnancy**
Excludes1 maternal care for viable fetus in abdominal pregnancy (O36.7-)
Coding Clinic: 2016, Q4, P49

O00.00 Abdominal pregnancy **without intrauterine pregnancy** ♀ 🔒 M
Abdominal pregnancy NOS

O00.01 Abdominal pregnancy **with intrauterine pregnancy** ♀ 🔒 M

● O00.1 **Tubal pregnancy**
Fallopian pregnancy
Rupture of (fallopian) tube due to pregnancy
Tubal abortion
Coding Clinic: 2016, Q4, P49

● O00.10 Tubal pregnancy **without intrauterine pregnancy**
Tubal pregnancy NOS

▶ O00.101 **Right tubal pregnancy without intrauterine pregnancy** ♀ 🔒 M

▶ O00.102 **Left tubal pregnancy without intrauterine pregnancy** ♀ 🔒 M

▶ O00.109 **Unspecified tubal pregnancy without intrauterine pregnancy** ♀ 🔒 M

● O00.11 Tubal pregnancy **with intrauterine pregnancy**

▶ O00.111 **Right tubal pregnancy with intrauterine pregnancy** ♀ 🔒 M

▶ O00.112 **Left tubal pregnancy with intrauterine pregnancy** ♀ 🔒 M

▶ O00.119 **Unspecified tubal pregnancy with intrauterine pregnancy** ♀ 🔒 M

● O00.2 **Ovarian pregnancy**
Coding Clinic: 2016, Q4, P49

● O00.20 Ovarian pregnancy **without intrauterine pregnancy**
Ovarian pregnancy NOS

▶ O00.201 **Right ovarian pregnancy without intrauterine pregnancy** ♀ 🔒 M

▶ O00.202 **Left ovarian pregnancy without intrauterine pregnancy** ♀ 🔒 M

▶ O00.209 **Unspecified ovarian pregnancy without intrauterine pregnancy** ♀ 🔒 M

● O00.21 Ovarian pregnancy **with intrauterine pregnancy**

▶ O00.211 **Right ovarian pregnancy with intrauterine pregnancy** ♀ 🔒 M

▶ O00.212 **Left ovarian pregnancy with intrauterine pregnancy** ♀ 🔒 M

▶ O00.219 **Unspecified ovarian pregnancy with intrauterine pregnancy** ♀ 🔒 M

● O00.8 **Other ectopic pregnancy**
Cervical pregnancy
Cornual pregnancy
Intraligamentous pregnancy
Mural pregnancy
Coding Clinic: 2016, Q4, P49

O00.80 Other ectopic pregnancy **without intrauterine pregnancy** ♀ 🔒 M
Other ectopic pregnancy NOS

O00.81 Other ectopic pregnancy **with intrauterine pregnancy** ♀ 🔒 M

▶ New ⟹ Revised ~~deleted~~ Deleted | Excludes 1 | Excludes 2 | Includes | Use additional | Code first | Code also | Key words
OGCR Official Guidelines ● Unacceptable Principal Diagnosis X Assign placeholder X ● Use Additional Character(s) ▶ Manifestation Code **Coding Clinic**

● **O00.9**   **Ectopic pregnancy, unspecified**
     Coding Clinic: 2016, Q4, P49

     O00.90   **Unspecified ectopic pregnancy without intrauterine pregnancy** ♀ 🦠   **M**
          Ectopic pregnancy NOS

     O00.91   **Unspecified ectopic pregnancy with intrauterine pregnancy** ♀ 🦠   **M**

● **O01**   **Hydatidiform mole**
     Use additional code from category O08 to identify any associated complication

     Excludes1   chorioadenoma (destruens) (D39.2)
               malignant hydatidiform mole (D39.2)

     O01.0   **Classical hydatidiform mole** ♀   **M**
          Complete hydatidiform mole

     O01.1   **Incomplete and partial hydatidiform mole** ♀   **M**

     O01.9   **Hydatidiform mole, unspecified** ♀   **M**
          Trophoblastic disease NOS
          Vesicular mole NOS

● **O02**   **Other abnormal products of conception**
     Use additional code from category O08 to identify any associated complication

     Excludes1   papyraceous fetus (O31.0-)

     O02.0   **Blighted ovum and nonhydatidiform mole** ♀   **M**
          Carneous mole   Molar pregnancy NEC
          Fleshy mole   Pathological ovum
          Intrauterine mole NOS

     O02.1   **Missed abortion** ♀   **M**
          Early fetal death, before completion of 20 weeks of gestation, with retention of dead fetus

          Excludes1   failed induced abortion (O07.-)
                 fetal death (intrauterine) (late) (O36.4)
                 missed abortion with blighted ovum (O02.0)
                 missed abortion with hydatidiform mole (O01.-)
                 missed abortion with nonhydatidiform (O02.0)
                 missed abortion with other abnormal products of conception (O02.8-)
                 missed delivery (O36.4)
                 stillbirth (P95)

● **O02.8**   **Other specified abnormal products of conception**
     Excludes1   abnormal products of conception with blighted ovum (O02.0)
                 abnormal products of conception with hydatidiform mole (O01.-)
                 abnormal products of conception with nonhydatidiform mole (O02.0)

     O02.81   **Inappropriate change in quantitative human chorionic gonadotropin (hCG) in early pregnancy** ♀   **M**
          Biochemical pregnancy
          Chemical pregnancy
          Inappropriate level of quantitative human chorionic gonadotropin (hCG) for gestational age in early pregnancy

     O02.89   **Other abnormal products of conception** ♀   **M**

     O02.9   **Abnormal product of conception, unspecified** ♀   **M**

● **O03**   **Spontaneous abortion**
     (Ex) For category O03 CC codes: See PDX Collection 954

     Note: Incomplete abortion includes retained products of conception following spontaneous abortion.

     Includes   miscarriage

     O03.0   **Genital tract and pelvic infection following incomplete spontaneous abortion** ♀ 🦠   **M**
          Endometritis following incomplete spontaneous abortion
          Oophoritis following incomplete spontaneous abortion
          Parametritis following incomplete spontaneous abortion
          Pelvic peritonitis following incomplete spontaneous abortion
          Salpingitis following incomplete spontaneous abortion
          Salpingo-oophoritis following incomplete spontaneous abortion

          Excludes1   sepsis following incomplete spontaneous abortion (O03.37)
                 urinary tract infection following incomplete spontaneous abortion (O03.38)

     O03.1   **Delayed or excessive hemorrhage following incomplete spontaneous abortion** ♀   **M**
          Afibrinogenemia following incomplete spontaneous abortion
          Defibrination syndrome following incomplete spontaneous abortion
          Hemolysis following incomplete spontaneous abortion
          Intravascular coagulation following incomplete spontaneous abortion

     O03.2   **Embolism following incomplete spontaneous abortion** ♀ 🦠   **M**
          Air embolism following incomplete spontaneous abortion
          Amniotic fluid embolism following incomplete spontaneous abortion
          Blood-clot embolism following incomplete spontaneous abortion
          Embolism NOS following incomplete spontaneous abortion
          Fat embolism following incomplete spontaneous abortion
          Pulmonary embolism following incomplete spontaneous abortion
          Pyemic embolism following incomplete spontaneous abortion
          Septic or septicopyemic embolism following incomplete spontaneous abortion
          Soap embolism following incomplete spontaneous abortion

● **O03.3**   **Other and unspecified complications following incomplete spontaneous abortion**

     O03.30   **Unspecified complication following incomplete spontaneous abortion** ♀ 🦠   **M**

     O03.31   **Shock following incomplete spontaneous abortion** ♀ 🦠   **M**
          Circulatory collapse following incomplete spontaneous abortion
          Shock (postprocedural) following incomplete spontaneous abortion

          Excludes1   shock due to infection following incomplete spontaneous abortion (O03.37)

     O03.32   **Renal failure following incomplete spontaneous abortion** ♀ 🦠   **M**
          Kidney failure (acute) following incomplete spontaneous abortion
          Oliguria following incomplete spontaneous abortion
          Renal shutdown following incomplete spontaneous abortion
          Renal tubular necrosis following incomplete spontaneous abortion
          Uremia following incomplete spontaneous abortion

Item 15-2 A **hydatidiform** mole is an overproduction of placental tissue. The tumor secretes a hormone, chorionic gonadotropic hormone (CGH), that indicates a positive pregnancy test. There is no viable fetus. More than 80% of hydatidiform moles are noncancerous.

N Newborn Age: 0   **P** Pediatric Age: 0–17   **M** Maternity DX: 12–55   **A** Adult Age: 15–124   ♀ Females Only   ♂ Males Only

 Complication\Comorbidity   Major C\C   (Ex) CC/MCC Exclusions   🦠 Hospital-Acquired Condition   **1119**

CHAPTER 15 (O00-O9A)

O03.33 **Metabolic disorder following incomplete spontaneous abortion** ♀ 🔍   M

O03.34 **Damage to pelvic organs following incomplete spontaneous abortion** ♀ 🔍   M

Laceration, perforation, tear or chemical damage of bladder following incomplete spontaneous abortion

Laceration, perforation, tear or chemical damage of bowel following incomplete spontaneous abortion

Laceration, perforation, tear or chemical damage of broad ligament following incomplete spontaneous abortion

Laceration, perforation, tear or chemical damage of cervix following incomplete spontaneous abortion

Laceration, perforation, tear or chemical damage of periurethral tissue following incomplete spontaneous abortion

Laceration, perforation, tear or chemical damage of uterus following incomplete spontaneous abortion

Laceration, perforation, tear or chemical damage of vagina following incomplete spontaneous abortion

O03.35 **Other venous complications following incomplete spontaneous abortion** ♀ 🔍   M

O03.36 **Cardiac arrest following incomplete spontaneous abortion** ♀ 🔍   M

O03.37 **Sepsis following incomplete spontaneous abortion** ♀ 🔍   M

Use additional code to identify infectious agent (B95-B97)

Use additional code to identify severe sepsis, if applicable (R65.2-)

Excludes1   septic or septicopyemic embolism following incomplete spontaneous abortion (O03.2)

O03.38 **Urinary tract infection following incomplete spontaneous abortion** ♀ 🔍   M

Cystitis following incomplete spontaneous abortion

O03.39 **Incomplete spontaneous abortion with other complications** ♀ 🔍   M

O03.4 **Incomplete spontaneous abortion without complication** ♀   M

O03.5 **Genital tract and pelvic infection following complete or unspecified spontaneous abortion** ♀ 🔍   M

Endometritis following complete or unspecified spontaneous abortion

Oophoritis following complete or unspecified spontaneous abortion

Parametritis following complete or unspecified spontaneous abortion

Pelvic peritonitis following complete or unspecified spontaneous abortion

Salpingitis following complete or unspecified spontaneous abortion

Salpingo-oophoritis following complete or unspecified spontaneous abortion

Excludes1   sepsis following complete or unspecified spontaneous abortion (O03.87)

urinary tract infection following complete or unspecified spontaneous abortion (O03.88)

O03.6 **Delayed or excessive hemorrhage following complete or unspecified spontaneous abortion** ♀   M

Afibrinogenemia following complete or unspecified spontaneous abortion

Defibrination syndrome following complete or unspecified spontaneous abortion

Hemolysis following complete or unspecified spontaneous abortion

Intravascular coagulation following complete or unspecified spontaneous abortion

O03.7 **Embolism following complete or unspecified spontaneous abortion** ♀ 🔍   M

Air embolism following complete or unspecified spontaneous abortion

Amniotic fluid embolism following complete or unspecified spontaneous abortion

Blood-clot embolism following complete or unspecified spontaneous abortion

Embolism NOS following complete or unspecified spontaneous abortion

Fat embolism following complete or unspecified spontaneous abortion

Pulmonary embolism following complete or unspecified spontaneous abortion

Pyemic embolism following complete or unspecified spontaneous abortion

Septic or septicopyemic embolism following complete or unspecified spontaneous abortion

Soap embolism following complete or unspecified spontaneous abortion

● **O03.8** **Other and unspecified complications following complete or unspecified spontaneous abortion**

O03.80 **Unspecified complication following complete or unspecified spontaneous abortion** ♀ 🔍   M

O03.81 **Shock following complete or unspecified spontaneous abortion** ♀ 🔍   M

Circulatory collapse following complete or unspecified spontaneous abortion

Shock (postprocedural) following complete or unspecified spontaneous abortion

Excludes1   shock due to infection following complete or unspecified spontaneous abortion (O03.87)

O03.82 **Renal failure following complete or unspecified spontaneous abortion** ♀ 🔍   M

Kidney failure (acute) following complete or unspecified spontaneous abortion

Oliguria following complete or unspecified spontaneous abortion

Renal shutdown following complete or unspecified spontaneous abortion

Renal tubular necrosis following complete or unspecified spontaneous abortion

Uremia following complete or unspecified spontaneous abortion

O03.83 **Metabolic disorder following complete or unspecified spontaneous abortion** ♀ 🔍   M

O03.84 **Damage to pelvic organs following complete or unspecified spontaneous abortion** ♀ 🔍   M

Laceration, perforation, tear or chemical damage of bladder following complete or unspecified spontaneous abortion

Laceration, perforation, tear or chemical damage of bowel following complete or unspecified spontaneous abortion

Laceration, perforation, tear or chemical damage of broad ligament following complete or unspecified spontaneous abortion

Laceration, perforation, tear or chemical damage of cervix following complete or unspecified spontaneous abortion

Laceration, perforation, tear or chemical damage of periurethral tissue following complete or unspecified spontaneous abortion

Laceration, perforation, tear or chemical damage of uterus following complete or unspecified spontaneous abortion

Laceration, perforation, tear or chemical damage of vagina following complete or unspecified spontaneous abortion

▶ New   ⇒ Revised   ~~deleted~~ Deleted   Excludes 1   Excludes 2   Includes   Use additional   Code first   Code also   Key words

OGCR Official Guidelines   ● Unacceptable Principal Diagnosis   X Assign placeholder X   ● Use Additional Character(s)   ▶ Manifestation Code   Coding Clinic

O03.85   **Other venous complications following complete or unspecified spontaneous abortion** ♀ 🦠   M

O03.86   **Cardiac arrest following complete or unspecified spontaneous abortion** ♀ 🦠   M

O03.87   **Sepsis following complete or unspecified spontaneous abortion** ♀ 🦠   M

Use additional code to identify infectious agent (B95-B97)

Use additional code to identify severe sepsis, if applicable (R65.2-)

Excludes1   septic or septicopyemic embolism following complete or unspecified spontaneous abortion (O03.7)

O03.88   **Urinary tract infection following complete or unspecified spontaneous abortion** ♀ 🦠   M

Cystitis following complete or unspecified spontaneous abortion

O03.89   **Complete or unspecified spontaneous abortion with other complications** ♀ 🦠   M

O03.9   **Complete or unspecified spontaneous abortion without complication** ♀   M

Miscarriage NOS

Spontaneous abortion NOS

● O04   **Complications following (induced) termination of pregnancy**

Includes   complications following (induced) termination of pregnancy

Excludes1   encounter for elective termination of pregnancy, uncomplicated (Z33.2)

failed attempted termination of pregnancy (O07.-)

(Ex) **For category O04 CC codes unless otherwise indicated:** See PDX Collection 954

O04.5   **Genital tract and pelvic infection following (induced) termination of pregnancy** ♀ 🦠   M

Endometritis following (induced) termination of pregnancy

Oophoritis following (induced) termination of pregnancy

Parametritis following (induced) termination of pregnancy

Pelvic peritonitis following (induced) termination of pregnancy

Salpingitis following (induced) termination of pregnancy

Salpingo-oophoritis following (induced) termination of pregnancy

Excludes1   sepsis following (induced) termination of pregnancy (O04.87)

urinary tract infection following (induced) termination of pregnancy (O04.88)

O04.6   **Delayed or excessive hemorrhage following (induced) termination of pregnancy** ♀   M

Afibrinogenemia following (induced) termination of pregnancy

Defibrination syndrome following (induced) termination of pregnancy

Hemolysis following (induced) termination of pregnancy

Intravascular coagulation following (induced) termination of pregnancy

O04.7   **Embolism following (induced) termination of pregnancy** ♀ 🦠   M

Air embolism following (induced) termination of pregnancy

Amniotic fluid embolism following (induced) termination of pregnancy

Blood-clot embolism following (induced) termination of pregnancy

Embolism NOS following (induced) termination of pregnancy

Fat embolism following (induced) termination of pregnancy

Pulmonary embolism following (induced) termination of pregnancy

Pyemic embolism following (induced) termination of pregnancy

Septic or septicopyemic embolism following (induced) termination of pregnancy

Soap embolism following (induced) termination of pregnancy

● O04.8   **(Induced) termination of pregnancy with other and unspecified complications**

O04.80   **(Induced) termination of pregnancy with unspecified complications** ♀ 🦠   M

O04.81   **Shock following (induced) termination of pregnancy** ♀ 🦠   M

Circulatory collapse following (induced) termination of pregnancy

Shock (postprocedural) following (induced) termination of pregnancy

Excludes1   shock due to infection following (induced) termination of pregnancy (O04.87)

O04.82   **Renal failure following (induced) termination of pregnancy** ♀ 🦠   M

Kidney failure (acute) following (induced) termination of pregnancy

Oliguria following (induced) termination of pregnancy

Renal shutdown following (induced) termination of pregnancy

Renal tubular necrosis following (induced) termination of pregnancy

Uremia following (induced) termination of pregnancy

O04.83   **Metabolic disorder following (induced) termination of pregnancy** ♀ 🦠   M

O04.84   **Damage to pelvic organs following (induced) termination of pregnancy** ♀ 🦠   M

Laceration, perforation, tear or chemical damage of bladder following (induced) termination of pregnancy

Laceration, perforation, tear or chemical damage of bowel following (induced) termination of pregnancy

Laceration, perforation, tear or chemical damage of broad ligament following (induced) termination of pregnancy

Laceration, perforation, tear or chemical damage of cervix following (induced) termination of pregnancy

Laceration, perforation, tear or chemical damage of periurethral tissue following (induced) termination of pregnancy

Laceration, perforation, tear or chemical damage of uterus following (induced) termination of pregnancy

Laceration, perforation, tear or chemical damage of vagina following (induced) termination of pregnancy

O04.85   **Other venous complications following (induced) termination of pregnancy** ♀ 🦠   M

O04.86   **Cardiac arrest following (induced) termination of pregnancy** ♀ 🦠   M

CHAPTER 15 (O00-O9A)

CHAPTER 15 (O00-O9A)

O04.87 Sepsis following (induced) termination of pregnancy ♀ ⊗   M

  Use additional code to identify infectious agent (B95-B97)

  Use additional code to identify severe sepsis, if applicable (R65.2-)

  Excludes1   septic or septicopyemic embolism following (induced) termination of pregnancy (O04.7)

  (Ex:) See PDX Collection 955

O04.88 Urinary tract infection following (induced) termination of pregnancy ♀ ⊗   M

  Cystitis following (induced) termination of pregnancy

O04.89 (Induced) termination of pregnancy with other complications ♀ ⊗   M

● **O07 Failed attempted termination of pregnancy**

  Includes   failure of attempted induction of termination of pregnancy
    incomplete elective abortion

  Excludes1   incomplete spontaneous abortion (O03.0-)

O07.0 Genital tract and pelvic infection following failed attempted termination of pregnancy ♀ ⊗   M

  Endometritis following failed attempted termination of pregnancy
  Oophoritis following failed attempted termination of pregnancy
  Parametritis following failed attempted termination of pregnancy
  Pelvic peritonitis following failed attempted termination of pregnancy
  Salpingitis following failed attempted termination of pregnancy
  Salpingo-oophoritis following failed attempted termination of pregnancy

  Excludes1   sepsis following failed attempted termination of pregnancy (O07.37)
    urinary tract infection following failed attempted termination of pregnancy (O07.38)

  (Ex:) See PDX Collection 956

O07.1 Delayed or excessive hemorrhage following failed attempted termination of pregnancy ♀ ⊗   M

  Afibrinogenemia following failed attempted termination of pregnancy
  Defibrination syndrome following failed attempted termination of pregnancy
  Hemolysis following failed attempted termination of pregnancy
  Intravascular coagulation following failed attempted termination of pregnancy

  (Ex:) See PDX Collection 957

O07.2 Embolism following failed attempted termination of pregnancy ♀ ⊗   M

  Air embolism following failed attempted termination of pregnancy
  Amniotic fluid embolism following failed attempted termination of pregnancy
  Blood-clot embolism following failed attempted termination of pregnancy
  Embolism NOS following failed attempted termination of pregnancy
  Fat embolism following failed attempted termination of pregnancy
  Pulmonary embolism following failed attempted termination of pregnancy
  Pyemic embolism following failed attempted termination of pregnancy
  Septic or septicopyemic embolism following failed attempted termination of pregnancy
  Soap embolism following failed attempted termination of pregnancy

  (Ex:) See PDX Collection 958

● **O07.3 Failed attempted termination of pregnancy with other and unspecified complications**

O07.30 Failed attempted termination of pregnancy with unspecified complications ♀ ⊗   M
  (Ex:) See PDX Collection 954

O07.31 Shock following failed attempted termination of pregnancy ♀ ⊗   M

  Circulatory collapse following failed attempted termination of pregnancy
  Shock (postprocedural) following failed attempted termination of pregnancy

  Excludes1   shock due to infection following failed attempted termination of pregnancy (O07.37)

  (Ex:) See PDX Collection 959

O07.32 Renal failure following failed attempted termination of pregnancy ♀ ⊗   M

  Kidney failure (acute) following failed attempted termination of pregnancy
  Oliguria following failed attempted termination of pregnancy
  Renal shutdown following failed attempted termination of pregnancy
  Renal tubular necrosis following failed attempted termination of pregnancy
  Uremia following failed attempted termination of pregnancy

  (Ex:) See PDX Collection 960

O07.33 Metabolic disorder following failed attempted termination of pregnancy ♀ ⊗   M
  (Ex:) See PDX Collection 954

O07.34 Damage to pelvic organs following failed attempted termination of pregnancy ♀ ⊗   M

  Laceration, perforation, tear or chemical damage of bladder following failed attempted termination of pregnancy
  Laceration, perforation, tear or chemical damage of bowel following failed attempted termination of pregnancy
  Laceration, perforation, tear or chemical damage of broad ligament following failed attempted termination of pregnancy
  Laceration, perforation, tear or chemical damage of cervix following failed attempted termination of pregnancy
  Laceration, perforation, tear or chemical damage of periurethral tissue following failed attempted termination of pregnancy
  Laceration, perforation, tear or chemical damage of uterus following failed attempted termination of pregnancy
  Laceration, perforation, tear or chemical damage of vagina following failed attempted termination of pregnancy

  (Ex:) See PDX Collection 961

O07.35 Other venous complications following failed attempted termination of pregnancy ♀ ⊗   M
  (Ex:) See PDX Collection 954

O07.36 Cardiac arrest following failed attempted termination of pregnancy ♀ ⊗   M
  (Ex:) See PDX Collection 954

O07.37 Sepsis following failed attempted termination of pregnancy ♀ ⊗   M

  Use additional code (B95-B97), to identify infectious agent
  Use additional code (R65.2-) to identify severe sepsis, if applicable

  Excludes1   septic or septicopyemic embolism following failed attempted termination of pregnancy (O07.2)

  (Ex:) See PDX Collection 956

▶ New   ⇒ Revised   ~~deleted~~ Deleted   Excludes 1   Excludes 2   Includes   Use additional   Code first   Code also   Key words

OGCR Official Guidelines   ● Unacceptable Principal Diagnosis   X Assign placeholder X   ● Use Additional Character(s)   ▶ Manifestation Code   **Coding Clinic**

O07.38　Urinary tract infection following failed attempted termination of pregnancy ♀ 🐾　　M

　　　　　Cystitis following failed attempted termination of pregnancy
　　　　　(Ex) See PDX Collection 954

O07.39　Failed attempted termination of pregnancy with other complications ♀ 🐾　　M
　　　　　(Ex) See PDX Collection 954

O07.4　Failed attempted termination of pregnancy without complication ♀　　M

● **O08　Complications following ectopic and molar pregnancy**
　　　This category is for use with categories O00-O02 to identify any associated complications.
　　　(Ex) For category O08 CC codes unless otherwise indicated: See PDX Collection 963

O08.0　Genital tract and pelvic infection following ectopic and molar pregnancy ♀ 🐾　　M
　　　　　Endometritis following ectopic and molar pregnancy
　　　　　Oophoritis following ectopic and molar pregnancy
　　　　　Parametritis following ectopic and molar pregnancy
　　　　　Pelvic peritonitis following ectopic and molar pregnancy
　　　　　Salpingitis following ectopic and molar pregnancy
　　　　　Salpingo-oophoritis following ectopic and molar pregnancy

　　　　　Excludes1　sepsis following ectopic and molar pregnancy (O08.82)
　　　　　　　　　　urinary tract infection (O08.83)
　　　　　(Ex) See PDX Collection 85

O08.1　Delayed or excessive hemorrhage following ectopic and molar pregnancy ♀ 🐾　　M
　　　　　Afibrinogenemia following ectopic and molar pregnancy
　　　　　Defibrination syndrome following ectopic and molar pregnancy
　　　　　Hemolysis following ectopic and molar pregnancy
　　　　　Intravascular coagulation following ectopic and molar pregnancy

　　　　　Excludes1　delayed or excessive hemorrhage due to incomplete abortion (O03.1)
　　　　　(Ex) See PDX Collection 962

O08.2　Embolism following ectopic and molar pregnancy ♀ 🐾 M
　　　　　Air embolism following ectopic and molar pregnancy
　　　　　Amniotic fluid embolism following ectopic and molar pregnancy
　　　　　Blood-clot embolism following ectopic and molar pregnancy
　　　　　Embolism NOS following ectopic and molar pregnancy
　　　　　Fat embolism following ectopic and molar pregnancy
　　　　　Pulmonary embolism following ectopic and molar pregnancy
　　　　　Pyemic embolism following ectopic and molar pregnancy
　　　　　Septic or septicopyemic embolism following ectopic and molar pregnancy
　　　　　Soap embolism following ectopic and molar pregnancy

O08.3　Shock following ectopic and molar pregnancy ♀ 🐾　　M
　　　　　Circulatory collapse following ectopic and molar pregnancy
　　　　　Shock (postprocedural) following ectopic and molar pregnancy

　　　　　Excludes1　shock due to infection following ectopic and molar pregnancy (O08.82)

O08.4　Renal failure following ectopic and molar pregnancy ♀ 🐾　　M
　　　　　Kidney failure (acute) following ectopic and molar pregnancy
　　　　　Oliguria following ectopic and molar pregnancy
　　　　　Renal shutdown following ectopic and molar pregnancy
　　　　　Renal tubular necrosis following ectopic and molar pregnancy
　　　　　Uremia following ectopic and molar pregnancy

O08.5　Metabolic disorders following an ectopic and molar pregnancy ♀ 🐾　　M

O08.6　Damage to pelvic organs and tissues following an ectopic and molar pregnancy ♀ 🐾　　M
　　　　　Laceration, perforation, tear or chemical damage of bladder following an ectopic and molar pregnancy
　　　　　Laceration, perforation, tear or chemical damage of bowel following an ectopic and molar pregnancy
　　　　　Laceration, perforation, tear or chemical damage of broad ligament following an ectopic and molar pregnancy
　　　　　Laceration, perforation, tear or chemical damage of cervix following an ectopic and molar pregnancy
　　　　　Laceration, perforation, tear or chemical damage of periurethral tissue following an ectopic and molar pregnancy
　　　　　Laceration, perforation, tear or chemical damage of uterus following an ectopic and molar pregnancy
　　　　　Laceration, perforation, tear or chemical damage of vagina following an ectopic and molar pregnancy

O08.7　Other venous complications following an ectopic and molar pregnancy ♀ 🐾　　M

● **O08.8　Other complications following an ectopic and molar pregnancy**

　　O08.81　Cardiac arrest following an ectopic and molar pregnancy ♀ 🐾　　M

　　O08.82　Sepsis following ectopic and molar pregnancy ♀ 🐾　　M
　　　　　Use additional code (B95-B97), to identify infectious agent
　　　　　Use additional code (R65.2-) to identify severe sepsis, if applicable
　　　　　Excludes1　septic or septicopyemic embolism following ectopic and molar pregnancy (O08.2)
　　　　　(Ex) See PDX Collection 85

　　O08.83　Urinary tract infection following an ectopic and molar pregnancy ♀ 🐾　　M
　　　　　Cystitis following an ectopic and molar pregnancy

　　O08.89　Other complications following an ectopic and molar pregnancy ♀ 🐾　　M

O08.9　Unspecified complication following an ectopic and molar pregnancy ♀ 🐾　　M

SUPERVISION OF HIGH RISK PREGNANCY (O09)

● **O09　Supervision of high risk pregnancy**
　　Coding Clinic: 2016, Q4, P125, 150

● **O09.0　Supervision of pregnancy with history of infertility**

　　● **O09.00　Supervision of pregnancy with history of infertility, unspecified trimester** ♀　　M

　　● **O09.01　Supervision of pregnancy with history of infertility, first trimester** ♀　　M

　　● **O09.02　Supervision of pregnancy with history of infertility, second trimester** ♀　　M

　　● **O09.03　Supervision of pregnancy with history of infertility, third trimester** ♀　　M

● **O09.1　Supervision of pregnancy with history of ectopic pregnancy**
　　Coding Clinic: 2016, Q4, P49-50

　　● **O09.10　Supervision of pregnancy with history of ectopic pregnancy, unspecified trimester** ♀　　M

　　● **O09.11　Supervision of pregnancy with history of ectopic pregnancy, first trimester** ♀　　M

　　● **O09.12　Supervision of pregnancy with history of ectopic pregnancy, second trimester** ♀　　M

　　● **O09.13　Supervision of pregnancy with history of ectopic pregnancy, third trimester** ♀　　M

● **O09.A   Supervision of pregnancy with history of molar pregnancy**
      Coding Clinic: 2016, Q4, P50

   ● **O09.A0   Supervision of pregnancy with history of molar pregnancy, unspecified trimester** ♀   M

   ● **O09.A1   Supervision of pregnancy with history of molar pregnancy, first trimester** ♀   M

   ● **O09.A2   Supervision of pregnancy with history of molar pregnancy, second trimester** ♀   M

   ● **O09.A3   Supervision of pregnancy with history of molar pregnancy, third trimester** ♀   M

● **O09.2   Supervision of pregnancy with other poor reproductive or obstetric history**
      Excludes2   pregnancy care for patient with history of recurrent pregnancy loss (O26.2-)

   ● **O09.21   Supervision of pregnancy with history of pre-term labor**

      ● **O09.211   Supervision of pregnancy with history of pre-term labor, first trimester** ♀   M

      ● **O09.212   Supervision of pregnancy with history of pre-term labor, second trimester** ♀ M

      ● **O09.213   Supervision of pregnancy with history of pre-term labor, third trimester** ♀   M

      ● **O09.219   Supervision of pregnancy with history of pre-term labor, unspecified trimester** ♀   M

   ● **O09.29   Supervision of pregnancy with other poor reproductive or obstetric history**
         Supervision of pregnancy with history of neonatal death
         Supervision of pregnancy with history of stillbirth

      ● **O09.291   Supervision of pregnancy with other poor reproductive or obstetric history, first trimester** ♀   M

      ● **O09.292   Supervision of pregnancy with other poor reproductive or obstetric history, second trimester** ♀   M

      ● **O09.293   Supervision of pregnancy with other poor reproductive or obstetric history, third trimester** ♀   M

      ● **O09.299   Supervision of pregnancy with other poor reproductive or obstetric history, unspecified trimester** ♀   M

● **O09.3   Supervision of pregnancy with insufficient antenatal care**
         Supervision of concealed pregnancy
         Supervision of hidden pregnancy

   ● **O09.30   Supervision of pregnancy with insufficient antenatal care, unspecified trimester** ♀   M

   ● **O09.31   Supervision of pregnancy with insufficient antenatal care, first trimester** ♀   M

   ● **O09.32   Supervision of pregnancy with insufficient antenatal care, second trimester** ♀   M

   ● **O09.33   Supervision of pregnancy with insufficient antenatal care, third trimester** ♀   M

● **O09.4   Supervision of pregnancy with grand multiparity**

   ● **O09.40   Supervision of pregnancy with grand multiparity, unspecified trimester** ♀   M

   ● **O09.41   Supervision of pregnancy with grand multiparity, first trimester** ♀   M

   ● **O09.42   Supervision of pregnancy with grand multiparity, second trimester** ♀   M

   ● **O09.43   Supervision of pregnancy with grand multiparity, third trimester** ♀   M

● **O09.5   Supervision of elderly primigravida and multigravida**
      Pregnancy for a female 35 years and older at expected date of delivery

   ● **O09.51   Supervision of elderly primigravida**

      ● **O09.511   Supervision of elderly primigravida, first trimester** ♀   M

      ● **O09.512   Supervision of elderly primigravida, second trimester** ♀   M

      ● **O09.513   Supervision of elderly primigravida, third trimester** ♀   M

      ● **O09.519   Supervision of elderly primigravida, unspecified trimester** ♀   M

   ● **O09.52   Supervision of elderly multigravida**

      ● **O09.521   Supervision of elderly multigravida, first trimester** ♀   M

      ● **O09.522   Supervision of elderly multigravida, second trimester** ♀   M

      ● **O09.523   Supervision of elderly multigravida, third trimester** ♀   M
            Coding Clinic: 2016, Q4, P150

      ● **O09.529   Supervision of elderly multigravida, unspecified trimester** ♀   M

● **O09.6   Supervision of young primigravida and multigravida**
      Supervision of pregnancy for a female less than 16 years old at expected date of delivery

   ● **O09.61   Supervision of young primigravida**

      ● **O09.611   Supervision of young primigravida, first trimester** ♀   M

      ● **O09.612   Supervision of young primigravida, second trimester** ♀   M

      ● **O09.613   Supervision of young primigravida, third trimester** ♀   M

      ● **O09.619   Supervision of young primigravida, unspecified trimester** ♀   M

   ● **O09.62   Supervision of young multigravida**

      ● **O09.621   Supervision of young multigravida, first trimester** ♀   M

      ● **O09.622   Supervision of young multigravida, second trimester** ♀   M

      ● **O09.623   Supervision of young multigravida, third trimester** ♀   M

      ● **O09.629   Supervision of young multigravida, unspecified trimester** ♀   M

● **O09.7   Supervision of high risk pregnancy due to social problems**

   ● **O09.70   Supervision of high risk pregnancy due to social problems, unspecified trimester** ♀   M

   ● **O09.71   Supervision of high risk pregnancy due to social problems, first trimester** ♀   M

   ● **O09.72   Supervision of high risk pregnancy due to social problems, second trimester** ♀   M

   ● **O09.73   Supervision of high risk pregnancy due to social problems, third trimester** ♀   M

● **O09.8   Supervision of other high risk pregnancies**

   ● **O09.81   Supervision of pregnancy resulting from assisted reproductive technology**
         Supervision of pregnancy resulting from in-vitro fertilization
         Excludes2   gestational carrier status (Z33.3)

      ● **O09.811   Supervision of pregnancy resulting from assisted reproductive technology, first trimester** ♀   M

      ● **O09.812   Supervision of pregnancy resulting from assisted reproductive technology, second trimester** ♀   M

▶ New   ⟹ Revised   ~~deleted~~ Deleted   Excludes 1   Excludes 2   Includes   Use additional   Code first   Code also   Key words
OGCR Official Guidelines   ● Unacceptable Principal Diagnosis   X Assign placeholder X   ● Use Additional Character(s)   ▶ Manifestation Code   Coding Clinic

● **O09.813**   **Supervision of pregnancy resulting from assisted reproductive technology, third trimester** ♀   M

● **O09.819**   **Supervision of pregnancy resulting from assisted reproductive technology, unspecified trimester** ♀   M

● **O09.82**   **Supervision of pregnancy with history of in utero procedure during previous pregnancy**

   ● **O09.821**   **Supervision of pregnancy with history of in utero procedure during previous pregnancy, first trimester** ♀   M

   ● **O09.822**   **Supervision of pregnancy with history of in utero procedure during previous pregnancy, second trimester** ♀   M

   ● **O09.823**   **Supervision of pregnancy with history of in utero procedure during previous pregnancy, third trimester** ♀   M

   ● **O09.829**   **Supervision of pregnancy with history of in utero procedure during previous pregnancy, unspecified trimester** ♀   M

     Excludes1   supervision of pregnancy affected by in utero procedure during current pregnancy (O35.7)

● **O09.89**   **Supervision of other high risk pregnancies**

   ● **O09.891**   **Supervision of other high risk pregnancies, first trimester** ♀   M

   ● **O09.892**   **Supervision of other high risk pregnancies, second trimester** ♀   M

   ● **O09.893**   **Supervision of other high risk pregnancies, third trimester** ♀   M

   ● **O09.899**   **Supervision of other high risk pregnancies, unspecified trimester** ♀   M

● **O09.9**   **Supervision of high risk pregnancy, unspecified**

   ● **O09.90**   **Supervision of high risk pregnancy, unspecified, unspecified trimester** ♀   M

   ● **O09.91**   **Supervision of high risk pregnancy, unspecified, first trimester** ♀   M

   ● **O09.92**   **Supervision of high risk pregnancy, unspecified, second trimester** ♀   M

   ● **O09.93**   **Supervision of high risk pregnancy, unspecified, third trimester** ♀   M

EDEMA, PROTEINURIA AND HYPERTENSIVE DISORDERS IN PREGNANCY, CHILDBIRTH AND THE PUERPERIUM (O10-O16)

● **O10**   **Pre-existing hypertension complicating pregnancy, childbirth and the puerperium**

   Includes   pre-existing hypertension with pre-existing proteinuria complicating pregnancy, childbirth and the puerperium

   Excludes2   pre-existing hypertension with superimposed pre-eclampsia complicating pregnancy, childbirth and the puerperium (O11.-)

   (Ex) **For category O10 CC codes: See PDX Collection 964**
   Coding Clinic: 2016, Q4, P50

● **O10.0**   **Pre-existing essential hypertension complicating pregnancy, childbirth and the puerperium**
     Any condition in I10 specified as a reason for obstetric care during pregnancy, childbirth or the puerperium

   ● **O10.01**   **Pre-existing essential hypertension complicating pregnancy**

     O10.011   **Pre-existing essential hypertension complicating pregnancy, first trimester** ♀   M

     O10.012   **Pre-existing essential hypertension complicating pregnancy, second trimester** ♀   M

     O10.013   **Pre-existing essential hypertension complicating pregnancy, third trimester** ♀   M

     O10.019   **Pre-existing essential hypertension complicating pregnancy, unspecified trimester** ♀   M

   O10.02   **Pre-existing essential hypertension complicating childbirth** ♀   M

   O10.03   **Pre-existing essential hypertension complicating the puerperium** ♀   M

● **O10.1**   **Pre-existing hypertensive heart disease complicating pregnancy, childbirth and the puerperium**
     Any condition in I11 specified as a reason for obstetric care during pregnancy, childbirth or the puerperium
     Use additional code from I11 to identify the type of hypertensive heart disease

   ● **O10.11**   **Pre-existing hypertensive heart disease complicating pregnancy**

     O10.111   **Pre-existing hypertensive heart disease complicating pregnancy, first trimester** ♀   M

     O10.112   **Pre-existing hypertensive heart disease complicating pregnancy, second trimester** ♀   M

     O10.113   **Pre-existing hypertensive heart disease complicating pregnancy, third trimester** ♀   M

     O10.119   **Pre-existing hypertensive heart disease complicating pregnancy, unspecified trimester** ♀   M

   O10.12   **Pre-existing hypertensive heart disease complicating childbirth** ♀   M

   O10.13   **Pre-existing hypertensive heart disease complicating the puerperium** ♀   M

● **O10.2**   **Pre-existing hypertensive chronic kidney disease complicating pregnancy, childbirth and the puerperium**
     Any condition in I12 specified as a reason for obstetric care during pregnancy, childbirth or the puerperium
     Use additional code from I12 to identify the type of hypertensive chronic kidney disease

   ● **O10.21**   **Pre-existing hypertensive chronic kidney disease complicating pregnancy**

     O10.211   **Pre-existing hypertensive chronic kidney disease complicating pregnancy, first trimester** ♀   M

     O10.212   **Pre-existing hypertensive chronic kidney disease complicating pregnancy, second trimester** ♀   M

     O10.213   **Pre-existing hypertensive chronic kidney disease complicating pregnancy, third trimester** ♀   M

     O10.219   **Pre-existing hypertensive chronic kidney disease complicating pregnancy, unspecified trimester** ♀   M

   O10.22   **Pre-existing hypertensive chronic kidney disease complicating childbirth** ♀   M

   O10.23   **Pre-existing hypertensive chronic kidney disease complicating the puerperium** ♀   M

CHAPTER 15 (O00-O9A)

● **O10.3** Pre-existing hypertensive heart and chronic kidney disease complicating pregnancy, childbirth and the puerperium
  Any condition in I13 specified as a reason for obstetric care during pregnancy, childbirth or the puerperium
  Use additional code from I13 to identify the type of hypertensive heart and chronic kidney disease

  ● **O10.31** Pre-existing hypertensive heart and chronic kidney disease complicating pregnancy
    O10.311 Pre-existing hypertensive heart and chronic kidney disease complicating pregnancy, first trimester ♀   M
    O10.312 Pre-existing hypertensive heart and chronic kidney disease complicating pregnancy, second trimester ♀   M
    O10.313 Pre-existing hypertensive heart and chronic kidney disease complicating pregnancy, third trimester ♀   M
    O10.319 Pre-existing hypertensive heart and chronic kidney disease complicating pregnancy, unspecified trimester ♀   M
  O10.32 Pre-existing hypertensive heart and chronic kidney disease complicating childbirth ♀   M
  O10.33 Pre-existing hypertensive heart and chronic kidney disease complicating the puerperium ♀   M

● **O10.4** Pre-existing secondary hypertension complicating pregnancy, childbirth and the puerperium
  Any condition in I15 specified as a reason for obstetric care during pregnancy, childbirth or the puerperium
  Use additional code from I15 to identify the type of secondary hypertension

  ● **O10.41** Pre-existing secondary hypertension complicating pregnancy
    O10.411 Pre-existing secondary hypertension complicating pregnancy, first trimester ♀   M
    O10.412 Pre-existing secondary hypertension complicating pregnancy, second trimester ♀   M
    O10.413 Pre-existing secondary hypertension complicating pregnancy, third trimester ♀   M
    O10.419 Pre-existing secondary hypertension complicating pregnancy, unspecified trimester ♀   M
  O10.42 Pre-existing secondary hypertension complicating childbirth ♀   M
  O10.43 Pre-existing secondary hypertension complicating the puerperium ♀   M

● **O10.9** Unspecified pre-existing hypertension complicating pregnancy, childbirth and the puerperium

  ● **O10.91** Unspecified pre-existing hypertension complicating pregnancy
    O10.911 Unspecified pre-existing hypertension complicating pregnancy, first trimester ♀   M
    O10.912 Unspecified pre-existing hypertension complicating pregnancy, second trimester ♀   M
    O10.913 Unspecified pre-existing hypertension complicating pregnancy, third trimester ♀   M
    O10.919 Unspecified pre-existing hypertension complicating pregnancy, unspecified trimester ♀   M
  O10.92 Unspecified pre-existing hypertension complicating childbirth ♀   M
  O10.93 Unspecified pre-existing hypertension complicating the puerperium ♀   M

● **O11** Pre-existing hypertension with pre-eclampsia
  Includes conditions in O10 complicated by pre-eclampsia pre-eclampsia superimposed pre-existing hypertension
  Use additional code from O10 to identify the type of hypertension
  (Ex) **For category O11 CC codes:** See PDX Collection 964
  Coding Clinic: 2016, Q4, P50

  O11.1 Pre-existing hypertension with pre-eclampsia, first trimester ♀   M
  O11.2 Pre-existing hypertension with pre-eclampsia, second trimester ♀   M
  O11.3 Pre-existing hypertension with pre-eclampsia, third trimester ♀   M
  O11.4 Pre-existing hypertension with pre-eclampsia, complicating childbirth ♀   M
  O11.5 Pre-existing hypertension with pre-eclampsia, complicating the puerperium ♀   M
  O11.9 Pre-existing hypertension with pre-eclampsia, unspecified trimester ♀   M

● **O12** Gestational [pregnancy-induced] edema and proteinuria without hypertension
  (Ex) **For category O12 CC codes:** See PDX Collection 965
  Coding Clinic: 2016, Q4, P50

  ● **O12.0** Gestational edema
    O12.00 Gestational edema, unspecified trimester ♀   M
    O12.01 Gestational edema, first trimester ♀   M
    O12.02 Gestational edema, second trimester ♀   M
    O12.03 Gestational edema, third trimester ♀   M
    O12.04 Gestational edema, complicating childbirth ♀   M
    O12.05 Gestational edema, complicating the puerperium ♀   M

  ● **O12.1** Gestational proteinuria
    O12.10 Gestational proteinuria, unspecified trimester ♀   M
    O12.11 Gestational proteinuria, first trimester ♀   M
    O12.12 Gestational proteinuria, second trimester ♀   M
    O12.13 Gestational proteinuria, third trimester ♀   M
    O12.14 Gestational proteinuria, complicating childbirth ♀   M
    O12.15 Gestational proteinuria, complicating the puerperium ♀   M

  ● **O12.2** Gestational edema with proteinuria
    O12.20 Gestational edema with proteinuria, unspecified trimester ♀   M
    O12.21 Gestational edema with proteinuria, first trimester ♀   M
      CC when PDx is its own CC
    O12.22 Gestational edema with proteinuria, second trimester ♀   M
      CC when PDx is its own CC
    O12.23 Gestational edema with proteinuria, third trimester ♀   M
      CC when PDx is its own CC
    O12.24 Gestational edema with proteinuria, complicating childbirth ♀   M
    O12.25 Gestational edema with proteinuria, complicating the puerperium ♀   M

▶ New   ⇒ Revised   ~~deleted~~ Deleted   Excludes 1   Excludes 2   Includes   Use additional   Code first   Code also   Key words
OGCR Official Guidelines   ● Unacceptable Principal Diagnosis   X Assign placeholder X   ● Use Additional Character(s)   ▶ Manifestation Code   **Coding Clinic**

● **O13** **Gestational [pregnancy-induced] hypertension without significant proteinuria**

     Includes   gestational hypertension NOS
                 transient hypertension of pregnancy
     Coding Clinic: 2016, Q4, P50

  O13.1 Gestational [pregnancy-induced] hypertension without significant proteinuria, **first trimester** ♀   M

  O13.2 Gestational [pregnancy-induced] hypertension without significant proteinuria, **second trimester** ♀   M

  O13.3 Gestational [pregnancy-induced] hypertension without significant proteinuria, **third trimester** ♀   M

  O13.4 Gestational [pregnancy-induced] hypertension without significant proteinuria, complicating **childbirth** ♀   M

  O13.5 Gestational [pregnancy-induced] hypertension without significant proteinuria, complicating the **puerperium** ♀   M

  O13.9 Gestational [pregnancy-induced] hypertension without significant proteinuria, **unspecified trimester** ♀   M

● **O14** **Pre-eclampsia**

     Excludes1   pre-existing hypertension with pre-eclampsia (O11)
     (Ex) For category O14 CC codes: See PDX Collection 964
     Coding Clinic: 2016, Q4, P50

  ● **O14.0** Mild to moderate pre-eclampsia

    O14.00 Mild to moderate pre-eclampsia, **unspecified trimester** ♀   M

    O14.02 Mild to moderate pre-eclampsia, **second trimester** ♀ 🐾   M

    O14.03 Mild to moderate pre-eclampsia, **third trimester** ♀ 🐾   M

    O14.04 Mild to moderate pre-eclampsia, complicating **childbirth** ♀   M

    O14.05 Mild to moderate pre-eclampsia, complicating the **puerperium** ♀   M

  ● **O14.1** Severe pre-eclampsia

     Excludes1   HELLP syndrome (O14.2-)

     H=hemolysis, EL=elevated liver enzymes, LP=low platelet count

    O14.10 Severe pre-eclampsia, **unspecified trimester** ♀   M

    O14.12 Severe pre-eclampsia, **second trimester** ♀ 🐾   M

    O14.13 Severe pre-eclampsia, **third trimester** ♀🐾   M

    O14.14 Severe pre-eclampsia complicating **childbirth** ♀   M

    O14.15 Severe pre-eclampsia, complicating the **puerperium** ♀   M

  ● **O14.2** HELLP syndrome

     Severe pre-eclampsia with hemolysis, elevated liver enzymes and low platelet count (HELLP)

    O14.20 HELLP syndrome (HELLP), **unspecified trimester** ♀   M

    O14.22 HELLP syndrome (HELLP), **second trimester** ♀ 🐾   M

    O14.23 HELLP syndrome (HELLP), **third trimester** ♀ 🐾   M

    O14.24 HELLP syndrome, complicating **childbirth** ♀   M

    O14.25 HELLP syndrome, complicating the **puerperium** ♀   M

  ● **O14.9** Unspecified pre-eclampsia

    O14.90 Unspecified pre-eclampsia, **unspecified trimester** ♀   M

    O14.92 Unspecified pre-eclampsia, **second trimester** ♀ 🐾   M

    O14.93 Unspecified pre-eclampsia, **third trimester** ♀ 🐾   M

    O14.94 Unspecified pre-eclampsia, complicating **childbirth** ♀   M

    O14.95 Unspecified pre-eclampsia, complicating the **puerperium** ♀   M

● **O15** **Eclampsia**

     Includes   convulsions following conditions in O10-O14 and O16
     (Ex) For category O15 CC codes: See PDX Collection 964

  ● **O15.0** Eclampsia complicating pregnancy
     Coding Clinic: 2016, Q4, P50

    O15.00 Eclampsia complicating pregnancy, **unspecified trimester** ♀   M

    O15.02 Eclampsia complicating pregnancy, **second trimester** ♀ 🐾   M

    O15.03 Eclampsia complicating pregnancy, **third trimester** ♀ 🐾   M

  O15.1 Eclampsia complicating **labor** ♀ 🐾   M

  O15.2 Eclampsia complicating the **puerperium** ♀ 🐾   M

  O15.9 Eclampsia, **unspecified** as to time period ♀   M
     Eclampsia NOS

● **O16** **Unspecified maternal hypertension**
     (Ex) For category O16 CC codes: See PDX Collection 964
     Coding Clinic: 2016, Q4, P50

  O16.1 Unspecified maternal hypertension, **first trimester** ♀ 🐾 M

  O16.2 Unspecified maternal hypertension, **second trimester** ♀ 🐾   M

  O16.3 Unspecified maternal hypertension, **third trimester** ♀ 🐾   M

  O16.4 Unspecified maternal hypertension, complicating **childbirth** ♀   M

  O16.5 Unspecified maternal hypertension, complicating the **puerperium** ♀   M

  O16.9 Unspecified maternal hypertension, **unspecified trimester** ♀   M

OTHER MATERNAL DISORDERS PREDOMINANTLY RELATED TO PREGNANCY (O20-O29)

     Excludes2   maternal care related to the fetus and amniotic cavity and possible delivery problems (O30-O48)
                 maternal diseases classifiable elsewhere but complicating pregnancy, labor and delivery, and the puerperium (O98-O99)

● **O20** **Hemorrhage in early pregnancy**

     Includes   hemorrhage before completion of 20 weeks gestation

     Excludes1   pregnancy with abortive outcome (O00-O08)
     (Ex) For category O20 CC codes: See PDX Collection 966

  O20.0 Threatened abortion ♀ 🐾   M
     Hemorrhage specified as due to threatened abortion

  O20.8 Other hemorrhage in early pregnancy ♀   M

  O20.9 Hemorrhage in early pregnancy, **unspecified** ♀ 🐾   M

● **O21** **Excessive vomiting in pregnancy**

  O21.0 Mild hyperemesis gravidarum ♀   M
     Hyperemesis gravidarum, mild or unspecified, starting before the end of the 20th week of gestation

  O21.1 Hyperemesis gravidarum with **metabolic disturbance** ♀   M
     Hyperemesis gravidarum, starting before the end of the 20th week of gestation, with metabolic disturbance such as carbohydrate depletion
     Hyperemesis gravidarum, starting before the end of the 20th week of gestation, with metabolic disturbance such as dehydration
     Hyperemesis gravidarum, starting before the end of the 20th week of gestation, with metabolic disturbance such as electrolyte imbalance

  O21.2 Late vomiting of pregnancy ♀   M
     Excessive vomiting starting after 20 completed weeks of gestation

  O21.8 Other vomiting complicating pregnancy ♀   M
     Vomiting due to diseases classified elsewhere, complicating pregnancy
     Use additional code, to identify cause

  O21.9 Vomiting of pregnancy, **unspecified** ♀   M

N Newborn Age: 0   **P** Pediatric Age: 0–17   **M** Maternity DX: 12–55   **A** Adult Age: 15–124   ♀ Females Only   ♂ Males Only

🐾 Complication\Comorbidity   🐾 Major C\C   (Ex) CC/MCC Exclusions   🐾 Hospital-Acquired Condition

1127

● **O22 Venous complications and hemorrhoids in pregnancy**

Excludes1 venous complications of:
abortion NOS (O03.9)
ectopic or molar pregnancy (O08.7)
failed attempted abortion (O07.35)
induced abortion (O04.85)
spontaneous abortion (O03.89)

Excludes2 obstetric pulmonary embolism (O88.-)
venous complications and hemorrhoids of childbirth and the puerperium (O87.-)

(Ex) For category O22 CC codes: See PDX Collection 967

● **O22.0 Varicose veins of lower extremity in pregnancy**
Varicose veins NOS in pregnancy

O22.00 Varicose veins of lower extremity in pregnancy, unspecified trimester ♀   M

O22.01 Varicose veins of lower extremity in pregnancy, first trimester ♀   M

O22.02 Varicose veins of lower extremity in pregnancy, second trimester ♀   M

O22.03 Varicose veins of lower extremity in pregnancy, third trimester ♀   M

● **O22.1 Genital varices in pregnancy**
Perineal varices in pregnancy
Vaginal varices in pregnancy
Vulval varices in pregnancy

O22.10 Genital varices in pregnancy, unspecified trimester ♀   M

O22.11 Genital varices in pregnancy, first trimester ♀ M

O22.12 Genital varices in pregnancy, second trimester ♀   M

O22.13 Genital varices in pregnancy, third trimester ♀ M

● **O22.2 Superficial thrombophlebitis in pregnancy**
Phlebitis in pregnancy NOS
Thrombophlebitis of legs in pregnancy
Thrombosis in pregnancy NOS

Use additional code to identify the superficial thrombophlebitis (I80.0-)

O22.20 Superficial thrombophlebitis in pregnancy, unspecified trimester ♀   M

O22.21 Superficial thrombophlebitis in pregnancy, first trimester ♀   M

O22.22 Superficial thrombophlebitis in pregnancy, second trimester ♀   M

O22.23 Superficial thrombophlebitis in pregnancy, third trimester ♀   M

● **O22.3 Deep phlebothrombosis in pregnancy**
Deep vein thrombosis, antepartum

Use additional code to identify the deep vein thrombosis (I82.4-, I82.5-, I82.62-. I82.72-)

Use additional code, if applicable, for associated long-term (current) use of anticoagulants (Z79.01)

O22.30 Deep phlebothrombosis in pregnancy, unspecified trimester ♀   M

O22.31 Deep phlebothrombosis in pregnancy, first trimester ♀   M

O22.32 Deep phlebothrombosis in pregnancy, second trimester ♀   M

O22.33 Deep phlebothrombosis in pregnancy, third trimester ♀   M

● **O22.4 Hemorrhoids in pregnancy**

O22.40 Hemorrhoids in pregnancy, unspecified trimester ♀   M

O22.41 Hemorrhoids in pregnancy, first trimester ♀   M

O22.42 Hemorrhoids in pregnancy, second trimester ♀   M

O22.43 Hemorrhoids in pregnancy, third trimester ♀   M

● **O22.5 Cerebral venous thrombosis in pregnancy**
Cerebrovenous sinus thrombosis in pregnancy

O22.50 Cerebral venous thrombosis in pregnancy, unspecified trimester ♀   M

O22.51 Cerebral venous thrombosis in pregnancy, first trimester ♀   M

O22.52 Cerebral venous thrombosis in pregnancy, second trimester ♀   M

O22.53 Cerebral venous thrombosis in pregnancy, third trimester ♀   M

● **O22.8 Other venous complications in pregnancy**

● **O22.8X Other venous complications in pregnancy**

O22.8X1 Other venous complications in pregnancy, first trimester ♀   M

O22.8X2 Other venous complications in pregnancy, second trimester ♀   M

O22.8X3 Other venous complications in pregnancy, third trimester ♀   M

O22.8X9 Other venous complications in pregnancy, unspecified trimester ♀   M

● **O22.9 Venous complication in pregnancy, unspecified**
Gestational phlebitis NOS
Gestational phlebopathy NOS
Gestational thrombosis NOS

O22.90 Venous complication in pregnancy, unspecified, unspecified trimester ♀   M

O22.91 Venous complication in pregnancy, unspecified, first trimester ♀   M

O22.92 Venous complication in pregnancy, unspecified, second trimester ♀   M

O22.93 Venous complication in pregnancy, unspecified, third trimester ♀   M

● **O23 Infections of genitourinary tract in pregnancy**

Use additional code to identify organism (B95.-, B96.-)

Excludes2 gonococcal infections complicating pregnancy, childbirth and the puerperium (O98.2)
infections with a predominantly sexual mode of transmission NOS complicating pregnancy, childbirth and the puerperium (O98.3)
syphilis complicating pregnancy, childbirth and the puerperium (O98.1)
tuberculosis of genitourinary system complicating pregnancy, childbirth and the puerperium (O98.0)
venereal disease NOS complicating pregnancy, childbirth and the puerperium (O98.3)

(Ex) For category O23 CC codes: See PDX Collection 968

● **O23.0 Infections of kidney in pregnancy**
Pyelonephritis in pregnancy

O23.00 Infections of kidney in pregnancy, unspecified trimester ♀   M

O23.01 Infections of kidney in pregnancy, first trimester ♀   M

O23.02 Infections of kidney in pregnancy, second trimester ♀   M

O23.03 Infections of kidney in pregnancy, third trimester ♀   M

● **O23.1 Infections of bladder in pregnancy**

O23.10 Infections of bladder in pregnancy, unspecified trimester ♀   M

O23.11 Infections of bladder in pregnancy, first trimester ♀   M

O23.12 Infections of bladder in pregnancy, second trimester ♀   M

O23.13 Infections of bladder in pregnancy, third trimester ♀   M

● **O23.2 Infections of urethra in pregnancy**

     O23.20 Infections of urethra in pregnancy, unspecified trimester ♀   M

     O23.21 Infections of urethra in pregnancy, first trimester ♀ 🖐   M

     O23.22 Infections of urethra in pregnancy, second trimester ♀ 🖐   M

     O23.23 Infections of urethra in pregnancy, third trimester ♀ 🖐   M

● **O23.3 Infections of other parts of urinary tract in pregnancy**

     O23.30 Infections of other parts of urinary tract in pregnancy, unspecified trimester ♀   M

     O23.31 Infections of other parts of urinary tract in pregnancy, first trimester ♀ 🖐   M

     O23.32 Infections of other parts of urinary tract in pregnancy, second trimester ♀ 🖐   M

     O23.33 Infections of other parts of urinary tract in pregnancy, third trimester ♀ 🖐   M

● **O23.4 Unspecified infection of urinary tract in pregnancy**

     O23.40 Unspecified infection of urinary tract in pregnancy, unspecified trimester ♀   M

     O23.41 Unspecified infection of urinary tract in pregnancy, first trimester ♀ 🖐   M

     O23.42 Unspecified infection of urinary tract in pregnancy, second trimester ♀ 🖐   M

     O23.43 Unspecified infection of urinary tract in pregnancy, third trimester ♀ 🖐   M

● **O23.5 Infections of the genital tract in pregnancy**

     ● O23.51 Infection of cervix in pregnancy

       O23.511 Infections of cervix in pregnancy, first trimester ♀ 🖐   M

       O23.512 Infections of cervix in pregnancy, second trimester ♀ 🖐   M

       O23.513 Infections of cervix in pregnancy, third trimester ♀ 🖐   M

       O23.519 Infections of cervix in pregnancy, unspecified trimester ♀   M

     ● O23.52 Salpingo-oophoritis in pregnancy
       Oophoritis = inflammation of ovary
       Salpingitis = inflammation of fallopian tube
       Oophoritis in pregnancy
       Salpingitis in pregnancy

       O23.521 Salpingo-oophoritis in pregnancy, first trimester ♀ 🖐   M

       O23.522 Salpingo-oophoritis in pregnancy, second trimester ♀ 🖐   M

       O23.523 Salpingo-oophoritis in pregnancy, third trimester ♀ 🖐   M

       O23.529 Salpingo-oophoritis in pregnancy, unspecified trimester ♀   M

     ● O23.59 Infection of other part of genital tract in pregnancy

       O23.591 Infection of other part of genital tract in pregnancy, first trimester ♀ 🖐   M

       O23.592 Infection of other part of genital tract in pregnancy, second trimester ♀ 🖐 M

       O23.593 Infection of other part of genital tract in pregnancy, third trimester ♀ 🖐 M

       O23.599 Infection of other part of genital tract in pregnancy, unspecified trimester ♀   M

● **O23.9 Unspecified genitourinary tract infection in pregnancy**
     Genitourinary tract infection in pregnancy NOS

     O23.90 Unspecified genitourinary tract infection in pregnancy, unspecified trimester ♀   M

     O23.91 Unspecified genitourinary tract infection in pregnancy, first trimester ♀ 🖐   M

     O23.92 Unspecified genitourinary tract infection in pregnancy, second trimester ♀ 🖐   M

     O23.93 Unspecified genitourinary tract infection in pregnancy, third trimester ♀ 🖐   M

OGCR Section I.C.15.g.

> Diabetes mellitus in pregnancy
>
> Diabetes mellitus is a significant complicating factor in pregnancy. Pregnant women who are diabetic should be assigned a code from category O24, Diabetes mellitus in pregnancy, childbirth, and the puerperium, first, followed by the appropriate diabetes code(s) (E08-E13) from Chapter 4.

● **O24 Diabetes mellitus in pregnancy, childbirth, and the puerperium**
     (Ex) **For category O24 CC codes:** See PDX Collection 969

     ● **O24.0 Pre-existing type 1 diabetes mellitus, in pregnancy, childbirth and the puerperium**
       Juvenile onset diabetes mellitus, in pregnancy, childbirth and the puerperium
       Ketosis-prone diabetes mellitus in pregnancy, childbirth and the puerperium
       Use additional code from category E10 to further identify any manifestations

       ● O24.01 Pre-existing type 1 diabetes mellitus, in pregnancy

         O24.011 Pre-existing type 1 diabetes mellitus, in pregnancy, first trimester ♀ 🖐   M

         O24.012 Pre-existing type 1 diabetes mellitus, in pregnancy, second trimester ♀ 🖐   M

         O24.013 Pre-existing type 1 diabetes mellitus, in pregnancy, third trimester ♀ 🖐   M

         O24.019 Pre-existing type 1 diabetes mellitus, in pregnancy, unspecified trimester ♀ 🖐   M

       O24.02 Pre-existing type 1 diabetes mellitus, in childbirth ♀ 🖐   M

       O24.03 Pre-existing type 1 diabetes mellitus, in the puerperium ♀ 🖐   M

     ● **O24.1 Pre-existing type 2 diabetes mellitus, in pregnancy, childbirth and the puerperium**
       Insulin-resistant diabetes mellitus in pregnancy, childbirth and the puerperium
       Use additional code (for):
         from category E11 to further identify any manifestations
         long-term (current) use of insulin (Z79.4)

       ● O24.11 Pre-existing type 2 diabetes mellitus, in pregnancy

         O24.111 Pre-existing type 2 diabetes mellitus, in pregnancy, first trimester ♀ 🖐   M

         O24.112 Pre-existing type 2 diabetes mellitus, in pregnancy, second trimester ♀ 🖐   M

         O24.113 Pre-existing type 2 diabetes mellitus, in pregnancy, third trimester ♀ 🖐   M

         O24.119 Pre-existing type 2 diabetes mellitus, in pregnancy, unspecified trimester ♀ 🖐   M

       O24.12 Pre-existing type 2 diabetes mellitus, in childbirth ♀ 🖐   M

       O24.13 Pre-existing type 2 diabetes mellitus, in the puerperium ♀ 🖐   M

N Newborn Age: 0   **P** Pediatric Age: 0–17   **M** Maternity DX: 12–55   **A** Adult Age: 15–124   ♀ Females Only   ♂ Males Only

🖐 Complication\Comorbidity   🖐 Major C\C   (Ex) CC/MCC Exclusions   🖐 Hospital-Acquired Condition

1129

CHAPTER 15 (O00–O9A)

CHAPTER 15 (O00-O9A)

- ● **O24.3** **Unspecified pre-existing diabetes mellitus in pregnancy, childbirth and the puerperium**
  Use additional code (for):
  from category E11 to further identify any manifestation
  long-term (current) use of insulin (Z79.4)
  - ● **O24.31** **Unspecified pre-existing diabetes mellitus in pregnancy**
    - O24.311 Unspecified pre-existing diabetes mellitus in pregnancy, first trimester ♀ 🔎   M
    - O24.312 Unspecified pre-existing diabetes mellitus in pregnancy, second trimester ♀ 🔎   M
    - O24.313 Unspecified pre-existing diabetes mellitus in pregnancy, third trimester ♀ 🔎   M
    - O24.319 Unspecified pre-existing diabetes mellitus in pregnancy, unspecified trimester ♀ 🔎   M
  - O24.32 Unspecified pre-existing diabetes mellitus in childbirth ♀ 🔎   M
  - O24.33 Unspecified pre-existing diabetes mellitus in the puerperium ♀ 🔎   M
- ● **O24.4** **Gestational diabetes mellitus**
  Diabetes mellitus arising in pregnancy
  Gestational diabetes mellitus NOS
  Coding Clinic: 2016, Q4, P50, 126
  - ● **O24.41** **Gestational diabetes mellitus in pregnancy**
    - O24.410 Gestational diabetes mellitus in pregnancy, diet controlled ♀   M
    - O24.414 Gestational diabetes mellitus in pregnancy, insulin controlled ♀   M
    - O24.415 Gestational diabetes mellitus in pregnancy, controlled by oral hypoglycemic drugs ♀   M
      Gestational diabetes mellitus in pregnancy, controlled by oral antidiabetic drugs
      Coding Clinic: 2016, Q4, P50
    - O24.419 Gestational diabetes mellitus in pregnancy, unspecified control ♀   M
      Coding Clinic: 2015, Q4, P34
  - ● **O24.42** **Gestational diabetes mellitus in childbirth**
    - O24.420 Gestational diabetes mellitus in childbirth, diet controlled ♀   M
    - O24.424 Gestational diabetes mellitus in childbirth, insulin controlled ♀   M
    - O24.425 Gestational diabetes mellitus in childbirth, controlled by oral hypoglycemic drugs ♀   M
      Gestational diabetes mellitus in childbirth, controlled by oral antidiabetic drugs
      Coding Clinic: 2016, Q4, P50
    - O24.429 Gestational diabetes mellitus in childbirth, unspecified control ♀   M

OGCR Section I.C.15.i.

Gestational (pregnancy induced) diabetes

Gestational (pregnancy induced) diabetes can occur during the second and third trimester of pregnancy in women who were not diabetic prior to pregnancy. Gestational diabetes can cause complications in the pregnancy similar to those of pre-existing diabetes mellitus. It also puts the woman at greater risk of developing diabetes after the pregnancy. Codes for gestational diabetes are in subcategory O24.4, Gestational diabetes mellitus. No other code from category O24, Diabetes mellitus in pregnancy, childbirth, and the puerperium, should be used with a code from O24.4

The codes under subcategory O24.4 include diet controlled, insulin controlled, **and controlled by oral hypoglycemic drugs.** If a patient with gestational diabetes is treated with both diet and insulin, only the code for insulin-controlled is required. **If a patient with gestational diabetes is treated with both diet and oral hypoglycemic medications, only the code for "controlled by oral hypoglycemic drugs" is required.** Code Z79.4, Long-term (current) use of insulin **or code Z79.84, Long-term (current) use of oral hypoglycemic drugs,** should not be assigned with codes from subcategory O24.4.

An abnormal glucose tolerance in pregnancy is assigned a code from subcategory O99.81, Abnormal glucose complicating pregnancy, childbirth, and the puerperium.

- ● **O24.43** **Gestational diabetes mellitus in the puerperium**
  - O24.430 Gestational diabetes mellitus in the puerperium, diet controlled ♀   M
  - O24.434 Gestational diabetes mellitus in the puerperium, insulin controlled ♀   M
  - O24.435 Gestational diabetes mellitus in puerperium, controlled by oral hypoglycemic drugs ♀   M
    Gestational diabetes mellitus in puerperium, controlled by oral antidiabetic drugs
    Coding Clinic: 2016, Q4, P50
  - O24.439 Gestational diabetes mellitus in the puerperium, unspecified control ♀   M
- ● **O24.8** **Other pre-existing diabetes mellitus in pregnancy, childbirth, and the puerperium**
  Use additional code (for):
  from categories E08, E09 and E13 to further identify any manifestation
  long-term (current) use of insulin (Z79.4)
  - ● **O24.81** **Other pre-existing diabetes mellitus in pregnancy**
    - O24.811 Other pre-existing diabetes mellitus in pregnancy, first trimester ♀ 🔎   M
    - O24.812 Other pre-existing diabetes mellitus in pregnancy, second trimester ♀ 🔎   M
    - O24.813 Other pre-existing diabetes mellitus in pregnancy, third trimester ♀ 🔎   M
    - O24.819 Other pre-existing diabetes mellitus in pregnancy, unspecified trimester ♀ 🔎   M
  - O24.82 Other pre-existing diabetes mellitus in childbirth ♀ 🔎   M
  - O24.83 Other pre-existing diabetes mellitus in the puerperium ♀ 🔎   M

▶ New   ⇒ Revised   ~~deleted~~ Deleted   Excludes 1   Excludes 2   Includes   Use additional   Code first   Code also   Key words
OGCR Official Guidelines   ● Unacceptable Principal Diagnosis   X Assign placeholder X   ● Use Additional Character(s)   ▶ Manifestation Code   Coding Clinic

● **O24.9 Unspecified diabetes mellitus in pregnancy, childbirth and the puerperium**

> Use additional code for long-term (current) use of insulin (Z79.4)
>
> *Unknown whether patient was diabetic before pregnancy occurred*

  ● **O24.91 Unspecified diabetes mellitus in pregnancy**

    O24.911 Unspecified diabetes mellitus in pregnancy, first trimester ♀ 🖐   M

    O24.912 Unspecified diabetes mellitus in pregnancy, second trimester ♀ 🖐   M

    O24.913 Unspecified diabetes mellitus in pregnancy, third trimester ♀ 🖐   M

    O24.919 Unspecified diabetes mellitus in pregnancy, unspecified trimester ♀ 🖐   M

  O24.92 Unspecified diabetes mellitus in childbirth ♀   M

  O24.93 Unspecified diabetes mellitus in the puerperium ♀ 🖐   M

● **O25 Malnutrition in pregnancy, childbirth and the puerperium**

  ● **O25.1 Malnutrition in pregnancy**

    O25.10 Malnutrition in pregnancy, unspecified trimester ♀   M

    O25.11 Malnutrition in pregnancy, first trimester ♀   M

    O25.12 Malnutrition in pregnancy, second trimester ♀ M

    O25.13 Malnutrition in pregnancy, third trimester ♀   M

  O25.2 Malnutrition in childbirth ♀   M

  O25.3 Malnutrition in the puerperium ♀   M

● **O26 Maternal care for other conditions predominantly related to pregnancy**

  ● **O26.0 Excessive weight gain in pregnancy**

    Excludes2   gestational edema (O12.0, O12.2)

    O26.00 Excessive weight gain in pregnancy, unspecified trimester ♀   M

    O26.01 Excessive weight gain in pregnancy, first trimester ♀   M

    O26.02 Excessive weight gain in pregnancy, second trimester ♀   M

    O26.03 Excessive weight gain in pregnancy, third trimester ♀   M

  ● **O26.1 Low weight gain in pregnancy**

    O26.10 Low weight gain in pregnancy, unspecified trimester ♀   M

    O26.11 Low weight gain in pregnancy, first trimester ♀   M

    O26.12 Low weight gain in pregnancy, second trimester ♀   M

    O26.13 Low weight gain in pregnancy, third trimester ♀   M

  ● **O26.2 Pregnancy care for patient with recurrent pregnancy loss**

    O26.20 Pregnancy care for patient with recurrent pregnancy loss, unspecified trimester ♀   M

    O26.21 Pregnancy care for patient with recurrent pregnancy loss, first trimester ♀   M

    O26.22 Pregnancy care for patient with recurrent pregnancy loss, second trimester ♀   M

    O26.23 Pregnancy care for patient with recurrent pregnancy loss, third trimester ♀   M

● **O26.3 Retained intrauterine contraceptive device in pregnancy**

  O26.30 Retained intrauterine contraceptive device in pregnancy, unspecified trimester ♀   M

  O26.31 Retained intrauterine contraceptive device in pregnancy, first trimester ♀   M

  O26.32 Retained intrauterine contraceptive device in pregnancy, second trimester ♀   M

  O26.33 Retained intrauterine contraceptive device in pregnancy, third trimester ♀   M

● **O26.4 Herpes gestationis**

  O26.40 Herpes gestationis, unspecified trimester ♀   M

  O26.41 Herpes gestationis, first trimester ♀   M

  O26.42 Herpes gestationis, second trimester ♀   M

  O26.43 Herpes gestationis, third trimester ♀   M

● **O26.5 Maternal hypotension syndrome**

> Supine hypotensive syndrome

  O26.50 Maternal hypotension syndrome, unspecified trimester ♀   M

  O26.51 Maternal hypotension syndrome, first trimester ♀   M

  O26.52 Maternal hypotension syndrome, second trimester ♀   M

  O26.53 Maternal hypotension syndrome, third trimester ♀   M

● **O26.6 Liver and biliary tract disorders in pregnancy, childbirth and the puerperium**

> Use additional code to identify the specific disorder

  Excludes2   hepatorenal syndrome following labor and delivery (O90.4)

  ● **O26.61 Liver and biliary tract disorders in pregnancy**

    (Ex:) **For category O26.61 CC codes: See PDX Collection 972**

    O26.611 Liver and biliary tract disorders in pregnancy, first trimester ♀ 🖐   M

    O26.612 Liver and biliary tract disorders in pregnancy, second trimester ♀ 🖐   M

    O26.613 Liver and biliary tract disorders in pregnancy, third trimester ♀ 🖐   M

    O26.619 Liver and biliary tract disorders in pregnancy, unspecified trimester ♀   M

  O26.62 Liver and biliary tract disorders in childbirth ♀ 🖐   M

    (Ex:) **See PDX Collection 972**

  O26.63 Liver and biliary tract disorders in the puerperium ♀   M

● **O26.7 Subluxation of symphysis (pubis) in pregnancy, childbirth and the puerperium**

  Excludes1   traumatic separation of symphysis (pubis) during childbirth (O71.6)

  ● **O26.71 Subluxation of symphysis (pubis) in pregnancy**

    O26.711 Subluxation of symphysis (pubis) in pregnancy, first trimester ♀   M

    O26.712 Subluxation of symphysis (pubis) in pregnancy, second trimester ♀   M

    O26.713 Subluxation of symphysis (pubis) in pregnancy, third trimester ♀   M

    O26.719 Subluxation of symphysis (pubis) in pregnancy, unspecified trimester ♀   M

  O26.72 Subluxation of symphysis (pubis) in childbirth ♀   M

  O26.73 Subluxation of symphysis (pubis) in the puerperium ♀   M

CHAPTER 15 (O00–O9A)

N Newborn Age: 0   **P** Pediatric Age: 0–17   **M** Maternity DX: 12–55   **A** Adult Age: 15–124   ♀ Females Only   ♂ Males Only

🖐 Complication\Comorbidity   🖐 Major C\C   (Ex:) CC/MCC Exclusions   🖐 Hospital-Acquired Condition

● O26.8   Other specified pregnancy related conditions
  ● O26.81   Pregnancy related exhaustion and fatigue
    O26.811   Pregnancy related exhaustion and fatigue, first trimester ♀   M
    O26.812   Pregnancy related exhaustion and fatigue, second trimester ♀   M
    O26.813   Pregnancy related exhaustion and fatigue, third trimester ♀   M
    O26.819   Pregnancy related exhaustion and fatigue, unspecified trimester ♀   M
  ● O26.82   Pregnancy related peripheral neuritis
    O26.821   Pregnancy related peripheral neuritis, first trimester ♀   M
    O26.822   Pregnancy related peripheral neuritis, second trimester ♀   M
    O26.823   Pregnancy related peripheral neuritis, third trimester ♀   M
    O26.829   Pregnancy related peripheral neuritis, unspecified trimester ♀   M
  ● O26.83   Pregnancy related renal disease
    Use additional code to identify the specific disorder
    (Ex) **For category O26.83 CC codes:** See PDX Collection 965
    O26.831   Pregnancy related renal disease, first trimester ♀ 🔊   M
    O26.832   Pregnancy related renal disease, second trimester ♀ 🔊   M
    O26.833   Pregnancy related renal disease, third trimester ♀ 🔊   M
    O26.839   Pregnancy related renal disease, unspecified trimester ♀   M
  ● O26.84   Uterine size-date discrepancy complicating pregnancy
    Excludes1   encounter for suspected problem with fetal growth ruled out (Z03.74)
    O26.841   Uterine size-date discrepancy, first trimester ♀   M
    O26.842   Uterine size-date discrepancy, second trimester ♀   M
    O26.843   Uterine size-date discrepancy, third trimester ♀   M
    O26.849   Uterine size-date discrepancy, unspecified trimester ♀   M
  ● O26.85   Spotting complicating pregnancy
    O26.851   Spotting complicating pregnancy, first trimester ♀   M
    O26.852   Spotting complicating pregnancy, second trimester ♀   M
    O26.853   Spotting complicating pregnancy, third trimester ♀   M
    O26.859   Spotting complicating pregnancy, unspecified trimester ♀   M
    O26.86   Pruritic urticarial papules and plaques of pregnancy (PUPPP) ♀   M
      Polymorphic eruption of pregnancy
  ● O26.87   Cervical shortening
    Excludes1   encounter for suspected cervical shortening ruled out (Z03.75)
    (Ex) **For category O26.87 CC codes:** See PDX Collection 973
    O26.872   Cervical shortening, second trimester ♀ 🔊   M
    O26.873   Cervical shortening, third trimester ♀ 🔊   M
    O26.879   Cervical shortening, unspecified trimester ♀ 🔊   M

  ● O26.89   Other specified pregnancy related conditions
    O26.891   Other specified pregnancy related conditions, first trimester ♀   M
    O26.892   Other specified pregnancy related conditions, second trimester ♀   M
    O26.893   Other specified pregnancy related conditions, third trimester ♀   M
      Coding Clinic: 2015, Q3, P40
    O26.899   Other specified pregnancy related conditions, unspecified trimester ♀   M
  ● O26.9   Pregnancy related conditions, unspecified
    O26.90   Pregnancy related conditions, unspecified, unspecified trimester ♀   M
    O26.91   Pregnancy related conditions, unspecified, first trimester ♀   M
    O26.92   Pregnancy related conditions, unspecified, second trimester ♀   M
    O26.93   Pregnancy related conditions, unspecified, third trimester ♀   M

● O28   Abnormal findings on antenatal screening of mother
  Excludes1   diagnostic findings classified elsewhere - see Alphabetical Index
  O28.0   Abnormal hematological finding on antenatal screening of mother ♀   M
  O28.1   Abnormal biochemical finding on antenatal screening of mother ♀   M
  O28.2   Abnormal cytological finding on antenatal screening of mother ♀   M
  O28.3   Abnormal ultrasonic finding on antenatal screening of mother ♀   M
    Coding Clinic: 2016, Q4, P5
  O28.4   Abnormal radiological finding on antenatal screening of mother ♀   M
  O28.5   Abnormal chromosomal and genetic finding on antenatal screening of mother ♀   M
  O28.8   Other abnormal findings on antenatal screening of mother ♀   M
  O28.9   Unspecified abnormal findings on antenatal screening of mother ♀   M

● O29   Complications of anesthesia during pregnancy
  Includes   maternal complications arising from the administration of a general, regional or local anesthetic, analgesic or other sedation during pregnancy
  Use additional code, if necessary, to identify the complication
  Excludes2   complications of anesthesia during labor and delivery (O74.-)
    complications of anesthesia during the puerperium (O89.-)
  ● O29.0   Pulmonary complications of anesthesia during pregnancy
    ● O29.01   Aspiration pneumonitis due to anesthesia during pregnancy
      Inhalation of stomach contents or secretions NOS due to anesthesia during pregnancy
      Mendelson's syndrome due to anesthesia during pregnancy
      O29.011   Aspiration pneumonitis due to anesthesia during pregnancy, first trimester ♀   M
      O29.012   Aspiration pneumonitis due to anesthesia during pregnancy, second trimester ♀   M
      O29.013   Aspiration pneumonitis due to anesthesia during pregnancy, third trimester ♀   M
      O29.019   Aspiration pneumonitis due to anesthesia during pregnancy, unspecified trimester ♀   M

▶ New   ⇒ Revised   ~~deleted~~ Deleted   Excludes 1   Excludes 2   Includes   Use additional   Code first   Code also   Key words
OGCR Official Guidelines   ● Unacceptable Principal Diagnosis   X Assign placeholder X   ● Use Additional Character(s)   ▶ Manifestation Code   Coding Clinic

● **O29.02   Pressure collapse of lung due to anesthesia during pregnancy**

    O29.021   Pressure collapse of lung due to anesthesia during pregnancy, first trimester ♀   M

    O29.022   Pressure collapse of lung due to anesthesia during pregnancy, second trimester ♀   M

    O29.023   Pressure collapse of lung due to anesthesia during pregnancy, third trimester ♀   M

    O29.029   Pressure collapse of lung due to anesthesia during pregnancy, unspecified trimester ♀   M

● **O29.09   Other pulmonary complications of anesthesia during pregnancy**

    O29.091   Other pulmonary complications of anesthesia during pregnancy, first trimester ♀   M

    O29.092   Other pulmonary complications of anesthesia during pregnancy, second trimester ♀   M

    O29.093   Other pulmonary complications of anesthesia during pregnancy, third trimester ♀   M

    O29.099   Other pulmonary complications of anesthesia during pregnancy, unspecified trimester ♀   M

● **O29.1   Cardiac complications of anesthesia during pregnancy**

● **O29.11   Cardiac arrest due to anesthesia during pregnancy**

    O29.111   Cardiac arrest due to anesthesia during pregnancy, first trimester ♀   M

    O29.112   Cardiac arrest due to anesthesia during pregnancy, second trimester ♀   M

    O29.113   Cardiac arrest due to anesthesia during pregnancy, third trimester ♀   M

    O29.119   Cardiac arrest due to anesthesia during pregnancy, unspecified trimester ♀   M

● **O29.12   Cardiac failure due to anesthesia during pregnancy**

    O29.121   Cardiac failure due to anesthesia during pregnancy, first trimester ♀   M

    O29.122   Cardiac failure due to anesthesia during pregnancy, second trimester ♀   M

    O29.123   Cardiac failure due to anesthesia during pregnancy, third trimester ♀   M

    O29.129   Cardiac failure due to anesthesia during pregnancy, unspecified trimester ♀   M

● **O29.19   Other cardiac complications of anesthesia during pregnancy**

    O29.191   Other cardiac complications of anesthesia during pregnancy, first trimester ♀   M

    O29.192   Other cardiac complications of anesthesia during pregnancy, second trimester ♀   M

    O29.193   Other cardiac complications of anesthesia during pregnancy, third trimester ♀   M

    O29.199   Other cardiac complications of anesthesia during pregnancy, unspecified trimester ♀   M

● **O29.2   Central nervous system complications of anesthesia during pregnancy**

● **O29.21   Cerebral anoxia due to anesthesia during pregnancy**

    O29.211   Cerebral anoxia due to anesthesia during pregnancy, first trimester ♀   M

    O29.212   Cerebral anoxia due to anesthesia during pregnancy, second trimester ♀   M

    O29.213   Cerebral anoxia due to anesthesia during pregnancy, third trimester ♀   M

    O29.219   Cerebral anoxia due to anesthesia during pregnancy, unspecified trimester ♀   M

● **O29.29   Other central nervous system complications of anesthesia during pregnancy**

    O29.291   Other central nervous system complications of anesthesia during pregnancy, first trimester ♀   M

    O29.292   Other central nervous system complications of anesthesia during pregnancy, second trimester ♀   M

    O29.293   Other central nervous system complications of anesthesia during pregnancy, third trimester ♀   M

    O29.299   Other central nervous system complications of anesthesia during pregnancy, unspecified trimester ♀   M

● **O29.3   Toxic reaction to local anesthesia during pregnancy**

● **O29.3X   Toxic reaction to local anesthesia during pregnancy**

    O29.3X1   Toxic reaction to local anesthesia during pregnancy, first trimester ♀   M

    O29.3X2   Toxic reaction to local anesthesia during pregnancy, second trimester ♀   M

    O29.3X3   Toxic reaction to local anesthesia during pregnancy, third trimester ♀   M

    O29.3X9   Toxic reaction to local anesthesia during pregnancy, unspecified trimester ♀   M

● **O29.4   Spinal and epidural anesthesia induced headache during pregnancy**

    O29.40   Spinal and epidural anesthesia induced headache during pregnancy, unspecified trimester ♀   M

    O29.41   Spinal and epidural anesthesia induced headache during pregnancy, first trimester ♀   M

    O29.42   Spinal and epidural anesthesia induced headache during pregnancy, second trimester ♀   M

    O29.43   Spinal and epidural anesthesia induced headache during pregnancy, third trimester ♀   M

● **O29.5   Other complications of spinal and epidural anesthesia during pregnancy**

● **O29.5X   Other complications of spinal and epidural anesthesia during pregnancy**

    O29.5X1   Other complications of spinal and epidural anesthesia during pregnancy, first trimester ♀   M

    O29.5X2   Other complications of spinal and epidural anesthesia during pregnancy, second trimester ♀   M

    O29.5X3   Other complications of spinal and epidural anesthesia during pregnancy, third trimester ♀   M

    O29.5X9   Other complications of spinal and epidural anesthesia during pregnancy, unspecified trimester ♀   M

CHAPTER 15 (O00-O9A)

- ● O29.6   **Failed or difficult intubation for anesthesia during pregnancy**
  - O29.60   Failed or difficult intubation for anesthesia during pregnancy, unspecified trimester ♀   M
  - O29.61   Failed or difficult intubation for anesthesia during pregnancy, first trimester ♀   M
  - O29.62   Failed or difficult intubation for anesthesia during pregnancy, second trimester ♀   M
  - O29.63   Failed or difficult intubation for anesthesia during pregnancy, third trimester ♀   M
- ● O29.8   **Other complications of anesthesia during pregnancy**
  - ● O29.8X   Other complications of anesthesia during pregnancy
    - O29.8X1   Other complications of anesthesia during pregnancy, first trimester ♀   M
    - O29.8X2   Other complications of anesthesia during pregnancy, second trimester ♀   M
    - O29.8X3   Other complications of anesthesia during pregnancy, third trimester ♀   M
    - O29.8X9   Other complications of anesthesia during pregnancy, unspecified trimester ♀   M
- ● O29.9   **Unspecified complication of anesthesia during pregnancy**
  - O29.90   Unspecified complication of anesthesia during pregnancy, unspecified trimester ♀   M
  - O29.91   Unspecified complication of anesthesia during pregnancy, first trimester ♀   M
  - O29.92   Unspecified complication of anesthesia during pregnancy, second trimester ♀   M
  - O29.93   Unspecified complication of anesthesia during pregnancy, third trimester ♀   M

MATERNAL CARE RELATED TO THE FETUS AND AMNIOTIC CAVITY AND POSSIBLE DELIVERY PROBLEMS (O30-O48)

- ● O30   **Multiple gestation**

  Code also any complications specific to multiple gestation

  Coding Clinic: 2016, Q4, P51

  - ● O30.0   **Twin pregnancy**
    - ● O30.00   Twin pregnancy, unspecified number of placenta and unspecified number of amniotic sacs
      - O30.001   Twin pregnancy, unspecified number of placenta and unspecified number of amniotic sacs, first trimester ♀   M
      - O30.002   Twin pregnancy, unspecified number of placenta and unspecified number of amniotic sacs, second trimester ♀   M
      - O30.003   Twin pregnancy, unspecified number of placenta and unspecified number of amniotic sacs, third trimester ♀   M
      - O30.009   Twin pregnancy, unspecified number of placenta and unspecified number of amniotic sacs, unspecified trimester ♀   M
    - ● O30.01   Twin pregnancy, monochorionic/monoamniotic

      Twin pregnancy, one placenta, one amniotic sac

      Excludes1   conjoined twins (O30.02-)
      - O30.011   Twin pregnancy, monochorionic/monoamniotic, first trimester ♀   M
      - O30.012   Twin pregnancy, monochorionic/monoamniotic, second trimester ♀   M
      - O30.013   Twin pregnancy, monochorionic/monoamniotic, third trimester ♀   M
      - O30.019   Twin pregnancy, monochorionic/monoamniotic, unspecified trimester ♀   M

- ● O30.02   Conjoined twin pregnancy
  - O30.021   Conjoined twin pregnancy, first trimester ♀   M
  - O30.022   Conjoined twin pregnancy, second trimester ♀   M
  - O30.023   Conjoined twin pregnancy, third trimester ♀   M
  - O30.029   Conjoined twin pregnancy, unspecified trimester ♀   M
- ● O30.03   Twin pregnancy, monochorionic/diamniotic

  Twin pregnancy, one placenta, two amniotic sacs
  - O30.031   Twin pregnancy, monochorionic/diamniotic, first trimester ♀   M
  - O30.032   Twin pregnancy, monochorionic/diamniotic, second trimester ♀   M
  - O30.033   Twin pregnancy, monochorionic/diamniotic, third trimester ♀   M
  - O30.039   Twin pregnancy, monochorionic/diamniotic, unspecified trimester ♀   M
- ● O30.04   Twin pregnancy, dichorionic/diamniotic

  Twin pregnancy, two placentae, two amniotic sacs
  - O30.041   Twin pregnancy, dichorionic/diamniotic, first trimester ♀   M
  - O30.042   Twin pregnancy, dichorionic/diamniotic, second trimester ♀   M
  - O30.043   Twin pregnancy, dichorionic/diamniotic, third trimester ♀   M
  - O30.049   Twin pregnancy, dichorionic/diamniotic, unspecified trimester ♀   M
- ● O30.09   Twin pregnancy, unable to determine number of placenta and number of amniotic sacs
  - O30.091   Twin pregnancy, unable to determine number of placenta and number of amniotic sacs, first trimester ♀   M
  - O30.092   Twin pregnancy, unable to determine number of placenta and number of amniotic sacs, second trimester ♀   M
  - O30.093   Twin pregnancy, unable to determine number of placenta and number of amniotic sacs, third trimester ♀   M
  - O30.099   Twin pregnancy, unable to determine number of placenta and number of amniotic sacs, unspecified trimester ♀   M
- ● O30.1   **Triplet pregnancy**

  (Ex) For category O30.1 CC codes: See PDX Collection 976
  - ● O30.10   Triplet pregnancy, unspecified number of placenta and unspecified number of amniotic sacs
    - O30.101   Triplet pregnancy, unspecified number of placenta and unspecified number of amniotic sacs, first trimester ♀   M
    - O30.102   Triplet pregnancy, unspecified number of placenta and unspecified number of amniotic sacs, second trimester ♀   M
    - O30.103   Triplet pregnancy, unspecified number of placenta and unspecified number of amniotic sacs, third trimester ♀   M

      Coding Clinic: 2016, Q2, P8
    - O30.109   Triplet pregnancy, unspecified number of placenta and unspecified number of amniotic sacs, unspecified trimester ♀   M

▶ New   ⇒ Revised   ~~deleted~~ Deleted   Excludes 1   Excludes 2   Includes   Use additional   Code first   Code also   Key words

OGCR Official Guidelines   ● Unacceptable Principal Diagnosis   X Assign placeholder X   ● Use Additional Character(s)   ▶ Manifestation Code   **Coding Clinic**

● **O30.11**   Triplet pregnancy with two or more monochorionic fetuses

     O30.111   Triplet pregnancy with two or more monochorionic fetuses, first trimester ♀ 🦠   M

     O30.112   Triplet pregnancy with two or more monochorionic fetuses, second trimester ♀ 🦠   M

     O30.113   Triplet pregnancy with two or more monochorionic fetuses, third trimester ♀ 🦠   M

     O30.119   Triplet pregnancy with two or more monochorionic fetuses, unspecified trimester ♀   M

● **O30.12**   Triplet pregnancy with two or more monoamniotic fetuses

     O30.121   Triplet pregnancy with two or more monoamniotic fetuses, first trimester ♀ 🦠   M

     O30.122   Triplet pregnancy with two or more monoamniotic fetuses, second trimester ♀ 🦠   M

     O30.123   Triplet pregnancy with two or more monoamniotic fetuses, third trimester ♀ 🦠   M

     O30.129   Triplet pregnancy with two or more monoamniotic fetuses, unspecified trimester ♀   M

● **O30.19**   Triplet pregnancy, unable to determine number of placenta and number of amniotic sacs

     O30.191   Triplet pregnancy, unable to determine number of placenta and number of amniotic sacs, first trimester ♀ 🦠   M

     O30.192   Triplet pregnancy, unable to determine number of placenta and number of amniotic sacs, second trimester ♀ 🦠   M

     O30.193   Triplet pregnancy, unable to determine number of placenta and number of amniotic sacs, third trimester ♀ 🦠   M

     O30.199   Triplet pregnancy, unable to determine number of placenta and number of amniotic sacs, unspecified trimester ♀   M

● **O30.2**   **Quadruplet pregnancy**
     (Ex) For category O30.2 CC codes: See PDX Collection 976

   ● **O30.20**   Quadruplet pregnancy, unspecified number of placenta and unspecified number of amniotic sacs

     O30.201   Quadruplet pregnancy, unspecified number of placenta and unspecified number of amniotic sacs, first trimester ♀ 🦠   M

     O30.202   Quadruplet pregnancy, unspecified number of placenta and unspecified number of amniotic sacs, second trimester ♀ 🦠   M

     O30.203   Quadruplet pregnancy, unspecified number of placenta and unspecified number of amniotic sacs, third trimester ♀ 🦠   M

     O30.209   Quadruplet pregnancy, unspecified number of placenta and unspecified number of amniotic sacs, unspecified trimester ♀   M

● **O30.21**   Quadruplet pregnancy with two or more monochorionic fetuses

     O30.211   Quadruplet pregnancy with two or more monochorionic fetuses, first trimester ♀ 🦠   M

     O30.212   Quadruplet pregnancy with two or more monochorionic fetuses, second trimester ♀ 🦠   M

     O30.213   Quadruplet pregnancy with two or more monochorionic fetuses, third trimester ♀ 🦠   M

     O30.219   Quadruplet pregnancy with two or more monochorionic fetuses, unspecified trimester ♀   M

● **O30.22**   Quadruplet pregnancy with two or more monoamniotic fetuses

     O30.221   Quadruplet pregnancy with two or more monoamniotic fetuses, first trimester ♀ 🦠   M

     O30.222   Quadruplet pregnancy with two or more monoamniotic fetuses, second trimester ♀ 🦠   M

     O30.223   Quadruplet pregnancy with two or more monoamniotic fetuses, third trimester ♀ 🦠   M

     O30.229   Quadruplet pregnancy with two or more monoamniotic fetuses, unspecified trimester ♀   M

● **O30.29**   Quadruplet pregnancy, unable to determine number of placenta and number of amniotic sacs

     O30.291   Quadruplet pregnancy, unable to determine number of placenta and number of amniotic sacs, first trimester ♀ 🦠   M

     O30.292   Quadruplet pregnancy, unable to determine number of placenta and number of amniotic sacs, second trimester ♀ 🦠   M

     O30.293   Quadruplet pregnancy, unable to determine number of placenta and number of amniotic sacs, third trimester ♀ 🦠   M

     O30.299   Quadruplet pregnancy, unable to determine number of placenta and number of amniotic sacs, unspecified trimester ♀   M

● **O30.8**   **Other specified multiple gestation**
     Multiple gestation pregnancy greater then quadruplets
     (Ex) For category O30.8 CC codes: See PDX Collection 976

   ● **O30.80**   Other specified multiple gestation, unspecified number of placenta and unspecified number of amniotic sacs

     O30.801   Other specified multiple gestation, unspecified number of placenta and unspecified number of amniotic sacs, first trimester ♀ 🦠   M

     O30.802   Other specified multiple gestation, unspecified number of placenta and unspecified number of amniotic sacs, second trimester ♀ 🦠   M

     O30.803   Other specified multiple gestation, unspecified number of placenta and unspecified number of amniotic sacs, third trimester ♀ 🦠   M

     O30.809   Other specified multiple gestation, unspecified number of placenta and unspecified number of amniotic sacs, unspecified trimester ♀   M

CHAPTER 15 (O00-O9A)

● **O30.81 Other specified multiple gestation with two or more monochorionic fetuses**

     O30.811 Other specified multiple gestation with two or more monochorionic fetuses, first trimester ♀ 🔒   M

     O30.812 Other specified multiple gestation with two or more monochorionic fetuses, second trimester ♀ 🔒   M

     O30.813 Other specified multiple gestation with two or more monochorionic fetuses, third trimester ♀ 🔒   M

     O30.819 Other specified multiple gestation with two or more monochorionic fetuses, unspecified trimester ♀   M

● **O30.82 Other specified multiple gestation with two or more monoamniotic fetuses**

     O30.821 Other specified multiple gestation with two or more monoamniotic fetuses, first trimester ♀ 🔒   M

     O30.822 Other specified multiple gestation with two or more monoamniotic fetuses, second trimester ♀ 🔒   M

     O30.823 Other specified multiple gestation with two or more monoamniotic fetuses, third trimester ♀ 🔒   M

     O30.829 Other specified multiple gestation with two or more monoamniotic fetuses, unspecified trimester ♀   M

● **O30.89 Other specified multiple gestation, unable to determine number of placenta and number of amniotic sacs**

     O30.891 Other specified multiple gestation, unable to determine number of placenta and number of amniotic sacs, first trimester ♀ 🔒   M

     O30.892 Other specified multiple gestation, unable to determine number of placenta and number of amniotic sacs, second trimester ♀ 🔒   M

     O30.893 Other specified multiple gestation, unable to determine number of placenta and number of amniotic sacs, third trimester ♀ 🔒   M

     O30.899 Other specified multiple gestation, unable to determine number of placenta and number of amniotic sacs, unspecified trimester ♀   M

● **O30.9 Multiple gestation, unspecified**
Multiple pregnancy NOS

     O30.90 Multiple gestation, unspecified, unspecified trimester ♀   M

     O30.91 Multiple gestation, unspecified, first trimester ♀   M

     O30.92 Multiple gestation, unspecified, second trimester ♀   M

     O30.93 Multiple gestation, unspecified, third trimester ♀   M

● **O31 Complications specific to multiple gestation**

     Excludes2   delayed delivery of second twin, triplet, etc. (O63.2)
                 malpresentation of one fetus or more (O32.9)
                 placental transfusion syndromes (O43.0-)

Coding Clinic: 2012, Q4, P107

One of the following 7th characters is to be assigned to each code under category O31. 7th character 0 is for single gestations and multiple gestations where the fetus is unspecified. 7th characters 1 through 9 are for cases of multiple gestations to identify the fetus for which the code applies. The appropriate code from category O30, Multiple gestation, must also be assigned when assigning a code from category O31 that has a 7th character of 1 through 9.

0	not applicable or unspecified
1	fetus 1
2	fetus 2
3	fetus 3
4	fetus 4
5	fetus 5
9	other fetus

● **O31.0 Papyraceous fetus**
Fetus compressus

     X ● **O31.00 Papyraceous fetus, unspecified trimester** ♀   M

     X ● **O31.01 Papyraceous fetus, first trimester** ♀   M

     X ● **O31.02 Papyraceous fetus, second trimester** ♀   M

     X ● **O31.03 Papyraceous fetus, third trimester** ♀   M

● **O31.1 Continuing pregnancy after spontaneous abortion of one fetus or more**

     X ● **O31.10 Continuing pregnancy after spontaneous abortion of one fetus or more, unspecified trimester** ♀   M

     X ● **O31.11 Continuing pregnancy after spontaneous abortion of one fetus or more, first trimester** ♀ M

     X ● **O31.12 Continuing pregnancy after spontaneous abortion of one fetus or more, second trimester** ♀   M

     X ● **O31.13 Continuing pregnancy after spontaneous abortion of one fetus or more, third trimester** ♀   M

● **O31.2 Continuing pregnancy after intrauterine death of one fetus or more**

     X ● **O31.20 Continuing pregnancy after intrauterine death of one fetus or more, unspecified trimester** ♀   M

     X ● **O31.21 Continuing pregnancy after intrauterine death of one fetus or more, first trimester** ♀   M

     X ● **O31.22 Continuing pregnancy after intrauterine death of one fetus or more, second trimester** ♀   M

     X ● **O31.23 Continuing pregnancy after intrauterine death of one fetus or more, third trimester** ♀   M

● **O31.3 Continuing pregnancy after elective fetal reduction of one fetus or more**
Continuing pregnancy after selective termination of one fetus or more

     X ● **O31.30 Continuing pregnancy after elective fetal reduction of one fetus or more, unspecified trimester** ♀   M

     X ● **O31.31 Continuing pregnancy after elective fetal reduction of one fetus or more, first trimester** ♀   M

     X ● **O31.32 Continuing pregnancy after elective fetal reduction of one fetus or more, second trimester** ♀   M

     X ● **O31.33 Continuing pregnancy after elective fetal reduction of one fetus or more, third trimester** ♀   M

● **O31.8** **Other complications specific to multiple gestation**
  (Ex) For category O31.8 CC codes: See PDX Collection 976

  ● **O31.8X** **Other complications specific to multiple gestation**

    ● **O31.8X1** **Other complications specific to multiple gestation, first trimester** ♀ 🔵   M

    ● **O31.8X2** **Other complications specific to multiple gestation, second trimester** ♀ 🔵   M

    ● **O31.8X3** **Other complications specific to multiple gestation, third trimester** ♀ 🔵   M

    ● **O31.8X9** **Other complications specific to multiple gestation, unspecified trimester** ♀   M

● **O32** **Maternal care for malpresentation of fetus**

  Includes   the listed conditions as a reason for observation, hospitalization or other obstetric care of the mother, or for cesarean delivery before onset of labor

  Excludes1   malpresentation of fetus with obstructed labor (O64.-)

  Coding Clinic: 2012, Q4, P107

  One of the following 7th characters is to be assigned to each code under category O32. 7th character Ø is for single gestations and multiple gestations where the fetus is unspecified. 7th characters 1 through 9 are for cases of multiple gestations to identify the fetus for which the code applies. The appropriate code from category O30, Multiple gestation, must also be assigned when assigning a code from category O32 that has a 7th character of 1 through 9.

Ø	not applicable or unspecified
1	fetus 1
2	fetus 2
3	fetus 3
4	fetus 4
5	fetus 5
9	other fetus

  X ● **O32.0** **Maternal care for unstable lie** ♀   M

  X ● **O32.1** **Maternal care for breech presentation** ♀   M
      Maternal care for buttocks presentation
      Maternal care for complete breech
      Maternal care for frank breech
      Excludes1   footling presentation (O32.8)
                      incomplete breech (O32.8)

  X ● **O32.2** **Maternal care for transverse and oblique lie** ♀   M
      Maternal care for oblique presentation
      Maternal care for transverse presentation

  X ● **O32.3** **Maternal care for face, brow and chin presentation** ♀   M

  X ● **O32.4** **Maternal care for high head at term** ♀   M
      Maternal care for failure of head to enter pelvic brim

  X ● **O32.6** **Maternal care for compound presentation** ♀   M

  X ● **O32.8** **Maternal care for other malpresentation of fetus** ♀   M
      Maternal care for footling presentation
      Maternal care for incomplete breech

  X ● **O32.9** **Maternal care for malpresentation of fetus, unspecified** ♀   M

● **O33** **Maternal care for disproportion**

  Includes   the listed conditions as a reason for observation, hospitalization or other obstetric care of the mother, or for cesarean delivery before onset of labor

  Excludes1   disproportion with obstructed labor (O65-O66)

  ● **O33.0** **Maternal care for disproportion due to deformity of maternal pelvic bones** ♀ 🔵   M
      Maternal care for disproportion due to pelvic deformity causing disproportion NOS
      (Ex) See PDX Collection 977

  ● **O33.1** **Maternal care for disproportion due to generally contracted pelvis** ♀   M
      Maternal care for disproportion due to contracted pelvis NOS causing disproportion

  ● **O33.2** **Maternal care for disproportion due to inlet contraction of pelvis** ♀   M
      Maternal care for disproportion due to inlet contraction (pelvis) causing disproportion

  X ● **O33.3** **Maternal care for disproportion due to outlet contraction of pelvis** ♀   M
      Maternal care for disproportion due to mid-cavity contraction (pelvis)
      Maternal care for disproportion due to outlet contraction (pelvis)

      One of the following 7th characters is to be assigned to code O33.3. 7th character Ø is for single gestations and multiple gestations where the fetus is unspecified. 7th characters 1 through 9 are for cases of multiple gestations to identify the fetus for which the code applies. The appropriate code from category O30, Multiple gestation, must also be assigned when assigning code O33.3 with a 7th character of 1 through 9.

Ø	not applicable or unspecified
1	fetus 1
2	fetus 2
3	fetus 3
4	fetus 4
5	fetus 5
9	other fetus

  X ● **O33.4** **Maternal care for disproportion of mixed maternal and fetal origin** ♀   M

      One of the following 7th characters is to be assigned to code O33.4. 7th character Ø is for single gestations and multiple gestations where the fetus is unspecified. 7th characters 1 through 9 are for cases of multiple gestations to identify the fetus for which the code applies. The appropriate code from category O30, Multiple gestation, must also be assigned when assigning code O33.4 with a 7th character of 1 through 9.

Ø	not applicable or unspecified
1	fetus 1
2	fetus 2
3	fetus 3
4	fetus 4
5	fetus 5
9	other fetus

CHAPTER 15 (O00-O9A)

X ● **O33.5 Maternal care for disproportion due to unusually large fetus ♀** M

Maternal care for disproportion due to disproportion of fetal origin with normally formed fetus
Maternal care for disproportion due to fetal disproportion NOS

One of the following 7th characters is to be assigned to code O33.5. 7th character Ø is for single gestations and multiple gestations where the fetus is unspecified. 7th characters 1 through 9 are for cases of multiple gestations to identify the fetus for which the code applies. The appropriate code from category O30, Multiple gestation, must also be assigned when assigning code O33.5 with a 7th character of 1 through 9.

Ø	not applicable or unspecified
1	fetus 1
2	fetus 2
3	fetus 3
4	fetus 4
5	fetus 5
9	other fetus

X ● **O33.6 Maternal care for disproportion due to hydrocephalic fetus ♀** M

One of the following 7th characters is to be assigned to code O33.6. 7th character Ø is for single gestations and multiple gestations where the fetus is unspecified. 7th characters 1 through 9 are for cases of multiple gestations to identify the fetus for which the code applies. The appropriate code from category O30, Multiple gestation, must also be assigned when assigning code O33.6 with a 7th character of 1 through 9.

Ø	not applicable or unspecified
1	fetus 1
2	fetus 2
3	fetus 3
4	fetus 4
5	fetus 5
9	other fetus

X ● **O33.7 Maternal care for disproportion due to other fetal deformities ♀** M

Maternal care for disproportion due to fetal ascites
Maternal care for disproportion due to fetal hydrops
Maternal care for disproportion due to fetal meningomyelocele
Maternal care for disproportion due to fetal sacral teratoma
Maternal care for disproportion due to fetal tumor

Excludes1 obstructed labor due to other fetal deformities (O66.3)

Coding Clinic: 2016, Q4, P51

One of the following 7th characters is to be assigned to code O33.7. 7th character Ø is for single gestations and multiple gestations where the fetus is unspecified. 7th characters 1 through 9 are for cases of multiple gestations to identify the fetus for which the code applies. The appropriate code from category O30, Multiple gestation, must also be assigned when assigning code O33.7 with a 7th character of 1 through 9.

Ø	not applicable or unspecified
1	fetus 1
2	fetus 2
3	fetus 3
4	fetus 4
5	fetus 5
9	other fetus

O33.8 Maternal care for disproportion of other origin ♀ M
O33.9 Maternal care for disproportion, unspecified ♀ M
Maternal care for disproportion due to cephalopelvic disproportion NOS
Maternal care for disproportion due to fetopelvic disproportion NOS

● **O34 Maternal care for abnormality of pelvic organs**

Includes the listed conditions as a reason for hospitalization or other obstetric care of the mother, or for cesarean delivery before onset of labor

Code first any associated obstructed labor (O65.5)
Use additional code for specific condition

● **O34.0 Maternal care for congenital malformation of uterus**
Maternal care for double uterus
Maternal care for uterus bicornis

O34.00 Maternal care for unspecified congenital malformation of uterus, unspecified trimester ♀ M

O34.01 Maternal care for unspecified congenital malformation of uterus, first trimester ♀ M

O34.02 Maternal care for unspecified congenital malformation of uterus, second trimester ♀ M

O34.03 Maternal care for unspecified congenital malformation of uterus, third trimester ♀ M

● **O34.1 Maternal care for benign tumor of corpus uteri**

Excludes2 maternal care for benign tumor of cervix (O34.4-)
maternal care for malignant neoplasm of uterus (O9A.1-)

O34.10 Maternal care for benign tumor of corpus uteri, unspecified trimester ♀ M

O34.11 Maternal care for benign tumor of corpus uteri, first trimester ♀ M

O34.12 Maternal care for benign tumor of corpus uteri, second trimester ♀ M

O34.13 Maternal care for benign tumor of corpus uteri, third trimester ♀ M

● **O34.2 Maternal care due to uterine scar from previous surgery**
Coding Clinic: 2016, Q4, P76

● **O34.21 Maternal care for scar from previous cesarean delivery**
Coding Clinic: 2016, Q4, P51

O34.211 Maternal care for low transverse scar from previous cesarean delivery ♀ M

O34.212 Maternal care for vertical scar from previous cesarean delivery ♀ M
Maternal care for classical scar from previous cesarean delivery

O34.219 Maternal care for unspecified type scar from previous cesarean delivery ♀ M

O34.29 Maternal care due to uterine scar from other previous surgery ♀ M
Maternal care due to uterine scar from other transmural uterine incision

● **O34.3 Maternal care for cervical incompetence**
Maternal care for cerclage with or without cervical incompetence
Maternal care for Shirodkar suture with or without cervical incompetence
Ⓔ**ⓍFor category O34.3 CC codes: See PDX Collection 973**

O34.30 Maternal care for cervical incompetence, unspecified trimester ♀ M

O34.31 Maternal care for cervical incompetence, first trimester ♀ M

O34.32 Maternal care for cervical incompetence, second trimester ♀ M

O34.33 Maternal care for cervical incompetence, third trimester ♀ M

▶ New　⟹ Revised　deleted Deleted　Excludes 1　Excludes 2　Includes　Use additional　Code first　Code also　Key words
OGCR Official Guidelines　● Unacceptable Principal Diagnosis　X Assign placeholder X　● Use Additional Character(s)　▷ Manifestation Code　Coding Clinic

● **O34.4 Maternal care for other abnormalities of cervix**
    O34.40 Maternal care for other abnormalities of cervix, unspecified trimester ♀   M
    O34.41 Maternal care for other abnormalities of cervix, first trimester ♀   M
    O34.42 Maternal care for other abnormalities of cervix, second trimester ♀   M
    O34.43 Maternal care for other abnormalities of cervix, third trimester ♀   M

● **O34.5 Maternal care for other abnormalities of gravid uterus**
  ● **O34.51 Maternal care for incarceration of gravid uterus**
    O34.511 Maternal care for incarceration of gravid uterus, first trimester ♀   M
    O34.512 Maternal care for incarceration of gravid uterus, second trimester ♀   M
    O34.513 Maternal care for incarceration of gravid uterus, third trimester ♀   M
    O34.519 Maternal care for incarceration of gravid uterus, unspecified trimester ♀   M

  ● **O34.52 Maternal care for prolapse of gravid uterus**
    O34.521 Maternal care for prolapse of gravid uterus, first trimester ♀   M
    O34.522 Maternal care for prolapse of gravid uterus, second trimester ♀   M
    O34.523 Maternal care for prolapse of gravid uterus, third trimester ♀   M
    O34.529 Maternal care for prolapse of gravid uterus, unspecified trimester ♀   M

  ● **O34.53 Maternal care for retroversion of gravid uterus**
    O34.531 Maternal care for retroversion of gravid uterus, first trimester ♀   M
    O34.532 Maternal care for retroversion of gravid uterus, second trimester ♀   M
    O34.533 Maternal care for retroversion of gravid uterus, third trimester ♀   M
    O34.539 Maternal care for retroversion of gravid uterus, unspecified trimester ♀   M

  ● **O34.59 Maternal care for other abnormalities of gravid uterus**
    O34.591 Maternal care for other abnormalities of gravid uterus, first trimester ♀   M
    O34.592 Maternal care for other abnormalities of gravid uterus, second trimester ♀ M
    O34.593 Maternal care for other abnormalities of gravid uterus, third trimester ♀   M
    O34.599 Maternal care for other abnormalities of gravid uterus, unspecified trimester ♀   M

● **O34.6 Maternal care for abnormality of vagina**
    Excludes2   maternal care for vaginal varices in pregnancy (O22.1-)
    O34.60 Maternal care for abnormality of vagina, unspecified trimester ♀   M
    O34.61 Maternal care for abnormality of vagina, first trimester ♀   M
    O34.62 Maternal care for abnormality of vagina, second trimester ♀   M
    O34.63 Maternal care for abnormality of vagina, third trimester ♀   M

● **O34.7 Maternal care for abnormality of vulva and perineum**
    Excludes2   maternal care for perineal and vulval varices in pregnancy (O22.1-)
    O34.70 Maternal care for abnormality of vulva and perineum, unspecified trimester ♀   M
    O34.71 Maternal care for abnormality of vulva and perineum, first trimester ♀   M
    O34.72 Maternal care for abnormality of vulva and perineum, second trimester ♀   M
    O34.73 Maternal care for abnormality of vulva and perineum, third trimester ♀   M

● **O34.8 Maternal care for other abnormalities of pelvic organs**
    O34.80 Maternal care for other abnormalities of pelvic organs, unspecified trimester ♀   M
    O34.81 Maternal care for other abnormalities of pelvic organs, first trimester ♀   M
    O34.82 Maternal care for other abnormalities of pelvic organs, second trimester ♀   M
    O34.83 Maternal care for other abnormalities of pelvic organs, third trimester ♀   M

● **O34.9 Maternal care for abnormality of pelvic organ, unspecified**
    O34.90 Maternal care for abnormality of pelvic organ, unspecified, unspecified trimester ♀   M
    O34.91 Maternal care for abnormality of pelvic organ, unspecified, first trimester ♀   M
    O34.92 Maternal care for abnormality of pelvic organ, unspecified, second trimester ♀   M
    O34.93 Maternal care for abnormality of pelvic organ, unspecified, third trimester ♀   M

● **O35 Maternal care for known or suspected fetal abnormality and damage**
    Includes   the listed conditions in the fetus as a reason for hospitalization or other obstetric care to the mother, or for termination of pregnancy
    Code also any associated maternal condition
    Excludes1   encounter for suspected maternal and fetal conditions ruled out (Z03.7-)

One of the following 7th characters is to be assigned to each code under category O35. 7th character Ø is for single gestations and multiple gestations where the fetus is unspecified. 7th characters 1 through 9 are for cases of multiple gestations to identify the fetus for which the code applies. The appropriate code from category O30, Multiple gestation, must also be assigned when assigning a code from category O35 that has a 7th character of 1 through 9.

Ø	not applicable or unspecified
1	fetus 1
2	fetus 2
3	fetus 3
4	fetus 4
5	fetus 5
9	other fetus

X ● **O35.0 Maternal care for (suspected) central nervous system malformation in fetus ♀**   M
    Maternal care for fetal anencephaly
    Maternal care for fetal hydrocephalus
    Maternal care for fetal spina bifida
    Excludes2   chromosomal abnormality in fetus (O35.1)

X ● **O35.1 Maternal care for (suspected) chromosomal abnormality in fetus ♀**   M

N Newborn Age: Ø   **P** Pediatric Age: Ø–17   **M** Maternity DX: 12–55   **A** Adult Age: 15–124   ♀ Females Only   ♂ Males Only

🖤 Complication\Comorbidity   🖤 Major C\C   (Ex) CC/MCC Exclusions   🖤 Hospital-Acquired Condition

1139

X ● **O35.2   Maternal care for (suspected) hereditary disease in fetus** ♀   M

       Excludes2   chromosomal abnormality in fetus (O35.1)

X ● **O35.3   Maternal care for (suspected) damage to fetus from viral disease in mother** ♀   M

       Maternal care for damage to fetus from maternal cytomegalovirus infection
       Maternal care for damage to fetus from maternal rubella
       Coding Clinic: 2016, Q4, P6

X ● **O35.4   Maternal care for (suspected) damage to fetus from alcohol** ♀   M

X ● **O35.5   Maternal care for (suspected) damage to fetus by drugs** ♀   M

       Maternal care for damage to fetus from drug addiction

X ● **O35.6   Maternal care for (suspected) damage to fetus by radiation** ♀   M

X ● **O35.7   Maternal care for (suspected) damage to fetus by other medical procedures** ♀   M

       Maternal care for damage to fetus by amniocentesis
       Maternal care for damage to fetus by biopsy procedures
       Maternal care for damage to fetus by hematological investigation
       Maternal care for damage to fetus by intrauterine contraceptive device
       Maternal care for damage to fetus by intrauterine surgery

X ● **O35.8   Maternal care for other (suspected) fetal abnormality and damage** ♀   M

       Maternal care for damage to fetus from maternal listeriosis
       Maternal care for damage to fetus from maternal toxoplasmosis

X ● **O35.9   Maternal care for (suspected) fetal abnormality and damage, unspecified** ♀   M

OGCR   Section I.C.15.e.l.

Fetal Conditions Affecting the Management of the Mother

1) Code from categories O35 and O36

Codes from categories O35, Maternal care for known or suspected fetal abnormality and damage, and O36, Maternal care for other fetal problems, are assigned only when the fetal condition is actually responsible for modifying the management of the mother, i.e., by requiring diagnostic studies, additional observation, special care, or termination of pregnancy. The fact that the fetal condition exists does not justify assigning a code from this series to the mother's record.

2) In utero surgery

In cases when surgery is performed on the fetus, a diagnosis code from category O35, Maternal care for known or suspected fetal abnormality and damage, should be assigned identifying the fetal condition. Assign the appropriate procedure code for the procedure performed.

No code from Chapter 16, the perinatal codes, should be used on the mother's record to identify fetal conditions. Surgery performed in utero on a fetus is still to be coded as an obstetric encounter.

● **O36   Maternal care for other fetal problems**

   Includes   the listed conditions in the fetus as a reason for hospitalization or other obstetric care of the mother, or for termination of pregnancy

   Excludes1   encounter for suspected maternal and fetal conditions ruled out (Z03.7-)
               placental transfusion syndromes (O43.0-)

   Excludes2   labor and delivery complicated by fetal stress (O77.-)

One of the following 7th characters is to be assigned to each code under category O36. 7th character 0 is for single gestations and multiple gestations where the fetus is unspecified. 7th characters 1 through 9 are for cases of multiple gestations to identify the fetus for which the code applies. The appropriate code from category O30, Multiple gestation, must also be assigned when assigning a code from category O36 that has a 7th character of 1 through 9.

0	not applicable or unspecified
1	fetus 1
2	fetus 2
3	fetus 3
4	fetus 4
5	fetus 5
9	other fetus

Coding Clinic: 2015, Q3, P40

● **O36.0   Maternal care for rhesus isoimmunization**
       Maternal care for Rh incompatibility (with hydrops fetalis)
       Ⓔₓ For category O36.0 CC codes: See PDX Collection 978

     ● **O36.01   Maternal care for anti-D [Rh] antibodies**

       ● **O36.011   Maternal care for anti-D [Rh] antibodies, first trimester** ♀ Ⓒ   M

       ● **O36.012   Maternal care for anti-D [Rh] antibodies, second trimester** ♀ Ⓒ   M

       ● **O36.013   Maternal care for anti-D [Rh] antibodies, third trimester** ♀ Ⓒ   M

       ● **O36.019   Maternal care for anti-D [Rh] antibodies, unspecified trimester** ♀   M

     ● **O36.09   Maternal care for other rhesus isoimmunization**

       ● **O36.091   Maternal care for other rhesus isoimmunization, first trimester** ♀ Ⓒ   M

       ● **O36.092   Maternal care for other rhesus isoimmunization, second trimester** ♀ Ⓒ   M

       ● **O36.093   Maternal care for other rhesus isoimmunization, third trimester** ♀ Ⓒ   M
               Coding Clinic: 2015, Q3, P40

       ● **O36.099   Maternal care for other rhesus isoimmunization, unspecified trimester** ♀   M

   ● **O36.1   Maternal care for other isoimmunization**
       Maternal care for ABO isoimmunization

     ● **O36.11   Maternal care for Anti-A sensitization**
       Maternal care for isoimmunization NOS (with hydrops fetalis)

       ● **O36.111   Maternal care for Anti-A sensitization, first trimester** ♀   M

       ● **O36.112   Maternal care for Anti-A sensitization, second trimester** ♀   M

       ● **O36.113   Maternal care for Anti-A sensitization, third trimester** ♀   M

       ● **O36.119   Maternal care for Anti-A sensitization, unspecified trimester** ♀   M

● O36.19 Maternal care for other isoimmunization
Maternal care for Anti-B sensitization
  ● O36.191 Maternal care for other
isoimmunization, first trimester ♀   M
  ● O36.192 Maternal care for other
isoimmunization, second
trimester ♀   M
  ● O36.193 Maternal care for other
isoimmunization, third trimester ♀ M
  ● O36.199 Maternal care for other
isoimmunization, unspecified
trimester ♀   M

● O36.2 Maternal care for hydrops fetalis
Maternal care for hydrops fetalis NOS
Maternal care for hydrops fetalis not associated with
isoimmunization
  Excludes1 hydrops fetalis associated with ABO
isoimmunization (O36.1-)
hydrops fetalis associated with rhesus
isoimmunization (O36.0-)
  ● O36.20 Maternal care for hydrops fetalis, unspecified
trimester ♀   M
  ● O36.21 Maternal care for hydrops fetalis, first
trimester ♀   M
  ● O36.22 Maternal care for hydrops fetalis, second
trimester ♀   M
  ● O36.23 Maternal care for hydrops fetalis, third
trimester ♀   M

● O36.4 Maternal care for intrauterine death ♀ 🅖   M
Maternal care for intrauterine fetal death NOS
Maternal care for intrauterine fetal death after
completion of 20 weeks of gestation
Maternal care for late fetal death
Maternal care for missed delivery
  Excludes1 missed abortion (O02.1)
stillbirth (P95)
  (Ex) See PDX Collection 979

● O36.5 Maternal care for known or suspected poor fetal growth
  ● O36.51 Maternal care for known or suspected placental
insufficiency
    ● O36.511 Maternal care for known or
suspected placental insufficiency, first
trimester ♀   M
    ● O36.512 Maternal care for known or suspected
placental insufficiency, second
trimester ♀   M
    ● O36.513 Maternal care for known or suspected
placental insufficiency, third
trimester ♀   M
    ● O36.519 Maternal care for known or suspected
placental insufficiency, unspecified
trimester ♀   M
  ● O36.59 Maternal care for other known or suspected
poor fetal growth
Maternal care for known or suspected light-
for-dates NOS
Maternal care for known or suspected small-
for-dates NOS
    ● O36.591 Maternal care for other known or
suspected poor fetal growth, first
trimester ♀   M
    ● O36.592 Maternal care for other known or
suspected poor fetal growth, second
trimester ♀   M
    ● O36.593 Maternal care for other known or
suspected poor fetal growth, third
trimester ♀   M
    ● O36.599 Maternal care for other known
or suspected poor fetal growth,
unspecified trimester ♀   M

● O36.6 Maternal care for excessive fetal growth
Maternal care for known or suspected large-for-dates
  X ● O36.60 Maternal care for excessive fetal growth,
unspecified trimester ♀   M
  X ● O36.61 Maternal care for excessive fetal growth, first
trimester ♀   M
  X ● O36.62 Maternal care for excessive fetal growth, second
trimester ♀   M
  X ● O36.63 Maternal care for excessive fetal growth, third
trimester ♀   M

● O36.7 Maternal care for viable fetus in abdominal pregnancy
  X ● O36.70 Maternal care for viable fetus in abdominal
pregnancy, unspecified trimester ♀   M
  X ● O36.71 Maternal care for viable fetus in abdominal
pregnancy, first trimester ♀   M
  X ● O36.72 Maternal care for viable fetus in abdominal
pregnancy, second trimester ♀   M
  X ● O36.73 Maternal care for viable fetus in abdominal
pregnancy, third trimester ♀   M

● O36.8 Maternal care for other specified fetal problems
  ● X ● O36.80 Pregnancy with inconclusive fetal viability ♀ M
Encounter to determine fetal viability of
pregnancy
  ● O36.81 Decreased fetal movements
    ● O36.812 Decreased fetal movements, second
trimester ♀   M
    ● O36.813 Decreased fetal movements, third
trimester ♀   M
    ● O36.819 Decreased fetal movements,
unspecified trimester ♀   M
  ● O36.82 Fetal anemia and thrombocytopenia
    ● O36.821 Fetal anemia and thrombocytopenia,
first trimester ♀   M
    ● O36.822 Fetal anemia and thrombocytopenia,
second trimester ♀   M
    ● O36.823 Fetal anemia and thrombocytopenia,
third trimester ♀   M
    ● O36.829 Fetal anemia and thrombocytopenia,
unspecified trimester ♀   M
  ▶● O36.83 Maternal care for abnormalities of the fetal
heart rate or rhythm
    ▶● O36.831 Maternal care for abnormalities of the
fetal heart rate or rhythm, first
trimester ♀   M
    ▶● O36.832 Maternal care for abnormalities of the
fetal heart rate or rhythm, second
trimester ♀   M
    ▶● O36.833 Maternal care for abnormalities of the
fetal heart rate or rhythm, third
trimester ♀   M
    ▶● O36.839 Maternal care for abnormalities of the
fetal heart rate or rhythm, unspecified
trimester ♀   M
  ● O36.89 Maternal care for other specified fetal problems
    ● O36.891 Maternal care for other specified fetal
problems, first trimester ♀   M
    ● O36.892 Maternal care for other specified fetal
problems, second trimester ♀   M
    ● O36.893 Maternal care for other specified fetal
problems, third trimester ♀   M
    ● O36.899 Maternal care for other specified fetal
problems, unspecified trimester ♀   M

CHAPTER 15 (O00–O9A)

● O36.9   **Maternal care for fetal problem, unspecified**

   X ● O36.90   Maternal care for fetal problem, unspecified, unspecified trimester ♀   M

   X ● O36.91   Maternal care for fetal problem, unspecified, first trimester ♀   M

   X ● O36.92   Maternal care for fetal problem, unspecified, second trimester ♀   M

   X ● O36.93   Maternal care for fetal problem, unspecified, third trimester ♀   M

● O40   **Polyhydramnios**
Overabundance of amniotic fluid

Includes	hydramnios
Excludes1	encounter for suspected maternal and fetal conditions ruled out (Z03.7-)

One of the following 7th characters is to be assigned to each code under category O40. 7th character 0 is for single gestations and multiple gestations where the fetus is unspecified. 7th characters 1 through 9 are for cases of multiple gestations to identify the fetus for which the code applies. The appropriate code from category O30, Multiple gestation, must also be assigned when assigning a code from category O40 that has a 7th character of 1 through 9.

0	not applicable or unspecified
1	fetus 1
2	fetus 2
3	fetus 3
4	fetus 4
5	fetus 5
9	other fetus

   X ● O40.1   Polyhydramnios, first trimester ♀   M

   X ● O40.2   Polyhydramnios, second trimester ♀   M

   X ● O40.3   Polyhydramnios, third trimester ♀   M

   X ● O40.9   Polyhydramnios, unspecified trimester ♀   M

● O41   **Other disorders of amniotic fluid and membranes**

Excludes1	encounter for suspected maternal and fetal conditions ruled out (Z03.7-)

One of the following 7th characters is to be assigned to each code under category O41. 7th character 0 is for single gestations and multiple gestations where the fetus is unspecified. 7th characters 1 through 9 are for cases of multiple gestations to identify the fetus for which the code applies. The appropriate code from category O30, Multiple gestation, must also be assigned when assigning a code from category O41 that has a 7th character of 1 through 9.

0	not applicable or unspecified
1	fetus 1
2	fetus 2
3	fetus 3
4	fetus 4
5	fetus 5
9	other fetus

● O41.0   **Oligohydramnios**
Scant volume of amniotic fluid
Oligohydramnios without rupture of membranes
Ⓔⓧ **For category O41.0 CC codes:** See PDX Collection 982

   X ● O41.00   Oligohydramnios, unspecified trimester ♀   M

   X ● O41.01   Oligohydramnios, first trimester ♀ 🐾   M

   X ● O41.02   Oligohydramnios, second trimester ♀ 🐾   M

   X ● O41.03   Oligohydramnios, third trimester ♀ 🐾   M

● O41.1   **Infection of amniotic sac and membranes**
Ⓔⓧ **For category O41.1 CC codes:** See PDX Collection 983

   ● O41.10   **Infection of amniotic sac and membranes, unspecified**

     ● O41.101   Infection of amniotic sac and membranes, unspecified, first trimester ♀ 🐾   M

     ● O41.102   Infection of amniotic sac and membranes, unspecified, second trimester ♀ 🐾   M

     ● O41.103   Infection of amniotic sac and membranes, unspecified, third trimester ♀ 🐾   M

     ● O41.109   Infection of amniotic sac and membranes, unspecified, unspecified trimester ♀   M

   ● O41.12   **Chorioamnionitis**

     ● O41.121   Chorioamnionitis, first trimester ♀ 🐾   M

     ● O41.122   Chorioamnionitis, second trimester ♀ 🐾   M

     ● O41.123   Chorioamnionitis, third trimester ♀ 🐾   M

     ● O41.129   Chorioamnionitis, unspecified trimester ♀   M

   ● O41.14   **Placentitis**

     ● O41.141   Placentitis, first trimester ♀ 🐾   M

     ● O41.142   Placentitis, second trimester ♀ 🐾   M

     ● O41.143   Placentitis, third trimester ♀ 🐾   M

     ● O41.149   Placentitis, unspecified trimester ♀   M

● O41.8   **Other specified disorders of amniotic fluid and membranes**

   ● O41.8X   **Other specified disorders of amniotic fluid and membranes**

     ● O41.8X1   Other specified disorders of amniotic fluid and membranes, first trimester ♀   M

     ● O41.8X2   Other specified disorders of amniotic fluid and membranes, second trimester ♀   M

     ● O41.8X3   Other specified disorders of amniotic fluid and membranes, third trimester ♀   M

     ● O41.8X9   Other specified disorders of amniotic fluid and membranes, unspecified trimester ♀   M

● O41.9   **Disorder of amniotic fluid and membranes, unspecified**

   X ● O41.90   Disorder of amniotic fluid and membranes, unspecified, unspecified trimester ♀   M

   X ● O41.91   Disorder of amniotic fluid and membranes, unspecified, first trimester ♀   M

   X ● O41.92   Disorder of amniotic fluid and membranes, unspecified, second trimester ♀   M

   X ● O41.93   Disorder of amniotic fluid and membranes, unspecified, third trimester ♀   M

▶ New   ⇒ Revised   ~~deleted~~ Deleted   Excludes 1   Excludes 2   Includes   Use additional   Code first   Code also   Key words

OGCR Official Guidelines   ● Unacceptable Principal Diagnosis   X Assign placeholder X   ▶ Use Additional Character(s)   ▶ Manifestation Code   **Coding Clinic**

● **O42　Premature rupture of membranes**

　● **O42.0　Premature rupture of membranes, onset of labor within 24 hours of rupture**

　　　O42.00　Premature rupture of membranes, onset of labor within 24 hours of rupture, unspecified weeks of gestation ♀　　M

　　● **O42.01　Preterm premature rupture of membranes, onset of labor within 24 hours of rupture**
　　　　Premature rupture of membranes before 37 completed weeks of gestation

　　　　　O42.011　Preterm premature rupture of membranes, onset of labor within 24 hours of rupture, first trimester ♀　　M

　　　　　O42.012　Preterm premature rupture of membranes, onset of labor within 24 hours of rupture, second trimester ♀ M

　　　　　O42.013　Preterm premature rupture of membranes, onset of labor within 24 hours of rupture, third trimester ♀　M

　　　　　O42.019　Preterm premature rupture of membranes, onset of labor within 24 hours of rupture, unspecified trimester ♀　　M

　　　O42.02　Full-term premature rupture of membranes, onset of labor within 24 hours of rupture ♀　M
　　　　Premature rupture of membranes at or after 37 completed weeks of gestation, onset of labor within 24 hours of rupture

　● **O42.1　Premature rupture of membranes, onset of labor more than 24 hours following rupture**

　　　O42.10　Premature rupture of membranes, onset of labor more than 24 hours following rupture, unspecified weeks of gestation ♀　　M

　　● **O42.11　Preterm premature rupture of membranes, onset of labor more than 24 hours following rupture**
　　　　Premature rupture of membranes before 37 completed weeks of gestation

　　　　　O42.111　Preterm premature rupture of membranes, onset of labor more than 24 hours following rupture, first trimester ♀　　M

　　　　　O42.112　Preterm premature rupture of membranes, onset of labor more than 24 hours following rupture, second trimester ♀　　M

　　　　　O42.113　Preterm premature rupture of membranes, onset of labor more than 24 hours following rupture, third trimester ♀　　M

　　　　　O42.119　Preterm premature rupture of membranes, onset of labor more than 24 hours following rupture, unspecified trimester ♀　　M

　　　O42.12　Full-term premature rupture of membranes, onset of labor more than 24 hours following rupture ♀　　M
　　　　Premature rupture of membranes at or after 37 completed weeks of gestation, onset of labor more than 24 hours following rupture

　● **O42.9　Premature rupture of membranes, unspecified as to length of time between rupture and onset of labor**

　　　O42.90　Premature rupture of membranes, unspecified as to length of time between rupture and onset of labor, unspecified weeks of gestation ♀　　M

　　● **O42.91　Preterm premature rupture of membranes, unspecified as to length of time between rupture and onset of labor**
　　　　Premature rupture of membranes before 37 completed weeks of gestation

　　　　　O42.911　Preterm premature rupture of membranes, unspecified as to length of time between rupture and onset of labor, first trimester ♀　　M

　　　　　O42.912　Preterm premature rupture of membranes, unspecified as to length of time between rupture and onset of labor, second trimester ♀　　M

　　　　　O42.913　Preterm premature rupture of membranes, unspecified as to length of time between rupture and onset of labor, third trimester ♀　　M

　　　　　O42.919　Preterm premature rupture of membranes, unspecified as to length of time between rupture and onset of labor, unspecified trimester ♀　　M

　　　O42.92　Full-term premature rupture of membranes, unspecified as to length of time between rupture and onset of labor ♀　　M
　　　　Premature rupture of membranes at or after 37 completed weeks of gestation, unspecified as to length of time between rupture and onset of labor

● **O43　Placental disorders**

　　Excludes2　maternal care for poor fetal growth due to placental insufficiency (O36.5-)
　　　　　placenta previa (O44.-)
　　　　　placental polyp (O90.89)
　　　　　placentitis (O41.14-)
　　　　　premature separation of placenta [abruptio placentae] (O45.-)

　● **O43.0　Placental transfusion syndromes**

　　● **O43.01　Fetomaternal placental transfusion syndrome**
　　　　Maternofetal placental transfusion syndrome

　　　　　O43.011　Fetomaternal placental transfusion syndrome, first trimester ♀　　M

　　　　　O43.012　Fetomaternal placental transfusion syndrome, second trimester ♀　　M

　　　　　O43.013　Fetomaternal placental transfusion syndrome, third trimester ♀　　M

　　　　　O43.019　Fetomaternal placental transfusion syndrome, unspecified trimester ♀　　M

　　● **O43.02　Fetus-to-fetus placental transfusion syndrome**

　　　　　O43.021　Fetus-to-fetus placental transfusion syndrome, first trimester ♀　　M

　　　　　O43.022　Fetus-to-fetus placental transfusion syndrome, second trimester ♀　　M

　　　　　O43.023　Fetus-to-fetus placental transfusion syndrome, third trimester ♀　　M

　　　　　O43.029　Fetus-to-fetus placental transfusion syndrome, unspecified trimester ♀　　M

CHAPTER 15 (O00-O9A)

N Newborn Age: 0　**P** Pediatric Age: 0–17　**M** Maternity DX: 12–55　**A** Adult Age: 15–124　♀ Females Only　♂ Males Only

🅒 Complication\Comorbidity　🅜 Major C\C　🅔🅧 CC/MCC Exclusions　🅗 Hospital-Acquired Condition

1143

- **O43.1   Malformation of placenta**
  - **O43.10   Malformation of placenta, unspecified**
    Abnormal placenta NOS
    - O43.101   Malformation of placenta, unspecified, first trimester ♀   M
    - O43.102   Malformation of placenta, unspecified, second trimester ♀   M
    - O43.103   Malformation of placenta, unspecified, third trimester ♀   M
    - O43.109   Malformation of placenta, unspecified, unspecified trimester ♀ M
  - **O43.11   Circumvallate placenta**
    - O43.111   Circumvallate placenta, first trimester ♀   M
    - O43.112   Circumvallate placenta, second trimester ♀   M
    - O43.113   Circumvallate placenta, third trimester ♀   M
    - O43.119   Circumvallate placenta, unspecified trimester ♀   M
  - **O43.12   Velamentous insertion of umbilical cord**
    - O43.121   Velamentous insertion of umbilical cord, first trimester ♀   M
    - O43.122   Velamentous insertion of umbilical cord, second trimester ♀
    - O43.123   Velamentous insertion of umbilical cord, third trimester ♀
    - O43.129   Velamentous insertion of umbilical cord, unspecified trimester ♀
  - **O43.19   Other malformation of placenta**
    - O43.191   Other malformation of placenta, first trimester ♀   M
    - O43.192   Other malformation of placenta, second trimester ♀   M
    - O43.193   Other malformation of placenta, third trimester ♀   M
    - O43.199   Other malformation of placenta, unspecified trimester ♀   M
- **O43.2   Morbidly adherent placenta**
    Code also associated third stage postpartum hemorrhage, if applicable (O72.0)
    Excludes1   retained placenta (O73.-)
  - **O43.21   Placenta accreta**
    - O43.211   Placenta accreta, first trimester ♀   M
    - O43.212   Placenta accreta, second trimester ♀   M
    - O43.213   Placenta accreta, third trimester ♀   M
    - O43.219   Placenta accreta, unspecified trimester ♀   M
  - **O43.22   Placenta increta**
    - O43.221   Placenta increta, first trimester ♀   M
    - O43.222   Placenta increta, second trimester ♀   M
    - O43.223   Placenta increta, third trimester ♀   M
    - O43.229   Placenta increta, unspecified trimester ♀   M
  - **O43.23   Placenta percreta**
    - O43.231   Placenta percreta, first trimester ♀   M
    - O43.232   Placenta percreta, second trimester ♀ M
    - O43.233   Placenta percreta, third trimester ♀   M
    - O43.239   Placenta percreta, unspecified trimester ♀   M

- **O43.8   Other placental disorders**
  - **O43.81   Placental infarction**
    - O43.811   Placental infarction, first trimester ♀ M
    - O43.812   Placental infarction, second trimester ♀   M
    - O43.813   Placental infarction, third trimester ♀   M
    - O43.819   Placental infarction, unspecified trimester ♀   M
  - **O43.89   Other placental disorders**
    Placental dysfunction
    - O43.891   Other placental disorders, first trimester ♀   M
    - O43.892   Other placental disorders, second trimester ♀   M
    - O43.893   Other placental disorders, third trimester ♀   M
    - O43.899   Other placental disorders, unspecified trimester ♀   M
- **O43.9   Unspecified placental disorder**
  - O43.90   Unspecified placental disorder, unspecified trimester ♀   M
  - O43.91   Unspecified placental disorder, first trimester ♀   M
  - O43.92   Unspecified placental disorder, second trimester ♀   M
  - O43.93   Unspecified placental disorder, third trimester ♀   M

- **O44   Placenta previa**
    (Ex) **For category O44 CC codes:** See PDX Collection 966
    Coding Clinic: 2016, Q4, P52
  - **O44.0   Complete placenta previa NOS or without hemorrhage**
    Placenta previa NOS
    - O44.00   Complete placenta previa NOS or without hemorrhage, unspecified trimester ♀   M
    - O44.01   Complete placenta previa NOS or without hemorrhage, first trimester ♀ 🐾   M
    - O44.02   Complete placenta previa NOS or without hemorrhage, second trimester ♀ 🐾   M
    - O44.03   Complete placenta previa NOS or without hemorrhage, third trimester ♀ 🐾   M
  - **O44.1   Complete placenta previa with hemorrhage**
    Excludes1   labor and delivery complicated by hemorrhage from vasa previa (O69.4)
    - O44.10   Complete placenta previa with hemorrhage, unspecified trimester ♀   M
    - O44.11   Complete placenta previa with hemorrhage, first trimester ♀ 🐾   M
    - O44.12   Complete placenta previa with hemorrhage, second trimester ♀ 🐾   M
    - O44.13   Complete placenta previa with hemorrhage, third trimester ♀ 🐾   M

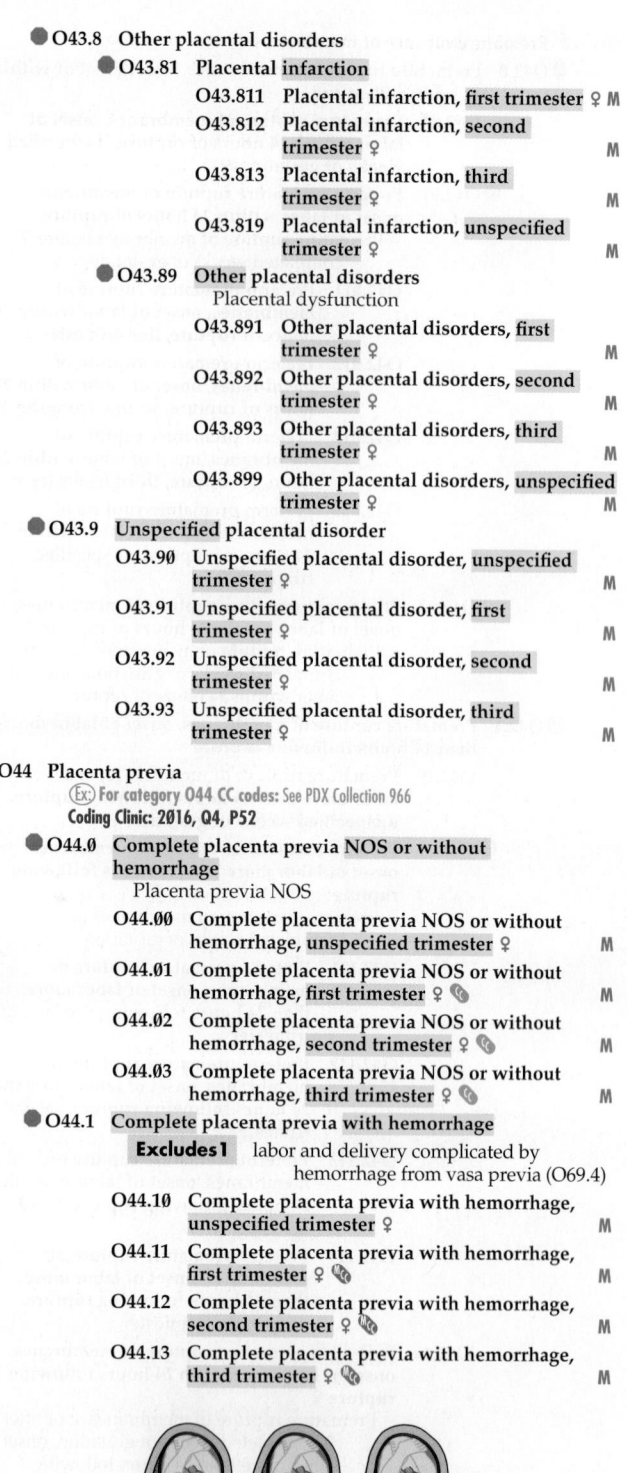

Figure 15-2   A. Marginal placento previa. **B.** Partial placenta previa. **C.** Total placento previa.

Item 15–3   Placenta previa is a condition in which the opening of the cervix is obstructed by the displaced placenta. The three types, marginal, partial, and total, are varying degrees of placenta displacement. Placenta abruption is the premature breaking away of the placenta from the site of the uterine implant before the delivery of the fetus.

▶ New   ⟹ Revised   ~~deleted~~ Deleted   Excludes 1   Excludes 2   Includes   Use additional   Code first   Code also   Key words

OGCR Official Guidelines   ● Unacceptable Principal Diagnosis   X Assign placeholder X   ● Use Additional Character(s)   ▶ Manifestation Code   **Coding Clinic**

- **O44.2** **Partial placenta previa without hemorrhage**
  Marginal placenta previa, NOS or without hemorrhage
  - O44.20 Partial placenta previa NOS or without hemorrhage, unspecified trimester ♀   M
  - O44.21 Partial placenta previa NOS or without hemorrhage, first trimester ♀ 🔖   M
  - O44.22 Partial placenta previa NOS or without hemorrhage, second trimester ♀ 🔖   M
  - O44.23 Partial placenta previa NOS or without hemorrhage, third trimester ♀ 🔖   M
- **O44.3** **Partial placenta previa with hemorrhage**
  Marginal placenta previa with hemorrhage
  - O44.30 Partial placenta previa with hemorrhage, unspecified trimester ♀   M
  - O44.31 Partial placenta previa with hemorrhage, first trimester ♀ 🔖   M
  - O44.32 Partial placenta previa with hemorrhage, second trimester ♀ 🔖   M
  - O44.33 Partial placenta previa with hemorrhage, third trimester ♀ 🔖   M
- **O44.4** **Low lying placenta NOS or without hemorrhage**
  Low implantation of placenta NOS or without hemorrhage
  - O44.40 Low lying placenta NOS or without hemorrhage, unspecified trimester ♀   M
  - O44.41 Low lying placenta NOS or without hemorrhage, first trimester ♀ 🔖   M
  - O44.42 Low lying placenta NOS or without hemorrhage, second trimester ♀ 🔖   M
  - O44.43 Low lying placenta NOS or without hemorrhage, third trimester ♀ 🔖   M
- **O44.5** **Low lying placenta with hemorrhage**
  Low implantation of placenta with hemorrhage
  - O44.50 Low lying placenta with hemorrhage, unspecified trimester ♀   M
  - O44.51 Low lying placenta with hemorrhage, first trimester ♀ 🔖   M
  - O44.52 Low lying placenta with hemorrhage, second trimester ♀ 🔖   M
  - O44.53 Low lying placenta with hemorrhage, third trimester ♀ 🔖   M
- **O45** **Premature separation of placenta [abruptio placentae]**
  - **O45.0** **Premature separation of placenta with coagulation defect**
    (Ex) For category O45.0 CC codes: See PDX Collection 985
    - O45.00 Premature separation of placenta with coagulation defect, unspecified
      - O45.001 Premature separation of placenta with coagulation defect, unspecified, first trimester ♀ 🔖   M
      - O45.002 Premature separation of placenta with coagulation defect, unspecified, second trimester ♀ 🔖   M
      - O45.003 Premature separation of placenta with coagulation defect, unspecified, third trimester ♀ 🔖   M
      - O45.009 Premature separation of placenta with coagulation defect, unspecified, unspecified trimester ♀   M

Figure 15-3 Abruptio placentae is classified according to the grade of separation of the placenta from the uterine wall. **A.** Mild separation in which hemorrhage is internal. **B.** Moderate separation in which there is external hemorrhage. **C.** Severe separation in which there is external hemorrhage and extreme separation.

- **O45.01** **Premature separation of placenta with afibrinogenemia**
  Premature separation of placenta with hypofibrinogenemia
  - O45.011 Premature separation of placenta with afibrinogenemia, first trimester ♀ 🔖 M
  - O45.012 Premature separation of placenta with afibrinogenemia, second trimester ♀ 🔖   M
  - O45.013 Premature separation of placenta with afibrinogenemia, third trimester ♀ 🔖   M
  - O45.019 Premature separation of placenta with afibrinogenemia, unspecified trimester ♀   M
- **O45.02** **Premature separation of placenta with disseminated intravascular coagulation**
  - O45.021 Premature separation of placenta with disseminated intravascular coagulation, first trimester ♀ 🔖   M
  - O45.022 Premature separation of placenta with disseminated intravascular coagulation, second trimester ♀ 🔖   M
  - O45.023 Premature separation of placenta with disseminated intravascular coagulation, third trimester ♀ 🔖   M
  - O45.029 Premature separation of placenta with disseminated intravascular coagulation, unspecified trimester ♀ M
- **O45.09** **Premature separation of placenta with other coagulation defect**
  - O45.091 Premature separation of placenta with other coagulation defect, first trimester ♀ 🔖   M
  - O45.092 Premature separation of placenta with other coagulation defect, second trimester ♀ 🔖   M
  - O45.093 Premature separation of placenta with other coagulation defect, third trimester ♀ 🔖   M
  - O45.099 Premature separation of placenta with other coagulation defect, unspecified trimester ♀   M
- **O45.8** **Other premature separation of placenta**
  (Ex) For category O45.8 CC codes: See PDX Collection 986
  - **O45.8X** **Other premature separation of placenta**
    - O45.8X1 Other premature separation of placenta, first trimester ♀ 🔖   M
    - O45.8X2 Other premature separation of placenta, second trimester ♀ 🔖   M
    - O45.8X3 Other premature separation of placenta, third trimester ♀ 🔖   M
    - O45.8X9 Other premature separation of placenta, unspecified trimester ♀   M

N Newborn Age: 0   **P** Pediatric Age: 0–17   **M** Maternity DX: 12–55   **A** Adult Age: 15–124   ♀ Females Only   ♂ Males Only

🔖 Complication\Comorbidity   🔖 Major C\C   (Ex) CC/MCC Exclusions   🔖 Hospital-Acquired Condition

1145

CHAPTER 15 (O00-O9A)

● **O45.9 Premature separation of placenta, unspecified**
Abruptio placentae NOS
(Ex) For category O45.9 CC codes: See PDX Collection 986

     O45.90 Premature separation of placenta, unspecified, unspecified trimester ♀   M

     O45.91 Premature separation of placenta, unspecified, first trimester ♀ 🔒   M

     O45.92 Premature separation of placenta, unspecified, second trimester ♀ 🔒   M

     O45.93 Premature separation of placenta, unspecified, third trimester ♀ 🔒   M

● **O46 Antepartum hemorrhage, not elsewhere classified**

     Excludes1   hemorrhage in early pregnancy (O20.-)
intrapartum hemorrhage NEC (O67.-)
placenta previa (O44.-)
premature separation of placenta [abruptio placentae] (O45.-)

● **O46.0 Antepartum hemorrhage with coagulation defect**
(Ex) For category O46.0 CC codes: See PDX Collection 985

     ● O46.00 Antepartum hemorrhage with coagulation defect, unspecified

         O46.001 Antepartum hemorrhage with coagulation defect, unspecified, first trimester ♀ 🔒   M

         O46.002 Antepartum hemorrhage with coagulation defect, unspecified, second trimester ♀ 🔒   M

         O46.003 Antepartum hemorrhage with coagulation defect, unspecified, third trimester ♀ 🔒   M

         O46.009 Antepartum hemorrhage with coagulation defect, unspecified, unspecified trimester ♀   M

     ● O46.01 Antepartum hemorrhage with afibrinogenemia
Antepartum hemorrhage with hypofibrinogenemia

         O46.011 Antepartum hemorrhage with afibrinogenemia, first trimester ♀ 🔒 M

         O46.012 Antepartum hemorrhage with afibrinogenemia, second trimester ♀ 🔒   M

         O46.013 Antepartum hemorrhage with afibrinogenemia, third trimester ♀ 🔒   M

         O46.019 Antepartum hemorrhage with afibrinogenemia, unspecified trimester ♀   M

     ● O46.02 Antepartum hemorrhage with disseminated intravascular coagulation

         O46.021 Antepartum hemorrhage with disseminated intravascular coagulation, first trimester ♀ 🔒   M

         O46.022 Antepartum hemorrhage with disseminated intravascular coagulation, second trimester ♀ 🔒   M

         O46.023 Antepartum hemorrhage with disseminated intravascular coagulation, third trimester ♀ 🔒   M

         O46.029 Antepartum hemorrhage with disseminated intravascular coagulation, unspecified trimester ♀ M

     ● O46.09 Antepartum hemorrhage with other coagulation defect

         O46.091 Antepartum hemorrhage with other coagulation defect, first trimester ♀ 🔒   M

         O46.092 Antepartum hemorrhage with other coagulation defect, second trimester ♀ 🔒   M

         O46.093 Antepartum hemorrhage with other coagulation defect, third trimester ♀ 🔒   M

         O46.099 Antepartum hemorrhage with other coagulation defect, unspecified trimester ♀   M

     ● O46.8 Other antepartum hemorrhage

         ● O46.8x Other antepartum hemorrhage

         O46.8x1 Other antepartum hemorrhage, first trimester ♀   M

         O46.8x2 Other antepartum hemorrhage, second trimester ♀   M

         O46.8x3 Other antepartum hemorrhage, third trimester ♀   M

         O46.8x9 Other antepartum hemorrhage, unspecified trimester ♀   M

     ● O46.9 Antepartum hemorrhage, unspecified

     O46.90 Antepartum hemorrhage, unspecified, unspecified trimester ♀   M

     O46.91 Antepartum hemorrhage, unspecified, first trimester ♀   M

     O46.92 Antepartum hemorrhage, unspecified, second trimester ♀   M

     O46.93 Antepartum hemorrhage, unspecified, third trimester ♀   M

● **O47 False labor**

     Includes   Braxton Hicks contractions
threatened labor

     Excludes1   preterm labor (O60.-)
(Ex) For category O47 CC codes: See PDX Collection 987

     ● O47.0 False labor before 37 completed weeks of gestation

     O47.00 False labor before 37 completed weeks of gestation, unspecified trimester ♀   M

     O47.02 False labor before 37 completed weeks of gestation, second trimester ♀ 🔒   M

     O47.03 False labor before 37 completed weeks of gestation, third trimester ♀ 🔒   M

     O47.1 False labor at or after 37 completed weeks of gestation ♀ 🔒   M

     O47.9 False labor, unspecified ♀   M

● **O48 Late pregnancy**

     O48.0 Post-term pregnancy ♀   M
Pregnancy over 40 completed weeks to 42 completed weeks gestation

     O48.1 Prolonged pregnancy ♀   M
Pregnancy which has advanced beyond 42 completed weeks gestation

▶ New   ⇒ Revised   ~~deleted~~ Deleted   Excludes 1   Excludes 2   Includes   Use additional   Code first   Code also   Key words

OGCR Official Guidelines   ● Unacceptable Principal Diagnosis   X Assign placeholder X   ● Use Additional Character(s)   ▷ Manifestation Code   **Coding Clinic**

COMPLICATIONS OF LABOR AND DELIVERY (O60-O77)

● **O60 Preterm labor**

| **Includes** | onset (spontaneous) of labor before 37 completed weeks of gestation |

| **Excludes1** | false labor (O47.0-) |
| | threatened labor NOS (O47.0-) |

(Ex) For category O60 CC codes: See PDX Collection 987

● **O60.0 Preterm labor without delivery**

    O60.00 Preterm labor without delivery, unspecified trimester ♀   M

    O60.02 Preterm labor without delivery, second trimester ♀ 🔵   M

    O60.03 Preterm labor without delivery, third trimester ♀ 🔵   M

● **O60.1 Preterm labor with preterm delivery**

One of the following 7th characters is to be assigned to each code under subcategory O60.1. 7th character 0 is for single gestations and multiple gestations where the fetus is unspecified. 7th characters 1 through 9 are for cases of multiple gestations to identify the fetus for which the code applies. The appropriate code from category O30, Multiple gestation, must also be assigned when assigning a code from subcategory O60.1 that has a 7th character of 1 through 9.

0	not applicable or unspecified
1	fetus 1
2	fetus 2
3	fetus 3
4	fetus 4
5	fetus 5
9	other fetus

Coding Clinic: 2016, Q2, P11

X● **O60.10 Preterm labor with preterm delivery, unspecified trimester** ♀ 🔵   M
    Preterm labor with delivery NOS

X● **O60.12 Preterm labor second trimester with preterm delivery second trimester** ♀ 🔵   M

X● **O60.13 Preterm labor second trimester with preterm delivery third trimester** ♀ 🔵   M

X● **O60.14 Preterm labor third trimester with preterm delivery third trimester** ♀ 🔵   M
    Coding Clinic: 2016, Q2, P10

● **O60.2 Term delivery with preterm labor**

One of the following 7th characters is to be assigned to each code under subcategory O60.2. 7th character 0 is for single gestations and multiple gestations where the fetus is unspecified. 7th characters 1 through 9 are for cases of multiple gestations to identify the fetus for which the code applies. The appropriate code from category O30, Multiple gestation, must also be assigned when assigning a code from subcategory O60.2 that has a 7th character of 1 through 9.

0	not applicable or unspecified
1	fetus 1
2	fetus 2
3	fetus 3
4	fetus 4
5	fetus 5
9	other fetus

X● **O60.20 Term delivery with preterm labor, unspecified trimester** ♀ 🔵   M

X● **O60.22 Term delivery with preterm labor, second trimester** ♀ 🔵   M

X● **O60.23 Term delivery with preterm labor, third trimester** ♀ 🔵   M

● **O61 Failed induction of labor**

    O61.0 Failed medical induction of labor ♀   M
      Failed induction (of labor) by oxytocin
      Failed induction (of labor) by prostaglandins

    O61.1 Failed instrumental induction of labor ♀   M
      Failed mechanical induction (of labor)
      Failed surgical induction (of labor)

    O61.8 Other failed induction of labor ♀   M

    O61.9 Failed induction of labor, unspecified ♀   M

● **O62 Abnormalities of forces of labor**

    O62.0 Primary inadequate contractions ♀   M
      Failure of cervical dilatation
      Primary hypotonic uterine dysfunction
      Uterine inertia during latent phase of labor

    O62.1 Secondary uterine inertia ♀   M
      Arrested active phase of labor
      Secondary hypotonic uterine dysfunction

    O62.2 Other uterine inertia ♀   M
      Atony of uterus without hemorrhage
      Atony of uterus NOS
      Desultory labor
      Hypotonic uterine dysfunction NOS
      Irregular labor
      Poor contractions
      Slow slope active phase of labor
      Uterine inertia NOS

| **Excludes1** | atony of uterus with hemorrhage (postpartum) (O72.1) |
| | postpartum atony of uterus without hemorrhage (O75.89) |

    O62.3 Precipitate labor ♀   M

    O62.4 Hypertonic, incoordinate, and prolonged uterine contractions ♀   M
      Cervical spasm
      Contraction ring dystocia
      Dyscoordinate labor
      Hour-glass contraction of uterus
      Hypertonic uterine dysfunction
      Incoordinate uterine action
      Tetanic contractions
      Uterine dystocia NOS
      Uterine spasm

| **Excludes1** | dystocia (fetal) (maternal) NOS (O66.9) |

    O62.8 Other abnormalities of forces of labor ♀   M

    O62.9 Abnormality of forces of labor, unspecified ♀   M

CHAPTER 15 (O00-O9A)

N Newborn Age: 0 **P** Pediatric Age: 0–17 **M** Maternity DX: 12–55 **A** Adult Age: 15–124 ♀ Females Only ♂ Males Only
🔵 Complication\Comorbidity 🔵 Major C\C (Ex) CC/MCC Exclusions 🔵 Hospital-Acquired Condition

1147

Figure 15-4 Five types of malposition and malpresentation of the fetus: **A.** Breech. **B.** Vertex. **C.** Face. **D.** Brow. **E.** Shoulder.

● O63   Long labor
   O63.0   Prolonged first stage (of labor) ♀   M
   O63.1   Prolonged second stage (of labor) ♀   M
   O63.2   Delayed delivery of second twin, triplet, etc. ♀   M
   O63.9   Long labor, unspecified ♀   M
     Prolonged labor NOS
     (Ex) See PDX Collection 988

● O64   Obstructed labor due to malposition and malpresentation of fetus

One of the following 7th characters is to be assigned to each code under category O64. 7th character 0 is for single gestations and multiple gestations where the fetus is unspecified. 7th characters 1 through 9 are for cases of multiple gestations to identify the fetus for which the code applies. The appropriate code from category O30, Multiple gestation, must also be assigned when assigning a code from category O64 that has a 7th character of 1 through 9.

   0   not applicable or unspecified
   1   fetus 1
   2   fetus 2
   3   fetus 3
   4   fetus 4
   5   fetus 5
   9   other fetus

X ● O64.0   Obstructed labor due to incomplete rotation of fetal head ♀   M
     Deep transverse arrest
     Obstructed labor due to persistent occipitoiliac (position)
     Obstructed labor due to persistent occipitoposterior (position)
     Obstructed labor due to persistent occipitosacral (position)
     Obstructed labor due to persistent occipitotransverse (position)
X ● O64.1   Obstructed labor due to breech presentation ♀   M
     Obstructed labor due to buttocks presentation
     Obstructed labor due to complete breech presentation
     Obstructed labor due to frank breech presentation
X ● O64.2   Obstructed labor due to face presentation ♀   M
     Obstructed labor due to chin presentation

X ● O64.3   Obstructed labor due to brow presentation ♀   M
X ● O64.4   Obstructed labor due to shoulder presentation ♀   M
     Prolapsed arm
     Excludes1   impacted shoulders (O66.0)
             shoulder dystocia (O66.0)
X ● O64.5   Obstructed labor due to compound presentation ♀   M
X ● O64.8   Obstructed labor due to other malposition and malpresentation ♀   M
     Obstructed labor due to footling presentation
     Obstructed labor due to incomplete breech presentation
X ● O64.9   Obstructed labor due to malposition and malpresentation, unspecified ♀   M

● O65   Obstructed labor due to maternal pelvic abnormality
   O65.0   Obstructed labor due to deformed pelvis ♀   M
   O65.1   Obstructed labor due to generally contracted pelvis ♀   M
   O65.2   Obstructed labor due to pelvic inlet contraction ♀   M
   O65.3   Obstructed labor due to pelvic outlet and mid-cavity contraction ♀   M
   O65.4   Obstructed labor due to fetopelvic disproportion, unspecified ♀   M
     Excludes1   dystocia due to abnormality of fetus (O66.2-O66.3)
   O65.5   Obstructed labor due to abnormality of maternal pelvic organs ♀   M
     Obstructed labor due to conditions listed in O34.-
     Use additional code to identify abnormality of pelvic organs O34.-
   O65.8   Obstructed labor due to other maternal pelvic abnormalities ♀   M
   O65.9   Obstructed labor due to maternal pelvic abnormality, unspecified ♀   M

● O66   Other obstructed labor
   O66.0   Obstructed labor due to shoulder dystocia ♀   M
     Impacted shoulders
   O66.1   Obstructed labor due to locked twins ♀   M
   O66.2   Obstructed labor due to unusually large fetus ♀   M
   O66.3   Obstructed labor due to other abnormalities of fetus ♀ M
     Dystocia due to fetal ascites
     Dystocia due to fetal hydrops
     Dystocia due to fetal meningomyelocele
     Dystocia due to fetal sacral teratoma
     Dystocia due to fetal tumor
     Dystocia due to hydrocephalic fetus
     Use additional code to identify cause of obstruction
   ● O66.4   Failed trial of labor
     O66.40   Failed trial of labor, unspecified ♀   M
     O66.41   Failed attempted vaginal birth after previous cesarean delivery ♀   M
        Code first rupture of uterus, if applicable (O71.0-, O71.1)
   O66.5   Attempted application of vacuum extractor and forceps ♀   M
     Attempted application of vacuum or forceps, with subsequent delivery by forceps or cesarean delivery
   O66.6   Obstructed labor due to other multiple fetuses ♀   M
   O66.8   Other specified obstructed labor ♀   M
     Use additional code to identify cause of obstruction
   O66.9   Obstructed labor, unspecified ♀   M
     Dystocia NOS
     Fetal dystocia NOS
     Maternal dystocia NOS

Figure 15-5 Hydrocephalic fetus causing disproportion.

▶ New   ⟹ Revised   ~~deleted~~ Deleted   Excludes 1   Excludes 2   Includes   Use additional   Code first   Code also   Key words
OGCR Official Guidelines   ● Unacceptable Principal Diagnosis   X Assign placeholder X   ● Use Additional Character(s)   ▷ Manifestation Code   **Coding Clinic**

● **O67   Labor and delivery complicated by intrapartum hemorrhage, not elsewhere classified**

 Excludes1   antepartum hemorrhage NEC (O46.-)
              placenta previa (O44.-)
              premature separation of placenta [abruptio placentae] (O45.-)

 Excludes2   postpartum hemorrhage (O72.-)

 O67.0   Intrapartum hemorrhage with coagulation defect ♀ 🦠 M
         Intrapartum hemorrhage (excessive) associated with afibrinogenemia
         Intrapartum hemorrhage (excessive) associated with disseminated intravascular coagulation
         Intrapartum hemorrhage (excessive) associated with hyperfibrinolysis
         Intrapartum hemorrhage (excessive) associated with hypofibrinogenemia
         Ex: See PDX Collection 985

 O67.8   Other intrapartum hemorrhage ♀   M
         Excessive intrapartum hemorrhage

 O67.9   Intrapartum hemorrhage, unspecified ♀   M

O68   Labor and delivery complicated by abnormality of fetal acid-base balance ♀ 🦠   M
      Fetal acidemia complicating labor and delivery
      Fetal acidosis complicating labor and delivery
      Fetal alkalosis complicating labor and delivery
      Fetal metabolic acidemia complicating labor and delivery

 Excludes1   fetal stress NOS (O77.9)
              labor and delivery complicated by electrocardiographic evidence of fetal stress (O77.8)
              labor and delivery complicated by ultrasonic evidence of fetal stress (O77.8)

 Excludes2   abnormality in fetal heart rate or rhythm (O76)
              labor and delivery complicated by meconium in amniotic fluid (O77.0)
         Ex: See PDX Collection 989

● **O69   Labor and delivery complicated by umbilical cord complications**
      One of the following 7th characters is to be assigned to each code under category O69. 7th character 0 is for single gestations and multiple gestations where the fetus is unspecified. 7th characters 1 through 9 are for cases of multiple gestations to identify the fetus for which the code applies. The appropriate code from category O30, Multiple gestation, must also be assigned when assigning a code from category O69 that has a 7th character of 1 through 9.

0	not applicable or unspecified
1	fetus 1
2	fetus 2
3	fetus 3
4	fetus 4
5	fetus 5
9	other fetus

 X ● **O69.0   Labor and delivery complicated by prolapse of cord** ♀   M
 X ● **O69.1   Labor and delivery complicated by cord around neck, with compression** ♀   M

 Excludes1   labor and delivery complicated by cord around neck, without compression (O69.81)

 X ● **O69.2   Labor and delivery complicated by other cord entanglement, with compression** ♀   M
         Labor and delivery complicated by compression of cord NOS
         Labor and delivery complicated by entanglement of cords of twins in monoamniotic sac
         Labor and delivery complicated by knot in cord

 Excludes1   labor and delivery complicated by other cord entanglement, without compression (O69.82)

 X ● **O69.3   Labor and delivery complicated by short cord** ♀   M
 X ● **O69.4   Labor and delivery complicated by vasa previa** ♀   M
         Labor and delivery complicated by hemorrhage from vasa previa

 X ● **O69.5   Labor and delivery complicated by vascular lesion of cord** ♀   M
         Labor and delivery complicated by cord bruising
         Labor and delivery complicated by cord hematoma
         Labor and delivery complicated by thrombosis of umbilical vessels

 ● **O69.8   Labor and delivery complicated by other cord complications**

   X ● **O69.81   Labor and delivery complicated by cord around neck, without compression** ♀   M
   X ● **O69.82   Labor and delivery complicated by other cord entanglement, without compression** ♀   M
   X ● **O69.89   Labor and delivery complicated by other cord complications** ♀   M

 X ● **O69.9   Labor and delivery complicated by cord complication, unspecified** ♀

● **O70   Perineal laceration during delivery**

 Includes   episiotomy extended by laceration

 Excludes1   obstetric high vaginal laceration alone (O71.4)

 O70.0   First degree perineal laceration during delivery ♀   M
         Perineal laceration, rupture or tear involving fourchette during delivery
         Perineal laceration, rupture or tear involving labia during delivery
         Perineal laceration, rupture or tear involving skin during delivery
         Perineal laceration, rupture or tear involving vagina during delivery
         Perineal laceration, rupture or tear involving vulva during delivery
         Slight perineal laceration, rupture or tear during delivery

 O70.1   Second degree perineal laceration during delivery ♀   M
         Perineal laceration, rupture or tear during delivery as in O70.0, also involving pelvic floor
         Perineal laceration, rupture or tear during delivery as in O70.0, also involving perineal muscles
         Perineal laceration, rupture or tear during delivery as in O70.0, also involving vaginal muscles

 Excludes1   perineal laceration involving anal sphincter (O70.2)

 Coding Clinic: 2016, CODING CIQ4, P53, Q2, P34

Figure 15-6   Perineal lacerations: **A.** First-degree is laceration of superficial tissues. **B.** Second-degree is limited to the pelvic floor and may involve the perineal or vaginal muscles. **C.** Third-degree involves the anal sphincter. **D.** Fourth-degree involves anal or rectal mucosa.

CHAPTER 15 (O00-O9A)

● **O70.2** **Third degree perineal laceration during delivery**
Perineal laceration, rupture or tear during delivery as in O70.1, also involving anal sphincter
Perineal laceration, rupture or tear during delivery as in O70.1, also involving rectovaginal septum
Perineal laceration, rupture or tear during delivery as in O70.1, also involving sphincter NOS

Excludes1   anal sphincter tear during delivery without third degree perineal laceration (O70.4)
perineal laceration involving anal or rectal mucosa (O70.3)

(Ex) For category O70.2 CC codes: See PDX Collection 990

O70.20 **Third degree perineal laceration during delivery, unspecified** ♀ 🅒   M

O70.21 **Third degree perineal laceration during delivery, IIIa** ♀ 🅒   M
Third degree perineal laceration during delivery with less than 50% of external anal sphincter (EAS) thickness torn

O70.22 **Third degree perineal laceration during delivery, IIIb** ♀ 🅒   M
Third degree perineal laceration during delivery with more than 50% external anal sphincter (EAS) thickness torn

O70.23 **Third degree perineal laceration during delivery, IIIc** ♀ 🅒   M
Third degree perineal laceration during delivery with both external anal sphincter (EAS) and internal anal sphincter (IAS) torn

O70.3 **Fourth degree perineal laceration during delivery** ♀ 🅒 M
Perineal laceration, rupture or tear during delivery as in O70.2, also involving anal mucosa
Perineal laceration, rupture or tear during delivery as in O70.2, also involving rectal mucosa
(Ex) See PDX Collection 991

O70.4 **Anal sphincter tear complicating delivery, not associated with third degree laceration** ♀ 🅒   M
Excludes1   anal sphincter tear with third degree perineal laceration (O70.2)
(Ex) See PDX Collection 992

O70.9 **Perineal laceration during delivery, unspecified** ♀   M

● **O71** **Other obstetric trauma**
Includes   obstetric damage from instruments

● **O71.0** **Rupture of uterus (spontaneous) before onset of labor**
Excludes1   disruption of (current) cesarean delivery wound (O90.0)
laceration of uterus, NEC (O71.81)
(Ex) For category O71.0 CC codes: See PDX Collection 993

O71.00 **Rupture of uterus before onset of labor, unspecified trimester** ♀   M

O71.02 **Rupture of uterus before onset of labor, second trimester** ♀ 🅒   M

O71.03 **Rupture of uterus before onset of labor, third trimester** ♀ 🅒   M

O71.1 **Rupture of uterus during labor** ♀ 🅒   M
Rupture of uterus not stated as occurring before onset of labor
Excludes1   disruption of cesarean delivery wound (O90.0)
laceration of uterus, NEC (O71.81)
(Ex) See PDX Collection 993

O71.2 **Postpartum inversion of uterus** ♀ 🅒   M
(Ex) See PDX Collection 994

O71.3 **Obstetric laceration of cervix** ♀ 🅒   M
Annular detachment of cervix
(Ex) See PDX Collection 995

O71.4 **Obstetric high vaginal laceration alone** ♀ 🅒   M
Laceration of vaginal wall without perineal laceration
Excludes1   obstetric high vaginal laceration with perineal laceration (O70.-)
(Ex) See PDX Collection 996

O71.5 **Other obstetric injury to pelvic organs** ♀ 🅒   M
Obstetric injury to bladder
Obstetric injury to urethra
Excludes2   obstetric periurethral trauma (O71.82)
(Ex) See PDX Collection 993

O71.6 **Obstetric damage to pelvic joints and ligaments** ♀ 🅒   M
Obstetric avulsion of inner symphyseal cartilage
Obstetric damage to coccyx
Obstetric traumatic separation of symphysis (pubis)
(Ex) See PDX Collection 997

O71.7 **Obstetric hematoma of pelvis** ♀ 🅒   M
Obstetric hematoma of perineum
Obstetric hematoma of vagina
Obstetric hematoma of vulva
(Ex) See PDX Collection 998

● **O71.8** **Other specified obstetric trauma**

O71.81 **Laceration of uterus, not elsewhere classified** ♀   M

O71.82 **Other specified trauma to perineum and vulva** ♀   M
Obstetric periurethral trauma

O71.89 **Other specified obstetric trauma** ♀   M

O71.9 **Obstetric trauma, unspecified** ♀   M

● **O72** **Postpartum hemorrhage**
Includes   hemorrhage after delivery of fetus or infant

O72.0 **Third-stage hemorrhage** ♀ 🅒   M
Hemorrhage associated with retained, trapped or adherent placenta
Retained placenta NOS
Code also type of adherent placenta (O43.2-)
(Ex) See PDX Collection 999

O72.1 **Other immediate postpartum hemorrhage** ♀ 🅒   M
Hemorrhage following delivery of placenta
Postpartum hemorrhage (atonic) NOS
Uterine atony with hemorrhage
Excludes1   uterine atony NOS (O62.2)
uterine atony without hemorrhage (O62.2)
postpartum atony of uterus without hemorrhage (O75.89)
(Ex) See PDX Collection 1000

O72.2 **Delayed and secondary postpartum hemorrhage** ♀ 🅒   M
Hemorrhage associated with retained portions of placenta or membranes after the first 24 hours following delivery of placenta
Retained products of conception NOS, following delivery
(Ex) See PDX Collection 1001

O72.3 **Postpartum coagulation defects** ♀   M
Postpartum afibrinogenemia
Postpartum fibrinolysis

● **O73** **Retained placenta and membranes, without hemorrhage**
Excludes1   placenta accreta (O43.21-)
placenta increta (O43.22-)
placenta percreta (O43.23-)

O73.0 **Retained placenta without hemorrhage** ♀   M
Adherent placenta, without hemorrhage
Trapped placenta without hemorrhage

O73.1 **Retained portions of placenta and membranes, without hemorrhage** ♀   M
Retained products of conception following delivery, without hemorrhage

▶ New   ⇒ Revised   ~~deleted~~ Deleted   Excludes 1   Excludes 2   Includes   Use additional   Code first   Code also   Key words
OGCR Official Guidelines   ● Unacceptable Principal Diagnosis   X Assign placeholder X   ● Use Additional Character(s)   ▶ Manifestation Code   **Coding Clinic**

● **O74   Complications of anesthesia during labor and delivery**

> **Includes**   maternal complications arising from the administration of a general, regional or local anesthetic, analgesic or other sedation during labor and delivery

> Use additional code, if applicable, to identify specific complication

O74.0   Aspiration pneumonitis due to anesthesia during labor and delivery ♀   M
> Inhalation of stomach contents or secretions NOS due to anesthesia during labor and delivery
> Mendelson's syndrome due to anesthesia during labor and delivery

O74.1   Other pulmonary complications of anesthesia during labor and delivery ♀   M

O74.2   Cardiac complications of anesthesia during labor and delivery ♀   M

O74.3   Central nervous system complications of anesthesia during labor and delivery ♀   M

O74.4   Toxic reaction to local anesthesia during labor and delivery ♀   M

O74.5   Spinal and epidural anesthesia-induced headache during labor and delivery ♀   M

O74.6   Other complications of spinal and epidural anesthesia during labor and delivery ♀   M

O74.7   Failed or difficult intubation for anesthesia during labor and delivery ♀   M

O74.8   Other complications of anesthesia during labor and delivery ♀   M

O74.9   Complication of anesthesia during labor and delivery, unspecified ♀   M

● **O75   Other complications of labor and delivery, not elsewhere classified**

> **Excludes2**   puerperal (postpartum) infection (O86.-)
> puerperal (postpartum) sepsis (O85)

O75.0   Maternal distress during labor and delivery ♀   M

O75.1   Shock during or following labor and delivery ♀ 🦠   M
> Obstetric shock following labor and delivery
> Ⓔⓧ See PDX Collection 1002

O75.2   Pyrexia during labor, not elsewhere classified ♀ 🦠   M
> Ⓔⓧ See PDX Collection 1003

O75.3   Other infection during labor ♀ 🦠   M
> Sepsis during labor
> Use additional code (B95-B97), to identify infectious agent
> Ⓔⓧ See PDX Collection 1004

O75.4   Other complications of obstetric surgery and procedures ♀   M
> Cardiac arrest following obstetric surgery or procedures
> Cardiac failure following obstetric surgery or procedures
> Cerebral anoxia following obstetric surgery or procedures
> Pulmonary edema following obstetric surgery or procedures
> Use additional code to identify specific complication
> **Excludes2**   complications of anesthesia during labor and delivery (O74.-)
> disruption of obstetrical (surgical) wound (O90.0-O90.1)
> hematoma of obstetrical (surgical) wound (O90.2)
> infection of obstetrical (surgical) wound (O86.0)

O75.5   Delayed delivery after artificial rupture of membranes ♀   M

● **O75.8   Other specified complications of labor and delivery**

O75.81   Maternal exhaustion complicating labor and delivery ♀   M

O75.82   Onset (spontaneous) of labor after 37 completed weeks of gestation but before 39 completed weeks gestation, with delivery by (planned) cesarean section ♀   M
> Delivery by (planned) cesarean section occurring after 37 completed weeks of gestation but before 39 completed weeks gestation due to (spontaneous) onset of labor
> *Code first to specify reason for planned cesarean section such as:*
> cephalopelvic disproportion (normally formed fetus) (O33.9)
> previous cesarean delivery (O34.21)

O75.89   Other specified complications of labor and delivery ♀   M

O75.9   Complication of labor and delivery, unspecified ♀   M

O76   Abnormality in fetal heart rate and rhythm complicating labor and delivery ♀   M
> Depressed fetal heart rate tones complicating labor and delivery
> Fetal bradycardia complicating labor and delivery
> Fetal heart rate decelerations complicating labor and delivery
> Fetal heart rate irregularity complicating labor and delivery
> Fetal heart rate abnormal variability complicating labor and delivery
> Fetal tachycardia complicating labor and delivery
> Non-reassuring fetal heart rate or rhythm complicating labor and delivery
> **Excludes1**   fetal stress NOS (O77.9)
> labor and delivery complicated by electrocardiographic evidence of fetal stress (O77.8)
> labor and delivery complicated by ultrasonic evidence of fetal stress (O77.8)
> **Excludes2**   fetal metabolic acidemia (O68)
> other fetal stress (O77.0-O77.1)

● **O77   Other fetal stress complicating labor and delivery**

O77.0   Labor and delivery complicated by meconium in amniotic fluid ♀   M

O77.1   Fetal stress in labor or delivery due to drug administration ♀   M

O77.8   Labor and delivery complicated by other evidence of fetal stress ♀   M
> Labor and delivery complicated by electrocardiographic evidence of fetal stress
> Labor and delivery complicated by ultrasonic evidence of fetal stress
> **Excludes1**   abnormality of fetal acid-base balance (O68)
> abnormality in fetal heart rate or rhythm (O76)
> fetal metabolic acidemia (O68)

O77.9   Labor and delivery complicated by fetal stress, unspecified ♀   M
> **Excludes1**   abnormality of fetal acid-base balance (O68)
> abnormality in fetal heart rate or rhythm (O76)
> fetal metabolic acidemia (O68)

CHAPTER 15 (O00-O9A)

Figure 15-7 The four stages of normal delivery: **I.** Lightening, which occurs 2 to 4 weeks before birth, at which time the fetus turns with head toward the vagina. **II.** Regular contractions begin, the amniotic sac ruptures, and dilation is complete. **III.** Delivery of the head and rotation. **IV.** Expulsion of placenta.

OGCR Section I.C., Chapter 15.n.

Normal Delivery, Code O80

1) Encounter for full term uncomplicated delivery

Code O80 should be assigned when a woman is admitted for a full-term normal delivery and delivers a single, healthy infant without any complications antepartum, during the delivery, or postpartum during the delivery episode. Code O80 is always a principal diagnosis. It is not to be used if any other code from chapter 15 is needed to describe a current complication of the antenatal, delivery, or perinatal period. Additional codes from other chapters may be used with code O80 if they are not related to or are in any way complicating the pregnancy.

2) Uncomplicated delivery with resolved antepartum complication

Code O80 may be used if the patient had a complication at some point during the pregnancy, but the complication is not present at the time of the admission for delivery.

3) Outcome of delivery for O80

Z37.0, Single live brith, is the only outcome of delivery code appropriate for use with O80.

ENCOUNTER FOR DELIVERY (O80-O82)

O80 **Encounter for full-term uncomplicated delivery** ♀   M
Delivery requiring minimal or no assistance, with or without episiotomy, without fetal manipulation [e.g., rotation version] or instrumentation [forceps] of a spontaneous, cephalic, vaginal, full-term, single, live-born infant. This code is for use as a single diagnosis code and is not to be used with any other code from chapter 15.
Use additional code to indicate outcome of delivery (Z37.0)
Coding Clinic: 2016, Q4, P124, 150

O82 **Encounter for cesarean delivery without indication** ♀   M
Use additional code to indicate outcome of delivery (Z37.0)

COMPLICATIONS PREDOMINANTLY RELATED TO THE PUERPERIUM (O85-O92)

Excludes2 mental and behavioral disorders associated with the puerperium (F53)
obstetrical tetanus (A34)
puerperal osteomalacia (M83.0)

O85 **Puerperal sepsis** ♀   M
Postpartum sepsis
Puerperal peritonitis
Puerperal pyemia
Use additional code (B95-B97), to identify infectious agent
Use additional code (R65.2-) to identify severe sepsis, if applicable
Excludes1 fever of unknown origin following delivery (O86.4)
genital tract infection following delivery (O86.1-)
obstetric pyemic and septic embolism (O88.3-)
puerperal septic thrombophlebitis (O86.81)
urinary tract infection following delivery (O86.2-)
Excludes2 sepsis during labor (O75.3)
Ex: See PDX Collection 1005

● O86 **Other puerperal infections**
Use additional code (B95-B97), to identify infectious agent
Excludes2 infection during labor (O75.3)
obstetrical tetanus (A34)
Ex: For category O86 CC codes unless otherwise indicated: See PDX Collection 968

O86.0 **Infection of obstetric surgical wound** ♀   M
Infected cesarean delivery wound following delivery
Infected perineal repair following delivery

● O86.1 **Other infection of genital tract following delivery**
O86.11 **Cervicitis following delivery** ♀   M
O86.12 **Endometritis following delivery** ♀   M
Ex: See PDX Collection 1005
O86.13 **Vaginitis following delivery** ♀   M
O86.19 **Other infection of genital tract following delivery** ♀   M

● O86.2 **Urinary tract infection following delivery**
O86.20 **Urinary tract infection following delivery, unspecified** ♀   M
Puerperal urinary tract infection NOS
O86.21 **Infection of kidney following delivery** ♀   M
O86.22 **Infection of bladder following delivery** ♀   M
Infection of urethra following delivery
O86.29 **Other urinary tract infection following delivery** ♀   M

O86.4 **Pyrexia of unknown origin following delivery** ♀   M
Puerperal infection NOS following delivery
Puerperal pyrexia NOS following delivery
Excludes2 pyrexia during labor (O75.2)
Ex: See PDX Collection 1006

● O86.8 **Other specified puerperal infections**
Ex: For category O86.8 CC codes: See PDX Collection 1005
O86.81 **Puerperal septic thrombophlebitis** ♀   M
O86.89 **Other specified puerperal infections** ♀   M

● O87 **Venous complications and hemorrhoids in the puerperium**

    Includes   venous complications in labor, delivery and the puerperium

    Excludes2   obstetric embolism (O88.-)
            puerperal septic thrombophlebitis (O86.81)
            venous complications in pregnancy (O22.-)

    (Ex:) **For category O87 CC codes:** See PDX Collection 967

    O87.0 **Superficial thrombophlebitis in the puerperium** ♀ 🏥   M
        Puerperal phlebitis NOS
        Puerperal thrombosis NOS

    O87.1 **Deep phlebothrombosis in the puerperium** ♀ 🏥   M
        Deep vein thrombosis, postpartum
        Pelvic thrombophlebitis, postpartum
        Use additional code to identify the deep vein thrombosis (I82.4-, I82.5-, I82.62-. I82.72-)
        Use additional code, if applicable, for associated long-term (current) use of anticoagulants (Z79.01)

    O87.2 **Hemorrhoids in the puerperium** ♀ 🏥   M

    O87.3 **Cerebral venous thrombosis in the puerperium** ♀ 🏥   M
        Cerebrovenous sinus thrombosis in the puerperium

    O87.4 **Varicose veins of lower extremity in the puerperium** ♀   M

    O87.8 **Other venous complications in the puerperium** ♀ 🏥   M
        Genital varices in the puerperium

    O87.9 **Venous complication in the puerperium, unspecified** ♀   M
        Puerperal phlebopathy NOS

O88 **Obstetric embolism**

    Excludes1   embolism complicating abortion NOS (O03.2)
            embolism complicating ectopic or molar pregnancy (O08.2)
            embolism complicating failed attempted abortion (O07.2)
            embolism complicating induced abortion (O04.7)
            embolism complicating spontaneous abortion (O03.2, O03.7)

    (Ex:) **For category O88 CC codes:** See PDX Collection 1007

  ● O88.0 **Obstetric air embolism**

    ● O88.01 **Obstetric air embolism in pregnancy**

      O88.011 **Air embolism in pregnancy, first trimester** ♀ 🏥   M

      O88.012 **Air embolism in pregnancy, second trimester** ♀ 🏥   M

      O88.013 **Air embolism in pregnancy, third trimester** ♀ 🏥   M

      O88.019 **Air embolism in pregnancy, unspecified trimester** ♀   M

    O88.02 **Air embolism in childbirth** ♀ 🏥   M

    O88.03 **Air embolism in the puerperium** ♀ 🏥   M

  ● O88.1 **Amniotic fluid embolism**
    Anaphylactoid syndrome in pregnancy

    ● O88.11 **Amniotic fluid embolism in pregnancy**

      O88.111 **Amniotic fluid embolism in pregnancy, first trimester** ♀ 🏥   M

      O88.112 **Amniotic fluid embolism in pregnancy, second trimester** ♀ 🏥   M

      O88.113 **Amniotic fluid embolism in pregnancy, third trimester** ♀ 🏥   M

      O88.119 **Amniotic fluid embolism in pregnancy, unspecified trimester** ♀   M

    O88.12 **Amniotic fluid embolism in childbirth** ♀ 🏥   M

    O88.13 **Amniotic fluid embolism in the puerperium** ♀ 🏥   M

  ● O88.2 **Obstetric thromboembolism**

    ● O88.21 **Thromboembolism in pregnancy**
      Obstetric (pulmonary) embolism NOS

      O88.211 **Thromboembolism in pregnancy, first trimester** ♀ 🏥   M

      O88.212 **Thromboembolism in pregnancy, second trimester** ♀ 🏥   M

      O88.213 **Thromboembolism in pregnancy, third trimester** ♀ 🏥   M

      O88.219 **Thromboembolism in pregnancy, unspecified trimester** ♀   M

    O88.22 **Thromboembolism in childbirth** ♀ 🏥   M

    O88.23 **Thromboembolism in the puerperium** ♀ 🏥   M
      Puerperal (pulmonary) embolism NOS

  ● O88.3 **Obstetric pyemic and septic embolism**

    ● O88.31 **Pyemic and septic embolism in pregnancy**

      O88.311 **Pyemic and septic embolism in pregnancy, first trimester** ♀ 🏥   M

      O88.312 **Pyemic and septic embolism in pregnancy, second trimester** ♀ 🏥   M

      O88.313 **Pyemic and septic embolism in pregnancy, third trimester** ♀ 🏥   M

      O88.319 **Pyemic and septic embolism in pregnancy, unspecified trimester** ♀ 🏥   M

    O88.32 **Pyemic and septic embolism in childbirth** ♀ 🏥   M

    O88.33 **Pyemic and septic embolism in the puerperium** ♀ 🏥   M

  ● O88.8 **Other obstetric embolism**
    Obstetric fat embolism

    ● O88.81 **Other embolism in pregnancy**

      O88.811 **Other embolism in pregnancy, first trimester** ♀ 🏥   M

      O88.812 **Other embolism in pregnancy, second trimester** ♀ 🏥   M

      O88.813 **Other embolism in pregnancy, third trimester** ♀ 🏥   M

      O88.819 **Other embolism in pregnancy, unspecified trimester** ♀   M

    O88.82 **Other embolism in childbirth** ♀ 🏥   M

    O88.83 **Other embolism in the puerperium** ♀ 🏥   M

● O89 **Complications of anesthesia during the puerperium**

    Includes   maternal complications arising from the administration of a general, regional or local anesthetic, analgesic or other sedation during the puerperium

    Use additional code, if applicable, to identify specific complication

  ● O89.0 **Pulmonary complications of anesthesia during the puerperium**

    O89.01 **Aspiration pneumonitis due to anesthesia during the puerperium** ♀   M
      Inhalation of stomach contents or secretions NOS due to anesthesia during the puerperium
      Mendelson's syndrome due to anesthesia during the puerperium

    O89.09 **Other pulmonary complications of anesthesia during the puerperium** ♀   M

    O89.1 **Cardiac complications of anesthesia during the puerperium** ♀   M

    O89.2 **Central nervous system complications of anesthesia during the puerperium** ♀   M

    O89.3 **Toxic reaction to local anesthesia during the puerperium** ♀   M

    O89.4 **Spinal and epidural anesthesia-induced headache during the puerperium** ♀   M

    O89.5 **Other complications of spinal and epidural anesthesia during the puerperium** ♀   M

    O89.6 **Failed or difficult intubation for anesthesia during the puerperium** ♀   M

    O89.8 **Other complications of anesthesia during the puerperium** ♀   M

    O89.9 **Complication of anesthesia during the puerperium, unspecified** ♀   M

CHAPTER 15 (O00–O9A)

N Newborn Age: 0   P Pediatric Age: 0–17   M Maternity DX: 12–55   A Adult Age: 15–124   ♀ Females Only   ♂ Males Only

🏥 Complication\Comorbidity   🏥 Major C\C   (Ex:) CC/MCC Exclusions   🏥 Hospital-Acquired Condition

CHAPTER 15 (O00-O9A)

● **O90**   **Complications of the puerperium, not elsewhere classified**

     O90.0   **Disruption of cesarean delivery wound** ♀   M
         Dehiscence of cesarean delivery wound
         Excludes1   rupture of uterus (spontaneous) before
                  onset of labor (O71.0-)
                  rupture of uterus during labor (O71.1)

     O90.1   **Disruption of perineal obstetric wound** ♀   M
         Disruption of wound of episiotomy
         Disruption of wound of perineal laceration
         Secondary perineal tear

     O90.2   **Hematoma of obstetric wound** ♀   M

     O90.3   **Peripartum cardiomyopathy** ♀ 🔖   M
         Conditions in I42.- arising during pregnancy and the
         puerperium
         Excludes1   pre-existing heart disease complicating
                  pregnancy and the puerperium
                  (O99.4-)
         (Ex) See PDX Collection 1008

     O90.4   **Postpartum acute kidney failure** ♀ 🔖   M
         Hepatorenal syndrome following labor and delivery
         (Ex) See PDX Collection 1009

     O90.5   **Postpartum thyroiditis** ♀   M

     O90.6   **Postpartum mood disturbance** ♀   M
         Postpartum blues   Postpartum sadness
         Postpartum dysphoria
         Excludes1   postpartum depression (F53)
                  puerperal psychosis (F53)

  ● **O90.8**   **Other complications of the puerperium, not elsewhere
         classified**
         O90.81   **Anemia of the puerperium** ♀   M
              Postpartum anemia NOS
              Excludes1   pre-existing anemia complicating
                      the puerperium (O99.03)

         O90.89   **Other complications of the puerperium, not
              elsewhere classified** ♀   M
              Placental polyp

     O90.9   **Complication of the puerperium, unspecified** ♀   M

● **O91**   **Infections of breast associated with pregnancy, the puerperium
and lactation**
     Use additional code to identify infection

  ● **O91.0**   **Infection of nipple associated with pregnancy, the
         puerperium and lactation**
    ● **O91.01**   **Infection of nipple associated with pregnancy**
              Gestational abscess of nipple
         O91.011   **Infection of nipple associated with
                 pregnancy, first trimester** ♀   M
         O91.012   **Infection of nipple associated with
                 pregnancy, second trimester** ♀   M
         O91.013   **Infection of nipple associated with
                 pregnancy, third trimester** ♀   M
         O91.019   **Infection of nipple associated with
                 pregnancy, unspecified trimester** ♀   M

         O91.02   **Infection of nipple associated with the
              puerperium** ♀   M
              Puerperal abscess of nipple

         O91.03   **Infection of nipple associated with lactation** ♀ M
              Abscess of nipple associated with lactation

  ● **O91.1**   **Abscess of breast associated with pregnancy, the
         puerperium and lactation**
    ● **O91.11**   **Abscess of breast associated with pregnancy**
              Gestational mammary abscess
              Gestational purulent mastitis
              Gestational subareolar abscess
         O91.111   **Abscess of breast associated with
                 pregnancy, first trimester** ♀   M
         O91.112   **Abscess of breast associated with
                 pregnancy, second trimester** ♀   M
         O91.113   **Abscess of breast associated with
                 pregnancy, third trimester** ♀   M
         O91.119   **Abscess of breast associated with
                 pregnancy, unspecified trimester** ♀   M

         O91.12   **Abscess of breast associated with the
              puerperium** ♀   M
              Puerperal mammary abscess
              Puerperal purulent mastitis
              Puerperal subareolar abscess

         O91.13   **Abscess of breast associated with lactation** ♀ M
              Mammary abscess associated with lactation
              Purulent mastitis associated with lactation
              Subareolar abscess associated with lactation

  ● **O91.2**   **Nonpurulent mastitis associated with pregnancy, the
         puerperium and lactation**
    ● **O91.21**   **Nonpurulent mastitis associated with
              pregnancy**
              Gestational interstitial mastitis
              Gestational lymphangitis of breast
              Gestational mastitis NOS
              Gestational parenchymatous mastitis
         O91.211   **Nonpurulent mastitis associated with
                 pregnancy, first trimester** ♀   M
         O91.212   **Nonpurulent mastitis associated with
                 pregnancy, second trimester** ♀   M
         O91.213   **Nonpurulent mastitis associated with
                 pregnancy, third trimester** ♀   M
         O91.219   **Nonpurulent mastitis associated with
                 pregnancy, unspecified trimester** ♀ M

         O91.22   **Nonpurulent mastitis associated with the
              puerperium** ♀   M
              Puerperal interstitial mastitis
              Puerperal lymphangitis of breast
              Puerperal mastitis NOS
              Puerperal parenchymatous mastitis

         O91.23   **Nonpurulent mastitis associated with
              lactation** ♀   M
              Interstitial mastitis associated with lactation
              Lymphangitis of breast associated with
              lactation
              Mastitis NOS associated with lactation
              Parenchymatous mastitis associated with
              lactation

● **O92**   **Other disorders of breast and disorders of lactation associated
with pregnancy and the puerperium**
  ● **O92.0**   **Retracted nipple associated with pregnancy, the
         puerperium, and lactation**
    ● **O92.01**   **Retracted nipple associated with pregnancy**
         O92.011   **Retracted nipple associated with
                 pregnancy, first trimester** ♀   M
         O92.012   **Retracted nipple associated with
                 pregnancy, second trimester** ♀   M
         O92.013   **Retracted nipple associated with
                 pregnancy, third trimester** ♀   M
         O92.019   **Retracted nipple associated with
                 pregnancy, unspecified trimester** ♀ M

         O92.02   **Retracted nipple associated with the
              puerperium** ♀   M

         O92.03   **Retracted nipple associated with lactation** ♀ M

  ● **O92.1**   **Cracked nipple associated with pregnancy, the
         puerperium, and lactation**
         Fissure of nipple, gestational or puerperal
    ● **O92.11**   **Cracked nipple associated with pregnancy**
         O92.111   **Cracked nipple associated with
                 pregnancy, first trimester** ♀   M
         O92.112   **Cracked nipple associated with
                 pregnancy, second trimester** ♀   M
         O92.113   **Cracked nipple associated with
                 pregnancy, third trimester** ♀   M
         O92.119   **Cracked nipple associated with
                 pregnancy, unspecified trimester** ♀ M

         O92.12   **Cracked nipple associated with the
              puerperium** ♀   M

         O92.13   **Cracked nipple associated with lactation** ♀   M

▶ New   ⇥ Revised   ~~deleted~~ Deleted   Excludes 1   Excludes 2   Includes   Use additional   Code first   Code also   Key words

OGCR Official Guidelines   ● Unacceptable Principal Diagnosis   X Assign placeholder X   ● Use Additional Character(s)   ▌ Manifestation Code   **Coding Clinic**

● **O92.2 Other and unspecified disorders of breast associated with pregnancy and the puerperium**

    O92.20 Unspecified disorder of breast associated with pregnancy and the puerperium ♀   M

    O92.29 Other disorders of breast associated with pregnancy and the puerperium ♀   M

O92.3 Agalactia ♀   M
    Primary agalactia

    Excludes1   elective agalactia (O92.5)
                   secondary agalactia (O92.5)
                   therapeutic agalactia (O92.5)

O92.4 Hypogalactia ♀   M

O92.5 Suppressed lactation ♀   M
    Elective agalactia   Therapeutic agalactia
    Secondary agalactia

    Excludes1   primary agalactia (O92.3)

O92.6 Galactorrhea ♀   M

● **O92.7 Other and unspecified disorders of lactation**

    O92.70 Unspecified disorders of lactation ♀   M

    O92.79 Other disorders of lactation ♀   M
           Puerperal galactocele

OTHER OBSTETRIC CONDITIONS, NOT ELSEWHERE CLASSIFIED (O94-O9A)

● **O94 Sequelae of complication of pregnancy, childbirth, and the puerperium** ♀   M

    Note: This category is to be used to indicate conditions in O00-O77.-, O85-O94 and O98-O9A.- as the cause of late effects. The 'sequelae' include conditions specified as such, or as late effects, which may occur at any time after the puerperium.

    Code first condition resulting from (sequela) of complication of pregnancy, childbirth, and the puerperium

O98 Maternal infectious and parasitic diseases classifiable elsewhere but complicating pregnancy, childbirth and the puerperium

    Includes   the listed conditions when complicating the pregnant state, when aggravated by the pregnancy, or as a reason for obstetric care

    Use additional code (Chapter 1), to identify specific infectious or parasitic disease

    Excludes2   herpes gestationis (O26.4-)
               infectious carrier state (O99.82-, O99.83-)
               obstetrical tetanus (A34)
               puerperal infection (O86.-)
               puerperal sepsis (O85)
               when the reason for maternal care is that the disease is known or suspected to have affected the fetus (O35-O36)

● **O98.0 Tuberculosis complicating pregnancy, childbirth and the puerperium**
    Conditions in A15-A19
    (Ex) **For category O98.0 CC codes:** See PDX Collection 1011

    ● **O98.01** Tuberculosis complicating pregnancy

        O98.011 Tuberculosis complicating pregnancy, first trimester ♀ 🗇   M

        O98.012 Tuberculosis complicating pregnancy, second trimester ♀ 🗇   M

        O98.013 Tuberculosis complicating pregnancy, third trimester ♀ 🗇   M

        O98.019 Tuberculosis complicating pregnancy, unspecified trimester ♀   M

    O98.02 Tuberculosis complicating childbirth ♀ 🗇   M

    O98.03 Tuberculosis complicating the puerperium ♀ 🗇   M

● **O98.1 Syphilis complicating pregnancy, childbirth and the puerperium**
    Conditions in A50-A53
    (Ex) **For category O98.1 CC codes:** See PDX Collection 1012

    ● **O98.11** Syphilis complicating pregnancy

        O98.111 Syphilis complicating pregnancy, first trimester ♀ 🗇   M

        O98.112 Syphilis complicating pregnancy, second trimester ♀ 🗇   M

        O98.113 Syphilis complicating pregnancy, third trimester ♀ 🗇   M

        O98.119 Syphilis complicating pregnancy, unspecified trimester ♀   M

    O98.12 Syphilis complicating childbirth ♀ 🗇   M

    O98.13 Syphilis complicating the puerperium ♀ 🗇   M

● **O98.2 Gonorrhea complicating pregnancy, childbirth and the puerperium**
    Conditions in A54.-
    (Ex) **For category O98.2 CC codes:** See PDX Collection 1012

    ● **O98.21** Gonorrhea complicating pregnancy

        O98.211 Gonorrhea complicating pregnancy, first trimester ♀ 🗇   M

        O98.212 Gonorrhea complicating pregnancy, second trimester ♀ 🗇   M

        O98.213 Gonorrhea complicating pregnancy, third trimester ♀ 🗇   M

        O98.219 Gonorrhea complicating pregnancy, unspecified trimester ♀   M

    O98.22 Gonorrhea complicating childbirth ♀ 🗇   M

    O98.23 Gonorrhea complicating the puerperium ♀ 🗇   M

● **O98.3 Other infections with a predominantly sexual mode of transmission complicating pregnancy, childbirth and the puerperium**
    Conditions in A55-A64
    (Ex) **For category O98.3 CC codes:** See PDX Collection 1012

    ● **O98.31** Other infections with a predominantly sexual mode of transmission complicating pregnancy

        O98.311 Other infections with a predominantly sexual mode of transmission complicating pregnancy, first trimester ♀ 🗇   M

        O98.312 Other infections with a predominantly sexual mode of transmission complicating pregnancy, second trimester ♀ 🗇   M

        O98.313 Other infections with a predominantly sexual mode of transmission complicating pregnancy, third trimester ♀ 🗇   M

        O98.319 Other infections with a predominantly sexual mode of transmission complicating pregnancy, unspecified trimester ♀   M

    O98.32 Other infections with a predominantly sexual mode of transmission complicating childbirth ♀ 🗇   M

    O98.33 Other infections with a predominantly sexual mode of transmission complicating the puerperium ♀ 🗇   M

N Newborn Age: 0   **P** Pediatric Age: 0–17   **M** Maternity DX: 12–55   **A** Adult Age: 15–124   ♀ Females Only   ♂ Males Only

🗇 Complication\Comorbidity   🗇 Major C\C   (Ex) CC/MCC Exclusions   🗇 Hospital-Acquired Condition

1155

● **O98.4   Viral hepatitis complicating pregnancy, childbirth and the puerperium**
Conditions in B15-B19
(Ex) **For category O98.4 CC codes:** See PDX Collection 1013

  ● **O98.41   Viral hepatitis complicating pregnancy**

    O98.411   Viral hepatitis complicating pregnancy, **first trimester** ♀   M

    O98.412   Viral hepatitis complicating pregnancy, **second trimester** ♀   M

    O98.413   Viral hepatitis complicating pregnancy, **third trimester** ♀   M

    O98.419   Viral hepatitis complicating pregnancy, **unspecified trimester** ♀   M

  O98.42   Viral hepatitis complicating **childbirth** ♀   M

  O98.43   Viral hepatitis complicating the **puerperium** ♀   M

● **O98.5   Other viral diseases complicating pregnancy, childbirth and the puerperium**
Conditions in A80-B09, B25-B34, R87.81-, R87.82-

  Excludes:1 human immunodeficiency virus [HIV] disease complicating pregnancy, childbirth and the puerperium (O98.7-)

(Ex) **For category O98.5 CC codes:** See PDX Collection 1013

  ● **O98.51   Other viral diseases complicating pregnancy**

    O98.511   Other viral diseases complicating pregnancy, **first trimester** ♀   M

    O98.512   Other viral diseases complicating pregnancy, **second trimester** ♀   M
    Coding Clinic: 2016, Q4, P5-6

    O98.513   Other viral diseases complicating pregnancy, **third trimester** ♀   M
    Coding Clinic: 2016, Q4, P6

    O98.519   Other viral diseases complicating pregnancy, **unspecified trimester** ♀   M

  O98.52   Other viral diseases complicating **childbirth** ♀   M

  O98.53   Other viral diseases complicating the **puerperium** ♀   M

● **O98.6   Protozoal diseases complicating pregnancy, childbirth and the puerperium**
Conditions in B50-B64

  ● **O98.61   Protozoal diseases complicating pregnancy**
    (Ex) **For category O98.61 CC codes:** See PDX Collection 1014

    O98.611   Protozoal diseases complicating pregnancy, **first trimester** ♀   M

    O98.612   Protozoal diseases complicating pregnancy, **second trimester** ♀   M

    O98.613   Protozoal diseases complicating pregnancy, **third trimester** ♀   M

    O98.619   Protozoal diseases complicating pregnancy, **unspecified trimester** ♀   M

  O98.62   Protozoal diseases complicating **childbirth** ♀   M
    (Ex) See PDX Collection 1015

  O98.63   Protozoal diseases complicating the **puerperium** ♀   M
    (Ex) See PDX Collection 1015

● **O98.7   Human immunodeficiency virus [HIV] disease complicating pregnancy, childbirth and the puerperium**
Use additional code to identify the type of HIV disease:
  Acquired immune deficiency syndrome (AIDS) (B20)
  Asymptomatic HIV status (Z21)
  HIV positive NOS (Z21)
  Symptomatic HIV disease (B20)

OGCR Section I.C.15.f.

HIV Infection in Pregnancy, Childbirth and the Puerperium

During pregnancy, childbirth or the puerperium, a patient admitted because of an HIV-related illness should receive a principal diagnosis from subcategory O98.7-. Human immunodeficiency [HIV] disease complicating pregnancy, childbirth and the puerperium, followed by the code(s) for the HIV-related illness(es).

Patients with asymptomatic HIV infection status admitted during pregnancy, childbirth, or the puerperium should receive codes of O98.7- and Z21, Asymptomatic human immunodeficiency virus [HIV] infection status.

(Ex) **For category O98.7 CC codes:** See PDX Collection 1013

  ● **O98.71   Human immunodeficiency virus [HIV] disease complicating pregnancy**

    O98.711   Human immunodeficiency virus [HIV] disease complicating pregnancy, **first trimester** ♀   M

    O98.712   Human immunodeficiency virus [HIV] disease complicating pregnancy, **second trimester** ♀   M

    O98.713   Human immunodeficiency virus [HIV] disease complicating pregnancy, **third trimester** ♀   M

    O98.719   Human immunodeficiency virus [HIV] disease complicating pregnancy, **unspecified trimester** ♀   M

  O98.72   Human immunodeficiency virus [HIV] disease complicating **childbirth** ♀   M

  O98.73   Human immunodeficiency virus [HIV] disease complicating the **puerperium** ♀   M

● **O98.8   Other maternal infectious and parasitic diseases complicating pregnancy, childbirth and the puerperium**
(Ex) **For category O98.8 CC codes:** See PDX Collection 1013

  ● **O98.81   Other maternal infectious and parasitic diseases complicating pregnancy**

    O98.811   Other maternal infectious and parasitic diseases complicating pregnancy, **first trimester** ♀   M

    O98.812   Other maternal infectious and parasitic diseases complicating pregnancy, **second trimester** ♀   M

    O98.813   Other maternal infectious and parasitic diseases complicating pregnancy, **third trimester** ♀   M

    O98.819   Other maternal infectious and parasitic diseases complicating pregnancy, **unspecified trimester** ♀   M

  O98.82   Other maternal infectious and parasitic diseases complicating **childbirth** ♀   M

  O98.83   Other maternal infectious and parasitic diseases complicating the **puerperium** ♀   M

● **O98.9** **Unspecified maternal infectious and parasitic disease complicating pregnancy, childbirth and the puerperium**
(Ex) For category O98.9 CC codes: See PDX Collection 1013

  ● **O98.91** Unspecified maternal infectious and parasitic disease complicating pregnancy

     O98.911 Unspecified maternal infectious and parasitic disease complicating pregnancy, first trimester ♀ 🦠   M

     O98.912 Unspecified maternal infectious and parasitic disease complicating pregnancy, second trimester ♀ 🦠   M

     O98.913 Unspecified maternal infectious and parasitic disease complicating pregnancy, third trimester ♀ 🦠   M

     O98.919 Unspecified maternal infectious and parasitic disease complicating pregnancy, unspecified trimester ♀   M

     O98.92 Unspecified maternal infectious and parasitic disease complicating childbirth ♀ 🦠   M

     O98.93 Unspecified maternal infectious and parasitic disease complicating the puerperium ♀ 🦠   M

● **O99** **Other maternal diseases classifiable elsewhere but complicating pregnancy, childbirth and the puerperium**

Includes: conditions which complicate the pregnant state, are aggravated by the pregnancy or are a main reason for obstetric care

Use additional code to identify specific condition

Excludes2 when the reason for maternal care is that the condition is known or suspected to have affected the fetus (O35-O36)

  ● **O99.0** Anemia complicating pregnancy, childbirth and the puerperium
Conditions in D50-D64

     Excludes1 anemia arising in the puerperium (O90.81)
postpartum anemia NOS (O90.81)

     ● **O99.01** Anemia complicating pregnancy

       O99.011 Anemia complicating pregnancy, first trimester ♀   M

       O99.012 Anemia complicating pregnancy, second trimester ♀   M

       O99.013 Anemia complicating pregnancy, third trimester ♀   M

       O99.019 Anemia complicating pregnancy, unspecified trimester ♀   M

     O99.02 Anemia complicating childbirth ♀   M

     O99.03 Anemia complicating the puerperium ♀   M

       Excludes1 postpartum anemia not pre-existing prior to delivery (O90.81)

  ● **O99.1** Other diseases of the blood and blood-forming organs and certain disorders involving the immune mechanism complicating pregnancy, childbirth and the puerperium
Conditions in D65-D89

     Excludes1 hemorrhage with coagulation defects (O45.-, O46.0-, O67.0, O72.3)
~~hemorrhage with coagulation defects (O45.-, O46.0-, O67.0, O72.3)~~

     (Ex) For category O99.1 CC codes unless otherwise indicated: See PDX Collection 1016

     ● **O99.11** Other diseases of the blood and blood-forming organs and certain disorders involving the immune mechanism complicating pregnancy

       O99.111 Other diseases of the blood and blood-forming organs and certain disorders involving the immune mechanism complicating pregnancy, first trimester ♀ 🦠   M

       O99.112 Other diseases of the blood and blood-forming organs and certain disorders involving the immune mechanism complicating pregnancy, second trimester ♀ 🦠   M

       O99.113 Other diseases of the blood and blood-forming organs and certain disorders involving the immune mechanism complicating pregnancy, third trimester ♀ 🦠   M

       O99.119 Other diseases of the blood and blood-forming organs and certain disorders involving the immune mechanism complicating pregnancy, unspecified trimester ♀ 🦠   M

       (Ex) See PDX Collection 1017

     O99.12 Other diseases of the blood and blood-forming organs and certain disorders involving the immune mechanism complicating childbirth ♀ 🦠   M

     O99.13 Other diseases of the blood and blood-forming organs and certain disorders involving the immune mechanism complicating the puerperium ♀ 🦠   M

  ● **O99.2** Endocrine, nutritional and metabolic diseases complicating pregnancy, childbirth and the puerperium
Conditions in E00-E88

     Excludes2 diabetes mellitus (O24.-)
malnutrition (O25.-)
postpartum thyroiditis (O90.5)

  ● **O99.21** Obesity complicating pregnancy, childbirth, and the puerperium

Use additional code to identify the type of obesity (E66.-)

     O99.210 Obesity complicating pregnancy, unspecified trimester ♀   M

     O99.211 Obesity complicating pregnancy, first trimester ♀   M

     O99.212 Obesity complicating pregnancy, second trimester ♀   M

     O99.213 Obesity complicating pregnancy, third trimester ♀   M

     O99.214 Obesity complicating childbirth ♀   M

     O99.215 Obesity complicating the puerperium ♀   M

  ● **O99.28** Other endocrine, nutritional and metabolic diseases complicating pregnancy, childbirth and the puerperium

     O99.280 Endocrine, nutritional and metabolic diseases complicating pregnancy, unspecified trimester ♀   M

     O99.281 Endocrine, nutritional and metabolic diseases complicating pregnancy, first trimester ♀   M

     O99.282 Endocrine, nutritional and metabolic diseases complicating pregnancy, second trimester ♀   M

     O99.283 Endocrine, nutritional and metabolic diseases complicating pregnancy, third trimester ♀   M

     O99.284 Endocrine, nutritional and metabolic diseases complicating childbirth ♀   M

     O99.285 Endocrine, nutritional and metabolic diseases complicating the puerperium ♀   M

CHAPTER 15 (O00-O9A)

N Newborn Age: 0   P Pediatric Age: 0–17   M Maternity DX: 12–55   A Adult Age: 15–124   ♀ Females Only   ♂ Males Only
🦠 Complication\Comorbidity   🦠 Major C\C   (Ex) CC/MCC Exclusions   🦠 Hospital-Acquired Condition
1157

● **O99.3 Mental disorders and diseases of the nervous system complicating pregnancy, childbirth and the puerperium**

● **O99.31 Alcohol use complicating pregnancy, childbirth, and the puerperium**

Use additional code(s) from F10 to identify manifestations of the alcohol use

O99.310 Alcohol use complicating pregnancy, unspecified trimester ♀ M

O99.311 Alcohol use complicating pregnancy, first trimester ♀ M

O99.312 Alcohol use complicating pregnancy, second trimester ♀ M

O99.313 Alcohol use complicating pregnancy, third trimester ♀ M

O99.314 Alcohol use complicating childbirth ♀ M

O99.315 Alcohol use complicating the puerperium ♀ M

● **O99.32 Drug use complicating pregnancy, childbirth, and the puerperium**

Use additional code(s) from F11-F16 and F18-F19 to identify manifestations of the drug use

(Ex:) For category O99.32 CC codes: See PDX Collection 1018

O99.320 Drug use complicating pregnancy, unspecified trimester ♀ M

O99.321 Drug use complicating pregnancy, first trimester ♀ 🏷 M

O99.322 Drug use complicating pregnancy, second trimester ♀ 🏷 M

O99.323 Drug use complicating pregnancy, third trimester ♀ 🏷 M

O99.324 Drug use complicating childbirth ♀ 🏷 M

O99.325 Drug use complicating the puerperium ♀ 🏷 M

● **O99.33 Tobacco use disorder complicating pregnancy, childbirth, and the puerperium**

Smoking complicating pregnancy, childbirth, and the puerperium

Use additional code from category F17 to identify type of tobacco nicotine dependence

O99.330 Smoking (tobacco) complicating pregnancy, unspecified trimester ♀ M

O99.331 Smoking (tobacco) complicating pregnancy, first trimester ♀ M

O99.332 Smoking (tobacco) complicating pregnancy, second trimester ♀ M

O99.333 Smoking (tobacco) complicating pregnancy, third trimester ♀ M

O99.334 Smoking (tobacco) complicating childbirth ♀ M

O99.335 Smoking (tobacco) complicating the puerperium ♀ M

● **O99.34 Other mental disorders complicating pregnancy, childbirth, and the puerperium**

Conditions in F01-F09 and F20-F99

Excludes2 postpartum mood disturbance (O90.6)
postnatal psychosis (F53)
puerperal psychosis (F53)

O99.340 Other mental disorders complicating pregnancy, unspecified trimester ♀ M

O99.341 Other mental disorders complicating pregnancy, first trimester ♀ M

O99.342 Other mental disorders complicating pregnancy, second trimester ♀ M

O99.343 Other mental disorders complicating pregnancy, third trimester ♀ M

O99.344 Other mental disorders complicating childbirth ♀ M

O99.345 Other mental disorders complicating the puerperium ♀ M

● **O99.35 Diseases of the nervous system complicating pregnancy, childbirth, and the puerperium**

Conditions in G00-G99

Excludes2 pregnancy related peripheral neuritis (O26.8-)

O99.350 Diseases of the nervous system complicating pregnancy, unspecified trimester ♀ M

O99.351 Diseases of the nervous system complicating pregnancy, first trimester ♀ M

O99.352 Diseases of the nervous system complicating pregnancy, second trimester ♀ M

O99.353 Diseases of the nervous system complicating pregnancy, third trimester ♀ M

O99.354 Diseases of the nervous system complicating childbirth ♀ 🏷 M

(Ex:) See PDX Collection 1016

O99.355 Diseases of the nervous system complicating the puerperium ♀ 🏷 M

(Ex:) See PDX Collection 1016

● **O99.4 Diseases of the circulatory system complicating pregnancy, childbirth and the puerperium**

Conditions in I00-I99

Excludes1 peripartum cardiomyopathy (O90.3)

Excludes2 hypertensive disorders (O10-O16)
obstetric embolism (O88.-)
venous complications and cerebrovenous sinus thrombosis in labor, childbirth and the puerperium (O87.-)
venous complications and cerebrovenous sinus thrombosis in pregnancy (O22.-)

(Ex:) For category O99.4 CC codes unless otherwise indicated: See PDX Collection 1019

● **O99.41 Diseases of the circulatory system complicating pregnancy**

Coding Clinic: 2016, Q2, P8

O99.411 Diseases of the circulatory system complicating pregnancy, first trimester ♀ 🏷 M

O99.412 Diseases of the circulatory system complicating pregnancy, second trimester ♀ 🏷 M

O99.413 Diseases of the circulatory system complicating pregnancy, third trimester ♀ 🏷 M

O99.419 Diseases of the circulatory system complicating pregnancy, unspecified trimester ♀ M

O99.42 Diseases of the circulatory system complicating childbirth ♀ 🏷 M

(Ex:) See PDX Collection 1008

O99.43 Diseases of the circulatory system complicating the puerperium ♀ 🏷 M

● **O99.5 Diseases of the respiratory system complicating pregnancy, childbirth and the puerperium**
Conditions in J00-J99

  ● **O99.51 Diseases of the respiratory system complicating pregnancy**

    O99.511 Diseases of the respiratory system complicating pregnancy, first trimester ♀   M

    O99.512 Diseases of the respiratory system complicating pregnancy, second trimester ♀   M

    O99.513 Diseases of the respiratory system complicating pregnancy, third trimester ♀   M

    O99.519 Diseases of the respiratory system complicating pregnancy, unspecified trimester ♀   M

  O99.52 Diseases of the respiratory system complicating childbirth ♀   M

  O99.53 Diseases of the respiratory system complicating the puerperium ♀   M

● **O99.6 Diseases of the digestive system complicating pregnancy, childbirth and the puerperium**
Conditions in K00-K93

  Excludes2   hemorrhoids in pregnancy (O22.4-)
      liver and biliary tract disorders in pregnancy, childbirth and the puerperium (O26.6-)

  ● **O99.61 Diseases of the digestive system complicating pregnancy**

    O99.611 Diseases of the digestive system complicating pregnancy, first trimester ♀   M

    O99.612 Diseases of the digestive system complicating pregnancy, second trimester ♀   M

    O99.613 Diseases of the digestive system complicating pregnancy, third trimester ♀   M

    O99.619 Diseases of the digestive system complicating pregnancy, unspecified trimester ♀   M

  O99.62 Diseases of the digestive system complicating childbirth ♀   M

  O99.63 Diseases of the digestive system complicating the puerperium ♀   M

● **O99.7 Diseases of the skin and subcutaneous tissue complicating pregnancy, childbirth and the puerperium**
Conditions in L00-L99

  Excludes2   herpes gestationis (O26.4)
      pruritic urticarial papules and plaques of pregnancy (PUPPP) (O26.86)

  ● **O99.71 Diseases of the skin and subcutaneous tissue complicating pregnancy**

    O99.711 Diseases of the skin and subcutaneous tissue complicating pregnancy, first trimester ♀   M

    O99.712 Diseases of the skin and subcutaneous tissue complicating pregnancy, second trimester ♀   M

    O99.713 Diseases of the skin and subcutaneous tissue complicating pregnancy, third trimester ♀   M

    O99.719 Diseases of the skin and subcutaneous tissue complicating pregnancy, unspecified trimester ♀   M

  O99.72 Diseases of the skin and subcutaneous tissue complicating childbirth ♀   M

  O99.73 Diseases of the skin and subcutaneous tissue complicating the puerperium ♀   M

● **O99.8 Other specified diseases and conditions complicating pregnancy, childbirth and the puerperium**
Conditions in D00-D48, H00-H95, M00-N99, and Q00-Q99

Use additional code to identify condition

  Excludes2   genitourinary infections in pregnancy (O23.-)
      infection of genitourinary tract following delivery (O86.1-O86.3)
      malignant neoplasm complicating pregnancy, childbirth and the puerperium (O9A.1-)
      maternal care for known or suspected abnormality of maternal pelvic organs (O34.-)
      postpartum acute kidney failure (O90.4)
      traumatic injuries in pregnancy (O9A.2-)

● **O99.81 Abnormal glucose complicating pregnancy, childbirth and the puerperium**

  Excludes1   gestational diabetes (O24.4-)

  O99.810 Abnormal glucose complicating pregnancy ♀   M

  O99.814 Abnormal glucose complicating childbirth ♀   M

  O99.815 Abnormal glucose complicating the puerperium ♀   M

● **O99.82 Streptococcus B carrier state complicating pregnancy, childbirth and the puerperium**

  Excludes1   Carrier of streptococcus group B (GBS) in a nonpregnant woman (Z22.330)

  ● **O99.820 Streptococcus B carrier state complicating pregnancy** ♀   M

  O99.824 Streptococcus B carrier state complicating childbirth ♀   M

  ● **O99.825 Streptococcus B carrier state complicating the puerperium** ♀   M

● **O99.83 Other infection carrier state complicating pregnancy, childbirth and the puerperium**

Use additional code to identify the carrier state (Z22.-)

  (Ex) **For category O99.83 CC codes:** See PDX Collection 1013

  O99.830 Other infection carrier state complicating pregnancy ♀ 🦠   M

  O99.834 Other infection carrier state complicating childbirth ♀ 🦠   M

  O99.835 Other infection carrier state complicating the puerperium ♀ 🦠   M

● **O99.84 Bariatric surgery status complicating pregnancy, childbirth and the puerperium**
Gastric banding status complicating pregnancy, childbirth and the puerperium
Gastric bypass status for obesity complicating pregnancy, childbirth and the puerperium
Obesity surgery status complicating pregnancy, childbirth and the puerperium

  O99.840 Bariatric surgery status complicating pregnancy, unspecified trimester ♀ M

  O99.841 Bariatric surgery status complicating pregnancy, first trimester ♀ M

  O99.842 Bariatric surgery status complicating pregnancy, second trimester ♀ M

  O99.843 Bariatric surgery status complicating pregnancy, third trimester ♀ M

  O99.844 Bariatric surgery status complicating childbirth ♀ M

  O99.845 Bariatric surgery status complicating the puerperium ♀ M

O99.89 Other specified diseases and conditions complicating pregnancy, childbirth and the puerperium ♀   M

N Newborn Age: 0   **P** Pediatric Age: 0–17   **M** Maternity DX: 12–55   **A** Adult Age: 15–124   ♀ Females Only   ♂ Males Only

🦠 Complication\Comorbidity   🦠 Major C\C   (Ex) CC/MCC Exclusions   🦠 Hospital-Acquired Condition

1159

CHAPTER 15 (O00-O9A)

OGCR Section I.C.2.l.3.

Malignant neoplasm in a pregnant patient
When a pregnant woman has a malignant neoplasm, a code from subcategory O9A.1-, Malignant neoplasm complicating pregnancy, childbirth, and the puerperium, should be sequenced first, followed by the appropriate code from Chapter 2 to indicate the type of neoplasm.

- O9A **Maternal malignant neoplasms, traumatic injuries and abuse classifiable elsewhere but complicating pregnancy, childbirth and the puerperium**
  - O9A.1 **Malignant neoplasm complicating pregnancy, childbirth and the puerperium**
    Conditions in C00-C96
    Use additional code to identify neoplasm
    Excludes2   maternal care for benign tumor of corpus uteri (O34.1-)
    maternal care for benign tumor of cervix (O34.4-)
    - O9A.11 **Malignant neoplasm complicating pregnancy**
      - O9A.111 **Malignant neoplasm complicating pregnancy, first trimester** ♀   M
      - O9A.112 **Malignant neoplasm complicating pregnancy, second trimester** ♀   M
      - O9A.113 **Malignant neoplasm complicating pregnancy, third trimester** ♀   M
      - O9A.119 **Malignant neoplasm complicating pregnancy, unspecified trimester** ♀   M
    - O9A.12 **Malignant neoplasm complicating childbirth** ♀   M
    - O9A.13 **Malignant neoplasm complicating the puerperium** ♀   M
      Coding Clinic: 2015, Q3, P19
  - O9A.2 **Injury, poisoning and certain other consequences of external causes complicating pregnancy, childbirth and the puerperium**
    Conditions in S00-T88, except T74 and T76
    Use additional code(s) to identify the injury or poisoning
    Excludes2   physical, sexual and psychological abuse complicating pregnancy, childbirth and the puerperium (O9A.3-, O9A.4-, O9A.5-)
    - O9A.21 **Injury, poisoning and certain other consequences of external causes complicating pregnancy**
      - O9A.211 **Injury, poisoning and certain other consequences of external causes complicating pregnancy, first trimester** ♀   M
      - O9A.212 **Injury, poisoning and certain other consequences of external causes complicating pregnancy, second trimester** ♀   M
      - O9A.213 **Injury, poisoning and certain other consequences of external causes complicating pregnancy, third trimester** ♀   M
      - O9A.219 **Injury, poisoning and certain other consequences of external causes complicating pregnancy, unspecified trimester** ♀   M
    - O9A.22 **Injury, poisoning and certain other consequences of external causes complicating childbirth** ♀   M
    - O9A.23 **Injury, poisoning and certain other consequences of external causes complicating the puerperium** ♀   M

- O9A.3 **Physical abuse complicating pregnancy, childbirth and the puerperium**
  Conditions in T74.11 or T76.11
  Use additional code (if applicable):
  to identify any associated current injury due to physical abuse
  to identify the perpetrator of abuse (Y07.-)
  Excludes2   sexual abuse complicating pregnancy, childbirth and the puerperium (O9A.4)
  - O9A.31 **Physical abuse complicating pregnancy**
    - O9A.311 **Physical abuse complicating pregnancy, first trimester** ♀   M
    - O9A.312 **Physical abuse complicating pregnancy, second trimester** ♀   M
    - O9A.313 **Physical abuse complicating pregnancy, third trimester** ♀   M
    - O9A.319 **Physical abuse complicating pregnancy, unspecified trimester** ♀   M
  - O9A.32 **Physical abuse complicating childbirth** ♀   M
  - O9A.33 **Physical abuse complicating the puerperium** ♀   M
- O9A.4 **Sexual abuse complicating pregnancy, childbirth and the puerperium**
  Conditions in T74.21 or T76.21
  Use additional code (if applicable):
  to identify any associated current injury due to sexual abuse
  to identify the perpetrator of abuse (Y07.-)
  - O9A.41 **Sexual abuse complicating pregnancy**
    - O9A.411 **Sexual abuse complicating pregnancy, first trimester** ♀   M
    - O9A.412 **Sexual abuse complicating pregnancy, second trimester** ♀   M
    - O9A.413 **Sexual abuse complicating pregnancy, third trimester** ♀   M
    - O9A.419 **Sexual abuse complicating pregnancy, unspecified trimester** ♀   M
  - O9A.42 **Sexual abuse complicating childbirth** ♀   M
  - O9A.43 **Sexual abuse complicating the puerperium** ♀   M
- O9A.5 **Psychological abuse complicating pregnancy, childbirth and the puerperium**
  Conditions in T74.31 or T76.31
  Use additional code to identify the perpetrator of abuse (Y07.-)
  - O9A.51 **Psychological abuse complicating pregnancy**
    - O9A.511 **Psychological abuse complicating pregnancy, first trimester** ♀   M
    - O9A.512 **Psychological abuse complicating pregnancy, second trimester** ♀   M
    - O9A.513 **Psychological abuse complicating pregnancy, third trimester** ♀   M
    - O9A.519 **Psychological abuse complicating pregnancy, unspecified trimester** ♀   M
  - O9A.52 **Psychological abuse complicating childbirth** ♀ M
  - O9A.53 **Psychological abuse complicating the puerperium** ♀   M

▶ New   ⇒ Revised   ~~deleted~~ Deleted   Excludes 1   Excludes 2   Includes   Use additional   Code first   Code also   Key words
OGCR Official Guidelines   ● Unacceptable Principal Diagnosis   X Assign placeholder X   ● Use Additional Character(s)   ▌ Manifestation Code   **Coding Clinic**

CHAPTER 16

CERTAIN CONDITIONS ORIGINATING IN THE PERINATAL PERIOD (P00-P96)

OGCR Chapter-Specific Coding Guidelines

16. **Chapter 16: Certain Conditions Originating in the Perinatal Period (P00-P96)**

For coding and reporting purposes the perinatal period is defined as before birth through the 28th day following birth. The following guidelines are provided for reporting purposes

a. **General Perinatal Rules**

1) **Use of Chapter 16 Codes**

Codes in this chapter are <u>never</u> for use on the maternal record. Codes from Chapter 15, the obstetric chapter, are never permitted on the newborn record. Chapter 16 codes may be used throughout the life of the patient if the condition is still present.

2) **Principal Diagnosis for Birth Record**

When coding the birth episode in a newborn record, assign a code from category Z38, Liveborn infants according to place of birth and type of delivery, as the principal diagnosis. A code from category Z38 is assigned only once, to a newborn at the time of birth. If a newborn is transferred to another institution, a code from category Z38 should not be used at the receiving hospital.

A code from category Z38 is used only on the newborn record, not on the mother's record.

3) **Use of Codes from other Chapters with Codes from Chapter 16**

Codes from other chapters may be used with codes from chapter 16 if the codes from the other chapters provide more specific detail. Codes for signs and symptoms may be assigned when a definitive diagnosis has not been established. If the reason for the encounter is a perinatal condition, the code from chapter 16 should be sequenced first.

4) **Use of Chapter 16 Codes after the Perinatal Period**

Should a condition originate in the perinatal period, and continue throughout the life of the patient, the perinatal code should continue to be used regardless of the patient's age.

5) **Birth process or community acquired conditions**

If a newborn has a condition that may be either due to the birth process or community acquired and the documentation does not indicate which it is, the default is due to the birth process and the code from Chapter 16 should be used. If the condition is community-acquired, a code from Chapter 16 should not be assigned.

6) **Code all clinically significant conditions**

All clinically significant conditions noted on routine newborn examination should be coded. A condition is clinically significant if it requires:

- clinical evaluation; or
- therapeutic treatment; or
- diagnostic procedures; or
- extended length of hospital stay; or
- increased nursing care and/or monitoring; or
- has implications for future health care needs

Note: The perinatal guidelines listed above are the same as the general coding guidelines for "additional diagnoses", except for the final point regarding implications for future health care needs. Codes should be assigned for conditions that have been specified by the provider as having implications for future health care needs.

b. **Observation and Evaluation of Newborns for Suspected Conditions not Found**

1) *Use of Z05 codes*

Assign a code from category Z05, Observation and evaluation of newborns and infants for suspected conditions ruled out, to identify those instances when a healthy newborn is evaluated for a suspected condition that is determined after study not to be present. Do not use a code from category Z05 when the patient has identified signs or symptoms of a suspected problem; in such cases code the sign or symptom.

2) *Z05 on Other than the Birth Record*

A code from category Z05 may also be assigned as a principal or first-listed code for readmissions or encounters when the code from category Z38 code no longer applies. Codes from category Z05 are for use only for healthy newborns and infants for which no condition after study is found to be present.

3) *Z05 on a birth record*

A code from category Z05 is to be used as a secondary code after the code from category Z38, Liveborn infants according to place of birth and type of delivery.

c. **Coding Additional Perinatal Diagnoses**

1) **Assigning codes for conditions that require treatment**

Assign codes for conditions that require treatment or further investigation, prolong the length of stay, or require resource utilization.

2) **Codes for conditions specified as having implications for future health care needs**

Assign codes for conditions that have been specified by the provider as having implications for future health care needs.

Note: This guideline should not be used for adult patients.

d. **Prematurity and Fetal Growth Retardation**

Providers utilize different criteria in determining prematurity. A code for prematurity should not be assigned unless it is documented. Assignment of codes in categories P05, Disorders of newborn related to slow fetal growth and fetal malnutrition, and P07, Disorders of newborn related to short gestation and low birth weight, not elsewhere classified, should be based on the recorded birth weight and estimated gestational age.

When both birth weight and gestational age are available, two codes from category P07 should be assigned, with the code for birth weight sequenced before the code for gestational age.

e. **Low birth weight and immaturity status**

Codes from category P07, Disorders of newborn related to short gestation and low birth weight, not elsewhere classified, are for use for a child or adult who was premature or had a low birth weight as a newborn and this is affecting the patient's current health status.

See Section I.C.21. Factors influencing health status and contact with health services, Status.

f. **Bacterial Sepsis of Newborn**

Category P36, Bacterial sepsis of newborn, includes congenital sepsis. If a perinate is documented as having sepsis without documentation of congenital or community acquired, the default is congenital and a code from category P36 should be assigned. If the P36 code includes the causal organism, an additional code from category B95, Streptococcus, Staphylococcus, and Enterococcus as the cause of diseases classified elsewhere, or B96, Other bacterial agents as the cause of diseases classified elsewhere, should not be assigned. If the P36 code does not include the causal organism, assign an additional code from category B96. If applicable, use additional codes to identify severe sepsis (R65.2-) and any associated acute organ dysfunction.

g. **Stillbirth**

Code P95, Stillbirth, is only for use in institutions that maintain separate records for stillbirths. No other code should be used with P95. Code P95 should not be used on the mother's record.

CHAPTER 16

CERTAIN CONDITIONS ORIGINATING IN THE PERINATAL PERIOD (P00-P96)

Note: Codes from this chapter are for use on newborn records only, never on maternal records.

> **Includes**   conditions that have their origin in the fetal or perinatal period (before birth through the first 28 days after birth) even if morbidity occurs later

> **Excludes2**   congenital malformations, deformations and chromosomal abnormalities (Q00-Q99)
> endocrine, nutritional and metabolic diseases (E00-E88)
> injury, poisoning and certain other consequences of external causes (S00-T88)
> neoplasms (C00-D49)
> tetanus neonatorum (A33)

This chapter contains the following blocks:

P00-P04	Newborn affected by maternal factors and by complications of pregnancy, labor, and delivery
P05-P08	Disorders of newborns related to length of gestation and fetal growth
P09	Abnormal findings on neonatal screening
P10-P15	Birth trauma
P19-P29	Respiratory and cardiovascular disorders specific to the perinatal period
P35-P39	Infections specific to the perinatal period
P50-P61	Hemorrhagic and hematological disorders of newborn
P70-P74	Transitory endocrine and metabolic disorders specific to newborn
P76-P78	Digestive system disorders of newborn
P80-P83	Conditions involving the integument and temperature regulation of newborn
P84	Other problems with newborn
P90-P96	Other disorders originating in the perinatal period

NEWBORN AFFECTED BY MATERNAL FACTORS AND BY COMPLICATIONS OF PREGNANCY, LABOR, AND DELIVERY (P00–P04)

Note: These codes are for use when the listed maternal conditions are specified as the cause of confirmed morbidity or potential morbidity which have their origin in the perinatal period (before birth through the first 28 days after birth).

● **P00**   Newborn affected by maternal conditions that may be unrelated to present pregnancy

Code first any current condition in newborn

> **Excludes2**   encounter for observation of newborn for suspected diseases and conditions ruled out (Z05.-)
> newborn affected by maternal complications of pregnancy (P01.-)
> newborn affected by maternal endocrine and metabolic disorders (P70–P74)
> newborn affected by noxious substances transmitted via placenta or breast milk (P04.-)

Coding Clinic: 2016, Q4, P54

P00.0   Newborn affected by maternal hypertensive disorders
Newborn affected by maternal conditions classifiable to O10-O11, O13-O16

P00.1   Newborn affected by maternal renal and urinary tract diseases
Newborn affected by maternal conditions classifiable to N00-N39

P00.2   Newborn affected by maternal infectious and parasitic diseases
Newborn affected by maternal infectious disease classifiable to A00-B99, J09 and J10

> **Excludes1**   ~~infections specific to the perinatal period (P35-P39)~~
> maternal genital tract or other localized infections (P00.8)

> ▶ **Excludes2**   infections specific to the perinatal period (P35-P39)

Coding Clinic: 2015, Q3, P21

P00.3   Newborn affected by other maternal circulatory and respiratory diseases
Newborn affected by maternal conditions classifiable to I00-I99, J00-J99, Q20-Q34 and not included in P00.0, P00.2

P00.4   Newborn affected by maternal nutritional disorders
Newborn affected by maternal disorders classifiable to E40-E64
Maternal malnutrition NOS

P00.5   Newborn affected by maternal injury
Newborn affected by maternal conditions classifiable to O9A.2-

P00.6   Newborn affected by surgical procedure on mother
Newborn affected by amniocentesis

> **Excludes1**   Cesarean delivery for present delivery (P03.4)
> damage to placenta from amniocentesis, cesarean delivery or surgical induction (P02.1)
> previous surgery to uterus or pelvic organs (P03.89)

> **Excludes2**   newborn affected by complication of (fetal) intrauterine procedure (P96.5)

P00.7   Newborn affected by other medical procedures on mother, not elsewhere classified
Newborn affected by radiation to mother

> **Excludes1**   damage to placenta from amniocentesis, cesarean delivery or surgical induction (P02.1)
> newborn affected by other complications of labor and delivery (P03.-)

● **P00.8**   Newborn affected by other maternal conditions

     P00.81   Newborn affected by periodontal disease in mother

     P00.89   Newborn affected by other maternal conditions
Newborn affected by conditions classifiable to T80-T88
Newborn affected by maternal genital tract or other localized infections
Newborn affected by maternal systemic lupus erythematosus

P00.9   Newborn affected by unspecified maternal condition

● **P01**   Newborn affected by maternal complications of pregnancy

Code first any current condition in newborn

> **Excludes2**   encounter for observation of newborn for suspected diseases and conditions ruled out (Z05.-)

Coding Clinic: 2016, Q4, P54

P01.0   Newborn affected by incompetent cervix

P01.1   Newborn affected by premature rupture of membranes

P01.2   Newborn affected by oligohydramnios

> **Excludes1**   oligohydramnios due to premature rupture of membranes (P01.1)

P01.3   Newborn affected by polyhydramnios
Excess of amniotic fluid, usually > 2000 mL
Newborn affected by hydramnios

P01.4   Newborn affected by ectopic pregnancy
Newborn affected by abdominal pregnancy

P01.5   **Newborn affected by multiple pregnancy**
    Newborn affected by triplet (pregnancy)
    Newborn affected by twin (pregnancy)

P01.6   **Newborn affected by maternal death**

P01.7   **Newborn affected by malpresentation before labor**
    Newborn affected by breech presentation before labor
    Newborn affected by external version before labor
    Newborn affected by face presentation before labor
    Newborn affected by transverse lie before labor
    Newborn affected by unstable lie before labor

P01.8   **Newborn affected by other maternal complications of pregnancy**

P01.9   **Newborn affected by maternal complication of pregnancy, unspecified**

● **P02**   **Newborn affected by complications of placenta, cord and membranes**
    Code first any current condition in newborn
    Excludes2   encounter for observation of newborn for suspected diseases and conditions ruled out (Z05.-)
    Coding Clinic: 2016, Q4, P54

P02.0   **Newborn affected by placenta previa**

P02.1   **Newborn affected by other forms of placental separation and hemorrhage**
    Newborn affected by abruptio placenta
    Newborn affected by accidental hemorrhage
    Newborn affected by antepartum hemorrhage
    Newborn affected by damage to placenta from amniocentesis, cesarean delivery or surgical induction
    Newborn affected by maternal blood loss
    Newborn affected by premature separation of placenta

● **P02.2**   **Newborn affected by other and unspecified morphological and functional abnormalities of placenta**

  P02.20   **Newborn affected by unspecified morphological and functional abnormalities of placenta**

  P02.29   **Newborn affected by other morphological and functional abnormalities of placenta**
      Newborn affected by placental dysfunction
      Newborn affected by placental infarction
      Newborn affected by placental insufficiency

P02.3   **Newborn affected by placental transfusion syndromes**
    Newborn affected by placental and cord abnormalities resulting in twin-to-twin or other transplacental transfusion

P02.4   **Newborn affected by prolapsed cord**

P02.5   **Newborn affected by other compression of umbilical cord**
    Newborn affected by umbilical cord (tightly) around neck
    Newborn affected by entanglement of umbilical cord
    Newborn affected by knot in umbilical cord

● **P02.6**   **Newborn affected by other and unspecified conditions of umbilical cord**

  P02.60   **Newborn affected by unspecified conditions of umbilical cord**

  P02.69   **Newborn affected by other conditions of umbilical cord**
      Newborn affected by short umbilical cord
      Newborn affected by vasa previa
      Excludes1   newborn affected by single umbilical artery (Q27.0)

P02.7   **Newborn affected by chorioamnionitis**
    Inflammation of chorion and amnion
    Newborn affected by amnionitis
    Newborn affected by membranitis
    Newborn affected by placentitis

P02.8   **Newborn affected by other abnormalities of membranes**

P02.9   **Newborn affected by abnormality of membranes, unspecified**

● **P03**   **Newborn affected by other complications of labor and delivery**
    Code first any current condition in newborn
    Excludes2   encounter for observation of newborn for suspected diseases and conditions ruled out (Z05.-)
    Coding Clinic: 2016, Q4, P54

P03.0   **Newborn affected by breech delivery and extraction**

P03.1   **Newborn affected by other malpresentation, malposition and disproportion during labor and delivery**
    Newborn affected by contracted pelvis
    Newborn affected by conditions classifiable to O64-O66
    Newborn affected by persistent occipitoposterior
    Newborn affected by transverse lie

P03.2   **Newborn affected by forceps delivery**

P03.3   **Newborn affected by delivery by vacuum extractor [ventouse]**

P03.4   **Newborn affected by Cesarean delivery**

P03.5   **Newborn affected by precipitate delivery**
    Newborn affected by rapid second stage

P03.6   **Newborn affected by abnormal uterine contractions**
    Newborn affected by conditions classifiable to O62.-, except O62.3
    Newborn affected by hypertonic labor
    Newborn affected by uterine inertia

● **P03.8**   **Newborn affected by other specified complications of labor and delivery**

  ● **P03.81**   **Newborn affected by abnormality in fetal (intrauterine) heart rate or rhythm**
      Excludes1   neonatal cardiac dysrhythmia (P29.1-)

    P03.810   **Newborn affected by abnormality in fetal (intrauterine) heart rate or rhythm before the onset of labor**

    P03.811   **Newborn affected by abnormality in fetal (intrauterine) heart rate or rhythm during labor**

    P03.819   **Newborn affected by abnormality in fetal (intrauterine) heart rate or rhythm, unspecified as to time of onset**

  P03.82   **Meconium passage during delivery**
      Excludes1   meconium aspiration (P24.00, P24.01)
              meconium staining (P96.83)

  P03.89   **Newborn affected by other specified complications of labor and delivery**
      Newborn affected by abnormality of maternal soft tissues
      Newborn affected by conditions classifiable to O60-O75 and by procedures used in labor and delivery not included in P02.- and P03.0-P03.6
      Newborn affected by induction of labor

P03.9   **Newborn affected by complication of labor and delivery, unspecified**

CHAPTER 16 (P00-P96)

N   Newborn Age: 0   P   Pediatric Age: 0–17   M   Maternity DX: 12–55   A   Adult Age: 15–124   ♀   Females Only   ♂   Males Only

🞕   Complication\Comorbidity   🞕   Major C\C   (Ex)   CC/MCC Exclusions   🞕   Hospital-Acquired Condition

● **P04 Newborn affected by noxious substances transmitted via placenta or breast milk**

    Includes   nonteratogenic effects of substances transmitted via placenta

    Excludes2   congenital malformations (Q00–Q99)

                 encounter for observation of newborn for suspected diseases and conditions ruled out (Z05.-)

                 neonatal jaundice from excessive hemolysis due to drugs or toxins transmitted from mother (P58.4)

                 newborn in contact with and (suspected) exposures hazardous to health not transmitted via placenta or breast milk (Z77.-)

Coding Clinic: 2016, Q4, P54

P04.0 Newborn affected by maternal anesthesia and analgesia in pregnancy, labor and delivery

     Newborn affected by reactions and intoxications from maternal opiates and tranquilizers administered during labor and delivery

P04.1 Newborn affected by other maternal medication

     Newborn affected by cancer chemotherapy

     Newborn affected by cytotoxic drugs

    Excludes1   dysmorphism due to warfarin (Q86.2)

                 fetal hydantoin syndrome (Q86.1)

                 maternal use of drugs of addiction (P04.4-)

Coding Clinic: 2016, Q4, P55

P04.2 Newborn affected by maternal use of tobacco

     Newborn affected by exposure in utero to tobacco smoke

    Excludes2   newborn exposure to environmental tobacco smoke (P96.81)

P04.3 Newborn affected by maternal use of alcohol

    Excludes1   fetal alcohol syndrome (Q86.0)

● **P04.4 Newborn affected by maternal use of drugs of addiction**

    P04.41 Newborn affected by maternal use of cocaine

         'Crack baby'

    P04.49 Newborn affected by maternal use of other drugs of addiction

        Excludes2   newborn affected by maternal anesthesia and analgesia (P04.0)

                      withdrawal symptoms from maternal use of drugs of addiction (P96.1)

P04.5 Newborn affected by maternal use of nutritional chemical substances

P04.6 Newborn affected by maternal exposure to environmental chemical substances

P04.8 Newborn affected by other maternal noxious substances

P04.9 Newborn affected by maternal noxious substance, unspecified

OGCR Section I.C.16.d.

Prematurity and Fetal Growth Retardation

Providers utilize different criteria in determining prematurity. A code for prematurity should not be assigned unless it is documented. Assignment of codes in categories P05, Disorders of newborn related to slow fetal growth and fetal malnutrition, and P07, Disorders of newborn related to short gestation and low birth weight, not elsewhere classified, should be based on the recorded birth weight and estimated gestational age.

When both birth weight and gestational age are available, two codes from category P07 should be assigned, with the code for birth weight sequenced before the code for gestational age.

DISORDERS OF NEWBORN RELATED TO LENGTH OF GESTATION AND FETAL GROWTH (P05–P08)

● **P05 Disorders of newborn related to slow fetal growth and fetal malnutrition**

    Coding Clinic: 2016, Q4, P56

● **P05.0 Newborn light for gestational age**

     Newborn light-for-dates

     Weight below but length above 10th percentile for gestational age

    P05.00 Newborn light for gestational age, unspecified weight

    P05.01 Newborn light for gestational age, less than 500 grams

    P05.02 Newborn light for gestational age, 500-749 grams

    P05.03 Newborn light for gestational age, 750-999 grams

    P05.04 Newborn light for gestational age, 1000-1249 grams

    P05.05 Newborn light for gestational age, 1250-1499 grams

    P05.06 Newborn light for gestational age, 1500-1749 grams

    P05.07 Newborn light for gestational age, 1750-1999 grams

    P05.08 Newborn light for gestational age, 2000-2499 grams

    P05.09 Newborn light for gestational age, 2500 grams and over

         Newborn light for gestational age, other

        Coding Clinic: 2016, Q4, P55

● **P05.1 Newborn small for gestational age**

     Newborn small-and-light-for-dates

     Newborn small-for-dates

     Weight and length below 10th percentile for gestational age

    P05.10 Newborn small for gestational age, unspecified weight

    P05.11 Newborn small for gestational age, less than 500 grams

    P05.12 Newborn small for gestational age, 500-749 grams

    P05.13 Newborn small for gestational age, 750-999 grams

    P05.14 Newborn small for gestational age, 1000-1249 grams

    P05.15 Newborn small for gestational age, 1250-1499 grams

    P05.16 Newborn small for gestational age, 1500-1749 grams

    P05.17 Newborn small for gestational age, 1750-1999 grams

    P05.18 Newborn small for gestational age, 2000-2499 grams

    P05.19 Newborn small for gestational age, other

         Newborn small for gestational age, 2500 grams and over

        Coding Clinic: 2016, Q4, P55

P05.2 Newborn affected by fetal (intrauterine) malnutrition not light or small for gestational age

     Infant, not light or small for gestational age, showing signs of fetal malnutrition, such as dry, peeling skin and loss of subcutaneous tissue

    Excludes1   newborn affected by fetal malnutrition with light for gestational age (P05.0-)

                 newborn affected by fetal malnutrition with small for gestational age (P05.1-)

P05.9 Newborn affected by slow intrauterine growth, unspecified

     Newborn affected by fetal growth retardation NOS

▶ New   ⟹ Revised   ~~deleted~~ Deleted   Excludes 1   Excludes 2   Includes   Use additional   Code first   Code also   Key words

OGCR Official Guidelines   ● Unacceptable Principal Diagnosis   X Assign placeholder X   ● Use Additional Character(s)   ▶ Manifestation Code   **Coding Clinic**

● **P07**   **Disorders of newborn related to short gestation and low birth weight, not elsewhere classified**

Note: When both birth weight and gestational age of the newborn are available, both should be coded with birth weight sequenced before gestational age.

   Includes   the listed conditions, without further specification, as the cause of morbidity or additional care, in newborn

● **P07.0**   **Extremely low birth weight newborn**
Newborn birth weight 999 g. or less

   Excludes1   low birth weight due to slow fetal growth and fetal malnutrition (P05.-)

   P07.00   **Extremely low birth weight newborn, unspecified weight**

   P07.01   **Extremely low birth weight newborn, less than 500 grams**

   P07.02   **Extremely low birth weight newborn, 500-749 grams**

   P07.03   **Extremely low birth weight newborn, 750-999 grams**

● **P07.1**   **Other low birth weight newborn**
Newborn birth weight 1000-2499 g.

   Excludes1   low birth weight due to slow fetal growth and fetal malnutrition (P05.-)

   P07.10   **Other low birth weight newborn, unspecified weight**

   P07.14   **Other low birth weight newborn, 1000-1249 grams**

   P07.15   **Other low birth weight newborn, 1250-1499 grams**

   P07.16   **Other low birth weight newborn, 1500-1749 grams**

   P07.17   **Other low birth weight newborn, 1750-1999 grams**

   P07.18   **Other low birth weight newborn, 2000-2499 grams**

● **P07.2**   **Extreme immaturity of newborn**
Less than 28 completed weeks (less than 196 completed days) of gestation

   P07.20   **Extreme immaturity of newborn, unspecified weeks of gestation**
Gestational age less than 28 completed weeks NOS

   P07.21   **Extreme immaturity of newborn, gestational age less than 23 completed weeks**
Extreme immaturity of newborn, gestational age less than 23 weeks, 0 days

   P07.22   **Extreme immaturity of newborn, gestational age 23 completed weeks**
Extreme immaturity of newborn, gestational age 23 weeks, 0 days through 23 weeks, 6 days

   P07.23   **Extreme immaturity of newborn, gestational age 24 completed weeks**
Extreme immaturity of newborn, gestational age 24 weeks, 0 days through 24 weeks, 6 days

   P07.24   **Extreme immaturity of newborn, gestational age 25 completed weeks**
Extreme immaturity of newborn, gestational age 25 weeks, 0 days through 25 weeks, 6 days

   P07.25   **Extreme immaturity of newborn, gestational age 26 completed weeks**
Extreme immaturity of newborn, gestational age 26 weeks, 0 days through 26 weeks, 6 days

   P07.26   **Extreme immaturity of newborn, gestational age 27 completed weeks**
Extreme immaturity of newborn, gestational age 27 weeks, 0 days through 27 weeks, 6 days

● **P07.3**   **Preterm [premature] newborn [other]**
28 completed weeks or more but less than 37 completed weeks (196 completed days but less than 259 completed days) of gestation
Prematurity NOS

   P07.30   **Preterm newborn, unspecified weeks of gestation**

   P07.31   **Preterm newborn, gestational age 28 completed weeks**
Preterm newborn, gestational age 28 weeks, 0 days through 28 weeks, 6 days

   P07.32   **Preterm newborn, gestational age 29 completed weeks**
Preterm newborn, gestational age 29 weeks, 0 days through 29 weeks, 6 days

   P07.33   **Preterm newborn, gestational age 30 completed weeks**
Preterm newborn, gestational age 30 weeks, 0 days through 30 weeks, 6 days

   P07.34   **Preterm newborn, gestational age 31 completed weeks**
Preterm newborn, gestational age 31 weeks, 0 days through 31 weeks, 6 days

   P07.35   **Preterm newborn, gestational age 32 completed weeks**
Preterm newborn, gestational age 32 weeks, 0 days through 32 weeks, 6 days

   P07.36   **Preterm newborn, gestational age 33 completed weeks**
Preterm newborn, gestational age 33 weeks, 0 days through 33 weeks, 6 days

   P07.37   **Preterm newborn, gestational age 34 completed weeks**
Preterm newborn, gestational age 34 weeks, 0 days through 34 weeks, 6 days
Coding Clinic: 2017, Q2, P7

   P07.38   **Preterm newborn, gestational age 35 completed weeks**
Preterm newborn, gestational age 35 weeks, 0 days through 35 weeks, 6 days

   P07.39   **Preterm newborn, gestational age 36 completed weeks**
Preterm newborn, gestational age 36 weeks, 0 days through 36 weeks, 6 days

● **P08**   **Disorders of newborn related to long gestation and high birth weight**

Note: When both birth weight and gestational age of the newborn are available, priority of assignment should be given to birth weight.

   Includes   the listed conditions, without further specification, as causes of morbidity or additional care, in newborn

P08.0   **Exceptionally large newborn baby**
Usually implies a birth weight of 4500 g. or more

   Excludes1   syndrome of infant of diabetic mother (P70.1)
syndrome of infant of mother with gestational diabetes (P70.0)

P08.1   **Other heavy for gestational age newborn**
Other newborn heavy- or large-for-dates regardless of period of gestation
Usually implies a birth weight of 4000 g. to 4499 g.

   Excludes1   newborn with a birth weight of 4500 or more (P08.0)
syndrome of infant of diabetic mother (P70.1)
syndrome of infant of mother with gestational diabetes (P70.0)

N Newborn Age: 0   **P** Pediatric Age: 0–17   **M** Maternity DX: 12–55   **A** Adult Age: 15–124   ♀ Females Only   ♂ Males Only

🅒 Complication\Comorbidity   🅜 Major C\C   (Ex) CC/MCC Exclusions   🅗 Hospital-Acquired Condition   **1165**

● **P08.2**   **Late newborn, not heavy for gestational age**
   P08.21   **Post-term newborn**
     Newborn with gestation period over 40
     completed weeks to 42 completed weeks
   P08.22   **Prolonged gestation of newborn**
     Newborn with gestation period over 42
     completed weeks (294 days or more), not
     heavy- or large-for-dates
     Postmaturity NOS

ABNORMAL FINDINGS ON NEONATAL SCREENING (P09)

P09   **Abnormal findings on neonatal screening**
   Use additional code to identify signs, symptoms and conditions
   associated with the screening
   Excludes2   nonspecific serologic evidence of human
     immunodeficiency virus [HIV] (R75)

BIRTH TRAUMA (P10-P15)

● **P10**   **Intracranial laceration and hemorrhage due to birth injury**
   Excludes1   intracranial hemorrhage of newborn NOS (P52.9)
     intracranial hemorrhage of newborn due to
     anoxia or hypoxia (P52.-)
     nontraumatic intracranial hemorrhage of
     newborn (P52.-)
   (Ex:) **For category P10 CC codes unless otherwise indicated:** See PDX Collection 1020

   P10.0   **Subdural hemorrhage due to birth injury** 🔖
     Subdural hematoma (localized) due to birth injury
     Excludes1   subdural hemorrhage accompanying
       tentorial tear (P10.4)
   P10.1   **Cerebral hemorrhage due to birth injury** 🔖
   P10.2   **Intraventricular hemorrhage due to birth injury** 🔖
     (Ex:) See PDX Collection 1021
   P10.3   **Subarachnoid hemorrhage due to birth injury** 🔖
     (Ex:) See PDX Collection 1022
   P10.4   **Tentorial tear due to birth injury** 🔖
     Pertaining to tentorium of cerebellum (extension of dura
     mater that separates cerebellum from inferior portion of
     occipital lobes)
   P10.8   **Other intracranial lacerations and hemorrhages due to**
     birth injury 🔖
   P10.9   **Unspecified intracranial laceration and hemorrhage due**
     to birth injury 🔖

● **P11**   **Other birth injuries to central nervous system**
   P11.0   **Cerebral edema due to birth injury** 🔖
     (Ex:) See PDX Collection 1020
   P11.1   **Other specified brain damage due to birth injury**
   P11.2   **Unspecified brain damage due to birth injury** 🔖
     (Ex:) See PDX Collection 1020
   P11.3   **Birth injury to facial nerve**
     Facial palsy due to birth injury
   P11.4   **Birth injury to other cranial nerves**
   P11.5   **Birth injury to spine and spinal cord**
     Fracture of spine due to birth injury
   P11.9   **Birth injury to central nervous system, unspecified** 🔖
     (Ex:) See PDX Collection 1020

● **P12**   **Birth injury to scalp**
   P12.0   **Cephalhematoma due to birth injury**
   P12.1   **Chignon (from vacuum extraction) due to birth injury**
   P12.2   **Epicranial subaponeurotic hemorrhage due to birth**
     injury 🔖
     Subgaleal hemorrhage
     (Ex:) See PDX Collection 1023
   P12.3   **Bruising of scalp due to birth injury**
   P12.4   **Injury of scalp of newborn due to monitoring**
     equipment
     Sampling incision of scalp of newborn
     Scalp clip (electrode) injury of newborn

● **P12.8**   **Other birth injuries to scalp**
   P12.81   **Caput succedaneum**
   P12.89   **Other birth injuries to scalp**
   P12.9   **Birth injury to scalp, unspecified**

● **P13**   **Birth injury to skeleton**
   Excludes2   birth injury to spine (P11.5)
   P13.0   **Fracture of skull due to birth injury**
   P13.1   **Other birth injuries to skull**
     Excludes1   cephalhematoma (P12.0)
   P13.2   **Birth injury to femur**
   P13.3   **Birth injury to other long bones**
   P13.4   **Fracture of clavicle due to birth injury**
   P13.8   **Birth injuries to other parts of skeleton**
   P13.9   **Birth injury to skeleton, unspecified**

● **P14**   **Birth injury to peripheral nervous system**
   P14.0   **Erb's paralysis due to birth injury**
   P14.1   **Klumpke's paralysis due to birth injury**
   P14.2   **Phrenic nerve paralysis due to birth injury**
   P14.3   **Other brachial plexus birth injuries**
   P14.8   **Birth injuries to other parts of peripheral nervous**
     system
   P14.9   **Birth injury to peripheral nervous system, unspecified**

Item 16-1   The **peripheral nervous system** consists of 31 pairs of
spinal nerves, 12 pairs of cranial nerves, and the autonomic nerves, which
are divided into the parasympathetic and sympathetic nerves. The cranial
nerves are: olfactory (I), optic (II), oculomotor (III), trochlear (IV), trigeminal
(V), abducens (VI), facial (VII), vestibulocochlear (VIII), glossopharyngeal (IX),
vagus (X), accessory (XI), and hypoglossal (XII).

Central Nervous System
- Brain
- Spinal cord

Peripheral Nervous System
- Cranial nerves (12)
- Spinal nerves
   cervical (8)
   thoracic (12)
   lumbar (5)
   sacral (5)
   coccyx (1)

Figure 16-1   The central nervous system consists of the brain and spinal
cord. The peripheral nervous system consists of nerves that lie outside
the skull and spinal cord. (From Stoy: Mosby's EMT-Basic Textbook, ed 2,
St. Louis, Mosby, 2007)

▶ New   ⇒ Revised   ~~deleted~~ Deleted   Excludes 1   Excludes 2   Includes   Use additional   Code first   Code also   Key words
OGCR Official Guidelines   ● Unacceptable Principal Diagnosis   X Assign placeholder X   ● Use Additional Character(s)   ▌ Manifestation Code   **Coding Clinic**

● **P15   Other birth injuries**

  P15.0   Birth injury to liver
      Rupture of liver due to birth injury

  P15.1   Birth injury to spleen
      Rupture of spleen due to birth injury

  P15.2   Sternomastoid injury due to birth injury

  P15.3   Birth injury to eye
      Subconjunctival hemorrhage due to birth injury
      Traumatic glaucoma due to birth injury

  P15.4   Birth injury to face
      Facial congestion due to birth injury

  P15.5   Birth injury to external genitalia

  P15.6   Subcutaneous fat necrosis due to birth injury

  P15.8   Other specified birth injuries

  P15.9   Birth injury, unspecified

RESPIRATORY AND CARDIOVASCULAR DISORDERS SPECIFIC TO THE PERINATAL PERIOD (P19-P29)

● **P19   Metabolic acidemia in newborn**
  Includes   metabolic acidemia in newborn

  P19.0   Metabolic acidemia in newborn first noted before onset of labor

  P19.1   Metabolic acidemia in newborn first noted during labor

  P19.2   Metabolic acidemia noted at birth

  P19.9   Metabolic acidemia, unspecified

● **P22   Respiratory distress of newborn**
  Excludes1   respiratory arrest of newborn (P28.81)
      respiratory failure of newborn NOS (P28.5)

  P22.0   Respiratory distress syndrome of newborn
      Cardiorespiratory distress syndrome of newborn
      Hyaline membrane disease
      Idiopathic respiratory distress syndrome [IRDS or RDS] of newborn
      Pulmonary hypoperfusion syndrome
      Respiratory distress syndrome, type I
      (Ex) See PDX Collection 748

  P22.1   Transient tachypnea of newborn
      Idiopathic tachypnea of newborn
      Respiratory distress syndrome, type II
      Wet lung syndrome

  P22.8   Other respiratory distress of newborn

  P22.9   Respiratory distress of newborn, unspecified

● **P23   Congenital pneumonia**
  Includes   infective pneumonia acquired in utero or during birth
  Excludes1   neonatal pneumonia resulting from aspiration (P24.-)
  (Ex) For category P23 CC codes: See PDX Collection 748

  P23.0   Congenital pneumonia due to viral agent
      Use additional code (B97) to identify organism
      Excludes1   congenital rubella pneumonitis (P35.0)

  P23.1   Congenital pneumonia due to Chlamydia

  P23.2   Congenital pneumonia due to staphylococcus

  P23.3   Congenital pneumonia due to streptococcus, group B

  P23.4   Congenital pneumonia due to Escherichia coli

  P23.5   Congenital pneumonia due to Pseudomonas

  P23.6   Congenital pneumonia due to other bacterial agents
      Congenital pneumonia due to Hemophilus influenzae
      Congenital pneumonia due to Klebsiella pneumoniae
      Congenital pneumonia due to Mycoplasma
      Congenital pneumonia due to Streptococcus, except group B
      Use additional code (B95-B96) to identify organism

  P23.8   Congenital pneumonia due to other organisms

  P23.9   Congenital pneumonia, unspecified

● **P24   Neonatal aspiration**
  Includes   aspiration in utero and during delivery

● **P24.0   Meconium aspiration**
  Excludes1   meconium passage (without aspiration) during delivery (P03.82)
      meconium staining (P96.83)

  P24.00   Meconium aspiration without respiratory symptoms
      Meconium aspiration NOS

  P24.01   Meconium aspiration with respiratory symptoms
      Meconium aspiration pneumonia
      Meconium aspiration pneumonitis
      Meconium aspiration syndrome NOS
      ⟹ Use additional code to identify any secondary pulmonary hypertension, if applicable (I27.2-)
      (Ex) See PDX Collection 748

● **P24.1   Neonatal aspiration of (clear) amniotic fluid and mucus**
      Neonatal aspiration of liquor (amnii)

  P24.10   Neonatal aspiration of (clear) amniotic fluid and mucus without respiratory symptoms
      Neonatal aspiration of amniotic fluid and mucus NOS

  P24.11   Neonatal aspiration of (clear) amniotic fluid and mucus with respiratory symptoms
      Neonatal aspiration of amniotic fluid and mucus with pneumonia
      Neonatal aspiration of amniotic fluid and mucus with pneumonitis
      ⟹ Use additional code to identify any secondary pulmonary hypertension, if applicable (I27.2-)
      (Ex) See PDX Collection 748

● **P24.2   Neonatal aspiration of blood**

  P24.20   Neonatal aspiration of blood without respiratory symptoms
      Neonatal aspiration of blood NOS

  P24.21   Neonatal aspiration of blood with respiratory symptoms
      Neonatal aspiration of blood with pneumonia
      Neonatal aspiration of blood with pneumonitis
      ⟹ Use additional code to identify any secondary pulmonary hypertension, if applicable (I27.2-)
      (Ex) See PDX Collection 748

● **P24.3   Neonatal aspiration of milk and regurgitated food**
      Neonatal aspiration of stomach contents

  P24.30   Neonatal aspiration of milk and regurgitated food without respiratory symptoms
      Neonatal aspiration of milk and regurgitated food NOS

  P24.31   Neonatal aspiration of milk and regurgitated food with respiratory symptoms
      Neonatal aspiration of milk and regurgitated food with pneumonia
      Neonatal aspiration of milk and regurgitated food with pneumonitis
      ⟹ Use additional code to identify any secondary pulmonary hypertension, if applicable (I27.2-)
      (Ex) See PDX Collection 748

CHAPTER 16 (P00-P96)

● **P24.8   Other neonatal aspiration**

    P24.80   Other neonatal aspiration without respiratory symptoms
        Neonatal aspiration NEC

    P24.81   Other neonatal aspiration with respiratory symptoms 🔒
        Neonatal aspiration pneumonia NEC
        Neonatal aspiration with pneumonitis NEC
        Neonatal aspiration with pneumonia NOS
        Neonatal aspiration with pneumonitis NOS
      ⟹ Use additional code to identify any secondary pulmonary hypertension, if applicable (I27.2-)
        (Ex:) See PDX Collection 748

    P24.9   Neonatal aspiration, unspecified

● **P25   Interstitial emphysema and related conditions originating in the perinatal period**
    (Ex:) For category P25 CC codes: See PDX Collection 748

    P25.0   Interstitial emphysema originating in the perinatal period 🔒

    P25.1   Pneumothorax originating in the perinatal period 🔒

    P25.2   Pneumomediastinum originating in the perinatal period 🔒

    P25.3   Pneumopericardium originating in the perinatal period 🔒

    P25.8   Other conditions related to interstitial emphysema originating in the perinatal period 🔒

● **P26   Pulmonary hemorrhage originating in the perinatal period**
    Excludes1   acute idiopathic hemorrhage in infants over 28 days old (R04.81)
    (Ex:) For category P26 CC codes: See PDX Collection 748

    P26.0   Tracheobronchial hemorrhage originating in the perinatal period 🔒

    P26.1   Massive pulmonary hemorrhage originating in the perinatal period 🔒

    P26.8   Other pulmonary hemorrhages originating in the perinatal period 🔒

    P26.9   Unspecified pulmonary hemorrhage originating in the perinatal period 🔒

● **P27   Chronic respiratory disease originating in the perinatal period**
    ~~Excludes1   respiratory distress of newborn (P22.0-P22.9)~~
    ▶ **Excludes2**   respiratory distress of newborn (P22.0-P22.9)
    (Ex:) For category P27 CC codes: See PDX Collection 748

    P27.0   Wilson-Mikity syndrome 🔒
        Pulmonary dysmaturity

    P27.1   Bronchopulmonary dysplasia originating in the perinatal period 🔒

    P27.8   Other chronic respiratory diseases originating in the perinatal period 🔒
        Congenital pulmonary fibrosis
        Ventilator lung in newborn

    P27.9   Unspecified chronic respiratory disease originating in the perinatal period 🔒

● **P28   Other respiratory conditions originating in the perinatal period**
    Excludes1   congenital malformations of the respiratory system (Q30-Q34)

    P28.0   Primary atelectasis of newborn 🔒
        Failure of lungs to expand properly at birth
        Primary failure to expand terminal respiratory units
        Pulmonary hypoplasia associated with short gestation
        Pulmonary immaturity NOS
        (Ex:) See PDX Collection 748

● **P28.1   Other and unspecified atelectasis of newborn**
    (Ex:) For category P28.1 CC codes: See PDX Collection 748

    P28.10   Unspecified atelectasis of newborn 🔒
        Atelectasis of newborn NOS

    P28.11   Resorption atelectasis without respiratory distress syndrome 🔒
        Excludes1   resorption atelectasis with respiratory distress syndrome (P22.0)

    P28.19   Other atelectasis of newborn
        Partial atelectasis of newborn
        Secondary atelectasis of newborn

    P28.2   Cyanotic attacks of newborn 🔒
        Excludes1   apnea of newborn (P28.3-P28.4)
        (Ex:) See PDX Collection 1024

    P28.3   Primary sleep apnea of newborn 🔒
        Central sleep apnea of newborn
        Obstructive sleep apnea of newborn
        Sleep apnea of newborn NOS
        (Ex:) See PDX Collection 1025

    P28.4   Other apnea of newborn 🔒
        Apnea of prematurity
        Obstructive apnea of newborn
        Excludes1   obstructive sleep apnea of newborn (P28.3)
        (Ex:) See PDX Collection 1026

    P28.5   Respiratory failure of newborn 🔒
        Excludes1   respiratory arrest of newborn (P28.81)
                 respiratory distress of newborn (P22.0-)
        (Ex:) See PDX Collection 748

● **P28.8   Other specified respiratory conditions of newborn**
    P28.81   Respiratory arrest of newborn 🔒
        (Ex:) See PDX Collection 1027
        Coding Clinic: 2017, Q2, P6

    P28.89   Other specified respiratory conditions of newborn
        Congenital laryngeal stridor
        Sniffles in newborn
        Snuffles in newborn
        Excludes1   early congenital syphilitic rhinitis (A50.05)

    P28.9   Respiratory condition of newborn, unspecified
        Respiratory depression in newborn

● **P29   Cardiovascular disorders originating in the perinatal period**
    Excludes1   congenital malformations of the circulatory system (Q20-Q28)

    P29.0   Neonatal cardiac failure

● **P29.1   Neonatal cardiac dysrhythmia**
    P29.11   Neonatal tachycardia
    P29.12   Neonatal bradycardia

    P29.2   Neonatal hypertension

● **P29.3   Persistent fetal circulation**
    ~~Delayed closure of ductus arteriosus~~
    ~~(Persistent) pulmonary hypertension of newborn~~
    (Ex:) For category P29.3 CC codes: See PDX Collection 1028

    ▶ **P29.30   Pulmonary hypertension of newborn** 🔒
        ▶Persistent pulmonary hypertension of newborn

    ▶ **P29.38   Other persistent fetal circulation** 🔒
        ▶Delayed closure of ductus arteriosus

    P29.4   Transient myocardial ischemia in newborn

● **P29.8   Other cardiovascular disorders originating in the perinatal period**
    P29.81   Cardiac arrest of newborn 🔒
        (Ex:) See PDX Collection 1029

    P29.89   Other cardiovascular disorders originating in the perinatal period

    P29.9   Cardiovascular disorder originating in the perinatal period, unspecified

▶ New ⟹ Revised ~~deleted~~ Deleted **Excludes 1** Excludes 2 Includes Use additional Code first Code also Key words
OGCR Official Guidelines ● Unacceptable Principal Diagnosis X Assign placeholder X ● Use Additional Character(s) ▸ Manifestation Code **Coding Clinic**

INFECTIONS SPECIFIC TO THE PERINATAL PERIOD (P35-P39)

Infections acquired in utero, during birth via the umbilicus, or during the first 28 days after birth

Excludes2 asymptomatic human immunodeficiency virus [HIV] infection status (Z21)
congenital gonococcal infection (A54.-)
congenital pneumonia (P23.-)
congenital syphilis (A50.-)
human immunodeficiency virus [HIV] disease (B20)
infant botulism (A48.51)
infectious diseases not specific to the perinatal period (A00-B99, J09, J10.-)
intestinal infectious disease (A00-A09)
laboratory evidence of human immunodeficiency virus [HIV] (R75)
tetanus neonatorum (A33)

● **P35   Congenital viral diseases**

Includes infections acquired in utero or during birth

(Ex) For category P35 CC codes unless otherwise indicated: See PDX Collection 562

P35.0   Congenital rubella syndrome 🔖
Congenital rubella pneumonitis
(Ex) See PDX Collection 1030

P35.1   Congenital cytomegalovirus infection 🔖
Viruses transmitted by multiple routes that cause mild/ subclinical infection
(Ex) See PDX Collection 1030

P35.2   Congenital herpesviral [herpes simplex] infection 🔖

P35.3   Congenital viral hepatitis 🔖

P35.8   Other congenital viral diseases 🔖
Congenital varicella [chickenpox]
Coding Clinic: 2016, Q4, P7

P35.9   Congenital viral disease, unspecified 🔖

● **P36   Bacterial sepsis of newborn**

Includes congenital sepsis

Use additional code(s), if applicable, to identify severe sepsis (R65.2-) and associated acute organ dysfunction(s)
(Ex) For category P36 CC codes: See PDX Collection 1031

P36.0   Sepsis of newborn due to streptococcus, group B 🔖

● **P36.1   Sepsis of newborn due to other and unspecified streptococci**

P36.10   Sepsis of newborn due to unspecified streptococci 🔖

P36.19   Sepsis of newborn due to other streptococci 🔖

P36.2   Sepsis of newborn due to Staphylococcus aureus 🔖

● **P36.3   Sepsis of newborn due to other and unspecified staphylococci**

P36.30   Sepsis of newborn due to unspecified staphylococci 🔖

P36.39   Sepsis of newborn due to other staphylococci 🔖

P36.4   Sepsis of newborn due to Escherichia coli 🔖

P36.5   Sepsis of newborn due to anaerobes 🔖

P36.8   Other bacterial sepsis of newborn 🔖
Use additional code from category B96 to identify organism

P36.9   Bacterial sepsis of newborn, unspecified 🔖

● **P37   Other congenital infectious and parasitic diseases**

Excludes2 congenital syphilis (A50.-)
infectious neonatal diarrhea (A00-A09)
necrotizing enterocolitis in newborn (P77.-)
noninfectious neonatal diarrhea (P78.3)
ophthalmia neonatorum due to gonococcus (A54.31)
tetanus neonatorum (A33)

(Ex) For category P37 CC codes: See PDX Collection 562

P37.0   Congenital tuberculosis 🔖

P37.1   Congenital toxoplasmosis 🔖
Parasitic infection, often causing mild flu-like illness
Hydrocephalus due to congenital toxoplasmosis

P37.2   Neonatal (disseminated) listeriosis 🔖
Acquired transplacentally or during/after parturition in which symptoms are those of sepsis

P37.3   Congenital falciparum malaria 🔖

P37.4   Other congenital malaria 🔖

P37.5   Neonatal candidiasis 🔖

P37.8   Other specified congenital infectious and parasitic diseases 🔖

P37.9   Congenital infectious or parasitic disease, unspecified 🔖

● **P38   Omphalitis of newborn**
Inflammation of umbilicus

Excludes1 omphalitis not of newborn (L08.82)
tetanus omphalitis (A33)
umbilical hemorrhage of newborn (P51.-)

(Ex) For category P38 CC codes: See PDX Collection 1032

P38.1   Omphalitis with mild hemorrhage 🔖

P38.9   Omphalitis without hemorrhage 🔖
Omphalitis of newborn NOS

● **P39   Other infections specific to the perinatal period**

Use additional code to identify organism or specific infection
(Ex) For category P39 CC codes unless otherwise indicated: See PDX Collection 1033

P39.0   Neonatal infective mastitis 🔖

Excludes1 breast engorgement of newborn (P83.4)
noninfective mastitis of newborn (P83.4)

(Ex) See PDX Collection 1032

P39.1   Neonatal conjunctivitis and dacryocystitis
Neonatal chlamydial conjunctivitis
Ophthalmia neonatorum NOS
Neonate = newborn

Excludes1 gonococcal conjunctivitis (A54.31)

P39.2   Intra-amniotic infection affecting newborn, not elsewhere classified 🔖

P39.3   Neonatal urinary tract infection 🔖
(Ex) See PDX Collection 1034

P39.4   Neonatal skin infection 🔖
Neonatal pyoderma

Excludes1 pemphigus neonatorum (L00)
staphylococcal scalded skin syndrome (L00)

P39.8   Other specified infections specific to the perinatal period 🔖

P39.9   Infection specific to the perinatal period, unspecified 🔖

CHAPTER 16 (P00-P96)

N Newborn Age: 0   P Pediatric Age: 0–17   M Maternity DX: 12–55   A Adult Age: 15–124   ♀ Females Only   ♂ Males Only

🔖 Complication\Comorbidity   🔖 Major C\C   (Ex) CC/MCC Exclusions   🔖 Hospital-Acquired Condition

HEMORRHAGIC AND HEMATOLOGICAL DISORDERS OF NEWBORN (P50-P61)

> **Excludes1**   congenital stenosis and stricture of bile ducts
> (Q44.3)
> Crigler-Najjar syndrome (E80.5)
> Dubin-Johnson syndrome (E80.6)
> Gilbert syndrome (E80.4)
> hereditary hemolytic anemias (D55-D58)

● **P50**   Newborn affected by intrauterine (fetal) blood loss

> **Excludes1**   congenital anemia from intrauterine (fetal) blood
> loss (P61.3)

P50.0   Newborn affected by intrauterine (fetal) blood loss from vasa previa

P50.1   Newborn affected by intrauterine (fetal) blood loss from ruptured cord

P50.2   Newborn affected by intrauterine (fetal) blood loss from placenta

P50.3   Newborn affected by hemorrhage into co-twin

P50.4   Newborn affected by hemorrhage into maternal circulation

P50.5   Newborn affected by intrauterine (fetal) blood loss from cut end of co-twin's cord

P50.8   Newborn affected by other intrauterine (fetal) blood loss

P50.9   Newborn affected by intrauterine (fetal) blood loss, unspecified
Newborn affected by fetal hemorrhage NOS

● **P51**   Umbilical hemorrhage of newborn

> **Excludes1**   omphalitis with mild hemorrhage (P38.1)
> umbilical hemorrhage from cut end of co-twins
> cord (P50.5)

P51.0   Massive umbilical hemorrhage of newborn

P51.8   Other umbilical hemorrhages of newborn
Slipped umbilical ligature NOS

P51.9   Umbilical hemorrhage of newborn, unspecified

● **P52**   Intracranial nontraumatic hemorrhage of newborn

> **Includes**   intracranial hemorrhage due to anoxia or hypoxia
> **Excludes1**   intracranial hemorrhage due to birth injury
> (P10.-)
> intracranial hemorrhage due to other injury
> (S06.-)

P52.0   Intraventricular (nontraumatic) hemorrhage, grade 1, of newborn 🔖
Subependymal hemorrhage (without intraventricular extension)
Bleeding into germinal matrix
(Ex:) See PDX Collection 1021

P52.1   Intraventricular (nontraumatic) hemorrhage, grade 2, of newborn 🔖
Subependymal hemorrhage with intraventricular extension
Bleeding into ventricle
(Ex:) See PDX Collection 1021

● **P52.2**   Intraventricular (nontraumatic) hemorrhage, grade 3 and grade 4, of newborn

P52.21   Intraventricular (nontraumatic) hemorrhage, grade 3, of newborn 🔖
Subependymal hemorrhage with intraventricular extension with enlargement of ventricle
(Ex:) See PDX Collection 1021

P52.22   Intraventricular (nontraumatic) hemorrhage, grade 4, of newborn 🔖
Bleeding into cerebral cortex
Subependymal hemorrhage with intracerebral extension
(Ex:) See PDX Collection 1021

P52.3   Unspecified intraventricular (nontraumatic) hemorrhage of newborn 🔖
(Ex:) See PDX Collection 1021

P52.4   Intracerebral (nontraumatic) hemorrhage of newborn 🔖
(Ex:) See PDX Collection 1020

P52.5   Subarachnoid (nontraumatic) hemorrhage of newborn 🔖
(Ex:) See PDX Collection 1022

P52.6   Cerebellar (nontraumatic) and posterior fossa hemorrhage of newborn 🔖
(Ex:) See PDX Collection 1020

P52.8   Other intracranial (nontraumatic) hemorrhages of newborn 🔖
(Ex:) See PDX Collection 1020

P52.9   Intracranial (nontraumatic) hemorrhage of newborn, unspecified 🔖
(Ex:) See PDX Collection 1020

● **P53**   Hemorrhagic disease of newborn 🔖
Vitamin K deficiency of newborn
(Ex:) See PDX Collection 1035

● **P54**   Other neonatal hemorrhages

> **Excludes1**   newborn affected by (intrauterine) blood loss
> (P50.-)
> pulmonary hemorrhage originating in the
> perinatal period (P26.-)

P54.0   Neonatal hematemesis
Vomiting of blood

> **Excludes1**   neonatal hematemesis due to swallowed
> maternal blood (P78.2)

P54.1   Neonatal melena 🔖
Dark-colored feces stained with blood pigments

> **Excludes1**   neonatal melena due to swallowed
> maternal blood (P78.2)

(Ex:) See PDX Collection 1036

P54.2   Neonatal rectal hemorrhage 🔖
(Ex:) See PDX Collection 1036

P54.3   Other neonatal gastrointestinal hemorrhage 🔖
(Ex:) See PDX Collection 1036

P54.4   Neonatal adrenal hemorrhage 🔖
(Ex:) See PDX Collection 1036

P54.5   Neonatal cutaneous hemorrhage
Neonatal bruising
Neonatal ecchymoses
Neonatal petechiae
Neonatal superficial hematomata

> **Excludes2**   bruising of scalp due to birth injury
> (P12.3)
> cephalhematoma due to birth injury
> (P12.0)

P54.6   Neonatal vaginal hemorrhage ♀
Neonatal pseudomenses

P54.8   Other specified neonatal hemorrhages

P54.9   Neonatal hemorrhage, unspecified

● **P55**   Hemolytic disease of newborn
*AKA erythroblastosis fetalis and is due to Rh isoimmunization,
result of Rh blood factor incompatibilities between mother (Rh
negative) and fetus (Rh positive)*

P55.0   Rh isoimmunization of newborn

P55.1   ABO isoimmunization of newborn
Coding Clinic: 2015, Q3, P20

P55.8   Other hemolytic diseases of newborn

P55.9   Hemolytic disease of newborn, unspecified

● **P56   Hydrops fetalis due to hemolytic disease**
Caused by maternal sensitization to fetal blood group antigen
> **Excludes1**   hydrops fetalis NOS (P83.2)
> (Ex) For category P56 CC codes: See PDX Collection 1037

   P56.0   Hydrops fetalis due to isoimmunization 🔖

● **P56.9   Hydrops fetalis due to other and unspecified hemolytic disease**

   P56.90   Hydrops fetalis due to unspecified hemolytic disease 🔖

   P56.99   Hydrops fetalis due to other hemolytic disease 🔖

● **P57   Kernicterus**
High levels of bilirubin in blood, with severe neural symptoms
(Ex) For category P57 CC codes unless otherwise indicated: See PDX Collection 1038

   P57.0   Kernicterus due to isoimmunization 🔖
   (Ex) See PDX Collection 1037

   P57.8   Other specified kernicterus 🔖
   > **Excludes1**   Crigler-Najjar syndrome (E80.5)

   P57.9   Kernicterus, unspecified 🔖

● **P58   Neonatal jaundice due to other excessive hemolysis**
> **Excludes1**   jaundice due to isoimmunization (P55-P57)

   P58.0   Neonatal jaundice due to bruising
   P58.1   Neonatal jaundice due to bleeding
   P58.2   Neonatal jaundice due to infection
   P58.3   Neonatal jaundice due to polycythemia

● **P58.4   Neonatal jaundice due to drugs or toxins transmitted from mother or given to newborn**
   Code first poisoning due to drug or toxin, if applicable (T36-T65 with fifth or sixth character 1-4 or 6)
   Use additional code for adverse effect, if applicable, to identify drug (T36-T50 with fifth or sixth character 5)

   ● **P58.41   Neonatal jaundice due to drugs or toxins transmitted from mother**

   ● **P58.42   Neonatal jaundice due to drugs or toxins given to newborn**

   P58.5   Neonatal jaundice due to swallowed maternal blood
   P58.8   Neonatal jaundice due to other specified excessive hemolysis
   P58.9   Neonatal jaundice due to excessive hemolysis, unspecified

● **P59   Neonatal jaundice from other and unspecified causes**
> **Excludes1**   jaundice due to inborn errors of metabolism (E70-E88)
> kernicterus (P57.-)

   P59.0   Neonatal jaundice associated with preterm delivery
   Hyperbilirubinemia of prematurity
   Jaundice due to delayed conjugation associated with preterm delivery

   P59.1   Inspissated bile syndrome 🔖
   (Ex) See PDX Collection 1038

● **P59.2   Neonatal jaundice from other and unspecified hepatocellular damage**
   > **Excludes1**   congenital viral hepatitis (P35.3)
   > (Ex) For category P59.2 CC codes unless otherwise indicated: See PDX Collection 1038

   P59.20   Neonatal jaundice from unspecified hepatocellular damage 🔖

   P59.29   Neonatal jaundice from other hepatocellular damage 🔖
   Neonatal giant cell hepatitis
   Neonatal (idiopathic) hepatitis

   P59.3   Neonatal jaundice from breast milk inhibitor
   P59.8   Neonatal jaundice from other specified causes
   P59.9   Neonatal jaundice, unspecified
   Neonatal physiological jaundice (intense)(prolonged) NOS
   Coding Clinic: 2015, Q3, P20

P60   Disseminated intravascular coagulation of newborn 🔖
   Defibrination syndrome of newborn
   (Ex) See PDX Collection 1035

● **P61   Other perinatal hematological disorders**
> **Excludes1**   transient hypogammaglobulinemia of infancy (D80.7)

   P61.0   Transient neonatal thrombocytopenia 🔖
   Lack of sufficient numbers of circulating thrombocytes (platelets)
   Neonatal thrombocytopenia due to exchange transfusion
   Neonatal thrombocytopenia due to idiopathic maternal thrombocytopenia
   Neonatal thrombocytopenia due to isoimmunization
   (Ex) See PDX Collection 1035

   P61.1   Polycythemia neonatorum
   Neonate = newborn

   P61.2   Anemia of prematurity 🔖
   (Ex) See PDX Collection 1039

   P61.3   Congenital anemia from fetal blood loss 🔖
   (Ex) See PDX Collection 1039

   P61.4   Other congenital anemias, not elsewhere classified 🔖
   Congenital anemia NOS
   (Ex) See PDX Collection 1039

   P61.5   Transient neonatal neutropenia 🔖
   Low levels of granulocytic neutrophilic white blood cells
   > **Excludes1**   congenital neutropenia (nontransient) (D70.0)
   (Ex) See PDX Collection 1040

   P61.6   Other transient neonatal disorders of coagulation 🔖
   (Ex) See PDX Collection 1035

   P61.8   Other specified perinatal hematological disorders
   P61.9   Perinatal hematological disorder, unspecified

TRANSITORY ENDOCRINE AND METABOLIC DISORDERS SPECIFIC TO NEWBORN (P70-P74)

> **Includes**   transitory endocrine and metabolic disturbances caused by the infant's response to maternal endocrine and metabolic factors, or its adjustment to extrauterine environment

● **P70   Transitory disorders of carbohydrate metabolism specific to newborn**

   P70.0   Syndrome of infant of mother with gestational diabetes
   Newborn (with hypoglycemia) affected by maternal gestational diabetes
   > **Excludes1**   newborn (with hypoglycemia) affected by maternal (pre-existing) diabetes mellitus (P70.1)
   > syndrome of infant of a diabetic mother (P70.1)

   P70.1   Syndrome of infant of a diabetic mother
   Newborn (with hypoglycemia) affected by maternal (pre-existing) diabetes mellitus
   > **Excludes1**   newborn (with hypoglycemia) affected by maternal gestational diabetes (P70.0)
   > syndrome of infant of mother with gestational diabetes (P70.0)

   P70.2   Neonatal diabetes mellitus 🔖
   (Ex) See PDX Collection 1041

   P70.3   Iatrogenic neonatal hypoglycemia
   P70.4   Other neonatal hypoglycemia
   Transitory neonatal hypoglycemia

   P70.8   Other transitory disorders of carbohydrate metabolism of newborn 🔖
   (Ex) See PDX Collection 1042

   P70.9   Transitory disorder of carbohydrate metabolism of newborn, unspecified

CHAPTER 16 (P00-P96)

P71 Transitory neonatal disorders of calcium and magnesium metabolism
> (Ex) For category P71 CC codes: See PDX Collection 1041

P71.0 Cow's milk hypocalcemia in newborn 🔖

P71.1 Other neonatal hypocalcemia 🔖
> **Excludes1** neonatal hypoparathyroidism (P71.4)

P71.2 Neonatal hypomagnesemia 🔖

P71.3 Neonatal tetany without calcium or magnesium deficiency 🔖
> Neonatal tetany NOS

P71.4 Transitory neonatal hypoparathyroidism 🔖

P71.8 Other transitory neonatal disorders of calcium and magnesium metabolism 🔖
> **Coding Clinic: 2016, Q4, P55**

P71.9 Transitory neonatal disorder of calcium and magnesium metabolism, unspecified 🔖

P72 Other transitory neonatal endocrine disorders
> **Excludes1** congenital hypothyroidism with or without goiter (E03.0-E03.1)
> dyshormonogenetic goiter (E07.1)
> Pendred's syndrome (E07.1)
> (Ex) For category P72 CC codes unless otherwise noted: See PDX Collection 1042

P72.0 Neonatal goiter, not elsewhere classified 🔖
> Transitory congenital goiter with normal functioning

P72.1 Transitory neonatal hyperthyroidism 🔖
> Neonatal thyrotoxicosis
> (Ex) See PDX Collection 1041

P72.2 Other transitory neonatal disorders of thyroid function, not elsewhere classified 🔖
> Transitory neonatal hypothyroidism

P72.8 Other specified transitory neonatal endocrine disorders 🔖

P72.9 Transitory neonatal endocrine disorder, unspecified

P74 Other transitory neonatal electrolyte and metabolic disturbances

P74.0 Late metabolic acidosis of newborn 🔖
> **Excludes1** (fetal) metabolic acidosis of newborn (P19)
> (Ex) See PDX Collection 1041

P74.1 Dehydration of newborn

P74.2 Disturbances of sodium balance of newborn

P74.3 Disturbances of potassium balance of newborn

P74.4 Other transitory electrolyte disturbances of newborn

P74.5 Transitory tyrosinemia of newborn 🔖
> (Ex) See PDX Collection 1042

P74.6 Transitory hyperammonemia of newborn 🔖
> (Ex) See PDX Collection 1042

P74.8 Other transitory metabolic disturbances of newborn 🔖
> Amino-acid metabolic disorders described as transitory
> (Ex) See PDX Collection 1042

P74.9 Transitory metabolic disturbance of newborn, unspecified

DIGESTIVE SYSTEM DISORDERS OF NEWBORN (P76-P78)

P76 Other intestinal obstruction of newborn

P76.0 Meconium plug syndrome
> *Fetal stool obstruction in large intestine, present at birth; may be symptom of organic disease.*
> Meconium ileus NOS
> **Excludes1** meconium ileus in cystic fibrosis (E84.11)

P76.1 Transitory ileus of newborn 🔖
> *Temporary obstruction of ileus (small intestine)*
> **Excludes1** Hirschsprung's disease (Q43.1)
> (Ex) See PDX Collection 1043

P76.2 Intestinal obstruction due to inspissated milk
> *Being thickened, dried, or made less fluid*

P76.8 Other specified intestinal obstruction of newborn
> **Excludes1** intestinal obstruction classifiable to K56.-

P76.9 Intestinal obstruction of newborn, unspecified

P77 Necrotizing enterocolitis of newborn
> (Ex) For category P77 CC codes: See PDX Collection 1044

P77.1 Stage 1 necrotizing enterocolitis in newborn 🔖
> Necrotizing enterocolitis without pneumatosis, without perforation

P77.2 Stage 2 necrotizing enterocolitis in newborn 🔖
> Necrotizing enterocolitis with pneumatosis, without perforation

P77.3 Stage 3 necrotizing enterocolitis in newborn 🔖
> Necrotizing enterocolitis with perforation
> Necrotizing enterocolitis with pneumatosis and perforation

P77.9 Necrotizing enterocolitis in newborn, unspecified 🔖
> Necrotizing enterocolitis in newborn, NOS

P78 Other perinatal digestive system disorders
> **Excludes1** cystic fibrosis (E84.0-E84.9)
> neonatal gastrointestinal hemorrhages (P54.0-P54.3)

P78.0 Perinatal intestinal perforation 🔖
> Meconium peritonitis
> (Ex) See PDX Collection 1044

P78.1 Other neonatal peritonitis
> Neonatal peritonitis NOS

P78.2 Neonatal hematemesis and melena due to swallowed maternal blood

P78.3 Noninfective neonatal diarrhea
> Neonatal diarrhea NOS

P78.8 Other specified perinatal digestive system disorders

P78.81 Congenital cirrhosis (of liver)

P78.82 Peptic ulcer of newborn

P78.83 Newborn esophageal reflux
> Neonatal esophageal reflux

▶ **P78.84 Gestational alloimmune liver disease**
> ▶GALD
> ▶Neonatal hemochromatosis
> ▶ **Excludes1** hemochromatosis (E83.11-)

P78.89 Other specified perinatal digestive system disorders

P78.9 Perinatal digestive system disorder, unspecified

▶ New   ⟹ Revised   ~~deleted~~ Deleted   Excludes 1   Excludes 2   Includes   Use additional   Code first   Code also   Key words
OGCR Official Guidelines   ● Unacceptable Principal Diagnosis   X Assign placeholder X   ● Use Additional Character(s)   ▶ Manifestation Code   **Coding Clinic**

CONDITIONS INVOLVING THE INTEGUMENT AND TEMPERATURE REGULATION OF NEWBORN (P80-P83)

● P80   **Hypothermia of newborn**

P80.0   **Cold injury syndrome**
Severe and usually chronic hypothermia associated with a pink flushed appearance, edema and neurological and biochemical abnormalities.

Excludes1   mild hypothermia of newborn (P80.8)

P80.8   **Other hypothermia of newborn**
Mild hypothermia of newborn

P80.9   **Hypothermia of newborn, unspecified**

● P81   **Other disturbances of temperature regulation of newborn**

P81.0   **Environmental hyperthermia of newborn**

P81.8   **Other specified disturbances of temperature regulation of newborn**

P81.9   **Disturbance of temperature regulation of newborn, unspecified**
Fever of newborn NOS

● P83   **Other conditions of integument specific to newborn**

Excludes1   congenital malformations of skin and integument (Q80-Q84)
hydrops fetalis due to hemolytic disease (P56.-)
neonatal skin infection (P39.4)
staphylococcal scalded skin syndrome (L00)

Excludes2   cradle cap (L21.0)
diaper [napkin] dermatitis (L22)

P83.0   **Sclerema neonatorum** 🅒
Neonate = newborn
(Ex) See PDX Collection 1045

P83.1   **Neonatal erythema toxicum**
Benign, generalized, transient pustules that become firm vesicles

P83.2   **Hydrops fetalis not due to hemolytic disease** 🅒
Severe, life-threatening problem of severe edema (swelling) as result of too much fluid leaving blood and entering tissue
Hydrops fetalis NOS
(Ex) See PDX Collection 1046

● P83.3   **Other and unspecified edema specific to newborn**
(Ex) For category P83.3 CC codes: See PDX Collection 1047

P83.30   **Unspecified edema specific to newborn** 🅒

P83.39   **Other edema specific to newborn** 🅒

P83.4   **Breast engorgement of newborn**
Noninfective mastitis of newborn

P83.5   **Congenital hydrocele** ♂

P83.6   **Umbilical polyp of newborn**

● P83.8   **Other specified conditions of integument specific to newborn**
~~Bronze baby syndrome~~
~~Neonatal scleroderma~~
~~Urticaria neonatorum~~

▶ P83.81   **Umbilical granuloma**
▶ **Excludes2**   Granulomatous disorder of the skin and subcutaneous tissue, unspecified (L92.9)

▶ P83.88   **Other specified conditions of integument specific to newborn**
▶Bronze baby syndrome
▶Neonatal scleroderma
▶Urticaria neonatorum

P83.9   **Condition of the integument specific to newborn, unspecified**

OTHER PROBLEMS WITH NEWBORN (P84)

P84   **Other problems with newborn**
Acidemia of newborn
Acidosis of newborn
Anoxia of newborn NOS
Asphyxia of newborn NOS
Hypercapnia of newborn
Hypoxemia of newborn
Hypoxia of newborn NOS
Mixed metabolic and respiratory acidosis of newborn

Excludes1   intracranial hemorrhage due to anoxia or hypoxia (P52.-)
hypoxic ischemic encephalopathy [HIE] (P91.6-)
late metabolic acidosis of newborn (P74.0)

OTHER DISORDERS ORIGINATING IN THE PERINATAL PERIOD (P90-P96)

● P90   **Convulsions of newborn** 🅒

Excludes1   benign myoclonic epilepsy in infancy (G40.3-)
benign neonatal convulsions (familial) (G40.3-)
(Ex) See PDX Collection 1048

● P91   **Other disturbances of cerebral status of newborn**

P91.0   **Neonatal cerebral ischemia** 🅒
(Ex) See PDX Collection 1049

P91.1   **Acquired periventricular cysts of newborn** 🅒
(Ex) See PDX Collection 1049

P91.2   **Neonatal cerebral leukomalacia** 🅒
Degeneration of white matter adjacent to cerebral ventricles following cerebral hypoxia or brain ischemia in neonates
Periventricular leukomalacia
(Ex) See PDX Collection 1022

P91.3   **Neonatal cerebral irritability** 🅒
(Ex) See PDX Collection 1049

P91.4   **Neonatal cerebral depression** 🅒
(Ex) See PDX Collection 1049

P91.5   **Neonatal coma** 🅒
(Ex) See PDX Collection 1049

● P91.6   **Hypoxic ischemic encephalopathy [HIE]**
▶ **Excludes1**   Neonatal cerebral depression (P91.4)
▶Neonatal cerebral irritability (P91.3)
▶Neonatal coma (P91.5)
(Ex) For category P91.6 CC codes: See PDX Collection 1050

P91.60   **Hypoxic ischemic encephalopathy [HIE], unspecified** 🅒

P91.61   **Mild hypoxic ischemic encephalopathy [HIE]** 🅒

P91.62   **Moderate hypoxic ischemic encephalopathy [HIE]** 🅒

P91.63   **Severe hypoxic ischemic encephalopathy [HIE]** 🅒

● P91.8   **Other specified disturbances of cerebral status of newborn**

▶● P91.81   **Neonatal encephalopathy**

▶▶ *P91.811   Neonatal encephalopathy in diseases classified elsewhere*
▶ *Code first underlying condition, if known, such as:*
▶congenital cirrhosis (of liver) (P78.71)
▶intracranial nontraumatic hemorrhage of newborn (P52.-)
▶kernicterus (P57.-)

▶ P91.819   **Neonatal encephalopathy, unspecified**

▶ P91.88   **Other specified disturbances of cerebral status of newborn**

P91.9   **Disturbance of cerebral status of newborn, unspecified**

N Newborn Age: 0   **P** Pediatric Age: 0–17   **M** Maternity DX: 12–55   **A** Adult Age: 15–124   ♀ Females Only   ♂ Males Only
🅒 Complication\Comorbidity   Major C\C   (Ex) CC/MCC Exclusions   Hospital-Acquired Condition

1173

P92   Feeding problems of newborn

> **Excludes1** ▶eating disorders (F50.-)
>   feeding problems in child over 28 days old
>   (R63.3)
> **Coding Clinic: 2017, Q1, P28; 2016, Q3, P19**

P92.0   Vomiting of newborn

> **Excludes1**   vomiting of child over 28 days old (R11.-)

P92.01   Bilious vomiting of newborn 🔖

> **Excludes1**   bilious vomiting in child over
>   28 days old (R11.14)
> (Ex:) See PDX Collection 1051

P92.09   Other vomiting of newborn

> **Excludes1**   regurgitation of food in newborn
>   (P92.1)

P92.1   Regurgitation and rumination of newborn

P92.2   Slow feeding of newborn

P92.3   Underfeeding of newborn

P92.4   Overfeeding of newborn

P92.5   Neonatal difficulty in feeding at breast
> **Coding Clinic: 2017, Q1, P28; 2016, Q3, P19**

P92.6   Failure to thrive in newborn

> **Excludes1**   failure to thrive in child over 28 days old
>   (R62.51)

P92.8   Other feeding problems of newborn

P92.9   Feeding problem of newborn, unspecified

P93   Reactions and intoxications due to drugs administered to newborn

> **Includes**   reactions and intoxications due to drugs
>   administered to fetus affecting newborn

> **Excludes1**   jaundice due to drugs or toxins transmitted from
>   mother or given to newborn (P58.4-)
>   reactions and intoxications from maternal
>   opiates, tranquilizers and other medication
>   (P04.0-P04.1, P04.4)
>   withdrawal symptoms from maternal use of
>   drugs of addiction (P96.1)
>   withdrawal symptoms from therapeutic use of
>   drugs in newborn (P96.2)
> (Ex:) For category P93 CC codes: See PDX Collection 1052

P93.0   Grey baby syndrome 🔖
>   Grey syndrome from chloramphenicol administration
>   in newborn

P93.8   Other reactions and intoxications due to drugs administered to newborn 🔖

>   Use additional code for adverse effect, if applicable,
>   to identify drug (T36-T50 with fifth or sixth
>   character 5)

P94   Disorders of muscle tone of newborn

P94.0   Transient neonatal myasthenia gravis 🔖

> **Excludes1**   myasthenia gravis (G70.0)
> (Ex:) See PDX Collection 1041

P94.1   Congenital hypertonia

P94.2   Congenital hypotonia
>   Floppy baby syndrome, unspecified

P94.8   Other disorders of muscle tone of newborn

P94.9   Disorder of muscle tone of newborn, unspecified

OGCR Section I.C.16.g.

Stillbirth

Code P95, Stillbirth, is only for use for institutions that maintain
separate records for stillbirths. No other code should be used with P95.
Code P95 should not be used on the mother's record.

P95   Stillbirth
>   Deadborn fetus NOS
>   Fetal death of unspecified cause
>   Stillbirth NOS

> **Excludes1**   maternal care for intrauterine death (O36.4)
>   missed abortion (O02.1)
>   outcome of delivery, stillbirth (Z37.1, Z37.3,
>   Z37.4, Z37.7)

P96   Other conditions originating in the perinatal period

P96.0   Congenital renal failure
>   Uremia of newborn

P96.1   Neonatal withdrawal symptoms from maternal use of drugs of addiction 🔖
>   Drug withdrawal syndrome in infant of dependent
>   mother
>   Neonatal abstinence syndrome

> **Excludes1**   reactions and intoxications from
>   maternal opiates and tranquilizers
>   administered during labor and
>   delivery (P04.0)
> (Ex:) See PDX Collection 1052

P96.2   Withdrawal symptoms from therapeutic use of drugs in newborn 🔖
> (Ex:) See PDX Collection 1052

P96.3   Wide cranial sutures of newborn
>   Neonatal craniotabes

P96.5   Complication to newborn due to (fetal) intrauterine procedure

> **Excludes2**   newborn affected by amniocentesis
>   (P00.6)

P96.8   Other specified conditions originating in the perinatal period

P96.81   Exposure to (parental) (environmental) tobacco smoke in the perinatal period

> **Excludes2**   newborn affected by in utero
>   exposure to tobacco (P04.2)
>   exposure to environmental
>   tobacco smoke after the
>   perinatal period (Z77.22)

P96.82   Delayed separation of umbilical cord

P96.83   Meconium staining

> **Excludes1**   meconium aspiration (P24.00,
>   P24.01)
>   meconium passage during
>   delivery (P03.82)

P96.89   Other specified conditions originating in the perinatal period
>   Use additional code to specify condition

P96.9   Condition originating in the perinatal period, unspecified
>   Congenital debility NOS

CHAPTER 16 (P00-P96)

▶ New   ⇒ Revised   ~~deleted~~ Deleted   Excludes 1   Excludes 2   Includes   Use additional   Code first   Code also   Key words
OGCR Official Guidelines   ● Unacceptable Principal Diagnosis   X Assign placeholder X   ● Use Additional Character(s)   ▌ Manifestation Code   **Coding Clinic**

CHAPTER 17

CONGENITAL MALFORMATIONS, DEFORMATIONS AND CHROMOSOMAL ABNORMALITIES (Q00-Q99)

OGCR Chapter-Specific Coding Guidelines

17. **Chapter 17: Congenital malformations, deformations, and chromosomal abnormalities (Q00-Q99)**

Assign an appropriate code(s) from categories Q00-Q99, Congenital malformations, deformations, and chromosomal abnormalities when a malformation/deformation or chromosomal abnormality is documented. A malformation/deformation/ or chromosomal abnormality may be the principal/first-listed diagnosis on a record or a secondary diagnosis.

When a malformation/deformation/or chromosomal abnormality does not have a unique code assignment, assign additional code(s) for any manifestations that may be present.

When the code assignment specifically identifies the malformation/deformation/or chromosomal abnormality, manifestations that are an inherent component of the anomaly should not be coded separately. Additional codes should be assigned for manifestations that are not an inherent component.

Codes from Chapter 17 may be used throughout the life of the patient. If a congenital malformation or deformity has been corrected, a personal history code should be used to identify the history of the malformation or deformity. Although present at birth, malformation/deformation/or chromosomal abnormality may not be identified until later in life. Whenever the condition is diagnosed by the physician, it is appropriate to assign a code from codes Q00-Q99.

For the birth admission, the appropriate code from category Z38, Liveborn infants, according to place of birth and type of delivery, should be sequenced as the principal diagnosis, followed by any congenital anomaly codes, Q00-Q99.

CHAPTER 17

CONGENITAL MALFORMATIONS, DEFORMATIONS AND CHROMOSOMAL ABNORMALITIES (Q00-Q99)

Note: Codes from this chapter are not for use on maternal or fetal records

Excludes2 inborn errors of metabolism (E70-E88)

This chapter contains the following blocks:

Q00-Q07	Congenital malformations of the nervous system
Q10-Q18	Congenital malformations of eye, ear, face and neck
Q20-Q28	Congenital malformations of the circulatory system
Q30-Q34	Congenital malformations of the respiratory system
Q35-Q37	Cleft lip and cleft palate
Q38-Q45	Other congenital malformations of the digestive system
Q50-Q56	Congenital malformations of genital organs
Q60-Q64	Congenital malformations of the urinary system
Q65-Q79	Congenital malformations and deformations of the musculoskeletal system
Q80-Q89	Other congenital malformations
Q90-Q99	Chromosomal abnormalities, not elsewhere classified

Figure 17-1 An infant with a large occipital encephalocele. The large skin-covered encephalocele is visible. (From Swaiman KF, Ashwal S, Ferriero DM: Pediatric Neurology: Principles and Practice, Philadelphia, Saunders, 2012)

CONGENITAL MALFORMATIONS OF THE NERVOUS SYSTEM (Q00–Q07)

● **Q00 Anencephaly and similar malformations**
Ⓔⓧ **For category Q00 CC codes:** See PDX Collection 1053

Q00.0 Anencephaly 🔖
Absence of skull with cerebral hemispheres missing or reduced to small masses attached to base of cranium
Acephaly
Acrania
Amyelencephaly
Hemianencephaly
Hemicephaly

Q00.1 Craniorachischisis 🔖
Developmental anomaly consisting of fissure of cranium and vertebral column

Q00.2 Iniencephaly 🔖
Developmental anomaly characterized by enlargement of foramen magnum and absence of laminae and spinous processes of cervical, dorsal

● **Q01 Encephalocele**
Sac-like protrusions of brain and membranes visible through an opening in skull

Includes	Arnold-Chiari syndrome, type III
	encephalocystocele
	encephalomyelocele
	hydroencephalocele
	hydromeningocele, cranial
	meningocele, cerebral
	meningoencephalocele
Excludes1	Meckel-Gruber syndrome (Q61.9)

Ⓔⓧ **For category Q01 CC codes:** See PDX Collection 1054

Q01.0 Frontal encephalocele 🔖
Q01.1 Nasofrontal encephalocele 🔖
Q01.2 Occipital encephalocele 🔖
Q01.8 Encephalocele of other sites 🔖
Q01.9 Encephalocele, unspecified 🔖

● **Q02 Microcephaly**
Head size measures significantly below normal based on standardized charts

Includes	hydromicrocephaly
	micrencephalon
Excludes1	Meckel-Gruber syndrome (Q61.9)

Coding Clinic: 2016, Q4, P7

● **Q03 Congenital hydrocephalus**
Accumulation of cerebrospinal fluid in ventricles resulting in swelling and enlargement

Includes	hydrocephalus in newborn
Excludes1	Arnold-Chiari syndrome, type II (Q07.0-)
	acquired hydrocephalus (G91.-)
	hydrocephalus due to congenital toxoplasmosis (P37.1)
	hydrocephalus with spina bifida (Q05.0-Q05.4)

Q03.0 Malformations of aqueduct of Sylvius
Anomaly of aqueduct of Sylvius
Obstruction of aqueduct of Sylvius, congenital
Stenosis of aqueduct of Sylvius

Q03.1 Atresia of foramina of Magendie and Luschka
Dandy-Walker syndrome

Q03.8 Other congenital hydrocephalus

Q03.9 Congenital hydrocephalus, unspecified

N Newborn Age: 0   **P** Pediatric Age: 0–17   **M** Maternity DX: 12–55   **A** Adult Age: 15–124   ♀ Females Only   ♂ Males Only

🔖 Complication\Comorbidity   🔖 Major C\C   Ⓔⓧ CC/MCC Exclusions   🔖 Hospital-Acquired Condition   **1175**

CHAPTER 17 (Q00-Q99)

CHAPTER 17 (Q00-Q99)

Q04 Other congenital malformations of brain

Excludes1 cyclopia (Q87.0)
          macrocephaly (Q75.3)

(Ex) **For category Q04 CC codes Q04.0-Q04.3:** See PDX Collection 1054
For category Q04 CC codes Q04.4-Q04.8: See PDX Collection 1055

Q04.0 Congenital malformations of corpus callosum
Agenesis of corpus callosum

Q04.1 Arhinencephaly
Congenital absence of olfactory bulbs, tract, or nerves

Q04.2 Holoprosencephaly
Failure of cleavage of forebrain (prosencephalon) resulting in incomplete or absent cortical separation and deficits in midline facial development

Q04.3 Other reduction deformities of brain
Absence of part of brain
Agenesis of part of brain
Cerebral cortex are not fully formed, brain surface is smooth
Agyria
Aplasia of part of brain
Hydranencephaly
Hypoplasia of part of brain
Lissencephaly
Congenital malformation or absence of convolutions of cerebral cortex
Microgyria
Malformation of brain characterized by excessive number of small convolutions (gyri) on surface
Pachygyria
Reduction in number of sulci of cerebrum

Excludes1 congenital malformations of corpus callosum (Q04.0)

Q04.4 Septo-optic dysplasia of brain

Q04.5 Megalencephaly
Abnormally large brain

Q04.6 Congenital cerebral cysts
Porencephaly   Schizencephaly

Excludes1 acquired porencephalic cyst (G93.0)

Q04.8 Other specified congenital malformations of brain
Arnold-Chiari syndrome, type IV
Macrogyria

Q04.9 Congenital malformation of brain, unspecified
Congenital anomaly NOS of brain
Congenital deformity NOS of brain
Congenital disease or lesion NOS of brain
Multiple anomalies NOS of brain, congenital

Q05 Spina bifida

Developmental anomaly characterized by defective closure of vertebral arch, through which spinal cord and meninges may protrude

Includes hydromeningocele (spinal)
          meningocele (spinal)
          meningomyelocele
          myelocele
          myelomeningocele
          rachischisis
          spina bifida (aperta)(cystica)
          syringomyelocele

Use additional code for any associated paraplegia (paraparesis) (G82.2-)

Excludes1 Arnold-Chiari syndrome, type II (Q07.0-)
          spina bifida occulta (Q76.0)

(Ex) **For category Q05 CC codes:** See PDX Collection 1056

Q05.0 Cervical spina bifida with hydrocephalus

Q05.1 Thoracic spina bifida with hydrocephalus
Dorsal spina bifida with hydrocephalus
Thoracolumbar spina bifida with hydrocephalus

Q05.2 Lumbar spina bifida with hydrocephalus
Lumbosacral spina bifida with hydrocephalus

Q05.3 Sacral spina bifida with hydrocephalus

Q05.4 Unspecified spina bifida with hydrocephalus

Q05.5 Cervical spina bifida without hydrocephalus

Q05.6 Thoracic spina bifida without hydrocephalus
Dorsal spina bifida NOS
Thoracolumbar spina bifida NOS

Q05.7 Lumbar spina bifida without hydrocephalus
Lumbosacral spina bifida NOS

Q05.8 Sacral spina bifida without hydrocephalus

Q05.9 Spina bifida, unspecified

Q06 Other congenital malformations of spinal cord

Q06.0 Amyelia
Congenital absence of spinal cord

Q06.1 Hypoplasia and dysplasia of spinal cord
Underdevelopment of spinal cord
Atelomyelia
Congenitally incomplete development of spinal cord
Myelatelia
Myelodysplasia of spinal cord
Defective development of spinal cord, especially lower segments

Q06.2 Diastematomyelia
Congenital anomaly, associated with spina bifida, in which spinal cord is split into halves and surrounded by dural sac

Q06.3 Other congenital cauda equina malformations

Q06.4 Hydromyelia
Dilation of central canal of spinal cord with increased fluid accumulation
Hydrorachis

Q06.8 Other specified congenital malformations of spinal cord

Q06.9 Congenital malformation of spinal cord, unspecified
Congenital anomaly NOS of spinal cord
Congenital deformity NOS of spinal cord
Congenital disease or lesion NOS of spinal cord

Q07 Other congenital malformations of nervous system

Excludes2 congenital central alveolar hypoventilation syndrome (G47.35)
          familial dysautonomia [Riley-Day] (G90.1)
          neurofibromatosis (nonmalignant) (Q85.0-)

Q07.0 Arnold-Chiari syndrome
Herniation of cerebellar tonsils and vermis through foramen magnum into spinal canal
Arnold-Chiari syndrome, type II

Excludes1 Arnold-Chiari syndrome, type III (Q01.-)
          Arnold-Chiari syndrome, type IV (Q04.8)

Q07.00 Arnold-Chiari syndrome without spina bifida or hydrocephalus

Q07.01 Arnold-Chiari syndrome with spina bifida

Q07.02 Arnold-Chiari syndrome with hydrocephalus
(Ex) See PDX Collection 1056

Q07.03 Arnold-Chiari syndrome with spina bifida and hydrocephalus
(Ex) See PDX Collection 1056

Q07.8 Other specified congenital malformations of nervous system
Agenesis of nerve
Displacement of brachial plexus
Jaw-winking syndrome
Marcus Gunn's syndrome

Q07.9 Congenital malformation of nervous system, unspecified
Congenital anomaly NOS of nervous system
Congenital deformity NOS of nervous system
Congenital disease or lesion NOS of nervous system

▶ New   ⇒ Revised   ~~deleted~~ Deleted   Excludes 1   Excludes 2   Includes   Use additional   Code first   Code also   Key words

OGCR Official Guidelines   ● Unacceptable Principal Diagnosis   X Assign placeholder X   ● Use Additional Character(s)   ▶ Manifestation Code   **Coding Clinic**

CONGENITAL MALFORMATIONS OF EYE, EAR, FACE AND NECK (Q10-Q18)

Excludes2   cleft lip and cleft palate (Q35-Q37)
congenital malformation of cervical spine (Q05.0, Q05.5, Q67.5, Q76.0-Q76.4)
congenital malformation of larynx (Q31.-)
congenital malformation of lip NEC (Q38.0)
congenital malformation of nose (Q30.-)
congenital malformation of parathyroid gland (Q89.2)
congenital malformation of thyroid gland (Q89.2)

● **Q10** **Congenital malformations of eyelid, lacrimal apparatus and orbit**

    Excludes1   cryptophthalmos NOS (Q11.2)
                    cryptophthalmos syndrome (Q87.0)

  Q10.0 **Congenital ptosis**
        Prolapse or drooping of upper eyelid from paralysis of third nerve or from sympathetic innervations

  Q10.1 **Congenital ectropion**
        Outward turning of eyelid

  Q10.2 **Congenital entropion**
        Inward turning of eyelid

  Q10.3 **Other congenital malformations of eyelid**
        Ablepharon
        Blepharophimosis, congenital
        Coloboma of eyelid
        Congenital absence or agenesis of cilia
        Congenital absence or agenesis of eyelid
        Congenital accessory eyelid
        Congenital accessory eye muscle
        Congenital malformation of eyelid NOS

  Q10.4 **Absence and agenesis of lacrimal apparatus**
        Congenital absence of punctum lacrimale

  Q10.5 **Congenital stenosis and stricture of lacrimal duct**

  Q10.6 **Other congenital malformations of lacrimal apparatus**
        Congenital malformation of lacrimal apparatus NOS

  Q10.7 **Congenital malformation of orbit**

● **Q11** **Anophthalmos, microphthalmos and macrophthalmos**
    Absence of eye and optic pit

  Q11.0 **Cystic eyeball**

  Q11.1 **Other anophthalmos**
        Anophthalmos NOS
        Agenesis of eye
           Absence of eye
        Aplasia of eye

  Q11.2 **Microphthalmos**
        Partial absence of eye and optic pit
        Cryptophthalmos NOS
        Dysplasia of eye
        Hypoplasia of eye
        Rudimentary eye
        Excludes1   cryptophthalmos syndrome (Q87.0)

  Q11.3 **Macrophthalmos**
        Congenital enlargement of eyes
        Excludes1   macrophthalmos in congenital glaucoma (Q15.0)

● **Q12** **Congenital lens malformations**

  Q12.0 **Congenital cataract**
  Q12.1 **Congenital displaced lens**
  Q12.2 **Coloboma of lens**
  Q12.3 **Congenital aphakia**
  Q12.4 **Spherophakia**
        Smaller, more spherical optic lens than normal
  Q12.8 **Other congenital lens malformations**
        Microphakia
  Q12.9 **Congenital lens malformation, unspecified**

Figure 17-2 Bilateral congenital **hydrophthalmia,** in which the eyes are very large in comparison to the other facial features due to glaucoma.

● **Q13** **Congenital malformations of anterior segment of eye**

  Q13.0 **Coloboma of iris**
        Coloboma NOS

  Q13.1 **Absence of iris**
        Aniridia
        Use additional code for associated glaucoma (H42)

  Q13.2 **Other congenital malformations of iris**
        Anisocoria, congenital
        Atresia of pupil
        Congenital malformation of iris NOS
        Corectopia

  Q13.3 **Congenital corneal opacity**

  Q13.4 **Other congenital corneal malformations**
        Congenital malformation of cornea NOS
        Microcornea
        Peter's anomaly

  Q13.5 **Blue sclera**
        Condition of unusual blueness of sclera; not harmful

● **Q13.8** **Other congenital malformations of anterior segment of eye**

    Q13.81 **Rieger's anomaly**
        Use additional code for associated glaucoma (H42)

    Q13.89 **Other congenital malformations of anterior segment of eye**

  Q13.9 **Congenital malformation of anterior segment of eye, unspecified**

● **Q14** **Congenital malformations of posterior segment of eye**

    Excludes2   optic nerve hypoplasia (H47.03-)

  Q14.0 **Congenital malformation of vitreous humor**
        Congenital vitreous opacity

  Q14.1 **Congenital malformation of retina**
        Congenital retinal aneurysm

  Q14.2 **Congenital malformation of optic disc**
        Coloboma of optic disc

  Q14.3 **Congenital malformation of choroid**

  Q14.8 **Other congenital malformations of posterior segment of eye**
        Coloboma of the fundus

  Q14.9 **Congenital malformation of posterior segment of eye, unspecified**

● **Q15** **Other congenital malformations of eye**

    Excludes1   congenital nystagmus (H55.01)
                   ocular albinism (E70.31-)
                   optic nerve hypoplasia (H47.03-)
                   retinitis pigmentosa (H35.52)

  Q15.0 **Congenital glaucoma**
        Axenfeld's anomaly
        Buphthalmos
        Congenital syndrome characterized by enlargement of the eye with symptoms of glaucoma.
        Glaucoma of childhood
        Glaucoma of newborn
        Hydrophthalmos
        Keratoglobus, congenital, with glaucoma
        Macrocornea with glaucoma
        Macrophthalmos in congenital glaucoma
        Megalocornea with glaucoma

CHAPTER 17 (Q00-Q99)

N Newborn Age: 0   **P** Pediatric Age: 0–17   **M** Maternity DX: 12–55   **A** Adult Age: 15–124   ♀ Females Only   ♂ Males Only

  Complication\Comorbidity   Major C\C   (Ex) CC/MCC Exclusions   Hospital-Acquired Condition

1177

Q15.8　Other specified congenital malformations of eye

Q15.9　Congenital malformation of eye, unspecified
　　　　Congenital anomaly of eye
　　　　Congenital deformity of eye

● **Q16　Congenital malformations of ear causing impairment of hearing**
　　Excludes1　congenital deafness (H90.-)

Q16.0　Congenital absence of (ear) auricle

Q16.1　Congenital absence, atresia and stricture of auditory canal (external)
　　　　Congenital atresia or stricture of osseous meatus

Q16.2　Absence of eustachian tube

Q16.3　Congenital malformation of ear ossicles
　　　　Congenital fusion of ear ossicles

Q16.4　Other congenital malformations of middle ear
　　　　Congenital malformation of middle ear NOS

Q16.5　Congenital malformation of inner ear
　　　　Congenital anomaly of membranous labyrinth
　　　　Congenital anomaly of organ of Corti

Q16.9　Congenital malformation of ear causing impairment of hearing, unspecified
　　　　Congenital absence of ear NOS

● **Q17　Other congenital malformations of ear**
　　Excludes1　congenital malformations of ear with impairment of hearing (Q16.0-Q16.9)
　　　　　　　preauricular sinus (Q18.1)

Q17.0　Accessory auricle
　　　　Accessory tragus
　　　　Polyotia
　　　　Preauricular appendage or tag
　　　　Supernumerary ear
　　　　Supernumerary lobule

Q17.1　Macrotia
　　　　Enlarged ears

Q17.2　Microtia
　　　　An abnormally small or underdeveloped external ear

Q17.3　Other misshapen ear
　　　　Pointed ear

Q17.4　Misplaced ear
　　　　Low-set ears
　　　　Excludes1　cervical auricle (Q18.2)

Q17.5　Prominent ear
　　　　Bat ear

Q17.8　Other specified congenital malformations of ear
　　　　Congenital absence of lobe of ear

Q17.9　Congenital malformation of ear, unspecified
　　　　Congenital anomaly of ear NOS

● **Q18　Other congenital malformations of face and neck**
　　Excludes1　cleft lip and cleft palate (Q35-Q37)
　　　　　　　conditions classified to Q67.0-Q67.4
　　　　　　　congenital malformations of skull and face bones (Q75.-)
　　　　　　　cyclopia (Q87.0)
　　　　　　　dentofacial anomalies [including malocclusion] (M26.-)
　　　　　　　malformation syndromes affecting facial appearance (Q87.0)
　　　　　　　persistent thyroglossal duct (Q89.2)

Q18.0　Sinus, fistula and cyst of branchial cleft
　　　　Branchial vestige
　　　　Branchial remnants (cysts, fistula, skin tags) that are developmental anomalies

Q18.1　Preauricular sinus and cyst
　　　　Fistula of auricle, congenital
　　　　Cervicoaural fistula
　　　　Abnormal passage in neck originating from first branchial cleft

Q18.2　Other branchial cleft malformations
　　　　Branchial cleft malformation NOS
　　　　Cervical auricle
　　　　Otocephaly

Q18.3　Webbing of neck
　　　　Pterygium colli
　　　　Thick fold of skin on side of neck

Q18.4　Macrostomia
　　　　Results from failure of union of maxillary and mandibular processes, results in abnormally large mouth

Q18.5　Microstomia

Q18.6　Macrocheilia
　　　　Excessive size of lips
　　　　Hypertrophy of lip, congenital

Q18.7　Microcheilia
　　　　Abnormal smallness of lips

Q18.8　Other specified congenital malformations of face and neck
　　　　Medial cyst of face and neck
　　　　Medial fistula of face and neck
　　　　Medial sinus of face and neck

Q18.9　Congenital malformation of face and neck, unspecified
　　　　Congenital anomaly NOS of face and neck

CONGENITAL MALFORMATIONS OF THE CIRCULATORY SYSTEM (Q20-Q28)

● **Q20　Congenital malformations of cardiac chambers and connections**
　　Excludes1　dextrocardia with situs inversus (Q89.3)
　　　　　　　mirror-image atrial arrangement with situs inversus (Q89.3)
　　Ⓔ **For category Q20 CC codes:** See PDX Collection 1057

Q20.0　Common arterial trunk 🔗
　　　　Persistent truncus arteriosus
　　　　Excludes1　aortic septal defect (Q21.4)

Q20.1　Double outlet right ventricle 🔗
　　　　Taussig-Bing syndrome

Q20.2　Double outlet left ventricle 🔗

Q20.3　Discordant ventriculoarterial connection 🔗
　　　　Dextrotransposition of aorta
　　　　Transposition of great vessels (complete)

Q20.4　Double inlet ventricle 🔗
　　　　Common ventricle
　　　　Cor triloculare biatriatum
　　　　Single ventricle

Q20.5　Discordant atrioventricular connection 🔗
　　　　Corrected transposition
　　　　Levotransposition
　　　　Ventricular inversion

Q20.6　Isomerism of atrial appendages
　　　　Isomerism of atrial appendages with asplenia or polysplenia

Q20.8　Other congenital malformations of cardiac chambers and connections
　　　　Cor binoculare

Q20.9　Congenital malformation of cardiac chambers and connections, unspecified

● **Q21　Congenital malformations of cardiac septa**
　　Excludes1　acquired cardiac septal defect (I51.0)

Q21.0　Ventricular septal defect 🔗
　　　　Roger's disease
　　　　Ⓔ See PDX Collection 1057

Q21.1　Atrial septal defect 🔗
　　　　Coronary sinus defect
　　　　Patent or persistent foramen ovale
　　　　Patent or persistent ostium secundum defect (type II)
　　　　Patent or persistent sinus venosus defect
　　　　Ⓔ See PDX Collection 1058

▶ New　　▶ Revised　　~~deleted~~ Deleted　　Excludes 1　　Excludes 2　　Includes　　Use additional　　Code first　　Code also　　Key words
OGCR Official Guidelines　● Unacceptable Principal Diagnosis　X Assign placeholder X　● Use Additional Character(s)　▶ Manifestation Code　　Coding Clinic

Q21.2 **Atrioventricular septal defect** 🏥
    Common atrioventricular canal
    Endocardial cushion defect
    Ostium primum atrial septal defect (type I)
    (Ex:) See PDX Collection 1057

Q21.3 **Tetralogy of Fallot** 🏥
    Ventricular septal defect with pulmonary stenosis or
    atresia, dextroposition of aorta and hypertrophy of
    right ventricle.
    (Ex:) See PDX Collection 1057

Q21.4 **Aortopulmonary septal defect**
    Aortic septal defect
    Aortopulmonary window

Q21.8 **Other congenital malformations of cardiac septa**
    Eisenmenger's defect
    Pentalogy of Fallot

    Excludes1 ~~Eisenmenger's complex (I27.8)~~
                  ~~Eisenmenger's syndrome (I27.8)~~

    ▶Code also if applicable:
      ▶Eisenmenger's complex (I27.83)
      ▶Eisenmenger's syndrome (I27.83)

Q21.9 **Congenital malformation of cardiac septum, unspecified**
    Septal (heart) defect NOS

● **Q22 Congenital malformations of pulmonary and tricuspid valves**
    (Ex:) For category Q22 CC codes unless otherwise indicated: See PDX Collection 1061

Q22.0 **Pulmonary valve atresia** 🏥
    (Ex:) See PDX Collection 1059

Q22.1 **Congenital pulmonary valve stenosis** 🏥
    (Ex:) See PDX Collection 1059

Q22.2 **Congenital pulmonary valve insufficiency** 🏥
    Congenital pulmonary valve regurgitation
    (Ex:) See PDX Collection 1060

Q22.3 **Other congenital malformations of pulmonary valve** 🏥
    Congenital malformation of pulmonary valve NOS
    Supernumerary cusps of pulmonary valve
    (Ex:) See PDX Collection 1060

Q22.4 **Congenital tricuspid stenosis** 🏥
    Congenital tricuspid atresia

Q22.5 **Ebstein's anomaly** 🏥
    Malformation of tricuspid valve

Q22.6 **Hypoplastic right heart syndrome** 🏥

Q22.8 **Other congenital malformations of tricuspid valve** 🏥

Q22.9 **Congenital malformation of tricuspid valve, unspecified** 🏥

● **Q23 Congenital malformations of aortic and mitral valves**
    (Ex:) For category Q23 CC codes unless otherwise indicated: See PDX Collection 1061

Q23.0 **Congenital stenosis of aortic valve** 🏥
    Congenital aortic atresia
    Congenital aortic stenosis NOS

    Excludes1 congenital stenosis of aortic valve in
               hypoplastic left heart syndrome
               (Q23.4)
               congenital subaortic stenosis (Q24.4)
               supravalvular aortic stenosis (congenital)
               (Q25.3)

Q23.1 **Congenital insufficiency of aortic valve** 🏥
    Bicuspid aortic valve
    Congenital aortic insufficiency

Q23.2 **Congenital mitral stenosis** 🏥
    Congenital mitral atresia

Q23.3 **Congenital mitral insufficiency** 🏥

Q23.4 **Hypoplastic left heart syndrome** 🏥

Q23.8 **Other congenital malformations of aortic and mitral valves**

Q23.9 **Congenital malformation of aortic and mitral valves, unspecified**

● Q24 **Other congenital malformations of heart**
    Excludes1 endocardial fibroelastosis (I42.4)

Q24.0 **Dextrocardia** 🏥
    Heart is located in right hemithorax

    Excludes1 dextrocardia with situs inversus (Q89.3)
               isomerism of atrial appendages (with
               asplenia or polysplenia) (Q20.6)
               mirror-image atrial arrangement with
               situs inversus (Q89.3)
    (Ex:) See PDX Collection 1062

Q24.1 **Levocardia** 🏥
    Normal position of heart but related structures on wrong side
    (Ex:) See PDX Collection 1062

Q24.2 **Cor triatriatum** 🏥
    Congenital heart defect; left atrium is subdivided
    (Ex:) See PDX Collection 1063

Q24.3 **Pulmonary infundibular stenosis** 🏥
    Subvalvular pulmonic stenosis
    (Ex:) See PDX Collection 1063

Q24.4 **Congenital subaortic stenosis** 🏥
    (Ex:) See PDX Collection 1063

Q24.5 **Malformation of coronary vessels** 🏥
    Congenital coronary (artery) aneurysm
    (Ex:) See PDX Collection 1064

Q24.6 **Congenital heart block** 🏥
    (Ex:) See PDX Collection 1065

Q24.8 **Other specified congenital malformations of heart**
    Congenital diverticulum of left ventricle
    Congenital malformation of myocardium
    Congenital malformation of pericardium
    Malposition of heart
    Uhl's disease

Q24.9 **Congenital malformation of heart, unspecified**
    Congenital anomaly of heart
    Congenital disease of heart

● Q25 **Congenital malformations of great arteries**

Q25.0 **Patent ductus arteriosus** 🏥
    Fetal blood vessel connecting left pulmonary artery directly
    to descending aorta
    Patent ductus Botallo
    Persistent ductus arteriosus
    (Ex:) See PDX Collection 1066

Q25.1 **Coarctation of aorta** 🏥
    Coarctation of aorta (preductal) (postductal)
    Stenosis of aorta
    (Ex:) See PDX Collection 1067
    Coding Clinic: 2016, Q4, P56-57

● Q25.2 **Atresia of aorta**
    (Ex:) For category Q25.2 CC codes: See PDX Collection 1068
    Coding Clinic: 2016, Q4, P56

    Q25.21 **Interruption of aortic arch** 🏥
             Atresia of aortic arch

    Q25.29 **Other atresia of aorta** 🏥
             Atresia of aorta

Q25.3 **Supravalvular aortic stenosis** 🏥
    Excludes1 congenital aortic stenosis NOS (Q23.0)
               congenital stenosis of aortic valve (Q23.0)
    (Ex:) See PDX Collection 1068

● Q25.4 **Other congenital malformations of aorta**
    Excludes1 hypoplasia of aorta in hypoplastic left
               heart syndrome (Q23.4)
    (Ex:) For category Q25.4 CC codes: See PDX Collection 1069
    Coding Clinic: 2016, Q4, P57

    Q25.40 **Congenital malformation of aorta unspecified** 🏥

    Q25.41 **Absence and aplasia of aorta** 🏥

    Q25.42 **Hypoplasia of aorta** 🏥

N Newborn Age: 0   **P** Pediatric Age: 0–17   **M** Maternity DX: 12–55   **A** Adult Age: 15–124   ♀ Females Only   ♂ Males Only

  🏥 Complication\Comorbidity   🏥 Major C\C   (Ex:) CC/MCC Exclusions   🏥 Hospital-Acquired Condition

CHAPTER 17 (Q00-Q99)

Q25.43 **Congenital aneurysm of aorta** 🔖
  Congenital aneurysm of aortic root
  Congenital aneurysm of aortic sinus

Q25.44 **Congenital dilation of aorta** 🔖

Q25.45 **Double aortic arch** 🔖
  Vascular ring of aorta

Q25.46 **Tortuous aortic arch** 🔖
  Persistent convolutions of aortic arch

Q25.47 **Right aortic arch** 🔖
  Persistent right aortic arch

Q25.48 **Anomalous origin of subclavian artery** 🔖

Q25.49 **Other congenital malformations of aorta** 🔖
  ▶ Aortic arch
  ▶ Bovine arch

Q25.5 **Atresia of pulmonary artery** 🔖
  (Ex:) See PDX Collection 1070

Q25.6 **Stenosis of pulmonary artery** 🔖
  Supravalvular pulmonary stenosis
  (Ex:) See PDX Collection 1070

● Q25.7 **Other congenital malformations of pulmonary artery**
  (Ex:) For category Q25.7 CC codes: See PDX Collection 1070

Q25.71 **Coarctation of pulmonary artery** 🔖

Q25.72 **Congenital pulmonary arteriovenous malformation** 🔖
  Congenital pulmonary arteriovenous aneurysm

Q25.79 **Other congenital malformations of pulmonary artery** 🔖
  Aberrant pulmonary artery
  Agenesis of pulmonary artery
  Congenital aneurysm of pulmonary artery
  Congenital anomaly of pulmonary artery
  Hypoplasia of pulmonary artery

Q25.8 **Other congenital malformations of other great arteries** 🔖
  (Ex:) See PDX Collection 1069

Q25.9 **Congenital malformation of great arteries, unspecified** 🔖
  (Ex:) See PDX Collection 1069

● Q26 **Congenital malformations of great veins**

Q26.0 **Congenital stenosis of vena cava** 🔖
  Congenital stenosis of vena cava (inferior)(superior)
  (Ex:) See PDX Collection 1071

Q26.1 **Persistent left superior vena cava** 🔖
  (Ex:) See PDX Collection 1071

Q26.2 **Total anomalous pulmonary venous connection** 🔖
  Total anomalous pulmonary venous return [TAPVR], subdiaphragmatic
  Total anomalous pulmonary venous return [TAPVR], supradiaphragmatic
  (Ex:) See PDX Collection 1072

Q26.3 **Partial anomalous pulmonary venous connection** 🔖
  Partial anomalous pulmonary venous return
  (Ex:) See PDX Collection 1073

Q26.4 **Anomalous pulmonary venous connection, unspecified** 🔖
  (Ex:) See PDX Collection 1073

Q26.5 **Anomalous portal venous connection**

Q26.6 **Portal vein-hepatic artery fistula**

Q26.8 **Other congenital malformations of great veins** 🔖
  Absence of vena cava (inferior) (superior)
  Azygos continuation of inferior vena cava
  Persistent left posterior cardinal vein
  Scimitar syndrome
  (Ex:) See PDX Collection 1071

Q26.9 **Congenital malformation of great vein, unspecified** 🔖
  Congenital anomaly of vena cava (inferior) (superior) NOS
  (Ex:) See PDX Collection 1074

● Q27 **Other congenital malformations of peripheral vascular system**
  Excludes2 anomalies of cerebral and precerebral vessels (Q28.0-Q28.3)
    anomalies of coronary vessels (Q24.5)
    anomalies of pulmonary artery (Q25.5-Q25.7)
    congenital retinal aneurysm (Q14.1)
    hemangioma and lymphangioma (D18.-)

Q27.0 **Congenital absence and hypoplasia of umbilical artery**
  Single umbilical artery

Q27.1 **Congenital renal artery stenosis**

Q27.2 **Other congenital malformations of renal artery**
  Congenital malformation of renal artery NOS
  Multiple renal arteries

● Q27.3 **Arteriovenous malformation (peripheral)**
  Arteriovenous aneurysm
  Excludes1 acquired arteriovenous aneurysm (I77.0)
  Excludes2 arteriovenous malformation of cerebral vessels (Q28.2)
    arteriovenous malformation of precerebral vessels (Q28.0)

Q27.30 **Arteriovenous malformation, site unspecified**
  (Ex:) See PDX Collection 1075

Q27.31 **Arteriovenous malformation of vessel of upper limb**

Q27.32 **Arteriovenous malformation of vessel of lower limb**

Q27.33 **Arteriovenous malformation of digestive system vessel**

Q27.34 **Arteriovenous malformation of renal vessel**

Q27.39 **Arteriovenous malformation, other site**

Q27.4 **Congenital phlebectasia** 🔖
  (Ex:) See PDX Collection 1075

Q27.8 **Other specified congenital malformations of peripheral vascular system**
  Absence of peripheral vascular system
  Atresia of peripheral vascular system
  Congenital aneurysm (peripheral)
  Congenital stricture, artery
  Congenital varix
  Excludes1 arteriovenous malformation (Q27.3-)

Q27.9 **Congenital malformation of peripheral vascular system, unspecified**
  Anomaly of artery or vein NOS

● Q28 **Other congenital malformations of circulatory system**
  Excludes1 congenital aneurysm NOS (Q27.8)
    congenital coronary aneurysm (Q24.5)
    ruptured cerebral arteriovenous malformation (I60.8)
    ruptured malformation of precerebral vessels (I72.0)
  Excludes2 congenital peripheral aneurysm (Q27.8)
    congenital pulmonary aneurysm (Q25.79)
    congenital retinal aneurysm (Q14.1)

Q28.0 **Arteriovenous malformation of precerebral vessels** 🔖
  Congenital arteriovenous precerebral aneurysm (nonruptured)
  (Ex:) See PDX Collection 1075

Q28.1 **Other malformations of precerebral vessels** 🔖
  Congenital malformation of precerebral vessels NOS
  Congenital precerebral aneurysm (nonruptured)
  (Ex:) See PDX Collection 1075

Q28.2 **Arteriovenous malformation of cerebral vessels** 🔖
  Arteriovenous malformation of brain NOS
  Congenital arteriovenous cerebral aneurysm (nonruptured)
  (Ex:) See PDX Collection 1076

Q28.3 **Other malformations of cerebral vessels** 🔖
  Congenital cerebral aneurysm (nonruptured)
  Congenital malformation of cerebral vessels NOS
  Developmental venous anomaly
  (Ex:) See PDX Collection 1076

▶ New   ⟹ Revised   ~~deleted~~ Deleted   Excludes 1   Excludes 2   Includes   Use additional   Code first   Code also   Key words

OGCR Official Guidelines   ● Unacceptable Principal Diagnosis   X Assign placeholder X   ● Use Additional Character(s)   ▸ Manifestation Code   **Coding Clinic**

Q28.8 Other specified congenital malformations of circulatory system 🖱
  Congenital aneurysm, specified site NEC
  Spinal vessel anomaly
  (Ex) See PDX Collection 1075

Q28.9 Congenital malformation of circulatory system, unspecified 🖱
  (Ex) See PDX Collection 1077

CONGENITAL MALFORMATIONS OF THE RESPIRATORY SYSTEM (Q30-Q34)

● **Q30 Congenital malformations of nose**
  Excludes1   congenital deviation of nasal septum (Q67.4)

  Q30.0 Choanal atresia
    Atresia of nares (anterior) (posterior)
    Congenital stenosis of nares (anterior) (posterior)

  Q30.1 Agenesis and underdevelopment of nose
    Congenital absent of nose

  Q30.2 Fissured, notched and cleft nose

  Q30.3 Congenital perforated nasal septum

  Q30.8 Other congenital malformations of nose
    Accessory nose
    Congenital anomaly of nasal sinus wall

  Q30.9 Congenital malformation of nose, unspecified

● **Q31 Congenital malformations of larynx**
  Excludes1   congenital laryngeal stridor NOS (P28.89)
  (Ex) For category Q31 CC codes: See PDX Collection 1078

  Q31.0 Web of larynx
    Glottic web of larynx
    Subglottic web of larynx
    Web of larynx NOS

  Q31.1 Congenital subglottic stenosis 🖱

  Q31.2 Laryngeal hypoplasia 🖱

  Q31.3 Laryngocele 🖱

  Q31.5 Congenital laryngomalacia 🖱

  Q31.8 Other congenital malformations of larynx 🖱
    Absence of larynx
    Agenesis of larynx
    Atresia of larynx
    Congenital cleft thyroid cartilage
    Congenital fissure of epiglottis
    Congenital stenosis of larynx NEC
    Posterior cleft of cricoid cartilage

  Q31.9 Congenital malformation of larynx, unspecified 🖱

● **Q32 Congenital malformations of trachea and bronchus**
  Excludes1   congenital bronchiectasis (Q33.4)
  (Ex) For category Q32 CC codes: See PDX Collection 1078

  Q32.0 Congenital tracheomalacia 🖱

  Q32.1 Other congenital malformations of trachea 🖱
    Atresia of trachea
    Congenital anomaly of tracheal cartilage
    Congenital dilatation of trachea
    Congenital malformation of trachea
    Congenital stenosis of trachea
    Congenital tracheocele

  Q32.2 Congenital bronchomalacia 🖱

  Q32.3 Congenital stenosis of bronchus 🖱

  Q32.4 Other congenital malformations of bronchus 🖱
    Absence of bronchus
    Agenesis of bronchus
    Atresia of bronchus
    Congenital diverticulum of bronchus
    Congenital malformation of bronchus NOS

● **Q33 Congenital malformations of lung**

  Q33.0 Congenital cystic lung 🖱
    Congenital cystic lung disease
    Congenital honeycomb lung
    Congenital polycystic lung disease
    Excludes1   cystic fibrosis (E84.0)
             cystic lung disease, acquired or
               unspecified (J98.4)
    (Ex) See PDX Collection 1079

  Q33.1 Accessory lobe of lung
    Azygos lobe (fissured), lung

  Q33.2 Sequestration of lung 🖱
    (Ex) See PDX Collection 1079

  Q33.3 Agenesis of lung 🖱
    Congenital absence of lung (lobe)
    (Ex) See PDX Collection 1079

  Q33.4 Congenital bronchiectasis 🖱
    (Ex) See PDX Collection 1080

  Q33.5 Ectopic tissue in lung

  Q33.6 Congenital hypoplasia and dysplasia of lung 🖱
    Excludes1   pulmonary hypoplasia associated with
               short gestation (P28.0)
    (Ex) See PDX Collection 1079

  Q33.8 Other congenital malformations of lung

  Q33.9 Congenital malformation of lung, unspecified

● **Q34 Other congenital malformations of respiratory system**
  Excludes2   congenital central alveolar hypoventilation
            syndrome (G47.35)

  Q34.0 Anomaly of pleura

  Q34.1 Congenital cyst of mediastinum

  Q34.8 Other specified congenital malformations of respiratory system
    Atresia of nasopharynx

  Q34.9 Congenital malformation of respiratory system, unspecified
    Congenital absence of respiratory system
    Congenital anomaly of respiratory system NOS

CLEFT LIP AND CLEFT PALATE (Q35-Q37)

  Use additional code to identify associated malformation of the
  nose (Q30.2)
  Excludes1   Robin's syndrome (Q87.0)

● **Q35 Cleft palate**
  Includes   fissure of palate
           palatoschisis
  Excludes1   cleft palate with cleft lip (Q37.-)

  Q35.1 Cleft hard palate

  Q35.3 Cleft soft palate

  Q35.5 Cleft hard palate with cleft soft palate

  Q35.7 Cleft uvula

  Q35.9 Cleft palate, unspecified
    Cleft palate NOS

Figure 17-3 Cleft palate.

N Newborn Age: 0   **P** Pediatric Age: 0–17   **M** Maternity DX: 12–55   **A** Adult Age: 15–124   ♀ Females Only   ♂ Males Only
🖱 Complication\Comorbidity   🖱 Major C\C   (Ex) CC/MCC Exclusions   🖱 Hospital-Acquired Condition

1181

CHAPTER 17 (Q00–Q99)

● **Q36   Cleft lip**

> **Includes**   cheiloschisis
> congenital fissure of lip
> harelip
> labium leporinum

> **Excludes1**   cleft lip with cleft palate (Q37.-)

   Q36.0   Cleft lip, bilateral

   Q36.1   Cleft lip, median

   Q36.9   Cleft lip, unilateral
> Cleft lip NOS

● **Q37   Cleft palate with cleft lip**

> **Includes**   cheilopalatoschisis

   Q37.0   Cleft hard palate with bilateral cleft lip

   Q37.1   Cleft hard palate with unilateral cleft lip
> Cleft hard palate with cleft lip NOS

   Q37.2   Cleft soft palate with bilateral cleft lip

   Q37.3   Cleft soft palate with unilateral cleft lip
> Cleft soft palate with cleft lip NOS

   Q37.4   Cleft hard and soft palate with bilateral cleft lip

   Q37.5   Cleft hard and soft palate with unilateral cleft lip
> Cleft hard and soft palate with cleft lip NOS

   Q37.8   Unspecified cleft palate with bilateral cleft lip

   Q37.9   Unspecified cleft palate with unilateral cleft lip
> Cleft palate with cleft lip NOS

OTHER CONGENITAL MALFORMATIONS OF THE DIGESTIVE SYSTEM (Q38–Q45)

● **Q38   Other congenital malformations of tongue, mouth and pharynx**

> **Excludes1**   dentofacial anomalies (M26.-)
> macrostomia (Q18.4)
> microstomia (Q18.5)

   Q38.0   Congenital malformations of lips, not elsewhere classified
> Congenital fistula of lip
> Congenital malformation of lip NOS
> Van der Woude's syndrome

> > **Excludes1**   cleft lip (Q36.-)
> > cleft lip with cleft palate (Q37.-)
> > macrocheilia (Q18.6)
> > microcheilia (Q18.7)

   Q38.1   Ankyloglossia
> *Restricted movement of tongue resulting in speech difficulty*
> Tongue tie

   Q38.2   Macroglossia
> *Excessive size of tongue*
> Congenital hypertrophy of tongue

   Q38.3   Other congenital malformations of tongue
> Aglossia
> Bifid tongue
> Congenital adhesion of tongue
> Congenital fissure of tongue
> Congenital malformation of tongue NOS
> Double tongue
> Hypoglossia
> Hypoplasia of tongue
> Microglossia

   Q38.4   Congenital malformations of salivary glands and ducts
> Atresia of salivary glands and ducts
> Congenital absence of salivary glands and ducts
> Congenital accessory salivary glands and ducts
> Congenital fistula of salivary gland

   Q38.5   Congenital malformations of palate, not elsewhere classified
> Congenital absence of uvula
> Congenital malformation of palate NOS
> Congenital high arched palate

> > **Excludes1**   cleft palate (Q35.-)
> > cleft palate with cleft lip (Q37.-)

   Q38.6   Other congenital malformations of mouth
> Congenital malformation of mouth NOS

   Q38.7   Congenital pharyngeal pouch
> Congenital diverticulum of pharynx

> > **Excludes1**   pharyngeal pouch syndrome (D82.1)

   Q38.8   Other congenital malformations of pharynx
> Congenital malformation of pharynx NOS
> Imperforate pharynx

● **Q39   Congenital malformations of esophagus**

> (Ex) For category Q39 CC codes Q39.0–Q39.4: See PDX Collection 1081
> For category Q39 CC codes Q39.5–Q39.9: See PDX Collection 1082

   Q39.0   Atresia of esophagus without fistula
> Atresia of esophagus NOS

   Q39.1   Atresia of esophagus with tracheo-esophageal fistula
> Atresia of esophagus with broncho-esophageal fistula

   Q39.2   Congenital tracheo-esophageal fistula without atresia
> Congenital tracheo-esophageal fistula NOS

   Q39.3   Congenital stenosis and stricture of esophagus

   Q39.4   Esophageal web

   Q39.5   Congenital dilatation of esophagus
> Congenital cardiospasm

   Q39.6   Congenital diverticulum of esophagus
> Congenital esophageal pouch

   Q39.8   Other congenital malformations of esophagus
> Congenital absence of esophagus
> Congenital displacement of esophagus
> Congenital duplication of esophagus

   Q39.9   Congenital malformation of esophagus, unspecified

● **Q40   Other congenital malformations of upper alimentary tract**

   Q40.0   Congenital hypertrophic pyloric stenosis
> Congenital or infantile constriction
> Congenital or infantile hypertrophy
> Congenital or infantile spasm
> Congenital or infantile stenosis
> Congenital or infantile stricture

   Q40.1   Congenital hiatus hernia
> Congenital displacement of cardia through esophageal hiatus

> > **Excludes1**   congenital diaphragmatic hernia (Q79.0)

   Q40.2   Other specified congenital malformations of stomach
> Congenital displacement of stomach
> Congenital diverticulum of stomach
> Congenital hourglass stomach
> Congenital duplication of stomach
> Megalogastria
> Microgastria

   Q40.3   Congenital malformation of stomach, unspecified

   Q40.8   Other specified congenital malformations of upper alimentary tract

   Q40.9   Congenital malformation of upper alimentary tract, unspecified
> Congenital anomaly of upper alimentary tract
> Congenital deformity of upper alimentary tract

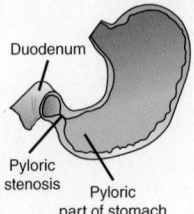

Duodenum

Pyloric stenosis

Pyloric part of stomach

Figure 17-4   Pyloric stenosis.

▶ New   ⇒ Revised   ~~deleted~~ Deleted   Excludes 1   Excludes 2   Includes   Use additional   Code first   Code also   Key words

OGCR Official Guidelines   ● Unacceptable Principal Diagnosis   X Assign placeholder X   ● Use Additional Character(s)   ▌ Manifestation Code   **Coding Clinic**

● **Q41 Congenital absence, atresia and stenosis of small intestine**

> **Includes**   congenital obstruction, occlusion or stricture of small intestine or intestine NOS

> **Excludes1**   cystic fibrosis with intestinal manifestation (E84.11)
> meconium ileus NOS (without cystic fibrosis) (P76.0)

> (Ex) **For category Q41 CC codes:** See PDX Collection 1083

> **Q41.0 Congenital absence, atresia and stenosis of duodenum** 🔖

> **Q41.1 Congenital absence, atresia and stenosis of jejunum** 🔖
> Apple peel syndrome
> Imperforate jejunum

> **Q41.2 Congenital absence, atresia and stenosis of ileum** 🔖

> **Q41.8 Congenital absence, atresia and stenosis of other specified parts of small intestine** 🔖

> **Q41.9 Congenital absence, atresia and stenosis of small intestine, part unspecified** 🔖
> Congenital absence, atresia and stenosis of intestine NOS

● **Q42 Congenital absence, atresia and stenosis of large intestine**

> **Includes**   congenital obstruction, occlusion and stricture of large intestine

> (Ex) **For category Q42 CC codes:** See PDX Collection 1084

> **Q42.0 Congenital absence, atresia and stenosis of rectum with fistula** 🔖

> **Q42.1 Congenital absence, atresia and stenosis of rectum without fistula** 🔖
> Imperforate rectum

> **Q42.2 Congenital absence, atresia and stenosis of anus with fistula** 🔖

> **Q42.3 Congenital absence, atresia and stenosis of anus without fistula** 🔖
> Imperforate anus

> **Q42.8 Congenital absence, atresia and stenosis of other parts of large intestine** 🔖

> **Q42.9 Congenital absence, atresia and stenosis of large intestine, part unspecified** 🔖

● **Q43 Other congenital malformations of intestine**

> (Ex) **For category Q43 CC codes unless otherwise indicated:** See PDX Collection 1087

> **Q43.0 Meckel's diverticulum (displaced) (hypertrophic)**
> *Congenital abnormality in which a pouch remains on the lower end of the small intestine*
> Persistent omphalomesenteric duct
> Persistent vitelline duct

> **Q43.1 Hirschsprung's disease** 🔖
> *Developmental disorder of enteric nervous system characterized by absence of ganglion cells in distal colon resulting in functional obstruction*
> Aganglionosis
> Congenital (aganglionic) megacolon
> (Ex) See PDX Collection 1085

> **Q43.2 Other congenital functional disorders of colon** 🔖
> Congenital dilatation of colon
> (Ex) See PDX Collection 1085

> **Q43.3 Congenital malformations of intestinal fixation** 🔖
> Congenital omental, anomalous adhesions [bands]
> Congenital peritoneal adhesions [bands]
> Incomplete rotation of cecum and colon
> Insufficient rotation of cecum and colon
> Jackson's membrane
> Malrotation of colon
> Rotation failure of cecum and colon
> Universal mesentery
> (Ex) See PDX Collection 1086

> **Q43.4 Duplication of intestine** 🔖

> **Q43.5 Ectopic anus** 🔖
> *Anal opening in abnormal location*

> **Q43.6 Congenital fistula of rectum and anus** 🔖

> > **Excludes1**   congenital fistula of anus with absence, atresia and stenosis (Q42.2)
> > congenital fistula of rectum with absence, atresia and stenosis (Q42.0)
> > congenital rectovaginal fistula (Q52.2)
> > congenital urethrorectal fistula (Q64.73)
> > pilonidal fistula or sinus (L05.-)

> **Q43.7 Persistent cloaca** 🔖
> *Malformation in which rectum, vagina, and urinary tract form one channel AKA congenital cloaca*
> Cloaca NOS

> **Q43.8 Other specified congenital malformations of intestine** 🔖
> Congenital blind loop syndrome
> Congenital diverticulitis, colon
> Congenital diverticulum, intestine
> Dolichocolon
> Megaloappendix
> Megaloduodenum
> Microcolon
> Transposition of appendix
> Transposition of colon
> Transposition of intestine

> **Q43.9 Congenital malformation of intestine, unspecified** 🔖

● **Q44 Congenital malformations of gallbladder, bile ducts and liver**

> (Ex) **For category Q44 CC codes unless otherwise indicated:** See PDX Collection 1088

> **Q44.0 Agenesis, aplasia and hypoplasia of gallbladder** 🔖
> Congenital absence of gallbladder

> **Q44.1 Other congenital malformations of gallbladder** 🔖
> Congenital malformation of gallbladder NOS
> Intrahepatic gallbladder

> **Q44.2 Atresia of bile ducts** 🔖
> (Ex) See PDX Collection 1089

> **Q44.3 Congenital stenosis and stricture of bile ducts** 🔖
> (Ex) See PDX Collection 1089

> **Q44.4 Choledochal cyst** 🔖

> **Q44.5 Other congenital malformations of bile ducts** 🔖
> Accessory hepatic duct
> Biliary duct duplication
> Congenital malformation of bile duct NOS
> Cystic duct duplication

> **Q44.6 Cystic disease of liver** 🔖
> Fibrocystic disease of liver
> (Ex) See PDX Collection 1090

> **Q44.7 Other congenital malformations of liver** 🔖
> Accessory liver
> Alagille's syndrome
> Congenital absence of liver
> Congenital hepatomegaly
> Congenital malformation of liver NOS

● **Q45 Other congenital malformations of digestive system**

> **Excludes2**   congenital diaphragmatic hernia (Q79.0)
> congenital hiatus hernia (Q40.1)

> (Ex) **For category Q45 CC codes:** See PDX Collection 1091

> **Q45.0 Agenesis, aplasia and hypoplasia of pancreas** 🔖
> Congenital absence of pancreas

> **Q45.1 Annular pancreas** 🔖

> **Q45.2 Congenital pancreatic cyst** 🔖

> **Q45.3 Other congenital malformations of pancreas and pancreatic duct** 🔖
> Accessory pancreas
> Congenital malformation of pancreas or pancreatic duct NOS

> > **Excludes1**   congenital diabetes mellitus (E10.-)
> > cystic fibrosis (E84.0-E84.9)
> > fibrocystic disease of pancreas (E84.-)
> > neonatal diabetes mellitus (P70.2)

CHAPTER 17 (Q00-Q99)

Q45.8 Other specified congenital malformations of digestive system
Absence (complete) (partial) of alimentary tract NOS
Duplication of digestive system
Malposition, congenital of digestive system

Q45.9 Congenital malformation of digestive system, unspecified
Congenital anomaly of digestive system
Congenital deformity of digestive system

CONGENITAL MALFORMATIONS OF GENITAL ORGANS (Q50-Q56)

Excludes1 androgen insensitivity syndrome (E34.5-)
syndromes associated with anomalies in the number and form of chromosomes (Q90-Q99)

- **Q50 Congenital malformations of ovaries, fallopian tubes and broad ligaments**
  - **Q50.0 Congenital absence of ovary**
    - **Excludes1** Turner's syndrome (Q96.-)
    - **Q50.01 Congenital absence of ovary, unilateral** ♀
    - **Q50.02 Congenital absence of ovary, bilateral** ♀
  - **Q50.1 Developmental ovarian cyst** ♀
  - **Q50.2 Congenital torsion of ovary** ♀
  - **Q50.3 Other congenital malformations of ovary**
    - **Q50.31 Accessory ovary** ♀
    - **Q50.32 Ovarian streak** ♀
      Inadequate ovaries with absent follicular and hormonal function
      46, XX with streak gonads
    - **Q50.39 Other congenital malformation of ovary** ♀
      Congenital malformation of ovary NOS
  - **Q50.4 Embryonic cyst of fallopian tube** ♀
    Fimbrial cyst
  - **Q50.5 Embryonic cyst of broad ligament** ♀
    Epoophoron cyst
    Parovarian cyst
  - **Q50.6 Other congenital malformations of fallopian tube and broad ligament** ♀
    Absence of fallopian tube and broad ligament
    Accessory fallopian tube and broad ligament
    Atresia of fallopian tube and broad ligament
    Congenital malformation of fallopian tube or broad ligament NOS
- **Q51 Congenital malformations of uterus and cervix**
  - **Q51.0 Agenesis and aplasia of uterus** ♀
    Congenital absence of uterus
  - **Q51.1 Doubling of uterus with doubling of cervix and vagina**
    - **Q51.10 Doubling of uterus with doubling of cervix and vagina without obstruction** ♀
      Doubling of uterus with doubling of cervix and vagina NOS
    - **Q51.11 Doubling of uterus with doubling of cervix and vagina with obstruction** ♀
  - **Q51.2 Other doubling of uterus** ♀
    Doubling of uterus NOS
    Septate uterus, complete or partial
  - **Q51.3 Bicornate uterus** ♀
    Bicornate uterus, complete or partial
    Birth defect in which uterus has two separate 'horns' that form top of uterus
  - **Q51.4 Unicornate uterus** ♀
    Unicornate uterus with or without a separate uterine horn
    Uterus with only one functioning horn
    Uterus with half being undeveloped
  - **Q51.5 Agenesis and aplasia of cervix** ♀
    Congenital absence of cervix
  - **Q51.6 Embryonic cyst of cervix** ♀
  - **Q51.7 Congenital fistulae between uterus and digestive and urinary tracts** ♀

- **Q51.8 Other congenital malformations of uterus and cervix**
  - **Q51.81 Other congenital malformations of uterus**
    - **Q51.810 Arcuate uterus** ♀
      Arcuatus uterus
    - **Q51.811 Hypoplasia of uterus** ♀
    - **Q51.818 Other congenital malformations of uterus** ♀
      Müllerian anomaly of uterus NEC
  - **Q51.82 Other congenital malformations of cervix**
    - **Q51.820 Cervical duplication** ♀
    - **Q51.821 Hypoplasia of cervix** ♀
    - **Q51.828 Other congenital malformations of cervix** ♀
  - **Q51.9 Congenital malformation of uterus and cervix, unspecified** ♀
- **Q52 Other congenital malformations of female genitalia**
  - **Q52.0 Congenital absence of vagina** ♀
    Vaginal agenesis, total or partial
  - **Q52.1 Doubling of vagina**
    - **Excludes1** doubling of vagina with doubling of uterus and cervix (Q51.1-)
    - **Q52.10 Doubling of vagina, unspecified** ♀
      Septate vagina NOS
    - **Q52.11 Transverse vaginal septum** ♀
    - **Q52.12 Longitudinal vaginal septum**
      Coding Clinic: 2016, Q4, P58
      - **Q52.120 Longitudinal vaginal septum, nonobstructing** ♀
      - **Q52.121 Longitudinal vaginal septum, obstructing, right side** ♀
      - **Q52.122 Longitudinal vaginal septum, obstructing, left side** ♀
      - **Q52.123 Longitudinal vaginal septum, microperforate, right side** ♀
      - **Q52.124 Longitudinal vaginal septum, microperforate, left side** ♀
        Coding Clinic: 2016, Q4, P59
      - **Q52.129 Other and unspecified longitudinal vaginal septum** ♀
  - **Q52.2 Congenital rectovaginal fistula** ♀
    - **Excludes1** cloaca (Q43.7)
  - **Q52.3 Imperforate hymen** ♀
    Membrane (hymen) completely closes vaginal orifice
  - **Q52.4 Other congenital malformations of vagina** ♀
    Canal of Nuck cyst, congenital
    Congenital malformation of vagina NOS
    Embryonic vaginal cyst
    Gartner's duct cyst
  - **Q52.5 Fusion of labia** ♀
  - **Q52.6 Congenital malformation of clitoris** ♀
  - **Q52.7 Other and unspecified congenital malformations of vulva**
    - **Q52.70 Unspecified congenital malformations of vulva** ♀
      Congenital malformation of vulva NOS
    - **Q52.71 Congenital absence of vulva** ♀
    - **Q52.79 Other congenital malformations of vulva** ♀
      Congenital cyst of vulva
  - **Q52.8 Other specified congenital malformations of female genitalia** ♀
  - **Q52.9 Congenital malformation of female genitalia, unspecified** ♀
- **Q53 Undescended and ectopic testicle**
  - **Q53.0 Ectopic testis**
    - **Q53.00 Ectopic testis, unspecified** ♂
    - **Q53.01 Ectopic testis, unilateral** ♂
    - **Q53.02 Ectopic testes, bilateral** ♂

▶ New ⇒ Revised ~~deleted~~ Deleted Excludes 1 Excludes 2 Includes Use additional Code first Code also Key words
OGCR Official Guidelines ● Unacceptable Principal Diagnosis X Assign placeholder X ● Use Additional Character(s) ▌ Manifestation Code Coding Clinic

Item 17-1 Testes form in the abdomen of the male and only descend into the scrotum during normal embryonic development. "Ectopic" testes are out of their normal place or "retained" (left behind) in the abdomen. Crypto (hidden) orchism (testicle) is a major risk factor for testicular cancer.

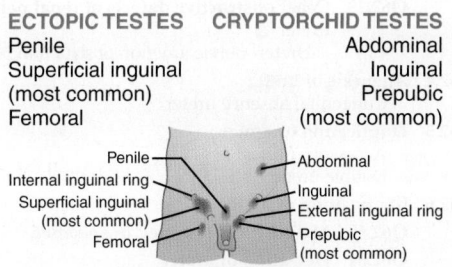

ECTOPIC TESTES	CRYPTORCHID TESTES
Penile	Abdominal
Superficial inguinal	Inguinal
(most common)	Prepubic
Femoral	(most common)

Figure 17-5 Undescended testes and the positions of the testes in various types of cryptorchidism or abnormal paths of descent.

- **Q53.1 Undescended testicle, unilateral**
  - Q53.10 Unspecified undescended testicle, unilateral ♂
  - **Q53.11 Abdominal testis, unilateral**
    - ▶ Q53.111 Unilateral intraabdominal testis ♂
    - ▶ Q53.112 Unilateral inguinal testis ♂
  - Q53.12 Ectopic perineal testis, unilateral ♂
  - ▶ Q53.13 Unilateral high scrotal testis ♂
- **Q53.2 Undescended testicle, bilateral**
  - Q53.20 Undescended testicle, unspecified, bilateral ♂
  - **Q53.21 Abdominal testis, bilateral**
    - ▶ Q53.211 Bilateral intraabdominal testes ♂
    - ▶ Q53.212 Bilateral inguinal testes ♂
  - Q53.22 Ectopic perineal testis, bilateral ♂
  - ▶ Q53.23 Bilateral high scrotal testes ♂
  - Q53.9 Undescended testicle, unspecified ♂
    - Cryptorchism NOS
- **Q54 Hypospadias**
  - *Birth defect of male; urethra opens in abnormal location on shaft*
  - **Excludes1** epispadias (Q64.0)
  - Q54.0 Hypospadias, balanic ♂
    - Hypospadias, coronal
    - Hypospadias, glandular
  - Q54.1 Hypospadias, penile ♂
  - Q54.2 Hypospadias, penoscrotal ♂
  - Q54.3 Hypospadias, perineal ♂
  - Q54.4 Congenital chordee ♂
    - Chordee without hypospadias
  - Q54.8 Other hypospadias ♂
    - Hypospadias with intersex state
  - Q54.9 Hypospadias, unspecified ♂
- **Q55 Other congenital malformations of male genital organs**
  - **Excludes1** congenital hydrocele (P83.5)
    - hypospadias (Q54.-)
  - Q55.0 Absence and aplasia of testis ♂
    - Monorchism
  - Q55.1 Hypoplasia of testis and scrotum ♂
    - Fusion of testes
  - **Q55.2 Other and unspecified congenital malformations of testis and scrotum**
    - Q55.20 Unspecified congenital malformations of testis and scrotum ♂
      - Congenital malformation of testis or scrotum NOS
    - Q55.21 **Polyorchism** ♂
      - *Developmental anomaly characterized by presence of more than two testes*

- Q55.22 **Retractile testis** ♂
- Q55.23 **Scrotal transposition** ♂
- Q55.29 **Other congenital malformations of testis and scrotum** ♂
- Q55.3 **Atresia of vas deferens** ♂
  - *Code first any associated cystic fibrosis (E84.-)*
- Q55.4 **Other congenital malformations of vas deferens, epididymis, seminal vesicles and prostate** ♂
  - Absence or aplasia of prostate
  - Absence or aplasia of spermatic cord
  - Congenital malformation of vas deferens, epididymis, seminal vesicles or prostate NOS
- Q55.5 **Congenital absence and aplasia of penis** ♂
- **Q55.6 Other congenital malformations of penis**
  - Q55.61 **Curvature of penis (lateral)** ♂
  - Q55.62 **Hypoplasia of penis** ♂
    - *Underdevelopment penis*
    - Micropenis
  - Q55.63 **Congenital torsion of penis** ♂
    - **Excludes1** acquired torsion of penis (N48.82)
  - Q55.64 **Hidden penis** ♂
    - Buried penis
    - Concealed penis
    - **Excludes1** acquired buried penis (N48.83)
  - Q55.69 **Other congenital malformation of penis** ♂
    - Congenital malformation of penis NOS
- Q55.7 **Congenital vasocutaneous fistula** ♂
  - *Abnormal opening between vas deferens and skin*
- Q55.8 **Other specified congenital malformations of male genital organs** ♂
- Q55.9 **Congenital malformation of male genital organ, unspecified** ♂
  - Congenital anomaly of male genital organ
  - Congenital deformity of male genital organ
- **Q56 Indeterminate sex and pseudohermaphroditism**
  - *Internal reproductive organs are opposite external physical characteristics.*
  - **Excludes1** 46,XX true hermaphrodite (Q99.1)
    - androgen insensitivity syndrome (E34.5-)
    - chimera 46,XX/46,XY true hermaphrodite (Q99.0)
    - female pseudohermaphroditism with adrenocortical disorder (E25.-)
    - pseudohermaphroditism with specified chromosomal anomaly (Q96-Q99)
    - pure gonadal dysgenesis (Q99.1)
  - Q56.0 **Hermaphroditism, not elsewhere classified**
    - Ovotestis
  - Q56.1 **Male pseudohermaphroditism, not elsewhere classified** ♂
    - 46, XY with streak gonads
    - Male pseudohermaphroditism NOS
  - Q56.2 **Female pseudohermaphroditism, not elsewhere classified** ♀
    - Female pseudohermaphroditism NOS
  - Q56.3 **Pseudohermaphroditism, unspecified**
  - Q56.4 **Indeterminate sex, unspecified**
    - Ambiguous genitalia

CHAPTER 17 (Q00-Q99)

CONGENITAL MALFORMATIONS OF THE URINARY SYSTEM (Q60-Q64)

● **Q60   Renal agenesis and other reduction defects of kidney**
　　Includes　congenital absence of kidney
　　　　　　　　congenital atrophy of kidney
　　　　　　　　infantile atrophy of kidney
　　Ex: For category Q60 CC codes: See PDX Collection 1092
　　Q60.0   Renal agenesis, unilateral
　　Q60.1   Renal agenesis, bilateral
　　Q60.2   Renal agenesis, unspecified
　　Q60.3   Renal hypoplasia, unilateral
　　Q60.4   Renal hypoplasia, bilateral
　　Q60.5   Renal hypoplasia, unspecified
　　Q60.6   Potter's syndrome

● **Q61   Cystic kidney disease**
　　Cysts that develop in failing kidney due to end-stage renal disease
　　Excludes1　acquired cyst of kidney (N28.1)
　　　　　　　　Potter's syndrome (Q60.6)
　● **Q61.0   Congenital renal cyst**
　　　Q61.00   Congenital renal cyst, unspecified
　　　　　　Cyst of kidney NOS (congenital)
　　　　　　Ex: See PDX Collection 1093
　　　Q61.01   Congenital single renal cyst
　　　　　　Ex: See PDX Collection 1094
　　　Q61.02   Congenital multiple renal cysts
　　　　　　Ex: See PDX Collection 1095
　　Q61.1   Polycystic kidney, infantile type
　　　　Polycystic kidney, autosomal recessive
　　　　Ex: For category Q61.1 CC codes: See PDX Collection 1096
　　　Q61.11   Cystic dilatation of collecting ducts
　　　Q61.19   Other polycystic kidney, infantile type
　　Q61.2   Polycystic kidney, adult type
　　　　Polycystic kidney, autosomal dominant
　　　　Ex: See PDX Collection 1096
　　Q61.3   Polycystic kidney, unspecified
　　　　Ex: See PDX Collection 1096
　　　　Coding Clinic: 2016, Q3, P23
　　Q61.4   Renal dysplasia
　　　　Multicystic dysplastic kidney
　　　　Multicystic kidney (development)
　　　　Multicystic kidney disease
　　　　Multicystic renal dysplasia
　　　　Excludes1　polycystic kidney disease (Q61.11-Q61.3)
　　　　Ex: See PDX Collection 1097
　　Q61.5   Medullary cystic kidney
　　　　Nephronopthisis
　　　　Sponge kidney NOS
　　　　Ex: See PDX Collection 1095
　　Q61.8   Other cystic kidney diseases
　　　　Fibrocystic kidney
　　　　Fibrocystic renal degeneration or disease
　　　　Ex: See PDX Collection 1095
　　Q61.9   Cystic kidney disease, unspecified
　　　　Meckel-Gruber syndrome
　　　　Ex: See PDX Collection 1093

● **Q62   Congenital obstructive defects of renal pelvis and congenital malformations of ureter**
　　Q62.0   Congenital hydronephrosis
　　　　Ex: See PDX Collection 1098
　● **Q62.1   Congenital occlusion of ureter**
　　　　Atresia and stenosis of ureter
　　　　Ex: For category Q62.1 CC codes: See PDX Collection 1098
　　　Q62.10   Congenital occlusion of ureter, unspecified
　　　Q62.11   Congenital occlusion of ureteropelvic junction
　　　Q62.12   Congenital occlusion of ureterovesical orifice
　　Q62.2   Congenital megaureter
　　　　Congenital dilatation of ureter
　　　　Ex: See PDX Collection 1098

● **Q62.3   Other obstructive defects of renal pelvis and ureter**
　　　Ex: For category Q62.3 CC codes: See PDX Collection 1098
　　　Q62.31   Congenital ureterocele, orthotopic
　　　Q62.32   Cecoureterocele
　　　　　　Ectopic ureterocele
　　　Q62.39   Other obstructive defects of renal pelvis and ureter
　　　　　　Ureteropelvic junction obstruction NOS
　　Q62.4   Agenesis of ureter
　　　　Congenital absence ureter
　　Q62.5   Duplication of ureter
　　　　Accessory ureter
　　　　Double ureter
　● **Q62.6   Malposition of ureter**
　　　Q62.60   Malposition of ureter, unspecified
　　　Q62.61   Deviation of ureter
　　　Q62.62   Displacement of ureter
　　　Q62.63   Anomalous implantation of ureter
　　　　　　Ectopia of ureter
　　　　　　Ectopic ureter
　　　Q62.69   Other malposition of ureter
　　Q62.7   Congenital vesico-uretero-renal reflux
　　Q62.8   Other congenital malformations of ureter
　　　　Anomaly of ureter NOS

● **Q63   Other congenital malformations of kidney**
　　Excludes1　congenital nephrotic syndrome (N04.-)
　　Q63.0   Accessory kidney
　　Q63.1   Lobulated, fused and horseshoe kidney
　　Q63.2   Ectopic kidney
　　　　Congenital displaced kidney
　　　　Malrotation of kidney
　　Q63.3   Hyperplastic and giant kidney
　　　　Compensatory hypertrophy of kidney
　　Q63.8   Other specified congenital malformations of kidney
　　　　Congenital renal calculi
　　Q63.9   Congenital malformation of kidney, unspecified

● **Q64   Other congenital malformations of urinary system**
　　Q64.0   Epispadias ♂
　　　　Urethral opening somewhere on dorsum of penis
　　　　Excludes1　hypospadias (Q54.-)
　● **Q64.1   Exstrophy of urinary bladder**
　　　　Bladder is exposed, inside out, and protrudes through abdominal wall
　　　　Ex: For category Q64.1 CC codes: See PDX Collection 1099
　　　Q64.10   Exstrophy of urinary bladder, unspecified
　　　　　　Ectopia vesicae
　　　Q64.11   Supravesical fissure of urinary bladder
　⇒　**Q64.12   Cloacal exstrophy of urinary bladder**
　　　Q64.19   Other exstrophy of urinary bladder
　　　　　　Extroversion of bladder
　　Q64.2   Congenital posterior urethral valves
　　　　Ex: See PDX Collection 1100
　● **Q64.3   Other atresia and stenosis of urethra and bladder neck**
　　　　Ex: For category Q64.3 CC codes: See PDX Collection 1100
　　　Q64.31   Congenital bladder neck obstruction
　　　　　　Congenital obstruction of vesicourethral orifice
　　　Q64.32   Congenital stricture of urethra
　　　Q64.33   Congenital stricture of urinary meatus
　　　Q64.39   Other atresia and stenosis of urethra and bladder neck
　　　　　　Atresia and stenosis of urethra and bladder neck NOS
　　Q64.4   Malformation of urachus
　　　　Cyst of urachus
　　　　Patent urachus
　　　　Prolapse of urachus
　　Q64.5   Congenital absence of bladder and urethra
　　Q64.6   Congenital diverticulum of bladder

▶ New　⇒ Revised　d̶e̶l̶e̶t̶e̶d̶ Deleted　Excludes 1　Excludes 2　Includes　Use additional　Code first　Code also　Key words
OGCR Official Guidelines　● Unacceptable Principal Diagnosis　X Assign placeholder X　● Use Additional Character(s)　▸ Manifestation Code　Coding Clinic

● **Q64.7 Other and unspecified congenital malformations of bladder and urethra**

> **Excludes1** congenital prolapse of bladder (mucosa) (Q79.4)

Q64.70 **Unspecified congenital malformation of bladder and urethra**
> Malformation of bladder or urethra NOS

Q64.71 **Congenital prolapse of urethra**

Q64.72 **Congenital prolapse of urinary meatus**

Q64.73 **Congenital urethrorectal fistula**

Q64.74 **Double urethra**

Q64.75 **Double urinary meatus**

Q64.79 **Other congenital malformations of bladder and urethra**

Q64.8 **Other specified congenital malformations of urinary system**

Q64.9 **Congenital malformation of urinary system, unspecified**
> Congenital anomaly NOS of urinary system
> Congenital deformity NOS of urinary system

CONGENITAL MALFORMATIONS AND DEFORMATIONS OF THE MUSCULOSKELETAL SYSTEM (Q65-Q79)

● **Q65 Congenital deformities of hip**

> **Excludes1** clicking hip (R29.4)

● Q65.0 **Congenital dislocation of hip, unilateral**

Q65.00 **Congenital dislocation of unspecified hip, unilateral**

Q65.01 **Congenital dislocation of right hip, unilateral**

Q65.02 **Congenital dislocation of left hip, unilateral**

Q65.1 **Congenital dislocation of hip, bilateral**

Q65.2 **Congenital dislocation of hip, unspecified**

● Q65.3 **Congenital partial dislocation of hip, unilateral**

Q65.30 **Congenital partial dislocation of unspecified hip, unilateral**

Q65.31 **Congenital partial dislocation of right hip, unilateral**

Q65.32 **Congenital partial dislocation of left hip, unilateral**

Q65.4 **Congenital partial dislocation of hip, bilateral**

Q65.5 **Congenital partial dislocation of hip, unspecified**

Q65.6 **Congenital unstable hip**
> Congenital dislocatable hip

● Q65.8 **Other congenital deformities of hip**

Q65.81 **Congenital coxa valga**

Q65.82 **Congenital coxa vara**

Q65.89 **Other specified congenital deformities of hip**
> Anteversion of femoral neck
> Congenital acetabular dysplasia

Q65.9 **Congenital deformity of hip, unspecified**

● **Q66 Congenital deformities of feet**

> **Excludes1** reduction defects of feet (Q72.-)
> valgus deformities (acquired) (M21.0-)
> varus deformities (acquired) (M21.1-)

Q66.0 **Congenital talipes equinovarus**
> *Heel is turned inward from midline and foot is plantar flexed; AKA clubfoot*

Q66.1 **Congenital talipes calcaneovarus**
> *Deformity of foot in which heel is turned toward midline of body and anterior of foot is elevated*

● Q66.2 **Congenital metatarsus (primus) varus**
> *Angulation of first metatarsal bone toward midline of body*
> **Coding Clinic: 2016, Q4, P59**

Q66.21 **Congenital metatarsus primus varus**

Q66.22 **Congenital metatarsus adductus**
> Congenital metatarsus varus

Q66.3 **Other congenital varus deformities of feet**
> Hallux varus, congenital

Q66.4 **Congenital talipes calcaneovalgus**

Item 17–2 Equinus foot is a term referring to the hoof of a horse. The deformity is usually congenital or spastic. **Talipes equinovarus** is referred to as clubfoot. The foot tends to be smaller than normal, with the heel pointing downward and the forefoot turning inward. The heel cord (Achilles tendon) is tight, causing the heel to be drawn up toward the leg.

Figure 17-6 Supination and cavus deformity of forefoot. (From Kliegman R, Nelson WE: Nelson Textbook of Pediatrics, Philadelphia, Saunders, 2007)

Figure 17-7 Talipes. (From Dorland: Dorland's Illustrated Medical Dictionary, ed 31, Saunders, 2007, p 1893)

● Q66.5 **Congenital pes planus**
> Congenital flat foot
> Congenital rigid flat foot
> Congenital spastic (everted) flat foot

> **Excludes1** pes planus, acquired (M21.4)

Q66.50 **Congenital pes planus, unspecified foot**

Q66.51 **Congenital pes planus, right foot**

Q66.52 **Congenital pes planus, left foot**

Q66.6 **Other congenital valgus deformities of feet**
> *Inward angulation*
> Congenital metatarsus valgus

Q66.7 **Congenital pes cavus**

● Q66.8 **Other congenital deformities of feet**

Q66.80 **Congenital vertical talus deformity, unspecified foot**

Q66.81 **Congenital vertical talus deformity, right foot**

Q66.82 **Congenital vertical talus deformity, left foot**

Q66.89 **Other specified congenital deformities of feet**
> Congenital asymmetric talipes
> Congenital clubfoot NOS
> Congenital talipes NOS
> Congenital tarsal coalition
> Hammer toe, congenital

Q66.9 **Congenital deformity of feet, unspecified**

N Newborn Age: 0   **P** Pediatric Age: 0–17   **M** Maternity DX: 12–55   **A** Adult Age: 15–124   ♀ Females Only   ♂ Males Only

🅒 Complication\Comorbidity   🅜 Major C\C   ⒺⓍ CC/MCC Exclusions   🅗 Hospital-Acquired Condition

● **Q67 Congenital musculoskeletal deformities of head, face, spine and chest**
> **Excludes1** congenital malformation syndromes classified to Q87.-
> Potter's syndrome (Q60.6)

Q67.0 Congenital facial asymmetry

Q67.1 Congenital compression facies

Q67.2 Dolichocephaly
Long head dimension

Q67.3 Plagiocephaly
Asymmetric shape of head resulting from irregular closure of cranial sutures

Q67.4 Other congenital deformities of skull, face and jaw
Congenital depressions in skull
Congenital hemifacial atrophy or hypertrophy
Deviation of nasal septum, congenital
Squashed or bent nose, congenital
> **Excludes1** dentofacial anomalies [including malocclusion] (M26.-)
> syphilitic saddle nose (A50.5)

Q67.5 Congenital deformity of spine
Congenital postural scoliosis
Congenital scoliosis NOS
> **Excludes1** infantile idiopathic scoliosis (M41.0)
> scoliosis due to congenital bony malformation (Q76.3)

(Ex:) See PDX Collection 1101

Q67.6 Pectus excavatum
Congenital funnel chest
Funnel-shaped chest depression

Q67.7 Pectus carinatum
Congenital pigeon chest

Q67.8 Other congenital deformities of chest
Congenital deformity of chest wall NOS
(Ex:) See PDX Collection 1102

● **Q68 Other congenital musculoskeletal deformities**
> **Excludes1** reduction defects of limb(s) (Q71-Q73)
> **Excludes2** congenital myotonic chondrodystrophy (G71.13)

Q68.0 Congenital deformity of sternocleidomastoid muscle
Congenital contracture of sternocleidomastoid (muscle)
Congenital (sternomastoid) torticollis
Sternomastoid tumor (congenital)

Q68.1 Congenital deformity of finger(s) and hand
Congenital clubfinger
Spade-like hand (congenital)
(Ex:) See PDX Collection 1102

Q68.2 Congenital deformity of knee
Congenital dislocation of knee
Congenital genu recurvatum
Hyperextension of knee resulting from hypermobility

Q68.3 Congenital bowing of femur
> **Excludes1** anteversion of femur (neck) (Q65.89)

Q68.4 Congenital bowing of tibia and fibula

Q68.5 Congenital bowing of long bones of leg, unspecified

Q68.6 Discoid meniscus

Figure 17-8 Mild to moderate inbowing of the lower leg. (From Lissauer T, Clayden G: Illustrated Textbook of Paediatrics, Edinburgh, Mosby, 2011)

Figure 17-9 Thumb and index finger. (From Chung K: Hand and Upper Extremity Reconstruction, 1e, Saunders, 2008)

Q68.8 Other specified congenital musculoskeletal deformities
Congenital deformity of clavicle
Congenital deformity of elbow
Congenital deformity of forearm
Congenital deformity of scapula
Congenital deformity of wrist
Congenital dislocation of elbow
Congenital dislocation of shoulder
Congenital dislocation of wrist

● **Q69 Polydactyly**
AKA hyperdactyly, consists of supernumerary fingers or toes

Q69.0 Accessory finger(s)

Q69.1 Accessory thumb(s)

Q69.2 Accessory toe(s)
Accessory hallux

Q69.9 Polydactyly, unspecified
Supernumerary digit(s) NOS

● **Q70 Syndactyly**
Webbing between distal phalanges of adjacent digits

● **Q70.0 Fused fingers**
Complex syndactyly of fingers with synostosis
  Q70.00 Fused fingers, unspecified hand
  Q70.01 Fused fingers, right hand
  Q70.02 Fused fingers, left hand
  Q70.03 Fused fingers, bilateral

● **Q70.1 Webbed fingers**
Simple syndactyly of fingers without synostosis
  Q70.10 Webbed fingers, unspecified hand
  Q70.11 Webbed fingers, right hand
  Q70.12 Webbed fingers, left hand
  Q70.13 Webbed fingers, bilateral

● **Q70.2 Fused toes**
Complex syndactyly of toes with synostosis
  Q70.20 Fused toes, unspecified foot
  Q70.21 Fused toes, right foot
  Q70.22 Fused toes, left foot
  Q70.23 Fused toes, bilateral

● **Q70.3 Webbed toes**
Simple syndactyly of toes without synostosis
  Q70.30 Webbed toes, unspecified foot
  Q70.31 Webbed toes, right foot
  Q70.32 Webbed toes, left foot
  Q70.33 Webbed toes, bilateral

Q70.4 Polysyndactyly, unspecified
> **Excludes1** specified syndactyly of hand and feet - code to specified conditions (Q70.0- -Q70.3-)

Extra and webbed digits

Q70.9 Syndactyly, unspecified
Symphalangy NOS

▶ New ⏵ Revised ~~deleted~~ Deleted Excludes 1 Excludes 2 Includes Use additional Code first Code also Key words

OGCR Official Guidelines ● Unacceptable Principal Diagnosis X Assign placeholder X ● Use Additional Character(s) ▶ Manifestation Code **Coding Clinic**

1188

- **Q71 Reduction defects of upper limb**
  - **Q71.0 Congenital complete absence of upper limb**
    - Q71.00 Congenital complete absence of unspecified upper limb
    - Q71.01 Congenital complete absence of right upper limb
    - Q71.02 Congenital complete absence of left upper limb
    - Q71.03 Congenital complete absence of upper limb, bilateral
  - **Q71.1 Congenital absence of upper arm and forearm with hand present**
    - Q71.10 Congenital absence of unspecified upper arm and forearm with hand present
    - Q71.11 Congenital absence of right upper arm and forearm with hand present
    - Q71.12 Congenital absence of left upper arm and forearm with hand present
    - Q71.13 Congenital absence of upper arm and forearm with hand present, bilateral
  - **Q71.2 Congenital absence of both forearm and hand**
    - Q71.20 Congenital absence of both forearm and hand, unspecified upper limb
    - Q71.21 Congenital absence of both forearm and hand, right upper limb
    - Q71.22 Congenital absence of both forearm and hand, left upper limb
    - Q71.23 Congenital absence of both forearm and hand, bilateral
  - **Q71.3 Congenital absence of hand and finger**
    - Q71.30 Congenital absence of unspecified hand and finger
    - Q71.31 Congenital absence of right hand and finger
    - Q71.32 Congenital absence of left hand and finger
    - Q71.33 Congenital absence of hand and finger, bilateral
  - **Q71.4 Longitudinal reduction defect of radius**
    Clubhand (congenital)
    Radial clubhand
    - Q71.40 Longitudinal reduction defect of unspecified radius
    - Q71.41 Longitudinal reduction defect of right radius
    - Q71.42 Longitudinal reduction defect of left radius
    - Q71.43 Longitudinal reduction defect of radius, bilateral
  - **Q71.5 Longitudinal reduction defect of ulna**
    - Q71.50 Longitudinal reduction defect of unspecified ulna
    - Q71.51 Longitudinal reduction defect of right ulna
    - Q71.52 Longitudinal reduction defect of left ulna
    - Q71.53 Longitudinal reduction defect of ulna, bilateral
  - **Q71.6 Lobster-claw hand**
    - Q71.60 Lobster-claw hand, unspecified hand
    - Q71.61 Lobster-claw right hand
    - Q71.62 Lobster-claw left hand
    - Q71.63 Lobster-claw hand, bilateral
  - **Q71.8 Other reduction defects of upper limb**
    - **Q71.81 Congenital shortening of upper limb**
      - Q71.811 Congenital shortening of right upper limb
      - Q71.812 Congenital shortening of left upper limb
      - Q71.813 Congenital shortening of upper limb, bilateral
      - Q71.819 Congenital shortening of unspecified upper limb
    - **Q71.89 Other reduction defects of upper limb**
      - Q71.891 Other reduction defects of right upper limb
      - Q71.892 Other reduction defects of left upper limb
      - Q71.893 Other reduction defects of upper limb, bilateral
      - Q71.899 Other reduction defects of unspecified upper limb
  - **Q71.9 Unspecified reduction defect of upper limb**
    - Q71.90 Unspecified reduction defect of unspecified upper limb
    - Q71.91 Unspecified reduction defect of right upper limb
    - Q71.92 Unspecified reduction defect of left upper limb
    - Q71.93 Unspecified reduction defect of upper limb, bilateral

- **Q72 Reduction defects of lower limb**
  - **Q72.0 Congenital complete absence of lower limb**
    - Q72.00 Congenital complete absence of unspecified lower limb
    - Q72.01 Congenital complete absence of right lower limb
    - Q72.02 Congenital complete absence of left lower limb
    - Q72.03 Congenital complete absence of lower limb, bilateral
  - **Q72.1 Congenital absence of thigh and lower leg with foot present**
    - Q72.10 Congenital absence of unspecified thigh and lower leg with foot present
    - Q72.11 Congenital absence of right thigh and lower leg with foot present
    - Q72.12 Congenital absence of left thigh and lower leg with foot present
    - Q72.13 Congenital absence of thigh and lower leg with foot present, bilateral
  - **Q72.2 Congenital absence of both lower leg and foot**
    - Q72.20 Congenital absence of both lower leg and foot, unspecified lower limb
    - Q72.21 Congenital absence of both lower leg and foot, right lower limb
    - Q72.22 Congenital absence of both left lower leg and foot, left lower limb
    - Q72.23 Congenital absence of both lower leg and foot, bilateral
  - **Q72.3 Congenital absence of foot and toe(s)**
    - Q72.30 Congenital absence of unspecified foot and toe(s)
    - Q72.31 Congenital absence of right foot and toe(s)
    - Q72.32 Congenital absence of left foot and toe(s)
    - Q72.33 Congenital absence of foot and toe(s), bilateral
  - **Q72.4 Longitudinal reduction defect of femur**
    Proximal femoral focal deficiency
    - Q72.40 Longitudinal reduction defect of unspecified femur
    - Q72.41 Longitudinal reduction defect of right femur
    - Q72.42 Longitudinal reduction defect of left femur
    - Q72.43 Longitudinal reduction defect of femur, bilateral
  - **Q72.5 Longitudinal reduction defect of tibia**
    - Q72.50 Longitudinal reduction defect of unspecified tibia
    - Q72.51 Longitudinal reduction defect of right tibia
    - Q72.52 Longitudinal reduction defect of left tibia
    - Q72.53 Longitudinal reduction defect of tibia, bilateral
  - **Q72.6 Longitudinal reduction defect of fibula**
    - Q72.60 Longitudinal reduction defect of unspecified fibula
    - Q72.61 Longitudinal reduction defect of right fibula
    - Q72.62 Longitudinal reduction defect of left fibula
    - Q72.63 Longitudinal reduction defect of fibula, bilateral

CHAPTER 17 (Q00–Q99)

CHAPTER 17 (Q00–Q99)

- Q72.7 **Split foot**
  - Q72.70 Split foot, unspecified lower limb
  - Q72.71 Split foot, right lower limb
  - Q72.72 Split foot, left lower limb
  - Q72.73 Split foot, bilateral
- Q72.8 **Other reduction defects of lower limb**
  - Q72.81 Congenital shortening of lower limb
    - Q72.811 Congenital shortening of right lower limb
    - Q72.812 Congenital shortening of left lower limb
    - Q72.813 Congenital shortening of lower limb, bilateral
    - Q72.819 Congenital shortening of unspecified lower limb
  - Q72.89 Other reduction defects of lower limb
    - Q72.891 Other reduction defects of right lower limb
    - Q72.892 Other reduction defects of left lower limb
    - Q72.893 Other reduction defects of lower limb, bilateral
    - Q72.899 Other reduction defects of unspecified lower limb
- Q72.9 **Unspecified reduction defect of lower limb**
  - Q72.90 Unspecified reduction defect of unspecified lower limb
  - Q72.91 Unspecified reduction defect of right lower limb
  - Q72.92 Unspecified reduction defect of left lower limb
  - Q72.93 Unspecified reduction defect of lower limb, bilateral
- Q73 **Reduction defects of unspecified limb**
  - Q73.0 **Congenital absence of unspecified limb(s)**
    Amelia NOS
  - Q73.1 **Phocomelia, unspecified limb(s)**
    Phocomelia NOS
    Absence/shortening of long bones primarily as a result of thalidomide
  - Q73.8 **Other reduction defects of unspecified limb(s)**
    Longitudinal reduction deformity of unspecified limb(s)
    Ectromelia of limb NOS
    Gross hypoplasia or aplasia of one or more long bones of limb(s)
    Hemimelia of limb NOS
    Absence of one-half of long bone
    Reduction defect of limb NOS
- Q74 **Other congenital malformations of limb(s)**
  - **Excludes1**   polydactyly (Q69.-)
    reduction defect of limb (Q71-Q73)
    syndactyly (Q70.-)
  - Q74.0 **Other congenital malformations of upper limb(s), including shoulder girdle**
    Accessory carpal bones
    Cleidocranial dysostosis
    Congenital pseudarthrosis of clavicle
    Macrodactylia (fingers)
    Madelung's deformity
    Radioulnar synostosis
    Sprengel's deformity
    Triphalangeal thumb
  - Q74.1 **Congenital malformation of knee**
    Congenital absence of patella
    Congenital dislocation of patella
    Congenital genu valgum
    Congenital genu varum
    Rudimentary patella
    - **Excludes1**   congenital dislocation of knee (Q68.2)
      congenital genu recurvatum (Q68.2)
      nail patella syndrome (Q87.2)

- Q74.2 **Other congenital malformations of lower limb(s), including pelvic girdle**
  Congenital fusion of sacroiliac joint
  Congenital malformation of ankle joint
  Congenital malformation of sacroiliac joint
  - **Excludes1**   anteversion of femur (neck) (Q65.89)
- Q74.3 **Arthrogryposis multiplex congenita** 🔖
- Q74.8 **Other specified congenital malformations of limb(s)**
- Q74.9 **Unspecified congenital malformation of limb(s)**
  Congenital anomaly of limb(s) NOS
- Q75 **Other congenital malformations of skull and face bones**
  - **Excludes1**   congenital malformation of face NOS (Q18.-)
    congenital malformation syndromes classified to Q87.-
    dentofacial anomalies [including malocclusion] (M26.-)
    musculoskeletal deformities of head and face (Q67.0-Q67.4)
    skull defects associated with congenital anomalies of brain such as:
      anencephaly (Q00.0)
      encephalocele (Q01.-)
      hydrocephalus (Q03.-)
      microcephaly (Q02)
  - Q75.0 **Craniosynostosis**
    Premature closure of sutures of skull
    Acrocephaly
    Imperfect fusion of skull
    Oxycephaly
    Trigonocephaly
  - Q75.1 **Craniofacial dysostosis**
    Congenital deformity of head
    Crouzon's disease
  - Q75.2 **Hypertelorism**
  - Q75.3 **Macrocephaly**
    Unusually large size of head; AKA megalocephaly
  - Q75.4 **Mandibulofacial dysostosis**
    Franceschetti syndrome
    Treacher Collins syndrome
  - Q75.5 **Oculomandibular dysostosis**
    Ossification of occular and mandibular bones
  - Q75.8 **Other specified congenital malformations of skull and face bones**
    Absence of skull bone, congenital
    Congenital deformity of forehead
    Platybasia
  - Q75.9 **Congenital malformation of skull and face bones, unspecified**
    Congenital anomaly of face bones NOS
    Congenital anomaly of skull NOS

Item 17–3 Anencephalus is a congenital deformity of the cranial vault. **Craniosynostosis,** also known as craniostenosis and stenocephaly, signifies any form of congenital deformity of the skull that results from the premature closing of the sutures of the skull. **Iniencephaly** is a deformity in which the head and neck are flexed backward to a great extent and the head is very large in comparison to the shortened body.

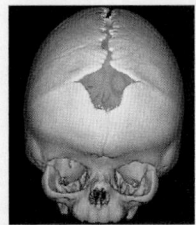

Figure 17-10 Generalized craniosynostosis without symptoms or signs of increased intracranial pressure. (From Goetz C: Textbook of Clinical Neurology, St. Louis, MO, Elsevier, 2007)

▶ New   ⇒ Revised   ~~deleted~~ Deleted   Excludes 1   Excludes 2   Includes   Use additional   Code first   Code also   Key words

OGCR Official Guidelines   ● Unacceptable Principal Diagnosis   X Assign placeholder X   ● Use Additional Character(s)   ▶ Manifestation Code   **Coding Clinic**

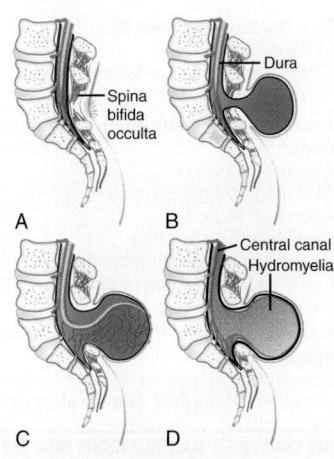

Figure 17-11 **A.** Spina bifida occulta. **B.** Meningocele.
C. Myelomeningocele. **D.** Myelocystocele (syringomyelocele)
or hydromyelia.

Item 17–4 **Spina bifida** is a midline spinal defect in which one or more
vertebrae fail to fuse, leaving an opening in the vertebral canal. When the
defect is not visible, it is called spina bifida occulta, and when it is visible, it is
called spina bifida cystica.

● **Q76** **Congenital malformations of spine and bony thorax**

  Excludes1 congenital musculoskeletal deformities of spine
  and chest (Q67.5-Q67.8)

  Q76.0 **Spina bifida occulta**

  Excludes1 meningocele (spinal) (Q05.-)
  spina bifida (aperta) (cystica) (Q05.-)

  Q76.1 **Klippel-Feil syndrome**
  Cervical fusion syndrome

  Q76.2 **Congenital spondylolisthesis**
  Congenital spondylolysis

  Excludes1 spondylolisthesis (acquired) (M43.1-)
  spondylolysis (acquired) (M43.0-)

  Q76.3 **Congenital scoliosis due to congenital bony
  malformation** 🔹
  Hemivertebra fusion or failure of segmentation with
  scoliosis
  (Ex) See PDX Collection 1101

  ● **Q76.4** **Other congenital malformations of spine, not associated
  with scoliosis**

    ● **Q76.41** **Congenital kyphosis**
    *Abnormal increase in convexity curvature of
    thoracic spinal column; AKA humpback*

      Q76.411 **Congenital kyphosis, occipito-atlanto-
      axial region**

      Q76.412 **Congenital kyphosis, cervical region**

      Q76.413 **Congenital kyphosis, cervicothoracic
      region**

      Q76.414 **Congenital kyphosis, thoracic region**

      Q76.415 **Congenital kyphosis, thoracolumbar
      region**

      Q76.419 **Congenital kyphosis, unspecified
      region**

  ● **Q76.42** **Congenital lordosis**
  *An abnormal increase in curvature of lumbar spine
  (sway back)*
  (Ex) For category **Q76.42** CC codes: See PDX Collection 1101

    Q76.425 **Congenital lordosis, thoracolumbar
    region** 🔹

    Q76.426 **Congenital lordosis, lumbar region** 🔹

    Q76.427 **Congenital lordosis, lumbosacral
    region** 🔹

    Q76.428 **Congenital lordosis, sacral and
    sacrococcygeal region** 🔹

    Q76.429 **Congenital lordosis, unspecified
    region** 🔹

  Q76.49 **Other congenital malformations of spine, not
  associated with scoliosis**
  Congenital absence of vertebra NOS
  Congenital fusion of spine NOS
  Congenital malformation of lumbosacral (joint)
  (region) NOS
  Congenital malformation of spine NOS
  Hemivertebra NOS
  Malformation of spine NOS
  Platyspondylisis NOS
  Supernumerary vertebra NOS

  Q76.5 **Cervical rib**
  Supernumerary rib in cervical region

  Q76.6 **Other congenital malformations of ribs** 🔹
  Accessory rib
  Congenital absence of rib
  Congenital fusion of ribs
  Congenital malformation of ribs NOS

  Excludes1 short rib syndrome (Q77.2)
  (Ex) See PDX Collection 1103

  Q76.7 **Congenital malformation of sternum** 🔹
  Congenital absence of sternum
  Sternum bifidum
  (Ex) See PDX Collection 1103

  Q76.8 **Other congenital malformations of bony thorax** 🔹
  (Ex) See PDX Collection 1103

  Q76.9 **Congenital malformation of bony thorax, unspecified** 🔹
  (Ex) See PDX Collection 1103

● **Q77** **Osteochondrodysplasia with defects of growth of tubular bones
and spine**

  Excludes1 mucopolysaccharidosis (E76.0-E76.3)
  Excludes2 congenital myotonic chondrodystrophy (G71.13)

  Q77.0 **Achondrogenesis**
  Hypochondrogenesis

  Q77.1 **Thanatophoric short stature**

  Q77.2 **Short rib syndrome** 🔹
  Asphyxiating thoracic dysplasia [Jeune]
  (Ex) See PDX Collection 1103

  Q77.3 **Chondrodysplasia punctata**
  Benign cartilaginous neoplasms

  Excludes1 rhizomelic chondrodysplasia punctata
  (E71.43)

  Q77.4 **Achondroplasia**
  *Disturbance of epiphyseal chondroblastic growth and
  maturation, results in dwarfism*
  Hypochondroplasia
  Osteosclerosis congenita

  Q77.5 **Diastrophic dysplasia**

  Q77.6 **Chondroectodermal dysplasia**
  *Defective development of skin, hair, teeth, with polydactyly
  and defect of cardiac septum*
  Ellis-van Creveld syndrome

  Q77.7 **Spondyloepiphyseal dysplasia**

  Q77.8 **Other osteochondrodysplasia with defects of growth of
  tubular bones and spine**

  Q77.9 **Osteochondrodysplasia with defects of growth of
  tubular bones and spine, unspecified**

CHAPTER 17 (Q00-Q99)

N Newborn Age: 0   **P** Pediatric Age: 0–17   **M** Maternity DX: 12–55   **A** Adult Age: 15–124   ♀ Females Only   ♂ Males Only

🔹 Complication\Comorbidity   🔹 Major C\C   (Ex) CC/MCC Exclusions   🔹 Hospital-Acquired Condition

1191

CHAPTER 17 (Q00-Q99)

● **Q78** **Other osteochondrodysplasias**
Disorder of development of bone and cartilage; common cause of dwarfism

     Excludes2   congenital myotonic chondrodystrophy (G71.13)

   Q78.0 **Osteogenesis imperfecta** 🔑
      Fragilitas ossium
      Osteopsathyrosis
      (Ex) See PDX Collection 1104

   Q78.1 **Polyostotic fibrous dysplasia**
      Albright(-McCune)(-Sternberg) syndrome

   Q78.2 **Osteopetrosis** 🔑
      Abnormally dense bone; AKA marble bones disease, ivory bones
      Albers-Schönberg syndrome
      Osteosclerosis NOS
      (Ex) See PDX Collection 1104

   Q78.3 **Progressive diaphyseal dysplasia**
      Camurati-Engelmann syndrome

   Q78.4 **Enchondromatosis**
      Thinning of overlying cortex of bone and distorted length
      Maffucci's syndrome
      Ollier's disease

   Q78.5 **Metaphyseal dysplasia**
      Disturbance in enchondral bone growth, causing ends of shafts to remain larger than normal in circumference
      Pyle's syndrome

   Q78.6 **Multiple congenital exostoses**
      Diaphyseal aclasis

   Q78.8 **Other specified osteochondrodysplasias**
      Osteopoikilosis

   Q78.9 **Osteochondrodysplasia, unspecified**
      Chondrodystrophy NOS
      AKA skeletal dysplasia (dwarfism) caused by genetic mutations affecting hyaline cartilage capping long bones and vertebrae
      Osteodystrophy NOS

● **Q79** **Congenital malformations of musculoskeletal system, not elsewhere classified**

     Excludes2   congenital (sternomastoid) torticollis (Q68.0)

   Q79.0 **Congenital diaphragmatic hernia** 🔑
      Excludes1   congenital hiatus hernia (Q40.1)
      (Ex) See PDX Collection 1105

   Q79.1 **Other congenital malformations of diaphragm** 🔑
      Absence of diaphragm
      Congenital malformation of diaphragm NOS
      Eventration of diaphragm
      (Ex) See PDX Collection 1105

   Q79.2 **Exomphalos** 🔑
      Abdominal hernia in which part of intestine protrudes at umbilicus; AKA exomphalos and exumbilication
      Omphalocele
      Excludes1   umbilical hernia (K42.-)
      (Ex) See PDX Collection 1106

   Q79.3 **Gastroschisis** 🔑
      Congenital fissure of anterior abdominal wall often with protrusion of small/large intestine
      (Ex) See PDX Collection 1106

   Q79.4 **Prune belly syndrome** 🔑
      Congenital prolapse of bladder mucosa
      Eagle-Barrett syndrome
      (Ex) See PDX Collection 1106

 ● **Q79.5** **Other congenital malformations of abdominal wall**
      Excludes1   umbilical hernia (K42.-)
      (Ex) For category Q79.5 CC codes: See PDX Collection 1106

     Q79.51 **Congenital hernia of bladder** 🔑

     Q79.59 **Other congenital malformations of abdominal wall** 🔑

   Q79.6 **Ehlers-Danlos syndrome** 🔑
      (Ex) See PDX Collection 1107
      Group of inherited disorders of connective tissue; AKA cutis hyperelastica

   Q79.8 **Other congenital malformations of musculoskeletal system**
      Absence of muscle
      Absence of tendon
      Accessory muscle
      Amyotrophia congenita
      Congenital constricting bands
      Congenital shortening of tendon
      Poland syndrome

   Q79.9 **Congenital malformation of musculoskeletal system, unspecified**
      Congenital anomaly of musculoskeletal system NOS
      Congenital deformity of musculoskeletal system NOS

OTHER CONGENITAL MALFORMATIONS (Q80-Q89)

● **Q80** **Congenital ichthyosis**
Characterized by increased keratinization, resulting in noninflammatory scaling of skin

     Excludes1   Refsum's disease (G60.1)

   Q80.0 **Ichthyosis vulgaris**

   Q80.1 **X-linked ichthyosis**

   Q80.2 **Lamellar ichthyosis**
      Collodion baby

   Q80.3 **Congenital bullous ichthyosiform erythroderma**

   Q80.4 **Harlequin fetus**

   Q80.8 **Other congenital ichthyosis**

   Q80.9 **Congenital ichthyosis, unspecified**

● **Q81** **Epidermolysis bullosa**
Loosening of epidermis

   Q81.0 **Epidermolysis bullosa simplex**
      Excludes1   Cockayne's syndrome (Q87.1)

   Q81.1 **Epidermolysis bullosa letalis**
      Herlitz' syndrome

   Q81.2 **Epidermolysis bullosa dystrophica**

   Q81.8 **Other epidermolysis bullosa**

   Q81.9 **Epidermolysis bullosa, unspecified**

● **Q82** **Other congenital malformations of skin**
     Excludes1   acrodermatitis enteropathica (E83.2)
                  congenital erythropoietic porphyria (E80.0)
                  pilonidal cyst or sinus (L05.-)
                  Sturge-Weber (-Dimitri) syndrome (Q85.8)

   Q82.0 **Hereditary lymphedema**
      Characterized by swelling of subcutaneous tissue caused by obstruction of lymphatic vessels and resulting edema of lymph fluid

   Q82.1 **Xeroderma pigmentosum**
      Extreme sensitivity to ultraviolet rays that most commonly affects the eyes and skin, but may also involve the nervous system

⇒ **Q82.2** **Congenital cutaneous mastocytosis**
      Characterized by infiltrates of mast cells in tissues/organs
      ~~Urticaria pigmentosa~~
      ▶Congenital diffuse cutaneous mastocytosis
      ▶Congenital maculopapular cutaneous mastocytosis
      ▶Congenital urticaria pigmentosa
      Excludes1   ~~malignant mastocytosis (C96.2)~~
                  ▶cutaneous mastocytosis NOS (D47.01)
                  ▶diffuse cutaneous mastocytosis (with onset after newborn period) (D47.01)
                  ▶malignant mastocytosis (C96.2-)
                  ▶systemic mastocytosis (D47.02)
                  ▶urticaria pigmentosa (non-congenital) (with onset after newborn period) (D47.01)

▶ New   ⇒ Revised   ~~deleted~~ Deleted   Excludes 1   Excludes 2   Includes   Use additional   Code first   Code also   Key words

OGCR Official Guidelines   ● Unacceptable Principal Diagnosis   X Assign placeholder X   ● Use Additional Character(s)   ⇒ Manifestation Code   **Coding Clinic**

Q82.3   Incontinentia pigmenti
Characterized by hypopigmented cutaneous in adults and early childhood

Q82.4   Ectodermal dysplasia (anhidrotic)
Absence/deficiency of tissues/structures, including teeth, hair, nails, and certain glands

> **Excludes1**   Ellis-van Creveld syndrome (Q77.6)

Q82.5   Congenital non-neoplastic nevus
Birthmark NOS
Flammeus Nevus
Portwine Nevus
Sanguineous Nevus
Strawberry Nevus
Vascular Nevus NOS
Verrucous Nevus

> **Excludes2**   Café au lait spots (L81.3)
> lentigo (L81.4)
> nevus NOS (D22.-)
> araneus nevus (I78.1)
> melanocytic nevus (D22.-)
> pigmented nevus (D22.-)
> spider nevus (I78.1)
> stellar nevus (I78.1)

Q82.6   Congenital sacral dimple
Parasacral dimple

> **Excludes2**   pilonidal cyst with abscess (L05.01)
> pilonidal cyst without abscess (L05.91)

Coding Clinic: 2016, Q4, P60

Q82.8   Other specified congenital malformations of skin
Abnormal palmar creases
Accessory skin tags
Benign familial pemphigus [Hailey-Hailey]
Congenital poikiloderma
Cutis laxa (hyperelastica)
Dermatoglyphic anomalies
Inherited keratosis palmaris et plantaris
Keratosis follicularis [Darier-White]

> **Excludes1**   Ehlers-Danlos syndrome (Q79.6)

Coding Clinic: 2016, Q1, P17

Q82.9   Congenital malformation of skin, unspecified

● **Q83   Congenital malformations of breast**

> **Excludes2**   absence of pectoral muscle (Q79.8)
> hypoplasia of breast (N64.82)
> micromastia (N64.82)

Q83.0   Congenital absence of breast with absent nipple

Q83.1   Accessory breast
Supernumerary breast

Q83.2   Absent nipple

Q83.3   Accessory nipple
Supernumerary nipple

Q83.8   Other congenital malformations of breast

Q83.9   Congenital malformation of breast, unspecified

● **Q84   Other congenital malformations of integument**

Q84.0   Congenital alopecia
Congenital atrichosis

Q84.1   Congenital morphological disturbances of hair, not elsewhere classified
Beaded hair
Monilethrix
Pili annulati

> **Excludes1**   Menkes' kinky hair syndrome (E83.0)

Q84.2   Other congenital malformations of hair
Congenital hypertrichosis
Congenital malformation of hair NOS
Persistent lanugo

Q84.3   Anonychia
Absence of nail

> **Excludes1**   nail patella syndrome (Q87.2)

Q84.4   Congenital leukonychia
Opaque, whitish discoloration of nails; AKA leukopathia unguium

Q84.5   Enlarged and hypertrophic nails
Congenital onychauxis
Pachyonychia

Q84.6   Other congenital malformations of nails
Congenital clubnail
Congenital koilonychia
Congenital malformation of nail NOS

Q84.8   Other specified congenital malformations of integument
Aplasia cutis congenita

Q84.9   Congenital malformation of integument, unspecified
Congenital anomaly of integument NOS
Congenital deformity of integument NOS

● **Q85   Phakomatoses, not elsewhere classified**

> **Excludes1**   ataxia telangiectasia [Louis-Bar] (G11.3)
> familial dysautonomia [Riley-Day] (G90.1)

● **Q85.0   Neurofibromatosis (nonmalignant)**
Developmental changes in nervous system and other structures, with formation of neurofibromas

Q85.00   Neurofibromatosis, unspecified

Q85.01   Neurofibromatosis, type 1
Von Recklinghausen disease

Q85.02   Neurofibromatosis, type 2
Acoustic neurofibromatosis

Q85.03   Schwannomatosis

Q85.09   Other neurofibromatosis

Q85.1   Tuberous sclerosis 🖚
Bourneville's disease
Epiloia
Ⓔ See PDX Collection 1108

Q85.8   Other phakomatoses, not elsewhere classified 🖚
Peutz-Jeghers Syndrome
Sturge-Weber(-Dimitri) syndrome
von Hippel-Lindau syndrome

> **Excludes1**   Meckel-Gruber syndrome (Q61.9)

Ⓔ See PDX Collection 1109

Q85.9   Phakomatosis, unspecified 🖚
Hamartosis NOS
Ⓔ See PDX Collection 1109

● **Q86   Congenital malformation syndromes due to known exogenous causes, not elsewhere classified**

> **Excludes2**   iodine-deficiency-related hypothyroidism (E00-E02)
> nonteratogenic effects of substances transmitted via placenta or breast milk (P04.-)

Q86.0   Fetal alcohol syndrome (dysmorphic)

Q86.1   Fetal hydantoin syndrome
Meadow's syndrome

Q86.2   Dysmorphism due to warfarin

Q86.8   Other congenital malformation syndromes due to known exogenous causes

● **Q87   Other specified congenital malformation syndromes affecting multiple systems**
Use additional code(s) to identify all associated manifestations

Q87.0   Congenital malformation syndromes predominantly affecting facial appearance
Acrocephalopolysyndactyly
Acrocephalosyndactyly [Apert]
Cryptophthalmos syndrome
Cyclopia
Goldenhar syndrome
Moebius syndrome
Oro-facial-digital syndrome
Robin syndrome
Whistling face

CHAPTER 17 (Q00-Q99)

N Newborn Age: 0   **P** Pediatric Age: 0–17   **M** Maternity DX: 12–55   **A** Adult Age: 15–124   ♀ Females Only   ♂ Males Only
🖚 Complication\Comorbidity   🖚 Major C\C   Ⓔ CC/MCC Exclusions   🖚 Hospital-Acquired Condition

1193

CHAPTER 17 (Q00-Q99)

Q87.1 Congenital malformation syndromes predominantly associated with short stature 🔖
Aarskog syndrome
Cockayne syndrome
De Lange syndrome
Dubowitz syndrome
Noonan syndrome
Prader-Willi syndrome
Robinow-Silverman-Smith syndrome
Russell-Silver syndrome
Seckel syndrome
> **Excludes1**   Ellis-van Creveld syndrome (Q77.6)
> Smith-Lemli-Opitz syndrome (E78.72)

Ⓔ See PDX Collection 1110

Q87.2 Congenital malformation syndromes predominantly involving limbs 🔖
Holt-Oram syndrome
Klippel-Trenaunay-Weber syndrome
Nail patella syndrome
Rubinstein-Taybi syndrome
Sirenomelia syndrome
Thrombocytopenia with absent radius [TAR] syndrome
VATER syndrome
Ⓔ See PDX Collection 540

Q87.3 Congenital malformation syndromes involving early overgrowth 🔖
Beckwith-Wiedemann syndrome
Sotos' syndrome
Weaver syndrome
Ⓔ See PDX Collection 540

● **Q87.4 Marfan's syndrome**
Ⓔ For category Q87.4 CC codes: See PDX Collection 1110

  Q87.40 Marfan's syndrome, unspecified 🔖

● **Q87.41 Marfan's syndrome with cardiovascular manifestations**
    Q87.410 Marfan's syndrome with aortic dilation 🔖
    Q87.418 Marfan's syndrome with other cardiovascular manifestations 🔖

  Q87.42 Marfan's syndrome with ocular manifestations 🔖

  Q87.43 Marfan's syndrome with skeletal manifestation 🔖

Q87.5 Other congenital malformation syndromes with other skeletal changes 🔖
Ⓔ See PDX Collection 540

● **Q87.8 Other specified congenital malformation syndromes, not elsewhere classified**
> **Excludes1**   Zellweger syndrome (E71.510)

Ⓔ For category Q87.8 CC codes: See PDX Collection 540

  Q87.81 Alport syndrome 🔖
Progressive sensorineural hearing loss, progressive pyelonephritis or glomerulonephritis, and ocular defects
Use additional code to identify stage of chronic kidney disease (N18.1-N18.6)

  Q87.82 Arterial tortuosity syndrome 🔖
Coding Clinic: 2016, Q4, P60-61

  Q87.89 Other specified congenital malformation syndromes, not elsewhere classified 🔖
Laurence-Moon (-Bardet)-Biedl syndrome

● **Q89 Other congenital malformations, not elsewhere classified**
 ● **Q89.0 Congenital absence and malformations of spleen**
> **Excludes1**   isomerism of atrial appendages (with asplenia or polysplenia) (Q20.6)

Ⓔ For category Q87.8 CC codes: See PDX Collection 1111

  Q89.01 Asplenia (congenital) 🔖

  Q89.09 Congenital malformations of spleen 🔖
Congenital splenomegaly

Q89.1 Congenital malformations of adrenal gland
> **Excludes1**   adrenogenital disorders (E25.-)
> congenital adrenal hyperplasia (E25.0)

Q89.2 Congenital malformations of other endocrine glands
Congenital malformation of parathyroid or thyroid gland
Persistent thyroglossal duct
Thyroglossal cyst
> **Excludes1**   congenital goiter (E03.0)
> congenital hypothyroidism (E03.1)

Q89.3 Situs inversus 🔖
Lateral transposition of viscera of thorax and abdomen
Dextrocardia with situs inversus
Mirror-image atrial arrangement with situs inversus
Situs inversus or transversus abdominalis
Situs inversus or transversus thoracis
Transposition of abdominal viscera
Transposition of thoracic viscera
> **Excludes1**   dextrocardia NOS (Q24.0)

Ⓔ See PDX Collection 1112

Q89.4 Conjoined twins 🔖
Craniopagus
Dicephaly
Pygopagus
Thoracopagus
Ⓔ See PDX Collection 1113

Q89.7 Multiple congenital malformations, not elsewhere classified 🔖
Multiple congenital anomalies NOS
Multiple congenital deformities NOS
> **Excludes1**   congenital malformation syndromes affecting multiple systems (Q87.-)

Ⓔ See PDX Collection 1112

Q89.8 Other specified congenital malformations 🔖
Use additional code(s) to identify all associated manifestations
Ⓔ See PDX Collection 540

Q89.9 Congenital malformation, unspecified
Congenital anomaly NOS
Congenital deformity NOS

CHROMOSOMAL ABNORMALITIES, NOT ELSEWHERE CLASSIFIED (Q90-Q99)

> **Excludes2**   mitochondrial metabolic disorders (E88.4-)

● **Q90 Down syndrome**
Use additional code(s) to identify any associated physical conditions and degree of intellectual disabilities (F70-F79)

Q90.0 Trisomy 21, nonmosaicism (meiotic nondisjunction)
Trisomy 21, nondisjunction, accounts for 95% of Downs syndrome cases

Q90.1 Trisomy 21, mosaicism (mitotic nondisjunction)

Q90.2 Trisomy 21, translocation

Q90.9 Down syndrome, unspecified
Trisomy 21 NOS

● **Q91 Trisomy 18 and Trisomy 13**
Ⓔ For category Q91 CC codes: See PDX Collection 1114

Q91.0 Trisomy 18, nonmosaicism (meiotic nondisjunction) 🔖
Q91.1 Trisomy 18, mosaicism (mitotic nondisjunction) 🔖
Q91.2 Trisomy 18, translocation 🔖
Q91.3 Trisomy 18, unspecified 🔖
Q91.4 Trisomy 13, nonmosaicism (meiotic nondisjunction) 🔖
Q91.5 Trisomy 13, mosaicism (mitotic nondisjunction) 🔖
Q91.6 Trisomy 13, translocation 🔖
Q91.7 Trisomy 13, unspecified 🔖

▶ New   ⇒ Revised   ~~deleted~~ Deleted   Excludes 1   Excludes 2   Includes   Use additional   Code first   Code also   Key words
OGCR Official Guidelines   ● Unacceptable Principal Diagnosis   X Assign placeholder X   ● Use Additional Character(s)   ▶ Manifestation Code   **Coding Clinic**

● **Q92   Other trisomies and partial trisomies of the autosomes, not elsewhere classified**

> **Includes**   unbalanced translocations and insertions
> **Excludes1**   trisomies of chromosomes 13, 18, 21 (Q90-Q91)

Q92.0   **Whole chromosome trisomy, nonmosaicism (meiotic nondisjunction)**

Q92.1   **Whole chromosome trisomy, mosaicism (mitotic nondisjunction)**

Q92.2   **Partial trisomy**
> Less than whole arm duplicated
> Whole arm or more duplicated
>> **Excludes1**   partial trisomy due to unbalanced translocation (Q92.5)

Q92.5   **Duplications with other complex rearrangements**
> Partial trisomy due to unbalanced translocations
> Code also any associated deletions due to unbalanced translocations, inversions and insertions (Q93.7)

● Q92.6   **Marker chromosomes**
> Trisomies due to dicentrics
> Trisomies due to extra rings
> Trisomies due to isochromosomes
> Individual with marker heterochromatin

Q92.61   **Marker chromosomes in normal individual**

Q92.62   **Marker chromosomes in abnormal individual**

Q92.7   **Triploidy and polyploidy**

Q92.8   **Other specified trisomies and partial trisomies of autosomes**
> Duplications identified by fluorescence in situ hybridization (FISH)
> Duplications identified by in situ hybridization (ISH)
> Duplications seen only at prometaphase

Q92.9   **Trisomy and partial trisomy of autosomes, unspecified**

● **Q93   Monosomies and deletions from the autosomes, not elsewhere classified**

> (Ex) **For category Q93 CC codes unless otherwise indicated:** See PDX Collection 1115

Q93.0   **Whole chromosome monosomy, nonmosaicism (meiotic nondisjunction)**

Q93.1   **Whole chromosome monosomy, mosaicism (mitotic nondisjunction)**

Q93.2   **Chromosome replaced with ring, dicentric or isochromosome**

Q93.3   **Deletion of short arm of chromosome 4** 🅒
> Wolff-Hirschorn syndrome

Q93.4   **Deletion of short arm of chromosome 5** 🅒
> Cri-du-chat syndrome
> (Ex) See PDX Collection 1116

Q93.5   **Other deletions of part of a chromosome** 🅒
> Angelman syndrome

Q93.7   **Deletions with other complex rearrangements** 🅒
> Deletions due to unbalanced translocations, inversions and insertions
> Code also any associated duplications due to unbalanced translocations, inversions and insertions (Q92.5)

● Q93.8   **Other deletions from the autosomes**

Q93.81   **Velo-cardio-facial syndrome** 🅜
> Deletion 22q11.2
> (Ex) See PDX Collection 1117

Q93.88   **Other microdeletions Miller-Dieker syndrome** 🅜
> Smith-Magenis syndrome
> (Ex) See PDX Collection 1118

Q93.89   **Other deletions from the autosomes** 🅜
> Deletions identified by fluorescence in situ hybridization (FISH)
> Deletions identified by in situ hybridization (ISH)
> Deletions seen only at prometaphase

Q93.9   **Deletion from autosomes, unspecified** 🅒

● **Q95   Balanced rearrangements and structural markers, not elsewhere classified**

> **Includes**   Robertsonian and balanced reciprocal translocations and insertions

Q95.0   **Balanced translocation and insertion in normal individual**

Q95.1   **Chromosome inversion in normal individual**

Q95.2   **Balanced autosomal rearrangement in abnormal individual**

Q95.3   **Balanced sex/autosomal rearrangement in abnormal individual**

Q95.5   **Individual with autosomal fragile site**

Q95.8   **Other balanced rearrangements and structural markers**

Q95.9   **Balanced rearrangement and structural marker, unspecified**

● **Q96   Turner's syndrome**
> *Caused by missing or incomplete X chromosome affecting growth and sexual development*
> **Excludes1**   Noonan syndrome (Q87.1)

Q96.0   **Karyotype 45, X** ♀

Q96.1   **Karyotype 46, X iso (Xq)** ♀
> Karyotype 46, isochromosome Xq

Q96.2   **Karyotype 46, X with abnormal sex chromosome, except iso (Xq)** ♀
> Karyotype 46, X with abnormal sex chromosome, except isochromosome Xq

Q96.3   **Mosaicism, 45, X/46, XX or XY** ♀

Q96.4   **Mosaicism, 45, X/other cell line(s) with abnormal sex chromosome** ♀

Q96.8   **Other variants of Turner's syndrome** ♀

Q96.9   **Turner's syndrome, unspecified** ♀

● **Q97   Other sex chromosome abnormalities, female phenotype, not elsewhere classified**
> **Excludes1**   Turner's syndrome (Q96.-)

Q97.0   **Karyotype 47, XXX** ♀

Q97.1   **Female with more than three X chromosomes** ♀

Q97.2   **Mosaicism, lines with various numbers of X chromosomes** ♀

Q97.3   **Female with 46, XY karyotype** ♀

Q97.8   **Other specified sex chromosome abnormalities, female phenotype** ♀

Q97.9   **Sex chromosome abnormality, female phenotype, unspecified** ♀

● **Q98   Other sex chromosome abnormalities, male phenotype, not elsewhere classified**

Q98.0   **Klinefelter syndrome karyotype 47, XXY** ♂

Q98.1   **Klinefelter syndrome, male with more than two X chromosomes** ♂

Q98.3   **Other male with 46, XX karyotype** ♂

Q98.4   **Klinefelter syndrome, unspecified** ♂

Q98.5   **Karyotype 47, XYY**

Q98.6   **Male with structurally abnormal sex chromosome** ♂

Q98.7   **Male with sex chromosome mosaicism** ♂

Q98.8   **Other specified sex chromosome abnormalities, male phenotype** ♂

Q98.9   **Sex chromosome abnormality, male phenotype, unspecified** ♂

● **Q99   Other chromosome abnormalities, not elsewhere classified**

Q99.0   **Chimera 46, XX/46, XY**
> Chimera 46, XX/46, XY true hermaphrodite

Q99.1   **46, XX true hermaphrodite**
> 46, XX with streak gonads
> 46, XY with streak gonads
> Pure gonadal dysgenesis

Q99.2   **Fragile X chromosome**
> Fragile X syndrome

Q99.8   **Other specified chromosome abnormalities**

Q99.9   **Chromosomal abnormality, unspecified**

CHAPTER 17 (Q00-Q99)

CHAPTER 18

SYMPTOMS, SIGNS AND ABNORMAL CLINICAL AND LABORATORY FINDINGS, NOT ELSEWHERE CLASSIFIED (R00-R99)

OGCR Chapter-Specific Coding Guidelines

18. **Chapter 18: Symptoms, signs, and abnormal clinical and laboratory findings, not elsewhere classified (R00-R99)**
Chapter 18 includes symptoms, signs, abnormal results of clinical or other investigative procedures, and ill-defined conditions regarding which no diagnosis classifiable elsewhere is recorded. Signs and symptoms that point to a specific diagnosis have been assigned to a category in other chapters of the classification.

a. Use of symptom codes
Codes that describe symptoms and signs are acceptable for reporting purposes when a related definitive diagnosis has not been established (confirmed) by the provider.

b. Use of a symptom code with a definitive diagnosis code
Codes for signs and symptoms may be reported in addition to a related definitive diagnosis when the sign or symptom is not routinely associated with that diagnosis, such as the various signs and symptoms associated with complex syndromes. The definitive diagnosis code should be sequenced before the symptom code.

Signs or symptoms that are associated routinely with a disease process should not be assigned as additional codes, unless otherwise instructed by the classification.

c. Combination codes that include symptoms
ICD-10-CM contains a number of combination codes that identify both the definitive diagnosis and common symptoms of that diagnosis. When using one of these combination codes, an additional code should not be assigned for the symptom.

d. Repeated falls
Code R29.6, Repeated falls, is for use for encounters when a patient has recently fallen and the reason for the fall is being investigated.

Code Z91.81, History of falling, is for use when a patient has fallen in the past and is at risk for future falls. When appropriate, both codes R29.6 and Z91.81 may be assigned together.

e. Coma scale
The coma scale codes (R40.2-) can be used in conjunction with traumatic brain injury codes, acute cerebrovascular disease or sequelae of cerebrovascular disease codes. These codes are primarily for use by trauma registries, but they may be used in any setting where this information is collected. The coma scale may also be used to assess the status of the central nervous system for other non-trauma conditions, such as monitoring patients in the intensive care unit regardless of medical condition. The coma scale codes should be sequenced after the diagnosis code(s).

These codes, one from each subcategory, are needed to complete the scale. The 7th character indicates when the scale was recorded. The 7th character should match for all three codes.

At a minimum, report the initial score documented on presentation at your facility. This may be a score from the emergency medicine technician (EMT) or in the emergency department. If desired, a facility may choose to capture multiple coma scale scores.

Assign code R40.24, Glasgow coma scale, total score, when only the total score is documented in the medical record and not the individual score(s).

f. Functional quadriplegia
GUIDELINE HAS BEEN DELETED EFFECTIVE OCTOBER 1, 2017

g. SIRS due to Non-Infectious Process
The systemic inflammatory response syndrome (SIRS) can develop as a result of certain non-infectious disease processes, such as trauma, malignant neoplasm, or pancreatitis. When SIRS is documented with a noninfectious condition, and no subsequent infection is documented, the code for the underlying condition, such as an injury, should be assigned, followed by code R65.10, Systemic inflammatory response syndrome (SIRS) of non-infectious origin without acute organ dysfunction, or code R65.11, Systemic inflammatory response syndrome (SIRS) of non-infectious origin with acute organ dysfunction. If an associated acute organ dysfunction is documented, the appropriate code(s) for the specific type of organ dysfunction(s) should be assigned in addition to code R65.11. If acute organ dysfunction is documented, but it cannot be determined if the acute organ dysfunction is associated with SIRS or due to another condition (e.g., directly due to the trauma), the provider should be queried.

h. Death NOS
Code R99, Ill-defined and unknown cause of mortality, is only for use in the very limited circumstance when a patient who has already died is brought into an emergency department or other healthcare facility and is pronounced dead upon arrival. It does not represent the discharge disposition of death.

i. NIHSS Stroke Scale
The NIH stroke scale (NIHSS) codes (R29.7- -) can be used in conjunction with acute stroke codes (I63) to identify the patient's neurological status and the severity of the stroke. The stroke scale codes should be sequenced after the acute stroke diagnosis code(s).

At a minimum, report the initial score documented. If desired, a facility may choose to capture multiple stroke scale scores.

See Section I.B.14. for information concerning the medical record documentation that may be used for assignment of the NIHSS codes.

Signs and symptoms
Codes that describe symptoms and signs, as opposed to diagnoses, are acceptable for reporting purposes when a related definitive diagnosis has not been established (confirmed) by the provider. Chapter 18 of ICD-10-CM, Symptoms, Signs, and Abnormal Clinical and Laboratory Findings, Not Elsewhere Classified (codes R00.0-R99) contains many, but not all codes for symptoms.

CHAPTER 18

SYMPTOMS, SIGNS AND ABNORMAL CLINICAL AND LABORATORY FINDINGS, NOT ELSEWHERE CLASSIFIED (R00-R99)

Note: This chapter includes symptoms, signs, abnormal results of clinical or other investigative procedures, and ill-defined conditions regarding which no diagnosis classifiable elsewhere is recorded.

Signs and symptoms that point rather definitely to a given diagnosis have been assigned to a category in other chapters of the classification. In general, categories in this chapter include the less well-defined conditions and symptoms that, without the necessary study of the case to establish a final diagnosis, point perhaps equally to two or more diseases or to two or more systems of the body. Practically all categories in the chapter could be designated 'not otherwise specified', 'unknown etiology' or 'transient'. The Alphabetical Index should be consulted to determine which symptoms and signs are to be allocated here and which to other chapters. The residual subcategories, numbered .8, are generally provided for other relevant symptoms that cannot be allocated elsewhere in the classification.

The conditions and signs or symptoms included in categories R00-R94 consist of:
(a) cases for which no more specific diagnosis can be made even after all the facts bearing on the case have been investigated;
(b) signs or symptoms existing at the time of initial encounter that proved to be transient and whose causes could not be determined;
(c) provisional diagnosis in a patient who failed to return for further investigation or care;
(d) cases referred elsewhere for investigation or treatment before the diagnosis was made;
(e) cases in which a more precise diagnosis was not available for any other reason;
(f) certain symptoms, for which supplementary information is provided, that represent important problems in medical care in their own right.

Excludes2 abnormal findings on antenatal screening of mother (O28.-)
certain conditions originating in the perinatal period (P04-P96)
signs and symptoms classified in the body system chapters
signs and symptoms of breast (N63, N64.5)

This chapter contains the following blocks:

R00-R09	Symptoms and signs involving the circulatory and respiratory systems
R10-R19	Symptoms and signs involving the digestive system and abdomen
R20-R23	Symptoms and signs involving the skin and subcutaneous tissue
R25-R29	Symptoms and signs involving the nervous and musculoskeletal systems
R30-R39	Symptoms and signs involving the genitourinary system
R40-R46	Symptoms and signs involving cognition, perception, emotional state and behavior
R47-R49	Symptoms and signs involving speech and voice
R50-R69	General symptoms and signs
R70-R79	Abnormal findings on examination of blood, without diagnosis
R80-R82	Abnormal findings on examination of urine, without diagnosis
R83-R89	Abnormal findings on examination of other body fluids, substances and tissues, without diagnosis
R90-R94	Abnormal findings on diagnostic imaging and in function studies, without diagnosis
R97	Abnormal tumor markers
R99	Ill-defined and unknown cause of mortality

SYMPTOMS AND SIGNS INVOLVING THE CIRCULATORY AND RESPIRATORY SYSTEMS (R00-R09)

● **R00** **Abnormalities of heart beat**
   Excludes1 abnormalities originating in the perinatal period (P29.1-)
   Excludes2 specified arrhythmias (I47-I49)
   R00.0 **Tachycardia, unspecified**
      Rapid heart rate >100 beats
      Rapid heart beat
      Sinoauricular tachycardia NOS
      Sinus [sinusal] tachycardia NOS
      Excludes1 neonatal tachycardia (P29.11)
         paroxysmal tachycardia (I47.-)
   R00.1 **Bradycardia, unspecified**
      Slow heart rate, <60
      Sinoatrial bradycardia
      Sinus bradycardia
      Slow heart beat
      Vagal bradycardia
      Use additional code for adverse effect, if applicable, to identify drug (T36-T50 with fifth or sixth character 5)
      Excludes1 neonatal bradycardia (P29.12)
   R00.2 **Palpitations**
      Awareness of heart beat
   R00.8 **Other abnormalities of heart beat**
   R00.9 **Unspecified abnormalities of heart beat**

CHAPTER 18 (R00-R99)

● **R01 Cardiac murmurs and other cardiac sounds**
> **Excludes1** cardiac murmurs and sounds originating in the perinatal period (P29.8)

R01.0 Benign and innocent cardiac murmurs
Functional cardiac murmur

R01.1 Cardiac murmur, unspecified
Cardiac bruit NOS
Heart murmur NOS
Systolic murmur NOS

R01.2 Other cardiac sounds
Cardiac dullness, increased or decreased
Precordial friction

OGCR Section I.C.9.a.7.

Hypertension, Transient
Assign code R03.0, Elevated blood pressure reading without diagnosis of hypertension, unless patient has an established diagnosis of hypertension. Assign code O13.-, Gestational [pregnancy-induced] hypertension with significant proteinuria, or O14.-, Pre-eclampsia, for transient hypertension of pregnancy.

● **R03 Abnormal blood-pressure reading, without diagnosis**

R03.0 Elevated blood-pressure reading, without diagnosis of hypertension
> **Note:** This category is to be used to record an episode of elevated blood pressure in a patient in whom no formal diagnosis of hypertension has been made, or as an isolated incidental finding.
> MCE: Questionable admission when principal dx

R03.1 Nonspecific low blood-pressure reading
> **Excludes1** hypotension (I95.-)
> maternal hypotension syndrome (O26.5-)
> neurogenic orthostatic hypotension (G90.3)

● **R04 Hemorrhage from respiratory passages**
(Ex) For category R04 CC codes: See PDX Collection 1119

R04.0 Epistaxis
Hemorrhage from nose
Nosebleed

R04.1 Hemorrhage from throat
> **Excludes2** hemoptysis (R04.2)

R04.2 Hemoptysis
Blood-stained sputum
Cough with hemorrhage

● **R04.8 Hemorrhage from other sites in respiratory passages**

R04.81 Acute idiopathic pulmonary hemorrhage in infants   P
AIPHI
Acute idiopathic hemorrhage in infants over 28 days old
> **Excludes1** perinatal pulmonary hemorrhage (P26.-)
> von Willebrand's disease (D68.0)

R04.89 Hemorrhage from other sites in respiratory passages
Pulmonary hemorrhage NOS

R04.9 Hemorrhage from respiratory passages, unspecified

R05 Cough
> **Excludes1** cough with hemorrhage (R04.2)
> smoker's cough (J41.0)

● **R06 Abnormalities of breathing**
> **Excludes1** acute respiratory distress syndrome (J80)
> respiratory arrest (R09.2)
> respiratory arrest of newborn (P28.81)
> respiratory distress syndrome of newborn (P22.-)
> respiratory failure (J96.-)
> respiratory failure of newborn (P28.5)

● **R06.0 Dyspnea**
> **Excludes1** tachypnea NOS (R06.82)
> transient tachypnea of newborn (P22.1)

R06.00 Dyspnea, unspecified
Coding Clinic: 2017, Q1, P26-27

R06.01 Orthopnea

R06.02 Shortness of breath

▶ **R06.03 Acute respiratory distress**

R06.09 Other forms of dyspnea

R06.1 Stridor
Harsh, high-pitched breath sound
> **Excludes1** congenital laryngeal stridor (P28.89)
> laryngismus (stridulus) (J38.5)

R06.2 Wheezing
> **Excludes1** Asthma (J45.-)
> Coding Clinic: 2016, Q2, P34

R06.3 Periodic breathing
Cheyne-Stokes breathing
An abnormal pattern of breathing with gradually increasing and decreasing tidal volume with some periods of apnea
(Ex) See PDX Collection 1120

R06.4 Hyperventilation
> **Excludes1** psychogenic hyperventilation (F45.8)

R06.5 Mouth breathing
> **Excludes2** dry mouth NOS (R68.2)

R06.6 Hiccough
> **Excludes1** psychogenic hiccough (F45.8)

R06.7 Sneezing

● **R06.8 Other abnormalities of breathing**

R06.81 Apnea, not elsewhere classified
Apnea NOS
> **Excludes1** apnea (of) newborn (P28.4)
> sleep apnea (G47.3-)
> sleep apnea of newborn (primary) (P28.3)

R06.82 Tachypnea, not elsewhere classified
Tachypnea NOS
> **Excludes1** transitory tachypnea of newborn (P22.1)

R06.83 Snoring

R06.89 Other abnormalities of breathing
Breath-holding (spells)
Sighing

R06.9 Unspecified abnormalities of breathing

● **R07 Pain in throat and chest**
> **Excludes1** epidemic myalgia (B33.0)
> **Excludes2** jaw pain R68.84
> pain in breast (N64.4)

R07.0 Pain in throat
> **Excludes1** chronic sore throat (J31.2)
> sore throat (acute) NOS (J02.9)
> **Excludes2** dysphagia (R13.1-)
> pain in neck (M54.2)

R07.1 Chest pain on breathing
Painful respiration

R07.2 Precordial pain

● **R07.8 Other chest pain**

R07.81 Pleurodynia
Pleurodynia NOS
> **Excludes1** epidemic pleurodynia (B33.0)

R07.82 Intercostal pain

R07.89 Other chest pain
Anterior chest-wall pain NOS

R07.9 Chest pain, unspecified

▶ New   ⟹ Revised   ~~deleted~~ Deleted   Excludes 1   Excludes 2   Includes   Use additional   Code first   Code also   Key words
OGCR Official Guidelines   ● Unacceptable Principal Diagnosis   X Assign placeholder X   ● Use Additional Character(s)   ▶ Manifestation Code   **Coding Clinic**

R09   **Other symptoms and signs involving the circulatory and respiratory system**

> **Excludes1**   acute respiratory distress syndrome (J80)
> respiratory arrest of newborn (P28.81)
> respiratory distress syndrome of newborn (P22.0)
> respiratory failure (J96.-)
> respiratory failure of newborn (P28.5)

● **R09.0**   **Asphyxia and hypoxemia**

> **Excludes1**   asphyxia due to carbon monoxide (T58.-)
> asphyxia due to foreign body in respiratory tract (T17.-)
> birth (intrauterine) asphyxia (P84)
> ~~hypercapnia (R06.4)~~
> hyperventilation (R06.4)
> traumatic asphyxia (T71.-)

> ▶ **Excludes2**   hypercapnia (R06.89)

     R09.01   **Asphyxia** 🔲
         (Ex) See PDX Collection 1121

     R09.02   **Hypoxemia**

R09.1   **Pleurisy**
     Occurs when double membrane (pleura) lining chest cavity and lung surface becomes inflamed causing sharp pain on inspiration/expiration

> **Excludes1**   pleurisy with effusion (J90)

R09.2   **Respiratory arrest** 🔲
     Cardiorespiratory failure

> **Excludes1**   cardiac arrest (I46.-)
> respiratory arrest of newborn (P28.81)
> respiratory distress of newborn (P22.0)
> respiratory failure (J96.-)
> respiratory failure of newborn (P28.5)
> respiratory insufficiency (R06.89)
> respiratory insufficiency of newborn (P28.5)

     MCC: Only if patient discharged alive
     (Ex) See PDX Collection 1121

R09.3   **Abnormal sputum**
     Abnormal amount of sputum
     Abnormal color of sputum
     Abnormal odor of sputum
     Excessive sputum

> **Excludes1**   blood-stained sputum (R04.2)

● **R09.8**   **Other specified symptoms and signs involving the circulatory and respiratory systems**

     R09.81   **Nasal congestion**

     R09.82   **Postnasal drip**

     R09.89   **Other specified symptoms and signs involving the circulatory and respiratory systems**
         Bruit (arterial)
         Abnormal chest percussion
         Feeling of foreign body in throat
         Friction sounds in chest
         Chest tympany
         Choking sensation
         Rales
         Wet rattling, clicking, crackling sounds on auscultation
         Weak pulse

> **Excludes2**   foreign body in throat (T17.2-)
> wheezing (R06.2)

SYMPTOMS AND SIGNS INVOLVING THE DIGESTIVE SYSTEM AND ABDOMEN (R10-R19)

> **Excludes2**   congenital or infantile pylorospasm (Q40.0)
> gastrointestinal hemorrhage (K92.0-K92.2)
> intestinal obstruction (K56.-)
> newborn gastrointestinal hemorrhage (P54.0-P54.3)
> newborn intestinal obstruction (P76.-)
> pylorospasm (K31.3)
> signs and symptoms involving the urinary system (R30-R39)
> symptoms referable to female genital organs (N94.-)
> symptoms referable to male genital organs (N48-N50)

● **R10**   **Abdominal and pelvic pain**

> **Excludes1**   renal colic (N23)
> **Excludes2**   dorsalgia (M54.-)
> flatulence and related conditions (R14.-)

R10.0   **Acute abdomen**
     Severe abdominal pain (generalized) (with abdominal rigidity)

> **Excludes1**   abdominal rigidity NOS (R19.3)
> generalized abdominal pain NOS (R10.84)
> localized abdominal pain (R10.1-R10.3-)

● **R10.1**   **Pain localized to upper abdomen**

     R10.10   **Upper abdominal pain, unspecified**

     R10.11   **Right upper quadrant pain**

     R10.12   **Left upper quadrant pain**

     R10.13   **Epigastric pain**
         Dyspepsia

> **Excludes1**   functional dyspepsia (K30)

R10.2   **Pelvic and perineal pain**

> **Excludes1**   vulvodynia (N94.81)

● **R10.3**   **Pain localized to other parts of lower abdomen**

     R10.30   **Lower abdominal pain, unspecified**

     R10.31   **Right lower quadrant pain**

     R10.32   **Left lower quadrant pain**

     R10.33   **Periumbilical pain**

● **R10.8**   **Other abdominal pain**

     ● **R10.81**   **Abdominal tenderness**
         Abdominal tenderness NOS

         R10.811   **Right upper quadrant abdominal tenderness**

         R10.812   **Left upper quadrant abdominal tenderness**

         R10.813   **Right lower quadrant abdominal tenderness**

         R10.814   **Left lower quadrant abdominal tenderness**

         R10.815   **Periumbilic abdominal tenderness**

         R10.816   **Epigastric abdominal tenderness**

         R10.817   **Generalized abdominal tenderness**

         R10.819   **Abdominal tenderness, unspecified site**

     ● **R10.82**   **Rebound abdominal tenderness**

         R10.821   **Right upper quadrant rebound abdominal tenderness**

         R10.822   **Left upper quadrant rebound abdominal tenderness**

         R10.823   **Right lower quadrant rebound abdominal tenderness**

N Newborn Age: 0   **P** Pediatric Age: 0–17   **M** Maternity DX: 12–55   **A** Adult Age: 15–124   ♀ Females Only   ♂ Males Only

🔲 Complication\Comorbidity   🔲 Major C\C   (Ex) CC/MCC Exclusions   🔲 Hospital-Acquired Condition

1199

R10.824   **Left lower quadrant rebound abdominal tenderness**

R10.825   **Periumbilic rebound abdominal tenderness**

R10.826   **Epigastric rebound abdominal tenderness**

R10.827   **Generalized rebound abdominal tenderness**

R10.829   **Rebound abdominal tenderness, unspecified site**

R10.83   **Colic**   P
Colic NOS
Infantile colic
Excludes1   colic in adult and child over 12 months old (R10.84)

R10.84   **Generalized abdominal pain**
Excludes1   generalized abdominal pain associated with acute abdomen (R10.0)

R10.9   **Unspecified abdominal pain**

● **R11   Nausea and vomiting**
Excludes1   cyclical vomiting associated with migraine (G43.A-)
excessive vomiting in pregnancy (O21.-)
hematemesis (K92.0)
neonatal hematemesis (P54.0)
newborn vomiting (P92.0-)
psychogenic vomiting (F50.89)
vomiting associated with bulimia nervosa (F50.2)
vomiting following gastrointestinal surgery (K91.0)
Coding Clinic: 2017, Q1, P27

● **R11.0   Nausea**
Nausea NOS
Nausea without vomiting

● **R11.1   Vomiting**
R11.10   **Vomiting, unspecified**
Vomiting NOS

R11.11   **Vomiting without nausea**

R11.12   **Projectile vomiting**

R11.13   **Vomiting of fecal matter**

R11.14   **Bilious vomiting**
Bilious emesis

R11.2   **Nausea with vomiting, unspecified**
Persistent nausea with vomiting NOS

R12   **Heartburn**
Excludes1   dyspepsia NOS (R10.13)
functional dyspepsia (K30)

● **R13   Aphagia and dysphagia**
R13.0   **Aphagia**
Inability to swallow
Excludes1   psychogenic aphagia (F50.9)

● **R13.1   Dysphagia**
Difficulty swallowing
Code first, if applicable, dysphagia following cerebrovascular disease (I69. with final characters -91)
Excludes1   psychogenic dysphagia (F45.8)

R13.10   **Dysphagia, unspecified**
Difficulty in swallowing NOS

R13.11   **Dysphagia, oral phase**

R13.12   **Dysphagia, oropharyngeal phase**

R13.13   **Dysphagia, pharyngeal phase**

R13.14   **Dysphagia, pharyngoesophageal phase**

R13.19   **Other dysphagia**
Cervical dysphagia
Neurogenic dysphagia

● **R14   Flatulence and related conditions**
Excludes1   psychogenic aerophagy (F45.8)

R14.0   **Abdominal distension (gaseous)**
Bloating
Tympanites (abdominal) (intestinal)

R14.1   **Gas pain**

R14.2   **Eructation**
Belching air from stomach through mouth

R14.3   **Flatulence**

● **R15   Fecal incontinence**
Includes   encopresis NOS
Excludes1   fecal incontinence of nonorganic origin (F98.1)

R15.0   **Incomplete defecation**
Excludes1   constipation (K59.0-)
fecal impaction (K56.41)

R15.1   **Fecal smearing**
Fecal soiling

R15.2   **Fecal urgency**

R15.9   **Full incontinence of feces**
Fecal incontinence NOS

● **R16   Hepatomegaly and splenomegaly, not elsewhere classified**
Enlargement of liver or spleen

R16.0   **Hepatomegaly, not elsewhere classified**
Hepatomegaly NOS

R16.1   **Splenomegaly, not elsewhere classified**
Splenomegaly NOS

R16.2   **Hepatomegaly with splenomegaly, not elsewhere classified**
Hepatosplenomegaly NOS

R17   **Unspecified jaundice** 🗝
Excludes1   neonatal jaundice (P55, P57-P59)
(Ex) See PDX Collection 1122

● **R18   Ascites**
Includes   fluid in peritoneal cavity
Excludes1   ascites in alcoholic cirrhosis (K70.31)
ascites in alcoholic hepatitis (K70.11)
ascites in toxic liver disease with chronic active hepatitis (K71.51)
(Ex) **For category R18 CC codes: See PDX Collection 1123**

● **R18.0   Malignant ascites** 🗝
Code first malignancy, such as:
malignant neoplasm of ovary (C56.-)
secondary malignant neoplasm of retroperitoneum and peritoneum (C78.6)

R18.8   **Other ascites** 🗝
Ascites NOS
Peritoneal effusion (chronic)

● **R19   Other symptoms and signs involving the digestive system and abdomen**
Excludes1   acute abdomen (R10.0)

● **R19.0   Intra-abdominal and pelvic swelling, mass and lump**
Excludes1   abdominal distension (gaseous) (R14.-)
ascites (R18.-)

R19.00   **Intra-abdominal and pelvic swelling, mass and lump, unspecified site**

R19.01   **Right upper quadrant abdominal swelling, mass and lump**

R19.02   **Left upper quadrant abdominal swelling, mass and lump**

R19.03   **Right lower quadrant abdominal swelling, mass and lump**

R19.04   **Left lower quadrant abdominal swelling, mass and lump**

R19.05 Periumbilic swelling, mass or lump
Diffuse or generalized umbilical swelling or mass

R19.06 Epigastric swelling, mass or lump

R19.07 Generalized intra-abdominal and pelvic swelling, mass and lump
Diffuse or generalized intra-abdominal swelling or mass NOS
Diffuse or generalized pelvic swelling or mass NOS

R19.09 Other intra-abdominal and pelvic swelling, mass and lump

● **R19.1 Abnormal bowel sounds**

R19.11 Absent bowel sounds

R19.12 Hyperactive bowel sounds

R19.15 Other abnormal bowel sounds
Abnormal bowel sounds NOS

R19.2 Visible peristalsis
Hyperperistalsis

● **R19.3 Abdominal rigidity**
Excludes1 abdominal rigidity with severe abdominal pain (R10.0)

R19.30 Abdominal rigidity, unspecified site

R19.31 Right upper quadrant abdominal rigidity

R19.32 Left upper quadrant abdominal rigidity

R19.33 Right lower quadrant abdominal rigidity

R19.34 Left lower quadrant abdominal rigidity

R19.35 Periumbilic abdominal rigidity

R19.36 Epigastric abdominal rigidity

R19.37 Generalized abdominal rigidity

R19.4 Change in bowel habit
Excludes1 constipation (K59.0-)
functional diarrhea (K59.1)

R19.5 Other fecal abnormalities
Abnormal stool color
Bulky stools
Mucus in stools
Occult blood in feces
Occult blood in stools
Excludes1 melena (K92.1)
neonatal melena (P54.1)

R19.6 Halitosis

R19.7 Diarrhea, unspecified
Diarrhea NOS
Excludes1 functional diarrhea (K59.1)
neonatal diarrhea (P78.3)
psychogenic diarrhea (F45.8)

R19.8 Other specified symptoms and signs involving the digestive system and abdomen

SYMPTOMS AND SIGNS INVOLVING THE SKIN AND SUBCUTANEOUS TISSUE (R20-R23)

Excludes2 symptoms relating to breast (N64.4-N64.5)

● **R20 Disturbances of skin sensation**
Excludes1 dissociative anesthesia and sensory loss (F44.6)
psychogenic disturbances (F45.8)

R20.0 Anesthesia of skin
Loss of sensation

R20.1 Hypoesthesia of skin
Unpleasant abnormal sensation

R20.2 Paresthesia of skin
Abnormal touch sensation, including burning, prickling, often in absence of external stimulus
Formication   Tingling skin
Pins and needles
Excludes1 acroparesthesia (I73.8)

R20.3 Hyperesthesia

R20.8 Other disturbances of skin sensation

R20.9 Unspecified disturbances of skin sensation

R21 Rash and other nonspecific skin eruption
Includes rash NOS
Excludes1 specified type of rash- code to condition
vesicular eruption (R23.8)

● **R22 Localized swelling, mass and lump of skin and subcutaneous tissue**
Includes subcutaneous nodules (localized) (superficial)
Excludes1 abnormal findings on diagnostic imaging (R90-R93)
edema (R60.-)
enlarged lymph nodes (R59.-)
localized adiposity (E65)
swelling of joint (M25.4-)

R22.0 Localized swelling, mass and lump, head

R22.1 Localized swelling, mass and lump, neck

R22.2 Localized swelling, mass and lump, trunk
Excludes1 intra-abdominal or pelvic mass and lump (R19.0-)
intra-abdominal or pelvic swelling (R19.0-)
Excludes2 breast mass and lump (N63)

● **R22.3 Localized swelling, mass and lump, upper limb**

R22.30 Localized swelling, mass and lump, unspecified upper limb

R22.31 Localized swelling, mass and lump, right upper limb

R22.32 Localized swelling, mass and lump, left upper limb

R22.33 Localized swelling, mass and lump, upper limb, bilateral

● **R22.4 Localized swelling, mass and lump, lower limb**

R22.40 Localized swelling, mass and lump, unspecified lower limb

R22.41 Localized swelling, mass and lump, right lower limb

R22.42 Localized swelling, mass and lump, left lower limb

R22.43 Localized swelling, mass and lump, lower limb, bilateral

R22.9 Localized swelling, mass and lump, unspecified

● **R23 Other skin changes**

R23.0 Cyanosis
Excludes1 acrocyanosis (I73.8)
cyanotic attacks of newborn (P28.2)

R23.1 Pallor
Clammy skin

R23.2 Flushing
Excessive blushing
Code first, if applicable, menopausal and female climacteric states (N95.1)

R23.3 Spontaneous ecchymoses
Small hemorrhagic spot of skin; AKA black and blue spot
Petechiae
Excludes1 ecchymoses of newborn (P54.5)
purpura (D69.-)

R23.4 Changes in skin texture
Desquamation of skin   Scaling of skin
Induration of skin
Excludes1 epidermal thickening NOS (L85.9)

R23.8 Other skin changes

R23.9 Unspecified skin changes

CHAPTER 18 (R00-R99)

SYMPTOMS AND SIGNS INVOLVING THE NERVOUS AND MUSCULOSKELETAL SYSTEMS (R25-R29)

● R25 **Abnormal involuntary movements**
Excludes1   specific movement disorders (G20-G26)
stereotyped movement disorders (F98.4)
tic disorders (F95.-)

R25.0 **Abnormal head movements**

R25.1 **Tremor, unspecified**
Excludes1   chorea NOS (G25.5)
essential tremor (G25.0)
hysterical tremor (F44.4)
intention tremor (G25.2)

R25.2 **Cramp and spasm**
Excludes2   carpopedal spasm (R29.0)
charley-horse (M62.831)
infantile spasms (G40.4-)
muscle spasm of back (M62.830)
muscle spasm of calf (M62.831)

R25.3 **Fasciculation**
Twitching NOS

R25.8 **Other abnormal involuntary movements**

R25.9 **Unspecified abnormal involuntary movements**

● R26 **Abnormalities of gait and mobility**
Excludes1   ataxia NOS (R27.0)
hereditary ataxia (G11.-)
locomotor (syphilitic) ataxia (A52.11)
immobility syndrome (paraplegic) (M62.3)

R26.0 **Ataxic gait**
Staggering gait

R26.1 **Paralytic gait**
Spastic gait

R26.2 **Difficulty in walking, not elsewhere classified**
Excludes1   falling (R29.6)
unsteadiness on feet (R26.81)
Coding Clinic: 2016, Q2, P7

● R26.8 **Other abnormalities of gait and mobility**
R26.81 **Unsteadiness on feet**
R26.89 **Other abnormalities of gait and mobility**

R26.9 **Unspecified abnormalities of gait and mobility**

● R27 **Other lack of coordination**
Excludes1   ataxic gait (R26.0)
hereditary ataxia (G11.-)
vertigo NOS (R42)

R27.0 **Ataxia, unspecified**
Excludes1   ataxia following cerebrovascular disease (I69. with final characters -93)

R27.8 **Other lack of coordination**

R27.9 **Unspecified lack of coordination**

● R29 **Other symptoms and signs involving the nervous and musculoskeletal systems**

R29.0 **Tetany** 🔖
Hyperexcitability of nerves and muscles characterized by spasm, twitching, and cramps
Carpopedal spasm
Excludes1   hysterical tetany (F44.5)
neonatal tetany (P71.3)
parathyroid tetany (E20.9)
post-thyroidectomy tetany (E89.2)
(Ex) See PDX Collection 1124

R29.1 **Meningismus** 🔖
(Ex) See PDX Collection 1125

R29.2 **Abnormal reflex**
Excludes2   abnormal pupillary reflex (H57.0)
hyperactive gag reflex (J39.2)
vasovagal reaction or syncope (R55)

R29.3 **Abnormal posture**

R29.4 **Clicking hip**
Excludes1   congenital deformities of hip (Q65.-)

R29.5 **Transient paralysis** 🔖
Code first any associated spinal cord injury (S14.0, S14.1-, S24.0, S24.1-, S34.0-, S34.1-)
Excludes1   transient ischemic attack (G45.9)
(Ex) See PDX Collection 1126

R29.6 **Repeated falls**
Falling
Tendency to fall
Excludes2   at risk for falling (Z91.81)
history of falling (Z91.81)

OGCR Section I.C.18.d.
Repeated falls
Code R29.6, Repeated falls, is for use for encounters when a patient has recently fallen and the reason for the fall is being investigated.
Code Z91.81, History of falling, is for use when a patient has fallen in the past and is at risk for future falls. When appropriate, both codes R29.6 and Z91.81 may be assigned together.

Coding Clinic: 2016, Q2, P7

● R29.7 **National Institutes of Health Stroke Scale (NIHSS) score**
Code first the type of cerebral infarction (I63-)
Coding Clinic: 2016, Q4, P61, 127

● R29.70 **NIHSS score 0-9**
● R29.700 **NIHSS score 0**
● R29.701 **NIHSS score 1**
● R29.702 **NIHSS score 2**
● R29.703 **NIHSS score 3**
● R29.704 **NIHSS score 4**
● R29.705 **NIHSS score 5**
● R29.706 **NIHSS score 6**
● R29.707 **NIHSS score 7**
● R29.708 **NIHSS score 8**
● R29.709 **NIHSS score 9**

● R29.71 **NIHSS score 10-19**
● R29.710 **NIHSS score 10**
● R29.711 **NIHSS score 11**
● R29.712 **NIHSS score 12**
● R29.713 **NIHSS score 13**
● R29.714 **NIHSS score 14**
● R29.715 **NIHSS score 15**
● R29.716 **NIHSS score 16**
● R29.717 **NIHSS score 17**
● R29.718 **NIHSS score 18**
● R29.719 **NIHSS score 19**

● R29.72 **NIHSS score 20-29**
● R29.720 **NIHSS score 20**
● R29.721 **NIHSS score 21**
● R29.722 **NIHSS score 22**
● R29.723 **NIHSS score 23**
● R29.724 **NIHSS score 24**
● R29.725 **NIHSS score 25**
● R29.726 **NIHSS score 26**
● R29.727 **NIHSS score 27**
● R29.728 **NIHSS score 28**
● R29.729 **NIHSS score 29**

OGCR Section I.C.18.i.
NIHSS Stroke Scale
The NIH stroke scale (NIHSS) codes (R29.7- -) can be used in conjunction with acute stroke codes (I63) to identify the patient's neurological status and the severity of the stroke. The stroke scale codes should be sequenced after the acute stroke diagnosis code(s).
At a minimum, report the initial score documented. If desired, a facility may choose to capture multiple stroke scale scores.

▶ New   ⇒ Revised   ~~deleted~~ Deleted   Excludes 1   Excludes 2   Includes   Use additional   Code first   Code also   Key words
OGCR Official Guidelines   ● Unacceptable Principal Diagnosis   X Assign placeholder X   ▌ Use Additional Character(s)   ▌ Manifestation Code   **Coding Clinic**

● R29.73   NIHSS score 30-39
- ● R29.730   NIHSS score 30
  Coding Clinic: 2016, Q4, P62
- ● R29.731   NIHSS score 31
- ● R29.732   NIHSS score 32
- ● R29.733   NIHSS score 33
- ● R29.734   NIHSS score 34
- ● R29.735   NIHSS score 35
- ● R29.736   NIHSS score 36
- ● R29.737   NIHSS score 37
- ● R29.738   NIHSS score 38
- ● R29.739   NIHSS score 39

● R29.74   NIHSS score 40-42
- ● R29.740   NIHSS score 40
- ● R29.741   NIHSS score 41
- ● R29.742   NIHSS score 42

● R29.8   **Other symptoms and signs involving the nervous and musculoskeletal systems**
- ● R29.81   **Other symptoms and signs involving the nervous system**
  - R29.810   **Facial weakness**
    Facial droop
    Excludes1   Bell's palsy (G51.0)
    facial weakness following cerebrovascular disease (I69. with final characters -92)
  - R29.818   **Other symptoms and signs involving the nervous system**
- ● R29.89   **Other symptoms and signs involving the musculoskeletal system**
  Excludes2   pain in limb (M79.6-)
  - R29.890   **Loss of height**
    Excludes1   osteoporosis (M80-M81)
  - R29.891   **Ocular torticollis**
    Excludes1   congenital (sterno-mastoid) torticollis Q68.0
    psychogenic torticollis (F45.8)
    spasmodic torticollis (G24.3)
    torticollis due to birth injury (P15.8)
    torticollis NOS M43.6
  - R29.898   **Other symptoms and signs involving the musculoskeletal system**

● R29.9   **Unspecified symptoms and signs involving the nervous and musculoskeletal systems**
- R29.90   Unspecified symptoms and signs involving the nervous system
- R29.91   Unspecified symptoms and signs involving the musculoskeletal system

SYMPTOMS AND SIGNS INVOLVING THE GENITOURINARY SYSTEM (R30-R39)

● R30   **Pain associated with micturition**
  Excludes1   psychogenic pain associated with micturition (F45.8)
- R30.0   **Dysuria**
  Painful urination
  Strangury
- R30.1   **Vesical tenesmus**
  Straining to urinate, with sensation of a full bladder even when empty
- R30.9   **Painful micturition, unspecified**
  Painful urination NOS

● R31   **Hematuria**
  Excludes1   hematuria included with underlying conditions, such as:
  acute cystitis with hematuria (N30.01)
  recurrent and persistent hematuria in glomerular diseases (N02.-)
- R31.0   **Gross hematuria**
  Coding Clinic: 2017, Q1, P17
- R31.1   **Benign essential microscopic hematuria**
- ● R31.2   **Other microscopic hematuria**
  Coding Clinic: 2016, Q4, P62
  - R31.21   **Asymptomatic microscopic hematuria**
    AMH
  - R31.29   **Other microscopic hematuria**
- R31.9   **Hematuria, unspecified**
  Coding Clinic: 2017, Q1, P6

● R32   **Unspecified urinary incontinence**
  Enuresis NOS
  Excludes1   functional urinary incontinence (R39.81)
  nonorganic enuresis (F98.0)
  stress incontinence and other specified urinary incontinence (N39.3-N39.4-)
  urinary incontinence associated with cognitive impairment (R39.81)

● R33   **Retention of urine**
  Excludes1   psychogenic retention of urine (F45.8)
- R33.0   **Drug induced retention of urine**
  Use additional code for adverse effect, if applicable, to identify drug (T36-T50 with fifth or sixth character 5)
- R33.8   **Other retention of urine**
  Code first, if applicable, any causal condition, such as:
  enlarged prostate (N40.1)
- R33.9   **Retention of urine, unspecified**

● R34   **Anuria and oliguria**
  Excludes1   anuria and oliguria complicating abortion or ectopic or molar pregnancy (O00-O07, O08.4)
  anuria and oliguria complicating pregnancy (O26.83-)
  anuria and oliguria complicating the puerperium (O90.4)

● R35   **Polyuria**
  Passage of excessive volume of urine
  Code first, if applicable, any causal condition, such as:
  enlarged prostate (N40.1)
  Excludes1   psychogenic polyuria (F45.8)
- R35.0   **Frequency of micturition**
  Discharge or passage of urine; AKA uresis
- R35.1   **Nocturia**
  Urinary frequency at night
- R35.8   **Other polyuria**
  Polyuria NOS

● R36   **Urethral discharge**
- R36.0   **Urethral discharge without blood**
- R36.1   **Hematospermia** ♂
  Presence of blood in semen
- R36.9   **Urethral discharge, unspecified**
  Penile discharge NOS
  Urethrorrhea

● R37   **Sexual dysfunction, unspecified**

CHAPTER 18 (R00-R99)

N   Newborn Age: 0   **P**   Pediatric Age: 0–17   **M**   Maternity DX: 12–55   **A**   Adult Age: 15–124   ♀   Females Only   ♂   Males Only

Complication\Comorbidity   Major C\C   (Ex)   CC/MCC Exclusions   Hospital-Acquired Condition

1203

R39   Other and unspecified symptoms and signs involving the genitourinary system

     R39.0   Extravasation of urine 🔖
         Leakage, discharge
         (Ex) See PDX Collection 1127

     ● **R39.1   Other difficulties with micturition**
         Code first, if applicable, any causal condition, such as:
         enlarged prostate (N40.1)

         R39.11   Hesitancy of micturition

         R39.12   Poor urinary stream
              Weak urinary steam

         R39.13   Splitting of urinary stream

         R39.14   Feeling of incomplete bladder emptying

         R39.15   Urgency of urination
            Excludes1   urge incontinence (N39.41, N39.46)

         R39.16   Straining to void

     ● **R39.19   Other difficulties with micturition**
            Coding Clinic: 2016, Q4, P63

            R39.191   Need to immediately re-void

            R39.192   Position dependent micturition

            R39.198   Other difficulties with micturition

     R39.2   Extrarenal uremia
         Prerenal uremia
         Excludes1   uremia NOS (N19)

     ● **R39.8   Other symptoms and signs involving the genitourinary system**

         R39.81   Functional urinary incontinence
            Urinary incontinence due to cognitive impairment, or severe physical disability or immobility
            Excludes1   stress incontinence and other specified urinary incontinence (N39.3-N39.4-) urinary incontinence NOS (R32)

         R39.82   Chronic bladder pain
            Coding Clinic: 2016, Q4, P64

     ▶ **R39.83   Unilateral non-palpable testicle** ♂

     ▶ **R39.84   Bilateral non-palpable testicles** ♂

         R39.89   Other symptoms and signs involving the genitourinary system
            Coding Clinic: 2016, Q4, P64

     R39.9   Unspecified symptoms and signs involving the genitourinary system

---

SYMPTOMS AND SIGNS INVOLVING COGNITION, PERCEPTION, EMOTIONAL STATE AND BEHAVIOR (R40-R46)

     Excludes2   symptoms and signs constituting part of a pattern of mental disorder (F01-F99)
            Coding Clinic: 2015, Q4, P40

● **R40   Somnolence, stupor and coma**
     Excludes1   neonatal coma (P91.5)
            somnolence, stupor and coma in diabetes (E08-E13)
            somnolence, stupor and coma in hepatic failure (K72.-)
            somnolence, stupor and coma in hypoglycemia (nondiabetic) (E15)

     R40.0   Somnolence
         Drowsiness
         Excludes1   coma (R40.2-)

     R40.1   Stupor
         Lowered level of consciousness
         Catatonic stupor
         Semicoma
         Excludes1   catatonic schizophrenia (F20.2)
                     coma (R40.2-)
                     depressive stupor (F31-F33)
                     dissociative stupor (F44.2)
                     manic stupor (F30.2)

OGCR Section I.C.18.e.

Coma scale

The coma scale codes (R40.2-) can be used in conjunction with traumatic brain injury codes, acute cerebrovascular disease or sequelae of cerebrovascular disease codes. These codes are primarily for use by trauma registries, but they may be used in any setting where this information is collected. **The coma scale may also be used to assess the status of the central nervous system for other non-trauma conditions, such as monitoring patients in the intensive care unit regardless of medical condition.** The coma scale codes should be sequenced after the diagnosis code(s).

These codes, one from each subcategory, are needed to complete the scale. The 7th character indicates when the scale was recorded. The 7th character should match for all three codes.

At a minimum, report the initial score documented on presentation at your facility. This may be a score from the emergency medicine technician (EMT) or in the emergency department. If desired, a facility may choose to capture multiple coma scale scores.

Assign code R40.24, Glasgow coma scale, total score, when only the total score is documented in the medical record and not the individual score(s).

● **R40.2   Coma**
     Code first any associated:
     fracture of skull (S02.-)
     intracranial injury (S06.-)
     Note: One code from each subcategory R40.21-R40-23 is required to complete the coma scale
     (Ex) **For category R40.2 CC codes:** See PDX Collection 515
         Coding Clinic: 2016, Q4, P127

     ● **R40.20   Unspecified coma** 🔖
         Coma NOS
         Unconsciousness NOS

     ● **R40.21   Coma scale, eyes open**

         The following appropriate 7th character is to be added to subcategory R40.21-:

0	unspecified time
1	in the field [EMT or ambulance]
2	at arrival to emergency department
3	at hospital admission
4	24 hours or more after hospital admission

         Coding Clinic: 2015, Q2, P18

     ●● **R40.211   Coma scale, eyes open, never** 🔖

     ●● **R40.212   Coma scale, eyes open, to pain** 🔖

     ●● **R40.213   Coma scale, eyes open, to sound**

     ●● **R40.214   Coma scale, eyes open, spontaneous**

     ● **R40.22   Coma scale, best verbal response**

         The following appropriate 7th character is to be added to subcategory R40.22-:

0	unspecified time
1	in the field [EMT or ambulance]
2	at arrival to emergency department
3	at hospital admission
4	24 hours or more after hospital admission

         Coding Clinic: 2015, Q2, P18

     ●● **R40.221   Coma scale, best verbal response, none** 🔖

     ●● **R40.222   Coma scale, best verbal response, incomprehensible words** 🔖
         ▶Incomprehensible sounds (2-5 years of age)
         ▶Moans/grunts to pain; restless (<2 years old)

▶ New   ⇒ Revised   ~~deleted~~ Deleted   Excludes 1   Excludes 2   Includes   Use additional   Code first   Code also   Key words

OGCR Official Guidelines   ● Unacceptable Principal Diagnosis   X Assign placeholder X   ● Use Additional Character(s)   ▶ Manifestation Code   **Coding Clinic**

Glasgow Coma Scale

Eye Opening Response	
• Spontaneous--open with blinking at baseline	4 points
• To verbal stimuli, command, speech	3 points
• To pain only (not applied to face)	2 points
• No response	1 point
Verbal Response	
• Oriented	5 points
• Confused conversation, but able to answer questions	4 points
• Inappropriate words	3 points
• Incomprehensible speech	2 points
• No response	1 point
Motor Response	
• Obeys commands for movement	6 points
• Purposeful movement to painful stimulus	5 points
• Withdraws in response to pain	4 points
• Flexion in response to pain (decorticate posturing)	3 points
• Extension response in response to pain (decerebrate posturing)	2 points
• No response	1 point
Categorization: Coma: No eye opening, no ability to follow commands, no word verbalizations (3-8)	
Head Injury Classification: Severe Head Injury--GCS score of 8 or less Moderate Head Injury--GCS score of 9 to 12 Mild head injury--GCS score of 13 to 15	
(Adapted from: Advanced Trauma Life Support: Course for Physicians, American College of Surgeons, 1993). http://www.bt.cdc.gov/masscasulatires/gscale.asp	

Figure 18-1

●● **R40.223** **Coma scale, best verbal response, inappropriate words**
▶ Inappropriate crying or screaming (< 2 years of age)
▶ Screaming (2-5 years of age)

●● **R40.224** **Coma scale, best verbal response, confused conversation**
▶ Inappropriate words (2-5 years of age)
▶ Irritable cries (< 2 years of age)

●● **R40.225** **Coma scale, best verbal response, oriented**
▶ Cooing or babbling or crying appropriately (< 2 years of age)
▶ Uses appropriate words (2- 5 years of age)

● **R40.23** Coma scale, **best motor response**
The following appropriate 7th character is to be added to subcategory R40.23-:

Ø	unspecified time
1	in the field [EMT or ambulance]
2	at arrival to emergency department
3	at hospital admission
4	24 hours or more after hospital admission

Coding Clinic: 2015, Q2, P18

●● **R40.231** **Coma scale, best motor response, none** 🔖

●● **R40.232** **Coma scale, best motor response, extension** 🔖
▶ Abnormal extensor posturing to pain or noxious stimuli (< 2 years of age)
▶ Extensor posturing to pain or noxious stimuli (2-5 years of age)

●● **R40.233** **Coma scale, best motor response, abnormal**
▶ Abnormal flexure posturing to pain or noxious stimuli (Ø-5 years of age)
▶ Flexion/decorticate posturing (< 2 years of age)

●● **R40.234** **Coma scale, best motor response, flexion withdrawal** 🔖
▶ Withdraws from pain or noxious stimuli (Ø-5 years of age)

●● **R40.235** **Coma scale, best motor response, localizes pain**
▶ Localizes pain (2-5 years of age)
▶ Withdraws to touch (< 2 years of age)

●● **R40.236** **Coma scale, best motor response, obeys commands**
▶ Normal or spontaneous movement (< 2 years of age)
▶ Obeys commands (2-5 years of age)

● **R40.24** Glasgow coma scale, **total score**
Note: Assign a code from subcategory R40.24, when only the total coma score is documented
The following appropriate 7th character is to be added to subcategory R40.24-:

Ø	unspecified time
1	in the field [EMT or ambulance]
2	at arrival to emergency department
3	at hospital admission
4	24 hours or more after hospital admission

Coding Clinic: 2016, Q4, P64; 2015, Q2, P18

●● **R40.241** Glasgow coma scale score 13-15
●● **R40.242** Glasgow coma scale score 9-12
●● **R40.243** Glasgow coma scale score 3-8
●● **R40.244** **Other coma, without documented Glasgow coma scale score, or with partial score reported**

R40.3 Persistent vegetative state 🔖
(Ex) See PDX Collection 515

R40.4 Transient alteration of awareness

● **R41** Other symptoms and signs involving cognitive functions and awareness
Excludes1 dissociative [conversion] disorders (F44.-)
mild cognitive impairment, so stated (G31.84)

R41.Ø Disorientation, **unspecified**
Confusion NOS   Delirium NOS
Coding Clinic: 2016, Q4, P71

R41.1 **Anterograde amnesia**

R41.2 **Retrograde amnesia**

R41.3 Other amnesia
Amnesia NOS
Memory loss NOS

Excludes1 amnestic disorder due to known physiologic condition (FØ4)
amnestic syndrome due to psychoactive substance use (F1Ø-F19 with 5th character .6)
mild memory disturbance due to known physiological condition (FØ6.8)
transient global amnesia (G45.4)

CHAPTER 18 (RØØ-R99)

N Newborn Age: Ø   **P** Pediatric Age: Ø–17   **M** Maternity DX: 12–55   **A** Adult Age: 15–124   ♀ Females Only   ♂ Males Only

🔖 Complication\Comorbidity   🔖 Major C\C   (Ex) CC/MCC Exclusions   🔖 Hospital-Acquired Condition

1205

R41.4　Neurologic neglect syndrome 🔗
　　Asomatognosia　　　　　　Left-sided neglect
　　Hemi-akinesia　　　　　　Sensory neglect
　　Hemi-inattention　　　　　Visuospatial neglect
　　Hemispatial neglect

　　　Excludes1　visuospatial deficit (R41.842)

　　　(Ex) See PDX Collection 1128

● **R41.8　Other symptoms and signs involving cognitive functions and awareness**

　　R41.81　Age-related cognitive decline　　　　　A
　　　　Senility NOS

　　R41.82　Altered mental status, unspecified
　　　　Change in mental status NOS

　　　　　Excludes1　altered level of consciousness
　　　　　　　　　　　(R40.-)
　　　　　　　　　　altered mental status due to
　　　　　　　　　　　known condition - code to
　　　　　　　　　　　condition
　　　　　　　　　　delirium NOS (R41.0)

　　　　Coding Clinic: 2012, Q4, P98

　● **R41.83　Borderline intellectual functioning**
　　　　IQ level 71 to 84

　　　　　Excludes1　intellectual disabilities (F70-F79)

　● **R41.84　Other specified cognitive deficit**

　　　　　Excludes1　cognitive deficits as sequelae of
　　　　　　　　　　cerebrovascular disease
　　　　　　　　　　(I69.01-, I69.11-, I69.21-,
　　　　　　　　　　I69.31-, I69.81-, I69.91-)

　　　R41.840　Attention and concentration deficit

　　　　　　Excludes1　attention-deficit
　　　　　　　　　　　hyperactivity
　　　　　　　　　　　disorders (F90.-)

　　　R41.841　Cognitive communication deficit

　　　R41.842　Visuospatial deficit

　　　R41.843　Psychomotor deficit

　　　R41.844　Frontal lobe and executive function deficit

　　R41.89　Other symptoms and signs involving cognitive functions and awareness
　　　　Anosognosia

R41.9　Unspecified symptoms and signs involving cognitive functions and awareness
　　▶Unspecified neurocognitive disorder

R42　Dizziness and giddiness
　　Light-headedness
　　Vertigo NOS

　　Excludes1　vertiginous syndromes (H81.-)
　　　　　　　vertigo from infrasound (T75.23)

　　Coding Clinic: 2015, Q4, P40

● **R43　Disturbances of smell and taste**

　　R43.0　Anosmia
　　　　Absence of sense of smell; AKA anosphresia and olfactory anesthesia

　　R43.1　Parosmia

　　R43.2　Parageusia
　　　　Perversion of sense of taste or bad taste in mouth; AKA dysgeusia

　　R43.8　Other disturbances of smell and taste
　　　　Mixed disturbance of smell and taste

　　R43.9　Unspecified disturbances of smell and taste

● **R44　Other symptoms and signs involving general sensations and perceptions**

　　　Excludes1　alcoholic hallucinations (F1.5)
　　　　　　　hallucinations in drug psychosis (F11-F19 with .5)
　　　　　　　hallucinations in mood disorders with psychotic
　　　　　　　　symptoms (F30.2, F31.5, F32.3, F33.3)
　　　　　　　hallucinations in schizophrenia, schizotypal and
　　　　　　　　delusional disorders (F20-F29)

　　　Excludes2　disturbances of skin sensation (R20.-)

　　R44.0　Auditory hallucinations 🔗
　　　　(Ex) See PDX Collection 1129

　　R44.1　Visual hallucinations

　　R44.2　Other hallucinations 🔗
　　　　(Ex) See PDX Collection 1129

　　R44.3　Hallucinations, unspecified 🔗
　　　　(Ex) See PDX Collection 1129

　　R44.8　Other symptoms and signs involving general sensations and perceptions

　　R44.9　Unspecified symptoms and signs involving general sensations and perceptions

● **R45　Symptoms and signs involving emotional state**

　　R45.0　Nervousness
　　　　Nervous tension

　　R45.1　Restlessness and agitation

　　R45.2　Unhappiness

　　R45.3　Demoralization and apathy

　　　　　Excludes1　anhedonia (R45.84)

　　R45.4　Irritability and anger

　　R45.5　Hostility

　　R45.6　Violent behavior

　　R45.7　State of emotional shock and stress, unspecified

　● **R45.8　Other symptoms and signs involving emotional state**

　　　R45.81　Low self-esteem

　　　R45.82　Worries

　　　R45.83　Excessive crying of child, adolescent or adult

　　　　　　Excludes1　excessive crying of infant (baby)
　　　　　　　　　　　R68.11

　　　R45.84　Anhedonia
　　　　　Total loss of feeling of pleasure in pleasurable acts

　　● **R45.85　Homicidal and suicidal ideations**

　　　　　Excludes1　suicide attempt (T14.91)

　　　　● **R45.850　Homicidal ideations**

　　　　　R45.851　Suicidal ideations 🔗
　　　　　　(Ex) See PDX Collection 1130

　　　R45.86　Emotional lability

　　　R45.87　Impulsiveness

　　　R45.89　Other symptoms and signs involving emotional state

● **R46　Symptoms and signs involving appearance and behavior**

　　　Excludes1　appearance and behavior in schizophrenia,
　　　　　　　schizotypal and delusional disorders
　　　　　　　(F20-F29)
　　　　　　　mental and behavioral disorders (F01-F99)

　　R46.0　Very low level of personal hygiene

　　R46.1　Bizarre personal appearance

　　R46.2　Strange and inexplicable behavior

　　R46.3　Overactivity

　　R46.4　Slowness and poor responsiveness

　　　　　Excludes1　stupor (R40.1)

　　R46.5　Suspiciousness and marked evasiveness

　　R46.6　Undue concern and preoccupation with stressful events

　　R46.7　Verbosity and circumstantial detail obscuring reason for contact

▶ New　⇒ Revised　~~deleted~~ Deleted　Excludes 1　Excludes 2　Includes　Use additional　Code first　Code also　Key words
OGCR Official Guidelines　● Unacceptable Principal Diagnosis　X Assign placeholder X　● Use Additional Character(s)　▌ Manifestation Code　**Coding Clinic**

● R46.8   **Other symptoms and signs involving appearance and behavior**
   ● R46.81   **Obsessive-compulsive behavior**
       Excludes1   obsessive-compulsive disorder (F42-)
   ● R46.89   **Other symptoms and signs involving appearance and behavior**

SYMPTOMS AND SIGNS INVOLVING SPEECH AND VOICE (R47-R49)

● R47   **Speech disturbances, not elsewhere classified**
   Excludes1   autism (F84.0)
          cluttering (F80.81)
          specific developmental disorders of speech and language (F80.-)
          stuttering (F80.81)

● R47.0   **Dysphasia and aphasia**
    R47.01   **Aphasia**
       Excludes1   aphasia following cerebrovascular disease (I69. with final characters -20)
            progressive isolated aphasia (G31.01)
       (Ex:) See PDX Collection 1131

    R47.02   **Dysphasia**
       Impairment in comprehension of speech, caused by left-sided brain damage
       Excludes1   dysphasia following cerebrovascular disease (I69. with final characters -21)

   R47.1   **Dysarthria and anarthria**
      Motor speech disorder
      Excludes1   dysarthria following cerebrovascular disease (I69. with final characters -22)

● R47.8   **Other speech disturbances**
   Excludes1   dysarthria following cerebrovascular disease (I69. with final characters -28)
    R47.81   **Slurred speech**
 ▷ R47.82   *Fluency disorder in conditions classified elsewhere*
       Stuttering in conditions classified elsewhere
       Code first underlying disease or condition, such as:
       Parkinson's disease (G20)
       Excludes1   adult onset fluency disorder (F98.5)
            childhood onset fluency disorder (F80.81)
            fluency disorder (stuttering) following cerebrovascular disease (I69. with final characters -23)
    R47.89   **Other speech disturbances**
   R47.9   **Unspecified speech disturbances**

● R48   **Dyslexia and other symbolic dysfunctions, not elsewhere classified**
   Excludes1   specific developmental disorders of scholastic skills (F81.-)

   R48.0   **Dyslexia and alexia**
   R48.1   **Agnosia**
      Loss of ability to recognize objects, persons, sounds, shapes, or smells
      Astereognosia (astereognosis)
      Autotopagnosia
      Excludes1   visual object agnosia (R48.3)
   R48.2   **Apraxia**
      Loss of ability to execute or carry out learned purposeful movements
      Excludes1   apraxia following cerebrovascular disease (I69. with final characters -90)

   R48.3   **Visual agnosia**
      Prosopagnosia
      Simultanagnosia (asimultagnosia)
   R48.8   **Other symbolic dysfunctions**
      Acalculia
      Difficulty performing simple mathematical tasks resulting from neurological injury
      Agraphia
      Coding Clinic: 2017, Q1, P27
   R48.9   **Unspecified symbolic dysfunctions**

● R49   **Voice and resonance disorders**
   Excludes1   psychogenic voice and resonance disorders (F44.4)
   R49.0   **Dysphonia**
      Hoarseness
   R49.1   **Aphonia**
      Loss of voice
● R49.2   **Hypernasality and hyponasality**
    R49.21   **Hypernasality**
    R49.22   **Hyponasality**
   R49.8   **Other voice and resonance disorders**
   R49.9   **Unspecified voice and resonance disorder**
      Change in voice NOS
      Resonance disorder NOS

GENERAL SYMPTOMS AND SIGNS (R50-R69)

● R50   **Fever of other and unknown origin**
   Excludes1   chills without fever (R68.83)
          febrile convulsions (R56.0-)
          fever of unknown origin during labor (O75.2)
          fever of unknown origin in newborn (P81.9)
          hypothermia due to illness (R68.0)
          malignant hyperthermia due to anesthesia (T88.3)
          puerperal pyrexia NOS (O86.4)

   R50.2   **Drug induced fever**
      Use additional code for adverse effect, if applicable, to identify drug (T36-T50 with fifth or sixth character 5)
      Excludes1   postvaccination (postimmunization) fever (R50.83)

● R50.8   **Other specified fever**
 ▷ R50.81   *Fever presenting with conditions classified elsewhere*
       Code first underlying condition when associated fever is present, such as with:
       leukemia (C91-C95)
       neutropenia (D70.-)
       sickle-cell disease (D57.-)
    R50.82   **Postprocedural fever**
       Excludes1   postprocedural infection (T81.4-)
            posttransfusion fever (R50.84)
            postvaccination (postimmunization) fever (R50.83)

    R50.83   **Postvaccination fever**
      Postimmunization fever
    R50.84   **Febrile nonhemolytic transfusion reaction**
      FNHTR
      Posttransfusion fever

   R50.9   **Fever, unspecified**
      Fever NOS
      Fever of unknown origin [FUO]
      Fever with chills
      Fever with rigors
      Hyperpyrexia NOS
      Persistent fever
      Pyrexia NOS

CHAPTER 18 (R00-R99)

R51   Headache
Facial pain NOS
Excludes1   atypical face pain (G50.1)
migraine and other headache syndromes
(G43-G44)
trigeminal neuralgia (G50.0)

R52   Pain, unspecified
Acute pain NOS   Pain NOS
Generalized pain NOS
Excludes1   acute and chronic pain, not elsewhere classified
(G89.-)
localized pain, unspecified type - code to pain by
site, such as:
abdomen pain (R10.-)
back pain (M54.9)
breast pain (N64.4)
chest pain (R07.1-R07.9)
ear pain (H92.0-)
eye pain (H57.1)
headache (R51)
joint pain (M25.5-)
limb pain (M79.6-)
lumbar region pain (M54.5)
pelvic and perineal pain (R10.2)
shoulder pain (M25.51-)
spine pain (M54.-)
throat pain (R07.0)
tongue pain (K14.6)
tooth pain (K08.8)
renal colic (N23)
pain disorders exclusively related to
psychological factors (F45.41)

● **R53   Malaise and fatigue**
R53.0   Neoplastic (malignant) related fatigue
Code first associated neoplasm

R53.1   Weakness
Asthenia NOS
Excludes1   age-related weakness (R54)
muscle weakness (M62.8-)
sarcopenia (M62.84)
senile asthenia (R54)
Coding Clinic: 2017, Q1, P7

R53.2   Functional quadriplegia 🔖
Complete immobility due to severe physical disability
or frailty
Excludes1   frailty NOS (R54)
hysterical paralysis (F44.4)
immobility syndrome (M62.3)
neurologic quadriplegia (G82.5-)
quadriplegia (G82.50)
(Ex) See PDX Collection 595
Coding Clinic: 2016, Q2, P6

● **R53.8   Other malaise and fatigue**
Excludes1   combat exhaustion and fatigue (F43.0)
congenital debility (P96.9)
~~exhaustion and fatigue due to depressive~~
~~episode (F32.-)~~
exhaustion and fatigue due to excessive
exertion (T73.3)
exhaustion and fatigue due to exposure
(T73.2)
exhaustion and fatigue due to heat (T67.-)
exhaustion and fatigue due to pregnancy
(O26.8-)
exhaustion and fatigue due to recurrent
depressive episode (F33)
exhaustion and fatigue due to senile
debility (R54)

R53.81   Other malaise
Chronic debility
Debility NOS
General physical deterioration
Malaise NOS
Nervous debility
Excludes1   age-related physical debility (R54)

R53.82   Chronic fatigue, unspecified
Chronic fatigue syndrome NOS
Excludes1   postviral fatigue syndrome
(G93.3)

R53.83   Other fatigue
Fatigue NOS   Lethargy
Lack of energy   Tiredness
▶ **Excludes2**   exhaustion and fatigue due to
depressive episode (F32.-)
Coding Clinic: 2017, Q1, P7

R54   Age-related physical debility   A
Frailty   Senile asthenia
Old age   Senile debility
Senescence
Excludes1   age-related cognitive decline (R41.81)
sarcopenia (M62.84)
senile psychosis (F03)
senility NOS (R41.81)

R55   Syncope and collapse
Blackout
Fainting
Vasovagal attack
Excludes1   cardiogenic shock (R57.0)
carotid sinus syncope (G90.01)
heat syncope (T67.1)
neurocirculatory asthenia (F45.8)
neurogenic orthostatic hypotension (G90.3)
orthostatic hypotension (I95.1)
postprocedural shock (T81.1-)
psychogenic syncope (F48.8)
shock NOS (R57.9)
shock complicating or following abortion or
ectopic or molar pregnancy (O00-O07, O08.3)
shock complicating or following labor and
delivery (O75.1)
Stokes-Adams attack (I45.9)
unconsciousness NOS (R40.2-)

● **R56   Convulsions, not elsewhere classified**
Excludes1   dissociative convulsions and seizures (F44.5)
epileptic convulsions and seizures (G40.-)
newborn convulsions and seizures (P90)

● **R56.0   Febrile convulsions**
(Ex) **For category R56.0 CC codes:** See PDX Collection 1132

R56.00   Simple febrile convulsions 🔖
Febrile convulsion NOS
Febrile seizure NOS

R56.01   Complex febrile convulsions 🔖
Atypical febrile seizure
Complex febrile seizure
Complicated febrile seizure
Excludes1   status epilepticus (G40.901)

R56.1   Post traumatic seizures 🔖
Excludes1   post traumatic epilepsy (G40.-)
(Ex) See PDX Collection 582

R56.9   Unspecified convulsions
Convulsion disorder   Recurrent convulsions
Fit NOS   Seizure(s) (convulsive) NOS

▶ New   ⟹ Revised   ~~deleted~~ Deleted   Excludes 1   Excludes 2   Includes   Use additional   Code first   Code also   Key words
OGCR Official Guidelines   ● Unacceptable Principal Diagnosis   X Assign placeholder X   ● Use Additional Character(s)   ▶ Manifestation Code   **Coding Clinic**

● **R57**   **Shock, not elsewhere classified**
     Excludes1   anaphylactic shock NOS (T78.2)
           anaphylactic reaction or shock due to adverse
              food reaction (T78.0-)
           anaphylactic shock due to adverse effect of
              correct drug or medicament properly
              administered (T88.6)
           anaphylactic shock due to serum (T80.5-)
           anesthetic shock (T88.3)
           electric shock (T75.4)
           obstetric shock (O75.1)
           postprocedural shock (T81.1-)
           psychic shock (F43.0)
           ~~septic shock (R65.21)~~
           shock complicating or following ectopic or molar
              pregnancy (O00-O07, O08.3)
           shock due to lightning (T75.01)
           traumatic shock (T79.4)
           toxic shock syndrome (A48.3)
     (Ex) **For category R57 CC codes:** See PDX Collection 1133

     R57.0   **Cardiogenic shock**
         ▶ **Excludes2**   septic shock (R65.21)
         MCC: Only if patient discharged alive

     R57.1   **Hypovolemic shock**
         Decreased blood volume (loss)
         MCC: Only if patient discharged alive

     R57.8   **Other shock**
         MCC: Only if patient discharged alive

     R57.9   **Shock, unspecified**
         Failure of peripheral circulation NOS
         Resulting in significant blood pressure drop

● **R58**   **Hemorrhage, not elsewhere classified**
     Hemorrhage NOS
     Excludes1   hemorrhage included with underlying
              conditions, such as:
           acute duodenal ulcer with hemorrhage (K26.0)
           acute gastritis with bleeding (K29.01)
           ulcerative enterocolitis with rectal bleeding
              (K51.01)

● **R59**   **Enlarged lymph nodes**
     Includes   swollen glands
     Excludes1   lymphadenitis NOS (I88.9)
           acute lymphadenitis (L04.-)
           chronic lymphadenitis (I88.1)
           mesenteric (acute) (chronic) lymphadenitis (I88.0)

     R59.0   **Localized enlarged lymph nodes**

     R59.1   **Generalized enlarged lymph nodes**
         Lymphadenopathy NOS

     R59.9   **Enlarged lymph nodes, unspecified**

● **R60**   **Edema, not elsewhere classified**
     Excludes1   angioneurotic edema (T78.3)
           ascites (R18.-)
           cerebral edema (G93.6)
           cerebral edema due to birth injury (P11.0)
           edema of larynx (J38.4)
           edema of nasopharynx (J39.2)
           edema of pharynx (J39.2)
           gestational edema (O12.0-)
           hereditary edema (Q82.0)
           hydrops fetalis NOS (P83.2)
           hydrothorax (J94.8)
           ~~nutritional edema (E40-E46)~~
           hydrops fetalis NOS (P83.2)
           newborn edema (P83.3)
           pulmonary edema (J81.-)

     R60.0   **Localized edema**

     R60.1   **Generalized edema**
         ▶ **Excludes2**   nutritional edema (E40-E46)

     R60.9   **Edema, unspecified**
         Fluid retention NOS

● **R61**   **Generalized hyperhidrosis**
     Excessive sweating
     Night sweats
     Secondary hyperhidrosis
     *Code first, if applicable, menopausal and female climacteric states
         (N95.1)*
     Excludes1   focal (primary) (secondary) hyperhidrosis (L74.5-)
           Frey's syndrome (L74.52)
           localized (primary) (secondary) hyperhidrosis
              (L74.5-)

● **R62**   **Lack of expected normal physiological development in**
     childhood and adults
     Excludes1   delayed puberty (E30.0)
           gonadal dysgenesis (Q99.1)
           hypopituitarism (E23.0)

     R62.0   **Delayed milestone in childhood**   P
         Delayed attainment of expected physiological
              developmental stage
         Late talker
         Late walker

     ● **R62.5**   **Other and unspecified lack of expected normal**
         physiological development in childhood
         Excludes1   HIV disease resulting in failure to thrive
              (B20)
              physical retardation due to malnutrition
                  (E45)

         R62.50   **Unspecified lack of expected normal**
              physiological development in childhood
              Infantilism NOS

         R62.51   **Failure to thrive (child)**   P
              Failure to gain weight
              Excludes1   failure to thrive in child under 28
                  days old (P92.6)

         R62.52   **Short stature (child)**
              Lack of growth   Short stature NOS
              Physical retardation
              Excludes1   short stature due to endocrine
                  disorder (E34.3)

         R62.59   **Other lack of expected normal physiological**
              development in childhood

     R62.7   **Adult failure to thrive**   A

● **R63**   **Symptoms and signs concerning food and fluid intake**
     Excludes1   bulimia NOS (F50.2)
           eating disorders of nonorganic origin (F50.-)
           malnutrition (E40-E46)

     R63.0   **Anorexia**
         Loss of appetite
         Excludes1   anorexia nervosa (F50.0-)
             loss of appetite of nonorganic origin
              (F50.89)

     R63.1   **Polydipsia**
         Excessive thirst

     R63.2   **Polyphagia**
         Excessive eating   Hyperalimentation NOS

     R63.3   **Feeding difficulties**
         Feeding problem (elderly) (infant) NOS
         ▶Picky eater
         Excludes1 ▶eating disorders (F50.-)
           feeding problems of newborn (P92.-)
           infant feeding disorder of nonorganic
              origin (F98.2-)
         Coding Clinic: 2017, Q1, P27; 2016, Q3, P19

     R63.4   **Abnormal weight loss**

     R63.5   **Abnormal weight gain**
         Excludes1   excessive weight gain in pregnancy
             (O26.0-)
           obesity (E66.-)

CHAPTER 18 (R00-R99)

N   Newborn Age: 0   **P**   Pediatric Age: 0–17   **M**   Maternity DX: 12–55   **A**   Adult Age: 15–124   ♀   Females Only   ♂   Males Only

 Complication\Comorbidity   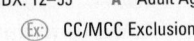 Major C\C   (Ex)   CC/MCC Exclusions   Hospital-Acquired Condition

1209

R63.6 Underweight

Use additional code to identify body mass index (BMI), if known (Z68.-)

Excludes1   abnormal weight loss (R63.4)
anorexia nervosa (F50.0-)
malnutrition (E40-E46)

R63.8 Other symptoms and signs concerning food and fluid intake

R64 Cachexia

Wasting syndrome

Code first underlying condition, if known

Excludes1   abnormal weight loss (R63.4)
nutritional marasmus (E41)

Ex: See PDX Collection 1134

R65 Symptoms and signs specifically associated with systemic inflammation and infection

Ex: For category R65 CC codes unless otherwise indicated: See PDX Collection 71

R65.1 Systemic inflammatory response syndrome (SIRS) of non-infectious origin

Code first underlying condition, such as:
heatstroke (T67.0)
injury and trauma (S00-T88)

Excludes1   sepsis - code to infection
severe sepsis (R65.2)

R65.10 Systemic inflammatory response syndrome (SIRS) of non-infectious origin without acute organ dysfunction

Systemic inflammatory response syndrome (SIRS) NOS

R65.11 Systemic inflammatory response syndrome (SIRS) of non-infectious origin with acute organ dysfunction

Use additional code to identify specific acute organ dysfunction, such as:
acute kidney failure (N17.-)
acute respiratory failure (J96.0-)
critical illness myopathy (G72.81)
critical illness polyneuropathy (G62.81)
disseminated intravascular coagulopathy [DIC] (D65)
encephalopathy (metabolic) (septic) (G93.41)
hepatic failure (K72.0-)

OGCR Section I.C.18.g.

SIRS due to Non-Infectious Process

The systemic inflammatory response syndrome (SIRS) can develop as a result of certain non-infectious disease processes, such as trauma, malignant neoplasm, or pancreatitis. When SIRS is documented with a noninfectious condition, and no subsequent infection is documented, the code for the underlying condition, such as an injury, should be assigned, followed by code R65.10, Systemic inflammatory response syndrome (SIRS) of non-infectious origin without acute organ dysfunction, or code R65.11, Systemic inflammatory response syndrome (SIRS) of non-infectious origin with acute organ dysfunction. If an associated acute organ dysfunction is documented, the appropriate code(s) for the specific type of organ dysfunction(s) should be assigned in addition to code R65.11. If acute organ dysfunction is documented, but it cannot be determined if the acute organ dysfunction is associated with SIRS or due to another condition (e.g., directly due to the trauma), the provider should be queried.

R65.2 Severe sepsis

Infection with associated acute organ dysfunction
Sepsis with acute organ dysfunction
Sepsis with multiple organ dysfunction
Systemic inflammatory response syndrome due to infectious process with acute organ dysfunction

Code first underlying infection, such as:
infection following a procedure (T81.4-)
infections following infusion, transfusion and therapeutic injection (T80.2-)
puerperal sepsis (O85)
sepsis following complete or unspecified spontaneous abortion (O03.87)
sepsis following ectopic and molar pregnancy (O08.82)
sepsis following incomplete spontaneous abortion (O03.37)
sepsis following (induced) termination of pregnancy (O04.87)
sepsis NOS (A41.9)

Use additional code to identify specific acute organ dysfunction, such as:
acute kidney failure (N17.-)
acute respiratory failure (J96.0-)
critical illness myopathy (G72.81)
critical illness polyneuropathy (G62.81)
disseminated intravascular coagulopathy [DIC] (D65)
encephalopathy (metabolic) (septic) (G93.41)
hepatic failure (K72.0-)
Coding Clinic: 2016, Q3, P8

R65.20 Severe sepsis without septic shock
Severe sepsis NOS
Coding Clinic: 2016, Q3, P14

R65.21 Severe sepsis with septic shock
MCC when PDx is its own MCC
Ex: See PDX Collection 1133

R68 Other general symptoms and signs

R68.0 Hypothermia, not associated with low environmental temperature

Excludes1   hypothermia NOS (accidental) (T68)
hypothermia due to anesthesia (T88.51)
hypothermia due to low environmental temperature (T68)
newborn hypothermia (P80.-)

R68.1 Nonspecific symptoms peculiar to infancy

Excludes1   colic, infantile (R10.83)
neonatal cerebral irritability (P91.3)
teething syndrome (K00.7)

R68.11 Excessive crying of infant (baby)   P

Excludes1   excessive crying of child, adolescent, or adult (R45.83)

R68.12 Fussy infant (baby)   P
Irritable infant

R68.13 Apparent life threatening event in infant (ALTE)   P

Apparent life threatening event in newborn
▶ Brief resolved unexplained event (BRUE)

Code first confirmed diagnosis, if known

Use additional code(s) for associated signs and symptoms if no confirmed diagnosis established, or if signs and symptoms are not associated routinely with confirmed diagnosis, or provide additional information for cause of ALTE

R68.19 Other nonspecific symptoms peculiar to infancy   P

R68.2 Dry mouth, unspecified

Excludes1   dry mouth due to dehydration (E86.0)
dry mouth due to sicca syndrome [Sjögren] (M35.0-)
salivary gland hyposecretion (K11.7)

R68.3 Clubbing of fingers
Clubbing of nails

Excludes1   congenital clubfinger (Q68.1)

▶ New   ⇒ Revised   ~~deleted~~ Deleted   Excludes 1   Excludes 2   Includes   Use additional   Code first   Code also   Key words
OGCR Official Guidelines   ● Unacceptable Principal Diagnosis   X Assign placeholder X   Use Additional Character(s)   ▶ Manifestation Code   **Coding Clinic**

● **R68.8 Other general symptoms and signs**
  R68.81 Early satiety
  R68.82 Decreased libido   A
    Decreased sexual desire
  R68.83 Chills (without fever)
    Chills NOS
    Excludes1   chills with fever (R50.9)
  R68.84 Jaw pain
    Mandibular pain
    Maxilla pain
    Excludes1   temporomandibular joint arthralgia (M26.62-)
  R68.89 Other general symptoms and signs

R69 Illness, unspecified
  Unknown and unspecified cases of morbidity

ABNORMAL FINDINGS ON EXAMINATION OF BLOOD, WITHOUT DIAGNOSIS (R70-R79)

Excludes2 abnormal findings on antenatal screening of mother (O28.-)
  abnormalities of lipids (E78.-)
  abnormalities of platelets and thrombocytes (D69.-)
  abnormalities of white blood cells classified elsewhere (D70-D72)
  coagulation hemorrhagic disorders (D65-D68)
  diagnostic abnormal findings classified elsewhere —see Alphabetical Index
  hemorrhagic and hematological disorders of newborn (P50-P61)

● **R70 Elevated erythrocyte sedimentation rate and abnormality of plasma viscosity**
  R70.0 Elevated erythrocyte sedimentation rate
  R70.1 Abnormal plasma viscosity

● **R71 Abnormality of red blood cells**
  Excludes1 anemias (D50-D64)
    anemia of premature infant (P61.2)
    benign (familial) polycythemia (D75.0)
    congenital anemias (P61.2-P61.4)
    newborn anemia due to isoimmunization (P55.-)
    polycythemia neonatorum (P61.1)
    polycythemia NOS (D75.1)
    polycythemia vera (D45)
    secondary polycythemia (D75.1)
  R71.0 Precipitous drop in hematocrit 🔲
    Drop (precipitous) in hemoglobin
    Drop in hematocrit
    Blood volume that has decreased red blood cells
    (Ex) See PDX Collection 1135
  R71.8 Other abnormality of red blood cells
    Abnormal red-cell morphology NOS
    Abnormal red-cell volume NOS
    Anisocytosis
    Red blood cells of unequal size
    Poikilocytosis
    Red blood cells of abnormal shape

● **R73 Elevated blood glucose level**
  Excludes1 diabetes mellitus (E08-E13)
    diabetes mellitus in pregnancy, childbirth and the puerperium (O24.-)
    neonatal disorders (P70.0-P70.2)
    postsurgical hypoinsulinemia (E89.1)
● **R73.0 Abnormal glucose**
  Excludes1 abnormal glucose in pregnancy (O99.81-)
    diabetes mellitus (E08-E13)
    dysmetabolic syndrome X (E88.81)
    gestational diabetes (O24.4-)
    glycosuria (R81)
    hypoglycemia (E16.2)
  R73.01 Impaired fasting glucose
    Elevated fasting glucose

  R73.02 Impaired glucose tolerance (oral)
    Elevated glucose tolerance
  R73.03 Prediabetes
    Latent diabetes
    Coding Clinic: 2016, Q4, P65
  R73.09 Other abnormal glucose
    Abnormal glucose NOS
    Abnormal non-fasting glucose tolerance
    Coding Clinic: 2016, Q4, P65
  R73.9 Hyperglycemia, unspecified

● **R74 Abnormal serum enzyme levels**
  R74.0 Nonspecific elevation of levels of transaminase and lactic acid dehydrogenase [LDH]
  R74.8 Abnormal levels of other serum enzymes
    Abnormal level of acid phosphatase
    Abnormal level of alkaline phosphatase
    Abnormal level of amylase
    Abnormal level of lipase [triacylglycerol lipase]
  R74.9 Abnormal serum enzyme level, unspecified

R75 Inconclusive laboratory evidence of human immunodeficiency virus [HIV]
  Nonconclusive HIV-test finding in infants
  Excludes1 asymptomatic human immunodeficiency virus [HIV] infection status (Z21)
    human immunodeficiency virus [HIV] disease (B20)

● **R76 Other abnormal immunological findings in serum**
  R76.0 Raised antibody titer
    Excludes1 isoimmunization in pregnancy (O36.0-O36.1)
    isoimmunization affecting newborn (P55.-)
● **R76.1 Nonspecific reaction to test for tuberculosis**
  R76.11 Nonspecific reaction to tuberculin skin test without active tuberculosis
    Abnormal result of Mantoux test
    PPD positive
    Tuberculin (skin test) positive
    Tuberculin (skin test) reactor
    Excludes1 nonspecific reaction to cell mediated immunity measurement of gamma interferon antigen response without active tuberculosis (R76.12)
  R76.12 Nonspecific reaction to cell mediated immunity measurement of gamma interferon antigen response without active tuberculosis
    Nonspecific reaction to QuantiFERON-TB test (QFT) without active tuberculosis
    Excludes1 nonspecific reaction to tuberculin skin test without active tuberculosis (R76.11)
    positive tuberculin skin test (R76.11)
  R76.8 Other specified abnormal immunological findings in serum
    Raised level of immunoglobulins NOS
  R76.9 Abnormal immunological finding in serum, unspecified

OGCR Section I.C.1.e and f.

Patients with inconclusive HIV serology

e. Patients with inconclusive HIV serology, but no definitive diagnosis or manifestations of the illness, may be assigned code R75, Inconclusive laboratory evidence of human immunodeficiency virus [HIV].

f. Previously diagnosed HIV-related illness

Patients with any known prior diagnosis of an HIV-related illness should be coded to B20. Once a patient has developed an HIV-related illness, the patient should always be assigned code B20 on every subsequent admission/encounter. Patients previously diagnosed with any HIV illness (B20) should never be assigned to R75 or Z21, Asymptomatic human immunodeficiency virus [HIV] infection status.

N Newborn Age: 0   P Pediatric Age: 0–17   M Maternity DX: 12–55   A Adult Age: 15–124   ♀ Females Only   ♂ Males Only
🔲 Complication\Comorbidity   Major C\C   (Ex) CC/MCC Exclusions   Hospital-Acquired Condition
1211

CHAPTER 18 (R00-R99)

● **R77** **Other abnormalities of plasma proteins**
> **Excludes1** disorders of plasma-protein metabolism (E88.0)

R77.0 **Abnormality of albumin**

R77.1 **Abnormality of globulin**
> Hyperglobulinemia NOS

R77.2 **Abnormality of alphafetoprotein**

R77.8 **Other specified abnormalities of plasma proteins**

R77.9 **Abnormality of plasma protein, unspecified**

● **R78** **Findings of drugs and other substances, not normally found in blood**
> Use additional code to identify any retained foreign body, if applicable (Z18.-)
> **Excludes1** mental or behavioral disorders due to psychoactive substance use (F10-F19)

R78.0 **Finding of alcohol in blood**
> Use additional external cause code (Y90.-), for detail regarding alcohol level.

R78.1 **Finding of opiate drug in blood**

R78.2 **Finding of cocaine in blood**

R78.3 **Finding of hallucinogen in blood**

R78.4 **Finding of other drugs of addictive potential in blood**

R78.5 **Finding of other psychotropic drug in blood**

R78.6 **Finding of steroid agent in blood**

● **R78.7** **Finding of abnormal level of heavy metals in blood**

> **R78.71** **Abnormal lead level in blood**
>> **Excludes1** lead poisoning (T56.0-)

> **R78.79** **Finding of abnormal level of heavy metals in blood**

● **R78.8** **Finding of other specified substances, not normally found in blood**

> **R78.81** **Bacteremia** 🔗
>> *Blood poisoning/bacteremia*
>> **Excludes1** sepsis-code to specified infection
>> (Ex) See PDX Collection 1136

> **R78.89** **Finding of other specified substances, not normally found in blood**
>> Finding of abnormal level of lithium in blood

R78.9 **Finding of unspecified substance, not normally found in blood**

● **R79** **Other abnormal findings of blood chemistry**
> Use additional code to identify any retained foreign body, if applicable (Z18.-)
> **Excludes1** ~~abnormality of fluid, electrolyte or acid-base balance (E86-E87)~~
> asymptomatic hyperuricemia (E79.0)
> hyperglycemia NOS (R73.9)
> hypoglycemia NOS (E16.2)
> neonatal hypoglycemia (P70.3-P70.4)
> specific findings indicating disorder of amino-acid metabolism (E70-E72)
> specific findings indicating disorder of carbohydrate metabolism (E73-E74)
> specific findings indicating disorder of lipid metabolism (E75.-)

R79.0 **Abnormal level of blood mineral**
> Abnormal blood level of cobalt
> Abnormal blood level of copper
> Abnormal blood level of iron
> Abnormal blood level of magnesium
> Abnormal blood level of mineral NEC
> Abnormal blood level of zinc
> **Excludes1** abnormal level of lithium (R78.89)
> disorders of mineral metabolism (E83.-)
> neonatal hypomagnesemia (P71.2)
> nutritional mineral deficiency (E58-E61)

R79.1 **Abnormal coagulation profile**
> Abnormal or prolonged bleeding time
> Abnormal or prolonged coagulation time
> Abnormal or prolonged partial thromboplastin time [PTT]
> Abnormal or prolonged prothrombin time [PT]
> **Excludes1** coagulation defects (D68.-)
> ▶ **Excludes2** abnormality of fluid, electrolyte or acid-base balance (E86-E87)

● **R79.8** **Other specified abnormal findings of blood chemistry**

R79.81 **Abnormal blood-gas level**

R79.82 **Elevated C-reactive protein (CRP)**

R79.89 **Other specified abnormal findings of blood chemistry**

R79.9 **Abnormal finding of blood chemistry, unspecified**

ABNORMAL FINDINGS ON EXAMINATION OF URINE, WITHOUT DIAGNOSIS (R80-R82)

> **Excludes1** abnormal findings on antenatal screening of mother (O28.-)
> diagnostic abnormal findings classified elsewhere - see Alphabetical Index
> specific findings indicating disorder of amino-acid metabolism (E70-E72)
> specific findings indicating disorder of carbohydrate metabolism (E73-E74)

● **R80** **Proteinuria**
> **Excludes1** gestational proteinuria (O12.1-)

R80.0 **Isolated proteinuria**
> Idiopathic proteinuria
> **Excludes1** isolated proteinuria with specific morphological lesion (N06.-)

R80.1 **Persistent proteinuria, unspecified**

R80.2 **Orthostatic proteinuria, unspecified**
> Postural proteinuria

R80.3 **Bence Jones proteinuria**

R80.8 **Other proteinuria**

R80.9 **Proteinuria, unspecified**
> Albuminuria NOS

○ **R81** **Glycosuria**
> **Excludes1** renal glycosuria (E74.8)

● **R82** **Other and unspecified abnormal findings in urine**
> **Includes** chromoabnormalities in urine
> Use additional code to identify any retained foreign body, if applicable (Z18.-)
> **Excludes2** hematuria (R31.-)

R82.0 **Chyluria** 🔗
> *White milky urine*
> **Excludes1** filarial chyluria (B74.-)
> (Ex) See PDX Collection 1137

R82.1 **Myoglobinuria** 🔗
> *Presence of myoglobin (iron containing protein) in urine*
> (Ex) See PDX Collection 1138

R82.2 **Biliuria**
> *Presence of bile pigments/salts in urine*

R82.3 **Hemoglobinuria**
> *Presence of hemoglobin in urine*
> **Excludes1** hemoglobinuria due to hemolysis from external causes NEC (D59.6)
> hemoglobinuria due to paroxysmal nocturnal [Marchiafava-Micheli] (D59.5)

▶ New　⇒ Revised　~~deleted~~ Deleted　Excludes 1　Excludes 2　Includes　Use additional　Code first　Code also　Key words
OGCR Official Guidelines　● Unacceptable Principal Diagnosis　X Assign placeholder X　● Use Additional Character(s)　▶ Manifestation Code　**Coding Clinic**

CHAPTER 18 (R00-R99)

R82.4   Acetonuria
     Ketonuria

R82.5   Elevated urine levels of drugs, medicaments and biological substances
     Elevated urine levels of catecholamines
     Elevated urine levels of indoleacetic acid
     Elevated urine levels of 17-ketosteroids
     Elevated urine levels of steroids

R82.6   Abnormal urine levels of substances chiefly nonmedicinal as to source
     Abnormal urine level of heavy metals

● **R82.7   Abnormal findings on microbiological examination of urine**

     Excludes1   colonization status (Z22.-)

     Coding Clinic: 2016, Q4, P65

     R82.71   Bacteriuria

     R82.79   Other abnormal findings on microbiological examination of urine
         Positive culture findings of urine

R82.8   Abnormal findings on cytological and histological examination of urine

● **R82.9   Other and unspecified abnormal findings in urine**

     R82.90   Unspecified abnormal findings in urine

     R82.91   Other chromoabnormalities of urine
         Chromoconversion (dipstick)
         Idiopathic dipstick converts positive for blood
             with no cellular forms in sediment

         Excludes1   hemoglobinuria (R82.3)
                   myoglobinuria (R82.1)

     R82.99   Other abnormal findings in urine
         Cells and casts in urine
         Crystalluria
         Melanuria

ABNORMAL FINDINGS ON EXAMINATION OF OTHER BODY FLUIDS, SUBSTANCES AND TISSUES, WITHOUT DIAGNOSIS (R83-R89)

     Excludes1   abnormal findings on antenatal screening of mother (O28.-)
         diagnostic abnormal findings classified elsewhere - see Alphabetical Index

     Excludes2   abnormal findings on examination of blood, without diagnosis (R70-R79)
         abnormal findings on examination of urine, without diagnosis (R80-R82)
         abnormal tumor markers (R97.-)

● **R83   Abnormal findings in cerebrospinal fluid**

     R83.0   Abnormal level of enzymes in cerebrospinal fluid

     R83.1   Abnormal level of hormones in cerebrospinal fluid

     R83.2   Abnormal level of other drugs, medicaments and biological substances in cerebrospinal fluid

     R83.3   Abnormal level of substances chiefly nonmedicinal as to source in cerebrospinal fluid

     R83.4   Abnormal immunological findings in cerebrospinal fluid

     R83.5   Abnormal microbiological findings in cerebrospinal fluid
         Positive culture findings in cerebrospinal fluid

         Excludes1   colonization status (Z22.-)

     R83.6   Abnormal cytological findings in cerebrospinal fluid

     R83.8   Other abnormal findings in cerebrospinal fluid
         Abnormal chromosomal findings in cerebrospinal fluid

     R83.9   Unspecified abnormal finding in cerebrospinal fluid

● **R84   Abnormal findings in specimens from respiratory organs and thorax**

     Includes   abnormal findings in bronchial washings
         abnormal findings in nasal secretions
         abnormal findings in pleural fluid
         abnormal findings in sputum
         abnormal findings in throat scrapings

     Excludes1   blood-stained sputum (R04.2)

     R84.0   Abnormal level of enzymes in specimens from respiratory organs and thorax

     R84.1   Abnormal level of hormones in specimens from respiratory organs and thorax

     R84.2   Abnormal level of other drugs, medicaments and biological substances in specimens from respiratory organs and thorax

     R84.3   Abnormal level of substances chiefly nonmedicinal as to source in specimens from respiratory organs and thorax

     R84.4   Abnormal immunological findings in specimens from respiratory organs and thorax

     R84.5   Abnormal microbiological findings in specimens from respiratory organs and thorax
         Positive culture findings in specimens from respiratory organs and thorax

         Excludes1   colonization status (Z22.-)

     R84.6   Abnormal cytological findings in specimens from respiratory organs and thorax

     R84.7   Abnormal histological findings in specimens from respiratory organs and thorax

     R84.8   Other abnormal findings in specimens from respiratory organs and thorax
         Abnormal chromosomal findings in specimens from respiratory organs and thorax

     R84.9   Unspecified abnormal finding in specimens from respiratory organs and thorax

● **R85   Abnormal findings in specimens from digestive organs and abdominal cavity**

     Includes   abnormal findings in peritoneal fluid
         abnormal findings in saliva

     Excludes1   cloudy peritoneal dialysis effluent (R88.0)
         fecal abnormalities (R19.5)

     R85.0   Abnormal level of enzymes in specimens from digestive organs and abdominal cavity

     R85.1   Abnormal level of hormones in specimens from digestive organs and abdominal cavity

     R85.2   Abnormal level of other drugs, medicaments and biological substances in specimens from digestive organs and abdominal cavity

     R85.3   Abnormal level of substances chiefly nonmedicinal as to source in specimens from digestive organs and abdominal cavity

     R85.4   Abnormal immunological findings in specimens from digestive organs and abdominal cavity

     R85.5   Abnormal microbiological findings in specimens from digestive organs and abdominal cavity
         Positive culture findings in specimens from digestive organs and abdominal cavity

         Excludes1   colonization status (Z22.-)

CHAPTER 18 (R00-R99)

N Newborn Age: 0   **P** Pediatric Age: 0–17   **M** Maternity DX: 12–55   **A** Adult Age: 15–124   ♀ Females Only   ♂ Males Only

🔖 Complication\Comorbidity   🔖 Major C\C   (Ex) CC/MCC Exclusions   🔖 Hospital-Acquired Condition

1213

● **R85.6** **Abnormal cytological findings in specimens from digestive organs and abdominal cavity**

  ● **R85.61** **Abnormal cytologic smear of anus**

     Excludes1   abnormal cytological findings in specimens from other digestive organs and abdominal cavity (R85.69)
carcinoma in situ of anus (histologically confirmed) (D01.3)
anal intraepithelial neoplasia I [AIN I] (K62.82)
anal intraepithelial neoplasia II [AIN II] (K62.82)
anal intraepithelial neoplasia III [AIN III] (D01.3)
dysplasia (mild) (moderate) of anus (histologically confirmed) (K62.82)
severe dysplasia of anus (histologically confirmed) (D01.3)

     Excludes2   anal high risk human papillomavirus (HPV) DNA test positive (R85.81)
anal low risk human papillomavirus (HPV) DNA test positive (R85.82)

     R85.610 **Atypical squamous cells of undetermined significance on cytologic smear of anus (ASC-US)**

     R85.611 **Atypical squamous cells cannot exclude high grade squamous intraepithelial lesion on cytologic smear of anus (ASC-H)**

     R85.612 **Low grade squamous intraepithelial lesion on cytologic smear of anus (LGSIL)**

     R85.613 **High grade squamous intraepithelial lesion on cytologic smear of anus (HGSIL)**

     R85.614 **Cytologic evidence of malignancy on smear of anus**

     R85.615 **Unsatisfactory cytologic smear of anus**
Inadequate sample of cytologic smear of anus

     R85.616 **Satisfactory anal smear but lacking transformation zone**

     R85.618 **Other abnormal cytological findings on specimens from anus**

     R85.619 **Unspecified abnormal cytological findings in specimens from anus**
Abnormal anal cytology NOS
Atypical glandular cells of anus NOS

  ● **R85.69** **Abnormal cytological findings in specimens from other digestive organs and abdominal cavity**

   R85.7 **Abnormal histological findings in specimens from digestive organs and abdominal cavity**

● **R85.8** **Other abnormal findings in specimens from digestive organs and abdominal cavity**

   R85.81 **Anal high risk human papillomavirus (HPV) DNA test positive**

     Excludes1   anogenital warts due to human papillomavirus (HPV) (A63.0)
condyloma acuminatum (A63.0)

   R85.82 **Anal low risk human papillomavirus (HPV) DNA test positive**
Use additional code for associated human papillomavirus (B97.7)

   R85.89 **Other abnormal findings in specimens from digestive organs and abdominal cavity**
Abnormal chromosomal findings in specimens from digestive organs and abdominal cavity

   R85.9 **Unspecified abnormal finding in specimens from digestive organs and abdominal cavity**

● **R86** **Abnormal findings in specimens from male genital organs**

   Includes   abnormal findings in prostatic secretions
abnormal findings in semen, seminal fluid
abnormal spermatozoa

   Excludes1   azoospermia (N46.0-)
oligospermia (N46.1-)

   R86.0 **Abnormal level of enzymes in specimens from male genital organs ♂**

   R86.1 **Abnormal level of hormones in specimens from male genital organs ♂**

   R86.2 **Abnormal level of other drugs, medicaments and biological substances in specimens from male genital organs ♂**

   R86.3 **Abnormal level of substances chiefly nonmedicinal as to source in specimens from male genital organs ♂**

   R86.4 **Abnormal immunological findings in specimens from male genital organs ♂**

   R86.5 **Abnormal microbiological findings in specimens from male genital organs ♂**
Positive culture findings in specimens from male genital organs

     Excludes1   colonization status (Z22.-)

   R86.6 **Abnormal cytological findings in specimens from male genital organs ♂**

   R86.7 **Abnormal histological findings in specimens from male genital organs ♂**

   R86.8 **Other abnormal findings in specimens from male genital organs ♂**
Abnormal chromosomal findings in specimens from male genital organs

   R86.9 **Unspecified abnormal finding in specimens from male genital organs ♂**

● **R87** **Abnormal findings in specimens from female genital organs**

   Includes   abnormal findings in secretion and smears from cervix uteri
abnormal findings in secretion and smears from vagina
abnormal findings in secretion and smears from vulva

   R87.0 **Abnormal level of enzymes in specimens from female genital organs ♀**

   R87.1 **Abnormal level of hormones in specimens from female genital organs ♀**

   R87.2 **Abnormal level of other drugs, medicaments and biological substances in specimens from female genital organs ♀**

   R87.3 **Abnormal level of substances chiefly nonmedicinal as to source in specimens from female genital organs ♀**

   R87.4 **Abnormal immunological findings in specimens from female genital organs ♀**

R87.5   **Abnormal microbiological findings in specimens from female genital organs** ♀
> Positive culture findings in specimens from female genital organs

>   **Excludes1**   colonization status (Z22.-)

● **R87.6**   **Abnormal cytological findings in specimens from female genital organs**

  ● **R87.61**   **Abnormal cytological findings in specimens from cervix uteri**

     Excludes1   abnormal cytological findings in specimens from other female genital organs (R87.69)
            abnormal cytological findings in specimens from vagina (R87.62-)
            carcinoma in situ of cervix uteri (histologically confirmed) (D06.-)
            cervical intraepithelial neoplasia I [CIN I] (N87.0)
            cervical intraepithelial neoplasia II [CIN II] (N87.1)
            cervical intraepithelial neoplasia III [CIN III] (D06.-)
            dysplasia (mild) (moderate) of cervix uteri (histologically confirmed) (N87.-)
            severe dysplasia of cervix uteri (histologically confirmed) (D06.-)

     Excludes2   cervical high risk human papillomavirus (HPV) DNA test positive (R87.810)
            cervical low risk human papillomavirus (HPV) DNA test positive (R87.820)

     R87.610   **Atypical squamous cells of undetermined significance on cytologic smear of cervix (ASC-US)** ♀

     R87.611   **Atypical squamous cells cannot exclude high grade squamous intraepithelial lesion on cytologic smear of cervix (ASC-H)** ♀

     R87.612   **Low grade squamous intraepithelial lesion on cytologic smear of cervix (LGSIL)** ♀

     R87.613   **High grade squamous intraepithelial lesion on cytologic smear of cervix (HGSIL)** ♀

     R87.614   **Cytologic evidence of malignancy on smear of cervix** ♀

     R87.615   **Unsatisfactory cytologic smear of cervix** ♀
> Inadequate sample of cytologic smear of cervix

     R87.616   **Satisfactory cervical smear but lacking transformation zone** ♀

     R87.618   **Other abnormal cytological findings on specimens from cervix uteri** ♀

     R87.619   **Unspecified abnormal cytological findings in specimens from cervix uteri** ♀
> Abnormal cervical cytology NOS
> Abnormal Papanicolaou smear of cervix NOS
> Abnormal thin preparation smear of cervix NOS
> Atypical endocervical cells of cervix NOS
> Atypical endometrial cells of cervix NOS
> Atypical glandular cells of cervix NOS

● **R87.62**   **Abnormal cytological findings in specimens from vagina**
> Use additional code to identify acquired absence of uterus and cervix, if applicable (Z90.71-)

     Excludes1   abnormal cytological findings in specimens from cervix uteri (R87.61-)
            abnormal cytological findings in specimens from other female genital organs (R87.69)
            carcinoma in situ of vagina (histologically confirmed) (D07.2)
            vaginal intraepithelial neoplasia I [VAIN I] (N89.0)
            vaginal intraepithelial neoplasia II [VAIN II] (N89.1)
            vaginal intraepithelial neoplasia III [VAIN III] (D07.2)
            dysplasia (mild) (moderate) of vagina (histologically confirmed) (N89.-)
            severe dysplasia of vagina (histologically confirmed) (D07.2)

     Excludes2   vaginal high risk human papillomavirus (HPV) DNA test positive (R87.811)
            vaginal low risk human papillomavirus (HPV) DNA test positive (R87.821)

     R87.620   **Atypical squamous cells of undetermined significance on cytologic smear of vagina (ASC-US)** ♀

     R87.621   **Atypical squamous cells cannot exclude high grade squamous intraepithelial lesion on cytologic smear of vagina (ASC-H)** ♀

     R87.622   **Low grade squamous intraepithelial lesion on cytologic smear of vagina (LGSIL)** ♀

     R87.623   **High grade squamous intraepithelial lesion on cytologic smear of vagina (HGSIL)** ♀

     R87.624   **Cytologic evidence of malignancy on smear of vagina** ♀

     R87.625   **Unsatisfactory cytologic smear of vagina** ♀
> Inadequate sample of cytologic smear of vagina

     R87.628   **Other abnormal cytological findings on specimens from vagina** ♀

     R87.629   **Unspecified abnormal cytological findings in specimens from vagina** ♀
> Abnormal Papanicolaou smear of vagina NOS
> Abnormal thin preparation smear of vagina NOS
> Abnormal vaginal cytology NOS
> Atypical endocervical cells of vagina NOS
> Atypical endometrial cells of vagina NOS
> Atypical glandular cells of vagina NOS

CHAPTER 18 (R00–R99)

R87.69   **Abnormal cytological findings in specimens from other female genital organs** ♀

     Abnormal cytological findings in specimens from female genital organs NOS

     Excludes1   dysplasia of vulva (histologically confirmed) (N90.0-N90.3)

R87.7   **Abnormal histological findings in specimens from female genital organs** ♀

     Excludes1   carcinoma in situ (histologically confirmed) of female genital organs (D06-D07.3)

           cervical intraepithelial neoplasia I [CIN I] (N87.0)

           cervical intraepithelial neoplasia II [CIN II] (N87.1)

           cervical intraepithelial neoplasia III [CIN III] (D06.-)

           dysplasia (mild) (moderate) of cervix uteri (histologically confirmed) (N87.-)

           dysplasia (mild) (moderate) of vagina (histologically confirmed) (N89.-)

           vaginal intraepithelial neoplasia I [VAIN I] (N89.0)

           vaginal intraepithelial neoplasia II [VAIN II] (N89.1)

           vaginal intraepithelial neoplasia III [VAIN III] (D07.2)

           severe dysplasia of cervix uteri (histologically confirmed) (D06.-)

           severe dysplasia of vagina (histologically confirmed) (D07.2)

● **R87.8**   **Other abnormal findings in specimens from female genital organs**

    ● **R87.81**   **High risk human papillomavirus (HPV) DNA test positive from female genital organs**

       Excludes1   anogenital warts due to human papillomavirus (HPV) (A63.0)

           condyloma acuminatum (A63.0)

       R87.810   **Cervical high risk human papillomavirus (HPV) DNA test positive** ♀

       R87.811   **Vaginal high risk human papillomavirus (HPV) DNA test positive** ♀

    ● **R87.82**   **Low risk human papillomavirus (HPV) DNA test positive from female genital organs**

       Use additional code for associated human papillomavirus (B97.7)

       R87.820   **Cervical low risk human papillomavirus (HPV) DNA test positive** ♀

       R87.821   **Vaginal low risk human papillomavirus (HPV) DNA test positive** ♀

     R87.89   **Other abnormal findings in specimens from female genital organs** ♀

       Abnormal chromosomal findings in specimens from female genital organs

    R87.9   **Unspecified abnormal finding in specimens from female genital organs** ♀

● **R88**   **Abnormal findings in other body fluids and substances**

    R88.0   **Cloudy (hemodialysis) (peritoneal) dialysis effluent**

    R88.8   **Abnormal findings in other body fluids and substances**

● **R89**   **Abnormal findings in specimens from other organs, systems and tissues**

    Includes   abnormal findings in nipple discharge

           abnormal findings in synovial fluid

           abnormal findings in wound secretions

    R89.0   **Abnormal level of enzymes in specimens from other organs, systems and tissues**

    R89.1   **Abnormal level of hormones in specimens from other organs, systems and tissues**

    R89.2   **Abnormal level of other drugs, medicaments and biological substances in specimens from other organs, systems and tissues**

    R89.3   **Abnormal level of substances chiefly nonmedicinal as to source in specimens from other organs, systems and tissues**

    R89.4   **Abnormal immunological findings in specimens from other organs, systems and tissues**

    R89.5   **Abnormal microbiological findings in specimens from other organs, systems and tissues**

       Positive culture findings in specimens from other organs, systems and tissues

       Excludes1   colonization status (Z22.-)

    R89.6   **Abnormal cytological findings in specimens from other organs, systems and tissues**

    R89.7   **Abnormal histological findings in specimens from other organs, systems and tissues**

    R89.8   **Other abnormal findings in specimens from other organs, systems and tissues**

       Abnormal chromosomal findings in specimens from other organs, systems and tissues

    R89.9   **Unspecified abnormal finding in specimens from other organs, systems and tissues**

ABNORMAL FINDINGS ON DIAGNOSTIC IMAGING AND IN FUNCTION STUDIES, WITHOUT DIAGNOSIS (R90-R94)

    Includes   nonspecific abnormal findings on diagnostic imaging by computerized axial tomography [CAT scan]

           nonspecific abnormal findings on diagnostic imaging by magnetic resonance imaging [MRI][NMR]

           nonspecific abnormal findings on diagnostic imaging by positron emission tomography [PET scan]

           nonspecific abnormal findings on diagnostic imaging by thermography

           nonspecific abnormal findings on diagnostic imaging by ultrasound [echogram]

           nonspecific abnormal findings on diagnostic imaging by X-ray examination

    Excludes1   abnormal findings on antenatal screening of mother (O28.-)

       diagnostic abnormal findings classified elsewhere - see Alphabetical Index

● **R90**   **Abnormal findings on diagnostic imaging of central nervous system**

    R90.0   **Intracranial space-occupying lesion found on diagnostic imaging of central nervous system**

    ● **R90.8**   **Other abnormal findings on diagnostic imaging of central nervous system**

       R90.81   **Abnormal echoencephalogram**

       R90.82   **White matter disease, unspecified**

       R90.89   **Other abnormal findings on diagnostic imaging of central nervous system**

           Other cerebrovascular abnormality found on diagnostic imaging of central nervous system

● **R91 Abnormal findings on diagnostic imaging of lung**

    R91.1 Solitary pulmonary nodule
        Coin lesion lung
        Solitary pulmonary nodule, subsegmental branch of the
           bronchial tree

    R91.8 Other nonspecific abnormal finding of lung field
        Lung mass NOS found on diagnostic imaging of lung
        Pulmonary infiltrate NOS
        Shadow, lung

● **R92 Abnormal and inconclusive findings on diagnostic imaging of breast**

    R92.0 Mammographic microcalcification found on diagnostic imaging of breast
        Excludes2 mammographic calcification (calculus) found on diagnostic imaging of breast (R92.1)

    R92.1 Mammographic calcification found on diagnostic imaging of breast
        Mammographic calculus found on diagnostic imaging of breast

    R92.2 Inconclusive mammogram
        Dense breasts NOS
        Inconclusive mammogram NEC
        Inconclusive mammography due to dense breasts
        Inconclusive mammography NEC
        Coding Clinic: 2015, Q1, P24

    R92.8 Other abnormal and inconclusive findings on diagnostic imaging of breast

● **R93 Abnormal findings on diagnostic imaging of other body structures**

    R93.0 Abnormal findings on diagnostic imaging of skull and head, not elsewhere classified
        Excludes1 intracranial space-occupying lesion found on diagnostic imaging (R90.0)

    R93.1 Abnormal findings on diagnostic imaging of heart and coronary circulation
        Abnormal echocardiogram NOS
        Abnormal heart shadow

    R93.2 Abnormal findings on diagnostic imaging of liver and biliary tract
        Nonvisualization of gallbladder

    R93.3 Abnormal findings on diagnostic imaging of other parts of digestive tract

    ● **R93.4 Abnormal findings on diagnostic imaging of urinary organs**
        Excludes2 hypertrophy of kidney (N28.81)
        Coding Clinic: 2016, Q4, P66

        R93.41 Abnormal radiologic findings on diagnostic imaging of renal pelvis, ureter, or bladder
            Filling defect of bladder found on diagnostic imaging
            Filling defect of renal pelvis found on diagnostic imaging
            Filling defect of ureter found on diagnostic imaging

      ● **R93.42 Abnormal radiologic findings on diagnostic imaging of kidney**
          R93.421 Abnormal radiologic findings on diagnostic imaging of right kidney
          R93.422 Abnormal radiologic findings on diagnostic imaging of left kidney
          R93.429 Abnormal radiologic findings on diagnostic imaging of unspecified kidney

        R93.49 Abnormal radiologic findings on diagnostic imaging of other urinary organs

    R93.5 Abnormal findings on diagnostic imaging of other abdominal regions, including retroperitoneum

    R93.6 Abnormal findings on diagnostic imaging of limbs
        Excludes2 abnormal finding in skin and subcutaneous tissue (R93.8)

    R93.7 Abnormal findings on diagnostic imaging of other parts of musculoskeletal system
        Excludes2 abnormal findings on diagnostic imaging of skull (R93.0)

    R93.8 Abnormal findings on diagnostic imaging of other specified body structures
        Abnormal finding by radioisotope localization of placenta
        Abnormal radiological finding in skin and subcutaneous tissue
        Mediastinal shift

    R93.9 Diagnostic imaging inconclusive due to excess body fat of patient

● **R94 Abnormal results of function studies**
    Includes abnormal results of radionuclide [radioisotope] uptake studies
              abnormal results of scintigraphy

    ● **R94.0 Abnormal results of function studies of central nervous system**
        R94.01 Abnormal electroencephalogram [EEG]
        R94.02 Abnormal brain scan
        R94.09 Abnormal results of other function studies of central nervous system

    ● **R94.1 Abnormal results of function studies of peripheral nervous system and special senses**
      ● **R94.11 Abnormal results of function studies of eye**
          R94.110 Abnormal electro-oculogram [EOG]
          R94.111 Abnormal electroretinogram [ERG]
             Abnormal retinal function study
          R94.112 Abnormal visually evoked potential [VEP]
          R94.113 Abnormal oculomotor study
          R94.118 Abnormal results of other function studies of eye

      ● **R94.12 Abnormal results of function studies of ear and other special senses**
          R94.120 Abnormal auditory function study
             Coding Clinic: 2016, Q3, P17
          R94.121 Abnormal vestibular function study
          R94.128 Abnormal results of other function studies of ear and other special senses

      ● **R94.13 Abnormal results of function studies of peripheral nervous system**
          R94.130 Abnormal response to nerve stimulation, unspecified
          R94.131 Abnormal electromyogram [EMG]
             Excludes1 electromyogram of eye (R94.113)
          R94.138 Abnormal results of other function studies of peripheral nervous system

Item 18–1 The **peripheral nervous system** consists of 31 pairs of spinal nerves, 12 pairs of cranial nerves, and the autonomic nerves, which are divided into the parasympathetic and sympathetic nerves. The cranial nerves are: olfactory (I), optic (II), oculomotor (III), trochlear (IV), trigeminal (V), abducens (VI), facial (VII), vestibulocochlear (VIII), glossopharyngeal (IX), vagus (X), accessory (XI), and hypoglossal (XII).

CHAPTER 18 (R00-R99)

Figure 18-2 Cranial nerves. (From Patton and Thibodeau: Anatomy and physiology, ed 7, St. Louis, Mosby, 2009)

Trochlear nerve (IV)
Optic nerve (II)
Olfactory nerve (I)
Abducens nerve (VI)
Oculomotor nerve (III)
Facial nerve (VII)
Trigeminal nerve (V)
Vestibulocochlear nerve (VIII)
Glossopharyngeal nerve (IX)
Vagus nerve (X)
Accessory nerve (XI)
Hypoglossal nerve (XII)

R94.2 Abnormal results of pulmonary function studies
Reduced ventilatory capacity
Reduced vital capacity

● **R94.3 Abnormal results of cardiovascular function studies**

  R94.30 Abnormal result of cardiovascular function study, unspecified

  R94.31 Abnormal electrocardiogram [ECG] [EKG]
  Excludes1 long QT syndrome (I45.81)

  R94.39 Abnormal result of other cardiovascular function study
  Abnormal electrophysiological intracardiac studies
  Abnormal phonocardiogram
  Abnormal vectorcardiogram

R94.4 Abnormal results of kidney function studies
Abnormal renal function test

R94.5 Abnormal results of liver function studies

R94.6 Abnormal results of thyroid function studies

R94.7 Abnormal results of other endocrine function studies
Excludes2 abnormal glucose (R73.0-)

R94.8 Abnormal results of function studies of other organs and systems
Abnormal basal metabolic rate [BMR]
Abnormal bladder function test
Abnormal splenic function test

ABNORMAL TUMOR MARKERS (R97)

● **R97 Abnormal tumor markers**
Elevated tumor associated antigens [TAA]
Elevated tumor specific antigens [TSA]

  R97.0 Elevated carcinoembryonic antigen [CEA]

  R97.1 Elevated cancer antigen 125 [CA 125]

● **R97.2 Elevated prostate specific antigen [PSA]**
  Coding Clinic: 2016, Q4, P66

  R97.20 Elevated prostate specific antigen [PSA] ♂ A
  MCE: Questionable admission when principal dx

  R97.21 Rising PSA following treatment for malignant neoplasm of prostate ♂ A
  MCE: Questionable admission when principal dx

  R97.8 Other abnormal tumor markers

ILL-DEFINED AND UNKNOWN CAUSE OF MORTALITY (R99)

R99 Ill-defined and unknown cause of mortality
Death (unexplained) NOS
Unspecified cause of mortality
OGCR Section I.C.18.h.

Death NOS
Code R99, Ill-defined and unknown cause of mortality, is only for use in the very limited circumstance when a patient who has already died is brought into the emergency department or other healthcare facility and is pronounced dead upon arrival. It does not represent the discharge disposition of death.

► New ⇒ Revised ~~deleted~~ Deleted Excludes 1 Excludes 2 Includes Use additional Code first Code also Key words
OGCR Official Guidelines ● Unacceptable Principal Diagnosis X Assign placeholder X ● Use Additional Character(s) ▸ Manifestation Code Coding Clinic

CHAPTER 19

INJURY, POISONING AND CERTAIN OTHER CONSEQUENCES OF EXTERNAL CAUSES (S00-T88)

OGCR Chapter-Specific Coding Guidelines

19. **Chapter 19: Injury, poisoning, and certain other consequences of external causes (S00-T88)**

a. **Application of 7th Characters in Chapter 19**

Most categories in chapter 19 have a 7th character requirement for each applicable code. Most categories in this chapter have three 7th character values (with the exception of fractures): A, initial encounter, D, subsequent encounter and S, sequela. Categories for traumatic fractures have additional 7th character values. While the patient may be seen by a new or different provider over the course of treatment for an injury, assignment of the 7th character is based on whether the patient is undergoing active treatment and not whether the provider is seeing the patient for the first time.

For complication codes, active treatment refers to treatment for the condition described by the code, even though it may be related to an earlier precipitating problem. For example, code T84.50XA, Infection and inflammatory reaction due to unspecified internal joint prosthesis, initial encounter, is used when active treatment is provided for the infection, even though the condition relates to the prosthetic device, implant or graft that was placed at a previous encounter.

7th character "A", initial encounter is used for each encounter where the patient is receiving active treatment for the condition.

7th character "D" subsequent encounter is used for encounters after the patient has completed active treatment of the condition and is receiving routine care for the condition during the healing or recovery phase.

The aftercare Z codes should not be used for aftercare for conditions such as injuries or poisonings, where 7th characters are provided to identify subsequent care. For example, for aftercare of an injury, assign the acute injury code with the 7th character "D" (subsequent encounter).

7th character "S", sequela, is for use for complications or conditions that arise as a direct result of a condition, such as scar formation after a burn. The scars are sequelae of the burn. When using 7th character "S", it is necessary to use both the injury code that precipitated the sequela and the code for the sequela itself. The "S" is added only to the injury code, not the sequela code. The 7th character "S" identifies the injury responsible for the sequela. The specific type of sequela (e.g. scar) is sequenced first, followed by the injury code.

See Section I.B.10. Sequelae, (Late Effects)

b. **Coding of Injuries**

When coding injuries, assign separate codes for each injury unless a combination code is provided, in which case the combination code is assigned. **Codes from category T07,** Unspecified multiple injuries should not be assigned in the inpatient setting unless information for a more specific code is not available. Traumatic injury codes (S00-T14.9) are not to be used for normal, healing surgical wounds or to identify complications of surgical wounds.

The code for the most serious injury, as determined by the provider and the focus of treatment, is sequenced first.

1) **Superficial injuries**

Superficial injuries such as abrasions or contusions are not coded when associated with more severe injuries of the same site.

2) **Primary injury with damage to nerves/blood vessels**

When a primary injury results in minor damage to peripheral nerves or blood vessels, the primary injury is sequenced first with additional code(s) for injuries to nerves and spinal cord (such as category S04), and/or injury to blood vessels (such as category S15). When the primary injury is to the blood vessels or nerves, that injury should be sequenced first.

c. **Coding of Traumatic Fractures**

The principles of multiple coding of injuries should be followed in coding fractures. Fractures of specified sites are coded individually by site in accordance with both the provisions within

categories S02, S12, S22, S32, S42, S49, S52, S59, S62, S72, S79, S82, S89, S92 and the level of detail furnished by medical record content.

A fracture not indicated as open or closed should be coded to closed. A fracture not indicated whether displaced or not displaced should be coded to displaced.

More specific guidelines are as follows:

1) **Initial vs. Subsequent Encounter for Fractures**

Traumatic fractures are coded using the appropriate 7th character for initial encounter (A, B, C) for each encounter where the patient is receiving active treatment for the fracture. The appropriate 7th character for initial encounter should also be assigned for a patient who delayed seeking treatment for the fracture or nonunion.

Fractures are coded using the appropriate 7th character for subsequent care for encounters after the patient has completed active treatment of the fracture and is receiving routine care for the fracture during the healing or recovery phase.

Care for complications of surgical treatment for fracture repairs during the healing or recovery phase should be coded with the appropriate complication codes.

Care of complications of fractures, such as malunion and nonunion, should be reported with the appropriate 7th character for subsequent care with nonunion (K, M, N,) or subsequent care with malunion (P, Q, R).

Malunion/nonunion: The appropriate 7th character for initial encounter should also be assigned for a patient who delayed seeking treatment for the fracture or nonunion.

The open fracture designations in the assignment of the 7th character for fractures of the forearm, femur and lower leg, including ankle are based on the Gustilo open fracture classification. When the Gustilo classification type is not specified for an open fracture, the 7th character for open fracture type I or II should be assigned (B, E, H, M, Q).

A code from category M80, not a traumatic fracture code, should be used for any patient with known osteoporosis who suffers a fracture, even if the patient had a minor fall or trauma, if that fall or trauma would not usually break a normal, healthy bone.

See Section I.C.13. Osteoporosis.

The aftercare Z codes should not be used for aftercare for traumatic fractures. For aftercare of a traumatic fracture, assign the acute fracture code with the appropriate 7th character.

2) **Multiple fractures sequencing**

Multiple fractures are sequenced in accordance with the severity of the fracture.

d. **Coding of Burns and Corrosions**

The ICD-10-CM makes a distinction between burns and corrosions. The burn codes are for thermal burns, except sunburns, that come from a heat source, such as a fire or hot appliance. The burn codes are also for burns resulting from electricity and radiation. Corrosions are burns due to chemicals. The guidelines are the same for burns and corrosions.

Current burns (T20-T25) are classified by depth, extent and by agent (X code). Burns are classified by depth as first degree (erythema), second degree (blistering), and third degree (full-thickness involvement). Burns of the eye and internal organs (T26-T28) are classified by site, but not by degree.

1) **Sequencing of burn and related condition codes**

Sequence first the code that reflects the highest degree of burn when more than one burn is present.

   a. When the reason for the admission or encounter is for treatment of external multiple burns, sequence first the code that reflects the burn of the highest degree.

   b. When a patient has both internal and external burns, the circumstances of admission govern the selection of the principal diagnosis or first-listed diagnosis.

   c. When a patient is admitted for burn injuries and other related conditions such as smoke inhalation and/or respiratory failure, the circumstances of admission govern the selection of the principal or first-listed diagnosis.

2) Burns of the same local site

Classify burns of the same local site (three-character category level, T2Ø-T28) but of different degrees to the subcategory identifying the highest degree recorded in the diagnosis.

3) Non-healing burns

Non-healing burns are coded as acute burns.

Necrosis of burned skin should be coded as a non-healed burn.

4) Infected Burn

For any documented infected burn site, use an additional code for the infection.

5) Assign separate codes for each burn site

When coding burns, assign separate codes for each burn site. Category T3Ø, Burn and corrosion, body region unspecified is extremely vague and should rarely be used.

6) Burns and Corrosions Classified According to Extent of Body Surface Involved

Assign codes from category T31, Burns classified according to extent of body surface involved, or T32, Corrosions classified according to extent of body surface involved, when the site of the burn is not specified or when there is a need for additional data. It is advisable to use category T31 as additional coding when needed to provide data for evaluating burn mortality, such as that needed by burn units. It is also advisable to use category T31 as an additional code for reporting purposes when there is mention of a third-degree burn involving 2Ø percent or more of the body surface.

Categories T31 and T32 are based on the classic "rule of nines" in estimating body surface involved: head and neck are assigned nine percent, each arm nine percent, each leg 18 percent, the anterior trunk 18 percent, posterior trunk 18 percent, and genitalia one percent. Providers may change these percentage assignments where necessary to accommodate infants and children who have proportionately larger heads than adults, and patients who have large buttocks, thighs, or abdomen that involve burns.

7) Encounters for treatment of sequela of burns

Encounters for the treatment of the late effects of burns or corrosions (i.e., scars or joint contractures) should be coded with a burn or corrosion code with the 7th character "S" for sequela.

8) Sequelae with a late effect code and current burn

When appropriate, both a code for a current burn or corrosion with 7th character "A" or "D" and a burn or corrosion code with 7th character "S" may be assigned on the same record (when both a current burn and sequelae of an old burn exist). Burns and corrosions do not heal at the same rate and a current healing wound may still exist with sequela of a healed burn or corrosion.

See Section I.B.1Ø. Sequela, (Late Effects)

9) Use of an external cause code with burns and corrosions

An external cause code should be used with burns and corrosions to identify the source and intent of the burn, as well as the place where it occurred.

e. Adverse Effects, Poisoning , Underdosing and Toxic Effects

Codes in categories T36-T65 are combination codes that include the substance that was taken as well as the intent. No additional external cause code is required for poisonings, toxic effects, adverse effects and underdosing codes.

1) Do not code directly from the Table of Drugs

Do not code directly from the Table of Drugs and Chemicals. Always refer back to the Tabular List.

2) Use as many codes as necessary to describe

Use as many codes as necessary to describe completely all drugs, medicinal or biological substances.

3) If the same code would describe the causative agent

If the same code would describe the causative agent for more than one adverse reaction, poisoning, toxic effect or underdosing, assign the code only once.

4) If two or more drugs, medicinal or biological substances

If two or more drugs, medicinal or biological substances are reported, code each individually unless a combination code is listed in the Table of Drugs and Chemicals.

5) The occurrence of drug toxicity is classified in ICD-10-CM as follows:

(a) Adverse Effect

When coding an adverse effect of a drug that has been correctly prescribed and properly administered, assign the appropriate code for the nature of the adverse effect followed by the appropriate code for the adverse effect of the drug (T36-T5Ø). The code for the drug should have a 5th or 6th character "5" (for example T36.ØX5-) Examples of the nature of an adverse effect are tachycardia, delirium, gastrointestinal hemorrhaging, vomiting, hypokalemia, hepatitis, renal failure, or respiratory failure.

(b) Poisoning

When coding a poisoning or reaction to the improper use of a medication (e.g., overdose, wrong substance given or taken in error, wrong route of administration), first assign the appropriate code from categories T36-T5Ø. The poisoning codes have an associated intent as their 5th or 6th character (accidental, intentional self-harm, assault and undetermined). If the intent of the poisoning is unknown or unspecified, code the intent as accidental intent. The undetermined intent is only for use if the documentation in the record specifies that the intent cannot be determined. Use additional code(s) for all manifestations of poisonings.

If there is also a diagnosis of abuse or dependence of the substance, the abuse or dependence is assigned as an additional code.

Examples of poisoning include:

(i) Error was made in drug prescription
Errors made in drug prescription or in the administration of the drug by provider, nurse, patient, or other person.

(ii) Overdose of a drug intentionally taken If an overdose of a drug was intentionally taken or administered and resulted in drug toxicity, it would be coded as a poisoning.

(iii) Nonprescribed drug taken with correctly prescribed and properly administered drug. If a nonprescribed drug or medicinal agent was taken in combination with a correctly prescribed and properly administered drug, any drug toxicity or other reaction resulting from the interaction of the two drugs would be classified as a poisoning.

(iv) Interaction of drug(s) and alcohol. When a reaction results from the interaction of a drug(s) and alcohol, this would be classified as poisoning.

See Section I.C.4. if poisoning is the result of insulin pump malfunctions.

(c) Underdosing

Underdosing refers to taking less of a medication than is prescribed by a provider or a manufacturer's instruction. For underdosing, assign the code from categories T36-T50 (fifth or sixth character "6").

Codes for underdosing should never be assigned as principal or first-listed codes. If a patient has a relapse or exacerbation of the medical condition for which the drug is prescribed because of the reduction in dose, then the medical condition itself should be coded.

Noncompliance (Z91.12-, Z91.13-) or complication of care (Y63.6-Y63.9) codes are to be used with an underdosing code to indicate intent, if known.

(d) Toxic Effects

When a harmful substance is ingested or comes in contact with a person, this is classified as a toxic effect. The toxic effect codes are in categories T51-T65.

Toxic effect codes have an associated intent: accidental, intentional self-harm, assault and undetermined.

f. Adult and child abuse, neglect and other maltreatment

Sequence first the appropriate code from categories T74 (Adult and child abuse, neglect and other maltreatment, confirmed) or T76 (Adult and child abuse, neglect and other maltreatment, suspected) for abuse, neglect and other maltreatment, followed by any accompanying mental health or injury code(s).

If the documentation in the medical record states abuse or neglect it is coded as confirmed (T74.-). It is coded as suspected if it is documented as suspected (T76.-).

For cases of confirmed abuse or neglect an external cause code from the assault section (X92-Y09) should be added to identify the cause of any physical injuries. A perpetrator code (Y07) should be added when the perpetrator of the abuse is known. For suspected cases of abuse or neglect, do not report external cause or perpetrator code.

If a suspected case of abuse, neglect or mistreatment is ruled out during an encounter code Z04.71, Encounter for examination and observation following alleged physical adult abuse, ruled out, or code Z04.72, Encounter for examination and observation following alleged child physical abuse, ruled out, should be used, not a code from T76.

If a suspected case of alleged rape or sexual abuse is ruled out during an encounter code Z04.41, Encounter for examination and observation following alleged adult rape or code Z04.42, Encounter for examination and observation following alleged child rape, should be used, not a code from T76.

See Section I.C.15. Abuse in a pregnant patient.

g. Complications of care

1) General guidelines for complications of care

(a) Documentation of complications of care

See Section I.B.16. for information on documentation of complications of care.

2) Pain due to medical devices

Pain associated with devices, implants or grafts left in a surgical site (for example painful hip prosthesis) is assigned to the appropriate code(s) found in Chapter 19, Injury, poisoning, and certain other consequences of external causes. Specific codes for pain due to medical devices are found in the T code section of the ICD-10-CM. Use additional code(s) from category G89 to identify acute or chronic pain due to presence of the device, implant or graft (G89.18 or G89.28).

3) Transplant complications

(a) Transplant complications other than kidney

Codes under category T86, Complications of transplanted organs and tissues, are for use for both complications and rejection of transplanted organs. A transplant complication code is only assigned if the complication affects the function of the transplanted organ. Two codes are required to fully describe a transplant complication: the appropriate code from category T86 and a secondary code that identifies the complication.

Pre-existing conditions or conditions that develop after the transplant are not coded as complications unless they affect the function of the transplanted organs.

See I.C.21. for transplant organ removal status
See I.C.2. for malignant neoplasm associated with transplanted organ.

(b) Kidney transplant complications

Patients who have undergone kidney transplant may still have some form of chronic kidney disease (CKD) because the kidney transplant may not fully restore kidney function. Code T86.1- should be assigned for documented complications of a kidney transplant, such as transplant failure or rejection or other transplant complication. Code T86.1- should not be assigned for post kidney transplant patients who have chronic kidney (CKD) unless a transplant complication such as transplant failure or rejection is documented. If the documentation is unclear as to whether the patient has a complication of the transplant, query the provider.

Conditions that affect the function of the transplanted kidney, other than CKD, should be assigned a code from subcategory T86.1, Complications of transplanted organ, Kidney, and a secondary code that identifies the complication.

For patients with CKD following a kidney transplant, but who do not have a complication such as failure or rejection, *see section I.C.14. Chronic kidney disease and kidney transplant status.*

4) Complication codes that include the external cause

As with certain other T codes, some of the complications of care codes have the external cause included in the code. The code includes the nature of the complication as well as the type of procedure that caused the complication. No external cause code indicating the type of procedure is necessary for these codes.

5) Complications of care codes within the body system chapters

Intraoperative and postprocedural complication codes are found within the body system chapters with codes specific to the organs and structures of that body system. These codes should be sequenced first, followed by a code(s) for the specific complication, if applicable.

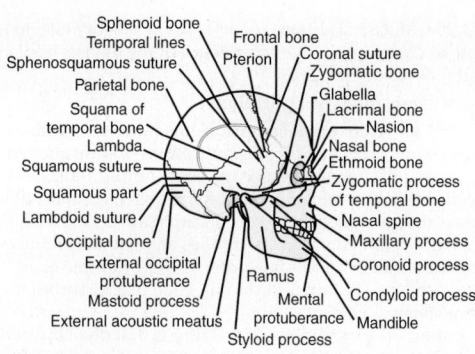

Figure 19-1 Lateral view of skull.

Figure 19-2 Frontal view of skull.

Figure 19-3 Anterior view of vertebral column.

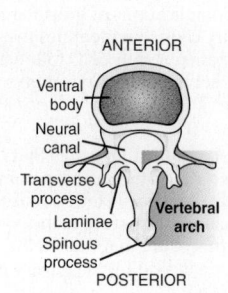

Figure 19-4 Vertebra viewed from above.

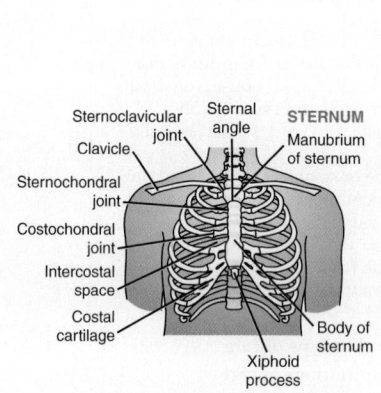

Figure 19-5 Anterior view of rib cage.

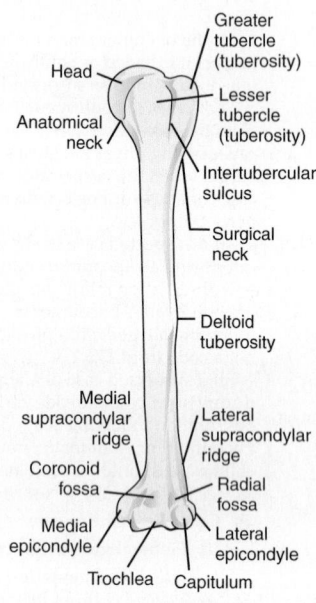

Figure 19-6 Anterior aspect of left humerus.

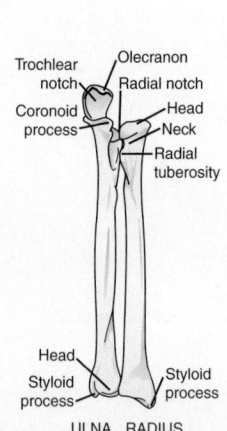

Figure 19-7 Anterior aspect of left radius and ulna.

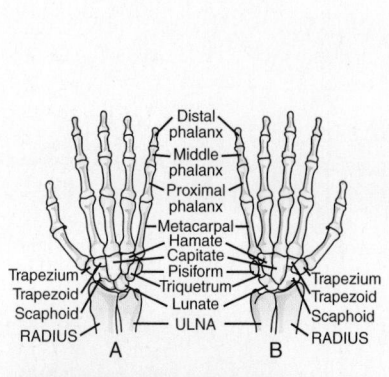

Figure 19-8 Right hand and wrist: **A.** Dorsal surface. **B.** Palmar surface.

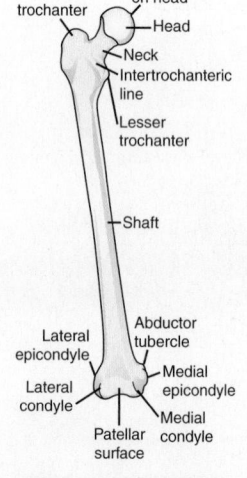

Figure 19-9 Anterior aspect of right femur.

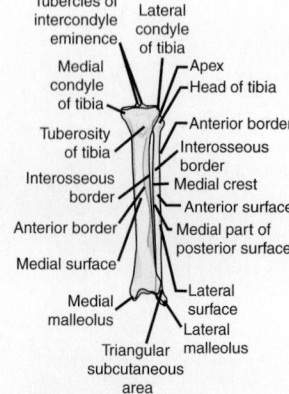

Figure 19-10 Anterior aspect of left tibia and fibula.

▶ New ⇒ Revised ~~deleted~~ Deleted ⬛ Excludes 1 ⬛ Excludes 2 ⬛ Includes ⬛ Use additional ⬛ Code first ⬛ Code also ⬛ Key words
OGCR Official Guidelines ● Unacceptable Principal Diagnosis X Assign placeholder X ● Use Additional Character(s) ▌ Manifestation Code **Coding Clinic**

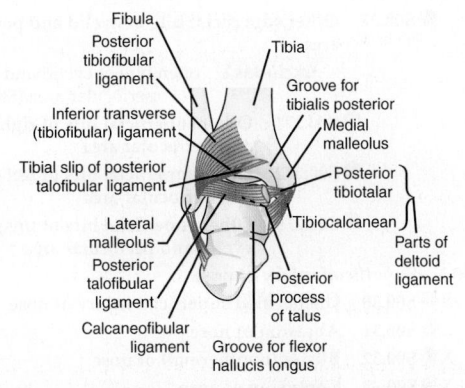

Figure 19-11   Posterior aspect of the left ankle joint.

Figure 19-12   Right foot viewed from above.

CHAPTER 19

INJURY, POISONING AND CERTAIN OTHER CONSEQUENCES OF EXTERNAL CAUSES (S00-T88)

Note: Use secondary code(s) from Chapter 20, External causes of morbidity, to indicate cause of injury. Codes within the T section that include the external cause do not require an additional external cause code.

Use additional code to identify any retained foreign body, if applicable (Z18.-)

Excludes1   birth trauma (P10-P15)
              obstetric trauma (O70-O71)

Note: The chapter uses the S-section for coding different types of injuries related to single body regions and the T-section to cover injuries to unspecified body regions as well as poisoning and certain other consequences of external causes.

This chapter contains the following blocks:

S00-S09	Injuries to the head
S10-S19	Injuries to the neck
S20-S29	Injuries to the thorax
S30-S39	Injuries to the abdomen, lower back, lumbar spine, pelvis and external genitals
S40-S49	Injuries to the shoulder and upper arm
S50-S59	Injuries to the elbow and forearm
S60-S69	Injuries to the wrist, hand, and fingers
S70-S79	Injuries to the hip and thigh
S80-S89	Injuries to the knee and lower leg
S90-S99	Injuries to the ankle and foot

T07	Injuries involving multiple body regions
T14	Injury of unspecified body region
T15-T19	Effects of foreign body entering through natural orifice
~~T20-T32~~	~~Burns and corrosions~~
T20-T25	Burns and corrosions of external body surface, specified by site
T26-T28	Burns and corrosions confined to eye and internal organs
T30-T32	Burns and corrosions of multiple and unspecified body regions
T33-T34	Frostbite
T36-T50	Poisoning by, adverse effect of and underdosing of drugs, medicaments and biological substances
T51-T65	Toxic effects of substances chiefly nonmedicinal as to source
T66-T78	Other and unspecified effects of external causes
T79	Certain early complications of trauma
T80-T88	Complications of surgical and medical care, not elsewhere classified

INJURIES TO THE HEAD (S00-S09)

Includes	injuries of ear
	injuries of eye
	injuries of face [any part]
	injuries of gum
	injuries of jaw
	injuries of oral cavity
	injuries of palate
	injuries of periocular area
	injuries of scalp
	injuries of temporomandibular joint area
	injuries of tongue
	injuries of tooth

Code also for any associated infection

Excludes2	burns and corrosions (T20-T32)
	effects of foreign body in ear (T16)
	effects of foreign body in larynx (T17.3)
	effects of foreign body in mouth NOS (T18.0)
	effects of foreign body in nose (T17.0-T17.1)
	effects of foreign body in pharynx (T17.2)
	effects of foreign body on external eye (T15.-)
	frostbite (T33-T34)
	insect bite or sting, venomous (T63.4)

● **S00   Superficial injury of head**

Excludes1	diffuse cerebral contusion (S06.2-)
	focal cerebral contusion (S06.3-)
	injury of eye and orbit (S05.-)
	open wound of head (S01.-)

The appropriate 7th character is to be added to each code from category S00

A	initial encounter
	All encounters involving diagnosis and treatment
D	subsequent encounter
	Encounters during the healing phase
S	sequela

● **S00.0   Superficial injury of scalp**

X● **S00.00   Unspecified superficial injury of scalp**

X● **S00.01   Abrasion of scalp**

X● **S00.02   Blister (nonthermal) of scalp**

X● **S00.03   Contusion of scalp**
            Bruise of scalp
            Hematoma of scalp

X● **S00.04   External constriction of part of scalp**

X● **S00.05   Superficial foreign body of scalp**
            Splinter in the scalp

X● **S00.06   Insect bite (nonvenomous) of scalp**

X● **S00.07   Other superficial bite of scalp**

            Excludes1   open bite of scalp (S01.05)

CHAPTER 19 (S00-T88)

- **S00.1** Contusion of eyelid and periocular area
  Black eye
  Excludes2   contusion of eyeball and orbital tissues (S05.1)
  - X **S00.10** Contusion of unspecified eyelid and periocular area
  - X **S00.11** Contusion of right eyelid and periocular area
  - X **S00.12** Contusion of left eyelid and periocular area
- **S00.2** Other and unspecified superficial injuries of eyelid and periocular area
  Excludes2   superficial injury of conjunctiva and cornea (S05.0-)
  - **S00.20** Unspecified superficial injury of eyelid and periocular area
    - **S00.201** Unspecified superficial injury of right eyelid and periocular area
    - **S00.202** Unspecified superficial injury of left eyelid and periocular area
    - **S00.209** Unspecified superficial injury of unspecified eyelid and periocular area
  - **S00.21** Abrasion of eyelid and periocular area
    - **S00.211** Abrasion of right eyelid and periocular area
    - **S00.212** Abrasion of left eyelid and periocular area
    - **S00.219** Abrasion of unspecified eyelid and periocular area
  - **S00.22** Blister (nonthermal) of eyelid and periocular area
    - **S00.221** Blister (nonthermal) of right eyelid and periocular area
    - **S00.222** Blister (nonthermal) of left eyelid and periocular area
    - **S00.229** Blister (nonthermal) of unspecified eyelid and periocular area
  - **S00.24** External constriction of eyelid and periocular area
    - **S00.241** External constriction of right eyelid and periocular area
    - **S00.242** External constriction of left eyelid and periocular area
    - **S00.249** External constriction of unspecified eyelid and periocular area
  - **S00.25** Superficial foreign body of eyelid and periocular area
    Splinter of eyelid and periocular area
    Excludes2   retained foreign body in eyelid (H02.81-)
    - **S00.251** Superficial foreign body of right eyelid and periocular area
    - **S00.252** Superficial foreign body of left eyelid and periocular area
    - **S00.259** Superficial foreign body of unspecified eyelid and periocular area
  - **S00.26** Insect bite (nonvenomous) of eyelid and periocular area
    - **S00.261** Insect bite (nonvenomous) of right eyelid and periocular area
    - **S00.262** Insect bite (nonvenomous) of left eyelid and periocular area
    - **S00.269** Insect bite (nonvenomous) of unspecified eyelid and periocular area

- **S00.27** Other superficial bite of eyelid and periocular area
  Excludes1   open bite of eyelid and periocular area (S01.15)
  - **S00.271** Other superficial bite of right eyelid and periocular area
  - **S00.272** Other superficial bite of left eyelid and periocular area
  - **S00.279** Other superficial bite of unspecified eyelid and periocular area
- **S00.3** Superficial injury of nose
  - X **S00.30** Unspecified superficial injury of nose
  - X **S00.31** Abrasion of nose
  - X **S00.32** Blister (nonthermal) of nose
  - X **S00.33** Contusion of nose
    Bruise of nose
    Hematoma of nose
  - X **S00.34** External constriction of nose
  - X **S00.35** Superficial foreign body of nose
    Splinter in the nose
  - X **S00.36** Insect bite (nonvenomous) of nose
  - X **S00.37** Other superficial bite of nose
    Excludes1   open bite of nose (S01.25)
- **S00.4** Superficial injury of ear
  - **S00.40** Unspecified superficial injury of ear
    - **S00.401** Unspecified superficial injury of right ear
    - **S00.402** Unspecified superficial injury of left ear
    - **S00.409** Unspecified superficial injury of unspecified ear
  - **S00.41** Abrasion of ear
    - **S00.411** Abrasion of right ear
    - **S00.412** Abrasion of left ear
    - **S00.419** Abrasion of unspecified ear
  - **S00.42** Blister (nonthermal) of ear
    - **S00.421** Blister (nonthermal) of right ear
    - **S00.422** Blister (nonthermal) of left ear
    - **S00.429** Blister (nonthermal) of unspecified ear
  - **S00.43** Contusion of ear
    Bruise of ear
    Hematoma of ear
    - **S00.431** Contusion of right ear
    - **S00.432** Contusion of left ear
    - **S00.439** Contusion of unspecified ear
  - **S00.44** External constriction of ear
    - **S00.441** External constriction of right ear
    - **S00.442** External constriction of left ear
    - **S00.449** External constriction of unspecified ear
  - **S00.45** Superficial foreign body of ear
    Splinter in the ear
    - **S00.451** Superficial foreign body of right ear
    - **S00.452** Superficial foreign body of left ear
    - **S00.459** Superficial foreign body of unspecified ear
  - **S00.46** Insect bite (nonvenomous) of ear
    - **S00.461** Insect bite (nonvenomous) of right ear
    - **S00.462** Insect bite (nonvenomous) of left ear
    - **S00.469** Insect bite (nonvenomous) of unspecified ear

▶ New   ⇒ Revised   ~~deleted~~ Deleted   Excludes 1   Excludes 2   Includes   Use additional   Code first   Code also   Key words
OGCR Official Guidelines   ● Unacceptable Principal Diagnosis   X Assign placeholder X   ● Use Additional Character(s)   ▌ Manifestation Code   **Coding Clinic**

● **S00.47   Other superficial bite of ear**
> **Excludes1**   open bite of ear (S01.35)
   ● S00.471   Other superficial bite of right ear
   ● S00.472   Other superficial bite of left ear
   ● S00.479   Other superficial bite of unspecified ear

● **S00.5   Superficial injury of lip and oral cavity**
  ● **S00.50   Unspecified superficial injury of lip and oral cavity**
   ● S00.501   Unspecified superficial injury of lip
   ● S00.502   Unspecified superficial injury of oral cavity
  ● **S00.51   Abrasion of lip and oral cavity**
   ● S00.511   Abrasion of lip
   ● S00.512   Abrasion of oral cavity
  ● **S00.52   Blister (nonthermal) of lip and oral cavity**
   ● S00.521   Blister (nonthermal) of lip
   ● S00.522   Blister (nonthermal) of oral cavity
  ● **S00.53   Contusion of lip and oral cavity**
   ● S00.531   Contusion of lip
       Bruise of lip
       ⟱ Hematoma of lip
   ● S00.532   Contusion of oral cavity
       ⟱ Bruise of oral cavity
       Hematoma of oral cavity
  ● **S00.54   External constriction of lip and oral cavity**
   ● S00.541   External constriction of lip
   ● S00.542   External constriction of oral cavity
  ● **S00.55   Superficial foreign body of lip and oral cavity**
   ● S00.551   Superficial foreign body of lip
       Splinter of lip and oral cavity
   ● S00.552   Superficial foreign body of oral cavity
       Splinter of lip and oral cavity
  ● **S00.56   Insect bite (nonvenomous) of lip and oral cavity**
   ● S00.561   Insect bite (nonvenomous) of lip
   ● S00.562   Insect bite (nonvenomous) of oral cavity
  ● **S00.57   Other superficial bite of lip and oral cavity**
   ● S00.571   Other superficial bite of lip
> **Excludes1**   open bite of lip (S01.551)
   ● S00.572   Other superficial bite of oral cavity
> **Excludes1**   open bite of oral cavity (S01.552)

● **S00.8   Superficial injury of other parts of head**
   Superficial injuries of face [any part]
  X ● **S00.80   Unspecified superficial injury of other part of head**
  X ● **S00.81   Abrasion of other part of head**
  X ● **S00.82   Blister (nonthermal) of other part of head**
  X ● **S00.83   Contusion of other part of head**
       Bruise of other part of head
       Hematoma of other part of head
  X ● **S00.84   External constriction of other part of head**
  X ● **S00.85   Superficial foreign body of other part of head**
       Splinter in other part of head
  X ● **S00.86   Insect bite (nonvenomous) of other part of head**
  X ● **S00.87   Other superficial bite of other part of head**
> **Excludes1**   open bite of other part of head (S01.85)

● **S00.9   Superficial injury of unspecified part of head**
  X ● **S00.90   Unspecified superficial injury of unspecified part of head**
  X ● **S00.91   Abrasion of unspecified part of head**
  X ● **S00.92   Blister (nonthermal) of unspecified part of head**
  X ● **S00.93   Contusion of unspecified part of head**
       Bruise of head
       Hematoma of head

X ● **S00.94   External constriction of unspecified part of head**
X ● **S00.95   Superficial foreign body of unspecified part of head**
       Splinter of head
X ● **S00.96   Insect bite (nonvenomous) of unspecified part of head**
X ● **S00.97   Other superficial bite of unspecified part of head**
> **Excludes1**   open bite of head (S01.95)

● **S01   Open wound of head**
   Code also any associated:
     injury of cranial nerve (S04.-)
     injury of muscle and tendon of head (S09.1-)
     intracranial injury (S06.-)
     wound infection
> **Excludes1**   open skull fracture (S02.- with 7th character B)
> **Excludes2**   injury of eye and orbit (S05.-)
>   traumatic amputation of part of head (S08.-)

The appropriate 7th character is to be added to each code from category S01

> | | |
> |---|---|
> | A | initial encounter |
> | D | subsequent encounter |
> | S | sequela |

● **S01.0   Open wound of scalp**
> **Excludes1**   avulsion of scalp (S08.0)
  X ● **S01.00   Unspecified open wound of scalp**
  X ● **S01.01   Laceration without foreign body of scalp**
  X ● **S01.02   Laceration with foreign body of scalp**
       Coding Clinic: 2015, Q1, P5-7
  X ● **S01.03   Puncture wound without foreign body of scalp**
  X ● **S01.04   Puncture wound with foreign body of scalp**
  X ● **S01.05   Open bite of scalp**
       Bite of scalp NOS
> **Excludes1**   superficial bite of scalp (S00.06, S00.07-)

● **S01.1   Open wound of eyelid and periocular area**
   Open wound of eyelid and periocular area with or without involvement of lacrimal passages
  ● **S01.10   Unspecified open wound of eyelid and periocular area**
       Ⓔ **For category S01.10 CC codes:** See PDX Collection 1139
   ● S01.101   Unspecified open wound of right eyelid and periocular area A 🅒
   ● S01.102   Unspecified open wound of left eyelid and periocular area A 🅒
   ● S01.109   Unspecified open wound of unspecified eyelid and periocular area A 🅒
  ● **S01.11   Laceration without foreign body of eyelid and periocular area**
   ● S01.111   Laceration without foreign body of right eyelid and periocular area
   ● S01.112   Laceration without foreign body of left eyelid and periocular area
   ● S01.119   Laceration without foreign body of unspecified eyelid and periocular area
  ● **S01.12   Laceration with foreign body of eyelid and periocular area**
   ● S01.121   Laceration with foreign body of right eyelid and periocular area
   ● S01.122   Laceration with foreign body of left eyelid and periocular area
   ● S01.129   Laceration with foreign body of unspecified eyelid and periocular area

N Newborn Age: 0   **P** Pediatric Age: 0–17   **M** Maternity DX: 12–55   **A** Adult Age: 15–124   ♀ Females Only   ♂ Males Only

🅒 Complication\Comorbidity   Ⓜ Major C\C   Ⓔ CC/MCC Exclusions   🅗 Hospital-Acquired Condition

1225

● S01.13   Puncture wound without foreign body of eyelid and periocular area
   ● S01.131   Puncture wound without foreign body of right eyelid and periocular area
   ● S01.132   Puncture wound without foreign body of left eyelid and periocular area
   ● S01.139   Puncture wound without foreign body of unspecified eyelid and periocular area

● S01.14   Puncture wound with foreign body of eyelid and periocular area
   ● S01.141   Puncture wound with foreign body of right eyelid and periocular area
   ● S01.142   Puncture wound with foreign body of left eyelid and periocular area
   ● S01.149   Puncture wound with foreign body of unspecified eyelid and periocular area

● S01.15   Open bite of eyelid and periocular area
    Bite of eyelid and periocular area NOS
    Excludes1   superficial bite of eyelid and periocular area (S00.26, S00.27)
   ● S01.151   Open bite of right eyelid and periocular area
   ● S01.152   Open bite of left eyelid and periocular area
   ● S01.159   Open bite of unspecified eyelid and periocular area

● S01.2   Open wound of nose
  X ● S01.20   Unspecified open wound of nose
  X ● S01.21   Laceration without foreign body of nose
    Coding Clinic: 2015, Q1, P5-6
  X ● S01.22   Laceration with foreign body of nose
  X ● S01.23   Puncture wound without foreign body of nose
  X ● S01.24   Puncture wound with foreign body of nose
  X ● S01.25   Open bite of nose
    Bite of nose NOS
    Excludes1   superficial bite of nose (S00.36, S00.37)

● S01.3   Open wound of ear
   ● S01.30   Unspecified open wound of ear
    ● S01.301   Unspecified open wound of right ear
    ● S01.302   Unspecified open wound of left ear
    ● S01.309   Unspecified open wound of unspecified ear
   ● S01.31   Laceration without foreign body of ear
    ● S01.311   Laceration without foreign body of right ear
    ● S01.312   Laceration without foreign body of left ear
    ● S01.319   Laceration without foreign body of unspecified ear
   ● S01.32   Laceration with foreign body of ear
    ● S01.321   Laceration with foreign body of right ear
    ● S01.322   Laceration with foreign body of left ear
    ● S01.329   Laceration with foreign body of unspecified ear

● S01.33   Puncture wound without foreign body of ear
   ● S01.331   Puncture wound without foreign body of right ear
   ● S01.332   Puncture wound without foreign body of left ear
   ● S01.339   Puncture wound without foreign body of unspecified ear

● S01.34   Puncture wound with foreign body of ear
   ● S01.341   Puncture wound with foreign body of right ear
   ● S01.342   Puncture wound with foreign body of left ear
   ● S01.349   Puncture wound with foreign body of unspecified ear

● S01.35   Open bite of ear
    Bite of ear NOS
    Excludes1   superficial bite of ear (S00.46, S00.47)
   ● S01.351   Open bite of right ear
   ● S01.352   Open bite of left ear
   ● S01.359   Open bite of unspecified ear

● S01.4   Open wound of cheek and temporomandibular area
   ● S01.40   Unspecified open wound of cheek and temporomandibular area
    ● S01.401   Unspecified open wound of right cheek and temporomandibular area
    ● S01.402   Unspecified open wound of left cheek and temporomandibular area
    ● S01.409   Unspecified open wound of unspecified cheek and temporomandibular area
   ● S01.41   Laceration without foreign body of cheek and temporomandibular area
    ● S01.411   Laceration without foreign body of right cheek and temporomandibular area
     Coding Clinic: 2015, Q1, P5-7
    ● S01.412   Laceration without foreign body of left cheek and temporomandibular area
    ● S01.419   Laceration without foreign body of unspecified cheek and temporomandibular area
   ● S01.42   Laceration with foreign body of cheek and temporomandibular area
    ● S01.421   Laceration with foreign body of right cheek and temporomandibular area
    ● S01.422   Laceration with foreign body of left cheek and temporomandibular area
    ● S01.429   Laceration with foreign body of unspecified cheek and temporomandibular area
   ● S01.43   Puncture wound without foreign body of cheek and temporomandibular area
    ● S01.431   Puncture wound without foreign body of right cheek and temporomandibular area
    ● S01.432   Puncture wound without foreign body of left cheek and temporomandibular area
    ● S01.439   Puncture wound without foreign body of unspecified cheek and temporomandibular area

▶ New   ⇒ Revised   ~~deleted~~ Deleted   Excludes 1   Excludes 2   Includes   Use additional   Code first   Code also   Key words
OGCR Official Guidelines   ● Unacceptable Principal Diagnosis   X Assign placeholder X   ● Use Additional Character(s)   ▍ Manifestation Code   Coding Clinic

● **S01.44** Puncture wound with foreign body of cheek and temporomandibular area
   ● **S01.441** Puncture wound with foreign body of right cheek and temporomandibular area
   ● **S01.442** Puncture wound with foreign body of left cheek and temporomandibular area
   ● **S01.449** Puncture wound with foreign body of unspecified cheek and temporomandibular area

● **S01.45** Open bite of cheek and temporomandibular area
   Bite of cheek and temporomandibular area NOS
   Excludes2 superficial bite of cheek and temporomandibular area (S00.86, S00.87)
   ● **S01.451** Open bite of right cheek and temporomandibular area
   ● **S01.452** Open bite of left cheek and temporomandibular area
   ● **S01.459** Open bite of unspecified cheek and temporomandibular area

● **S01.5** Open wound of lip and oral cavity
   Excludes2 tooth dislocation (S03.2)
   tooth fracture (S02.5)

  ● **S01.50** Unspecified open wound of lip and oral cavity
   ● **S01.501** Unspecified open wound of lip
   ● **S01.502** Unspecified open wound of oral cavity

  ● **S01.51** Laceration of lip and oral cavity without foreign body
   ● **S01.511** Laceration without foreign body of lip
   ● **S01.512** Laceration without foreign body of oral cavity

  ● **S01.52** Laceration of lip and oral cavity with foreign body
   ● **S01.521** Laceration with foreign body of lip
   ● **S01.522** Laceration with foreign body of oral cavity

  ● **S01.53** Puncture wound of lip and oral cavity without foreign body
   ● **S01.531** Puncture wound without foreign body of lip
   ● **S01.532** Puncture wound without foreign body of oral cavity

  ● **S01.54** Puncture wound of lip and oral cavity with foreign body
   ● **S01.541** Puncture wound with foreign body of lip
   ● **S01.542** Puncture wound with foreign body of oral cavity

  ● **S01.55** Open bite of lip and oral cavity
   ● **S01.551** Open bite of lip
    Bite of lip NOS
    Excludes1 superficial bite of lip (S00.571)
   ● **S01.552** Open bite of oral cavity
    Bite of oral cavity NOS
    Excludes1 superficial bite of oral cavity (S00.572)

● **S01.8** Open wound of other parts of head
  X ● **S01.80** Unspecified open wound of other part of head
  X ● **S01.81** Laceration without foreign body of other part of head
  X ● **S01.82** Laceration with foreign body of other part of head
  X ● **S01.83** Puncture wound without foreign body of other part of head
  X ● **S01.84** Puncture wound with foreign body of other part of head
  X ● **S01.85** Open bite of other part of head
   Bite of other part of head NOS
   ➡ **Excludes1** superficial bite of other part of head (S00.87)

● **S01.9** Open wound of unspecified part of head
  X ● **S01.90** Unspecified open wound of unspecified part of head
  X ● **S01.91** Laceration without foreign body of unspecified part of head
  X ● **S01.92** Laceration with foreign body of unspecified part of head
  X ● **S01.93** Puncture wound without foreign body of unspecified part of head
  X ● **S01.94** Puncture wound with foreign body of unspecified part of head
  X ● **S01.95** Open bite of unspecified part of head
   Bite of head NOS
   Excludes1 superficial bite of head NOS (S00.97)

● **S02** Fracture of skull and facial bones
  Note: A fracture not indicated as open or closed should be coded to closed
  The appropriate 7th character is to be added to each code from category S02

A	initial encounter for closed fracture
B	initial encounter for open fracture
D	subsequent encounter for fracture with routine healing
G	subsequent encounter for fracture with delayed healing
K	subsequent encounter for fracture with nonunion
S	sequela

  Code also any associated intracranial injury (S06.-)

X ● **S02.0** Fracture of vault of skull A, K 🦠, B 🦠, A, B 🦠
  Fracture of frontal bone
  Fracture of parietal bone
  (Ex) For category S02.0 CC codes S02.0[A,B]: See PDX Collection 1140
  For S02.0[K]: See PDX Collection 897

● **S02.1** Fracture of base of skull
  Excludes1 orbit NOS (S02.8)
  Excludes2 orbital floor (S02.3-)
  (Ex) For category S02.1 CC codes: For S02.1[A,B] CC codes: See PDX Collection 1140 For S02.1[K] CC codes: See PDX Collection 897
  Coding Clinic: 2016, Q4, P66
  ● **S02.10** Unspecified fracture of base of skull
   ● **S02.101** Fracture of base of skull, right side A, K 🦠, B 🦠, A, B 🦠
   ● **S02.102** Fracture of base of skull, left side A, K 🦠, B 🦠, A, B 🦠
   ● **S02.109** Fracture of base of skull, unspecified side A, K 🦠, B 🦠, A, B 🦠

N Newborn Age: 0   **P** Pediatric Age: 0–17   **M** Maternity DX: 12–55   **A** Adult Age: 15–124   ♀ Females Only   ♂ Males Only

🦠 Complication\Comorbidity   🦠 Major C\C   (Ex) CC/MCC Exclusions   🦠 Hospital-Acquired Condition

1227

● **S02.11**   Fracture of occiput

    ● **S02.110**   Type I occipital condyle fracture, unspecified side A, K , B , A, B

    ● **S02.111**   Type II occipital condyle fracture, unspecified side A, K , B , A, B

    ● **S02.112**   Type III occipital condyle fracture, unspecified side A, K , B , A, B

    ● **S02.113**   Unspecified occipital condyle fracture A, K , B , A, B

    ● **S02.118**   Other fracture of occiput, unspecified side A, K , B , A, B

    ● **S02.119**   Unspecified fracture of occiput A, K , B , A, B

    ● **S02.11A**   Type I occipital condyle fracture, right side A, K , B , A, B

    ● **S02.11B**   Type I occipital condyle fracture, left side A, K , B , A, B

    ● **S02.11C**   Type II occipital condyle fracture, right side A, K , B , A, B

    ● **S02.11D**   Type II occipital condyle fracture, left side A, K , B , A, B

    ● **S02.11E**   Type III occipital condyle fracture, right side A, K , B , A, B

    ● **S02.11F**   Type III occipital condyle fracture, left side A, K , B , A, B

    ● **S02.11G**   Other fracture of occiput, right side A, K , B , A, B

    ● **S02.11H**   Other fracture of occiput, left side A, K , B , A, B

X ● **S02.19**   Other fracture of base of skull A, K , B , A, B

        Fracture of anterior fossa of base of skull
        Fracture of ethmoid sinus
        Fracture of frontal sinus
        Fracture of middle fossa of base of skull
        Fracture of orbital roof
        Fracture of posterior fossa of base of skull
        Fracture of sphenoid
        Fracture of temporal bone

X ● **S02.2**   Fracture of nasal bones B, K , B

       (Ex:) For category S02.2 CC codes S02.2[B]: See PDX Collection 1141
          For S02.2[K]: See PDX Collection 897

● **S02.3**   Fracture of orbital floor

      Excludes1   orbit NOS (S02.8)
      Excludes2   orbital roof (S02.1-)

       (Ex:) For category S02.3 CC codes S02.3[A,B]: See PDX Collection 1142
          For S02.3[K]: See PDX Collection 897
       Coding Clinic: 2016, Q4, P66

X ● **S02.30**   Fracture of orbital floor, unspecified side A, B, K , A, B

X ● **S02.31**   Fracture of orbital floor, right side A, B, K , A, B

X ● **S02.32**   Fracture of orbital floor, left side A, B, K , A, B

● **S02.4**   Fracture of malar, maxillary and zygoma bones

        Fracture of superior maxilla
        Fracture of upper jaw (bone)
        Fracture of zygomatic process of temporal bone

       (Ex:) For category S02.4 CC codes S02.4[A,B] unless otherwise indicated:
          See PDX Collection 1143 For S02.4[K]: See PDX Collection 897
       Coding Clinic: 2016, Q4, P66

    ● **S02.40**   Fracture of malar, maxillary and zygoma bones, unspecified

      ● **S02.400**   Malar fracture unspecified side A, B, K , A, B

      ● **S02.401**   Maxillary fracture, unspecified side A, B, K , A, B

      ● **S02.402**   Zygomatic fracture, unspecified side A, B, K , A, B

      ● **S02.40A**   Malar fracture, right side A, B, K , A, B

      ● **S02.40B**   Malar fracture, left side A, B, K , A, B

      ● **S02.40C**   Maxillary fracture, right side A, B, K , A, B

      ● **S02.40D**   Maxillary fracture, left side A, B, K , A, B

      ● **S02.40E**   Zygomatic fracture, right side A, B, K , A, B

      ● **S02.40F**   Zygomatic fracture, left side A, B, K , A, B

    ● **S02.41**   LeFort fracture

      ● **S02.411**   LeFort I fracture A, B, K , A, B

      ● **S02.412**   LeFort II fracture A, B, K , A, B

      ● **S02.413**   LeFort III fracture A, B, K , A, B

X ● **S02.42**   Fracture of alveolus of maxilla A, B, K , A, B

       (Ex:) For S02.42[A,B]: See PDX Collection 1142 For S02.42[K]: See PDX Collection 897

X ● **S02.5**   Fracture of tooth (traumatic) Broken tooth K

      Excludes1   cracked tooth (nontraumatic) (K03.81)
       (Ex:) See PDX Collection 897

● **S02.6**   Fracture of mandible

        Fracture of lower jaw (bone)

       (Ex:) For category S02.6 CC codes S02.6[A,B]: See PDX Collection 1143
          For S02.6[K]: See PDX Collection 897
       Coding Clinic: 2016, Q4, P66

    ● **S02.60**   Fracture of mandible of unspecified site

      ● **S02.600**   Fracture of unspecified part of body of mandible, unspecified side A, B, K , A, B

      ● **S02.601**   Fracture of unspecified part of body of right mandible A, B, K , A, B

      ● **S02.602**   Fracture of unspecified part of body of left mandible A, B, K , A, B

      ● **S02.609**   Fracture of mandible, unspecified A, B, K , A, B

    ● **S02.61**   Fracture of condylar process of mandible

      ● **S02.610**   Fracture of condylar process of mandible, unspecified side A, B, K , A, B

      ● **S02.611**   Fracture of condylar process of right mandible A, B, K , A, B

      ● **S02.612**   Fracture of condylar process of left mandible A, B, K , A, B

    ● **S02.62**   Fracture of subcondylar process of mandible

      ● **S02.620**   Fracture of subcondylar process of mandible, unspecified side A, B, K , A, B

      ● **S02.621**   Fracture of subcondylar process of right mandible A, B, K , A, B

      ● **S02.622**   Fracture of subcondylar process of left mandible A, B, K , A, B

    ● **S02.63**   Fracture of coronoid process of mandible

      ● **S02.630**   Fracture of coronoid process of mandible, unspecified side A, B, K , A, B

      ● **S02.631**   Fracture of coronoid process of right mandible A, B, K , A, B

      ● **S02.632**   Fracture of coronoid process of left mandible A, B, K , A, B

    ● **S02.64**   Fracture of ramus of mandible

      ● **S02.640**   Fracture of ramus of mandible, unspecified side A, B, K , A, B

      ● **S02.641**   Fracture of ramus of right mandible A, B, K , A, B

      ● **S02.642**   Fracture of ramus of left mandible A, B, K , A, B

▶ New   ⟹ Revised   ~~deleted~~ Deleted   Excludes 1   Excludes 2   Includes   Use additional   Code first   Code also   Key words

OGCR Official Guidelines   ● Unacceptable Principal Diagnosis   X Assign placeholder X   ● Use Additional Character(s)   ▶ Manifestation Code   **Coding Clinic**

1228

● **S02.65**　Fracture of angle of mandible

   ● **S02.650**　Fracture of angle of mandible, unspecified side A, B, K 🔵, A, B 🔵

   ● **S02.651**　Fracture of angle of right mandible A, B, K 🔵, A, B 🔵

   ● **S02.652**　Fracture of angle of left mandible A, B, K 🔵, A, B 🔵

X ● **S02.66**　Fracture of symphysis of mandible A, B, K 🔵, A, B 🔵

● **S02.67**　Fracture of alveolus of mandible

   ● **S02.670**　Fracture of alveolus of mandible, unspecified side A, B, K 🔵, A, B 🔵

   ● **S02.671**　Fracture of alveolus of right mandible A, B, K 🔵, A, B 🔵

   ● **S02.672**　Fracture of alveolus of left mandible A, B, K 🔵, A, B 🔵

X ● **S02.69**　Fracture of mandible of other specified site A, B, K 🔵, A, B 🔵

● **S02.8**　Fractures of other specified skull and facial bones

   Fracture of orbit NOS
   Fracture of palate

   Excludes1　fracture of orbital floor (S02.3-)
           fracture of orbital roof (S02.1-)

   (Ex) For category S02.8 CC codes S02.8[A,B]: See PDX Collection 1142
   For S02.8[K]: See PDX Collection 897

   Coding Clinic: 2016, Q4, P66

X ● **S02.80**　Fracture of other specified skull and facial bones, unspecified side A, B, K 🔵, A, B 🔵

X ● **S02.81**　Fracture of other specified skull and facial bones, right side A, B, K 🔵, A, B 🔵

X ● **S02.82**　Fracture of other specified skull and facial bones, left side A, B, K 🔵, A, B 🔵

● **S02.9**　Fracture of unspecified skull and facial bones

X ● **S02.91**　Unspecified fracture of skull A, K 🔵, B 🔵, A, B 🔵

   (Ex) For category S02.91 CC codes S02.91[A,B]: See PDX Collection 1140 For S02.91[K]: See PDX Collection 897

X ● **S02.92**　Unspecified fracture of facial bones A, B, K 🔵, A, B 🔵

   (Ex) For category S02.92 CC codes S02.92[A,B]: See PDX Collection 1142 For S02.92[K]: See PDX Collection 897

● **S03**　Dislocation and sprain of joints and ligaments of head

   Includes　avulsion of joint (capsule) or ligament of head
          laceration of cartilage, joint (capsule) or ligament of head
          sprain of cartilage, joint (capsule) or ligament of head
          traumatic hemarthrosis of joint or ligament of head
          traumatic rupture of joint or ligament of head
          traumatic subluxation of joint or ligament of head
          traumatic tear of joint or ligament of head

   Code also any associated open wound

   Excludes2　Strain of muscle or tendon of head (S09.1)

   The appropriate 7th character is to be added to each code from category S03

A	initial encounter
D	subsequent encounter
S	sequela

● **S03.0**　Dislocation of jaw

   Dislocation of jaw (cartilage) (meniscus)
   Dislocation of mandible
   Dislocation of temporomandibular (joint)
   Coding Clinic: 2016, Q4, P67

X ● **S03.00**　Dislocation of jaw, unspecified side

X ● **S03.01**　Dislocation of jaw, right side

X ● **S03.02**　Dislocation of jaw, left side

X ● **S03.03**　Dislocation of jaw, bilateral side

X ● **S03.1**　Dislocation of septal cartilage of nose

X ● **S03.2**　Dislocation of tooth

X ● **S03.4**　Sprain of jaw

   Sprain of temporomandibular (joint) (ligament)
   Coding Clinic: 2016, Q4, P67

X ● **S03.40**　Sprain of jaw, unspecified side

X ● **S03.41**　Sprain of jaw, right side

X ● **S03.42**　Sprain of jaw, left side

X ● **S03.43**　Sprain of jaw, bilateral side

X ● **S03.8**　Sprain of joints and ligaments of other parts of head

X ● **S03.9**　Sprain of joints and ligaments of unspecified parts of head

● **S04**　Injury of cranial nerve

   The selection of side should be based on the side of the body being affected

   Code first any associated intracranial injury (S06.-)

   Code also any associated:
     open wound of head (S01.-)
     skull fracture (S02.-)

   The appropriate 7th character is to be added to each code from category S04

A	initial encounter
D	subsequent encounter
S	sequela

● **S04.0**　Injury of optic nerve and pathways

   ➡ Use additional code to identify any visual field defect or blindness (H53.4-, H54.-)
   (Ex) For category S04.0 CC codes: See PDX Collection 1144

   ● **S04.01**　Injury of optic nerve
     Injury of 2nd cranial nerve

     ● **S04.011**　Injury of optic nerve, right eye A 🔵

     ● **S04.012**　Injury of optic nerve, left eye A 🔵

     ● **S04.019**　Injury of optic nerve, unspecified eye A 🔵
        Injury of optic nerve NOS

   X ● **S04.02**　Injury of optic chiasm A 🔵

   ● **S04.03**　Injury of optic tract and pathways
     Injury of optic radiation

     ➡● **S04.031**　Injury of optic tract and pathways, right side A 🔵

     ➡● **S04.032**　Injury of optic tract and pathways, left side A 🔵

     ➡● **S04.039**　Injury of optic tract and pathways, unspecified side A 🔵
        Injury of optic tract and pathways NOS

   ● **S04.04**　Injury of visual cortex

     ➡● **S04.041**　Injury of visual cortex, right side A 🔵

     ➡● **S04.042**　Injury of visual cortex, left side A 🔵

     ➡● **S04.049**　Injury of visual cortex, unspecified side A 🔵
        Injury of visual cortex NOS

● **S04.1**　Injury of oculomotor nerve
   Injury of 3rd cranial nerve
   (Ex) For category S04.1 CC codes: See PDX Collection 1145

   X ● **S04.10**　Injury of oculomotor nerve, unspecified side A 🔵

   X ● **S04.11**　Injury of oculomotor nerve, right side A 🔵

   X ● **S04.12**　Injury of oculomotor nerve, left side A 🔵

● **S04.2**　Injury of trochlear nerve
   Injury of 4th cranial nerve
   (Ex) For category S04.2 CC codes: See PDX Collection 1146

   X ● **S04.20**　Injury of trochlear nerve, unspecified side A 🔵

   X ● **S04.21**　Injury of trochlear nerve, right side A 🔵

   X ● **S04.22**　Injury of trochlear nerve, left side A 🔵

CHAPTER 19 (S00-T88)

Figure 19-13 Cranial nerves. (From Patton and Thibodeau: Anatomy and physiology, ed 7, St. Louis, Mosby, 2009)

Trochlear nerve (IV)
Optic nerve (II)
Olfactory nerve (I)
Abducens nerve (VI)
Oculomotor nerve (III)
Facial nerve (VII)
Trigeminal nerve (V)
Vestibulocochlear nerve (VIII)
Glossopharyngeal nerve (IX)
Vagus nerve (X)
Accessory nerve (XI)
Hypoglossal nerve (XII)

● **S04.3   Injury of trigeminal nerve**
      Injury of 5th cranial nerve
      Ⓔⓧ **For category S04.3 CC codes:** See PDX Collection 1147

   X● **S04.30   Injury of trigeminal nerve, unspecified side** A 🔊
   X● **S04.31   Injury of trigeminal nerve, right side** A 🔊
   X● **S04.32   Injury of trigeminal nerve, left side** A 🔊

● **S04.4   Injury of abducent nerve**
      Injury of 6th cranial nerve
      Ⓔⓧ **For category S04.4 CC codes:** See PDX Collection 1148

   X● **S04.40   Injury of abducent nerve, unspecified side** A 🔊
   X● **S04.41   Injury of abducent nerve, right side** A 🔊
   X● **S04.42   Injury of abducent nerve, left side** A 🔊

● **S04.5   Injury of facial nerve**
      Injury of 7th cranial nerve
      Ⓔⓧ **For category S04.5 CC codes:** See PDX Collection 1149

   X● **S04.50   Injury of facial nerve, unspecified side** A 🔊
   X● **S04.51   Injury of facial nerve, right side** A 🔊
   X● **S04.52   Injury of facial nerve, left side** A 🔊

● **S04.6   Injury of acoustic nerve**
      Injury of auditory nerve
      Injury of 8th cranial nerve
      Ⓔⓧ **For category S04.6 CC codes:** See PDX Collection 1150

   X● **S04.60   Injury of acoustic nerve, unspecified side** A 🔊
   X● **S04.61   Injury of acoustic nerve, right side** A 🔊
   X● **S04.62   Injury of acoustic nerve, left side** A 🔊

● **S04.7   Injury of accessory nerve**
      Injury of 11th cranial nerve
      Ⓔⓧ **For category S04.7 CC codes:** See PDX Collection 1151

   X● **S04.70   Injury of accessory nerve, unspecified side** A 🔊
   X● **S04.71   Injury of accessory nerve, right side** A 🔊
   X● **S04.72   Injury of accessory nerve, left side** A 🔊

● **S04.8   Injury of other cranial nerves**
      Ⓔⓧ **For category S04.8 CC codes:** See PDX Collection 1152

   ● **S04.81   Injury of olfactory [1st] nerve**
      ● **S04.811   Injury of olfactory [1st] nerve, right side** A 🔊
      ● **S04.812   Injury of olfactory [1st] nerve, left side** A 🔊
      ● **S04.819   Injury of olfactory [1st] nerve, unspecified side** A 🔊

   ● **S04.89   Injury of other cranial nerves**
      Injury of vagus [10th] nerve
      ● **S04.891   Injury of other cranial nerves, right side** A 🔊
      ● **S04.892   Injury of other cranial nerves, left side** A 🔊
      ● **S04.899   Injury of other cranial nerves, unspecified side** A 🔊

   X● **S04.9   Injury of unspecified cranial nerve** A 🔊
      Ⓔⓧ See PDX Collection 1152

▶ New   ⇒ Revised   ~~deleted~~ Deleted   Excludes 1   Excludes 2   Includes   Use additional   Code first   Code also   Key words
OGCR Official Guidelines   ● Unacceptable Principal Diagnosis   X Assign placeholder X   ● Use Additional Character(s)   ▸ Manifestation Code   **Coding Clinic**

● **S05   Injury of eye and orbit**

Includes   open wound of eye and orbit

Excludes2   2nd cranial [optic] nerve injury (S04.0-)
3rd cranial [oculomotor] nerve injury (S04.1-)
open wound of eyelid and periocular area (S01.1-)
orbital bone fracture (S02.1-, S02.3-, S02.8-)
superficial injury of eyelid (S00.1-S00.2)

The appropriate 7th character is to be added to each code from category S05

A	initial encounter
D	subsequent encounter
S	sequela

● **S05.0   Injury of conjunctiva and corneal abrasion without foreign body**

Excludes1   foreign body in conjunctival sac (T15.1)
foreign body in cornea (T15.0)

(Ex) **For category S05 CC codes unless otherwise indicated:** See PDX Collection 1139

X● **S05.00   Injury of conjunctiva and corneal abrasion without foreign body, unspecified eye**

X● **S05.01   Injury of conjunctiva and corneal abrasion without foreign body, right eye**

X● **S05.02   Injury of conjunctiva and corneal abrasion without foreign body, left eye**

● **S05.1   Contusion of eyeball and orbital tissues**
Traumatic hyphema

Excludes2   black eye NOS (S00.1)
contusion of eyelid and periocular area (S00.1)

X● **S05.10   Contusion of eyeball and orbital tissues, unspecified eye**

X● **S05.11   Contusion of eyeball and orbital tissues, right eye**

X● **S05.12   Contusion of eyeball and orbital tissues, left eye**

● **S05.2   Ocular laceration and rupture with prolapse or loss of intraocular tissue**

X● **S05.20   Ocular laceration and rupture with prolapse or loss of intraocular tissue, unspecified eye** A 🕭

X● **S05.21   Ocular laceration and rupture with prolapse or loss of intraocular tissue, right eye** A 🕭

X● **S05.22   Ocular laceration and rupture with prolapse or loss of intraocular tissue, left eye** A 🕭

● **S05.3   Ocular laceration without prolapse or loss of intraocular tissue**
Laceration of eye NOS

X● **S05.30   Ocular laceration without prolapse or loss of intraocular tissue, unspecified eye** A 🕭

X● **S05.31   Ocular laceration without prolapse or loss of intraocular tissue, right eye** A 🕭

X● **S05.32   Ocular laceration without prolapse or loss of intraocular tissue, left eye** A 🕭

● **S05.4   Penetrating wound of orbit with or without foreign body**

Excludes2   retained (old) foreign body following penetrating wound in orbit (H05.5-)

X● **S05.40   Penetrating wound of orbit with or without foreign body, unspecified eye** A 🕭

X● **S05.41   Penetrating wound of orbit with or without foreign body, right eye** A 🕭

X● **S05.42   Penetrating wound of orbit with or without foreign body, left eye** A 🕭

● **S05.5   Penetrating wound with foreign body of eyeball**

Excludes2   retained (old) intraocular foreign body (H44.6-, H44.7)

(Ex) **For category S05.5 CC codes:** See PDX Collection 1153

X● **S05.50   Penetrating wound with foreign body of unspecified eyeball** A 🕭

X● **S05.51   Penetrating wound with foreign body of right eyeball** A 🕭

X● **S05.52   Penetrating wound with foreign body of left eyeball** A 🕭

● **S05.6   Penetrating wound without foreign body of eyeball**
Ocular penetration NOS

X● **S05.60   Penetrating wound without foreign body of unspecified eyeball**

X● **S05.61   Penetrating wound without foreign body of right eyeball**

X● **S05.62   Penetrating wound without foreign body of left eyeball**

● **S05.7   Avulsion of eye**
Traumatic enucleation

X● **S05.70   Avulsion of unspecified eye** A 🕭

X● **S05.71   Avulsion of right eye** A 🕭

X● **S05.72   Avulsion of left eye** A 🕭

● **S05.8   Other injuries of eye and orbit**
Lacrimal duct injury

● **S05.8X   Other injuries of eye and orbit**

● **S05.8X1   Other injuries of right eye and orbit** A 🕭

● **S05.8X2   Other injuries of left eye and orbit** A 🕭

● **S05.8X9   Other injuries of unspecified eye and orbit** A 🕭

● **S05.9   Unspecified injury of eye and orbit**
Injury of eye NOS

X● **S05.90   Unspecified injury of unspecified eye and orbit**

X● **S05.91   Unspecified injury of right eye and orbit** A 🕭

X● **S05.92   Unspecified injury of left eye and orbit** A 🕭

● **S06   Intracranial injury**

Includes   traumatic brain injury

Code also any associated:
open wound of head (S01.-)
skull fracture (S02.-)

Excludes1   head injury NOS (S09.90)

The appropriate 7th character is to be added to each code from category S06

A	initial encounter
D	subsequent encounter
S	sequela

▶**Note:** 7th characters D and S do not apply to codes in category S06 with 6th character 7 - death due to brain injury prior to regaining consciousness, or 8 - death due to other cause prior to regaining consciousness.

(Ex) **For category S06 CC codes unless otherwise indicated:** See PDX Collection 1154

Coding Clinic: 2015, Q4, P40

● **S06.0   Concussion**
Commotio cerebri

Excludes1   concussion with other intracranial injuries classified in subcategories S06.1- to S06.6- , S06.81- and S06.82- code to specified intracranial injury

Coding Clinic: 2016, Q4, P67

● **S06.0X   Concussion**

● **S06.0X0   Concussion without loss of consciousness**

● **S06.0X1   Concussion with loss of consciousness of 30 minutes or less** A 🕭, A 🕭

● **S06.0X9   Concussion with loss of consciousness of unspecified duration** A 🕭, A 🕭
Concussion NOS
Coding Clinic: 2016, Q4, P68

N Newborn Age: 0   **P** Pediatric Age: 0–17   **M** Maternity DX: 12–55   **A** Adult Age: 15–124   ♀ Females Only   ♂ Males Only

🕭 Complication\Comorbidity   🕭 Major C\C   (Ex) CC/MCC Exclusions   🕭 Hospital-Acquired Condition

1231

● **S06.1 Traumatic cerebral edema**
Diffuse traumatic cerebral edema
Focal traumatic cerebral edema
Coding Clinic: 2016, Q4, P67

  ● **S06.1X Traumatic cerebral edema**

    ● **S06.1X0 Traumatic cerebral edema without loss of consciousness** A 🔹
MCC when PDx is its own MCC
(Ex:) See PDX Collection 612
Coding Clinic: 2015, Q1, P12

    ● **S06.1X1 Traumatic cerebral edema with loss of consciousness of 30 minutes or less** A 🔹, A 🔹
MCC when PDx is its own MCC
(Ex:) See PDX Collection 1155

    ● **S06.1X2 Traumatic cerebral edema with loss of consciousness of 31 minutes to 59 minutes** A 🔹, A 🔹
MCC when PDx is its own MCC
(Ex:) See PDX Collection 1155

    ● **S06.1X3 Traumatic cerebral edema with loss of consciousness of 1 hour to 5 hours 59 minutes** A 🔹, A 🔹
MCC when PDx is its own MCC
(Ex:) See PDX Collection 1155

    ● **S06.1X4 Traumatic cerebral edema with loss of consciousness of 6 hours to 24 hours** A 🔹, A 🔹
MCC when PDx is its own MCC
(Ex:) See PDX Collection 1155

    ● **S06.1X5 Traumatic cerebral edema with loss of consciousness greater than 24 hours with return to pre-existing conscious level** A 🔹, A 🔹
MCC when PDx is its own MCC
(Ex:) See PDX Collection 1155

    ● **S06.1X6 Traumatic cerebral edema with loss of consciousness greater than 24 hours without return to pre-existing conscious level with patient surviving** A 🔹, A 🔹
MCC when PDx is its own MCC

    ● **S06.1X7 Traumatic cerebral edema with loss of consciousness of any duration with death due to brain injury prior to regaining consciousness** A 🔹, A 🔹
MCC when PDx is its own MCC

    ● **S06.1X8 Traumatic cerebral edema with loss of consciousness of any duration with death due to other cause prior to regaining consciousness** A 🔹, A 🔹
MCC when PDx is its own MCC

    ● **S06.1X9 Traumatic cerebral edema with loss of consciousness of unspecified duration** A 🔹, A 🔹
Traumatic cerebral edema NOS
MCC when PDx is its own MCC
(Ex:) See PDX Collection 1155

● **S06.2 Diffuse traumatic brain injury**
Diffuse axonal brain injury
Excludes1   traumatic diffuse cerebral edema (S06.1X-)

  ● **S06.2X Diffuse traumatic brain injury**

    ● **S06.2X0 Diffuse traumatic brain injury without loss of consciousness**

    ● **S06.2X1 Diffuse traumatic brain injury with loss of consciousness of 30 minutes or less** A 🔹, A 🔹

    ● **S06.2X2 Diffuse traumatic brain injury with loss of consciousness of 31 minutes to 59 minutes** A 🔹, A 🔹

    ● **S06.2X3 Diffuse traumatic brain injury with loss of consciousness of 1 hour to 5 hours 59 minutes** A 🔹, A 🔹

    ● **S06.2X4 Diffuse traumatic brain injury with loss of consciousness of 6 hours to 24 hours** A 🔹, A 🔹

    ● **S06.2X5 Diffuse traumatic brain injury with loss of consciousness greater than 24 hours with return to pre-existing conscious levels** A 🔹, A 🔹

    ● **S06.2X6 Diffuse traumatic brain injury with loss of consciousness greater than 24 hours without return to pre-existing conscious level with patient surviving** A 🔹, A 🔹

    ● **S06.2X7 Diffuse traumatic brain injury with loss of consciousness of any duration with death due to brain injury prior to regaining consciousness** A 🔹, A 🔹

    ● **S06.2X8 Diffuse traumatic brain injury with loss of consciousness of any duration with death due to other cause prior to regaining consciousness** A 🔹, A 🔹

    ● **S06.2X9 Diffuse traumatic brain injury with loss of consciousness of unspecified duration** A 🔹, A 🔹
Diffuse traumatic brain injury NOS

● **S06.3 Focal traumatic brain injury**
Excludes1   any condition classifiable to S06.4-S06.6
focal cerebral edema (S06.1)

  ● **S06.30 Unspecified focal traumatic brain injury**

    ● **S06.300 Unspecified focal traumatic brain injury without loss of consciousness**

    ● **S06.301 Unspecified focal traumatic brain injury with loss of consciousness of 30 minutes or less** A 🔹, A 🔹

    ● **S06.302 Unspecified focal traumatic brain injury with loss of consciousness of 31 minutes to 59 minutes** A 🔹, A 🔹

    ● **S06.303 Unspecified focal traumatic brain injury with loss of consciousness of 1 hour to 5 hours 59 minutes** A 🔹, A 🔹

    ● **S06.304 Unspecified focal traumatic brain injury with loss of consciousness of 6 hours to 24 hours** A 🔹, A 🔹

    ● **S06.305 Unspecified focal traumatic brain injury with loss of consciousness greater than 24 hours with return to pre-existing conscious level** A 🔹, A 🔹

    ● **S06.306 Unspecified focal traumatic brain injury with loss of consciousness greater than 24 hours without return to pre-existing conscious level with patient surviving** A 🔹, A 🔹

    ● **S06.307 Unspecified focal traumatic brain injury with loss of consciousness of any duration with death due to brain injury prior to regaining consciousness** A 🔹, A 🔹

    ● **S06.308 Unspecified focal traumatic brain injury with loss of consciousness of any duration with death due to other cause prior to regaining consciousness** A 🔹, A 🔹

    ● **S06.309 Unspecified focal traumatic brain injury with loss of consciousness of unspecified duration** A 🔹, A 🔹
Unspecified focal traumatic brain injury NOS

▶ New   ⇒ Revised   ~~deleted~~ Deleted   Excludes 1   Excludes 2   Includes   Use additional   Code first   Code also   Key words
OGCR Official Guidelines   ● Unacceptable Principal Diagnosis   X Assign placeholder X   ● Use Additional Character(s)   ▌Manifestation Code   **Coding Clinic**

● **S06.31**   Contusion and laceration of right cerebrum

   ● **S06.310**   Contusion and laceration of right cerebrum without loss of consciousness A 🐾, A 🐾

   ● **S06.311**   Contusion and laceration of right cerebrum with loss of consciousness of 30 minutes or less A 🐾, A 🐾

   ● **S06.312**   Contusion and laceration of right cerebrum with loss of consciousness of 31 minutes to 59 minutes A 🐾, A 🐾

   ● **S06.313**   Contusion and laceration of right cerebrum with loss of consciousness of 1 hour to 5 hours 59 minutes A 🐾, A 🐾

   ● **S06.314**   Contusion and laceration of right cerebrum with loss of consciousness of 6 hours to 24 hours A 🐾, A 🐾

   ● **S06.315**   Contusion and laceration of right cerebrum with loss of consciousness greater than 24 hours with return to pre-existing conscious level A 🐾, A 🐾

   ● **S06.316**   Contusion and laceration of right cerebrum with loss of consciousness greater than 24 hours without return to pre-existing conscious level with patient surviving A 🐾, A 🐾

   ● **S06.317**   Contusion and laceration of right cerebrum with loss of consciousness of any duration with death due to brain injury prior to regaining consciousness A 🐾, A 🐾

   ● **S06.318**   Contusion and laceration of right cerebrum with loss of consciousness of any duration with death due to other cause prior to regaining consciousness A 🐾, A 🐾

   ● **S06.319**   Contusion and laceration of right cerebrum with loss of consciousness of unspecified duration A 🐾, A 🐾
        Contusion and laceration of right cerebrum NOS

● **S06.32**   Contusion and laceration of left cerebrum

   ● **S06.320**   Contusion and laceration of left cerebrum without loss of consciousness A 🐾, A 🐾

   ● **S06.321**   Contusion and laceration of left cerebrum with loss of consciousness of 30 minutes or less A 🐾, A 🐾

   ● **S06.322**   Contusion and laceration of left cerebrum with loss of consciousness of 31 minutes to 59 minutes A 🐾, A 🐾

   ● **S06.323**   Contusion and laceration of left cerebrum with loss of consciousness of 1 hour to 5 hours 59 minutes A 🐾, A 🐾

   ● **S06.324**   Contusion and laceration of left cerebrum with loss of consciousness of 6 hours to 24 hours A 🐾, A 🐾

   ● **S06.325**   Contusion and laceration of left cerebrum with loss of consciousness greater than 24 hours with return to pre-existing conscious level A 🐾, A 🐾

   ● **S06.326**   Contusion and laceration of left cerebrum with loss of consciousness greater than 24 hours without return to pre-existing conscious level with patient surviving A 🐾, A 🐾

   ● **S06.327**   Contusion and laceration of left cerebrum with loss of consciousness of any duration with death due to brain injury prior to regaining consciousness A 🐾, A 🐾

   ● **S06.328**   Contusion and laceration of left cerebrum with loss of consciousness of any duration with death due to other cause prior to regaining consciousness A 🐾, A 🐾

   ● **S06.329**   Contusion and laceration of left cerebrum with loss of consciousness of unspecified duration A 🐾, A 🐾
        Contusion and laceration of left cerebrum NOS

● **S06.33**   Contusion and laceration of cerebrum, unspecified

   ● **S06.330**   Contusion and laceration of cerebrum, unspecified, without loss of consciousness A 🐾, A 🐾

   ● **S06.331**   Contusion and laceration of cerebrum, unspecified, with loss of consciousness of 30 minutes or less A 🐾, A 🐾

   ● **S06.332**   Contusion and laceration of cerebrum, unspecified, with loss of consciousness of 31 minutes to 59 minutes A 🐾, A 🐾

   ● **S06.333**   Contusion and laceration of cerebrum, unspecified, with loss of consciousness of 1 hour to 5 hours 59 minutes A 🐾, A 🐾

   ● **S06.334**   Contusion and laceration of cerebrum, unspecified, with loss of consciousness of 6 hours to 24 hours A 🐾, A 🐾

   ● **S06.335**   Contusion and laceration of cerebrum, unspecified, with loss of consciousness greater than 24 hours with return to pre-existing conscious level A 🐾, A 🐾

   ● **S06.336**   Contusion and laceration of cerebrum, unspecified, with loss of consciousness greater than 24 hours without return to pre-existing conscious level with patient surviving A 🐾, A 🐾

   ● **S06.337**   Contusion and laceration of cerebrum, unspecified, with loss of consciousness of any duration with death due to brain injury prior to regaining consciousness A 🐾, A 🐾

   ● **S06.338**   Contusion and laceration of cerebrum, unspecified, with loss of consciousness of any duration with death due to other cause prior to regaining consciousness A 🐾, A 🐾

   ● **S06.339**   Contusion and laceration of cerebrum, unspecified, with loss of consciousness of unspecified duration A 🐾, A 🐾
        Contusion and laceration of cerebrum NOS

CHAPTER 19 (S00-T88)

CHAPTER 19 (S00-T88)

● **S06.34   Traumatic hemorrhage of right cerebrum**
Traumatic intracerebral hemorrhage and
hematoma of right cerebrum

● **S06.340   Traumatic hemorrhage of right
cerebrum without loss of
consciousness** A 🔍, A 🔍
Coding Clinic: 2015, Q1, P12

● **S06.341   Traumatic hemorrhage of right
cerebrum with loss of consciousness
of 30 minutes or less** A 🔍, A 🔍

● **S06.342   Traumatic hemorrhage of right
cerebrum with loss of consciousness
of 31 minutes to 59 minutes** A 🔍,
A 🔍

● **S06.343   Traumatic hemorrhage of right
cerebrum with loss of consciousness
of 1 hours to 5 hours 59 minutes** A 🔍,
A 🔍

● **S06.344   Traumatic hemorrhage of right
cerebrum with loss of consciousness
of 6 hours to 24 hours** A 🔍, A 🔍

● **S06.345   Traumatic hemorrhage of right
cerebrum with loss of consciousness
greater than 24 hours with return to
pre-existing conscious level** A 🔍,
A 🔍

● **S06.346   Traumatic hemorrhage of right
cerebrum with loss of consciousness
greater than 24 hours without return
to pre-existing conscious level with
patient surviving** A 🔍, A 🔍

● **S06.347   Traumatic hemorrhage of right
cerebrum with loss of consciousness
of any duration with death due to
brain injury prior to regaining
consciousness** A 🔍, A 🔍

● **S06.348   Traumatic hemorrhage of right
cerebrum with loss of consciousness
of any duration with death due to
other cause prior to regaining
consciousness** A 🔍, A 🔍

● **S06.349   Traumatic hemorrhage of right
cerebrum with loss of consciousness
of unspecified duration** A 🔍, A 🔍
Traumatic hemorrhage of right
cerebrum NOS

● **S06.35   Traumatic hemorrhage of left cerebrum**
Traumatic intracerebral hemorrhage and
hematoma of left cerebrum

● **S06.350   Traumatic hemorrhage of left
cerebrum without loss of
consciousness** A 🔍, A 🔍

● **S06.351   Traumatic hemorrhage of left
cerebrum with loss of consciousness
of 30 minutes or less** A 🔍, A 🔍

● **S06.352   Traumatic hemorrhage of left
cerebrum with loss of consciousness
of 31 minutes to 59 minutes** A 🔍,
A 🔍

● **S06.353   Traumatic hemorrhage of left
cerebrum with loss of consciousness
of 1 hours to 5 hours 59 minutes** A 🔍,
A 🔍

● **S06.354   Traumatic hemorrhage of left
cerebrum with loss of consciousness
of 6 hours to 24 hours** A 🔍, A 🔍

● **S06.355   Traumatic hemorrhage of left
cerebrum with loss of consciousness
greater than 24 hours with return to
pre-existing conscious level** A 🔍,
A 🔍

● **S06.356   Traumatic hemorrhage of left
cerebrum with loss of consciousness
greater than 24 hours without return
to pre-existing conscious level with
patient surviving** A 🔍, A 🔍

● **S06.357   Traumatic hemorrhage of left
cerebrum with loss of consciousness
of any duration with death due to
brain injury prior to regaining
consciousness** A 🔍, A 🔍

● **S06.358   Traumatic hemorrhage of left
cerebrum with loss of consciousness
of any duration with death due to
other cause prior to regaining
consciousness** A 🔍, A 🔍

● **S06.359   Traumatic hemorrhage of left
cerebrum with loss of consciousness
of unspecified duration** A 🔍, A 🔍
Traumatic hemorrhage of left
cerebrum NOS

● **S06.36   Traumatic hemorrhage of cerebrum, unspecified**
Traumatic intracerebral hemorrhage and
hematoma, unspecified

● **S06.360   Traumatic hemorrhage of cerebrum,
unspecified, without loss of
consciousness** A 🔍, A 🔍

● **S06.361   Traumatic hemorrhage of cerebrum,
unspecified, with loss of
consciousness of 30 minutes or less**
A 🔍, A 🔍

● **S06.362   Traumatic hemorrhage of cerebrum,
unspecified, with loss of
consciousness of 31 minutes to
59 minutes** A 🔍, A 🔍

● **S06.363   Traumatic hemorrhage of cerebrum,
unspecified, with loss of
consciousness of 1 hours to 5 hours
59 minutes** A 🔍, A 🔍

● **S06.364   Traumatic hemorrhage of cerebrum,
unspecified, with loss of
consciousness of 6 hours to 24 hours**
A 🔍, A 🔍

● **S06.365   Traumatic hemorrhage of cerebrum,
unspecified, with loss of
consciousness greater than 24 hours
with return to pre-existing conscious
level** A 🔍, A 🔍

● **S06.366   Traumatic hemorrhage of cerebrum,
unspecified, with loss of
consciousness greater than 24 hours
without return to pre-existing
conscious level with patient surviving**
A 🔍, A 🔍

● **S06.367   Traumatic hemorrhage of cerebrum,
unspecified, with loss of
consciousness of any duration with
death due to brain injury prior to
regaining consciousness** A 🔍, A 🔍

● **S06.368   Traumatic hemorrhage of cerebrum,
unspecified, with loss of
consciousness of any duration with
death due to other cause prior to
regaining consciousness** A 🔍, A 🔍

● **S06.369   Traumatic hemorrhage of cerebrum,
unspecified, with loss of
consciousness of unspecified duration**
A 🔍, A 🔍
Traumatic hemorrhage of cerebrum
NOS

▶ New   ⟹ Revised   ~~deleted~~ Deleted   Excludes 1   Excludes 2   Includes   Use additional   Code first   Code also   Key words
OGCR Official Guidelines   ● Unacceptable Principal Diagnosis   X Assign placeholder X   ● Use Additional Character(s)   ⟩ Manifestation Code   Coding Clinic

● **S06.37** Contusion, laceration, and hemorrhage of cerebellum
- ● **S06.370** Contusion, laceration, and hemorrhage of cerebellum without loss of consciousness A 🔵, A 🔵
  - (Ex) No exclusions
- ● **S06.371** Contusion, laceration, and hemorrhage of cerebellum with loss of consciousness of 30 minutes or less A 🔵, A 🔵
- ● **S06.372** Contusion, laceration, and hemorrhage of cerebellum with loss of consciousness of 31 minutes to 59 minutes A 🔵, A 🔵
- ● **S06.373** Contusion, laceration, and hemorrhage of cerebellum with loss of consciousness of 1 hour to 5 hours 59 minutes A 🔵, A 🔵
- ● **S06.374** Contusion, laceration, and hemorrhage of cerebellum with loss of consciousness of 6 hours to 24 hours A 🔵, A 🔵
- ● **S06.375** Contusion, laceration, and hemorrhage of cerebellum with loss of consciousness greater than 24 hours with return to pre-existing conscious level A 🔵, A 🔵
- ● **S06.376** Contusion, laceration, and hemorrhage of cerebellum with loss of consciousness greater than 24 hours without return to pre-existing conscious level with patient surviving A 🔵, A 🔵
- ● **S06.377** Contusion, laceration, and hemorrhage of cerebellum with loss of consciousness of any duration with death due to brain injury prior to regaining consciousness A 🔵, A 🔵
- ● **S06.378** Contusion, laceration, and hemorrhage of cerebellum with loss of consciousness of any duration with death due to other cause prior to regaining consciousness A 🔵, A 🔵
- ● **S06.379** Contusion, laceration, and hemorrhage of cerebellum with loss of consciousness of unspecified duration A 🔵, A 🔵
  - Contusion, laceration, and hemorrhage of cerebellum NOS

● **S06.38** Contusion, laceration, and hemorrhage of brainstem
- ● **S06.380** Contusion, laceration, and hemorrhage of brainstem without loss of consciousness A 🔵, A 🔵
  - (Ex) No exclusions
- ● **S06.381** Contusion, laceration, and hemorrhage of brainstem with loss of consciousness of 30 minutes or less A 🔵, A 🔵
- ● **S06.382** Contusion, laceration, and hemorrhage of brainstem with loss of consciousness of 31 minutes to 59 minutes A 🔵, A 🔵
- ● **S06.383** Contusion, laceration, and hemorrhage of brainstem with loss of consciousness of 1 hour to 5 hours 59 minutes A 🔵, A 🔵
- ● **S06.384** Contusion, laceration, and hemorrhage of brainstem with loss of consciousness of 6 hours to 24 hours A 🔵, A 🔵

- ● **S06.385** Contusion, laceration, and hemorrhage of brainstem with loss of consciousness greater than 24 hours with return to pre-existing conscious level A 🔵, A 🔵
- ● **S06.386** Contusion, laceration, and hemorrhage of brainstem with loss of consciousness greater than 24 hours without return to pre-existing conscious level with patient surviving A 🔵, A 🔵
- ● **S06.387** Contusion, laceration, and hemorrhage of brainstem with loss of consciousness of any duration with death due to brain injury prior to regaining consciousness A 🔵, A 🔵
- ● **S06.388** Contusion, laceration, and hemorrhage of brainstem with loss of consciousness of any duration with death due to other cause prior to regaining consciousness A 🔵, A 🔵
- ● **S06.389** Contusion, laceration, and hemorrhage of brainstem with loss of consciousness of unspecified duration A 🔵, A 🔵
  - Contusion, laceration, and hemorrhage of brainstem NOS

● **S06.4** Epidural hemorrhage
- *Situated outside dura mater*
- Extradural hemorrhage NOS
- *Intracranial hemorrhage due to trauma*
- Extradural hemorrhage (traumatic)

- ● **S06.4X** Epidural hemorrhage
  - ● **S06.4X0** Epidural hemorrhage without loss of consciousness A 🔵, A 🔵
  - ● **S06.4X1** Epidural hemorrhage with loss of consciousness of 30 minutes or less A 🔵, A 🔵
  - ● **S06.4X2** Epidural hemorrhage with loss of consciousness of 31 minutes to 59 minutes A 🔵, A 🔵
  - ● **S06.4X3** Epidural hemorrhage with loss of consciousness of 1 hour to 5 hours 59 minutes A 🔵, A 🔵
  - ● **S06.4X4** Epidural hemorrhage with loss of consciousness of 6 hours to 24 hours A 🔵, A 🔵
  - ● **S06.4X5** Epidural hemorrhage with loss of consciousness greater than 24 hours with return to pre-existing conscious level A 🔵, A 🔵
  - ● **S06.4X6** Epidural hemorrhage with loss of consciousness greater than 24 hours without return to pre-existing conscious level with patient surviving A 🔵, A 🔵
  - ● **S06.4X7** Epidural hemorrhage with loss of consciousness of any duration with death due to brain injury prior to regaining consciousness A 🔵, A 🔵
  - ● **S06.4X8** Epidural hemorrhage with loss of consciousness of any duration with death due to other causes prior to regaining consciousness A 🔵, A 🔵
  - ● **S06.4X9** Epidural hemorrhage with loss of consciousness of unspecified duration A 🔵, A 🔵
    - Epidural hemorrhage NOS

N Newborn Age: 0　　**P** Pediatric Age: 0–17　　**M** Maternity DX: 12–55　　**A** Adult Age: 15–124　　♀ Females Only　　♂ Males Only

🔵 Complication\Comorbidity　　🔵 Major C\C　　(Ex) CC/MCC Exclusions　　🔵 Hospital-Acquired Condition

● S06.5   **Traumatic subdural hemorrhage**
   ● S06.5X   **Traumatic subdural hemorrhage**
     ● S06.5X0   Traumatic subdural hemorrhage without loss of consciousness A 🔍, A 🔍
         Coding Clinic: 2015, Q3, P37
     ● S06.5X1   Traumatic subdural hemorrhage with loss of consciousness of 30 minutes or less A 🔍, A 🔍
     ● S06.5X2   Traumatic subdural hemorrhage with loss of consciousness of 31 minutes to 59 minutes A 🔍, A 🔍
     ● S06.5X3   Traumatic subdural hemorrhage with loss of consciousness of 1 hour to 5 hours 59 minutes A 🔍, A 🔍
     ● S06.5X4   Traumatic subdural hemorrhage with loss of consciousness of 6 hours to 24 hours A 🔍, A 🔍
     ● S06.5X5   Traumatic subdural hemorrhage with loss of consciousness greater than 24 hours with return to pre-existing conscious level A 🔍, A 🔍
     ● S06.5X6   Traumatic subdural hemorrhage with loss of consciousness greater than 24 hours without return to pre-existing conscious level with patient surviving A 🔍, A 🔍
     ● S06.5X7   Traumatic subdural hemorrhage with loss of consciousness of any duration with death due to brain injury before regaining consciousness A 🔍, A 🔍
     ● S06.5X8   Traumatic subdural hemorrhage with loss of consciousness of any duration with death due to other cause before regaining consciousness A 🔍, A 🔍
     ● S06.5X9   Traumatic subdural hemorrhage with loss of consciousness of unspecified duration A 🔍, A 🔍
         Traumatic subdural hemorrhage NOS

● S06.6   **Traumatic subarachnoid hemorrhage**
     Between arachnoid and pia mater
     Coding Clinic: 2016, Q4, P67
   ● S06.6X   **Traumatic subarachnoid hemorrhage**
     ● S06.6X0   Traumatic subarachnoid hemorrhage without loss of consciousness A 🔍, A 🔍
         Coding Clinic: 2015, Q3, P37
     ● S06.6X1   Traumatic subarachnoid hemorrhage with loss of consciousness of 30 minutes or less A 🔍, A 🔍
     ● S06.6X2   Traumatic subarachnoid hemorrhage with loss of consciousness of 31 minutes to 59 minutes A 🔍, A 🔍
     ● S06.6X3   Traumatic subarachnoid hemorrhage with loss of consciousness of 1 hour to 5 hours 59 minutes A 🔍, A 🔍
     ● S06.6X4   Traumatic subarachnoid hemorrhage with loss of consciousness of 6 hours to 24 hours A 🔍, A 🔍
     ● S06.6X5   Traumatic subarachnoid hemorrhage with loss of consciousness greater than 24 hours with return to pre-existing conscious level A 🔍, A 🔍
     ● S06.6X6   Traumatic subarachnoid hemorrhage with loss of consciousness greater than 24 hours without return to pre-existing conscious level with patient surviving A 🔍, A 🔍

● S06.6X7   Traumatic subarachnoid hemorrhage with loss of consciousness of any duration with death due to brain injury prior to regaining consciousness A 🔍, A 🔍
● S06.6X8   Traumatic subarachnoid hemorrhage with loss of consciousness of any duration with death due to other cause prior to regaining consciousness A 🔍, A 🔍
● S06.6X9   Traumatic subarachnoid hemorrhage with loss of consciousness of unspecified duration A 🔍, A 🔍
       Traumatic subarachnoid hemorrhage NOS

● S06.8   **Other specified intracranial injuries**
   ● S06.81   Injury of right internal carotid artery, intracranial portion, not elsewhere classified
     Coding Clinic: 2016, Q4, P67
     ● S06.810   Injury of right internal carotid artery, intracranial portion, not elsewhere classified without loss of consciousness
     ● S06.811   Injury of right internal carotid artery, intracranial portion, not elsewhere classified with loss of consciousness of 30 minutes or less A 🔍, A 🔍
     ● S06.812   Injury of right internal carotid artery, intracranial portion, not elsewhere classified with loss of consciousness of 31 minutes to 59 minutes A 🔍, A 🔍
     ● S06.813   Injury of right internal carotid artery, intracranial portion, not elsewhere classified with loss of consciousness of 1 hour to 5 hours 59 minutes A 🔍, A 🔍
     ● S06.814   Injury of right internal carotid artery, intracranial portion, not elsewhere classified with loss of consciousness of 6 hours to 24 hours A 🔍, A 🔍
     ● S06.815   Injury of right internal carotid artery, intracranial portion, not elsewhere classified with loss of consciousness greater than 24 hours with return to pre-existing conscious level A 🔍, A 🔍
     ● S06.816   Injury of right internal carotid artery, intracranial portion, not elsewhere classified with loss of consciousness greater than 24 hours without return to pre-existing conscious level with patient surviving A 🔍, A 🔍
     ● S06.817   Injury of right internal carotid artery, intracranial portion, not elsewhere classified with loss of consciousness of any duration with death due to brain injury prior to regaining consciousness A 🔍, A 🔍
     ● S06.818   Injury of right internal carotid artery, intracranial portion, not elsewhere classified with loss of consciousness of any duration with death due to other cause prior to regaining consciousness A 🔍, A 🔍
     ● S06.819   Injury of right internal carotid artery, intracranial portion, not elsewhere classified with loss of consciousness of unspecified duration A 🔍, A 🔍
         Injury of right internal carotid artery, intracranial portion, not elsewhere classified NOS

● **S06.82** Injury of left internal carotid artery, intracranial portion, not elsewhere classified
Coding Clinic: 2016, Q4, P67

● **S06.820** Injury of left internal carotid artery, intracranial portion, not elsewhere classified without loss of consciousness

● **S06.821** Injury of left internal carotid artery, intracranial portion, not elsewhere classified with loss of consciousness of 30 minutes or less A 🔹, A 🔹

● **S06.822** Injury of left internal carotid artery, intracranial portion, not elsewhere classified with loss of consciousness of 31 minutes to 59 minutes A 🔹, A 🔹

● **S06.823** Injury of left internal carotid artery, intracranial portion, not elsewhere classified with loss of consciousness of 1 hour to 5 hours 59 minutes A 🔹, A 🔹

● **S06.824** Injury of left internal carotid artery, intracranial portion, not elsewhere classified with loss of consciousness of 6 hours to 24 hours A 🔹, A 🔹

● **S06.825** Injury of left internal carotid artery, intracranial portion, not elsewhere classified with loss of consciousness greater than 24 hours with return to pre-existing conscious level A 🔹, A 🔹

● **S06.826** Injury of left internal carotid artery, intracranial portion, not elsewhere classified with loss of consciousness greater than 24 hours without return to pre-existing conscious level with patient surviving A 🔹, A 🔹

● **S06.827** Injury of left internal carotid artery, intracranial portion, not elsewhere classified with loss of consciousness of any duration with death due to brain injury prior to regaining consciousness A 🔹, A 🔹

● **S06.828** Injury of left internal carotid artery, intracranial portion, not elsewhere classified with loss of consciousness of any duration with death due to other cause prior to regaining consciousness A 🔹, A 🔹

● **S06.829** Injury of left internal carotid artery, intracranial portion, not elsewhere classified with loss of consciousness of unspecified duration A 🔹, A 🔹
Injury of left internal carotid artery, intracranial portion, not elsewhere classified NOS

● **S06.89** Other specified intracranial injury
Excludes1 concussion (S06.0X-)

● **S06.890** Other specified intracranial injury without loss of consciousness

● **S06.891** Other specified intracranial injury with loss of consciousness of 30 minutes or less A 🔹, A 🔹

● **S06.892** Other specified intracranial injury with loss of consciousness of 31 minutes to 59 minutes A 🔹, A 🔹

● **S06.893** Other specified intracranial injury with loss of consciousness of 1 hour to 5 hours 59 minutes A 🔹, A 🔹

● **S06.894** Other specified intracranial injury with loss of consciousness of 6 hours to 24 hours A 🔹, A 🔹

● **S06.895** Other specified intracranial injury with loss of consciousness greater than 24 hours with return to pre-existing conscious level A 🔹, A 🔹

● **S06.896** Other specified intracranial injury with loss of consciousness greater than 24 hours without return to pre-existing conscious level with patient surviving A 🔹, A 🔹

● **S06.897** Other specified intracranial injury with loss of consciousness of any duration with death due to brain injury prior to regaining consciousness A 🔹, A 🔹

● **S06.898** Other specified intracranial injury with loss of consciousness of any duration with death due to other cause prior to regaining consciousness A 🔹, A 🔹

● **S06.899** Other specified intracranial injury with loss of consciousness of unspecified duration A 🔹, A 🔹

● **S06.9** Unspecified intracranial injury
Brain injury NOS
Head injury NOS with loss of consciousness
Traumatic brain injury NOS
Excludes1 conditions classifiable to S06.0- to S06.8-code to specified intracranial injury
head injury NOS (S09.90)

● **S06.9X** Unspecified intracranial injury

● **S06.9X0** Unspecified intracranial injury without loss of consciousness

● **S06.9X1** Unspecified intracranial injury with loss of consciousness of 30 minutes or less A 🔹, A 🔹

● **S06.9X2** Unspecified intracranial injury with loss of consciousness of 31 minutes to 59 minutes A 🔹, A 🔹

● **S06.9X3** Unspecified intracranial injury with loss of consciousness of 1 hour to 5 hours 59 minutes A 🔹, A 🔹

● **S06.9X4** Unspecified intracranial injury with loss of consciousness of 6 hours to 24 hours A 🔹, A 🔹

● **S06.9X5** Unspecified intracranial injury with loss of consciousness greater than 24 hours with return to pre-existing conscious level A 🔹, A 🔹

● **S06.9X6** Unspecified intracranial injury with loss of consciousness greater than 24 hours without return to pre-existing conscious level with patient surviving A 🔹, A 🔹

● **S06.9X7** Unspecified intracranial injury with loss of consciousness of any duration with death due to brain injury prior to regaining consciousness A 🔹, A 🔹

● **S06.9X8** Unspecified intracranial injury with loss of consciousness of any duration with death due to other cause prior to regaining consciousness A 🔹, A 🔹

● **S06.9X9** Unspecified intracranial injury with loss of consciousness of unspecified duration A 🔹, A 🔹

CHAPTER 19 (S00-T88)

N Newborn Age: 0   **P** Pediatric Age: 0–17   **M** Maternity DX: 12–55   **A** Adult Age: 15–124   ♀ Females Only   ♂ Males Only

🔹 Complication\Comorbidity   🔹 Major C\C   (Ex) CC/MCC Exclusions   🔹 Hospital-Acquired Condition

1237

CHAPTER 19 (S00-T88)

● **S07   Crushing injury of head**

Use additional code for all associated injuries, such as:
intracranial injuries (S06.-)
skull fractures (S02.-)

The appropriate 7th character is to be added to each code from category S07

> A   initial encounter
> D   subsequent encounter
> S   sequela

(Ex:) **For category S07 CC codes:** See PDX Collection 1156

X ● **S07.0   Crushing injury of face** A 🔓, A 🔒

X ● **S07.1   Crushing injury of skull** A 🔓, A 🔒

X ● **S07.8   Crushing injury of other parts of head** A 🔓, A 🔒

X ● **S07.9   Crushing injury of head, part unspecified** A 🔓, A 🔒

● **S08   Avulsion and traumatic amputation of part of head**

An amputation not identified as partial or complete should be coded to complete

The appropriate 7th character is to be added to each code from category S08

> A   initial encounter
> D   subsequent encounter
> S   sequela

X ● **S08.0   Avulsion of scalp**

● **S08.1   Traumatic amputation of ear**

  ● **S08.11   Complete traumatic amputation of ear**

    ● **S08.111   Complete traumatic amputation of right ear**

    ● **S08.112   Complete traumatic amputation of left ear**

    ● **S08.119   Complete traumatic amputation of unspecified ear**

  ● **S08.12   Partial traumatic amputation of ear**

    ● **S08.121   Partial traumatic amputation of right ear**

    ● **S08.122   Partial traumatic amputation of left ear**

    ● **S08.129   Partial traumatic amputation of unspecified ear**

● **S08.8   Traumatic amputation of other parts of head**

  ● **S08.81   Traumatic amputation of nose**

    ● **S08.811   Complete traumatic amputation of nose**

    ● **S08.812   Partial traumatic amputation of nose**

  X ● **S08.89   Traumatic amputation of other parts of head**

● **S09   Other and unspecified injuries of head**

The appropriate 7th character is to be added to each code from category S09

> A   initial encounter
> D   subsequent encounter
> S   sequela

X ● **S09.0   Injury of blood vessels of head, not elsewhere classified** A 🔒

> **Excludes1**   injury of cerebral blood vessels (S06.-)
> injury of precerebral blood vessels (S15.-)

(Ex:) See PDX Collection 1157

● **S09.1   Injury of muscle and tendon of head**

Code also any associated open wound (S01.-)

> **Excludes2**   sprain to joints and ligament of head (S03.9)

X ● **S09.10   Unspecified injury of muscle and tendon of head**

Injury of muscle and tendon of head NOS

X ● **S09.11   Strain of muscle and tendon of head**

X ● **S09.12   Laceration of muscle and tendon of head**

X ● **S09.19   Other specified injury of muscle and tendon of head**

● **S09.2   Traumatic rupture of ear drum**

> **Excludes1**   traumatic rupture of ear drum due to blast injury (S09.31-)

(Ex:) **For category S09.2 CC codes:** See PDX Collection 1158

X ● **S09.20   Traumatic rupture of unspecified ear drum** A 🔒

X ● **S09.21   Traumatic rupture of right ear drum** A 🔒

X ● **S09.22   Traumatic rupture of left ear drum** A 🔒

● **S09.3   Other specified and unspecified injury of middle and inner ear**

> **Excludes1**   injury to ear NOS (S09.91-)
> **Excludes2**   injury to external ear (S00.4-, S01.3-, S08.1-)

(Ex:) **For category S09.3 CC codes:** See PDX Collection 1158

● **S09.30   Unspecified injury of middle and inner ear**

  ● **S09.301   Unspecified injury of right middle and inner ear** A 🔒

  ● **S09.302   Unspecified injury of left middle and inner ear** A 🔒

  ● **S09.309   Unspecified injury of unspecified middle and inner ear** A 🔒

● **S09.31   Primary blast injury of ear**

Blast injury of ear NOS

  ● **S09.311   Primary blast injury of right ear** A 🔒

  ● **S09.312   Primary blast injury of left ear** A 🔒

  ● **S09.313   Primary blast injury of ear, bilateral** A 🔒

  ● **S09.319   Primary blast injury of unspecified ear** A 🔒

● **S09.39   Other specified injury of middle and inner ear**

Secondary blast injury to ear

  ● **S09.391   Other specified injury of right middle and inner ear** A 🔒

  ● **S09.392   Other specified injury of left middle and inner ear** A 🔒

  ● **S09.399   Other specified injury of unspecified middle and inner ear** A 🔒

X ● **S09.8   Other specified injuries of head**

● **S09.9   Unspecified injury of face and head**

X ● **S09.90   Unspecified injury of head**

Head injury NOS

> **Excludes1**   brain injury NOS (S06.9-)
> head injury NOS with loss of consciousness (S06.9-)
> intracranial injury NOS (S06.9-)

X ● **S09.91   Unspecified injury of ear**

Injury of ear NOS

X ● **S09.92   Unspecified injury of nose**

Injury of nose NOS

X ● **S09.93   Unspecified injury of face**

Injury of face NOS

▶ New   ⇒ Revised   ~~deleted~~ Deleted   Excludes 1   Excludes 2   Includes   Use additional   Code first   Code also   Key words

OGCR Official Guidelines   ● Unacceptable Principal Diagnosis   X Assign placeholder X   ● Use Additional Character(s)   ▶ Manifestation Code   **Coding Clinic**

INJURIES TO THE NECK (S10-S19)

Includes	injuries of nape
	injuries of supraclavicular region
	injuries of throat
Excludes2	burns and corrosions (T20-T32)
	effects of foreign body in esophagus (T18.1)
	effects of foreign body in larynx (T17.3)
	effects of foreign body in pharynx (T17.2)
	effects of foreign body in trachea (T17.4)
	frostbite (T33-T34)
	insect bite or sting, venomous (T63.4)

● **S10   Superficial injury of neck**

The appropriate 7th character is to be added to each code from category S10

A	initial encounter
D	subsequent encounter
S	sequela

X● **S10.0   Contusion of throat**
         Contusion of cervical esophagus
         Contusion of larynx
         Contusion of pharynx
         Contusion of trachea

● **S10.1   Other and unspecified superficial injuries of throat**

   X● **S10.10   Unspecified superficial injuries of throat**

   X● **S10.11   Abrasion of throat**

   X● **S10.12   Blister (nonthermal) of throat**

   X● **S10.14   External constriction of part of throat**

   X● **S10.15   Superficial foreign body of throat**
         Splinter in the throat

   X● **S10.16   Insect bite (nonvenomous) of throat**

   X● **S10.17   Other superficial bite of throat**
         Excludes1   open bite of throat (S11.85)

● **S10.8   Superficial injury of other specified parts of neck**

   X● **S10.80   Unspecified superficial injury of other specified part of neck**

   X● **S10.81   Abrasion of other specified part of neck**

   X● **S10.82   Blister (nonthermal) of other specified part of neck**

   X● **S10.83   Contusion of other specified part of neck**

   X● **S10.84   External constriction of other specified part of neck**

   X● **S10.85   Superficial foreign body of other specified part of neck**
         Splinter in other part of neck

   X● **S10.86   Insect bite of other specified part of neck**

   X● **S10.87   Other superficial bite of other specified part of neck**
         Excludes1   open bite of other specified parts of neck (S11.85)

● **S10.9   Superficial injury of unspecified part of neck**

   X● **S10.90   Unspecified superficial injury of unspecified part of neck**

   X● **S10.91   Abrasion of unspecified part of neck**

   X● **S10.92   Blister (nonthermal) of unspecified part of neck**

   X● **S10.93   Contusion of unspecified part of neck**

   X● **S10.94   External constriction of unspecified part of neck**

   X● **S10.95   Superficial foreign body of unspecified part of neck**

   X● **S10.96   Insect bite of unspecified part of neck**

   X● **S10.97   Other superficial bite of unspecified part of neck**

● **S11   Open wound of neck**

Code also any associated:
    spinal cord injury (S14.0, S14.1-)
    wound infection

    Excludes2   open fracture of vertebra (S12.- with 7th character B)

The appropriate 7th character is to be added to each code from category S11

A	initial encounter
D	subsequent encounter
S	sequela

● **S11.0   Open wound of larynx and trachea**
     (Ex) For category S11.0 CC codes: See PDX Collection 1159

   ● **S11.01   Open wound of larynx**
       Excludes2   open wound of vocal cord (S11.03)

     ● **S11.011   Laceration without foreign body of larynx A** 🏥

     ● **S11.012   Laceration with foreign body of larynx A** 🏥

     ● **S11.013   Puncture wound without foreign body of larynx A** 🏥

     ● **S11.014   Puncture wound with foreign body of larynx A** 🏥

     ● **S11.015   Open bite of larynx A** 🏥
         Bite of larynx NOS

     ● **S11.019   Unspecified open wound of larynx A** 🏥

   ● **S11.02   Open wound of trachea**
       Open wound of cervical trachea
       Open wound of trachea NOS
       Excludes2   open wound of thoracic trachea (S27.5-)

     ● **S11.021   Laceration without foreign body of trachea A** 🏥

     ● **S11.022   Laceration with foreign body of trachea A** 🏥

     ● **S11.023   Puncture wound without foreign body of trachea A** 🏥

     ● **S11.024   Puncture wound with foreign body of trachea A** 🏥

     ● **S11.025   Open bite of trachea A** 🏥
         Bite of trachea NOS

     ● **S11.029   Unspecified open wound of trachea A** 🏥

   ● **S11.03   Open wound of vocal cord**

     ● **S11.031   Laceration without foreign body of vocal cord A** 🏥

     ● **S11.032   Laceration with foreign body of vocal cord A** 🏥

     ● **S11.033   Puncture wound without foreign body of vocal cord A** 🏥

     ● **S11.034   Puncture wound with foreign body of vocal cord A** 🏥

     ● **S11.035   Open bite of vocal cord A** 🏥
         Bite of vocal cord NOS

     ● **S11.039   Unspecified open wound of vocal cord A** 🏥

● **S11.1**   **Open wound of thyroid gland**
   (Ex) **For category S11.1 CC codes unless otherwise indicated:** See PDX Collection 1160

X ● **S11.10**   **Unspecified open wound of thyroid gland** A 🔖

X ● **S11.11**   **Laceration without foreign body of thyroid gland** A 🔖

X ● **S11.12**   **Laceration with foreign body of thyroid gland** A 🔖
      (Ex) See PDX Collection 1161

X ● **S11.13**   **Puncture wound without foreign body of thyroid gland** A 🔖

X ● **S11.14**   **Puncture wound with foreign body of thyroid gland** A 🔖
      (Ex) See PDX Collection 1161

X ● **S11.15**   **Open bite of thyroid gland** A 🔖
      Bite of thyroid gland NOS

● **S11.2**   **Open wound of pharynx and cervical esophagus**
   Excludes1   open wound of esophagus NOS (S27.8-)
   (Ex) **For category S11.2 CC codes unless otherwise indicated:** See PDX Collection 1162

X ● **S11.20**   **Unspecified open wound of pharynx and cervical esophagus** A 🔖

X ● **S11.21**   **Laceration without foreign body of pharynx and cervical esophagus** A 🔖

X ● **S11.22**   **Laceration with foreign body of pharynx and cervical esophagus** A 🔖
      (Ex) See PDX Collection 1163

X ● **S11.23**   **Puncture wound without foreign body of pharynx and cervical esophagus** A 🔖

X ● **S11.24**   **Puncture wound with foreign body of pharynx and cervical esophagus** A 🔖
      (Ex) See PDX Collection 1163

X ● **S11.25**   **Open bite of pharynx and cervical esophagus** A 🔖
      Bite of pharynx and cervical esophagus NOS

● **S11.8**   **Open wound of other specified parts of neck**

X ● **S11.80**   **Unspecified open specified wound of other part of neck**

X ● **S11.81**   **Laceration without foreign body of other specified part of neck**

X ● **S11.82**   **Laceration with foreign body of other specified part of neck**

X ● **S11.83**   **Puncture wound without foreign body of other specified part of neck**

X ● **S11.84**   **Puncture wound with foreign body of other specified part of neck**

X ● **S11.85**   **Open bite of other specified part of neck**
      Bite of other part of neck NOS
      Excludes1   superficial bite of other specified part of neck (S10.87)

X ● **S11.89**   **Other open wound of other part of neck**

● **S11.9**   **Open wound of unspecified part of neck**

X ● **S11.90**   **Unspecified open wound of unspecified part of neck**

X ● **S11.91**   **Laceration without foreign body of unspecified part of neck**

X ● **S11.92**   **Laceration with foreign body of unspecified part of neck**

X ● **S11.93**   **Puncture wound without foreign body of unspecified part of neck**

X ● **S11.94**   **Puncture wound with foreign body of unspecified part of neck**

X ● **S11.95**   **Open bite of unspecified part of neck**
      Bite of neck NOS
      Excludes1   superficial bite of neck (S10.97)

● **S12**   **Fracture of cervical vertebra and other parts of neck**
   Note: A fracture not indicated as displaced or nondisplaced should be coded to displaced
      A fracture not indicated as open or closed should be coded to closed

   Includes   fracture of cervical neural arch
              fracture of cervical spine
              fracture of cervical spinous process
              fracture of cervical transverse process
              fracture of cervical vertebral arch
              fracture of neck

Code first any associated cervical spinal cord injury (S14.0, S14.1-)

The appropriate 7th character is to be added to all codes from subcategories S12.0-S12.6

A	initial encounter for closed fracture
B	initial encounter for open fracture
D	subsequent encounter for fracture with routine healing
G	subsequent encounter for fracture with delayed healing
K	subsequent encounter for fracture with nonunion
S	sequela

   (Ex) **For category S12 CC codes S12[A,B]:** See PDX Collection 1164
      For S12[K]: See PDX Collection 897 **unless otherwise indicated**

● **S12.0**   **Fracture of first cervical vertebra**
   Atlas

   ● **S12.00**   **Unspecified fracture of first cervical vertebra**

      ● **S12.000**   **Unspecified displaced fracture of first cervical vertebra** A, K 🔖, B 🔖, A, B 🔖

      ● **S12.001**   **Unspecified nondisplaced fracture of first cervical vertebra** A, K 🔖, B 🔖, A, B 🔖

   X ● **S12.01**   **Stable burst fracture of first cervical vertebra** A, K 🔖, B 🔖, A, B 🔖

   X ● **S12.02**   **Unstable burst fracture of first cervical vertebra** A, K 🔖, B 🔖, A, B 🔖

   ● **S12.03**   **Posterior arch fracture of first cervical vertebra**

      ● **S12.030**   **Displaced posterior arch fracture of first cervical vertebra** A, K 🔖, B 🔖, A, B 🔖

      ● **S12.031**   **Nondisplaced posterior arch fracture of first cervical vertebra** A, K 🔖, B 🔖, A, B 🔖

   ● **S12.04**   **Lateral mass fracture of first cervical vertebra**

      ● **S12.040**   **Displaced lateral mass fracture of first cervical vertebra** A, K 🔖, B 🔖, A, B 🔖

      ● **S12.041**   **Nondisplaced lateral mass fracture of first cervical vertebra** A, K 🔖, B 🔖, A, B 🔖

   ● **S12.09**   **Other fracture of first cervical vertebra**

      ● **S12.090**   **Other displaced fracture of first cervical vertebra** A, K 🔖, B 🔖, A, B 🔖

      ● **S12.091**   **Other nondisplaced fracture of first cervical vertebra** A, K 🔖, B 🔖, A, B 🔖

● **S12.1**   **Fracture of second cervical vertebra**
   Axis

   ● **S12.10**   **Unspecified fracture of second cervical vertebra**

      ● **S12.100**   **Unspecified displaced fracture of second cervical vertebra** A, K 🔖, B 🔖, A, B 🔖

      ● **S12.101**   **Unspecified nondisplaced fracture of second cervical vertebra** A, K 🔖, B 🔖, A, B 🔖

● **S12.11** Type II dens fracture
   ● **S12.110** Anterior displaced Type II dens fracture A, K ▨ B ▨, A, B ▨
   ● **S12.111** Posterior displaced Type II dens fracture A, K ▨ B ▨, A, B ▨
   ● **S12.112** Nondisplaced Type II dens fracture A, K ▨ B ▨, A, B ▨
● **S12.12** Other dens fracture
   ● **S12.120** Other displaced dens fracture A, K ▨ B ▨, A, B ▨
   ● **S12.121** Other nondisplaced dens fracture A, K ▨ B ▨, A, B ▨
● **S12.13** Unspecified traumatic spondylolisthesis of second cervical vertebra
   ● **S12.130** Unspecified traumatic displaced spondylolisthesis of second cervical vertebra A, K ▨ B ▨, A, B ▨
   ● **S12.131** Unspecified traumatic nondisplaced spondylolisthesis of second cervical vertebra A, K ▨ B ▨, A, B ▨
X ● **S12.14** Type III traumatic spondylolisthesis of second cervical vertebra A, K ▨ B ▨, A, B ▨
● **S12.15** Other traumatic spondylolisthesis of second cervical vertebra
   ● **S12.150** Other traumatic displaced spondylolisthesis of second cervical vertebra A, K ▨ B ▨, A, B ▨
   ● **S12.151** Other traumatic nondisplaced spondylolisthesis of second cervical vertebra A, K ▨ B ▨, A, B ▨
● **S12.19** Other fracture of second cervical vertebra
   ● **S12.190** Other displaced fracture of second cervical vertebra A, K ▨ B ▨, A, B ▨
   ● **S12.191** Other nondisplaced fracture of second cervical vertebra A, K ▨ B ▨, A, B ▨
● **S12.2** Fracture of third cervical vertebra
  ● **S12.20** Unspecified fracture of third cervical vertebra
   ● **S12.200** Unspecified displaced fracture of third cervical vertebra A, K ▨ B ▨, A, B ▨
   ● **S12.201** Unspecified nondisplaced fracture of third cervical vertebra A, K ▨ B ▨, A, B ▨
  ● **S12.23** Unspecified traumatic spondylolisthesis of third cervical vertebra
   ● **S12.230** Unspecified traumatic displaced spondylolisthesis of third cervical vertebra A, K ▨ B ▨, A, B ▨
   ● **S12.231** Unspecified traumatic nondisplaced spondylolisthesis of third cervical vertebra A, K ▨ B ▨, A, B ▨
X ● **S12.24** Type III traumatic spondylolisthesis of third cervical vertebra A, K ▨ B ▨, A, B ▨
  ● **S12.25** Other traumatic spondylolisthesis of third cervical vertebra
   ● **S12.250** Other traumatic displaced spondylolisthesis of third cervical vertebra A, K ▨ B ▨, A, B ▨
   ● **S12.251** Other traumatic nondisplaced spondylolisthesis of third cervical vertebra A, K ▨ B ▨, A, B ▨
  ● **S12.29** Other fracture of third cervical vertebra
   ● **S12.290** Other displaced fracture of third cervical vertebra A, K ▨ B ▨, A, B ▨
   ● **S12.291** Other nondisplaced fracture of third cervical vertebra A, K ▨ B ▨, A, B ▨

● **S12.3** Fracture of fourth cervical vertebra
  ● **S12.30** Unspecified fracture of fourth cervical vertebra
   ● **S12.300** Unspecified displaced fracture of fourth cervical vertebra A, K ▨ B ▨, A, B ▨
   ● **S12.301** Unspecified nondisplaced fracture of fourth cervical vertebra A, K ▨ B ▨, A, B ▨
  ● **S12.33** Unspecified traumatic spondylolisthesis of fourth cervical vertebra
   ● **S12.330** Unspecified traumatic displaced spondylolisthesis of fourth cervical vertebra A, K ▨ B ▨, A, B ▨
   ● **S12.331** Unspecified traumatic nondisplaced spondylolisthesis of fourth cervical vertebra A, K ▨ B ▨, A, B ▨
X ● **S12.34** Type III traumatic spondylolisthesis of fourth cervical vertebra A, K ▨ B ▨, A, B ▨
  ● **S12.35** Other traumatic spondylolisthesis of fourth cervical vertebra
   ● **S12.350** Other traumatic displaced spondylolisthesis of fourth cervical vertebra A, K ▨ B ▨, A, B ▨
   ● **S12.351** Other traumatic nondisplaced spondylolisthesis of fourth cervical vertebra A, K ▨ B ▨, A, B ▨
  ● **S12.39** Other fracture of fourth cervical vertebra
   ● **S12.390** Other displaced fracture of fourth cervical vertebra A, K ▨ B ▨, A, B ▨
   ● **S12.391** Other nondisplaced fracture of fourth cervical vertebra A, K ▨ B ▨, A, B ▨
● **S12.4** Fracture of fifth cervical vertebra
  ● **S12.40** Unspecified fracture of fifth cervical vertebra
   ● **S12.400** Unspecified displaced fracture of fifth cervical vertebra A, K ▨ B ▨, A, B ▨
   ● **S12.401** Unspecified nondisplaced fracture of fifth cervical vertebra A, K ▨ B ▨, A, B ▨
  ● **S12.43** Unspecified traumatic spondylolisthesis of fifth cervical vertebra
   ● **S12.430** Unspecified traumatic displaced spondylolisthesis of fifth cervical vertebra A, K ▨ B ▨, A, B ▨
   ● **S12.431** Unspecified traumatic nondisplaced spondylolisthesis of fifth cervical vertebra A, K ▨ B ▨, A, B ▨
X ● **S12.44** Type III traumatic spondylolisthesis of fifth cervical vertebra A, K ▨ B ▨, A, B ▨
  ● **S12.45** Other traumatic spondylolisthesis of fifth cervical vertebra
   ● **S12.450** Other traumatic displaced spondylolisthesis of fifth cervical vertebra A, K ▨ B ▨, A, B ▨
   ● **S12.451** Other traumatic nondisplaced spondylolisthesis of fifth cervical vertebra A, K ▨ B ▨, A, B ▨
  ● **S12.49** Other fracture of fifth cervical vertebra
   ● **S12.490** Other displaced fracture of fifth cervical vertebra A, K ▨ B ▨, A, B ▨
   ● **S12.491** Other nondisplaced fracture of fifth cervical vertebra A, K ▨ B ▨, A, B ▨

CHAPTER 19 (S00-T88)

N   Newborn Age: 0   P   Pediatric Age: 0–17   M   Maternity DX: 12–55   A   Adult Age: 15–124   ♀   Females Only   ♂   Males Only
▨   Complication\Comorbidity   ▨   Major C\C   (Ex)   CC/MCC Exclusions   ▨   Hospital-Acquired Condition

CHAPTER 19 (S00-T88)

● **S12.5**   Fracture of sixth cervical vertebra
   ● **S12.50**   Unspecified fracture of sixth cervical vertebra
     ● **S12.500**   Unspecified displaced fracture of sixth cervical vertebra A, K 🔒, B 🔒, A, B 🔒
     ● **S12.501**   Unspecified nondisplaced fracture of sixth cervical vertebra A, K 🔒, B 🔒, A, B 🔒
   ● **S12.53**   Unspecified traumatic spondylolisthesis of sixth cervical vertebra
     ● **S12.530**   Unspecified traumatic displaced spondylolisthesis of sixth cervical vertebra A, K 🔒, B 🔒, A, B 🔒
     ● **S12.531**   Unspecified traumatic nondisplaced spondylolisthesis of sixth cervical vertebra A, K 🔒, B 🔒, A, B 🔒
  X ● **S12.54**   Type III traumatic spondylolisthesis of sixth cervical vertebra A, K 🔒, B 🔒, A, B 🔒
   ● **S12.55**   Other traumatic spondylolisthesis of sixth cervical vertebra
     ● **S12.550**   Other traumatic displaced spondylolisthesis of sixth cervical vertebra A, K 🔒, B 🔒, A, B 🔒
     ● **S12.551**   Other traumatic nondisplaced spondylolisthesis of sixth cervical vertebra A, K 🔒, B 🔒, A, B 🔒
   ● **S12.59**   Other fracture of sixth cervical vertebra
     ● **S12.590**   Other displaced fracture of sixth cervical vertebra A, K 🔒, B 🔒, A, B 🔒
     ● **S12.591**   Other nondisplaced fracture of sixth cervical vertebra A, K 🔒, B 🔒, A, B 🔒
● **S12.6**   Fracture of seventh cervical vertebra
   S12.60   Unspecified fracture of seventh cervical vertebra
     ● **S12.600**   Unspecified displaced fracture of seventh cervical vertebra A, K 🔒, B 🔒, A, B 🔒
     ● **S12.601**   Unspecified nondisplaced fracture of seventh cervical vertebra A, K 🔒, B 🔒, A, B 🔒
   ● **S12.63**   Unspecified traumatic spondylolisthesis of seventh cervical vertebra
     ● **S12.630**   Unspecified traumatic displaced spondylolisthesis of seventh cervical vertebra A, K 🔒, B 🔒, A, B 🔒
     ● **S12.631**   Unspecified traumatic nondisplaced spondylolisthesis of seventh cervical vertebra A, K 🔒, B 🔒, A, B 🔒
  X ● **S12.64**   Type III traumatic spondylolisthesis of seventh cervical vertebra A, K 🔒, B 🔒, A, B 🔒
   ● **S12.65**   Other traumatic spondylolisthesis of seventh cervical vertebra
     ● **S12.650**   Other traumatic displaced spondylolisthesis of seventh cervical vertebra A, K 🔒, B 🔒, A, B 🔒
     ● **S12.651**   Other traumatic nondisplaced spondylolisthesis of seventh cervical vertebra A, K 🔒, B 🔒, A, B 🔒
   ● **S12.69**   Other fracture of seventh cervical vertebra
     ● **S12.690**   Other displaced fracture of seventh cervical vertebra A, K 🔒, B 🔒, A, B 🔒
     ● **S12.691**   Other nondisplaced fracture of seventh cervical vertebra A, K 🔒, B 🔒, A, B 🔒

X ● **S12.8**   Fracture of other parts of neck A 🔒, A 🔒

Hyoid bone	Thyroid cartilage
Larynx	Trachea

   The appropriate 7th character is to be added to code S12.8

A	initial encounter
D	subsequent encounter
S	sequela

   (Ex:) See PDX Collection 1165

X ● **S12.9**   Fracture of neck, unspecified A 🔒, A 🔒
   Fracture of neck NOS
   Fracture of cervical spine NOS
   Fracture of cervical vertebra NOS
   The appropriate 7th character is to be added to code S12.9

A	initial encounter
D	subsequent encounter
S	sequela

● **S13**   Dislocation and sprain of joints and ligaments at neck level
   Includes   avulsion of joint or ligament at neck level
     laceration of cartilage, joint or ligament at neck level
     sprain of cartilage, joint or ligament at neck level
     traumatic hemarthrosis of joint or ligament at neck level
     traumatic rupture of joint or ligament at neck level
     traumatic subluxation of joint or ligament at neck level
     traumatic tear of joint or ligament at neck level
   Code also any associated open wound
   Excludes2   strain of muscle or tendon at neck level (S16.1)
   The appropriate 7th character is to be added to each code from category S13

A	initial encounter
D	subsequent encounter
S	sequela

   (Ex:) **For category S13 CC codes:** See PDX Collection 913

X ● **S13.0**   Traumatic rupture of cervical intervertebral disc A 🔒, A 🔒
     Excludes1   rupture or displacement (nontraumatic) of cervical intervertebral disc NOS (M50.-)

● **S13.1**   Subluxation and dislocation of cervical vertebrae
   Code also any associated:
     open wound of neck (S11.-)
     spinal cord injury (S14.1-)
   Excludes2   fracture of cervical vertebrae (S12.0-S12.3-)
   ● **S13.10**   Subluxation and dislocation of unspecified cervical vertebrae
     ● **S13.100**   Subluxation of unspecified cervical vertebrae A 🔒, A 🔒
     ● **S13.101**   Dislocation of unspecified cervical vertebrae A 🔒, A 🔒
   ● **S13.11**   Subluxation and dislocation of C0/C1 cervical vertebrae
     Subluxation and dislocation of atlantooccipital joint
     Subluxation and dislocation of atloidooccipital joint
     Subluxation and dislocation of occipitoatloid joint
     ● **S13.110**   Subluxation of C0/C1 cervical vertebrae A 🔒, A 🔒
     ● **S13.111**   Dislocation of C0/C1 cervical vertebrae A 🔒, A 🔒

▶ New   ⇒ Revised   ~~deleted~~ Deleted   Excludes 1   Excludes 2   Includes   Use additional   Code first   Code also   Key words
OGCR Official Guidelines   ● Unacceptable Principal Diagnosis   X Assign placeholder X   ● Use Additional Character(s)   ▶ Manifestation Code   Coding Clinic

● S13.12 **Subluxation and dislocation of C1/C2 cervical vertebrae**
  Subluxation and dislocation of atlantoaxial joint

  ● S13.120 **Subluxation of C1/C2 cervical vertebrae** A 🔾, A 🔾
  ● S13.121 **Dislocation of C1/C2 cervical vertebrae** A 🔾, A 🔾

● S13.13 **Subluxation and dislocation of C2/C3 cervical vertebrae**

  ● S13.130 **Subluxation of C2/C3 cervical vertebrae** A 🔾, A 🔾
  ● S13.131 **Dislocation of C2/C3 cervical vertebrae** A 🔾, A 🔾

● S13.14 **Subluxation and dislocation of C3/C4 cervical vertebrae**

  ● S13.140 **Subluxation of C3/C4 cervical vertebrae** A 🔾, A 🔾
  ● S13.141 **Dislocation of C3/C4 cervical vertebrae** A 🔾, A 🔾

● S13.15 **Subluxation and dislocation of C4/C5 cervical vertebrae**

  ● S13.150 **Subluxation of C4/C5 cervical vertebrae** A 🔾, A 🔾
  ● S13.151 **Dislocation of C4/C5 cervical vertebrae** A 🔾, A 🔾

● S13.16 **Subluxation and dislocation of C5/C6 cervical vertebrae**

  ● S13.160 **Subluxation of C5/C6 cervical vertebrae** A 🔾, A 🔾
  ● S13.161 **Dislocation of C5/C6 cervical vertebrae** A 🔾, A 🔾

● S13.17 **Subluxation and dislocation of C6/C7 cervical vertebrae**

  ● S13.170 **Subluxation of C6/C7 cervical vertebrae** A 🔾, A 🔾
  ● S13.171 **Dislocation of C6/C7 cervical vertebrae** A 🔾, A 🔾

● S13.18 **Subluxation and dislocation of C7/T1 cervical vertebrae**

  ● S13.180 **Subluxation of C7/T1 cervical vertebrae** A 🔾, A 🔾
  ● S13.181 **Dislocation of C7/T1 cervical vertebrae** A 🔾, A 🔾

● S13.2 **Dislocation of other and unspecified parts of neck**
  X ● S13.20 **Dislocation of unspecified parts of neck** A 🔾, A 🔾
  X ● S13.29 **Dislocation of other parts of neck** A 🔾, A 🔾

X ● S13.4 **Sprain of ligaments of cervical spine**
  Sprain of anterior longitudinal (ligament), cervical
  Sprain of atlanto-axial (joints)
  Sprain of atlanto-occipital (joints)
  Whiplash injury of cervical spine

X ● S13.5 **Sprain of thyroid region**
  Sprain of cricoarytenoid (joint) (ligament)
  Sprain of cricothyroid (joint) (ligament)
  Sprain of thyroid cartilage

X ● S13.8 **Sprain of joints and ligaments of other parts of neck**

X ● S13.9 **Sprain of joints and ligaments of unspecified parts of neck**

● S14 **Injury of nerves and spinal cord at neck level**
  Note: Code to highest level of cervical cord injury
  Code also any associated:
    fracture of cervical vertebra (S12.0--S12.6.-)
    open wound of neck (S11.-)
    transient paralysis (R29.5)
  The appropriate 7th character is to be added to each code from category S14

A	initial encounter
D	subsequent encounter
S	sequela

  (Ex) **For category S14 CC codes:** See PDX Collection 1166

X ● S14.0 **Concussion and edema of cervical spinal cord** A 🔾
● S14.1 **Other and unspecified injuries of cervical spinal cord**
  ● S14.10 **Unspecified injury of cervical spinal cord**
    ● S14.101 **Unspecified injury at C1 level of cervical spinal cord** A 🔾, A 🔾
    ● S14.102 **Unspecified injury at C2 level of cervical spinal cord** A 🔾, A 🔾
    ● S14.103 **Unspecified injury at C3 level of cervical spinal cord** A 🔾, A 🔾
    ● S14.104 **Unspecified injury at C4 level of cervical spinal cord** A 🔾, A 🔾
    ● S14.105 **Unspecified injury at C5 level of cervical spinal cord** A 🔾, A 🔾
    ● S14.106 **Unspecified injury at C6 level of cervical spinal cord** A 🔾, A 🔾
    ● S14.107 **Unspecified injury at C7 level of cervical spinal cord** A 🔾, A 🔾
    ● S14.108 **Unspecified injury at C8 level of cervical spinal cord** A 🔾
    ● S14.109 **Unspecified injury at unspecified level of cervical spinal cord**
      Injury of cervical spinal cord NOS
  ● S14.11 **Complete lesion of cervical spinal cord**
    ● S14.111 **Complete lesion at C1 level of cervical spinal cord** A 🔾, A 🔾
    ● S14.112 **Complete lesion at C2 level of cervical spinal cord** A 🔾, A 🔾
    ● S14.113 **Complete lesion at C3 level of cervical spinal cord** A 🔾, A 🔾
    ● S14.114 **Complete lesion at C4 level of cervical spinal cord** A 🔾, A 🔾
    ● S14.115 **Complete lesion at C5 level of cervical spinal cord** A 🔾, A 🔾
    ● S14.116 **Complete lesion at C6 level of cervical spinal cord** A 🔾, A 🔾
    ● S14.117 **Complete lesion at C7 level of cervical spinal cord** A 🔾, A 🔾
    ● S14.118 **Complete lesion at C8 level of cervical spinal cord** A 🔾
    ● S14.119 **Complete lesion at unspecified level of cervical spinal cord**

N Newborn Age: 0   **P** Pediatric Age: 0–17   **M** Maternity DX: 12–55   **A** Adult Age: 15–124   ♀ Females Only   ♂ Males Only
🔾 Complication\Comorbidity   🔾 Major C\C   (Ex) CC/MCC Exclusions   🔾 Hospital-Acquired Condition

1243

● **S14.12**   Central cord syndrome of cervical spinal cord

    ● **S14.121**   Central cord syndrome at C1 level of cervical spinal cord A 🔖, A 🔖

    ● **S14.122**   Central cord syndrome at C2 level of cervical spinal cord A 🔖, A 🔖

    ● **S14.123**   Central cord syndrome at C3 level of cervical spinal cord A 🔖, A 🔖

    ● **S14.124**   Central cord syndrome at C4 level of cervical spinal cord A 🔖, A 🔖

    ● **S14.125**   Central cord syndrome at C5 level of cervical spinal cord A 🔖, A 🔖

    ● **S14.126**   Central cord syndrome at C6 level of cervical spinal cord A 🔖, A 🔖

    ● **S14.127**   Central cord syndrome at C7 level of cervical spinal cord A 🔖, A 🔖

    ● **S14.128**   Central cord syndrome at C8 level of cervical spinal cord A 🔖

    ● **S14.129**   Central cord syndrome at unspecified level of cervical spinal cord

● **S14.13**   Anterior cord syndrome of cervical spinal cord

    ● **S14.131**   Anterior cord syndrome at C1 level of cervical spinal cord A 🔖, A 🔖

    ● **S14.132**   Anterior cord syndrome at C2 level of cervical spinal cord A 🔖, A 🔖

    ● **S14.133**   Anterior cord syndrome at C3 level of cervical spinal cord A 🔖, A 🔖

    ● **S14.134**   Anterior cord syndrome at C4 level of cervical spinal cord A 🔖, A 🔖

    ● **S14.135**   Anterior cord syndrome at C5 level of cervical spinal cord A 🔖, A 🔖

    ● **S14.136**   Anterior cord syndrome at C6 level of cervical spinal cord A 🔖, A 🔖

    ● **S14.137**   Anterior cord syndrome at C7 level of cervical spinal cord A 🔖, A 🔖

    ● **S14.138**   Anterior cord syndrome at C8 level of cervical spinal cord A 🔖

    ● **S14.139**   Anterior cord syndrome at unspecified level of cervical spinal cord

● **S14.14**   Brown-Séquard syndrome of cervical spinal cord

    ● **S14.141**   Brown-Séquard syndrome at C1 level of cervical spinal cord A 🔖

    ● **S14.142**   Brown-Séquard syndrome at C2 level of cervical spinal cord A 🔖

    ● **S14.143**   Brown-Séquard syndrome at C3 level of cervical spinal cord A 🔖

    ● **S14.144**   Brown-Séquard syndrome at C4 level of cervical spinal cord A 🔖

    ● **S14.145**   Brown-Séquard syndrome at C5 level of cervical spinal cord A 🔖

    ● **S14.146**   Brown-Séquard syndrome at C6 level of cervical spinal cord A 🔖

    ● **S14.147**   Brown-Séquard syndrome at C7 level of cervical spinal cord A 🔖

    ● **S14.148**   Brown-Séquard syndrome at C8 level of cervical spinal cord A 🔖

    ● **S14.149**   Brown-Séquard syndrome at unspecified level of cervical spinal cord

● **S14.15**   Other incomplete lesions of cervical spinal cord
     Incomplete lesion of cervical spinal cord NOS
     Posterior cord syndrome of cervical spinal cord

    ● **S14.151**   Other incomplete lesion at C1 level of cervical spinal cord A 🔖, A 🔖

    ● **S14.152**   Other incomplete lesion at C2 level of cervical spinal cord A 🔖, A 🔖

    ● **S14.153**   Other incomplete lesion at C3 level of cervical spinal cord A 🔖, A 🔖

    ● **S14.154**   Other incomplete lesion at C4 level of cervical spinal cord A 🔖, A 🔖

    ● **S14.155**   Other incomplete lesion at C5 level of cervical spinal cord A 🔖, A 🔖

    ● **S14.156**   Other incomplete lesion at C6 level of cervical spinal cord A 🔖, A 🔖

    ● **S14.157**   Other incomplete lesion at C7 level of cervical spinal cord A 🔖, A 🔖

    ● **S14.158**   Other incomplete lesion at C8 level of cervical spinal cord A 🔖

    ● **S14.159**   Other incomplete lesion at unspecified level of cervical spinal cord

X ● **S14.2**   Injury of nerve root of cervical spine

X ● **S14.3**   Injury of brachial plexus

X ● **S14.4**   Injury of peripheral nerves of neck

X ● **S14.5**   Injury of cervical sympathetic nerves

X ● **S14.8**   Injury of other specified nerves of neck

X ● **S14.9**   Injury of unspecified nerves of neck

● **S15**   **Injury of blood vessels at neck level**
     Code also any associated open wound (S11.-)
     The appropriate 7th character is to be added to each code from category S15

     | | |
     A   initial encounter
     D   subsequent encounter
     S   sequela

   ● **S15.0**   Injury of carotid artery of neck
     Injury of carotid artery (common) (external) (internal, extracranial portion)
     Injury of carotid artery NOS

     Excludes1   injury of internal carotid artery, intracranial portion (S06.8)

     (Ex) For category S15.0 CC codes: See PDX Collection 1167

    ● **S15.00**   Unspecified injury of carotid artery

      ● **S15.001**   Unspecified injury of right carotid artery A 🔖

      ● **S15.002**   Unspecified injury of left carotid artery A 🔖

      ● **S15.009**   Unspecified injury of unspecified carotid artery A 🔖

    ● **S15.01**   Minor laceration of carotid artery
     Incomplete transection of carotid artery
     Laceration of carotid artery NOS
     Superficial laceration of carotid artery

      ● **S15.011**   Minor laceration of right carotid artery A 🔖

      ● **S15.012**   Minor laceration of left carotid artery A 🔖

      ● **S15.019**   Minor laceration of unspecified carotid artery A 🔖

    ● **S15.02**   Major laceration of carotid artery
     Complete transection of carotid artery
     Traumatic rupture of carotid artery

      ● **S15.021**   Major laceration of right carotid artery A 🔖

      ● **S15.022**   Major laceration of left carotid artery A 🔖

      ● **S15.029**   Major laceration of unspecified carotid artery A 🔖

    ● **S15.09**   Other specified injury of carotid artery

      ● **S15.091**   Other specified injury of right carotid artery A 🔖

      ● **S15.092**   Other specified injury of left carotid artery A 🔖

      ● **S15.099**   Other specified injury of unspecified carotid artery A 🔖

▶ New   ⇒ Revised   ~~deleted~~ Deleted   Excludes 1   Excludes 2   Includes   Use additional   Code first   Code also   Key words
OGCR Official Guidelines   ● Unacceptable Principal Diagnosis   X Assign placeholder X   ● Use Additional Character(s)   ▶ Manifestation Code   **Coding Clinic**

● **S15.1**   **Injury of vertebral artery**
    (Ex:) **For category S15.1 CC codes:** See PDX Collection 1157
  ● **S15.10**   **Unspecified injury of vertebral artery**
    ● **S15.101**   Unspecified injury of **right vertebral artery** A (⬡)
    ● **S15.102**   Unspecified injury of **left vertebral artery** A (⬡)
    ● **S15.109**   Unspecified injury of **unspecified vertebral artery** A (⬡)
  ● **S15.11**   **Minor laceration of vertebral artery**
    Incomplete transection of vertebral artery
    Laceration of vertebral artery NOS
    Superficial laceration of vertebral artery
    ● **S15.111**   Minor laceration of **right vertebral artery** A (⬡)
    ● **S15.112**   Minor laceration of **left vertebral artery** A (⬡)
    ● **S15.119**   Minor laceration of **unspecified vertebral artery** A (⬡)
  ● **S15.12**   **Major laceration of vertebral artery**
    Complete transection of vertebral artery
    Traumatic rupture of vertebral artery
    ● **S15.121**   Major laceration of **right vertebral artery** A (⬡)
    ● **S15.122**   Major laceration of **left vertebral artery** A (⬡)
    ● **S15.129**   Major laceration of **unspecified vertebral artery** A (⬡)
  ● **S15.19**   **Other specified injury of vertebral artery**
    ● **S15.191**   Other specified injury of **right vertebral artery** A (⬡)
    ● **S15.192**   Other specified injury of **left vertebral artery** A (⬡)
    ● **S15.199**   Other specified injury of **unspecified vertebral artery** A (⬡)

● **S15.2**   **Injury of external jugular vein**
    (Ex:) **For category S15.2 CC codes:** See PDX Collection 1157
  ● **S15.20**   **Unspecified injury of external jugular vein**
    ● **S15.201**   Unspecified injury of **right external jugular vein** A (⬡)
    ● **S15.202**   Unspecified injury of **left external jugular vein** A (⬡)
    ● **S15.209**   Unspecified injury of **unspecified external jugular vein** A (⬡)
  ● **S15.21**   **Minor laceration of external jugular vein**
    Incomplete transection of external jugular vein
    Laceration of external jugular vein NOS
    Superficial laceration of external jugular vein
    ● **S15.211**   Minor laceration of **right external jugular vein** A (⬡)
    ● **S15.212**   Minor laceration of **left external jugular vein** A (⬡)
    ● **S15.219**   Minor laceration of **unspecified external jugular vein** A (⬡)
  ● **S15.22**   **Major laceration of external jugular vein**
    Complete transection of external jugular vein
    Traumatic rupture of external jugular vein
    ● **S15.221**   Major laceration of **right external jugular vein** A (⬡)
    ● **S15.222**   Major laceration of **left external jugular vein** A (⬡)
    ● **S15.229**   Major laceration of **unspecified external jugular vein** A (⬡)

  ● **S15.29**   **Other specified injury of external jugular vein**
    ● **S15.291**   Other specified injury of **right external jugular vein** A (⬡)
    ● **S15.292**   Other specified injury of **left external jugular vein** A (⬡)
    ● **S15.299**   Other specified injury of **unspecified external jugular vein** A (⬡)

● **S15.3**   **Injury of internal jugular vein**
    (Ex:) **For category S15.3 CC codes:** See PDX Collection 1157
  ● **S15.30**   **Unspecified injury of internal jugular vein**
    ● **S15.301**   Unspecified injury of **right internal jugular vein** A (⬡)
    ● **S15.302**   Unspecified injury of **left internal jugular vein** A (⬡)
    ● **S15.309**   Unspecified injury of **unspecified internal jugular vein** A (⬡)
  ● **S15.31**   **Minor laceration of internal jugular vein**
    Incomplete transection of internal jugular vein
    Laceration of internal jugular vein NOS
    Superficial laceration of internal jugular vein
    ● **S15.311**   Minor laceration of **right internal jugular vein** A (⬡)
    ● **S15.312**   Minor laceration of **left internal jugular vein** A (⬡)
    ● **S15.319**   Minor laceration of **unspecified internal jugular vein** A (⬡)
  ● **S15.32**   **Major laceration of internal jugular vein**
    Complete transection of internal jugular vein
    Traumatic rupture of internal jugular vein
    ● **S15.321**   Major laceration of **right internal jugular vein** A (⬡)
    ● **S15.322**   Major laceration of **left internal jugular vein** A (⬡)
    ● **S15.329**   Major laceration of **unspecified internal jugular vein** A (⬡)
  ● **S15.39**   **Other specified injury of internal jugular vein**
    ● **S15.391**   Other specified injury of **right internal jugular vein** A (⬡)
    ● **S15.392**   Other specified injury of **left internal jugular vein** A (⬡)
    ● **S15.399**   Other specified injury of **unspecified internal jugular vein** A (⬡)

X● **S15.8**   **Injury of other specified blood vessels at neck level** A (⬡)
    (Ex:) See PDX Collection 1157
X● **S15.9**   **Injury of unspecified blood vessel at neck level** A (⬡)
    (Ex:) See PDX Collection 1157

● **S16**   **Injury of muscle, fascia and tendon at neck level**
    Code also any associated open wound (S11.-)
    Excludes2   sprain of joint or ligament at neck level (S13.9)
    The appropriate 7th character is to be added to each code from category S16

A	initial encounter
D	subsequent encounter
S	sequela

X● **S16.1**   **Strain of muscle, fascia and tendon at neck level**
X● **S16.2**   **Laceration of muscle, fascia and tendon at neck level**
X● **S16.8**   **Other specified injury of muscle, fascia and tendon at neck level**
X● **S16.9**   **Unspecified injury of muscle, fascia and tendon at neck level**

CHAPTER 19 (S00-T88)

● **S17**   **Crushing injury of neck**

> Use additional code for all associated injuries, such as:
> injury of blood vessels (S15.-)
> open wound of neck (S11.-)
> spinal cord injury (S14.0, S14.1-)
> vertebral fracture (S12.0--S12.3-)

> The appropriate 7th character is to be added to each code from category S17

> | A | initial encounter |
> |---|---|
> | D | subsequent encounter |
> | S | sequela |

> ⒺⓍ **For category S17 CC codes:** See PDX Collection 1156

X ● **S17.0**   Crushing injury of **larynx and trachea** A 🔹, A 🔹

X ● **S17.8**   Crushing injury of **other specified parts of neck** A 🔹, A 🔹

X ● **S17.9**   Crushing injury of neck, part **unspecified** A 🔹, A 🔹

● **S19**   **Other and unspecified injuries of neck**

> The appropriate 7th character is to be added to each code from category S19

> | A | initial encounter |
> |---|---|
> | D | subsequent encounter |
> | S | sequela |

●   **S19.8**   **Other specified injuries of neck**

    X ● **S19.80**   Other specified injuries of **unspecified** part of neck

    X ● **S19.81**   Other specified injuries of **larynx**

    X ● **S19.82**   Other specified injuries of **cervical trachea**

>   **Excludes2**   other specified injury of thoracic trachea (S27.5-)

    X ● **S19.83**   Other specified injuries of **vocal cord**

    X ● **S19.84**   Other specified injuries of **thyroid gland**

    X ● **S19.85**   Other specified injuries of **pharynx and cervical esophagus**

    X ● **S19.89**   Other specified injuries of other specified part of neck

X ● **S19.9**   **Unspecified injury of neck**

INJURIES TO THE THORAX (S20-S29)

Includes	injuries of breast
	injuries of chest (wall)
	injuries of interscapular area
Excludes2	burns and corrosions (T20-T32)
	effects of foreign body in bronchus (T17.5)
	effects of foreign body in esophagus (T18.1)
	effects of foreign body in lung (T17.8)
	effects of foreign body in trachea (T17.4)
	frostbite (T33-T34)
	injuries of axilla
	injuries of clavicle
	injuries of scapular region
	injuries of shoulder
	insect bite or sting, venomous (T63.4)

● **S20**   **Superficial injury of thorax**

> The appropriate 7th character is to be added to each code from category S20

> | A | initial encounter |
> |---|---|
> | D | subsequent encounter |
> | S | sequela |

●   **S20.0**   **Contusion of breast**

    X ● **S20.00**   Contusion of breast, **unspecified** breast

    X ● **S20.01**   Contusion of **right** breast

    X ● **S20.02**   Contusion of **left** breast

●   **S20.1**   **Other and unspecified superficial injuries of breast**

   ● **S20.10**   **Unspecified superficial injuries of breast**

     ● **S20.101**   Unspecified superficial injuries of breast, **right breast**

     ● **S20.102**   Unspecified superficial injuries of breast, **left breast**

     ● **S20.109**   Unspecified superficial injuries of breast, **unspecified breast**

   ● **S20.11**   **Abrasion of breast**

     ● **S20.111**   Abrasion of breast, **right breast**

     ● **S20.112**   Abrasion of breast, **left breast**

     ● **S20.119**   Abrasion of breast, **unspecified breast**

   ● **S20.12**   **Blister (nonthermal) of breast**

     ● **S20.121**   Blister (nonthermal) of breast, **right breast**

     ● **S20.122**   Blister (nonthermal) of breast, **left breast**

     ● **S20.129**   Blister (nonthermal) of breast, **unspecified breast**

   ● **S20.14**   **External constriction of part of breast**

     ● **S20.141**   External constriction of part of breast, **right breast**

     ● **S20.142**   External constriction of part of breast, **left breast**

     ● **S20.149**   External constriction of part of breast, **unspecified breast**

   ● **S20.15**   **Superficial foreign body of breast**
> Splinter in the breast

     ● **S20.151**   Superficial foreign body of breast, **right breast**

     ● **S20.152**   Superficial foreign body of breast, **left breast**

     ● **S20.159**   Superficial foreign body of breast, **unspecified breast**

   ● **S20.16**   **Insect bite (nonvenomous) of breast**

     ● **S20.161**   Insect bite (nonvenomous) of breast, **right breast**

     ● **S20.162**   Insect bite (nonvenomous) of breast, **left breast**

     ● **S20.169**   Insect bite (nonvenomous) of breast, **unspecified breast**

   ● **S20.17**   **Other superficial bite of breast**

>   **Excludes1**   open bite of breast (S21.05-)

     ● **S20.171**   Other superficial bite of breast, **right breast**

     ● **S20.172**   Other superficial bite of breast, **left breast**

     ● **S20.179**   Other superficial bite of breast, **unspecified breast**

●   **S20.2**   **Contusion of thorax**

   X ● **S20.20**   Contusion of thorax, **unspecified**

   ● **S20.21**   **Contusion of front wall of thorax**

     ● **S20.211**   Contusion of **right** front wall of thorax

     ● **S20.212**   Contusion of **left** front wall of thorax

     ● **S20.219**   Contusion of **unspecified** front wall of thorax

   ● **S20.22**   **Contusion of back wall of thorax**

     ● **S20.221**   Contusion of **right** back wall of thorax

     ● **S20.222**   Contusion of **left** back wall of thorax

     ● **S20.229**   Contusion of **unspecified** back wall of thorax

● **S20.3**   Other and unspecified superficial injuries of front wall of thorax
  ● **S20.30**   Unspecified superficial injuries of front wall of thorax
    ● **S20.301**   Unspecified superficial injuries of right front wall of thorax
    ● **S20.302**   Unspecified superficial injuries of left front wall of thorax
    ● **S20.309**   Unspecified superficial injuries of unspecified front wall of thorax
  ● **S20.31**   Abrasion of front wall of thorax
    ● **S20.311**   Abrasion of right front wall of thorax
    ● **S20.312**   Abrasion of left front wall of thorax
    ● **S20.319**   Abrasion of unspecified front wall of thorax
  ● **S20.32**   Blister (nonthermal) of front wall of thorax
    ● **S20.321**   Blister (nonthermal) of right front wall of thorax
    ● **S20.322**   Blister (nonthermal) of left front wall of thorax
    ● **S20.329**   Blister (nonthermal) of unspecified front wall of thorax
  ● **S20.34**   External constriction of front wall of thorax
    ● **S20.341**   External constriction of right front wall of thorax
    ● **S20.342**   External constriction of left front wall of thorax
    ● **S20.349**   External constriction of unspecified front wall of thorax
  ● **S20.35**   Superficial foreign body of front wall of thorax
     Splinter in front wall of thorax
    ● **S20.351**   Superficial foreign body of right front wall of thorax
    ● **S20.352**   Superficial foreign body of left front wall of thorax
    ● **S20.359**   Superficial foreign body of unspecified front wall of thorax
  ● **S20.36**   Insect bite (nonvenomous) of front wall of thorax
    ● **S20.361**   Insect bite (nonvenomous) of right front wall of thorax
    ● **S20.362**   Insect bite (nonvenomous) of left front wall of thorax
    ● **S20.369**   Insect bite (nonvenomous) of unspecified front wall of thorax
  ● **S20.37**   Other superficial bite of front wall of thorax
     Excludes1   open bite of front wall of thorax (S21.14)
    ● **S20.371**   Other superficial bite of right front wall of thorax
    ● **S20.372**   Other superficial bite of left front wall of thorax
    ● **S20.379**   Other superficial bite of unspecified front wall of thorax
● **S20.4**   Other and unspecified superficial injuries of back wall of thorax
  ● **S20.40**   Unspecified superficial injuries of back wall of thorax
    ● **S20.401**   Unspecified superficial injuries of right back wall of thorax
    ● **S20.402**   Unspecified superficial injuries of left back wall of thorax
    ● **S20.409**   Unspecified superficial injuries of unspecified back wall of thorax

● **S20.41**   Abrasion of back wall of thorax
  ● **S20.411**   Abrasion of right back wall of thorax
  ● **S20.412**   Abrasion of left back wall of thorax
  ● **S20.419**   Abrasion of unspecified back wall of thorax
● **S20.42**   Blister (nonthermal) of back wall of thorax
  ● **S20.421**   Blister (nonthermal) of right back wall of thorax
  ● **S20.422**   Blister (nonthermal) of left back wall of thorax
  ● **S20.429**   Blister (nonthermal) of unspecified back wall of thorax
● **S20.44**   External constriction of back wall of thorax
  ● **S20.441**   External constriction of right back wall of thorax
  ● **S20.442**   External constriction of left back wall of thorax
  ● **S20.449**   External constriction of unspecified back wall of thorax
● **S20.45**   Superficial foreign body of back wall of thorax
   Splinter of back wall of thorax
  ● **S20.451**   Superficial foreign body of right back wall of thorax
  ● **S20.452**   Superficial foreign body of left back wall of thorax
  ● **S20.459**   Superficial foreign body of unspecified back wall of thorax
● **S20.46**   Insect bite (nonvenomous) of back wall of thorax
  ● **S20.461**   Insect bite (nonvenomous) of right back wall of thorax
  ● **S20.462**   Insect bite (nonvenomous) of left back wall of thorax
  ● **S20.469**   Insect bite (nonvenomous) of unspecified back wall of thorax
● **S20.47**   Other superficial bite of back wall of thorax
   Excludes1   open bite of back wall of thorax (S21.24)
  ● **S20.471**   Other superficial bite of right back wall of thorax
  ● **S20.472**   Other superficial bite of left back wall of thorax
  ● **S20.479**   Other superficial bite of unspecified back wall of thorax
● **S20.9**   Superficial injury of unspecified parts of thorax
   Excludes1   contusion of thorax NOS (S20.20)
X ● **S20.90**   Unspecified superficial injury of unspecified parts of thorax
   Superficial injury of thoracic wall NOS
X ● **S20.91**   Abrasion of unspecified parts of thorax
X ● **S20.92**   Blister (nonthermal) of unspecified parts of thorax
X ● **S20.94**   External constriction of unspecified parts of thorax
X ● **S20.95**   Superficial foreign body of unspecified parts of thorax
   Splinter in thorax NOS
X ● **S20.96**   Insect bite (nonvenomous) of unspecified parts of thorax
X ● **S20.97**   Other superficial bite of unspecified parts of thorax
   Excludes1   open bite of thorax NOS (S21.95)

N Newborn Age: 0   **P** Pediatric Age: 0–17   **M** Maternity DX: 12–55   **A** Adult Age: 15–124   ♀ Females Only   ♂ Males Only

🅒 Complication\Comorbidity   🅜 Major C\C   (Ex) CC/MCC Exclusions   🅗 Hospital-Acquired Condition

1247

CHAPTER 19 (S00–T88)

Item 19–1   Pneumothorax is a collection of gas (positive air pressure) in the pleural space resulting in the lung collapsing. A **tension pneumothorax** is life-threatening and is a result of air in the pleural space causing a displacement in the mediastinal structures and cardiopulmonary function compromise. A **traumatic pneumothorax** results from blunt or penetrating injury that disrupts the parietal/visceral pleura. **Hemothorax** is blood or bloody fluid in the pleural cavity as a result of traumatic blood vessel rupture or inflammation of the lungs from pneumonia.

● **S21   Open wound of thorax**

> Code also any associated injury such as:
> injury of heart (S26.-)
> injury of intrathoracic organs (S27.-)
> rib fracture (S22.3-, S22.4-)
> spinal cord injury (S24.0-, S24.1-)
> traumatic hemothorax (S27.1)
> traumatic hemopneumothorax (S27.3)
> traumatic pneumothorax (S27.0)
> wound infection

> **Excludes1**   traumatic amputation (partial) of thorax (S28.1)

> The appropriate 7th character is to be added to each code from category S21

> | | |
> |---|---|
> | A | initial encounter |
> | D | subsequent encounter |
> | S | sequela |

● **S21.0   Open wound of breast**

   ● **S21.00   Unspecified** open wound of breast

      ● **S21.001   Unspecified** open wound of **right** breast

      ● **S21.002   Unspecified** open wound of **left** breast

      ● **S21.009   Unspecified** open wound of **unspecified** breast

   ● **S21.01   Laceration without foreign body** of breast

      ● **S21.011   Laceration without foreign body** of **right** breast

      ● **S21.012   Laceration without foreign body** of **left** breast

      ● **S21.019   Laceration without foreign body** of **unspecified** breast

   ● **S21.02   Laceration with foreign body** of breast

      ● **S21.021   Laceration with foreign body** of **right** breast

      ● **S21.022   Laceration with foreign body** of **left** breast

      ● **S21.029   Laceration with foreign body** of **unspecified** breast

   ● **S21.03   Puncture wound without foreign body** of breast

      ● **S21.031   Puncture wound without foreign body** of **right** breast

      ● **S21.032   Puncture wound without foreign body** of **left** breast

      ● **S21.039   Puncture wound without foreign body** of **unspecified** breast

   ● **S21.04   Puncture wound with foreign body** of breast

      ● **S21.041   Puncture wound with foreign body** of **right** breast

      ● **S21.042   Puncture wound with foreign body** of **left** breast

      ● **S21.049   Puncture wound with foreign body** of **unspecified** breast

   ● **S21.05   Open bite** of breast
      Bite of breast NOS

      Excludes1   superficial bite of breast (S20.17)

      ● **S21.051   Open bite** of **right** breast

      ● **S21.052   Open bite** of **left** breast

      ● **S21.059   Open bite** of **unspecified** breast

● **S21.1   Open wound of front wall of thorax without penetration into thoracic cavity**

> Open wound of chest without penetration into thoracic cavity

> (Ex) **For category S21.1 CC codes:** See PDX Collection 1168

   ● **S21.10   Unspecified** open wound of front wall of thorax **without penetration into thoracic cavity**

      ● **S21.101   Unspecified** open wound of **right** front wall of thorax without penetration into thoracic cavity A 🕭

      ● **S21.102   Unspecified** open wound of **left** front wall of thorax without penetration into thoracic cavity A 🕭

      ● **S21.109   Unspecified** open wound of **unspecified** front wall of thorax without penetration into thoracic cavity A 🕭

   ● **S21.11   Laceration without foreign body** of front wall of thorax without penetration into thoracic cavity

      ● **S21.111   Laceration without foreign body** of **right** front wall of thorax without penetration into thoracic cavity A 🕭

      ● **S21.112   Laceration without foreign body** of **left** front wall of thorax without penetration into thoracic cavity A 🕭

      ● **S21.119   Laceration without foreign body** of **unspecified** front wall of thorax without penetration into thoracic cavity A 🕭

   ● **S21.12   Laceration with foreign body** of front wall of thorax without penetration into thoracic cavity

      ● **S21.121   Laceration with foreign body** of **right** front wall of thorax without penetration into thoracic cavity A 🕭

      ● **S21.122   Laceration with foreign body** of **left** front wall of thorax without penetration into thoracic cavity A 🕭

      ● **S21.129   Laceration with foreign body** of **unspecified** front wall of thorax without penetration into thoracic cavity A 🕭

   ● **S21.13   Puncture wound without foreign body** of front wall of thorax without penetration into thoracic cavity

      ● **S21.131   Puncture wound without foreign body** of **right** front wall of thorax without penetration into thoracic cavity A 🕭

      ● **S21.132   Puncture wound without foreign body** of **left** front wall of thorax without penetration into thoracic cavity A 🕭

      ● **S21.139   Puncture wound without foreign body** of **unspecified** front wall of thorax without penetration into thoracic cavity A 🕭

   ● **S21.14   Puncture wound with foreign body** of front wall of thorax without penetration into thoracic cavity

      ● **S21.141   Puncture wound with foreign body** of **right** front wall of thorax without penetration into thoracic cavity A 🕭

      ● **S21.142   Puncture wound with foreign body** of **left** front wall of thorax without penetration into thoracic cavity A 🕭

      ● **S21.149   Puncture wound with foreign body** of **unspecified** front wall of thorax without penetration into thoracic cavity A 🕭

● **S21.15** **Open bite of front wall of thorax without penetration into thoracic cavity**
  Bite of front wall of thorax NOS

  Excludes1   superficial bite of front wall of thorax (S20.37)

  ● **S21.151** Open bite of right front wall of thorax without penetration into thoracic cavity A ✪

  ● **S21.152** Open bite of left front wall of thorax without penetration into thoracic cavity A ✪

  ● **S21.159** Open bite of unspecified front wall of thorax without penetration into thoracic cavity A ✪

● **S21.2** **Open wound of back wall of thorax without penetration into thoracic cavity**

  ● **S21.20** **Unspecified open wound of back wall of thorax without penetration into thoracic cavity**

    ● **S21.201** Unspecified open wound of right back wall of thorax without penetration into thoracic cavity

    ● **S21.202** Unspecified open wound of left back wall of thorax without penetration into thoracic cavity

    ● **S21.209** Unspecified open wound of unspecified back wall of thorax without penetration into thoracic cavity

  ● **S21.21** **Laceration without foreign body of back wall of thorax without penetration into thoracic cavity**

    ● **S21.211** Laceration without foreign body of right back wall of thorax without penetration into thoracic cavity

    ● **S21.212** Laceration without foreign body of left back wall of thorax without penetration into thoracic cavity

    ● **S21.219** Laceration without foreign body of unspecified back wall of thorax without penetration into thoracic cavity

  ● **S21.22** **Laceration with foreign body of back wall of thorax without penetration into thoracic cavity**

    ● **S21.221** Laceration with foreign body of right back wall of thorax without penetration into thoracic cavity

    ● **S21.222** Laceration with foreign body of left back wall of thorax without penetration into thoracic cavity

    ● **S21.229** Laceration with foreign body of unspecified back wall of thorax without penetration into thoracic cavity

  ● **S21.23** **Puncture wound without foreign body of back wall of thorax without penetration into thoracic cavity**

    ● **S21.231** Puncture wound without foreign body of right back wall of thorax without penetration into thoracic cavity

    ● **S21.232** Puncture wound without foreign body of left back wall of thorax without penetration into thoracic cavity

    ● **S21.239** Puncture wound without foreign body of unspecified back wall of thorax without penetration into thoracic cavity

● **S21.24** **Puncture wound with foreign body of back wall of thorax without penetration into thoracic cavity**

  ● **S21.241** Puncture wound with foreign body of right back wall of thorax without penetration into thoracic cavity

  ● **S21.242** Puncture wound with foreign body of left back wall of thorax without penetration into thoracic cavity

  ● **S21.249** Puncture wound with foreign body of unspecified back wall of thorax without penetration into thoracic cavity

● **S21.25** **Open bite of back wall of thorax without penetration into thoracic cavity**
  Bite of back wall of thorax NOS

  Excludes1   superficial bite of back wall of thorax (S20.47)

  ● **S21.251** Open bite of right back wall of thorax without penetration into thoracic cavity

  ● **S21.252** Open bite of left back wall of thorax without penetration into thoracic cavity

  ● **S21.259** Open bite of unspecified back wall of thorax without penetration into thoracic cavity

● **S21.3** **Open wound of front wall of thorax with penetration into thoracic cavity**
  Open wound of chest with penetration into thoracic cavity
  Ⓔ⅍ **For category S21.3 CC codes unless otherwise indicated:** See PDX Collection 1169

  ● **S21.30** **Unspecified open wound of front wall of thorax with penetration into thoracic cavity**

    ● **S21.301** Unspecified open wound of right front wall of thorax with penetration into thoracic cavity A ✪

    ● **S21.302** Unspecified open wound of left front wall of thorax with penetration into thoracic cavity A ✪

    ● **S21.309** Unspecified open wound of unspecified front wall of thorax with penetration into thoracic cavity A ✪
      Ⓔ⅍ See PDX Collection 1170

  ● **S21.31** **Laceration without foreign body of front wall of thorax with penetration into thoracic cavity**

    ● **S21.311** Laceration without foreign body of right front wall of thorax with penetration into thoracic cavity A ✪

    ● **S21.312** Laceration without foreign body of left front wall of thorax with penetration into thoracic cavity A ✪

    ● **S21.319** Laceration without foreign body of unspecified front wall of thorax with penetration into thoracic cavity A ✪

  ● **S21.32** **Laceration with foreign body of front wall of thorax with penetration into thoracic cavity**

    ● **S21.321** Laceration with foreign body of right front wall of thorax with penetration into thoracic cavity A ✪

    ● **S21.322** Laceration with foreign body of left front wall of thorax with penetration into thoracic cavity A ✪

    ● **S21.329** Laceration with foreign body of unspecified front wall of thorax with penetration into thoracic cavity A ✪

N Newborn Age: 0   **P** Pediatric Age: 0–17   **M** Maternity DX: 12–55   **A** Adult Age: 15–124   ♀ Females Only   ♂ Males Only

✪ Complication\Comorbidity   ✪ Major C\C   Ⓔ⅍ CC/MCC Exclusions   ✪ Hospital-Acquired Condition

1249

● **S21.33**   Puncture wound without foreign body of front wall of thorax with penetration into thoracic cavity

    ● **S21.331**   Puncture wound without foreign body of right front wall of thorax with penetration into thoracic cavity A 🐾

    ● **S21.332**   Puncture wound without foreign body of left front wall of thorax with penetration into thoracic cavity A 🐾

    ● **S21.339**   Puncture wound without foreign body of unspecified front wall of thorax with penetration into thoracic cavity A 🐾

● **S21.34**   Puncture wound with foreign body of front wall of thorax with penetration into thoracic cavity

    ● **S21.341**   Puncture wound with foreign body of right front wall of thorax with penetration into thoracic cavity A 🐾

    ● **S21.342**   Puncture wound with foreign body of left front wall of thorax with penetration into thoracic cavity A 🐾

    ● **S21.349**   Puncture wound with foreign body of unspecified front wall of thorax with penetration into thoracic cavity A 🐾

● **S21.35**   Open bite of front wall of thorax with penetration into thoracic cavity

    Excludes1   superficial bite of front wall of thorax (S20.37)

    ● **S21.351**   Open bite of right front wall of thorax with penetration into thoracic cavity A 🐾

    ● **S21.352**   Open bite of left front wall of thorax with penetration into thoracic cavity A 🐾

    ● **S21.359**   Open bite of unspecified front wall of thorax with penetration into thoracic cavity A 🐾

● **S21.4**   Open wound of back wall of thorax with penetration into thoracic cavity

    (Ex) For category S21.4 CC codes: See PDX Collection 1169

    ● **S21.40**   Unspecified open wound of back wall of thorax with penetration into thoracic cavity

      ● **S21.401**   Unspecified open wound of right back wall of thorax with penetration into thoracic cavity A 🐾

      ● **S21.402**   Unspecified open wound of left back wall of thorax with penetration into thoracic cavity A 🐾

      ● **S21.409**   Unspecified open wound of unspecified back wall of thorax with penetration into thoracic cavity A 🐾

    ● **S21.41**   Laceration without foreign body of back wall of thorax with penetration into thoracic cavity

      ● **S21.411**   Laceration without foreign body of right back wall of thorax with penetration into thoracic cavity A 🐾

      ● **S21.412**   Laceration without foreign body of left back wall of thorax with penetration into thoracic cavity A 🐾

      ● **S21.419**   Laceration without foreign body of unspecified back wall of thorax with penetration into thoracic cavity A 🐾

● **S21.42**   Laceration with foreign body of back wall of thorax with penetration into thoracic cavity

    ● **S21.421**   Laceration with foreign body of right back wall of thorax with penetration into thoracic cavity A 🐾

    ● **S21.422**   Laceration with foreign body of left back wall of thorax with penetration into thoracic cavity A 🐾

    ● **S21.429**   Laceration with foreign body of unspecified back wall of thorax with penetration into thoracic cavity A 🐾

● **S21.43**   Puncture wound without foreign body of back wall of thorax with penetration into thoracic cavity

    ● **S21.431**   Puncture wound without foreign body of right back wall of thorax with penetration into thoracic cavity A 🐾

    ● **S21.432**   Puncture wound without foreign body of left back wall of thorax with penetration into thoracic cavity A 🐾

    ● **S21.439**   Puncture wound without foreign body of unspecified back wall of thorax with penetration into thoracic cavity A 🐾

● **S21.44**   Puncture wound with foreign body of back wall of thorax with penetration into thoracic cavity

    ● **S21.441**   Puncture wound with foreign body of right back wall of thorax with penetration into thoracic cavity A 🐾

    ● **S21.442**   Puncture wound with foreign body of left back wall of thorax with penetration into thoracic cavity A 🐾

    ● **S21.449**   Puncture wound with foreign body of unspecified back wall of thorax with penetration into thoracic cavity A 🐾

● **S21.45**   Open bite of back wall of thorax with penetration into thoracic cavity

    Bite of back wall of thorax NOS

    Excludes1   superficial bite of back wall of thorax (S20.47)

    ● **S21.451**   Open bite of right back wall of thorax with penetration into thoracic cavity A 🐾

    ● **S21.452**   Open bite of left back wall of thorax with penetration into thoracic cavity A 🐾

    ● **S21.459**   Open bite of unspecified back wall of thorax with penetration into thoracic cavity A 🐾

● **S21.9**   Open wound of unspecified part of thorax

    Open wound of thoracic wall NOS

    (Ex) For category S21.9 CC codes: See PDX Collection 1168

X ● **S21.90**   Unspecified open wound of unspecified part of thorax A 🐾

X ● **S21.91**   Laceration without foreign body of unspecified part of thorax A 🐾

X ● **S21.92**   Laceration with foreign body of unspecified part of thorax A 🐾

X ● **S21.93**   Puncture wound without foreign body of unspecified part of thorax A 🐾

X ● **S21.94**   Puncture wound with foreign body of unspecified part of thorax A 🐾

X ● **S21.95**   Open bite of unspecified part of thorax A 🐾

    Excludes1   superficial bite of thorax (S20.97)

CHAPTER 19 (S00–T88)

▶ New   ⇒ Revised   ~~deleted~~ Deleted   Excludes 1   Excludes 2   Includes   Use additional   Code first   Code also   Key words

OGCR Official Guidelines   ● Unacceptable Principal Diagnosis   X Assign placeholder X   ● Use Additional Character(s)   ▶ Manifestation Code   **Coding Clinic**

● **S22   Fracture of rib(s), sternum and thoracic spine**

Note: A fracture not indicated as displaced or nondisplaced should be coded to displaced

A fracture not indicated as open or closed should be coded to closed

Includes   fracture of thoracic neural arch
fracture of thoracic spinous process
fracture of thoracic transverse process
fracture of thoracic vertebra
fracture of thoracic vertebral arch

Code first any associated:
injury of intrathoracic organ (S27.-)
spinal cord injury (S24.0-, S24.1-)

Excludes1   transection of thorax (S28.1)

Excludes2   fracture of clavicle (S42.0-)
fracture of scapula (S42.1-)

The appropriate 7th character is to be added to each code from category S22

> A   initial encounter for closed fracture
> B   initial encounter for open fracture
> D   subsequent encounter for fracture with routine healing
> G   subsequent encounter for fracture with delayed healing
> K   subsequent encounter for fracture with nonunion
> S   sequela

● **S22.0   Fracture of thoracic vertebra**
(Ex) **For category S22.0 CC codes S22.0[A,B]:** See PDX Collection 1171
For S22.0[K]: See PDX Collection 897

● **S22.00   Fracture of unspecified thoracic vertebra**
● **S22.000   Wedge compression** fracture of unspecified thoracic vertebra A, K 🖤, B 🖤, A, B 🖤
● **S22.001   Stable burst fracture** of unspecified thoracic vertebra A, K 🖤, B 🖤, A, B 🖤
● **S22.002   Unstable burst fracture** of unspecified thoracic vertebra A, K 🖤, B 🖤, A, B 🖤
● **S22.008   Other fracture** of unspecified thoracic vertebra A, K 🖤, B 🖤, A, B 🖤
● **S22.009   Unspecified fracture** of unspecified thoracic vertebra A, K 🖤, B 🖤, A, B 🖤

● **S22.01   Fracture of first thoracic vertebra**
● **S22.010   Wedge compression** fracture of first thoracic vertebra A, K 🖤, B 🖤, A, B 🖤
● **S22.011   Stable burst fracture** of first thoracic vertebra A, K 🖤, B 🖤, A, B 🖤
● **S22.012   Unstable burst fracture** of first thoracic vertebra A, K 🖤, B 🖤, A, B 🖤
● **S22.018   Other fracture** of first thoracic vertebra A, K 🖤, B 🖤, A, B 🖤
● **S22.019   Unspecified fracture** of first thoracic vertebra A, K 🖤, B 🖤, A, B 🖤

● **S22.02   Fracture of second thoracic vertebra**
● **S22.020   Wedge compression** fracture of second thoracic vertebra A, K 🖤, B 🖤, A, B 🖤
● **S22.021   Stable burst fracture** of second thoracic vertebra A, K 🖤, B 🖤, A, B 🖤

● **S22.022   Unstable burst fracture** of second thoracic vertebra A, K 🖤, B 🖤, A, B 🖤
● **S22.028   Other fracture** of second thoracic vertebra A, K 🖤, B 🖤, A, B 🖤
● **S22.029   Unspecified fracture** of second thoracic vertebra A, K 🖤, B 🖤, A, B 🖤

● **S22.03   Fracture of third thoracic vertebra**
● **S22.030   Wedge compression** fracture of third thoracic vertebra A, K 🖤, B 🖤, A, B 🖤
● **S22.031   Stable burst fracture** of third thoracic vertebra A, K 🖤, B 🖤, A, B 🖤
● **S22.032   Unstable burst fracture** of third thoracic vertebra A, K 🖤, B 🖤, A, B 🖤
● **S22.038   Other fracture** of third thoracic vertebra A, K 🖤, B 🖤, A, B 🖤
● **S22.039   Unspecified fracture** of third thoracic vertebra A, K 🖤, B 🖤, A, B 🖤

● **S22.04   Fracture of fourth thoracic vertebra**
● **S22.040   Wedge compression** fracture of fourth thoracic vertebra A, K 🖤, B 🖤, A, B 🖤
● **S22.041   Stable burst fracture** of fourth thoracic vertebra A, K 🖤, B 🖤, A, B 🖤
● **S22.042   Unstable burst fracture** of fourth thoracic vertebra A, K 🖤, B 🖤, A, B 🖤
● **S22.048   Other fracture** of fourth thoracic vertebra A, K 🖤, B 🖤, A, B 🖤
● **S22.049   Unspecified fracture** of fourth thoracic vertebra A, K 🖤, B 🖤, A, B 🖤

● **S22.05   Fracture of T5-T6 vertebra**
● **S22.050   Wedge compression** fracture of T5-T6 vertebra A, K 🖤, B 🖤, A, B 🖤
● **S22.051   Stable burst fracture** of T5-T6 vertebra A, K 🖤, B 🖤, A, B 🖤
● **S22.052   Unstable burst fracture** of T5-T6 vertebra A, K 🖤, B 🖤, A, B 🖤
● **S22.058   Other fracture** of T5-T6 vertebra A, K 🖤, B 🖤, A, B 🖤
● **S22.059   Unspecified fracture** of T5-T6 vertebra A, K 🖤, B 🖤, A, B 🖤

● **S22.06   Fracture of T7-T8 vertebra**
● **S22.060   Wedge compression** fracture of T7-T8 vertebra A, K 🖤, B 🖤, A, B 🖤
● **S22.061   Stable burst fracture** of T7-T8 vertebra A, K 🖤, B 🖤, A, B 🖤
● **S22.062   Unstable burst fracture** of T7-T8 vertebra A, K 🖤, B 🖤, A, B 🖤
● **S22.068   Other fracture** of T7-T8 thoracic vertebra A, K 🖤, B 🖤, A, B 🖤
● **S22.069   Unspecified fracture** of T7-T8 vertebra A, K 🖤, B 🖤, A, B 🖤

● **S22.07**   Fracture of T9-T10 vertebra
  ● **S22.070**   Wedge compression fracture of T9-T10 vertebra A, K 🖐, B 🖐, A, B 🖐
  ● **S22.071**   Stable burst fracture of T9-T10 vertebra A, K 🖐, B 🖐, A, B 🖐
  ● **S22.072**   Unstable burst fracture of T9-T10 vertebra A, K 🖐, B 🖐, A, B 🖐
  ● **S22.078**   Other fracture of T9-T10 vertebra A, K 🖐, B 🖐, A, B 🖐
  ● **S22.079**   Unspecified fracture of T9-T10 vertebra A, K 🖐, B 🖐, A, B 🖐

● **S22.08**   Fracture of T11-T12 vertebra
  ● **S22.080**   Wedge compression fracture of T11-T12 vertebra A, K 🖐, B 🖐, A, B 🖐
  ● **S22.081**   Stable burst fracture of T11-T12 vertebra A, K 🖐, B 🖐, A, B 🖐
  ● **S22.082**   Unstable burst fracture of T11-T12 vertebra A, K 🖐, B 🖐, A, B 🖐
  ● **S22.088**   Other fracture of T11-T12 vertebra A, K 🖐, B 🖐, A, B 🖐
  ● **S22.089**   Unspecified fracture of T11-T12 vertebra A, K 🖐, B 🖐, A, B 🖐

● **S22.2**   Fracture of sternum
  (Ex) For category S22.2 CC codes S22.2[A,B]: See PDX Collection 1172
  For S22.2[K]: See PDX Collection 897

X ● **S22.20**   Unspecified fracture of sternum A, K 🖐, B 🖐, A, B 🖐
X ● **S22.21**   Fracture of manubrium A, K 🖐, B 🖐, A, B 🖐
X ● **S22.22**   Fracture of body of sternum A, K 🖐, B 🖐, A, B 🖐
X ● **S22.23**   Sternal manubrial dissociation A, K 🖐, B 🖐, A, B 🖐
X ● **S22.24**   Fracture of xiphoid process A, K 🖐, B 🖐, A, B 🖐

● **S22.3**   Fracture of one rib
  (Ex) For category S22.3 CC codes S22.3[A]: See PDX Collection 1173
  For S22.3[B]: See PDX Collection 1174 For S22.3[K]: See PDX Collection 897

X ● **S22.31**   Fracture of one rib, right side A, K 🖐, B 🖐, A, B 🖐
X ● **S22.32**   Fracture of one rib, left side A, K 🖐, B 🖐, A, B 🖐
X ● **S22.39**   Fracture of one rib, unspecified side A, K 🖐, B 🖐, A, B 🖐

● **S22.4**   Multiple fractures of ribs
  Fractures of two or more ribs
  Excludes1   flail chest (S22.5-)
  (Ex) For category S22.4 CC codes S22.4[A,B]: See PDX Collection 1174
  For S22.49[B]: No exclusions For S22.4[K]: See PDX Collection 897

X ● **S22.41**   Multiple fractures of ribs, right side A, K 🖐, B 🖐, A, B 🖐
X ● **S22.42**   Multiple fractures of ribs, left side A, K 🖐, B 🖐, A, B 🖐
X ● **S22.43**   Multiple fractures of ribs, bilateral A, K 🖐, B 🖐, A, B 🖐
X ● **S22.49**   Multiple fractures of ribs, unspecified side A, K 🖐, B 🖐, A, B 🖐

X ● **S22.5**   Flail chest K 🖐, A, B 🖐, A, B 🖐
  Unstable chest due to sternum and/or rib fracture
  (Ex) For category S22.5 CC codes S22.5[A,B]: See PDX Collection 1175
  For S22.5[K]: See PDX Collection 897

X ● **S22.9**   Fracture of bony thorax, part unspecified A, K 🖐, B 🖐, A, B 🖐
  (Ex) For category S22.9 CC codes S22.9[A,B]: See PDX Collection 1176
  For S22.9[K]: See PDX Collection 897

● **S23**   Dislocation and sprain of joints and ligaments of thorax
  Includes   avulsion of joint or ligament of thorax
     laceration of cartilage, joint or ligament of thorax
     sprain of cartilage, joint or ligament of thorax
     traumatic hemarthrosis of joint or ligament of thorax
     traumatic rupture of joint or ligament of thorax
     traumatic subluxation of joint or ligament of thorax
     traumatic tear of joint or ligament of thorax
  Code also any associated open wound
  Excludes2   dislocation, sprain of sternoclavicular joint (S43.2, S43.6)
     strain of muscle or tendon of thorax (S29.01-)
  The appropriate 7th character is to be added to each code from category S23

> A   initial encounter
> D   subsequent encounter
> S   sequela

X ● **S23.0**   Traumatic rupture of thoracic intervertebral disc
  Excludes1   rupture or displacement (nontraumatic) of thoracic intervertebral disc NOS (M51.- with fifth character 4)

● **S23.1**   Subluxation and dislocation of thoracic vertebra
  Code also any associated
     open wound of thorax (S21.-)
     spinal cord injury (S24.0-, S24.1-)
  Excludes2   fracture of thoracic vertebrae (S22.0-)

  ● **S23.10**   Subluxation and dislocation of unspecified thoracic vertebra
    ● **S23.100**   Subluxation of unspecified thoracic vertebra
    ● **S23.101**   Dislocation of unspecified thoracic vertebra

  ● **S23.11**   Subluxation and dislocation of T1/T2 thoracic vertebra
    ● **S23.110**   Subluxation of T1/T2 thoracic vertebra
    ● **S23.111**   Dislocation of T1/T2 thoracic vertebra

  ● **S23.12**   Subluxation and dislocation of T2/T3-T3/T4 thoracic vertebra
    ● **S23.120**   Subluxation of T2/T3 thoracic vertebra
    ● **S23.121**   Dislocation of T2/T3 thoracic vertebra
    ● **S23.122**   Subluxation of T3/T4 thoracic vertebra
    ● **S23.123**   Dislocation of T3/T4 thoracic vertebra

  ● **S23.13**   Subluxation and dislocation of T4/T5-T5/T6 thoracic vertebra
    ● **S23.130**   Subluxation of T4/T5 thoracic vertebra
    ● **S23.131**   Dislocation of T4/T5 thoracic vertebra
    ● **S23.132**   Subluxation of T5/T6 thoracic vertebra
    ● **S23.133**   Dislocation of T5/T6 thoracic vertebra

  ● **S23.14**   Subluxation and dislocation of T6/T7-T7/T8 thoracic vertebra
    ● **S23.140**   Subluxation of T6/T7 thoracic vertebra
    ● **S23.141**   Dislocation of T6/T7 thoracic vertebra
    ● **S23.142**   Subluxation of T7/T8 thoracic vertebra
    ● **S23.143**   Dislocation of T7/T8 thoracic vertebra

▶ New   ⇒ Revised   ~~deleted~~ Deleted   Excludes 1   Excludes 2   Includes   Use additional   Code first   Code also   Key words
OGCR Official Guidelines   ● Unacceptable Principal Diagnosis   X Assign placeholder X   ● Use Additional Character(s)   ▶ Manifestation Code   Coding Clinic

● S23.15   Subluxation and dislocation of T8/T9-T9/T10 thoracic vertebra
  ● S23.150   **Subluxation of T8/T9 thoracic vertebra**
  ● S23.151   **Dislocation of T8/T9 thoracic vertebra**
  ● S23.152   **Subluxation of T9/T10 thoracic vertebra**
  ● S23.153   **Dislocation of T9/T10 thoracic vertebra**
● S23.16   Subluxation and dislocation of T10/T11-T11/T12 thoracic vertebra
  ● S23.160   **Subluxation of T10/T11 thoracic vertebra**
  ● S23.161   **Dislocation of T10/T11 thoracic vertebra**
  ● S23.162   **Subluxation of T11/T12 thoracic vertebra**
  ● S23.163   **Dislocation of T11/T12 thoracic vertebra**
● S23.17   Subluxation and dislocation of T12/L1 thoracic vertebra
  ● S23.170   **Subluxation of T12/L1 thoracic vertebra**
  ● S23.171   **Dislocation of T12/L1 thoracic vertebra**

● S23.2   Dislocation of other and unspecified parts of thorax
  X● S23.20   **Dislocation of unspecified part of thorax**
  X● S23.29   **Dislocation of other parts of thorax**
X● S23.3   Sprain of ligaments of thoracic spine
● S23.4   Sprain of ribs and sternum
  X● S23.41   **Sprain of ribs**
  ● S23.42   **Sprain of sternum**
    ● S23.420   Sprain of sternoclavicular (joint) (ligament)
    ● S23.421   Sprain of chondrosternal joint
    ● S23.428   Other sprain of sternum
    ● S23.429   Unspecified sprain of sternum
X● S23.8   Sprain of other specified parts of thorax
X● S23.9   Sprain of unspecified parts of thorax

● S24   Injury of nerves and spinal cord at thorax level

Note: Code to highest level of thoracic spinal cord injury.

Injuries to the spinal cord (S24.0 and S24.1) refer to the cord level and not bone level injury, and can affect nerve roots at and below the level given.

Code also any associated:
  fracture of thoracic vertebra (S22.0-)
  open wound of thorax (S21.-)
  transient paralysis (R29.5)

Excludes2   injury of brachial plexus (S14.3)

The appropriate 7th character is to be added to each code from category S24

  A   initial encounter
  D   subsequent encounter
  S   sequela

(Ex) **For category S24 CC codes:** See PDX Collection 1177

X● S24.0   Concussion and edema of thoracic spinal cord A 🐾
● S24.1   Other and unspecified injuries of thoracic spinal cord
  ● S24.10   Unspecified injury of thoracic spinal cord
    ● S24.101   Unspecified injury at T1 level of thoracic spinal cord A 🐾, A 🐾
    ● S24.102   Unspecified injury at T2-T6 level of thoracic spinal cord A 🐾, A 🐾
    ● S24.103   Unspecified injury at T7-T10 level of thoracic spinal cord A 🐾, A 🐾

    ● S24.104   Unspecified injury at T11-T12 level of thoracic spinal cord A 🐾, A 🐾
    ● S24.109   Unspecified injury at unspecified level of thoracic spinal cord
                Injury of thoracic spinal cord NOS
● S24.11   Complete lesion of thoracic spinal cord
    ● S24.111   Complete lesion at T1 level of thoracic spinal cord A 🐾, A 🐾
    ● S24.112   Complete lesion at T2-T6 level of thoracic spinal cord A 🐾, A 🐾
    ● S24.113   Complete lesion at T7-T10 level of thoracic spinal cord A 🐾, A 🐾
    ● S24.114   Complete lesion at T11-T12 level of thoracic spinal cord A 🐾, A 🐾
    ● S24.119   Complete lesion at unspecified level of thoracic spinal cord
● S24.13   Anterior cord syndrome of thoracic spinal cord
    ● S24.131   Anterior cord syndrome at T1 level of thoracic spinal cord A 🐾, A 🐾
    ● S24.132   Anterior cord syndrome at T2-T6 level of thoracic spinal cord A 🐾, A 🐾
    ● S24.133   Anterior cord syndrome at T7-T10 level of thoracic spinal cord A 🐾, A 🐾
    ● S24.134   Anterior cord syndrome at T11-T12 level of thoracic spinal cord A 🐾, A 🐾
    ● S24.139   Anterior cord syndrome at unspecified level of thoracic spinal cord
● S24.14   Brown-Séquard syndrome of thoracic spinal cord
    ● S24.141   Brown-Séquard syndrome at T1 level of thoracic spinal cord A 🐾
    ● S24.142   Brown-Séquard syndrome at T2-T6 level of thoracic spinal cord A 🐾
    ● S24.143   Brown-Séquard syndrome at T7-T10 level of thoracic spinal cord A 🐾
    ● S24.144   Brown-Séquard syndrome at T11-T12 level of thoracic spinal cord A 🐾
    ● S24.149   Brown-Séquard syndrome at unspecified level of thoracic spinal cord
● S24.15   Other incomplete lesions of thoracic spinal cord
            Incomplete lesion of thoracic spinal cord NOS
            Posterior cord syndrome of thoracic spinal cord
    ● S24.151   Other incomplete lesion at T1 level of thoracic spinal cord A 🐾, A 🐾
    ● S24.152   Other incomplete lesion at T2-T6 level of thoracic spinal cord A 🐾, A 🐾
    ● S24.153   Other incomplete lesion at T7-T10 level of thoracic spinal cord A 🐾, A 🐾
    ● S24.154   Other incomplete lesion at T11-T12 level of thoracic spinal cord A 🐾, A 🐾
    ● S24.159   Other incomplete lesion at unspecified level of thoracic spinal cord

X● S24.2   Injury of nerve root of thoracic spine
X● S24.3   Injury of peripheral nerves of thorax
X● S24.4   Injury of thoracic sympathetic nervous system
            Injury of cardiac plexus
            Injury of esophageal plexus
            Injury of pulmonary plexus
            Injury of stellate ganglion
            Injury of thoracic sympathetic ganglion
X● S24.8   Injury of other specified nerves of thorax
X● S24.9   Injury of unspecified nerve of thorax

N Newborn Age: 0   **P** Pediatric Age: 0–17   **M** Maternity DX: 12–55   **A** Adult Age: 15–124   ♀ Females Only   ♂ Males Only

🐾 Complication\Comorbidity   🐾 Major C\C   (Ex) CC/MCC Exclusions   🐾 Hospital-Acquired Condition

1253

CHAPTER 19 (S00-T88)

● **S25   Injury of blood vessels of thorax**

The appropriate 7th character is to be added to each code from category S25

A	initial encounter
D	subsequent encounter
S	sequela

Code also any associated open wound (S21.-)

● **S25.0   Injury of thoracic aorta**

Injury of aorta NOS

(Ex) For category S25.0 CC codes: See PDX Collection 1178

X● **S25.00   Unspecified injury of thoracic aorta** A 🔖

X● **S25.01   Minor laceration of thoracic aorta** A 🔖

Incomplete transection of thoracic aorta

Laceration of thoracic aorta NOS

Superficial laceration of thoracic aorta

X● **S25.02   Major laceration of thoracic aorta** A 🔖

Complete transection of thoracic aorta

Traumatic rupture of thoracic aorta

X● **S25.09   Other specified injury of thoracic aorta** A 🔖

● **S25.1   Injury of innominate or subclavian artery**

(Ex) For category S25.1 CC codes: See PDX Collection 1179

● **S25.10   Unspecified injury of innominate or subclavian artery**

● **S25.101   Unspecified injury of right innominate or subclavian artery** A 🔖

● **S25.102   Unspecified injury of left innominate or subclavian artery** A 🔖

● **S25.109   Unspecified injury of unspecified innominate or subclavian artery** A 🔖

● **S25.11   Minor laceration of innominate or subclavian artery**

Incomplete transection of innominate or subclavian artery

Laceration of innominate or subclavian artery NOS

Superficial laceration of innominate or subclavian artery

● **S25.111   Minor laceration of right innominate or subclavian artery** A 🔖

● **S25.112   Minor laceration of left innominate or subclavian artery** A 🔖

● **S25.119   Minor laceration of unspecified innominate or subclavian artery** A 🔖

● **S25.12   Major laceration of innominate or subclavian artery**

Complete transection of innominate or subclavian artery

Traumatic rupture of innominate or subclavian artery

● **S25.121   Major laceration of right innominate or subclavian artery** A 🔖

● **S25.122   Major laceration of left innominate or subclavian artery** A 🔖

● **S25.129   Major laceration of unspecified innominate or subclavian artery** A 🔖

● **S25.19   Other specified injury of innominate or subclavian artery**

● **S25.191   Other specified injury of right innominate or subclavian artery** A 🔖

● **S25.192   Other specified injury of left innominate or subclavian artery** A 🔖

● **S25.199   Other specified injury of unspecified innominate or subclavian artery** A 🔖

● **S25.2   Injury of superior vena cava**

Injury of vena cava NOS

(Ex) For category S25.2 CC codes: See PDX Collection 1180

X● **S25.20   Unspecified injury of superior vena cava** A 🔖

X● **S25.21   Minor laceration of superior vena cava** A 🔖

Incomplete transection of superior vena cava

Laceration of superior vena cava NOS

Superficial laceration of superior vena cava

X● **S25.22   Major laceration of superior vena cava** A 🔖

Complete transection of superior vena cava

Traumatic rupture of superior vena cava

X● **S25.29   Other specified injury of superior vena cava** A 🔖

● **S25.3   Injury of innominate or subclavian vein**

(Ex) For category S25.3 CC codes: See PDX Collection 1181

● **S25.30   Unspecified injury of innominate or subclavian vein**

● **S25.301   Unspecified injury of right innominate or subclavian vein** A 🔖

● **S25.302   Unspecified injury of left innominate or subclavian vein** A 🔖

● **S25.309   Unspecified injury of unspecified innominate or subclavian vein** A 🔖

● **S25.31   Minor laceration of innominate or subclavian vein**

Incomplete transection of innominate or subclavian vein

Laceration of innominate or subclavian vein NOS

Superficial laceration of innominate or subclavian vein

● **S25.311   Minor laceration of right innominate or subclavian vein** A 🔖

● **S25.312   Minor laceration of left innominate or subclavian vein** A 🔖

● **S25.319   Minor laceration of unspecified innominate or subclavian vein** A 🔖

● **S25.32   Major laceration of innominate or subclavian vein**

Complete transection of innominate or subclavian vein

Traumatic rupture of innominate or subclavian vein

● **S25.321   Major laceration of right innominate or subclavian vein** A 🔖

● **S25.322   Major laceration of left innominate or subclavian vein** A 🔖

● **S25.329   Major laceration of unspecified innominate or subclavian vein** A 🔖

● **S25.39   Other specified injury of innominate or subclavian vein**

● **S25.391   Other specified injury of right innominate or subclavian vein** A 🔖

● **S25.392   Other specified injury of left innominate or subclavian vein** A 🔖

● **S25.399   Other specified injury of unspecified innominate or subclavian vein** A 🔖

▶ New   ⇒ Revised   ~~deleted~~ Deleted   Excludes 1   Excludes 2   Includes   Use additional   Code first   Code also   Key words

OGCR Official Guidelines   ● Unacceptable Principal Diagnosis   X Assign placeholder X   ● Use Additional Character(s)   ▌ Manifestation Code   **Coding Clinic**

● **S25.4   Injury of pulmonary blood vessels**
     (Ex) **For category S25.4 CC codes unless otherwise indicated:** See PDX Collection 1182

   ● **S25.40   Unspecified injury of pulmonary blood vessels**

     ● **S25.401   Unspecified injury of right pulmonary blood vessels** A 🦠

     ● **S25.402   Unspecified injury of left pulmonary blood vessels** A 🦠

     ● **S25.409   Unspecified injury of unspecified pulmonary blood vessels** A 🦠

   ● **S25.41   Minor laceration of pulmonary blood vessels**
     Incomplete transection of pulmonary blood vessels
     Laceration of pulmonary blood vessels NOS
     Superficial laceration of pulmonary blood vessels

     ● **S25.411   Minor laceration of right pulmonary blood vessels** A 🦠

     ● **S25.412   Minor laceration of left pulmonary blood vessels** A 🦠

     ● **S25.419   Minor laceration of unspecified pulmonary blood vessels** A 🦠

   ● **S25.42   Major laceration of pulmonary blood vessels**
     Complete transection of pulmonary blood vessels
     Traumatic rupture of pulmonary blood vessels

     ● **S25.421   Major laceration of right pulmonary blood vessels** A 🦠
       (Ex) See PDX Collection 1183

     ● **S25.422   Major laceration of left pulmonary blood vessels** A 🦠

     ● **S25.429   Major laceration of unspecified pulmonary blood vessels** A 🦠

   ● **S25.49   Other specified injury of pulmonary blood vessels**

     ● **S25.491   Other specified injury of right pulmonary blood vessels** A 🦠

     ● **S25.492   Other specified injury of left pulmonary blood vessels** A 🦠

     ● **S25.499   Other specified injury of unspecified pulmonary blood vessels** A 🦠

● **S25.5   Injury of intercostal blood vessels**
     (Ex) **For category S25.5 CC codes:** See PDX Collection 1184

   ● **S25.50   Unspecified injury of intercostal blood vessels**

     ● **S25.501   Unspecified injury of intercostal blood vessels, right side** A 🦠

     ● **S25.502   Unspecified injury of intercostal blood vessels, left side** A 🦠

     ● **S25.509   Unspecified injury of intercostal blood vessels, unspecified side** A 🦠

   ● **S25.51   Laceration of intercostal blood vessels**

     ● **S25.511   Laceration of intercostal blood vessels, right side** A 🦠

     ● **S25.512   Laceration of intercostal blood vessels, left side** A 🦠

     ● **S25.519   Laceration of intercostal blood vessels, unspecified side** A 🦠

   ● **S25.59   Other specified injury of intercostal blood vessels**

     ● **S25.591   Other specified injury of intercostal blood vessels, right side** A 🦠

     ● **S25.592   Other specified injury of intercostal blood vessels, left side** A 🦠

     ● **S25.599   Other specified injury of intercostal blood vessels, unspecified side** A 🦠

● **S25.8   Injury of other blood vessels of thorax**
     Injury of azygos vein
     Injury of mammary artery or vein
     (Ex) **For category S25.8 CC codes:** See PDX Collection 1185

   ● **S25.80   Unspecified injury of other blood vessels of thorax**

     ● **S25.801   Unspecified injury of other blood vessels of thorax, right side** A 🦠

     ● **S25.802   Unspecified injury of other blood vessels of thorax, left side** A 🦠

     ● **S25.809   Unspecified injury of other blood vessels of thorax, unspecified side** A 🦠

   ● **S25.81   Laceration of other blood vessels of thorax**

     ● **S25.811   Laceration of other blood vessels of thorax, right side** A 🦠

     ● **S25.812   Laceration of other blood vessels of thorax, left side** A 🦠

     ● **S25.819   Laceration of other blood vessels of thorax, unspecified side** A 🦠

   ● **S25.89   Other specified injury of other blood vessels of thorax**

     ● **S25.891   Other specified injury of other blood vessels of thorax, right side** A 🦠

     ● **S25.892   Other specified injury of other blood vessels of thorax, left side** A 🦠

     ● **S25.899   Other specified injury of other blood vessels of thorax, unspecified side** A 🦠

● **S25.9   Injury of unspecified blood vessel of thorax**
     (Ex) **For category S25.9 CC codes:** See PDX Collection 1185

   X ● **S25.90   Unspecified injury of unspecified blood vessel of thorax** A 🦠

   X ● **S25.91   Laceration of unspecified blood vessel of thorax** A 🦠

   X ● **S25.99   Other specified injury of unspecified blood vessel of thorax** A 🦠

● **S26   Injury of heart**

     The appropriate 7th character is to be added to each code from category S26

A	initial encounter
D	subsequent encounter
S	sequela

     Code also any associated:
       open wound of thorax (S21.-)
       traumatic hemopneumothorax (S27.2)
       traumatic hemothorax (S27.1)
       traumatic pneumothorax (S27.0)
     (Ex) **For category S26 CC codes unless otherwise indicated:** See PDX Collection 1187

   ● **S26.0   Injury of heart with hemopericardium**
     Hemopericardium: effusion of blood within pericardium

     X ● **S26.00   Unspecified injury of heart with hemopericardium** A 🦠
       (Ex) See PDX Collection 1186

     X ● **S26.01   Contusion of heart with hemopericardium** A 🦠

CHAPTER 19 (S00–T88)

N   Newborn Age: 0   **P**   Pediatric Age: 0–17   **M**   Maternity DX: 12–55   **A**   Adult Age: 15–124   ♀   Females Only   ♂   Males Only

🦠   Complication\Comorbidity   🦠   Major C\C   (Ex)   CC/MCC Exclusions   🦠   Hospital-Acquired Condition

1255

CHAPTER 19 (S00-T88)

- **S26.02**   **Laceration of heart with hemopericardium**
  - **S26.020**   **Mild laceration of heart with hemopericardium** A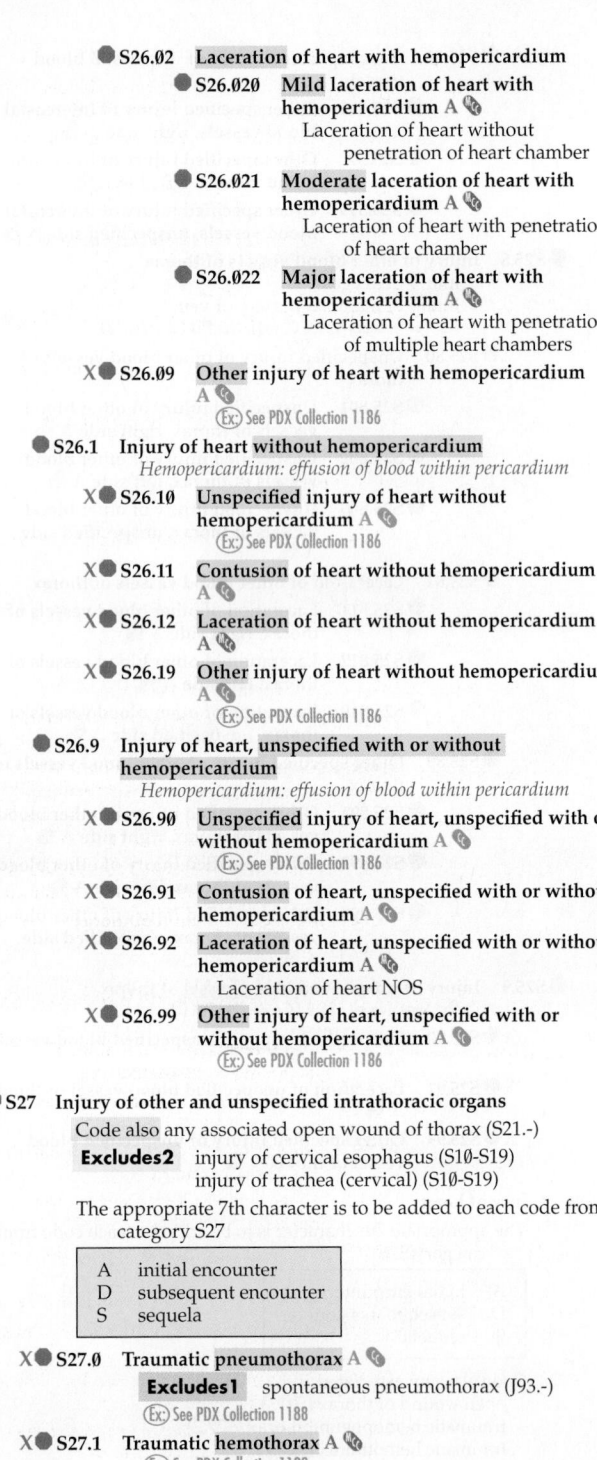
    Laceration of heart without penetration of heart chamber
  - **S26.021**   **Moderate laceration of heart with hemopericardium** A
    Laceration of heart with penetration of heart chamber
  - **S26.022**   **Major laceration of heart with hemopericardium** A
    Laceration of heart with penetration of multiple heart chambers
  - X **S26.09**   **Other injury of heart with hemopericardium** A
    Ex: See PDX Collection 1186
- **S26.1**   **Injury of heart without hemopericardium**
  Hemopericardium: effusion of blood within pericardium
  - X **S26.10**   **Unspecified injury of heart without hemopericardium** A
    Ex: See PDX Collection 1186
  - X **S26.11**   **Contusion of heart without hemopericardium** A
  - X **S26.12**   **Laceration of heart without hemopericardium** A
  - X **S26.19**   **Other injury of heart without hemopericardium** A
    Ex: See PDX Collection 1186
- **S26.9**   **Injury of heart, unspecified with or without hemopericardium**
  Hemopericardium: effusion of blood within pericardium
  - X **S26.90**   **Unspecified injury of heart, unspecified with or without hemopericardium** A
    Ex: See PDX Collection 1186
  - X **S26.91**   **Contusion of heart, unspecified with or without hemopericardium** A
  - X **S26.92**   **Laceration of heart, unspecified with or without hemopericardium** A
    Laceration of heart NOS
  - X **S26.99**   **Other injury of heart, unspecified with or without hemopericardium** A
    Ex: See PDX Collection 1186

- **S27**   **Injury of other and unspecified intrathoracic organs**
  Code also any associated open wound of thorax (S21.-)
  Excludes2   injury of cervical esophagus (S10-S19)
  injury of trachea (cervical) (S10-S19)
  The appropriate 7th character is to be added to each code from category S27

A	initial encounter
D	subsequent encounter
S	sequela

  - X **S27.0**   **Traumatic pneumothorax** A
    Excludes1   spontaneous pneumothorax (J93.-)
    Ex: See PDX Collection 1188
  - X **S27.1**   **Traumatic hemothorax** A
    Ex: See PDX Collection 1188
  - X **S27.2**   **Traumatic hemopneumothorax** A
    Ex: See PDX Collection 1188

- **S27.3**   **Other and unspecified injuries of lung**
  Ex: For category S27.3 CC codes unless otherwise indicated: See PDX Collection 1189
  - **S27.30**   **Unspecified injury of lung**
    - **S27.301**   **Unspecified injury of lung, unilateral** A
    - **S27.302**   **Unspecified injury of lung, bilateral** A
    - **S27.309**   **Unspecified injury of lung, unspecified** A
  - **S27.31**   **Primary blast injury of lung**
    Blast injury of lung NOS
    - **S27.311**   **Primary blast injury of lung, unilateral** A
    - **S27.312**   **Primary blast injury of lung, bilateral** A
    - **S27.319**   **Primary blast injury of lung, unspecified** A
  - **S27.32**   **Contusion of lung**
    - **S27.321**   **Contusion of lung, unilateral** A
    - **S27.322**   **Contusion of lung, bilateral** A
    - **S27.329**   **Contusion of lung, unspecified** A
  - **S27.33**   **Laceration of lung**
    Ex: For category S27.33 CC codes: See PDX Collection 1190
    - **S27.331**   **Laceration of lung, unilateral** A
    - **S27.332**   **Laceration of lung, bilateral** A
    - **S27.339**   **Laceration of lung, unspecified** A
  - **S27.39**   **Other injuries of lung**
    Secondary blast injury of lung
    - **S27.391**   **Other injuries of lung, unilateral** A
    - **S27.392**   **Other injuries of lung, bilateral** A
    - **S27.399**   **Other injuries of lung, unspecified** A
- **S27.4**   **Injury of bronchus**
  Ex: For category S27.4 CC codes: See PDX Collection 1191
  - **S27.40**   **Unspecified injury of bronchus**
    - **S27.401**   **Unspecified injury of bronchus, unilateral** A
    - **S27.402**   **Unspecified injury of bronchus, bilateral** A
    - **S27.409**   **Unspecified injury of bronchus, unspecified** A
  - **S27.41**   **Primary blast injury of bronchus**
    Blast injury of bronchus NOS
    - **S27.411**   **Primary blast injury of bronchus, unilateral** A
    - **S27.412**   **Primary blast injury of bronchus, bilateral** A
    - **S27.419**   **Primary blast injury of bronchus, unspecified** A
  - **S27.42**   **Contusion of bronchus**
    - **S27.421**   **Contusion of bronchus, unilateral** A
    - **S27.422**   **Contusion of bronchus, bilateral** A
    - **S27.429**   **Contusion of bronchus, unspecified** A
  - **S27.43**   **Laceration of bronchus**
    - **S27.431**   **Laceration of bronchus, unilateral** A
    - **S27.432**   **Laceration of bronchus, bilateral** A
    - **S27.439**   **Laceration of bronchus, unspecified** A

Item 19–2   Pneumothorax is a collection of gas (positive air pressure) in the pleural space resulting in the lung collapsing. A **tension pneumothorax** is life-threatening and is a result of air in the pleural space causing a displacement in the mediastinal structures and cardiopulmonary function compromise. A **traumatic pneumothorax** results from blunt or penetrating injury that disrupts the parietal/visceral pleura. **Hemothorax** is blood or bloody fluid in the pleural cavity as a result of traumatic blood vessel rupture or inflammation of the lungs from pneumonia.

▶ New   ➡ Revised   ~~deleted~~ Deleted   Excludes 1   Excludes 2   Includes   Use additional   Code first   Code also   Key words

OGCR Official Guidelines   ● Unacceptable Principal Diagnosis   X Assign placeholder X   ● Use Additional Character(s)   ▶ Manifestation Code   **Coding Clinic**

- **S27.49** **Other injury of bronchus**
  Secondary blast injury of bronchus
  - **S27.491** **Other injury of bronchus, unilateral** A
  - **S27.492** **Other injury of bronchus, bilateral** A
  - **S27.499** **Other injury of bronchus, unspecified** A
- **S27.5** **Injury of thoracic trachea**
  (Ex) *For category S27.5 CC codes:* See PDX Collection 1169
  - X **S27.50** **Unspecified injury of thoracic trachea** A
  - X **S27.51** **Primary blast injury of thoracic trachea** A
    Blast injury of thoracic trachea NOS
  - X **S27.52** **Contusion of thoracic trachea** A
  - X **S27.53** **Laceration of thoracic trachea** A
  - X **S27.59** **Other injury of thoracic trachea** A
    Secondary blast injury of thoracic trachea
- **S27.6** **Injury of pleura**
  (Ex) *For category S27.6 CC codes:* See PDX Collection 1169
  - X **S27.60** **Unspecified injury of pleura** A
  - X **S27.63** **Laceration of pleura** A
  - X **S27.69** **Other injury of pleura** A
- **S27.8** **Injury of other specified intrathoracic organs**
  - **S27.80** **Injury of diaphragm**
    (Ex) *For category S27.80 CC codes:* See PDX Collection 1192
    - **S27.802** **Contusion of diaphragm** A
    - **S27.803** **Laceration of diaphragm** A
    - **S27.808** **Other injury of diaphragm** A
    - **S27.809** **Unspecified injury of diaphragm** A
  - **S27.81** **Injury of esophagus (thoracic part)**
    (Ex) *For category S27.81 CC codes:* See PDX Collection 1193
    - **S27.812** **Contusion of esophagus (thoracic part)** A
    - **S27.813** **Laceration of esophagus (thoracic part)** A
    - **S27.818** **Other injury of esophagus (thoracic part)** A
    - **S27.819** **Unspecified injury of esophagus (thoracic part)** A
  - **S27.89** **Injury of other specified intrathoracic organs**
    Injury of lymphatic thoracic duct
    Injury of thymus gland
    (Ex) *For category S27.89 CC codes:* See PDX Collection 1169
    - **S27.892** **Contusion of other specified intrathoracic organs** A
    - **S27.893** **Laceration of other specified intrathoracic organs** A
    - **S27.898** **Other injury of other specified intrathoracic organs** A
    - **S27.899** **Unspecified injury of other specified intrathoracic organs** A
  - X **S27.9** **Injury of unspecified intrathoracic organ** A
    (Ex) See PDX Collection 1194
- **S28** **Crushing injury of thorax, and traumatic amputation of part of thorax**
  The appropriate 7th character is to be added to each code from category S28

A	initial encounter
D	subsequent encounter
S	sequela

  - X **S28.0** **Crushed chest**
    Use additional code for all associated injuries
    Excludes1 flail chest (S22.5)
  - X **S28.1** **Traumatic amputation (partial) of part of thorax, except breast** A
    (Ex) *For category S28.1 CC codes:* See PDX Collection 1168

- **S28.2** **Traumatic amputation of breast**
  - **S28.21** **Complete traumatic amputation of breast**
    Traumatic amputation of breast NOS
    - **S28.211** **Complete traumatic amputation of right breast**
    - **S28.212** **Complete traumatic amputation of left breast**
    - **S28.219** **Complete traumatic amputation of unspecified breast**
  - **S28.22** **Partial traumatic amputation of breast**
    - **S28.221** **Partial traumatic amputation of right breast**
    - **S28.222** **Partial traumatic amputation of left breast**
    - **S28.229** **Partial traumatic amputation of unspecified breast**
- **S29** **Other and unspecified injuries of thorax**
  Code also any associated open wound (S21.-)
  The appropriate 7th character is to be added to each code from category S29

A	initial encounter
D	subsequent encounter
S	sequela

  - **S29.0** **Injury of muscle and tendon at thorax level**
    - **S29.00** **Unspecified injury of muscle and tendon of thorax**
      - **S29.001** **Unspecified injury of muscle and tendon of front wall of thorax**
      - **S29.002** **Unspecified injury of muscle and tendon of back wall of thorax**
      - **S29.009** **Unspecified injury of muscle and tendon of unspecified wall of thorax**
    - **S29.01** **Strain of muscle and tendon of thorax**
      - **S29.011** **Strain of muscle and tendon of front wall of thorax**
      - **S29.012** **Strain of muscle and tendon of back wall of thorax**
      - **S29.019** **Strain of muscle and tendon of unspecified wall of thorax**
    - **S29.02** **Laceration of muscle and tendon of thorax**
      (Ex) *For category S29.02 CC codes:* See PDX Collection 1168
      - **S29.021** **Laceration of muscle and tendon of front wall of thorax** A
      - **S29.022** **Laceration of muscle and tendon of back wall of thorax**
      - **S29.029** **Laceration of muscle and tendon of unspecified wall of thorax** A
    - **S29.09** **Other injury of muscle and tendon of thorax**
      - **S29.091** **Other injury of muscle and tendon of front wall of thorax**
      - **S29.092** **Other injury of muscle and tendon of back wall of thorax**
      - **S29.099** **Other injury of muscle and tendon of unspecified wall of thorax**
  - X **S29.8** **Other specified injuries of thorax**
  - X **S29.9** **Unspecified injury of thorax**

CHAPTER 19 (S00-T88)

N Newborn Age: 0   P Pediatric Age: 0–17   M Maternity DX: 12–55   A Adult Age: 15–124   ♀ Females Only   ♂ Males Only

Complication\Comorbidity   Major C\C   (Ex) CC/MCC Exclusions   Hospital-Acquired Condition

CHAPTER 19 (S00-T88)

INJURIES TO THE ABDOMEN, LOWER BACK, LUMBAR SPINE PELVIS AND EXTERNAL GENITALS (S30-S39)

Includes   injuries to the abdominal wall
injuries to the anus
injuries to the buttock
injuries to the external genitalia
injuries to the flank
injuries to the groin

Excludes2   burns and corrosions (T20-T32)
effects of foreign body in anus and rectum (T18.5)
effects of foreign body in genitourinary tract (T19.-)
effects of foreign body in stomach, small intestine and colon (T18.2-T18.4)
frostbite (T33-T34)
insect bite or sting, venomous (T63.4)

● **S30   Superficial injury of abdomen, lower back, pelvis and external genitals**

Excludes2   superficial injury of hip (S70.-)

The appropriate 7th character is to be added to each code from category S30

A	initial encounter
D	subsequent encounter
S	sequela

X● **S30.0   Contusion of lower back and pelvis**
Contusion of buttock

X● **S30.1   Contusion of abdominal wall**
Contusion of flank
Contusion of groin

● **S30.2   Contusion of external genital organs**

   ● **S30.20   Contusion of unspecified external genital organ**

      ● **S30.201   Contusion of unspecified external genital organ, male ♂**

      ● **S30.202   Contusion of unspecified external genital organ, female ♀**

   X● **S30.21   Contusion of penis ♂**

   X● **S30.22   Contusion of scrotum and testes ♂**

   X● **S30.23   Contusion of vagina and vulva ♀**

X● **S30.3   Contusion of anus**

● **S30.8   Other superficial injuries of abdomen, lower back, pelvis and external genitals**

   ● **S30.81   Abrasion of abdomen, lower back, pelvis and external genitals**

      ● **S30.810   Abrasion of lower back and pelvis**

      ● **S30.811   Abrasion of abdominal wall**

      ● **S30.812   Abrasion of penis ♂**

      ● **S30.813   Abrasion of scrotum and testes ♂**

      ● **S30.814   Abrasion of vagina and vulva ♀**

      ● **S30.815   Abrasion of unspecified external genital organs, male ♂**

      ● **S30.816   Abrasion of unspecified external genital organs, female ♀**

      ● **S30.817   Abrasion of anus**

   ● **S30.82   Blister (nonthermal) of abdomen, lower back, pelvis and external genitals**

      ● **S30.820   Blister (nonthermal) of lower back and pelvis**

      ● **S30.821   Blister (nonthermal) of abdominal wall**

      ● **S30.822   Blister (nonthermal) of penis ♂**

      ● **S30.823   Blister (nonthermal) of scrotum and testes ♂**

      ● **S30.824   Blister (nonthermal) of vagina and vulva ♀**

      ● **S30.825   Blister (nonthermal) of unspecified external genital organs, male ♂**

      ● **S30.826   Blister (nonthermal) of unspecified external genital organs, female ♀**

      ● **S30.827   Blister (nonthermal) of anus**

   ● **S30.84   External constriction of abdomen, lower back, pelvis and external genitals**

      ● **S30.840   External constriction of lower back and pelvis**

      ● **S30.841   External constriction of abdominal wall**

      ● **S30.842   External constriction of penis ♂**
Hair tourniquet syndrome of penis
Use additional cause code to identify the constricting item (W49.0-)

      ● **S30.843   External constriction of scrotum and testes ♂**

      ● **S30.844   External constriction of vagina and vulva ♀**

      ● **S30.845   External constriction of unspecified external genital organs, male ♂**

      ● **S30.846   External constriction of unspecified external genital organs, female ♀**

● **S30.85   Superficial foreign body of abdomen, lower back, pelvis and external genitals**
Splinter in the abdomen, lower back, pelvis and external genitals

   ● **S30.850   Superficial foreign body of lower back and pelvis**

   ● **S30.851   Superficial foreign body of abdominal wall**

   ● **S30.852   Superficial foreign body of penis ♂**

   ● **S30.853   Superficial foreign body of scrotum and testes ♂**

   ● **S30.854   Superficial foreign body of vagina and vulva ♀**

   ● **S30.855   Superficial foreign body of unspecified external genital organs, male ♂**

   ● **S30.856   Superficial foreign body of unspecified external genital organs, female ♀**

   ● **S30.857   Superficial foreign body of anus**

● **S30.86   Insect bite (nonvenomous) of abdomen, lower back, pelvis and external genitals**

   ● **S30.860   Insect bite (nonvenomous) of lower back and pelvis**

   ● **S30.861   Insect bite (nonvenomous) of abdominal wall**

   ● **S30.862   Insect bite (nonvenomous) of penis ♂**

   ● **S30.863   Insect bite (nonvenomous) of scrotum and testes ♂**

   ● **S30.864   Insect bite (nonvenomous) of vagina and vulva ♀**

   ● **S30.865   Insect bite (nonvenomous) of unspecified external genital organs, male ♂**

   ● **S30.866   Insect bite (nonvenomous) of unspecified external genital organs, female ♀**

   ● **S30.867   Insect bite (nonvenomous) of anus**

▶ New   ⇒ Revised   ~~deleted~~ Deleted   Excludes 1   Excludes 2   Includes   Use additional   Code first   Code also   Key words
OGCR Official Guidelines   ● Unacceptable Principal Diagnosis   X Assign placeholder X   ● Use Additional Character(s)   ▶ Manifestation Code   **Coding Clinic**

● S30.87   Other superficial bite of abdomen, lower back, pelvis and external genitals

> **Excludes1**   open bite of abdomen, lower back, pelvis and external genitals (S31.05, S31.15, S31.25, S31.35, S31.45, S31.55)

  ● S30.870   Other superficial bite of lower back and pelvis
  ● S30.871   Other superficial bite of abdominal wall
  ● S30.872   Other superficial bite of penis ♂
  ● S30.873   Other superficial bite of scrotum and testes ♂
  ● S30.874   Other superficial bite of vagina and vulva ♀
  ● S30.875   Other superficial bite of unspecified external genital organs, male ♂
  ● S30.876   Other superficial bite of unspecified external genital organs, female ♀
  ● S30.877   Other superficial bite of anus

● S30.9   Unspecified superficial injury of abdomen, lower back, pelvis and external genitals

  X ● S30.91   Unspecified superficial injury of lower back and pelvis
  X ● S30.92   Unspecified superficial injury of abdominal wall
  X ● S30.93   Unspecified superficial injury of penis ♂
  X ● S30.94   Unspecified superficial injury of scrotum and testes ♂
  X ● S30.95   Unspecified superficial injury of vagina and vulva ♀
  X ● S30.96   Unspecified superficial injury of unspecified external genital organs, male ♂
  X ● S30.97   Unspecified superficial injury of unspecified external genital organs, female ♀
  X ● S30.98   Unspecified superficial injury of anus

● S31   Open wound of abdomen, lower back, pelvis and external genitals

> Code also any associated:
> spinal cord injury (S24.0, S24.1-, S34.0-, S34.1-)
> wound infection

> **Excludes1**   traumatic amputation of part of abdomen, lower back and pelvis (S38.2-, S38.3)

> **Excludes2**   open wound of hip (S71.00-S71.02)
> open fracture of pelvis (S32.1--S32.9 with 7th character B)

> The appropriate 7th character is to be added to each code from category S31

> | A | initial encounter |
> | D | subsequent encounter |
> | S | sequela |

● S31.0   Open wound of lower back and pelvis

> (Ex) For category S31.0 CC codes: See PDX Collection 1195

  ● S31.00   Unspecified open wound of lower back and pelvis
    ● S31.000   Unspecified open wound of lower back and pelvis without penetration into retroperitoneum
      Unspecified open wound of lower back and pelvis NOS
    ● S31.001   Unspecified open wound of lower back and pelvis with penetration into retroperitoneum A 🐾

● S31.01   Laceration without foreign body of lower back and pelvis
  ● S31.010   Laceration without foreign body of lower back and pelvis without penetration into retroperitoneum
    Laceration without foreign body of lower back and pelvis NOS
  ● S31.011   Laceration without foreign body of lower back and pelvis with penetration into retroperitoneum A 🐾

● S31.02   Laceration with foreign body of lower back and pelvis
  ● S31.020   Laceration with foreign body of lower back and pelvis without penetration into retroperitoneum
    Laceration with foreign body of lower back and pelvis NOS
  ● S31.021   Laceration with foreign body of lower back and pelvis with penetration into retroperitoneum A 🐾

● S31.03   Puncture wound without foreign body of lower back and pelvis
  ● S31.030   Puncture wound without foreign body of lower back and pelvis without penetration into retroperitoneum
    Puncture wound without foreign body of lower back and pelvis NOS
  ● S31.031   Puncture wound without foreign body of lower back and pelvis with penetration into retroperitoneum A 🐾

● S31.04   Puncture wound with foreign body of lower back and pelvis
  ● S31.040   Puncture wound with foreign body of lower back and pelvis without penetration into retroperitoneum
    Puncture wound with foreign body of lower back and pelvis NOS
  ● S31.041   Puncture wound with foreign body of lower back and pelvis with penetration into retroperitoneum A 🐾

● S31.05   Open bite of lower back and pelvis
  Bite of lower back and pelvis NOS

> **Excludes1**   superficial bite of lower back and pelvis (S30.860, S30.870)

  ● S31.050   Open bite of lower back and pelvis without penetration into retroperitoneum
    Open bite of lower back and pelvis NOS
  ● S31.051   Open bite of lower back and pelvis with penetration into retroperitoneum A 🐾

● S31.1   Open wound of abdominal wall without penetration into peritoneal cavity
  Open wound of abdominal wall NOS

> **Excludes2**   open wound of abdominal wall with penetration into peritoneal cavity (S31.6-)

  ● S31.10   Unspecified open wound of abdominal wall without penetration into peritoneal cavity
    ● S31.100   Unspecified open wound of abdominal wall, right upper quadrant without penetration into peritoneal cavity
    ● S31.101   Unspecified open wound of abdominal wall, left upper quadrant without penetration into peritoneal cavity

N Newborn Age: 0   **P** Pediatric Age: 0–17   **M** Maternity DX: 12–55   **A** Adult Age: 15–124   ♀ Females Only   ♂ Males Only

🐾 Complication\Comorbidity   🐾 Major C\C   (Ex) CC/MCC Exclusions   🐾 Hospital-Acquired Condition

1259

● S31.102   Unspecified open wound of abdominal wall, epigastric region without penetration into peritoneal cavity

● S31.103   Unspecified open wound of abdominal wall, right lower quadrant without penetration into peritoneal cavity

● S31.104   Unspecified open wound of abdominal wall, left lower quadrant without penetration into peritoneal cavity

● S31.105   Unspecified open wound of abdominal wall, periumbilic region without penetration into peritoneal cavity

● S31.109   Unspecified open wound of abdominal wall, unspecified quadrant without penetration into peritoneal cavity
  Unspecified open wound of abdominal wall NOS

● S31.11   Laceration without foreign body of abdominal wall without penetration into peritoneal cavity

● S31.110   Laceration without foreign body of abdominal wall, right upper quadrant without penetration into peritoneal cavity

● S31.111   Laceration without foreign body of abdominal wall, left upper quadrant without penetration into peritoneal cavity

● S31.112   Laceration without foreign body of abdominal wall, epigastric region without penetration into peritoneal cavity

● S31.113   Laceration without foreign body of abdominal wall, right lower quadrant without penetration into peritoneal cavity

● S31.114   Laceration without foreign body of abdominal wall, left lower quadrant without penetration into peritoneal cavity

● S31.115   Laceration without foreign body of abdominal wall, periumbilic region without penetration into peritoneal cavity

● S31.119   Laceration without foreign body of abdominal wall, unspecified quadrant without penetration into peritoneal cavity

● S31.12   Laceration with foreign body of abdominal wall without penetration into peritoneal cavity

● S31.120   Laceration of abdominal wall with foreign body, right upper quadrant without penetration into peritoneal cavity

● S31.121   Laceration of abdominal wall with foreign body, left upper quadrant without penetration into peritoneal cavity

● S31.122   Laceration of abdominal wall with foreign body, epigastric region without penetration into peritoneal cavity

● S31.123   Laceration of abdominal wall with foreign body, right lower quadrant without penetration into peritoneal cavity

● S31.124   Laceration of abdominal wall with foreign body, left lower quadrant without penetration into peritoneal cavity

● S31.125   Laceration of abdominal wall with foreign body, periumbilic region without penetration into peritoneal cavity

● S31.129   Laceration of abdominal wall with foreign body, unspecified quadrant without penetration into peritoneal cavity

● S31.13   Puncture wound of abdominal wall without foreign body without penetration into peritoneal cavity

● S31.130   Puncture wound of abdominal wall without foreign body, right upper quadrant without penetration into peritoneal cavity

● S31.131   Puncture wound of abdominal wall without foreign body, left upper quadrant without penetration into peritoneal cavity

● S31.132   Puncture wound of abdominal wall without foreign body, epigastric region without penetration into peritoneal cavity

● S31.133   Puncture wound of abdominal wall without foreign body, right lower quadrant without penetration into peritoneal cavity

● S31.134   Puncture wound of abdominal wall without foreign body, left lower quadrant without penetration into peritoneal cavity

● S31.135   Puncture wound of abdominal wall without foreign body, periumbilic region without penetration into peritoneal cavity

● S31.139   Puncture wound of abdominal wall without foreign body, unspecified quadrant without penetration into peritoneal cavity

● S31.14   Puncture wound of abdominal wall with foreign body without penetration into peritoneal cavity

● S31.140   Puncture wound of abdominal wall with foreign body, right upper quadrant without penetration into peritoneal cavity

● S31.141   Puncture wound of abdominal wall with foreign body, left upper quadrant without penetration into peritoneal cavity

● S31.142   Puncture wound of abdominal wall with foreign body, epigastric region without penetration into peritoneal cavity

● S31.143   Puncture wound of abdominal wall with foreign body, right lower quadrant without penetration into peritoneal cavity

● S31.144   Puncture wound of abdominal wall with foreign body, left lower quadrant without penetration into peritoneal cavity

● S31.145   Puncture wound of abdominal wall with foreign body, periumbilic region without penetration into peritoneal cavity

● S31.149   Puncture wound of abdominal wall with foreign body, unspecified quadrant without penetration into peritoneal cavity

● **S31.15**   Open bite of abdominal wall without penetration into peritoneal cavity
Bite of abdominal wall NOS

Excludes1   superficial bite of abdominal wall (S30.871)

    ● **S31.150**   Open bite of abdominal wall, right upper quadrant without penetration into peritoneal cavity

    ● **S31.151**   Open bite of abdominal wall, left upper quadrant without penetration into peritoneal cavity

    ● **S31.152**   Open bite of abdominal wall, epigastric region without penetration into peritoneal cavity

    ● **S31.153**   Open bite of abdominal wall, right lower quadrant without penetration into peritoneal cavity

    ● **S31.154**   Open bite of abdominal wall, left lower quadrant without penetration into peritoneal cavity

    ● **S31.155**   Open bite of abdominal wall, periumbilic region without penetration into peritoneal cavity

    ● **S31.159**   Open bite of abdominal wall, unspecified quadrant without penetration into peritoneal cavity

● **S31.2**   Open wound of penis

  X ● **S31.20**   Unspecified open wound of penis ♂

  X ● **S31.21**   Laceration without foreign body of penis ♂

  X ● **S31.22**   Laceration with foreign body of penis ♂

  X ● **S31.23**   Puncture wound without foreign body of penis ♂

  X ● **S31.24**   Puncture wound with foreign body of penis ♂

  X ● **S31.25**   Open bite of penis ♂
Bite of penis NOS

Excludes1   superficial bite of penis (S30.862, S30.872)

● **S31.3**   Open wound of scrotum and testes

  X ● **S31.30**   Unspecified open wound of scrotum and testes ♂

  X ● **S31.31**   Laceration without foreign body of scrotum and testes ♂

  X ● **S31.32**   Laceration with foreign body of scrotum and testes ♂

  X ● **S31.33**   Puncture wound without foreign body of scrotum and testes ♂

  X ● **S31.34**   Puncture wound with foreign body of scrotum and testes ♂

  X ● **S31.35**   Open bite of scrotum and testes ♂
Bite of scrotum and testes NOS

Excludes1   superficial bite of scrotum and testes (S30.863, S30.873)

● **S31.4**   Open wound of vagina and vulva

Excludes1   injury to vagina and vulva during delivery (O70.-, O71.4)

  X ● **S31.40**   Unspecified open wound of vagina and vulva ♀

  X ● **S31.41**   Laceration without foreign body of vagina and vulva ♀

  X ● **S31.42**   Laceration with foreign body of vagina and vulva ♀

  X ● **S31.43**   Puncture wound without foreign body of vagina and vulva ♀

  X ● **S31.44**   Puncture wound with foreign body of vagina and vulva ♀

  X ● **S31.45**   Open bite of vagina and vulva ♀
Bite of vagina and vulva NOS

Excludes1   superficial bite of vagina and vulva (S30.864, S30.874)

● **S31.5**   Open wound of unspecified external genital organs

Excludes1   traumatic amputation of external genital organs (S38.21, S38.22)

    ● **S31.50**   Unspecified open wound of unspecified external genital organs

      ● **S31.501**   Unspecified open wound of unspecified external genital organs, male ♂

      ● **S31.502**   Unspecified open wound of unspecified external genital organs, female ♀

    ● **S31.51**   Laceration without foreign body of unspecified external genital organs

      ● **S31.511**   Laceration without foreign body of unspecified external genital organs, male ♂

      ● **S31.512**   Laceration without foreign body of unspecified external genital organs, female ♀

    ● **S31.52**   Laceration with foreign body of unspecified external genital organs

      ● **S31.521**   Laceration with foreign body of unspecified external genital organs, male ♂

      ● **S31.522**   Laceration with foreign body of unspecified external genital organs, female ♀

    ● **S31.53**   Puncture wound without foreign body of unspecified external genital organs

      ● **S31.531**   Puncture wound without foreign body of unspecified external genital organs, male ♂

      ● **S31.532**   Puncture wound without foreign body of unspecified external genital organs, female ♀

    ● **S31.54**   Puncture wound with foreign body of unspecified external genital organs

      ● **S31.541**   Puncture wound with foreign body of unspecified external genital organs, male ♂

      ● **S31.542**   Puncture wound with foreign body of unspecified external genital organs, female ♀

    ● **S31.55**   Open bite of unspecified external genital organs
Bite of unspecified external genital organs NOS

Excludes1   superficial bite of unspecified external genital organs (S30.865, S30.866, S30.875, S30.876)

      ● **S31.551**   Open bite of unspecified external genital organs, male ♂

      ● **S31.552**   Open bite of unspecified external genital organs, female ♀

● **S31.6**   Open wound of abdominal wall with penetration into peritoneal cavity

   (Ex) **For category S31.6 CC codes: See PDX Collection 1195**

    ● **S31.60**   Unspecified open wound of abdominal wall with penetration into peritoneal cavity

      ● **S31.600**   Unspecified open wound of abdominal wall, right upper quadrant with penetration into peritoneal cavity A ⬢

      ● **S31.601**   Unspecified open wound of abdominal wall, left upper quadrant with penetration into peritoneal cavity A ⬢

      ● **S31.602**   Unspecified open wound of abdominal wall, epigastric region with penetration into peritoneal cavity A ⬢

N   Newborn Age: 0   **P**   Pediatric Age: 0–17   **M**   Maternity DX: 12–55   **A**   Adult Age: 15–124   ♀   Females Only   ♂   Males Only

⬢   Complication\Comorbidity   ⬢   Major C\C   (Ex)   CC/MCC Exclusions   ⬢   Hospital-Acquired Condition

1261

● S31.603   Unspecified open wound of abdominal wall, right lower quadrant with penetration into peritoneal cavity A 🔾

● S31.604   Unspecified open wound of abdominal wall, left lower quadrant with penetration into peritoneal cavity A 🔾

● S31.605   Unspecified open wound of abdominal wall, periumbilic region with penetration into peritoneal cavity A 🔾

● S31.609   Unspecified open wound of abdominal wall, unspecified quadrant with penetration into peritoneal cavity A 🔾

● S31.61   Laceration without foreign body of abdominal wall with penetration into peritoneal cavity

● S31.610   Laceration without foreign body of abdominal wall, right upper quadrant with penetration into peritoneal cavity A 🔾

● S31.611   Laceration without foreign body of abdominal wall, left upper quadrant with penetration into peritoneal cavity A 🔾

● S31.612   Laceration without foreign body of abdominal wall, epigastric region with penetration into peritoneal cavity A 🔾

● S31.613   Laceration without foreign body of abdominal wall, right lower quadrant with penetration into peritoneal cavity A 🔾,
     Coding Clinic: 2015, Q4, P37

● S31.614   Laceration without foreign body of abdominal wall, left lower quadrant with penetration into peritoneal cavity A 🔾

● S31.615   Laceration without foreign body of abdominal wall, periumbilic region with penetration into peritoneal cavity A 🔾

● S31.619   Laceration without foreign body of abdominal wall, unspecified quadrant with penetration into peritoneal cavity A 🔾

● S31.62   Laceration with foreign body of abdominal wall with penetration into peritoneal cavity

● S31.620   Laceration with foreign body of abdominal wall, right upper quadrant with penetration into peritoneal cavity A 🔾

● S31.621   Laceration with foreign body of abdominal wall, left upper quadrant with penetration into peritoneal cavity A 🔾

● S31.622   Laceration with foreign body of abdominal wall, epigastric region with penetration into peritoneal cavity A 🔾

● S31.623   Laceration with foreign body of abdominal wall, right lower quadrant with penetration into peritoneal cavity A 🔾

● S31.624   Laceration with foreign body of abdominal wall, left lower quadrant with penetration into peritoneal cavity A 🔾

● S31.625   Laceration with foreign body of abdominal wall, periumbilic region with penetration into peritoneal cavity A 🔾

● S31.629   Laceration with foreign body of abdominal wall, unspecified quadrant with penetration into peritoneal cavity A 🔾

● S31.63   Puncture wound without foreign body of abdominal wall with penetration into peritoneal cavity

● S31.630   Puncture wound without foreign body of abdominal wall, right upper quadrant with penetration into peritoneal cavity A 🔾

● S31.631   Puncture wound without foreign body of abdominal wall, left upper quadrant with penetration into peritoneal cavity A 🔾

● S31.632   Puncture wound without foreign body of abdominal wall, epigastric region with penetration into peritoneal cavity A 🔾

● S31.633   Puncture wound without foreign body of abdominal wall, right lower quadrant with penetration into peritoneal cavity A 🔾

● S31.634   Puncture wound without foreign body of abdominal wall, left lower quadrant with penetration into peritoneal cavity A 🔾

● S31.635   Puncture wound without foreign body of abdominal wall, periumbilic region with penetration into peritoneal cavity A 🔾

● S31.639   Puncture wound without foreign body of abdominal wall, unspecified quadrant with penetration into peritoneal cavity A 🔾

● S31.64   Puncture wound with foreign body of abdominal wall with penetration into peritoneal cavity

● S31.640   Puncture wound with foreign body of abdominal wall, right upper quadrant with penetration into peritoneal cavity A 🔾

● S31.641   Puncture wound with foreign body of abdominal wall, left upper quadrant with penetration into peritoneal cavity A 🔾

● S31.642   Puncture wound with foreign body of abdominal wall, epigastric region with penetration into peritoneal cavity A 🔾

● S31.643   Puncture wound with foreign body of abdominal wall, right lower quadrant with penetration into peritoneal cavity A 🔾

● S31.644   Puncture wound with foreign body of abdominal wall, left lower quadrant with penetration into peritoneal cavity A 🔾

● S31.645   Puncture wound with foreign body of abdominal wall, periumbilic region with penetration into peritoneal cavity A 🔾

● S31.649   Puncture wound with foreign body of abdominal wall, unspecified quadrant with penetration into peritoneal cavity A 🔾

▶ New   ⇒ Revised   ~~deleted~~ Deleted   Excludes 1   Excludes 2   Includes   Use additional   Code first   Code also   Key words
OGCR Official Guidelines   ● Unacceptable Principal Diagnosis   X Assign placeholder X   ● Use Additional Character(s)   ▌ Manifestation Code   **Coding Clinic**

● **S31.65**   **Open bite of abdominal wall with penetration into peritoneal cavity**
> **Excludes1**   superficial bite of abdominal wall (S30.861, S30.871)

   ● **S31.650**   **Open bite of abdominal wall, right upper quadrant with penetration into peritoneal cavity** A 🗞

   ● **S31.651**   **Open bite of abdominal wall, left upper quadrant with penetration into peritoneal cavity** A 🗞

   ● **S31.652**   **Open bite of abdominal wall, epigastric region with penetration into peritoneal cavity** A 🗞

   ● **S31.653**   **Open bite of abdominal wall, right lower quadrant with penetration into peritoneal cavity** A 🗞

   ● **S31.654**   **Open bite of abdominal wall, left lower quadrant with penetration into peritoneal cavity** A 🗞

   ● **S31.655**   **Open bite of abdominal wall, periumbilic region with penetration into peritoneal cavity** A 🗞

   ● **S31.659**   **Open bite of abdominal wall, unspecified quadrant with penetration into peritoneal cavity** A 🗞

● **S31.8**   **Open wound of other parts of abdomen, lower back and pelvis**

   ● **S31.80**   **Open wound of unspecified buttock**

    ● **S31.801**   **Laceration without foreign body of unspecified buttock**

    ● **S31.802**   **Laceration with foreign body of unspecified buttock**

    ● **S31.803**   **Puncture wound without foreign body of unspecified buttock**

    ● **S31.804**   **Puncture wound with foreign body of unspecified buttock**

    ● **S31.805**   **Open bite of unspecified buttock**
> Bite of buttock NOS
> **Excludes1**   superficial bite of buttock (S30.870)

    ● **S31.809**   **Unspecified open wound of unspecified buttock**

   ● **S31.81**   **Open wound of right buttock**

    ● **S31.811**   **Laceration without foreign body of right buttock**

    ● **S31.812**   **Laceration with foreign body of right buttock**

    ● **S31.813**   **Puncture wound without foreign body of right buttock**

    ● **S31.814**   **Puncture wound with foreign body of right buttock**

    ● **S31.815**   **Open bite of right buttock**
> Bite of right buttock NOS
> **Excludes1**   superficial bite of buttock (S30.870)

    ● **S31.819**   **Unspecified open wound of right buttock**

   ● **S31.82**   **Open wound of left buttock**

    ● **S31.821**   **Laceration without foreign body of left buttock**

    ● **S31.822**   **Laceration with foreign body of left buttock**

    ● **S31.823**   **Puncture wound without foreign body of left buttock**

    ● **S31.824**   **Puncture wound with foreign body of left buttock**

    ● **S31.825**   **Open bite of left buttock**
> Bite of left buttock NOS
> **Excludes1**   superficial bite of buttock (S30.870)

    ● **S31.829**   **Unspecified open wound of left buttock**

● **S31.83**   **Open wound of anus**

   ● **S31.831**   **Laceration without foreign body of anus**

   ● **S31.832**   **Laceration with foreign body of anus**

   ● **S31.833**   **Puncture wound without foreign body of anus**

   ● **S31.834**   **Puncture wound with foreign body of anus**

   ● **S31.835**   **Open bite of anus**
> Bite of anus NOS
> **Excludes1**   superficial bite of anus (S30.877)

   ● **S31.839**   **Unspecified open wound of anus**

● **S32**   **Fracture of lumbar spine and pelvis**

> **Note:** A fracture not indicated as displaced or nondisplaced should be coded to displaced
>
> A fracture not indicated as opened or closed should be coded to closed

> **Includes**   fracture of lumbosacral neural arch
> fracture of lumbosacral spinous process
> fracture of lumbosacral transverse process
> fracture of lumbosacral vertebra
> fracture of lumbosacral vertebral arch

Code first any associated spinal cord and spinal nerve injury (S34.-)

> **Excludes1**   transection of abdomen (S38.3)
>
> **Excludes2**   fracture of hip NOS (S72.0-)

The appropriate 7th character is to be added to each code from category S32

A	initial encounter for closed fracture
B	initial encounter for open fracture
D	subsequent encounter for fracture with routine healing
G	subsequent encounter for fracture with delayed healing
K	subsequent encounter for fracture with nonunion
S	sequela

● **S32.0**   **Fracture of lumbar vertebra**
> Fracture of lumbar spine NOS
> (Ex) For category S32.0 CC codes S32.0[A,B]: See PDX Collection 1196
> For S32.0[K]: See PDX Collection 897

   ● **S32.00**   **Fracture of unspecified lumbar vertebra**

    ● **S32.000**   **Wedge compression fracture of unspecified lumbar vertebra** A, K 🗞, B 🗞, A, B 🗞

    ● **S32.001**   **Stable burst fracture of unspecified lumbar vertebra** A, K 🗞, B 🗞, A, B 🗞

    ● **S32.002**   **Unstable burst fracture of unspecified lumbar vertebra** A, K 🗞, B 🗞, A, B 🗞

    ● **S32.008**   **Other fracture of unspecified lumbar vertebra** A, K 🗞, B 🗞, A, B 🗞

    ● **S32.009**   **Unspecified fracture of unspecified lumbar vertebra** A, K 🗞, B 🗞, A, B 🗞

   ● **S32.01**   **Fracture of first lumbar vertebra**

    ● **S32.010**   **Wedge compression fracture of first lumbar vertebra** A, K 🗞, B 🗞, A, B 🗞

    ● **S32.011**   **Stable burst fracture of first lumbar vertebra** A, K 🗞, B 🗞, A, B 🗞

    ● **S32.012**   **Unstable burst fracture of first lumbar vertebra** A, K 🗞, B 🗞, A, B 🗞

    ● **S32.018**   **Other fracture of first lumbar vertebra** A, K 🗞, B 🗞, A, B 🗞

    ● **S32.019**   **Unspecified fracture of first lumbar vertebra** A, K 🗞, B 🗞, A, B 🗞

N Newborn Age: 0	**P** Pediatric Age: 0–17	**M** Maternity DX: 12–55	**A** Adult Age: 15–124	♀ Females Only	♂ Males Only

🗞 Complication\Comorbidity   🗞 Major C\C   (Ex) CC/MCC Exclusions   🗞 Hospital-Acquired Condition

1263

CHAPTER 19 (S00–T88)

● **S32.02**   **Fracture of second lumbar vertebra**

    ● **S32.020**   **Wedge compression** fracture of second lumbar vertebra A, K 🔹, B 🔹, A, B 🔹

    ● **S32.021**   **Stable burst** fracture of second lumbar vertebra A, K 🔹, B 🔹, A, B 🔹

    ● **S32.022**   **Unstable burst** fracture of second lumbar vertebra A, K 🔹, B 🔹, A, B 🔹

    ● **S32.028**   **Other** fracture of second lumbar vertebra A, K 🔹, B 🔹, A, B 🔹

    ● **S32.029**   **Unspecified** fracture of second lumbar vertebra A, K 🔹, B 🔹, A, B 🔹

● **S32.03**   **Fracture of third lumbar vertebra**

    ● **S32.030**   **Wedge compression** fracture of third lumbar vertebra A, K 🔹, B 🔹, A, B 🔹

    ● **S32.031**   **Stable burst** fracture of third lumbar vertebra A, K 🔹, B 🔹, A, B 🔹

    ● **S32.032**   **Unstable burst** fracture of third lumbar vertebra A, K 🔹, B 🔹, A, B 🔹

    ● **S32.038**   **Other** fracture of third lumbar vertebra A, K 🔹, B 🔹, A, B 🔹

    ● **S32.039**   **Unspecified** fracture of third lumbar vertebra A, K 🔹, B 🔹, A, B 🔹

● **S32.04**   **Fracture of fourth lumbar vertebra**

    ● **S32.040**   **Wedge compression** fracture of fourth lumbar vertebra A, K 🔹, B 🔹, A, B 🔹

    ● **S32.041**   **Stable burst** fracture of fourth lumbar vertebra A, K 🔹, B 🔹, A, B 🔹

    ● **S32.042**   **Unstable burst** fracture of fourth lumbar vertebra A, K 🔹, B 🔹, A, B 🔹

    ● **S32.048**   **Other** fracture of fourth lumbar vertebra A, K 🔹, B 🔹, A, B 🔹

    ● **S32.049**   **Unspecified** fracture of fourth lumbar vertebra A, K 🔹, B 🔹, A, B 🔹

● **S32.05**   **Fracture of fifth lumbar vertebra**

    ● **S32.050**   **Wedge compression** fracture of fifth lumbar vertebra A, K 🔹, B 🔹, A, B 🔹

    ● **S32.051**   **Stable burst** fracture of fifth lumbar vertebra A, K 🔹, B 🔹, A, B 🔹

    ● **S32.052**   **Unstable burst** fracture of fifth lumbar vertebra A, K 🔹, B 🔹, A, B 🔹

    ● **S32.058**   **Other** fracture of fifth lumbar vertebra A, K 🔹, B 🔹, A, B 🔹

    ● **S32.059**   **Unspecified** fracture of fifth lumbar vertebra A, K 🔹, B 🔹, A, B 🔹

● **S32.1**   **Fracture of sacrum**

    For vertical fractures, code to most medial fracture extension

    Use two codes if both a vertical and transverse fracture are present

    Code also any associated fracture of pelvic ring (S32.8-)

    (Ex) **For category S32.1 CC codes S32.1[A,B]:** See PDX Collection 1197
    For S32.1[K]: See PDX Collection 897

  X ● **S32.10**   **Unspecified** fracture of sacrum A, K 🔹, B 🔹, A, B 🔹

    ● **S32.11**   **Zone I fracture of sacrum**
      Vertical sacral ala fracture of sacrum

      ● **S32.110**   **Nondisplaced Zone I** fracture of sacrum A, K 🔹, B 🔹, A, B 🔹

      ● **S32.111**   **Minimally displaced Zone I** fracture of sacrum A, K 🔹, B 🔹, A, B 🔹

      ● **S32.112**   **Severely displaced Zone I** fracture of sacrum A, K 🔹, B 🔹, A, B 🔹

      ● **S32.119**   **Unspecified Zone I** fracture of sacrum A, K 🔹, B 🔹, A, B 🔹

● **S32.12**   **Zone II fracture of sacrum**
    Vertical foraminal region fracture of sacrum

    ● **S32.120**   **Nondisplaced Zone II** fracture of sacrum A, K 🔹, B 🔹, A, B 🔹

    ● **S32.121**   **Minimally displaced Zone II** fracture of sacrum A, K 🔹, B 🔹, A, B 🔹

    ● **S32.122**   **Severely displaced Zone II** fracture of sacrum A, K 🔹, B 🔹, A, B 🔹

    ● **S32.129**   **Unspecified Zone II** fracture of sacrum A, K 🔹, B 🔹, A, B 🔹

● **S32.13**   **Zone III fracture of sacrum**
    Vertical fracture into spinal canal region of sacrum

    ● **S32.130**   **Nondisplaced Zone III** fracture of sacrum A, K 🔹, B 🔹, A, B 🔹

    ● **S32.131**   **Minimally displaced Zone III** fracture of sacrum A, K 🔹, B 🔹, A, B 🔹

    ● **S32.132**   **Severely displaced Zone III** fracture of sacrum A, K 🔹, B 🔹, A, B 🔹

    ● **S32.139**   **Unspecified Zone III** fracture of sacrum A, K 🔹, B 🔹, A, B 🔹

X ● **S32.14**   **Type 1 fracture of sacrum** A, K 🔹, B 🔹, A, B 🔹
    Transverse flexion fracture of sacrum without displacement

X ● **S32.15**   **Type 2 fracture of sacrum** A, K 🔹, B 🔹, A, B 🔹
    Transverse flexion fracture of sacrum with posterior displacement

X ● **S32.16**   **Type 3 fracture of sacrum** A, K 🔹, B 🔹, A, B 🔹
    Transverse extension fracture of sacrum with anterior displacement

X ● **S32.17**   **Type 4 fracture of sacrum** A, K 🔹, B 🔹, A, B 🔹
    Transverse segmental comminution of upper sacrum

X ● **S32.19**   **Other fracture of sacrum** A, K 🔹, B 🔹, A, B 🔹

X ● **S32.2**   **Fracture of coccyx** A, K 🔹, B 🔹, A, B 🔹

    (Ex) **For category S32.2 CC codes S32.2[A,B]:** See PDX Collection 1197
    For S32.2[K]: See PDX Collection 897

● **S32.3**   **Fracture of ilium**

    Excludes1   fracture of ilium with associated disruption of pelvic ring (S32.8-)

    (Ex) **For category S32.3 CC codes S32.3[A]:** See PDX Collection 1176
    For S32.3[B]: See PDX Collection 1198 **For S32.3[K]:** See PDX Collection 897

    ● **S32.30**   **Unspecified fracture of ilium**

      ● **S32.301**   **Unspecified fracture of right** ilium A, K 🔹, B 🔹, A, B 🔹

      ● **S32.302**   **Unspecified fracture of left** ilium A, K 🔹, B 🔹, A, B 🔹

      ● **S32.309**   **Unspecified fracture of unspecified** ilium A, K 🔹, B 🔹, A, B 🔹

    ● **S32.31**   **Avulsion fracture of ilium**

      ● **S32.311**   **Displaced avulsion fracture of right** ilium A, K 🔹, B 🔹, A, B 🔹

      ● **S32.312**   **Displaced avulsion fracture of left** ilium A, K 🔹, B 🔹, A, B 🔹

      ● **S32.313**   **Displaced avulsion fracture of unspecified** ilium A, K 🔹, B 🔹, A, B 🔹

      ● **S32.314**   **Nondisplaced avulsion fracture of right** ilium A, K 🔹, B 🔹, A, B 🔹

      ● **S32.315**   **Nondisplaced avulsion fracture of left** ilium A, K 🔹, B 🔹, A, B 🔹

      ● **S32.316**   **Nondisplaced avulsion fracture of unspecified** ilium A, K 🔹, B 🔹, A, B 🔹

▶ New   ⇒ Revised   ~~deleted~~ Deleted   Excludes 1   Excludes 2   Includes   Use additional   Code first   Code also   Key words

OGCR Official Guidelines   ● Unacceptable Principal Diagnosis   X Assign placeholder X   ● Use Additional Character(s)   ▶ Manifestation Code   **Coding Clinic**

- **S32.39   Other fracture of ilium**
  - **S32.391   Other fracture of right ilium** A, K, B, A, B
  - **S32.392   Other fracture of left ilium** A, K, B, A, B
  - **S32.399   Other fracture of unspecified ilium** A, K, B, A, B
- **S32.4   Fracture of acetabulum**

  Code also any associated fracture of pelvic ring (S32.8-)

  (Ex) **For category S32.4 CC codes S32.4[A]:** See PDX Collection 1199 **For S32.4[B]:** See PDX Collection 1200 **For S32.4[K]:** See PDX Collection 897

  - **S32.40   Unspecified fracture of acetabulum**
    - **S32.401   Unspecified fracture of right acetabulum** K, A, B, A, B
    - **S32.402   Unspecified fracture of left acetabulum** K, A, B, A, B
    - **S32.409   Unspecified fracture of unspecified acetabulum** K, A, B, A, B
  - **S32.41   Fracture of anterior wall of acetabulum**
    - **S32.411   Displaced fracture of anterior wall of right acetabulum** K, A, B, A, B
    - **S32.412   Displaced fracture of anterior wall of left acetabulum** K, A, B, A, B
    - **S32.413   Displaced fracture of anterior wall of unspecified acetabulum** K, A, B, A, B
    - **S32.414   Nondisplaced fracture of anterior wall of right acetabulum** K, A, B, A, B
    - **S32.415   Nondisplaced fracture of anterior wall of left acetabulum** K, A, B, A, B
    - **S32.416   Nondisplaced fracture of anterior wall of unspecified acetabulum** K, A, B, A, B
  - **S32.42   Fracture of posterior wall of acetabulum**
    - **S32.421   Displaced fracture of posterior wall of right acetabulum** K, A, B, A, B
    - **S32.422   Displaced fracture of posterior wall of left acetabulum** K, A, B, A, B
    - **S32.423   Displaced fracture of posterior wall of unspecified acetabulum** K, A, B, A, B
    - **S32.424   Nondisplaced fracture of posterior wall of right acetabulum** K, A, B, A, B
    - **S32.425   Nondisplaced fracture of posterior wall of left acetabulum** K, A, B, A, B
    - **S32.426   Nondisplaced fracture of posterior wall of unspecified acetabulum** K, A, B, A, B
  - **S32.43   Fracture of anterior column [iliopubic] of acetabulum**
    - **S32.431   Displaced fracture of anterior column [iliopubic] of right acetabulum** K, A, B, A, B
    - **S32.432   Displaced fracture of anterior column [iliopubic] of left acetabulum** K, A, B, A, B
    - **S32.433   Displaced fracture of anterior column [iliopubic] of unspecified acetabulum** K, A, B, A, B
  - **S32.434   Nondisplaced fracture of anterior column [iliopubic] of right acetabulum** K, A, B, A, B
  - **S32.435   Nondisplaced fracture of anterior column [iliopubic] of left acetabulum** K, A, B, A, B
  - **S32.436   Nondisplaced fracture of anterior column [iliopubic] of unspecified acetabulum** K, A, B, A, B
  - **S32.44   Fracture of posterior column [ilioischial] of acetabulum**
    - **S32.441   Displaced fracture of posterior column [ilioischial] of right acetabulum** K, A, B, A, B
    - **S32.442   Displaced fracture of posterior column [ilioischial] of left acetabulum** K, A, B, A, B
    - **S32.443   Displaced fracture of posterior column [ilioischial] of unspecified acetabulum** K, A, B, A, B
    - **S32.444   Nondisplaced fracture of posterior column [ilioischial] of right acetabulum** K, A, B, A, B
    - **S32.445   Nondisplaced fracture of posterior column [ilioischial] of left acetabulum** K, A, B, A, B
    - **S32.446   Nondisplaced fracture of posterior column [ilioischial] of unspecified acetabulum** K, A, B, A, B
  - **S32.45   Transverse fracture of acetabulum**
    - **S32.451   Displaced transverse fracture of right acetabulum** K, A, B, A, B
    - **S32.452   Displaced transverse fracture of left acetabulum** K, A, B, A, B
    - **S32.453   Displaced transverse fracture of unspecified acetabulum** K, A, B, A, B
    - **S32.454   Nondisplaced transverse fracture of right acetabulum** K, A, B, A, B
    - **S32.455   Nondisplaced transverse fracture of left acetabulum** K, A, B, A, B
    - **S32.456   Nondisplaced transverse fracture of unspecified acetabulum** K, A, B, A, B
  - **S32.46   Associated transverse-posterior fracture of acetabulum**
    - **S32.461   Displaced associated transverse-posterior fracture of right acetabulum** K, A, B, A, B
    - **S32.462   Displaced associated transverse-posterior fracture of left acetabulum** K, A, B, A, B
    - **S32.463   Displaced associated transverse-posterior fracture of unspecified acetabulum** K, A, B, A, B
    - **S32.464   Nondisplaced associated transverse-posterior fracture of right acetabulum** K, A, B, A, B
    - **S32.465   Nondisplaced associated transverse-posterior fracture of left acetabulum** K, A, B, A, B
    - **S32.466   Nondisplaced associated transverse-posterior fracture of unspecified acetabulum** K, A, B, A, B

N Newborn Age: 0   **P** Pediatric Age: 0–17   **M** Maternity DX: 12–55   **A** Adult Age: 15–124   ♀ Females Only   ♂ Males Only

Complication\Comorbidity   Major C\C   (Ex) CC/MCC Exclusions   Hospital-Acquired Condition

1265

CHAPTER 19 (S00-T88)

CHAPTER 19 (S00-T88)

● **S32.47**   Fracture of medial wall of acetabulum
- ● **S32.471**   Displaced fracture of medial wall of right acetabulum K, A, B, A, B
- ● **S32.472**   Displaced fracture of medial wall of left acetabulum K, A, B, A, B
- ● **S32.473**   Displaced fracture of medial wall of unspecified acetabulum K, A, B, A, B
- ● **S32.474**   Nondisplaced fracture of medial wall of right acetabulum K, A, B, A, B
- ● **S32.475**   Nondisplaced fracture of medial wall of left acetabulum K, A, B, A, B
- ● **S32.476**   Nondisplaced fracture of medial wall of unspecified acetabulum K, A, B, A, B

● **S32.48**   Dome fracture of acetabulum
- ● **S32.481**   Displaced dome fracture of right acetabulum K, A, B, A, B
- ● **S32.482**   Displaced dome fracture of left acetabulum K, A, B, A, B
- ● **S32.483**   Displaced dome fracture of unspecified acetabulum K, A, B, A, B
- ● **S32.484**   Nondisplaced dome fracture of right acetabulum K, A, B, A, B
- ● **S32.485**   Nondisplaced dome fracture of left acetabulum K, A, B, A, B
- ● **S32.486**   Nondisplaced dome fracture of unspecified acetabulum K, A, B, A, B

● **S32.49**   Other fracture of acetabulum
- ● **S32.491**   Other fracture of right acetabulum K, A, B, A, B
- ● **S32.492**   Other fracture of left acetabulum K, A, B, A, B
- ● **S32.499**   Other fracture of unspecified acetabulum K, A, B, A, B

● **S32.5**   Fracture of pubis
> **Excludes1**   fracture of pubis with associated disruption of pelvic ring (S32.8-)
>
> Ex: For category S32.5 CC codes S32.5[A,B]: See PDX Collection 1201 For S32.5[K]: See PDX Collection 897

● **S32.50**   Unspecified fracture of pubis
- ● **S32.501**   Unspecified fracture of right pubis A, K, B, A, B
- ● **S32.502**   Unspecified fracture of left pubis A, K, B, A, B
- ● **S32.509**   Unspecified fracture of unspecified pubis A, K, B, A, B

● **S32.51**   Fracture of superior rim of pubis
- ● **S32.511**   Fracture of superior rim of right pubis A, K, B, A, B
- ● **S32.512**   Fracture of superior rim of left pubis A, K, B, A, B
- ● **S32.519**   Fracture of superior rim of unspecified pubis A, K, B, A, B

● **S32.59**   Other specified fracture of pubis
- ● **S32.591**   Other specified fracture of right pubis A, K, B, A, B
- ● **S32.592**   Other specified fracture of left pubis A, K, B, A, B
- ● **S32.599**   Other specified fracture of unspecified pubis A, K, B, A, B

● **S32.6**   Fracture of ischium
> **Excludes1**   fracture of ischium with associated disruption of pelvic ring (S32.8-)
>
> Ex: For category S32.6 CC codes S32.6[A]: See PDX Collection 1202 For S32.6[B]: See PDX Collection 1203 For S32.5[K]: See PDX Collection 897

● **S32.60**   Unspecified fracture of ischium
- ● **S32.601**   Unspecified fracture of right ischium A, K, B, A, B
- ● **S32.602**   Unspecified fracture of left ischium A, K, B, A, B
- ● **S32.609**   Unspecified fracture of unspecified ischium A, K, B, A, B

● **S32.61**   Avulsion fracture of ischium
- ● **S32.611**   Displaced avulsion fracture of right ischium A, K, B, A, B
- ● **S32.612**   Displaced avulsion fracture of left ischium A, K, B, A, B
- ● **S32.613**   Displaced avulsion fracture of unspecified ischium A, K, B, A, B
- ● **S32.614**   Nondisplaced avulsion fracture of right ischium A, K, B, A, B
- ● **S32.615**   Nondisplaced avulsion fracture of left ischium A, K, B, A, B
- ● **S32.616**   Nondisplaced avulsion fracture of unspecified ischium A, K, B, A, B

● **S32.69**   Other specified fracture of ischium
- ● **S32.691**   Other specified fracture of right ischium A, K, B, A, B
- ● **S32.692**   Other specified fracture of left ischium A, K, B, A, B
- ● **S32.699**   Other specified fracture of unspecified ischium A, K, B, A, B

● **S32.8**   Fracture of other parts of pelvis
> Code also any associated:
> fracture of acetabulum (S32.4-)
> sacral fracture (S32.1-)

● **S32.81**   Multiple fractures of pelvis with disruption of pelvic ring
> Multiple pelvic fractures with disruption of pelvic circle
>
> Ex: For category S32.81 CC codes S32.81[A,B]: See PDX Collection 1204 For S32.81[K]: See PDX Collection 897
- ● **S32.810**   Multiple fractures of pelvis with stable disruption of pelvic ring A, K, B, A, B
- ● **S32.811**   Multiple fractures of pelvis with unstable disruption of pelvic ring A, K, B, A, B

X ● **S32.82**   Multiple fractures of pelvis without disruption of pelvic ring A, K, B, A, B
> Multiple pelvic fractures without disruption of pelvic circle
>
> Ex: For category S32.82 CC codes S32.82[A,B]: See PDX Collection 1205 For S32.81[K]: See PDX Collection 897

X ● **S32.89**   Fracture of other parts of pelvis A, K, B, A, B
> Ex: For category S32.89 CC codes S32.89[A,B]: See PDX Collection 1206 For S32.89[K]: See PDX Collection 897

X ● **S32.9**   Fracture of unspecified parts of lumbosacral spine and pelvis A, K, B, A, B
> Fracture of lumbosacral spine NOS
> Fracture of pelvis NOS
>
> Ex: For category S32.9 CC codes S32.9[A,B]: See PDX Collection 1204 For S32.9[K]: See PDX Collection 897
>
> **Coding Clinic: 2012, Q4, P93**

▶ New   ⇒ Revised   ~~deleted~~ Deleted   Excludes 1   Excludes 2   Includes   Use additional   Code first   Code also   Key words

OGCR Official Guidelines   ● Unacceptable Principal Diagnosis   X Assign placeholder X   ● Use Additional Character(s)   ▷ Manifestation Code   **Coding Clinic**

● **S33 Dislocation and sprain of joints and ligaments of lumbar spine and pelvis**

Includes   avulsion of joint or ligament of lumbar spine and pelvis
laceration of cartilage, joint or ligament of lumbar spine and pelvis
sprain of cartilage, joint or ligament of lumbar spine and pelvis
traumatic hemarthrosis of joint or ligament of lumbar spine and pelvis
traumatic rupture of joint or ligament of lumbar spine and pelvis
traumatic subluxation of joint or ligament of lumbar spine and pelvis
traumatic tear of joint or ligament of lumbar spine and pelvis

Code also any associated open wound

Excludes1   nontraumatic rupture or displacement of lumbar intervertebral disc NOS (M51.-)
obstetric damage to pelvic joints and ligaments (O71.6)

Excludes2   dislocation and sprain of joints and ligaments of hip (S73.-)
strain of muscle of lower back and pelvis (S39.01-)

The appropriate 7th character is to be added to each code from category S33

> A   initial encounter
> D   subsequent encounter
> S   sequela

X● **S33.0 Traumatic rupture of lumbar intervertebral disc**
Excludes1   rupture or displacement (nontraumatic) of lumbar intervertebral disc NOS (M51.- with fifth character 6)

● **S33.1 Subluxation and dislocation of lumbar vertebra**
Code also any associated:
open wound of abdomen, lower back and pelvis (S31)
spinal cord injury (S24.0, S24.1-, S34.0-, S34.1-)
Excludes2   fracture of lumbar vertebrae (S32.0-)

● S33.10 Subluxation and dislocation of unspecified lumbar vertebra
● S33.100 Subluxation of unspecified lumbar vertebra
● S33.101 Dislocation of unspecified lumbar vertebra
● S33.11 Subluxation and dislocation of L1/L2 lumbar vertebra
● S33.110 Subluxation of L1/L2 lumbar vertebra
● S33.111 Dislocation of L1/L2 lumbar vertebra
● S33.12 Subluxation and dislocation of L2/L3 lumbar vertebra
● S33.120 Subluxation of L2/L3 lumbar vertebra
● S33.121 Dislocation of L2/L3 lumbar vertebra
● S33.13 Subluxation and dislocation of L3/L4 lumbar vertebra
● S33.130 Subluxation of L3/L4 lumbar vertebra
● S33.131 Dislocation of L3/L4 lumbar vertebra
● S33.14 Subluxation and dislocation of L4/L5 lumbar vertebra
● S33.140 Subluxation of L4/L5 lumbar vertebra
● S33.141 Dislocation of L4/L5 lumbar vertebra

X● S33.2 Dislocation of sacroiliac and sacrococcygeal joint
● S33.3 Dislocation of other and unspecified parts of lumbar spine and pelvis
X● S33.30 Dislocation of unspecified parts of lumbar spine and pelvis
X● S33.39 Dislocation of other parts of lumbar spine and pelvis
X● S33.4 Traumatic rupture of symphysis pubis
X● S33.5 Sprain of ligaments of lumbar spine
X● S33.6 Sprain of sacroiliac joint
X● S33.8 Sprain of other parts of lumbar spine and pelvis
X● S33.9 Sprain of unspecified parts of lumbar spine and pelvis

● **S34 Injury of lumbar and sacral spinal cord and nerves at abdomen, lower back and pelvis level**
Note: Code to highest level of lumbar cord injury
Injuries to the spinal cord (S34.0 and S34.1) refer to the cord level and not bone level injury, and can affect nerve roots at and below the level given.
The appropriate 7th character is to be added to each code from category S34

> A   initial encounter
> D   subsequent encounter
> S   sequela

Code also any associated:
fracture of vertebra (S22.0-, S32.0-)
open wound of abdomen, lower back and pelvis (S31.-)
transient paralysis (R29.5)
(Ex) **For category S34 CC codes unless otherwise indicated:** See PDX Collection 1207

● **S34.0 Concussion and edema of lumbar and sacral spinal cord**
X● S34.01 Concussion and edema of lumbar spinal cord A 🐾
X● S34.02 Concussion and edema of sacral spinal cord A 🐾
Concussion and edema of conus medullaris
(Ex) See PDX Collection 1208

● **S34.1 Other and unspecified injury of lumbar and sacral spinal cord**
● S34.10 Unspecified injury to lumbar spinal cord
● S34.101 Unspecified injury to L₁ level of lumbar spinal cord A 🐾, A 🐾
Unspecified injury to lumbar spinal cord level 1
● S34.102 Unspecified injury to L₂ level of lumbar spinal cord A 🐾, A 🐾
Unspecified injury to lumbar spinal cord level 2
● S34.103 Unspecified injury to L₃ level of lumbar spinal cord A 🐾, A 🐾
Unspecified injury to lumbar spinal cord level 3
● S34.104 Unspecified injury to L₄ level of lumbar spinal cord A 🐾, A 🐾
Unspecified injury to lumbar spinal cord level 4
● S34.105 Unspecified injury to L₅ level of lumbar spinal cord A 🐾, A 🐾
Unspecified injury to lumbar spinal cord level 5
● S34.109 Unspecified injury to unspecified level of lumbar spinal cord A 🐾, A 🐾

N Newborn Age: 0   P Pediatric Age: 0–17   M Maternity DX: 12–55   A Adult Age: 15–124   ♀ Females Only   ♂ Males Only   🐾 Complication\Comorbidity   🐾 Major C\C   (Ex) CC/MCC Exclusions   🐾 Hospital-Acquired Condition

1267

● S34.11 **Complete lesion** of lumbar spinal cord

   ● S34.111 **Complete lesion of L$_1$ level of lumbar spinal cord** A 🔖, A 🔖
      Complete lesion of lumbar spinal cord level 1

   ● S34.112 **Complete lesion of L$_2$ level of lumbar spinal cord** A 🔖, A 🔖
      Complete lesion of lumbar spinal cord level 2

   ● S34.113 **Complete lesion of L$_3$ level of lumbar spinal cord** A 🔖, A 🔖
      Complete lesion of lumbar spinal cord level 3

   ● S34.114 **Complete lesion of L$_4$ level of lumbar spinal cord** A 🔖, A 🔖
      Complete lesion of lumbar spinal cord level 4

   ● S34.115 **Complete lesion of L$_5$ level of lumbar spinal cord** A 🔖, A 🔖
      Complete lesion of lumbar spinal cord level 5

   ● S34.119 **Complete lesion of unspecified level of lumbar spinal cord** A 🔖, A 🔖

● S34.12 **Incomplete lesion** of lumbar spinal cord

   ● S34.121 **Incomplete lesion of L$_1$ level of lumbar spinal cord** A 🔖, A 🔖
      Incomplete lesion of lumbar spinal cord level 1

   ● S34.122 **Incomplete lesion of L$_2$ level of lumbar spinal cord** A 🔖, A 🔖
      Incomplete lesion of lumbar spinal cord level 2

   ● S34.123 **Incomplete lesion of L$_3$ level of lumbar spinal cord** A 🔖, A 🔖
      Incomplete lesion of lumbar spinal cord level 3

   ● S34.124 **Incomplete lesion of L$_4$ level of lumbar spinal cord** A 🔖, A 🔖
      Incomplete lesion of lumbar spinal cord level 4

   ● S34.125 **Incomplete lesion of L$_5$ level of lumbar spinal cord** A 🔖, A 🔖
      Incomplete lesion of lumbar spinal cord level 5

   ● S34.129 **Incomplete lesion of unspecified level of lumbar spinal cord** A 🔖, A 🔖

● S34.13 **Other and unspecified injury to sacral** spinal cord
   Other injury to conus medullaris
   (Ex) For category S34.13 CC codes: See PDX Collection 1208

   ● S34.131 **Complete lesion of sacral spinal cord** A 🔖, A 🔖
      Complete lesion of conus medullaris

   ● S34.132 **Incomplete lesion of sacral spinal cord** A 🔖, A 🔖
      Incomplete lesion of conus medullaris

   ● S34.139 **Unspecified injury to sacral spinal cord** A 🔖, A 🔖
      Unspecified injury of conus medullaris

● S34.2 **Injury of nerve root** of lumbar and sacral spine

   X ● S34.21 **Injury of nerve root of lumbar spine**

   X ● S34.22 **Injury of nerve root of sacral spine**

X ● S34.3 **Injury of cauda equina** A 🔖, A 🔖
   (Ex) See PDX Collection 1208

X ● S34.4 **Injury of lumbosacral plexus**

X ● S34.5 **Injury of lumbar, sacral and pelvic sympathetic nerves**
   Injury of celiac ganglion or plexus
   Injury of hypogastric plexus
   Injury of mesenteric plexus (inferior) (superior)
   Injury of splanchnic nerve

X ● S34.6 **Injury of peripheral nerve(s) at abdomen, lower back and pelvis level**

X ● S34.8 **Injury of other nerves at abdomen, lower back and pelvis level**

X ● S34.9 **Injury of unspecified nerves at abdomen, lower back and pelvis level**

● S35 **Injury of blood vessels at abdomen, lower back and pelvis level**
   The appropriate 7th character is to be added to each code from category S35

A	initial encounter
D	subsequent encounter
S	sequela

   Code also any associated open wound (S31.-)

● S35.0 **Injury of abdominal aorta**
   Excludes1 injury of aorta NOS (S25.0)
   (Ex) For category S35.0 CC codes: See PDX Collection 1209

   X ● S35.00 **Unspecified injury of abdominal aorta** A 🔖

   X ● S35.01 **Minor laceration of abdominal aorta** A 🔖
      Incomplete transection of abdominal aorta
      Laceration of abdominal aorta NOS
      Superficial laceration of abdominal aorta

   X ● S35.02 **Major laceration of abdominal aorta** A 🔖
      Complete transection of abdominal aorta
      Traumatic rupture of abdominal aorta

   X ● S35.09 **Other injury of abdominal aorta** A 🔖

● S35.1 **Injury of inferior vena cava**
   Injury of hepatic vein
   Excludes1 injury of vena cava NOS (S25.2)
   (Ex) For category S35.1 CC codes: See PDX Collection 1210

   X ● S35.10 **Unspecified injury of inferior vena cava** A 🔖

   X ● S35.11 **Minor laceration of inferior vena cava** A 🔖
      Incomplete transection of inferior vena cava
      Laceration of inferior vena cava NOS
      Superficial laceration of inferior vena cava

   X ● S35.12 **Major laceration of inferior vena cava** A 🔖
      Complete transection of inferior vena cava
      Traumatic rupture of inferior vena cava

   X ● S35.19 **Other injury of inferior vena cava** A 🔖

● S35.2 **Injury of celiac or mesenteric artery and branches**

   ● S35.21 **Injury of celiac artery**
   (Ex) For category S35.21 CC codes: See PDX Collection 1211

      ● S35.211 **Minor laceration of celiac artery** A 🔖
         Incomplete transection of celiac artery
         Laceration of celiac artery NOS
         Superficial laceration of celiac artery

      ● S35.212 **Major laceration of celiac artery** A 🔖
         Complete transection of celiac artery
         Traumatic rupture of celiac artery

      ● S35.218 **Other injury of celiac artery** A 🔖

      ● S35.219 **Unspecified injury of celiac artery** A 🔖

- **S35.22　Injury of superior mesenteric artery**
  - (Ex) For category S35.22 CC codes: See PDX Collection 1212
  - **S35.221　Minor laceration of superior mesenteric artery A** 🔖
    - Incomplete transection of superior mesenteric artery
    - Laceration of superior mesenteric artery NOS
    - Superficial laceration of superior mesenteric artery
  - **S35.222　Major laceration of superior mesenteric artery A** 🔖
    - Complete transection of superior mesenteric artery
    - Traumatic rupture of superior mesenteric artery
  - **S35.228　Other injury of superior mesenteric artery A** 🔖
  - **S35.229　Unspecified injury of superior mesenteric artery A** 🔖
- **S35.23　Injury of inferior mesenteric artery**
  - (Ex) For category S35.23 CC codes: See PDX Collection 1213
  - **S35.231　Minor laceration of inferior mesenteric artery A** 🔖
    - Incomplete transection of inferior mesenteric artery
    - Laceration of inferior mesenteric artery NOS
    - Superficial laceration of inferior mesenteric artery
  - **S35.232　Major laceration of inferior mesenteric artery A** 🔖
    - Complete transection of inferior mesenteric artery
    - Traumatic rupture of inferior mesenteric artery
  - **S35.238　Other injury of inferior mesenteric artery A** 🔖
  - **S35.239　Unspecified injury of inferior mesenteric artery A** 🔖
- **S35.29　Injury of branches of celiac and mesenteric artery**
  - Injury of gastric artery
  - Injury of gastroduodenal artery
  - Injury of hepatic artery
  - Injury of splenic artery
  - (Ex) For category S35.29 CC codes unless otherwise indicated: See PDX Collection 1215
  - **S35.291　Minor laceration of branches of celiac and mesenteric artery A** 🔖
    - Incomplete transection of branches of celiac and mesenteric artery
    - Laceration of branches of celiac and mesenteric artery NOS
    - Superficial laceration of branches of celiac and mesenteric artery
    - (Ex) See PDX Collection 1214
  - **S35.292　Major laceration of branches of celiac and mesenteric artery A** 🔖
    - Complete transection of branches of celiac and mesenteric artery
    - Traumatic rupture of branches of celiac and mesenteric artery
  - **S35.298　Other injury of branches of celiac and mesenteric artery A** 🔖
  - **S35.299　Unspecified injury of branches of celiac and mesenteric artery A** 🔖
    - (Ex) See PDX Collection 1216

- **S35.3　Injury of portal or splenic vein and branches**
  - **S35.31　Injury of portal vein**
    - (Ex) For category S35.31 CC codes: See PDX Collection 1217
    - **S35.311　Laceration of portal vein A** 🔖
    - **S35.318　Other specified injury of portal vein A** 🔖
    - **S35.319　Unspecified injury of portal vein A** 🔖
  - **S35.32　Injury of splenic vein**
    - (Ex) For category S35.32 CC codes: See PDX Collection 1218
    - **S35.321　Laceration of splenic vein A** 🔖
    - **S35.328　Other specified injury of splenic vein A** 🔖
    - **S35.329　Unspecified injury of splenic vein A** 🔖
  - **S35.33　Injury of superior mesenteric vein**
    - (Ex) For category S35.33 CC codes: See PDX Collection 1219
    - **S35.331　Laceration of superior mesenteric vein A** 🔖
    - **S35.338　Other specified injury of superior mesenteric vein A** 🔖
    - **S35.339　Unspecified injury of superior mesenteric vein A** 🔖
  - **S35.34　Injury of inferior mesenteric vein**
    - (Ex) For category S35.34 CC codes: See PDX Collection 1220
    - **S35.341　Laceration of inferior mesenteric vein A** 🔖
    - **S35.348　Other specified injury of inferior mesenteric vein A** 🔖
    - **S35.349　Unspecified injury of inferior mesenteric vein A** 🔖
- **S35.4　Injury of renal blood vessels**
  - **S35.40　Unspecified injury of renal blood vessel**
    - (Ex) For category S35.40 CC codes S35.401-S35.403: See PDX Collection 1221
    - For category S35.40 CC codes S35.404-S35.406: See PDX Collection 1222
    - **S35.401　Unspecified injury of right renal artery A** 🔖
    - **S35.402　Unspecified injury of left renal artery A** 🔖
    - **S35.403　Unspecified injury of unspecified renal artery A** 🔖
    - **S35.404　Unspecified injury of right renal vein A** 🔖
    - **S35.405　Unspecified injury of left renal vein A** 🔖
    - **S35.406　Unspecified injury of unspecified renal vein A** 🔖
  - **S35.41　Laceration of renal blood vessel**
    - (Ex) For category S35.41 CC codes S35.411-S35.413: See PDX Collection 1221
    - For category S35.41 CC codes S35.414-S35.416: See PDX Collection 1222
    - **S35.411　Laceration of right renal artery A** 🔖
    - **S35.412　Laceration of left renal artery A** 🔖
    - **S35.413　Laceration of unspecified renal artery A** 🔖
    - **S35.414　Laceration of right renal vein A** 🔖
    - **S35.415　Laceration of left renal vein A** 🔖
    - **S35.416　Laceration of unspecified renal vein A** 🔖

CHAPTER 19 (S00-T88)

● **S35.49**   **Other specified injury of renal blood vessel**
Ex: For category S35.49 CC codes S35.491-S35.493:
See PDX Collection 1221
For category S35.49 CC codes S35.494-S35.496:
See PDX Collection 1222

● **S35.491**   Other specified injury of right renal artery A 🔖

● **S35.492**   Other specified injury of left renal artery A 🔖

● **S35.493**   Other specified injury of unspecified renal artery A 🔖

● **S35.494**   Other specified injury of right renal vein A 🔖

● **S35.495**   Other specified injury of left renal vein A 🔖

● **S35.496**   Other specified injury of unspecified renal vein A 🔖

● **S35.5**   **Injury of iliac blood vessels**

X ● **S35.50**   Injury of unspecified iliac blood vessel(s) A 🔖
Ex: See PDX Collection 1223

● **S35.51**   Injury of iliac artery or vein
Injury of hypogastric artery or vein
Ex: For category S35.51 CC codes S35.511-S35.513:
See PDX Collection 1224
For category S35.51 CC codes S35.514-S35.516:
See PDX Collection 1225

● **S35.511**   Injury of right iliac artery A 🔖

● **S35.512**   Injury of left iliac artery A 🔖

● **S35.513**   Injury of unspecified iliac artery A 🔖

● **S35.514**   Injury of right iliac vein A 🔖

● **S35.515**   Injury of left iliac vein A 🔖

● **S35.516**   Injury of unspecified iliac vein A 🔖

● **S35.53**   Injury of uterine artery or vein
Ex: For category S35.53 CC codes S35.531-S35.533:
See PDX Collection 1226
For category S35.53 CC codes S35.534-S35.536:
See PDX Collection 1227

● **S35.531**   Injury of right uterine artery ♀ A 🔖

● **S35.532**   Injury of left uterine artery ♀ A 🔖

● **S35.533**   Injury of unspecified uterine artery ♀ A 🔖

● **S35.534**   Injury of right uterine vein ♀ A 🔖

● **S35.535**   Injury of left uterine vein ♀ A 🔖

● **S35.536**   Injury of unspecified uterine vein ♀ A 🔖

X ● **S35.59**   Injury of other iliac blood vessels A 🔖
Ex: See PDX Collection 1223

● **S35.8**   **Injury of other blood vessels at abdomen, lower back and pelvis level**
Injury of ovarian artery or vein
Ex: For category S35.8 CC codes: See PDX Collection 1228

● **S35.8X**   Injury of other blood vessels at abdomen, lower back and pelvis level

● **S35.8X1**   Laceration of other blood vessels at abdomen, lower back and pelvis level A 🔖

● **S35.8X8**   Other specified injury of other blood vessels at abdomen, lower back and pelvis level A 🔖

● **S35.8X9**   Unspecified injury of other blood vessels at abdomen, lower back and pelvis level A 🔖

● **S35.9**   **Injury of unspecified blood vessel at abdomen, lower back and pelvis level**
Ex: For category S35.9 CC codes: See PDX Collection 1229

X ● **S35.90**   Unspecified injury of unspecified blood vessel at abdomen, lower back and pelvis level A 🔖

X ● **S35.91**   Laceration of unspecified blood vessel at abdomen, lower back and pelvis level A 🔖

X ● **S35.99**   Other specified injury of unspecified blood vessel at abdomen, lower back and pelvis level A 🔖

● **S36**   **Injury of intra-abdominal organs**
The appropriate 7th character is to be added to each code from category S36

A	initial encounter
D	subsequent encounter
S	sequela

Code also any associated open wound (S31.-)

● **S36.0**   **Injury of spleen**
Ex: For category S36.0 CC codes: See PDX Collection 1230

X ● **S36.00**   Unspecified injury of spleen A 🔖

● **S36.02**   Contusion of spleen

● **S36.020**   Minor contusion of spleen A 🔖
Contusion of spleen less than 2 cm

● **S36.021**   Major contusion of spleen A 🔖
Contusion of spleen greater than 2 cm

● **S36.029**   Unspecified contusion of spleen A 🔖
Coding Clinic: 2015, Q2, P36, Q1, P11

● **S36.03**   Laceration of spleen

● **S36.030**   Superficial (capsular) laceration of spleen A 🔖
Laceration of spleen less than 1 cm
Minor laceration of spleen

● **S36.031**   Moderate laceration of spleen A 🔖
Laceration of spleen 1 to 3 cm
Coding Clinic: 2015, Q2, P36, Q1, P11

● **S36.032**   Major laceration of spleen A 🔖
Avulsion of spleen
Laceration of spleen greater than 3 cm
Massive laceration of spleen
Multiple moderate lacerations of spleen
Stellate laceration of spleen

● **S36.039**   Unspecified laceration of spleen A 🔖

X ● **S36.09**   Other injury of spleen A 🔖

● **S36.1**   **Injury of liver and gallbladder and bile duct**

● **S36.11**   Injury of liver
Ex: For category S36.11 CC codes: See PDX Collection 1231

● **S36.112**   Contusion of liver A 🔖

● **S36.113**   Laceration of liver, unspecified degree A 🔖

● **S36.114**   Minor laceration of liver A 🔖
Laceration involving capsule only, or, without significant involvement of hepatic parenchyma [i.e., less than 1 cm deep]

● **S36.115**   Moderate laceration of liver A 🔖
Laceration involving parenchyma but without major disruption of parenchyma [i.e., less than 10 cm long and less than 3 cm deep]

● **S36.116**   Major laceration of liver A 🔖
Laceration with significant disruption of hepatic parenchyma [i.e., greater than 10 cm long and 3 cm deep]
Multiple moderate lacerations, with or without hematoma
Stellate laceration of liver

● **S36.118**   Other injury of liver A 🔖

● **S36.119**   Unspecified injury of liver A 🔖
Coding Clinic: 2015, Q2, P17

▶ New   ⇒ Revised   ~~deleted~~ Deleted   Excludes 1   Excludes 2   Includes   Use additional   Code first   Code also   Key words

OGCR Official Guidelines   ● Unacceptable Principal Diagnosis   X Assign placeholder X   ● Use Additional Character(s)   ) Manifestation Code   Coding Clinic

● S36.12   Injury of gallbladder
   (Ex) **For category S36.12 CC codes:** See PDX Collection 1232
   ● S36.122   Contusion of gallbladder A %
   ● S36.123   Laceration of gallbladder A %
   ● S36.128   Other injury of gallbladder A %
   ● S36.129   Unspecified injury of gallbladder A %
X ● S36.13   Injury of bile duct A %
   (Ex) See PDX Collection 1232
● S36.2   Injury of pancreas
   (Ex) **For category S36.2 CC codes:** See PDX Collection 1233
   ● S36.20   Unspecified injury of pancreas
      ● S36.200   Unspecified injury of head of pancreas A %
      ● S36.201   Unspecified injury of body of pancreas A %
      ● S36.202   Unspecified injury of tail of pancreas A %
      ● S36.209   Unspecified injury of unspecified part of pancreas A %
   ● S36.22   Contusion of pancreas
      ● S36.220   Contusion of head of pancreas A %
      ● S36.221   Contusion of body of pancreas A %
      ● S36.222   Contusion of tail of pancreas A %
      ● S36.229   Contusion of unspecified part of pancreas A %
   ● S36.23   Laceration of pancreas, unspecified degree
      ● S36.230   Laceration of head of pancreas, unspecified degree A %
      ● S36.231   Laceration of body of pancreas, unspecified degree A %
      ● S36.232   Laceration of tail of pancreas, unspecified degree A %
      ● S36.239   Laceration of unspecified part of pancreas, unspecified degree A %
   ● S36.24   Minor laceration of pancreas
      ● S36.240   Minor laceration of head of pancreas A %
      ● S36.241   Minor laceration of body of pancreas A %
      ● S36.242   Minor laceration of tail of pancreas A %
      ● S36.249   Minor laceration of unspecified part of pancreas A %
   ● S36.25   Moderate laceration of pancreas
      ● S36.250   Moderate laceration of head of pancreas A %
      ● S36.251   Moderate laceration of body of pancreas A %
      ● S36.252   Moderate laceration of tail of pancreas A %
      ● S36.259   Moderate laceration of unspecified part of pancreas A %
   ● S36.26   Major laceration of pancreas
      ● S36.260   Major laceration of head of pancreas A %
      ● S36.261   Major laceration of body of pancreas A %
      ● S36.262   Major laceration of tail of pancreas A %
      ● S36.269   Major laceration of unspecified part of pancreas A %

● S36.29   Other injury of pancreas
   ● S36.290   Other injury of head of pancreas A %
   ● S36.291   Other injury of body of pancreas A %
   ● S36.292   Other injury of tail of pancreas A %
   ● S36.299   Other injury of unspecified part of pancreas A %
● S36.3   Injury of stomach
   (Ex) **For category S36.3 CC codes:** See PDX Collection 1234
X ● S36.30   Unspecified injury of stomach A %
X ● S36.32   Contusion of stomach A %
X ● S36.33   Laceration of stomach A %
X ● S36.39   Other injury of stomach A %
● S36.4   Injury of small intestine
   (Ex) **For category S36.4 CC codes:** See PDX Collection 1235
   ● S36.40   Unspecified injury of small intestine
      ● S36.400   Unspecified injury of duodenum A %
      ● S36.408   Unspecified injury of other part of small intestine A %
      ● S36.409   Unspecified injury of unspecified part of small intestine A %
   ● S36.41   Primary blast injury of small intestine
      Blast injury of small intestine NOS
      ● S36.410   Primary blast injury of duodenum A %
      ● S36.418   Primary blast injury of other part of small intestine A %
      ● S36.419   Primary blast injury of unspecified part of small intestine A %
   ● S36.42   Contusion of small intestine
      ● S36.420   Contusion of duodenum A %
      ● S36.428   Contusion of other part of small intestine A %
      ● S36.429   Contusion of unspecified part of small intestine A %
   ● S36.43   Laceration of small intestine
      ● S36.430   Laceration of duodenum A %
      ● S36.438   Laceration of other part of small intestine A %
      ● S36.439   Laceration of unspecified part of small intestine A %
   ● S36.49   Other injury of small intestine
      ● S36.490   Other injury of duodenum A %
      ● S36.498   Other injury of other part of small intestine A %
      ● S36.499   Other injury of unspecified part of small intestine A %
● S36.5   Injury of colon
   Excludes2   injury of rectum (S36.6-)
   (Ex) **For category S36.5 CC codes:** See PDX Collection 1236
   ● S36.50   Unspecified injury of colon
      ● S36.500   Unspecified injury of ascending [right] colon A %
      ● S36.501   Unspecified injury of transverse colon A %
      ● S36.502   Unspecified injury of descending [left] colon A %
      ● S36.503   Unspecified injury of sigmoid colon A %
      ● S36.508   Unspecified injury of other part of colon A %
      ● S36.509   Unspecified injury of unspecified part of colon A %

CHAPTER 19 (S00-T88)

N Newborn Age: 0   P Pediatric Age: 0–17   M Maternity DX: 12–55   A Adult Age: 15–124   ♀ Females Only   ♂ Males Only
% Complication\Comorbidity   % Major C\C   (Ex) CC/MCC Exclusions   % Hospital-Acquired Condition

1271

● S36.51   **Primary blast injury of colon**
           Blast injury of colon NOS
   ● S36.510   **Primary blast injury of ascending [right] colon** A 🔾
   ● S36.511   **Primary blast injury of transverse colon** A 🔾
   ● S36.512   **Primary blast injury of descending [left] colon** A 🔾
   ● S36.513   **Primary blast injury of sigmoid colon** A 🔾
   ● S36.518   **Primary blast injury of other part of colon** A 🔾
   ● S36.519   **Primary blast injury of unspecified part of colon** A 🔾

● S36.52   **Contusion of colon**
   ● S36.520   **Contusion of ascending [right] colon** A 🔾
   ● S36.521   **Contusion of transverse colon** A 🔾
   ● S36.522   **Contusion of descending [left] colon** A 🔾
   ● S36.523   **Contusion of sigmoid colon** A 🔾
   ● S36.528   **Contusion of other part of colon** A 🔾
   ● S36.529   **Contusion of unspecified part of colon** A 🔾

● S36.53   **Laceration of colon**
   ● S36.530   **Laceration of ascending [right] colon** A 🔾
   ● S36.531   **Laceration of transverse colon** A 🔾
   ● S36.532   **Laceration of descending [left] colon** A 🔾
   ● S36.533   **Laceration of sigmoid colon** A 🔾
   ● S36.538   **Laceration of other part of colon** A 🔾
     S36.539   **Laceration of unspecified part of colon** A 🔾

● S36.59   **Other injury of colon**
           Secondary blast injury of colon
   ● S36.590   **Other injury of ascending [right] colon** A 🔾
   ● S36.591   **Other injury of transverse colon** A 🔾
   ● S36.592   **Other injury of descending [left] colon** A 🔾
   ● S36.593   **Other injury of sigmoid colon** A 🔾
   ● S36.598   **Other injury of other part of colon** A 🔾
   ● S36.599   **Other injury of unspecified part of colon** A 🔾

● S36.6   **Injury of rectum**
          (Ex) **For category S36.6 CC codes:** See PDX Collection 1236
   X ● S36.60   **Unspecified injury of rectum** A 🔾
   X ● S36.61   **Primary blast injury of rectum** A 🔾
             Blast injury of rectum NOS
   X ● S36.62   **Contusion of rectum** A 🔾
   X ● S36.63   **Laceration of rectum** A 🔾
   X ● S36.69   **Other injury of rectum** A 🔾
             Secondary blast injury of rectum

● S36.8   **Injury of other intra-abdominal organs**
          (Ex) **For category S36.8 CC codes:** See PDX Collection 1195
   X ● S36.81   **Injury of peritoneum** A 🔾
   ● S36.89   **Injury of other intra-abdominal organs**
             Injury of retroperitoneum
   ● S36.892   **Contusion of other intra-abdominal organs** A 🔾
   ● S36.893   **Laceration of other intra-abdominal organs** A 🔾
   ● S36.898   **Other injury of other intra-abdominal organs** A 🔾
     S36.899   **Unspecified injury of other intra-abdominal organs** A 🔾

● S36.9   **Injury of unspecified intra-abdominal organ**
          (Ex) **For category S36.9 CC codes:** See PDX Collection 1195
   X ● S36.90   **Unspecified injury of unspecified intra-abdominal organ** A 🔾
   X ● S36.92   **Contusion of unspecified intra-abdominal organ** A 🔾
   X ● S36.93   **Laceration of unspecified intra-abdominal organ** A 🔾
   X ● S36.99   **Other injury of unspecified intra-abdominal organ** A 🔾

● S37   **Injury of urinary and pelvic organs**
        Code also any associated open wound (S31.-)
        Excludes1   obstetric trauma to pelvic organs (O71.-)
        Excludes2   injury of peritoneum (S36.81)
                        injury of retroperitoneum (S36.89-)
        The appropriate 7th character is to be added to each code from category S37

        ┌─────────────────────────────────────┐
        │ A   initial encounter   │
        │ D   subsequent encounter   │
        │ S   sequela   │
        └─────────────────────────────────────┘

● S37.0   **Injury of kidney**
          Excludes2   acute kidney injury (nontraumatic) (N17.9)
          (Ex) **For category S37.0 CC codes:** See PDX Collection 1237
   ● S37.00   **Unspecified injury of kidney**
      ● S37.001   **Unspecified injury of right kidney** A 🔾
      ● S37.002   **Unspecified injury of left kidney** A 🔾
      ● S37.009   **Unspecified injury of unspecified kidney** A 🔾
   ● S37.01   **Minor contusion of kidney**
             Contusion of kidney less than 2 cm
             Contusion of kidney NOS
      ● S37.011   **Minor contusion of right kidney** A 🔾
      ● S37.012   **Minor contusion of left kidney** A 🔾
      ● S37.019   **Minor contusion of unspecified kidney** A 🔾
   ● S37.02   **Major contusion of kidney**
             Contusion of kidney greater than 2 cm
      ● S37.021   **Major contusion of right kidney** A 🔾
      ● S37.022   **Major contusion of left kidney** A 🔾
      ● S37.029   **Major contusion of unspecified kidney** A 🔾
   ● S37.03   **Laceration of kidney, unspecified degree**
      ● S37.031   **Laceration of right kidney, unspecified degree** A 🔾
      ● S37.032   **Laceration of left kidney, unspecified degree** A 🔾
      ● S37.039   **Laceration of unspecified kidney, unspecified degree** A 🔾
   ● S37.04   **Minor laceration of kidney**
             Laceration of kidney less than 1 cm
      ● S37.041   **Minor laceration of right kidney** A 🔾
      ● S37.042   **Minor laceration of left kidney** A 🔾
      ● S37.049   **Minor laceration of unspecified kidney** A 🔾
   ● S37.05   **Moderate laceration of kidney**
             Laceration of kidney 1 to 3 cm
      ● S37.051   **Moderate laceration of right kidney** A 🔾
      ● S37.052   **Moderate laceration of left kidney** A 🔾
      ● S37.059   **Moderate laceration of unspecified kidney** A 🔾

▶ New   ⟹ Revised   ~~deleted~~ Deleted | Excludes 1 | | Excludes 2 | | Includes | | Use additional | | Code first | | Code also | | Key words |

OGCR Official Guidelines   ● Unacceptable Principal Diagnosis   X Assign placeholder X   ● Use Additional Character(s)   ▶ Manifestation Code   **Coding Clinic**

● **S37.06**   **Major laceration of kidney**
    Avulsion of kidney
    Laceration of kidney greater than 3 cm
    Massive laceration of kidney
    Multiple moderate lacerations of kidney
    Stellate laceration of kidney
    ● **S37.061**   Major laceration of right kidney A 🦠
    ● **S37.062**   Major laceration of left kidney A 🦠
    ● **S37.069**   Major laceration of unspecified kidney A 🦠
● **S37.09**   **Other injury of kidney**
    ● **S37.091**   Other injury of right kidney A 🦠
    ● **S37.092**   Other injury of left kidney A 🦠
    ● **S37.099**   Other injury of unspecified kidney A 🦠

● **S37.1**   **Injury of ureter**
    Ⓔ **For category S37.1 CC codes:** See PDX Collection 1238
X ● **S37.10**   Unspecified injury of ureter A 🦠
X ● **S37.12**   Contusion of ureter A 🦠
X ● **S37.13**   Laceration of ureter A 🦠
X ● **S37.19**   Other injury of ureter A 🦠

● **S37.2**   **Injury of bladder**
    Ⓔ **For category S37.2 CC codes:** See PDX Collection 1239
X ● **S37.20**   Unspecified injury of bladder A 🦠
X ● **S37.22**   Contusion of bladder A 🦠
X ● **S37.23**   Laceration of bladder A 🦠
X ● **S37.29**   Other injury of bladder A 🦠

● **S37.3**   **Injury of urethra**
    Ⓔ **For category S37.3 CC codes:** See PDX Collection 1239
X ● **S37.30**   Unspecified injury of urethra A 🦠
X ● **S37.32**   Contusion of urethra A 🦠
X ● **S37.33**   Laceration of urethra A 🦠
X ● **S37.39**   Other injury of urethra A 🦠

● **S37.4**   **Injury of ovary**
    ● **S37.40**   **Unspecified injury of ovary**
        ● **S37.401**   Unspecified injury of ovary, unilateral ♀
        ● **S37.402**   Unspecified injury of ovary, bilateral ♀
        ● **S37.409**   Unspecified injury of ovary, unspecified ♀
    ● **S37.42**   **Contusion of ovary**
        ● **S37.421**   Contusion of ovary, unilateral ♀
        ● **S37.422**   Contusion of ovary, bilateral ♀
        ● **S37.429**   Contusion of ovary, unspecified ♀
    ● **S37.43**   **Laceration of ovary**
        ● **S37.431**   Laceration of ovary, unilateral ♀
        ● **S37.432**   Laceration of ovary, bilateral ♀
        ● **S37.439**   Laceration of ovary, unspecified ♀
    ● **S37.49**   **Other injury of ovary**
        ● **S37.491**   Other injury of ovary, unilateral ♀
        ● **S37.492**   Other injury of ovary, bilateral ♀
        ● **S37.499**   Other injury of ovary, unspecified ♀

● **S37.5**   **Injury of fallopian tube**
    ● **S37.50**   **Unspecified injury of fallopian tube**
        ● **S37.501**   Unspecified injury of fallopian tube, unilateral ♀
        ● **S37.502**   Unspecified injury of fallopian tube, bilateral ♀
        ● **S37.509**   Unspecified injury of fallopian tube, unspecified ♀

● **S37.51**   **Primary blast injury of fallopian tube**
    Blast injury of fallopian tube NOS
    ● **S37.511**   Primary blast injury of fallopian tube, unilateral ♀
    ● **S37.512**   Primary blast injury of fallopian tube, bilateral ♀
    ● **S37.519**   Primary blast injury of fallopian tube, unspecified ♀
● **S37.52**   **Contusion of fallopian tube**
    ● **S37.521**   Contusion of fallopian tube, unilateral ♀
    ● **S37.522**   Contusion of fallopian tube, bilateral ♀
    ● **S37.529**   Contusion of fallopian tube, unspecified ♀
● **S37.53**   **Laceration of fallopian tube**
    ● **S37.531**   Laceration of fallopian tube, unilateral ♀
    ● **S37.532**   Laceration of fallopian tube, bilateral ♀
    ● **S37.539**   Laceration of fallopian tube, unspecified ♀
● **S37.59**   **Other injury of fallopian tube**
    Secondary blast injury of fallopian tube
    ● **S37.591**   Other injury of fallopian tube, unilateral ♀
    ● **S37.592**   Other injury of fallopian tube, bilateral ♀
    ● **S37.599**   Other injury of fallopian tube, unspecified ♀

● **S37.6**   **Injury of uterus**
    Excludes1   injury to gravid uterus (O9A.2-)
                  injury to uterus during delivery (O71.-)
    Ⓔ **For category S37.6 CC codes:** See PDX Collection 1240
X ● **S37.60**   Unspecified injury of uterus ♀ A 🦠
X ● **S37.62**   Contusion of uterus ♀ A 🦠
X ● **S37.63**   Laceration of uterus ♀ A 🦠
X ● **S37.69**   Other injury of uterus ♀ A 🦠

● **S37.8**   **Injury of other urinary and pelvic organs**
    ● **S37.81**   **Injury of adrenal gland**
        Ⓔ **For category S37.81 CC codes:** See PDX Collection 1241
        ● **S37.812**   Contusion of adrenal gland A 🦠
        ● **S37.813**   Laceration of adrenal gland A 🦠
        ● **S37.818**   Other injury of adrenal gland A 🦠
        ● **S37.819**   Unspecified injury of adrenal gland A 🦠
    ● **S37.82**   **Injury of prostate**
        ● **S37.822**   Contusion of prostate ♂
        ● **S37.823**   Laceration of prostate ♂
        ● **S37.828**   Other injury of prostate ♂
        ● **S37.829**   Unspecified injury of prostate ♂
    ● **S37.89**   **Injury of other urinary and pelvic organ**
        Ⓔ **For category S37.89 CC codes:** See PDX Collection 1242
        ● **S37.892**   Contusion of other urinary and pelvic organ A 🦠
        ● **S37.893**   Laceration of other urinary and pelvic organ A 🦠
        ● **S37.898**   Other injury of other urinary and pelvic organ A 🦠
        ● **S37.899**   Unspecified injury of other urinary and pelvic organ A 🦠

CHAPTER 19 (S00–T88)

N   Newborn Age: 0   P   Pediatric Age: 0–17   M   Maternity DX: 12–55   A   Adult Age: 15–124   ♀   Females Only   ♂   Males Only
🦠   Complication\Comorbidity   🦠   Major C\C   Ⓔ   CC/MCC Exclusions   🦠   Hospital-Acquired Condition

1273

CHAPTER 19 (S00-T88)

● **S37.9**   **Injury of unspecified urinary and pelvic organ**
     Ex: For category S37.9 CC codes: See PDX Collection 1242

X● **S37.90**   Unspecified injury of unspecified urinary and pelvic organ A 🔖

X● **S37.92**   Contusion of unspecified urinary and pelvic organ A 🔖

X● **S37.93**   Laceration of unspecified urinary and pelvic organ A 🔖

X● **S37.99**   Other injury of unspecified urinary and pelvic organ A 🔖

● **S38**   **Crushing injury and traumatic amputation of abdomen, lower back, pelvis and external genitals**
     An amputation not identified as partial or complete should be coded to complete
     The appropriate 7th character is to be added to each code from category S38

     A   initial encounter
     D   subsequent encounter
     S   sequela

● **S38.0**   **Crushing injury of external genital organs**
     Use additional code for any associated injuries

● **S38.00**   Crushing injury of unspecified external genital organs

● **S38.001**   Crushing injury of unspecified external genital organs, male ♂

● **S38.002**   Crushing injury of unspecified external genital organs, female ♀

X● **S38.01**   Crushing injury of penis ♂

X● **S38.02**   Crushing injury of scrotum and testis ♂

X● **S38.03**   Crushing injury of vulva ♀

X● **S38.1**   **Crushing injury of abdomen, lower back, and pelvis**
     Use additional code for all associated injuries, such as:
     fracture of thoracic or lumbar spine and pelvis (S22.0-, S32.-)
     injury to intra-abdominal organs (S36.-)
     injury to urinary and pelvic organs (S37.-)
     open wound of abdominal wall (S31.-)
     spinal cord injury (S34.0, S34.1-)

     Excludes2   crushing injury of external genital organs (S38.0-)

● **S38.2**   **Traumatic amputation of external genital organs**

● **S38.21**   Traumatic amputation of female external genital organs
     Traumatic amputation of clitoris
     Traumatic amputation of labium (majus) (minus)
     Traumatic amputation of vulva

● **S38.211**   Complete traumatic amputation of female external genital organs ♀

● **S38.212**   Partial traumatic amputation of female external genital organs ♀

● **S38.22**   Traumatic amputation of penis

● **S38.221**   Complete traumatic amputation of penis ♂

● **S38.222**   Partial traumatic amputation of penis ♂

● **S38.23**   Traumatic amputation of scrotum and testis

● **S38.231**   Complete traumatic amputation of scrotum and testis ♂

● **S38.232**   Partial traumatic amputation of scrotum and testis ♂

X● **S38.3**   **Transection (partial) of abdomen**

● **S39**   **Other and unspecified injuries of abdomen, lower back, pelvis and external genitals**
     Code also any associated open wound (S31.-)

     Excludes2   sprain of joints and ligaments of lumbar spine and pelvis (S33.-)

     The appropriate 7th character is to be added to each code from category S39

     A   initial encounter
     D   subsequent encounter
     S   sequela

● **S39.0**   **Injury of muscle, fascia and tendon of abdomen, lower back and pelvis**

● **S39.00**   Unspecified injury of muscle, fascia and tendon of abdomen, lower back and pelvis

● **S39.001**   Unspecified injury of muscle, fascia and tendon of abdomen

● **S39.002**   Unspecified injury of muscle, fascia and tendon of lower back

● **S39.003**   Unspecified injury of muscle, fascia and tendon of pelvis

● **S39.01**   Strain of muscle, fascia and tendon of abdomen, lower back and pelvis

● **S39.011**   Strain of muscle, fascia and tendon of abdomen

● **S39.012**   Strain of muscle, fascia and tendon of lower back
     Coding Clinic: 2016, Q4, P74

● **S39.013**   Strain of muscle, fascia and tendon of pelvis

● **S39.02**   Laceration of muscle, fascia and tendon of abdomen, lower back and pelvis

● **S39.021**   Laceration of muscle, fascia and tendon of abdomen

● **S39.022**   Laceration of muscle, fascia and tendon of lower back

● **S39.023**   Laceration of muscle, fascia and tendon of pelvis

● **S39.09**   Other injury of muscle, fascia and tendon of abdomen, lower back and pelvis

● **S39.091**   Other injury of muscle, fascia and tendon of abdomen

● **S39.092**   Other injury of muscle, fascia and tendon of lower back

● **S39.093**   Other injury of muscle, fascia and tendon of pelvis

● **S39.8**   **Other specified injuries of abdomen, lower back, pelvis and external genitals**

X● **S39.81**   Other specified injuries of abdomen

X● **S39.82**   Other specified injuries of lower back

X● **S39.83**   Other specified injuries of pelvis

● **S39.84**   Other specified injuries of external genitals

● **S39.840**   Fracture of corpus cavernosum penis ♂

● **S39.848**   Other specified injuries of external genitals

● **S39.9**   **Unspecified injury of abdomen, lower back, pelvis and external genitals**

X● **S39.91**   Unspecified injury of abdomen

X● **S39.92**   Unspecified injury of lower back

X● **S39.93**   Unspecified injury of pelvis

X● **S39.94**   Unspecified injury of external genitals

▶ New   ⇒ Revised   ~~deleted~~ Deleted   Excludes 1   Excludes 2   Includes   Use additional   Code first   Code also   Key words
OGCR Official Guidelines   ● Unacceptable Principal Diagnosis   X Assign placeholder X   ● Use Additional Character(s)   ▶ Manifestation Code   **Coding Clinic**

INJURIES TO THE SHOULDER AND UPPER ARM (S40-S49)

Includes	injuries of axilla injuries of scapular region
Excludes2	burns and corrosions (T20-T32)
	frostbite (T33-T34)
	injuries of elbow (S50-S59)
	insect bite or sting, venomous (T63.4)

● **S40**   **Superficial injury of shoulder and upper arm**

The appropriate 7th character is to be added to each code from category S40

A	initial encounter
D	subsequent encounter
S	sequela

● **S40.0**   Contusion of shoulder and upper arm
  ● **S40.01**   Contusion of shoulder
    ● S40.011   Contusion of right shoulder
    ● S40.012   Contusion of left shoulder
    ● S40.019   Contusion of unspecified shoulder
  ● **S40.02**   Contusion of upper arm
    ● S40.021   Contusion of right upper arm
    ● S40.022   Contusion of left upper arm
    ● S40.029   Contusion of unspecified upper arm
● **S40.2**   Other superficial injuries of shoulder
  ● **S40.21**   Abrasion of shoulder
    ● S40.211   Abrasion of right shoulder
    ● S40.212   Abrasion of left shoulder
    ● S40.219   Abrasion of unspecified shoulder
  ● **S40.22**   Blister (nonthermal) of shoulder
    ● S40.221   Blister (nonthermal) of right shoulder
    ● S40.222   Blister (nonthermal) of left shoulder
    ● S40.229   Blister (nonthermal) of unspecified shoulder
  ● **S40.24**   External constriction of shoulder
    ● S40.241   External constriction of right shoulder
    ● S40.242   External constriction of left shoulder
    ● S40.249   External constriction of unspecified shoulder
  ● **S40.25**   Superficial foreign body of shoulder
    Splinter in the shoulder
    ● S40.251   Superficial foreign body of right shoulder
    ● S40.252   Superficial foreign body of left shoulder
    ● S40.259   Superficial foreign body of unspecified shoulder
  ● **S40.26**   Insect bite (nonvenomous) of shoulder
    ● S40.261   Insect bite (nonvenomous) of right shoulder
    ● S40.262   Insect bite (nonvenomous) of left shoulder
    ● S40.269   Insect bite (nonvenomous) of unspecified shoulder
  ● **S40.27**   Other superficial bite of shoulder
    Excludes1   open bite of shoulder (S41.05)
    ● S40.271   Other superficial bite of right shoulder
    ● S40.272   Other superficial bite of left shoulder
    ● S40.279   Other superficial bite of unspecified shoulder

● **S40.8**   Other superficial injuries of upper arm
  ● **S40.81**   Abrasion of upper arm
    ● S40.811   Abrasion of right upper arm
    ● S40.812   Abrasion of left upper arm
    ● S40.819   Abrasion of unspecified upper arm
  ● **S40.82**   Blister (nonthermal) of upper arm
    ● S40.821   Blister (nonthermal) of right upper arm
    ● S40.822   Blister (nonthermal) of left upper arm
    ● S40.829   Blister (nonthermal) of unspecified upper arm
  ● **S40.84**   External constriction of upper arm
    ● S40.841   External constriction of right upper arm
    ● S40.842   External constriction of left upper arm
    ● S40.849   External constriction of unspecified upper arm
  ● **S40.85**   Superficial foreign body of upper arm
    Splinter in the upper arm
    ● S40.851   Superficial foreign body of right upper arm
    ● S40.852   Superficial foreign body of left upper arm
    ● S40.859   Superficial foreign body of unspecified upper arm
  ● **S40.86**   Insect bite (nonvenomous) of upper arm
    ● S40.861   Insect bite (nonvenomous) of right upper arm
    ● S40.862   Insect bite (nonvenomous) of left upper arm
    ● S40.869   Insect bite (nonvenomous) of unspecified upper arm
  ● **S40.87**   Other superficial bite of upper arm
    Excludes1   open bite of upper arm (S41.14)
    Excludes2   other superficial bite of shoulder (S40.27-)
    ● S40.871   Other superficial bite of right upper arm
    ● S40.872   Other superficial bite of left upper arm
    ● S40.879   Other superficial bite of unspecified upper arm
● **S40.9**   Unspecified superficial injury of shoulder and upper arm
  ● **S40.91**   Unspecified superficial injury of shoulder
    ● S40.911   Unspecified superficial injury of right shoulder
    ● S40.912   Unspecified superficial injury of left shoulder
    ● S40.919   Unspecified superficial injury of unspecified shoulder
  ● **S40.92**   Unspecified superficial injury of upper arm
    ● S40.921   Unspecified superficial injury of right upper arm
    ● S40.922   Unspecified superficial injury of left upper arm
    ● S40.929   Unspecified superficial injury of unspecified upper arm

CHAPTER 19 (S00-T88)

S41   Open wound of shoulder and upper arm

Code also any associated wound infection

Excludes1   traumatic amputation of shoulder and upper arm (S48.-)

Excludes2   open fracture of shoulder and upper arm (S42.- with 7th character B or C)

The appropriate 7th character is to be added to each code from category S41

> A   initial encounter
> D   subsequent encounter
> S   sequela

● **S41.0   Open wound of shoulder**

  ● **S41.00   Unspecified open wound of shoulder**

    ● S41.001   Unspecified open wound of right shoulder
    ● S41.002   Unspecified open wound of left shoulder
    ● S41.009   Unspecified open wound of unspecified shoulder

  ● **S41.01   Laceration without foreign body of shoulder**

    ● S41.011   Laceration without foreign body of right shoulder
    ● S41.012   Laceration without foreign body of left shoulder
    ● S41.019   Laceration without foreign body of unspecified shoulder

  ● **S41.02   Laceration with foreign body of shoulder**

    ● S41.021   Laceration with foreign body of right shoulder
    ● S41.022   Laceration with foreign body of left shoulder
    ● S41.029   Laceration with foreign body of unspecified shoulder

  ● **S41.03   Puncture wound without foreign body of shoulder**

    ● S41.031   Puncture wound without foreign body of right shoulder
    ● S41.032   Puncture wound without foreign body of left shoulder
    ● S41.039   Puncture wound without foreign body of unspecified shoulder

  ● **S41.04   Puncture wound with foreign body of shoulder**

    ● S41.041   Puncture wound with foreign body of right shoulder
    ● S41.042   Puncture wound with foreign body of left shoulder
    ● S41.049   Puncture wound with foreign body of unspecified shoulder

  ● **S41.05   Open bite of shoulder**

    Bite of shoulder NOS

    Excludes1   superficial bite of shoulder (S40.27)

    ● S41.051   Open bite of right shoulder
    ● S41.052   Open bite of left shoulder
    ● S41.059   Open bite of unspecified shoulder

● **S41.1   Open wound of upper arm**

  ● **S41.10   Unspecified open wound of upper arm**

    ● S41.101   Unspecified open wound of right upper arm
    ● S41.102   Unspecified open wound of left upper arm
    ● S41.109   Unspecified open wound of unspecified upper arm

  ● **S41.11   Laceration without foreign body of upper arm**

    ● S41.111   Laceration without foreign body of right upper arm
    ● S41.112   Laceration without foreign body of left upper arm
    ● S41.119   Laceration without foreign body of unspecified upper arm

  ● **S41.12   Laceration with foreign body of upper arm**

    ● S41.121   Laceration with foreign body of right upper arm
    ● S41.122   Laceration with foreign body of left upper arm
    ● S41.129   Laceration with foreign body of unspecified upper arm

  ● **S41.13   Puncture wound without foreign body of upper arm**

    ● S41.131   Puncture wound without foreign body of right upper arm
    ● S41.132   Puncture wound without foreign body of left upper arm
    ● S41.139   Puncture wound without foreign body of unspecified upper arm

  ● **S41.14   Puncture wound with foreign body of upper arm**

    ● S41.141   Puncture wound with foreign body of right upper arm
    ● S41.142   Puncture wound with foreign body of left upper arm
    ● S41.149   Puncture wound with foreign body of unspecified upper arm

  ● **S41.15   Open bite of upper arm**

    Bite of upper arm NOS

    Excludes1   superficial bite of upper arm (S40.87)

    ● S41.151   Open bite of right upper arm
    ● S41.152   Open bite of left upper arm
    ● S41.159   Open bite of unspecified upper arm

● **S42   Fracture of shoulder and upper arm**

Note: A fracture not indicated as displaced or nondisplaced should be coded to displaced

A fracture not indicated as open or closed should be coded to closed

Excludes1   traumatic amputation of shoulder and upper arm (S48.-)

The appropriate 7th character is to be added to all codes from category S42

> A   initial encounter for closed fracture
> B   initial encounter for open fracture
> D   subsequent encounter for fracture with routine healing
> G   subsequent encounter for fracture with delayed healing
> K   subsequent encounter for fracture with nonunion
> P   subsequent encounter for fracture with malunion
> S   sequela

● **S42.0   Fracture of clavicle**

  (Ex) For S42.0[B]: See PDX Collection 1243 For S42.0[K,P]: See PDX Collection 897

  ● **S42.00   Fracture of unspecified part of clavicle**

    ● S42.001   Fracture of unspecified part of right clavicle B, K, P ✎, B ✎
    ● S42.002   Fracture of unspecified part of left clavicle B, K, P ✎, B ✎
    ● S42.009   Fracture of unspecified part of unspecified clavicle B, K, P ✎, B ✎
      Coding Clinic: 2012, Q4, P3

▶ New   ⇒ Revised   ~~deleted~~ Deleted   Excludes 1   Excludes 2   Includes   Use additional   Code first   Code also   Key words

OGCR Official Guidelines   ● Unacceptable Principal Diagnosis   X Assign placeholder X   ▶ Use Additional Character(s)   ▶ Manifestation Code   **Coding Clinic**

● **S42.01**   Fracture of sternal end of clavicle
  - ● **S42.011**   Anterior displaced fracture of sternal end of right clavicle B, K, P 🔹, B 🔹
  - ● **S42.012**   Anterior displaced fracture of sternal end of left clavicle B, K, P 🔹, B 🔹
  - ● **S42.013**   Anterior displaced fracture of sternal end of unspecified clavicle B, K, P 🔹, B 🔹
    > Displaced fracture of sternal end of clavicle NOS
  - ● **S42.014**   Posterior displaced fracture of sternal end of right clavicle B, K, P 🔹, B 🔹
  - ● **S42.015**   Posterior displaced fracture of sternal end of left clavicle B, K, P 🔹, B 🔹
  - ● **S42.016**   Posterior displaced fracture of sternal end of unspecified clavicle B, K, P 🔹, B 🔹
  - ● **S42.017**   Nondisplaced fracture of sternal end of right clavicle B, K, P 🔹, B 🔹
  - ● **S42.018**   Nondisplaced fracture of sternal end of left clavicle B, K, P 🔹, B 🔹
  - ● **S42.019**   Nondisplaced fracture of sternal end of unspecified clavicle B, K, P 🔹, B 🔹

● **S42.02**   Fracture of shaft of clavicle
  - ● **S42.021**   Displaced fracture of shaft of right clavicle B, K, P 🔹, B 🔹
  - ● **S42.022**   Displaced fracture of shaft of left clavicle B, K, P 🔹, B 🔹
  - ● **S42.023**   Displaced fracture of shaft of unspecified clavicle B, K, P 🔹, B 🔹
  - ● **S42.024**   Nondisplaced fracture of shaft of right clavicle B, K, P 🔹, B 🔹
  - ● **S42.025**   Nondisplaced fracture of shaft of left clavicle B, K, P 🔹, B 🔹
  - ● **S42.026**   Nondisplaced fracture of shaft of unspecified clavicle B, K, P 🔹, B 🔹

● **S42.03**   Fracture of lateral end of clavicle
  > Fracture of acromial end of clavicle
  - ● **S42.031**   Displaced fracture of lateral end of right clavicle B, K, P 🔹, B 🔹
  - ● **S42.032**   Displaced fracture of lateral end of left clavicle B, K, P 🔹, B 🔹
  - ● **S42.033**   Displaced fracture of lateral end of unspecified clavicle B, K, P 🔹, B 🔹
  - ● **S42.034**   Nondisplaced fracture of lateral end of right clavicle B, K, P 🔹, B 🔹
  - ● **S42.035**   Nondisplaced fracture of lateral end of left clavicle B, K, P 🔹, B 🔹
  - ● **S42.036**   Nondisplaced fracture of lateral end of unspecified clavicle B, K, P 🔹, B 🔹

● **S42.1**   Fracture of scapula
  > (Ex) **For S42.1[B]:** See PDX Collection 1244 **For S42.1[K,P]:** See PDX Collection 897

  ● **S42.10**   Fracture of unspecified part of scapula
  - ● **S42.101**   Fracture of unspecified part of scapula, right shoulder B, K, P 🔹, B 🔹
  - ● **S42.102**   Fracture of unspecified part of scapula, left shoulder B, K, P 🔹, B 🔹
  - ● **S42.109**   Fracture of unspecified part of scapula, unspecified shoulder B, K, P 🔹, B 🔹

● **S42.11**   Fracture of body of scapula
  - ● **S42.111**   Displaced fracture of body of scapula, right shoulder B, K, P 🔹, B 🔹
  - ● **S42.112**   Displaced fracture of body of scapula, left shoulder B, K, P 🔹, B 🔹
  - ● **S42.113**   Displaced fracture of body of scapula, unspecified shoulder B, K, P 🔹, B 🔹
  - ● **S42.114**   Nondisplaced fracture of body of scapula, right shoulder B, K, P 🔹, B 🔹
  - ● **S42.115**   Nondisplaced fracture of body of scapula, left shoulder B, K, P 🔹, B 🔹
  - ● **S42.116**   Nondisplaced fracture of body of scapula, unspecified shoulder B, K, P 🔹, B 🔹

● **S42.12**   Fracture of acromial process
  - ● **S42.121**   Displaced fracture of acromial process, right shoulder B, K, P 🔹, B 🔹
  - ● **S42.122**   Displaced fracture of acromial process, left shoulder B, K, P 🔹, B 🔹
  - ● **S42.123**   Displaced fracture of acromial process, unspecified shoulder B, K, P 🔹, B 🔹
  - ● **S42.124**   Nondisplaced fracture of acromial process, right shoulder B, K, P 🔹, B 🔹
  - ● **S42.125**   Nondisplaced fracture of acromial process, left shoulder B, K, P 🔹, B 🔹
  - ● **S42.126**   Nondisplaced fracture, of acromial process, unspecified shoulder B, K, P 🔹, B 🔹

● **S42.13**   Fracture of coracoid process
  - ● **S42.131**   Displaced fracture of coracoid process, right shoulder B, K, P 🔹, B 🔹
  - ● **S42.132**   Displaced fracture of coracoid process, left shoulder B, K, P 🔹, B 🔹
  - ● **S42.133**   Displaced fracture of coracoid process, unspecified shoulder B, K, P 🔹, B 🔹
  - ● **S42.134**   Nondisplaced fracture of coracoid process, right shoulder B, K, P 🔹, B 🔹
  - ● **S42.135**   Nondisplaced fracture of coracoid process, left shoulder B, K, P 🔹, B 🔹
  - ● **S42.136**   Nondisplaced fracture of coracoid process, unspecified shoulder B, K, P 🔹, B 🔹

● **S42.14**   Fracture of glenoid cavity of scapula
  - ● **S42.141**   Displaced fracture of glenoid cavity of scapula, right shoulder B, K, P 🔹, B 🔹
  - ● **S42.142**   Displaced fracture of glenoid cavity of scapula, left shoulder B, K, P 🔹, B 🔹
  - ● **S42.143**   Displaced fracture of glenoid cavity of scapula, unspecified shoulder B, K, P 🔹, B 🔹
  - ● **S42.144**   Nondisplaced fracture of glenoid cavity of scapula, right shoulder B, K, P 🔹, B 🔹
  - ● **S42.145**   Nondisplaced fracture of glenoid cavity of scapula, left shoulder B, K, P 🔹, B 🔹
  - ● **S42.146**   Nondisplaced fracture of glenoid cavity of scapula, unspecified shoulder B, K, P 🔹, B 🔹

CHAPTER 19 (S00–T88)

CHAPTER 19 (S00–T88)

● **S42.15**   Fracture of neck of scapula

  ● **S42.151**   Displaced fracture of neck of scapula, right shoulder B, K, P 🔖, B 🔖

  ● **S42.152**   Displaced fracture of neck of scapula, left shoulder B, K, P 🔖, B 🔖

  ● **S42.153**   Displaced fracture of neck of scapula, unspecified shoulder B, K, P 🔖, B 🔖

  ● **S42.154**   Nondisplaced fracture of neck of scapula, right shoulder B, K, P 🔖, B 🔖

  ● **S42.155**   Nondisplaced fracture of neck of scapula, left shoulder B, K, P 🔖, B 🔖

  ● **S42.156**   Nondisplaced fracture of neck of scapula, unspecified shoulder B, K, P 🔖, B 🔖

● **S42.19**   Fracture of other part of scapula

  ● **S42.191**   Fracture of other part of scapula, right shoulder B, K, P 🔖, B 🔖

  ● **S42.192**   Fracture of other part of scapula, left shoulder B, K, P 🔖, B 🔖

  ● **S42.199**   Fracture of other part of scapula, unspecified shoulder B, K, P 🔖, B 🔖

● **S42.2**   Fracture of upper end of humerus

     Fracture of proximal end of humerus

     Excludes2   fracture of shaft of humerus (S42.3-)
                physeal fracture of upper end of humerus (S49.0-)

  ● **S42.20**   Unspecified fracture of upper end of humerus

    ● **S42.201**   Unspecified fracture of upper end of right humerus A, K, P 🔖, B 🔖, A, B 🔖

       (Ex:) For S42.201[A]: See PDX Collection 1245
            For S42.201[B]: See PDX Collection 1246
            For S42.201[K,P]: See PDX Collection 897

    ● **S42.202**   Unspecified fracture of upper end of left humerus A, K, P 🔖, B 🔖, A, B 🔖

       (Ex:) For category S42.202 CC codes
            S42.202[A]: See PDX Collection 1247
            For S42.202[B]: See PDX Collection 1246
            For S42.202[K,P]: See PDX Collection 897

    ● **S42.209**   Unspecified fracture of upper end of unspecified humerus A, K, P 🔖, B 🔖, A, B 🔖

       (Ex:) For S42.209[A]: See PDX Collection 1248
            For S42.202[B]: See PDX Collection 1246
            For S42.202[K,P]: See PDX Collection 897

  ● **S42.21**   Unspecified fracture of surgical neck of humerus

       Fracture of neck of humerus NOS

    ● **S42.211**   Unspecified displaced fracture of surgical neck of right humerus A, K, P 🔖, B 🔖, A, B 🔖

       (Ex:) For S42.211[A]: See PDX Collection 1245
            For S42.211[B]: See PDX Collection 1246
            For S42.211[K,P]: See PDX Collection 897

    ● **S42.212**   Unspecified displaced fracture of surgical neck of left humerus A, K, P 🔖, B 🔖, A, B 🔖

       (Ex:) For S42.212[A]: See PDX Collection 1247
            For S42.212[B]: See PDX Collection 1246
            For S42.212[K,P]: See PDX Collection 897

    ● **S42.213**   Unspecified displaced fracture of surgical neck of unspecified humerus A, K, P 🔖, B 🔖, A, B 🔖

       (Ex:) For S42.213[A]: See PDX Collection 1248
            For S42.213[B]: See PDX Collection 1246
            For S42.213[K,P]: See PDX Collection 897

    ● **S42.214**   Unspecified nondisplaced fracture of surgical neck of right humerus A, K, P 🔖, B 🔖, A, B 🔖

       (Ex:) For S42.214[A]: See PDX Collection 1245
            For S42.214[B]: See PDX Collection 1246
            For S42.214[K,P]: See PDX Collection 897

    ● **S42.215**   Unspecified nondisplaced fracture of surgical neck of left humerus A, K, P 🔖, B 🔖, A, B 🔖

       (Ex:) For S42.215[A]: See PDX Collection 1247
            For S42.215[B]: See PDX Collection 1246
            For S42.215[K,P]: See PDX Collection 897

    ● **S42.216**   Unspecified nondisplaced fracture of surgical neck of unspecified humerus A, K, P 🔖, B 🔖, A, B 🔖

       (Ex:) For S42.216[A]: See PDX Collection 1248
            For S42.216[B]: See PDX Collection 1246
            For S42.216[K,P]: See PDX Collection 897

  ● **S42.22**   2-part fracture of surgical neck of humerus

    ● **S42.221**   2-part displaced fracture of surgical neck of right humerus A, K, P 🔖, B 🔖, A, B 🔖

       (Ex:) For S42.221[A]: See PDX Collection 1245
            For S42.221[B]: See PDX Collection 1246
            For S42.221[K,P]: See PDX Collection 897

    ● **S42.222**   2-part displaced fracture of surgical neck of left humerus A, K, P 🔖, B 🔖, A, B 🔖

       (Ex:) For S42.222[A]: See PDX Collection 1247
            For S42.222[B]: See PDX Collection 1246
            For S42.222[K,P]: See PDX Collection 897

    ● **S42.223**   2-part displaced fracture of surgical neck of unspecified humerus A, K, P 🔖, B 🔖, A, B 🔖

       (Ex:) For S42.223[A]: See PDX Collection 1248
            For S42.223[B]: See PDX Collection 1246
            For S42.223[K,P]: See PDX Collection 897

    ● **S42.224**   2-part nondisplaced fracture of surgical neck of right humerus A, K, P 🔖, B 🔖, A, B 🔖

       (Ex:) For S42.224[A]: See PDX Collection 1245
            For S42.224[B]: See PDX Collection 1246
            For S42.224[K,P]: See PDX Collection 897

    ● **S42.225**   2-part nondisplaced fracture of surgical neck of left humerus A, K, P 🔖, B 🔖, A, B 🔖

       (Ex:) For S42.225[A]: See PDX Collection 1247
            For S42.225[B]: See PDX Collection 1246
            For S42.225[K,P]: See PDX Collection 897

    ● **S42.226**   2-part nondisplaced fracture of surgical neck of unspecified humerus A, K, P 🔖, B 🔖, A, B 🔖

       (Ex:) For S42.226[A]: See PDX Collection 1248
            For S42.226[B]: See PDX Collection 1246
            For S42.226[K,P]: See PDX Collection 897

▶ New   ⇒ Revised   ~~deleted~~ Deleted   Excludes 1   Excludes 2   Includes   Use additional   Code first   Code also   Key words

OGCR Official Guidelines   ● Unacceptable Principal Diagnosis   X Assign placeholder X   ● Use Additional Character(s)   ▌ Manifestation Code   **Coding Clinic**

● **S42.23**   **3-part fracture of surgical neck of humerus**

  ● **S42.231**   **3-part fracture of surgical neck of right humerus** A, K, P 🦠, B 🦠, A, B 🦠
     Ⓔ **For S42.231[A]:** See PDX Collection 1245
       For S42.231[B]: See PDX Collection 1246
       For S42.231[K,P]: See PDX Collection 897

  ● **S42.232**   **3-part fracture of surgical neck of left humerus** A, K, P 🦠, B 🦠, A, B
     Ⓔ **For S42.232[A]:** See PDX Collection 1247
       For S42.232[B]: See PDX Collection 1246
       For S42.232[K,P]: See PDX Collection 897

  ● **S42.239**   **3-part fracture of surgical neck of unspecified humerus** A, K, P 🦠, B 🦠, A, B
     Ⓔ **For S42.239[A]:** See PDX Collection 1248
       For S42.239[B]: See PDX Collection 1246
       For S42.239[K,P]: See PDX Collection 897

● **S42.24**   **4-part fracture of surgical neck of humerus**

  ● **S42.241**   **4-part fracture of surgical neck of right humerus** A, K, P 🦠, B 🦠, A, B 🦠
     Ⓔ **For S42.241[A]:** See PDX Collection 1245
       For S42.241[B]: See PDX Collection 1246
       For S42.241[K,P]: See PDX Collection 897

  ● **S42.242**   **4-part fracture of surgical neck of left humerus** A, K, P 🦠, B 🦠, A, B 🦠
     Ⓔ **For S42.242[A]:** See PDX Collection 1247
       For S42.242[B]: See PDX Collection 1246
       For S42.242[K,P]: See PDX Collection 897

  ● **S42.249**   **4-part fracture of surgical neck of unspecified humerus** A, K, P 🦠, B 🦠, A, B 🦠
     Ⓔ **For S42.249[A]:** See PDX Collection 1248
       For S42.249[B]: See PDX Collection 1246
       For S42.249[K,P]: See PDX Collection 897

● **S42.25**   **Fracture of greater tuberosity of humerus**

  ● **S42.251**   **Displaced fracture of greater tuberosity of right humerus** A, K, P 🦠, B 🦠, A, B
     Ⓔ **For S42.251[A]:** See PDX Collection 1245
       For S42.251[B]: See PDX Collection 1246
       For S42.251[K,P]: See PDX Collection 897

  ● **S42.252**   **Displaced fracture of greater tuberosity of left humerus** A, K, P 🦠, B 🦠, A, B
     Ⓔ **For S42.252[A]:** See PDX Collection 1247
       For S42.252[B]: See PDX Collection 1246
       For S42.252[K,P]: See PDX Collection 897

  ● **S42.253**   **Displaced fracture of greater tuberosity of unspecified humerus** A, K, P 🦠, B 🦠, A, B 🦠
     Ⓔ **For S42.253[A]:** See PDX Collection 1248
       For S42.253[B]: See PDX Collection 1246
       For S42.253[K,P]: See PDX Collection 897

  ● **S42.254**   **Nondisplaced fracture of greater tuberosity of right humerus** A, K, P 🦠, B 🦠, A, B
     Ⓔ **For S42.254[A]:** See PDX Collection 1245
       For S42.254[B]: See PDX Collection 1246
       For S42.254[K,P]: See PDX Collection 897

  ● **S42.255**   **Nondisplaced fracture of greater tuberosity of left humerus** A, K, P 🦠, B 🦠, A, B
     Ⓔ **For S42.255[A]:** See PDX Collection 1247
       For S42.255[B]: See PDX Collection 1246
       For S42.255[K,P]: See PDX Collection 897

  ● **S42.256**   **Nondisplaced fracture of greater tuberosity of unspecified humerus** A, K, P 🦠, B 🦠, A, B 🦠
     Ⓔ **For S42.256[A]:** See PDX Collection 1248
       For S42.256[B]: See PDX Collection 1246
       For S42.256[K,P]: See PDX Collection 897

● **S42.26**   **Fracture of lesser tuberosity of humerus**

  ● **S42.261**   **Displaced fracture of lesser tuberosity of right humerus** A, K, P 🦠, B 🦠, A, B
     Ⓔ **For S42.261[A]:** See PDX Collection 1245
       For S42.261[B]: See PDX Collection 1246
       For S42.261[K,P]: See PDX Collection 897

  ● **S42.262**   **Displaced fracture of lesser tuberosity of left humerus** A, K, P 🦠, B 🦠, A, B
     Ⓔ **For S42.262[A]:** See PDX Collection 1247
       For S42.262[B]: See PDX Collection 1246
       For S42.262[K,P]: See PDX Collection 897

  ● **S42.263**   **Displaced fracture of lesser tuberosity of unspecified humerus** A, K, P 🦠, B 🦠, A, B 🦠
     Ⓔ **For S42.263[A]:** See PDX Collection 1248
       For S42.263[B]: See PDX Collection 1246
       For S42.263[K,P]: See PDX Collection 897

  ● **S42.264**   **Nondisplaced fracture of lesser tuberosity of right humerus** A, K, P 🦠, B 🦠, A, B 🦠
     Ⓔ **For S42.264[A]:** See PDX Collection 1245
       For S42.264[B]: See PDX Collection 1246
       For S42.264[K,P]: See PDX Collection 897

  ● **S42.265**   **Nondisplaced fracture of lesser tuberosity of left humerus** A, K, P 🦠, B 🦠, A, B 🦠
     Ⓔ **For S42.265[A]:** See PDX Collection 1247
       For S42.265[B]: See PDX Collection 1246
       For S42.265[K,P]: See PDX Collection 897

  ● **S42.266**   **Nondisplaced fracture of lesser tuberosity of unspecified humerus** A, K, P 🦠, B 🦠, A, B 🦠
     Ⓔ **For S42.266[A]:** See PDX Collection 1248
       For S42.266[B]: See PDX Collection 1246
       For S42.266[K,P]: See PDX Collection 897

● **S42.27**   **Torus fracture of upper end of humerus**

The appropriate 7th character is to be added to all codes in subcategory S42.27

A	initial encounter for closed fracture
D	subsequent encounter for fracture with routine healing
G	subsequent encounter for fracture with delayed healing
K	subsequent encounter for fracture with nonunion
P	subsequent encounter for fracture with malunion
S	sequela

  ● **S42.271**   **Torus fracture of upper end of right humerus** A, K, P 🦠, A 🦠
     Ⓔ **For S42.271[A]:** See PDX Collection 1245
       For S42.271[K,P]: See PDX Collection 897

  ● **S42.272**   **Torus fracture of upper end of left humerus** A, K, P 🦠, A 🦠
     Ⓔ **For S42.272[A]:** See PDX Collection 1247
       For S42.272[K,P]: See PDX Collection 897

  ● **S42.279**   **Torus fracture of upper end of unspecified humerus** A, K, P 🦠, A 🦠
     Ⓔ **For S42.279[A]:** See PDX Collection 1248
       For S42.279[K,P]: See PDX Collection 897

CHAPTER 19 (S00–T88)

N Newborn Age: 0   **P** Pediatric Age: 0–17   **M** Maternity DX: 12–55   **A** Adult Age: 15–124   ♀ Females Only   ♂ Males Only

🦠 Complication\Comorbidity   🦠 Major C\C   Ⓔ CC/MCC Exclusions   🦠 Hospital-Acquired Condition

1279

CHAPTER 19 (S00–T88)

● **S42.29**   **Other fracture of upper end of humerus**
Fracture of anatomical neck of humerus
Fracture of articular head of humerus

    ● **S42.291**   **Other displaced fracture of upper end of right humerus** A, K, P 🔳, B 🔳, A, B 🔳
       (Ex:) **For S42.291[A]:** See PDX Collection 1245
       For S42.291[B]: See PDX Collection 1246
       For S42.291[K,P]: See PDX Collection 897

    ● **S42.292**   **Other displaced fracture of upper end of left humerus** A, K, P 🔳, B 🔳, A, B 🔳
       (Ex:) **For S42.292[A]:** See PDX Collection 1247
       For S42.292[B]: See PDX Collection 1246
       For S42.292[K,P]: See PDX Collection 897

    ● **S42.293**   **Other displaced fracture of upper end of unspecified humerus** A, K, P 🔳, B 🔳, A, B 🔳
       (Ex:) **For S42.293[A]:** See PDX Collection 1248
       For S42.293[B]: See PDX Collection 1246
       For S42.293[K,P]: See PDX Collection 897

    ● **S42.294**   **Other nondisplaced fracture of upper end of right humerus** A, K, P 🔳, B 🔳, A, B 🔳
       (Ex:) **For S42.294[A]:** See PDX Collection 1245
       For S42.294[B]: See PDX Collection 1246
       For S42.294[K,P]: See PDX Collection 897

    ● **S42.295**   **Other nondisplaced fracture of upper end of left humerus** A, K, P 🔳, B 🔳, A, B 🔳
       (Ex:) **For S42.295[A]:** See PDX Collection 1247
       For S42.295[B]: See PDX Collection 1246
       For S42.295[K,P]: See PDX Collection 897

    ● **S42.296**   **Other nondisplaced fracture of upper end of unspecified humerus** A, K, P 🔳, B 🔳, A, B 🔳
       (Ex:) **For S42.296[A]:** See PDX Collection 1248
       For S42.296[B]: See PDX Collection 1246
       For S42.296[K,P]: See PDX Collection 897

● **S42.3**   **Fracture of shaft of humerus**
Fracture of humerus NOS
Fracture of upper arm NOS

   Excludes2   physeal fractures of upper end of humerus (S49.0-)
       physeal fractures of lower end of humerus (S49.1-)

   ● **S42.30**   **Unspecified fracture of shaft of humerus**

    ● **S42.301**   **Unspecified fracture of shaft of humerus, right arm** A, K, P 🔳, B 🔳, A, B 🔳
       (Ex:) **For S42.301[A]:** See PDX Collection 1245
       For S42.301[B]: See PDX Collection 1246
       For S42.301[K,P]: See PDX Collection 897

    ● **S42.302**   **Unspecified fracture of shaft of humerus, left arm** A, K, P 🔳, B 🔳, A, B 🔳
       (Ex:) **For S42.302[A]:** See PDX Collection 1247
       For S42.302[B]: See PDX Collection 1246
       For S42.302[K,P]: See PDX Collection 897

    ● **S42.309**   **Unspecified fracture of shaft of humerus, unspecified arm** A, K, P 🔳, B 🔳, A, B 🔳
       (Ex:) **For S42.309[A]:** See PDX Collection 1248
       For S42.309[B]: See PDX Collection 1246
       For S42.309[K,P]: See PDX Collection 897

● **S42.31**   **Greenstick fracture of shaft of humerus**
The appropriate 7th character is to be added to all codes in subcategory S42.31

A	initial encounter for closed fracture
D	subsequent encounter for fracture with routine healing
G	subsequent encounter for fracture with delayed healing
K	subsequent encounter for fracture with nonunion
P	subsequent encounter for fracture with malunion
S	sequela

   ● **S42.311**   **Greenstick fracture of shaft of humerus, right arm** A, K, P 🔳, A 🔳
       (Ex:) **For S42.311[A]:** See PDX Collection 1249
       For S42.311[K,P]: See PDX Collection 897

   ● **S42.312**   **Greenstick fracture of shaft of humerus, left arm** A, K, P 🔳, A 🔳
       (Ex:) **For S42.312[A]:** See PDX Collection 1250
       For S42.312[K,P]: See PDX Collection 897

   ● **S42.319**   **Greenstick fracture of shaft of humerus, unspecified arm** A, K, P 🔳, A 🔳
       (Ex:) **For S42.319[A]:** See PDX Collection 1251
       For S42.319[K,P]: See PDX Collection 897

● **S42.32**   **Transverse fracture of shaft of humerus**

   ● **S42.321**   **Displaced transverse fracture of shaft of humerus, right arm** A, K, P 🔳, B 🔳, A, B 🔳
       (Ex:) **For S42.321[A]:** See PDX Collection 1250
       For S42.321[B]: See PDX Collection 1246
       For S42.321[K,P]: See PDX Collection 897

   ● **S42.322**   **Displaced transverse fracture of shaft of humerus, left arm** A, K, P 🔳, B 🔳, A, B 🔳
       (Ex:) **For S42.322[A]:** See PDX Collection 1250
       For S42.322[B]: See PDX Collection 1246
       For S42.322[K,P]: See PDX Collection 897

   ● **S42.323**   **Displaced transverse fracture of shaft of humerus, unspecified arm** A, K, P 🔳, B 🔳, A, B 🔳
       (Ex:) **For S42.323[A]:** See PDX Collection 1251
       For S42.323[B]: See PDX Collection 1246
       For S42.313[K,P]: See PDX Collection 897

   ● **S42.324**   **Nondisplaced transverse fracture of shaft of humerus, right arm** A, K, P 🔳, B 🔳, A, B 🔳
       (Ex:) **For S42.324[A]:** See PDX Collection 1249
       For S42.324[B]: See PDX Collection 1246
       For S42.324[K,P]: See PDX Collection 897

   ● **S42.325**   **Nondisplaced transverse fracture of shaft of humerus, left arm** A, K, P 🔳, B 🔳, A, B 🔳
       (Ex:) **For S42.325[A]:** See PDX Collection 1250
       For S42.325[B]: See PDX Collection 1246
       For S42.325[K,P]: See PDX Collection 897

   ● **S42.326**   **Nondisplaced transverse fracture of shaft of humerus, unspecified arm** A, K, P 🔳, B 🔳, A, B 🔳
       (Ex:) **For S42.326[A]:** See PDX Collection 1251
       For S42.326[B]: See PDX Collection 1246
       For S42.316[K,P]: See PDX Collection 897

▶ New   ⇒ Revised   ~~deleted~~ Deleted   Excludes 1   Excludes 2   Includes   Use additional   Code first   Code also   Key words
OGCR Official Guidelines   ● Unacceptable Principal Diagnosis   X Assign placeholder X   ● Use Additional Character(s)   ▌ Manifestation Code   **Coding Clinic**

● **S42.33**   Oblique fracture of shaft of humerus

  ● **S42.331**   Displaced oblique fracture of shaft of humerus, right arm A, K, P 🦠, B 🦠, A, B 🦠

    Ex: For S42.331[A]: See PDX Collection 1249
    For S42.331[B]: See PDX Collection 1246
    For S42.331[K,P]: See PDX Collection 897

  ● **S42.332**   Displaced oblique fracture of shaft of humerus, left arm A, K, P 🦠, B 🦠, A, B 🦠

    Ex: For S42.332[A]: See PDX Collection 1250
    For S42.332[B]: See PDX Collection 1246
    For S42.332[K,P]: See PDX Collection 897

  ● **S42.333**   Displaced oblique fracture of shaft of humerus, unspecified arm A, K, P 🦠, B 🦠, A, B 🦠

    Ex: For S42.333[A]: See PDX Collection 1251
    For S42.333[B]: See PDX Collection 1246
    For S42.333[K,P]: See PDX Collection 897

  ● **S42.334**   Nondisplaced oblique fracture of shaft of humerus, right arm A, K, P 🦠, B 🦠, A, B 🦠

    Ex: For S42.334[A]: See PDX Collection 1249
    For S42.334[B]: See PDX Collection 1246
    For S42.334[K,P]: See PDX Collection 897

  ● **S42.335**   Nondisplaced oblique fracture of shaft of humerus, left arm A, K, P 🦠, B 🦠, A, B 🦠

    Ex: For S42.335[A]: See PDX Collection 1250
    For S42.335[B]: See PDX Collection 1246
    For S42.335[K,P]: See PDX Collection 897

  ● **S42.336**   Nondisplaced oblique fracture of shaft of humerus, unspecified arm A, K, P 🦠, B 🦠, A, B 🦠

    Ex: For S42.336[A]: See PDX Collection 1251
    For S42.336[B]: See PDX Collection 1246
    For S42.336[K,P]: See PDX Collection 897

● **S42.34**   Spiral fracture of shaft of humerus

  ● **S42.341**   Displaced spiral fracture of shaft of humerus, right arm A, K, P 🦠, B 🦠, A, B 🦠

    Ex: For S42.341[A]: See PDX Collection 1249
    For S42.341[B]: See PDX Collection 1246
    For S42.341[K,P]: See PDX Collection 897

  ● **S42.342**   Displaced spiral fracture of shaft of humerus, left arm A, K, P 🦠, B 🦠, A, B 🦠

    Ex: For S42.342[A]: See PDX Collection 1250
    For S42.342[B]: See PDX Collection 1246
    For S42.342[K,P]: See PDX Collection 897

  ● **S42.343**   Displaced spiral fracture of shaft of humerus, unspecified arm A, K, P 🦠, B 🦠, A, B 🦠

    Ex: For S42.343[A]: See PDX Collection 1251
    For S42.343[B]: See PDX Collection 1246
    For S42.343[K,P]: See PDX Collection 897

  ● **S42.344**   Nondisplaced spiral fracture of shaft of humerus, right arm A, K, P 🦠, B 🦠, A, B 🦠

    Ex: For S42.344[A]: See PDX Collection 1249
    For S42.344[B]: See PDX Collection 1246
    For S42.344[K,P]: See PDX Collection 897

  ● **S42.345**   Nondisplaced spiral fracture of shaft of humerus, left arm A, K, P 🦠, B 🦠, A, B 🦠

    Ex: For S42.345[A]: See PDX Collection 1250
    For S42.345[B]: See PDX Collection 1246
    For S42.345[K,P]: See PDX Collection 897

  ● **S42.346**   Nondisplaced spiral fracture of shaft of humerus, unspecified arm A, K, P 🦠, B 🦠, A, B 🦠

    Ex: For S42.346[A]: See PDX Collection 1251
    For S42.346[B]: See PDX Collection 1246
    For S42.346[K,P]: See PDX Collection 897

● **S42.35**   Comminuted fracture of shaft of humerus

  ● **S42.351**   Displaced comminuted fracture of shaft of humerus, right arm A, K, P 🦠, B 🦠, A, B 🦠

    Ex: For S42.351[A]: See PDX Collection 1249
    For S42.351[B]: See PDX Collection 1246
    For S42.351[K,P]: See PDX Collection 897

  ● **S42.352**   Displaced comminuted fracture of shaft of humerus, left arm A, K, P 🦠, B 🦠, A, B 🦠

    Ex: For S42.352[A]: See PDX Collection 1250
    For S42.352[B]: See PDX Collection 1246
    For S42.352[K,P]: See PDX Collection 897

  ● **S42.353**   Displaced comminuted fracture of shaft of humerus, unspecified arm A, K, P 🦠, B 🦠, A, B 🦠

    Ex: For S42.353[A]: See PDX Collection 1251
    For S42.353[B]: See PDX Collection 1246
    For S42.353[K,P]: See PDX Collection 897

  ● **S42.354**   Nondisplaced comminuted fracture of shaft of humerus, right arm A, K, P 🦠, B 🦠, A, B 🦠

    Ex: For S42.354[A]: See PDX Collection 1249
    For S42.354[B]: See PDX Collection 1246
    For S42.354[K,P]: See PDX Collection 897

  ● **S42.355**   Nondisplaced comminuted fracture of shaft of humerus, left arm A, K, P 🦠, B 🦠, A, B 🦠

    Ex: For S42.355[A]: See PDX Collection 1250
    For S42.355[B]: See PDX Collection 1246
    For S42.355[K,P]: See PDX Collection 897

  ● **S42.356**   Nondisplaced comminuted fracture of shaft of humerus, unspecified arm A, K, P 🦠, B 🦠, A, B 🦠

    Ex: For S42.356[A]: See PDX Collection 1251
    For S42.356[B]: See PDX Collection 1246
    For S42.356[K,P]: See PDX Collection 897

● **S42.36**   Segmental fracture of shaft of humerus

  ● **S42.361**   Displaced segmental fracture of shaft of humerus, right arm A, K, P 🦠, B 🦠, A, B 🦠

    Ex: For S42.361[A]: See PDX Collection 1249
    For S42.361[B]: See PDX Collection 1246
    For S42.361[K,P]: See PDX Collection 897

  ● **S42.362**   Displaced segmental fracture of shaft of humerus, left arm A, K, P 🦠, B 🦠, A, B 🦠

    Ex: For S42.362[A]: See PDX Collection 1250
    For S42.362[B]: See PDX Collection 1246
    For S42.362[K,P]: See PDX Collection 897

  ● **S42.363**   Displaced segmental fracture of shaft of humerus, unspecified arm A, K, P 🦠, B 🦠, A, B 🦠

    Ex: For S42.363[A]: See PDX Collection 1251
    For S42.363[B]: See PDX Collection 1246
    For S42.363[K,P]: See PDX Collection 897

  ● **S42.364**   Nondisplaced segmental fracture of shaft of humerus, right arm A, K, P 🦠, B 🦠, A, B 🦠

    Ex: For S42.364[A]: See PDX Collection 1249
    For S42.364[B]: See PDX Collection 1246
    For S42.364[K,P]: See PDX Collection 897

  ● **S42.365**   Nondisplaced segmental fracture of shaft of humerus, left arm A, K, P 🦠, B 🦠, A, B 🦠

    Ex: For S42.365[A]: See PDX Collection 1250
    For S42.365[B]: See PDX Collection 1246
    For S42.365[K,P]: See PDX Collection 897

  ● **S42.366**   Nondisplaced segmental fracture of shaft of humerus, unspecified arm A, K, P 🦠, B 🦠, A, B 🦠

    Ex: For S42.366[A]: See PDX Collection 1251
    For S42.366[B]: See PDX Collection 1246
    For S42.366[K,P]: See PDX Collection 897

CHAPTER 19 (S00-T88)

N   Newborn Age: 0   P   Pediatric Age: 0–17   M   Maternity DX: 12–55   A   Adult Age: 15–124   ♀   Females Only   ♂   Males Only

🦠   Complication\Comorbidity   🦠   Major C\C   Ex: CC/MCC Exclusions   🦠   Hospital-Acquired Condition

● **S42.39**   **Other fracture of shaft of humerus**

     ● **S42.391**   **Other fracture of shaft of right humerus** A, K, P 🔵, B 🔵, A, B 🔵
         (Ex:) For S42.391[A]: See PDX Collection 1249
         For S42.391[B]: See PDX Collection 1246
         For S42.391[K,P]: See PDX Collection 897

     ● **S42.392**   **Other fracture of shaft of left humerus** A, K, P 🔵, B 🔵, A, B 🔵
         (Ex:) For S42.392[A]: See PDX Collection 1250
         For S42.392[B]: See PDX Collection 1246
         For S42.392[K,P]: See PDX Collection 897

     ● **S42.399**   **Other fracture of shaft of unspecified humerus** A, K, P 🔵, B 🔵, A, B 🔵
         (Ex:) For S42.399[A]: See PDX Collection 1251
         For S42.399[B]: See PDX Collection 1246
         For S42.399[K,P]: See PDX Collection 897

● **S42.4**   **Fracture of lower end of humerus**
     Fracture of distal end of humerus

     Excludes2   fracture of shaft of humerus (S42.3-)
         physeal fracture of lower end of humerus (S49.1-)

     ● **S42.40**   **Unspecified fracture of lower end of humerus**
         Fracture of elbow NOS

     ● **S42.401**   **Unspecified fracture of lower end of right humerus** A, K, P 🔵, B 🔵, A, B 🔵
         (Ex:) For S42.401[A]: See PDX Collection 1245
         For S42.401[B]: See PDX Collection 1246
         For S42.401[K,P]: See PDX Collection 897

     ● **S42.402**   **Unspecified fracture of lower end of left humerus** A, K, P 🔵, B 🔵, A, B 🔵
         (Ex:) For S42.402[A]: See PDX Collection 1247
         For S42.402[B]: See PDX Collection 1246
         For S42.402[K,P]: See PDX Collection 897

     ● **S42.409**   **Unspecified fracture of lower end of unspecified humerus** A, K, P 🔵, B 🔵, A, B 🔵
         (Ex:) For S42.409[A]: See PDX Collection 1248
         For S42.409[B]: See PDX Collection 1246
         For S42.409[K,P]: See PDX Collection 897

     ● **S42.41**   **Simple supracondylar fracture without intercondylar fracture of humerus**

     ● **S42.411**   **Displaced simple supracondylar fracture without intercondylar fracture of right humerus** A, K, P 🔵, B 🔵, A, B 🔵
         (Ex:) For S42.411[A]: See PDX Collection 1245
         For S42.411[B]: See PDX Collection 1246
         For S42.411[K,P]: See PDX Collection 897

     ● **S42.412**   **Displaced simple supracondylar fracture without intercondylar fracture of left humerus** A, K, P 🔵, B 🔵, A, B 🔵
         (Ex:) For S42.412[A]: See PDX Collection 1247
         For S42.412[B]: See PDX Collection 1246
         For S42.412[K,P]: See PDX Collection 897

     ● **S42.413**   **Displaced simple supracondylar fracture without intercondylar fracture of unspecified humerus** A, K, P 🔵, B 🔵, A, B 🔵
         (Ex:) For S42.413[A]: See PDX Collection 1248
         For S42.413[B]: See PDX Collection 1246
         For S42.413[K,P]: See PDX Collection 897

     ● **S42.414**   **Nondisplaced simple supracondylar fracture without intercondylar fracture of right humerus** A, K, P 🔵, B 🔵, A, B 🔵
         (Ex:) For S42.414[A]: See PDX Collection 1245
         For S42.414[B]: See PDX Collection 1246
         For S42.414[K,P]: See PDX Collection 897

     ● **S42.415**   **Nondisplaced simple supracondylar fracture without intercondylar fracture of left humerus** A, K, P 🔵, B 🔵, A, B 🔵
         (Ex:) For S42.415[A]: See PDX Collection 1247
         For S42.415[B]: See PDX Collection 1246
         For S42.415[K,P]: See PDX Collection 897

     ● **S42.416**   **Nondisplaced simple supracondylar fracture without intercondylar fracture of unspecified humerus** A, K, P 🔵, B 🔵, A, B 🔵
         (Ex:) For S42.416[A]: See PDX Collection 1248
         For S42.416[B]: See PDX Collection 1246
         For S42.416[K,P]: See PDX Collection 897

● **S42.42**   **Comminuted supracondylar fracture without intercondylar fracture of humerus**

     ● **S42.421**   **Displaced comminuted supracondylar fracture without intercondylar fracture of right humerus** A, K, P 🔵, B 🔵, A, B 🔵
         (Ex:) For S42.421[A]: See PDX Collection 1245
         For S42.421[B]: See PDX Collection 1246
         For S42.421[K,P]: See PDX Collection 897

     ● **S42.422**   **Displaced comminuted supracondylar fracture without intercondylar fracture of left humerus** A, K, P 🔵, B 🔵, A, B 🔵
         (Ex:) For S42.422[A]: See PDX Collection 1247
         For S42.422[B]: See PDX Collection 1246
         For S42.422[K,P]: See PDX Collection 897

     ● **S42.423**   **Displaced comminuted supracondylar fracture without intercondylar fracture of unspecified humerus** A, K, P 🔵, B 🔵, A, B 🔵
         (Ex:) For S42.423[A]: See PDX Collection 1248
         For S42.423[B]: See PDX Collection 1246
         For S42.423[K,P]: See PDX Collection 897

     ● **S42.424**   **Nondisplaced comminuted supracondylar fracture without intercondylar fracture of right humerus** A, K, P 🔵, B 🔵, A, B 🔵
         (Ex:) For S42.424[A]: See PDX Collection 1245
         For S42.424[B]: See PDX Collection 1246
         For S42.424[K,P]: See PDX Collection 897

     ● **S42.425**   **Nondisplaced comminuted supracondylar fracture without intercondylar fracture of left humerus** A, K, P 🔵, B 🔵, A, B 🔵
         (Ex:) For S42.425[A]: See PDX Collection 1247
         For S42.425[B]: See PDX Collection 1246
         For S42.425[K,P]: See PDX Collection 897

     ● **S42.426**   **Nondisplaced comminuted supracondylar fracture without intercondylar fracture of unspecified humerus** A, K, P 🔵, B 🔵, A, B 🔵
         (Ex:) For S42.426[A]: See PDX Collection 1248
         For S42.426[B]: See PDX Collection 1246
         For S42.426[K,P]: See PDX Collection 897

● **S42.43** Fracture (avulsion) of lateral epicondyle of humerus

  ● **S42.431** Displaced fracture (avulsion) of lateral epicondyle of right humerus
  A, K, P 🐾, B 🐾, A, B 🐾
  (Ex:) **For S42.431[A]:** See PDX Collection 1245
  For S42.431[B]: See PDX Collection 1246
  For S42.431[K,P]: See PDX Collection 897

  ● **S42.432** Displaced fracture (avulsion) of lateral epicondyle of left humerus A, K, P 🐾, B 🐾, A, B 🐾
  (Ex:) **For S42.432[A]:** See PDX Collection 1247
  For S42.432[B]: See PDX Collection 1246
  For S42.432[K,P]: See PDX Collection 897

  ● **S42.433** Displaced fracture (avulsion) of lateral epicondyle of unspecified humerus A, K, P 🐾, B 🐾, A, B 🐾
  (Ex:) **For S42.433[A]:** See PDX Collection 1248
  For S42.433[B]: See PDX Collection 1246
  For S42.433[K,P]: See PDX Collection 897

  ● **S42.434** Nondisplaced fracture (avulsion) of lateral epicondyle of right humerus
  A, K, P 🐾, B 🐾, A, B 🐾
  (Ex:) **For S42.434[A]:** See PDX Collection 1245
  For S42.434[B]: See PDX Collection 1246
  For S42.434[K,P]: See PDX Collection 897

  ● **S42.435** Nondisplaced fracture (avulsion) of lateral epicondyle of left humerus
  A, K, P 🐾, B 🐾, A, B 🐾
  (Ex:) **For S42.435[A]:** See PDX Collection 1247
  For S42.435[B]: See PDX Collection 1246
  For S42.435[K,P]: See PDX Collection 897

  ● **S42.436** Nondisplaced fracture (avulsion) of lateral epicondyle of unspecified humerus A, K, P 🐾, B 🐾, A, B 🐾
  (Ex:) **For S42.436[A]:** See PDX Collection 1248
  For S42.436[B]: See PDX Collection 1246
  For S42.436[K,P]: See PDX Collection 897

● **S42.44** Fracture (avulsion) of medial epicondyle of humerus

  ● **S42.441** Displaced fracture (avulsion) of medial epicondyle of right humerus
  A, K, P 🐾, B 🐾, A, B 🐾
  (Ex:) **For S42.441[A]:** See PDX Collection 1245
  For S42.441[B]: See PDX Collection 1246
  For S42.441[K,P]: See PDX Collection 897

  ● **S42.442** Displaced fracture (avulsion) of medial epicondyle of left humerus
  A, K, P 🐾, B 🐾, A, B 🐾
  (Ex:) **For S42.442[A]:** See PDX Collection 1247
  For S42.442[B]: See PDX Collection 1246
  For S42.442[K,P]: See PDX Collection 897

  ● **S42.443** Displaced fracture (avulsion) of medial epicondyle of unspecified humerus A, K, P 🐾, B 🐾, A, B 🐾
  (Ex:) **For S42.443[A]:** See PDX Collection 1248
  For S42.443[B]: See PDX Collection 1246
  For S42.443[K,P]: See PDX Collection 897

  ● **S42.444** Nondisplaced fracture (avulsion) of medial epicondyle of right humerus
  A, K, P 🐾, B 🐾, A, B 🐾
  (Ex:) **For S42.444[A]:** See PDX Collection 1245
  For S42.444[B]: See PDX Collection 1246
  For S42.444[K,P]: See PDX Collection 897

  ● **S42.445** Nondisplaced fracture (avulsion) of medial epicondyle of left humerus
  A, K, P 🐾, B 🐾, A, B 🐾
  (Ex:) **For S42.445[A]:** See PDX Collection 1247
  For S42.445[B]: See PDX Collection 1246
  For S42.445[K,P]: See PDX Collection 897

  ● **S42.446** Nondisplaced fracture (avulsion) of medial epicondyle of unspecified humerus A, K, P 🐾, B 🐾, A, B 🐾
  (Ex:) **For S42.446[A]:** See PDX Collection 1248
  For S42.446[B]: See PDX Collection 1246
  For S42.446[K,P]: See PDX Collection 897

  ● **S42.447** Incarcerated fracture (avulsion) of medial epicondyle of right humerus
  A, K, P 🐾, B 🐾, A, B 🐾
  (Ex:) **For S42.447[A]:** See PDX Collection 1245
  For S42.447[B]: See PDX Collection 1246
  For S42.447[K,P]: See PDX Collection 897

  ● **S42.448** Incarcerated fracture (avulsion) of medial epicondyle of left humerus
  A, K, P 🐾, B 🐾, A, B 🐾
  (Ex:) **For S42.448[A]:** See PDX Collection 1247
  For S42.448[B]: See PDX Collection 1246
  For S42.448[K,P]: See PDX Collection 897

  ● **S42.449** Incarcerated fracture (avulsion) of medial epicondyle of unspecified humerus A, K, P 🐾, B 🐾, A, B 🐾
  (Ex:) **For S42.449[A]:** See PDX Collection 1248
  For S42.449[B]: See PDX Collection 1246
  For S42.449[K,P]: See PDX Collection 897

● **S42.45** Fracture of lateral condyle of humerus
  Fracture of capitellum of humerus

  ● **S42.451** Displaced fracture of lateral condyle of right humerus A, K, P 🐾, B 🐾, A, B 🐾
  (Ex:) **For S42.451[A]:** See PDX Collection 1245
  For S42.451[B]: See PDX Collection 1246
  For S42.451[K,P]: See PDX Collection 897

  ● **S42.452** Displaced fracture of lateral condyle of left humerus A, K, P 🐾, B 🐾, A, B 🐾
  (Ex:) **For S42.452[A]:** See PDX Collection 1247
  For S42.452[B]: See PDX Collection 1246
  For S42.452[K,P]: See PDX Collection 897

  ● **S42.453** Displaced fracture of lateral condyle of unspecified humerus A, K, P 🐾, B 🐾, A, B 🐾
  (Ex:) **For S42.453[A]:** See PDX Collection 1248
  For S42.453[B]: See PDX Collection 1246
  For S42.453[K,P]: See PDX Collection 897

  ● **S42.454** Nondisplaced fracture of lateral condyle of right humerus A, K, P 🐾, B 🐾, A, B 🐾
  (Ex:) **For S42.454[A]:** See PDX Collection 1245
  For S42.454[B]: See PDX Collection 1246
  For S42.454[K,P]: See PDX Collection 897

  ● **S42.455** Nondisplaced fracture of lateral condyle of left humerus A, K, P 🐾, B 🐾, A, B 🐾
  (Ex:) **For S42.455[A]:** See PDX Collection 1247
  For S42.455[B]: See PDX Collection 1246
  For S42.455[K,P]: See PDX Collection 897

  ● **S42.456** Nondisplaced fracture of lateral condyle of unspecified humerus
  A, K, P 🐾, B 🐾, A, B 🐾
  (Ex:) **For S42.456[A]:** See PDX Collection 1248
  For S42.456[B]: See PDX Collection 1246
  For S42.456[K,P]: See PDX Collection 897

CHAPTER 19 (S00-T88)

N Newborn Age: 0   **P** Pediatric Age: 0–17   **M** Maternity DX: 12–55   **A** Adult Age: 15–124   ♀ Females Only   ♂ Males Only

🐾 Complication\Comorbidity   🐾 Major C\C   (Ex:) CC/MCC Exclusions   🐾 Hospital-Acquired Condition

1283

● S42.46   Fracture of medial condyle of humerus
Trochlea fracture of humerus

   ● S42.461   Displaced fracture of medial condyle
of right humerus A, K, P 🔁, B 🔁,
A, B 🔁
      Ex: For S42.461[A]: PDX Collection 1245
      For S42.461[B]: See PDX Collection 1246
      For S42.461[K,P]: See PDX Collection 897

   ● S42.462   Displaced fracture of medial condyle
of left humerus A, K, P 🔁, B 🔁,
A, B 🔁
      Ex: For S42.462[A]: PDX Collection 1247
      For S42.462[B]: See PDX Collection 1246
      For S42.462[K,P]: See PDX Collection 897

   ● S42.463   Displaced fracture of medial condyle
of unspecified humerus A, K, P 🔁,
B 🔁, A, B 🔁
      Ex: For S42.463[A]: PDX Collection 1248
      For S42.463[B]: See PDX Collection 1246
      For S42.463[K,P]: See PDX Collection 897

   ● S42.464   Nondisplaced fracture of medial
condyle of right humerus A, K, P 🔁,
B 🔁, A, B 🔁
      Ex: For S42.464[A]: PDX Collection 1245
      For S42.464[B]: See PDX Collection 1246
      For S42.464[K,P]: See PDX Collection 897

   ● S42.465   Nondisplaced fracture of medial
condyle of left humerus A, K, P 🔁,
B 🔁, A, B 🔁
      Ex: For S42.465[A]: PDX Collection 1247
      For S42.465[B]: See PDX Collection 1246
      For S42.465[K,P]: See PDX Collection 897

   ● S42.466   Nondisplaced fracture of medial
condyle of unspecified humerus
A, K, P 🔁, B 🔁, A, B 🔁
      Ex: For S42.466[A]: PDX Collection 1248
      For S42.466[B]: See PDX Collection 1246
      For S42.466[K,P]: See PDX Collection 897

● S42.47   Transcondylar fracture of humerus

   ● S42.471   Displaced transcondylar fracture of
right humerus A, K, P 🔁, B 🔁, A, B 🔁
      Ex: For S42.471[A]: See PDX Collection 1245
      For S42.471[B]: See PDX Collection 1246
      For S42.471[K,P]: See PDX Collection 897

   ● S42.472   Displaced transcondylar fracture of
left humerus A, K, P 🔁, B 🔁, A, B 🔁
      Ex: For S42.472[A]: See PDX Collection 1247
      For S42.472[B]: See PDX Collection 1246
      For S42.472[K,P]: See PDX Collection 897

   ● S42.473   Displaced transcondylar fracture of
unspecified humerus A, K, P 🔁, B 🔁,
A, B 🔁
      Ex: For S42.473[A]: See PDX Collection 1248
      For S42.473[B]: See PDX Collection 1246
      For S42.473[K,P]: See PDX Collection 897

   ● S42.474   Nondisplaced transcondylar fracture
of right humerus A, K, P 🔁, B 🔁,
A, B 🔁
      Ex: For S42.474[A]: See PDX Collection 1245
      For S42.474[B]: See PDX Collection 1246
      For S42.474[K,P]: See PDX Collection 897

   ● S42.475   Nondisplaced transcondylar fracture
of left humerus A, K, P 🔁, B 🔁,
A, B 🔁
      Ex: For S42.475[A]: See PDX Collection 1247
      For S42.475[B]: See PDX Collection 1246
      For S42.475[K,P]: See PDX Collection 897

   ● S42.476   Nondisplaced transcondylar fracture
of unspecified humerus A, K, P 🔁,
B 🔁, A, B 🔁
      Ex: For S42.476[A]: See PDX Collection 1248
      For S42.476[B]: See PDX Collection 1246
      For S42.476[K,P]: See PDX Collection 897

● S42.48   Torus fracture of lower end of humerus

The appropriate 7th character is to be added to
all codes in subcategory S42.48

A	initial encounter for closed fracture
D	subsequent encounter for fracture with routine healing
G	subsequent encounter for fracture with delayed healing
K	subsequent encounter for fracture with nonunion
P	subsequent encounter for fracture with malunion
S	sequela

   ● S42.481   Torus fracture of lower end of right
humerus A, K, P 🔁, A 🔁
      Ex: For S42.481[A]: See PDX Collection 1245
      For S42.481[K,P]: See PDX Collection 897

   ● S42.482   Torus fracture of lower end of left
humerus A, K, P 🔁, A 🔁
      Ex: For S42.482[A]: See PDX Collection 1247
      For S42.482[K,P]: See PDX Collection 897

   ● S42.489   Torus fracture of lower end of
unspecified humerus A, K, P 🔁, A 🔁
      Ex: For S42.489[A]: See PDX Collection 1248
      For S42.489[K,P]: See PDX Collection 897

● S42.49   Other fracture of lower end of humerus

   ● S42.491   Other displaced fracture of lower end
of right humerus A, K, P 🔁, B 🔁,
A, B 🔁
      Ex: For S42.491[A]: See PDX Collection 1245
      For S42.491[B]: See PDX Collection 1246
      For S42.491[K,P]: See PDX Collection 897

   ● S42.492   Other displaced fracture of lower end
of left humerus A, K, P 🔁, B 🔁,
A, B 🔁
      Ex: For S42.492[A]: See PDX Collection 1247
      For S42.492[B]: See PDX Collection 1246
      For S42.492[K,P]: See PDX Collection 897

   ● S42.493   Other displaced fracture of lower end
of unspecified humerus A, K, P 🔁,
B 🔁, A, B 🔁
      Ex: For S42.493[A]: See PDX Collection 1248
      For S42.493[B]: See PDX Collection 1246
      For S42.493[K,P]: See PDX Collection 897

   ● S42.494   Other nondisplaced fracture of lower
end of right humerus A, K, P 🔁, B 🔁,
A, B 🔁
      Ex: For S42.494[A]: See PDX Collection 1245
      For S42.494[B]: See PDX Collection 1246
      For S42.494[K,P]: See PDX Collection 897

   ● S42.495   Other nondisplaced fracture of lower
end of left humerus A, K, P 🔁, B 🔁,
A, B 🔁
      Ex: For S42.495[A]: See PDX Collection 1247
      For S42.495[B]: See PDX Collection 1246
      For S42.495[K,P]: See PDX Collection 897

   ● S42.496   Other nondisplaced fracture of lower
end of unspecified humerus
A, K, P 🔁, B 🔁, A, B 🔁
      Ex: For S42.496[A]: See PDX Collection 1248
      For S42.496[B]: See PDX Collection 1246
      For S42.496[K,P]: See PDX Collection 897

● S42.9   Fracture of shoulder girdle, part unspecified
Fracture of shoulder NOS
   Ex: For category S42.9 CC codes S42.9[A]: See PDX Collection 1248
   For S42.9[B]: See PDX Collection 1246 For S42.9[K,P]: See PDX
   Collection 897

X ● S42.90   Fracture of unspecified shoulder girdle, part
unspecified A, K, P 🔁, B 🔁, A, B 🔁

X ● S42.91   Fracture of right shoulder girdle, part
unspecified A, K, P 🔁, B 🔁, A, B 🔁

X ● S42.92   Fracture of left shoulder girdle, part unspecified
A, K, P 🔁, B 🔁, A, B 🔁

▶ New   ⇨ Revised   d̶e̶l̶e̶t̶e̶d̶ Deleted   Excludes 1   Excludes 2   Includes   Use additional   Code first   Code also   Key words
OGCR Official Guidelines   ● Unacceptable Principal Diagnosis   X Assign placeholder X   ● Use Additional Character(s)   ▶ Manifestation Code   Coding Clinic

● **S43**   **Dislocation and sprain of joints and ligaments of shoulder girdle**

     Includes   avulsion of joint or ligament of shoulder girdle

              laceration of cartilage, joint or ligament of shoulder girdle

              sprain of cartilage, joint or ligament of shoulder girdle

              traumatic hemarthrosis of joint or ligament of shoulder girdle

              traumatic rupture of joint or ligament of shoulder girdle

              traumatic subluxation of joint or ligament of shoulder girdle

              traumatic tear of joint or ligament of shoulder girdle

     Code also any associated open wound

     Excludes2   strain of muscle, fascia and tendon of shoulder and upper arm (S46.-)

     The appropriate 7th character is to be added to each code from category S43

A	initial encounter
D	subsequent encounter
S	sequela

● **S43.0**   **Subluxation and dislocation of shoulder joint**

     Dislocation of glenohumeral joint

     Subluxation of glenohumeral joint

     ● **S43.00**   **Unspecified subluxation and dislocation of shoulder joint**

         Dislocation of humerus NOS

         Subluxation of humerus NOS

         ● **S43.001**   Unspecified subluxation of right shoulder joint

         ● **S43.002**   Unspecified subluxation of left shoulder joint

         ● **S43.003**   Unspecified subluxation of unspecified shoulder joint

         ● **S43.004**   Unspecified dislocation of right shoulder joint

         ● **S43.005**   Unspecified dislocation of left shoulder joint

         ● **S43.006**   Unspecified dislocation of unspecified shoulder joint

     ● **S43.01**   **Anterior subluxation and dislocation of humerus**

         ● **S43.011**   Anterior subluxation of right humerus

         ● **S43.012**   Anterior subluxation of left humerus

         ● **S43.013**   Anterior subluxation of unspecified humerus

         ● **S43.014**   Anterior dislocation of right humerus

         ● **S43.015**   Anterior dislocation of left humerus

         ● **S43.016**   Anterior dislocation of unspecified humerus

     ● **S43.02**   **Posterior subluxation and dislocation of humerus**

         ● **S43.021**   Posterior subluxation of right humerus

         ● **S43.022**   Posterior subluxation of left humerus

         ● **S43.023**   Posterior subluxation of unspecified humerus

         ● **S43.024**   Posterior dislocation of right humerus

         ● **S43.025**   Posterior dislocation of left humerus

         ● **S43.026**   Posterior dislocation of unspecified humerus

● **S43.03**   **Inferior subluxation and dislocation of humerus**

     ● **S43.031**   Inferior subluxation of right humerus

     ● **S43.032**   Inferior subluxation of left humerus

     ● **S43.033**   Inferior subluxation of unspecified humerus

     ● **S43.034**   Inferior dislocation of right humerus

     ● **S43.035**   Inferior dislocation of left humerus

     ● **S43.036**   Inferior dislocation of unspecified humerus

● **S43.08**   **Other subluxation and dislocation of shoulder joint**

     ● **S43.081**   Other subluxation of right shoulder joint

     ● **S43.082**   Other subluxation of left shoulder joint

     ● **S43.083**   Other subluxation of unspecified shoulder joint

     ● **S43.084**   Other dislocation of right shoulder joint

     ● **S43.085**   Other dislocation of left shoulder joint

     ● **S43.086**   Other dislocation of unspecified shoulder joint

● **S43.1**   **Subluxation and dislocation of acromioclavicular joint**

     ● **S43.10**   **Unspecified dislocation of acromioclavicular joint**

         ● **S43.101**   Unspecified dislocation of right acromioclavicular joint

         ● **S43.102**   Unspecified dislocation of left acromioclavicular joint

         ● **S43.109**   Unspecified dislocation of unspecified acromioclavicular joint

     ● **S43.11**   **Subluxation of acromioclavicular joint**

         ● **S43.111**   Subluxation of right acromioclavicular joint

         ● **S43.112**   Subluxation of left acromioclavicular joint

         ● **S43.119**   Subluxation of unspecified acromioclavicular joint

     ● **S43.12**   **Dislocation of acromioclavicular joint, 100%-200% displacement**

         ● **S43.121**   Dislocation of right acromioclavicular joint, 100%-200% displacement

         ● **S43.122**   Dislocation of left acromioclavicular joint, 100%-200% displacement

         ● **S43.129**   Dislocation of unspecified acromioclavicular joint, 100%-200% displacement

     ● **S43.13**   **Dislocation of acromioclavicular joint, greater than 200% displacement**

         ● **S43.131**   Dislocation of right acromioclavicular joint, greater than 200% displacement

         ● **S43.132**   Dislocation of left acromioclavicular joint, greater than 200% displacement

         ● **S43.139**   Dislocation of unspecified acromioclavicular joint, greater than 200% displacement

     ● **S43.14**   **Inferior dislocation of acromioclavicular joint**

         ● **S43.141**   Inferior dislocation of right acromioclavicular joint

         ● **S43.142**   Inferior dislocation of left acromioclavicular joint

         ● **S43.149**   Inferior dislocation of unspecified acromioclavicular joint

CHAPTER 19 (S00-T88)

N Newborn Age: 0   **P** Pediatric Age: 0–17   **M** Maternity DX: 12–55   **A** Adult Age: 15–124   ♀ Females Only   ♂ Males Only

🔖 Complication\Comorbidity   🔖 Major C\C   (Ex) CC/MCC Exclusions   🔖 Hospital-Acquired Condition

1285

● S43.15 Posterior dislocation of acromioclavicular joint
   ● S43.151 Posterior dislocation of right acromioclavicular joint
   ● S43.152 Posterior dislocation of left acromioclavicular joint
   ● S43.159 Posterior dislocation of unspecified acromioclavicular joint
● S43.2 Subluxation and dislocation of sternoclavicular joint
  ● S43.20 Unspecified subluxation and dislocation of sternoclavicular joint
   ● S43.201 Unspecified subluxation of right sternoclavicular joint A 🖇, A 🖇
    Ex: See PDX Collection 1252
   ● S43.202 Unspecified subluxation of left sternoclavicular joint A 🖇, A 🖇
    Ex: See PDX Collection 1253
   ● S43.203 Unspecified subluxation of unspecified sternoclavicular joint A 🖇, A 🖇
    Ex: See PDX Collection 914
   ● S43.204 Unspecified dislocation of right sternoclavicular joint A 🖇, A 🖇
    Ex: See PDX Collection 1252
   ● S43.205 Unspecified dislocation of left sternoclavicular joint A 🖇, A 🖇
    Ex: See PDX Collection 1253
   ● S43.206 Unspecified dislocation of unspecified sternoclavicular joint A 🖇, A 🖇
    Ex: See PDX Collection 914
  ● S43.21 Anterior subluxation and dislocation of sternoclavicular joint
   ● S43.211 Anterior subluxation of right sternoclavicular joint A 🖇, A 🖇
    Ex: See PDX Collection 1252
   ● S43.212 Anterior subluxation of left sternoclavicular joint A 🖇, A 🖇
    Ex: See PDX Collection 1253
   ● S43.213 Anterior subluxation of unspecified sternoclavicular joint A 🖇, A 🖇
    Ex: See PDX Collection 914
   ● S43.214 Anterior dislocation of right sternoclavicular joint A 🖇, A 🖇
    Ex: See PDX Collection 1252
   ● S43.215 Anterior dislocation of left sternoclavicular joint A 🖇, A 🖇
    Ex: See PDX Collection 1253
   ● S43.216 Anterior dislocation of unspecified sternoclavicular joint A 🖇, A 🖇
    Ex: See PDX Collection 914
  ● S43.22 Posterior subluxation and dislocation of sternoclavicular joint
   ● S43.221 Posterior subluxation of right sternoclavicular joint A 🖇, A 🖇
    Ex: See PDX Collection 1252
   ● S43.222 Posterior subluxation of left sternoclavicular joint A 🖇, A 🖇
    Ex: See PDX Collection 1253
   ● S43.223 Posterior subluxation of unspecified sternoclavicular joint A 🖇, A 🖇
    Ex: See PDX Collection 914
   ● S43.224 Posterior dislocation of right sternoclavicular joint A 🖇, A 🖇
    Ex: See PDX Collection 1252
   ● S43.225 Posterior dislocation of left sternoclavicular joint A 🖇, A 🖇
    Ex: See PDX Collection 1253
   ● S43.226 Posterior dislocation of unspecified sternoclavicular joint A 🖇, A 🖇
    Ex: See PDX Collection 914

● S43.3 Subluxation and dislocation of other and unspecified parts of shoulder girdle
  ● S43.30 Subluxation and dislocation of unspecified parts of shoulder girdle
    Dislocation of shoulder girdle NOS
    Subluxation of shoulder girdle NOS
   ● S43.301 Subluxation of unspecified parts of right shoulder girdle
   ● S43.302 Subluxation of unspecified parts of left shoulder girdle
   ● S43.303 Subluxation of unspecified parts of unspecified shoulder girdle
   ● S43.304 Dislocation of unspecified parts of right shoulder girdle
   ● S43.305 Dislocation of unspecified parts of left shoulder girdle
   ● S43.306 Dislocation of unspecified parts of unspecified shoulder girdle
  ● S43.31 Subluxation and dislocation of scapula
   ● S43.311 Subluxation of right scapula
   ● S43.312 Subluxation of left scapula
   ● S43.313 Subluxation of unspecified scapula
   ● S43.314 Dislocation of right scapula
   ● S43.315 Dislocation of left scapula
   ● S43.316 Dislocation of unspecified scapula
  ● S43.39 Subluxation and dislocation of other parts of shoulder girdle
   ● S43.391 Subluxation of other parts of right shoulder girdle
   ● S43.392 Subluxation of other parts of left shoulder girdle
   ● S43.393 Subluxation of other parts of unspecified shoulder girdle
   ● S43.394 Dislocation of other parts of right shoulder girdle
   ● S43.395 Dislocation of other parts of left shoulder girdle
   ● S43.396 Dislocation of other parts of unspecified shoulder girdle
● S43.4 Sprain of shoulder joint
  ● S43.40 Unspecified sprain of shoulder joint
   ● S43.401 Unspecified sprain of right shoulder joint
   ● S43.402 Unspecified sprain of left shoulder joint
   ● S43.409 Unspecified sprain of unspecified shoulder joint
  ● S43.41 Sprain of coracohumeral (ligament)
   ● S43.411 Sprain of right coracohumeral (ligament)
   ● S43.412 Sprain of left coracohumeral (ligament)
   ● S43.419 Sprain of unspecified coracohumeral (ligament)
  ● S43.42 Sprain of rotator cuff capsule
    Encounters during the healing phase
    Excludes1 rotator cuff syndrome (complete) (incomplete), not specified as traumatic (M75.1-)
    Excludes2 injury of tendon of rotator cuff (S46.0-)
   ● S43.421 Sprain of right rotator cuff capsule
   ● S43.422 Sprain of left rotator cuff capsule
   ● S43.429 Sprain of unspecified rotator cuff capsule

▶ New   ⇒ Revised   ~~deleted~~ Deleted   Excludes 1   Excludes 2   Includes   Use additional   Code first   Code also   Key words

OGCR Official Guidelines   ● Unacceptable Principal Diagnosis   X Assign placeholder X   ● Use Additional Character(s)   🖇 Manifestation Code   **Coding Clinic**

● **S43.43** **Superior glenoid labrum lesion**
SLAP lesion

   ● **S43.431** Superior glenoid labrum lesion of right shoulder

   ● **S43.432** Superior glenoid labrum lesion of left shoulder

   ● **S43.439** Superior glenoid labrum lesion of unspecified shoulder

● **S43.49** **Other sprain of shoulder joint**

   ● **S43.491** Other sprain of right shoulder joint

   ● **S43.492** Other sprain of left shoulder joint

   ● **S43.499** Other sprain of unspecified shoulder joint

● **S43.5** **Sprain of acromioclavicular joint**
Sprain of acromioclavicular ligament

   X ● **S43.50** Sprain of unspecified acromioclavicular joint

   X ● **S43.51** Sprain of right acromioclavicular joint

   X ● **S43.52** Sprain of left acromioclavicular joint

● **S43.6** **Sprain of sternoclavicular joint**

   X ● **S43.60** Sprain of unspecified sternoclavicular joint

   X ● **S43.61** Sprain of right sternoclavicular joint

   X ● **S43.62** Sprain of left sternoclavicular joint

● **S43.8** **Sprain of other specified parts of shoulder girdle**

   X ● **S43.80** Sprain of other specified parts of unspecified shoulder girdle

   X ● **S43.81** Sprain of other specified parts of right shoulder girdle

   X ● **S43.82** Sprain of other specified parts of left shoulder girdle

● **S43.9** **Sprain of unspecified parts of shoulder girdle**

   X ● **S43.90** Sprain of unspecified parts of unspecified shoulder girdle
Sprain of shoulder girdle NOS

   X ● **S43.91** Sprain of unspecified parts of right shoulder girdle

   X ● **S43.92** Sprain of unspecified parts of left shoulder girdle

● **S44** **Injury of nerves at shoulder and upper arm level**
Code also any associated open wound (S41.-)

   Excludes2 injury of brachial plexus (S14.3-)

The appropriate 7th character is to be added to each code from category S44

A	initial encounter
D	subsequent encounter
S	sequela

● **S44.0** **Injury of ulnar nerve at upper arm level**

   Excludes1 ulnar nerve NOS (S54.0)

   X ● **S44.00** Injury of ulnar nerve at upper arm level, unspecified arm

   X ● **S44.01** Injury of ulnar nerve at upper arm level, right arm

   X ● **S44.02** Injury of ulnar nerve at upper arm level, left arm

● **S44.1** **Injury of median nerve at upper arm level**

   Excludes1 median nerve NOS (S54.1)

   X ● **S44.10** Injury of median nerve at upper arm level, unspecified arm

   X ● **S44.11** Injury of median nerve at upper arm level, right arm

   X ● **S44.12** Injury of median nerve at upper arm level, left arm

● **S44.2** **Injury of radial nerve at upper arm level**

   Excludes1 radial nerve NOS (S54.2)

   X ● **S44.20** Injury of radial nerve at upper arm level, unspecified arm

   X ● **S44.21** Injury of radial nerve at upper arm level, right arm

   X ● **S44.22** Injury of radial nerve at upper arm level, left arm

● **S44.3** **Injury of axillary nerve**

   X ● **S44.30** Injury of axillary nerve, unspecified arm

   X ● **S44.31** Injury of axillary nerve, right arm

   X ● **S44.32** Injury of axillary nerve, left arm

● **S44.4** **Injury of musculocutaneous nerve**

   X ● **S44.40** Injury of musculocutaneous nerve, unspecified arm

   X ● **S44.41** Injury of musculocutaneous nerve, right arm

   X ● **S44.42** Injury of musculocutaneous nerve, left arm

● **S44.5** **Injury of cutaneous sensory nerve at shoulder and upper arm level**

   X ● **S44.50** Injury of cutaneous sensory nerve at shoulder and upper arm level, unspecified arm

   X ● **S44.51** Injury of cutaneous sensory nerve at shoulder and upper arm level, right arm

   X ● **S44.52** Injury of cutaneous sensory nerve at shoulder and upper arm level, left arm

● **S44.8** **Injury of other nerves at shoulder and upper arm level**

   ● **S44.8X** Injury of other nerves at shoulder and upper arm level

      ● **S44.8X1** Injury of other nerves at shoulder and upper arm level, right arm

      ● **S44.8X2** Injury of other nerves at shoulder and upper arm level, left arm

      ● **S44.8X9** Injury of other nerves at shoulder and upper arm level, unspecified arm

● **S44.9** **Injury of unspecified nerve at shoulder and upper arm level**

   X ● **S44.90** Injury of unspecified nerve at shoulder and upper arm level, unspecified arm

   X ● **S44.91** Injury of unspecified nerve at shoulder and upper arm level, right arm

   X ● **S44.92** Injury of unspecified nerve at shoulder and upper arm level, left arm

● **S45** **Injury of blood vessels at shoulder and upper arm level**
Code also any associated open wound (S41.-)

   Excludes2 injury of subclavian artery (S25.1)
   injury of subclavian vein (S25.3)

The appropriate 7th character is to be added to each code from category S45

A	initial encounter
D	subsequent encounter
S	sequela

● **S45.0** **Injury of axillary artery**

   ● **S45.00** Unspecified injury of axillary artery

      ● **S45.001** Unspecified injury of axillary artery, right side A 🔖
      Ex: See PDX Collection 1254

      ● **S45.002** Unspecified injury of axillary artery, left side A 🔖
      Ex: See PDX Collection 1255

      ● **S45.009** Unspecified injury of axillary artery, unspecified side A 🔖
      Ex: See PDX Collection 1256

CHAPTER 19 (SØØ-T88)

CHAPTER 19 (S00-T88)

- ● **S45.01**   Laceration of axillary artery
  - ● **S45.011**   Laceration of axillary artery, right side A 🔁
    - Ex: See PDX Collection 1254
  - ● **S45.012**   Laceration of axillary artery, left side A 🔁
    - Ex: See PDX Collection 1255
  - ● **S45.019**   Laceration of axillary artery, unspecified side A 🔁
    - Ex: See PDX Collection 1256
- ● **S45.09**   Other specified injury of axillary artery
  - ● **S45.091**   Other specified injury of axillary artery, right side A 🔁
    - Ex: See PDX Collection 1254
  - ● **S45.092**   Other specified injury of axillary artery, left side A 🔁
    - Ex: See PDX Collection 1255
  - ● **S45.099**   Other specified injury of axillary artery, unspecified side A 🔁
    - Ex: See PDX Collection 1256
- ● **S45.1**   Injury of brachial artery
  - ● **S45.10**   Unspecified injury of brachial artery
    - ● **S45.101**   Unspecified injury of brachial artery, right side A 🔁
      - Ex: See PDX Collection 1257
    - ● **S45.102**   Unspecified injury of brachial artery, left side A 🔁
      - Ex: See PDX Collection 1258
    - ● **S45.109**   Unspecified injury of brachial artery, unspecified side A 🔁
      - Ex: See PDX Collection 1259
  - ● **S45.11**   Laceration of brachial artery
    - ● **S45.111**   Laceration of brachial artery, right side A 🔁
      - Ex: See PDX Collection 1257
    - ● **S45.112**   Laceration of brachial artery, left side A 🔁
      - Ex: See PDX Collection 1258
    - ● **S45.119**   Laceration of brachial artery, unspecified side A 🔁
      - Ex: See PDX Collection 1259
  - ● **S45.19**   Other specified injury of brachial artery
    - ● **S45.191**   Other specified injury of brachial artery, right side A 🔁
      - Ex: See PDX Collection 1257
    - ● **S45.192**   Other specified injury of brachial artery, left side A 🔁
      - Ex: See PDX Collection 1258
    - ● **S45.199**   Other specified injury of brachial artery, unspecified side A 🔁
- ● **S45.2**   Injury of axillary or brachial vein
  - ● **S45.20**   Unspecified injury of axillary or brachial vein
    - ● **S45.201**   Unspecified injury of axillary or brachial vein, right side A 🔁
      - Ex: See PDX Collection 1257
    - ● **S45.202**   Unspecified injury of axillary or brachial vein, left side A 🔁
      - Ex: See PDX Collection 1258
    - ● **S45.209**   Unspecified injury of axillary or brachial vein, unspecified side A 🔁
      - Ex: See PDX Collection 1259
  - ● **S45.21**   Laceration of axillary or brachial vein
    - ● **S45.211**   Laceration of axillary or brachial vein, right side A 🔁
      - Ex: See PDX Collection 1257
    - ● **S45.212**   Laceration of axillary or brachial vein, left side A 🔁
      - Ex: See PDX Collection 1258
    - ● **S45.219**   Laceration of axillary or brachial vein, unspecified side A 🔁
      - Ex: See PDX Collection 1259

- ● **S45.29**   Other specified injury of axillary or brachial vein
  - ● **S45.291**   Other specified injury of axillary or brachial vein, right side A 🔁
    - Ex: See PDX Collection 1257
  - ● **S45.292**   Other specified injury of axillary or brachial vein, left side A 🔁
    - Ex: See PDX Collection 1258
  - ● **S45.299**   Other specified injury of axillary or brachial vein, unspecified side A 🔁
    - Ex: See PDX Collection 1259
- ● **S45.3**   Injury of superficial vein at shoulder and upper arm level
  - ● **S45.30**   Unspecified injury of superficial vein at shoulder and upper arm level
    - ● **S45.301**   Unspecified injury of superficial vein at shoulder and upper arm level, right arm A 🔁
      - Ex: See PDX Collection 1260
    - ● **S45.302**   Unspecified injury of superficial vein at shoulder and upper arm level, left arm A 🔁
      - Ex: See PDX Collection 1261
    - ● **S45.309**   Unspecified injury of superficial vein at shoulder and upper arm level, unspecified arm A 🔁
      - Ex: See PDX Collection 1262
  - ● **S45.31**   Laceration of superficial vein at shoulder and upper arm level
    - ● **S45.311**   Laceration of superficial vein at shoulder and upper arm level, right arm A 🔁
      - Ex: See PDX Collection 1260
    - ● **S45.312**   Laceration of superficial vein at shoulder and upper arm level, left arm A 🔁
      - Ex: See PDX Collection 1261
    - ● **S45.319**   Laceration of superficial vein at shoulder and upper arm level, unspecified arm A 🔁
      - Ex: See PDX Collection 1262
  - ● **S45.39**   Other specified injury of superficial vein at shoulder and upper arm level
    - ● **S45.391**   Other specified injury of superficial vein at shoulder and upper arm level, right arm A 🔁
      - Ex: See PDX Collection 1260
    - ● **S45.392**   Other specified injury of superficial vein at shoulder and upper arm level, left arm A 🔁
      - Ex: See PDX Collection 1261
    - ● **S45.399**   Other specified injury of superficial vein at shoulder and upper arm level, unspecified arm A 🔁
      - Ex: See PDX Collection 1262
- ● **S45.8**   Injury of other specified blood vessels at shoulder and upper arm level
  - ● **S45.80**   Unspecified injury of other specified blood vessels at shoulder and upper arm level
    - ● **S45.801**   Unspecified injury of other specified blood vessels at shoulder and upper arm level, right arm A 🔁
      - Ex: See PDX Collection 1260
    - ● **S45.802**   Unspecified injury of other specified blood vessels at shoulder and upper arm level, left arm A 🔁
      - Ex: See PDX Collection 1261
    - ● **S45.809**   Unspecified injury of other specified blood vessels at shoulder and upper arm level, unspecified arm A 🔁
      - Ex: See PDX Collection 1262

▶ New   ⟫ Revised   ~~deleted~~ Deleted   Excludes 1   Excludes 2   Includes   Use additional   Code first   Code also   Key words

OGCR Official Guidelines   ● Unacceptable Principal Diagnosis   X Assign placeholder X   ▶ Use Additional Character(s)   ▌ Manifestation Code   **Coding Clinic**

● S45.81 Laceration of other specified blood vessels at shoulder and upper arm level
  ● S45.811 Laceration of other specified blood vessels at shoulder and upper arm level, right arm A 🦠
    (Ex:) See PDX Collection 1260
  ● S45.812 Laceration of other specified blood vessels at shoulder and upper arm level, left arm A 🦠
    (Ex:) See PDX Collection 1261
  ● S45.819 Laceration of other specified blood vessels at shoulder and upper arm level, unspecified arm A 🦠
    (Ex:) See PDX Collection 1262
● S45.89 Other specified injury of other specified blood vessels at shoulder and upper arm level
  ● S45.891 Other specified injury of other specified blood vessels at shoulder and upper arm level, right arm A 🦠
    (Ex:) See PDX Collection 1260
  ● S45.892 Other specified injury of other specified blood vessels at shoulder and upper arm level, left arm A 🦠
    (Ex:) See PDX Collection 1261
  ● S45.899 Other specified injury of other specified blood vessels at shoulder and upper arm level, unspecified arm A 🦠
    (Ex:) See PDX Collection 1262
● S45.9 Injury of unspecified blood vessel at shoulder and upper arm level
  ● S45.90 Unspecified injury of unspecified blood vessel at shoulder and upper arm level
    ● S45.901 Unspecified injury of unspecified blood vessel at shoulder and upper arm level, right arm A 🦠
      (Ex:) See PDX Collection 1260
    ● S45.902 Unspecified injury of unspecified blood vessel at shoulder and upper arm level, left arm A 🦠
      (Ex:) See PDX Collection 1261
    ● S45.909 Unspecified injury of unspecified blood vessel at shoulder and upper arm level, unspecified arm A 🦠
      (Ex:) See PDX Collection 1262
  ● S45.91 Laceration of unspecified blood vessel at shoulder and upper arm level
    ● S45.911 Laceration of unspecified blood vessel at shoulder and upper arm level, right arm A 🦠
      (Ex:) See PDX Collection 1260
    ● S45.912 Laceration of unspecified blood vessel at shoulder and upper arm level, left arm A 🦠
      (Ex:) See PDX Collection 1261
    ● S45.919 Laceration of unspecified blood vessel at shoulder and upper arm level, unspecified arm A 🦠
      (Ex:) See PDX Collection 1262
  ● S45.99 Other specified injury of unspecified blood vessel at shoulder and upper arm level
    ● S45.991 Other specified injury of unspecified blood vessel at shoulder and upper arm level, right arm A 🦠
      (Ex:) See PDX Collection 1260
    ● S45.992 Other specified injury of unspecified blood vessel at shoulder and upper arm level, left arm A 🦠
      (Ex:) See PDX Collection 1261
    ● S45.999 Other specified injury of unspecified blood vessel at shoulder and upper arm level, unspecified arm A 🦠
      (Ex:) See PDX Collection 1262

● S46 Injury of muscle, fascia and tendon at shoulder and upper arm level
  Code also any associated open wound (S41.-)
  Excludes2 injury of muscle, fascia and tendon at elbow (S56.-)
              sprain of joints and ligaments of shoulder girdle (S43.9)
  The appropriate 7th character is to be added to each code from category S46

A	initial encounter
D	subsequent encounter
S	sequela

● S46.0 Injury of muscle(s) and tendon(s) of the rotator cuff of shoulder
  ● S46.00 Unspecified injury of muscle(s) and tendon(s) of the rotator cuff of shoulder
    ● S46.001 Unspecified injury of muscle(s) and tendon(s) of the rotator cuff of right shoulder
    ● S46.002 Unspecified injury of muscle(s) and tendon(s) of the rotator cuff of left shoulder
    ● S46.009 Unspecified injury of muscle(s) and tendon(s) of the rotator cuff of unspecified shoulder
  ● S46.01 Strain of muscle(s) and tendon(s) of the rotator cuff of shoulder
    Acute onset due to trauma to rotator cuff muscle/tendon
    ● S46.011 Strain of muscle(s) and tendon(s) of the rotator cuff of right shoulder
    ● S46.012 Strain of muscle(s) and tendon(s) of the rotator cuff of left shoulder
    ● S46.019 Strain of muscle(s) and tendon(s) of the rotator cuff of unspecified shoulder
  ● S46.02 Laceration of muscle(s) and tendon(s) of the rotator cuff of shoulder
    ● S46.021 Laceration of muscle(s) and tendon(s) of the rotator cuff of right shoulder A 🦠
      (Ex:) See PDX Collection 1263
    ● S46.022 Laceration of muscle(s) and tendon(s) of the rotator cuff of left shoulder A 🦠
      (Ex:) See PDX Collection 1264
    ● S46.029 Laceration of muscle(s) and tendon(s) of the rotator cuff of unspecified shoulder A 🦠
      (Ex:) See PDX Collection 1265
  ● S46.09 Other injury of muscle(s) and tendon(s) of the rotator cuff of shoulder
    ● S46.091 Other injury of muscle(s) and tendon(s) of the rotator cuff of right shoulder
    ● S46.092 Other injury of muscle(s) and tendon(s) of the rotator cuff of left shoulder
    ● S46.099 Other injury of muscle(s) and tendon(s) of the rotator cuff of unspecified shoulder

CHAPTER 19 (S00–T88)

● **S46.1**   Injury of muscle, fascia and tendon of long head of biceps

  ● **S46.10**   Unspecified injury of muscle, fascia and tendon of long head of biceps

    ● **S46.101**   Unspecified injury of muscle, fascia and tendon of long head of biceps, right arm

    ● **S46.102**   Unspecified injury of muscle, fascia and tendon of long head of biceps, left arm

    ● **S46.109**   Unspecified injury of muscle, fascia and tendon of long head of biceps, unspecified arm

  ● **S46.11**   Strain of muscle, fascia and tendon of long head of biceps

    ● **S46.111**   Strain of muscle, fascia and tendon of long head of biceps, right arm

    ● **S46.112**   Strain of muscle, fascia and tendon of long head of biceps, left arm

    ● **S46.119**   Strain of muscle, fascia and tendon of long head of biceps, unspecified arm

  ● **S46.12**   Laceration of muscle, fascia and tendon of long head of biceps

    ● **S46.121**   Laceration of muscle, fascia and tendon of long head of biceps, right arm A 🔒
       (Ex) See PDX Collection 1263

    ● **S46.122**   Laceration of muscle, fascia and tendon of long head of biceps, left arm A 🔒
       (Ex) See PDX Collection 1264

    ● **S46.129**   Laceration of muscle, fascia and tendon of long head of biceps, unspecified arm A 🔒
       (Ex) See PDX Collection 1265

  ● **S46.19**   Other injury of muscle, fascia and tendon of long head of biceps

    ● **S46.191**   Other injury of muscle, fascia and tendon of long head of biceps, right arm

    ● **S46.192**   Other injury of muscle, fascia and tendon of long head of biceps, left arm

    ● **S46.199**   Other injury of muscle, fascia and tendon of long head of biceps, unspecified arm

● **S46.2**   Injury of muscle, fascia and tendon of other parts of biceps

  ● **S46.20**   Unspecified injury of muscle, fascia and tendon of other parts of biceps

    ● **S46.201**   Unspecified injury of muscle, fascia and tendon of other parts of biceps, right arm

    ● **S46.202**   Unspecified injury of muscle, fascia and tendon of other parts of biceps, left arm

    ● **S46.209**   Unspecified injury of muscle, fascia and tendon of other parts of biceps, unspecified arm

  ● **S46.21**   Strain of muscle, fascia and tendon of other parts of biceps

    ● **S46.211**   Strain of muscle, fascia and tendon of other parts of biceps, right arm

    ● **S46.212**   Strain of muscle, fascia and tendon of other parts of biceps, left arm

    ● **S46.219**   Strain of muscle, fascia and tendon of other parts of biceps, unspecified arm

  ● **S46.22**   Laceration of muscle, fascia and tendon of other parts of biceps

    ● **S46.221**   Laceration of muscle, fascia and tendon of other parts of biceps, right arm A 🔒
       (Ex) See PDX Collection 1263

    ● **S46.222**   Laceration of muscle, fascia and tendon of other parts of biceps, left arm A 🔒
       (Ex) See PDX Collection 1264

    ● **S46.229**   Laceration of muscle, fascia and tendon of other parts of biceps, unspecified arm A 🔒
       (Ex) See PDX Collection 1265

  ● **S46.29**   Other injury of muscle, fascia and tendon of other parts of biceps

    ● **S46.291**   Other injury of muscle, fascia and tendon of other parts of biceps, right arm

    ● **S46.292**   Other injury of muscle, fascia and tendon of other parts of biceps, left arm

    ● **S46.299**   Other injury of muscle, fascia and tendon of other parts of biceps, unspecified arm

● **S46.3**   Injury of muscle, fascia and tendon of triceps

  ● **S46.30**   Unspecified injury of muscle, fascia and tendon of triceps

    ● **S46.301**   Unspecified injury of muscle, fascia and tendon of triceps, right arm

    ● **S46.302**   Unspecified injury of muscle, fascia and tendon of triceps, left arm

    ● **S46.309**   Unspecified injury of muscle, fascia and tendon of triceps, unspecified arm

  ● **S46.31**   Strain of muscle, fascia and tendon of triceps

    ● **S46.311**   Strain of muscle, fascia and tendon of triceps, right arm

    ● **S46.312**   Strain of muscle, fascia and tendon of triceps, left arm

    ● **S46.319**   Strain of muscle, fascia and tendon of triceps, unspecified arm

  ● **S46.32**   Laceration of muscle, fascia and tendon of triceps

    ● **S46.321**   Laceration of muscle, fascia and tendon of triceps, right arm A 🔒
       (Ex) See PDX Collection 1263

    ● **S46.322**   Laceration of muscle, fascia and tendon of triceps, left arm A 🔒
       (Ex) See PDX Collection 1264

    ● **S46.329**   Laceration of muscle, fascia and tendon of triceps, unspecified arm A 🔒
       (Ex) See PDX Collection 1265

  ● **S46.39**   Other injury of muscle, fascia and tendon of triceps

    ● **S46.391**   Other injury of muscle, fascia and tendon of triceps, right arm

    ● **S46.392**   Other injury of muscle, fascia and tendon of triceps, left arm

    ● **S46.399**   Other injury of muscle, fascia and tendon of triceps, unspecified arm

● **S46.8**   Injury of other muscles, fascia and tendons at shoulder and upper arm level

  ● **S46.80**   Unspecified injury of other muscles, fascia and tendons at shoulder and upper arm level

    ● **S46.801**   Unspecified injury of other muscles, fascia and tendons at shoulder and upper arm level, right arm

    ● **S46.802**   Unspecified injury of other muscles, fascia and tendons at shoulder and upper arm level, left arm

    ● **S46.809**   Unspecified injury of other muscles, fascia and tendons at shoulder and upper arm level, unspecified arm

▶ New   ⇒ Revised   ~~deleted~~ Deleted   Excludes 1   Excludes 2   Includes   Use additional   Code first   Code also   Key words

OGCR Official Guidelines   ● Unacceptable Principal Diagnosis   X Assign placeholder X   ● Use Additional Character(s)   ▌ Manifestation Code   **Coding Clinic**

● **S46.81** Strain of other muscles, fascia and tendons at shoulder and upper arm level

  ● **S46.811** Strain of other muscles, fascia and tendons at shoulder and upper arm level, right arm

  ● **S46.812** Strain of other muscles, fascia and tendons at shoulder and upper arm level, left arm

  ● **S46.819** Strain of other muscles, fascia and tendons at shoulder and upper arm level, unspecified arm

● **S46.82** Laceration of other muscles, fascia and tendons at shoulder and upper arm level

  ● **S46.821** Laceration of other muscles, fascia and tendons at shoulder and upper arm level, right arm A ⬡
       (Ex:) See PDX Collection 1263

  ● **S46.822** Laceration of other muscles, fascia and tendons at shoulder and upper arm level, left arm A ⬡
       (Ex:) See PDX Collection 1264

  ● **S46.829** Laceration of other muscles, fascia and tendons at shoulder and upper arm level, unspecified arm A ⬡
       (Ex:) See PDX Collection 1265

● **S46.89** Other injury of other muscles, fascia and tendons at shoulder and upper arm level

  ● **S46.891** Other injury of other muscles, fascia and tendons at shoulder and upper arm level, right arm

  ● **S46.892** Other injury of other muscles, fascia and tendons at shoulder and upper arm level, left arm

  ● **S46.899** Other injury of other muscles, fascia and tendons at shoulder and upper arm level, unspecified arm

● **S46.9** Injury of unspecified muscle, fascia and tendon at shoulder and upper arm level

  ● **S46.90** Unspecified injury of unspecified muscle, fascia and tendon at shoulder and upper arm level

    ● **S46.901** Unspecified injury of unspecified muscle, fascia and tendon at shoulder and upper arm level, right arm

    ● **S46.902** Unspecified injury of unspecified muscle, fascia and tendon at shoulder and upper arm level, left arm

    ● **S46.909** Unspecified injury of unspecified muscle, fascia and tendon at shoulder and upper arm level, unspecified arm

  ● **S46.91** Strain of unspecified muscle, fascia and tendon at shoulder and upper arm level

    ● **S46.911** Strain of unspecified muscle, fascia and tendon at shoulder and upper arm level, right arm

    ● **S46.912** Strain of unspecified muscle, fascia and tendon at shoulder and upper arm level, left arm

    ● **S46.919** Strain of unspecified muscle, fascia and tendon at shoulder and upper arm level, unspecified arm

● **S46.92** Laceration of unspecified muscle, fascia and tendon at shoulder and upper arm level

  ● **S46.921** Laceration of unspecified muscle, fascia and tendon at shoulder and upper arm level, right arm A ⬡
       (Ex:) See PDX Collection 1263

  ● **S46.922** Laceration of unspecified muscle, fascia and tendon at shoulder and upper arm level, left arm A ⬡
       (Ex:) See PDX Collection 1264

  ● **S46.929** Laceration of unspecified muscle, fascia and tendon at shoulder and upper arm level, unspecified arm A ⬡
       (Ex:) See PDX Collection 1265

● **S46.99** Other injury of unspecified muscle, fascia and tendon at shoulder and upper arm level

  ● **S46.991** Other injury of unspecified muscle, fascia and tendon at shoulder and upper arm level, right arm

  ● **S46.992** Other injury of unspecified muscle, fascia and tendon at shoulder and upper arm level, left arm

  ● **S46.999** Other injury of unspecified muscle, fascia and tendon at shoulder and upper arm level, unspecified arm

● **S47** **Crushing injury of shoulder and upper arm**

Use additional code for all associated injuries

Excludes2   crushing injury of elbow (S57.0-)

The appropriate 7th character is to be added to each code from category S47

A	initial encounter
D	subsequent encounter
S	sequela

X ● **S47.1** Crushing injury of right shoulder and upper arm

X ● **S47.2** Crushing injury of left shoulder and upper arm

X ● **S47.9** Crushing injury of shoulder and upper arm, unspecified arm

● **S48** **Traumatic amputation of shoulder and upper arm**

An amputation not identified as partial or complete should be coded to complete

Excludes1   traumatic amputation at elbow level (S58.0)

The appropriate 7th character is to be added to each code from category S48

A	initial encounter
D	subsequent encounter
S	sequela

● **S48.0** Traumatic amputation at shoulder joint

  ● **S48.01** Complete traumatic amputation at shoulder joint

    ● **S48.011** Complete traumatic amputation at right shoulder joint A ⬡
       (Ex:) See PDX Collection 1266

    ● **S48.012** Complete traumatic amputation at left shoulder joint A ⬡
       (Ex:) See PDX Collection 1267

    ● **S48.019** Complete traumatic amputation at unspecified shoulder joint A ⬡
       (Ex:) See PDX Collection 1268

N Newborn Age: 0   **P** Pediatric Age: 0–17   **M** Maternity DX: 12–55   **A** Adult Age: 15–124   ♀ Females Only   ♂ Males Only

⬡ Complication\Comorbidity   ⬡ Major C\C   (Ex:) CC/MCC Exclusions   ⬡ Hospital-Acquired Condition

1291

● S48.02　Partial traumatic amputation at shoulder joint
　　● S48.021　Partial traumatic amputation at right shoulder joint A 🐾
　　　　　(Ex) See PDX Collection 1266
　　● S48.022　Partial traumatic amputation at left shoulder joint A 🐾
　　　　　(Ex) See PDX Collection 1267
　　● S48.029　Partial traumatic amputation at unspecified shoulder joint A 🐾
　　　　　(Ex) See PDX Collection 1268
● S48.1　Traumatic amputation at level between shoulder and elbow
　● S48.11　Complete traumatic amputation at level between shoulder and elbow
　　● S48.111　Complete traumatic amputation at level between right shoulder and elbow A 🐾
　　　　　(Ex) See PDX Collection 1266
　　● S48.112　Complete traumatic amputation at level between left shoulder and elbow A 🐾
　　　　　(Ex) See PDX Collection 1267
　　● S48.119　Complete traumatic amputation at level between unspecified shoulder and elbow A 🐾
　　　　　(Ex) See PDX Collection 1268
　● S48.12　Partial traumatic amputation at level between shoulder and elbow
　　● S48.121　Partial traumatic amputation at level between right shoulder and elbow A 🐾
　　　　　(Ex) See PDX Collection 1266
　　● S48.122　Partial traumatic amputation at level between left shoulder and elbow A 🐾
　　　　　(Ex) See PDX Collection 1267
　　● S48.129　Partial traumatic amputation at level between unspecified shoulder and elbow A 🐾
　　　　　(Ex) See PDX Collection 1268
● S48.9　Traumatic amputation of shoulder and upper arm, level unspecified
　● S48.91　Complete traumatic amputation of shoulder and upper arm, level unspecified
　　● S48.911　Complete traumatic amputation of right shoulder and upper arm, level unspecified A 🐾
　　　　　(Ex) See PDX Collection 1266
　　● S48.912　Complete traumatic amputation of left shoulder and upper arm, level unspecified A 🐾
　　　　　(Ex) See PDX Collection 1267
　　● S48.919　Complete traumatic amputation of unspecified shoulder and upper arm, level unspecified A 🐾
　　　　　(Ex) See PDX Collection 1268
　● S48.92　Partial traumatic amputation of shoulder and upper arm, level unspecified
　　● S48.921　Partial traumatic amputation of right shoulder and upper arm, level unspecified A 🐾
　　　　　(Ex) See PDX Collection 1266
　　● S48.922　Partial traumatic amputation of left shoulder and upper arm, level unspecified A 🐾
　　　　　(Ex) See PDX Collection 1267
　　● S48.929　Partial traumatic amputation of unspecified shoulder and upper arm, level unspecified A 🐾
　　　　　(Ex) See PDX Collection 1268

Item 19-3　SALTER-HARRIS TYPE 1: epiphysis is completely separated from end of bone, or metaphysic growth plate remains attached to epiphysis
SALTER-HARRIS TYPE 2: epiphysis and growth plate are partially separated from metaphysis, which is cracked—most common type
SALTER-HARRIS TYPE 3: fracture occurring through epiphysis and separates part of epiphysis and growth plate from metaphysis fracture, usually at distal end of tibia
SALTER-HARRIS TYPE 4: fracture runs through epiphysis, across growth plate, into metaphysic, surgery is required to restore joint surface to normal and align growth plate

● S49　Other and unspecified injuries of shoulder and upper arm
　　The appropriate 7th character is to be added to each code from subcategories S49.0 and S49.1

A	initial encounter for closed fracture
D	subsequent encounter for fracture with routine healing
G	subsequent encounter for fracture with delayed healing
K	subsequent encounter for fracture with nonunion
P	subsequent encounter for fracture with malunion
S	sequela

● S49.0　Physeal fracture of upper end of humerus
　● S49.00　Unspecified physeal fracture of upper end of humerus
　　● S49.001　Unspecified physeal fracture of upper end of humerus, right arm A, K, P 🐾, A 🐾
　　　　　(Ex) For S49.001[A]: See PDX Collection 1245
　　　　　For S49.001[K,P]: See PDX Collection 897
　　● S49.002　Unspecified physeal fracture of upper end of humerus, left arm A, K, P 🐾, A 🐾
　　　　　(Ex) For S49.002[A]: See PDX Collection 1247
　　　　　For S49.002[K,P]: See PDX Collection 897
　　● S49.009　Unspecified physeal fracture of upper end of humerus, unspecified arm A, K, P 🐾, A 🐾
　　　　　(Ex) For S49.009[A]: See PDX Collection 1248
　　　　　For S49.009[K,P]: See PDX Collection 897
　● S49.01　Salter-Harris Type I physeal fracture of upper end of humerus
　　● S49.011　Salter-Harris Type I physeal fracture of upper end of humerus, right arm A, K, P 🐾, A 🐾
　　　　　(Ex) For S49.011[A]: See PDX Collection 1245
　　　　　For S49.011[K,P]: See PDX Collection 897
　　● S49.012　Salter-Harris Type I physeal fracture of upper end of humerus, left arm A, K, P 🐾, A 🐾
　　　　　(Ex) For S49.012[A]: See PDX Collection 1247
　　　　　For S49.012[K,P]: See PDX Collection 897
　　● S49.019　Salter-Harris Type I physeal fracture of upper end of humerus, unspecified arm A, K, P 🐾, A 🐾
　　　　　(Ex) For S49.019[A]: See PDX Collection 1248
　　　　　For S49.019[K,P]: See PDX Collection 897
　● S49.02　Salter-Harris Type II physeal fracture of upper end of humerus
　　● S49.021　Salter-Harris Type II physeal fracture of upper end of humerus, right arm A, K, P 🐾, A 🐾
　　　　　(Ex) For S49.021[A]: See PDX Collection 1245
　　　　　For S49.021[K,P]: See PDX Collection 897
　　● S49.022　Salter-Harris Type II physeal fracture of upper end of humerus, left arm A, K, P 🐾, A 🐾
　　　　　(Ex) For S49.022[A]: See PDX Collection 1247
　　　　　For S49.022[K,P]: See PDX Collection 897
　　● S49.029　Salter-Harris Type II physeal fracture of upper end of humerus, unspecified arm A, K, P 🐾, A 🐾
　　　　　(Ex) For S49.029[A]: See PDX Collection 1248
　　　　　For S49.029[K,P]: See PDX Collection 897

▶ New　⇒ Revised　~~deleted~~ Deleted　Excludes 1　Excludes 2　Includes　Use additional　Code first　Code also　Key words
OGCR Official Guidelines　● Unacceptable Principal Diagnosis　X Assign placeholder X　● Use Additional Character(s)　▌ Manifestation Code　**Coding Clinic**

● **S49.03　Salter-Harris Type III physeal fracture of upper end of humerus**

　● S49.031　Salter-Harris Type III physeal fracture of upper end of humerus, **right arm**
　　　A, K, P 🩹, A 🩹
　　　(Ex) **For S49.031[A]:** See PDX Collection 1245
　　　　　　For S49.031[K,P]: See PDX Collection 897

　● S49.032　Salter-Harris Type III physeal fracture of upper end of humerus, **left arm**
　　　A, K, P 🩹, A 🩹
　　　(Ex) **For S49.032[A]:** See PDX Collection 1247
　　　　　　For S49.032[K,P]: See PDX Collection 897

　● S49.039　Salter-Harris Type III physeal fracture of upper end of humerus, **unspecified arm** A, K, P 🩹, A 🩹
　　　(Ex) **For S49.039[A]:** See PDX Collection 1248
　　　　　　For S49.039[K,P]: See PDX Collection 897

● **S49.04　Salter-Harris Type IV physeal fracture of upper end of humerus**

　● S49.041　Salter-Harris Type IV physeal fracture of upper end of humerus, **right arm**
　　　A, K, P 🩹, A 🩹
　　　(Ex) **For S49.041[A]:** See PDX Collection 1245
　　　　　　For S49.041[K,P]: See PDX Collection 897

　● S49.042　Salter-Harris Type IV physeal fracture of upper end of humerus, **left arm**
　　　A, K, P 🩹, A 🩹
　　　(Ex) **For S49.042[A]:** See PDX Collection 1247
　　　　　　For S49.042[K,P]: See PDX Collection 897

　● S49.049　Salter-Harris Type IV physeal fracture of upper end of humerus, **unspecified arm** A, K, P 🩹, A 🩹
　　　(Ex) **For S49.049[A]:** See PDX Collection 1248
　　　　　　For S49.049[K,P]: See PDX Collection 897

● **S49.09　Other physeal fracture of upper end of humerus**

　● S49.091　Other physeal fracture of upper end of humerus, **right arm** A, K, P 🩹, A 🩹
　　　(Ex) **For S49.091[A]:** See PDX Collection 1245
　　　　　　For S49.091[K,P]: See PDX Collection 897

　● S49.092　Other physeal fracture of upper end of humerus, **left arm** A, K, P 🩹, A 🩹
　　　(Ex) **For S49.092[A]:** See PDX Collection 1247
　　　　　　For S49.092[K,P]: See PDX Collection 897

　● S49.099　Other physeal fracture of upper end of humerus, **unspecified arm**
　　　A, K, P 🩹, A 🩹
　　　(Ex) **For S49.099[A]:** See PDX Collection 1248
　　　　　　For S49.099[K,P]: See PDX Collection 897

● **S49.1　Physeal fracture of lower end of humerus**

　● **S49.10　Unspecified physeal fracture of lower end of humerus**

　　● S49.101　Unspecified physeal fracture of lower end of humerus, **right arm** A, K, P 🩹, A 🩹
　　　　(Ex) **For S49.101[A]:** See PDX Collection 1245
　　　　　　　For S49.101[K,P]: See PDX Collection 897

　　● S49.102　Unspecified physeal fracture of lower end of humerus, **left arm** A, K, P 🩹, A 🩹
　　　　(Ex) **For S49.102[A]:** See PDX Collection 1247
　　　　　　　For S49.102[K,P]: See PDX Collection 897

　　● S49.109　Unspecified physeal fracture of lower end of humerus, **unspecified arm**
　　　　A, K, P 🩹, A 🩹
　　　　(Ex) **For S49.109[A]:** See PDX Collection 1248
　　　　　　　For S49.109[K,P]: See PDX Collection 897

● **S49.11　Salter-Harris Type I physeal fracture of lower end of humerus**

　● S49.111　Salter-Harris Type I physeal fracture of lower end of humerus, **right arm**
　　　A, K, P 🩹, A 🩹
　　　(Ex) **For S49.111[A]:** See PDX Collection 1245
　　　　　　For S49.111[K,P]: See PDX Collection 897

　● S49.112　Salter-Harris Type I physeal fracture of lower end of humerus, **left arm**
　　　A, K, P 🩹, A 🩹
　　　(Ex) **For S49.112[A]:** See PDX Collection 1247
　　　　　　For S49.112[K,P]: See PDX Collection 897

　● S49.119　Salter-Harris Type I physeal fracture of lower end of humerus, **unspecified arm** A, K, P 🩹, A 🩹
　　　(Ex) **For S49.119[A]:** See PDX Collection 1248
　　　　　　For S49.119[K,P]: See PDX Collection 897

● **S49.12　Salter-Harris Type II physeal fracture of lower end of humerus**

　● S49.121　Salter-Harris Type II physeal fracture of lower end of humerus, **right arm**
　　　A, K, P 🩹, A 🩹
　　　(Ex) **For S49.121[A]:** See PDX Collection 1245
　　　　　　For S49.121[K,P]: See PDX Collection 897

　● S49.122　Salter-Harris Type II physeal fracture of lower end of humerus, **left arm**
　　　A, K, P 🩹, A 🩹
　　　(Ex) **For S49.122[A]:** See PDX Collection 1247
　　　　　　For S49.122[K,P]: See PDX Collection 897

　● S49.129　Salter-Harris Type II physeal fracture of lower end of humerus, **unspecified arm** A, K, P 🩹, A 🩹
　　　(Ex) **For S49.129[A]:** See PDX Collection 1248
　　　　　　For S49.129[K,P]: See PDX Collection 897

● **S49.13　Salter-Harris Type III physeal fracture of lower end of humerus**

　● S49.131　Salter-Harris Type III physeal fracture of lower end of humerus, **right arm**
　　　A, K, P 🩹, A 🩹
　　　(Ex) **For S49.131[A]:** See PDX Collection 1245
　　　　　　For S49.131[K,P]: See PDX Collection 897

　● S49.132　Salter-Harris Type III physeal fracture of lower end of humerus, **left arm**
　　　A, K, P 🩹, A 🩹
　　　(Ex) **For S49.132[A]:** See PDX Collection 1247
　　　　　　For S49.132[K,P]: See PDX Collection 897

　● S49.139　Salter-Harris Type III physeal fracture of lower end of humerus, **unspecified arm** A, K, P 🩹, A 🩹
　　　(Ex) **For S49.139[A]:** See PDX Collection 1248
　　　　　　For S49.139[K,P]: See PDX Collection 897

● **S49.14　Salter-Harris Type IV physeal fracture of lower end of humerus**

　● S49.141　Salter-Harris Type IV physeal fracture of lower end of humerus, **right arm**
　　　A, K, P 🩹, A 🩹
　　　(Ex) **For S49.141[A]:** See PDX Collection 1245
　　　　　　For S49.141[K,P]: See PDX Collection 897

　● S49.142　Salter-Harris Type IV physeal fracture of lower end of humerus, **left arm**
　　　A, K, P 🩹, A 🩹
　　　(Ex) **For S49.142[A]:** See PDX Collection 1247
　　　　　　For S49.142[K,P]: See PDX Collection 897

　● S49.149　Salter-Harris Type IV physeal fracture of lower end of humerus, **unspecified arm** A, K, P 🩹, A 🩹
　　　(Ex) **For S49.149[A]:** See PDX Collection 1248
　　　　　　For S49.149[K,P]: See PDX Collection 897

N Newborn Age: 0　　**P** Pediatric Age: 0–17　　**M** Maternity DX: 12–55　　**A** Adult Age: 15–124　　♀ Females Only　　♂ Males Only

🩹 Complication\Comorbidity　　🩹 Major C\C　　(Ex) CC/MCC Exclusions　　🩹 Hospital-Acquired Condition

1293

CHAPTER 19 (S00-T88)

● S49.19   Other physeal fracture of lower end of humerus
  ● S49.191   Other physeal fracture of lower end
             of humerus, right arm A, K, P 🔘, A 🔘
                  (Ex:) For S49.191[A]: See PDX Collection 1245
                       For S49.191[K,P]: See PDX Collection 897
  ● S49.192   Other physeal fracture of lower end
             of humerus, left arm A, K, P 🔘, A 🔘
                  (Ex:) For S49.192[A]: See PDX Collection 1247
                       For S49.192[K,P]: See PDX Collection 897
  ● S49.199   Other physeal fracture of lower end
             of humerus, unspecified arm
             A, K, P 🔘, A 🔘
                  (Ex:) For S49.199[A]: See PDX Collection 1248
                       For S49.199[K,P]: See PDX Collection 897
● S49.8   Other specified injuries of shoulder and upper arm
        The appropriate 7th character is to be added to each
        code in subcategory S49.8

A	initial encounter
D	subsequent encounter
S	sequela

  X ● S49.80   Other specified injuries of shoulder and upper
             arm, unspecified arm
  X ● S49.81   Other specified injuries of right shoulder and
             upper arm
  X ● S49.82   Other specified injuries of left shoulder and
             upper arm
● S49.9   Unspecified injury of shoulder and upper arm
        The appropriate 7th character is to be added to each
        code in subcategory S49.9

A	initial encounter
D	subsequent encounter
S	sequela

  X ● S49.90   Unspecified injury of shoulder and upper arm,
             unspecified arm
  X ● S49.91   Unspecified injury of right shoulder and upper
             arm
  X ● S49.92   Unspecified injury of left shoulder and upper
             arm

INJURIES TO THE ELBOW AND FOREARM (S50-S59)

Excludes2   burns and corrosions (T20-T32)
            frostbite (T33-T34)
            injuries of wrist and hand (S60-S69)
            insect bite or sting, venomous (T63.4)

● S50   Superficial injury of elbow and forearm
        Excludes2   superficial injury of wrist and hand (S60.-)
        The appropriate 7th character is to be added to each code from
        category S50

A	initial encounter
D	subsequent encounter
S	sequela

  ● S50.0   Contusion of elbow
    X ● S50.00   Contusion of unspecified elbow
    X ● S50.01   Contusion of right elbow
    X ● S50.02   Contusion of left elbow
  ● S50.1   Contusion of forearm
    X ● S50.10   Contusion of unspecified forearm
    X ● S50.11   Contusion of right forearm
    X ● S50.12   Contusion of left forearm

● S50.3   Other superficial injuries of elbow
  ● S50.31   Abrasion of elbow
    ● S50.311   Abrasion of right elbow
    ● S50.312   Abrasion of left elbow
    ● S50.319   Abrasion of unspecified elbow
  ● S50.32   Blister (nonthermal) of elbow
    ● S50.321   Blister (nonthermal) of right elbow
    ● S50.322   Blister (nonthermal) of left elbow
    ● S50.329   Blister (nonthermal) of unspecified
               elbow
  ● S50.34   External constriction of elbow
    ● S50.341   External constriction of right elbow
    ● S50.342   External constriction of left elbow
    ● S50.349   External constriction of unspecified
               elbow
  ● S50.35   Superficial foreign body of elbow
             Splinter in the elbow
    ● S50.351   Superficial foreign body of right
               elbow
    ● S50.352   Superficial foreign body of left elbow
    ● S50.359   Superficial foreign body of
               unspecified elbow
  ● S50.36   Insect bite (nonvenomous) of elbow
    ● S50.361   Insect bite (nonvenomous) of right
               elbow
    ● S50.362   Insect bite (nonvenomous) of left
               elbow
    ● S50.369   Insect bite (nonvenomous) of
               unspecified elbow
  ● S50.37   Other superficial bite of elbow
             Excludes1   open bite of elbow (S51.04)
    ● S50.371   Other superficial bite of right elbow
    ● S50.372   Other superficial bite of left elbow
    ● S50.379   Other superficial bite of unspecified
               elbow
● S50.8   Other superficial injuries of forearm
  ● S50.81   Abrasion of forearm
    ● S50.811   Abrasion of right forearm
    ● S50.812   Abrasion of left forearm
    ● S50.819   Abrasion of unspecified forearm
  ● S50.82   Blister (nonthermal) of forearm
    ● S50.821   Blister (nonthermal) of right forearm
    ● S50.822   Blister (nonthermal) of left forearm
    ● S50.829   Blister (nonthermal) of unspecified
               forearm
  ● S50.84   External constriction of forearm
    ● S50.841   External constriction of right forearm
    ● S50.842   External constriction of left forearm
    ● S50.849   External constriction of unspecified
               forearm
  ● S50.85   Superficial foreign body of forearm
             Splinter in the forearm
    ● S50.851   Superficial foreign body of right
               forearm
    ● S50.852   Superficial foreign body of left
               forearm
    ● S50.859   Superficial foreign body of
               unspecified forearm

▶ New   ⇒ Revised   ~~deleted~~ Deleted   Excludes 1   Excludes 2   Includes   Use additional   Code first   Code also   Key words

OGCR Official Guidelines   ● Unacceptable Principal Diagnosis   X Assign placeholder X   ▶ Use Additional Character(s)   ▶ Manifestation Code   **Coding Clinic**

● **S50.86**   Insect bite (nonvenomous) of forearm
   ● **S50.861**   Insect bite (nonvenomous) of right forearm
   ● **S50.862**   Insect bite (nonvenomous) of left forearm
   ● **S50.869**   Insect bite (nonvenomous) of unspecified forearm
● **S50.87**   Other superficial bite of forearm
   Excludes1   open bite of forearm (S51.84)
   ● **S50.871**   Other superficial bite of right forearm
   ● **S50.872**   Other superficial bite of left forearm
   ● **S50.879**   Other superficial bite of unspecified forearm
● **S50.9**   Unspecified superficial injury of elbow and forearm
   ● **S50.90**   Unspecified superficial injury of elbow
     ● **S50.901**   Unspecified superficial injury of right elbow
     ● **S50.902**   Unspecified superficial injury of left elbow
     ● **S50.909**   Unspecified superficial injury of unspecified elbow
   ● **S50.91**   Unspecified superficial injury of forearm
     ● **S50.911**   Unspecified superficial injury of right forearm
     ● **S50.912**   Unspecified superficial injury of left forearm
     ● **S50.919**   Unspecified superficial injury of unspecified forearm

● **S51**   Open wound of elbow and forearm
   Code also any associated wound infection
   Excludes1   open fracture of elbow and forearm (S52.- with open fracture 7th character)
     traumatic amputation of elbow and forearm (S58.-)
   Excludes2   open wound of wrist and hand (S61.-)
   The appropriate 7th character is to be added to each code from category S51

> A   initial encounter
> D   subsequent encounter
> S   sequela

   ● **S51.0**   Open wound of elbow
     ● **S51.00**   Unspecified open wound of elbow
       ● **S51.001**   Unspecified open wound of right elbow
         Coding Clinic: 2012, Q4, P108
       ● **S51.002**   Unspecified open wound of left elbow
       ● **S51.009**   Unspecified open wound of unspecified elbow
         Open wound of elbow NOS
     ● **S51.01**   Laceration without foreign body of elbow
       ● **S51.011**   Laceration without foreign body of right elbow
       ● **S51.012**   Laceration without foreign body of left elbow
       ● **S51.019**   Laceration without foreign body of unspecified elbow
     ● **S51.02**   Laceration with foreign body of elbow
       ● **S51.021**   Laceration with foreign body of right elbow
       ● **S51.022**   Laceration with foreign body of left elbow
       ● **S51.029**   Laceration with foreign body of unspecified elbow

   ● **S51.03**   Puncture wound without foreign body of elbow
     ● **S51.031**   Puncture wound without foreign body of right elbow
     ● **S51.032**   Puncture wound without foreign body of left elbow
     ● **S51.039**   Puncture wound without foreign body of unspecified elbow
   ● **S51.04**   Puncture wound with foreign body of elbow
     ● **S51.041**   Puncture wound with foreign body of right elbow
     ● **S51.042**   Puncture wound with foreign body of left elbow
     ● **S51.049**   Puncture wound with foreign body of unspecified elbow
   ● **S51.05**   Open bite of elbow
     Bite of elbow NOS
     Excludes1   superficial bite of elbow (S50.36, S50.37)
     ● **S51.051**   Open bite, right elbow
     ● **S51.052**   Open bite, left elbow
     ● **S51.059**   Open bite, unspecified elbow
● **S51.8**   Open wound of forearm
   Excludes2   open wound of elbow (S51.0-)
   ● **S51.80**   Unspecified open wound of forearm
     ● **S51.801**   Unspecified open wound of right forearm
     ● **S51.802**   Unspecified open wound of left forearm
     ● **S51.809**   Unspecified open wound of unspecified forearm
       Open wound of forearm NOS
   ● **S51.81**   Laceration without foreign body of forearm
     ● **S51.811**   Laceration without foreign body of right forearm
     ● **S51.812**   Laceration without foreign body of left forearm
     ● **S51.819**   Laceration without foreign body of unspecified forearm
   ● **S51.82**   Laceration with foreign body of forearm
     ● **S51.821**   Laceration with foreign body of right forearm
     ● **S51.822**   Laceration with foreign body of left forearm
     ● **S51.829**   Laceration with foreign body of unspecified forearm
   ● **S51.83**   Puncture wound without foreign body of forearm
     ● **S51.831**   Puncture wound without foreign body of right forearm
     ● **S51.832**   Puncture wound without foreign body of left forearm
     ● **S51.839**   Puncture wound without foreign body of unspecified forearm
   ● **S51.84**   Puncture wound with foreign body of forearm
     ● **S51.841**   Puncture wound with foreign body of right forearm
     ● **S51.842**   Puncture wound with foreign body of left forearm
     ● **S51.849**   Puncture wound with foreign body of unspecified forearm
   ● **S51.85**   Open bite of forearm
     Bite of forearm NOS
     Excludes1   superficial bite of forearm (S50.86, S50.87)
     ● **S51.851**   Open bite of right forearm
     ● **S51.852**   Open bite of left forearm
     ● **S51.859**   Open bite of unspecified forearm

CHAPTER 19 (S00-T88)

N Newborn Age: 0   **P** Pediatric Age: 0–17   **M** Maternity DX: 12–55   **A** Adult Age: 15–124   ♀ Females Only   ♂ Males Only

🐾 Complication\Comorbidity   🐾 Major C\C   (Ex) CC/MCC Exclusions   🐾 Hospital-Acquired Condition

1295

● **S52   Fracture of forearm**

Note: A fracture not identified as displaced or nondisplaced should be coded to displaced

A fracture not designated as open or closed should be coded to closed

The open fracture designations are based on the Gustilo open fracture classification

Excludes1   traumatic amputation of forearm (S58.-)

Excludes2   fracture at wrist and hand level (S62.-)

The appropriate 7th character is to be added to all codes from category S52

A	initial encounter for closed fracture
B	initial encounter for open fracture type I or II
	initial encounter for open fracture NOS
C	initial encounter for open fracture type IIIA, IIIB, or IIIC
D	subsequent encounter for closed fracture with routine healing
E	subsequent encounter for open fracture type I or II with routine healing
F	subsequent encounter for open fracture type IIIA, IIIB, or IIIC with routine healing
G	subsequent encounter for closed fracture with delayed healing
H	subsequent encounter for open fracture type I or II with delayed healing
J	subsequent encounter for open fracture type IIIA, IIIB, or IIIC with delayed healing
K	subsequent encounter for closed fracture with nonunion
M	subsequent encounter for open fracture type I or II with nonunion
N	subsequent encounter for open fracture type IIIA, IIIB, or IIIC with nonunion
P	subsequent encounter for closed fracture with malunion
Q	subsequent encounter for open fracture type I or II with malunion
R	subsequent encounter for open fracture type IIIA, IIIB, or IIIC with malunion
S	sequela

Coding Clinic: 2016, Q1, P33

● **S52.0   Fracture of upper end of ulna**

Fracture of proximal end of ulna

Excludes2   fracture of elbow NOS (S42.40-)
fractures of shaft of ulna (S52.2-)

● **S52.00   Unspecified fracture of upper end of ulna**

(Ex:) For category S52.00 CC codes S52.00[B,C]:
See PDX Collection 1269 For S52.00[K,M,N,P,Q,R]:
See PDX Collection 897

● **S52.001   Unspecified fracture of upper end of right ulna** K, M, N, P, Q, R 🔒, B, C 🔒, B, C 🔒

● **S52.002   Unspecified fracture of upper end of left ulna** K, M, N, P, Q, R 🔒, B, C 🔒, B, C 🔒

● **S52.009   Unspecified fracture of upper end of unspecified ulna** K, M, N, P, Q, R 🔒, B, C 🔒, B, C 🔒

● **S52.01   Torus fracture of upper end of ulna**

The appropriate 7th character is to be added to all codes in subcategory S52.01

A	initial encounter for closed fracture
D	subsequent encounter for fracture with routine healing
G	subsequent encounter for fracture with delayed healing
K	subsequent encounter for fracture with nonunion
P	subsequent encounter for fracture with malunion
S	sequela

● **S52.011   Torus fracture of upper end of right ulna** A, K, P 🔒, A 🔒

(Ex:) For code S52.011[A]: See PDX Collection 1270
For S52.011[K,P]: See PDX Collection 897

● **S52.012   Torus fracture of upper end of left ulna** A, K, P 🔒, A 🔒

(Ex:) For code S52.012[A]: See PDX Collection 1271
For S52.012[K,P]: See PDX Collection 897

● **S52.019   Torus fracture of upper end of unspecified ulna** A, K, P 🔒, A 🔒

(Ex:) For code S52.019[A]: See PDX Collection 1272
For S52.019[K,P]: See PDX Collection 897

● **S52.02   Fracture of olecranon process without intraarticular extension of ulna**

(Ex:) For category S52.02 CC codes S52.02[B,C]: See PDX Collection 1273 For S52.02[K,M,N,P,Q,R]: See PDX Collection 897

● **S52.021   Displaced fracture of olecranon process without intraarticular extension of right ulna** K, M, N, P, Q, R 🔒, B, C 🔒, B, C 🔒

● **S52.022   Displaced fracture of olecranon process without intraarticular extension of left ulna** K, M, N, P, Q, R 🔒, B, C 🔒, B, C 🔒

● **S52.023   Displaced fracture of olecranon process without intraarticular extension of unspecified ulna** K, M, N, P, Q, R 🔒, B, C 🔒, B, C 🔒

● **S52.024   Nondisplaced fracture of olecranon process without intraarticular extension of right ulna** K, M, N, P, Q, R 🔒, B, C 🔒, B, C 🔒

● **S52.025   Nondisplaced fracture of olecranon process without intraarticular extension of left ulna** K, M, N, P, Q, R 🔒, B, C 🔒, B, C 🔒

● **S52.026   Nondisplaced fracture of olecranon process without intraarticular extension of unspecified ulna** K, M, N, P, Q, R 🔒, B, C 🔒, B, C 🔒

● **S52.03** Fracture of olecranon process with intraarticular extension of ulna

    (Ex) **For category S52.03 CC codes S52.03[B,C]:** See PDX Collection 1273 **For S52.03[K,M,N,P,Q,R]:** See PDX Collection 897

  ● **S52.031** Displaced fracture of olecranon process with intraarticular extension of right ulna K, M, N, P, Q, R 🔹, B, C 🔹, B, C 🔹

  ● **S52.032** Displaced fracture of olecranon process with intraarticular extension of left ulna K, M, N, P, Q, R 🔹, B, C 🔹, B, C 🔹

  ● **S52.033** Displaced fracture of olecranon process with intraarticular extension of unspecified ulna K, M, N, P, Q, R 🔹, B, C 🔹, B, C 🔹

  ● **S52.034** Nondisplaced fracture of olecranon process with intraarticular extension of right ulna K, M, N, P, Q, R 🔹, B, C 🔹, B, C 🔹

  ● **S52.035** Nondisplaced fracture of olecranon process with intraarticular extension of left ulna K, M, N, P, Q, R 🔹, B, C 🔹, B, C 🔹

  ● **S52.036** Nondisplaced fracture of olecranon process with intraarticular extension of unspecified ulna K, M, N, P, Q, R 🔹, B, C 🔹, B, C 🔹

● **S52.04** Fracture of coronoid process of ulna

    (Ex) **For category S52.04 CC codes S52.04[B,C]:** See PDX Collection 1269 **For S52.04[K,M,N,P,Q,R]:** See PDX Collection 897

  ● **S52.041** Displaced fracture of coronoid process of right ulna K, M, N, P, Q, R 🔹, B, C 🔹, B, C 🔹

  ● **S52.042** Displaced fracture of coronoid process of left ulna K, M, N, P, Q, R 🔹, B, C 🔹, B, C 🔹

  ● **S52.043** Displaced fracture of coronoid process of unspecified ulna K, M, N, P, Q, R 🔹, B, C 🔹, B, C 🔹

  ● **S52.044** Nondisplaced fracture of coronoid process of right ulna K, M, N, P, Q, R 🔹, B, C 🔹, B, C 🔹

  ● **S52.045** Nondisplaced fracture of coronoid process of left ulna K, M, N, P, Q, R 🔹, B, C 🔹, B, C 🔹

  ● **S52.046** Nondisplaced fracture of coronoid process of unspecified ulna K, M, N, P, Q, R 🔹, B, C 🔹, B, C 🔹

● **S52.09** Other fracture of upper end of ulna

    (Ex) **For category S52.09 CC codes S52.09[B,C]:** See PDX Collection 1269 **For S52.09[K,M,N,P,Q,R]:** See PDX Collection 897

  ● **S52.091** Other fracture of upper end of right ulna K, M, N, P, Q, R 🔹, B, C 🔹, B, C 🔹

  ● **S52.092** Other fracture of upper end of left ulna K, M, N, P, Q, R 🔹, B, C 🔹, B, C 🔹

  ● **S52.099** Other fracture of upper end of unspecified ulna K, M, N, P, Q, R 🔹, B, C 🔹, B, C 🔹

● **S52.1** Fracture of upper end of radius

    Fracture of proximal end of radius

    Excludes2 physeal fractures of upper end of radius (S59.2-)
        fracture of shaft of radius (S52.3-)

● **S52.10** Unspecified fracture of upper end of radius

    (Ex) **For category S52.10 CC codes S52.10[B,C]:** See PDX Collection 1269 **For S52.10[K,M,N,P,Q,R]:** See PDX Collection 897

  ● **S52.101** Unspecified fracture of upper end of right radius K, M, N, P, Q, R 🔹, B, C 🔹, B, C 🔹

  ● **S52.102** Unspecified fracture of upper end of left radius K, M, N, P, Q, R 🔹, B, C 🔹, B, C 🔹

  ● **S52.109** Unspecified fracture of upper end of unspecified radius K, M, N, P, Q, R 🔹, B, C 🔹, B, C 🔹

● **S52.11** Torus fracture of upper end of radius

    The appropriate 7th character is to be added to all codes in subcategory S52.11

A	initial encounter for closed fracture
D	subsequent encounter for fracture with routine healing
G	subsequent encounter for fracture with delayed healing
K	subsequent encounter for fracture with nonunion
P	subsequent encounter for fracture with malunion
S	sequela

  ● **S52.111** Torus fracture of upper end of right radius A, K, P 🔹, A 🔹

    (Ex) **For code S52.111[A]:** See PDX Collection 1270 **For S52.111[K,P]:** See PDX Collection 897

  ● **S52.112** Torus fracture of upper end of left radius A, K, P 🔹, A 🔹

    (Ex) **For code S52.112[A]:** See PDX Collection 1271 **For S52.112[K,P]:** See PDX Collection 897

  ● **S52.119** Torus fracture of upper end of unspecified radius A, K, P 🔹, A 🔹

    (Ex) **For code S52.119[A]:** See PDX Collection 1272 **For S52.119[K,P]:** See PDX Collection 897

● **S52.12** Fracture of head of radius

    (Ex) **For category S52.12 CC codes S52.12[B,C]:** See PDX Collection 1269 **For S52.12[K,M,N,P,Q,R]:** See PDX Collection 897

  ● **S52.121** Displaced fracture of head of right radius K, M, N, P, Q, R 🔹, B, C 🔹, B, C 🔹

  ● **S52.122** Displaced fracture of head of left radius K, M, N, P, Q, R 🔹, B, C 🔹, B, C 🔹

  ● **S52.123** Displaced fracture of head of unspecified radius K, M, N, P, Q, R 🔹, B, C 🔹, B, C 🔹

  ● **S52.124** Nondisplaced fracture of head of right radius K, M, N, P, Q, R 🔹, B, C 🔹, B, C 🔹

  ● **S52.125** Nondisplaced fracture of head of left radius K, M, N, P, Q, R 🔹, B, C 🔹, B, C 🔹

  ● **S52.126** Nondisplaced fracture of head of unspecified radius K, M, N, P, Q, R 🔹, B, C 🔹, B, C 🔹

N Newborn Age: 0   **P** Pediatric Age: 0–17   **M** Maternity DX: 12–55   **A** Adult Age: 15–124   ♀ Females Only   ♂ Males Only

🔹 Complication\Comorbidity   🔹 Major C\C   (Ex) CC/MCC Exclusions   🔹 Hospital-Acquired Condition

1297

CHAPTER 19 (S00–T88)

- **S52.13** **Fracture of neck of radius**
  (Ex:) For category S52.13 CC codes S52.13[B,C]: See PDX Collection 1269 For S52.13[K,M,N,P,Q,R]: See PDX Collection 897
  - **S52.131** **Displaced fracture of neck of right radius** K, M, N, P, Q, R, B, C, B, C
  - **S52.132** **Displaced fracture of neck of left radius** K, M, N, P, Q, R, B, C, B, C
  - **S52.133** **Displaced fracture of neck of unspecified radius** K, M, N, P, Q, R, B, C, B, C
  - **S52.134** **Nondisplaced fracture of neck of right radius** K, M, N, P, Q, R, B, C, B, C
  - **S52.135** **Nondisplaced fracture of neck of left radius** K, M, N, P, Q, R, B, C, B, C
  - **S52.136** **Nondisplaced fracture of neck of unspecified radius** K, M, N, P, Q, R, B, C, B, C
- **S52.18** **Other fracture of upper end of radius**
  (Ex:) For category S52.18 CC codes S52.18[B,C]: See PDX Collection 1269 For S52.18[K,M,N,P,Q,R]: See PDX Collection 897
  - **S52.181** **Other fracture of upper end of right radius** K, M, N, P, Q, R, B, C, B, C
  - **S52.182** **Other fracture of upper end of left radius** K, M, N, P, Q, R, B, C, B, C
  - **S52.189** **Other fracture of upper end of unspecified radius** K, M, N, P, Q, R, B, C, B, C
- **S52.2** **Fracture of shaft of ulna**
  - **S52.20** **Unspecified fracture of shaft of ulna**
    Fracture of ulna NOS
    - **S52.201** **Unspecified fracture of shaft of right ulna** A, K, M, N, P, Q, R, B, C, A, B, C
      (Ex:) For code S52.201[A]: See PDX Collection 1270 For S52.201[B,C]: See PDX Collection 1269 For S52.201[K,M,N,P,Q,R]: See PDX Collection 897
    - **S52.202** **Unspecified fracture of shaft of left ulna** A, K, M, N, P, Q, R, B, C, A, B, C
      (Ex:) For code S52.202[A]: See PDX Collection 1271 For S52.202[B,C]: See PDX Collection 1269 For S52.202[K,M,N,P,Q,R]: See PDX Collection 897
    - **S52.209** **Unspecified fracture of shaft of unspecified ulna** A, K, M, N, P, Q, R, B, C, A, B, C
      (Ex:) For code S52.209[A]: See PDX Collection 1272 For code S52.209[B,C]: See PDX Collection 1269 For S52.209[K,M,N,P,Q,R]: See PDX Collection 897

- **S52.21** **Greenstick fracture of shaft of ulna**
  The appropriate 7th character is to be added to all codes in subcategory S52.21

A	initial encounter for closed fracture
D	subsequent encounter for fracture with routine healing
G	subsequent encounter for fracture with delayed healing
K	subsequent encounter for fracture with nonunion
P	subsequent encounter for fracture with malunion
S	sequela

  - **S52.211** **Greenstick fracture of shaft of right ulna** A, K, P, A
    (Ex:) For code S52.211[A]: See PDX Collection 1270 For S52.211[K,P]: See PDX Collection 897
  - **S52.212** **Greenstick fracture of shaft of left ulna** A, K, P, A
    (Ex:) For code S52.212[A]: See PDX Collection 1271 For S52.202[K,P]: See PDX Collection 897
  - **S52.219** **Greenstick fracture of shaft of unspecified ulna** A, K, P, A
    (Ex:) For code S52.219[A]: See PDX Collection 1272 For S52.219[K,P]: See PDX Collection 897
- **S52.22** **Transverse fracture of shaft of ulna**
  - **S52.221** **Displaced transverse fracture of shaft of right ulna** A, K, M, N, P, Q, R, B, C, A, B, C
    (Ex:) For code S52.221[A]: See PDX Collection 1270 For S52.221[B,C]: See PDX Collection 1269 For S52.221[K,M,N,P,Q,R]: See PDX Collection 897
  - **S52.222** **Displaced transverse fracture of shaft of left ulna** A, K, M, N, P, Q, R, B, C, A, B, C
    (Ex:) For code S52.222[A]: See PDX Collection 1271 For code S52.222[B,C]: See PDX Collection 1269 For S52.222[K,M,N,P,Q,R]: See PDX Collection 897
  - **S52.223** **Displaced transverse fracture of shaft of unspecified ulna** A, K, M, N, P, Q, R, B, C, A, B, C
    (Ex:) For code S52.223[A]: See PDX Collection 1272 For S52.223[B,C]: See PDX Collection 1269 For S52.223[K,M,N,P,Q,R]: See PDX Collection 897
  - **S52.224** **Nondisplaced transverse fracture of shaft of right ulna** A, K, M, N, P, Q, R, B, C, A, B, C
    (Ex:) For code S52.224[A]: See PDX Collection 1270 For S52.224[B,C]: See PDX Collection 1269 For S52.224[K,M,N,P,Q,R]: See PDX Collection 897
  - **S52.225** **Nondisplaced transverse fracture of shaft of left ulna** A, K, M, N, P, Q, R, B, C, A, B, C
    (Ex:) For code S52.225[A]: See PDX Collection 1271 For S52.225[B,C]: See PDX Collection 1269 For S52.225[K,M,N,P,Q,R]: See PDX Collection 897
  - **S52.226** **Nondisplaced transverse fracture of shaft of unspecified ulna** A, K, M, N, P, Q, R, B, C, A, B, C
    (Ex:) For code S52.226[A]: See PDX Collection 1272 For code S52.226[B,C]: See PDX Collection 1269 For S52.226[K,M,N,P,Q,R]: See PDX Collection 897

▶ New   ⇒ Revised   ~~deleted~~ Deleted   Excludes 1   Excludes 2   Includes   Use additional   Code first   Code also   Key words
OGCR Official Guidelines   ● Unacceptable Principal Diagnosis   X Assign placeholder X   ● Use Additional Character(s)   ▶ Manifestation Code   **Coding Clinic**

- ● S52.23   Oblique fracture of shaft of ulna
  - ● S52.231   Displaced oblique fracture of shaft of right ulna A, K, M, N, P, Q, R 🖫, B, C 🖫, A, B, C 🖫
    - (Ex:) **For code S52.231[A]:** See PDX Collection 1270
      For S52.231[B,C]: See PDX Collection 1269
      For S52.231[K,M,N,P,Q,R]: See PDX Collection 897
  - ● S52.232   Displaced oblique fracture of shaft of left ulna A, K, M, N, P, Q, R 🖫, B, C 🖫, A, B, C 🖫
    - (Ex:) **For code S52.232[A]:** See PDX Collection 1271
      For code S52.232[B,C]: See PDX Collection 1269 **For S52.232[K,M,N,P,Q,R]:** See PDX Collection 897
  - ● S52.233   Displaced oblique fracture of shaft of unspecified ulna A, K, M, N, P, Q, R 🖫, B, C 🖫, A, B, C 🖫
    - (Ex:) **For code S52.233[A]:** See PDX Collection 1272
      For code S52.233[B,C]: See PDX Collection 1269 **For S52.233[K,M,N,P,Q,R]:** See PDX Collection 897
  - ● S52.234   Nondisplaced oblique fracture of shaft of right ulna A, K, M, N, P, Q, R 🖫, B, C 🖫, A, B, C 🖫
    - (Ex:) **For code S52.234[A]:** See PDX Collection 1270
      For S52.234[B,C]: See PDX Collection 1269
      For S52.234[K,M,N,P,Q,R]: See PDX Collection 897
  - ● S52.235   Nondisplaced oblique fracture of shaft of left ulna A, K, M, N, P, Q, R 🖫, B, C 🖫, A, B, C 🖫
    - (Ex:) **For code S52.235[A]:** See PDX Collection 1271
      For code S52.235[B,C]: See PDX Collection 1269 **For S52.235[K,M,N,P,Q,R]:** See PDX Collection 897
  - ● S52.236   Nondisplaced oblique fracture of shaft of unspecified ulna A, K, M, N, P, Q, R 🖫, B, C 🖫, A, B, C 🖫
    - (Ex:) **For code S52.236[A]:** See PDX Collection 1272
      For code S52.236[B,C]: See PDX Collection 1269 **For S52.236[K,M,N,P,Q,R]:** See PDX Collection 897
- ● S52.24   Spiral fracture of shaft of ulna
  - ● S52.241   Displaced spiral fracture of shaft of ulna, right arm A, K, M, N, P, Q, R 🖫, B, C 🖫, A, B, C 🖫
    - (Ex:) **For code S52.241[A]:** See PDX Collection 1270
      For S52.241[B,C]: See PDX Collection 1269
      For S52.241[K,M,N,P,Q,R]: See PDX Collection 897
  - ● S52.242   Displaced spiral fracture of shaft of ulna, left arm A, K, M, N, P, Q, R 🖫, B, C 🖫, A, B, C 🖫
    - (Ex:) **For code S52.242[A]:** See PDX Collection 1271
      For code S52.242[B,C]: See PDX Collection 1269 **For S52.242[K,M,N,P,Q,R]:** See PDX Collection 897
  - ● S52.243   Displaced spiral fracture of shaft of ulna, unspecified arm A, K, M, N, P, Q, R 🖫, B, C 🖫, A, B, C 🖫
    - (Ex:) **For code S52.243[A]:** See PDX Collection 1272
      For code S52.243[B,C]: See PDX Collection 1269 **For S52.243[K,M,N,P,Q,R]:** See PDX Collection 897

- ● S52.244   Nondisplaced spiral fracture of shaft of ulna, right arm A, K, M, N, P, Q, R 🖫, B, C 🖫, A, B, C 🖫
  - (Ex:) **For code S52.244[A]:** See PDX Collection 1270
    For S52.244[B,C]: See PDX Collection 1269
    For S52.244[K,M,N,P,Q,R]: See PDX Collection 897
- ● S52.245   Nondisplaced spiral fracture of shaft of ulna, left arm A, K, M, N, P, Q, R 🖫, B, C 🖫, A, B, C 🖫
  - (Ex:) **For code S52.245[A]:** See PDX Collection 1271
    For code S52.245[B,C]: See PDX Collection 1269 **For S52.245[K,M,N,P,Q,R]:** See PDX Collection 897
- ● S52.246   Nondisplaced spiral fracture of shaft of ulna, unspecified arm A, K, M, N, P, Q, R 🖫, B, C 🖫, A, B, C 🖫
  - (Ex:) **For code S52.246[A]:** See PDX Collection 1272
    For code S52.246[B,C]: See PDX Collection 1269 **For S52.246[K,M,N,P,Q,R]:** See PDX Collection 897
- ● S52.25   Comminuted fracture of shaft of ulna
  - ● S52.251   Displaced comminuted fracture of shaft of ulna, right arm A, K, M, N, P, Q, R 🖫, B, C 🖫, A, B, C 🖫
    - (Ex:) **For code S52.251[A]:** See PDX Collection 1270
      For S52.251[B,C]: See PDX Collection 1269
      For S52.251[K,M,N,P,Q,R]: See PDX Collection 897
  - ● S52.252   Displaced comminuted fracture of shaft of ulna, left arm A, K, M, N, P, Q, R 🖫, B, C 🖫, A, B, C 🖫
    - (Ex:) **For code S52.252[A]:** See PDX Collection 1271
      For code S52.252[B,C]: See PDX Collection 1269 **For S52.252[K,M,N,P,Q,R]:** See PDX Collection 897
  - ● S52.253   Displaced comminuted fracture of shaft of ulna, unspecified arm A, K, M, N, P, Q, R 🖫, B, C 🖫, A, B, C 🖫
    - (Ex:) **For code S52.253[A]:** See PDX Collection 1272
      For code S52.253[B,C]: See PDX Collection 1269 **For S52.253[K,M,N,P,Q,R]:** See PDX Collection 897
  - ● S52.254   Nondisplaced comminuted fracture of shaft of ulna, right arm A, K, M, N, P, Q, R 🖫, B, C 🖫, A, B, C 🖫
    - (Ex:) **For code S52.254[A]:** See PDX Collection 1270
      For S52.254[B,C]: See PDX Collection 1269
      For S52.254[K,M,N,P,Q,R]: See PDX Collection 897
  - ● S52.255   Nondisplaced comminuted fracture of shaft of ulna, left arm A, K, M, N, P, Q, R 🖫, B, C 🖫, A, B, C 🖫
    - (Ex:) **For code S52.255[A]:** See PDX Collection 1271
      For code S52.255[B,C]: See PDX Collection 1269 **For S52.255[K,M,N,P,Q,R]:** See PDX Collection 897
  - ● S52.256   Nondisplaced comminuted fracture of shaft of ulna, unspecified arm A, K, M, N, P, Q, R 🖫, B, C 🖫, A, B, C 🖫
    - (Ex:) **For code S52.256[A]:** See PDX Collection 1272
      For code S52.256[B,C]: See PDX Collection 1269 **For S52.256[K,M,N,P,Q,R]:** See PDX Collection 897

N Newborn Age: 0   **P** Pediatric Age: 0–17   **M** Maternity DX: 12–55   **A** Adult Age: 15–124   ♀ Females Only   ♂ Males Only

🖫 Complication\Comorbidity   🖫 Major C\C   (Ex:) CC/MCC Exclusions   🖫 Hospital-Acquired Condition

1299

CHAPTER 19 (S00–T88)

● S52.26   Segmental fracture of shaft of ulna
  ● S52.261   Displaced segmental fracture of shaft
              of ulna, right arm
              A, K, M, N, P, Q, R 🔒, B, C 🔒,
              A, B, C 🔒
              (Ex:) For code S52.261[A]: See PDX Collection 1270
                   For S52.261[B,C]: See PDX Collection 1269
                   For S52.261[K,M,N,P,Q,R]: See PDX
                   Collection 897

  ● S52.262   Displaced segmental fracture of shaft
              of ulna, left arm A, K, M, N, P, Q, R 🔒,
              B, C 🔒, A, B, C 🔒
              (Ex:) For code S52.262[A]: See PDX Collection 1271
                   For code S52.262[B,C]: See PDX
                   Collection 1269 For S52.262[K,M,N,P,Q,R]:
                   See PDX Collection 897

  ● S52.263   Displaced segmental fracture of shaft
              of ulna, unspecified arm
              A, K, M, N, P, Q, R 🔒, B, C 🔒,
              A, B, C 🔒
              (Ex:) For code S52.263[A]: See PDX Collection 1272
                   For code S52.263[B,C]: See PDX
                   Collection 1269 For S52.263[K,M,N,P,Q,R]:
                   See PDX Collection 897

  ● S52.264   Nondisplaced segmental fracture of
              shaft of ulna, right arm
              A, K, M, N, P, Q, R 🔒, B, C 🔒,
              A, B, C 🔒
              (Ex:) For code S52.264[A]: See PDX Collection 1270
                   For S52.264[B,C]: See PDX Collection 1269
                   For S52.264[K,M,N,P,Q,R]: See PDX
                   Collection 897

  ● S52.265   Nondisplaced segmental fracture of
              shaft of ulna, left arm
              A, K, M, N, P, Q, R 🔒, B, C 🔒,
              A, B, C 🔒
              (Ex:) For code S52.265[A]: See PDX Collection 1271
                   For code S52.265[B,C]: See PDX
                   Collection 1269 For S52.265[K,M,N,P,Q,R]:
                   See PDX Collection 897

  ● S52.266   Nondisplaced segmental fracture of
              shaft of ulna, unspecified arm
              A, K, M, N, P, Q, R 🔒, B, C 🔒,
              A, B, C 🔒
              (Ex:) For code S52.266[A]: See PDX Collection 1272
                   For code S52.266[B,C]: See PDX
                   Collection 1269 For S52.266[K,M,N,P,Q,R]:
                   See PDX Collection 897

● S52.27   Monteggia's fracture of ulna
            Fracture of upper shaft of ulna with dislocation
            of radial head
            (Ex:) For category S52.27 CC codes S52.27[B,C]: See PDX
                 Collection 1269 For S52.27[K,M,N,P,Q,R]: See PDX
                 Collection 897

  ● S52.271   Monteggia's fracture of right ulna
              K, M, N, P, Q, R 🔒, B, C 🔒, B, C 🔒
  ● S52.272   Monteggia's fracture of left ulna
              K, M, N, P, Q, R 🔒, B, C 🔒, B, C 🔒
  ● S52.279   Monteggia's fracture of unspecified
              ulna K, M, N, P, Q, R 🔒, B, C 🔒,
              B, C 🔒

● S52.28   Bent bone of ulna
  ● S52.281   Bent bone of right ulna
              A, K, M, N, P, Q, R 🔒, B, C 🔒,
              A, B, C 🔒
              (Ex:) For code S52.281[A]: See PDX Collection 1270
                   For S52.281[B,C]: See PDX Collection 1269
                   For S52.281[K,M,N,P,Q,R]: See PDX
                   Collection 897

  ● S52.282   Bent bone of left ulna
              A, K, M, N, P, Q, R 🔒, B, C 🔒,
              A, B, C 🔒
              (Ex:) For code S52.282[A]: See PDX Collection 1271
                   For code S52.282[B,C]: See PDX
                   Collection 1269 For S52.282[K,M,N,P,Q,R]:
                   See PDX Collection 897

  ● S52.283   Bent bone of unspecified ulna
              A, K, M, N, P, Q, R 🔒, B, C 🔒,
              A, B, C 🔒
              (Ex:) For code S52.283[A]: See PDX Collection 1272
                   For code S52.283[B,C]: See PDX
                   Collection 1269 For S52.283[K,M,N,P,Q,R]:
                   See PDX Collection 897

● S52.29   Other fracture of shaft of ulna
  ● S52.291   Other fracture of shaft of right ulna
              A, K, M, N, P, Q, R 🔒, B, C 🔒,
              A, B, C 🔒
              (Ex:) For code S52.291[A]: See PDX Collection 1270
                   For S52.291[B,C]: See PDX Collection 1269
                   For S52.291[K,M,N,P,Q,R]: See PDX
                   Collection 897

  ● S52.292   Other fracture of shaft of left ulna
              A, K, M, N, P, Q, R 🔒, B, C 🔒,
              A, B, C 🔒
              (Ex:) For code S52.292[A]: See PDX Collection 1271
                   For code S52.292[B,C]: See PDX
                   Collection 1269 For S52.292[K,M,N,P,Q,R]:
                   See PDX Collection 897

  ● S52.299   Other fracture of shaft of unspecified
              ulna A, K, M, N, P, Q, R 🔒, B, C 🔒,
              A, B, C 🔒
              (Ex:) For code S52.299[A]: See PDX Collection 1272
                   For code S52.299[B,C]: See PDX
                   Collection 1269 For S52.299[K,M,N,P,Q,R]:
                   See PDX Collection 897

● S52.3   Fracture of shaft of radius
  ● S52.30   Unspecified fracture of shaft of radius
    ● S52.301   Unspecified fracture of shaft of right
                radius A, K, M, N, P, Q, R 🔒, B, C 🔒,
                A, B, C 🔒
                (Ex:) For code S52.301[A]: See PDX Collection 1270
                     For S52.301[B,C]: See PDX Collection 1269
                     For S52.301[K,M,N,P,Q,R]: See PDX
                     Collection 897

    ● S52.302   Unspecified fracture of shaft of left
                radius A, K, M, N, P, Q, R 🔒, B, C 🔒,
                A, B, C 🔒
                (Ex:) For code S52.302[A]: See PDX Collection 1271
                     For code S52.302[B,C]: See PDX
                     Collection 1269 For S52.302[K,M,N,P,Q,R]:
                     See PDX Collection 897

    ● S52.309   Unspecified fracture of shaft of
                unspecified radius
                A, K, M, N, P, Q, R 🔒, B, C 🔒,
                A, B, C 🔒
                (Ex:) For code S52.309[A]: See PDX Collection 1272
                     For code S52.309[B,C]: See PDX
                     Collection 1269 For S52.309[K,M,N,P,Q,R]:
                     See PDX Collection 897

▶ New   ➡ Revised   ~~deleted~~ Deleted   Excludes 1   Excludes 2   Includes   Use additional   Code first   Code also   Key words
OGCR Official Guidelines   ● Unacceptable Principal Diagnosis   X Assign placeholder X   ● Use Additional Character(s)   ▶ Manifestation Code   Coding Clinic

● **S52.31**   Greenstick fracture of shaft of radius

The appropriate 7th character is to be added to all codes in subcategory S52.31

A	initial encounter for closed fracture
D	subsequent encounter for fracture with routine healing
G	subsequent encounter for fracture with delayed healing
K	subsequent encounter for fracture with nonunion
P	subsequent encounter for fracture with malunion
S	sequela

● **S52.311**   **Greenstick fracture of shaft of radius, right arm** A, K, P 🏷, A 🏷
  - (Ex) For code S52.311[A]: See PDX Collection 1270
  - For S52.311[K,P]: See PDX Collection 897

● **S52.312**   **Greenstick fracture of shaft of radius, left arm** A, K, P 🏷, A 🏷
  - (Ex) For code S52.312[A]: See PDX Collection 1271
  - For S52.312[K,P]: See PDX Collection 897

● **S52.319**   **Greenstick fracture of shaft of radius, unspecified arm** A, K, P 🏷, A 🏷
  - (Ex) For code S52.319[A]: See PDX Collection 1272
  - For S52.319[K,P]: See PDX Collection 897

● **S52.32**   Transverse fracture of shaft of radius

● **S52.321**   **Displaced transverse fracture of shaft of right radius** A, K, M, N, P, Q, R 🏷, B, C 🏷, A, B, C 🏷
  - (Ex) For code S52.321[A]: See PDX Collection 1270
  - For S52.321[B,C]: See PDX Collection 1269
  - For S52.321[K,M,N,P,Q,R]: See PDX Collection 897

● **S52.322**   **Displaced transverse fracture of shaft of left radius** A, K, M, N, P, Q, R 🏷, B, C 🏷, A, B, C 🏷
  - (Ex) For code S52.322[A]: See PDX Collection 1271
  - For code S52.322[B,C]: See PDX Collection 1269 For S52.322[K,M,N,P,Q,R]: See PDX Collection 897

● **S52.323**   **Displaced transverse fracture of shaft of unspecified radius** A, K, M, N, P, Q, R 🏷, B, C 🏷, A, B, C 🏷
  - (Ex) For code S52.323[A]: See PDX Collection 1272
  - For S52.323[B,C]: See PDX Collection 1269 For S52.323[K,M,N,P,Q,R]: See PDX Collection 897

● **S52.324**   **Nondisplaced transverse fracture of shaft of right radius** A, K, M, N, P, Q, R 🏷, B, C 🏷, A, B, C 🏷
  - (Ex) For code S52.324[A]: See PDX Collection 1270
  - For S52.324[B,C]: See PDX Collection 1269
  - For S52.324[K,M,N,P,Q,R]: See PDX Collection 897

● **S52.325**   **Nondisplaced transverse fracture of shaft of left radius** A, K, M, N, P, Q, R 🏷, B, C 🏷, A, B, C 🏷
  - (Ex) For code S52.325[A]: See PDX Collection 1271
  - For code S52.325[B,C]: See PDX Collection 1269 For S52.325[K,M,N,P,Q,R]: See PDX Collection 897

● **S52.326**   **Nondisplaced transverse fracture of shaft of unspecified radius** A, K, M, N, P, Q, R 🏷, B, C 🏷, A, B, C 🏷
  - (Ex) For code S52.326[A]: See PDX Collection 1272
  - For code S52.326[B,C]: See PDX Collection 1269 For S52.326[K,M,N,P,Q,R]: See PDX Collection 897

● **S52.33**   Oblique fracture of shaft of radius

● **S52.331**   **Displaced oblique fracture of shaft of right radius** A, K, M, N, P, Q, R 🏷, B, C 🏷, A, B, C 🏷
  - (Ex) For code S52.331[A]: See PDX Collection 1270
  - For S52.331[B,C]: See PDX Collection 1269
  - For S52.331[K,M,N,P,Q,R]: See PDX Collection 897

● **S52.332**   **Displaced oblique fracture of shaft of left radius** A, K, M, N, P, Q, R 🏷, B, C 🏷, A, B, C 🏷
  - (Ex) For code S52.332[A]: See PDX Collection 1271
  - For code S52.332[B,C]: See PDX Collection 1269 For S52.332[K,M,N,P,Q,R]: See PDX Collection 897

● **S52.333**   **Displaced oblique fracture of shaft of unspecified radius** A, K, M, N, P, Q, R 🏷, B, C 🏷, A, B, C 🏷
  - (Ex) For code S52.333[A]: See PDX Collection 1272
  - For S52.333[B,C]: See PDX Collection 1269 For S52.333[K,M,N,P,Q,R]: See PDX Collection 897

● **S52.334**   **Nondisplaced oblique fracture of shaft of right radius** A, K, M, N, P, Q, R 🏷, B, C 🏷, A, B, C 🏷
  - (Ex) For code S52.334[A]: See PDX Collection 1270
  - For S52.334[B,C]: See PDX Collection 1269
  - For S52.334[K,M,N,P,Q,R]: See PDX Collection 897

● **S52.335**   **Nondisplaced oblique fracture of shaft of left radius** A, K, M, N, P, Q, R 🏷, B, C 🏷, A, B, C 🏷
  - (Ex) For code S52.335[A]: See PDX Collection 1271
  - For S52.335[B,C]: See PDX Collection 1269 For S52.335[K,M,N,P,Q,R]: See PDX Collection 897

● **S52.336**   **Nondisplaced oblique fracture of shaft of unspecified radius** A, K, M, N, P, Q, R 🏷, B, C 🏷, A, B, C 🏷
  - (Ex) For code S52.336[A]: See PDX Collection 1272
  - For S52.336[B,C]: See PDX Collection 1269 For S52.336[K,M,N,P,Q,R]: See PDX Collection 897

● **S52.34**   Spiral fracture of shaft of radius

● **S52.341**   **Displaced spiral fracture of shaft of radius, right arm** A, K, M, N, P, Q, R 🏷, B, C 🏷, A, B, C 🏷
  - (Ex) For code S52.341[A]: See PDX Collection 1270
  - For S52.341[B,C]: See PDX Collection 1269
  - For S52.341[K,M,N,P,Q,R]: See PDX Collection 897

● **S52.342**   **Displaced spiral fracture of shaft of radius, left arm** A, K, M, N, P, Q, R 🏷, B, C 🏷, A, B, C 🏷
  - (Ex) For code S52.342[A]: See PDX Collection 1271
  - For code S52.342[B,C]: See PDX Collection 1269 For S52.342[K,M,N,P,Q,R]: See PDX Collection 897

● **S52.343**   **Displaced spiral fracture of shaft of radius, unspecified arm** A, K, M, N, P, Q, R 🏷, B, C 🏷, A, B, C 🏷
  - (Ex) For code S52.343[A]: See PDX Collection 1272
  - For S52.343[B,C]: See PDX Collection 1269 For S52.343[K,M,N,P,Q,R]: See PDX Collection 897

CHAPTER 19 (S00-T88)

● **S52.344** **Nondisplaced spiral fracture of shaft of radius, right arm**
A, K, M, N, P, Q, R 🔖, B, C 🔖,
A, B, C 🔖
(Ex:) For code S52.344[A]: See PDX Collection 1270
For S52.344[B,C]: See PDX Collection 1269
For S52.344[K,M,N,P,Q,R]: See PDX Collection 897

● **S52.345** **Nondisplaced spiral fracture of shaft of radius, left arm**
A, K, M, N, P, Q, R 🔖, B, C 🔖,
A, B, C 🔖
(Ex:) For code S52.345[A]: See PDX Collection 1271
For code S52.345[B,C]: See PDX Collection 1269 For S52.345[K,M,N,P,Q,R]: See PDX Collection 897

● **S52.346** **Nondisplaced spiral fracture of shaft of radius, unspecified arm**
A, K, M, N, P, Q, R 🔖, B, C 🔖,
A, B, C 🔖
(Ex:) For code S52.346[A]: See PDX Collection 1272
For code S52.346[B,C]: See PDX Collection 1269 For S52.346[K,M,N,P,Q,R]: See PDX Collection 897

● **S52.35** **Comminuted fracture of shaft of radius**

● **S52.351** **Displaced comminuted fracture of shaft of radius, right arm**
A, K, M, N, P, Q, R 🔖, B, C 🔖,
A, B, C 🔖
(Ex:) For code S52.351[A]: See PDX Collection 1270
For S52.351[B,C]: See PDX Collection 1269
For S52.351[K,M,N,P,Q,R]: See PDX Collection 897

● **S52.352** **Displaced comminuted fracture of shaft of radius, left arm**
A, K, M, N, P, Q, R 🔖, B, C 🔖,
A, B, C 🔖
(Ex:) For code S52.352[A]: See PDX Collection 1271
For code S52.352[B,C]: See PDX Collection 1269 For S52.352[K,M,N,P,Q,R]: See PDX Collection 897

● **S52.353** **Displaced comminuted fracture of shaft of radius, unspecified arm**
A, K, M, N, P, Q, R 🔖, B, C 🔖,
A, B, C 🔖
(Ex:) For code S52.353[A]: See PDX Collection 1272
For code S52.353[B,C]: See PDX Collection 1269 For S52.353[K,M,N,P,Q,R]: See PDX Collection 897

● **S52.354** **Nondisplaced comminuted fracture of shaft of radius, right arm**
A, K, M, N, P, Q, R 🔖, B, C 🔖,
A, B, C 🔖
(Ex:) For code S52.354[A]: See PDX Collection 1270
For S52.354[B,C]: See PDX Collection 1269
For S52.354[K,M,N,P,Q,R]: See PDX Collection 897

● **S52.355** **Nondisplaced comminuted fracture of shaft of radius, left arm**
A, K, M, N, P, Q, R 🔖, B, C 🔖,
A, B, C 🔖
(Ex:) For code S52.355[A]: See PDX Collection 1271
For code S52.355[B,C]: See PDX Collection 1269 For S52.355[K,M,N,P,Q,R]: See PDX Collection 897

● **S52.356** **Nondisplaced comminuted fracture of shaft of radius, unspecified arm**
A, K, M, N, P, Q, R 🔖, B, C 🔖,
A, B, C 🔖
(Ex:) For code S52.356[A]: See PDX Collection 1272
For code S52.356[B,C]: See PDX Collection 1269 For S52.356[K,M,N,P,Q,R]: See PDX Collection 897

● **S52.36** **Segmental fracture of shaft of radius**

● **S52.361** **Displaced segmental fracture of shaft of radius, right arm**
A, K, M, N, P, Q, R 🔖, B, C 🔖,
A, B, C 🔖
(Ex:) For code S52.361[A]: See PDX Collection 1270
For S52.361[B,C]: See PDX Collection 1269
For S52.361[K,M,N,P,Q,R]: See PDX Collection 897

● **S52.362** **Displaced segmental fracture of shaft of radius, left arm**
A, K, M, N, P, Q, R 🔖, B, C 🔖,
A, B, C 🔖
(Ex:) For code S52.362[A]: See PDX Collection 1271
For code S52.362[B,C]: See PDX Collection 1269 For S52.362[K,M,N,P,Q,R]: See PDX Collection 897

● **S52.363** **Displaced segmental fracture of shaft of radius, unspecified arm**
A, K, M, N, P, Q, R 🔖, B, C 🔖,
A, B, C 🔖
(Ex:) For code S52.363[A]: See PDX Collection 1272
For code S52.363[B,C]: See PDX Collection 1269 For S52.363[K,M,N,P,Q,R]: See PDX Collection 897

● **S52.364** **Nondisplaced segmental fracture of shaft of radius, right arm**
A, K, M, N, P, Q, R 🔖, B, C 🔖,
A, B, C 🔖
(Ex:) For code S52.364[A]: See PDX Collection 1270
For S52.364[B,C]: See PDX Collection 1269
For S52.364[K,M,N,P,Q,R]: See PDX Collection 897

● **S52.365** **Nondisplaced segmental fracture of shaft of radius, left arm**
A, K, M, N, P, Q, R 🔖, B, C 🔖,
A, B, C 🔖
(Ex:) For code S52.365[A]: See PDX Collection 1271
For code S52.365[B,C]: See PDX Collection 1269 For S52.365[K,M,N,P,Q,R]: See PDX Collection 897

● **S52.366** **Nondisplaced segmental fracture of shaft of radius, unspecified arm**
A, K, M, N, P, Q, R 🔖, B, C 🔖,
A, B, C 🔖
(Ex:) For code S52.366[A]: See PDX Collection 1272
For code S52.366[B,C]: See PDX Collection 1269 For S52.366[K,M,N,P,Q,R]: See PDX Collection 897

● **S52.37** **Galeazzi's fracture**
Fracture of lower shaft of radius with radioulnar joint dislocation

● **S52.371** **Galeazzi's fracture of right radius**
A, K, M, N, P, Q, R 🔖, B, C 🔖,
A, B, C 🔖
(Ex:) For code S52.371[A]: See PDX Collection 1270
For S52.371[B,C]: See PDX Collection 1269
For S52.371[K,M,N,P,Q,R]: See PDX Collection 897

● **S52.372** **Galeazzi's fracture of left radius**
A, K, M, N, P, Q, R 🔖, B, C 🔖,
A, B, C 🔖
(Ex:) For code S52.372[A]: See PDX Collection 1271
For code S52.372[B,C]: See PDX Collection 1269 For S52.372[K,M,N,P,Q,R]: See PDX Collection 897

● **S52.379** **Galeazzi's fracture of unspecified radius** A, K, M, N, P, Q, R 🔖, B, C 🔖,
A, B, C 🔖
(Ex:) For code S52.379[A]: See PDX Collection 1272
For code S52.379[B,C]: See PDX Collection 1269 For S52.379[K,M,N,P,Q,R]: See PDX Collection 897

▶ New   ⇒ Revised   ~~deleted~~ Deleted   Excludes 1   Excludes 2   Includes   Use additional   Code first   Code also   Key words
OGCR Official Guidelines   ● Unacceptable Principal Diagnosis   X Assign placeholder X   ● Use Additional Character(s)   ▶ Manifestation Code   Coding Clinic

● S52.38   **Bent bone of radius**
　　● S52.381   **Bent bone of right radius**
　　　　A, K, M, N, P, Q, R 🅒, B, C 🅒,
　　　　A, B, C 🅒
　　　　　Ⓔⓧ **For code S52.381[A]:** See PDX Collection 1270
　　　　　　　 For S52.381[B,C]: See PDX Collection 1269
　　　　　　　 For S52.381[K,M,N,P,Q,R]: See PDX
　　　　　　　 Collection 897

　　● S52.382   **Bent bone of left radius**
　　　　A, K, M, N, P, Q, R 🅒, B, C 🅒,
　　　　A, B, C 🅒
　　　　　Ⓔⓧ **For code S52.382[A]:** See PDX Collection 1271
　　　　　　　 For code S52.382[B,C]: See PDX
　　　　　　　 Collection 1269 **For S52.382[K,M,N,P,Q,R]:**
　　　　　　　 See PDX Collection 897

　　● S52.389   **Bent bone of unspecified radius**
　　　　A, K, M, N, P, Q, R 🅒, B, C 🅒,
　　　　A, B, C 🅒
　　　　　Ⓔⓧ **For code S52.389[A]:** See PDX Collection 1272
　　　　　　　 For code S52.389[B,C]: See PDX
　　　　　　　 Collection 1269 **For S52.389[K,M,N,P,Q,R]:**
　　　　　　　 See PDX Collection 897

● S52.39   **Other fracture of shaft of radius**
　　● S52.391   **Other fracture of shaft of radius, right**
　　　　arm A, K, M, N, P, Q, R 🅒, B, C 🅒,
　　　　A, B, C 🅒
　　　　　Ⓔⓧ **For code S52.391[A]:** See PDX Collection 1270
　　　　　　　 For S52.391[B,C]: See PDX Collection 1269
　　　　　　　 For S52.391[K,M,N,P,Q,R]: See PDX
　　　　　　　 Collection 897

　　● S52.392   **Other fracture of shaft of radius, left**
　　　　arm A, K, M, N, P, Q, R 🅒, B, C 🅒,
　　　　A, B, C 🅒
　　　　　Ⓔⓧ **For code S52.392[A]:** See PDX Collection 1271
　　　　　　　 For code S52.392[B,C]: See PDX
　　　　　　　 Collection 1269 **For S52.392[K,M,N,P,Q,R]:**
　　　　　　　 See PDX Collection 897

　　● S52.399   **Other fracture of shaft of radius,**
　　　　unspecified arm A, K, M, N, P, Q, R 🅒,
　　　　B, C 🅒, A, B, C 🅒
　　　　　Ⓔⓧ **For code S52.399[A]:** See PDX Collection 1272
　　　　　　　 For code S52.399[B,C]: See PDX
　　　　　　　 Collection 1269 **For S52.399[K,M,N,P,Q,R]:**
　　　　　　　 See PDX Collection 897

● S52.5   **Fracture of lower end of radius**
　　　　Fracture of distal end of radius
　　　　Excludes2　physeal fractures of lower end of radius
　　　　　　　　　(S59.2-)

　● S52.50   **Unspecified fracture of the lower end of radius**
　　● S52.501   **Unspecified fracture of the lower end**
　　　　of right radius A, K, M, N, P, Q, R 🅒,
　　　　B, C 🅒, A, B, C 🅒
　　　　　Ⓔⓧ **For code S52.501[A]:** See PDX Collection 1270
　　　　　　　 For S52.501[B,C]: See PDX Collection 1269
　　　　　　　 For S52.501[K,M,N,P,Q,R]: See PDX
　　　　　　　 Collection 897

　　● S52.502   **Unspecified fracture of the lower end**
　　　　of left radius A, K, M, N, P, Q, R 🅒,
　　　　B, C 🅒, A, B, C 🅒
　　　　　Ⓔⓧ **For code S52.502[A]:** See PDX Collection 1271
　　　　　　　 For code S52.502[B,C]: See PDX
　　　　　　　 Collection 1269 **For S52.502[K,M,N,P,Q,R]:**
　　　　　　　 See PDX Collection 897

　　● S52.509   **Unspecified fracture of the lower end**
　　　　of unspecified radius
　　　　A, K, M, N, P, Q, R 🅒, B, C 🅒,
　　　　A, B, C 🅒
　　　　　Ⓔⓧ **For code S52.509[A]:** See PDX Collection 1272
　　　　　　　 For code S52.509[B,C]: See PDX
　　　　　　　 Collection 1269 **For S52.509[K,M,N,P,Q,R]:**
　　　　　　　 See PDX Collection 897

● S52.51   **Fracture of radial styloid process**
　　● S52.511   **Displaced fracture of right radial**
　　　　styloid process A, K, M, N, P, Q, R 🅒,
　　　　B, C 🅒, A, B, C 🅒
　　　　　Ⓔⓧ **For code S52.511[A]:** See PDX Collection 1270
　　　　　　　 For S52.511[B,C]: See PDX Collection 1269
　　　　　　　 For S52.511[K,M,N,P,Q,R]: See PDX
　　　　　　　 Collection 897

　　● S52.512   **Displaced fracture of left radial**
　　　　styloid process A, K, M, N, P, Q, R 🅒,
　　　　B, C 🅒, A, B, C 🅒
　　　　　Ⓔⓧ **For code S52.512[A]:** See PDX Collection 1271
　　　　　　　 For S52.512[B,C]: See PDX
　　　　　　　 Collection 1269 **For S52.512[K,M,N,P,Q,R]:**
　　　　　　　 See PDX Collection 897

　　● S52.513   **Displaced fracture of unspecified**
　　　　radial styloid process
　　　　A, K, M, N, P, Q, R 🅒, B, C 🅒,
　　　　A, B, C 🅒
　　　　　Ⓔⓧ **For code S52.513[A]:** See PDX Collection 1272
　　　　　　　 For S52.513[B,C]: See PDX
　　　　　　　 Collection 1269 **For S52.513[K,M,N,P,Q,R]:**
　　　　　　　 See PDX Collection 897

　　● S52.514   **Nondisplaced fracture of right radial**
　　　　styloid process A, K, M, N, P, Q, R 🅒,
　　　　B, C 🅒, A, B, C 🅒
　　　　　Ⓔⓧ **For code S52.514[A]:** See PDX Collection 1270
　　　　　　　 For S52.514[B,C]: See PDX Collection 1269
　　　　　　　 For S52.514[K,M,N,P,Q,R]: See PDX
　　　　　　　 Collection 897

　　● S52.515   **Nondisplaced fracture of left radial**
　　　　styloid process A, K, M, N, P, Q, R 🅒,
　　　　B, C 🅒, A, B, C 🅒
　　　　　Ⓔⓧ **For code S52.515[A]:** See PDX Collection 1271
　　　　　　　 For code S52.515[B,C]: See PDX
　　　　　　　 Collection 1269 **For S52.515[K,M,N,P,Q,R]:**
　　　　　　　 See PDX Collection 897

　　● S52.516   **Nondisplaced fracture of unspecified**
　　　　radial styloid process
　　　　A, K, M, N, P, Q, R 🅒, B, C 🅒,
　　　　A, B, C 🅒
　　　　　Ⓔⓧ **For code S52.516[A]:** See PDX Collection 1272
　　　　　　　 For code S52.516[B,C]: See PDX
　　　　　　　 Collection 1269 **For S52.516[K,M,N,P,Q,R]:**
　　　　　　　 See PDX Collection 897

● S52.52   **Torus fracture of lower end of radius**
　　　　The appropriate 7th character is to be added to
　　　　all codes in subcategory S52.52

A	initial encounter for closed fracture
D	subsequent encounter for fracture with routine healing
G	subsequent encounter for fracture with delayed healing
K	subsequent encounter for fracture with nonunion
P	subsequent encounter for fracture with malunion
S	sequela

　　● S52.521   **Torus fracture of lower end of right**
　　　　radius A, K, P 🅒, A 🅒
　　　　　Ⓔⓧ **For code S52.521[A]:** See PDX Collection 1270
　　　　　　　 For S52.521[K,P]: See PDX Collection 897

　　● S52.522   **Torus fracture of lower end of left**
　　　　radius A, K, P 🅒, A 🅒
　　　　　Ⓔⓧ **For code S52.522[A]:** See PDX Collection 1271
　　　　　　　 For S52.522[K,P]: See PDX Collection 897

　　● S52.529   **Torus fracture of lower end of**
　　　　unspecified radius A, K, P 🅒, A 🅒
　　　　　Ⓔⓧ **For code S52.529[A]:** See PDX Collection 1272
　　　　　　　 For S52.529[K,P]: See PDX Collection 897

CHAPTER 19 (S00-T88)

N Newborn Age: 0   **P** Pediatric Age: 0–17   **M** Maternity DX: 12–55   **A** Adult Age: 15–124   ♀ Females Only   ♂ Males Only

🅒 Complication\Comorbidity   🅜 Major C\C   Ⓔⓧ CC/MCC Exclusions   🅗 Hospital-Acquired Condition

1303

● S52.53   Colles' fracture
    ● S52.531   Colles' fracture of right radius
                 A, K, M, N, P, Q, R 🔟, B, C 🔟,
                 A, B, C 🔟
                 Ⓔ For code S52.531[A]: See PDX Collection 1270
                       For S52.531[B,C]: See PDX Collection 1269
                       For S52.531[K,M,N,P,Q,R]: See PDX
                       Collection 897

    ● S52.532   Colles' fracture of left radius
                 A, K, M, N, P, Q, R 🔟, B, C 🔟,
                 A, B, C 🔟
                 Ⓔ For code S52.532[A]: See PDX Collection 1271
                       For code S52.532[B,C]: See PDX
                       Collection 1269 For S52.532[K,M,N,P,Q,R]:
                       See PDX Collection 897
                 Coding Clinic: 2016, Q2, P5

    ● S52.539   Colles' fracture of unspecified radius
                 A, K, M, N, P, Q, R 🔟, B, C 🔟,
                 A, B, C 🔟
                 Ⓔ For code S52.539[A]: See PDX Collection 1272
                       For code S52.539[B,C]: See PDX
                       Collection 1269 For S52.539[K,M,N,P,Q,R]:
                       See PDX Collection 897

● S52.54   Smith's fracture
    ● S52.541   Smith's fracture of right radius
                 A, K, M, N, P, Q, R 🔟, B, C 🔟,
                 A, B, C 🔟
                 Ⓔ For code S52.541[A]: See PDX Collection 1270
                       For S52.541[B,C]: See PDX Collection 1269
                       For S52.541[K,M,N,P,Q,R]: See PDX
                       Collection 897

    ● S52.542   Smith's fracture of left radius
                 A, K, M, N, P, Q, R 🔟, B, C 🔟,
                 A, B, C 🔟
                 Ⓔ For code S52.542[A]: See PDX Collection 1271
                       For code S52.542[B,C]: See PDX
                       Collection 1269 For S52.542[K,M,N,P,Q,R]:
                       See PDX Collection 897

    ● S52.549   Smith's fracture of unspecified radius
                 A, K, M, N, P, Q, R 🔟, B, C 🔟,
                 A, B, C 🔟
                 Ⓔ For code S52.549[A]: See PDX Collection 1272
                       For code S52.549[B,C]: See PDX
                       Collection 1269 For S52.549[K,M,N,P,Q,R]:
                       See PDX Collection 897

● S52.55   Other extraarticular fracture of lower end of
            radius
    ● S52.551   Other extraarticular fracture of lower
                 end of right radius
                 A, K, M, N, P, Q, R 🔟, B, C 🔟,
                 A, B, C 🔟
                 Ⓔ For code S52.551[A]: See PDX Collection 1270
                       For S52.551[B,C]: See PDX Collection 1269
                       For S52.551[K,M,N,P,Q,R]: See PDX
                       Collection 897

    ● S52.552   Other extraarticular fracture of lower
                 end of left radius
                 A, K, M, N, P, Q, R 🔟, B, C 🔟,
                 A, B, C 🔟
                 Ⓔ For code S52.552[A]: See PDX Collection 1271
                       For code S52.552[B,C]: See PDX
                       Collection 1269 For S52.552[K,M,N,P,Q,R]:
                       See PDX Collection 897

    ● S52.559   Other extraarticular fracture of lower
                 end of unspecified radius
                 A, K, M, N, P, Q, R 🔟, B, C 🔟,
                 A, B, C 🔟
                 Ⓔ For code S52.559[A]: See PDX Collection 1272
                       For code S52.559[B,C]: See PDX
                       Collection 1269 For S52.559[K,M,N,P,Q,R]:
                       See PDX Collection 897

● S52.56   Barton's fracture
    ● S52.561   Barton's fracture of right radius
                 A, K, M, N, P, Q, R 🔟, B, C 🔟,
                 A, B, C 🔟
                 Ⓔ For code S52.561[A]: See PDX Collection 1270
                       For S52.561[B,C]: See PDX Collection 1269
                       For S52.561[K,M,N,P,Q,R]: See PDX
                       Collection 897

    ● S52.562   Barton's fracture of left radius
                 A, K, M, N, P, Q, R 🔟, B, C 🔟,
                 A, B, C 🔟
                 Ⓔ For code S52.562[A]: See PDX Collection 1271
                       For code S52.562[B,C]: See PDX
                       Collection 1269 For S52.562[K,M,N,P,Q,R]:
                       See PDX Collection 897

    ● S52.569   Barton's fracture of unspecified radius
                 A, K, M, N, P, Q, R 🔟, B, C 🔟,
                 A, B, C 🔟
                 Ⓔ For code S52.569[A]: See PDX Collection 1272
                       For code S52.569[B,C]: See PDX
                       Collection 1269 For S52.569[K,M,N,P,Q,R]:
                       See PDX Collection 897

● S52.57   Other intraarticular fracture of lower end of
            radius
    ● S52.571   Other intraarticular fracture of lower
                 end of right radius
                 A, K, M, N, P, Q, R 🔟, B, C 🔟,
                 A, B, C 🔟
                 Ⓔ For code S52.571[A]: See PDX Collection 1270
                       For S52.571[B,C]: See PDX Collection 1269
                       For S52.571[K,M,N,P,Q,R]: See PDX
                       Collection 897

    ● S52.572   Other intraarticular fracture of lower
                 end of left radius
                 A, K, M, N, P, Q, R 🔟, B, C 🔟,
                 A, B, C 🔟
                 Ⓔ For code S52.572[A]: See PDX Collection 1271
                       For code S52.572[B,C]: See PDX
                       Collection 1269 For S52.572[K,M,N,P,Q,R]:
                       See PDX Collection 897

    ● S52.579   Other intraarticular fracture of lower
                 end of unspecified radius
                 A, K, M, N, P, Q, R 🔟, B, C 🔟,
                 A, B, C 🔟
                 Ⓔ For code S52.579[A]: See PDX Collection 1272
                       For code S52.579[B,C]: See PDX
                       Collection 1269 For S52.579[K,M,N,P,Q,R]:
                       See PDX Collection 897

● S52.59   Other fractures of lower end of radius
    ● S52.591   Other fractures of lower end of right
                 radius A, K, M, N, P, Q, R 🔟, B, C 🔟,
                 A, B, C 🔟
                 Ⓔ For code S52.591[A]: See PDX Collection 1270
                       For S52.591[B,C]: See PDX Collection 1269
                       For S52.591[K,M,N,P,Q,R]: See PDX
                       Collection 897

    ● S52.592   Other fractures of lower end of left
                 radius A, K, M, N, P, Q, R 🔟, B, C 🔟,
                 A, B, C 🔟
                 Ⓔ For code S52.592[A]: See PDX Collection 1271
                       For code S52.592[B,C]: See PDX
                       Collection 1269 For S52.592[K,M,N,P,Q,R]:
                       See PDX Collection 897

    ● S52.599   Other fractures of lower end of
                 unspecified radius
                 A, K, M, N, P, Q, R 🔟, B, C 🔟,
                 A, B, C 🔟
                 Ⓔ For code S52.599[A]: See PDX Collection 1272
                       For code S52.599[B,C]: See PDX
                       Collection 1269 For S52.599[K,M,N,P,Q,R]:
                       See PDX Collection 897

▶ New   ⇒ Revised   ~~deleted~~ Deleted   Excludes 1   Excludes 2   Includes   Use additional   Code first   Code also   Key words
OGCR Official Guidelines   ● Unacceptable Principal Diagnosis   X Assign placeholder X   ● Use Additional Character(s)   ▶ Manifestation Code   Coding Clinic

● S52.6   Fracture of lower end of ulna
  ● S52.60   Unspecified fracture of lower end of ulna
    ● S52.601   Unspecified fracture of lower end of right ulna A, K, M, N, P, Q, R 🦠, B, C 🦠, A, B, C 🦠
       (Ex) For code S52.601[A]: See PDX Collection 1270
            For S52.601[B,C]: See PDX Collection 1269
            For S52.601[K,M,N,P,Q,R]: See PDX Collection 897
    ● S52.602   Unspecified fracture of lower end of left ulna A, K, M, N, P, Q, R 🦠, B, C 🦠, A, B, C 🦠
       (Ex) For code S52.602[A]: See PDX Collection 1271
            For code S52.602[B,C]: See PDX Collection 1269 For S52.602[K,M,N,P,Q,R]: See PDX Collection 897
    ● S52.609   Unspecified fracture of lower end of unspecified ulna A, K, M, N, P, Q, R 🦠, B, C 🦠, A, B, C 🦠
       (Ex) For code S52.609[A]: See PDX Collection 1272
            For code S52.609[B,C]: See PDX Collection 1269 For S52.609[K,M,N,P,Q,R]: See PDX Collection 897

  ● S52.61   Fracture of ulna styloid process
    ● S52.611   Displaced fracture of right ulna styloid process A, K, M, N, P, Q, R 🦠, B, C 🦠, A, B, C 🦠
       (Ex) For code S52.611[A]: See PDX Collection 1270
            For S52.611[B,C]: See PDX Collection 1269
            For S52.611[K,M,N,P,Q,R]: See PDX Collection 897
    ● S52.612   Displaced fracture of left ulna styloid process A, K, M, N, P, Q, R 🦠, B, C 🦠, A, B, C 🦠
       (Ex) For code S52.612[A]: See PDX Collection 1271
            For code S52.612[B,C]: See PDX Collection 1269 For S52.612[K,M,N,P,Q,R]: See PDX Collection 897
    ● S52.613   Displaced fracture of unspecified ulna styloid process A, K, M, N, P, Q, R 🦠, B, C 🦠, A, B, C 🦠
       (Ex) For code S52.613[A]: See PDX Collection 1272
            For code S52.613[B,C]: See PDX Collection 1269 For S52.613[K,M,N,P,Q,R]: See PDX Collection 897
    ● S52.614   Nondisplaced fracture of right ulna styloid process A, K, M, N, P, Q, R 🦠, B, C 🦠, A, B, C 🦠
       (Ex) For code S52.614[A]: See PDX Collection 1270
            For S52.614[B,C]: See PDX Collection 1269
            For S52.614[K,M,N,P,Q,R]: See PDX Collection 897
    ● S52.615   Nondisplaced fracture of left ulna styloid process A, K, M, N, P, Q, R 🦠, B, C 🦠, A, B, C 🦠
       (Ex) For code S52.615[A]: See PDX Collection 1271
            For code S52.615[B,C]: See PDX Collection 1269 For S52.615[K,M,N,P,Q,R]: See PDX Collection 897
    ● S52.616   Nondisplaced fracture of unspecified ulna styloid process A, K, M, N, P, Q, R 🦠, B, C 🦠, A, B, C 🦠
       (Ex) For code S52.616[A]: See PDX Collection 1272
            For code S52.616[B,C]: See PDX Collection 1269 For S52.616[K,M,N,P,Q,R]: See PDX Collection 897

● S52.62   Torus fracture of lower end of ulna
   The appropriate 7th character is to be added to all codes in subcategory S52.62

A	initial encounter for closed fracture
D	subsequent encounter for fracture with routine healing
G	subsequent encounter for fracture with delayed healing
K	subsequent encounter for fracture with nonunion
P	subsequent encounter for fracture with malunion
S	sequela

    ● S52.621   Torus fracture of lower end of right ulna A, K, P 🦠, A 🦠
       (Ex) For code S52.621[A]: See PDX Collection 1270
            For S52.621[K,P]: See PDX Collection 897
    ● S52.622   Torus fracture of lower end of left ulna A, K, P 🦠, A 🦠
       (Ex) For code S52.622[A]: See PDX Collection 1271
            For S52.622[K,P]: See PDX Collection 897
    ● S52.629   Torus fracture of lower end of unspecified ulna A, K, P 🦠, A 🦠
       (Ex) For code S52.629[A]: See PDX Collection 1272
            For S52.629[K,P]: See PDX Collection 897

  ● S52.69   Other fracture of lower end of ulna
    ● S52.691   Other fracture of lower end of right ulna A, K, M, N, P, Q, R 🦠, B, C 🦠, A, B, C 🦠
       (Ex) For code S52.691[A]: See PDX Collection 1270
            For S52.691[B,C]: See PDX Collection 1269
            For S52.691[K,M,N,P,Q,R]: See PDX Collection 897
    ● S52.692   Other fracture of lower end of left ulna A, K, M, N, P, Q, R 🦠, B, C 🦠, A, B, C 🦠
       (Ex) For code S52.692[A]: See PDX Collection 1271
            For code S52.692[B,C]: See PDX Collection 1269 For S52.692[K,M,N,P,Q,R]: See PDX Collection 897
    ● S52.699   Other fracture of lower end of unspecified ulna A, K, M, N, P, Q, R 🦠, B, C 🦠, A, B, C 🦠
       (Ex) For code S52.699[A]: See PDX Collection 1272
            For code S52.699[B,C]: See PDX Collection 1269 For S52.699[K,M,N,P,Q,R]: See PDX Collection 897

● S52.9   Unspecified fracture of forearm
   (Ex) For category S52.9 CC codes S52.9[A]: See PDX Collection 1272
        For code S52.9[B,C]: See PDX Collection 1269 For S52.9[K,M,N,P,Q,R]: See PDX Collection 897
  X ● S52.90   Unspecified fracture of unspecified forearm A, K, M, N, P, Q, R 🦠, B, C 🦠, A, B, C 🦠
  X ● S52.91   Unspecified fracture of right forearm A, K, M, N, P, Q, R 🦠, B, C 🦠, A, B, C 🦠
  X ● S52.92   Unspecified fracture of left forearm A, K, M, N, P, Q, R 🦠, B, C 🦠, A, B, C 🦠

CHAPTER 19 (S00-T88)

● **S53**   **Dislocation and sprain of joints and ligaments of elbow**

Includes   avulsion of joint or ligament of elbow
laceration of cartilage, joint or ligament of elbow
sprain of cartilage, joint or ligament of elbow
traumatic hemarthrosis of joint or ligament of elbow
traumatic rupture of joint or ligament of elbow
traumatic subluxation of joint or ligament of elbow
traumatic tear of joint or ligament of elbow

Code also any associated open wound

Excludes2   strain of muscle, fascia and tendon at forearm level (S56.-)

The appropriate 7th character is to be added to each code from category S53

> A   initial encounter
> D   subsequent encounter
> S   sequela

● **S53.0**   **Subluxation and dislocation of radial head**
Dislocation of radiohumeral joint
Subluxation of radiohumeral joint

Excludes1   Monteggia's fracture-dislocation (S52.27-)

● **S53.00**   **Unspecified subluxation and dislocation of radial head**

● **S53.001**   Unspecified subluxation of right radial head

● **S53.002**   Unspecified subluxation of left radial head

● **S53.003**   Unspecified subluxation of unspecified radial head

● **S53.004**   Unspecified dislocation of right radial head

● **S53.005**   Unspecified dislocation of left radial head

● **S53.006**   Unspecified dislocation of unspecified radial head

● **S53.01**   **Anterior subluxation and dislocation of radial head**
Anteriomedial subluxation and dislocation of radial head

● **S53.011**   Anterior subluxation of right radial head

● **S53.012**   Anterior subluxation of left radial head

● **S53.013**   Anterior subluxation of unspecified radial head

● **S53.014**   Anterior dislocation of right radial head

● **S53.015**   Anterior dislocation of left radial head

● **S53.016**   Anterior dislocation of unspecified radial head

● **S53.02**   **Posterior subluxation and dislocation of radial head**
Posteriolateral subluxation and dislocation of radial head

● **S53.021**   Posterior subluxation of right radial head

● **S53.022**   Posterior subluxation of left radial head

● **S53.023**   Posterior subluxation of unspecified radial head

● **S53.024**   Posterior dislocation of right radial head

● **S53.025**   Posterior dislocation of left radial head

● **S53.026**   Posterior dislocation of unspecified radial head

● **S53.03**   **Nursemaid's elbow**

● **S53.031**   Nursemaid's elbow, right elbow
Coding Clinic: 2015, Q1, P7-8

● **S53.032**   Nursemaid's elbow, left elbow

● **S53.033**   Nursemaid's elbow, unspecified elbow

● **S53.09**   **Other subluxation and dislocation of radial head**

● **S53.091**   Other subluxation of right radial head

● **S53.092**   Other subluxation of left radial head

● **S53.093**   Other subluxation of unspecified radial head

● **S53.094**   Other dislocation of right radial head

● **S53.095**   Other dislocation of left radial head

● **S53.096**   Other dislocation of unspecified radial head

● **S53.1**   **Subluxation and dislocation of ulnohumeral joint**
Subluxation and dislocation of elbow NOS

Excludes1   dislocation of radial head alone (S53.0-)

● **S53.10**   **Unspecified subluxation and dislocation of ulnohumeral joint**

● **S53.101**   Unspecified subluxation of right ulnohumeral joint

● **S53.102**   Unspecified subluxation of left ulnohumeral joint

● **S53.103**   Unspecified subluxation of unspecified ulnohumeral joint

● **S53.104**   Unspecified dislocation of right ulnohumeral joint

● **S53.105**   Unspecified dislocation of left ulnohumeral joint

● **S53.106**   Unspecified dislocation of unspecified ulnohumeral joint

● **S53.11**   **Anterior subluxation and dislocation of ulnohumeral joint**

● **S53.111**   Anterior subluxation of right ulnohumeral joint

● **S53.112**   Anterior subluxation of left ulnohumeral joint

● **S53.113**   Anterior subluxation of unspecified ulnohumeral joint

● **S53.114**   Anterior dislocation of right ulnohumeral joint
Coding Clinic: 2012, Q4, P108

● **S53.115**   Anterior dislocation of left ulnohumeral joint

● **S53.116**   Anterior dislocation of unspecified ulnohumeral joint

● **S53.12**   **Posterior subluxation and dislocation of ulnohumeral joint**

● **S53.121**   Posterior subluxation of right ulnohumeral joint

● **S53.122**   Posterior subluxation of left ulnohumeral joint

● **S53.123**   Posterior subluxation of unspecified ulnohumeral joint

● **S53.124**   Posterior dislocation of right ulnohumeral joint

● **S53.125**   Posterior dislocation of left ulnohumeral joint

● **S53.126**   Posterior dislocation of unspecified ulnohumeral joint

● S53.13   **Medial subluxation and dislocation of ulnohumeral joint**
- ● S53.131   Medial subluxation of right ulnohumeral joint
- ● S53.132   Medial subluxation of left ulnohumeral joint
- ● S53.133   Medial subluxation of unspecified ulnohumeral joint
- ● S53.134   Medial dislocation of right ulnohumeral joint
- ● S53.135   Medial dislocation of left ulnohumeral joint
- ● S53.136   Medial dislocation of unspecified ulnohumeral joint

● S53.14   **Lateral subluxation and dislocation of ulnohumeral joint**
- ● S53.141   Lateral subluxation of right ulnohumeral joint
- ● S53.142   Lateral subluxation of left ulnohumeral joint
- ● S53.143   Lateral subluxation of unspecified ulnohumeral joint
- ● S53.144   Lateral dislocation of right ulnohumeral joint
- ● S53.145   Lateral dislocation of left ulnohumeral joint
- ● S53.146   Lateral dislocation of unspecified ulnohumeral joint

● S53.19   **Other subluxation and dislocation of ulnohumeral joint**
- ● S53.191   Other subluxation of right ulnohumeral joint
- ● S53.192   Other subluxation of left ulnohumeral joint
- ● S53.193   Other subluxation of unspecified ulnohumeral joint
- ● S53.194   Other dislocation of right ulnohumeral joint
- ● S53.195   Other dislocation of left ulnohumeral joint
- ● S53.196   Other dislocation of unspecified ulnohumeral joint

● S53.2   **Traumatic rupture of radial collateral ligament**

    Excludes1   sprain of radial collateral ligament NOS (S53.43-)

- X ● S53.20   Traumatic rupture of unspecified radial collateral ligament
- X ● S53.21   Traumatic rupture of right radial collateral ligament
- X ● S53.22   Traumatic rupture of left radial collateral ligament

● S53.3   **Traumatic rupture of ulnar collateral ligament**

    Excludes1   sprain of ulnar collateral ligament (S53.44-)

- X ● S53.30   Traumatic rupture of unspecified ulnar collateral ligament
- X ● S53.31   Traumatic rupture of right ulnar collateral ligament
- X ● S53.32   Traumatic rupture of left ulnar collateral ligament

● S53.4   **Sprain of elbow**

    Excludes2   traumatic rupture of radial collateral ligament (S53.2-)
              traumatic rupture of ulnar collateral ligament (S53.3-)

● S53.40   **Unspecified sprain of elbow**
- ● S53.401   Unspecified sprain of right elbow
- ● S53.402   Unspecified sprain of left elbow
- ● S53.409   Unspecified sprain of unspecified elbow
  - Sprain of elbow NOS

● S53.41   **Radiohumeral (joint) sprain**
- ● S53.411   Radiohumeral (joint) sprain of right elbow
- ● S53.412   Radiohumeral (joint) sprain of left elbow
- ● S53.419   Radiohumeral (joint) sprain of unspecified elbow

● S53.42   **Ulnohumeral (joint) sprain**
- ● S53.421   Ulnohumeral (joint) sprain of right elbow
- ● S53.422   Ulnohumeral (joint) sprain of left elbow
- ● S53.429   Ulnohumeral (joint) sprain of unspecified elbow

● S53.43   **Radial collateral ligament sprain**
- ● S53.431   Radial collateral ligament sprain of right elbow
- ● S53.432   Radial collateral ligament sprain of left elbow
- ● S53.439   Radial collateral ligament sprain of unspecified elbow

● S53.44   **Ulnar collateral ligament sprain**
- ● S53.441   Ulnar collateral ligament sprain of right elbow
- ● S53.442   Ulnar collateral ligament sprain of left elbow
- ● S53.449   Ulnar collateral ligament sprain of unspecified elbow

● S53.49   **Other sprain of elbow**
- ● S53.491   Other sprain of right elbow
- ● S53.492   Other sprain of left elbow
- ● S53.499   Other sprain of unspecified elbow

● S54   **Injury of nerves at forearm level**

    Code also any associated open wound (S51.-)

    Excludes2   injury of nerves at wrist and hand level (S64.-)

    The appropriate 7th character is to be added to each code from category S54

A	initial encounter
D	subsequent encounter
S	sequela

● S54.0   **Injury of ulnar nerve at forearm level**
    Injury of ulnar nerve NOS
- X ● S54.00   Injury of ulnar nerve at forearm level, unspecified arm
- X ● S54.01   Injury of ulnar nerve at forearm level, right arm
- X ● S54.02   Injury of ulnar nerve at forearm level, left arm

● S54.1   **Injury of median nerve at forearm level**
    Injury of median nerve NOS
- X ● S54.10   Injury of median nerve at forearm level, unspecified arm
- X ● S54.11   Injury of median nerve at forearm level, right arm
- X ● S54.12   Injury of median nerve at forearm level, left arm

● **S54.2 Injury of radial nerve at forearm level**
    Injury of radial nerve NOS

X● **S54.20 Injury of radial nerve at forearm level, unspecified arm**

X● **S54.21 Injury of radial nerve at forearm level, right arm**

X● **S54.22 Injury of radial nerve at forearm level, left arm**

● **S54.3 Injury of cutaneous sensory nerve at forearm level**

X● **S54.30 Injury of cutaneous sensory nerve at forearm level, unspecified arm**

X● **S54.31 Injury of cutaneous sensory nerve at forearm level, right arm**

X● **S54.32 Injury of cutaneous sensory nerve at forearm level, left arm**

● **S54.8 Injury of other nerves at forearm level**

● **S54.8X Injury of other nerves at forearm level**

● **S54.8X1 Injury of other nerves at forearm level, right arm**

● **S54.8X2 Injury of other nerves at forearm level, left arm**

● **S54.8X9 Injury of other nerves at forearm level, unspecified arm**

● **S54.9 Injury of unspecified nerve at forearm level**

X● **S54.90 Injury of unspecified nerve at forearm level, unspecified arm**

X● **S54.91 Injury of unspecified nerve at forearm level, right arm**

X● **S54.92 Injury of unspecified nerve at forearm level, left arm**

● **S55 Injury of blood vessels at forearm level**
    Code also any associated open wound (S51.-)
    Excludes2 injury of blood vessels at wrist and hand level (S65.-)
              injury of brachial vessels (S45.1-S45.2)
    The appropriate 7th character is to be added to each code from category S55

> | A | initial encounter |
> | D | subsequent encounter |
> | S | sequela |

● **S55.0 Injury of ulnar artery at forearm level**

● **S55.00 Unspecified injury of ulnar artery at forearm level**

● **S55.001 Unspecified injury of ulnar artery at forearm level, right arm** A ℗
    (Ex) See PDX Collection 1274

● **S55.002 Unspecified injury of ulnar artery at forearm level, left arm** A ℗
    (Ex) See PDX Collection 1275

● **S55.009 Unspecified injury of ulnar artery at forearm level, unspecified arm** A ℗
    (Ex) See PDX Collection 1276

● **S55.01 Laceration of ulnar artery at forearm level**

● **S55.011 Laceration of ulnar artery at forearm level, right arm** A ℗
    (Ex) See PDX Collection 1274

● **S55.012 Laceration of ulnar artery at forearm level, left arm** A ℗
    (Ex) See PDX Collection 1275

● **S55.019 Laceration of ulnar artery at forearm level, unspecified arm** A ℗
    (Ex) See PDX Collection 1276

● **S55.09 Other specified injury of ulnar artery at forearm level**

● **S55.091 Other specified injury of ulnar artery at forearm level, right arm** A ℗
    (Ex) See PDX Collection 1274

● **S55.092 Other specified injury of ulnar artery at forearm level, left arm** A ℗
    (Ex) See PDX Collection 1275

● **S55.099 Other specified injury of ulnar artery at forearm level, unspecified arm** A ℗
    (Ex) See PDX Collection 1276

● **S55.1 Injury of radial artery at forearm level**

● **S55.10 Unspecified injury of radial artery at forearm level**

● **S55.101 Unspecified injury of radial artery at forearm level, right arm** A ℗
    (Ex) See PDX Collection 1277

● **S55.102 Unspecified injury of radial artery at forearm level, left arm** A ℗
    (Ex) See PDX Collection 1278

● **S55.109 Unspecified injury of radial artery at forearm level, unspecified arm** A ℗
    (Ex) See PDX Collection 1279

● **S55.11 Laceration of radial artery at forearm level**

● **S55.111 Laceration of radial artery at forearm level, right arm** A ℗
    (Ex) See PDX Collection 1277

● **S55.112 Laceration of radial artery at forearm level, left arm** A ℗
    (Ex) See PDX Collection 1278

● **S55.119 Laceration of radial artery at forearm level, unspecified arm** A ℗
    (Ex) See PDX Collection 1279

● **S55.19 Other specified injury of radial artery at forearm level**

● **S55.191 Other specified injury of radial artery at forearm level, right arm** A ℗
    (Ex) See PDX Collection 1277

● **S55.192 Other specified injury of radial artery at forearm level, left arm** A ℗
    (Ex) See PDX Collection 1278

● **S55.199 Other specified injury of radial artery at forearm level, unspecified arm** A ℗
    (Ex) See PDX Collection 1279

● **S55.2 Injury of vein at forearm level**

● **S55.20 Unspecified injury of vein at forearm level**

● **S55.201 Unspecified injury of vein at forearm level, right arm** A ℗
    (Ex) See PDX Collection 1260

● **S55.202 Unspecified injury of vein at forearm level, left arm** A ℗
    (Ex) See PDX Collection 1261

● **S55.209 Unspecified injury of vein at forearm level, unspecified arm** A ℗
    (Ex) See PDX Collection 1262

● **S55.21 Laceration of vein at forearm level**

● **S55.211 Laceration of vein at forearm level, right arm** A ℗
    (Ex) See PDX Collection 1260

● **S55.212 Laceration of vein at forearm level, left arm** A ℗
    (Ex) See PDX Collection 1261

● **S55.219 Laceration of vein at forearm level, unspecified arm** A ℗
    (Ex) See PDX Collection 1262

▶ New   ⇒ Revised   ~~deleted~~ Deleted   Excludes 1   Excludes 2   Includes   Use additional   Code first   Code also   Key words
OGCR Official Guidelines   ● Unacceptable Principal Diagnosis   X Assign placeholder X   ● Use Additional Character(s)   ▶ Manifestation Code   **Coding Clinic**

● **S55.29**   Other specified injury of vein at forearm level
- ● **S55.291**   Other specified injury of vein at forearm level, right arm A 🔗
  - (Ex:) See PDX Collection 1260
- ● **S55.292**   Other specified injury of vein at forearm level, left arm A 🔗
  - (Ex:) See PDX Collection 1261
- ● **S55.299**   Other specified injury of vein at forearm level, unspecified arm A 🔗
  - (Ex:) See PDX Collection 1262

● **S55.8**   Injury of other blood vessels at forearm level
- ● **S55.80**   Unspecified injury of other blood vessels at forearm level
  - ● **S55.801**   Unspecified injury of other blood vessels at forearm level, right arm A 🔗
    - (Ex:) See PDX Collection 1260
  - ● **S55.802**   Unspecified injury of other blood vessels at forearm level, left arm A 🔗
    - (Ex:) See PDX Collection 1261
  - ● **S55.809**   Unspecified injury of other blood vessels at forearm level, unspecified arm A 🔗
    - (Ex:) See PDX Collection 1262
- ● **S55.81**   Laceration of other blood vessels at forearm level
  - ● **S55.811**   Laceration of other blood vessels at forearm level, right arm A 🔗
    - (Ex:) See PDX Collection 1260
  - ● **S55.812**   Laceration of other blood vessels at forearm level, left arm A 🔗
    - (Ex:) See PDX Collection 1261
  - ● **S55.819**   Laceration of other blood vessels at forearm level, unspecified arm A 🔗
    - (Ex:) See PDX Collection 1262
- ● **S55.89**   Other specified injury of other blood vessels at forearm level
  - ● **S55.891**   Other specified injury of other blood vessels at forearm level, right arm A 🔗
    - (Ex:) See PDX Collection 1260
  - ● **S55.892**   Other specified injury of other blood vessels at forearm level, left arm A 🔗
    - (Ex:) See PDX Collection 1261
  - ● **S55.899**   Other specified injury of other blood vessels at forearm level, unspecified arm A 🔗
    - (Ex:) See PDX Collection 1262

● **S55.9**   Injury of unspecified blood vessel at forearm level
- ● **S55.90**   Unspecified injury of unspecified blood vessel at forearm level
  - ● **S55.901**   Unspecified injury of unspecified blood vessel at forearm level, right arm A 🔗
    - (Ex:) See PDX Collection 1260
  - ● **S55.902**   Unspecified injury of unspecified blood vessel at forearm level, left arm A 🔗
    - (Ex:) See PDX Collection 1261
  - ● **S55.909**   Unspecified injury of unspecified blood vessel at forearm level, unspecified arm A 🔗
    - (Ex:) See PDX Collection 1262

● **S55.91**   Laceration of unspecified blood vessel at forearm level
- ● **S55.911**   Laceration of unspecified blood vessel at forearm level, right arm A 🔗
  - (Ex:) See PDX Collection 1260
- ● **S55.912**   Laceration of unspecified blood vessel at forearm level, left arm A 🔗
  - (Ex:) See PDX Collection 1261
- ● **S55.919**   Laceration of unspecified blood vessel at forearm level, unspecified arm A 🔗
  - (Ex:) See PDX Collection 1262

● **S55.99**   Other specified injury of unspecified blood vessel at forearm level
- ● **S55.991**   Other specified injury of unspecified blood vessel at forearm level, right arm A 🔗
  - (Ex:) See PDX Collection 1260
- ● **S55.992**   Other specified injury of unspecified blood vessel at forearm level, left arm A 🔗
  - (Ex:) See PDX Collection 1261
- ● **S55.999**   Other specified injury of unspecified blood vessel at forearm level, unspecified arm A 🔗
  - (Ex:) See PDX Collection 1262

● **S56**   **Injury of muscle, fascia and tendon at forearm level**

Code also any associated open wound (S51.-)

Excludes2   injury of muscle, fascia and tendon at or below wrist (S66.-)

sprain of joints and ligaments of elbow (S53.4-)

The appropriate 7th character is to be added to each code from category S56

A	initial encounter
D	subsequent encounter
S	sequela

● **S56.0**   Injury of flexor muscle, fascia and tendon of thumb at forearm level
- ● **S56.00**   Unspecified injury of flexor muscle, fascia and tendon of thumb at forearm level
  - ● **S56.001**   Unspecified injury of flexor muscle, fascia and tendon of right thumb at forearm level
  - ● **S56.002**   Unspecified injury of flexor muscle, fascia and tendon of left thumb at forearm level
  - ● **S56.009**   Unspecified injury of flexor muscle, fascia and tendon of unspecified thumb at forearm level
- ● **S56.01**   Strain of flexor muscle, fascia and tendon of thumb at forearm level
  - ● **S56.011**   Strain of flexor muscle, fascia and tendon of right thumb at forearm level
  - ● **S56.012**   Strain of flexor muscle, fascia and tendon of left thumb at forearm level
  - ● **S56.019**   Strain of flexor muscle, fascia and tendon of unspecified thumb at forearm level

CHAPTER 19 (S00-T88)

- S56.02 **Laceration** of flexor muscle, fascia and tendon of thumb at forearm level
  - S56.021 Laceration of flexor muscle, fascia and tendon of **right thumb** at forearm level A 🔖
    (Ex) See PDX Collection 1280
  - S56.022 Laceration of flexor muscle, fascia and tendon of **left thumb** at forearm level A 🔖
    (Ex) See PDX Collection 1281
  - S56.029 Laceration of flexor muscle, fascia and tendon of **unspecified thumb** at forearm level A 🔖
    (Ex) See PDX Collection 1282
- S56.09 **Other injury** of flexor muscle, fascia and tendon of thumb at forearm level
  - S56.091 Other injury of flexor muscle, fascia and tendon of **right thumb** at forearm level
  - S56.092 Other injury of flexor muscle, fascia and tendon of **left thumb** at forearm level
  - S56.099 Other injury of flexor muscle, fascia and tendon of **unspecified thumb** at forearm level
- S56.1 Injury of flexor muscle, fascia and tendon of **other and unspecified finger** at forearm level
  - S56.10 **Unspecified** injury of flexor muscle, fascia and tendon of other and unspecified finger at forearm level
    - S56.101 Unspecified injury of flexor muscle, fascia and tendon of **right index** finger at forearm level
    - S56.102 Unspecified injury of flexor muscle, fascia and tendon of **left index** finger at forearm level
    - S56.103 Unspecified injury of flexor muscle, fascia and tendon of **right middle** finger at forearm level
    - S56.104 Unspecified injury of flexor muscle, fascia and tendon of **left middle** finger at forearm level
    - S56.105 Unspecified injury of flexor muscle, fascia and tendon of **right ring** finger at forearm level
    - S56.106 Unspecified injury of flexor muscle, fascia and tendon of **left ring** finger at forearm level
    - S56.107 Unspecified injury of flexor muscle, fascia and tendon of **right little** finger at forearm level
    - S56.108 Unspecified injury of flexor muscle, fascia and tendon of **left little** finger at forearm level
    - S56.109 Unspecified injury of flexor muscle, fascia and tendon of **unspecified** finger at forearm level
  - S56.11 **Strain** of flexor muscle, fascia and tendon of other and unspecified finger at forearm level
    - S56.111 Strain of flexor muscle, fascia and tendon of **right index** finger at forearm level
    - S56.112 Strain of flexor muscle, fascia and tendon of **left index** finger at forearm level
    - S56.113 Strain of flexor muscle, fascia and tendon of **right middle** finger at forearm level
    - S56.114 Strain of flexor muscle, fascia and tendon of **left middle** finger at forearm level

- S56.115 Strain of flexor muscle, fascia and tendon of **right ring** finger at forearm level
- S56.116 Strain of flexor muscle, fascia and tendon of **left ring** finger at forearm level
- S56.117 Strain of flexor muscle, fascia and tendon of **right little** finger at forearm level
- S56.118 Strain of flexor muscle, fascia and tendon of **left little** finger at forearm level
- S56.119 Strain of flexor muscle, fascia and tendon of finger of **unspecified** finger at forearm level
- S56.12 **Laceration** of flexor muscle, fascia and tendon of other and unspecified finger at forearm level
  - S56.121 Laceration of flexor muscle, fascia and tendon of **right index** finger at forearm level A 🔖
    (Ex) See PDX Collection 1280
  - S56.122 Laceration of flexor muscle, fascia and tendon of **left index** finger at forearm level A 🔖
    (Ex) See PDX Collection 1281
  - S56.123 Laceration of flexor muscle, fascia and tendon of **right middle** finger at forearm level A 🔖
    (Ex) See PDX Collection 1280
  - S56.124 Laceration of flexor muscle, fascia and tendon of **left middle** finger at forearm level A 🔖
    (Ex) See PDX Collection 1281
  - S56.125 Laceration of flexor muscle, fascia and tendon of **right ring** finger at forearm level A 🔖
    (Ex) See PDX Collection 1280
  - S56.126 Laceration of flexor muscle, fascia and tendon of **left ring** finger at forearm level A 🔖
    (Ex) See PDX Collection 1281
  - S56.127 Laceration of flexor muscle, fascia and tendon of **right little** finger at forearm level A 🔖
    (Ex) See PDX Collection 1280
  - S56.128 Laceration of flexor muscle, fascia and tendon of **left little** finger at forearm level A 🔖
    (Ex) See PDX Collection 1281
  - S56.129 Laceration of flexor muscle, fascia and tendon of **unspecified** finger at forearm level A 🔖
    (Ex) See PDX Collection 1282
- S56.19 **Other injury** of flexor muscle, fascia and tendon of other and unspecified finger at forearm level
  - S56.191 Other injury of flexor muscle, fascia and tendon of **right index** finger at forearm level
  - S56.192 Other injury of flexor muscle, fascia and tendon of **left index** finger at forearm level
  - S56.193 Other injury of flexor muscle, fascia and tendon of **right middle** finger at forearm level
  - S56.194 Other injury of flexor muscle, fascia and tendon of **left middle** finger at forearm level
  - S56.195 Other injury of flexor muscle, fascia and tendon of **right ring** finger at forearm level

▶ New ➡ Revised ~~deleted~~ Deleted | Excludes 1 | Excludes 2 | Includes | Use additional | Code first | Code also | Key words

OGCR Official Guidelines ● Unacceptable Principal Diagnosis X Assign placeholder X ● Use Additional Character(s) ▶ Manifestation Code **Coding Clinic**

● S56.196   Other injury of flexor muscle, fascia and tendon of left ring finger at forearm level

● S56.197   Other injury of flexor muscle, fascia and tendon of right little finger at forearm level

● S56.198   Other injury of flexor muscle, fascia and tendon of left little finger at forearm level

● S56.199   Other injury of flexor muscle, fascia and tendon of unspecified finger at forearm level

● S56.2   Injury of other flexor muscle, fascia and tendon at forearm level

  ● S56.20   Unspecified injury of other flexor muscle, fascia and tendon at forearm level

    ● S56.201   Unspecified injury of other flexor muscle, fascia and tendon at forearm level, right arm

    ● S56.202   Unspecified injury of other flexor muscle, fascia and tendon at forearm level, left arm

    ● S56.209   Unspecified injury of other flexor muscle, fascia and tendon at forearm level, unspecified arm

  ● S56.21   Strain of other flexor muscle, fascia and tendon at forearm level

    ● S56.211   Strain of other flexor muscle, fascia and tendon at forearm level, right arm

    ● S56.212   Strain of other flexor muscle, fascia and tendon at forearm level, left arm

    ● S56.219   Strain of other flexor muscle, fascia and tendon at forearm level, unspecified arm

  ● S56.22   Laceration of other flexor muscle, fascia and tendon at forearm level

    ● S56.221   Laceration of other flexor muscle, fascia and tendon at forearm level, right arm A 🦠
        (Ex) See PDX Collection 1280

    ● S56.222   Laceration of other flexor muscle, fascia and tendon at forearm level, left arm A 🦠
        (Ex) See PDX Collection 1281

    ● S56.229   Laceration of other flexor muscle, fascia and tendon at forearm level, unspecified arm A 🦠
        (Ex) See PDX Collection 1282

  ● S56.29   Other injury of other flexor muscle, fascia and tendon at forearm level

    ● S56.291   Other injury of other flexor muscle, fascia and tendon at forearm level, right arm

    ● S56.292   Other injury of other flexor muscle, fascia and tendon at forearm level, left arm

    ● S56.299   Other injury of other flexor muscle, fascia and tendon at forearm level, unspecified arm

● S56.3   Injury of extensor or abductor muscles, fascia and tendons of thumb at forearm level

  ● S56.30   Unspecified injury of extensor or abductor muscles, fascia and tendons of thumb at forearm level

    ● S56.301   Unspecified injury of extensor or abductor muscles, fascia and tendons of right thumb at forearm level

    ● S56.302   Unspecified injury of extensor or abductor muscles, fascia and tendons of left thumb at forearm level

    ● S56.309   Unspecified injury of extensor or abductor muscles, fascia and tendons of unspecified thumb at forearm level

● S56.31   Strain of extensor or abductor muscles, fascia and tendons of thumb at forearm level

  ● S56.311   Strain of extensor or abductor muscles, fascia and tendons of right thumb at forearm level

  ● S56.312   Strain of extensor or abductor muscles, fascia and tendons of left thumb at forearm level

  ● S56.319   Strain of extensor or abductor muscles, fascia and tendons of unspecified thumb at forearm level

● S56.32   Laceration of extensor or abductor muscles, fascia and tendons of thumb at forearm level

  ● S56.321   Laceration of extensor or abductor muscles, fascia and tendons of right thumb at forearm level A 🦠
    (Ex) See PDX Collection 1280

  ● S56.322   Laceration of extensor or abductor muscles, fascia and tendons of left thumb at forearm level A 🦠
    (Ex) See PDX Collection 1281

  ● S56.329   Laceration of extensor or abductor muscles, fascia and tendons of unspecified thumb at forearm level A 🦠
    (Ex) See PDX Collection 1282

● S56.39   Other injury of extensor or abductor muscles, fascia and tendons of thumb at forearm level

  ● S56.391   Other injury of extensor or abductor muscles, fascia and tendons of right thumb at forearm level

  ● S56.392   Other injury of extensor or abductor muscles, fascia and tendons of left thumb at forearm level

  ● S56.399   Other injury of extensor or abductor muscles, fascia and tendons of unspecified thumb at forearm level

● S56.4   Injury of extensor muscle, fascia and tendon of other and unspecified finger at forearm level

  ● S56.40   Unspecified injury of extensor muscle, fascia and tendon of other and unspecified finger at forearm level

    ● S56.401   Unspecified injury of extensor muscle, fascia and tendon of right index finger at forearm level

    ● S56.402   Unspecified injury of extensor muscle, fascia and tendon of left index finger at forearm level

    ● S56.403   Unspecified injury of extensor muscle, fascia and tendon of right middle finger at forearm level

    ● S56.404   Unspecified injury of extensor muscle, fascia and tendon of left middle finger at forearm level

    ● S56.405   Unspecified injury of extensor muscle, fascia and tendon of right ring finger at forearm level

    ● S56.406   Unspecified injury of extensor muscle, fascia and tendon of left ring finger at forearm level

    ● S56.407   Unspecified injury of extensor muscle, fascia and tendon of right little finger at forearm level

    ● S56.408   Unspecified injury of extensor muscle, fascia and tendon of left little finger at forearm level

    ● S56.409   Unspecified injury of extensor muscle, fascia and tendon of unspecified finger at forearm level

● S56.41   Strain of extensor muscle, fascia and tendon of other and unspecified finger at forearm level

   ● S56.411   Strain of extensor muscle, fascia and tendon of right index finger at forearm level

   ● S56.412   Strain of extensor muscle, fascia and tendon of left index finger at forearm level

   ● S56.413   Strain of extensor muscle, fascia and tendon of right middle finger at forearm level

   ● S56.414   Strain of extensor muscle, fascia and tendon of left middle finger at forearm level

   ● S56.415   Strain of extensor muscle, fascia and tendon of right ring finger at forearm level

   ● S56.416   Strain of extensor muscle, fascia and tendon of left ring finger at forearm level

   ● S56.417   Strain of extensor muscle, fascia and tendon of right little finger at forearm level

   ● S56.418   Strain of extensor muscle, fascia and tendon of left little finger at forearm level

   ● S56.419   Strain of extensor muscle, fascia and tendon of finger, unspecified finger at forearm level

● S56.42   Laceration of extensor muscle, fascia and tendon of other and unspecified finger at forearm level

   ● S56.421   Laceration of extensor muscle, fascia and tendon of right index finger at forearm level A 🗞
      (Ex) See PDX Collection 1280

   ● S56.422   Laceration of extensor muscle, fascia and tendon of left index finger at forearm level A 🗞
      (Ex) See PDX Collection 1281

   ● S56.423   Laceration of extensor muscle, fascia and tendon of right middle finger at forearm level A 🗞
      (Ex) See PDX Collection 1280

   ● S56.424   Laceration of extensor muscle, fascia and tendon of left middle finger at forearm level A 🗞
      (Ex) See PDX Collection 1281

   ● S56.425   Laceration of extensor muscle, fascia and tendon of right ring finger at forearm level A 🗞
      (Ex) See PDX Collection 1280

   ● S56.426   Laceration of extensor muscle, fascia and tendon of left ring finger at forearm level A 🗞
      (Ex) See PDX Collection 1281

   ● S56.427   Laceration of extensor muscle, fascia and tendon of right little finger at forearm level A 🗞
      (Ex) See PDX Collection 1280

   ● S56.428   Laceration of extensor muscle, fascia and tendon of left little finger at forearm level A 🗞
      (Ex) See PDX Collection 1281

   ● S56.429   Laceration of extensor muscle, fascia and tendon of unspecified finger at forearm level A 🗞
      (Ex) See PDX Collection 1282

● S56.49   Other injury of extensor muscle, fascia and tendon of other and unspecified finger at forearm level

   ● S56.491   Other injury of extensor muscle, fascia and tendon of right index finger at forearm level

   ● S56.492   Other injury of extensor muscle, fascia and tendon of left index finger at forearm level

   ● S56.493   Other injury of extensor muscle, fascia and tendon of right middle finger at forearm level

   ● S56.494   Other injury of extensor muscle, fascia and tendon of left middle finger at forearm level

   ● S56.495   Other injury of extensor muscle, fascia and tendon of right ring finger at forearm level

   ● S56.496   Other injury of extensor muscle, fascia and tendon of left ring finger at forearm level

   ● S56.497   Other injury of extensor muscle, fascia and tendon of right little finger at forearm level

   ● S56.498   Other injury of extensor muscle, fascia and tendon of left little finger at forearm level

   ● S56.499   Other injury of extensor muscle, fascia and tendon of unspecified finger at forearm level

● S56.5   Injury of other extensor muscle, fascia and tendon at forearm level

   ● S56.50   Unspecified injury of other extensor muscle, fascia and tendon at forearm level

      ● S56.501   Unspecified injury of other extensor muscle, fascia and tendon at forearm level, right arm

      ● S56.502   Unspecified injury of other extensor muscle, fascia and tendon at forearm level, left arm

      ● S56.509   Unspecified injury of other extensor muscle, fascia and tendon at forearm level, unspecified arm

   ● S56.51   Strain of other extensor muscle, fascia and tendon at forearm level

      ● S56.511   Strain of other extensor muscle, fascia and tendon at forearm level, right arm

      ● S56.512   Strain of other extensor muscle, fascia and tendon at forearm level, left arm

      ● S56.519   Strain of other extensor muscle, fascia and tendon at forearm level, unspecified arm

   ● S56.52   Laceration of other extensor muscle, fascia and tendon at forearm level

      ● S56.521   Laceration of other extensor muscle, fascia and tendon at forearm level, right arm A 🗞
         (Ex) See PDX Collection 1280

      ● S56.522   Laceration of other extensor muscle, fascia and tendon at forearm level, left arm A 🗞
         (Ex) See PDX Collection 1281

      ● S56.529   Laceration of other extensor muscle, fascia and tendon at forearm level, unspecified arm A 🗞
         (Ex) See PDX Collection 1282

▶ New   ⮕ Revised   ~~deleted~~ Deleted   Excludes 1   Excludes 2   Includes   Use additional   Code first   Code also   Key words

OGCR Official Guidelines   ● Unacceptable Principal Diagnosis   X Assign placeholder X   ● Use Additional Character(s)   ▶ Manifestation Code   **Coding Clinic**

● S56.59   Other injury of other extensor muscle, fascia and tendon at forearm level

  ● S56.591   Other injury of other extensor muscle, fascia and tendon at forearm level, right arm

  ● S56.592   Other injury of other extensor muscle, fascia and tendon at forearm level, left arm

  ● S56.599   Other injury of other extensor muscle, fascia and tendon at forearm level, unspecified arm

● S56.8   Injury of other muscles, fascia and tendons at forearm level

  ● S56.80   Unspecified injury of other muscles, fascia and tendons at forearm level

    ● S56.801   Unspecified injury of other muscles, fascia and tendons at forearm level, right arm

    ● S56.802   Unspecified injury of other muscles, fascia and tendons at forearm level, left arm

    ● S56.809   Unspecified injury of other muscles, fascia and tendons at forearm level, unspecified arm

  ● S56.81   Strain of other muscles, fascia and tendons at forearm level

    ● S56.811   Strain of other muscles, fascia and tendons at forearm level, right arm

    ● S56.812   Strain of other muscles, fascia and tendons at forearm level, left arm

    ● S56.819   Strain of other muscles, fascia and tendons at forearm level, unspecified arm

  ● S56.82   Laceration of other muscles, fascia and tendons at forearm level

    ● S56.821   Laceration of other muscles, fascia and tendons at forearm level, right arm A 🔖
      (Ex:) See PDX Collection 1280

    ● S56.822   Laceration of other muscles, fascia and tendons at forearm level, left arm A 🔖
      (Ex:) See PDX Collection 1281

    ● S56.829   Laceration of other muscles, fascia and tendons at forearm level, unspecified arm A 🔖
      (Ex:) See PDX Collection 1282

  ● S56.89   Other injury of other muscles, fascia and tendons at forearm level

    ● S56.891   Other injury of other muscles, fascia and tendons at forearm level, right arm

    ● S56.892   Other injury of other muscles, fascia and tendons at forearm level, left arm

    ● S56.899   Other injury of other muscles, fascia and tendons at forearm level, unspecified arm

● S56.9   Injury of unspecified muscles, fascia and tendons at forearm level

  ● S56.90   Unspecified injury of unspecified muscles, fascia and tendons at forearm level

    ● S56.901   Unspecified injury of unspecified muscles, fascia and tendons at forearm level, right arm

    ● S56.902   Unspecified injury of unspecified muscles, fascia and tendons at forearm level, left arm

    ● S56.909   Unspecified injury of unspecified muscles, fascia and tendons at forearm level, unspecified arm

● S56.91   Strain of unspecified muscles, fascia and tendons at forearm level

  ● S56.911   Strain of unspecified muscles, fascia and tendons at forearm level, right arm

  ● S56.912   Strain of unspecified muscles, fascia and tendons at forearm level, left arm

  ● S56.919   Strain of unspecified muscles, fascia and tendons at forearm level, unspecified arm

● S56.92   Laceration of unspecified muscles, fascia and tendons at forearm level

  ● S56.921   Laceration of unspecified muscles, fascia and tendons at forearm level, right arm A 🔖
    (Ex:) See PDX Collection 1280

  ● S56.922   Laceration of unspecified muscles, fascia and tendons at forearm level, left arm A 🔖
    (Ex:) See PDX Collection 1281

  ● S56.929   Laceration of unspecified muscles, fascia and tendons at forearm level, unspecified arm A 🔖
    (Ex:) See PDX Collection 1282

● S56.99   Other injury of unspecified muscles, fascia and tendons at forearm level

  ● S56.991   Other injury of unspecified muscles, fascia and tendons at forearm level, right arm

  ● S56.992   Other injury of unspecified muscles, fascia and tendons at forearm level, left arm

  ● S56.999   Other injury of unspecified muscles, fascia and tendons at forearm level, unspecified arm

● S57   **Crushing injury of elbow and forearm**

  Use additional code(s) for all associated injuries

  Excludes2   crushing injury of wrist and hand (S67.-)

  The appropriate 7th character is to be added to each code from category S57

A	initial encounter
D	subsequent encounter
S	sequela

● S57.0   Crushing injury of elbow

  X ● S57.00   Crushing injury of unspecified elbow

  X ● S57.01   Crushing injury of right elbow

  X ● S57.02   Crushing injury of left elbow

● S57.8   Crushing injury of forearm

  X ● S57.80   Crushing injury of unspecified forearm

  X ● S57.81   Crushing injury of right forearm

  X ● S57.82   Crushing injury of left forearm

N Newborn Age: Ø   **P** Pediatric Age: Ø–17   **M** Maternity DX: 12–55   **A** Adult Age: 15–124   ♀ Females Only   ♂ Males Only

🔖 Complication\Comorbidity   🔖 Major C\C   (Ex:) CC/MCC Exclusions   🔖 Hospital-Acquired Condition

1313

● **S58**   **Traumatic amputation of elbow and forearm**
An amputation not identified as partial or complete should be coded to complete

   Excludes1   traumatic amputation of wrist and hand (S68.-)

The appropriate 7th character is to be added to each code from category S58

> A   initial encounter
> D   subsequent encounter
> S   sequela

● **S58.0**   **Traumatic amputation at elbow level**
   ● **S58.01**   **Complete traumatic amputation at elbow level**
     ● **S58.011**   **Complete traumatic amputation at elbow level, right arm** A 🔗
       (Ex:) See PDX Collection 1266
     ● **S58.012**   **Complete traumatic amputation at elbow level, left arm** A 🔗
       (Ex:) See PDX Collection 1267
     ● **S58.019**   **Complete traumatic amputation at elbow level, unspecified arm** A 🔗
       (Ex:) See PDX Collection 1268

   ● **S58.02**   **Partial traumatic amputation at elbow level**
     ● **S58.021**   **Partial traumatic amputation at elbow level, right arm** A 🔗
       (Ex:) See PDX Collection 1266
     ● **S58.022**   **Partial traumatic amputation at elbow level, left arm** A 🔗
       (Ex:) See PDX Collection 1267
     ● **S58.029**   **Partial traumatic amputation at elbow level, unspecified arm** A 🔗
       (Ex:) See PDX Collection 1268

● **S58.1**   **Traumatic amputation at level between elbow and wrist**
   ● **S58.11**   **Complete traumatic amputation at level between elbow and wrist**
     ● **S58.111**   **Complete traumatic amputation at level between elbow and wrist, right arm** A 🔗
       (Ex:) See PDX Collection 1266
     ● **S58.112**   **Complete traumatic amputation at level between elbow and wrist, left arm** A 🔗
       (Ex:) See PDX Collection 1267
     ● **S58.119**   **Complete traumatic amputation at level between elbow and wrist, unspecified arm** A 🔗
       (Ex:) See PDX Collection 1268

   ● **S58.12**   **Partial traumatic amputation at level between elbow and wrist**
     ● **S58.121**   **Partial traumatic amputation at level between elbow and wrist, right arm** A 🔗
       (Ex:) See PDX Collection 1266
     ● **S58.122**   **Partial traumatic amputation at level between elbow and wrist, left arm** A 🔗
       (Ex:) See PDX Collection 1267
     ● **S58.129**   **Partial traumatic amputation at level between elbow and wrist, unspecified arm** A 🔗
       (Ex:) See PDX Collection 1268

● **S58.9**   **Traumatic amputation of forearm, level unspecified**
   Excludes1   traumatic amputation of wrist (S68.-)
   ● **S58.91**   **Complete traumatic amputation of forearm, level unspecified**
     ● **S58.911**   **Complete traumatic amputation of right forearm, level unspecified** A 🔗
       (Ex:) See PDX Collection 1266
     ● **S58.912**   **Complete traumatic amputation of left forearm, level unspecified** A 🔗
       (Ex:) See PDX Collection 1267
     ● **S58.919**   **Complete traumatic amputation of unspecified forearm, level unspecified** A 🔗
       (Ex:) See PDX Collection 1268

   ● **S58.92**   **Partial traumatic amputation of forearm, level unspecified**
     ● **S58.921**   **Partial traumatic amputation of right forearm, level unspecified** A 🔗
       (Ex:) See PDX Collection 1266
     ● **S58.922**   **Partial traumatic amputation of left forearm, level unspecified** A 🔗
       (Ex:) See PDX Collection 1267
     ● **S58.929**   **Partial traumatic amputation of unspecified forearm, level unspecified** A 🔗
       (Ex:) See PDX Collection 1268

● **S59**   **Other and unspecified injuries of elbow and forearm**
   Excludes2   other and unspecified injuries of wrist and hand (S69.-)

The appropriate 7th character is to be added to each code from subcategories S59.0, S59.1, and S59.2

> A   initial encounter for closed fracture
> D   subsequent encounter for fracture with routine healing
> G   subsequent encounter for fracture with delayed healing
> K   subsequent encounter for fracture with nonunion
> P   subsequent encounter for fracture with malunion
> S   sequela

● **S59.0**   **Physeal fracture of lower end of ulna**
   ● **S59.00**   **Unspecified physeal fracture of lower end of ulna**
     ● **S59.001**   **Unspecified physeal fracture of lower end of ulna, right arm** A, K, P 🔗, A 🔗
       (Ex:) For code S59.001[A]: See PDX Collection 1270
       For S59.001[K,P]: See PDX Collection 897
     ● **S59.002**   **Unspecified physeal fracture of lower end of ulna, left arm** A, K, P 🔗, A 🔗
       (Ex:) For code S59.002[A]: See PDX Collection 1271
       For S59.002[K,P]: See PDX Collection 897
     ● **S59.009**   **Unspecified physeal fracture of lower end of ulna, unspecified arm** A, K, P 🔗, A 🔗
       (Ex:) For code S59.009[A]: See PDX Collection 1272
       For S59.009[K,P]: See PDX Collection 897

   ● **S59.01**   **Salter-Harris Type I physeal fracture of lower end of ulna**
     ● **S59.011**   **Salter-Harris Type I physeal fracture of lower end of ulna, right arm** A, K, P 🔗, A 🔗
       (Ex:) For code S59.011[A]: See PDX Collection 1270
       For S59.011[K,P]: See PDX Collection 897
     ● **S59.012**   **Salter-Harris Type I physeal fracture of lower end of ulna, left arm** A, K, P 🔗, A 🔗
       (Ex:) For code S59.012[A]: See PDX Collection 1271
       For S59.012[K,P]: See PDX Collection 897
     ● **S59.019**   **Salter-Harris Type I physeal fracture of lower end of ulna, unspecified arm** A, K, P 🔗, A 🔗
       (Ex:) For code S59.019[A]: See PDX Collection 1272
       For S59.019[K,P]: See PDX Collection 897

▶ New   ⏩ Revised   ~~deleted~~ Deleted   Excludes 1   Excludes 2   Includes   Use additional   Code first   Code also   Key words
OGCR Official Guidelines   ● Unacceptable Principal Diagnosis   X Assign placeholder X   🔗 Use Additional Character(s)   ▶ Manifestation Code   **Coding Clinic**

Item 19–4 SALTER-HARRIS TYPE 1: epiphysis is completely separated from end of bone, or metaphysic growth plate remains attached to epiphysis

SALTER-HARRIS TYPE 2: epiphysis and growth plate are partially separated from metaphysis, which is cracked—most common type

SALTER-HARRIS TYPE 3: fracture occurring through epiphysis and separates part of epiphysis and growth plate from metaphysis fracture, usually at distal end of tibia

SALTER-HARRIS TYPE 4: fracture runs through epiphysis, across growth plate, into metaphysic, surgery is required to restore joint surface to normal and align growth plate

● **S59.02** **Salter-Harris Type II physeal fracture of lower end of ulna**

    ● **S59.021** **Salter-Harris Type II physeal fracture of lower end of ulna, right arm** A, K, P 🔹, A 🔸
       (Ex) **For code S59.021[A]:** See PDX Collection 1270
       For S59.021[K,P]: See PDX Collection 897

    ● **S59.022** **Salter-Harris Type II physeal fracture of lower end of ulna, left arm** A, K, P 🔹, A 🔸
       (Ex) **For code S59.022[A]:** See PDX Collection 1271
       For S59.022[K,P]: See PDX Collection 897

    ● **S59.029** **Salter-Harris Type II physeal fracture of lower end of ulna, unspecified arm** A, K, P 🔹, A 🔸
       (Ex) **For code S59.029[A]:** See PDX Collection 1272
       For S59.029[K,P]: See PDX Collection 897

● **S59.03** **Salter-Harris Type III physeal fracture of lower end of ulna**

    ● **S59.031** **Salter-Harris Type III physeal fracture of lower end of ulna, right arm** A, K, P 🔹, A 🔸
       (Ex) **For code S59.031[A]:** See PDX Collection 1270
       For S59.031[K,P]: See PDX Collection 897

    ● **S59.032** **Salter-Harris Type III physeal fracture of lower end of ulna, left arm** A, K, P 🔹, A 🔸
       (Ex) **For code S59.032[A]:** See PDX Collection 1271
       For S59.032[K,P]: See PDX Collection 897

    ● **S59.039** **Salter-Harris Type III physeal fracture of lower end of ulna, unspecified arm** A, K, P 🔹, A 🔸
       (Ex) **For code S59.039[A]:** See PDX Collection 1272
       For S59.039[K,P]: See PDX Collection 897

● **S59.04** **Salter-Harris Type IV physeal fracture of lower end of ulna**

    ● **S59.041** **Salter-Harris Type IV physeal fracture of lower end of ulna, right arm** A, K, P 🔹, A 🔸
       (Ex) **For code S59.041[A]:** See PDX Collection 1270
       For S59.041[K,P]: See PDX Collection 897

    ● **S59.042** **Salter-Harris Type IV physeal fracture of lower end of ulna, left arm** A, K, P 🔹, A 🔸
       (Ex) **For code S59.042[A]:** See PDX Collection 1271
       For S59.042[K,P]: See PDX Collection 897

    ● **S59.049** **Salter-Harris Type IV physeal fracture of lower end of ulna, unspecified arm** A, K, P 🔹, A 🔸
       (Ex) **For code S59.049[A]:** See PDX Collection 1272
       For S59.049[K,P]: See PDX Collection 897

● **S59.09** **Other physeal fracture of lower end of ulna**

    ● **S59.091** **Other physeal fracture of lower end of ulna, right arm** A, K, P 🔹, A 🔸
       (Ex) **For code S59.091[A]:** See PDX Collection 1270
       For S59.091[K,P]: See PDX Collection 897

    ● **S59.092** **Other physeal fracture of lower end of ulna, left arm** A, K, P 🔹, A 🔸
       (Ex) **For code S59.092[A]:** See PDX Collection 1271
       For S59.092[K,P]: See PDX Collection 897

    ● **S59.099** **Other physeal fracture of lower end of ulna, unspecified arm** A, K, P 🔹, A 🔸
       (Ex) **For code S59.099[A]:** See PDX Collection 1272
       For S59.099[K,P]: See PDX Collection 897

● **S59.1** **Physeal fracture of upper end of radius**
     (Ex) **For category S59.1 CC codes:** See PDX Collection 897

    ● **S59.10** **Unspecified physeal fracture of upper end of radius**

       ● **S59.101** **Unspecified physeal fracture of upper end of radius, right arm** K, P 🔹

       ● **S59.102** **Unspecified physeal fracture of upper end of radius, left arm** K, P 🔹

       ● **S59.109** **Unspecified physeal fracture of upper end of radius, unspecified arm** K, P 🔹

    ● **S59.11** **Salter-Harris Type I physeal fracture of upper end of radius**

       ● **S59.111** **Salter-Harris Type I physeal fracture of upper end of radius, right arm** K, P 🔹

       ● **S59.112** **Salter-Harris Type I physeal fracture of upper end of radius, left arm** K, P 🔹

       ● **S59.119** **Salter-Harris Type I physeal fracture of upper end of radius, unspecified arm** K, P 🔹

    ● **S59.12** **Salter-Harris Type II physeal fracture of upper end of radius**

       ● **S59.121** **Salter-Harris Type II physeal fracture of upper end of radius, right arm** K, P 🔹

       ● **S59.122** **Salter-Harris Type II physeal fracture of upper end of radius, left arm** K, P 🔹

       ● **S59.129** **Salter-Harris Type II physeal fracture of upper end of radius, unspecified arm** K, P 🔹

    ● **S59.13** **Salter-Harris Type III physeal fracture of upper end of radius**

       ● **S59.131** **Salter-Harris Type III physeal fracture of upper end of radius, right arm** K, P 🔹

       ● **S59.132** **Salter-Harris Type III physeal fracture of upper end of radius, left arm** K, P 🔹

       ● **S59.139** **Salter-Harris Type III physeal fracture of upper end of radius, unspecified arm** K, P 🔹

    ● **S59.14** **Salter-Harris Type IV physeal fracture of upper end of radius**

       ● **S59.141** **Salter-Harris Type IV physeal fracture of upper end of radius, right arm** K, P 🔹

       ● **S59.142** **Salter-Harris Type IV physeal fracture of upper end of radius, left arm** K, P 🔹

       ● **S59.149** **Salter-Harris Type IV physeal fracture of upper end of radius, unspecified arm** K, P 🔹

CHAPTER 19 (S00-T88)

N Newborn Age: 0   **P** Pediatric Age: 0–17   **M** Maternity DX: 12–55   **A** Adult Age: 15–124   ♀ Females Only   ♂ Males Only

🔹 Complication\Comorbidity   🔸 Major C\C   (Ex) CC/MCC Exclusions   🔹 Hospital-Acquired Condition

1315

● S59.19   Other physeal fracture of upper end of radius
     ● S59.191   Other physeal fracture of upper end of radius, right arm K, P 🖉
     ● S59.192   Other physeal fracture of upper end of radius, left arm K, P 🖉
     ● S59.199   Other physeal fracture of upper end of radius, unspecified arm K, P 🖉

● S59.2   Physeal fracture of lower end of radius
   ● S59.20   Unspecified physeal fracture of lower end of radius
     ● S59.201   Unspecified physeal fracture of lower end of radius, right arm A, K, P 🖉, A 🖉
       Ⓔⓧ **For code S59.201[A]:** See PDX Collection 1270
       For S59.201[K,P]: See PDX Collection 897
     ● S59.202   Unspecified physeal fracture of lower end of radius, left arm A, K, P 🖉, A 🖉
       Ⓔⓧ **For code S59.202[A]:** See PDX Collection 1271
       For S59.202[K,P]: See PDX Collection 897
     ● S59.209   Unspecified physeal fracture of lower end of radius, unspecified arm A, K, P 🖉, A 🖉
       Ⓔⓧ **For code S59.209[A]:** See PDX Collection 1272
       For S59.209[K,P]: See PDX Collection 897
   ● S59.21   Salter-Harris Type I physeal fracture of lower end of radius
     ● S59.211   Salter-Harris Type I physeal fracture of lower end of radius, right arm A, K, P 🖉, A 🖉
       Ⓔⓧ **For code S59.211[A]:** See PDX Collection 1270
       For S59.211[K,P]: See PDX Collection 897
     ● S59.212   Salter-Harris Type I physeal fracture of lower end of radius, left arm A, K, P 🖉, A 🖉
       Ⓔⓧ **For code S59.212[A]:** See PDX Collection 1271
       For S59.212[K,P]: See PDX Collection 897
     ● S59.219   Salter-Harris Type I physeal fracture of lower end of radius, unspecified arm A, K, P 🖉, A 🖉
       Ⓔⓧ **For code S59.219[A]:** See PDX Collection 1272
       For S59.219[K,P]: See PDX Collection 897
   ● S59.22   Salter-Harris Type II physeal fracture of lower end of radius
     ● S59.221   Salter-Harris Type II physeal fracture of lower end of radius, right arm A, K, P 🖉, A 🖉
       Ⓔⓧ **For code S59.221[A]:** See PDX Collection 1270
       For S59.221[K,P]: See PDX Collection 897
     ● S59.222   Salter-Harris Type II physeal fracture of lower end of radius, left arm A, K, P 🖉, A 🖉
       Ⓔⓧ **For code S59.222[A]:** See PDX Collection 1271
       For S59.222[K,P]: See PDX Collection 897
     ● S59.229   Salter-Harris Type II physeal fracture of lower end of radius, unspecified arm A, K, P 🖉, A 🖉
       Ⓔⓧ **For code S59.229[A]:** See PDX Collection 1272
       For S59.229[K,P]: See PDX Collection 897
   ● S59.23   Salter-Harris Type III physeal fracture of lower end of radius
     ● S59.231   Salter-Harris Type III physeal fracture of lower end of radius, right arm A, K, P 🖉, A 🖉
       Ⓔⓧ **For code S59.231[A]:** See PDX Collection 1270
       For S59.231[K,P]: See PDX Collection 897
     ● S59.232   Salter-Harris Type III physeal fracture of lower end of radius, left arm A, K, P 🖉, A 🖉
       Ⓔⓧ **For code S59.232[A]:** See PDX Collection 1271
       For S59.232[K,P]: See PDX Collection 897
     ● S59.239   Salter-Harris Type III physeal fracture of lower end of radius, unspecified arm A, K, P 🖉, A 🖉
       Ⓔⓧ **For code S59.239[A]:** See PDX Collection 1272
       For S59.239[K,P]: See PDX Collection 897

● S59.24   Salter-Harris Type IV physeal fracture of lower end of radius
     ● S59.241   Salter-Harris Type IV physeal fracture of lower end of radius, right arm A, K, P 🖉, A 🖉
       Ⓔⓧ **For code S59.241[A]:** See PDX Collection 1270
       For S59.241[K,P]: See PDX Collection 897
     ● S59.242   Salter-Harris Type IV physeal fracture of lower end of radius, left arm A, K, P 🖉, A 🖉
       Ⓔⓧ **For code S59.242[A]:** See PDX Collection 1271
       For S59.242[K,P]: See PDX Collection 897
     ● S59.249   Salter-Harris Type IV physeal fracture of lower end of radius, unspecified arm A, K, P 🖉, A 🖉
       Ⓔⓧ **For code S59.249[A]:** See PDX Collection 1272
       For S59.249[K,P]: See PDX Collection 897
   ● S59.29   Other physeal fracture of lower end of radius
     ● S59.291   Other physeal fracture of lower end of radius, right arm A, K, P 🖉, A 🖉
       Ⓔⓧ **For code S59.291[A]:** See PDX Collection 1270
       For S59.291[K,P]: See PDX Collection 897
     ● S59.292   Other physeal fracture of lower end of radius, left arm A, K, P 🖉, A 🖉
       Ⓔⓧ **For code S59.292[A]:** See PDX Collection 1271
       For S59.292[K,P]: See PDX Collection 897
     ● S59.299   Other physeal fracture of lower end of radius, unspecified arm A, K, P 🖉, A 🖉
       Ⓔⓧ **For code S59.299[A]:** See PDX Collection 1272
       For S59.299[K,P]: See PDX Collection 897

● S59.8   **Other specified injuries of elbow and forearm**
     The appropriate 7th character is to be added to each code in subcategory S59.8

A	initial encounter
D	subsequent encounter
S	sequela

   ● S59.80   Other specified injuries of elbow
     ● S59.801   Other specified injuries of right elbow
     ● S59.802   Other specified injuries of left elbow
     ● S59.809   Other specified injuries of unspecified elbow
   ● S59.81   Other specified injuries of forearm
     ● S59.811   Other specified injuries right forearm
     ● S59.812   Other specified injuries left forearm
     ● S59.819   Other specified injuries unspecified forearm

● S59.9   **Unspecified injury of elbow and forearm**
     The appropriate 7th character is to be added to each code in subcategory S59.9

A	initial encounter
D	subsequent encounter
S	sequela

   ● S59.90   Unspecified injury of elbow
     ● S59.901   Unspecified injury of right elbow
     ● S59.902   Unspecified injury of left elbow
     ● S59.909   Unspecified injury of unspecified elbow
   ● S59.91   Unspecified injury of forearm
     ● S59.911   Unspecified injury of right forearm
     ● S59.912   Unspecified injury of left forearm
     ● S59.919   Unspecified injury of unspecified forearm

▶ New   ⇒ Revised   ~~deleted~~ Deleted   Excludes 1   Excludes 2   Includes   Use additional   Code first   Code also   Key words
OGCR Official Guidelines   ● Unacceptable Principal Diagnosis   X Assign placeholder X   🖉 Use Additional Character(s)   ▌ Manifestation Code   **Coding Clinic**

INJURIES TO THE WRIST, HAND AND FINGERS (S60-S69)

> **Excludes2**   burns and corrosions (T20-T32)
> frostbite (T33-T34)
> insect bite or sting, venomous (T63.4)

● **S60**   **Superficial injury of wrist, hand and fingers**

The appropriate 7th character is to be added to each code from category S60

> A   initial encounter
> D   subsequent encounter
> S   sequela

● **S60.0**   **Contusion of finger without damage to nail**

> **Excludes1**   contusion involving nail (matrix) (S60.1)

X ● **S60.00**   Contusion of unspecified finger without damage to nail
Contusion of finger(s) NOS

● **S60.01**   Contusion of thumb without damage to nail
  ● **S60.011**   Contusion of right thumb without damage to nail
  ● **S60.012**   Contusion of left thumb without damage to nail
  ● **S60.019**   Contusion of unspecified thumb without damage to nail

● **S60.02**   Contusion of index finger without damage to nail
  ● **S60.021**   Contusion of right index finger without damage to nail
  ● **S60.022**   Contusion of left index finger without damage to nail
  ● **S60.029**   Contusion of unspecified index finger without damage to nail

● **S60.03**   Contusion of middle finger without damage to nail
  ● **S60.031**   Contusion of right middle finger without damage to nail
  ● **S60.032**   Contusion of left middle finger without damage to nail
  ● **S60.039**   Contusion of unspecified middle finger without damage to nail

● **S60.04**   Contusion of ring finger without damage to nail
  ● **S60.041**   Contusion of right ring finger without damage to nail
  ● **S60.042**   Contusion of left ring finger without damage to nail
  ● **S60.049**   Contusion of unspecified ring finger without damage to nail

● **S60.05**   Contusion of little finger without damage to nail
  ● **S60.051**   Contusion of right little finger without damage to nail
  ● **S60.052**   Contusion of left little finger without damage to nail
  ● **S60.059**   Contusion of unspecified little finger without damage to nail

● **S60.1**   **Contusion of finger with damage to nail**

X ● **S60.10**   Contusion of unspecified finger with damage to nail

● **S60.11**   Contusion of thumb with damage to nail
  ● **S60.111**   Contusion of right thumb with damage to nail
  ● **S60.112**   Contusion of left thumb with damage to nail
  ● **S60.119**   Contusion of unspecified thumb with damage to nail

● **S60.12**   Contusion of index finger with damage to nail
  ● **S60.121**   Contusion of right index finger with damage to nail
  ● **S60.122**   Contusion of left index finger with damage to nail
  ● **S60.129**   Contusion of unspecified index finger with damage to nail

● **S60.13**   Contusion of middle finger with damage to nail
  ● **S60.131**   Contusion of right middle finger with damage to nail
  ● **S60.132**   Contusion of left middle finger with damage to nail
  ● **S60.139**   Contusion of unspecified middle finger with damage to nail

● **S60.14**   Contusion of ring finger with damage to nail
  ● **S60.141**   Contusion of right ring finger with damage to nail
  ● **S60.142**   Contusion of left ring finger with damage to nail
  ● **S60.149**   Contusion of unspecified ring finger with damage to nail

● **S60.15**   Contusion of little finger with damage to nail
  ● **S60.151**   Contusion of right little finger with damage to nail
  ● **S60.152**   Contusion of left little finger with damage to nail
  ● **S60.159**   Contusion of unspecified little finger with damage to nail

● **S60.2**   **Contusion of wrist and hand**

> **Excludes2**   contusion of fingers (S60.0-, S60.1-)

● **S60.21**   Contusion of wrist
  ● **S60.211**   Contusion of right wrist
  ● **S60.212**   Contusion of left wrist
  ● **S60.219**   Contusion of unspecified wrist

● **S60.22**   Contusion of hand
  ● **S60.221**   Contusion of right hand
  ● **S60.222**   Contusion of left hand
  ● **S60.229**   Contusion of unspecified hand

● **S60.3**   **Other superficial injuries of thumb**

● **S60.31**   Abrasion of thumb
  ● **S60.311**   Abrasion of right thumb
  ● **S60.312**   Abrasion of left thumb
  ● **S60.319**   Abrasion of unspecified thumb

● **S60.32**   Blister (nonthermal) of thumb
  ● **S60.321**   Blister (nonthermal) of right thumb
  ● **S60.322**   Blister (nonthermal) of left thumb
  ● **S60.329**   Blister (nonthermal) of unspecified thumb

● **S60.34**   External constriction of thumb
  Hair tourniquet syndrome of thumb
  Use additional cause code to identify the constricting item (W49.0-)
  ● **S60.341**   External constriction of right thumb
  ● **S60.342**   External constriction of left thumb
  ● **S60.349**   External constriction of unspecified thumb

● **S60.35**   Superficial foreign body of thumb
  Splinter in the thumb
  ● **S60.351**   Superficial foreign body of right thumb
  ● **S60.352**   Superficial foreign body of left thumb
  ● **S60.359**   Superficial foreign body of unspecified thumb

● **S60.36**   Insect bite (nonvenomous) of thumb
     ● **S60.361**   Insect bite (nonvenomous) of right thumb
     ● **S60.362**   Insect bite (nonvenomous) of left thumb
     ● **S60.369**   Insect bite (nonvenomous) of unspecified thumb
● **S60.37**   Other superficial bite of thumb
     Excludes1   open bite of thumb (S61.05-, S61.15-)
     ● **S60.371**   Other superficial bite of right thumb
     ● **S60.372**   Other superficial bite of left thumb
     ● **S60.379**   Other superficial bite of unspecified thumb
● **S60.39**   Other superficial injuries of thumb
     ● **S60.391**   Other superficial injuries of right thumb
     ● **S60.392**   Other superficial injuries of left thumb
     ● **S60.399**   Other superficial injuries of unspecified thumb
● **S60.4**   Other superficial injuries of other fingers
     ● **S60.41**   Abrasion of fingers
         ● **S60.410**   Abrasion of right index finger
         ● **S60.411**   Abrasion of left index finger
         ● **S60.412**   Abrasion of right middle finger
         ● **S60.413**   Abrasion of left middle finger
         ● **S60.414**   Abrasion of right ring finger
         ● **S60.415**   Abrasion of left ring finger
         ● **S60.416**   Abrasion of right little finger
         ● **S60.417**   Abrasion of left little finger
         ● **S60.418**   Abrasion of other finger
             Abrasion of specified finger with unspecified laterality
         ● **S60.419**   Abrasion of unspecified finger
     ● **S60.42**   Blister (nonthermal) of fingers
         ● **S60.420**   Blister (nonthermal) of right index finger
         ● **S60.421**   Blister (nonthermal) of left index finger
         ● **S60.422**   Blister (nonthermal) of right middle finger
         ● **S60.423**   Blister (nonthermal) of left middle finger
         ● **S60.424**   Blister (nonthermal) of right ring finger
         ● **S60.425**   Blister (nonthermal) of left ring finger
         ● **S60.426**   Blister (nonthermal) of right little finger
         ● **S60.427**   Blister (nonthermal) of left little finger
         ● **S60.428**   Blister (nonthermal) of other finger
             Blister (nonthermal) of specified finger with unspecified laterality
         ● **S60.429**   Blister (nonthermal) of unspecified finger
     ● **S60.44**   External constriction of fingers
         Hair tourniquet syndrome of finger
         Use additional cause code to identify the constricting item (W49.0-)
         ● **S60.440**   External constriction of right index finger
         ● **S60.441**   External constriction of left index finger

         ● **S60.442**   External constriction of right middle finger
         ● **S60.443**   External constriction of left middle finger
         ● **S60.444**   External constriction of right ring finger
         ● **S60.445**   External constriction of left ring finger
         ● **S60.446**   External constriction of right little finger
         ● **S60.447**   External constriction of left little finger
         ● **S60.448**   External constriction of other finger
             External constriction of specified finger with unspecified laterality
         ● **S60.449**   External constriction of unspecified finger
     ● **S60.45**   Superficial foreign body of fingers
         Splinter in the finger(s)
         ● **S60.450**   Superficial foreign body of right index finger
         ● **S60.451**   Superficial foreign body of left index finger
         ● **S60.452**   Superficial foreign body of right middle finger
         ● **S60.453**   Superficial foreign body of left middle finger
         ● **S60.454**   Superficial foreign body of right ring finger
         ● **S60.455**   Superficial foreign body of left ring finger
         ● **S60.456**   Superficial foreign body of right little finger
         ● **S60.457**   Superficial foreign body of left little finger
         ● **S60.458**   Superficial foreign body of other finger
             Superficial foreign body of specified finger with unspecified laterality
         ● **S60.459**   Superficial foreign body of unspecified finger
     ● **S60.46**   Insect bite (nonvenomous) of fingers
         ● **S60.460**   Insect bite (nonvenomous) of right index finger
         ● **S60.461**   Insect bite (nonvenomous) of left index finger
         ● **S60.462**   Insect bite (nonvenomous) of right middle finger
         ● **S60.463**   Insect bite (nonvenomous) of left middle finger
         ● **S60.464**   Insect bite (nonvenomous) of right ring finger
         ● **S60.465**   Insect bite (nonvenomous) of left ring finger
         ● **S60.466**   Insect bite (nonvenomous) of right little finger
         ● **S60.467**   Insect bite (nonvenomous) of left little finger
         ● **S60.468**   Insect bite (nonvenomous) of other finger
             Insect bite (nonvenomous) of specified finger with unspecified laterality
         ● **S60.469**   Insect bite (nonvenomous) of unspecified finger

● S60.47   **Other superficial bite of fingers**
     Excludes1   open bite of fingers (S61.25-, S61.35-)
   ● S60.470   Other superficial bite of right index finger
   ● S60.471   Other superficial bite of left index finger
   ● S60.472   Other superficial bite of right middle finger
   ● S60.473   Other superficial bite of left middle finger
   ● S60.474   Other superficial bite of right ring finger
   ● S60.475   Other superficial bite of left ring finger
   ● S60.476   Other superficial bite of right little finger
   ● S60.477   Other superficial bite of left little finger
   ● S60.478   Other superficial bite of other finger
       Other superficial bite of specified finger with unspecified laterality
   ● S60.479   Other superficial bite of unspecified finger

● S60.5   **Other superficial injuries of hand**
     Excludes2   superficial injuries of fingers (S60.3-, S60.4-)
 ● S60.51   **Abrasion of hand**
   ● S60.511   Abrasion of right hand
   ● S60.512   Abrasion of left hand
   ● S60.519   Abrasion of unspecified hand
 ● S60.52   **Blister (nonthermal) of hand**
   ● S60.521   Blister (nonthermal) of right hand
   ● S60.522   Blister (nonthermal) of left hand
   ● S60.529   Blister (nonthermal) of unspecified hand
 ● S60.54   **External constriction of hand**
   ● S60.541   External constriction of right hand
   ● S60.542   External constriction of left hand
   ● S60.549   External constriction of unspecified hand
 ● S60.55   **Superficial foreign body of hand**
     Splinter in the hand
   ● S60.551   Superficial foreign body of right hand
   ● S60.552   Superficial foreign body of left hand
   ● S60.559   Superficial foreign body of unspecified hand
 ● S60.56   **Insect bite (nonvenomous) of hand**
   ● S60.561   Insect bite (nonvenomous) of right hand
   ● S60.562   Insect bite (nonvenomous) of left hand
   ● S60.569   Insect bite (nonvenomous) of unspecified hand
 ● S60.57   **Other superficial bite of hand**
     Excludes1   open bite of hand (S61.45-)
   ● S60.571   Other superficial bite of hand of right hand
   ● S60.572   Other superficial bite of hand of left hand
   ● S60.579   Other superficial bite of hand of unspecified hand

● S60.8   **Other superficial injuries of wrist**
 ● S60.81   **Abrasion of wrist**
   ● S60.811   Abrasion of right wrist
   ● S60.812   Abrasion of left wrist
   ● S60.819   Abrasion of unspecified wrist
 ● S60.82   **Blister (nonthermal) of wrist**
   ● S60.821   Blister (nonthermal) of right wrist
   ● S60.822   Blister (nonthermal) of left wrist
   ● S60.829   Blister (nonthermal) of unspecified wrist
 ● S60.84   **External constriction of wrist**
   ● S60.841   External constriction of right wrist
   ● S60.842   External constriction of left wrist
   ● S60.849   External constriction of unspecified wrist
 ● S60.85   **Superficial foreign body of wrist**
     Splinter in the wrist
   ● S60.851   Superficial foreign body of right wrist
   ● S60.852   Superficial foreign body of left wrist
   ● S60.859   Superficial foreign body of unspecified wrist
 ● S60.86   **Insect bite (nonvenomous) of wrist**
   ● S60.861   Insect bite (nonvenomous) of right wrist
   ● S60.862   Insect bite (nonvenomous) of left wrist
   ● S60.869   Insect bite (nonvenomous) of unspecified wrist
 ● S60.87   **Other superficial bite of wrist**
     Excludes1   open bite of wrist (S61.55)
   ● S60.871   Other superficial bite of right wrist
   ● S60.872   Other superficial bite of left wrist
   ● S60.879   Other superficial bite of unspecified wrist

● S60.9   **Unspecified superficial injury of wrist, hand and fingers**
 ● S60.91   **Unspecified superficial injury of wrist**
   ● S60.911   Unspecified superficial injury of right wrist
   ● S60.912   Unspecified superficial injury of left wrist
   ● S60.919   Unspecified superficial injury of unspecified wrist
 ● S60.92   **Unspecified superficial injury of hand**
   ● S60.921   Unspecified superficial injury of right hand
   ● S60.922   Unspecified superficial injury of left hand
   ● S60.929   Unspecified superficial injury of unspecified hand
 ● S60.93   **Unspecified superficial injury of thumb**
   ● S60.931   Unspecified superficial injury of right thumb
   ● S60.932   Unspecified superficial injury of left thumb
   ● S60.939   Unspecified superficial injury of unspecified thumb

CHAPTER 19 (S00-T88)

N Newborn Age: 0   P Pediatric Age: 0–17   M Maternity DX: 12–55   A Adult Age: 15–124   ♀ Females Only   ♂ Males Only
  Complication\Comorbidity   Major C\C   Ⓔₓ CC/MCC Exclusions   Hospital-Acquired Condition

1319

● **S60.94** Unspecified superficial injury of other fingers

● **S60.940** Unspecified superficial injury of right index finger

● **S60.941** Unspecified superficial injury of left index finger

● **S60.942** Unspecified superficial injury of right middle finger

● **S60.943** Unspecified superficial injury of left middle finger

● **S60.944** Unspecified superficial injury of right ring finger

● **S60.945** Unspecified superficial injury of left ring finger

● **S60.946** Unspecified superficial injury of right little finger

● **S60.947** Unspecified superficial injury of left little finger

● **S60.948** Unspecified superficial injury of other finger

Unspecified superficial injury of specified finger with unspecified laterality

● **S60.949** Unspecified superficial injury of unspecified finger

● **S61** Open wound of wrist, hand and fingers

Code also any associated wound infection

Excludes1 open fracture of wrist, hand and finger (S62.- with 7th character B)

traumatic amputation of wrist and hand (S68.-)

The appropriate 7th character is to be added to each code from category S61

A initial encounter
D subsequent encounter
S sequela

● **S61.0** Open wound of thumb without damage to nail

Excludes1 open wound of thumb with damage to nail (S61.1-)

● **S61.00** Unspecified open wound of thumb without damage to nail

● **S61.001** Unspecified open wound of right thumb without damage to nail

● **S61.002** Unspecified open wound of left thumb without damage to nail

● **S61.009** Unspecified open wound of unspecified thumb without damage to nail

● **S61.01** Laceration without foreign body of thumb without damage to nail

● **S61.011** Laceration without foreign body of right thumb without damage to nail

● **S61.012** Laceration without foreign body of left thumb without damage to nail

● **S61.019** Laceration without foreign body of unspecified thumb without damage to nail

● **S61.02** Laceration with foreign body of thumb without damage to nail

● **S61.021** Laceration with foreign body of right thumb without damage to nail

● **S61.022** Laceration with foreign body of left thumb without damage to nail

● **S61.029** Laceration with foreign body of unspecified thumb without damage to nail

● **S61.03** Puncture wound without foreign body of thumb without damage to nail

● **S61.031** Puncture wound without foreign body of right thumb without damage to nail

● **S61.032** Puncture wound without foreign body of left thumb without damage to nail

● **S61.039** Puncture wound without foreign body of unspecified thumb without damage to nail

● **S61.04** Puncture wound with foreign body of thumb without damage to nail

● **S61.041** Puncture wound with foreign body of right thumb without damage to nail

● **S61.042** Puncture wound with foreign body of left thumb without damage to nail

● **S61.049** Puncture wound with foreign body of unspecified thumb without damage to nail

● **S61.05** Open bite of thumb without damage to nail

Bite of thumb NOS

Excludes1 superficial bite of thumb (S60.36-, S60.37-)

● **S61.051** Open bite of right thumb without damage to nail

● **S61.052** Open bite of left thumb without damage to nail

● **S61.059** Open bite of unspecified thumb without damage to nail

● **S61.1** Open wound of thumb with damage to nail

● **S61.10** Unspecified open wound of thumb with damage to nail

● **S61.101** Unspecified open wound of right thumb with damage to nail

● **S61.102** Unspecified open wound of left thumb with damage to nail

● **S61.109** Unspecified open wound of unspecified thumb with damage to nail

● **S61.11** Laceration without foreign body of thumb with damage to nail

● **S61.111** Laceration without foreign body of right thumb with damage to nail

● **S61.112** Laceration without foreign body of left thumb with damage to nail

● **S61.119** Laceration without foreign body of unspecified thumb with damage to nail

● **S61.12** Laceration with foreign body of thumb with damage to nail

● **S61.121** Laceration with foreign body of right thumb with damage to nail

● **S61.122** Laceration with foreign body of left thumb with damage to nail

● **S61.129** Laceration with foreign body of unspecified thumb with damage to nail

● **S61.13** Puncture wound without foreign body of thumb with damage to nail

● **S61.131** Puncture wound without foreign body of right thumb with damage to nail

● **S61.132** Puncture wound without foreign body of left thumb with damage to nail

● **S61.139** Puncture wound without foreign body of unspecified thumb with damage to nail

● **S61.14**   **Puncture wound with foreign body of thumb with damage to nail**

   ● **S61.141**   Puncture wound with foreign body of right thumb with damage to nail

   ● **S61.142**   Puncture wound with foreign body of left thumb with damage to nail

   ● **S61.149**   Puncture wound with foreign body of unspecified thumb with damage to nail

● **S61.15**   **Open bite of thumb with damage to nail**
      Bite of thumb with damage to nail NOS

     Excludes1   superficial bite of thumb (S60.36-, S60.37-)

   ● **S61.151**   Open bite of right thumb with damage to nail

   ● **S61.152**   Open bite of left thumb with damage to nail

   ● **S61.159**   Open bite of unspecified thumb with damage to nail

● **S61.2**   **Open wound of other finger without damage to nail**

     Excludes1   open wound of finger involving nail (matrix) (S61.3-)

     Excludes2   open wound of thumb without damage to nail (S61.0-)

  ● **S61.20**   **Unspecified open wound of other finger without damage to nail**

   ● **S61.200**   Unspecified open wound of right index finger without damage to nail

   ● **S61.201**   Unspecified open wound of left index finger without damage to nail

   ● **S61.202**   Unspecified open wound of right middle finger without damage to nail

   ● **S61.203**   Unspecified open wound of left middle finger without damage to nail

   ● **S61.204**   Unspecified open wound of right ring finger without damage to nail

   ● **S61.205**   Unspecified open wound of left ring finger without damage to nail

   ● **S61.206**   Unspecified open wound of right little finger without damage to nail

   ● **S61.207**   Unspecified open wound of left little finger without damage to nail

   ● **S61.208**   Unspecified open wound of other finger without damage to nail
      Unspecified open wound of specified finger with unspecified laterality without damage to nail

   ● **S61.209**   Unspecified open wound of unspecified finger without damage to nail

  ● **S61.21**   **Laceration without foreign body of finger without damage to nail**

   ● **S61.210**   Laceration without foreign body of right index finger without damage to nail

   ● **S61.211**   Laceration without foreign body of left index finger without damage to nail

   ● **S61.212**   Laceration without foreign body of right middle finger without damage to nail

   ● **S61.213**   Laceration without foreign body of left middle finger without damage to nail

   ● **S61.214**   Laceration without foreign body of right ring finger without damage to nail

   ● **S61.215**   Laceration without foreign body of left ring finger without damage to nail

   ● **S61.216**   Laceration without foreign body of right little finger without damage to nail

   ● **S61.217**   Laceration without foreign body of left little finger without damage to nail

   ● **S61.218**   Laceration without foreign body of other finger without damage to nail
      Laceration without foreign body of specified finger with unspecified laterality without damage to nail

   ● **S61.219**   Laceration without foreign body of unspecified finger without damage to nail

  ● **S61.22**   **Laceration with foreign body of finger without damage to nail**

   ● **S61.220**   Laceration with foreign body of right index finger without damage to nail

   ● **S61.221**   Laceration with foreign body of left index finger without damage to nail

   ● **S61.222**   Laceration with foreign body of right middle finger without damage to nail

   ● **S61.223**   Laceration with foreign body of left middle finger without damage to nail

   ● **S61.224**   Laceration with foreign body of right ring finger without damage to nail

   ● **S61.225**   Laceration with foreign body of left ring finger without damage to nail

   ● **S61.226**   Laceration with foreign body of right little finger without damage to nail

   ● **S61.227**   Laceration with foreign body of left little finger without damage to nail

   ● **S61.228**   Laceration with foreign body of other finger without damage to nail
      Laceration with foreign body of specified finger with unspecified laterality without damage to nail

   ● **S61.229**   Laceration with foreign body of unspecified finger without damage to nail

  ● **S61.23**   **Puncture wound without foreign body of finger without damage to nail**

   ● **S61.230**   Puncture wound without foreign body of right index finger without damage to nail

   ● **S61.231**   Puncture wound without foreign body of left index finger without damage to nail

   ● **S61.232**   Puncture wound without foreign body of right middle finger without damage to nail

   ● **S61.233**   Puncture wound without foreign body of left middle finger without damage to nail

   ● **S61.234**   Puncture wound without foreign body of right ring finger without damage to nail

   ● **S61.235**   Puncture wound without foreign body of left ring finger without damage to nail

   ● **S61.236**   Puncture wound without foreign body of right little finger without damage to nail

   ● **S61.237**   Puncture wound without foreign body of left little finger without damage to nail

   ● **S61.238**   Puncture wound without foreign body of other finger without damage to nail
      Puncture wound without foreign body of specified finger with unspecified laterality without damage to nail

   ● **S61.239**   Puncture wound without foreign body of unspecified finger without damage to nail

CHAPTER 19 (S00-T88)

● **S61.24** **Puncture wound with foreign body of finger without damage to nail**

   ● **S61.240** Puncture wound with foreign body of **right index** finger without damage to nail

   ● **S61.241** Puncture wound with foreign body of **left index** finger without damage to nail

   ● **S61.242** Puncture wound with foreign body of **right middle** finger without damage to nail

   ● **S61.243** Puncture wound with foreign body of **left middle** finger without damage to nail

   ● **S61.244** Puncture wound with foreign body of **right ring** finger without damage to nail

   ● **S61.245** Puncture wound with foreign body of **left ring** finger without damage to nail

   ● **S61.246** Puncture wound with foreign body of **right little** finger without damage to nail

   ● **S61.247** Puncture wound with foreign body of **left little** finger without damage to nail

   ● **S61.248** Puncture wound with foreign body of **other** finger without damage to nail

      Puncture wound with foreign body of specified finger with unspecified laterality without damage to nail

   ● **S61.249** Puncture wound with foreign body of **unspecified** finger without damage to nail

● **S61.25** **Open bite of finger without damage to nail**

   Bite of finger without damage to nail NOS

   Excludes1 superficial bite of finger (S60.46-, S60.47-)

   ● **S61.250** Open bite of **right index** finger without damage to nail

   ● **S61.251** Open bite of **left index** finger without damage to nail

   ● **S61.252** Open bite of **right middle** finger without damage to nail

   ● **S61.253** Open bite of **left middle** finger without damage to nail

   ● **S61.254** Open bite of **right ring** finger without damage to nail

   ● **S61.255** Open bite of **left ring** finger without damage to nail

   ● **S61.256** Open bite of **right little** finger without damage to nail

   ● **S61.257** Open bite of **left little** finger without damage to nail

   ● **S61.258** Open bite of **other** finger without damage to nail

      Open bite of specified finger with unspecified laterality without damage to nail

   ● **S61.259** Open bite of **unspecified** finger without damage to nail

● **S61.3** **Open wound of other finger with damage to nail**

   ● **S61.30** **Unspecified open wound of finger with damage to nail**

      ● **S61.300** Unspecified open wound of **right index** finger with damage to nail

      ● **S61.301** Unspecified open wound of **left index** finger with damage to nail

      ● **S61.302** Unspecified open wound of **right middle** finger with damage to nail

      ● **S61.303** Unspecified open wound of **left middle** finger with damage to nail

      ● **S61.304** Unspecified open wound of **right ring** finger with damage to nail

      ● **S61.305** Unspecified open wound of **left ring** finger with damage to nail

      ● **S61.306** Unspecified open wound of **right little** finger with damage to nail

      ● **S61.307** Unspecified open wound of **left little** finger with damage to nail

      ● **S61.308** Unspecified open wound of **other** finger with damage to nail

         Unspecified open wound of specified finger with unspecified laterality with damage to nail

      ● **S61.309** Unspecified open wound of **unspecified** finger with damage to nail

   ● **S61.31** **Laceration without foreign body of finger with damage to nail**

      ● **S61.310** Laceration without foreign body of **right index** finger with damage to nail

      ● **S61.311** Laceration without foreign body of **left index** finger with damage to nail

      ● **S61.312** Laceration without foreign body of **right middle** finger with damage to nail

      ● **S61.313** Laceration without foreign body of **left middle** finger with damage to nail

      ● **S61.314** Laceration without foreign body of **right ring** finger with damage to nail

      ● **S61.315** Laceration without foreign body of **left ring** finger with damage to nail

      ● **S61.316** Laceration without foreign body of **right little** finger with damage to nail

      ● **S61.317** Laceration without foreign body of **left little** finger with damage to nail

      ● **S61.318** Laceration without foreign body of **other** finger with damage to nail

         Laceration without foreign body of specified finger with unspecified laterality with damage to nail

      ● **S61.319** Laceration without foreign body of **unspecified** finger with damage to nail

   ● **S61.32** **Laceration with foreign body of finger with damage to nail**

      ● **S61.320** Laceration with foreign body of **right index** finger with damage to nail

      ● **S61.321** Laceration with foreign body of **left index** finger with damage to nail

      ● **S61.322** Laceration with foreign body of **right middle** finger with damage to nail

● S61.323   Laceration with foreign body of left middle finger with damage to nail

● S61.324   Laceration with foreign body of right ring finger with damage to nail

● S61.325   Laceration with foreign body of left ring finger with damage to nail

● S61.326   Laceration with foreign body of right little finger with damage to nail

● S61.327   Laceration with foreign body of left little finger with damage to nail

● S61.328   Laceration with foreign body of other finger with damage to nail
Laceration with foreign body of specified finger with unspecified laterality with damage to nail

● S61.329   Laceration with foreign body of unspecified finger with damage to nail

● S61.33   **Puncture wound without foreign body of finger with damage to nail**

● S61.330   Puncture wound without foreign body of right index finger with damage to nail

● S61.331   Puncture wound without foreign body of left index finger with damage to nail

● S61.332   Puncture wound without foreign body of right middle finger with damage to nail

● S61.333   Puncture wound without foreign body of left middle finger with damage to nail

● S61.334   Puncture wound without foreign body of right ring finger with damage to nail

● S61.335   Puncture wound without foreign body of left ring finger with damage to nail

● S61.336   Puncture wound without foreign body of right little finger with damage to nail

● S61.337   Puncture wound without foreign body of left little finger with damage to nail

● S61.338   Puncture wound without foreign body of other finger with damage to nail
Puncture wound without foreign body of specified finger with unspecified laterality with damage to nail

● S61.339   Puncture wound without foreign body of unspecified finger with damage to nail

● S61.34   **Puncture wound with foreign body of finger with damage to nail**

● S61.340   Puncture wound with foreign body of right index finger with damage to nail

● S61.341   Puncture wound with foreign body of left index finger with damage to nail

● S61.342   Puncture wound with foreign body of right middle finger with damage to nail

● S61.343   Puncture wound with foreign body of left middle finger with damage to nail

● S61.344   Puncture wound with foreign body of right ring finger with damage to nail

● S61.345   Puncture wound with foreign body of left ring finger with damage to nail

● S61.346   Puncture wound with foreign body of right little finger with damage to nail

● S61.347   Puncture wound with foreign body of left little finger with damage to nail

● S61.348   Puncture wound with foreign body of other finger with damage to nail
Puncture wound with foreign body of specified finger with unspecified laterality with damage to nail

● S61.349   Puncture wound with foreign body of unspecified finger with damage to nail

● S61.35   **Open bite of finger with damage to nail**
Bite of finger with damage to nail NOS

    Excludes1   superficial bite of finger (S60.46-, S60.47-)

● S61.350   Open bite of right index finger with damage to nail

● S61.351   Open bite of left index finger with damage to nail

● S61.352   Open bite of right middle finger with damage to nail

● S61.353   Open bite of left middle finger with damage to nail

● S61.354   Open bite of right ring finger with damage to nail

● S61.355   Open bite of left ring finger with damage to nail

● S61.356   Open bite of right little finger with damage to nail

● S61.357   Open bite of left little finger with damage to nail

● S61.358   Open bite of other finger with damage to nail
Open bite of specified finger with unspecified laterality with damage to nail

● S61.359   Open bite of unspecified finger with damage to nail

● S61.4   **Open wound of hand**

● S61.40   **Unspecified open wound of hand**

● S61.401   Unspecified open wound of right hand

● S61.402   Unspecified open wound of left hand

● S61.409   Unspecified open wound of unspecified hand

● S61.41   **Laceration without foreign body of hand**

● S61.411   Laceration without foreign body of right hand

● S61.412   Laceration without foreign body of left hand

● S61.419   Laceration without foreign body of unspecified hand

● S61.42   **Laceration with foreign body of hand**

● S61.421   Laceration with foreign body of right hand

● S61.422   Laceration with foreign body of left hand

● S61.429   Laceration with foreign body of unspecified hand

● S61.43   **Puncture wound without foreign body of hand**
  ● S61.431   Puncture wound without foreign body of **right** hand
  ● S61.432   Puncture wound without foreign body of **left** hand
  ● S61.439   Puncture wound without foreign body of **unspecified** hand
● S61.44   **Puncture wound with foreign body of hand**
  ● S61.441   Puncture wound with foreign body of **right** hand
  ● S61.442   Puncture wound with foreign body of **left** hand
  ● S61.449   Puncture wound with foreign body of **unspecified** hand
● S61.45   **Open bite of hand**
    Bite of hand NOS
    Excludes1   superficial bite of hand (S60.56-, S60.57-)
  ● S61.451   Open bite of **right** hand
  ● S61.452   Open bite of **left** hand
  ● S61.459   Open bite of **unspecified** hand
● S61.5   **Open wound of wrist**
  ● S61.50   **Unspecified open wound of wrist**
    ● S61.501   Unspecified open wound of **right** wrist
    ● S61.502   Unspecified open wound of **left** wrist
    ● S61.509   Unspecified open wound of **unspecified** wrist
  ● S61.51   **Laceration without foreign body of wrist**
    ● S61.511   Laceration without foreign body of **right** wrist
    ● S61.512   Laceration without foreign body of **left** wrist
    ● S61.519   Laceration without foreign body of **unspecified** wrist
  ● S61.52   **Laceration with foreign body of wrist**
    ● S61.521   Laceration with foreign body of **right** wrist
    ● S61.522   Laceration with foreign body of **left** wrist
    ● S61.529   Laceration with foreign body of **unspecified** wrist
  ● S61.53   **Puncture wound without foreign body of wrist**
    ● S61.531   Puncture wound without foreign body of **right** wrist
    ● S61.532   Puncture wound without foreign body of **left** wrist
    ● S61.539   Puncture wound without foreign body of **unspecified** wrist
  ● S61.54   **Puncture wound with foreign body of wrist**
    ● S61.541   Puncture wound with foreign body of **right** wrist
    ● S61.542   Puncture wound with foreign body of **left** wrist
    ● S61.549   Puncture wound with foreign body of **unspecified** wrist
  ● S61.55   **Open bite of wrist**
    Bite of wrist NOS
    Excludes1   superficial bite of wrist (S60.86-, S60.87-)
    ● S61.551   Open bite of **right** wrist
    ● S61.552   Open bite of **left** wrist
    ● S61.559   Open bite of **unspecified** wrist

● S62   **Fracture at wrist and hand level**
  Note: A fracture not indicated as displaced or nondisplaced should be coded to displaced
    A fracture not indicated as open or closed should be coded to closed
  Excludes1   traumatic amputation of wrist and hand (S68.-)
  Excludes2   fracture of distal parts of ulna and radius (S52.-)
  The appropriate 7th character is to be added to each code from category S62

> A   initial encounter for closed fracture
> B   initial encounter for open fracture
> D   subsequent encounter for fracture with routine healing
> G   subsequent encounter for fracture with delayed healing
> K   subsequent encounter for fracture with nonunion
> P   subsequent encounter for fracture with malunion
> S   sequela

● S62.0   **Fracture of navicular [scaphoid] bone of wrist**
  (Ex) For category S62.0 CC codes S62.0[B]: See PDX Collection 1283
    For S62.0[K,P]: See PDX Collection 897
  ● S62.00   **Unspecified fracture of navicular [scaphoid] bone of wrist**
    ● S62.001   Unspecified fracture of navicular [scaphoid] bone of **right** wrist B, K, P ● B ●
    ● S62.002   Unspecified fracture of navicular [scaphoid] bone of **left** wrist B, K, P ● B ●
        Coding Clinic: 2012, Q4, P106
    ● S62.009   Unspecified fracture of navicular [scaphoid] bone of **unspecified** wrist B, K, P ● B ●
  ● S62.01   **Fracture of distal pole of navicular [scaphoid] bone of wrist**
    Fracture of volar tuberosity of navicular [scaphoid] bone of wrist
    ● S62.011   Displaced fracture of distal pole of navicular [scaphoid] bone of **right** wrist B, K, P ● B ●
    ● S62.012   Displaced fracture of distal pole of navicular [scaphoid] bone of **left** wrist B, K, P ● B ●
    ● S62.013   Displaced fracture of distal pole of navicular [scaphoid] bone of **unspecified** wrist B, K, P ● B ●
    ● S62.014   Nondisplaced fracture of distal pole of navicular [scaphoid] bone of **right** wrist B, K, P ● B ●
    ● S62.015   Nondisplaced fracture of distal pole of navicular [scaphoid] bone of **left** wrist B, K, P ● B ●
    ● S62.016   Nondisplaced fracture of distal pole of navicular [scaphoid] bone of **unspecified** wrist B, K, P ● B ●
  ● S62.02   **Fracture of middle third of navicular [scaphoid] bone of wrist**
    ● S62.021   Displaced fracture of middle third of navicular [scaphoid] bone of **right** wrist B, K, P ● B ●
    ● S62.022   Displaced fracture of middle third of navicular [scaphoid] bone of **left** wrist B, K, P ● B ●
    ● S62.023   Displaced fracture of middle third of navicular [scaphoid] bone of **unspecified** wrist B, K, P ● B ●
    ● S62.024   Nondisplaced fracture of middle third of navicular [scaphoid] bone of **right** wrist B, K, P ● B ●
    ● S62.025   Nondisplaced fracture of middle third of navicular [scaphoid] bone of **left** wrist B, K, P ● B ●
    ● S62.026   Nondisplaced fracture of middle third of navicular [scaphoid] bone of **unspecified** wrist B, K, P ● B ●

▶ New   ⇒ Revised   ~~deleted~~ Deleted   Excludes 1   Excludes 2   Includes   Use additional   Code first   Code also   Key words
OGCR Official Guidelines   ● Unacceptable Principal Diagnosis   X Assign placeholder X   ● Use Additional Character(s)   ▲ Manifestation Code   **Coding Clinic**

● S62.03　Fracture of proximal third of navicular [scaphoid] bone of wrist

　● S62.031　Displaced fracture of proximal third of navicular [scaphoid] bone of right wrist B, K, P 🔿, B 🔿

　● S62.032　Displaced fracture of proximal third of navicular [scaphoid] bone of left wrist B, K, P 🔿, B 🔿

　● S62.033　Displaced fracture of proximal third of navicular [scaphoid] bone of unspecified wrist B, K, P 🔿, B 🔿

　● S62.034　Nondisplaced fracture of proximal third of navicular [scaphoid] bone of right wrist B, K, P 🔿, B 🔿

　● S62.035　Nondisplaced fracture of proximal third of navicular [scaphoid] bone of left wrist B, K, P 🔿, B 🔿

　● S62.036　Nondisplaced fracture of proximal third of navicular [scaphoid] bone of unspecified wrist B, K, P 🔿, B 🔿

● S62.1　Fracture of other and unspecified carpal bone(s)

　　Excludes2　fracture of scaphoid of wrist (S62.0-)

　　Ⓔⓧ **For category S62.1 CC codes S62.1[B]:** See PDX Collection 1283
　　For S62.0[K,P]: See PDX Collection 897

　● S62.10　Fracture of unspecified carpal bone
　　　Fracture of wrist NOS

　　● S62.101　Fracture of unspecified carpal bone, right wrist B, K, P 🔿, B 🔿

　　● S62.102　Fracture of unspecified carpal bone, left wrist B, K, P 🔿, B 🔿
　　　　Coding Clinic: 2012, Q4, P95

　　● S62.109　Fracture of unspecified carpal bone, unspecified wrist B, K, P 🔿, B 🔿

　● S62.11　Fracture of triquetrum [cuneiform] bone of wrist

　　● S62.111　Displaced fracture of triquetrum [cuneiform] bone, right wrist B, K, P 🔿, B 🔿

　　● S62.112　Displaced fracture of triquetrum [cuneiform] bone, left wrist B, K, P 🔿, B 🔿

　　● S62.113　Displaced fracture of triquetrum [cuneiform] bone, unspecified wrist B, K, P 🔿, B 🔿

　　● S62.114　Nondisplaced fracture of triquetrum [cuneiform] bone, right wrist B, K, P 🔿, B 🔿

　　● S62.115　Nondisplaced fracture of triquetrum [cuneiform] bone, left wrist B, K, P 🔿, B 🔿

　　● S62.116　Nondisplaced fracture of triquetrum [cuneiform] bone, unspecified wrist B, K, P 🔿, B 🔿

　● S62.12　Fracture of lunate [semilunar]

　　● S62.121　Displaced fracture of lunate [semilunar], right wrist B, K, P 🔿, B 🔿

　　● S62.122　Displaced fracture of lunate [semilunar], left wrist B, K, P 🔿, B 🔿

　　● S62.123　Displaced fracture of lunate [semilunar], unspecified wrist B, K, P 🔿, B 🔿

　　● S62.124　Nondisplaced fracture of lunate [semilunar], right wrist B, K, P 🔿, B 🔿

　　● S62.125　Nondisplaced fracture of lunate [semilunar], left wrist B, K, P 🔿, B 🔿

　　● S62.126　Nondisplaced fracture of lunate [semilunar], unspecified wrist B, K, P 🔿, B 🔿

● S62.13　Fracture of capitate [os magnum] bone

　● S62.131　Displaced fracture of capitate [os magnum] bone, right wrist B, K, P 🔿, B 🔿

　● S62.132　Displaced fracture of capitate [os magnum] bone, left wrist B, K, P 🔿, B 🔿

　● S62.133　Displaced fracture of capitate [os magnum] bone, unspecified wrist B, K, P 🔿, B 🔿

　● S62.134　Nondisplaced fracture of capitate [os magnum] bone, right wrist B, K, P 🔿, B 🔿

　● S62.135　Nondisplaced fracture of capitate [os magnum] bone, left wrist B, K, P 🔿, B 🔿

　● S62.136　Nondisplaced fracture of capitate [os magnum] bone, unspecified wrist B, K, P 🔿, B 🔿

● S62.14　Fracture of body of hamate [unciform] bone
　　Fracture of hamate [unciform] bone NOS

　● S62.141　Displaced fracture of body of hamate [unciform] bone, right wrist B, K, P 🔿, B 🔿

　● S62.142　Displaced fracture of body of hamate [unciform] bone, left wrist B, K, P 🔿, B 🔿

　● S62.143　Displaced fracture of body of hamate [unciform] bone, unspecified wrist B, K, P 🔿, B 🔿

　● S62.144　Nondisplaced fracture of body of hamate [unciform] bone, right wrist B, K, P 🔿, B 🔿

　● S62.145　Nondisplaced fracture of body of hamate [unciform] bone, left wrist B, K, P 🔿, B 🔿

　● S62.146　Nondisplaced fracture of body of hamate [unciform] bone, unspecified wrist B, K, P 🔿, B 🔿

● S62.15　Fracture of hook process of hamate [unciform] bone
　　Fracture of unciform process of hamate [unciform] bone

　● S62.151　Displaced fracture of hook process of hamate [unciform] bone, right wrist B, K, P 🔿, B 🔿

　● S62.152　Displaced fracture of hook process of hamate [unciform] bone, left wrist B, K, P 🔿, B 🔿

　● S62.153　Displaced fracture of hook process of hamate [unciform] bone, unspecified wrist B, K, P 🔿, B 🔿

　● S62.154　Nondisplaced fracture of hook process of hamate [unciform] bone, right wrist B, K, P 🔿, B 🔿

　● S62.155　Nondisplaced fracture of hook process of hamate [unciform] bone, left wrist B, K, P 🔿, B 🔿

　● S62.156　Nondisplaced fracture of hook process of hamate [unciform] bone, unspecified wrist B, K, P 🔿, B 🔿

● S62.16　Fracture of pisiform

　● S62.161　Displaced fracture of pisiform, right wrist B, K, P 🔿, B 🔿

　● S62.162　Displaced fracture of pisiform, left wrist B, K, P 🔿, B 🔿

　● S62.163　Displaced fracture of pisiform, unspecified wrist B, K, P 🔿, B 🔿

　● S62.164　Nondisplaced fracture of pisiform, right wrist B, K, P 🔿, B 🔿

　● S62.165　Nondisplaced fracture of pisiform, left wrist B, K, P 🔿, B 🔿

　● S62.166　Nondisplaced fracture of pisiform, unspecified wrist B, K, P 🔿, B 🔿

CHAPTER 19 (S00-T88)

N　Newborn Age: 0　　P　Pediatric Age: 0–17　　M　Maternity DX: 12–55　　A　Adult Age: 15–124　　♀　Females Only　　♂　Males Only

🔿　Complication\Comorbidity　　🔿　Major C\C　　Ⓔⓧ　CC/MCC Exclusions　　🔿　Hospital-Acquired Condition

● **S62.17**   Fracture of trapezium [larger multangular]

    ● **S62.171**   Displaced fracture of trapezium [larger multangular], right wrist
      B, K, P ☟, B ☟

    ● **S62.172**   Displaced fracture of trapezium [larger multangular], left wrist
      B, K, P ☟, B ☟

    ● **S62.173**   Displaced fracture of trapezium [larger multangular], unspecified wrist B, K, P ☟, B ☟

    ● **S62.174**   Nondisplaced fracture of trapezium [larger multangular], right wrist
      B, K, P ☟, B ☟

    ● **S62.175**   Nondisplaced fracture of trapezium [larger multangular], left wrist
      B, K, P ☟, B ☟

    ● **S62.176**   Nondisplaced fracture of trapezium [larger multangular], unspecified wrist B, K, P ☟, B ☟

● **S62.18**   Fracture of trapezoid [smaller multangular]

    ● **S62.181**   Displaced fracture of trapezoid [smaller multangular], right wrist
      B, K, P ☟, B ☟

    ● **S62.182**   Displaced fracture of trapezoid [smaller multangular], left wrist
      B, K, P ☟, B ☟

    ● **S62.183**   Displaced fracture of trapezoid [smaller multangular], unspecified wrist B, K, P ☟, B ☟

    ● **S62.184**   Nondisplaced fracture of trapezoid [smaller multangular], right wrist
      B, K, P ☟, B ☟

    ● **S62.185**   Nondisplaced fracture of trapezoid [smaller multangular], left wrist
      B, K, P ☟, B ☟

    ● **S62.186**   Nondisplaced fracture of trapezoid [smaller multangular], unspecified wrist B, K, P ☟, B ☟

● **S62.2**   Fracture of first metacarpal bone

    Ex⃝ For category S62.2 CC codes S62.2[B]: See PDX Collection 1284
    For S62.2[K,P]: See PDX Collection 897

    ● **S62.20**   Unspecified fracture of first metacarpal bone

      ● **S62.201**   Unspecified fracture of first metacarpal bone, right hand
        B, K, P ☟, B ☟

      ● **S62.202**   Unspecified fracture of first metacarpal bone, left hand B, K, P ☟, B ☟

      ● **S62.209**   Unspecified fracture of first metacarpal bone, unspecified hand
        B, K, P ☟, B ☟

    ● **S62.21**   Bennett's fracture

      ● **S62.211**   Bennett's fracture, right hand
        B, K, P ☟, B ☟

      ● **S62.212**   Bennett's fracture, left hand B, K, P ☟, B ☟

      ● **S62.213**   Bennett's fracture, unspecified hand
        B, K, P ☟, B ☟

    ● **S62.22**   Rolando's fracture

      ● **S62.221**   Displaced Rolando's fracture, right hand B, K, P ☟, B ☟

      ● **S62.222**   Displaced Rolando's fracture, left hand B, K, P ☟, B ☟

      ● **S62.223**   Displaced Rolando's fracture, unspecified hand B, K, P ☟, B ☟

      ● **S62.224**   Nondisplaced Rolando's fracture, right hand B, K, P ☟, B ☟

      ● **S62.225**   Nondisplaced Rolando's fracture, left hand B, K, P ☟, B ☟

      ● **S62.226**   Nondisplaced Rolando's fracture, unspecified hand B, K, P ☟, B ☟

● **S62.23**   Other fracture of base of first metacarpal bone

    ● **S62.231**   Other displaced fracture of base of first metacarpal bone, right hand
      B, K, P ☟, B ☟

    ● **S62.232**   Other displaced fracture of base of first metacarpal bone, left hand
      B, K, P ☟, B ☟

    ● **S62.233**   Other displaced fracture of base of first metacarpal bone, unspecified hand B, K, P ☟, B ☟

    ● **S62.234**   Other nondisplaced fracture of base of first metacarpal bone, right hand
      B, K, P ☟, B ☟

    ● **S62.235**   Other nondisplaced fracture of base of first metacarpal bone, left hand
      B, K, P ☟, B ☟

    ● **S62.236**   Other nondisplaced fracture of base of first metacarpal bone, unspecified hand B, K, P ☟, B ☟

● **S62.24**   Fracture of shaft of first metacarpal bone

    ● **S62.241**   Displaced fracture of shaft of first metacarpal bone, right hand
      B, K, P ☟, B ☟

    ● **S62.242**   Displaced fracture of shaft of first metacarpal bone, left hand B, K, P ☟,
      B ☟

    ● **S62.243**   Displaced fracture of shaft of first metacarpal bone, unspecified hand
      B, K, P ☟, B ☟

    ● **S62.244**   Nondisplaced fracture of shaft of first metacarpal bone, right hand
      B, K, P ☟, B ☟

    ● **S62.245**   Nondisplaced fracture of shaft of first metacarpal bone, left hand B, K, P ☟,
      B ☟

    ● **S62.246**   Nondisplaced fracture of shaft of first metacarpal bone, unspecified hand
      B, K, P ☟, B ☟

● **S62.25**   Fracture of neck of first metacarpal bone

    ● **S62.251**   Displaced fracture of neck of first metacarpal bone, right hand
      B, K, P ☟, B ☟

    ● **S62.252**   Displaced fracture of neck of first metacarpal bone, left hand B, K, P ☟,
      B ☟

    ● **S62.253**   Displaced fracture of neck of first metacarpal bone, unspecified hand
      B, K, P ☟, B ☟

    ● **S62.254**   Nondisplaced fracture of neck of first metacarpal bone, right hand
      B, K, P ☟, B ☟

    ● **S62.255**   Nondisplaced fracture of neck of first metacarpal bone, left hand B, K, P ☟,
      B ☟

    ● **S62.256**   Nondisplaced fracture of neck of first metacarpal bone, unspecified hand
      B, K, P ☟, B ☟

● **S62.29**   Other fracture of first metacarpal bone

    ● **S62.291**   Other fracture of first metacarpal bone, right hand B, K, P ☟, B ☟

    ● **S62.292**   Other fracture of first metacarpal bone, left hand B, K, P ☟, B ☟

    ● **S62.299**   Other fracture of first metacarpal bone, unspecified hand B, K, P ☟,
      B ☟

▶ New   ⇒ Revised   ~~deleted~~ Deleted   Excludes 1   Excludes 2   Includes   Use additional   Code first   Code also   Key words

OGCR Official Guidelines   ● Unacceptable Principal Diagnosis   X Assign placeholder X   ☟ Use Additional Character(s)   ▶ Manifestation Code   **Coding Clinic**

● S62.3   Fracture of other and unspecified metacarpal bone
    Excludes2   fracture of first metacarpal bone (S62.2-)
    (Ex) **For category S62.3 CC codes S62.3[B]:** See PDX Collection 1284
        For S62.3[K,P]: See PDX Collection 897

● S62.30   Unspecified fracture of other metacarpal bone
    ● S62.300   Unspecified fracture of second metacarpal bone, right hand B, K, P 🔓, B 🔓
    ● S62.301   Unspecified fracture of second metacarpal bone, left hand B, K, P 🔓, B 🔓
    ● S62.302   Unspecified fracture of third metacarpal bone, right hand B, K, P 🔓, B 🔓
    ● S62.303   Unspecified fracture of third metacarpal bone, left hand B, K, P 🔓, B 🔓
    ● S62.304   Unspecified fracture of fourth metacarpal bone, right hand B, K, P 🔓, B 🔓
    ● S62.305   Unspecified fracture of fourth metacarpal bone, left hand B, K, P 🔓, B 🔓
    ● S62.306   Unspecified fracture of fifth metacarpal bone, right hand B, K, P 🔓, B 🔓
    ● S62.307   Unspecified fracture of fifth metacarpal bone, left hand B, K, P 🔓, B 🔓
    ● S62.308   Unspecified fracture of other metacarpal bone B, K, P 🔓, B 🔓
        Unspecified fracture of specified metacarpal bone with unspecified laterality
    ● S62.309   Unspecified fracture of unspecified metacarpal bone B, K, P 🔓, B 🔓

● S62.31   Displaced fracture of base of other metacarpal bone
    ● S62.310   Displaced fracture of base of second metacarpal bone, right hand B, K, P 🔓, B 🔓
    ⇒● S62.311   Displaced fracture of base of second metacarpal bone, left hand B, K, P 🔓, B 🔓
    ● S62.312   Displaced fracture of base of third metacarpal bone, right hand B, K, P 🔓, B 🔓
    ● S62.313   Displaced fracture of base of third metacarpal bone, left hand B, K, P 🔓, B 🔓
    ● S62.314   Displaced fracture of base of fourth metacarpal bone, right hand B, K, P 🔓, B 🔓
    ● S62.315   Displaced fracture of base of fourth metacarpal bone, left hand B, K, P 🔓, B 🔓
    ● S62.316   Displaced fracture of base of fifth metacarpal bone, right hand B, K, P 🔓, B 🔓
    ⇒● S62.317   Displaced fracture of base of fifth metacarpal bone, left hand B, K, P 🔓, B 🔓
    ● S62.318   Displaced fracture of base of other metacarpal bone B, K, P 🔓, B 🔓
        Displaced fracture of base of specified metacarpal bone with unspecified laterality
    ● S62.319   Displaced fracture of base of unspecified metacarpal bone B, K, P 🔓, B 🔓

● S62.32   Displaced fracture of shaft of other metacarpal bone
    ● S62.320   Displaced fracture of shaft of second metacarpal bone, right hand B, K, P 🔓, B 🔓
    ● S62.321   Displaced fracture of shaft of second metacarpal bone, left hand B, K, P 🔓, B 🔓
    ● S62.322   Displaced fracture of shaft of third metacarpal bone, right hand B, K, P 🔓, B 🔓
    ● S62.323   Displaced fracture of shaft of third metacarpal bone, left hand B, K, P 🔓, B 🔓
    ● S62.324   Displaced fracture of shaft of fourth metacarpal bone, right hand B, K, P 🔓, B 🔓
    ● S62.325   Displaced fracture of shaft of fourth metacarpal bone, left hand B, K, P 🔓, B 🔓
    ● S62.326   Displaced fracture of shaft of fifth metacarpal bone, right hand B, K, P 🔓, B 🔓
    ● S62.327   Displaced fracture of shaft of fifth metacarpal bone, left hand B, K, P 🔓, B 🔓
    ● S62.328   Displaced fracture of shaft of other metacarpal bone B, K, P 🔓, B 🔓
        Displaced fracture of shaft of specified metacarpal bone with unspecified laterality
    ● S62.329   Displaced fracture of shaft of unspecified metacarpal bone B, K, P 🔓, B 🔓

● S62.33   Displaced fracture of neck of other metacarpal bone
    ● S62.330   Displaced fracture of neck of second metacarpal bone, right hand B, K, P 🔓, B 🔓
    ● S62.331   Displaced fracture of neck of second metacarpal bone, left hand B, K, P 🔓, B 🔓
    ● S62.332   Displaced fracture of neck of third metacarpal bone, right hand B, K, P 🔓, B 🔓
    ● S62.333   Displaced fracture of neck of third metacarpal bone, left hand B, K, P 🔓, B 🔓
    ● S62.334   Displaced fracture of neck of fourth metacarpal bone, right hand B, K, P 🔓, B 🔓
    ● S62.335   Displaced fracture of neck of fourth metacarpal bone, left hand B, K, P 🔓, B 🔓
    ● S62.336   Displaced fracture of neck of fifth metacarpal bone, right hand B, K, P 🔓, B 🔓
    ● S62.337   Displaced fracture of neck of fifth metacarpal bone, left hand B, K, P 🔓, B 🔓
    ● S62.338   Displaced fracture of neck of other metacarpal bone B, K, P 🔓, B 🔓
        Displaced fracture of neck of specified metacarpal bone with unspecified laterality
    ● S62.339   Displaced fracture of neck of unspecified metacarpal bone B, K, P 🔓, B 🔓

CHAPTER 19 (S00-T88)

CHAPTER 19 (S00-T88)

● S62.34   Nondisplaced fracture of base of other metacarpal bone

  ● S62.340   Nondisplaced fracture of base of second metacarpal bone, right hand B, K, P 🖎, B 🖎

  ⇒● S62.341   Nondisplaced fracture of base of second metacarpal bone, left hand B, K, P 🖎, B 🖎

  ● S62.342   Nondisplaced fracture of base of third metacarpal bone, right hand B, K, P 🖎, B 🖎

  ● S62.343   Nondisplaced fracture of base of third metacarpal bone, left hand B, K, P 🖎, B 🖎

  ● S62.344   Nondisplaced fracture of base of fourth metacarpal bone, right hand B, K, P 🖎, B 🖎

  ● S62.345   Nondisplaced fracture of base of fourth metacarpal bone, left hand B, K, P 🖎, B 🖎

  ● S62.346   Nondisplaced fracture of base of fifth metacarpal bone, right hand B, K, P 🖎, B 🖎

  ⇒● S62.347   Nondisplaced fracture of base of fifth metacarpal bone, left hand B, K, P 🖎, B 🖎

  ● S62.348   Nondisplaced fracture of base of other metacarpal bone B, K, P 🖎, B 🖎
     Nondisplaced fracture of base of specified metacarpal bone with unspecified laterality

  ● S62.349   Nondisplaced fracture of base of unspecified metacarpal bone B, K, P 🖎, B 🖎

● S62.35   Nondisplaced fracture of shaft of other metacarpal bone

  ● S62.350   Nondisplaced fracture of shaft of second metacarpal bone, right hand B, K, P 🖎, B 🖎

  ● S62.351   Nondisplaced fracture of shaft of second metacarpal bone, left hand B, K, P 🖎, B 🖎

  ● S62.352   Nondisplaced fracture of shaft of third metacarpal bone, right hand B, K, P 🖎, B 🖎

  ● S62.353   Nondisplaced fracture of shaft of third metacarpal bone, left hand B, K, P 🖎, B 🖎

  ● S62.354   Nondisplaced fracture of shaft of fourth metacarpal bone, right hand B, K, P 🖎, B 🖎

  ● S62.355   Nondisplaced fracture of shaft of fourth metacarpal bone, left hand B, K, P 🖎, B 🖎

  ● S62.356   Nondisplaced fracture of shaft of fifth metacarpal bone, right hand B, K, P 🖎, B 🖎

  ● S62.357   Nondisplaced fracture of shaft of fifth metacarpal bone, left hand B, K, P 🖎, B 🖎

  ● S62.358   Nondisplaced fracture of shaft of other metacarpal bone B, K, P 🖎, B 🖎
     Nondisplaced fracture of shaft of specified metacarpal bone with unspecified laterality

  ● S62.359   Nondisplaced fracture of shaft of unspecified metacarpal bone B, K, P 🖎, B 🖎

● S62.36   Nondisplaced fracture of neck of other metacarpal bone

  ● S62.360   Nondisplaced fracture of neck of second metacarpal bone, right hand B, K, P 🖎, B 🖎

  ● S62.361   Nondisplaced fracture of neck of second metacarpal bone, left hand B, K, P 🖎, B 🖎

  ● S62.362   Nondisplaced fracture of neck of third metacarpal bone, right hand B, K, P 🖎, B 🖎

  ● S62.363   Nondisplaced fracture of neck of third metacarpal bone, left hand B, K, P 🖎, B 🖎

  ● S62.364   Nondisplaced fracture of neck of fourth metacarpal bone, right hand B, K, P 🖎, B 🖎

  ● S62.365   Nondisplaced fracture of neck of fourth metacarpal bone, left hand B, K, P 🖎, B 🖎

  ● S62.366   Nondisplaced fracture of neck of fifth metacarpal bone, right hand B, K, P 🖎, B 🖎

  ● S62.367   Nondisplaced fracture of neck of fifth metacarpal bone, left hand B, K, P 🖎, B 🖎

  ● S62.368   Nondisplaced fracture of neck of other metacarpal bone B, K, P 🖎, B 🖎
     Nondisplaced fracture of neck of specified metacarpal bone with unspecified laterality

  ● S62.369   Nondisplaced fracture of neck of unspecified metacarpal bone B, K, P 🖎, B 🖎

● S62.39   Other fracture of other metacarpal bone

  ● S62.390   Other fracture of second metacarpal bone, right hand B, K, P 🖎, B 🖎

  ● S62.391   Other fracture of second metacarpal bone, left hand B, K, P 🖎, B 🖎

  ● S62.392   Other fracture of third metacarpal bone, right hand B, K, P 🖎, B 🖎

  ● S62.393   Other fracture of third metacarpal bone, left hand B, K, P 🖎, B 🖎

  ● S62.394   Other fracture of fourth metacarpal bone, right hand B, K, P 🖎, B 🖎

  ● S62.395   Other fracture of fourth metacarpal bone, left hand B, K, P 🖎, B 🖎

  ● S62.396   Other fracture of fifth metacarpal bone, right hand B, K, P 🖎, B 🖎

  ● S62.397   Other fracture of fifth metacarpal bone, left hand B, K, P 🖎, B 🖎

  ● S62.398   Other fracture of other metacarpal bone B, K, P 🖎, B 🖎
     Other fracture of specified metacarpal bone with unspecified laterality

  ● S62.399   Other fracture of unspecified metacarpal bone B, K, P 🖎, B 🖎

● S62.5   Fracture of thumb
  (Ex) For category S62.5 CC codes S62.5[B]: See PDX Collection 1285
  For S62.5[K,P]: See PDX Collection 897

● S62.50   Fracture of unspecified phalanx of thumb

  ● S62.501   Fracture of unspecified phalanx of right thumb B, K, P 🖎, B 🖎

  ● S62.502   Fracture of unspecified phalanx of left thumb B, K, P 🖎, B 🖎

  ● S62.509   Fracture of unspecified phalanx of unspecified thumb B, K, P 🖎, B 🖎

▶ New   ⇒ Revised   ~~deleted~~ Deleted   Excludes 1   Excludes 2   Includes   Use additional   Code first   Code also   Key words

OGCR Official Guidelines   ● Unacceptable Principal Diagnosis   X Assign placeholder X   ▌ Use Additional Character(s)   ▌ Manifestation Code   **Coding Clinic**

● S62.51 Fracture of proximal phalanx of thumb
  ● S62.511 Displaced fracture of proximal phalanx of right thumb B, K, P 🔹, B 🔹
  ● S62.512 Displaced fracture of proximal phalanx of left thumb B, K, P 🔹, B 🔹
  ● S62.513 Displaced fracture of proximal phalanx of unspecified thumb B, K, P 🔹, B 🔹
  ● S62.514 Nondisplaced fracture of proximal phalanx of right thumb B, K, P 🔹, B 🔹
  ● S62.515 Nondisplaced fracture of proximal phalanx of left thumb B, K, P 🔹, B 🔹
  ● S62.516 Nondisplaced fracture of proximal phalanx of unspecified thumb B, K, P 🔹, B 🔹

● S62.52 Fracture of distal phalanx of thumb
  ● S62.521 Displaced fracture of distal phalanx of right thumb B, K, P 🔹, B 🔹
  ● S62.522 Displaced fracture of distal phalanx of left thumb B, K, P 🔹, B 🔹
  ● S62.523 Displaced fracture of distal phalanx of unspecified thumb B, K, P 🔹, B 🔹
  ● S62.524 Nondisplaced fracture of distal phalanx of right thumb B, K, P 🔹, B 🔹
  ● S62.525 Nondisplaced fracture of distal phalanx of left thumb B, K, P 🔹, B 🔹
  ● S62.526 Nondisplaced fracture of distal phalanx of unspecified thumb B, K, P 🔹, B 🔹

● S62.6 Fracture of other and unspecified finger(s)
  Excludes2 fracture of thumb (S62.5-)
  (Ex) For category S62.6 CC codes S62.6[B]: See PDX Collection 1285
  For S62.5[K,P]: See PDX Collection 897

  ● S62.60 Fracture of unspecified phalanx of finger
    ● S62.600 Fracture of unspecified phalanx of right index finger B, K, P 🔹, B 🔹
    ● S62.601 Fracture of unspecified phalanx of left index finger B, K, P 🔹, B 🔹
    ● S62.602 Fracture of unspecified phalanx of right middle finger B, K, P 🔹, B 🔹
    ● S62.603 Fracture of unspecified phalanx of left middle finger B, K, P 🔹, B 🔹
    ● S62.604 Fracture of unspecified phalanx of right ring finger B, K, P 🔹, B 🔹
    ● S62.605 Fracture of unspecified phalanx of left ring finger B, K, P 🔹, B 🔹
    ● S62.606 Fracture of unspecified phalanx of right little finger B, K, P 🔹, B 🔹
    ● S62.607 Fracture of unspecified phalanx of left little finger B, K, P 🔹, B 🔹
    ● S62.608 Fracture of unspecified phalanx of other finger B, K, P 🔹, B 🔹
      Fracture of unspecified phalanx of specified finger with unspecified laterality
    ● S62.609 Fracture of unspecified phalanx of unspecified finger B, K, P 🔹, B 🔹

  ● S62.61 Displaced fracture of proximal phalanx of finger
    ● S62.610 Displaced fracture of proximal phalanx of right index finger B, K, P 🔹, B 🔹
    ● S62.611 Displaced fracture of proximal phalanx of left index finger B, K, P 🔹, B 🔹
    ● S62.612 Displaced fracture of proximal phalanx of right middle finger B, K, P 🔹, B 🔹

    ● S62.613 Displaced fracture of proximal phalanx of left middle finger B, K, P 🔹, B 🔹
    ● S62.614 Displaced fracture of proximal phalanx of right ring finger B, K, P 🔹, B 🔹
    ● S62.615 Displaced fracture of proximal phalanx of left ring finger B, K, P 🔹, B 🔹
    ● S62.616 Displaced fracture of proximal phalanx of right little finger B, K, P 🔹, B 🔹
    ● S62.617 Displaced fracture of proximal phalanx of left little finger B, K, P 🔹, B 🔹
    ● S62.618 Displaced fracture of proximal phalanx of other finger B, K, P 🔹, B 🔹
      Displaced fracture of proximal phalanx of specified finger with unspecified laterality
    ● S62.619 Displaced fracture of proximal phalanx of unspecified finger B, K, P 🔹, B 🔹

⇒ ● S62.62 Displaced fracture of middle phalanx of finger
  ⇒ ● S62.620 Displaced fracture of middle phalanx of right index finger B, K, P 🔹, B 🔹
  ⇒ ● S62.621 Displaced fracture of middle phalanx of left index finger B, K, P 🔹, B 🔹
  ⇒ ● S62.622 Displaced fracture of middle phalanx of right middle finger B, K, P 🔹, B 🔹
  ⇒ ● S62.623 Displaced fracture of middle phalanx of left middle finger B, K, P 🔹, B 🔹
  ⇒ ● S62.624 Displaced fracture of middle phalanx of right ring finger B, K, P 🔹, B 🔹
  ⇒ ● S62.625 Displaced fracture of middle phalanx of left ring finger B, K, P 🔹, B 🔹
  ● S62.626 Displaced fracture of medial phalanx of right little finger B, K, P 🔹, B 🔹
  ● S62.627 Displaced fracture of medial phalanx of left little finger B, K, P 🔹, B 🔹
  ● S62.628 Displaced fracture of medial phalanx of other finger B, K, P 🔹, B 🔹
    Displaced fracture of medial phalanx of specified finger with unspecified laterality
  ● S62.629 Displaced fracture of medial phalanx of unspecified finger B, K, P 🔹, B 🔹

● S62.63 Displaced fracture of distal phalanx of finger
  ● S62.630 Displaced fracture of distal phalanx of right index finger B, K, P 🔹, B 🔹
  ● S62.631 Displaced fracture of distal phalanx of left index finger B, K, P 🔹, B 🔹
  ● S62.632 Displaced fracture of distal phalanx of right middle finger B, K, P 🔹, B 🔹
  ● S62.633 Displaced fracture of distal phalanx of left middle finger B, K, P 🔹, B 🔹
  ● S62.634 Displaced fracture of distal phalanx of right ring finger B, K, P 🔹, B 🔹
  ● S62.635 Displaced fracture of distal phalanx of left ring finger B, K, P 🔹, B 🔹
  ● S62.636 Displaced fracture of distal phalanx of right little finger B, K, P 🔹, B 🔹
  ● S62.637 Displaced fracture of distal phalanx of left little finger B, K, P 🔹, B 🔹
  ● S62.638 Displaced fracture of distal phalanx of other finger B, K, P 🔹, B 🔹
    Displaced fracture of distal phalanx of specified finger with unspecified laterality
  ● S62.639 Displaced fracture of distal phalanx of unspecified finger B, K, P 🔹, B 🔹

N Newborn Age: 0   P Pediatric Age: 0–17   M Maternity DX: 12–55   A Adult Age: 15–124   ♀ Females Only   ♂ Males Only
🔹 Complication\Comorbidity   🔹 Major C\C   (Ex) CC/MCC Exclusions   🔹 Hospital-Acquired Condition

● **S62.64**   Nondisplaced fracture of proximal phalanx of finger

   ● **S62.640**   Nondisplaced fracture of proximal phalanx of right index finger B, K, P 🖐, B 🖐

   ● **S62.641**   Nondisplaced fracture of proximal phalanx of left index finger B, K, P 🖐, B 🖐

   ● **S62.642**   Nondisplaced fracture of proximal phalanx of right middle finger B, K, P 🖐, B 🖐

   ● **S62.643**   Nondisplaced fracture of proximal phalanx of left middle finger B, K, P 🖐, B 🖐

   ● **S62.644**   Nondisplaced fracture of proximal phalanx of right ring finger B, K, P 🖐, B 🖐

   ● **S62.645**   Nondisplaced fracture of proximal phalanx of left ring finger B, K, P 🖐, B 🖐

   ● **S62.646**   Nondisplaced fracture of proximal phalanx of right little finger B, K, P 🖐, B 🖐

   ● **S62.647**   Nondisplaced fracture of proximal phalanx of left little finger B, K, P 🖐, B 🖐

   ● **S62.648**   Nondisplaced fracture of proximal phalanx of other finger B, K, P 🖐, B 🖐
       Nondisplaced fracture of proximal phalanx of specified finger with unspecified laterality

   ● **S62.649**   Nondisplaced fracture of proximal phalanx of unspecified finger B, K, P 🖐, B 🖐

➡● **S62.65**   Nondisplaced fracture of middle phalanx of finger

   ➡● **S62.650**   Nondisplaced fracture of middle phalanx of right index finger B, K, P 🖐, B 🖐

   ➡● **S62.651**   Nondisplaced fracture of middle phalanx of left index finger B, K, P 🖐, B 🖐

   ➡● **S62.652**   Nondisplaced fracture of middle phalanx of right middle finger B, K, P 🖐, B 🖐

   ➡● **S62.653**   Nondisplaced fracture of middle phalanx of left middle finger B, K, P 🖐, B 🖐

   ● **S62.654**   Nondisplaced fracture of medial phalanx of right ring finger B, K, P 🖐, B 🖐

   ● **S62.655**   Nondisplaced fracture of medial phalanx of left ring finger B, K, P 🖐, B 🖐

   ● **S62.656**   Nondisplaced fracture of medial phalanx of right little finger B, K, P 🖐, B 🖐

   ● **S62.657**   Nondisplaced fracture of medial phalanx of left little finger B, K, P 🖐, B 🖐

   ● **S62.658**   Nondisplaced fracture of medial phalanx of other finger B, K, P 🖐, B 🖐
       Nondisplaced fracture of medial phalanx of specified finger with unspecified laterality

   ● **S62.659**   Nondisplaced fracture of medial phalanx of unspecified finger B, K, P 🖐, B 🖐

Figure 19-14   Dorsal dislocation of the distal phalanx of the index finger. (From Hardy M, Snaith B: Musculoskeletal Trauma: A Guide to Assessment and Diagnosis, 1e, Elsevier, 2011)

  ● **S62.66**   Nondisplaced fracture of distal phalanx of finger

   ● **S62.660**   Nondisplaced fracture of distal phalanx of right index finger B, K, P 🖐, B 🖐

   ● **S62.661**   Nondisplaced fracture of distal phalanx of left index finger B, K, P 🖐, B 🖐

   ● **S62.662**   Nondisplaced fracture of distal phalanx of right middle finger B, K, P 🖐, B 🖐

   ● **S62.663**   Nondisplaced fracture of distal phalanx of left middle finger B, K, P 🖐, B 🖐

   ● **S62.664**   Nondisplaced fracture of distal phalanx of right ring finger B, K, P 🖐, B 🖐

   ● **S62.665**   Nondisplaced fracture of distal phalanx of left ring finger B, K, P 🖐, B 🖐

   ● **S62.666**   Nondisplaced fracture of distal phalanx of right little finger B, K, P 🖐, B 🖐

   ● **S62.667**   Nondisplaced fracture of distal phalanx of left little finger B, K, P 🖐, B 🖐

   ● **S62.668**   Nondisplaced fracture of distal phalanx of other finger B, K, P 🖐, B 🖐
       Nondisplaced fracture of distal phalanx of specified finger with unspecified laterality

   ● **S62.669**   Nondisplaced fracture of distal phalanx of unspecified finger B, K, P 🖐, B 🖐

● **S62.9**   Unspecified fracture of wrist and hand

  X● **S62.90**   Unspecified fracture of unspecified wrist and hand B, K, P 🖐, B 🖐
      (Ex) For S62.90[B]: See PDX Collection 1286 For S62.90[K,P]: See PDX Collection 897

  X● **S62.91**   Unspecified fracture of right wrist and hand B, K, P 🖐, B 🖐
      (Ex) For S62.91[B]: See PDX Collection 1287 For S62.91[K,P]: See PDX Collection 897

  X● **S62.92**   Unspecified fracture of left wrist and hand B, K, P 🖐, B 🖐
      (Ex) For S62.92[B]: See PDX Collection 1287 For S62.92[K,P]: See PDX Collection 897

CHAPTER 19 (S00-T88)

1330

▶ New   ⟹ Revised   ~~deleted~~ Deleted   Excludes 1   Excludes 2   Includes   Use additional   Code first   Code also   Key words
OGCR Official Guidelines   ● Unacceptable Principal Diagnosis   X Assign placeholder X   ● Use Additional Character(s)   ▶ Manifestation Code   **Coding Clinic**

● S63 **Dislocation and sprain of joints and ligaments at wrist and hand level**

    Includes   avulsion of joint or ligament at wrist and hand level

        laceration of cartilage, joint or ligament at wrist and hand level

        sprain of cartilage, joint or ligament at wrist and hand level

        traumatic hemarthrosis of joint or ligament at wrist and hand level

        traumatic rupture of joint or ligament at wrist and hand level

        traumatic subluxation of joint or ligament at wrist and hand level

        traumatic tear of joint or ligament at wrist and hand level

    Code also any associated open wound

    Excludes2   strain of muscle, fascia and tendon of wrist and hand (S66.-)

    The appropriate 7th character is to be added to each code from category S63

> A   initial encounter
> D   subsequent encounter
> S   sequela

● S63.0 **Subluxation and dislocation of wrist and hand joints**

  ● S63.00 **Unspecified subluxation and dislocation of wrist and hand**
      Dislocation of carpal bone NOS
      Dislocation of distal end of radius NOS
      Subluxation of carpal bone NOS
      Subluxation of distal end of radius NOS

    ● S63.001 **Unspecified subluxation of right wrist and hand**

    ● S63.002 **Unspecified subluxation of left wrist and hand**

    ● S63.003 **Unspecified subluxation of unspecified wrist and hand**

    ● S63.004 **Unspecified dislocation of right wrist and hand**

    ● S63.005 **Unspecified dislocation of left wrist and hand**

    ● S63.006 **Unspecified dislocation of unspecified wrist and hand**

  ● S63.01 **Subluxation and dislocation of distal radioulnar joint**

    ● S63.011 **Subluxation of distal radioulnar joint of right wrist**

    ● S63.012 **Subluxation of distal radioulnar joint of left wrist**

    ● S63.013 **Subluxation of distal radioulnar joint of unspecified wrist**

    ● S63.014 **Dislocation of distal radioulnar joint of right wrist**

    ● S63.015 **Dislocation of distal radioulnar joint of left wrist**

    ● S63.016 **Dislocation of distal radioulnar joint of unspecified wrist**

  ● S63.02 **Subluxation and dislocation of radiocarpal joint**

    ● S63.021 **Subluxation of radiocarpal joint of right wrist**

    ● S63.022 **Subluxation of radiocarpal joint of left wrist**

    ● S63.023 **Subluxation of radiocarpal joint of unspecified wrist**

    ● S63.024 **Dislocation of radiocarpal joint of right wrist**

    ● S63.025 **Dislocation of radiocarpal joint of left wrist**

    ● S63.026 **Dislocation of radiocarpal joint of unspecified wrist**

● S63.03 **Subluxation and dislocation of midcarpal joint**

  ● S63.031 **Subluxation of midcarpal joint of right wrist**

  ● S63.032 **Subluxation of midcarpal joint of left wrist**

  ● S63.033 **Subluxation of midcarpal joint of unspecified wrist**

  ● S63.034 **Dislocation of midcarpal joint of right wrist**

  ● S63.035 **Dislocation of midcarpal joint of left wrist**

  ● S63.036 **Dislocation of midcarpal joint of unspecified wrist**

● S63.04 **Subluxation and dislocation of carpometacarpal joint of thumb**

    Excludes2   interphalangeal subluxation and dislocation of thumb (S63.1-)

  ● S63.041 **Subluxation of carpometacarpal joint of right thumb**

  ● S63.042 **Subluxation of carpometacarpal joint of left thumb**

  ● S63.043 **Subluxation of carpometacarpal joint of unspecified thumb**

  ● S63.044 **Dislocation of carpometacarpal joint of right thumb**

  ● S63.045 **Dislocation of carpometacarpal joint of left thumb**

  ● S63.046 **Dislocation of carpometacarpal joint of unspecified thumb**

● S63.05 **Subluxation and dislocation of other carpometacarpal joint**

    Excludes2   subluxation and dislocation of carpometacarpal joint of thumb (S63.04-)

  ● S63.051 **Subluxation of other carpometacarpal joint of right hand**

  ● S63.052 **Subluxation of other carpometacarpal joint of left hand**

  ● S63.053 **Subluxation of other carpometacarpal joint of unspecified hand**

  ● S63.054 **Dislocation of other carpometacarpal joint of right hand**

  ● S63.055 **Dislocation of other carpometacarpal joint of left hand**

  ● S63.056 **Dislocation of other carpometacarpal joint of unspecified hand**

● S63.06 **Subluxation and dislocation of metacarpal (bone), proximal end**

  ● S63.061 **Subluxation of metacarpal (bone), proximal end of right hand**

  ● S63.062 **Subluxation of metacarpal (bone), proximal end of left hand**

  ● S63.063 **Subluxation of metacarpal (bone), proximal end of unspecified hand**

  ● S63.064 **Dislocation of metacarpal (bone), proximal end of right hand**

  ● S63.065 **Dislocation of metacarpal (bone), proximal end of left hand**

  ● S63.066 **Dislocation of metacarpal (bone), proximal end of unspecified hand**

CHAPTER 19 (S00-T88)

● S63.07   Subluxation and dislocation of distal end of ulna
   ● S63.071   Subluxation of distal end of right ulna
   ● S63.072   Subluxation of distal end of left ulna
   ● S63.073   Subluxation of distal end of unspecified ulna
   ● S63.074   Dislocation of distal end of right ulna
   ● S63.075   Dislocation of distal end of left ulna
   ● S63.076   Dislocation of distal end of unspecified ulna

● S63.09   Other subluxation and dislocation of wrist and hand
   ● S63.091   Other subluxation of right wrist and hand
   ● S63.092   Other subluxation of left wrist and hand
   ● S63.093   Other subluxation of unspecified wrist and hand
   ● S63.094   Other dislocation of right wrist and hand
   ● S63.095   Other dislocation of left wrist and hand
   ● S63.096   Other dislocation of unspecified wrist and hand

● S63.1   Subluxation and dislocation of thumb
  ● S63.10   Unspecified subluxation and dislocation of thumb
   ● S63.101   Unspecified subluxation of right thumb
   ● S63.102   Unspecified subluxation of left thumb
   ● S63.103   Unspecified subluxation of unspecified thumb
   ● S63.104   Unspecified dislocation of right thumb
   ● S63.105   Unspecified dislocation of left thumb
   ● S63.106   Unspecified dislocation of unspecified thumb

  ● S63.11   Subluxation and dislocation of metacarpophalangeal joint of thumb
   ● S63.111   Subluxation of metacarpophalangeal joint of right thumb
   ● S63.112   Subluxation of metacarpophalangeal joint of left thumb
   ● S63.113   Subluxation of metacarpophalangeal joint of unspecified thumb
   ● S63.114   Dislocation of metacarpophalangeal joint of right thumb
   ● S63.115   Dislocation of metacarpophalangeal joint of left thumb
   ● S63.116   Dislocation of metacarpophalangeal joint of unspecified thumb

➡️● S63.12   Subluxation and dislocation of interphalangeal joint of thumb
  ➡️● S63.121   Subluxation of interphalangeal joint of right thumb
  ➡️● S63.122   Subluxation of interphalangeal joint of left thumb
  ➡️● S63.123   Subluxation of interphalangeal joint of unspecified thumb
  ➡️● S63.124   Dislocation of interphalangeal joint of right thumb
  ➡️● S63.125   Dislocation of interphalangeal joint of left thumb
  ➡️● S63.126   Dislocation of interphalangeal joint of unspecified thumb

● S63.2   Subluxation and dislocation of other finger(s)
  Excludes2   subluxation and dislocation of thumb (S63.1-)

● S63.20   Unspecified subluxation of other finger
   ● S63.200   Unspecified subluxation of right index finger
   ● S63.201   Unspecified subluxation of left index finger
   ● S63.202   Unspecified subluxation of right middle finger
   ● S63.203   Unspecified subluxation of left middle finger
   ● S63.204   Unspecified subluxation of right ring finger
   ● S63.205   Unspecified subluxation of left ring finger
   ● S63.206   Unspecified subluxation of right little finger
   ● S63.207   Unspecified subluxation of left little finger
   ● S63.208   Unspecified subluxation of other finger
     Unspecified subluxation of specified finger with unspecified laterality
   ● S63.209   Unspecified subluxation of unspecified finger

● S63.21   Subluxation of metacarpophalangeal joint of finger
   ● S63.210   Subluxation of metacarpophalangeal joint of right index finger
   ● S63.211   Subluxation of metacarpophalangeal joint of left index finger
   ● S63.212   Subluxation of metacarpophalangeal joint of right middle finger
   ● S63.213   Subluxation of metacarpophalangeal joint of left middle finger
   ● S63.214   Subluxation of metacarpophalangeal joint of right ring finger
   ● S63.215   Subluxation of metacarpophalangeal joint of left ring finger
   ● S63.216   Subluxation of metacarpophalangeal joint of right little finger
   ● S63.217   Subluxation of metacarpophalangeal joint of left little finger
   ● S63.218   Subluxation of metacarpophalangeal joint of other finger
     Subluxation of metacarpophalangeal joint of specified finger with unspecified laterality
   ● S63.219   Subluxation of metacarpophalangeal joint of unspecified finger

● S63.22   Subluxation of unspecified interphalangeal joint of finger
   ● S63.220   Subluxation of unspecified interphalangeal joint of right index finger
   ● S63.221   Subluxation of unspecified interphalangeal joint of left index finger
   ● S63.222   Subluxation of unspecified interphalangeal joint of right middle finger
   ● S63.223   Subluxation of unspecified interphalangeal joint of left middle finger

▶ New   ➡️ Revised   ~~deleted~~ Deleted   Excludes 1   Excludes 2   Includes   Use additional   Code first   Code also   Key words
OGCR Official Guidelines   ● Unacceptable Principal Diagnosis   X Assign placeholder X   ● Use Additional Character(s)   ▶ Manifestation Code   Coding Clinic

● S63.224   Subluxation of unspecified interphalangeal joint of right ring finger

● S63.225   Subluxation of unspecified interphalangeal joint of left ring finger

● S63.226   Subluxation of unspecified interphalangeal joint of right little finger

● S63.227   Subluxation of unspecified interphalangeal joint of left little finger

● S63.228   Subluxation of unspecified interphalangeal joint of other finger
  Subluxation of unspecified interphalangeal joint of specified finger with unspecified laterality

● S63.229   Subluxation of unspecified interphalangeal joint of unspecified finger

● S63.23   Subluxation of proximal interphalangeal joint of finger

● S63.230   Subluxation of proximal interphalangeal joint of right index finger

● S63.231   Subluxation of proximal interphalangeal joint of left index finger

● S63.232   Subluxation of proximal interphalangeal joint of right middle finger

● S63.233   Subluxation of proximal interphalangeal joint of left middle finger

● S63.234   Subluxation of proximal interphalangeal joint of right ring finger

● S63.235   Subluxation of proximal interphalangeal joint of left ring finger

● S63.236   Subluxation of proximal interphalangeal joint of right little finger

● S63.237   Subluxation of proximal interphalangeal joint of left little finger

● S63.238   Subluxation of proximal interphalangeal joint of other finger
  Subluxation of proximal interphalangeal joint of specified finger with unspecified laterality

● S63.239   Subluxation of proximal interphalangeal joint of unspecified finger

● S63.24   Subluxation of distal interphalangeal joint of finger

● S63.240   Subluxation of distal interphalangeal joint of right index finger

● S63.241   Subluxation of distal interphalangeal joint of left index finger

● S63.242   Subluxation of distal interphalangeal joint of right middle finger

● S63.243   Subluxation of distal interphalangeal joint of left middle finger

● S63.244   Subluxation of distal interphalangeal joint of right ring finger

● S63.245   Subluxation of distal interphalangeal joint of left ring finger

● S63.246   Subluxation of distal interphalangeal joint of right little finger

● S63.247   Subluxation of distal interphalangeal joint of left little finger

● S63.248   Subluxation of distal interphalangeal joint of other finger
  Subluxation of distal interphalangeal joint of specified finger with unspecified laterality

● S63.249   Subluxation of distal interphalangeal joint of unspecified finger

● S63.25   Unspecified dislocation of other finger

● S63.250   Unspecified dislocation of right index finger

● S63.251   Unspecified dislocation of left index finger

● S63.252   Unspecified dislocation of right middle finger

● S63.253   Unspecified dislocation of left middle finger

● S63.254   Unspecified dislocation of right ring finger

● S63.255   Unspecified dislocation of left ring finger

● S63.256   Unspecified dislocation of right little finger

● S63.257   Unspecified dislocation of left little finger

● S63.258   Unspecified dislocation of other finger
  Unspecified dislocation of specified finger with unspecified laterality

● S63.259   Unspecified dislocation of unspecified finger
  ⇛ Unspecified dislocation of unspecified finger with unspecified laterality

● S63.26   Dislocation of metacarpophalangeal joint of finger

● S63.260   Dislocation of metacarpophalangeal joint of right index finger

● S63.261   Dislocation of metacarpophalangeal joint of left index finger

● S63.262   Dislocation of metacarpophalangeal joint of right middle finger

● S63.263   Dislocation of metacarpophalangeal joint of left middle finger

● S63.264   Dislocation of metacarpophalangeal joint of right ring finger

● S63.265   Dislocation of metacarpophalangeal joint of left ring finger

● S63.266   Dislocation of metacarpophalangeal joint of right little finger

● S63.267   Dislocation of metacarpophalangeal joint of left little finger

● S63.268   Dislocation of metacarpophalangeal joint of other finger
  Dislocation of metacarpophalangeal joint of specified finger with unspecified laterality

● S63.269   Dislocation of metacarpophalangeal joint of unspecified finger

CHAPTER 19 (S00-T88)

● **S63.27** **Dislocation of unspecified interphalangeal joint of finger**

   ● **S63.270** Dislocation of unspecified interphalangeal joint of **right index finger**

   ● **S63.271** Dislocation of unspecified interphalangeal joint of **left index finger**

   ● **S63.272** Dislocation of unspecified interphalangeal joint of **right middle finger**

   ● **S63.273** Dislocation of unspecified interphalangeal joint of **left middle finger**

   ● **S63.274** Dislocation of unspecified interphalangeal joint of **right ring finger**

   ● **S63.275** Dislocation of unspecified interphalangeal joint of **left ring finger**

   ● **S63.276** Dislocation of unspecified interphalangeal joint of **right little finger**

   ● **S63.277** Dislocation of unspecified interphalangeal joint of **left little finger**

   ● **S63.278** Dislocation of unspecified interphalangeal joint of **other finger**
           Dislocation of unspecified interphalangeal joint of specified finger with unspecified laterality

   ● **S63.279** Dislocation of unspecified interphalangeal joint of **unspecified finger**
          ⟶Dislocation of unspecified interphalangeal joint of unspecified finger without specified laterality

● **S63.28** **Dislocation of proximal interphalangeal joint of finger**

   ● **S63.280** Dislocation of proximal interphalangeal joint of **right index finger**

   ● **S63.281** Dislocation of proximal interphalangeal joint of **left index finger**

   ● **S63.282** Dislocation of proximal interphalangeal joint of **right middle finger**

   ● **S63.283** Dislocation of proximal interphalangeal joint of **left middle finger**

   ● **S63.284** Dislocation of proximal interphalangeal joint of **right ring finger**

   ● **S63.285** Dislocation of proximal interphalangeal joint of **left ring finger**

   ● **S63.286** Dislocation of proximal interphalangeal joint of **right little finger**

   ● **S63.287** Dislocation of proximal interphalangeal joint of **left little finger**

   ● **S63.288** Dislocation of proximal interphalangeal joint of **other finger**
           Dislocation of proximal interphalangeal joint of specified finger with unspecified laterality

   ● **S63.289** Dislocation of proximal interphalangeal joint of **unspecified finger**

● **S63.29** **Dislocation of distal interphalangeal joint of finger**

   ● **S63.290** Dislocation of distal interphalangeal joint of **right index finger**

   ● **S63.291** Dislocation of distal interphalangeal joint of **left index finger**

   ● **S63.292** Dislocation of distal interphalangeal joint of **right middle finger**

   ● **S63.293** Dislocation of distal interphalangeal joint of **left middle finger**

   ● **S63.294** Dislocation of distal interphalangeal joint of **right ring finger**

   ● **S63.295** Dislocation of distal interphalangeal joint of **left ring finger**

   ● **S63.296** Dislocation of distal interphalangeal joint of **right little finger**

   ● **S63.297** Dislocation of distal interphalangeal joint of **left little finger**

   ● **S63.298** Dislocation of distal interphalangeal joint of **other finger**
           Dislocation of distal interphalangeal joint of specified finger with unspecified laterality

   ● **S63.299** Dislocation of distal interphalangeal joint of **unspecified finger**

● **S63.3** **Traumatic rupture of ligament of wrist**

   ● **S63.30** Traumatic rupture of **unspecified ligament of wrist**

      ● **S63.301** Traumatic rupture of unspecified ligament of **right wrist**

      ● **S63.302** Traumatic rupture of unspecified ligament of **left wrist**

      ● **S63.309** Traumatic rupture of unspecified ligament of **unspecified wrist**

   ● **S63.31** Traumatic rupture of **collateral ligament of wrist**

      ● **S63.311** Traumatic rupture of collateral ligament of **right wrist**

      ● **S63.312** Traumatic rupture of collateral ligament of **left wrist**

      ● **S63.319** Traumatic rupture of collateral ligament of **unspecified wrist**

   ● **S63.32** Traumatic rupture of **radiocarpal ligament**

      ● **S63.321** Traumatic rupture of **right radiocarpal ligament**

      ● **S63.322** Traumatic rupture of **left radiocarpal ligament**

      ● **S63.329** Traumatic rupture of **unspecified radiocarpal ligament**

   ● **S63.33** Traumatic rupture of **ulnocarpal (palmar) ligament**

      ● **S63.331** Traumatic rupture of **right ulnocarpal (palmar) ligament**

      ● **S63.332** Traumatic rupture of **left ulnocarpal (palmar) ligament**

      ● **S63.339** Traumatic rupture of **unspecified ulnocarpal (palmar) ligament**

   ● **S63.39** Traumatic rupture of **other ligament of wrist**

      ● **S63.391** Traumatic rupture of other ligament of **right wrist**

      ● **S63.392** Traumatic rupture of other ligament of **left wrist**

      ● **S63.399** Traumatic rupture of other ligament of **unspecified wrist**

▶ New   ⟹ Revised   ~~deleted~~ Deleted | Excludes 1 | | Excludes 2 | | Includes | | Use additional | | Code first | | Code also | | Key words |

OGCR Official Guidelines   ● Unacceptable Principal Diagnosis   X Assign placeholder X   ● Use Additional Character(s)   ▌ Manifestation Code   **Coding Clinic**

- **S63.4** Traumatic rupture of ligament of finger at metacarpophalangeal and interphalangeal joint(s)
  - **S63.40** Traumatic rupture of unspecified ligament of finger at metacarpophalangeal and interphalangeal joint
    - **S63.400** Traumatic rupture of unspecified ligament of right index finger at metacarpophalangeal and interphalangeal joint
    - **S63.401** Traumatic rupture of unspecified ligament of left index finger at metacarpophalangeal and interphalangeal joint
    - **S63.402** Traumatic rupture of unspecified ligament of right middle finger at metacarpophalangeal and interphalangeal joint
    - **S63.403** Traumatic rupture of unspecified ligament of left middle finger at metacarpophalangeal and interphalangeal joint
    - **S63.404** Traumatic rupture of unspecified ligament of right ring finger at metacarpophalangeal and interphalangeal joint
    - **S63.405** Traumatic rupture of unspecified ligament of left ring finger at metacarpophalangeal and interphalangeal joint
    - **S63.406** Traumatic rupture of unspecified ligament of right little finger at metacarpophalangeal and interphalangeal joint
    - **S63.407** Traumatic rupture of unspecified ligament of left little finger at metacarpophalangeal and interphalangeal joint
    - **S63.408** Traumatic rupture of unspecified ligament of other finger at metacarpophalangeal and interphalangeal joint
      Traumatic rupture of unspecified ligament of specified finger with unspecified laterality at metacarpophalangeal and interphalangeal joint
    - **S63.409** Traumatic rupture of unspecified ligament of unspecified finger at metacarpophalangeal and interphalangeal joint
  - **S63.41** Traumatic rupture of collateral ligament of finger at metacarpophalangeal and interphalangeal joint
    - **S63.410** Traumatic rupture of collateral ligament of right index finger at metacarpophalangeal and interphalangeal joint
    - **S63.411** Traumatic rupture of collateral ligament of left index finger at metacarpophalangeal and interphalangeal joint
    - **S63.412** Traumatic rupture of collateral ligament of right middle finger at metacarpophalangeal and interphalangeal joint
    - **S63.413** Traumatic rupture of collateral ligament of left middle finger at metacarpophalangeal and interphalangeal joint
    - **S63.414** Traumatic rupture of collateral ligament of right ring finger at metacarpophalangeal and interphalangeal joint

- **S63.415** Traumatic rupture of collateral ligament of left ring finger at metacarpophalangeal and interphalangeal joint
- **S63.416** Traumatic rupture of collateral ligament of right little finger at metacarpophalangeal and interphalangeal joint
- **S63.417** Traumatic rupture of collateral ligament of left little finger at metacarpophalangeal and interphalangeal joint
- **S63.418** Traumatic rupture of collateral ligament of other finger at metacarpophalangeal and interphalangeal joint
  Traumatic rupture of collateral ligament of specified finger with unspecified laterality at metacarpophalangeal and interphalangeal joint
- **S63.419** Traumatic rupture of collateral ligament of unspecified finger at metacarpophalangeal and interphalangeal joint
- **S63.42** Traumatic rupture of palmar ligament of finger at metacarpophalangeal and interphalangeal joint
  - **S63.420** Traumatic rupture of palmar ligament of right index finger at metacarpophalangeal and interphalangeal joint
  - **S63.421** Traumatic rupture of palmar ligament of left index finger at metacarpophalangeal and interphalangeal joint
  - **S63.422** Traumatic rupture of palmar ligament of right middle finger at metacarpophalangeal and interphalangeal joint
  - **S63.423** Traumatic rupture of palmar ligament of left middle finger at metacarpophalangeal and interphalangeal joint
  - **S63.424** Traumatic rupture of palmar ligament of right ring finger at metacarpophalangeal and interphalangeal joint
  - **S63.425** Traumatic rupture of palmar ligament of left ring finger at metacarpophalangeal and interphalangeal joint
  - **S63.426** Traumatic rupture of palmar ligament of right little finger at metacarpophalangeal and interphalangeal joint
  - **S63.427** Traumatic rupture of palmar ligament of left little finger at metacarpophalangeal and interphalangeal joint
  - **S63.428** Traumatic rupture of palmar ligament of other finger at metacarpophalangeal and interphalangeal joint
    Traumatic rupture of palmar ligament of specified finger with unspecified laterality at metacarpophalangeal and interphalangeal joint
  - **S63.429** Traumatic rupture of palmar ligament of unspecified finger at metacarpophalangeal and interphalangeal joint

CHAPTER 19 (S00–T88)

● **S63.43**   Traumatic rupture of volar plate of finger at metacarpophalangeal and interphalangeal joint

  ● **S63.430**   Traumatic rupture of volar plate of right index finger at metacarpophalangeal and interphalangeal joint

  ● **S63.431**   Traumatic rupture of volar plate of left index finger at metacarpophalangeal and interphalangeal joint

  ● **S63.432**   Traumatic rupture of volar plate of right middle finger at metacarpophalangeal and interphalangeal joint

  ● **S63.433**   Traumatic rupture of volar plate of left middle finger at metacarpophalangeal and interphalangeal joint

  ● **S63.434**   Traumatic rupture of volar plate of right ring finger at metacarpophalangeal and interphalangeal joint

  ● **S63.435**   Traumatic rupture of volar plate of left ring finger at metacarpophalangeal and interphalangeal joint

  ● **S63.436**   Traumatic rupture of volar plate of right little finger at metacarpophalangeal and interphalangeal joint

  ● **S63.437**   Traumatic rupture of volar plate of left little finger at metacarpophalangeal and interphalangeal joint

  ● **S63.438**   Traumatic rupture of volar plate of other finger at metacarpophalangeal and interphalangeal joint
       Traumatic rupture of volar plate of specified finger with unspecified laterality at metacarpophalangeal and interphalangeal joint

  ● **S63.439**   Traumatic rupture of volar plate of unspecified finger at metacarpophalangeal and interphalangeal joint

● **S63.49**   Traumatic rupture of other ligament of finger at metacarpophalangeal and interphalangeal joint

  ● **S63.490**   Traumatic rupture of other ligament of right index finger at metacarpophalangeal and interphalangeal joint

  ● **S63.491**   Traumatic rupture of other ligament of left index finger at metacarpophalangeal and interphalangeal joint

  ● **S63.492**   Traumatic rupture of other ligament of right middle finger at metacarpophalangeal and interphalangeal joint

  ● **S63.493**   Traumatic rupture of other ligament of left middle finger at metacarpophalangeal and interphalangeal joint

  ● **S63.494**   Traumatic rupture of other ligament of right ring finger at metacarpophalangeal and interphalangeal joint

  ● **S63.495**   Traumatic rupture of other ligament of left ring finger at metacarpophalangeal and interphalangeal joint

  ● **S63.496**   Traumatic rupture of other ligament of right little finger at metacarpophalangeal and interphalangeal joint

  ● **S63.497**   Traumatic rupture of other ligament of left little finger at metacarpophalangeal and interphalangeal joint

  ● **S63.498**   Traumatic rupture of other ligament of other finger at metacarpophalangeal and interphalangeal joint
       Traumatic rupture of ligament of specified finger with unspecified laterality at metacarpophalangeal and interphalangeal joint

  ● **S63.499**   Traumatic rupture of other ligament of unspecified finger at metacarpophalangeal and interphalangeal joint

● **S63.5**   Other and unspecified sprain of wrist

  ● **S63.50**   Unspecified sprain of wrist

    ● **S63.501**   Unspecified sprain of right wrist

    ● **S63.502**   Unspecified sprain of left wrist

    ● **S63.509**   Unspecified sprain of unspecified wrist

  ● **S63.51**   Sprain of carpal (joint)

    ● **S63.511**   Sprain of carpal joint of right wrist

    ● **S63.512**   Sprain of carpal joint of left wrist

    ● **S63.519**   Sprain of carpal joint of unspecified wrist

  ● **S63.52**   Sprain of radiocarpal joint

     Excludes1   traumatic rupture of radiocarpal ligament (S63.32-)

    ● **S63.521**   Sprain of radiocarpal joint of right wrist

    ● **S63.522**   Sprain of radiocarpal joint of left wrist

    ● **S63.529**   Sprain of radiocarpal joint of unspecified wrist

  ● **S63.59**   Other specified sprain of wrist

    ● **S63.591**   Other specified sprain of right wrist

    ● **S63.592**   Other specified sprain of left wrist

    ● **S63.599**   Other specified sprain of unspecified wrist

▶ New   ⇒ Revised   ~~deleted~~ Deleted   Excludes 1   Excludes 2   Includes   Use additional   Code first   Code also   Key words

OGCR Official Guidelines   ● Unacceptable Principal Diagnosis   X Assign placeholder X   ● Use Additional Character(s)   ▸ Manifestation Code   **Coding Clinic**

● S63.6   Other and unspecified sprain of finger(s)

> **Excludes1**   traumatic rupture of ligament of finger at metacarpophalangeal and interphalangeal joint(s) (S63.4-)

● S63.60   Unspecified sprain of thumb

● S63.601   Unspecified sprain of right thumb

● S63.602   Unspecified sprain of left thumb

● S63.609   Unspecified sprain of unspecified thumb

● S63.61   Unspecified sprain of other and unspecified finger(s)

● S63.610   Unspecified sprain of right index finger

● S63.611   Unspecified sprain of left index finger

● S63.612   Unspecified sprain of right middle finger

● S63.613   Unspecified sprain of left middle finger

● S63.614   Unspecified sprain of right ring finger

● S63.615   Unspecified sprain of left ring finger

● S63.616   Unspecified sprain of right little finger

● S63.617   Unspecified sprain of left little finger

● S63.618   Unspecified sprain of other finger

> Unspecified sprain of specified finger with unspecified laterality

● S63.619   Unspecified sprain of unspecified finger

● S63.62   Sprain of interphalangeal joint of thumb

● S63.621   Sprain of interphalangeal joint of right thumb

● S63.622   Sprain of interphalangeal joint of left thumb

● S63.629   Sprain of interphalangeal joint of unspecified thumb

● S63.63   Sprain of interphalangeal joint of other and unspecified finger(s)

● S63.630   Sprain of interphalangeal joint of right index finger

● S63.631   Sprain of interphalangeal joint of left index finger

● S63.632   Sprain of interphalangeal joint of right middle finger

● S63.633   Sprain of interphalangeal joint of left middle finger

● S63.634   Sprain of interphalangeal joint of right ring finger

● S63.635   Sprain of interphalangeal joint of left ring finger

● S63.636   Sprain of interphalangeal joint of right little finger

● S63.637   Sprain of interphalangeal joint of left little finger

● S63.638   Sprain of interphalangeal joint of other finger

● S63.639   Sprain of interphalangeal joint of unspecified finger

● S63.64   Sprain of metacarpophalangeal joint of thumb

● S63.641   Sprain of metacarpophalangeal joint of right thumb

● S63.642   Sprain of metacarpophalangeal joint of left thumb

● S63.649   Sprain of metacarpophalangeal joint of unspecified thumb

● S63.65   Sprain of metacarpophalangeal joint of other and unspecified finger(s)

● S63.650   Sprain of metacarpophalangeal joint of right index finger

● S63.651   Sprain of metacarpophalangeal joint of left index finger

● S63.652   Sprain of metacarpophalangeal joint of right middle finger

● S63.653   Sprain of metacarpophalangeal joint of left middle finger

● S63.654   Sprain of metacarpophalangeal joint of right ring finger

● S63.655   Sprain of metacarpophalangeal joint of left ring finger

● S63.656   Sprain of metacarpophalangeal joint of right little finger

● S63.657   Sprain of metacarpophalangeal joint of left little finger

● S63.658   Sprain of metacarpophalangeal joint of other finger

> Sprain of metacarpophalangeal joint of specified finger with unspecified laterality

● S63.659   Sprain of metacarpophalangeal joint of unspecified finger

● S63.68   Other sprain of thumb

● S63.681   Other sprain of right thumb

● S63.682   Other sprain of left thumb

● S63.689   Other sprain of unspecified thumb

● S63.69   Other sprain of other and unspecified finger(s)

● S63.690   Other sprain of right index finger

● S63.691   Other sprain of left index finger

● S63.692   Other sprain of right middle finger

● S63.693   Other sprain of left middle finger

● S63.694   Other sprain of right ring finger

● S63.695   Other sprain of left ring finger

● S63.696   Other sprain of right little finger

● S63.697   Other sprain of left little finger

● S63.698   Other sprain of other finger

> Other sprain of specified finger with unspecified laterality

● S63.699   Other sprain of unspecified finger

● S63.8   Sprain of other part of wrist and hand

● S63.8X   Sprain of other part of wrist and hand

● S63.8X1   Sprain of other part of right wrist and hand

● S63.8X2   Sprain of other part of left wrist and hand

● S63.8X9   Sprain of other part of unspecified wrist and hand

● S63.9   Sprain of unspecified part of wrist and hand

X ● S63.90   Sprain of unspecified part of unspecified wrist and hand

X ● S63.91   Sprain of unspecified part of right wrist and hand

X ● S63.92   Sprain of unspecified part of left wrist and hand

S64   Injury of nerves at wrist and hand level

The appropriate 7th character is to be added to each code from category S64

A	initial encounter
D	subsequent encounter
S	sequela

Code also any associated open wound (S61.-)

● **S64.0**   Injury of ulnar nerve at wrist and hand level

X ● **S64.00**   Injury of ulnar nerve at wrist and hand level of unspecified arm

X ● **S64.01**   Injury of ulnar nerve at wrist and hand level of right arm

X ● **S64.02**   Injury of ulnar nerve at wrist and hand level of left arm

● **S64.1**   Injury of median nerve at wrist and hand level

X ● **S64.10**   Injury of median nerve at wrist and hand level of unspecified arm

X ● **S64.11**   Injury of median nerve at wrist and hand level of right arm

X ● **S64.12**   Injury of median nerve at wrist and hand level of left arm

● **S64.2**   Injury of radial nerve at wrist and hand level

X ● **S64.20**   Injury of radial nerve at wrist and hand level of unspecified arm

X ● **S64.21**   Injury of radial nerve at wrist and hand level of right arm

X ● **S64.22**   Injury of radial nerve at wrist and hand level of left arm

● **S64.3**   Injury of digital nerve of thumb

X ● **S64.30**   Injury of digital nerve of unspecified thumb

X ● **S64.31**   Injury of digital nerve of right thumb

X ● **S64.32**   Injury of digital nerve of left thumb

● **S64.4**   Injury of digital nerve of other and unspecified finger

X ● **S64.40**   Injury of digital nerve of unspecified finger

● **S64.49**   Injury of digital nerve of other finger

● **S64.490**   Injury of digital nerve of right index finger

● **S64.491**   Injury of digital nerve of left index finger

● **S64.492**   Injury of digital nerve of right middle finger

● **S64.493**   Injury of digital nerve of left middle finger

● **S64.494**   Injury of digital nerve of right ring finger

● **S64.495**   Injury of digital nerve of left ring finger

● **S64.496**   Injury of digital nerve of right little finger

● **S64.497**   Injury of digital nerve of left little finger

● **S64.498**   Injury of digital nerve of other finger

Injury of digital nerve of specified finger with unspecified laterality

● **S64.8**   Injury of other nerves at wrist and hand level

● **S64.8X**   Injury of other nerves at wrist and hand level

● **S64.8X1**   Injury of other nerves at wrist and hand level of right arm

● **S64.8X2**   Injury of other nerves at wrist and hand level of left arm

● **S64.8X9**   Injury of other nerves at wrist and hand level of unspecified arm

● **S64.9**   Injury of unspecified nerve at wrist and hand level

X ● **S64.90**   Injury of unspecified nerve at wrist and hand level of unspecified arm

X ● **S64.91**   Injury of unspecified nerve at wrist and hand level of right arm

X ● **S64.92**   Injury of unspecified nerve at wrist and hand level of left arm

S65   Injury of blood vessels at wrist and hand level

The appropriate 7th character is to be added to each code from category S65

A	initial encounter
D	subsequent encounter
S	sequela

Code also any associated open wound (S61.-)

● **S65.0**   Injury of ulnar artery at wrist and hand level

● **S65.00**   Unspecified injury of ulnar artery at wrist and hand level

● **S65.001**   Unspecified injury of ulnar artery at wrist and hand level of right arm A
(Ex) See PDX Collection 1274

● **S65.002**   Unspecified injury of ulnar artery at wrist and hand level of left arm A
(Ex) See PDX Collection 1275

● **S65.009**   Unspecified injury of ulnar artery at wrist and hand level of unspecified arm A
(Ex) See PDX Collection 1276

● **S65.01**   Laceration of ulnar artery at wrist and hand level

● **S65.011**   Laceration of ulnar artery at wrist and hand level of right arm A
(Ex) See PDX Collection 1274

● **S65.012**   Laceration of ulnar artery at wrist and hand level of left arm A
(Ex) See PDX Collection 1275

● **S65.019**   Laceration of ulnar artery at wrist and hand level of unspecified arm A
(Ex) See PDX Collection 1276

● **S65.09**   Other specified injury of ulnar artery at wrist and hand level

● **S65.091**   Other specified injury of ulnar artery at wrist and hand level of right arm A
(Ex) See PDX Collection 1274

● **S65.092**   Other specified injury of ulnar artery at wrist and hand level of left arm A
(Ex) See PDX Collection 1275

● **S65.099**   Other specified injury of ulnar artery at wrist and hand level of unspecified arm A
(Ex) See PDX Collection 1276

▶ New   ⇥ Revised   ~~deleted~~ Deleted   Excludes 1   Excludes 2   Includes   Use additional   Code first   Code also   Key words

OGCR Official Guidelines   ● Unacceptable Principal Diagnosis   X Assign placeholder X   ● Use Additional Character(s)   ▶ Manifestation Code   **Coding Clinic**

● S65.1   Injury of radial artery at wrist and hand level
   ● S65.10   Unspecified injury of radial artery at wrist and hand level
      ● S65.101   Unspecified injury of radial artery at wrist and hand level of right arm A 🦠
         Ex) See PDX Collection 1277
      ● S65.102   Unspecified injury of radial artery at wrist and hand level of left arm A 🦠
         Ex) See PDX Collection 1278
      ● S65.109   Unspecified injury of radial artery at wrist and hand level of unspecified arm A 🦠
         Ex) See PDX Collection 1279
   ● S65.11   Laceration of radial artery at wrist and hand level
      ● S65.111   Laceration of radial artery at wrist and hand level of right arm A 🦠
         Ex) See PDX Collection 1277
      ● S65.112   Laceration of radial artery at wrist and hand level of left arm A 🦠
         Ex) See PDX Collection 1278
      ● S65.119   Laceration of radial artery at wrist and hand level of unspecified arm A 🦠
         Ex) See PDX Collection 1279
   ● S65.19   Other specified injury of radial artery at wrist and hand level
      ● S65.191   Other specified injury of radial artery at wrist and hand level of right arm A 🦠
         Ex) See PDX Collection 1277
      ● S65.192   Other specified injury of radial artery at wrist and hand level of left arm A 🦠
         Ex) See PDX Collection 1278
      ● S65.199   Other specified injury of radial artery at wrist and hand level of unspecified arm A 🦠
         Ex) See PDX Collection 1279

● S65.2   Injury of superficial palmar arch
   ● S65.20   Unspecified injury of superficial palmar arch
      ● S65.201   Unspecified injury of superficial palmar arch of right hand A 🦠
         Ex) See PDX Collection 1288
      ● S65.202   Unspecified injury of superficial palmar arch of left hand A 🦠
         Ex) See PDX Collection 1289
      ● S65.209   Unspecified injury of superficial palmar arch of unspecified hand A 🦠
         Ex) See PDX Collection 1290
   ● S65.21   Laceration of superficial palmar arch
      ● S65.211   Laceration of superficial palmar arch of right hand A 🦠
         Ex) See PDX Collection 1288
      ● S65.212   Laceration of superficial palmar arch of left hand A 🦠
         Ex) See PDX Collection 1289
      ● S65.219   Laceration of superficial palmar arch of unspecified hand A 🦠
         Ex) See PDX Collection 1290
   ● S65.29   Other specified injury of superficial palmar arch
      ● S65.291   Other specified injury of superficial palmar arch of right hand A 🦠
         Ex) See PDX Collection 1288
      ● S65.292   Other specified injury of superficial palmar arch of left hand A 🦠
         Ex) See PDX Collection 1289
      ● S65.299   Other specified injury of superficial palmar arch of unspecified hand A 🦠
         Ex) See PDX Collection 1290

● S65.3   Injury of deep palmar arch
   ● S65.30   Unspecified injury of deep palmar arch
      ● S65.301   Unspecified injury of deep palmar arch of right hand A 🦠
         Ex) See PDX Collection 1288
      ● S65.302   Unspecified injury of deep palmar arch of left hand A 🦠
         Ex) See PDX Collection 1289
      ● S65.309   Unspecified injury of deep palmar arch of unspecified hand A 🦠
         Ex) See PDX Collection 1290
   ● S65.31   Laceration of deep palmar arch
      ● S65.311   Laceration of deep palmar arch of right hand A 🦠
         Ex) See PDX Collection 1288
      ● S65.312   Laceration of deep palmar arch of left hand A 🦠
         Ex) See PDX Collection 1289
      ● S65.319   Laceration of deep palmar arch of unspecified hand A 🦠
         Ex) See PDX Collection 1290
   ● S65.39   Other specified injury of deep palmar arch
      ● S65.391   Other specified injury of deep palmar arch of right hand A 🦠
         Ex) See PDX Collection 1288
      ● S65.392   Other specified injury of deep palmar arch of left hand A 🦠
         Ex) See PDX Collection 1289
      ● S65.399   Other specified injury of deep palmar arch of unspecified hand A 🦠
         Ex) See PDX Collection 1290

● S65.4   Injury of blood vessel of thumb
   ● S65.40   Unspecified injury of blood vessel of thumb
      ● S65.401   Unspecified injury of blood vessel of right thumb A 🦠
         Ex) See PDX Collection 1291
      ● S65.402   Unspecified injury of blood vessel of left thumb A 🦠
         Ex) See PDX Collection 1292
      ● S65.409   Unspecified injury of blood vessel of unspecified thumb A 🦠
         Ex) See PDX Collection 1293
   ● S65.41   Laceration of blood vessel of thumb
      ● S65.411   Laceration of blood vessel of right thumb A 🦠
         Ex) See PDX Collection 1291
      ● S65.412   Laceration of blood vessel of left thumb A 🦠
         Ex) See PDX Collection 1292
      ● S65.419   Laceration of blood vessel of unspecified thumb A 🦠
         Ex) See PDX Collection 1293
   ● S65.49   Other specified injury of blood vessel of thumb
      ● S65.491   Other specified injury of blood vessel of right thumb A 🦠
         Ex) See PDX Collection 1291
      ● S65.492   Other specified injury of blood vessel of left thumb A 🦠
         Ex) See PDX Collection 1292
      ● S65.499   Other specified injury of blood vessel of unspecified thumb A 🦠
         Ex) See PDX Collection 1293

CHAPTER 19 (S00-T88)

N   Newborn Age: 0   P   Pediatric Age: 0–17   M   Maternity DX: 12–55   A   Adult Age: 15–124   ♀   Females Only   ♂   Males Only
🦠   Complication\Comorbidity   🦠   Major C\C   Ex)   CC/MCC Exclusions   🦠   Hospital-Acquired Condition

CHAPTER 19 (S00-T88)

● S65.5 Injury of blood vessel of other and unspecified finger

  ● S65.50 Unspecified injury of blood vessel of other and unspecified finger

    ● S65.500 Unspecified injury of blood vessel of right index finger A 🖉
      (Ex:) See PDX Collection 1291

    ● S65.501 Unspecified injury of blood vessel of left index finger A 🖉
      (Ex:) See PDX Collection 1292

    ● S65.502 Unspecified injury of blood vessel of right middle finger A 🖉
      (Ex:) See PDX Collection 1291

    ● S65.503 Unspecified injury of blood vessel of left middle finger A 🖉
      (Ex:) See PDX Collection 1292

    ● S65.504 Unspecified injury of blood vessel of right ring finger A 🖉
      (Ex:) See PDX Collection 1291

    ● S65.505 Unspecified injury of blood vessel of left ring finger A 🖉
      (Ex:) See PDX Collection 1292

    ● S65.506 Unspecified injury of blood vessel of right little finger A 🖉
      (Ex:) See PDX Collection 1291

    ● S65.507 Unspecified injury of blood vessel of left little finger A 🖉
      (Ex:) See PDX Collection 1292

    ● S65.508 Unspecified injury of blood vessel of other finger A 🖉
      Unspecified injury of blood vessel of specified finger with unspecified laterality
      (Ex:) See PDX Collection 1293

    ● S65.509 Unspecified injury of blood vessel of unspecified finger A 🖉
      (Ex:) See PDX Collection 1293

  ● S65.51 Laceration of blood vessel of other and unspecified finger

    ● S65.510 Laceration of blood vessel of right index finger A 🖉
      (Ex:) See PDX Collection 1291

    ● S65.511 Laceration of blood vessel of left index finger A 🖉
      (Ex:) See PDX Collection 1292

    ● S65.512 Laceration of blood vessel of right middle finger A 🖉
      (Ex:) See PDX Collection 1291

    ● S65.513 Laceration of blood vessel of left middle finger A 🖉
      (Ex:) See PDX Collection 1292

    ● S65.514 Laceration of blood vessel of right ring finger A 🖉
      (Ex:) See PDX Collection 1291

    ● S65.515 Laceration of blood vessel of left ring finger A 🖉
      (Ex:) See PDX Collection 1292

    ● S65.516 Laceration of blood vessel of right little finger A 🖉
      (Ex:) See PDX Collection 1291

    ● S65.517 Laceration of blood vessel of left little finger A 🖉
      (Ex:) See PDX Collection 1292

    ● S65.518 Laceration of blood vessel of other finger A 🖉
      Laceration of blood vessel of specified finger with unspecified laterality
      (Ex:) See PDX Collection 1293

    ● S65.519 Laceration of blood vessel of unspecified finger A 🖉
      (Ex:) See PDX Collection 1293

  ● S65.59 Other specified injury of blood vessel of other and unspecified finger

    ● S65.590 Other specified injury of blood vessel of right index finger A 🖉
      (Ex:) See PDX Collection 1291

    ● S65.591 Other specified injury of blood vessel of left index finger A 🖉
      (Ex:) See PDX Collection 1292

    ● S65.592 Other specified injury of blood vessel of right middle finger A 🖉
      (Ex:) See PDX Collection 1291

    ● S65.593 Other specified injury of blood vessel of left middle finger A 🖉
      (Ex:) See PDX Collection 1292

    ● S65.594 Other specified injury of blood vessel of right ring finger A 🖉
      (Ex:) See PDX Collection 1291

    ● S65.595 Other specified injury of blood vessel of left ring finger A 🖉
      (Ex:) See PDX Collection 1292

    ● S65.596 Other specified injury of blood vessel of right little finger A 🖉
      (Ex:) See PDX Collection 1291

    ● S65.597 Other specified injury of blood vessel of left little finger A 🖉
      (Ex:) See PDX Collection 1292

    ● S65.598 Other specified injury of blood vessel of other finger A 🖉
      Other specified injury of blood vessel of specified finger with unspecified laterality
      (Ex:) See PDX Collection 1293

    ● S65.599 Other specified injury of blood vessel of unspecified finger A 🖉
      (Ex:) See PDX Collection 1293

● S65.8 Injury of other blood vessels at wrist and hand level

  ● S65.80 Unspecified injury of other blood vessels at wrist and hand level

    ● S65.801 Unspecified injury of other blood vessels at wrist and hand level of right arm A 🖉
      (Ex:) See PDX Collection 1260

    ● S65.802 Unspecified injury of other blood vessels at wrist and hand level of left arm A 🖉
      (Ex:) See PDX Collection 1261

    ● S65.809 Unspecified injury of other blood vessels at wrist and hand level of unspecified arm A 🖉
      (Ex:) See PDX Collection 1262

  ● S65.81 Laceration of other blood vessels at wrist and hand level

    ● S65.811 Laceration of other blood vessels at wrist and hand level of right arm A 🖉
      (Ex:) See PDX Collection 1260

    ● S65.812 Laceration of other blood vessels at wrist and hand level of left arm A 🖉
      (Ex:) See PDX Collection 1261

    ● S65.819 Laceration of other blood vessels at wrist and hand level of unspecified arm A 🖉
      (Ex:) See PDX Collection 1262

▶ New   ➠ Revised   ~~deleted~~ Deleted   Excludes 1   Excludes 2   Includes   Use additional   Code first   Code also   Key words

OGCR Official Guidelines   ● Unacceptable Principal Diagnosis   X Assign placeholder X   ● Use Additional Character(s)   ▶ Manifestation Code   **Coding Clinic**

● S65.89   Other specified injury of other blood vessels at wrist and hand level

   ● S65.891   Other specified injury of other blood vessels at wrist and hand level of **right arm** A ⬡
                   (Ex:) See PDX Collection 1260

   ● S65.892   Other specified injury of other blood vessels at wrist and hand level of **left arm** A ⬡
                   (Ex:) See PDX Collection 1261

   ● S65.899   Other specified injury of other blood vessels at wrist and hand level of **unspecified arm** A ⬡
                   (Ex:) See PDX Collection 1262

● S65.9   Injury of **unspecified blood vessel** at wrist and hand level

   ● S65.90   **Unspecified** injury of unspecified blood vessel at wrist and hand level

      ● S65.901   Unspecified injury of unspecified blood vessel at wrist and hand level of **right arm** A ⬡
                      (Ex:) See PDX Collection 1260

      ● S65.902   Unspecified injury of unspecified blood vessel at wrist and hand level of **left arm** A ⬡
                      (Ex:) See PDX Collection 1261

      ● S65.909   Unspecified injury of unspecified blood vessel at wrist and hand level of **unspecified arm** A ⬡
                      (Ex:) See PDX Collection 1262

   ● S65.91   Laceration of **unspecified blood vessel** at wrist and hand level

      ● S65.911   Laceration of **unspecified blood vessel** at wrist and hand level of **right arm** A ⬡
                      (Ex:) See PDX Collection 1260

      ● S65.912   Laceration of **unspecified** blood vessel at wrist and hand level of **left arm** A ⬡
                      (Ex:) See PDX Collection 1261

      ● S65.919   Laceration of **unspecified** blood vessel at wrist and hand level of **unspecified arm** A ⬡
                      (Ex:) See PDX Collection 1262

   ● S65.99   Other specified injury of unspecified blood vessel at wrist and hand level

      ● S65.991   Other specified injury of **unspecified** blood vessel at wrist and hand of **right arm** A ⬡
                      (Ex:) See PDX Collection 1260

      ● S65.992   Other specified injury of **unspecified** blood vessel at wrist and hand of **left arm** A ⬡
                      (Ex:) See PDX Collection 1261

      ● S65.999   Other specified injury of **unspecified** blood vessel at wrist and hand of **unspecified arm** A ⬡
                      (Ex:) See PDX Collection 1262

● S66   **Injury of muscle, fascia and tendon at wrist and hand level**

   Code also any associated open wound (S61.-)

   Excludes2   sprain of joints and ligaments of wrist and hand (S63.-)

   The appropriate 7th character is to be added to each code from category S66

A	initial encounter
D	subsequent encounter
S	sequela

● S66.0   Injury of **long flexor** muscle, fascia and tendon of **thumb** at wrist and hand level

   ● S66.00   **Unspecified** injury of long flexor muscle, fascia and tendon of thumb at wrist and hand level

      ● S66.001   Unspecified injury of long flexor muscle, fascia and tendon of **right** thumb at wrist and hand level

      ● S66.002   Unspecified injury of long flexor muscle, fascia and tendon of **left** thumb at wrist and hand level

      ● S66.009   Unspecified injury of long flexor muscle, fascia and tendon of **unspecified** thumb at wrist and hand level

   ● S66.01   **Strain** of long flexor muscle, fascia and tendon of thumb at wrist and hand level

      ● S66.011   Strain of long flexor muscle, fascia and tendon of **right** thumb at wrist and hand level

      ● S66.012   Strain of long flexor muscle, fascia and tendon of **left** thumb at wrist and hand level

      ● S66.019   Strain of long flexor muscle, fascia and tendon of **unspecified** thumb at wrist and hand level

   ● S66.02   **Laceration** of long flexor muscle, fascia and tendon of thumb at wrist and hand level

      ● S66.021   Laceration of long flexor muscle, fascia and tendon of **right** thumb at wrist and hand level A ⬡
                      (Ex:) See PDX Collection 1294

      ● S66.022   Laceration of long flexor muscle, fascia and tendon of **left** thumb at wrist and hand level A ⬡
                      (Ex:) See PDX Collection 1295

      ● S66.029   Laceration of long flexor muscle, fascia and tendon of **unspecified** thumb at wrist and hand level A ⬡
                      (Ex:) See PDX Collection 1296

   ● S66.09   Other specified injury of long flexor muscle, fascia and tendon of thumb at wrist and hand level

      ● S66.091   Other specified injury of long flexor muscle, fascia and tendon of **right** thumb at wrist and hand level

      ● S66.092   Other specified injury of long flexor muscle, fascia and tendon of **left** thumb at wrist and hand level

      ● S66.099   Other specified injury of long flexor muscle, fascia and tendon of **unspecified** thumb at wrist and hand level

● **S66.1**   **Injury of flexor muscle, fascia and tendon of other and unspecified finger at wrist and hand level**

> **Excludes2**   injury of long flexor muscle, fascia and tendon of thumb at wrist and hand level (S66.0-)

● **S66.10**   Unspecified injury of flexor muscle, fascia and tendon of other and unspecified finger at wrist and hand level

   ● **S66.100**   Unspecified injury of flexor muscle, fascia and tendon of right index finger at wrist and hand level

   ● **S66.101**   Unspecified injury of flexor muscle, fascia and tendon of left index finger at wrist and hand level

   ● **S66.102**   Unspecified injury of flexor muscle, fascia and tendon of right middle finger at wrist and hand level

   ● **S66.103**   Unspecified injury of flexor muscle, fascia and tendon of left middle finger at wrist and hand level

   ● **S66.104**   Unspecified injury of flexor muscle, fascia and tendon of right ring finger at wrist and hand level

   ● **S66.105**   Unspecified injury of flexor muscle, fascia and tendon of left ring finger at wrist and hand level

   ● **S66.106**   Unspecified injury of flexor muscle, fascia and tendon of right little finger at wrist and hand level

   ● **S66.107**   Unspecified injury of flexor muscle, fascia and tendon of left little finger at wrist and hand level

   ● **S66.108**   Unspecified injury of flexor muscle, fascia and tendon of other finger at wrist and hand level

> Unspecified injury of flexor muscle, fascia and tendon of specified finger with unspecified laterality at wrist and hand level

   ● **S66.109**   Unspecified injury of flexor muscle, fascia and tendon of unspecified finger at wrist and hand level

● **S66.11**   Strain of flexor muscle, fascia and tendon of other and unspecified finger at wrist and hand level

   ● **S66.110**   Strain of flexor muscle, fascia and tendon of right index finger at wrist and hand level

   ● **S66.111**   Strain of flexor muscle, fascia and tendon of left index finger at wrist and hand level

   ● **S66.112**   Strain of flexor muscle, fascia and tendon of right middle finger at wrist and hand level

   ● **S66.113**   Strain of flexor muscle, fascia and tendon of left middle finger at wrist and hand level

   ● **S66.114**   Strain of flexor muscle, fascia and tendon of right ring finger at wrist and hand level

   ● **S66.115**   Strain of flexor muscle, fascia and tendon of left ring finger at wrist and hand level

   ● **S66.116**   Strain of flexor muscle, fascia and tendon of right little finger at wrist and hand level

   ● **S66.117**   Strain of flexor muscle, fascia and tendon of left little finger at wrist and hand level

   ● **S66.118**   Strain of flexor muscle, fascia and tendon of other finger at wrist and hand level

> Strain of flexor muscle, fascia and tendon of specified finger with unspecified laterality at wrist and hand level

   ● **S66.119**   Strain of flexor muscle, fascia and tendon of unspecified finger at wrist and hand level

● **S66.12**   Laceration of flexor muscle, fascia and tendon of other and unspecified finger at wrist and hand level

   ● **S66.120**   Laceration of flexor muscle, fascia and tendon of right index finger at wrist and hand level A ✎
> Ex: See PDX Collection 1294

   ● **S66.121**   Laceration of flexor muscle, fascia and tendon of left index finger at wrist and hand level A ✎
> Ex: See PDX Collection 1295

   ● **S66.122**   Laceration of flexor muscle, fascia and tendon of right middle finger at wrist and hand level A ✎
> Ex: See PDX Collection 1294

   ● **S66.123**   Laceration of flexor muscle, fascia and tendon of left middle finger at wrist and hand level A ✎
> Ex: See PDX Collection 1295

   ● **S66.124**   Laceration of flexor muscle, fascia and tendon of right ring finger at wrist and hand level A ✎
> Ex: See PDX Collection 1294

   ● **S66.125**   Laceration of flexor muscle, fascia and tendon of left ring finger at wrist and hand level A ✎
> Ex: See PDX Collection 1295

   ● **S66.126**   Laceration of flexor muscle, fascia and tendon of right little finger at wrist and hand level A ✎
> Ex: See PDX Collection 1294

   ● **S66.127**   Laceration of flexor muscle, fascia and tendon of left little finger at wrist and hand level A ✎
> Ex: See PDX Collection 1295

   ● **S66.128**   Laceration of flexor muscle, fascia and tendon of other finger at wrist and hand level A ✎

> Laceration of flexor muscle, fascia and tendon of specified finger with unspecified laterality at wrist and hand level
> Ex: See PDX Collection 1296

   ● **S66.129**   Laceration of flexor muscle, fascia and tendon of unspecified finger at wrist and hand level A ✎
> Ex: See PDX Collection 1296

▶ New   ➟ Revised   ~~deleted~~ Deleted   Excludes 1   Excludes 2   Includes   Use additional   Code first   Code also   Key words

OGCR Official Guidelines   ● Unacceptable Principal Diagnosis   X Assign placeholder X   ● Use Additional Character(s)   ▶ Manifestation Code   **Coding Clinic**

● S66.19   Other injury of flexor muscle, fascia and tendon of other and unspecified finger at wrist and hand level

   ● S66.190   Other injury of flexor muscle, fascia and tendon of right index finger at wrist and hand level

   ● S66.191   Other injury of flexor muscle, fascia and tendon of left index finger at wrist and hand level

   ● S66.192   Other injury of flexor muscle, fascia and tendon of right middle finger at wrist and hand level

   ● S66.193   Other injury of flexor muscle, fascia and tendon of left middle finger at wrist and hand level

   ● S66.194   Other injury of flexor muscle, fascia and tendon of right ring finger at wrist and hand level

   ● S66.195   Other injury of flexor muscle, fascia and tendon of left ring finger at wrist and hand level

   ● S66.196   Other injury of flexor muscle, fascia and tendon of right little finger at wrist and hand level

   ● S66.197   Other injury of flexor muscle, fascia and tendon of left little finger at wrist and hand level

   ● S66.198   Other injury of flexor muscle, fascia and tendon of other finger at wrist and hand level

       Other injury of flexor muscle, fascia and tendon of specified finger with unspecified laterality at wrist and hand level

   ● S66.199   Other injury of flexor muscle, fascia and tendon of unspecified finger at wrist and hand level

● S66.2   Injury of extensor muscle, fascia and tendon of thumb at wrist and hand level

   ● S66.20   Unspecified injury of extensor muscle, fascia and tendon of thumb at wrist and hand level

      ● S66.201   Unspecified injury of extensor muscle, fascia and tendon of right thumb at wrist and hand level

      ● S66.202   Unspecified injury of extensor muscle, fascia and tendon of left thumb at wrist and hand level

      ● S66.209   Unspecified injury of extensor muscle, fascia and tendon of unspecified thumb at wrist and hand level

   ● S66.21   Strain of extensor muscle, fascia and tendon of thumb at wrist and hand level

      ● S66.211   Strain of extensor muscle, fascia and tendon of right thumb at wrist and hand level

      ● S66.212   Strain of extensor muscle, fascia and tendon of left thumb at wrist and hand level

      ● S66.219   Strain of extensor muscle, fascia and tendon of unspecified thumb at wrist and hand level

● S66.22   Laceration of extensor muscle, fascia and tendon of thumb at wrist and hand level

   ● S66.221   Laceration of extensor muscle, fascia and tendon of right thumb at wrist and hand level A ⓒ
       Ⓔⓧ See PDX Collection 1294

   ● S66.222   Laceration of extensor muscle, fascia and tendon of left thumb at wrist and hand level A ⓒ
       Ⓔⓧ See PDX Collection 1295

   ● S66.229   Laceration of extensor muscle, fascia and tendon of unspecified thumb at wrist and hand level A ⓒ
       Ⓔⓧ See PDX Collection 1296

● S66.29   Other specified injury of extensor muscle, fascia and tendon of thumb at wrist and hand level

   ● S66.291   Other specified injury of extensor muscle, fascia and tendon of right thumb at wrist and hand level

   ● S66.292   Other specified injury of extensor muscle, fascia and tendon of left thumb at wrist and hand level

   ● S66.299   Other specified injury of extensor muscle, fascia and tendon of unspecified thumb at wrist and hand level

● S66.3   Injury of extensor muscle, fascia and tendon of other and unspecified finger at wrist and hand level

   Excludes2   injury of extensor muscle, fascia and tendon of thumb at wrist and hand level (S66.2-)

   ● S66.30   Unspecified injury of extensor muscle, fascia and tendon of other and unspecified finger at wrist and hand level

      ● S66.300   Unspecified injury of extensor muscle, fascia and tendon of right index finger at wrist and hand level

      ● S66.301   Unspecified injury of extensor muscle, fascia and tendon of left index finger at wrist and hand level

      ● S66.302   Unspecified injury of extensor muscle, fascia and tendon of right middle finger at wrist and hand level

      ● S66.303   Unspecified injury of extensor muscle, fascia and tendon of left middle finger at wrist and hand level

      ● S66.304   Unspecified injury of extensor muscle, fascia and tendon of right ring finger at wrist and hand level

      ● S66.305   Unspecified injury of extensor muscle, fascia and tendon of left ring finger at wrist and hand level

      ● S66.306   Unspecified injury of extensor muscle, fascia and tendon of right little finger at wrist and hand level

      ● S66.307   Unspecified injury of extensor muscle, fascia and tendon of left little finger at wrist and hand level

      ● S66.308   Unspecified injury of extensor muscle, fascia and tendon of other finger at wrist and hand level

         Unspecified injury of extensor muscle, fascia and tendon of specified finger with unspecified laterality at wrist and hand level

      ● S66.309   Unspecified injury of extensor muscle, fascia and tendon of unspecified finger at wrist and hand level

CHAPTER 19 (S00–T88)

CHAPTER 19 (S00-T88)

● S66.31   **Strain** of extensor muscle, fascia and tendon of **other and unspecified** finger at wrist and hand level

    ● S66.310   Strain of extensor muscle, fascia and tendon of **right index** finger at wrist and hand level

    ● S66.311   Strain of extensor muscle, fascia and tendon of **left index** finger at wrist and hand level

    ● S66.312   Strain of extensor muscle, fascia and tendon of **right middle** finger at wrist and hand level

    ● S66.313   Strain of extensor muscle, fascia and tendon of **left middle** finger at wrist and hand level

    ● S66.314   Strain of extensor muscle, fascia and tendon of **right ring** finger at wrist and hand level

    ● S66.315   Strain of extensor muscle, fascia and tendon of **left ring** finger at wrist and hand level

    ● S66.316   Strain of extensor muscle, fascia and tendon of **right little** finger at wrist and hand level

    ● S66.317   Strain of extensor muscle, fascia and tendon of **left little** finger at wrist and hand level

    ● S66.318   Strain of extensor muscle, fascia and tendon of **other** finger at wrist and hand level

         Strain of extensor muscle, fascia and tendon of specified finger with unspecified laterality at wrist and hand level

    ● S66.319   Strain of extensor muscle, fascia and tendon of **unspecified** finger at wrist and hand level

● S66.32   **Laceration** of extensor muscle, fascia and tendon of **other and unspecified** finger at wrist and hand level

    ● S66.320   Laceration of extensor muscle, fascia and tendon of **right index** finger at wrist and hand level A
         (Ex:) See PDX Collection 1294

    ● S66.321   Laceration of extensor muscle, fascia and tendon of **left index** finger at wrist and hand level A
         (Ex:) See PDX Collection 1295

    ● S66.322   Laceration of extensor muscle, fascia and tendon of **right middle** finger at wrist and hand level A
         (Ex:) See PDX Collection 1294

    ● S66.323   Laceration of extensor muscle, fascia and tendon of **left middle** finger at wrist and hand level A
         (Ex:) See PDX Collection 1295

    ● S66.324   Laceration of extensor muscle, fascia and tendon of **right ring** finger at wrist and hand level A
         (Ex:) See PDX Collection 1294

    ● S66.325   Laceration of extensor muscle, fascia and tendon of **left ring** finger at wrist and hand level A
         (Ex:) See PDX Collection 1295

    ● S66.326   Laceration of extensor muscle, fascia and tendon of **right little** finger at wrist and hand level A
         (Ex:) See PDX Collection 1294

    ● S66.327   Laceration of extensor muscle, fascia and tendon of **left little** finger at wrist and hand level A
         (Ex:) See PDX Collection 1295

    ● S66.328   Laceration of extensor muscle, fascia and tendon of **other** finger at wrist and hand level A
         Laceration of extensor muscle, fascia and tendon of specified finger with unspecified laterality at wrist and hand level
         (Ex:) See PDX Collection 1296

    ● S66.329   Laceration of extensor muscle, fascia and tendon of **unspecified** finger at wrist and hand level A
         (Ex:) See PDX Collection 1296

● S66.39   **Other injury** of extensor muscle, fascia and tendon of other and unspecified finger at wrist and hand level

    ● S66.390   Other injury of extensor muscle, fascia and tendon of **right index** finger at wrist and hand level

    ● S66.391   Other injury of extensor muscle, fascia and tendon of **left index** finger at wrist and hand level

    ● S66.392   Other injury of extensor muscle, fascia and tendon of **right middle** finger at wrist and hand level

    ● S66.393   Other injury of extensor muscle, fascia and tendon of **left middle** finger at wrist and hand level

    ● S66.394   Other injury of extensor muscle, fascia and tendon of **right ring** finger at wrist and hand level

    ● S66.395   Other injury of extensor muscle, fascia and tendon of **left ring** finger at wrist and hand level

    ● S66.396   Other injury of extensor muscle, fascia and tendon of **right little** finger at wrist and hand level

    ● S66.397   Other injury of extensor muscle, fascia and tendon of **left little** finger at wrist and hand level

    ● S66.398   Other injury of extensor muscle, fascia and tendon of **other** finger at wrist and hand level

         Other injury of extensor muscle, fascia and tendon of specified finger with unspecified laterality at wrist and hand level

    ● S66.399   Other injury of extensor muscle, fascia and tendon of **unspecified** finger at wrist and hand level

● S66.4   **Injury of intrinsic** muscle, fascia and tendon of **thumb** at wrist and hand level

    ● S66.40   **Unspecified injury** of intrinsic muscle, fascia and tendon of thumb at wrist and hand level

      ● S66.401   Unspecified injury of intrinsic muscle, fascia and tendon of **right** thumb at wrist and hand level

      ● S66.402   Unspecified injury of intrinsic muscle, fascia and tendon of **left** thumb at wrist and hand level

      ● S66.409   Unspecified injury of intrinsic muscle, fascia and tendon of **unspecified** thumb at wrist and hand level

    ● S66.41   **Strain** of intrinsic muscle, fascia and tendon of thumb at wrist and hand level

      ● S66.411   Strain of intrinsic muscle, fascia and tendon of **right** thumb at wrist and hand level

      ● S66.412   Strain of intrinsic muscle, fascia and tendon of **left** thumb at wrist and hand level

      ● S66.419   Strain of intrinsic muscle, fascia and tendon of **unspecified** thumb at wrist and hand level

● S66.42 Laceration of intrinsic muscle, fascia and tendon of thumb at wrist and hand level

   ● S66.421 Laceration of intrinsic muscle, fascia and tendon of right thumb at wrist and hand level A 🦠
        (Ex) See PDX Collection 1294

   ● S66.422 Laceration of intrinsic muscle, fascia and tendon of left thumb at wrist and hand level A 🦠
        (Ex) See PDX Collection 1295

   ● S66.429 Laceration of intrinsic muscle, fascia and tendon of unspecified thumb at wrist and hand level A 🦠
        (Ex) See PDX Collection 1296

● S66.49 Other specified injury of intrinsic muscle, fascia and tendon of thumb at wrist and hand level

   ● S66.491 Other specified injury of intrinsic muscle, fascia and tendon of right thumb at wrist and hand level

   ● S66.492 Other specified injury of intrinsic muscle, fascia and tendon of left thumb at wrist and hand level

   ● S66.499 Other specified injury of intrinsic muscle, fascia and tendon of unspecified thumb at wrist and hand level

● S66.5 Injury of intrinsic muscle, fascia and tendon of other and unspecified finger at wrist and hand level

   Excludes2 injury of intrinsic muscle, fascia and tendon of thumb at wrist and hand level (S66.4-)

   ● S66.50 Unspecified injury of intrinsic muscle, fascia and tendon of other and unspecified finger at wrist and hand level

      ● S66.500 Unspecified injury of intrinsic muscle, fascia and tendon of right index finger at wrist and hand level

      ● S66.501 Unspecified injury of intrinsic muscle, fascia and tendon of left index finger at wrist and hand level

      ● S66.502 Unspecified injury of intrinsic muscle, fascia and tendon of right middle finger at wrist and hand level

      ● S66.503 Unspecified injury of intrinsic muscle, fascia and tendon of left middle finger at wrist and hand level

      ● S66.504 Unspecified injury of intrinsic muscle, fascia and tendon of right ring finger at wrist and hand level

      ● S66.505 Unspecified injury of intrinsic muscle, fascia and tendon of left ring finger at wrist and hand level

      ● S66.506 Unspecified injury of intrinsic muscle, fascia and tendon of right little finger at wrist and hand level

      ● S66.507 Unspecified injury of intrinsic muscle, fascia and tendon of left little finger at wrist and hand level

      ● S66.508 Unspecified injury of intrinsic muscle, fascia and tendon of other finger at wrist and hand level
           Unspecified injury of intrinsic muscle, fascia and tendon of specified finger with unspecified laterality at wrist and hand level

      ● S66.509 Unspecified injury of intrinsic muscle, fascia and tendon of unspecified finger at wrist and hand level

● S66.51 Strain of intrinsic muscle, fascia and tendon of other and unspecified finger at wrist and hand level

   ● S66.510 Strain of intrinsic muscle, fascia and tendon of right index finger at wrist and hand level

   ● S66.511 Strain of intrinsic muscle, fascia and tendon of left index finger at wrist and hand level

   ● S66.512 Strain of intrinsic muscle, fascia and tendon of right middle finger at wrist and hand level

   ● S66.513 Strain of intrinsic muscle, fascia and tendon of left middle finger at wrist and hand level

   ● S66.514 Strain of intrinsic muscle, fascia and tendon of right ring finger at wrist and hand level

   ● S66.515 Strain of intrinsic muscle, fascia and tendon of left ring finger at wrist and hand level

   ● S66.516 Strain of intrinsic muscle, fascia and tendon of right little finger at wrist and hand level

   ● S66.517 Strain of intrinsic muscle, fascia and tendon of left little finger at wrist and hand level

   ● S66.518 Strain of intrinsic muscle, fascia and tendon of other finger at wrist and hand level
        Strain of intrinsic muscle, fascia and tendon of specified finger with unspecified laterality at wrist and hand level

   ● S66.519 Strain of intrinsic muscle, fascia and tendon of unspecified finger at wrist and hand level

● S66.52 Laceration of intrinsic muscle, fascia and tendon of other and unspecified finger at wrist and hand level

   ● S66.520 Laceration of intrinsic muscle, fascia and tendon of right index finger at wrist and hand level A 🦠
        (Ex) See PDX Collection 1294

   ● S66.521 Laceration of intrinsic muscle, fascia and tendon of left index finger at wrist and hand level A 🦠
        (Ex) See PDX Collection 1295

   ● S66.522 Laceration of intrinsic muscle, fascia and tendon of right middle finger at wrist and hand level A 🦠
        (Ex) See PDX Collection 1294

   ● S66.523 Laceration of intrinsic muscle, fascia and tendon of left middle finger at wrist and hand level A 🦠
        (Ex) See PDX Collection 1295

   ● S66.524 Laceration of intrinsic muscle, fascia and tendon of right ring finger at wrist and hand level A 🦠
        (Ex) See PDX Collection 1294

   ● S66.525 Laceration of intrinsic muscle, fascia and tendon of left ring finger at wrist and hand level A 🦠
        (Ex) See PDX Collection 1295

   ● S66.526 Laceration of intrinsic muscle, fascia and tendon of right little finger at wrist and hand level A 🦠
        (Ex) See PDX Collection 1294

   ● S66.527 Laceration of intrinsic muscle, fascia and tendon of left little finger at wrist and hand level A 🦠
        (Ex) See PDX Collection 1295

CHAPTER 19 (S00-T88)

● S66.528   Laceration of intrinsic muscle, fascia and tendon of other finger at wrist and hand level A
> Laceration of intrinsic muscle, fascia and tendon of specified finger with unspecified laterality at wrist and hand level
> (Ex:) See PDX Collection 1296

● S66.529   Laceration of intrinsic muscle, fascia and tendon of unspecified finger at wrist and hand level A
> (Ex:) See PDX Collection 1296

● S66.59   Other injury of intrinsic muscle, fascia and tendon of other and unspecified finger at wrist and hand level

● S66.590   Other injury of intrinsic muscle, fascia and tendon of right index finger at wrist and hand level

● S66.591   Other injury of intrinsic muscle, fascia and tendon of left index finger at wrist and hand level

● S66.592   Other injury of intrinsic muscle, fascia and tendon of right middle finger at wrist and hand level

● S66.593   Other injury of intrinsic muscle, fascia and tendon of left middle finger at wrist and hand level

● S66.594   Other injury of intrinsic muscle, fascia and tendon of right ring finger at wrist and hand level

● S66.595   Other injury of intrinsic muscle, fascia and tendon of left ring finger at wrist and hand level

● S66.596   Other injury of intrinsic muscle, fascia and tendon of right little finger at wrist and hand level

● S66.597   Other injury of intrinsic muscle, fascia and tendon of left little finger at wrist and hand level

● S66.598   Other injury of intrinsic muscle, fascia and tendon of other finger at wrist and hand level
> Other injury of intrinsic muscle, fascia and tendon of specified finger with unspecified laterality at wrist and hand level

● S66.599   Other injury of intrinsic muscle, fascia and tendon of unspecified finger at wrist and hand level

● S66.8   Injury of other specified muscles, fascia and tendons at wrist and hand level

● S66.80   Unspecified injury of other specified muscles, fascia and tendons at wrist and hand level

● S66.801   Unspecified injury of other specified muscles, fascia and tendons at wrist and hand level, right hand

● S66.802   Unspecified injury of other specified muscles, fascia and tendons at wrist and hand level, left hand

● S66.809   Unspecified injury of other specified muscles, fascia and tendons at wrist and hand level, unspecified hand

● S66.81   Strain of other specified muscles, fascia and tendons at wrist and hand level

● S66.811   Strain of other specified muscles, fascia and tendons at wrist and hand level, right hand

● S66.812   Strain of other specified muscles, fascia and tendons at wrist and hand level, left hand

● S66.819   Strain of other specified muscles, fascia and tendons at wrist and hand level, unspecified hand

● S66.82   Laceration of other specified muscles, fascia and tendons at wrist and hand level

● S66.821   Laceration of other specified muscles, fascia and tendons at wrist and hand level, right hand A
> (Ex:) See PDX Collection 1294

● S66.822   Laceration of other specified muscles, fascia and tendons at wrist and hand level, left hand A
> (Ex:) See PDX Collection 1295

● S66.829   Laceration of other specified muscles, fascia and tendons at wrist and hand level, unspecified hand A
> (Ex:) See PDX Collection 1296

● S66.89   Other injury of other specified muscles, fascia and tendons at wrist and hand level

● S66.891   Other injury of other specified muscles, fascia and tendons at wrist and hand level, right hand

● S66.892   Other injury of other specified muscles, fascia and tendons at wrist and hand level, left hand

● S66.899   Other injury of other specified muscles, fascia and tendons at wrist and hand level, unspecified hand

● S66.9   Injury of unspecified muscle, fascia and tendon at wrist and hand level

● S66.90   Unspecified injury of unspecified muscle, fascia and tendon at wrist and hand level

● S66.901   Unspecified injury of unspecified muscle, fascia and tendon at wrist and hand level, right hand

● S66.902   Unspecified injury of unspecified muscle, fascia and tendon at wrist and hand level, left hand

● S66.909   Unspecified injury of unspecified muscle, fascia and tendon at wrist and hand level, unspecified hand

● S66.91   Strain of unspecified muscle, fascia and tendon at wrist and hand level

● S66.911   Strain of unspecified muscle, fascia and tendon at wrist and hand level, right hand

● S66.912   Strain of unspecified muscle, fascia and tendon at wrist and hand level, left hand

● S66.919   Strain of unspecified muscle, fascia and tendon at wrist and hand level, unspecified hand

● **S66.92** Laceration of unspecified muscle, fascia and tendon at wrist and hand level
    ● **S66.921** Laceration of unspecified muscle, fascia and tendon at wrist and hand level, **right hand** A 🔹
         (Ex) See PDX Collection 1294
    ● **S66.922** Laceration of unspecified muscle, fascia and tendon at wrist and hand level, **left hand** A 🔹
         (Ex) See PDX Collection 1295
    ● **S66.929** Laceration of unspecified muscle, fascia and tendon at wrist and hand level, **unspecified hand** A 🔹
         (Ex) See PDX Collection 1296
● **S66.99** Other injury of unspecified muscle, fascia and tendon at wrist and hand level
    ● **S66.991** Other injury of unspecified muscle, fascia and tendon at wrist and hand level, **right hand**
    ● **S66.992** Other injury of unspecified muscle, fascia and tendon at wrist and hand level, **left hand**
    ● **S66.999** Other injury of unspecified muscle, fascia and tendon at wrist and hand level, **unspecified hand**

● **S67** **Crushing injury of wrist, hand and fingers**
Use additional code for all associated injuries, such as:
    fracture of wrist and hand (S62.-)
    open wound of wrist and hand (S61.-)
The appropriate 7th character is to be added to each code from category S67

A	initial encounter
D	subsequent encounter
S	sequela

● **S67.0** Crushing injury of **thumb**
   X ● **S67.00** Crushing injury of **unspecified** thumb
   X ● **S67.01** Crushing injury of **right** thumb
   X ● **S67.02** Crushing injury of **left** thumb
● **S67.1** Crushing injury of other and unspecified **finger(s)**
     Excludes2 crushing injury of thumb (S67.0-)
   X ● **S67.10** Crushing injury of **unspecified** finger(s)
   ● **S67.19** Crushing injury of other finger(s)
    ● **S67.190** Crushing injury of **right index finger**
    ● **S67.191** Crushing injury of **left index finger**
    ● **S67.192** Crushing injury of **right middle finger**
    ● **S67.193** Crushing injury of **left middle finger**
    ● **S67.194** Crushing injury of **right ring finger**
    ● **S67.195** Crushing injury of **left ring finger**
    ● **S67.196** Crushing injury of **right little finger**
    ● **S67.197** Crushing injury of **left little finger**
    ● **S67.198** Crushing injury of **other finger**
         Crushing injury of specified finger with unspecified laterality
● **S67.2** Crushing injury of **hand**
     Excludes2 crushing injury of fingers (S67.1-)
                  crushing injury of thumb (S67.0-)
   X ● **S67.20** Crushing injury of **unspecified** hand
   X ● **S67.21** Crushing injury of **right** hand
   X ● **S67.22** Crushing injury of **left** hand
● **S67.3** Crushing injury of **wrist**
   X ● **S67.30** Crushing injury of **unspecified** wrist
   X ● **S67.31** Crushing injury of **right** wrist
   X ● **S67.32** Crushing injury of **left** wrist

● **S67.4** Crushing injury of **wrist and hand**
     Excludes1 crushing injury of hand alone (S67.2-)
                  crushing injury of wrist alone (S67.3-)
     Excludes2 crushing injury of fingers (S67.1-)
                  crushing injury of thumb (S67.0-)
   X ● **S67.40** Crushing injury of **unspecified** wrist and hand
   X ● **S67.41** Crushing injury of **right** wrist and hand
   X ● **S67.42** Crushing injury of **left** wrist and hand
● **S67.9** Crushing injury of **unspecified** part(s) of wrist, hand and fingers
   X ● **S67.90** Crushing injury of unspecified part(s) of **unspecified** wrist, hand and fingers
   X ● **S67.91** Crushing injury of unspecified part(s) of **right** wrist, hand and fingers
   X ● **S67.92** Crushing injury of unspecified part(s) of **left** wrist, hand and fingers

● **S68** **Traumatic amputation of wrist, hand and fingers**
An amputation not identified as partial or complete should be coded to complete
The appropriate 7th character is to be added to each code from category S68

A	initial encounter
D	subsequent encounter
S	sequela

● **S68.0** Traumatic **metacarpophalangeal** amputation of **thumb**
     Traumatic amputation of thumb NOS
   ● **S68.01** Complete traumatic metacarpophalangeal amputation of thumb
    ● **S68.011** Complete traumatic metacarpophalangeal amputation of **right thumb**
    ● **S68.012** Complete traumatic metacarpophalangeal amputation of **left thumb**
    ● **S68.019** Complete traumatic metacarpophalangeal amputation of **unspecified thumb**
   ● **S68.02** Partial traumatic metacarpophalangeal amputation of thumb
    ● **S68.021** Partial traumatic metacarpophalangeal amputation of **right thumb**
    ● **S68.022** Partial traumatic metacarpophalangeal amputation of **left thumb**
    ● **S68.029** Partial traumatic metacarpophalangeal amputation of **unspecified thumb**
● **S68.1** Traumatic **metacarpophalangeal** amputation of other and unspecified finger
     Traumatic amputation of finger NOS
     Excludes2 traumatic metacarpophalangeal amputation of thumb (S68.0-)
   ● **S68.11** Complete traumatic metacarpophalangeal amputation of other and unspecified finger
    ● **S68.110** Complete traumatic metacarpophalangeal amputation of **right index finger**
    ● **S68.111** Complete traumatic metacarpophalangeal amputation of **left index finger**
    ● **S68.112** Complete traumatic metacarpophalangeal amputation of **right middle finger**
    ● **S68.113** Complete traumatic metacarpophalangeal amputation of **left middle finger**

CHAPTER 19 (S00-T88)

N Newborn Age: 0   P Pediatric Age: 0–17   M Maternity DX: 12–55   A Adult Age: 15–124   ♀ Females Only   ♂ Males Only
🔹 Complication\Comorbidity   🔹 Major C\C   (Ex) CC/MCC Exclusions   🔹 Hospital-Acquired Condition
1347

● **S68.114** Complete traumatic metacarpophalangeal amputation of right ring finger

● **S68.115** Complete traumatic metacarpophalangeal amputation of left ring finger

● **S68.116** Complete traumatic metacarpophalangeal amputation of right little finger

● **S68.117** Complete traumatic metacarpophalangeal amputation of left little finger

● **S68.118** Complete traumatic metacarpophalangeal amputation of other finger

     Complete traumatic metacarpophalangeal amputation of specified finger with unspecified laterality

● **S68.119** Complete traumatic metacarpophalangeal amputation of unspecified finger

● **S68.12** Partial traumatic metacarpophalangeal amputation of other and unspecified finger

● **S68.120** Partial traumatic metacarpophalangeal amputation of right index finger

● **S68.121** Partial traumatic metacarpophalangeal amputation of left index finger

● **S68.122** Partial traumatic metacarpophalangeal amputation of right middle finger

● **S68.123** Partial traumatic metacarpophalangeal amputation of left middle finger

● **S68.124** Partial traumatic metacarpophalangeal amputation of right ring finger

● **S68.125** Partial traumatic metacarpophalangeal amputation of left ring finger

● **S68.126** Partial traumatic metacarpophalangeal amputation of right little finger

● **S68.127** Partial traumatic metacarpophalangeal amputation of left little finger

● **S68.128** Partial traumatic metacarpophalangeal amputation of other finger

     Partial traumatic metacarpophalangeal amputation of specified finger with unspecified laterality

● **S68.129** Partial traumatic metacarpophalangeal amputation of unspecified finger

● **S68.4** Traumatic amputation of hand at wrist level

     Traumatic amputation of hand NOS

     Traumatic amputation of wrist

● **S68.41** Complete traumatic amputation of hand at wrist level

● **S68.411** Complete traumatic amputation of right hand at wrist level A 🔖

     (Ex:) See PDX Collection 1266

● **S68.412** Complete traumatic amputation of left hand at wrist level A 🔖

     (Ex:) See PDX Collection 1267

● **S68.419** Complete traumatic amputation of unspecified hand at wrist level A 🔖

     (Ex:) See PDX Collection 1268

● **S68.42** Partial traumatic amputation of hand at wrist level

● **S68.421** Partial traumatic amputation of right hand at wrist level A 🔖

     (Ex:) See PDX Collection 1266

● **S68.422** Partial traumatic amputation of left hand at wrist level A 🔖

     (Ex:) See PDX Collection 1267

● **S68.429** Partial traumatic amputation of unspecified hand at wrist level A 🔖

     (Ex:) See PDX Collection 1268

● **S68.5** Traumatic transphalangeal amputation of thumb

     Traumatic interphalangeal joint amputation of thumb

● **S68.51** Complete traumatic transphalangeal amputation of thumb

● **S68.511** Complete traumatic transphalangeal amputation of right thumb

● **S68.512** Complete traumatic transphalangeal amputation of left thumb

● **S68.519** Complete traumatic transphalangeal amputation of unspecified thumb

● **S68.52** Partial traumatic transphalangeal amputation of thumb

● **S68.521** Partial traumatic transphalangeal amputation of right thumb

● **S68.522** Partial traumatic transphalangeal amputation of left thumb

● **S68.529** Partial traumatic transphalangeal amputation of unspecified thumb

● **S68.6** Traumatic transphalangeal amputation of other and unspecified finger

● **S68.61** Complete traumatic transphalangeal amputation of other and unspecified finger(s)

● **S68.610** Complete traumatic transphalangeal amputation of right index finger

● **S68.611** Complete traumatic transphalangeal amputation of left index finger

● **S68.612** Complete traumatic transphalangeal amputation of right middle finger

● **S68.613** Complete traumatic transphalangeal amputation of left middle finger

● **S68.614** Complete traumatic transphalangeal amputation of right ring finger

● **S68.615** Complete traumatic transphalangeal amputation of left ring finger

● **S68.616** Complete traumatic transphalangeal amputation of right little finger

● **S68.617** Complete traumatic transphalangeal amputation of left little finger

● **S68.618** Complete traumatic transphalangeal amputation of other finger

     Complete traumatic transphalangeal amputation of specified finger with unspecified laterality

● **S68.619** Complete traumatic transphalangeal amputation of unspecified finger

● **S68.62** Partial traumatic transphalangeal amputation of other and unspecified finger

● **S68.620** Partial traumatic transphalangeal amputation of right index finger

● **S68.621** Partial traumatic transphalangeal amputation of left index finger

● **S68.622** Partial traumatic transphalangeal amputation of right middle finger

● **S68.623** Partial traumatic transphalangeal amputation of left middle finger

▶ New   ⇒ Revised   ~~deleted~~ Deleted   Excludes 1   Excludes 2   Includes   Use additional   Code first   Code also   Key words

OGCR Official Guidelines   ● Unacceptable Principal Diagnosis   X Assign placeholder X   ● Use Additional Character(s)   ▶ Manifestation Code   **Coding Clinic**

S68.624   **Partial** traumatic transphalangeal amputation of **right ring** finger

S68.625   **Partial** traumatic transphalangeal amputation of **left ring** finger

S68.626   **Partial** traumatic transphalangeal amputation of **right little** finger

S68.627   **Partial** traumatic transphalangeal amputation of **left little** finger

S68.628   **Partial** traumatic transphalangeal amputation of **other** finger
  Partial traumatic transphalangeal amputation of specified finger with unspecified laterality

S68.629   **Partial** traumatic transphalangeal amputation of **unspecified** finger

S68.7   Traumatic **transmetacarpal amputation of hand**

S68.71   **Complete** traumatic transmetacarpal amputation of hand

S68.711   Complete traumatic transmetacarpal amputation of **right hand** A 🦠
  (Ex) See PDX Collection 1266

S68.712   Complete traumatic transmetacarpal amputation of **left hand** A 🦠
  (Ex) See PDX Collection 1267

S68.719   Complete traumatic transmetacarpal amputation of **unspecified hand** A 🦠
  (Ex) See PDX Collection 1268

S68.72   **Partial** traumatic transmetacarpal amputation of hand

S68.721   Partial traumatic transmetacarpal amputation of **right hand** A 🦠
  (Ex) See PDX Collection 1266

S68.722   Partial traumatic transmetacarpal amputation of **left hand** A 🦠
  (Ex) See PDX Collection 1267

S68.729   Partial traumatic transmetacarpal amputation of **unspecified hand** A 🦠
  (Ex) See PDX Collection 1268

S69   Other and unspecified injuries of wrist, hand and finger(s)
  The appropriate 7th character is to be added to each code from category S69

A	initial encounter
D	subsequent encounter
S	sequela

S69.8   Other specified injuries of wrist, hand and finger(s)

X S69.80   Other specified injuries of **unspecified** wrist, hand and finger(s)

X S69.81   Other specified injuries of **right** wrist, hand and finger(s)

X S69.82   Other specified injuries of **left** wrist, hand and finger(s)

S69.9   **Unspecified** injury of wrist, hand and finger(s)

X S69.90   Unspecified injury of **unspecified** wrist, hand and finger(s)

X S69.91   Unspecified injury of **right** wrist, hand and finger(s)

X S69.92   Unspecified injury of **left** wrist, hand and finger(s)

INJURIES TO THE HIP AND THIGH (S70-S79)

Excludes2   burns and corrosions (T20-T32)
  frostbite (T33-T34)
  snake bite (T63.0-)
  venomous insect bite or sting (T63.4-)

S70   Superficial injury of hip and thigh
  The appropriate 7th character is to be added to each code from category S70

A	initial encounter
D	subsequent encounter
S	sequela

S70.0   Contusion of **hip**

X S70.00   Contusion of **unspecified** hip

X S70.01   Contusion of **right** hip

X S70.02   Contusion of **left** hip

S70.1   Contusion of **thigh**

X S70.10   Contusion of **unspecified** thigh

X S70.11   Contusion of **right** thigh

X S70.12   Contusion of **left** thigh

S70.2   Other superficial injuries of hip

S70.21   **Abrasion** of hip

S70.211   Abrasion, **right hip**

S70.212   Abrasion, **left hip**

S70.219   Abrasion, **unspecified** hip

S70.22   **Blister** (nonthermal) of hip

S70.221   Blister (nonthermal), **right hip**

S70.222   Blister (nonthermal), **left hip**

S70.229   Blister (nonthermal), **unspecified** hip

S70.24   **External constriction** of hip

S70.241   External constriction, **right hip**

S70.242   External constriction, **left hip**

S70.249   External constriction, **unspecified** hip

S70.25   **Superficial foreign body** of hip
  Splinter in the hip

S70.251   Superficial foreign body, **right hip**

S70.252   Superficial foreign body, **left hip**

S70.259   Superficial foreign body, **unspecified** hip

S70.26   **Insect bite** (nonvenomous) of hip

S70.261   Insect bite (nonvenomous), **right hip**

S70.262   Insect bite (nonvenomous), **left hip**

S70.269   Insect bite (nonvenomous), **unspecified** hip

S70.27   **Other superficial bite** of hip
  Excludes1   open bite of hip (S71.05-)

S70.271   Other superficial bite of hip, **right hip**

S70.272   Other superficial bite of hip, **left hip**

S70.279   Other superficial bite of hip, **unspecified** hip

S70.3   Other superficial injuries of **thigh**

S70.31   **Abrasion** of thigh

S70.311   Abrasion, **right thigh**

S70.312   Abrasion, **left thigh**

S70.319   Abrasion, **unspecified** thigh

S70.32   **Blister** (nonthermal) of thigh

S70.321   Blister (nonthermal), **right thigh**

S70.322   Blister (nonthermal), **left thigh**

S70.329   Blister (nonthermal), **unspecified** thigh

CHAPTER 19 (S00-T88)

N Newborn Age: 0   **P** Pediatric Age: 0–17   **M** Maternity DX: 12–55   **A** Adult Age: 15–124   ♀ Females Only   ♂ Males Only

🦠 Complication\Comorbidity   🦠 Major C\C   (Ex) CC/MCC Exclusions   🦠 Hospital-Acquired Condition

1349

- S70.34   **External constriction** of thigh
  - S70.341   External constriction, **right** thigh
  - S70.342   External constriction, **left** thigh
  - S70.349   External constriction, **unspecified** thigh
- S70.35   **Superficial foreign body of thigh**
  Splinter in the thigh
  - S70.351   Superficial foreign body, **right** thigh
  - S70.352   Superficial foreign body, **left** thigh
  - S70.359   Superficial foreign body, **unspecified** thigh
- S70.36   Insect bite (nonvenomous) of thigh
  - S70.361   Insect bite (nonvenomous), **right** thigh
  - S70.362   Insect bite (nonvenomous), **left** thigh
  - S70.369   Insect bite (nonvenomous), **unspecified** thigh
- S70.37   **Other superficial bite of thigh**
  - **Excludes1**   open bite of thigh (S71.15)
  - S70.371   Other superficial bite of **right** thigh
  - S70.372   Other superficial bite of **left** thigh
  - S70.379   Other superficial bite of **unspecified** thigh
- S70.9   **Unspecified superficial injury of hip and thigh**
  - S70.91   Unspecified superficial injury of hip
    - S70.911   Unspecified superficial injury of **right** hip
    - S70.912   Unspecified superficial injury of **left** hip
    - S70.919   Unspecified superficial injury of **unspecified** hip
  - S70.92   Unspecified superficial injury of thigh
    - S70.921   Unspecified superficial injury of **right** thigh
    - S70.922   Unspecified superficial injury of **left** thigh
    - S70.929   Unspecified superficial injury of **unspecified** thigh
- S71   **Open wound of hip and thigh**
  Code also any associated wound infection
  - **Excludes1**   open fracture of hip and thigh (S72.-)
                traumatic amputation of hip and thigh (S78.-)
  - **Excludes2**   bite of venomous animal (T63.-)
                open wound of ankle, foot and toes (S91.-)
                open wound of knee and lower leg (S81.-)

  The appropriate 7th character is to be added to each code from category S71

A	initial encounter
D	subsequent encounter
S	sequela

  - S71.0   **Open wound of hip**
    - S71.00   **Unspecified** open wound of hip
      - S71.001   Unspecified open wound, **right** hip
      - S71.002   Unspecified open wound, **left** hip
      - S71.009   Unspecified open wound, **unspecified** hip
    - S71.01   **Laceration without foreign body of hip**
      - S71.011   Laceration without foreign body, **right** hip
      - S71.012   Laceration without foreign body, **left** hip
      - S71.019   Laceration without foreign body, **unspecified** hip

- S71.02   **Laceration with foreign body of hip**
  - S71.021   Laceration with foreign body, **right** hip
  - S71.022   Laceration with foreign body, **left** hip
  - S71.029   Laceration with foreign body, **unspecified** hip
- S71.03   **Puncture wound without foreign** body of hip
  - S71.031   Puncture wound without foreign body, **right** hip
  - S71.032   Puncture wound without foreign body, **left** hip
  - S71.039   Puncture wound without foreign body, **unspecified** hip
- S71.04   **Puncture wound with foreign body of hip**
  - S71.041   Puncture wound with foreign body, **right** hip
  - S71.042   Puncture wound with foreign body, **left** hip
  - S71.049   Puncture wound with foreign body, **unspecified** hip
- S71.05   **Open bite of hip**
  Bite of hip NOS
  - **Excludes1**   superficial bite of hip (S70.26, S70.27)
  - S71.051   Open bite, **right** hip
  - S71.052   Open bite, **left** hip
  - S71.059   Open bite, **unspecified** hip
- S71.1   **Open wound of thigh**
  - S71.10   **Unspecified** open wound of thigh
    - S71.101   Unspecified open wound, **right** thigh
    - S71.102   Unspecified open wound, **left** thigh
    - S71.109   Unspecified open wound, **unspecified** thigh
  - S71.11   **Laceration without foreign body of thigh**
    - S71.111   Laceration without foreign body, **right** thigh
    - S71.112   Laceration without foreign body, **left** thigh
    - S71.119   Laceration without foreign body, **unspecified** thigh
  - S71.12   **Laceration with foreign body of thigh**
    - S71.121   Laceration with foreign body, **right** thigh
    - S71.122   Laceration with foreign body, **left** thigh
    - S71.129   Laceration with foreign body, **unspecified** thigh
  - S71.13   **Puncture wound without foreign** body of thigh
    - S71.131   Puncture wound without foreign body, **right** thigh
    - S71.132   Puncture wound without foreign body, **left** thigh
    - S71.139   Puncture wound without foreign body, **unspecified** thigh
  - S71.14   **Puncture wound with foreign body of thigh**
    - S71.141   Puncture wound with foreign body, **right** thigh
    - S71.142   Puncture wound with foreign body, **left** thigh
    - S71.149   Puncture wound with foreign body, **unspecified** thigh
  - S71.15   **Open bite of thigh**
    Bite of thigh NOS
    - **Excludes1**   superficial bite of thigh (S70.37-)
    - S71.151   Open bite, **right** thigh
    - S71.152   Open bite, **left** thigh
    - S71.159   Open bite, **unspecified** thigh

▶ New   ➠ Revised   ~~deleted~~ Deleted   Excludes 1   Excludes 2   Includes   Use additional   Code first   Code also   Key words

OGCR Official Guidelines   ● Unacceptable Principal Diagnosis   **X** Assign placeholder X   ● Use Additional Character(s)   ▶ Manifestation Code   **Coding Clinic**

● **S72**   **Fracture of femur**

> **Note:** A fracture not indicated as displaced or nondisplaced should be coded to displaced
>
> A fracture not indicated as open or closed should be coded to closed
>
> The open fracture designations are based on the Gustilo open fracture classification

> **Excludes1**   traumatic amputation of hip and thigh (S78.-)
>
> **Excludes2**   fracture of lower leg and ankle (S82.-)
>
>   fracture of foot (S92.-)
>
> ➧ periprosthetic fracture of prosthetic implant of hip (M97.0-)

> The appropriate 7th character is to be added to all codes from category S72

> | | |
> |---|---|
> | A | initial encounter for closed fracture |
> | B | initial encounter for open fracture type I or II |
> | | initial encounter for open fracture NOS |
> | C | initial encounter for open fracture type IIIA, IIIB, or IIIC |
> | D | subsequent encounter for closed fracture with routine healing |
> | E | subsequent encounter for open fracture type I or II with routine healing |
> | F | subsequent encounter for open fracture type IIIA, IIIB, or IIIC with routine healing |
> | G | subsequent encounter for closed fracture with delayed healing |
> | H | subsequent encounter for open fracture type I or II with delayed healing |
> | J | subsequent encounter for open fracture type IIIA, IIIB, or IIIC with delayed healing |
> | K | subsequent encounter for closed fracture with nonunion |
> | M | subsequent encounter for open fracture type I or II with nonunion |
> | N | subsequent encounter for open fracture type IIIA, IIIB, or IIIC with nonunion |
> | P | subsequent encounter for closed fracture with malunion |
> | Q | subsequent encounter for open fracture type I or II with malunion |
> | R | subsequent encounter for open fracture type IIIA, IIIB, or IIIC with malunion |
> | S | sequela |

● **S72.0**   **Fracture of head and neck of femur**

> **Excludes2**   physeal fracture of upper end of femur (S79.0-)

● **S72.00**   **Fracture of unspecified part of neck of femur**
> Fracture of hip NOS
> Fracture of neck of femur NOS

● **S72.001**   **Fracture of unspecified part of neck of right femur** K, M, N, P, Q, R 🔾, A, B, C 🔾, A, B, C 🔾
> (Ex) **For S72.001[A]:** See PDX Collection 1297
> **For S72.001[B,C]:** See PDX Collection 1298
> **For S72.001[K,M,N,P,Q,R]:** See PDX Collection 897

● **S72.002**   **Fracture of unspecified part of neck of left femur** K, M, N, P, Q, R 🔾, A, B, C 🔾, A, B, C 🔾
> (Ex) **For S72.002[A]:** See PDX Collection 1299
> **For S72.002[B,C]:** See PDX Collection 1298
> **For S72.002[K,M,N,P,Q,R]:** See PDX Collection 897

> **Coding Clinic: 2015, Q4, P37, Q1, P17**

● **S72.009**   **Fracture of unspecified part of neck of unspecified femur** K, M, N, P, Q, R 🔾, A, B, C 🔾, A, B, C 🔾
> (Ex) **For S72.009[A,B,C]:** See PDX Collection 1298
> **For S72.009[K,M,N,P,Q,R]:** See PDX Collection 897

● **S72.01**   **Unspecified intracapsular fracture of femur**
> Subcapital fracture of femur

● **S72.011**   **Unspecified intracapsular fracture of right femur** K, M, N, P, Q, R 🔾, A, B, C 🔾, A, B, C 🔾
> (Ex) **For S72.011[A]:** See PDX Collection 1297
> **For S72.011[B,C]:** See PDX Collection 1298
> **For S72.011[K,M,N,P,Q,R]:** See PDX Collection 897

● **S72.012**   **Unspecified intracapsular fracture of left femur** K, M, N, P, Q, R 🔾, A, B, C 🔾, A, B, C 🔾
> (Ex) **For S72.012[A]:** See PDX Collection 1299
> **For S72.012[B,C]:** See PDX Collection 1298
> **For S72.012[K,M,N,P,Q,R]:** See PDX Collection 897

● **S72.019**   **Unspecified intracapsular fracture of unspecified femur** K, M, N, P, Q, R 🔾, A, B, C 🔾, A, B, C 🔾
> (Ex) **For S72.019[A,B,C]:** See PDX Collection 1298
> **For S72.019[K,M,N,P,Q,R]:** See PDX Collection 897

● **S72.02**   **Fracture of epiphysis (separation) (upper) of femur**
> Transepiphyseal fracture of femur
> *Fracture and separation across growth plate*

> **Excludes1**   capital femoral epiphyseal fracture (pediatric) of femur (S79.01-)
> Salter-Harris Type I physeal fracture of upper end of femur (S79.01-)

● **S72.021**   **Displaced fracture of epiphysis (separation) (upper) of right femur** K, M, N, P, Q, R 🔾, A, B, C 🔾, A, B, C 🔾
> (Ex) **For S72.021[A]:** See PDX Collection 1297
> **For S72.021[B,C]:** See PDX Collection 1298
> **For S72.021[K,M,N,P,Q,R]:** See PDX Collection 897

● **S72.022**   **Displaced fracture of epiphysis (separation) (upper) of left femur** K, M, N, P, Q, R 🔾, A, B, C 🔾, A, B, C 🔾
> (Ex) **For S72.022[A]:** See PDX Collection 1299
> **For S72.022[B,C]:** See PDX Collection 1298
> **For S72.022[K,M,N,P,Q,R]:** See PDX Collection 897

● **S72.023**   **Displaced fracture of epiphysis (separation) (upper) of unspecified femur** K, M, N, P, Q, R 🔾, A, B, C 🔾, A, B, C 🔾
> (Ex) **For S72.023[A,B,C]:** See PDX Collection 1298
> **For S72.023[K,M,N,P,Q,R]:** See PDX Collection 897

● **S72.024**   **Nondisplaced fracture of epiphysis (separation) (upper) of right femur** K, M, N, P, Q, R 🔾, A, B, C 🔾, A, B, C 🔾
> (Ex) **For S72.024[A]:** See PDX Collection 1297
> **For S72.024[B,C]:** See PDX Collection 1298
> **For S72.024[K,M,N,P,Q,R]:** See PDX Collection 897

● **S72.025**   **Nondisplaced fracture of epiphysis (separation) (upper) of left femur** K, M, N, P, Q, R 🔾, A, B, C 🔾, A, B, C 🔾
> (Ex) **For S72.025[A]:** See PDX Collection 1299
> **For S72.025[B,C]:** See PDX Collection 1298
> **For S72.025[K,M,N,P,Q,R]:** See PDX Collection 897

● **S72.026**   **Nondisplaced fracture of epiphysis (separation) (upper) of unspecified femur** K, M, N, P, Q, R 🔾, A, B, C 🔾, A, B, C 🔾
> (Ex) **For S72.026[A,B,C]:** See PDX Collection 1298
> **For S72.026[K,M,N,P,Q,R]:** See PDX Collection 897

CHAPTER 19 (S00-T88)

● **S72.03** **Midcervical fracture of femur**
Transcervical fracture of femur NOS

● **S72.031** **Displaced midcervical fracture of right femur** K, M, N, P, Q, R 🪙, A, B, C 🪙, A, B, C 🪙
(Ex) For S72.031[A]: See PDX Collection 1297
For S72.031[B,C]: See PDX Collection 1298
For S72.031[K,M,N,P,Q,R]: See PDX Collection 897

● **S72.032** **Displaced midcervical fracture of left femur** K, M, N, P, Q, R 🪙, A, B, C 🪙, A, B, C 🪙
(Ex) For S72.032[A]: See PDX Collection 1299
For S72.032[B,C]: See PDX Collection 1298
For S72.032[K,M,N,P,Q,R]: See PDX Collection 897

● **S72.033** **Displaced midcervical fracture of unspecified femur** K, M, N, P, Q, R 🪙, A, B, C 🪙, A, B, C 🪙
(Ex) For S72.033[A,B,C]: See PDX Collection 1298
For S72.033[K,M,N,P,Q,R]: See PDX Collection 897

● **S72.034** **Nondisplaced midcervical fracture of right femur** K, M, N, P, Q, R 🪙, A, B, C 🪙, A, B, C 🪙
(Ex) For S72.034[A]: See PDX Collection 1297
For S72.034[B,C]: See PDX Collection 1298
For S72.034[K,M,N,P,Q,R]: See PDX Collection 897

● **S72.035** **Nondisplaced midcervical fracture of left femur** K, M, N, P, Q, R 🪙, A, B, C 🪙, A, B, C 🪙
(Ex) For S72.035[A]: See PDX Collection 1299
For S72.035[B,C]: See PDX Collection 1298
For S72.035[K,M,N,P,Q,R]: See PDX Collection 897

● **S72.036** **Nondisplaced midcervical fracture of unspecified femur** K, M, N, P, Q, R 🪙, A, B, C 🪙, A, B, C 🪙
(Ex) For S72.036[A,B,C]: See PDX Collection 1298
For S72.036[K,M,N,P,Q,R]: See PDX Collection 897

● **S72.04** **Fracture of base of neck of femur**
Cervicotrochanteric fracture of femur

● **S72.041** **Displaced fracture of base of neck of right femur** K, M, N, P, Q, R 🪙, A, B, C 🪙, A, B, C 🪙
(Ex) For S72.041[A]: See PDX Collection 1297
For S72.041[B,C]: See PDX Collection 1298
For S72.041[K,M,N,P,Q,R]: See PDX Collection 897

● **S72.042** **Displaced fracture of base of neck of left femur** K, M, N, P, Q, R 🪙, A, B, C 🪙, A, B, C 🪙
(Ex) For S72.042[A]: See PDX Collection 1299
For S72.042[B,C]: See PDX Collection 1298
For S72.042[K,M,N,P,Q,R]: See PDX Collection 897

● **S72.043** **Displaced fracture of base of neck of unspecified femur** K, M, N, P, Q, R 🪙, A, B, C 🪙, A, B, C 🪙
(Ex) For S72.043[A,B,C]: See PDX Collection 1298
For S72.043[K,M,N,P,Q,R]: See PDX Collection 897

● **S72.044** **Nondisplaced fracture of base of neck of right femur** K, M, N, P, Q, R 🪙, A, B, C 🪙
(Ex) For S72.044[A]: See PDX Collection 1297
For S72.044[B,C]: See PDX Collection 1298
For S72.044[K,M,N,P,Q,R]: See PDX Collection 897

● **S72.045** **Nondisplaced fracture of base of neck of left femur** K, M, N, P, Q, R 🪙, A, B, C 🪙
(Ex) For S72.045[A]: See PDX Collection 1299
For S72.045[B,C]: See PDX Collection 1298
For S72.045[K,M,N,P,Q,R]: See PDX Collection 897

● **S72.046** **Nondisplaced fracture of base of neck of unspecified femur** K, M, N, P, Q, R 🪙, A, B, C 🪙
(Ex) For S72.046[A,B,C]: See PDX Collection 1298
For S72.046[K,M,N,P,Q,R]: See PDX Collection 897

● **S72.05** **Unspecified fracture of head of femur**
Fracture of head of femur NOS

● **S72.051** **Unspecified fracture of head of right femur** K, M, N, P, Q, R 🪙, A, B, C 🪙, A, B, C 🪙
(Ex) For S72.051[A]: See PDX Collection 1297
For S72.051[B,C]: See PDX Collection 1298
For S72.051[K,M,N,P,Q,R]: See PDX Collection 897

● **S72.052** **Unspecified fracture of head of left femur** K, M, N, P, Q, R 🪙, A, B, C 🪙
(Ex) For S72.052[A]: See PDX Collection 1299
For S72.052[B,C]: See PDX Collection 1298
For S72.052[K,M,N,P,Q,R]: See PDX Collection 897

● **S72.059** **Unspecified fracture of head of unspecified femur** K, M, N, P, Q, R 🪙, A, B, C 🪙, A, B, C 🪙
(Ex) For S72.059[A,B,C]: See PDX Collection 1298
For S72.059[K,M,N,P,Q,R]: See PDX Collection 897

● **S72.06** **Articular fracture of head of femur**

● **S72.061** **Displaced articular fracture of head of right femur** K, M, N, P, Q, R 🪙, A, B, C 🪙, A, B, C 🪙
(Ex) For S72.061[A]: See PDX Collection 1297
For S72.061[B,C]: See PDX Collection 1298
For S72.061[K,M,N,P,Q,R]: See PDX Collection 897

● **S72.062** **Displaced articular fracture of head of left femur** K, M, N, P, Q, R 🪙, A, B, C 🪙, A, B, C 🪙
(Ex) For S72.062[A]: See PDX Collection 1299
For S72.062[B,C]: See PDX Collection 1298
For S72.062[K,M,N,P,Q,R]: See PDX Collection 897

● **S72.063** **Displaced articular fracture of head of unspecified femur** K, M, N, P, Q, R 🪙, A, B, C 🪙, A, B, C 🪙
(Ex) For S72.063[A,B,C]: See PDX Collection 1298
For S72.063[K,M,N,P,Q,R]: See PDX Collection 897

● **S72.064** **Nondisplaced articular fracture of head of right femur** K, M, N, P, Q, R 🪙, A, B, C 🪙, A, B, C 🪙
(Ex) For S72.064[A]: See PDX Collection 1297
For S72.064[B,C]: See PDX Collection 1298
For S72.064[K,M,N,P,Q,R]: See PDX Collection 897

● **S72.065** **Nondisplaced articular fracture of head of left femur** K, M, N, P, Q, R 🪙, A, B, C 🪙, A, B, C 🪙
(Ex) For S72.065[A]: See PDX Collection 1299
For S72.065[B,C]: See PDX Collection 1298
For S72.065[K,M,N,P,Q,R]: See PDX Collection 897

● **S72.066** **Nondisplaced articular fracture of head of unspecified femur** K, M, N, P, Q, R 🪙, A, B, C 🪙, A, B, C 🪙
(Ex) For S72.066[A,B,C]: See PDX Collection 1298
For S72.066[K,M,N,P,Q,R]: See PDX Collection 897

▶ New   ⇒ Revised   ~~deleted~~ Deleted   Excludes 1   Excludes 2   Includes   Use additional   Code first   Code also   Key words
OGCR Official Guidelines   ● Unacceptable Principal Diagnosis   X Assign placeholder X   ● Use Additional Character(s)   ▶ Manifestation Code   **Coding Clinic**

● **S72.09   Other fracture of head and neck of femur**
   ● **S72.091   Other fracture of head and neck of right femur** K, M, N, P, Q, R , A, B, C , A, B, C
      (Ex:) **For S72.091[A]:** See PDX Collection 1297
      For S72.091[B,C]: See PDX Collection 1298
      For S72.091[K,M,N,P,Q,R]: See PDX Collection 897

   ● **S72.092   Other fracture of head and neck of left femur** K, M, N, P, Q, R , A, B, C , A, B, C
      (Ex:) **For S72.092[A]:** See PDX Collection 1299
      For S72.092[B,C]: See PDX Collection 1298
      For S72.092[K,M,N,P,Q,R]: See PDX Collection 897

   ● **S72.099   Other fracture of head and neck of unspecified femur** K, M, N, P, Q, R , A, B, C , A, B, C
      (Ex:) **For S72.099[A,B,C]:** See PDX Collection 1298
      For S72.099[K,M,N,P,Q,R]: See PDX Collection 897

● **S72.1   Pertrochanteric fracture**
   Fracture extending close to, but not into, joint
   ● **S72.10   Unspecified trochanteric fracture of femur**
      Fracture of trochanter NOS
      ● **S72.101   Unspecified trochanteric fracture of right femur** K, M, N, P, Q, R , A, B, C , A, B, C
         (Ex:) **For S72.101[A]:** See PDX Collection 1297
         For S72.101[B,C]: See PDX Collection 1298
         For S72.101[K,M,N,P,Q,R]: See PDX Collection 897

      ● **S72.102   Unspecified trochanteric fracture of left femur** K, M, N, P, Q, R , A, B, C , A, B, C
         (Ex:) **For S72.102[A]:** See PDX Collection 1299
         For S72.102[B,C]: See PDX Collection 1298
         For S72.102[K,M,N,P,Q,R]: See PDX Collection 897

      ● **S72.109   Unspecified trochanteric fracture of unspecified femur** K, M, N, P, Q, R , A, B, C , A, B, C
         (Ex:) **For S72.109[A,B,C]:** See PDX Collection 1298
         For S72.109[K,M,N,P,Q,R]: See PDX Collection 897

   ● **S72.11   Fracture of greater trochanter of femur**
      ● **S72.111   Displaced fracture of greater trochanter of right femur** K, M, N, P, Q, R , A, B, C , A, B, C
         (Ex:) **For S72.111[A]:** See PDX Collection 1297
         For S72.111[B,C]: See PDX Collection 1298
         For S72.111[K,M,N,P,Q,R]: See PDX Collection 897

      ● **S72.112   Displaced fracture of greater trochanter of left femur** K, M, N, P, Q, R , A, B, C , A, B, C
         (Ex:) **For S72.112[A]:** See PDX Collection 1299
         For S72.112[B,C]: See PDX Collection 1298
         For S72.112[K,M,N,P,Q,R]: See PDX Collection 897

      ● **S72.113   Displaced fracture of greater trochanter of unspecified femur** K, M, N, P, Q, R , A, B, C , A, B, C
         (Ex:) **For S72.113[A,B,C]:** See PDX Collection 1298
         For S72.113[K,M,N,P,Q,R]: See PDX Collection 897

      ● **S72.114   Nondisplaced fracture of greater trochanter of right femur** K, M, N, P, Q, R , A, B, C , A, B, C
         (Ex:) **For S72.114[A]:** See PDX Collection 1297
         For S72.114[B,C]: See PDX Collection 1298
         For S72.114[K,M,N,P,Q,R]: See PDX Collection 897

● **S72.115   Nondisplaced fracture of greater trochanter of left femur** K, M, N, P, Q, R , A, B, C , A, B, C
   (Ex:) **For S72.115[A]:** See PDX Collection 1299
   For S72.115[B,C]: See PDX Collection 1298
   For S72.115[K,M,N,P,Q,R]: See PDX Collection 897

● **S72.116   Nondisplaced fracture of greater trochanter of unspecified femur** K, M, N, P, Q, R , A, B, C , A, B, C
   (Ex:) **For S72.116[A,B,C]:** See PDX Collection 1298
   For S72.116[K,M,N,P,Q,R]: See PDX Collection 897

● **S72.12   Fracture of lesser trochanter of femur**
   ● **S72.121   Displaced fracture of lesser trochanter of right femur** K, M, N, P, Q, R , A, B, C , A, B, C
      (Ex:) **For S72.121[A]:** See PDX Collection 1297
      For S72.121[B,C]: See PDX Collection 1298
      For S72.121[K,M,N,P,Q,R]: See PDX Collection 897

   ● **S72.122   Displaced fracture of lesser trochanter of left femur** K, M, N, P, Q, R , A, B, C , A, B, C
      (Ex:) **For S72.122[A]:** See PDX Collection 1299
      For S72.122[B,C]: See PDX Collection 1298
      For S72.122[K,M,N,P,Q,R]: See PDX Collection 897

   ● **S72.123   Displaced fracture of lesser trochanter of unspecified femur** K, M, N, P, Q, R , A, B, C , A, B, C
      (Ex:) **For S72.123[A,B,C]:** See PDX Collection 1298
      For S72.123[K,M,N,P,Q,R]: See PDX Collection 897

   ● **S72.124   Nondisplaced fracture of lesser trochanter of right femur** K, M, N, P, Q, R , A, B, C , A, B, C
      (Ex:) **For S72.124[A]:** See PDX Collection 1297
      For S72.124[B,C]: See PDX Collection 1298
      For S72.124[K,M,N,P,Q,R]: See PDX Collection 897

   ● **S72.125   Nondisplaced fracture of lesser trochanter of left femur** K, M, N, P, Q, R , A, B, C , A, B, C
      (Ex:) **For S72.125[A]:** See PDX Collection 1299
      For S72.125[B,C]: See PDX Collection 1298
      For S72.125[K,M,N,P,Q,R]: See PDX Collection 897

   ● **S72.126   Nondisplaced fracture of lesser trochanter of unspecified femur** K, M, N, P, Q, R , A, B, C , A, B, C
      (Ex:) **For S72.126[A,B,C]:** See PDX Collection 1298
      For S72.126[K,M,N,P,Q,R]: See PDX Collection 897

● **S72.13   Apophyseal fracture of femur**
   Pertaining to articulations between articular facets of adjacent vertebrae
   Excludes 1   chronic (nontraumatic) slipped upper femoral epiphysis (M93.0-)
   ● **S72.131   Displaced apophyseal fracture of right femur** K, M, N, P, Q, R , A, B, C , A, B, C
      (Ex:) **For S72.131[A]:** See PDX Collection 1297
      For S72.131[B,C]: See PDX Collection 1298
      For S72.131[K,M,N,P,Q,R]: See PDX Collection 897

   ● **S72.132   Displaced apophyseal fracture of left femur** K, M, N, P, Q, R , A, B, C , A, B, C
      (Ex:) **For S72.132[A]:** See PDX Collection 1299
      For S72.132[B,C]: See PDX Collection 1298
      For S72.132[K,M,N,P,Q,R]: See PDX Collection 897

N Newborn Age: 0   **P** Pediatric Age: 0–17   **M** Maternity DX: 12–55   **A** Adult Age: 15–124   ♀ Females Only   ♂ Males Only
 Complication\Comorbidity   Major C\C   (Ex:) CC/MCC Exclusions   Hospital-Acquired Condition

1353

CHAPTER 19 (S00-T88)

CHAPTER 19 (S00-T88)

● **S72.133** Displaced apophyseal fracture of unspecified femur K, M, N, P, Q, R 🔵, A, B, C 🔵, A, B, C 🔵
> (Ex) For S72.133[A,B,C]: See PDX Collection 1298
> For S72.133[K,M,N,P,Q,R]: See PDX Collection 897

● **S72.134** Nondisplaced apophyseal fracture of right femur K, M, N, P, Q, R 🔵, A, B, C 🔵, A, B, C 🔵
> (Ex) For S72.134[A]: See PDX Collection 1297
> For S72.134[B,C]: See PDX Collection 1298
> For S72.134[K,M,N,P,Q,R]: See PDX Collection 897

● **S72.135** Nondisplaced apophyseal fracture of left femur K, M, N, P, Q, R 🔵, A, B, C 🔵, A, B, C 🔵
> (Ex) For S72.135[A]: See PDX Collection 1299
> For S72.135[B,C]: See PDX Collection 1298
> For S72.135[K,M,N,P,Q,R]: See PDX Collection 897

● **S72.136** Nondisplaced apophyseal fracture of unspecified femur K, M, N, P, Q, R 🔵, A, B, C 🔵, A, B, C 🔵
> (Ex) For S72.136[A,B,C]: See PDX Collection 1298
> For S72.136[K,M,N,P,Q,R]: See PDX Collection 897

● **S72.14** Intertrochanteric fracture of femur

● **S72.141** Displaced intertrochanteric fracture of right femur K, M, N, P, Q, R 🔵, A, B, C 🔵, A, B, C 🔵
> (Ex) For S72.141[A]: See PDX Collection 1297
> For S72.141[B,C]: See PDX Collection 1298
> For S72.141[K,M,N,P,Q,R]: See PDX Collection 897

Coding Clinic: 2016, Q3, P17

● **S72.142** Displaced intertrochanteric fracture of left femur K, M, N, P, Q, R 🔵, A, B, C 🔵, A, B, C 🔵
> (Ex) For S72.142[A]: See PDX Collection 1299
> For S72.142[B,C]: See PDX Collection 1298
> For S72.142[K,M,N,P,Q,R]: See PDX Collection 897

● **S72.143** Displaced intertrochanteric fracture of unspecified femur K, M, N, P, Q, R 🔵, A, B, C 🔵, A, B, C 🔵
> (Ex) For S72.143[A,B,C]: See PDX Collection 1298
> For S72.143[K,M,N,P,Q,R]: See PDX Collection 897

● **S72.144** Nondisplaced intertrochanteric fracture of right femur K, M, N, P, Q, R 🔵, A, B, C 🔵, A, B, C 🔵
> (Ex) For S72.144[A]: See PDX Collection 1297
> For S72.144[B,C]: See PDX Collection 1298
> For S72.144[K,M,N,P,Q,R]: See PDX Collection 897

● **S72.145** Nondisplaced intertrochanteric fracture of left femur K, M, N, P, Q, R 🔵, A, B, C 🔵, A, B, C 🔵
> (Ex) For S72.145[A]: See PDX Collection 1299
> For S72.145[B,C]: See PDX Collection 1298
> For S72.145[K,M,N,P,Q,R]: See PDX Collection 897

● **S72.146** Nondisplaced intertrochanteric fracture of unspecified femur K, M, N, P, Q, R 🔵, A, B, C 🔵, A, B, C 🔵
> (Ex) For S72.146[A,B,C]: See PDX Collection 1298
> For S72.146[K,M,N,P,Q,R]: See PDX Collection 897

● **S72.2** Subtrochanteric fracture of femur
Subtrochanteric: inferior to trochanter
> (Ex) For category S72.2 CC codes S72.2[A,B,C]: See PDX Collection 1298
> For S72.2[K,M,N,P,Q,R]: See PDX Collection 897

X ● **S72.21** Displaced subtrochanteric fracture of right femur K, M, N, P, Q, R 🔵, A, B, C 🔵, A, B, C 🔵

X ● **S72.22** Displaced subtrochanteric fracture of left femur K, M, N, P, Q, R 🔵, A, B, C 🔵, A, B, C 🔵

X ● **S72.23** Displaced subtrochanteric fracture of unspecified femur K, M, N, P, Q, R 🔵, A, B, C 🔵, A, B, C 🔵

X ● **S72.24** Nondisplaced subtrochanteric fracture of right femur K, M, N, P, Q, R 🔵, A, B, C 🔵, A, B, C 🔵

X ● **S72.25** Nondisplaced subtrochanteric fracture of left femur K, M, N, P, Q, R 🔵, A, B, C 🔵, A, B, C 🔵

X ● **S72.26** Nondisplaced subtrochanteric fracture of unspecified femur K, M, N, P, Q, R 🔵, A, B, C 🔵, A, B, C 🔵

● **S72.3** Fracture of shaft of femur

● **S72.30** Unspecified fracture of shaft of femur

● **S72.301** Unspecified fracture of shaft of right femur K, M, N, P, Q, R 🔵, A, B, C 🔵, A, B, C 🔵
> (Ex) For S72.301[A]: See PDX Collection 1297
> For S72.301[B,C]: See PDX Collection 1298
> For S72.301[K,M,N,P,Q,R]: See PDX Collection 897

● **S72.302** Unspecified fracture of shaft of left femur K, M, N, P, Q, R 🔵, A, B, C 🔵, A, B, C 🔵
> (Ex) For S72.302[A]: See PDX Collection 1299
> For S72.302[B,C]: See PDX Collection 1298
> For S72.302[K,M,N,P,Q,R]: See PDX Collection 897

● **S72.309** Unspecified fracture of shaft of unspecified femur K, M, N, P, Q, R 🔵, A, B, C 🔵, A, B, C 🔵
> (Ex) For S72.309[A,B,C]: See PDX Collection 1298
> For S72.309[K,M,N,P,Q,R]: See PDX Collection 897

● **S72.32** Transverse fracture of shaft of femur

● **S72.321** Displaced transverse fracture of shaft of right femur K, M, N, P, Q, R 🔵, A, B, C 🔵, A, B, C 🔵
> (Ex) For S72.321[A]: See PDX Collection 1297
> For S72.321[B,C]: See PDX Collection 1298
> For S72.321[K,M,N,P,Q,R]: See PDX Collection 897

● **S72.322** Displaced transverse fracture of shaft of left femur K, M, N, P, Q, R 🔵, A, B, C 🔵, A, B, C 🔵
> (Ex) For S72.322[A]: See PDX Collection 1299
> For S72.322[B,C]: See PDX Collection 1298
> For S72.322[K,M,N,P,Q,R]: See PDX Collection 897

● **S72.323** Displaced transverse fracture of shaft of unspecified femur K, M, N, P, Q, R 🔵, A, B, C 🔵, A, B, C 🔵
> (Ex) For S72.323[A,B,C]: See PDX Collection 1298
> For S72.323[K,M,N,P,Q,R]: See PDX Collection 897

● **S72.324** Nondisplaced transverse fracture of shaft of right femur K, M, N, P, Q, R 🔵, A, B, C 🔵, A, B, C 🔵
> (Ex) For S72.324[A]: See PDX Collection 1297
> For S72.324[B,C]: See PDX Collection 1298
> For S72.324[K,M,N,P,Q,R]: See PDX Collection 897

▶ New   ⟹ Revised   ~~deleted~~ Deleted   Excludes 1   Excludes 2   Includes   Use additional   Code first   Code also   Key words
OGCR Official Guidelines   ● Unacceptable Principal Diagnosis   X Assign placeholder X   ● Use Additional Character(s)   ⟩ Manifestation Code   **Coding Clinic**

● **S72.325** **Nondisplaced** transverse fracture of shaft of **left** femur K, M, N, P, Q, R 🗲, A, B, C 🗲, A, B, C 🗲

    (Ex:) **For S72.325[A]:** See PDX Collection 1299
    For S72.325[B,C]: See PDX Collection 1298
    For S72.325[K,M,N,P,Q,R]: See PDX
    Collection 897

● **S72.326** **Nondisplaced** transverse fracture of shaft of **unspecified** femur K, M, N, P, Q, R 🗲, A, B, C 🗲, A, B, C 🗲

    (Ex:) **For S72.326[A,B,C]:** See PDX Collection 1298
    For S72.326[K,M,N,P,Q,R]: See PDX
    Collection 897

● **S72.33** Oblique fracture of shaft of femur

  ● **S72.331** **Displaced** oblique fracture of shaft of **right** femur K, M, N, P, Q, R 🗲, A, B, C 🗲, A, B, C 🗲

    (Ex:) **For S72.331[A]:** See PDX Collection 1297
    For S72.331[B,C]: See PDX Collection 1298
    For S72.331[K,M,N,P,Q,R]: See PDX
    Collection 897

  ● **S72.332** **Displaced** oblique fracture of shaft of **left** femur K, M, N, P, Q, R 🗲, A, B, C 🗲, A, B, C 🗲

    (Ex:) **For S72.332[A]:** See PDX Collection 1299
    For S72.332[B,C]: See PDX Collection 1298
    For S72.332[K,M,N,P,Q,R]: See PDX
    Collection 897

  ● **S72.333** **Displaced** oblique fracture of shaft of **unspecified** femur K, M, N, P, Q, R 🗲, A, B, C 🗲, A, B, C 🗲

    (Ex:) **For S72.333[A,B,C]:** See PDX Collection 1298
    For S72.333[K,M,N,P,Q,R]: See PDX
    Collection 897

  ● **S72.334** **Nondisplaced** oblique fracture of shaft of **right** femur K, M, N, P, Q, R 🗲, A, B, C 🗲, A, B, C 🗲

    (Ex:) **For S72.334[A]:** See PDX Collection 1297
    For S72.334[B,C]: See PDX Collection 1298
    For S72.334[K,M,N,P,Q,R]: See PDX
    Collection 897

  ● **S72.335** **Nondisplaced** oblique fracture of shaft of **left** femur K, M, N, P, Q, R 🗲, A, B, C 🗲, A, B, C 🗲

    (Ex:) **For S72.335[A]:** See PDX Collection 1299
    For S72.335[B,C]: See PDX Collection 1298
    For S72.335[K,M,N,P,Q,R]: See PDX
    Collection 897

  ● **S72.336** **Nondisplaced** oblique fracture of shaft of **unspecified** femur K, M, N, P, Q, R 🗲, A, B, C 🗲, A, B, C 🗲

    (Ex:) **For S72.336[A,B,C]:** See PDX Collection 1298
    For S72.336[K,M,N,P,Q,R]: See PDX
    Collection 897

● **S72.34** Spiral fracture of shaft of femur

  ● **S72.341** **Displaced** spiral fracture of shaft of **right** femur K, M, N, P, Q, R 🗲, A, B, C 🗲, A, B, C 🗲

    (Ex:) **For S72.341[A]:** See PDX Collection 1297
    For S72.341[B,C]: See PDX Collection 1298
    For S72.341[K,M,N,P,Q,R]: See PDX
    Collection 897

  ● **S72.342** **Displaced** spiral fracture of shaft of **left** femur K, M, N, P, Q, R 🗲, A, B, C 🗲, A, B, C 🗲

    (Ex:) **For S72.342[A]:** See PDX Collection 1299
    For S72.342[B,C]: See PDX Collection 1298
    For S72.342[K,M,N,P,Q,R]: See PDX
    Collection 897

● **S72.343** **Displaced** spiral fracture of shaft of **unspecified** femur K, M, N, P, Q, R 🗲, A, B, C 🗲, A, B, C 🗲

    (Ex:) **For S72.343[A,B,C]:** See PDX Collection 1298
    For S72.343[K,M,N,P,Q,R]: See PDX
    Collection 897

● **S72.344** **Nondisplaced** spiral fracture of shaft of **right** femur K, M, N, P, Q, R 🗲, A, B, C 🗲, A, B, C 🗲

    (Ex:) **For S72.344[A]:** See PDX Collection 1297
    For S72.344[B,C]: See PDX Collection 1298
    For S72.344[K,M,N,P,Q,R]: See PDX
    Collection 897

● **S72.345** **Nondisplaced** spiral fracture of shaft of **left** femur K, M, N, P, Q, R 🗲, A, B, C 🗲, A, B, C 🗲

    (Ex:) **For S72.345[A]:** See PDX Collection 1299
    For S72.345[B,C]: See PDX Collection 1298
    For S72.345[K,M,N,P,Q,R]: See PDX
    Collection 897

● **S72.346** **Nondisplaced** spiral fracture of shaft of **unspecified** femur K, M, N, P, Q, R 🗲, A, B, C 🗲, A, B, C 🗲

    (Ex:) **For S72.346[A,B,C]:** See PDX Collection 1298
    For S72.346[K,M,N,P,Q,R]: See PDX
    Collection 897

● **S72.35** Comminuted fracture of shaft of femur

  ● **S72.351** **Displaced** comminuted fracture of shaft of **right** femur K, M, N, P, Q, R 🗲, A, B, C 🗲, A, B, C 🗲

    (Ex:) **For S72.351[A]:** See PDX Collection 1297
    For S72.351[B,C]: See PDX Collection 1298
    For S72.351[K,M,N,P,Q,R]: See PDX
    Collection 897

  ● **S72.352** **Displaced** comminuted fracture of shaft of **left** femur K, M, N, P, Q, R 🗲, A, B, C 🗲, A, B, C 🗲

    (Ex:) **For S72.352[A]:** See PDX Collection 1299
    For S72.352[B,C]: See PDX Collection 1298
    For S72.352[K,M,N,P,Q,R]: See PDX
    Collection 897

  ● **S72.353** **Displaced** comminuted fracture of shaft of **unspecified** femur K, M, N, P, Q, R 🗲, A, B, C 🗲, A, B, C 🗲

    (Ex:) **For S72.353[A,B,C]:** See PDX Collection 1298
    For S72.353[K,M,N,P,Q,R]: See PDX
    Collection 897

  ● **S72.354** **Nondisplaced** comminuted fracture of shaft of **right** femur K, M, N, P, Q, R 🗲, A, B, C 🗲, A, B, C 🗲

    (Ex:) **For S72.354[A]:** See PDX Collection 1297
    For S72.354[B,C]: See PDX Collection 1298
    For S72.354[K,M,N,P,Q,R]: See PDX
    Collection 897

  ● **S72.355** **Nondisplaced** comminuted fracture of shaft of **left** femur K, M, N, P, Q, R 🗲, A, B, C 🗲, A, B, C 🗲

    (Ex:) **For S72.355[A]:** See PDX Collection 1299
    For S72.355[B,C]: See PDX Collection 1298
    For S72.355[K,M,N,P,Q,R]: See PDX
    Collection 897

  ● **S72.356** **Nondisplaced** comminuted fracture of shaft of **unspecified** femur K, M, N, P, Q, R 🗲, A, B, C 🗲, A, B, C 🗲

    (Ex:) **For S72.356[A,B,C]:** See PDX Collection 1298
    For S72.356[K,M,N,P,Q,R]: See PDX
    Collection 897

CHAPTER 19 (S00-T88)

N Newborn Age: 0   **P** Pediatric Age: 0–17   **M** Maternity DX: 12–55   **A** Adult Age: 15–124   ♀ Females Only   ♂ Males Only

🗲 Complication\Comorbidity   🗲 Major C\C   (Ex:) CC/MCC Exclusions   🗲 Hospital-Acquired Condition

1355

● S72.36   Segmental fracture of shaft of femur
   ● S72.361   Displaced segmental fracture of shaft of right femur K, M, N, P, Q, R 🔲, A, B, C 🔲, A, B, C 🔲
      (Ex:) For S72.361[A]: See PDX Collection 1297
      For S72.361[B,C]: See PDX Collection 1298
      For S72.361[K,M,N,P,Q,R]: See PDX Collection 897

   ● S72.362   Displaced segmental fracture of shaft of left femur K, M, N, P, Q, R 🔲, A, B, C 🔲, A, B, C 🔲
      (Ex:) For S72.362[A]: See PDX Collection 1299
      For S72.362[B,C]: See PDX Collection 1298
      For S72.362[K,M,N,P,Q,R]: See PDX Collection 897

   ● S72.363   Displaced segmental fracture of shaft of unspecified femur K, M, N, P, Q, R 🔲, A, B, C 🔲, A, B, C 🔲
      (Ex:) For S72.363[A,B,C]: See PDX Collection 1298
      For S72.363[K,M,N,P,Q,R]: See PDX Collection 897

   ● S72.364   Nondisplaced segmental fracture of shaft of right femur K, M, N, P, Q, R 🔲, A, B, C 🔲, A, B, C 🔲
      (Ex:) For S72.364[A]: See PDX Collection 1297
      For S72.364[B,C]: See PDX Collection 1298
      For S72.364[K,M,N,P,Q,R]: See PDX Collection 897

   ● S72.365   Nondisplaced segmental fracture of shaft of left femur K, M, N, P, Q, R 🔲, A, B, C 🔲, A, B, C 🔲
      (Ex:) For S72.365[A]: See PDX Collection 1299
      For S72.365[B,C]: See PDX Collection 1298
      For S72.365[K,M,N,P,Q,R]: See PDX Collection 897

   ● S72.366   Nondisplaced segmental fracture of shaft of unspecified femur K, M, N, P, Q, R 🔲, A, B, C 🔲, A, B, C 🔲
      (Ex:) For S72.366[A,B,C]: See PDX Collection 1298
      For S72.366[K,M,N,P,Q,R]: See PDX Collection 897

● S72.39   Other fracture of shaft of femur
   ● S72.391   Other fracture of shaft of right femur K, M, N, P, Q, R 🔲, A, B, C 🔲, A, B, C 🔲
      (Ex:) For S72.391[A]: See PDX Collection 1297
      For S72.391[B,C]: See PDX Collection 1298
      For S72.391[K,M,N,P,Q,R]: See PDX Collection 897

   ● S72.392   Other fracture of shaft of left femur K, M, N, P, Q, R 🔲, A, B, C 🔲, A, B, C 🔲
      (Ex:) For S72.392[A]: See PDX Collection 1299
      For S72.392[B,C]: See PDX Collection 1298
      For S72.392[K,M,N,P,Q,R]: See PDX Collection 897

   ● S72.399   Other fracture of shaft of unspecified femur K, M, N, P, Q, R 🔲, A, B, C 🔲, A, B, C 🔲
      (Ex:) For S72.399[A,B,C]: See PDX Collection 1298
      For S72.399[K,M,N,P,Q,R]: See PDX Collection 897

● S72.4   Fracture of lower end of femur
Fracture of distal end of femur
Excludes2   fracture of shaft of femur (S72.3-)
physeal fracture of lower end of femur (S79.1-)

● S72.40   Unspecified fracture of lower end of femur
   ● S72.401   Unspecified fracture of lower end of right femur A, K, M, N, P, Q, R 🔲, B, C 🔲, A, B, C 🔲
      (Ex:) For S72.401[A]: See PDX Collection 1300
      For S72.401[B,C]: See PDX Collection 1301
      For S72.401[K,M,N,P,Q,R]: See PDX Collection 897
      Coding Clinic: 2016, Q4, P43

   ● S72.402   Unspecified fracture of lower end of left femur A, K, M, N, P, Q, R 🔲, B, C 🔲, A, B, C 🔲
      (Ex:) For S72.402[A]: See PDX Collection 1302
      For S72.402[B,C]: See PDX Collection 1301
      For S72.401[K,M,N,P,Q,R]: See PDX Collection 897

   ● S72.409   Unspecified fracture of lower end of unspecified femur A, K, M, N, P, Q, R 🔲, B, C 🔲, A, B, C 🔲
      (Ex:) For S72.409[A,B,C]: See PDX Collection 1301
      For S72.401[K,M,N,P,Q,R]: See PDX Collection 897

● S72.41   Unspecified condyle fracture of lower end of femur
Condyle fracture of femur NOS
   ● S72.411   Displaced unspecified condyle fracture of lower end of right femur A, K, M, N, P, Q, R 🔲, B, C 🔲, A, B, C 🔲
      (Ex:) For S72.411[A]: See PDX Collection 1300
      For S72.411[B,C]: See PDX Collection 1301
      For S72.411[K,M,N,P,Q,R]: See PDX Collection 897

   ● S72.412   Displaced unspecified condyle fracture of lower end of left femur A, K, M, N, P, Q, R 🔲, B, C 🔲, A, B, C 🔲
      (Ex:) For S72.412[A]: See PDX Collection 1302
      For S72.412[B,C]: See PDX Collection 1301
      For S72.411[K,M,N,P,Q,R]: See PDX Collection 897

   ● S72.413   Displaced unspecified condyle fracture of lower end of unspecified femur A, K, M, N, P, Q, R 🔲, B, C 🔲, A, B, C 🔲
      (Ex:) For S72.413[A,B,C]: See PDX Collection 1301
      For S72.413[K,M,N,P,Q,R]: See PDX Collection 897

   ● S72.414   Nondisplaced unspecified condyle fracture of lower end of right femur A, K, M, N, P, Q, R 🔲, B, C 🔲, A, B, C 🔲
      (Ex:) For S72.414[A]: See PDX Collection 1300
      For S72.414[B,C]: See PDX Collection 1301
      For S72.414[K,M,N,P,Q,R]: See PDX Collection 897

   ● S72.415   Nondisplaced unspecified condyle fracture of lower end of left femur A, K, M, N, P, Q, R 🔲, B, C 🔲, A, B, C 🔲
      (Ex:) For S72.415[A]: See PDX Collection 1302
      For S72.415[B,C]: See PDX Collection 1301
      For S72.415[K,M,N,P,Q,R]: See PDX Collection 897

   ● S72.416   Nondisplaced unspecified condyle fracture of lower end of unspecified femur A, K, M, N, P, Q, R 🔲, B, C 🔲, A, B, C 🔲
      (Ex:) For S72.416[A,B,C]: See PDX Collection 1301
      For S72.416[K,M,N,P,Q,R]: See PDX Collection 897

▶ New   ⇒ Revised   ~~deleted~~ Deleted   Excludes 1   Excludes 2   Includes   Use additional   Code first   Code also   Key words
OGCR Official Guidelines   ● Unacceptable Principal Diagnosis   X Assign placeholder X   ● Use Additional Character(s)   ▌ Manifestation Code   Coding Clinic

● S72.42　Fracture of lateral condyle of femur
　　● S72.421　Displaced fracture of lateral condyle of right femur A, K, M, N, P, Q, R 🅒, B, C 🅜, A, B, C 🅗
　　　　ⒺⓍ For S72.421[A]: See PDX Collection 1300
　　　　　　For S72.421[B,C]: See PDX Collection 1301
　　　　　　For S72.421[K,M,N,P,Q,R]: See PDX Collection 897
　　● S72.422　Displaced fracture of lateral condyle of left femur A, K, M, N, P, Q, R 🅒, B, C 🅜, A, B, C 🅗
　　　　ⒺⓍ For S72.422[A]: See PDX Collection 1302
　　　　　　For S72.422[B,C]: See PDX Collection 1301
　　　　　　For S72.422[K,M,N,P,Q,R]: See PDX Collection 897
　　● S72.423　Displaced fracture of lateral condyle of unspecified femur
　　　　A, K, M, N, P, Q, R 🅒, B, C 🅜, A, B, C 🅗
　　　　ⒺⓍ For S72.423[A,B,C]: See PDX Collection 1301
　　　　　　For S72.423[K,M,N,P,Q,R]: See PDX Collection 897
　　● S72.424　Nondisplaced fracture of lateral condyle of right femur
　　　　A, K, M, N, P, Q, R 🅒, B, C 🅜, A, B, C 🅗
　　　　ⒺⓍ For S72.424[A]: See PDX Collection 1300
　　　　　　For S72.424[B,C]: See PDX Collection 1301
　　　　　　For S72.424[K,M,N,P,Q,R]: See PDX Collection 897
　　● S72.425　Nondisplaced fracture of lateral condyle of left femur
　　　　A, K, M, N, P, Q, R 🅒, B, C 🅜, A, B, C 🅗
　　　　ⒺⓍ For S72.425[A]: See PDX Collection 1302
　　　　　　For S72.425[B,C]: See PDX Collection 1301
　　　　　　For S72.425[K,M,N,P,Q,R]: See PDX Collection 897
　　● S72.426　Nondisplaced fracture of lateral condyle of unspecified femur
　　　　A, K, M, N, P, Q, R 🅒, B, C 🅜, A, B, C 🅗
　　　　ⒺⓍ For S72.426[A,B,C]: See PDX Collection 1301
　　　　　　For S72.426[K,M,N,P,Q,R]: See PDX Collection 897
● S72.43　Fracture of medial condyle of femur
　　● S72.431　Displaced fracture of medial condyle of right femur A, K, M, N, P, Q, R 🅒, B, C 🅜, A, B, C 🅗
　　　　ⒺⓍ For S72.431[A]: See PDX Collection 1300
　　　　　　For S72.431[B,C]: See PDX Collection 1301
　　　　　　For S72.431[K,M,N,P,Q,R]: See PDX Collection 897
　　● S72.432　Displaced fracture of medial condyle of left femur A, K, M, N, P, Q, R 🅒, B, C 🅜, A, B, C 🅗
　　　　ⒺⓍ For S72.432[A]: See PDX Collection 1302
　　　　　　For S72.432[B,C]: See PDX Collection 1301
　　　　　　For S72.432[K,M,N,P,Q,R]: See PDX Collection 897
　　● S72.433　Displaced fracture of medial condyle of unspecified femur
　　　　A, K, M, N, P, Q, R 🅒, B, C 🅜, A, B, C 🅗
　　　　ⒺⓍ For S72.433[A,B,C]: See PDX Collection 1301
　　　　　　For S72.433[K,M,N,P,Q,R]: See PDX Collection 897
　　● S72.434　Nondisplaced fracture of medial condyle of right femur
　　　　A, K, M, N, P, Q, R 🅒, B, C 🅜, A, B, C 🅗
　　　　ⒺⓍ For S72.434[A]: See PDX Collection 1300
　　　　　　For S72.434[B,C]: See PDX Collection 1301
　　　　　　For S72.434[K,M,N,P,Q,R]: See PDX Collection 897

　　● S72.435　Nondisplaced fracture of medial condyle of left femur
　　　　A, K, M, N, P, Q, R 🅒, B, C 🅜, A, B, C 🅗
　　　　ⒺⓍ For S72.435[A]: See PDX Collection 1302
　　　　　　For S72.435[B,C]: See PDX Collection 1301
　　　　　　For S72.435[K,M,N,P,Q,R]: See PDX Collection 897
　　● S72.436　Nondisplaced fracture of medial condyle of unspecified femur
　　　　A, K, M, N, P, Q, R 🅒, B, C 🅜, A, B, C 🅗
　　　　ⒺⓍ For S72.436[A,B,C]: See PDX Collection 1301
　　　　　　For S72.436[K,M,N,P,Q,R]: See PDX Collection 897
● S72.44　Fracture of lower epiphysis (separation) of femur
　　　Excludes1　Salter-Harris Type I physeal fracture of lower end of femur (S79.11-)
　　● S72.441　Displaced fracture of lower epiphysis (separation) of right femur
　　　　A, K, M, N, P, Q, R 🅒, B, C 🅜, A, B, C 🅗
　　　　ⒺⓍ For S72.441[A]: See PDX Collection 1300
　　　　　　For S72.441[B,C]: See PDX Collection 1301
　　　　　　For S72.441[K,M,N,P,Q,R]: See PDX Collection 897
　　● S72.442　Displaced fracture of lower epiphysis (separation) of left femur
　　　　A, K, M, N, P, Q, R 🅒, B, C 🅜, A, B, C 🅗
　　　　ⒺⓍ For S72.442[A]: See PDX Collection 1302
　　　　　　For S72.442[B,C]: See PDX Collection 1301
　　　　　　For S72.442[K,M,N,P,Q,R]: See PDX Collection 897
　　● S72.443　Displaced fracture of lower epiphysis (separation) of unspecified femur
　　　　A, K, M, N, P, Q, R 🅒, B, C 🅜, A, B, C 🅗
　　　　ⒺⓍ For S72.443[A,B,C]: See PDX Collection 1301
　　　　　　For S72.443[K,M,N,P,Q,R]: See PDX Collection 897
　　● S72.444　Nondisplaced fracture of lower epiphysis (separation) of right femur
　　　　A, K, M, N, P, Q, R 🅒, B, C 🅜, A, B, C 🅗
　　　　ⒺⓍ For S72.444[A]: See PDX Collection 1300
　　　　　　For S72.444[B,C]: See PDX Collection 1301
　　　　　　For S72.444[K,M,N,P,Q,R]: See PDX Collection 897
　　● S72.445　Nondisplaced fracture of lower epiphysis (separation) of left femur
　　　　A, K, M, N, P, Q, R 🅒, B, C 🅜, A, B, C 🅗
　　　　ⒺⓍ For S72.445[A]: See PDX Collection 1302
　　　　　　For S72.445[B,C]: See PDX Collection 1301
　　　　　　For S72.445[K,M,N,P,Q,R]: See PDX Collection 897
　　● S72.446　Nondisplaced fracture of lower epiphysis (separation) of unspecified femur A, K, M, N, P, Q, R 🅒, B, C 🅜, A, B, C 🅗
　　　　ⒺⓍ For S72.446[A,B,C]: See PDX Collection 1301
　　　　　　For S72.446[K,M,N,P,Q,R]: See PDX Collection 897

CHAPTER 19 (S00-T88)

● **S72.45** **Supracondylar fracture without intracondylar extension of lower end of femur**
Supracondylar fracture of lower end of femur NOS

　Excludes1 supracondylar fracture with intracondylar extension of lower end of femur (S72.46-)

● **S72.451** **Displaced supracondylar fracture without intracondylar extension of lower end of right femur**
A, K, M, N, P, Q, R 🔁, B, C 🔁, A, B, C 🔁
　(Ex:) **For S72.451[A]:** See PDX Collection 1300
　　For S72.451[B,C]: See PDX Collection 1301
　　For S72.451[K,M,N,P,Q,R]: See PDX Collection 897

● **S72.452** **Displaced supracondylar fracture without intracondylar extension of lower end of left femur**
A, K, M, N, P, Q, R 🔁, B, C 🔁, A, B, C 🔁
　(Ex:) **For S72.452[A]:** See PDX Collection 1302
　　For S72.452[B,C]: See PDX Collection 1301
　　For S72.452[K,M,N,P,Q,R]: See PDX Collection 897

● **S72.453** **Displaced supracondylar fracture without intracondylar extension of lower end of unspecified femur**
A, K, M, N, P, Q, R 🔁, B, C 🔁, A, B, C 🔁
　(Ex:) **For S72.453[A,B,C]:** See PDX Collection 1301
　　For S72.453[K,M,N,P,Q,R]: See PDX Collection 897

● **S72.454** **Nondisplaced supracondylar fracture without intracondylar extension of lower end of right femur**
A, K, M, N, P, Q, R 🔁, B, C 🔁, A, B, C 🔁
　(Ex:) **For S72.454[A]:** See PDX Collection 1300
　　For S72.454[B,C]: See PDX Collection 1301
　　For S72.454[K,M,N,P,Q,R]: See PDX Collection 897

● **S72.455** **Nondisplaced supracondylar fracture without intracondylar extension of lower end of left femur**
A, K, M, N, P, Q, R 🔁, B, C 🔁, A, B, C 🔁
　(Ex:) **For S72.455[A]:** See PDX Collection 1302
　　For S72.455[B,C]: See PDX Collection 1301
　　For S72.455[K,M,N,P,Q,R]: See PDX Collection 897

● **S72.456** **Nondisplaced supracondylar fracture without intracondylar extension of lower end of unspecified femur**
A, K, M, N, P, Q, R 🔁, B, C 🔁, A, B, C 🔁
　(Ex:) **For S72.456[A,B,C]:** See PDX Collection 1301
　　For S72.456[K,M,N,P,Q,R]: See PDX Collection 897

● **S72.46** **Supracondylar fracture with intracondylar extension of lower end of femur**

　Excludes1 supracondylar fracture without intracondylar extension of lower end of femur (S72.45-)

● **S72.461** **Displaced supracondylar fracture with intracondylar extension of lower end of right femur**
A, K, M, N, P, Q, R 🔁, B, C 🔁, A, B, C 🔁
　(Ex:) **For S72.461[A]:** See PDX Collection 1300
　　For S72.461[B,C]: See PDX Collection 1301
　　For S72.461[K,M,N,P,Q,R]: See PDX Collection 897

● **S72.462** **Displaced supracondylar fracture with intracondylar extension of lower end of left femur**
A, K, M, N, P, Q, R 🔁, B, C 🔁, A, B, C 🔁
　(Ex:) **For S72.462[A]:** See PDX Collection 1302
　　For S72.462[B,C]: See PDX Collection 1301
　　For S72.462[K,M,N,P,Q,R]: See PDX Collection 897

● **S72.463** **Displaced supracondylar fracture with intracondylar extension of lower end of unspecified femur**
A, K, M, N, P, Q, R 🔁, B, C 🔁, A, B, C 🔁
　(Ex:) **For S72.463[A,B,C]:** See PDX Collection 1301
　　For S72.463[K,M,N,P,Q,R]: See PDX Collection 897

● **S72.464** **Nondisplaced supracondylar fracture with intracondylar extension of lower end of right femur**
A, K, M, N, P, Q, R 🔁, B, C 🔁, A, B, C 🔁
　(Ex:) **For S72.464[A]:** See PDX Collection 1300
　　For S72.464[B,C]: See PDX Collection 1301
　　For S72.464[K,M,N,P,Q,R]: See PDX Collection 897

● **S72.465** **Nondisplaced supracondylar fracture with intracondylar extension of lower end of left femur**
A, K, M, N, P, Q, R 🔁, B, C 🔁, A, B, C 🔁
　(Ex:) **For S72.465[A]:** See PDX Collection 1302
　　For S72.465[B,C]: See PDX Collection 1301
　　For S72.465[K,M,N,P,Q,R]: See PDX Collection 897

● **S72.466** **Nondisplaced supracondylar fracture with intracondylar extension of lower end of unspecified femur**
A, K, M, N, P, Q, R 🔁, B, C 🔁, A, B, C 🔁
　(Ex:) **For S72.466[A,B,C]:** See PDX Collection 1301
　　For S72.466[K,M,N,P,Q,R]: See PDX Collection 897

▶ New　⇒ Revised　~~deleted~~ Deleted　Excludes 1　Excludes 2　Includes　Use additional　Code first　Code also　Key words
OGCR Official Guidelines　● Unacceptable Principal Diagnosis　X Assign placeholder X　● Use Additional Character(s)　▶ Manifestation Code　**Coding Clinic**

● **S72.47**   **Torus fracture of lower end of femur**
The appropriate 7th character is to be added to all codes in subcategory S72.47

A	initial encounter for closed fracture
D	subsequent encounter for fracture with routine healing
G	subsequent encounter for fracture with delayed healing
K	subsequent encounter for fracture with nonunion
P	subsequent encounter for fracture with malunion
S	sequela

● **S72.471**   **Torus fracture of lower end of right femur** A, K, P 🦠, A 🦠
(Ex) **For S72.471[A]:** See PDX Collection 1300
For S72.471[K,P]: See PDX Collection 897

● **S72.472**   **Torus fracture of lower end of left femur** A, K, P 🦠, A 🦠
(Ex) **For S72.472[A]:** See PDX Collection 1302
For S72.472[K,P]: See PDX Collection 897

● **S72.479**   **Torus fracture of lower end of unspecified femur** A, K, P 🦠, A 🦠
(Ex) **For S72.479[A]:** See PDX Collection 1301
For S72.479[K,P]: See PDX Collection 897

● **S72.49**   **Other fracture of lower end of femur**

● **S72.491**   **Other fracture of lower end of right femur** A, K, M, N, P, Q, R 🦠, B, C 🦠, A, B, C 🦠
(Ex) **For S72.491[A]:** See PDX Collection 1300
For S72.491[B,C]: See PDX Collection 1303
For S72.491[K,M,N,P,Q,R]: See PDX Collection 897

● **S72.492**   **Other fracture of lower end of left femur** A, K, M, N, P, Q, R 🦠, B, C 🦠, A, B, C 🦠
(Ex) **For S72.492[A]:** See PDX Collection 1302
For S72.492[B,C]: See PDX Collection 1303
For S72.492[K,M,N,P,Q,R]: See PDX Collection 897

● **S72.499**   **Other fracture of lower end of unspecified femur**
A, K, M, N, P, Q, R 🦠, B, C 🦠, A, B, C 🦠
(Ex) **For S72.499[A]:** See PDX Collection 1301
For S72.499[B,C]: See PDX Collection 1303
For S72.499[K,M,N,P,Q,R]: See PDX Collection 897

● **S72.8**   **Other fracture of femur**
(Ex) **For category S72.8 CC codes S72.8[A,B,C]:** See PDX Collection 1298
For S72.8[K,M,N,P,Q,R]: See PDX Collection 897

● **S72.8X**   **Other fracture of femur**

● **S72.8X1**   **Other fracture of right femur** K, M, N, P, Q, R 🦠, A, B, C 🦠, A, B, C 🦠

● **S72.8X2**   **Other fracture of left femur** K, M, N, P, Q, R 🦠, A, B, C 🦠, A, B, C 🦠

● **S72.8X9**   **Other fracture of unspecified femur** K, M, N, P, Q, R 🦠, A, B, C 🦠, A, B, C 🦠

● **S72.9**   **Unspecified fracture of femur**
Fracture of thigh NOS
Fracture of upper leg NOS
Excludes1   fracture of hip NOS (S72.00-, S72.01-)
(Ex) **For category S72.9 CC codes S72.9[A,B,C]:** See PDX Collection 1298
For S72.9[K,M,N,P,Q,R]: See PDX Collection 897

X● **S72.90**   **Unspecified fracture of unspecified femur**
K, M, N, P, Q, R 🦠, A, B, C 🦠, A, B, C 🦠
Coding Clinic: 2012, Q4, P94

X● **S72.91**   **Unspecified fracture of right femur** K, M, N, P, Q, R 🦠, A, B, C 🦠, A, B, C 🦠

X● **S72.92**   **Unspecified fracture of left femur** K, M, N, P, Q, R 🦠, A, B, C 🦠, A, B, C 🦠

● **S73**   **Dislocation and sprain of joint and ligaments of hip**
Includes   avulsion of joint or ligament of hip
laceration of cartilage, joint or ligament of hip
sprain of cartilage, joint or ligament of hip
traumatic hemarthrosis of joint or ligament of hip
traumatic rupture of joint or ligament of hip
traumatic subluxation of joint or ligament of hip
traumatic tear of joint or ligament of hip
Code also any associated open wound
Excludes2   strain of muscle, fascia and tendon of hip and thigh (S76.-)
The appropriate 7th character is to be added to each code from category S73

A	initial encounter
D	subsequent encounter
S	sequela

● **S73.0**   **Subluxation and dislocation of hip**
Out of position
Excludes2   dislocation and subluxation of hip prosthesis (T84.020, T84.021)

● **S73.00**   **Unspecified subluxation and dislocation of hip**
Dislocation of hip NOS
Subluxation of hip NOS

● **S73.001**   **Unspecified subluxation of right hip** A 🦠, A 🦠
(Ex) See PDX Collection 1304

● **S73.002**   **Unspecified subluxation of left hip** A 🦠, A 🦠
(Ex) See PDX Collection 1305

● **S73.003**   **Unspecified subluxation of unspecified hip** A 🦠, A 🦠
(Ex) See PDX Collection 1306

● **S73.004**   **Unspecified dislocation of right hip** A 🦠, A 🦠
(Ex) See PDX Collection 1304

● **S73.005**   **Unspecified dislocation of left hip** A 🦠, A 🦠
(Ex) See PDX Collection 1305

● **S73.006**   **Unspecified dislocation of unspecified hip** A 🦠, A 🦠
(Ex) See PDX Collection 1306

● **S73.01**   **Posterior subluxation and dislocation of hip**

● **S73.011**   **Posterior subluxation of right hip** A 🦠, A 🦠
(Ex) See PDX Collection 1307

● **S73.012**   **Posterior subluxation of left hip** A 🦠, A 🦠
(Ex) See PDX Collection 1308

● **S73.013**   **Posterior subluxation of unspecified hip** A 🦠, A 🦠
(Ex) See PDX Collection 1309

● **S73.014**   **Posterior dislocation of right hip** A 🦠, A 🦠
(Ex) See PDX Collection 1307

● **S73.015**   **Posterior dislocation of left hip** A 🦠, A 🦠
(Ex) See PDX Collection 1308

● **S73.016**   **Posterior dislocation of unspecified hip** A 🦠, A 🦠
(Ex) See PDX Collection 1309

CHAPTER 19 (S00-T88)

- **S73.02** Obturator subluxation and dislocation of hip
  - **S73.021** Obturator subluxation of right hip A, A
    - (Ex:) See PDX Collection 1310
  - **S73.022** Obturator subluxation of left hip A, A
    - (Ex:) See PDX Collection 1311
  - **S73.023** Obturator subluxation of unspecified hip A, A
    - (Ex:) See PDX Collection 1312
  - **S73.024** Obturator dislocation of right hip A, A
    - (Ex:) See PDX Collection 1310
  - **S73.025** Obturator dislocation of left hip A, A
    - (Ex:) See PDX Collection 1311
  - **S73.026** Obturator dislocation of unspecified hip A, A
    - (Ex:) See PDX Collection 1312
- **S73.03** Other anterior subluxation and dislocation of hip
  - **S73.031** Other anterior subluxation of right hip A, A
    - (Ex:) See PDX Collection 1313
  - **S73.032** Other anterior subluxation of left hip A, A
    - (Ex:) See PDX Collection 1314
  - **S73.033** Other anterior subluxation of unspecified hip A, A
    - (Ex:) See PDX Collection 1315
  - **S73.034** Other anterior dislocation of right hip A, A
    - (Ex:) See PDX Collection 1313
  - **S73.035** Other anterior dislocation of left hip A, A
    - (Ex:) See PDX Collection 1314
  - **S73.036** Other anterior dislocation of unspecified hip A, A
    - (Ex:) See PDX Collection 1315
- **S73.04** Central subluxation and dislocation of hip
  - **S73.041** Central subluxation of right hip A, A
    - (Ex:) See PDX Collection 1304
  - **S73.042** Central subluxation of left hip A, A
    - (Ex:) See PDX Collection 1305
  - **S73.043** Central subluxation of unspecified hip A, A
    - (Ex:) See PDX Collection 1306
  - **S73.044** Central dislocation of right hip A, A
    - (Ex:) See PDX Collection 1304
  - **S73.045** Central dislocation of left hip A, A
    - (Ex:) See PDX Collection 1305
  - **S73.046** Central dislocation of unspecified hip A, A
    - (Ex:) See PDX Collection 1306
- **S73.1** Sprain of hip
  - **S73.10** Unspecified sprain of hip
    - **S73.101** Unspecified sprain of right hip
    - **S73.102** Unspecified sprain of left hip
    - **S73.109** Unspecified sprain of unspecified hip

- **S73.11** Iliofemoral ligament sprain of hip
  - **S73.111** Iliofemoral ligament sprain of right hip
  - **S73.112** Iliofemoral ligament sprain of left hip
  - **S73.119** Iliofemoral ligament sprain of unspecified hip
- **S73.12** Ischiocapsular (ligament) sprain of hip
  - **S73.121** Ischiocapsular ligament sprain of right hip
  - **S73.122** Ischiocapsular ligament sprain of left hip
  - **S73.129** Ischiocapsular ligament sprain of unspecified hip
- **S73.19** Other sprain of hip
  - **S73.191** Other sprain of right hip
  - **S73.192** Other sprain of left hip
  - **S73.199** Other sprain of unspecified hip

- **S74** Injury of nerves at hip and thigh level
  Code also any associated open wound (S71.-)
  Excludes2 injury of nerves at ankle and foot level (S94.-)
  injury of nerves at lower leg level (S84.-)

  The appropriate 7th character is to be added to each code from category S74

A	initial encounter
D	subsequent encounter
S	sequela

  - **S74.0** Injury of sciatic nerve at hip and thigh level
    - X **S74.00** Injury of sciatic nerve at hip and thigh level, unspecified leg
    - X **S74.01** Injury of sciatic nerve at hip and thigh level, right leg
    - X **S74.02** Injury of sciatic nerve at hip and thigh level, left leg
  - **S74.1** Injury of femoral nerve at hip and thigh level
    - X **S74.10** Injury of femoral nerve at hip and thigh level, unspecified leg
    - X **S74.11** Injury of femoral nerve at hip and thigh level, right leg
    - X **S74.12** Injury of femoral nerve at hip and thigh level, left leg
  - **S74.2** Injury of cutaneous sensory nerve at hip and thigh level
    - X **S74.20** Injury of cutaneous sensory nerve at hip and thigh level, unspecified leg
    - X **S74.21** Injury of cutaneous sensory nerve at hip and high level, right leg
    - X **S74.22** Injury of cutaneous sensory nerve at hip and thigh level, left leg
  - **S74.8** Injury of other nerves at hip and thigh level
    - **S74.8X** Injury of other nerves at hip and thigh level
      - **S74.8X1** Injury of other nerves at hip and thigh level, right leg
      - **S74.8X2** Injury of other nerves at hip and thigh level, left leg
      - **S74.8X9** Injury of other nerves at hip and thigh level, unspecified leg
  - **S74.9** Injury of unspecified nerve at hip and thigh level
    - X **S74.90** Injury of unspecified nerve at hip and thigh level, unspecified leg
    - X **S74.91** Injury of unspecified nerve at hip and thigh level, right leg
    - X **S74.92** Injury of unspecified nerve at hip and thigh level, left leg

▶ New   ⇒ Revised   ~~deleted~~ Deleted   Excludes 1   Excludes 2   Includes   Use additional   Code first   Code also   Key words
OGCR Official Guidelines   ● Unacceptable Principal Diagnosis   X Assign placeholder X   ● Use Additional Character(s)   ▶ Manifestation Code   **Coding Clinic**

● **S75 Injury of blood vessels at hip and thigh level**

    Code also any associated open wound (S71.-)

    Excludes2 injury of blood vessels at lower leg level (S85.-)
                  injury of popliteal artery (S85.0)

    The appropriate 7th character is to be added to each code from
        category S75

> A   initial encounter
> D   subsequent encounter
> S   sequela

● **S75.0 Injury of femoral artery**

  ● **S75.00 Unspecified injury of femoral artery**

    ● **S75.001 Unspecified injury of femoral artery, right leg** A 🐾
        Ⓔⓧ See PDX Collection 1316

    ● **S75.002 Unspecified injury of femoral artery, left leg** A 🐾
        Ⓔⓧ See PDX Collection 1317

    ● **S75.009 Unspecified injury of femoral artery, unspecified leg** A 🐾
        Ⓔⓧ See PDX Collection 1318

  ● **S75.01 Minor laceration of femoral artery**
    Incomplete transection of femoral artery
    Laceration of femoral artery NOS
    Superficial laceration of femoral artery

    ● **S75.011 Minor laceration of femoral artery, right leg** A 🐾
        Ⓔⓧ See PDX Collection 1316

    ● **S75.012 Minor laceration of femoral artery, left leg** A 🐾
        Ⓔⓧ See PDX Collection 1317

    ● **S75.019 Minor laceration of femoral artery, unspecified leg** A 🐾
        Ⓔⓧ See PDX Collection 1318

  ● **S75.02 Major laceration of femoral artery**
    Complete transection of femoral artery
    Traumatic rupture of femoral artery

    ● **S75.021 Major laceration of femoral artery, right leg** A 🐾
        Ⓔⓧ See PDX Collection 1316

    ● **S75.022 Major laceration of femoral artery, left leg** A 🐾
        Ⓔⓧ See PDX Collection 1317

    ● **S75.029 Major laceration of femoral artery, unspecified leg** A 🐾
        Ⓔⓧ See PDX Collection 1318

  ● **S75.09 Other specified injury of femoral artery**

    ● **S75.091 Other specified injury of femoral artery, right leg** A 🐾
        Ⓔⓧ See PDX Collection 1316

    ● **S75.092 Other specified injury of femoral artery, left leg** A 🐾
        Ⓔⓧ See PDX Collection 1317

    ● **S75.099 Other specified injury of femoral artery, unspecified leg** A 🐾
        Ⓔⓧ See PDX Collection 1318

● **S75.1 Injury of femoral vein at hip and thigh level**

  ● **S75.10 Unspecified injury of femoral vein at hip and thigh level**

    ● **S75.101 Unspecified injury of femoral vein at hip and thigh level, right leg** A 🐾
        Ⓔⓧ See PDX Collection 1319

    ● **S75.102 Unspecified injury of femoral vein at hip and thigh level, left leg** A 🐾
        Ⓔⓧ See PDX Collection 1320

    ● **S75.109 Unspecified injury of femoral vein at hip and thigh level, unspecified leg** A 🐾
        Ⓔⓧ See PDX Collection 1321

● **S75.11 Minor laceration of femoral vein at hip and thigh level**
    Incomplete transection of femoral vein at hip
      and thigh level
    Laceration of femoral vein at hip and thigh
      level NOS
    Superficial laceration of femoral vein at hip
      and thigh level

    ● **S75.111 Minor laceration of femoral vein at hip and thigh level, right leg** A 🐾
        Ⓔⓧ See PDX Collection 1319

    ● **S75.112 Minor laceration of femoral vein at hip and thigh level, left leg** A 🐾
        Ⓔⓧ See PDX Collection 1320

    ● **S75.119 Minor laceration of femoral vein at hip and thigh level, unspecified leg** A 🐾
        Ⓔⓧ See PDX Collection 1321

  ● **S75.12 Major laceration of femoral vein at hip and thigh level**
    Complete transection of femoral vein at hip
      and thigh level
    Traumatic rupture of femoral vein at hip and
      thigh level

    ● **S75.121 Major laceration of femoral vein at hip and thigh level, right leg** A 🐾
        Ⓔⓧ See PDX Collection 1319

    ● **S75.122 Major laceration of femoral vein at hip and thigh level, left leg** A 🐾
        Ⓔⓧ See PDX Collection 1320

    ● **S75.129 Major laceration of femoral vein at hip and thigh level, unspecified leg** A 🐾
        Ⓔⓧ See PDX Collection 1321

  ● **S75.19 Other specified injury of femoral vein at hip and thigh level**

    ● **S75.191 Other specified injury of femoral vein at hip and thigh level, right leg** A 🐾
        Ⓔⓧ See PDX Collection 1319

    ● **S75.192 Other specified injury of femoral vein at hip and thigh level, left leg** A 🐾
        Ⓔⓧ See PDX Collection 1320

    ● **S75.199 Other specified injury of femoral vein at hip and thigh level, unspecified leg** A 🐾
        Ⓔⓧ See PDX Collection 1321

● **S75.2 Injury of greater saphenous vein at hip and thigh level**
    Excludes1 greater saphenous vein NOS (S85.3)

  ● **S75.20 Unspecified injury of greater saphenous vein at hip and thigh level**

    ● **S75.201 Unspecified injury of greater saphenous vein at hip and thigh level, right leg** A 🐾
        Ⓔⓧ See PDX Collection 1322

    ● **S75.202 Unspecified injury of greater saphenous vein at hip and thigh level, left leg** A 🐾
        Ⓔⓧ See PDX Collection 1323

    ● **S75.209 Unspecified injury of greater saphenous vein at hip and thigh level, unspecified leg** A 🐾
        Ⓔⓧ See PDX Collection 1324

CHAPTER 19 (S00–T88)

● **S75.21**   Minor laceration of greater saphenous vein at hip and thigh level
　　　Incomplete transection of greater saphenous vein at hip and thigh level
　　　Laceration of greater saphenous vein at hip and thigh level NOS
　　　Superficial laceration of greater saphenous vein at hip and thigh level

　　● **S75.211**   Minor laceration of greater saphenous vein at hip and thigh level, right leg A ⊜
　　　　(Ex:) See PDX Collection 1322

　　● **S75.212**   Minor laceration of greater saphenous vein at hip and thigh level, left leg A ⊜
　　　　(Ex:) See PDX Collection 1323

　　● **S75.219**   Minor laceration of greater saphenous vein at hip and thigh level, unspecified leg A ⊜
　　　　(Ex:) See PDX Collection 1324

● **S75.22**   Major laceration of greater saphenous vein at hip and thigh level
　　　Complete transection of greater saphenous vein at hip and thigh level
　　　Traumatic rupture of greater saphenous vein at hip and thigh level

　　● **S75.221**   Major laceration of greater saphenous vein at hip and thigh level, right leg A ⊜
　　　　(Ex:) See PDX Collection 1322

　　● **S75.222**   Major laceration of greater saphenous vein at hip and thigh level, left leg A ⊜
　　　　(Ex:) See PDX Collection 1323

　　● **S75.229**   Major laceration of greater saphenous vein at hip and thigh level, unspecified leg A ⊜
　　　　(Ex:) See PDX Collection 1324

● **S75.29**   Other specified injury of greater saphenous vein at hip and thigh level

　　● **S75.291**   Other specified injury of greater saphenous vein at hip and thigh level, right leg A ⊜
　　　　(Ex:) See PDX Collection 1322

　　● **S75.292**   Other specified injury of greater saphenous vein at hip and thigh level, left leg A ⊜
　　　　(Ex:) See PDX Collection 1323

　　● **S75.299**   Other specified injury of greater saphenous vein at hip and thigh level, unspecified leg A ⊜
　　　　(Ex:) See PDX Collection 1324

● **S75.8**   Injury of other blood vessels at hip and thigh level

　● **S75.80**   Unspecified injury of other blood vessels at hip and thigh level

　　● **S75.801**   Unspecified injury of other blood vessels at hip and thigh level, right leg A ⊜
　　　　(Ex:) See PDX Collection 1325

　　● **S75.802**   Unspecified injury of other blood vessels at hip and thigh level, left leg A ⊜
　　　　(Ex:) See PDX Collection 1326

　　● **S75.809**   Unspecified injury of other blood vessels at hip and thigh level, unspecified leg A ⊜
　　　　(Ex:) See PDX Collection 1327

　● **S75.81**   Laceration of other blood vessels at hip and thigh level

　　● **S75.811**   Laceration of other blood vessels at hip and thigh level, right leg A ⊜
　　　　(Ex:) See PDX Collection 1325

　　● **S75.812**   Laceration of other blood vessels at hip and thigh level, left leg A ⊜
　　　　(Ex:) See PDX Collection 1326

　　● **S75.819**   Laceration of other blood vessels at hip and thigh level, unspecified leg A ⊜
　　　　(Ex:) See PDX Collection 1327

　● **S75.89**   Other specified injury of other blood vessels at hip and thigh level

　　● **S75.891**   Other specified injury of other blood vessels at hip and thigh level, right leg A ⊜
　　　　(Ex:) See PDX Collection 1325

　　● **S75.892**   Other specified injury of other blood vessels at hip and thigh level, left leg A ⊜
　　　　(Ex:) See PDX Collection 1326

　　● **S75.899**   Other specified injury of other blood vessels at hip and thigh level, unspecified leg A ⊜
　　　　(Ex:) See PDX Collection 1327

● **S75.9**   Injury of unspecified blood vessel at hip and thigh level

　● **S75.90**   Unspecified injury of unspecified blood vessel at hip and thigh level

　　● **S75.901**   Unspecified injury of unspecified blood vessel at hip and thigh level, right leg A ⊜
　　　　(Ex:) See PDX Collection 1325

　　● **S75.902**   Unspecified injury of unspecified blood vessel at hip and thigh level, left leg A ⊜
　　　　(Ex:) See PDX Collection 1326

　　● **S75.909**   Unspecified injury of unspecified blood vessel at hip and thigh level, unspecified leg A ⊜
　　　　(Ex:) See PDX Collection 1327

　● **S75.91**   Laceration of unspecified blood vessel at hip and thigh level

　　● **S75.911**   Laceration of unspecified blood vessel at hip and thigh level, right leg A ⊜
　　　　(Ex:) See PDX Collection 1325

　　● **S75.912**   Laceration of unspecified blood vessel at hip and thigh level, left leg A ⊜
　　　　(Ex:) See PDX Collection 1326

　　● **S75.919**   Laceration of unspecified blood vessel at hip and thigh level, unspecified leg A ⊜
　　　　(Ex:) See PDX Collection 1327

　● **S75.99**   Other specified injury of unspecified blood vessel at hip and thigh level

　　● **S75.991**   Other specified injury of unspecified blood vessel at hip and thigh level, right leg A ⊜
　　　　(Ex:) See PDX Collection 1325

　　● **S75.992**   Other specified injury of unspecified blood vessel at hip and thigh level, left leg A ⊜
　　　　(Ex:) See PDX Collection 1326

　　● **S75.999**   Other specified injury of unspecified blood vessel at hip and thigh level, unspecified leg A ⊜
　　　　(Ex:) See PDX Collection 1327

● S76 **Injury of muscle, fascia and tendon at hip and thigh level**

Code also any associated open wound (S71.-)

Excludes2   injury of muscle, fascia and tendon at lower leg level (S86)

sprain of joint and ligament of hip (S73.1)

The appropriate 7th character is to be added to each code from category S76

A	initial encounter
D	subsequent encounter
S	sequela

● S76.0 **Injury of muscle, fascia and tendon of hip**

● S76.00 **Unspecified** injury of muscle, fascia and tendon of hip

● S76.001 Unspecified injury of muscle, fascia and tendon of **right** hip

● S76.002 Unspecified injury of muscle, fascia and tendon of **left** hip

● S76.009 Unspecified injury of muscle, fascia and tendon of **unspecified** hip

● S76.01 **Strain** of muscle, fascia and tendon of hip

● S76.011 Strain of muscle, fascia and tendon of **right** hip

● S76.012 Strain of muscle, fascia and tendon of **left** hip

● S76.019 Strain of muscle, fascia and tendon of **unspecified** hip

● S76.02 **Laceration** of muscle, fascia and tendon of hip

● S76.021 Laceration of muscle, fascia and tendon of **right** hip A 🦠
(Ex) See PDX Collection 1328

● S76.022 Laceration of muscle, fascia and tendon of **left** hip A 🦠
(Ex) See PDX Collection 1329

● S76.029 Laceration of muscle, fascia and tendon of **unspecified** hip A 🦠
(Ex) See PDX Collection 1330

● S76.09 **Other** specified injury of muscle, fascia and tendon of hip

● S76.091 Other specified injury of muscle, fascia and tendon of **right** hip

● S76.092 Other specified injury of muscle, fascia and tendon of **left** hip

● S76.099 Other specified injury of muscle, fascia and tendon of **unspecified** hip

● S76.1 **Injury of quadriceps muscle, fascia and tendon**
Injury of patellar ligament (tendon)

● S76.10 **Unspecified** injury of quadriceps muscle, fascia and tendon

● S76.101 Unspecified injury of **right** quadriceps muscle, fascia and tendon

● S76.102 Unspecified injury of **left** quadriceps muscle, fascia and tendon

● S76.109 Unspecified injury of **unspecified** quadriceps muscle, fascia and tendon

● S76.11 **Strain** of quadriceps muscle, fascia and tendon

● S76.111 Strain of **right** quadriceps muscle, fascia and tendon

● S76.112 Strain of **left** quadriceps muscle, fascia and tendon

● S76.119 Strain of **unspecified** quadriceps muscle, fascia and tendon

● S76.12 **Laceration** of quadriceps muscle, fascia and tendon

● S76.121 Laceration of **right** quadriceps muscle, fascia and tendon A 🦠
(Ex) See PDX Collection 1328

● S76.122 Laceration of **left** quadriceps muscle, fascia and tendon A 🦠
(Ex) See PDX Collection 1329

● S76.129 Laceration of **unspecified** quadriceps muscle, fascia and tendon A 🦠
(Ex) See PDX Collection 1330

● S76.19 **Other** specified injury of quadriceps muscle, fascia and tendon

● S76.191 Other specified injury of **right** quadriceps muscle, fascia and tendon

● S76.192 Other specified injury of **left** quadriceps muscle, fascia and tendon

● S76.199 Other specified injury of **unspecified** quadriceps muscle, fascia and tendon

● S76.2 **Injury of adductor muscle, fascia and tendon of thigh**

● S76.20 **Unspecified** injury of adductor muscle, fascia and tendon of thigh

● S76.201 Unspecified injury of adductor muscle, fascia and tendon of **right** thigh

● S76.202 Unspecified injury of adductor muscle, fascia and tendon of **left** thigh

● S76.209 Unspecified injury of adductor muscle, fascia and tendon of **unspecified** thigh

● S76.21 **Strain** of adductor muscle, fascia and tendon of thigh

● S76.211 Strain of adductor muscle, fascia and tendon of **right** thigh

● S76.212 Strain of adductor muscle, fascia and tendon of **left** thigh

● S76.219 Strain of adductor muscle, fascia and tendon of **unspecified** thigh

● S76.22 **Laceration** of adductor muscle, fascia and tendon of thigh

● S76.221 Laceration of adductor muscle, fascia and tendon of **right** thigh A 🦠
(Ex) See PDX Collection 1328

● S76.222 Laceration of adductor muscle, fascia and tendon of **left** thigh A 🦠
(Ex) See PDX Collection 1329

● S76.229 Laceration of adductor muscle, fascia and tendon of **unspecified** thigh A 🦠
(Ex) See PDX Collection 1330

● S76.29 **Other** injury of adductor muscle, fascia and tendon of thigh

● S76.291 Other injury of adductor muscle, fascia and tendon of **right** thigh

● S76.292 Other injury of adductor muscle, fascia and tendon of **left** thigh

● S76.299 Other injury of adductor muscle, fascia and tendon of **unspecified** thigh

CHAPTER 19 (S00–T88)

● **S76.3** Injury of muscle, fascia and tendon of the posterior muscle group at thigh level

   ● **S76.30** Unspecified injury of muscle, fascia and tendon of the posterior muscle group at thigh level

      ● **S76.301** Unspecified injury of muscle, fascia and tendon of the posterior muscle group at thigh level, right thigh

      ● **S76.302** Unspecified injury of muscle, fascia and tendon of the posterior muscle group at thigh level, left thigh

      ● **S76.309** Unspecified injury of muscle, fascia and tendon of the posterior muscle group at thigh level, unspecified thigh

   ● **S76.31** Strain of muscle, fascia and tendon of the posterior muscle group at thigh level

      ● **S76.311** Strain of muscle, fascia and tendon of the posterior muscle group at thigh level, right thigh

      ● **S76.312** Strain of muscle, fascia and tendon of the posterior muscle group at thigh level, left thigh

      ● **S76.319** Strain of muscle, fascia and tendon of the posterior muscle group at thigh level, unspecified thigh

   ● **S76.32** Laceration of muscle, fascia and tendon of the posterior muscle group at thigh level

      ● **S76.321** Laceration of muscle, fascia and tendon of the posterior muscle group at thigh level, right thigh A 🔖
         Ex: See PDX Collection 1328

      ● **S76.322** Laceration of muscle, fascia and tendon of the posterior muscle group at thigh level, left thigh A 🔖
         Ex: See PDX Collection 1329

      ● **S76.329** Laceration of muscle, fascia and tendon of the posterior muscle group at thigh level, unspecified thigh A 🔖
         Ex: See PDX Collection 1330

   ● **S76.39** Other specified injury of muscle, fascia and tendon of the posterior muscle group at thigh level

      ● **S76.391** Other specified injury of muscle, fascia and tendon of the posterior muscle group at thigh level, right thigh

      ● **S76.392** Other specified injury of muscle, fascia and tendon of the posterior muscle group at thigh level, left thigh

      ● **S76.399** Other specified injury of muscle, fascia and tendon of the posterior muscle group at thigh level, unspecified thigh

● **S76.8** Injury of other specified muscles, fascia and tendons at thigh level

   ● **S76.80** Unspecified injury of other specified muscles, fascia and tendons at thigh level

      ● **S76.801** Unspecified injury of other specified muscles, fascia and tendons at thigh level, right thigh

      ● **S76.802** Unspecified injury of other specified muscles, fascia and tendons at thigh level, left thigh

      ● **S76.809** Unspecified injury of other specified muscles, fascia and tendons at thigh level, unspecified thigh

● **S76.81** Strain of other specified specified muscles, fascia and tendons at thigh level

      ● **S76.811** Strain of other specified muscles, fascia and tendons at thigh level, right thigh

      ● **S76.812** Strain of other specified muscles, fascia and tendons at thigh level, left thigh

      ● **S76.819** Strain of other specified muscles, fascia and tendons at thigh level, unspecified thigh

   ● **S76.82** Laceration of other specified muscles, fascia and tendons at thigh level

      ● **S76.821** Laceration of other specified muscles, fascia and tendons at thigh level, right thigh A 🔖
         Ex: See PDX Collection 1328

      ● **S76.822** Laceration of other specified muscles, fascia and tendons at thigh level, left thigh A 🔖
         Ex: See PDX Collection 1329

      ● **S76.829** Laceration of other specified muscles, fascia and tendons at thigh level, unspecified thigh A 🔖
         Ex: See PDX Collection 1330

   ● **S76.89** Other injury of other specified muscles, fascia and tendons at thigh level

      ● **S76.891** Other injury of other specified muscles, fascia and tendons at thigh level, right thigh

      ● **S76.892** Other injury of other specified muscles, fascia and tendons at thigh level, left thigh

      ● **S76.899** Other injury of other specified muscles, fascia and tendons at thigh level, unspecified thigh

● **S76.9** Injury of unspecified muscles, fascia and tendons at thigh level

   ● **S76.90** Unspecified injury of unspecified muscles, fascia and tendons at thigh level

      ● **S76.901** Unspecified injury of unspecified muscles, fascia and tendons at thigh level, right thigh

      ● **S76.902** Unspecified injury of unspecified muscles, fascia and tendons at thigh level, left thigh

      ● **S76.909** Unspecified injury of unspecified muscles, fascia and tendons at thigh level, unspecified thigh

   ● **S76.91** Strain of unspecified muscles, fascia and tendons at thigh level

      ● **S76.911** Strain of unspecified muscles, fascia and tendons at thigh level, right thigh

      ● **S76.912** Strain of unspecified muscles, fascia and tendons at thigh level, left thigh

      ● **S76.919** Strain of unspecified muscles fascia and tendons at thigh level, unspecified thigh

   ● **S76.92** Laceration of unspecified muscles, fascia and tendons at thigh level

      ● **S76.921** Laceration of unspecified muscles, fascia and tendons at thigh level, right thigh A 🔖
         Ex: See PDX Collection 1328

      ● **S76.922** Laceration of unspecified muscles, fascia and tendons at thigh level, left thigh A 🔖
         Ex: See PDX Collection 1329

      ● **S76.929** Laceration of unspecified muscles, fascia and tendons at thigh level, unspecified thigh A 🔖
         Ex: See PDX Collection 1330

▶ New   ⇒ Revised   ~~deleted~~ Deleted   Excludes 1   Excludes 2   Includes   Use additional   Code first   Code also   Key words

OGCR Official Guidelines   ● Unacceptable Principal Diagnosis   X Assign placeholder X   ● Use Additional Character(s)   ▶ Manifestation Code   **Coding Clinic**

S76.99   **Other specified injury of unspecified muscles, fascia and tendons at thigh level**

S76.991   Other specified injury of unspecified muscles, fascia and tendons at thigh level, **right** thigh

S76.992   Other specified injury of unspecified muscles, fascia and tendons at thigh level, **left** thigh

S76.999   Other specified injury of unspecified muscles, fascia and tendons at thigh level, **unspecified** thigh

S77   **Crushing injury of hip and thigh**
Use additional code(s) for all associated injuries

Excludes2   crushing injury of ankle and foot (S97.-)
crushing injury of lower leg (S87.-)

The appropriate 7th character is to be added to each code from category S77

A   initial encounter
D   subsequent encounter
S   sequela

S77.0   **Crushing injury of hip**
(Ex:) For category S77.0 CC codes: See PDX Collection 1331

X   S77.00   Crushing injury of **unspecified** hip A 🦠, A 🦠
X   S77.01   Crushing injury of **right** hip A 🦠, A 🦠
X   S77.02   Crushing injury of **left** hip A 🦠, A 🦠

S77.1   **Crushing injury of thigh**
(Ex:) For category S77.1 CC codes: See PDX Collection 1332

X   S77.10   Crushing injury of **unspecified** thigh A 🦠, A 🦠
X   S77.11   Crushing injury of **right** thigh A 🦠, A 🦠
X   S77.12   Crushing injury of **left** thigh A 🦠, A 🦠

S77.2   **Crushing injury of hip with thigh**

X   S77.20   Crushing injury of **unspecified** hip with thigh
X   S77.21   Crushing injury of **right** hip with thigh
X   S77.22   Crushing injury of **left** hip with thigh

S78   **Traumatic amputation of hip and thigh**
An amputation not identified as partial or complete should be coded to complete

Excludes1   traumatic amputation of knee (S88.0-)

The appropriate 7th character is to be added to each code from category S78

A   initial encounter
D   subsequent encounter
S   sequela

S78.0   **Traumatic amputation at hip joint**

S78.01   **Complete** traumatic amputation at hip joint

S78.011   Complete traumatic amputation at **right** hip joint A 🦠
(Ex:) See PDX Collection 1333

S78.012   Complete traumatic amputation at **left** hip joint A 🦠
(Ex:) See PDX Collection 1334

S78.019   Complete traumatic amputation at **unspecified** hip joint A 🦠
(Ex:) See PDX Collection 1335

S78.02   **Partial** traumatic amputation at hip joint

S78.021   Partial traumatic amputation at **right** hip joint A 🦠
(Ex:) See PDX Collection 1333

S78.022   Partial traumatic amputation at **left** hip joint A 🦠
(Ex:) See PDX Collection 1334

S78.029   Partial traumatic amputation at **unspecified** hip joint A 🦠
(Ex:) See PDX Collection 1335

S78.1   **Traumatic amputation at level between hip and knee**

Excludes1   traumatic amputation of knee (S88.0-)

S78.11   **Complete** traumatic amputation at level between hip and knee

S78.111   Complete traumatic amputation at level between **right** hip and knee A 🦠
(Ex:) See PDX Collection 1333

S78.112   Complete traumatic amputation at level between **left** hip and knee A 🦠
(Ex:) See PDX Collection 1334

S78.119   Complete traumatic amputation at level between **unspecified** hip and knee A 🦠
(Ex:) See PDX Collection 1335

S78.12   **Partial** traumatic amputation at level between hip and knee

S78.121   Partial traumatic amputation at level between **right** hip and knee A 🦠
(Ex:) See PDX Collection 1333

S78.122   Partial traumatic amputation at level between **left** hip and knee A 🦠
(Ex:) See PDX Collection 1334

S78.129   Partial traumatic amputation at level between **unspecified** hip and knee A 🦠
(Ex:) See PDX Collection 1335

S78.9   **Traumatic amputation of hip and thigh, level unspecified**

S78.91   **Complete** traumatic amputation of hip and thigh, level unspecified

S78.911   Complete traumatic amputation of **right** hip and thigh, level unspecified A 🦠
(Ex:) See PDX Collection 1333

S78.912   Complete traumatic amputation of **left** hip and thigh, level unspecified A 🦠
(Ex:) See PDX Collection 1334

S78.919   Complete traumatic amputation of **unspecified** hip and thigh, level unspecified A 🦠
(Ex:) See PDX Collection 1335

S78.92   **Partial** traumatic amputation of hip and thigh, level unspecified

S78.921   Partial traumatic amputation of **right** hip and thigh, level unspecified A 🦠
(Ex:) See PDX Collection 1333

S78.922   Partial traumatic amputation of **left** hip and thigh, level unspecified A 🦠
(Ex:) See PDX Collection 1334

S78.929   Partial traumatic amputation of **unspecified** hip and thigh, level unspecified A 🦠
(Ex:) See PDX Collection 1335

CHAPTER 19 (S00-T88)

● **S79**   **Other and unspecified injuries of hip and thigh**

Note: A fracture not indicated as open or closed should be coded to closed

The appropriate 7th character is to be added to each code from subcategories S79.0 and S79.1

> A   initial encounter for closed fracture
> D   subsequent encounter for fracture with routine healing
> G   subsequent encounter for fracture with delayed healing
> K   subsequent encounter for fracture with nonunion
> P   subsequent encounter for fracture with malunion
> S   sequela

● **S79.0**   **Physeal fracture of upper end of femur**

    Excludes1   apophyseal fracture of upper end of femur (S72.13-)
                     nontraumatic slipped upper femoral epiphysis (M93.0-)

● **S79.00**   **Unspecified physeal fracture of upper end of femur**

   ● **S79.001**   **Unspecified physeal fracture of upper end of right femur** K, P 🔷, A 🔷, A 🔷
        (Ex:) For S79.001[A]: See PDX Collection 1297
              For S79.001[K,P]: See PDX Collection 897

   ● **S79.002**   **Unspecified physeal fracture of upper end of left femur** K, P 🔷, A 🔷, A 🔷
        (Ex:) For S79.002[A]: See PDX Collection 1299
              For S79.002[K,P]: See PDX Collection 897

   ● **S79.009**   **Unspecified physeal fracture of upper end of unspecified femur** K, P 🔷, A 🔷, A 🔷
        (Ex:) For S79.009[A]: See PDX Collection 1298
              For S79.009[K,P]: See PDX Collection 897

● **S79.01**   **Salter-Harris Type I physeal fracture of upper end of femur**

    Acute on chronic slipped capital femoral epiphysis (traumatic)
    Acute slipped capital femoral epiphysis (traumatic)
    Capital femoral epiphyseal fracture

    Excludes1   chronic slipped upper femoral epiphysis (nontraumatic) (M93.02-)

   ● **S79.011**   **Salter-Harris Type I physeal fracture of upper end of right femur** K, P 🔷, A 🔷, A 🔷
        (Ex:) For S79.011[A]: See PDX Collection 1297
              For S79.011[K,P]: See PDX Collection 897

   ● **S79.012**   **Salter-Harris Type I physeal fracture of upper end of left femur** K, P 🔷, A 🔷, A 🔷
        (Ex:) For S79.012[A]: See PDX Collection 1299
              For S79.012[K,P]: See PDX Collection 897

   ● **S79.019**   **Salter-Harris Type I physeal fracture of upper end of unspecified femur** K, P 🔷, A 🔷, A 🔷
        (Ex:) For S79.019[A]: See PDX Collection 1298
              For S79.019[K,P]: See PDX Collection 897

● **S79.09**   **Other physeal fracture of upper end of femur**

   ● **S79.091**   **Other physeal fracture of upper end of right femur** K, P 🔷, A 🔷, A 🔷
        (Ex:) For S79.091[A]: See PDX Collection 1297
              For S79.091[K,P]: See PDX Collection 897

   ● **S79.092**   **Other physeal fracture of upper end of left femur** K, P 🔷, A 🔷, A 🔷
        (Ex:) For S79.092[A]: See PDX Collection 1299
              For S79.092[K,P]: See PDX Collection 897

   ● **S79.099**   **Other physeal fracture of upper end of unspecified femur** K, P 🔷, A 🔷, A 🔷
        (Ex:) For S79.099[A]: See PDX Collection 1298
              For S79.099[K,P]: See PDX Collection 897

● **S79.1**   **Physeal fracture of lower end of femur**

● **S79.10**   **Unspecified physeal fracture of lower end of femur**

   ● **S79.101**   **Unspecified physeal fracture of lower end of right femur** A, K, P 🔷, A 🔷
        (Ex:) For S79.101[A]: See PDX Collection 1300
              For S79.101[K,P]: See PDX Collection 897

   ● **S79.102**   **Unspecified physeal fracture of lower end of left femur** A, K, P 🔷, A 🔷
        (Ex:) For S79.102[A]: See PDX Collection 1302
              For S72.102[K,P]: See PDX Collection 897

   ● **S79.109**   **Unspecified physeal fracture of lower end of unspecified femur** A, K, P 🔷, A 🔷
        (Ex:) For S79.109[A]: See PDX Collection 1301
              For S79.109[K,P]: See PDX Collection 897

● **S79.11**   **Salter-Harris Type I physeal fracture of lower end of femur**

   ● **S79.111**   **Salter-Harris Type I physeal fracture of lower end of right femur** A, K, P 🔷, A 🔷
        (Ex:) For S79.111[A]: See PDX Collection 1300
              For S79.111[K,P]: See PDX Collection 897

   ● **S79.112**   **Salter-Harris Type I physeal fracture of lower end of left femur** A, K, P 🔷, A 🔷
        (Ex:) For S79.112[A]: See PDX Collection 1302
              For S72.112[K,P]: See PDX Collection 897

   ● **S79.119**   **Salter-Harris Type I physeal fracture of lower end of unspecified femur** A, K, P 🔷, A 🔷
        (Ex:) For S79.119[A]: See PDX Collection 1301
              For S79.119[K,P]: See PDX Collection 897

● **S79.12**   **Salter-Harris Type II physeal fracture of lower end of femur**

   ● **S79.121**   **Salter-Harris Type II physeal fracture of lower end of right femur** A, K, P 🔷, A 🔷
        (Ex:) For S79.121[A]: See PDX Collection 1300
              For S79.121[K,P]: See PDX Collection 897

   ● **S79.122**   **Salter-Harris Type II physeal fracture of lower end of left femur** A, K, P 🔷, A 🔷
        (Ex:) For S79.122[A]: See PDX Collection 1302
              For S72.122[K,P]: See PDX Collection 897

   ● **S79.129**   **Salter-Harris Type II physeal fracture of lower end of unspecified femur** A, K, P 🔷, A 🔷
        (Ex:) For S79.129[A]: See PDX Collection 1301
              For S79.129[K,P]: See PDX Collection 897

Item 19–5   SALTER-HARRIS TYPE 1: epiphysis is completely separated from end of bone, or metaphysic growth plate remains attached to epiphysis

SALTER-HARRIS TYPE 2: epiphysis and growth plate are partially separated from metaphysis, which is cracked—most common type

SALTER-HARRIS TYPE 3: fracture occurring through epiphysis and separates part of epiphysis and growth plate from metaphysis fracture, usually at distal end of tibia

SALTER-HARRIS TYPE 4: fracture runs through epiphysis, across growth plate, into metaphysic, surgery is required to restore joint surface to normal and align growth plate

▶ New   ➡ Revised   ~~deleted~~ Deleted   Excludes 1   Excludes 2   Includes   Use additional   Code first   Code also   Key words

OGCR Official Guidelines   ● Unacceptable Principal Diagnosis   X Assign placeholder X   ● Use Additional Character(s)   ▶ Manifestation Code   **Coding Clinic**

● **S79.13**   **Salter-Harris Type III physeal fracture of lower end of femur**

  ● **S79.131**   Salter-Harris Type III physeal fracture of lower end of **right** femur A, K, P 🔖, A 🔖
     (Ex) **For S79.131[A]:** See PDX Collection 1300
     For S79.131[K,P]: See PDX Collection 897

  ● **S79.132**   Salter-Harris Type III physeal fracture of lower end of **left** femur A, K, P 🔖, A 🔖
     (Ex) **For S79.132[A]:** See PDX Collection 1302
     For S72.132[K,P]: See PDX Collection 897

  ● **S79.139**   Salter-Harris Type III physeal fracture of lower end of **unspecified** femur A, K, P 🔖, A 🔖
     (Ex) **For S79.139[A]:** See PDX Collection 1301
     For S79.139[K,P]: See PDX Collection 897

● **S79.14**   **Salter-Harris Type IV physeal fracture of lower end of femur**

  ● **S79.141**   Salter-Harris Type IV physeal fracture of lower end of **right** femur A, K, P 🔖, A 🔖
     (Ex) **For S79.141[A]:** See PDX Collection 1300
     For S79.141[K,P]: See PDX Collection 897

  ● **S79.142**   Salter-Harris Type IV physeal fracture of lower end of **left** femur A, K, P 🔖, A 🔖
     (Ex) **For S79.142[A]:** See PDX Collection 1302
     For S72.142[K,P]: See PDX Collection 897

  ● **S79.149**   Salter-Harris Type IV physeal fracture of lower end of **unspecified** femur A, K, P 🔖, A 🔖
     (Ex) **For S79.149[A]:** See PDX Collection 1301
     For S79.149[K,P]: See PDX Collection 897

● **S79.19**   **Other physeal fracture of lower end of femur**

  ● **S79.191**   Other physeal fracture of lower end of **right** femur A, K, P 🔖, A 🔖
     (Ex) **For S79.191[A]:** See PDX Collection 1300
     For S79.191[K,P]: See PDX Collection 897

  ● **S79.192**   Other physeal fracture of lower end of **left** femur A, K, P 🔖, A 🔖
     (Ex) **For S79.192[A]:** See PDX Collection 1302
     For S72.192[K,P]: See PDX Collection 897

  ● **S79.199**   Other physeal fracture of lower end of **unspecified** femur A, K, P 🔖, A 🔖
     (Ex) **For S79.199[A]:** See PDX Collection 1301
     For S79.199[K,P]: See PDX Collection 897

● **S79.8**   **Other specified injuries of hip and thigh**

The appropriate 7th character is to be added to each code in subcategory S79.8

A	initial encounter
D	subsequent encounter
S	sequela

 ● **S79.81**   **Other specified injuries of hip**

  ● **S79.811**   Other specified injuries of **right** hip
  ● **S79.812**   Other specified injuries of **left** hip
  ● **S79.819**   Other specified injuries of **unspecified** hip

 ● **S79.82**   **Other specified injuries of thigh**

  ● **S79.821**   Other specified injuries of **right** thigh
  ● **S79.822**   Other specified injuries of **left** thigh
  ● **S79.829**   Other specified injuries of **unspecified** thigh

● **S79.9**   **Unspecified injury of hip and thigh**

The appropriate 7th character is to be added to each code in subcategory S79.9

A	initial encounter
D	subsequent encounter
S	sequela

 ● **S79.91**   **Unspecified injury of hip**

  ● **S79.911**   Unspecified injury of **right** hip
  ● **S79.912**   Unspecified injury of **left** hip
  ● **S79.919**   Unspecified injury of **unspecified** hip

 ● **S79.92**   **Unspecified injury of thigh**

  ● **S79.921**   Unspecified injury of **right** thigh
  ● **S79.922**   Unspecified injury of **left** thigh
  ● **S79.929**   Unspecified injury of **unspecified** thigh

---

INJURIES TO THE KNEE AND LOWER LEG (S80-S89)

Excludes2   burns and corrosions (T20-T32)
     frostbite (T33-T34)
     injuries of ankle and foot, except fracture of ankle and malleolus (S90-S99)
     insect bite or sting, venomous (T63.4)

● **S80**   **Superficial injury of knee and lower leg**

Excludes2   superficial injury of ankle and foot (S90.-)

The appropriate 7th character is to be added to each code from category S80

A	initial encounter
D	subsequent encounter
S	sequela

● **S80.0**   **Contusion of knee**

  ✕ ● **S80.00**   Contusion of **unspecified** knee
  ✕ ● **S80.01**   Contusion of **right** knee
  ✕ ● **S80.02**   Contusion of **left** knee

● **S80.1**   **Contusion of lower leg**

  ✕ ● **S80.10**   Contusion of **unspecified** lower leg
  ✕ ● **S80.11**   Contusion of **right** lower leg
  ✕ ● **S80.12**   Contusion of **left** lower leg

● **S80.2**   **Other superficial injuries of knee**

 ● **S80.21**   **Abrasion of knee**
  ● **S80.211**   Abrasion, **right** knee
  ● **S80.212**   Abrasion, **left** knee
  ● **S80.219**   Abrasion, **unspecified** knee

 ● **S80.22**   **Blister (nonthermal) of knee**
  ● **S80.221**   Blister (nonthermal), **right** knee
  ● **S80.222**   Blister (nonthermal), **left** knee
  ● **S80.229**   Blister (nonthermal), **unspecified** knee

 ● **S80.24**   **External constriction of knee**
  ● **S80.241**   External constriction, **right** knee
  ● **S80.242**   External constriction, **left** knee
  ● **S80.249**   External constriction, **unspecified** knee

 ● **S80.25**   **Superficial foreign body of knee**
     Splinter in the knee
  ● **S80.251**   Superficial foreign body, **right** knee
  ● **S80.252**   Superficial foreign body, **left** knee
  ● **S80.259**   Superficial foreign body, **unspecified** knee

N Newborn Age: 0   **P** Pediatric Age: 0–17   **M** Maternity DX: 12–55   **A** Adult Age: 15–124   ♀ Females Only   ♂ Males Only

🔖 Complication\Comorbidity   🔖 Major C\C   (Ex) CC/MCC Exclusions   🔖 Hospital-Acquired Condition

1367

● **S80.26   Insect bite (nonvenomous) of knee**
   ● S80.261   Insect bite (nonvenomous), **right** knee
   ● S80.262   Insect bite (nonvenomous), **left** knee
   ● S80.269   Insect bite (nonvenomous), **unspecified** knee
● **S80.27   Other superficial bite of knee**
     Excludes1   open bite of knee (S81.05-)
   ● S80.271   Other superficial bite of **right** knee
   ● S80.272   Other superficial bite of **left** knee
   ● S80.279   Other superficial bite of **unspecified** knee

● **S80.8   Other superficial injuries of lower leg**
 ● **S80.81   Abrasion of lower leg**
   ● S80.811   Abrasion, **right** lower leg
   ● S80.812   Abrasion, **left** lower leg
   ● S80.819   Abrasion, **unspecified** lower leg
 ● **S80.82   Blister (nonthermal) of lower leg**
   ● S80.821   Blister (nonthermal), **right** lower leg
   ● S80.822   Blister (nonthermal), **left** lower leg
   ● S80.829   Blister (nonthermal), **unspecified** lower leg
 ● **S80.84   External constriction of lower leg**
   ● S80.841   External constriction, **right** lower leg
   ● S80.842   External constriction, **left** lower leg
   ● S80.849   External constriction, **unspecified** lower leg
 ● **S80.85   Superficial foreign body of lower leg**
     Splinter in the lower leg
   ● S80.851   Superficial foreign body, **right** lower leg
   ● S80.852   Superficial foreign body, **left** lower leg
   ● S80.859   Superficial foreign body, **unspecified** lower leg
 ● **S80.86   Insect bite (nonvenomous) of lower leg**
   ● S80.861   Insect bite (nonvenomous), **right** lower leg
   ● S80.862   Insect bite (nonvenomous), **left** lower leg
   ● S80.869   Insect bite (nonvenomous), **unspecified** lower leg
 ● **S80.87   Other superficial bite of lower leg**
     Excludes1   open bite of lower leg (S81.85-)
   ● S80.871   Other superficial bite, **right** lower leg
   ● S80.872   Other superficial bite, **left** lower leg
   ● S80.879   Other superficial bite, **unspecified** lower leg

● **S80.9   Unspecified superficial injury of knee and lower leg**
 ● **S80.91   Unspecified superficial injury of knee**
   ● S80.911   Unspecified superficial injury of **right** knee
   ● S80.912   Unspecified superficial injury of **left** knee
   ● S80.919   Unspecified superficial injury of **unspecified** knee

 ● **S80.92   Unspecified superficial injury of lower leg**
   ● S80.921   Unspecified superficial injury of **right** lower leg
   ● S80.922   Unspecified superficial injury of **left** lower leg
   ● S80.929   Unspecified superficial injury of **unspecified** lower leg

● **S81   Open wound of knee and lower leg**
   Code also any associated wound infection
   Excludes1   open fracture of knee and lower leg (S82.-)
            traumatic amputation of lower leg (S88.-)
   Excludes2   open wound of ankle and foot (S91.-)
   The appropriate 7th character is to be added to each code from category S81

A	initial encounter
D	subsequent encounter
S	sequela

 ● **S81.0   Open wound of knee**
  ● **S81.00   Unspecified open wound of knee**
   ● S81.001   Unspecified open wound, **right** knee
   ● S81.002   Unspecified open wound, **left** knee
   ● S81.009   Unspecified open wound, **unspecified** knee
  ● **S81.01   Laceration without foreign body of knee**
   ● S81.011   Laceration without foreign body, **right** knee
   ● S81.012   Laceration without foreign body, **left** knee
   ● S81.019   Laceration without foreign body, **unspecified** knee
  ● **S81.02   Laceration with foreign body of knee**
   ● S81.021   Laceration with foreign body, **right** knee
   ● S81.022   Laceration with foreign body, **left** knee
   ● S81.029   Laceration with foreign body, **unspecified** knee
  ● **S81.03   Puncture wound without foreign body of knee**
   ● S81.031   Puncture wound without foreign body, **right** knee
   ● S81.032   Puncture wound without foreign body, **left** knee
   ● S81.039   Puncture wound without foreign body, **unspecified** knee
  ● **S81.04   Puncture wound with foreign body of knee**
   ● S81.041   Puncture wound with foreign body, **right** knee
   ● S81.042   Puncture wound with foreign body, **left** knee
   ● S81.049   Puncture wound with foreign body, **unspecified** knee

● **S81.05**   **Open bite of knee**
    Bite of knee NOS

    Excludes1 superficial bite of knee (S80.27-)

  ● **S81.051**   **Open bite, right knee**

  ● **S81.052**   **Open bite, left knee**

  ● **S81.059**   **Open bite, unspecified knee**

● **S81.8**   **Open wound of lower leg**

  ● **S81.80**   **Unspecified open wound of lower leg**

    ● **S81.801**   **Unspecified open wound, right lower leg**

    ● **S81.802**   **Unspecified open wound, left lower leg**

    ● **S81.809**   **Unspecified open wound, unspecified lower leg**

  ● **S81.81**   **Laceration without foreign body of lower leg**

    ● **S81.811**   **Laceration without foreign body, right lower leg**

    ● **S81.812**   **Laceration without foreign body, left lower leg**

    ● **S81.819**   **Laceration without foreign body, unspecified lower leg**

  ● **S81.82**   **Laceration with foreign body of lower leg**

    ● **S81.821**   **Laceration with foreign body, right lower leg**

    ● **S81.822**   **Laceration with foreign body, left lower leg**

    ● **S81.829**   **Laceration with foreign body, unspecified lower leg**

  ● **S81.83**   **Puncture wound without foreign body of lower leg**

    ● **S81.831**   **Puncture wound without foreign body, right lower leg**

    ● **S81.832**   **Puncture wound without foreign body, left lower leg**

    ● **S81.839**   **Puncture wound without foreign body, unspecified lower leg**

  ● **S81.84**   **Puncture wound with foreign body of lower leg**

    ● **S81.841**   **Puncture wound with foreign body, right lower leg**
          Coding Clinic: 2016, Q3, P46

    ● **S81.842**   **Puncture wound with foreign body, left lower leg**

    ● **S81.849**   **Puncture wound with foreign body, unspecified lower leg**

  ● **S81.85**   **Open bite of lower leg**
    Bite of lower leg NOS

    Excludes1 superficial bite of lower leg (S80.86-, S80.87-)

    ● **S81.851**   **Open bite, right lower leg**

    ● **S81.852**   **Open bite, left lower leg**

    ● **S81.859**   **Open bite, unspecified lower leg**

● **S82**   **Fracture of lower leg, including ankle**

  Note: A fracture not indicated as displaced or nondisplaced should be coded to displaced

  A fracture not indicated as open or closed should be coded to closed

  The open fracture designations are based on the Gustilo open fracture classification

  Includes   fracture of malleolus

  Excludes1 traumatic amputation of lower leg (S88.-)

  Excludes2 fracture of foot, except ankle (S92.-)
    ➡ periprosthetic fracture of prosthetic implant of knee (M97.0-)

The appropriate 7th character is to be added to all codes from category S82

A	initial encounter for closed fracture
B	initial encounter for open fracture type I or II initial encounter for open fracture NOS
C	initial encounter for open fracture type IIIA, IIIB, or IIIC
D	subsequent encounter for closed fracture with routine healing
E	subsequent encounter for open fracture type I or II with routine healing
F	subsequent encounter for open fracture type IIIA, IIIB, or IIIC with routine healing
G	subsequent encounter for closed fracture with delayed healing
H	subsequent encounter for open fracture type I or II with delayed healing
J	subsequent encounter for open fracture type IIIA, IIIB, or IIIC with delayed healing
K	subsequent encounter for closed fracture with nonunion
M	subsequent encounter for open fracture type I or II with nonunion
N	subsequent encounter for open fracture type IIIA, IIIB, or IIIC with nonunion
P	subsequent encounter for closed fracture with malunion
Q	subsequent encounter for open fracture type I or II with malunion
R	subsequent encounter for open fracture type IIIA, IIIB, or IIIC with malunion
S	sequela

● **S82.0**   **Fracture of patella**
    Knee cap

  ● **S82.00**   **Unspecified fracture of patella**

    ● **S82.001**   **Unspecified fracture of right patella**
        A, B, C,K,M, N, P, Q, R 🔖, A, B, C 🔖
        (Ex) For S82.001[A]: See PDX Collection 1336
        For S82.001[B,C]: See PDX Collection 1337
        For S82.001[K,M,N,P,Q,R]: See PDX Collection 897

    ● **S82.002**   **Unspecified fracture of left patella**
        A, B, C,K,M, N, P, Q, R 🔖, A, B, C 🔖
        (Ex) For S82.002[A]: See PDX Collection 1338
        For S82.002[B,C]: See PDX Collection 1337
        For S82.002[K,M,N,P,Q,R]: See PDX Collection 897

    ● **S82.009**   **Unspecified fracture of unspecified patella** A, B, C,K,M, N, P, Q, R 🔖, A, B, C 🔖
        (Ex) For S82.009[A]: See PDX Collection 1339
        For S82.009[B,C]: See PDX Collection 1337
        For S82.009[K,M,N,P,Q,R]: See PDX Collection 897

● **S82.Ø1**   Osteochondral fracture of patella

  ● **S82.Ø11**   **Displaced osteochondral fracture of right patella** A, B, C,K,M, N, P, Q, R 🔒, A, B, C 🔒
    Ex: **For S82.Ø11[A]:** See PDX Collection 1336
      For S82.Ø11[B,C]: See PDX Collection 1337
      For S82.Ø11[K,M,N,P,Q,R]: See PDX Collection 897

  ● **S82.Ø12**   **Displaced osteochondral fracture of left patella** A, B, C,K,M, N, P, Q, R 🔒, A, B, C 🔒
    Ex: **For S82.Ø12[A]:** See PDX Collection 1338
      For S82.Ø12[B,C]: See PDX Collection 1337
      For S82.Ø12[K,M,N,P,Q,R]: See PDX Collection 897

  ● **S82.Ø13**   **Displaced osteochondral fracture of unspecified patella** A, B, C,K,M, N, P, Q, R 🔒, A, B, C 🔒
    Ex: **For S82.Ø13[A]:** See PDX Collection 1339
      For S82.Ø13[B,C]: See PDX Collection 1337
      For S82.Ø13[K,M,N,P,Q,R]: See PDX Collection 897

  ● **S82.Ø14**   **Nondisplaced osteochondral fracture of right patella** A, B, C,K,M, N, P, Q, R 🔒, A, B, C 🔒
    Ex: **For S82.Ø14[A]:** See PDX Collection 1336
      For S82.Ø14[B,C]: See PDX Collection 1337
      For S82.Ø14[K,M,N,P,Q,R]: See PDX Collection 897

  ● **S82.Ø15**   **Nondisplaced osteochondral fracture of left patella** A, B, C,K,M, N, P, Q, R 🔒, A, B, C 🔒
    Ex: **For S82.Ø15[A]:** See PDX Collection 1338
      For S82.Ø15[B,C]: See PDX Collection 1337
      For S82.Ø15[K,M,N,P,Q,R]: See PDX Collection 897

  ● **S82.Ø16**   **Nondisplaced osteochondral fracture of unspecified patella** A, B, C,K,M, N, P, Q, R 🔒, A, B, C 🔒
    Ex: **For S82.Ø16[A]:** See PDX Collection 1339
      For S82.Ø16[B,C]: See PDX Collection 1337
      For S82.Ø16[K,M,N,P,Q,R]: See PDX Collection 897

● **S82.Ø2**   Longitudinal fracture of patella

  ● **S82.Ø21**   **Displaced longitudinal fracture of right patella** A, B, C,K,M, N, P, Q, R 🔒, A, B, C 🔒
    Ex: **For S82.Ø21[A]:** See PDX Collection 1336
      For S82.Ø21[B,C]: See PDX Collection 1337
      For S82.Ø21[K,M,N,P,Q,R]: See PDX Collection 897

  ● **S82.Ø22**   **Displaced longitudinal fracture of left patella** A, B, C,K,M, N, P, Q, R 🔒, A, B, C 🔒
    Ex: **For S82.Ø22[A]:** See PDX Collection 1338
      For S82.Ø22[B,C]: See PDX Collection 1337
      For S82.Ø22[K,M,N,P,Q,R]: See PDX Collection 897

  ● **S82.Ø23**   **Displaced longitudinal fracture of unspecified patella** A, B, C,K,M, N, P, Q, R 🔒, A, B, C 🔒
    Ex: **For S82.Ø23[A]:** See PDX Collection 1339
      For S82.Ø23[B,C]: See PDX Collection 1337
      For S82.Ø23[K,M,N,P,Q,R]: See PDX Collection 897

  ● **S82.Ø24**   **Nondisplaced longitudinal fracture of right patella** A, B, C,K,M, N, P, Q, R 🔒, A, B, C 🔒
    Ex: **For S82.Ø24[A]:** See PDX Collection 1336
      For S82.Ø24[B,C]: See PDX Collection 1337
      For S82.Ø24[K,M,N,P,Q,R]: See PDX Collection 897

  ● **S82.Ø25**   **Nondisplaced longitudinal fracture of left patella** A, B, C,K,M, N, P, Q, R 🔒, A, B, C 🔒
    Ex: **For S82.Ø25[A]:** See PDX Collection 1338
      For S82.Ø25[B,C]: See PDX Collection 1337
      For S82.Ø25[K,M,N,P,Q,R]: See PDX Collection 897

  ● **S82.Ø26**   **Nondisplaced longitudinal fracture of unspecified patella** A, B, C,K,M, N, P, Q, R 🔒, A, B, C 🔒
    Ex: **For S82.Ø26[A]:** See PDX Collection 1339
      For S82.Ø26[B,C]: See PDX Collection 1337
      For S82.Ø26[K,M,N,P,Q,R]: See PDX Collection 897

● **S82.Ø3**   Transverse fracture of patella

  ● **S82.Ø31**   **Displaced transverse fracture of right patella** A, B, C,K,M, N, P, Q, R 🔒, A, B, C 🔒
    Ex: **For S82.Ø31[A]:** See PDX Collection 1336
      For S82.Ø31[B,C]: See PDX Collection 1337
      For S82.Ø31[K,M,N,P,Q,R]: See PDX Collection 897

  ● **S82.Ø32**   **Displaced transverse fracture of left patella** A, B, C,K,M, N, P, Q, R 🔒, A, B, C 🔒
    Ex: **For S82.Ø32[A]:** See PDX Collection 1338
      For S82.Ø32[B,C]: See PDX Collection 1337
      For S82.Ø32[K,M,N,P,Q,R]: See PDX Collection 897

  ● **S82.Ø33**   **Displaced transverse fracture of unspecified patella** A, B, C,K,M, N, P, Q, R 🔒, A, B, C 🔒
    Ex: **For S82.Ø33[A]:** See PDX Collection 1339
      For S82.Ø33[B,C]: See PDX Collection 1337
      For S82.Ø33[K,M,N,P,Q,R]: See PDX Collection 897

  ● **S82.Ø34**   **Nondisplaced transverse fracture of right patella** A, B, C,K,M, N, P, Q, R 🔒, A, B, C 🔒
    Ex: **For S82.Ø34[A]:** See PDX Collection 1336
      For S82.Ø34[B,C]: See PDX Collection 1337
      For S82.Ø34[K,M,N,P,Q,R]: See PDX Collection 897

  ● **S82.Ø35**   **Nondisplaced transverse fracture of left patella** A, B, C,K,M, N, P, Q, R 🔒, A, B, C 🔒
    Ex: **For S82.Ø35[A]:** See PDX Collection 1338
      For S82.Ø35[B,C]: See PDX Collection 1337
      For S82.Ø35[K,M,N,P,Q,R]: See PDX Collection 897

  ● **S82.Ø36**   **Nondisplaced transverse fracture of unspecified patella** A, B, C,K,M, N, P, Q, R 🔒, A, B, C 🔒
    Ex: **For S82.Ø36[A]:** See PDX Collection 1339
      For S82.Ø36[B,C]: See PDX Collection 1337
      For S82.Ø36[K,M,N,P,Q,R]: See PDX Collection 897

▶ New   ⇒ Revised   ~~deleted~~ Deleted   Excludes 1   Excludes 2   Includes   Use additional   Code first   Code also   Key words
OGCR Official Guidelines   ● Unacceptable Principal Diagnosis   X Assign placeholder X   ● Use Additional Character(s)   ▶ Manifestation Code   **Coding Clinic**

● **S82.04**   Comminuted fracture of patella

  ● **S82.041**   Displaced comminuted fracture of right patella A, B, C,K,M, N, P, Q, R 🦠, A, B, C 🦠
      Ⓔⓧ **For S82.041[A]:** See PDX Collection 1336
        For S82.041[B,C]: See PDX Collection 1337
        For S82.041[K,M,N,P,Q,R]: See PDX Collection 897

  ● **S82.042**   Displaced comminuted fracture of left patella A, B, C,K,M, N, P, Q, R 🦠, A, B, C 🦠
      Ⓔⓧ **For S82.042[A]:** See PDX Collection 1338
        For S82.042[B,C]: See PDX Collection 1337
        For S82.042[K,M,N,P,Q,R]: See PDX Collection 897

  ● **S82.043**   Displaced comminuted fracture of unspecified patella A, B, C,K,M, N, P, Q, R 🦠, A, B, C 🦠
      Ⓔⓧ **For S82.043[A]:** See PDX Collection 1339
        For S82.043[B,C]: See PDX Collection 1337
        For S82.043[K,M,N,P,Q,R]: See PDX Collection 897

  ● **S82.044**   Nondisplaced comminuted fracture of right patella A, B, C,K,M, N, P, Q, R 🦠, A, B, C 🦠
      Ⓔⓧ **For S82.044[A]:** See PDX Collection 1336
        For S82.044[B,C]: See PDX Collection 1337
        For S82.044[K,M,N,P,Q,R]: See PDX Collection 897

  ● **S82.045**   Nondisplaced comminuted fracture of left patella A, B, C,K,M, N, P, Q, R 🦠, A, B, C 🦠
      Ⓔⓧ **For S82.045[A]:** See PDX Collection 1338
        For S82.045[B,C]: See PDX Collection 1337
        For S82.045[K,M,N,P,Q,R]: See PDX Collection 897

  ● **S82.046**   Nondisplaced comminuted fracture of unspecified patella A, B, C,K,M, N, P, Q, R 🦠, A, B, C 🦠
      Ⓔⓧ **For S82.046[A]:** See PDX Collection 1339
        For S82.046[B,C]: See PDX Collection 1337
        For S82.046[K,M,N,P,Q,R]: See PDX Collection 897

● **S82.09**   Other fracture of patella

  ● **S82.091**   Other fracture of right patella A, B, C,K,M, N, P, Q, R 🦠, A, B, C 🦠
      Ⓔⓧ **For S82.091[A]:** See PDX Collection 1336
        For S82.091[B,C]: See PDX Collection 1337
        For S82.091[K,M,N,P,Q,R]: See PDX Collection 897

  ● **S82.092**   Other fracture of left patella A, B, C,K,M, N, P, Q, R 🦠, A, B, C 🦠
      Ⓔⓧ **For S82.092[A]:** See PDX Collection 1338
        For S82.092[B,C]: See PDX Collection 1337
        For S82.092[K,M,N,P,Q,R]: See PDX Collection 897

  ● **S82.099**   Other fracture of unspecified patella A, B, C,K,M, N, P, Q, R 🦠, A, B, C 🦠
      Ⓔⓧ **For S82.099[A]:** See PDX Collection 1339
        For S82.099[B,C]: See PDX Collection 1337
        For S82.099[K,M,N,P,Q,R]: See PDX Collection 897

● **S82.1**   Fracture of upper end of tibia
    Fracture of proximal end of tibia
    Excludes2   fracture of shaft of tibia (S82.2-)
             physeal fracture of upper end of tibia (S89.0-)

● **S82.10**   Unspecified fracture of upper end of tibia

  ● **S82.101**   Unspecified fracture of upper end of right tibia A, K, M, N, P, Q, R 🦠, B, C 🦠, A, B, C 🦠
      Ⓔⓧ **For S82.101[A]:** See PDX Collection 1340
        For S82.101[B,C]: See PDX Collection 1341
        For S82.101[K,M,N,P,Q,R]: See PDX Collection 897

  ● **S82.102**   Unspecified fracture of upper end of left tibia A, K, M, N, P, Q, R 🦠, B, C 🦠, A, B, C 🦠
      Ⓔⓧ **For S82.102[A]:** See PDX Collection 1342
        For S82.102[B,C]: See PDX Collection 1341
        For S82.102[K,M,N,P,Q,R]: See PDX Collection 897

  ● **S82.109**   Unspecified fracture of upper end of unspecified tibia A, K, M, N, P, Q, R 🦠, B, C 🦠, A, B, C 🦠
      Ⓔⓧ **For S82.109[A,B,C]:** See PDX Collection 1341
        For S82.109[K,M,N,P,Q,R]: See PDX Collection 897

● **S82.11**   Fracture of tibial spine

  ● **S82.111**   Displaced fracture of right tibial spine A, K, M, N, P, Q, R 🦠, B, C 🦠, A, B, C 🦠
      Ⓔⓧ **For S82.111[A]:** See PDX Collection 1340
        For S82.111[B,C]: See PDX Collection 1341
        For S82.111[K,M,N,P,Q,R]: See PDX Collection 897

  ● **S82.112**   Displaced fracture of left tibial spine A, K, M, N, P, Q, R 🦠, B, C 🦠, A, B, C 🦠
      Ⓔⓧ **For S82.112[A]:** See PDX Collection 1342
        For S82.112[B,C]: See PDX Collection 1341
        For S82.112[K,M,N,P,Q,R]: See PDX Collection 897

  ● **S82.113**   Displaced fracture of unspecified tibial spine A, K, M, N, P, Q, R 🦠, B, C 🦠, A, B, C 🦠
      Ⓔⓧ **For S82.113 [A,B,C]:** See PDX Collection 1341
        For S82.113[K,M,N,P,Q,R]: See PDX Collection 897

  ● **S82.114**   Nondisplaced fracture of right tibial spine A, K, M, N, P, Q, R 🦠, B, C 🦠, A, B, C 🦠
      Ⓔⓧ **For S82.114[A]:** See PDX Collection 1340
        For S82.114[B,C]: See PDX Collection 1341
        For S82.114[K,M,N,P,Q,R]: See PDX Collection 897

  ● **S82.115**   Nondisplaced fracture of left tibial spine A, K, M, N, P, Q, R 🦠, B, C 🦠, A, B, C 🦠
      Ⓔⓧ **For S82.115[A]:** See PDX Collection 1342
        For S82.115[B,C]: See PDX Collection 1341
        For S82.115[K,M,N,P,Q,R]: See PDX Collection 897

  ● **S82.116**   Nondisplaced fracture of unspecified tibial spine A, K, M, N, P, Q, R 🦠, B, C 🦠, A, B, C 🦠
      Ⓔⓧ **For S82.116[A,B,C]:** See PDX Collection 1341
        For S82.116[K,M,N,P,Q,R]: See PDX Collection 897

CHAPTER 19 (S00-T88)

N Newborn Age: 0   **P** Pediatric Age: 0–17   **M** Maternity DX: 12–55   **A** Adult Age: 15–124   ♀ Females Only   ♂ Males Only

🦠 Complication\Comorbidity   🦠 Major C\C   Ⓔⓧ CC/MCC Exclusions   🦠 Hospital-Acquired Condition

1371

CHAPTER 19 (S00-T88)

● **S82.12　Fracture of lateral condyle of tibia**

  ● **S82.121　Displaced fracture of lateral condyle of right tibia** A, K, M, N, P, Q, R 🔒, B, C 🔒, A, B, C 🔒
    (Ex:) For S82.121[A]: See PDX Collection 1340
    For S82.121[B,C]: See PDX Collection 1341
    For S82.121[K,M,N,P,Q,R]: See PDX Collection 897

  ● **S82.122　Displaced fracture of lateral condyle of left tibia** A, K, M, N, P, Q, R 🔒, B, C 🔒, A, B, C 🔒
    (Ex:) For S82.122[A]: See PDX Collection 1342
    For S82.122[B,C]: See PDX Collection 1341
    For S82.122[K,M,N,P,Q,R]: See PDX Collection 897

  ● **S82.123　Displaced fracture of lateral condyle of unspecified tibia** A, K, M, N, P, Q, R 🔒, B, C 🔒, A, B, C 🔒
    (Ex:) For S82.123[A,B,C]: See PDX Collection 1341
    For S82.123[K,M,N,P,Q,R]: See PDX Collection 897

  ● **S82.124　Nondisplaced fracture of lateral condyle of right tibia** A, K, M, N, P, Q, R 🔒, B, C 🔒, A, B, C 🔒
    (Ex:) For S82.124[A]: See PDX Collection 1340
    For S82.124[B,C]: See PDX Collection 1341
    For S82.124[K,M,N,P,Q,R]: See PDX Collection 897

  ● **S82.125　Nondisplaced fracture of lateral condyle of left tibia** A, K, M, N, P, Q, R 🔒, B, C 🔒, A, B, C 🔒
    (Ex:) For S82.125[A]: See PDX Collection 1342
    For S82.125[B,C]: See PDX Collection 1341
    For S82.125[K,M,N,P,Q,R]: See PDX Collection 897

  ● **S82.126　Nondisplaced fracture of lateral condyle of unspecified tibia** A, K, M, N, P, Q, R 🔒, B, C 🔒, A, B, C 🔒
    (Ex:) For S82.126[A,B,C]: See PDX Collection 1341
    For S82.126[K,M,N,P,Q,R]: See PDX Collection 897

● **S82.13　Fracture of medial condyle of tibia**

  ● **S82.131　Displaced fracture of medial condyle of right tibia** A, K, M, N, P, Q, R 🔒, B, C 🔒, A, B, C 🔒
    (Ex:) For S82.131[A]: See PDX Collection 1340
    For S82.131[B,C]: See PDX Collection 1341
    For S82.131[K,M,N,P,Q,R]: See PDX Collection 897

  ● **S82.132　Displaced fracture of medial condyle of left tibia** A, K, M, N, P, Q, R 🔒, B, C 🔒, A, B, C 🔒
    (Ex:) For S82.132[A]: See PDX Collection 1342
    For S82.132[B,C]: See PDX Collection 1341
    For S82.132[K,M,N,P,Q,R]: See PDX Collection 897

  ● **S82.133　Displaced fracture of medial condyle of unspecified tibia** A, K, M, N, P, Q, R 🔒, B, C 🔒, A, B, C 🔒
    (Ex:) For S82.133[A,B,C]: See PDX Collection 1341
    For S82.133[K,M,N,P,Q,R]: See PDX Collection 897

  ● **S82.134　Nondisplaced fracture of medial condyle of right tibia** A, K, M, N, P, Q, R 🔒, B, C 🔒, A, B, C 🔒
    (Ex:) For S82.134[A]: See PDX Collection 1340
    For S82.134[B,C]: See PDX Collection 1341
    For S82.134[K,M,N,P,Q,R]: See PDX Collection 897

  ● **S82.135　Nondisplaced fracture of medial condyle of left tibia** A, K, M, N, P, Q, R 🔒, B, C 🔒, A, B, C 🔒
    (Ex:) For S82.135[A]: See PDX Collection 1342
    For S82.135[B,C]: See PDX Collection 1341
    For S82.135[K,M,N,P,Q,R]: See PDX Collection 897

  ● **S82.136　Nondisplaced fracture of medial condyle of unspecified tibia** A, K, M, N, P, Q, R 🔒, B, C 🔒, A, B, C 🔒
    (Ex:) For S82.136[A,B,C]: See PDX Collection 1341
    For S82.136[K,M,N,P,Q,R]: See PDX Collection 897

● **S82.14　Bicondylar fracture of tibia**
  Fracture of tibial plateau NOS

  ● **S82.141　Displaced bicondylar fracture of right tibia** A, K, M, N, P, Q, R 🔒, B, C 🔒, A, B, C 🔒
    (Ex:) For S82.141[A]: See PDX Collection 1340
    For S82.141[B,C]: See PDX Collection 1341
    For S82.141[K,M,N,P,Q,R]: See PDX Collection 897

  ● **S82.142　Displaced bicondylar fracture of left tibia** A, K, M, N, P, Q, R 🔒, B, C 🔒, A, B, C 🔒
    (Ex:) For S82.142[A]: See PDX Collection 1342
    For S82.142[B,C]: See PDX Collection 1341
    For S82.142[K,M,N,P,Q,R]: See PDX Collection 897

  ● **S82.143　Displaced bicondylar fracture of unspecified tibia** A, K, M, N, P, Q, R 🔒, B, C 🔒, A, B, C 🔒
    (Ex:) For S82.143[A,B,C]: See PDX Collection 1341
    For S82.143[K,M,N,P,Q,R]: See PDX Collection 897

  ● **S82.144　Nondisplaced bicondylar fracture of right tibia** A, K, M, N, P, Q, R 🔒, B, C 🔒, A, B, C 🔒
    (Ex:) For S82.144[A]: See PDX Collection 1340
    For S82.144[B,C]: See PDX Collection 1341
    For S82.144[K,M,N,P,Q,R]: See PDX Collection 897

  ● **S82.145　Nondisplaced bicondylar fracture of left tibia** A, K, M, N, P, Q, R 🔒, B, C 🔒, A, B, C 🔒
    (Ex:) For S82.145[A]: See PDX Collection 1342
    For S82.145[B,C]: See PDX Collection 1341
    For S82.145[K,M,N,P,Q,R]: See PDX Collection 897

  ● **S82.146　Nondisplaced bicondylar fracture of unspecified tibia** A, K, M, N, P, Q, R 🔒, B, C 🔒, A, B, C 🔒
    (Ex:) For S82.146[A,B,C]: See PDX Collection 1341
    For S82.146[K,M,N,P,Q,R]: See PDX Collection 897

● **S82.15　Fracture of tibial tuberosity**

  ● **S82.151　Displaced fracture of right tibial tuberosity** A, K, M, N, P, Q, R 🔒, B, C 🔒, A, B, C 🔒
    (Ex:) For S82.151[A]: See PDX Collection 1340
    For S82.151[B,C]: See PDX Collection 1341
    For S82.151[K,M,N,P,Q,R]: See PDX Collection 897

  ● **S82.152　Displaced fracture of left tibial tuberosity** A, K, M, N, P, Q, R 🔒, B, C 🔒, A, B, C 🔒
    (Ex:) For S82.152[A]: See PDX Collection 1342
    For S82.152[B,C]: See PDX Collection 1341
    For S82.152[K,M,N,P,Q,R]: See PDX Collection 897

▶ New　➠ Revised　~~deleted~~ Deleted　Excludes 1　Excludes 2　Includes　Use additional　Code first　Code also　Key words
OGCR Official Guidelines　● Unacceptable Principal Diagnosis　X Assign placeholder X　● Use Additional Character(s)　▶ Manifestation Code　Coding Clinic

● **S82.153** **Displaced** fracture of **unspecified tibial tuberosity** A, K, M, N, P, Q, R 🔹, B, C 🔹, A, B, C 🔹
　　Ⓔ For S82.153[A,B,C]: See PDX Collection 1341
　　For S82.153[K,M,N,P,Q,R]: See PDX Collection 897

● **S82.154** **Nondisplaced** fracture of **right tibial tuberosity** A, K, M, N, P, Q, R 🔹, B, C 🔹, A, B, C 🔹
　　Ⓔ For S82.154[A]: See PDX Collection 1340
　　For S82.154[B,C]: See PDX Collection 1341
　　For S82.154[K,M,N,P,Q,R]: See PDX Collection 897

● **S82.155** **Nondisplaced** fracture of **left tibial tuberosity** A, K, M, N, P, Q, R 🔹, B, C 🔹, A, B, C 🔹
　　Ⓔ For S82.155[A]: See PDX Collection 1342
　　For S82.155[B,C]: See PDX Collection 1341
　　For S82.155[K,M,N,P,Q,R]: See PDX Collection 897

● **S82.156** **Nondisplaced** fracture of **unspecified tibial tuberosity** A, K, M, N, P, Q, R 🔹, B, C 🔹, A, B, C 🔹
　　Ⓔ For S82.156[A,B,C]: See PDX Collection 1341
　　For S82.156[K,M,N,P,Q,R]: See PDX Collection 897

● **S82.16** **Torus fracture of upper end of tibia**
　　The appropriate 7th character is to be added to all codes in subcategory S82.16

A	initial encounter for closed fracture
D	subsequent encounter for fracture with routine healing
G	subsequent encounter for fracture with delayed healing
K	subsequent encounter for fracture with nonunion
P	subsequent encounter for fracture with malunion
S	sequela

● **S82.161** **Torus fracture of upper end of right tibia** A, K, P 🔹, A 🔹
　　Ⓔ For S82.161[A]: See PDX Collection 1343
　　For S82.161[K,P]: See PDX Collection 897

● **S82.162** **Torus fracture of upper end of left tibia** A, K, P 🔹, A 🔹
　　Ⓔ For S82.162[A]: See PDX Collection 1344
　　For S82.162[K,P]: See PDX Collection 897

● **S82.169** **Torus fracture of upper end of unspecified tibia** A, K, P 🔹, A 🔹
　　Ⓔ For S82.169[A]: See PDX Collection 1345
　　For S82.169[K,P]: See PDX Collection 897

● **S82.19** **Other fracture of upper end of tibia**

● **S82.191** **Other fracture of upper end of right tibia** A, K, M, N, P, Q, R 🔹, B, C 🔹, A, B, C 🔹
　　Ⓔ For S82.191[A]: See PDX Collection 1340
　　For S82.191[B,C]: See PDX Collection 1341
　　For S82.191[K,M,N,P,Q,R]: See PDX Collection 897

● **S82.192** **Other fracture of upper end of left tibia** A, K, M, N, P, Q, R 🔹, B, C 🔹, A, B, C 🔹
　　Ⓔ For S82.192[A]: See PDX Collection 1342
　　For S82.192[B,C]: See PDX Collection 1341
　　For S82.192[K,M,N,P,Q,R]: See PDX Collection 897

● **S82.199** **Other fracture of upper end of unspecified tibia** A, K, M, N, P, Q, R 🔹, B, C 🔹, A, B, C 🔹
　　Ⓔ For S82.199[A,B,C]: See PDX Collection 1341
　　For S82.199[K,M,N,P,Q,R]: See PDX Collection 897

● **S82.2** **Fracture of shaft of tibia**

● **S82.20** **Unspecified fracture of shaft of tibia**
　　Fracture of tibia NOS

● **S82.201** **Unspecified fracture of shaft of right tibia** A, K, M, N, P, Q, R 🔹, B, C 🔹, A, B, C 🔹
　　Ⓔ For S82.201[A]: See PDX Collection 1346
　　For S82.201[B,C]: See PDX Collection 1341
　　For S82.201[K,M,N,P,Q,R]: See PDX Collection 897

● **S82.202** **Unspecified fracture of shaft of left tibia** A, K, M, N, P, Q, R 🔹, B, C 🔹, A, B, C 🔹
　　Ⓔ For S82.202[A]: See PDX Collection 1342
　　For S82.202[B,C]: See PDX Collection 1341
　　For S82.202[K,M,N,P,Q,R]: See PDX Collection 897

● **S82.209** **Unspecified fracture of shaft of unspecified tibia** A, K, M, N, P, Q, R 🔹, B, C 🔹, A, B, C 🔹
　　Ⓔ For S82.209[A,B,C]: See PDX Collection 1341
　　For S82.209[K,M,N,P,Q,R]: See PDX Collection 897

● **S82.22** **Transverse fracture of shaft of tibia**

● **S82.221** **Displaced transverse fracture of shaft of right tibia** A, K, M, N, P, Q, R 🔹, B, C 🔹, A, B, C 🔹
　　Ⓔ For S82.221[A]: See PDX Collection 1340
　　For S82.221[B,C]: See PDX Collection 1341
　　For S82.221[K,M,N,P,Q,R]: See PDX Collection 897

● **S82.222** **Displaced transverse fracture of shaft of left tibia** A, K, M, N, P, Q, R 🔹, B, C 🔹, A, B, C 🔹
　　Ⓔ For S82.222[A]: See PDX Collection 1342
　　For S82.222[B,C]: See PDX Collection 1341
　　For S82.222[K,M,N,P,Q,R]: See PDX Collection 897

● **S82.223** **Displaced transverse fracture of shaft of unspecified tibia** A, K, M, N, P, Q, R 🔹, B, C 🔹, A, B, C 🔹
　　Ⓔ For S82.223[A,B,C]: See PDX Collection 1341
　　For S82.223[K,M,N,P,Q,R]: See PDX Collection 897

● **S82.224** **Nondisplaced transverse fracture of shaft of right tibia** A, K, M, N, P, Q, R 🔹, B, C 🔹, A, B, C 🔹
　　Ⓔ For S82.224[A]: See PDX Collection 1340
　　For S82.224[B,C]: See PDX Collection 1341
　　For S82.224[K,M,N,P,Q,R]: See PDX Collection 897

● **S82.225** **Nondisplaced transverse fracture of shaft of left tibia** A, K, M, N, P, Q, R 🔹, B, C 🔹, A, B, C 🔹
　　Ⓔ For S82.225[A]: See PDX Collection 1342
　　For S82.225[B,C]: See PDX Collection 1341
　　For S82.225[K,M,N,P,Q,R]: See PDX Collection 897

● **S82.226** **Nondisplaced transverse fracture of shaft of unspecified tibia** A, K, M, N, P, Q, R 🔹, B, C 🔹, A, B, C 🔹
　　Ⓔ For S82.226[A,B,C]: See PDX Collection 1341
　　For S82.226[K,M,N,P,Q,R]: See PDX Collection 897

CHAPTER 19 (S00-T88)

- ● S82.23   **Oblique fracture of shaft of tibia**
  - ● S82.231   **Displaced oblique fracture of shaft of right tibia** A, K, M, N, P, Q, R 🔖, B, C 🔖, A, B, C 🔖
    - (Ex:) **For S82.231[A]:** See PDX Collection 1340
      For S82.231[B,C]: See PDX Collection 1341
      For S82.231[K,M,N,P,Q,R]: See PDX Collection 897
  - ● S82.232   **Displaced oblique fracture of shaft of left tibia** A, K, M, N, P, Q, R 🔖, B, C 🔖, A, B, C 🔖
    - (Ex:) **For S82.232[A]:** See PDX Collection 1342
      For S82.232[B,C]: See PDX Collection 1341
      For S82.232[K,M,N,P,Q,R]: See PDX Collection 897
  - ● S82.233   **Displaced oblique fracture of shaft of unspecified tibia** A, K, M, N, P, Q, R 🔖, B, C 🔖, A, B, C 🔖
    - (Ex:) **For S82.233[A,B,C]:** See PDX Collection 1341
      For S82.233[K,M,N,P,Q,R]: See PDX Collection 897
  - ● S82.234   **Nondisplaced oblique fracture of shaft of right tibia** A, K, M, N, P, Q, R 🔖, B, C 🔖, A, B, C 🔖
    - (Ex:) **For S82.234[A]:** See PDX Collection 1340
      For S82.234[B,C]: See PDX Collection 1341
      For S82.234[K,M,N,P,Q,R]: See PDX Collection 897
    - **Coding Clinic: 2015, Q1, P9-10**
  - ● S82.235   **Nondisplaced oblique fracture of shaft of left tibia** A, K, M, N, P, Q, R 🔖, B, C 🔖, A, B, C 🔖
    - (Ex:) **For S82.235[A]:** See PDX Collection 1342
      For S82.235[B,C]: See PDX Collection 1341
      For S82.235[K,M,N,P,Q,R]: See PDX Collection 897
  - ● S82.236   **Nondisplaced oblique fracture of shaft of unspecified tibia** A, K, M, N, P, Q, R 🔖, B, C 🔖, A, B, C 🔖
    - (Ex:) **For S82.236[A,B,C]:** See PDX Collection 1341
      For S82.236[K,M,N,P,Q,R]: See PDX Collection 897
- ● S82.24   **Spiral fracture of shaft of tibia**
  Toddler fracture
  - ● S82.241   **Displaced spiral fracture of shaft of right tibia** A, K, M, N, P, Q, R 🔖, B, C 🔖, A, B, C 🔖
    - (Ex:) **For S82.241[A]:** See PDX Collection 1340
      For S82.241[B,C]: See PDX Collection 1341
      For S82.241[K,M,N,P,Q,R]: See PDX Collection 897
  - ● S82.242   **Displaced spiral fracture of shaft of left tibia** A, K, M, N, P, Q, R 🔖, B, C 🔖, A, B, C 🔖
    - (Ex:) **For S82.242[A]:** See PDX Collection 1342
      For S82.242[B,C]: See PDX Collection 1341
      For S82.242[K,M,N,P,Q,R]: See PDX Collection 897
  - ● S82.243   **Displaced spiral fracture of shaft of unspecified tibia** A, K, M, N, P, Q, R 🔖, B, C 🔖, A, B, C 🔖
    - (Ex:) **For S82.243[A,B,C]:** See PDX Collection 1341
      For S82.243[K,M,N,P,Q,R]: See PDX Collection 897
  - ● S82.244   **Nondisplaced spiral fracture of shaft of right tibia** A, K, M, N, P, Q, R 🔖, B, C 🔖, A, B, C 🔖
    - (Ex:) **For S82.244[A]:** See PDX Collection 1340
      For S82.244[B,C]: See PDX Collection 1341
      For S82.244[K,M,N,P,Q,R]: See PDX Collection 897

- ● S82.245   **Nondisplaced spiral fracture of shaft of left tibia** A, K, M, N, P, Q, R 🔖, B, C 🔖, A, B, C 🔖
  - (Ex:) **For S82.245[A]:** See PDX Collection 1342
    For S82.245[B,C]: See PDX Collection 1341
    For S82.245[K,M,N,P,Q,R]: See PDX Collection 897
- ● S82.246   **Nondisplaced spiral fracture of shaft of unspecified tibia** A, K, M, N, P, Q, R 🔖, B, C 🔖, A, B, C 🔖
  - (Ex:) **For S82.246[A,B,C]:** See PDX Collection 1341
    For S82.246[K,M,N,P,Q,R]: See PDX Collection 897
- ● S82.25   **Comminuted fracture of shaft of tibia**
  - ● S82.251   **Displaced comminuted fracture of shaft of right tibia** A, K, M, N, P, Q, R 🔖, B, C 🔖, A, B, C 🔖
    - (Ex:) **For S82.251[A]:** See PDX Collection 1340
      For S82.251[B,C]: See PDX Collection 1341
      For S82.251[K,M,N,P,Q,R]: See PDX Collection 897
    - **Coding Clinic: 2015, Q2, P6**
  - ● S82.252   **Displaced comminuted fracture of shaft of left tibia** A, K, M, N, P, Q, R 🔖, B, C 🔖, A, B, C 🔖
    - (Ex:) **For S82.252[A]:** See PDX Collection 1342
      For S82.252[B,C]: See PDX Collection 1341
      For S82.252[K,M,N,P,Q,R]: See PDX Collection 897
  - ● S82.253   **Displaced comminuted fracture of shaft of unspecified tibia** A, K, M, N, P, Q, R 🔖, B, C 🔖, A, B, C 🔖
    - (Ex:) **For S82.253[A,B,C]:** See PDX Collection 1341
      For S82.253[K,M,N,P,Q,R]: See PDX Collection 897
  - ● S82.254   **Nondisplaced comminuted fracture of shaft of right tibia** A, K, M, N, P, Q, R 🔖, B, C 🔖, A, B, C 🔖
    - (Ex:) **For S82.254[A]:** See PDX Collection 1340
      For S82.254[B,C]: See PDX Collection 1341
      For S82.254[K,M,N,P,Q,R]: See PDX Collection 897
  - ● S82.255   **Nondisplaced comminuted fracture of shaft of left tibia** A, K, M, N, P, Q, R 🔖, B, C 🔖, A, B, C 🔖
    - (Ex:) **For S82.255[A]:** See PDX Collection 1342
      For S82.255[B,C]: See PDX Collection 1341
      For S82.255[K,M,N,P,Q,R]: See PDX Collection 897
  - ● S82.256   **Nondisplaced comminuted fracture of shaft of unspecified tibia** A, K, M, N, P, Q, R 🔖, B, C 🔖, A, B, C 🔖
    - (Ex:) **For S82.256[A,B,C]:** See PDX Collection 1341
      For S82.256[K,M,N,P,Q,R]: See PDX Collection 897
- ● S82.26   **Segmental fracture of shaft of tibia**
  - ● S82.261   **Displaced segmental fracture of shaft of right tibia** A, K, M, N, P, Q, R 🔖, B, C 🔖, A, B, C 🔖
    - (Ex:) **For S82.261[A]:** See PDX Collection 1340
      For S82.261[B,C]: See PDX Collection 1341
      For S82.261[K,M,N,P,Q,R]: See PDX Collection 897
  - ● S82.262   **Displaced segmental fracture of shaft of left tibia** A, K, M, N, P, Q, R 🔖, B, C 🔖, A, B, C 🔖
    - (Ex:) **For S82.262[A]:** See PDX Collection 1342
      For S82.262[B,C]: See PDX Collection 1341
      For S82.262[K,M,N,P,Q,R]: See PDX Collection 897

▶ New   ⇶ Revised   ~~deleted~~ Deleted   Excludes 1   Excludes 2   Includes   Use additional   Code first   Code also   Key words
OGCR Official Guidelines   ● Unacceptable Principal Diagnosis   X Assign placeholder X   ● Use Additional Character(s)   ▶ Manifestation Code   **Coding Clinic**

● S82.263 **Displaced segmental fracture of shaft of unspecified tibia** A, K, M, N, P, Q, R 🪙, B, C 🪙, A, B, C 🪙
   (Ex) **For S82.263[A,B,C]:** See PDX Collection 1341
   For S82.263[K,M,N,P,Q,R]: See PDX Collection 897

● S82.264 **Nondisplaced segmental fracture of shaft of right tibia** A, K, M, N, P, Q, R 🪙, B, C 🪙, A, B, C 🪙
   (Ex) **For S82.264[A]:** See PDX Collection 1340
   For S82.264[B,C]: See PDX Collection 1341
   For S82.264[K,M,N,P,Q,R]: See PDX Collection 897

● S82.265 **Nondisplaced segmental fracture of shaft of left tibia** A, K, M, N, P, Q, R 🪙, B, C 🪙, A, B, C 🪙
   (Ex) **For S82.265[A]:** See PDX Collection 1342
   For S82.265[B,C]: See PDX Collection 1341
   For S82.265[K,M,N,P,Q,R]: See PDX Collection 897

● S82.266 **Nondisplaced segmental fracture of shaft of unspecified tibia** A, K, M, N, P, Q, R 🪙, B, C 🪙, A, B, C 🪙
   (Ex) **For S82.266[A,B,C]:** See PDX Collection 1341
   For S82.266[K,M,N,P,Q,R]: See PDX Collection 897

● S82.29 **Other fracture of shaft of tibia**

● S82.291 **Other fracture of shaft of right tibia** A, K, M, N, P, Q, R 🪙, B, C 🪙, A, B, C 🪙
   (Ex) **For S82.291[A]:** See PDX Collection 1340
   For S82.291[B,C]: See PDX Collection 1341
   For S82.291[K,M,N,P,Q,R]: See PDX Collection 897

● S82.292 **Other fracture of shaft of left tibia** A, K, M, N, P, Q, R 🪙, B, C 🪙, A, B, C 🪙
   (Ex) **For S82.292[A]:** See PDX Collection 1342
   For S82.292[B,C]: See PDX Collection 1341
   For S82.292[K,M,N,P,Q,R]: See PDX Collection 897

● S82.299 **Other fracture of shaft of unspecified tibia** A, K, M, N, P, Q, R 🪙, B, C 🪙, A, B, C 🪙
   (Ex) **For S82.299[A,B,C]:** See PDX Collection 1341
   For S82.299[K,M,N,P,Q,R]: See PDX Collection 897

● S82.3 **Fracture of lower end of tibia**
   Excludes1 bimalleolar fracture of lower leg (S82.84-)
   fracture of medial malleolus alone (S82.5-)
   Maisonneuve's fracture (S82.86-)
   pilon fracture of distal tibia (S82.87-)
   trimalleolar fractures of lower leg (S82.85-)

● S82.30 **Unspecified fracture of lower end of tibia**
   (Ex) **For category S82.30 CC codes S82.30[B,C]:** See PDX Collection 1347 **For S82.30[K,M,N,P,Q,R]:** See PDX Collection 897

● S82.301 **Unspecified fracture of lower end of right tibia** B, C, K, M, N, P, Q, R 🪙, B, C 🪙

● S82.302 **Unspecified fracture of lower end of left tibia** B, C, K, M, N, P, Q, R 🪙, B, C 🪙

● S82.309 **Unspecified fracture of lower end of unspecified tibia** B, C, K, M, N, P, Q, R 🪙, B, C 🪙

● S82.31 **Torus fracture of lower end of tibia**
   The appropriate 7th character is to be added to all codes in subcategory S82.31

A	initial encounter for closed fracture
D	subsequent encounter for fracture with routine healing
G	subsequent encounter for fracture with delayed healing
K	subsequent encounter for fracture with nonunion
P	subsequent encounter for fracture with malunion
S	sequela

● S82.311 **Torus fracture of lower end of right tibia** A, K, P 🪙, A 🪙
   (Ex) **For S82.311[A]:** See PDX Collection 1343
   For S82.311[K,P]: See PDX Collection 897

● S82.312 **Torus fracture of lower end of left tibia** A, K, P 🪙, A 🪙
   (Ex) **For S82.312[A]:** See PDX Collection 1344
   For S82.312[K,P]: See PDX Collection 897

● S82.319 **Torus fracture of lower end of unspecified tibia** A, K, P 🪙, A 🪙
   (Ex) **For S82.319[A]:** See PDX Collection 1345
   S82.319[K,P]: See PDX Collection 897

● S82.39 **Other fracture of lower end of tibia**
   (Ex) **For category S82.39 CC codes S82.39[B,C]:** See PDX Collection 1347 **For S82.39[K,M,N,P,Q,R]:** See PDX Collection 897

● S82.391 **Other fracture of lower end of right tibia** B, C, K, M, N, P, Q, R 🪙, B, C 🪙

● S82.392 **Other fracture of lower end of left tibia** B, C, K, M, N, P, Q, R 🪙, B, C 🪙
   Coding Clinic: 2015, Q1, P25

● S82.399 **Other fracture of lower end of unspecified tibia** B, C, K, M, N, P, Q, R 🪙, B, C 🪙

● S82.4 **Fracture of shaft of fibula**
   Excludes2 fracture of lateral malleolus alone (S82.6-)
   (Ex) **For category S82.4 CC codes S82.4[B,C]:** See PDX Collection 1341
   For S82.4[K,M,N,P,Q,R]: See PDX Collection 897

● S82.40 **Unspecified fracture of shaft of fibula**

● S82.401 **Unspecified fracture of shaft of right fibula** K, M, N, P, Q, R 🪙, B, C 🪙, B, C 🪙

● S82.402 **Unspecified fracture of shaft of left fibula** K, M, N, P, Q, R 🪙, B, C 🪙, B, C 🪙

● S82.409 **Unspecified fracture of shaft of unspecified fibula** K, M, N, P, Q, R 🪙, B, C 🪙, B, C 🪙

● S82.42 **Transverse fracture of shaft of fibula**

● S82.421 **Displaced transverse fracture of shaft of right fibula** K, M, N, P, Q, R 🪙, B, C 🪙, B, C 🪙

● S82.422 **Displaced transverse fracture of shaft of left fibula** K, M, N, P, Q, R 🪙, B, C 🪙, B, C 🪙

● S82.423 **Displaced transverse fracture of shaft of unspecified fibula** K, M, N, P, Q, R 🪙, B, C 🪙, B, C 🪙

● S82.424 **Nondisplaced transverse fracture of shaft of right fibula** K, M, N, P, Q, R 🪙, B, C 🪙, B, C 🪙

● S82.425 **Nondisplaced transverse fracture of shaft of left fibula** K, M, N, P, Q, R 🪙, B, C 🪙, B, C 🪙

● S82.426 **Nondisplaced transverse fracture of shaft of unspecified fibula** K, M, N, P, Q, R 🪙, B, C 🪙, B, C 🪙

CHAPTER 19 (S00-T88)

● S82.43   **Oblique fracture of shaft of fibula**

    ● S82.431   **Displaced oblique fracture of shaft of right fibula** K, M, N, P, Q, R 🔲, B, C 🔲, B, C 🔲

    ● S82.432   **Displaced oblique fracture of shaft of left fibula** K, M, N, P, Q, R 🔲, B, C 🔲, B, C 🔲

    ● S82.433   **Displaced oblique fracture of shaft of unspecified fibula** K, M, N, P, Q, R 🔲, B, C 🔲, B, C 🔲

    ● S82.434   **Nondisplaced oblique fracture of shaft of right fibula** K, M, N, P, Q, R 🔲, B, C 🔲, B, C 🔲

    ● S82.435   **Nondisplaced oblique fracture of shaft of left fibula** K, M, N, P, Q, R 🔲, B, C 🔲, B, C 🔲

    ● S82.436   **Nondisplaced oblique fracture of shaft of unspecified fibula** K, M, N, P, Q, R 🔲, B, C 🔲, B, C 🔲

● S82.44   **Spiral fracture of shaft of fibula**

    ● S82.441   **Displaced spiral fracture of shaft of right fibula** K, M, N, P, Q, R 🔲, B, C 🔲, B, C 🔲

    ● S82.442   **Displaced spiral fracture of shaft of left fibula** K, M, N, P, Q, R 🔲, B, C 🔲, B, C 🔲

    ● S82.443   **Displaced spiral fracture of shaft of unspecified fibula** K, M, N, P, Q, R 🔲, B, C 🔲, B, C 🔲

    ● S82.444   **Nondisplaced spiral fracture of shaft of right fibula** K, M, N, P, Q, R 🔲, B, C 🔲, B, C 🔲

    ● S82.445   **Nondisplaced spiral fracture of shaft of left fibula** K, M, N, P, Q, R 🔲, B, C 🔲, B, C 🔲

    ● S82.446   **Nondisplaced spiral fracture of shaft of unspecified fibula** K, M, N, P, Q, R 🔲, B, C 🔲, B, C 🔲

● S82.45   **Comminuted fracture of shaft of fibula**

    ● S82.451   **Displaced comminuted fracture of shaft of right fibula** K, M, N, P, Q, R 🔲, B, C 🔲, B, C 🔲

    ● S82.452   **Displaced comminuted fracture of shaft of left fibula** K, M, N, P, Q, R 🔲, B, C 🔲, B, C 🔲

    ● S82.453   **Displaced comminuted fracture of shaft of unspecified fibula** K, M, N, P, Q, R 🔲, B, C 🔲, B, C 🔲

    ● S82.454   **Nondisplaced comminuted fracture of shaft of right fibula** K, M, N, P, Q, R 🔲, B, C 🔲, B, C 🔲

    ● S82.455   **Nondisplaced comminuted fracture of shaft of left fibula** K, M, N, P, Q, R 🔲, B, C 🔲, B, C 🔲

    ● S82.456   **Nondisplaced comminuted fracture of shaft of unspecified fibula** K, M, N, P, Q, R 🔲, B, C 🔲, B, C 🔲

● S82.46   **Segmental fracture of shaft of fibula**

    ● S82.461   **Displaced segmental fracture of shaft of right fibula** K, M, N, P, Q, R 🔲, B, C 🔲, B, C 🔲

    ● S82.462   **Displaced segmental fracture of shaft of left fibula** K, M, N, P, Q, R 🔲, B, C 🔲, B, C 🔲

    ● S82.463   **Displaced segmental fracture of shaft of unspecified fibula** K, M, N, P, Q, R 🔲, B, C 🔲, B, C 🔲

    ● S82.464   **Nondisplaced segmental fracture of shaft of right fibula** K, M, N, P, Q, R 🔲, B, C 🔲, B, C 🔲

    ● S82.465   **Nondisplaced segmental fracture of shaft of left fibula** K, M, N, P, Q, R 🔲, B, C 🔲, B, C 🔲

    ● S82.466   **Nondisplaced segmental fracture of shaft of unspecified fibula** K, M, N, P, Q, R 🔲, B, C 🔲, B, C 🔲

● S82.49   **Other fracture of shaft of fibula**

    ● S82.491   **Other fracture of shaft of right fibula** K, M, N, P, Q, R 🔲, B, C 🔲, B, C 🔲

    ● S82.492   **Other fracture of shaft of left fibula** K, M, N, P, Q, R 🔲, B, C 🔲, B, C 🔲

    ● S82.499   **Other fracture of shaft of unspecified fibula** K, M, N, P, Q, R 🔲, B, C 🔲, B, C 🔲

● S82.5   **Fracture of medial malleolus**

    Excludes1   pilon fracture of distal tibia (S82.87-)
                 Salter-Harris type III of lower end of tibia (S89.13-)
                 Salter-Harris type IV of lower end of tibia (S89.14-)

    (Ex) **For category S82.5 CC codes S82.5[B,C]:** See PDX Collection 1347
        For S82.5[K,M,N,P,Q,R]: See PDX Collection 897

    X ● S82.51   **Displaced fracture of medial malleolus of right tibia** B, C, K, M, N, P, Q, R 🔲, B, C 🔲

    X ● S82.52   **Displaced fracture of medial malleolus of left tibia** B, C, K, M, N, P, Q, R 🔲, B, C 🔲

    X ● S82.53   **Displaced fracture of medial malleolus of unspecified tibia** B, C, K, M, N, P, Q, R 🔲, B, C 🔲

    X ● S82.54   **Nondisplaced fracture of medial malleolus of right tibia** B, C, K, M, N, P, Q, R 🔲, B, C 🔲

    X ● S82.55   **Nondisplaced fracture of medial malleolus of left tibia** B, C, K, M, N, P, Q, R 🔲, B, C 🔲

    X ● S82.56   **Nondisplaced fracture of medial malleolus of unspecified tibia** B, C, K, M, N, P, Q, R 🔲, B, C 🔲

● S82.6   **Fracture of lateral malleolus**

    Excludes1   pilon fracture of distal tibia (S82.87-)

    (Ex) **For category S82.6 CC codes S82.6[B,C]:** See PDX Collection 1347
        For S82.6[K,M,N,P,Q,R]: See PDX Collection 897

    X ● S82.61   **Displaced fracture of lateral malleolus of right fibula** B, C, K, M, N, P, Q, R 🔲, B, C 🔲

    X ● S82.62   **Displaced fracture of lateral malleolus of left fibula** B, C, K, M, N, P, Q, R 🔲, B, C 🔲

    X ● S82.63   **Displaced fracture of lateral malleolus of unspecified fibula** B, C, K, M, N, P, Q, R 🔲, B, C 🔲

    X ● S82.64   **Nondisplaced fracture of lateral malleolus of right fibula** B, C, K, M, N, P, Q, R 🔲, B, C 🔲

    X ● S82.65   **Nondisplaced fracture of lateral malleolus of left fibula** B, C, K, M, N, P, Q, R 🔲, B, C 🔲

    X ● S82.66   **Nondisplaced fracture of lateral malleolus of unspecified fibula** B, C, K, M, N, P, Q, R 🔲, B, C 🔲

▶ New   ⟹ Revised   ~~deleted~~ Deleted   Excludes 1   Excludes 2   Includes   Use additional   Code first   Code also   Key words

OGCR Official Guidelines   ● Unacceptable Principal Diagnosis   X Assign placeholder X   ● Use Additional Character(s)   ▶ Manifestation Code   **Coding Clinic**

● **S82.8   Other fractures of lower leg**
  ● **S82.81   Torus fracture of upper end of fibula**

The appropriate 7th character is to be added to all codes in subcategory S82.81

A	initial encounter for closed fracture
D	subsequent encounter for fracture with routine healing
G	subsequent encounter for fracture with delayed healing
K	subsequent encounter for fracture with nonunion
P	subsequent encounter for fracture with malunion
S	sequela

(Ex) **For category S82.81 CC codes:** See PDX Collection 897

  ● **S82.811   Torus fracture of upper end of right fibula** K, P 🔵
  ● **S82.812   Torus fracture of upper end of left fibula** K, P 🔵
  ● **S82.819   Torus fracture of upper end of unspecified fibula** K, P 🔵

  ● **S82.82   Torus fracture of lower end of fibula**

The appropriate 7th character is to be added to all codes in subcategory S82.82

A	initial encounter for closed fracture
D	subsequent encounter for fracture with routine healing
G	subsequent encounter for fracture with delayed healing
K	subsequent encounter for fracture with nonunion
P	subsequent encounter for fracture with malunion
S	sequela

(Ex) **For category S82.82 CC codes:** See PDX Collection 897

  ● **S82.821   Torus fracture of lower end of right fibula** K, P 🔵
  ● **S82.822   Torus fracture of lower end of left fibula** K, P 🔵
  ● **S82.829   Torus fracture of lower end of unspecified fibula** K, P 🔵

  ● **S82.83   Other fracture of upper and lower end of fibula**
    (Ex) **For category S82.83 CC codes S82.83[B,C]:** See PDX Collection 1341 **For S82.83[K,M,N,P,Q,R]:** See PDX Collection 897

  ● **S82.831   Other fracture of upper and lower end of right fibula** K, M, N, P, Q, R 🔵, B, C 🔴, B, C 🔵
  ● **S82.832   Other fracture of upper and lower end of left fibula** K, M, N, P, Q, R 🔵, B, C 🔴, B, C 🔵
      Coding Clinic: 2015, Q1, P9-10
  ● **S82.839   Other fracture of upper and lower end of unspecified fibula** K, M, N, P, Q, R 🔵, B, C 🔴, B, C 🔵

  ● **S82.84   Bimalleolar fracture of lower leg**
    (Ex) **For category S82.84 CC codes S82.84[B,C]:** See PDX Collection 1347 **For S82.84[K,M,N,P,Q,R]:** See PDX Collection 897

  ● **S82.841   Displaced bimalleolar fracture of right lower leg** B, C, K, M, N, P, Q, R 🔵, B, C 🔵
  ● **S82.842   Displaced bimalleolar fracture of left lower leg** B, C, K, M, N, P, Q, R 🔵, B, C 🔵
  ● **S82.843   Displaced bimalleolar fracture of unspecified lower leg** B, C, K, M, N, P, Q, R 🔵, B, C 🔵

  ● **S82.844   Nondisplaced bimalleolar fracture of right lower leg** B, C, K, M, N, P, Q, R 🔵, B, C 🔵
  ● **S82.845   Nondisplaced bimalleolar fracture of left lower leg** B, C, K, M, N, P, Q, R 🔵, B, C 🔵
  ● **S82.846   Nondisplaced bimalleolar fracture of unspecified lower leg** B, C, K, M, N, P, Q, R 🔵, B, C 🔵

  ● **S82.85   Trimalleolar fracture of lower leg**
    (Ex) **For category S82.85 CC codes S82.85[B,C]:** See PDX Collection 1347 **For S82.85[K,M,N,P,Q,R]:** See PDX Collection 897

  ● **S82.851   Displaced trimalleolar fracture of right lower leg** B, C, K, M, N, P, Q, R 🔵, B, C 🔵
  ● **S82.852   Displaced trimalleolar fracture of left lower leg** B, C, K, M, N, P, Q, R 🔵, B, C 🔵
  ● **S82.853   Displaced trimalleolar fracture of unspecified lower leg** B, C, K, M, N, P, Q, R 🔵, B, C 🔵
  ● **S82.854   Nondisplaced trimalleolar fracture of right lower leg** B, C, K, M, N, P, Q, R 🔵, B, C 🔵
  ● **S82.855   Nondisplaced trimalleolar fracture of left lower leg** B, C, K, M, N, P, Q, R 🔵, B, C 🔵
  ● **S82.856   Nondisplaced trimalleolar fracture of unspecified lower leg** B, C, K, M, N, P, Q, R 🔵, B, C 🔵

  ● **S82.86   Maisonneuve's fracture**
    (Ex) **For category S82.86 CC codes S82.86[B,C]:** See PDX Collection 1341 **For S82.86[K,M,N,P,Q,R]:** See PDX Collection 897

  ● **S82.861   Displaced Maisonneuve's fracture of right leg** K, M, N, P, Q, R 🔵, B, C 🔵, B, C 🔵
  ● **S82.862   Displaced Maisonneuve's fracture of left leg** K, M, N, P, Q, R 🔵, B, C 🔵, B, C 🔵
  ● **S82.863   Displaced Maisonneuve's fracture of unspecified leg** K, M, N, P, Q, R 🔵, B, C 🔵, B, C 🔵
  ● **S82.864   Nondisplaced Maisonneuve's fracture of right leg** K, M, N, P, Q, R 🔵, B, C 🔵, B, C 🔵
  ● **S82.865   Nondisplaced Maisonneuve's fracture of left leg** K, M, N, P, Q, R 🔵, B, C 🔵, B, C 🔵
  ● **S82.866   Nondisplaced Maisonneuve's fracture of unspecified leg** K, M, N, P, Q, R 🔵, B, C 🔵, B, C 🔵

  ● **S82.87   Pilon fracture of tibia**
    (Ex) **For category S82.87 CC codes S82.87[B,C]:** See PDX Collection 1347 **For S82.87[K,M,N,P,Q,R]:** See PDX Collection 897

  ● **S82.871   Displaced pilon fracture of right tibia** B, C, K, M, N, P, Q, R 🔵, B, C 🔵
  ● **S82.872   Displaced pilon fracture of left tibia** B, C, K, M, N, P, Q, R 🔵, B, C 🔵
  ● **S82.873   Displaced pilon fracture of unspecified tibia** B, C, K, M, N, P, Q, R 🔵, B, C 🔵
  ● **S82.874   Nondisplaced pilon fracture of right tibia** B, C, K, M, N, P, Q, R 🔵, B, C 🔵
  ● **S82.875   Nondisplaced pilon fracture of left tibia** B, C, K, M, N, P, Q, R 🔵, B, C 🔵
  ● **S82.876   Nondisplaced pilon fracture of unspecified tibia** B, C, K, M, N, P, Q, R 🔵, B, C 🔵

N Newborn Age: 0   **P** Pediatric Age: 0–17   **M** Maternity DX: 12–55   **A** Adult Age: 15–124   ♀ Females Only   ♂ Males Only

🔵 Complication\Comorbidity   🔴 Major C\C   (Ex) CC/MCC Exclusions   🔵 Hospital-Acquired Condition

1377

CHAPTER 19 (S00–T88)

● **S82.89**   **Other fractures of lower leg**
Fracture of ankle NOS
(Ex) **For category S82.89 CC codes S82.89[B,C]:** See PDX Collection 1347 **For S82.89[K,M,N,P,Q,R]:** See PDX Collection 897

     ● **S82.891**   **Other fracture of right lower leg**
B, C, K, M, N, P, Q, R ✎, B, C ✎

     ● **S82.892**   **Other fracture of left lower leg**
B, C, K, M, N, P, Q, R ✎, B, C ✎

     ● **S82.899**   **Other fracture of unspecified lower leg** B, C, K, M, N, P, Q, R ✎, B, C ✎

● **S82.9**   **Unspecified fracture of lower leg**
(Ex) **For category S82.9 CC codes S82.9[B,C]:** See PDX Collection 1348 **For S82.9[K,M,N,P,Q,R]:** See PDX Collection 897

X ● **S82.90**   **Unspecified fracture of unspecified lower leg** A, K, M, N, P, Q, R ✎, B, C ✎

X ● **S82.91**   **Unspecified fracture of right lower leg** A, K, M, N, P, Q, R ✎, B, C ✎

X ● **S82.92**   **Unspecified fracture of left lower leg** A, K, M, N, P, Q, R ✎, B, C ✎

● **S83**   **Dislocation and sprain of joints and ligaments of knee**

Includes   avulsion of joint or ligament of knee
laceration of cartilage, joint or ligament of knee
sprain of cartilage, joint or ligament of knee
traumatic hemarthrosis of joint or ligament of knee
traumatic rupture of joint or ligament of knee
traumatic subluxation of joint or ligament of knee
traumatic tear of joint or ligament of knee

Code also any associated open wound

Excludes1   derangement of patella (M22.0-M22.3)
injury of patellar ligament (tendon) (S76.1-)
internal derangement of knee (M23.-)
old dislocation of knee (M24.36)
pathological dislocation of knee (M24.36)
recurrent dislocation of knee (M22.0)

Excludes2   strain of muscle, fascia and tendon of lower leg (S86.-)

The appropriate 7th character is to be added to each code from category S83

   A   initial encounter
   D   subsequent encounter
   S   sequela

● **S83.0**   **Subluxation and dislocation of patella**

   ● **S83.00**   **Unspecified subluxation and dislocation of patella**

     ● **S83.001**   **Unspecified subluxation of right patella**

     ● **S83.002**   **Unspecified subluxation of left patella**

     ● **S83.003**   **Unspecified subluxation of unspecified patella**

     ● **S83.004**   **Unspecified dislocation of right patella**

     ● **S83.005**   **Unspecified dislocation of left patella**

     ● **S83.006**   **Unspecified dislocation of unspecified patella**

   ● **S83.01**   **Lateral subluxation and dislocation of patella**

     ● **S83.011**   **Lateral subluxation of right patella**

     ● **S83.012**   **Lateral subluxation of left patella**

     ● **S83.013**   **Lateral subluxation of unspecified patella**

     ● **S83.014**   **Lateral dislocation of right patella**

     ● **S83.015**   **Lateral dislocation of left patella**

     ● **S83.016**   **Lateral dislocation of unspecified patella**

● **S83.09**   **Other subluxation and dislocation of patella**

     ● **S83.091**   **Other subluxation of right patella**

     ● **S83.092**   **Other subluxation of left patella**

     ● **S83.093**   **Other subluxation of unspecified patella**

     ● **S83.094**   **Other dislocation of right patella**

     ● **S83.095**   **Other dislocation of left patella**

     ● **S83.096**   **Other dislocation of unspecified patella**

● **S83.1**   **Subluxation and dislocation of knee**

Excludes2   instability of knee prosthesis (T84.022, T84.023)

   ● **S83.10**   **Unspecified subluxation and dislocation of knee**

     ● **S83.101**   **Unspecified subluxation of right knee**

     ● **S83.102**   **Unspecified subluxation of left knee**

     ● **S83.103**   **Unspecified subluxation of unspecified knee**

     ● **S83.104**   **Unspecified dislocation of right knee**

     ● **S83.105**   **Unspecified dislocation of left knee**

     ● **S83.106**   **Unspecified dislocation of unspecified knee**

   ● **S83.11**   **Anterior subluxation and dislocation of proximal end of tibia**
Posterior subluxation and dislocation of distal end of femur

     ● **S83.111**   **Anterior subluxation of proximal end of tibia, right knee**

     ● **S83.112**   **Anterior subluxation of proximal end of tibia, left knee**

     ● **S83.113**   **Anterior subluxation of proximal end of tibia, unspecified knee**

     ● **S83.114**   **Anterior dislocation of proximal end of tibia, right knee**

     ● **S83.115**   **Anterior dislocation of proximal end of tibia, left knee**

     ● **S83.116**   **Anterior dislocation of proximal end of tibia, unspecified knee**

   ● **S83.12**   **Posterior subluxation and dislocation of proximal end of tibia**
Anterior dislocation of distal end of femur

     ● **S83.121**   **Posterior subluxation of proximal end of tibia, right knee**

     ● **S83.122**   **Posterior subluxation of proximal end of tibia, left knee**

     ● **S83.123**   **Posterior subluxation of proximal end of tibia, unspecified knee**

     ● **S83.124**   **Posterior dislocation of proximal end of tibia, right knee**

     ● **S83.125**   **Posterior dislocation of proximal end of tibia, left knee**

     ● **S83.126**   **Posterior dislocation of proximal end of tibia, unspecified knee**

   ● **S83.13**   **Medial subluxation and dislocation of proximal end of tibia**

     ● **S83.131**   **Medial subluxation of proximal end of tibia, right knee**

     ● **S83.132**   **Medial subluxation of proximal end of tibia, left knee**

     ● **S83.133**   **Medial subluxation of proximal end of tibia, unspecified knee**

     ● **S83.134**   **Medial dislocation of proximal end of tibia, right knee**

     ● **S83.135**   **Medial dislocation of proximal end of tibia, left knee**

     ● **S83.136**   **Medial dislocation of proximal end of tibia, unspecified knee**

▶ New   ➠ Revised   ~~deleted~~ Deleted   Excludes 1   Excludes 2   Includes   Use additional   Code first   Code also   Key words
OGCR Official Guidelines   ● Unacceptable Principal Diagnosis   X Assign placeholder X   ● Use Additional Character(s)   ▶ Manifestation Code   **Coding Clinic**

● **S83.14**   Lateral subluxation and dislocation of proximal end of tibia
- ● **S83.141**   Lateral subluxation of proximal end of tibia, right knee
- ● **S83.142**   Lateral subluxation of proximal end of tibia, left knee
- ● **S83.143**   Lateral subluxation of proximal end of tibia, unspecified knee
- ● **S83.144**   Lateral dislocation of proximal end of tibia, right knee
- ● **S83.145**   Lateral dislocation of proximal end of tibia, left knee
- ● **S83.146**   Lateral dislocation of proximal end of tibia, unspecified knee

● **S83.19**   Other subluxation and dislocation of knee
- ● **S83.191**   Other subluxation of right knee
- ● **S83.192**   Other subluxation of left knee
- ● **S83.193**   Other subluxation of unspecified knee
- ● **S83.194**   Other dislocation of right knee
- ● **S83.195**   Other dislocation of left knee
- ● **S83.196**   Other dislocation of unspecified knee

● **S83.2**   Tear of meniscus, current injury

> **Excludes1**   old bucket-handle tear (M23.2)

● **S83.20**   Tear of unspecified meniscus, current injury
Tear of meniscus of knee NOS
- ● **S83.200**   Bucket-handle tear of unspecified meniscus, current injury, right knee
- ● **S83.201**   Bucket-handle tear of unspecified meniscus, current injury, left knee
- ● **S83.202**   Bucket-handle tear of unspecified meniscus, current injury, unspecified knee
- ● **S83.203**   Other tear of unspecified meniscus, current injury, right knee
- ● **S83.204**   Other tear of unspecified meniscus, current injury, left knee
- ● **S83.205**   Other tear of unspecified meniscus, current injury, unspecified knee
- ● **S83.206**   Unspecified tear of unspecified meniscus, current injury, right knee
- ● **S83.207**   Unspecified tear of unspecified meniscus, current injury, left knee
- ● **S83.209**   Unspecified tear of unspecified meniscus, current injury, unspecified knee

● **S83.21**   Bucket-handle tear of medial meniscus, current injury
- ● **S83.211**   Bucket-handle tear of medial meniscus, current injury, right knee
- ● **S83.212**   Bucket-handle tear of medial meniscus, current injury, left knee
- ● **S83.219**   Bucket-handle tear of medial meniscus, current injury, unspecified knee

● **S83.22**   Peripheral tear of medial meniscus, current injury
- ● **S83.221**   Peripheral tear of medial meniscus, current injury, right knee
- ● **S83.222**   Peripheral tear of medial meniscus, current injury, left knee
- ● **S83.229**   Peripheral tear of medial meniscus, current injury, unspecified knee

● **S83.23**   Complex tear of medial meniscus, current injury
- ● **S83.231**   Complex tear of medial meniscus, current injury, right knee
- ● **S83.232**   Complex tear of medial meniscus, current injury, left knee
- ● **S83.239**   Complex tear of medial meniscus, current injury, unspecified knee

● **S83.24**   Other tear of medial meniscus, current injury
- ● **S83.241**   Other tear of medial meniscus, current injury, right knee
- ● **S83.242**   Other tear of medial meniscus, current injury, left knee
- ● **S83.249**   Other tear of medial meniscus, current injury, unspecified knee

● **S83.25**   Bucket-handle tear of lateral meniscus, current injury
- ● **S83.251**   Bucket-handle tear of lateral meniscus, current injury, right knee
- ● **S83.252**   Bucket-handle tear of lateral meniscus, current injury, left knee
- ● **S83.259**   Bucket-handle tear of lateral meniscus, current injury, unspecified knee

● **S83.26**   Peripheral tear of lateral meniscus, current injury
- ● **S83.261**   Peripheral tear of lateral meniscus, current injury, right knee
- ● **S83.262**   Peripheral tear of lateral meniscus, current injury, left knee
- ● **S83.269**   Peripheral tear of lateral meniscus, current injury, unspecified knee

● **S83.27**   Complex tear of lateral meniscus, current injury
- ● **S83.271**   Complex tear of lateral meniscus, current injury, right knee
- ● **S83.272**   Complex tear of lateral meniscus, current injury, left knee
- ● **S83.279**   Complex tear of lateral meniscus, current injury, unspecified knee

● **S83.28**   Other tear of lateral meniscus, current injury
- ● **S83.281**   Other tear of lateral meniscus, current injury, right knee
- ● **S83.282**   Other tear of lateral meniscus, current injury, left knee
- ● **S83.289**   Other tear of lateral meniscus, current injury, unspecified knee

● **S83.3**   Tear of articular cartilage of knee, current
- X● **S83.30**   Tear of articular cartilage of unspecified knee, current
- X● **S83.31**   Tear of articular cartilage of right knee, current
- X● **S83.32**   Tear of articular cartilage of left knee, current

● **S83.4**   Sprain of collateral ligament of knee
- ● **S83.40**   Sprain of unspecified collateral ligament of knee
  - ● **S83.401**   Sprain of unspecified collateral ligament of right knee
  - ● **S83.402**   Sprain of unspecified collateral ligament of left knee
  - ● **S83.409**   Sprain of unspecified collateral ligament of unspecified knee
- ● **S83.41**   Sprain of medial collateral ligament of knee
  Sprain of tibial collateral ligament
  - ● **S83.411**   Sprain of medial collateral ligament of right knee
  - ● **S83.412**   Sprain of medial collateral ligament of left knee
  - ● **S83.419**   Sprain of medial collateral ligament of unspecified knee

N Newborn Age: 0   **P** Pediatric Age: 0–17   **M** Maternity DX: 12–55   **A** Adult Age: 15–124   ♀ Females Only   ♂ Males Only

🅒 Complication\Comorbidity   🅜 Major C\C   (Ex) CC/MCC Exclusions   🅗 Hospital-Acquired Condition

1379

CHAPTER 19 (SØØ-T88)

● S83.42　Sprain of lateral collateral ligament of knee
　　　　　Sprain of fibular collateral ligament
　　● S83.421　Sprain of lateral collateral ligament of right knee
　　● S83.422　Sprain of lateral collateral ligament of left knee
　　● S83.429　Sprain of lateral collateral ligament of unspecified knee
● S83.5　Sprain of cruciate ligament of knee
　● S83.50　Sprain of unspecified cruciate ligament of knee
　　● S83.501　Sprain of unspecified cruciate ligament of right knee
　　● S83.502　Sprain of unspecified cruciate ligament of left knee
　　● S83.509　Sprain of unspecified cruciate ligament of unspecified knee
　● S83.51　Sprain of anterior cruciate ligament of knee
　　● S83.511　Sprain of anterior cruciate ligament of right knee
　　　　　　Coding Clinic: 2Ø16, Q2, P4
　　● S83.512　Sprain of anterior cruciate ligament of left knee
　　● S83.519　Sprain of anterior cruciate ligament of unspecified knee
　● S83.52　Sprain of posterior cruciate ligament of knee
　　● S83.521　Sprain of posterior cruciate ligament of right knee
　　● S83.522　Sprain of posterior cruciate ligament of left knee
　　● S83.529　Sprain of posterior cruciate ligament of unspecified knee
● S83.6　Sprain of the superior tibiofibular joint and ligament
　X● S83.60　Sprain of the superior tibiofibular joint and ligament, unspecified knee
　X● S83.61　Sprain of the superior tibiofibular joint and ligament, right knee
　X● S83.62　Sprain of the superior tibiofibular joint and ligament, left knee
● S83.8　Sprain of other specified parts of knee
　● S83.8X　Sprain of other specified parts of knee
　　● S83.8X1　Sprain of other specified parts of right knee
　　● S83.8X2　Sprain of other specified parts of left knee
　　● S83.8X9　Sprain of other specified parts of unspecified knee
● S83.9　Sprain of unspecified site of knee
　X● S83.90　Sprain of unspecified site of unspecified knee
　X● S83.91　Sprain of unspecified site of right knee
　X● S83.92　Sprain of unspecified site of left knee

● S84　Injury of nerves at lower leg level
　　Code also any associated open wound (S81.-)
　　Excludes2　injury of nerves at ankle and foot level (S94.-)
　　The appropriate 7th character is to be added to each code from category S84

A	initial encounter
D	subsequent encounter
S	sequela

● S84.0　Injury of tibial nerve at lower leg level
　X● S84.00　Injury of tibial nerve at lower leg level, unspecified leg
　X● S84.01　Injury of tibial nerve at lower leg level, right leg
　X● S84.02　Injury of tibial nerve at lower leg level, left leg

● S84.1　Injury of peroneal nerve at lower leg level
　X● S84.10　Injury of peroneal nerve at lower leg level, unspecified leg
　X● S84.11　Injury of peroneal nerve at lower leg level, right leg
　X● S84.12　Injury of peroneal nerve at lower leg level, left leg
● S84.2　Injury of cutaneous sensory nerve at lower leg level
　X● S84.20　Injury of cutaneous sensory nerve at lower leg level, unspecified leg
　X● S84.21　Injury of cutaneous sensory nerve at lower leg level, right leg
　X● S84.22　Injury of cutaneous sensory nerve at lower leg level, left leg
● S84.8　Injury of other nerves at lower leg level
　● S84.80　Injury of other nerves at lower leg level
　　● S84.801　Injury of other nerves at lower leg level, right leg
　　● S84.802　Injury of other nerves at lower leg level, left leg
　　● S84.809　Injury of other nerves at lower leg level, unspecified leg
● S84.9　Injury of unspecified nerve at lower leg level
　X● S84.90　Injury of unspecified nerve at lower leg level, unspecified leg
　X● S84.91　Injury of unspecified nerve at lower leg level, right leg
　X● S84.92　Injury of unspecified nerve at lower leg level, left leg

● S85　Injury of blood vessels at lower leg level
　　Code also any associated open wound (S81.-)
　　Excludes2　injury of blood vessels at ankle and foot level (S95.-)
　　The appropriate 7th character is to be added to each code from category S85

A	initial encounter
D	subsequent encounter
S	sequela

● S85.0　Injury of popliteal artery
　● S85.00　Unspecified injury of popliteal artery
　　● S85.001　Unspecified injury of popliteal artery, right leg A ⬡
　　　　　　(Ex) See PDX Collection 1349
　　● S85.002　Unspecified injury of popliteal artery, left leg A ⬡
　　　　　　(Ex) See PDX Collection 135Ø
　　● S85.009　Unspecified injury of popliteal artery, unspecified leg A ⬡
　　　　　　(Ex) See PDX Collection 1351
　● S85.01　Laceration of popliteal artery
　　● S85.011　Laceration of popliteal artery, right leg A ⬡
　　　　　　(Ex) See PDX Collection 1349
　　● S85.012　Laceration of popliteal artery, left leg A ⬡
　　　　　　(Ex) See PDX Collection 135Ø
　　● S85.019　Laceration of popliteal artery, unspecified leg A ⬡
　　　　　　(Ex) See PDX Collection 1351

▶ New　⇒ Revised　d̶e̶l̶e̶t̶e̶d̶ Deleted　Excludes 1　Excludes 2　Includes　Use additional　Code first　Code also　Key words
OGCR Official Guidelines　● Unacceptable Principal Diagnosis　X Assign placeholder X　● Use Additional Character(s)　▶ Manifestation Code　**Coding Clinic**

● **S85.09**   Other specified injury of popliteal artery
    ● **S85.091**   Other specified injury of popliteal artery, right leg A 🅒
         (Ex:) See PDX Collection 1349
    ● **S85.092**   Other specified injury of popliteal artery, left leg A 🅒
         (Ex:) See PDX Collection 1350
    ● **S85.099**   Other specified injury of popliteal artery, unspecified leg A 🅒
         (Ex:) See PDX Collection 1351

● **S85.1**   Injury of tibial artery
    ● **S85.10**   Unspecified injury of unspecified tibial artery
        Injury of tibial artery NOS
       ● **S85.101**   Unspecified injury of unspecified tibial artery, right leg A 🅒
           (Ex:) See PDX Collection 1352
       ● **S85.102**   Unspecified injury of unspecified tibial artery, left leg A 🅒
           (Ex:) See PDX Collection 1353
       ● **S85.109**   Unspecified injury of unspecified tibial artery, unspecified leg A 🅒
           (Ex:) See PDX Collection 1354
    ● **S85.11**   Laceration of unspecified tibial artery
       ● **S85.111**   Laceration of unspecified tibial artery, right leg A 🅒
           (Ex:) See PDX Collection 1352
       ● **S85.112**   Laceration of unspecified tibial artery, left leg A 🅒
           (Ex:) See PDX Collection 1353
       ● **S85.119**   Laceration of unspecified tibial artery, unspecified leg A 🅒
           (Ex:) See PDX Collection 1354
    ● **S85.12**   Other specified injury of unspecified tibial artery
       ● **S85.121**   Other specified injury of unspecified tibial artery, right leg A 🅒
           (Ex:) See PDX Collection 1352
       ● **S85.122**   Other specified injury of unspecified tibial artery, left leg A 🅒
           (Ex:) See PDX Collection 1353
       ● **S85.129**   Other specified injury of unspecified tibial artery, unspecified leg A 🅒
           (Ex:) See PDX Collection 1354
    ● **S85.13**   Unspecified injury of anterior tibial artery
       ● **S85.131**   Unspecified injury of anterior tibial artery, right leg A 🅒
           (Ex:) See PDX Collection 1355
       ● **S85.132**   Unspecified injury of anterior tibial artery, left leg A 🅒
           (Ex:) See PDX Collection 1356
       ● **S85.139**   Unspecified injury of anterior tibial artery, unspecified leg A 🅒
           (Ex:) See PDX Collection 1357
    ● **S85.14**   Laceration of anterior tibial artery
       ● **S85.141**   Laceration of anterior tibial artery, right leg A 🅒
           (Ex:) See PDX Collection 1355
       ● **S85.142**   Laceration of anterior tibial artery, left leg A 🅒
           (Ex:) See PDX Collection 1356
       ● **S85.149**   Laceration of anterior tibial artery, unspecified leg A 🅒
           (Ex:) See PDX Collection 1357

● **S85.15**   Other specified injury of anterior tibial artery
    ● **S85.151**   Other specified injury of anterior tibial artery, right leg A 🅒
         (Ex:) See PDX Collection 1355
    ● **S85.152**   Other specified injury of anterior tibial artery, left leg A 🅒
         (Ex:) See PDX Collection 1356
    ● **S85.159**   Other specified injury of anterior tibial artery, unspecified leg A 🅒
         (Ex:) See PDX Collection 1357

● **S85.16**   Unspecified injury of posterior tibial artery
    ● **S85.161**   Unspecified injury of posterior tibial artery, right leg A 🅒
         (Ex:) See PDX Collection 1358
    ● **S85.162**   Unspecified injury of posterior tibial artery, left leg A 🅒
         (Ex:) See PDX Collection 1359
    ● **S85.169**   Unspecified injury of posterior tibial artery, unspecified leg A 🅒
         (Ex:) See PDX Collection 1360

● **S85.17**   Laceration of posterior tibial artery
    ● **S85.171**   Laceration of posterior tibial artery, right leg A 🅒
         (Ex:) See PDX Collection 1358
    ● **S85.172**   Laceration of posterior tibial artery, left leg A 🅒
         (Ex:) See PDX Collection 1359
    ● **S85.179**   Laceration of posterior tibial artery, unspecified leg A 🅒
         (Ex:) See PDX Collection 1360

● **S85.18**   Other specified injury of posterior tibial artery
    ● **S85.181**   Other specified injury of posterior tibial artery, right leg A 🅒
         (Ex:) See PDX Collection 1358
    ● **S85.182**   Other specified injury of posterior tibial artery, left leg A 🅒
         (Ex:) See PDX Collection 1359
    ● **S85.189**   Other specified injury of posterior tibial artery, unspecified leg A 🅒
         (Ex:) See PDX Collection 1360

● **S85.2**   Injury of peroneal artery
    ● **S85.20**   Unspecified injury of peroneal artery
       ● **S85.201**   Unspecified injury of peroneal artery, right leg A 🅒
           (Ex:) See PDX Collection 1325
       ● **S85.202**   Unspecified injury of peroneal artery, left leg A 🅒
           (Ex:) See PDX Collection 1326
       ● **S85.209**   Unspecified injury of peroneal artery, unspecified leg A 🅒
           (Ex:) See PDX Collection 1327
    ● **S85.21**   Laceration of peroneal artery
       ● **S85.211**   Laceration of peroneal artery, right leg A 🅒
           (Ex:) See PDX Collection 1325
       ● **S85.212**   Laceration of peroneal artery, left leg A 🅒
           (Ex:) See PDX Collection 1326
       ● **S85.219**   Laceration of peroneal artery, unspecified leg A 🅒
           (Ex:) See PDX Collection 1327

CHAPTER 19 (S00–T88)

● S85.29   Other specified injury of peroneal artery
   ● S85.291   Other specified injury of peroneal artery, right leg A 🦶
      Ex: See PDX Collection 1325
   ● S85.292   Other specified injury of peroneal artery, left leg A 🦶
      Ex: See PDX Collection 1326
   ● S85.299   Other specified injury of peroneal artery, unspecified leg A 🦶
      Ex: See PDX Collection 1327

● S85.3   Injury of greater saphenous vein at lower leg level
   Injury of greater saphenous vein NOS
   Injury of saphenous vein NOS
  ● S85.30   Unspecified injury of greater saphenous vein at lower leg level
    ● S85.301   Unspecified injury of greater saphenous vein at lower leg level, right leg A 🦶
      Ex: See PDX Collection 1322
    ● S85.302   Unspecified injury of greater saphenous vein at lower leg level, left leg A 🦶
      Ex: See PDX Collection 1323
    ● S85.309   Unspecified injury of greater saphenous vein at lower leg level, unspecified leg A 🦶
      Ex: See PDX Collection 1324
  ● S85.31   Laceration of greater saphenous vein at lower leg level
    ● S85.311   Laceration of greater saphenous vein at lower leg level, right leg A 🦶
      Ex: See PDX Collection 1322
    ● S85.312   Laceration of greater saphenous vein at lower leg level, left leg A 🦶
      Ex: See PDX Collection 1323
    ● S85.319   Laceration of greater saphenous vein at lower leg level, unspecified leg A 🦶
      Ex: See PDX Collection 1324
  ● S85.39   Other specified injury of greater saphenous vein at lower leg level
    ● S85.391   Other specified injury of greater saphenous vein at lower leg level, right leg A 🦶
      Ex: See PDX Collection 1322
    ● S85.392   Other specified injury of greater saphenous vein at lower leg level, left leg A 🦶
      Ex: See PDX Collection 1323
    ● S85.399   Other specified injury of greater saphenous vein at lower leg level, unspecified leg A 🦶
      Ex: See PDX Collection 1324

● S85.4   Injury of lesser saphenous vein at lower leg level
  ● S85.40   Unspecified injury of lesser saphenous vein at lower leg level
    ● S85.401   Unspecified injury of lesser saphenous vein at lower leg level, right leg A 🦶
      Ex: See PDX Collection 1322
    ● S85.402   Unspecified injury of lesser saphenous vein at lower leg level, left leg A 🦶
      Ex: See PDX Collection 1323
    ● S85.409   Unspecified injury of lesser saphenous vein at lower leg level, unspecified leg A 🦶
      Ex: See PDX Collection 1324

● S85.41   Laceration of lesser saphenous vein at lower leg level
   ● S85.411   Laceration of lesser saphenous vein at lower leg level, right leg A 🦶
      Ex: See PDX Collection 1322
   ● S85.412   Laceration of lesser saphenous vein at lower leg level, left leg A 🦶
      Ex: See PDX Collection 1323
   ● S85.419   Laceration of lesser saphenous vein at lower leg level, unspecified leg A 🦶
      Ex: See PDX Collection 1324

● S85.49   Other specified injury of lesser saphenous vein at lower leg level
   ● S85.491   Other specified injury of lesser saphenous vein at lower leg level, right leg A 🦶
      Ex: See PDX Collection 1322
   ● S85.492   Other specified injury of lesser saphenous vein at lower leg level, left leg A 🦶
      Ex: See PDX Collection 1323
   ● S85.499   Other specified injury of lesser saphenous vein at lower leg level, unspecified leg A 🦶
      Ex: See PDX Collection 1324

● S85.5   Injury of popliteal vein
  ● S85.50   Unspecified injury of popliteal vein
    ● S85.501   Unspecified injury of popliteal vein, right leg A 🦶
      Ex: See PDX Collection 1361
    ● S85.502   Unspecified injury of popliteal vein, left leg A 🦶
      Ex: See PDX Collection 1362
    ● S85.509   Unspecified injury of popliteal vein, unspecified leg A 🦶
      Ex: See PDX Collection 1363
  ● S85.51   Laceration of popliteal vein
    ● S85.511   Laceration of popliteal vein, right leg A 🦶
      Ex: See PDX Collection 1361
    ● S85.512   Laceration of popliteal vein, left leg A 🦶
      Ex: See PDX Collection 1362
    ● S85.519   Laceration of popliteal vein, unspecified leg A 🦶
      Ex: See PDX Collection 1363
  ● S85.59   Other specified injury of popliteal vein
    ● S85.591   Other specified injury of popliteal vein, right leg A 🦶
      Ex: See PDX Collection 1361
    ● S85.592   Other specified injury of popliteal vein, left leg A 🦶
      Ex: See PDX Collection 1362
    ● S85.599   Other specified injury of popliteal vein, unspecified leg A 🦶
      Ex: See PDX Collection 1363

● S85.8   Injury of other blood vessels at lower leg level
  ● S85.80   Unspecified injury of other blood vessels at lower leg level
    ● S85.801   Unspecified injury of other blood vessels at lower leg level, right leg A 🦶
      Ex: See PDX Collection 1325
    ● S85.802   Unspecified injury of other blood vessels at lower leg level, left leg A 🦶
      Ex: See PDX Collection 1326
    ● S85.809   Unspecified injury of other blood vessels at lower leg level, unspecified leg A 🦶
      Ex: See PDX Collection 1327

CHAPTER 19 (S00-T88)

▶ New   ⟫ Revised   ~~deleted~~ Deleted   Excludes 1   Excludes 2   Includes   Use additional   Code first   Code also   Key words

OGCR Official Guidelines   ● Unacceptable Principal Diagnosis   X Assign placeholder X   ▶ Use Additional Character(s)   ❱ Manifestation Code   **Coding Clinic**

● **S85.81** Laceration of other blood vessels at lower leg level
 ● **S85.811** Laceration of other blood vessels at lower leg level, right leg A 🦠
  (Ex:) See PDX Collection 1325
 ● **S85.812** Laceration of other blood vessels at lower leg level, left leg A 🦠
  (Ex:) See PDX Collection 1326
 ● **S85.819** Laceration of other blood vessels at lower leg level, unspecified leg A 🦠
  (Ex:) See PDX Collection 1327
● **S85.89** Other specified injury of other blood vessels at lower leg level
 ● **S85.891** Other specified injury of other blood vessels at lower leg level, right leg A 🦠
  (Ex:) See PDX Collection 1325
 ● **S85.892** Other specified injury of other blood vessels at lower leg level, left leg A 🦠
  (Ex:) See PDX Collection 1326
 ● **S85.899** Other specified injury of other blood vessels at lower leg level, unspecified leg A 🦠
  (Ex:) See PDX Collection 1327

● **S85.9** Injury of unspecified blood vessel at lower leg level
 ● **S85.90** Unspecified injury of unspecified blood vessel at lower leg level
  ● **S85.901** Unspecified injury of unspecified blood vessel at lower leg level, right leg A 🦠
   (Ex:) See PDX Collection 1325
  ● **S85.902** Unspecified injury of unspecified blood vessel at lower leg level, left leg A 🦠
   (Ex:) See PDX Collection 1326
  ● **S85.909** Unspecified injury of unspecified blood vessel at lower leg level, unspecified leg A 🦠
   (Ex:) See PDX Collection 1327
 ● **S85.91** Laceration of unspecified blood vessel at lower leg level
  ● **S85.911** Laceration of unspecified blood vessel at lower leg level, right leg A 🦠
   (Ex:) See PDX Collection 1325
  ● **S85.912** Laceration of unspecified blood vessel at lower leg level, left leg A 🦠
   (Ex:) See PDX Collection 1326
  ● **S85.919** Laceration of unspecified blood vessel at lower leg level, unspecified leg A 🦠
   (Ex:) See PDX Collection 1327
 ● **S85.99** Other specified injury of unspecified blood vessel at lower leg level
  ● **S85.991** Other specified injury of unspecified blood vessel at lower leg level, right leg A 🦠
   (Ex:) See PDX Collection 1325
  ● **S85.992** Other specified injury of unspecified blood vessel at lower leg level, left leg A 🦠
   (Ex:) See PDX Collection 1326
  ● **S85.999** Other specified injury of unspecified blood vessel at lower leg level, unspecified leg A 🦠
   (Ex:) See PDX Collection 1327

● **S86** Injury of muscle, fascia and tendon at lower leg level
 Code also any associated open wound (S81.-)
 Excludes2 injury of muscle, fascia and tendon at ankle (S96.-)
     injury of patellar ligament (tendon) (S76.1-)
     sprain of joints and ligaments of knee (S83.-)
 The appropriate 7th character is to be added to each code from category S86

A	initial encounter
D	subsequent encounter
S	sequela

● **S86.0** Injury of Achilles tendon
 ● **S86.00** Unspecified injury of Achilles tendon
  ● **S86.001** Unspecified injury of right Achilles tendon
  ● **S86.002** Unspecified injury of left Achilles tendon
  ● **S86.009** Unspecified injury of unspecified Achilles tendon
 ● **S86.01** Strain of Achilles tendon
  ● **S86.011** Strain of right Achilles tendon
  ● **S86.012** Strain of left Achilles tendon
  ● **S86.019** Strain of unspecified Achilles tendon
 ● **S86.02** Laceration of Achilles tendon
  ● **S86.021** Laceration of right Achilles tendon A 🦠
   (Ex:) See PDX Collection 1364
  ● **S86.022** Laceration of left Achilles tendon A 🦠
   (Ex:) See PDX Collection 1365
  ● **S86.029** Laceration of unspecified Achilles tendon A 🦠
   (Ex:) See PDX Collection 1366
 ● **S86.09** Other specified injury of Achilles tendon
  ● **S86.091** Other specified injury of right Achilles tendon
  ● **S86.092** Other specified injury of left Achilles tendon
  ● **S86.099** Other specified injury of unspecified Achilles tendon
● **S86.1** Injury of other muscle(s) and tendon(s) of posterior muscle group at lower leg level
 ● **S86.10** Unspecified injury of other muscle(s) and tendon(s) of posterior muscle group at lower leg level
  ● **S86.101** Unspecified injury of other muscle(s) and tendon(s) of posterior muscle group at lower leg level, right leg
  ● **S86.102** Unspecified injury of other muscle(s) and tendon(s) of posterior muscle group at lower leg level, left leg
  ● **S86.109** Unspecified injury of other muscle(s) and tendon(s) of posterior muscle group at lower leg level, unspecified leg
 ● **S86.11** Strain of other muscle(s) and tendon(s) of posterior muscle group at lower leg level
  ● **S86.111** Strain of other muscle(s) and tendon(s) of posterior muscle group at lower leg level, right leg
  ● **S86.112** Strain of other muscle(s) and tendon(s) of posterior muscle group at lower leg level, left leg
  ● **S86.119** Strain of other muscle(s) and tendon(s) of posterior muscle group at lower leg level, unspecified leg

CHAPTER 19 (S00-T88)

N Newborn Age: 0 P Pediatric Age: 0–17 M Maternity DX: 12–55 A Adult Age: 15–124 ♀ Females Only ♂ Males Only
🦠 Complication\Comorbidity 🦠 Major C\C (Ex:) CC/MCC Exclusions 🦠 Hospital-Acquired Condition

1383

● **S86.12** Laceration of other muscle(s) and tendon(s) of posterior muscle group at lower leg level

  ● **S86.121** Laceration of other muscle(s) and tendon(s) of posterior muscle group at lower leg level, right leg A €

    (Ex) See PDX Collection 1364

  ● **S86.122** Laceration of other muscle(s) and tendon(s) of posterior muscle group at lower leg level, left leg A €

    (Ex) See PDX Collection 1365

  ● **S86.129** Laceration of other muscle(s) and tendon(s) of posterior muscle group at lower leg level, unspecified leg A €

    (Ex) See PDX Collection 1366

● **S86.19** Other injury of other muscle(s) and tendon(s) of posterior muscle group at lower leg level

  ● **S86.191** Other injury of other muscle(s) and tendon(s) of posterior muscle group at lower leg level, right leg

  ● **S86.192** Other injury of other muscle(s) and tendon(s) of posterior muscle group at lower leg level, left leg

  ● **S86.199** Other injury of other muscle(s) and tendon(s) of posterior muscle group at lower leg level, unspecified leg

● **S86.2** Injury of muscle(s) and tendon(s) of anterior muscle group at lower leg level

  ● **S86.20** Unspecified injury of muscle(s) and tendon(s) of anterior muscle group at lower leg level

    ● **S86.201** Unspecified injury of muscle(s) and tendon(s) of anterior muscle group at lower leg level, right leg

    ● **S86.202** Unspecified injury of muscle(s) and tendon(s) of anterior muscle group at lower leg level, left leg

    ● **S86.209** Unspecified injury of muscle(s) and tendon(s) of anterior muscle group at lower leg level, unspecified leg

  ● **S86.21** Strain of muscle(s) and tendon(s) of anterior muscle group at lower leg level

    ● **S86.211** Strain of muscle(s) and tendon(s) of anterior muscle group at lower leg level, right leg

    ● **S86.212** Strain of muscle(s) and tendon(s) of anterior muscle group at lower leg level, left leg

    ● **S86.219** Strain of muscle(s) and tendon(s) of anterior muscle group at lower leg level, unspecified leg

  ● **S86.22** Laceration of muscle(s) and tendon(s) of anterior muscle group at lower leg level

    ● **S86.221** Laceration of muscle(s) and tendon(s) of anterior muscle group at lower leg level, right leg A €

      (Ex) See PDX Collection 1364

    ● **S86.222** Laceration of muscle(s) and tendon(s) of anterior muscle group at lower leg level, left leg A €

      (Ex) See PDX Collection 1365

    ● **S86.229** Laceration of muscle(s) and tendon(s) of anterior muscle group at lower leg level, unspecified leg A €

      (Ex) See PDX Collection 1366

● **S86.29** Other injury of muscle(s) and tendon(s) of anterior muscle group at lower leg level

  ● **S86.291** Other injury of muscle(s) and tendon(s) of anterior muscle group at lower leg level, right leg

  ● **S86.292** Other injury of muscle(s) and tendon(s) of anterior muscle group at lower leg level, left leg

  ● **S86.299** Other injury of muscle(s) and tendon(s) of anterior muscle group at lower leg level, unspecified leg

● **S86.3** Injury of muscle(s) and tendon(s) of peroneal muscle group at lower leg level

  ● **S86.30** Unspecified injury of muscle(s) and tendon(s) of peroneal muscle group at lower leg level

    ● **S86.301** Unspecified injury of muscle(s) and tendon(s) of peroneal muscle group at lower leg level, right leg

    ● **S86.302** Unspecified injury of muscle(s) and tendon(s) of peroneal muscle group at lower leg level, left leg

    ● **S86.309** Unspecified injury of muscle(s) and tendon(s) of peroneal muscle group at lower leg level, unspecified leg

  ● **S86.31** Strain of muscle(s) and tendon(s) of peroneal muscle group at lower leg level

    ● **S86.311** Strain of muscle(s) and tendon(s) of peroneal muscle group at lower leg level, right leg

    ● **S86.312** Strain of muscle(s) and tendon(s) of peroneal muscle group at lower leg level, left leg

    ● **S86.319** Strain of muscle(s) and tendon(s) of peroneal muscle group at lower leg level, unspecified leg

  ● **S86.32** Laceration of muscle(s) and tendon(s) of peroneal muscle group at lower leg level

    ● **S86.321** Laceration of muscle(s) and tendon(s) of peroneal muscle group at lower leg level, right leg A €

      (Ex) See PDX Collection 1364

    ● **S86.322** Laceration of muscle(s) and tendon(s) of peroneal muscle group at lower leg level, left leg A €

      (Ex) See PDX Collection 1365

    ● **S86.329** Laceration of muscle(s) and tendon(s) of peroneal muscle group at lower leg level, unspecified leg A €

      (Ex) See PDX Collection 1366

  ● **S86.39** Other injury of muscle(s) and tendon(s) of peroneal muscle group at lower leg level

    ● **S86.391** Other injury of muscle(s) and tendon(s) of peroneal muscle group at lower leg level, right leg

    ● **S86.392** Other injury of muscle(s) and tendon(s) of peroneal muscle group at lower leg level, left leg

    ● **S86.399** Other injury of muscle(s) and tendon(s) of peroneal muscle group at lower leg level, unspecified leg

● S86.8   Injury of other muscles and tendons at lower leg level
 ● S86.80   Unspecified injury of other muscles and tendons at lower leg level
  ● S86.801   Unspecified injury of other muscle(s) and tendon(s) at lower leg level, right leg
  ● S86.802   Unspecified injury of other muscle(s) and tendon(s) at lower leg level, left leg
  ● S86.809   Unspecified injury of other muscle(s) and tendon(s) at lower leg level, unspecified leg
 ● S86.81   Strain of other muscles and tendons at lower leg level
  ● S86.811   Strain of other muscle(s) and tendon(s) at lower leg level, right leg
  ● S86.812   Strain of other muscle(s) and tendon(s) at lower leg level, left leg
  ● S86.819   Strain of other muscle(s) and tendon(s) at lower leg level, unspecified leg
 ● S86.82   Laceration of other muscles and tendons at lower leg level
  ● S86.821   Laceration of other muscle(s) and tendon(s) at lower leg level, right leg A ⦶
             (Ex:) See PDX Collection 1364
  ● S86.822   Laceration of other muscle(s) and tendon(s) at lower leg level, left leg A ⦶
             (Ex:) See PDX Collection 1365
  ● S86.829   Laceration of other muscle(s) and tendon(s) at lower leg level, unspecified leg A ⦶
             (Ex:) See PDX Collection 1366
 ● S86.89   Other injury of other muscles and tendons at lower leg level
  ● S86.891   Other injury of other muscle(s) and tendon(s) at lower leg level, right leg
  ● S86.892   Other injury of other muscle(s) and tendon(s) at lower leg level, left leg
  ● S86.899   Other injury of other muscle(s) and tendon(s) at lower leg level, unspecified leg
● S86.9   Injury of unspecified muscle and tendon at lower leg level
 ● S86.90   Unspecified injury of unspecified muscle and tendon at lower leg level
  ● S86.901   Unspecified injury of unspecified muscle(s) and tendon(s) at lower leg level, right leg
  ● S86.902   Unspecified injury of unspecified muscle(s) and tendon(s) at lower leg level, left leg
  ● S86.909   Unspecified injury of unspecified muscle(s) and tendon(s) at lower leg level, unspecified leg
 ● S86.91   Strain of unspecified muscle and tendon at lower leg level
  ● S86.911   Strain of unspecified muscle(s) and tendon(s) at lower leg level, right leg
  ● S86.912   Strain of unspecified muscle(s) and tendon(s) at lower leg level, left leg
  ● S86.919   Strain of unspecified muscle(s) and tendon(s) at lower leg level, unspecified leg

 ● S86.92   Laceration of unspecified muscle and tendon at lower leg level
  ● S86.921   Laceration of unspecified muscle(s) and tendon(s) at lower leg level, right leg A ⦶
             (Ex:) See PDX Collection 1364
  ● S86.922   Laceration of unspecified muscle(s) and tendon(s) at lower leg level, left leg A ⦶
             (Ex:) See PDX Collection 1365
  ● S86.929   Laceration of unspecified muscle(s) and tendon(s) at lower leg level, unspecified leg A ⦶
             (Ex:) See PDX Collection 1366
 ● S86.99   Other injury of unspecified muscle and tendon at lower leg level
  ● S86.991   Other injury of unspecified muscle(s) and tendon(s) at lower leg level, right leg
  ● S86.992   Other injury of unspecified muscle(s) and tendon(s) at lower leg level, left leg
  ● S86.999   Other injury of unspecified muscle(s) and tendon(s) at lower leg level, unspecified leg

● S87   Crushing injury of lower leg
       Use additional code(s) for all associated injuries
       Excludes2   crushing injury of ankle and foot (S97.-)
       The appropriate 7th character is to be added to each code from category S87

A	initial encounter
D	subsequent encounter
S	sequela

 ● S87.0   Crushing injury of knee
  X ● S87.00   Crushing injury of unspecified knee
  X ● S87.01   Crushing injury of right knee
  X ● S87.02   Crushing injury of left knee
 ● S87.8   Crushing injury of lower leg
  X ● S87.80   Crushing injury of unspecified lower leg
  X ● S87.81   Crushing injury of right lower leg
  X ● S87.82   Crushing injury of left lower leg

● S88   Traumatic amputation of lower leg
       An amputation not identified as partial or complete should be coded to complete
       Excludes1   traumatic amputation of ankle and foot (S98.-)
       The appropriate 7th character is to be added to each code from category S88

A	initial encounter
D	subsequent encounter
S	sequela

 ● S88.0   Traumatic amputation at knee level
  ● S88.01   Complete traumatic amputation at knee level
   ● S88.011   Complete traumatic amputation at knee level, right lower leg A ⦶
              (Ex:) See PDX Collection 1333
   ● S88.012   Complete traumatic amputation at knee level, left lower leg A ⦶
              (Ex:) See PDX Collection 1334
   ● S88.019   Complete traumatic amputation at knee level, unspecified lower leg A ⦶
              (Ex:) See PDX Collection 1335

CHAPTER 19 (S00–T88)

● S88.02　Partial traumatic amputation at knee level

　　● S88.021　Partial traumatic amputation at knee level, **right** lower leg A 🔗
　　　　Ex: See PDX Collection 1333

　　● S88.022　Partial traumatic amputation at knee level, **left** lower leg A 🔗
　　　　Ex: See PDX Collection 1334

　　● S88.029　Partial traumatic amputation at knee level, **unspecified** lower leg A 🔗
　　　　Ex: See PDX Collection 1335

● S88.1　Traumatic amputation at level between knee and ankle

　● S88.11　Complete traumatic amputation at level between knee and ankle

　　● S88.111　Complete traumatic amputation at level between knee and ankle, **right** lower leg A 🔗
　　　　Ex: See PDX Collection 1333

　　● S88.112　Complete traumatic amputation at level between knee and ankle, **left** lower leg A 🔗
　　　　Ex: See PDX Collection 1334

　　● S88.119　Complete traumatic amputation at level between knee and ankle, **unspecified** lower leg A 🔗
　　　　Ex: See PDX Collection 1335

　● S88.12　Partial traumatic amputation at level between knee and ankle

　　● S88.121　Partial traumatic amputation at level between knee and ankle, **right** lower leg A 🔗
　　　　Ex: See PDX Collection 1333

　　● S88.122　Partial traumatic amputation at level between knee and ankle, **left** lower leg A 🔗
　　　　Ex: See PDX Collection 1334

　　● S88.129　Partial traumatic amputation at level between knee and ankle, **unspecified** lower leg A 🔗
　　　　Ex: See PDX Collection 1335

● S88.9　Traumatic amputation of lower leg, **level unspecified**

　● S88.91　Complete traumatic amputation of lower leg, level unspecified

　　● S88.911　Complete traumatic amputation of **right** lower leg, level unspecified A 🔗
　　　　Ex: See PDX Collection 1333

　　● S88.912　Complete traumatic amputation of **left** lower leg, level unspecified A 🔗
　　　　Ex: See PDX Collection 1334

　　● S88.919　Complete traumatic amputation of **unspecified** lower leg, level unspecified A 🔗
　　　　Ex: See PDX Collection 1335

　● S88.92　Partial traumatic amputation of lower leg, level unspecified

　　● S88.921　Partial traumatic amputation of **right** lower leg, level **unspecified** A 🔗
　　　　Ex: See PDX Collection 1333

　　● S88.922　Partial traumatic amputation of **left** lower leg, level unspecified A 🔗
　　　　Ex: See PDX Collection 1334

　　● S88.929　Partial traumatic amputation of **unspecified** lower leg, level unspecified A 🔗
　　　　Ex: See PDX Collection 1335

● S89　Other and unspecified injuries of lower leg

　Note: A fracture not indicated as open or closed should be coded to closed

　Excludes2　other and unspecified injuries of ankle and foot (S99.-)

　The appropriate 7th character is to be added to each code from subcategories S89.0, S89.1, S89.2, and S89.3

A	initial encounter for closed fracture
D	subsequent encounter for fracture with routine healing
G	subsequent encounter for fracture with delayed healing
K	subsequent encounter for fracture with nonunion
P	subsequent encounter for fracture with malunion
S	sequela

● S89.0　Physeal fracture of **upper end** of tibia

　● S89.00　Unspecified physeal fracture of upper end of tibia

　　● S89.001　Unspecified physeal fracture of upper end of **right** tibia A, K, P 🔗, A 🔗
　　　　Ex: For S89.001[A]: See PDX Collection 1340
　　　　　　For S89.001[K,P]: See PDX Collection 897

　　● S89.002　Unspecified physeal fracture of upper end of **left** tibia A, K, P 🔗, A 🔗
　　　　Ex: For S89.002[A]: See PDX Collection 1342
　　　　　　For S89.002[K,P]: See PDX Collection 897

　　● S89.009　Unspecified physeal fracture of upper end of **unspecified** tibia A, K, P 🔗, A 🔗
　　　　Ex: For S89.009[A]: See PDX Collection 1341
　　　　　　For S89.009[K,P]: See PDX Collection 897

　● S89.01　Salter-Harris Type I physeal fracture of upper end of tibia

　　● S89.011　Salter-Harris Type I physeal fracture of upper end of **right** tibia A, K, P 🔗, A 🔗
　　　　Ex: For S89.011[A]: See PDX Collection 1340
　　　　　　For S89.011[K,P]: See PDX Collection 897

　　● S89.012　Salter-Harris Type I physeal fracture of upper end of **left** tibia A, K, P 🔗, A 🔗
　　　　Ex: For S89.012[A]: See PDX Collection 1342
　　　　　　For S89.012[K,P]: See PDX Collection 897

　　● S89.019　Salter-Harris Type I physeal fracture of upper end of **unspecified** tibia A, K, P 🔗, A 🔗
　　　　Ex: For S89.019[A]: See PDX Collection 1341
　　　　　　For S89.019[K,P]: See PDX Collection 897

　● S89.02　Salter-Harris Type II physeal fracture of upper end of tibia

　　● S89.021　Salter-Harris Type II physeal fracture of upper end of **right** tibia A, K, P 🔗, A 🔗
　　　　Ex: For S89.021[A]: See PDX Collection 1340
　　　　　　For S89.021[K,P]: See PDX Collection 897

　　● S89.022　Salter-Harris Type II physeal fracture of upper end of **left** tibia A, K, P 🔗, A 🔗
　　　　Ex: For S89.022[A]: See PDX Collection 1342
　　　　　　For S89.022[K,P]: See PDX Collection 897

　　● S89.029　Salter-Harris Type II physeal fracture of upper end of **unspecified** tibia A, K, P 🔗, A 🔗
　　　　Ex: For S89.029[A]: See PDX Collection 1341
　　　　　　For S89.029[K,P]: See PDX Collection 897

▶ New　➡ Revised　~~deleted~~ Deleted　Excludes 1　Excludes 2　Includes　Use additional　Code first　Code also　Key words

OGCR Official Guidelines　● Unacceptable Principal Diagnosis　X Assign placeholder X　● Use Additional Character(s)　▶ Manifestation Code　**Coding Clinic**

● **S89.03**　Salter-Harris Type III physeal fracture of upper end of tibia

　　● **S89.031**　Salter-Harris Type III physeal fracture of upper end of right tibia A, K, P 🅒, A 🅜
　　　　Ⓔ **For S89.031[A]:** See PDX Collection 1340
　　　　　　For S89.031[K,P]: See PDX Collection 897

　　● **S89.032**　Salter-Harris Type III physeal fracture of upper end of left tibia A, K, P 🅒, A 🅜
　　　　Ⓔ **For S89.032[A]:** See PDX Collection 1342
　　　　　　For S89.032[K,P]: See PDX Collection 897

　　● **S89.039**　Salter-Harris Type III physeal fracture of upper end of unspecified tibia A, K, P 🅒, A 🅜
　　　　Ⓔ **For S89.039[A]:** See PDX Collection 1341
　　　　　　For S89.039[K,P]: See PDX Collection 897

● **S89.04**　Salter-Harris Type IV physeal fracture of upper end of tibia

　　● **S89.041**　Salter-Harris Type IV physeal fracture of upper end of right tibia A, K, P 🅒, A 🅜
　　　　Ⓔ **For S89.041[A]:** See PDX Collection 1340
　　　　　　For S89.041[K,P]: See PDX Collection 897

　　● **S89.042**　Salter-Harris Type IV physeal fracture of upper end of left tibia A, K, P 🅒, A 🅜
　　　　Ⓔ **For S89.042[A]:** See PDX Collection 1342
　　　　　　For S89.042[K,P]: See PDX Collection 897

　　● **S89.049**　Salter-Harris Type IV physeal fracture of upper end of unspecified tibia A, K, P 🅒, A 🅜
　　　　Ⓔ **For S89.049[A]:** See PDX Collection 1341
　　　　　　For S89.049[K,P]: See PDX Collection 897

● **S89.09**　Other physeal fracture of upper end of tibia

　　● **S89.091**　Other physeal fracture of upper end of right tibia A, K, P 🅒, A 🅜
　　　　Ⓔ **For S89.091[A]:** See PDX Collection 1340
　　　　　　For S89.091[K,P]: See PDX Collection 897

　　● **S89.092**　Other physeal fracture of upper end of left tibia A, K, P 🅒, A 🅜
　　　　Ⓔ **For S89.092[A]:** See PDX Collection 1342
　　　　　　For S89.092[K,P]: See PDX Collection 897

　　● **S89.099**　Other physeal fracture of upper end of unspecified tibia A, K, P 🅒, A 🅜
　　　　Ⓔ **For S89.099[A]:** See PDX Collection 1341
　　　　　　For S89.099[K,P]: See PDX Collection 897

● **S89.1**　Physeal fracture of lower end of tibia
　　Ⓔ **For category S89.1 CC codes:** See PDX Collection 897

● **S89.10**　Unspecified physeal fracture of lower end of tibia

　　● **S89.101**　Unspecified physeal fracture of lower end of right tibia K, P 🅒

　　● **S89.102**　Unspecified physeal fracture of lower end of left tibia K, P 🅒

　　● **S89.109**　Unspecified physeal fracture of lower end of unspecified tibia K, P 🅒

● **S89.11**　Salter-Harris Type I physeal fracture of lower end of tibia

　　● **S89.111**　Salter-Harris Type I physeal fracture of lower end of right tibia K, P 🅒

　　● **S89.112**　Salter-Harris Type I physeal fracture of lower end of left tibia K, P 🅒

　　● **S89.119**　Salter-Harris Type I physeal fracture of lower end of unspecified tibia K, P 🅒

● **S89.12**　Salter-Harris Type II physeal fracture of lower end of tibia

　　● **S89.121**　Salter-Harris Type II physeal fracture of lower end of right tibia K, P 🅒

　　● **S89.122**　Salter-Harris Type II physeal fracture of lower end of left tibia K, P 🅒

　　● **S89.129**　Salter-Harris Type II physeal fracture of lower end of unspecified tibia K, P 🅒

● **S89.13**　Salter-Harris Type III physeal fracture of lower end of tibia
　　Excludes1　fracture of medial malleolus (adult) (S82.5-)

　　● **S89.131**　Salter-Harris Type III physeal fracture of lower end of right tibia K, P 🅒

　　● **S89.132**　Salter-Harris Type III physeal fracture of lower end of left tibia K, P 🅒

　　● **S89.139**　Salter-Harris Type III physeal fracture of lower end of unspecified tibia K, P 🅒

● **S89.14**　Salter-Harris Type IV physeal fracture of lower end of tibia
　　Excludes1　fracture of medial malleolus (adult) (S82.5-)

　　● **S89.141**　Salter-Harris Type IV physeal fracture of lower end of right tibia K, P 🅒

　　● **S89.142**　Salter-Harris Type IV physeal fracture of lower end of left tibia K, P 🅒

　　● **S89.149**　Salter-Harris Type IV physeal fracture of lower end of unspecified tibia K, P 🅒

● **S89.19**　Other physeal fracture of lower end of tibia

　　● **S89.191**　Other physeal fracture of lower end of right tibia K, P 🅒

　　● **S89.192**　Other physeal fracture of lower end of left tibia K, P 🅒

　　● **S89.199**　Other physeal fracture of lower end of unspecified tibia K, P 🅒

● **S89.2**　Physeal fracture of upper end of fibula
　　Ⓔ **For category S89.2 CC codes:** See PDX Collection 897

● **S89.20**　Unspecified physeal fracture of upper end of fibula

　　● **S89.201**　Unspecified physeal fracture of upper end of right fibula K, P 🅒

　　● **S89.202**　Unspecified physeal fracture of upper end of left fibula K, P 🅒

　　● **S89.209**　Unspecified physeal fracture of upper end of unspecified fibula K, P 🅒

● **S89.21**　Salter-Harris Type I physeal fracture of upper end of fibula

　　● **S89.211**　Salter-Harris Type I physeal fracture of upper end of right fibula K, P 🅒

　　● **S89.212**　Salter-Harris Type I physeal fracture of upper end of left fibula K, P 🅒

　　● **S89.219**　Salter-Harris Type I physeal fracture of upper end of unspecified fibula K, P 🅒

● **S89.22**　Salter-Harris Type II physeal fracture of upper end of fibula

　　● **S89.221**　Salter-Harris Type II physeal fracture of upper end of right fibula K, P 🅒

　　● **S89.222**　Salter-Harris Type II physeal fracture of upper end of left fibula K, P 🅒

　　● **S89.229**　Salter-Harris Type II physeal fracture of upper end of unspecified fibula K, P 🅒

N Newborn Age: 0　　**P** Pediatric Age: 0–17　　**M** Maternity DX: 12–55　　**A** Adult Age: 15–124　　♀ Females Only　　♂ Males Only

🅒 Complication\Comorbidity　　🅜 Major C\C　　Ⓔ CC/MCC Exclusions　　🅗 Hospital-Acquired Condition

1387

S89.29 **Other** physeal fracture of upper end of fibula

● S89.291 Other physeal fracture of upper end of **right** fibula K, P 🔾

● S89.292 Other physeal fracture of upper end of **left** fibula K, P 🔾

● S89.299 Other physeal fracture of upper end of **unspecified** fibula K, P 🔾

● S89.3 **Physeal** fracture of lower end of fibula

Ex: For category **S89.3** CC codes: See PDX Collection 897

● S89.30 **Unspecified** physeal fracture of lower end of fibula

● S89.301 Unspecified physeal fracture of lower end of **right** fibula K, P 🔾

● S89.302 Unspecified physeal fracture of lower end of **left** fibula K, P 🔾

● S89.309 Unspecified physeal fracture of lower end of **unspecified** fibula K, P 🔾

● S89.31 **Salter-Harris Type I** physeal fracture of lower end of fibula

● S89.311 Salter-Harris Type I physeal fracture of lower end of **right** fibula K, P 🔾

● S89.312 Salter-Harris Type I physeal fracture of lower end of **left** fibula K, P 🔾

● S89.319 Salter-Harris Type I physeal fracture of lower end of **unspecified** fibula K, P 🔾

● S89.32 **Salter-Harris Type II** physeal fracture of lower end of fibula

● S89.321 Salter-Harris Type II physeal fracture of lower end of **right** fibula K, P 🔾

● S89.322 Salter-Harris Type II physeal fracture of lower end of **left** fibula K, P 🔾

● S89.329 Salter-Harris Type II physeal fracture of lower end of **unspecified** fibula K, P 🔾

● S89.39 **Other** physeal fracture of lower end of fibula

● S89.391 Other physeal fracture of lower end of **right** fibula K, P 🔾

● S89.392 Other physeal fracture of lower end of **left** fibula K, P 🔾

● S89.399 Other physeal fracture of lower end of **unspecified** fibula K, P 🔾

● S89.8 **Other specified** injuries of lower leg

The appropriate 7th character is to be added to each code in subcategory S89.8

A	initial encounter
D	subsequent encounter
S	sequela

X ● S89.80 Other specified injuries of **unspecified** lower leg

X ● S89.81 Other specified injuries of **right** lower leg

X ● S89.82 Other specified injuries of **left** lower leg

● S89.9 **Unspecified** injury of lower leg

The appropriate 7th character is to be added to each code in subcategory S89.9

A	initial encounter
D	subsequent encounter
S	sequela

X ● S89.90 Unspecified injury of **unspecified** lower leg

X ● S89.91 Unspecified injury of **right** lower leg

X ● S89.92 Unspecified injury of **left** lower leg

INJURIES TO THE ANKLE AND FOOT (S90-S99)

Excludes2 burns and corrosions (T20-T32)
fracture of ankle and malleolus (S82.-)
frostbite (T33-T34)
insect bite or sting, venomous (T63.4)

● S90 **Superficial injury of ankle, foot and toes**

The appropriate 7th character is to be added to each code from category S90

A	initial encounter
D	subsequent encounter
S	sequela

● S90.0 **Contusion of ankle**

X ● S90.00 Contusion of **unspecified** ankle

X ● S90.01 Contusion of **right** ankle

X ● S90.02 Contusion of **left** ankle

● S90.1 **Contusion of toe without damage to nail**

● S90.11 Contusion of **great** toe without damage to nail

● S90.111 Contusion of **right** great toe without damage to nail

● S90.112 Contusion of **left** great toe without damage to nail

● S90.119 Contusion of **unspecified** great toe without damage to nail

● S90.12 Contusion of **lesser** toe without damage to nail

● S90.121 Contusion of **right** lesser toe(s) without damage to nail

● S90.122 Contusion of **left** lesser toe(s) without damage to nail

● S90.129 Contusion of **unspecified** lesser toe(s) without damage to nail
Contusion of toe NOS

● S90.2 **Contusion of toe with damage to nail**

● S90.21 Contusion of **great** toe with damage to nail

● S90.211 Contusion of **right** great toe with damage to nail

● S90.212 Contusion of **left** great toe with damage to nail

● S90.219 Contusion of **unspecified** great toe with damage to nail

● S90.22 Contusion of **lesser** toe with damage to nail

● S90.221 Contusion of **right** lesser toe(s) with damage to nail

● S90.222 Contusion of **left** lesser toe(s) with damage to nail

● S90.229 Contusion of **unspecified** lesser toe(s) with damage to nail

● S90.3 **Contusion of foot**

Excludes2 contusion of toes (S90.1-, S90.2-)

X ● S90.30 Contusion of **unspecified** foot
Contusion of foot NOS

X ● S90.31 Contusion of **right** foot

X ● S90.32 Contusion of **left** foot

● S90.4 **Other superficial injuries of toe**

● S90.41 **Abrasion** of toe

● S90.411 Abrasion, **right** great toe

● S90.412 Abrasion, **left** great toe

● S90.413 Abrasion, **unspecified** great toe

● S90.414 Abrasion, **right** lesser toe(s)

● S90.415 Abrasion, **left** lesser toe(s)

● S90.416 Abrasion, **unspecified** lesser toe(s)

▶ New   ➡ Revised   ~~deleted~~ Deleted   Excludes 1   Excludes 2   Includes   Use additional   Code first   Code also   Key words

OGCR Official Guidelines   ● Unacceptable Principal Diagnosis   X Assign placeholder X   ● Use Additional Character(s)   ▶ Manifestation Code   Coding Clinic

● S90.42 Blister (nonthermal) of toe
   ● S90.421 Blister (nonthermal), right great toe
   ● S90.422 Blister (nonthermal), left great toe
   ● S90.423 Blister (nonthermal), unspecified great toe
   ● S90.424 Blister (nonthermal), right lesser toe(s)
   ● S90.425 Blister (nonthermal), left lesser toe(s)
   ● S90.426 Blister (nonthermal), unspecified lesser toe(s)

● S90.44 External constriction of toe
   Hair tourniquet syndrome of toe
   ● S90.441 External constriction, right great toe
   ● S90.442 External constriction, left great toe
   ● S90.443 External constriction, unspecified great toe
   ● S90.444 External constriction, right lesser toe(s)
   ● S90.445 External constriction, left lesser toe(s)
   ● S90.446 External constriction, unspecified lesser toe(s)

● S90.45 Superficial foreign body of toe
   Splinter in the toe
   ● S90.451 Superficial foreign body, right great toe
   ● S90.452 Superficial foreign body, left great toe
   ● S90.453 Superficial foreign body, unspecified great toe
   ● S90.454 Superficial foreign body, right lesser toe(s)
   ● S90.455 Superficial foreign body, left lesser toe(s)
   ● S90.456 Superficial foreign body, unspecified lesser toe(s)

● S90.46 Insect bite (nonvenomous) of toe
   ● S90.461 Insect bite (nonvenomous), right great toe
   ● S90.462 Insect bite (nonvenomous), left great toe
   ● S90.463 Insect bite (nonvenomous), unspecified great toe
   ● S90.464 Insect bite (nonvenomous), right lesser toe(s)
   ● S90.465 Insect bite (nonvenomous), left lesser toe(s)
   ● S90.466 Insect bite (nonvenomous), unspecified lesser toe(s)

● S90.47 Other superficial bite of toe
   Excludes1   open bite of toe (S91.15-, S91.25-)
   ● S90.471 Other superficial bite of right great toe
   ● S90.472 Other superficial bite of left great toe
   ● S90.473 Other superficial bite of unspecified great toe
   ● S90.474 Other superficial bite of right lesser toe(s)
   ● S90.475 Other superficial bite of left lesser toe(s)
   ● S90.476 Other superficial bite of unspecified lesser toe(s)

● S90.5 Other superficial injuries of ankle
  ● S90.51 Abrasion of ankle
   ● S90.511 Abrasion, right ankle
   ● S90.512 Abrasion, left ankle
   ● S90.519 Abrasion, unspecified ankle

● S90.52 Blister (nonthermal) of ankle
   ● S90.521 Blister (nonthermal), right ankle
   ● S90.522 Blister (nonthermal), left ankle
   ● S90.529 Blister (nonthermal), unspecified ankle

● S90.54 External constriction of ankle
   ● S90.541 External constriction, right ankle
   ● S90.542 External constriction, left ankle
   ● S90.549 External constriction, unspecified ankle

● S90.55 Superficial foreign body of ankle
   Splinter in the ankle
   ● S90.551 Superficial foreign body, right ankle
   ● S90.552 Superficial foreign body, left ankle
   ● S90.559 Superficial foreign body, unspecified ankle

● S90.56 Insect bite (nonvenomous) of ankle
   ● S90.561 Insect bite (nonvenomous), right ankle
   ● S90.562 Insect bite (nonvenomous), left ankle
   ● S90.569 Insect bite (nonvenomous), unspecified ankle

● S90.57 Other superficial bite of ankle
   Excludes1   open bite of ankle (S91.05-)
   ● S90.571 Other superficial bite of ankle, right ankle
   ● S90.572 Other superficial bite of ankle, left ankle
   ● S90.579 Other superficial bite of ankle, unspecified ankle

● S90.8 Other superficial injuries of foot
  ● S90.81 Abrasion of foot
   ● S90.811 Abrasion, right foot
   ● S90.812 Abrasion, left foot
   ● S90.819 Abrasion, unspecified foot

  ● S90.82 Blister (nonthermal) of foot
   ● S90.821 Blister (nonthermal), right foot
   ● S90.822 Blister (nonthermal), left foot
   ● S90.829 Blister (nonthermal), unspecified foot

  ● S90.84 External constriction of foot
   ● S90.841 External constriction, right foot
   ● S90.842 External constriction, left foot
   ● S90.849 External constriction, unspecified foot

  ● S90.85 Superficial foreign body of foot
   Splinter in the foot
   ● S90.851 Superficial foreign body, right foot
   ● S90.852 Superficial foreign body, left foot
   ● S90.859 Superficial foreign body, unspecified foot

  ● S90.86 Insect bite (nonvenomous) of foot
   ● S90.861 Insect bite (nonvenomous), right foot
   ● S90.862 Insect bite (nonvenomous), left foot
   ● S90.869 Insect bite (nonvenomous), unspecified foot

  ● S90.87 Other superficial bite of foot
   Excludes1   open bite of foot (S91.35-)
   ● S90.871 Other superficial bite of right foot
   ● S90.872 Other superficial bite of left foot
   ● S90.879 Other superficial bite of unspecified foot

CHAPTER 19 (S00-T88)

N Newborn Age: 0   P Pediatric Age: 0–17   M Maternity DX: 12–55   A Adult Age: 15–124   ♀ Females Only   ♂ Males Only
    🝔 Complication\Comorbidity   🝔 Major C\C   Ⓔ CC/MCC Exclusions   🝔 Hospital-Acquired Condition

- **S90.9 Unspecified superficial injury of ankle, foot and toe**
  - **S90.91 Unspecified superficial injury of ankle**
    - S90.911 Unspecified superficial injury of right ankle
    - S90.912 Unspecified superficial injury of left ankle
    - S90.919 Unspecified superficial injury of unspecified ankle
  - **S90.92 Unspecified superficial injury of foot**
    - S90.921 Unspecified superficial injury of right foot
    - S90.922 Unspecified superficial injury of left foot
    - S90.929 Unspecified superficial injury of unspecified foot
  - **S90.93 Unspecified superficial injury of toes**
    - S90.931 Unspecified superficial injury of right great toe
    - S90.932 Unspecified superficial injury of left great toe
    - S90.933 Unspecified superficial injury of unspecified great toe
    - S90.934 Unspecified superficial injury of right lesser toe(s)
    - S90.935 Unspecified superficial injury of left lesser toe(s)
    - S90.936 Unspecified superficial injury of unspecified lesser toe(s)

- **S91 Open wound of ankle, foot and toes**

  Code also any associated wound infection

  Excludes1   open fracture of ankle, foot and toes (S92.-with 7th character B)
               traumatic amputation of ankle and foot (S98.-)

  The appropriate 7th character is to be added to each code from category S91

A	initial encounter
D	subsequent encounter
S	sequela

  - **S91.0 Open wound of ankle**
    - **S91.00 Unspecified open wound of ankle**
      - S91.001 Unspecified open wound, right ankle
      - S91.002 Unspecified open wound, left ankle
      - S91.009 Unspecified open wound, unspecified ankle
    - **S91.01 Laceration without foreign body of ankle**
      - S91.011 Laceration without foreign body, right ankle
      - S91.012 Laceration without foreign body, left ankle
      - S91.019 Laceration without foreign body, unspecified ankle
    - **S91.02 Laceration with foreign body of ankle**
      - S91.021 Laceration with foreign body, right ankle
      - S91.022 Laceration with foreign body, left ankle
      - S91.029 Laceration with foreign body, unspecified ankle
    - **S91.03 Puncture wound without foreign body of ankle**
      - S91.031 Puncture wound without foreign body, right ankle
      - S91.032 Puncture wound without foreign body, left ankle
      - S91.039 Puncture wound without foreign body, unspecified ankle

  - **S91.04 Puncture wound with foreign body of ankle**
    - S91.041 Puncture wound with foreign body, right ankle
    - S91.042 Puncture wound with foreign body, left ankle
    - S91.049 Puncture wound with foreign body, unspecified ankle
  - **S91.05 Open bite of ankle**
    Excludes1   superficial bite of ankle (S90.56-, S90.57-)
    - S91.051 Open bite, right ankle
    - S91.052 Open bite, left ankle
    - S91.059 Open bite, unspecified ankle

  - **S91.1 Open wound of toe without damage to nail**
    - **S91.10 Unspecified open wound of toe without damage to nail**
      - S91.101 Unspecified open wound of right great toe without damage to nail
      - S91.102 Unspecified open wound of left great toe without damage to nail
      - S91.103 Unspecified open wound of unspecified great toe without damage to nail
      - S91.104 Unspecified open wound of right lesser toe(s) without damage to nail
      - S91.105 Unspecified open wound of left lesser toe(s) without damage to nail
      - S91.106 Unspecified open wound of unspecified lesser toe(s) without damage to nail
      - S91.109 Unspecified open wound of unspecified toe(s) without damage to nail
    - **S91.11 Laceration without foreign body of toe without damage to nail**
      - S91.111 Laceration without foreign body of right great toe without damage to nail
      - S91.112 Laceration without foreign body of left great toe without damage to nail
      - S91.113 Laceration without foreign body of unspecified great toe without damage to nail
      - S91.114 Laceration without foreign body of right lesser toe(s) without damage to nail
      - S91.115 Laceration without foreign body of left lesser toe(s) without damage to nail
      - S91.116 Laceration without foreign body of unspecified lesser toe(s) without damage to nail
      - S91.119 Laceration without foreign body of unspecified toe without damage to nail
    - **S91.12 Laceration with foreign body of toe without damage to nail**
      - S91.121 Laceration with foreign body of right great toe without damage to nail
      - S91.122 Laceration with foreign body of left great toe without damage to nail
      - S91.123 Laceration with foreign body of unspecified great toe without damage to nail
      - S91.124 Laceration with foreign body of right lesser toe(s) without damage to nail

▶ New   ⇒ Revised   deleted Deleted   Excludes 1   Excludes 2   Includes   Use additional   Code first   Code also   Key words

OGCR Official Guidelines   ● Unacceptable Principal Diagnosis   X Assign placeholder X   ● Use Additional Character(s)   ▶ Manifestation Code   **Coding Clinic**

● S91.125   Laceration with foreign body of left lesser toe(s) without damage to nail

● S91.126   Laceration with foreign body of unspecified lesser toe(s) without damage to nail

● S91.129   Laceration with foreign body of unspecified toe(s) without damage to nail

● S91.13   Puncture wound without foreign body of toe without damage to nail

  ● S91.131   Puncture wound without foreign body of right great toe without damage to nail

  ● S91.132   Puncture wound without foreign body of left great toe without damage to nail

  ● S91.133   Puncture wound without foreign body of unspecified great toe without damage to nail

  ● S91.134   Puncture wound without foreign body of right lesser toe(s) without damage to nail

  ● S91.135   Puncture wound without foreign body of left lesser toe(s) without damage to nail

  ● S91.136   Puncture wound without foreign body of unspecified lesser toe(s) without damage to nail

  ● S91.139   Puncture wound without foreign body of unspecified toe(s) without damage to nail

● S91.14   Puncture wound with foreign body of toe without damage to nail

  ● S91.141   Puncture wound with foreign body of right great toe without damage to nail

  ● S91.142   Puncture wound with foreign body of left great toe without damage to nail

  ● S91.143   Puncture wound with foreign body of unspecified great toe without damage to nail

  ● S91.144   Puncture wound with foreign body of right lesser toe(s) without damage to nail

  ● S91.145   Puncture wound with foreign body of left lesser toe(s) without damage to nail

  ● S91.146   Puncture wound with foreign body of unspecified lesser toe(s) without damage to nail

  ● S91.149   Puncture wound with foreign body of unspecified toe(s) without damage to nail

● S91.15   Open bite of toe without damage to nail
Bite of toe NOS

> **Excludes1**   superficial bite of toe (S90.46-, S90.47-)

  ● S91.151   Open bite of right great toe without damage to nail

  ● S91.152   Open bite of left great toe without damage to nail

  ● S91.153   Open bite of unspecified great toe without damage to nail

  ● S91.154   Open bite of right lesser toe(s) without damage to nail

  ● S91.155   Open bite of left lesser toe(s) without damage to nail

  ● S91.156   Open bite of unspecified lesser toe(s) without damage to nail

  ● S91.159   Open bite of unspecified toe(s) without damage to nail

● S91.2   Open wound of toe with damage to nail

● S91.20   Unspecified open wound of toe with damage to nail

  ● S91.201   Unspecified open wound of right great toe with damage to nail

  ● S91.202   Unspecified open wound of left great toe with damage to nail

  ● S91.203   Unspecified open wound of unspecified great toe with damage to nail

  ● S91.204   Unspecified open wound of right lesser toe(s) with damage to nail

  ● S91.205   Unspecified open wound of left lesser toe(s) with damage to nail

  ● S91.206   Unspecified open wound of unspecified lesser toe(s) with damage to nail

  ● S91.209   Unspecified open wound of unspecified toe(s) with damage to nail

● S91.21   Laceration without foreign body of toe with damage to nail

  ● S91.211   Laceration without foreign body of right great toe with damage to nail

  ● S91.212   Laceration without foreign body of left great toe with damage to nail

  ● S91.213   Laceration without foreign body of unspecified great toe with damage to nail

  ● S91.214   Laceration without foreign body of right lesser toe(s) with damage to nail

  ● S91.215   Laceration without foreign body of left lesser toe(s) with damage to nail

  ● S91.216   Laceration without foreign body of unspecified lesser toe(s) with damage to nail

  ● S91.219   Laceration without foreign body of unspecified toe(s) with damage to nail

● S91.22   Laceration with foreign body of toe with damage to nail

  ● S91.221   Laceration with foreign body of right great toe with damage to nail

  ● S91.222   Laceration with foreign body of left great toe with damage to nail

  ● S91.223   Laceration with foreign body of unspecified great toe with damage to nail

  ● S91.224   Laceration with foreign body of right lesser toe(s) with damage to nail

  ● S91.225   Laceration with foreign body of left lesser toe(s) with damage to nail

  ● S91.226   Laceration with foreign body of unspecified lesser toe(s) with damage to nail

  ● S91.229   Laceration with foreign body of unspecified toe(s) with damage to nail

CHAPTER 19 (S00-T88)

● **S91.23** **Puncture wound without foreign body** of toe with damage to nail

    ● **S91.231** Puncture wound without foreign body of **right great** toe with damage to nail

    ● **S91.232** Puncture wound without foreign body of **left great** toe with damage to nail

    ● **S91.233** Puncture wound without foreign body of **unspecified great** toe with damage to nail

    ● **S91.234** Puncture wound without foreign body of **right lesser** toe(s) with damage to nail

    ● **S91.235** Puncture wound without foreign body of **left lesser** toe(s) with damage to nail

    ● **S91.236** Puncture wound without foreign body of **unspecified lesser** toe(s) with damage to nail

    ● **S91.239** Puncture wound without foreign body of **unspecified** toe(s) with damage to nail

● **S91.24** **Puncture wound with foreign body** of toe with damage to nail

    ● **S91.241** Puncture wound with foreign body of **right great** toe with damage to nail

    ● **S91.242** Puncture wound with foreign body of **left great** toe with damage to nail

    ● **S91.243** Puncture wound with foreign body of **unspecified great** toe with damage to nail

    ● **S91.244** Puncture wound with foreign body of **right lesser** toe(s) with damage to nail

    ● **S91.245** Puncture wound with foreign body of **left lesser** toe(s) with damage to nail

    ● **S91.246** Puncture wound with foreign body of **unspecified lesser** toe(s) with damage to nail

    ● **S91.249** Puncture wound with foreign body of **unspecified** toe(s) with damage to nail

● **S91.25** **Open bite** of toe with damage to nail

    Bite of toe with damage to nail NOS

    Excludes1 superficial bite of toe (S90.46-, S90.47-)

    ● **S91.251** Open bite of **right great** toe with damage to nail

    ● **S91.252** Open bite of **left great** toe with damage to nail

    ● **S91.253** Open bite of **unspecified great** toe with damage to nail

    ● **S91.254** Open bite of **right lesser** toe(s) with damage to nail

    ● **S91.255** Open bite of **left lesser** toe(s) with damage to nail

    ● **S91.256** Open bite of **unspecified lesser** toe(s) with damage to nail

    ● **S91.259** Open bite of **unspecified** toe(s) with damage to nail

● **S91.3** **Open wound** of foot

  ● **S91.30** **Unspecified open wound** of foot

    ● **S91.301** Unspecified open wound, **right foot**

    ● **S91.302** Unspecified open wound, **left foot**

    ● **S91.309** Unspecified open wound, **unspecified** foot

● **S91.31** **Laceration without foreign body** of foot

    ● **S91.311** Laceration without foreign body, **right** foot

    ● **S91.312** Laceration without foreign body, **left** foot

    ● **S91.319** Laceration without foreign body, **unspecified** foot

● **S91.32** **Laceration with foreign body** of foot

    ● **S91.321** Laceration with foreign body, **right** foot

    ● **S91.322** Laceration with foreign body, **left foot**

    ● **S91.329** Laceration with foreign body, **unspecified** foot

● **S91.33** **Puncture wound without foreign body** of foot

    ● **S91.331** Puncture wound without foreign body, **right foot**

    ● **S91.332** Puncture wound without foreign body, **left foot**

    ● **S91.339** Puncture wound without foreign body, **unspecified** foot

● **S91.34** **Puncture wound with foreign body** of foot

    ● **S91.341** Puncture wound with foreign body, **right foot**

    ● **S91.342** Puncture wound with foreign body, **left foot**

    ● **S91.349** Puncture wound with foreign body, **unspecified** foot

● **S91.35** **Open bite** of foot

    Excludes1 superficial bite of foot (S90.86-, S90.87-)

    ● **S91.351** Open bite, **right foot**

    ● **S91.352** Open bite, **left foot**

    ● **S91.359** Open bite, **unspecified foot**

● **S92** **Fracture of foot and toe, except ankle**

  Note: A fracture not indicated as displaced or nondisplaced should be coded to displaced

      A fracture not indicated as open or closed should be coded to closed

  Excludes1 traumatic amputation of ankle and foot (S98.-)

  Excludes2 fracture of ankle (S82.-)

                 fracture of malleolus (S82.-)

  The appropriate 7th character is to be added to each code from category S92

A	initial encounter for closed fracture
B	initial encounter for open fracture
D	subsequent encounter for fracture with routine healing
G	subsequent encounter for fracture with delayed healing
K	subsequent encounter for fracture with nonunion
P	subsequent encounter for fracture with malunion
S	sequela

● **S92.0** **Fracture of calcaneus**

    Heel bone   Os calcis

    Excludes2 Physeal fracture of calcaneus (S99.0-)

    Ⓔⓧ **For category S92.0 CC codes S92.0[B]:** See PDX Collection 1367

             For S92.0[K,P]: See PDX Collection 897

  ● **S92.00** **Unspecified fracture of calcaneus**

    ● **S92.001** Unspecified fracture of **right** calcaneus
             B, K, P 🔖, B 🔖

    ● **S92.002** Unspecified fracture of **left** calcaneus
             B, K, P 🔖, B 🔖

    ● **S92.009** Unspecified fracture of **unspecified** calcaneus B, K, P 🔖, B 🔖

● **S92.01   Fracture of body of calcaneus**
    ● S92.011   Displaced fracture of body of right calcaneus B, K, P 🔹, B 🔸
    ● S92.012   Displaced fracture of body of left calcaneus B, K, P 🔹, B 🔸
    ● S92.013   Displaced fracture of body of unspecified calcaneus B, K, P 🔹, B 🔸
    ● S92.014   Nondisplaced fracture of body of right calcaneus B, K, P 🔹, B 🔸
    ● S92.015   Nondisplaced fracture of body of left calcaneus B, K, P 🔹, B 🔸
    ● S92.016   Nondisplaced fracture of body of unspecified calcaneus B, K, P 🔹, B 🔸

● **S92.02   Fracture of anterior process of calcaneus**
    ● S92.021   Displaced fracture of anterior process of right calcaneus B, K, P 🔹, B 🔸
    ● S92.022   Displaced fracture of anterior process of left calcaneus B, K, P 🔹, B 🔸
    ● S92.023   Displaced fracture of anterior process of unspecified calcaneus B, K, P 🔹, B 🔸
    ● S92.024   Nondisplaced fracture of anterior process of right calcaneus B, K, P 🔹, B 🔸
    ● S92.025   Nondisplaced fracture of anterior process of left calcaneus B, K, P 🔹, B 🔸
    ● S92.026   Nondisplaced fracture of anterior process of unspecified calcaneus B, K, P 🔹, B 🔸

● **S92.03   Avulsion fracture of tuberosity of calcaneus**
    ● S92.031   Displaced avulsion fracture of tuberosity of right calcaneus B, K, P 🔹, B 🔸
    ● S92.032   Displaced avulsion fracture of tuberosity of left calcaneus B, K, P 🔹, B 🔸
    ● S92.033   Displaced avulsion fracture of tuberosity of unspecified calcaneus B, K, P 🔹, B 🔸
    ● S92.034   Nondisplaced avulsion fracture of tuberosity of right calcaneus B, K, P 🔹, B 🔸
    ● S92.035   Nondisplaced avulsion fracture of tuberosity of left calcaneus B, K, P 🔹, B 🔸
    ● S92.036   Nondisplaced avulsion fracture of tuberosity of unspecified calcaneus B, K, P 🔹, B 🔸

● **S92.04   Other fracture of tuberosity of calcaneus**
    ● S92.041   Displaced other fracture of tuberosity of right calcaneus B, K, P 🔹, B 🔸
    ● S92.042   Displaced other fracture of tuberosity of left calcaneus B, K, P 🔹, B 🔸
    ● S92.043   Displaced other fracture of tuberosity of unspecified calcaneus B, K, P 🔹, B 🔸
    ● S92.044   Nondisplaced other fracture of tuberosity of right calcaneus B, K, P 🔹, B 🔸
    ● S92.045   Nondisplaced other fracture of tuberosity of left calcaneus B, K, P 🔹, B 🔸
    ● S92.046   Nondisplaced other fracture of tuberosity of unspecified calcaneus B, K, P 🔹, B 🔸

● **S92.05   Other extraarticular fracture of calcaneus**
    ● S92.051   Displaced other extraarticular fracture of right calcaneus B, K, P 🔹, B 🔸
    ● S92.052   Displaced other extraarticular fracture of left calcaneus B, K, P 🔹, B 🔸
    ● S92.053   Displaced other extraarticular fracture of unspecified calcaneus B, K, P 🔹, B 🔸
    ● S92.054   Nondisplaced other extraarticular fracture of right calcaneus B, K, P 🔹, B 🔸
    ● S92.055   Nondisplaced other extraarticular fracture of left calcaneus B, K, P 🔹, B 🔸
    ● S92.056   Nondisplaced other extraarticular fracture of unspecified calcaneus B, K, P 🔹, B 🔸

● **S92.06   Intraarticular fracture of calcaneus**
    ● S92.061   Displaced intraarticular fracture of right calcaneus B, K, P 🔹, B 🔸
    ● S92.062   Displaced intraarticular fracture of left calcaneus B, K, P 🔹, B 🔸
    ● S92.063   Displaced intraarticular fracture of unspecified calcaneus B, K, P 🔹, B 🔸
    ● S92.064   Nondisplaced intraarticular fracture of right calcaneus B, K, P 🔹, B 🔸
    ● S92.065   Nondisplaced intraarticular fracture of left calcaneus B, K, P 🔹, B 🔸
    ● S92.066   Nondisplaced intraarticular fracture of unspecified calcaneus B, K, P 🔹, B 🔸

● **S92.1   Fracture of talus**
    Astragalus
    (Ex) For category S92.1 CC codes S92.1[B]: See PDX Collection 1368
        For S92.1[K,P]: See PDX Collection 897

    ● **S92.10   Unspecified fracture of talus**
       ● S92.101   Unspecified fracture of right talus B, K, P 🔹, B 🔸
       ● S92.102   Unspecified fracture of left talus B, K, P 🔹, B 🔸
       ● S92.109   Unspecified fracture of unspecified talus B, K, P 🔹, B 🔸

    ● **S92.11   Fracture of neck of talus**
       ● S92.111   Displaced fracture of neck of right talus B, K, P 🔹, B 🔸
       ● S92.112   Displaced fracture of neck of left talus B, K, P 🔹, B 🔸
       ● S92.113   Displaced fracture of neck of unspecified talus B, K, P 🔹, B 🔸
       ● S92.114   Nondisplaced fracture of neck of right talus B, K, P 🔹, B 🔸
       ● S92.115   Nondisplaced fracture of neck of left talus B, K, P 🔹, B 🔸
       ● S92.116   Nondisplaced fracture of neck of unspecified talus B, K, P 🔹, B 🔸

    ● **S92.12   Fracture of body of talus**
       ● S92.121   Displaced fracture of body of right talus B, K, P 🔹, B 🔸
       ● S92.122   Displaced fracture of body of left talus B, K, P 🔹, B 🔸
       ● S92.123   Displaced fracture of body of unspecified talus B, K, P 🔹, B 🔸
       ● S92.124   Nondisplaced fracture of body of right talus B, K, P 🔹, B 🔸
       ● S92.125   Nondisplaced fracture of body of left talus B, K, P 🔹, B 🔸
       ● S92.126   Nondisplaced fracture of body of unspecified talus B, K, P 🔹, B 🔸

CHAPTER 19 (S00–T88)

N   Newborn Age: 0   P   Pediatric Age: 0–17   M   Maternity DX: 12–55   A   Adult Age: 15–124   ♀   Females Only   ♂   Males Only
🔹   Complication\Comorbidity   🔸   Major C\C   (Ex)   CC/MCC Exclusions   🔹   Hospital-Acquired Condition
1393

CHAPTER 19 (S00-T88)

- S92.13 Fracture of posterior process of talus
  - S92.131 Displaced fracture of posterior process of right talus B, K, P, B
  - S92.132 Displaced fracture of posterior process of left talus B, K, P, B
  - S92.133 Displaced fracture of posterior process of unspecified talus B, K, P, B
  - S92.134 Nondisplaced fracture of posterior process of right talus B, K, P, B
  - S92.135 Nondisplaced fracture of posterior process of left talus B, K, P, B
  - S92.136 Nondisplaced fracture of posterior process of unspecified talus B, K, P, B
- S92.14 Dome fracture of talus
  - **Excludes1** osteochondritis dissecans (M93.2)
  - S92.141 Displaced dome fracture of right talus B, K, P, B
  - S92.142 Displaced dome fracture of left talus B, K, P, B
  - S92.143 Displaced dome fracture of unspecified talus B, K, P, B
  - S92.144 Nondisplaced dome fracture of right talus B, K, P, B
  - S92.145 Nondisplaced dome fracture of left talus B, K, P, B
  - S92.146 Nondisplaced dome fracture of unspecified talus B, K, P, B
- S92.15 Avulsion fracture (chip fracture) of talus
  - S92.151 Displaced avulsion fracture (chip fracture) of right talus B, K, P, B
  - S92.152 Displaced avulsion fracture (chip fracture) of left talus B, K, P, B
  - S92.153 Displaced avulsion fracture (chip fracture) of unspecified talus B, K, P, B
  - S92.154 Nondisplaced avulsion fracture (chip fracture) of right talus B, K, P, B
  - S92.155 Nondisplaced avulsion fracture (chip fracture) of left talus B, K, P, B
  - S92.156 Nondisplaced avulsion fracture (chip fracture) of unspecified talus B, K, P, B
- S92.19 Other fracture of talus
  - S92.191 Other fracture of right talus B, K, P, B
  - S92.192 Other fracture of left talus B, K, P, B
  - S92.199 Other fracture of unspecified talus B, K, P, B
- S92.2 Fracture of other and unspecified tarsal bone(s)
  - (Ex) For category S92.2 CC codes S92.2[B]: See PDX Collection 1368
    For S92.2[K,P]: See PDX Collection 897 unless otherwise indicated
  - S92.20 Fracture of unspecified tarsal bone(s)
    - (Ex) For category S92.20 CC codes S92.20[B]: See PDX Collection 1369 For S92.20[K,P]: See PDX Collection 897
    - S92.201 Fracture of unspecified tarsal bone(s) of right foot B, K, P, B
    - S92.202 Fracture of unspecified tarsal bone(s) of left foot B, K, P, B
    - S92.209 Fracture of unspecified tarsal bone(s) of unspecified foot B, K, P, B

- S92.21 Fracture of cuboid bone
  - S92.211 Displaced fracture of cuboid bone of right foot B, K, P, B
  - S92.212 Displaced fracture of cuboid bone of left foot B, K, P, B
  - S92.213 Displaced fracture of cuboid bone of unspecified foot B, K, P, B
  - S92.214 Nondisplaced fracture of cuboid bone of right foot B, K, P, B
  - S92.215 Nondisplaced fracture of cuboid bone of left foot B, K, P, B
  - S92.216 Nondisplaced fracture of cuboid bone of unspecified foot B, K, P, B
- S92.22 Fracture of lateral cuneiform
  - S92.221 Displaced fracture of lateral cuneiform of right foot B, K, P, B
  - S92.222 Displaced fracture of lateral cuneiform of left foot B, K, P, B
  - S92.223 Displaced fracture of lateral cuneiform of unspecified foot B, K, P, B
  - S92.224 Nondisplaced fracture of lateral cuneiform of right foot B, K, P, B
  - S92.225 Nondisplaced fracture of lateral cuneiform of left foot B, K, P, B
  - S92.226 Nondisplaced fracture of lateral cuneiform of unspecified foot B, K, P, B
- S92.23 Fracture of intermediate cuneiform
  - S92.231 Displaced fracture of intermediate cuneiform of right foot B, K, P, B
  - S92.232 Displaced fracture of intermediate cuneiform of left foot B, K, P, B
  - S92.233 Displaced fracture of intermediate cuneiform of unspecified foot B, K, P, B
  - S92.234 Nondisplaced fracture of intermediate cuneiform of right foot B, K, P, B
  - S92.235 Nondisplaced fracture of intermediate cuneiform of left foot B, K, P, B
  - S92.236 Nondisplaced fracture of intermediate cuneiform of unspecified foot B, K, P, B
- S92.24 Fracture of medial cuneiform
  - S92.241 Displaced fracture of medial cuneiform of right foot B, K, P, B
  - S92.242 Displaced fracture of medial cuneiform of left foot B, K, P, B
  - S92.243 Displaced fracture of medial cuneiform of unspecified foot B, K, P, B
  - S92.244 Nondisplaced fracture of medial cuneiform of right foot B, K, P, B
  - S92.245 Nondisplaced fracture of medial cuneiform of left foot B, K, P, B
  - S92.246 Nondisplaced fracture of medial cuneiform of unspecified foot B, K, P, B

▶ New ⇒ Revised ~~deleted~~ Deleted | Excludes 1 | Excludes 2 | Includes | Use additional | Code first | Code also | Key words | OGCR Official Guidelines ● Unacceptable Principal Diagnosis X Assign placeholder X ● Use Additional Character(s) ▮ Manifestation Code **Coding Clinic**

● **S92.25   Fracture of navicular [scaphoid] of foot**
  ● S92.251   Displaced fracture of navicular [scaphoid] of right foot B, K, P 🅒, B 🅜
  ● S92.252   Displaced fracture of navicular [scaphoid] of left foot B, K, P 🅒, B 🅜
  ● S92.253   Displaced fracture of navicular [scaphoid] of unspecified foot B, K, P 🅒, B 🅜
  ● S92.254   Nondisplaced fracture of navicular [scaphoid] of right foot B, K, P 🅒, B 🅜
  ● S92.255   Nondisplaced fracture of navicular [scaphoid] of left foot B, K, P 🅒, B 🅜
  ● S92.256   Nondisplaced fracture of navicular [scaphoid] of unspecified foot B, K, P 🅒, B 🅜

● **S92.3   Fracture of metatarsal bone(s)**
  Excludes2   Physeal fracture of metatarsal (S99.1-)
  (Ex) For category S92.3 CC codes S92.3[B]: See PDX Collection 1368
       For S92.3[K,P]: See PDX Collection 897
  ● **S92.30   Fracture of unspecified metatarsal bone(s)**
    ● S92.301   Fracture of unspecified metatarsal bone(s), right foot B, K, P 🅒, B 🅜
    ● S92.302   Fracture of unspecified metatarsal bone(s), left foot B, K, P 🅒, B 🅜
    ● S92.309   Fracture of unspecified metatarsal bone(s), unspecified foot B, K, P 🅒, B 🅜
  ● **S92.31   Fracture of first metatarsal bone**
    ● S92.311   Displaced fracture of first metatarsal bone, right foot B, K, P 🅒, B 🅜
    ● S92.312   Displaced fracture of first metatarsal bone, left foot B, K, P 🅒, B 🅜
    ● S92.313   Displaced fracture of first metatarsal bone, unspecified foot B, K, P 🅒, B 🅜
    ● S92.314   Nondisplaced fracture of first metatarsal bone, right foot B, K, P 🅒, B 🅜
    ● S92.315   Nondisplaced fracture of first metatarsal bone, left foot B, K, P 🅒, B 🅜
    ● S92.316   Nondisplaced fracture of first metatarsal bone, unspecified foot B, K, P 🅒, B 🅜
  ● **S92.32   Fracture of second metatarsal bone**
    ● S92.321   Displaced fracture of second metatarsal bone, right foot B, K, P 🅒, B 🅜
    ● S92.322   Displaced fracture of second metatarsal bone, left foot B, K, P 🅒, B 🅜
    ● S92.323   Displaced fracture of second metatarsal bone, unspecified foot B, K, P 🅒, B 🅜
    ● S92.324   Nondisplaced fracture of second metatarsal bone, right foot B, K, P 🅒, B 🅜
    ● S92.325   Nondisplaced fracture of second metatarsal bone, left foot B, K, P 🅒, B 🅜
    ● S92.326   Nondisplaced fracture of second metatarsal bone, unspecified foot B, K, P 🅒, B 🅜

● **S92.33   Fracture of third metatarsal bone**
  ● S92.331   Displaced fracture of third metatarsal bone, right foot B, K, P 🅒, B 🅜
  ● S92.332   Displaced fracture of third metatarsal bone, left foot B, K, P 🅒, B 🅜
  ● S92.333   Displaced fracture of third metatarsal bone, unspecified foot B, K, P 🅒, B 🅜
  ● S92.334   Nondisplaced fracture of third metatarsal bone, right foot B, K, P 🅒, B 🅜
  ● S92.335   Nondisplaced fracture of third metatarsal bone, left foot B, K, P 🅒, B 🅜
  ● S92.336   Nondisplaced fracture of third metatarsal bone, unspecified foot B, K, P 🅒, B 🅜
● **S92.34   Fracture of fourth metatarsal bone**
  ● S92.341   Displaced fracture of fourth metatarsal bone, right foot B, K, P 🅒, B 🅜
  ● S92.342   Displaced fracture of fourth metatarsal bone, left foot B, K, P 🅒, B 🅜
  ● S92.343   Displaced fracture of fourth metatarsal bone, unspecified foot B, K, P 🅒, B 🅜
  ● S92.344   Nondisplaced fracture of fourth metatarsal bone, right foot B, K, P 🅒, B 🅜
  ● S92.345   Nondisplaced fracture of fourth metatarsal bone, left foot B, K, P 🅒, B 🅜
  ● S92.346   Nondisplaced fracture of fourth metatarsal bone, unspecified foot B, K, P 🅒, B 🅜
● **S92.35   Fracture of fifth metatarsal bone**
  ● S92.351   Displaced fracture of fifth metatarsal bone, right foot B, K, P 🅒, B 🅜
  ● S92.352   Displaced fracture of fifth metatarsal bone, left foot B, K, P 🅒, B 🅜
  ● S92.353   Displaced fracture of fifth metatarsal bone, unspecified foot B, K, P 🅒, B 🅜
  ● S92.354   Nondisplaced fracture of fifth metatarsal bone, right foot B, K, P 🅒, B 🅜
  ● S92.355   Nondisplaced fracture of fifth metatarsal bone, left foot B, K, P 🅒, B 🅜
  ● S92.356   Nondisplaced fracture of fifth metatarsal bone, unspecified foot B, K, P 🅒, B 🅜
● **S92.4   Fracture of great toe**
  Excludes2   Physeal fracture of phalanx of toe (S99.2-)
  (Ex) For category S92.4 CC codes: See PDX Collection 897
  ● **S92.40   Unspecified fracture of great toe**
    ● S92.401   Displaced unspecified fracture of right great toe K, P 🅒
    ● S92.402   Displaced unspecified fracture of left great toe K, P 🅒
    ● S92.403   Displaced unspecified fracture of unspecified great toe K, P 🅒
    ● S92.404   Nondisplaced unspecified fracture of right great toe K, P 🅒
    ● S92.405   Nondisplaced unspecified fracture of left great toe K, P 🅒
    ● S92.406   Nondisplaced unspecified fracture of unspecified great toe K, P 🅒

CHAPTER 19 (S00-T88)

● S92.41   Fracture of proximal phalanx of great toe
- ● S92.411   Displaced fracture of proximal phalanx of right great toe K, P ⓒ
- ● S92.412   Displaced fracture of proximal phalanx of left great toe K, P ⓒ
- ● S92.413   Displaced fracture of proximal phalanx of unspecified great toe K, P ⓒ
- ● S92.414   Nondisplaced fracture of proximal phalanx of right great toe K, P ⓒ
- ● S92.415   Nondisplaced fracture of proximal phalanx of left great toe K, P ⓒ
- ● S92.416   Nondisplaced fracture of proximal phalanx of unspecified great toe K, P ⓒ

● S92.42   Fracture of distal phalanx of great toe
- ● S92.421   Displaced fracture of distal phalanx of right great toe K, P ⓒ
- ● S92.422   Displaced fracture of distal phalanx of left great toe K, P ⓒ
- ● S92.423   Displaced fracture of distal phalanx of unspecified great toe K, P ⓒ
- ● S92.424   Nondisplaced fracture of distal phalanx of right great toe K, P ⓒ
- ● S92.425   Nondisplaced fracture of distal phalanx of left great toe K, P ⓒ
- ● S92.426   Nondisplaced fracture of distal phalanx of unspecified great toe K, P ⓒ

● S92.49   Other fracture of great toe
- ● S92.491   Other fracture of right great toe K, P ⓒ
- ● S92.492   Other fracture of left great toe K, P ⓒ
- ● S92.499   Other fracture of unspecified great toe K, P ⓒ

● S92.5   Fracture of lesser toe(s)
> **Excludes2**   Physeal fracture of phalanx of toe (S99.2-)
>
> ⒺⓍ **For category S92.5 CC codes: See PDX Collection 897**

- ● S92.50   Unspecified fracture of lesser toe(s)
  - ● S92.501   Displaced unspecified fracture of right lesser toe(s) K, P ⓒ
  - ● S92.502   Displaced unspecified fracture of left lesser toe(s) K, P ⓒ
  - ● S92.503   Displaced unspecified fracture of unspecified lesser toe(s) K, P ⓒ
  - ● S92.504   Nondisplaced unspecified fracture of right lesser toe(s) K, P ⓒ
  - ● S92.505   Nondisplaced unspecified fracture of left lesser toe(s) K, P ⓒ
  - ● S92.506   Nondisplaced unspecified fracture of unspecified lesser toe(s) K, P ⓒ

- ● S92.51   Fracture of proximal phalanx of lesser toe(s)
  - ● S92.511   Displaced fracture of proximal phalanx of right lesser toe(s) K, P ⓒ
  - ● S92.512   Displaced fracture of proximal phalanx of left lesser toe(s) K, P ⓒ
  - ● S92.513   Displaced fracture of proximal phalanx of unspecified lesser toe(s) K, P ⓒ
  - ● S92.514   Nondisplaced fracture of proximal phalanx of right lesser toe(s) K, P ⓒ
  - ● S92.515   Nondisplaced fracture of proximal phalanx of left lesser toe(s) K, P ⓒ
  - ● S92.516   Nondisplaced fracture of proximal phalanx of unspecified lesser toe(s) K, P ⓒ

⇨● S92.52   Fracture of middle phalanx of lesser toe(s)
- ⇨● S92.521   Displaced fracture of middle phalanx of right lesser toe(s) K, P ⓒ
- ⇨● S92.522   Displaced fracture of middle phalanx of left lesser toe(s) K, P ⓒ
- ⇨● S92.523   Displaced fracture of middle phalanx of unspecified lesser toe(s) K, P ⓒ
- ⇨● S92.524   Nondisplaced fracture of middle phalanx of right lesser toe(s) K, P ⓒ
- ⇨● S92.525   Nondisplaced fracture of middle phalanx of left lesser toe(s) K, P ⓒ
- ⇨● S92.526   Nondisplaced fracture of middle phalanx of unspecified lesser toe(s) K, P ⓒ

● S92.53   Fracture of distal phalanx of lesser toe(s)
- ● S92.531   Displaced fracture of distal phalanx of right lesser toe(s) K, P ⓒ
- ● S92.532   Displaced fracture of distal phalanx of left lesser toe(s) K, P ⓒ
- ● S92.533   Displaced fracture of distal phalanx of unspecified lesser toe(s) K, P ⓒ
- ● S92.534   Nondisplaced fracture of distal phalanx of right lesser toe(s) K, P ⓒ
- ● S92.535   Nondisplaced fracture of distal phalanx of left lesser toe(s) K, P ⓒ
- ● S92.536   Nondisplaced fracture of distal phalanx of unspecified lesser toe(s) K, P ⓒ

● S92.59   Other fracture of lesser toe(s)
- ● S92.591   Other fracture of right lesser toe(s) K, P ⓒ
- ● S92.592   Other fracture of left lesser toe(s) K, P ⓒ
- ● S92.599   Other fracture of unspecified lesser toe(s) K, P ⓒ

● S92.8   Other fracture of foot, except ankle
> ⒺⓍ **For category S92.8 CC codes S92.8[B]: See PDX Collection 1369**
> **For S92.90[K,P]: See PDX Collection 897**

- ● S92.81   Other fracture of foot
  Sesamoid fracture of foot
  Coding Clinic: 2016, Q4, P68
  - ● S92.811   Other fracture of right foot B, K, P ⓒ, B ⓒ
  - ● S92.812   Other fracture of left foot B, K, P ⓒ, B ⓒ
  - ● S92.819   Other fracture of unspecified foot B, K, P ⓒ, B ⓒ

● S92.9   Unspecified fracture of foot and toe
- ● S92.90   Unspecified fracture of foot
  > ⒺⓍ **For category S92.90 CC codes S92.90[B]: See PDX Collection 1369 For S92.90[K,P]: See PDX Collection 897**
  - ● S92.901   Unspecified fracture of right foot B, K, P ⓒ, B ⓒ
  - ● S92.902   Unspecified fracture of left foot B, K, P ⓒ, B ⓒ
  - ● S92.909   Unspecified fracture of unspecified foot B, K, P ⓒ, B ⓒ

- ● S92.91   Unspecified fracture of toe
  > ⒺⓍ **For category S92.91 CC codes: See PDX Collection 897**
  - ● S92.911   Unspecified fracture of right toe(s) K, P ⓒ
  - ● S92.912   Unspecified fracture of left toe(s) K, P ⓒ
  - ● S92.919   Unspecified fracture of unspecified toe(s) K, P ⓒ

▶ New   ⇨ Revised   ~~deleted~~ Deleted   Excludes 1   Excludes 2   Includes   Use additional   Code first   Code also   Key words
OGCR Official Guidelines   ● Unacceptable Principal Diagnosis   X Assign placeholder X   ● Use Additional Character(s)   ▶ Manifestation Code   **Coding Clinic**

● S93   **Dislocation and sprain of joints and ligaments at ankle, foot and toe level**

   Includes   avulsion of joint or ligament of ankle, foot and toe

   laceration of cartilage, joint or ligament of ankle, foot and toe

   sprain of cartilage, joint or ligament of ankle, foot and toe

   traumatic hemarthrosis of joint or ligament of ankle, foot and toe

   traumatic rupture of joint or ligament of ankle, foot and toe

   traumatic subluxation of joint or ligament of ankle, foot and toe

   traumatic tear of joint or ligament of ankle, foot and toe

   Code also any associated open wound

   Excludes2   strain of muscle and tendon of ankle and foot (S96.-)

   The appropriate 7th character is to be added to each code from category S93

A	initial encounter
D	subsequent encounter
S	sequela

● **S93.0**   **Subluxation and dislocation of ankle joint**
   Subluxation and dislocation of astragalus
   Subluxation and dislocation of fibula, lower end
   Subluxation and dislocation of talus
   Subluxation and dislocation of tibia, lower end

   X ● **S93.01**   **Subluxation of right ankle joint**
   X ● **S93.02**   **Subluxation of left ankle joint**
   X ● **S93.03**   **Subluxation of unspecified ankle joint**
   X ● **S93.04**   **Dislocation of right ankle joint**
   X ● **S93.05**   **Dislocation of left ankle joint**
   X ● **S93.06**   **Dislocation of unspecified ankle joint**

● **S93.1**   **Subluxation and dislocation of toe**

   ● **S93.10**   **Unspecified subluxation and dislocation of toe**
   Dislocation of toe NOS
   Subluxation of toe NOS

   ● **S93.101**   **Unspecified subluxation of right toe(s)**
   ● **S93.102**   **Unspecified subluxation of left toe(s)**
   ● **S93.103**   **Unspecified subluxation of unspecified toe(s)**
   ● **S93.104**   **Unspecified dislocation of right toe(s)**
   ● **S93.105**   **Unspecified dislocation of left toe(s)**
   ● **S93.106**   **Unspecified dislocation of unspecified toe(s)**

   ● **S93.11**   **Dislocation of interphalangeal joint**
   ● **S93.111**   **Dislocation of interphalangeal joint of right great toe**
   ● **S93.112**   **Dislocation of interphalangeal joint of left great toe**
   ● **S93.113**   **Dislocation of interphalangeal joint of unspecified great toe**
   ● **S93.114**   **Dislocation of interphalangeal joint of right lesser toe(s)**
   ● **S93.115**   **Dislocation of interphalangeal joint of left lesser toe(s)**
   ● **S93.116**   **Dislocation of interphalangeal joint of unspecified lesser toe(s)**
   ● **S93.119**   **Dislocation of interphalangeal joint of unspecified toe(s)**

● **S93.12**   **Dislocation of metatarsophalangeal joint**
   ● **S93.121**   **Dislocation of metatarsophalangeal joint of right great toe**
   ● **S93.122**   **Dislocation of metatarsophalangeal joint of left great toe**
   ● **S93.123**   **Dislocation of metatarsophalangeal joint of unspecified great toe**
   ● **S93.124**   **Dislocation of metatarsophalangeal joint of right lesser toe(s)**
   ● **S93.125**   **Dislocation of metatarsophalangeal joint of left lesser toe(s)**
   ● **S93.126**   **Dislocation of metatarsophalangeal joint of unspecified lesser toe(s)**
   ● **S93.129**   **Dislocation of metatarsophalangeal joint of unspecified toe(s)**

● **S93.13**   **Subluxation of interphalangeal joint**
   ● **S93.131**   **Subluxation of interphalangeal joint of right great toe**
   ● **S93.132**   **Subluxation of interphalangeal joint of left great toe**
   ● **S93.133**   **Subluxation of interphalangeal joint of unspecified great toe**
   ● **S93.134**   **Subluxation of interphalangeal joint of right lesser toe(s)**
   ● **S93.135**   **Subluxation of interphalangeal joint of left lesser toe(s)**
   ● **S93.136**   **Subluxation of interphalangeal joint of unspecified lesser toe(s)**
   ● **S93.139**   **Subluxation of interphalangeal joint of unspecified toe(s)**

● **S93.14**   **Subluxation of metatarsophalangeal joint**
   ● **S93.141**   **Subluxation of metatarsophalangeal joint of right great toe**
   ● **S93.142**   **Subluxation of metatarsophalangeal joint of left great toe**
   ● **S93.143**   **Subluxation of metatarsophalangeal joint of unspecified great toe**
   ● **S93.144**   **Subluxation of metatarsophalangeal joint of right lesser toe(s)**
   ● **S93.145**   **Subluxation of metatarsophalangeal joint of left lesser toe(s)**
   ● **S93.146**   **Subluxation of metatarsophalangeal joint of unspecified lesser toe(s)**
   ● **S93.149**   **Subluxation of metatarsophalangeal joint of unspecified toe(s)**

● **S93.3**   **Subluxation and dislocation of foot**

   Excludes2   dislocation of toe (S93.1-)

   ● **S93.30**   **Unspecified subluxation and dislocation of foot**
   Dislocation of foot NOS
   Subluxation of foot NOS

   ● **S93.301**   **Unspecified subluxation of right foot**
   ● **S93.302**   **Unspecified subluxation of left foot**
   ● **S93.303**   **Unspecified subluxation of unspecified foot**
   ● **S93.304**   **Unspecified dislocation of right foot**
   ● **S93.305**   **Unspecified dislocation of left foot**
   ● **S93.306**   **Unspecified dislocation of unspecified foot**

   ● **S93.31**   **Subluxation and dislocation of tarsal joint**
   ● **S93.311**   **Subluxation of tarsal joint of right foot**
   ● **S93.312**   **Subluxation of tarsal joint of left foot**
   ● **S93.313**   **Subluxation of tarsal joint of unspecified foot**
   ● **S93.314**   **Dislocation of tarsal joint of right foot**
   ● **S93.315**   **Dislocation of tarsal joint of left foot**
   ● **S93.316**   **Dislocation of tarsal joint of unspecified foot**

N Newborn Age: 0   **P** Pediatric Age: 0–17   **M** Maternity DX: 12–55   **A** Adult Age: 15–124   ♀ Females Only   ♂ Males Only

🐷 Complication\Comorbidity   🐷 Major C\C   (Ex) CC/MCC Exclusions   🐷 Hospital-Acquired Condition

1397

CHAPTER 19 (S00-T88)

● S93.32　Subluxation and dislocation of tarsometatarsal joint
- ● S93.321　Subluxation of tarsometatarsal joint of right foot
- ● S93.322　Subluxation of tarsometatarsal joint of left foot
- ● S93.323　Subluxation of tarsometatarsal joint of unspecified foot
- ● S93.324　Dislocation of tarsometatarsal joint of right foot
- ● S93.325　Dislocation of tarsometatarsal joint of left foot
- ● S93.326　Dislocation of tarsometatarsal joint of unspecified foot

● S93.33　Other subluxation and dislocation of foot
- ● S93.331　Other subluxation of right foot
- ● S93.332　Other subluxation of left foot
- ● S93.333　Other subluxation of unspecified foot
- ● S93.334　Other dislocation of right foot
- ● S93.335　Other dislocation of left foot
- ● S93.336　Other dislocation of unspecified foot

● S93.4　Sprain of ankle
　Injury to ligaments when one or more is stretched/torn
　Excludes2　injury of Achilles tendon (S86.0-)

● S93.40　Sprain of unspecified ligament of ankle
　Sprain of ankle NOS
　Sprained ankle NOS
- ● S93.401　Sprain of unspecified ligament of right ankle
- ● S93.402　Sprain of unspecified ligament of left ankle
- ● S93.409　Sprain of unspecified ligament of unspecified ankle

● S93.41　Sprain of calcaneofibular ligament
- ● S93.411　Sprain of calcaneofibular ligament of right ankle
- ● S93.412　Sprain of calcaneofibular ligament of left ankle
- ● S93.419　Sprain of calcaneofibular ligament of unspecified ankle

● S93.42　Sprain of deltoid ligament
- ● S93.421　Sprain of deltoid ligament of right ankle
- ● S93.422　Sprain of deltoid ligament of left ankle
- ● S93.429　Sprain of deltoid ligament of unspecified ankle

● S93.43　Sprain of tibiofibular ligament
- ● S93.431　Sprain of tibiofibular ligament of right ankle
- ● S93.432　Sprain of tibiofibular ligament of left ankle
- ● S93.439　Sprain of tibiofibular ligament of unspecified ankle

● S93.49　Sprain of other ligament of ankle
　Sprain of internal collateral ligament
　Sprain of talofibular ligament
- ● S93.491　Sprain of other ligament of right ankle
- ● S93.492　Sprain of other ligament of left ankle
- ● S93.499　Sprain of other ligament of unspecified ankle

● S93.5　Sprain of toe
● S93.50　Unspecified sprain of toe
- ● S93.501　Unspecified sprain of right great toe
- ● S93.502　Unspecified sprain of left great toe
- ● S93.503　Unspecified sprain of unspecified great toe
- ● S93.504　Unspecified sprain of right lesser toe(s)
- ● S93.505　Unspecified sprain of left lesser toe(s)
- ● S93.506　Unspecified sprain of unspecified lesser toe(s)
- ● S93.509　Unspecified sprain of unspecified toe(s)

● S93.51　Sprain of interphalangeal joint of toe
- ● S93.511　Sprain of interphalangeal joint of right great toe
- ● S93.512　Sprain of interphalangeal joint of left great toe
- ● S93.513　Sprain of interphalangeal joint of unspecified great toe
- ● S93.514　Sprain of interphalangeal joint of right lesser toe(s)
- ● S93.515　Sprain of interphalangeal joint of left lesser toe(s)
- ● S93.516　Sprain of interphalangeal joint of unspecified lesser toe(s)
- ● S93.519　Sprain of interphalangeal joint of unspecified toe(s)

● S93.52　Sprain of metatarsophalangeal joint of toe
- ● S93.521　Sprain of metatarsophalangeal joint of right great toe
- ● S93.522　Sprain of metatarsophalangeal joint of left great toe
- ● S93.523　Sprain of metatarsophalangeal joint of unspecified great toe
- ● S93.524　Sprain of metatarsophalangeal joint of right lesser toe(s)
- ● S93.525　Sprain of metatarsophalangeal joint of left lesser toe(s)
- ● S93.526　Sprain of metatarsophalangeal joint of unspecified lesser toe(s)
- ● S93.529　Sprain of metatarsophalangeal joint of unspecified toe(s)

● S93.6　Sprain of foot
　Excludes2　sprain of metatarsophalangeal joint of toe (S93.52-)
　　sprain of toe (S93.5-)

● S93.60　Unspecified sprain of foot
- ● S93.601　Unspecified sprain of right foot
- ● S93.602　Unspecified sprain of left foot
- ● S93.609　Unspecified sprain of unspecified foot

● S93.61　Sprain of tarsal ligament of foot
- ● S93.611　Sprain of tarsal ligament of right foot
- ● S93.612　Sprain of tarsal ligament of left foot
- ● S93.619　Sprain of tarsal ligament of unspecified foot

● S93.62　Sprain of tarsometatarsal ligament of foot
- ● S93.621　Sprain of tarsometatarsal ligament of right foot
- ● S93.622　Sprain of tarsometatarsal ligament of left foot
- ● S93.629　Sprain of tarsometatarsal ligament of unspecified foot

● S93.69　Other sprain of foot
- ● S93.691　Other sprain of right foot
- ● S93.692　Other sprain of left foot
- ● S93.699　Other sprain of unspecified foot

▶ New　⇒ Revised　~~deleted~~ Deleted　Excludes 1　Excludes 2　Includes　Use additional　Code first　Code also　Key words
OGCR Official Guidelines　● Unacceptable Principal Diagnosis　X Assign placeholder X　● Use Additional Character(s)　▶ Manifestation Code　**Coding Clinic**

● S94 **Injury of nerves at ankle and foot level**

The appropriate 7th character is to be added to each code from category S94

> A   initial encounter
> D   subsequent encounter
> S   sequela

Code also any associated open wound (S91.-)

● **S94.0 Injury of lateral plantar nerve**
- X● S94.00   Injury of lateral plantar nerve, unspecified leg
- X● S94.01   Injury of lateral plantar nerve, right leg
- X● S94.02   Injury of lateral plantar nerve, left leg

● **S94.1 Injury of medial plantar nerve**
- X● S94.10   Injury of medial plantar nerve, unspecified leg
- X● S94.11   Injury of medial plantar nerve, right leg
- X● S94.12   Injury of medial plantar nerve, left leg

● **S94.2 Injury of deep peroneal nerve at ankle and foot level**
  Injury of terminal, lateral branch of deep peroneal nerve
- X● S94.20   Injury of deep peroneal nerve at ankle and foot level, unspecified leg
- X● S94.21   Injury of deep peroneal nerve at ankle and foot level, right leg
- X● S94.22   Injury of deep peroneal nerve at ankle and foot level, left leg

● **S94.3 Injury of cutaneous sensory nerve at ankle and foot level**
- X● S94.30   Injury of cutaneous sensory nerve at ankle and foot level, unspecified leg
- X● S94.31   Injury of cutaneous sensory nerve at ankle and foot level, right leg
- X● S94.32   Injury of cutaneous sensory nerve at ankle and foot level, left leg

● **S94.8 Injury of other nerves at ankle and foot level**
  ● S94.8X   Injury of other nerves at ankle and foot level
  - ● S94.8X1   Injury of other nerves at ankle and foot level, right leg
  - ● S94.8X2   Injury of other nerves at ankle and foot level, left leg
  - ● S94.8X9   Injury of other nerves at ankle and foot level, unspecified leg

● **S94.9 Injury of unspecified nerve at ankle and foot level**
- X● S94.90   Injury of unspecified nerve at ankle and foot level, unspecified leg
- X● S94.91   Injury of unspecified nerve at ankle and foot level, right leg
- X● S94.92   Injury of unspecified nerve at ankle and foot level, left leg

● S95 **Injury of blood vessels at ankle and foot level**

Code also any associated open wound (S91.-)

Excludes2   injury of posterior tibial artery and vein (S85.1-, S85.8-)

The appropriate 7th character is to be added to each code from category S95

> A   initial encounter
> D   subsequent encounter
> S   sequela

● **S95.0 Injury of dorsal artery of foot**
  ● S95.00   Unspecified injury of dorsal artery of foot
  - ● S95.001   Unspecified injury of dorsal artery of right foot A 🔧
    (Ex:) See PDX Collection 1325
  - ● S95.002   Unspecified injury of dorsal artery of left foot A 🔧
    (Ex:) See PDX Collection 1326
  - ● S95.009   Unspecified injury of dorsal artery of unspecified foot A 🔧
    (Ex:) See PDX Collection 1327

  ● S95.01   Laceration of dorsal artery of foot
  - ● S95.011   Laceration of dorsal artery of right foot A 🔧
    (Ex:) See PDX Collection 1325
  - ● S95.012   Laceration of dorsal artery of left foot A 🔧
    (Ex:) See PDX Collection 1326
  - ● S95.019   Laceration of dorsal artery of unspecified foot A 🔧
    (Ex:) See PDX Collection 1327

  ● S95.09   Other specified injury of dorsal artery of foot
  - ● S95.091   Other specified injury of dorsal artery of right foot A 🔧
    (Ex:) See PDX Collection 1325
  - ● S95.092   Other specified injury of dorsal artery of left foot A 🔧
    (Ex:) See PDX Collection 1326
  - ● S95.099   Other specified injury of dorsal artery of unspecified foot A 🔧
    (Ex:) See PDX Collection 1327

● **S95.1 Injury of plantar artery of foot**
  ● S95.10   Unspecified injury of plantar artery of foot
  - ● S95.101   Unspecified injury of plantar artery of right foot A 🔧
    (Ex:) See PDX Collection 1370
  - ● S95.102   Unspecified injury of plantar artery of left foot A 🔧
    (Ex:) See PDX Collection 1371
  - ● S95.109   Unspecified injury of plantar artery of unspecified foot A 🔧
    (Ex:) See PDX Collection 1372

  ● S95.11   Laceration of plantar artery of foot
  - ● S95.111   Laceration of plantar artery of right foot A 🔧
    (Ex:) See PDX Collection 1370
  - ● S95.112   Laceration of plantar artery of left foot A 🔧
    (Ex:) See PDX Collection 1371
  - ● S95.119   Laceration of plantar artery of unspecified foot A 🔧
    (Ex:) See PDX Collection 1372

  ● S95.19   Other specified injury of plantar artery of foot
  - ● S95.191   Other specified injury of plantar artery of right foot A 🔧
    (Ex:) See PDX Collection 1370
  - ● S95.192   Other specified injury of plantar artery of left foot A 🔧
    (Ex:) See PDX Collection 1371
  - ● S95.199   Other specified injury of plantar artery of unspecified foot A 🔧
    (Ex:) See PDX Collection 1372

● **S95.2 Injury of dorsal vein of foot**
  ● S95.20   Unspecified injury of dorsal vein of foot
  - ● S95.201   Unspecified injury of dorsal vein of right foot A 🔧
    (Ex:) See PDX Collection 1325
  - ● S95.202   Unspecified injury of dorsal vein of left foot A 🔧
    (Ex:) See PDX Collection 1326
  - ● S95.209   Unspecified injury of dorsal vein of unspecified foot A 🔧
    (Ex:) See PDX Collection 1327

  ● S95.21   Laceration of dorsal vein of foot
  - ● S95.211   Laceration of dorsal vein of right foot A 🔧
    (Ex:) See PDX Collection 1325
  - ● S95.212   Laceration of dorsal vein of left foot A 🔧
    (Ex:) See PDX Collection 1326
  - ● S95.219   Laceration of dorsal vein of unspecified foot A 🔧
    (Ex:) See PDX Collection 1327

N Newborn Age: 0   P Pediatric Age: 0–17   M Maternity DX: 12–55   A Adult Age: 15–124   ♀ Females Only   ♂ Males Only
🔧 Complication\Comorbidity   🔧 Major C\C   (Ex:) CC/MCC Exclusions   🔧 Hospital-Acquired Condition

● S95.29   Other specified injury of dorsal vein of foot
   ● S95.291   Other specified injury of dorsal vein
              of right foot A 🔗
              (Ex:) See PDX Collection 1325
   ● S95.292   Other specified injury of dorsal vein
              of left foot A 🔗
              (Ex:) See PDX Collection 1326
   ● S95.299   Other specified injury of dorsal vein
              of unspecified foot A 🔗
              (Ex:) See PDX Collection 1327

● S95.8   Injury of other blood vessels at ankle and foot level
   ● S95.80   Unspecified injury of other blood vessels at
             ankle and foot level
      ● S95.801   Unspecified injury of other blood
                 vessels at ankle and foot level, right
                 leg A 🔗
                 (Ex:) See PDX Collection 1325
      ● S95.802   Unspecified injury of other blood
                 vessels at ankle and foot level, left leg
                 A 🔗
                 (Ex:) See PDX Collection 1326
      ● S95.809   Unspecified injury of other blood
                 vessels at ankle and foot level,
                 unspecified leg A 🔗
                 (Ex:) See PDX Collection 1327
   ● S95.81   Laceration of other blood vessels at ankle and
             foot level
      ● S95.811   Laceration of other blood vessels at
                 ankle and foot level, right leg A 🔗
                 (Ex:) See PDX Collection 1325
      ● S95.812   Laceration of other blood vessels at
                 ankle and foot level, left leg A 🔗
                 (Ex:) See PDX Collection 1326
      ● S95.819   Laceration of other blood vessels at
                 ankle and foot level, unspecified leg
                 A 🔗
                 (Ex:) See PDX Collection 1327
   ● S95.89   Other specified injury of other blood vessels at
             ankle and foot level
      ● S95.891   Other specified injury of other blood
                 vessels at ankle and foot level, right
                 leg A 🔗
                 (Ex:) See PDX Collection 1325
      ● S95.892   Other specified injury of other blood
                 vessels at ankle and foot level, left leg
                 A 🔗
                 (Ex:) See PDX Collection 1326
      ● S95.899   Other specified injury of other blood
                 vessels at ankle and foot level,
                 unspecified leg A 🔗
                 (Ex:) See PDX Collection 1327

● S95.9   Injury of unspecified blood vessel at ankle and foot
         level
   ● S95.90   Unspecified injury of unspecified blood vessel
             at ankle and foot level
      ● S95.901   Unspecified injury of unspecified
                 blood vessel at ankle and foot level,
                 right leg A 🔗
                 (Ex:) See PDX Collection 1325
      ● S95.902   Unspecified injury of unspecified
                 blood vessel at ankle and foot level,
                 left leg A 🔗
                 (Ex:) See PDX Collection 1326
      ● S95.909   Unspecified injury of unspecified
                 blood vessel at ankle and foot level,
                 unspecified leg A 🔗
                 (Ex:) See PDX Collection 1327

● S95.91   Laceration of unspecified blood vessel at ankle
          and foot level
   ● S95.911   Laceration of unspecified blood vessel
              at ankle and foot level, right leg A 🔗
              (Ex:) See PDX Collection 1325
   ● S95.912   Laceration of unspecified blood vessel
              at ankle and foot level, left leg A 🔗
              (Ex:) See PDX Collection 1326
   ● S95.919   Laceration of unspecified blood vessel
              at ankle and foot level, unspecified
              leg A 🔗
              (Ex:) See PDX Collection 1327
● S95.99   Other specified injury of unspecified blood
          vessel at ankle and foot level
   ● S95.991   Other specified injury of unspecified
              blood vessel at ankle and foot level,
              right leg A 🔗
              (Ex:) See PDX Collection 1325
   ● S95.992   Other specified injury of unspecified
              blood vessel at ankle and foot level,
              left leg A 🔗
              (Ex:) See PDX Collection 1326
   ● S95.999   Other specified injury of unspecified
              blood vessel at ankle and foot level,
              unspecified leg A 🔗
              (Ex:) See PDX Collection 1327

● S96   Injury of muscle and tendon at ankle and foot level
       Code also any associated open wound (S91.-)
       Excludes2   injury of Achilles tendon (S86.Ø-)
                    sprain of joints and ligaments of ankle and foot
                    (S93.-)
       The appropriate 7th character is to be added to each code from
          category S96

       | A   initial encounter |
       | D   subsequent encounter |
       | S   sequela |

   ● S96.Ø   Injury of muscle and tendon of long flexor muscle of toe
            at ankle and foot level
      ● S96.ØØ   Unspecified injury of muscle and tendon of
                long flexor muscle of toe at ankle and foot level
         ● S96.ØØ1   Unspecified injury of muscle and
                    tendon of long flexor muscle of toe at
                    ankle and foot level, right foot
         ● S96.ØØ2   Unspecified injury of muscle and
                    tendon of long flexor muscle of toe at
                    ankle and foot level, left foot
         ● S96.ØØ9   Unspecified injury of muscle and
                    tendon of long flexor muscle of toe at
                    ankle and foot level, unspecified foot
      ● S96.Ø1   Strain of muscle and tendon of long flexor
                muscle of toe at ankle and foot level
         ● S96.Ø11   Strain of muscle and tendon of long
                    flexor muscle of toe at ankle and foot
                    level, right foot
         ● S96.Ø12   Strain of muscle and tendon of long
                    flexor muscle of toe at ankle and foot
                    level, left foot
         ● S96.Ø19   Strain of muscle and tendon of long
                    flexor muscle of toe at ankle and foot
                    level, unspecified foot

● **S96.02**   Laceration of muscle and tendon of long flexor muscle of toe at ankle and foot level
   ● **S96.021**   Laceration of muscle and tendon of long flexor muscle of toe at ankle and foot level, right foot A 🗫
     Ex: See PDX Collection 1364
   ● **S96.022**   Laceration of muscle and tendon of long flexor muscle of toe at ankle and foot level, left foot A 🗫
     Ex: See PDX Collection 1365
   ● **S96.029**   Laceration of muscle and tendon of long flexor muscle of toe at ankle and foot level, unspecified foot A 🗫
     Ex: See PDX Collection 1366

● **S96.09**   Other injury of muscle and tendon of long flexor muscle of toe at ankle and foot level
   ● **S96.091**   Other injury of muscle and tendon of long flexor muscle of toe at ankle and foot level, right foot
   ● **S96.092**   Other injury of muscle and tendon of long flexor muscle of toe at ankle and foot level, left foot
   ● **S96.099**   Other injury of muscle and tendon of long flexor muscle of toe at ankle and foot level, unspecified foot

● **S96.1**   Injury of muscle and tendon of long extensor muscle of toe at ankle and foot level
   ● **S96.10**   Unspecified injury of muscle and tendon of long extensor muscle of toe at ankle and foot level
     ● **S96.101**   Unspecified injury of muscle and tendon of long extensor muscle of toe at ankle and foot level, right foot
     ● **S96.102**   Unspecified injury of muscle and tendon of long extensor muscle of toe at ankle and foot level, left foot
     ● **S96.109**   Unspecified injury of muscle and tendon of long extensor muscle of toe at ankle and foot level, unspecified foot

   ● **S96.11**   Strain of muscle and tendon of long extensor muscle of toe at ankle and foot level
     ● **S96.111**   Strain of muscle and tendon of long extensor muscle of toe at ankle and foot level, right foot
     ● **S96.112**   Strain of muscle and tendon of long extensor muscle of toe at ankle and foot level, left foot
     ● **S96.119**   Strain of muscle and tendon of long extensor muscle of toe at ankle and foot level, unspecified foot

   ● **S96.12**   Laceration of muscle and tendon of long extensor muscle of toe at ankle and foot level
     ● **S96.121**   Laceration of muscle and tendon of long extensor muscle of toe at ankle and foot level, right foot A 🗫
      Ex: See PDX Collection 1364
     ● **S96.122**   Laceration of muscle and tendon of long extensor muscle of toe at ankle and foot level, left foot A 🗫
      Ex: See PDX Collection 1365
     ● **S96.129**   Laceration of muscle and tendon of long extensor muscle of toe at ankle and foot level, unspecified foot A 🗫
      Ex: See PDX Collection 1366

● **S96.19**   Other specified injury of muscle and tendon of long extensor muscle of toe at ankle and foot level
   ● **S96.191**   Other specified injury of muscle and tendon of long extensor muscle of toe at ankle and foot level, right foot
   ● **S96.192**   Other specified injury of muscle and tendon of long extensor muscle of toe at ankle and foot level, left foot
   ● **S96.199**   Other specified injury of muscle and tendon of long extensor muscle of toe at ankle and foot level, unspecified foot

● **S96.2**   Injury of intrinsic muscle and tendon at ankle and foot level
   ● **S96.20**   Unspecified injury of intrinsic muscle and tendon at ankle and foot level
     ● **S96.201**   Unspecified injury of intrinsic muscle and tendon at ankle and foot level, right foot
     ● **S96.202**   Unspecified injury of intrinsic muscle and tendon at ankle and foot level, left foot
     ● **S96.209**   Unspecified injury of intrinsic muscle and tendon at ankle and foot level, unspecified foot

   ● **S96.21**   Strain of intrinsic muscle and tendon at ankle and foot level
     ● **S96.211**   Strain of intrinsic muscle and tendon at ankle and foot level, right foot
     ● **S96.212**   Strain of intrinsic muscle and tendon at ankle and foot level, left foot
     ● **S96.219**   Strain of intrinsic muscle and tendon at ankle and foot level, unspecified foot

   ● **S96.22**   Laceration of intrinsic muscle and tendon at ankle and foot level
     ● **S96.221**   Laceration of intrinsic muscle and tendon at ankle and foot level, right foot A 🗫
      Ex: See PDX Collection 1364
     ● **S96.222**   Laceration of intrinsic muscle and tendon at left ankle and foot level, left foot A 🗫
      Ex: See PDX Collection 1365
     ● **S96.229**   Laceration of intrinsic muscle and tendon at ankle and foot level, unspecified foot A 🗫
      Ex: See PDX Collection 1366

   ● **S96.29**   Other specified injury of intrinsic muscle and tendon at ankle and foot level
     ● **S96.291**   Other specified injury of intrinsic muscle and tendon at ankle and foot level, right foot
     ● **S96.292**   Other specified injury of intrinsic muscle and tendon at ankle and foot level, left foot
     ● **S96.299**   Other specified injury of intrinsic muscle and tendon at ankle and foot level, unspecified foot

---

N   Newborn Age: 0   P   Pediatric Age: 0–17   M   Maternity DX: 12–55   A   Adult Age: 15–124   ♀   Females Only   ♂   Males Only
🗫   Complication\Comorbidity   🗫   Major C\C   Ex: CC/MCC Exclusions   🗫   Hospital-Acquired Condition

● **S96.8** **Injury of other** specified muscles and tendons at ankle and foot level

  ● **S96.80** Unspecified injury of other specified muscles and tendons at ankle and foot level

    ● **S96.801** Unspecified injury of other specified muscles and tendons at ankle and foot level, **right foot**

    ● **S96.802** Unspecified injury of other specified muscles and tendons at ankle and foot level, **left foot**

    ● **S96.809** Unspecified injury of other specified muscles and tendons at ankle and foot level, **unspecified** foot

  ● **S96.81** **Strain of other** specified muscles and tendons at ankle and foot level

    ● **S96.811** Strain of other specified muscles and tendons at ankle and foot level, **right foot**

    ● **S96.812** Strain of other specified muscles and tendons at ankle and foot level, **left foot**

    ● **S96.819** Strain of other specified muscles and tendons at ankle and foot level, **unspecified** foot

  ● **S96.82** **Laceration** of other specified muscles and tendons at ankle and foot level

    ● **S96.821** Laceration of other specified muscles and tendons at ankle and foot level, **right foot** A ⟨🔗⟩
       Ex: See PDX Collection 1364

    ● **S96.822** Laceration of other specified muscles and tendons at ankle and foot level, **left foot** A ⟨🔗⟩
       Ex: See PDX Collection 1365

    ● **S96.829** Laceration of other specified muscles and tendons at ankle and foot level, **unspecified** foot A ⟨🔗⟩
       Ex: See PDX Collection 1366

  ● **S96.89** **Other** specified injury of other specified muscles and tendons at ankle and foot level

    ● **S96.891** Other specified injury of other specified muscles and tendons at ankle and foot level, **right foot**

    ● **S96.892** Other specified injury of other specified muscles and tendons at ankle and foot level, **left foot**

    ● **S96.899** Other specified injury of other specified muscles and tendons at ankle and foot level, **unspecified foot**

● **S96.9** **Injury of** unspecified muscle and tendon at ankle and foot level

  ● **S96.90** Unspecified injury of unspecified muscle and tendon at ankle and foot level

    ● **S96.901** Unspecified injury of unspecified muscle and tendon at ankle and foot level, **right foot**

    ● **S96.902** Unspecified injury of unspecified muscle and tendon at ankle and foot level, **left foot**

    ● **S96.909** Unspecified injury of unspecified muscle and tendon at ankle and foot level, **unspecified foot**

  ● **S96.91** **Strain of** unspecified muscle and tendon at ankle and foot level

    ● **S96.911** Strain of unspecified muscle and tendon at ankle and foot level, **right foot**

    ● **S96.912** Strain of unspecified muscle and tendon at ankle and foot level, **left foot**

    ● **S96.919** Strain of unspecified muscle and tendon at ankle and foot level, **unspecified foot**

● **S96.92** **Laceration** of unspecified muscle and tendon at ankle and foot level

  ● **S96.921** Laceration of unspecified muscle and tendon at ankle and foot level, **right foot** A ⟨🔗⟩
    Ex: See PDX Collection 1364

  ● **S96.922** Laceration of unspecified muscle and tendon at ankle and foot level, **left foot** A ⟨🔗⟩
    Ex: See PDX Collection 1365

  ● **S96.929** Laceration of unspecified muscle and tendon at ankle and foot level, **unspecified foot** A ⟨🔗⟩
    Ex: See PDX Collection 1366

● **S96.99** **Other** specified injury of unspecified muscle and tendon at ankle and foot level

  ● **S96.991** Other specified injury of unspecified muscle and tendon at ankle and foot level, **right foot**

  ● **S96.992** Other specified injury of unspecified muscle and tendon at ankle and foot level, **left foot**

  ● **S96.999** Other specified injury of unspecified muscle and tendon at ankle and foot level, **unspecified foot**

● **S97** **Crushing injury of ankle and foot**

  Use additional code(s) for all associated injuries

  The appropriate 7th character is to be added to each code from category S97

A	initial encounter
D	subsequent encounter
S	sequela

● **S97.0** **Crushing injury of ankle**

  X ● **S97.00** Crushing injury of **unspecified** ankle
  X ● **S97.01** Crushing injury of **right** ankle
  X ● **S97.02** Crushing injury of **left** ankle

● **S97.1** **Crushing injury of toe**

  ● **S97.10** Crushing injury of **unspecified** toe(s)

    ● **S97.101** Crushing injury of unspecified **right** toe(s)

    ● **S97.102** Crushing injury of unspecified **left** toe(s)

    ● **S97.109** Crushing injury of **unspecified** toe(s)
      Crushing injury of toe NOS

  ● **S97.11** Crushing injury of **great toe**

    ● **S97.111** Crushing injury of **right** great toe
    ● **S97.112** Crushing injury of **left** great toe
    ● **S97.119** Crushing injury of **unspecified** great toe

  ● **S97.12** Crushing injury of **lesser** toe(s)

    ● **S97.121** Crushing injury of **right** lesser toe(s)
    ● **S97.122** Crushing injury of **left** lesser toe(s)
    ● **S97.129** Crushing injury of lesser toe(s), **unspecified** toe(s)

● **S97.8** **Crushing injury of foot**

  X ● **S97.80** Crushing injury of foot, **unspecified** side
    Crushing injury of foot NOS

  X ● **S97.81** Crushing injury of **right** foot
  X ● **S97.82** Crushing injury of **left** foot

▶ New   ⟱ Revised   ~~deleted~~ Deleted   Excludes 1   Excludes 2   Includes   Use additional   Code first   Code also   Key words

OGCR Official Guidelines   ● Unacceptable Principal Diagnosis   X Assign placeholder X   ● Use Additional Character(s)   ▶ Manifestation Code   **Coding Clinic**

● **S98**   **Traumatic amputation of ankle and foot**

> An amputation not identified as partial or complete should be coded to complete
>
> The appropriate 7th character is to be added to each code from category S98

> | A | initial encounter |
> | D | subsequent encounter |
> | S | sequela |

  ● **S98.0**   **Traumatic amputation of foot at ankle level**

    ● **S98.01**   **Complete** traumatic amputation of foot at ankle level

      ● **S98.011**   **Complete traumatic amputation of right foot at ankle level** A 🖘
        (Ex:) See PDX Collection 1333

      ● **S98.012**   **Complete traumatic amputation of left foot at ankle level** A 🖘
        (Ex:) See PDX Collection 1334

      ● **S98.019**   **Complete traumatic amputation of unspecified foot at ankle level** A 🖘
        (Ex:) See PDX Collection 1335

    ● **S98.02**   **Partial** traumatic amputation of foot at ankle level

      ● **S98.021**   **Partial traumatic amputation of right foot at ankle level** A 🖘
        (Ex:) See PDX Collection 1333

      ● **S98.022**   **Partial traumatic amputation of left foot at ankle level** A 🖘
        (Ex:) See PDX Collection 1334

      ● **S98.029**   **Partial traumatic amputation of unspecified foot at ankle level** A 🖘
        (Ex:) See PDX Collection 1335

  ● **S98.1**   **Traumatic amputation of one toe**

    ● **S98.11**   **Complete** traumatic amputation of great toe

      ● **S98.111**   **Complete traumatic amputation of right great toe**

      ● **S98.112**   **Complete traumatic amputation of left great toe**

      ● **S98.119**   **Complete traumatic amputation of unspecified great toe**

    ● **S98.12**   **Partial** traumatic amputation of great toe

      ● **S98.121**   **Partial traumatic amputation of right great toe**

      ● **S98.122**   **Partial traumatic amputation of left great toe**

      ● **S98.129**   **Partial traumatic amputation of unspecified great toe**

    ● **S98.13**   **Complete traumatic amputation of one lesser toe**

      Traumatic amputation of toe NOS

      ● **S98.131**   **Complete traumatic amputation of one right lesser toe**

      ● **S98.132**   **Complete traumatic amputation of one left lesser toe**

      ● **S98.139**   **Complete traumatic amputation of one unspecified lesser toe**

    ● **S98.14**   **Partial traumatic amputation of one lesser toe**

      ● **S98.141**   **Partial traumatic amputation of one right lesser toe**

      ● **S98.142**   **Partial traumatic amputation of one left lesser toe**

      ● **S98.149**   **Partial traumatic amputation of one unspecified lesser toe**

  ● **S98.2**   **Traumatic amputation of two or more lesser toes**

    ● **S98.21**   **Complete** traumatic amputation of two or more lesser toes

      ● **S98.211**   **Complete traumatic amputation of two or more right lesser toes**

      ● **S98.212**   **Complete traumatic amputation of two or more left lesser toes**

      ● **S98.219**   **Complete traumatic amputation of two or more unspecified lesser toes**

    ● **S98.22**   **Partial** traumatic amputation of two or more lesser toes

      ● **S98.221**   **Partial traumatic amputation of two or more right lesser toes**

      ● **S98.222**   **Partial traumatic amputation of two or more left lesser toes**

      ● **S98.229**   **Partial traumatic amputation of two or more unspecified lesser toes**

  ● **S98.3**   **Traumatic amputation of midfoot**

    ● **S98.31**   **Complete** traumatic amputation of midfoot

      ● **S98.311**   **Complete traumatic amputation of right midfoot** A 🖘
        (Ex:) See PDX Collection 1333

      ● **S98.312**   **Complete traumatic amputation of left midfoot** A 🖘
        (Ex:) See PDX Collection 1334

      ● **S98.319**   **Complete traumatic amputation of unspecified midfoot** A 🖘
        (Ex:) See PDX Collection 1335

    ● **S98.32**   **Partial** traumatic amputation of midfoot

      ● **S98.321**   **Partial traumatic amputation of right midfoot** A 🖘
        (Ex:) See PDX Collection 1333

      ● **S98.322**   **Partial traumatic amputation of left midfoot** A 🖘
        (Ex:) See PDX Collection 1334

      ● **S98.329**   **Partial traumatic amputation of unspecified midfoot** A 🖘
        (Ex:) See PDX Collection 1335

  ● **S98.9**   **Traumatic amputation of foot, level unspecified**

    ● **S98.91**   **Complete** traumatic amputation of foot, level unspecified

      ● **S98.911**   **Complete traumatic amputation of right foot, level unspecified** A 🖘
        (Ex:) See PDX Collection 1333

      ● **S98.912**   **Complete traumatic amputation of left foot, level unspecified** A 🖘
        (Ex:) See PDX Collection 1334

      ● **S98.919**   **Complete traumatic amputation of unspecified foot, level unspecified** A 🖘
        (Ex:) See PDX Collection 1335

    ● **S98.92**   **Partial** traumatic amputation of foot, level unspecified

      ● **S98.921**   **Partial traumatic amputation of right foot, level unspecified** A 🖘
        (Ex:) See PDX Collection 1333

      ● **S98.922**   **Partial traumatic amputation of left foot, level unspecified** A 🖘
        (Ex:) See PDX Collection 1334

      ● **S98.929**   **Partial traumatic amputation of unspecified foot, level unspecified** A 🖘
        (Ex:) See PDX Collection 1335

CHAPTER 19 (S00-T88)

S99   **Other and unspecified injuries of ankle and foot**
Coding Clinic: 2016, Q4, P68

     S99.0   Physeal fracture of calcaneus

         The appropriate 7th character is to be added to each code from subcategories S99.0

A	initial encounter for closed fracture
B	initial encounter for open fracture
D	subsequent encounter for fracture with routine healing
G	subsequent encounter for fracture with delayed healing
K	subsequent encounter for fracture with nonunion
P	subsequent encounter for fracture with malunion
S	sequela

         S99.00   Unspecified physeal fracture of calcaneus

            S99.001   Unspecified physeal fracture of right calcaneus

            S99.002   Unspecified physeal fracture of left calcaneus

            S99.009   Unspecified physeal fracture of unspecified calcaneus

         S99.01   Salter-Harris Type I physeal fracture of calcaneus
Coding Clinic: 2016, Q4, P69

            S99.011   Salter-Harris Type I physeal fracture of right calcaneus

            S99.012   Salter-Harris Type I physeal fracture of left calcaneus

            S99.019   Salter-Harris Type I physeal fracture of unspecified calcaneus

         S99.02   Salter-Harris Type II physeal fracture of calcaneus
Coding Clinic: 2016, Q4, P69

            S99.021   Salter-Harris Type II physeal fracture of right calcaneus

            S99.022   Salter-Harris Type II physeal fracture of left calcaneus

            S99.029   Salter-Harris Type II physeal fracture of unspecified calcaneus

         S99.03   Salter-Harris Type III physeal fracture of calcaneus
Coding Clinic: 2016, Q4, P69

            S99.031   Salter-Harris Type III physeal fracture of right calcaneus

            S99.032   Salter-Harris Type III physeal fracture of left calcaneus

            S99.039   Salter-Harris Type III physeal fracture of unspecified calcaneus

         S99.04   Salter-Harris Type IV physeal fracture of calcaneus
Coding Clinic: 2016, Q4, P69

            S99.041   Salter-Harris Type IV physeal fracture of right calcaneus

            S99.042   Salter-Harris Type IV physeal fracture of left calcaneus

            S99.049   Salter-Harris Type IV physeal fracture of unspecified calcaneus

         S99.09   Other physeal fracture of calcaneus
Coding Clinic: 2016, Q4, P69

            S99.091   Other physeal fracture of right calcaneus

            S99.092   Other physeal fracture of left calcaneus

            S99.099   Other physeal fracture of unspecified calcaneus

     S99.1   Physeal fracture of metatarsal

         The appropriate 7th character is to be added to each code from subcategories S99.1

A	initial encounter for closed fracture
B	initial encounter for open fracture
D	subsequent encounter for fracture with routine healing
G	subsequent encounter for fracture with delayed healing
K	subsequent encounter for fracture with nonunion
P	subsequent encounter for fracture with malunion
S	sequela

         S99.10   Unspecified physeal fracture of metatarsal

            S99.101   Unspecified physeal fracture of right metatarsal

            S99.102   Unspecified physeal fracture of left metatarsal

            S99.109   Unspecified physeal fracture of unspecified metatarsal

         S99.11   Salter-Harris Type I physeal fracture of metatarsal
Coding Clinic: 2016, Q4, P69

            S99.111   Salter-Harris Type I physeal fracture of right metatarsal

            S99.112   Salter-Harris Type I physeal fracture of left metatarsal

            S99.119   Salter-Harris Type I physeal fracture of unspecified metatarsal

         S99.12   Salter-Harris Type II physeal fracture of metatarsal
Coding Clinic: 2016, Q4, P69

            S99.121   Salter-Harris Type II physeal fracture of right metatarsal

            S99.122   Salter-Harris Type II physeal fracture of left metatarsal

            S99.129   Salter-Harris Type II physeal fracture of unspecified metatarsal

         S99.13   Salter-Harris Type III physeal fracture of metatarsal
Coding Clinic: 2016, Q4, P69

            S99.131   Salter-Harris Type III physeal fracture of right metatarsal

            S99.132   Salter-Harris Type III physeal fracture of left metatarsal

            S99.139   Salter-Harris Type III physeal fracture of unspecified metatarsal

         S99.14   Salter-Harris Type IV physeal fracture of metatarsal
Coding Clinic: 2016, Q4, P69

            S99.141   Salter-Harris Type IV physeal fracture of right metatarsal

            S99.142   Salter-Harris Type IV physeal fracture of left metatarsal

            S99.149   Salter-Harris Type IV physeal fracture of unspecified metatarsal

         S99.19   Other physeal fracture of metatarsal
Coding Clinic: 2016, Q4, P69

            S99.191   Other physeal fracture of right metatarsal

            S99.192   Other physeal fracture of left metatarsal

            S99.199   Other physeal fracture of unspecified metatarsal

● **S99.2**   **Physeal fracture of phalanx of toe**

The appropriate 7th character is to be added to each code from subcategories S99.2

A	initial encounter for closed fracture
B	initial encounter for open fracture
D	subsequent encounter for fracture with routine healing
G	subsequent encounter for fracture with delayed healing
K	subsequent encounter for fracture with nonunion
P	subsequent encounter for fracture with malunion
S	sequela

● **S99.20**   **Unspecified physeal fracture of phalanx of toe**

    ● **S99.201**   Unspecified physeal fracture of phalanx of **right** toe

    ● **S99.202**   Unspecified physeal fracture of phalanx of **right** toe

    ● **S99.209**   Unspecified physeal fracture of phalanx of **unspecified** toe

● **S99.21**   **Salter-Harris Type I physeal fracture of phalanx of toe**
     Coding Clinic: 2016, Q4, P69

    ● **S99.211**   Salter-Harris Type I physeal fracture of phalanx of **right** toe

    ● **S99.212**   Salter-Harris Type I physeal fracture of phalanx of **left** toe

    ● **S99.219**   Salter-Harris Type I physeal fracture of phalanx of **unspecified** toe

● **S99.22**   **Salter-Harris Type II physeal fracture of phalanx of toe**
     Coding Clinic: 2016, Q4, P69

    ● **S99.221**   Salter-Harris Type II physeal fracture of phalanx of **right** toe

    ● **S99.222**   Salter-Harris Type II physeal fracture of phalanx of **left** toe

    ● **S99.229**   Salter-Harris Type II physeal fracture of phalanx of **unspecified** toe

● **S99.23**   **Salter-Harris Type III physeal fracture of phalanx of toe**
     Coding Clinic: 2016, Q4, P69

    ● **S99.231**   Salter-Harris Type III physeal fracture of phalanx of **right** toe

    ● **S99.232**   Salter-Harris Type III physeal fracture of phalanx of **left** toe

    ● **S99.239**   Salter-Harris Type III physeal fracture of phalanx of **unspecified** toe

● **S99.24**   **Salter-Harris Type IV physeal fracture of phalanx of toe**
     Coding Clinic: 2016, Q4, P69

    ● **S99.241**   Salter-Harris Type IV physeal fracture of phalanx of **right** toe

    ● **S99.242**   Salter-Harris Type IV physeal fracture of phalanx of **left** toe

    ● **S99.249**   Salter-Harris Type IV physeal fracture of phalanx of **unspecified** toe

● **S99.29**   **Other physeal fracture of phalanx of toe**
     Coding Clinic: 2016, Q4, P69

    ● **S99.291**   Other physeal fracture of phalanx of **right** toe

    ● **S99.292**   Other physeal fracture of phalanx of **left** toe

    ● **S99.299**   Other physeal fracture of phalanx of **unspecified** toe

● **S99.8**   **Other specified injuries of ankle and foot**

The appropriate 7th character is to be added to each code from subcategory S99.8

A	initial encounter
D	subsequent encounter
S	sequela

● **S99.81**   **Other specified injuries of ankle**

    ● **S99.811**   Other specified injuries of **right** ankle

    ● **S99.812**   Other specified injuries of **left** ankle

    ● **S99.819**   Other specified injuries of **unspecified** ankle

● **S99.82**   **Other specified injuries of foot**

    ● **S99.821**   Other specified injuries of **right** foot

    ● **S99.822**   Other specified injuries of **left** foot

    ● **S99.829**   Other specified injuries of **unspecified** foot

● **S99.9**   **Unspecified injury of ankle and foot**

The appropriate 7th character is to be added to each code from subcategory S99.9

A	initial encounter
D	subsequent encounter
S	sequela

● **S99.91**   **Unspecified injury of ankle**

    ● **S99.911**   Unspecified injury of **right** ankle

    ● **S99.912**   Unspecified injury of **left** ankle

    ● **S99.919**   Unspecified injury of **unspecified** ankle

● **S99.92**   **Unspecified injury of foot**

    ● **S99.921**   Unspecified injury of **right** foot

    ● **S99.922**   Unspecified injury of **left** foot

    ● **S99.929**   Unspecified injury of **unspecified** foot

---

INJURY, POISONING AND CERTAIN OTHER CONSEQUENCES OF EXTERNAL CAUSES (T07-T88)

INJURIES INVOLVING MULTIPLE BODY REGIONS (T07)

Excludes1   burns and corrosions (T20-T32)
         frostbite (T33-T34)
         insect bite or sting, venomous (T63.4)
         sunburn (L55.-)

X ● **T07**   **Unspecified multiple injuries**

▶ The appropriate 7th character is to be added to code T07

▶A	initial encounter
▶D	subsequent encounter
▶S	sequela

➡ **Excludes1**   injury NOS (T14.90)

INJURY OF UNSPECIFIED BODY REGION (T14)

● **T14**   **Injury of unspecified body region**

▶ The appropriate 7th character is to be added to each code from category T14

▶A	initial encounter
▶D	subsequent encounter
▶S	sequela

Excludes1   multiple unspecified injuries (T07)

X ● **T14.8**   **Other injury of unspecified body region**

    Abrasion NOS   Skin injury NOS
    Contusion NOS   Vascular injury NOS
    Crush injury NOS   ▶Wound NOS
    Fracture NOS

● **T14.9**   **Unspecified injury**

    X ● **T14.90**   **Injury, unspecified**
         Injury NOS

    X ● **T14.91**   **Suicide attempt**
         Attempted suicide NOS

CHAPTER 19 (S00-T88)

 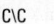

EFFECTS OF FOREIGN BODY ENTERING THROUGH NATURAL ORIFICE (T15-T19)

Excludes2   foreign body accidentally left in operation wound (T81.5-)
foreign body in penetrating wound - see open wound by body region
residual foreign body in soft tissue (M79.5)
splinter, without open wound - see superficial injury by body region

● **T15   Foreign body on external eye**

Excludes2   foreign body in penetrating wound of orbit and eye ball (S05.4-, S05.5-)
open wound of eyelid and periocular area (S01.1-)
retained foreign body in eyelid (H02.8-)
retained (old) foreign body in penetrating wound of orbit and eye ball (H05.5-, H44.6-, H44.7-)
superficial foreign body of eyelid and periocular area (S00.25-)

The appropriate 7th character is to be added to each code from category T15

> A   initial encounter
> D   subsequent encounter
> S   sequela

● **T15.0   Foreign body in cornea**
   X● **T15.00   Foreign body in cornea, unspecified eye**
   X● **T15.01   Foreign body in cornea, right eye**
   X● **T15.02   Foreign body in cornea, left eye**

● **T15.1   Foreign body in conjunctival sac**
   X● **T15.10   Foreign body in conjunctival sac, unspecified eye**
   X● **T15.11   Foreign body in conjunctival sac, right eye**
   X● **T15.12   Foreign body in conjunctival sac, left eye**

● **T15.8   Foreign body in other and multiple parts of external eye**
   Foreign body in lacrimal punctum
   X● **T15.80   Foreign body in other and multiple parts of external eye, unspecified eye**
   X● **T15.81   Foreign body in other and multiple parts of external eye, right eye**
   X● **T15.82   Foreign body in other and multiple parts of external eye, left eye**

● **T15.9   Foreign body on external eye, part unspecified**
   X● **T15.90   Foreign body on external eye, part unspecified, unspecified eye**
   X● **T15.91   Foreign body on external eye, part unspecified, right eye**
   X● **T15.92   Foreign body on external eye, part unspecified, left eye**

● **T16   Foreign body in ear**
Includes   foreign body in auditory canal

The appropriate 7th character is to be added to each code from category T16

> A   initial encounter
> D   subsequent encounter
> S   sequela

X● **T16.1   Foreign body in right ear**
X● **T16.2   Foreign body in left ear**
X● **T16.9   Foreign body in ear, unspecified ear**

● **T17   Foreign body in respiratory tract**
The appropriate 7th character is to be added to each code from category T17

> A   initial encounter
> D   subsequent encounter
> S   sequela

X● **T17.0   Foreign body in nasal sinus**
X● **T17.1   Foreign body in nostril**
   Foreign body in nose NOS

● **T17.2   Foreign body in pharynx**
   Foreign body in nasopharynx
   Foreign body in throat NOS
   ● **T17.20   Unspecified foreign body in pharynx**
     ● **T17.200   Unspecified foreign body in pharynx causing asphyxiation**
     ● **T17.208   Unspecified foreign body in pharynx causing other injury**
   ● **T17.21   Gastric contents in pharynx**
     Aspiration of gastric contents into pharynx
     Vomitus in pharynx
     ● **T17.210   Gastric contents in pharynx causing asphyxiation**
     ● **T17.218   Gastric contents in pharynx causing other injury**
   ● **T17.22   Food in pharynx**
     Bones in pharynx
     Seeds in pharynx
     ● **T17.220   Food in pharynx causing asphyxiation**
     ● **T17.228   Food in pharynx causing other injury**
   ● **T17.29   Other foreign object in pharynx**
     ● **T17.290   Other foreign object in pharynx causing asphyxiation**
     ● **T17.298   Other foreign object in pharynx causing other injury**

● **T17.3   Foreign body in larynx**
   ● **T17.30   Unspecified foreign body in larynx**
     ● **T17.300   Unspecified foreign body in larynx causing asphyxiation**
     ● **T17.308   Unspecified foreign body in larynx causing other injury**
   ● **T17.31   Gastric contents in larynx**
     Aspiration of gastric contents into larynx
     Vomitus in larynx
     ● **T17.310   Gastric contents in larynx causing asphyxiation**
     ● **T17.318   Gastric contents in larynx causing other injury**
   ● **T17.32   Food in larynx**
     Bones in larynx
     Seeds in larynx
     ● **T17.320   Food in larynx causing asphyxiation**
     ● **T17.328   Food in larynx causing other injury**
   ● **T17.39   Other foreign object in larynx**
     ● **T17.390   Other foreign object in larynx causing asphyxiation**
     ● **T17.398   Other foreign object in larynx causing other injury**

● **T17.4   Foreign body in trachea**
   (Ex) For category T17.4 CC codes: See PDX Collection 1373
   ● **T17.40   Unspecified foreign body in trachea**
     ● **T17.400   Unspecified foreign body in trachea causing asphyxiation** A 🦠
     ● **T17.408   Unspecified foreign body in trachea causing other injury** A 🦠

▶ New   ⇒ Revised   ~~deleted~~ Deleted   Excludes 1   Excludes 2   Includes   Use additional   Code first   Code also   Key words

OGCR Official Guidelines   ● Unacceptable Principal Diagnosis   X Assign placeholder X   ● Use Additional Character(s)   ▶ Manifestation Code   **Coding Clinic**

● **T17.41**   Gastric contents in trachea
    Aspiration of gastric contents into trachea
    Vomitus in trachea
    ● **T17.410**   Gastric contents in trachea causing asphyxiation A 🔹
    ● **T17.418**   Gastric contents in trachea causing other injury A 🔹

● **T17.42**   Food in trachea
    Bones in trachea
    Seeds in trachea
    ● **T17.420**   Food in trachea causing asphyxiation A 🔹
    ● **T17.428**   Food in trachea causing other injury A 🔹

● **T17.49**   Other foreign object in trachea
    ● **T17.490**   Other foreign object in trachea causing asphyxiation A 🔹
    ● **T17.498**   Other foreign object in trachea causing other injury A 🔹

● **T17.5**   Foreign body in bronchus
    (Ex) For category T17.5 CC codes: See PDX Collection 1374
    ● **T17.50**   Unspecified foreign body in bronchus
      ● **T17.500**   Unspecified foreign body in bronchus causing asphyxiation A 🔹
      ● **T17.508**   Unspecified foreign body in bronchus causing other injury A 🔹

    ● **T17.51**   Gastric contents in bronchus
      Aspiration of gastric contents into bronchus
      Vomitus in bronchus
      ● **T17.510**   Gastric contents in bronchus causing asphyxiation A 🔹
      ● **T17.518**   Gastric contents in bronchus causing other injury A 🔹

    ● **T17.52**   Food in bronchus
      Bones in bronchus
      Seeds in bronchus
      ● **T17.520**   Food in bronchus causing asphyxiation A 🔹
      ● **T17.528**   Food in bronchus causing other injury A 🔹

    ● **T17.59**   Other foreign object in bronchus
      ● **T17.590**   Other foreign object in bronchus causing asphyxiation A 🔹
      ● **T17.598**   Other foreign object in bronchus causing other injury A 🔹

● **T17.8**   Foreign body in other parts of respiratory tract
    Foreign body in bronchioles
    Foreign body in lung
    (Ex) For category T17.8 CC codes: See PDX Collection 1374
    ● **T17.80**   Unspecified foreign body in other parts of respiratory tract
      ● **T17.800**   Unspecified foreign body in other parts of respiratory tract causing asphyxiation A 🔹
      ● **T17.808**   Unspecified foreign body in other parts of respiratory tract causing other injury A 🔹

    ● **T17.81**   Gastric contents in other parts of respiratory tract
      Aspiration of gastric contents into other parts of respiratory tract
      Vomitus in other parts of respiratory tract
      ● **T17.810**   Gastric contents in other parts of respiratory tract causing asphyxiation A 🔹
      ● **T17.818**   Gastric contents in other parts of respiratory tract causing other injury A 🔹

● **T17.82**   Food in other parts of respiratory tract
    Bones in other parts of respiratory tract
    Seeds in other parts of respiratory tract
    ● **T17.820**   Food in other parts of respiratory tract causing asphyxiation A 🔹
    ● **T17.828**   Food in other parts of respiratory tract causing other injury A 🔹

● **T17.89**   Other foreign object in other parts of respiratory tract
    ● **T17.890**   Other foreign object in other parts of respiratory tract causing asphyxiation
    ● **T17.898**   Other foreign object in other parts of respiratory tract causing other injury A 🔹

● **T17.9**   Foreign body in respiratory tract, part unspecified
    ● **T17.90**   Unspecified foreign body in respiratory tract, part unspecified
      ● **T17.900**   Unspecified foreign body in respiratory tract, part unspecified causing asphyxiation
      ● **T17.908**   Unspecified foreign body in respiratory tract, part unspecified causing other injury

    ● **T17.91**   Gastric contents in respiratory tract, part unspecified
      Aspiration of gastric contents into respiratory tract, part unspecified
      Vomitus in trachea respiratory tract, part unspecified
      ● **T17.910**   Gastric contents in respiratory tract, part unspecified causing asphyxiation
      ● **T17.918**   Gastric contents in respiratory tract, part unspecified causing other injury

    ● **T17.92**   Food in respiratory tract, part unspecified
      Bones in respiratory tract, part unspecified
      Seeds in respiratory tract, part unspecified
      ● **T17.920**   Food in respiratory tract, part unspecified causing asphyxiation
      ● **T17.928**   Food in respiratory tract, part unspecified causing other injury

    ● **T17.99**   Other foreign object in respiratory tract, part unspecified
      ● **T17.990**   Other foreign object in respiratory tract, part unspecified in causing asphyxiation
      ● **T17.998**   Other foreign object in respiratory tract, part unspecified causing other injury

● **T18**   Foreign body in alimentary tract
    Excludes2   foreign body in pharynx (T17.2-)

    The appropriate 7th character is to be added to each code from category T18

      | | |
      A   initial encounter
      D   subsequent encounter
      S   sequela

X ● **T18.0**   Foreign body in mouth
X ● **T18.1**   Foreign body in esophagus
    Excludes2   foreign body in respiratory tract (T17.-)
    ● **T18.10**   Unspecified foreign body in esophagus
      ● **T18.100**   Unspecified foreign body in esophagus causing compression of trachea
        Unspecified foreign body in esophagus causing obstruction of respiration
      ● **T18.108**   Unspecified foreign body in esophagus causing other injury

CHAPTER 19 (S00-T88)

CHAPTER 19 (S00-T88)

● T18.11 **Gastric contents in esophagus**
Vomitus in esophagus

● T18.110 **Gastric contents in esophagus causing compression of trachea**
Gastric contents in esophagus causing obstruction of respiration

● T18.118 **Gastric contents in esophagus causing other injury**

● T18.12 **Food in esophagus**
Bones in esophagus
Seeds in esophagus

● T18.120 **Food in esophagus causing compression of trachea**
Food in esophagus causing obstruction of respiration

● T18.128 **Food in esophagus causing other injury**

● T18.19 **Other foreign object in esophagus**

● T18.190 **Other foreign object in esophagus causing compression of trachea**
Other foreign body in esophagus causing obstruction of respiration
Coding Clinic: 2015, Q1, P24

● T18.198 **Other foreign object in esophagus causing other injury**
Coding Clinic: 2015, Q1, P24

X ● T18.2 **Foreign body in stomach**

X ● T18.3 **Foreign body in small intestine**

X ● T18.4 **Foreign body in colon**

X ● T18.5 **Foreign body in anus and rectum**
Foreign body in rectosigmoid (junction)

X ● T18.8 **Foreign body in other parts of alimentary tract**

X ● T18.9 **Foreign body of alimentary tract, part unspecified**
Foreign body in digestive system NOS
Swallowed foreign body NOS

● T19 **Foreign body in genitourinary tract**

Excludes2 complications due to implanted mesh (T83.7-)
mechanical complications of contraceptive device (intrauterine) (vaginal) (T83.3-)
presence of contraceptive device (intrauterine) (vaginal) (Z97.5)

The appropriate 7th character is to be added to each code from category T19

> A   initial encounter
> D   subsequent encounter
> S   sequela

X ● T19.0 **Foreign body in urethra**

X ● T19.1 **Foreign body in bladder**

X ● T19.2 **Foreign body in vulva and vagina** ♀

X ● T19.3 **Foreign body in uterus** ♀

X ● T19.4 **Foreign body in penis** ♂

X ● T19.8 **Foreign body in other parts of genitourinary tract**

X ● T19.9 **Foreign body in genitourinary tract, part unspecified**

BURNS AND CORROSIONS (T20-T32)

Includes burns (thermal) from electrical heating appliances
burns (thermal) from electricity
burns (thermal) from flame
burns (thermal) from friction
burns (thermal) from hot air and hot gases
burns (thermal) from hot objects
burns (thermal) from lightning
burns (thermal) from radiation chemical
burn [corrosion] (external) (internal) scalds

Excludes2 erythema [dermatitis] ab igne (L59.0)
radiation-related disorders of the skin and subcutaneous tissue (L55-L59)
sunburn (L55.-)

OGCR Section I.C.19.d.

Burns and Corrosions
The ICD-10-CM makes a distinction between burn and corrosions. The burn codes are for thermal burns, except sunburns, that come from a heat source, such as a fire or hot appliance. The burn codes are also for burns resulting from electricity and radiation. Corrosions are burns due to chemicals. The guidelines for burns and corrosions are the same.

Current burns (T20-T25) are classified by depth, extent and by agent (X code). Burns are classified by depth as first degree (erythema), second degree (blistering), and third degree (full-thickness involvement). Burns of the eye and internal organs (T26-T28) are classified by site, but not by degree.

1) Sequencing of burn and related condition codes
Sequence first the code that reflects the highest degree of burn when more than one burn is present.

a. When the reason for the admission or encounter is for treatment of external multiple burns, sequence first the code that reflects the burn of the highest degree.

b. When a patient has both internal and external burns, the circumstances of admission govern the selection of the principal diagnosis or first-listed diagnosis.

c. When a patient is admitted for burn injuries and other related conditions such as smoke inhalation and/or respiratory failure, the circumstances of admission govern the selection of the principal or first-listed diagnosis.

2) Burns of the same local site
Classify burns of the same local site (three-character category level, T20-T28) but of different degrees to the subcategory identifying the highest degree recorded in the diagnosis.

BURNS AND CORROSIONS OF EXTERNAL BODY SURFACE, SPECIFIED BY SITE (T20-T25)

Includes burns and corrosions of first degree [erythema]
burns and corrosions of second degree [blisters] [epidermal loss]
burns and corrosions of third degree [deep necrosis of underlying tissue] [full-thickness skin loss]

Use additional code from category T31 or T32 to identify extent of body surface involved

● T20 **Burn and corrosion of head, face, and neck**

Excludes2 burn and corrosion of ear drum (T28.41, T28.91)
burn and corrosion of eye and adnexa (T26.-)
burn and corrosion of mouth and pharynx (T28.0)

The appropriate 7th character is to be added to each code from category T20

> A   initial encounter
> D   subsequent encounter
> S   sequela

● T20.0 **Burn of unspecified degree of head, face, and neck**
Use additional external cause code to identify the source, place and intent of the burn (X00-X19, X75-X77, X96-X98, Y92)

X ● T20.00 **Burn of unspecified degree of head, face, and neck, unspecified site**

● T20.01 **Burn of unspecified degree of ear [any part, except ear drum]**

Excludes2 burn of ear drum (T28.41-)

● T20.011 **Burn of unspecified degree of right ear [any part, except ear drum]**

● T20.012 **Burn of unspecified degree of left ear [any part, except ear drum]**

● T20.019 **Burn of unspecified degree of unspecified ear [any part, except ear drum]**

▶ New   ⇒ Revised   ~~deleted~~ Deleted | Excludes 1 | | Excludes 2 | | Includes | | Use additional | | Code first | | Code also | | Key words |

OGCR Official Guidelines   ● Unacceptable Principal Diagnosis   X Assign placeholder X   ● Use Additional Character(s)   ▶ Manifestation Code   **Coding Clinic**

Figure 19-15 A. Second-degree burn. **B.** Third-degree burn. (A. From Black J, Hawks J: Medical-Surgical Nursing: Clinical Management for Positive Outcomes, 8e, Saunders, 2008. B. From Marx J, Hockberger R, Walls R: Rosen's Emergency Medicine - Concepts and Clinical Practice, 7e, Mosby, 2009)

X● **T20.02**   Burn of unspecified degree of lip(s)

X● **T20.03**   Burn of unspecified degree of chin

X● **T20.04**   Burn of unspecified degree of nose (septum)

X● **T20.05**   Burn of unspecified degree of scalp [any part]

X● **T20.06**   Burn of unspecified degree of forehead and cheek

X● **T20.07**   Burn of unspecified degree of neck

X● **T20.09**   Burn of unspecified degree of multiple sites of head, face, and neck

● **T20.1**   Burn of first degree of head, face, and neck

Use additional external cause code to identify the source, place and intent of the burn (X00-X19, X75-X77, X96-X98, Y92)

X● **T20.10**   Burn of first degree of head, face, and neck, unspecified site

● **T20.11**   Burn of first degree of ear [any part, except ear drum]

Excludes2   burn of ear drum (T28.41-)

● **T20.111**   Burn of first degree of right ear [any part, except ear drum]

● **T20.112**   Burn of first degree of left ear [any part, except ear drum]

● **T20.119**   Burn of first degree of unspecified ear [any part, except ear drum]

X● **T20.12**   Burn of first degree of lip(s)

X● **T20.13**   Burn of first degree of chin

X● **T20.14**   Burn of first degree of nose (septum)

X● **T20.15**   Burn of first degree of scalp [any part]

X● **T20.16**   Burn of first degree of forehead and cheek

X● **T20.17**   Burn of first degree of neck

X● **T20.19**   Burn of first degree of multiple sites of head, face, and neck

● **T20.2**   Burn of second degree of head, face, and neck

Use additional external cause code to identify the source, place and intent of the burn (X00-X19, X75-X77, X96-X98, Y92)

X● **T20.20**   Burn of second degree of head, face, and neck, unspecified site

● **T20.21**   Burn of second degree of ear [any part, except ear drum]

Excludes2   burn of ear drum (T28.41-)

● **T20.211**   Burn of second degree of right ear [any part, except ear drum]

● **T20.212**   Burn of second degree of left ear [any part, except ear drum]

● **T20.219**   Burn of second degree of unspecified ear [any part, except ear drum]

X● **T20.22**   Burn of second degree of lip(s)

X● **T20.23**   Burn of second degree of chin

X● **T20.24**   Burn of second degree of nose (septum)

X● **T20.25**   Burn of second degree of scalp [any part]
Coding Clinic: 2015, Q1, P19

X● **T20.26**   Burn of second degree of forehead and cheek

X● **T20.27**   Burn of second degree of neck

X● **T20.29**   Burn of second degree of multiple sites of head, face, and neck

● **T20.3**   Burn of third degree of head, face, and neck

Use additional external cause code to identify the source, place and intent of the burn (X00-X19, X75-X77, X96-X98, Y92)

X● **T20.30**   Burn of third degree of head, face, and neck, unspecified site A ✪, A ✪
(Ex) See PDX Collection 1375

● **T20.31**   Burn of third degree of ear [any part, except ear drum]

Excludes2   burn of ear drum (T28.41-)

(Ex) For category T20.31 CC codes: See PDX Collection 1376

● **T20.311**   Burn of third degree of right ear [any part, except ear drum] A ✪, A ✪

● **T20.312**   Burn of third degree of left ear [any part, except ear drum] A ✪, A ✪
Coding Clinic: 2015, Q1, P18

● **T20.319**   Burn of third degree of unspecified ear [any part, except ear drum] A ✪, A ✪

X● **T20.32**   Burn of third degree of lip(s) A ✪, A ✪
(Ex) See PDX Collection 1377

X● **T20.33**   Burn of third degree of chin A ✪, A ✪
(Ex) See PDX Collection 1378

X● **T20.34**   Burn of third degree of nose (septum) A ✪, A ✪
(Ex) See PDX Collection 1379

X● **T20.35**   Burn of third degree of scalp [any part] A ✪, A ✪
(Ex) See PDX Collection 1380

X● **T20.36**   Burn of third degree of forehead and cheek A ✪, A ✪
(Ex) See PDX Collection 1381

X● **T20.37**   Burn of third degree of neck A ✪, A ✪
(Ex) See PDX Collection 1382

X● **T20.39**   Burn of third degree of multiple sites of head, face, and neck A ✪, A ✪
(Ex) See PDX Collection 1383

● **T20.4**   Corrosion of unspecified degree of head, face, and neck

Code first (T51-T65) to identify chemical and intent

Use additional external cause code to identify place (Y92)

X● **T20.40**   Corrosion of unspecified degree of head, face, and neck, unspecified site

● **T20.41**   Corrosion of unspecified degree of ear [any part, except ear drum]

Excludes2   corrosion of ear drum (T28.91-)

● **T20.411**   Corrosion of unspecified degree of right ear [any part, except ear drum]

● **T20.412**   Corrosion of unspecified degree of left ear [any part, except ear drum]

● **T20.419**   Corrosion of unspecified degree of unspecified ear [any part, except ear drum]

X● **T20.42**   Corrosion of unspecified degree of lip(s)

X● **T20.43**   Corrosion of unspecified degree of chin

X● **T20.44**   Corrosion of unspecified degree of nose (septum)

X● **T20.45**   Corrosion of unspecified degree of scalp [any part]

X● **T20.46**   Corrosion of unspecified degree of forehead and cheek

X● **T20.47**   Corrosion of unspecified degree of neck

X● **T20.49**   Corrosion of unspecified degree of multiple sites of head, face, and neck

N Newborn Age: 0   **P** Pediatric Age: 0–17   **M** Maternity DX: 12–55   **A** Adult Age: 15–124   ♀ Females Only   ♂ Males Only

✪ Complication\Comorbidity   ✪ Major C\C   (Ex) CC/MCC Exclusions   ✪ Hospital-Acquired Condition

1409

CHAPTER 19 (S00-T88)

CHAPTER 19 (S00–T88)

● **T20.5**   **Corrosion of first degree of head, face, and neck**
Code first (T51-T65) to identify chemical and intent
Use additional external cause code to identify place (Y92)

X ● **T20.50**   Corrosion of first degree of head, face, and neck, unspecified site

● **T20.51**   Corrosion of first degree of ear [any part, except ear drum]
>**Excludes2**   corrosion of ear drum (T28.91-)
>
> ● **T20.511**   Corrosion of first degree of right ear [any part, except ear drum]
> ● **T20.512**   Corrosion of first degree of left ear [any part, except ear drum]
> ● **T20.519**   Corrosion of first degree of unspecified ear [any part, except ear drum]

X ● **T20.52**   Corrosion of first degree of lip(s)
X ● **T20.53**   Corrosion of first degree of chin
X ● **T20.54**   Corrosion of first degree of nose (septum)
X ● **T20.55**   Corrosion of first degree of scalp [any part]
X ● **T20.56**   Corrosion of first degree of forehead and cheek
X ● **T20.57**   Corrosion of first degree of neck
X ● **T20.59**   Corrosion of first degree of multiple sites of head, face, and neck

● **T20.6**   **Corrosion of second degree of head, face, and neck**
Code first (T51-T65) to identify chemical and intent
Use additional external cause code to identify place (Y92)

X ● **T20.60**   Corrosion of second degree of head, face, and neck, unspecified site

● **T20.61**   Corrosion of second degree of ear [any part, except ear drum]
>**Excludes2**   corrosion of ear drum (T28.91-)
>
> ● **T20.611**   Corrosion of second degree of right ear [any part, except ear drum]
> ● **T20.612**   Corrosion of second degree of left ear [any part, except ear drum]
> ● **T20.619**   Corrosion of second degree of unspecified ear [any part, except ear drum]

X ● **T20.62**   Corrosion of second degree of lip(s)
X ● **T20.63**   Corrosion of second degree of chin
X ● **T20.64**   Corrosion of second degree of nose (septum)
X ● **T20.65**   Corrosion of second degree of scalp [any part]
X ● **T20.66**   Corrosion of second degree of forehead and cheek
X ● **T20.67**   Corrosion of second degree of neck
X ● **T20.69**   Corrosion of second degree of multiple sites of head, face, and neck

● **T20.7**   **Corrosion of third degree of head, face, and neck**
Code first (T51-T65) to identify chemical and intent
Use additional external cause code to identify place (Y92)

X ● **T20.70**   Corrosion of third degree of head, face, and neck, unspecified site A, A
(Ex) See PDX Collection 1375

● **T20.71**   Corrosion of third degree of ear [any part, except ear drum]
>**Excludes2**   corrosion of ear drum (T28.91-)
>(Ex) For category T20.71 CC codes: See PDX Collection 1376
>
> ● **T20.711**   Corrosion of third degree of right ear [any part, except ear drum] A, A
> ● **T20.712**   Corrosion of third degree of left ear [any part, except ear drum] A, A
> ● **T20.719**   Corrosion of third degree of unspecified ear [any part, except ear drum] A, A

X ● **T20.72**   Corrosion of third degree of lip(s) A, A
(Ex) See PDX Collection 1377
X ● **T20.73**   Corrosion of third degree of chin A, A
(Ex) See PDX Collection 1378
X ● **T20.74**   Corrosion of third degree of nose (septum) A, A
(Ex) See PDX Collection 1379
X ● **T20.75**   Corrosion of third degree of scalp [any part] A, A
(Ex) See PDX Collection 1380
X ● **T20.76**   Corrosion of third degree of forehead and cheek A, A
(Ex) See PDX Collection 1381
X ● **T20.77**   Corrosion of third degree of neck A, A
(Ex) See PDX Collection 1382
X ● **T20.79**   Corrosion of third degree of multiple sites of head, face, and neck A, A
(Ex) See PDX Collection 1383

● **T21**   **Burn and corrosion of trunk**
>**Includes**   burns and corrosion of hip region
>**Excludes2**   burns and corrosion of axilla (T22.- with fifth character 4)
>burns and corrosion of scapular region (T22.- with fifth character 6)
>burns and corrosion of shoulder (T22.- with fifth character 5)

The appropriate 7th character is to be added to each code from category T21

A	initial encounter
D	subsequent encounter
S	sequela

● **T21.0**   **Burn of unspecified degree of trunk**
Use additional external cause code to identify the source, place and intent of the burn (X00-X19, X75-X77, X96-X98, Y92)

X ● **T21.00**   Burn of unspecified degree of trunk, unspecified site
X ● **T21.01**   Burn of unspecified degree of chest wall
Burn of of unspecified degree of breast
X ● **T21.02**   Burn of unspecified degree of abdominal wall
Burn of unspecified degree of flank
Burn of unspecified degree of groin
X ● **T21.03**   Burn of unspecified degree of upper back
Burn of unspecified degree of interscapular region
X ● **T21.04**   Burn of unspecified degree of lower back
X ● **T21.05**   Burn of unspecified degree of buttock
Burn of unspecified degree of anus
X ● **T21.06**   Burn of unspecified degree of male genital region ♂
Burn of unspecified degree of penis
Burn of unspecified degree of scrotum
Burn of unspecified degree of testis
X ● **T21.07**   Burn of unspecified degree of female genital region ♀
Burn of unspecified degree of labium (majus) (minus)
Burn of unspecified degree of perineum
Burn of unspecified degree of vulva
>**Excludes2**   burn of vagina (T28.3)
X ● **T21.09**   Burn of unspecified degree of other site of trunk

▶ New   ⇒ Revised   ~~deleted~~ Deleted   Excludes 1   Excludes 2   Includes   Use additional   Code first   Code also   Key words
OGCR Official Guidelines   ● Unacceptable Principal Diagnosis   X Assign placeholder X   ▶ Use Additional Character(s)   ▶ Manifestation Code   **Coding Clinic**

● **T21.1** **Burn of first degree of trunk**

　　Use additional external cause code to identify the source, place and intent of the burn (X00-X19, X75-X77, X96-X98, Y92)

　X ● **T21.10** **Burn of first degree of trunk, unspecified site**

　X ● **T21.11** **Burn of first degree of chest wall**
　　　　　Burn of first degree of breast

　X ● **T21.12** **Burn of first degree of abdominal wall**
　　　　　Burn of first degree of flank
　　　　　Burn of first degree of groin

　X ● **T21.13** **Burn of first degree of upper back**
　　　　　Burn of first degree of interscapular region

　X ● **T21.14** **Burn of first degree of lower back**

　X ● **T21.15** **Burn of first degree of buttock**
　　　　　Burn of first degree of anus

　X ● **T21.16** **Burn of first degree of male genital region** ♂
　　　　　Burn of first degree of penis
　　　　　Burn of first degree of scrotum
　　　　　Burn of first degree of testis

　X ● **T21.17** **Burn of first degree of female genital region** ♀
　　　　　Burn of first degree of labium (majus) (minus)
　　　　　Burn of first degree of perineum
　　　　　Burn of first degree of vulva
　　　　　Excludes2 burn of vagina (T28.3)

　X ● **T21.19** **Burn of first degree of other site of trunk**

● **T21.2** **Burn of second degree of trunk**

　　Use additional external cause code to identify the source, place and intent of the burn (X00-X19, X75-X77, X96-X98, Y92)

　X ● **T21.20** **Burn of second degree of trunk, unspecified site**

　X ● **T21.21** **Burn of second degree of chest wall**
　　　　　Burn of second degree of breast

　X ● **T21.22** **Burn of second degree of abdominal wall**
　　　　　Burn of second degree of flank
　　　　　Burn of second degree of groin

　X ● **T21.23** **Burn of second degree of upper back**
　　　　　Burn of second degree of interscapular region

　X ● **T21.24** **Burn of second degree of lower back**

　X ● **T21.25** **Burn of second degree of buttock**
　　　　　Burn of second degree of anus

　X ● **T21.26** **Burn of second degree of male genital region** ♂
　　　　　Burn of second degree of penis
　　　　　Burn of second degree of scrotum
　　　　　Burn of second degree of testis

　X ● **T21.27** **Burn of second degree of female genital region** ♀
　　　　　Burn of second degree of labium (majus) (minus)
　　　　　Burn of second degree of perineum
　　　　　Burn of second degree of vulva
　　　　　Excludes2 burn of vagina (T28.3)

　X ● **T21.29** **Burn of second degree of other site of trunk**

● **T21.3** **Burn of third degree of trunk**

　　Use additional external cause code to identify the source, place and intent of the burn (X00-X19, X75-X77, X96-X98, Y92)

　X ● **T21.30** **Burn of third degree of trunk, unspecified site** A 🅒, A 🅗
　　　　　Ⓔ See PDX Collection 1384

　X ● **T21.31** **Burn of third degree of chest wall** A 🅒, A 🅗
　　　　　Burn of third degree of breast
　　　　　Ⓔ See PDX Collection 1385
　　　　　Coding Clinic: 2016, Q2, P6

　X ● **T21.32** **Burn of third degree of abdominal wall** A 🅒, A 🅗
　　　　　Burn of third degree of flank
　　　　　Burn of third degree of groin
　　　　　Ⓔ See PDX Collection 1386

　X ● **T21.33** **Burn of third degree of upper back** A 🅒, A 🅗
　　　　　Burn of third degree of interscapular region
　　　　　Ⓔ See PDX Collection 1387

　X ● **T21.34** **Burn of third degree of lower back** A 🅒, A 🅗
　　　　　Ⓔ See PDX Collection 1387

　X ● **T21.35** **Burn of third degree of buttock** A 🅒, A 🅗
　　　　　Burn of third degree of anus
　　　　　Ⓔ See PDX Collection 1387

　X ● **T21.36** **Burn of third degree of male genital region** ♂ A 🅒, A 🅗
　　　　　Burn of third degree of penis
　　　　　Burn of third degree of scrotum
　　　　　Burn of third degree of testis
　　　　　Ⓔ See PDX Collection 1388

　X ● **T21.37** **Burn of third degree of female genital region** ♀ A 🅒, A 🅗
　　　　　Burn of third degree of labium (majus) (minus)
　　　　　Burn of third degree of perineum
　　　　　Burn of third degree of vulva
　　　　　Excludes2 burn of vagina (T28.3)
　　　　　Ⓔ See PDX Collection 1388

　X ● **T21.39** **Burn of third degree of other site of trunk** A 🅒, A 🅗
　　　　　Ⓔ See PDX Collection 1384

● **T21.4** **Corrosion of unspecified degree of trunk**

　　Code first (T51-T65) to identify chemical and intent
　　Use additional external cause code to identify place (Y92)

　X ● **T21.40** **Corrosion of unspecified degree of trunk, unspecified site**

　X ● **T21.41** **Corrosion of unspecified degree of chest wall**
　　　　　Corrosion of unspecified degree of breast

　X ● **T21.42** **Corrosion of unspecified degree of abdominal wall**
　　　　　Corrosion of unspecified degree of flank
　　　　　Corrosion of unspecified degree of groin

　X ● **T21.43** **Corrosion of unspecified degree of upper back**
　　　　　Corrosion of unspecified degree of interscapular region

　X ● **T21.44** **Corrosion of unspecified degree of lower back**

　X ● **T21.45** **Corrosion of unspecified degree of buttock**
　　　　　Corrosion of unspecified degree of anus

　X ● **T21.46** **Corrosion of unspecified degree of male genital region** ♂
　　　　　Corrosion of unspecified degree of penis
　　　　　Corrosion of unspecified degree of scrotum
　　　　　Corrosion of unspecified degree of testis

　X ● **T21.47** **Corrosion of unspecified degree of female genital region** ♀
　　　　　Corrosion of unspecified degree of labium (majus) (minus)
　　　　　Corrosion of unspecified degree of perineum
　　　　　Corrosion of unspecified degree of vulva
　　　　　Excludes2 corrosion of vagina (T28.8)

　X ● **T21.49** **Corrosion of unspecified degree of other site of trunk**

CHAPTER 19 (S00-T88)

● **T21.5 Corrosion of first degree of trunk**
    Code first (T51-T65) to identify chemical and intent
    Use additional external cause code to identify place (Y92)

  X● **T21.5Ø Corrosion of first degree of trunk, unspecified site**

  X● **T21.51 Corrosion of first degree of chest wall**
      Corrosion of first degree of breast

  X● **T21.52 Corrosion of first degree of abdominal wall**
      Corrosion of first degree of flank
      Corrosion of first degree of groin

  X● **T21.53 Corrosion of first degree of upper back**
      Corrosion of first degree of interscapular region

  X● **T21.54 Corrosion of first degree of lower back**

  X● **T21.55 Corrosion of first degree of buttock**
      Corrosion of first degree of anus

  X● **T21.56 Corrosion of first degree of male genital region ♂**
      Corrosion of first degree of penis
      Corrosion of first degree of scrotum
      Corrosion of first degree of testis

  X● **T21.57 Corrosion of first degree of female genital region ♀**
      Corrosion of first degree of labium (majus) (minus)
      Corrosion of first degree of perineum
      Corrosion of first degree of vulva
      Excludes2   corrosion of vagina (T28.8)

  X● **T21.59 Corrosion of first degree of other site of trunk**

● **T21.6 Corrosion of second degree of trunk**
    Code first (T51-T65) to identify chemical and intent
    Use additional external cause code to identify place (Y92)

  X● **T21.6Ø Corrosion of second degree of trunk, unspecified site**

  X● **T21.61 Corrosion of second degree of chest wall**
      Corrosion of second degree of breast

  X● **T21.62 Corrosion of second degree of abdominal wall**
      Corrosion of second degree of flank
      Corrosion of second degree of groin

  X● **T21.63 Corrosion of second degree of upper back**
      Corrosion of second degree of interscapular region

  X● **T21.64 Corrosion of second degree of lower back**

  X● **T21.65 Corrosion of second degree of buttock**
      Corrosion of second degree of anus

  X● **T21.66 Corrosion of second degree of male genital region ♂**
      Corrosion of second degree of penis
      Corrosion of second degree of scrotum
      Corrosion of second degree of testis

  X● **T21.67 Corrosion of second degree of female genital region ♀**
      Corrosion of second degree of labium (majus) (minus)
      Corrosion of second degree of perineum
      Corrosion of second degree of vulva
      Excludes2   corrosion of vagina (T28.8)

  X● **T21.69 Corrosion of second degree of other site of trunk**

● **T21.7 Corrosion of third degree of trunk**
    Code first (T51-T65) to identify chemical and intent
    Use additional external cause code to identify place (Y92)

  X● **T21.7Ø Corrosion of third degree of trunk, unspecified site** A ⬡, A ⬡
      (Ex:) See PDX Collection 1384

  X● **T21.71 Corrosion of third degree of chest wall** A ⬡, A ⬡
      Corrosion of third degree of breast
      (Ex:) See PDX Collection 1385

  X● **T21.72 Corrosion of third degree of abdominal wall** A ⬡, A ⬡
      Corrosion of third degree of flank
      Corrosion of third degree of groin
      (Ex:) See PDX Collection 1386

  X● **T21.73 Corrosion of third degree of upper back** A ⬡, A ⬡
      Corrosion of third degree of interscapular region
      (Ex:) See PDX Collection 1387

  X● **T21.74 Corrosion of third degree of lower back** A ⬡, A ⬡
      (Ex:) See PDX Collection 1387

  X● **T21.75 Corrosion of third degree of buttock** A ⬡, A ⬡
      Corrosion of third degree of anus
      (Ex:) See PDX Collection 1387

  X● **T21.76 Corrosion of third degree of male genital region ♂** A ⬡, A ⬡
      Corrosion of third degree of penis
      Corrosion of third degree of scrotum
      Corrosion of third degree of testis
      (Ex:) See PDX Collection 1388

  X● **T21.77 Corrosion of third degree of female genital region ♀** A ⬡, A ⬡
      Corrosion of third degree of labium (majus) (minus)
      Corrosion of third degree of perineum
      Corrosion of third degree of vulva
      Excludes2   corrosion of vagina (T28.8)
      (Ex:) See PDX Collection 1388

  X● **T21.79 Corrosion of third degree of other site of trunk** A ⬡, A ⬡
      (Ex:) See PDX Collection 1384

● **T22 Burn and corrosion of shoulder and upper limb, except wrist and hand**
    Excludes2   burn and corrosion of interscapular region (T21.-)
                 burn and corrosion of wrist and hand (T23.-)
    The appropriate 7th character is to be added to each code from category T22

    | A | initial encounter |
    | D | subsequent encounter |
    | S | sequela |

● **T22.Ø Burn of unspecified degree of shoulder and upper limb, except wrist and hand**
    Use additional external cause code to identify the source, place and intent of the burn (XØØ-X19, X75-X77, X96-X98, Y92)

  X● **T22.ØØ Burn of unspecified degree of shoulder and upper limb, except wrist and hand, unspecified site**

  ● **T22.Ø1 Burn of unspecified degree of forearm**

    ● **T22.Ø11 Burn of unspecified degree of right forearm**

    ● **T22.Ø12 Burn of unspecified degree of left forearm**

    ● **T22.Ø19 Burn of unspecified degree of unspecified forearm**

▶ New   ⬛▶ Revised   ~~deleted~~ Deleted   Excludes 1   Excludes 2   Includes   Use additional   Code first   Code also   Key words
OGCR Official Guidelines   ● Unacceptable Principal Diagnosis   X Assign placeholder X   ● Use Additional Character(s)   ▶ Manifestation Code   **Coding Clinic**

● **T22.02** Burn of unspecified degree of elbow
   ● **T22.021** Burn of unspecified degree of right elbow
   ● **T22.022** Burn of unspecified degree of left elbow
   ● **T22.029** Burn of unspecified degree of unspecified elbow
● **T22.03** Burn of unspecified degree of upper arm
   ● **T22.031** Burn of unspecified degree of right upper arm
   ● **T22.032** Burn of unspecified degree of left upper arm
   ● **T22.039** Burn of unspecified degree of unspecified upper arm
● **T22.04** Burn of unspecified degree of axilla
   ● **T22.041** Burn of unspecified degree of right axilla
   ● **T22.042** Burn of unspecified degree of left axilla
   ● **T22.049** Burn of unspecified degree of unspecified axilla
● **T22.05** Burn of unspecified degree of shoulder
   ● **T22.051** Burn of unspecified degree of right shoulder
   ● **T22.052** Burn of unspecified degree of left shoulder
   ● **T22.059** Burn of unspecified degree of unspecified shoulder
● **T22.06** Burn of unspecified degree of scapular region
   ● **T22.061** Burn of unspecified degree of right scapular region
   ● **T22.062** Burn of unspecified degree of left scapular region
   ● **T22.069** Burn of unspecified degree of unspecified scapular region
● **T22.09** Burn of unspecified degree of multiple sites of shoulder and upper limb, except wrist and hand
   ● **T22.091** Burn of unspecified degree of multiple sites of right shoulder and upper limb, except wrist and hand
   ● **T22.092** Burn of unspecified degree of multiple sites of left shoulder and upper limb, except wrist and hand
   ● **T22.099** Burn of unspecified degree of multiple sites of unspecified shoulder and upper limb, except wrist and hand
● **T22.1** Burn of first degree of shoulder and upper limb, except wrist and hand
   Use additional external cause code to identify the source, place and intent of the burn (X00-X19, X75-X77, X96-X98, Y92)
  X ● **T22.10** Burn of first degree of shoulder and upper limb, except wrist and hand, unspecified site
● **T22.11** Burn of first degree of forearm
   ● **T22.111** Burn of first degree of right forearm
   ● **T22.112** Burn of first degree of left forearm
   ● **T22.119** Burn of first degree of unspecified forearm
● **T22.12** Burn of first degree of elbow
   ● **T22.121** Burn of first degree of right elbow
   ● **T22.122** Burn of first degree of left elbow
   ● **T22.129** Burn of first degree of unspecified elbow

● **T22.13** Burn of first degree of upper arm
   ● **T22.131** Burn of first degree of right upper arm
   ● **T22.132** Burn of first degree of left upper arm
   ● **T22.139** Burn of first degree of unspecified upper arm
● **T22.14** Burn of first degree of axilla
   ● **T22.141** Burn of first degree of right axilla
   ● **T22.142** Burn of first degree of left axilla
   ● **T22.149** Burn of first degree of unspecified axilla
● **T22.15** Burn of first degree of shoulder
   ● **T22.151** Burn of first degree of right shoulder
   ● **T22.152** Burn of first degree of left shoulder
   ● **T22.159** Burn of first degree of unspecified shoulder
● **T22.16** Burn of first degree of scapular region
   ● **T22.161** Burn of first degree of right scapular region
   ● **T22.162** Burn of first degree of left scapular region
   ● **T22.169** Burn of first degree of unspecified scapular region
● **T22.19** Burn of first degree of multiple sites of shoulder and upper limb, except wrist and hand
   ● **T22.191** Burn of first degree of multiple sites of right shoulder and upper limb, except wrist and hand
   ● **T22.192** Burn of first degree of multiple sites of left shoulder and upper limb, except wrist and hand
   ● **T22.199** Burn of first degree of multiple sites of unspecified shoulder and upper limb, except wrist and hand
● **T22.2** Burn of second degree of shoulder and upper limb, except wrist and hand
   Use additional external cause code to identify the source, place and intent of the burn (X00-X19, X75-X77, X96-X98, Y92)
  X ● **T22.20** Burn of second degree of shoulder and upper limb, except wrist and hand, unspecified site
● **T22.21** Burn of second degree of forearm
   ● **T22.211** Burn of second degree of right forearm
   ● **T22.212** Burn of second degree of left forearm
   ● **T22.219** Burn of second degree of unspecified forearm
● **T22.22** Burn of second degree of elbow
   ● **T22.221** Burn of second degree of right elbow
   ● **T22.222** Burn of second degree of left elbow
   ● **T22.229** Burn of second degree of unspecified elbow
● **T22.23** Burn of second degree of upper arm
   ● **T22.231** Burn of second degree of right upper arm
   ● **T22.232** Burn of second degree of left upper arm
   ● **T22.239** Burn of second degree of unspecified upper arm
● **T22.24** Burn of second degree of axilla
   ● **T22.241** Burn of second degree of right axilla
   ● **T22.242** Burn of second degree of left axilla
   ● **T22.249** Burn of second degree of unspecified axilla

CHAPTER 19 (S00-T88)

N Newborn Age: 0   **P** Pediatric Age: 0–17   **M** Maternity DX: 12–55   **A** Adult Age: 15–124   ♀ Females Only   ♂ Males Only

🖤 Complication\Comorbidity   🖤 Major C\C   (Ex) CC/MCC Exclusions   🖤 Hospital-Acquired Condition

1413

● T22.25　Burn of second degree of shoulder
  ● T22.251　Burn of second degree of right shoulder
  ● T22.252　Burn of second degree of left shoulder
  ● T22.259　Burn of second degree of unspecified shoulder
● T22.26　Burn of second degree of scapular region
  ● T22.261　Burn of second degree of right scapular region
  ● T22.262　Burn of second degree of left scapular region
  ● T22.269　Burn of second degree of unspecified scapular region
● T22.29　Burn of second degree of multiple sites of shoulder and upper limb, except wrist and hand
  ● T22.291　Burn of second degree of multiple sites of right shoulder and upper limb, except wrist and hand
  ● T22.292　Burn of second degree of multiple sites of left shoulder and upper limb, except wrist and hand
  ● T22.299　Burn of second degree of multiple sites of unspecified shoulder and upper limb, except wrist and hand
● T22.3　Burn of third degree of shoulder and upper limb, except wrist and hand
  Use additional external cause code to identify the source, place and intent of the burn (X00-X19, X75-X77, X96-X98, Y92)
X ● T22.30　Burn of third degree of shoulder and upper limb, except wrist and hand, unspecified site A ⊗, A ⊗
  Ⓔ See PDX Collection 1389
● T22.31　Burn of third degree of forearm
  Ⓔ For category T22.31 CC codes: See PDX Collection 1390
  ● T22.311　Burn of third degree of right forearm A ⊗, A ⊗
  ● T22.312　Burn of third degree of left forearm A ⊗, A ⊗
  ● T22.319　Burn of third degree of unspecified forearm A ⊗, A ⊗
● T22.32　Burn of third degree of elbow
  Ⓔ For category T22.32 CC codes: See PDX Collection 1391
  ● T22.321　Burn of third degree of right elbow A ⊗, A ⊗
  ● T22.322　Burn of third degree of left elbow A ⊗, A ⊗
  ● T22.329　Burn of third degree of unspecified elbow A ⊗, A ⊗
● T22.33　Burn of third degree of upper arm
  Ⓔ For category T22.33 CC codes: See PDX Collection 1392
  ● T22.331　Burn of third degree of right upper arm A ⊗, A ⊗
  ● T22.332　Burn of third degree of left upper arm A ⊗, A ⊗
  ● T22.339　Burn of third degree of unspecified upper arm A ⊗, A ⊗
● T22.34　Burn of third degree of axilla
  Ⓔ For category T22.34 CC codes: See PDX Collection 1393
  ● T22.341　Burn of third degree of right axilla A ⊗, A ⊗
  ● T22.342　Burn of third degree of left axilla A ⊗, A ⊗
  ● T22.349　Burn of third degree of unspecified axilla A ⊗, A ⊗

● T22.35　Burn of third degree of shoulder
  Ⓔ For category T22.35 CC codes: See PDX Collection 1394
  ● T22.351　Burn of third degree of right shoulder A ⊗, A ⊗
  ● T22.352　Burn of third degree of left shoulder A ⊗, A ⊗
  ● T22.359　Burn of third degree of unspecified shoulder A ⊗, A ⊗
● T22.36　Burn of third degree of scapular region
  Ⓔ For category T22.36 CC codes: See PDX Collection 1395
  ● T22.361　Burn of third degree of right scapular region A ⊗, A ⊗
  ● T22.362　Burn of third degree of left scapular region A ⊗, A ⊗
  ● T22.369　Burn of third degree of unspecified scapular region A ⊗, A ⊗
● T22.39　Burn of third degree of multiple sites of shoulder and upper limb, except wrist and hand
  Ⓔ For category T22.39 CC codes: See PDX Collection 1389
  ● T22.391　Burn of third degree of multiple sites of right shoulder and upper limb, except wrist and hand A ⊗, A ⊗
  ● T22.392　Burn of third degree of multiple sites of left shoulder and upper limb, except wrist and hand A ⊗, A ⊗
  ● T22.399　Burn of third degree of multiple sites of unspecified shoulder and upper limb, except wrist and hand A ⊗, A ⊗
● T22.4　Corrosion of unspecified degree of shoulder and upper limb, except wrist and hand
  Code first (T51-T65) to identify chemical and intent
  Use additional external cause code to identify place (Y92)
X ● T22.40　Corrosion of unspecified degree of shoulder and upper limb, except wrist and hand, unspecified site
● T22.41　Corrosion of unspecified degree of forearm
  ● T22.411　Corrosion of unspecified degree of right forearm
  ● T22.412　Corrosion of unspecified degree of left forearm
  ● T22.419　Corrosion of unspecified degree of unspecified forearm
● T22.42　Corrosion of unspecified degree of elbow
  ● T22.421　Corrosion of unspecified degree of right elbow
  ● T22.422　Corrosion of unspecified degree of left elbow
  ● T22.429　Corrosion of unspecified degree of unspecified elbow
● T22.43　Corrosion of unspecified degree of upper arm
  ● T22.431　Corrosion of unspecified degree of right upper arm
  ● T22.432　Corrosion of unspecified degree of left upper arm
  ● T22.439　Corrosion of unspecified degree of unspecified upper arm
● T22.44　Corrosion of unspecified degree of axilla
  ● T22.441　Corrosion of unspecified degree of right axilla
  ● T22.442　Corrosion of unspecified degree of left axilla
  ● T22.449　Corrosion of unspecified degree of unspecified axilla

▶ New　⟹ Revised　~~deleted~~ Deleted　Excludes 1　Excludes 2　Includes　Use additional　Code first　Code also　Key words
OGCR Official Guidelines　● Unacceptable Principal Diagnosis　X Assign placeholder X　● Use Additional Character(s)　▶ Manifestation Code　Coding Clinic

● T22.45   Corrosion of unspecified degree of shoulder
    ● T22.451   Corrosion of unspecified degree of right shoulder
    ● T22.452   Corrosion of unspecified degree of left shoulder
    ● T22.459   Corrosion of unspecified degree of unspecified shoulder
● T22.46   Corrosion of unspecified degree of scapular region
    ● T22.461   Corrosion of unspecified degree of right scapular region
    ● T22.462   Corrosion of unspecified degree of left scapular region
    ● T22.469   Corrosion of unspecified degree of unspecified scapular region
● T22.49   Corrosion of unspecified degree of multiple sites of shoulder and upper limb, except wrist and hand
    ● T22.491   Corrosion of unspecified degree of multiple sites of right shoulder and upper limb, except wrist and hand
    ● T22.492   Corrosion of unspecified degree of multiple sites of left shoulder and upper limb, except wrist and hand
    ● T22.499   Corrosion of unspecified degree of multiple sites of unspecified shoulder and upper limb, except wrist and hand

● T22.5   Corrosion of first degree of shoulder and upper limb, except wrist and hand
    Code first (T51-T65) to identify chemical and intent
    Use additional external cause code to identify place (Y92)
    X ● T22.50   Corrosion of first degree of shoulder and upper limb, except wrist and hand unspecified site
    ● T22.51   Corrosion of first degree of forearm
      ● T22.511   Corrosion of first degree of right forearm
      ● T22.512   Corrosion of first degree of left forearm
      ● T22.519   Corrosion of first degree of unspecified forearm
    ● T22.52   Corrosion of first degree of elbow
      ● T22.521   Corrosion of first degree of right elbow
      ● T22.522   Corrosion of first degree of left elbow
      ● T22.529   Corrosion of first degree of unspecified elbow
    ● T22.53   Corrosion of first degree of upper arm
      ● T22.531   Corrosion of first degree of right upper arm
      ● T22.532   Corrosion of first degree of left upper arm
      ● T22.539   Corrosion of first degree of unspecified upper arm
    ● T22.54   Corrosion of first degree of axilla
      ● T22.541   Corrosion of first degree of right axilla
      ● T22.542   Corrosion of first degree of left axilla
      ● T22.549   Corrosion of first degree of unspecified axilla

● T22.55   Corrosion of first degree of shoulder
    ● T22.551   Corrosion of first degree of right shoulder
    ● T22.552   Corrosion of first degree of left shoulder
    ● T22.559   Corrosion of first degree of unspecified shoulder
● T22.56   Corrosion of first degree of scapular region
    ● T22.561   Corrosion of first degree of right scapular region
    ● T22.562   Corrosion of first degree of left scapular region
    ● T22.569   Corrosion of first degree of unspecified scapular region
● T22.59   Corrosion of first degree of multiple sites of shoulder and upper limb, except wrist and hand
    ● T22.591   Corrosion of first degree of multiple sites of right shoulder and upper limb, except wrist and hand
    ● T22.592   Corrosion of first degree of multiple sites of left shoulder and upper limb, except wrist and hand
    ● T22.599   Corrosion of first degree of multiple sites of unspecified shoulder and upper limb, except wrist and hand

● T22.6   Corrosion of second degree of shoulder and upper limb, except wrist and hand
    Code first (T51-T65) to identify chemical and intent
    Use additional external cause code to identify place (Y92)
    X ● T22.60   Corrosion of second degree of shoulder and upper limb, except wrist and hand, unspecified site
    ● T22.61   Corrosion of second degree of forearm
      ● T22.611   Corrosion of second degree of right forearm
      ● T22.612   Corrosion of second degree of left forearm
      ● T22.619   Corrosion of second degree of unspecified forearm
    ● T22.62   Corrosion of second degree of elbow
      ● T22.621   Corrosion of second degree of right elbow
      ● T22.622   Corrosion of second degree of left elbow
      ● T22.629   Corrosion of second degree of unspecified elbow
    ● T22.63   Corrosion of second degree of upper arm
      ● T22.631   Corrosion of second degree of right upper arm
      ● T22.632   Corrosion of second degree of left upper arm
      ● T22.639   Corrosion of second degree of unspecified upper arm
    ● T22.64   Corrosion of second degree of axilla
      ● T22.641   Corrosion of second degree of right axilla
      ● T22.642   Corrosion of second degree of left axilla
      ● T22.649   Corrosion of second degree of unspecified axilla

CHAPTER 19 (S00-T88)

CHAPTER 19 (SØØ-T88)

● T22.65   Corrosion of second degree of shoulder
    ● T22.651   Corrosion of second degree of right shoulder
    ● T22.652   Corrosion of second degree of left shoulder
    ● T22.659   Corrosion of second degree of unspecified shoulder

● T22.66   Corrosion of second degree of scapular region
    ● T22.661   Corrosion of second degree of right scapular region
    ● T22.662   Corrosion of second degree of left scapular region
    ● T22.669   Corrosion of second degree of unspecified scapular region

● T22.69   Corrosion of second degree of multiple sites of shoulder and upper limb, except wrist and hand
    ● T22.691   Corrosion of second degree of multiple sites of right shoulder and upper limb, except wrist and hand
    ● T22.692   Corrosion of second degree of multiple sites of left shoulder and upper limb, except wrist and hand
    ● T22.699   Corrosion of second degree of multiple sites of unspecified shoulder and upper limb, except wrist and hand

● T22.7   Corrosion of third degree of shoulder and upper limb, except wrist and hand
Code first (T51-T65) *to identify chemical and intent*
Use additional external cause code to identify place (Y92)

X ● T22.70   Corrosion of third degree of shoulder and upper limb, except wrist and hand, unspecified site A 🔾, A 🔾
    (Ex) See PDX Collection 1389

● T22.71   Corrosion of third degree of forearm
    (Ex) For category T22.71 CC codes: See PDX Collection 139Ø
    ● T22.711   Corrosion of third degree of right forearm A 🔾, A 🔾
    ● T22.712   Corrosion of third degree of left forearm A 🔾, A 🔾
    ● T22.719   Corrosion of third degree of unspecified forearm A 🔾, A 🔾

● T22.72   Corrosion of third degree of elbow
    (Ex) For category T22.72 CC codes: See PDX Collection 1391
    ● T22.721   Corrosion of third degree of right elbow A 🔾, A 🔾
    ● T22.722   Corrosion of third degree of left elbow A 🔾, A 🔾
    ● T22.729   Corrosion of third degree of unspecified elbow A 🔾, A 🔾

● T22.73   Corrosion of third degree of upper arm
    (Ex) For category T22.73 CC codes: See PDX Collection 1392
    ● T22.731   Corrosion of third degree of right upper arm A 🔾, A 🔾
    ● T22.732   Corrosion of third degree of left upper arm A 🔾, A 🔾
    ● T22.739   Corrosion of third degree of unspecified upper arm A 🔾, A 🔾

● T22.74   Corrosion of third degree of axilla
    (Ex) For category T22.74 CC codes: See PDX Collection 1393
    ● T22.741   Corrosion of third degree of right axilla A 🔾, A 🔾
    ● T22.742   Corrosion of third degree of left axilla A 🔾, A 🔾
    ● T22.749   Corrosion of third degree of unspecified axilla A 🔾, A 🔾

● T22.75   Corrosion of third degree of shoulder
    (Ex) For category T22.75 CC codes: See PDX Collection 1394
    ● T22.751   Corrosion of third degree of right shoulder A 🔾, A 🔾
    ● T22.752   Corrosion of third degree of left shoulder A 🔾, A 🔾
    ● T22.759   Corrosion of third degree of unspecified shoulder A 🔾, A 🔾

● T22.76   Corrosion of third degree of scapular region
    (Ex) For category T22.76 CC codes: See PDX Collection 1395
    ● T22.761   Corrosion of third degree of right scapular region A 🔾, A 🔾
    ● T22.762   Corrosion of third degree of left scapular region A 🔾, A 🔾
    ● T22.769   Corrosion of third degree of unspecified scapular region A 🔾, A 🔾

● T22.79   Corrosion of third degree of multiple sites of shoulder and upper limb, except wrist and hand
    (Ex) For category T22.79 CC codes: See PDX Collection 1389
    ● T22.791   Corrosion of third degree of multiple sites of right shoulder and upper limb, except wrist and hand A 🔾, A 🔾
    ● T22.792   Corrosion of third degree of multiple sites of left shoulder and upper limb, except wrist and hand A 🔾, A 🔾
    ● T22.799   Corrosion of third degree of multiple sites of unspecified shoulder and upper limb, except wrist and hand A 🔾, A 🔾

● T23   Burn and corrosion of wrist and hand
The appropriate 7th character is to be added to each code from category T23

A	initial encounter
D	subsequent encounter
S	sequela

● T23.Ø   Burn of unspecified degree of wrist and hand
Use additional external cause code to identify the source, place and intent of the burn (XØØ-X19, X75-X77, X96-X98, Y92)
    ● T23.ØØ   Burn of unspecified degree of hand, unspecified site
        ● T23.ØØ1   Burn of unspecified degree of right hand, unspecified site
        ● T23.ØØ2   Burn of unspecified degree of left hand, unspecified site
        ● T23.ØØ9   Burn of unspecified degree of unspecified hand, unspecified site

    ● T23.Ø1   Burn of unspecified degree of thumb (nail)
        ● T23.Ø11   Burn of unspecified degree of right thumb (nail)
        ● T23.Ø12   Burn of unspecified degree of left thumb (nail)
        ● T23.Ø19   Burn of unspecified degree of unspecified thumb (nail)

    ● T23.Ø2   Burn of unspecified degree of single finger (nail) except thumb
        ● T23.Ø21   Burn of unspecified degree of single right finger (nail) except thumb
        ● T23.Ø22   Burn of unspecified degree of single left finger (nail) except thumb
        ● T23.Ø29   Burn of unspecified degree of unspecified single finger (nail) except thumb

▶ New   ⇒ Revised   ~~deleted~~ Deleted   Excludes 1   Excludes 2   Includes   Use additional   Code first   Code also   Key words
OGCR Official Guidelines   ● Unacceptable Principal Diagnosis   X Assign placeholder X   ● Use Additional Character(s)   ▷ Manifestation Code   Coding Clinic

- T23.03   Burn of unspecified degree of multiple fingers (nail), not including thumb
  - T23.031   Burn of unspecified degree of multiple right fingers (nail), not including thumb
  - T23.032   Burn of unspecified degree of multiple left fingers (nail), not including thumb
  - T23.039   Burn of unspecified degree of unspecified multiple fingers (nail), not including thumb
- T23.04   Burn of unspecified degree of multiple fingers (nail), including thumb
  - T23.041   Burn of unspecified degree of multiple right fingers (nail), including thumb
  - T23.042   Burn of unspecified degree of multiple left fingers (nail), including thumb
  - T23.049   Burn of unspecified degree of unspecified multiple fingers (nail), including thumb
- T23.05   Burn of unspecified degree of palm
  - T23.051   Burn of unspecified degree of right palm
  - T23.052   Burn of unspecified degree of left palm
  - T23.059   Burn of unspecified degree of unspecified palm
- T23.06   Burn of unspecified degree of back of hand
  - T23.061   Burn of unspecified degree of back of right hand
  - T23.062   Burn of unspecified degree of back of left hand
  - T23.069   Burn of unspecified degree of back of unspecified hand
- T23.07   Burn of unspecified degree of wrist
  - T23.071   Burn of unspecified degree of right wrist
  - T23.072   Burn of unspecified degree of left wrist
  - T23.079   Burn of unspecified degree of unspecified wrist
- T23.09   Burn of unspecified degree of multiple sites of wrist and hand
  - T23.091   Burn of unspecified degree of multiple sites of right wrist and hand
  - T23.092   Burn of unspecified degree of multiple sites of left wrist and hand
  - T23.099   Burn of unspecified degree of multiple sites of unspecified wrist and hand
- T23.1   Burn of first degree of wrist and hand
  Use additional external cause code to identify the source, place and intent of the burn (X00-X19, X75-X77, X96-X98, Y92)
  - T23.10   Burn of first degree of hand, unspecified site
    - T23.101   Burn of first degree of right hand, unspecified site
    - T23.102   Burn of first degree of left hand, unspecified site
    - T23.109   Burn of first degree of unspecified hand, unspecified site

- T23.11   Burn of first degree of thumb (nail)
  - T23.111   Burn of first degree of right thumb (nail)
  - T23.112   Burn of first degree of left thumb (nail)
  - T23.119   Burn of first degree of unspecified thumb (nail)
- T23.12   Burn of first degree of single finger (nail) except thumb
  - T23.121   Burn of first degree of single right finger (nail) except thumb
  - T23.122   Burn of first degree of single left finger (nail) except thumb
  - T23.129   Burn of first degree of unspecified single finger (nail) except thumb
- T23.13   Burn of first degree of multiple fingers (nail), not including thumb
  - T23.131   Burn of first degree of multiple right fingers (nail), not including thumb
  - T23.132   Burn of first degree of multiple left fingers (nail), not including thumb
  - T23.139   Burn of first degree of unspecified multiple fingers (nail), not including thumb
- T23.14   Burn of first degree of multiple fingers (nail), including thumb
  - T23.141   Burn of first degree of multiple right fingers (nail), including thumb
  - T23.142   Burn of first degree of multiple left fingers (nail), including thumb
  - T23.149   Burn of first degree of unspecified multiple fingers (nail), including thumb
- T23.15   Burn of first degree of palm
  - T23.151   Burn of first degree of right palm
  - T23.152   Burn of first degree of left palm
  - T23.159   Burn of first degree of unspecified palm
- T23.16   Burn of first degree of back of hand
  - T23.161   Burn of first degree of back of right hand
  - T23.162   Burn of first degree of back of left hand
  - T23.169   Burn of first degree of back of unspecified hand
- T23.17   Burn of first degree of wrist
  - T23.171   Burn of first degree of right wrist
  - T23.172   Burn of first degree of left wrist
  - T23.179   Burn of first degree of unspecified wrist
- T23.19   Burn of first degree of multiple sites of wrist and hand
  - T23.191   Burn of first degree of multiple sites of right wrist and hand
  - T23.192   Burn of first degree of multiple sites of left wrist and hand
  - T23.199   Burn of first degree of multiple sites of unspecified wrist and hand

T23.2 Burn of second degree of wrist and hand

Use additional external cause code to identify the source, place and intent of the burn (X00-X19, X75-X77, X96-X98, Y92)

- **T23.20** Burn of second degree of hand, unspecified site
  - **T23.201** Burn of second degree of right hand, unspecified site
  - **T23.202** Burn of second degree of left hand, unspecified site
  - **T23.209** Burn of second degree of unspecified hand, unspecified site
- **T23.21** Burn of second degree of thumb (nail)
  - **T23.211** Burn of second degree of right thumb (nail)
  - **T23.212** Burn of second degree of left thumb (nail)
  - **T23.219** Burn of second degree of unspecified thumb (nail)
- **T23.22** Burn of second degree of single finger (nail) except thumb
  - **T23.221** Burn of second degree of single right finger (nail) except thumb
  - **T23.222** Burn of second degree of single left finger (nail) except thumb
  - **T23.229** Burn of second degree of unspecified single finger (nail) except thumb
- **T23.23** Burn of second degree of multiple fingers (nail), not including thumb
  - **T23.231** Burn of second degree of multiple right fingers (nail), not including thumb
  - **T23.232** Burn of second degree of multiple left fingers (nail), not including thumb
  - **T23.239** Burn of second degree of unspecified multiple fingers (nail), not including thumb
- **T23.24** Burn of second degree of multiple fingers (nail), including thumb
  - **T23.241** Burn of second degree of multiple right fingers (nail), including thumb
  - **T23.242** Burn of second degree of multiple left fingers (nail), including thumb
  - **T23.249** Burn of second degree of unspecified multiple fingers (nail), including thumb
- **T23.25** Burn of second degree of palm
  - **T23.251** Burn of second degree of right palm
  - **T23.252** Burn of second degree of left palm
  - **T23.259** Burn of second degree of unspecified palm
- **T23.26** Burn of second degree of back of hand
  - **T23.261** Burn of second degree of back of right hand
  - **T23.262** Burn of second degree of back of left hand
  - **T23.269** Burn of second degree of back of unspecified hand
- **T23.27** Burn of second degree of wrist
  - **T23.271** Burn of second degree of right wrist
  - **T23.272** Burn of second degree of left wrist
  - **T23.279** Burn of second degree of unspecified wrist
- **T23.29** Burn of second degree of multiple sites of wrist and hand
  - **T23.291** Burn of second degree of multiple sites of right wrist and hand
  - **T23.292** Burn of second degree of multiple sites of left wrist and hand
  - **T23.299** Burn of second degree of multiple sites of unspecified wrist and hand

T23.3 Burn of third degree of wrist and hand

Use additional external cause code to identify the source, place and intent of the burn (X00-X19, X75-X77, X96-X98, Y92)

- **T23.30** Burn of third degree of hand, unspecified site
  - For category T23.30 CC codes: See PDX Collection 1396
  - **T23.301** Burn of third degree of right hand, unspecified site A, A
    - Coding Clinic: 2015, Q1, P19
  - **T23.302** Burn of third degree of left hand, unspecified site A, A
    - Coding Clinic: 2016, Q2, P5
  - **T23.309** Burn of third degree of unspecified hand, unspecified site A, A
- **T23.31** Burn of third degree of thumb (nail)
  - For category T23.31 CC codes: See PDX Collection 1397
  - **T23.311** Burn of third degree of right thumb (nail) A, A
  - **T23.312** Burn of third degree of left thumb (nail) A, A
  - **T23.319** Burn of third degree of unspecified thumb (nail) A, A
- **T23.32** Burn of third degree of single finger (nail) except thumb
  - For category T23.32 CC codes: See PDX Collection 1398
  - **T23.321** Burn of third degree of single right finger (nail) except thumb A, A
  - **T23.322** Burn of third degree of single left finger (nail) except thumb A, A
  - **T23.329** Burn of third degree of unspecified single finger (nail) except thumb A, A
- **T23.33** Burn of third degree of multiple fingers (nail), not including thumb
  - For category T23.33 CC codes: See PDX Collection 1399
  - **T23.331** Burn of third degree of multiple right fingers (nail), not including thumb A, A
  - **T23.332** Burn of third degree of multiple left fingers (nail), not including thumb A, A
  - **T23.339** Burn of third degree of unspecified multiple fingers (nail), not including thumb A, A
- **T23.34** Burn of third degree of multiple fingers (nail), including thumb
  - For category T23.34 CC codes: See PDX Collection 1400
  - **T23.341** Burn of third degree of multiple right fingers (nail), including thumb A, A
  - **T23.342** Burn of third degree of multiple left fingers (nail), including thumb A, A
  - **T23.349** Burn of third degree of unspecified multiple fingers (nail), including thumb A, A
- **T23.35** Burn of third degree of palm
  - For category T23.35 CC codes: See PDX Collection 1401
  - **T23.351** Burn of third degree of right palm A, A
  - **T23.352** Burn of third degree of left palm A, A
  - **T23.359** Burn of third degree of unspecified palm A, A
- **T23.36** Burn of third degree of back of hand
  - For category T23.36 CC codes: See PDX Collection 1402
  - **T23.361** Burn of third degree of back of right hand A, A
  - **T23.362** Burn of third degree of back of left hand A, A
  - **T23.369** Burn of third degree of back of unspecified hand A, A

▶ New ▷ Revised ~~deleted~~ Deleted | Excludes 1 | Excludes 2 | Includes | Use additional | Code first | Code also | Key words

OGCR Official Guidelines ● Unacceptable Principal Diagnosis X Assign placeholder X ● Use Additional Character(s) ▷ Manifestation Code **Coding Clinic**

● **T23.37**   Burn of third degree of wrist
  (Ex) **For category T23.37 CC codes:** See PDX Collection 1403
 ● **T23.371** Burn of third degree of right wrist
   A 🪙, A 🪙
 ● **T23.372** Burn of third degree of left wrist A 🪙,
   A 🪙
 ● **T23.379** Burn of third degree of unspecified
   wrist A 🪙, A 🪙
● **T23.39** Burn of third degree of multiple sites of wrist
  and hand
  (Ex) **For category T23.39 CC codes:** See PDX Collection 1396
 ● **T23.391** Burn of third degree of multiple sites
   of right wrist and hand A 🪙, A 🪙
 ● **T23.392** Burn of third degree of multiple sites
   of left wrist and hand A 🪙, A 🪙
 ● **T23.399** Burn of third degree of multiple sites
   of unspecified wrist and hand A 🪙,
   A 🪙

● **T23.4** Corrosion of unspecified degree of wrist and hand
  Code first (T51-T65) to identify chemical and intent
  Use additional external cause code to identify
   place (Y92)
 ● **T23.40** Corrosion of unspecified degree of hand,
   unspecified site
  ● **T23.401** Corrosion of unspecified degree of
    right hand, unspecified site
  ● **T23.402** Corrosion of unspecified degree of
    left hand, unspecified site
  ● **T23.409** Corrosion of unspecified degree of
    unspecified hand, unspecified site
 ● **T23.41** Corrosion of unspecified degree of thumb (nail)
  ● **T23.411** Corrosion of unspecified degree of
    right thumb (nail)
  ● **T23.412** Corrosion of unspecified degree of
    left thumb (nail)
  ● **T23.419** Corrosion of unspecified degree of
    unspecified thumb (nail)
 ● **T23.42** Corrosion of unspecified degree of single finger
   (nail) except thumb
  ● **T23.421** Corrosion of unspecified degree of
    single right finger (nail) except thumb
  ● **T23.422** Corrosion of unspecified degree of
    single left finger (nail) except thumb
  ● **T23.429** Corrosion of unspecified degree of
    unspecified single finger (nail) except
    thumb
 ● **T23.43** Corrosion of unspecified degree of multiple
   fingers (nail), not including thumb
  ● **T23.431** Corrosion of unspecified degree
    of multiple right fingers (nail), not
    including thumb
  ● **T23.432** Corrosion of unspecified degree
    of multiple left fingers (nail), not
    including thumb
  ● **T23.439** Corrosion of unspecified degree of
    unspecified multiple fingers (nail),
    not including thumb
 ● **T23.44** Corrosion of unspecified degree of multiple
   fingers (nail), including thumb
  ● **T23.441** Corrosion of unspecified degree of
    multiple right fingers (nail), including
    thumb
  ● **T23.442** Corrosion of unspecified degree of
    multiple left fingers (nail), including
    thumb
  ● **T23.449** Corrosion of unspecified degree of
    unspecified multiple fingers (nail),
    including thumb

● **T23.45** Corrosion of unspecified degree of palm
 ● **T23.451** Corrosion of unspecified degree of
   right palm
 ● **T23.452** Corrosion of unspecified degree of
   left palm
 ● **T23.459** Corrosion of unspecified degree of
   unspecified palm
● **T23.46** Corrosion of unspecified degree of back of
  hand
 ● **T23.461** Corrosion of unspecified degree of
   back of right hand
 ● **T23.462** Corrosion of unspecified degree of
   back of left hand
 ● **T23.469** Corrosion of unspecified degree of
   back of unspecified hand
● **T23.47** Corrosion of unspecified degree of wrist
 ● **T23.471** Corrosion of unspecified degree of
   right wrist
 ● **T23.472** Corrosion of unspecified degree of
   left wrist
 ● **T23.479** Corrosion of unspecified degree of
   unspecified wrist
● **T23.49** Corrosion of unspecified degree of multiple
  sites of wrist and hand
 ● **T23.491** Corrosion of unspecified degree of
   multiple sites of right wrist and hand
 ● **T23.492** Corrosion of unspecified degree of
   multiple sites of left wrist and hand
 ● **T23.499** Corrosion of unspecified degree of
   multiple sites of unspecified wrist
   and hand

● **T23.5** Corrosion of first degree of wrist and hand
  Code first (T51-T65) to identify chemical and intent
  Use additional external cause code to identify
   place (Y92)
 ● **T23.50** Corrosion of first degree of hand, unspecified
   site
  ● **T23.501** Corrosion of first degree of right
    hand, unspecified site
  ● **T23.502** Corrosion of first degree of left hand,
    unspecified site
  ● **T23.509** Corrosion of first degree of
    unspecified hand, unspecified site
 ● **T23.51** Corrosion of first degree of thumb (nail)
  ● **T23.511** Corrosion of first degree of right
    thumb (nail)
  ● **T23.512** Corrosion of first degree of left thumb
    (nail)
  ● **T23.519** Corrosion of first degree of
    unspecified thumb (nail)
 ● **T23.52** Corrosion of first degree of single finger (nail)
   except thumb
  ● **T23.521** Corrosion of first degree of single
    right finger (nail) except thumb
  ● **T23.522** Corrosion of first degree of single left
    finger (nail) except thumb
  ● **T23.529** Corrosion of first degree of
    unspecified single finger (nail) except
    thumb
 ● **T23.53** Corrosion of first degree of multiple fingers
   (nail), not including thumb
  ● **T23.531** Corrosion of first degree of multiple
    right fingers (nail), not including
    thumb
  ● **T23.532** Corrosion of first degree of multiple
    left fingers (nail), not including
    thumb
  ● **T23.539** Corrosion of first degree of
    unspecified multiple fingers (nail),
    not including thumb

N Newborn Age: 0 **P** Pediatric Age: 0–17 **M** Maternity DX: 12–55 **A** Adult Age: 15–124 ♀ Females Only ♂ Males Only

🪙 Complication\Comorbidity 🪙 Major C\C (Ex) CC/MCC Exclusions 🪙 Hospital-Acquired Condition

1419

CHAPTER 19 (S00-T88)

● **T23.54** Corrosion of first degree of multiple fingers (nail), including thumb
  ● **T23.541** Corrosion of first degree of multiple right fingers (nail), including thumb
  ● **T23.542** Corrosion of first degree of multiple left fingers (nail), including thumb
  ● **T23.549** Corrosion of first degree of unspecified multiple fingers (nail), including thumb

● **T23.55** Corrosion of first degree of palm
  ● **T23.551** Corrosion of first degree of right palm
  ● **T23.552** Corrosion of first degree of left palm
  ● **T23.559** Corrosion of first degree of unspecified palm

● **T23.56** Corrosion of first degree of back of hand
  ● **T23.561** Corrosion of first degree of back of right hand
  ● **T23.562** Corrosion of first degree of back of left hand
  ● **T23.569** Corrosion of first degree of back of unspecified hand

● **T23.57** Corrosion of first degree of wrist
  ● **T23.571** Corrosion of first degree of right wrist
  ● **T23.572** Corrosion of first degree of left wrist
  ● **T23.579** Corrosion of first degree of unspecified wrist

● **T23.59** Corrosion of first degree of multiple sites of wrist and hand
  ● **T23.591** Corrosion of first degree of multiple sites of right wrist and hand
  ● **T23.592** Corrosion of first degree of multiple sites of left wrist and hand
  ● **T23.599** Corrosion of first degree of multiple sites of unspecified wrist and hand

● **T23.6** Corrosion of second degree of wrist and hand
Code first (T51-T65) to identify chemical and intent
Use additional external cause code to identify place (Y92)

● **T23.60** Corrosion of second degree of hand, unspecified site
  ● **T23.601** Corrosion of second degree of right hand, unspecified site
  ● **T23.602** Corrosion of second degree of left hand, unspecified site
  ● **T23.609** Corrosion of second degree of unspecified hand, unspecified site

● **T23.61** Corrosion of second degree of thumb (nail)
  ● **T23.611** Corrosion of second degree of right thumb (nail)
  ● **T23.612** Corrosion of second degree of left thumb (nail)
  ● **T23.619** Corrosion of second degree of unspecified thumb (nail)

● **T23.62** Corrosion of second degree of single finger (nail) except thumb
  ● **T23.621** Corrosion of second degree of single right finger (nail) except thumb
  ● **T23.622** Corrosion of second degree of single left finger (nail) except thumb
  ● **T23.629** Corrosion of second degree of unspecified single finger (nail) except thumb

● **T23.63** Corrosion of second degree of multiple fingers (nail), not including thumb
  ● **T23.631** Corrosion of second degree of multiple right fingers (nail), not including thumb
  ● **T23.632** Corrosion of second degree of multiple left fingers (nail), not including thumb
  ● **T23.639** Corrosion of second degree of unspecified multiple fingers (nail), not including thumb

● **T23.64** Corrosion of second degree of multiple fingers (nail), including thumb
  ● **T23.641** Corrosion of second degree of multiple right fingers (nail), including thumb
  ● **T23.642** Corrosion of second degree of multiple left fingers (nail), including thumb
  ● **T23.649** Corrosion of second degree of unspecified multiple fingers (nail), including thumb

● **T23.65** Corrosion of second degree of palm
  ● **T23.651** Corrosion of second degree of right palm
  ● **T23.652** Corrosion of second degree of left palm
  ● **T23.659** Corrosion of second degree of unspecified palm

● **T23.66** Corrosion of second degree of back of hand
  ● **T23.661** Corrosion of second degree back of right hand
  ● **T23.662** Corrosion of second degree back of left hand
  ● **T23.669** Corrosion of second degree back of unspecified hand

● **T23.67** Corrosion of second degree of wrist
  ● **T23.671** Corrosion of second degree of right wrist
  ● **T23.672** Corrosion of second degree of left wrist
  ● **T23.679** Corrosion of second degree of unspecified wrist

● **T23.69** Corrosion of second degree of multiple sites of wrist and hand
  ● **T23.691** Corrosion of second degree of multiple sites of right wrist and hand
  ● **T23.692** Corrosion of second degree of multiple sites of left wrist and hand
  ● **T23.699** Corrosion of second degree of multiple sites of unspecified wrist and hand

● **T23.7** Corrosion of third degree of wrist and hand
Code first (T51-T65) to identify chemical and intent
Use additional external cause code to identify place (Y92)

● **T23.70** Corrosion of third degree of hand, unspecified site
  Ⓔ **For category T23.70 CC codes:** See PDX Collection 1396
  ● **T23.701** Corrosion of third degree of right hand, unspecified site A, A
  ● **T23.702** Corrosion of third degree of left hand, unspecified site A, A
  ● **T23.709** Corrosion of third degree of unspecified hand, unspecified site A, A

● T23.71   Corrosion of third degree of thumb (nail)
　　　　(Ex) For category T23.71 CC codes: See PDX Collection 1397
　　● T23.711   Corrosion of third degree of right
　　　　　　thumb (nail) A 🔖, A 🔖
　　● T23.712   Corrosion of third degree of left
　　　　　　thumb (nail) A 🔖, A 🔖
　　● T23.719   Corrosion of third degree of
　　　　　　unspecified thumb (nail) A 🔖, A 🔖

● T23.72   Corrosion of third degree of single finger (nail)
　　　　except thumb
　　　　(Ex) For category T23.72 CC codes: See PDX Collection 1398
　　● T23.721   Corrosion of third degree of single
　　　　　　right finger (nail) except thumb A 🔖,
　　　　　　A 🔖
　　● T23.722   Corrosion of third degree of single
　　　　　　left finger (nail) except thumb A 🔖,
　　　　　　A 🔖
　　● T23.729   Corrosion of third degree of
　　　　　　unspecified single finger (nail) except
　　　　　　thumb A 🔖, A 🔖

● T23.73   Corrosion of third degree of multiple fingers
　　　　(nail), not including thumb
　　　　(Ex) For category T23.73 CC codes: See PDX Collection 1399
　　● T23.731   Corrosion of third degree of multiple
　　　　　　right fingers (nail), not including
　　　　　　thumb A 🔖, A 🔖
　　● T23.732   Corrosion of third degree of multiple
　　　　　　left fingers (nail), not including
　　　　　　thumb A 🔖, A 🔖
　　● T23.739   Corrosion of third degree of
　　　　　　unspecified multiple fingers (nail),
　　　　　　not including thumb A 🔖, A 🔖

● T23.74   Corrosion of third degree of multiple fingers
　　　　(nail), including thumb
　　　　(Ex) For category T23.74 CC codes: See PDX Collection 1400
　　● T23.741   Corrosion of third degree of multiple
　　　　　　right fingers (nail), including thumb
　　　　　　A 🔖, A 🔖
　　● T23.742   Corrosion of third degree of multiple
　　　　　　left fingers (nail), including thumb
　　　　　　A 🔖, A 🔖
　　● T23.749   Corrosion of third degree of
　　　　　　unspecified multiple fingers (nail),
　　　　　　including thumb A 🔖, A 🔖

● T23.75   Corrosion of third degree of palm
　　　　(Ex) For category T23.75 CC codes: See PDX Collection 1401
　　● T23.751   Corrosion of third degree of right
　　　　　　palm A 🔖, A 🔖
　　● T23.752   Corrosion of third degree of left palm
　　　　　　A 🔖, A 🔖
　　● T23.759   Corrosion of third degree of
　　　　　　unspecified palm A 🔖, A 🔖

● T23.76   Corrosion of third degree of back of hand
　　　　(Ex) For category T23.76 CC codes: See PDX Collection 1402
　　● T23.761   Corrosion of third degree of back of
　　　　　　right hand A 🔖, A 🔖
　　● T23.762   Corrosion of third degree of back of
　　　　　　left hand A 🔖, A 🔖
　　● T23.769   Corrosion of third degree of back of
　　　　　　unspecified hand A 🔖, A 🔖

● T23.77   Corrosion of third degree of wrist
　　　　(Ex) For category T23.77 CC codes: See PDX Collection 1403
　　● T23.771   Corrosion of third degree of right
　　　　　　wrist A 🔖, A 🔖
　　● T23.772   Corrosion of third degree of left wrist
　　　　　　A 🔖, A 🔖
　　● T23.779   Corrosion of third degree of
　　　　　　unspecified wrist A 🔖, A 🔖

● T23.79   Corrosion of third degree of multiple sites of
　　　　wrist and hand
　　　　(Ex) For category T23.79 CC codes: See PDX Collection 1396
　　● T23.791   Corrosion of third degree of multiple
　　　　　　sites of right wrist and hand A 🔖,
　　　　　　A 🔖
　　● T23.792   Corrosion of third degree of multiple
　　　　　　sites of left wrist and hand A 🔖, A 🔖
　　● T23.799   Corrosion of third degree of multiple
　　　　　　sites of unspecified wrist and hand
　　　　　　A 🔖, A 🔖

● T24   Burn and corrosion of lower limb, except ankle and foot
　　　Excludes2   burn and corrosion of ankle and foot (T25.-)
　　　　　　　　burn and corrosion of hip region (T21.-)
　　　The appropriate 7th character is to be added to each code from
　　　category T24

A	initial encounter
D	subsequent encounter
S	sequela

● T24.Ø   Burn of unspecified degree of lower limb, except ankle
　　　　and foot
　　　　Use additional external cause code to identify the
　　　　source, place and intent of the burn (XØØ-X19,
　　　　X75-X77, X96-X98, Y92)
　　● T24.ØØ   Burn of unspecified degree of unspecified site
　　　　　　of lower limb, except ankle and foot
　　　　● T24.ØØ1   Burn of unspecified degree of
　　　　　　　　unspecified site of right lower limb,
　　　　　　　　except ankle and foot
　　　　● T24.ØØ2   Burn of unspecified degree of
　　　　　　　　unspecified site of left lower limb,
　　　　　　　　except ankle and foot
　　　　● T24.ØØ9   Burn of unspecified degree of
　　　　　　　　unspecified site of unspecified lower
　　　　　　　　limb, except ankle and foot
　　● T24.Ø1   Burn of unspecified degree of thigh
　　　　● T24.Ø11   Burn of unspecified degree of right
　　　　　　　　thigh
　　　　● T24.Ø12   Burn of unspecified degree of left
　　　　　　　　thigh
　　　　● T24.Ø19   Burn of unspecified degree of
　　　　　　　　unspecified thigh
　　● T24.Ø2   Burn of unspecified degree of knee
　　　　● T24.Ø21   Burn of unspecified degree of right
　　　　　　　　knee
　　　　● T24.Ø22   Burn of unspecified degree of left
　　　　　　　　knee
　　　　● T24.Ø29   Burn of unspecified degree of
　　　　　　　　unspecified knee
　　● T24.Ø3   Burn of unspecified degree of lower leg
　　　　● T24.Ø31   Burn of unspecified degree of right
　　　　　　　　lower leg
　　　　● T24.Ø32   Burn of unspecified degree of left
　　　　　　　　lower leg
　　　　● T24.Ø39   Burn of unspecified degree of
　　　　　　　　unspecified lower leg
　　● T24.Ø9   Burn of unspecified degree of multiple sites of
　　　　　　lower limb, except ankle and foot
　　　　● T24.Ø91   Burn of unspecified degree of
　　　　　　　　multiple sites of right lower limb,
　　　　　　　　except ankle and foot
　　　　● T24.Ø92   Burn of unspecified degree of
　　　　　　　　multiple sites of left lower limb,
　　　　　　　　except ankle and foot
　　　　● T24.Ø99   Burn of unspecified degree of
　　　　　　　　multiple sites of unspecified lower
　　　　　　　　limb, except ankle and foot

CHAPTER 19 (SØØ-T88)

● **T24.1**   Burn of first degree of lower limb, except ankle and foot

> Use additional external cause code to identify the source, place and intent of the burn (X00-X19, X75-X77, X96-X98, Y92)

  ● **T24.10**   Burn of first degree of unspecified site of lower limb, except ankle and foot

    ● **T24.101**   Burn of first degree of unspecified site of right lower limb, except ankle and foot

    ● **T24.102**   Burn of first degree of unspecified site of left lower limb, except ankle and foot

    ● **T24.109**   Burn of first degree of unspecified site of unspecified lower limb, except ankle and foot

  ● **T24.11**   Burn of first degree of thigh

    ● **T24.111**   Burn of first degree of right thigh

    ● **T24.112**   Burn of first degree of left thigh

    ● **T24.119**   Burn of first degree of unspecified thigh

  ● **T24.12**   Burn of first degree of knee

    ● **T24.121**   Burn of first degree of right knee

    ● **T24.122**   Burn of first degree of left knee

    ● **T24.129**   Burn of first degree of unspecified knee

  ● **T24.13**   Burn of first degree of lower leg

    ● **T24.131**   Burn of first degree of right lower leg

    ● **T24.132**   Burn of first degree of left lower leg

    ● **T24.139**   Burn of first degree of unspecified lower leg

  ● **T24.19**   Burn of first degree of multiple sites of lower limb, except ankle and foot

    ● **T24.191**   Burn of first degree of multiple sites of right lower limb, except ankle and foot

    ● **T24.192**   Burn of first degree of multiple sites of left lower limb, except ankle and foot

    ● **T24.199**   Burn of first degree of multiple sites of unspecified lower limb, except ankle and foot

● **T24.2**   Burn of second degree of lower limb, except ankle and foot

> Use additional external cause code to identify the source, place and intent of the burn (X00-X19, X75-X77, X96-X98, Y92)

  ● **T24.20**   Burn of second degree of unspecified site of lower limb, except ankle and foot

    ● **T24.201**   Burn of second degree of unspecified site of right lower limb, except ankle and foot

    ● **T24.202**   Burn of second degree of unspecified site of left lower limb, except ankle and foot

    ● **T24.209**   Burn of second degree of unspecified site of unspecified lower limb, except ankle and foot

  ● **T24.21**   Burn of second degree of thigh

    ● **T24.211**   Burn of second degree of right thigh

    ● **T24.212**   Burn of second degree of left thigh

    ● **T24.219**   Burn of second degree of unspecified thigh

  ● **T24.22**   Burn of second degree of knee

    ● **T24.221**   Burn of second degree of right knee

    ● **T24.222**   Burn of second degree of left knee

    ● **T24.229**   Burn of second degree of unspecified knee

● **T24.23**   Burn of second degree of lower leg

    ● **T24.231**   Burn of second degree of right lower leg

    ● **T24.232**   Burn of second degree of left lower leg

    ● **T24.239**   Burn of second degree of unspecified lower leg

  ● **T24.29**   Burn of second degree of multiple sites of lower limb, except ankle and foot

    ● **T24.291**   Burn of second degree of multiple sites of right lower limb, except ankle and foot

    ● **T24.292**   Burn of second degree of multiple sites of left lower limb, except ankle and foot

    ● **T24.299**   Burn of second degree of multiple sites of unspecified lower limb, except ankle and foot

● **T24.3**   Burn of third degree of lower limb, except ankle and foot

> Use additional external cause code to identify the source, place and intent of the burn (X00-X19, X75-X77, X96-X98, Y92)

  ● **T24.30**   Burn of third degree of unspecified site of lower limb, except ankle and foot

> Ⓔₓ For category T24.30 CC codes: See PDX Collection 1404

    ● **T24.301**   Burn of third degree of unspecified site of right lower limb, except ankle and foot A 🖉, A 🖉

    ● **T24.302**   Burn of third degree of unspecified site of left lower limb, except ankle and foot A 🖉, A 🖉

    ● **T24.309**   Burn of third degree of unspecified site of unspecified lower limb, except ankle and foot A 🖉, A 🖉

  ● **T24.31**   Burn of third degree of thigh

> Ⓔₓ For category T24.31 CC codes: See PDX Collection 1405

    ● **T24.311**   Burn of third degree of right thigh A 🖉, A 🖉

    ● **T24.312**   Burn of third degree of left thigh A 🖉, A 🖉

    ● **T24.319**   Burn of third degree of unspecified thigh A 🖉, A 🖉

  ● **T24.32**   Burn of third degree of knee

> Ⓔₓ For category T24.32 CC codes: See PDX Collection 1406

    ● **T24.321**   Burn of third degree of right knee A 🖉, A 🖉

    ● **T24.322**   Burn of third degree of left knee A 🖉, A 🖉

    ● **T24.329**   Burn of third degree of unspecified knee A 🖉, A 🖉

  ● **T24.33**   Burn of third degree of lower leg

> Ⓔₓ For category T24.33 CC codes: See PDX Collection 1407

    ● **T24.331**   Burn of third degree of right lower leg A 🖉, A 🖉

    ● **T24.332**   Burn of third degree of left lower leg A 🖉, A 🖉

    ● **T24.339**   Burn of third degree of unspecified lower leg A 🖉, A 🖉

  ● **T24.39**   Burn of third degree of multiple sites of lower limb, except ankle and foot

> Ⓔₓ For category T24.39 CC codes: See PDX Collection 1404

    ● **T24.391**   Burn of third degree of multiple sites of right lower limb, except ankle and foot A 🖉, A 🖉

> **Coding Clinic: 2016, Q2, P5**

    ● **T24.392**   Burn of third degree of multiple sites of left lower limb, except ankle and foot A 🖉, A 🖉

    ● **T24.399**   Burn of third degree of multiple sites of unspecified lower limb, except ankle and foot A 🖉, A 🖉

▶ New   ⇒ Revised   ~~deleted~~ Deleted   Excludes 1   Excludes 2   Includes   Use additional   Code first   Code also   Key words

OGCR Official Guidelines   ● Unacceptable Principal Diagnosis   X Assign placeholder X   ▶ Use Additional Character(s)   ▶ Manifestation Code   **Coding Clinic**

● **T24.4**   **Corrosion of unspecified degree of lower limb, except ankle and foot**

     Code first (T51-T65) *to identify chemical and intent*

     Use additional external cause code to identify place (Y92)

     ● **T24.40**   **Corrosion of unspecified degree of unspecified site of lower limb, except ankle and foot**

         ● **T24.401**   Corrosion of unspecified degree of unspecified site of right lower limb, except ankle and foot

         ● **T24.402**   Corrosion of unspecified degree of unspecified site of left lower limb, except ankle and foot

         ● **T24.409**   Corrosion of unspecified degree of unspecified site of unspecified lower limb, except ankle and foot

     ● **T24.41**   **Corrosion of unspecified degree of thigh**

         ● **T24.411**   Corrosion of unspecified degree of right thigh

         ● **T24.412**   Corrosion of unspecified degree of left thigh

         ● **T24.419**   Corrosion of unspecified degree of unspecified thigh

     ● **T24.42**   **Corrosion of unspecified degree of knee**

         ● **T24.421**   Corrosion of unspecified degree of right knee

         ● **T24.422**   Corrosion of unspecified degree of left knee

         ● **T24.429**   Corrosion of unspecified degree of unspecified knee

     ● **T24.43**   **Corrosion of unspecified degree of lower leg**

         ● **T24.431**   Corrosion of unspecified degree of right lower leg

         ● **T24.432**   Corrosion of unspecified degree of left lower leg

         ● **T24.439**   Corrosion of unspecified degree of unspecified lower leg

     ● **T24.49**   **Corrosion of unspecified degree of multiple sites of lower limb, except ankle and foot**

         ● **T24.491**   Corrosion of unspecified degree of multiple sites of right lower limb, except ankle and foot

         ● **T24.492**   Corrosion of unspecified degree of multiple sites of left lower limb, except ankle and foot

         ● **T24.499**   Corrosion of unspecified degree of multiple sites of unspecified lower limb, except ankle and foot

● **T24.5**   **Corrosion of first degree of lower limb, except ankle and foot**

     Code first (T51-T65) *to identify chemical and intent*

     Use additional external cause code to identify place (Y92)

     ● **T24.50**   **Corrosion of first degree of unspecified site of lower limb, except ankle and foot**

         ● **T24.501**   Corrosion of first degree of unspecified site of right lower limb, except ankle and foot

         ● **T24.502**   Corrosion of first degree of unspecified site of left lower limb, except ankle and foot

         ● **T24.509**   Corrosion of first degree of unspecified site of unspecified lower limb, except ankle and foot

● **T24.51**   **Corrosion of first degree of thigh**

     ● **T24.511**   Corrosion of first degree of right thigh

     ● **T24.512**   Corrosion of first degree of left thigh

     ● **T24.519**   Corrosion of first degree of unspecified thigh

● **T24.52**   **Corrosion of first degree of knee**

     ● **T24.521**   Corrosion of first degree of right knee

     ● **T24.522**   Corrosion of first degree of left knee

     ● **T24.529**   Corrosion of first degree of unspecified knee

● **T24.53**   **Corrosion of first degree of lower leg**

     ● **T24.531**   Corrosion of first degree of right lower leg

     ● **T24.532**   Corrosion of first degree of left lower leg

     ● **T24.539**   Corrosion of first degree of unspecified lower leg

● **T24.59**   **Corrosion of first degree of multiple sites of lower limb, except ankle and foot**

     ● **T24.591**   Corrosion of first degree of multiple sites of right lower limb, except ankle and foot

     ● **T24.592**   Corrosion of first degree of multiple sites of left lower limb, except ankle and foot

     ● **T24.599**   Corrosion of first degree of multiple sites of unspecified lower limb, except ankle and foot

● **T24.6**   **Corrosion of second degree of lower limb, except ankle and foot**

     Code first (T51-T65) *to identify chemical and intent*

     Use additional external cause code to identify place (Y92)

     ● **T24.60**   **Corrosion of second degree of unspecified site of lower limb, except ankle and foot**

         ● **T24.601**   Corrosion of second degree of unspecified site of right lower limb, except ankle and foot

         ● **T24.602**   Corrosion of second degree of unspecified site of left lower limb, except ankle and foot

         ● **T24.609**   Corrosion of second degree of unspecified site of unspecified lower limb, except ankle and foot

     ● **T24.61**   **Corrosion of second degree of thigh**

         ● **T24.611**   Corrosion of second degree of right thigh

         ● **T24.612**   Corrosion of second degree of left thigh

         ● **T24.619**   Corrosion of second degree of unspecified thigh

     ● **T24.62**   **Corrosion of second degree of knee**

         ● **T24.621**   Corrosion of second degree of right knee

         ● **T24.622**   Corrosion of second degree of left knee

         ● **T24.629**   Corrosion of second degree of unspecified knee

     ● **T24.63**   **Corrosion of second degree of lower leg**

         ● **T24.631**   Corrosion of second degree of right lower leg

         ● **T24.632**   Corrosion of second degree of left lower leg

         ● **T24.639**   Corrosion of second degree of unspecified lower leg

CHAPTER 19 (S00-T88)

- **T24.69** Corrosion of second degree of multiple sites of lower limb, except ankle and foot
  - **T24.691** Corrosion of second degree of multiple sites of right lower limb, except ankle and foot
  - **T24.692** Corrosion of second degree of multiple sites of left lower limb, except ankle and foot
  - **T24.699** Corrosion of second degree of multiple sites of unspecified lower limb, except ankle and foot
- **T24.7** Corrosion of third degree of lower limb, except ankle and foot

  Code first (T51-T65) to identify chemical and intent

  Use additional external cause code to identify place (Y92)
  - **T24.70** Corrosion of third degree of unspecified site of lower limb, except ankle and foot

    (Ex) For category T24.70 CC codes: See PDX Collection 1404
    - **T24.701** Corrosion of third degree of unspecified site of right lower limb, except ankle and foot A 🔾, A 🔾
    - **T24.702** Corrosion of third degree of unspecified site of left lower limb, except ankle and foot A 🔾, A 🔾
    - **T24.709** Corrosion of third degree of unspecified site of unspecified lower limb, except ankle and foot A 🔾, A 🔾
  - **T24.71** Corrosion of third degree of thigh

    (Ex) For category T24.71 CC codes: See PDX Collection 1405
    - **T24.711** Corrosion of third degree of right thigh A 🔾, A 🔾
    - **T24.712** Corrosion of third degree of left thigh A 🔾, A 🔾
    - **T24.719** Corrosion of third degree of unspecified thigh A 🔾, A 🔾
  - **T24.72** Corrosion of third degree of knee

    (Ex) For category T24.72 CC codes: See PDX Collection 1406
    - **T24.721** Corrosion of third degree of right knee A 🔾, A 🔾
    - **T24.722** Corrosion of third degree of left knee A 🔾, A 🔾
    - **T24.729** Corrosion of third degree of unspecified knee A 🔾, A 🔾
  - **T24.73** Corrosion of third degree of lower leg

    (Ex) For category T24.73 CC codes: See PDX Collection 1407
    - **T24.731** Corrosion of third degree of right lower leg A 🔾, A 🔾
    - **T24.732** Corrosion of third degree of left lower leg A 🔾, A 🔾
    - **T24.739** Corrosion of third degree of unspecified lower leg A 🔾, A 🔾
  - **T24.79** Corrosion of third degree of multiple sites of lower limb, except ankle and foot

    (Ex) For category T24.79 CC codes: See PDX Collection 1404
    - **T24.791** Corrosion of third degree of multiple sites of right lower limb, except ankle and foot A 🔾, A 🔾
    - **T24.792** Corrosion of third degree of multiple sites of left lower limb, except ankle and foot A 🔾, A 🔾
    - **T24.799** Corrosion of third degree of multiple sites of unspecified lower limb, except ankle and foot A 🔾, A 🔾

- **T25** Burn and corrosion of ankle and foot

  The appropriate 7th character is to be added to each code from category T25

A	initial encounter
D	subsequent encounter
S	sequela

  - **T25.0** Burn of unspecified degree of ankle and foot

    Use additional external cause code to identify the source, place and intent of the burn (X00-X19, X75-X77, X96-X98, Y92)
    - **T25.01** Burn of unspecified degree of ankle
      - **T25.011** Burn of unspecified degree of right ankle
      - **T25.012** Burn of unspecified degree of left ankle
      - **T25.019** Burn of unspecified degree of unspecified ankle
    - **T25.02** Burn of unspecified degree of foot

      Excludes2 burn of unspecified degree of toe(s) (nail) (T25.03-)
      - **T25.021** Burn of unspecified degree of right foot
      - **T25.022** Burn of unspecified degree of left foot
      - **T25.029** Burn of unspecified degree of unspecified foot
    - **T25.03** Burn of unspecified degree of toe(s) (nail)
      - **T25.031** Burn of unspecified degree of right toe(s) (nail)
      - **T25.032** Burn of unspecified degree of left toe(s) (nail)
      - **T25.039** Burn of unspecified degree of unspecified toe(s) (nail)
    - **T25.09** Burn of unspecified degree of multiple sites of ankle and foot
      - **T25.091** Burn of unspecified degree of multiple sites of right ankle and foot
      - **T25.092** Burn of unspecified degree of multiple sites of left ankle and foot
      - **T25.099** Burn of unspecified degree of multiple sites of unspecified ankle and foot
  - **T25.1** Burn of first degree of ankle and foot

    Use additional external cause code to identify the source, place and intent of the burn (X00-X19, X75-X77, X96-X98, Y92)
    - **T25.11** Burn of first degree of ankle
      - **T25.111** Burn of first degree of right ankle
      - **T25.112** Burn of first degree of left ankle
      - **T25.119** Burn of first degree of unspecified ankle
    - **T25.12** Burn of first degree of foot

      Excludes2 burn of first degree of toe(s) (nail) (T25.13-)
      - **T25.121** Burn of first degree of right foot
      - **T25.122** Burn of first degree of left foot
      - **T25.129** Burn of first degree of unspecified foot
    - **T25.13** Burn of first degree of toe(s) (nail)
      - **T25.131** Burn of first degree of right toe(s) (nail)
      - **T25.132** Burn of first degree of left toe(s) (nail)
      - **T25.139** Burn of first degree of unspecified toe(s) (nail)

▶ New   ⇒ Revised   ~~deleted~~ Deleted   Excludes 1   Excludes 2   Includes   Use additional   Code first   Code also   Key words

OGCR Official Guidelines   ● Unacceptable Principal Diagnosis   X Assign placeholder X   ● Use Additional Character(s)   ▶ Manifestation Code   **Coding Clinic**

● **T25.19** Burn of first degree of multiple sites of ankle and foot

- ● **T25.191** Burn of first degree of multiple sites of right ankle and foot
- ● **T25.192** Burn of first degree of multiple sites of left ankle and foot
- ● **T25.199** Burn of first degree of multiple sites of unspecified ankle and foot

● **T25.2** Burn of second degree of ankle and foot

Use additional external cause code to identify the source, place and intent of the burn (X00-X19, X75-X77, X96-X98, Y92)

● **T25.21** Burn of second degree of ankle
- ● **T25.211** Burn of second degree of right ankle
- ● **T25.212** Burn of second degree of left ankle
- ● **T25.219** Burn of second degree of unspecified ankle

● **T25.22** Burn of second degree of foot

Excludes2 burn of second degree of toe(s) (nail) (T25.23-)

- ● **T25.221** Burn of second degree of right foot
- ● **T25.222** Burn of second degree of left foot
- ● **T25.229** Burn of second degree of unspecified foot

● **T25.23** Burn of second degree of toe(s) (nail)
- ● **T25.231** Burn of second degree of right toe(s) (nail)
- ● **T25.232** Burn of second degree of left toe(s) (nail)
- ● **T25.239** Burn of second degree of unspecified toe(s) (nail)

● **T25.29** Burn of second degree of multiple sites of ankle and foot
- ● **T25.291** Burn of second degree of multiple sites of right ankle and foot
- ● **T25.292** Burn of second degree of multiple sites of left ankle and foot
- ● **T25.299** Burn of second degree of multiple sites of unspecified ankle and foot

● **T25.3** Burn of third degree of ankle and foot

Use additional external cause code to identify the source, place and intent of the burn (X00-X19, X75-X77, X96-X98, Y92)

● **T25.31** Burn of third degree of ankle
ⒺⓍ **For category T25.31 CC codes:** See PDX Collection 1408
- ● **T25.311** Burn of third degree of right ankle A 🟡, A 🟡
- ● **T25.312** Burn of third degree of left ankle A 🟡, A 🟡
- ● **T25.319** Burn of third degree of unspecified ankle A 🟡, A 🟡

● **T25.32** Burn of third degree of foot

Excludes2 burn of third degree of toe(s) (nail) (T25.33-)
ⒺⓍ **For category T25.32 CC codes:** See PDX Collection 1409
- ● **T25.321** Burn of third degree of right foot A 🟡, A 🟡
- ● **T25.322** Burn of third degree of left foot A 🟡, A 🟡
- ● **T25.329** Burn of third degree of unspecified foot A 🟡, A 🟡

● **T25.33** Burn of third degree of toe(s) (nail)
ⒺⓍ **For category T25.33 CC codes:** See PDX Collection 1410
- ● **T25.331** Burn of third degree of right toe(s) (nail) A 🟡, A 🟡
- ● **T25.332** Burn of third degree of left toe(s) (nail) A 🟡, A 🟡
- ● **T25.339** Burn of third degree of unspecified toe(s) (nail) A 🟡, A 🟡

● **T25.39** Burn of third degree of multiple sites of ankle and foot
ⒺⓍ **For category T25.39 CC codes:** See PDX Collection 1404
- ● **T25.391** Burn of third degree of multiple sites of right ankle and foot A 🟡, A 🟡
- ● **T25.392** Burn of third degree of multiple sites of left ankle and foot A 🟡, A 🟡
- ● **T25.399** Burn of third degree of multiple sites of unspecified ankle and foot A 🟡, A 🟡

● **T25.4** Corrosion of unspecified degree of ankle and foot

Code first (T51-T65) to identify chemical and intent
Use additional external cause code to identify place (Y92)

● **T25.41** Corrosion of unspecified degree of ankle
- ● **T25.411** Corrosion of unspecified degree of right ankle
- ● **T25.412** Corrosion of unspecified degree of left ankle
- ● **T25.419** Corrosion of unspecified degree of unspecified ankle

● **T25.42** Corrosion of unspecified degree of foot

Excludes2 corrosion of unspecified degree of toe(s) (nail) (T25.43-)

- ● **T25.421** Corrosion of unspecified degree of right foot
- ● **T25.422** Corrosion of unspecified degree of left foot
- ● **T25.429** Corrosion of unspecified degree of unspecified foot

● **T25.43** Corrosion of unspecified degree of toe(s) (nail)
- ● **T25.431** Corrosion of unspecified degree of right toe(s) (nail)
- ● **T25.432** Corrosion of unspecified degree of left toe(s) (nail)
- ● **T25.439** Corrosion of unspecified degree of unspecified toe(s) (nail)

● **T25.49** Corrosion of unspecified degree of multiple sites of ankle and foot
- ● **T25.491** Corrosion of unspecified degree of multiple sites of right ankle and foot
- ● **T25.492** Corrosion of unspecified degree of multiple sites of left ankle and foot
- ● **T25.499** Corrosion of unspecified degree of multiple sites of unspecified ankle and foot

● **T25.5** Corrosion of first degree of ankle and foot

Code first (T51-T65) to identify chemical and intent
Use additional external cause code to identify place (Y92)

● **T25.51** Corrosion of first degree of ankle
- ● **T25.511** Corrosion of first degree of right ankle
- ● **T25.512** Corrosion of first degree of left ankle
- ● **T25.519** Corrosion of first degree of unspecified ankle

CHAPTER 19 (S00-T88)

● **T25.52　Corrosion of first degree of foot**
　　　Excludes2　corrosion of first degree of toe(s) (nail) (T25.53-)
　　● T25.521　Corrosion of first degree of right foot
　　● T25.522　Corrosion of first degree of left foot
　　● T25.529　Corrosion of first degree of unspecified foot
● **T25.53　Corrosion of first degree of toe(s) (nail)**
　　● T25.531　Corrosion of first degree of right toe(s) (nail)
　　● T25.532　Corrosion of first degree of left toe(s) (nail)
　　● T25.539　Corrosion of first degree of unspecified toe(s) (nail)
● **T25.59　Corrosion of first degree of multiple sites of ankle and foot**
　　● T25.591　Corrosion of first degree of multiple sites of right ankle and foot
　　● T25.592　Corrosion of first degree of multiple sites of left ankle and foot
　　● T25.599　Corrosion of first degree of multiple sites of unspecified ankle and foot

● **T25.6　Corrosion of second degree of ankle and foot**
　　Code first (T51-T65) to identify chemical and intent
　　Use additional external cause code to identify place (Y92)
　● **T25.61　Corrosion of second degree of ankle**
　　● T25.611　Corrosion of second degree of right ankle
　　● T25.612　Corrosion of second degree of left ankle
　　● T25.619　Corrosion of second degree of unspecified ankle
　● **T25.62　Corrosion of second degree of foot**
　　　Excludes2　corrosion of second degree of toe(s) (nail) (T25.63-)
　　● T25.621　Corrosion of second degree of right foot
　　● T25.622　Corrosion of second degree of left foot
　　● T25.629　Corrosion of second degree of unspecified foot
　● **T25.63　Corrosion of second degree of toe(s) (nail)**
　　● T25.631　Corrosion of second degree of right toe(s) (nail)
　　● T25.632　Corrosion of second degree of left toe(s) (nail)
　　● T25.639　Corrosion of second degree of unspecified toe(s) (nail)
　● **T25.69　Corrosion of second degree of multiple sites of ankle and foot**
　　● T25.691　Corrosion of second degree of right ankle and foot
　　● T25.692　Corrosion of second degree of left ankle and foot
　　● T25.699　Corrosion of second degree of unspecified ankle and foot

● **T25.7　Corrosion of third degree of ankle and foot**
　　Code first (T51-T65) to identify chemical and intent
　　Use additional external cause code to identify place (Y92)
　● **T25.71　Corrosion of third degree of ankle**
　　　Ⓔ For category T25.71 CC codes: See PDX Collection 1408
　　● T25.711　Corrosion of third degree of right ankle A 🔄, A 🔄
　　● T25.712　Corrosion of third degree of left ankle A 🔄, A 🔄
　　● T25.719　Corrosion of third degree of unspecified ankle A 🔄, A 🔄

● **T25.72　Corrosion of third degree of foot**
　　　Excludes2　corrosion of third degree of toe(s) (nail) (T25.73-)
　　　Ⓔ For category T25.72 CC codes: See PDX Collection 1409
　　● T25.721　Corrosion of third degree of right foot A 🔄, A 🔄
　　● T25.722　Corrosion of third degree of left foot A 🔄, A 🔄
　　● T25.729　Corrosion of third degree of unspecified foot A 🔄, A 🔄
● **T25.73　Corrosion of third degree of toe(s) (nail)**
　　　Ⓔ For category T25.73 CC codes: See PDX Collection 1410
　　● T25.731　Corrosion of third degree of right toe(s) (nail) A 🔄, A 🔄
　　● T25.732　Corrosion of third degree of left toe(s) (nail) A 🔄, A 🔄
　　● T25.739　Corrosion of third degree of unspecified toe(s) (nail) A 🔄, A 🔄
● **T25.79　Corrosion of third degree of multiple sites of ankle and foot**
　　　Ⓔ For category T25.79 CC codes: See PDX Collection 1404
　　● T25.791　Corrosion of third degree of multiple sites of right ankle and foot A 🔄, A 🔄
　　● T25.792　Corrosion of third degree of multiple sites of left ankle and foot A 🔄, A 🔄
　　● T25.799　Corrosion of third degree of multiple sites of unspecified ankle and foot A 🔄, A 🔄

BURNS AND CORROSIONS CONFINED TO EYE AND INTERNAL ORGANS (T26-T28)

● **T26　Burn and corrosion confined to eye and adnexa**
　　The appropriate 7th character is to be added to each code from category T26

A	initial encounter
D	subsequent encounter
S	sequela

　● **T26.0　Burn of eyelid and periocular area**
　　Use additional external cause code to identify the source, place and intent of the burn (X00-X19, X75-X77, X96-X98, Y92)
　　X● T26.00　Burn of unspecified eyelid and periocular area
　　X● T26.01　Burn of right eyelid and periocular area
　　X● T26.02　Burn of left eyelid and periocular area
　● **T26.1　Burn of cornea and conjunctival sac**
　　Use additional external cause code to identify the source, place and intent of the burn (X00-X19, X75-X77, X96-X98, Y92)
　　X● T26.10　Burn of cornea and conjunctival sac, unspecified eye
　　X● T26.11　Burn of cornea and conjunctival sac, right eye
　　X● T26.12　Burn of cornea and conjunctival sac, left eye
　● **T26.2　Burn with resulting rupture and destruction of eyeball**
　　Use additional external cause code to identify the source, place and intent of the burn (X00-X19, X75-X77, X96-X98, Y92)
　　　Ⓔ For category T26.2 CC codes: No exclusions
　　X● T26.20　Burn with resulting rupture and destruction of unspecified eyeball A 🔄, A 🔄
　　X● T26.21　Burn with resulting rupture and destruction of right eyeball A 🔄, A 🔄
　　X● T26.22　Burn with resulting rupture and destruction of left eyeball A 🔄, A 🔄

▶ New　⇒ Revised　~~deleted~~ Deleted　Excludes 1　Excludes 2　Includes　Use additional　Code first　Code also　Key words
OGCR Official Guidelines　● Unacceptable Principal Diagnosis　X Assign placeholder X　● Use Additional Character(s)　▶ Manifestation Code　**Coding Clinic**

● **T26.3**   Burns of other specified parts of eye and adnexa

Use additional external cause code to identify the source, place and intent of the burn (X00-X19, X75-X77, X96-X98, Y92)

X● **T26.30**   Burns of other specified parts of unspecified eye and adnexa

X● **T26.31**   Burns of other specified parts of right eye and adnexa

X● **T26.32**   Burns of other specified parts of left eye and adnexa

● **T26.4**   Burn of eye and adnexa, part unspecified

Use additional external cause code to identify the source, place and intent of the burn (X00-X19, X75-X77, X96-X98, Y92)

X● **T26.40**   Burn of unspecified eye and adnexa, part unspecified

X● **T26.41**   Burn of right eye and adnexa, part unspecified

X● **T26.42**   Burn of left eye and adnexa, part unspecified

● **T26.5**   Corrosion of eyelid and periocular area

Code first (T51-T65) *to identify chemical and intent*
Use additional external cause code to identify place (Y92)

X● **T26.50**   Corrosion of unspecified eyelid and periocular area

X● **T26.51**   Corrosion of right eyelid and periocular area

X● **T26.52**   Corrosion of left eyelid and periocular area

● **T26.6**   Corrosion of cornea and conjunctival sac

Code first (T51-T65) *to identify chemical and intent*
Use additional external cause code to identify place (Y92)

X● **T26.60**   Corrosion of cornea and conjunctival sac, unspecified eye

X● **T26.61**   Corrosion of cornea and conjunctival sac, right eye

X● **T26.62**   Corrosion of cornea and conjunctival sac, left eye

● **T26.7**   Corrosion with resulting rupture and destruction of eyeball

Code first (T51-T65) *to identify chemical and intent*
Use additional external cause code to identify place (Y92)

(Ex:) **For category T26.7 CC codes:** No exclusions

X● **T26.70**   Corrosion with resulting rupture and destruction of unspecified eyeball A 🦠, A 🦠

X● **T26.71**   Corrosion with resulting rupture and destruction of right eyeball A 🦠, A 🦠

X● **T26.72**   Corrosion with resulting rupture and destruction of left eyeball A 🦠, A 🦠

● **T26.8**   Corrosions of other specified parts of eye and adnexa

Code first (T51-T65) *to identify chemical and intent*
Use additional external cause code to identify place (Y92)

X● **T26.80**   Corrosions of other specified parts of unspecified eye and adnexa

X● **T26.81**   Corrosions of other specified parts of right eye and adnexa

X● **T26.82**   Corrosions of other specified parts of left eye and adnexa

● **T26.9**   Corrosion of eye and adnexa, part unspecified

Code first (T51-T65) *to identify chemical and intent*
Use additional external cause code to identify place (Y92)

X● **T26.90**   Corrosion of unspecified eye and adnexa, part unspecified

X● **T26.91**   Corrosion of right eye and adnexa, part unspecified

X● **T26.92**   Corrosion of left eye and adnexa, part unspecified

● **T27**   Burn and corrosion of respiratory tract

Use additional external cause code to identify the source and intent of the burn (X00-X19, X75-X77, X96-X98)
Use additional external cause code to identify place (Y92)
The appropriate 7th character is to be added to each code from category T27

A	initial encounter
D	subsequent encounter
S	sequela

(Ex:) **For category T27 CC codes:** See PDX Collection 1411

X● **T27.0**   Burn of larynx and trachea A 🦠, A 🦠

X● **T27.1**   Burn involving larynx and trachea with lung A 🦠, A 🦠

X● **T27.2**   Burn of other parts of respiratory tract A 🦠, A 🦠
Burn of thoracic cavity

X● **T27.3**   Burn of respiratory tract, part unspecified A 🦠, A 🦠

Code first (T51-T65) to identify chemical and intent for codes T27.4-T27.7

X● **T27.4**   Corrosion of larynx and trachea A 🦠, A 🦠
▶ *Code first* (T51-T65) *to identify chemical and intent*

X● **T27.5**   Corrosion involving larynx and trachea with lung A 🦠,

X● **T27.6**   Corrosion of other parts of respiratory tract A 🦠, A 🦠
▶ *Code first* (T51-T65) *to identify chemical and intent*

X● **T27.7**   Corrosion of respiratory tract, part unspecified A 🦠, A 🦠
▶ *Code first* (T51-T65) *to identify chemical and intent*

● **T28**   Burn and corrosion of other internal organs

Use additional external cause code to identify the source and intent of the burn (X00-X19, X75-X77, X96-X98)
Use additional external cause code to identify place (Y92)
The appropriate 7th character is to be added to each code from category T28

A	initial encounter
D	subsequent encounter
S	sequela

X● **T28.0**   Burn of mouth and pharynx

X● **T28.1**   Burn of esophagus A 🦠, A 🦠
(Ex:) See PDX Collection 1412

X● **T28.2**   Burn of other parts of alimentary tract A 🦠, A 🦠
(Ex:) See PDX Collection 1413

X● **T28.3**   Burn of internal genitourinary organs

X● **T28.4**   Burns of other and unspecified internal organs
▶ *Code first* (T51-T65) *to identify chemical and intent*

X● **T28.40**   Burn of unspecified internal organ

● **T28.41**   Burn of ear drum

● **T28.411**   Burn of right ear drum

● **T28.412**   Burn of left ear drum

● **T28.419**   Burn of unspecified ear drum

X● **T28.49**   Burn of other internal organ

Code first (T51-T65) to identify chemical and intent for T28.5-T28.9

X● **T28.5**   Corrosion of mouth and pharynx
▶ *Code first* (T51-T65) *to identify chemical and intent*

X● **T28.6**   Corrosion of esophagus A 🦠, A 🦠
▶ *Code first* (T51-T65) *to identify chemical and intent*
(Ex:) See PDX Collection 1412

X● **T28.7**   Corrosion of other parts of alimentary tract A 🦠, A 🦠
▶ *Code first* (T51-T65) *to identify chemical and intent*
(Ex:) See PDX Collection 1413

X● **T28.8**   Corrosion of internal genitourinary organs
▶ *Code first* (T51-T65) *to identify chemical and intent*

N Newborn Age: 0   **P** Pediatric Age: 0-17   **M** Maternity DX: 12-55   **A** Adult Age: 15-124   ♀ Females Only   ♂ Males Only

🦠 Complication\Comorbidity   🦠 Major C\C   (Ex:) CC/MCC Exclusions   🦠 Hospital-Acquired Condition

1427

CHAPTER 19 (S00-T88)

CHAPTER 19 (S00-T88)

● **T28.9**   **Corrosions of other and unspecified internal organs**
▶ *Code first (T51-T65) to identify chemical and intent*
X● **T28.90**   **Corrosions of unspecified internal organs**
● **T28.91**   **Corrosions of ear drum**
     ● **T28.911**   **Corrosions of right ear drum**
     ● **T28.912**   **Corrosions of left ear drum**
     ● **T28.919**   **Corrosions of unspecified ear drum**
X● **T28.99**   **Corrosions of other internal organs**

OGCR Section I.C.19.d.5.

Assign separate code for each burn site
When coding burns, assign separate codes for each burn site. Category T30, Burn and corrosion, body region unspecified is extremely vague and should rarely be used.

BURNS AND CORROSIONS OF MULTIPLE AND UNSPECIFIED BODY REGIONS (T30-T32)

● **T30**   **Burn and corrosion, body region unspecified**
     T30.0   **Burn of unspecified body region, unspecified degree**
           This code is not for inpatient use. Code to specified site and degree of burns
           Burn NOS
           Multiple burns NOS
     T30.4   **Corrosion of unspecified body region, unspecified degree**
           This code is not for inpatient use. Code to specified site and degree of corrosion
           Corrosion NOS
           Multiple corrosion NOS

● **T31**   **Burns classified according to extent of body surface involved**
     Note: This category is to be used as the primary code only when the site of the burn is unspecified. It should be used as a supplementary code with categories T20-T25 when the site is specified.
     Ⓔⓧ **For category T31 CC codes:** See PDX Collection 1414
     T31.0   **Burns involving less than 10% of body surface**
●   **T31.1**   **Burns involving 10-19% of body surface**
        T31.10   **Burns involving 10-19% of body surface with 0% to 9% third degree burns** 🔖 🔖
             Burns involving 10-19% of body surface NOS
        T31.11   **Burns involving 10-19% of body surface with 10-19% third degree burns** 🔖 🔖
●   **T31.2**   **Burns involving 20-29% of body surface**
        T31.20   **Burns involving 20-29% of body surface with 0% to 9% third degree burns** 🔖 🔖
             Burns involving 20-29% of body surface NOS
        T31.21   **Burns involving 20-29% of body surface with 10-19% third degree burns** 🔖 🔖
        T31.22   **Burns involving 20-29% of body surface with 20-29% third degree burns** 🔖 🔖

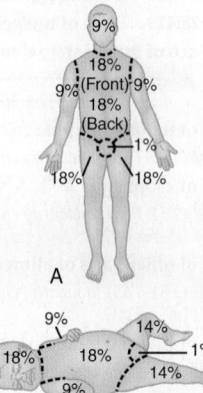

A

B

Figure 19-16   Rule of nines: percentages of total body area. (From Marx: *Rosen's Emergency Medicine: Concepts and Clinical Practice,* ed 6, Mosby, 2006)

● **T31.3**   **Burns involving 30-39% of body surface**
     T31.30   **Burns involving 30-39% of body surface with 0% to 9% third degree burns** 🔖 🔖
          Burns involving 30-39% of body surface NOS
     T31.31   **Burns involving 30-39% of body surface with 10-19% third degree burns** 🔖 🔖
     T31.32   **Burns involving 30-39% of body surface with 20-29% third degree burns** 🔖 🔖
     T31.33   **Burns involving 30-39% of body surface with 30-39% third degree burns** 🔖 🔖
● **T31.4**   **Burns involving 40-49% of body surface**
     T31.40   **Burns involving 40-49% of body surface with 0% to 9% third degree burns** 🔖 🔖
          Burns involving 40-49% of body surface NOS
     T31.41   **Burns involving 40-49% of body surface with 10-19% third degree burns** 🔖 🔖
     T31.42   **Burns involving 40-49% of body surface with 20-29% third degree burns** 🔖 🔖
     T31.43   **Burns involving 40-49% of body surface with 30-39% third degree burns** 🔖 🔖
     T31.44   **Burns involving 40-49% of body surface with 40-49% third degree burns** 🔖 🔖
● **T31.5**   **Burns involving 50-59% of body surface**
     T31.50   **Burns involving 50-59% of body surface with 0% to 9% third degree burns** 🔖 🔖
          Burns involving 50-59% of body surface NOS
     T31.51   **Burns involving 50-59% of body surface with 10-19% third degree burns** 🔖 🔖
     T31.52   **Burns involving 50-59% of body surface with 20-29% third degree burns** 🔖 🔖
     T31.53   **Burns involving 50-59% of body surface with 30-39% third degree burns** 🔖 🔖
     T31.54   **Burns involving 50-59% of body surface with 40-49% third degree burns** 🔖 🔖
     T31.55   **Burns involving 50-59% of body surface with 50-59% third degree burns** 🔖 🔖
● **T31.6**   **Burns involving 60-69% of body surface**
     T31.60   **Burns involving 60-69% of body surface with 0% to 9% third degree burns** 🔖 🔖
          Burns involving 60-69% of body surface NOS
     T31.61   **Burns involving 60-69% of body surface with 10-19% third degree burns** 🔖 🔖
     T31.62   **Burns involving 60-69% of body surface with 20-29% third degree burns** 🔖 🔖
     T31.63   **Burns involving 60-69% of body surface with 30-39% third degree burns** 🔖 🔖
     T31.64   **Burns involving 60-69% of body surface with 40-49% third degree burns** 🔖 🔖
     T31.65   **Burns involving 60-69% of body surface with 50-59% third degree burns** 🔖 🔖
     T31.66   **Burns involving 60-69% of body surface with 60-69% third degree burns** 🔖 🔖
● **T31.7**   **Burns involving 70-79% of body surface**
     T31.70   **Burns involving 70-79% of body surface with 0% to 9% third degree burns** 🔖 🔖
          Burns involving 70-79% of body surface NOS
     T31.71   **Burns involving 70-79% of body surface with 10-19% third degree burns** 🔖 🔖
     T31.72   **Burns involving 70-79% of body surface with 20-29% third degree burns** 🔖 🔖
     T31.73   **Burns involving 70-79% of body surface with 30-39% third degree burns** 🔖 🔖
     T31.74   **Burns involving 70-79% of body surface with 40-49% third degree burns** 🔖 🔖
     T31.75   **Burns involving 70-79% of body surface with 50-59% third degree burns** 🔖 🔖
     T31.76   **Burns involving 70-79% of body surface with 60-69% third degree burns** 🔖 🔖
     T31.77   **Burns involving 70-79% of body surface with 70-79% third degree burns** 🔖 🔖

▶ New   ⇒ Revised   ~~deleted~~ Deleted   Excludes 1   Excludes 2   Includes   Use additional   Code first   Code also   Key words
OGCR Official Guidelines   ● Unacceptable Principal Diagnosis   X Assign placeholder X   ● Use Additional Character(s)   ▌ Manifestation Code   **Coding Clinic**

● **T31.8**   Burns involving 80-89% of body surface

   T31.80   **Burns involving 80-89% of body surface with 0% to 9% third degree burns** 🝙 🝙
      Burns involving 80-89% of body surface NOS

   T31.81   **Burns involving 80-89% of body surface with 10-19% third degree burns** 🝙 🝙

   T31.82   **Burns involving 80-89% of body surface with 20-29% third degree burns** 🝙 🝙

   T31.83   **Burns involving 80-89% of body surface with 30-39% third degree burns** 🝙 🝙

   T31.84   **Burns involving 80-89% of body surface with 40-49% third degree burns** 🝙 🝙

   T31.85   **Burns involving 80-89% of body surface with 50-59% third degree burns** 🝙 🝙

   T31.86   **Burns involving 80-89% of body surface with 60-69% third degree burns** 🝙 🝙

   T31.87   **Burns involving 80-89% of body surface with 70-79% third degree burns** 🝙 🝙

   T31.88   **Burns involving 80-89% of body surface with 80-89% third degree burns** 🝙 🝙

● **T31.9**   Burns involving 90% or more of body surface

   T31.90   **Burns involving 90% or more of body surface with 0% to 9% third degree burns** 🝙 🝙
      Burns involving 90% or more of body surface NOS

   T31.91   **Burns involving 90% or more of body surface with 10-19% third degree burns** 🝙 🝙

   T31.92   **Burns involving 90% or more of body surface with 20-29% third degree burns** 🝙 🝙

   T31.93   **Burns involving 90% or more of body surface with 30-39% third degree burns** 🝙 🝙

   T31.94   **Burns involving 90% or more of body surface with 40-49% third degree burns** 🝙 🝙

   T31.95   **Burns involving 90% or more of body surface with 50-59% third degree burns** 🝙 🝙

   T31.96   **Burns involving 90% or more of body surface with 60-69% third degree burns** 🝙 🝙

   T31.97   **Burns involving 90% or more of body surface with 70-79% third degree burns** 🝙 🝙

   T31.98   **Burns involving 90% or more of body surface with 80-89% third degree burns** 🝙 🝙

   T31.99   **Burns involving 90% or more of body surface with 90% or more third degree burns** 🝙 🝙

● **T32**   **Corrosions classified according to extent of body surface involved**

   Note: This category is to be used as the primary code only when the site of the corrosion is unspecified. It may be used as a supplementary code with categories T20-T25 when the site is specified.

   Ⓔⓧ **For category T32 CC codes:** See PDX Collection 1414

   T32.0   Corrosions involving less than 10% of body surface

● **T32.1**   Corrosions involving 10-19% of body surface

   T32.10   **Corrosions involving 10-19% of body surface with 0% to 9% third degree corrosion** 🝙 🝙
      Corrosions involving 10-19% of body surface NOS

   T32.11   **Corrosions involving 10-19% of body surface with 10-19% third degree corrosion** 🝙 🝙

● **T32.2**   Corrosions involving 20-29% of body surface

   T32.20   **Corrosions involving 20-29% of body surface with 0% to 9% third degree corrosion** 🝙 🝙

   T32.21   **Corrosions involving 20-29% of body surface with 10-19% third degree corrosion** 🝙 🝙

   T32.22   **Corrosions involving 20-29% of body surface with 20-29% third degree corrosion** 🝙 🝙

● **T32.3**   Corrosions involving 30-39% of body surface

   T32.30   **Corrosions involving 30-39% of body surface with 0% to 9% third degree corrosion** 🝙 🝙

   T32.31   **Corrosions involving 30-39% of body surface with 10-19% third degree corrosion** 🝙 🝙

   T32.32   **Corrosions involving 30-39% of body surface with 20-29% third degree corrosion** 🝙 🝙

   T32.33   **Corrosions involving 30-39% of body surface with 30-39% third degree corrosion** 🝙 🝙

● **T32.4**   Corrosions involving 40-49% of body surface

   T32.40   **Corrosions involving 40-49% of body surface with 0% to 9% third degree corrosion** 🝙 🝙

   T32.41   **Corrosions involving 40-49% of body surface with 10-19% third degree corrosion** 🝙 🝙

   T32.42   **Corrosions involving 40-49% of body surface with 20-29% third degree corrosion** 🝙 🝙

   T32.43   **Corrosions involving 40-49% of body surface with 30-39% third degree corrosion** 🝙 🝙

   T32.44   **Corrosions involving 40-49% of body surface with 40-49% third degree corrosion** 🝙 🝙

● **T32.5**   Corrosions involving 50-59% of body surface

   T32.50   **Corrosions involving 50-59% of body surface with 0% to 9% third degree corrosion** 🝙 🝙

   T32.51   **Corrosions involving 50-59% of body surface with 10-19% third degree corrosion** 🝙 🝙

   T32.52   **Corrosions involving 50-59% of body surface with 20-29% third degree corrosion** 🝙 🝙

   T32.53   **Corrosions involving 50-59% of body surface with 30-39% third degree corrosion** 🝙 🝙

   T32.54   **Corrosions involving 50-59% of body surface with 40-49% third degree corrosion** 🝙 🝙

   T32.55   **Corrosions involving 50-59% of body surface with 50-59% third degree corrosion** 🝙 🝙

● **T32.6**   Corrosions involving 60-69% of body surface

   T32.60   **Corrosions involving 60-69% of body surface with 0% to 9% third degree corrosion** 🝙 🝙

   T32.61   **Corrosions involving 60-69% of body surface with 10-19% third degree corrosion** 🝙 🝙

   T32.62   **Corrosions involving 60-69% of body surface with 20-29% third degree corrosion** 🝙 🝙

   T32.63   **Corrosions involving 60-69% of body surface with 30-39% third degree corrosion** 🝙 🝙

   T32.64   **Corrosions involving 60-69% of body surface with 40-49% third degree corrosion** 🝙 🝙

   T32.65   **Corrosions involving 60-69% of body surface with 50-59% third degree corrosion** 🝙 🝙

   T32.66   **Corrosions involving 60-69% of body surface with 60-69% third degree corrosion** 🝙 🝙

● **T32.7**   Corrosions involving 70-79% of body surface

   T32.70   **Corrosions involving 70-79% of body surface with 0% to 9% third degree corrosion** 🝙 🝙

   T32.71   **Corrosions involving 70-79% of body surface with 10-19% third degree corrosion** 🝙 🝙

   T32.72   **Corrosions involving 70-79% of body surface with 20-29% third degree corrosion** 🝙 🝙

   T32.73   **Corrosions involving 70-79% of body surface with 30-39% third degree corrosion** 🝙 🝙

   T32.74   **Corrosions involving 70-79% of body surface with 40-49% third degree corrosion** 🝙 🝙

   T32.75   **Corrosions involving 70-79% of body surface with 50-59% third degree corrosion** 🝙 🝙

   T32.76   **Corrosions involving 70-79% of body surface with 60-69% third degree corrosion** 🝙 🝙

   T32.77   **Corrosions involving 70-79% of body surface with 70-79% third degree corrosion** 🝙 🝙

N Newborn Age: 0   **P** Pediatric Age: 0–17   **M** Maternity DX: 12–55   **A** Adult Age: 15–124   ♀ Females Only   ♂ Males Only

🝙 Complication\Comorbidity   🝙 Major C\C   Ⓔⓧ CC/MCC Exclusions   🝙 Hospital-Acquired Condition

1429

● **T32.8**   Corrosions involving 80-89% of body surface

     T32.80   Corrosions involving 80-89% of body surface with 0% to 9% third degree corrosion 🔖 🔖

     T32.81   Corrosions involving 80-89% of body surface with 10-19% third degree corrosion 🔖 🔖

     T32.82   Corrosions involving 80-89% of body surface with 20-29% third degree corrosion 🔖 🔖

     T32.83   Corrosions involving 80-89% of body surface with 30-39% third degree corrosion 🔖 🔖

     T32.84   Corrosions involving 80-89% of body surface with 40-49% third degree corrosion 🔖 🔖

     T32.85   Corrosions involving 80-89% of body surface with 50-59% third degree corrosion 🔖 🔖

     T32.86   Corrosions involving 80-89% of body surface with 60-69% third degree corrosion 🔖 🔖

     T32.87   Corrosions involving 80-89% of body surface with 70-79% third degree corrosion 🔖 🔖

     T32.88   Corrosions involving 80-89% of body surface with 80-89% third degree corrosion 🔖 🔖

● **T32.9**   Corrosions involving 90% or more of body surface

     T32.90   Corrosions involving 90% or more of body surface with 0% to 9% third degree corrosion 🔖 🔖

     T32.91   Corrosions involving 90% or more of body surface with 10-19% third degree corrosion 🔖 🔖

     T32.92   Corrosions involving 90% or more of body surface with 20-29% third degree corrosion 🔖 🔖

     T32.93   Corrosions involving 90% or more of body surface with 30-39% third degree corrosion 🔖 🔖

     T32.94   Corrosions involving 90% or more of body surface with 40-49% third degree corrosion 🔖 🔖

     T32.95   Corrosions involving 90% or more of body surface with 50-59% third degree corrosion 🔖 🔖

     T32.96   Corrosions involving 90% or more of body surface with 60-69% third degree corrosion 🔖 🔖

     T32.97   Corrosions involving 90% or more of body surface with 70-79% third degree corrosion 🔖 🔖

     T32.98   Corrosions involving 90% or more of body surface with 80-89% third degree corrosion 🔖 🔖

     T32.99   Corrosions involving 90% or more of body surface with 90% or more third degree corrosion 🔖 🔖

FROSTBITE (T33-T34)

Excludes2   hypothermia and other effects of reduced temperature (T68, T69.-)

● **T33**   **Superficial frostbite**

   Includes   frostbite with partial thickness skin loss

   The appropriate 7th character is to be added to each code from category T33

A	initial encounter
D	subsequent encounter
S	sequela

● **T33.0**   Superficial frostbite of head

    (Ex) **For category T33.0 CC codes:** See PDX Collection 1415

   ● **T33.01**   Superficial frostbite of ear

     ● **T33.011**   Superficial frostbite of right ear A 🔖, A 🔖

     ● **T33.012**   Superficial frostbite of left ear A 🔖, A 🔖

     ● **T33.019**   Superficial frostbite of unspecified ear A 🔖, A 🔖

X ● **T33.02**   Superficial frostbite of nose A 🔖, A 🔖

X ● **T33.09**   Superficial frostbite of other part of head A 🔖, A 🔖

X ● **T33.1**   Superficial frostbite of neck A 🔖, A 🔖

   (Ex) See PDX Collection 1415

X ● **T33.2**   Superficial frostbite of thorax A 🔖, A 🔖

   (Ex) See PDX Collection 1416

X ● **T33.3**   Superficial frostbite of abdominal wall, lower back and pelvis A 🔖, A 🔖

   (Ex) See PDX Collection 1416

● **T33.4**   Superficial frostbite of arm

   Excludes2   superficial frostbite of wrist and hand (T33.5-)

   (Ex) **For category T33.4 CC codes:** See PDX Collection 1416

X ● **T33.40**   Superficial frostbite of unspecified arm A 🔖, A 🔖

X ● **T33.41**   Superficial frostbite of right arm A 🔖, A 🔖

X ● **T33.42**   Superficial frostbite of left arm A 🔖, A 🔖

● **T33.5**   Superficial frostbite of wrist, hand, and fingers

   (Ex) **For category T33.5 CC codes:** See PDX Collection 1417

   ● **T33.51**   Superficial frostbite of wrist

     ● **T33.511**   Superficial frostbite of right wrist A 🔖, A 🔖

     ● **T33.512**   Superficial frostbite of left wrist A 🔖, A 🔖

     ● **T33.519**   Superficial frostbite of unspecified wrist A 🔖, A 🔖

   ● **T33.52**   Superficial frostbite of hand

    Excludes2   superficial frostbite of fingers (T33.53-)

     ● **T33.521**   Superficial frostbite of right hand A 🔖, A 🔖

     ● **T33.522**   Superficial frostbite of left hand A 🔖, A 🔖

     ● **T33.529**   Superficial frostbite of unspecified hand A 🔖, A 🔖

   ● **T33.53**   Superficial frostbite of finger(s)

     ● **T33.531**   Superficial frostbite of right finger(s) A 🔖, A 🔖

     ● **T33.532**   Superficial frostbite of left finger(s) A 🔖, A 🔖

     ● **T33.539**   Superficial frostbite of unspecified finger(s) A 🔖, A 🔖

● **T33.6**   Superficial frostbite of hip and thigh

   (Ex) **For category T33.6 CC codes:** See PDX Collection 1416

X ● **T33.60**   Superficial frostbite of unspecified hip and thigh A 🔖, A 🔖

X ● **T33.61**   Superficial frostbite of right hip and thigh A 🔖, A 🔖

X ● **T33.62**   Superficial frostbite of left hip and thigh A 🔖, A 🔖

● **T33.7**   Superficial frostbite of knee and lower leg

   Excludes2   superficial frostbite of ankle and foot (T33.8-)

   (Ex) **For category T33.7 CC codes:** See PDX Collection 1416

X ● **T33.70**   Superficial frostbite of unspecified knee and lower leg A 🔖, A 🔖

X ● **T33.71**   Superficial frostbite of right knee and lower leg A 🔖, A 🔖

X ● **T33.72**   Superficial frostbite of left knee and lower leg A 🔖, A 🔖

● **T33.8**   Superficial frostbite of ankle, foot, and toe(s)

   (Ex) **For category T33.8 CC codes:** See PDX Collection 1418

   ● **T33.81**   Superficial frostbite of ankle

     ● **T33.811**   Superficial frostbite of right ankle A 🔖, A 🔖

     ● **T33.812**   Superficial frostbite of left ankle A 🔖, A 🔖

     ● **T33.819**   Superficial frostbite of unspecified ankle A 🔖, A 🔖

▶ New   ⇒ Revised   ~~deleted~~ Deleted   Excludes 1   Excludes 2   Includes   Use additional   Code first   Code also   Key words

OGCR Official Guidelines   ● Unacceptable Principal Diagnosis   X Assign placeholder X   ● Use Additional Character(s)   ▶ Manifestation Code   **Coding Clinic**

● **T33.82** Superficial frostbite of foot
    ● **T33.821** Superficial frostbite of right foot A 🦠, A 🦠
    ● **T33.822** Superficial frostbite of left foot A 🦠, A 🦠
    ● **T33.829** Superficial frostbite of unspecified foot A 🦠, A 🦠

● **T33.83** Superficial frostbite of toe(s)
    ● **T33.831** Superficial frostbite of right toe(s) A 🦠, A 🦠
    ● **T33.832** Superficial frostbite of left toe(s) A 🦠, A 🦠
    ● **T33.839** Superficial frostbite of unspecified toe(s) A 🦠, A 🦠

● **T33.9** Superficial frostbite of other and unspecified sites
    (Ex) **For category T33.9 CC codes:** See PDX Collection 1416

X ● **T33.90** Superficial frostbite of unspecified sites A 🦠, A 🦠
    Superficial frostbite NOS

X ● **T33.99** Superficial frostbite of other sites A 🦠, A 🦠
    Superficial frostbite of leg NOS
    Superficial frostbite of trunk NOS

● **T34** Frostbite with tissue necrosis
    The appropriate 7th character is to be added to each code from category T34

> A   initial encounter
> D   subsequent encounter
> S   sequela

● **T34.0** Frostbite with tissue necrosis of head
    (Ex) **For category T34.0 CC codes:** See PDX Collection 1415

    ● **T34.01** Frostbite with tissue necrosis of ear
        ● **T34.011** Frostbite with tissue necrosis of right ear A 🦠, A 🦠
        ● **T34.012** Frostbite with tissue necrosis of left ear A 🦠, A 🦠
        ● **T34.019** Frostbite with tissue necrosis of unspecified ear A 🦠, A 🦠
    X ● **T34.02** Frostbite with tissue necrosis of nose A 🦠, A 🦠
    X ● **T34.09** Frostbite with tissue necrosis of other part of head A 🦠, A 🦠

X ● **T34.1** Frostbite with tissue necrosis of neck A 🦠, A 🦠
    (Ex) See PDX Collection 1415

X ● **T34.2** Frostbite with tissue necrosis of thorax A 🦠, A 🦠
    (Ex) See PDX Collection 1416

X ● **T34.3** Frostbite with tissue necrosis of abdominal wall, lower back and pelvis A 🦠, A 🦠
    (Ex) See PDX Collection 1416

● **T34.4** Frostbite with tissue necrosis of arm
    Excludes2 frostbite with tissue necrosis of wrist and hand (T34.5-)
    (Ex) **For category T34.4 CC codes:** See PDX Collection 1416

X ● **T34.40** Frostbite with tissue necrosis of unspecified arm A 🦠, A 🦠

X ● **T34.41** Frostbite with tissue necrosis of right arm A 🦠, A 🦠

X ● **T34.42** Frostbite with tissue necrosis of left arm A 🦠, A 🦠

● **T34.5** Frostbite with tissue necrosis of wrist, hand, and finger(s)
    (Ex) **For category T34.5 CC codes:** See PDX Collection 1417

    ● **T34.51** Frostbite with tissue necrosis of wrist
        ● **T34.511** Frostbite with tissue necrosis of right wrist A 🦠, A 🦠
        ● **T34.512** Frostbite with tissue necrosis of left wrist A 🦠, A 🦠
        ● **T34.519** Frostbite with tissue necrosis of unspecified wrist A 🦠, A 🦠

● **T34.52** Frostbite with tissue necrosis of hand
    Excludes2 frostbite with tissue necrosis of finger(s) (T34.53-)
    ● **T34.521** Frostbite with tissue necrosis of right hand A 🦠, A 🦠
    ● **T34.522** Frostbite with tissue necrosis of left hand A 🦠, A 🦠
    ● **T34.529** Frostbite with tissue necrosis of unspecified hand A 🦠, A 🦠

● **T34.53** Frostbite with tissue necrosis of finger(s)
    ● **T34.531** Frostbite with tissue necrosis of right finger(s) A 🦠, A 🦠
    ● **T34.532** Frostbite with tissue necrosis of left finger(s) A 🦠, A 🦠
    ● **T34.539** Frostbite with tissue necrosis of unspecified finger(s) A 🦠, A 🦠

● **T34.6** Frostbite with tissue necrosis of hip and thigh
    (Ex) **For category T34.6 CC codes:** See PDX Collection 1416

X ● **T34.60** Frostbite with tissue necrosis of unspecified hip and thigh A 🦠, A 🦠

X ● **T34.61** Frostbite with tissue necrosis of right hip and thigh A 🦠, A 🦠

X ● **T34.62** Frostbite with tissue necrosis of left hip and thigh A 🦠, A 🦠

● **T34.7** Frostbite with tissue necrosis of knee and lower leg
    Excludes2 frostbite with tissue necrosis of ankle and foot (T34.8-)
    (Ex) **For category T34.7 CC codes:** See PDX Collection 1416

X ● **T34.70** Frostbite with tissue necrosis of unspecified knee and lower leg A 🦠, A 🦠

X ● **T34.71** Frostbite with tissue necrosis of right knee and lower leg A 🦠, A 🦠

X ● **T34.72** Frostbite with tissue necrosis of left knee and lower leg A 🦠, A 🦠

● **T34.8** Frostbite with tissue necrosis of ankle, foot, and toe(s)
    (Ex) **For category T34.8 CC codes:** See PDX Collection 1418

    ● **T34.81** Frostbite with tissue necrosis of ankle
        ● **T34.811** Frostbite with tissue necrosis of right ankle A 🦠, A 🦠
        ● **T34.812** Frostbite with tissue necrosis of left ankle A 🦠, A 🦠
        ● **T34.819** Frostbite with tissue necrosis of unspecified ankle A 🦠, A 🦠

    ● **T34.82** Frostbite with tissue necrosis of foot
        ● **T34.821** Frostbite with tissue necrosis of right foot A 🦠, A 🦠
        ● **T34.822** Frostbite with tissue necrosis of left foot A 🦠, A 🦠
        ● **T34.829** Frostbite with tissue necrosis of unspecified foot A 🦠, A 🦠

    ● **T34.83** Frostbite with tissue necrosis of toe(s)
        ● **T34.831** Frostbite with tissue necrosis of right toe(s) A 🦠, A 🦠
        ● **T34.832** Frostbite with tissue necrosis of left toe(s) A 🦠, A 🦠
        ● **T34.839** Frostbite with tissue necrosis of unspecified toe(s) A 🦠, A 🦠

● **T34.9** Frostbite with tissue necrosis of other and unspecified sites
    (Ex) **For category T34.9 CC codes:** See PDX Collection 1416

X ● **T34.90** Frostbite with tissue necrosis of unspecified sites A 🦠, A 🦠
    Frostbite with tissue necrosis NOS

X ● **T34.99** Frostbite with tissue necrosis of other sites A 🦠, A 🦠
    Frostbite with tissue necrosis of leg NOS
    Frostbite with tissue necrosis of trunk NOS

CHAPTER 19 (S00–T88)

OGCR See Section I.C.19.e.

Adverse Effects, Poisoning , Underdosing and Toxic Effects
Codes in categories T36-T65 are combination codes that include the
substance that was taken as well as the intent. No additional external
cause code is required for poisonings, toxic effects, adverse effects and
underdosing codes.

POISONING BY, ADVERSE EFFECTS OF AND UNDERDOSING OF DRUGS MEDICAMENTS AND BIOLOGICAL SUBSTANCES (T36-T50)

Includes   adverse effect of correct substance properly
                    administered
               poisoning by overdose of substance
               poisoning by wrong substance given or taken in
                    error
               underdosing by (inadvertently) (deliberately)
                    taking less substance than prescribed or
                    instructed

Code first, for adverse effects, the nature of the adverse effect, such as:
   adverse effect NOS (T88.7)
   aspirin gastritis (K29.-)
   blood disorders (D56-D76)
   contact dermatitis (L23-L25)
   dermatitis due to substances taken internally (L27.-)
   nephropathy (N14.0-N14.2)

Note: The drug giving rise to the adverse effect should be
            identified by use of codes from categories T36-T50 with
            fifth or sixth character 5.

Use additional code(s) to specify:
   manifestations of poisoning
   underdosing or failure in dosage during medical and surgical
        care (Y63.6, Y63.8-Y63.9)
   underdosing of medication regimen (Z91.12-, Z91.13-)

Excludes1 toxic reaction to local anesthesia in pregnancy
                    (O29.3-)

Excludes2 abuse and dependence of psychoactive
                    substances (F10-F19)
               abuse of non-dependence-producing substances
                    (F55.-)
               drug reaction and poisoning affecting newborn
                    (P00-P96)
               pathological drug intoxication (inebriation)
                    (F10-F19)

● **T36** **Poisoning by, adverse effect of and underdosing of systemic
         antibiotics**
         Excludes1 antineoplastic antibiotics (T45.1-)
                      locally applied antibiotic NEC (T49.0)
                      topically used antibiotic for ear, nose and throat
                           (T49.6)
                      topically used antibiotic for eye (T49.5)
         The appropriate 7th character is to be added to each code from
              category T36

A	initial encounter
D	subsequent encounter
S	sequela

   ● **T36.0** **Poisoning by, adverse effect of and underdosing of
              penicillins**
         ● **T36.0X** **Poisoning by, adverse effect of and
                    underdosing of penicillins**
               ● **T36.0X1** **Poisoning by penicillins, accidental
                            (unintentional)**
                                 Poisoning by penicillins NOS
               ● **T36.0X2** **Poisoning by penicillins, intentional
                            self-harm**
               ● **T36.0X3** **Poisoning by penicillins, assault**
               ● **T36.0X4** **Poisoning by penicillins,
                            undetermined**
               ●● **T36.0X5** **Adverse effect of penicillins**
               ●● **T36.0X6** **Underdosing of penicillins**

● **T36.1** **Poisoning by, adverse effect of and underdosing of
           cephalosporins and other betalactam antibiotics**
      ● **T36.1X** **Poisoning by, adverse effect of and
                 underdosing of cephalosporins and other beta-
                 lactam antibiotics**
            ● **T36.1X1** **Poisoning by cephalosporins and
                         other beta-lactam antibiotics,
                         accidental (unintentional)**
                              Poisoning by cephalosporins and
                                 other beta-lactam antibiotics
                                 NOS
            ● **T36.1X2** **Poisoning by cephalosporins and
                         other beta-lactam antibiotics,
                         intentional self-harm**
            ● **T36.1X3** **Poisoning by cephalosporins and
                         other beta-lactam antibiotics, assault**
            ● **T36.1X4** **Poisoning by cephalosporins and
                         other beta-lactam antibiotics,
                         undetermined**
            ●● **T36.1X5** **Adverse effect of cephalosporins and
                         other beta-lactam antibiotics**
            ●● **T36.1X6** **Underdosing of cephalosporins and
                         other beta-lactam antibiotics**

● **T36.2** **Poisoning by, adverse effect of and underdosing of
           chloramphenicol group**
      ● **T36.2X** **Poisoning by, adverse effect of and
                 underdosing of chloramphenicol group**
            ● **T36.2X1** **Poisoning by chloramphenicol group,
                         accidental (unintentional)**
                              Poisoning by chloramphenicol
                                 group NOS
            ● **T36.2X2** **Poisoning by chloramphenicol group,
                         intentional self-harm**
            ● **T36.2X3** **Poisoning by chloramphenicol group,
                         assault**
            ● **T36.2X4** **Poisoning by chloramphenicol group,
                         undetermined**
            ●● **T36.2X5** **Adverse effect of chloramphenicol
                         group**
            ●● **T36.2X6** **Underdosing of chloramphenicol
                         group**

● **T36.3** **Poisoning by, adverse effect of and underdosing of
           macrolides**
      ● **T36.3X** **Poisoning by, adverse effect of and
                 underdosing of macrolides**
            ● **T36.3X1** **Poisoning by macrolides, accidental
                         (unintentional)**
                              Poisoning by macrolides NOS
            ● **T36.3X2** **Poisoning by macrolides, intentional
                         self-harm**
            ● **T36.3X3** **Poisoning by macrolides, assault**
            ● **T36.3X4** **Poisoning by macrolides,
                         undetermined**
            ●● **T36.3X5** **Adverse effect of macrolides**
            ●● **T36.3X6** **Underdosing of macrolides**

● **T36.4** **Poisoning by, adverse effect of and underdosing of
           tetracyclines**
      ● **T36.4X** **Poisoning by, adverse effect of and
                 underdosing of tetracyclines**
            ● **T36.4X1** **Poisoning by tetracyclines, accidental
                         (unintentional)**
                              Poisoning by tetracyclines NOS
            ● **T36.4X2** **Poisoning by tetracyclines,
                         intentional self-harm**
            ● **T36.4X3** **Poisoning by tetracyclines, assault**
            ● **T36.4X4** **Poisoning by tetracyclines,
                         undetermined**
            ●● **T36.4X5** **Adverse effect of tetracyclines**
            ●● **T36.4X6** **Underdosing of tetracyclines**

● **T36.5**   Poisoning by, adverse effect of and underdosing of aminoglycosides
> Poisoning by, adverse effect of and underdosing of streptomycin

   ● **T36.5X**   Poisoning by, adverse effect of and underdosing of aminoglycosides

     ● **T36.5X1**   Poisoning by aminoglycosides, accidental (unintentional)
> Poisoning by aminoglycosides NOS

     ● **T36.5X2**   Poisoning by aminoglycosides, intentional self-harm

     ● **T36.5X3**   Poisoning by aminoglycosides, assault

     ● **T36.5X4**   Poisoning by aminoglycosides, undetermined

     ●● **T36.5X5**   Adverse effect of aminoglycosides

     ●● **T36.5X6**   Underdosing of aminoglycosides

● **T36.6**   Poisoning by, adverse effect of and underdosing of rifampicins

   ● **T36.6X**   Poisoning by, adverse effect of and underdosing of rifampicins

     ● **T36.6X1**   Poisoning by rifampicins, accidental (unintentional)
> Poisoning by rifampicins NOS

     ● **T36.6X2**   Poisoning by rifampicins, intentional self-harm

     ● **T36.6X3**   Poisoning by rifampicins, assault

     ● **T36.6X4**   Poisoning by rifampicins, undetermined

     ●● **T36.6X5**   Adverse effect of rifampicins

     ●● **T36.6X6**   Underdosing of rifampicins

● **T36.7**   Poisoning by, adverse effect of and underdosing of antifungal antibiotics, systemically used

   ● **T36.7X**   Poisoning by, adverse effect of and underdosing of antifungal antibiotics, systemically used

     ● **T36.7X1**   Poisoning by antifungal antibiotics, systemically used, accidental (unintentional)
> Poisoning by antifungal antibiotics, systemically used NOS

     ● **T36.7X2**   Poisoning by antifungal antibiotics, systemically used, intentional self-harm

     ● **T36.7X3**   Poisoning by antifungal antibiotics, systemically used, assault

     ● **T36.7X4**   Poisoning by antifungal antibiotics, systemically used, undetermined

     ●● **T36.7X5**   Adverse effect of antifungal antibiotics, systemically used

     ●● **T36.7X6**   Underdosing of antifungal antibiotics, systemically used

● **T36.8**   Poisoning by, adverse effect of and underdosing of other systemic antibiotics

   ● **T36.8X**   Poisoning by, adverse effect of and underdosing of other systemic antibiotics

     ● **T36.8X1**   Poisoning by other systemic antibiotics, accidental (unintentional)
> Poisoning by other systemic antibiotics NOS

     ● **T36.8X2**   Poisoning by other systemic antibiotics, intentional self-harm

     ● **T36.8X3**   Poisoning by other systemic antibiotics, assault

     ● **T36.8X4**   Poisoning by other systemic antibiotics, undetermined

     ●● **T36.8X5**   Adverse effect of other systemic antibiotics
> **Coding Clinic: 2017, Q1, P39**

     ●● **T36.8X6**   Underdosing of other systemic antibiotics

● **T36.9**   Poisoning by, adverse effect of and underdosing of unspecified systemic antibiotic

   X● **T36.91**   Poisoning by unspecified systemic antibiotic, accidental (unintentional)
> Poisoning by systemic antibiotic NOS

   X● **T36.92**   Poisoning by unspecified systemic antibiotic, intentional self-harm

   X● **T36.93**   Poisoning by unspecified systemic antibiotic, assault

   X● **T36.94**   Poisoning by unspecified systemic antibiotic, undetermined

   ●X● **T36.95**   Adverse effect of unspecified systemic antibiotic

   ●X● **T36.96**   Underdosing of unspecified systemic antibiotic

● **T37**   Poisoning by, adverse effect of and underdosing of other systemic anti-infectives and antiparasitics

   Excludes1   anti-infectives topically used for ear, nose and throat (T49.6-)
> anti-infectives topically used for eye (T49.5-)
> locally applied anti-infectives NEC (T49.0-)

   The appropriate 7th character is to be added to each code from category T37

> A   initial encounter
> D   subsequent encounter
> S   sequela

● **T37.0**   Poisoning by, adverse effect of and underdosing of sulfonamides

   ● **T37.0X**   Poisoning by, adverse effect of and underdosing of sulfonamides

     ● **T37.0X1**   Poisoning by sulfonamides, accidental (unintentional)
> Poisoning by sulfonamides NOS

     ● **T37.0X2**   Poisoning by sulfonamides, intentional self-harm

     ● **T37.0X3**   Poisoning by sulfonamides, assault

     ● **T37.0X4**   Poisoning by sulfonamides, undetermined

     ●● **T37.0X5**   Adverse effect of sulfonamides

     ●● **T37.0X6**   Underdosing of sulfonamides

● **T37.1**   Poisoning by, adverse effect of and underdosing of antimycobacterial drugs

   Excludes1   rifampicins (T36.6-) streptomycin (T36.5-)

   ● **T37.1X**   Poisoning by, adverse effect of and underdosing of antimycobacterial drugs

     ● **T37.1X1**   Poisoning by antimycobacterial drugs, accidental (unintentional)
> Poisoning by antimycobacterial drugs NOS

     ● **T37.1X2**   Poisoning by antimycobacterial drugs, intentional self-harm

     ● **T37.1X3**   Poisoning by antimycobacterial drugs, assault

     ● **T37.1X4**   Poisoning by antimycobacterial drugs, undetermined

     ●● **T37.1X5**   Adverse effect of antimycobacterial drugs

     ●● **T37.1X6**   Underdosing of antimycobacterial drugs

● **T37.2** **Poisoning by, adverse effect of and underdosing of antimalarials and drugs acting on other blood protozoa**

   Excludes1 hydroxyquinoline derivatives (T37.8-)

  ● **T37.2X** **Poisoning by, adverse effect of and underdosing of** antimalarials and drugs acting on other blood protozoa

    ● **T37.2X1** **Poisoning by antimalarials and drugs acting on other blood protozoa, accidental (unintentional)**

      Poisoning by antimalarials and drugs acting on other blood protozoa NOS

    ● **T37.2X2** **Poisoning by antimalarials and drugs acting on other blood protozoa, intentional self-harm**

    ● **T37.2X3** **Poisoning by antimalarials and drugs acting on other blood protozoa, assault**

    ● **T37.2X4** **Poisoning by antimalarials and drugs acting on other blood protozoa, undetermined**

    ●● **T37.2X5** **Adverse effect of antimalarials and drugs acting on other blood protozoa**

    ●● **T37.2X6** **Underdosing of antimalarials and drugs acting on other blood protozoa**

● **T37.3** **Poisoning by, adverse effect of and underdosing of other antiprotozoal drugs**

  ● **T37.3X** **Poisoning by, adverse effect of and underdosing of** other antiprotozoal drugs

    ● **T37.3X1** **Poisoning by other antiprotozoal drugs, accidental (unintentional)**

      Poisoning by other antiprotozoal drugs NOS

    ● **T37.3X2** **Poisoning by other antiprotozoal drugs, intentional self-harm**

    ● **T37.3X3** **Poisoning by other antiprotozoal drugs, assault**

    ● **T37.3X4** **Poisoning by other antiprotozoal drugs, undetermined**

    ●● **T37.3X5** **Adverse effect of other antiprotozoal drugs**

    ●● **T37.3X6** **Underdosing of other antiprotozoal drugs**

● **T37.4** **Poisoning by, adverse effect of and underdosing of anthelminthics**

  ● **T37.4X** **Poisoning by, adverse effect of and underdosing of** anthelminthics

    ● **T37.4X1** **Poisoning by anthelminthics, accidental (unintentional)**

      Poisoning by anthelminthics NOS

    ● **T37.4X2** **Poisoning by anthelminthics, intentional self-harm**

    ● **T37.4X3** **Poisoning by anthelminthics, assault**

    ● **T37.4X4** **Poisoning by anthelminthics, undetermined**

    ●● **T37.4X5** **Adverse effect of anthelminthics**

    ●● **T37.4X6** **Underdosing of anthelminthics**

● **T37.5** **Poisoning by, adverse effect of and underdosing of antiviral drugs**

   Excludes1 amantadine (T42.8-)

      cytarabine (T45.1-)

  ● **T37.5X** **Poisoning by, adverse effect of and underdosing of** antiviral drugs

    ● **T37.5X1** **Poisoning by antiviral drugs, accidental (unintentional)**

      Poisoning by antiviral drugs NOS

    ● **T37.5X2** **Poisoning by antiviral drugs, intentional self-harm**

    ● **T37.5X3** **Poisoning by antiviral drugs, assault**

    ● **T37.5X4** **Poisoning by antiviral drugs, undetermined**

    ●● **T37.5X5** **Adverse effect of antiviral drugs**

    ●● **T37.5X6** **Underdosing of antiviral drugs**

● **T37.8** **Poisoning by, adverse effect of and underdosing of other specified systemic anti-infectives and antiparasitics**

  Poisoning by, adverse effect of and underdosing of hydroxyquinoline derivatives

   Excludes1 antimalarial drugs (T37.2-)

  ● **T37.8X** **Poisoning by, adverse effect of and underdosing of** other specified systemic anti-infectives and antiparasitics

    ● **T37.8X1** **Poisoning by other specified systemic anti-infectives and antiparasitics, accidental (unintentional)**

      Poisoning by other specified systemic anti-infectives and antiparasitics NOS

    ● **T37.8X2** **Poisoning by other specified systemic anti-infectives and antiparasitics, intentional self-harm**

    ● **T37.8X3** **Poisoning by other specified systemic anti-infectives and antiparasitics, assault**

    ● **T37.8X4** **Poisoning by other specified systemic anti-infectives and antiparasitics, undetermined**

    ●● **T37.8X5** **Adverse effect of other specified systemic anti-infectives and antiparasitics**

    ●● **T37.8X6** **Underdosing of other specified systemic anti-infectives and antiparasitics**

● **T37.9** **Poisoning by, adverse effect of and underdosing of unspecified systemic anti-infective and antiparasitics**

  X● **T37.91** **Poisoning by unspecified systemic anti-infective and antiparasitics, accidental (unintentional)**

    Poisoning by, adverse effect of and underdosing of systemic anti-infective and antiparasitics NOS

  X● **T37.92** **Poisoning by unspecified systemic anti-infective and antiparasitics, intentional self-harm**

  X● **T37.93** **Poisoning by unspecified systemic anti-infective and antiparasitics, assault**

  X● **T37.94** **Poisoning by unspecified systemic anti-infective and antiparasitics, undetermined**

  ●X● **T37.95** **Adverse effect of unspecified systemic anti-infective and antiparasitic**

  ●X● **T37.96** **Underdosing of unspecified systemic anti-infectives and antiparasitics**

▶ New   ⇒ Revised   ~~deleted~~ Deleted   Excludes 1   Excludes 2   Includes   Use additional   Code first   Code also   Key words

1434   OGCR Official Guidelines   ● Unacceptable Principal Diagnosis   X Assign placeholder X   ● Use Additional Character(s)   ▌ Manifestation Code   **Coding Clinic**

● **T38** **Poisoning by, adverse effect of and underdosing of hormones and their synthetic substitutes and antagonists, not elsewhere classified**

> **Excludes1**   mineralocorticoids and their antagonists (T50.0-)
> oxytocic hormones (T48.0-)
> parathyroid hormones and derivatives (T50.9-)

> The appropriate 7th character is to be added to each code from category T38

> | | |
> |---|---|
> | A | initial encounter |
> | D | subsequent encounter |
> | S | sequela |

● **T38.0** **Poisoning by, adverse effect of and underdosing of glucocorticoids and synthetic analogues**

> **Excludes1**   glucocorticoids, topically used (T49.-)

● **T38.0X** **Poisoning by, adverse effect of and underdosing of glucocorticoids and synthetic analogues**

● **T38.0X1** **Poisoning by glucocorticoids and synthetic analogues, accidental (unintentional)**
Poisoning by glucocorticoids and synthetic analogues NOS

● **T38.0X2** **Poisoning by glucocorticoids and synthetic analogues, intentional self-harm**

● **T38.0X3** **Poisoning by glucocorticoids and synthetic analogues, assault**

● **T38.0X4** **Poisoning by glucocorticoids and synthetic analogues, undetermined**

●● **T38.0X5** **Adverse effect of glucocorticoids and synthetic analogues**

●● **T38.0X6** **Underdosing of glucocorticoids and synthetic analogues**

● **T38.1** **Poisoning by, adverse effect of and underdosing of thyroid hormones and substitutes**

● **T38.1X** **Poisoning by, adverse effect of and underdosing of thyroid hormones and substitutes**

● **T38.1X1** **Poisoning by thyroid hormones and substitutes, accidental (unintentional)**
Poisoning by thyroid hormones and substitutes NOS

● **T38.1X2** **Poisoning by thyroid hormones and substitutes, intentional self-harm**

● **T38.1X3** **Poisoning by thyroid hormones and substitutes, assault**

● **T38.1X4** **Poisoning by thyroid hormones and substitutes, undetermined**

●● **T38.1X5** **Adverse effect of thyroid hormones and substitutes**

●● **T38.1X6** **Underdosing of thyroid hormones and substitutes**

● **T38.2** **Poisoning by, adverse effect of and underdosing of antithyroid drugs**

● **T38.2X** **Poisoning by, adverse effect of and underdosing of antithyroid drugs**

● **T38.2X1** **Poisoning by antithyroid drugs, accidental (unintentional)**
Poisoning by antithyroid drugs NOS

● **T38.2X2** **Poisoning by antithyroid drugs, intentional self-harm**

● **T38.2X3** **Poisoning by antithyroid drugs, assault**

● **T38.2X4** **Poisoning by antithyroid drugs, undetermined**

●● **T38.2X5** **Adverse effect of antithyroid drugs**

●● **T38.2X6** **Underdosing of antithyroid drugs**

● **T38.3** **Poisoning by, adverse effect of and underdosing of insulin and oral hypoglycemic [antidiabetic] drugs**

● **T38.3X** **Poisoning by, adverse effect of and underdosing of insulin and oral hypoglycemic [antidiabetic] drugs**

● **T38.3X1** **Poisoning by insulin and oral hypoglycemic [antidiabetic] drugs, accidental (unintentional)**
Poisoning by insulin and oral hypoglycemic [antidiabetic] drugs NOS

● **T38.3X2** **Poisoning by insulin and oral hypoglycemic [antidiabetic] drugs, intentional self-harm**

● **T38.3X3** **Poisoning by insulin and oral hypoglycemic [antidiabetic] drugs, assault**

● **T38.3X4** **Poisoning by insulin and oral hypoglycemic [antidiabetic] drugs, undetermined**

●● **T38.3X5** **Adverse effect of insulin and oral hypoglycemic [antidiabetic] drugs**

●● **T38.3X6** **Underdosing of insulin and oral hypoglycemic [antidiabetic] drugs**

● **T38.4** **Poisoning by, adverse effect of and underdosing of oral contraceptives**
Poisoning by, adverse effect of and underdosing of multiple- and single-ingredient oral contraceptive preparations

● **T38.4X** **Poisoning by, adverse effect of and underdosing of oral contraceptives**

● **T38.4X1** **Poisoning by oral contraceptives, accidental (unintentional)**
Poisoning by oral contraceptives NOS

● **T38.4X2** **Poisoning by oral contraceptives, intentional self-harm**

● **T38.4X3** **Poisoning by oral contraceptives, assault**

● **T38.4X4** **Poisoning by oral contraceptives, undetermined**

●● **T38.4X5** **Adverse effect of oral contraceptives**

●● **T38.4X6** **Underdosing of oral contraceptives**

● **T38.5** **Poisoning by, adverse effect of and underdosing of other estrogens and progestogens**
Poisoning by, adverse effect of and underdosing of estrogens and progestogens mixtures and substitutes

● **T38.5X** **Poisoning by, adverse effect of and underdosing of other estrogens and progestogens**

● **T38.5X1** **Poisoning by other estrogens and progestogens, accidental (unintentional)**
Poisoning by other estrogens and progestogens NOS

● **T38.5X2** **Poisoning by other estrogens and progestogens, intentional self-harm**

● **T38.5X3** **Poisoning by other estrogens and progestogens, assault**

● **T38.5X4** **Poisoning by other estrogens and progestogens, undetermined**

●● **T38.5X5** **Adverse effect of other estrogens and progestogens**

●● **T38.5X6** **Underdosing of other estrogens and progestogens**

N Newborn Age: 0   **P** Pediatric Age: 0–17   **M** Maternity DX: 12–55   **A** Adult Age: 15–124   ♀ Females Only   ♂ Males Only

🐾 Complication\Comorbidity   🐾 Major C\C   Ⓔⓧ CC/MCC Exclusions   🐾 Hospital-Acquired Condition

1435

CHAPTER 19 (S00-T88)

● **T38.6** **Poisoning by, adverse effect of and underdosing of antigonadotrophins, antiestrogens, antiandrogens, not elsewhere classified**
    Poisoning by, adverse effect of and underdosing of tamoxifen

  ● **T38.6X** **Poisoning by, adverse effect of and underdosing of antigonadotrophins, antiestrogens, antiandrogens, not elsewhere classified**

    ● **T38.6X1** **Poisoning by antigonadotrophins, antiestrogens, antiandrogens, not elsewhere classified, accidental (unintentional)**
        Poisoning by antigonadotrophins, antiestrogens, antiandrogens, not elsewhere classified NOS

    ● **T38.6X2** **Poisoning by antigonadotrophins, antiestrogens, antiandrogens, not elsewhere classified, intentional self-harm**

    ● **T38.6X3** **Poisoning by antigonadotrophins, antiestrogens, antiandrogens, not elsewhere classified, assault**

    ● **T38.6X4** **Poisoning by antigonadotrophins, antiestrogens, antiandrogens, not elsewhere classified, undetermined**

    ●● **T38.6X5** **Adverse effect of antigonadotrophins, antiestrogens, antiandrogens, not elsewhere classified**

    ●● **T38.6X6** **Underdosing of antigonadotrophins, antiestrogens, antiandrogens, not elsewhere classified**

● **T38.7** **Poisoning by, adverse effect of and underdosing of androgens and anabolic congeners**

  ● **T38.7X** **Poisoning by, adverse effect of and underdosing of androgens and anabolic congeners**

    ● **T38.7X1** **Poisoning by androgens and anabolic congeners, accidental (unintentional)**
        Poisoning by androgens and anabolic congeners NOS

    ● **T38.7X2** **Poisoning by androgens and anabolic congeners, intentional self-harm**

    ● **T38.7X3** **Poisoning by androgens and anabolic congeners, assault**

    ● **T38.7X4** **Poisoning by androgens and anabolic congeners, undetermined**

    ●● **T38.7X5** **Adverse effect of androgens and anabolic congeners**

    ●● **T38.7X6** **Underdosing of androgens and anabolic congeners**

● **T38.8** **Poisoning by, adverse effect of and underdosing of other and unspecified hormones and synthetic substitutes**

  ● **T38.80** **Poisoning by, adverse effect of and underdosing of unspecified hormones and synthetic substitutes**

    ● **T38.801** **Poisoning by unspecified hormones and synthetic substitutes, accidental (unintentional)**
        Poisoning by unspecified hormones and synthetic substitutes NOS

    ● **T38.802** **Poisoning by unspecified hormones and synthetic substitutes, intentional self-harm**

    ● **T38.803** **Poisoning by unspecified hormones and synthetic substitutes, assault**

    ● **T38.804** **Poisoning by unspecified hormones and synthetic substitutes, undetermined**

    ●● **T38.805** **Adverse effect of unspecified hormones and synthetic substitutes**

    ●● **T38.806** **Underdosing of unspecified hormones and synthetic substitutes**

  ● **T38.81** **Poisoning by, adverse effect of and underdosing of anterior pituitary [adenohypophyseal] hormones**

    ● **T38.811** **Poisoning by anterior pituitary [adenohypophyseal] hormones, accidental (unintentional)**
        Poisoning by anterior pituitary [adenohypophyseal] hormones NOS

    ● **T38.812** **Poisoning by anterior pituitary [adenohypophyseal] hormones, intentional self-harm**

    ● **T38.813** **Poisoning by anterior pituitary [adenohypophyseal] hormones, assault**

    ● **T38.814** **Poisoning by anterior pituitary [adenohypophyseal] hormones, undetermined**

    ●● **T38.815** **Adverse effect of anterior pituitary [adenohypophyseal] hormones**

    ●● **T38.816** **Underdosing of anterior pituitary [adenohypophyseal] hormones**

  ● **T38.89** **Poisoning by, adverse effect of and underdosing of other hormones and synthetic substitutes**

    ● **T38.891** **Poisoning by other hormones and synthetic substitutes, accidental (unintentional)**
        Poisoning by other hormones and synthetic substitutes NOS

    ● **T38.892** **Poisoning by other hormones and synthetic substitutes, intentional self-harm**

    ● **T38.893** **Poisoning by other hormones and synthetic substitutes, assault**

    ● **T38.894** **Poisoning by other hormones and synthetic substitutes, undetermined**

    ●● **T38.895** **Adverse effect of other hormones and synthetic substitutes**

    ●● **T38.896** **Underdosing of other hormones and synthetic substitutes**

● **T38.9** **Poisoning by, adverse effect of and underdosing of other and unspecified hormone antagonists**

  ● **T38.90** **Poisoning by, adverse effect of and underdosing of unspecified hormone antagonists**

    ● **T38.901** **Poisoning by unspecified hormone antagonists, accidental (unintentional)**
        Poisoning by unspecified hormone antagonists NOS

    ● **T38.902** **Poisoning by unspecified hormone antagonists, intentional self-harm**

    ● **T38.903** **Poisoning by unspecified hormone antagonists, assault**

    ● **T38.904** **Poisoning by unspecified hormone antagonists, undetermined**

    ●● **T38.905** **Adverse effect of unspecified hormone antagonists**

    ●● **T38.906** **Underdosing of unspecified hormone antagonists**

▶ New   ⇒ Revised   ~~deleted~~ Deleted   Excludes 1   Excludes 2   Includes   Use additional   Code first   Code also   Key words
OGCR Official Guidelines   ● Unacceptable Principal Diagnosis   X Assign placeholder X   ● Use Additional Character(s)   ▶ Manifestation Code   **Coding Clinic**

● T38.99   Poisoning by, adverse effect of and underdosing of other hormone antagonists
  ● T38.991   Poisoning by other hormone antagonists, accidental (unintentional)
              Poisoning by other hormone antagonists NOS
  ● T38.992   Poisoning by other hormone antagonists, intentional self-harm
  ● T38.993   Poisoning by other hormone antagonists, assault
  ● T38.994   Poisoning by other hormone antagonists, undetermined
  ●● T38.995   Adverse effect of other hormone antagonists
  ●● T38.996   Underdosing of other hormone antagonists

● T39   Poisoning by, adverse effect of and underdosing of nonopioid analgesics, antipyretics and antirheumatics

The appropriate 7th character is to be added to each code from category T39

A	initial encounter
D	subsequent encounter
S	sequela

● T39.0   Poisoning by, adverse effect of and underdosing of salicylates
  ● T39.01   Poisoning by, adverse effect of and underdosing of aspirin
              Poisoning by, adverse effect of and underdosing of acetylsalicylic acid
    ● T39.011   Poisoning by aspirin, accidental (unintentional)
    ● T39.012   Poisoning by aspirin, intentional self-harm
    ● T39.013   Poisoning by aspirin, assault
    ● T39.014   Poisoning by aspirin, undetermined
    ●● T39.015   Adverse effect of aspirin
                 Coding Clinic: 2016, Q1, P15
    ●● T39.016   Underdosing of aspirin
  ● T39.09   Poisoning by, adverse effect of and underdosing of other salicylates
    ● T39.091   Poisoning by salicylates, accidental (unintentional)
                Poisoning by salicylates NOS
    ● T39.092   Poisoning by salicylates, intentional self-harm
    ● T39.093   Poisoning by salicylates, assault
    ● T39.094   Poisoning by salicylates, undetermined
    ●● T39.095   Adverse effect of salicylates
    ●● T39.096   Underdosing of salicylates

● T39.1   Poisoning by, adverse effect of and underdosing of 4-Aminophenol derivatives
  ● T39.1X   Poisoning by, adverse effect of and underdosing of 4-Aminophenol derivatives
    ● T39.1X1   Poisoning by 4-Aminophenol derivatives, accidental (unintentional)
                Poisoning by 4-Aminophenol derivatives NOS
    ● T39.1X2   Poisoning by 4-Aminophenol derivatives, intentional self-harm
    ● T39.1X3   Poisoning by 4-Aminophenol derivatives, assault
    ● T39.1X4   Poisoning by 4-Aminophenol derivatives, undetermined
    ●● T39.1X5   Adverse effect of 4-Aminophenol derivatives
    ●● T39.1X6   Underdosing of 4-Aminophenol derivatives

● T39.2   Poisoning by, adverse effect of and underdosing of pyrazolone derivatives
  ● T39.2X   Poisoning by, adverse effect of and underdosing of pyrazolone derivatives
    ● T39.2X1   Poisoning by pyrazolone derivatives, accidental (unintentional)
                Poisoning by pyrazolone derivatives NOS
    ● T39.2X2   Poisoning by pyrazolone derivatives, intentional self-harm
    ● T39.2X3   Poisoning by pyrazolone derivatives, assault
    ● T39.2X4   Poisoning by pyrazolone derivatives, undetermined
    ●● T39.2X5   Adverse effect of pyrazolone derivatives
    ●● T39.2X6   Underdosing of pyrazolone derivatives

● T39.3   Poisoning by, adverse effect of and underdosing of other nonsteroidal anti-inflammatory drugs [NSAID]
  ● T39.31   Poisoning by, adverse effect of and underdosing of propionic acid derivatives
              Poisoning by, adverse effect of and underdosing of fenoprofen
              Poisoning by, adverse effect of and underdosing of flurbiprofen
              Poisoning by, adverse effect of and underdosing of ibuprofen
              Poisoning by, adverse effect of and underdosing of ketoprofen
              Poisoning by, adverse effect of and underdosing of naproxen
              Poisoning by, adverse effect of and underdosing of oxaprozin
    ● T39.311   Poisoning by propionic acid derivatives, accidental (unintentional)
    ● T39.312   Poisoning by propionic acid derivatives, intentional self-harm
    ● T39.313   Poisoning by propionic acid derivatives, assault
    ● T39.314   Poisoning by propionic acid derivatives, undetermined
    ●● T39.315   Adverse effect of propionic acid derivatives
    ●● T39.316   Underdosing of propionic acid derivatives
  ● T39.39   Poisoning by, adverse effect of and underdosing of other nonsteroidal anti-inflammatory drugs [NSAID]
    ● T39.391   Poisoning by other nonsteroidal anti-inflammatory drugs [NSAID], accidental (unintentional)
                Poisoning by other nonsteroidal anti-inflammatory drugs NOS
    ● T39.392   Poisoning by other nonsteroidal anti-inflammatory drugs [NSAID], intentional self-harm
    ● T39.393   Poisoning by other nonsteroidal anti-inflammatory drugs [NSAID], assault
    ● T39.394   Poisoning by other nonsteroidal anti-inflammatory drugs [NSAID], undetermined
    ●● T39.395   Adverse effect of other nonsteroidal anti-inflammatory drugs [NSAID]
    ●● T39.396   Underdosing of other nonsteroidal anti-inflammatory drugs [NSAID]

CHAPTER 19 (S00-T88)

● **T39.4** **Poisoning by, adverse effect of and underdosing of antirheumatics, not elsewhere classified**

> **Excludes1**   poisoning by, adverse effect of and underdosing of glucocorticoids (T38.0-)
> poisoning by, adverse effect of and underdosing of salicylates (T39.0-)

● **T39.4X** **Poisoning by, adverse effect of and underdosing of antirheumatics, not elsewhere classified**

   ● **T39.4X1** **Poisoning by antirheumatics, not elsewhere classified, accidental (unintentional)**
     Poisoning by antirheumatics, not elsewhere classified NOS

   ● **T39.4X2** **Poisoning by antirheumatics, not elsewhere classified, intentional self-harm**

   ● **T39.4X3** **Poisoning by antirheumatics, not elsewhere classified, assault**

   ● **T39.4X4** **Poisoning by antirheumatics, not elsewhere classified, undetermined**

   ●● **T39.4X5** **Adverse effect of antirheumatics, not elsewhere classified**

   ●● **T39.4X6** **Underdosing of antirheumatics, not elsewhere classified**

● **T39.8** **Poisoning by, adverse effect of and underdosing of other nonopioid analgesics and antipyretics, not elsewhere classified**

● **T39.8X** **Poisoning by, adverse effect of and underdosing of other nonopioid analgesics and antipyretics, not elsewhere classified**

   ● **T39.8X1** **Poisoning by other nonopioid analgesics and antipyretics, not elsewhere classified, accidental (unintentional)**
     Poisoning by other nonopioid analgesics and antipyretics, not elsewhere classified NOS

   ● **T39.8X2** **Poisoning by other nonopioid analgesics and antipyretics, not elsewhere classified, intentional self-harm**

   ● **T39.8X3** **Poisoning by other nonopioid analgesics and antipyretics, not elsewhere classified, assault**

   ● **T39.8X4** **Poisoning by other nonopioid analgesics and antipyretics, not elsewhere classified, undetermined**

   ●● **T39.8X5** **Adverse effect of other nonopioid analgesics and antipyretics, not elsewhere classified**

   ●● **T39.8X6** **Underdosing of other nonopioid analgesics and antipyretics, not elsewhere classified**

● **T39.9** **Poisoning by, adverse effect of and underdosing of unspecified nonopioid analgesic, antipyretic and antirheumatic**

  X ● **T39.91** **Poisoning by unspecified nonopioid analgesic, antipyretic and antirheumatic, accidental (unintentional)**
     Poisoning by nonopioid analgesic, antipyretic and antirheumatic NOS

  X ● **T39.92** **Poisoning by unspecified nonopioid analgesic, antipyretic and antirheumatic, intentional self-harm**

  X ● **T39.93** **Poisoning by unspecified nonopioid analgesic, antipyretic and antirheumatic, assault**

  X ● **T39.94** **Poisoning by unspecified nonopioid analgesic, antipyretic and antirheumatic, undetermined**

  ● X ● **T39.95** **Adverse effect of unspecified nonopioid analgesic, antipyretic and antirheumatic**

  ● X ● **T39.96** **Underdosing of unspecified nonopioid analgesic, antipyretic and antirheumatic**

● **T40** **Poisoning by, adverse effect of and underdosing of narcotics and psychodysleptics [hallucinogens]**

> **Excludes2**   drug dependence and related mental and behavioral disorders due to psychoactive substance use (F10.-F19.-)

The appropriate 7th character is to be added to each code from category T40

A	initial encounter
D	subsequent encounter
S	sequela

● **T40.0** **Poisoning by, adverse effect of and underdosing of opium**

● **T40.0X** **Poisoning by, adverse effect of and underdosing of opium**

   ● **T40.0X1** **Poisoning by opium, accidental (unintentional)**
     Poisoning by opium NOS

   ● **T40.0X2** **Poisoning by opium, intentional self-harm**

   ● **T40.0X3** **Poisoning by opium, assault**

   ● **T40.0X4** **Poisoning by opium, undetermined**

   ●● **T40.0X5** **Adverse effect of opium**

   ●● **T40.0X6** **Underdosing of opium**

● **T40.1** **Poisoning by and adverse effect of heroin**

● **T40.1X** **Poisoning by and adverse effect of heroin**

   ● **T40.1X1** **Poisoning by heroin, accidental (unintentional)**
     Poisoning by heroin NOS

   ● **T40.1X2** **Poisoning by heroin, intentional self-harm**

   ● **T40.1X3** **Poisoning by heroin, assault**

   ● **T40.1X4** **Poisoning by heroin, undetermined**

● **T40.2** **Poisoning by, adverse effect of and underdosing of other opioids**

● **T40.2X** **Poisoning by, adverse effect of and underdosing of other opioids**

   ● **T40.2X1** **Poisoning by other opioids, accidental (unintentional)**
     Poisoning by other opioids NOS

   ● **T40.2X2** **Poisoning by other opioids, intentional self-harm**

   ● **T40.2X3** **Poisoning by other opioids, assault**

   ● **T40.2X4** **Poisoning by other opioids, undetermined**

   ●● **T40.2X5** **Adverse effect of other opioids**

   ●● **T40.2X6** **Underdosing of other opioids**

● **T40.3** **Poisoning by, adverse effect of and underdosing of methadone**

● **T40.3X** **Poisoning by, adverse effect of and underdosing of methadone**

   ● **T40.3X1** **Poisoning by methadone, accidental (unintentional)**
     Poisoning by methadone NOS

   ● **T40.3X2** **Poisoning by methadone, intentional self-harm**

   ● **T40.3X3** **Poisoning by methadone, assault**

   ● **T40.3X4** **Poisoning by methadone, undetermined**

   ●● **T40.3X5** **Adverse effect of methadone**

   ●● **T40.3X6** **Underdosing of methadone**

▶ New   ⇒ Revised   ~~deleted~~ Deleted   Excludes 1   Excludes 2   Includes   Use additional   Code first   Code also   Key words

OGCR Official Guidelines   ● Unacceptable Principal Diagnosis   X Assign placeholder X   ● Use Additional Character(s)   ▶ Manifestation Code   **Coding Clinic**

● **T40.4** Poisoning by, adverse effect of and underdosing of other synthetic narcotics

   ● **T40.4X** Poisoning by, adverse effect of and underdosing of other synthetic narcotics

      ● **T40.4X1** Poisoning by other synthetic narcotics, accidental (unintentional)
         Poisoning by other synthetic narcotics NOS

      ● **T40.4X2** Poisoning by other synthetic narcotics, intentional self-harm

      ● **T40.4X3** Poisoning by other synthetic narcotics, assault

      ● **T40.4X4** Poisoning by other synthetic narcotics, undetermined

      ●● **T40.4X5** Adverse effect of other synthetic narcotics

      ●● **T40.4X6** Underdosing of other synthetic narcotics

● **T40.5** Poisoning by, adverse effect of and underdosing of cocaine

   ● **T40.5X** Poisoning by, adverse effect of and underdosing of cocaine

      ● **T40.5X1** Poisoning by cocaine, accidental (unintentional)
         Poisoning by cocaine NOS
         Coding Clinic: 2016, Q2, P9

      ● **T40.5X2** Poisoning by cocaine, intentional self-harm

      ● **T40.5X3** Poisoning by cocaine, assault

      ● **T40.5X4** Poisoning by cocaine, undetermined

      ●● **T40.5X5** Adverse effect of cocaine

      ●● **T40.5X6** Underdosing of cocaine

● **T40.6** Poisoning by, adverse effect of and underdosing of other and unspecified narcotics

   ● **T40.60** Poisoning by, adverse effect of and underdosing of unspecified narcotics

      ● **T40.601** Poisoning by unspecified narcotics, accidental (unintentional)
         Poisoning by narcotics NOS

      ● **T40.602** Poisoning by unspecified narcotics, intentional self-harm

      ● **T40.603** Poisoning by unspecified narcotics, assault

      ● **T40.604** Poisoning by unspecified narcotics, undetermined

      ●● **T40.605** Adverse effect of unspecified narcotics

      ●● **T40.606** Underdosing of unspecified narcotics

   ● **T40.69** Poisoning by, adverse effect of and underdosing of other narcotics

      ● **T40.691** Poisoning by other narcotics, accidental (unintentional)
         Poisoning by other narcotics NOS

      ● **T40.692** Poisoning by other narcotics, intentional self-harm

      ● **T40.693** Poisoning by other narcotics, assault

      ● **T40.694** Poisoning by other narcotics, undetermined

      ●● **T40.695** Adverse effect of other narcotics

      ●● **T40.696** Underdosing of other narcotics

● **T40.7** Poisoning by, adverse effect of and underdosing of cannabis (derivatives)

   ● **T40.7X** Poisoning by, adverse effect of and underdosing of cannabis (derivatives)

      ● **T40.7X1** Poisoning by cannabis (derivatives), accidental (unintentional)
         Poisoning by cannabis NOS

      ● **T40.7X2** Poisoning by cannabis (derivatives), intentional self-harm

      ● **T40.7X3** Poisoning by cannabis (derivatives), assault

      ● **T40.7X4** Poisoning by cannabis (derivatives), undetermined

      ●● **T40.7X5** Adverse effect of cannabis (derivatives)

      ●● **T40.7X6** Underdosing of cannabis (derivatives)

● **T40.8** Poisoning by and adverse effect of lysergide [LSD]

   ● **T40.8X** Poisoning by and adverse effect of lysergide [LSD]

      ● **T40.8X1** Poisoning by lysergide [LSD], accidental (unintentional)
         Poisoning by lysergide [LSD] NOS

      ● **T40.8X2** Poisoning by lysergide [LSD], intentional self-harm

      ● **T40.8X3** Poisoning by lysergide [LSD], assault

      ● **T40.8X4** Poisoning by lysergide [LSD], undetermined

● **T40.9** Poisoning by, adverse effect of and underdosing of other and unspecified psychodysleptics [hallucinogens]

   ● **T40.90** Poisoning by, adverse effect of and underdosing of unspecified psychodysleptics [hallucinogens]

      ● **T40.901** Poisoning by unspecified psychodysleptics [hallucinogens], accidental (unintentional)

      ● **T40.902** Poisoning by unspecified psychodysleptics [hallucinogens], intentional self-harm

      ● **T40.903** Poisoning by unspecified psychodysleptics [hallucinogens], assault

      ● **T40.904** Poisoning by unspecified psychodysleptics [hallucinogens], undetermined

      ●● **T40.905** Adverse effect of unspecified psychodysleptics [hallucinogens]

      ●● **T40.906** Underdosing of unspecified psychodysleptics

   ● **T40.99** Poisoning by, adverse effect of and underdosing of other psychodysleptics [hallucinogens]

      ● **T40.991** Poisoning by other psychodysleptics [hallucinogens], accidental (unintentional)
         Poisoning by other psychodysleptics [hallucinogens] NOS

      ● **T40.992** Poisoning by other psychodysleptics [hallucinogens], intentional self-harm

      ● **T40.993** Poisoning by other psychodysleptics [hallucinogens], assault

      ● **T40.994** Poisoning by other psychodysleptics [hallucinogens], undetermined

      ●● **T40.995** Adverse effect of other psychodysleptics [hallucinogens]

      ●● **T40.996** Underdosing of other psychodysleptics

CHAPTER 19 (S00-T88)

● **T41   Poisoning by, adverse effect of and underdosing of anesthetics and therapeutic gases**

> **Excludes1**   benzodiazepines (T42.4-)
> cocaine (T40.5-)
> complications of anesthesia during pregnancy (O29.-)
> complications of anesthesia during labor and delivery (O74.-)
> complications of anesthesia during the puerperium (O89.-) opioids (T40.0-T40.2-)

> The appropriate 7th character is to be added to each code from category T41

> | | |
> |---|---|
> | A | initial encounter |
> | D | subsequent encounter |
> | S | sequela |

● **T41.0   Poisoning by, adverse effect of and underdosing of inhaled anesthetics**

> **Excludes1**   oxygen (T41.5-)

> ● **T41.0X   Poisoning by, adverse effect of and underdosing of inhaled anesthetics**

>> ● **T41.0X1   Poisoning by inhaled anesthetics, accidental (unintentional)**
>> Poisoning by inhaled anesthetics NOS

>> ● **T41.0X2   Poisoning by inhaled anesthetics, intentional self-harm**

>> ● **T41.0X3   Poisoning by inhaled anesthetics, assault**

>> ● **T41.0X4   Poisoning by inhaled anesthetics, undetermined**

>> ●● **T41.0X5   Adverse effect of inhaled anesthetics**

>> ●● **T41.0X6   Underdosing of inhaled anesthetics**

● **T41.1   Poisoning by, adverse effect of and underdosing of intravenous anesthetics**
> Poisoning by, adverse effect of and underdosing of thiobarbiturates

> ● **T41.1X   Poisoning by, adverse effect of and underdosing of intravenous anesthetics**

>> ● **T41.1X1   Poisoning by intravenous anesthetics, accidental (unintentional)**
>> Poisoning by intravenous anesthetics NOS

>> ● **T41.1X2   Poisoning by intravenous anesthetics, intentional self-harm**

>> ● **T41.1X3   Poisoning by intravenous anesthetics, assault**

>> ● **T41.1X4   Poisoning by intravenous anesthetics, undetermined**

>> ●● **T41.1X5   Adverse effect of intravenous anesthetics**

>> ●● **T41.1X6   Underdosing of intravenous anesthetics**

● **T41.2   Poisoning by, adverse effect of and underdosing of other and unspecified general anesthetics**

> ● **T41.20   Poisoning by, adverse effect of and underdosing of unspecified general anesthetics**

>> ● **T41.201   Poisoning by unspecified general anesthetics, accidental (unintentional)**
>> Poisoning by general anesthetics NOS

>> ● **T41.202   Poisoning by unspecified general anesthetics, intentional self-harm**

>> ● **T41.203   Poisoning by unspecified general anesthetics, assault**

>> ● **T41.204   Poisoning by unspecified general anesthetics, undetermined**

>> ●● **T41.205   Adverse effect of unspecified general anesthetics**
>> **Coding Clinic: 2016, Q4, P73**

>> ●● **T41.206   Underdosing of unspecified general anesthetics**

● **T41.29   Poisoning by, adverse effect of and underdosing of other general anesthetics**

>> ● **T41.291   Poisoning by other general anesthetics, accidental (unintentional)**
>> Poisoning by other general anesthetics NOS

>> ● **T41.292   Poisoning by other general anesthetics, intentional self-harm**

>> ● **T41.293   Poisoning by other general anesthetics, assault**

>> ● **T41.294   Poisoning by other general anesthetics, undetermined**

>> ●● **T41.295   Adverse effect of other general anesthetics**

>> ●● **T41.296   Underdosing of other general anesthetics**

● **T41.3   Poisoning by, adverse effect of and underdosing of local anesthetics**
> Cocaine (topical)

> **Excludes2**   poisoning by cocaine used as a central nervous system stimulant (T40.5X1-T40.5X4)

> ● **T41.3X   Poisoning by, adverse effect of and underdosing of local anesthetics**

>> ● **T41.3X1   Poisoning by local anesthetics, accidental (unintentional)**
>> Poisoning by local anesthetics NOS

>> ● **T41.3X2   Poisoning by local anesthetics, intentional self-harm**

>> ● **T41.3X3   Poisoning by local anesthetics, assault**

>> ● **T41.3X4   Poisoning by local anesthetics, undetermined**

>> ●● **T41.3X5   Adverse effect of local anesthetics**

>> ●● **T41.3X6   Underdosing of local anesthetics**

● **T41.4   Poisoning by, adverse effect of and underdosing of unspecified anesthetic**

> X ● **T41.41   Poisoning by unspecified anesthetic, accidental (unintentional)**
> Poisoning by anesthetic NOS

> X ● **T41.42   Poisoning by unspecified anesthetic, intentional self-harm**

> X ● **T41.43   Poisoning by unspecified anesthetic, assault**

> X ● **T41.44   Poisoning by unspecified anesthetic, undetermined**

> ●X ● **T41.45   Adverse effect of unspecified anesthetic**

> ●X ● **T41.46   Underdosing of unspecified anesthetics**

● **T41.5   Poisoning by, adverse effect of and underdosing of therapeutic gases**

> ● **T41.5X   Poisoning by, adverse effect of and underdosing of therapeutic gases**

>> ● **T41.5X1   Poisoning by therapeutic gases, accidental (unintentional)**
>> Poisoning by therapeutic gases NOS

>> ● **T41.5X2   Poisoning by therapeutic gases, intentional self-harm**

>> ● **T41.5X3   Poisoning by therapeutic gases, assault**

>> ● **T41.5X4   Poisoning by therapeutic gases, undetermined**

>> ●● **T41.5X5   Adverse effect of therapeutic gases**

>> ●● **T41.5X6   Underdosing of therapeutic gases**

▶ New   ⇒ Revised   ~~deleted~~ Deleted   Excludes 1   Excludes 2   Includes   Use additional   Code first   Code also   Key words

OGCR Official Guidelines   ● Unacceptable Principal Diagnosis   X Assign placeholder X   ● Use Additional Character(s)   ▶ Manifestation Code   **Coding Clinic**

● **T42   Poisoning by, adverse effect of and underdosing of antiepileptic, sedative-hypnotic and antiparkinsonism drugs**

> **Excludes2**   drug dependence and related mental and behavioral disorders due to psychoactive substance use (F1Ø.--F19.-)

> The appropriate 7th character is to be added to each code from category T42

> | A | initial encounter |
> |---|---|
> | D | subsequent encounter |
> | S | sequela |

● **T42.Ø   Poisoning by, adverse effect of and underdosing of hydantoin derivatives**

  ● **T42.ØX   Poisoning by, adverse effect of and underdosing of hydantoin derivatives**

   ● **T42.ØX1   Poisoning by hydantoin derivatives, accidental (unintentional)**
   > Poisoning by hydantoin derivatives NOS

   ● **T42.ØX2   Poisoning by hydantoin derivatives, intentional self-harm**

   ● **T42.ØX3   Poisoning by hydantoin derivatives, assault**

   ● **T42.ØX4   Poisoning by hydantoin derivatives, undetermined**

   ●● **T42.ØX5   Adverse effect of hydantoin derivatives**

   ●● **T42.ØX6   Underdosing of hydantoin derivatives**

● **T42.1   Poisoning by, adverse effect of and underdosing of iminostilbenes**
  > Poisoning by, adverse effect of and underdosing of carbamazepine

  ● **T42.1X   Poisoning by, adverse effect of and underdosing of iminostilbenes**

   ● **T42.1X1   Poisoning by iminostilbenes, accidental (unintentional)**
   > Poisoning by iminostilbenes NOS

   ● **T42.1X2   Poisoning by iminostilbenes, intentional self-harm**

   ● **T42.1X3   Poisoning by iminostilbenes, assault**

   ● **T42.1X4   Poisoning by iminostilbenes, undetermined**

   ●● **T42.1X5   Adverse effect of iminostilbenes**

   ●● **T42.1X6   Underdosing of iminostilbenes**

● **T42.2   Poisoning by, adverse effect of and underdosing of succinimides and oxazolidinediones**

  ● **T42.2X   Poisoning by, adverse effect of and underdosing of succinimides and oxazolidinediones**

   ● **T42.2X1   Poisoning by succinimides and oxazolidinediones, accidental (unintentional)**
   > Poisoning by succinimides and oxazolidinediones NOS

   ● **T42.2X2   Poisoning by succinimides and oxazolidinediones, intentional self-harm**

   ● **T42.2X3   Poisoning by succinimides and oxazolidinediones, assault**

   ● **T42.2X4   Poisoning by succinimides and oxazolidinediones, undetermined**

   ●● **T42.2X5   Adverse effect of succinimides and oxazolidinediones**

   ●● **T42.2X6   Underdosing of succinimides and oxazolidinediones**

● **T42.3   Poisoning by, adverse effect of and underdosing of barbiturates**

> **Excludes1**   poisoning by, adverse effect of and underdosing of thiobarbiturates (T41.1-)

  ● **T42.3X   Poisoning by, adverse effect of and underdosing of barbiturates**

   ● **T42.3X1   Poisoning by barbiturates, accidental (unintentional)**
   > Poisoning by barbiturates NOS

   ● **T42.3X2   Poisoning by barbiturates, intentional self-harm**

   ● **T42.3X3   Poisoning by barbiturates, assault**

   ● **T42.3X4   Poisoning by barbiturates, undetermined**

   ●● **T42.3X5   Adverse effect of barbiturates**

   ●● **T42.3X6   Underdosing of barbiturates**

● **T42.4   Poisoning by, adverse effect of and underdosing of benzodiazepines**

  ● **T42.4X   Poisoning by, adverse effect of and underdosing of benzodiazepines**

   ● **T42.4X1   Poisoning by benzodiazepines, accidental (unintentional)**
   > Poisoning by benzodiazepines NOS

   ● **T42.4X2   Poisoning by benzodiazepines, intentional self-harm**

   ● **T42.4X3   Poisoning by benzodiazepines, assault**

   ● **T42.4X4   Poisoning by benzodiazepines, undetermined**

   ●● **T42.4X5   Adverse effect of benzodiazepines**

   ●● **T42.4X6   Underdosing of benzodiazepines**

● **T42.5   Poisoning by, adverse effect of and underdosing of mixed antiepileptics**

  ● **T42.5X   Poisoning by, adverse effect of and underdosing of antiepileptics**

   ● **T42.5X1   Poisoning by mixed antiepileptics, accidental (unintentional)**
   > Poisoning by mixed antiepileptics NOS

   ● **T42.5X2   Poisoning by mixed antiepileptics, intentional self-harm**

   ● **T42.5X3   Poisoning by mixed antiepileptics, assault**

   ● **T42.5X4   Poisoning by mixed antiepileptics, undetermined**

   ●● **T42.5X5   Adverse effect of mixed antiepileptics**

   ●● **T42.5X6   Underdosing of mixed antiepileptics**

CHAPTER 19 (SØØ-T88)

N Newborn Age: Ø   **P** Pediatric Age: Ø–17   **M** Maternity DX: 12–55   **A** Adult Age: 15–124   ♀ Females Only   ♂ Males Only

Complication\Comorbidity   Major C\C   (Ex) CC/MCC Exclusions   Hospital-Acquired Condition

1441

● **T42.6 Poisoning by, adverse effect of and underdosing of other antiepileptic and sedative-hypnotic drugs**
Poisoning by, adverse effect of and underdosing of methaqualone
Poisoning by, adverse effect of and underdosing of valproic acid
Excludes1 poisoning by, adverse effect of and underdosing of carbamazepine (T42.1-)
● **T42.6X Poisoning by, adverse effect of and underdosing of other antiepileptic and sedative-hypnotic drugs**
● **T42.6X1 Poisoning by other antiepileptic and sedative-hypnotic drugs, accidental (unintentional)**
Poisoning by other antiepileptic and sedative-hypnotic drugs NOS
● **T42.6X2 Poisoning by other antiepileptic and sedative-hypnotic drugs, intentional self-harm**
● **T42.6X3 Poisoning by other antiepileptic and sedative-hypnotic drugs, assault**
● **T42.6X4 Poisoning by other antiepileptic and sedative-hypnotic drugs, undetermined**
●● **T42.6X5 Adverse effect of other antiepileptic and sedative-hypnotic drugs**
●● **T42.6X6 Underdosing of other antiepileptic and sedative-hypnotic drugs**
● **T42.7 Poisoning by, adverse effect of and underdosing of unspecified antiepileptic and sedative-hypnotic drugs**
X● **T42.71 Poisoning by unspecified antiepileptic and sedative-hypnotic drugs, accidental (unintentional)**
Poisoning by antiepileptic and sedative-hypnotic drugs NOS
X● **T42.72 Poisoning by unspecified antiepileptic and sedative-hypnotic drugs, intentional self-harm**
X● **T42.73 Poisoning by unspecified antiepileptic and sedative-hypnotic drugs, assault**
X● **T42.74 Poisoning by unspecified antiepileptic and sedative-hypnotic drugs, undetermined**
●X● **T42.75 Adverse effect of unspecified antiepileptic and sedative-hypnotic drugs**
●X● **T42.76 Underdosing of unspecified antiepileptic and sedative-hypnotic drugs**
● **T42.8 Poisoning by, adverse effect of and underdosing of antiparkinsonism drugs and other central muscle-tone depressants**
Poisoning by, adverse effect of and underdosing of amantadine
● **T42.8X Poisoning by, adverse effect of and underdosing of antiparkinsonism drugs and other central muscle-tone depressants**
● **T42.8X1 Poisoning by antiparkinsonism drugs and other central muscle-tone depressants, accidental (unintentional)**
Poisoning by antiparkinsonism drugs and other central muscle-tone depressants NOS
● **T42.8X2 Poisoning by antiparkinsonism drugs and other central muscle-tone depressants, intentional self-harm**
● **T42.8X3 Poisoning by antiparkinsonism drugs and other central muscle-tone depressants, assault**
● **T42.8X4 Poisoning by antiparkinsonism drugs and other central muscle-tone depressants, undetermined**

●● **T42.8X5 Adverse effect of antiparkinsonism drugs and other central muscle-tone depressants**
●● **T42.8X6 Underdosing of antiparkinsonism drugs and other central muscle-tone depressants**
● **T43 Poisoning by, adverse effect of and underdosing of psychotropic drugs, not elsewhere classified**
Excludes1 appetite depressants (T50.5-)
barbiturates (T42.3-)
benzodiazepines (T42.4-)
methaqualone (T42.6-)
psychodysleptics [hallucinogens] (T40.7-T40.9-)
Excludes2 drug dependence and related mental and behavioral disorders due to psychoactive substance use (F10.--F19.-)
The appropriate 7th character is to be added to each code from category T43
A	initial encounter
D	subsequent encounter
S	sequela
● **T43.0 Poisoning by, adverse effect of and underdosing of tricyclic and tetracyclic antidepressants**
● **T43.01 Poisoning by, adverse effect of and underdosing of tricyclic antidepressants**
● **T43.011 Poisoning by tricyclic antidepressants, accidental (unintentional)**
Poisoning by tricyclic antidepressants NOS
● **T43.012 Poisoning by tricyclic antidepressants, intentional self-harm**
● **T43.013 Poisoning by tricyclic antidepressants, assault**
● **T43.014 Poisoning by tricyclic antidepressants, undetermined**
●● **T43.015 Adverse effect of tricyclic antidepressants**
●● **T43.016 Underdosing of tricyclic antidepressants**
● **T43.02 Poisoning by, adverse effect of and underdosing of tetracyclic antidepressants**
● **T43.021 Poisoning by tetracyclic antidepressants, accidental (unintentional)**
Poisoning by tetracyclic antidepressants NOS
● **T43.022 Poisoning by tetracyclic antidepressants, intentional self-harm**
● **T43.023 Poisoning by tetracyclic antidepressants, assault**
● **T43.024 Poisoning by tetracyclic antidepressants, undetermined**
●● **T43.025 Adverse effect of tetracyclic antidepressants**
●● **T43.026 Underdosing of tetracyclic antidepressants**
● **T43.1 Poisoning by, adverse effect of and underdosing of monoamine-oxidase-inhibitor antidepressants**
● **T43.1X Poisoning by, adverse effect of and underdosing of monoamine-oxidase-inhibitor antidepressants**
● **T43.1X1 Poisoning by monoamine-oxidase-inhibitor antidepressants, accidental (unintentional)**
Poisoning by monoamine-oxidase-inhibitor antidepressants NOS
● **T43.1X2 Poisoning by monoamine-oxidase-inhibitor antidepressants, intentional self-harm**

● T43.1X3   Poisoning by monoamine-oxidase-inhibitor antidepressants, assault

● T43.1X4   Poisoning by monoamine-oxidase-inhibitor antidepressants, undetermined

●● T43.1X5   Adverse effect of monoamine-oxidase-inhibitor antidepressants

●● T43.1X6   Underdosing of monoamine-oxidase-inhibitor antidepressants

● T43.2   Poisoning by, adverse effect of and underdosing of other and unspecified antidepressants

  ● T43.20   Poisoning by, adverse effect of and underdosing of unspecified antidepressants

    ● T43.201   Poisoning by unspecified antidepressants, accidental (unintentional)
          Poisoning by antidepressants NOS

    ● T43.202   Poisoning by unspecified antidepressants, intentional self-harm

    ● T43.203   Poisoning by unspecified antidepressants, assault

    ● T43.204   Poisoning by unspecified antidepressants, undetermined

    ●● T43.205   Adverse effect of unspecified antidepressants
         ▶Antidepressant discontinuation syndrome

    ●● T43.206   Underdosing of unspecified antidepressants

  ● T43.21   Poisoning by, adverse effect of and underdosing of selective serotonin and norepinephrine reuptake inhibitors
       Poisoning by, adverse effect of and underdosing of SSNRI antidepressants

    ● T43.211   Poisoning by selective serotonin and norepinephrine reuptake inhibitors, accidental (unintentional)

    ● T43.212   Poisoning by selective serotonin and norepinephrine reuptake inhibitors, intentional self-harm

    ● T43.213   Poisoning by selective serotonin and norepinephrine reuptake inhibitors, assault

    ● T43.214   Poisoning by selective serotonin and norepinephrine reuptake inhibitors, undetermined

    ●● T43.215   Adverse effect of selective serotonin and norepinephrine reuptake inhibitors

    ●● T43.216   Underdosing of selective serotonin and norepinephrine reuptake inhibitors

  ● T43.22   Poisoning by, adverse effect of and underdosing of selective serotonin reuptake inhibitors
       Poisoning by, adverse effect of and underdosing of SSRI antidepressants

    ● T43.221   Poisoning by selective serotonin reuptake inhibitors, accidental (unintentional)

    ● T43.222   Poisoning by selective serotonin reuptake inhibitors, intentional self-harm

    ● T43.223   Poisoning by selective serotonin reuptake inhibitors, assault

    ● T43.224   Poisoning by selective serotonin reuptake inhibitors, undetermined

    ●● T43.225   Adverse effect of selective serotonin reuptake inhibitors

    ●● T43.226   Underdosing of selective serotonin reuptake inhibitors

● T43.29   Poisoning by, adverse effect of and underdosing of other antidepressants

  ● T43.291   Poisoning by other antidepressants, accidental (unintentional)
         Poisoning by other antidepressants NOS

  ● T43.292   Poisoning by other antidepressants, intentional self-harm

  ● T43.293   Poisoning by other antidepressants, assault

  ● T43.294   Poisoning by other antidepressants, undetermined

  ●● T43.295   Adverse effect of other antidepressants

  ●● T43.296   Underdosing of other antidepressants

● T43.3   Poisoning by, adverse effect of and underdosing of phenothiazine antipsychotics and neuroleptics

  ● T43.3X   Poisoning by, adverse effect of and underdosing of phenothiazine antipsychotics and neuroleptics

    ● T43.3X1   Poisoning by phenothiazine antipsychotics and neuroleptics, accidental (unintentional)
         Poisoning by phenothiazine antipsychotics and neuroleptics NOS

    ● T43.3X2   Poisoning by phenothiazine antipsychotics and neuroleptics, intentional self-harm

    ● T43.3X3   Poisoning by phenothiazine antipsychotics and neuroleptics, assault

    ● T43.3X4   Poisoning by phenothiazine antipsychotics and neuroleptics, undetermined

    ●● T43.3X5   Adverse effect of phenothiazine antipsychotics and neuroleptics

    ●● T43.3X6   Underdosing of phenothiazine antipsychotics and neuroleptics

● T43.4   Poisoning by, adverse effect of and underdosing of butyrophenone and thiothixene neuroleptics

  ● T43.4X   Poisoning by, adverse effect of and underdosing of butyrophenone and thiothixene neuroleptics

    ● T43.4X1   Poisoning by butyrophenone and thiothixene neuroleptics, accidental (unintentional)
         Poisoning by butyrophenone and thiothixene neuroleptics NOS

    ● T43.4X2   Poisoning by butyrophenone and thiothixene neuroleptics, intentional self-harm

    ● T43.4X3   Poisoning by butyrophenone and thiothixene neuroleptics, assault

    ● T43.4X4   Poisoning by butyrophenone and thiothixene neuroleptics, undetermined

    ●● T43.4X5   Adverse effect of butyrophenone and thiothixene neuroleptics

    ●● T43.4X6   Underdosing of butyrophenone and thiothixene neuroleptics

N Newborn Age: 0   **P** Pediatric Age: 0–17   **M** Maternity DX: 12–55   **A** Adult Age: 15–124   ♀ Females Only   ♂ Males Only

🅒 Complication\Comorbidity   🅜 Major C\C   (Exc) CC/MCC Exclusions   🅗 Hospital-Acquired Condition

1443

● T43.5 Poisoning by, adverse effect of and underdosing of other and unspecified antipsychotics and neuroleptics

Excludes1 poisoning by, adverse effect of and underdosing of rauwolfia (T46.5-)

● T43.50 Poisoning by, adverse effect of and underdosing of unspecified antipsychotics and neuroleptics

● T43.501 Poisoning by unspecified antipsychotics and neuroleptics, accidental (unintentional)
Poisoning by antipsychotics and neuroleptics NOS

● T43.502 Poisoning by unspecified antipsychotics and neuroleptics, intentional self-harm

● T43.503 Poisoning by unspecified antipsychotics and neuroleptics, assault

● T43.504 Poisoning by unspecified antipsychotics and neuroleptics, undetermined

●● T43.505 Adverse effect of unspecified antipsychotics and neuroleptics

●● T43.506 Underdosing of unspecified antipsychotics and neuroleptics

● T43.59 Poisoning by, adverse effect of and underdosing of other antipsychotics and neuroleptics

● T43.591 Poisoning by other antipsychotics and neuroleptics, accidental (unintentional)
Poisoning by other antipsychotics and neuroleptics NOS

● T43.592 Poisoning by other antipsychotics and neuroleptics, intentional self-harm
Coding Clinic: 2017, Q1, P40

● T43.593 Poisoning by other antipsychotics and neuroleptics, assault

● T43.594 Poisoning by other antipsychotics and neuroleptics, undetermined

●● T43.595 Adverse effect of other antipsychotics and neuroleptics

●● T43.596 Underdosing of other antipsychotics and neuroleptics

● T43.6 Poisoning by, adverse effect of and underdosing of psychostimulants

Excludes1 poisoning by, adverse effect of and underdosing of cocaine (T40.5-)

● T43.60 Poisoning by, adverse effect of and underdosing of unspecified psychostimulant

● T43.601 Poisoning by unspecified psychostimulants, accidental (unintentional)
Poisoning by psychostimulants NOS

● T43.602 Poisoning by unspecified psychostimulants, intentional self-harm

● T43.603 Poisoning by unspecified psychostimulants, assault

● T43.604 Poisoning by unspecified psychostimulants, undetermined

●● T43.605 Adverse effect of unspecified psychostimulants

●● T43.606 Underdosing of unspecified psychostimulants

● T43.61 Poisoning by, adverse effect of and underdosing of caffeine

● T43.611 Poisoning by caffeine, accidental (unintentional)
Poisoning by caffeine NOS

● T43.612 Poisoning by caffeine, intentional self-harm

● T43.613 Poisoning by caffeine, assault

● T43.614 Poisoning by caffeine, undetermined

●● T43.615 Adverse effect of caffeine

●● T43.616 Underdosing of caffeine

● T43.62 Poisoning by, adverse effect of and underdosing of amphetamines
Poisoning by, adverse effect of and underdosing of methamphetamines

● T43.621 Poisoning by amphetamines, accidental (unintentional)
Poisoning by amphetamines NOS

● T43.622 Poisoning by amphetamines, intentional self-harm

● T43.623 Poisoning by amphetamines, assault

● T43.624 Poisoning by amphetamines, undetermined

●● T43.625 Adverse effect of amphetamines

●● T43.626 Underdosing of amphetamines

● T43.63 Poisoning by, adverse effect of and underdosing of methylphenidate

● T43.631 Poisoning by methylphenidate, accidental (unintentional)
Poisoning by methylphenidate NOS

● T43.632 Poisoning by methylphenidate, intentional self-harm

● T43.633 Poisoning by methylphenidate, assault

● T43.634 Poisoning by methylphenidate, undetermined

●● T43.635 Adverse effect of methylphenidate

●● T43.636 Underdosing of methylphenidate

● T43.69 Poisoning by, adverse effect of and underdosing of other psychostimulants

● T43.691 Poisoning by other psychostimulants, accidental (unintentional)
Poisoning by other psychostimulants NOS

● T43.692 Poisoning by other psychostimulants, intentional self-harm

● T43.693 Poisoning by other psychostimulants, assault

● T43.694 Poisoning by other psychostimulants, undetermined

●● T43.695 Adverse effect of other psychostimulants

●● T43.696 Underdosing of other psychostimulants

● T43.8 Poisoning by, adverse effect of and underdosing of other psychotropic drugs

● T43.8X Poisoning by, adverse effect of and underdosing of other psychotropic drugs

● T43.8X1 Poisoning by other psychotropic drugs, accidental (unintentional)
Poisoning by other psychotropic drugs NOS

● T43.8X2 Poisoning by other psychotropic drugs, intentional self-harm

● T43.8X3 Poisoning by other psychotropic drugs, assault

● T43.8X4 Poisoning by other psychotropic drugs, undetermined

●● T43.8X5 Adverse effect of other psychotropic drugs

●● T43.8X6 Underdosing of other psychotropic drugs

▶ New   ⟹ Revised   deleted Deleted   Excludes 1   Excludes 2   Includes   Use additional   Code first   Code also   Key words
OGCR Official Guidelines   ● Unacceptable Principal Diagnosis   X Assign placeholder X   ● Use Additional Character(s)   ▶ Manifestation Code   Coding Clinic

● T43.9　Poisoning by, adverse effect of and underdosing of unspecified psychotropic drug

  X ● T43.91　Poisoning by unspecified psychotropic drug, accidental (unintentional)
      Poisoning by psychotropic drug NOS

  X ● T43.92　Poisoning by unspecified psychotropic drug, intentional self-harm

  X ● T43.93　Poisoning by unspecified psychotropic drug, assault

  X ● T43.94　Poisoning by unspecified psychotropic drug, undetermined

  ● X ● T43.95　Adverse effect of unspecified psychotropic drug

  ● X ● T43.96　Underdosing of unspecified psychotropic drug

● T44　Poisoning by, adverse effect of and underdosing of drugs primarily affecting the autonomic nervous system

  The appropriate 7th character is to be added to each code from category T44

A	initial encounter
D	subsequent encounter
S	sequela

● T44.0　Poisoning by, adverse effect of and underdosing of anticholinesterase agents

  ● T44.0X　Poisoning by, adverse effect of and underdosing of anticholinesterase agents

    ● T44.0X1　Poisoning by anticholinesterase agents, accidental (unintentional)
      Poisoning by anticholinesterase agents NOS

    ● T44.0X2　Poisoning by anticholinesterase agents, intentional self-harm

    ● T44.0X3　Poisoning by anticholinesterase agents, assault

    ● T44.0X4　Poisoning by anticholinesterase agents, undetermined

    ● ● T44.0X5　Adverse effect of anticholinesterase agents

    ● ● T44.0X6　Underdosing of anticholinesterase agents

● T44.1　Poisoning by, adverse effect of and underdosing of other parasympathomimetics [cholinergics]

  ● T44.1X　Poisoning by, adverse effect of and underdosing of other parasympathomimetics [cholinergics]

    ● T44.1X1　Poisoning by other parasympathomimetics [cholinergics], accidental (unintentional)
      Poisoning by other parasympathomimetics [cholinergics] NOS

    ● T44.1X2　Poisoning by other parasympathomimetics [cholinergics], intentional self-harm

    ● T44.1X3　Poisoning by other parasympathomimetics [cholinergics], assault

    ● T44.1X4　Poisoning by other parasympathomimetics [cholinergics], undetermined

    ● ● T44.1X5　Adverse effect of other parasympathomimetics [cholinergics]

    ● ● T44.1X6　Underdosing of other parasympathomimetics

● T44.2　Poisoning by, adverse effect of and underdosing of ganglionic blocking drugs

  ● T44.2X　Poisoning by, adverse effect of and underdosing of ganglionic blocking drugs

    ● T44.2X1　Poisoning by ganglionic blocking drugs, accidental (unintentional)
      Poisoning by ganglionic blocking drugs NOS

    ● T44.2X2　Poisoning by ganglionic blocking drugs, intentional self-harm

    ● T44.2X3　Poisoning by ganglionic blocking drugs, assault

    ● T44.2X4　Poisoning by ganglionic blocking drugs, undetermined

    ● ● T44.2X5　Adverse effect of ganglionic blocking drugs

    ● ● T44.2X6　Underdosing of ganglionic blocking drugs

● T44.3　Poisoning by, adverse effect of and underdosing of other parasympatholytics [anticholinergics and antimuscarinics] and spasmolytics
  Poisoning by, adverse effect of and underdosing of papaverine

  ● T44.3X　Poisoning by, adverse effect of and underdosing of other parasympatholytics [anticholinergics and antimuscarinics] and spasmolytics

    ● T44.3X1　Poisoning by other parasympatholytics [anticholinergics and antimuscarinics] and spasmolytics, accidental (unintentional)
      Poisoning by other parasympatholytics [anticholinergics and antimuscarinics] and spasmolytics NOS

    ● T44.3X2　Poisoning by other parasympatholytics [anticholinergics and antimuscarinics] and spasmolytics, intentional self-harm

    ● T44.3X3　Poisoning by other parasympatholytics [anticholinergics and antimuscarinics] and spasmolytics, assault

    ● T44.3X4　Poisoning by other parasympatholytics [anticholinergics and antimuscarinics] and spasmolytics, undetermined

    ● ● T44.3X5　Adverse effect of other parasympatholytics [anticholinergics and antimuscarinics] and spasmolytics

    ● ● T44.3X6　Underdosing of other parasympatholytics [anticholinergics and antimuscarinics] and spasmolytics

● **T44.4 Poisoning by, adverse effect of and underdosing of predominantly alpha-adrenoreceptor agonists**
Poisoning by, adverse effect of and underdosing of metaraminol

  ● **T44.4X Poisoning by, adverse effect of and underdosing of predominantly alpha-adrenoreceptor agonists**

    ● **T44.4X1 Poisoning by predominantly alpha-adrenoreceptor agonists, accidental (unintentional)**
Poisoning by predominantly alpha-adrenoreceptor agonists NOS

    ● **T44.4X2 Poisoning by predominantly alpha-adrenoreceptor agonists, intentional self-harm**

    ● **T44.4X3 Poisoning by predominantly alpha-adrenoreceptor agonists, assault**

    ● **T44.4X4 Poisoning by predominantly alpha-adrenoreceptor agonists, undetermined**

    ●● **T44.4X5 Adverse effect of predominantly alpha-adrenoreceptor agonists**

    ●● **T44.4X6 Underdosing of predominantly alpha-adrenoreceptor agonists**

● **T44.5 Poisoning by, adverse effect of and underdosing of predominantly beta-adrenoreceptor agonists**

  Excludes1   poisoning by, adverse effect of and underdosing of beta-adrenoreceptor agonists used in asthma therapy (T48.6-)

  ● **T44.5X Poisoning by, adverse effect of and underdosing of predominantly beta-adrenoreceptor agonists**

    ● **T44.5X1 Poisoning by predominantly beta-adrenoreceptor agonists, accidental (unintentional)**
Poisoning by predominantly beta-adrenoreceptor agonists NOS

    ● **T44.5X2 Poisoning by predominantly beta-adrenoreceptor agonists, intentional self-harm**

    ● **T44.5X3 Poisoning by predominantly beta-adrenoreceptor agonists, assault**

    ● **T44.5X4 Poisoning by predominantly beta-adrenoreceptor agonists, undetermined**

    ●● **T44.5X5 Adverse effect of predominantly beta-adrenoreceptor agonists**

    ●● **T44.5X6 Underdosing of predominantly beta-adrenoreceptor agonists**

● **T44.6 Poisoning by, adverse effect of and underdosing of alpha-adrenoreceptor antagonists**

  Excludes1   poisoning by, adverse effect of and underdosing of ergot alkaloids (T48.0)

  ● **T44.6X Poisoning by, adverse effect of and underdosing of alpha-adrenoreceptor antagonists**

    ● **T44.6X1 Poisoning by alpha-adrenoreceptor antagonists, accidental (unintentional)**
Poisoning by alpha-adrenoreceptor antagonists NOS

    ● **T44.6X2 Poisoning by alpha-adrenoreceptor antagonists, intentional self-harm**

    ● **T44.6X3 Poisoning by alpha-adrenoreceptor antagonists, assault**

    ● **T44.6X4 Poisoning by alpha-adrenoreceptor antagonists, undetermined**

    ●● **T44.6X5 Adverse effect of alpha-adrenoreceptor antagonists**

    ●● **T44.6X6 Underdosing of alpha-adrenoreceptor antagonists**

● **T44.7 Poisoning by, adverse effect of and underdosing of beta-adrenoreceptor antagonists**

  ● **T44.7X Poisoning by, adverse effect of and underdosing of beta-adrenoreceptor antagonists**

    ● **T44.7X1 Poisoning by beta-adrenoreceptor antagonists, accidental (unintentional)**
Poisoning by beta-adrenoreceptor antagonists NOS

    ● **T44.7X2 Poisoning by beta-adrenoreceptor antagonists, intentional self-harm**

    ● **T44.7X3 Poisoning by beta-adrenoreceptor antagonists, assault**

    ● **T44.7X4 Poisoning by beta-adrenoreceptor antagonists, undetermined**

    ●● **T44.7X5 Adverse effect of beta-adrenoreceptor antagonists**

    ●● **T44.7X6 Underdosing of beta-adrenoreceptor antagonists**

● **T44.8 Poisoning by, adverse effect of and underdosing of centrally-acting and adrenergic-neuron-blocking agents**

  Excludes1   poisoning by, adverse effect of and underdosing of clonidine (T46.5)
poisoning by, adverse effect of and underdosing of guanethidine (T46.5)

  ● **T44.8X Poisoning by, adverse effect of and underdosing of centrally-acting and adrenergic-neuron-blocking agents**

    ● **T44.8X1 Poisoning by centrally-acting and adrenergic-neuron-blocking agents, accidental (unintentional)**
Poisoning by centrally-acting and adrenergic-neuron-blocking agents NOS

    ● **T44.8X2 Poisoning by centrally-acting and adrenergic-neuron-blocking agents, intentional self-harm**

    ● **T44.8X3 Poisoning by centrally-acting and adrenergic-neuron-blocking agents, assault**

    ● **T44.8X4 Poisoning by centrally-acting and adrenergic-neuron-blocking agents, undetermined**

    ●● **T44.8X5 Adverse effect of centrally-acting and adrenergic-neuron-blocking agents**

    ●● **T44.8X6 Underdosing of centrally-acting and adrenergic-neuron-blocking agents**

● **T44.9 Poisoning by, adverse effect of and underdosing of other and unspecified drugs primarily affecting the autonomic nervous system**
Poisoning by, adverse effect of and underdosing of drug stimulating both alpha and beta-adrenoreceptors

  ● **T44.90 Poisoning by, adverse effect of and underdosing of unspecified drugs primarily affecting the autonomic nervous system**

    ● **T44.901 Poisoning by unspecified drugs primarily affecting the autonomic nervous system, accidental (unintentional)**
Poisoning by unspecified drugs primarily affecting the autonomic nervous system NOS

    ● **T44.902 Poisoning by unspecified drugs primarily affecting the autonomic nervous system, intentional self-harm**

    ● **T44.903 Poisoning by unspecified drugs primarily affecting the autonomic nervous system, assault**

● T44.904 **Poisoning by unspecified drugs primarily affecting the autonomic nervous system, undetermined**

●● T44.905 **Adverse effect of unspecified drugs primarily affecting the autonomic nervous system**

●● T44.906 **Underdosing of unspecified drugs primarily affecting the autonomic nervous system**

● T44.99 **Poisoning by, adverse effect of and underdosing of other drugs primarily affecting the autonomic nervous system**

　● T44.991 **Poisoning by other drug primarily affecting the autonomic nervous system, accidental (unintentional)**
　　Poisoning by other drugs primarily affecting the autonomic nervous system NOS

　● T44.992 **Poisoning by other drug primarily affecting the autonomic nervous system, intentional self-harm**

　● T44.993 **Poisoning by other drug primarily affecting the autonomic nervous system, assault**

　● T44.994 **Poisoning by other drug primarily affecting the autonomic nervous system, undetermined**

　●● T44.995 **Adverse effect of other drug primarily affecting the autonomic nervous system**

　●● T44.996 **Underdosing of other drug primarily affecting the autonomic nervous system**

● T45 **Poisoning by, adverse effect of and underdosing of primarily systemic and hematological agents, not elsewhere classified**

The appropriate 7th character is to be added to each code from category T45

A	initial encounter
D	subsequent encounter
S	sequela

● T45.0 **Poisoning by, adverse effect of and underdosing of antiallergic and antiemetic drugs**

Excludes1　poisoning by, adverse effect of and underdosing of phenothiazine-based neuroleptics (T43.3)

　● T45.0X **Poisoning by, adverse effect of and underdosing of antiallergic and antiemetic drugs**

　　● T45.0X1 **Poisoning by antiallergic and antiemetic drugs, accidental (unintentional)**
　　　Poisoning by antiallergic and antiemetic drugs NOS

　　● T45.0X2 **Poisoning by antiallergic and antiemetic drugs, intentional self-harm**

　　● T45.0X3 **Poisoning by antiallergic and antiemetic drugs, assault**

　　● T45.0X4 **Poisoning by antiallergic and antiemetic drugs, undetermined**

　　●● T45.0X5 **Adverse effect of antiallergic and antiemetic drugs**

　　●● T45.0X6 **Underdosing of antiallergic and antiemetic drugs**

● T45.1 **Poisoning by, adverse effect of and underdosing of antineoplastic and immunosuppressive drugs**

Excludes1　poisoning by, adverse effect of and underdosing of tamoxifen (T38.6)

　● T45.1X **Poisoning by, adverse effect of and underdosing of antineoplastic and immunosuppressive drugs**

　　● T45.1X1 **Poisoning by antineoplastic and immunosuppressive drugs, accidental (unintentional)**
　　　Poisoning by antineoplastic and immunosuppressive drugs NOS

　　● T45.1X2 **Poisoning by antineoplastic and immunosuppressive drugs, intentional self-harm**

　　● T45.1X3 **Poisoning by antineoplastic and immunosuppressive drugs, assault**

　　● T45.1X4 **Poisoning by antineoplastic and immunosuppressive drugs, undetermined**

　　●● T45.1X5 **Adverse effect of antineoplastic and immunosuppressive drugs**

　　●● T45.1X6 **Underdosing of antineoplastic and immunosuppressive drugs**

● T45.2 **Poisoning by, adverse effect of and underdosing of vitamins**

Excludes2　poisoning by, adverse effect of and underdosing of nicotinic acid (derivatives) (T46.7)
poisoning by, adverse effect of and underdosing of iron (T45.4)
poisoning by, adverse effect of and underdosing of vitamin K (T45.7)

　● T45.2X **Poisoning by, adverse effect of and underdosing of vitamins**

　　● T45.2X1 **Poisoning by vitamins, accidental (unintentional)**
　　　Poisoning by vitamins NOS

　　● T45.2X2 **Poisoning by vitamins, intentional self-harm**

　　● T45.2X3 **Poisoning by vitamins, assault**

　　● T45.2X4 **Poisoning by vitamins, undetermined**

　　●● T45.2X5 **Adverse effect of vitamins**

　　●● T45.2X6 **Underdosing of vitamins**

Excludes1　vitamin deficiencies (E50-E56)

● T45.3 **Poisoning by, adverse effect of and underdosing of enzymes**

　● T45.3X **Poisoning by, adverse effect of and underdosing of enzymes**

　　● T45.3X1 **Poisoning by enzymes, accidental (unintentional)**
　　　Poisoning by enzymes NOS

　　● T45.3X2 **Poisoning by enzymes, intentional self-harm**

　　● T45.3X3 **Poisoning by enzymes, assault**

　　● T45.3X4 **Poisoning by enzymes, undetermined**

　　●● T45.3X5 **Adverse effect of enzymes**

　　●● T45.3X6 **Underdosing of enzymes**

CHAPTER 19 (S00-T88)

CHAPTER 19 (S00-T88)

- T45.4 **Poisoning by, adverse effect of and underdosing of iron and its compounds**
  - T45.4X **Poisoning by, adverse effect of and underdosing of iron and its compounds**
    - T45.4X1 **Poisoning by iron and its compounds, accidental (unintentional)**
      Poisoning by iron and its compounds NOS
    - T45.4X2 **Poisoning by iron and its compounds, intentional self-harm**
    - T45.4X3 **Poisoning by iron and its compounds, assault**
    - T45.4X4 **Poisoning by iron and its compounds, undetermined**
    - T45.4X5 **Adverse effect of iron and its compounds**
    - T45.4X6 **Underdosing of iron and its compounds**
      Excludes1   iron deficiency (E61.1)
- T45.5 **Poisoning by, adverse effect of and underdosing of anticoagulants and antithrombotic drugs**
  - T45.51 **Poisoning by, adverse effect of and underdosing of anticoagulants**
    - T45.511 **Poisoning by anticoagulants, accidental (unintentional)**
      Poisoning by anticoagulants NOS
    - T45.512 **Poisoning by anticoagulants, intentional self-harm**
    - T45.513 **Poisoning by anticoagulants, assault**
    - T45.514 **Poisoning by anticoagulants, undetermined**
    - T45.515 **Adverse effect of anticoagulants**
      Coding Clinic: 2016, Q1, P14; 2013, Q2, P35
    - T45.516 **Underdosing of anticoagulants**
  - T45.52 **Poisoning by, adverse effect of and underdosing of antithrombotic drugs**
    Poisoning by, adverse effect of and underdosing of antiplatelet drugs
    Excludes2   poisoning by, adverse effect of and underdosing of aspirin (T39.01-)
    poisoning by, adverse effect of and underdosing of acetylsalicylic acid (T39.01-)
    - T45.521 **Poisoning by antithrombotic drugs, accidental (unintentional)**
      Poisoning by antithrombotic drug NOS
    - T45.522 **Poisoning by antithrombotic drugs, intentional self-harm**
    - T45.523 **Poisoning by antithrombotic drugs, assault**
    - T45.524 **Poisoning by antithrombotic drugs, undetermined**
    - T45.525 **Adverse effect of antithrombotic drugs**
      Coding Clinic: 2016, Q1, P15
    - T45.526 **Underdosing of antithrombotic drugs**

- T45.6 **Poisoning by, adverse effect of and underdosing of fibrinolysis-affecting drugs**
  - T45.60 **Poisoning by, adverse effect of and underdosing of unspecified fibrinolysis-affecting drugs**
    - T45.601 **Poisoning by unspecified fibrinolysis-affecting drugs, accidental (unintentional)**
      Poisoning by fibrinolysis-affecting drug NOS
    - T45.602 **Poisoning by unspecified fibrinolysis-affecting drugs, intentional self-harm**
    - T45.603 **Poisoning by unspecified fibrinolysis-affecting drugs, assault**
    - T45.604 **Poisoning by unspecified fibrinolysis-affecting drugs, undetermined**
    - T45.605 **Adverse effect of unspecified fibrinolysis-affecting drugs**
    - T45.606 **Underdosing of unspecified fibrinolysis-affecting drugs**
  - T45.61 **Poisoning by, adverse effect of and underdosing of thrombolytic drugs**
    - T45.611 **Poisoning by thrombolytic drug, accidental (unintentional)**
      Poisoning by thrombolytic drug NOS
    - T45.612 **Poisoning by thrombolytic drug, intentional self-harm**
    - T45.613 **Poisoning by thrombolytic drug, assault**
    - T45.614 **Poisoning by thrombolytic drug, undetermined**
    - T45.615 **Adverse effect of thrombolytic drugs**
      Coding Clinic: 2017, Q2, P10
    - T45.616 **Underdosing of thrombolytic drugs**
  - T45.62 **Poisoning by, adverse effect of and underdosing of hemostatic drugs**
    - T45.621 **Poisoning by hemostatic drug, accidental (unintentional)**
      Poisoning by hemostatic drug NOS
    - T45.622 **Poisoning by hemostatic drug, intentional self-harm**
    - T45.623 **Poisoning by hemostatic drug, assault**
    - T45.624 **Poisoning by hemostatic drug, undetermined**
    - T45.625 **Adverse effect of hemostatic drug**
    - T45.626 **Underdosing of hemostatic drugs**
  - T45.69 **Poisoning by, adverse effect of and underdosing of other fibrinolysis-affecting drugs**
    - T45.691 **Poisoning by other fibrinolysis-affecting drugs, accidental (unintentional)**
      Poisoning by other fibrinolysis-affecting drug NOS
    - T45.692 **Poisoning by other fibrinolysis-affecting drugs, intentional self-harm**
    - T45.693 **Poisoning by other fibrinolysis-affecting drugs, assault**
    - T45.694 **Poisoning by other fibrinolysis-affecting drugs, undetermined**
    - T45.695 **Adverse effect of other fibrinolysis-affecting drugs**
    - T45.696 **Underdosing of other fibrinolysis-affecting drugs**

▶ New   ⇒ Revised   ~~deleted~~ Deleted   Excludes 1   Excludes 2   Includes   Use additional   Code first   Code also   Key words
OGCR Official Guidelines   ● Unacceptable Principal Diagnosis   X Assign placeholder X   ● Use Additional Character(s)   ▶ Manifestation Code   Coding Clinic

● T45.7   Poisoning by, adverse effect of and underdosing
           of anticoagulant antagonists, vitamin K and other
           coagulants
    ● T45.7X   Poisoning by, adverse effect of and
              underdosing of anticoagulant antagonists,
              vitamin K and other coagulants
        ● T45.7X1   Poisoning by anticoagulant
                   antagonists, vitamin K and other
                   coagulants, accidental (unintentional)
                       Poisoning by anticoagulant
                           antagonists, vitamin K and
                           other coagulants NOS
        ● T45.7X2   Poisoning by anticoagulant
                   antagonists, vitamin K and other
                   coagulants, intentional self-harm
        ● T45.7X3   Poisoning by anticoagulant
                   antagonists, vitamin K and other
                   coagulants, assault
        ● T45.7X4   Poisoning by anticoagulant
                   antagonists, vitamin K and other
                   coagulants, undetermined
        ●● T45.7X5 Adverse effect of anticoagulant
                   antagonists, vitamin K and other
                   coagulants
        ●● T45.7X6 Underdosing of anticoagulant
                   antagonist, vitamin K and other
                   coagulants
                   Excludes1   vitamin K deficiency
                                    (E56.1)

● T45.8   Poisoning by, adverse effect of and underdosing of other
           primarily systemic and hematological agents
           Poisoning by, adverse effect of and underdosing of liver
               preparations and other antianemic agents
           Poisoning by, adverse effect of and underdosing of
               natural blood and blood products
           Poisoning by, adverse effect of and underdosing of
               plasma substitute
           Excludes2   poisoning by, adverse effect of and
                            underdosing of immunoglobulin
                            (T50.Z1)
                            poisoning by, adverse effect of and
                            underdosing of iron (T45.4)
                            transfusion reactions (T80.-)
    ● T45.8X   Poisoning by, adverse effect of and
              underdosing of other primarily systemic and
              hematological agents
        ● T45.8X1   Poisoning by other primarily systemic
                   and hematological agents, accidental
                   (unintentional)
                       Poisoning by other primarily
                           systemic and hematological
                           agents NOS
        ● T45.8X2   Poisoning by other primarily systemic
                   and hematological agents, intentional
                   self-harm
        ● T45.8X3   Poisoning by other primarily systemic
                   and hematological agents, assault
        ● T45.8X4   Poisoning by other primarily
                   systemic and hematological agents,
                   undetermined
        ●● T45.8X5 Adverse effect of other primarily
                   systemic and hematological agents
                   Coding Clinic: 2016, Q4, P42
        ●● T45.8X6 Underdosing of other primarily
                   systemic and hematological agents

● T45.9   Poisoning by, adverse effect of and underdosing of
           unspecified primarily systemic and hematological agent
    X● T45.91   Poisoning by unspecified primarily systemic
              and hematological agent, accidental
              (unintentional)
                  Poisoning by primarily systemic and
                      hematological agent NOS
    X● T45.92   Poisoning by unspecified primarily systemic
              and hematological agent, intentional self-harm
    X● T45.93   Poisoning by unspecified primarily systemic
              and hematological agent, assault
    X● T45.94   Poisoning by unspecified primarily systemic
              and hematological agent, undetermined
    ●X● T45.95 Adverse effect of unspecified primarily
              systemic and hematological agent
    ●X● T45.96 Underdosing of unspecified primarily systemic
              and hematological agent

● T46   Poisoning by, adverse effect of and underdosing of agents
         primarily affecting the cardiovascular system
         Excludes1   poisoning by, adverse effect of and underdosing
                          of metaraminol (T44.4)
         The appropriate 7th character is to be added to each code from
         category T46

A	initial encounter
D	subsequent encounter
S	sequela

● T46.0   Poisoning by, adverse effect of and underdosing of
           cardiac-stimulant glycosides and drugs of similar action
    ● T46.0X   Poisoning by, adverse effect of and
              underdosing of cardiac-stimulant glycosides
              and drugs of similar action
        ● T46.0X1   Poisoning by cardiac-stimulant
                   glycosides and drugs of similar
                   action, accidental (unintentional)
                       Poisoning by cardiac-stimulant
                           glycosides and drugs of similar
                           action NOS
        ● T46.0X2   Poisoning by cardiac-stimulant
                   glycosides and drugs of similar
                   action, intentional self-harm
        ● T46.0X3   Poisoning by cardiac-stimulant
                   glycosides and drugs of similar
                   action, assault
        ● T46.0X4   Poisoning by cardiac-stimulant
                   glycosides and drugs of similar
                   action, undetermined
        ●● T46.0X5 Adverse effect of cardiac-stimulant
                   glycosides and drugs of similar action
        ●● T46.0X6 Underdosing of cardiac-stimulant
                   glycosides and drugs of similar action

● T46.1   Poisoning by, adverse effect of and underdosing of
           calcium-channel blockers
    ● T46.1X   Poisoning by, adverse effect of and
              underdosing of calcium-channel blockers
        ● T46.1X1   Poisoning by calcium-channel
                   blockers, accidental (unintentional)
                       Poisoning by calcium-channel
                           blockers NOS
        ● T46.1X2   Poisoning by calcium-channel
                   blockers, intentional self-harm
        ● T46.1X3   Poisoning by calcium-channel
                   blockers, assault
        ● T46.1X4   Poisoning by calcium-channel
                   blockers, undetermined
        ●● T46.1X5 Adverse effect of calcium-channel
                   blockers
        ●● T46.1X6 Underdosing of calcium-channel
                   blockers

CHAPTER 19 (S00–T88)

● **T46.2** **Poisoning by, adverse effect of and underdosing of other antidysrhythmic drugs, not elsewhere classified**

> **Excludes1** poisoning by, adverse effect of and underdosing of beta-adrenoreceptor antagonists (T44.7-)

● **T46.2X** **Poisoning by, adverse effect of and underdosing of other antidysrhythmic drugs**

● **T46.2X1** **Poisoning by other antidysrhythmic drugs, accidental (unintentional)**
Poisoning by other antidysrhythmic drugs NOS

● **T46.2X2** **Poisoning by other antidysrhythmic drugs, intentional self-harm**

● **T46.2X3** **Poisoning by other antidysrhythmic drugs, assault**

● **T46.2X4** **Poisoning by other antidysrhythmic drugs, undetermined**

●● **T46.2X5** **Adverse effect of other antidysrhythmic drugs**

●● **T46.2X6** **Underdosing of other antidysrhythmic drugs**

● **T46.3** **Poisoning by, adverse effect of and underdosing of coronary vasodilators**
Poisoning by, adverse effect of and underdosing of dipyridamole

> **Excludes1** poisoning by, adverse effect of and underdosing of calcium-channel blockers (T46.1)

● **T46.3X** **Poisoning by, adverse effect of and underdosing of coronary vasodilators**

● **T46.3X1** **Poisoning by coronary vasodilators, accidental (unintentional)**
Poisoning by coronary vasodilators NOS

● **T46.3X2** **Poisoning by coronary vasodilators, intentional self-harm**

● **T46.3X3** **Poisoning by coronary vasodilators, assault**

● **T46.3X4** **Poisoning by coronary vasodilators, undetermined**

●● **T46.3X5** **Adverse effect of coronary vasodilators**

●● **T46.3X6** **Underdosing of coronary vasodilators**

● **T46.4** **Poisoning by, adverse effect of and underdosing of angiotensin-converting-enzyme inhibitors**

● **T46.4X** **Poisoning by, adverse effect of and underdosing of angiotensin-converting-enzyme inhibitors**

● **T46.4X1** **Poisoning by angiotensin-converting-enzyme inhibitors, accidental (unintentional)**
Poisoning by angiotensin-converting-enzyme inhibitors NOS

● **T46.4X2** **Poisoning by angiotensin-converting-enzyme inhibitors, intentional self-harm**

● **T46.4X3** **Poisoning by angiotensin-converting-enzyme inhibitors, assault**

● **T46.4X4** **Poisoning by angiotensin-converting-enzyme inhibitors, undetermined**

●● **T46.4X5** **Adverse effect of angiotensin-converting-enzyme inhibitors**

●● **T46.4X6** **Underdosing of angiotensin-converting-enzyme inhibitors**

● **T46.5** **Poisoning by, adverse effect of and underdosing of other antihypertensive drugs**

> **Excludes2** poisoning by, adverse effect of and underdosing of beta-adrenoreceptor antagonists (T44.7)
> poisoning by, adverse effect of and underdosing of calcium-channel blockers (T46.1)
> poisoning by, adverse effect of and underdosing of diuretics (T50.0-T50.2)

● **T46.5X** **Poisoning by, adverse effect of and underdosing of other antihypertensive drugs**

● **T46.5X1** **Poisoning by other antihypertensive drugs, accidental (unintentional)**
Poisoning by other antihypertensive drugs NOS

● **T46.5X2** **Poisoning by other antihypertensive drugs, intentional self-harm**

● **T46.5X3** **Poisoning by other antihypertensive drugs, assault**

● **T46.5X4** **Poisoning by other antihypertensive drugs, undetermined**

●● **T46.5X5** **Adverse effect of other antihypertensive drugs**

●● **T46.5X6** **Underdosing of other antihypertensive drugs**

● **T46.6** **Poisoning by, adverse effect of and underdosing of antihyperlipidemic and antiarteriosclerotic drugs**

● **T46.6X** **Poisoning by, adverse effect of and underdosing of antihyperlipidemic and antiarteriosclerotic drugs**

● **T46.6X1** **Poisoning by antihyperlipidemic and antiarteriosclerotic drugs, accidental (unintentional)**
Poisoning by antihyperlipidemic and antiarteriosclerotic drugs NOS

● **T46.6X2** **Poisoning by antihyperlipidemic and antiarteriosclerotic drugs, intentional self-harm**

● **T46.6X3** **Poisoning by antihyperlipidemic and antiarteriosclerotic drugs, assault**

● **T46.6X4** **Poisoning by antihyperlipidemic and antiarteriosclerotic drugs, undetermined**

●● **T46.6X5** **Adverse effect of antihyperlipidemic and antiarteriosclerotic drugs**

●● **T46.6X6** **Underdosing of antihyperlipidemic and antiarteriosclerotic drugs**

● **T46.7** **Poisoning by, adverse effect of and underdosing of peripheral vasodilators**
Poisoning by, adverse effect of and underdosing of nicotinic acid (derivatives)

> **Excludes1** poisoning by, adverse effect of and underdosing of papaverine (T44.3)

● **T46.7X** **Poisoning by, adverse effect of and underdosing of peripheral vasodilators**

● **T46.7X1** **Poisoning by peripheral vasodilators, accidental (unintentional)**
Poisoning by peripheral vasodilators NOS

● **T46.7X2** **Poisoning by peripheral vasodilators, intentional self-harm**

● **T46.7X3** **Poisoning by peripheral vasodilators, assault**

● **T46.7X4** **Poisoning by peripheral vasodilators, undetermined**

●● **T46.7X5** **Adverse effect of peripheral vasodilators**

●● **T46.7X6** **Underdosing of peripheral vasodilators**

▶ New   ⟹ Revised   ~~deleted~~ Deleted   Excludes 1   Excludes 2   Includes   Use additional   Code first   Code also   Key words

OGCR Official Guidelines   ● Unacceptable Principal Diagnosis   X Assign placeholder X   ● Use Additional Character(s)   ▌ Manifestation Code   **Coding Clinic**

● **T46.8**　Poisoning by, adverse effect of and underdosing of antivaricose drugs, including sclerosing agents
　　● **T46.8X**　Poisoning by, adverse effect of and underdosing of antivaricose drugs, including sclerosing agents
　　　　● **T46.8X1**　Poisoning by antivaricose drugs, including sclerosing agents, accidental (unintentional)
　　　　　　　　Poisoning by antivaricose drugs, including sclerosing agents NOS
　　　　● **T46.8X2**　Poisoning by antivaricose drugs, including sclerosing agents, intentional self-harm
　　　　● **T46.8X3**　Poisoning by antivaricose drugs, including sclerosing agents, assault
　　　　● **T46.8X4**　Poisoning by antivaricose drugs, including sclerosing agents, undetermined
　　　　●● **T46.8X5**　Adverse effect of antivaricose drugs, including sclerosing agents
　　　　●● **T46.8X6**　Underdosing of antivaricose drugs, including sclerosing agents
● **T46.9**　Poisoning by, adverse effect of and underdosing of other and unspecified agents primarily affecting the cardiovascular system
　　● **T46.90**　Poisoning by, adverse effect of and underdosing of unspecified agents primarily affecting the cardiovascular system
　　　　● **T46.901**　Poisoning by unspecified agents primarily affecting the cardiovascular system, accidental (unintentional)
　　　　● **T46.902**　Poisoning by unspecified agents primarily affecting the cardiovascular system, intentional self-harm
　　　　● **T46.903**　Poisoning by unspecified agents primarily affecting the cardiovascular system, assault
　　　　● **T46.904**　Poisoning by unspecified agents primarily affecting the cardiovascular system, undetermined
　　　　●● **T46.905**　Adverse effect of unspecified agents primarily affecting the cardiovascular system
　　　　●● **T46.906**　Underdosing of unspecified agents primarily affecting the cardiovascular system
　　● **T46.99**　Poisoning by, adverse effect of and underdosing of other agents primarily affecting the cardiovascular system
　　　　● **T46.991**　Poisoning by other agents primarily affecting the cardiovascular system, accidental (unintentional)
　　　　● **T46.992**　Poisoning by other agents primarily affecting the cardiovascular system, intentional self-harm
　　　　● **T46.993**　Poisoning by other agents primarily affecting the cardiovascular system, assault
　　　　● **T46.994**　Poisoning by other agents primarily affecting the cardiovascular system, undetermined
　　　　●● **T46.995**　Adverse effect of other agents primarily affecting the cardiovascular system
　　　　●● **T46.996**　Underdosing of other agents primarily affecting the cardiovascular system

● **T47**　Poisoning by, adverse effect of and underdosing of agents primarily affecting the gastrointestinal system
　　The appropriate 7th character is to be added to each code from category T47

A	initial encounter
D	subsequent encounter
S	sequela

● **T47.0**　Poisoning by, adverse effect of and underdosing of histamine H2-receptor blockers
　　● **T47.0X**　Poisoning by, adverse effect of and underdosing of histamine H2-receptor blockers
　　　　● **T47.0X1**　Poisoning by histamine H2-receptor blockers, accidental (unintentional)
　　　　　　　　Poisoning by histamine H2-receptor blockers NOS
　　　　● **T47.0X2**　Poisoning by histamine H2-receptor blockers, intentional self-harm
　　　　● **T47.0X3**　Poisoning by histamine H2-receptor blockers, assault
　　　　● **T47.0X4**　Poisoning by histamine H2-receptor blockers, undetermined
　　　　●● **T47.0X5**　Adverse effect of histamine H2-receptor blockers
　　　　●● **T47.0X6**　Underdosing of histamine H2-receptor blockers
● **T47.1**　Poisoning by, adverse effect of and underdosing of other antacids and anti-gastric-secretion drugs
　　● **T47.1X**　Poisoning by, adverse effect of and underdosing of other antacids and anti-gastric-secretion drugs
　　　　● **T47.1X1**　Poisoning by other antacids and anti-gastric-secretion drugs, accidental (unintentional)
　　　　　　　　Poisoning by other antacids and anti-gastric-secretion drugs NOS
　　　　● **T47.1X2**　Poisoning by other antacids and anti-gastric-secretion drugs, intentional self-harm
　　　　● **T47.1X3**　Poisoning by other antacids and anti-gastric-secretion drugs, assault
　　　　● **T47.1X4**　Poisoning by other antacids and anti-gastric-secretion drugs, undetermined
　　　　●● **T47.1X5**　Adverse effect of other antacids and anti-gastric-secretion drugs
　　　　●● **T47.1X6**　Underdosing of other antacids and anti-gastric-secretion drugs
● **T47.2**　Poisoning by, adverse effect of and underdosing of stimulant laxatives
　　● **T47.2X**　Poisoning by, adverse effect of and underdosing of stimulant laxatives
　　　　● **T47.2X1**　Poisoning by stimulant laxatives, accidental (unintentional)
　　　　　　　　Poisoning by stimulant laxatives NOS
　　　　● **T47.2X2**　Poisoning by stimulant laxatives, intentional self-harm
　　　　● **T47.2X3**　Poisoning by stimulant laxatives, assault
　　　　● **T47.2X4**　Poisoning by stimulant laxatives, undetermined
　　　　●● **T47.2X5**　Adverse effect of stimulant laxatives
　　　　●● **T47.2X6**　Underdosing of stimulant laxatives

CHAPTER 19 (S00-T88)

N Newborn Age: 0　　**P** Pediatric Age: 0–17　　**M** Maternity DX: 12–55　　**A** Adult Age: 15–124　　♀ Females Only　　♂ Males Only

🗣 Complication\Comorbidity　　🗣 Major C\C　　(Ex) CC/MCC Exclusions　　🗣 Hospital-Acquired Condition

1451

● **T47.3** Poisoning by, adverse effect of and underdosing of saline and osmotic laxatives
  ● **T47.3X** Poisoning by and adverse effect of saline and osmotic laxatives
    ● **T47.3X1** Poisoning by saline and osmotic laxatives, accidental (unintentional)
      Poisoning by saline and osmotic laxatives NOS
    ● **T47.3X2** Poisoning by saline and osmotic laxatives, intentional self-harm
    ● **T47.3X3** Poisoning by saline and osmotic laxatives, assault
    ● **T47.3X4** Poisoning by saline and osmotic laxatives, undetermined
    ●● **T47.3X5** Adverse effect of saline and osmotic laxatives
    ●● **T47.3X6** Underdosing of saline and osmotic laxatives

● **T47.4** Poisoning by, adverse effect of and underdosing of other laxatives
  ● **T47.4X** Poisoning by, adverse effect of and underdosing of other laxatives
    ● **T47.4X1** Poisoning by other laxatives, accidental (unintentional)
      Poisoning by other laxatives NOS
    ● **T47.4X2** Poisoning by other laxatives, intentional self-harm
    ● **T47.4X3** Poisoning by other laxatives, assault
    ● **T47.4X4** Poisoning by other laxatives, undetermined
    ●● **T47.4X5** Adverse effect of other laxatives
    ●● **T47.4X6** Underdosing of other laxatives

● **T47.5** Poisoning by, adverse effect of and underdosing of digestants
  ● **T47.5X** Poisoning by, adverse effect of and underdosing of digestants
    ● **T47.5X1** Poisoning by digestants, accidental (unintentional)
      Poisoning by digestants NOS
    ● **T47.5X2** Poisoning by digestants, intentional self-harm
    ● **T47.5X3** Poisoning by digestants, assault
    ● **T47.5X4** Poisoning by digestants, undetermined
    ●● **T47.5X5** Adverse effect of digestants
    ●● **T47.5X6** Underdosing of digestants

● **T47.6** Poisoning by, adverse effect of and underdosing of antidiarrheal drugs
  Excludes2 poisoning by, adverse effect of and underdosing of systemic antibiotics and other anti-infectives (T36-T37)
  ● **T47.6X** Poisoning by, adverse effect of and underdosing of antidiarrheal drugs
    ● **T47.6X1** Poisoning by antidiarrheal drugs, accidental (unintentional)
      Poisoning by antidiarrheal drugs NOS
    ● **T47.6X2** Poisoning by antidiarrheal drugs, intentional self-harm
    ● **T47.6X3** Poisoning by antidiarrheal drugs, assault
    ● **T47.6X4** Poisoning by antidiarrheal drugs, undetermined
    ●● **T47.6X5** Adverse effect of antidiarrheal drugs
    ●● **T47.6X6** Underdosing of antidiarrheal drugs

● **T47.7** Poisoning by, adverse effect of and underdosing of emetics
  ● **T47.7X** Poisoning by, adverse effect of and underdosing of emetics
    ● **T47.7X1** Poisoning by emetics, accidental (unintentional)
      Poisoning by emetics NOS
    ● **T47.7X2** Poisoning by emetics, intentional self-harm
    ● **T47.7X3** Poisoning by emetics, assault
    ● **T47.7X4** Poisoning by emetics, undetermined
    ●● **T47.7X5** Adverse effect of emetics
    ●● **T47.7X6** Underdosing of emetics

● **T47.8** Poisoning by, adverse effect of and underdosing of other agents primarily affecting gastrointestinal system
  ● **T47.8X** Poisoning by, adverse effect of and underdosing of other agents primarily affecting gastrointestinal system
    ● **T47.8X1** Poisoning by other agents primarily affecting gastrointestinal system, accidental (unintentional)
      Poisoning by other agents primarily affecting gastrointestinal system NOS
    ● **T47.8X2** Poisoning by other agents primarily affecting gastrointestinal system, intentional self-harm
    ● **T47.8X3** Poisoning by other agents primarily affecting gastrointestinal system, assault
    ● **T47.8X4** Poisoning by other agents primarily affecting gastrointestinal system, undetermined
    ●● **T47.8X5** Adverse effect of other agents primarily affecting gastrointestinal system
    ●● **T47.8X6** Underdosing of other agents primarily affecting gastrointestinal system

● **T47.9** Poisoning by, adverse effect of and underdosing of unspecified agents primarily affecting the gastrointestinal system
  X ● **T47.91** Poisoning by unspecified agents primarily affecting the gastrointestinal system, accidental (unintentional)
    Poisoning by agents primarily affecting the gastrointestinal system NOS
  X ● **T47.92** Poisoning by unspecified agents primarily affecting the gastrointestinal system, intentional self-harm
  X ● **T47.93** Poisoning by unspecified agents primarily affecting the gastrointestinal system, assault
  X ● **T47.94** Poisoning by unspecified agents primarily affecting the gastrointestinal system, undetermined
  ● X ● **T47.95** Adverse effect of unspecified agents primarily affecting the gastrointestinal system
  ● X ● **T47.96** Underdosing of unspecified agents primarily affecting the gastrointestinal system

▶ New   ⇒ Revised   ~~deleted~~ Deleted   Excludes 1   Excludes 2   Includes   Use additional   Code first   Code also   Key words
OGCR Official Guidelines   ● Unacceptable Principal Diagnosis   X Assign placeholder X   ● Use Additional Character(s)   ▶ Manifestation Code   **Coding Clinic**

● **T48** **Poisoning by, adverse effect of and underdosing of agents primarily acting on smooth and skeletal muscles and the respiratory system**

> The appropriate 7th character is to be added to each code from category T48

> | | |
> |---|---|
> | A | initial encounter |
> | D | subsequent encounter |
> | S | sequela |

● **T48.0** **Poisoning by, adverse effect of and underdosing of oxytocic drugs**

> **Excludes1**   poisoning by, adverse effect of and underdosing of estrogens, progestogens and antagonists (T38.4-T38.6)

  ● **T48.0X** **Poisoning by, adverse effect of and underdosing of oxytocic drugs**

    ● **T48.0X1** **Poisoning by oxytocic drugs, accidental (unintentional)**
> Poisoning by oxytocic drugs NOS

    ● **T48.0X2** **Poisoning by oxytocic drugs, intentional self-harm**

    ● **T48.0X3** **Poisoning by oxytocic drugs, assault**

    ● **T48.0X4** **Poisoning by oxytocic drugs, undetermined**

    ●● **T48.0X5** **Adverse effect of oxytocic drugs**

    ●● **T48.0X6** **Underdosing of oxytocic drugs**

● **T48.1** **Poisoning by, adverse effect of and underdosing of skeletal muscle relaxants [neuromuscular blocking agents]**

  ● **T48.1X** **Poisoning by, adverse effect of and underdosing of skeletal muscle relaxants [neuromuscular blocking agents]**

    ● **T48.1X1** **Poisoning by skeletal muscle relaxants [neuromuscular blocking agents], accidental (unintentional)**
> Poisoning by skeletal muscle relaxants [neuromuscular blocking agents] NOS

    ● **T48.1X2** **Poisoning by skeletal muscle relaxants [neuromuscular blocking agents], intentional self-harm**

    ● **T48.1X3** **Poisoning by skeletal muscle relaxants [neuromuscular blocking agents], assault**

    ● **T48.1X4** **Poisoning by skeletal muscle relaxants [neuromuscular blocking agents], undetermined**

    ●● **T48.1X5** **Adverse effect of skeletal muscle relaxants [neuromuscular blocking agents]**

    ●● **T48.1X6** **Underdosing of skeletal muscle relaxants [neuromuscular blocking agents]**

● **T48.2** **Poisoning by, adverse effect of and underdosing of other and unspecified drugs acting on muscles**

  ● **T48.20** **Poisoning by, adverse effect of and underdosing of unspecified drugs acting on muscles**

    ● **T48.201** **Poisoning by unspecified drugs acting on muscles, accidental (unintentional)**
> Poisoning by unspecified drugs acting on muscles NOS

    ● **T48.202** **Poisoning by unspecified drugs acting on muscles, intentional self-harm**

    ● **T48.203** **Poisoning by unspecified drugs acting on muscles, assault**

    ● **T48.204** **Poisoning by unspecified drugs acting on muscles, undetermined**

    ●● **T48.205** **Adverse effect of unspecified drugs acting on muscles**

    ●● **T48.206** **Underdosing of unspecified drugs acting on muscles**

  ● **T48.29** **Poisoning by, adverse effect of and underdosing of other drugs acting on muscles**

    ● **T48.291** **Poisoning by other drugs acting on muscles, accidental (unintentional)**
> Poisoning by other drugs acting on muscles NOS

    ● **T48.292** **Poisoning by other drugs acting on muscles, intentional self-harm**

    ● **T48.293** **Poisoning by other drugs acting on muscles, assault**

    ● **T48.294** **Poisoning by other drugs acting on muscles, undetermined**

    ●● **T48.295** **Adverse effect of other drugs acting on muscles**

    ●● **T48.296** **Underdosing of other drugs acting on muscles**

● **T48.3** **Poisoning by, adverse effect of and underdosing of antitussives**

  ● **T48.3X** **Poisoning by, adverse effect of and underdosing of antitussives**

    ● **T48.3X1** **Poisoning by antitussives, accidental (unintentional)**
> Poisoning by antitussives NOS

    ● **T48.3X2** **Poisoning by antitussives, intentional self-harm**

    ● **T48.3X3** **Poisoning by antitussives, assault**

    ● **T48.3X4** **Poisoning by antitussives, undetermined**

    ●● **T48.3X5** **Adverse effect of antitussives**

    ●● **T48.3X6** **Underdosing of antitussives**

● **T48.4** **Poisoning by, adverse effect of and underdosing of expectorants**

  ● **T48.4X** **Poisoning by, adverse effect of and underdosing of expectorants**

    ● **T48.4X1** **Poisoning by expectorants, accidental (unintentional)**
> Poisoning by expectorants NOS

    ● **T48.4X2** **Poisoning by expectorants, intentional self-harm**

    ● **T48.4X3** **Poisoning by expectorants, assault**

    ● **T48.4X4** **Poisoning by expectorants, undetermined**

    ●● **T48.4X5** **Adverse effect of expectorants**

    ●● **T48.4X6** **Underdosing of expectorants**

● **T48.5** **Poisoning by, adverse effect of and underdosing of other anti-common-cold drugs**

> Poisoning by, adverse effect of and underdosing of decongestants

> **Excludes2**   poisoning by, adverse effect of and underdosing of antipyretics, NEC (T39.9-)
> poisoning by, adverse effect of and underdosing of non-steroidal antiinflammatory drugs (T39.3-)
> poisoning by, adverse effect of and underdosing of salicylates (T39.0-)

  ● **T48.5X** **Poisoning by, adverse effect of and underdosing of other anti-common-cold drugs**

    ● **T48.5X1** **Poisoning by other anti-common-cold drugs, accidental (unintentional)**
> Poisoning by other anti-common-cold drugs NOS

    ● **T48.5X2** **Poisoning by other anti-common-cold drugs, intentional self-harm**

    ● **T48.5X3** **Poisoning by other anti-common-cold drugs, assault**

    ● **T48.5X4** **Poisoning by other anti-common-cold drugs, undetermined**

    ●● **T48.5X5** **Adverse effect of other anti-common-cold drugs**

    ●● **T48.5X6** **Underdosing of other anti-common-cold drugs**

N Newborn Age: Ø   **P** Pediatric Age: Ø–17   **M** Maternity DX: 12–55   **A** Adult Age: 15–124   ♀ Females Only   ♂ Males Only

 Complication\Comorbidity   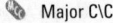 Major C\C   (Ⓔ) CC/MCC Exclusions   Hospital-Acquired Condition

1453

CHAPTER 19 (SØØ-T88)

● **T48.6　Poisoning by, adverse effect of and underdosing of antiasthmatics, not elsewhere classified**
　　Poisoning by, adverse effect of and underdosing of beta-adrenoreceptor agonists used in asthma therapy
　　Excludes1　poisoning by, adverse effect of and underdosing of beta-adrenoreceptor agonists not used in asthma therapy (T44.5)
　　　　poisoning by, adverse effect of and underdosing of anterior pituitary [adenohypophyseal] hormones (T38.8)

● **T48.6X　Poisoning by, adverse effect of and underdosing of antiasthmatics**
● **T48.6X1　Poisoning by antiasthmatics, accidental (unintentional)**
　　Poisoning by antiasthmatics NOS
● **T48.6X2　Poisoning by antiasthmatics, intentional self-harm**
● **T48.6X3　Poisoning by antiasthmatics, assault**
● **T48.6X4　Poisoning by antiasthmatics, undetermined**
●● **T48.6X5　Adverse effect of antiasthmatics**
●● **T48.6X6　Underdosing of antiasthmatics**

● **T48.9　Poisoning by, adverse effect of and underdosing of other and unspecified agents primarily acting on the respiratory system**

● **T48.90　Poisoning by, adverse effect of and underdosing of unspecified agents primarily acting on the respiratory system**
● **T48.901　Poisoning by unspecified agents primarily acting on the respiratory system, accidental (unintentional)**
● **T48.902　Poisoning by unspecified agents primarily acting on the respiratory system, intentional self-harm**
● **T48.903　Poisoning by unspecified agents primarily acting on the respiratory system, assault**
● **T48.904　Poisoning by unspecified agents primarily acting on the respiratory system, undetermined**
●● **T48.905　Adverse effect of unspecified agents primarily acting on the respiratory system**
●● **T48.906　Underdosing of unspecified agents primarily acting on the respiratory system**

● **T48.99　Poisoning by, adverse effect of and underdosing of other agents primarily acting on the respiratory system**
● **T48.991　Poisoning by other agents primarily acting on the respiratory system, accidental (unintentional)**
● **T48.992　Poisoning by other agents primarily acting on the respiratory system, intentional self-harm**
● **T48.993　Poisoning by other agents primarily acting on the respiratory system, assault**
● **T48.994　Poisoning by other agents primarily acting on the respiratory system, undetermined**
●● **T48.995　Adverse effect of other agents primarily acting on the respiratory system**
●● **T48.996　Underdosing of other agents primarily acting on the respiratory system**

● **T49　Poisoning by, adverse effect of and underdosing of topical agents primarily affecting skin and mucous membrane and by ophthalmological, otorhinolaryngological and dental drugs**
　　Includes　poisoning by, adverse effect of and underdosing of glucocorticoids, topically used
　　The appropriate 7th character is to be added to each code from category T49

　　A　initial encounter
　　D　subsequent encounter
　　S　sequela

● **T49.0　Poisoning by, adverse effect of and underdosing of local antifungal, anti-infective and anti-inflammatory drugs**
● **T49.0X　Poisoning by, adverse effect of and underdosing of local antifungal, anti-infective and anti-inflammatory drugs**
● **T49.0X1　Poisoning by local antifungal, anti-infective and anti-inflammatory drugs, accidental (unintentional)**
　　Poisoning by local antifungal, anti-infective and anti-inflammatory drugs NOS
● **T49.0X2　Poisoning by local antifungal, anti-infective and anti-inflammatory drugs, intentional self-harm**
● **T49.0X3　Poisoning by local antifungal, anti-infective and anti-inflammatory drugs, assault**
● **T49.0X4　Poisoning by local antifungal, anti-infective and anti-inflammatory drugs, undetermined**
●● **T49.0X5　Adverse effect of local antifungal, anti-infective and anti-inflammatory drugs**
●● **T49.0X6　Underdosing of local antifungal, anti-infective and anti-inflammatory drugs**

● **T49.1　Poisoning by, adverse effect of and underdosing of antipruritics**
● **T49.1X　Poisoning by, adverse effect of and underdosing of antipruritics**
● **T49.1X1　Poisoning by antipruritics, accidental (unintentional)**
　　Poisoning by antipruritics NOS
● **T49.1X2　Poisoning by antipruritics, intentional self-harm**
● **T49.1X3　Poisoning by antipruritics, assault**
● **T49.1X4　Poisoning by antipruritics, undetermined**
●● **T49.1X5　Adverse effect of antipruritics**
●● **T49.1X6　Underdosing of antipruritics**

● **T49.2　Poisoning by, adverse effect of and underdosing of local astringents and local detergents**
● **T49.2X　Poisoning by, adverse effect of and underdosing of local astringents and local detergents**
● **T49.2X1　Poisoning by local astringents and local detergents, accidental (unintentional)**
　　Poisoning by local astringents and local detergents NOS
● **T49.2X2　Poisoning by local astringents and local detergents, intentional self-harm**
● **T49.2X3　Poisoning by local astringents and local detergents, assault**
● **T49.2X4　Poisoning by local astringents and local detergents, undetermined**
●● **T49.2X5　Adverse effect of local astringents and local detergents**
●● **T49.2X6　Underdosing of local astringents and local detergents**

CHAPTER 19 (S00-T88)

● T49.3   Poisoning by, adverse effect of and underdosing of emollients, demulcents and protectants
   ● T49.3X   Poisoning by, adverse effect of and underdosing of emollients, demulcents and protectants
      ● T49.3X1   Poisoning by emollients, demulcents and protectants, accidental (unintentional)
         Poisoning by emollients, demulcents and protectants NOS
      ● T49.3X2   Poisoning by emollients, demulcents and protectants, intentional self-harm
      ● T49.3X3   Poisoning by emollients, demulcents and protectants, assault
      ● T49.3X4   Poisoning by emollients, demulcents and protectants, undetermined
      ●● T49.3X5   Adverse effect of emollients, demulcents and protectants
      ●● T49.3X6   Underdosing of emollients, demulcents and protectants

● T49.4   Poisoning by, adverse effect of and underdosing of keratolytics, keratoplastics, and other hair treatment drugs and preparations
   ● T49.4X   Poisoning by, adverse effect of and underdosing of keratolytics, keratoplastics, and other hair treatment drugs and preparations
      ● T49.4X1   Poisoning by keratolytics, keratoplastics, and other hair treatment drugs and preparations, accidental (unintentional)
         Poisoning by keratolytics, keratoplastics, and other hair treatment drugs and preparations NOS
      ● T49.4X2   Poisoning by keratolytics, keratoplastics, and other hair treatment drugs and preparations, intentional self-harm
      ● T49.4X3   Poisoning by keratolytics, keratoplastics, and other hair treatment drugs and preparations, assault
      ● T49.4X4   Poisoning by keratolytics, keratoplastics, and other hair treatment drugs and preparations, undetermined
      ●● T49.4X5   Adverse effect of keratolytics, keratoplastics, and other hair treatment drugs and preparations
      ●● T49.4X6   Underdosing of keratolytics, keratoplastics, and other hair treatment drugs and preparations

● T49.5   Poisoning by, adverse effect of and underdosing of ophthalmological drugs and preparations
   ● T49.5X   Poisoning by, adverse effect of and underdosing of ophthalmological drugs and preparations
      ● T49.5X1   Poisoning by ophthalmological drugs and preparations, accidental (unintentional)
         Poisoning by ophthalmological drugs and preparations NOS
      ● T49.5X2   Poisoning by ophthalmological drugs and preparations, intentional self-harm
      ● T49.5X3   Poisoning by ophthalmological drugs and preparations, assault
      ● T49.5X4   Poisoning by ophthalmological drugs and preparations, undetermined
      ●● T49.5X5   Adverse effect of ophthalmological drugs and preparations
      ●● T49.5X6   Underdosing of ophthalmological drugs and preparations

● T49.6   Poisoning by, adverse effect of and underdosing of otorhinolaryngological drugs and preparations
   ● T49.6X   Poisoning by, adverse effect of and underdosing of otorhinolaryngological drugs and preparations
      ● T49.6X1   Poisoning by otorhinolaryngological drugs and preparations, accidental (unintentional)
         Poisoning by otorhinolaryngological drugs and preparations NOS
      ● T49.6X2   Poisoning by otorhinolaryngological drugs and preparations, intentional self-harm
      ● T49.6X3   Poisoning by otorhinolaryngological drugs and preparations, assault
      ● T49.6X4   Poisoning by otorhinolaryngological drugs and preparations, undetermined
      ●● T49.6X5   Adverse effect of otorhinolaryngological drugs and preparations
      ●● T49.6X6   Underdosing of otorhinolaryngological drugs and preparations

● T49.7   Poisoning by, adverse effect of and underdosing of dental drugs, topically applied
   ● T49.7X   Poisoning by, adverse effect of and underdosing of dental drugs, topically applied
      ● T49.7X1   Poisoning by dental drugs, topically applied, accidental (unintentional)
         Poisoning by dental drugs, topically applied NOS
      ● T49.7X2   Poisoning by dental drugs, topically applied, intentional self-harm
      ● T49.7X3   Poisoning by dental drugs, topically applied, assault
      ● T49.7X4   Poisoning by dental drugs, topically applied, undetermined
      ●● T49.7X5   Adverse effect of dental drugs, topically applied
      ●● T49.7X6   Underdosing of dental drugs, topically applied

● T49.8   Poisoning by, adverse effect of and underdosing of other topical agents
      Poisoning by, adverse effect of and underdosing of spermicides
   ● T49.8X   Poisoning by, adverse effect of and underdosing of other topical agents
      ● T49.8X1   Poisoning by other topical agents, accidental (unintentional)
         Poisoning by other topical agents NOS
      ● T49.8X2   Poisoning by other topical agents, intentional self-harm
      ● T49.8X3   Poisoning by other topical agents, assault
      ● T49.8X4   Poisoning by other topical agents, undetermined
      ●● T49.8X5   Adverse effect of other topical agents
      ●● T49.8X6   Underdosing of other topical agents

● T49.9   Poisoning by, adverse effect of and underdosing of unspecified topical agent
   X● T49.91   Poisoning by unspecified topical agent, accidental (unintentional)
   X● T49.92   Poisoning by unspecified topical agent, intentional self-harm
   X● T49.93   Poisoning by unspecified topical agent, assault
   X● T49.94   Poisoning by unspecified topical agent, undetermined
   ●X● T49.95   Adverse effect of unspecified topical agent
   ●X● T49.96   Underdosing of unspecified topical agent

CHAPTER 19 (S00-T88)

● T50   Poisoning by, adverse effect of and underdosing of diuretics and other and unspecified drugs, medicaments and biological substances

The appropriate 7th character is to be added to each code from category T50

> A   initial encounter
> D   subsequent encounter
> S   sequela

● T50.0   Poisoning by, adverse effect of and underdosing of mineralocorticoids and their antagonists

   ● T50.0X   Poisoning by, adverse effect of and underdosing of mineralocorticoids and their antagonists

     ● T50.0X1   Poisoning by mineralocorticoids and their antagonists, accidental (unintentional)

> Poisoning by mineralocorticoids and their antagonists NOS

     ● T50.0X2   Poisoning by mineralocorticoids and their antagonists, intentional self-harm

     ● T50.0X3   Poisoning by mineralocorticoids and their antagonists, assault

     ● T50.0X4   Poisoning by mineralocorticoids and their antagonists, undetermined

     ●● T50.0X5   Adverse effect of mineralocorticoids and their antagonists

     ●● T50.0X6   Underdosing of mineralocorticoids and their antagonists

● T50.1   Poisoning by, adverse effect of and underdosing of loop [high-ceiling] diuretics

   ● T50.1X   Poisoning by, adverse effect of and underdosing of loop [high-ceiling] diuretics

     ● T50.1X1   Poisoning by loop [high-ceiling] diuretics, accidental (unintentional)

> Poisoning by loop [high-ceiling] diuretics NOS

     ● T50.1X2   Poisoning by loop [high-ceiling] diuretics, intentional self-harm

     ● T50.1X3   Poisoning by loop [high-ceiling] diuretics, assault

     ● T50.1X4   Poisoning by loop [high-ceiling] diuretics, undetermined

     ●● T50.1X5   Adverse effect of loop [high-ceiling] diuretics

     ●● T50.1X6   Underdosing of loop [high-ceiling] diuretics

● T50.2   Poisoning by, adverse effect of and underdosing of carbonic-anhydrase inhibitors, benzothiadiazides and other diuretics

> Poisoning by, adverse effect of and underdosing of acetazolamide

   ● T50.2X   Poisoning by, adverse effect of and underdosing of carbonic-anhydrase inhibitors, benzothiadiazides and other diuretics

     ● T50.2X1   Poisoning by carbonic-anhydrase inhibitors, benzothiadiazides and other diuretics, accidental (unintentional)

> Poisoning by carbonic-anhydrase inhibitors, benzothiadiazides and other diuretics NOS

     ● T50.2X2   Poisoning by carbonic-anhydrase inhibitors, benzothiadiazides and other diuretics, intentional self-harm

     ● T50.2X3   Poisoning by carbonic-anhydrase inhibitors, benzothiadiazides and other diuretics, assault

     ● T50.2X4   Poisoning by carbonic-anhydrase inhibitors, benzothiadiazides and other diuretics, undetermined

     ●● T50.2X5   Adverse effect of carbonic-anhydrase inhibitors, benzothiadiazides and other diuretics

     ●● T50.2X6   Underdosing of carbonic-anhydrase inhibitors, benzothiadiazides and other diuretics

● T50.3   Poisoning by, adverse effect of and underdosing of electrolytic, caloric and water-balance agents

> Poisoning by, adverse effect of and underdosing of oral rehydration salts

   ● T50.3X   Poisoning by, adverse effect of and underdosing of electrolytic, caloric and water-balance agents

     ● T50.3X1   Poisoning by electrolytic, caloric and water-balance agents, accidental (unintentional)

> Poisoning by electrolytic, caloric and water-balance agents NOS

     ● T50.3X2   Poisoning by electrolytic, caloric and water-balance agents, intentional self-harm

     ● T50.3X3   Poisoning by electrolytic, caloric and water-balance agents, assault

     ● T50.3X4   Poisoning by electrolytic, caloric and water-balance agents, undetermined

     ●● T50.3X5   Adverse effect of electrolytic, caloric and water-balance agents

     ●● T50.3X6   Underdosing of electrolytic, caloric and water-balance agents

● T50.4   Poisoning by, adverse effect of and underdosing of drugs affecting uric acid metabolism

   ● T50.4X   Poisoning by, adverse effect of and underdosing of drugs affecting uric acid metabolism

     ● T50.4X1   Poisoning by drugs affecting uric acid metabolism, accidental (unintentional)

> Poisoning by drugs affecting uric acid metabolism NOS

     ● T50.4X2   Poisoning by drugs affecting uric acid metabolism, intentional self-harm

     ● T50.4X3   Poisoning by drugs affecting uric acid metabolism, assault

     ● T50.4X4   Poisoning by drugs affecting uric acid metabolism, undetermined

     ●● T50.4X5   Adverse effect of drugs affecting uric acid metabolism

     ●● T50.4X6   Underdosing of drugs affecting uric acid metabolism

● T50.5   Poisoning by, adverse effect of and underdosing of appetite depressants

   ● T50.5X   Poisoning by, adverse effect of and underdosing of appetite depressants

     ● T50.5X1   Poisoning by appetite depressants, accidental (unintentional)

> Poisoning by appetite depressants NOS

     ● T50.5X2   Poisoning by appetite depressants, intentional self-harm

     ● T50.5X3   Poisoning by appetite depressants, assault

     ● T50.5X4   Poisoning by appetite depressants, undetermined

     ●● T50.5X5   Adverse effect of appetite depressants

     ●● T50.5X6   Underdosing of appetite depressants

▶ New   ⇒ Revised   ~~deleted~~ Deleted   Excludes 1   Excludes 2   Includes   Use additional   Code first   Code also   Key words

OGCR Official Guidelines   ● Unacceptable Principal Diagnosis   X Assign placeholder X   ● Use Additional Character(s)   ▶ Manifestation Code   **Coding Clinic**

● T50.6   Poisoning by, adverse effect of and underdosing of
          antidotes and chelating agents
            Poisoning by, adverse effect of and underdosing of
            alcohol deterrents
    ● T50.6X   Poisoning by, adverse effect of and
              underdosing of antidotes and chelating agents
        ● T50.6X1   Poisoning by antidotes and chelating
                    agents, accidental (unintentional)
                      Poisoning by antidotes and chelating
                      agents NOS
        ● T50.6X2   Poisoning by antidotes and chelating
                    agents, intentional self-harm
        ● T50.6X3   Poisoning by antidotes and chelating
                    agents, assault
        ● T50.6X4   Poisoning by antidotes and chelating
                    agents, undetermined
        ●● T50.6X5 Adverse effect of antidotes and
                    chelating agents
        ●● T50.6X6 Underdosing of antidotes and
                    chelating agents
● T50.7   Poisoning by, adverse effect of and underdosing of
          analeptics and opioid receptor antagonists
    ● T50.7X   Poisoning by, adverse effect of and
              underdosing of analeptics and opioid receptor
              antagonists
        ● T50.7X1   Poisoning by analeptics and opioid
                    receptor antagonists, accidental
                    (unintentional)
                      Poisoning by analeptics and opioid
                      receptor antagonists NOS
        ● T50.7X2   Poisoning by analeptics and opioid
                    receptor antagonists, intentional
                    self-harm
        ● T50.7X3   Poisoning by analeptics and opioid
                    receptor antagonists, assault
        ● T50.7X4   Poisoning by analeptics and opioid
                    receptor antagonists, undetermined
        ●● T50.7X5 Adverse effect of analeptics and
                    opioid receptor antagonists
        ●● T50.7X6 Underdosing of analeptics and opioid
                    receptor antagonists
● T50.8   Poisoning by, adverse effect of and underdosing of
          diagnostic agents
    ● T50.8X   Poisoning by, adverse effect of and
              underdosing of diagnostic agents
        ● T50.8X1   Poisoning by diagnostic agents,
                    accidental (unintentional)
                      Poisoning by diagnostic agents NOS
        ● T50.8X2   Poisoning by diagnostic agents,
                    intentional self-harm
        ● T50.8X3   Poisoning by diagnostic agents,
                    assault
        ● T50.8X4   Poisoning by diagnostic agents,
                    undetermined
        ●● T50.8X5 Adverse effect of diagnostic agents
        ●● T50.8X6 Underdosing of diagnostic agents
● T50.A   Poisoning by, adverse effect of and underdosing of
          bacterial vaccines
    ● T50.A1   Poisoning by, adverse effect of and
              underdosing of pertussis vaccine, including
              combinations with a pertussis component
        ● T50.A11   Poisoning by pertussis vaccine,
                    including combinations with a
                    pertussis component, accidental
                    (unintentional)
        ● T50.A12   Poisoning by pertussis vaccine,
                    including combinations with a
                    pertussis component, intentional
                    self-harm

        ● T50.A13   Poisoning by pertussis vaccine,
                    including combinations with a
                    pertussis component, assault
        ● T50.A14   Poisoning by pertussis vaccine,
                    including combinations with a
                    pertussis component, undetermined
        ●● T50.A15 Adverse effect of pertussis vaccine,
                    including combinations with a
                    pertussis component
        ●● T50.A16 Underdosing of pertussis vaccine,
                    including combinations with a
                    pertussis component
    ● T50.A2   Poisoning by, adverse effect of and
              underdosing of mixed bacterial vaccines
              without a pertussis component
        ● T50.A21   Poisoning by mixed bacterial vaccines
                    without a pertussis component,
                    accidental (unintentional)
        ● T50.A22   Poisoning by mixed bacterial vaccines
                    without a pertussis component,
                    intentional self-harm
        ● T50.A23   Poisoning by mixed bacterial vaccines
                    without a pertussis component,
                    assault
        ● T50.A24   Poisoning by mixed bacterial vaccines
                    without a pertussis component,
                    undetermined
        ●● T50.A25 Adverse effect of mixed bacterial
                    vaccines without a pertussis
                    component
        ●● T50.A26 Underdosing of mixed bacterial
                    vaccines without a pertussis
                    component
    ● T50.A9   Poisoning by, adverse effect of and
              underdosing of other bacterial vaccines
        ● T50.A91   Poisoning by other bacterial vaccines,
                    accidental (unintentional)
        ● T50.A92   Poisoning by other bacterial vaccines,
                    intentional self-harm
        ● T50.A93   Poisoning by other bacterial vaccines,
                    assault
        ● T50.A94   Poisoning by other bacterial vaccines,
                    undetermined
        ●● T50.A95 Adverse effect of other bacterial
                    vaccines
        ●● T50.A96 Underdosing of other bacterial
                    vaccines
● T50.B   Poisoning by, adverse effect of and underdosing of viral
          vaccines
    ● T50.B1   Poisoning by, adverse effect of and
              underdosing of smallpox vaccines
        ● T50.B11   Poisoning by smallpox vaccines,
                    accidental (unintentional)
        ● T50.B12   Poisoning by smallpox vaccines,
                    intentional self-harm
        ● T50.B13   Poisoning by smallpox vaccines,
                    assault
        ● T50.B14   Poisoning by smallpox vaccines,
                    undetermined
        ●● T50.B15 Adverse effect of smallpox vaccines
        ●● T50.B16 Underdosing of smallpox vaccines

CHAPTER 19 (S00-T88)

T50.B9 **Poisoning by, adverse effect of and underdosing of other viral vaccines**
- T50.B91 Poisoning by other viral vaccines, accidental (unintentional)
- T50.B92 Poisoning by other viral vaccines, intentional self-harm
- T50.B93 Poisoning by other viral vaccines, assault
- T50.B94 Poisoning by other viral vaccines, undetermined
- T50.B95 Adverse effect of other viral vaccines
- T50.B96 Underdosing of other viral vaccines

T50.Z **Poisoning by, adverse effect of and underdosing of other vaccines and biological substances**
- T50.Z1 Poisoning by, adverse effect of and underdosing of immunoglobulin
  - T50.Z11 Poisoning by immunoglobulin, accidental (unintentional)
  - T50.Z12 Poisoning by immunoglobulin, intentional self-harm
  - T50.Z13 Poisoning by immunoglobulin, assault
  - T50.Z14 Poisoning by immunoglobulin, undetermined
  - T50.Z15 Adverse effect of immunoglobulin
  - T50.Z16 Underdosing of immunoglobulin
- T50.Z9 Poisoning by, adverse effect of and underdosing of other vaccines and biological substances
  - T50.Z91 Poisoning by other vaccines and biological substances, accidental (unintentional)
  - T50.Z92 Poisoning by other vaccines and biological substances, intentional self-harm
  - T50.Z93 Poisoning by other vaccines and biological substances, assault
  - T50.Z94 Poisoning by other vaccines and biological substances, undetermined
  - T50.Z95 Adverse effect of other vaccines and biological substances
  - T50.Z96 Underdosing of other vaccines and biological substances

T50.9 **Poisoning by, adverse effect of and underdosing of other and unspecified drugs, medicaments and biological substances**
- T50.90 Poisoning by, adverse effect of and underdosing of unspecified drugs, medicaments and biological substances
  - T50.901 Poisoning by unspecified drugs, medicaments and biological substances, accidental (unintentional)
    Coding Clinic: 2015, Q1, P21
  - T50.902 Poisoning by unspecified drugs, medicaments and biological substances, intentional self-harm
  - T50.903 Poisoning by unspecified drugs, medicaments and biological substances, assault
  - T50.904 Poisoning by unspecified drugs, medicaments and biological substances, undetermined
  - T50.905 Adverse effect of unspecified drugs, medicaments and biological substances
  - T50.906 Underdosing of unspecified drugs, medicaments and biological substances

T50.99 **Poisoning by, adverse effect of and underdosing of other drugs, medicaments and biological substances**
- T50.991 Poisoning by other drugs, medicaments and biological substances, accidental (unintentional)
- T50.992 Poisoning by other drugs, medicaments and biological substances, intentional self-harm
- T50.993 Poisoning by other drugs, medicaments and biological substances, assault
- T50.994 Poisoning by other drugs, medicaments and biological substances, undetermined
- T50.995 Adverse effect of other drugs, medicaments and biological substances
- T50.996 Underdosing of other drugs, medicaments and biological substances

TOXIC EFFECTS OF SUBSTANCES CHIEFLY NONMEDICINAL AS TO SOURCE (T51-T65)

Note: When no intent is indicated code to accidental. Undetermined intent is only for use when there is specific documentation in the record that the intent of the toxic effect cannot be determined.

Use additional code(s): for all associated manifestations of toxic effect, such as:
respiratory conditions due to external agents (J60-J70)
personal history of foreign body fully removed (Z87.821)
to identify any retained foreign body, if applicable (Z18.-)

Excludes1 contact with and (suspected) exposure to toxic substances (Z77.-)

T51 **Toxic effect of alcohol**
The appropriate 7th character is to be added to each code from category T51

A initial encounter
D subsequent encounter
S sequela

T51.0 **Toxic effect of ethanol**
Toxic effect of ethyl alcohol
Excludes2 acute alcohol intoxication or 'hangover' effects (F10.129, F10.229, F10.929)
drunkenness (F10.129, F10.229, F10.929)
pathological alcohol intoxication (F10.129, F10.229, F10.929)
- T51.0X Toxic effect of ethanol
  - T51.0X1 Toxic effect of ethanol, accidental (unintentional)
    Toxic effect of ethanol NOS
  - T51.0X2 Toxic effect of ethanol, intentional self-harm
  - T51.0X3 Toxic effect of ethanol, assault
  - T51.0X4 Toxic effect of ethanol, undetermined

T51.1 **Toxic effect of methanol**
Toxic effect of methyl alcohol
- T51.1X Toxic effect of methanol
  - T51.1X1 Toxic effect of methanol, accidental (unintentional)
    Toxic effect of methanol NOS
  - T51.1X2 Toxic effect of methanol, intentional self-harm
  - T51.1X3 Toxic effect of methanol, assault
  - T51.1X4 Toxic effect of methanol, undetermined

New | Revised | deleted Deleted | Excludes 1 | Excludes 2 | Includes | Use additional | Code first | Code also | Key words
OGCR Official Guidelines | Unacceptable Principal Diagnosis | X Assign placeholder X | Use Additional Character(s) | Manifestation Code | Coding Clinic

● **T51.2**   **Toxic effect of 2-Propanol**
Toxic effect of isopropyl alcohol

  ● **T51.2X**   **Toxic effect of 2-Propanol**

    ● **T51.2X1**   **Toxic effect of 2-Propanol, accidental (unintentional)**
Toxic effect of 2-Propanol NOS

    ● **T51.2X2**   **Toxic effect of 2-Propanol, intentional self-harm**

    ● **T51.2X3**   **Toxic effect of 2-Propanol, assault**

    ● **T51.2X4**   **Toxic effect of 2-Propanol, undetermined**

● **T51.3**   **Toxic effect of fusel oil**
Toxic effect of amyl alcohol
Toxic effect of butyl [1-butanol] alcohol
Toxic effect of propyl [1-propanol] alcohol

  ● **T51.3X**   **Toxic effect of fusel oil**

    ● **T51.3X1**   **Toxic effect of fusel oil, accidental (unintentional)**
Toxic effect of fusel oil NOS

    ● **T51.3X2**   **Toxic effect of fusel oil, intentional self-harm**

    ● **T51.3X3**   **Toxic effect of fusel oil, assault**

    ● **T51.3X4**   **Toxic effect of fusel oil, undetermined**

● **T51.8**   **Toxic effect of other alcohols**

  ● **T51.8X**   **Toxic effect of other alcohols**

    ● **T51.8X1**   **Toxic effect of other alcohols, accidental (unintentional)**
Toxic effect of other alcohols NOS

    ● **T51.8X2**   **Toxic effect of other alcohols, intentional self-harm**

    ● **T51.8X3**   **Toxic effect of other alcohols, assault**

    ● **T51.8X4**   **Toxic effect of other alcohols, undetermined**

● **T51.9**   **Toxic effect of unspecified alcohol**

  X ● **T51.91**   **Toxic effect of unspecified alcohol, accidental (unintentional)**

  X ● **T51.92**   **Toxic effect of unspecified alcohol, intentional self-harm**

  X ● **T51.93**   **Toxic effect of unspecified alcohol, assault**

  X ● **T51.94**   **Toxic effect of unspecified alcohol, undetermined**

● **T52**   **Toxic effect of organic solvents**

  Excludes1   halogen derivatives of aliphatic and aromatic hydrocarbons (T53.-)

The appropriate 7th character is to be added to each code from category T52

A	initial encounter
D	subsequent encounter
S	sequela

● **T52.0**   **Toxic effects of petroleum products**
Toxic effects of gasoline [petrol]
Toxic effects of kerosene [paraffin oil]
Toxic effects of paraffin wax
Toxic effects of ether petroleum
Toxic effects of naphtha petroleum
Toxic effects of spirit petroleum

  ● **T52.0X**   **Toxic effects of petroleum products**

    ● **T52.0X1**   **Toxic effect of petroleum products, accidental (unintentional)**
Toxic effects of petroleum products NOS

    ● **T52.0X2**   **Toxic effect of petroleum products, intentional self-harm**

    ● **T52.0X3**   **Toxic effect of petroleum products, assault**

    ● **T52.0X4**   **Toxic effect of petroleum products, undetermined**

● **T52.1**   **Toxic effects of benzene**

  Excludes1   homologues of benzene (T52.2)
nitroderivatives and aminoderivatives of benzene and its homologues (T65.3)

  ● **T52.1X**   **Toxic effects of benzene**

    ● **T52.1X1**   **Toxic effect of benzene, accidental (unintentional)**
Toxic effects of benzene NOS

    ● **T52.1X2**   **Toxic effect of benzene, intentional self-harm**

    ● **T52.1X3**   **Toxic effect of benzene, assault**

    ● **T52.1X4**   **Toxic effect of benzene, undetermined**

● **T52.2**   **Toxic effects of homologues of benzene**
Toxic effects of toluene [methylbenzene]
Toxic effects of xylene [dimethylbenzene]

  ● **T52.2X**   **Toxic effects of homologues of benzene**

    ● **T52.2X1**   **Toxic effect of homologues of benzene, accidental (unintentional)**
Toxic effects of homologues of benzene NOS

    ● **T52.2X2**   **Toxic effect of homologues of benzene, intentional self-harm**

    ● **T52.2X3**   **Toxic effect of homologues of benzene, assault**

    ● **T52.2X4**   **Toxic effect of homologues of benzene, undetermined**

● **T52.3**   **Toxic effects of glycols**

  ● **T52.3X**   **Toxic effects of glycols**

    ● **T52.3X1**   **Toxic effect of glycols, accidental (unintentional)**
Toxic effects of glycols NOS

    ● **T52.3X2**   **Toxic effect of glycols, intentional self-harm**

    ● **T52.3X3**   **Toxic effect of glycols, assault**

    ● **T52.3X4**   **Toxic effect of glycols, undetermined**

● **T52.4**   **Toxic effects of ketones**

  ● **T52.4X**   **Toxic effects of ketones**

    ● **T52.4X1**   **Toxic effect of ketones, accidental (unintentional)**
Toxic effects of ketones NOS

    ● **T52.4X2**   **Toxic effect of ketones, intentional self-harm**

    ● **T52.4X3**   **Toxic effect of ketones, assault**

    ● **T52.4X4**   **Toxic effect of ketones, undetermined**

● **T52.8**   **Toxic effects of other organic solvents**

  ● **T52.8X**   **Toxic effects of other organic solvents**

    ● **T52.8X1**   **Toxic effect of other organic solvents, accidental (unintentional)**
Toxic effects of other organic solvents NOS

    ● **T52.8X2**   **Toxic effect of other organic solvents, intentional self-harm**

    ● **T52.8X3**   **Toxic effect of other organic solvents, assault**

    ● **T52.8X4**   **Toxic effect of other organic solvents, undetermined**

● **T52.9**   **Toxic effects of unspecified organic solvent**

  X ● **T52.91**   **Toxic effect of unspecified organic solvent, accidental (unintentional)**

  X ● **T52.92**   **Toxic effect of unspecified organic solvent, intentional self-harm**

  X ● **T52.93**   **Toxic effect of unspecified organic solvent, assault**

  X ● **T52.94**   **Toxic effect of unspecified organic solvent, undetermined**

CHAPTER 19 (S00-T88)

N   Newborn Age: 0   **P**   Pediatric Age: 0–17   **M**   Maternity DX: 12–55   **A**   Adult Age: 15–124   ♀   Females Only   ♂   Males Only

🅒   Complication\Comorbidity   🅜   Major C\C   (Ex)   CC/MCC Exclusions   🅗   Hospital-Acquired Condition

1459

● **T53**   **Toxic effect of halogen derivatives of aliphatic and aromatic hydrocarbons**

The appropriate 7th character is to be added to each code from category T53

> A   initial encounter
> D   subsequent encounter
> S   sequela

● **T53.0**   **Toxic effects of carbon tetrachloride**
Toxic effects of tetrachloromethane

  ● **T53.0X**   **Toxic effects of carbon tetrachloride**

    ● **T53.0X1**   **Toxic effect of carbon tetrachloride, accidental (unintentional)**
Toxic effects of carbon tetrachloride NOS

    ● **T53.0X2**   **Toxic effect of carbon tetrachloride, intentional self-harm**

    ● **T53.0X3**   **Toxic effect of carbon tetrachloride, assault**

    ● **T53.0X4**   **Toxic effect of carbon tetrachloride, undetermined**

● **T53.1**   **Toxic effects of chloroform**
Toxic effects of trichloromethane

  ● **T53.1X**   **Toxic effects of chloroform**

    ● **T53.1X1**   **Toxic effect of chloroform, accidental (unintentional)**
Toxic effects of chloroform NOS

    ● **T53.1X2**   **Toxic effect of chloroform, intentional self-harm**

    ● **T53.1X3**   **Toxic effect of chloroform, assault**

    ● **T53.1X4**   **Toxic effect of chloroform, undetermined**

● **T53.2**   **Toxic effects of trichloroethylene**
Toxic effects of trichloroethene

  ● **T53.2X**   **Toxic effects of trichloroethylene**

    ● **T53.2X1**   **Toxic effect of trichloroethylene, accidental (unintentional)**
Toxic effects of trichloroethylene NOS

    ● **T53.2X2**   **Toxic effect of trichloroethylene, intentional self-harm**

    ● **T53.2X3**   **Toxic effect of trichloroethylene, assault**

    ● **T53.2X4**   **Toxic effect of trichloroethylene, undetermined**

● **T53.3**   **Toxic effects of tetrachloroethylene**
Toxic effects of perchloroethylene
Toxic effect of tetrachloroethene

  ● **T53.3X**   **Toxic effects of tetrachloroethylene**

    ● **T53.3X1**   **Toxic effect of tetrachloroethylene, accidental (unintentional)**
Toxic effects of tetrachloroethylene NOS

    ● **T53.3X2**   **Toxic effect of tetrachloroethylene, intentional self-harm**

    ● **T53.3X3**   **Toxic effect of tetrachloroethylene, assault**

    ● **T53.3X4**   **Toxic effect of tetrachloroethylene, undetermined**

● **T53.4**   **Toxic effects of dichloromethane**
Toxic effects of methylene chloride

  ● **T53.4X**   **Toxic effects of dichloromethane**

    ● **T53.4X1**   **Toxic effect of dichloromethane, accidental (unintentional)**
Toxic effects of dichloromethane NOS

    ● **T53.4X2**   **Toxic effect of dichloromethane, intentional self-harm**

    ● **T53.4X3**   **Toxic effect of dichloromethane, assault**

    ● **T53.4X4**   **Toxic effect of dichloromethane, undetermined**

● **T53.5**   **Toxic effects of chlorofluorocarbons**

  ● **T53.5X**   **Toxic effects of chlorofluorocarbons**

    ● **T53.5X1**   **Toxic effect of chlorofluorocarbons, accidental (unintentional)**
Toxic effects of chlorofluorocarbons NOS

    ● **T53.5X2**   **Toxic effect of chlorofluorocarbons, intentional self-harm**

    ● **T53.5X3**   **Toxic effect of chlorofluorocarbons, assault**

    ● **T53.5X4**   **Toxic effect of chlorofluorocarbons, undetermined**

● **T53.6**   **Toxic effects of other halogen derivatives of aliphatic hydrocarbons**

  ● **T53.6X**   **Toxic effects of other halogen derivatives of aliphatic hydrocarbons**

    ● **T53.6X1**   **Toxic effect of other halogen derivatives of aliphatic hydrocarbons, accidental (unintentional)**
Toxic effects of other halogen derivatives of aliphatic hydrocarbons NOS

    ● **T53.6X2**   **Toxic effect of other halogen derivatives of aliphatic hydrocarbons, intentional self-harm**

    ● **T53.6X3**   **Toxic effect of other halogen derivatives of aliphatic hydrocarbons, assault**

    ● **T53.6X4**   **Toxic effect of other halogen derivatives of aliphatic hydrocarbons, undetermined**

● **T53.7**   **Toxic effects of other halogen derivatives of aromatic hydrocarbons**

  ● **T53.7X**   **Toxic effects of other halogen derivatives of aromatic hydrocarbons**

    ● **T53.7X1**   **Toxic effect of other halogen derivatives of aromatic hydrocarbons, accidental (unintentional)**
Toxic effects of other halogen derivatives of aromatic hydrocarbons NOS

    ● **T53.7X2**   **Toxic effect of other halogen derivatives of aromatic hydrocarbons, intentional self-harm**

    ● **T53.7X3**   **Toxic effect of other halogen derivatives of aromatic hydrocarbons, assault**

    ● **T53.7X4**   **Toxic effect of other halogen derivatives of aromatic hydrocarbons, undetermined**

▶ New   ⇒ Revised   ~~deleted~~ Deleted | Excludes 1 | | Excludes 2 | | Includes | | Use additional | | Code first | | Code also | | Key words |
OGCR Official Guidelines   ● Unacceptable Principal Diagnosis   X Assign placeholder X   ● Use Additional Character(s)   ▶ Manifestation Code   **Coding Clinic**

● **T53.9** Toxic effects of unspecified halogen derivatives of aliphatic and aromatic hydrocarbons

   X ● **T53.91** Toxic effect of unspecified halogen derivatives of aliphatic and aromatic hydrocarbons, accidental (unintentional)

   X ● **T53.92** Toxic effect of unspecified halogen derivatives of aliphatic and aromatic hydrocarbons, intentional self-harm

   X ● **T53.93** Toxic effect of unspecified halogen derivatives of aliphatic and aromatic hydrocarbons, assault

   X ● **T53.94** Toxic effect of unspecified halogen derivatives of aliphatic and aromatic hydrocarbons, undetermined

● **T54** Toxic effect of corrosive substances

The appropriate 7th character is to be added to each code from category T54

> A   initial encounter
> D   subsequent encounter
> S   sequela

● **T54.0** Toxic effects of phenol and phenol homologues

   ● **T54.0X** Toxic effects of phenol and phenol homologues

     ● **T54.0X1** Toxic effect of phenol and phenol homologues, accidental (unintentional)
Toxic effects of phenol and phenol homologues NOS

     ● **T54.0X2** Toxic effect of phenol and phenol homologues, intentional self-harm

     ● **T54.0X3** Toxic effect of phenol and phenol homologues, assault

     ● **T54.0X4** Toxic effect of phenol and phenol homologues, undetermined

● **T54.1** Toxic effects of other corrosive organic compounds

   ● **T54.1X** Toxic effects of other corrosive organic compounds

     ● **T54.1X1** Toxic effect of other corrosive organic compounds, accidental (unintentional)
Toxic effects of other corrosive organic compounds NOS

     ● **T54.1X2** Toxic effect of other corrosive organic compounds, intentional self-harm

     ● **T54.1X3** Toxic effect of other corrosive organic compounds, assault

     ● **T54.1X4** Toxic effect of other corrosive organic compounds, undetermined

● **T54.2** Toxic effects of corrosive acids and acid-like substances
Toxic effects of hydrochloric acid
Toxic effects of sulfuric acid

   ● **T54.2X** Toxic effects of corrosive acids and acid-like substances

     ● **T54.2X1** Toxic effect of corrosive acids and acid-like substances, accidental (unintentional)
Toxic effects of corrosive acids and acid-like substances NOS

     ● **T54.2X2** Toxic effect of corrosive acids and acid-like substances, intentional self-harm

     ● **T54.2X3** Toxic effect of corrosive acids and acid-like substances, assault

     ● **T54.2X4** Toxic effect of corrosive acids and acid-like substances, undetermined

● **T54.3** Toxic effects of corrosive alkalis and alkali-like substances
Toxic effects of potassium hydroxide
Toxic effects of sodium hydroxide

   ● **T54.3X** Toxic effects of corrosive alkalis and alkali-like substances

     ● **T54.3X1** Toxic effect of corrosive alkalis and alkali-like substances, accidental (unintentional)
Toxic effects of corrosive alkalis and alkali-like substances NOS

     ● **T54.3X2** Toxic effect of corrosive alkalis and alkali-like substances, intentional self-harm

     ● **T54.3X3** Toxic effect of corrosive alkalis and alkali-like substances, assault

     ● **T54.3X4** Toxic effect of corrosive alkalis and alkali-like substances, undetermined

● **T54.9** Toxic effects of unspecified corrosive substance

   X ● **T54.91** Toxic effect of unspecified corrosive substance, accidental (unintentional)

   X ● **T54.92** Toxic effect of unspecified corrosive substance, intentional self-harm

   X ● **T54.93** Toxic effect of unspecified corrosive substance, assault

   X ● **T54.94** Toxic effect of unspecified corrosive substance, undetermined

● **T55** Toxic effect of soaps and detergents

The appropriate 7th character is to be added to each code from category T55

> A   initial encounter
> D   subsequent encounter
> S   sequela

● **T55.0** Toxic effect of soaps

   ● **T55.0X** Toxic effect of soaps

     ● **T55.0X1** Toxic effect of soaps, accidental (unintentional)
Toxic effect of soaps NOS

     ● **T55.0X2** Toxic effect of soaps, intentional self-harm

     ● **T55.0X3** Toxic effect of soaps, assault

     ● **T55.0X4** Toxic effect of soaps, undetermined

● **T55.1** Toxic effect of detergents

   ● **T55.1X** Toxic effect of detergents

     ● **T55.1X1** Toxic effect of detergents, accidental (unintentional)
Toxic effect of detergents NOS

     ● **T55.1X2** Toxic effect of detergents, intentional self-harm

     ● **T55.1X3** Toxic effect of detergents, assault

     ● **T55.1X4** Toxic effect of detergents, undetermined

CHAPTER 19 (S00-T88)

● **T56** **Toxic effect of metals**

Includes   toxic effects of fumes and vapors of metals
toxic effects of metals from all sources, except medicinal substances

Use additional code to identify any retained metal foreign body, if applicable (Z18.0-, T18.1-)

Excludes1   arsenic and its compounds (T57.0)
manganese and its compounds (T57.2)

The appropriate 7th character is to be added to each code from category T56

A	initial encounter
D	subsequent encounter
S	sequela

● **T56.0**   Toxic effects of lead and its compounds
   ● **T56.0X** Toxic effects of lead and its compounds
      ● **T56.0X1** **Toxic effect of lead and its compounds, accidental (unintentional)**
           Toxic effects of lead and its compounds NOS
      ● **T56.0X2** **Toxic effect of lead and its compounds, intentional self-harm**
      ● **T56.0X3** **Toxic effect of lead and its compounds, assault**
      ● **T56.0X4** **Toxic effect of lead and its compounds, undetermined**

● **T56.1**   Toxic effects of mercury and its compounds
   ● **T56.1X** Toxic effects of mercury and its compounds
      ● **T56.1X1** **Toxic effect of mercury and its compounds, accidental (unintentional)**
           Toxic effects of mercury and its compounds NOS
      ● **T56.1X2** **Toxic effect of mercury and its compounds, intentional self-harm**
      ● **T56.1X3** **Toxic effect of mercury and its compounds, assault**
      ● **T56.1X4** **Toxic effect of mercury and its compounds, undetermined**

● **T56.2**   Toxic effects of chromium and its compounds
   ● **T56.2X** Toxic effects of chromium and its compounds
      ● **T56.2X1** **Toxic effect of chromium and its compounds, accidental (unintentional)**
           Toxic effects of chromium and its compounds NOS
      ● **T56.2X2** **Toxic effect of chromium and its compounds, intentional self-harm**
      ● **T56.2X3** **Toxic effect of chromium and its compounds, assault**
      ● **T56.2X4** **Toxic effect of chromium and its compounds, undetermined**

● **T56.3**   Toxic effects of cadmium and its compounds
   ● **T56.3X** Toxic effects of cadmium and its compounds
      ● **T56.3X1** **Toxic effect of cadmium and its compounds, accidental (unintentional)**
           Toxic effects of cadmium and its compounds NOS
      ● **T56.3X2** **Toxic effect of cadmium and its compounds, intentional self-harm**
      ● **T56.3X3** **Toxic effect of cadmium and its compounds, assault**
      ● **T56.3X4** **Toxic effect of cadmium and its compounds, undetermined**

● **T56.4**   Toxic effects of copper and its compounds
   ● **T56.4X** Toxic effects of copper and its compounds
      ● **T56.4X1** **Toxic effect of copper and its compounds, accidental (unintentional)**
           Toxic effects of copper and its compounds NOS
      ● **T56.4X2** **Toxic effect of copper and its compounds, intentional self-harm**
      ● **T56.4X3** **Toxic effect of copper and its compounds, assault**
      ● **T56.4X4** **Toxic effect of copper and its compounds, undetermined**

● **T56.5**   Toxic effects of zinc and its compounds
   ● **T56.5X** Toxic effects of zinc and its compounds
      ● **T56.5X1** **Toxic effect of zinc and its compounds, accidental (unintentional)**
           Toxic effects of zinc and its compounds NOS
      ● **T56.5X2** **Toxic effect of zinc and its compounds, intentional self-harm**
      ● **T56.5X3** **Toxic effect of zinc and its compounds, assault**
      ● **T56.5X4** **Toxic effect of zinc and its compounds, undetermined**

● **T56.6**   Toxic effects of tin and its compounds
   ● **T56.6X** Toxic effects of tin and its compounds
      ● **T56.6X1** **Toxic effect of tin and its compounds, accidental (unintentional)**
           Toxic effects of tin and its compounds NOS
      ● **T56.6X2** **Toxic effect of tin and its compounds, intentional self-harm**
      ● **T56.6X3** **Toxic effect of tin and its compounds, assault**
      ● **T56.6X4** **Toxic effect of tin and its compounds, undetermined**

● **T56.7**   Toxic effects of beryllium and its compounds
   ● **T56.7X** Toxic effects of beryllium and its compounds
      ● **T56.7X1** **Toxic effect of beryllium and its compounds, accidental (unintentional)**
           Toxic effects of beryllium and its compounds NOS
      ● **T56.7X2** **Toxic effect of beryllium and its compounds, intentional self-harm**
      ● **T56.7X3** **Toxic effect of beryllium and its compounds, assault**
      ● **T56.7X4** **Toxic effect of beryllium and its compounds, undetermined**

● **T56.8**   Toxic effects of other metals
   ● **T56.81** Toxic effect of thallium
      ● **T56.811** **Toxic effect of thallium, accidental (unintentional)**
           Toxic effect of thallium NOS
      ● **T56.812** **Toxic effect of thallium, intentional self-harm**
      ● **T56.813** **Toxic effect of thallium, assault**
      ● **T56.814** **Toxic effect of thallium, undetermined**
   ● **T56.89** Toxic effects of other metals
      ● **T56.891** **Toxic effect of other metals, accidental (unintentional)**
           Toxic effects of other metals NOS
      ● **T56.892** **Toxic effect of other metals, intentional self-harm**
      ● **T56.893** **Toxic effect of other metals, assault**
      ● **T56.894** **Toxic effect of other metals, undetermined**

▶ New   ⇒ Revised   ~~deleted~~ Deleted   Excludes 1   Excludes 2   Includes   Use additional   Code first   Code also   Key words

OGCR Official Guidelines   ● Unacceptable Principal Diagnosis   X Assign placeholder X   ● Use Additional Character(s)   ▶ Manifestation Code   **Coding Clinic**

● **T56.9**　Toxic effects of unspecified metal
　　X● **T56.91**　Toxic effect of unspecified metal, accidental (unintentional)
　　X● **T56.92**　Toxic effect of unspecified metal, intentional self-harm
　　X● **T56.93**　Toxic effect of unspecified metal, assault
　　X● **T56.94**　Toxic effect of unspecified metal, undetermined

● **T57**　Toxic effect of other inorganic substances
　　The appropriate 7th character is to be added to each code from category T57

> | A | initial encounter |
> | D | subsequent encounter |
> | S | sequela |

　● **T57.0**　Toxic effect of arsenic and its compounds
　　● **T57.0X**　Toxic effect of arsenic and its compounds
　　　● **T57.0X1**　Toxic effect of arsenic and its compounds, accidental (unintentional)
　　　　　　Toxic effect of arsenic and its compounds NOS
　　　● **T57.0X2**　Toxic effect of arsenic and its compounds, intentional self-harm
　　　● **T57.0X3**　Toxic effect of arsenic and its compounds, assault
　　　● **T57.0X4**　Toxic effect of arsenic and its compounds, undetermined

　● **T57.1**　Toxic effect of phosphorus and its compounds
　　　Excludes1　organophosphate insecticides (T60.0)
　　● **T57.1X**　Toxic effect of phosphorus and its compounds
　　　● **T57.1X1**　Toxic effect of phosphorus and its compounds, accidental (unintentional)
　　　　　　Toxic effect of phosphorus and its compounds NOS
　　　● **T57.1X2**　Toxic effect of phosphorus and its compounds, intentional self-harm
　　　● **T57.1X3**　Toxic effect of phosphorus and its compounds, assault
　　　● **T57.1X4**　Toxic effect of phosphorus and its compounds, undetermined

　● **T57.2**　Toxic effect of manganese and its compounds
　　● **T57.2X**　Toxic effect of manganese and its compounds
　　　● **T57.2X1**　Toxic effect of manganese and its compounds, accidental (unintentional)
　　　　　　Toxic effect of manganese and its compounds NOS
　　　● **T57.2X2**　Toxic effect of manganese and its compounds, intentional self-harm
　　　● **T57.2X3**　Toxic effect of manganese and its compounds, assault
　　　● **T57.2X4**　Toxic effect of manganese and its compounds, undetermined

　● **T57.3**　Toxic effect of hydrogen cyanide
　　● **T57.3X**　Toxic effect of hydrogen cyanide
　　　● **T57.3X1**　Toxic effect of hydrogen cyanide, accidental (unintentional)
　　　　　　Toxic effect of hydrogen cyanide NOS
　　　● **T57.3X2**　Toxic effect of hydrogen cyanide, intentional self-harm
　　　● **T57.3X3**　Toxic effect of hydrogen cyanide, assault
　　　● **T57.3X4**　Toxic effect of hydrogen cyanide, undetermined

● **T57.8**　Toxic effect of other specified inorganic substances
　　● **T57.8X**　Toxic effect of other specified inorganic substances
　　　● **T57.8X1**　Toxic effect of other specified inorganic substances, accidental (unintentional)
　　　　　　Toxic effect of other specified inorganic substances NOS
　　　● **T57.8X2**　Toxic effect of other specified inorganic substances, intentional self-harm
　　　● **T57.8X3**　Toxic effect of other specified inorganic substances, assault
　　　● **T57.8X4**　Toxic effect of other specified inorganic substances, undetermined

　● **T57.9**　Toxic effect of unspecified inorganic substance
　　X● **T57.91**　Toxic effect of unspecified inorganic substance, accidental (unintentional)
　　X● **T57.92**　Toxic effect of unspecified inorganic substance, intentional self-harm
　　X● **T57.93**　Toxic effect of unspecified inorganic substance, assault
　　X● **T57.94**　Toxic effect of unspecified inorganic substance, undetermined

● **T58**　Toxic effect of carbon monoxide
　　Includes　asphyxiation from carbon monoxide
　　　　　　toxic effect of carbon monoxide from all sources
　　The appropriate 7th character is to be added to each code from category T58

> | A | initial encounter |
> | D | subsequent encounter |
> | S | sequela |

　● **T58.0**　Toxic effect of carbon monoxide from motor vehicle exhaust
　　　Toxic effect of exhaust gas from gas engine
　　　Toxic effect of exhaust gas from motor pump
　　X● **T58.01**　Toxic effect of carbon monoxide from motor vehicle exhaust, accidental (unintentional)
　　X● **T58.02**　Toxic effect of carbon monoxide from motor vehicle exhaust, intentional self-harm
　　X● **T58.03**　Toxic effect of carbon monoxide from motor vehicle exhaust, assault
　　X● **T58.04**　Toxic effect of carbon monoxide from motor vehicle exhaust, undetermined

　● **T58.1**　Toxic effect of carbon monoxide from utility gas
　　　Toxic effect of acetylene
　　　Toxic effect of gas NOS used for lighting, heating, cooking
　　　Toxic effect of water gas
　　X● **T58.11**　Toxic effect of carbon monoxide from utility gas, accidental (unintentional)
　　X● **T58.12**　Toxic effect of carbon monoxide from utility gas, intentional self-harm
　　X● **T58.13**　Toxic effect of carbon monoxide from utility gas, assault
　　X● **T58.14**　Toxic effect of carbon monoxide from utility gas, undetermined

CHAPTER 19 (S00-T88)

● **T58.2** **Toxic effect of carbon monoxide from incomplete combustion of other domestic fuels**
Toxic effect of carbon monoxide from incomplete combustion of coal, coke, kerosene, wood

  ● **T58.2X** **Toxic effect of carbon monoxide from incomplete combustion of other domestic fuels**

    ● **T58.2X1** Toxic effect of carbon monoxide from incomplete combustion of other domestic fuels, **accidental (unintentional)**

    ● **T58.2X2** Toxic effect of carbon monoxide from incomplete combustion of other domestic fuels, **intentional self-harm**

    ● **T58.2X3** Toxic effect of carbon monoxide from incomplete combustion of other domestic fuels, **assault**

    ● **T58.2X4** Toxic effect of carbon monoxide from incomplete combustion of other domestic fuels, **undetermined**

● **T58.8** **Toxic effect of carbon monoxide from other source**
Toxic effect of carbon monoxide from blast furnace gas
Toxic effect of carbon monoxide from fuels in industrial use
Toxic effect of carbon monoxide from kiln vapor

  ● **T58.8X** **Toxic effect of carbon monoxide from other source**

    ● **T58.8X1** Toxic effect of carbon monoxide from other source, **accidental (unintentional)**

    ● **T58.8X2** Toxic effect of carbon monoxide from other source, **intentional self-harm**

    ● **T58.8X3** Toxic effect of carbon monoxide from other source, **assault**

    ● **T58.8X4** Toxic effect of carbon monoxide from other source, **undetermined**

● **T58.9** **Toxic effect of carbon monoxide from unspecified source**

  X ● **T58.91** Toxic effect of carbon monoxide from unspecified source, **accidental (unintentional)**

  X ● **T58.92** Toxic effect of carbon monoxide from unspecified source, **intentional self-harm**

  X ● **T58.93** Toxic effect of carbon monoxide from unspecified source, **assault**

  X ● **T58.94** Toxic effect of carbon monoxide from unspecified source, **undetermined**

● **T59** **Toxic effect of other gases, fumes and vapors**

Includes	aerosol propellants
Excludes1	chlorofluorocarbons (T53.5)

The appropriate 7th character is to be added to each code from category T59

> A   initial encounter
> D   subsequent encounter
> S   sequela

● **T59.0** **Toxic effect of nitrogen oxides**

  ● **T59.0X** **Toxic effect of nitrogen oxides**

    ● **T59.0X1** Toxic effect of nitrogen oxides, **accidental (unintentional)**
Toxic effect of nitrogen oxides NOS

    ● **T59.0X2** Toxic effect of nitrogen oxides, **intentional self-harm**

    ● **T59.0X3** Toxic effect of nitrogen oxides, **assault**

    ● **T59.0X4** Toxic effect of nitrogen oxides, **undetermined**

● **T59.1** **Toxic effect of sulfur dioxide**

  ● **T59.1X** **Toxic effect of sulfur dioxide**

    ● **T59.1X1** Toxic effect of sulfur dioxide, **accidental (unintentional)**
Toxic effect of sulfur dioxide NOS

    ● **T59.1X2** Toxic effect of sulfur dioxide, **intentional self-harm**

    ● **T59.1X3** Toxic effect of sulfur dioxide, **assault**

    ● **T59.1X4** Toxic effect of sulfur dioxide, **undetermined**

● **T59.2** **Toxic effect of formaldehyde**

  ● **T59.2X** **Toxic effect of formaldehyde**

    ● **T59.2X1** Toxic effect of formaldehyde, **accidental (unintentional)**
Toxic effect of formaldehyde NOS

    ● **T59.2X2** Toxic effect of formaldehyde, **intentional self-harm**

    ● **T59.2X3** Toxic effect of formaldehyde, **assault**

    ● **T59.2X4** Toxic effect of formaldehyde, **undetermined**

● **T59.3** **Toxic effect of lacrimogenic gas**
Toxic effect of tear gas

  ● **T59.3X** **Toxic effect of lacrimogenic gas**

    ● **T59.3X1** Toxic effect of lacrimogenic gas, **accidental (unintentional)**
Toxic effect of lacrimogenic gas NOS

    ● **T59.3X2** Toxic effect of lacrimogenic gas, **intentional self-harm**

    ● **T59.3X3** Toxic effect of lacrimogenic gas, **assault**

    ● **T59.3X4** Toxic effect of lacrimogenic gas, **undetermined**

● **T59.4** **Toxic effect of chlorine gas**

  ● **T59.4X** **Toxic effect of chlorine gas**

    ● **T59.4X1** Toxic effect of chlorine gas, **accidental (unintentional)**
Toxic effect of chlorine gas NOS

    ● **T59.4X2** Toxic effect of chlorine gas, **intentional self-harm**

    ● **T59.4X3** Toxic effect of chlorine gas, **assault**

    ● **T59.4X4** Toxic effect of chlorine gas, **undetermined**

● **T59.5** **Toxic effect of fluorine gas and hydrogen fluoride**

  ● **T59.5X** **Toxic effect of fluorine gas and hydrogen fluoride**

    ● **T59.5X1** Toxic effect of fluorine gas and hydrogen fluoride, **accidental (unintentional)**
Toxic effect of fluorine gas and hydrogen fluoride NOS

    ● **T59.5X2** Toxic effect of fluorine gas and hydrogen fluoride, **intentional self-harm**

    ● **T59.5X3** Toxic effect of fluorine gas and hydrogen fluoride, **assault**

    ● **T59.5X4** Toxic effect of fluorine gas and hydrogen fluoride, **undetermined**

● **T59.6** **Toxic effect of hydrogen sulfide**

  ● **T59.6X** **Toxic effect of hydrogen sulfide**

    ● **T59.6X1** Toxic effect of hydrogen sulfide, **accidental (unintentional)**
Toxic effect of hydrogen sulfide NOS

    ● **T59.6X2** Toxic effect of hydrogen sulfide, **intentional self-harm**

    ● **T59.6X3** Toxic effect of hydrogen sulfide, **assault**

    ● **T59.6X4** Toxic effect of hydrogen sulfide, **undetermined**

▶ New   ⇒ Revised   ~~deleted~~ Deleted   Excludes 1   Excludes 2   Includes   Use additional   Code first   Code also   Key words
OGCR Official Guidelines   ● Unacceptable Principal Diagnosis   X Assign placeholder X   ● Use Additional Character(s)   ▷ Manifestation Code   **Coding Clinic**

● **T59.7**   Toxic effect of carbon dioxide
  ● **T59.7X**   Toxic effect of carbon dioxide
    ● **T59.7X1**   Toxic effect of carbon dioxide, accidental (unintentional)
           Toxic effect of carbon dioxide NOS
    ● **T59.7X2**   Toxic effect of carbon dioxide, intentional self-harm
    ● **T59.7X3**   Toxic effect of carbon dioxide, assault
    ● **T59.7X4**   Toxic effect of carbon dioxide, undetermined
● **T59.8**   Toxic effect of other specified gases, fumes and vapors
  ● **T59.81**   Toxic effect of smoke
           Smoke inhalation
         Excludes2   toxic effect of cigarette (tobacco) smoke (T65.22-)
    ● **T59.811**   Toxic effect of smoke, accidental (unintentional)
           Toxic effect of smoke NOS
    ● **T59.812**   Toxic effect of smoke, intentional self-harm
    ● **T59.813**   Toxic effect of smoke, assault
    ● **T59.814**   Toxic effect of smoke, undetermined
  ● **T59.89**   Toxic effect of other specified gases, fumes and vapors
    ● **T59.891**   Toxic effect of other specified gases, fumes and vapors, accidental (unintentional)
    ● **T59.892**   Toxic effect of other specified gases, fumes and vapors, intentional self-harm
    ● **T59.893**   Toxic effect of other specified gases, fumes and vapors, assault
    ● **T59.894**   Toxic effect of other specified gases, fumes and vapors, undetermined
● **T59.9**   Toxic effect of unspecified gases, fumes and vapors
  X ● **T59.91**   Toxic effect of unspecified gases, fumes and vapors, accidental (unintentional)
  X ● **T59.92**   Toxic effect of unspecified gases, fumes and vapors, intentional self-harm
  X ● **T59.93**   Toxic effect of unspecified gases, fumes and vapors, assault
  X ● **T59.94**   Toxic effect of unspecified gases, fumes and vapors, undetermined

● **T60**   Toxic effect of pesticides
         Includes   toxic effect of wood preservatives
         The appropriate 7th character is to be added to each code from category T60

A	initial encounter
D	subsequent encounter
S	sequela

  ● **T60.0**   Toxic effect of organophosphate and carbamate insecticides
    ● **T60.0X**   Toxic effect of organophosphate and carbamate insecticides
      ● **T60.0X1**   Toxic effect of organophosphate and carbamate insecticides, accidental (unintentional)
             Toxic effect of organophosphate and carbamate insecticides NOS
      ● **T60.0X2**   Toxic effect of organophosphate and carbamate insecticides, intentional self-harm
      ● **T60.0X3**   Toxic effect of organophosphate and carbamate insecticides, assault
      ● **T60.0X4**   Toxic effect of organophosphate and carbamate insecticides, undetermined

● **T60.1**   Toxic effect of halogenated insecticides
       Excludes1   chlorinated hydrocarbon (T53.-)
  ● **T60.1X**   Toxic effect of halogenated insecticides
    ● **T60.1X1**   Toxic effect of halogenated insecticides, accidental (unintentional)
           Toxic effect of halogenated insecticides NOS
    ● **T60.1X2**   Toxic effect of halogenated insecticides, intentional self-harm
    ● **T60.1X3**   Toxic effect of halogenated insecticides, assault
    ● **T60.1X4**   Toxic effect of halogenated insecticides, undetermined
● **T60.2**   Toxic effect of other insecticides
  ● **T60.2X**   Toxic effect of other insecticides
    ● **T60.2X1**   Toxic effect of other insecticides, accidental (unintentional)
           Toxic effect of other insecticides NOS
    ● **T60.2X2**   Toxic effect of other insecticides, intentional self-harm
    ● **T60.2X3**   Toxic effect of other insecticides, assault
    ● **T60.2X4**   Toxic effect of other insecticides, undetermined
● **T60.3**   Toxic effect of herbicides and fungicides
  ● **T60.3X**   Toxic effect of herbicides and fungicides
    ● **T60.3X1**   Toxic effect of herbicides and fungicides, accidental (unintentional)
           Toxic effect of herbicides and fungicides NOS
    ● **T60.3X2**   Toxic effect of herbicides and fungicides, intentional self-harm
    ● **T60.3X3**   Toxic effect of herbicides and fungicides, assault
    ● **T60.3X4**   Toxic effect of herbicides and fungicides, undetermined
● **T60.4**   Toxic effect of rodenticides
       Excludes1   strychnine and its salts (T65.1)
                  thallium (T56.81-)
  ● **T60.4X**   Toxic effect of rodenticides
    ● **T60.4X1**   Toxic effect of rodenticides, accidental (unintentional)
           Toxic effect of rodenticides NOS
    ● **T60.4X2**   Toxic effect of rodenticides, intentional self-harm
    ● **T60.4X3**   Toxic effect of rodenticides, assault
    ● **T60.4X4**   Toxic effect of rodenticides, undetermined
● **T60.8**   Toxic effect of other pesticides
  ● **T60.8X**   Toxic effect of other pesticides
    ● **T60.8X1**   Toxic effect of other pesticides, accidental (unintentional)
           Toxic effect of other pesticides NOS
    ● **T60.8X2**   Toxic effect of other pesticides, intentional self-harm
    ● **T60.8X3**   Toxic effect of other pesticides, assault
    ● **T60.8X4**   Toxic effect of other pesticides, undetermined
● **T60.9**   Toxic effect of unspecified pesticide
  X ● **T60.91**   Toxic effect of unspecified pesticide, accidental (unintentional)
  X ● **T60.92**   Toxic effect of unspecified pesticide, intentional self-harm
  X ● **T60.93**   Toxic effect of unspecified pesticide, assault
  X ● **T60.94**   Toxic effect of unspecified pesticide, undetermined

CHAPTER 19 (S00-T88)

● **T61   Toxic effect of noxious substances eaten as seafood**

Excludes1   allergic reaction to food, such as:
    anaphylactic reaction or shock due to adverse
        food reaction (T78.0-)
    bacterial foodborne intoxications (A05.-)
    dermatitis (L23.6, L25.4, L27.2)
    food protein-induced enterocolitis syndrome
        (K52.21)
    food protein-induced enteropathy (K52.22)
    gastroenteritis (noninfective) (K52.29)
    toxic effect of aflatoxin and other mycotoxins
        (T64)
    toxic effect of cyanides (T65.0-)
    toxic effect of harmful algae bloom (T65.82-)
    toxic effect of hydrogen cyanide (T57.3-)
    toxic effect of mercury (T56.1-)
    toxic effect of red tide (T65.82-)

The appropriate 7th character is to be added to each code from
    category T61

A	initial encounter
D	subsequent encounter
S	sequela

● **T61.0   Ciguatera fish poisoning**

X● **T61.01   Ciguatera fish poisoning, accidental
(unintentional)**

X● **T61.02   Ciguatera fish poisoning, intentional self-harm**

X● **T61.03   Ciguatera fish poisoning, assault**

X● **T61.04   Ciguatera fish poisoning, undetermined**

● **T61.1   Scombroid fish poisoning**
Histamine-like syndrome

X● **T61.11   Scombroid fish poisoning, accidental
(unintentional)**

X● **T61.12   Scombroid fish poisoning, intentional
self-harm**

X● **T61.13   Scombroid fish poisoning, assault**

X● **T61.14   Scombroid fish poisoning, undetermined**

● **T61.7   Other fish and shellfish poisoning**

● **T61.77   Other fish poisoning**

● **T61.771   Other fish poisoning, accidental
(unintentional)**

● **T61.772   Other fish poisoning, intentional
self-harm**

● **T61.773   Other fish poisoning, assault**

● **T61.774   Other fish poisoning, undetermined**

● **T61.78   Other shellfish poisoning**

● **T61.781   Other shellfish poisoning, accidental
(unintentional)**

● **T61.782   Other shellfish poisoning, intentional
self-harm**

● **T61.783   Other shellfish poisoning, assault**

● **T61.784   Other shellfish poisoning,
undetermined**

● **T61.8   Toxic effect of other seafood**

● **T61.8X   Toxic effect of other seafood**

● **T61.8X1   Toxic effect of other seafood,
accidental (unintentional)**

● **T61.8X2   Toxic effect of other seafood,
intentional self-harm**

● **T61.8X3   Toxic effect of other seafood, assault**

● **T61.8X4   Toxic effect of other seafood,
undetermined**

● **T61.9   Toxic effect of unspecified seafood**

X● **T61.91   Toxic effect of unspecified seafood, accidental
(unintentional)**

X● **T61.92   Toxic effect of unspecified seafood, intentional
self-harm**

X● **T61.93   Toxic effect of unspecified seafood, assault**

X● **T61.94   Toxic effect of unspecified seafood,
undetermined**

● **T62   Toxic effect of other noxious substances eaten as food**

Excludes1   allergic reaction to food, such as:
    anaphylactic shock (reaction) due to adverse
        food reaction (T78.0-)
    dermatitis (L23.6, L25.4, L27.2)
    food protein-induced enterocolitis syndrome
        (K52.21)
    food protein-induced enteropathy (K52.22)
    gastroenteritis (noninfective) (K52.29)
    bacterial food borne intoxications (A05.-)
toxic effect of aflatoxin and other mycotoxins
    (T64)
toxic effect of cyanides (T65.0-)
toxic effect of hydrogen cyanide (T57.3-)
toxic effect of mercury (T56.1-)

The appropriate 7th character is to be added to each code from
    category T62

A	initial encounter
D	subsequent encounter
S	sequela

● **T62.0   Toxic effect of ingested mushrooms**

● **T62.0X   Toxic effect of ingested mushrooms**

● **T62.0X1   Toxic effect of ingested mushrooms,
accidental (unintentional)**
Toxic effect of ingested mushrooms
NOS

● **T62.0X2   Toxic effect of ingested mushrooms,
intentional self-harm**

● **T62.0X3   Toxic effect of ingested mushrooms,
assault**

● **T62.0X4   Toxic effect of ingested mushrooms,
undetermined**

● **T62.1   Toxic effect of ingested berries**

● **T62.1X   Toxic effect of ingested berries**

● **T62.1X1   Toxic effect of ingested berries,
accidental (unintentional)**
Toxic effect of ingested berries NOS

● **T62.1X2   Toxic effect of ingested berries,
intentional self-harm**

● **T62.1X3   Toxic effect of ingested berries,
assault**

● **T62.1X4   Toxic effect of ingested berries,
undetermined**

● **T62.2   Toxic effect of other ingested (parts of) plant(s)**

● **T62.2X   Toxic effect of other ingested (parts of) plant(s)**

● **T62.2X1   Toxic effect of other ingested (parts
of) plant(s), accidental (unintentional)**
Toxic effect of other ingested (parts
of) plant(s) NOS

● **T62.2X2   Toxic effect of other ingested (parts
of) plant(s), intentional self-harm**

● **T62.2X3   Toxic effect of other ingested (parts
of) plant(s), assault**

● **T62.2X4   Toxic effect of other ingested (parts
of) plant(s), undetermined**

▶ New   ⇒ Revised   ~~deleted~~ Deleted   Excludes 1   Excludes 2   Includes   Use additional   Code first   Code also   Key words

OGCR Official Guidelines   ● Unacceptable Principal Diagnosis   X Assign placeholder X   ● Use Additional Character(s)   ▶ Manifestation Code   **Coding Clinic**

● **T62.8** Toxic effect of other specified noxious substances eaten as food

● **T62.8X** Toxic effect of other specified noxious substances eaten as food

● **T62.8X1** Toxic effect of other specified noxious substances eaten as food, accidental (unintentional)
Toxic effect of other specified noxious substances eaten as food NOS

● **T62.8X2** Toxic effect of other specified noxious substances eaten as food, intentional self-harm

● **T62.8X3** Toxic effect of other specified noxious substances eaten as food, assault

● **T62.8X4** Toxic effect of other specified noxious substances eaten as food, undetermined

● **T62.9** Toxic effect of unspecified noxious substance eaten as food

X ● **T62.91** Toxic effect of unspecified noxious substance eaten as food, accidental (unintentional)
Toxic effect of unspecified noxious substance eaten as food NOS

X ● **T62.92** Toxic effect of unspecified noxious substance eaten as food, intentional self-harm

X ● **T62.93** Toxic effect of unspecified noxious substance eaten as food, assault

X ● **T62.94** Toxic effect of unspecified noxious substance eaten as food, undetermined

● **T63** Toxic effect of contact with venomous animals and plants

Includes bite or touch of venomous animal
pricked or stuck by thorn or leaf

Excludes2 ingestion of toxic animal or plant (T61.-, T62.-)

The appropriate 7th character is to be added to each code from category T63

A	initial encounter
D	subsequent encounter
S	sequela

● **T63.0** Toxic effect of snake venom

● **T63.00** Toxic effect of unspecified snake venom

● **T63.001** Toxic effect of unspecified snake venom, accidental (unintentional)
Toxic effect of unspecified snake venom NOS

● **T63.002** Toxic effect of unspecified snake venom, intentional self-harm

● **T63.003** Toxic effect of unspecified snake venom, assault

● **T63.004** Toxic effect of unspecified snake venom, undetermined

● **T63.01** Toxic effect of rattlesnake venom

● **T63.011** Toxic effect of rattlesnake venom, accidental (unintentional)
Toxic effect of rattlesnake venom NOS

● **T63.012** Toxic effect of rattlesnake venom, intentional self-harm

● **T63.013** Toxic effect of rattlesnake venom, assault

● **T63.014** Toxic effect of rattlesnake venom, undetermined

● **T63.02** Toxic effect of coral snake venom

● **T63.021** Toxic effect of coral snake venom, accidental (unintentional)
Toxic effect of coral snake venom NOS

● **T63.022** Toxic effect of coral snake venom, intentional self-harm

● **T63.023** Toxic effect of coral snake venom, assault

● **T63.024** Toxic effect of coral snake venom, undetermined

● **T63.03** Toxic effect of taipan venom

● **T63.031** Toxic effect of taipan venom, accidental (unintentional)
Toxic effect of taipan venom NOS

● **T63.032** Toxic effect of taipan venom, intentional self-harm

● **T63.033** Toxic effect of taipan venom, assault

● **T63.034** Toxic effect of taipan venom, undetermined

● **T63.04** Toxic effect of cobra venom

● **T63.041** Toxic effect of cobra venom, accidental (unintentional)
Toxic effect of cobra venom NOS

● **T63.042** Toxic effect of cobra venom, intentional self-harm

● **T63.043** Toxic effect of cobra venom, assault

● **T63.044** Toxic effect of cobra venom, undetermined

● **T63.06** Toxic effect of venom of other North and South American snake

● **T63.061** Toxic effect of venom of other North and South American snake, accidental (unintentional)
Toxic effect of venom of other North and South American snake NOS

● **T63.062** Toxic effect of venom of other North and South American snake, intentional self-harm

● **T63.063** Toxic effect of venom of other North and South American snake, assault

● **T63.064** Toxic effect of venom of other North and South American snake, undetermined

● **T63.07** Toxic effect of venom of other Australian snake

● **T63.071** Toxic effect of venom of other Australian snake, accidental (unintentional)
Toxic effect of venom of other Australian snake NOS

● **T63.072** Toxic effect of venom of other Australian snake, intentional self-harm

● **T63.073** Toxic effect of venom of other Australian snake, assault

● **T63.074** Toxic effect of venom of other Australian snake, undetermined

● **T63.08** Toxic effect of venom of other African and Asian snake

● **T63.081** Toxic effect of venom of other African and Asian snake, accidental (unintentional)
Toxic effect of venom of other African and Asian snake NOS

● **T63.082** Toxic effect of venom of other African and Asian snake, intentional self-harm

● **T63.083** Toxic effect of venom of other African and Asian snake, assault

● **T63.084** Toxic effect of venom of other African and Asian snake, undetermined

CHAPTER 19 (S00-T88)

● T63.09   Toxic effect of venom of other snake
- ● T63.091   Toxic effect of venom of other snake, accidental (unintentional)
  Toxic effect of venom of other snake NOS
- ● T63.092   Toxic effect of venom of other snake, intentional self-harm
- ● T63.093   Toxic effect of venom of other snake, assault
- ● T63.094   Toxic effect of venom of other snake, undetermined

● T63.1   Toxic effect of venom of other reptiles
- ● T63.11   Toxic effect of venom of gila monster
  - ● T63.111   Toxic effect of venom of gila monster, accidental (unintentional)
    Toxic effect of venom of gila monster NOS
  - ● T63.112   Toxic effect of venom of gila monster, intentional self-harm
  - ● T63.113   Toxic effect of venom of gila monster, assault
  - ● T63.114   Toxic effect of venom of gila monster, undetermined
- ● T63.12   Toxic effect of venom of other venomous lizard
  - ● T63.121   Toxic effect of venom of other venomous lizard, accidental (unintentional)
    Toxic effect of venom of other venomous lizard NOS
  - ● T63.122   Toxic effect of venom of other venomous lizard, intentional self-harm
  - ● T63.123   Toxic effect of venom of other venomous lizard, assault
  - ● T63.124   Toxic effect of venom of other venomous lizard, undetermined
- ● T63.19   Toxic effect of venom of other reptiles
  - ● T63.191   Toxic effect of venom of other reptiles, accidental (unintentional)
    Toxic effect of venom of other reptiles NOS
  - ● T63.192   Toxic effect of venom of other reptiles, intentional self-harm
  - ● T63.193   Toxic effect of venom of other reptiles, assault
  - ● T63.194   Toxic effect of venom of other reptiles, undetermined

● T63.2   Toxic effect of venom of scorpion
- ● T63.2X   Toxic effect of venom of scorpion
  - ● T63.2X1   Toxic effect of venom of scorpion, accidental (unintentional)
    Toxic effect of venom of scorpion NOS
  - ● T63.2X2   Toxic effect of venom of scorpion, intentional self-harm
  - ● T63.2X3   Toxic effect of venom of scorpion, assault
  - ● T63.2X4   Toxic effect of venom of scorpion, undetermined

● T63.3   Toxic effect of venom of spider
- ● T63.30   Toxic effect of unspecified spider venom
  - ● T63.301   Toxic effect of unspecified spider venom, accidental (unintentional)
  - ● T63.302   Toxic effect of unspecified spider venom, intentional self-harm
  - ● T63.303   Toxic effect of unspecified spider venom, assault
  - ● T63.304   Toxic effect of unspecified spider venom, undetermined

● T63.31   Toxic effect of venom of black widow spider
- ● T63.311   Toxic effect of venom of black widow spider, accidental (unintentional)
- ● T63.312   Toxic effect of venom of black widow spider, intentional self-harm
- ● T63.313   Toxic effect of venom of black widow spider, assault
- ● T63.314   Toxic effect of venom of black widow spider, undetermined

● T63.32   Toxic effect of venom of tarantula
- ● T63.321   Toxic effect of venom of tarantula, accidental (unintentional)
- ● T63.322   Toxic effect of venom of tarantula, intentional self-harm
- ● T63.323   Toxic effect of venom of tarantula, assault
- ● T63.324   Toxic effect of venom of tarantula, undetermined

● T63.33   Toxic effect of venom of brown recluse spider
- ● T63.331   Toxic effect of venom of brown recluse spider, accidental (unintentional)
- ● T63.332   Toxic effect of venom of brown recluse spider, intentional self-harm
- ● T63.333   Toxic effect of venom of brown recluse spider, assault
- ● T63.334   Toxic effect of venom of brown recluse spider, undetermined

● T63.39   Toxic effect of venom of other spider
- ● T63.391   Toxic effect of venom of other spider, accidental (unintentional)
- ● T63.392   Toxic effect of venom of other spider, intentional self-harm
- ● T63.393   Toxic effect of venom of other spider, assault
- ● T63.394   Toxic effect of venom of other spider, undetermined

● T63.4   Toxic effect of venom of other arthropods
- ● T63.41   Toxic effect of venom of centipedes and venomous millipedes
  - ● T63.411   Toxic effect of venom of centipedes and venomous millipedes, accidental (unintentional)
  - ● T63.412   Toxic effect of venom of centipedes and venomous millipedes, intentional self-harm
  - ● T63.413   Toxic effect of venom of centipedes and venomous millipedes, assault
  - ● T63.414   Toxic effect of venom of centipedes and venomous millipedes, undetermined
- ● T63.42   Toxic effect of venom of ants
  - ● T63.421   Toxic effect of venom of ants, accidental (unintentional)
  - ● T63.422   Toxic effect of venom of ants, intentional self-harm
  - ● T63.423   Toxic effect of venom of ants, assault
  - ● T63.424   Toxic effect of venom of ants, undetermined
- ● T63.43   Toxic effect of venom of caterpillars
  - ● T63.431   Toxic effect of venom of caterpillars, accidental (unintentional)
  - ● T63.432   Toxic effect of venom of caterpillars, intentional self-harm
  - ● T63.433   Toxic effect of venom of caterpillars, assault
  - ● T63.434   Toxic effect of venom of caterpillars, undetermined

● **T63.44**   Toxic effect of venom of bees
  ● **T63.441**   Toxic effect of venom of bees, accidental (unintentional)
  ● **T63.442**   Toxic effect of venom of bees, intentional self-harm
  ● **T63.443**   Toxic effect of venom of bees, assault
  ● **T63.444**   Toxic effect of venom of bees, undetermined

● **T63.45**   Toxic effect of venom of hornets
  ● **T63.451**   Toxic effect of venom of hornets, accidental (unintentional)
  ● **T63.452**   Toxic effect of venom of hornets, intentional self-harm
  ● **T63.453**   Toxic effect of venom of hornets, assault
  ● **T63.454**   Toxic effect of venom of hornets, undetermined

● **T63.46**   Toxic effect of venom of wasps
    Toxic effect of yellow jacket
  ● **T63.461**   Toxic effect of venom of wasps, accidental (unintentional)
  ● **T63.462**   Toxic effect of venom of wasps, intentional self-harm
  ● **T63.463**   Toxic effect of venom of wasps, assault
  ● **T63.464**   Toxic effect of venom of wasps, undetermined

● **T63.48**   Toxic effect of venom of other arthropod
  ● **T63.481**   Toxic effect of venom of other arthropod, accidental (unintentional)
  ● **T63.482**   Toxic effect of venom of other arthropod, intentional self-harm
  ● **T63.483**   Toxic effect of venom of other arthropod, assault
  ● **T63.484**   Toxic effect of venom of other arthropod, undetermined

● **T63.5**   Toxic effect of contact with venomous fish
    Excludes2   poisoning by ingestion of fish (T61.-)
  ● **T63.51**   Toxic effect of contact with stingray
    ● **T63.511**   Toxic effect of contact with stingray, accidental (unintentional)
    ● **T63.512**   Toxic effect of contact with stingray, intentional self-harm
    ● **T63.513**   Toxic effect of contact with stingray, assault
    ● **T63.514**   Toxic effect of contact with stingray, undetermined
  ● **T63.59**   Toxic effect of contact with other venomous fish
    ● **T63.591**   Toxic effect of contact with other venomous fish, accidental (unintentional)
    ● **T63.592**   Toxic effect of contact with other venomous fish, intentional self-harm
    ● **T63.593**   Toxic effect of contact with other venomous fish, assault
    ● **T63.594**   Toxic effect of contact with other venomous fish, undetermined

● **T63.6**   Toxic effect of contact with other venomous marine animals
    Excludes1   sea-snake venom (T63.09)
    Excludes2   poisoning by ingestion of shellfish (T61.78-)
  ● **T63.61**   Toxic effect of contact with Portugese Man-o-war
    Toxic effect of contact with bluebottle
    ● **T63.611**   Toxic effect of contact with Portugese Man-o-war, accidental (unintentional)
    ● **T63.612**   Toxic effect of contact with Portugese Man-o-war, intentional self-harm

    ● **T63.613**   Toxic effect of contact with Portugese Man-o-war, assault
    ● **T63.614**   Toxic effect of contact with Portugese Man-o-war, undetermined
  ● **T63.62**   Toxic effect of contact with other jellyfish
    ● **T63.621**   Toxic effect of contact with other jellyfish, accidental (unintentional)
    ● **T63.622**   Toxic effect of contact with other jellyfish, intentional self-harm
    ● **T63.623**   Toxic effect of contact with other jellyfish, assault
    ● **T63.624**   Toxic effect of contact with other jellyfish, undetermined
  ● **T63.63**   Toxic effect of contact with sea anemone
    ● **T63.631**   Toxic effect of contact with sea anemone, accidental (unintentional)
    ● **T63.632**   Toxic effect of contact with sea anemone, intentional self-harm
    ● **T63.633**   Toxic effect of contact with sea anemone, assault
    ● **T63.634**   Toxic effect of contact with sea anemone, undetermined
  ● **T63.69**   Toxic effect of contact with other venomous marine animals
    ● **T63.691**   Toxic effect of contact with other venomous marine animals, accidental (unintentional)
    ● **T63.692**   Toxic effect of contact with other venomous marine animals, intentional self-harm
    ● **T63.693**   Toxic effect of contact with other venomous marine animals, assault
    ● **T63.694**   Toxic effect of contact with other venomous marine animals, undetermined

● **T63.7**   Toxic effect of contact with venomous plant
  ● **T63.71**   Toxic effect of contact with venomous marine plant
    ● **T63.711**   Toxic effect of contact with venomous marine plant, accidental (unintentional)
    ● **T63.712**   Toxic effect of contact with venomous marine plant, intentional self-harm
    ● **T63.713**   Toxic effect of contact with venomous marine plant, assault
    ● **T63.714**   Toxic effect of contact with venomous marine plant, undetermined
  ● **T63.79**   Toxic effect of contact with other venomous plant
    ● **T63.791**   Toxic effect of contact with other venomous plant, accidental (unintentional)
    ● **T63.792**   Toxic effect of contact with other venomous plant, intentional self-harm
    ● **T63.793**   Toxic effect of contact with other venomous plant, assault
    ● **T63.794**   Toxic effect of contact with other venomous plant, undetermined

● **T63.8**   Toxic effect of contact with other venomous animals
  ● **T63.81**   Toxic effect of contact with venomous frog
    Excludes1   contact with nonvenomous frog (W62.0)
    ● **T63.811**   Toxic effect of contact with venomous frog, accidental (unintentional)
    ● **T63.812**   Toxic effect of contact with venomous frog, intentional self-harm
    ● **T63.813**   Toxic effect of contact with venomous frog, assault
    ● **T63.814**   Toxic effect of contact with venomous frog, undetermined

N Newborn Age: 0   **P** Pediatric Age: 0–17   **M** Maternity DX: 12–55   **A** Adult Age: 15–124   ♀ Females Only   ♂ Males Only

 Complication\Comorbidity   Major C\C   (Ex) CC/MCC Exclusions   Hospital-Acquired Condition

1469

● **T63.82** Toxic effect of contact with venomous toad
  Excludes1 contact with nonvenomous toad (W62.1)
  ● **T63.821** Toxic effect of contact with venomous toad, accidental (unintentional)
  ● **T63.822** Toxic effect of contact with venomous toad, intentional self-harm
  ● **T63.823** Toxic effect of contact with venomous toad, assault
  ● **T63.824** Toxic effect of contact with venomous toad, undetermined
● **T63.83** Toxic effect of contact with other venomous amphibian
  Excludes1 contact with nonvenomous amphibian (W62.9)
  ● **T63.831** Toxic effect of contact with other venomous amphibian, accidental (unintentional)
  ● **T63.832** Toxic effect of contact with other venomous amphibian, intentional self-harm
  ● **T63.833** Toxic effect of contact with other venomous amphibian, assault
  ● **T63.834** Toxic effect of contact with other venomous amphibian, undetermined
● **T63.89** Toxic effect of contact with other venomous animals
  ● **T63.891** Toxic effect of contact with other venomous animals, accidental (unintentional)
  ● **T63.892** Toxic effect of contact with other venomous animals, intentional self-harm
  ● **T63.893** Toxic effect of contact with other venomous animals, assault
  ● **T63.894** Toxic effect of contact with other venomous animals, undetermined
● **T63.9** Toxic effect of contact with unspecified venomous animal
  X ● **T63.91** Toxic effect of contact with unspecified venomous animal, accidental (unintentional)
  X ● **T63.92** Toxic effect of contact with unspecified venomous animal, intentional self-harm
  X ● **T63.93** Toxic effect of contact with unspecified venomous animal, assault
  X ● **T63.94** Toxic effect of contact with unspecified venomous animal, undetermined

● **T64** Toxic effect of aflatoxin and other mycotoxin food contaminants
  The appropriate 7th character is to be added to each code from category T64

A	initial encounter
D	subsequent encounter
S	sequela

  ● **T64.0** Toxic effect of aflatoxin
    X ● **T64.01** Toxic effect of aflatoxin, accidental (unintentional)
    X ● **T64.02** Toxic effect of aflatoxin, intentional self-harm
    X ● **T64.03** Toxic effect of aflatoxin, assault
    X ● **T64.04** Toxic effect of aflatoxin, undetermined
  ● **T64.8** Toxic effect of other mycotoxin food contaminants
    X ● **T64.81** Toxic effect of other mycotoxin food contaminants, accidental (unintentional)
    X ● **T64.82** Toxic effect of other mycotoxin food contaminants, intentional self-harm
    X ● **T64.83** Toxic effect of other mycotoxin food contaminants, assault
    X ● **T64.84** Toxic effect of other mycotoxin food contaminants, undetermined

● **T65** Toxic effect of other and unspecified substances
  The appropriate 7th character is to be added to each code from category T65

A	initial encounter
D	subsequent encounter
S	sequela

● **T65.0** Toxic effect of cyanides
  Excludes1 hydrogen cyanide (T57.3-)
  ● **T65.0X** Toxic effect of cyanides
    ● **T65.0X1** Toxic effect of cyanides, accidental (unintentional)
      Toxic effect of cyanides NOS
    ● **T65.0X2** Toxic effect of cyanides, intentional self-harm
    ● **T65.0X3** Toxic effect of cyanides, assault
    ● **T65.0X4** Toxic effect of cyanides, undetermined
● **T65.1** Toxic effect of strychnine and its salts
  ● **T65.1X** Toxic effect of strychnine and its salts
    ● **T65.1X1** Toxic effect of strychnine and its salts, accidental (unintentional)
      Toxic effect of strychnine and its salts NOS
    ● **T65.1X2** Toxic effect of strychnine and its salts, intentional self-harm
    ● **T65.1X3** Toxic effect of strychnine and its salts, assault
    ● **T65.1X4** Toxic effect of strychnine and its salts, undetermined
● **T65.2** Toxic effect of tobacco and nicotine
  Excludes2 nicotine dependence (F17.-)
  ● **T65.21** Toxic effect of chewing tobacco
    ● **T65.211** Toxic effect of chewing tobacco, accidental (unintentional)
      Toxic effect of chewing tobacco NOS
    ● **T65.212** Toxic effect of chewing tobacco, intentional self-harm
    ● **T65.213** Toxic effect of chewing tobacco, assault
    ● **T65.214** Toxic effect of chewing tobacco, undetermined
  ● **T65.22** Toxic effect of tobacco cigarettes
    Toxic effect of tobacco smoke
    Use additional code for exposure to second hand tobacco smoke (Z57.31, Z77.22)
    ● **T65.221** Toxic effect of tobacco cigarettes, accidental (unintentional)
      Toxic effect of tobacco cigarettes NOS
    ● **T65.222** Toxic effect of tobacco cigarettes, intentional self-harm
    ● **T65.223** Toxic effect of tobacco cigarettes, assault
    ● **T65.224** Toxic effect of tobacco cigarettes, undetermined
  ● **T65.29** Toxic effect of other tobacco and nicotine
    ● **T65.291** Toxic effect of other tobacco and nicotine, accidental (unintentional)
      Toxic effect of other tobacco and nicotine NOS
    ● **T65.292** Toxic effect of other tobacco and nicotine, intentional self-harm
    ● **T65.293** Toxic effect of other tobacco and nicotine, assault
    ● **T65.294** Toxic effect of other tobacco and nicotine, undetermined

▶ New   ⇒ Revised   ~~deleted~~ Deleted   Excludes 1   Excludes 2   Includes   Use additional   Code first   Code also   Key words
OGCR Official Guidelines   ● Unacceptable Principal Diagnosis   X Assign placeholder X   ● Use Additional Character(s)   ▌ Manifestation Code   **Coding Clinic**

● **T65.3   Toxic effect of nitroderivatives and aminoderivatives of benzene and its homologues**
  Toxic effect of anilin [benzenamine]
  Toxic effect of nitrobenzene
  Toxic effect of trinitrotoluene

  ● **T65.3X   Toxic effect of nitroderivatives and aminoderivatives of benzene and its homologues**

    ● **T65.3X1   Toxic effect of nitroderivatives and aminoderivatives of benzene and its homologues, accidental (unintentional)**
      Toxic effect of nitroderivatives and aminoderivatives of benzene and its homologues NOS

    ● **T65.3X2   Toxic effect of nitroderivatives and aminoderivatives of benzene and its homologues, intentional self-harm**

    ● **T65.3X3   Toxic effect of nitroderivatives and aminoderivatives of benzene and its homologues, assault**

    ● **T65.3X4   Toxic effect of nitroderivatives and aminoderivatives of benzene and its homologues, undetermined**

● **T65.4   Toxic effect of carbon disulfide**

  ● **T65.4X   Toxic effect of carbon disulfide**

    ● **T65.4X1   Toxic effect of carbon disulfide, accidental (unintentional)**
      Toxic effect of carbon disulfide NOS

    ● **T65.4X2   Toxic effect of carbon disulfide, intentional self-harm**

    ● **T65.4X3   Toxic effect of carbon disulfide, assault**

    ● **T65.4X4   Toxic effect of carbon disulfide, undetermined**

● **T65.5   Toxic effect of nitroglycerin and other nitric acids and esters**
  Toxic effect of 1,2,3-Propanetriol trinitrate

  ● **T65.5X   Toxic effect of nitroglycerin and other nitric acids and esters**

    ● **T65.5X1   Toxic effect of nitroglycerin and other nitric acids and esters, accidental (unintentional)**
      Toxic effect of nitroglycerin and other nitric acids and esters NOS

    ● **T65.5X2   Toxic effect of nitroglycerin and other nitric acids and esters, intentional self-harm**

    ● **T65.5X3   Toxic effect of nitroglycerin and other nitric acids and esters, assault**

    ● **T65.5X4   Toxic effect of nitroglycerin and other nitric acids and esters, undetermined**

● **T65.6   Toxic effect of paints and dyes, not elsewhere classified**

  ● **T65.6X   Toxic effect of paints and dyes, not elsewhere classified**

    ● **T65.6X1   Toxic effect of paints and dyes, not elsewhere classified, accidental (unintentional)**
      Toxic effect of paints and dyes NOS

    ● **T65.6X2   Toxic effect of paints and dyes, not elsewhere classified, intentional self-harm**

    ● **T65.6X3   Toxic effect of paints and dyes, not elsewhere classified, assault**

    ● **T65.6X4   Toxic effect of paints and dyes, not elsewhere classified, undetermined**

● **T65.8   Toxic effect of other specified substances**

  ● **T65.81   Toxic effect of latex**

    ● **T65.811   Toxic effect of latex, accidental (unintentional)**
      Toxic effect of latex NOS

    ● **T65.812   Toxic effect of latex, intentional self-harm**

    ● **T65.813   Toxic effect of latex, assault**

    ● **T65.814   Toxic effect of latex, undetermined**

  ● **T65.82   Toxic effect of harmful algae and algae toxins**
    Toxic effect of (harmful) algae bloom NOS
    Toxic effect of blue-green algae bloom
    Toxic effect of brown tide
    Toxic effect of cyanobacteria bloom
    Toxic effect of Florida red tide
    Toxic effect of pfiesteria piscicida
    Toxic effect of red tide

    ● **T65.821   Toxic effect of harmful algae and algae toxins, accidental (unintentional)**
      Toxic effect of harmful algae and algae toxins NOS

    ● **T65.822   Toxic effect of harmful algae and algae toxins, intentional self-harm**

    ● **T65.823   Toxic effect of harmful algae and algae toxins, assault**

    ● **T65.824   Toxic effect of harmful algae and algae toxins, undetermined**

  ● **T65.83   Toxic effect of fiberglass**

    ● **T65.831   Toxic effect of fiberglass, accidental (unintentional)**
      Toxic effect of fiberglass NOS

    ● **T65.832   Toxic effect of fiberglass, intentional self-harm**

    ● **T65.833   Toxic effect of fiberglass, assault**

    ● **T65.834   Toxic effect of fiberglass, undetermined**

  ● **T65.89   Toxic effect of other specified substances**

    ● **T65.891   Toxic effect of other specified substances, accidental (unintentional)**
      Toxic effect of other specified substances NOS

    ● **T65.892   Toxic effect of other specified substances, intentional self-harm**

    ● **T65.893   Toxic effect of other specified substances, assault**

    ● **T65.894   Toxic effect of other specified substances, undetermined**

● **T65.9   Toxic effect of unspecified substance**

  X ● **T65.91   Toxic effect of unspecified substance, accidental (unintentional)**
      Poisoning NOS

  X ● **T65.92   Toxic effect of unspecified substance, intentional self-harm**

  X ● **T65.93   Toxic effect of unspecified substance, assault**

  X ● **T65.94   Toxic effect of unspecified substance, undetermined**

N Newborn Age: 0   **P** Pediatric Age: 0–17   **M** Maternity DX: 12–55   **A** Adult Age: 15–124   ♀ Females Only   ♂ Males Only

🔵 Complication\Comorbidity   🔵 Major C\C   (Ex:) CC/MCC Exclusions   🔵 Hospital-Acquired Condition

CHAPTER 19 (S00-T88)

OTHER AND UNSPECIFIED EFFECTS OF EXTERNAL CAUSES (T66-T78)

● **T66**   **Radiation sickness, unspecified**

     Excludes1   specified adverse effects of radiation, such as:
           burns (T20-T31)
           leukemia (C91-C95)
           radiation gastroenteritis and colitis (K52.0)
           radiation pneumonitis (J70.0)
           radiation related disorders of the skin and
             subcutaneous tissue (L55-L59)
           sunburn (L55.-)

     The appropriate 7th character is to be added to code T66

     | | |
     A   initial encounter
     D   subsequent encounter
     S   sequela

● **T67**   **Effects of heat and light**

     Excludes1   erythema [dermatitis] ab igne (L59.0)
           malignant hyperpyrexia due to anesthesia (T88.3)
           radiation-related disorders of the skin and
             subcutaneous tissue (L55-L59)

     Excludes2   burns (T20-T31)
           sunburn (L55.-)
           sweat disorder due to heat (L74-L75)

     The appropriate 7th character is to be added to each code from
       category T67

     A   initial encounter
     D   subsequent encounter
     S   sequela

X ● **T67.0**   **Heatstroke and sunstroke** A 🖐, A 🖐
         Heat apoplexy
         Heat pyrexia
         Siriasis
         Thermoplegia
         Use additional code(s) to identify any associated
           complications of heatstroke, such as:
         coma and stupor (R40.-)
         systemic inflammatory response syndrome (R65.1-)
         (Ex) See PDX Collection 1419

X ● **T67.1**   **Heat syncope**
         Heat collapse

X ● **T67.2**   **Heat cramp**

X ● **T67.3**   **Heat exhaustion, anhydrotic**
         Heat prostration due to water depletion
         Excludes1   heat exhaustion due to salt depletion
                (T67.4)

X ● **T67.4**   **Heat exhaustion due to salt depletion**
         Heat prostration due to salt (and water) depletion

X ● **T67.5**   **Heat exhaustion, unspecified**
         Heat prostration NOS

X ● **T67.6**   **Heat fatigue, transient**

X ● **T67.7**   **Heat edema**

X ● **T67.8**   **Other effects of heat and light**

X ● **T67.9**   **Effect of heat and light, unspecified**

X ● **T68**   **Hypothermia**
     Accidental hypothermia
     Hypothermia NOS
     Use additional code to identify source of exposure:
       Exposure to excessive cold of man-made origin (W93)
       Exposure to excessive cold of natural origin (X31)

     Excludes1   hypothermia following anesthesia (T88.51)
           hypothermia not associated with low
             environmental temperature (R68.0)
           hypothermia of newborn (P80.-)

     Excludes2   frostbite (T33-T34)

     The appropriate 7th character is to be added to code T68

     A   initial encounter
     D   subsequent encounter
     S   sequela

● **T69**   **Other effects of reduced temperature**
     Use additional code to identify source of exposure:
       Exposure to excessive cold of man-made origin (W93)
       Exposure to excessive cold of natural origin (X31)

     Excludes2   frostbite (T33-T34)

     The appropriate 7th character is to be added to each code from
       category T69

     A   initial encounter
     D   subsequent encounter
     S   sequela

   ● **T69.0**   **Immersion hand and foot**

     ● **T69.01**   **Immersion hand**

       ● **T69.011**   **Immersion hand, right hand**

       ● **T69.012**   **Immersion hand, left hand**

       ● **T69.019**   **Immersion hand, unspecified hand**

     ● **T69.02**   **Immersion foot**
         Trench foot
         (Ex) For category T69.02 CC codes: See PDX Collection 1420

       ● **T69.021**   **Immersion foot, right foot** A 🖐, A 🖐

       ● **T69.022**   **Immersion foot, left foot** A 🖐, A 🖐

       ● **T69.029**   **Immersion foot, unspecified foot** A 🖐,
           A 🖐

X ● **T69.1**   **Chilblains**

X ● **T69.8**   **Other specified effects of reduced temperature**

X ● **T69.9**   **Effect of reduced temperature, unspecified**

● **T70**   **Effects of air pressure and water pressure**
     The appropriate 7th character is to be added to each code from
       category T70

     A   initial encounter
     D   subsequent encounter
     S   sequela

X ● **T70.0**   **Otitic barotrauma**
         Aero-otitis media
         Effects of change in ambient atmospheric pressure or
           water pressure on ears

X ● **T70.1**   **Sinus barotrauma**
         Aerosinusitis
         Effects of change in ambient atmospheric pressure on
           sinuses

   ● **T70.2**   **Other and unspecified effects of high altitude**
     Excludes2   polycythemia due to high altitude (D75.1)

X ● **T70.20**   **Unspecified effects of high altitude**

X ● **T70.29**   **Other effects of high altitude**
         Alpine sickness
         Anoxia due to high altitude
         Barotrauma NOS
         Hypobaropathy
         Mountain sickness

X ● **T70.3**   **Caisson disease [decompression sickness]** A 🖐, A 🖐
         Compressed-air disease
         Diver's palsy or paralysis
         (Ex) See PDX Collection 1421

X ● **T70.4**   **Effects of high-pressure fluids**
         Hydraulic jet injection (industrial)
         Pneumatic jet injection (industrial)
         Traumatic jet injection (industrial)

X ● **T70.8**   **Other effects of air pressure and water pressure**

X ● **T70.9**   **Effect of air pressure and water pressure, unspecified**

▶ New   ⇒ Revised   ~~deleted~~ Deleted   Excludes 1   Excludes 2   Includes   Use additional   Code first   Code also   Key words

OGCR Official Guidelines   ● Unacceptable Principal Diagnosis   X Assign placeholder X   ● Use Additional Character(s)   ▶ Manifestation Code   **Coding Clinic**

1472

● **T71   Asphyxiation**
Mechanical suffocation
Traumatic suffocation

Excludes1   acute respiratory distress (syndrome) (J80)
anoxia due to high altitude (T70.2)
asphyxia NOS (R09.01)
asphyxia from carbon monoxide (T58.-)
asphyxia from inhalation of food or foreign body
(T17.-)
asphyxia from other gases, fumes and vapors
(T59.-)
respiratory distress (syndrome) in newborn
(P22.-)

The appropriate 7th character is to be added to each code from
category T71

A	initial encounter
D	subsequent encounter
S	sequela

(Ex:) For category T71 CC codes: See PDX Collection 1422

● **T71.1   Asphyxiation due to mechanical threat to breathing**
Suffocation due to mechanical threat to breathing

● **T71.11   Asphyxiation due to smothering under pillow**

● **T71.111   Asphyxiation due to smothering
under pillow, accidental** A 🔾, A 🔾
Asphyxiation due to smothering
under pillow NOS

● **T71.112   Asphyxiation due to smothering
under pillow, intentional self-harm**
A 🔾, A 🔾

● **T71.113   Asphyxiation due to smothering
under pillow, assault** A 🔾, A 🔾

● **T71.114   Asphyxiation due to smothering
under pillow, undetermined** A 🔾,
A 🔾

● **T71.12   Asphyxiation due to plastic bag**

● **T71.121   Asphyxiation due to plastic bag,
accidental** A 🔾, A 🔾
Asphyxiation due to plastic bag
NOS

● **T71.122   Asphyxiation due to plastic bag,
intentional self-harm** A 🔾, A 🔾

● **T71.123   Asphyxiation due to plastic bag,
assault** A 🔾, A 🔾

● **T71.124   Asphyxiation due to plastic bag,
undetermined** A 🔾, A 🔾

● **T71.13   Asphyxiation due to being trapped in bed
linens**

● **T71.131   Asphyxiation due to being trapped in
bed linens, accidental** A 🔾, A 🔾
Asphyxiation due to being trapped
in bed linens NOS

● **T71.132   Asphyxiation due to being trapped in
bed linens, intentional self-harm**
A 🔾, A 🔾

● **T71.133   Asphyxiation due to being trapped in
bed linens, assault** A 🔾, A 🔾

● **T71.134   Asphyxiation due to being trapped in
bed linens, undetermined** A 🔾, A 🔾

● **T71.14   Asphyxiation due to smothering under another
person's body (in bed)**

● **T71.141   Asphyxiation due to smothering
under another person's body (in bed),
accidental** A 🔾, A 🔾
Asphyxiation due to smothering
under another person's body
(in bed) NOS

● **T71.143   Asphyxiation due to smothering
under another person's body (in bed),
assault** A 🔾, A 🔾

● **T71.144   Asphyxiation due to smothering
under another person's body (in bed),
undetermined** A 🔾, A 🔾

● **T71.15   Asphyxiation due to smothering in furniture**

● **T71.151   Asphyxiation due to smothering in
furniture, accidental** A 🔾, A 🔾
Asphyxiation due to smothering in
furniture NOS

● **T71.152   Asphyxiation due to smothering in
furniture, intentional self-harm** A 🔾,
A 🔾

● **T71.153   Asphyxiation due to smothering in
furniture, assault** A 🔾, A 🔾

● **T71.154   Asphyxiation due to smothering in
furniture, undetermined** A 🔾, A 🔾

● **T71.16   Asphyxiation due to hanging**
Hanging by window shade cord
Use additional code for any associated injuries,
such as:
crushing injury of neck (S17.-)
fracture of cervical vertebrae (S12.0-S12.2-)
open wound of neck (S11.-)

● **T71.161   Asphyxiation due to hanging,
accidental** A 🔾, A 🔾
Asphyxiation due to hanging NOS
Hanging NOS

● **T71.162   Asphyxiation due to hanging,
intentional self-harm** A 🔾, A 🔾

● **T71.163   Asphyxiation due to hanging, assault**
A 🔾, A 🔾

● **T71.164   Asphyxiation due to hanging,
undetermined** A 🔾, A 🔾

● **T71.19   Asphyxiation due to mechanical**
Threat to breathing due to other causes

● **T71.191   Asphyxiation due to mechanical
threat to breathing due to other
causes, accidental** A 🔾, A 🔾
Asphyxiation due to other causes
NOS
Coding Clinic: 2016, Q4, P76

● **T71.192   Asphyxiation due to mechanical
threat to breathing due to other
causes, intentional self-harm** A 🔾,
A 🔾

● **T71.193   Asphyxiation due to mechanical
threat to breathing due to other
causes, assault** A 🔾, A 🔾

● **T71.194   Asphyxiation due to mechanical
threat to breathing due to other
causes, undetermined** A 🔾, A 🔾

● **T71.2 Asphyxiation due to systemic oxygen deficiency due to low oxygen content in ambient air**
     Suffocation due to systemic oxygen deficiency due to low oxygen content in ambient air

X ● **T71.20 Asphyxiation due to systemic oxygen deficiency due to low oxygen content in ambient air due to unspecified cause** A 🖉, A 🖉

X ● **T71.21 Asphyxiation due to cave-in or falling earth** A 🖉, A 🖉
         Use additional code for any associated cataclysm (X34-X38)

● **T71.22 Asphyxiation due to being trapped in a car trunk**

     ● **T71.221 Asphyxiation due to being trapped in a car trunk, accidental** A 🖉

     ● **T71.222 Asphyxiation due to being trapped in a car trunk, intentional self-harm** A 🖉

     ● **T71.223 Asphyxiation due to being trapped in a car trunk, assault** A 🖉

     ● **T71.224 Asphyxiation due to being trapped in a car trunk, undetermined** A 🖉

● **T71.23 Asphyxiation due to being trapped in a (discarded) refrigerator**

     ● **T71.231 Asphyxiation due to being trapped in a (discarded) refrigerator, accidental** A 🖉

     ● **T71.232 Asphyxiation due to being trapped in a (discarded) refrigerator, intentional self-harm** A 🖉

     ● **T71.233 Asphyxiation due to being trapped in a (discarded) refrigerator, assault** A 🖉

     ● **T71.234 Asphyxiation due to being trapped in a (discarded) refrigerator, undetermined** A 🖉

X ● **T71.29 Asphyxiation due to being trapped in other low oxygen environment** A 🖉, A 🖉

X ● **T71.9 Asphyxiation due to unspecified cause** A 🖉, A 🖉
     Suffocation (by strangulation) due to unspecified cause
     Suffocation NOS
     Systemic oxygen deficiency due to low oxygen content in ambient air due to unspecified cause
     Systemic oxygen deficiency due to mechanical threat to breathing due to unspecified cause
     Traumatic asphyxia NOS

● **T73 Effects of other deprivation**

     The appropriate 7th character is to be added to each code from category T73

A	initial encounter
D	subsequent encounter
S	sequela

X ● **T73.0 Starvation**
     Deprivation of food

X ● **T73.1 Deprivation of water**

X ● **T73.2 Exhaustion due to exposure**

X ● **T73.3 Exhaustion due to excessive exertion**
     Exhaustion due to overexertion

X ● **T73.8 Other effects of deprivation**

X ● **T73.9 Effect of deprivation, unspecified**

● **T74 Adult and child abuse, neglect and other maltreatment, confirmed**
     Use additional code, if applicable, to identify any associated current injury
     Use additional external cause code to identify perpetrator, if known (Y07.-)

     Excludes1 abuse and maltreatment in pregnancy (O9A.3-, O9A.4-, O9A.5-)
           adult and child maltreatment, suspected (T76.-)

     The appropriate 7th character is to be added to each code from category T74

A	initial encounter
D	subsequent encounter
S	sequela

Ⓔⓧ For category T74 CC codes unless otherwise indicated: See PDX Collection 1423

● **T74.0 Neglect or abandonment, confirmed**

X ● **T74.01 Adult neglect or abandonment, confirmed** A 🖉   A

X ● **T74.02 Child neglect or abandonment, confirmed** A 🖉   P

● **T74.1 Physical abuse, confirmed**
     Excludes2 sexual abuse (T74.2-)

X ● **T74.11 Adult physical abuse, confirmed** A 🖉   A

X ● **T74.12 Child physical abuse, confirmed** A 🖉   P
     Excludes2 shaken infant syndrome (T74.4)

● **T74.2 Sexual abuse, confirmed**
     Rape, confirmed
     Sexual assault, confirmed

X ● **T74.21 Adult sexual abuse, confirmed** A 🖉   A

X ● **T74.22 Child sexual abuse, confirmed** A 🖉   P

● **T74.3 Psychological abuse, confirmed**

X ● **T74.31 Adult psychological abuse, confirmed**   A

X ● **T74.32 Child psychological abuse, confirmed** A 🖉   P

X ● **T74.4 Shaken infant syndrome** A 🖉   P

● **T74.9 Unspecified maltreatment, confirmed**

X ● **T74.91 Unspecified adult maltreatment, confirmed** A 🖉   A
     Ⓔⓧ See PDX Collection 1424

X ● **T74.92 Unspecified child maltreatment, confirmed** A 🖉   P

● **T75 Other and unspecified effects of other external causes**
     Excludes1 adverse effects NEC (T78.-)
     Excludes2 burns (electric) (T20-T31)

     The appropriate 7th character is to be added to each code from category T75

A	initial encounter
D	subsequent encounter
S	sequela

● **T75.0 Effects of lightning**
     Struck by lightning

X ● **T75.00 Unspecified effects of lightning**
     Struck by lightning NOS

X ● **T75.01 Shock due to being struck by lightning**

X ● **T75.09 Other effects of lightning**
     Use additional code for other effects of lightning

X ● **T75.1 Unspecified effects of drowning and nonfatal submersion** A 🖉, A 🖉
     Immersion
     Excludes1 specified effects of drowning code to effects
     Ⓔⓧ See PDX Collection 1425

▶ New   ⇒ Revised   ~~deleted~~ Deleted   Excludes 1   Excludes 2   Includes   Use additional   Code first   Code also   Key words

OGCR Official Guidelines   ● Unacceptable Principal Diagnosis   X Assign placeholder X   ● Use Additional Character(s)   ▶ Manifestation Code   **Coding Clinic**

● **T75.2   Effects of vibration**
   X● **T75.20   Unspecified effects of vibration**
   X● **T75.21   Pneumatic hammer syndrome**
   X● **T75.22   Traumatic vasospastic syndrome**
   X● **T75.23   Vertigo from infrasound**
       Excludes1   vertigo NOS (R42)
   X● **T75.29   Other effects of vibration**
X● **T75.3   Motion sickness**
     Airsickness   Travel sickness
     Seasickness
     Use additional external cause code to identify vehicle or type of motion (Y92.81-, Y93.5-)
X● **T75.4   Electrocution**
     Shock from electric current
     Shock from electroshock gun (taser)
● **T75.8   Other specified effects of external causes**
   X● **T75.81   Effects of abnormal gravitation [G] forces**
   X● **T75.82   Effects of weightlessness**
   X● **T75.89   Other specified effects of external causes**

● **T76   Adult and child abuse, neglect and other maltreatment, suspected**
     Use additional code, if applicable, to identify any associated current injury
     Excludes1   adult and child maltreatment, confirmed (T74.-)
           suspected abuse and maltreatment in pregnancy (O9A.3-, O9A.4-, O9A.5-)
           suspected adult physical abuse, ruled out (Z04.71)
           suspected adult sexual abuse, ruled out (Z04.41)
           suspected child physical abuse, ruled out (Z04.72)
           suspected child sexual abuse, ruled out (Z04.42)
     The appropriate 7th character is to be added to each code from category T76

A	initial encounter
D	subsequent encounter
S	sequela

Ⓔ⒳ **For category T76 CC codes unless otherwise indicated:** See PDX Collection 1423
Coding Clinic: 2016, Q4, P129

● **T76.0   Neglect or abandonment, suspected**
   X● **T76.01   Adult neglect or abandonment, suspected** A 🔒   A
   X● **T76.02   Child neglect or abandonment, suspected** A 🔒   P
● **T76.1   Physical abuse, suspected**
   X● **T76.11   Adult physical abuse, suspected** A 🔒   A
   X● **T76.12   Child physical abuse, suspected** A 🔒   P
● **T76.2   Sexual abuse, suspected**
     Rape, suspected
     ~~Sexual abuse, suspected~~
     Excludes1   alleged abuse, ruled out (Z04.7)
   X● **T76.21   Adult sexual abuse, suspected** A 🔒   A
   X● **T76.22   Child sexual abuse, suspected** A 🔒   P
● **T76.3   Psychological abuse, suspected**
   X● **T76.31   Adult psychological abuse, suspected**   A
   X● **T76.32   Child psychological abuse, suspected** A 🔒   P
● **T76.9   Unspecified maltreatment, suspected**
   X● **T76.91   Unspecified adult maltreatment, suspected** A 🔒   A
           Ⓔ⒳ See PDX Collection 1424
   X● **T76.92   Unspecified child maltreatment, suspected** A 🔒   P

● **T78   Adverse effects, not elsewhere classified**
     Excludes2   complications of surgical and medical care NEC (T80-T88)
     The appropriate 7th character is to be added to each code from category T78

A	initial encounter
D	subsequent encounter
S	sequela

Ⓔ⒳ **For category T78 CC codes:** See PDX Collection 1426

● **T78.0   Anaphylactic reaction due to food**
     Anaphylactic reaction due to adverse food reaction
     Anaphylactic shock or reaction due to nonpoisonous foods
     Anaphylactoid reaction due to food
   X● **T78.00   Anaphylactic reaction due to unspecified food** A 🔒
   X● **T78.01   Anaphylactic reaction due to peanuts** A 🔒
   X● **T78.02   Anaphylactic reaction due to shellfish (crustaceans)** A 🔒
   X● **T78.03   Anaphylactic reaction due to other fish** A 🔒
   X● **T78.04   Anaphylactic reaction due to fruits and vegetables** A 🔒
   X● **T78.05   Anaphylactic reaction due to tree nuts and seeds** A 🔒
       Excludes2   anaphylactic reaction due to peanuts (T78.01)
   X● **T78.06   Anaphylactic reaction due to food additives** A 🔒
   X● **T78.07   Anaphylactic reaction due to milk and dairy products** A 🔒
   X● **T78.08   Anaphylactic reaction due to eggs** A 🔒
   X● **T78.09   Anaphylactic reaction due to other food products** A 🔒
X● **T78.1   Other adverse food reactions, not elsewhere classified**
     Use additional code to identify the type of reaction, if applicable
     Excludes1   anaphylactic reaction or shock due to adverse food reaction (T78.0-)
           anaphylactic reaction due to food (T78.0-)
           bacterial food borne intoxications (A05.-)
     Excludes2   allergic and dietetic gastroenteritis and colitis (K52.29)
           allergic rhinitis due to food (J30.5)
           dermatitis due to food in contact with skin (L23.6, L24.6, L25.4)
           dermatitis due to ingested food (L27.2)
           food protein-induced enterocolitis syndrome (K52.21)
           food protein-induced enteropathy (K52.22)
X● **T78.2   Anaphylactic shock, unspecified** A 🔒
     Occurs when allergic response triggers large quantities of histamines, prostaglandins, leukotrienes resulting in systemic vasodilation
     Allergic shock
     Anaphylactic reaction
     Anaphylaxis
     Excludes1   anaphylactic reaction or shock due to adverse effect of correct medicinal substance properly administered (T88.6)
           anaphylactic reaction or shock due to adverse food reaction (T78.0-)
           anaphylactic reaction or shock due to serum (T80.5-)

CHAPTER 19 (S00-T88)

X ● **T78.3　Angioneurotic edema**
　　Allergic angioedema
　　Giant urticaria
　　Vascular disorder resulting from abnormalities of autonomic
　　　nervous system fibers supplying blood vessels
　　Quincke's edema
　　Excludes1　serum urticaria (T80.6-)
　　　　　　　　urticaria (L50.-)

● **T78.4　Other and unspecified allergy**
　　Excludes1　specified types of allergic reaction
　　　　　　　　such as:
　　　　　　　　allergic diarrhea (K52.29)
　　　　　　　　allergic gastroenteritis and colitis
　　　　　　　　　(K52.29)
　　　　　　　　dermatitis (L23-L25, L27.-)
　　　　　　　　food protein-induced enterocolitis
　　　　　　　　　syndrome (K52.21)
　　　　　　　　food protein-induced enteropathy
　　　　　　　　　(K52.22)
　　　　　　　　hay fever (J30.1)

　X ● **T78.40　Allergy, unspecified**
　　　　Allergic reaction NOS
　　　　Hypersensitivity NOS

　X ● **T78.41　Arthus phenomenon**
　　　　Arthus reaction

　X ● **T78.49　Other allergy**

X ● **T78.8　Other adverse effects, not elsewhere classified**

CERTAIN EARLY COMPLICATIONS OF TRAUMA (T79)

● **T79　Certain early complications of trauma, not elsewhere classified**
　　Excludes2　acute respiratory distress syndrome (J80)
　　　　　　　　complications occurring during or following
　　　　　　　　　medical procedures (T80-T88)
　　　　　　　　complications of surgical and medical care NEC
　　　　　　　　　(T80-T88)
　　　　　　　　newborn respiratory distress syndrome (P22.0)
　　The appropriate 7th character is to be added to each code from
　　category T79

A	initial encounter
D	subsequent encounter
S	sequela

X ● **T79.0　Air embolism (traumatic) A 🐾**
　　Excludes1　air embolism complicating abortion
　　　　　　　　or ectopic or molar pregnancy
　　　　　　　　　(O00-O07, O08.2)
　　　　　　　　air embolism complicating pregnancy,
　　　　　　　　　childbirth and the puerperium
　　　　　　　　　(O88.0)
　　　　　　　　air embolism following infusion,
　　　　　　　　　transfusion, and therapeutic injection
　　　　　　　　　(T80.0)
　　　　　　　　air embolism following procedure NEC
　　　　　　　　　(T81.7-)
　　　(Ex:) See PDX Collection 1427

X ● **T79.1　Fat embolism (traumatic) A 🐾**
　　Excludes1　fat embolism complicating:
　　　　　　　　abortion or ectopic or molar pregnancy
　　　　　　　　　(O00-O07, O08.2)
　　　　　　　　pregnancy, childbirth and the
　　　　　　　　　puerperium (O88.8)
　　　(Ex:) See PDX Collection 1428

X ● **T79.2　Traumatic secondary and recurrent hemorrhage and seroma A 🐾**
　　　(Ex:) See PDX Collection 1429

X ● **T79.4　Traumatic shock A 🐾**
　　Shock (immediate) (delayed) following injury
　　Excludes1　anaphylactic shock due to adverse
　　　　　　　　food reaction (T78.0-)
　　　　　　　　anaphylactic shock due to correct
　　　　　　　　　medicinal substance properly
　　　　　　　　　administered (T88.6)
　　　　　　　　anaphylactic shock due to serum
　　　　　　　　　(T80.5-)
　　　　　　　　anaphylactic shock NOS (T78.2)
　　　　　　　　anesthetic shock (T88.2)
　　　　　　　　electric shock (T75.4)
　　　　　　　　nontraumatic shock NEC (R57.-)
　　　　　　　　obstetric shock (O75.1)
　　　　　　　　postprocedural shock (T81.1-)
　　　　　　　　septic shock (R65.21)
　　　　　　　　shock complicating abortion or
　　　　　　　　　ectopic or molar pregnancy
　　　　　　　　　(O00-O07, O08.3)
　　　　　　　　shock due to lightning (T75.01)
　　　　　　　　shock NOS (R57.9)
　　　(Ex:) See PDX Collection 1430

X ● **T79.5　Traumatic anuria A 🐾**
　　Crush syndrome
　　Renal failure following crushing
　　　(Ex:) See PDX Collection 1431

X ● **T79.6　Traumatic ischemia of muscle**
　　Traumatic rhabdomyolysis
　　Volkmann's ischemic contracture
　　Excludes2　anterior tibial syndrome (M76.8)
　　　　　　　　compartment syndrome
　　　　　　　　　(traumatic) (T79.A-)
　　　　　　　　nontraumatic ischemia of muscle
　　　　　　　　　(M62.2-)

X ● **T79.7　Traumatic subcutaneous emphysema A 🐾**
　　Excludes1　emphysema NOS (J43)
　　　　　　　　emphysema (subcutaneous)
　　　　　　　　　resulting from a procedure
　　　　　　　　　(T81.82)
　　　(Ex:) See PDX Collection 1432

● **T79.A　Traumatic compartment syndrome**
　　Excludes1　fibromyalgia (M79.7)
　　　　　　　　nontraumatic compartment
　　　　　　　　　syndrome (M79.A-)
　　　　　　　　traumatic ischemic infarction of
　　　　　　　　　muscle (T79.6)
　　　(Ex:) **For category T79.A CC codes unless otherwise indicated:** See
　　　　PDX Collection 1433

　X ● **T79.A0　Compartment syndrome, unspecified**
　　　　A 🐾
　　　　Compartment syndrome NOS
　　　　(Ex:) See PDX Collection 896

　● **T79.A1　Traumatic compartment syndrome of upper extremity**
　　　　Traumatic compartment syndrome
　　　　　of shoulder, arm, forearm, wrist,
　　　　　hand, and fingers

　　　● **T79.A11　Traumatic compartment
　　　　　　syndrome of right upper
　　　　　　extremity A 🐾**

　　　● **T79.A12　Traumatic compartment
　　　　　　syndrome of left upper
　　　　　　extremity A 🐾**

　　　● **T79.A19　Traumatic compartment
　　　　　　syndrome of unspecified upper
　　　　　　extremity A 🐾**

▶ New　➡ Revised　~~deleted~~ Deleted　Excludes 1　Excludes 2　Includes　Use additional　Code first　Code also　Key words
OGCR Official Guidelines　● Unacceptable Principal Diagnosis　X Assign placeholder X　● Use Additional Character(s)　▶ Manifestation Code　**Coding Clinic**

● **T79.A2** **Traumatic compartment syndrome of lower extremity**
     Traumatic compartment syndrome of hip, buttock, thigh, leg, foot, and toes

     ● **T79.A21** **Traumatic compartment syndrome of right lower extremity A** 🔹

     ● **T79.A22** **Traumatic compartment syndrome of left lower extremity A** 🔹

     ● **T79.A29** **Traumatic compartment syndrome of unspecified lower extremity A** 🔹

X● **T79.A3** **Traumatic compartment syndrome of abdomen A** 🔹
     Ⓔⓧ See PDX Collection 1434

X● **T79.A9** **Traumatic compartment syndrome of other sites A** 🔹
     Ⓔⓧ See PDX Collection 896

X● **T79.8** **Other early complications of trauma**

X● **T79.9** **Unspecified early complication of trauma**

COMPLICATIONS OF SURGICAL AND MEDICAL CARE NOT ELSEWHERE CLASSIFIED (T80-T88)

Use additional code for adverse effect, if applicable, to identify drug (T36-T50 with fifth or sixth character 5)

Use additional code(s) to identify the specified condition resulting from the complication.

Use additional code to identify devices involved and details of circumstances (Y62-Y82)

Excludes2   any encounters with medical care for postprocedural conditions in which no complications are present, such as:
     artificial opening status (Z93.-)
     closure of external stoma (Z43.-)
     fitting and adjustment of external prosthetic device (Z44.-)
     burns and corrosions from local applications and irradiation (T20-T32)
     complications of surgical procedures during pregnancy, childbirth and the puerperium (O00-O9A)
     mechanical complication of respirator [ventilator] (J95.850)
     poisoning and toxic effects of drugs and chemicals (T36-T65 with fifth or sixth character 1-4 or 6)
     postprocedural fever (R50.82)
     specified complications classified elsewhere, such as:
       cerebrospinal fluid leak from spinal puncture (G97.0)
       colostomy malfunction (K94.0-)
       disorders of fluid and electrolyte imbalance (E86-E87)
       functional disturbances following cardiac surgery (I97.0-I97.1)
       intraoperative and postprocedural complications of specified body systems (D78.-, E36.-, E89.-, G97.3-, G97.4, H59.3-, H59.-, H95.2-, H95.3, I97.4-, I97.5, J95.6-, J95.7, K91.6-, L76.-, M96.-, N99.-)
       ostomy complications (J95.0-, K94.-, N99.5-)
       postgastric surgery syndromes (K91.1)
       postlaminectomy syndrome NEC (M96.1)
       postmastectomy lymphedema syndrome (I97.2)
       postsurgical blind-loop syndrome (K91.2)
       ventilator associated pneumonia (J95.851)

● **T80** **Complications following infusion, transfusion and therapeutic injection**

   Includes   complications following perfusion

   Excludes2   bone marrow transplant rejection (T86.01)
     febrile nonhemolytic transfusion reaction (R50.84)
     fluid overload due to transfusion (E87.71)
     posttransfusion purpura (D69.51)
     transfusion associated circulatory overload (TACO) (E87.71)
     transfusion (red blood cell) associated hemochromatosis (E83.111)
     transfusion related acute lung injury (TRALI) (J95.84)

The appropriate 7th character is to be added to each code from category T80

A	initial encounter
D	subsequent encounter
S	sequela

X● **T80.0** **Air embolism following infusion, transfusion and therapeutic injection A** 🔹, **A** 🔹
     Ⓔⓧ See PDX Collection 1435

X● **T80.1** **Vascular complications following infusion, transfusion and therapeutic injection A** 🔹

     Use additional code to identify the vascular complication

     Excludes2   extravasation of vesicant agent (T80.81-)
       infiltration of vesicant agent (T80.81-)
       vascular complications specified as due to prosthetic devices, implants and grafts (T82.8- T83.8-, T84.8-, T85.8-)
       postprocedural vascular complications (T81.7-)
     Ⓔⓧ See PDX Collection 1436

● **T80.2** **Infections following infusion, transfusion and therapeutic injection**

     Use additional code to identify the specific infection, such as:
       sepsis (A41.9)

     Use additional code (R65.2-) to identify severe sepsis, if applicable

     Excludes2   infections specified as due to prosthetic devices, implants and grafts (T82.6-T82.7, T83.5-T83.6, T84.5-T84.7, T85.7)
       postprocedural infections (T81.4-)
     Ⓔⓧ **For category T80.2 CC codes:** See PDX Collection 948

     ● **T80.21** **Infection due to central venous catheter**
       Infection due to pulmonary artery catheter (Swan-Ganz catheter)

       ● **T80.211** **Bloodstream infection due to central venous catheter A** 🔹, **A** 🔹
         Catheter-related bloodstream infection (CRBSI) NOS
         Central line-associated bloodstream infection (CLABSI)
         Bloodstream infection due to Hickman catheter
         Bloodstream infection due to peripherally inserted central catheter (PICC)
         Bloodstream infection due to portacath (port-a-cath)
         Bloodstream infection due to pulmonary artery catheter
         Bloodstream infection due to triple lumen catheter
         Bloodstream infection due to umbilical venous catheter

CHAPTER 19 (S00-T88)

N Newborn Age: 0   **P** Pediatric Age: 0–17   **M** Maternity DX: 12–55   **A** Adult Age: 15–124   ♀ Females Only   ♂ Males Only

🔹 Complication\Comorbidity   🔹 Major C\C   Ⓔⓧ CC/MCC Exclusions   🔹 Hospital-Acquired Condition

1477

CHAPTER 19 (S00-T88)

● T80.212 Local infection due to central venous
catheter A 🔒, A 🔒
Exit or insertion site infection
Local infection due to Hickman
catheter
Local infection due to peripherally
inserted central catheter (PICC)
Local infection due to portacath
(port-a-cath)
Local infection due to pulmonary
artery catheter
Local infection due to triple lumen
catheter
Local infection due to umbilical
venous catheter
Port or reservoir infection
Tunnel infection

● T80.218 Other infection due to central venous
catheter A 🔒, A 🔒
Other central line-associated infection
Other infection due to Hickman
catheter
Other infection due to peripherally
inserted central catheter (PICC)
Other infection due to portacath
(port-a-cath)
Other infection due to pulmonary
artery catheter
Other infection due to triple lumen
catheter
Other infection due to umbilical
venous catheter

● T80.219 Unspecified infection due to central
venous catheter A 🔒, A 🔒
Central line-associated infection
NOS
Unspecified infection due to
Hickman catheter
Unspecified infection due to
peripherally inserted central
catheter (PICC)
Unspecified infection due to
portacath (port-a-cath)
Unspecified infection due to
pulmonary artery catheter
Unspecified infection due to triple
lumen catheter
Unspecified infection due to
umbilical venous catheter

X ● T80.22 Acute infection following transfusion, infusion,
or injection of blood and blood products A 🔒

X ● T80.29 Infection following other infusion, transfusion
and therapeutic injection A 🔒

● T80.3 ABO incompatibility reaction due to transfusion of
blood or blood products
Excludes1   minor blood group antigens reactions
(Duffy) (E) (K(ell)) (Kidd) (Lewis)
(M) (N) (P) (S) (T80.A)
(Ex:) For category T80.3 CC codes: See PDX Collection 1437

X ● T80.30 ABO incompatibility reaction due to
transfusion of blood or blood products,
unspecified A 🔒, A 🔒
ABO incompatibility blood transfusion NOS
Reaction to ABO incompatibility from
transfusion NOS

● T80.31 ABO incompatibility with hemolytic
transfusion reaction

● T80.310 ABO incompatibility with acute
hemolytic transfusion reaction A 🔒,
A 🔒
ABO incompatibility with hemolytic
transfusion reaction less than 24
hours after transfusion
Acute hemolytic transfusion
reaction (AHTR) due to ABO
incompatibility

● T80.311 ABO incompatibility with delayed
hemolytic transfusion reaction A 🔒,
A 🔒
ABO incompatibility with hemolytic
transfusion reaction 24 hours or
more after transfusion
Delayed hemolytic transfusion
reaction (DHTR) due to ABO
incompatibility

● T80.319 ABO incompatibility with hemolytic
transfusion reaction, unspecified A 🔒,
A 🔒
ABO incompatibility with
hemolytic transfusion reaction
at unspecified time after
transfusion
Hemolytic transfusion reaction
(HTR) due to ABO
incompatibility NOS

X ● T80.39 Other ABO incompatibility reaction due to
transfusion of blood or blood products A 🔒,
A 🔒
Delayed serologic transfusion reaction (DSTR)
from ABO incompatibility
Other ABO incompatible blood transfusion
Other reaction to ABO incompatible blood
transfusion

● T80.4 Rh incompatibility reaction due to transfusion of blood
or blood products
Reaction due to incompatibility of Rh antigens (C) (c)
(D) (E) (e)
(Ex:) For category T80.4 CC codes unless otherwise indicated: See PDX
Collection 1437

X ● T80.40 Rh incompatibility reaction due to transfusion
of blood or blood products, unspecified A 🔒
Reaction due to Rh factor in transfusion NOS
Rh incompatible blood transfusion NOS

● T80.41 Rh incompatibility with hemolytic transfusion
reaction

● T80.410 Rh incompatibility with acute
hemolytic transfusion reaction A 🔒
Acute hemolytic transfusion
reaction (AHTR) due to Rh
incompatibility
Rh incompatibility with hemolytic
transfusion reaction less than 24
hours after transfusion

● T80.411 Rh incompatibility with delayed
hemolytic transfusion reaction A 🔒
Delayed hemolytic transfusion
reaction (DHTR) due to Rh
incompatibility
Rh incompatibility with hemolytic
transfusion reaction 24 hours or
more after transfusion

● T80.419 Rh incompatibility with hemolytic
transfusion reaction, unspecified A 🔒
Rh incompatibility with hemolytic
transfusion reaction at
unspecified time after
transfusion
Hemolytic transfusion
reaction (HTR) due to Rh
incompatibility NOS

X ● T80.49 Other Rh incompatibility reaction due to
transfusion of blood or blood products A 🔒
Delayed serologic transfusion reaction (DSTR)
from Rh incompatibility
Other reaction to Rh incompatible blood
transfusion
(Ex:) See PDX Collection 1438

▶ New   ➡ Revised   ~~deleted~~ Deleted   Excludes 1   Excludes 2   Includes   Use additional   Code first   Code also   Key words
OGCR Official Guidelines   ● Unacceptable Principal Diagnosis   X Assign placeholder X   ● Use Additional Character(s)   ▶ Manifestation Code   Coding Clinic

●T80.A **Non-ABO incompatibility** reaction due to transfusion of blood or blood products
Reaction due to incompatibility of minor antigens (Duffy) (Kell) (Kidd) (Lewis) (M) (N) (P) (S)
(Ex) For category T80.A CC codes unless otherwise indicated: See PDX Collection 1438

X●T80.A0 **Non-ABO incompatibility reaction due to transfusion of blood or blood products, unspecified** A ⬡
Non-ABO antigen incompatibility reaction from transfusion NOS

●T80.A1 Non-ABO incompatibility with **hemolytic transfusion reaction**

●T80.A10 Non-ABO incompatibility with **acute hemolytic transfusion reaction** A ⬡
Acute hemolytic transfusion reaction (AHTR) due to non-ABO incompatibility
Non-ABO incompatibility with hemolytic transfusion reaction less than 24 hours after transfusion

●T80.A11 Non-ABO incompatibility with **delayed hemolytic transfusion reaction** A ⬡
Delayed hemolytic transfusion reaction (DHTR) due to non-ABO incompatibility
Non-ABO incompatibility with hemolytic transfusion reaction 24 or more hours after transfusion

●T80.A19 Non-ABO incompatibility with **hemolytic transfusion reaction, unspecified** A ⬡
Hemolytic transfusion reaction (HTR) due to non-ABO incompatibility NOS
Non-ABO incompatibility with hemolytic transfusion reaction at unspecified time after transfusion

X●T80.A9 **Other non-ABO incompatibility reaction due to transfusion of blood or blood products** A ⬡
Delayed serologic transfusion reaction (DSTR) from non-ABO incompatibility
Other reaction to non-ABO incompatible blood transfusion
(Ex) See PDX Collection 1437

●T80.5 **Anaphylactic reaction due to serum**
Allergic reaction due to serum
Anaphylactic shock due to serum
Anaphylactoid reaction due to serum
Anaphylaxis due to serum

Excludes1 ABO incompatibility reaction due to transfusion of blood or blood products (T80.3-)
allergic reaction or shock NOS (T78.2)
anaphylactic reaction or shock NOS (T78.2)
anaphylactic reaction or shock due to adverse effect of correct medicinal substance properly administered (T88.6)
other serum reaction (T80.6-)
(Ex) For category T80.5 CC codes: See PDX Collection 1439

X●T80.51 Anaphylactic reaction due to **administration of blood and blood products** A ⬡

X●T80.52 Anaphylactic reaction due to **vaccination** A ⬡

X●T80.59 Anaphylactic reaction due to **other serum** A ⬡

●T80.6 **Other serum reactions**
Intoxication by serum   Serum sickness
Protein sickness   Serum urticaria
Serum rash

Excludes2 serum hepatitis (B16-B19)
(Ex) For category T80.6 CC codes unless otherwise indicated: See PDX Collection 1439

X●T80.61 Other serum reaction due to **administration of blood and blood products** A ⬡

X●T80.62 Other serum reaction due to **vaccination** A ⬡

X●T80.69 Other serum reaction due to **other serum** A ⬡
▶ Code also, if applicable, arthropathy in hypersensitivity reactions classified elsewhere (M36.4)
(Ex) See PDX Collection 1440

●T80.8 **Other complications following infusion, transfusion and therapeutic injection**

●T80.81 **Extravasation of vesicant agent**
Infiltration of vesicant agent
(Ex) For category T80.81 CC codes: See PDX Collection 1439

●T80.810 **Extravasation of vesicant antineoplastic chemotherapy** A ⬡
Infiltration of vesicant antineoplastic chemotherapy

●T80.818 **Extravasation of other vesicant agent** A ⬡
Infiltration of other vesicant agent

X●T80.89 **Other complications following infusion, transfusion and therapeutic injection**
Delayed serologic transfusion reaction (DSTR), unspecified incompatibility
Use additional code to identify graft-versus-host reaction, if applicable, (D89.81-)

●T80.9 **Unspecified complication following infusion, transfusion and therapeutic injection**

X●T80.90 Unspecified complication **following infusion and therapeutic injection**

●T80.91 **Hemolytic transfusion reaction, unspecified incompatibility**
Excludes1 ABO incompatibility with hemolytic transfusion reaction (T80.31-)
Non-ABO incompatibility with hemolytic transfusion reaction (T80.A1-)
Rh incompatibility with hemolytic transfusion reaction (T80.41-)
(Ex) For category T80.91 CC codes: See PDX Collection 1437

●T80.910 **Acute hemolytic transfusion reaction, unspecified incompatibility** A ⬡

●T80.911 **Delayed hemolytic transfusion reaction, unspecified incompatibility** A ⬡

●T80.919 **Hemolytic transfusion reaction, unspecified incompatibility, unspecified as acute or delayed** A ⬡
Hemolytic transfusion reaction NOS

X●T80.92 **Unspecified transfusion reaction**

CHAPTER 19 (SØØ-T88)

Transfusion reaction NOS

● **T81   Complications of procedures, not elsewhere classified**

Use additional code for adverse effect, if applicable, to identify drug (T36-T50 with fifth or sixth character 5)

Excludes2   complications following immunization (T88.Ø-T88.1)

complications following infusion, transfusion and therapeutic injection (T80.-)

complications of transplanted organs and tissue (T86.-)

poisoning and toxic effects of drugs and chemicals (T36-T65 with fifth or sixth character 1-4 or 6)

specified complications classified elsewhere, such as:

complication of prosthetic devices, implants and grafts (T82-T85)

dermatitis due to drugs and medicaments (L23.3, L24.4, L25.1, L27.Ø-L27.1)

endosseous dental implant failure (M27.6-)

floppy iris syndrome (IFIS) (intraoperative) H21.81

intraoperative and postprocedural complications of specific body system (D78.-, E36.-, E89.-, G97.3-, G97.4, H59.3-, H59.-, H95.2-, H95.3, I97.4-, I97.5, J95, K91.-, L76.-, M96.-, N99.-)

ostomy complications (J95.Ø-, K94.-, N99.5-)

plateau iris syndrome (post-iridectomy) (postprocedural) H21.82

Coding Clinic: 2016, Q4, P29

The appropriate 7th character is to be added to each code from category T81

A	initial encounter
D	subsequent encounter
S	sequela

● **T81.1   Postprocedural shock**

Shock during or resulting from a procedure, not elsewhere classified

Excludes1   anaphylactic shock NOS (T78.2)

anaphylactic shock due to correct substance properly administered (T88.6)

anaphylactic shock due to serum (T80.5-)

anesthetic shock (T88.2)

electric shock (T75.4)

obstetric shock (O75.1)

septic shock (R65.21)

shock following abortion or ectopic or molar pregnancy (O00-O07, O08.3)

traumatic shock (T79.4)

(Ex) **For category T81.1 CC codes:** See PDX Collection 1441

X● **T81.10   Postprocedural shock unspecified** A 🔖

Collapse NOS during or resulting from a procedure, not elsewhere classified

Postprocedural failure of peripheral circulation

Postprocedural shock NOS

X● **T81.11   Postprocedural cardiogenic shock** A 🔖

●X● **T81.12   Postprocedural septic shock** A 🔖

Postprocedural endotoxic shock resulting from a procedure, not elsewhere classified

Postprocedural gram-negative shock resulting from a procedure, not elsewhere classified

Code first underlying infection

Use additional code, to identify any associated acute organ dysfunction, if applicable

X● **T81.19   Other postprocedural shock** A 🔖

Postprocedural hypovolemic shock

● **T81.3   Disruption of wound, not elsewhere classified**

Disruption of any suture materials or other closure methods

Excludes1   breakdown (mechanical) of permanent sutures (T85.612)

displacement of permanent sutures (T85.622)

disruption of cesarean delivery wound (O90.Ø)

disruption of perineal obstetric wound (O90.1)

mechanical complication of permanent sutures NEC (T85.692)

(Ex) **For category T81.3 CC codes:** See PDX Collection 1442

X● **T81.30   Disruption of wound, unspecified** A 🔖

Disruption of wound NOS

X● **T81.31   Disruption of external operation (surgical) wound, not elsewhere classified** A 🔖

Excludes1   dehiscence of amputation stump (T87.81)

Dehiscence of operation wound NOS

Disruption of operation wound NOS

Disruption or dehiscence of closure of cornea

Disruption or dehiscence of closure of mucosa

Disruption or dehiscence of closure of skin and subcutaneous tissue

Full-thickness skin disruption or dehiscence

Superficial disruption or dehiscence of operation wound

Coding Clinic: 2015, Q1, P20

X● **T81.32   Disruption of internal operation (surgical) wound, not elsewhere classified** A 🔖

Deep disruption or dehiscence of operation wound NOS

Disruption or dehiscence of closure of internal organ or other internal tissue

Disruption or dehiscence of closure of muscle or muscle flap

Disruption or dehiscence of closure of ribs or rib cage

Disruption or dehiscence of closure of skull or craniotomy

Disruption or dehiscence of closure of sternum or sternotomy

Disruption or dehiscence of closure of tendon or ligament

Disruption or dehiscence of closure of superficial or muscular fascia

X● **T81.33   Disruption of traumatic injury wound repair** A 🔖

Disruption or dehiscence of closure of traumatic laceration (external) (internal)

▶ New   ⟹ Revised   ~~deleted~~ Deleted   Excludes 1   Excludes 2   Includes   Use additional   Code first   Code also   Key words

OGCR Official Guidelines   ● Unacceptable Principal Diagnosis   X Assign placeholder X   ● Use Additional Character(s)   ▷ Manifestation Code   **Coding Clinic**

X⬤ **T81.4**   **Infection following a procedure** A 🅒, A 🅜

     Intra-abdominal abscess following a procedure
     Postprocedural infection, not elsewhere classified
     Sepsis following a procedure
     Stitch abscess following a procedure
     Subphrenic abscess following a procedure
     Wound abscess following a procedure

     Use additional code to identify infection

     Use additional code (R65.2-) to identify severe sepsis, if applicable

     Excludes1   obstetric surgical wound infection (O86.0)
                       postprocedural fever NOS (R50.82)
                       postprocedural retroperitoneal abscess (K68.11)

     Excludes2   bleb associated endophthalmitis (H59.4-)
                       infection due to infusion, transfusion and therapeutic injection (T80.2-)
                       infection due to prosthetic devices, implants and grafts (T82.6-T82.7, T83.5-T83.6, T84.5-T84.7, T85.7)

     Ⓔˣ See PDX Collection 805

     Coding Clinic: 2015, Q4, P37

⬤ **T81.5**   **Complications of foreign body accidentally left in body following procedure**

     Ⓔˣ For category T81.5 CC codes: See PDX Collection 1443

   ⬤ **T81.50**   Unspecified complication of foreign body accidentally left in body following procedure

     ⬤ **T81.500**   Unspecified complication of foreign body accidentally left in body following surgical operation A 🅒, A 🅜

     ⬤ **T81.501**   Unspecified complication of foreign body accidentally left in body following infusion or transfusion A 🅒, A 🅜

     ⬤ **T81.502**   Unspecified complication of foreign body accidentally left in body following kidney dialysis A 🅒, A 🅜

     ⬤ **T81.503**   Unspecified complication of foreign body accidentally left in body following injection or immunization A 🅒, A 🅜

     ⬤ **T81.504**   Unspecified complication of foreign body accidentally left in body following endoscopic examination A 🅒, A 🅜

     ⬤ **T81.505**   Unspecified complication of foreign body accidentally left in body following heart catheterization A 🅒, A 🅜

     ⬤ **T81.506**   Unspecified complication of foreign body accidentally left in body following aspiration, puncture or other catheterization A 🅒, A 🅜

     ⬤ **T81.507**   Unspecified complication of foreign body accidentally left in body following removal of catheter or packing A 🅒, A 🅜

     ⬤ **T81.508**   Unspecified complication of foreign body accidentally left in body following other procedure A 🅒, A 🅜

     ⬤ **T81.509**   Unspecified complication of foreign body accidentally left in body following unspecified procedure A 🅒, A 🅜

⬤ **T81.51**   **Adhesions due to foreign body accidentally left in body following procedure**

     ⬤ **T81.510**   Adhesions due to foreign body accidentally left in body following surgical operation A 🅒, A 🅜

     ⬤ **T81.511**   Adhesions due to foreign body accidentally left in body following infusion or transfusion A 🅒, A 🅜

     ⬤ **T81.512**   Adhesions due to foreign body accidentally left in body following kidney dialysis A 🅒, A 🅜

     ⬤ **T81.513**   Adhesions due to foreign body accidentally left in body following injection or immunization A 🅒, A 🅜

     ⬤ **T81.514**   Adhesions due to foreign body accidentally left in body following endoscopic examination A 🅒, A 🅜

     ⬤ **T81.515**   Adhesions due to foreign body accidentally left in body following heart catheterization A 🅒, A 🅜

     ⬤ **T81.516**   Adhesions due to foreign body accidentally left in body following aspiration, puncture or other catheterization A 🅒, A 🅜

     ⬤ **T81.517**   Adhesions due to foreign body accidentally left in body following removal of catheter or packing A 🅒, A 🅜

     ⬤ **T81.518**   Adhesions due to foreign body accidentally left in body following other procedure A 🅒, A 🅜

     ⬤ **T81.519**   Adhesions due to foreign body accidentally left in body following unspecified procedure A 🅒, A 🅜

   ⬤ **T81.52**   Obstruction due to foreign body accidentally left in body following procedure

     ⬤ **T81.520**   Obstruction due to foreign body accidentally left in body following surgical operation A 🅒, A 🅜

     ⬤ **T81.521**   Obstruction due to foreign body accidentally left in body following infusion or transfusion A 🅒, A 🅜

     ⬤ **T81.522**   Obstruction due to foreign body accidentally left in body following kidney dialysis A 🅒, A 🅜

     ⬤ **T81.523**   Obstruction due to foreign body accidentally left in body following injection or immunization A 🅒, A 🅜

     ⬤ **T81.524**   Obstruction due to foreign body accidentally left in body following endoscopic examination A 🅒, A 🅜

     ⬤ **T81.525**   Obstruction due to foreign body accidentally left in body following heart catheterization A 🅒, A 🅜

     ⬤ **T81.526**   Obstruction due to foreign body accidentally left in body following aspiration, puncture or other catheterization A 🅒, A 🅜

     ⬤ **T81.527**   Obstruction due to foreign body accidentally left in body following removal of catheter or packing A 🅒, A 🅜

     ⬤ **T81.528**   Obstruction due to foreign body accidentally left in body following other procedure A 🅒, A 🅜

     ⬤ **T81.529**   Obstruction due to foreign body accidentally left in body following unspecified procedure A 🅒, A 🅜

● **T81.53** Perforation due to foreign body accidentally left in body following procedure

  ● **T81.530** Perforation due to foreign body accidentally left in body following surgical operation A 🐾, A 🐾

  ● **T81.531** Perforation due to foreign body accidentally left in body following infusion or transfusion A 🐾, A 🐾

  ● **T81.532** Perforation due to foreign body accidentally left in body following kidney dialysis A 🐾, A 🐾

  ● **T81.533** Perforation due to foreign body accidentally left in body following injection or immunization A 🐾, A 🐾

  ● **T81.534** Perforation due to foreign body accidentally left in body following endoscopic examination A 🐾, A 🐾

  ● **T81.535** Perforation due to foreign body accidentally left in body following heart catheterization A 🐾, A 🐾

  ● **T81.536** Perforation due to foreign body accidentally left in body following aspiration, puncture or other catheterization A 🐾, A 🐾

  ● **T81.537** Perforation due to foreign body accidentally left in body following removal of catheter or packing A 🐾, A 🐾

  ● **T81.538** Perforation due to foreign body accidentally left in body following other procedure A 🐾, A 🐾

  ● **T81.539** Perforation due to foreign body accidentally left in body following unspecified procedure A 🐾, A 🐾

● **T81.59** Other complications of foreign body accidentally left in body following procedure

  Excludes2 obstruction or perforation due to prosthetic devices and implants intentionally left in body (T82.0-T82.5, T83.0-T83.4, T83.7, T84.0-T84.4, T85.0-T85.6)

  ● **T81.590** Other complications of foreign body accidentally left in body following surgical operation A 🐾, A 🐾

  ● **T81.591** Other complications of foreign body accidentally left in body following infusion or transfusion A 🐾, A 🐾

  ● **T81.592** Other complications of foreign body accidentally left in body following kidney dialysis A 🐾, A 🐾

  ● **T81.593** Other complications of foreign body accidentally left in body following injection or immunization A 🐾, A 🐾

  ● **T81.594** Other complications of foreign body accidentally left in body following endoscopic examination A 🐾, A 🐾

  ● **T81.595** Other complications of foreign body accidentally left in body following heart catheterization A 🐾, A 🐾

  ● **T81.596** Other complications of foreign body accidentally left in body following aspiration, puncture or other catheterization A 🐾, A 🐾

  ● **T81.597** Other complications of foreign body accidentally left in body following removal of catheter or packing A 🐾, A 🐾

  ● **T81.598** Other complications of foreign body accidentally left in body following other procedure A 🐾, A 🐾

  ● **T81.599** Other complications of foreign body accidentally left in body following unspecified procedure A 🐾, A 🐾

● **T81.6** Acute reaction to foreign substance accidentally left during a procedure

  Excludes2 complications of foreign body accidentally left in body cavity or operation wound following procedure (T81.5-)

  Ⓔ For category T81.6 CC codes: See PDX Collection 1444

X ● **T81.60** Unspecified acute reaction to foreign substance accidentally left during a procedure A 🐾, A 🐾

X ● **T81.61** Aseptic peritonitis due to foreign substance accidentally left during a procedure A 🐾, A 🐾
    Chemical peritonitis

X ● **T81.69** Other acute reaction to foreign substance accidentally left during a procedure A 🐾, A 🐾

● **T81.7** Vascular complications following a procedure, not elsewhere classified
  Air embolism following procedure NEC
  Phlebitis or thrombophlebitis resulting from a procedure

  Excludes1 embolism complicating abortion or ectopic or molar pregnancy (O00-O07, O08.2)
    embolism complicating pregnancy, childbirth and the puerperium (O88.-)
    traumatic embolism (T79.0)

  Excludes2 embolism due to prosthetic devices, implants and grafts (T82.8, T83.81, T84.8-, T85.1-)
    embolism following infusion, transfusion and therapeutic injection (T80.0)

  ● **T81.71** Complication of artery following a procedure, not elsewhere classified

    ● **T81.710** Complication of mesenteric artery following a procedure, not elsewhere classified A 🐾
      Ⓔ See PDX Collection 1445

    ● **T81.711** Complication of renal artery following a procedure, not elsewhere classified A 🐾
      Ⓔ See PDX Collection 1445

    ● **T81.718** Complication of other artery following a procedure, not elsewhere classified A 🐾
      Ⓔ See PDX Collection 1446

    ● **T81.719** Complication of unspecified artery following a procedure, not elsewhere classified A 🐾
      Ⓔ See PDX Collection 1446

X ● **T81.72** Complication of vein following a procedure, not elsewhere classified A 🐾
    Ⓔ See PDX Collection 1446

● **T81.8**   **Other complications of procedures, not elsewhere classified**

     Excludes2   hypothermia following anesthesia (T88.51)
                 malignant hyperpyrexia due to anesthesia (T88.3)

X ● **T81.81**   **Complication of inhalation therapy**

X ● **T81.82**   **Emphysema (subcutaneous) resulting from a procedure**

X ● **T81.83**   **Persistent postprocedural fistula** A 🦠
       (Ex) See PDX Collection 1447

X ● **T81.89**   **Other complications of procedures, not elsewhere classified**
       Use additional code to specify complication, such as:
           postprocedural delirium (F05)

X ● **T81.9**   **Unspecified complication of procedure**

● **T82**   **Complications of cardiac and vascular prosthetic devices, implants and grafts**

     Excludes2   failure and rejection of transplanted organs and tissue (T86.-)

     The appropriate 7th character is to be added to each code from category T82

> A   initial encounter
> D   subsequent encounter
> S   sequela

● **T82.0**   **Mechanical complication of heart valve prosthesis**
     Mechanical complication of artificial heart valve

     Excludes1   mechanical complication of biological heart valve graft (T82.22-)

     (Ex) For category T82.0 CC codes: See PDX Collection 1448

X ● **T82.01**   **Breakdown (mechanical) of heart valve prosthesis** A 🦠

X ● **T82.02**   **Displacement of heart valve prosthesis** A 🦠
       Malposition of heart valve prosthesis

X ● **T82.03**   **Leakage of heart valve prosthesis** A 🦠

X ● **T82.09**   **Other mechanical complication of heart valve prosthesis** A 🦠
       Obstruction (mechanical) of heart valve prosthesis
       Perforation of heart valve prosthesis
       Protrusion of heart valve prosthesis

● **T82.1**   **Mechanical complication of cardiac electronic device**
     (Ex) For category T82.1 CC codes unless otherwise indicated: See PDX Collection 1449

   ● **T82.11**   **Breakdown (mechanical) of cardiac electronic device**

     ● **T82.110**   **Breakdown (mechanical) of cardiac electrode** A 🦠

     ● **T82.111**   **Breakdown (mechanical) of cardiac pulse generator (battery)** A 🦠

     ● **T82.118**   **Breakdown (mechanical) of other cardiac electronic device** A 🦠
         (Ex) See PDX Collection 1450

     ● **T82.119**   **Breakdown (mechanical) of unspecified cardiac electronic device** A 🦠
         (Ex) No Exclusions

   ● **T82.12**   **Displacement of cardiac electronic device**
     Malposition of cardiac electronic device

     ● **T82.120**   **Displacement of cardiac electrode** A 🦠

     ● **T82.121**   **Displacement of cardiac pulse generator (battery)** A 🦠

     ● **T82.128**   **Displacement of other cardiac electronic device** A 🦠
         (Ex) See PDX Collection 1450

     ● **T82.129**   **Displacement of unspecified cardiac electronic device** A 🦠
         (Ex) No Exclusions

   ● **T82.19**   **Other mechanical complication of cardiac electronic device**
     Leakage of cardiac electronic device
     Obstruction of cardiac electronic device
     Perforation of cardiac electronic device
     Protrusion of cardiac electronic device

     ● **T82.190**   **Other mechanical complication of cardiac electrode** A 🦠

     ● **T82.191**   **Other mechanical complication of cardiac pulse generator (battery)** A 🦠

     ● **T82.198**   **Other mechanical complication of other cardiac electronic device** A 🦠
         (Ex) See PDX Collection 1450

     ● **T82.199**   **Other mechanical complication of unspecified cardiac device** A 🦠
         (Ex) No Exclusions

● **T82.2**   **Mechanical complication of coronary artery bypass graft and biological heart valve graft**

     Excludes1   mechanical complication of artificial heart valve prosthesis (T82.0-)

   ● **T82.21**   **Mechanical complication of coronary artery bypass graft**
     (Ex) For category T82.21 CC codes: See PDX Collection 1451

     ● **T82.211**   **Breakdown (mechanical) of coronary artery bypass graft** A 🦠

     ● **T82.212**   **Displacement of coronary artery bypass graft** A 🦠
         Malposition of coronary artery bypass graft

     ● **T82.213**   **Leakage of coronary artery bypass graft** A 🦠

     ● **T82.218**   **Other mechanical complication of coronary artery bypass graft** A 🦠
         Obstruction, mechanical of coronary artery bypass graft
         Perforation of coronary artery bypass graft
         Protrusion of coronary artery bypass graft

   ● **T82.22**   **Mechanical complication of biological heart valve graft**
     (Ex) For category T82.22 CC codes: See PDX Collection 1450

     ● **T82.221**   **Breakdown (mechanical) of biological heart valve graft** A 🦠

     ● **T82.222**   **Displacement of biological heart valve graft** A 🦠
         Malposition of biological heart valve graft

     ● **T82.223**   **Leakage of biological heart valve graft** A 🦠

     ● **T82.228**   **Other mechanical complication of biological heart valve graft** A 🦠
         Obstruction of biological heart valve graft
         Perforation of biological heart valve graft
         Protrusion of biological heart valve graft

CHAPTER 19 (S00-T88)

● **T82.3** **Mechanical complication of other vascular grafts**
   (Ex) For category T82.3 CC codes: See PDX Collection 1452

  ● **T82.31** **Breakdown (mechanical) of other vascular grafts**

    ● **T82.310** **Breakdown (mechanical) of aortic (bifurcation) graft (replacement)** A 🦠

    ● **T82.311** **Breakdown (mechanical) of carotid arterial graft (bypass)** A 🦠

    ● **T82.312** **Breakdown (mechanical) of femoral arterial graft (bypass)** A 🦠

    ● **T82.318** **Breakdown (mechanical) of other vascular grafts** A 🦠

    ● **T82.319** **Breakdown (mechanical) of unspecified vascular grafts** A 🦠

  ● **T82.32** **Displacement of other vascular grafts**
    Malposition of other vascular grafts

    ● **T82.320** **Displacement of aortic (bifurcation) graft (replacement)** A 🦠

    ● **T82.321** **Displacement of carotid arterial graft (bypass)** A 🦠

    ● **T82.322** **Displacement of femoral arterial graft (bypass)** A 🦠

    ● **T82.328** **Displacement of other vascular grafts** A 🦠

    ● **T82.329** **Displacement of unspecified vascular grafts** A 🦠

  ● **T82.33** **Leakage of other vascular grafts**

    ● **T82.330** **Leakage of aortic (bifurcation) graft (replacement)** A 🦠

    ● **T82.331** **Leakage of carotid arterial graft (bypass)** A 🦠

    ● **T82.332** **Leakage of femoral arterial graft (bypass)** A 🦠

    ● **T82.338** **Leakage of other vascular grafts** A 🦠

    ● **T82.339** **Leakage of unspecified vascular graft** A 🦠

  ● **T82.39** **Other mechanical complication of other vascular grafts**
    Obstruction (mechanical) of other vascular grafts
    Perforation of other vascular grafts
    Protrusion of other vascular grafts

    ● **T82.390** **Other mechanical complication of aortic (bifurcation) graft (replacement)** A 🦠

    ● **T82.391** **Other mechanical complication of carotid arterial graft (bypass)** A 🦠

    ● **T82.392** **Other mechanical complication of femoral arterial graft (bypass)** A 🦠

    ● **T82.398** **Other mechanical complication of other vascular grafts** A 🦠

    ● **T82.399** **Other mechanical complication of unspecified vascular grafts** A 🦠

● **T82.4** **Mechanical complication of vascular dialysis catheter**
   Mechanical complication of hemodialysis catheter

   Excludes1   mechanical complication of intraperitoneal dialysis catheter (T85.62)
   (Ex) For category T82.4 CC codes: See PDX Collection 1452

  X ● **T82.41** **Breakdown (mechanical) of vascular dialysis catheter** A 🦠

  X ● **T82.42** **Displacement of vascular dialysis catheter** A 🦠
    Malposition of vascular dialysis catheter

  X ● **T82.43** **Leakage of vascular dialysis catheter** A 🦠

  X ● **T82.49** **Other complication of vascular dialysis catheter** A 🦠
    Obstruction (mechanical) of vascular dialysis catheter
    Perforation of vascular dialysis catheter
    Protrusion of vascular dialysis catheter

● **T82.5** **Mechanical complication of other cardiac and vascular devices and implants**

   Excludes2   mechanical complication of epidural and subdural infusion catheter (T85.61)
   (Ex) For category T82.5 CC codes unless otherwise indicated: See PDX Collection 1452

  ● **T82.51** **Breakdown (mechanical) of other cardiac and vascular devices and implants**

    ● **T82.510** **Breakdown (mechanical) of surgically created arteriovenous fistula** A 🦠

    ● **T82.511** **Breakdown (mechanical) of surgically created arteriovenous shunt** A 🦠

    ● **T82.512** **Breakdown (mechanical) of artificial heart** A 🦠
      (Ex) See PDX Collection 1450

    ● **T82.513** **Breakdown (mechanical) of balloon (counterpulsation) device** A 🦠

    ● **T82.514** **Breakdown (mechanical) of infusion catheter** A 🦠

    ● **T82.515** **Breakdown (mechanical) of umbrella device** A 🦠

    ● **T82.518** **Breakdown (mechanical) of other cardiac and vascular devices and implants** A 🦠

    ● **T82.519** **Breakdown (mechanical) of unspecified cardiac and vascular devices and implants** A 🦠
      (Ex) See PDX Collection 1453

  ● **T82.52** **Displacement of other cardiac and vascular devices and implants**
    Malposition of other cardiac and vascular devices and implants

    ● **T82.520** **Displacement of surgically created arteriovenous fistula** A 🦠

    ● **T82.521** **Displacement of surgically created arteriovenous shunt** A 🦠

    ● **T82.522** **Displacement of artificial heart** A 🦠
      (Ex) See PDX Collection 1450

    ● **T82.523** **Displacement of balloon (counterpulsation) device** A 🦠

    ● **T82.524** **Displacement of infusion catheter** A 🦠

    ● **T82.525** **Displacement of umbrella device** A 🦠

    ● **T82.528** **Displacement of other cardiac and vascular devices and implants** A 🦠

    ● **T82.529** **Displacement of unspecified cardiac and vascular devices and implants** A 🦠

  ● **T82.53** **Leakage of other cardiac and vascular devices and implants**

    ● **T82.530** **Leakage of surgically created arteriovenous fistula** A 🦠

    ● **T82.531** **Leakage of surgically created arteriovenous shunt** A 🦠

    ● **T82.532** **Leakage of artificial heart** A 🦠
      (Ex) See PDX Collection 1450

    ● **T82.533** **Leakage of balloon (counterpulsation) device** A 🦠

    ● **T82.534** **Leakage of infusion catheter** A 🦠

    ● **T82.535** **Leakage of umbrella device** A 🦠

    ● **T82.538** **Leakage of other cardiac and vascular devices and implants** A 🦠

    ● **T82.539** **Leakage of unspecified cardiac and vascular devices and implants** A 🦠
      (Ex) See PDX Collection 1453

▶ New   ⇒ Revised   ~~deleted~~ Deleted   Excludes 1   Excludes 2   Includes   Use additional   Code first   Code also   Key words

OGCR Official Guidelines   ● Unacceptable Principal Diagnosis   X Assign placeholder X   ● Use Additional Character(s)   ▸ Manifestation Code   **Coding Clinic**

● **T82.59** Other mechanical complication of other cardiac and vascular devices and implants
Obstruction (mechanical) of other cardiac and vascular devices and implants
Perforation of other cardiac and vascular devices and implants
Protrusion of other cardiac and vascular devices and implants

● **T82.590** Other mechanical complication of surgically created arteriovenous fistula A 🖐

● **T82.591** Other mechanical complication of surgically created arteriovenous shunt A 🖐

● **T82.592** Other mechanical complication of artificial heart A 🖐
(Ex) See PDX Collection 1450

● **T82.593** Other mechanical complication of balloon (counterpulsation) device

● **T82.594** Other mechanical complication of infusion catheter A 🖐
(Ex) See PDX Collection 1450

● **T82.595** Other mechanical complication of umbrella device A 🖐

● **T82.598** Other mechanical complication of other cardiac and vascular devices and implants A 🖐
(Ex) See PDX Collection 1450

● **T82.599** Other mechanical complication of unspecified cardiac and vascular devices and implants A 🖐
(Ex) See PDX Collection 1453

X ● **T82.6** Infection and inflammatory reaction due to cardiac valve prosthesis A 🖐, A 🖐
Use additional code to identify infection
(Ex) See PDX Collection 1454

X ● **T82.7** Infection and inflammatory reaction due to other cardiac and vascular devices, implants and grafts A 🖐, A 🖐
Use additional code to identify infection
(Ex) See PDX Collection 1454

● **T82.8** Other specified complications of cardiac and vascular prosthetic devices, implants and grafts

● **T82.81** Embolism due to cardiac and vascular prosthetic devices, implants and grafts
Coding Clinic: 2016, Q4, P70

● **T82.817** Embolism due to cardiac prosthetic devices, implants and grafts A 🖐
(Ex) See PDX Collection 1455
Coding Clinic: 2016, Q4, P70; 2015, Q1, P20

● **T82.818** Embolism due to vascular prosthetic devices, implants and grafts A 🖐
(Ex) See PDX Collection 1454

● **T82.82** Fibrosis due to cardiac and vascular prosthetic devices, implants and grafts
Coding Clinic: 2016, Q4, P70

● **T82.827** Fibrosis due to cardiac prosthetic devices, implants and grafts A 🖐
(Ex) See PDX Collection 1455

● **T82.828** Fibrosis due to vascular prosthetic devices, implants and grafts A 🖐
(Ex) See PDX Collection 1454

● **T82.83** Hemorrhage due to cardiac and vascular prosthetic devices, implants and grafts
Coding Clinic: 2016, Q4, P70

● **T82.837** Hemorrhage due to cardiac prosthetic devices, implants and grafts A 🖐
(Ex) See PDX Collection 1455

● **T82.838** Hemorrhage due to vascular prosthetic devices, implants and grafts A 🖐
(Ex) See PDX Collection 1454

● **T82.84** Pain due to cardiac and vascular prosthetic devices, implants and grafts
Coding Clinic: 2016, Q4, P70

● **T82.847** Pain due to cardiac prosthetic devices, implants and grafts A 🖐
(Ex) See PDX Collection 1455

● **T82.848** Pain due to vascular prosthetic devices, implants and grafts A 🖐
(Ex) See PDX Collection 1454

● **T82.85** Stenosis due to cardiac and vascular prosthetic devices, implants and grafts

● **T82.855** Stenosis of coronary artery stent A 🖐
In-stent stenosis (restenosis) of coronary artery stent
Restenosis of coronary artery stent
(Ex) See PDX Collection 1455
Coding Clinic: 2016, Q4, P70

● **T82.856** Stenosis of peripheral vascular stent A 🖐
In-stent stenosis (restenosis) of peripheral vascular stent
Restenosis of peripheral vascular stent
(Ex) See PDX Collection 1454
Coding Clinic: 2016, Q4, P70

● **T82.857** Stenosis of other cardiac prosthetic devices, implants and grafts A 🖐
(Ex) See PDX Collection 1455
Coding Clinic: 2016, Q4, P70

● **T82.858** Stenosis of other vascular prosthetic devices, implants and grafts A 🖐
(Ex) See PDX Collection 1454
Coding Clinic: 2016, Q4, P70

● **T82.86** Thrombosis of cardiac and vascular prosthetic devices, implants and grafts

● **T82.867** Thrombosis due to cardiac prosthetic devices, implants and grafts A 🖐
(Ex) See PDX Collection 1455

● **T82.868** Thrombosis due to vascular prosthetic devices, implants and grafts A 🖐
(Ex) See PDX Collection 1454

● **T82.89** Other specified complication of cardiac and vascular prosthetic devices, implants and grafts

● **T82.897** Other specified complication of cardiac prosthetic devices, implants and grafts A 🖐
(Ex) See PDX Collection 1455

● **T82.898** Other specified complication of vascular prosthetic devices, implants and grafts A 🖐
(Ex) See PDX Collection 1454

X ● **T82.9** Unspecified complication of cardiac and vascular prosthetic device, implant and graft A 🖐
(Ex) See PDX Collection 1455

CHAPTER 19 (S00-T88)

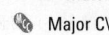

CHAPTER 19 (S00-T88)

● **T83** **Complications of genitourinary prosthetic devices, implants and grafts**

    Excludes2   failure and rejection of transplanted organs and tissue (T86.-)

    The appropriate 7th character is to be added to each code from category T83

      | | |
    A   initial encounter
    D   subsequent encounter
    S   sequela

    (Ex) For category T83 CC codes: See PDX Collection 1456
    Coding Clinic: 2016, Q4, P70-71

  ● **T83.0** **Mechanical complication of urinary catheter**

      Excludes2   complications of stoma of urinary tract (N99.5-)

      Coding Clinic: 2016, Q4, P70

    ● **T83.01** **Breakdown (mechanical) of urinary catheter**

      ● **T83.010** **Breakdown (mechanical) of cystostomy catheter** A 🔓

      ● **T83.011** **Breakdown (mechanical) of indwelling urethral catheter**

      ● **T83.012** **Breakdown (mechanical) of nephrostomy catheter**

      ● **T83.018** **Breakdown (mechanical) of other urinary catheter**
          Breakdown (mechanical) of Hopkins catheter
          Breakdown (mechanical) of ileostomy catheter
          Breakdown (mechanical) urostomy catheter

    ● **T83.02** **Displacement of urinary catheter**
      Malposition of urinary catheter

      ● **T83.020** **Displacement of cystostomy catheter** A 🔓

      ● **T83.021** **Displacement of indwelling urethral catheter**

      ● **T83.022** **Displacement of nephrostomy catheter**

      ● **T83.028** **Displacement of other urinary catheter**
          Displacement of Hopkins catheter
          Displacement of ileostomy catheter
          Displacement of urostomy catheter

    ● **T83.03** **Leakage of urinary catheter**

      ● **T83.030** **Leakage of cystostomy catheter** A 🔓

      ● **T83.031** **Leakage of indwelling urethral catheter**

      ● **T83.032** **Leakage of nephrostomy catheter**

      ● **T83.038** **Leakage of other urinary catheter**
          Leakage of Hopkins catheter
          Leakage of ileostomy catheter
          Leakage of urostomy catheter

    ● **T83.09** **Other mechanical complication of urinary catheter**
      Obstruction (mechanical) of urinary catheter
      Perforation of urinary catheter
      Protrusion of urinary catheter

      ● **T83.090** **Other mechanical complication of cystostomy catheter** A 🔓

      ● **T83.091** **Other mechanical complication of indwelling urethral catheter**

      ● **T83.092** **Other mechanical complication of nephrostomy catheter**

      ● **T83.098** **Other mechanical complication of other urinary catheter**
          Other mechanical complication of Hopkins catheter
          Other mechanical complication of ileostomy catheter
          Other mechanical complication of urostomy catheter

  ● **T83.1** **Mechanical complication of other urinary devices and implants**
    Coding Clinic: 2016, Q4, P70

    ● **T83.11** **Breakdown (mechanical) of other urinary devices and implants**

      ● **T83.110** **Breakdown (mechanical) of urinary electronic stimulator device** A 🔓

        Excludes2   Breakdown (mechanical) of electrode (lead) for sacral nerve neurostimulator (T85.111)
                Breakdown (mechanical) of implanted electronic sacral neurostimulator, pulse generator or receiver (T85.113)

      ● **T83.111** **Breakdown (mechanical) of implanted urinary sphincter** A 🔓

      ● **T83.112** **Breakdown (mechanical) of indwelling ureteral stent** A 🔓

      ● **T83.113** **Breakdown (mechanical) of other urinary stents** A 🔓
          Breakdown (mechanical) of ileal conduit stent
          Breakdown (mechanical) of nephroureteral stent

      ● **T83.118** **Breakdown (mechanical) of other urinary devices and implants** A 🔓

    ● **T83.12** **Displacement of other urinary devices and implants**
      Malposition of other urinary devices and implants

      ● **T83.120** **Displacement of urinary electronic stimulator device** A 🔓

        Excludes2   Displacement of electrode (lead) for sacral nerve neurostimulator (T85.121)
                Displacement of implanted electronic sacral neurostimulator, pulse generator or receiver (T85.123)

      ● **T83.121** **Displacement of implanted urinary sphincter** A 🔓

      ● **T83.122** **Displacement of indwelling ureteral stent** A 🔓

      ● **T83.123** **Displacement of other urinary stents** A 🔓
          Displacement of ileal conduit stent
          Displacement of nephroureteral stent

      ● **T83.128** **Displacement of other urinary devices and implants** A 🔓

● **T83.19 Other mechanical complication of other urinary devices and implants**
     Leakage of other urinary devices and implants
     Obstruction (mechanical) of other urinary devices and implants
     Perforation of other urinary devices and implants
     Protrusion of other urinary devices and implants

  ● **T83.190 Other mechanical complication of urinary electronic stimulator device** A 🦠

        Excludes2   Other mechanical complication of electrode (lead) for sacral nerve neurostimulator (T85.191)
                Other mechanical complication of implanted electronic sacral neurostimulator, pulse generator or receiver (T85.193)

  ● **T83.191 Other mechanical complication of implanted urinary sphincter** A 🦠

  ● **T83.192 Other mechanical complication of indwelling ureteral stent** A 🦠

  ● **T83.193 Other mechanical complication of other urinary stent** A 🦠
      Other mechanical complication of ileal conduit stent
      Other mechanical complication of nephroureteral stent

  ● **T83.198 Other mechanical complication of other urinary devices and implants** A 🦠

● **T83.2 Mechanical complication of graft of urinary organ**
    Coding Clinic: 2016, Q4, P70

  X ● **T83.21 Breakdown (mechanical) of graft of urinary organ** A 🦠

  X ● **T83.22 Displacement of graft of urinary organ** A 🦠
      Malposition of graft of urinary organ

  X ● **T83.23 Leakage of graft of urinary organ** A 🦠

  X ● **T83.24 Erosion of graft of urinary organ** A 🦠
      Coding Clinic: 2016, Q4, P70

  X ● **T83.25 Exposure of graft of urinary organ** A 🦠
      Coding Clinic: 2016, Q4, P70

  X ● **T83.29 Other mechanical complication of graft of urinary organ** A 🦠
      Obstruction (mechanical) of graft of urinary organ
      Perforation of graft of urinary organ
      Protrusion of graft of urinary organ

● **T83.3 Mechanical complication of intrauterine contraceptive device**

  X ● **T83.31 Breakdown (mechanical) of intrauterine contraceptive device** ♀

  X ● **T83.32 Displacement of intrauterine contraceptive device** ♀
      Malposition of intrauterine contraceptive device
      Missing string of intrauterine contraceptive device

  X ● **T83.39 Other mechanical complication of intrauterine contraceptive device** ♀
      Leakage of intrauterine contraceptive device
      Obstruction (mechanical) of intrauterine contraceptive device
      Perforation of intrauterine contraceptive device
      Protrusion of intrauterine contraceptive device

● **T83.4 Mechanical complication of other prosthetic devices, implants and grafts of genital tract**
    Coding Clinic: 2016, Q4, P71

  ● **T83.41 Breakdown (mechanical) of other prosthetic devices, implants and grafts of genital tract**

    ● **T83.410 Breakdown (mechanical) of implanted penile prosthesis** ♂ A 🦠
       Breakdown (mechanical) of penile prosthesis cylinder
       Breakdown (mechanical) of penile prosthesis pump
       Breakdown (mechanical) of penile prosthesis reservoir

    ● **T83.411 Breakdown (mechanical) of implanted testicular prosthesis** A 🦠

    ● **T83.418 Breakdown (mechanical) of other prosthetic devices, implants and grafts of genital tract** A 🦠

  ● **T83.42 Displacement of other prosthetic devices, implants and grafts of genital tract**
      Malposition of other prosthetic devices, implants and grafts of genital tract

    ● **T83.420 Displacement of implanted penile prosthesis** ♂ A 🦠
       Displacement of penile prosthesis cylinder
       Displacement of penile prosthesis pump
       Displacement of penile prosthesis reservoir

    ● **T83.421 Displacement of implanted testicular prosthesis** A 🦠

    ● **T83.428 Displacement of other prosthetic devices, implants and grafts of genital tract** A 🦠

  ● **T83.49 Other mechanical complication of other prosthetic devices, implants and grafts of genital tract**
      Leakage of other prosthetic devices, implants and grafts of genital tract
      Obstruction, mechanical of other prosthetic devices, implants and grafts of genital tract
      Perforation of other prosthetic devices, implants and grafts of genital tract
      Protrusion of other prosthetic devices, implants and grafts of genital tract

    ● **T83.490 Other mechanical complication of implanted penile prosthesis** ♂ A 🦠
       Other mechanical complication of penile prosthesis cylinder
       Other mechanical complication of penile prosthesis pump
       Other mechanical complication of penile prosthesis reservoir

    ● **T83.491 Other mechanical complication of implanted testicular prosthesis** A 🦠

    ● **T83.498 Other mechanical complication of other prosthetic devices, implants and grafts of genital tract** A 🦠

N Newborn Age: 0   **P** Pediatric Age: 0–17   **M** Maternity DX: 12–55   **A** Adult Age: 15–124   ♀ Females Only   ♂ Males Only

🦠 Complication\Comorbidity   🦠 Major C\C   (Ex) CC/MCC Exclusions   🦠 Hospital-Acquired Condition

● **T83.5   Infection and inflammatory reaction due to prosthetic device, implant and graft in urinary system**

Use additional code to identify infection

(Ex:) For category T83.5 CC codes unless otherwise indicated: See PDX Collection 1458

Coding Clinic: 2016, Q4, P71

● **T83.51   Infection and inflammatory reaction due to urinary catheter**

Excludes2   complications of stoma of urinary tract (N99.5-)

● **T83.510   Infection and inflammatory reaction due to cystostomy catheter** A 🔌

● **T83.511   Infection and inflammatory reaction due to indwelling urethral catheter** A 🔌, 🔌

(Ex:) See PDX Collection 1457

● **T83.512   Infection and inflammatory reaction due to nephrostomy catheter** A 🔌

● **T83.518   Infection and inflammatory reaction due to other urinary catheter** A 🔌, 🔌

Infection and inflammatory reaction due to Hopkins catheter

Infection and inflammatory reaction due to ileostomy catheter

Infection and inflammatory reaction due to urostomy catheter

● **T83.59   Infection and inflammatory reaction due to prosthetic device, implant and graft in urinary system**

● **T83.590   Infection and inflammatory reaction due to implanted urinary neurostimulation device** A 🔌

Excludes2   Infection and inflammatory reaction due to electrode lead of sacral nerve neurostimulator (T85.732)

Infection and inflammatory reaction due to pulse generator or receiver of sacral nerve neurostimulator (T85.734)

● **T83.591   Infection and inflammatory reaction due to implanted urinary sphincter** A 🔌

● **T83.592   Infection and inflammatory reaction due to indwelling ureteral stent** A 🔌

● **T83.593   Infection and inflammatory reaction due to other urinary stents** A 🔌

Infection and inflammatory reaction due to ileal conduit stents

Infection and inflammatory reaction due to nephroureteral stent

● **T83.598   Infection and inflammatory reaction due to other prosthetic device, implant and graft in urinary system** A 🔌

● **T83.6   Infection and inflammatory reaction due to prosthetic device, implant and graft in genital tract**

Use additional code to identify infection

(Ex:) For category T83.6: See PDX Collection 1458

Coding Clinic: 2016, Q4, P71

● **T83.61   Infection and inflammatory reaction due to implanted penile prosthesis** A 🔌

Infection and inflammatory reaction due to penile prosthesis cylinder

Infection and inflammatory reaction due to penile prosthesis pump

Infection and inflammatory reaction due to penile prosthesis reservoir

● **T83.62   Infection and inflammatory reaction due to implanted testicular prosthesis** A 🔌

● **T83.69   Infection and inflammatory reaction due to other prosthetic device, implant and graft in genital tract** A 🔌

● **T83.7   Complications due to implanted mesh and other prosthetic materials**

(Ex:) For Category T83.7 CC codes unless otherwise indicated: See PDX Collection 1456

Coding Clinic: 2016, Q4, P71

● **T83.71   Erosion of implanted mesh and other prosthetic materials to surrounding organ or tissue**

Coding Clinic: 2016, Q4, P71

● **T83.711   Erosion of implanted vaginal mesh to surrounding organ or tissue** ♀

Erosion of implanted vaginal mesh into pelvic floor muscles

Coding Clinic: 2016, Q4, P71

● **T83.712   Erosion of implanted urethral mesh to surrounding organ or tissue** A 🔌

Erosion of implanted female urethral sling

Erosion of implanted male urethral sling

Erosion of implanted urethral mesh into pelvic floor muscles

● **T83.713   Erosion of implanted urethral bulking agent to surrounding organ or tissue** A 🔌

● **T83.714   Erosion of implanted ureteral bulking agent to surrounding organ or tissue** A 🔌

● **T83.718   Erosion of other implanted mesh to organ or tissue** A 🔌

Coding Clinic: 2016, Q4, P71

● **T83.719   Erosion of other prosthetic materials to surrounding organ or tissue** A 🔌

Coding Clinic: 2016, Q4, P71

● **T83.72   Exposure of implanted mesh and other prosthetic materials into surrounding organ or tissue**

Extrusion of implanted mesh

Coding Clinic: 2016, Q4, P71

● **T83.721   Exposure of implanted vaginal mesh into vagina** ♀

Exposure of implanted vaginal mesh through vaginal wall

● **T83.722   Exposure of implanted urethral mesh into urethra** A 🔌

Exposure of implanted female urethral sling

Exposure of implanted male urethral sling

Exposure of implanted urethral mesh through urethral wall

▶ New   ➡ Revised   ~~deleted~~ Deleted   Excludes 1   Excludes 2   Includes   Use additional   Code first   Code also   Key words

OGCR Official Guidelines   ● Unacceptable Principal Diagnosis   X Assign placeholder X   ● Use Additional Character(s)   ▶ Manifestation Code   Coding Clinic

● **T83.723** **Exposure of implanted urethral bulking agent into urethra** A 🦠

● **T83.724** **Exposure of implanted ureteral bulking agent into ureter** A 🦠

● **T83.728** **Exposure of other implanted mesh into organ or tissue** A 🦠
     Coding Clinic: 2016, Q4, P71

● **T83.729** **Exposure of other prosthetic materials into organ or tissue** A 🦠
     Coding Clinic: 2016, Q4, P71

X ● **T83.79** **Other specified complications due to other genitourinary prosthetic materials** A 🦠
     (Ex) See PDX Collection 1458

● **T83.8** **Other specified complications of genitourinary prosthetic devices, implants and grafts**
     (Ex) For category T83.8 CC codes: See PDX Collection 1458

X ● **T83.81** **Embolism due to genitourinary prosthetic devices, implants and grafts** A 🦠

X ● **T83.82** **Fibrosis due to genitourinary prosthetic devices, implants and grafts** A 🦠

X ● **T83.83** **Hemorrhage due to genitourinary prosthetic devices, implants and grafts** A 🦠

X ● **T83.84** **Pain due to genitourinary prosthetic devices, implants and grafts** A 🦠

X ● **T83.85** **Stenosis due to genitourinary prosthetic devices, implants and grafts** A 🦠

X ● **T83.86** **Thrombosis due to genitourinary prosthetic devices, implants and grafts** A 🦠

X ● **T83.89** **Other specified complication of genitourinary prosthetic devices, implants and grafts** A 🦠

X ● **T83.9** **Unspecified complication of genitourinary prosthetic device, implant and graft** A 🦠
     (Ex) See PDX Collection 1458

● **T84** **Complications of internal orthopedic prosthetic devices, implants and grafts**

     Excludes2 failure and rejection of transplanted organs and tissues (T86.-)
         fracture of bone following insertion of orthopedic implant, joint prosthesis or bone plate (M96.6)

     The appropriate 7th character is to be added to each code from category T84

A	initial encounter
D	subsequent encounter
S	sequela

     (Ex) For category T84 CC codes unless otherwise indicated: See PDX Collection 911

● **T84.0** **Mechanical complication of internal joint prosthesis**

● **T84.01** **Broken internal joint prosthesis**
     Breakage (fracture) of prosthetic joint
     Broken prosthetic joint implant

     ➡ **Excludes1** periprosthetic joint implant fracture (M97-)
     Coding Clinic: 2016, Q4, P42

● **T84.010** **Broken internal right hip prosthesis** A 🦠

● **T84.011** **Broken internal left hip prosthesis** A 🦠

● **T84.012** **Broken internal right knee prosthesis** A 🦠

● **T84.013** **Broken internal left knee prosthesis** A 🦠

● **T84.018** **Broken internal joint prosthesis, other site** A 🦠
     Use additional code to identify the joint (Z96.6-)

● **T84.019** **Broken internal joint prosthesis, unspecified site** A 🦠

● **T84.02** **Dislocation of internal joint prosthesis**
     Instability of internal joint prosthesis
     Subluxation of internal joint prosthesis

● **T84.020** **Dislocation of internal right hip prosthesis** A 🦠

● **T84.021** **Dislocation of internal left hip prosthesis** A 🦠

● **T84.022** **Instability of internal right knee prosthesis** A 🦠

● **T84.023** **Instability of internal left knee prosthesis** A 🦠

● **T84.028** **Dislocation of other internal joint prosthesis** A 🦠
     Use additional code to identify the joint (Z96.6-)

● **T84.029** **Dislocation of unspecified internal joint prosthesis** A 🦠

● **T84.03** **Mechanical loosening of internal prosthetic joint**
     Aseptic loosening of prosthetic joint

● **T84.030** **Mechanical loosening of internal right hip prosthetic joint** A 🦠

● **T84.031** **Mechanical loosening of internal left hip prosthetic joint** A 🦠

● **T84.032** **Mechanical loosening of internal right knee prosthetic joint** A 🦠

● **T84.033** **Mechanical loosening of internal left knee prosthetic joint** A 🦠

● **T84.038** **Mechanical loosening of other internal prosthetic joint** A 🦠
     Use additional code to identify the joint (Z96.6-)

● **T84.039** **Mechanical loosening of unspecified internal prosthetic joint** A 🦠

● **T84.05** **Periprosthetic osteolysis of internal prosthetic joint**
     Use additional code to identify major osseous defect, if applicable (M89.7-)

● **T84.050** **Periprosthetic osteolysis of internal prosthetic right hip joint** A 🦠

● **T84.051** **Periprosthetic osteolysis of internal prosthetic left hip joint** A 🦠

● **T84.052** **Periprosthetic osteolysis of internal prosthetic right knee joint** A 🦠

● **T84.053** **Periprosthetic osteolysis of internal prosthetic left knee joint** A 🦠

● **T84.058** **Periprosthetic osteolysis of other internal prosthetic joint** A 🦠
     Use additional code to identify the joint (Z96.6-)

● **T84.059** **Periprosthetic osteolysis of unspecified internal prosthetic joint** A 🦠

● **T84.06** **Wear of articular bearing surface of internal prosthetic joint**

● **T84.060** **Wear of articular bearing surface of internal prosthetic right hip joint** A 🦠

● **T84.061** **Wear of articular bearing surface of internal prosthetic left hip joint** A 🦠

● **T84.062** **Wear of articular bearing surface of internal prosthetic right knee joint** A 🦠

● **T84.063** **Wear of articular bearing surface of internal prosthetic left knee joint** A 🦠

● **T84.068** **Wear of articular bearing surface of other internal prosthetic joint** A 🦠
     Use additional code to identify the joint (Z96.6-)

● **T84.069** **Wear of articular bearing surface of unspecified internal prosthetic joint** A 🦠

CHAPTER 19 (S00–T88)

● **T84.09** Other mechanical complication of internal joint prosthesis
Prosthetic joint implant failure NOS

● **T84.090** Other mechanical complication of internal right hip prosthesis A ⊘

● **T84.091** Other mechanical complication of internal left hip prosthesis A ⊘

● **T84.092** Other mechanical complication of internal right knee prosthesis A ⊘

● **T84.093** Other mechanical complication of internal left knee prosthesis A ⊘

● **T84.098** Other mechanical complication of other internal joint prosthesis A ⊘
Use additional code to identify the joint (Z96.6-)

● **T84.099** Other mechanical complication of unspecified internal joint prosthesis A ⊘

● **T84.1** Mechanical complication of internal fixation device of bones of limb

Excludes2 mechanical complication of internal fixation device of bones of feet (T84.2-)
mechanical complication of internal fixation device of bones of fingers (T84.2-)
mechanical complication of internal fixation device of bones of hands (T84.2-)
mechanical complication of internal fixation device of bones of toes (T84.2-)

● **T84.11** Breakdown (mechanical) of internal fixation device of bones of limb

● **T84.110** Breakdown (mechanical) of internal fixation device of right humerus A ⊘

● **T84.111** Breakdown (mechanical) of internal fixation device of left humerus A ⊘

● **T84.112** Breakdown (mechanical) of internal fixation device of bone of right forearm A ⊘

● **T84.113** Breakdown (mechanical) of internal fixation device of bone of left forearm A ⊘

● **T84.114** Breakdown (mechanical) of internal fixation device of right femur A ⊘

● **T84.115** Breakdown (mechanical) of internal fixation device of left femur A ⊘

● **T84.116** Breakdown (mechanical) of internal fixation device of bone of right lower leg A ⊘

● **T84.117** Breakdown (mechanical) of internal fixation device of bone of left lower leg A ⊘

● **T84.119** Breakdown (mechanical) of internal fixation device of unspecified bone of limb A ⊘

● **T84.12** Displacement of internal fixation device of bones of limb
Malposition of internal fixation device of bones of limb

● **T84.120** Displacement of internal fixation device of right humerus A ⊘

● **T84.121** Displacement of internal fixation device of left humerus A ⊘

● **T84.122** Displacement of internal fixation device of bone of right forearm A ⊘

● **T84.123** Displacement of internal fixation device of bone of left forearm A ⊘

● **T84.124** Displacement of internal fixation device of right femur A ⊘

● **T84.125** Displacement of internal fixation device of left femur A ⊘

● **T84.126** Displacement of internal fixation device of bone of right lower leg A ⊘

● **T84.127** Displacement of internal fixation device of bone of left lower leg A ⊘

● **T84.129** Displacement of internal fixation device of unspecified bone of limb A ⊘

● **T84.19** Other mechanical complication of internal fixation device of bones of limb
Obstruction (mechanical) of internal fixation device of bones of limb
Perforation of internal fixation device of bones of limb
Protrusion of internal fixation device of bones of limb

● **T84.190** Other mechanical complication of internal fixation device of right humerus A ⊘

● **T84.191** Other mechanical complication of internal fixation device of left humerus A ⊘

● **T84.192** Other mechanical complication of internal fixation device of bone of right forearm A ⊘

● **T84.193** Other mechanical complication of internal fixation device of bone of left forearm A ⊘

● **T84.194** Other mechanical complication of internal fixation device of right femur A ⊘

● **T84.195** Other mechanical complication of internal fixation device of left femur A ⊘

● **T84.196** Other mechanical complication of internal fixation device of bone of right lower leg A ⊘

● **T84.197** Other mechanical complication of internal fixation device of bone of left lower leg A ⊘

● **T84.199** Other mechanical complication of internal fixation device of unspecified bone of limb A ⊘

● **T84.2** Mechanical complication of internal fixation device of other bones

● **T84.21** Breakdown (mechanical) of internal fixation device of other bones

● **T84.210** Breakdown (mechanical) of internal fixation device of bones of hand and fingers A ⊘

● **T84.213** Breakdown (mechanical) of internal fixation device of bones of foot and toes A ⊘

● **T84.216** Breakdown (mechanical) of internal fixation device of vertebrae A ⊘

● **T84.218** Breakdown (mechanical) of internal fixation device of other bones A ⊘

● **T84.22** Displacement of internal fixation device of other bones
Malposition of internal fixation device of other bones

● **T84.220** Displacement of internal fixation device of bones of hand and fingers A ⊘

● **T84.223** Displacement of internal fixation device of bones of foot and toes A ⊘

● **T84.226** Displacement of internal fixation device of vertebrae A ⊘

● **T84.228** Displacement of internal fixation device of other bones A ⊘

▶ New ⟹ Revised ~~deleted~~ Deleted | Excludes 1 | Excludes 2 | Includes | Use additional | Code first | Code also | Key words |
OGCR Official Guidelines ● Unacceptable Principal Diagnosis X Assign placeholder X ● Use Additional Character(s) ▌Manifestation Code **Coding Clinic**

● **T84.29** **Other mechanical complication of internal fixation device of other bones**
      Obstruction (mechanical) of internal fixation device of other bones
      Perforation of internal fixation device of other bones
      Protrusion of internal fixation device of other bones

  ● **T84.290** **Other mechanical complication of internal fixation device of bones of hand and fingers** A 🦠

  ● **T84.293** **Other mechanical complication of internal fixation device of bones of foot and toes** A 🦠

  ● **T84.296** **Other mechanical complication of internal fixation device of vertebrae** A 🦠

  ● **T84.298** **Other mechanical complication of internal fixation device of other bones** A 🦠

● **T84.3** **Mechanical complication of other bone devices, implants and grafts**
    Excludes2   other complications of bone graft (T86.83-)

  ● **T84.31** **Breakdown (mechanical) of other bone devices, implants and grafts**

    ● **T84.310** **Breakdown (mechanical) of electronic bone stimulator** A 🦠

    ● **T84.318** **Breakdown (mechanical) of other bone devices, implants and grafts** A 🦠

  ● **T84.32** **Displacement of other bone devices, implants and grafts**
      Malposition of other bone devices, implants and grafts

    ● **T84.320** **Displacement of electronic bone stimulator** A 🦠

    ● **T84.328** **Displacement of other bone devices, implants and grafts** A 🦠

  ● **T84.39** **Other mechanical complication of other bone devices, implants and grafts**
      Obstruction (mechanical) of other bone devices, implants and grafts
      Perforation of other bone devices, implants and grafts
      Protrusion of other bone devices, implants and grafts

    ● **T84.390** **Other mechanical complication of electronic bone stimulator** A 🦠

    ● **T84.398** **Other mechanical complication of other bone devices, implants and grafts** A 🦠

● **T84.4** **Mechanical complication of other internal orthopedic devices, implants and grafts**

  ● **T84.41** **Breakdown (mechanical) of other internal orthopedic devices, implants and grafts**

    ● **T84.410** **Breakdown (mechanical) of muscle and tendon graft** A 🦠

    ● **T84.418** **Breakdown (mechanical) of other internal orthopedic devices, implants and grafts** A 🦠

  ● **T84.42** **Displacement of other internal orthopedic devices, implants and grafts**
      Malposition of other internal orthopedic devices, implants and grafts

    ● **T84.420** **Displacement of muscle and tendon graft** A 🦠

    ● **T84.428** **Displacement of other internal orthopedic devices, implants and grafts** A 🦠

● **T84.49** **Other mechanical complication of other internal orthopedic devices, implants and grafts**
      Mechanical complication of other internal orthopedic devices, implants and grafts NOS
      Obstruction (mechanical) of other internal orthopedic devices, implants and grafts
      Perforation of other internal orthopedic devices, implants and grafts
      Protrusion of other internal orthopedic devices, implants and grafts

  ● **T84.490** **Other mechanical complication of muscle and tendon graft** A 🦠

  ● **T84.498** **Other mechanical complication of other internal orthopedic devices, implants and grafts** A 🦠

● **T84.5** **Infection and inflammatory reaction due to internal joint prosthesis**
    Use additional code to identify infection
    (Ex) For category T84.5 CC codes: See PDX Collection 1459
    Coding Clinic: 2015, Q1, P16

  X ● **T84.50** **Infection and inflammatory reaction due to unspecified internal joint prosthesis** A 🦠
      Coding Clinic: 2015, Q1, P3

  X ● **T84.51** **Infection and inflammatory reaction due to internal right hip prosthesis** A 🦠
      Coding Clinic: 2015, Q4, P36

  X ● **T84.52** **Infection and inflammatory reaction due to internal left hip prosthesis** A 🦠
      Coding Clinic: 2015, Q1, P16-17

  X ● **T84.53** **Infection and inflammatory reaction due to internal right knee prosthesis** A 🦠

  X ● **T84.54** **Infection and inflammatory reaction due to internal left knee prosthesis** A 🦠

  X ● **T84.59** **Infection and inflammatory reaction due to other internal joint prosthesis** A 🦠

● **T84.6** **Infection and inflammatory reaction due to internal fixation device**
    Use additional code to identify infection
    (Ex) For category T84.6 CC codes: See PDX Collection 1459

  X ● **T84.60** **Infection and inflammatory reaction due to internal fixation device of unspecified site** A 🦠, A 🦠

  ● **T84.61** **Infection and inflammatory reaction due to internal fixation device of arm**

    ● **T84.610** **Infection and inflammatory reaction due to internal fixation device of right humerus** A 🦠, A 🦠

    ● **T84.611** **Infection and inflammatory reaction due to internal fixation device of left humerus** A 🦠, A 🦠

    ● **T84.612** **Infection and inflammatory reaction due to internal fixation device of right radius** A 🦠, A 🦠

    ● **T84.613** **Infection and inflammatory reaction due to internal fixation device of left radius** A 🦠, A 🦠

    ● **T84.614** **Infection and inflammatory reaction due to internal fixation device of right ulna** A 🦠, A 🦠

    ● **T84.615** **Infection and inflammatory reaction due to internal fixation device of left ulna** A 🦠, A 🦠

    ● **T84.619** **Infection and inflammatory reaction due to internal fixation device of unspecified bone of arm** A 🦠, A 🦠

N Newborn Age: 0   **P** Pediatric Age: 0–17   **M** Maternity DX: 12–55   **A** Adult Age: 15–124   ♀ Females Only   ♂ Males Only

🦠 Complication\Comorbidity   🦠 Major C\C   (Ex) CC/MCC Exclusions   🦠 Hospital-Acquired Condition

1491

● T84.62 **Infection and inflammatory reaction due to internal fixation device of leg**

  ● T84.620 **Infection and inflammatory reaction due to internal fixation device of right femur** A ⚖

  ● T84.621 **Infection and inflammatory reaction due to internal fixation device of left femur** A ⚖

  ● T84.622 **Infection and inflammatory reaction due to internal fixation device of right tibia** A ⚖

  ● T84.623 **Infection and inflammatory reaction due to internal fixation device of left tibia** A ⚖

  ● T84.624 **Infection and inflammatory reaction due to internal fixation device of right fibula** A ⚖

  ● T84.625 **Infection and inflammatory reaction due to internal fixation device of left fibula** A ⚖

  ● T84.629 **Infection and inflammatory reaction due to internal fixation device of unspecified bone of leg** A ⚖

X● T84.63 **Infection and inflammatory reaction due to internal fixation device of spine** A ⚖, A ⚖

X● T84.69 **Infection and inflammatory reaction due to internal fixation device of other site** A ⚖, A ⚖

● T84.7 **Infection and inflammatory reaction due to other internal orthopedic prosthetic devices, implants and grafts** A ⚖, A ⚖

  Use additional code to identify infection
  (Ex:) See PDX Collection 1459

● T84.8 **Other specified complications of internal orthopedic prosthetic devices, implants and grafts**
  (Ex:) For category T84.8 CC codes: See PDX Collection 1459

X● T84.81 **Embolism due to internal orthopedic prosthetic devices, implants and grafts** A ⚖

X● T84.82 **Fibrosis due to internal orthopedic prosthetic devices, implants and grafts** A ⚖

X● T84.83 **Hemorrhage due to internal orthopedic prosthetic devices, implants and grafts** A ⚖

X● T84.84 **Pain due to internal orthopedic prosthetic devices, implants and grafts** A ⚖

X● T84.85 **Stenosis due to internal orthopedic prosthetic devices, implants and grafts** A ⚖

X● T84.86 **Thrombosis due to internal orthopedic prosthetic devices, implants and grafts** A ⚖

X● T84.89 **Other specified complication of internal orthopedic prosthetic devices, implants and grafts** A ⚖

X● T84.9 **Unspecified complication of internal orthopedic prosthetic device, implant and graft** A ⚖
  (Ex:) See PDX Collection 1459

● T85 **Complications of other internal prosthetic devices, implants and grafts**

  Excludes2 failure and rejection of transplanted organs and tissue (T86.-)

  The appropriate 7th character is to be added to each code from category T85

A	initial encounter
D	subsequent encounter
S	sequela

Coding Clinic: 2016, Q4, P71

● T85.0 **Mechanical complication of ventricular intracranial (communicating) shunt**
  (Ex:) For category T85.0 CC codes: See PDX Collection 1460

X● T85.01 **Breakdown (mechanical) of ventricular intracranial (communicating) shunt** A ⚖

X● T85.02 **Displacement of ventricular intracranial (communicating) shunt** A ⚖
  Malposition of ventricular intracranial (communicating) shunt

X● T85.03 **Leakage of ventricular intracranial (communicating) shunt** A ⚖

X● T85.09 **Other mechanical complication of ventricular intracranial (communicating) shunt** A ⚖
  Obstruction (mechanical) of ventricular intracranial (communicating) shunt
  Perforation of ventricular intracranial (communicating) shunt
  Protrusion of ventricular intracranial (communicating) shunt

● T85.1 **Mechanical complication of implanted electronic stimulator of nervous system**
  (Ex:) For category T85.1 CC codes: See PDX Collection 1460
  Coding Clinic: 2016, Q4, P71

  ● T85.11 **Breakdown (mechanical) of implanted electronic stimulator of nervous system**

    ● T85.110 **Breakdown (mechanical) of implanted electronic neurostimulator of brain electrode (lead)** A ⚖

    ● T85.111 **Breakdown (mechanical) of implanted electronic neurostimulator of peripheral nerve electrode (lead)** A ⚖
    Breakdown of electrode (lead) for cranial nerve neurostimulators
    Breakdown of electrode (lead) for gastric neurostimulator
    Breakdown of electrode (lead) for sacral nerve neurostimulator
    Breakdown of electrode (lead) for vagal nerve neurostimulators

    ● T85.112 **Breakdown (mechanical) of implanted electronic neurostimulator of spinal cord electrode (lead)** A ⚖

    ● T85.113 **Breakdown (mechanical) of implanted electronic neurostimulator, generator** A ⚖
    Breakdown (mechanical) of implanted electronic neurostimuator generator, brain, peripheral, gastric, spinal
    Breakdown (mechanical) of implanted electronic sacral neurostimulator, pulse generator or receiver

    ● T85.118 **Breakdown (mechanical) of other implanted electronic stimulator of nervous system** A ⚖

CHAPTER 19 (S00-T88)

● **T85.12** **Displacement of implanted electronic stimulator of nervous system**
Malposition of implanted electronic stimulator of nervous system

  ● **T85.120** **Displacement of implanted electronic neurostimulator of brain electrode (lead)** A 🔖

  ● **T85.121** **Displacement of implanted electronic neurostimulator of peripheral nerve electrode (lead)** A 🔖
Displacement of electrode (lead) for cranial nerve neurostimulators
Displacement of electrode (lead) for gastric neurostimulator
Displacement of electrode (lead) for sacral nerve neurostimulator
Displacement of electrode (lead) for vagal nerve neurostimulators

  ● **T85.122** **Displacement of implanted electronic neurostimulator of spinal cord electrode (lead)** A 🔖

  ● **T85.123** **Displacement of implanted electronic neurostimulator, generator** A 🔖
Displacement of implanted electronic neurostimulator generator, brain, peripheral, gastric, spinal
Displacement of implanted electronic sacral neurostimulator, pulse generator or receiver

  ● **T85.128** **Displacement of other implanted electronic stimulator of nervous system** A 🔖

● **T85.19** **Other mechanical complication of implanted electronic stimulator of nervous system**
Leakage of implanted electronic stimulator of nervous system
Obstruction (mechanical) of implanted electronic stimulator of nervous system
Perforation of implanted electronic stimulator of nervous system
Protrusion of implanted electronic stimulator of nervous system

  ● **T85.190** **Other mechanical complication of implanted electronic neurostimulator of brain electrode (lead)** A 🔖

  ● **T85.191** **Other mechanical complication of implanted electronic neurostimulator of peripheral nerve electrode (lead)** A 🔖
Other mechanical complication of electrode (lead) for cranial nerve neurostimulators
Other mechanical complication of electrode (lead) for gastric neurostimulator
Other mechanical complication of electrode (lead) for sacral nerve neurostimulator
Other mechanical complication of electrode (lead) for vagal nerve neurostimulators

  ● **T85.192** **Other mechanical complication of implanted electronic neurostimulator of spinal cord electrode (lead)** A 🔖

  ● **T85.193** **Other mechanical complication of implanted electronic neurostimulator, generator** A 🔖
Other mechanical complication of implanted electronic neurostimulator generator, brain, peripheral, gastric, spinal
Other mechanical complication of implanted electronic sacral neurostimulator, pulse generator or receiver

  ● **T85.199** **Other mechanical complication of other implanted electronic stimulator of nervous system** A 🔖

● **T85.2** **Mechanical complication of intraocular lens**
  (Ex) **For category T85.2 CC codes:** See PDX Collection 1461

  X ● **T85.21** **Breakdown (mechanical) of intraocular lens** A 🔖

  X ● **T85.22** **Displacement of intraocular lens** A 🔖
Malposition of intraocular lens

  X ● **T85.29** **Other mechanical complication of intraocular lens** A 🔖
Obstruction (mechanical) of intraocular lens
Perforation of intraocular lens
Protrusion of intraocular lens

● **T85.3** **Mechanical complication of other ocular prosthetic devices, implants and grafts**
Excludes2 other complications of corneal graft (T86.84-)
  (Ex) **For category T85.3 CC codes:** See PDX Collection 1462

  ● **T85.31** **Breakdown (mechanical) of other ocular prosthetic devices, implants and grafts**

    ● **T85.310** **Breakdown (mechanical) of prosthetic orbit of right eye** A 🔖

    ● **T85.311** **Breakdown (mechanical) of prosthetic orbit of left eye** A 🔖

    ● **T85.318** **Breakdown (mechanical) of other ocular prosthetic devices, implants and grafts**

  ● **T85.32** **Displacement of other ocular prosthetic devices, implants and grafts**
Malposition of other ocular prosthetic devices, implants and grafts

    ● **T85.320** **Displacement of prosthetic orbit of right eye** A 🔖

    ● **T85.321** **Displacement of prosthetic orbit of left eye** A 🔖

    ● **T85.328** **Displacement of other ocular prosthetic devices, implants and grafts**

  ● **T85.39** **Other mechanical complication of other ocular prosthetic devices, implants and grafts**
Obstruction (mechanical) of other ocular prosthetic devices, implants and grafts
Perforation of other ocular prosthetic devices, implants and grafts
Protrusion of other ocular prosthetic devices, implants and grafts

    ● **T85.390** **Other mechanical complication of prosthetic orbit of right eye** A 🔖

    ● **T85.391** **Other mechanical complication of prosthetic orbit of left eye** A 🔖

    ● **T85.398** **Other mechanical complication of other ocular prosthetic devices, implants and grafts**

CHAPTER 19 (S00-T88)

N Newborn Age: Ø   **P** Pediatric Age: Ø–17   **M** Maternity DX: 12–55   **A** Adult Age: 15–124   ♀ Females Only   ♂ Males Only
🔖 Complication\Comorbidity   🔖 Major C\C   (Ex) CC/MCC Exclusions   🔖 Hospital-Acquired Condition

1493

CHAPTER 19 (S00-T88)

● **T85.4**   **Mechanical complication of breast prosthesis and implant**
> (Ex:) For category T85.4 CC codes: See PDX Collection 1463

   X● **T85.41**   **Breakdown (mechanical) of breast prosthesis and implant** A 🔖

   X● **T85.42**   **Displacement of breast prosthesis and implant** A 🔖
> Malposition of breast prosthesis and implant

   X● **T85.43**   **Leakage of breast prosthesis and implant** A 🔖

   X● **T85.44**   **Capsular contracture of breast implant** A 🔖

   X● **T85.49**   **Other mechanical complication of breast prosthesis and implant** A 🔖
> Obstruction (mechanical) of breast prosthesis and implant
> Perforation of breast prosthesis and implant
> Protrusion of breast prosthesis and implant

● **T85.5**   **Mechanical complication of gastrointestinal prosthetic devices, implants and grafts**
> (Ex:) For category T85.5 CC codes: See PDX Collection 1464

   ● **T85.51**   **Breakdown (mechanical) of gastrointestinal prosthetic devices, implants and grafts**

     ● **T85.510**   **Breakdown (mechanical) of bile duct prosthesis** A 🔖

     ● **T85.511**   **Breakdown (mechanical) of esophageal anti-reflux device** A 🔖

     ● **T85.518**   **Breakdown (mechanical) of other gastrointestinal prosthetic devices, implants and grafts** A 🔖

   ● **T85.52**   **Displacement of gastrointestinal prosthetic devices, implants and grafts**
> Malposition of gastrointestinal prosthetic devices, implants and grafts

     ● **T85.520**   **Displacement of bile duct prosthesis** A 🔖

     ● **T85.521**   **Displacement of esophageal anti-reflux device** A 🔖

     ● **T85.528**   **Displacement of other gastrointestinal prosthetic devices, implants and grafts** A 🔖

   ● **T85.59**   **Other mechanical complication of gastrointestinal prosthetic devices, implants and**
> Obstruction, mechanical of gastrointestinal prosthetic devices, implants and grafts
> Perforation of gastrointestinal prosthetic devices, implants and grafts
> Protrusion of gastrointestinal prosthetic devices, implants and grafts

     ● **T85.590**   **Other mechanical complication of bile duct prosthesis** A 🔖

     ● **T85.591**   **Other mechanical complication of esophageal anti-reflux device** A 🔖

     ● **T85.598**   **Other mechanical complication of other gastrointestinal prosthetic devices, implants and grafts** A 🔖

● **T85.6**   **Mechanical complication of other specified internal and external prosthetic devices, implants and grafts**
> Coding Clinic: 2016, Q4, P71

   ● **T85.61**   **Breakdown (mechanical) of other specified internal prosthetic devices, implants and grafts**

     ● **T85.610**   **Breakdown (mechanical) of cranial or spinal infusion catheter** A 🔖
> Breakdown (mechanical) of epidural infusion catheter
> Breakdown (mechanical) of intrathecal infusion catheter
> Breakdown (mechanical) of subarachnoid infusion catheter
> Breakdown (mechanical) of subdural infusion catheter
> (Ex:) See PDX Collection 1465

     ● **T85.611**   **Breakdown (mechanical) of intraperitoneal dialysis catheter** A 🔖
>> **Excludes1**   mechanical complication of vascular dialysis catheter (T82.4-)
> (Ex:) See PDX Collection 1466

     ● **T85.612**   **Breakdown (mechanical) of permanent sutures** A 🔖
>> **Excludes1**   mechanical complication of permanent (wire) suture used in bone repair (T84.1-T84.2)
> (Ex:) See PDX Collection 1467

     ● **T85.613**   **Breakdown (mechanical) of artificial skin graft and decellularized allodermis** A 🔖
> Failure of artificial skin graft and decellularized allodermis
> Non-adherence of artificial skin graft and decellularized allodermis
> Poor incorporation of artificial skin graft and decellularized allodermis
> Shearing of artificial skin graft and decellularized allodermis
> (Ex:) See PDX Collection 1468

     ● **T85.614**   **Breakdown (mechanical) of insulin pump** A 🔖
> (Ex:) See PDX Collection 1469

     ● **T85.615**   **Breakdown (mechanical) of other nervous system device, implant or graft** A 🔖
> Breakdown (mechanical) of intrathecal infusion pump
> (Ex:) See PDX Collection 1467

     ● **T85.618**   **Breakdown (mechanical) of other specified internal prosthetic devices, implants and grafts** A 🔖
> (Ex:) See PDX Collection 1467

▶ New   ⇒ Revised   ~~deleted~~ Deleted   Excludes 1   Excludes 2   Includes   Use additional   Code first   Code also   Key words

OGCR Official Guidelines   ● Unacceptable Principal Diagnosis   X Assign placeholder X   ● Use Additional Character(s)   ▶ Manifestation Code   **Coding Clinic**

● **T85.62 Displacement of other specified internal prosthetic devices, implants and grafts**
Malposition of other specified internal prosthetic devices, implants and grafts

● **T85.620 Displacement of cranial or spinal infusion catheter** A
Displacement of epidural infusion catheter
Displacement of intrathecal infusion catheter
Displacement of subarachnoid infusion catheter
Displacement of subdural infusion catheter
(Ex.) See PDX Collection 1465

● **T85.621 Displacement of intraperitoneal dialysis catheter** A
Excludes1 mechanical complication of vascular dialysis catheter (T82.4-)
(Ex.) See PDX Collection 1466

● **T85.622 Displacement of permanent sutures** A
Excludes1 mechanical complication of permanent (wire) suture used in bone repair (T84.1-T84.2)
(Ex.) See PDX Collection 1467

● **T85.623 Displacement of artificial skin graft and decellularized allodermis** A
Dislodgement of artificial skin graft and decellularized allodermis
~~Displacement of artificial skin graft and decellularized allodermis~~
(Ex.) See PDX Collection 1468

● **T85.624 Displacement of insulin pump** A
(Ex.) See PDX Collection 1469

● **T85.625 Displacement of other nervous system device, implant or graft** A
Displacement of intrathecal infusion pump
(Ex.) See PDX Collection 1467

● **T85.628 Displacement of other specified internal prosthetic devices, implants and grafts** A
(Ex.) See PDX Collection 1467
Coding Clinic: 2015, Q1, P15

● **T85.63 Leakage of other specified internal prosthetic devices, implants and grafts**

● **T85.630 Leakage of cranial or spinal infusion catheter** A
Leakage of epidural infusion catheter
Leakage of intrathecal infusion catheter
Leakage of subdural infusion catheter
Leakage of subarachnoid infusion catheter
(Ex.) See PDX Collection 1465

● **T85.631 Leakage of intraperitoneal dialysis catheter** A
Excludes1 mechanical complication of vascular dialysis catheter (T82.4)
(Ex.) See PDX Collection 1466

● **T85.633 Leakage of insulin pump** A
(Ex.) See PDX Collection 1469

● **T85.635 Leakage of other nervous system device, implant or graft** A
Leakage of intrathecal infusion pump
(Ex.) See PDX Collection 1467

● **T85.638 Leakage of other specified internal prosthetic devices, implants and grafts** A
(Ex.) See PDX Collection 1467

● **T85.69 Other mechanical complication of other specified internal prosthetic devices, implants and grafts**
Obstruction, mechanical of other specified internal prosthetic devices, implants and grafts
Perforation of other specified internal prosthetic devices, implants and grafts
Protrusion of other specified internal prosthetic devices, implants and grafts

● **T85.690 Other mechanical complication of cranial or spinal infusion catheter** A
Other mechanical complication of epidural infusion catheter
Other mechanical complication of intrathecal infusion catheter
Other mechanical complication of subarachnoid infusion catheter
Other mechanical complication of subdural infusion catheter
(Ex.) See PDX Collection 1465

● **T85.691 Other mechanical complication of intraperitoneal dialysis catheter** A
Excludes1 mechanical complication of vascular dialysis catheter (T82.4)
(Ex.) See PDX Collection 1466

● **T85.692 Other mechanical complication of permanent sutures** A
Excludes1 mechanical complication of permanent (wire) suture used in bone repair (T84.1-T84.2)
(Ex.) See PDX Collection 1467

● **T85.693 Other mechanical complication of artificial skin graft and decellularized allodermis** A
(Ex.) See PDX Collection 1468

● **T85.694 Other mechanical complication of insulin pump** A
(Ex.) See PDX Collection 1469

● **T85.695 Other mechanical complication of other nervous system device, implant or graft** A
Other mechanical complication of intrathecal infusion pump
(Ex.) See PDX Collection 1467

● **T85.698 Other mechanical complication of other specified internal prosthetic devices, implants and grafts** A
Mechanical complication of nonabsorbable surgical material NOS
(Ex.) See PDX Collection 1467

CHAPTER 19 (S00-T88)

● **T85.7   Infection and inflammatory reaction due to other internal prosthetic devices, implants and grafts**

Use additional code to identify infection

(Ex) For category T85.7 CC codes unless otherwise indicated: See PDX Collection 1470

Coding Clinic: 2016, Q4, P72

X● **T85.71   Infection and inflammatory reaction due to peritoneal dialysis catheter** A 🔧

(Ex) See PDX Collection 1467

X● **T85.72   Infection and inflammatory reaction due to insulin pump** A 🔧

● **T85.73   Infection and inflammatory reaction due to nervous system devices, implants and graft**

● **T85.730   Infection and inflammatory reaction due to ventricular intracranial (communicating) shunt** A 🔧

● **T85.731   Infection and inflammatory reaction due to implanted electronic neurostimulator of brain, electrode (lead)** A 🔧

● **T85.732   Infection and inflammatory reaction due to implanted electronic neurostimulator of peripheral nerve, electrode (lead)** A 🔧

Infection and inflammatory reaction due to electrode (lead) for cranial nerve neurostimulators

Infection and inflammatory reaction due to electrode (lead) for gastric neurostimulator

Infection and inflammatory reaction due to electrode (lead) for sacral nerve neurostimulator

Infection and inflammatory reaction due to electrode (lead) for vagal nerve neurostimulators

● **T85.733   Infection and inflammatory reaction due to implanted electronic neurostimulator of spinal cord, electrode (lead)** A 🔧

● **T85.734   Infection and inflammatory reaction due to implanted electronic neurostimulator, generator** A 🔧

Generator pocket infection

● **T85.735   Infection and inflammatory reaction due to cranial or spinal infusion catheter** A 🔧

Infection and inflammatory reaction due to epidural catheter

Infection and inflammatory reaction due to intrathecal infusion catheter

Infection and inflammatory reaction due to subarachnoid catheter

Infection and inflammatory reaction due to subdural catheter

● **T85.738   Infection and inflammatory reaction due to other nervous system device, implant or graft** A 🔧

Infection and inflammatory reaction due to intrathecal infusion pump

X● **T85.79   Infection and inflammatory reaction due to other internal prosthetic devices, implants and grafts** A 🔧

Coding Clinic: 2016, Q4, P72

● **T85.8   Other specified complications of internal prosthetic devices, implants and grafts, not elsewhere classified**

(Ex) For category T85.8 CC codes: See PDX Collection 1470

Coding Clinic: 2016, Q4, P72

● **T85.81   Embolism due to internal prosthetic devices, implants and grafts, not elsewhere classified**

● **T85.810   Embolism due to nervous system prosthetic devices, implants and grafts** A, D 🔧

● **T85.818   Embolism due to other internal prosthetic devices, implants and grafts**

● **T85.82   Fibrosis due to internal prosthetic devices, implants and grafts, not elsewhere classified**

● **T85.820   Fibrosis due to nervous system prosthetic devices, implants and grafts** A, D 🔧

● **T85.828   Fibrosis due to other internal prosthetic devices, implants and grafts**

● **T85.83   Hemorrhage due to internal prosthetic devices, implants and grafts, not elsewhere classified**

● **T85.830   Hemorrhage due to nervous system prosthetic devices, implants and grafts** A, D 🔧

● **T85.838   Hemorrhage due to other internal prosthetic devices, implants and grafts**

● **T85.84   Pain due to internal prosthetic devices, implants and grafts, not elsewhere classified**

● **T85.840   Pain due to nervous system prosthetic devices, implants and grafts** A, D 🔧

● **T85.848   Pain due to other internal prosthetic devices, implants and grafts**

● **T85.85   Stenosis due to internal prosthetic devices, implants and grafts, not elsewhere classified**

● **T85.850   Stenosis due to nervous system prosthetic devices, implants and grafts** A, D 🔧

● **T85.858   Stenosis due to other internal prosthetic devices, implants and grafts**

● **T85.86   Thrombosis due to internal prosthetic devices, implants and grafts, not elsewhere classified**

● **T85.860   Thrombosis due to nervous system prosthetic devices, implants and grafts** A, D 🔧

● **T85.868   Thrombosis due to other internal prosthetic devices, implants and grafts**

● **T85.89   Other specified complication of internal prosthetic devices, implants and grafts, not elsewhere classified**

Coding Clinic: 2016, Q4, P72

● **T85.890   Other specified complication of nervous system prosthetic devices, implants and grafts** A, D 🔧

● **T85.898   Other specified complication of other internal prosthetic devices, implants and grafts**

X● **T85.9   Unspecified complication of internal prosthetic device, implant and graft**

Complication of internal prosthetic device, implant and graft NOS

▶ New   ⇒ Revised   ~~deleted~~ Deleted | Excludes 1 | | Excludes 2 | | Includes | | Use additional | | Code first | | Code also | | Key words |

OGCR Official Guidelines   ● Unacceptable Principal Diagnosis   X Assign placeholder X   ● Use Additional Character(s)   ▶ Manifestation Code   **Coding Clinic**

● **T86   Complications of transplanted organs and tissue**

Use additional code to identify other transplant complications, such as:
graft-versus-host disease (D89.81-)
malignancy associated with organ transplant (C80.2)
post-transplant lymphoproliferative disorders (PTLD) (D47.Z1)

● **T86.0   Complications of bone marrow transplant**

(Ex:) **For category T86.0 CC codes:** See PDX Collection 514

T86.00   **Unspecified complication of bone marrow transplant**🔖

T86.01   **Bone marrow transplant rejection**🔖

T86.02   **Bone marrow transplant failure**🔖

T86.03   **Bone marrow transplant infection**🔖

T86.09   **Other complications of bone marrow transplant**🔖

● **T86.1   Complications of kidney transplant**

(Ex:) **For category T86.1 CC codes:** See PDX Collection 1471

T86.10   **Unspecified complication of kidney transplant**🔖

T86.11   **Kidney transplant rejection**🔖

T86.12   **Kidney transplant failure**🔖
     Coding Clinic: 2013, Q1, P24

T86.13   **Kidney transplant infection**🔖

Use additional code to specify infection

T86.19   **Other complication of kidney transplant**🔖

● **T86.2   Complications of heart transplant**

Excludes1   complication of:
artificial heart device (T82.5)
heart-lung transplant (T86.3)

(Ex:) **For category T86.2 CC codes:** See PDX Collection 1472

T86.20   **Unspecified complication of heart transplant**🔖

T86.21   **Heart transplant rejection**🔖

T86.22   **Heart transplant failure**🔖

T86.23   **Heart transplant infection**🔖

Use additional code to specify infection

● T86.29   **Other complications of heart transplant**

T86.290   **Cardiac allograft vasculopathy**🔖

Excludes1   atherosclerosis of coronary arteries (I25.75-, I25.76-, I25.81-)

T86.298   **Other complications of heart transplant**🔖

● **T86.3   Complications of heart-lung transplant**

(Ex:) **For category T86.3 CC codes:** See PDX Collection 1472

T86.30   **Unspecified complication of heart-lung transplant**🔖
     CC when PDx is its own CC

T86.31   **Heart-lung transplant rejection**🔖
     CC when PDx is its own CC

T86.32   **Heart-lung transplant failure**🔖
     CC when PDx is its own CC

T86.33   **Heart-lung transplant infection**🔖

Use additional code to specify infection
CC when PDx is its own CC

T86.39   **Other complications of heart-lung transplant**🔖
     CC when PDx is its own CC

● **T86.4   Complications of liver transplant**

(Ex:) **For category T86.4 CC codes:** See PDX Collection 1473

T86.40   **Unspecified complication of liver transplant**🔖

T86.41   **Liver transplant rejection**🔖

T86.42   **Liver transplant failure**🔖

T86.43   **Liver transplant infection**🔖

Use additional code to identify infection, such as:
Cytomegalovirus (CMV) infection (B25.-)

T86.49   **Other complications of liver transplant**🔖

● **T86.5   Complications of stem cell transplant**🔖
Complications from stem cells from peripheral blood
Complications from stem cells from umbilical cord

(Ex:) See PDX Collection 1474

● **T86.8   Complications of other transplanted organs and tissues**

● **T86.81   Complications of lung transplant**

Excludes1   complication of heart-lung transplant (T86.3-)

(Ex:) **For category T86.81 CC codes:** See PDX Collection 1475

T86.810   **Lung transplant rejection**🔖

T86.811   **Lung transplant failure**🔖

T86.812   **Lung transplant infection**🔖

Use additional code to specify infection

T86.818   **Other complications of lung transplant**🔖

T86.819   **Unspecified complication of lung transplant**🔖

● **T86.82   Complications of skin graft (allograft) (autograft)**

Excludes2   complication of artificial skin graft (T85.693)

(Ex:) **For category T86.82 CC codes:** See PDX Collection 1476

T86.820   **Skin graft (allograft) rejection**🔖

T86.821   **Skin graft (allograft) (autograft) failure**🔖

T86.822   **Skin graft (allograft) (autograft) infection**🔖

Use additional code to specify infection

T86.828   **Other complications of skin graft (allograft) (autograft)**🔖

T86.829   **Unspecified complication of skin graft (allograft) (autograft)**🔖

CHAPTER 19 (S00-T88)

N   Newborn Age: 0   **P**   Pediatric Age: 0–17   **M**   Maternity DX: 12–55   **A**   Adult Age: 15–124   ♀   Females Only   ♂   Males Only

🔖   Complication\Comorbidity   🔖   Major C\C   (Ex:)   CC/MCC Exclusions   🔖   Hospital-Acquired Condition

1497

● T86.83   **Complications of bone graft**
      Excludes2   mechanical complications of
           bone graft (T84.3-)
      (Ex) For category T86.83 CC codes: See PDX Collection 1477

    T86.830   **Bone graft rejection**
    T86.831   **Bone graft failure**
    T86.832   **Bone graft infection**
        Use additional code to specify
        infection
    T86.838   **Other complications of bone graft**
    T86.839   **Unspecified complication of bone
           graft**

● T86.84   **Complications of corneal transplant**
      Excludes2   mechanical complications of
           corneal graft (T85.3-)
      (Ex) For category T86.84 CC codes unless otherwise indicated:
        See PDX Collection 1479

    T86.840   **Corneal transplant rejection**
        (Ex) See PDX Collection 1478
    T86.841   **Corneal transplant failure**
        (Ex) See PDX Collection 1478
    T86.842   **Corneal transplant infection**
        Use additional code to specify
        infection
    T86.848   **Other complications of corneal
           transplant**
    T86.849   **Unspecified complication of corneal
           transplant**

● T86.85   **Complication of intestine transplant**
      (Ex) For category T86.85 CC codes: See PDX Collection 495

    T86.850   **Intestine transplant rejection**
    T86.851   **Intestine transplant failure**
    T86.852   **Intestine transplant infection**
        Use additional code to specify
        infection
    T86.858   **Other complications of intestine
           transplant**
    T86.859   **Unspecified complication of intestine
           transplant**

● T86.89   **Complications of other transplanted tissue**
      Transplant failure or rejection of pancreas
      (Ex) For category T86.89 CC codes: See PDX Collection 1480

    T86.890   **Other transplanted tissue rejection**
    T86.891   **Other transplanted tissue failure**
    T86.892   **Other transplanted tissue infection**
        Use additional code to specify
        infection
    T86.898   **Other complications of other
           transplanted tissue**
    T86.899   **Unspecified complication of other
           transplanted tissue**

● T86.9   **Complication of unspecified transplanted organ and tissue**
      (Ex) For category T86.9 CC codes: See PDX Collection 495

    T86.90   **Unspecified complication of unspecified
          transplanted organ and tissue**
    T86.91   **Unspecified transplanted organ and tissue
          rejection**
    T86.92   **Unspecified transplanted organ and tissue
          failure**
    T86.93   **Unspecified transplanted organ and tissue
          infection**
        Use additional code to specify infection
    T86.99   **Other complications of unspecified
          transplanted organ and tissue**

● T87   **Complications peculiar to reattachment and amputation**

● T87.0   **Complications of reattached (part of) upper extremity**
      (Ex) For category T87.0 CC codes: See PDX Collection 1481

  ● T87.0X   **Complications of reattached (part of) upper
         extremity**
    T87.0X1   **Complications of reattached (part of)
        right upper extremity**
    T87.0X2   **Complications of reattached (part of)
        left upper extremity**
    T87.0X9   **Complications of reattached (part of)
        unspecified upper extremity**

● T87.1   **Complications of reattached (part of) lower extremity**
      (Ex) For category T87.1 CC codes: See PDX Collection 1482

  ● T87.1X   **Complications of reattached (part of) lower
         extremity**
    T87.1X1   **Complications of reattached (part of)
        right lower extremity**
    T87.1X2   **Complications of reattached (part of)
        left lower extremity**
    T87.1X9   **Complications of reattached (part of)
        unspecified lower extremity**

  T87.2   **Complications of other reattached body part**
      (Ex) See PDX Collection 1483

● T87.3   **Neuroma of amputation stump**
    T87.30   **Neuroma of amputation stump, unspecified
          extremity**
    T87.31   **Neuroma of amputation stump, right upper
          extremity**
    T87.32   **Neuroma of amputation stump, left upper
          extremity**
    T87.33   **Neuroma of amputation stump, right lower
          extremity**
    T87.34   **Neuroma of amputation stump, left lower
          extremity**

● T87.4   **Infection of amputation stump**
      (Ex) For category T87.4 CC codes: See PDX Collection 1484

    T87.40   **Infection of amputation stump, unspecified
          extremity**
    T87.41   **Infection of amputation stump, right upper
          extremity**
    T87.42   **Infection of amputation stump, left upper
          extremity**
    T87.43   **Infection of amputation stump, right lower
          extremity**
    T87.44   **Infection of amputation stump, left lower
          extremity**

● T87.5   **Necrosis of amputation stump**
    T87.50   **Necrosis of amputation stump, unspecified
          extremity**
    T87.51   **Necrosis of amputation stump, right upper
          extremity**
    T87.52   **Necrosis of amputation stump, left upper
          extremity**
    T87.53   **Necrosis of amputation stump, right lower
          extremity**
    T87.54   **Necrosis of amputation stump, left lower
          extremity**

● T87.8   **Other complications of amputation stump**
    T87.81   **Dehiscence of amputation stump**
    T87.89   **Other complications of amputation stump**
        Amputation stump contracture
        Amputation stump contracture of next
          proximal joint
        Amputation stump flexion
        Amputation stump edema
        Amputation stump hematoma
        Excludes2   phantom limb syndrome
           (G54.6-G54.7)

  T87.9   **Unspecified complications of amputation stump**

▶ New   ⟹ Revised   ~~deleted~~ Deleted   Excludes 1   Excludes 2   Includes   Use additional   Code first   Code also   Key words

OGCR Official Guidelines   ● Unacceptable Principal Diagnosis   X Assign placeholder X   ● Use Additional Character(s)   ▌ Manifestation Code   **Coding Clinic**

● **T88** **Other complications of surgical and medical care, not elsewhere classified**

> **Excludes2** complication following infusion, transfusion and therapeutic injection (T80.-)
> complication following procedure NEC (T81.-)
> complications of anesthesia in labor and delivery (O74.-)
> complications of anesthesia in pregnancy (O29.-)
> complications of anesthesia in puerperium (O89.-)
> complications of devices, implants and grafts (T82-T85)
> complications of obstetric surgery and procedure (O75.4)
> dermatitis due to drugs and medicaments (L23.3, L24.4, L25.1, L27.0-L27.1)
> poisoning and toxic effects of drugs and chemicals (T36-T65 with fifth or sixth character 1-4 or 6)
> specified complications classified elsewhere

The appropriate 7th character is to be added to each code from category T88

A	initial encounter
D	subsequent encounter
S	sequela

X ● **T88.0** **Infection following immunization** A 🔹
> Sepsis following immunization
> (Ex) See PDX Collection 948

X ● **T88.1** **Other complications following immunization, not elsewhere classified** A 🔹
> Generalized vaccinia
> Rash following immunization
>> **Excludes1** vaccinia not from vaccine (B08.011)
>> **Excludes2** anaphylactic shock due to serum (T80.5-)
>> other serum reactions (T80.6-)
>> postimmunization arthropathy (M02.2)
>> postimmunization encephalitis (G04.02)
>> postimmunization fever (R50.83)
> (Ex) See PDX Collection 1485

X ● **T88.2** **Shock due to anesthesia** A 🔹
> Use additional code for adverse effect, if applicable, to identify drug (T41.- with fifth or sixth character 5)
>> **Excludes1** complications of anesthesia (in):
>> labor and delivery (O74.-)
>> pregnancy (O29.-)
>> puerperium (O89.-)
>> postprocedural shock NOS (T81.1-)
> (Ex) See PDX Collection 1441

X ● **T88.3** **Malignant hyperthermia due to anesthesia** A 🔹
> Use additional code for adverse effect, if applicable, to identify drug (T41.- with fifth or sixth character 5)
> (Ex) See PDX Collection 1486

X ● **T88.4** **Failed or difficult intubation**

● **T88.5** **Other complications of anesthesia**
> Use additional code for adverse effect, if applicable, to identify drug (T41.- with fifth or sixth character 5)
> **Coding Clinic: 2016, Q4, P72**

X ● **T88.51** **Hypothermia following anesthesia**

X ● **T88.52** **Failed moderate sedation during procedure**
> Failed conscious sedation during procedure
>> **Excludes2** personal history of failed moderate sedation (Z92.83)

X ● **T88.53** **Unintended awareness under general anesthesia during procedure**
>> **Excludes2** personal history of unintended awareness under general anesthesia (Z92.84)
> **Coding Clinic: 2016, Q4, P72-73**

X ● **T88.59** **Other complications of anesthesia**

X ● **T88.6** **Anaphylactic reaction due to adverse effect of correct drug or medicament properly administered** A 🔹
> Anaphylactic shock due to adverse effect of correct drug or medicament properly administered
> Anaphylactoid reaction NOS
> Use additional code for adverse effect, if applicable, to identify drug (T36-T50 with fifth or sixth character 5)
>> **Excludes1** anaphylactic reaction due to serum (T80.5-)
>> anaphylactic shock or reaction due to adverse food reaction (T78.0-)
> (Ex) See PDX Collection 1426

X ● **T88.7** **Unspecified adverse effect of drug or medicament**
> Drug hypersensitivity NOS
> Drug reaction NOS
> Use additional code for adverse effect, if applicable, to identify drug (T36-T50 with fifth or sixth character 5)
>> **Excludes1** specified adverse effects of drugs and medicaments (A00-R94 and T80-T88.6, T88.8)

X ● **T88.8** **Other specified complications of surgical and medical care, not elsewhere classified**
> Use additional code to identify the complication

X ● **T88.9** **Complication of surgical and medical care, unspecified**

CHAPTER 20

EXTERNAL CAUSES OF MORBIDITY (V00-Y99)

OGCR Chapter-Specific Coding Guidelines

20. **Chapter 20: External Causes of Morbidity (V00-Y99)**

The external causes of morbidity codes should never be sequenced as the first-listed or principal diagnosis.

External cause codes are intended to provide data for injury research and evaluation of injury prevention strategies. These codes capture how the injury or health condition happened (cause), the intent (unintentional or accidental; or intentional, such as suicide or assault), the place where the event occurred the activity of the patient at the time of the event, and the person's status (e.g., civilian, military).

There is no national requirement for mandatory ICD-10-CM external cause code reporting. Unless a provider is subject to a state-based external cause code reporting mandate or these codes are required by a particular payer, reporting of ICD-10-CM codes in Chapter 20, External Causes of Morbidity, is not required. In the absence of a mandatory reporting requirement, providers are encouraged to voluntarily report external cause codes, as they provide valuable data for injury research and evaluation of injury prevention strategies.

a. **General External Cause Coding Guidelines**

1) **Used with any code in the range of A00.0-T88.9, Z00-Z99**

An external cause code may be used with any code in the range of A00.0-T88.9, Z00-Z99, classification that **represents** a health condition due to an external cause. Though they are most applicable to injuries, they are also valid for use with such things as infections or diseases due to an external source, and other health conditions, such as a heart attack that occurs during strenuous physical activity.

2) **External cause code used for length of treatment**

Assign the external cause code, with the appropriate 7th character (initial encounter, subsequent encounter or sequela) for each encounter for which the injury or condition is being treated.

Most categories in chapter 20 have a 7th character requirement for each applicable code. Most categories in this chapter have three 7th character values: A, initial encounter, D, subsequent encounter and S, sequela. While the patient may be seen by a new or different provider over the course of treatment for an injury or condition, assignment of the 7th character for external cause should match the 7th character of the code assigned for the associated injury or condition for the encounter.

3) **Use the full range of external cause codes**

Use the full range of external cause codes to completely describe the cause, the intent, the place of occurrence and if applicable, the activity of the patient at the time of the event, and the patient's status, for all injuries, and other health conditions due to an external cause.

4) **Assign as many external cause codes as necessary**

Assign as many external cause codes as necessary to fully explain each cause. If only one external code can be recorded, assign the code most related to the principal diagnosis.

5) **The selection of the appropriate external cause code**

The selection of the appropriate external cause code is guided by the Alphabetic Index of External Causes and by Inclusion and Exclusion notes in the Tabular List.

6) **External cause code can never be a principal diagnosis**

An external cause code can never be a principal (first-listed) diagnosis.

7) **Combination external cause codes**

Certain of the external cause codes are combination codes that identify sequential events that result in an injury, such as a fall which results in striking against an object. The injury may be due to either event or both. The combination external cause code used should correspond to the sequence of events regardless of which caused the most serious injury.

8) **No external cause code needed in certain circumstances**

No external cause code from Chapter 20 is needed if the external cause and intent are included in a code from another chapter (e.g. T36.0X1- Poisoning by penicillins, accidental (unintentional)).

b. **Place of Occurrence Guideline**

Codes from category Y92, Place of occurrence of the external cause, are secondary codes for use after other external cause codes to identify the location of the patient at the time of injury or other condition.

Generally, a place of occurrence code is assigned only once, at the initial encounter for treatment. However, in the rare instance that a new injury occurs during hospitalization, an additional place of occurrence code may be assigned. No 7th characters are used for Y92. Only one code from Y92 should be recorded on a medical record.

Do not use place of occurrence code Y92.9 if the place is not stated or is not applicable.

c. **Activity Code**

Assign a code from category Y93, Activity code, to describe the activity of the patient at the time the injury or other health condition occurred.

An activity code is used only once, at the initial encounter for treatment. Only one code from Y93 should be recorded on a medical record.

The activity codes are not applicable to poisonings, adverse effects, misadventures or sequela.

Do not assign Y93.9, Unspecified activity, if the activity is not stated.

A code from category Y93 is appropriate for use with external cause and intent codes if identifying the activity provides additional information about the event.

d. **Place of Occurrence, Activity, and Status Codes Used with other External Cause Code**

When applicable, place of occurrence, activity, and external cause status codes are sequenced after the main external cause code(s). Regardless of the number of external cause codes assigned, there should be only one place of occurrence code, one activity code, and one external cause status code assigned to an encounter.

e. If the Reporting Format Limits the Number of External Cause Codes

If the reporting format limits the number of external cause codes that can be used in reporting clinical data, report the code for the cause/intent most related to the principal diagnosis. If the format permits capture of additional external cause codes, the cause/intent, including medical misadventures, of the additional events should be reported rather than the codes for place, activity, or external status.

f. Multiple External Cause Coding Guidelines

More than one external cause code is required to fully describe the external cause of an illness or injury. The assignment of external cause codes should be sequenced in the following priority:

If two or more events cause separate injuries, an external cause code should be assigned for each cause. The first-listed external cause code will be selected in the following order:

External codes for child and adult abuse take priority over all other external cause codes.

See Section I.C.19., Child and Adult abuse guidelines.

External codes for terrorism events take priority over all other external cause codes except child and adult abuse.

External cause codes for cataclysmic events take priority over all other external cause codes except child and adult abuse and terrorism.

External cause codes for transport accidents take priority over all other external cause codes except cataclysmic events, child and adult abuse and terrorism.

Activity and external cause status codes are assigned following all causal (intent) external cause codes.

The first-listed external cause code should correspond to the cause of the most serious diagnosis due to an assault, accident, or self-harm, following the order of hierarchy listed above.

g. Child and Adult Abuse Guideline

Adult and child abuse, neglect and maltreatment are classified as assault. Any of the assault codes may be used to indicate the external cause of any injury resulting from the confirmed abuse.

For confirmed cases of abuse, neglect and maltreatment, when the perpetrator is known, a code from Y07, Perpetrator of maltreatment and neglect, should accompany any other assault codes.

See Section I.C.19. Adult and child abuse, neglect and other maltreatment

h. Unknown or Undetermined Intent Guideline

If the intent (accident, self-harm, assault) of the cause of an injury or other condition is unknown or unspecified, code the intent as accidental intent. All transport accident categories assume accidental intent.

1) Use of undetermined intent

External cause codes for events of undetermined intent are only for use if the documentation in the record specifies that the intent cannot be determined.

i. Sequelae (Late Effects) of External Cause Guidelines

1) Sequelae external cause codes

Sequela are reported using the external cause code with the 7th character "S" for sequela. These codes should be used with any report of a late effect or sequela resulting from a previous injury.

See Section I.B.10. Sequela, (Late Effects)

2) Sequela external cause code with a related current injury

A sequela external cause code should never be used with a related current nature of injury code.

3) Use of sequela external cause codes for subsequent visits

Use a late effect external cause code for subsequent visits when a late effect of the initial injury is being treated. Do not use a late effect external cause code for subsequent visits for follow-up care (e.g., to assess healing, to receive rehabilitative therapy) of the injury when no late effect of the injury has been documented.

j. Terrorism Guidelines

1) Cause of injury identified by the Federal Government (FBI) as terrorism

When the cause of an injury is identified by the Federal Government (FBI) as terrorism, the first-listed external cause code should be a code from category Y38, Terrorism. The definition of terrorism employed by the FBI is found at the inclusion note at the beginning of category Y38. Use additional code for place of occurrence (Y92.-). More than one Y38 code may be assigned if the injury is the result of more than one mechanism of terrorism.

2) Cause of an injury is suspected to be the result of terrorism

When the cause of an injury is suspected to be the result of terrorism a code from category Y38 should not be assigned. Suspected cases should be classified as assault.

3) Code Y38.9, Terrorism, secondary effects

Assign code Y38.9, Terrorism, secondary effects, for conditions occurring subsequent to the terrorist event. This code should not be assigned for conditions that are due to the initial terrorist act.

It is acceptable to assign code Y38.9 with another code from Y38 if there is an injury due to the initial terrorist event and an injury that is a subsequent result of the terrorist event.

k. External cause status

A code from category Y99, External cause status, should be assigned whenever any other external cause code is assigned for an encounter, including an Activity code, except for the events noted below. Assign a code from category Y99, External cause status, to indicate the work status of the person at the time the event occurred. The status code indicates whether the event occurred during military activity, whether a non-military person was at work, whether an individual including a student or volunteer was involved in a non-work activity at the time of the causal event.

A code from Y99, External cause status, should be assigned, when applicable, with other external cause codes, such as transport accidents and falls. The external cause status codes are not applicable to poisonings, adverse effects, misadventures or late effects.

Do not assign a code from category Y99 if no other external cause codes (cause, activity) are applicable for the encounter.

An external cause status code is used only once, at the initial encounter for treatment. Only one code from Y99 should be recorded on a medical record.

Do not assign code Y99.9, Unspecified external cause status, if the status is not stated.

CHAPTER 20

EXTERNAL CAUSES OF MORBIDITY (V00-Y99)

Note: This chapter permits the classification of environmental events and circumstances as the cause of injury, and other adverse effects. Where a code from this section is applicable, it is intended that it shall be used secondary to a code from another chapter of the Classification indicating the nature of the condition. Most often, the condition will be classifiable to Chapter 19, Injury, poisoning and certain other consequences of external causes (S00-T88). Other conditions that may be stated to be due to external causes are classified in Chapters I to XVIII. For these conditions, codes from Chapter 20 should be used to provide additional information as to the cause of the condition.

This chapter contains the following blocks:

V00-X58	Accidents
V00-V99	Transport accidents
V00-V09	Pedestrian injured in transport accident
V10-V19	Pedal cycle rider injured in transport accident
V20-V29	Motorcycle rider injured in transport accident
V30-V39	Occupant of three-wheeled motor vehicle injured in transport accident
V40-V49	Car occupant injured in transport accident
V50-V59	Occupant of pick-up truck or van injured in transport accident
V60-V69	Occupant of heavy transport vehicle injured in transport accident
V70-V79	Bus occupant injured in transport accident
V80-V89	Other land transport accidents
V90-V94	Water transport accidents
V95-V97	Air and space transport accidents
V98-V99	Other and unspecified transport accidents
W00-X58	Other external causes of accidental injury
W00-W19	Slipping, tripping, stumbling and falls
W20-W49	Exposure to inanimate mechanical forces
W50-W64	Exposure to animate mechanical forces
W65-W74	Accidental non-transport drowning and submersion
W85-W99	Exposure to electric current, radiation and extreme ambient air temperature and pressure
X00-X08	Exposure to smoke, fire and flames
X10-X19	Contact with heat and hot substances
X30-X39	Exposure to forces of nature
~~X50~~	~~Overexertion and strenuous or repetitive movements~~
X52, X58	Accidental exposure to other specified factors
X71-X83	Intentional self-harm
X92-Y09	Assault
Y21-Y33	Event of undetermined intent
Y35-Y38	Legal intervention, operations of war, military operations, and terrorism
Y62-Y84	Complications of medical and surgical care
Y62-Y69	Misadventures to patients during surgical and medical care
Y70-Y82	Medical devices associated with adverse incidents in diagnostic and therapeutic use
Y83-Y84	Surgical and other medical procedures as the cause of abnormal reaction of the patient, or of later complication, without mention of misadventure at the time of the procedure
Y90-Y99	Supplementary factors related to causes of morbidity classified elsewhere

ACCIDENTS (V00-X58)

TRANSPORT ACCIDENTS (V00-V99)

Note: This section is structured in 12 groups. Those relating to land transport accidents (V00-V89) reflect the victim's mode of transport and are subdivided to identify the victim's 'counterpart' or the type of event. The vehicle of which the injured person is an occupant is identified in the first two characters since it is seen as the most important factor to identify for prevention purposes. A transport accident is one in which the vehicle involved must be moving or running or in use for transport purposes at the time of the accident.

Use additional code to identify:
Airbag injury (W22.1)
Type of street or road (Y92.4-)
Use of cellular telephone and other electronic equipment at the time of the transport accident (Y93.C-)

Excludes1 agricultural vehicles in stationary use or maintenance (W31.-)
assault by crashing of motor vehicle (Y03.-)
automobile or motor cycle in stationary use or maintenance - code to type of accident
crashing of motor vehicle, undetermined intent (Y32)
intentional self-harm by crashing of motor vehicle (X82)

Excludes2 transport accidents due to cataclysm (X34-X38)

Note: Definitions related to transport accidents:

(a) A transport accident (V00-V99) is any accident involving a device designed primarily for, or used at the time primarily for, conveying persons or good from one place to another.

(b) A public highway [trafficway] or street is the entire width between property lines (or other boundary lines) of land open to the public as a matter of right or custom for purposes of moving persons or property from one place to another. A roadway is that part of the public highway designed, improved and customarily used for vehicular traffic.

(c) A traffic accident is any vehicle accident occurring on the public highway [i.e., originating on, terminating on, or involving a vehicle partially on the highway]. A vehicle accident is assumed to have occurred on the public highway unless another place is specified, except in the case of accidents involving only off-road motor vehicles, which are classified as nontraffic accidents unless the contrary is stated.

(d) A nontraffic accident is any vehicle accident that occurs entirely in any place other than a public highway.

(e) A pedestrian is any person involved in an accident who was not at the time of the accident riding in or on a motor vehicle, railway train, streetcar or animal-drawn or other vehicle, or on a pedal cycle or animal. This includes, a person changing a tire, working on a parked car, or a person on foot. It also includes the user of a pedestrian conveyance such as a baby-stroller, ice-skates, skis, sled, roller skates, a skateboard, nonmotorized or motorized wheelchair, motorized mobility scooter, or nonmotorized scooter.

(f) A driver is an occupant of a transport vehicle who is operating or intending to operate it.

(g) A passenger is any occupant of a transport vehicle other than the driver, except a person traveling on the outside of the vehicle.

(h) A person on the outside of a vehicle is any person being transported by a vehicle but not occupying the space normally reserved for the driver or passengers, or the space intended for the transport of property. This includes a person travelling on the bodywork, bumper, fender, roof, running board or step of a vehicle, as well as, hanging on the outside of the vehicle.

(i) A pedal cycle is any land transport vehicle operated solely by nonmotorized pedals including a bicycle or tricycle.

(j) A pedal cyclist is any person riding a pedal cycle or in a sidecar or trailer attached to a pedal cycle.

▶ New   ⇒ Revised   ~~deleted~~ Deleted   Excludes 1   Excludes 2   Includes   Use additional   Code first   Code also   Key words

OGCR Official Guidelines   ● Unacceptable Principal Diagnosis   X Assign placeholder X   ● Use Additional Character(s)   ▶ Manifestation Code   **Coding Clinic**

(k) A motorcycle is a two-wheeled motor vehicle with one or two riding saddles and sometimes with a third wheel for the support of a sidecar. The sidecar is considered part of the motorcycle. This includes a moped, motor scooter, or motorized bicycle.

(l) A motorcycle rider is any person riding a motorcycle or in a sidecar or trailer attached to the motorcycle.

(m) A three-wheeled motor vehicle is a motorized tricycle designed primarily for on-road use. This includes a motor-driven tricycle, a motorized rickshaw, or a three-wheeled motor car.

(n) A car [automobile] is a four-wheeled motor vehicle designed primarily for carrying up to 7 persons. A trailer being towed by the car is considered part of the car. It does not include a van or minivan—see definition (o)

(o) A pick-up truck or van is a four or six-wheeled motor vehicle designed for carrying passengers as well as property or cargo weighing less than the local limit for classification as a heavy goods vehicle, and not requiring a special driver's license. This includes a minivan and a sport-utility vehicle (SUV).

(p) A heavy transport vehicle is a motor vehicle designed primarily for carrying property, meeting local criteria for classification as a heavy goods vehicle in terms of weight and requiring a special driver's license.

(q) A bus (coach) is a motor vehicle designed or adapted primarily for carrying more than 10 passengers, and requiring a special driver's license.

(r) A railway train or railway vehicle is any device, with or without freight or passenger cars coupled to it, designed for traffic on a railway track. This includes subterranean (subways) or elevated trains.

(s) A streetcar is a device designed and used primarily for transporting passengers within a municipality, running on rails, usually subject to normal traffic control signals, and operated principally on a right-of-way that forms part of the roadway. This includes a tram or trolley that runs on rails. A trailer being towed by a streetcar is considered part of the streetcar.

(t) A special vehicle mainly used on industrial premises is a motor vehicle designed primarily for use within the buildings and premises of industrial or commercial establishments. This includes battery-powered airport passenger vehicles or baggage/mail trucks, forklifts, coal-cars in a coal mine, logging cars and trucks used in mines or quarries.

(u) A special vehicle mainly used in agriculture is a motor vehicle designed specifically for use in farming and agriculture (horticulture), to work the land, tend and harvest crops and transport materials on the farm. This includes harvesters, farm machinery and tractor and trailers.

(v) A special construction vehicle is a motor vehicle designed specifically for use on construction and demolition sites. This includes bulldozers, diggers, earth levellers, dump trucks, backhoes, front-end loaders, pavers, and mechanical shovels.

(w) A special all-terrain vehicle is a motor vehicle of special design to enable it to negotiate over rough or soft terrain, snow or sand. Examples of special design are high construction, special wheels and tires, tracks, and support on a cushion of air. This includes snow mobiles, all-terrain vehicles (ATV), and dune buggies. It does not include passenger vehicle designated as sport utility vehicles (SUV).

(x) A watercraft is any device designed for transporting passengers or goods on water. This includes motor or sail boats, ships, and hovercraft.

(y) An aircraft is any device for transporting passengers or goods in the air. This includes hot-air balloons, gliders, helicopters and airplanes.

(z) A military vehicle is any motorized vehicle operating on a public roadway owned by the military and being operated by a member of the military.

PEDESTRIAN INJURED IN TRANSPORT ACCIDENT (VØØ-VØ9)

Includes person changing tire on transport vehicle
person examining engine of vehicle broken down in (on side of) road

Excludes1 fall due to non-transport collision with other person (W03)
pedestrian on foot falling (slipping) on ice and snow (W00.-)
struck or bumped by another person (W51)

● VØØ Pedestrian conveyance accident
Use additional place of occurrence and activity external cause codes, if known (Y92.-, Y93.-)

Excludes1 collision with another person without fall (W51)
fall due to person on foot colliding with another person on foot (W03)
fall from non-moving wheelchair, nonmotorized scooter and motorized mobility scooter without collision (W05.-)
pedestrian (conveyance) collision with other land transport vehicle (V01-V09)
pedestrian on foot falling (slipping) on ice and snow (W00.-)

The appropriate 7th character is to be added to each code from category VØØ

A initial encounter
D subsequent encounter
S sequela

● VØØ.Ø Pedestrian on foot injured in collision with pedestrian conveyance
X● VØØ.Ø1 Pedestrian on foot injured in collision with roller-skater
X● VØØ.Ø2 Pedestrian on foot injured in collision with skateboarder
X● VØØ.Ø9 Pedestrian on foot injured in collision with other pedestrian conveyance

● VØØ.1 Rolling-type pedestrian conveyance accident
Excludes1 accident with babystroller (V00.82-)
accident with wheelchair (powered) (V00.81-)
accident with motorized mobility scooter (V00.83-)

● VØØ.11 In-line roller-skate accident
● VØØ.111 Fall from in-line roller-skates
● VØØ.112 In-line roller-skater colliding with stationary object
● VØØ.118 Other in-line roller-skate accident
Excludes1 roller-skater collision with other land transport vehicle (V01-V09 with 5th character 1)

● VØØ.12 Non-in-line roller-skate accident
● VØØ.121 Fall from non-in-line roller-skates
● VØØ.122 Non-in-line roller-skater colliding with stationary object
● VØØ.128 Other non-in-line roller-skating accident
Excludes1 roller-skater collision with other land transport vehicle (V01-V09 with 5th character 1)

N Newborn Age: Ø P Pediatric Age: Ø–17 M Maternity DX: 12–55 A Adult Age: 15–124 ♀ Females Only ♂ Males Only
Complication\Comorbidity Major C\C CC/MCC Exclusions Hospital-Acquired Condition

CHAPTER 2Ø (VØ1-Y99)

1503

- ● V00.13 **Skateboard accident**
  - ● V00.131 **Fall from skateboard**
  - ● V00.132 **Skateboarder colliding with stationary object**
  - ● V00.138 **Other skateboard accident**
    - **Excludes1** skateboarder collision with other land transport vehicle (V01-V09 with 5th character 2)
- ● V00.14 **Scooter (nonmotorized) accident**
  - **Excludes1** motorscooter accident (V20-V29)
  - ● V00.141 **Fall from scooter (nonmotorized)**
  - ● V00.142 **Scooter (nonmotorized) colliding with stationary object**
  - ● V00.148 **Other scooter (nonmotorized) accident**
    - **Excludes1** scooter (non-motorized) collision with other land transport vehicle (V01-V09 with fifth character 9)
- ● V00.15 **Heelies accident**
  - Rolling shoe
  - Wheeled shoe
  - Wheelies accident
  - ● V00.151 **Fall from heelies**
  - ● V00.152 **Heelies colliding with stationary object**
  - ● V00.158 **Other heelies accident**
- ● V00.18 **Accident on other rolling-type pedestrian conveyance**
  - ● V00.181 **Fall from other rolling-type pedestrian conveyance**
  - ● V00.182 **Pedestrian on other rolling-type pedestrian conveyance colliding with stationary object**
  - ● V00.188 **Other accident on other rolling-type pedestrian conveyance**
- ● V00.2 **Gliding-type pedestrian conveyance accident**
  - ● V00.21 **Ice-skates accident**
    - ● V00.211 **Fall from ice-skates**
    - ● V00.212 **Ice-skater colliding with stationary object**
    - ● V00.218 **Other ice-skates accident**
      - **Excludes1** ice-skater collision with other land transport vehicle (V01-V09 with 5th digit 9)
  - ● V00.22 **Sled accident**
    - ● V00.221 **Fall from sled**
    - ● V00.222 **Sledder colliding with stationary object**
    - ● V00.228 **Other sled accident**
      - **Excludes1** sled collision with other land transport vehicle (V01-V09 with 5th digit 9)

- ● V00.28 **Other gliding-type pedestrian conveyance accident**
  - ● V00.281 **Fall from other gliding-type pedestrian conveyance**
  - ● V00.282 **Pedestrian on other gliding-type pedestrian conveyance colliding with stationary object**
  - ● V00.288 **Other accident on other gliding-type pedestrian conveyance**
    - **Excludes1** gliding-type pedestrian conveyance collision with other land transport vehicle (V01-V09 with 5th digit 9)
- ● V00.3 **Flat-bottomed pedestrian conveyance accident**
  - ● V00.31 **Snowboard accident**
    - ● V00.311 **Fall from snowboard**
    - ● V00.312 **Snowboarder colliding with stationary object**
    - ● V00.318 **Other snowboard accident**
      - **Excludes1** snowboarder collision with other land transport vehicle (V01-V09 with 5th digit 9)
  - ● V00.32 **Snow-ski accident**
    - ● V00.321 **Fall from snow-skis**
      - **Coding Clinic: 2015, Q1, P12**
    - ● V00.322 **Snow-skier colliding with stationary object**
    - ● V00.328 **Other snow-ski accident**
      - **Excludes1** snow-skier collision with other land transport vehicle (V01-V09 with 5th digit 9)
  - ● V00.38 **Other flat-bottomed pedestrian conveyance accident**
    - ● V00.381 **Fall from other flat-bottomed pedestrian conveyance**
    - ● V00.382 **Pedestrian on other flat-bottomed pedestrian conveyance colliding with stationary object**
    - ● V00.388 **Other accident on other flat-bottomed pedestrian conveyance**
- ● V00.8 **Accident on other pedestrian conveyance**
  - ● V00.81 **Accident with wheelchair (powered)**
    - ● V00.811 **Fall from moving wheelchair (powered)**
      - **Excludes1** fall from non-moving wheelchair (W05.0)
    - ● V00.812 **Wheelchair (powered) colliding with stationary object**
    - ● V00.818 **Other accident with wheelchair (powered)**
  - ● V00.82 **Accident with babystroller**
    - ● V00.821 **Fall from babystroller**
    - ● V00.822 **Babystroller colliding with stationary object**
    - ● V00.828 **Other accident with babystroller**

▶ New   ⇨ Revised   ~~deleted~~ Deleted   Excludes 1   Excludes 2   Includes   Use additional   Code first   Code also   Key words

OGCR Official Guidelines   ● Unacceptable Principal Diagnosis   X Assign placeholder X   ● Use Additional Character(s)   ▶ Manifestation Code   **Coding Clinic**

- ● **V00.83** **Accident with** motorized mobility scooter
  - ● **V00.831** **Fall from motorized mobility scooter**
    - **Excludes1** fall from non-moving motorized mobility scooter (W05.2)
  - ● **V00.832** **Motorized mobility scooter colliding with stationary object**
  - ● **V00.838** **Other accident with motorized mobility scooter**
- ● **V00.89** **Accident on other pedestrian conveyance**
  - ● **V00.891** **Fall from other pedestrian conveyance**
  - ● **V00.892** **Pedestrian on other pedestrian conveyance colliding with stationary object**
  - ● **V00.898** **Other accident on other pedestrian conveyance**
    - **Excludes1** other pedestrian (conveyance) collision with other land transport vehicle (V01-V09 with 5th digit 9)

- ● **V01** **Pedestrian injured in collision with pedal cycle**

  The appropriate 7th character is to be added to each code from category V01

A	initial encounter
D	subsequent encounter
S	sequela

  - ● **V01.0** **Pedestrian injured in collision with pedal cycle in nontraffic accident**
    - X ● **V01.00** **Pedestrian on foot injured in collision with pedal cycle in nontraffic accident**
      Pedestrian NOS injured in collision with pedal cycle in nontraffic accident
    - X ● **V01.01** **Pedestrian on roller-skates injured in collision with pedal cycle in nontraffic accident**
    - X ● **V01.02** **Pedestrian on skateboard injured in collision with pedal cycle in nontraffic accident**
    - X ● **V01.09** **Pedestrian with other conveyance injured in collision with pedal cycle in nontraffic accident**
      Pedestrian with babystroller injured in collision with pedal cycle in nontraffic accident
      Pedestrian in wheelchair (powered) injured in collision with pedal cycle in nontraffic accident
      Pedestrian in motorized mobility scooter injured in collision with pedal cycle in nontraffic accident
      Pedestrian on ice-skates injured in collision with pedal cycle in nontraffic accident
      Pedestrian on nonmotorized scooter injured in collision with pedal cycle in nontraffic accident
      Pedestrian on sled injured in collision with pedal cycle in nontraffic accident
      Pedestrian on snowboard injured in collision with pedal cycle in nontraffic accident
      Pedestrian on snow-skis injured in collision with pedal cycle in nontraffic accident

- ● **V01.1** **Pedestrian injured in collision with pedal cycle in traffic accident**
  - X ● **V01.10** **Pedestrian on foot injured in collision with pedal cycle in traffic accident**
    Pedestrian NOS injured in collision with pedal cycle in traffic accident
  - X ● **V01.11** **Pedestrian on roller-skates injured in collision with pedal cycle in traffic accident**
  - X ● **V01.12** **Pedestrian on skateboard injured in collision with pedal cycle in traffic accident**
  - X ● **V01.19** **Pedestrian with other conveyance injured in collision with pedal cycle in traffic accident**
    Pedestrian with babystroller injured in collision with pedal cycle in traffic accident
    Pedestrian in wheelchair (powered) injured in collision with pedal cycle in traffic accident
    Pedestrian in motorized mobility scooter injured in collision with pedal cycle in traffic accident
    Pedestrian on ice-skates injured in collision with pedal cycle in traffic accident
    Pedestrian on nonmotorized scooter injured in collision with pedal cycle in traffic accident
    Pedestrian on sled injured in collision with pedal cycle in traffic accident
    Pedestrian on snowboard injured in collision with pedal cycle in traffic accident
    Pedestrian on snow-skis injured in collision with pedal cycle in traffic accident

- ● **V01.9** **Pedestrian injured in collision with pedal cycle, unspecified whether traffic or nontraffic accident**
  - X ● **V01.90** **Pedestrian on foot injured in collision with pedal cycle, unspecified whether traffic or nontraffic accident**
    Pedestrian NOS injured in collision with pedal cycle, unspecified whether traffic or nontraffic accident
  - X ● **V01.91** **Pedestrian on roller-skates injured in collision with pedal cycle, unspecified whether traffic or nontraffic accident**
  - X ● **V01.92** **Pedestrian on skateboard injured in collision with pedal cycle, unspecified whether traffic or nontraffic accident**
  - X ● **V01.99** **Pedestrian with other conveyance injured in collision with pedal cycle, unspecified whether traffic or nontraffic accident**
    Pedestrian with babystroller injured in collision with pedal cycle, unspecified whether traffic or nontraffic accident
    Pedestrian in wheelchair (powered) injured in collision with pedal cycle, unspecified whether traffic or nontraffic accident
    Pedestrian in motorized mobility scooter injured in collision with pedal cycle, unspecified whether traffic or nontraffic accident
    Pedestrian on ice-skates injured in collision with pedal cycle unspecified, whether traffic or nontraffic accident
    Pedestrian on nonmotorized scooter injured in collision with pedal cycle, unspecified whether traffic or nontraffic accident
    Pedestrian on sled injured in collision with pedal cycle unspecified, whether traffic or nontraffic accident
    Pedestrian on snowboard injured in collision with pedal cycle, unspecified whether traffic or nontraffic accident
    Pedestrian on snow-skis injured in collision with pedal cycle, unspecified whether traffic or nontraffic accident

● V02   Pedestrian injured in collision with two- or three-wheeled motor vehicle

The appropriate 7th character is to be added to each code from category V02

> A   initial encounter
> D   subsequent encounter
> S   sequela

● V02.0   Pedestrian injured in collision with two- or three-wheeled motor vehicle in nontraffic accident

X ● V02.00   Pedestrian on foot injured in collision with two- or three-wheeled motor vehicle in nontraffic accident
> Pedestrian NOS injured in collision with two- or three-wheeled motor vehicle in nontraffic accident

X ● V02.01   Pedestrian on roller-skates injured in collision with two- or three-wheeled motor vehicle in nontraffic accident

X ● V02.02   Pedestrian on skateboard injured in collision with two- or three-wheeled motor vehicle in nontraffic accident

X ● V02.09   Pedestrian with other conveyance injured in collision with two- or three-wheeled motor vehicle in nontraffic accident
> Pedestrian with babystroller injured in collision with two- or three-wheeled motor vehicle in nontraffic accident
> Pedestrian on ice-skates injured in collision with two- or three-wheeled motor vehicle in nontraffic accident
> Pedestrian in wheelchair (powered) injured in collision with two- or three-wheeled motor vehicle in nontraffic accident
> Pedestrian in motorized mobility scooter injured in collision with two- or three-wheeled motor vehicle in nontraffic accident
> Pedestrian on nonmotorized scooter injured in collision with two- or three-wheeled motor vehicle in nontraffic accident
> Pedestrian on sled injured in collision with two- or three-wheeled motor vehicle in nontraffic accident
> Pedestrian on snowboard injured in collision with two- or three-wheeled motor vehicle in nontraffic accident
> Pedestrian on snow-skis injured in collision with two- or three-wheeled motor vehicle in nontraffic accident

● V02.1   Pedestrian injured in collision with two- or three-wheeled motor vehicle in traffic accident

X ● V02.10   Pedestrian on foot injured in collision with two- or three-wheeled motor vehicle in traffic accident
> Pedestrian NOS injured in collision with two- or three-wheeled motor vehicle in traffic accident

X ● V02.11   Pedestrian on roller-skates injured in collision with two- or three-wheeled motor vehicle in traffic accident

X ● V02.12   Pedestrian on skateboard injured in collision with two- or three-wheeled motor vehicle in traffic accident

X ● V02.19   Pedestrian with other conveyance injured in collision with two- or three-wheeled motor vehicle in traffic accident
> Pedestrian with babystroller injured in collision with two- or three-wheeled motor vehicle in traffic accident
> Pedestrian in wheelchair (powered) injured in collision with two- or three-wheeled motor vehicle in traffic accident
> Pedestrian in motorized mobility scooter injured in collision with two- or three-wheeled motor vehicle in traffic accident
> Pedestrian on ice-skates injured in collision with two- or three-wheeled motor vehicle in traffic accident
> Pedestrian on nonmotorized scooter injured in collision with two- or three-wheeled motor vehicle in traffic accident
> Pedestrian on sled injured in collision with two- or three-wheeled motor vehicle in traffic accident
> Pedestrian on snowboard injured in collision with two- or three-wheeled motor vehicle in traffic accident
> Pedestrian on snow-skis injured in collision with two- or three-wheeled motor vehicle in traffic accident

● V02.9   Pedestrian injured in collision with two- or three-wheeled motor vehicle, unspecified whether traffic or nontraffic accident

X ● V02.90   Pedestrian on foot injured in collision with two- or three-wheeled motor vehicle, unspecified whether traffic or nontraffic accident
> Pedestrian NOS injured in collision with two- or three-wheeled motor vehicle, unspecified whether traffic or nontraffic accident

X ● V02.91   Pedestrian on roller-skates injured in collision with two- or three-wheeled motor vehicle, unspecified whether traffic or nontraffic accident

X ● V02.92   Pedestrian on skateboard injured in collision with two- or three-wheeled motor vehicle, unspecified whether traffic or nontraffic accident

▶ New   ⇒ Revised   ~~deleted~~ Deleted   Excludes 1   Excludes 2   Includes   Use additional   Code first   Code also   Key words
OGCR Official Guidelines   ● Unacceptable Principal Diagnosis   X Assign placeholder X   ● Use Additional Character(s)   ▶ Manifestation Code   Coding Clinic

X● **V02.99   Pedestrian with other conveyance injured in collision with two- or three-wheeled motor vehicle, unspecified whether traffic or nontraffic accident**
> Pedestrian with babystroller injured in collision with two- or three-wheeled motor vehicle, unspecified whether traffic or nontraffic accident
> Pedestrian in wheelchair (powered) injured in collision with two- or three-wheeled motor vehicle, unspecified whether traffic or nontraffic accident
> Pedestrian in motorized mobility scooter injured in collision with two- or three-wheeled motor vehicle, unspecified whether traffic or nontraffic accident
> Pedestrian on ice-skates injured in collision with two- or three-wheeled motor vehicle, unspecified whether traffic or nontraffic accident
> Pedestrian on nonmotorized scooter injured in collision with two- or three-wheeled motor vehicle, unspecified whether traffic or nontraffic accident
> Pedestrian on sled injured in collision with two- or three-wheeled motor vehicle, unspecified whether traffic or nontraffic accident
> Pedestrian on snowboard injured in collision with two- or three-wheeled motor vehicle, unspecified whether traffic or nontraffic accident
> Pedestrian on snow-skis injured in collision with two- or three-wheeled motor vehicle, unspecified whether traffic or nontraffic accident

●**V03   Pedestrian injured in collision with car, pick-up truck or van**
> The appropriate 7th character is to be added to each code from category V03

A	initial encounter
D	subsequent encounter
S	sequela

●**V03.0   Pedestrian injured in collision with car, pick-up truck or van in nontraffic accident**

X● **V03.00   Pedestrian on foot injured in collision with car, pick-up truck or van in nontraffic accident**
> Pedestrian NOS injured in collision with car, pick-up truck or van in nontraffic accident

X● **V03.01   Pedestrian on roller-skates injured in collision with car, pick-up truck or van in nontraffic accident**

X● **V03.02   Pedestrian on skateboard injured in collision with car, pick-up truck or van in nontraffic accident**

X● **V03.09   Pedestrian with other conveyance injured in collision with car, pick-up truck or van in nontraffic accident**
> Pedestrian with babystroller injured in collision with car, pick-up truck or van in nontraffic accident
> Pedestrian in wheelchair (powered) injured in collision with car, pick-up truck or van in nontraffic accident
> Pedestrian in motorized mobility scooter injured in collision with car, pick-up truck or van in nontraffic accident
> Pedestrian on ice-skates injured in collision with car, pick-up truck or van in nontraffic accident
> Pedestrian on nonmotorized scooter injured in collision with car, pick-up truck or van in nontraffic accident
> Pedestrian on sled injured in collision with car, pick-up truck or van in nontraffic accident
> Pedestrian on snowboard injured in collision with car, pick-up truck or van in nontraffic accident
> Pedestrian on snow-skis injured in collision with car, pick-up truck or van in nontraffic accident

●**V03.1   Pedestrian injured in collision with car, pick-up truck or van in traffic accident**

X● **V03.10   Pedestrian on foot injured in collision with car, pick-up truck or van in traffic accident**
> Pedestrian NOS injured in collision with car, pick-up truck or van in traffic accident

X● **V03.11   Pedestrian on roller-skates injured in collision with car, pick-up truck or van in traffic accident**

X● **V03.12   Pedestrian on skateboard injured in collision with car, pick-up truck or van in traffic accident**

X● **V03.19   Pedestrian with other conveyance injured in collision with car, pick-up truck or van in traffic accident**
> Pedestrian with babystroller injured in collision with car, pick-up truck or van in traffic accident
> Pedestrian in wheelchair (powered) injured in collision with car, pick-up truck or van in traffic accident
> Pedestrian in motorized mobility scooter injured in collision with car, pick-up truck or van in traffic accident
> Pedestrian on ice-skates injured in collision with car, pick-up truck or van in traffic accident
> Pedestrian on nonmotorized scooter injured in collision with car, pick-up truck or van in traffic accident
> Pedestrian on sled injured in collision with car, pick-up truck or van in traffic accident
> Pedestrian on snowboard injured in collision with car, pick-up truck or van in traffic accident
> Pedestrian on snow-skis injured in collision with car, pick-up truck or van in traffic accident

N Newborn Age: 0   **P** Pediatric Age: 0–17   **M** Maternity DX: 12–55   **A** Adult Age: 15–124   ♀ Females Only   ♂ Males Only

Complication\Comorbidity   Major C\C   (Ex) CC/MCC Exclusions   Hospital-Acquired Condition   **1507**

● **V03.9**   **Pedestrian injured in collision with car, pick-up truck or van, unspecified whether traffic or nontraffic accident**

   X● **V03.90**   **Pedestrian on foot injured in collision with car, pick-up truck or van, unspecified whether traffic or nontraffic accident**
       Pedestrian NOS injured in collision with car, pick-up truck or van, unspecified whether traffic or nontraffic accident

   X● **V03.91**   **Pedestrian on roller-skates injured in collision with car, pick-up truck or van, unspecified whether traffic or nontraffic accident**

   X● **V03.92**   **Pedestrian on skateboard injured in collision with car, pick-up truck or van, unspecified whether traffic or nontraffic accident**

   X● **V03.99**   **Pedestrian with other conveyance injured in collision with car, pick-up truck or van, unspecified whether traffic or nontraffic accident**
       Pedestrian with babystroller injured in collision with car, pick-up truck or van, unspecified whether traffic or nontraffic accident
       Pedestrian in wheelchair (powered) injured in collision with car, pick-up truck or van, unspecified whether traffic or nontraffic accident
       Pedestrian in motorized mobility scooter injured in collision with car, pick-up truck or van, unspecified whether traffic or nontraffic accident
       Pedestrian on ice-skates injured in collision with car, pick-up truck or van, unspecified whether traffic or nontraffic accident
       Pedestrian on nonmotorized scooter injured in collision with car, pick-up truck or van, unspecified whether traffic or nontraffic accident
       Pedestrian on sled injured in collision with car, pick-up truck or van in nontraffic accident
       Pedestrian on snowboard injured in collision with car, pick-up truck or van, unspecified whether traffic or nontraffic accident
       Pedestrian on snow-skis injured in collision with car, pick-up truck or van, unspecified whether traffic or nontraffic accident

● **V04**   **Pedestrian injured in collision with heavy transport vehicle or bus**

   Excludes1   pedestrian injured in collision with military vehicle (V09.01, V09.21)

   The appropriate 7th character is to be added to each code from category V04

     | A | initial encounter |
     | D | subsequent encounter |
     | S | sequela |

● **V04.0**   **Pedestrian injured in collision with heavy transport vehicle or bus in nontraffic accident**

   X● **V04.00**   **Pedestrian on foot injured in collision with heavy transport vehicle or bus in nontraffic accident**
       Pedestrian NOS injured in collision with heavy transport vehicle or bus in nontraffic accident

   X● **V04.01**   **Pedestrian on roller-skates injured in collision with heavy transport vehicle or bus in nontraffic accident**

   X● **V04.02**   **Pedestrian on skateboard injured in collision with heavy transport vehicle or bus in nontraffic accident**

   X● **V04.09**   **Pedestrian with other conveyance injured in collision with heavy transport vehicle or bus in nontraffic accident**
       Pedestrian with babystroller injured in collision with heavy transport vehicle or bus in nontraffic accident
       Pedestrian in wheelchair (powered) injured in collision with heavy transport vehicle or bus in nontraffic accident
       Pedestrian in motorized mobility scooter injured in collision with heavy transport vehicle or bus in nontraffic accident
       Pedestrian on ice-skates injured in collision with heavy transport vehicle or bus in nontraffic accident
       Pedestrian on nonmotorized scooter injured in collision with heavy transport vehicle or bus in nontraffic accident
       Pedestrian on sled injured in collision with heavy transport vehicle or bus in nontraffic accident
       Pedestrian on snowboard injured in collision with heavy transport vehicle or bus in nontraffic accident
       Pedestrian on snow-skis injured in collision with heavy transport vehicle or bus in nontraffic accident

● **V04.1**   **Pedestrian injured in collision with heavy transport vehicle or bus in traffic accident**

   X● **V04.10**   **Pedestrian on foot injured in collision with heavy transport vehicle or bus in traffic accident**
       Pedestrian NOS injured in collision with heavy transport vehicle or bus in traffic accident

   X● **V04.11**   **Pedestrian on roller-skates injured in collision with heavy transport vehicle or bus in traffic accident**

   X● **V04.12**   **Pedestrian on skateboard injured in collision with heavy transport vehicle or bus in traffic accident**

   X● **V04.19**   **Pedestrian with other conveyance injured in collision with heavy transport vehicle or bus in traffic accident**
       Pedestrian with babystroller injured in collision with heavy transport vehicle or bus in traffic accident
       Pedestrian in wheelchair (powered) injured in collision with heavy transport vehicle or bus in traffic accident
       Pedestrian in motorized mobility scooter injured in collision with heavy transport vehicle or bus in traffic accident
       Pedestrian on ice-skates injured in collision with heavy transport vehicle or bus in traffic accident
       Pedestrian on nonmotorized scooter injured in collision with heavy transport vehicle or bus in traffic accident
       Pedestrian on sled injured in collision with heavy transport vehicle or bus in traffic accident
       Pedestrian on snowboard injured in collision with heavy transport vehicle or bus in traffic accident
       Pedestrian on snow-skis injured in collision with heavy transport vehicle or bus in traffic accident

● **V04.9** Pedestrian injured in collision with heavy transport vehicle or bus, unspecified whether traffic or nontraffic accident

X● **V04.90** Pedestrian on foot injured in collision with heavy transport vehicle or bus, unspecified whether traffic or nontraffic accident
Pedestrian NOS injured in collision with heavy transport vehicle or bus, unspecified whether traffic or nontraffic accident

X● **V04.91** Pedestrian on roller-skates injured in collision with heavy transport vehicle or bus, unspecified whether traffic or nontraffic accident

X● **V04.92** Pedestrian on skateboard injured in collision with heavy transport vehicle or bus, unspecified whether traffic or nontraffic accident

X● **V04.99** Pedestrian with other conveyance injured in collision with heavy transport vehicle or bus, unspecified whether traffic or nontraffic accident
Pedestrian with babystroller injured in collision with heavy transport vehicle or bus, unspecified whether traffic or nontraffic accident
Pedestrian in wheelchair (powered) injured in collision with heavy transport vehicle or bus, unspecified whether traffic or nontraffic accident
Pedestrian in motorized mobility scooter injured in collision with heavy transport vehicle or bus, unspecified whether traffic or nontraffic accident
Pedestrian on ice-skates injured in collision with heavy transport vehicle or bus, unspecified whether traffic or nontraffic accident
Pedestrian on nonmotorized scooter injured in collision with heavy transport vehicle or bus, unspecified whether traffic or nontraffic accident
Pedestrian on sled injured in collision with heavy transport vehicle or bus, unspecified whether traffic or nontraffic accident
Pedestrian on snowboard injured in collision with heavy transport vehicle or bus, unspecified whether traffic or nontraffic accident
Pedestrian on snow-skis injured in collision with heavy transport vehicle or bus, unspecified whether traffic or nontraffic accident

● **V05** Pedestrian injured in collision with railway train or railway vehicle

The appropriate 7th character is to be added to each code from category V05

A	initial encounter
D	subsequent encounter
S	sequela

● **V05.0** Pedestrian injured in collision with railway train or railway vehicle in nontraffic accident

X● **V05.00** Pedestrian on foot injured in collision with railway train or railway vehicle in nontraffic accident
Pedestrian NOS injured in collision with railway train or railway vehicle in nontraffic accident

X● **V05.01** Pedestrian on roller-skates injured in collision with railway train or railway vehicle in nontraffic accident

X● **V05.02** Pedestrian on skateboard injured in collision with railway train or railway vehicle in nontraffic accident

X● **V05.09** Pedestrian with other conveyance injured in collision with railway train or railway vehicle in nontraffic accident
Pedestrian with babystroller injured in collision with railway train or railway vehicle in nontraffic accident
Pedestrian in wheelchair (powered) injured in collision with railway train or railway vehicle in nontraffic accident
Pedestrian in motorized mobility scooter injured in collision with railway train or railway vehicle in nontraffic accident
Pedestrian on ice-skates injured in collision with railway train or railway vehicle in nontraffic accident
Pedestrian on nonmotorized scooter injured in collision with railway train or railway vehicle in nontraffic accident
Pedestrian on sled injured in collision with railway train or railway vehicle in nontraffic accident
Pedestrian on snowboard injured in collision with railway train or railway vehicle in nontraffic accident
Pedestrian on snow-skis injured in collision with railway train or railway vehicle in nontraffic accident

● **V05.1** Pedestrian injured in collision with railway train or railway vehicle in traffic accident

X● **V05.10** Pedestrian on foot injured in collision with railway train or railway vehicle in traffic accident
Pedestrian NOS injured in collision with railway train or railway vehicle in traffic accident

X● **V05.11** Pedestrian on roller-skates injured in collision with railway train or railway vehicle in traffic accident

X● **V05.12** Pedestrian on skateboard injured in collision with railway train or railway vehicle in traffic accident

X● **V05.19** Pedestrian with other conveyance injured in collision with railway train or railway vehicle in traffic accident
Pedestrian with babystroller injured in collision with railway train or railway vehicle in traffic accident
Pedestrian in wheelchair (powered) injured in collision with railway train or railway vehicle in traffic accident
Pedestrian in motorized mobility scooter injured in collision with railway train or railway vehicle in traffic accident
Pedestrian on ice-skates injured in collision with railway train or railway vehicle in traffic accident
Pedestrian on nonmotorized scooter injured in collision with railway train or railway vehicle in traffic accident
Pedestrian on sled injured in collision with railway train or railway vehicle in traffic accident
Pedestrian on snowboard injured in collision with railway train or railway vehicle in traffic accident
Pedestrian on snow-skis injured in collision with railway train or railway vehicle in traffic accident

CHAPTER 20 (V01-Y99)

- **V05.9** Pedestrian injured in collision with railway train or railway vehicle, unspecified whether traffic or nontraffic accident
  - X● **V05.90** Pedestrian on foot injured in collision with railway train or railway vehicle, unspecified whether traffic or nontraffic accident

    Pedestrian NOS injured in collision with railway train or railway vehicle, unspecified whether traffic or nontraffic accident
  - X● **V05.91** Pedestrian on roller-skates injured in collision with railway train or railway vehicle, unspecified whether traffic or nontraffic accident
  - X● **V05.92** Pedestrian on skateboard injured in collision with railway train or railway vehicle, unspecified whether traffic or nontraffic accident
  - X● **V05.99** Pedestrian with other conveyance injured in collision with railway train or railway vehicle, unspecified whether traffic or nontraffic accident

    Pedestrian with babystroller injured in collision with railway train or railway vehicle, unspecified whether traffic or nontraffic

    Pedestrian in wheelchair (powered) injured in collision with railway train or railway vehicle, unspecified whether traffic or nontraffic

    Pedestrian in motorized mobility scooter injured in collision with railway train or railway vehicle, unspecified whether traffic or nontraffic

    Pedestrian on ice-skates injured in collision with railway train or railway vehicle, unspecified whether traffic or nontraffic

    Pedestrian on nonmotorized scooter injured in collision with railway train or railway vehicle, unspecified whether traffic or nontraffic

    Pedestrian on sled injured in collision with railway train or railway vehicle, unspecified whether traffic or nontraffic

    Pedestrian on snowboard injured in collision with railway train or railway vehicle, unspecified whether traffic or nontraffic

    Pedestrian on snow-skis injured in collision with railway train or railway vehicle, unspecified whether traffic or nontraffic

- ● **V06** Pedestrian injured in collision with other nonmotor vehicle

  | Includes | collision with animal-drawn vehicle, animal being ridden, nonpowered streetcar |
  | Excludes1 | pedestrian injured in collision with pedestrian conveyance (V00.0-) |

  The appropriate 7th character is to be added to each code from category V06

A	initial encounter
D	subsequent encounter
S	sequela

  - ● **V06.0** Pedestrian injured in collision with other nonmotor vehicle in nontraffic accident
    - X● **V06.00** Pedestrian on foot injured in collision with other nonmotor vehicle in nontraffic accident

      Pedestrian NOS injured in collision with other nonmotor vehicle in nontraffic accident
    - X● **V06.01** Pedestrian on roller-skates injured in collision with other nonmotor vehicle in nontraffic accident
    - X● **V06.02** Pedestrian on skateboard injured in collision with other nonmotor vehicle in nontraffic accident

  - X● **V06.09** Pedestrian with other conveyance injured in collision with other nonmotor vehicle in nontraffic accident

    Pedestrian with babystroller injured in collision with other nonmotor vehicle in nontraffic accident

    Pedestrian in wheelchair (powered) injured in collision with other nonmotor vehicle in nontraffic accident

    Pedestrian in motorized mobility scooter injured in collision with other nonmotor vehicle in nontraffic accident

    Pedestrian on ice-skates injured in collision with other nonmotor vehicle in nontraffic accident

    Pedestrian on nonmotorized scooter injured in collision with other nonmotor vehicle in nontraffic accident

    Pedestrian on sled injured in collision with other nonmotor vehicle in nontraffic accident

    Pedestrian on snowboard injured in collision with other nonmotor vehicle in nontraffic accident

    Pedestrian on snow-skis injured in collision with other nonmotor vehicle in nontraffic accident

  - ● **V06.1** Pedestrian injured in collision with other nonmotor vehicle in traffic accident
    - X● **V06.10** Pedestrian on foot injured in collision with other nonmotor vehicle in traffic accident

      Pedestrian NOS injured in collision with other nonmotor vehicle in traffic accident
    - X● **V06.11** Pedestrian on roller-skates injured in collision with other nonmotor vehicle in traffic accident
    - X● **V06.12** Pedestrian on skateboard injured in collision with other nonmotor vehicle in traffic accident
    - X● **V06.19** Pedestrian with other conveyance injured in collision with other nonmotor vehicle in traffic accident

      Pedestrian with babystroller injured in collision with other nonmotor vehicle in nontraffic accident

      Pedestrian in wheelchair (powered) injured in collision with other nonmotor vehicle in traffic accident

      Pedestrian in motorized mobility scooter injured in collision with other nonmotor vehicle in traffic accident

      Pedestrian on ice-skates injured in collision with other nonmotor vehicle in traffic accident

      Pedestrian on nonmotorized scooter injured in collision with other nonmotor vehicle in traffic accident

      Pedestrian on sled injured in collision with other nonmotor vehicle in traffic accident

      Pedestrian on snowboard injured in collision with other nonmotor vehicle in traffic accident

      Pedestrian on snow-skis injured in collision with other nonmotor vehicle in traffic accident

  - ● **V06.9** Pedestrian injured in collision with other nonmotor vehicle, unspecified whether traffic or nontraffic accident
    - X● **V06.90** Pedestrian on foot injured in collision with other nonmotor vehicle, unspecified whether traffic or nontraffic accident

      Pedestrian NOS injured in collision with other nonmotor vehicle, unspecified whether traffic or nontraffic accident
    - X● **V06.91** Pedestrian on roller-skates injured in collision with other nonmotor vehicle, unspecified whether traffic or nontraffic accident

▶ New   ⇒ Revised   ~~deleted~~ Deleted   Excludes 1   Excludes 2   Includes   Use additional   Code first   Code also   Key words

1510

OGCR Official Guidelines   ● Unacceptable Principal Diagnosis   X Assign placeholder X   ● Use Additional Character(s)   ▶ Manifestation Code   **Coding Clinic**

X ● **V06.92**   **Pedestrian on skateboard injured in collision with other nonmotor vehicle, unspecified whether traffic or nontraffic accident**

X ● **V06.99**   **Pedestrian with other conveyance injured in collision with other nonmotor vehicle, unspecified whether traffic or nontraffic accident**

Pedestrian with babystroller injured in collision with other nonmotor vehicle, unspecified whether traffic or nontraffic accident

Pedestrian in wheelchair (powered) injured in collision with other nonmotor vehicle, unspecified whether traffic or nontraffic accident

Pedestrian in motorized mobility scooter injured in collision with other nonmotor vehicle, unspecified whether traffic or nontraffic accident

Pedestrian on ice-skates injured in collision with other nonmotor vehicle, unspecified whether traffic or nontraffic accident

Pedestrian on nonmotorized scooter injured in collision with other nonmotor vehicle, unspecified whether traffic or nontraffic accident

Pedestrian on sled injured in collision with other nonmotor vehicle, unspecified whether traffic or nontraffic accident

Pedestrian on snowboard injured in collision with other nonmotor vehicle, unspecified whether traffic or nontraffic accident

Pedestrian on snow-skis injured in collision with other nonmotor vehicle, unspecified whether traffic or nontraffic accident

● **V09**   **Pedestrian injured in other and unspecified transport accidents**

The appropriate 7th character is to be added to each code from category V09

A	initial encounter
D	subsequent encounter
S	sequela

● **V09.0**   **Pedestrian injured in nontraffic accident involving other and unspecified motor vehicles**

X ● **V09.00**   **Pedestrian injured in nontraffic accident involving unspecified motor vehicles**

X ● **V09.01**   **Pedestrian injured in nontraffic accident involving military vehicle**

X ● **V09.09**   **Pedestrian injured in nontraffic accident involving other motor vehicles**

Pedestrian injured in nontraffic accident by special vehicle

X ● **V09.1**   **Pedestrian injured in unspecified nontraffic accident**

● **V09.2**   **Pedestrian injured in traffic accident involving other and unspecified motor vehicles**

X ● **V09.20**   **Pedestrian injured in traffic accident involving unspecified motor vehicles**

X ● **V09.21**   **Pedestrian injured in traffic accident involving military vehicle**

X ● **V09.29**   **Pedestrian injured in traffic accident involving other motor vehicles**

X ● **V09.3**   **Pedestrian injured in unspecified traffic accident**

X ● **V09.9**   **Pedestrian injured in unspecified transport accident**

PEDAL CYCLE RIDER INJURED IN TRANSPORT ACCIDENT (V10-V19)

Includes	any non-motorized vehicle, excluding an animal-drawn vehicle, or a sidecar or trailer attached to the pedal cycle
Excludes2	rupture of pedal cycle tire (W37.0)

● **V10**   **Pedal cycle rider injured in collision with pedestrian or animal**

Excludes1	pedal cycle rider collision with animal-drawn vehicle or animal being ridden (V16.-)

The appropriate 7th character is to be added to each code from category V10

A	initial encounter
D	subsequent encounter
S	sequela

X ● **V10.0**   **Pedal cycle driver injured in collision with pedestrian or animal in nontraffic accident**

X ● **V10.1**   **Pedal cycle passenger injured in collision with pedestrian or animal in nontraffic accident**

X ● **V10.2**   **Unspecified pedal cyclist injured in collision with pedestrian or animal in nontraffic accident**

X ● **V10.3**   **Person boarding or alighting a pedal cycle injured in collision with pedestrian or animal**

X ● **V10.4**   **Pedal cycle driver injured in collision with pedestrian or animal in traffic accident**

X ● **V10.5**   **Pedal cycle passenger injured in collision with pedestrian or animal in traffic accident**

X ● **V10.9**   **Unspecified pedal cyclist injured in collision with pedestrian or animal in traffic accident**

● **V11**   **Pedal cycle rider injured in collision with other pedal cycle**

The appropriate 7th character is to be added to each code from category V11

A	initial encounter
D	subsequent encounter
S	sequela

X ● **V11.0**   **Pedal cycle driver injured in collision with other pedal cycle in nontraffic accident**

X ● **V11.1**   **Pedal cycle passenger injured in collision with other pedal cycle in nontraffic accident**

X ● **V11.2**   **Unspecified pedal cyclist injured in collision with other pedal cycle in nontraffic accident**

X ● **V11.3**   **Person boarding or alighting a pedal cycle injured in collision with other pedal cycle**

X ● **V11.4**   **Pedal cycle driver injured in collision with other pedal cycle in traffic accident**

X ● **V11.5**   **Pedal cycle passenger injured in collision with other pedal cycle in traffic accident**

X ● **V11.9**   **Unspecified pedal cyclist injured in collision with other pedal cycle in traffic accident**

CHAPTER 20 (V01-Y99)

● **V12   Pedal cycle rider injured in collision with two- or three-wheeled motor vehicle**

The appropriate 7th character is to be added to each code from category V12

> A   initial encounter
> D   subsequent encounter
> S   sequela

X● **V12.0**   Pedal cycle driver injured in collision with two- or three-wheeled motor vehicle in nontraffic accident

X● **V12.1**   Pedal cycle passenger injured in collision with two- or three-wheeled motor vehicle in nontraffic accident

X● **V12.2**   Unspecified pedal cyclist injured in collision with two- or three-wheeled motor vehicle in nontraffic accident

X● **V12.3**   Person boarding or alighting a pedal cycle injured in collision with two- or three-wheeled motor vehicle

X● **V12.4**   Pedal cycle driver injured in collision with two- or three-wheeled motor vehicle in traffic accident

X● **V12.5**   Pedal cycle passenger injured in collision with two- or three-wheeled motor vehicle in traffic accident

X● **V12.9**   Unspecified pedal cyclist injured in collision with two- or three-wheeled motor vehicle in traffic accident

● **V13   Pedal cycle rider injured in collision with car, pick-up truck or van**

The appropriate 7th character is to be added to each code from category V13

> A   initial encounter
> D   subsequent encounter
> S   sequela

X● **V13.0**   Pedal cycle driver injured in collision with car, pick-up truck or van in nontraffic accident

X● **V13.1**   Pedal cycle passenger injured in collision with car, pick-up truck or van in nontraffic accident

X● **V13.2**   Unspecified pedal cyclist injured in collision with car, pick-up truck or van in nontraffic accident

X● **V13.3**   Person boarding or alighting a pedal cycle injured in collision with car, pick-up truck or van

X● **V13.4**   Pedal cycle driver injured in collision with car, pick-up truck or van in traffic accident

X● **V13.5**   Pedal cycle passenger injured in collision with car, pick-up truck or van in traffic accident

X● **V13.9**   Unspecified pedal cyclist injured in collision with car, pick-up truck or van in traffic accident

● **V14   Pedal cycle rider injured in collision with heavy transport vehicle or bus**

> **Excludes1**   pedal cycle rider injured in collision with military vehicle (V19.81)

The appropriate 7th character is to be added to each code from category V14

> A   initial encounter
> D   subsequent encounter
> S   sequela

X● **V14.0**   Pedal cycle driver injured in collision with heavy transport vehicle or bus in nontraffic accident

X● **V14.1**   Pedal cycle passenger injured in collision with heavy transport vehicle or bus in nontraffic accident

X● **V14.2**   Unspecified pedal cyclist injured in collision with heavy transport vehicle or bus in nontraffic accident

X● **V14.3**   Person boarding or alighting a pedal cycle injured in collision with heavy transport vehicle or bus

X● **V14.4**   Pedal cycle driver injured in collision with heavy transport vehicle or bus in traffic accident

X● **V14.5**   Pedal cycle passenger injured in collision with heavy transport vehicle or bus in traffic accident

X● **V14.9**   Unspecified pedal cyclist injured in collision with heavy transport vehicle or bus in traffic accident

● **V15   Pedal cycle rider injured in collision with railway train or railway vehicle**

The appropriate 7th character is to be added to each code from category V15

> A   initial encounter
> D   subsequent encounter
> S   sequela

X● **V15.0**   Pedal cycle driver injured in collision with railway train or railway vehicle in nontraffic accident

X● **V15.1**   Pedal cycle passenger injured in collision with railway train or railway vehicle in nontraffic accident

X● **V15.2**   Unspecified pedal cyclist injured in collision with railway train or railway vehicle in nontraffic accident

X● **V15.3**   Person boarding or alighting a pedal cycle injured in collision with railway train or railway vehicle

X● **V15.4**   Pedal cycle driver injured in collision with railway train or railway vehicle in traffic accident

X● **V15.5**   Pedal cycle passenger injured in collision with railway train or railway vehicle in traffic accident

X● **V15.9**   Unspecified pedal cyclist injured in collision with railway train or railway vehicle in traffic accident

● **V16   Pedal cycle rider injured in collision with other nonmotor vehicle**

> **Includes**   collision with animal-drawn vehicle, animal being ridden, streetcar

The appropriate 7th character is to be added to each code from category V16

> A   initial encounter
> D   subsequent encounter
> S   sequela

X● **V16.0**   Pedal cycle driver injured in collision with other nonmotor vehicle in nontraffic accident

X● **V16.1**   Pedal cycle passenger injured in collision with other nonmotor vehicle in nontraffic accident

X● **V16.2**   Unspecified pedal cyclist injured in collision with other nonmotor vehicle in nontraffic accident

X● **V16.3**   Person boarding or alighting a pedal cycle injured in collision with other nonmotor vehicle in nontraffic accident

X● **V16.4**   Pedal cycle driver injured in collision with other nonmotor vehicle in traffic accident

X● **V16.5**   Pedal cycle passenger injured in collision with other nonmotor vehicle in traffic accident

X● **V16.9**   Unspecified pedal cyclist injured in collision with other nonmotor vehicle in traffic accident

● **V17   Pedal cycle rider injured in collision with fixed or stationary object**

The appropriate 7th character is to be added to each code from category V17

> A   initial encounter
> D   subsequent encounter
> S   sequela

X● **V17.0**   Pedal cycle driver injured in collision with fixed or stationary object in nontraffic accident

X● **V17.1**   Pedal cycle passenger injured in collision with fixed or stationary object in nontraffic accident

X● **V17.2**   Unspecified pedal cyclist injured in collision with fixed or stationary object in nontraffic accident

X● **V17.3**   Person boarding or alighting a pedal cycle injured in collision with fixed or stationary object

X● **V17.4**   Pedal cycle driver injured in collision with fixed or stationary object in traffic accident

X● **V17.5**   Pedal cycle passenger injured in collision with fixed or stationary object in traffic accident

X● **V17.9**   Unspecified pedal cyclist injured in collision with fixed or stationary object in traffic accident

▶ New   ⇒ Revised   ~~deleted~~ Deleted   Excludes 1   Excludes 2   Includes   Use additional   Code first   Code also   Key words

1512   OGCR Official Guidelines   ● Unacceptable Principal Diagnosis   X Assign placeholder X   ● Use Additional Character(s)   ▶ Manifestation Code   **Coding Clinic**

● **V18**   **Pedal cycle rider injured in noncollision transport accident**

     Includes   fall or thrown from pedal cycle (without antecedent collision)
                         overturning pedal cycle NOS
                         overturning pedal cycle without collision

     The appropriate 7th character is to be added to each code from category V18

A	initial encounter
D	subsequent encounter
S	sequela

X● **V18.0**   Pedal cycle **driver** injured in noncollision transport accident in **nontraffic accident**

X● **V18.1**   Pedal cycle **passenger** injured in noncollision transport accident in **nontraffic accident**

X● **V18.2**   Unspecified pedal cyclist injured in noncollision transport accident in **nontraffic accident**

X● **V18.3**   Person boarding or alighting a pedal cycle injured in noncollision transport accident

X● **V18.4**   Pedal cycle **driver** injured in noncollision transport accident in **traffic accident**

X● **V18.5**   Pedal cycle **passenger** injured in noncollision transport accident in **traffic accident**

X● **V18.9**   Unspecified pedal cyclist injured in noncollision transport accident in **traffic accident**

● **V19**   **Pedal cycle rider injured in other and unspecified transport accidents**

     The appropriate 7th character is to be added to each code from category V19

A	initial encounter
D	subsequent encounter
S	sequela

● **V19.0**   Pedal cycle **driver** injured in collision with other and unspecified motor vehicles in **nontraffic accident**

     X● **V19.00**   Pedal cycle driver injured in collision with **unspecified** motor vehicles in nontraffic accident

     X● **V19.09**   Pedal cycle driver injured in collision with **other** motor vehicles in nontraffic accident

● **V19.1**   Pedal cycle **passenger** injured in collision with other and unspecified motor vehicles in **nontraffic accident**

     X● **V19.10**   Pedal cycle passenger injured in collision with **unspecified** motor vehicles in nontraffic accident

     X● **V19.19**   Pedal cycle passenger injured in collision with **other** motor vehicles in nontraffic accident

● **V19.2**   Unspecified pedal cyclist injured in collision with other and unspecified motor vehicles in nontraffic accident

     X● **V19.20**   Unspecified pedal cyclist injured in collision with **unspecified** motor vehicles in nontraffic accident
                   Pedal cycle collision NOS, nontraffic

     X● **V19.29**   Unspecified pedal cyclist injured in collision with **other** motor vehicles in nontraffic accident

X● **V19.3**   Pedal cyclist (driver) (passenger) injured in **unspecified** nontraffic accident
           Pedal cycle accident NOS, nontraffic
           Pedal cyclist injured in nontraffic accident NOS

● **V19.4**   Pedal cycle **driver** injured in collision with other and unspecified motor vehicles in **traffic accident**

     X● **V19.40**   Pedal cycle driver injured in collision with **unspecified** motor vehicles in traffic accident

     X● **V19.49**   Pedal cycle driver injured in collision with **other** motor vehicles in traffic accident

● **V19.5**   Pedal cycle **passenger** injured in collision with other and unspecified motor vehicles in **traffic accident**

     X● **V19.50**   Pedal cycle passenger injured in collision with **unspecified** motor vehicles in traffic accident

     X● **V19.59**   Pedal cycle passenger injured in collision with **other** motor vehicles in traffic accident

● **V19.6**   Unspecified pedal cyclist injured in collision with other and unspecified motor vehicles in traffic accident

     X● **V19.60**   Unspecified pedal cyclist injured in collision with **unspecified** motor vehicles in traffic accident
                   Pedal cycle collision NOS (traffic)

     X● **V19.69**   Unspecified pedal cyclist injured in collision with **other** motor vehicles in traffic accident

● **V19.8**   Pedal cyclist (driver) (passenger) injured in other specified transport accidents

     X● **V19.81**   Pedal cyclist (driver) (passenger) injured in transport accident with **military** vehicle

     X● **V19.88**   Pedal cyclist (driver) (passenger) injured in **other** specified transport accidents

X● **V19.9**   Pedal cyclist (driver) (passenger) injured in **unspecified** traffic accident
           Pedal cycle accident NOS

MOTORCYCLE RIDER INJURED IN TRANSPORT ACCIDENT (V20-V29)

     Includes   moped motorcycle with sidecar motorized bicycle motor scooter

     Excludes1   three-wheeled motor vehicle (V30-V39)

● **V20**   **Motorcycle rider injured in collision with pedestrian or animal**

     Excludes1   motorcycle rider collision with animal-drawn vehicle or animal being ridden (V26.-)

     The appropriate 7th character is to be added to each code from category V20

A	initial encounter
D	subsequent encounter
S	sequela

X● **V20.0**   Motorcycle **driver** injured in collision with pedestrian or animal in **nontraffic accident**

X● **V20.1**   Motorcycle **passenger** injured in collision with pedestrian or animal in **nontraffic accident**

X● **V20.2**   Unspecified motorcycle rider injured in collision with pedestrian or animal in **nontraffic accident**

X● **V20.3**   Person boarding or alighting a motorcycle injured in collision with pedestrian or animal

X● **V20.4**   Motorcycle **driver** injured in collision with pedestrian or animal in **traffic accident**

X● **V20.5**   Motorcycle **passenger** injured in collision with pedestrian or animal in **traffic accident**

X● **V20.9**   Unspecified motorcycle rider injured in collision with pedestrian or animal in **traffic accident**

● **V21**   **Motorcycle rider injured in collision with pedal cycle**

     The appropriate 7th character is to be added to each code from category V21

A	initial encounter
D	subsequent encounter
S	sequela

X● **V21.0**   Motorcycle **driver** injured in collision with pedal cycle in **nontraffic accident**

X● **V21.1**   Motorcycle **passenger** injured in collision with pedal cycle in **nontraffic accident**

X● **V21.2**   Unspecified motorcycle rider injured in collision with pedal cycle in **nontraffic accident**

X● **V21.3**   Person boarding or alighting a motorcycle injured in collision with pedal cycle

X● **V21.4**   Motorcycle **driver** injured in collision with pedal cycle in **traffic accident**

X● **V21.5**   Motorcycle **passenger** injured in collision with pedal cycle in **traffic accident**

X● **V21.9**   Unspecified motorcycle rider injured in collision with pedal cycle in **traffic accident**

N Newborn Age: 0   **P** Pediatric Age: 0–17   **M** Maternity DX: 12–55   **A** Adult Age: 15–124   ♀ Females Only   ♂ Males Only

Complication\Comorbidity   Major C\C   (Ex) CC/MCC Exclusions   Hospital-Acquired Condition

1513

● **V22** **Motorcycle rider injured in collision with two- or three-wheeled motor vehicle**

The appropriate 7th character is to be added to each code from category V22

> A   initial encounter
> D   subsequent encounter
> S   sequela

X● **V22.0** Motorcycle driver injured in collision with two- or three-wheeled motor vehicle in nontraffic accident

X● **V22.1** Motorcycle passenger injured in collision with two- or three-wheeled motor vehicle in nontraffic accident

X● **V22.2** Unspecified motorcycle rider injured in collision with two- or three-wheeled motor vehicle in nontraffic accident

X● **V22.3** Person boarding or alighting a motorcycle injured in collision with two- or three-wheeled motor vehicle

X● **V22.4** Motorcycle driver injured in collision with two- or three-wheeled motor vehicle in traffic accident

X● **V22.5** Motorcycle passenger injured in collision with two- or three-wheeled motor vehicle in traffic accident

X● **V22.9** Unspecified motorcycle rider injured in collision with two- or three-wheeled motor vehicle in traffic accident

● **V23** **Motorcycle rider injured in collision with car, pick-up truck or van**

The appropriate 7th character is to be added to each code from category V23

> A   initial encounter
> D   subsequent encounter
> S   sequela

X● **V23.0** Motorcycle driver injured in collision with car, pick-up truck or van in nontraffic accident

X● **V23.1** Motorcycle passenger injured in collision with car, pick-up truck or van in nontraffic accident

X● **V23.2** Unspecified motorcycle rider injured in collision with car, pick-up truck or van in nontraffic accident

X● **V23.3** Person boarding or alighting a motorcycle injured in collision with car, pick-up truck or van

X● **V23.4** Motorcycle driver injured in collision with car, pick-up truck or van in traffic accident

X● **V23.5** Motorcycle passenger injured in collision with car, pick-up truck or van in traffic accident

X● **V23.9** Unspecified motorcycle rider injured in collision with car, pick-up truck or van in traffic accident

● **V24** **Motorcycle rider injured in collision with heavy transport vehicle or bus**

Excludes1   motorcycle rider injured in collision with military vehicle (V29.81)

The appropriate 7th character is to be added to each code from category V24

> A   initial encounter
> D   subsequent encounter
> S   sequela

X● **V24.0** Motorcycle driver injured in collision with heavy transport vehicle or bus in nontraffic accident

X● **V24.1** Motorcycle passenger injured in collision with heavy transport vehicle or bus in nontraffic accident

X● **V24.2** Unspecified motorcycle rider injured in collision with heavy transport vehicle or bus in nontraffic accident

X● **V24.3** Person boarding or alighting a motorcycle injured in collision with heavy transport vehicle or bus

X● **V24.4** Motorcycle driver injured in collision with heavy transport vehicle or bus in traffic accident

X● **V24.5** Motorcycle passenger injured in collision with heavy transport vehicle or bus in traffic accident

X● **V24.9** Unspecified motorcycle rider injured in collision with heavy transport vehicle or bus in traffic accident

● **V25** **Motorcycle rider injured in collision with railway train or railway vehicle**

The appropriate 7th character is to be added to each code from category V25

> A   initial encounter
> D   subsequent encounter
> S   sequela

X● **V25.0** Motorcycle driver injured in collision with railway train or railway vehicle in nontraffic accident

X● **V25.1** Motorcycle passenger injured in collision with railway train or railway vehicle in nontraffic accident

X● **V25.2** Unspecified motorcycle rider injured in collision with railway train or railway vehicle in nontraffic accident

X● **V25.3** Person boarding or alighting a motorcycle injured in collision with railway train or railway vehicle

X● **V25.4** Motorcycle driver injured in collision with railway train or railway vehicle in traffic accident

X● **V25.5** Motorcycle passenger injured in collision with railway train or railway vehicle in traffic accident

X● **V25.9** Unspecified motorcycle rider injured in collision with railway train or railway vehicle in traffic accident

● **V26** **Motorcycle rider injured in collision with other nonmotor vehicle**

Includes   collision with animal-drawn vehicle, animal being ridden, streetcar

The appropriate 7th character is to be added to each code from category V26

> A   initial encounter
> D   subsequent encounter
> S   sequela

X● **V26.0** Motorcycle driver injured in collision with other nonmotor vehicle in nontraffic accident

X● **V26.1** Motorcycle passenger injured in collision with other nonmotor vehicle in nontraffic accident

X● **V26.2** Unspecified motorcycle rider injured in collision with other nonmotor vehicle in nontraffic accident

X● **V26.3** Person boarding or alighting a motorcycle injured in collision with other nonmotor vehicle

X● **V26.4** Motorcycle driver injured in collision with other nonmotor vehicle in traffic accident

X● **V26.5** Motorcycle passenger injured in collision with other nonmotor vehicle in traffic accident

X● **V26.9** Unspecified motorcycle rider injured in collision with other nonmotor vehicle in traffic accident

● **V27** **Motorcycle rider injured in collision with fixed or stationary object**

The appropriate 7th character is to be added to each code from category V27

> A   initial encounter
> D   subsequent encounter
> S   sequela

X● **V27.0** Motorcycle driver injured in collision with fixed or stationary object in nontraffic accident

X● **V27.1** Motorcycle passenger injured in collision with fixed or stationary object in nontraffic accident

X● **V27.2** Unspecified motorcycle rider injured in collision with fixed or stationary object in nontraffic accident

X● **V27.3** Person boarding or alighting a motorcycle injured in collision with fixed or stationary object

X● **V27.4** Motorcycle driver injured in collision with fixed or stationary object in traffic accident

X● **V27.5** Motorcycle passenger injured in collision with fixed or stationary object in traffic accident

X● **V27.9** Unspecified motorcycle rider injured in collision with fixed or stationary object in traffic accident

▶ New   ⟹ Revised   ~~deleted~~ Deleted   Excludes 1   Excludes 2   Includes   Use additional   Code first   Code also   Key words

OGCR Official Guidelines   ● Unacceptable Principal Diagnosis   X Assign placeholder X   ● Use Additional Character(s)   ▶ Manifestation Code   **Coding Clinic**

●V28 **Motorcycle rider injured in noncollision transport accident**

| Includes | fall or thrown from motorcycle (without antecedent collision) overturning motorcycle NOS overturning motorcycle without collision |

The appropriate 7th character is to be added to each code from category V28

A	initial encounter
D	subsequent encounter
S	sequela

X● V28.0 Motorcycle driver injured in noncollision transport accident in nontraffic accident

X● V28.1 Motorcycle passenger injured in noncollision transport accident in nontraffic accident

X● V28.2 Unspecified motorcycle rider injured in noncollision transport accident in nontraffic accident

X● V28.3 Person boarding or alighting a motorcycle injured in noncollision transport accident

X● V28.4 Motorcycle driver injured in noncollision transport accident in traffic accident

X● V28.5 Motorcycle passenger injured in noncollision transport accident in traffic accident

X● V28.9 Unspecified motorcycle rider injured in noncollision transport accident in traffic accident

●V29 **Motorcycle rider injured in other and unspecified transport accidents**

The appropriate 7th character is to be added to each code from category V29

A	initial encounter
D	subsequent encounter
S	sequela

Coding Clinic: 2015, Q3, P20

●V29.0 Motorcycle driver injured in collision with other and unspecified motor vehicles in nontraffic accident

X● V29.00 Motorcycle driver injured in collision with unspecified motor vehicles in nontraffic accident

X● V29.09 Motorcycle driver injured in collision with other motor vehicles in nontraffic accident

●V29.1 Motorcycle passenger injured in collision with other and unspecified motor vehicles in nontraffic accident

X● V29.10 Motorcycle passenger injured in collision with unspecified motor vehicles in nontraffic accident

X● V29.19 Motorcycle passenger injured in collision with other motor vehicles in nontraffic accident

●V29.2 Unspecified motorcycle rider injured in collision with other and unspecified motor vehicles in nontraffic accident

X● V29.20 Unspecified motorcycle rider injured in collision with unspecified motor vehicles in nontraffic accident
Motorcycle collision NOS, nontraffic

X● V29.29 Unspecified motorcycle rider injured in collision with other motor vehicles in nontraffic accident

X● V29.3 Motorcycle rider (driver) (passenger) injured in unspecified nontraffic accident
Motorcycle accident NOS, nontraffic
Motorcycle rider injured in nontraffic accident NOS

●V29.4 Motorcycle driver injured in collision with other and unspecified motor vehicles in traffic accident

X● V29.40 Motorcycle driver injured in collision with unspecified motor vehicles in traffic accident

X● V29.49 Motorcycle driver injured in collision with other motor vehicles in traffic accident

●V29.5 Motorcycle passenger injured in collision with other and unspecified motor vehicles in traffic accident

X● V29.50 Motorcycle passenger injured in collision with unspecified motor vehicles in traffic accident

X● V29.59 Motorcycle passenger injured in collision with other motor vehicles in traffic accident

●V29.6 Unspecified motorcycle rider injured in collision with other and unspecified motor vehicles in traffic accident

X● V29.60 Unspecified motorcycle rider injured in collision with unspecified motor vehicles in traffic accident
Motorcycle collision NOS (traffic)

X● V29.69 Unspecified motorcycle rider injured in collision with other motor vehicles in traffic accident

●V29.8 Motorcycle rider (driver) (passenger) injured in other specified transport accidents

X● V29.81 Motorcycle rider (driver) (passenger) injured in transport accident with military vehicle

X● V29.88 Motorcycle rider (driver) (passenger) injured in other specified transport accidents

X● V29.9 Motorcycle rider (driver) (passenger) injured in unspecified traffic accident
Motorcycle accident NOS

OCCUPANT OF THREE-WHEELED MOTOR VEHICLE INJURED IN TRANSPORT ACCIDENT (V30-V39)

| Includes | motorized tricycle motorized rickshaw three-wheeled motor car |
| Excludes1 | all-terrain vehicles (V86.-) motorcycle with sidecar (V20-V29) vehicle designed primarily for off-road use (V86.-) |

●V30 **Occupant of three-wheeled motor vehicle injured in collision with pedestrian or animal**

| Excludes1 | three-wheeled motor vehicle collision with animal-drawn vehicle or animal being ridden (V36.-) |

The appropriate 7th character is to be added to each code from category V30

A	initial encounter
D	subsequent encounter
S	sequela

X● V30.0 Driver of three-wheeled motor vehicle injured in collision with pedestrian or animal in nontraffic accident

X● V30.1 Passenger in three-wheeled motor vehicle injured in collision with pedestrian or animal in nontraffic accident

X● V30.2 Person on outside of three-wheeled motor vehicle injured in collision with pedestrian or animal in nontraffic accident

X● V30.3 Unspecified occupant of three-wheeled motor vehicle injured in collision with pedestrian or animal in nontraffic accident

X● V30.4 Person boarding or alighting a three-wheeled motor vehicle injured in collision with pedestrian or animal

X● V30.5 Driver of three-wheeled motor vehicle injured in collision with pedestrian or animal in traffic accident

X● V30.6 Passenger in three-wheeled motor vehicle injured in collision with pedestrian or animal in traffic accident

X● V30.7 Person on outside of three-wheeled motor vehicle injured in collision with pedestrian or animal in traffic accident

X● V30.9 Unspecified occupant of three-wheeled motor vehicle injured in collision with pedestrian or animal in traffic accident

CHAPTER 20 (V01-Y99)

● **V31 Occupant of three-wheeled motor vehicle injured in collision with pedal cycle**

The appropriate 7th character is to be added to each code from category V31

> A initial encounter
> D subsequent encounter
> S sequela

X● **V31.0** Driver of three-wheeled motor vehicle injured in collision with pedal cycle in nontraffic accident

X● **V31.1** Passenger in three-wheeled motor vehicle injured in collision with pedal cycle in nontraffic accident

X● **V31.2** Person on outside of three-wheeled motor vehicle injured in collision with pedal cycle in nontraffic accident

X● **V31.3** Unspecified occupant of three-wheeled motor vehicle injured in collision with pedal cycle in nontraffic accident

X● **V31.4** Person boarding or alighting a three-wheeled motor vehicle injured in collision with pedal cycle

X● **V31.5** Driver of three-wheeled motor vehicle injured in collision with pedal cycle in traffic accident

X● **V31.6** Passenger in three-wheeled motor vehicle injured in collision with pedal cycle in traffic accident

X● **V31.7** Person on outside of three-wheeled motor vehicle injured in collision with pedal cycle in traffic accident

X● **V31.9** Unspecified occupant of three-wheeled motor vehicle injured in collision with pedal cycle in traffic accident

● **V32 Occupant of three-wheeled motor vehicle injured in collision with two- or three-wheeled motor vehicle**

The appropriate 7th character is to be added to each code from category V32

> A initial encounter
> D subsequent encounter
> S sequela

X● **V32.0** Driver of three-wheeled motor vehicle injured in collision with two- or three-wheeled motor vehicle in nontraffic accident

X● **V32.1** Passenger in three-wheeled motor vehicle injured in collision with two- or three-wheeled motor vehicle in nontraffic accident

X● **V32.2** Person on outside of three-wheeled motor vehicle injured in collision with two- or three-wheeled motor vehicle in nontraffic accident

X● **V32.3** Unspecified occupant of three-wheeled motor vehicle injured in collision with two- or three-wheeled motor vehicle in nontraffic accident

X● **V32.4** Person boarding or alighting a three-wheeled motor vehicle injured in collision with two- or three-wheeled motor vehicle

X● **V32.5** Driver of three-wheeled motor vehicle injured in collision with two- or three-wheeled motor vehicle in traffic accident

X● **V32.6** Passenger in three-wheeled motor vehicle injured in collision with two- or three-wheeled motor vehicle in traffic accident

X● **V32.7** Person on outside of three-wheeled motor vehicle injured in collision with two- or three-wheeled motor vehicle in traffic accident

X● **V32.9** Unspecified occupant of three-wheeled motor vehicle injured in collision with two- or three-wheeled motor vehicle in traffic accident

● **V33 Occupant of three-wheeled motor vehicle injured in collision with car, pick-up truck or van**

The appropriate 7th character is to be added to each code from category V33

> A initial encounter
> D subsequent encounter
> S sequela

X● **V33.0** Driver of three-wheeled motor vehicle injured in collision with car, pick-up truck or van in nontraffic accident

X● **V33.1** Passenger in three-wheeled motor vehicle injured in collision with car, pick-up truck or van in nontraffic accident

X● **V33.2** Person on outside of three-wheeled motor vehicle injured in collision with car, pick-up truck or van in nontraffic accident

X● **V33.3** Unspecified occupant of three-wheeled motor vehicle injured in collision with car, pick-up truck or van in nontraffic accident

X● **V33.4** Person boarding or alighting a three-wheeled motor vehicle injured in collision with car, pick-up truck or van

X● **V33.5** Driver of three-wheeled motor vehicle injured in collision with car, pick-up truck or van in traffic accident

X● **V33.6** Passenger in three-wheeled motor vehicle injured in collision with car, pick-up truck or van in traffic accident

X● **V33.7** Person on outside of three-wheeled motor vehicle injured in collision with car, pick-up truck or van in traffic accident

X● **V33.9** Unspecified occupant of three-wheeled motor vehicle injured in collision with car, pick-up truck or van in traffic accident

● **V34 Occupant of three-wheeled motor vehicle injured in collision with heavy transport vehicle or bus**

Excludes1 occupant of three-wheeled motor vehicle injured in collision with military vehicle (V39.81)

The appropriate 7th character is to be added to each code from category V34

> A initial encounter
> D subsequent encounter
> S sequela

X● **V34.0** Driver of three-wheeled motor vehicle injured in collision with heavy transport vehicle or bus in nontraffic accident

X● **V34.1** Passenger in three-wheeled motor vehicle injured in collision with heavy transport vehicle or bus in nontraffic accident

X● **V34.2** Person on outside of three-wheeled motor vehicle injured in collision with heavy transport vehicle or bus in nontraffic accident

X● **V34.3** Unspecified occupant of three-wheeled motor vehicle injured in collision with heavy transport vehicle or bus in nontraffic accident

X● **V34.4** Person boarding or alighting a three-wheeled motor vehicle injured in collision with heavy transport vehicle or bus

X● **V34.5** Driver of three-wheeled motor vehicle injured in collision with heavy transport vehicle or bus in traffic accident

X● **V34.6** Passenger in three-wheeled motor vehicle injured in collision with heavy transport vehicle or bus in traffic accident

X● **V34.7** Person on outside of three-wheeled motor vehicle injured in collision with heavy transport vehicle or bus in traffic accident

X● **V34.9** Unspecified occupant of three-wheeled motor vehicle injured in collision with heavy transport vehicle or bus in traffic accident

▶ New ⇒ Revised ~~deleted~~ Deleted Excludes 1 Excludes 2 Includes Use additional Code first Code also Key words
OGCR Official Guidelines ● Unacceptable Principal Diagnosis X Assign placeholder X ● Use Additional Character(s) ▶ Manifestation Code **Coding Clinic**

● **V35**   **Occupant of three-wheeled motor vehicle injured in collision with railway train or railway vehicle**

The appropriate 7th character is to be added to each code from category V35

> A   initial encounter
> D   subsequent encounter
> S   sequela

X● **V35.0**   Driver of three-wheeled motor vehicle injured in collision with railway train or railway vehicle in nontraffic accident

X● **V35.1**   Passenger in three-wheeled motor vehicle injured in collision with railway train or railway vehicle in nontraffic accident

X● **V35.2**   Person on outside of three-wheeled motor vehicle injured in collision with railway train or railway vehicle in nontraffic accident

X● **V35.3**   Unspecified occupant of three-wheeled motor vehicle injured in collision with railway train or railway vehicle in nontraffic accident

X● **V35.4**   Person boarding or alighting a three-wheeled motor vehicle injured in collision with railway train or railway vehicle

X● **V35.5**   Driver of three-wheeled motor vehicle injured in collision with railway train or railway vehicle in traffic accident

X● **V35.6**   Passenger in three-wheeled motor vehicle injured in collision with railway train or railway vehicle in traffic accident

X● **V35.7**   Person on outside of three-wheeled motor vehicle injured in collision with railway train or railway vehicle in traffic accident

X● **V35.9**   Unspecified occupant of three-wheeled motor vehicle injured in collision with railway train or railway vehicle in traffic accident

● **V36**   **Occupant of three-wheeled motor vehicle injured in collision with other nonmotor vehicle**

> **Includes**   collision with animal-drawn vehicle, animal being ridden, streetcar

The appropriate 7th character is to be added to each code from category V36

> A   initial encounter
> D   subsequent encounter
> S   sequela

X● **V36.0**   Driver of three-wheeled motor vehicle injured in collision with other nonmotor vehicle in nontraffic accident

X● **V36.1**   Passenger in three-wheeled motor vehicle injured in collision with other nonmotor vehicle in nontraffic accident

X● **V36.2**   Person on outside of three-wheeled motor vehicle injured in collision with other nonmotor vehicle in nontraffic accident

X● **V36.3**   Unspecified occupant of three-wheeled motor vehicle injured in collision with other nonmotor vehicle in nontraffic accident

X● **V36.4**   Person boarding or alighting a three-wheeled motor vehicle injured in collision with other nonmotor vehicle

X● **V36.5**   Driver of three-wheeled motor vehicle injured in collision with other nonmotor vehicle in traffic accident

X● **V36.6**   Passenger in three-wheeled motor vehicle injured in collision with other nonmotor vehicle in traffic accident

X● **V36.7**   Person on outside of three-wheeled motor vehicle injured in collision with other nonmotor vehicle in traffic accident

X● **V36.9**   Unspecified occupant of three-wheeled motor vehicle injured in collision with other nonmotor vehicle in traffic accident

● **V37**   **Occupant of three-wheeled motor vehicle injured in collision with fixed or stationary object**

The appropriate 7th character is to be added to each code from category V37

> A   initial encounter
> D   subsequent encounter
> S   sequela

X● **V37.0**   Driver of three-wheeled motor vehicle injured in collision with fixed or stationary object in nontraffic accident

X● **V37.1**   Passenger in three-wheeled motor vehicle injured in collision with fixed or stationary object in nontraffic accident

X● **V37.2**   Person on outside of three-wheeled motor vehicle injured in collision with fixed or stationary object in nontraffic accident

X● **V37.3**   Unspecified occupant of three-wheeled motor vehicle injured in collision with fixed or stationary object in nontraffic accident

X● **V37.4**   Person boarding or alighting a three-wheeled motor vehicle injured in collision with fixed or stationary object

X● **V37.5**   Driver of three-wheeled motor vehicle injured in collision with fixed or stationary object in traffic accident

X● **V37.6**   Passenger in three-wheeled motor vehicle injured in collision with fixed or stationary object in traffic accident

X● **V37.7**   Person on outside of three-wheeled motor vehicle injured in collision with fixed or stationary object in traffic accident

X● **V37.9**   Unspecified occupant of three-wheeled motor vehicle injured in collision with fixed or stationary object in traffic accident

● **V38**   **Occupant of three-wheeled motor vehicle injured in noncollision transport accident**

> **Includes**   fall or thrown from three-wheeled motor vehicle
> overturning of three-wheeled motor vehicle NOS
> overturning of three-wheeled motor vehicle without collision

The appropriate 7th character is to be added to each code from category V38

> A   initial encounter
> D   subsequent encounter
> S   sequela

X● **V38.0**   Driver of three-wheeled motor vehicle injured in noncollision transport accident in nontraffic accident

X● **V38.1**   Passenger in three-wheeled motor vehicle injured in noncollision transport accident in nontraffic accident

X● **V38.2**   Person on outside of three-wheeled motor vehicle injured in noncollision transport accident in nontraffic accident

X● **V38.3**   Unspecified occupant of three-wheeled motor vehicle injured in noncollision transport accident in nontraffic accident

X● **V38.4**   Person boarding or alighting a three-wheeled motor vehicle injured in noncollision transport accident

X● **V38.5**   Driver of three-wheeled motor vehicle injured in noncollision transport accident in traffic accident

X● **V38.6**   Passenger in three-wheeled motor vehicle injured in noncollision transport accident in traffic accident

X● **V38.7**   Person on outside of three-wheeled motor vehicle injured in noncollision transport accident in traffic accident

X● **V38.9**   Unspecified occupant of three-wheeled motor vehicle injured in noncollision transport accident in traffic accident

CHAPTER 20 (V01-Y99)

V39   **Occupant of three-wheeled motor vehicle injured in other and unspecified transport accidents**

The appropriate 7th character is to be added to each code from category V39

A	initial encounter
D	subsequent encounter
S	sequela

● **V39.0**   **Driver of three-wheeled motor vehicle injured in collision with other and unspecified motor vehicles in nontraffic accident**

    X● **V39.00**   Driver of three-wheeled motor vehicle injured in collision with unspecified motor vehicles in nontraffic accident

    X● **V39.09**   Driver of three-wheeled motor vehicle injured in collision with other motor vehicles in nontraffic accident

● **V39.1**   **Passenger in three-wheeled motor vehicle injured in collision with other and unspecified motor vehicles in nontraffic accident**

    X● **V39.10**   Passenger in three-wheeled motor vehicle injured in collision with unspecified motor vehicles in nontraffic accident

    X● **V39.19**   Passenger in three-wheeled motor vehicle injured in collision with other motor vehicles in nontraffic accident

● **V39.2**   **Unspecified occupant of three-wheeled motor vehicle injured in collision with other and unspecified motor vehicles in nontraffic accident**

    X● **V39.20**   Unspecified occupant of three-wheeled motor vehicle injured in collision with unspecified motor vehicles in nontraffic accident
        Collision NOS involving three-wheeled motor vehicle, nontraffic

    X● **V39.29**   Unspecified occupant of three-wheeled motor vehicle injured in collision with other motor vehicles in nontraffic accident

X● **V39.3**   **Occupant (driver) (passenger) of three-wheeled motor vehicle injured in unspecified nontraffic accident**
      Accident NOS involving three-wheeled motor vehicle, nontraffic
      Occupant of three-wheeled motor vehicle injured in nontraffic accident NOS

● **V39.4**   **Driver of three-wheeled motor vehicle injured in collision with other and unspecified motor vehicles in traffic accident**

    X● **V39.40**   Driver of three-wheeled motor vehicle injured in collision with unspecified motor vehicles in traffic accident

    X● **V39.49**   Driver of three-wheeled motor vehicle injured in collision with other motor vehicles in traffic accident

● **V39.5**   **Passenger in three-wheeled motor vehicle injured in collision with other and unspecified motor vehicles in traffic accident**

    X● **V39.50**   Passenger in three-wheeled motor vehicle injured in collision with unspecified motor vehicles in traffic accident

    X● **V39.59**   Passenger in three-wheeled motor vehicle injured in collision with other motor vehicles in traffic accident

● **V39.6**   **Unspecified occupant of three-wheeled motor vehicle injured in collision with other and unspecified motor vehicles in traffic accident**

    X● **V39.60**   Unspecified occupant of three-wheeled motor vehicle injured in collision with unspecified motor vehicles in traffic accident
        Collision NOS involving three-wheeled motor vehicle (traffic)

    X● **V39.69**   Unspecified occupant of three-wheeled motor vehicle injured in collision with other motor vehicles in traffic accident

● **V39.8**   **Occupant (driver) (passenger) of three-wheeled motor vehicle injured in other specified transport accidents**

    X● **V39.81**   Occupant (driver) (passenger) of three-wheeled motor vehicle injured in transport accident with military vehicle

    X● **V39.89**   Occupant (driver) (passenger) of three-wheeled motor vehicle injured in other specified transport accidents

X● **V39.9**   **Occupant (driver) (passenger) of three-wheeled motor vehicle injured in unspecified traffic accident**
      Accident NOS involving three-wheeled motor vehicle

CAR OCCUPANT INJURED IN TRANSPORT ACCIDENT (V40-V49)

Includes	a four-wheeled motor vehicle designed primarily for carrying passengers
	automobile (pulling a trailer or camper)

Excludes 1	bus (V50-V59)
	minibus (V50-V59)
	minivan (V50-V59)
	motorcoach (V70-V79)
	pick-up truck (V50-V59)
	sport utility vehicle (SUV) (V50-V59)

● **V40**   **Car occupant injured in collision with pedestrian or animal**

Excludes 1	car collision with animal-drawn vehicle or animal being ridden (V46.-)

The appropriate 7th character is to be added to each code from category V40

A	initial encounter
D	subsequent encounter
S	sequela

  X● **V40.0**   Car driver injured in collision with pedestrian or animal in nontraffic accident

  X● **V40.1**   Car passenger injured in collision with pedestrian or animal in nontraffic accident

  X● **V40.2**   Person on outside of car injured in collision with pedestrian or animal in nontraffic accident

  X● **V40.3**   Unspecified car occupant injured in collision with pedestrian or animal in nontraffic accident

  X● **V40.4**   Person boarding or alighting a car injured in collision with pedestrian or animal

  X● **V40.5**   Car driver injured in collision with pedestrian or animal in traffic accident

  X● **V40.6**   Car passenger injured in collision with pedestrian or animal in traffic accident

  X● **V40.7**   Person on outside of car injured in collision with pedestrian or animal in traffic accident

  X● **V40.9**   Unspecified car occupant injured in collision with pedestrian or animal in traffic accident

● **V41**   **Car occupant injured in collision with pedal cycle**

The appropriate 7th character is to be added to each code from category V41

A	initial encounter
D	subsequent encounter
S	sequela

  X● **V41.0**   Car driver injured in collision with pedal cycle in nontraffic accident

  X● **V41.1**   Car passenger injured in collision with pedal cycle in nontraffic accident

  X● **V41.2**   Person on outside of car injured in collision with pedal cycle in nontraffic accident

  X● **V41.3**   Unspecified car occupant injured in collision with pedal cycle in nontraffic accident

  X● **V41.4**   Person boarding or alighting a car injured in collision with pedal cycle

  X● **V41.5**   Car driver injured in collision with pedal cycle in traffic accident

  X● **V41.6**   Car passenger injured in collision with pedal cycle in traffic accident

▶ New   ⇒ Revised   ~~deleted~~ Deleted   Excludes 1   Excludes 2   Includes   Use additional   Code first   Code also   Key words

OGCR Official Guidelines   ● Unacceptable Principal Diagnosis   X Assign placeholder X   ● Use Additional Character(s)   ▶ Manifestation Code   **Coding Clinic**

X● **V41.7** Person on outside of car injured in collision with pedal cycle in traffic accident

X● **V41.9** Unspecified car occupant injured in collision with pedal cycle in traffic accident

● **V42** Car occupant injured in collision with two- or three-wheeled motor vehicle

The appropriate 7th character is to be added to each code from category V42

A	initial encounter
D	subsequent encounter
S	sequela

X● **V42.0** Car driver injured in collision with two- or three-wheeled motor vehicle in nontraffic accident

X● **V42.1** Car passenger injured in collision with two- or three-wheeled motor vehicle in nontraffic accident

X● **V42.2** Person on outside of car injured in collision with two- or three-wheeled motor vehicle in nontraffic accident

X● **V42.3** Unspecified car occupant injured in collision with two- or three-wheeled motor vehicle in nontraffic accident

X● **V42.4** Person boarding or alighting a car injured in collision with two- or three-wheeled motor vehicle

X● **V42.5** Car driver injured in collision with two- or three-wheeled motor vehicle in traffic accident

X● **V42.6** Car passenger injured in collision with two- or three-wheeled motor vehicle in traffic accident

X● **V42.7** Person on outside of car injured in collision with two- or three-wheeled motor vehicle in traffic accident

X● **V42.9** Unspecified car occupant injured in collision with two- or three-wheeled motor vehicle in traffic accident

● **V43** Car occupant injured in collision with car, pick-up truck or van

The appropriate 7th character is to be added to each code from category V43

A	initial encounter
D	subsequent encounter
S	sequela

● **V43.0** Car driver injured in collision with car, pick-up truck or van in nontraffic accident

X● **V43.01** Car driver injured in collision with sport utility vehicle in nontraffic accident

X● **V43.02** Car driver injured in collision with other type car in nontraffic accident

X● **V43.03** Car driver injured in collision with pick-up truck in nontraffic accident

X● **V43.04** Car driver injured in collision with van in nontraffic accident

● **V43.1** Car passenger injured in collision with car, pick-up truck or van in nontraffic accident

X● **V43.11** Car passenger injured in collision with sport utility vehicle in nontraffic accident

X● **V43.12** Car passenger injured in collision with other type car in nontraffic accident

X● **V43.13** Car passenger injured in collision with pick-up in nontraffic accident

X● **V43.14** Car passenger injured in collision with van in nontraffic accident

● **V43.2** Person on outside of car injured in collision with car, pick-up truck or van in nontraffic accident

X● **V43.21** Person on outside of car injured in collision with sport utility vehicle in nontraffic accident

X● **V43.22** Person on outside of car injured in collision with other type car in nontraffic accident

X● **V43.23** Person on outside of car injured in collision with pick-up truck in nontraffic accident

X● **V43.24** Person on outside of car injured in collision with van in nontraffic accident

● **V43.3** Unspecified car occupant injured in collision with car, pick-up truck or van in nontraffic accident

X● **V43.31** Unspecified car occupant injured in collision with sport utility vehicle in nontraffic accident

X● **V43.32** Unspecified car occupant injured in collision with other type car in nontraffic accident

X● **V43.33** Unspecified car occupant injured in collision with pick-up truck in nontraffic accident

X● **V43.34** Unspecified car occupant injured in collision with van in nontraffic accident

● **V43.4** Person boarding or alighting a car injured in collision with car, pick-up truck or van

X● **V43.41** Person boarding or alighting a car injured in collision with sport utility vehicle

X● **V43.42** Person boarding or alighting a car injured in collision with other type car

X● **V43.43** Person boarding or alighting a car injured in collision with pick-up truck

X● **V43.44** Person boarding or alighting a car injured in collision with van

● **V43.5** Car driver injured in collision with car, pick-up truck or van in traffic accident

X● **V43.51** Car driver injured in collision with sport utility vehicle in traffic accident

X● **V43.52** Car driver injured in collision with other type car in traffic accident

X● **V43.53** Car driver injured in collision with pick-up truck in traffic accident

X● **V43.54** Car driver injured in collision with van in traffic accident

● **V43.6** Car passenger injured in collision with car, pick-up truck or van in traffic accident

X● **V43.61** Car passenger injured in collision with sport utility vehicle in traffic accident
Coding Clinic: 2015, Q1, P5-7

X● **V43.62** Car passenger injured in collision with other type car in traffic accident

X● **V43.63** Car passenger injured in collision with pick-up truck in traffic accident

X● **V43.64** Car passenger injured in collision with van in traffic accident

● **V43.7** Person on outside of car injured in collision with car, pick-up truck or van in traffic accident

X● **V43.71** Person on outside of car injured in collision with sport utility vehicle in traffic accident

X● **V43.72** Person on outside of car injured in collision with other type car in traffic accident

X● **V43.73** Person on outside of car injured in collision with pick-up truck in traffic accident

X● **V43.74** Person on outside of car injured in collision with van in traffic accident

● **V43.9** Unspecified car occupant injured in collision with car, pick-up truck or van in traffic accident

X● **V43.91** Unspecified car occupant injured in collision with sport utility vehicle in traffic accident

X● **V43.92** Unspecified car occupant injured in collision with other type car in traffic accident

X● **V43.93** Unspecified car occupant injured in collision with pick-up truck in traffic accident

X● **V43.94** Unspecified car occupant injured in collision with van in traffic accident

CHAPTER 20 (V01-Y99)

N Newborn Age: 0   **P** Pediatric Age: 0–17   **M** Maternity DX: 12–55   **A** Adult Age: 15–124   ♀ Females Only   ♂ Males Only

🔧 Complication\Comorbidity   🔧 Major C\C   (Ex) CC/MCC Exclusions   🔧 Hospital-Acquired Condition

1519

● **V44   Car occupant injured in collision with heavy transport vehicle or bus**

> **Excludes1**   car occupant injured in collision with military vehicle (V49.81)

> The appropriate 7th character is to be added to each code from category V44

> | A | initial encounter |
> |---|---|
> | D | subsequent encounter |
> | S | sequela |

X ● **V44.0   Car driver injured in collision with heavy transport vehicle or bus in nontraffic accident**

X ● **V44.1   Car passenger injured in collision with heavy transport vehicle or bus in nontraffic accident**

X ● **V44.2   Person on outside of car injured in collision with heavy transport vehicle or bus in nontraffic accident**

X ● **V44.3   Unspecified car occupant injured in collision with heavy transport vehicle or bus in nontraffic accident**

X ● **V44.4   Person boarding or alighting a car injured in collision with heavy transport vehicle or bus**

X ● **V44.5   Car driver injured in collision with heavy transport vehicle or bus in traffic accident**

X ● **V44.6   Car passenger injured in collision with heavy transport vehicle or bus in traffic accident**

X ● **V44.7   Person on outside of car injured in collision with heavy transport vehicle or bus in traffic accident**

X ● **V44.9   Unspecified car occupant injured in collision with heavy transport vehicle or bus in traffic accident**

● **V45   Car occupant injured in collision with railway train or railway vehicle**

> The appropriate 7th character is to be added to each code from category V45

> | A | initial encounter |
> |---|---|
> | D | subsequent encounter |
> | S | sequela |

X ● **V45.0   Car driver injured in collision with railway train or railway vehicle in nontraffic accident**

X ● **V45.1   Car passenger injured in collision with railway train or railway vehicle in nontraffic accident**

X ● **V45.2   Person on outside of car injured in collision with railway train or railway vehicle in nontraffic accident**

X ● **V45.3   Unspecified car occupant injured in collision with railway train or railway vehicle in nontraffic accident**

X ● **V45.4   Person boarding or alighting a car injured in collision with railway train or railway vehicle**

X ● **V45.5   Car driver injured in collision with railway train or railway vehicle in traffic accident**

X ● **V45.6   Car passenger injured in collision with railway train or railway vehicle in traffic accident**

X ● **V45.7   Person on outside of car injured in collision with railway train or railway vehicle in traffic accident**

X ● **V45.9   Unspecified car occupant injured in collision with railway train or railway vehicle in traffic accident**

● **V46   Car occupant injured in collision with other nonmotor vehicle**

> **Includes**   collision with animal-drawn vehicle, animal being ridden, streetcar

> The appropriate 7th character is to be added to each code from category V46

> | A | initial encounter |
> |---|---|
> | D | subsequent encounter |
> | S | sequela |

X ● **V46.0   Car driver injured in collision with other nonmotor vehicle in nontraffic accident**

X ● **V46.1   Car passenger injured in collision with other nonmotor vehicle in nontraffic accident**

X ● **V46.2   Person on outside of car injured in collision with other nonmotor vehicle in nontraffic accident**

X ● **V46.3   Unspecified car occupant injured in collision with other nonmotor vehicle in nontraffic accident**

X ● **V46.4   Person boarding or alighting a car injured in collision with other nonmotor vehicle**

X ● **V46.5   Car driver injured in collision with other nonmotor vehicle in traffic accident**

X ● **V46.6   Car passenger injured in collision with other nonmotor vehicle in traffic accident**

X ● **V46.7   Person on outside of car injured in collision with other nonmotor vehicle in traffic accident**

X ● **V46.9   Unspecified car occupant injured in collision with other nonmotor vehicle in traffic accident**

● **V47   Car occupant injured in collision with fixed or stationary object**

> The appropriate 7th character is to be added to each code from category V47

> | A | initial encounter |
> |---|---|
> | D | subsequent encounter |
> | S | sequela |

Coding Clinic: 2016, Q4, P73

X ● **V47.0   Car driver injured in collision with fixed or stationary object in nontraffic accident**

X ● **V47.1   Car passenger injured in collision with fixed or stationary object in nontraffic accident**

X ● **V47.2   Person on outside of car injured in collision with fixed or stationary object in nontraffic accident**

X ● **V47.3   Unspecified car occupant injured in collision with fixed or stationary object in nontraffic accident**

X ● **V47.4   Person boarding or alighting a car injured in collision with fixed or stationary object**

X ● **V47.5   Car driver injured in collision with fixed or stationary object in traffic accident**

X ● **V47.6   Car passenger injured in collision with fixed or stationary object in traffic accident**

X ● **V47.7   Person on outside of car injured in collision with fixed or stationary object in traffic accident**

X ● **V47.9   Unspecified car occupant injured in collision with fixed or stationary object in traffic accident**

● **V48   Car occupant injured in noncollision transport accident**

> **Includes**   overturning car NOS
> overturning car without collision

> The appropriate 7th character is to be added to each code from category V48

> | A | initial encounter |
> |---|---|
> | D | subsequent encounter |
> | S | sequela |

X ● **V48.0   Car driver injured in noncollision transport accident in nontraffic accident**

X ● **V48.1   Car passenger injured in noncollision transport accident in nontraffic accident**

X ● **V48.2   Person on outside of car injured in noncollision transport accident in nontraffic accident**

X ● **V48.3   Unspecified car occupant injured in noncollision transport accident in nontraffic accident**

X ● **V48.4   Person boarding or alighting a car injured in noncollision transport accident**

X ● **V48.5   Car driver injured in noncollision transport accident in traffic accident**

X ● **V48.6   Car passenger injured in noncollision transport accident in traffic accident**

X ● **V48.7   Person on outside of car injured in noncollision transport accident in traffic accident**

X ● **V48.9   Unspecified car occupant injured in noncollision transport accident in traffic accident**

▶ New   ⇒ Revised   ~~deleted~~ Deleted   Excludes 1   Excludes 2   Includes   Use additional   Code first   Code also   Key words

OGCR Official Guidelines   ● Unacceptable Principal Diagnosis   X Assign placeholder X   ● Use Additional Character(s)   ▶ Manifestation Code   **Coding Clinic**

● **V49 Car occupant injured in other and unspecified transport accidents**

> The appropriate 7th character is to be added to each code from category V49

> | | |
> |---|---|
> | A | initial encounter |
> | D | subsequent encounter |
> | S | sequela |

● **V49.0 Driver injured in collision with other and unspecified motor vehicles in nontraffic accident**

X● **V49.00 Driver injured in collision with unspecified motor vehicles in nontraffic accident**

X● **V49.09 Driver injured in collision with other motor vehicles in nontraffic accident**

● **V49.1 Passenger injured in collision with other and unspecified motor vehicles in nontraffic accident**

X● **V49.10 Passenger injured in collision with unspecified motor vehicles in nontraffic accident**

X● **V49.19 Passenger injured in collision with other motor vehicles in nontraffic accident**

● **V49.2 Unspecified car occupant injured in collision with other and unspecified motor vehicles in nontraffic accident**

X● **V49.20 Unspecified car occupant injured in collision with unspecified motor vehicles in nontraffic accident**
    Car collision NOS, nontraffic

X● **V49.29 Unspecified car occupant injured in collision with other motor vehicles in nontraffic accident**

X● **V49.3 Car occupant (driver) (passenger) injured in unspecified nontraffic accident**
    Car accident NOS, nontraffic
    Car occupant injured in nontraffic accident NOS

● **V49.4 Driver injured in collision with other and unspecified motor vehicles in traffic accident**

X● **V49.40 Driver injured in collision with unspecified motor vehicles in traffic accident**

X● **V49.49 Driver injured in collision with other motor vehicles in traffic accident**

● **V49.5 Passenger injured in collision with other and unspecified motor vehicles in traffic accident**

X● **V49.50 Passenger injured in collision with unspecified motor vehicles in traffic accident**

X● **V49.59 Passenger injured in collision with other motor vehicles in traffic accident**

● **V49.6 Unspecified car occupant injured in collision with other and unspecified motor vehicles in traffic accident**

X● **V49.60 Unspecified car occupant injured in collision with unspecified motor vehicles in traffic accident**
    Car collision NOS (traffic)

X● **V49.69 Unspecified car occupant injured in collision with other motor vehicles in traffic accident**

● **V49.8 Car occupant (driver) (passenger) injured in other specified transport accidents**

X● **V49.81 Car occupant (driver) (passenger) injured in transport accident with military vehicle**

X● **V49.88 Car occupant (driver) (passenger) injured in other specified transport accidents**

X● **V49.9 Car occupant (driver) (passenger) injured in unspecified traffic accident**
    Car accident NOS
    Coding Clinic: 2015, Q1, P11

OCCUPANT OF PICK-UP TRUCK OR VAN INJURED IN TRANSPORT ACCIDENT (V50-V59)

> | | |
> |---|---|
> | **Includes** | a four- or six-wheel motor vehicle designed primarily for carrying passengers and property but weighing less than the local limit for classification as a heavy goods vehicle |
> | | minibus |
> | | minivan |
> | | sport utility vehicle (SUV) |
> | | truck |
> | | van |
> | **Excludes1** | heavy transport vehicle (V60-V69) |

● **V50 Occupant of pick-up truck or van injured in collision with pedestrian or animal**

> | | |
> |---|---|
> | **Excludes1** | pick-up truck or van collision with animal-drawn vehicle or animal being ridden (V56.-) |

> The appropriate 7th character is to be added to each code from category V50

> | | |
> |---|---|
> | A | initial encounter |
> | D | subsequent encounter |
> | S | sequela |

X● **V50.0 Driver of pick-up truck or van injured in collision with pedestrian or animal in nontraffic accident**

X● **V50.1 Passenger in pick-up truck or van injured in collision with pedestrian or animal in nontraffic accident**

X● **V50.2 Person on outside of pick-up truck or van injured in collision with pedestrian or animal in nontraffic accident**

X● **V50.3 Unspecified occupant of pick-up truck or van injured in collision with pedestrian or animal in nontraffic accident**

X● **V50.4 Person boarding or alighting a pick-up truck or van injured in collision with pedestrian or animal**

X● **V50.5 Driver of pick-up truck or van injured in collision with pedestrian or animal in traffic accident**

X● **V50.6 Passenger in pick-up truck or van injured in collision with pedestrian or animal in traffic accident**

X● **V50.7 Person on outside of pick-up truck or van injured in collision with pedestrian or animal in traffic accident**

X● **V50.9 Unspecified occupant of pick-up truck or van injured in collision with pedestrian or animal in traffic accident**

● **V51 Occupant of pick-up truck or van injured in collision with pedal cycle**

> The appropriate 7th character is to be added to each code from category V51

> | | |
> |---|---|
> | A | initial encounter |
> | D | subsequent encounter |
> | S | sequela |

X● **V51.0 Driver of pick-up truck or van injured in collision with pedal cycle in nontraffic accident**

X● **V51.1 Passenger in pick-up truck or van injured in collision with pedal cycle in nontraffic accident**

X● **V51.2 Person on outside of pick-up truck or van injured in collision with pedal cycle in nontraffic accident**

X● **V51.3 Unspecified occupant of pick-up truck or van injured in collision with pedal cycle in nontraffic accident**

X● **V51.4 Person boarding or alighting a pick-up truck or van injured in collision with pedal cycle**

X● **V51.5 Driver of pick-up truck or van injured in collision with pedal cycle in traffic accident**

X● **V51.6 Passenger in pick-up truck or van injured in collision with pedal cycle in traffic accident**

X● **V51.7 Person on outside of pick-up truck or van injured in collision with pedal cycle in traffic accident**

X● **V51.9 Unspecified occupant of pick-up truck or van injured in collision with pedal cycle in traffic accident**

● **V52 Occupant of pick-up truck or van injured in collision with two- or three-wheeled motor vehicle**

The appropriate 7th character is to be added to each code from category V52

> A initial encounter
> D subsequent encounter
> S sequela

X● **V52.Ø** Driver of pick-up truck or van injured in collision with two- or three-wheeled motor vehicle in nontraffic accident

X● **V52.1** Passenger in pick-up truck or van injured in collision with two- or three-wheeled motor vehicle in nontraffic accident

X● **V52.2** Person on outside of pick-up truck or van injured in collision with two- or three-wheeled motor vehicle in nontraffic accident

X● **V52.3** Unspecified occupant of pick-up truck or van injured in collision with two- or three-wheeled motor vehicle in nontraffic accident

X● **V52.4** Person boarding or alighting a pick-up truck or van injured in collision with two- or three-wheeled motor vehicle

X● **V52.5** Driver of pick-up truck or van injured in collision with two- or three-wheeled motor vehicle in traffic accident

X● **V52.6** Passenger in pick-up truck or van injured in collision with two- or three-wheeled motor vehicle in traffic accident

X● **V52.7** Person on outside of pick-up truck or van injured in collision with two- or three-wheeled motor vehicle in traffic accident

X● **V52.9** Unspecified occupant of pick-up truck or van injured in collision with two- or three-wheeled motor vehicle in traffic accident

● **V53 Occupant of pick-up truck or van injured in collision with car, pick-up truck or van**

The appropriate 7th character is to be added to each code from category V53

> A initial encounter
> D subsequent encounter
> S sequela

X● **V53.Ø** Driver of pick-up truck or van injured in collision with car, pick-up truck or van in nontraffic accident

X● **V53.1** Passenger in pick-up truck or van injured in collision with car, pick-up truck or van in nontraffic accident

X● **V53.2** Person on outside of pick-up truck or van injured in collision with car, pick-up truck or van in nontraffic accident

X● **V53.3** Unspecified occupant of pick-up truck or van injured in collision with car, pick-up truck or van in nontraffic accident

X● **V53.4** Person boarding or alighting a pick-up truck or van injured in collision with car, pick-up truck or van

X● **V53.5** Driver of pick-up truck or van injured in collision with car, pick-up truck or van in traffic accident

X● **V53.6** Passenger in pick-up truck or van injured in collision with car, pick-up truck or van in traffic accident

X● **V53.7** Person on outside of pick-up truck or van injured in collision with car, pick-up truck or van in traffic accident

X● **V53.9** Unspecified occupant of pick-up truck or van injured in collision with car, pick-up truck or van in traffic accident

● **V54 Occupant of pick-up truck or van injured in collision with heavy transport vehicle or bus**

Excludes1 occupant of pick-up truck or van injured in collision with military vehicle (V59.81)

The appropriate 7th character is to be added to each code from category V54

> A initial encounter
> D subsequent encounter
> S sequela

X● **V54.Ø** Driver of pick-up truck or van injured in collision with heavy transport vehicle or bus in nontraffic accident

X● **V54.1** Passenger in pick-up truck or van injured in collision with heavy transport vehicle or bus in nontraffic accident

X● **V54.2** Person on outside of pick-up truck or van injured in collision with heavy transport vehicle or bus in nontraffic accident

X● **V54.3** Unspecified occupant of pick-up truck or van injured in collision with heavy transport vehicle or bus in nontraffic accident

X● **V54.4** Person boarding or alighting a pick-up truck or van injured in collision with heavy transport vehicle or bus

X● **V54.5** Driver of pick-up truck or van injured in collision with heavy transport vehicle or bus in traffic accident

X● **V54.6** Passenger in pick-up truck or van injured in collision with heavy transport vehicle or bus in traffic accident

X● **V54.7** Person on outside of pick-up truck or van injured in collision with heavy transport vehicle or bus in traffic accident

X● **V54.9** Unspecified occupant of pick-up truck or van injured in collision with heavy transport vehicle or bus in traffic accident

● **V55 Occupant of pick-up truck or van injured in collision with railway train or railway vehicle**

The appropriate 7th character is to be added to each code from category V55

> A initial encounter
> D subsequent encounter
> S sequela

X● **V55.Ø** Driver of pick-up truck or van injured in collision with railway train or railway vehicle in nontraffic accident

X● **V55.1** Passenger in pick-up truck or van injured in collision with railway train or railway vehicle in nontraffic accident

X● **V55.2** Person on outside of pick-up truck or van injured in collision with railway train or railway vehicle in nontraffic accident

X● **V55.3** Unspecified occupant of pick-up truck or van injured in collision with railway train or railway vehicle in nontraffic accident

X● **V55.4** Person boarding or alighting a pick-up truck or van injured in collision with railway train or railway vehicle

X● **V55.5** Driver of pick-up truck or van injured in collision with railway train or railway vehicle in traffic accident

X● **V55.6** Passenger in pick-up truck or van injured in collision with railway train or railway vehicle in traffic accident

X● **V55.7** Person on outside of pick-up truck or van injured in collision with railway train or railway vehicle in traffic accident

X● **V55.9** Unspecified occupant of pick-up truck or van injured in collision with railway train or railway vehicle in traffic accident

● **V56 Occupant of pick-up truck or van injured in collision with other nonmotor vehicle**

> **Includes** collision with animal-drawn vehicle, animal being ridden, streetcar

> The appropriate 7th character is to be added to each code from category V56

> | A | initial encounter |
> |---|---|
> | D | subsequent encounter |
> | S | sequela |

X● **V56.0** Driver of pick-up truck or van injured in collision with other nonmotor vehicle in nontraffic accident

X● **V56.1** Passenger in pick-up truck or van injured in collision with other nonmotor vehicle in nontraffic accident

X● **V56.2** Person on outside of pick-up truck or van injured in collision with other nonmotor vehicle in nontraffic accident

X● **V56.3** Unspecified occupant of pick-up truck or van injured in collision with other nonmotor vehicle in nontraffic accident

X● **V56.4** Person boarding or alighting a pick-up truck or van injured in collision with other nonmotor vehicle

X● **V56.5** Driver of pick-up truck or van injured in collision with other nonmotor vehicle in traffic accident

X● **V56.6** Passenger in pick-up truck or van injured in collision with other nonmotor vehicle in traffic accident

X● **V56.7** Person on outside of pick-up truck or van injured in collision with other nonmotor vehicle in traffic accident

X● **V56.9** Unspecified occupant of pick-up truck or van injured in collision with other nonmotor vehicle in traffic accident

● **V57 Occupant of pick-up truck or van injured in collision with fixed or stationary object**

> The appropriate 7th character is to be added to each code from category V57

> | A | initial encounter |
> |---|---|
> | D | subsequent encounter |
> | S | sequela |

X● **V57.0** Driver of pick-up truck or van injured in collision with fixed or stationary object in nontraffic accident

X● **V57.1** Passenger in pick-up truck or van injured in collision with fixed or stationary object in nontraffic accident

X● **V57.2** Person on outside of pick-up truck or van injured in collision with fixed or stationary object in nontraffic accident

X● **V57.3** Unspecified occupant of pick-up truck or van injured in collision with fixed or stationary object in nontraffic accident

X● **V57.4** Person boarding or alighting a pick-up truck or van injured in collision with fixed or stationary object

X● **V57.5** Driver of pick-up truck or van injured in collision with fixed or stationary object in traffic accident

X● **V57.6** Passenger in pick-up truck or van injured in collision with fixed or stationary object in traffic accident

X● **V57.7** Person on outside of pick-up truck or van injured in collision with fixed or stationary object in traffic accident

X● **V57.9** Unspecified occupant of pick-up truck or van injured in collision with fixed or stationary object in traffic accident

● **V58 Occupant of pick-up truck or van injured in noncollision transport accident**

> **Includes** overturning pick-up truck or van NOS
> overturning pick-up truck or van without collision

> The appropriate 7th character is to be added to each code from category V58

> | A | initial encounter |
> |---|---|
> | D | subsequent encounter |
> | S | sequela |

X● **V58.0** Driver of pick-up truck or van injured in noncollision transport accident in nontraffic accident

X● **V58.1** Passenger in pick-up truck or van injured in noncollision transport accident in nontraffic accident

X● **V58.2** Person on outside of pick-up truck or van injured in noncollision transport accident in nontraffic accident

X● **V58.3** Unspecified occupant of pick-up truck or van injured in noncollision transport accident in nontraffic accident

X● **V58.4** Person boarding or alighting a pick-up truck or van injured in noncollision transport accident

X● **V58.5** Driver of pick-up truck or van injured in noncollision transport accident in traffic accident

X● **V58.6** Passenger in pick-up truck or van injured in noncollision transport accident in traffic accident

X● **V58.7** Person on outside of pick-up truck or van injured in noncollision transport accident in traffic accident

X● **V58.9** Unspecified occupant of pick-up truck or van injured in noncollision transport accident in traffic accident

● **V59 Occupant of pick-up truck or van injured in other and unspecified transport accidents**

> The appropriate 7th character is to be added to each code from category V59

> | A | initial encounter |
> |---|---|
> | D | subsequent encounter |
> | S | sequela |

● **V59.0** Driver of pick-up truck or van injured in collision with other and unspecified motor vehicles in nontraffic accident

   X● **V59.00** Driver of pick-up truck or van injured in collision with unspecified motor vehicles in nontraffic accident

   X● **V59.09** Driver of pick-up truck or van injured in collision with other motor vehicles in nontraffic accident

● **V59.1** Passenger in pick-up truck or van injured in collision with other and unspecified motor vehicles in nontraffic accident

   X● **V59.10** Passenger in pick-up truck or van injured in collision with unspecified motor vehicles in nontraffic accident

   X● **V59.19** Passenger in pick-up truck or van injured in collision with other motor vehicles in nontraffic accident

● **V59.2** Unspecified occupant of pick-up truck or van injured in collision with other and unspecified motor vehicles in nontraffic accident

   X● **V59.20** Unspecified occupant of pick-up truck or van injured in collision with unspecified motor vehicles in nontraffic accident
> Collision NOS involving pick-up truck or van, nontraffic

   X● **V59.29** Unspecified occupant of pick-up truck or van injured in collision with other motor vehicles in nontraffic accident

N Newborn Age: 0   **P** Pediatric Age: 0–17   **M** Maternity DX: 12–55   **A** Adult Age: 15–124   ♀ Females Only   ♂ Males Only

Complication\Comorbidity   Major C\C   (Ex) CC/MCC Exclusions   Hospital-Acquired Condition   1523

X● **V59.3** **Occupant (driver) (passenger) of pick-up truck or van injured in unspecified nontraffic accident**
> Accident NOS involving pick-up truck or van, nontraffic
> Occupant of pick-up truck or van injured in nontraffic accident NOS

● **V59.4** **Driver of pick-up truck or van injured in collision with other and unspecified motor vehicles in traffic accident**

  X● **V59.40** **Driver of pick-up truck or van injured in collision with unspecified motor vehicles in traffic accident**

  X● **V59.49** **Driver of pick-up truck or van injured in collision with other motor vehicles in traffic accident**

● **V59.5** **Passenger in pick-up truck or van injured in collision with other and unspecified motor vehicles in traffic accident**

  X● **V59.50** **Passenger in pick-up truck or van injured in collision with unspecified motor vehicles in traffic accident**

  X● **V59.59** **Passenger in pick-up truck or van injured in collision with other motor vehicles in traffic accident**

● **V59.6** **Unspecified occupant of pick-up truck or van injured in collision with other and unspecified motor vehicles in traffic accident**

  X● **V59.60** **Unspecified occupant of pick-up truck or van injured in collision with unspecified motor vehicles in traffic accident**
> Collision NOS involving pick-up truck or van (traffic)

  X● **V59.69** **Unspecified occupant of pick-up truck or van injured in collision with other motor vehicles in traffic accident**

● **V59.8** **Occupant (driver) (passenger) of pick-up truck or van injured in other specified transport accidents**

  X● **V59.81** **Occupant (driver) (passenger) of pick-up truck or van injured in transport accident with military vehicle**

  X● **V59.88** **Occupant (driver) (passenger) of pick-up truck or van injured in other specified transport accidents**

X● **V59.9** **Occupant (driver) (passenger) of pick-up truck or van injured in unspecified traffic accident**
> Accident NOS involving pick-up truck or van

OCCUPANT OF HEAVY TRANSPORT VEHICLE INJURED IN TRANSPORT ACCIDENT (V60-V69)

Includes   18 wheeler
              armored car
              panel truck

Excludes1   bus
              motorcoach

● **V60** **Occupant of heavy transport vehicle injured in collision with pedestrian or animal**

  Excludes1   heavy transport vehicle collision with animal-drawn vehicle or animal being ridden (V66.-)

The appropriate 7th character is to be added to each code from category V60

> A   initial encounter
> D   subsequent encounter
> S   sequela

X● **V60.0** **Driver of heavy transport vehicle injured in collision with pedestrian or animal in nontraffic accident**

X● **V60.1** **Passenger in heavy transport vehicle injured in collision with pedestrian or animal in nontraffic accident**

X● **V60.2** **Person on outside of heavy transport vehicle injured in collision with pedestrian or animal in nontraffic accident**

X● **V60.3** **Unspecified occupant of heavy transport vehicle injured in collision with pedestrian or animal in nontraffic accident**

X● **V60.4** **Person boarding or alighting a heavy transport vehicle injured in collision with pedestrian or animal**

X● **V60.5** **Driver of heavy transport vehicle injured in collision with pedestrian or animal in traffic accident**

X● **V60.6** **Passenger in heavy transport vehicle injured in collision with pedestrian or animal in traffic accident**

X● **V60.7** **Person on outside of heavy transport vehicle injured in collision with pedestrian or animal in traffic accident**

X● **V60.9** **Unspecified occupant of heavy transport vehicle injured in collision with pedestrian or animal in traffic accident**

● **V61** **Occupant of heavy transport vehicle injured in collision with pedal cycle**

The appropriate 7th character is to be added to each code from category V61

> A   initial encounter
> D   subsequent encounter
> S   sequela

X● **V61.0** **Driver of heavy transport vehicle injured in collision with pedal cycle in nontraffic accident**

X● **V61.1** **Passenger in heavy transport vehicle injured in collision with pedal cycle in nontraffic accident**

X● **V61.2** **Person on outside of heavy transport vehicle injured in collision with pedal cycle in nontraffic accident**

X● **V61.3** **Unspecified occupant of heavy transport vehicle injured in collision with pedal cycle in nontraffic accident**

X● **V61.4** **Person boarding or alighting a heavy transport vehicle injured in collision with pedal cycle while boarding or alighting**

X● **V61.5** **Driver of heavy transport vehicle injured in collision with pedal cycle in traffic accident**

X● **V61.6** **Passenger in heavy transport vehicle injured in collision with pedal cycle in traffic accident**

X● **V61.7** **Person on outside of heavy transport vehicle injured in collision with pedal cycle in traffic accident**

X● **V61.9** **Unspecified occupant of heavy transport vehicle injured in collision with pedal cycle in traffic accident**

● **V62** **Occupant of heavy transport vehicle injured in collision with two- or three-wheeled motor vehicle**

The appropriate 7th character is to be added to each code from category V62

> A   initial encounter
> D   subsequent encounter
> S   sequela

X● **V62.0** **Driver of heavy transport vehicle injured in collision with two- or three-wheeled motor vehicle in nontraffic accident**

X● **V62.1** **Passenger in heavy transport vehicle injured in collision with two- or three-wheeled motor vehicle in nontraffic accident**

X● **V62.2** **Person on outside of heavy transport vehicle injured in collision with two- or three-wheeled motor vehicle in nontraffic accident**

X● **V62.3** **Unspecified occupant of heavy transport vehicle injured in collision with two- or three-wheeled motor vehicle in nontraffic accident**

X● **V62.4** **Person boarding or alighting a heavy transport vehicle injured in collision with two- or three-wheeled motor vehicle**

X● **V62.5** **Driver of heavy transport vehicle injured in collision with two- or three-wheeled motor vehicle in traffic accident**

X● **V62.6** **Passenger in heavy transport vehicle injured in collision with two- or three-wheeled motor vehicle in traffic accident**

▶ New   ⮕ Revised   ~~deleted~~ Deleted   Excludes 1   Excludes 2   Includes   Use additional   Code first   Code also   Key words
OGCR Official Guidelines   ● Unacceptable Principal Diagnosis   X Assign placeholder X   ● Use Additional Character(s)   ▶ Manifestation Code   **Coding Clinic**

X ● **V62.7**   Person on outside of heavy transport vehicle injured in collision with two- or three-wheeled motor vehicle in traffic accident

X ● **V62.9**   Unspecified occupant of heavy transport vehicle injured in collision with two- or three-wheeled motor vehicle in traffic accident

● **V63**   Occupant of heavy transport vehicle injured in collision with car, pick-up truck or van

The appropriate 7th character is to be added to each code from category V63

> A   initial encounter
> D   subsequent encounter
> S   sequela

X ● **V63.0**   Driver of heavy transport vehicle injured in collision with car, pick-up truck or van in nontraffic accident

X ● **V63.1**   Passenger in heavy transport vehicle injured in collision with car, pick-up truck or van in nontraffic accident

X ● **V63.2**   Person on outside of heavy transport vehicle injured in collision with car, pick-up truck or van in nontraffic accident

X ● **V63.3**   Unspecified occupant of heavy transport vehicle injured in collision with car, pick-up truck or van in nontraffic accident

X ● **V63.4**   Person boarding or alighting a heavy transport vehicle injured in collision with car, pick-up truck or van

X ● **V63.5**   Driver of heavy transport vehicle injured in collision with car, pick-up truck or van in traffic accident

X ● **V63.6**   Passenger in heavy transport vehicle injured in collision with car, pick-up truck or van in traffic accident

X ● **V63.7**   Person on outside of heavy transport vehicle injured in collision with car, pick-up truck or van in traffic accident

X ● **V63.9**   Unspecified occupant of heavy transport vehicle injured in collision with car, pick-up truck or van in traffic accident

● **V64**   Occupant of heavy transport vehicle injured in collision with heavy transport vehicle or bus

Excludes1   occupant of heavy transport vehicle injured in collision with military vehicle (V69.81)

The appropriate 7th character is to be added to each code from category V64

> A   initial encounter
> D   subsequent encounter
> S   sequela

X ● **V64.0**   Driver of heavy transport vehicle injured in collision with heavy transport vehicle or bus in nontraffic accident

X ● **V64.1**   Passenger in heavy transport vehicle injured in collision with heavy transport vehicle or bus in nontraffic accident

X ● **V64.2**   Person on outside of heavy transport vehicle injured in collision with heavy transport vehicle or bus in nontraffic accident

X ● **V64.3**   Unspecified occupant of heavy transport vehicle injured in collision with heavy transport vehicle or bus in nontraffic accident

X ● **V64.4**   Person boarding or alighting a heavy transport vehicle injured in collision with heavy transport vehicle or bus while boarding or alighting

X ● **V64.5**   Driver of heavy transport vehicle injured in collision with heavy transport vehicle or bus in traffic accident

X ● **V64.6**   Passenger in heavy transport vehicle injured in collision with heavy transport vehicle or bus in traffic accident

X ● **V64.7**   Person on outside of heavy transport vehicle injured in collision with heavy transport vehicle or bus in traffic accident

X ● **V64.9**   Unspecified occupant of heavy transport vehicle injured in collision with heavy transport vehicle or bus in traffic accident

● **V65**   Occupant of heavy transport vehicle injured in collision with railway train or railway vehicle

The appropriate 7th character is to be added to each code from category V65

> A   initial encounter
> D   subsequent encounter
> S   sequela

X ● **V65.0**   Driver of heavy transport vehicle injured in collision with railway train or railway vehicle in nontraffic accident

X ● **V65.1**   Passenger in heavy transport vehicle injured in collision with railway train or railway vehicle in nontraffic accident

X ● **V65.2**   Person on outside of heavy transport vehicle injured in collision with railway train or railway vehicle in nontraffic accident

X ● **V65.3**   Unspecified occupant of heavy transport vehicle injured in collision with railway train or railway vehicle in nontraffic accident

X ● **V65.4**   Person boarding or alighting a heavy transport vehicle injured in collision with railway train or railway vehicle

X ● **V65.5**   Driver of heavy transport vehicle injured in collision with railway train or railway vehicle in traffic accident

X ● **V65.6**   Passenger in heavy transport vehicle injured in collision with railway train or railway vehicle in traffic accident

X ● **V65.7**   Person on outside of heavy transport vehicle injured in collision with railway train or railway vehicle in traffic accident

X ● **V65.9**   Unspecified occupant of heavy transport vehicle injured in collision with railway train or railway vehicle in traffic accident

● **V66**   Occupant of heavy transport vehicle injured in collision with other nonmotor vehicle

Includes   collision with animal-drawn vehicle, animal being ridden, streetcar

The appropriate 7th character is to be added to each code from category V66

> A   initial encounter
> D   subsequent encounter
> S   sequela

X ● **V66.0**   Driver of heavy transport vehicle injured in collision with other nonmotor vehicle in nontraffic accident

X ● **V66.1**   Passenger in heavy transport vehicle injured in collision with other nonmotor vehicle in nontraffic accident

X ● **V66.2**   Person on outside of heavy transport vehicle injured in collision with other nonmotor vehicle in nontraffic accident

X ● **V66.3**   Unspecified occupant of heavy transport vehicle injured in collision with other nonmotor vehicle in nontraffic accident

X ● **V66.4**   Person boarding or alighting a heavy transport vehicle injured in collision with other nonmotor vehicle

X ● **V66.5**   Driver of heavy transport vehicle injured in collision with other nonmotor vehicle in traffic accident

X ● **V66.6**   Passenger in heavy transport vehicle injured in collision with other nonmotor vehicle in traffic accident

X ● **V66.7**   Person on outside of heavy transport vehicle injured in collision with other nonmotor vehicle in traffic accident

X ● **V66.9**   Unspecified occupant of heavy transport vehicle injured in collision with other nonmotor vehicle in traffic accident

CHAPTER 20 (V01-Y99)

- **V67 Occupant of heavy transport vehicle injured in collision with fixed or stationary object**

  The appropriate 7th character is to be added to each code from category V67

A	initial encounter
D	subsequent encounter
S	sequela

  X● **V67.0** Driver of heavy transport vehicle injured in collision with fixed or stationary object in nontraffic accident

  X● **V67.1** Passenger in heavy transport vehicle injured in collision with fixed or stationary object in nontraffic accident

  X● **V67.2** Person on outside of heavy transport vehicle injured in collision with fixed or stationary object in nontraffic accident

  X● **V67.3** Unspecified occupant of heavy transport vehicle injured in collision with fixed or stationary object in nontraffic accident

  X● **V67.4** Person boarding or alighting a heavy transport vehicle injured in collision with fixed or stationary object

  X● **V67.5** Driver of heavy transport vehicle injured in collision with fixed or stationary object in traffic accident

  X● **V67.6** Passenger in heavy transport vehicle injured in collision with fixed or stationary object in traffic accident

  X● **V67.7** Person on outside of heavy transport vehicle injured in collision with fixed or stationary object in traffic accident

  X● **V67.9** Unspecified occupant of heavy transport vehicle injured in collision with fixed or stationary object in traffic accident

- **V68 Occupant of heavy transport vehicle injured in noncollision transport accident**

  Includes overturning heavy transport vehicle NOS
  overturning heavy transport vehicle without collision

  The appropriate 7th character is to be added to each code from category V68

A	initial encounter
D	subsequent encounter
S	sequela

  X● **V68.0** Driver of heavy transport vehicle injured in noncollision transport accident in nontraffic accident

  X● **V68.1** Passenger in heavy transport vehicle injured in noncollision transport accident in nontraffic accident

  X● **V68.2** Person on outside of heavy transport vehicle injured in noncollision transport accident in nontraffic accident

  X● **V68.3** Unspecified occupant of heavy transport vehicle injured in noncollision transport accident in nontraffic accident

  X● **V68.4** Person boarding or alighting a heavy transport vehicle injured in noncollision transport accident

  X● **V68.5** Driver of heavy transport vehicle injured in noncollision transport accident in traffic accident

  X● **V68.6** Passenger in heavy transport vehicle injured in noncollision transport accident in traffic accident

  X● **V68.7** Person on outside of heavy transport vehicle injured in noncollision transport accident in traffic accident

  X● **V68.9** Unspecified occupant of heavy transport vehicle injured in noncollision transport accident in traffic accident

- **V69 Occupant of heavy transport vehicle injured in other and unspecified transport accidents**

  The appropriate 7th character is to be added to each code from category V69

A	initial encounter
D	subsequent encounter
S	sequela

- ● **V69.0** Driver of heavy transport vehicle injured in collision with other and unspecified motor vehicles in nontraffic accident

  X● **V69.00** Driver of heavy transport vehicle injured in collision with unspecified motor vehicles in nontraffic accident

  X● **V69.09** Driver of heavy transport vehicle injured in collision with other motor vehicles in nontraffic accident

- ● **V69.1** Passenger in heavy transport vehicle injured in collision with other and unspecified motor vehicles in nontraffic accident

  X● **V69.10** Passenger in heavy transport vehicle injured in collision with unspecified motor vehicles in nontraffic accident

  X● **V69.19** Passenger in heavy transport vehicle injured in collision with other motor vehicles in nontraffic accident

- ● **V69.2** Unspecified occupant of heavy transport vehicle injured in collision with other and unspecified motor vehicles in nontraffic accident

  X● **V69.20** Unspecified occupant of heavy transport vehicle injured in collision with unspecified motor vehicles in nontraffic accident
  Collision NOS involving heavy transport vehicle, nontraffic

  X● **V69.29** Unspecified occupant of heavy transport vehicle injured in collision with other motor vehicles in nontraffic accident

  X● **V69.3** Occupant (driver) (passenger) of heavy transport vehicle injured in unspecified nontraffic accident
  Accident NOS involving heavy transport vehicle, nontraffic
  Occupant of heavy transport vehicle injured in nontraffic accident NOS

- ● **V69.4** Driver of heavy transport vehicle injured in collision with other and unspecified motor vehicles in traffic accident

  X● **V69.40** Driver of heavy transport vehicle injured in collision with unspecified motor vehicles in traffic accident

  X● **V69.49** Driver of heavy transport vehicle injured in collision with other motor vehicles in traffic accident

- ● **V69.5** Passenger in heavy transport vehicle injured in collision with other and unspecified motor vehicles in traffic accident

  X● **V69.50** Passenger in heavy transport vehicle injured in collision with unspecified motor vehicles in traffic accident

  X● **V69.59** Passenger in heavy transport vehicle injured in collision with other motor vehicles in traffic accident

▶ New   ⟹ Revised   ~~deleted~~ Deleted   Excludes 1   Excludes 2   Includes   Use additional   Code first   Code also   Key words
OGCR Official Guidelines   ● Unacceptable Principal Diagnosis   X Assign placeholder X   ● Use Additional Character(s)   ▶ Manifestation Code   **Coding Clinic**

X● **V69.6** Unspecified occupant of heavy transport vehicle injured in collision with other and unspecified motor vehicles in traffic accident

    X● **V69.60** Unspecified occupant of heavy transport vehicle injured in collision with unspecified motor vehicles in traffic accident

      Collision NOS involving heavy transport vehicle (traffic)

    X● **V69.69** Unspecified occupant of heavy transport vehicle injured in collision with other motor vehicles in traffic accident

● **V69.8** Occupant (driver) (passenger) of heavy transport vehicle injured in other specified transport accidents

    X● **V69.81** Occupant (driver) (passenger) of heavy transport vehicle injured in transport accidents with military vehicle

    X● **V69.88** Occupant (driver) (passenger) of heavy transport vehicle injured in other specified transport accidents

X● **V69.9** Occupant (driver) (passenger) of heavy transport vehicle injured in unspecified traffic accident

      Accident NOS involving heavy transport vehicle

BUS OCCUPANT INJURED IN TRANSPORT ACCIDENT (V70-V79)

Includes	motorcoach
Excludes1	minibus (V50-V59)

● **V70** Bus occupant injured in collision with pedestrian or animal

    Excludes1 bus collision with animal-drawn vehicle or animal being ridden (V76.-)

    The appropriate 7th character is to be added to each code from category V70

A	initial encounter
D	subsequent encounter
S	sequela

X● **V70.0** Driver of bus injured in collision with pedestrian or animal in nontraffic accident

X● **V70.1** Passenger on bus injured in collision with pedestrian or animal in nontraffic accident

X● **V70.2** Person on outside of bus injured in collision with pedestrian or animal in nontraffic accident

X● **V70.3** Unspecified occupant of bus injured in collision with pedestrian or animal in nontraffic accident

X● **V70.4** Person boarding or alighting from bus injured in collision with pedestrian or animal

X● **V70.5** Driver of bus injured in collision with pedestrian or animal in traffic accident

X● **V70.6** Passenger on bus injured in collision with pedestrian or animal in traffic accident

X● **V70.7** Person on outside of bus injured in collision with pedestrian or animal in traffic accident

X● **V70.9** Unspecified occupant of bus injured in collision with pedestrian or animal in traffic accident

● **V71** Bus occupant injured in collision with pedal cycle

    The appropriate 7th character is to be added to each code from category V71

A	initial encounter
D	subsequent encounter
S	sequela

X● **V71.0** Driver of bus injured in collision with pedal cycle in nontraffic accident

X● **V71.1** Passenger on bus injured in collision with pedal cycle in nontraffic accident

X● **V71.2** Person on outside of bus injured in collision with pedal cycle in nontraffic accident

X● **V71.3** Unspecified occupant of bus injured in collision with pedal cycle in nontraffic accident

X● **V71.4** Person boarding or alighting from bus injured in collision with pedal cycle

X● **V71.5** Driver of bus injured in collision with pedal cycle in traffic accident

X● **V71.6** Passenger on bus injured in collision with pedal cycle in traffic accident

X● **V71.7** Person on outside of bus injured in collision with pedal cycle in traffic accident

X● **V71.9** Unspecified occupant of bus injured in collision with pedal cycle in traffic accident

● **V72** Bus occupant injured in collision with two- or three-wheeled motor vehicle

    The appropriate 7th character is to be added to each code from category V72

A	initial encounter
D	subsequent encounter
S	sequela

X● **V72.0** Driver of bus injured in collision with two- or three-wheeled motor vehicle in nontraffic accident

X● **V72.1** Passenger on bus injured in collision with two- or three-wheeled motor vehicle in nontraffic accident

X● **V72.2** Person on outside of bus injured in collision with two- or three-wheeled motor vehicle in nontraffic accident

X● **V72.3** Unspecified occupant of bus injured in collision with two- or three-wheeled motor vehicle in nontraffic accident

X● **V72.4** Person boarding or alighting from bus injured in collision with two- or three-wheeled motor vehicle

X● **V72.5** Driver of bus injured in collision with two- or three-wheeled motor vehicle in traffic accident

X● **V72.6** Passenger on bus injured in collision with two- or three-wheeled motor vehicle in traffic accident

X● **V72.7** Person on outside of bus injured in collision with two- or three-wheeled motor vehicle in traffic accident

X● **V72.9** Unspecified occupant of bus injured in collision with two- or three-wheeled motor vehicle in traffic accident

● **V73** Bus occupant injured in collision with car, pick-up truck or van

    The appropriate 7th character is to be added to each code from category V73

A	initial encounter
D	subsequent encounter
S	sequela

X● **V73.0** Driver of bus injured in collision with car, pick-up truck or van in nontraffic accident

X● **V73.1** Passenger on bus injured in collision with car, pick-up truck or van in nontraffic accident

X● **V73.2** Person on outside of bus injured in collision with car, pick-up truck or van in nontraffic accident

X● **V73.3** Unspecified occupant of bus injured in collision with car, pick-up truck or van in nontraffic accident

X● **V73.4** Person boarding or alighting from bus injured in collision with car, pick-up truck or van

X● **V73.5** Driver of bus injured in collision with car, pick-up truck or van in traffic accident

X● **V73.6** Passenger on bus injured in collision with car, pick-up truck or van in traffic accident

X● **V73.7** Person on outside of bus injured in collision with car, pick-up truck or van in traffic accident

X● **V73.9** Unspecified occupant of bus injured in collision with car, pick-up truck or van in traffic accident

N Newborn Age: 0   **P** Pediatric Age: 0–17   **M** Maternity DX: 12–55   **A** Adult Age: 15–124   ♀ Females Only   ♂ Males Only

Complication\Comorbidity   Major C\C   (Ex) CC/MCC Exclusions   Hospital-Acquired Condition

1527

CHAPTER 20 (V01-Y99)

● **V74** **Bus occupant injured in collision with heavy transport vehicle or bus**

> **Excludes1** bus occupant injured in collision with military vehicle (V79.81)

> The appropriate 7th character is to be added to each code from category V74

> | A | initial encounter |
> |---|---|
> | D | subsequent encounter |
> | S | sequela |

X● **V74.0** Driver of bus injured in collision with heavy transport vehicle or bus in nontraffic accident

X● **V74.1** Passenger on bus injured in collision with heavy transport vehicle or bus in nontraffic accident

X● **V74.2** Person on outside of bus injured in collision with heavy transport vehicle or bus in nontraffic accident

X● **V74.3** Unspecified occupant of bus injured in collision with heavy transport vehicle or bus in nontraffic accident

X● **V74.4** Person boarding or alighting from bus injured in collision with heavy transport vehicle or bus

X● **V74.5** Driver of bus injured in collision with heavy transport vehicle or bus in traffic accident

X● **V74.6** Passenger on bus injured in collision with heavy transport vehicle or bus in traffic accident

X● **V74.7** Person on outside of bus injured in collision with heavy transport vehicle or bus in traffic accident

X● **V74.9** Unspecified occupant of bus injured in collision with heavy transport vehicle or bus in traffic accident

● **V75** **Bus occupant injured in collision with railway train or railway vehicle**

> The appropriate 7th character is to be added to each code from category V75

> | A | initial encounter |
> |---|---|
> | D | subsequent encounter |
> | S | sequela |

X● **V75.0** Driver of bus injured in collision with railway train or railway vehicle in nontraffic accident

X● **V75.1** Passenger on bus injured in collision with railway train or railway vehicle in nontraffic accident

X● **V75.2** Person on outside of bus injured in collision with railway train or railway vehicle in nontraffic accident

X● **V75.3** Unspecified occupant of bus injured in collision with railway train or railway vehicle in nontraffic accident

X● **V75.4** Person boarding or alighting from bus injured in collision with railway train or railway vehicle

X● **V75.5** Driver of bus injured in collision with railway train or railway vehicle in traffic accident

X● **V75.6** Passenger on bus injured in collision with railway train or railway vehicle in traffic accident

X● **V75.7** Person on outside of bus injured in collision with railway train or railway vehicle in traffic accident

X● **V75.9** Unspecified occupant of bus injured in collision with railway train or railway vehicle in traffic accident

● **V76** **Bus occupant injured in collision with other nonmotor vehicle**

> **Includes** collision with animal-drawn vehicle, animal being ridden, streetcar

> The appropriate 7th character is to be added to each code from category V76

> | A | initial encounter |
> |---|---|
> | D | subsequent encounter |
> | S | sequela |

X● **V76.0** Driver of bus injured in collision with other nonmotor vehicle in nontraffic accident

X● **V76.1** Passenger on bus injured in collision with other nonmotor vehicle in nontraffic accident

X● **V76.2** Person on outside of bus injured in collision with other nonmotor vehicle in nontraffic accident

X● **V76.3** Unspecified occupant of bus injured in collision with other nonmotor vehicle in nontraffic accident

X● **V76.4** Person boarding or alighting from bus injured in collision with other nonmotor vehicle

X● **V76.5** Driver of bus injured in collision with other nonmotor vehicle in traffic accident

X● **V76.6** Passenger on bus injured in collision with other nonmotor vehicle in traffic accident

X● **V76.7** Person on outside of bus injured in collision with other nonmotor vehicle in traffic accident

X● **V76.9** Unspecified occupant of bus injured in collision with other nonmotor vehicle in traffic accident

● **V77** **Bus occupant injured in collision with fixed or stationary object**

> The appropriate 7th character is to be added to each code from category V77

> | A | initial encounter |
> |---|---|
> | D | subsequent encounter |
> | S | sequela |

X● **V77.0** Driver of bus injured in collision with fixed or stationary object in nontraffic accident

X● **V77.1** Passenger on bus injured in collision with fixed or stationary object in nontraffic accident

X● **V77.2** Person on outside of bus injured in collision with fixed or stationary object in nontraffic accident

X● **V77.3** Unspecified occupant of bus injured in collision with fixed or stationary object in nontraffic accident

X● **V77.4** Person boarding or alighting from bus injured in collision with fixed or stationary object

X● **V77.5** Driver of bus injured in collision with fixed or stationary object in traffic accident

X● **V77.6** Passenger on bus injured in collision with fixed or stationary object in traffic accident

X● **V77.7** Person on outside of bus injured in collision with fixed or stationary object in traffic accident

X● **V77.9** Unspecified occupant of bus injured in collision with fixed or stationary object in traffic accident

● **V78** **Bus occupant injured in noncollision transport accident**

> **Includes** overturning bus NOS
> overturning bus without collision

> The appropriate 7th character is to be added to each code from category V78

> | A | initial encounter |
> |---|---|
> | D | subsequent encounter |
> | S | sequela |

X● **V78.0** Driver of bus injured in noncollision transport accident in nontraffic accident

X● **V78.1** Passenger on bus injured in noncollision transport accident in nontraffic accident

X● **V78.2** Person on outside of bus injured in noncollision transport accident in nontraffic accident

X● **V78.3** Unspecified occupant of bus injured in noncollision transport accident in nontraffic accident

X● **V78.4** Person boarding or alighting from bus injured in noncollision transport accident

X● **V78.5** Driver of bus injured in noncollision transport accident in traffic accident

X● **V78.6** Passenger on bus injured in noncollision transport accident in traffic accident

X● **V78.7** Person on outside of bus injured in noncollision transport accident in traffic accident

X● **V78.9** Unspecified occupant of bus injured in noncollision transport accident in traffic accident

▶ New   ⇒ Revised   ~~deleted~~ Deleted   Excludes 1   Excludes 2   Includes   Use additional   Code first   Code also   Key words
OGCR Official Guidelines   ● Unacceptable Principal Diagnosis   X Assign placeholder X   ● Use Additional Character(s)   ▶ Manifestation Code   **Coding Clinic**

● **V79** **Bus occupant injured in other and unspecified transport accidents**

> The appropriate 7th character is to be added to each code from category V79

A	initial encounter
D	subsequent encounter
S	sequela

● **V79.0** **Driver of bus injured in collision with other and unspecified motor vehicles in nontraffic accident**

  X● **V79.00** Driver of bus injured in collision with unspecified motor vehicles in nontraffic accident

  X● **V79.09** Driver of bus injured in collision with other motor vehicles in nontraffic accident

● **V79.1** **Passenger on bus injured in collision with other and unspecified motor vehicles in nontraffic accident**

  X● **V79.10** Passenger on bus injured in collision with unspecified motor vehicles in nontraffic accident

  X● **V79.19** Passenger on bus injured in collision with other motor vehicles in nontraffic accident

● **V79.2** **Unspecified bus occupant injured in collision with other and unspecified motor vehicles in nontraffic accident**

  X● **V79.20** Unspecified bus occupant injured in collision with unspecified motor vehicles in nontraffic accident
  > Bus collision NOS, nontraffic

  X● **V79.29** Unspecified bus occupant injured in collision with other motor vehicles in nontraffic accident

X● **V79.3** **Bus occupant (driver) (passenger) injured in unspecified nontraffic accident**
  > Bus accident NOS, nontraffic
  > Bus occupant injured in nontraffic accident NOS

● **V79.4** **Driver of bus injured in collision with other and unspecified motor vehicles in traffic accident**

  X● **V79.40** Driver of bus injured in collision with unspecified motor vehicles in traffic accident

  X● **V79.49** Driver of bus injured in collision with other motor vehicles in traffic accident

● **V79.5** **Passenger on bus injured in collision with other and unspecified motor vehicles in traffic accident**

  X● **V79.50** Passenger on bus injured in collision with unspecified motor vehicles in traffic accident

  X● **V79.59** Passenger on bus injured in collision with other motor vehicles in traffic accident

● **V79.6** **Unspecified bus occupant injured in collision with other and unspecified motor vehicles in traffic accident**

  X● **V79.60** Unspecified bus occupant injured in collision with unspecified motor vehicles in traffic accident
  > Bus collision NOS (traffic)

  X● **V79.69** Unspecified bus occupant injured in collision with other motor vehicles in traffic accident

● **V79.8** **Bus occupant (driver) (passenger) injured in other specified transport accidents**

  X● **V79.81** Bus occupant (driver) (passenger) injured in transport accidents with military vehicle

  X● **V79.88** Bus occupant (driver) (passenger) injured in other specified transport accidents

X● **V79.9** **Bus occupant (driver) (passenger) injured in unspecified traffic accident**
  > Bus accident NOS

OTHER LAND TRANSPORT ACCIDENTS (V80-V89)

● **V80** **Animal-rider or occupant of animal-drawn vehicle injured in transport accident**

> The appropriate 7th character is to be added to each code from category V80

A	initial encounter
D	subsequent encounter
S	sequela

● **V80.0** **Animal-rider or occupant of animal drawn vehicle injured by fall from or being thrown from animal or animal-drawn vehicle in noncollision accident**

  ● **V80.01** Animal-rider injured by fall from or being thrown from animal in noncollision accident

    ● **V80.010** Animal-rider injured by fall from or being thrown from horse in noncollision accident

    ● **V80.018** Animal-rider injured by fall from or being thrown from other animal in noncollision accident

  X● **V80.02** Occupant of animal-drawn vehicle injured by fall from or being thrown from animal-drawn vehicle in noncollision accident
  > Overturning animal-drawn vehicle NOS
  > Overturning animal-drawn vehicle without collision

● **V80.1** **Animal-rider or occupant of animal-drawn vehicle injured in collision with pedestrian or animal**

  Excludes1 animal-rider or animal-drawn vehicle collision with animal-drawn vehicle or animal being ridden (V80.7)

  X● **V80.11** Animal-rider injured in collision with pedestrian or animal

  X● **V80.12** Occupant of animal-drawn vehicle injured in collision with pedestrian or animal

● **V80.2** **Animal-rider or occupant of animal-drawn vehicle injured in collision with pedal cycle**

  X● **V80.21** Animal-rider injured in collision with pedal cycle

  X● **V80.22** Occupant of animal-drawn vehicle injured in collision with pedal cycle

● **V80.3** **Animal-rider or occupant of animal-drawn vehicle injured in collision with two- or three-wheeled motor vehicle**

  X● **V80.31** Animal-rider injured in collision with two- or three-wheeled motor vehicle

  X● **V80.32** Occupant of animal-drawn vehicle injured in collision with two- or three-wheeled motor vehicle

● **V80.4** **Animal-rider or occupant of animal-drawn vehicle injured in collision with car, pick-up truck, van, heavy transport vehicle or bus**

  Excludes1 animal-rider injured in collision with military vehicle (V80.910)
  occupant of animal-drawn vehicle injured in collision with military vehicle (V80.920)

  X● **V80.41** Animal-rider injured in collision with car, pick-up truck, van, heavy transport vehicle or bus

  X● **V80.42** Occupant of animal-drawn vehicle injured in collision with car, pick-up truck, van, heavy transport vehicle or bus

CHAPTER 20 (V01-Y99)

● **V80.5** Animal-rider or occupant of animal-drawn vehicle injured in collision with other specified motor vehicle

X● **V80.51** Animal-rider injured in collision with other specified motor vehicle

X● **V80.52** Occupant of animal-drawn vehicle injured in collision with other specified motor vehicle

● **V80.6** Animal-rider or occupant of animal-drawn vehicle injured in collision with railway train or railway vehicle

X● **V80.61** Animal-rider injured in collision with railway train or railway vehicle

X● **V80.62** Occupant of animal-drawn vehicle injured in collision with railway train or railway vehicle

● **V80.7** Animal-rider or occupant of animal-drawn vehicle injured in collision with other nonmotor vehicles

● **V80.71** Animal-rider or occupant of animal-drawn vehicle injured in collision with animal being ridden

● **V80.710** Animal-rider injured in collision with other animal being ridden

● **V80.711** Occupant of animal-drawn vehicle injured in collision with animal being ridden

● **V80.72** Animal-rider or occupant of animal-drawn vehicle injured in collision with other animal-drawn vehicle

● **V80.720** Animal-rider injured in collision with animal-drawn vehicle

● **V80.721** Occupant of animal-drawn vehicle injured in collision with other animal-drawn vehicle

● **V80.73** Animal-rider or occupant of animal-drawn vehicle injured in collision with streetcar

● **V80.730** Animal-rider injured in collision with streetcar

● **V80.731** Occupant of animal-drawn vehicle injured in collision with streetcar

● **V80.79** Animal-rider or occupant of animal-drawn vehicle injured in collision with other nonmotor vehicles

● **V80.790** Animal-rider injured in collision with other nonmotor vehicles

● **V80.791** Occupant of animal-drawn vehicle injured in collision with other nonmotor vehicles

● **V80.8** Animal-rider or occupant of animal-drawn vehicle injured in collision with fixed or stationary object

X● **V80.81** Animal-rider injured in collision with fixed or stationary object

X● **V80.82** Occupant of animal-drawn vehicle injured in collision with fixed or stationary object

● **V80.9** Animal-rider or occupant of animal-drawn vehicle injured in other and unspecified transport accidents

● **V80.91** Animal-rider injured in other and unspecified transport accidents

● **V80.910** Animal-rider injured in transport accident with military vehicle

● **V80.918** Animal-rider injured in other transport accident

● **V80.919** Animal-rider injured in unspecified transport accident
Animal rider accident NOS

● **V80.92** Occupant of animal-drawn vehicle injured in other and unspecified transport accidents

● **V80.920** Occupant of animal-drawn vehicle injured in transport accident with military vehicle

● **V80.928** Occupant of animal-drawn vehicle injured in other transport accident

● **V80.929** Occupant of animal-drawn vehicle injured in unspecified transport accident
Animal-drawn vehicle accident NOS

● **V81** Occupant of railway train or railway vehicle injured in transport accident

Includes derailment of railway train or railway vehicle
person on outside of train

Excludes1 streetcar (V82.-)

The appropriate 7th character is to be added to each code from category V81

A	initial encounter
D	subsequent encounter
S	sequela

X● **V81.0** Occupant of railway train or railway vehicle injured in collision with motor vehicle in nontraffic accident

Excludes1 occupant of railway train or railway vehicle injured due to collision with military vehicle (V81.83)

X● **V81.1** Occupant of railway train or railway vehicle injured in collision with motor vehicle in traffic accident

Excludes1 occupant of railway train or railway vehicle injured due to collision with military vehicle (V81.83)

X● **V81.2** Occupant of railway train or railway vehicle injured in collision with or hit by rolling stock

X● **V81.3** Occupant of railway train or railway vehicle injured in collision with other object
Railway collision NOS

X● **V81.4** Person injured while boarding or alighting from railway train or railway vehicle

X● **V81.5** Occupant of railway train or railway vehicle injured by fall in railway train or railway vehicle

X● **V81.6** Occupant of railway train or railway vehicle injured by fall from railway train or railway vehicle

X● **V81.7** Occupant of railway train or railway vehicle injured in derailment without antecedent collision

● **V81.8** Occupant of railway train or railway vehicle injured in other specified railway accidents

X● **V81.81** Occupant of railway train or railway vehicle injured due to explosion or fire on train

X● **V81.82** Occupant of railway train or railway vehicle injured due to object falling onto train
Occupant of railway train or railway vehicle injured due to falling earth onto train
Occupant of railway train or railway vehicle injured due to falling rocks onto train
Occupant of railway train or railway vehicle injured due to falling snow onto train
Occupant of railway train or railway vehicle injured due to falling trees onto train

X● **V81.83** Occupant of railway train or railway vehicle injured due to collision with military vehicle

X● **V81.89** Occupant of railway train or railway vehicle injured due to other specified railway accident

X● **V81.9** Occupant of railway train or railway vehicle injured in unspecified railway accident
Railway accident NOS

● **V82   Occupant of powered streetcar injured in transport accident**

> **Includes**   interurban electric car
> person on outside of streetcar
> tram (car)
> trolley (car)

> **Excludes1**   bus (V70-V79)
> motorcoach (V70-V79)
> nonpowered streetcar (V76.-)
> train (V81.-)

The appropriate 7th character is to be added to each code from category V82

> A   initial encounter
> D   subsequent encounter
> S   sequela

X● **V82.0   Occupant of streetcar injured in collision with motor vehicle in nontraffic accident**

X● **V82.1   Occupant of streetcar injured in collision with motor vehicle in traffic accident**

X● **V82.2   Occupant of streetcar injured in collision with or hit by rolling stock**

X● **V82.3   Occupant of streetcar injured in collision with other object**

> **Excludes1**   collision with animal-drawn vehicle or animal being ridden (V82.8)

X● **V82.4   Person injured while boarding or alighting from streetcar**

X● **V82.5   Occupant of streetcar injured by fall in streetcar**

> **Excludes1**   fall in streetcar:
> while boarding or alighting (V82.4)
> with antecedent collision (V82.0-V82.3)

X● **V82.6   Occupant of streetcar injured by fall from streetcar**

> **Excludes1**   fall from streetcar:
> while boarding or alighting (V82.4)
> with antecedent collision (V82.0-V82.3)

X● **V82.7   Occupant of streetcar injured in derailment without antecedent collision**

> **Excludes1**   occupant of streetcar injured in derailment with antecedent collision (V82.0-V82.3)

X● **V82.8   Occupant of streetcar injured in other specified transport accidents**
> Streetcar collision with military vehicle
> Streetcar collision with train or nonmotor vehicles

X● **V82.9   Occupant of streetcar injured in unspecified traffic accident**
> Streetcar accident NOS

● **V83   Occupant of special vehicle mainly used on industrial premises injured in transport accident**

> **Includes**   battery-powered airport passenger vehicle
> battery-powered truck (baggage) (mail)
> coal-car in mine
> forklift (truck)
> logging car
> self-propelled industrial truck
> station baggage truck (powered)
> tram, truck, or tub (powered) in mine or quarry

> **Excludes1**   special construction vehicles (V85.-)
> special industrial vehicle in stationary use or maintenance (W31.-)

The appropriate 7th character is to be added to each code from category V83

> A   initial encounter
> D   subsequent encounter
> S   sequela

X● **V83.0   Driver of special industrial vehicle injured in traffic accident**

X● **V83.1   Passenger of special industrial vehicle injured in traffic accident**

X● **V83.2   Person on outside of special industrial vehicle injured in traffic accident**

X● **V83.3   Unspecified occupant of special industrial vehicle injured in traffic accident**

X● **V83.4   Person injured while boarding or alighting from special industrial vehicle**

X● **V83.5   Driver of special industrial vehicle injured in nontraffic accident**

X● **V83.6   Passenger of special industrial vehicle injured in nontraffic accident**

X● **V83.7   Person on outside of special industrial vehicle injured in nontraffic accident**

X● **V83.9   Unspecified occupant of special industrial vehicle injured in nontraffic accident**
> Special-industrial-vehicle accident NOS

● **V84   Occupant of special vehicle mainly used in agriculture injured in transport accident**

> **Includes**   self-propelled farm machinery
> tractor (and trailer)

> **Excludes1**   animal-powered farm machinery accident (W30.8-)
> contact with combine harvester (W30.0)
> special agricultural vehicle in stationary use or maintenance (W30.-)

The appropriate 7th character is to be added to each code from category V84

> A   initial encounter
> D   subsequent encounter
> S   sequela

X● **V84.0   Driver of special agricultural vehicle injured in traffic accident**

X● **V84.1   Passenger of special agricultural vehicle injured in traffic accident**

X● **V84.2   Person on outside of special agricultural vehicle injured in traffic accident**

X● **V84.3   Unspecified occupant of special agricultural vehicle injured in traffic accident**

X● **V84.4   Person injured while boarding or alighting from special agricultural vehicle**

X● **V84.5   Driver of special agricultural vehicle injured in nontraffic accident**

X● **V84.6   Passenger of special agricultural vehicle injured in nontraffic accident**

X● **V84.7   Person on outside of special agricultural vehicle injured in nontraffic accident**

X● **V84.9   Unspecified occupant of special agricultural vehicle injured in nontraffic accident**
> Special-agricultural vehicle accident NOS

● **V85   Occupant of special construction vehicle injured in transport accident**

> **Includes**   bulldozer
> digger
> dump truck
> earth-leveller
> mechanical shovel
> road-roller

> **Excludes1**   special industrial vehicle (V83.-)
> special construction vehicle in stationary use or maintenance (W31.-)

The appropriate 7th character is to be added to each code from category V85

> A   initial encounter
> D   subsequent encounter
> S   sequela

X● **V85.0   Driver of special construction vehicle injured in traffic accident**

X● **V85.1   Passenger of special construction vehicle injured in traffic accident**

X● **V85.2** **Person on outside of special construction vehicle injured in traffic accident**

X● **V85.3** **Unspecified occupant of special construction vehicle injured in traffic accident**

X● **V85.4** **Person injured while boarding or alighting from special construction vehicle**

X● **V85.5** **Driver of special construction vehicle injured in nontraffic accident**

X● **V85.6** **Passenger of special construction vehicle injured in nontraffic accident**

X● **V85.7** **Person on outside of special construction vehicle injured in nontraffic accident**

X● **V85.9** **Unspecified occupant of special construction vehicle injured in nontraffic accident**
    Special-construction-vehicle accident NOS

● **V86** **Occupant of special all-terrain or other off-road motor vehicle, injured in transport accident**

     Excludes1   special all-terrain vehicle in stationary use or maintenance (W31.-)
    sport-utility vehicle (V50-V59)
    three-wheeled motor vehicle designed for on-road use (V30-V39)

The appropriate 7th character is to be added to each code from category V86

> A   initial encounter
> D   subsequent encounter
> S   sequela

● **V86.0** **Driver of special all-terrain or other off-road motor vehicle injured in traffic accident**

   X● **V86.01** **Driver of ambulance or fire engine injured in traffic accident**

   X● **V86.02** **Driver of snowmobile injured in traffic accident**

   X● **V86.03** **Driver of dune buggy injured in traffic accident**

   X● **V86.04** **Driver of military vehicle injured in traffic accident**

▶X● **V86.05** **Driver of 3- or 4-wheeled all-terrain vehicle (ATV) injured in traffic accident**

▶X● **V86.06** **Driver of dirt bike or motor/cross bike injured in traffic accident**

   X● **V86.09** **Driver of other off-road special all-terrain or other off-road vehicle injured in traffic accident**
    Driver of dirt bike injured in traffic accident
    Driver of go cart injured in traffic accident
    Driver of golf cart injured in traffic accident

● **V86.1** **Passenger of special all-terrain or other off-road motor vehicle injured in traffic accident**

   X● **V86.11** **Passenger of ambulance or fire engine injured in traffic accident**

   X● **V86.12** **Passenger of snowmobile injured in traffic accident**

   X● **V86.13** **Passenger of dune buggy injured in traffic accident**

   X● **V86.14** **Passenger of military vehicle injured in traffic accident**

▶X● **V86.15** **Passenger of 3- or 4-wheeled all-terrain vehicle (ATV) injured in traffic accident**

▶X● **V86.16** **Passenger of dirt bike or motor/cross bike injured in traffic accident**

   X● **V86.19** **Passenger of other off-road special all-terrain or other off-road off-road motor vehicle injured in traffic accident**
    Passenger of dirt bike injured in traffic accident
    Passenger of go cart injured in traffic accident
    Passenger of golf cart injured in traffic accident

● **V86.2** **Person on outside of special all-terrain or other off-road motor vehicle injured in traffic accident**

   X● **V86.21** **Person on outside of ambulance or fire engine injured in traffic accident**

   X● **V86.22** **Person on outside of snowmobile injured in traffic accident**

   X● **V86.23** **Person on outside of dune buggy injured in traffic accident**

   X● **V86.24** **Person on outside of military vehicle injured in traffic accident**

▶X● **V86.25** **Person on outside of 3- or 4-wheeled all-terrain vehicle (ATV) injured in traffic accident**

▶X● **V86.26** **Person on outside of dirt bike or motor/cross bike injured in traffic accident**

   X● **V86.29** **Person on outside of other special all-terrain or other off-road motor vehicle injured in traffic accident**
    Person on outside of dirt bike injured in traffic accident
    Person on outside of go cart in traffic accident
    Person on outside of golf cart injured in traffic accident

● **V86.3** **Unspecified occupant of special all-terrain or other off-road motor vehicle injured in traffic accident**

   X● **V86.31** **Unspecified occupant of ambulance or fire engine injured in traffic accident**

   X● **V86.32** **Unspecified occupant of snowmobile injured in traffic accident**

   X● **V86.33** **Unspecified occupant of dune buggy injured in traffic accident**

   X● **V86.34** **Unspecified occupant of military vehicle injured in traffic accident**

▶X● **V86.35** **Unspecified occupant of 3- or 4-wheeled all-terrain vehicle (ATV) injured in traffic accident**

▶X● **V86.36** **Unspecified occupant of dirt bike or motor/cross bike injured in traffic accident**

   X● **V86.39** **Unspecified occupant of other special all-terrain or other off-road motor vehicle injured in traffic accident**
    Unspecified occupant of dirt bike injured in traffic accident
    Unspecified occupant of go cart injured in traffic accident
    Unspecified occupant of golf cart injured in traffic accident

● **V86.4** **Person injured while boarding or alighting from special all-terrain or other off-road motor vehicle**

   X● **V86.41** **Person injured while boarding or alighting from ambulance or fire engine**

   X● **V86.42** **Person injured while boarding or alighting from snowmobile**

   X● **V86.43** **Person injured while boarding or alighting from dune buggy**

   X● **V86.44** **Person injured while boarding or alighting from military vehicle**

▶X● **V86.45** **Person injured while boarding or alighting from a 3- or 4-wheeled all-terrain vehicle (ATV)**

▶X● **V86.46** **Person injured while boarding or alighting from a dirt bike or motor/cross bike**

   X● **V86.49** **Person injured while boarding or alighting from other special all-terrain or other off-road motor vehicle**
    Person injured while boarding or alighting from dirt bike
    Person injured while boarding or alighting from go cart
    Person injured while boarding or alighting from golf cart

CHAPTER 20 (V01-Y99)

1532

▶ New   ⇒ Revised   ~~deleted~~ Deleted   Excludes 1   Excludes 2   Includes   Use additional   Code first   Code also   Key words

OGCR Official Guidelines   ● Unacceptable Principal Diagnosis   X Assign placeholder X   ● Use Additional Character(s)   ▶ Manifestation Code   **Coding Clinic**

● **V86.5** Driver of special all-terrain or other off-road motor vehicle injured in nontraffic accident

   X● **V86.51** Driver of ambulance or fire engine injured in nontraffic accident

   X● **V86.52** Driver of snowmobile injured in nontraffic accident

   X● **V86.53** Driver of dune buggy injured in nontraffic accident

   X● **V86.54** Driver of military vehicle injured in nontraffic accident

  ▶X● **V86.55** Driver of 3- or 4-wheeled all-terrain vehicle (ATV) injured in nontraffic accident

  ▶X● **V86.56** Driver of dirt bike or motor/cross bike injured in nontraffic accident

   X● **V86.59** Driver of other off-road special all-terrain or other off-road motor vehicle injured in nontraffic accident

       Driver of dirt bike injured in nontraffic accident

       Driver of go cart injured in nontraffic accident

       Driver of golf cart injured in nontraffic accident

● **V86.6** Passenger of special all-terrain or other off-road motor vehicle injured in nontraffic accident

   X● **V86.61** Passenger of ambulance or fire engine injured in nontraffic accident

   X● **V86.62** Passenger of snowmobile injured in nontraffic accident

   X● **V86.63** Passenger of dune buggy injured in nontraffic accident

   X● **V86.64** Passenger of military vehicle injured in nontraffic accident

  ▶X● **V86.65** Passenger of 3- or 4-wheeled all-terrain vehicle (ATV) injured in nontraffic accident

  ▶X● **V86.66** Passenger of dirt bike or motor/cross bike injured in nontraffic accident

   X● **V86.69** Passenger of other special all-terrain or other off-road vehicle injured in nontraffic accident

       Passenger of dirt bike injured in nontraffic accident

       Passenger of go cart injured in nontraffic accident

       Passenger of golf cart injured in nontraffic accident

● **V86.7** Person on outside of special all-terrain or other off-road motor vehicle injured in nontraffic accident

   X● **V86.71** Person on outside of ambulance or fire engine injured in nontraffic accident

   X● **V86.72** Person on outside of snowmobile injured in nontraffic accident

   X● **V86.73** Person on outside of dune buggy injured in nontraffic accident

   X● **V86.74** Person on outside of military vehicle injured in nontraffic accident

  ▶X● **V86.75** Person on outside of 3- or 4-wheeled all-terrain vehicle (ATV) injured in nontraffic accident

  ▶X● **V86.76** Person on outside of dirt bike or motor/cross bike injured in nontraffic accident

   X● **V86.79** Person on outside of other special all-terrain or other off-road motor vehicles injured in nontraffic accident

       Person on outside of dirt bike injured in nontraffic accident

       Person on outside of go cart injured in nontraffic accident

       Person on outside of golf cart injured in nontraffic accident

● **V86.9** Unspecified occupant of special all-terrain or other off-road motor vehicle injured in nontraffic accident

   X● **V86.91** Unspecified occupant of ambulance or fire engine injured in nontraffic accident

   X● **V86.92** Unspecified occupant of snowmobile injured in nontraffic accident

   X● **V86.93** Unspecified occupant of dune buggy injured in nontraffic accident

   X● **V86.94** Unspecified occupant of military vehicle injured in nontraffic accident

  ▶X● **V86.95** Unspecified occupant of 3- or 4-wheeled all-terrain vehicle (ATV) injured in nontraffic accident

  ▶X● **V86.96** Unspecified occupant of dirt bike or motor/cross bike injured in nontraffic accident

   X● **V86.99** Unspecified occupant of other special all-terrain or other off-road motor vehicle injured in nontraffic accident

       ~~All-terrain motor-vehicle accident NOS~~

       Off-road motor-vehicle accident NOS

       Other motor-vehicle accident NOS

       ~~Unspecified occupant of dirt bike injured in nontraffic accident~~

       Unspecified occupant of go cart injured in nontraffic accident

       Unspecified occupant of golf cart injured in nontraffic accident

       Unspecified occupant of race car injured in nontraffic accident

● **V87** Traffic accident of specified type but victim's mode of transport unknown

   Excludes1   collision involving:

          pedal cycle (V10-V19)

          pedestrian (V01-V09)

   The appropriate 7th character is to be added to each code from category V87

A	initial encounter
D	subsequent encounter
S	sequela

   X● **V87.0** Person injured in collision between car and two- or three-wheeled powered vehicle (traffic)

   X● **V87.1** Person injured in collision between other motor vehicle and two- or three-wheeled motor vehicle (traffic)

   X● **V87.2** Person injured in collision between car and pick-up truck or van (traffic)

   X● **V87.3** Person injured in collision between car and bus (traffic)

   X● **V87.4** Person injured in collision between car and heavy transport vehicle (traffic)

   X● **V87.5** Person injured in collision between heavy transport vehicle and bus (traffic)

   X● **V87.6** Person injured in collision between railway train or railway vehicle and car (traffic)

   X● **V87.7** Person injured in collision between other specified motor vehicles (traffic)

   X● **V87.8** Person injured in other specified noncollision transport accidents involving motor vehicle (traffic)

   X● **V87.9** Person injured in other specified (collision) (noncollision) transport accidents involving nonmotor vehicle (traffic)

● **V88** Nontraffic accident of specified type but victim's mode of transport unknown

   Excludes1   collision involving:

          pedal cycle (V10-V19)

          pedestrian (V01-V09)

   The appropriate 7th character is to be added to each code from category V88

A	initial encounter
D	subsequent encounter
S	sequela

   X● **V88.0** Person injured in collision between car and two- or three-wheeled motor vehicle, nontraffic

   X● **V88.1** Person injured in collision between other motor vehicle and two- or three-wheeled motor vehicle, nontraffic

   X● **V88.2** Person injured in collision between car and pick-up truck or van, nontraffic

---

N Newborn Age: 0   **P** Pediatric Age: 0–17   **M** Maternity DX: 12–55   **A** Adult Age: 15–124   ♀ Females Only   ♂ Males Only

● Complication\Comorbidity   ● Major C\C   Ⓔⓧ CC/MCC Exclusions   ● Hospital-Acquired Condition

1533

CHAPTER 20 (V01-Y99)

X● **V88.3**   **Person injured in collision between car and bus, nontraffic**

X● **V88.4**   **Person injured in collision between car and heavy transport vehicle, nontraffic**

X● **V88.5**   **Person injured in collision between heavy transport vehicle and bus, nontraffic**

X● **V88.6**   **Person injured in collision between railway train or railway vehicle and car, nontraffic**

X● **V88.7**   **Person injured in collision between other specified motor vehicle, nontraffic**

X● **V88.8**   **Person injured in other specified noncollision transport accidents involving motor vehicle, nontraffic**

X● **V88.9**   **Person injured in other specified (collision) (noncollision) transport accidents involving nonmotor vehicle, nontraffic**

● **V89**   **Motor- or nonmotor-vehicle accident, type of vehicle unspecified**

> The appropriate 7th character is to be added to each code from category V89
>
> | | |
> |---|---|
> | A | initial encounter |
> | D | subsequent encounter |
> | S | sequela |

X● **V89.0**   **Person injured in unspecified motor-vehicle accident, nontraffic**
Motor-vehicle accident NOS, nontraffic

X● **V89.1**   **Person injured in unspecified nonmotor-vehicle accident, nontraffic**
Nonmotor-vehicle accident NOS (nontraffic)

X● **V89.2**   **Person injured in unspecified motor-vehicle accident, traffic**
Motor-vehicle accident [MVA] NOS
Road (traffic) accident [RTA] NOS

X● **V89.3**   **Person injured in unspecified nonmotor-vehicle accident, traffic**
Nonmotor-vehicle traffic accident NOS

X● **V89.9**   **Person injured in unspecified vehicle accident**
Collision NOS

WATER TRANSPORT ACCIDENTS (V90-V94)

● **V90**   **Drowning and submersion due to accident to watercraft**

> **Excludes1**   civilian water transport accident involving military watercraft (V94.81-)
> fall into water not from watercraft (W16.-)
> military watercraft accident in military or war operations (Y36.0-, Y37.0-)
> water-transport–related drowning or submersion without accident to watercraft (V92.-)

> The appropriate 7th character is to be added to each code from category V90
>
> | | |
> |---|---|
> | A | initial encounter |
> | D | subsequent encounter |
> | S | sequela |

● **V90.0**   **Drowning and submersion due to watercraft overturning**

X● **V90.00**   **Drowning and submersion due to merchant ship overturning**

X● **V90.01**   **Drowning and submersion due to passenger ship overturning**
Drowning and submersion due to ferry-boat overturning
Drowning and submersion due to liner overturning

X● **V90.02**   **Drowning and submersion due to fishing boat overturning**

X● **V90.03**   **Drowning and submersion due to other powered watercraft overturning**
Drowning and submersion due to hovercraft (on open water) overturning
Drowning and submersion due to jet ski overturning

X● **V90.04**   **Drowning and submersion due to sailboat overturning**

X● **V90.05**   **Drowning and submersion due to canoe or kayak overturning**

X● **V90.06**   **Drowning and submersion due to (nonpowered) inflatable craft overturning**

X● **V90.08**   **Drowning and submersion due to other unpowered watercraft overturning**
Drowning and submersion due to windsurfer overturning

X● **V90.09**   **Drowning and submersion due to unspecified watercraft overturning**
Drowning and submersion due to boat NOS overturning
Drowning and submersion due to ship NOS overturning
Drowning and submersion due to watercraft NOS overturning

● **V90.1**   **Drowning and submersion due to watercraft sinking**

X● **V90.10**   **Drowning and submersion due to merchant ship sinking**

X● **V90.11**   **Drowning and submersion due to passenger ship sinking**
Drowning and submersion due to ferry-boat sinking
Drowning and submersion due to liner sinking

X● **V90.12**   **Drowning and submersion due to fishing boat sinking**

X● **V90.13**   **Drowning and submersion due to other powered watercraft sinking**
Drowning and submersion due to hovercraft (on open water) sinking
Drowning and submersion due to jet ski sinking

X● **V90.14**   **Drowning and submersion due to sailboat sinking**

X● **V90.15**   **Drowning and submersion due to canoe or kayak sinking**

X● **V90.16**   **Drowning and submersion due to (nonpowered) inflatable craft sinking**

X● **V90.18**   **Drowning and submersion due to other unpowered watercraft sinking**

X● **V90.19**   **Drowning and submersion due to unspecified watercraft sinking**
Drowning and submersion due to boat NOS sinking
Drowning and submersion due to ship NOS sinking
Drowning and submersion due to watercraft NOS sinking

● **V90.2**   **Drowning and submersion due to falling or jumping from burning watercraft**

X● **V90.20**   **Drowning and submersion due to falling or jumping from burning merchant ship**

X● **V90.21**   **Drowning and submersion due to falling or jumping from burning passenger ship**
Drowning and submersion due to falling or jumping from burning ferry-boat
Drowning and submersion due to falling or jumping from burning liner

X● **V90.22**   **Drowning and submersion due to falling or jumping from burning fishing boat**

X● **V90.23**   **Drowning and submersion due to falling or jumping from other burning powered watercraft**
Drowning and submersion due to falling and jumping from burning hovercraft (on open water)
Drowning and submersion due to falling and jumping from burning jet ski

X● **V90.24**   **Drowning and submersion due to falling or jumping from burning sailboat**

▶ New   ⇒ Revised   ~~deleted~~ Deleted   Excludes 1   Excludes 2   Includes   Use additional   Code first   Code also   Key words

OGCR Official Guidelines   ● Unacceptable Principal Diagnosis   X Assign placeholder X   ● Use Additional Character(s)   ▶ Manifestation Code   **Coding Clinic**

X● **V90.25**   **Drowning and submersion due to falling or jumping from burning canoe or kayak**

X● **V90.26**   **Drowning and submersion due to falling or jumping from burning (nonpowered) inflatable craft**

X● **V90.27**   **Drowning and submersion due to falling or jumping from burning water-skis**

X● **V90.28**   **Drowning and submersion due to falling or jumping from other burning unpowered watercraft**
Drowning and submersion due to falling and jumping from burning surf-board
Drowning and submersion due to falling and jumping from burning windsurfer

X● **V90.29**   **Drowning and submersion due to falling or jumping from unspecified burning watercraft**
Drowning and submersion due to falling or jumping from burning boat NOS
Drowning and submersion due to falling or jumping from burning ship NOS
Drowning and submersion due to falling or jumping from burning watercraft NOS

● **V90.3**   **Drowning and submersion due to falling or jumping from crushed watercraft**

X● **V90.30**   **Drowning and submersion due to falling or jumping from crushed merchant ship**

X● **V90.31**   **Drowning and submersion due to falling or jumping from crushed passenger ship**
Drowning and submersion due to falling and jumping from crushed ferry-boat
Drowning and submersion due to falling and jumping from crushed liner

X● **V90.32**   **Drowning and submersion due to falling or jumping from crushed fishing boat**

X● **V90.33**   **Drowning and submersion due to falling or jumping from other crushed powered watercraft**
Drowning and submersion due to falling and jumping from crushed hovercraft
Drowning and submersion due to falling and jumping from crushed jet ski

X● **V90.34**   **Drowning and submersion due to falling or jumping from crushed sailboat**

X● **V90.35**   **Drowning and submersion due to falling or jumping from crushed canoe or kayak**

X● **V90.36**   **Drowning and submersion due to falling or jumping from crushed (nonpowered) inflatable craft**

X● **V90.37**   **Drowning and submersion due to falling or jumping from crushed water-skis**

X● **V90.38**   **Drowning and submersion due to falling or jumping from other crushed unpowered watercraft**
Drowning and submersion due to falling and jumping from crushed surf-board
Drowning and submersion due to falling and jumping from crushed windsurfer

X● **V90.39**   **Drowning and submersion due to falling or jumping from crushed unspecified watercraft**
Drowning and submersion due to falling and jumping from crushed boat NOS
Drowning and submersion due to falling and jumping from crushed ship NOS
Drowning and submersion due to falling and jumping from crushed watercraft NOS

● **V90.8**   **Drowning and submersion due to other accident to watercraft**

X● **V90.80**   **Drowning and submersion due to other accident to merchant ship**

X● **V90.81**   **Drowning and submersion due to other accident to passenger ship**
Drowning and submersion due to other accident to ferry-boat
Drowning and submersion due to other accident to liner

X● **V90.82**   **Drowning and submersion due to other accident to fishing boat**

X● **V90.83**   **Drowning and submersion due to other accident to other powered watercraft**
Drowning and submersion due to other accident to hovercraft (on open water)
Drowning and submersion due to other accident to jet ski

X● **V90.84**   **Drowning and submersion due to other accident to sailboat**

X● **V90.85**   **Drowning and submersion due to other accident to canoe or kayak**

X● **V90.86**   **Drowning and submersion due to other accident to (nonpowered) inflatable craft**

X● **V90.87**   **Drowning and submersion due to other accident to water-skis**

X● **V90.88**   **Drowning and submersion due to other accident to other unpowered watercraft**
Drowning and submersion due to other accident to surf-board
Drowning and submersion due to other accident to windsurfer

X● **V90.89**   **Drowning and submersion due to other accident to unspecified watercraft**
Drowning and submersion due to other accident to boat NOS
Drowning and submersion due to other accident to ship NOS
Drowning and submersion due to other accident to watercraft NOS

● **V91**   **Other injury due to accident to watercraft**

Includes   any injury except drowning and submersion as a result of an accident to watercraft

Excludes1   civilian water transport accident involving military watercraft (V94.81-)
military watercraft accident in military or war operations (Y36, Y37.-)

Excludes2   drowning and submersion due to accident to watercraft (V90.-)

The appropriate 7th character is to be added to each code from category V91

A	initial encounter
D	subsequent encounter
S	sequela

● **V91.0**   **Burn due to watercraft on fire**

Excludes1   burn from localized fire or explosion on board ship without accident to watercraft (V93.-)

X● **V91.00**   **Burn due to merchant ship on fire**

X● **V91.01**   **Burn due to passenger ship on fire**
Burn due to ferry-boat on fire
Burn due to liner on fire

X● **V91.02**   **Burn due to fishing boat on fire**

X● **V91.03**   **Burn due to other powered watercraft on fire**
Burn due to hovercraft (on open water) on fire
Burn due to jet ski on fire

X● **V91.04**   **Burn due to sailboat on fire**

X● **V91.05**   **Burn due to canoe or kayak on fire**

X● **V91.06**   **Burn due to (nonpowered) inflatable craft on fire**

X● **V91.07**   **Burn due to water-skis on fire**

X● **V91.08**   **Burn due to other unpowered watercraft on fire**

X● **V91.09**   **Burn due to unspecified watercraft on fire**
Burn due to boat NOS on fire
Burn due to ship NOS on fire
Burn due to watercraft NOS on fire

CHAPTER 20 (V01-Y99)

CHAPTER 20 (V01-Y99)

● **V91.1**   **Crushed between watercraft and other watercraft or other object due to collision**

Crushed by lifeboat after abandoning ship in a collision

Note: Select the specified type of watercraft that the victim was on at the time of the collision.

X ● **V91.10**   **Crushed between merchant ship and other watercraft or other object due to collision**

X ● **V91.11**   **Crushed between passenger ship and other watercraft or other object due to collision**

Crushed between ferry-boat and other watercraft or other object due to collision

Crushed between liner and other watercraft or other object due to collision

X ● **V91.12**   **Crushed between fishing boat and other watercraft or other object due to collision**

X ● **V91.13**   **Crushed between other powered watercraft and other watercraft or other object due to collision**

Crushed between hovercraft (on open water) and other watercraft or other object due to collision

Crushed between jet ski and other watercraft or other object due to collision

X ● **V91.14**   **Crushed between sailboat and other watercraft or other object due to collision**

X ● **V91.15**   **Crushed between canoe or kayak and other watercraft or other object due to collision**

X ● **V91.16**   **Crushed between (nonpowered) inflatable craft and other watercraft or other object due to collision**

X ● **V91.18**   **Crushed between other unpowered watercraft and other watercraft or other object due to collision**

Crushed between surfboard and other watercraft or other object due to collision

Crushed between windsurfer and other watercraft or other object due to collision

X ● **V91.19**   **Crushed between unspecified watercraft and other watercraft or other object due to collision**

Crushed between boat NOS and other watercraft or other object due to collision

Crushed between ship NOS and other watercraft or other object due to collision

Crushed between watercraft NOS and other watercraft or other object due to collision

● **V91.2**   **Fall due to collision between watercraft and other watercraft or other object**

Fall while remaining on watercraft after collision

Note: Select the specified type of watercraft that the victim was on at the time of the collision.

Excludes1   crushed between watercraft and other watercraft and other object due to collision (V91.1-)

drowning and submersion due to falling from crushed watercraft (V90.3-)

X ● **V91.20**   **Fall due to collision between merchant ship and other watercraft or other object**

X ● **V91.21**   **Fall due to collision between passenger ship and other watercraft or other object**

Fall due to collision between ferry-boat and other watercraft or other object

Fall due to collision between liner and other watercraft or other object

X ● **V91.22**   **Fall due to collision between fishing boat and other watercraft or other object**

X ● **V91.23**   **Fall due to collision between other powered watercraft and other watercraft or other object**

Fall due to collision between hovercraft (on open water) and other watercraft or other object

Fall due to collision between jet ski and other watercraft or other object

X ● **V91.24**   **Fall due to collision between sailboat and other watercraft or other object**

X ● **V91.25**   **Fall due to collision between canoe or kayak and other watercraft or other object**

X ● **V91.26**   **Fall due to collision between (nonpowered) inflatable craft and other watercraft or other object**

X ● **V91.29**   **Fall due to collision between unspecified watercraft and other watercraft or other object**

Fall due to collision between boat NOS and other watercraft or other object

Fall due to collision between ship NOS and other watercraft or other object

Fall due to collision between watercraft NOS and other watercraft or other object

● **V91.3**   **Hit or struck by falling object due to accident to watercraft**

Hit or struck by falling object (part of damaged watercraft or other object) after falling or jumping from damaged watercraft

Excludes2   drowning or submersion due to fall or jumping from damaged watercraft (V90.2-, V90.3-)

X ● **V91.30**   **Hit or struck by falling object due to accident to merchant ship**

X ● **V91.31**   **Hit or struck by falling object due to accident to passenger ship**

Hit or struck by falling object due to accident to ferry-boat

Hit or struck by falling object due to accident to liner

X ● **V91.32**   **Hit or struck by falling object due to accident to fishing boat**

X ● **V91.33**   **Hit or struck by falling object due to accident to other powered watercraft**

Hit or struck by falling object due to accident to hovercraft (on open water)

Hit or struck by falling object due to accident to jet ski

X ● **V91.34**   **Hit or struck by falling object due to accident to sailboat**

X ● **V91.35**   **Hit or struck by falling object due to accident to canoe or kayak**

X ● **V91.36**   **Hit or struck by falling object due to accident to (nonpowered) inflatable craft**

X ● **V91.37**   **Hit or struck by falling object due to accident to water-skis**

Hit by water-skis after jumping off of waterskis

X ● **V91.38**   **Hit or struck by falling object due to accident to other unpowered watercraft**

Hit or struck by surf-board after falling off damaged surf-board

Hit or struck by object after falling off damaged windsurfer

X ● **V91.39**   **Hit or struck by falling object due to accident to unspecified watercraft**

Hit or struck by falling object due to accident to boat NOS

Hit or struck by falling object due to accident to ship NOS

Hit or struck by falling object due to accident to watercraft NOS

▶ New   ⇒ Revised   ~~deleted~~ Deleted   Excludes 1   Excludes 2   Includes   Use additional   Code first   Code also   Key words

OGCR Official Guidelines   ● Unacceptable Principal Diagnosis   X Assign placeholder X   ● Use Additional Character(s)   ▌ Manifestation Code   **Coding Clinic**

X● **V91.8   Other injury due to other accident to watercraft**

X● **V91.80   Other injury due to other accident to merchant ship**

X● **V91.81   Other injury due to other accident to passenger ship**
  Other injury due to other accident to ferry-boat
  Other injury due to other accident to liner

X● **V91.82   Other injury due to other accident to fishing boat**

X● **V91.83   Other injury due to other accident to other powered watercraft**
  Other injury due to other accident to hovercraft (on open water)
  Other injury due to other accident to jet ski

X● **V91.84   Other injury due to other accident to sailboat**

X● **V91.85   Other injury due to other accident to canoe or kayak**

X● **V91.86   Other injury due to other accident to (nonpowered) inflatable craft**

X● **V91.87   Other injury due to other accident to water-skis**

X● **V91.88   Other injury due to other accident to other unpowered watercraft**
  Other injury due to other accident to surf-board
  Other injury due to other accident to windsurfer

X● **V91.89   Other injury due to other accident to unspecified watercraft**
  Other injury due to other accident to boat NOS
  Other injury due to other accident to ship NOS
  Other injury due to other accident to watercraft NOS

● **V92   Drowning and submersion due to accident on board watercraft, without accident to watercraft**

Excludes1	civilian water transport accident involving military watercraft (V94.81-)
	drowning or submersion due to accident to watercraft (V90-V91)
	drowning or submersion of diver who voluntarily jumps from boat not involved in an accident (W16.711, W16.721)
	fall into water without watercraft (W16.-)
	military watercraft accident in military or war operations (Y36, Y37)

The appropriate 7th character is to be added to each code from category V92

A	initial encounter
D	subsequent encounter
S	sequela

● **V92.0   Drowning and submersion due to fall off watercraft**
  Drowning and submersion due to fall from gangplank of watercraft
  Drowning and submersion due to fall overboard watercraft

Excludes2	hitting head on object or bottom of body of water due to fall from watercraft (V94.0-)

X● **V92.00   Drowning and submersion due to fall off merchant ship**

X● **V92.01   Drowning and submersion due to fall off passenger ship**
  Drowning and submersion due to fall off ferry-boat
  Drowning and submersion due to fall off liner

X● **V92.02   Drowning and submersion due to fall off fishing boat**

X● **V92.03   Drowning and submersion due to fall off other powered watercraft**
  Drowning and submersion due to fall off hovercraft (on open water)
  Drowning and submersion due to fall off jet ski

X● **V92.04   Drowning and submersion due to fall off sailboat**

X● **V92.05   Drowning and submersion due to fall off canoe or kayak**

X● **V92.06   Drowning and submersion due to fall off (nonpowered) inflatable craft**

X● **V92.07   Drowning and submersion due to fall off water-skis**

Excludes1	drowning and submersion due to falling off burning water-skis (V90.27)
	drowning and submersion due to falling off crushed water-skis (V90.37)
	hit by boat while water-skiing NOS (V94.X)

X● **V92.08   Drowning and submersion due to fall off other unpowered watercraft**
  Drowning and submersion due to fall off surf-board
  Drowning and submersion due to fall off windsurfer

Excludes1	drowning and submersion due to fall off burning unpowered watercraft (V90.28)
	drowning and submersion due to fall off crushed unpowered watercraft (V90.38)
	drowning and submersion due to fall off damaged unpowered watercraft (V90.88)
	drowning and submersion due to rider of nonpowered watercraft being hit by other watercraft (V94.-)
	other injury due to rider of nonpowered watercraft being hit by other watercraft (V94.-)

X● **V92.09   Drowning and submersion due to fall off unspecified watercraft**
  Drowning and submersion due to fall off boat NOS
  Drowning and submersion due to fall off ship
  Drowning and submersion due to fall off watercraft NOS

● **V92.1   Drowning and submersion due to being thrown overboard by motion of watercraft**

Excludes1	drowning and submersion due to fall off surf-board (V92.08)
	drowning and submersion due to fall off water-skis (V92.07)
	drowning and submersion due to fall off windsurfer (V92.08)

X● **V92.10   Drowning and submersion due to being thrown overboard by motion of merchant ship**

X● **V92.11   Drowning and submersion due to being thrown overboard by motion of passenger ship**
  Drowning and submersion due to being thrown overboard by motion of ferry-boat
  Drowning and submersion due to being thrown overboard by motion of liner

CHAPTER 20 (V01-Y99)

X ● **V92.12** **Drowning and submersion due to being thrown overboard by motion of fishing boat**

X ● **V92.13** **Drowning and submersion due to being thrown overboard by motion of other powered watercraft**

Drowning and submersion due to being thrown overboard by motion of hovercraft

X ● **V92.14** **Drowning and submersion due to being thrown overboard by motion of sailboat**

X ● **V92.15** **Drowning and submersion due to being thrown overboard by motion of canoe or kayak**

X ● **V92.16** **Drowning and submersion due to being thrown overboard by motion of (nonpowered) inflatable craft**

X ● **V92.19** **Drowning and submersion due to being thrown overboard by motion of unspecified watercraft**

Drowning and submersion due to being thrown overboard by motion of boat NOS

Drowning and submersion due to being thrown overboard by motion of ship NOS

Drowning and submersion due to being thrown overboard by motion of watercraft NOS

● **V92.2** **Drowning and submersion due to being washed overboard from watercraft**

Code first any associated cataclysm (X37.0-)

X ● **V92.20** **Drowning and submersion due to being washed overboard from merchant ship**

X ● **V92.21** **Drowning and submersion due to being washed overboard from passenger ship**

Drowning and submersion due to being washed overboard from ferry-boat

Drowning and submersion due to being washed overboard from liner

X ● **V92.22** **Drowning and submersion due to being washed overboard from fishing boat**

X ● **V92.23** **Drowning and submersion due to being washed overboard from other powered watercraft**

Drowning and submersion due to being washed overboard from hovercraft (on open water)

Drowning and submersion due to being washed overboard from jet ski

X ● **V92.24** **Drowning and submersion due to being washed overboard from sailboat**

X ● **V92.25** **Drowning and submersion due to being washed overboard from canoe or kayak**

X ● **V92.26** **Drowning and submersion due to being washed overboard from (nonpowered) inflatable craft**

X ● **V92.27** **Drowning and submersion due to being washed overboard from water-skis**

Excludes1   drowning and submersion due to fall off water-skis (V92.07)

X ● **V92.28** **Drowning and submersion due to being washed overboard from other unpowered watercraft**

Drowning and submersion due to being washed overboard from surf-board

Drowning and submersion due to being washed overboard from windsurfer

X ● **V92.29** **Drowning and submersion due to being washed overboard from unspecified watercraft**

Drowning and submersion due to being washed overboard from boat NOS

Drowning and submersion due to being washed overboard from ship NOS

Drowning and submersion due to being washed overboard from watercraft NOS

● **V93** **Other injury due to accident on board watercraft, without accident to watercraft**

Excludes1   civilian water transport accident involving military watercraft (V94.81-)

other injury due to accident to watercraft (V91.-)

military watercraft accident in military or war operations (Y36, Y37.-)

Excludes2   drowning and submersion due to accident on board watercraft, without accident to watercraft (V92.-)

The appropriate 7th character is to be added to each code from category V93

> A   initial encounter
> D   subsequent encounter
> S   sequela

● **V93.0** **Burn due to localized fire on board watercraft**

Excludes1   burn due to watercraft on fire (V91.0-)

X ● **V93.00** **Burn due to localized fire on board merchant vessel**

X ● **V93.01** **Burn due to localized fire on board passenger vessel**

Burn due to localized fire on board ferry-boat

Burn due to localized fire on board liner

X ● **V93.02** **Burn due to localized fire on board fishing boat**

X ● **V93.03** **Burn due to localized fire on board other powered watercraft**

Burn due to localized fire on board hovercraft

Burn due to localized fire on board jet ski

X ● **V93.04** **Burn due to localized fire on board sailboat**

X ● **V93.09** **Burn due to localized fire on board unspecified watercraft**

Burn due to localized fire on board boat NOS

Burn due to localized fire on board ship NOS

Burn due to localized fire on board watercraft NOS

● **V93.1** **Other burn on board watercraft**

Burn due to source other than fire on board watercraft

Excludes1   burn due to watercraft on fire (V91.0-)

X ● **V93.10** **Other burn on board merchant vessel**

X ● **V93.11** **Other burn on board passenger vessel**

Other burn on board ferry-boat

Other burn on board liner

X ● **V93.12** **Other burn on board fishing boat**

X ● **V93.13** **Other burn on board other powered watercraft**

Other burn on board hovercraft

Other burn on board jet ski

X ● **V93.14** **Other burn on board sailboat**

X ● **V93.19** **Other burn on board unspecified watercraft**

Other burn on board boat NOS

Other burn on board ship NOS

Other burn on board watercraft NOS

● **V93.2** **Heat exposure on board watercraft**

Excludes1   exposure to man-made heat not aboard watercraft (W92)

exposure to natural heat while on board watercraft (X30)

exposure to sunlight while on board watercraft (X32)

Excludes2   burn due to fire on board watercraft (V93.0-)

X ● **V93.20** **Heat exposure on board merchant ship**

X ● **V93.21** **Heat exposure on board passenger ship**

Heat exposure on board ferry-boat

Heat exposure on board liner

X ● **V93.22** **Heat exposure on board fishing boat**

X ● **V93.23** **Heat exposure on board other powered watercraft**

Heat exposure on board hovercraft

X ● **V93.24** **Heat exposure on board sailboat**

X ● **V93.29** **Heat exposure on board unspecified watercraft**

Heat exposure on board boat NOS

Heat exposure on board ship NOS

Heat exposure on board watercraft NOS

▶ New   ⇒ Revised   ~~deleted~~ Deleted   Excludes 1   Excludes 2   Includes   Use additional   Code first   Code also   Key words

OGCR Official Guidelines   ● Unacceptable Principal Diagnosis   X Assign placeholder X   ● Use Additional Character(s)   ▌ Manifestation Code   **Coding Clinic**

● **V93.3 Fall on board watercraft**
>
> **Excludes1**   fall due to collision of watercraft (V91.2-)

X● **V93.30 Fall on board merchant ship**

X● **V93.31 Fall on board passenger ship**
> Fall on board ferry-boat
> Fall on board liner

X● **V93.32 Fall on board fishing boat**

X● **V93.33 Fall on board other powered watercraft**
> Fall on board hovercraft (on open water)
> Fall on board jet ski

X● **V93.34 Fall on board sailboat**

X● **V93.35 Fall on board canoe or kayak**

X● **V93.36 Fall on board (nonpowered) inflatable craft**

X● **V93.38 Fall on board other unpowered watercraft**

X● **V93.39 Fall on board unspecified watercraft**
> Fall on board boat NOS
> Fall on board ship NOS
> Fall on board watercraft NOS

● **V93.4 Struck by falling object on board watercraft**
> Hit by falling object on board watercraft
>
> **Excludes1**   struck by falling object due to accident to watercraft (V91.3)

X● **V93.40 Struck by falling object on merchant ship**

X● **V93.41 Struck by falling object on passenger ship**
> Struck by falling object on ferry-boat
> Struck by falling object on liner

X● **V93.42 Struck by falling object on fishing boat**

X● **V93.43 Struck by falling object on other powered watercraft**
> Struck by falling object on hovercraft

X● **V93.44 Struck by falling object on sailboat**

X● **V93.48 Struck by falling object on other unpowered watercraft**

X● **V93.49 Struck by falling object on unspecified watercraft**

● **V93.5 Explosion on board watercraft**
> Boiler explosion on steamship
>
> **Excludes2**   fire on board watercraft (V93.0-)

X● **V93.50 Explosion on board merchant ship**

X● **V93.51 Explosion on board passenger ship**
> Explosion on board ferry-boat
> Explosion on board liner

X● **V93.52 Explosion on board fishing boat**

X● **V93.53 Explosion on board other powered watercraft**
> Explosion on board hovercraft
> Explosion on board jet ski

X● **V93.54 Explosion on board sailboat**

X● **V93.59 Explosion on board unspecified watercraft**
> Explosion on board boat NOS
> Explosion on board ship NOS
> Explosion on board watercraft NOS

● **V93.6 Machinery accident on board watercraft**
>
> **Excludes1**   machinery explosion on board watercraft (V93.4-)
>   machinery fire on board watercraft (V93.0-)

X● **V93.60 Machinery accident on board merchant ship**

X● **V93.61 Machinery accident on board passenger ship**
> Machinery accident on board ferry-boat
> Machinery accident on board liner

X● **V93.62 Machinery accident on board fishing boat**

X● **V93.63 Machinery accident on board other powered watercraft**
> Machinery accident on board hovercraft

X● **V93.64 Machinery accident on board sailboat**

X● **V93.69 Machinery accident on board unspecified watercraft**
> Machinery accident on board boat NOS
> Machinery accident on board ship NOS
> Machinery accident on board watercraft NOS

● **V93.8 Other injury due to other accident on board watercraft**
> Accidental poisoning by gases or fumes on watercraft

X● **V93.80 Other injury due to other accident on board merchant ship**

X● **V93.81 Other injury due to other accident on board passenger ship**
> Other injury due to other accident on board ferry-boat
> Other injury due to other accident on board liner

X● **V93.82 Other injury due to other accident on board fishing boat**

X● **V93.83 Other injury due to other accident on board other powered watercraft**
> Other injury due to other accident on board hovercraft
> Other injury due to other accident on board jet ski

X● **V93.84 Other injury due to other accident on board sailboat**

X● **V93.85 Other injury due to other accident on board canoe or kayak**

X● **V93.86 Other injury due to other accident on board (nonpowered) inflatable craft**

X● **V93.87 Other injury due to other accident on board water-skis**
> Hit or struck by object while waterskiing

X● **V93.88 Other injury due to other accident on board other unpowered watercraft**
> Hit or struck by object while surfing
> Hit or struck by object while on board windsurfer

X● **V93.89 Other injury due to other accident on board unspecified watercraft**
> Other injury due to other accident on board boat NOS
> Other injury due to other accident on board ship NOS
> Other injury due to other accident on board watercraft NOS

● **V94 Other and unspecified water transport accidents**
>
> **Excludes1**   military watercraft accidents in military or war operations (Y36, Y37)

The appropriate 7th character is to be added to each code from category V94

> | | |
> |---|---|
> | A | initial encounter |
> | D | subsequent encounter |
> | S | sequela |

X● **V94.0 Hitting object or bottom of body of water due to fall from watercraft**
>
> **Excludes2**   drowning and submersion due to fall from watercraft (V92.0-)

● **V94.1 Bather struck by watercraft**
> Swimmer hit by watercraft

X● **V94.11 Bather struck by powered watercraft**

X● **V94.12 Bather struck by nonpowered watercraft**

● **V94.2 Rider of nonpowered watercraft struck by other watercraft**

X● **V94.21 Rider of nonpowered watercraft struck by other nonpowered watercraft**
> Canoer hit by other nonpowered watercraft
> Surfer hit by other nonpowered watercraft
> Windsurfer hit by other nonpowered watercraft

X● **V94.22 Rider of nonpowered watercraft struck by powered watercraft**
> Canoer hit by motorboat
> Surfer hit by motorboat
> Windsurfer hit by motorboat

N Newborn Age: 0   **P** Pediatric Age: 0–17   **M** Maternity DX: 12–55   **A** Adult Age: 15–124   ♀ Females Only   ♂ Males Only

🔘 Complication\Comorbidity   🔘 Major C\C   (Ex) CC/MCC Exclusions   🔘 Hospital-Acquired Condition

1539

CHAPTER 20 (V01-Y99)

CHAPTER 20 (V01-Y99)

- ● **V94.3** **Injury to rider of (inflatable) watercraft being pulled behind other watercraft**
  - X● **V94.31** **Injury to rider of (inflatable) recreational watercraft being pulled behind other watercraft**
    Injury to rider of inner-tube pulled behind motor boat
  - X● **V94.32** **Injury to rider of non-recreational watercraft being pulled behind other watercraft**
    Injury to occupant of dingy being pulled behind boat or ship
    Injury to occupant of life-raft being pulled behind boat or ship
- X● **V94.4** **Injury to barefoot water-skier**
    Injury to person being pulled behind boat or ship
- ● **V94.8** **Other water transport accident**
  - ● **V94.81** **Water transport accident involving military watercraft**
    - ● **V94.810** **Civilian watercraft involved in water transport accident with military watercraft**
      Passenger on civilian watercraft injured due to accident with military watercraft
    - ● **V94.811** **Civilian in water injured by military watercraft**
    - ● **V94.818** **Other water transport accident involving military watercraft**
  - X● **V94.89** **Other water transport accident**
- X● **V94.9** **Unspecified water transport accident**
    Water transport accident NOS

AIR AND SPACE TRANSPORT ACCIDENTS (V95-V97)

Excludes1   military aircraft accidents in military or war operations (Y36, Y37)

- ● **V95** **Accident to powered aircraft causing injury to occupant**
  The appropriate 7th character is to be added to each code from category V95

A	initial encounter
D	subsequent encounter
S	sequela

  - ● **V95.0** **Helicopter accident injuring occupant**
    - X● **V95.00** **Unspecified helicopter accident injuring occupant**
    - X● **V95.01** **Helicopter crash injuring occupant**
    - X● **V95.02** **Forced landing of helicopter injuring occupant**
    - X● **V95.03** **Helicopter collision injuring occupant**
      Helicopter collision with any object, fixed, movable or moving
    - X● **V95.04** **Helicopter fire injuring occupant**
    - X● **V95.05** **Helicopter explosion injuring occupant**
    - X● **V95.09** **Other helicopter accident injuring occupant**
  - ● **V95.1** **Ultralight, microlight or powered-glider accident injuring occupant**
    - X● **V95.10** **Unspecified ultralight, microlight or powered-glider accident injuring occupant**
    - X● **V95.11** **Ultralight, microlight or powered-glider crash injuring occupant**
    - X● **V95.12** **Forced landing of ultralight, microlight or powered-glider injuring occupant**

- X● **V95.13** **Ultralight, microlight or powered-glider collision injuring occupant**
    Ultralight, microlight or powered-glider collision with any object, fixed, movable or moving
  - X● **V95.14** **Ultralight, microlight or powered-glider fire injuring occupant**
  - X● **V95.15** **Ultralight, microlight or powered-glider explosion injuring occupant**
  - X● **V95.19** **Other ultralight, microlight or powered-glider accident injuring occupant**
- ● **V95.2** **Other private fixed-wing aircraft accident injuring occupant**
  - X● **V95.20** **Unspecified accident to other private fixed-wing aircraft, injuring occupant**
  - X● **V95.21** **Other private fixed-wing aircraft crash injuring occupant**
  - X● **V95.22** **Forced landing of other private fixed-wing aircraft injuring occupant**
  - X● **V95.23** **Other private fixed-wing aircraft collision injuring occupant**
    Other private fixed-wing aircraft collision with any object, fixed, movable or moving
  - X● **V95.24** **Other private fixed-wing aircraft fire injuring occupant**
  - X● **V95.25** **Other private fixed-wing aircraft explosion injuring occupant**
  - X● **V95.29** **Other accident to other private fixed-wing aircraft injuring occupant**
- ● **V95.3** **Commercial fixed-wing aircraft accident injuring occupant**
  - X● **V95.30** **Unspecified accident to commercial fixed-wing aircraft injuring occupant**
  - X● **V95.31** **Commercial fixed-wing aircraft crash injuring occupant**
  - X● **V95.32** **Forced landing of commercial fixed-wing aircraft injuring occupant**
  - X● **V95.33** **Commercial fixed-wing aircraft collision injuring occupant**
    Commercial fixed-wing aircraft collision with any object, fixed, movable or moving
  - X● **V95.34** **Commercial fixed-wing aircraft fire injuring occupant**
  - X● **V95.35** **Commercial fixed-wing aircraft explosion injuring occupant**
  - X● **V95.39** **Other accident to commercial fixed-wing aircraft injuring occupant**
- ● **V95.4** **Spacecraft accident injuring occupant**
  - X● **V95.40** **Unspecified spacecraft accident injuring occupant**
  - X● **V95.41** **Spacecraft crash injuring occupant**
  - X● **V95.42** **Forced landing of spacecraft injuring occupant**
  - X● **V95.43** **Spacecraft collision injuring occupant**
    Spacecraft collision with any object, fixed, moveable or moving
  - X● **V95.44** **Spacecraft fire injuring occupant**
  - X● **V95.45** **Spacecraft explosion injuring occupant**
  - X● **V95.49** **Other spacecraft accident injuring occupant**
- X● **V95.8** **Other powered aircraft accidents injuring occupant**
- X● **V95.9** **Unspecified aircraft accident injuring occupant**
    Aircraft accident NOS
    Air transport accident NOS

▶ New   ⇒ Revised   ~~deleted~~ Deleted   Excludes 1   Excludes 2   Includes   Use additional   Code first   Code also   Key words

OGCR Official Guidelines   ● Unacceptable Principal Diagnosis   X Assign placeholder X   ● Use Additional Character(s)   ▶ Manifestation Code   **Coding Clinic**

● **V96**   **Accident to nonpowered aircraft causing injury to occupant**

The appropriate 7th character is to be added to each code from category V96

A	initial encounter
D	subsequent encounter
S	sequela

  ● **V96.0**   **Balloon** accident injuring occupant

    X● **V96.00**   **Unspecified** balloon accident injuring occupant

    X● **V96.01**   Balloon **crash** injuring occupant

    X● **V96.02**   **Forced landing** of balloon injuring occupant

    X● **V96.03**   Balloon **collision** injuring occupant

          Balloon collision with any object, fixed, moveable or moving

    X● **V96.04**   Balloon **fire** injuring occupant

    X● **V96.05**   Balloon **explosion** injuring occupant

    X● **V96.09**   **Other** balloon accident injuring occupant

  ● **V96.1**   **Hang-glider** accident injuring occupant

    X● **V96.10**   **Unspecified** hang-glider accident injuring occupant

    X● **V96.11**   Hang-glider **crash** injuring occupant

    X● **V96.12**   **Forced landing** of hang-glider injuring occupant

    X● **V96.13**   Hang-glider **collision** injuring occupant

          Hang-glider collision with any object, fixed, moveable or moving

    X● **V96.14**   Hang-glider **fire** injuring occupant

    X● **V96.15**   Hang-glider **explosion** injuring occupant

    X● **V96.19**   **Other** hang-glider accident injuring occupant

  ● **V96.2**   **Glider** (nonpowered) accident injuring occupant

    X● **V96.20**   **Unspecified** glider (nonpowered) accident injuring occupant

    X● **V96.21**   Glider (nonpowered) **crash** injuring occupant

    X● **V96.22**   **Forced landing** of glider (nonpowered) injuring occupant

    X● **V96.23**   Glider (nonpowered) **collision** injuring occupant

          Glider (nonpowered) collision with any object, fixed, moveable or moving

    X● **V96.24**   Glider (nonpowered) **fire** injuring occupant

    X● **V96.25**   Glider (nonpowered) **explosion** injuring occupant

    X● **V96.29**   **Other** glider (nonpowered) accident injuring occupant

  X● **V96.8**   **Other** nonpowered-aircraft accidents injuring occupant

        Kite carrying a person accident injuring occupant

  X● **V96.9**   **Unspecified** nonpowered-aircraft accident injuring occupant

        Nonpowered-aircraft accident NOS

● **V97**   **Other specified air transport accidents**

The appropriate 7th character is to be added to each code from category V97

A	initial encounter
D	subsequent encounter
S	sequela

  X● **V97.0**   **Occupant of aircraft injured in other specified air transport accidents**

        Fall in, on or from aircraft in air transport accident

    Excludes1   accident while boarding or alighting aircraft (V97.1)

  X● **V97.1**   **Person injured while boarding or alighting from aircraft**

● **V97.2**   **Parachutist accident**

  X● **V97.21**   **Parachutist entangled in object**

        Parachutist landing in tree

  X● **V97.22**   **Parachutist injured on landing**

  X● **V97.29**   **Other** parachutist accident

● **V97.3**   **Person on ground injured in air transport accident**

  X● **V97.31**   **Hit by object falling from aircraft**

        Hit by crashing aircraft

        Injured by aircraft hitting house

        Injured by aircraft hitting car

  X● **V97.32**   **Injured by rotating propeller**

  X● **V97.33**   **Sucked into jet engine**

  X● **V97.39**   **Other** injury to person on ground due to air transport accident

● **V97.8**   **Other air transport accidents, not elsewhere classified**

  Excludes1   aircraft accident NOS (V95.9)

        exposure to changes in air pressure during ascent or descent (W94.-)

  ● **V97.81**   **Air transport accident involving military aircraft**

    ● **V97.810**   **Civilian aircraft involved in air transport accident with military aircraft**

          Passenger in civilian aircraft injured due to accident with military aircraft

    ● **V97.811**   **Civilian injured by military aircraft**

    ● **V97.818**   **Other air transport accident involving military aircraft**

  X● **V97.89**   **Other air transport accidents, not elsewhere classified**

        Injury from machinery on aircraft

OTHER AND UNSPECIFIED TRANSPORT ACCIDENTS (V98-V99)

Excludes1   vehicle accident, type of vehicle unspecified (V89.-)

● **V98**   **Other specified transport accidents**

The appropriate 7th character is to be added to each code from category V98

A	initial encounter
D	subsequent encounter
S	sequela

  X● **V98.0**   **Accident to, on or involving cable-car, not on rails**

        Caught or dragged by cable-car, not on rails

        Fall or jump from cable-car, not on rails

        Object thrown from or in cable-car, not on rails

  X● **V98.1**   **Accident to, on or involving land-yacht**

  X● **V98.2**   **Accident to, on or involving ice yacht**

  X● **V98.3**   **Accident to, on or involving ski lift**

        Accident to, on or involving ski chair-lift

        Accident to, on or involving ski-lift with gondola

  X● **V98.8**   **Other specified transport accidents**

X● **V99**   **Unspecified transport accident**

The appropriate 7th character is to be added to code V99

A	initial encounter
D	subsequent encounter
S	sequela

OTHER EXTERNAL CAUSES OF ACCIDENTAL INJURY (W00-X58)

SLIPPING, TRIPPING, STUMBLING AND FALLS (W00-W19)

Excludes1   assault involving a fall (Y01-Y02)
      fall from animal (V80.-)
      fall (in) (from) machinery (in operation) (W28-W31)
      fall (in) (from) transport vehicle (V01-V99)
      intentional self-harm involving a fall (X80-X81)

Excludes2   at risk for fall (history of fall) Z91.81
      fall (in) (from) burning building (X00.-)
      ➡ fall into fire (X00-X04, X08)

● **W00   Fall due to ice and snow**

Includes   pedestrian on foot falling (slipping) on ice and snow

Excludes1   fall on (from) ice and snow involving pedestrian conveyance (V00.-)
      fall from stairs and steps not due to ice and snow (W10.-)

The appropriate 7th character is to be added to each code from category W00

A	initial encounter
D	subsequent encounter
S	sequela

X ● **W00.0   Fall on same level due to ice and snow**
      Coding Clinic: 2016, Q2, P5

X ● **W00.1   Fall from stairs and steps due to ice and snow**

X ● **W00.2   Other fall from one level to another due to ice and snow**

X ● **W00.9   Unspecified fall due to ice and snow**

● **W01   Fall on same level from slipping, tripping and stumbling**

Includes   fall on moving sidewalk

Excludes1   fall due to bumping (striking) against object (W18.0-)
      fall in shower or bathtub (W18.2-)
      fall on same level NOS (W18.30)
      fall on same level from slipping, tripping and stumbling due to ice or snow (W00.0)
      fall off or from toilet (W18.1-)
      slipping, tripping and stumbling NOS (W18.40)
      slipping, tripping and stumbling without falling (W18.4-)

The appropriate 7th character is to be added to each code from category W01

A	initial encounter
D	subsequent encounter
S	sequela

X ● **W01.0   Fall on same level from slipping, tripping and stumbling without subsequent striking against object**
      Falling over animal

● **W01.1   Fall on same level from slipping, tripping and stumbling with subsequent striking against object**

X ● **W01.10   Fall on same level from slipping, tripping and stumbling with subsequent striking against unspecified object**

● **W01.11   Fall on same level from slipping, tripping and stumbling with subsequent striking against sharp object**

● **W01.110   Fall on same level from slipping, tripping and stumbling with subsequent striking against sharp glass**

● **W01.111   Fall on same level from slipping, tripping and stumbling with subsequent striking against power tool or machine**

● **W01.118   Fall on same level from slipping, tripping and stumbling with subsequent striking against other sharp object**

● **W01.119   Fall on same level from slipping, tripping and stumbling with subsequent striking against unspecified sharp object**

● **W01.19   Fall on same level from slipping, tripping and stumbling with subsequent striking against other object**

● **W01.190   Fall on same level from slipping, tripping and stumbling with subsequent striking against furniture**

● **W01.198   Fall on same level from slipping, tripping and stumbling with subsequent striking against other object**

X ● **W03   Other fall on same level due to collision with another person**
      Fall due to non-transport collision with other person

Excludes1   collision with another person without fall (W51)
      crushed or pushed by a crowd or human stampede (W52)
      fall involving pedestrian conveyance (V00-V09)
      fall due to ice or snow (W00)
      fall on same level NOS (W18.30)

The appropriate 7th character is to be added to code W03

A	initial encounter
D	subsequent encounter
S	sequela

Coding Clinic: 2015, Q1, P9-10; 2012, Q4, P108

X ● **W04   Fall while being carried or supported by other persons**
      Accidentally dropped while being carried

The appropriate 7th character is to be added to code W04

A	initial encounter
D	subsequent encounter
S	sequel

● **W05   Fall from non-moving wheelchair, nonmotorized scooter and motorized mobility scooter**

Excludes1   fall from moving wheelchair (powered) (V00.811)
      fall from moving motorized mobility scooter (V00.831)
      fall from nonmotorized scooter (V00.141)

The appropriate 7th character is to be added to each code from category W05

A	initial encounter
D	subsequent encounter
S	sequela

X ● **W05.0   Fall from non-moving wheelchair**

X ● **W05.1   Fall from non-moving nonmotorized scooter**

X ● **W05.2   Fall from non-moving motorized mobility scooter**

X ● **W06   Fall from bed**

The appropriate 7th character is to be added to code W06

A	initial encounter
D	subsequent encounter
S	sequela

X ● **W07   Fall from chair**

The appropriate 7th character is to be added to code W07

A	initial encounter
D	subsequent encounter
S	sequela

▶ New   ⟴ Revised   ~~deleted~~ Deleted   Excludes 1   Excludes 2   Includes   Use additional   Code first   Code also   Key words

OGCR Official Guidelines   ● Unacceptable Principal Diagnosis   X Assign placeholder X   ● Use Additional Character(s)   ▌ Manifestation Code   **Coding Clinic**

X ● **W08**   **Fall from other furniture**

> The appropriate 7th character is to be added to code W08

> | | |
> |---|---|
> | A | initial encounter |
> | D | subsequent encounter |
> | S | sequela |

● **W09**   **Fall on and from playground equipment**

> **Excludes1**   fall involving recreational machinery (W31)

> The appropriate 7th character is to be added to each code from category W09

> | | |
> |---|---|
> | A | initial encounter |
> | D | subsequent encounter |
> | S | sequela |

X ● **W09.0**   Fall on or from playground slide

X ● **W09.1**   Fall from playground swing

X ● **W09.2**   Fall on or from jungle gym

X ● **W09.8**   Fall on or from other playground equipment

● **W10**   **Fall on and from stairs and steps**

> **Excludes1**   fall from stairs and steps due to ice and snow (W00.1)

> The appropriate 7th character is to be added to each code from category W10

> | | |
> |---|---|
> | A | initial encounter |
> | D | subsequent encounter |
> | S | sequela |

X ● **W10.0**   Fall (on) (from) escalator

X ● **W10.1**   Fall (on) (from) sidewalk curb

X ● **W10.2**   Fall (on) (from) incline
> Fall (on) (from) ramp

X ● **W10.8**   Fall (on) (from) other stairs and steps

X ● **W10.9**   Fall (on) (from) unspecified stairs and steps

X ● **W11**   **Fall on and from ladder**

> The appropriate 7th character is to be added to code W11

> | | |
> |---|---|
> | A | initial encounter |
> | D | subsequent encounter |
> | S | sequela |

X ● **W12**   **Fall on and from scaffolding**

> The appropriate 7th character is to be added to code W12

> | | |
> |---|---|
> | A | initial encounter |
> | D | subsequent encounter |
> | S | sequela |

● **W13**   **Fall from, out of or through building or structure**

> The appropriate 7th character is to be added to each code from category W13

> | | |
> |---|---|
> | A | initial encounter |
> | D | subsequent encounter |
> | S | sequela |

X ● **W13.0**   Fall from, out of or through balcony
> Fall from, out of or through railing

X ● **W13.1**   Fall from, out of or through bridge

X ● **W13.2**   Fall from, out of or through roof

X ● **W13.3**   Fall through floor

X ● **W13.4**   Fall from, out of or through window

> **Excludes2**   fall with subsequent striking against sharp glass (W01.110)

X ● **W13.8**   Fall from, out of or through other building or structure
> Fall from, out of or through viaduct
> Fall from, out of or through wall
> Fall from, out of or through flag-pole

X ● **W13.9**   Fall from, out of or through building, not otherwise specified

> **Excludes1**   collapse of a building or structure (W20.-)
> fall or jump from burning building or structure (X00.-)

X ● **W14**   **Fall from tree**

> The appropriate 7th character is to be added to code W14

> | | |
> |---|---|
> | A | initial encounter |
> | D | subsequent encounter |
> | S | sequela |

X ● **W15**   **Fall from cliff**

> The appropriate 7th character is to be added to code W15

> | | |
> |---|---|
> | A | initial encounter |
> | D | subsequent encounter |
> | S | sequela |

● **W16**   **Fall, jump or diving into water**

> **Excludes1**   accidental non-watercraft drowning and submersion not involving fall (W65-W74)
> effects of air pressure from diving (W94.-)
> fall into water from watercraft (V90-V94)
> hitting an object or against bottom when falling from watercraft (V94.0)

> **Excludes2**   striking or hitting diving board (W21.4)

> The appropriate 7th character is to be added to each code from category W16

> | | |
> |---|---|
> | A | initial encounter |
> | D | subsequent encounter |
> | S | sequela |

● **W16.0**   **Fall into swimming pool**
> Fall into swimming pool NOS

> **Excludes1**   fall into empty swimming pool (W17.3)

● **W16.01**   **Fall into swimming pool striking water surface**

● **W16.011**   **Fall into swimming pool striking water surface causing drowning and submersion**

> **Excludes1**   drowning and submersion while in swimming pool without fall (W67)

● **W16.012**   **Fall into swimming pool striking water surface causing other injury**

● W16.02 **Fall into swimming pool striking bottom**
  ● W16.021 **Fall into swimming pool striking bottom causing drowning and submersion**
    Excludes1 drowning and submersion while in swimming pool without fall (W67)
  ● W16.022 **Fall into swimming pool striking bottom causing other injury**
● W16.03 **Fall into swimming pool striking wall**
  ● W16.031 **Fall into swimming pool striking wall causing drowning and submersion**
    Excludes1 drowning and submersion while in swimming pool without fall (W67)
  ● W16.032 **Fall into swimming pool striking wall causing other injury**
● W16.1 **Fall into natural body of water**
  Fall into lake
  Fall into open sea
  Fall into river
  Fall into stream
  ● W16.11 **Fall into natural body of water striking water surface**
    ● W16.111 **Fall into natural body of water striking water surface causing drowning and submersion**
      Excludes1 drowning and submersion while in natural body of water without fall (W69)
    ● W16.112 **Fall into natural body of water striking water surface causing other injury**
  ● W16.12 **Fall into natural body of water striking bottom**
    ● W16.121 **Fall into natural body of water striking bottom causing drowning and submersion**
      Excludes1 drowning and submersion while in natural body of water without fall (W69)
    ● W16.122 **Fall into natural body of water striking bottom causing other injury**
  ● W16.13 **Fall into natural body of water striking side**
    ● W16.131 **Fall into natural body of water striking side causing drowning and submersion**
      Excludes1 drowning and submersion while in natural body of water without fall (W69)
    ● W16.132 **Fall into natural body of water striking side causing other injury**
● W16.2 **Fall in (into) filled bathtub or bucket of water**
  ● W16.21 **Fall in (into) filled bathtub**
    Excludes1 fall into empty bathtub (W18.2)
    ● W16.211 **Fall in (into) filled bathtub causing drowning and submersion**
      Excludes1 drowning and submersion while in filled bathtub without fall (W65)
    ● W16.212 **Fall in (into) filled bathtub causing other injury**

● W16.22 **Fall in (into) bucket of water**
  ● W16.221 **Fall in (into) bucket of water causing drowning and submersion**
  ● W16.222 **Fall in (into) bucket of water causing other injury**
● W16.3 **Fall into other water**
  Fall into fountain
  Fall into reservoir
  ● W16.31 **Fall into other water striking water surface**
    ● W16.311 **Fall into other water striking water surface causing drowning and submersion**
      Excludes1 drowning and submersion while in other water without fall (W73)
    ● W16.312 **Fall into other water striking water surface causing other injury**
  ● W16.32 **Fall into other water striking bottom**
    ● W16.321 **Fall into other water striking bottom causing drowning and submersion**
      Excludes1 drowning and submersion while in other water without fall (W73)
    ● W16.322 **Fall into other water striking bottom causing other injury**
  ● W16.33 **Fall into other water striking wall**
    ● W16.331 **Fall into other water striking wall causing drowning and submersion**
      Excludes1 drowning and submersion while in other water without fall (W73)
    ● W16.332 **Fall into other water striking wall causing other injury**
● W16.4 **Fall into unspecified water**
  X ● W16.41 **Fall into unspecified water causing drowning and submersion**
  X ● W16.42 **Fall into unspecified water causing other injury**
● W16.5 **Jumping or diving into swimming pool**
  ● W16.51 **Jumping or diving into swimming pool striking water surface**
    ● W16.511 **Jumping or diving into swimming pool striking water surface causing drowning and submersion**
      Excludes1 drowning and submersion while in swimming pool without jumping or diving (W67)
    ● W16.512 **Jumping or diving into swimming pool striking water surface causing other injury**
  ● W16.52 **Jumping or diving into swimming pool striking bottom**
    ● W16.521 **Jumping or diving into swimming pool striking bottom causing drowning and submersion**
      Excludes1 drowning and submersion while in swimming pool without jumping or diving (W67)
    ● W16.522 **Jumping or diving into swimming pool striking bottom causing other injury**

▶ New   ⇒ Revised   ~~deleted~~ Deleted   Excludes 1   Excludes 2   Includes   Use additional   Code first   Code also   Key words
OGCR Official Guidelines   ● Unacceptable Principal Diagnosis   X Assign placeholder X   ● Use Additional Character(s)   ▶ Manifestation Code   Coding Clinic

● **W16.53** Jumping or diving into swimming pool striking wall

  ● **W16.531** Jumping or diving into swimming pool striking wall causing drowning and submersion

    Excludes1 drowning and submersion while in swimming pool without jumping or diving (W67)

  ● **W16.532** Jumping or diving into swimming pool striking wall causing other injury

● **W16.6** Jumping or diving into natural body of water

Jumping or diving into lake
Jumping or diving into open sea
Jumping or diving into river
Jumping or diving into stream

  ● **W16.61** Jumping or diving into natural body of water striking water surface

    ● **W16.611** Jumping or diving into natural body of water striking water surface causing drowning and submersion

      Excludes1 drowning and submersion while in natural body of water without jumping or diving (W69)

    ● **W16.612** Jumping or diving into natural body of water striking water surface causing other injury

  ● **W16.62** Jumping or diving into natural body of water striking bottom

    ● **W16.621** Jumping or diving into natural body of water striking bottom causing drowning and submersion

      Excludes1 drowning and submersion while in natural body of water without jumping or diving (W69)

    ● **W16.622** Jumping or diving into natural body of water striking bottom causing other injury

● **W16.7** Jumping or diving from boat

  Excludes1 fall from boat into water - see watercraft accident (V90-V94)

  ● **W16.71** Jumping or diving from boat striking water surface

    ● **W16.711** Jumping or diving from boat striking water surface causing drowning and submersion

    ● **W16.712** Jumping or diving from boat striking water surface causing other injury

  ● **W16.72** Jumping or diving from boat striking bottom

    ● **W16.721** Jumping or diving from boat striking bottom causing drowning and submersion

    ● **W16.722** Jumping or diving from boat striking bottom causing other injury

● **W16.8** Jumping or diving into other water

Jumping or diving into fountain
Jumping or diving into reservoir

  ● **W16.81** Jumping or diving into other water striking water surface

    ● **W16.811** Jumping or diving into other water striking water surface causing drowning and submersion

      Excludes1 drowning and submersion while in other water without jumping or diving (W73)

    ● **W16.812** Jumping or diving into other water striking water surface causing other injury

  ● **W16.82** Jumping or diving into other water striking bottom

    ● **W16.821** Jumping or diving into other water striking bottom causing drowning and submersion

      Excludes1 drowning and submersion while in other water without jumping or diving (W73)

    ● **W16.822** Jumping or diving into other water striking bottom causing other injury

  ● **W16.83** Jumping or diving into other water striking wall

    ● **W16.831** Jumping or diving into other water striking wall causing drowning and submersion

      Excludes1 drowning and submersion while in other water without jumping or diving (W73)

    ● **W16.832** Jumping or diving into other water striking wall causing other injury

● **W16.9** Jumping or diving into unspecified water

  X● **W16.91** Jumping or diving into unspecified water causing drowning and submersion

  X● **W16.92** Jumping or diving into unspecified water causing other injury

● **W17** Other fall from one level to another

The appropriate 7th character is to be added to each code from category W17

A	initial encounter
D	subsequent encounter
S	sequela

X● **W17.0** Fall into well

X● **W17.1** Fall into storm drain or manhole

X● **W17.2** Fall into hole

Fall into pit

X● **W17.3** Fall into empty swimming pool

  Excludes1 fall into filled swimming pool (W16.0-)

X● **W17.4** Fall from dock

● **W17.8** Other fall from one level to another

  X● **W17.81** Fall down embankment (hill)

  X● **W17.82** Fall from (out of) grocery cart

Fall due to grocery cart tipping over

  X● **W17.89** Other fall from one level to another

Fall from cherry picker
Fall from lifting device
Fall from mobile elevated work platform [MEWP]
Fall from sky lift

Coding Clinic: 2015, Q2, P6

N Newborn Age: 0   **P** Pediatric Age: 0–17   **M** Maternity DX: 12–55   **A** Adult Age: 15–124   ♀ Females Only   ♂ Males Only

🏀 Complication\Comorbidity   🏀 Major C\C   Ⓔⓧ CC/MCC Exclusions   🏀 Hospital-Acquired Condition

1545

CHAPTER 20 (V01-Y99)

● **W18   Other slipping, tripping and stumbling and falls**

The appropriate 7th character is to be added to each code from category W18

A	initial encounter
D	subsequent encounter
S	sequela

● **W18.0   Fall due to bumping against object**

Striking against object with subsequent fall

> **Excludes1**   fall on same level due to slipping, tripping, or stumbling with subsequent striking against object (W01.1-)

X ● **W18.00   Striking against unspecified object with subsequent fall**

X ● **W18.01   Striking against sports equipment with subsequent fall**

X ● **W18.02   Striking against glass with subsequent fall**

X ● **W18.09   Striking against other object with subsequent fall**

● **W18.1   Fall from or off toilet**

X ● **W18.11   Fall from or off toilet without subsequent striking against object**

Fall from (off) toilet NOS

X ● **W18.12   Fall from or off toilet with subsequent striking against object**

X ● **W18.2   Fall in (into) shower or empty bathtub**

> **Excludes1**   fall in full bathtub causing drowning or submersion (W16.21-)

● **W18.3   Other and unspecified fall on same level**

X ● **W18.30   Fall on same level, unspecified**

X ● **W18.31   Fall on same level due to stepping on an object**

Fall on same level due to stepping on an animal

> **Excludes1**   slipping, tripping and stumbling without fall due to stepping on animal (W18.41)

X ● **W18.39   Other fall on same level**

● **W18.4   Slipping, tripping and stumbling without falling**

> **Excludes1**   collision with another person without fall (W51)

X ● **W18.40   Slipping, tripping and stumbling without falling, unspecified**

X ● **W18.41   Slipping, tripping and stumbling without falling due to stepping on object**

Slipping, tripping and stumbling without falling due to stepping on animal

> **Excludes1**   slipping, tripping and stumbling with fall due to stepping on animal (W18.31)

X ● **W18.42   Slipping, tripping and stumbling without falling due to stepping into hole or opening**

X ● **W18.43   Slipping, tripping and stumbling without falling due to stepping from one level to another**

X ● **W18.49   Other slipping, tripping and stumbling without falling**

X ● **W19   Unspecified fall**

Accidental fall NOS

The appropriate 7th character is to be added to code W19

A	initial encounter
D	subsequent encounter
S	sequela

Coding Clinic: 2012, Q4, P95

EXPOSURE TO INANIMATE MECHANICAL FORCES (W20-W49)

> **Excludes1**   assault (X92-Y09)
> contact or collision with animals or persons (W50-W64)
> exposure to inanimate mechanical forces involving military or war operations (Y36.-, Y37.-)
> intentional self-harm (X71-X83)

Coding Clinic: 2016, Q4, P129

● **W20   Struck by thrown, projected or falling object**

Code first any associated:
cataclysm (X34-X39)
lightning strike (T75.00)

> **Excludes1**   falling object in machinery accident (W24, W28-W31)
> falling object in transport accident (V01-V99)
> object set in motion by explosion (W35-W40)
> object set in motion by firearm (W32-W34)
> struck by thrown sports equipment (W21.-)

The appropriate 7th character is to be added to each code from category W20

A	initial encounter
D	subsequent encounter
S	sequela

X ● **W20.0   Struck by falling object in cave-in**

> **Excludes2**   asphyxiation due to cave-in (T71.21)

X ● **W20.1   Struck by object due to collapse of building**

> **Excludes1**   struck by object due to collapse of burning building (X00.2, X02.2)

X ● **W20.8   Other cause of strike by thrown, projected or falling object**

> **Excludes1**   struck by thrown sports equipment (W21.-)

● **W21   Striking against or struck by sports equipment**

> **Excludes1**   assault with sports equipment (Y08.0-)
> striking against or struck by sports equipment with subsequent fall (W18.01)

The appropriate 7th character is to be added to each code from category W21

A	initial encounter
D	subsequent encounter
S	sequela

● **W21.0   Struck by hit or thrown ball**

X ● **W21.00   Struck by hit or thrown ball, unspecified type**

X ● **W21.01   Struck by football**

X ● **W21.02   Struck by soccer ball**

X ● **W21.03   Struck by baseball**

X ● **W21.04   Struck by golf ball**

X ● **W21.05   Struck by basketball**

X ● **W21.06   Struck by volleyball**

X ● **W21.07   Struck by softball**

X ● **W21.09   Struck by other hit or thrown ball**

● **W21.1   Struck by bat, racquet or club**

X ● **W21.11   Struck by baseball bat**

X ● **W21.12   Struck by tennis racquet**

X ● **W21.13   Struck by golf club**

X ● **W21.19   Struck by other bat, racquet or club**

● **W21.2   Struck by hockey stick or puck**

● **W21.21   Struck by hockey stick**

● **W21.210   Struck by ice hockey stick**

● **W21.211   Struck by field hockey stick**

● **W21.22   Struck by hockey puck**

● **W21.220   Struck by ice hockey puck**

● **W21.221   Struck by field hockey puck**

▶ New   ▶ Revised   ~~deleted~~ Deleted   Excludes 1   Excludes 2   Includes   Use additional   Code first   Code also   Key words

OGCR Official Guidelines   ● Unacceptable Principal Diagnosis   X Assign placeholder X   ● Use Additional Character(s)   ▶ Manifestation Code   Coding Clinic

- **W21.3 Struck by sports foot wear**
  - X **W21.31 Struck by shoe cleats**
    - Stepped on by shoe cleats
  - X **W21.32 Struck by skate blades**
    - Skated over by skate blades
  - X **W21.39 Struck by other sports foot wear**
- X **W21.4 Striking against diving board**
  - Use additional code for subsequent falling into water, if applicable (W16.-)
- **W21.8 Striking against or struck by other sports equipment**
  - X **W21.81 Striking against or struck by football helmet**
  - X **W21.89 Striking against or struck by other sports equipment**
- X **W21.9 Striking against or struck by unspecified sports equipment**

- **W22 Striking against or struck by other objects**
  - **Excludes1**   striking against or struck by object with subsequent fall (W18.09)

  The appropriate 7th character is to be added to each code from category W22

A	initial encounter
D	subsequent encounter
S	sequela

  - **W22.0 Striking against stationary object**
    - **Excludes1**   striking against stationary sports equipment (W21.8)
    - X **W22.01 Walked into wall**
    - X **W22.02 Walked into lamppost**
    - X **W22.03 Walked into furniture**
    - **W22.04 Striking against wall of swimming pool**
      - **W22.041 Striking against wall of swimming pool causing drowning and submersion**
        - **Excludes1**   drowning and submersion while swimming without striking against wall (W67)
      - **W22.042 Striking against wall of swimming pool causing other injury**
    - X **W22.09 Striking against other stationary object**
  - **W22.1 Striking against or struck by automobile airbag**
    - X **W22.10 Striking against or struck by unspecified automobile airbag**
    - X **W22.11 Striking against or struck by driver side automobile airbag**
    - X **W22.12 Striking against or struck by front passenger side automobile airbag**
    - X **W22.19 Striking against or struck by other automobile airbag**
  - X **W22.8 Striking against or struck by other objects**
    - Striking against or struck by object NOS
    - **Excludes1**   struck by thrown, projected or falling object (W20.-)

- **W23 Caught, crushed, jammed or pinched in or between objects**
  - **Excludes1**   injury caused by cutting or piercing instruments (W25-W27)
    - injury caused by firearms malfunction (W32.1, W33.1-, W34.1-)
    - injury caused by lifting and transmission devices (W24.-)
    - injury caused by machinery (W28-W31)
    - injury caused by nonpowered hand tools (W27.-)
    - injury caused by transport vehicle being used as a means of transportation (V01-V99)
    - injury caused by struck by thrown, projected or falling object (W20.-)

  The appropriate 7th character is to be added to each code from category W23

A	initial encounter
D	subsequent encounter
S	sequela

  - X **W23.0 Caught, crushed, jammed, or pinched between moving objects**
  - X **W23.1 Caught, crushed, jammed, or pinched between stationary objects**

- **W24 Contact with lifting and transmission devices, not elsewhere classified**
  - **Excludes1**   transport accidents (V01-V99)

  The appropriate 7th character is to be added to each code from category W24

A	initial encounter
D	subsequent encounter
S	sequela

  - X **W24.0 Contact with lifting devices, not elsewhere classified**
    - Contact with chain hoist
    - Contact with drive belt
    - Contact with pulley (block)
  - X **W24.1 Contact with transmission devices, not elsewhere classified**
    - Contact with transmission belt or cable

- X **W25 Contact with sharp glass**
  - *Code first any associated:*
    - injury due to flying glass from explosion or firearm discharge (W32-W40)
    - transport accident (V00-V99)
  - **Excludes1**   fall on same level due to slipping, tripping and stumbling with subsequent striking against sharp glass (W01.10)
    - striking against sharp glass with subsequent fall (W18.02)
  - **Excludes2**   glass embedded in skin (W45)

  The appropriate 7th character is to be added to code W25

A	initial encounter
D	subsequent encounter
S	sequela

● **W26   Contact with other sharp objects**

     Excludes2   sharp object(s) embedded in skin (W45)

     The appropriate 7th character is to be added to each code from category W26

A	initial encounter
D	subsequent encounter
S	sequela

     Coding Clinic: 2016, Q4, P73

X● **W26.0   Contact with knife**

       Excludes1   contact with electric knife (W29.1)

X● **W26.1   Contact with sword or dagger**

X● **W26.2   Contact with edge of stiff paper**

       Paper cut

       Coding Clinic: 2016, Q4, P73

X● **W26.8   Contact with other sharp object(s), not elsewhere classified**

       Contact with tin can lid

       Coding Clinic: 2016, Q4, P73

X● **W26.9   Contact with unspecified sharp object(s)**

       Coding Clinic: 2016, Q4, P73

● **W27   Contact with nonpowered hand tool**

     The appropriate 7th character is to be added to each code from category W27

A	initial encounter
D	subsequent encounter
S	sequela

X● **W27.0   Contact with workbench tool**

       Contact with auger

       Contact with axe

       Contact with chisel

       Contact with handsaw

       Contact with screwdriver

X● **W27.1   Contact with garden tool**

       Contact with hoe

       Contact with nonpowered lawn mower

       Contact with pitchfork

       Contact with rake

X● **W27.2   Contact with scissors**

X● **W27.3   Contact with needle (sewing)**

       Excludes1   contact with hypodermic needle (W46.-)

X● **W27.4   Contact with kitchen utensil**

       Contact with fork

       Contact with ice-pick

       Contact with can-opener NOS

X● **W27.5   Contact with paper-cutter**

X● **W27.8   Contact with other nonpowered hand tool**

       Contact with nonpowered sewing machine

       Contact with shovel

X● **W28   Contact with powered lawn mower**

     Powered lawn mower (commercial) (residential)

     Excludes1   contact with nonpowered lawn mower (W27.1)

     Excludes2   exposure to electric current (W86.-)

     The appropriate 7th character is to be added to code W28

A	initial encounter
D	subsequent encounter
S	sequela

● **W29   Contact with other powered hand tools and household machinery**

     Excludes1   contact with commercial machinery (W31.82)

                    contact with hot household appliance (X15)

                    contact with nonpowered hand tool (W27.-)

                    exposure to electric current (W86)

     The appropriate 7th character is to be added to each code from category W29

A	initial encounter
D	subsequent encounter
S	sequela

X● **W29.0   Contact with powered kitchen appliance**

       Contact with blender

       Contact with can-opener

       Contact with garbage disposal

       Contact with mixer

X● **W29.1   Contact with electric knife**

X● **W29.2   Contact with other powered household machinery**

       Contact with electric fan

       Contact with powered dryer (clothes) (powered) (spin)

       Contact with washing-machine

       Contact with sewing machine

X● **W29.3   Contact with powered garden and outdoor hand tools and machinery**

       Contact with chainsaw

       Contact with edger

       Contact with garden cultivator (tiller)

       Contact with hedge trimmer

       Contact with other powered garden tool

       Excludes1   contact with powered lawn mower (W28)

X● **W29.4   Contact with nail gun**

➡X● **W29.8   Contact with other powered hand tools and household machinery**

       Contact with do-it-yourself tool NOS

● **W30   Contact with agricultural machinery**

     Includes   animal-powered farm machine

     Excludes1   agricultural transport vehicle accident (V01-V99)

                    explosion of grain store (W40.8)

                    exposure to electric current (W86.-)

     The appropriate 7th character is to be added to each code from category W30

A	initial encounter
D	subsequent encounter
S	sequela

X● **W30.0   Contact with combine harvester**

       Contact with reaper

       Contact with thresher

X● **W30.1   Contact with power take-off devices (PTO)**

X● **W30.2   Contact with hay derrick**

X● **W30.3   Contact with grain storage elevator**

       Excludes1   explosion of grain store (W40.8)

● **W30.8   Contact with other specified agricultural machinery**

X● **W30.81   Contact with agricultural transport vehicle in stationary use**

       Contact with agricultural transport vehicle under repair, not on public roadway

       Excludes1   agricultural transport vehicle accident (V01-V99)

X● **W30.89   Contact with other specified agricultural machinery**

X● **W30.9   Contact with unspecified agricultural machinery**

       Contact with farm machinery NOS

▶ New   ⇒ Revised   ~~deleted~~ Deleted   Excludes 1   Excludes 2   Includes   Use additional   Code first   Code also   Key words

OGCR Official Guidelines   ● Unacceptable Principal Diagnosis   X Assign placeholder X   ● Use Additional Character(s)   ▶ Manifestation Code   **Coding Clinic**

● **W31   Contact with other and unspecified machinery**

> **Excludes1**   contact with agricultural machinery (W30.-)
> contact with machinery in transport under
>   own power or being towed by a vehicle
>   (VØ1-V99)
> exposure to electric current (W86)

The appropriate 7th character is to be added to each code from
category W31

> | | |
> |---|---|
> | A | initial encounter |
> | D | subsequent encounter |
> | S | sequela |

X● **W31.Ø   Contact with mining and earth-drilling machinery**
> Contact with bore or drill (land) (seabed)
> Contact with shaft hoist
> Contact with shaft lift
> Contact with undercutter

X● **W31.1   Contact with metalworking machines**
> Contact with abrasive wheel
> Contact with forging machine
> Contact with lathe
> Contact with mechanical shears
> Contact with metal drilling machine
> Contact with milling machine
> Contact with power press
> Contact with rolling-mill
> Contact with metal sawing machine

X● **W31.2   Contact with powered woodworking and forming
machines**
> Contact with band saw
> Contact with bench saw
> Contact with circular saw
> Contact with molding machine
> Contact with overhead plane
> Contact with powered saw
> Contact with radial saw
> Contact with sander
>
> > **Excludes1**   nonpowered woodworking tools (W27.Ø)

X● **W31.3   Contact with prime movers**
> Contact with gas turbine
> Contact with internal combustion engine
> Contact with steam engine
> Contact with water driven turbine

● **W31.8   Contact with other specified machinery**

X● **W31.81   Contact with recreational machinery**
> Contact with roller-coaster

X● **W31.82   Contact with other commercial machinery**
> Contact with commercial electric fan
> Contact with commercial kitchen appliances
> Contact with commercial powered dryer
>   (clothes) (powered) (spin)
> Contact with commercial washing-machine
> Contact with commercial sewing machine
>
> > **Excludes1**   contact with household
> >   machinery (W29.-)
> >   contact with powered lawn
> >   mower (W28)

X● **W31.83   Contact with special construction vehicle in
stationary use**
> Contact with special construction vehicle
>   under repair, not on public roadway
>
> > **Excludes1**   special construction vehicle
> >   accident (VØ1-V99)

X● **W31.89   Contact with other specified machinery**

X● **W31.9   Contact with unspecified machinery**
> Contact with machinery NOS

● **W32   Accidental handgun discharge and malfunction**

> **Includes**   accidental discharge and malfunction of gun for
>   single hand use
> accidental discharge and malfunction of pistol
> accidental discharge and malfunction of revolver
> handgun discharge and malfunction NOS

> **Excludes1**   accidental airgun discharge and malfunction
>   (W34.Ø1Ø, W34.11Ø)
> accidental BB gun discharge and malfunction
>   (W34.Ø1Ø, W34.11Ø)
> accidental pellet gun discharge and malfunction
>   (W34.Ø1Ø, W34.11Ø)
> accidental shotgun discharge and malfunction
>   (W33.Ø1, W33.11)
> assault by handgun discharge (X93)
> handgun discharge involving legal intervention
>   (Y35.Ø-)
> handgun discharge involving military or war
>   operations (Y36.4-)
> intentional self-harm by handgun discharge (X72)
> Very pistol discharge and malfunction (W34.Ø9,
>   W34.19)

The appropriate 7th character is to be added to each code from
category W32

> | | |
> |---|---|
> | A | initial encounter |
> | D | subsequent encounter |
> | S | sequela |

X● **W32.Ø   Accidental handgun discharge**
X● **W32.1   Accidental handgun malfunction**
> Injury due to explosion of handgun (parts)
> Injury due to malfunction of mechanism or component
>   of handgun
> Injury due to recoil of handgun
> Powder burn from handgun

● **W33   Accidental rifle, shotgun and larger firearm discharge and
malfunction**

> **Includes**   rifle, shotgun and larger firearm discharge and
>   malfunction NOS

> **Excludes1**   accidental airgun discharge and malfunction
>   (W34.Ø1Ø, W34.11Ø)
> accidental BB gun discharge and malfunction
>   (W34.Ø1Ø, W34.11Ø)
> accidental handgun discharge and malfunction
>   (W32.-)
> accidental pellet gun discharge and malfunction
>   (W34.Ø1Ø, W34.11Ø)
> assault by rifle, shotgun and larger firearm
>   discharge (X94)
> firearm discharge involving legal intervention
>   (Y35.Ø-)
> firearm discharge involving military or war
>   operations (Y36.4-)
> intentional self-harm by rifle, shotgun and larger
>   firearm discharge (X73)

The appropriate 7th character is to be added to each code from
category W33

> | | |
> |---|---|
> | A | initial encounter |
> | D | subsequent encounter |
> | S | sequela |

● **W33.Ø   Accidental rifle, shotgun and larger firearm discharge**

X● **W33.ØØ   Accidental discharge of unspecified larger
firearm**
> Discharge of unspecified larger firearm NOS

X● **W33.Ø1   Accidental discharge of shotgun**
> Discharge of shotgun NOS

X● **W33.Ø2   Accidental discharge of hunting rifle**
> Discharge of hunting rifle NOS

X● **W33.Ø3   Accidental discharge of machine gun**
> Discharge of machine gun NOS

X● **W33.Ø9   Accidental discharge of other larger firearm**
> Discharge of other larger firearm NOS

● **W33.1 Accidental rifle, shotgun and larger firearm malfunction**
Injury due to explosion of rifle, shotgun and larger firearm (parts)
Injury due to malfunction of mechanism or component of rifle, shotgun and larger firearm
Injury due to piercing, cutting, crushing or pinching due to (by) slide trigger mechanism, scope or other gun part
Injury due to recoil of rifle, shotgun and larger firearm
Powder burn from rifle, shotgun and larger firearm

X● **W33.10 Accidental malfunction of unspecified larger firearm**
Malfunction of unspecified larger firearm NOS

X● **W33.11 Accidental malfunction of shotgun**
Malfunction of shotgun NOS

X● **W33.12 Accidental malfunction of hunting rifle**
Malfunction of hunting rifle NOS

X● **W33.13 Accidental malfunction of machine gun**
Malfunction of machine gun NOS

X● **W33.19 Accidental malfunction of other larger firearm**
Malfunction of other larger firearm NOS

● **W34 Accidental discharge and malfunction from other and unspecified firearms and guns**
The appropriate 7th character is to be added to each code from category W34

A	initial encounter
D	subsequent encounter
S	sequela

● **W34.0 Accidental discharge from other and unspecified firearms and guns**

X● **W34.00 Accidental discharge from unspecified firearms or gun**
Discharge from firearm NOS
Gunshot wound NOS
Shot NOS
Coding Clinic: 2015, Q1, P17

● **W34.01 Accidental discharge of gas, air or spring-operated guns**

● **W34.010 Accidental discharge of airgun**
Accidental discharge of BB gun
Accidental discharge of pellet gun

● **W34.011 Accidental discharge of paintball gun**
Accidental injury due to paintball discharge

● **W34.018 Accidental discharge of other gas, air or spring-operated gun**

X● **W34.09 Accidental discharge from other specified firearms**
Accidental discharge from Very pistol [flare]

● **W34.1 Accidental malfunction from other and unspecified firearms and guns**

X● **W34.10 Accidental malfunction from unspecified firearms or gun**
Firearm malfunction NOS

● **W34.11 Accidental malfunction of gas, air or spring-operated guns**

● **W34.110 Accidental malfunction of airgun**
Accidental malfunction of BB gun
Accidental malfunction of pellet gun

● **W34.111 Accidental malfunction of paintball gun**
Accidental injury due to paintball gun malfunction

● **W34.118 Accidental malfunction of other gas, air or spring-operated gun**

X● **W34.19 Accidental malfunction from other specified firearms**
Accidental malfunction from Very pistol [flare]

X● **W35 Explosion and rupture of boiler**
Excludes1   explosion and rupture of boiler on watercraft (V93.4)

The appropriate 7th character is to be added to code W35

A	initial encounter
D	subsequent encounter
S	sequela

● **W36 Explosion and rupture of gas cylinder**
The appropriate 7th character is to be added to each code from category W36

A	initial encounter
D	subsequent encounter
S	sequela

X● **W36.1 Explosion and rupture of aerosol can**
X● **W36.2 Explosion and rupture of air tank**
X● **W36.3 Explosion and rupture of pressurized-gas tank**
X● **W36.8 Explosion and rupture of other gas cylinder**
X● **W36.9 Explosion and rupture of unspecified gas cylinder**

● **W37 Explosion and rupture of pressurized tire, pipe or hose**
The appropriate 7th character is to be added to each code from category W37

A	initial encounter
D	subsequent encounter
S	sequela

X● **W37.0 Explosion of bicycle tire**
X● **W37.8 Explosion and rupture of other pressurized tire, pipe or hose**

X● **W38 Explosion and rupture of other specified pressurized devices**
The appropriate 7th character is to be added to code W38

A	initial encounter
D	subsequent encounter
S	sequela

X● **W39 Discharge of firework**
The appropriate 7th character is to be added to code W39

A	initial encounter
D	subsequent encounter
S	sequela

● **W40 Explosion of other materials**
Excludes1   assault by explosive material (X96)
explosion involving legal intervention (Y35.1-)
explosion involving military or war operations (Y36.0-, Y36.2-)
intentional self-harm by explosive material (X75)

The appropriate 7th character is to be added to each code from category W40

A	initial encounter
D	subsequent encounter
S	sequela

X● **W40.0 Explosion of blasting material**
Explosion of blasting cap
Explosion of detonator
Explosion of dynamite
Explosion of explosive (any) used in blasting operations

X● **W40.1 Explosion of explosive gases**
Explosion of acetylene
Explosion of butane
Explosion of coal gas
Explosion in mine NOS
Explosion of explosive gas
Explosion of fire damp
Explosion of gasoline fumes
Explosion of methane
Explosion of propane

▶ New   ⇛ Revised   ~~deleted~~ Deleted   Excludes 1   Excludes 2   Includes   Use additional   Code first   Code also   Key words
OGCR Official Guidelines   ● Unacceptable Principal Diagnosis   X Assign placeholder X   ● Use Additional Character(s)   ▶ Manifestation Code   **Coding Clinic**

X● W40.8　**Explosion of other specified explosive materials**
　　　　　Explosion in dump NOS
　　　　　Explosion in factory NOS
　　　　　Explosion in grain store
　　　　　Explosion in munitions
　　　　　　Excludes1　explosion involving legal intervention
　　　　　　　　　　　(Y35.1-)
　　　　　　　　　　explosion involving military or war
　　　　　　　　　　　operations (Y36.0-, Y36.2-)

X● W40.9　**Explosion of unspecified explosive materials**
　　　　　Explosion NOS

● W42　**Exposure to noise**
　　　The appropriate 7th character is to be added to each code from
　　　category W42

A	initial encounter
D	subsequent encounter
S	sequela

X● W42.0　**Exposure to supersonic waves**
X● W42.9　**Exposure to other noise**
　　　　　Exposure to sound waves NOS

● W45　**Foreign body or object entering through skin**
　　　　Includes　foreign body or object embedded in skin
　　　　　　　　　nail embedded in skin
　　　　Excludes2　contact with hand tools (nonpowered) (powered)
　　　　　　　　　(W27-W29)
　　　　　　　　　contact with other sharp object(s) (W26.-)
　　　　　　　　　contact with sharp glass (W25.-)
　　　　　　　　　struck by objects (W20-W22)
　　　The appropriate 7th character is to be added to each code from
　　　category W45

A	initial encounter
D	subsequent encounter
S	sequela

X● W45.0　**Nail entering through skin**
X● W45.8　**Other foreign body or object entering through skin**
　　　　　Splinter in skin NOS

● W46　**Contact with hypodermic needle**
　　　The appropriate 7th character is to be added to each code from
　　　category W46

A	initial encounter
D	subsequent encounter
S	sequela

X● W46.0　**Contact with hypodermic needle**
　　　　　Hypodermic needle stick NOS
X● W46.1　**Contact with contaminated hypodermic needle**

● W49　**Exposure to other inanimate mechanical forces**
　　　　Includes　exposure to abnormal gravitational [G] forces
　　　　　　　　　exposure to inanimate mechanical forces NEC
　　　　Excludes1　exposure to inanimate mechanical forces
　　　　　　　　　involving military or war operations (Y36.-,
　　　　　　　　　Y37.-)
　　　The appropriate 7th character is to be added to each code from
　　　category W49

A	initial encounter
D	subsequent encounter
S	sequela

● W49.0　**Item causing external constriction**
　　X● W49.01　**Hair causing external constriction**
　　X● W49.02　**String or thread causing external constriction**
　　X● W49.03　**Rubber band causing external constriction**
　　X● W49.04　**Ring or other jewelry causing external
　　　　　　　constriction**
　　X● W49.09　**Other item causing external constriction**
X● W49.9　**Exposure to other inanimate mechanical forces**

EXPOSURE TO ANIMATE MECHANICAL FORCES (W50-W64)
　　　Excludes1　toxic effect of contact with venomous animals
　　　　　　　　and plants (T63.-)

● W50　**Accidental hit, strike, kick, twist, bite or scratch by another person**
　　　　Includes　hit, strike, kick, twist, bite, or scratch by another
　　　　　　　　　person NOS
　　　　Excludes1　assault by bodily force (Y04)
　　　　　　　　　struck by objects (W20-W22)
　　　The appropriate 7th character is to be added to each code from
　　　category W50

A	initial encounter
D	subsequent encounter
S	sequela

X● W50.0　**Accidental hit or strike by another person**
　　　　　Hit or strike by another person NOS
X● W50.1　**Accidental kick by another person**
　　　　　Kick by another person NOS
X● W50.2　**Accidental twist by another person**
　　　　　Twist by another person NOS
　　　　　Coding Clinic: 2015, Q1, P8
X● W50.3　**Accidental bite by another person**
　　　　　Human bite
　　　　　Bite by another person NOS
X● W50.4　**Accidental scratch by another person**
　　　　　Scratch by another person NOS

X● W51　**Accidental striking against or bumped into by another person**
　　　　Excludes1　assault by striking against or bumping into by
　　　　　　　　　another person (Y04.2)
　　　　　　　　　fall due to collision with another person (W03)
　　　The appropriate 7th character is to be added to code W51

A	initial encounter
D	subsequent encounter
S	sequela

X● W52　**Crushed, pushed or stepped on by crowd or human stampede**
　　　　　Crushed, pushed or stepped on by crowd or human stampede
　　　　　　with or without fall
　　　The appropriate 7th character is to be added to code W52

A	initial encounter
D	subsequent encounter
S	sequela

● W53　**Contact with rodent**
　　　　Includes　contact with saliva, feces or urine of rodent
　　　The appropriate 7th character is to be added to each code from
　　　category W53

A	initial encounter
D	subsequent encounter
S	sequela

● W53.0　**Contact with mouse**
　　X● W53.01　**Bitten by mouse**
　　X● W53.09　**Other contact with mouse**
● W53.1　**Contact with rat**
　　X● W53.11　**Bitten by rat**
　　X● W53.19　**Other contact with rat**
● W53.2　**Contact with squirrel**
　　X● W53.21　**Bitten by squirrel**
　　X● W53.29　**Other contact with squirrel**
● W53.8　**Contact with other rodent**
　　X● W53.81　**Bitten by other rodent**
　　X● W53.89　**Other contact with other rodent**

CHAPTER 20 (V01-Y99)

CHAPTER 20 (V01-Y99)

● W54   **Contact with dog**

> **Includes**   contact with saliva, feces or urine of dog
>
> The appropriate 7th character is to be added to each code from category W54

A	initial encounter
D	subsequent encounter
S	sequela

X● **W54.0**   **Bitten by dog**

X● **W54.1**   **Struck by dog**
> Knocked over by dog

X● **W54.8**   **Other contact with dog**

● W55   **Contact with other mammals**

> **Includes**   contact with saliva, feces or urine of mammal
>
> **Excludes1**   animal being ridden - see transport accidents
> bitten or struck by dog (W54)
> bitten or struck by rodent (W53.-)
> contact with marine mammals (W56.X-)
>
> The appropriate 7th character is to be added to each code from category W55

A	initial encounter
D	subsequent encounter
S	sequela

● **W55.0**   **Contact with cat**

     X● **W55.01**   **Bitten by cat**

     X● **W55.03**   **Scratched by cat**

     X● **W55.09**   **Other contact with cat**

● **W55.1**   **Contact with horse**

     X● **W55.11**   **Bitten by horse**

     X● **W55.12**   **Struck by horse**

     X● **W55.19**   **Other contact with horse**

● **W55.2**   **Contact with cow**
> Contact with bull

     X● **W55.21**   **Bitten by cow**

     X● **W55.22**   **Struck by cow**
> Gored by bull

     X● **W55.29**   **Other contact with cow**

● **W55.3**   **Contact with other hoof stock**
> Contact with goats
> Contact with sheep

     X● **W55.31**   **Bitten by other hoof stock**

     X● **W55.32**   **Struck by other hoof stock**
> Gored by goat
> Gored by ram

     X● **W55.39**   **Other contact with other hoof stock**

● **W55.4**   **Contact with pig**

     X● **W55.41**   **Bitten by pig**

     X● **W55.42**   **Struck by pig**

     X● **W55.49**   **Other contact with pig**

● **W55.5**   **Contact with raccoon**

     X● **W55.51**   **Bitten by raccoon**

     X● **W55.52**   **Struck by raccoon**

     X● **W55.59**   **Other contact with raccoon**

● **W55.8**   **Contact with other mammals**

     X● **W55.81**   **Bitten by other mammals**

     X● **W55.82**   **Struck by other mammals**

     X● **W55.89**   **Other contact with other mammals**

● W56   **Contact with nonvenomous marine animal**

> **Excludes1**   contact with venomous marine animal (T63.-)
>
> The appropriate 7th character is to be added to each code from category W56

A	initial encounter
D	subsequent encounter
S	sequela

● **W56.0**   **Contact with dolphin**

     X● **W56.01**   **Bitten by dolphin**

     X● **W56.02**   **Struck by dolphin**

     X● **W56.09**   **Other contact with dolphin**

● **W56.1**   **Contact with sea lion**

     X● **W56.11**   **Bitten by sea lion**

     X● **W56.12**   **Struck by sea lion**

     X● **W56.19**   **Other contact with sea lion**

● **W56.2**   **Contact with orca**
> Contact with killer whale

     X● **W56.21**   **Bitten by orca**

     X● **W56.22**   **Struck by orca**

     X● **W56.29**   **Other contact with orca**

● **W56.3**   **Contact with other marine mammals**

     X● **W56.31**   **Bitten by other marine mammals**

     X● **W56.32**   **Struck by other marine mammals**

     X● **W56.39**   **Other contact with other marine mammals**

● **W56.4**   **Contact with shark**

     X● **W56.41**   **Bitten by shark**

     X● **W56.42**   **Struck by shark**

     X● **W56.49**   **Other contact with shark**

● **W56.5**   **Contact with other fish**

     X● **W56.51**   **Bitten by other fish**

     X● **W56.52**   **Struck by other fish**

     X● **W56.59**   **Other contact with other fish**

● **W56.8**   **Contact with other nonvenomous marine animals**

     X● **W56.81**   **Bitten by other nonvenomous marine animals**

     X● **W56.82**   **Struck by other nonvenomous marine animals**

     X● **W56.89**   **Other contact with other nonvenomous marine animals**

X● W57   **Bitten or stung by nonvenomous insect and other nonvenomous arthropods**

> **Excludes1**   contact with venomous insects and arthropods (T63.2-, T63.3-, T63.4-)
>
> The appropriate 7th character is to be added to code W57

A	initial encounter
D	subsequent encounter
S	sequela

● W58   **Contact with crocodile or alligator**

> The appropriate 7th character is to be added to each code from category W58

A	initial encounter
D	subsequent encounter
S	sequela

● **W58.0**   **Contact with alligator**

     X● **W58.01**   **Bitten by alligator**

     X● **W58.02**   **Struck by alligator**

     X● **W58.03**   **Crushed by alligator**

     X● **W58.09**   **Other contact with alligator**

● **W58.1**   **Contact with crocodile**

     X● **W58.11**   **Bitten by crocodile**

     X● **W58.12**   **Struck by crocodile**

     X● **W58.13**   **Crushed by crocodile**

     X● **W58.19**   **Other contact with crocodile**

▶ New   ⇒ Revised   ~~deleted~~ Deleted   Excludes 1   Excludes 2   Includes   Use additional   Code first   Code also   Key words

OGCR Official Guidelines   ● Unacceptable Principal Diagnosis   X Assign placeholder X   ● Use Additional Character(s)   ▶ Manifestation Code   **Coding Clinic**

● W59   Contact with other nonvenomous reptiles

> Excludes1   contact with venomous reptile (T63.0-, T63.1-)

The appropriate 7th character is to be added to each code from category W59

> A   initial encounter
> D   subsequent encounter
> S   sequela

● W59.0   Contact with nonvenomous lizards
X ● W59.01   Bitten by nonvenomous lizards
X ● W59.02   Struck by nonvenomous lizards
X ● W59.09   Other contact with nonvenomous lizards
> Exposure to nonvenomous lizards

● W59.1   Contact with nonvenomous snakes
X ● W59.11   Bitten by nonvenomous snake
X ● W59.12   Struck by nonvenomous snake
X ● W59.13   Crushed by nonvenomous snake
X ● W59.19   Other contact with nonvenomous snake

● W59.2   Contact with turtles

> Excludes1   contact with tortoises (W59.8-)

X ● W59.21   Bitten by turtle
X ● W59.22   Struck by turtle
X ● W59.29   Other contact with turtle
> Exposure to turtles

● W59.8   Contact with other nonvenomous reptiles
X ● W59.81   Bitten by other nonvenomous reptiles
X ● W59.82   Struck by other nonvenomous reptiles
X ● W59.83   Crushed by other nonvenomous reptiles
X ● W59.89   Other contact with other nonvenomous reptiles

X ● W60   Contact with nonvenomous plant thorns and spines and sharp leaves

> Excludes1   contact with venomous plants (T63.X7-)

The appropriate 7th character is to be added to code W60

> A   initial encounter
> D   subsequent encounter
> S   sequela

● W61   Contact with birds (domestic) (wild)

> Includes   contact with excreta of birds

The appropriate 7th character is to be added to each code from category W61

> A   initial encounter
> D   subsequent encounter
> S   sequela

● W61.0   Contact with parrot
X ● W61.01   Bitten by parrot
X ● W61.02   Struck by parrot
X ● W61.09   Other contact with parrot
> Exposure to parrots

● W61.1   Contact with macaw
X ● W61.11   Bitten by macaw
X ● W61.12   Struck by macaw
X ● W61.19   Other contact with macaw
> Exposure to macaws

● W61.2   Contact with other psittacines
X ● W61.21   Bitten by other psittacines
X ● W61.22   Struck by other psittacines
X ● W61.29   Other contact with other psittacines
> Exposure to other psittacines

● W61.3   Contact with chicken
X ● W61.32   Struck by chicken
X ● W61.33   Pecked by chicken
X ● W61.39   Other contact with chicken
> Exposure to chickens

● W61.4   Contact with turkey
X ● W61.42   Struck by turkey
X ● W61.43   Pecked by turkey
X ● W61.49   Other contact with turkey

● W61.5   Contact with goose
X ● W61.51   Bitten by goose
X ● W61.52   Struck by goose
X ● W61.59   Other contact with goose

● W61.6   Contact with duck
X ● W61.61   Bitten by duck
X ● W61.62   Struck by duck
X ● W61.69   Other contact with duck

● W61.9   Contact with other birds
X ● W61.91   Bitten by other birds
X ● W61.92   Struck by other birds
X ● W61.99   Other contact with other birds
> Contact with bird NOS

● W62   Contact with nonvenomous amphibians

> Excludes1   contact with venomous amphibians (T63.81-R63.83)

The appropriate 7th character is to be added to each code from category W62

> A   initial encounter
> D   subsequent encounter
> S   sequela

X ● W62.0   Contact with nonvenomous frogs
X ● W62.1   Contact with nonvenomous toads
X ● W62.9   Contact with other nonvenomous amphibians

X ● W64   Exposure to other animate mechanical forces

> Includes   exposure to nonvenomous animal NOS
> Excludes1   contact with venomous animal (T63.-)

The appropriate 7th character is to be added to code W64

> A   initial encounter
> D   subsequent encounter
> S   sequela

ACCIDENTAL NON-TRANSPORT DROWNING AND SUBMERSION (W65-W74)

> Excludes1   accidental drowning and submersion due to fall into water (W16.-)
> accidental drowning and submersion due to water transport accident (V90.-, V92.-)
> Excludes2   accidental drowning and submersion due to cataclysm (X34-X39)

X ● W65   Accidental drowning and submersion while in bathtub

> Excludes1   accidental drowning and submersion due to fall in (into) bathtub (W16.211)

The appropriate 7th character is to be added to code W65

> A   initial encounter
> D   subsequent encounter
> S   sequela

X ● W67   Accidental drowning and submersion while in swimming pool

> Excludes1   accidental drowning and submersion due to fall into swimming pool (W16.011, W16.021, W16.031)
> accidental drowning and submersion due to striking into wall of swimming pool (W22.041)

The appropriate 7th character is to be added to code W67

> A   initial encounter
> D   subsequent encounter
> S   sequela

CHAPTER 20 (V01-Y99)

N   Newborn Age: 0   P   Pediatric Age: 0–17   M   Maternity DX: 12–55   A   Adult Age: 15–124   ♀   Females Only   ♂   Males Only
🍂 Complication\Comorbidity   🍂 Major C\C   (Ex) CC/MCC Exclusions   🍂 Hospital-Acquired Condition

1553

X● **W69 Accidental drowning and submersion while in natural water**
Accidental drowning and submersion while in lake
Accidental drowning and submersion while in open sea
Accidental drowning and submersion while in river
Accidental drowning and submersion while in stream

     Excludes1   accidental drowning and submersion due to fall into natural body of water (W16.111, W16.121, W16.131)

The appropriate 7th character is to be added to code W69

A	initial encounter
D	subsequent encounter
S	sequela

X● **W73 Other specified cause of accidental non-transport drowning and submersion**
Accidental drowning and submersion while in quenching tank
Accidental drowning and submersion while in reservoir

     Excludes1   accidental drowning and submersion due to fall into other water (W16.311, W16.321, W16.331)

The appropriate 7th character is to be added to code W73

A	initial encounter
D	subsequent encounter
S	sequela

X● **W74 Unspecified cause of accidental drowning and submersion**
Drowning NOS

The appropriate 7th character is to be added to code W74

A	initial encounter
D	subsequent encounter
S	sequela

EXPOSURE TO ELECTRIC CURRENT, RADIATION AND EXTREME AMBIENT AIR TEMPERATURE AND PRESSURE (W85-W99)

     Excludes1   exposure to:
                 failure in dosage of radiation or temperature during surgical and medical care (Y63.2-Y63.5)
                 lightning (T75.Ø-)
                 natural cold (X31)
                 natural heat (X3Ø)
                 natural radiation NOS (X39)
                 radiological procedure and radiotherapy (Y84.2)
                 sunlight (X32)

X● **W85 Exposure to electric transmission lines**
Broken power line

The appropriate 7th character is to be added to code W85

A	initial encounter
D	subsequent encounter
S	sequela

● **W86 Exposure to other specified electric current**

The appropriate 7th character is to be added to each code from category W86

A	initial encounter
D	subsequent encounter
S	sequela

X● **W86.Ø Exposure to domestic wiring and appliances**
X● **W86.1 Exposure to industrial wiring, appliances and electrical machinery**
Exposure to conductors
Exposure to control apparatus
Exposure to electrical equipment and machinery
Exposure to transformers

X● **W86.8 Exposure to other electric current**
Exposure to wiring and appliances in or on farm (not farmhouse)
Exposure to wiring and appliances outdoors
Exposure to wiring and appliances in or on public building
Exposure to wiring and appliances in or on residential institutions
Exposure to wiring and appliances in or on schools

● **W88 Exposure to ionizing radiation**
     Excludes1   exposure to sunlight (X32)

The appropriate 7th character is to be added to each code from category W88

A	initial encounter
D	subsequent encounter
S	sequela

X● **W88.Ø Exposure to X-rays**
X● **W88.1 Exposure to radioactive isotopes**
X● **W88.8 Exposure to other ionizing radiation**

● **W89 Exposure to man-made visible and ultraviolet light**
     Includes   exposure to welding light (arc)
     Excludes1   exposure to sunlight (X32)

The appropriate 7th character is to be added to each code from category W89

A	initial encounter
D	subsequent encounter
S	sequela

X● **W89.Ø Exposure to welding light (arc)**
X● **W89.1 Exposure to tanning bed**
X● **W89.8 Exposure to other man-made visible and ultraviolet light**
X● **W89.9 Exposure to unspecified man-made visible and ultraviolet light**

● **W9Ø Exposure to other nonionizing radiation**
     Excludes1   exposure to sunlight (X32)

The appropriate 7th character is to be added to each code from category W9Ø

A	initial encounter
D	subsequent encounter
S	sequela

X● **W9Ø.Ø Exposure to radiofrequency**
X● **W9Ø.1 Exposure to infrared radiation**
X● **W9Ø.2 Exposure to laser radiation**
X● **W9Ø.8 Exposure to other nonionizing radiation**

X● **W92 Exposure to excessive heat of man-made origin**
The appropriate 7th character is to be added to code W92

A	initial encounter
D	subsequent encounter
S	sequela

● **W93 Exposure to excessive cold of man-made origin**
The appropriate 7th character is to be added to each code from category W93

A	initial encounter
D	subsequent encounter
S	sequela

● **W93.Ø Contact with or inhalation of dry ice**
X● **W93.Ø1 Contact with dry ice**
X● **W93.Ø2 Inhalation of dry ice**

▶ New   ⇒ Revised   ~~deleted~~ Deleted   Excludes 1   Excludes 2   Includes   Use additional   Code first   Code also   Key words
OGCR Official Guidelines   ● Unacceptable Principal Diagnosis   X Assign placeholder X   ● Use Additional Character(s)   ▶ Manifestation Code   **Coding Clinic**

X● W93.1 Contact with or inhalation of liquid air
   X● W93.11 Contact with liquid air
      Contact with liquid hydrogen
      Contact with liquid nitrogen
   X● W93.12 Inhalation of liquid air
      Inhalation of liquid hydrogen
      Inhalation of liquid nitrogen
X● W93.2 Prolonged exposure in deep freeze unit or refrigerator
X● W93.8 Exposure to other excessive cold of man-made origin

● W94 Exposure to high and low air pressure and changes in air pressure

The appropriate 7th character is to be added to each code from category W94

> A initial encounter
> D subsequent encounter
> S sequela

X● W94.0 Exposure to prolonged high air pressure
● W94.1 Exposure to prolonged low air pressure
   X● W94.11 Exposure to residence or prolonged visit at high altitude
   X● W94.12 Exposure to other prolonged low air pressure
● W94.2 Exposure to rapid changes in air pressure during ascent
   X● W94.21 Exposure to reduction in atmospheric pressure while surfacing from deep-water diving
   X● W94.22 Exposure to reduction in atmospheric pressure while surfacing from underground
   X● W94.23 Exposure to sudden change in air pressure in aircraft during ascent
   X● W94.29 Exposure to other rapid changes in air pressure during ascent
● W94.3 Exposure to rapid changes in air pressure during descent
   X● W94.31 Exposure to sudden change in air pressure in aircraft during descent
   X● W94.32 Exposure to high air pressure from rapid descent in water
   X● W94.39 Exposure to other rapid changes in air pressure during descent

X● W99 Exposure to other man-made environmental factors

The appropriate 7th character is to be added to code W99

> A initial encounter
> D subsequent encounter
> S sequela

EXPOSURE TO SMOKE, FIRE AND FLAMES (X00-X08)

Excludes1 arson (X97)
Excludes2 explosions (W35-W40)
      lightning (T75.0-)
      transport accident (V01-V99)

● X00 Exposure to uncontrolled fire in building or structure
Includes conflagration in building or structure
Code first any associated cataclysm
Excludes2 exposure to ignition or melting of nightwear (X05)
      exposure to ignition or melting of other clothing and apparel (X06.-)
      exposure to other specified smoke, fire and flames (X08.-)

The appropriate 7th character is to be added to each code from category X00

> A initial encounter
> D subsequent encounter
> S sequela

X● X00.0 Exposure to flames in uncontrolled fire in building or structure
     Coding Clinic: 2016, Q2, P5-6; 2015, Q1, P19
X● X00.1 Exposure to smoke in uncontrolled fire in building or structure

X● X00.2 Injury due to collapse of burning building or structure in uncontrolled fire
    Excludes1 injury due to collapse of building not on fire (W20.1)
X● X00.3 Fall from burning building or structure in uncontrolled fire
X● X00.4 Hit by object from burning building or structure in uncontrolled fire
X● X00.5 Jump from burning building or structure in uncontrolled fire
X● X00.8 Other exposure to uncontrolled fire in building or structure

● X01 Exposure to uncontrolled fire, not in building or structure
Includes exposure to forest fire
The appropriate 7th character is to be added to each code from category X01

> A initial encounter
> D subsequent encounter
> S sequela

X● X01.0 Exposure to flames in uncontrolled fire, not in building or structure
X● X01.1 Exposure to smoke in uncontrolled fire, not in building or structure
X● X01.3 Fall due to uncontrolled fire, not in building or structure
X● X01.4 Hit by object due to uncontrolled fire, not in building or structure
X● X01.8 Other exposure to uncontrolled fire, not in building or structure

● X02 Exposure to controlled fire in building or structure
Includes exposure to fire in fireplace exposure to fire in stove
The appropriate 7th character is to be added to each code from category X02

> A initial encounter
> D subsequent encounter
> S sequela

X● X02.0 Exposure to flames in controlled fire in building or structure
X● X02.1 Exposure to smoke in controlled fire in building or structure
X● X02.2 Injury due to collapse of burning building or structure in controlled fire
    Excludes1 injury due to collapse of building not on fire (W20.1)
X● X02.3 Fall from burning building or structure in controlled fire
X● X02.4 Hit by object from burning building or structure in controlled fire
X● X02.5 Jump from burning building or structure in controlled fire
X● X02.8 Other exposure to controlled fire in building or structure

● X03 Exposure to controlled fire, not in building or structure
Includes exposure to bon fire exposure to camp fire exposure to trash fire
The appropriate 7th character is to be added to each code from category X03

> A initial encounter
> D subsequent encounter
> S sequela

X● X03.0 Exposure to flames in controlled fire, not in building or structure
     Coding Clinic: 2015, Q1, P19
X● X03.1 Exposure to smoke in controlled fire, not in building or structure
X● X03.3 Fall due to controlled fire, not in building or structure
X● X03.4 Hit by object due to controlled fire, not in building or structure
X● X03.8 Other exposure to controlled fire, not in building or structure

X ● **X04 Exposure to ignition of highly flammable material**
Exposure to ignition of gasoline
Exposure to ignition of kerosene
Exposure to ignition of petrol
     Excludes2   exposure to ignition or melting of nightwear
                (X05)
            exposure to ignition or melting of other clothing
                and apparel (X06)
The appropriate 7th character is to be added to code X04

A	initial encounter
D	subsequent encounter
S	sequela

Coding Clinic: 2016, Q2, P4

X ● **X05 Exposure to ignition or melting of nightwear**
     Excludes2   exposure to uncontrolled fire in building or
                structure (X00.-)
            exposure to uncontrolled fire, not in building or
                structure (X01.-)
            exposure to controlled fire in building or
                structure (X02.-)
            exposure to controlled fire, not in building or
                structure (X03.-)
            exposure to ignition of highly flammable
                materials (X04.-)
The appropriate 7th character is to be added to code X05

A	initial encounter
D	subsequent encounter
S	sequela

X ● **X06 Exposure to ignition or melting of other clothing and apparel**
     Excludes2   exposure to uncontrolled fire in building or
                structure (X00.-)
            exposure to uncontrolled fire, not in building or
                structure (X01.-)
            exposure to controlled fire in building or
                structure (X02.-)
            exposure to controlled fire, not in building or
                structure (X03.-)
            exposure to ignition of highly flammable
                materials (X04.-)
The appropriate 7th character is to be added to each code from
     category X06

A	initial encounter
D	subsequent encounter
S	sequela

X ● **X06.0 Exposure to ignition of plastic jewelry**
X ● **X06.1 Exposure to melting of plastic jewelry**
X ● **X06.2 Exposure to ignition of other clothing and apparel**
X ● **X06.3 Exposure to melting of other clothing and apparel**

● **X08 Exposure to other specified smoke, fire and flames**
The appropriate 7th character is to be added to each code from
     category X08

A	initial encounter
D	subsequent encounter
S	sequela

● **X08.0 Exposure to bed fire**
Exposure to mattress fire
X ● **X08.00 Exposure to bed fire due to unspecified burning material**
X ● **X08.01 Exposure to bed fire due to burning cigarette**
       Coding Clinic: 2015, Q1, P19
X ● **X08.09 Exposure to bed fire due to other burning material**

● **X08.1 Exposure to sofa fire**
X ● **X08.10 Exposure to sofa fire due to unspecified burning material**
X ● **X08.11 Exposure to sofa fire due to burning cigarette**
X ● **X08.19 Exposure to sofa fire due to other burning material**
● **X08.2 Exposure to other furniture fire**
X ● **X08.20 Exposure to other furniture fire due to unspecified burning material**
X ● **X08.21 Exposure to other furniture fire due to burning cigarette**
X ● **X08.29 Exposure to other furniture fire due to other burning material**
X ● **X08.8 Exposure to other specified smoke, fire and flames**

CONTACT WITH HEAT AND HOT SUBSTANCES (X10-X19)

     Excludes1   exposure to excessive natural heat (X30)
           ➡ exposure to fire and flames (X00-X08)

● **X10 Contact with hot drinks, food, fats and cooking oils**
The appropriate 7th character is to be added to each code from
     category X10

A	initial encounter
D	subsequent encounter
S	sequela

X ● **X10.0 Contact with hot drinks**
X ● **X10.1 Contact with hot food**
X ● **X10.2 Contact with fats and cooking oils**

● **X11 Contact with hot tap-water**
     Includes   contact with boiling tap-water
               contact with boiling water NOS
     Excludes1   contact with water heated on stove (X12)
The appropriate 7th character is to be added to each code from
     category X11

A	initial encounter
D	subsequent encounter
S	sequela

X ● **X11.0 Contact with hot water in bath or tub**
       Excludes1   contact with running hot water in bath or
                   tub (X11.1)
X ● **X11.1 Contact with running hot water**
Contact with hot water running out of hose
Contact with hot water running out of tap
X ● **X11.8 Contact with other hot tap-water**
Contact with hot water in bucket
Contact with hot tap-water NOS

X ● **X12 Contact with other hot fluids**
Contact with water heated on stove
     Excludes1   hot (liquid) metals (X18)
The appropriate 7th character is to be added to code X12

A	initial encounter
D	subsequent encounter
S	sequela

● **X13 Contact with steam and other hot vapors**
The appropriate 7th character is to be added to each code from
     category X13

A	initial encounter
D	subsequent encounter
S	sequela

X ● **X13.0 Inhalation of steam and other hot vapors**
X ● **X13.1 Other contact with steam and other hot vapors**

● **X14**   **Contact with hot air and other hot gases**

The appropriate 7th character is to be added to each code from category X14

A	initial encounter
D	subsequent encounter
S	sequela

X● **X14.0**   **Inhalation of hot air and gases**

X● **X14.1**   **Other contact with hot air and other hot gases**

● **X15**   **Contact with hot household appliances**

> **Excludes1**   contact with heating appliances (X16)
> contact with powered household appliances (W29.-)
> exposure to controlled fire in building or structure due to household appliance (X02.8)
> exposure to household appliances electrical current (W86.0)

The appropriate 7th character is to be added to each code from category X15

A	initial encounter
D	subsequent encounter
S	sequela

X● **X15.0**   **Contact with hot stove (kitchen)**

X● **X15.1**   **Contact with hot toaster**

X● **X15.2**   **Contact with hotplate**

X● **X15.3**   **Contact with hot saucepan or skillet**

X● **X15.8**   **Contact with other hot household appliances**
> Contact with cooker
> Contact with kettle
> Contact with light bulbs

X● **X16**   **Contact with hot heating appliances, radiators and pipes**

> **Excludes1**   contact with powered appliances (W29.-)
> exposure to controlled fire in building or structure due to appliance (X02.8)
> exposure to industrial appliances electrical current (W86.1)

The appropriate 7th character is to be added to code X16

A	initial encounter
D	subsequent encounter
S	sequela

X● **X17**   **Contact with hot engines, machinery and tools**

> **Excludes1**   contact with hot heating appliances, radiators and pipes (X16)
> contact with hot household appliances (X15)

The appropriate 7th character is to be added to code X17

A	initial encounter
D	subsequent encounter
S	sequela

X● **X18**   **Contact with other hot metals**
> Contact with liquid metal

The appropriate 7th character is to be added to code X18

A	initial encounter
D	subsequent encounter
S	sequela

X● **X19**   **Contact with other heat and hot substances**

> **Excludes1** ▸ objects that are not normally hot, e.g., an object made hot by a house fire (X00-X08)

The appropriate 7th character is to be added to code X19

A	initial encounter
D	subsequent encounter
S	sequela

EXPOSURE TO FORCES OF NATURE (X30-X39)

X● **X30**   **Exposure to excessive natural heat**
> Exposure to excessive heat as the cause of sunstroke
> Exposure to heat NOS

> **Excludes1**   excessive heat of man-made origin (W92)
> exposure to man-made radiation (W89)
> exposure to sunlight (X32)
> exposure to tanning bed (W89)

The appropriate 7th character is to be added to code X30

A	initial encounter
D	subsequent encounter
S	sequela

X● **X31**   **Exposure to excessive natural cold**
> Excessive cold as the cause of chilblains NOS
> Excessive cold as the cause of immersion foot or hand
> Exposure to cold NOS
> Exposure to weather conditions

> **Excludes1**   cold of man-made origin (W93.-)
> contact with or inhalation of dry ice (W93.-)
> contact with or inhalation of liquefied gas (W93.-)

The appropriate 7th character is to be added to code X31

A	initial encounter
D	subsequent encounter
S	sequela

X● **X32**   **Exposure to sunlight**

> **Excludes1**   man-made radiation (tanning bed) (W89)

> ▸ **Excludes2**   radiation-related disorders of the skin and subcutaneous tissue (L55-L59)

The appropriate 7th character is to be added to code X32

A	initial encounter
D	subsequent encounter
S	sequela

X● **X34**   **Earthquake**

> **Excludes2**   tidal wave (tsunami) due to earthquake (X37.41)

The appropriate 7th character is to be added to code X34

A	initial encounter
D	subsequent encounter
S	sequela

X● **X35**   **Volcanic eruption**

> **Excludes2**   tidal wave (tsunami) due to volcanic eruption (X37.41)

The appropriate 7th character is to be added to code X35

A	initial encounter
D	subsequent encounter
S	sequela

● **X36**   **Avalanche, landslide and other earth movements**

> **Includes**   victim of mudslide of cataclysmic nature

> **Excludes1**   earthquake (X34)

> **Excludes2**   transport accident involving collision with avalanche or landslide not in motion (V01-V99)

The appropriate 7th character is to be added to each code from category X36

A	initial encounter
D	subsequent encounter
S	sequela

X● **X36.0**   **Collapse of dam or man-made structure causing earth movement**

X● **X36.1**   **Avalanche, landslide, or mudslide**

N Newborn Age: 0   **P** Pediatric Age: 0–17   **M** Maternity DX: 12–55   **A** Adult Age: 15–124   ♀ Females Only   ♂ Males Only

🔖 Complication\Comorbidity   🔖 Major C\C   (Ex) CC/MCC Exclusions   🔖 Hospital-Acquired Condition

1557

CHAPTER 20 (V01-Y99)

CHAPTER 20 (V01-Y99)

● **X37   Cataclysmic storm**

The appropriate 7th character is to be added to each code from category X37

A	initial encounter
D	subsequent encounter
S	sequela

X● **X37.0   Hurricane**
Storm surge   Typhoon

X● **X37.1   Tornado**
Cyclone   Twister

X● **X37.2   Blizzard (snow) (ice)**

X● **X37.3   Dust storm**

● **X37.4   Tidalwave**

     X● **X37.41   Tidal wave due to earthquake or volcanic eruption**
         Tidal wave NOS
         Tsunami

     X● **X37.42   Tidal wave due to storm**

     X● **X37.43   Tidal wave due to landslide**

X● **X37.8   Other cataclysmic storms**
Cloudburst
Torrential rain

> **Excludes2**   flood (X38)

X● **X37.9   Unspecified cataclysmic storm**
Storm NOS

> **Excludes1**   collapse of dam or man-made structure causing earth movement (X39.0)

X● **X38   Flood**
Flood arising from remote storm
Flood of cataclysmic nature arising from melting snow
Flood resulting directly from storm

> **Excludes1**   collapse of dam or man-made structure causing earth movement (X39.0)
> tidal wave NOS (X37.41)
> tidal wave caused by storm (X37.2)

The appropriate 7th character is to be added to code X38

A	initial encounter
D	subsequent encounter
S	sequela

● **X39   Exposure to other forces of nature**

The appropriate 7th character is to be added to each code from category X39

A	initial encounter
D	subsequent encounter
S	sequela

● **X39.0   Exposure to natural radiation**

> **Excludes1**   contact with and (suspected) exposure to radon and other naturally occuring radiation (Z77.123)
> exposure to man-made radiation (W88-W90)
> exposure to sunlight (X32)

     X● **X39.01   Exposure to radon**

     X● **X39.08   Exposure to other natural radiation**

X● **X39.8   Other exposure to forces of nature**

OVEREXERTION AND STRENUOUS OR REPETITIVE MOVEMENTS (X50)

● **X50   Overexertion and strenuous or repetitive movements**

The appropriate 7th character is to be added to each code from category X50

A	initial encounter
D	subsequent encounter
S	sequela

Coding Clinic: 2016, Q4, P73-74

X● **X50.0   Overexertion from strenuous movement or load**
Lifting heavy objects
Lifting weights
Coding Clinic: 2016, Q4, P74

X● **X50.1   Overexertion from prolonged static or awkward postures**
Prolonged bending
Prolonged kneeling
Prolonged reaching
Prolonged sitting
Prolonged standing
Prolonged twisting
Static bending
Static kneeling
Static reaching
Static sitting
Static standing
Static twisting

X● **X50.3   Overexertion from repetitive movements**
Use of hand as hammer

> **Excludes2**   Overuse from prolonged static or awkward postures (X50.1)

Coding Clinic: 2016, Q4, P74

X● **X50.9   Other and unspecified overexertion or strenuous movements or postures**
Contact pressure
Contact stress

ACCIDENTAL EXPOSURE TO OTHER SPECIFIED FACTORS (X52, X58)

X● **X52   Prolonged stay in weightless environment**
Weightlessness in spacecraft (simulator)

The appropriate 7th character is to be added to code X52

A	initial encounter
D	subsequent encounter
S	sequela

X● **X58   Exposure to other specified factors**
Accident NOS
Exposure NOS

The appropriate 7th character is to be added to code X58

A	initial encounter
D	subsequent encounter
S	sequela

INTENTIONAL SELF-HARM (X71-X83)

Purposely self-inflicted injury
Suicide (attempted)

● **X71   Intentional self-harm by drowning and submersion**

The appropriate 7th character is to be added to each code from category X71

A	initial encounter
D	subsequent encounter
S	sequela

X● **X71.0   Intentional self-harm by drowning and submersion while in bathtub**

X● **X71.1   Intentional self-harm by drowning and submersion while in swimming pool**

X● **X71.2   Intentional self-harm by drowning and submersion after jump into swimming pool**

▶ New   ⇒ Revised   ~~deleted~~ Deleted   Excludes 1   Excludes 2   Includes   Use additional   Code first   Code also   Key words

OGCR Official Guidelines   ● Unacceptable Principal Diagnosis   X Assign placeholder X   ● Use Additional Character(s)   ▶ Manifestation Code   Coding Clinic

X⬤ **X71.3**   **Intentional self-harm by drowning and submersion in natural water**

X⬤ **X71.8**   **Other intentional self-harm by drowning and submersion**

X⬤ **X71.9**   **Intentional self-harm by drowning and submersion, unspecified**

X⬤ **X72**   **Intentional self-harm by handgun discharge**
Intentional self-harm by gun for single hand use
Intentional self-harm by pistol
Intentional self-harm by revolver

> **Excludes1**   Very pistol (X74.8)

The appropriate 7th character is to be added to code X72

A	initial encounter
D	subsequent encounter
S	sequela

⬤ **X73**   **Intentional self-harm by rifle, shotgun and larger firearm discharge**

> **Excludes1**   airgun (X74.Ø1)

The appropriate 7th character is to be added to each code from category X73

A	initial encounter
D	subsequent encounter
S	sequela

X⬤ **X73.Ø**   **Intentional self-harm by shotgun discharge**
X⬤ **X73.1**   **Intentional self-harm by hunting rifle discharge**
X⬤ **X73.2**   **Intentional self-harm by machine gun discharge**
X⬤ **X73.8**   **Intentional self-harm by other larger firearm discharge**
X⬤ **X73.9**   **Intentional self-harm by unspecified larger firearm discharge**

⬤ **X74**   **Intentional self-harm by other and unspecified firearm and gun discharge**

The appropriate 7th character is to be added to each code from category X74

A	initial encounter
D	subsequent encounter
S	sequela

⬤ **X74.Ø**   **Intentional self-harm by gas, air or spring-operated guns**
   X⬤ **X74.Ø1**   **Intentional self-harm by airgun**
     Intentional self-harm by BB gun discharge
     Intentional self-harm by pellet gun discharge
   X⬤ **X74.Ø2**   **Intentional self-harm by paintball gun**
   X⬤ **X74.Ø9**   **Intentional self-harm by other gas, air or spring-operated gun**
X⬤ **X74.8**   **Intentional self-harm by other firearm discharge**
     Intentional self-harm by Very pistol [flare] discharge
X⬤ **X74.9**   **Intentional self-harm by unspecified firearm discharge**

X⬤ **X75**   **Intentional self-harm by explosive material**

The appropriate 7th character is to be added to code X75

A	initial encounter
D	subsequent encounter
S	sequela

X⬤ **X76**   **Intentional self-harm by smoke, fire and flames**

The appropriate 7th character is to be added to code X76

A	initial encounter
D	subsequent encounter
S	sequela

⬤ **X77**   **Intentional self-harm by steam, hot vapors and hot objects**

The appropriate 7th character is to be added to each code from category X77

A	initial encounter
D	subsequent encounter
S	sequela

X⬤ **X77.Ø**   **Intentional self-harm by steam or hot vapors**
X⬤ **X77.1**   **Intentional self-harm by hot tap water**
X⬤ **X77.2**   **Intentional self-harm by other hot fluids**
X⬤ **X77.3**   **Intentional self-harm by hot household appliances**
X⬤ **X77.8**   **Intentional self-harm by other hot objects**
X⬤ **X77.9**   **Intentional self-harm by unspecified hot objects**

⬤ **X78**   **Intentional self-harm by sharp object**

The appropriate 7th character is to be added to each code from category X78

A	initial encounter
D	subsequent encounter
S	sequela

X⬤ **X78.Ø**   **Intentional self-harm by sharp glass**
X⬤ **X78.1**   **Intentional self-harm by knife**
X⬤ **X78.2**   **Intentional self-harm by sword or dagger**
X⬤ **X78.8**   **Intentional self-harm by other sharp object**
X⬤ **X78.9**   **Intentional self-harm by unspecified sharp object**

X⬤ **X79**   **Intentional self-harm by blunt object**

The appropriate 7th character is to be added to code X79

A	initial encounter
D	subsequent encounter
S	sequela

X⬤ **X80**   **Intentional self-harm by jumping from a high place**
Intentional fall from one level to another

The appropriate 7th character is to be added to code X80

A	initial encounter
D	subsequent encounter
S	sequela

⬤ **X81**   **Intentional self-harm by jumping or lying in front of moving object**

The appropriate 7th character is to be added to each code from category X81

A	initial encounter
D	subsequent encounter
S	sequela

X⬤ **X81.Ø**   **Intentional self-harm by jumping or lying in front of motor vehicle**
X⬤ **X81.1**   **Intentional self-harm by jumping or lying in front of (subway) train**
X⬤ **X81.8**   **Intentional self-harm by jumping or lying in front of other moving object**

⬤ **X82**   **Intentional self-harm by crashing of motor vehicle**

The appropriate 7th character is to be added to each code from category X82

A	initial encounter
D	subsequent encounter
S	sequela

X⬤ **X82.Ø**   **Intentional collision of motor vehicle with other motor vehicle**
X⬤ **X82.1**   **Intentional collision of motor vehicle with train**
X⬤ **X82.2**   **Intentional collision of motor vehicle with tree**
X⬤ **X82.8**   **Other intentional self-harm by crashing of motor vehicle**

CHAPTER 2Ø (VØ1-Y99)

● **X83**   **Intentional self-harm by other specified means**
> **Excludes1**   intentional self-harm by poisoning or contact with toxic substance - see Table of Drugs and Chemicals
>
> The appropriate 7th character is to be added to each code from category X83
>
> | A | initial encounter |
> | D | subsequent encounter |
> | S | sequela |

X● **X83.0**   **Intentional self-harm by crashing of aircraft**
X● **X83.1**   **Intentional self-harm by electrocution**
X● **X83.2**   **Intentional self-harm by exposure to extremes of cold**
X● **X83.8**   **Intentional self-harm by other specified means**

ASSAULT (X92-Y09)

> **Includes**   homicide injuries inflicted by another person with intent to injure or kill, by any means
>
> **Excludes1**   injuries due to legal intervention (Y35.-)
> injuries due to operations of war (Y36.-)
> injuries due to terrorism (Y38.-)

● **X92**   **Assault by drowning and submersion**
> The appropriate 7th character is to be added to each code from category X92
>
> | A | initial encounter |
> | D | subsequent encounter |
> | S | sequela |

X● **X92.0**   **Assault by drowning and submersion while in bathtub**
X● **X92.1**   **Assault by drowning and submersion while in swimming pool**
X● **X92.2**   **Assault by drowning and submersion after push into swimming pool**
X● **X92.3**   **Assault by drowning and submersion in natural water**
X● **X92.8**   **Other assault by drowning and submersion**
X● **X92.9**   **Assault by drowning and submersion, unspecified**

X● **X93**   **Assault by handgun discharge**
> Assault by discharge of gun for single hand use
> Assault by discharge of pistol
> Assault by discharge of revolver
>
> **Excludes1**   Very pistol (X95.8)
>
> The appropriate 7th character is to be added to code X93
>
> | A | initial encounter |
> | D | subsequent encounter |
> | S | sequela |

● **X94**   **Assault by rifle, shotgun and larger firearm discharge**
> **Excludes1**   airgun (X95.01)
>
> The appropriate 7th character is to be added to each code from category X94
>
> | A | initial encounter |
> | D | subsequent encounter |
> | S | sequela |

X● **X94.0**   **Assault by shotgun**
X● **X94.1**   **Assault by hunting rifle**
X● **X94.2**   **Assault by machine gun**
X● **X94.8**   **Assault by other larger firearm discharge**
X● **X94.9**   **Assault by unspecified larger firearm discharge**

● **X95**   **Assault by other and unspecified firearm and gun discharge**
> The appropriate 7th character is to be added to each code from category X95
>
> | A | initial encounter |
> | D | subsequent encounter |
> | S | sequela |

● **X95.0**   **Assault by gas, air or spring-operated guns**
X● **X95.01**   **Assault by airgun discharge**
> Assault by BB gun discharge
> Assault by pellet gun discharge
X● **X95.02**   **Assault by paintball gun discharge**
X● **X95.09**   **Assault by other gas, air or spring-operated gun**
X● **X95.8**   **Assault by other firearm discharge**
> Assault by very pistol [flare] discharge
X● **X95.9**   **Assault by unspecified firearm discharge**
> Coding Clinic: 2016, Q3, P24

● **X96**   **Assault by explosive material**
> **Excludes1**   incendiary device (X97)
> terrorism involving explosive material (Y38.2-)
>
> The appropriate 7th character is to be added to each code from category X96
>
> | A | initial encounter |
> | D | subsequent encounter |
> | S | sequela |

X● **X96.0**   **Assault by antipersonnel bomb**
> **Excludes1**   antipersonnel bomb use in military or war (Y36.2-)
X● **X96.1**   **Assault by gasoline bomb**
X● **X96.2**   **Assault by letter bomb**
X● **X96.3**   **Assault by fertilizer bomb**
X● **X96.4**   **Assault by pipe bomb**
X● **X96.8**   **Assault by other specified explosive**
X● **X96.9**   **Assault by unspecified explosive**

X● **X97**   **Assault by smoke, fire and flames**
> Assault by arson
> Assault by cigarettes
> Assault by incendiary device
>
> The appropriate 7th character is to be added to code X97
>
> | A | initial encounter |
> | D | subsequent encounter |
> | S | sequela |

● **X98**   **Assault by steam, hot vapors and hot objects**
> The appropriate 7th character is to be added to each code from category X98
>
> | A | initial encounter |
> | D | subsequent encounter |
> | S | sequela |

X● **X98.0**   **Assault by steam or hot vapors**
X● **X98.1**   **Assault by hot tap water**
X● **X98.2**   **Assault by hot fluids**
X● **X98.3**   **Assault by hot household appliances**
X● **X98.8**   **Assault by other hot objects**
X● **X98.9**   **Assault by unspecified hot objects**

● **X99**   **Assault by sharp object**

> **Excludes1**   assault by strike by sports equipment (Y08.0-)
>
> The appropriate 7th character is to be added to each code from category X99

> | | |
> |---|---|
> | A | initial encounter |
> | D | subsequent encounter |
> | S | sequela |

   X● **X99.0**   **Assault by sharp glass**
   X● **X99.1**   **Assault by knife**
   X● **X99.2**   **Assault by sword or dagger**
   X● **X99.8**   **Assault by other sharp object**
   X● **X99.9**   **Assault by unspecified sharp object**
         Assault by stabbing NOS

X● **Y00**   **Assault by blunt object**

> **Excludes1**   assault by strike by sports equipment (Y08.0)
>
> The appropriate 7th character is to be added to code Y00

> | | |
> |---|---|
> | A | initial encounter |
> | D | subsequent encounter |
> | S | sequela |

X● **Y01**   **Assault by pushing from high place**

> The appropriate 7th character is to be added to code Y01

> | | |
> |---|---|
> | A | initial encounter |
> | D | subsequent encounter |
> | S | sequela |

● **Y02**   **Assault by pushing or placing victim in front of moving object**

> The appropriate 7th character is to be added to each code from category Y02

> | | |
> |---|---|
> | A | initial encounter |
> | D | subsequent encounter |
> | S | sequela |

   X● **Y02.0**   **Assault by pushing or placing victim in front of motor vehicle**
   X● **Y02.1**   **Assault by pushing or placing victim in front of (subway) train**
   X● **Y02.8**   **Assault by pushing or placing victim in front of other moving object**

● **Y03**   **Assault by crashing of motor vehicle**

> The appropriate 7th character is to be added to each code from category Y03

> | | |
> |---|---|
> | A | initial encounter |
> | D | subsequent encounter |
> | S | sequela |

   X● **Y03.0**   **Assault by being hit or run over by motor vehicle**
   X● **Y03.8**   **Other assault by crashing of motor vehicle**

● **Y04**   **Assault by bodily force**

> **Excludes1**   assault by:
>   submersion (X92.-)
>   use of weapon (X93-X95, X99, Y00)
>
> The appropriate 7th character is to be added to each code from category Y04

> | | |
> |---|---|
> | A | initial encounter |
> | D | subsequent encounter |
> | S | sequela |

   X● **Y04.0**   **Assault by unarmed brawl or fight**
   X● **Y04.1**   **Assault by human bite**
   X● **Y04.2**   **Assault by strike against or bumped into by another person**
   X● **Y04.8**   **Assault by other bodily force**
         Assault by bodily force NOS

OGCR Section I.C.19.f.

> Adult and child abuse, neglect and other maltreatment
>
> Sequence first the appropriate code from categories T74 or T76 for abuse, neglect and other maltreatment, followed by any accompanying mental health or injury code(s).
>
> If the documentation in the medical record states abuse or neglect it is coded as confirmed (T74.-). It is coded as suspected if it is documented as suspected (T76.-).
>
> For cases of confirmed abuse or neglect an external cause code from the assault section (X92-Y09) should be added to identify the cause of any physical injuries. A perpetrator code (Y07) should be added when the perpetrator of the abuse is known. For suspected cases of abuse or neglect, do not report external cause or perpetrator code.
>
> If a suspected case of abuse, neglect or mistreatment is ruled out during an encounter code Z04.71, Encounter for examination and observation following alleged physical adult abuse, ruled out, or code Z04.72, Encounter for examination and observation following alleged adult rape, should be used, not a code from T76.
>
> If a suspected case of alleged rape or sexual abuse is ruled out during an encounter code Z04.41, Encounter for examination and observation following alleged adult rape or code Z04.42, Encounter for examination and observation following alleged child rape should be used, not a code from T76.

● **Y07**   **Perpetrator of assault, maltreatment and neglect**

> **Note:** Codes from this category are for use only in cases of confirmed abuse (T74.-)
>
> > Selection of the correct perpetrator code is based on the relationship between the perpetrator and the victim
>
> **Includes**   perpetrator of abandonment
>   perpetrator of emotional neglect
>   perpetrator of mental cruelty
>   perpetrator of physical abuse
>   perpetrator of physical neglect
>   perpetrator of sexual abuse
>   perpetrator of torture

Coding Clinic: 2016, Q4, P129

● **Y07.0**   **Spouse or partner, perpetrator of maltreatment and neglect**
> Spouse or partner, perpetrator of maltreatment and neglect against spouse or partner

     Y07.01   **Husband, perpetrator of maltreatment and neglect**
     Y07.02   **Wife, perpetrator of maltreatment and neglect**
     Y07.03   **Male partner, perpetrator of maltreatment and neglect**
     Y07.04   **Female partner, perpetrator of maltreatment and neglect**

● **Y07.1**   **Parent (adoptive) (biological), perpetrator of maltreatment and neglect**

     Y07.11   **Biological father, perpetrator of maltreatment and neglect**
     Y07.12   **Biological mother, perpetrator of maltreatment and neglect**
     Y07.13   **Adoptive father, perpetrator of maltreatment and neglect**
     Y07.14   **Adoptive mother, perpetrator of maltreatment and neglect**

● **Y07.4**   **Other family member, perpetrator of maltreatment and neglect**

   ● **Y07.41**   **Sibling, perpetrator of maltreatment and neglect**

> > **Excludes1**   stepsibling, perpetrator of maltreatment and neglect (Y07.435, Y07.436)

       Y07.410   **Brother, perpetrator of maltreatment and neglect**
       Y07.411   **Sister, perpetrator of maltreatment and neglect**

N Newborn Age: 0   **P** Pediatric Age: 0–17   **M** Maternity DX: 12–55   **A** Adult Age: 15–124   ♀ Females Only   ♂ Males Only

● Complication\Comorbidity   Major C\C   (Ex) CC/MCC Exclusions   Hospital-Acquired Condition

1561

● **Y07.42 Foster parent,** perpetrator of maltreatment and neglect

    Y07.420 Foster father, perpetrator of maltreatment and neglect

    Y07.421 Foster mother, perpetrator of maltreatment and neglect

● **Y07.43 Stepparent or stepsibling,** perpetrator of maltreatment and neglect

    Y07.430 Stepfather, perpetrator of maltreatment and neglect

    Y07.432 Male friend of parent (co-residing in household), perpetrator of maltreatment and neglect

    Y07.433 Stepmother, perpetrator of maltreatment and neglect

    Y07.434 Female friend of parent (co-residing in household), perpetrator of maltreatment and neglect

    Y07.435 Stepbrother, perpetrator or maltreatment and neglect

    Y07.436 Stepsister, perpetrator of maltreatment and neglect

● **Y07.49 Other family member,** perpetrator of maltreatment and neglect

    Y07.490 Male cousin, perpetrator of maltreatment and neglect

    Y07.491 Female cousin, perpetrator of maltreatment and neglect

    Y07.499 Other family member, perpetrator of maltreatment and neglect

● **Y07.5 Non-family member,** perpetrator of maltreatment and neglect

    Y07.50 Unspecified non-family member, perpetrator of maltreatment and neglect

● **Y07.51 Daycare provider,** perpetrator of maltreatment and neglect

    Y07.510 At-home childcare provider, perpetrator of maltreatment and neglect

    Y07.511 Daycare center childcare provider, perpetrator of maltreatment and neglect

    Y07.512 At-home adultcare provider, perpetrator of maltreatment and neglect

    Y07.513 Adultcare center provider, perpetrator of maltreatment and neglect

    Y07.519 Unspecified daycare provider, perpetrator of maltreatment and neglect

● **Y07.52 Healthcare provider,** perpetrator of maltreatment and neglect

    Y07.521 Mental health provider, perpetrator of maltreatment and neglect

    Y07.528 Other therapist or healthcare provider, perpetrator of maltreatment and neglect

       Nurse perpetrator of maltreatment and neglect

       Occupational therapist perpetrator of maltreatment and neglect

       Physical therapist perpetrator of maltreatment and neglect

       Speech therapist perpetrator of maltreatment and neglect

    Y07.529 Unspecified healthcare provider, perpetrator of maltreatment and neglect

    Y07.53 Teacher or instructor, perpetrator of maltreatment and neglect

       Coach, perpetrator of maltreatment and neglect

    Y07.59 Other non-family member, perpetrator of maltreatment and neglect

    Y07.9 Unspecified perpetrator of maltreatment and neglect

● **Y08 Assault by other specified means**

The appropriate 7th character is to be added to each code from category Y08

A	initial encounter
D	subsequent encounter
S	sequela

● **Y08.0 Assault by strike by sport equipment**

  X● **Y08.01 Assault by strike by hockey stick**

  X● **Y08.02 Assault by strike by baseball bat**

  X● **Y08.09 Assault by strike by other specified type of sport equipment**

● **Y08.8 Assault by other specified means**

  X● **Y08.81 Assault by crashing of aircraft**

  X● **Y08.89 Assault by other specified means**

● **Y09 Assault by unspecified means**

  Assassination (attempted) NOS
  Homicide (attempted) NOS
  Manslaughter (attempted) NOS
  Murder (attempted) NOS

EVENT OF UNDETERMINED INTENT (Y21-Y33)

Undetermined intent is only for use when there is specific documentation in the record that the intent of the injury cannot be determined. If no such documentation is present, code to accidental (unintentional)

● **Y21 Drowning and submersion, undetermined intent**

The appropriate 7th character is to be added to each code from category Y21

A	initial encounter
D	subsequent encounter
S	sequela

  X● **Y21.0 Drowning and submersion while in bathtub, undetermined intent**

  X● **Y21.1 Drowning and submersion after fall into bathtub, undetermined intent**

  X● **Y21.2 Drowning and submersion while in swimming pool, undetermined intent**

  X● **Y21.3 Drowning and submersion after fall into swimming pool, undetermined intent**

  X● **Y21.4 Drowning and submersion in natural water, undetermined intent**

  X● **Y21.8 Other drowning and submersion, undetermined intent**

  X● **Y21.9 Unspecified drowning and submersion, undetermined intent**

X● **Y22 Handgun discharge, undetermined intent**

  Discharge of gun for single hand use, undetermined intent
  Discharge of pistol, undetermined intent
  Discharge of revolver, undetermined intent

  Excludes2 very pistol (Y24.8)

The appropriate 7th character is to be added to code Y22

A	initial encounter
D	subsequent encounter
S	sequela

● **Y23 Rifle, shotgun and larger firearm discharge, undetermined intent**

> **Excludes2** airgun (Y24.0)

> The appropriate 7th character is to be added to each code from category Y23

A	initial encounter
D	subsequent encounter
S	sequela

X● **Y23.0 Shotgun discharge, undetermined intent**
X● **Y23.1 Hunting rifle discharge, undetermined intent**
X● **Y23.2 Military firearm discharge, undetermined intent**
X● **Y23.3 Machine gun discharge, undetermined intent**
X● **Y23.8 Other larger firearm discharge, undetermined intent**
X● **Y23.9 Unspecified larger firearm discharge, undetermined intent**

● **Y24 Other and unspecified firearm discharge, undetermined intent**

> The appropriate 7th character is to be added to each code from category Y24

A	initial encounter
D	subsequent encounter
S	sequela

X● **Y24.0 Airgun discharge, undetermined intent**
> BB gun discharge, undetermined intent
> Pellet gun discharge, undetermined intent
X● **Y24.8 Other firearm discharge, undetermined intent**
> Paintball gun discharge, undetermined intent
> Very pistol [flare] discharge, undetermined intent
X● **Y24.9 Unspecified firearm discharge, undetermined intent**

X● **Y25 Contact with explosive material, undetermined intent**

> The appropriate 7th character is to be added to code Y25

A	initial encounter
D	subsequent encounter
S	sequela

X● **Y26 Exposure to smoke, fire and flames, undetermined intent**

> The appropriate 7th character is to be added to code Y26

A	initial encounter
D	subsequent encounter
S	sequela

● **Y27 Contact with steam, hot vapors and hot objects, undetermined intent**

> The appropriate 7th character is to be added to each code from category Y27

A	initial encounter
D	subsequent encounter
S	sequela

X● **Y27.0 Contact with steam and hot vapors, undetermined intent**
X● **Y27.1 Contact with hot tap water, undetermined intent**
X● **Y27.2 Contact with hot fluids, undetermined intent**
X● **Y27.3 Contact with hot household appliance, undetermined intent**
X● **Y27.8 Contact with other hot objects, undetermined intent**
X● **Y27.9 Contact with unspecified hot objects, undetermined intent**

● **Y28 Contact with sharp object, undetermined intent**

> The appropriate 7th character is to be added to each code from category Y28

A	initial encounter
D	subsequent encounter
S	sequela

X● **Y28.0 Contact with sharp glass, undetermined intent**
X● **Y28.1 Contact with knife, undetermined intent**
X● **Y28.2 Contact with sword or dagger, undetermined intent**
X● **Y28.8 Contact with other sharp object, undetermined intent**
X● **Y28.9 Contact with unspecified sharp object, undetermined intent**

X● **Y29 Contact with blunt object, undetermined intent**

> The appropriate 7th character is to be added to code Y29

A	initial encounter
D	subsequent encounter
S	sequela

X● **Y30 Falling, jumping or pushed from a high place, undetermined intent**

> Victim falling from one level to another, undetermined intent
> The appropriate 7th character is to be added to code Y30

A	initial encounter
D	subsequent encounter
S	sequela

X● **Y31 Falling, lying or running before or into moving object, undetermined intent**

> The appropriate 7th character is to be added to code Y31

A	initial encounter
D	subsequent encounter
S	sequela

X● **Y32 Crashing of motor vehicle, undetermined intent**

> The appropriate 7th character is to be added to code Y32

A	initial encounter
D	subsequent encounter
S	sequela

X● **Y33 Other specified events, undetermined intent**

> The appropriate 7th character is to be added to code Y33

A	initial encounter
D	subsequent encounter
S	sequela

CHAPTER 20 (V01-Y99)

LEGAL INTERVENTION, OPERATIONS OF WAR, MILITARY OPERATIONS, AND TERRORISM (Y35-Y38)

● **Y35   Legal intervention**

     Includes   any injury sustained as a result of an encounter with any law enforcement official, serving in any capacity at the time of the encounter, whether on-duty or off-duty. Includes: injury to law enforcement official, suspect and bystander

     The appropriate 7th character is to be added to each code from category Y35

       A   initial encounter
       D   subsequent encounter
       S   sequela

● **Y35.0   Legal intervention involving firearm discharge**

   ● **Y35.00   Legal intervention involving unspecified firearm discharge**
            Legal intervention involving gunshot wound
            Legal intervention involving shot NOS

     ● **Y35.001   Legal intervention involving unspecified firearm discharge, law enforcement official injured**

     ● **Y35.002   Legal intervention involving unspecified firearm discharge, bystander injured**

     ● **Y35.003   Legal intervention involving unspecified firearm discharge, suspect injured**

   ● **Y35.01   Legal intervention involving injury by machine gun**

     ● **Y35.011   Legal intervention involving injury by machine gun, law enforcement official injured**

     ● **Y35.012   Legal intervention involving injury by machine gun, bystander injured**

     ● **Y35.013   Legal intervention involving injury by machine gun, suspect injured**

   ● **Y35.02   Legal intervention involving injury by handgun**

     ● **Y35.021   Legal intervention involving injury by handgun, law enforcement official injured**

     ● **Y35.022   Legal intervention involving injury by handgun, bystander injured**

     ● **Y35.023   Legal intervention involving injury by handgun, suspect injured**

   ● **Y35.03   Legal intervention involving injury by rifle pellet**

     ● **Y35.031   Legal intervention involving injury by rifle pellet, law enforcement official injured**

     ● **Y35.032   Legal intervention involving injury by rifle pellet, bystander injured**

     ● **Y35.033   Legal intervention involving injury by rifle pellet, suspect injured**

   ● **Y35.04   Legal intervention involving injury by rubber bullet**

     ● **Y35.041   Legal intervention involving injury by rubber bullet, law enforcement official injured**

     ● **Y35.042   Legal intervention involving injury by rubber bullet, bystander injured**

     ● **Y35.043   Legal intervention involving injury by rubber bullet, suspect injured**

   ● **Y35.09   Legal intervention involving other firearm discharge**

     ● **Y35.091   Legal intervention involving other firearm discharge, law enforcement official injured**

     ● **Y35.092   Legal intervention involving other firearm discharge, bystander injured**

     ● **Y35.093   Legal intervention involving other firearm discharge, suspect injured**

● **Y35.1   Legal intervention involving explosives**

   ● **Y35.10   Legal intervention involving unspecified explosives**

     ● **Y35.101   Legal intervention involving unspecified explosives, law enforcement official injured**

     ● **Y35.102   Legal intervention involving unspecified explosives, bystander injured**

     ● **Y35.103   Legal intervention involving unspecified explosives, suspect injured**

   ● **Y35.11   Legal intervention involving injury by dynamite**

     ● **Y35.111   Legal intervention involving injury by dynamite, law enforcement official injured**

     ● **Y35.112   Legal intervention involving injury by dynamite, bystander injured**

     ● **Y35.113   Legal intervention involving injury by dynamite, suspect injured**

   ● **Y35.12   Legal intervention involving injury by explosive shell**

     ● **Y35.121   Legal intervention involving injury by explosive shell, law enforcement official injured**

     ● **Y35.122   Legal intervention involving injury by explosive shell, bystander injured**

     ● **Y35.123   Legal intervention involving injury by explosive shell, suspect injured**

   ● **Y35.19   Legal intervention involving other explosives**
            Legal intervention involving injury by grenade
            Legal intervention involving injury by mortar bomb

     ● **Y35.191   Legal intervention involving other explosives, law enforcement official injured**

     ● **Y35.192   Legal intervention involving other explosives, bystander injured**

     ● **Y35.193   Legal intervention involving other explosives, suspect injured**

● **Y35.2   Legal intervention involving gas**
       Legal intervention involving asphyxiation by gas
       Legal intervention involving poisoning by gas

   ● **Y35.20   Legal intervention involving unspecified gas**

     ● **Y35.201   Legal intervention involving unspecified gas, law enforcement official injured**

     ● **Y35.202   Legal intervention involving unspecified gas, bystander injured**

     ● **Y35.203   Legal intervention involving unspecified gas, suspect injured**

▶ New   ⇒ Revised   ~~deleted~~ Deleted   Excludes 1   Excludes 2   Includes   Use additional   Code first   Code also   Key words

OGCR Official Guidelines   ● Unacceptable Principal Diagnosis   X Assign placeholder X   ● Use Additional Character(s)   ▶ Manifestation Code   **Coding Clinic**

- **Y35.21** Legal intervention involving injury by tear gas
  - **Y35.211** Legal intervention involving injury by tear gas, law enforcement official injured
  - **Y35.212** Legal intervention involving injury by tear gas, bystander injured
  - **Y35.213** Legal intervention involving injury by tear gas, suspect injured
- **Y35.29** Legal intervention involving other gas
  - **Y35.291** Legal intervention involving other gas, law enforcement official injured
  - **Y35.292** Legal intervention involving other gas, bystander injured
  - **Y35.293** Legal intervention involving other gas, suspect injured
- **Y35.3** Legal intervention involving blunt objects

  Legal intervention involving being hit or struck by blunt object
  - **Y35.30** Legal intervention involving unspecified blunt objects
    - **Y35.301** Legal intervention involving unspecified blunt objects, law enforcement official injured
    - **Y35.302** Legal intervention involving unspecified blunt objects, bystander injured
    - **Y35.303** Legal intervention involving unspecified blunt objects, suspect injured
  - **Y35.31** Legal intervention involving baton
    - **Y35.311** Legal intervention involving baton, law enforcement official injured
    - **Y35.312** Legal intervention involving baton, bystander injured
    - **Y35.313** Legal intervention involving baton, suspect injured
  - **Y35.39** Legal intervention involving other blunt objects
    - **Y35.391** Legal intervention involving other blunt objects, law enforcement official injured
    - **Y35.392** Legal intervention involving other blunt objects, bystander injured
    - **Y35.393** Legal intervention involving other blunt objects, suspect injured
- **Y35.4** Legal intervention involving sharp objects

  Legal intervention involving being cut by sharp objects

  Legal intervention involving being stabbed by sharp objects
  - **Y35.40** Legal intervention involving unspecified sharp objects
    - **Y35.401** Legal intervention involving unspecified sharp objects, law enforcement official injured
    - **Y35.402** Legal intervention involving unspecified sharp objects, bystander injured
    - **Y35.403** Legal intervention involving unspecified sharp objects, suspect injured
  - **Y35.41** Legal intervention involving bayonet
    - **Y35.411** Legal intervention involving bayonet, law enforcement official injured
    - **Y35.412** Legal intervention involving bayonet, bystander injured
    - **Y35.413** Legal intervention involving bayonet, suspect injured

- **Y35.49** Legal intervention involving other sharp objects
  - **Y35.491** Legal intervention involving other sharp objects, law enforcement official injured
  - **Y35.492** Legal intervention involving other sharp objects, bystander injured
  - **Y35.493** Legal intervention involving other sharp objects, suspect injured
- **Y35.8** Legal intervention involving other specified means
  - **Y35.81** Legal intervention involving manhandling
    - **Y35.811** Legal intervention involving manhandling, law enforcement official injured
    - **Y35.812** Legal intervention involving manhandling, bystander injured
    - **Y35.813** Legal intervention involving manhandling, suspect injured
  - **Y35.89** Legal intervention involving other specified means
    - **Y35.891** Legal intervention involving other specified means, law enforcement official injured
    - **Y35.892** Legal intervention involving other specified means, bystander injured
    - **Y35.893** Legal intervention involving other specified means, suspect injured
- **Y35.9** Legal intervention, means unspecified
  - X **Y35.91** Legal intervention, means unspecified, law enforcement official injured
  - X **Y35.92** Legal intervention, means unspecified, bystander injured
  - X **Y35.93** Legal intervention, means unspecified, suspect injured
- **Y36** Operations of war
  - **Includes** injuries to military personnel and civilians caused by war, civil insurrection, and peacekeeping missions
  - **Excludes1** injury to military personnel occurring during peacetime military operations (Y37.-)

    military vehicles involved in transport accidents with non-military vehicle during peacetime (V09.01, V09.21, V19.81, V29.81, V39.81, V49.81, V59.81, V69.81, V79.81)

  The appropriate 7th character is to be added to each code from category Y36

A	initial encounter
D	subsequent encounter
S	sequela

  - **Y36.0** War operations involving explosion of marine weapons

    Weapons and military watercraft
    - **Y36.00** War operations involving explosion of unspecified marine weapon

      War operations involving underwater blast NOS
      - **Y36.000** War operations involving explosion of unspecified marine weapon, military personnel
      - **Y36.001** War operations involving explosion of unspecified marine weapon, civilian
    - **Y36.01** War operations involving explosion of depth-charge
      - **Y36.010** War operations involving explosion of depth-charge, military personnel
      - **Y36.011** War operations involving explosion of depth-charge, civilian

● **Y36.02**   **War operations involving explosion of marine mine**
War operations involving explosion of marine mine, at sea or in harbor

● **Y36.020**   War operations involving explosion of marine mine, military personnel

● **Y36.021**   War operations involving explosion of marine mine, civilian

● **Y36.03**   **War operations involving explosion of sea-based artillery shell**

● **Y36.030**   War operations involving explosion of sea-based artillery shell, military personnel

● **Y36.031**   War operations involving explosion of sea-based artillery shell, civilian

● **Y36.04**   **War operations involving explosion of torpedo**

● **Y36.040**   War operations involving explosion of torpedo, military personnel

● **Y36.041**   War operations involving explosion of torpedo, civilian

● **Y36.05**   **War operations involving accidental detonation of onboard marine weapons**

● **Y36.050**   War operations involving accidental detonation of onboard marine weapons, military personnel

● **Y36.051**   War operations involving accidental detonation of onboard marine weapons, civilian

● **Y36.09**   **War operations involving explosion of other marine weapons**

● **Y36.090**   War operations involving explosion of other marine weapons, military personnel

● **Y36.091**   War operations involving explosion of other marine weapons, civilian

● **Y36.1**   **War operations involving destruction of aircraft**

● **Y36.10**   **War operations involving unspecified destruction of aircraft**

● **Y36.100**   War operations involving unspecified destruction of aircraft, military personnel

● **Y36.101**   War operations involving unspecified destruction of aircraft, civilian

● **Y36.11**   **War operations involving destruction of aircraft due to enemy fire or explosives**
War operations involving destruction of aircraft due to air to air missile
War operations involving destruction of aircraft due to explosive placed on aircraft
War operations involving destruction of aircraft due to rocket propelled grenade [RPG]
War operations involving destruction of aircraft due to small arms fire
War operations involving destruction of aircraft due to surface to air missile

● **Y36.110**   War operations involving destruction of aircraft due to enemy fire or explosives, military personnel

● **Y36.111**   War operations involving destruction of aircraft due to enemy fire or explosives, civilian

● **Y36.12**   **War operations involving destruction of aircraft due to collision with other aircraft**

● **Y36.120**   War operations involving destruction of aircraft due to collision with other aircraft, military personnel

● **Y36.121**   War operations involving destruction of aircraft due to collision with other aircraft, civilian

● **Y36.13**   **War operations involving destruction of aircraft due to onboard fire**

● **Y36.130**   War operations involving destruction of aircraft due to onboard fire, military personnel

● **Y36.131**   War operations involving destruction of aircraft due to onboard fire, civilian

● **Y36.14**   **War operations involving destruction of aircraft due to accidental detonation of onboard munitions and explosives**

● **Y36.140**   War operations involving destruction of aircraft due to accidental detonation of onboard munitions and explosives, military personnel

● **Y36.141**   War operations involving destruction of aircraft due to accidental detonation of onboard munitions and explosives, civilian

● **Y36.19**   **War operations involving other destruction of aircraft**

● **Y36.190**   War operations involving other destruction of aircraft, military personnel

● **Y36.191**   War operations involving other destruction of aircraft, civilian

● **Y36.2**   **War operations involving other explosions and fragments**

Excludes1   war operations involving explosion of aircraft (Y36.1-)
war operations involving explosion of marine weapons (Y36.0-)
war operations involving explosion of nuclear weapons (Y36.5-)
war operations involving explosion occurring after cessation of hostilities (Y36.8-)

● **Y36.20**   **War operations involving unspecified explosion and fragments**
War operations involving air blast NOS
War operations involving blast NOS
War operations involving blast fragments NOS
War operations involving blast wave NOS
War operations involving blast wind NOS
War operations involving explosion NOS
War operations involving explosion of bomb NOS

● **Y36.200**   War operations involving unspecified explosion and fragments, military personnel

● **Y36.201**   War operations involving unspecified explosion and fragments, civilian

● **Y36.21**   **War operations involving explosion of aerial bomb**

● **Y36.210**   War operations involving explosion of aerial bomb, military personnel

● **Y36.211**   War operations involving explosion of aerial bomb, civilian

● **Y36.22**   **War operations involving explosion of guided missile**

● **Y36.220**   War operations involving explosion of guided missile, military personnel

● **Y36.221**   War operations involving explosion of guided missile, civilian

● **Y36.23 War operations involving explosion of improvised explosive device [IED]**
War operations involving explosion of person-borne improvised explosive device [IED]
War operations involving explosion of vehicle-borne improvised explosive device [IED]
War operations involving explosion of roadside improvised explosive device [IED]

● **Y36.230 War operations involving explosion of improvised explosive device [IED], military personnel**

● **Y36.231 War operations involving explosion of improvised explosive device [IED], civilian**

● **Y36.24 War operations involving explosion due to accidental detonation and discharge of own munitions or munitions launch device**

● **Y36.240 War operations involving explosion due to accidental detonation and discharge of own munitions or munitions launch device, military personnel**

● **Y36.241 War operations involving explosion due to accidental detonation and discharge of own munitions or munitions launch device, civilian**

● **Y36.25 War operations involving fragments from munitions**

● **Y36.250 War operations involving fragments from munitions, military personnel**

● **Y36.251 War operations involving fragments from munitions, civilian**

● **Y36.26 War operations involving fragments of improvised explosive device [IED]**
War operations involving fragments of person-borne improvised explosive device [IED]
War operations involving fragments of vehicle-borne improvised explosive device [IED]
War operations involving fragments of roadside improvised explosive device [IED]

● **Y36.260 War operations involving fragments of improvised explosive device [IED], military personnel**

● **Y36.261 War operations involving fragments of improvised explosive device [IED], civilian**

● **Y36.27 War operations involving fragments from weapons**

● **Y36.270 War operations involving fragments from weapons, military personnel**

● **Y36.271 War operations involving fragments from weapons, civilian**

● **Y36.29 War operations involving other explosions and fragments**
War operations involving explosion of grenade
War operations involving explosions of land mine
War operations involving shrapnel NOS

● **Y36.290 War operations involving other explosions and fragments, military personnel**

● **Y36.291 War operations involving other explosions and fragments, civilian**

● **Y36.3 War operations involving fires, conflagrations and hot substances**
War operations involving smoke, fumes, and heat from fires, conflagrations and hot substances

Excludes1 war operations involving fires and conflagrations aboard military aircraft (Y36.1-)
war operations involving fires and conflagrations aboard military watercraft (Y36.0-)
war operations involving fires and conflagrations caused indirectly by conventional weapons (Y36.2-)
war operations involving fires and thermal effects of nuclear weapons (Y36.53-)

● **Y36.30 War operations involving unspecified fire, conflagration and hot substance**

● **Y36.300 War operations involving unspecified fire, conflagration and hot substance, military personnel**

● **Y36.301 War operations involving unspecified fire, conflagration and hot substance, civilian**

● **Y36.31 War operations involving gasoline bomb**
War operations involving incendiary bomb
War operations involving petrol bomb

● **Y36.310 War operations involving gasoline bomb, military personnel**

● **Y36.311 War operations involving gasoline bomb, civilian**

● **Y36.32 War operations involving incendiary bullet**

● **Y36.320 War operations involving incendiary bullet, military personnel**

● **Y36.321 War operations involving incendiary bullet, civilian**

● **Y36.33 War operations involving flamethrower**

● **Y36.330 War operations involving flamethrower, military personnel**

● **Y36.331 War operations involving flamethrower, civilian**

● **Y36.39 War operations involving other fires, conflagrations and hot substances**

● **Y36.390 War operations involving other fires, conflagrations and hot substances, military personnel**

● **Y36.391 War operations involving other fires, conflagrations and hot substances, civilian**

● **Y36.4 War operations involving firearm discharge and other forms of conventional warfare**

● **Y36.41 War operations involving rubber bullets**

● **Y36.410 War operations involving rubber bullets, military personnel**

● **Y36.411 War operations involving rubber bullets, civilian**

● **Y36.42 War operations involving firearms pellets**

● **Y36.420 War operations involving firearms pellets, military personnel**

● **Y36.421 War operations involving firearms pellets, civilian**

● **Y36.43**   **War operations involving other firearms discharge**
War operations involving bullets NOS

> **Excludes1**   war operations involving munitions fragments (Y36.25-)
> war operations involving incendiary bullets (Y36.32-)

● **Y36.430**   War operations involving other firearms discharge, military personnel

● **Y36.431**   War operations involving other firearms discharge, civilian

● **Y36.44**   **War operations involving unarmed hand to hand combat**

> **Excludes1**   war operations involving combat using blunt or piercing object (Y36.45-)
> war operations involving intentional restriction of air and airway (Y36.46-)
> war operations involving unintentional restriction of air and airway (Y36.47-)

● **Y36.440**   War operations involving unarmed hand to hand combat, military personnel

● **Y36.441**   War operations involving unarmed hand to hand combat, civilian

● **Y36.45**   **War operations involving combat using blunt or piercing object**

● **Y36.450**   War operations involving combat using blunt or piercing object, military personnel

● **Y36.451**   War operations involving combat using blunt or piercing object, civilian

● **Y36.46**   **War operations involving intentional restriction of air and airway**

● **Y36.460**   War operations involving intentional restriction of air and airway, military personnel

● **Y36.461**   War operations involving intentional restriction of air and airway, civilian

● **Y36.47**   **War operations involving unintentional restriction of air and airway**

● **Y36.470**   War operations involving unintentional restriction of air and airway, military personnel

● **Y36.471**   War operations involving unintentional restriction of air and airway, civilian

● **Y36.49**   **War operations involving other forms of conventional warfare**

● **Y36.490**   War operations involving other forms of conventional warfare, military personnel

● **Y36.491**   War operations involving other forms of conventional warfare, civilian

● **Y36.5**   **War operations involving nuclear weapons**
War operations involving dirty bomb NOS

● **Y36.50**   **War operations involving unspecified effect of nuclear weapon**

● **Y36.500**   War operations involving unspecified effect of nuclear weapon, military personnel

● **Y36.501**   War operations involving unspecified effect of nuclear weapon, civilian

● **Y36.51**   **War operations involving direct blast effect of nuclear weapon**
War operations involving blast pressure of nuclear weapon

● **Y36.510**   War operations involving direct blast effect of nuclear weapon, military personnel

● **Y36.511**   War operations involving direct blast effect of nuclear weapon, civilian

● **Y36.52**   **War operations involving indirect blast effect of nuclear weapon**
War operations involving being thrown by blast of nuclear weapon
War operations involving being struck or crushed by blast debris of nuclear weapon

● **Y36.520**   War operations involving indirect blast effect of nuclear weapon, military personnel

● **Y36.521**   War operations involving indirect blast effect of nuclear weapon, civilian

● **Y36.53**   **War operations involving thermal radiation effect of nuclear weapon**
War operations involving direct heat from nuclear weapon
War operation involving fireball effects from nuclear weapon

● **Y36.530**   War operations involving thermal radiation effect of nuclear weapon, military personnel

● **Y36.531**   War operations involving thermal radiation effect of nuclear weapon, civilian

● **Y36.54**   **War operation involving nuclear radiation effects of nuclear weapon**
War operation involving acute radiation exposure from nuclear weapon
War operation involving exposure to immediate ionizing radiation from nuclear weapon
War operation involving fallout exposure from nuclear weapon
War operation involving secondary effects of nuclear weapons

● **Y36.540**   War operation involving nuclear radiation effects of nuclear weapon, military personnel

● **Y36.541**   War operation involving nuclear radiation effects of nuclear weapon, civilian

● **Y36.59**   **War operation involving other effects of nuclear weapons**

● **Y36.590**   War operation involving other effects of nuclear weapons, military personnel

● **Y36.591**   War operation involving other effects of nuclear weapons, civilian

● **Y36.6**   **War operations involving biological weapons**

● **Y36.6X**   **War operations involving biological weapons**

● **Y36.6X0**   War operations involving biological weapons, military personnel

● **Y36.6X1**   War operations involving biological weapons, civilian

---

▶ New   ⇒ Revised   ~~deleted~~ Deleted   Excludes 1   Excludes 2   Includes   Use additional   Code first   Code also   Key words

OGCR Official Guidelines   ● Unacceptable Principal Diagnosis   X Assign placeholder X   ● Use Additional Character(s)   ▌ Manifestation Code   **Coding Clinic**

● Y36.7 **War operations involving chemical weapons and other forms of unconventional warfare**
  Excludes1   war operations involving incendiary devices (Y36.3-, Y36.5-)
  ● Y36.7X **War operations involving chemical weapons and other forms of unconventional warfare**
    ● Y36.7X0 **War operations involving chemical weapons and other forms of unconventional warfare, military personnel**
    ● Y36.7X1 **War operations involving chemical weapons and other forms of unconventional warfare, civilian**
● Y36.8 **War operations occurring after cessation of hostilities**
  War operations classifiable to categories Y36.0-Y36.8 but occurring after cessation of hostilities
  ● Y36.81 **Explosion of mine placed during war operations but exploding after cessation of hostilities**
    ● Y36.810 **Explosion of mine placed during war operations but exploding after cessation of hostilities, military personnel**
    ● Y36.811 **Explosion of mine placed during war operations but exploding after cessation of hostilities, civilian**
  ● Y36.82 **Explosion of bomb placed during war operations but exploding after cessation of hostilities**
    ● Y36.820 **Explosion of bomb placed during war operations but exploding after cessation of hostilities, military personnel**
    ● Y36.821 **Explosion of bomb placed during war operations but exploding after cessation of hostilities, civilian**
  ● Y36.88 **Other war operations occurring after cessation of hostilities**
    ● Y36.880 **Other war operations occurring after cessation of hostilities, military personnel**
    ● Y36.881 **Other war operations occurring after cessation of hostilities, civilian**
  ● Y36.89 **Unspecified war operations occurring after cessation of hostilities**
    ● Y36.890 **Unspecified war operations occurring after cessation of hostilities, military personnel**
    ● Y36.891 **Unspecified war operations occurring after cessation of hostilities, civilian**
● Y36.9 **Other and unspecified war operations**
  X ● Y36.90 **War operations, unspecified**
  X ● Y36.91 **War operations involving unspecified weapon of mass destruction [WMD]**
  X ● Y36.92 **War operations involving friendly fire**

● Y37 **Military operations**
  Includes   Injuries to military personnel and civilians occurring during peacetime on military property and during routine military exercises and operations
  Excludes1   military aircraft involved in aircraft accident with civilian aircraft (V97.81-)
  military vehicles involved in transport accident with civilian vehicle (V09.01, V09.21, V19.81, V29.81, V39.81, V49.81, V59.81, V69.81, V79.81)
  military watercraft involved in water transport accident with civilian watercraft (V94.81-)
  war operations (Y36.-)
  The appropriate 7th character is to be added to each code from category Y37

A	initial encounter
D	subsequent encounter
S	sequela

● Y37.0 **Military operations involving explosion of marine weapons**
  ● Y37.00 **Military operations involving explosion of unspecified marine weapon**
    Military operations involving underwater blast NOS
    ● Y37.000 **Military operations involving explosion of unspecified marine weapon, military personnel**
    ● Y37.001 **Military operations involving explosion of unspecified marine weapon, civilian**
  ● Y37.01 **Military operations involving explosion of depth-charge**
    ● Y37.010 **Military operations involving explosion of depth-charge, military personnel**
    ● Y37.011 **Military operations involving explosion of depth-charge, civilian**
  ● Y37.02 **Military operations involving explosion of marine mine**
    Military operations involving explosion of marine mine, at sea or in harbor
    ● Y37.020 **Military operations involving explosion of marine mine, military personnel**
    ● Y37.021 **Military operations involving explosion of marine mine, civilian**
  ● Y37.03 **Military operations involving explosion of sea-based artillery shell**
    ● Y37.030 **Military operations involving explosion of sea-based artillery shell, military personnel**
    ● Y37.031 **Military operations involving explosion of sea-based artillery shell, civilian**
  ● Y37.04 **Military operations involving explosion of torpedo**
    ● Y37.040 **Military operations involving explosion of torpedo, military personnel**
    ● Y37.041 **Military operations involving explosion of torpedo, civilian**
  ● Y37.05 **Military operations involving accidental detonation of onboard marine weapons**
    ● Y37.050 **Military operations involving accidental detonation of onboard marine weapons, military personnel**
    ● Y37.051 **Military operations involving accidental detonation of onboard marine weapons, civilian**

● **Y37.09** Military operations involving explosion of other marine weapons
- ● **Y37.090** Military operations involving explosion of other marine weapons, military personnel
- ● **Y37.091** Military operations involving explosion of other marine weapons, civilian

● **Y37.1** Military operations involving destruction of aircraft
- ● **Y37.10** Military operations involving unspecified destruction of aircraft
  - ● **Y37.100** Military operations involving unspecified destruction of aircraft, military personnel
  - ● **Y37.101** Military operations involving unspecified destruction of aircraft, civilian
- ● **Y37.11** Military operations involving destruction of aircraft due to enemy fire or explosives
  Military operations involving destruction of aircraft due to air to air missile
  Military operations involving destruction of aircraft due to explosive placed on aircraft
  Military operations involving destruction of aircraft due to rocket propelled grenade [RPG]
  Military operations involving destruction of aircraft due to small arms fire
  Military operations involving destruction of aircraft due to surface to air missile
  - ● **Y37.110** Military operations involving destruction of aircraft due to enemy fire or explosives, military personnel
  - ● **Y37.111** Military operations involving destruction of aircraft due to enemy fire or explosives, civilian
- ● **Y37.12** Military operations involving destruction of aircraft due to collision with other aircraft
  - ● **Y37.120** Military operations involving destruction of aircraft due to collision with other aircraft, military personnel
  - ● **Y37.121** Military operations involving destruction of aircraft due to collision with other aircraft, civilian
- ● **Y37.13** Military operations involving destruction of aircraft due to onboard fire
  - ● **Y37.130** Military operations involving destruction of aircraft due to onboard fire, military personnel
  - ● **Y37.131** Military operations involving destruction of aircraft due to onboard fire, civilian
- ● **Y37.14** Military operations involving destruction of aircraft due to accidental detonation of onboard munitions and explosives
  - ● **Y37.140** Military operations involving destruction of aircraft due to accidental detonation of onboard munitions and explosives, military personnel
  - ● **Y37.141** Military operations involving destruction of aircraft due to accidental detonation of onboard munitions and explosives, civilian
- ● **Y37.19** Military operations involving other destruction of aircraft
  - ● **Y37.190** Military operations involving other destruction of aircraft, military personnel
  - ● **Y37.191** Military operations involving other destruction of aircraft, civilian

● **Y37.2** Military operations involving other explosions and fragments
  Excludes1 military operations involving explosion of aircraft (Y37.1-)
  military operations involving explosion of marine weapons (Y37.0-)
  military operations involving explosion of nuclear weapons (Y37.5-)
- ● **Y37.20** Military operations involving unspecified explosion and fragments
  Military operations involving air blast NOS
  Military operations involving blast NOS
  Military operations involving blast fragments NOS
  Military operations involving blast wave NOS
  Military operations involving blast wind NOS
  Military operations involving explosion NOS
  Military operations involving explosion of bomb NOS
  - ● **Y37.200** Military operations involving unspecified explosion and fragments, military personnel
  - ● **Y37.201** Military operations involving unspecified explosion and fragments, civilian
- ● **Y37.21** Military operations involving explosion of aerial bomb
  - ● **Y37.210** Military operations involving explosion of aerial bomb, military personnel
  - ● **Y37.211** Military operations involving explosion of aerial bomb, civilian
- ● **Y37.22** Military operations involving explosion of guided missile
  - ● **Y37.220** Military operations involving explosion of guided missile, military personnel
  - ● **Y37.221** Military operations involving explosion of guided missile, civilian
- ● **Y37.23** Military operations involving explosion of improvised explosive device [IED]
  Military operations involving explosion of person-borne improvised explosive device [IED]
  Military operations involving explosion of vehicle-borne improvised explosive device [IED]
  Military operations involving explosion of roadside improvised explosive device [IED]
  - ● **Y37.230** Military operations involving explosion of improvised explosive device [IED], military personnel
  - ● **Y37.231** Military operations involving explosion of improvised explosive device [IED], civilian
- ● **Y37.24** Military operations involving explosion due to accidental detonation and discharge of own munitions or munitions launch device
  - ● **Y37.240** Military operations involving explosion due to accidental detonation and discharge of own munitions or munitions launch device, military personnel
  - ● **Y37.241** Military operations involving explosion due to accidental detonation and discharge of own munitions or munitions launch device, civilian

▶ New   ➡ Revised   ~~deleted~~ Deleted   Excludes 1   Excludes 2   Includes   Use additional   Code first   Code also   Key words
OGCR Official Guidelines   ● Unacceptable Principal Diagnosis   X Assign placeholder X   ● Use Additional Character(s)   ▶ Manifestation Code   Coding Clinic

● **Y37.25** **Military operations involving fragments from munitions**
    ● **Y37.250** **Military operations involving fragments from munitions, military personnel**
    ● **Y37.251** **Military operations involving fragments from munitions, civilian**

● **Y37.26** **Military operations involving fragments of improvised explosive device [IED]**
    Military operations involving fragments of person-borne improvised explosive device [IED]
    Military operations involving fragments of vehicle-borne improvised explosive device [IED]
    Military operations involving fragments of roadside improvised explosive device [IED]
    ● **Y37.260** **Military operations involving fragments of improvised explosive device [IED], military personnel**
    ● **Y37.261** **Military operations involving fragments of improvised explosive device [IED], civilian**

● **Y37.27** **Military operations involving fragments from weapons**
    ● **Y37.270** **Military operations involving fragments from weapons, military personnel**
    ● **Y37.271** **Military operations involving fragments from weapons, civilian**

● **Y37.29** **Military operations involving other explosions and fragments**
    Military operations involving explosion of grenade
    Military operations involving explosions of land mine
    Military operations involving shrapnel NOS
    ● **Y37.290** **Military operations involving other explosions and fragments, military personnel**
    ● **Y37.291** **Military operations involving other explosions and fragments, civilian**

● **Y37.3** **Military operations involving fires, conflagrations and hot substances**
    Military operations involving smoke, fumes, and heat from fires, conflagrations and hot substances
    Excludes1 military operations involving fires and conflagrations aboard military aircraft (Y37.1-)
        military operations involving fires and conflagrations aboard military watercraft (Y37.0-)
        military operations involving fires and conflagrations caused indirectly by conventional weapons (Y37.2-)
        military operations involving fires and thermal effects of nuclear weapons (Y36.53-)
    ● **Y37.30** **Military operations involving unspecified fire, conflagration and hot substance**
        ● **Y37.300** **Military operations involving unspecified fire, conflagration and hot substance, military personnel**
        ● **Y37.301** **Military operations involving unspecified fire, conflagration and hot substance, civilian**
    ● **Y37.31** **Military operations involving gasoline bomb**
        Military operations involving incendiary bomb
        Military operations involving petrol bomb
        ● **Y37.310** **Military operations involving gasoline bomb, military personnel**
        ● **Y37.311** **Military operations involving gasoline bomb, civilian**

● **Y37.32** **Military operations involving incendiary bullet**
    ● **Y37.320** **Military operations involving incendiary bullet, military personnel**
    ● **Y37.321** **Military operations involving incendiary bullet, civilian**

● **Y37.33** **Military operations involving flamethrower**
    ● **Y37.330** **Military operations involving flamethrower, military personnel**
    ● **Y37.331** **Military operations involving flamethrower, civilian**

● **Y37.39** **Military operations involving other fires, conflagrations and hot substances**
    ● **Y37.390** **Military operations involving other fires, conflagrations and hot substances, military personnel**
    ● **Y37.391** **Military operations involving other fires, conflagrations and hot substances, civilian**

● **Y37.4** **Military operations involving firearm discharge and other forms of conventional warfare**
    ● **Y37.41** **Military operations involving rubber bullets**
        ● **Y37.410** **Military operations involving rubber bullets, military personnel**
        ● **Y37.411** **Military operations involving rubber bullets, civilian**
    ● **Y37.42** **Military operations involving firearms pellets**
        ● **Y37.420** **Military operations involving firearms pellets, military personnel**
        ● **Y37.421** **Military operations involving firearms pellets, civilian**
    ● **Y37.43** **Military operations involving other firearms discharge**
        Military operations involving bullets NOS
        Excludes1 military operations involving munitions fragments (Y37.25-)
            military operations involving incendiary bullets (Y37.32-)
        ● **Y37.430** **Military operations involving other firearms discharge, military personnel**
        ● **Y37.431** **Military operations involving other firearms discharge, civilian**
    ● **Y37.44** **Military operations involving unarmed hand to hand combat**
        Excludes1 military operations involving combat using blunt or piercing object (Y37.45-)
            military operations involving intentional restriction of air and airway (Y37.46-)
            military operations involving unintentional restriction of air and airway (Y37.47-)
        ● **Y37.440** **Military operations involving unarmed hand to hand combat, military personnel**
        ● **Y37.441** **Military operations involving unarmed hand to hand combat, civilian**
    ● **Y37.45** **Military operations involving combat using blunt or piercing object**
        ● **Y37.450** **Military operations involving combat using blunt or piercing object, military personnel**
        ● **Y37.451** **Military operations involving combat using blunt or piercing object, civilian**

N Newborn Age: 0   **P** Pediatric Age: 0–17   **M** Maternity DX: 12–55   **A** Adult Age: 15–124   ♀ Females Only   ♂ Males Only

🅒 Complication\Comorbidity   🅜 Major C\C   ⒺⓍ CC/MCC Exclusions   🅗 Hospital-Acquired Condition

● **Y37.46** **Military operations involving intentional restriction of air and airway**

  ● **Y37.460** **Military operations involving intentional restriction of air and airway, military personnel**

  ● **Y37.461** **Military operations involving intentional restriction of air and airway, civilian**

● **Y37.47** **Military operations involving unintentional restriction of air and airway**

  ● **Y37.470** **Military operations involving unintentional restriction of air and airway, military personnel**

  ● **Y37.471** **Military operations involving unintentional restriction of air and airway, civilian**

● **Y37.49** **Military operations involving other forms of conventional warfare**

  ● **Y37.490** **Military operations involving other forms of conventional warfare, military personnel**

  ● **Y37.491** **Military operations involving other forms of conventional warfare, civilian**

● **Y37.5** **Military operations involving nuclear weapons**
    Military operation involving dirty bomb NOS

● **Y37.50** **Military operations involving unspecified effect of nuclear weapon**

  ● **Y37.500** **Military operations involving unspecified effect of nuclear weapon, military personnel**

  ● **Y37.501** **Military operations involving unspecified effect of nuclear weapon, civilian**

● **Y37.51** **Military operations involving direct blast effect of nuclear weapon**
    Military operations involving blast pressure of nuclear weapon

  ● **Y37.510** **Military operations involving direct blast effect of nuclear weapon, military personnel**

  ● **Y37.511** **Military operations involving direct blast effect of nuclear weapon, civilian**

● **Y37.52** **Military operations involving indirect blast effect of nuclear weapon**
    Military operations involving being thrown by blast of nuclear weapon
    Military operations involving being struck or crushed by blast debris of nuclear weapon

  ● **Y37.520** **Military operations involving indirect blast effect of nuclear weapon, military personnel**

  ● **Y37.521** **Military operations involving indirect blast effect of nuclear weapon, civilian**

● **Y37.53** **Military operations involving thermal radiation effect of nuclear weapon**
    Military operations involving direct heat from nuclear weapon
    Military operation involving fireball effects from nuclear weapon

  ● **Y37.530** **Military operations involving thermal radiation effect of nuclear weapon, military personnel**

  ● **Y37.531** **Military operations involving thermal radiation effect of nuclear weapon, civilian**

● **Y37.54** **Military operation involving nuclear radiation effects of nuclear weapon**
    Military operation involving acute radiation exposure from nuclear weapon
    Military operation involving exposure to immediate ionizing radiation from nuclear weapon
    Military operation involving fallout exposure from nuclear weapon
    Military operation involving secondary effects of nuclear weapons

  ● **Y37.540** **Military operation involving nuclear radiation effects of nuclear weapon, military personnel**

  ● **Y37.541** **Military operation involving nuclear radiation effects of nuclear weapon, civilian**

● **Y37.59** **Military operation involving other effects of nuclear weapons**

  ● **Y37.590** **Military operation involving other effects of nuclear weapons, military personnel**

  ● **Y37.591** **Military operation involving other effects of nuclear weapons, civilian**

● **Y37.6** **Military operations involving biological weapons**

  ● **Y37.6X** **Military operations involving biological weapons**

    ● **Y37.6X0** **Military operations involving biological weapons, military personnel**

    ● **Y37.6X1** **Military operations involving biological weapons, civilian**

● **Y37.7** **Military operations involving chemical weapons and other forms of unconventional warfare**

  Excludes1 military operations involving incendiary devices (Y36.3-, Y36.5-)

  ● **Y37.7X** **Military operations involving chemical weapons and other forms of unconventional warfare**

    ● **Y37.7X0** **Military operations involving chemical weapons and other forms of unconventional warfare, military personnel**

    ● **Y37.7X1** **Military operations involving chemical weapons and other forms of unconventional warfare, civilian**

● **Y37.9** **Other and unspecified military operations**

  X ● **Y37.90** **Military operations, unspecified**

  X ● **Y37.91** **Military operations involving unspecified weapon of mass destruction [WMD]**

  X ● **Y37.92** **Military operations involving friendly fire**

▶ New   ⇒ Revised   deleted Deleted   Excludes 1   Excludes 2   Includes   Use additional   Code first   Code also   Key words

OGCR Official Guidelines   ● Unacceptable Principal Diagnosis   X Assign placeholder X   ▶ Use Additional Character(s)   ▶ Manifestation Code   Coding Clinic

- **Y38   Terrorism**

  These codes are for use to identify injuries resulting from the unlawful use of force or violence against persons or property to intimidate or coerce a government, the civilian population, or any segment thereof, in furtherance of political or social objective

  Use additional code for place of occurrence (Y92.-)

  The appropriate 7th character is to be added to each code from category Y38

  > A   initial encounter
  > D   subsequent encounter
  > S   sequela

  - **Y38.0   Terrorism involving explosion of marine weapons**
    Terrorism involving depth-charge
    Terrorism involving marine mine
    Terrorism involving mine NOS, at sea or in harbor
    Terrorism involving sea-based artillery shell
    Terrorism involving torpedo
    Terrorism involving underwater blast

    - **Y38.0X   Terrorism involving explosion of marine weapons**
      - **Y38.0X1   Terrorism involving explosion of marine weapons, public safety official injured**
      - **Y38.0X2   Terrorism involving explosion of marine weapons, civilian injured**
      - **Y38.0X3   Terrorism involving explosion of marine weapons, terrorist injured**

  - **Y38.1   Terrorism involving destruction of aircraft**
    Terrorism involving aircraft burned
    Terrorism involving aircraft exploded
    Terrorism involving aircraft being shot down
    Terrorism involving aircraft used as a weapon

    - **Y38.1X   Terrorism involving destruction of aircraft**
      - **Y38.1X1   Terrorism involving destruction of aircraft, public safety official injured**
      - **Y38.1X2   Terrorism involving destruction of aircraft, civilian injured**
      - **Y38.1X3   Terrorism involving destruction of aircraft, terrorist injured**

  - **Y38.2   Terrorism involving other explosions and fragments**
    Terrorism involving antipersonnel (fragments) bomb
    Terrorism involving blast NOS
    Terrorism involving explosion NOS
    Terrorism involving explosion of breech block
    Terrorism involving explosion of cannon block
    Terrorism involving explosion (fragments) of artillery shell
    Terrorism involving explosion (fragments) of bomb
    Terrorism involving explosion (fragments) of grenade
    Terrorism involving explosion (fragments) of guided missile
    Terrorism involving explosion (fragments) of land mine
    Terrorism involving explosion of mortar bomb
    Terrorism involving explosion of munitions
    Terrorism involving explosion (fragments) of rocket
    Terrorism involving explosion (fragments) of shell
    Terrorism involving shrapnel
    Terrorism involving mine NOS, on land

    Excludes1   terrorism involving explosion of nuclear weapon (Y38.5)
    terrorism involving suicide bomber (Y38.81)

    - **Y38.2X   Terrorism involving other explosions and fragments**
      - **Y38.2X1   Terrorism involving other explosions and fragments, public safety official injured**
      - **Y38.2X2   Terrorism involving other explosions and fragments, civilian injured**
      - **Y38.2X3   Terrorism involving other explosions and fragments, terrorist injured**

- **Y38.3   Terrorism involving fires, conflagration and hot substances**
  Terrorism involving conflagration NOS
  Terrorism involving fire NOS
  Terrorism involving petrol bomb

  Excludes1   terrorism involving fire or heat of nuclear weapon (Y38.5)

  - **Y38.3X   Terrorism involving fires, conflagration and hot substances**
    - **Y38.3X1   Terrorism involving fires, conflagration and hot substances, public safety official injured**
    - **Y38.3X2   Terrorism involving fires, conflagration and hot substances, civilian injured**
    - **Y38.3X3   Terrorism involving fires, conflagration and hot substances, terrorist injured**

- **Y38.4   Terrorism involving firearms**
  Terrorism involving carbine bullet
  Terrorism involving machine gun bullet
  Terrorism involving pellets (shotgun)
  Terrorism involving pistol bullet
  Terrorism involving rifle bullet
  Terrorism involving rubber (rifle) bullet

  - **Y38.4X   Terrorism involving firearms**
    - **Y38.4X1   Terrorism involving firearms, public safety official injured**
    - **Y38.4X2   Terrorism involving firearms, civilian injured**
    - **Y38.4X3   Terrorism involving firearms, terrorist injured**

- **Y38.5   Terrorism involving nuclear weapons**
  Terrorism involving blast effects of nuclear weapon
  Terrorism involving exposure to ionizing radiation from nuclear weapon
  Terrorism involving fireball effect of nuclear weapon
  Terrorism involving heat from nuclear weapon

  - **Y38.5X   Terrorism involving nuclear weapons**
    - **Y38.5X1   Terrorism involving nuclear weapons, public safety official injured**
    - **Y38.5X2   Terrorism involving nuclear weapons, civilian injured**
    - **Y38.5X3   Terrorism involving nuclear weapons, terrorist injured**

- **Y38.6   Terrorism involving biological weapons**
  Terrorism involving anthrax
  Terrorism involving cholera
  A serious, often deadly, infectious disease of small intestine
  Terrorism involving smallpox

  - **Y38.6X   Terrorism involving biological weapons**
    - **Y38.6X1   Terrorism involving biological weapons, public safety official injured**
    - **Y38.6X2   Terrorism involving biological weapons, civilian injured**
    - **Y38.6X3   Terrorism involving biological weapons, terrorist injured**

- **Y38.7   Terrorism involving chemical weapons**
  Terrorism involving gases, fumes, chemicals
  Terrorism involving hydrogen cyanide
  Terrorism involving phosgene
  Terrorism involving sarin

  - **Y38.7X   Terrorism involving chemical weapons**
    - **Y38.7X1   Terrorism involving chemical weapons, public safety official injured**
    - **Y38.7X2   Terrorism involving chemical weapons, civilian injured**
    - **Y38.7X3   Terrorism involving chemical weapons, terrorist injured**

CHAPTER 20 (V01-Y99)

● **Y38.8 Terrorism involving other and unspecified means**
  ● **Y38.80 Terrorism involving unspecified means**
      Terrorism NOS
  ● **Y38.81 Terrorism involving suicide bomber**
    ● **Y38.811 Terrorism involving suicide bomber, public safety official injured**
    ● **Y38.812 Terrorism involving suicide bomber, civilian injured**
  ● **Y38.89 Terrorism involving other means**
      Terrorism involving drowning and submersion
      Terrorism involving lasers
      Terrorism involving piercing or stabbing instruments
    ● **Y38.891 Terrorism involving other means, public safety official injured**
    ● **Y38.892 Terrorism involving other means, civilian injured**
    ● **Y38.893 Terrorism involving other means, terrorist injured**
● **Y38.9 Terrorism, secondary effects**
    Note: This code is for use to identify conditions occurring subsequent to a terrorist attack not those that are due to the initial terrorist attack.
  ● **Y38.9X Terrorism, secondary effects**
    ● **Y38.9X1 Terrorism, secondary effects, public safety official injured**
    ● **Y38.9X2 Terrorism, secondary effects, civilian injured categories**

COMPLICATIONS OF MEDICAL AND SURGICAL CARE (Y62-Y84)

Includes   complications of medical devices surgical and medical procedures as the cause of abnormal reaction of the patient, or of later complication, without mention of misadventure at the time of the procedure

MISADVENTURES TO PATIENTS DURING SURGICAL AND MEDICAL CARE (Y62-Y69)

Excludes1   surgical and medical procedures as the cause of abnormal reaction of the patient, without mention of misadventure at the time of the procedure (Y83-Y84)
Excludes2   breakdown or malfunctioning of medical device (during procedure) (after implantation) (ongoing use) (Y70-Y82)

● **Y62 Failure of sterile precautions during surgical and medical care**
  Y62.0 Failure of sterile precautions during surgical operation
  Y62.1 Failure of sterile precautions during infusion or transfusion
  Y62.2 Failure of sterile precautions during kidney dialysis and other perfusion
  Y62.3 Failure of sterile precautions during injection or immunization
  Y62.4 Failure of sterile precautions during endoscopic examination
  Y62.5 Failure of sterile precautions during heart catheterization
  Y62.6 Failure of sterile precautions during aspiration, puncture and other catheterization
  Y62.8 Failure of sterile precautions during other surgical and medical care
  Y62.9 Failure of sterile precautions during unspecified surgical and medical care

● **Y63 Failure in dosage during surgical and medical care**
  Excludes2   accidental overdose of drug or wrong drug given in error (T36-T50)
  Y63.0 Excessive amount of blood or other fluid given during transfusion or infusion
  Y63.1 Incorrect dilution of fluid used during infusion
  Y63.2 Overdose of radiation given during therapy
  Y63.3 Inadvertent exposure of patient to radiation during medical care
  Y63.4 Failure in dosage in electroshock or insulin-shock therapy
  Y63.5 Inappropriate temperature in local application and packing
  Y63.6 Underdosing and nonadministration of necessary drug, medicament or biological substance
  Y63.8 Failure in dosage during other surgical and medical care
  Y63.9 Failure in dosage during unspecified surgical and medical care

● **Y64 Contaminated medical or biological substances**
  Y64.0 Contaminated medical or biological substance, transfused or infused
  Y64.1 Contaminated medical or biological substance, injected or used for immunization
  Y64.8 Contaminated medical or biological substance administered by other means
  Y64.9 Contaminated medical or biological substance administered by unspecified means
      Administered contaminated medical or biological substance NOS

● **Y65 Other misadventures during surgical and medical care**
  Y65.0 Mismatched blood in transfusion
  Y65.1 Wrong fluid used in infusion
  Y65.2 Failure in suture or ligature during surgical operation
  Y65.3 Endotracheal tube wrongly placed during anesthetic procedure
  Y65.4 Failure to introduce or to remove other tube or instrument
  ● **Y65.5 Performance of wrong procedure (operation)**
    ● **Y65.51 Performance of wrong procedure (operation) on correct patient**
      Wrong device implanted into correct surgical site
      Excludes1   performance of correct procedure (operation) on wrong side or body part (Y65.53)
      MCE: Wrong procedure performed
    ● **Y65.52 Performance of procedure (operation) on patient not scheduled for surgery**
      Performance of procedure (operation) intended for another patient
      Performance of procedure (operation) on wrong patient
      MCE: Wrong procedure performed
    ● **Y65.53 Performance of correct procedure (operation) on wrong side or body part**
      Performance of correct procedure (operation) on wrong side
      Performance of correct procedure (operation) on wrong site
      MCE: Wrong procedure performed
  Y65.8 Other specified misadventures during surgical and medical care

Y66 Nonadministration of surgical and medical care
  Premature cessation of surgical and medical care
  Excludes1   DNR status (Z66)
      palliative care (Z51.5)

Y69 Unspecified misadventure during surgical and medical care

MEDICAL DEVICES ASSOCIATED WITH ADVERSE INCIDENTS IN DIAGNOSTIC AND THERAPEUTIC USE (Y70-Y82)

Includes breakdown or malfunction of medical devices (during use) (after implantation) (ongoing use)

Excludes2 breakdown or malfunctioning of medical device (after implantation) (during procedure) (ongoing use) (Y70-Y82)
later complications following use of medical devices without breakdown or malfunctioning of device (Y83-Y84)
misadventure to patients during surgical and medical care, classifiable to (Y62-Y69)
surgical and other medical procedures as the cause of abnormal reaction of the patient, or of later complication, without mention of misadventure at the time of the procedure (Y83-Y84)

● Y70 Anesthesiology devices associated with adverse incidents
  Y70.0 Diagnostic and monitoring anesthesiology devices associated with adverse incidents
  Y70.1 Therapeutic (nonsurgical) and rehabilitative anesthesiology devices associated with adverse incidents
  Y70.2 Prosthetic and other implants, materials and accessory anesthesiology devices associated with adverse incidents
  Y70.3 Surgical instruments, materials and anesthesiology devices (including sutures) associated with adverse incidents
  Y70.8 Miscellaneous anesthesiology devices associated with adverse incidents, not elsewhere classified

● Y71 Cardiovascular devices associated with adverse incidents
  Y71.0 Diagnostic and monitoring cardiovascular devices associated with adverse incidents
  Y71.1 Therapeutic (nonsurgical) and rehabilitative cardiovascular devices associated with adverse incidents
  Y71.2 Prosthetic and other implants, materials and accessory cardiovascular devices associated with adverse incidents
  Y71.3 Surgical instruments, materials and cardiovascular devices (including sutures) associated with adverse incidents
  Y71.8 Miscellaneous cardiovascular devices associated with adverse incidents, not elsewhere classified

● Y72 Otorhinolaryngological devices associated with adverse incidents
  Y72.0 Diagnostic and monitoring otorhinolaryngological devices associated with adverse incidents
  Y72.1 Therapeutic (nonsurgical) and rehabilitative otorhinolaryngological devices associated with adverse incidents
  Y72.2 Prosthetic and other implants, materials and accessory otorhinolaryngological devices associated with adverse incidents
  Y72.3 Surgical instruments, materials and otorhinolaryngological devices (including sutures) associated with adverse incidents
  Y72.8 Miscellaneous otorhinolaryngological devices associated with adverse incidents, not elsewhere classified

● Y73 Gastroenterology and urology devices associated with adverse incidents
  Y73.0 Diagnostic and monitoring gastroenterology and urology devices associated with adverse incidents
  Y73.1 Therapeutic (nonsurgical) and rehabilitative gastroenterology and urology devices associated with adverse incidents
  Y73.2 Prosthetic and other implants, materials and accessory gastroenterology and urology devices associated with adverse incidents
  Y73.3 Surgical instruments, materials and gastroenterology and urology devices (including sutures) associated with adverse incidents
  Y73.8 Miscellaneous gastroenterology and urology devices associated with adverse incidents, not elsewhere classified

● Y74 General hospital and personal-use devices associated with adverse incidents
  Y74.0 Diagnostic and monitoring general hospital and personal-use devices associated with adverse incidents
  Y74.1 Therapeutic (nonsurgical) and rehabilitative general hospital and personal-use devices associated with adverse incidents
  Y74.2 Prosthetic and other implants, materials and accessory general hospital and personal-use devices associated with adverse incidents
  Y74.3 Surgical instruments, materials and general hospital and personal-use devices (including sutures) associated with adverse incidents
  Y74.8 Miscellaneous general hospital and personal-use devices associated with adverse incidents, not elsewhere classified

● Y75 Neurological devices associated with adverse incidents
  Y75.0 Diagnostic and monitoring neurological devices associated with adverse incidents
  Y75.1 Therapeutic (nonsurgical) and rehabilitative neurological devices associated with adverse incidents
  Y75.2 Prosthetic and other implants, materials and neurological devices associated with adverse incidents
  Y75.3 Surgical instruments, materials and neurological devices (including sutures) associated with adverse incidents
  Y75.8 Miscellaneous neurological devices associated with adverse incidents, not elsewhere classified

● Y76 Obstetric and gynecological devices associated with adverse incidents
  Y76.0 Diagnostic and monitoring obstetric and gynecological devices associated with adverse incidents ♀
  Y76.1 Therapeutic (nonsurgical) and rehabilitative obstetric and gynecological devices associated with adverse incidents ♀
  Y76.2 Prosthetic and other implants, materials and accessory obstetric and gynecological devices associated with adverse incidents ♀
  Y76.3 Surgical instruments, materials and obstetric and gynecological devices (including sutures) associated with adverse incidents ♀
  Y76.8 Miscellaneous obstetric and gynecological devices associated with adverse incidents, not elsewhere classified ♀

CHAPTER 20 (V01-Y99)

● Y77 **Ophthalmic devices associated with adverse incidents**

    Y77.0 **Diagnostic and monitoring ophthalmic devices associated with adverse incidents**

    Y77.1 **Therapeutic (nonsurgical) and rehabilitative ophthalmic devices associated with adverse incidents**

    Y77.2 **Prosthetic and other implants, materials and accessory ophthalmic devices associated with adverse incidents**

    Y77.3 **Surgical instruments, materials and ophthalmic devices (including sutures) associated with adverse incidents**

    Y77.8 **Miscellaneous ophthalmic devices associated with adverse incidents, not elsewhere classified**

● Y78 **Radiological devices associated with adverse incidents**

    Y78.0 **Diagnostic and monitoring radiological devices associated with adverse incidents**

    Y78.1 **Therapeutic (nonsurgical) and rehabilitative radiological devices associated with adverse incidents**

    Y78.2 **Prosthetic and other implants, materials and accessory radiological devices associated with adverse incidents**

    Y78.3 **Surgical instruments, materials and radiological devices (including sutures) associated with adverse incidents**

    Y78.8 **Miscellaneous radiological devices associated with adverse incidents, not elsewhere classified**

● Y79 **Orthopedic devices associated with adverse incidents**

    Y79.0 **Diagnostic and monitoring orthopedic devices associated with adverse incidents**

    Y79.1 **Therapeutic (nonsurgical) and rehabilitative orthopedic devices associated with adverse incidents**

    Y79.2 **Prosthetic and other implants, materials and accessory orthopedic devices associated with adverse incidents**

    Y79.3 **Surgical instruments, materials and orthopedic devices (including sutures) associated with adverse incidents**

    Y79.8 **Miscellaneous orthopedic devices associated with adverse incidents, not elsewhere classified**

● Y80 **Physical medicine devices associated with adverse incidents**

    Y80.0 **Diagnostic and monitoring physical medicine devices associated with adverse incidents**

    Y80.1 **Therapeutic (nonsurgical) and rehabilitative physical medicine devices associated with adverse incidents**

    Y80.2 **Prosthetic and other implants, materials and accessory physical medicine devices associated with adverse incidents**

    Y80.3 **Surgical instruments, materials and physical medicine devices (including sutures) associated with adverse incidents**

    Y80.8 **Miscellaneous physical medicine devices associated with adverse incidents, not elsewhere classified**

● Y81 **General- and plastic-surgery devices associated with adverse incidents**

    Y81.0 **Diagnostic and monitoring general- and plastic-surgery devices associated with adverse incidents**

    Y81.1 **Therapeutic (nonsurgical) and rehabilitative general- and plastic-surgery devices associated with adverse incidents**

    Y81.2 **Prosthetic and other implants, materials and accessory general- and plastic-surgery devices associated with adverse incidents**

    Y81.3 **Surgical instruments, materials and general- and plastic-surgery devices (including sutures) associated with adverse incidents**

    Y81.8 **Miscellaneous general- and plastic-surgery devices associated with adverse incidents, not elsewhere classified**

● Y82 **Other and unspecified medical devices associated with adverse incidents**

    Y82.8 **Other medical devices associated with adverse incidents**

    Y82.9 **Unspecified medical devices associated with adverse incidents**

SURGICAL AND OTHER MEDICAL PROCEDURES AS THE CAUSE OF ABNORMAL REACTION OF THE PATIENT, OR OF LATER COMPLICATION, WITHOUT MENTION OF MISADVENTURE AT THE TIME OF THE PROCEDURE (Y83-Y84)

> **Excludes1** misadventures to patients during surgical and medical care, classifiable to (Y62-Y69)
>
> **Excludes2** breakdown or malfunctioning of medical device (after implantation) (during procedure) (ongoing use) (Y70-Y82)

● Y83 **Surgical operation and other surgical procedures as the cause of abnormal reaction of the patient, or of later complication, without mention of misadventure at the time of the procedure**

    Y83.0 **Surgical operation with transplant of whole organ as the cause of abnormal reaction of the patient, or of later complication, without mention of misadventure at the time of the procedure**

    Y83.1 **Surgical operation with implant of artificial internal device as the cause of abnormal reaction of the patient, or of later complication, without mention of misadventure at the time of the procedure**

    Y83.2 **Surgical operation with anastomosis, bypass or graft as the cause of abnormal reaction of the patient, or of later complication, without mention of misadventure at the time of the procedure**

    Y83.3 **Surgical operation with formation of external stoma as the cause of abnormal reaction of the patient, or of later complication, without mention of misadventure at the time of the procedure**

    Y83.4 **Other reconstructive surgery as the cause of abnormal reaction of the patient, or of later complication, without mention of misadventure at the time of the procedure**

    Y83.5 **Amputation of limb(s) as the cause of abnormal reaction of the patient, or of later complication, without mention of misadventure at the time of the procedure**

    Y83.6 **Removal of other organ (partial) (total) as the cause of abnormal reaction of the patient, or of later complication, without mention of misadventure at the time of the procedure**

    Y83.8 **Other surgical procedures as the cause of abnormal reaction of the patient, or of later complication, without mention of misadventure at the time of the procedure**

    Y83.9 **Surgical procedure, unspecified as the cause of abnormal reaction of the patient, or of later complication, without mention of misadventure at the time of the procedure**

● Y84 **Other medical procedures as the cause of abnormal reaction of the patient, or of later complication, without mention of misadventure at the time of the procedure**

    Y84.0 **Cardiac catheterization as the cause of abnormal reaction of the patient, or of later complication, without mention of misadventure at the time of the procedure**

    Y84.1 **Kidney dialysis as the cause of abnormal reaction of the patient, or of later complication, without mention of misadventure at the time of the procedure**

    Y84.2 **Radiological procedure and radiotherapy as the cause of abnormal reaction of the patient, or of later complication, without mention of misadventure at the time of the procedure**
        Coding Clinic: 2017, Q1, P34

    Y84.3 **Shock therapy as the cause of abnormal reaction of the patient, or of later complication, without mention of misadventure at the time of the procedure**

    Y84.4 **Aspiration of fluid as the cause of abnormal reaction of the patient, or of later complication, without mention of misadventure at the time of the procedure**

    Y84.5 **Insertion of gastric or duodenal sound as the cause of abnormal reaction of the patient, or of later complication, without mention of misadventure at the time of the procedure**

    Y84.6 **Urinary catheterization as the cause of abnormal reaction of the patient, or of later complication, without mention of misadventure at the time of the procedure**

▶ New   ⟹ Revised   ~~deleted~~ Deleted   Excludes 1   Excludes 2   Includes   Use additional   Code first   Code also   Key words
OGCR Official Guidelines   ● Unacceptable Principal Diagnosis   X Assign placeholder X   ● Use Additional Character(s)   ▶ Manifestation Code   Coding Clinic

Y84.7   **Blood-sampling** as the cause of abnormal reaction of the patient, or of later complication, without mention of misadventure at the time of the procedure

Y84.8   **Other medical procedures** as the cause of abnormal reaction of the patient, or of later complication, without mention of misadventure at the time of the procedure

Y84.9   **Medical procedure, unspecified** as the cause of abnormal reaction of the patient, or of later complication, without mention of misadventure at the time of the procedure

SUPPLEMENTARY FACTORS RELATED TO CAUSES OF MORBIDITY CLASSIFIED ELSEWHERE (Y90-Y99)

Note: These categories may be used to provide supplementary information concerning causes of morbidity. They are not to be used for single-condition coding.

● **Y90**   **Evidence of alcohol involvement determined by blood alcohol level**

Code first any associated alcohol related disorders (F10)

Y90.0   Blood alcohol level of **less than 20 mg/100 ml**

Y90.1   Blood alcohol level of **20-39 mg/100 ml**

Y90.2   Blood alcohol level of **40-59 mg/100 ml**

Y90.3   Blood alcohol level of **60-79 mg/100 ml**

Y90.4   Blood alcohol level of **80-99 mg/100 ml**

Y90.5   Blood alcohol level of **100-119 mg/100 ml**

Y90.6   Blood alcohol level of **120-199 mg/100 ml**

Y90.7   Blood alcohol level of **200-239 mg/100 ml**

Y90.8   Blood alcohol level of **240 mg/100 ml or more**

Y90.9   **Presence of alcohol in blood, level not specified**

OGCR Section I.C.20.b.

Place of Occurrence Guideline

Codes from category Y92, Place of occurrence of the external cause, are secondary codes for use after other external cause codes to identify the location of the patient at the time of injury or other condition.

Generally, a place of occurrence code is assigned only once, at the initial encounter for treatment. However, in the rare instance that a new injury occurs during hospitalization, an additional place of occurrence code may be assigned. No 7th characters are used for Y92. Only one code from Y92 should be recorded on a medical record.

Do not use place of occurrence code Y92.9 if the place is not stated or is not applicable.

● **Y92**   **Place of occurrence of the external cause**

The following category is for use, when relevant, to identify the place of occurrence of the external cause. Use in conjunction with an activity code.

Place of occurrence should be recorded only at the initial encounter for treatment

● **Y92.0**   **Non-institutional (private) residence** as the place of occurrence of the external cause

Excludes1   abandoned or derelict house (Y92.89)
home under construction but not yet occupied (Y92.6-)
institutional place of residence (Y92.1-)

● **Y92.00**   **Unspecified** non-institutional (private) residence as the place of occurrence of the external cause

Y92.000   **Kitchen** of unspecified non-institutional (private) residence as the place of occurrence of the external cause

Y92.001   **Dining room** of unspecified non-institutional (private) residence as the place of occurrence of the external cause

Y92.002   **Bathroom** of unspecified non-institutional (private) residence single-family (private) house as the place of occurrence of the external cause

Y92.003   **Bedroom** of unspecified non-institutional (private) residence as the place of occurrence of the external cause

Y92.007   **Garden or yard** of unspecified non-institutional (private) residence as the place of occurrence of the external cause

Y92.008   **Other place** in unspecified non-institutional (private) residence as the place of occurrence of the external cause

Y92.009   **Unspecified place** in unspecified non-institutional (private) residence as the place of occurrence of the external cause

Home (NOS) as the place of occurrence of the external cause

● **Y92.01**   **Single-family non-institutional (private) house as the place of occurrence of the external cause**

Farmhouse as the place of occurrence of the external cause

Excludes1   barn (Y92.71)
chicken coop or hen house (Y92.72)
farm field (Y92.73)
orchard (Y92.74)
single family mobile home or trailer (Y92.02-)
slaughter house (Y92.86)

Y92.010   **Kitchen** of single-family (private) house as the place of occurrence of the external cause

Y92.011   **Dining room** of single-family (private) house as the place of occurrence of the external cause

Y92.012   **Bathroom** of single-family (private) house as the place of occurrence of the external cause

Y92.013   **Bedroom** of single-family (private) house as the place of occurrence of the external cause

Y92.014   **Private driveway** to single-family (private) house as the place of occurrence of the external cause

Y92.015   **Private garage** of single-family (private) house as the place of occurrence of the external cause

Y92.016   **Swimming pool** in single-family (private) house or garden as the place of occurrence of the external cause

Y92.017   **Garden or yard** in single-family (private) house as the place of occurrence of the external cause

Y92.018   **Other place** in single-family (private) house as the place of occurrence of the external cause

Y92.019   **Unspecified place** in single-family (private) house as the place of occurrence of the external cause

● **Y92.02** **Mobile home** as the place of occurrence of the external cause

  Y92.020 **Kitchen** in mobile home as the place of occurrence of the external cause

  Y92.021 **Dining room** in mobile home as the place of occurrence of the external cause

  Y92.022 **Bathroom** in mobile home as the place of occurrence of the external cause

  Y92.023 **Bedroom** in mobile home as the place of occurrence of the external cause

  Y92.024 **Driveway** of mobile home as the place of occurrence of the external cause

  Y92.025 **Garage** of mobile home as the place of occurrence of the external cause

  Y92.026 **Swimming pool** of mobile home as the place of occurrence of the external cause

  Y92.027 **Garden or yard** of mobile home as the place of occurrence of the external cause

  Y92.028 **Other place** in mobile home as the place of occurrence of the external cause

  Y92.029 **Unspecified** place in mobile home as the place of occurrence of the external cause

● **Y92.03** **Apartment** as the place of occurrence of the external cause
  Condominium as the place of occurrence of the external cause
  Co-op apartment as the place of occurrence of the external cause

  Y92.030 **Kitchen** in apartment as the place of occurrence of the external cause

  Y92.031 **Bathroom** in apartment as the place of occurrence of the external cause

  Y92.032 **Bedroom** in apartment as the place of occurrence of the external cause

  Y92.038 **Other place** in apartment as the place of occurrence of the external cause

  Y92.039 **Unspecified** place in apartment as the place of occurrence of the external cause

● **Y92.04** **Boarding-house** as the place of occurrence of the external cause

  Y92.040 **Kitchen** in boarding-house as the place of occurrence of the external cause

  Y92.041 **Bathroom** in boarding-house as the place of occurrence of the external cause

  Y92.042 **Bedroom** in boarding-house as the place of occurrence of the external cause

  Y92.043 **Driveway** of boarding-house as the place of occurrence of the external cause

  Y92.044 **Garage** of boarding-house as the place of occurrence of the external cause

  Y92.045 **Swimming pool** of boarding-house as the place of occurrence of the external cause

  Y92.046 **Garden or yard** of boarding-house as the place of occurrence of the external cause

  Y92.048 **Other place** in boarding-house as the place of occurrence of the external cause

  Y92.049 **Unspecified** place in boarding-house as the place of occurrence of the external cause

● **Y92.09** **Other non-institutional residence** as the place of occurrence of the external cause

  Y92.090 **Kitchen** in other non-institutional residence as the place of occurrence of the external cause

  Y92.091 **Bathroom** in other non-institutional residence as the place of occurrence of the external cause

  Y92.092 **Bedroom** in other non-institutional residence as the place of occurrence of the external cause

  Y92.093 **Driveway** of other non-institutional residence as the place of occurrence of the external cause

  Y92.094 **Garage** of other non-institutional residence as the place of occurrence of the external cause

  Y92.095 **Swimming pool** of other non-institutional residence as the place of occurrence of the external cause

  Y92.096 **Garden or yard** of other non-institutional residence as the place of occurrence of the external cause

  Y92.098 **Other place** in other non-institutional residence as the place of occurrence of the external cause

  Y92.099 **Unspecified** place in other non-institutional residence as the place of occurrence of the external cause
  Coding Clinic: 2017, Q2, P10

● **Y92.1** **Institutional (nonprivate) residence** as the place of occurrence of the external cause

  Y92.10 **Unspecified** residential institution as the place of occurrence of the external cause

● **Y92.11** **Children's home and orphanage** as the place of occurrence of the external cause

  Y92.110 **Kitchen** in children's home and orphanage as the place of occurrence of the external cause

  Y92.111 **Bathroom** in children's home and orphanage as the place of occurrence of the external cause

  Y92.112 **Bedroom** in children's home and orphanage as the place of occurrence of the external cause

  Y92.113 **Driveway** of children's home and orphanage as the place of occurrence of the external cause

  Y92.114 **Garage** of children's home and orphanage as the place of occurrence of the external cause

  Y92.115 **Swimming pool** of children's home and orphanage as the place of occurrence of the external cause

  Y92.116 **Garden or yard** of children's home and orphanage as the place of occurrence of the external cause

  Y92.118 **Other place** in children's home and orphanage as the place of occurrence of the external cause

  Y92.119 **Unspecified** place in children's home and orphanage as the place of occurrence of the external cause

● **Y92.12   Nursing home** as the place of occurrence of the external cause
　　　　Home for the sick as the place of occurrence of the external cause
　　　　Hospice as the place of occurrence of the external cause

Y92.120   Kitchen in nursing home as the place of occurrence of the external cause

Y92.121   Bathroom in nursing home as the place of occurrence of the external cause

Y92.122   Bedroom in nursing home as the place of occurrence of the external cause

Y92.123   Driveway of nursing home as the place of occurrence of the external cause

Y92.124   Garage of nursing home as the place of occurrence of the external cause

Y92.125   Swimming pool of nursing home as the place of occurrence of the external cause

Y92.126   Garden or yard of nursing home as the place of occurrence of the external cause

Y92.128   Other place in nursing home as the place of occurrence of the external cause

Y92.129   Unspecified place in nursing home as the place of occurrence of the external cause

　　　　　Coding Clinic: 2017, Q2, P10

● **Y92.13   Military base** as the place of occurrence of the external cause

　　Excludes1   military training grounds (Y92.83)

Y92.130   Kitchen on military base as the place of occurrence of the external cause

Y92.131   Mess hall on military base as the place of occurrence of the external cause

Y92.133   Barracks on military base as the place of occurrence of the external cause

Y92.135   Garage on military base as the place of occurrence of the external cause

Y92.136   Swimming pool on military base as the place of occurrence of the external cause

Y92.137   Garden or yard on military base as the place of occurrence of the external cause

Y92.138   Other place on military base as the place of occurrence of the external cause

Y92.139   Unspecified place military base as the place of occurrence of the external cause

● **Y92.14   Prison** as the place of occurrence of the external cause

Y92.140   Kitchen in prison as the place of occurrence of the external cause

Y92.141   Dining room in prison as the place of occurrence of the external cause

Y92.142   Bathroom in prison as the place of occurrence of the external cause

Y92.143   Cell of prison as the place of occurrence of the external cause

Y92.146   Swimming pool of prison as the place of occurrence of the external cause

Y92.147   Courtyard of prison as the place of occurrence of the external cause

Y92.148   Other place in prison as the place of occurrence of the external cause

Y92.149   Unspecified place in prison as the place of occurrence of the external cause

● **Y92.15   Reform school** as the place of occurrence of the external cause

Y92.150   Kitchen in reform school as the place of occurrence of the external cause

Y92.151   Dining room in reform school as the place of occurrence of the external cause

Y92.152   Bathroom in reform school as the place of occurrence of the external cause

Y92.153   Bedroom in reform school as the place of occurrence of the external cause

Y92.154   Driveway of reform school as the place of occurrence of the external cause

Y92.155   Garage of reform school as the place of occurrence of the external cause

Y92.156   Swimming pool of reform school as the place of occurrence of the external cause

Y92.157   Garden or yard of reform school as the place of occurrence of the external cause

Y92.158   Other place in reform school as the place of occurrence of the external cause

Y92.159   Unspecified place in reform school as the place of occurrence of the external cause

● **Y92.16   School dormitory** as the place of occurrence of the external cause

　　Excludes1   reform school as the place of occurrence of the external cause (Y92.15-)
　　　　school buildings and grounds as the place of occurrence of the external cause (Y92.2-)
　　　　school sports and athletic areas as the place of occurrence of the external cause (Y92.3-)

Y92.160   Kitchen in school dormitory as the place of occurrence of the external cause

Y92.161   Dining room in school dormitory as the place of occurrence of the external cause

Y92.162   Bathroom in school dormitory as the place of occurrence of the external cause

Y92.163   Bedroom in school dormitory as the place of occurrence of the external cause

Y92.168   Other place in school dormitory as the place of occurrence of the external cause

Y92.169   Unspecified place in school dormitory as the place of occurrence of the external cause

N Newborn Age: 0　　**P** Pediatric Age: 0–17　　**M** Maternity DX: 12–55　　**A** Adult Age: 15–124　　♀ Females Only　　♂ Males Only

🅒 Complication\Comorbidity　　🅜 Major C\C　　🄴🄭 CC/MCC Exclusions　　🅗 Hospital-Acquired Condition

1579

● **Y92.19** **Other specified residential institution** as the place of occurrence of the external cause

Y92.190 **Kitchen** in other specified residential institution as the place of occurrence of the external cause

Y92.191 **Dining room** in other specified residential institution as the place of occurrence of the external cause

Y92.192 **Bathroom** in other specified residential institution as the place of occurrence of the external cause

Y92.193 **Bedroom** in other specified residential institution as the place of occurrence of the external cause

Y92.194 **Driveway** of other specified residential institution as the place of occurrence of the external cause

Y92.195 **Garage** of other specified residential institution as the place of occurrence of the external cause

Y92.196 **Pool** of other specified residential institution as the place of occurrence of the external cause

Y92.197 **Garden or yard** of other specified residential institution as the place of occurrence of the external cause

Y92.198 **Other place** in other specified residential institution as the place of occurrence of the external cause
Coding Clinic: 2017, Q2, P11

Y92.199 **Unspecified place** in other specified residential institution as the place of occurrence of the external cause
Coding Clinic: 2017, Q2, P10

● **Y92.2** **School, other institution and public administrative area** as the place of occurrence of the external cause
Building and adjacent grounds used by the general public or by a particular group of the public

Excludes1 building under construction as the place of occurrence of the external cause (Y92.6)
residential institution as the place of occurrence of the external cause (Y92.1)
school dormitory as the place of occurrence of the external cause (Y92.16-)
sports and athletics area of schools as the place of occurrence of the external cause (Y92.3-)

● **Y92.21** **School (private) (public) (state)** as the place of occurrence of the external cause

Y92.210 **Daycare center** as the place of occurrence of the external cause

Y92.211 **Elementary school** as the place of occurrence of the external cause
Kindergarten as the place of occurrence of the external cause

Y92.212 **Middle school** as the place of occurrence of the external cause

Y92.213 **High school** as the place of occurrence of the external cause
Coding Clinic: 2012, Q4, P108

Y92.214 **College** as the place of occurrence of the external cause
University as the place of occurrence of the external cause

Y92.215 **Trade school** as the place of occurrence of the external cause

Y92.218 **Other school** as the place of occurrence of the external cause

Y92.219 **Unspecified school** as the place of occurrence of the external cause

Y92.22 **Religious institution** as the place of occurrence of the external cause
Church as the place of occurrence of the external cause
Mosque as the place of occurrence of the external cause
Synagogue as the place of occurrence of the external cause

● **Y92.23** **Hospital** as the place of occurrence of the external cause

Excludes1 ambulatory (outpatient) health services establishments (Y92.53-)
home for the sick as the place of occurrence of the external cause (Y92.12-)
hospice as the place of occurrence of the external cause (Y92.12-)
nursing home as the place of occurrence of the external cause (Y92.12-)

Y92.230 **Patient room** in hospital as the place of occurrence of the external cause

Y92.231 **Patient bathroom** in hospital as the place of occurrence of the external cause

Y92.232 **Corridor** of hospital as the place of occurrence of the external cause

Y92.233 **Cafeteria** of hospital as the place of occurrence of the external cause

Y92.234 **Operating room** of hospital as the place of occurrence of the external cause

Y92.238 **Other place** in hospital as the place of occurrence of the external cause

Y92.239 **Unspecified place** in hospital as the place of occurrence of the external cause

● **Y92.24** **Public administrative building** as the place of occurrence of the external cause

Y92.240 **Courthouse** as the place of occurrence of the external cause

Y92.241 **Library** as the place of occurrence of the external cause

Y92.242 **Post office** as the place of occurrence of the external cause

Y92.243 **City hall** as the place of occurrence of the external cause

Y92.248 **Other public administrative building** as the place of occurrence of the external cause

● **Y92.25** **Cultural building** as the place of occurrence of the external cause

Y92.250 **Art gallery** as the place of occurrence of the external cause

Y92.251 **Museum** as the place of occurrence of the external cause

Y92.252 **Music hall** as the place of occurrence of the external cause

Y92.253 **Opera house** as the place of occurrence of the external cause

Y92.254 **Theater (live)** as the place of occurrence of the external cause

Y92.258 **Other cultural public building** as the place of occurrence of the external cause

Y92.26 **Movie house or cinema** as the place of occurrence of the external cause

Y92.29 **Other specified public building** as the place of occurrence of the external cause
Assembly hall as the place of occurrence of the external cause
Clubhouse as the place of occurrence of the external cause

▶ New ⇒ Revised ~~deleted~~ Deleted Excludes 1 Excludes 2 Includes Use additional Code first Code also Key words
OGCR Official Guidelines ● Unacceptable Principal Diagnosis X Assign placeholder X ● Use Additional Character(s) ▶ Manifestation Code **Coding Clinic**

● **Y92.3**   **Sports and athletics area as the place of occurrence of the external cause**

    ● **Y92.31**   **Athletic court as the place of occurrence of the external cause**

       Excludes1   tennis court in private home or garden (Y92.09)

       Y92.310   **Basketball court as the place of occurrence of the external cause**

       Y92.311   **Squash court as the place of occurrence of the external cause**

       Y92.312   **Tennis court as the place of occurrence of the external cause**

       Y92.318   **Other athletic court as the place of occurrence of the external cause**

    ● **Y92.32**   **Athletic field as the place of occurrence of the external cause**

       Y92.320   **Baseball field as the place of occurrence of the external cause**

       Y92.321   **Football field as the place of occurrence of the external cause**

       Y92.322   **Soccer field as the place of occurrence of the external cause**

       Y92.328   **Other athletic field as the place of occurrence of the external cause**

          Cricket field as the place of occurrence of the external cause

          Hockey field as the place of occurrence of the external cause

    ● **Y92.33**   **Skating rink as the place of occurrence of the external cause**

       Y92.330   **Ice skating rink (indoor) (outdoor) as the place of occurrence of the external cause**

       Y92.331   **Roller skating rink as the place of occurrence of the external cause**

    Y92.34   **Swimming pool (public) as the place of occurrence of the external cause**

       Excludes1   swimming pool in private home or garden (Y92.016)

    Y92.39   **Other specified sports and athletic area as the place of occurrence of the external cause**

       Golf-course as the place of occurrence of the external cause

       Gymnasium as the place of occurrence of the external cause

       Riding-school as the place of occurrence of the external cause

       Stadium as the place of occurrence of the external cause

● **Y92.4**   **Street, highway and other paved roadways as the place of occurrence of the external cause**

       Excludes1   private driveway of residence (Y92.014, Y92.024, Y92.043, Y92.093, Y92.113, Y92.123, Y92.154, Y92.194)

    ● **Y92.41**   **Street and highway as the place of occurrence of the external cause**

       Y92.410   **Unspecified street and highway as the place of occurrence of the external cause**

          Road NOS as the place of occurrence of the external cause

       Y92.411   **Interstate highway as the place of occurrence of the external cause**

          Freeway as the place of occurrence of the external cause

          Motorway as the place of occurrence of the external cause

       Y92.412   **Parkway as the place of occurrence of the external cause**

       Y92.413   **State road as the place of occurrence of the external cause**

       Y92.414   **Local residential or business street as the place of occurrence of the external cause**

       Y92.415   **Exit ramp or entrance ramp of street or highway as the place of occurrence of the external cause**

    ● **Y92.48**   **Other paved roadways as the place of occurrence of the external cause**

       Y92.480   **Sidewalk as the place of occurrence of the external cause**

       Y92.481   **Parking lot as the place of occurrence of the external cause**

       Y92.482   **Bike path as the place of occurrence of the external cause**

       Y92.488   **Other paved roadways as the place of occurrence of the external cause**

● **Y92.5**   **Trade and service area as the place of occurrence of the external cause**

       Excludes1   garage in private home (Y92.015) schools and other public administration buildings (Y92.2-)

    ● **Y92.51**   **Private commercial establishments as the place of occurrence of the external cause**

       Y92.510   **Bank as the place of occurrence of the external cause**

       Y92.511   **Restaurant or café as the place of occurrence of the external cause**

       Y92.512   **Supermarket, store or market as the place of occurrence of the external cause**

       Y92.513   **Shop (commercial) as the place of occurrence of the external cause**

    ● **Y92.52**   **Service areas as the place of occurrence of the external cause**

       Y92.520   **Airport as the place of occurrence of the external cause**

       Y92.521   **Bus station as the place of occurrence of the external cause**

       Y92.522   **Railway station as the place of occurrence of the external cause**

       Y92.523   **Highway rest stop as the place of occurrence of the external cause**

       Y92.524   **Gas station as the place of occurrence of the external cause**

          Petroleum station as the place of occurrence of the external cause

          Service station as the place of occurrence of the external cause

    ● **Y92.53**   **Ambulatory health services establishments as the place of occurrence of the external cause**

       Y92.530   **Ambulatory surgery center as the place of occurrence of the external cause**

          Outpatient surgery center, including that connected with a hospital as the place of occurrence of the external cause

          Same day surgery center, including that connected with a hospital as the place of occurrence of the external cause

       Y92.531   **Health care provider office as the place of occurrence of the external cause**

          Physician office as the place of occurrence of the external cause

       Y92.532   **Urgent care center as the place of occurrence of the external cause**

       Y92.538   **Other ambulatory health services establishments as the place of occurrence of the external cause**

CHAPTER 20 (V01-Y99)

N Newborn Age: 0   **P** Pediatric Age: 0–17   **M** Maternity DX: 12–55   **A** Adult Age: 15–124   ♀ Females Only   ♂ Males Only

Complication\Comorbidity   Major C\C   (Ex) CC/MCC Exclusions   Hospital-Acquired Condition

1581

Y92.59   **Other trade areas** as the place of occurrence of the external cause

     Office building as the place of occurrence of the external cause

     Casino as the place of occurrence of the external cause

     Garage (commercial) as the place of occurrence of the external cause

     Hotel as the place of occurrence of the external cause

     Radio or television station as the place of occurrence of the external cause

     Shopping mall as the place of occurrence of the external cause

     Warehouse as the place of occurrence of the external cause

● Y92.6   **Industrial and construction area** as the place of occurrence of the external cause

Y92.61   **Building [any] under construction** as the place of occurrence of the external cause

Y92.62   **Dock or shipyard** as the place of occurrence of the external cause

     Dockyard as the place of occurrence of the external cause

     Dry dock as the place of occurrence of the external cause

     Shipyard as the place of occurrence of the external cause

Y92.63   **Factory** as the place of occurrence of the external cause

     Factory building as the place of occurrence of the external cause

     Factory premises as the place of occurrence of the external cause

     Industrial yard as the place of occurrence of the external cause

Y92.64   **Mine or pit** as the place of occurrence of the external cause

     Mine as the place of occurrence of the external cause

Y92.65   **Oil rig** as the place of occurrence of the external cause

     Pit (coal) (gravel) (sand) as the place of occurrence of the external cause

Y92.69   **Other specified industrial and construction area** as the place of occurrence of the external cause

     Gasworks as the place of occurrence of the external cause

     Power-station (coal) (nuclear) (oil) as the place of occurrence of the external cause

     Tunnel under construction as the place of occurrence of the external cause

     Workshop as the place of occurrence of the external cause

● Y92.7   **Farm** as the place of occurrence of the external cause

     Ranch as the place of occurrence of the external cause

     Excludes1   farmhouse and home premises of farm (Y92.01-)

Y92.71   **Barn** as the place of occurrence of the external cause

Y92.72   **Chicken coop** as the place of occurrence of the external cause

     Hen house as the place of occurrence of the external cause

Y92.73   **Farm field** as the place of occurrence of the external cause

Y92.74   **Orchard** as the place of occurrence of the external cause

Y92.79   **Other farm location** as the place of occurrence of the external cause

● Y92.8   **Other places** as the place of occurrence of the external cause

● Y92.81   **Transport vehicle** as the place of occurrence of the external cause

     Excludes1   transport accidents (V00-V99)

Y92.810   **Car** as the place of occurrence of the external cause

Y92.811   **Bus** as the place of occurrence of the external cause

Y92.812   **Truck** as the place of occurrence of the external cause

Y92.813   **Airplane** as the place of occurrence of the external cause

Y92.814   **Boat** as the place of occurrence of the external cause

Y92.815   **Train** as the place of occurrence of the external cause

Y92.816   **Subway** car as the place of occurrence of the external cause

Y92.818   **Other transport vehicle** as the place of occurrence of the external cause

● Y92.82   **Wilderness area**

Y92.820   **Desert** as the place of occurrence of the external cause

Y92.821   **Forest** as the place of occurrence of the external cause

Y92.828   **Other wilderness area** as the place of occurrence of the external cause

     Swamp as the place of occurrence of the external cause

     Mountain as the place of occurrence of the external cause

     Marsh as the place of occurrence of the external cause

     Prairie as the place of occurrence of the external cause

● Y92.83   **Recreation area** as the place of occurrence of the external cause

Y92.830   **Public park** as the place of occurrence of the external cause

Y92.831   **Amusement park** as the place of occurrence of the external cause

Y92.832   **Beach** as the place of occurrence of the external cause

     Seashore as the place of occurrence of the external cause

Y92.833   **Campsite** as the place of occurrence of the external cause

Y92.834   **Zoological garden (zoo)** as the place of occurrence of the external cause

Y92.838   **Other recreation area** as the place of occurrence of the external cause

Y92.84   **Military training ground** as the place of occurrence of the external cause

Y92.85   **Railroad track** as the place of occurrence of the external cause

Y92.86   **Slaughter house** as the place of occurrence of the external cause

Y92.89   **Other specified places** as the place of occurrence of the external cause

     Derelict house as the place of occurrence of the external cause

OGCR   Section I.C.20.b.

Do not use place of occurrence code Y92.9 if the place is not stated or is not applicable.

Y92.9   **Unspecified place or not applicable**

▶ New   ⇒ Revised   ~~deleted~~ Deleted   Excludes 1   Excludes 2   Includes   Use additional   Code first   Code also   Key words

OGCR Official Guidelines   ● Unacceptable Principal Diagnosis   X Assign placeholder X   ● Use Additional Character(s)   ▶ Manifestation Code   **Coding Clinic**

Activity Code

Assign a code from category Y93, Activity code, to describe the activity of the patient at the time the injury or other health condition occurred.

An activity code is used only once, at the initial encounter for treatment. Only one code from Y93 should be recorded on a medical record.

The activity codes are not applicable to poisonings, adverse effects, misadventures or sequela.

Do not assign Y93.9, Unspecified activity, if the activity is not stated.

A code from category Y93 is appropriate for use with external cause and intent codes if identifying the activity provides additional information about the event.

● **Y93 Activity codes**

> **Note:** Category Y93 is provided for use to indicate the activity of the person seeking healthcare for an injury or health condition, such as a heart attack while shoveling snow, which resulted from, or was contributed to, by the activity. These codes are appropriate for use for both acute injuries, such as those from chapter 19, and conditions that are due to the long-term, cumulative effects of an activity, such as those from chapter 13. They are also appropriate for use with external cause codes for cause and intent if identifying the activity provides additional information on the event. These codes should be used in conjunction with codes for external cause status (Y99) and place of occurrence (Y92).
>
> This section contains the following broad activity categories:

Y93.0	Activities involving walking and running
Y93.1	Activities involving water and water craft
Y93.2	Activities involving ice and snow
Y93.3	Activities involving climbing, rappelling, and jumping off
Y93.4	Activities involving dancing and other rhythmic movement
Y93.5	Activities involving other sports and athletics played individually
Y93.6	Activities involving other sports and athletics played as a team or group
Y93.7	Activities involving other specified sports and athletics
Y93.A	Activities involving other cardiorespiratory exercise
Y93.B	Activities involving other muscle strengthening exercises
Y93.C	Activities involving computer technology and electronic devices
Y93.D	Activities involving arts and handcrafts
Y93.E	Activities involving personal hygiene and interior property and clothing maintenance
Y93.F	Activities involving caregiving
Y93.G	Activities involving food preparation, cooking and grilling
Y93.H	Activities involving exterior property and land maintenance, building and construction
Y93.I	Activities involving roller coasters and other types of external motion
Y93.J	Activities involving playing musical instrument
Y93.K	Activities involving animal care
Y93.8	Activities, other specified
Y93.9	Activity, unspecified

● **Y93.0 Activities involving walking and running**
> **Excludes1**   Activity, walking an animal (Y93.K1)
> Activity, walking or running on a treadmill (Y93.A1)

Y93.01 Activity, walking, marching and hiking
Activity, walking, marching and hiking on level or elevated terrain
> **Excludes1**   activity, mountain climbing (Y93.31)

Y93.02 Activity, running

● **Y93.1 Activities involving water and water craft**
> **Excludes1**   activities involving ice (Y93.2-)

Y93.11 Activity, swimming

Y93.12 Activity, springboard and platform diving

Y93.13 Activity, water polo

Y93.14 Activity, water aerobics and water exercise

Y93.15 Activity, underwater diving and snorkeling
Activity, SCUBA diving

Y93.16 Activity, rowing, canoeing, kayaking, rafting and tubing
Activity, canoeing, kayaking, rafting and tubing in calm and turbulent water

Y93.17 Activity, water skiing and wake boarding

Y93.18 Activity, surfing, windsurfing and boogie boarding
Activity, water sliding

Y93.19 Activity, other involving water and watercraft
Activity involving water NOS
Activity, parasailing
Activity, water survival training and testing

● **Y93.2 Activities involving ice and snow**
> **Excludes1**   activity, shoveling ice and snow (Y93.H1)

Y93.21 Activity, ice skating
Activity, figure skating (singles) (pairs)
Activity, ice dancing
> **Excludes1**   activity, ice hockey (Y93.22)

Y93.22 Activity, ice hockey

Y93.23 Activity, snow (alpine) (downhill) skiing, snow boarding, sledding, tobogganing and snow tubing
> **Excludes1**   activity, cross country skiing (Y93.24)

Y93.24 Activity, cross country skiing
Activity, nordic skiing

Y93.29 Activity, other activity involving ice and snow
Activity, activity involving ice and snow NOS

● **Y93.3 Activities involving climbing, rappelling and jumping off**
> **Excludes1**   activity, hiking on level or elevated terrain (Y93.01)
> activity, jumping rope (Y93.56)
> activity, trampoline jumping (Y93.44)

Y93.31 Activity, mountain climbing, rock climbing and wall climbing

Y93.32 Activity, rappelling

Y93.33 Activity, BASE jumping
Activity, building, Antenna, Span, Earth jumping

Y93.34 Activity, bungee jumping

Y93.35 Activity, hang gliding

Y93.39 Activity, other activity involving climbing, rappelling and jumping off

● **Y93.4 Activities involving dancing and other rhythmic movement**
> **Excludes1**   activity, martial arts (Y93.75)

Y93.41 Activity, dancing
Coding Clinic: 2012, Q4, P108

Y93.42 Activity, yoga

Y93.43 Activity, gymnastics
Activity, rhythmic gymnastics
> **Excludes1**   activity, trampolining (Y93.44)

Y93.44 Activity, trampolining

Y93.45 Activity, cheerleading

Y93.49 Activity, other involving dancing and other rhythmic movements

● **Y93.5**   **Activities involving other sports and athletics played individually**

> **Excludes1**   activity, dancing (Y93.41)
> activity, gymnastic (Y93.43)
> activity, trampolining (Y93.44)
> activity, yoga (Y93.42)

Y93.51   **Activity, roller skating (inline) and skateboarding**

Y93.52   **Activity, horseback riding**

Y93.53   **Activity, golf**

Y93.54   **Activity, bowling**

Y93.55   **Activity, bike riding**

Y93.56   **Activity, jumping rope**

Y93.57   **Activity, non-running track and field events**

> **Excludes1**   activity, running (any form) (Y93.02)

Y93.59   **Activity, other involving other sports and athletics played individually**

> **Excludes1**   activities involving climbing, rappelling, and jumping (Y93.3-)
> activities involving ice and snow (Y93.2-)
> activities involving walking and running (Y93.0-)
> activities involving water and watercraft (Y93.1-)

● **Y93.6**   **Activities involving other sports and athletics played as a team or group**

> **Excludes1**   activity, ice hockey (Y93.22)
> activity, water polo (Y93.13)

Y93.61   **Activity, American tackle football**
Activity, football NOS

Y93.62   **Activity, American flag or touch football**

Y93.63   **Activity, rugby**

Y93.64   **Activity, baseball**
Activity, softball

Y93.65   **Activity, lacrosse and field hockey**
Coding Clinic: 2015, Q1, P9

Y93.66   **Activity, soccer**

Y93.67   **Activity, basketball**

Y93.68   **Activity, volleyball (beach) (court)**

Y93.6A   **Activity, physical games generally associated with school recess, summer camp and children**
Activity, capture the flag
Activity, dodge ball
Activity, four square
Activity, kickball

Y93.69   **Activity, other involving other sports and athletics played as a team or group**
Cricket

● **Y93.7**   **Activities involving other specified sports and athletics**

Y93.71   **Activity, boxing**

Y93.72   **Activity, wrestling**

Y93.73   **Activity, racquet and hand sports**
Activity, handball
Activity, racquetball
Activity, squash
Activity, tennis

Y93.74   **Activity, frisbee**
Activity, ultimate frisbee

Y93.75   **Activity, martial arts**
Activity, combatives

Y93.79   **Activity, other specified sports and athletics**

> **Excludes1**   sports and athletics activities specified in categories Y93.0-Y93.6

● **Y93.A**   **Activities involving other cardiorespiratory exercise**
Activities involving physical training

Y93.A1   **Activity, exercise machines primarily for cardiorespiratory conditioning**
Activity, elliptical and stepper machines
Activity, stationary bike
Activity, treadmill

Y93.A2   **Activity, calisthenics**
Activity, jumping jacks
Activity, warm up and cool down

Y93.A3   **Activity, aerobic and step exercise**

Y93.A4   **Activity, circuit training**

Y93.A5   **Activity, obstacle course**
Activity, challenge course
Activity, confidence course

Y93.A6   **Activity, grass drills**
Activity, guerilla drills

Y93.A9   **Activity, other involving other cardiorespiratory exercise**

> **Excludes1**   activities involving cardiorespiratory exercise specified in categories Y93.0-Y93.7

● **Y93.B**   **Activity involving other muscle strengthening exercises**

Y93.B1   **Activity, exercise machines primarily for muscle strengthening**

Y93.B2   **Activity, push-ups, pull-ups, sit-ups**

Y93.B3   **Activity, free weights**
Activity, barbells
Activity, dumbbells

Y93.B4   **Activity, pilates**

Y93.B9   **Activity, other involving other muscle strengthening exercises**

> **Excludes1**   activities involving muscle strengthening specified in categories Y93.0-Y93.A

● **Y93.C**   **Activities involving computer technology and electronic devices**

> **Excludes1**   activity, electronic musical keyboard or instruments (Y93.J-)

Y93.C1   **Activity, computer keyboarding**
Activity, electronic game playing using keyboard or other stationary device

Y93.C2   **Activity, hand held interactive electronic device**
Activity, cellular telephone and communication device
Activity, electronic game playing using interactive device

> **Excludes1**   activity, electronic game playing using keyboard or other stationary device (Y93.C1)

Y93.C9   **Activity, other involving computer technology and electronic devices**

● **Y93.D**   **Activities involving arts and handcrafts**

> **Excludes1**   activities involving playing musical instrument (Y93.J-)

Y93.D1   **Knitting and crocheting**

Y93.D2   **Sewing**

Y93.D3   **Furniture building and finishing**
Furniture repair

Y93.D9   **Activity, other involving arts and handcrafts**

▶ New   ⇒ Revised   ~~deleted~~ Deleted   Excludes 1   Excludes 2   Includes   Use additional   Code first   Code also   Key words

OGCR Official Guidelines   ● Unacceptable Principal Diagnosis   X Assign placeholder X   ● Use Additional Character(s)   ▶ Manifestation Code   Coding Clinic

- **Y93.E Activities involving personal hygiene and interior property and clothing maintenance**
  - **Excludes1** activities involving cooking and grilling (Y93.G-)
    activities involving exterior property and land maintenance, building and construction (Y93.H-)
    activity involving caregiving (Y93.F-)
    activity, dishwashing (Y93.G1)
    activity, food preparation (Y93.G1)
    activity, gardening (Y93.H2)
  - Y93.E1 **Activity, personal bathing and showering**
  - Y93.E2 **Activity, laundry**
  - Y93.E3 **Activity, vacuuming**
  - Y93.E4 **Activity, ironing**
  - Y93.E5 **Activity, floor mopping and cleaning**
  - Y93.E6 **Activity, residential relocation**
    Activity, packing up and unpacking involved in moving to a new residence
  - Y93.E8 **Activity, other personal hygiene activity**
  - Y93.E9 **Activity, other household maintenance**
- **Y93.F Activities involving person providing caregiving**
  Activity involving the provider of caregiving
  - Y93.F1 **Activity, caregiving involving bathing**
  - Y93.F2 **Activity, caregiving involving lifting**
    Coding Clinic: 2016, Q4, P74
  - Y93.F9 **Activity, other caregiving**
- **Y93.G Activities involving food preparation, cooking and grilling**
  - Y93.G1 **Activity, food preparation and clean up**
    Activity, dishwashing
  - Y93.G2 **Activity, grilling and smoking food**
  - Y93.G3 **Activity, cooking and baking**
    Activity, use of stove, oven and microwave oven
  - Y93.G9 **Activity, other activity involving cooking and grilling**
- **Y93.H Activities involving property and land maintenance, building and construction**
  - Y93.H1 **Activity, digging, shoveling and raking**
    Activity, dirt digging
    Activity, raking leaves
    Activity, snow shoveling
  - Y93.H2 **Activity, gardening and landscaping**
    Activity, pruning, trimming shrubs, weeding
  - Y93.H3 **Activity, building and construction**
  - Y93.H9 **Activity, other activity involving property and land maintenance, building and construction**
- **Y93.I Activities involving roller coasters and other types of external motion**
  - Y93.I1 **Activity, rollercoaster riding**
  - Y93.I9 **Activity, other involving external motion**
- **Y93.J Activities involving playing musical instrument**
  Activity involving playing electric musical instrument
  - Y93.J1 **Activity, piano playing**
    Activity, musical keyboard (electronic) playing
  - Y93.J2 **Activity, drum and other percussion instrument playing**
  - Y93.J3 **Activity, string instrument playing**
  - Y93.J4 **Activity, winds and brass instrument playing**

- **Y93.K Activities involving animal care**
  - **Excludes1** activity, horseback riding (Y93.52)
  - Y93.K1 **Activity, walking an animal**
  - Y93.K2 **Activity, milking an animal**
  - Y93.K3 **Activity, grooming and shearing an animal**
  - Y93.K9 **Activity, other activity involving animal care**
- **Y93.8 Other activity**
  Coding Clinic: 2016, Q4, P74
  - Y93.81 **Activity, refereeing a sports activity**
  - Y93.82 **Activity, spectator at an event**
  - Y93.83 **Activity, rough housing and horseplay**
    Coding Clinic: 2015, Q1, P8
  - Y93.84 **Activity, sleeping**
  - Y93.85 **Activity, choking game**
    Activity, blackout game
    Activity, fainting game
    Activity, pass out game
    Coding Clinic: 2016, Q4, P74-76
  - Y93.89 **Activity, other specified**
  - **OGCR** See Section I.C.20.c.
    Do not assign Y93.9, Unspecified activity, if the activity is not stated.
- **Y93.9 Activity, unspecified**

- Y95 **Nosocomial condition**

- **Y99 External cause status**
  Note: A single code from category Y99 should be used in conjunction with the external cause code(s) assigned to a record to indicate the status of the person at the time the event occurred.
  Coding Clinic: 2016, Q4, P74
  - Y99.0 **Civilian activity done for income or pay**
    Civilian activity done for financial or other compensation
    - **Excludes1** military activity (Y99.1)
      volunteer activity (Y99.2)
  - Y99.1 **Military activity**
    - **Excludes1** activity of off duty military personnel (Y99.8)
  - Y99.2 **Volunteer activity**
    - **Excludes1** activity of child or other family member assisting in compensated work of other family member (Y99.8)
  - Y99.8 **Other external cause status**
    Activity NEC
    Activity of child or other family member assisting in compensated work of other family member
    Hobby not done for income
    Leisure activity
    Off-duty activity of military personnel
    Recreation or sport not for income or while a student
    Student activity
    - **Excludes1** civilian activity done for income or compensation (Y99.0)
      military activity (Y99.1)
    Coding Clinic: 2012, Q4, P108
  - Y99.9 **Unspecified external cause status**

N Newborn Age: 0   **P** Pediatric Age: 0–17   **M** Maternity DX: 12–55   **A** Adult Age: 15–124   ♀ Females Only   ♂ Males Only

🔗 Complication\Comorbidity   🔗 Major C\C   (Ex.) CC/MCC Exclusions   🔗 Hospital-Acquired Condition

1585

CHAPTER 21

FACTORS INFLUENCING HEALTH STATUS AND CONTACT WITH HEALTH SERVICES (Z00-Z99)

OGCR Chapter-Specific Coding Guidelines

21. **Chapter 21: Factors influencing health status and contact with health services (Z00-Z99)**
Note: The chapter specific guidelines provide additional information about the use of Z codes for specified encounters.

a. **Use of Z codes in any healthcare setting**
Z codes are for use in any healthcare setting. Z codes may be used as either a first-listed (principal diagnosis code in the inpatient setting) or secondary code, depending on the circumstances of the encounter. Certain Z codes may only be used as first-listed or principal diagnosis.

b. **Z Codes indicate a reason for an encounter**
Z codes are not procedure codes. A corresponding procedure code must accompany a Z code to describe any procedure performed.

c. **Categories of Z Codes**

1) **Contact/Exposure**
Category Z20 indicates contact with, and suspected exposure to, communicable diseases. These codes are for patients who do not show any sign or symptom of a disease but are suspected to have been exposed to it by close personal contact with an infected individual or are in an area where a disease is epidemic.

Category Z77, Other contact with and (suspected) exposures hazardous to health, indicates contact with and suspected exposures hazardous to health.

Contact/exposure codes may be used as a first-listed code to explain an encounter for testing, or, more commonly, as a secondary code to identify a potential risk.

2) **Inoculations and vaccinations**
Code Z23 is for encounters for inoculations and vaccinations. It indicates that a patient is being seen to receive a prophylactic inoculation against a disease. Procedure codes are required to identify the actual administration of the injection and the type(s) of immunizations given. Code Z23 may be used as a secondary code if the inoculation is given as a routine part of preventive health care, such as a well-baby visit.

3) **Status**
Status codes indicate that a patient is either a carrier of a disease or has the sequelae or residual of a past disease or condition. This includes such things as the presence of prosthetic or mechanical devices resulting from past treatment. A status code is informative, because the status may affect the course of treatment and its outcome. A status code is distinct from a history code. The history code indicates that the patient no longer has the condition.

A status code should not be used with a diagnosis code from one of the body system chapters, if the diagnosis code includes the information provided by the status code. For example, code Z94.1, Heart transplant status, should not be used with a code from subcategory T86.2, Complications of heart transplant. The status code does not provide additional information. The complication code indicates that the patient is a heart transplant patient.

For encounters for weaning from a mechanical ventilator, assign a code from subcategory J96.1, Chronic respiratory failure, followed by code Z99.11, Dependence on respirator [ventilator] status.

The status Z codes/categories are:

Z14	Genetic carrier
	Genetic carrier status indicates that a person carries a gene, associated with a particular disease, which may be passed to offspring who may develop that disease. The person does not have the disease and is not at risk of developing the disease.
Z15	Genetic susceptibility to disease Genetic susceptibility indicates that a person has a gene that increases the risk of that person developing the disease.

Codes from category Z15 should not be used as principal or first-listed codes. If the patient has the condition to which he/she is susceptible, and that condition is the reason for the encounter, the code for the current condition should be sequenced first. If the patient is being seen for follow-up after completed treatment for this condition, and the condition no longer exists, a follow-up

code should be sequenced first, followed by the appropriate personal history and genetic susceptibility codes. If the purpose of the encounter is genetic counseling associated with procreative management, code Z31.5, Encounter for genetic counseling, should be assigned as the first-listed code, followed by a code from category Z15. Additional codes should be assigned for any applicable family or personal history.

Z16	Resistance to antimicrobial drugs
	This code indicates that a patient has a condition that is resistant to antimicrobial drug treatment. Sequence the infection code first.
Z17	Estrogen receptor status
Z18	Retained foreign body fragments
Z19	Hormone sensitivity malignancy status
Z21	Asymptomatic HIV infection status This code indicates that a patient has tested positive for HIV but has manifested no signs or symptoms of the disease.
Z22	Carrier of infectious disease Carrier status indicates that a person harbors the specific organisms of a disease without manifest symptoms and is capable of transmitting the infection.
Z28.3	Underimmunization status
Z33.1	Pregnant state, incidental This code is a secondary code only for use when the pregnancy is in no way complicating the reason for visit. Otherwise, a code from the obstetric chapter is required.
Z66	Do not resuscitate

This code may be used when it is documented by the provider that a patient is on do not resuscitate status at any time during the stay.

Z67	Blood type
Z68	Body mass index (BMI)
	As with all other secondary diagnosis codes, the BMI codes should only be assigned when they meet the definition of a reportable diagnosis (see Section III, Reporting Additional Diagnoses).
Z74.01	Bed confinement status
Z76.82	Awaiting organ transplant status
Z78	Other specified health status

Code Z78.1, Physical restraint status, may be used when it is documented by the provider that a patient has been put in restraints during the current encounter. Please note that this code should not be reported when it is documented by the provider that a patient is temporarily restrained during a procedure.

Z79	Long-term (current) drug therapy

Codes from this category indicate a patient's continuous use of a prescribed drug (including such things as aspirin therapy) for the long-term treatment of a condition or for prophylactic use. It is not for use for patients who have addictions to drugs. This subcategory is not for use of medications for detoxification or maintenance programs to prevent withdrawal symptoms in patients with drug dependence (e.g., methadone maintenance for opiate dependence). Assign the appropriate code for the drug dependence instead.

Assign a code from Z79 if the patient is receiving a medication for an extended period as a prophylactic measure (such as for the prevention of deep vein thrombosis) or as treatment of a chronic condition (such as arthritis) or a disease requiring a lengthy course of treatment (such as cancer). Do not assign a code from category Z79 for medication being administered for a brief period of time to treat an acute illness or injury (such as a course of antibiotics to treat acute bronchitis).

Z88	Allergy status to drugs, medicaments and biological substances Except: Z88.9, Allergy status to unspecified drugs, medicaments and biological substances status
Z89	Acquired absence of limb
Z90	Acquired absence of organs, not elsewhere classified
Z91.0-	Allergy status, other than to drugs and biological substances
Z92.82	Status post administration of tPA (rtPA) in a different facility within the last 24 hours prior to admission to a current facility Assign code Z92.82, Status post administration of tPA (rtPA) in a different facility within the last 24 hours prior to admission to current facility, as a secondary diagnosis when a patient is received by transfer into a facility and documentation indicates they were administered tissue plasminogen activator (tPA) within the last 24 hours prior to

admission to the current facility. This guideline applies even if the patient is still receiving the tPA at the time they are received into the current facility. The appropriate code for the condition for which the tPA was administered (such as cerebrovascular disease or myocardial infarction) should be assigned first. Code Z92.82 is only applicable to the receiving facility record and not to the transferring facility record.

Z93	Artificial opening status
Z94	Transplanted organ and tissue status
Z95	Presence of cardiac and vascular implants and grafts
Z96	Presence of other functional implants
Z97	Presence of other devices
Z98	Other postprocedural states

Assign code Z98.85, Transplanted organ removal status, to indicate that a transplanted organ has been previously removed. This code should not be assigned for the encounter in which the transplanted organ is removed. The complication necessitating removal of the transplant organ should be assigned for that encounter.

See section I.C.19. for information on the coding of organ transplant complications.

Z99	Dependence on enabling machines and devices, not elsewhere classified

Note: Categories Z89-Z90 and Z93-Z99 are for use only if there are no complications or malfunctions of the organ or tissue replaced, the amputation site or the equipment on which the patient is dependent.

4) History (of)

There are two types of history Z codes, personal and family. Personal history codes explain a patient's past medical condition that no longer exists and is not receiving any treatment, but that has the potential for recurrence, and therefore may require continued monitoring.

Family history codes are for use when a patient has a family member(s) who has had a particular disease that causes the patient to be at higher risk of also contracting the disease.

Personal history codes may be used in conjunction with follow-up codes and family history codes may be used in conjunction with screening codes to explain the need for a test or procedure. History codes are also acceptable on any medical record regardless of the reason for visit. A history of an illness, even if no longer present, is important information that may alter the type of treatment ordered.

The history Z code categories are:

Z80	Family history of primary malignant neoplasm
Z81	Family history of mental and behavioral disorders
Z82	Family history of certain disabilities and chronic diseases (leading to disablement)
Z83	Family history of other specific disorders
Z84	Family history of other conditions
Z85	Personal history of malignant neoplasm
Z86	Personal history of certain other diseases
Z87	Personal history of other diseases and conditions
Z91.4-	Personal history of psychological trauma, not elsewhere classified
Z91.5	Personal history of self-harm
Z91.81	**History of falling**
Z91.82	**Personal history of military deployment**
Z92	Personal history of medical treatment Except: Z92.0, Personal history of contraception Except: Z92.82, Status post administration of tPA (rtPA) in a different facility within the last 24 hours prior to admission to a current facility

5) Screening

Screening is the testing for disease or disease precursors in seemingly well individuals so that early detection and treatment can be provided for those who test positive for the disease (e.g., screening mammogram).

The testing of a person to rule out or confirm a suspected diagnosis because the patient has some sign or symptom is a diagnostic examination, not a screening. In these cases, the sign or symptom is used to explain the reason for the test.

A screening code may be a first-listed code if the reason for the visit is specifically the screening exam. It may also be used as an additional code if the screening is done during an office visit for other health problems. A screening code is

not necessary if the screening is inherent to a routine examination, such as a pap smear done during a routine pelvic examination.

Should a condition be discovered during the screening then the code for the condition may be assigned as an additional diagnosis.

The Z code indicates that a screening exam is planned. A procedure code is required to confirm that the screening was performed.

The screening Z codes/categories:

Z11	Encounter for screening for infectious and parasitic diseases
Z12	Encounter for screening for malignant neoplasms
Z13	Encounter for screening for other diseases and disorders Except: Z13.9, Encounter for screening, unspecified
Z36	Encounter for antenatal screening for mother

6) Observation

There are three observation Z code categories. They are for use in very limited circumstances when a person is being observed for a suspected condition that is ruled out. The observation codes are not for use if an injury or illness or any signs or symptoms related to the suspected condition are present. In such cases the diagnosis/symptom code is used with the corresponding external cause code.

The observation codes are to be used as principal diagnosis only. The only exception to this is when the principal diagnosis is required to be a code from category Z38, Liveborn infants according to place of birth and type of delivery. Then a code from category Z05, Encounter for observation and evaluation of newborn for suspected diseases and conditions ruled out, is sequenced after the Z38 code. Additional codes may be used in addition to the observation code but only if they are unrelated to the suspected condition being observed.

Codes from subcategory Z03.7 Encounter for suspected maternal and fetal conditions ruled out, may either be used as a first-listed or as an additional code assignment depending on the case. They are for use in very limited circumstances on a maternal record when an encounter is for a suspected maternal or fetal condition that is ruled out during that encounter (for example, a maternal or fetal condition may be suspected due to an abnormal test result). These codes should not be used when the condition is confirmed. In those cases, the confirmed condition should be coded. In addition, these codes are not for use if an illness or any signs or symptoms related to the suspected condition or problem are present. In such cases the diagnosis/symptom code is used.

Additional codes may be used in addition to the code from subcategory Z03.7, but only if they are unrelated to the suspected condition being evaluated.

Codes from subcategory Z03.7 may not be used for encounters for antenatal screening of mother. *See Section I.C.21. Screening.*

For encounters for suspected fetal condition that are inconclusive following testing and evaluation, assign the appropriate code from category O35, O36, O40 or O41.

The observation Z code categories:

Z03	Encounter for medical observation for suspected diseases and conditions ruled out
Z04	Encounter for examination and observation for other reasons Except: Z04.9, Encounter for examination and observation for unspecified reason
Z05	Encounter for observation and evaluation of newborn for suspected diseases and conditions ruled out

7) Aftercare

Aftercare visit codes cover situations when the initial treatment of a disease has been performed and the patient requires continued care during the healing or recovery phase, or for the long-term consequences of the disease. The aftercare Z code should not be used if treatment is directed at a current, acute disease. The diagnosis code is to be used in these cases.

Exceptions to this rule are codes Z51.0, Encounter for antineoplastic radiation therapy, and codes from subcategory Z51.1, Encounter for antineoplastic chemotherapy and immunotherapy. These codes are to be first-listed, followed by the diagnosis code when a patient's encounter is solely to receive radiation therapy, chemotherapy, or immunotherapy for the treatment of a neoplasm. If the reason for the encounter is more than one type of antineoplastic therapy, code Z51.0 and a code from subcategory Z51.1 may be assigned together, in which case one of these codes would be reported as a secondary diagnosis.

The aftercare Z codes should also not be used for aftercare for injuries. For aftercare of an injury, assign the acute injury code with the appropriate 7th character (for subsequent encounter).

The aftercare codes are generally first-listed to explain the specific reason for the encounter. An aftercare code may be used as an additional code when some type of aftercare is provided in addition to the reason for admission and no diagnosis code is applicable. An example of this would be the closure of a colostomy during an encounter for treatment of another condition.

Aftercare codes should be used in conjunction with other aftercare codes or diagnosis codes to provide better detail on the specifics of an aftercare encounter visit, unless otherwise directed by the classification. Should a patient receive multiple types of antineoplastic therapy during the same encounter, code Z51.0, Encounter for antineoplastic radiation therapy, and codes from subcategory Z51.1, Encounter for antineoplastic chemotherapy and immunotherapy, may be used together on a record. The sequencing of multiple aftercare codes depends on the circumstances of the encounter.

Certain aftercare Z code categories need a secondary diagnosis code to describe the resolving condition or sequelae. For others, the condition is included in the code title.

Additional Z code aftercare category terms include fitting and adjustment, and attention to artificial openings.

Status Z codes may be used with aftercare Z codes to indicate the nature of the aftercare. For example code Z95.1, Presence of aortocoronary bypass graft, may be used with code Z48.812, Encounter for surgical aftercare following surgery on the circulatory system, to indicate the surgery for which the aftercare is being performed. A status code should not be used when the aftercare code indicates the type of status, such as using Z43.0, Encounter for attention to tracheostomy, with Z93.0, Tracheostomy status.

The aftercare Z category/codes:

Z42	Encounter for plastic and reconstructive surgery following medical procedure or healed injury
Z43	Encounter for attention to artificial openings
Z44	Encounter for fitting and adjustment of external prosthetic device
Z45	Encounter for adjustment and management of implanted device
Z46	Encounter for fitting and adjustment of other devices
Z47	Orthopedic aftercare
Z48	Encounter for other postprocedural aftercare
Z49	Encounter for care involving renal dialysis
Z51	Encounter for other aftercare and medical care

8) Follow-up

The follow-up codes are used to explain continuing surveillance following completed treatment of a disease, condition, or injury. They imply that the condition has been fully treated and no longer exists. They should not be confused with aftercare codes, or injury codes with a 7th character for subsequent encounter, that explain ongoing care of a healing condition or its sequelae. Follow-up codes may be used in conjunction with history codes to provide the full picture of the healed condition and its treatment. The follow-up code is sequenced first, followed by the history code.

A follow-up code may be used to explain multiple visits. Should a condition be found to have recurred on the follow-up visit, then the diagnosis code for the condition should be assigned in place of the follow-up code.

The follow-up Z code categories:

Z08	Encounter for follow-up examination after completed treatment for malignant neoplasm
Z09	Encounter for follow-up examination after completed treatment for conditions other than malignant neoplasm
Z39	Encounter for maternal postpartum care and examination

9) Donor

Codes in category Z52, Donors of organs and tissues, are used for living individuals who are donating blood or other body tissue.

These codes are only for individuals donating for others, not for self-donations. They are not used to identify cadaveric donations.

10) Counseling

Counseling Z codes are used when a patient or family member receives assistance in the aftermath of an illness or injury, or when support is required in coping with family or social problems.

The counseling Z codes/categories:

Z30.0-	Encounter for general counseling and advice on contraception
Z31.5	Encounter for **procreative** genetic counseling
Z31.6-	Encounter for general counseling and advice on procreation
Z32.2	Encounter for childbirth instruction
Z32.3	Encounter for childcare instruction
Z69	Encounter for mental health services for victim and perpetrator of abuse
Z70	Counseling related to sexual attitude, behavior and orientation
Z71	Persons encountering health services for other counseling and medical advice, not elsewhere classified
Z76.81	Expectant mother prebirth pediatrician visit

11) Encounters for Obstetrical and Reproductive Services

See Section I.C.15. Pregnancy, Childbirth, and the Puerperium, for further instruction on the use of these codes.

Z codes for pregnancy are for use in those circumstances when none of the problems or complications included in the codes from the Obstetrics chapter exist (a routine prenatal visit or postpartum care). Codes in category Z34, Encounter for supervision of normal pregnancy, are always first listed and are not to be used with any other code from the OB chapter.

Codes in category Z3A, Weeks of gestation, may be assigned to provide additional information about the pregnancy. Category Z3A codes should not be assigned for pregnancies with abortive outcomes (categories O00-O08), elective termination of pregnancy (code Z33.2), nor for postpartum conditions, as category Z3A is not applicable to these conditions. The date of the admission should be used to determine weeks of gestation for inpatient admissions that encompass more than one gestational week.

The outcome of delivery, category Z37, should be included on all maternal delivery records. It is always a secondary code. Codes in category Z37 should not be used on the newborn record.

Z codes for family planning (contraceptive) or procreative management and counseling should be included on an obstetric record either during the pregnancy or the postpartum stage, if applicable.

Z codes/categories for obstetrical and reproductive services:

Z30	Encounter for contraceptive management
Z31	Encounter for procreative management
Z32.2	Encounter for childbirth instruction
Z32.3	Encounter for childcare instruction
Z33	Pregnant state
Z34	Encounter for supervision of normal pregnancy
Z36	Encounter for antenatal screening of mother
Z3A	Weeks of gestation
Z37	Outcome of delivery
Z39	Encounter for maternal postpartum care and examination
Z76.81	Expectant mother prebirth pediatrician visit

12) Newborns and Infants

See Section I.C.16. Newborn (Perinatal) Guidelines, for further instruction on the use of these codes.

Newborn Z codes/categories:

Z76.1	Encounter for health supervision and care of foundling
Z00.1-	Encounter for routine child health examination
Z38	Liveborn infants according to place of birth and type of delivery

13) Routine and administrative examinations

The Z codes allow for the description of encounters for routine examinations, such as, a general check-up, or, examinations for administrative purposes, such as, a pre-employment physical. The codes are not to be used if the examination is for diagnosis of a suspected condition or for treatment purposes. In such cases the diagnosis code is used. During a routine exam, should a diagnosis or condition be discovered, it should be coded as an additional code. Pre-existing and chronic conditions and history codes may also be included as additional codes as long as the examination is for administrative purposes and not focused on any particular condition.

Some of the codes for routine health examinations distinguish between "with" and "without" abnormal findings. Code assignment depends on the information that is known at the time the encounter is being coded. For example, if no abnormal findings were found during the examination, but the encounter is being coded before test results are back, it is acceptable to assign the code for "without abnormal findings." When assigning a code for "with abnormal findings," additional code(s) should be assigned to identify the specific abnormal finding(s).

Pre-operative examination and pre-procedural laboratory examination Z codes are for use only in those situations when a patient is being cleared for a procedure or surgery and no treatment is given.

The Z codes/categories for routine and administrative examinations:

Z00	Encounter for general examination without complaint, suspected or reported diagnosis
Z01	Encounter for other special examination without complaint, suspected or reported diagnosis
Z02	Encounter for administrative examination Except: Z02.9, Encounter for administrative examinations, unspecified
Z32.0-	Encounter for pregnancy test

14) Miscellaneous Z codes

The miscellaneous Z codes capture a number of other health care encounters that do not fall into one of the other categories. Certain of these codes identify the reason for the encounter; others are for use as additional codes that provide useful information on circumstances that may affect a patient's care and treatment.

Prophylactic Organ Removal

For encounters specifically for prophylactic removal of an organ (such as prophylactic removal of breasts due to a genetic susceptibility to cancer or a family history of cancer), the principal or first-listed code should be a code from category Z40, Encounter for prophylactic surgery, followed by the appropriate codes to identify the associated risk factor (such as genetic susceptibility or family history).

If the patient has a malignancy of one site and is having prophylactic removal at another site to prevent either a new primary malignancy or metastatic disease, a code for the malignancy should also be assigned in addition to a code from subcategory Z40.0, Encounter for prophylactic surgery for risk factors related to malignant neoplasms. A Z40.0 code should not be assigned if the patient is having organ removal for treatment of a malignancy, such as the removal of the testes for the treatment of prostate cancer.

Miscellaneous Z codes/categories:

Z28	Immunization not carried out Except: Z28.3, Underimmunization status
Z29	Encounter for other prophylactic measures
Z40	Encounter for prophylactic surgery
Z41	Encounter for procedures for purposes other than remedying health state Except: Z41.9, Encounter for procedure for purposes other than remedying health state, unspecified
Z53	Persons encountering health services for specific procedures and treatment, not carried out
Z55	Problems related to education and literacy
Z56	Problems related to employment and unemployment
Z57	Occupational exposure to risk factors
Z58	Problems related to physical environment
Z59	Problems related to housing and economic circumstances
Z60	Problems related to social environment
Z62	Problems related to upbringing
Z63	Other problems related to primary support group, including family circumstances
Z64	Problems related to certain psychosocial circumstances
Z65	Problems related to other psychosocial circumstances
Z72	Problems related to lifestyle Note: These codes should be assigned only when the documentation specifies that the patient has an associated problem
Z73	Problems related to life-management difficulty
Z74	Problems related to care provider dependency Except: Z74.01, Bed confinement status
Z75	Problems related to medical facilities and other health care
Z76.0	Encounter for issue of repeat prescription
Z76.3	Healthy person accompanying sick person
Z76.4	Other boarder to healthcare facility
Z76.5	Malingerer [conscious simulation]
Z91.1-	Patient's noncompliance with medical treatment and regimen
Z91.83	Wandering in diseases classified elsewhere
Z91.84-	**Oral health risk factors**
Z91.89	Other specified personal risk factors, not elsewhere classified

15) Nonspecific Z codes

Certain Z codes are so non-specific, or potentially redundant with other codes in the classification, that there can be little justification for their use in the inpatient setting. Their use in the outpatient setting should be limited to those instances when there is no further documentation to permit more precise coding. Otherwise, any sign or symptom or any other reason for visit that is captured in another code should be used.

Nonspecific Z codes/categories:

Z02.9	Encounter for administrative examinations, unspecified
Z04.9	Encounter for examination and observation for unspecified reason
Z13.9	Encounter for screening, unspecified
Z41.9	Encounter for procedure for purposes other than remedying health state, unspecified
Z52.9	Donor of unspecified organ or tissue
Z86.59	Personal history of other mental and behavioral disorders
Z88.9	Allergy status to unspecified drugs, medicaments and biological substances status
Z92.0	Personal history of contraception

16) Z Codes That May Only be Principal/First-Listed Diagnosis

The following Z codes/categories may only be reported as the principal/first-listed diagnosis, except when there are multiple encounters on the same day and the medical records for the encounters are combined:

Z00	Encounter for general examination without complaint, suspected or reported diagnosis Except: Z00.6
Z01	Encounter for other special examination without complaint, suspected or reported diagnosis
Z02	Encounter for administrative examination
Z03	Encounter for medical observation for suspected diseases and conditions ruled out
Z04	Encounter for examination and observation for other reasons
Z33.2	Encounter for elective termination of pregnancy
Z31.81	Encounter for male factor infertility in female patient
Z31.83	Encounter for assisted reproductive fertility procedure cycle
Z31.84	Encounter for fertility preservation procedure
Z34	Encounter for supervision of normal pregnancy
Z39	Encounter for maternal postpartum care and examination
Z38	Liveborn infants according to place of birth and type of delivery
Z40	**Encounter for prophylactic surgery**
Z42	Encounter for plastic and reconstructive surgery following medical procedure or healed injury
Z51.0	Encounter for antineoplastic radiation therapy
Z51.1-	Encounter for antineoplastic chemotherapy and immunotherapy
Z52	Donors of organs and tissues Except: Z52.9, Donor of unspecified organ or tissue
Z76.1	Encounter for health supervision and care of foundling
Z76.2	Encounter for health supervision and care of other healthy infant and child
Z99.12	Encounter for respirator [ventilator] dependence during power failure

CHAPTER 21

FACTORS INFLUENCING HEALTH STATUS AND CONTACT WITH HEALTH SERVICES (ZØØ-Z99)

Note: Z codes represent reasons for encounters. A corresponding procedure code must accompany a Z code if a procedure is performed. Categories ZØØ-Z99 are provided for occasions when circumstances other than a disease, injury or external cause classifiable to categories AØØ-Y89 are recorded as 'diagnoses' or 'problems.' This can arise in two main ways:

(a) When a person who may or may not be sick encounters the health services for some specific purpose, such as to receive limited care or service for a current condition, to donate an organ or tissue, to receive prophylactic vaccination (immunization), or to discuss a problem which is in itself not a disease or injury.

(b) When some circumstance or problem is present which influences the person's health status but is not in itself a current illness or injury.

This chapter contains the following blocks:

ZØØ-Z13	Persons encountering health services for examination
Z14-Z15	Genetic carrier and genetic susceptibility to disease
Z16	Resistance to antimicrobial drugs
Z17	Estrogen receptor status
Z18	Retained foreign body fragments
~~Z19~~	~~Hormone sensitivity malignancy status~~
Z20-Z29	Persons with potential health hazards related to communicable diseases
Z30-Z39	Persons encountering health services in circumstances related to reproduction
Z40-Z53	Encounters for other specific health care
Z55-Z65	Persons with potential health hazards related to socioeconomic and psychosocial circumstances
Z66	Do not resuscitate status
Z67	Blood type
Z68	Body mass index (BMI)
Z69-Z76	Persons encountering health services in other circumstances
Z77-Z99	Persons with potential health hazards related to family and personal history and certain conditions influencing health status

PERSONS ENCOUNTERING HEALTH SERVICES FOR EXAMINATIONS (ZØØ-Z13)

Note: Nonspecific abnormal findings disclosed at the time of these examinations are classified to categories R70-R94.

> **Excludes1**   examinations related to pregnancy and reproduction (Z30-Z36, Z39.-)

● **ZØØ**   **Encounter for general examination without complaint, suspected or reported diagnosis**

> **Excludes1**   encounter for examination for administrative purposes (ZØ2.-)

> **Excludes2**   encounter for pre-procedural examinations (ZØ1.81-)
> special screening examinations (Z11-Z13)

● **ZØØ.Ø**   **Encounter for general adult medical examination**
Encounter for adult periodic examination (annual) (physical) and any associated laboratory and radiologic examinations

> **Excludes1**   encounter for examination of sign or symptom - code to sign or symptom
> general health check-up of infant or child (ZØØ.12.-)
> Coding Clinic: 2016, Q4, P131

● **ZØØ.ØØ**   **Encounter for general adult medical examination without abnormal findings**   A
Encounter for adult health check-up NOS
Coding Clinic: 2016, Q1, P37

● **ZØØ.Ø1**   **Encounter for general adult medical examination with abnormal findings**   A
Use additional code to identify abnormal findings
Coding Clinic: 2016, Q1, P36

● **ZØØ.1**   **Encounter for newborn, infant and child health examinations**

● **ZØØ.11**   **Newborn health examination**
Health check for child under 29 days old
Use additional code to identify any abnormal findings

> **Excludes1**   health check for child over 28 days old (ZØØ.12-)

● **ZØØ.110**   **Health examination for newborn under 8 days old**   N
Health check for newborn under 8 days old

● **ZØØ.111**   **Health examination for newborn 8 to 28 days old**   N
Health check for newborn 8 to 28 days old
Newborn weight check

● **ZØØ.12**   **Encounter for routine child health examination**
Encounter for development testing of infant or child
Health check (routine) for child over 28 days old

> **Excludes1**   health check for child under 29 days old (ZØØ.11-)
> health supervision of foundling or other healthy infant or child (Z76.1-Z76.2)
> newborn health examination (ZØØ.11-)

● **ZØØ.121**   **Encounter for routine child health examination with abnormal findings**   P
Use additional code to identify abnormal findings
Coding Clinic: 2016, Q1, P34-35

● **ZØØ.129**   **Encounter for routine child health examination without abnormal findings**   P
Encounter for routine child health examination NOS
Coding Clinic: 2016, Q1, P34

● **ZØØ.2**   **Encounter for examination for period of rapid growth in childhood**   P

● **ZØØ.3**   **Encounter for examination for adolescent development state**   P
Encounter for puberty development state

● **ZØØ.5**   **Encounter for examination of potential donor of organ and tissue**

ZØØ.6   **Encounter for examination for normal comparison and control in clinical research program**
Examination of participant or control in clinical research program

● **ZØØ.7**   **Encounter for examination for period of delayed growth in childhood**

● **ZØØ.70**   **Encounter for examination for period of delayed growth in childhood without abnormal findings**   P

● **ZØØ.71**   **Encounter for examination for period of delayed growth in childhood with abnormal findings**   P
Use additional code to identify abnormal findings

● **ZØØ.8**   **Encounter for other general examination**
Encounter for health examination in population surveys

▶ New   ⟾ Revised   ~~deleted~~ Deleted   Excludes 1   Excludes 2   Includes   Use additional   Code first   Code also   Key words
OGCR Official Guidelines   ● Unacceptable Principal Diagnosis   X Assign placeholder X   ● Use Additional Character(s)   ▶ Manifestation Code   Coding Clinic

● **Z01   Encounter for other special examination without complaint, suspected or reported diagnosis**

> **Includes**   routine examination of specific system

> **Note:** Codes from category Z01 represent the reason for the encounter. A separate procedure code is required to identify any examinations or procedures performed.

> **Excludes1**   encounter for examination for administrative purposes (Z02.-)
> encounter for examination for suspected conditions, proven not to exist (Z03.-)
> encounter for laboratory and radiologic examinations as a component of general medical examinations (Z00.0-)
> encounter for laboratory, radiologic and imaging examinations for sign(s) and symptom(s) - code to the sign(s) or symptom(s)

> **Excludes2**   screening examinations (Z11-Z13)

● **Z01.0   Encounter for examination of eyes and vision**

> **Excludes1**   examination for driving license (Z02.4)

> **Z01.00   Encounter for examination of eyes and vision without abnormal findings**
> Encounter for examination of eyes and vision NOS

> **Z01.01   Encounter for examination of eyes and vision with abnormal findings**
> Use additional code to identify abnormal findings
> **Coding Clinic: 2016, Q4, P21**

● **Z01.1   Encounter for examination of ears and hearing**

> ● **Z01.10   Encounter for examination of ears and hearing without abnormal findings**
> Encounter for examination of ears and hearing NOS
> **Coding Clinic: 2016, Q4, P25**

> ● **Z01.11   Encounter for examination of ears and hearing with abnormal findings**
> **Coding Clinic: 2016, Q3, P18**

>> ● **Z01.110   Encounter for hearing examination following failed hearing screening**
>> **Coding Clinic: 2016, Q3, P18-19**

>> ● **Z01.118   Encounter for examination of ears and hearing with other abnormal findings**
>> Use additional code to identify abnormal findings
>> **Coding Clinic: 2016, Q3, P17**

> ● **Z01.12   Encounter for hearing conservation and treatment**

● **Z01.2   Encounter for dental examination and cleaning**

> ● **Z01.20   Encounter for dental examination and cleaning without abnormal findings**
> Encounter for dental examination and cleaning NOS

> ● **Z01.21   Encounter for dental examination and cleaning with abnormal findings**
> Use additional code to identify abnormal findings

● **Z01.3   Encounter for examination of blood pressure**

> ● **Z01.30   Encounter for examination of blood pressure without abnormal findings**
> Encounter for examination of blood pressure NOS

> ● **Z01.31   Encounter for examination of blood pressure with abnormal findings**
> Use additional code to identify abnormal findings

● **Z01.4   Encounter for gynecological examination**

> **Excludes2**   pregnancy examination or test (Z32.0-)
> routine examination for contraceptive maintenance (Z30.4-)

● **Z01.41   Encounter for routine gynecological examination**
> Encounter for general gynecological examination with or without cervical smear
> Encounter for gynecological examination (general) (routine) NOS
> Encounter for pelvic examination (annual) (periodic)

> Use additional code:
> for screening for human papillomavirus, if applicable (Z11.51)
> for screening vaginal pap smear, if applicable (Z12.72)
> to identify acquired absence of uterus, if applicable (Z90.71-)

> **Excludes1**   gynecologic examination status-post hysterectomy for malignant condition (Z08)
> screening cervical pap smear not a part of a routine gynecological examination (Z12.4)

> **Z01.411   Encounter for gynecological examination (general) (routine) with abnormal findings ♀**
> Use additional code to identify any abnormal findings

> **Z01.419   Encounter for gynecological examination (general) (routine) without abnormal findings ♀**

> **Z01.42   Encounter for cervical smear to confirm findings of recent normal smear following initial abnormal smear ♀**

● **Z01.8   Encounter for other specified special examinations**

> ● **Z01.81   Encounter for preprocedural examinations**
> Encounter for preoperative examinations
> Encounter for radiological and imaging examinations as part of preprocedural examination

> **Z01.810   Encounter for preprocedural cardiovascular examination**

> **Z01.811   Encounter for preprocedural respiratory examination**

> ● **Z01.812   Encounter for preprocedural laboratory examination**
> Blood and urine tests prior to treatment or procedure

> ● **Z01.818   Encounter for other preprocedural examination**
> Encounter for preprocedural examination NOS
> Encounter for examinations prior to antineoplastic chemotherapy

> ● **Z01.82   Encounter for allergy testing**
>> **Excludes1**   encounter for antibody response examination (Z01.84)

> ● **Z01.83   Encounter for blood typing**
> Encounter for Rh typing

> ● **Z01.84   Encounter for antibody response examination**
> Encounter for immunity status testing
>> **Excludes1**   encounter for allergy testing (Z01.82)

> ● **Z01.89   Encounter for other specified special examinations**

CHAPTER 21 (Z00-Z99)

● **Z02** **Encounter for administrative examination**
  ● **Z02.0** **Encounter for examination for admission to educational institution**
      Encounter for examination for admission to preschool (education)
      Encounter for examination for re-admission to school following illness or medical treatment
  Z02.1 **Encounter for pre-employment examination**
  ● **Z02.2** **Encounter for examination for admission to residential institution**
      Excludes1 examination for admission to prison (Z02.89)
  Z02.3 **Encounter for examination for recruitment to armed forces**
  ● **Z02.4** **Encounter for examination for driving license**
  ● **Z02.5** **Encounter for examination for participation in sport**
      Excludes1 blood-alcohol and blood-drug test (Z02.83)
  ● **Z02.6** **Encounter for examination for insurance purposes**
  ● **Z02.7** **Encounter for issue of medical certificate**
      Excludes1 encounter for general medical examination (Z00-Z01, Z02.0-Z02.6, Z02.8-Z02.9)
    ● **Z02.71** **Encounter for disability determination**
      Encounter for issue of medical certificate of incapacity
      Encounter for issue of medical certificate of invalidity
    ● **Z02.79** **Encounter for issue of other medical certificate**
  ● **Z02.8** **Encounter for other administrative examinations**
    Z02.81 **Encounter for paternity testing**
    ● **Z02.82** **Encounter for adoption services**
    Z02.83 **Encounter for blood-alcohol and blood-drug test**
      Use additional code for findings of alcohol or drugs in blood (R78.-)
    ● **Z02.89** **Encounter for other administrative examinations**
      Encounter for examination for admission to prison
      Encounter for examination for admission to summer camp
      Encounter for immigration examination
      Encounter for naturalization examination
      Encounter for premarital examination
      Excludes1 health supervision of foundling or other healthy infant or child (Z76.1-Z76.2)
  ● **Z02.9** **Encounter for administrative examinations, unspecified**

OGCR Section II.C.21.c.6.

Observation

There are **three** observation Z code categories. They are for use in very limited circumstances when a person is being observed for a suspected condition that is ruled out. The observation codes are not for use if an injury or illnesses or any signs or symptoms related to the suspected condition are present. In such cases the diagnosis/symptom code is used with the corresponding external cause code.

The observation codes are to be used as principal diagnosis only. **The only exception to this is when the principal diagnosis is required to be a code from category Z38, Liveborn infants according to place of birth and type of delivery. Then a code from category Z05, Encounter for observation and evaluation of newborn for suspected diseases and conditions ruled out, is sequenced after the Z38 code.** Additional codes may be used in addition to the observation code but only if they are unrelated to the suspected condition being observed.

Codes from subcategory Z03.7 Encounter for suspected maternal and fetal conditions ruled out, may either be used as a first listed or as an additional code assignment depending on the case. They are for use in very limited circumstances on a maternal record when an encounter is for a suspected maternal or fetal condition that is ruled out during that encounter (for example, a maternal or fetal condition may be suspected due to an abnormal test result). These codes should not be used when the condition is confirmed. In those cases, the confirmed condition should be coded. In addition, these codes are not for use if an illness or any signs or symptoms related to the suspected condition or problem are present. In such cases the diagnosis/symptom code is used.

Additional codes may be used in addition to the code from subcategory Z03.7, but only if they are unrelated to the suspected condition being evaluated.

Codes from subcategory Z03.7 may not be used for encounters for antenatal screening of mother. *See Section I.C.21. Screening.*

For encounters for suspected fetal condition that are inconclusive following testing and evaluation, assign the appropriate code from category O35, O36, O40 or O41.

The observation Z code categories:

Z03 Encounter for medical observation for suspected diseases and conditions ruled out

Z04 Encounter for examination and observation for other reasons
    Except: Z04.9, Encounter for examination and observation for unspecified reason

Z05 Encounter for observation and evaluation of newborn for suspected diseases and conditions ruled out

● **Z03** **Encounter for medical observation for suspected diseases and conditions ruled out**
    This category is to be used when a person without a diagnosis is suspected of having an abnormal condition, without signs or symptoms, which requires study, but after examination and observation, is ruled out. This category is also for use for administrative and legal observation status.
    Excludes1 contact with and (suspected) exposures hazardous to health (Z77.-)
      ▶encounter for observation and evaluation of newborn for suspected diseases and conditions ruled out (Z05.0-)
      newborn observation for suspected condition, ruled out (P00-P04)
      person with feared complaint in whom no diagnosis is made (Z71.1)
      signs or symptoms under study - code to signs or symptoms
    Z03.6 **Encounter for observation for suspected toxic effect from ingested substance ruled out**
      Encounter for observation for suspected adverse effect from drug
      Encounter for observation for suspected poisoning

▶ New   ⇒ Revised   ~~deleted~~ Deleted   Excludes 1   Excludes 2   Includes   Use additional   Code first   Code also   Key words
OGCR Official Guidelines   ● Unacceptable Principal Diagnosis   X Assign placeholder X   ● Use Additional Character(s)   ▶ Manifestation Code   Coding Clinic

● **Z03.7 Encounter for suspected maternal and fetal conditions ruled out**

Encounter for suspected maternal and fetal conditions not found

> **Excludes1** known or suspected fetal anomalies affecting management of mother, not ruled out (O26.-, O35.-, O36.-, O40.-, O41.-)

● **Z03.71 Encounter for suspected problem with amniotic cavity and membrane ruled out ♀**   **M**

Encounter for suspected oligohydramnios ruled out

Encounter for suspected polyhydramnios ruled out

● **Z03.72 Encounter for suspected placental problem ruled out ♀**   **M**

● **Z03.73 Encounter for suspected fetal anomaly ruled out ♀**   **M**

Coding Clinic: 2016, Q4, P6

● **Z03.74 Encounter for suspected problem with fetal growth ruled out ♀**   **M**

● **Z03.75 Encounter for suspected cervical shortening ruled out ♀**   **M**

● **Z03.79 Encounter for other suspected maternal and fetal conditions ruled out ♀**   **M**

Coding Clinic: 2016, Q4, P7

● **Z03.8 Encounter for observation for other suspected diseases and conditions ruled out**

● **Z03.81 Encounter for observation for suspected exposure to biological agents ruled out**

Z03.810 Encounter for observation for suspected exposure to anthrax ruled out

Z03.818 Encounter for observation for suspected exposure to other biological agents ruled out

Z03.89 Encounter for observation for other suspected diseases and conditions ruled out

● **Z04 Encounter for examination and observation for other reasons**

> **Includes** encounter for examination for medicolegal reasons
>
> This category is to be used when a person without a diagnosis is suspected of having an abnormal condition, without signs or symptoms, which requires study, but after examination and observation, is ruled-out. This category is also for use for administrative and legal observation status.

Z04.1 Encounter for examination and observation following transport accident

> **Excludes1** encounter for examination and observation following work accident (Z04.2)

Z04.2 Encounter for examination and observation following work accident

Z04.3 Encounter for examination and observation following other accident

● **Z04.4 Encounter for examination and observation following alleged rape**

Encounter for examination and observation of victim following alleged rape

Encounter for examination and observation of victim following alleged sexual abuse

Coding Clinic: 2016, Q4, P129

Z04.41 Encounter for examination and observation following alleged adult rape   **A**

Suspected adult rape, ruled out

Suspected adult sexual abuse, ruled out

Z04.42 Encounter for examination and observation following alleged child rape   **P**

Suspected child rape, ruled out

Suspected child sexual abuse, ruled out

Z04.6 Encounter for general psychiatric examination, requested by authority

● **Z04.7 Encounter for examination and observation following alleged physical abuse**

Z04.71 Encounter for examination and observation following alleged adult physical abuse   **A**

Suspected adult physical abuse, ruled out

> **Excludes1** confirmed case of adult physical abuse (T74.-)
>
> encounter for examination and observation following alleged adult sexual abuse (Z04.41)
>
> suspected case of adult physical abuse, not ruled out (T76.-)

Z04.72 Encounter for examination and observation following alleged child physical abuse   **P**

Suspected child physical abuse, ruled out

> **Excludes1** confirmed case of child physical abuse (T74.-)
>
> encounter for examination and observation following alleged child sexual abuse (Z04.42)
>
> suspected case of child physical abuse, not ruled out (T76.-)

Z04.8 Encounter for examination and observation for other specified reasons

Encounter for examination and observation for request for expert evidence

● **Z04.9 Encounter for examination and observation for unspecified reason**

Encounter for observation NOS

● **Z05 Encounter for observation and evaluation of newborn for suspected diseases and conditions ruled out**

➠ This category is to be used for newborns, within the neonatal period (the first 28 days of life), who are suspected of having an abnormal condition, but without signs or symptoms, and which, after examination and observation, is ruled out.

> ~~**Excludes1** newborn observation for suspected condition, related to exposure from the mother or birth process (P00-P04)~~

Coding Clinic: 2016, Q4, P54, 77, 126-127, 130

Z05.0 Observation and evaluation of newborn for suspected cardiac condition ruled out

Z05.1 Observation and evaluation of newborn for suspected infectious condition ruled out

Z05.2 Observation and evaluation of newborn for suspected neurological condition ruled out

Z05.3 Observation and evaluation of newborn for suspected respiratory condition ruled out

● **Z05.4 Observation and evaluation of newborn for suspected genetic, metabolic or immunologic condition ruled out**

Z05.41 Observation and evaluation of newborn for suspected genetic condition ruled out

Coding Clinic: 2016, Q4, P55

Z05.42 Observation and evaluation of newborn for suspected metabolic condition ruled out

Z05.43 Observation and evaluation of newborn for suspected immunologic condition ruled out

Z05.5 Observation and evaluation of newborn for suspected gastrointestinal condition ruled out

Z05.6 Observation and evaluation of newborn for suspected genitourinary condition ruled out

CHAPTER 21 (Z00-Z99)

N Newborn Age: 0   **P** Pediatric Age: 0–17   **M** Maternity DX: 12–55   **A** Adult Age: 15–124   ♀ Females Only   ♂ Males Only

🅒 Complication\Comorbidity   🅜 Major C\C   (Ex) CC/MCC Exclusions   🅗 Hospital-Acquired Condition

1593

● **Z05.7** **Observation and evaluation of newborn for suspected skin, subcutaneous, musculoskeletal and connective tissue condition ruled out**

     Z05.71 **Observation and evaluation of newborn for suspected skin and subcutaneous tissue condition ruled out**

     Z05.72 **Observation and evaluation of newborn for suspected musculoskeletal condition ruled out**

     Z05.73 **Observation and evaluation of newborn for suspected connective tissue condition ruled out**

   Z05.8 **Observation and evaluation of newborn for other specified suspected condition ruled out**

   Z05.9 **Observation and evaluation of newborn for unspecified suspected condition ruled out**

OGCR See Section II.C.21.c.8.

The follow-up codes are used to explain continuing surveillance following completed treatment of a disease, condition, or injury. They imply that the condition has been fully treated and no longer exists. They should not be confused with aftercare codes, or injury codes with 7th character "D," that explain ongoing care of a healing condition or its sequelae. Follow-up codes may be used in conjunction with history codes to provide the full picture of the healed condition and its treatment. The follow-up code is sequenced first, followed by the history code.

A follow-up code may be used to explain multiple visits. Should a condition be found to have recurred on the follow-up visit, then the diagnosis code for the condition should be assigned in place of the follow-up code.

The follow-up Z code categories:

Z08   Encounter for follow-up examination after completed treatment for malignant neoplasm

Z09   Encounter for follow-up examination after completed treatment for conditions other than malignant neoplasm

Z39   Encounter for maternal postpartum care and examination

● **Z08** **Encounter for follow-up examination after completed treatment for malignant neoplasm**

Medical surveillance following completed treatment

Use additional code to identify any acquired absence of organs (Z90.-)

Use additional code to identify the personal history of malignant neoplasm (Z85.-)

Excludes1 aftercare following medical care (Z43-Z49, Z51)

● **Z09** **Encounter for follow-up examination after completed treatment for conditions other than malignant neoplasm**

Medical surveillance following completed treatment

Use additional code to identify any applicable history of disease code (Z86.-. Z87.-)

Excludes1 aftercare following medical care (Z43-Z49, Z51)
surveillance of contraception (Z30.4-)
surveillance of prosthetic and other medical devices (Z44-Z46)

Coding Clinic: 2017, Q1, P9; 2015, Q1, P8

OGCR Section II.C.21.c.5.

Screening

Screening is the testing for disease or disease precursors in seemingly well individuals so that early detection and treatment can be provided for those who test positive for the disease (e.g., screening mammogram).

The testing of a person to rule out or confirm a suspected diagnosis because the patient has some sign or symptom is a diagnostic examination, not a screening. In these cases, the sign or symptom is used to explain the reason for the test.

A screening code may be a first listed code if the reason for the visit is specifically the screening exam. It may also be used as an additional code if the screening is done during an office visit for other health problems. A screening code is not necessary if the screening is inherent to a routine examination, such as a pap smear done during a routine pelvic examination.

Should a condition be discovered during the screening then the code for the condition may be assigned as an additional diagnosis.

The Z code indicates that a screening exam is planned. A procedure code is required to confirm that the screening was performed.

The screening Z codes /categories:

Z11   Encounter for screening for infectious and parasitic diseases

Z12   Encounter for screening for malignant neoplasms

Z13   Encounter for screening for other diseases and disorders
Except: Z13.9, Encounter for screening, unspecified

Z36   Encounter for antenatal screening for mother

● **Z11** **Encounter for screening for infectious and parasitic diseases**

Screening is the testing for disease or disease precursors in asymptomatic individuals so that early detection and treatment can be provided for those who test positive for the disease.

Excludes1 encounter for diagnostic examination - code to sign or symptom

● **Z11.0** **Encounter for screening for intestinal infectious diseases**

● **Z11.1** **Encounter for screening for respiratory tuberculosis**

● **Z11.2** **Encounter for screening for other bacterial diseases**

● **Z11.3** **Encounter for screening for infections with a predominantly sexual mode of transmission**

Excludes2 encounter for screening for human immunodeficiency virus [HIV] (Z11.4)
encounter for screening for human papillomavirus (Z11.51)

● **Z11.4** **Encounter for screening for human immunodeficiency virus [HIV]**

● **Z11.5** **Encounter for screening for other viral diseases**

Excludes2 encounter for screening for viral intestinal disease (Z11.0)

   ● **Z11.51** **Encounter for screening for human papillomavirus (HPV)**

   ● **Z11.59** **Encounter for screening for other viral diseases**

● **Z11.6** **Encounter for screening for other protozoal diseases and helminthiases**

Diseases or infestations caused by parasitic worms

Excludes2 encounter for screening for protozoal intestinal disease (Z11.0)

● **Z11.8** **Encounter for screening for other infectious and parasitic diseases**

Encounter for screening for chlamydia
Encounter for screening for rickettsial
Encounter for screening for spirochetal
Encounter for screening for mycoses

● **Z11.9** **Encounter for screening for infectious and parasitic diseases, unspecified**

CHAPTER 21 (Z00-Z99)

● **Z12   Encounter for screening for malignant neoplasms**
     Screening is the testing for disease or disease precursors in asymptomatic individuals so that early detection and treatment can be provided for those who test positive for the disease.

     Use additional code to identify any family history of malignant neoplasm (Z80.-)

     Excludes1   encounter for diagnostic examination - code to sign or symptom

   ● **Z12.0   Encounter for screening for malignant neoplasm of stomach**

   ● **Z12.1   Encounter for screening for malignant neoplasm of intestinal tract**

     ● **Z12.10   Encounter for screening for malignant neoplasm of intestinal tract, unspecified**

     ● **Z12.11   Encounter for screening for malignant neoplasm of colon**
       Encounter for screening colonoscopy NOS
       Coding Clinic: 2017, Q1, P8-9

     ● **Z12.12   Encounter for screening for malignant neoplasm of rectum**

     ● **Z12.13   Encounter for screening for malignant neoplasm of small intestine**

   ● **Z12.2   Encounter for screening for malignant neoplasm of respiratory organs**

   ● **Z12.3   Encounter for screening for malignant neoplasm of breast**

     ● **Z12.31   Encounter for screening mammogram for malignant neoplasm of breast**
       Excludes1   inconclusive mammogram (R92.2)
       Coding Clinic: 2015, Q1, P24

     ● **Z12.39   Encounter for other screening for malignant neoplasm of breast**

   ● **Z12.4   Encounter for screening for malignant neoplasm of cervix ♀**
     Encounter for screening pap smear for malignant neoplasm of cervix
     Excludes1   when screening is part of general gynecological examination (Z01.4-)
     Excludes2   encounter for screening for human papillomavirus (Z11.51)

   Z12.5   Encounter for screening for malignant neoplasm of prostate ♂

   ● **Z12.6   Encounter for screening for malignant neoplasm of bladder**

   ● **Z12.7   Encounter for screening for malignant neoplasm of other genitourinary organs**

     ● **Z12.71   Encounter for screening for malignant neoplasm of testis ♂**

     ● **Z12.72   Encounter for screening for malignant neoplasm of vagina ♀**
       Vaginal pap smear status - post hysterectomy for non-malignant condition
       Use additional code to identify acquired absence of uterus (Z90.71-)
       Excludes1   vaginal pap smear status - post hysterectomy for malignant conditions (Z08)

     ● **Z12.73   Encounter for screening for malignant neoplasm of ovary ♀**

     ● **Z12.79   Encounter for screening for malignant neoplasm of other genitourinary organs**

   ● **Z12.8   Encounter for screening for malignant neoplasm of other sites**

     ● **Z12.81   Encounter for screening for malignant neoplasm of oral cavity**

     ● **Z12.82   Encounter for screening for malignant neoplasm of nervous system**

     ● **Z12.83   Encounter for screening for malignant neoplasm of skin**

     ● **Z12.89   Encounter for screening for malignant neoplasm of other sites**

   ● **Z12.9   Encounter for screening for malignant neoplasm, site unspecified**

● **Z13   Encounter for screening for other diseases and disorders**
     Screening is the testing for disease or disease precursors in asymptomatic individuals so that early detection and treatment can be provided for those who test positive for the disease.

     Excludes1   encounter for diagnostic examination - code to sign or symptom

   ● **Z13.0   Encounter for screening for diseases of the blood and blood-forming organs and certain disorders involving the immune mechanism**

   ● **Z13.1   Encounter for screening for diabetes mellitus**

   ● **Z13.2   Encounter for screening for nutritional, metabolic and other endocrine disorders**

     ● **Z13.21   Encounter for screening for nutritional disorder**

     ● **Z13.22   Encounter for screening for metabolic disorder**

       ● **Z13.220   Encounter for screening for lipoid disorders**
         Encounter for screening for cholesterol level
         Encounter for screening for hypercholesterolemia
         Encounter for screening for hyperlipidemia

       ● **Z13.228   Encounter for screening for other metabolic disorders**

     ● **Z13.29   Encounter for screening for other suspected endocrine disorder**
       Excludes1   encounter for screening for diabetes mellitus (Z13.1)

   ● **Z13.4   Encounter for screening for certain developmental disorders in childhood**   P
     Encounter for screening for developmental handicaps in early childhood
     Excludes1   routine development testing of infant or child (Z00.1-)

   ● **Z13.5   Encounter for screening for eye and ear disorders**
     Excludes2   encounter for general hearing examination (Z01.1-)
       encounter for general vision examination (Z01.0-)
     Coding Clinic: 2016, Q3, P17

   ● **Z13.6   Encounter for screening for cardiovascular disorders**

   ● **Z13.7   Encounter for screening for genetic and chromosomal anomalies**
     Excludes1   genetic testing for procreative management (Z31.4-)

     ● **Z13.71   Encounter for nonprocreative screening for genetic disease carrier status**

     ● **Z13.79   Encounter for other screening for genetic and chromosomal anomalies**

CHAPTER 21 (Z00-Z99)

● **Z13.8** Encounter for screening for other specified diseases and disorders

    Excludes2 screening for malignant neoplasms (Z12.-)

  ● **Z13.81** Encounter for screening for digestive system disorders

    ● **Z13.810** Encounter for screening for upper gastrointestinal disorder

    ● **Z13.811** Encounter for screening for lower gastrointestinal disorder

      Excludes1 encounter for screening for intestinal infectious disease (Z11.0)

    ● **Z13.818** Encounter for screening for other digestive system disorders

  ● **Z13.82** Encounter for screening for musculoskeletal disorder

    ● **Z13.820** Encounter for screening for osteoporosis

    ● **Z13.828** Encounter for screening for other musculoskeletal disorder

  ● **Z13.83** Encounter for screening for respiratory disorder NEC

    Excludes1 encounter for screening for respiratory tuberculosis (Z11.1)

  ● **Z13.84** Encounter for screening for dental disorders

  ● **Z13.85** Encounter for screening for nervous system disorders

    ● **Z13.850** Encounter for screening for traumatic brain injury

    ● **Z13.858** Encounter for screening for other nervous system disorders

  ● **Z13.88** Encounter for screening for disorder due to exposure to contaminants

    Excludes1 those exposed to contaminants without suspected disorders (Z57-Z77.-)

  ● **Z13.89** Encounter for screening for other disorder

    Encounter for screening for genitourinary disorders

● **Z13.9** Encounter for screening, unspecified

GENETIC CARRIER AND GENETIC SUSCEPTIBILITY TO DISEASE (Z14-Z15)

● **Z14** Genetic carrier

  ● **Z14.0** Hemophilia A carrier

    ● **Z14.01** Asymptomatic hemophilia A carrier

    ● **Z14.02** Symptomatic hemophilia A carrier

  ● **Z14.1** Cystic fibrosis carrier

  ● **Z14.8** Genetic carrier of other disease

● **Z15** Genetic susceptibility to disease

  Excludes1 chromosomal anomalies (Q90-Q99)

  Includes confirmed abnormal gene

  Use additional code, if applicable, for any associated family history of the disease (Z80-Z84)

  ● **Z15.0** Genetic susceptibility to malignant neoplasm

    Code first if applicable, any current malignant neoplasm (C00-C75, C81-C96)

    Use additional code, if applicable, for any personal history of malignant neoplasm (Z85.-)

    ● **Z15.01** Genetic susceptibility to malignant neoplasm of breast

    ● **Z15.02** Genetic susceptibility to malignant neoplasm of ovary ♀

    ● **Z15.03** Genetic susceptibility to malignant neoplasm of prostate ♂

    ● **Z15.04** Genetic susceptibility to malignant neoplasm of endometrium ♀

    ● **Z15.09** Genetic susceptibility to other malignant neoplasm

  ● **Z15.8** Genetic susceptibility to other disease

    ● **Z15.81** Genetic susceptibility to multiple endocrine neoplasia [MEN]

      Excludes1 multiple endocrine neoplasia [MEN] syndromes (E31.2-)

    ● **Z15.89** Genetic susceptibility to other disease

RESISTANCE TO ANTIMICROBIAL DRUGS (Z16)

● **Z16** Resistance to antimicrobial drugs

  Note: The codes in this category are provided for use as additional codes to identify the resistance and non-responsiveness of a condition to antimicrobial drugs.

  Code first the infection

  Excludes1 Methicillin resistant Staphylococcus aureus infection (A49.02)

    ~~Methicillin resistant Staphylococcus aureus infection in diseases classified elsewhere (B95.62)~~

    Methicillin resistant Staphylococcus aureus pneumonia (J15.212)

    Sepsis due to Methicillin resistant Staphylococcus aureus (A41.02)

  ● **Z16.1** Resistance to beta lactam antibiotics

    ● **Z16.10** Resistance to unspecified beta lactam antibiotics

    ● **Z16.11** Resistance to penicillins

      Resistance to amoxicillin

      Resistance to ampicillin

    ● **Z16.12** Extended spectrum beta lactamase (ESBL) resistance

      ▶ **Excludes2** Methicillin resistant Staphylococcus aureus infection in diseases classified elsewhere (B95.62)

    ● **Z16.19** Resistance to other specified beta lactam antibiotics

      Resistance to cephalosporins

  ● **Z16.2** Resistance to other antibiotics

    ● **Z16.20** Resistance to unspecified antibiotic

      Resistance to antibiotics NOS

    ● **Z16.21** Resistance to vancomycin

    ● **Z16.22** Resistance to vancomycin related antibiotics

    ● **Z16.23** Resistance to quinolones and fluoroquinolones

    ● **Z16.24** Resistance to multiple antibiotics

    ● **Z16.29** Resistance to other single specified antibiotic

      Resistance to aminoglycosides

      Resistance to macrolides

      Resistance to sulfonamides

      Resistance to tetracyclines

  ● **Z16.3** Resistance to other antimicrobial drugs

    Excludes1 resistance to antibiotics (Z16.1-, Z16.2-)

    ● **Z16.30** Resistance to unspecified antimicrobial drugs

      Drug resistance NOS

    ● **Z16.31** Resistance to antiparasitic drug(s)

      Resistance to quinine and related compounds

    ● **Z16.32** Resistance to antifungal drug(s)

    ● **Z16.33** Resistance to antiviral drug(s)

    ● **Z16.34** Resistance to antimycobacterial drug(s)

      Resistance to tuberculostatics

      ● **Z16.341** Resistance to single antimycobacterial drug

        Resistance to antimycobacterial drug NOS

      ● **Z16.342** Resistance to multiple antimycobacterial drugs

---

▶ New   ⮕ Revised   ~~deleted~~ Deleted   Excludes 1   Excludes 2   Includes   Use additional   Code first   Code also   Key words

OGCR Official Guidelines   ● Unacceptable Principal Diagnosis   X Assign placeholder X   ● Use Additional Character(s)   ▶ Manifestation Code   **Coding Clinic**

● Z16.35   Resistance to multiple antimicrobial drugs
     Excludes1   Resistance to multiple antibiotics only (Z16.24)
● Z16.39   Resistance to other specified antimicrobial drug

ESTROGEN RECEPTOR STATUS (Z17)

● Z17   Estrogen receptor status
     Code first malignant neoplasm of breast (C50.-)
   ● Z17.0   Estrogen receptor positive status [ER+]
   ● Z17.1   Estrogen receptor negative status [ER-]

RETAINED FOREIGN BODY FRAGMENTS (Z18)

● Z18   Retained foreign body fragments
     Includes   embedded fragment (status)
                  embedded splinter (status)
                  retained foreign body status
     Excludes1   artificial joint prosthesis status (Z96.6-)
                  foreign body accidentally left during a procedure (T81.5-)
                  foreign body entering through orifice (T15-T19)
                  in situ cardiac device (Z95.-)
                  organ or tissue replaced by means other than transplant (Z96.-, Z97.-)
                  organ or tissue replaced by transplant (Z94.-)
                  personal history of retained foreign body fully removed Z87.821
                  superficial foreign body (non-embedded splinter) - code to superficial foreign body, by site
   ● Z18.0   Retained radioactive fragments
     ● Z18.01   Retained depleted uranium fragments
     ● Z18.09   Other retained radioactive fragments
           Other retained depleted isotope fragments
           Retained nontherapeutic radioactive fragments
   ● Z18.1   Retained metal fragments
     Excludes1   retained radioactive metal fragments (Z18.01-Z18.09)
     ● Z18.10   Retained metal fragments, unspecified
           Retained metal fragment NOS
     ● Z18.11   Retained magnetic metal fragments
     ● Z18.12   Retained nonmagnetic metal fragments
   ● Z18.2   Retained plastic fragments
         Acrylics fragments
         Diethylhexylphthalates fragments
         Isocyanate fragments
   ● Z18.3   Retained organic fragments
     ● Z18.31   Retained animal quills or spines
     ● Z18.32   Retained tooth
     ● Z18.33   Retained wood fragments
     ● Z18.39   Other retained organic fragments
   ● Z18.8   Other specified retained foreign body
     ● Z18.81   Retained glass fragments
     ● Z18.83   Retained stone or crystalline fragments
           Retained concrete or cement fragments
     ● Z18.89   Other specified retained foreign body fragments
           Coding Clinic: 2016, Q3, P24
   ● Z18.9   Retained foreign body fragments, unspecified material

HORMONE SENSITIVITY MALIGNANCY STATUS (Z19)

● Z19   Hormone sensitivity malignancy status
     Code first malignant neoplasm —see Table of Neoplasms, by site, malignant
     Coding Clinic: 2016, Q4, P129
   Z19.1   Hormone sensitive malignancy status
     Coding Clinic: 2016, Q4, P76
   Z19.2   Hormone resistant malignancy status
     Castrate resistant prostate malignancy status
     Coding Clinic: 2016, Q4, P76

PERSONS WITH POTENTIAL HEALTH HAZARDS RELATED TO COMMUNICABLE DISEASES (Z20-Z29)

● Z20   Contact with and (suspected) exposure to communicable diseases
     Excludes1   carrier of infectious disease (Z22.-)
                  diagnosed current infectious or parasitic disease - see Alphabetic Index
     Excludes2   personal history of infectious and parasitic diseases (Z86.1-)
   ● Z20.0   Contact with and (suspected) exposure to intestinal infectious diseases
     Z20.01   Contact with and (suspected) exposure to intestinal infectious diseases due to Escherichia coli (E. coli)
     ● Z20.09   Contact with and (suspected) exposure to other intestinal infectious diseases
   ● Z20.1   Contact with and (suspected) exposure to tuberculosis
   ● Z20.2   Contact with and (suspected) exposure to infections with a predominantly sexual mode of transmission
   ● Z20.3   Contact with and (suspected) exposure to rabies
   ● Z20.4   Contact with and (suspected) exposure to rubella
   Z20.5   Contact with and (suspected) exposure to viral hepatitis
   Z20.6   Contact with and (suspected) exposure to human immunodeficiency virus [HIV]
     Excludes1   asymptomatic human immunodeficiency virus [HIV]
                  HIV infection status (Z21)
   ● Z20.7   Contact with and (suspected) exposure to pediculosis, acariasis and other infestations
   ● Z20.8   Contact with and (suspected) exposure to other communicable diseases
     ● Z20.81   Contact with and (suspected) exposure to other bacterial communicable diseases
       ● Z20.810   Contact with and (suspected) exposure to anthrax
       Z20.811   Contact with and (suspected) exposure to meningococcus
       ● Z20.818   Contact with and (suspected) exposure to other bacterial communicable diseases
     ● Z20.82   Contact with and (suspected) exposure to other viral communicable diseases
       Z20.820   Contact with and (suspected) exposure to varicella
       Z20.828   Contact with and (suspected) exposure to other viral communicable diseases
           Coding Clinic: 2016, Q4, P6-7, 121
     ● Z20.89   Contact with and (suspected) exposure to other communicable diseases
   ● Z20.9   Contact with and (suspected) exposure to unspecified communicable disease

Z21   Asymptomatic human immunodeficiency virus [HIV] infection status
     HIV positive NOS
     Code first Human immunodeficiency virus [HIV] disease complicating pregnancy, childbirth and the puerperium, if applicable (O98.7-)
     Excludes1   acquired immunodeficiency syndrome (B20)
                  contact with human immunodeficiency virus [HIV] (Z20.6)
                  exposure to human immunodeficiency virus [HIV] (Z20.6)
                  human immunodeficiency virus [HIV] disease (B20)
                  inconclusive laboratory evidence of human immunodeficiency virus [HIV] (R75)
     MCE: Questionable admission when principal dx

CHAPTER 21 (Z00-Z99)

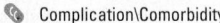 N   Newborn Age: 0   P   Pediatric Age: 0-17   M   Maternity DX: 12-55   A   Adult Age: 15-124   ♀   Females Only   ♂   Males Only

 Complication\Comorbidity   Major C\C   (Ex)   CC/MCC Exclusions   Hospital-Acquired Condition

● **Z22   Carrier of infectious disease**

Includes   colonization status
suspected carrier

Excludes2   carrier of viral hepatitis (B18.-)

● **Z22.0   Carrier of typhoid**

● **Z22.1   Carrier of other intestinal infectious diseases**

● **Z22.2   Carrier of diphtheria**

● **Z22.3   Carrier of other specified bacterial diseases**

● **Z22.31   Carrier of bacterial disease due to meningococci**

● **Z22.32   Carrier of bacterial disease due to staphylococci**

● **Z22.321   Carrier or suspected carrier of Methicillin susceptible Staphylococcus aureus**
MSSA colonization

● **Z22.322   Carrier or suspected carrier of Methicillin resistant Staphylococcus aureus**
MRSA colonization

● **Z22.33   Carrier of bacterial disease due to streptococci**

● **Z22.330   Carrier of Group B streptococcus**

Excludes1   Carrier of streptococcus group B (GBS) complicating pregnancy, childbirth and the puerperium (O99.82-)

● **Z22.338   Carrier of other streptococcus**

● **Z22.39   Carrier of other specified bacterial diseases**

● **Z22.4   Carrier of infections with a predominantly sexual mode of transmission**

● **Z22.6   Carrier of human T-lymphotropic virus type-1 [HTLV-1] infection**

● **Z22.8   Carrier of other infectious diseases**

● **Z22.9   Carrier of infectious disease, unspecified**

● **Z23   Encounter for immunization**

Code first any routine childhood examination

Note: Procedure codes are required to identify the types of immunizations given.

● **Z28   Immunization not carried out and underimmunization status**

Includes   vaccination not carried out

● **Z28.0   Immunization not carried out because of contraindication**

● **Z28.01   Immunization not carried out because of acute illness of patient**

● **Z28.02   Immunization not carried out because of chronic illness or condition of patient**

● **Z28.03   Immunization not carried out because of immune compromised state of patient**

● **Z28.04   Immunization not carried out because of patient allergy to vaccine or component**

● **Z28.09   Immunization not carried out because of other contraindication**

● **Z28.1   Immunization not carried out because of patient decision for reasons of belief or group pressure**
Immunization not carried out because of religious belief

● **Z28.2   Immunization not carried out because of patient decision for other and unspecified reason**

● **Z28.20   Immunization not carried out because of patient decision for unspecified reason**

● **Z28.21   Immunization not carried out because of patient refusal**

● **Z28.29   Immunization not carried out because of patient decision for other reason**

● **Z28.3   Underimmunization status**
Delinquent immunization status
Lapsed immunization schedule status

● **Z28.8   Immunization not carried out for other reason**

● **Z28.81   Immunization not carried out due to patient having had the disease**

● **Z28.82   Immunization not carried out because of caregiver refusal**
Immunization not carried out because of guardian refusal
Immunization not carried out because of parent refusal

Excludes1   immunization not carried out because of caregiver refusal because of religious belief (Z28.1)

● **Z28.89   Immunization not carried out for other reason**

● **Z28.9   Immunization not carried out for unspecified reason**

● **Z29   Encounter for other prophylactic measures**

Excludes1   desensitization to allergens (Z51.6)
prophylactic surgery (Z40.-)
Coding Clinic: 2016, Q4, P130

● **Z29.1   Encounter for prophylactic immunotherapy**
Encounter for administration of immunoglobulin
Coding Clinic: 2016, Q4, P78-79

● **Z29.11   Encounter for prophylactic immunotherapy for respiratory syncytial virus (RSV)**

● **Z29.12   Encounter for prophylactic antivenin**

● **Z29.13   Encounter for prophylactic Rho(D) immune globulin**

● **Z29.14   Encounter for prophylactic rabies immune globin**

● **Z29.3   Encounter for prophylactic fluoride administration**
Coding Clinic: 2016, Q4, P79

● **Z29.8   Encounter for other specified prophylactic measures**
Coding Clinic: 2016, Q4, P79

● **Z29.9   Encounter for prophylactic measures, unspecified**
Coding Clinic: 2016, Q4, P79

PERSONS ENCOUNTERING HEALTH SERVICES IN CIRCUMSTANCES RELATED TO REPRODUCTION (Z30-Z39)

● **Z30   Encounter for contraceptive management**

● **Z30.0   Encounter for general counseling and advice on contraception**

● **Z30.01   Encounter for initial prescription of contraceptives**

Excludes1   encounter for surveillance of contraceptives (Z30.4-)

● **Z30.011   Encounter for initial prescription of contraceptive pills ♀**

● **Z30.012   Encounter for prescription of emergency contraception ♀**
Encounter for postcoital contraception

● **Z30.013   Encounter for initial prescription of injectable contraceptive ♀**

● **Z30.014   Encounter for initial prescription of intrauterine contraceptive device ♀**

Excludes1   encounter for insertion of intrauterine contraceptive device (Z30.430, Z30.432)

▶ New   ⮕ Revised   ~~deleted~~ Deleted   Excludes 1   Excludes 2   Includes   Use additional   Code first   Code also   Key words
OGCR Official Guidelines   ● Unacceptable Principal Diagnosis   X Assign placeholder X   ● Use Additional Character(s)   ▌ Manifestation Code   **Coding Clinic**

● **Z30.015**   Encounter for initial prescription of vaginal ring hormonal contraceptive ♀
     Coding Clinic: 2016, Q4, P78

● **Z30.016**   Encounter for initial prescription of transdermal patch hormonal contraceptive device
     Coding Clinic: 2016, Q4, P78

● **Z30.017**   Encounter for initial prescription of implantable subdermal contraceptive
     Coding Clinic: 2016, Q4, P78

● **Z30.018**   Encounter for initial prescription of other contraceptives ♀
     Encounter for initial prescription of barrier contraception
     Encounter for initial prescription of diaphragm

● **Z30.019**   Encounter for initial prescription of contraceptives, unspecified ♀

● **Z30.02**   Counseling and instruction in natural family planning to avoid pregnancy

● **Z30.09**   Encounter for other general counseling and advice on contraception
     Encounter for family planning advice NOS

Z30.2   Encounter for sterilization

● **Z30.4**   Encounter for surveillance of contraceptives

● **Z30.40**   Encounter for surveillance of contraceptives, unspecified

● **Z30.41**   Encounter for surveillance of contraceptive pills ♀
     Encounter for repeat prescription for contraceptive pill

● **Z30.42**   Encounter for surveillance of injectable contraceptive ♀

● **Z30.43**   Encounter for surveillance of intrauterine contraceptive device

  ● **Z30.430**   Encounter for insertion of intrauterine contraceptive device ♀

  ● **Z30.431**   Encounter for routine checking of intrauterine contraceptive device ♀

  ● **Z30.432**   Encounter for removal of intrauterine contraceptive device ♀

  ● **Z30.433**   Encounter for removal and reinsertion of intrauterine contraceptive device ♀
     Encounter for replacement of intrauterine contraceptive device

● **Z30.44**   Encounter for surveillance of vaginal ring hormonal contraceptive device ♀
     Coding Clinic: 2016, Q4, P78

● **Z30.45**   Encounter for surveillance of transdermal patch hormonal contraceptive device ♀
     Coding Clinic: 2016, Q4, P78

● **Z30.46**   Encounter for surveillance of implantable subdermal contraceptive ♀
     Encounter for checking, reinsertion or removal of implantable subdermal contraceptive
     Coding Clinic: 2016, Q4, P78

● **Z30.49**   Encounter for surveillance of other contraceptives ♀
     Encounter for surveillance of barrier contraception
     Encounter for surveillance of diaphragm

● **Z30.8**   Encounter for other contraceptive management
     Encounter for postvasectomy sperm count
     Encounter for routine examination for contraceptive maintenance
     Excludes1   sperm count following sterilization reversal (Z31.42)
       sperm count for fertility testing (Z31.41)

● **Z30.9**   Encounter for contraceptive management, unspecified

● **Z31**   Encounter for procreative management
     Excludes1   complications associated with artificial fertilization (N98.-)
       female infertility (N97.-)
       male infertility (N46.-)

Z31.0   Encounter for reversal of previous sterilization

● **Z31.4**   Encounter for procreative investigation and testing
     Excludes1   postvasectomy sperm count (Z30.8)

● **Z31.41**   Encounter for fertility testing
     Encounter for fallopian tube patency testing
     Encounter for sperm count for fertility testing

● **Z31.42**   Aftercare following sterilization reversal
     Sperm count following sterilization reversal

● **Z31.43**   Encounter for genetic testing of female for procreative management
     Use additional code for recurrent pregnancy loss, if applicable (N96, O26.2-)
     Excludes1   nonprocreative genetic testing (Z13.7-)

  ● **Z31.430**   Encounter of female for testing for genetic disease carrier status for procreative management ♀

  ● **Z31.438**   Encounter for other genetic testing of female for procreative management ♀

● **Z31.44**   Encounter for genetic testing of male for procreative management
     Excludes1   nonprocreative genetic testing (Z13.7-)

  ● **Z31.440**   Encounter of male for testing for genetic disease carrier status for procreative management ♂

  ● **Z31.441**   Encounter for testing of male partner of patient with recurrent pregnancy loss ♂   A

  ● **Z31.448**   Encounter for other genetic testing of male for procreative management ♂   A

● **Z31.49**   Encounter for other procreative investigation and testing

➡● **Z31.5**   Encounter for procreative genetic counseling

● **Z31.6**   Encounter for general counseling and advice on procreation

● **Z31.61**   Procreative counseling and advice using natural family planning

● **Z31.62**   Encounter for fertility preservation counseling
     Encounter for fertility preservation counseling prior to cancer therapy
     Encounter for fertility preservation counseling prior to surgical removal of gonads

● **Z31.69**   Encounter for other general counseling and advice on procreation

● **Z31.7**   Encounter for procreative management and counseling for gestational carrier
     Excludes1   pregnant state, gestational carrier (Z33.3)
     Coding Clinic: 2016, Q4, P78

N Newborn Age: 0   **P** Pediatric Age: 0–17   **M** Maternity DX: 12–55   **A** Adult Age: 15–124   ♀ Females Only   ♂ Males Only
🅒 Complication\Comorbidity   🅜 Major C\C   ⒺⓍ CC/MCC Exclusions   🅗 Hospital-Acquired Condition

1599

● **Z31.8** **Encounter for other procreative management**
   ● **Z31.81** Encounter for male factor infertility in female patient ♀
   ● **Z31.82** Encounter for Rh incompatibility status ♀
      Coding Clinic: 2015, Q3, P40
   ● **Z31.83** Encounter for assisted reproductive fertility procedure cycle ♀
      Patient undergoing in vitro fertilization cycle
      Use additional code to identify the type of infertility
      Excludes1 pre-cycle diagnosis and testing - code to reason for encounter
   ● **Z31.84** Encounter for fertility preservation procedure
      Encounter for fertility preservation procedure prior to cancer therapy
      Encounter for fertility preservation procedure prior to surgical removal of gonads
   ● **Z31.89** Encounter for other procreative management
● **Z31.9** Encounter for procreative management, unspecified

● **Z32** **Encounter for pregnancy test and childbirth and childcare instruction**
   ● **Z32.0** Encounter for pregnancy test
      Z32.00 Encounter for pregnancy test, result unknown ♀
         Encounter for pregnancy test NOS
      Z32.01 Encounter for pregnancy test, result positive ♀   M
      Z32.02 Encounter for pregnancy test, result negative ♀
   ● **Z32.2** Encounter for childbirth instruction
   ● **Z32.3** Encounter for childcare instruction
      Encounter for prenatal or postpartum childcare instruction

● **Z33** **Pregnant state**
   ● **Z33.1** Pregnant state, incidental ♀   M
      Pregnant state NOS
      Excludes1 complications of pregnancy (O00-O9A)
         pregnant state, gestational carrier (Z33.3)
   Z33.2 Encounter for elective termination of pregnancy ♀   M
      Excludes1 early fetal death with retention of dead fetus (O02.1)
         late fetal death (O36.4)
         spontaneous abortion (O03)
      Coding Clinic: 2016, Q4, P130
   ● **Z33.3** Pregnant state, gestational carrier ♀
      Excludes1 encounter for procreative management and counseling for gestational carrier (Z31.7)
      Coding Clinic: 2016, Q4, P78

● **Z34** **Encounter for supervision of normal pregnancy**
   Excludes1 any complication of pregnancy (O00-O9A)
      encounter for pregnancy test (Z32.0-)
      encounter for supervision of high risk pregnancy (O09.-)
   Coding Clinic: 2016, Q4, P6
   ● **Z34.0** Encounter for supervision of normal first pregnancy
      ● **Z34.00** Encounter for supervision of normal first pregnancy, unspecified trimester ♀   M
      ● **Z34.01** Encounter for supervision of normal first pregnancy, first trimester ♀   M
      ● **Z34.02** Encounter for supervision of normal first pregnancy, second trimester ♀   M
      ● **Z34.03** Encounter for supervision of normal first pregnancy, third trimester ♀   M
   ● **Z34.8** Encounter for supervision of other normal pregnancy
      ● **Z34.80** Encounter for supervision of other normal pregnancy, unspecified trimester ♀   M
      ● **Z34.81** Encounter for supervision of other normal pregnancy, first trimester ♀   M

First trimester (0 to 14 weeks) | Second trimester (14 to 28 weeks) | Third trimester (28 weeks to delivery)

Figure 21-1 Trimesters. (From Shiland, Betsy J. Medical Terminology & Anatomy for ICD-10 Coding, ed 2, Mosby, 2015)

      ● **Z34.82** Encounter for supervision of other normal pregnancy, second trimester ♀   M
      ● **Z34.83** Encounter for supervision of other normal pregnancy, third trimester ♀   M
   ● **Z34.9** Encounter for supervision of normal pregnancy, unspecified
      ● **Z34.90** Encounter for supervision of normal pregnancy, unspecified, unspecified trimester ♀   M
      ● **Z34.91** Encounter for supervision of normal pregnancy, unspecified, first trimester ♀   M
      ● **Z34.92** Encounter for supervision of normal pregnancy, unspecified, second trimester ♀   M
      ● **Z34.93** Encounter for supervision of normal pregnancy, unspecified, third trimester ♀   M

● **Z36** **Encounter for antenatal screening of mother** ♀
   ▶ **Includes** Encounter for placental sample (taken vaginally)
      ▶ Screening is the testing for disease or disease precursors in asymptomatic individuals so that early detection and treatment can be provided for those who test positive for the disease.
   Excludes1 ~~abnormal findings on antenatal screening of mother (O28.-)~~
      diagnostic examination - code to sign or symptom
      encounter for suspected maternal and fetal conditions ruled out (Z03.7-)
      suspected fetal condition affecting management of pregnancy - code to condition in Chapter 15
   Excludes2 ▶ abnormal findings on antenatal screening of mother (O28.-)
      genetic counseling and testing (Z31.43-, Z31.5)
      routine prenatal care (Z34)
   ▶ **Z36.0** Encounter for antenatal screening for chromosomal anomalies ♀   M
   ▶ **Z36.1** Encounter for antenatal screening for raised alphafetoprotein level ♀   M
      ▶ Encounter for antenatal screening for elevated maternal serum alphafetoprotein level
   ▶ **Z36.2** Encounter for other antenatal screening follow-up ♀   M
      ▶ Non-visualized anatomy on a previous scan
   ▶ **Z36.3** Encounter for antenatal screening for malformations ♀ M
      ▶ Screening for a suspected anomaly
   ▶ **Z36.4** Encounter for antenatal screening for fetal growth retardation ♀   M
      ▶ Intrauterine growth restriction (IUGR)/small-for-dates
   ▶ **Z36.5** Encounter for antenatal screening for isoimmunization ♀   M
   ▶● **Z36.8** Encounter for other antenatal screening
      ▶ **Z36.81** Encounter for antenatal screening for hydrops fetalis ♀   M
      ▶ **Z36.82** Encounter for antenatal screening for nuchal translucency ♀   M
      ▶ **Z36.83** Encounter for fetal screening for congenital cardiac abnormalities ♀   M
      ▶ **Z36.84** Encounter for antenatal screening for fetal lung maturity ♀   M

▶ New   ⇒ Revised   ~~deleted~~ Deleted   Excludes 1   Excludes 2   Includes   Use additional   Code first   Code also   Key words
OGCR Official Guidelines   ● Unacceptable Principal Diagnosis   X Assign placeholder X   ● Use Additional Character(s)   ▶ Manifestation Code   **Coding Clinic**

▶ **Z36.85**   Encounter for antenatal screening for Streptococcus B ♀   M

▶ **Z36.86**   Encounter for antenatal screening for cervical length ♀   M
     ▶ Screening for risk of pre-term labor

▶ **Z36.87**   Encounter for antenatal screening for uncertain dates ♀

▶ **Z36.88**   Encounter for antenatal screening for fetal macrosomia ♀   M
     ▶ Screening for large-for-dates

▶ **Z36.89**   Encounter for other specified antenatal screening ♀   M

▶ **Z36.8A**   Encounter for antenatal screening for other genetic defects ♀   M

▶ **Z36.9**   Encounter for antenatal screening, unspecified ♀   M

● **Z3A**   **Weeks of gestation**
     Note: Codes from category Z3A are for use, only on the maternal record, to indicate the weeks of gestation of the pregnancy, if known.
     ⟹ *Code first complications of pregnancy, childbirth and the puerperium (O09-O9A)*
     Coding Clinic: 2016, Q4, P130; 2013, Q2, P33

● **Z3A.0**   Weeks of gestation of pregnancy, unspecified or less than 10 weeks
   ● **Z3A.00**   Weeks of gestation of pregnancy not specified ♀   M
   ● **Z3A.01**   Less than 8 weeks gestation of pregnancy ♀   M
   ● **Z3A.08**   8 weeks gestation of pregnancy ♀   M
   ● **Z3A.09**   9 weeks gestation of pregnancy ♀   M

● **Z3A.1**   Weeks of gestation of pregnancy, weeks 10-19
   ● **Z3A.10**   10 weeks gestation of pregnancy ♀   M
   ● **Z3A.11**   11 weeks gestation of pregnancy ♀   M
   ● **Z3A.12**   12 weeks gestation of pregnancy ♀   M
   ● **Z3A.13**   13 weeks gestation of pregnancy ♀   M
   ● **Z3A.14**   14 weeks gestation of pregnancy ♀   M
   ● **Z3A.15**   15 weeks gestation of pregnancy ♀   M
   ● **Z3A.16**   16 weeks gestation of pregnancy ♀   M
     Coding Clinic: 2016, Q4, P5
   ● **Z3A.17**   17 weeks gestation of pregnancy ♀   M
   ● **Z3A.18**   18 weeks gestation of pregnancy ♀   M
   ● **Z3A.19**   19 weeks gestation of pregnancy ♀   M

● **Z3A.2**   Weeks of gestation of pregnancy, weeks 20-29
   ● **Z3A.20**   20 weeks gestation of pregnancy ♀   M
     Coding Clinic: 2016, Q4, P6
   ● **Z3A.21**   21 weeks gestation of pregnancy ♀   M
   ● **Z3A.22**   22 weeks gestation of pregnancy ♀   M
     Coding Clinic: 2016, Q4, P6
   ● **Z3A.23**   23 weeks gestation of pregnancy ♀   M
   ● **Z3A.24**   24 weeks gestation of pregnancy ♀   M
   ● **Z3A.25**   25 weeks gestation of pregnancy ♀   M
   ● **Z3A.26**   26 weeks gestation of pregnancy ♀   M
   ● **Z3A.27**   27 weeks gestation of pregnancy ♀   M
   ● **Z3A.28**   28 weeks gestation of pregnancy ♀   M
   ● **Z3A.29**   29 weeks gestation of pregnancy ♀   M

● **Z3A.3**   Weeks of gestation of pregnancy, weeks 30-39
   ● **Z3A.30**   30 weeks gestation of pregnancy ♀   M
   ● **Z3A.31**   31 weeks gestation of pregnancy ♀   M
   ● **Z3A.32**   32 weeks gestation of pregnancy ♀   M
     Coding Clinic: 2016, Q4, P6
   ● **Z3A.33**   33 weeks gestation of pregnancy ♀   M
   ● **Z3A.34**   34 weeks gestation of pregnancy ♀   M
   ● **Z3A.35**   35 weeks gestation of pregnancy ♀   M
   ● **Z3A.36**   36 weeks gestation of pregnancy ♀   M
   ● **Z3A.37**   37 weeks gestation of pregnancy ♀   M
   ● **Z3A.38**   38 weeks gestation of pregnancy ♀   M
     Coding Clinic: 2016, Q2, P34
   ● **Z3A.39**   39 weeks gestation of pregnancy ♀

● **Z3A.4**   Weeks of gestation of pregnancy, weeks 40 or greater
   ● **Z3A.40**   40 weeks gestation of pregnancy ♀   M
   ● **Z3A.41**   41 weeks gestation of pregnancy ♀   M
   ● **Z3A.42**   42 weeks gestation of pregnancy ♀   M
   ● **Z3A.49**   Greater than 42 weeks gestation of pregnancy ♀   M

● **Z37**   **Outcome of delivery**
     This category is intended for use as an additional code to identify the outcome of delivery on the mother's record. It is not for use on the newborn record.
     Excludes1   stillbirth (P95)
● **Z37.0**   Single live birth ♀   M
     Coding Clinic: 2016, Q2, P34
● **Z37.1**   Single stillbirth ♀   M
● **Z37.2**   Twins, both liveborn ♀   M
● **Z37.3**   Twins, one liveborn and one stillborn ♀   M
● **Z37.4**   Twins, both stillborn ♀   M
● **Z37.5**   Other multiple births, all liveborn
   ● **Z37.50**   Multiple births, unspecified, all liveborn ♀   M
   ● **Z37.51**   Triplets, all liveborn ♀   M
   ● **Z37.52**   Quadruplets, all liveborn ♀   M
   ● **Z37.53**   Quintuplets, all liveborn ♀   M
   ● **Z37.54**   Sextuplets, all liveborn ♀   M
   ● **Z37.59**   Other multiple births, all liveborn ♀   M
● **Z37.6**   Other multiple births, some liveborn
   ● **Z37.60**   Multiple births, unspecified, some liveborn ♀   M
   ● **Z37.61**   Triplets, some liveborn ♀   M
   ● **Z37.62**   Quadruplets, some liveborn ♀   M
   ● **Z37.63**   Quintuplets, some liveborn ♀   M
   ● **Z37.64**   Sextuplets, some liveborn ♀   M
   ● **Z37.69**   Other multiple births, some liveborn ♀   M
● **Z37.7**   Other multiple births, all stillborn ♀   M
● **Z37.9**   Outcome of delivery, unspecified ♀   M
     Multiple birth NOS
     Single birth NOS

● **Z38**   **Liveborn infants according to place of birth and type of delivery**
     This category is for use as the principal code on the initial record of a newborn baby. It is to be used for the initial birth record only. It is not to be used on the mother's record.
     Coding Clinic: 2017, Q2, P6-7; 2016, Q4, P126-127, 130; 2015, Q2, P15
● **Z38.0**   Single liveborn infant, born in hospital
     Single liveborn infant, born in birthing center or other health care facility
     Coding Clinic: 2017, Q2, P5-7
   Z38.00   Single liveborn infant, delivered vaginally   N
     Coding Clinic: 2016, Q4, P7, 55
   Z38.01   Single liveborn infant, delivered by cesarean   N
     Coding Clinic: 2017, Q2, P7; 2016, Q3, P18
  Z38.1   Single liveborn infant, born outside hospital   N
  Z38.2   Single liveborn infant, unspecified as to place of birth   N
     Single liveborn infant NOS
● **Z38.3**   Twin liveborn infant, born in hospital
   Z38.30   Twin liveborn infant, delivered vaginally   N
   Z38.31   Twin liveborn infant, delivered by cesarean   N
  Z38.4   Twin liveborn infant, born outside hospital   N
  Z38.5   Twin liveborn infant, unspecified as to place of birth   N
● **Z38.6**   Other multiple liveborn infant, born in hospital
   Z38.61   Triplet liveborn infant, delivered vaginally   N
   Z38.62   Triplet liveborn infant, delivered by cesarean   N
   Z38.63   Quadruplet liveborn infant, delivered vaginally   N
   Z38.64   Quadruplet liveborn infant, delivered by cesarean   N
   Z38.65   Quintuplet liveborn infant, delivered vaginally   N

N Newborn Age: 0   **P** Pediatric Age: 0–17   **M** Maternity DX: 12–55   **A** Adult Age: 15–124   ♀ Females Only   ♂ Males Only

🅒 Complication\Comorbidity   🅜 Major C\C   (Ex) CC/MCC Exclusions   🅗 Hospital-Acquired Condition

1601

CHAPTER 21 (Z00-Z99)

Z38.66	Quintuplet liveborn infant, delivered by cesarean	N
Z38.68	Other multiple liveborn infant, delivered vaginally	N
Z38.69	Other multiple liveborn infant, delivered by cesarean	N
Z38.7	Other multiple liveborn infant, born outside hospital	N
Z38.8	Other multiple liveborn infant, unspecified as to place of birth	N

● **Z39**   **Encounter for maternal postpartum care and examination**

Z39.0   Encounter for care and examination of mother immediately after delivery ♀   M

Care and observation in uncomplicated cases when the delivery occurs outside a healthcare facility

> **Excludes1**   care for postpartum complication - see Alphabetic index

● **Z39.1**   Encounter for care and examination of lactating mother ♀   M

Encounter for supervision of lactation

> **Excludes1**   disorders of lactation (O92.-)

● **Z39.2**   Encounter for routine postpartum follow-up ♀   M

ENCOUNTERS FOR OTHER SPECIFIC HEALTH CARE (Z40-Z53)

Categories Z40-Z53 are intended for use to indicate a reason for care. They may be used for patients who have already been treated for a disease or injury, but who are receiving aftercare or prophylactic care, or care to consolidate the treatment, or to deal with a residual state

> **Excludes2**   follow-up examination for medical surveillance after treatment (Z08-Z09)

● **Z40**   **Encounter for prophylactic surgery**

> **Excludes1**   organ donations (Z52.-)
> therapeutic organ removal - code to condition

Coding Clinic: 2016, Q4, P79

● **Z40.0**   Encounter for prophylactic surgery for risk factors related to malignant neoplasms

Admission for prophylactic organ removal

Use additional code to identify risk factor

Z40.00   Encounter for prophylactic removal of unspecified organ

Z40.01   Encounter for prophylactic removal of breast

⇒ **Z40.02**   Encounter for prophylactic removal of ovary(s) ♀

> ▶Encounter for prophylactic removal of ovary(s) and fallopian tube(s)

▶ **Z40.03**   Encounter for prophylactic removal of fallopian tube(s) ♀

Z40.09   Encounter for prophylactic removal of other organ

● **Z40.8**   Encounter for other prophylactic surgery

● **Z40.9**   Encounter for prophylactic surgery, unspecified

● **Z41**   **Encounter for procedures for purposes other than remedying health state**

Z41.1   Encounter for cosmetic surgery

Encounter for cosmetic breast implant

Encounter for cosmetic procedure

> **Excludes1**   encounter for plastic and reconstructive surgery following medical procedure or healed injury (Z42.-)
> encounter for post-mastectomy breast implantation (Z42.1)

Z41.2   Encounter for routine and ritual male circumcision ♂

● **Z41.3**   Encounter for ear piercing

Z41.8   Encounter for other procedures for purposes other than remedying health state

● **Z41.9**   Encounter for procedure for purposes other than remedying health state, unspecified

● **Z42**   **Encounter for plastic and reconstructive surgery following medical procedure or healed injury**

> **Excludes1**   encounter for cosmetic plastic surgery (Z41.1)
> encounter for plastic surgery for treatment of current injury - code to relevent injury

Z42.1   Encounter for breast reconstruction following mastectomy   A

> **Excludes1**   deformity and disproportion of reconstructed breast (N65.1-)

Z42.8   Encounter for other plastic and reconstructive surgery following medical procedure or healed injury

Coding Clinic: 2017, Q1, P42

● **Z43**   **Encounter for attention to artificial openings**

> **Includes**   closure of artificial openings
> passage of sounds or bougies through artificial openings
> reforming artificial openings
> removal of catheter from artificial openings
> toilet or cleansing of artificial openings

> **Excludes1**   ~~artificial opening status only, without need for care (Z93.-)~~
> complications of external stoma (J95.0-, K94.-, N99.5-)

> **Excludes2**   fitting and adjustment of prosthetic and other devices (Z44-Z46)

Z43.0   Encounter for attention to tracheostomy

Z43.1   Encounter for attention to gastrostomy

> ▶ **Excludes2**   artificial opening status only, without need for care (Z93.-)

Ex: See PDX Collection 1487

Z43.2   Encounter for attention to ileostomy

Coding Clinic: 2016, Q3, P5

Z43.3   Encounter for attention to colostomy

Z43.4   Encounter for attention to other artificial openings of digestive tract

Z43.5   Encounter for attention to cystostomy

Z43.6   Encounter for attention to other artificial openings of urinary tract

Encounter for attention to nephrostomy

Encounter for attention to ureterostomy

Encounter for attention to urethrostomy

Z43.7   Encounter for attention to artificial vagina

Z43.8   Encounter for attention to other artificial openings

● **Z43.9**   Encounter for attention to unspecified artificial opening

● **Z44**   **Encounter for fitting and adjustment of external prosthetic device**

> **Includes**   removal or replacement of external prosthetic device

> **Excludes1**   malfunction or other complications of device - see Alphabetical Index presence of prosthetic device (Z97.-)

● **Z44.0**   Encounter for fitting and adjustment of artificial arm

● **Z44.00**   Encounter for fitting and adjustment of unspecified artificial arm

Z44.001   Encounter for fitting and adjustment of unspecified right artificial arm

Z44.002   Encounter for fitting and adjustment of unspecified left artificial arm

Z44.009   Encounter for fitting and adjustment of unspecified artificial arm, unspecified arm

● **Z44.01**   Encounter for fitting and adjustment of complete artificial arm

Z44.011   Encounter for fitting and adjustment of complete right artificial arm

Z44.012   Encounter for fitting and adjustment of complete left artificial arm

Z44.019   Encounter for fitting and adjustment of complete artificial arm, unspecified arm

---

▶ New   ⇒ Revised   ~~deleted~~ Deleted   Excludes 1   Excludes 2   Includes   Use additional   Code first   Code also   Key words

OGCR Official Guidelines   ● Unacceptable Principal Diagnosis   X Assign placeholder X   ▌Use Additional Character(s)   ▌Manifestation Code   **Coding Clinic**

Z44.02　Encounter for fitting and adjustment of partial artificial arm

　　Z44.021　Encounter for fitting and adjustment of partial artificial right arm

　　Z44.022　Encounter for fitting and adjustment of partial artificial left arm

　　Z44.029　Encounter for fitting and adjustment of partial artificial arm, unspecified arm

Z44.1　Encounter for fitting and adjustment of artificial leg

　Z44.10　Encounter for fitting and adjustment of unspecified artificial leg

　　Z44.101　Encounter for fitting and adjustment of unspecified right artificial leg

　　Z44.102　Encounter for fitting and adjustment of unspecified left artificial leg

　　Z44.109　Encounter for fitting and adjustment of unspecified artificial leg, unspecified leg

　Z44.11　Encounter for fitting and adjustment of complete artificial leg

　　Z44.111　Encounter for fitting and adjustment of complete right artificial leg

　　Z44.112　Encounter for fitting and adjustment of complete left artificial leg

　　Z44.119　Encounter for fitting and adjustment of complete artificial leg, unspecified leg

　Z44.12　Encounter for fitting and adjustment of partial artificial leg

　　Z44.121　Encounter for fitting and adjustment of partial artificial right leg

　　Z44.122　Encounter for fitting and adjustment of partial artificial left leg

　　Z44.129　Encounter for fitting and adjustment of partial artificial leg, unspecified leg

Z44.2　Encounter for fitting and adjustment of artificial eye

　Excludes1　mechanical complication of ocular prosthesis (T85.3)

　Z44.20　Encounter for fitting and adjustment of artificial eye, unspecified

　Z44.21　Encounter for fitting and adjustment of artificial right eye

　Z44.22　Encounter for fitting and adjustment of artificial left eye

Z44.3　Encounter for fitting and adjustment of external breast prosthesis

　Excludes1　complications of breast implant (T85.4-)
　　　　　encounter for adjustment or removal of breast implant (Z45.81-)
　　　　　encounter for initial breast implant insertion for cosmetic breast augmentation (Z41.1)
　　　　　encounter for breast reconstruction following mastectomy (Z42.1)

　Z44.30　Encounter for fitting and adjustment of external breast prosthesis, unspecified breast

　Z44.31　Encounter for fitting and adjustment of external right breast prosthesis

　Z44.32　Encounter for fitting and adjustment of external left breast prosthesis

Z44.8　Encounter for fitting and adjustment of other external prosthetic devices

Z44.9　Encounter for fitting and adjustment of unspecified external prosthetic device

Z45　Encounter for adjustment and management of implanted device

　Includes　removal or replacement of implanted device

　Excludes1　malfunction or other complications of device - see Alphabetical Index
~~presence of prosthetic and other devices (Z95-Z97)~~

　Excludes2　encounter for fitting and adjustment of non-implanted device (Z46.-)

Z45.0　Encounter for adjustment and management of cardiac device

　Z45.01　Encounter for adjustment and management of cardiac pacemaker

　　Encounter for adjustment and management of cardiac resynchronization therapy pacemaker (CRT-P)

　　Excludes1　encounter for adjustment and management of automatic implantable cardiac defibrillator with synchronous cardiac pacemaker (Z45.02)

　　Z45.010　Encounter for checking and testing of cardiac pacemaker pulse generator [battery]

　　　　Encounter for replacing cardiac pacemaker pulse generator [battery]

　　　　MCE: Questionable admission when principal dx

　　Z45.018　Encounter for adjustment and management of other part of cardiac pacemaker

　　　▶ **Excludes2**　presence of prosthetic and other devices (Z95-Z97)

　　　　MCE: Questionable admission when principal dx

　Z45.02　Encounter for adjustment and management of automatic implantable cardiac defibrillator

　　　Encounter for adjustment and management of automatic implantable cardiac defibrillator with synchronous cardiac pacemaker

　　　Encounter for adjustment and management of cardiac resynchronization therapy defibrillator (CRT-D)

　　　MCE: Questionable admission when principal dx

　Z45.09　Encounter for adjustment and management of other cardiac device

　　　MCE: Questionable admission when principal dx

Z45.1　Encounter for adjustment and management of infusion pump

Z45.2　Encounter for adjustment and management of vascular access device

　　Encounter for adjustment and management of vascular catheters

　　Excludes1　encounter for adjustment and management of renal dialysis catheter (Z49.01)

Z45.3　Encounter for adjustment and management of implanted devices of the special senses

　Z45.31　Encounter for adjustment and management of implanted visual substitution device

　Z45.32　Encounter for adjustment and management of implanted hearing device

　　Excludes1　encounter for fitting and adjustment of hearing aide (Z46.1)

　　Z45.320　Encounter for adjustment and management of bone conduction device

　　Z45.321　Encounter for adjustment and management of cochlear device

　　Z45.328　Encounter for adjustment and management of other implanted hearing device

N Newborn Age: Ø　　**P** Pediatric Age: Ø–17　　**M** Maternity DX: 12–55　　**A** Adult Age: 15–124　　♀ Females Only　　♂ Males Only

🅒 Complication\Comorbidity　　🅜 Major C\C　　(Ex) CC/MCC Exclusions　　🅗 Hospital-Acquired Condition

1603

CHAPTER 21 (ZØØ-Z99)

● **Z45.4**　**Encounter for adjustment and management of implanted nervous system device**

　　Z45.41　**Encounter for adjustment and management of cerebrospinal fluid drainage device**
　　　　Encounter for adjustment and management of cerebral ventricular (communicating) shunt

　　Z45.42　**Encounter for adjustment and management of neuropacemaker (brain) (peripheral nerve) (spinal cord)**

　　Z45.49　**Encounter for adjustment and management of other implanted nervous system device**

● **Z45.8**　**Encounter for adjustment and management of other implanted devices**

　　● **Z45.81**　**Encounter for adjustment or removal of breast implant**
　　　　Encounter for elective implant exchange (different material) (different size)
　　　　Encounter for removal of tissue expander without synchronous insertion of permanent implant

　　　　Excludes1　complications of breast implant (T85.4-)
　　　　　　encounter for initial breast implant insertion for cosmetic breast augmentation (Z41.1)
　　　　　　encounter for breast reconstruction following mastectomy (Z42.1)

　　　　Z45.811　**Encounter for adjustment or removal of right breast implant**

　　　　Z45.812　**Encounter for adjustment or removal of left breast implant**

　　　　Z45.819　**Encounter for adjustment or removal of unspecified breast implant**

　　● **Z45.82**　**Encounter for adjustment or removal of myringotomy device (stent) (tube)**

　　● **Z45.89**　**Encounter for adjustment and management of other implanted devices**

● **Z45.9**　**Encounter for adjustment and management of unspecified implanted device**

● **Z46**　**Encounter for fitting and adjustment of other devices**

　　Includes　removal or replacement of other device

　　Excludes1　malfunction or other complications of device - see Alphabetical Index

　　Excludes2　encounter for fitting and management of implanted devices (Z45.-)
　　　　issue of repeat prescription only (Z76.0)
　　　　presence of prosthetic and other devices (Z95-Z97)

● **Z46.0**　**Encounter for fitting and adjustment of spectacles and contact lenses**

● **Z46.1**　**Encounter for fitting and adjustment of hearing aid**
　　　　Excludes1　encounter for adjustment and management of implanted hearing device (Z45.32-)

　　Z46.2　**Encounter for fitting and adjustment of other devices related to nervous system and special senses**
　　　　Excludes2　encounter for adjustment and management of implanted nervous system device (Z45.4-)
　　　　　　encounter for adjustment and management of implanted visual substitution device (Z45.31)

　　Z46.3　**Encounter for fitting and adjustment of dental prosthetic device**
　　　　Encounter for fitting and adjustment of dentures

● **Z46.4**　**Encounter for fitting and adjustment of orthodontic device**

● **Z46.5**　**Encounter for fitting and adjustment of other gastrointestinal appliance and device**
　　　　Excludes1　encounter for attention to artificial openings of digestive tract (Z43.1-Z43.4)

　　● **Z46.51**　**Encounter for fitting and adjustment of gastric lap band**

　　● **Z46.59**　**Encounter for fitting and adjustment of other gastrointestinal appliance and device**

● **Z46.6**　**Encounter for fitting and adjustment of urinary device**
　　　　Excludes2　attention to artificial openings of urinary tract (Z43.5, Z43.6)

● **Z46.8**　**Encounter for fitting and adjustment of other specified devices**

　　● **Z46.81**　**Encounter for fitting and adjustment of insulin pump**
　　　　Encounter for insulin pump instruction and training
　　　　Encounter for insulin pump titration

　　Z46.82　**Encounter for fitting and adjustment of non-vascular catheter**

　　● **Z46.89**　**Encounter for fitting and adjustment of other specified devices**
　　　　Encounter for fitting and adjustment of wheelchair

● **Z46.9**　**Encounter for fitting and adjustment of unspecified device**

● **Z47**　**Orthopedic aftercare**
　　Excludes1　aftercare for healing fracture - code to fracture with 7th character D

　　Z47.1　**Aftercare following joint replacement surgery**
　　　　Use additional code to identify the joint (Z96.6-)

　　Z47.2　**Encounter for removal of internal fixation device**
　　　　Excludes1　encounter for adjustment of internal fixation device for fracture treatment - code to fracture with appropriate 7th character
　　　　　　encounter for removal of external fixation device - code to fracture with 7th character D
　　　　　　infection or inflammatory reaction to internal fixation device (T84.6-)
　　　　　　mechanical complication of internal fixation device (T84.1-)

● **Z47.3**　**Aftercare following explantation of joint prosthesis**
　　　　Aftercare following explantation of joint prosthesis, staged procedure
　　　　Encounter for joint prosthesis insertion following prior explantation of joint prosthesis
　　　　Coding Clinic: 2015, Q1, P17

　　Z47.31　**Aftercare following explantation of shoulder joint prosthesis**
　　　　Excludes1　acquired absence of shoulder joint following prior explantation of shoulder joint prosthesis (Z89.23-)
　　　　　　shoulder joint prosthesis explantation status (Z89.23-)

　　Z47.32　**Aftercare following explantation of hip joint prosthesis**
　　　　Excludes1　acquired absence of hip joint following prior explantation of hip joint prosthesis (Z89.62-)
　　　　　　hip joint prosthesis explantation status (Z89.62-)
　　　　Coding Clinic: 2015, Q1, P17

　　Z47.33　**Aftercare following explantation of knee joint prosthesis**
　　　　Excludes1　acquired absence of knee joint following prior explantation of knee prosthesis (Z89.52-)
　　　　　　knee joint prosthesis explantation status (Z89.52-)

▶ New　⇒ Revised　~~deleted~~ Deleted　Excludes 1　Excludes 2　Includes　Use additional　Code first　Code also　Key words
OGCR Official Guidelines　● Unacceptable Principal Diagnosis　X Assign placeholder X　● Use Additional Character(s)　▶ Manifestation Code　**Coding Clinic**

● **Z47.8   Encounter for other orthopedic aftercare**

    Z47.81   Encounter for orthopedic aftercare following surgical amputation

        Use additional code to identify the limb amputated (Z89.-)

    Z47.82   Encounter for orthopedic aftercare following scoliosis surgery

    Z47.89   Encounter for other orthopedic aftercare
        Coding Clinic: 2015, Q1, P8

● **Z48   Encounter for other postprocedural aftercare**

    Excludes1 ▶ encounter for aftercare following injury - code to Injury, by site, with appropriate 7th character for subsequent encounter

        encounter for follow-up examination after completed treatment (Z08-Z09)

    Excludes2   encounter for attention to artificial openings (Z43.-)

        encounter for fitting and adjustment of prosthetic and other devices (Z44-Z46)

● **Z48.0   Encounter for attention to dressings, sutures and drains**

    Excludes1   encounter for planned postprocedural wound closure (Z48.1)

    ● **Z48.00   Encounter for change or removal of nonsurgical wound dressing**

        Encounter for change or removal of wound dressing NOS

    ● **Z48.01   Encounter for change or removal of surgical wound dressing**
        Coding Clinic: 2015, Q4, P38

    ● **Z48.02   Encounter for removal of sutures**
        Encounter for removal of staples
        Coding Clinic: 2015, Q1, P6

    Z48.03   Encounter for change or removal of drains

  Z48.1   Encounter for planned postprocedural wound closure

    Excludes1   encounter for attention to dressings and sutures (Z48.0-)

● **Z48.2   Encounter for aftercare following organ transplant**

    Z48.21   Encounter for aftercare following heart transplant 🦠
        CC when PDx is its own CC
        (Ex.) See PDX Collection 1488

    Z48.22   Encounter for aftercare following kidney transplant 🦠
        CC when PDx is its own CC
        (Ex.) See PDX Collection 1489

    Z48.23   Encounter for aftercare following liver transplant 🦠
        CC when PDx is its own CC
        (Ex.) See PDX Collection 1490

    Z48.24   Encounter for aftercare following lung transplant 🦠
        CC when PDx is its own CC
        (Ex.) See PDX Collection 1491

    ● **Z48.28   Encounter for aftercare following multiple organ transplant**

        Z48.280   Encounter for aftercare following heart-lung transplant 🦠
            CC when PDx is its own CC
            (Ex.) See PDX Collection 1488

        Z48.288   Encounter for aftercare following multiple organ transplant

    ● **Z48.29   Encounter for aftercare following other organ transplant**

        Z48.290   Encounter for aftercare following bone marrow transplant 🦠
            CC when PDx is its own CC
            (Ex.) See PDX Collection 1492

        Z48.298   Encounter for aftercare following other organ transplant

  Z48.3   Aftercare following surgery for neoplasm
    Use additional code to identify the neoplasm

● **Z48.8   Encounter for other specified postprocedural aftercare**

    ● **Z48.81   Encounter for surgical aftercare following surgery on specified body systems**

        These codes identify the body system requiring aftercare. They are for use in conjunction with other aftercare codes to fully explain the aftercare encounter. The condition treated should also be coded if still present.

        Excludes1   aftercare for injury - code the injury with 7th character D

            aftercare following surgery for neoplasm (Z48.3)

        Excludes2   aftercare following organ transplant (Z48.2-)

            orthopedic aftercare (Z47.-)

        Z48.810   Encounter for surgical aftercare following surgery on the sense organs

        Z48.811   Encounter for surgical aftercare following surgery on the nervous system

            Excludes2   encounter for surgical aftercare following surgery on the sense organs (Z48.810)

        Z48.812   Encounter for surgical aftercare following surgery on the circulatory system
            Coding Clinic: 2012, Q4, P96

        Z48.813   Encounter for surgical aftercare following surgery on the respiratory system

        Z48.814   Encounter for surgical aftercare following surgery on the teeth or oral cavity

        Z48.815   Encounter for surgical aftercare following surgery on the digestive system
            Coding Clinic: 2015, Q4, P38

        Z48.816   Encounter for surgical aftercare following surgery on the genitourinary system

            Excludes1   encounter for aftercare following sterilization reversal (Z31.42)

        Z48.817   Encounter for surgical aftercare following surgery on the skin and subcutaneous tissue
            Coding Clinic: 2015, Q1, P6

    Z48.89   Encounter for other specified surgical aftercare

● **Z49   Encounter for care involving renal dialysis**
    Code also associated end stage renal disease (N18.6)

● **Z49.0   Preparatory care for renal dialysis**
    Encounter for dialysis instruction and training

    Z49.01   Encounter for fitting and adjustment of extracorporeal dialysis catheter
        Removal or replacement of renal dialysis catheter
        Toilet or cleansing of renal dialysis catheter

    ● **Z49.02   Encounter for fitting and adjustment of peritoneal dialysis catheter**

● **Z49.3   Encounter for adequacy testing for dialysis**

    ● **Z49.31   Encounter for adequacy testing for hemodialysis**

    ● **Z49.32   Encounter for adequacy testing for peritoneal dialysis**
        Encounter for peritoneal equilibration test

CHAPTER 21 (Z00-Z99)

CHAPTER 21 (Z00-Z99)

● **Z51**   **Encounter for other aftercare and medical care**
     Code also condition requiring care
     Excludes1   follow-up examination after treatment (Z08-Z09)
     Coding Clinic: 2017, Q1, P49; 2016, Q4, P130

    Z51.0   Encounter for antineoplastic radiation therapy
● **Z51.1**   Encounter for antineoplastic chemotherapy and immunotherapy
     Excludes2   encounter for chemotherapy and immunotherapy for nonneoplastic condition-code to condition

     Z51.11   Encounter for antineoplastic chemotherapy
        Coding Clinic: 2015, Q3, P19

     Z51.12   Encounter for antineoplastic immunotherapy

    Z51.5   Encounter for palliative care
       Coding Clinic: 2017, Q1, P48-49

● **Z51.6**   Encounter for desensitization to allergens
       Coding Clinic: 2016, Q4, P77-79

● **Z51.8**   Encounter for other specified aftercare
     Excludes1   holiday relief care (Z75.5)

     Z51.81   Encounter for therapeutic drug level monitoring
       Code also any long-term (current) drug therapy (Z79.-)
       Excludes1   encounter for blood-drug test for administrative or medicolegal reasons (Z02.83)

    ● **Z51.89**   Encounter for other specified aftercare
       MCE: This code may be considered "acceptable" when a secondary diagnosis is also coded on the record.
       Coding Clinic: 2012, Q4, P96-97

● **Z52**   **Donors of organs and tissues**
     Includes   autologous and other living donors
     Excludes1   cadaveric donor - omit code examination of potential donor (Z00.5)
     Coding Clinic: 2012, Q4, P100

● **Z52.0**   Blood donor
   ● **Z52.00**   Unspecified blood donor
     ● **Z52.000**   Unspecified donor, whole blood
     ● **Z52.001**   Unspecified donor, stem cells
     ● **Z52.008**   Unspecified donor, other blood

   ● **Z52.01**   Autologous blood donor
     ● **Z52.010**   Autologous donor, whole blood
     ● **Z52.011**   Autologous donor, stem cells
     ● **Z52.018**   Autologous donor, other blood

   ● **Z52.09**   Other blood donor
     Volunteer donor
     ● **Z52.090**   Other blood donor, whole blood
     ● **Z52.091**   Other blood donor, stem cells
     ● **Z52.098**   Other blood donor, other blood

● **Z52.1**   Skin donor
    Z52.10   Skin donor, unspecified
    Z52.11   Skin donor, autologous
    Z52.19   Skin donor, other

● **Z52.2**   Bone donor
    Z52.20   Bone donor, unspecified
    Z52.21   Bone donor, autologous
    Z52.29   Bone donor, other

    Z52.3   Bone marrow donor
    Z52.4   Kidney donor
    Z52.5   Cornea donor
    Z52.6   Liver donor
       Coding Clinic: 2012, Q4, P100

● **Z52.8**   Donor of other specified organs or tissues
   ● **Z52.81**   Egg (Oocyte) donor
     ● **Z52.810**   Egg (Oocyte) donor under age 35, anonymous recipient ♀
       Egg donor under age 35 NOS
     ● **Z52.811**   Egg (Oocyte) donor under age 35, designated recipient ♀
     ● **Z52.812**   Egg (Oocyte) donor age 35 and over, anonymous recipient ♀
       Egg donor age 35 and over NOS
     ● **Z52.813**   Egg (Oocyte) donor age 35 and over, designated recipient ♀
     ● **Z52.819**   Egg (Oocyte) donor, unspecified ♀

    Z52.89   Donor of other specified organs or tissues

    Z52.9   Donor of unspecified organ or tissue
     Donor NOS

● **Z53**   **Persons encountering health services for specific procedures and treatment, not carried out**
● **Z53.0**   Procedure and treatment not carried out because of contraindication
   ● **Z53.01**   Procedure and treatment not carried out due to patient smoking
   ● **Z53.09**   Procedure and treatment not carried out because of other contraindication

● **Z53.1**   Procedure and treatment not carried out because of patient's decision for reasons of belief and group pressure

● **Z53.2**   Procedure and treatment not carried out because of patient's decision for other and unspecified reasons
   ● **Z53.20**   Procedure and treatment not carried out because of patient's decision for unspecified reasons
   ● **Z53.21**   Procedure and treatment not carried out due to patient leaving prior to being seen by health care provider
   ● **Z53.29**   Procedure and treatment not carried out because of patient's decision for other reasons

● **Z53.3**   Procedure converted to open procedure
     Coding Clinic: 2016, Q4, P79
   ● **Z53.31**   Laparoscopic surgical procedure converted to open procedure
       Coding Clinic: 2016, Q4, P100
   ● **Z53.32**   Thoracoscopic surgical procedure converted to open procedure
   ● **Z53.33**   Arthroscopic surgical procedure converted to open procedure
   ● **Z53.39**   Other specified procedure converted to open procedure

● **Z53.8**   Procedure and treatment not carried out for other reasons

● **Z53.9**   Procedure and treatment not carried out, unspecified reason

---

PERSONS WITH POTENTIAL HEALTH HAZARDS RELATED TO SOCIOECONOMIC AND PSYCHOSOCIAL CIRCUMSTANCES (Z55-Z65)

● **Z55**   **Problems related to education and literacy**
     Excludes1   disorders of psychological development (F80-F89)
● **Z55.0**   Illiteracy and low-level literacy
● **Z55.1**   Schooling unavailable and unattainable
● **Z55.2**   Failed school examinations
● **Z55.3**   Underachievement in school
● **Z55.4**   Educational maladjustment and discord with teachers and classmates
● **Z55.8**   Other problems related to education and literacy
     Problems related to inadequate teaching
● **Z55.9**   Problems related to education and literacy, unspecified
     Academic problems NOS

▶ New   ⇒ Revised   ~~deleted~~ Deleted   Excludes 1   Excludes 2   Includes   Use additional   Code first   Code also   Key words
OGCR Official Guidelines   ● Unacceptable Principal Diagnosis   X Assign placeholder X   ● Use Additional Character(s)   ▶ Manifestation Code   Coding Clinic

● **Z56 Problems related to employment and unemployment**

> **Excludes2** occupational exposure to risk factors (Z57.-)
> problems related to housing and economic
> circumstances (Z59.-)

● **Z56.0 Unemployment, unspecified**

● **Z56.1 Change of job**   A

● **Z56.2 Threat of job loss**

● **Z56.3 Stressful work schedule**

● **Z56.4 Discord with boss and workmates**

● **Z56.5 Uncongenial work environment**
> Difficult conditions at work

● **Z56.6 Other physical and mental strain related to work**

● **Z56.8 Other problems related to employment**

> ● **Z56.81 Sexual harassment on the job**

> ● **Z56.82 Military deployment status**
> > Individual (civilian or military) currently
> > deployed in theater or in support
> > of military war, peacekeeping and
> > humanitarian operations

> ● **Z56.89 Other problems related to employment**

● **Z56.9 Unspecified problems related to employment**
> Occupational problems NOS

● **Z57 Occupational exposure to risk factors**

● **Z57.0 Occupational exposure to noise**

● **Z57.1 Occupational exposure to radiation**

● **Z57.2 Occupational exposure to dust**

● **Z57.3 Occupational exposure to other air contaminants**

> ● **Z57.31 Occupational exposure to environmental
> tobacco smoke**

> > **Excludes2** exposure to environmental
> > tobacco smoke (Z77.22)

> ● **Z57.39 Occupational exposure to other air
> contaminants**

● **Z57.4 Occupational exposure to toxic agents in agriculture**
> Occupational exposure to solids, liquids, gases or
> vapors in agriculture

● **Z57.5 Occupational exposure to toxic agents in other industries**
> Occupational exposure to solids, liquids, gases or
> vapors in other industries

● **Z57.6 Occupational exposure to extreme temperature**

● **Z57.7 Occupational exposure to vibration**

● **Z57.8 Occupational exposure to other risk factors**

● **Z57.9 Occupational exposure to unspecified risk factor**

● **Z59 Problems related to housing and economic circumstances**

> **Excludes2** problems related to upbringing (Z62.-)

● **Z59.0 Homelessness**

● **Z59.1 Inadequate housing**
> Lack of heating
> Restriction of space
> Technical defects in home preventing adequate care
> Unsatisfactory surroundings

> > **Excludes1** problems related to the natural and
> > physical environment (Z77.1-)

● **Z59.2 Discord with neighbors, lodgers and landlord**

● **Z59.3 Problems related to living in residential institution**
> Boarding-school resident

> > **Excludes1** institutional upbringing (Z62.2)

● **Z59.4 Lack of adequate food and safe drinking water**
> Inadequate drinking water supply

> > **Excludes1** effects of hunger (T73.0)
> > inappropriate diet or eating habits (Z72.4)
> > malnutrition (E40-E46)

● **Z59.5 Extreme poverty**

● **Z59.6 Low income**

● **Z59.7 Insufficient social insurance and welfare support**

● **Z59.8 Other problems related to housing and economic
circumstances**
> Foreclosure on loan
> Isolated dwelling
> Problems with creditors

● **Z59.9 Problem related to housing and economic circumstances,
unspecified**

● **Z60 Problems related to social environment**

● **Z60.0 Problems of adjustment to life-cycle transitions**
> Empty nest syndrome
> Phase of life problem
> Problem with adjustment to retirement [pension]

● **Z60.2 Problems related to living alone**

● **Z60.3 Acculturation difficulty**
> Problem with migration
> Problem with social transplantation

● **Z60.4 Social exclusion and rejection**
> Exclusion and rejection on the basis of personal
> characteristics, such as unusual physical
> appearance, illness or behavior.

> > **Excludes1** target of adverse discrimination such as
> > for racial or religious reasons (Z60.5)

● **Z60.5 Target of (perceived) adverse discrimination and
persecution**

> > **Excludes1** social exclusion and rejection (Z60.4)

● **Z60.8 Other problems related to social environment**

● **Z60.9 Problem related to social environment, unspecified**

● **Z62 Problems related to upbringing**

> **Includes** current and past negative life events in childhood
> current and past problems of a child related to
> upbringing

> **Excludes2** maltreatment syndrome (T74.-)
> problems related to housing and economic
> circumstances (Z59.-)

● **Z62.0 Inadequate parental supervision and control**

● **Z62.1 Parental overprotection**

● **Z62.2 Upbringing away from parents**

> > **Excludes1** problems with boarding school (Z59.3)

> ● **Z62.21 Child in welfare custody**   P
> > Child in care of non-parental family member
> > Child in foster care

> > **Excludes2** problem for parent due to child
> > in welfare custody (Z63.5)

> ● **Z62.22 Institutional upbringing**
> > Child living in orphanage or group home

> ● **Z62.29 Other upbringing away from parents**

● **Z62.3 Hostility towards and scapegoating of child**   P

● **Z62.6 Inappropriate (excessive) parental pressure**

CHAPTER 21 (Z00-Z99)

N Newborn Age: 0   P Pediatric Age: 0–17   M Maternity DX: 12–55   A Adult Age: 15–124   ♀ Females Only   ♂ Males Only

🔹 Complication\Comorbidity   🔹 Major C\C   Ⓔ CC/MCC Exclusions   🔹 Hospital-Acquired Condition

● **Z62.8   Other specified problems related to upbringing**

● **Z62.81   Personal history of abuse in childhood**

● **Z62.810   Personal history of physical and sexual abuse in childhood**

> **Excludes1**   current child physical abuse (T74.12, T76.12)
> current child sexual abuse (T74.22, T76.22)

● **Z62.811   Personal history of psychological abuse in childhood**

> **Excludes1**   current child psychological abuse (T74.32, T76.32)

● **Z62.812   Personal history of neglect in childhood**

> **Excludes1**   current child neglect (T74.02, T76.02)

● **Z62.819   Personal history of unspecified abuse in childhood**

> **Excludes1**   current child abuse NOS (T74.92, T76.92)

● **Z62.82   Parent-child conflict**

● **Z62.820   Parent-biological child conflict**
Parent-child problem NOS

● **Z62.821   Parent-adopted child conflict**

● **Z62.822   Parent-foster child conflict**

● **Z62.89   Other specified problems related to upbringing**

● **Z62.890   Parent-child estrangement NEC**

● **Z62.891   Sibling rivalry**

● **Z62.898   Other specified problems related to upbringing**

● **Z62.9   Problem related to upbringing, unspecified**

● **Z63   Other problems related to primary support group, including family circumstances**

> **Excludes2**   maltreatment syndrome (T74.-, T76)
> parent-child problems (Z62.-)
> problems related to negative life events in childhood (Z62.-)
> problems related to upbringing (Z62.-)

● **Z63.0   Problems in relationship with spouse or partner**

▶ Relationship distress with spouse or intimate partner

> **Excludes1**   counseling for spousal or partner abuse problems (Z69.1)
> counseling related to sexual attitude, behavior, and orientation (Z70.-)

● **Z63.1   Problems in relationship with in-laws**

● **Z63.3   Absence of family member**

> **Excludes1**   absence of family member due to disappearance and death (Z63.4)
> absence of family member due to separation and divorce (Z63.5)

● **Z63.31   Absence of family member due to military deployment**
Individual or family affected by other family member being on military deployment

> **Excludes1**   family disruption due to return of family member from military deployment (Z63.71)

● **Z63.32   Other absence of family member**

● **Z63.4   Disappearance and death of family member**
Assumed death of family member
Bereavement

● **Z63.5   Disruption of family by separation and divorce**
Marital estrangement

● **Z63.6   Dependent relative needing care at home**

● **Z63.7   Other stressful life events affecting family and household**

● **Z63.71   Stress on family due to return of family member from military deployment**
Individual or family affected by family member having returned from military deployment (current or past conflict)

● **Z63.72   Alcoholism and drug addiction in family**

● **Z63.79   Other stressful life events affecting family and household**
Anxiety (normal) about sick person in family
Health problems within family
Ill or disturbed family member
Isolated family

● **Z63.8   Other specified problems related to primary support group**
Family discord NOS
Family estrangement NOS
High expressed emotional level within family
Inadequate family support NOS
Inadequate or distorted communication within family

● **Z63.9   Problem related to primary support group, unspecified**
Relationship disorder NOS

● **Z64   Problems related to certain psychosocial circumstances**

● **Z64.0   Problems related to unwanted pregnancy** ♀

● **Z64.1   Problems related to multiparity** ♀

● **Z64.4   Discord with counselors**
Discord with probation officer
Discord with social worker

● **Z65   Problems related to other psychosocial circumstances**

● **Z65.0   Conviction in civil and criminal proceedings without imprisonment**

● **Z65.1   Imprisonment and other incarceration**

● **Z65.2   Problems related to release from prison**

● **Z65.3   Problems related to other legal circumstances**
Arrest
Child custody or support proceedings
Litigation
Prosecution

● **Z65.4   Victim of crime and terrorism**
Victim of torture

● **Z65.5   Exposure to disaster, war and other hostilities**

> **Excludes1**   target of perceived discrimination or persecution (Z60.5)

● **Z65.8   Other specified problems related to psychosocial circumstances**
▶ Religious or spiritual problem

● **Z65.9   Problem related to unspecified psychosocial circumstances**

DO NOT RESUSCITATE STATUS (Z66)

● **Z66   Do not resuscitate**
DNR status

▶ New   ⇒ Revised   ~~deleted~~ Deleted   Excludes 1   Excludes 2   Includes   Use additional   Code first   Code also   Key words

OGCR Official Guidelines   ● Unacceptable Principal Diagnosis   X Assign placeholder X   ● Use Additional Character(s)   ▶ Manifestation Code   **Coding Clinic**

BLOOD TYPE (Z67)

● **Z67**   **Blood type**
     Coding Clinic: 2015, Q3, P40
   ● **Z67.1**   Type A blood
     ● Z67.10   Type A blood, Rh positive
     ● Z67.11   Type A blood, Rh negative
   ● **Z67.2**   Type B blood
     ● Z67.20   Type B blood, Rh positive
     ● Z67.21   Type B blood, Rh negative
   ● **Z67.3**   Type AB blood
     ● Z67.30   Type AB blood, Rh positive
     ● Z67.31   Type AB blood, Rh negative
   ● **Z67.4**   Type O blood
     ● Z67.40   Type O blood, Rh positive
     ● Z67.41   Type O blood, Rh negative
   ● **Z67.9**   Unspecified blood type
     ● Z67.90   Unspecified blood type, Rh positive
     ● Z67.91   Unspecified blood type, Rh negative
           Coding Clinic: 2015, Q3, P40

BODY MASS INDEX [BMI] (Z68)

OGCR   Section I.B.14.

General Coding Guidelines

14. Documentation for BMI, Depth of Non-pressure ulcers, Pressure Ulcer Stages, Coma Scale, and NIH Stroke Scale

For the Body Mass Index (BMI), depth of non-pressure chronic ulcers, pressure ulcer stage, coma scale, and NIH stroke scale (NIHSS) codes, code assignment may be based on medical record documentation from clinicians who are not the patient's provider (i.e., physician or other qualified healthcare practitioner legally accountable for establishing the patient's diagnosis), since this information is typically documented by other clinicians involved in the care of the patient (e.g., a dietitian often documents the BMI, a nurse often documents the pressure ulcer stages, and an emergency medical technician often documents the coma scale). However, the associated diagnosis (such as overweight, obesity, acute stroke, or pressure ulcer) must be documented by the patient's provider. If there is conflicting medical record documentation, either from the same clinician or different clinicians, the patient's attending provider should be queried for clarification.

The BMI, coma scale, and NIHSS codes should only be reported as secondary diagnoses.

● **Z68**   **Body mass index [BMI]**
     Kilograms per meters squared
     Note: BMI adult codes are for use for persons 21 years of age or older.
        BMI pediatric codes are for use for persons 2-20 years of age. These percentiles are based on the growth charts published by the Centers for Disease Control and Prevention (CDC)
     Coding Clinic: 2016, Q4, P129
 ⇒● **Z68.1**   Body mass index (BMI) 19.9 or less, adult 🦠   A
       (Ex) See PDX Collection 1493
       Coding Clinic: 2017, Q1, P39
   ● **Z68.2**   Body mass index (BMI) 20-29, adult
     ● Z68.20   Body mass index (BMI) 20.0-20.9, adult   A
     ● Z68.21   Body mass index (BMI) 21.0-21.9, adult   A
     ● Z68.22   Body mass index (BMI) 22.0-22.9, adult   A
     ● Z68.23   Body mass index (BMI) 23.0-23.9, adult   A
     ● Z68.24   Body mass index (BMI) 24.0-24.9, adult   A
     ● Z68.25   Body mass index (BMI) 25.0-25.9, adult   A
     ● Z68.26   Body mass index (BMI) 26.0-26.9, adult   A
     ● Z68.27   Body mass index (BMI) 27.0-27.9, adult   A
     ● Z68.28   Body mass index (BMI) 28.0-28.9, adult   A
     ● Z68.29   Body mass index (BMI) 29.0-29.9, adult   A

● **Z68.3**   Body mass index (BMI) 30-39, adult
   ● Z68.30   Body mass index (BMI) 30.0-30.9, adult   A
   ● Z68.31   Body mass index (BMI) 31.0-31.9, adult   A
   ● Z68.32   Body mass index (BMI) 32.0-32.9, adult   A
   ● Z68.33   Body mass index (BMI) 33.0-33.9, adult   A
   ● Z68.34   Body mass index (BMI) 34.0-34.9, adult   A
   ● Z68.35   Body mass index (BMI) 35.0-35.9, adult   A
   ● Z68.36   Body mass index (BMI) 36.0-36.9, adult   A
   ● Z68.37   Body mass index (BMI) 37.0-37.9, adult   A
   ● Z68.38   Body mass index (BMI) 38.0-38.9, adult   A
   ● Z68.39   Body mass index (BMI) 39.0-39.9, adult   A
● **Z68.4**   Body mass index (BMI) 40 or greater, adult
     (Ex) For category Z68.4 CC codes: See PDX Collection 1494
   ● Z68.41   Body mass index (BMI) 40.0-44.9, adult 🦠   A
   ● Z68.42   Body mass index (BMI) 45.0-49.9, adult 🦠   A
   ● Z68.43   Body mass index (BMI) 50-59.9, adult 🦠   A
   ● Z68.44   Body mass index (BMI) 60.0-69.9, adult 🦠   A
   ● Z68.45   Body mass index (BMI) 70 or greater, adult 🦠   A
● **Z68.5**   Body mass index (BMI) pediatric
   ● Z68.51   Body mass index (BMI) pediatric, less than 5th percentile for age
   ● Z68.52   Body mass index (BMI) pediatric, 5th percentile to less than 85th percentile for age
   ● Z68.53   Body mass index (BMI) pediatric, 85th percentile to less than 95th percentile for age
   ● Z68.54   Body mass index (BMI) pediatric, greater than or equal to 95th percentile for age

PERSONS ENCOUNTERING HEALTH SERVICES IN OTHER CIRCUMSTANCES (Z69-Z76)

● **Z69**   **Encounter for mental health services for victim and perpetrator of abuse**
     Includes   counseling for victims and perpetrators of abuse
   ● **Z69.0**   Encounter for mental health services for child abuse problems
     ● **Z69.01**   Encounter for mental health services for parental child abuse
       Z69.010   **Encounter for mental health services for victim of parental child abuse**   P
         ▶Encounter for mental health services for victim of child abuse by parent
         ▶Encounter for mental health services for victim of child neglect by parent
         ▶Encounter for mental health services for victim of child psychological abuse by parent
         ▶Encounter for mental health services for victim of child sexual abuse by parent
      ● Z69.011   **Encounter for mental health services for perpetrator of parental child abuse**
         ▶Encounter for mental health services for perpetrator of parental child neglect
         ▶Encounter for mental health services for perpetrator of parental child psychological abuse
         ▶Encounter for mental health services for perpetrator of parental child sexual abuse
         Excludes1   encounter for mental health services for non-parental child abuse (Z69.02-)

CHAPTER 21 (Z00-Z99)

CHAPTER 21 (Z00-Z99)

● **Z69.02** **Encounter for mental health services for non-parental child abuse**

Z69.020 **Encounter for mental health services for victim of non-parental child abuse** P
  ▶Encounter for mental health services for victim of non-parental child neglect
  ▶Encounter for mental health services for victim of non-parental child psychological abuse
  ▶Encounter for mental health services for victim of non-parental child sexual abuse

● **Z69.021** **Encounter for mental health services for perpetrator of non- parental child abuse**
  ▶Encounter for mental health services for perpetrator of non-parental child neglect
  ▶Encounter for mental health services for perpetrator of non-parental child psychological abuse
  ▶Encounter for mental health services for perpetrator of non-parental child sexual abuse

● **Z69.1** **Encounter for mental health services for spousal or partner abuse problems**

● **Z69.11** **Encounter for mental health services for victim of spousal or partner abuse**
  ▶Encounter for mental health services for victim of spouse or partner neglect
  ▶Encounter for mental health services for victim of spouse or partner psychological abuse
  ▶Encounter for mental health services for victim of spouse or partner violence, physical

● **Z69.12** **Encounter for mental health services for perpetrator of spousal or partner abuse**
  ▶Encounter for mental health services for perpetrator of spouse or partner neglect
  ▶Encounter for mental health services for perpetrator of spouse or partner psychological abuse
  ▶Encounter for mental health services for perpetrator of spouse or partner violence, physical
  ▶Encounter for mental health services for perpetrator of spouse or partner violence, sexual

● **Z69.8** **Encounter for mental health services for victim or perpetrator of other abuse**

● **Z69.81** **Encounter for mental health services for victim of other abuse**
  ▶Encounter for mental health services for perpetrator of non-spousal adult abuse
  ▶Encounter for mental health services for victim of non-spousal adult abuse
  ▶Encounter for mental health services for victim of spouse or partner violence, sexual
  Encounter for rape victim counseling

● **Z69.82** **Encounter for mental health services for perpetrator of other abuse**

● **Z70** **Counseling related to sexual attitude, behavior and orientation**
  Includes encounter for mental health services for sexual attitude, behavior and orientation
  Excludes2 contraceptive or procreative counseling (Z30-Z31)

● **Z70.0** **Counseling related to sexual attitude**

● **Z70.1** **Counseling related to patient's sexual behavior and orientation**
  Patient concerned regarding impotence
  Patient concerned regarding non-responsiveness
  Patient concerned regarding promiscuity
  Patient concerned regarding sexual orientation

● **Z70.2** **Counseling related to sexual behavior and orientation of third party**
  Advice sought regarding sexual behavior and orientation of child
  Advice sought regarding sexual behavior and orientation of partner
  Advice sought regarding sexual behavior and orientation of spouse

● **Z70.3** **Counseling related to combined concerns regarding sexual attitude, behavior and orientation**

● **Z70.8** **Other sex counseling**
  Encounter for sex education

● **Z70.9** **Sex counseling, unspecified**

● **Z71** **Persons encountering health services for other counseling and medical advice, not elsewhere classified**
  Excludes2 contraceptive or procreation counseling (Z30-Z31)
  sex counseling (Z70.-)

● **Z71.0** **Person encountering health services to consult on behalf of another person**
  Person encountering health services to seek advice or treatment for non-attending third party
  Excludes2 anxiety (normal) about sick person in family (Z63.7)
  expectant (adoptive) parent(s) pre-birth pediatrician visit (Z76.81)

● **Z71.1** **Person with feared health complaint in whom no diagnosis is made**
  Person encountering health services with feared condition which was not demonstrated
  Person encountering health services in which problem was normal state
  'Worried well'
  Excludes1 medical observation for suspected diseases and conditions proven not to exist (Z03.-)
  Coding Clinic: 2016, Q4, P7

● **Z71.2** **Person consulting for explanation of examination or test findings**

● **Z71.3** **Dietary counseling and surveillance**
  Use additional code for any associated underlying medical condition
  Use additional code to identify body mass index (BMI), if known (Z68.-)

● **Z71.4** **Alcohol abuse counseling and surveillance**
  Use additional code for alcohol abuse or dependence (F10.-)

● **Z71.41** **Alcohol abuse counseling and surveillance of alcoholic**

● **Z71.42** **Counseling for family member of alcoholic**
  Counseling for significant other, partner, or friend of alcoholic

▶ New ⇒ Revised ~~deleted~~ Deleted Excludes 1 Excludes 2 Includes Use additional Code first Code also Key words
OGCR Official Guidelines ● Unacceptable Principal Diagnosis X Assign placeholder X ● Use Additional Character(s) ▶ Manifestation Code Coding Clinic

● **Z71.5**   **Drug abuse counseling and surveillance**
Use additional code for drug abuse or dependence (F11-F16, F18-F19)

    ● **Z71.51**   **Drug abuse counseling and surveillance of drug abuser**

    ● **Z71.52**   **Counseling for family member of drug abuser**
Counseling for significant other, partner, or friend of drug abuser

● **Z71.6**   **Tobacco abuse counseling**
Use additional code for nicotine dependence (F17.-)

● **Z71.7**   **Human immunodeficiency virus [HIV] counseling**

● **Z71.8**   **Other specified counseling**

    Excludes2   counseling for contraception (Z30.0-)
counseling for genetics (Z31.5)
counseling for procreative management (Z31.6)

    ● **Z71.81**   **Spiritual or religious counseling**

    ▶● **Z71.82**   **Exercise counseling**

    ▶ **Z71.83**   **Encounter for nonprocreative genetic counseling**

       Excludes1   ▶counseling for procreative genetics (Z31.5)
▶counseling for procreative management (Z31.6)

    ● **Z71.89**   **Other specified counseling**

● **Z71.9**   **Counseling, unspecified**
Encounter for medical advice NOS

● **Z72**   **Problems related to lifestyle**

    Excludes2   problems related to life-management difficulty (Z73.-)
problems related to socioeconomic and psychosocial circumstances (Z55-Z65)

    Coding Clinic: 2016, Q4, P130

● **Z72.0**   **Tobacco use**
Tobacco use NOS

    Excludes1   history of tobacco dependence (Z87.891)
nicotine dependence (F17.2-)
tobacco dependence (F17.2-)
tobacco use during pregnancy (O99.33-)

● **Z72.3**   **Lack of physical exercise**

● **Z72.4**   **Inappropriate diet and eating habits**

    Excludes1   behavioral eating disorders of infancy or childhood (F98.2.-F98.3)
eating disorders (F50.-)
lack of adequate food (Z59.4)
malnutrition and other nutritional deficiencies (E40-E64)

● **Z72.5**   **High risk sexual behavior**
Promiscuity

    Excludes1   paraphilias (F65)

    ● **Z72.51**   **High risk heterosexual behavior**

    ● **Z72.52**   **High risk homosexual behavior**

    ● **Z72.53**   **High risk bisexual behavior**

● **Z72.6**   **Gambling and betting**

    Excludes1   compulsive or pathological gambling (F63.0)

● **Z72.8**   **Other problems related to lifestyle**

    ● **Z72.81**   **Antisocial behavior**

       Excludes1   conduct disorders (F91.-)

       Z72.810   **Child and adolescent antisocial behavior**   P
Antisocial behavior (child) (adolescent) without manifest psychiatric disorder
Delinquency NOS
Group delinquency
Offenses in the context of gang membership
Stealing in company with others
Truancy from school

       Z72.811   **Adult antisocial behavior**   A
Adult antisocial behavior without manifest psychiatric disorder

    ● **Z72.82**   **Problems related to sleep**

       Z72.820   **Sleep deprivation**
Lack of adequate sleep

         Excludes1   insomnia (G47.0-)

       ● **Z72.821**   **Inadequate sleep hygiene**
Bad sleep habits
Irregular sleep habits
Unhealthy sleep wake schedule

         Excludes1   insomnia (F51.0-, G47.0-)

    ● **Z72.89**   **Other problems related to lifestyle**
Self-damaging behavior

● **Z72.9**   **Problem related to lifestyle, unspecified**

● **Z73**   **Problems related to life management difficulty**

    Excludes2   problems related to socioeconomic and psychosocial circumstances (Z55-Z65)

● **Z73.0**   **Burn-out**

● **Z73.1**   **Type A behavior pattern**

● **Z73.2**   **Lack of relaxation and leisure**

● **Z73.3**   **Stress, not elsewhere classified**
Physical and mental strain NOS

    Excludes1   stress related to employment or unemployment (Z56.-)

● **Z73.4**   **Inadequate social skills, not elsewhere classified**

● **Z73.5**   **Social role conflict, not elsewhere classified**

● **Z73.6**   **Limitation of activities due to disability**

    Excludes1   care-provider dependency (Z74.-)

● **Z73.8**   **Other problems related to life management difficulty**

    ● **Z73.81**   **Behavioral insomnia of childhood**

       ● **Z73.810**   **Behavioral insomnia of childhood, sleep-onset association type**   P

       ● **Z73.811**   **Behavioral insomnia of childhood, limit setting type**   P

       ● **Z73.812**   **Behavioral insomnia of childhood, combined type**   P

       ● **Z73.819**   **Behavioral insomnia of childhood, unspecified type**   P

    ● **Z73.82**   **Dual sensory impairment**

    ● **Z73.89**   **Other problems related to life management difficulty**

● **Z73.9**   **Problem related to life management difficulty, unspecified**

CHAPTER 21 (Z00-Z99)

Z74   Problems related to care provider dependency

> **Excludes2**   dependence on enabling machines or devices NEC (Z99.-)

- **Z74.0   Reduced mobility**
  - **Z74.01   Bed confinement status**
    Bedridden
  - **Z74.09   Other reduced mobility**
    Chairridden
    Reduced mobility NOS
    > **Excludes2**   wheelchair dependence (Z99.3)
- **Z74.1   Need for assistance with personal care**
- **Z74.2   Need for assistance at home and no other household member able to render care**
- **Z74.3   Need for continuous supervision**
- **Z74.8   Other problems related to care provider dependency**
- **Z74.9   Problem related to care provider dependency, unspecified**

Z75   Problems related to medical facilities and other health care

- **Z75.0   Medical services not available in home**
  > **Excludes1**   no other household member able to render care (Z74.2)
- **Z75.1   Person awaiting admission to adequate facility elsewhere**
- **Z75.2   Other waiting period for investigation and treatment**
- **Z75.3   Unavailability and inaccessibility of health care facilities**
  > **Excludes1**   bed unavailable (Z75.1)
- **Z75.4   Unavailability and inaccessibility of other helping agencies**
- **Z75.5   Holiday relief care**
- **Z75.8   Other problems related to medical facilities and other health care**
- **Z75.9   Unspecified problem related to medical facilities and other health care**

Z76   Persons encountering health services in other circumstances

- **Z76.0   Encounter for issue of repeat prescription**
  Encounter for issue of repeat prescription for appliance
  Encounter for issue of repeat prescription for medicaments
  Encounter for issue of repeat prescription for spectacles
  > **Excludes2**   issue of medical certificate (Z02.7)
  > repeat prescription for contraceptive (Z30.4-)
- **Z76.1   Encounter for health supervision and care of foundling**
- **Z76.2   Encounter for health supervision and care of other healthy infant and child**   P
  Encounter for medical or nursing care or supervision of healthy infant under circumstances such as adverse socioeconomic conditions at home
  Encounter for medical or nursing care or supervision of healthy infant under circumstances such as awaiting foster or adoptive placement
  Encounter for medical or nursing care or supervision of healthy infant under circumstances such as maternal illness
  Encounter for medical or nursing care or supervision of healthy infant under circumstances such as number of children at home preventing or interfering with normal care
- **Z76.3   Healthy person accompanying sick person**
- **Z76.4   Other boarder to healthcare facility**
  > **Excludes1**   homelessness (Z59.0)

Z76.5   Malingerer [conscious simulation]
Person feigning illness (with obvious motivation)
> **Excludes1**   factitious disorder (F68.1-)
> peregrinating patient (F68.1-)

- **Z76.8   Persons encountering health services in other specified circumstances**
  - **Z76.81   Expectant parent(s) prebirth pediatrician visit**
    Pre-adoption pediatrician visit for adoptive parent(s)
  - **Z76.82   Awaiting organ transplant status**
    Patient waiting for organ availability
  - **Z76.89   Persons encountering health services in other specified circumstances**
    Persons encountering health services NOS

PERSONS WITH POTENTIAL HEALTH HAZARDS RELATED TO FAMILY AND PERSONAL HISTORY AND CERTAIN CONDITIONS INFLUENCING HEALTH STATUS (Z77-Z99)

Code also any follow-up examination (Z08-Z09)

Z77   Other contact with and (suspected) exposures hazardous to health

> **Includes**   contact with and (suspected) exposures to potential hazards to health

> **Excludes2**   contact with and (suspected) exposure to communicable diseases (Z20.-)
> exposure to (parental) (environmental) tobacco smoke in the perinatal period (P96.81)
> newborn affected by noxious substances transmitted via placenta or breast milk (P04.-)
> occupational exposure to risk factors (Z57.-)
> retained foreign body (Z18.-)
> retained foreign body fully removed (Z87.821)
> toxic effects of substances chiefly nonmedicinal as to source (T51-T65)

- **Z77.0   Contact with and (suspected) exposure to hazardous, chiefly nonmedicinal, chemicals**
  - **Z77.01   Contact with and (suspected) exposure to hazardous metals**
    - **Z77.010   Contact with and (suspected) exposure to arsenic**
    - **Z77.011   Contact with and (suspected) exposure to lead**
    - **Z77.012   Contact with and (suspected) exposure to uranium**
      > **Excludes1**   retained depleted uranium fragments (Z18.01)
    - **Z77.018   Contact with and (suspected) exposure to other hazardous metals**
      Contact with and (suspected) exposure to chromium compounds
      Contact with and (suspected) exposure to nickel dust
  - **Z77.02   Contact with and (suspected) exposure to hazardous aromatic compounds**
    - **Z77.020   Contact with and (suspected) exposure to aromatic amines**
    - **Z77.021   Contact with and (suspected) exposure to benzene**
    - **Z77.028   Contact with and (suspected) exposure to other hazardous aromatic compounds**
      Aromatic dyes NOS
      Polycyclic aromatic hydrocarbons

▶ New   ⇒ Revised   ~~deleted~~ Deleted   Excludes 1   Excludes 2   Includes   Use additional   Code first   Code also   Key words
OGCR Official Guidelines   ● Unacceptable Principal Diagnosis   X Assign placeholder X   ● Use Additional Character(s)   ▌ Manifestation Code   Coding Clinic

- ● **Z77.09** **Contact with and (suspected) exposure to other hazardous, chiefly nonmedicinal, chemicals**
  - ● **Z77.090** **Contact with and (suspected) exposure to asbestos**
  - ● **Z77.098** **Contact with and (suspected) exposure to other hazardous, chiefly nonmedicinal, chemicals**
    Dyes NOS
- ● **Z77.1** **Contact with and (suspected) exposure to environmental pollution and hazards in the physical environment**
  - ● **Z77.11** **Contact with and (suspected) exposure to environmental pollution**
    - ● **Z77.110** **Contact with and (suspected) exposure to air pollution**
    - ● **Z77.111** **Contact with and (suspected) exposure to water pollution**
    - ● **Z77.112** **Contact with and (suspected) exposure to soil pollution**
    - ● **Z77.118** **Contact with and (suspected) exposure to other environmental pollution**
  - ● **Z77.12** **Contact with and (suspected) exposure to hazards in the physical environment**
    - ● **Z77.120** **Contact with and (suspected) exposure to mold (toxic)**
    - ● **Z77.121** **Contact with and (suspected) exposure to harmful algae and algae toxins**
      Contact with and (suspected) exposure to (harmful) algae bloom NOS
      Contact with and (suspected) exposure to blue-green algae bloom
      Contact with and (suspected) exposure to brown tide
      Contact with and (suspected) exposure to cyanobacteria bloom
      Contact with and (suspected) exposure to Florida red tide
      Contact with and (suspected) exposure to pfiesteria piscicida
      Contact with and (suspected) exposure to red tide
    - ● **Z77.122** **Contact with and (suspected) exposure to noise**
    - ● **Z77.123** **Contact with and (suspected) exposure to radon and other naturally occuring radiation**
      Excludes2   radiation exposure as the cause of a confirmed condition (W88-W90, X39.0-)
      radiation sickness NOS (T66)
    - ● **Z77.128** **Contact with and (suspected) exposure to other hazards in the physical environment**

- ● **Z77.2** **Contact with and (suspected) exposure to other hazardous substances**
  - ● **Z77.21** **Contact with and (suspected) exposure to potentially hazardous body fluids**
  - ● **Z77.22** **Contact with and (suspected) exposure to environmental tobacco smoke (acute) (chronic)**
    Exposure to second hand tobacco smoke (acute) (chronic)
    Passive smoking (acute) (chronic)
    Excludes1   nicotine dependence (F17.-)
    tobacco use (Z72.0)
    Excludes2   occupational exposure to environmental tobacco smoke (Z57.31)
  - ● **Z77.29** **Contact with and (suspected) exposure to other hazardous substances**
    Coding Clinic: 2016, Q2, P34
- ● **Z77.9** **Other contact with and (suspected) exposures hazardous to health**

- ● **Z78** **Other specified health status**
  Excludes2   asymptomatic human immunodeficiency virus [HIV] infection status (Z21)
  postprocedural status (Z93-Z99)
  sex reassignment status (Z87.890)
  - ● **Z78.0** **Asymptomatic menopausal state** ♀   A
    Menopausal state NOS
    Postmenopausal status NOS
    Excludes2   symptomatic menopausal state (N95.1)
  - ● **Z78.1** **Physical restraint status**
    Excludes1   physical restraint due to a procedure - omit code
  - ● **Z78.9** **Other specified health status**

- ● **Z79** **Long term (current) drug therapy**
  Includes   long term (current) drug use for prophylactic purposes
  Code also any therapeutic drug level monitoring (Z51.81)
  Excludes2   drug abuse and dependence (F11-F19)
  drug use complicating pregnancy, childbirth, and the puerperium (O99.32-)
  long term (current) use of oral antidiabetic drugs (Z79.84)
  long term (current) use of oral hypoglycemic drugs (Z79.84)
  - ● **Z79.0** **Long term (current) use of anticoagulants and antithrombotics/antiplatelets**
    Excludes2   long term (current) use of aspirin (Z79.82)
    - **Z79.01** **Long term (current) use of anticoagulants**
    - ● **Z79.02** **Long term (current) use of antithrombotics/antiplatelets**
  - ● **Z79.1** **Long term (current) use of non-steroidal anti-inflammatories (NSAID)**
    Excludes2   long term (current) use of aspirin (Z79.82)
  - ● **Z79.2** **Long term (current) use of antibiotics**
  - **Z79.3** **Long term (current) use of hormonal contraceptives**
    Long term (current) use of birth control pill or patch
  - **Z79.4** **Long term (current) use of insulin**
    Coding Clinic: 2016, Q4, P121-122, 126
  - ● **Z79.5** **Long term (current) use of steroids**
    - ● **Z79.51** **Long term (current) use of inhaled steroids**
    - ● **Z79.52** **Long term (current) use of systemic steroids**

CHAPTER 21 (Z00-Z99)

N Newborn Age: 0   **P** Pediatric Age: 0–17   **M** Maternity DX: 12–55   **A** Adult Age: 15–124   ♀ Females Only   ♂ Males Only

🔵 Complication\Comorbidity   🔵 Major C\C   (Ex) CC/MCC Exclusions   🔵 Hospital-Acquired Condition

1613

CHAPTER 21 (Z00-Z99)

- **Z79.8 Other long term (current) drug therapy**
  - **Z79.81 Long term (current) use of agents affecting estrogen receptors and estrogen levels**

    Code first, if applicable:
    malignant neoplasm of breast (C50.-)
    malignant neoplasm of prostate (C61)

    Use additional code, if applicable, to identify:
    estrogen receptor positive status (Z17.0)
    family history of breast cancer (Z80.3)
    genetic susceptibility to malignant neoplasm (cancer) (Z15.0-)
    personal history of breast cancer (Z85.3)
    personal history of prostate cancer (Z85.46)
    postmenopausal status (Z78.0)

    Excludes1 ⟹ hormone replacement therapy (Z79.890)

    - **Z79.810 Long term (current) use of selective estrogen receptor modulators (SERMs)**
      Long term (current) use of raloxifene (Evista)
      Long term (current) use of tamoxifen (Nolvadex)
      Long term (current) use of toremifene (Fareston)

    - **Z79.811 Long term (current) use of aromatase inhibitors**
      Long term (current) use of anastrozole (Arimidex)
      Long term (current) use of exemestane (Aromasin)
      Long term (current) use of letrozole (Femara)

    - **Z79.818 Long term (current) use of other agents affecting estrogen receptors and estrogen levels**
      Long term (current) use of estrogen receptor downregulators
      Long term (current) use of fulvestrant (Faslodex)
      Long term (current) use of gonadotropin-releasing hormone (GnRH) agonist
      Long term (current) use of goserelin acetate (Zoladex)
      Long term (current) use of leuprolide acetate (leuprorelin) (Lupron)
      Long term (current) use of megestrol acetate (Megace)

  - **Z79.82 Long term (current) use of aspirin**
  - **Z79.83 Long term (current) use of bisphosphonates**
    Coding Clinic: 2016, Q4, P42
  - **Z79.84 Long term (current) use of oral hypoglycemic drugs**
    Long term (current) use of oral antidiabetic drugs

    Excludes2 long term (current) use of insulin (Z79.4)

    Coding Clinic: 2016, Q4, P76, 121-122, 126

- **Z79.89 Other long term (current) drug therapy**
  - ⟹ **Z79.890 Hormone replacement therapy**
  - **Z79.891 Long term (current) use of opiate analgesic**
    Long term (current) use of methadone for pain management

    Excludes1 methadone use NOS (F11.9-)
    use of methadone for treatment of heroin addiction (F11.2-)

  - **Z79.899 Other long term (current) drug therapy**
    Coding Clinic: 2015, Q4, P34, Q3, P21

- **Z80 Family history of primary malignant neoplasm**
  - **Z80.0 Family history of malignant neoplasm of digestive organs**
    Conditions classifiable to C15-C26
  - **Z80.1 Family history of malignant neoplasm of trachea, bronchus and lung**
    Conditions classifiable to C33-C34
  - **Z80.2 Family history of malignant neoplasm of other respiratory and intrathoracic organs**
    Conditions classifiable to C30-C32, C37-C39
  - **Z80.3 Family history of malignant neoplasm of breast**
    Conditions classifiable to C50.-
  - **Z80.4 Family history of malignant neoplasm of genital organs**
    Conditions classifiable to C51-C63
    - **Z80.41 Family history of malignant neoplasm of ovary**
    - **Z80.42 Family history of malignant neoplasm of prostate**
    - **Z80.43 Family history of malignant neoplasm of testis**
    - **Z80.49 Family history of malignant neoplasm of other genital organs**
  - **Z80.5 Family history of malignant neoplasm of urinary tract**
    Conditions classifiable to C64-C68
    - **Z80.51 Family history of malignant neoplasm of kidney**
    - **Z80.52 Family history of malignant neoplasm of bladder**
    - **Z80.59 Family history of malignant neoplasm of other urinary tract organ**
  - **Z80.6 Family history of leukemia**
    Conditions classifiable to C91-C95
  - **Z80.7 Family history of other malignant neoplasms of lymphoid, hematopoietic and related tissues**
    Conditions classifiable to C81-C90, C96.-
  - **Z80.8 Family history of malignant neoplasm of other organs or systems**
    Conditions classifiable to C00-C14, C40-C49, C69-C79
  - **Z80.9 Family history of malignant neoplasm, unspecified**
    Conditions classifiable to C80.1

- **Z81 Family history of mental and behavioral disorders**
  - **Z81.0 Family history of intellectual disabilities**
    Conditions classifiable to F70-F79
  - **Z81.1 Family history of alcohol abuse and dependence**
    Conditions classifiable to F10.-
  - **Z81.2 Family history of tobacco abuse and dependence**
    Conditions classifiable to F17.-
  - **Z81.3 Family history of other psychoactive substance abuse and dependence**
    Conditions classifiable to F11-F16, F18-F19
  - **Z81.4 Family history of other substance abuse and dependence**
    Conditions classifiable to F55
  - **Z81.8 Family history of other mental and behavioral disorders**
    Conditions classifiable elsewhere in F01-F99

▶ New   ⟹ Revised   ~~deleted~~ Deleted   Excludes 1   Excludes 2   Includes   Use additional   Code first   Code also   Key words
OGCR Official Guidelines   ● Unacceptable Principal Diagnosis   X Assign placeholder X   ● Use Additional Character(s)   ▮ Manifestation Code   Coding Clinic

● **Z82 Family history of certain disabilities and chronic diseases (leading to disablement)**

　● **Z82.0 Family history of epilepsy and other diseases of the nervous system**
　　　Conditions classifiable to G00-G99

　● **Z82.1 Family history of blindness and visual loss**
　　　Conditions classifiable to H54.-

　● **Z82.2 Family history of deafness and hearing loss**
　　　Conditions classifiable to H90-H91

　● **Z82.3 Family history of stroke**
　　　Conditions classifiable to I60-I64

　● **Z82.4 Family history of ischemic heart disease and other diseases of the circulatory system**
　　　Conditions classifiable to I00-I52, I65-I99

　　● **Z82.41 Family history of sudden cardiac death**

　　● **Z82.49 Family history of ischemic heart disease and other diseases of the circulatory system**

　● **Z82.5 Family history of asthma and other chronic lower respiratory diseases**
　　　Conditions classifiable to J40-J47
　　　Excludes2　family history of other diseases of the respiratory system (Z83.6)

　● **Z82.6 Family history of arthritis and other diseases of the musculoskeletal system and connective tissue**
　　　Conditions classifiable to M00-M99

　　● **Z82.61 Family history of arthritis**

　　● **Z82.62 Family history of osteoporosis**

　　● **Z82.69 Family history of other diseases of the musculoskeletal system and connective tissue**

　● **Z82.7 Family history of congenital malformations, deformations and chromosomal abnormalities**
　　　Conditions classifiable to Q00-Q99

　　● **Z82.71 Family history of polycystic kidney**

　　● **Z82.79 Family history of other congenital malformations, deformations and chromosomal abnormalities**

　● **Z82.8 Family history of other disabilities and chronic diseases leading to disablement, not elsewhere classified**

● **Z83 Family history of other specific disorders**
　　Excludes2　contact with and (suspected) exposure to communicable disease in the family (Z20.-)

　● **Z83.0 Family history of human immunodeficiency virus [HIV] disease**
　　　Conditions classifiable to B20

　● **Z83.1 Family history of other infectious and parasitic diseases**
　　　Conditions classifiable to A00-B19, B25-B94, B99

　● **Z83.2 Family history of diseases of the blood and blood-forming organs and certain disorders involving the immune mechanism**
　　　Conditions classifiable to D50-D89

　● **Z83.3 Family history of diabetes mellitus**
　　　Conditions classifiable to E08-E13

　● **Z83.4 Family history of other endocrine, nutritional and metabolic diseases**
　　　Conditions classifiable to E00-E07, E15-E88

　　● **Z83.41 Family history of multiple endocrine neoplasia [MEN] syndrome**

　　● **Z83.42 Family history of familial hypercholesterolemia**
　　　　Coding Clinic: 2016, Q4, P77

　　● **Z83.49 Family history of other endocrine, nutritional and metabolic diseases**

● **Z83.5 Family history of eye and ear disorders**

　● **Z83.51 Family history of eye disorders**
　　　Conditions classifiable to H00-H53, H55-H59
　　　Excludes2　family history of blindness and visual loss (Z82.1)

　　● **Z83.511 Family history of glaucoma**

　　● **Z83.518 Family history of other specified eye disorder**

　● **Z83.52 Family history of ear disorders**
　　　Conditions classifiable to H60-H83, H92-H95
　　　Excludes2　family history of deafness and hearing loss (Z82.2)

● **Z83.6 Family history of other diseases of the respiratory system**
　　　Conditions classifiable to J00-J39, J60-J99
　　　Excludes2　family history of asthma and other chronic lower respiratory diseases (Z82.5)

● **Z83.7 Family history of diseases of the digestive system**
　　　Conditions classifiable to K00-K93

　● **Z83.71 Family history of colonic polyps**
　　　~~Excludes1~~　~~family history of malignant neoplasm of digestive organs (Z80.0)~~

　　▶ **Excludes2**　family history of malignant neoplasm of digestive organs (Z80.0)

　● **Z83.79 Family history of other diseases of the digestive system**

● **Z84 Family history of other conditions**

　● **Z84.0 Family history of diseases of the skin and subcutaneous tissue**
　　　Conditions classifiable to L00-L99

　● **Z84.1 Family history of disorders of kidney and ureter**
　　　Conditions classifiable to N00-N29

　● **Z84.2 Family history of other diseases of the genitourinary system**
　　　Conditions classifiable to N30-N99
　　　Coding Clinic: 2016, Q4, P77

　● **Z84.3 Family history of consanguinity**

　● **Z84.8 Family history of other specified conditions**

　　● **Z84.81 Family history of carrier of genetic disease**

　　● **Z84.82 Family history of sudden infant death syndrome**
　　　　Family history of SIDS

　　● **Z84.89 Family history of other specified conditions**

● **Z85 Personal history of malignant neoplasm**
　　Code first any follow-up examination after treatment of malignant neoplasm (Z08)
　　Use additional code to identify:
　　　alcohol use and dependence (F10.-)
　　　exposure to environmental tobacco smoke (Z77.22)
　　　history of tobacco dependence (Z87.891)
　　　occupational exposure to environmental tobacco smoke (Z57.31)
　　　tobacco dependence (F17.-)
　　　tobacco use (Z72.0)
　　Excludes2　personal history of benign neoplasm (Z86.01-)
　　　　personal history of carcinoma-in-situ (Z86.00-)

CHAPTER 21 (Z00-Z99)

● **Z85.0** **Personal history of malignant neoplasm of digestive organs**

  ● **Z85.00** Personal history of malignant neoplasm of unspecified digestive organ

  ● **Z85.01** Personal history of malignant neoplasm of esophagus
    Conditions classifiable to C15

  ● **Z85.02** Personal history of malignant neoplasm of stomach

    ● **Z85.020** Personal history of malignant carcinoid tumor of stomach
      Conditions classifiable to C7A.092

    ● **Z85.028** Personal history of other malignant neoplasm of stomach
      Conditions classifiable to C16

  ● **Z85.03** Personal history of malignant neoplasm of large intestine

    ● **Z85.030** Personal history of malignant carcinoid tumor of large intestine
      Conditions classifiable to C7A.022-C7A.025, C7A.029

    ● **Z85.038** Personal history of other malignant neoplasm of large intestine
      Conditions classifiable to C18

  ● **Z85.04** Personal history of malignant neoplasm of rectum, rectosigmoid junction, and anus

    ● **Z85.040** Personal history of malignant carcinoid tumor of rectum
      Conditions classifiable to C7A.026

    ● **Z85.048** Personal history of other malignant neoplasm of rectum, rectosigmoid junction, and anus
      Conditions classifiable to C19-C21

  ● **Z85.05** Personal history of malignant neoplasm of liver
    Conditions classifiable to C22

  ● **Z85.06** Personal history of malignant neoplasm of small intestine

    ● **Z85.060** Personal history of malignant carcinoid tumor of small intestine
      Conditions classifiable to C7A.01-

    ● **Z85.068** Personal history of other malignant neoplasm of small intestine
      Conditions classifiable to C17

  ● **Z85.07** Personal history of malignant neoplasm of pancreas
    Conditions classifiable to C25

  ● **Z85.09** Personal history of malignant neoplasm of other digestive organs

● **Z85.1** **Personal history of malignant neoplasm of trachea, bronchus and lung**

  ● **Z85.11** Personal history of malignant neoplasm of bronchus and lung

    ● **Z85.110** Personal history of malignant carcinoid tumor of bronchus and lung
      Conditions classifiable to C7A.090

    ● **Z85.118** Personal history of other malignant neoplasm of bronchus and lung
      Conditions classifiable to C34

  ● **Z85.12** Personal history of malignant neoplasm of trachea
    Conditions classifiable to C33

● **Z85.2** **Personal history of malignant neoplasm of other respiratory and intrathoracic organs**

  ● **Z85.20** Personal history of malignant neoplasm of unspecified respiratory organ

  ● **Z85.21** Personal history of malignant neoplasm of larynx
    Conditions classifiable to C32

  ● **Z85.22** Personal history of malignant neoplasm of nasal cavities, middle ear, and accessory sinuses
    Conditions classifiable to C30-C31

  ● **Z85.23** Personal history of malignant neoplasm of thymus

    ● **Z85.230** Personal history of malignant carcinoid tumor of thymus
      Conditions classifiable to C7A.091

    ● **Z85.238** Personal history of other malignant neoplasm of thymus
      Conditions classifiable to C37

  ● **Z85.29** Personal history of malignant neoplasm of other respiratory and intrathoracic organs

● **Z85.3** **Personal history of malignant neoplasm of breast**
  Conditions classifiable to C50.-

● **Z85.4** **Personal history of malignant neoplasm of genital organs**
  Conditions classifiable to C51-C63

  ● **Z85.40** Personal history of malignant neoplasm of unspecified female genital organ ♀

  ● **Z85.41** Personal history of malignant neoplasm of cervix uteri ♀

  ● **Z85.42** Personal history of malignant neoplasm of other parts of uterus ♀

  ● **Z85.43** Personal history of malignant neoplasm of ovary ♀

  ● **Z85.44** Personal history of malignant neoplasm of other female genital organs ♀

  ● **Z85.45** Personal history of malignant neoplasm of unspecified male genital organ ♂

  ● **Z85.46** Personal history of malignant neoplasm of prostate ♂

  ● **Z85.47** Personal history of malignant neoplasm of testis ♂

  ● **Z85.48** Personal history of malignant neoplasm of epididymis ♂

  ● **Z85.49** Personal history of malignant neoplasm of other male genital organs ♂

● **Z85.5** **Personal history of malignant neoplasm of urinary tract**
  Conditions classifiable to C64-C68

  ● **Z85.50** Personal history of malignant neoplasm of unspecified urinary tract organ

  ● **Z85.51** Personal history of malignant neoplasm of bladder

  ● **Z85.52** Personal history of malignant neoplasm of kidney

    Excludes1 personal history of malignant neoplasm of renal pelvis (Z85.53)

    ● **Z85.520** Personal history of malignant carcinoid tumor of kidney
      Conditions classifiable to C7A.093

    ● **Z85.528** Personal history of other malignant neoplasm of kidney
      Conditions classifiable to C64

  ● **Z85.53** Personal history of malignant neoplasm of renal pelvis

  ● **Z85.54** Personal history of malignant neoplasm of ureter

  ● **Z85.59** Personal history of malignant neoplasm of other urinary tract organ

● **Z85.6 Personal history of leukemia**
Conditions classifiable to C91-C95

> **Excludes1** leukemia in remission C91.0-C95.9 with 5th character 1

● **Z85.7 Personal history of other malignant neoplasms of lymphoid, hematopoietic and related tissues**

● **Z85.71 Personal history of Hodgkin lymphoma**
Conditions classifiable to C81

● **Z85.72 Personal history of non-Hodgkin lymphomas**
Conditions classifiable to C82-C85

● **Z85.79 Personal history of other malignant neoplasms of lymphoid, hematopoietic and related tissues**
Conditions classifiable to C88-C90, C96

> **Excludes1** multiple myeloma in remission (C90.01)
> plasma cell leukemia in remission (C90.11)
> plasmacytoma in remission (C90.21)

● **Z85.8 Personal history of malignant neoplasms of other organs and systems**
Conditions classifiable to C00-C14, C40-C49, C69-C75, C7A.098, C76-C79

● **Z85.81 Personal history of malignant neoplasm of lip, oral cavity, and pharynx**

● **Z85.810 Personal history of malignant neoplasm of tongue**

● **Z85.818 Personal history of malignant neoplasm of other sites of lip, oral cavity, and pharynx**

● **Z85.819 Personal history of malignant neoplasm of unspecified site of lip, oral cavity, and pharynx**

● **Z85.82 Personal history of malignant neoplasm of skin**

● **Z85.820 Personal history of malignant melanoma of skin**
Conditions classifiable to C43

● **Z85.821 Personal history of Merkel cell carcinoma**
Conditions classifiable to C4A

● **Z85.828 Personal history of other malignant neoplasm of skin**
Conditions classifiable to C44

● **Z85.83 Personal history of malignant neoplasm of bone and soft tissue**

● **Z85.830 Personal history of malignant neoplasm of bone**

● **Z85.831 Personal history of malignant neoplasm of soft tissue**

> **Excludes2** personal history of malignant neoplasm of skin (Z85.82-)

● **Z85.84 Personal history of malignant neoplasm of eye and nervous tissue**

● **Z85.840 Personal history of malignant neoplasm of eye**

● **Z85.841 Personal history of malignant neoplasm of brain**

● **Z85.848 Personal history of malignant neoplasm of other parts of nervous tissue**

● **Z85.85 Personal history of malignant neoplasm of endocrine glands**

● **Z85.850 Personal history of malignant neoplasm of thyroid**

● **Z85.858 Personal history of malignant neoplasm of other endocrine glands**

● **Z85.89 Personal history of malignant neoplasm of other organs and systems**

● **Z85.9 Personal history of malignant neoplasm, unspecified**
Conditions classifiable to C7A.00, C80.1

● **Z86 Personal history of certain other diseases**
Code first any follow-up examination after treatment (Z09)

● **Z86.0 Personal history of in-situ and benign neoplasms and neoplasms of uncertain behavior**

> **Excludes2** personal history of malignant neoplasms (Z85.-)

● **Z86.00 Personal history of in-situ neoplasm**
Conditions classifiable to D00-D09

● **Z86.000 Personal history of in-situ neoplasm of breast**

● **Z86.001 Personal history of in-situ neoplasm of cervix uteri ♀**
Personal history of cervical intraepithelial neoplasia III [CIN III]

● **Z86.008 Personal history of in-situ neoplasm of other site**
Personal history of vaginal intraepithelial neoplasia III [VAIN III]
Personal history of vulvar intraepithelial neoplasia III [VIN III]

● **Z86.01 Personal history of benign neoplasm**
Coding Clinic: 2017, Q1, P14

● **Z86.010 Personal history of colonic polyps**
Coding Clinic: 2017, Q1, P9, P14

● **Z86.011 Personal history of benign neoplasm of the brain**

● **Z86.012 Personal history of benign carcinoid tumor**

● **Z86.018 Personal history of other benign neoplasm**
Coding Clinic: 2017, Q1, P14

● **Z86.03 Personal history of neoplasm of uncertain behavior**

● **Z86.1 Personal history of infectious and parasitic diseases**
Conditions classifiable to A00-B89, B99

> **Excludes1** personal history of infectious diseases specific to a body system sequelae of infectious and parasitic diseases (B90-B94)

Coding Clinic: 2016, Q4, P5

● **Z86.11 Personal history of tuberculosis**

● **Z86.12 Personal history of poliomyelitis**

● **Z86.13 Personal history of malaria**

● **Z86.14 Personal history of Methicillin resistant Staphylococcus aureus infection**
Personal history of MRSA infection

● **Z86.19 Personal history of other infectious and parasitic diseases**

● **Z86.2 Personal history of diseases of the blood and blood-forming organs and certain disorders involving the immune mechanism**
Conditions classifiable to D50-D89

● **Z86.3 Personal history of endocrine, nutritional and metabolic diseases**
Conditions classifiable to E00-E88

● **Z86.31 Personal history of diabetic foot ulcer**

> **Excludes2** current diabetic foot ulcer (E08.621, E09.621, E10.621, E11.621, E13.621)

● **Z86.32 Personal history of gestational diabetes ♀**
Personal history of conditions classifiable to O24.4-

> **Excludes1** gestational diabetes mellitus in current pregnancy (O24.4-)

● **Z86.39 Personal history of other endocrine, nutritional and metabolic disease**

CHAPTER 21 (Z00-Z99)

● **Z86.5 Personal history of mental and behavioral disorders**
Conditions classifiable to F40–F59

  ● **Z86.51 Personal history of combat and operational stress reaction**   A

  ● **Z86.59 Personal history of other mental and behavioral disorders**

● **Z86.6 Personal history of diseases of the nervous system and sense organs**
Conditions classifiable to G00–G99, H00–H95

  ● **Z86.61 Personal history of infections of the central nervous system**
Personal history of encephalitis
Personal history of meningitis

  ● **Z86.69 Personal history of other diseases of the nervous system and sense organs**
Coding Clinic: 2016, Q4, P25

● **Z86.7 Personal history of diseases of the circulatory system**
Conditions classifiable to I00–I99

  Excludes2   old myocardial infarction (I25.2)
personal history of anaphylactic shock (Z87.892)
postmyocardial infarction syndrome (I24.1)

  ● **Z86.71 Personal history of venous thrombosis and embolism**

    ● **Z86.711 Personal history of pulmonary embolism**

    ● **Z86.718 Personal history of other venous thrombosis and embolism**

  ● **Z86.72 Personal history of thrombophlebitis**

  ● **Z86.73 Personal history of transient ischemic attack (TIA), and cerebral infarction without residual deficits**
Personal history of prolonged reversible ischemic neurological deficit (PRIND)
Personal history of stroke NOS without residual deficits

    Excludes1   personal history of traumatic brain injury (Z87.820)
sequelae of cerebrovascular disease (I69.-)

    Coding Clinic: 2012, Q4, P3

  ● **Z86.74 Personal history of sudden cardiac arrest**
Personal history of sudden cardiac death successfully resuscitated

  ● **Z86.79 Personal history of other diseases of the circulatory system**

● **Z87 Personal history of other diseases and conditions**
Code first any follow-up examination after treatment (Z09)

● **Z87.0 Personal history of diseases of the respiratory system**
Conditions classifiable to J00–J99

  ● **Z87.01 Personal history of pneumonia (recurrent)**

  ● **Z87.09 Personal history of other diseases of the respiratory system**

● **Z87.1 Personal history of diseases of the digestive system**
Conditions classifiable to K00–K93

  ● **Z87.11 Personal history of peptic ulcer disease**

  ● **Z87.19 Personal history of other diseases of the digestive system**
Coding Clinic: 2017, Q1, P14

● **Z87.2 Personal history of diseases of the skin and subcutaneous tissue**
Conditions classifiable to L00–L99

  Excludes2   personal history of diabetic foot ulcer (Z86.31)

● **Z87.3 Personal history of diseases of the musculoskeletal system and connective tissue**
Conditions classifiable to M00–M99

  Excludes2   personal history of (healed) traumatic fracture (Z87.81)

  ● **Z87.31 Personal history of (healed) nontraumatic fracture**

    ● **Z87.310 Personal history of (healed) osteoporosis fracture**
Personal history of (healed) fragility fracture
Personal history of (healed) collapsed vertebra due to osteoporosis

    ● **Z87.311 Personal history of (healed) other pathological fracture**
Personal history of (healed) collapsed vertebra NOS

      Excludes2   personal history of osteoporosis fracture (Z87.310)

    ● **Z87.312 Personal history of (healed) stress fracture**
Personal history of (healed) fatigue fracture

  ● **Z87.39 Personal history of other diseases of the musculoskeletal system and connective tissue**

● **Z87.4 Personal history of diseases of genitourinary system**
Conditions classifiable to N00–N99

  ● **Z87.41 Personal history of dysplasia of the female genital tract**

    Excludes1 ⟹ personal history of intraepithelial neoplasia III of female genital tract (Z86.001, Z86.008)
personal history of malignant neoplasm of female genital tract (Z85.40–Z85.44)

    ● **Z87.410 Personal history of cervical dysplasia ♀**

    ● **Z87.411 Personal history of vaginal dysplasia ♀**

    ● **Z87.412 Personal history of vulvar dysplasia ♀**

  ● **Z87.42 Personal history of other diseases of the female genital tract ♀**

  ● **Z87.43 Personal history of diseases of male genital organs**

    ● **Z87.430 Personal history of prostatic dysplasia ♂**

      Excludes1   personal history of malignant neoplasm of prostate (Z85.46)

    ● **Z87.438 Personal history of other diseases of male genital organs ♂**

▶ New   ⟹ Revised   ~~deleted~~ Deleted   Excludes 1   Excludes 2   Includes   Use additional   Code first   Code also   Key words

OGCR Official Guidelines   ● Unacceptable Principal Diagnosis   X Assign placeholder X   ● Use Additional Character(s)   ▌ Manifestation Code   **Coding Clinic**

● **Z87.44 Personal history of diseases of urinary system**

> **Excludes1** personal history of malignant neoplasm of cervix uteri (Z85.41)

> ● **Z87.440 Personal history of urinary (tract) infections**

> ● **Z87.441 Personal history of nephrotic syndrome**

> ● **Z87.442 Personal history of urinary calculi**
>> Personal history of kidney stones

> ● **Z87.448 Personal history of other diseases of urinary system**

● **Z87.5 Personal history of complications of pregnancy, childbirth and the puerperium**
> Conditions classifiable to O00-O9A

> **Excludes2** recurrent pregnancy loss (N96)

> ● **Z87.51 Personal history of pre-term labor ♀**

>> **Excludes1** current pregnancy with history of pre-term labor (O09.21-)

> ● **Z87.59 Personal history of other complications of pregnancy, childbirth and the puerperium ♀**
>> Personal history of trophoblastic disease

● **Z87.7 Personal history of (corrected) congenital malformations**
> Conditions classifiable to Q00-Q89 that have been repaired or corrected

> **Excludes1** congenital malformations that have been partially corrected or repair but which still require medical treatment - code to condition

> **Excludes2** other postprocedural states (Z98.-)
> personal history of medical treatment (Z92.-)
> presence of cardiac and vascular implants and grafts (Z95.-)
> presence of other devices (Z97.-)
> presence of other functional implants (Z96.-)
> transplanted organ and tissue status (Z94.-)

> ● **Z87.71 Personal history of (corrected) congenital malformations of genitourinary system**

>> ● **Z87.710 Personal history of (corrected) hypospadias ♂**

>> ● **Z87.718 Personal history of other specified (corrected) congenital malformations of genitourinary system**

> ● **Z87.72 Personal history of (corrected) congenital malformations of nervous system and sense organs**

>> ● **Z87.720 Personal history of (corrected) congenital malformations of eye**

>> ● **Z87.721 Personal history of (corrected) congenital malformations of ear**

>> ● **Z87.728 Personal history of other specified (corrected) congenital malformations of nervous system and sense organs**

> ● **Z87.73 Personal history of (corrected) congenital malformations of digestive system**

>> ● **Z87.730 Personal history of (corrected) cleft lip and palate**

>> ● **Z87.738 Personal history of other specified (corrected) congenital malformations of digestive system**

> ● **Z87.74 Personal history of (corrected) congenital malformations of heart and circulatory system**

> ● **Z87.75 Personal history of (corrected) congenital malformations of respiratory system**

> ● **Z87.76 Personal history of (corrected) congenital malformations of integument, limbs and musculoskeletal system**

> ● **Z87.79 Personal history of other (corrected) congenital malformations**

>> ● **Z87.790 Personal history of (corrected) congenital malformations of face and neck**

>> ● **Z87.798 Personal history of other (corrected) congenital malformations**

● **Z87.8 Personal history of other specified conditions**

> **Excludes2** personal history of self harm (Z91.5)

> ● **Z87.81 Personal history of (healed) traumatic fracture**

>> **Excludes2** personal history of (healed) nontraumatic fracture (Z87.31-)

> ● **Z87.82 Personal history of other (healed) physical injury and trauma**
>> Conditions classifiable to S00-T88, except traumatic fractures

>> ● **Z87.820 Personal history of traumatic brain injury**

>>> **Excludes1** personal history of transient ischemic attack (TIA), and cerebral infarction without residual deficits (Z86.73)

>> ● **Z87.821 Personal history of retained foreign body fully removed**

>> ● **Z87.828 Personal history of other (healed) physical injury and trauma**

> ● **Z87.89 Personal history of other specified conditions**

>> **Z87.890 Personal history of sex reassignment**

>> ● **Z87.891 Personal history of nicotine dependence**

>>> **Excludes1** current nicotine dependence (F17.2-)

>>> Coding Clinic: 2017, Q2, P27

>> ● **Z87.892 Personal history of anaphylaxis**
>>> Code also allergy status such as:
>>> allergy status to drugs, medicaments and biological substances (Z88.-)
>>> allergy status, other than to drugs and biological substances (Z91.0-)

>> ● **Z87.898 Personal history of other specified conditions**
>>> Coding Clinic: 2013, Q1, P21

CHAPTER 21 (Z00-Z99)

Z88 **Allergy status to drugs, medicaments and biological substances**

> **Excludes2** allergy status, other than to drugs and biological substances (Z91.0-)

- **Z88.0** Allergy status to penicillin
- **Z88.1** Allergy status to other antibiotic agents status
- **Z88.2** Allergy status to sulfonamides status
  Coding Clinic: 2015, Q3, P23
- **Z88.3** Allergy status to other anti-infective agents status
- **Z88.4** Allergy status to anesthetic agent status
- **Z88.5** Allergy status to narcotic agent status
- **Z88.6** Allergy status to analgesic agent status
- **Z88.7** Allergy status to serum and vaccine status
- **Z88.8** Allergy status to other drugs, medicaments and biological substances status
- **Z88.9** Allergy status to unspecified drugs, medicaments and biological substances status

Z89 Acquired absence of limb

> **Includes** amputation status
> postprocedural loss of limb
> post-traumatic loss of limb

> **Excludes1** acquired deformities of limbs (M20-M21)
> congenital absence of limbs (Q71-Q73)

- **Z89.0** Acquired absence of thumb and other finger(s)
  - **Z89.01** Acquired absence of thumb
    - **Z89.011** Acquired absence of right thumb
    - **Z89.012** Acquired absence of left thumb
    - **Z89.019** Acquired absence of unspecified thumb
  - **Z89.02** Acquired absence of other finger(s)
    > **Excludes2** acquired absence of thumb (Z89.01-)
    - **Z89.021** Acquired absence of right finger(s)
    - **Z89.022** Acquired absence of left finger(s)
    - **Z89.029** Acquired absence of unspecified finger(s)
- **Z89.1** Acquired absence of hand and wrist
  - **Z89.11** Acquired absence of hand
    - **Z89.111** Acquired absence of right hand
    - **Z89.112** Acquired absence of left hand
    - **Z89.119** Acquired absence of unspecified hand
  - **Z89.12** Acquired absence of wrist
    Disarticulation at wrist
    - **Z89.121** Acquired absence of right wrist
    - **Z89.122** Acquired absence of left wrist
    - **Z89.129** Acquired absence of unspecified wrist
- **Z89.2** Acquired absence of upper limb above wrist
  - **Z89.20** Acquired absence of upper limb, unspecified level
    - **Z89.201** Acquired absence of right upper limb, unspecified level
    - **Z89.202** Acquired absence of left upper limb, unspecified level
    - **Z89.209** Acquired absence of unspecified upper limb, unspecified level
      Acquired absence of arm NOS
  - **Z89.21** Acquired absence of upper limb below elbow
    - **Z89.211** Acquired absence of right upper limb below elbow
    - **Z89.212** Acquired absence of left upper limb below elbow
    - **Z89.219** Acquired absence of unspecified upper limb below elbow

- **Z89.22** Acquired absence of upper limb above elbow
  Disarticulation at elbow
  - **Z89.221** Acquired absence of right upper limb above elbow
  - **Z89.222** Acquired absence of left upper limb above elbow
  - **Z89.229** Acquired absence of unspecified upper limb above elbow
- **Z89.23** Acquired absence of shoulder
  Acquired absence of shoulder joint following explantation of shoulder joint prosthesis, with or without presence of antibiotic-impregnated cement spacer
  - **Z89.231** Acquired absence of right shoulder
  - **Z89.232** Acquired absence of left shoulder
  - **Z89.239** Acquired absence of unspecified shoulder
- **Z89.4** Acquired absence of toe(s), foot, and ankle
  - **Z89.41** Acquired absence of great toe
    - **Z89.411** Acquired absence of right great toe
    - **Z89.412** Acquired absence of left great toe
    - **Z89.419** Acquired absence of unspecified great toe
  - **Z89.42** Acquired absence of other toe(s)
    > **Excludes2** acquired absence of great toe (Z89.41-)
    - **Z89.421** Acquired absence of other right toe(s)
    - **Z89.422** Acquired absence of other left toe(s)
    - **Z89.429** Acquired absence of other toe(s), unspecified side
  - **Z89.43** Acquired absence of foot
    - **Z89.431** Acquired absence of right foot
    - **Z89.432** Acquired absence of left foot
    - **Z89.439** Acquired absence of unspecified foot
  - **Z89.44** Acquired absence of ankle
    Disarticulation of ankle
    - **Z89.441** Acquired absence of right ankle
    - **Z89.442** Acquired absence of left ankle
    - **Z89.449** Acquired absence of unspecified ankle
- **Z89.5** Acquired absence of leg below knee
  - **Z89.51** Acquired absence of leg below knee
    - **Z89.511** Acquired absence of right leg below knee
    - **Z89.512** Acquired absence of left leg below knee
    - **Z89.519** Acquired absence of unspecified leg below knee
  - **Z89.52** Acquired absence of knee
    Acquired absence of knee joint following explantation of knee joint prosthesis, with or without presence of antibiotic-impregnated cement spacer
    - **Z89.521** Acquired absence of right knee
    - **Z89.522** Acquired absence of left knee
    - **Z89.529** Acquired absence of unspecified knee

▶ New ⇒ Revised ~~deleted~~ Deleted | Excludes 1 | Excludes 2 | Includes | Use additional | Code first | Code also | Key words

OGCR Official Guidelines ● Unacceptable Principal Diagnosis X Assign placeholder X ● Use Additional Character(s) ▶ Manifestation Code **Coding Clinic**

- **Z89.6** Acquired absence of leg above knee
  - **Z89.61** Acquired absence of leg above knee
    Acquired absence of leg NOS
    Disarticulation at knee
    - **Z89.611** Acquired absence of right leg above knee
    - **Z89.612** Acquired absence of left leg above knee
    - **Z89.619** Acquired absence of unspecified leg above knee
  - **Z89.62** Acquired absence of hip
    Acquired absence of hip joint following explantation of hip joint prosthesis, with or without presence of antibiotic-impregnated cement spacer
    Disarticulation at hip
    - **Z89.621** Acquired absence of right hip joint
    - **Z89.622** Acquired absence of left hip joint
    - **Z89.629** Acquired absence of unspecified hip joint
  - **Z89.9** Acquired absence of limb, unspecified
- **Z90** Acquired absence of organs, not elsewhere classified
  - **Includes** postprocedural or post-traumatic loss of body part NEC
  - **Excludes1** congenital absence - see Alphabetical Index
  - **Excludes2** postprocedural absence of endocrine glands (E89.-)
  - **Z90.0** Acquired absence of part of head and neck
    - **Z90.01** Acquired absence of eye
    - **Z90.02** Acquired absence of larynx
    - **Z90.09** Acquired absence of other part of head and neck
      Acquired absence of nose
      - **Excludes2** teeth (K08.1)
  - **Z90.1** Acquired absence of breast and nipple
    - **Z90.10** Acquired absence of unspecified breast and nipple
    - **Z90.11** Acquired absence of right breast and nipple
    - **Z90.12** Acquired absence of left breast and nipple
    - **Z90.13** Acquired absence of bilateral breasts and nipples
  - **Z90.2** Acquired absence of lung [part of]
  - **Z90.3** Acquired absence of stomach [part of]
  - **Z90.4** Acquired absence of other specified parts of digestive tract
    - **Z90.41** Acquired absence of pancreas
      Code also exocrine pancreatic insufficiency (K86.81)
      Use additional code to identify any associated:
      insulin use (Z79.4)
      diabetes mellitus, postpancreatectomy (E13.-)
      - **Z90.410** Acquired total absence of pancreas
        Acquired absence of pancreas NOS
      - **Z90.411** Acquired partial absence of pancreas
    - **Z90.49** Acquired absence of other specified parts of digestive tract
  - **Z90.5** Acquired absence of kidney
  - **Z90.6** Acquired absence of other parts of urinary tract
    Acquired absence of bladder

- **Z90.7** Acquired absence of genital organ(s)
  - **Excludes1** personal history of sex reassignment (Z87.890)
  - **Excludes2** female genital mutilation status (N90.81-)
  - **Z90.71** Acquired absence of cervix and uterus
    - **Z90.710** Acquired absence of both cervix and uterus ♀
      Acquired absence of uterus NOS
      Status post total hysterectomy
    - **Z90.711** Acquired absence of uterus with remaining cervical stump ♀
      Status post partial hysterectomy with remaining cervical stump
    - **Z90.712** Acquired absence of cervix with remaining uterus ♀
  - **Z90.72** Acquired absence of ovaries
    - **Z90.721** Acquired absence of ovaries, unilateral ♀
    - **Z90.722** Acquired absence of ovaries, bilateral ♀
  - **Z90.79** Acquired absence of other genital organ(s)
- **Z90.8** Acquired absence of other organs
  - **Z90.81** Acquired absence of spleen
  - **Z90.89** Acquired absence of other organs
- **Z91** Personal risk factors, not elsewhere classified
  - **Excludes2** contact with and (suspected) exposures hazardous to health (Z77.-)
    exposure to pollution and other problems related to physical environment (Z77.1-)
    ▶female genital mutilation status (N90.81-)
    occupational exposure to risk factors (Z57.-)
    personal history of physical injury and trauma (Z87.81, Z87.82)
  - **Z91.0** Allergy status, other than to drugs and biological substances
    - **Excludes2** allergy status to drugs, medicaments, and biological substances (Z88.-)
    - **Z91.01** Food allergy status
      - **Excludes2** food additives allergy status (Z91.02)
      - **Z91.010** Allergy to peanuts
      - **Z91.011** Allergy to milk products
        - **Excludes1** lactose intolerance (E73.-)
      - **Z91.012** Allergy to eggs
      - **Z91.013** Allergy to seafood
        Allergy to shellfish
        Allergy to octopus or squid ink
      - **Z91.018** Allergy to other foods
        Allergy to nuts other than peanuts
    - **Z91.02** Food additives allergy status
    - **Z91.03** Insect allergy status
      - **Z91.030** Bee allergy status
      - **Z91.038** Other insect allergy status
    - **Z91.04** Nonmedicinal substance allergy status
      - **Z91.040** Latex allergy status
        Latex sensitivity status
      - **Z91.041** Radiographic dye allergy status
        Allergy status to contrast media used for diagnostic X-ray procedure
      - **Z91.048** Other nonmedicinal substance allergy status
    - **Z91.09** Other allergy status, other than to drugs and biological substances

N Newborn Age: 0   **P** Pediatric Age: 0–17   **M** Maternity DX: 12–55   **A** Adult Age: 15–124   ♀ Females Only   ♂ Males Only

Complication\Comorbidity   Major C\C   (Ex) CC/MCC Exclusions   Hospital-Acquired Condition   **1621**

CHAPTER 21 (Z00-Z99)

- **Z91.1 Patient's noncompliance with medical treatment and regimen**
  - **Z91.11 Patient's noncompliance with dietary regimen**
  - **Z91.12 Patient's intentional underdosing of medication regimen**

    Code first underdosing of medication (T36-T50) with fifth or sixth character 6

    Excludes1 adverse effect of prescribed drug taken as directed - code to adverse effect

    poisoning (overdose) - code to poisoning
    - **Z91.120 Patient's intentional underdosing of medication regimen due to financial hardship**
    - **Z91.128 Patient's intentional underdosing of medication regimen for other reason**
  - **Z91.13 Patient's unintentional underdosing of medication regimen**

    Code first underdosing of medication (T36-T50) with fifth or sixth character 6

    Excludes1 adverse effect of prescribed drug taken as directed - code to adverse effect

    poisoning (overdose) - code to poisoning
    - **Z91.130 Patient's unintentional underdosing of medication regimen due to age-related debility**
    - **Z91.138 Patient's unintentional underdosing of medication regimen for other reason**
  - **Z91.14 Patient's other noncompliance with medication regimen**

    Patient's underdosing of medication NOS
  - **Z91.15 Patient's noncompliance with renal dialysis**
  - **Z91.19 Patient's noncompliance with other medical treatment and regimen**

    ▶Nonadherence to medical treatment
- **Z91.4 Personal history of psychological trauma, not elsewhere classified**
  - **Z91.41 Personal history of adult abuse**

    Excludes2 personal history of abuse in childhood (Z62.81-)
    - **Z91.410 Personal history of adult physical and sexual abuse** A

      Excludes1 current adult physical abuse (T74.11, T76.11)

      current adult sexual abuse (T74.21, T76.11)
    - **Z91.411 Personal history of adult psychological abuse** A
    - **Z91.412 Personal history of adult neglect** A

      Excludes1 current adult neglect (T74.01, T76.01)
    - **Z91.419 Personal history of unspecified adult abuse** A
  - **Z91.49 Other personal history of psychological trauma, not elsewhere classified**

- **Z91.5 Personal history of self-harm**

  Personal history of parasuicide

  Personal history of self-poisoning

  Personal history of suicide attempt
- **Z91.8 Other specified personal risk factors, not elsewhere classified**
  - **Z91.81 History of falling**

    At risk for falling
  - **Z91.82 Personal history of military deployment** A

    Individual (civilian or military) with past history of military war, peacekeeping and humanitarian deployment (current or past conflict)

    Returned from military deployment
  - ▷ **Z91.83 Wandering in diseases classified elsewhere**

    Code first underlying disorder such as:

    Alzheimer's disease (G30.-)

    autism or pervasive developmental disorder (F84.-)

    intellectual disabilities (F70-F79)

    unspecified dementia with behavioral disturbance (F03.9-)
  - ▶● **Z91.84 Oral health risk factors**
    - ▶● **Z91.841 Risk for dental caries, low**
    - ▶● **Z91.842 Risk for dental caries, moderate**
    - ▶● **Z91.843 Risk for dental caries, high**
    - ▶● **Z91.849 Unspecified risk for dental caries**
  - **Z91.89 Other specified personal risk factors, not elsewhere classified**

    Coding Clinic: 2017, Q1, P46
- **Z92 Personal history of medical treatment**

  Excludes2 postprocedural states (Z98.-)
  - **Z92.0 Personal history of contraception**

    Excludes1 counseling or management of current contraceptive practices (Z30.-)

    long term (current) use of contraception (Z79.3)

    presence of (intrauterine) contraceptive device (Z97.5)
  - **Z92.2 Personal history of drug therapy**

    Excludes2 long term (current) drug therapy (Z79.-)
    - **Z92.21 Personal history of antineoplastic chemotherapy**
    - **Z92.22 Personal history of monoclonal drug therapy**
    - **Z92.23 Personal history of estrogen therapy**
    - **Z92.24 Personal history of steroid therapy**
      - **Z92.240 Personal history of inhaled steroid therapy**
      - **Z92.241 Personal history of systemic steroid therapy**

        Personal history of steroid therapy NOS
    - **Z92.25 Personal history of immunosupression therapy**

      Excludes2 personal history of steroid therapy (Z92.24)
    - **Z92.29 Personal history of other drug therapy**
  - **Z92.3 Personal history of irradiation**

    Personal history of exposure to therapeutic radiation

    Excludes1 exposure to radiation in the physical environment (Z77.12)

    occupational exposure to radiation (Z57.1)

CHAPTER 21 (Z00-Z99)

● **Z92.8   Personal history of other medical treatment**
Coding Clinic: 2016, Q4, P72

    ● **Z92.81   Personal history of extracorporeal membrane oxygenation (ECMO)**

    ● **Z92.82   Status post administration of tPA (rtPA) in a different facility within the last 24 hours prior to admission to current facility**

        Code first condition requiring tPA administration, such as:
        acute cerebral infarction (I63.-)
        acute myocardial infarction (I21.-, I22.-)

    ● **Z92.83   Personal history of failed moderate sedation**
        Personal history of failed conscious sedation

        Excludes2   failed moderate sedation during procedure (T88.52)

    ● **Z92.84   Personal history of unintended awareness under general anesthesia**

        Excludes2   unintended awareness under general anesthesia during procedure (T88.53)

        Coding Clinic: 2016, Q4, P72, 77

    ● **Z92.89   Personal history of other medical treatment**

● **Z93   Artificial opening status**

    Excludes1   artificial openings requiring attention or management (Z43.-)
        complications of external stoma (J95.0-, K94.-, N99.5-)

    ● **Z93.0   Tracheostomy status**
    ● **Z93.1   Gastrostomy status**
    ● **Z93.2   Ileostomy status**
    ● **Z93.3   Colostomy status**
    ● **Z93.4   Other artificial openings of gastrointestinal tract status**
    ● **Z93.5   Cystostomy status**

        ● **Z93.50   Unspecified cystostomy status**
        ● **Z93.51   Cutaneous-vesicostomy status**
        ● **Z93.52   Appendico-vesicostomy status**
        ● **Z93.59   Other cystostomy status**

    ● **Z93.6   Other artificial openings of urinary tract status**
        Nephrostomy status
        Ureterostomy status
        Urethrostomy status

    ● **Z93.8   Other artificial opening status**
    ● **Z93.9   Artificial opening status, unspecified**

● **Z94   Transplanted organ and tissue status**

    Includes   organ or tissue replaced by heterogenous or homogenous transplant

    Excludes1   complications of transplanted organ or tissue - see Alphabetical Index

    Excludes2   presence of vascular grafts (Z95.-)

    ● **Z94.0   Kidney transplant status** 🔖
        (Ex) See PDX Collection 1489

    ● **Z94.1   Heart transplant status** 🔖

        Excludes1   artificial heart status (Z95.812)
        heart-valve replacement status (Z95.2-Z95.4)

        (Ex) See PDX Collection 1488

    ● **Z94.2   Lung transplant status** 🔖
        (Ex) See PDX Collection 1491

    ● **Z94.3   Heart and lungs transplant status** 🔖
        CC when PDx is its own CC
        (Ex) See PDX Collection 1488

● **Z94.4   Liver transplant status** 🔖
    (Ex) See PDX Collection 1490

● **Z94.5   Skin transplant status**
    Autogenous skin transplant status

● **Z94.6   Bone transplant status**
● **Z94.7   Corneal transplant status**
● **Z94.8   Other transplanted organ and tissue status**

    ● **Z94.81   Bone marrow transplant status** 🔖
        (Ex) See PDX Collection 1492

    ● **Z94.82   Intestine transplant status** 🔖
        (Ex) See PDX Collection 1495

    ● **Z94.83   Pancreas transplant status** 🔖
        (Ex) See PDX Collection 1496

    ● **Z94.84   Stem cells transplant status** 🔖
        (Ex) See PDX Collection 1497

    ● **Z94.89   Other transplanted organ and tissue status**

● **Z94.9   Transplanted organ and tissue status, unspecified**

● **Z95   Presence of cardiac and vascular implants and grafts**

    ~~Excludes1   complications of cardiac and vascular devices, implants and grafts (T82.-)~~

    ▶ **Excludes2**   complications of cardiac and vascular devices, implants and grafts (T82.-)

    ● **Z95.0   Presence of cardiac pacemaker**
        Presence of cardiac resynchronization therapy (CRT-P) pacemaker

        Excludes1   adjustment or management of cardiac device (Z45.0-)
        adjustment or management of cardiac pacemaker (Z45.0)
        presence of automatic (implantable) cardiac defibrillator with synchronous cardiac pacemaker (Z95.810)

    ● **Z95.1   Presence of aortocoronary bypass graft**
        Presence of coronary artery bypass graft

    ● **Z95.2   Presence of prosthetic heart valve**
        Presence of heart valve NOS

    ● **Z95.3   Presence of xenogenic heart valve**
    ● **Z95.4   Presence of other heart-valve replacement**
    ● **Z95.5   Presence of coronary angioplasty implant and graft**

        Excludes1   coronary angioplasty status without implant and graft (Z98.61)

    ● **Z95.8   Presence of other cardiac and vascular implants and grafts**

        ● **Z95.81   Presence of other cardiac implants and grafts**
            (Ex) For category Z95.81 CC codes: See PDX Collection 1498

            ● **Z95.810   Presence of automatic (implantable) cardiac defibrillator**
                Presence of automatic (implantable) cardiac defibrillator with synchronous cardiac pacemaker
                Presence of cardiac resynchronization therapy defibrillator (CRT-D)
                Presence of cardioverter-defibrillator (ICD)

            ● **Z95.811   Presence of heart assist device** 🔖
            ● **Z95.812   Presence of fully implantable artificial heart** 🔖
            ● **Z95.818   Presence of other cardiac implants and grafts**

CHAPTER 21 (Z00-Z99)

● **Z95.82**   Presence of other vascular implants and grafts
  ● **Z95.820**   Peripheral vascular angioplasty status with implants and grafts
        Excludes1   peripheral vascular angioplasty without implant and graft (Z98.62)
  ● **Z95.828**   Presence of other vascular implants and grafts
        Presence of intravascular prosthesis NEC
● **Z95.9**   Presence of cardiac and vascular implant and graft, unspecified

● **Z96**   Presence of other functional implants
    Excludes2   complications of internal prosthetic devices, implants and grafts (T82-T85)
              fitting and adjustment of prosthetic and other devices (Z44-Z46)
● **Z96.0**   Presence of urogenital implants
● **Z96.1**   Presence of intraocular lens
        Presence of pseudophakia
● **Z96.2**   Presence of otological and audiological implants
  ● **Z96.20**   Presence of otological and audiological implant, unspecified
  ● **Z96.21**   Cochlear implant status
  ● **Z96.22**   Myringotomy tube(s) status
  ● **Z96.29**   Presence of other otological and audiological implants
        Presence of bone-conduction hearing device
        Presence of eustachian tube stent
        Stapes replacement
● **Z96.3**   Presence of artificial larynx
● **Z96.4**   Presence of endocrine implants
  ● **Z96.41**   Presence of insulin pump (external) (internal)
  ● **Z96.49**   Presence of other endocrine implants
● **Z96.5**   Presence of tooth-root and mandibular implants
● **Z96.6**   Presence of orthopedic joint implants
  ● **Z96.60**   Presence of unspecified orthopedic joint implant
  ● **Z96.61**   Presence of artificial shoulder joint
    ● **Z96.611**   Presence of right artificial shoulder joint
    ● **Z96.612**   Presence of left artificial shoulder joint
    ● **Z96.619**   Presence of unspecified artificial shoulder joint
  ● **Z96.62**   Presence of artificial elbow joint
    ● **Z96.621**   Presence of right artificial elbow joint
    ● **Z96.622**   Presence of left artificial elbow joint
    ● **Z96.629**   Presence of unspecified artificial elbow joint
  ● **Z96.63**   Presence of artificial wrist joint
    ● **Z96.631**   Presence of right artificial wrist joint
    ● **Z96.632**   Presence of left artificial wrist joint
    ● **Z96.639**   Presence of unspecified artificial wrist joint

● **Z96.64**   Presence of artificial hip joint
        Hip-joint replacement (partial) (total)
    ● **Z96.641**   Presence of right artificial hip joint
          Coding Clinic: 2016, Q3, P17
    ● **Z96.642**   Presence of left artificial hip joint
          Coding Clinic: 2015, Q1, P16
    ● **Z96.643**   Presence of artificial hip joint, bilateral
    ● **Z96.649**   Presence of unspecified artificial hip joint
● **Z96.65**   Presence of artificial knee joint
    ● **Z96.651**   Presence of right artificial knee joint
    ● **Z96.652**   Presence of left artificial knee joint
    ● **Z96.653**   Presence of artificial knee joint, bilateral
    ● **Z96.659**   Presence of unspecified artificial knee joint
● **Z96.66**   Presence of artificial ankle joint
    ● **Z96.661**   Presence of right artificial ankle joint
    ● **Z96.662**   Presence of left artificial ankle joint
    ● **Z96.669**   Presence of unspecified artificial ankle joint
● **Z96.69**   Presence of other orthopedic joint implants
    ● **Z96.691**   Finger-joint replacement of right hand
    ● **Z96.692**   Finger-joint replacement of left hand
    ● **Z96.693**   Finger-joint replacement, bilateral
    ● **Z96.698**   Presence of other orthopedic joint implants
● **Z96.7**   Presence of other bone and tendon implants
        Presence of skull plate
● **Z96.8**   Presence of other specified functional implants
    ● **Z96.81**   Presence of artificial skin
    ● **Z96.89**   Presence of other specified functional implants
● **Z96.9**   Presence of functional implant, unspecified

● **Z97**   Presence of other devices
    Excludes1   complications of internal prosthetic devices, implants and grafts (T82-T85)
              fitting and adjustment of prosthetic and other devices (Z44-Z46)
    Excludes2   presence of cerebrospinal fluid drainage device (Z98.2)
● **Z97.0**   Presence of artificial eye
● **Z97.1**   Presence of artificial limb (complete) (partial)
    ● **Z97.10**   Presence of artificial limb (complete) (partial), unspecified
    ● **Z97.11**   Presence of artificial right arm (complete) (partial)
    ● **Z97.12**   Presence of artificial left arm (complete) (partial)
    ● **Z97.13**   Presence of artificial right leg (complete) (partial)
    ● **Z97.14**   Presence of artificial left leg (complete) (partial)
    ● **Z97.15**   Presence of artificial arms, bilateral (complete) (partial)
    ● **Z97.16**   Presence of artificial legs, bilateral (complete) (partial)

● **Z97.2**   **Presence of dental prosthetic device (complete) (partial)**
Presence of dentures (complete) (partial)

● **Z97.3**   **Presence of spectacles and contact lenses**

● **Z97.4**   **Presence of external hearing-aid**

● **Z97.5**   **Presence of (intrauterine) contraceptive device ♀**

     Excludes1   checking, reinsertion or removal of implantable subdermal contraceptive (Z30.46)

                    checking, reinsertion or removal of intrauterine contraceptive device (Z30.43-)

● **Z97.8**   **Presence of other specified devices**

● **Z98**   **Other postprocedural states**

     Excludes2   aftercare (Z43-Z49, Z51)
                    follow-up medical care (Z08-Z09)
                    postprocedural complication - see Alphabetical Index

● **Z98.0**   **Intestinal bypass and anastomosis status**

     Excludes2   bariatric surgery status (Z98.84)
                    gastric bypass status (Z98.84)
                    obesity surgery status (Z98.84)

● **Z98.1**   **Arthrodesis status**

● **Z98.2**   **Presence of cerebrospinal fluid drainage device**
Presence of CSF shunt

● **Z98.3**   **Post therapeutic collapse of lung status**

     Code first underlying disease

● **Z98.4**   **Cataract extraction status**

     Use additional code to identify intraocular lens implant status (Z96.1)

     Excludes1   aphakia (H27.0)

   ● **Z98.41**   **Cataract extraction status, right eye**

   ● **Z98.42**   **Cataract extraction status, left eye**

   ● **Z98.49**   **Cataract extraction status, unspecified eye**

● **Z98.5**   **Sterilization status**

     Excludes1   female infertility (N97.-)
                    male infertility (N46.-)

   ● **Z98.51**   **Tubal ligation status ♀**

   ● **Z98.52**   **Vasectomy status ♂**   A

● **Z98.6**   **Angioplasty status**

   ● **Z98.61**   **Coronary angioplasty status**

       Excludes1   coronary angioplasty status with implant and graft (Z95.5)

   ● **Z98.62**   **Peripheral vascular angioplasty status**

       Excludes1   peripheral vascular angioplasty status with implant and graft (Z95.820)

● **Z98.8**   **Other specified postprocedural states**
     Coding Clinic: 2016, Q4, P76

   ● **Z98.81**   **Dental procedure status**

     ● **Z98.810**   **Dental sealant status**

     ● **Z98.811**   **Dental restoration status**
                 Dental crown status
                 Dental fillings status

     ● **Z98.818**   **Other dental procedure status**

● **Z98.82**   **Breast implant status**

     Excludes1   breast implant removal status (Z98.86)

● **Z98.83**   **Filtering (vitreous) bleb after glaucoma surgery status**

     Excludes1   inflammation (infection) of postprocedural bleb (H59.4-)

● **Z98.84**   **Bariatric surgery status**
     Gastric banding status
     Gastric bypass status for obesity
     Obesity surgery status

     Excludes1   bariatric surgery status complicating pregnancy, childbirth, or the puerperium (O99.84)

     Excludes2   intestinal bypass and anastomosis status (Z98.0)

● **Z98.85**   **Transplanted organ removal status**
     Transplanted organ previously removed due to complication, failure, rejection or infection

     Excludes1   encounter for removal of transplanted organ -code to complication of transplanted organ (T86.-)

● **Z98.86**   **Personal history of breast implant removal**

● **Z98.87**   **Personal history of in utero procedure**

   ● **Z98.870**   **Personal history of in utero procedure during pregnancy ♀**

       Excludes2   complications from in utero procedure for current pregnancy (O35.7)
                    supervision of current pregnancy with history of in utero procedure during previous pregnancy (O09.82-)

   ● **Z98.871**   **Personal history of in utero procedure while a fetus**

●● **Z98.89**   **Other specified postprocedural states**
     Coding Clinic: 2016, Q4, P76

   ● **Z98.890**   **Other specified postprocedural states**
             Personal history of surgery, not elsewhere classified

   ● **Z98.891**   **History of uterine scar from previous surgery**

       Excludes1   Maternal care due to uterine scar from previous surgery (O34.2-)
       Coding Clinic: 2016, Q4, P52, P76

N Newborn Age: 0   **P** Pediatric Age: 0–17   **M** Maternity DX: 12–55   **A** Adult Age: 15–124   ♀ Females Only   ♂ Males Only

   Complication\Comorbidity   Major C\C   (Ex:) CC/MCC Exclusions   Hospital-Acquired Condition

1625

● **Z99　Dependence on enabling machines and devices, not elsewhere classified**

　　Excludes1　cardiac pacemaker status (Z95.Ø)

● **Z99.Ø　Dependence on aspirator**

● **Z99.1　Dependence on respirator**

　　Dependence on ventilator

　　(Ex) **For category Z99.1 CC codes:** See PDX Collection 759

　　Z99.11　Dependence on respirator [ventilator] status 🔄

　　　　Coding Clinic: 2Ø15, Q1, P21

　　Z99.12　Encounter for respirator [ventilator] dependence during power failure 🔄

　　　　Excludes1　mechanical complication of respirator [ventilator] (J95.85Ø)

● **Z99.2　Dependence on renal dialysis**

　　Hemodialysis status

　　Peritoneal dialysis status

　　Presence of arteriovenous shunt for dialysis

　　Renal dialysis status NOS

　　Excludes1　encounter for fitting and adjustment of dialysis catheter (Z49.Ø-)

　　Excludes2　noncompliance with renal dialysis (Z91.15)

　　Coding Clinic: 2Ø16, Q1, P13

● **Z99.3　Dependence on wheelchair**

　　Wheelchair confinement status

　　Code first cause of dependence, such as:

　　　muscular dystrophy (G71.Ø)

　　　obesity (E66.-)

● **Z99.8　Dependence on other enabling machines and devices**

● **Z99.81　Dependence on supplemental oxygen**

　　Dependence on long-term oxygen

● **Z99.89　Dependence on other enabling machines and devices**

　　Dependence on machine or device NOS

PDX Collections
for CC/MCC Exclusions

FY 2018 MS-DRG Version 35

PDX Collection 2
A00.0-A00.9

PDX Collection 3
A01.00-A01.4

PDX Collection 4
A01.00-A01.09, A01.4-A02.0, A03.9-A05.2, A07.4,
A08.0-A09, A48.51-A48.52, K30, K52.1-K52.3, K52.82-K52.9,
K58.0-K58.9, K65.0, K65.2, K65.8, K68.12-K68.9,
P76.8-P77.9, P78.1, P78.3-P78.89

PDX Collection 5
A02.1, A20.7, A22.7, A26.7, A32.7, A39.2-A39.4, A40.0-A40.1,
A40.8-A41.9, A42.7, A48.2-A48.4, A48.8-A49.9, A54.86,
B00.7, B37.7, B92, B94.2-B96.89, P36.0-P36.9, P39.2,
P39.4-P39.9, R65.10-R65.20, Z16.10-Z16.39

PDX Collection 6
A02.21, A17.0-A17.1, A27.81, A39.0, A50.41, A51.41, A52.13,
A54.82, A54.84, A54.89-A54.9, A74.81-A74.9, A87.0-A87.9,
A96.2, A98.3-A98.4, B26.1, B33.24, B33.4-B33.8,
B34.1-B34.2, B34.4-B34.8, B37.5, B38.4, B45.1, B58.2,
B92, B94.2-94.9, B97.10, B97.19, B97.29, B97.5-B97.6,
B97.81-B97.89, G00.0-G03.9, G04.2, G32.89, G96.8-G96.9,
G98.0-G98.8, G99.8

PDX Collection 7
A02.22, A15.0-A15.6, A15.8-A15.9, A17.9, A18.82, A18.84,
A18.89, A20.2, A21.1, A22.1, A31.0, A37.01, A37.11, A37.81,
A37.91, A42.0, A43.0, A48.1, B25.0, B39.0-B39.2, B44.0,
B58.3, B59, B67.1, J09.X1-J09.X2, J10.00-J10.1, J11.00-J11.1,
J12.0-J12.3, J12.89-J18.1, J18.8-J18.9, J22, J60, J62.0-J67.7,
J68.0-J70.4, J70.8-J70.9, J98.4, J98.8-J99, R91.1

PDX Collection 8
A02.23, A18.02, A18.09, A39.83-A39.84, A54.40,
A54.42-A54.43, A54.82, A54.84, A54.89-A54.9, B06.82,
M00.00-M02.30, M02.319, M02.329, M02.339, M02.349,
M02.359, M02.369, M02.379-M02.9, M05.40-M05.59,

M05.70-M06.09, M06.20-M06.39, M06.80-M07.69,
M11.00-M11.9, M12.10-M15.0, M15.3-M15.9, M16.2-M16.9,
M17.2-M17.9, M18.2-M18.9, M19.111-M19.93,
M24.10-M24.176, M25.00, M25.08-M25.18, M25.40-M25.676,
M25.80-M25.9, M35.2, M36.1-M36.4, R29.4

PDX Collection 9
A02.24, A18.03-A18.09, M46.20-M46.39, M86.00-M86.9

PDX Collection 10
A02.25-A02.29

PDX Collection 11
A02.8

PDX Collection 12
A02.9

PDX Collection 13
A00.1, A01.00-A01.09, A01.4-A02.0, A03.0, A03.9,
A04.9-A05.2, A06.0-A06.2, A06.9, A07.1-A07.9, A08.4-A09,
A18.32-A18.39, A18.83, A48.51-A48.52, B37.82, B82.9,
J09.X3-J09.X9, J10.2-J10.89, J11.2-J11.89, K30, K31.84,
K50.00-K51.919, K52.1-K52.3, K52.82-K55.1, K55.30-K55.33,
K55.8-K55.9, K58.0-K58.9, P70.0-P70.4, P70.9-P71.9, P72.1,
P72.9-P74.4, P74.9, P76.8-P77.9, P78.1, P78.3-P78.89, P94.0

PDX Collection 14
A02.0, A03.9-A05.0, A05.2, A07.4, A08.0-A09, J09.X3-J09.X9,
J10.2-J10.89, J11.2-J11.89, K30, K31.84, K52.1-K52.3,
K52.82-K52.9, K58.0-K58.9, K65.0, K65.2, K65.8,
K68.12-K68.9, P76.8-P77.9, P78.1, P78.3-P78.89

PDX Collection 15
A00.1, A01.00-A01.09, A01.4-A02.0, A03.9, A04.0-A04.8,
A04.9-A05.2, A06.0-A06.2, A06.9, A07.1-A09, A18.32-A18.39,
A18.83, A48.51-A48.52, B37.82, B82.9, J09.X3-J09.X9,
J10.2-J10.89, J11.2-J11.89, K30, K31.84, K50.00-K51.919,
K52.1-K52.3, K52.82-K55.1, K55.30-K55.33, K55.8-K55.9,
K58.0-K58.9, P70.0-P70.4, P70.9-P71.9, P72.1, P72.9-P74.4,
P74.9, P76.8-P77.9, P78.1, P78.3-P78.89, P94.0

PDX Collection 16
A00.1, A01.00-A01.09, A01.4-A02.0, A03.9-A05.0, A05.2,
A06.0-A06.2, A06.9, A07.1-A09, A18.32-A18.39, A18.83,
B37.82, B82.9, J09.X3-J09.X9, J10.2-J10.89, J11.2-J11.89,
K30, K31.84, K52.1-K52.3, K52.82-K52.9, K58.0-K58.9,
K65.0, K65.2, K65.8, K68.12-K68.9, P76.8-P77.9, P78.1,
P78.3-P78.89

PDX Collection 17
A00.0-A09, A48.51-A48.52

PDX Collection 18
A04.71-A04.72, A05.0-A05.2, A48.51-A48.52

PDX Collection 19
A02.0, A03.9-A05.2, A07.4, A08.0-A09, A48.51-A48.52,
J09.X3-J09.X9, J10.2-J10.89, J11.2-J11.89, K30, K31.84,
K52.1-K52.3, K52.82-K52.9, K58.0-K58.9, K65.0, K65.2,
K65.8, K68.12-K68.9, P76.8-P77.9, P78.1, P78.3-P78.89

PDX Collection 20
A06.0-A06.1, A07.4

PDX Collection 21
A02.0, A03.9-A05.0, A05.2, A06.0-A06.2, A06.9, A07.1-A09,
B82.9, J09.X3-J09.X9, J10.2-J10.89, J11.2-J11.89, K30,
K31.84, K50.00-K51.919, K52.1-K52.3, K52.82-K55.1,
K55.30-K55.33, K55.8-K55.9, K58.0-K58.9, P76.8-P77.9,
P78.1, P78.3, P78.81-P78.89

PDX Collection 22
A06.0-A06.6, A06.81-A06.89

PDX Collection 23
A06.4, K75.0

PDX Collection 24
A06.5, J85.0-J85.2

PDX Collection 25
A06.6, G06.0

PDX Collection 26
A02.0, A03.9-A05.0, A05.2, A06.0-A06.2, A06.9, A07.1-A09, B82.9, J09.X3-J09.X9, J10.2-J10.89, J11.2-J11.89, K30, K31.84, K52.1-K52.3, K52.82-K52.9, K58.0-K58.9

PDX Collection 27
A02.0, A03.9-A05.0, A05.2, A06.0-A06.2, A06.9, A07.1-A09, B82.9, J09.X3-J09.X9, J10.2-J10.89, J11.2-J11.89, K30, K31.84, K52.1-K52.3, K52.82-K52.9, K58.0-K58.9, K65.0, K65.2, K65.8, K68.12-K68.9

PDX Collection 28
A02.0, A03.9-A05.0, A05.2, A06.0-A06.2, A06.9, A07.1-A09, A18.32-A18.39, A18.83, B37.82, B82.9, J09.X3-J09.X9, J10.2-J10.89, J11.2-J11.89, K30, K31.84, K52.1-K52.3, K52.82-K52.9, K58.0-K58.9, K65.0, K65.2, K65.8, K68.12-K68.9, P76.8-P77.9, P78.1, P78.3-P78.89

PDX Collection 29
A15.0-A15.9, A17.9, A18.82, A18.84, A18.89-A19.9, A22.1, A31.0, A31.2-A31.9, A37.01, A37.11, A37.81, A37.91, A48.1, A49.3-A49.9, B25.0, B44.0, B90.9, B92, B94.2-B94.9, B96.0, B96.6-B96.89, J09.X1-J09.X2, J10.00-J10.1, J11.00-J11.1, J12.0-J12.3, J12.89-J18.1, J18.8-J18.9, J44.9, J47.0-J70.4, J70.8-J70.9, J98.4, R91.1

PDX Collection 30
A15.0-A17.82, A17.89-A19.9

PDX Collection 31
A15.0-A17.82, A17.89, A18.31-A18.39, A18.83, A19.0-A19.9

PDX Collection 32
A02.21, A17.0-A17.1, A17.89-A17.9, A18.82, A18.84, A18.89, A27.81, A31.2-A31.9, A39.0, A49.3-A49.9, A50.41, A51.41, A52.13, A54.82, A54.84, A54.89-A54.9, A87.0-A87.9, B00.3, B02.1, B26.1, B37.5, B38.4, B45.1, B58.2, B90.0, B92, B94.2-B94.9, B96.0, B96.6-B96.89, G00.0-G03.9, G04.2, G32.89, G61.0, G96.8-G96.9, G98.0-G98.8, G99.8

PDX Collection 33
A17.81-A17.82, A17.89-A17.9, A18.82, A18.84, A18.89, A31.2-A31.9, A49.3-A49.9, B90.0, B92, B94.2-B94.9, B96.0, B96.6-B96.89

PDX Collection 34
A17.89-A17.9, A18.82, A18.84, A18.89, A31.2-A31.9, A49.3-A49.9, B90.0, B92, B94.2-B94.9, B96.0, B96.6-B96.89

PDX Collection 35
A17.9, A18.82, A18.84, A18.89, A31.2-A31.9, A49.3-A49.9, B92, B94.2-B94.9, B96.0, B96.6-B96.89

PDX Collection 36
A18.01

PDX Collection 37
A18.02

PDX Collection 38
A18.01, A18.03

PDX Collection 39
A18.01-A18.02, A18.09

PDX Collection 40
A17.9, A18.10, A18.82, A18.84, A18.89, A31.2-A31.9, A49.3-A49.9, B90.1, B92, B94.2-B94.9, B96.0, B96.6-B96.89

PDX Collection 41
A17.9, A18.10-A18.13, A18.82, A18.84, A18.89, A31.2-A31.9, A49.3-A49.9, B90.1, B92, B94.2-B94.9, B96.0, B96.6-B96.89

PDX Collection 42
A17.9, A18.10, A18.82, A18.84, A18.89, A31.2-A31.9, A49.3-A49.9, B90.1, B92, B94.2-B94.9, B96.0, B96.6-B96.89

PDX Collection 43
A17.9, A18.0, A18.16-A18.18, A18.82, A18.84, A18.89, A31.2-A31.9, A49.3-A49.9, B90.1, B92, B94.2-B94.9, B96.0, B96.6-B96.89

PDX Collection 44
A17.9, A18.2, A18.82, A18.84, A18.89, A31.2-A31.9, A49.3-A49.9, B92, B94.2-B94.9, B96.0, B96.6-B96.89

PDX Collection 45
A17.9, A18.31-A18.39, A18.82-A18.84, A18.89, A31.2-A31.9, A49.3-A49.9, B92, B94.2-B94.9, B96.0, B96.6-B96.89

PDX Collection 46
A17.9, A18.50-A18.59, A18.82, A18.84, A18.89, A31.2-A31.9, A49.3-A49.9, B92, B94.2-B94.9, B96.0, B96.6-B96.89

PDX Collection 47
A17.9, A18.6, A18.82, A18.84, A18.89, A31.2-A31.9, A49.3-A49.9, B92, B94.2-B94.9, B96.0, B96.6-B96.89

PDX Collection 48
A17.9, A18.7, A18.82, A18.84, A18.89, A31.2-A31.9, A49.3-A49.9, B92, B94.2-B94.9, B96.0, B96.6-B96.89

PDX Collection 49
A17.9, A18.81-A18.82, A18.84, A18.89, A31.2-A31.9, A49.3-A49.9, B92, B94.2-B94.9, B96.0, B96.6-B96.89

PDX Collection 50
A17.9, A18.82, A18.84-A18.85 A18.89, A31.2-A31.9, A49.3-A49.9, B92, B94.2-B94.9, B96.0, B96.6-B96.89

PDX Collection 51
A17.9, A18.82, A18.84, A18.89, A19.0-A19.9, A31.2-A31.9, A49.3-A49.9, B92, B94.2-B94.9, B96.0, B96.6-B96.89

PDX Collection 52
A20.0-A20.9

PDX Collection 53
A20.2, J12.81

PDX Collection 54
A20.3, A20.8

PDX Collection 55
A02.1, A20.0-A20.9, A22.7, A26.7, A32.7, A40.0-A40.1, A40.8-A41.9, A42.7, A54.86, B37.7, P36.0-P36.9, P39.2, P39.4-P39.9, R65.10-R65.20

PDX Collection 56
A20.9

PDX Collection 57
A21.0

PDX Collection 58
A21.1, J12.81

PDX Collection 59
A22.1, A37.01, A37.11, A37.81, A37.91, A48.1, B25.0, B44.0, J09.X1-J09.X2, J10.00-J10.1, J11.00-J11.1, J15.29, J15.5-J18.0, J18.8-J18.9, J22, J60-J70.4, J70.8-J70.9, J98.4, J98.8-J99, R91.1

PDX Collection 60
A21.3

PDX Collection 61
A21.0-A21.9

PDX Collection 62
A22.0

PDX Collection 63
A15.0-A15.9, A17.9, A18.82, A18.84, A18.89, A20.2, A21.1-A21.2, A22.1, A31.0, A37.01, A37.11, A37.81, A37.91, A42.0, A43.0, A48.1, B25.0, B39.0-B39.2, B44.0, B58.3, B59, B67.1, J09.X1-J09.X2, J10.00-J10.1, J11.00-J11.1, J12.0-J12.3, J12.81-J18.1, J18.8-J18.9, J22, J44.9, J47.0-J70.4, J70.8-J70.9, J98.4, J98.8-J99, R91.1

PDX Collection 64
A22.2

PDX Collection 65
A22.8

PDX Collection 66
A22.0-A22.9

PDX Collection 67
A23.0-A23.9

PDX Collection 68
A24.0

PDX Collection 69
A24.1-A24.9

PDX Collection 70
A25.0-A25.9

PDX Collection 71
A02.1, A20.7, A22.7, A26.7, A32.7, A39.2-A39.4, A40.0-A40.1, A40.8-A41.9, A42.7, A48.2-A48.4, A48.8-A49.9, A54.86, B00.7, B3.77, B92, B94.2-B96.89, R65.10-R65.20, Z16.10-Z16.39

PDX Collection 72
A27.0-A27.9

PDX Collection 73
A02.21, A17.0-A17.1, A27.0-A27.9, A39.0, A50.41, A51.41, A52.13, A54.82, A54.84, A54.89-A54.9, A74.81-A74.9, A87.0-A87.9, A96.2, A98.3-A98.4, B26.1, B33.24, B33.4-B33.8, B34.1-B34.2, B34.4-B34.8, B37.5, B38.4, B45.1, B58.2, B92, B94.2-B94.9, B97.10, B97.19, B97.29, B97.5-B97.6, B97.81-B97.89, G00.0-G03.9, G04.2, G32.89, G61.0, G96.8-G96.9, G98.0-G98.8, G99.8

PDX Collection 74
A26.0, A26.8-A26.9, A28.0, A28.2-A28.9, A32.0-A32.12, A32.81-A32.9

PDX Collection 75
A28.1, B97.21

PDX Collection 76
A30.0

PDX Collection 77
A30.1

PDX Collection 78
A30.2-A30.4

PDX Collection 79
A30.5

PDX Collection 80
A30.8

PDX Collection 81
A30.9

PDX Collection 82
A15.0-A15.9, A17.9, A18.82, A18.84, A18.89, A22.1, A31.0, A31.2-A31.9, A37.01, A37.11, A37.81, A37.91, A48.1, A49.3-A49.9, B25.0, B44.0, B90.0, B92, B94.2-B94.9, B96.0, B96.6-B96.89, J09.X1-J09.X2, J10.00-J10.1, J11.00-J11.1, J12.0-J12.3, J12.89-J18.1, J18.8-J18.9, J44.9, J47.0-J70.4, J70.8-J70.9, J98.4, R91.1

PDX Collection 83
A31.0-A31.9

PDX Collection 84
A33, P29.0-P29.2, P29.4, P29.89-P29.9, P94.1-P94.9, P96.0, P96.3-P96.5, P96.82-P96.89

PDX Collection 85
A34, O08.0, O08.2-O08.9, O11.4, O11.5, O12.04, O12.05, O12.14, O12.15, O12.24, O12.25, O13.4, O13.5, O14.04, O14.05, O14.14, O14.15, O14.24, O14.25, O14.94, O14.95, O16.4, O16.5, O20.0-O20.9, O25.10-O25.3, O26.10-O26.13, O26.30-O26.43, O26.63-O26.819, O26.841-O26.86, O26.891-O26.93, O29.011-O29.93, O35.7XX0-O35.7XX9, O44.00-O44.13, O44.20-O44.53, O45.8X1-O45.93, O75.4,

075.81, 075.89-075.9, O80, O90.89, O99.111-O99.285,
O99.330-O99.335, O99.350-O99.355, O99.511-O99.73,
O99.820-O99.825, O99.840-O9A.53

PDX Collection 86

A35, B92, B94.2-B94.9

PDX Collection 87

A36.0-A36.9

PDX Collection 88

A36.81, A52.06, B33.20-B33.22, I00, I01.2-I01.9, I09.0, I09.9,
I23.0-I23.3, I23.6-I23.8, I40.0-I41, I51.0, I51.4, I87.8-I87.9,
I99.8-I99.9

PDX Collection 89

A37.00-A37.91

PDX Collection 90

A15.0-A15.9, A17.9, A18.82, A18.84, A18.89, A21.2,
A22.1, A31.0, A37.00-A37.91, A42.0, A43.0, A48.1, B25.0,
B39.0-B39.2, B44.0, B58.3, B59, B67.1, J09.X1-J09.X2,
J10.00-J10.1, J11.00-J11.1, J12.0-J12.3, J12.89-J18.1,
J18.8-J18.9, J22, J44.9, J47.0-J70.4, J70.8-J70.9, J98.4,
J98.8-J98.9, Q33.4, R91.1

PDX Collection 91

A38.0-A38.9, A46, J02.0, J03.00-J03.01

PDX Collection 92

A02.21, A17.0-A17.1, A27.81, A39.0, A39.89-A39.9,
A49.3-A49.9, A50.41, A51.41, A52.13, A54.82, A54.84,
A54.89-A54.9, A87.0-A87.9, B00.3, B02.1, B26.1, B37.5,
B38.4, B45.1, B58.2, B92, B94.2-B94.9, B96.0, B96.6-B96.89,
G00.0-G03.9, G04.2, G32.89, G61.0, G96.8-G96.9,
G98.0-G98.8, G99.8

PDX Collection 93

A39.1, A39.89-A39.9, A49.3-A49.9, B92, B94.2-B94.9, B96.0,
B96.6-B96.89

PDX Collection 94

A02.1, A20.7, A22.7, A26.7, A32.7, A39.2-A39.4,
A39.89-A41.9, A42.7, A49.3-A49.9, A54.86, B00.7, B37.7,
B92, B94.2-B94.9, B96.0, B96.6-B96.89, R65.10-R65.20

PDX Collection 95

A39.50, A39.89-A39.9, A49.3-A49.9, B92, B94.2-B94.9, B96.0,
B96.6-B96.89

PDX Collection 96

A39.51, A39.89-A39.9, A49.3-A49.9, B92, B94.2-B94.9, B96.0,
B96.6-B96.89

PDX Collection 97

A39.52, A49.3-A49.9, B92, B94.2-B94.9, B96.0, B96.6-B96.89

PDX Collection 98

A39.53, A39.89-A39.9, A49.3-A49.9, B92, B94.2-B94.9, B96.0,
B96.6-B96.89

PDX Collection 99

A39.81, A39.89-A39.9, A49.3-A49.9, B92, B94.2-B94.9, B96.0,
B96.6-B96.89

PDX Collection 100

A39.82, A39.89-A39.9, A49.3-A49.9, B92, B94.2-B94.9, B96.0,
B96.6-B96.89

PDX Collection 101

A39.83-A39.9, A49.3-A49.9, B92, B94.2-B94.9, B96.0,
B96.6-B96.89

PDX Collection 102

A39.89-A39.9, A49.3-A49.9, B92, B94.2-B94.9, B96.0,
B96.6-B96.89

PDX Collection 103

A42.0, A42.81-A43.0, A43.8-A43.9, B47.1, J12.81

PDX Collection 104

A42.1, A42.81-A42.9, A43.8-A43.9, B47.1

PDX Collection 105

A42.2, A42.81-A42.9, A43.8-A43.9, B47.1

PDX Collection 106

A42.0-A42.2, A42.81-A43.9, B47.1-B47.9, L08.1

PDX Collection 107

A42.81-A42.9, A43.1-A43.9, B47.1, L08.1

PDX Collection 108

A44.0-A44.9, A68.0-A68.9, A69.20-A69.29, A75.0-A79.9,
B55.0-B57.5, B60.0

PDX Collection 109

A48.0, B92, B94.2-B94.9

PDX Collection 110

A15.0-A15.9, A17.9, A18.82, A18.84, A18.89, A21.2, A22.1,
A31.0, A37.01, A37.11, A37.81, A37.91, A42.0, A43.0, A48.1,
B25.0, B39.0-B39.2, B44.0, B58.3, B59, B67.1, J09.X1-J09.X2,
J10.00-J10.1, J11.00-J11.1, J12.0-J12.3, J12.89-J18.1,
J18.8-J18.9, J22, J44.9, J47.0-J70.4, J70.8-J70.9, J98.4,
J98.8-J98.9, Q33.4, R91.1

PDX Collection 111

A48.3, G89.0-G89.4, R09.89, R29.700-R29.742, R41.0-R41.3,
R41.82, R41.9, R44.8-R44.9, R45.83-R45.84, R46.0-R46.89,
R52, R57.0-R57.9, R65.21, R68.0-R68.19, R68.81-R68.89, R69

PDX Collection 112

A50.01-A51.46, A51.5-A53.9

PDX Collection 113

A50.01-A51.46, A51.5-A54.85, A54.89-A58, A63.8, A64, B92,
B94.2-B94.9, M02.30-M02.39, N34.1

PDX Collection 114

A50.01-A51.46, A51.5-A53.9, A56.00-A56.8, A63.8-A64, B92,
B94.2-B94.9, N34.1

PDX Collection 115

A02.21, A17.0-A17.1, A27.81, A39.0, A50.01-A51.46,
A51.5-A53.9, A54.82, A54.84, A54.89-A54.9, A56.00-A56.8,
A63.8-A64, A87.0-A87.9, B00.3, B02.1, B26.1, B37.5, B38.4,
B45.1, B58.2, B92, B94.2-B94.9, G00.0-G03.9, G04.2, G32.89,
G61.0, G96.8-G96.9, G98.0-G98.8, G99.8, N34.1

PDX Collection 116

A50.01-A51.46, A51.5-A54.85, A54.89-A58, A63.8, A64,
M02.30-M02.39, N34.1

PDX Collection 117

A02.21, A17.0-A17.1, A27.81, A39.0, A50.01-A51.46,
A51.5-A54.49, A54.5-A54.85, A54.89-A58, A63.8-A64,
A74.81-A74.9, A87.0-A87.9, A96.2, A98.3-A98.4, B26.1, B33.24,
B33.4-B33.8, B34.1-B34.2, B34.4-B34.8, B37.5, B38.4, B45.1,
B58.2, B92, B94.2-B94.9, B97.10, B97.19, B97.29, B97.5-B97.6,
B97.81-B97.89, G00.0-G03.9, G04.2, G32.89, G61.0,
G96.8-G96.9, G98.0-G98.8, G99.8, M02.30-M02.39, N34.1

PDX Collection 118

A50.01-A51.46, A51.5-A54.85, A54.89-A58, A63.8, A64,
K71.0-K71.9, K73.1-K73.8, K74.0-K74.69, K75.2-K76.0,
K76.4-K76.5, K76.89-K76.9, M02.30-M02.39, N34.1

PDX Collection 119

A18.09, A50.01-A51.46, A51.5-A54.85, A54.89-A58,
A63.8, A64, A66.6, M02.30-M02.39, M84.80-M84.9,
M85.10-M85.19, M85.80-M85.89, M86.30-M86.8X9,
M89.20-M89.39, M89.50-M89.59, M89.8X0-M89.8X9, M94.1,
M94.351-M94.8X9, N34.1

PDX Collection 120

A18.50-A18.59, A50.01-A51.46, A51.5-A54.85, A54.89-A58,
A63.8-A64, H15.001-H15.009, H15.091-H15.129,
M02.30-M02.39, N34.1

PDX Collection 121

A54.00-A54.29, A54.82, A54.84, A54.89, A54.9, A56.00-A56.8,
A63.8-A64, B92, B94.-B94.9, N34.1

PDX Collection 122

A02.23, A17.9, A18.02, A18.09, A18.82, A18.84, A18.89,
A39.83-A39.84, A50.01-A51.9, A52.00-A54.89, A54.9-A58,
A63.8, A64, B06.82, M00.00-M02.9, M05.40-M05.59,
M05.70-M06.09, M06.20-M06.39, M06.80-M07.69,
M11.00-M11.9, M12.10-M15.0, M15.3-M15.9, M16.2-M16.9,
M17.2-M17.9, M18.2-M18.9, M19.111-M19.93,
M24.10-M24.176, M25.00, M25.08, M25.10-M25.18,
M25.40-M25.676, M25.80-M25.9, M35.2, M36.1-M36.4,
N34.1, R29.4

PDX Collection 123

A50.01-A51.46, A51.5-A54.85, A54.89-A58, A63.8, A64,
M02.30-M02.39, N25.81-N25.89, N34.1

PDX Collection 124

A01.00-A01.09, A39.51, A50.01-A58, A63.8-A64, A78,
B33.20-B33.22, B37.6, B40.0-B40.9, I00, I01.1-I02.0,
I05.0-I05.1, I05.2, I05.8-I08.3, I08.9-I09.1, I09.89-I09.9,
I23.0-I23.3, I23.6-I23.8, I33.0-I41, I42.4, I51.0, I51.4,
I87.8-I87.9, I99.8-I99.9, M00.00, M00.08-M00.10,
M00.18-M00.20, M00.28-M00.80, M00.88-M00.9,
M02.30-M02.39, N34.1, Q22.2, Q23.8, Q23.9, Q24.8,
T82.6XX[A]

PDX Collection 125

A18.31, A34, A50.01-A58, A63.8, A64, K35.2-K35.3, K63.4,
K63.89-K63.9, K65.1, K65.3, K65.9, K67, K86.81-K86.89,
K92.89-K92.9, M02.30-M02.39, N34.1, N73.3-N73.4, N73.6,
O08.0, O08.82, O85, O86.12, O86.81, O86.89, P78.0, R11.13,
T81.60X[A]-T81.69X[A]

PDX Collection 126

A69.1

PDX Collection 127

A70

PDX Collection 128

A17.82, A44.0-A44.9, A50.42, A52.14, A68.0-A68.9,
A69.20-A69.29, A75.0-A79.9, A81.1, A81.82-A81.89,
A83.0-A85.8, A87.2, A88.0, A88.8, A92.1-A92.8, A93.0, B00.4,
B00.82, B01.11-B01.12, B04, B06.01, B08.09, B08.20-B08.22,
B08.60-B08.79, B09, B10.01-B10.09, B26.2, B33.1, B45.0,
B45.2-B45.9, B50.9, B55.0-B57.5, B58.2, B60.0, B75, B97.10,
B97.21, G04.00-G04.01, G04.31, G04.81-G05.4, G37.0,
G37.4-G37.5, J09.X3-J09.X9, J10.2-J10.89, J11.2-J11.89,
L44.4, M1A.10X0-M1A.19X1, P35.2-P35.9, P37.0-P37.4,
P37.8-P37.9, T56.0X1-T56.0X4[A]

PDX Collection 129

A77.0-A79.9

PDX Collection 130

A80.0-A80.39

PDX Collection 131

A17.82, A50.42, A52.14, A75.9, A79.9, A81.00-A81.9,
A83.0-A85.8, A87.2, A88.0, A88.8, A92.1-A92.2, A92.4-A92.8,
A93.0, B00.4, B00.82, B01.11-B01.12, B04, B06.01, B08.09,
B08.20-B08.22, B08.60-B08.79, B09, B10.01-B10.09,
B26.2, B33.1, B45.0, B45.2-B45.9, B58.2, B75, B97.10,
G04.00-G04.01, G04.31, G04.81-G05.4, G37.0, G37.4-G37.5,
I67.3, J09.X3-J09.X9, J10.2-J10.89, J11.2-J11.89, L44.4,
M1A.10X0-M1A.19X1, P35.2-P35.9, P37.0-P37.4, P37.8-P37.9,
T56.0X1-T56.0X4[A]

PDX Collection 132

A81.1, B92, B94.2-B94.9

PDX Collection 133
A17.82, A50.42, A52.14, A75.9, A79.9, A81.00-A81.9, A83.0-A85.8, A87.2, A88.0, A88.8, A92.1-A92.2, A92.4-A92.8, A93.0, B00.4, B00.82, B01.11-B01.12, B04, B06.01, B08.09, B08.20-B08.22, B08.60-B08.79, B09, B10.01-B10.09, B26.2, B27.00-B27.99, B33.1, B45.0, B45.2-B45.9, B58.2, B75, G04.00-G04.01, G04.31, G04.81-G05.4, G37.0, G37.4-G37.5, I67.3, J09.X3-J09.X9, J10.2-J10.89, J11.2-J11.89, L44.4, M1A.10X0-M1A.19X1, P35.2-P35.9, P37.0-P37.4, P37.8-P37.9, T56.0X1-T56.0X4[A]

PDX Collection 134
A81.00-A81.9, I67.3

PDX Collection 135
A81.00-A81.9, A92.30-A92.39, B97.21, I67.3

PDX Collection 136
A82.0-A82.9

PDX Collection 137
A17.82, A50.42, A52.14, A75.9, A79.9, A81.1, A81.82-A81.89, A83.0-A85.8, A87.2, A88.0, A88.8, A92.1-A92.8, A93.0, B00.4, B00.82, B01.11-B01.12, B04, B06.01, B08.09, B08.20-B08.22, B08.60-B08.79, B09, B10.01-B10.09, B26.2, B27.00-B27.99, B33.1, B45.0, B45.2-B45.9, B58.2, B75, B97.10-B97.21, G04.00-G04.01, G04.31, G04.81-G04.91, G05.3-G05.4, G37.0, G37.4-G37.5, J09.X3-J09.X9, J10.2-J10.89, J11.2-J11.89, L44.4, M1A.10X0-M1A.19X1, P35.2-P35.9, P37.0-P37.9, T56.0X1-T56.0X4[A]

PDX Collection 138
A17.82, A50.42, A52.14, A75.9, A79.9, A81.1, A81.82-A81.89, A83.0-A85.8, A87.2, A88.0, A88.8, A92.1-A92.8, A93.0, B00.4, B00.82, B01.11-B01.12, B04, B06.01, B08.09, B08.20-B08.22, B08.60-B08.79, B09, B10.01-B10.09, B26.2, B27.00-B27.99, B33.1, B45.0, B45.2-B45.9, B58.2, B75, B97.10-B97.21, G04.00-G04.01, G04.31, G04.81-G04.91, G05.3-G05.4, G37.0, G37.4-G37.5, H66.40-H66.43, J09.X3-J09.X9, J10.2-J10.89, J11.2-J11.89, L44.4, M1A.10X0-M1A.19X1, M32.0-M32.9, P35.2-P35.9, P37.0-P37.9, T56.0X1-T56.0X4[A]

PDX Collection 139
A17.82, A50.42, A52.14, A75.9, A79.9, A81.1, A81.82-A81.89, A83.0-A86, A87.2, A88.0, A88.8-A89, A92.1-A92.2, A92.4-A92.8, A93.0, B00.4, B00.82, B01.11-B01.12, B04, B06.01, B08.09, B08.20-B08.22, B08.60-B08.79, B09, B10.01-B10.09, B26.2, B27.00-B27.99, B33.1, B45.0, B45.2-B45.9, B58.2, B75, B97.10, G04.00-G04.01, G04.31, G04.81-G04.91, G05.3-G05.4, G37.0, G37.4-G37.5, H66.40-H66.43, J09. X3-J09.X9, J10.2-J10.89, J11.2-J11.89, L44.4, M1A.10X0-M1A.19X1, M32.0-M32.9, P35.2-P35.9, P37.0-P37.9, T56.0X1-T56.0X4[A]

PDX Collection 140
A02.21, A17.0-A17.1, A27.81, A39.0, A50.41, A51.41, A52.13, A54.82-A54.84, A54.89-A54.9, A74.81-A74.9, A87.0-A87.9, A96.2, A98.3-A98.4, B26.1, B33.24, B33.4-B33.8, B34.1-B34.8, B37.5, B38.4, B45.1, B58.2, B92, B94.2-B94.9, B97.10, B97.19, B97.29, B97.5-B97.6, B97.81-B97.89, G00.0-G03.9, G04.2, G32.89, G61.0, G96.8-G96.9, G98.0-G98.8, G99.8

PDX Collection 141
A02.21, A17.0-A17.1, A27.81, A39.0, A50.41, A51.41, A52.13, A54.82-A54.84, A54.89-A54.9, A74.81-A74.9, A87.0-A87.9, A92.30-A92.39, A96.2, A98.3-A98.4, B26.1, B33.24, B33.4-B33.8, B34.1-B34.8, B37.5, B38.4, B45.1, B58.2, B92, B94.2-B94.9, B97.10, B97.19, B97.21-B97.29, B97.5-B97.6, B97.81-B97.89, G00.0-G03.9, G04.2, G32.89, G61.0, G96.8-G96.9, G98.0-G98.8, G99.8

PDX Collection 142
A90

PDX Collection 143
A91, A92.0-A94, A98.0-A98.2, A98.8-A99, B33.1

PDX Collection 144
A17.82, A50.42, A52.14, A75.9, A79.9, A81.1, A81.82-A81.89, A83.0-A85.8, A87.2, A88.0, A88.8, A91-A94, A98.0-A98.2, A98.8-A99, B00.4, B00.82, B01.11-B01.12, B04, B06.01, B08.09, B08.20-B08.22, B08.60-B08.79, B09, B10.01-B10.09, B26.2, B27.00-B27.99, B33.1, B45.0, B45.2-B45.9, B58.2, B75, B97.10, B97.21, G04.00-G04.01, G04.31, G04.81-G04.91, G05.3-G05.4, G37.0, G37.4-G37.5, J09.X3-J09.X9, J10.2-J10.89, J11.2-J11.89, L44.4, M1A.10X0-M1A.19X1, P35.2-P35.9, P37.0-P37.9, T56.0X1-T56.0X4[A]

PDX Collection 145
A17.82, A50.42, A52.14, A75.9, A79.9, A81.1, A81.82-A81.89, A83.0-A85.8, A87.2, A88.0, A88.8, A91, A92.0-A92.2, A92.4-A94, A98.0-A98.2, A98.8-A99, B00.4, B00.82, B01.11-B01.12, B04, B06.01, B08.09, B08.20-B08.22, B08.60-B08.79, B09, B10.01-B10.09, B26.2, B27.00-B27.99, B33.1, B45.0, B45.2-B45.9, B58.2, B75, B97.10, G04.00-G04.01, G04.31, G04.81-G04.91, G05.3-G05.4, G37.0, G37.4-G37.5, J09.X3-J09.X9, J10.2-J10.89, J11.2-J11.89, L44.4, P35.2-P35.9, P37.0-P37.9

PDX Collection 146
A95.0-A95.9

PDX Collection 147
A74.81-A74.9, A88.1, A96.0-A96.9, A98.3-A98.5, B25.8-B25.9, B33.24-B34.2, B34.4-B34.8, B97.0-B97.89

PDX Collection 148
A17.9, A18.10-A18.11, A18.13, A18.82, A18.84, A18.89, A54.21, A54.29, A54.82, A54.84, A54.89-A54.9, A59.00, A59.8-A59.9, A98.5, B37.41-B37.49, B97.21, E08.21-E08.29, E08.618-E08.638, E08.649-E08.8, E09.21-E09.29, E09.618-E09.638, E09.649-E09.8, E10.21-E10.29, E10.618-E10.638, E10.649, E10.69-E10.8, E11.21-E11.29, E11.618-E11.638, E11.649, E11.69-E11.8, E13.21-E13.29, E13.618-E13.638, E13.649-E13.8, M10.30-M10.39, N00.0-N11.0, N11.8-N13.39, N13.6, N14.0-N17.9, N19, N25.0-N26.1, N26.9-N27.9, N28.1-N29, N36.41-N36.43, N36.8-N36.9, N39.8-N39.9, R31.0-R31.9

PDX Collection 149
B00.2

PDX Collection 150
A02.21, A17.0-A17.1, A27.81, A39.0, A50.41, A51.41, A52.13, A54.82, A54.84, A54.89-A54.9, A87.0-A87.9, B00.3, B00.82-B00.9, B02.1, B10.81-B10.89, B26.1, B37.5, B38.4, B45.1, B58.2, B92, B94.2-B94.9, G00.0-G03.9, G04.2, G32.89, G61.0, G96.8-G96.9, G98.0-G98.8, G99.8

PDX Collection 151
B00.4, B00.82-B00.9, B10.01-B10.89, B92, B94.2-B94.9

PDX Collection 152
B00.50-B00.59, B00.89-B00.9, B10.81-B10.89

PDX Collection 153
A02.1, A20.7, A22.7, A26.7, A32.7, A39.2-A39.4, A40.0-A41.9, A42.7, A54.86, B00.7, B00.82-B00.9, B10.81-B10.89, B37.7, B92, B94.2-B94.9, R65.10-R65.20

PDX Collection 154
B00.3, B00.81-B00.9, B10.81-B10.89, B92, B94.2-B94.9

PDX Collection 155
A74.81-A74.9, A96.2, A98.3-A98.4, B00.82-B00.9, B01.12, B02.24, B10.81-B10.89, B33.24, B33.4-B33.8, B34.1-B34.2, B34.4-B34.8, B92, B94.2-B94.9, B97.10, B97.19, B97.29, B97.5-B97.6, B97.81-B97.89, G04.00-G04.01, G04.31, G04.81-G04.89, G05.3-G05.4, G37.3

PDX Collection 156
A74.81-A74.9, A96.2, A98.3-A98.4, B00.82-B00.9, B10.81-B10.89, B33.24, B33.4-B33.8, B34.1-B34.2, B34.4-B34.8, B92, B94.2-B94.9, B97.10, B97.19, B97.29, B97.5-B97.6, B97.81-B97.89

PDX Collection 157
A74.81-A74.9, A96.2, A98.3-A98.4, B01.0, B01.12, B01.81-B01.9, B08.04, B33.24, B33.4-B33.8, B34.1-B34.2, B34.4-B34.8, B92, B94.2-B94.9, B97.10, B97.19, B97.29, B97.5-B97.6, B97.81-B97.89

PDX Collection 158
A74.81-A74.9, A96.2, A98.3-A98.4, B01.0-B01.12, B01.81-B01.9, B08.04, B33.24, B33.4-B33.8, B34.1-B34.2, B34.4-B34.8, B92, B94.2-B94.9, B97.10, B97.19, B97.29, B97.5-B97.6, B97.81-B97.89

PDX Collection 159
A74.81-A74.9, A96.2, A98.3-A98.4, B00.82, B01.0, B01.12, B01.81-B01.9, B02.24, B08.04, B33.24, B33.4-B33.8, B34.1-B34.2, B34.4-B34.8, B92, B94.2-B94.9, B97.10, B97.19, B97.29, B97.5-B97.6, B97.81-B97.89, G04.00-G04.01, G04.31, G04.81-G04.89, G05.3-G05.4, G37.3

PDX Collection 160
A74.81-A74.9, A96.2, A98.3-A98.4, B01.0, B01.12-B01.9, B08.04, B33.24, B33.4-B33.8, B34.1-B34.2, B34.4-B34.8, B92, B94.2-B94.9, B97.10, B97.19, B97.29, B97.5-B97.6, B97.81-B97.89

PDX Collection 161
A74.81-A74.9, A96.2, A98.3-A98.4, B00.3, B00.82-B00.9, B02.0-B02.29, B02.7-B02.9, B10.81-B10.89, B33.24, B33.4-B33.8, B34.1-B34.2, B34.4-B34.8, B92, B94.2-B94.9, B97.10, B97.19, B97.29, B97.5-B97.6, B97.81-B97.89

PDX Collection 162
A02.21, A17.0-A17.1, A27.81, A39.0, A50.41, A51.41, A52.13, A54.82, A54.84, A54.89-A54.9, A74.81-A74.9, A87.0-A87.9, A96.2, A98.3-A98.4, B00.3, B00.82-B00.9, B02.0-B02.29, B02.7-B02.9, B10.81-B10.89, B26.1, B33.24, B33.4, B33.8, B34.1-B34.2, B34.4-B34.8, B37.5, B38.4, B45.1, B58.2, B92, B94.2-B94.9, B97.10, B97.19, B97.29, B97.5-B97.6, B97.81-B97.89, G00.0-G03.9, G04.2, G32.89, G61.0, G96.8-G96.9, G98.0-G98.8, G99.8

PDX Collection 163
A74.81-A74.9, A96.2, A98.3-A98.4, B00.3, B00.82-B00.9, B01.12, B02.0-B02.29, B02.7-B02.9, B10.81-B10.89, B33.24, B33.4-B33.8, B34.1-B34.2, B34.4-B34.8, B92, B94.2-B94.9, B97.10, B97.19, B97.29, B97.5-B97.6, B97.81-B97.89, G04.00-G04.01, G04.31, G04.81-G04.89, G05.3-G05.4, G37.3

PDX Collection 164
B02.30-B02.39

PDX Collection 165
A60.00-A60.9, A74.81-A74.9, A96.2, A98.3-A98.4, B00.0-B00.2, B00.4-B00.9, B02.0-B02.9, B10.01-B10.89, B33.24, B33.4-B33.8, B34.1-B34.2, B34.4, B34.8, B92, B94.2-B94.9, B97.10, B97.19, B97.29, B97.5-B97.6, B97.81-B97.89

PDX Collection 166
B01.0-B01.9, B03, B08.010-B08.04

PDX Collection 167
B04, B08.010-B08.011, B08.09, B08.3, B08.60-B08.79, B09, L44.4

PDX Collection 168
A74.81-A74.9, A96.2, A98.3-A98.4, B05.0-B05.1, B05.4, B05.89-B05.9, B33.24, B33.4-B33.8, B34.1-B34.2, B34.4-B34.8, B92, B94.2-B94.9, B97.10, B97.19, B97.29, B97.5-B97.6, B97.81-B97.89

PDX Collection 169
A74.81-A74.9, A96.2, A98.3-A98.4, B05.1, B05.4,
B05.89-B05.9, B33.24, B33.4-B33.8, B34.1-B34.2,
B34.4-B34.8, B92, B94.2-B94.9, B97.10, B97.19, B97.29,
B97.5-B97.6, B97.81-B97.89

PDX Collection 170
A74.81-A74.9, A96.2, A98.3-A98.4, B05.1-B05.2, B05.4,
B05.89-B05.9, B33.24, B33.4-B33.8, B34.1-B34.2,
B34.4-B34.8, B92, B94.2-B94.9, B97.10, B97.19, B97.29,
B97.5-B97.6, B97.81-B97.89

PDX Collection 171
A74.81-A74.9, A96.2, A98.3-A98.4, B05.1, B05.4,
B05.81-B05.9, B33.24, B33.4-B33.8, B34.1-B34.2,
B34.4-B34.8, B92, B94.2-B94.9, B97.10, B97.19, B97.29,
B97.5-B97.6, B97.81-B97.89

PDX Collection 172
A74.81-A74.9, A96.2, A98.3-A98.4, B05.1, B05.4,
B05.81-B05.9, B06.00-B06.81, B06.89-B06.9, B33.24,
B33.4-B33.8, B34.1-B34.2, B34.4-B34.8, B92, B94.2-B94.9,
B97.10, B97.19, B97.29, B97.5-B97.6, B97.81-B97.89

PDX Collection 173
A74.81-A74.9, A96.2, A98.3-A98.4, B05.1, B05.4,
B05.81-B05.9, B06.81-B06.82, B06.89-B06.9, B33.24,
B33.4-B33.8, B34.1-B34.2, B34.4-B34.8, B92, B94.2-B94.9,
B97.10, B97.19, B97.29, B97.5-B97.6, B97.81-B97.89

PDX Collection 174
B08.3, B34.3

PDX Collection 175
A74.81-A74.9, A96.2, A98.3-A98.4, B15.0-B19.9, B33.24,
B33.4-B33.8, B34.1-B34.2, B34.4-B34.8, B92, B94.2-B94.9,
B97.10, B97.19, B97.29, B97.5-B97.6, B97.81-B97.89

PDX Collection 176
B20, B92, B94.2-B94.9

PDX Collection 177
B25.2, K85.00-K86.1, K86.81-K86.9

PDX Collection 178
A96.0-A96.9, A98.3-A98.5, B25.8-B25.9, B33.24-B34.2,
B34.4-B34.8, B97.0-B97.32, B97.39, B97.5-B97.89

PDX Collection 179
A74.81-A74.9, A96.2, A98.3-A98.4, B26.0, B26.82-B26.83,
B26.85-B26.9, B33.24, B33.4-B33.8, B34.1-B34.8, B92,
B94.2-B94.9, B97.10, B97.19, B97.29, B97.5-B97.6,
B97.81-B97.89

PDX Collection 180
A02.21, A17.0-A17.1, A27.81, A39.0, A50.41, A51.41,
A52.13, A54.82, A54.84, A54.89-A54.9, A74.81-A74.9,
A87.0-A87.9, A96.2, A98.3-A98.4, B00.3, B02.1, B26.1,
B26.82-B26.83, B26.85-B26.9, B33.24, B33.4-B33.8,
B34.1-B34.2, B34.4-B34.8, B37.5, B38.4, B45.1, B58.2, B92,
B94.2, B94.8-B94.9, B97.10, B97.19, B97.29, B97.5-B97.6,
B97.81-B97.89, G00.0-G03.9, G04.2, G32.89, G61.0,
G96.8-G96.9, G98.0-G98.8, G99.8

PDX Collection 181
A74.81-A74.9, A96.2, A98.3-A98.4, B26.2, B26.82-B26.83,
B26.85-B26.9, B33.24, B33.4, B33.8, B34.1-B34.2,
B34.4-B34.8, B92, B94.2, B94.8-B94.9, B97.10, B97.19,
B97.29, B97.5-B97.6, B97.81-B97.89

PDX Collection 182
A74.81-A74.9, A96.2, A98.3-A98.4, B26.3, B26.82-B26.83,
B26.85-B26.9, B33.24, B33.4, B33.8, B34.1-B34.2,
B34.4-B34.8, B92, B94.2, B94.8-B94.9, B97.10, B97.19,
B97.29, B97.5-B97.6, B97.81-B97.89

PDX Collection 183
A74.81-A74.9, A96.2, A98.3-A98.4, B26.81-B26.83,
B26.85-B26.9, B33.24, B33.4, B33.8, B34.1-B34.2,

B34.4-B34.8, B92, B94.2, B94.8-B94.9, B97.10, B97.19,
B97.29, B97.5-B97.6, B97.81-B97.89

PDX Collection 184
A74.81-A74.9, A96.2, A98.3-A98.4, B26.82-B26.83,
B26.85-B26.9, B33.24, B33.4, B33.8, B34.1-B34.2,
B34.4-B34.8, B92, B94.2, B94.8-B94.9, B97.10, B97.19,
B97.29, B97.5-B97.6, B97.81-B97.89

PDX Collection 185
A74.81-A74.9, A96.2, A98.3-A98.4, B26.82-B26.9, B33.24,
B33.4, B33.8, B34.1-B34.2, B34.4-B34.8, B92, B94.2,
B94.8-B94.9, B97.10, B97.19, B97.29, B97.5-B97.6,
B97.81-B97.89

PDX Collection 186
A52.06, B33.20-B33.22, I00, I01.2-I01.9, I09.0, I09.9,
I23.0-I23.3, I23.6-I23.8, I40.0-I41, I51.0, I51.4, I87.8-I87.9,
I99.8-I99.9

PDX Collection 187
A01.00-A01.09, A39.51, A52.03, A78, B33.21, B37.6,
B40.0-B40.9, I00, I01.1, I01.8-I02.0, I05.0-I07.9, I08.1-I08.3,
I08.9, I09.1, I09.89-I09.9, I33.0-I39, I42.4, I87.8-I87.9,
I99.8-I99.9, Q22.2, Q23.8-Q23.9, Q24.8, T82.6XXA

PDX Collection 188
B33.23, I01.0, I09.2, I30.0-I30.9, I31.3-I32, I87.8-I87.9,
I99.8-I99.9

PDX Collection 189
A74.81-A74.9, A88.1, A96.0-A96.9, A98.3-A98.5,
B19.20-B19.21, B25.8-B25.9, B33.24, B33.3-B34.2,
B34.4-B34.8, B97.0-B97.89

PDX Collection 190
B37.0-B37.9, B48.3, B49, B92, B94.2-B94.9

PDX Collection 191
B37.1, B37.41-B37.82, B37.84-B37.9, N25.81-N25.89

PDX Collection 192
A02.21, A17.0-A17.1, A27.81, A39.0, A50.41, A51.41,
A52.13, A54.82, A54.84, A54.89-A54.9, A87.0-A87.9, B00.3,
B02.1, B26.1, B37.0-B38.4, B45.1, B48.3, B49, B58.2,
B92, B94.2-B94.9, G00.0-G03.9, G04.2, G32.89, G61.0,
G96.8-G96.9, G98.0, G98.8-G99.8

PDX Collection 193
A02.1, A20.7, A22.7, A26.7, A32.7, A39.2-A39.4, A40.0-A40.1,
A40.8-A41.9, A42.7, A48.2-A48.4, A48.8-A49.9, A54.86,
B00.7, B37.0-B37.9, B48.3, B49, B92, B94.2-B96.89,
R65.10-R65.20, Z16.10-Z16.39

PDX Collection 194
B37.1, B37.5-B37.82, B37.84-B37.9

PDX Collection 195
B38.0-B38.2, B38.7, B38.89-B38.9, B48.3, B49, B92,
B94.2-B94.9

PDX Collection 196
B38.0-B39.9

PDX Collection 197
B38.0-B38.9

PDX Collection 198
A02.21, A17.0-A17.1, A39.0, A50.41, A51.41, A52.13,
A54.82, A54.84, A54.89-A54.9, A87.0-A87.9, B00.3, B02.1,
B26.1, B37.5, B38.4-B38.87, B38.89-B38.9, B45.1, B48.3,
B49, B58.2, B92, B94.2-B94.9, G00.0-G03.9, G04.2, G32.89,
G61.0, G96.8-G96.9, G98.0, G98.8-G99.8

PDX Collection 199
B38.7, B38.89-B38.9, B48.3, B49, B92, B94.2-B94.9

PDX Collection 200
A22.1, A37.01-A37.11, A37.81, A37.9, A48.1, B25.0,
B39.0-B39.4, B39.9-B44.0, B48.3, B49, B92, B94.2-B94.9,
J09.X1-J09.X2, J10.00-J10.1, J11.00-J11.1, J12.0-J12.3,

J12.89-J18.1, J18.8-J18.9, J44.9, J47.0-J47.9, J60-J70.4,
J70.8-J70.9, J98.4, R91.1

PDX Collection 201
B38.0-B39.4

PDX Collection 202
B40.0-B40.9, B48.3, B49, B92, B94.2-B94.9

PDX Collection 203
B41.0-B41.9, B48.3, B49, B92, B94.2-B94.9

PDX Collection 204
B44.1-B44.7, B44.89-B44.9, B48.3-B48.4, B49, B92,
B94.2-B94.9

PDX Collection 205
B44.81, J22, J98.8-J98.9

PDX Collection 206
B45.0, B45.2-B45.9, B48.3, B49, B92, B94.2-B94.9

PDX Collection 207
A02.21, A17.0-A17.1, A27.81, A39.0, A50.41, A51.41,
A52.13, A54.82, A54.84, A54.89-A54.9, A87.0-A87.9, B00.3,
B02.1, B26.1, B37.5, B38.4, B45.1, B58.2, E08.40-E08.49,
E08.618-E08.638, E08.649-E08.8, E09.40-E09.49,
E09.618-E09.638, E09.649-E09.8, E10.40-E10.49,
E10.618-E10.638, E10.649, E10.69, E10.8, E11.40-E11.49,
E11.618-E11.638, E11.649, E11.69-E11.8, E13.40-E13.49,
E13.618-E13.638, E13.649-E13.69, E13.8, G00.0-G03.9,
G04.2, G32.89, G61.0, G96.8-G96.9, G98.0-G98.8, G99.8

PDX Collection 208
B46.0-B46.9, B48.3, B49, B92, B94.2-B94.9

PDX Collection 209
B47.0, B48.3, B49, B92, B94.2-B94.9

PDX Collection 210
A42.81-A42.9, A43.8-A43.9, B47.1-B47.9

PDX Collection 211
B48.2-B48.3, B49, B92, B94.2-B94.9

PDX Collection 212
B48.3, B49

PDX Collection 213
B48.3, B48.8-B49, B92, B94.2-B94.9

PDX Collection 214
B50.0-B57.5

PDX Collection 215
A44.0-A44.9, A68.0-A68.9, A69.20-A69.29, B50.0-B57.5,
B60.0

PDX Collection 216
A17.9, A18.10-A18.13, A18.82, A18.84, A18.89, A54.21,
A54.29, A54.82, A54.84, A54.89-A54.9, A59.00, A59.8-A59.9,
B37.41-B37.49, B50.0-B57.5, E08.21-E08.29, E08.618,
E08.620-E08.638, E08.649-E08.8, E09.21-E09.29,
E09.618-E09.638, E09.649-E09.8, E10.21-E10.29,
E10.618-E10.638, E10.649, E10.69-E10.8, E11.21-E11.29,
E11.618-E11.638, E11.649, E11.69-E11.8, E13.21-E13.29,
E13.618-E13.638, E13.649-E13.8, E88.3, M10.30-M10.39,
N00.0-N11.0, N11.8-N13.39, N13.6, N14.0-N19, N25.0-N26.1,
N26.9-N27.9, N28.1-N29, N36.41-N36.43, N36.8-N36.9,
N39.8-N39.9, R31.0-R31.9

PDX Collection 217
B50.0-B57.5, B97.21

PDX Collection 218
A44.0-A44.9, A68.0-A68.9, A69.20-A69.29, A75.0-A79.9,
B50.0-B57.5, B60.0

PDX Collection 219
B57.0, B57.2, B92, B94.2-B94.9

PDX Collection 220
B58.00, B58.82-B58.9, B92, B94.2-B94.9

1631

PDX Collection 221
B58.00-B58.01, B58.82-B58.9, B92, B94.2-B94.4

PDX Collection 222
B58.00, B58.09, B58.82-B58.9, B92, B94.2-B94.9

PDX Collection 223
B58.00, B58.1, B58.82-B58.9, B92, B94.2-B94.9

PDX Collection 224
B58.00, B58.2, B58.82-B58.9, B92, B94.2-B94.9

PDX Collection 225
A22.1, A37.01, A37.11, A37.81, A37.91, A48.1, B25.0,
B44.0, B58.00, B58.3, B58.82-B58.9, B92, B94.2-B94.9,
J09.X1-J09.X2, J10.00-J10.1, J11.00-J11.1, J12.0-J12.3,
J12.89-J18.1, J18.8-J18.9, J44.9, J47.0-J70.4, J70.8-J70.9,
J98.4, R91.1

PDX Collection 226
B58.00, B58.81-B58.9, B92, B94.2-B94.9

PDX Collection 227
B58.9

PDX Collection 228
A22.1, A37.01, A37.11, A37.81, A37.91, A48.1, B25.0,
B44.0, B59, B92, B94.2-B94.9, J09.X1-J09.X2, J10.00-J10.1,
J11.00-J11.1, J12.0-J12.3, J12.89-J15.20, J15.211-J18.1,
J18.8-J18.9, J44.9, J47.0-J70.4, J70.8-J70.9, J98.4, R91.1

PDX Collection 229
B59, B60.10-B60.11, B60.19-B64, B89, B99.8-B99.9, L94.6,
M35.2

PDX Collection 230
B65.0-B65.9

PDX Collection 231
B66.0-B66.9

PDX Collection 232
B67.0, B67.8-B67.99

PDX Collection 233
B67.1, B67.8-B67.99, J12.81

PDX Collection 234
B67.2, B67.32-B67.39, B67.8-B67.99

PDX Collection 235
B67.31, B67.8-B67.99

PDX Collection 236
B67.4, B67.8-B67.99

PDX Collection 237
B67.5, B67.8-B67.99

PDX Collection 238
B67.61-B67.69, B67.8-B67.99

PDX Collection 239
B67.7-B67.99

PDX Collection 240
B67.8-B67.99

PDX Collection 241
A00.1, A01.00-A01.09, A01.4-A02.0, A03.9-A05.2,
A06.0-A06.2, A06.9, A07.1-A09, A18.32-A18.39, A18.83,
A48.51-A48.52, B37.82, B68.0-B71.9, B82.9, J09.X3-J09.X9,
J10.2-J10.89, J11.2-J11.89, K30, K31.84, K52.1-K52.3,
K52.82-K52.9, K58.0-K58.9, P76.8-P77.9, P78.1, P78.3-P78.89

PDX Collection 242
B68.0-B71.9

PDX Collection 243
B72-B74.9

PDX Collection 244
A17.82, A50.42, A52.14, A75.9, A79.9, A81.1, A81.82-A81.89,
A83.0-A85.8, A87.2, A88.0, A88.8, A92.1-A92.8, A93.0, B00.4,
B00.82, B01.11-B01.12, B04, B06.01, B08.09, B08.20-B08.22,
B08.60-B08.79, B09, B10.01-B10.09, B26.2, B33.1, B45.0,

B45.2-B45.9, B58.2, B75, B97.10, B97.21, G04.00-G04.01,
G04.31, G04.81-G05.4, G37.0, G37.4-G37.5, J09.X3-J09.X9,
J10.2-J10.89, J11.2-J11.89, L44.4, M1A.10X0-M1A.10X1,
M1A.1110-M1A.19X1, P35.2-P35.9, P37.0-P37.4, P37.8-P37.9,
T56.0X1-T56.0X4[A]

PDX Collection 245
B76.0-B76.9

PDX Collection 246
B77.0-B78.0, B78.7-B82.0

PDX Collection 247
A15.0-A15.6, A15.8-A15.9, A17.9, A18.82, A18.84, A18.89,
A21.2, A22.1, A31.0, A37.01, A37.11, A37.81, A37.91, A42.0,
A43.0, A48.1, B25.0, B39.0-B39.2, B44.0, B58.3, B59, B67.1,
B77.0-B78.0, B78.7-B82.0, J09.X1-J09.X2, J10.00-J10.1,
J11.00-J11.1, J12.0-J12.3, J12.89-J18.1, J18.8-J18.9, J22,
J44.9, J47.0-J70.4, J70.8-J70.9, J98.4, J98.8-J99, Q33.4,
R91.1

PDX Collection 248
B77.0-B78.0, B78.7-B83.3, B83.8-B83.9

PDX Collection 249
A15.0-A15.6, A15.8-A15.9, A17.9, A18.82, A18.84, A18.89,
A21.2, A22.1, A31.0, A37.01, A37.11, A37.81, A37.91, A42.0,
A43.0, A48.1, B25.0, B34.1-B34.2, B34.4-B34.8, B39.0-B39.2,
B44.0, B58.3, B59, B67.1, B97.19-B97.29, B97.5-B97.6,
B97.81-B97.89, J09.X1-J09.X2, J10.00-J10.1, J11.00-J11.1,
J12.0-J12.3, J12.89-J15.20, J15.211-J18.1, J18.8-J18.9, J22,
J44.9, J47.0-J70.4, J70.8-J70.9, J98.4, J98.8-J99, Q33.4,
R91.1

PDX Collection 250
A74.81, A74.9, B33.3-B33.4, B34.1-B34.2, B34.4-B34.8,
B97.10, B97.19-B97.29, B97.31-B97.39, B97.5-B97.6,
B97.81-B97.89

PDX Collection 251
A74.81, A74.9, B33.3-B33.4, B34.1-B34.2, B34.4-B34.8,
B97.10, B97.19-B97.39, B97.5-B97.6, B97.81, B97.89

PDX Collection 252
A74.81, A74.9, B20, B33.3-B33.4, B34.1-B34.2, B34.4, B34.8,
B97.10, B97.19-B97.39, B97.5-B97.6, B97.81, B97.89

PDX Collection 253
C15.3-C15.9, C26.0, C26.9, C45.7-C45.9, C46.4, C76.8, C7A.00,
C7A.098-C7B.00, C7B.1, C80.0-C80.2, D49.0, D49.81-D49.9

PDX Collection 254
C16.0-C16.9, C26.0, C26.9, C45.7-C45.9, C46.4, C49.A2, C76.8,
C7A.00, C7A.092, C7A.094-C7B.00, C7B.1, C80.0-C80.2, D49.0,
D49.81-D49.9

PDX Collection 255
C17.0, C17.8-C17.9, C26.0, C26.9, C45.7-C45.9, C46.4,
C76.8, C7A.00-C7A.010, C7A.019, C7A.098-C7B.00, C7B.1,
C80.0-C80.2, D49.0, D49.81-D49.9

PDX Collection 256
C17.1, C17.8-C17.9, C26.0, C26.9, C45.7-C45.9, C46.4, C76.8,
C7A.00, C7A.011, C7A.019, C7A.098, C7A.1-C7B.00, C7B.1,
C80.0-C80.2, D49.0, D49.81-D49.9

PDX Collection 257
C17.2, C17.8-C17.9, C26.0, C26.9, C45.7-C45.9, C46.4, C76.8,
C7A.00, C7A.012-C7A.019, C7A.098, C7A.1-C7B.00, C7B.1,
C80.0-C80.2, D49.0, D49.81-D49.9

PDX Collection 258
C17.3-C17.9, C26.0, C26.9, C45.7-C45.9, C46.4, C76.8,
C7A.00, C7A.019, C7A.098-C7B.00, C7B.1, C80.0-C80.2, D49.0,
D49.81-D49.9

PDX Collection 259
C17.8-C17.9, C26.0, C26.9, C45.7-C45.9, C46.4, C76.8, C7A.00,
C7A.019, C7A.098, C7A.1-C7B.00, C7B.1, C80.0-C80.2, D49.0,
D49.81-D49.9

PDX Collection 260
C18.0, C18.8-C18.9, C26.0-C26.9, C45.7-C45.9, C46.4,
C76.8, C7A.00, C7A.021, C7A.029, C7A.098-C7B.00, C7B.1,
C80.0-C80.2, D49.0, D49.81-D49.9

PDX Collection 261
C18.1, C18.8-C18.9, C26.0, C26.9, C45.7-C45.9, C46.4, C76.8,
C7A.00, C7A.020, C7A.029, C7A.098, C7A.1-C7B.00, C7B.1,
C80.0-C80.2, D49.0, D49.81-D49.9

PDX Collection 262
C18.2, C18.8-C18.9, C26.0, C26.9, C45.7-C45.9, C46.4, C76.8,
C7A.00, C7A.022, C7A.029, C7A.098, C7A.1-C7B.00, C7B.1,
C80.0-C80.2, D49.0, D49.81-D49.9

PDX Collection 263
C18.3, C18.8-C18.9, C26.0, C26.9, C45.7-C45.9, C46.4, C76.8,
C7A.00, C7A.029, C7A.098-C7B.00, C7B.1, C80.0-C80.2, D49.0,
D49.81-D49.9

PDX Collection 264
C18.4, C18.8-C18.9, C26.0, C26.9, C45.7-C45.9, C46.4, C76.8,
C7A.00, C7A.023, C7A.029, C7A.098, C7A.1-C7B.00, C7B.1,
C80.0-C80.2, D49.0, D49.81-D49.9

PDX Collection 265
C18.5, C18.8-C18.9, C26.0, C26.9, C45.7-C45.9, C46.4, C76.8,
C7A.00, C7A.029, C7A.098-C7B.00, C7B.1, C80.0-C80.2, D49.0,
D49.81-D49.9

PDX Collection 266
C18.6, C18.8-C18.9, C26.0, C26.9, C45.7-C45.9, C46.4,
C76.8, C7A.00, C7A.024, C7A.029, C7A.098-C7B.00, C7B.1,
C80.0-C80.2, D49.0, D49.81-D49.9

PDX Collection 267
C18.7-C18.9, C26.0, C26.9, C45.7-C45.9, C46.4, C76.8,
C7A.00, C7A.025, C7A.029, C7A.098, C7A.1-C7B.00, C7B.1,
C80.0-C80.2, D49.0, D49.81-D49.9

PDX Collection 268
C18.8-C18.9, C26.0, C26.9, C45.7-C45.9, C46.4, C76.8, C7A.00,
C7A.029, C7A.098, C7A.1-C7B.00, C7B.1, C80.0-C80.2, D49.0,
D49.81-D49.9

PDX Collection 269
C19, C21.2-C21.8, C26.0, C26.9, C45.7-C45.9, C46.4, C76.8,
C7A.00, C7A.098, C7A.1-C7B.00, C7B.1, C80.0-C80.2, D49.0,
D49.81-D49.9

PDX Collection 270
C20, C21.2-C21.8, C26.0, C26.9, C45.7-C45.9, C46.4, C76.8,
C7A.00, C7A.026, C7A.098, C7A.1-C7B.00, C7B.1, C80.0-C80.2,
D49.0, D49.81-D49.9

PDX Collection 271
C21.0-C21.8, C26.0, C26.9, C45.7-C45.9, C46.4, C76.8,
C7A.00, C7A.098, C7A.1-C7B.00, C7B.1, C80.0-C80.2, D49.0,
D49.81-D49.9

PDX Collection 272
C21.2-C21.8, C26.0, C26.9, C45.7-C45.9, C46.4, C76.8,
C7A.00, C7A.098, C7A.1-C7B.00, C7B.1, C80.0-C80.2, D49.0,
D49.81-D49.9

PDX Collection 273
C22.0-C22.9, C26.0, C26.9, C45.7-C45.9, C46.4, C76.8,
C7A.00, C7A.098, C7A.1-C7B.00, C7B.1, C80.0-C80.2, D49.0,
D49.81-D49.9

PDX Collection 274
C23, C24.8-C24.9, C26.0, C26.9, C45.7-C45.9, C46.4, C76.8,
C7A.00, C7A.098, C7A.1-C7B.00, C7B.1, C8.00-C8.02, D49.0,
D49.81-D49.9

PDX Collection 275
C24.0, C24.8-C24.9, C26.0, C26.9, C45.7-C45.9, C46.4,
C76.8, C7A.00, C7A.098-C7B.00, C7B.1, C80.0-C80.2, D49.0,
D49.81-D49.9

PDX Collection 276
C24.1, C24.8-C24.9, C26.0, C26.9, C45.7-C45.9, C46.4, C76.8, C7A.00, C7A.098, C7A.1, C7A.8, C7B.00, C7B.1, C80.0-C80.2, D49.0, D49.81-D49.9

PDX Collection 277
C24.8-C24.9, C26.0, C26.9, C45.7-C45.9, C46.4, C76.8, C7A.00, C7A.098-C7A.8, C7B.00, C7B.1, C80.0-C80.2, D49.0, D49.81-D49.9

PDX Collection 278
C25.0-C26.0, C26.9, C45.7-C45.9, C46.4, C76.8, C7A.00, C7A.098, C7A.1-C7B.00, C7B.1, C8.00-C80.2, D49.0, D49.81-D49.9

PDX Collection 279
C33, C34.00-C34.92, C39.9, C45.7-C45.9, C46.50-C46.52, C76.1, C76.8, C78.00-C78.1, C78.30-C78.39, C7A.00, C7A.090, C7A.098-C7B.00, C7B.1, C80.0-C80.2, D49.1, D49.81-D49.9

PDX Collection 280
C34.00-C34.02, C34.80-C34.92, C39.9, C45.7-C45.9, C46.50-C46.52, C76.8, C7A.00, C7A.090, C7A.098, C7A.1-C7B.00, C7B.1, C80.0-C80.2, D49.1, D49.81-D49.9

PDX Collection 281
C34.10-C34.12, C34.80-C34.92, C39.9, C45.7-C45.9, C46.50-C46.52, C76.8, C7A.00, C7A.090, C7A.098-C7B.00, C7B.1, C80.0-C80.2, D49.1, D49.81-D49.9

PDX Collection 282
C34.2, C34.80-C34.92, C39.9, C45.7-C45.9, C46.50-C46.52, C76.8, C7A.00, C7A.090, C7A.098-C7B.00, C7B.1, C80.0-C80.2, D49.1, D49.81-D49.9

PDX Collection 283
C34.30-C34.92, C39.9, C45.7-C45.9, C46.50-C46.52, C76.8, C7A.00, C7A.090, C7A.098-C7B.00, C7B.1, C80.0-C80.2, D49.1, D49.81-D49.9

PDX Collection 284
C34.80-C34.92, C39.9, C45.7-C45.9, C46.50-C46.52, C76.8, C7A.00, C7A.090, C7A.098-C7B.00, C7B.1, C80.0-C80.2, D49.1, D49.81-D49.9

PDX Collection 285
C37, C7A.091

PDX Collection 286
C38.0, C45.2

PDX Collection 287
C38.1-C38.3, C38.8, C39.9, C45.7-C45.9, C76.8, C7A.00, C7A.098-C7B.00, C7B.1, C80.0-C80.2, D49.1, D49.81-D49.9

PDX Collection 288
C38.4, C39.9, C45.0, C45.7-C45.9, C76.8, C7A.00, C7A.098, C7A.1-C7B.00, C7B.1, C80.0-C80.2, D49.1, D49.81-D49.9

PDX Collection 289
C40.00-C40.02, C40.80-C40.92, C41.9, Z51.0

PDX Collection 290
C40.10-C40.12, C40.80-C40.92, C41.9, Z51.0

PDX Collection 291
C40.20-C40.22, C40.80-C40.92, C41.9, Z51.0

PDX Collection 292
C40.30-C40.92, C41.9, Z51.0

PDX Collection 293
C40.00-C41.9, Z51.0

PDX Collection 294
C40.80-C41.0, C41.9, Z51.0

PDX Collection 295
C40.80-C40.92, C41.1, C41.9, Z51.0

PDX Collection 296
C40.80-C40.9, C41.2, C41.9, Z51.0

PDX Collection 297
C40.80-C40.92, C41.3, C41.9, Z51.0

PDX Collection 298
C40.80-C40.92, C41.4-C41.9, Z51.0

PDX Collection 299
C45.1, C48.0-C48.8, Z51.0

PDX Collection 300
C46.0, C46.7-C46.9, Z51.0

PDX Collection 301
C46.1, C46.7-C46.9, Z51.0

PDX Collection 302
C46.2, C46.7-C46.9, Z51.0

PDX Collection 303
C45.7-C45.9, C46.3, C76.8-C77.9, C7A.00, C7A.098-C7B.01, C7B.1, C80.0-C80.2, D49.81-D49.9

PDX Collection 304
C46.4, C46.7-C46.9, Z51.0

PDX Collection 305
C46.0-C46.9, Z51.0

PDX Collection 306
C45.7-C46.9, C51.0-C72.9, C76.0-C79.9, C7A.00, C7A.093, C7A.098-C7B.8, C80.0-C80.2, D00.00-D02.4, D04.0-D09.9, D37.01-D44.9, D48.0-D49.9, Z51.0

PDX Collection 307
Z51.0

PDX Collection 308
C48.0, Z51.0

PDX Collection 309
C45.9, C56.1-C57.4, C76.3, C79.60-C79.62, C7A.00, C7A.098-C7B.00, C7B.1, C80.0-C80.2

PDX Collection 310
C45.7-C45.9, C64.1-C65.9, C68.8-C68.9, C76.8, C7A.00, C7A.093, C7A.098-C7B.00, C7B.1, C80.0-C80.2, D49.511-D49.59, D49.81-D49.9

PDX Collection 311
C45.7-C45.9, C66.1-C66.9, C68.8-C68.9, C76.8, C7A.00, C7A.098, C7A.1-C7B.00, C7B.1, C80.0-C80.2, D49.511-D49.59, D49.81-D49.9

PDX Collection 312
C68.0-C68.9, C79.82

PDX Collection 313
C6.41-C66.9, C68.0-C68.9, C76.3, C79.00-C79.19, C7A.093

PDX Collection 314
C45.7-C45.9, C70.0, C70.9, C72.9, C76.8, C7A.00, C7A.098-C7B.00, C7B.1, C80.0-C80.2, D49.6-D49.9

PDX Collection 315
C45.7-C45.9, C70.1, C72.9, C76.8, C7A.00, C7A.098-C7B.00, C7B.1, C80.0-C80.2, D49.6-D49.9

PDX Collection 316
C45.7-C45.9, C70.0, C70.9-C71.9, C72.20-C72.9, C76.8, C7A.00, C7A.098-C7B.00, C7B.1, C80.0-C80.2, D49.6-D49.9

PDX Collection 317
C45.7-C45.9, C72.0-C72.1, C72.9, C76.8, C7A.00, C7A.098, C7A.1-C7B.00, C7B.1, C80.0-C80.2, D49.6-D49.9

PDX Collection 318
C45.7-C45.9, C72.20-C72.9, C76.8, C7A.00, C7A.098-C7B.00, C7B.1, C80.0-C80.2, D49.6-D49.9

PDX Collection 319
C45.7-C45.9, C70.0-C72.9, C76.8, C79.31-C79.49, C7A.00, C7A.098-C7B.00, C7B.1, C80.0-C80.2, D49.6-D49.9

PDX Collection 320
C45.7-C45.9, C74.00-C74.92, C75.9, C76.2, C76.8, C79.70-C79.72, C7A.00, C7A.098-C7B.00, C7B.1, C80.0-C80.2

PDX Collection 321
C75.0, C75.8-C75.9

PDX Collection 322
C75.1-C75.2, Z51.0

PDX Collection 323
C75.3, Z51.0

PDX Collection 324
C75.4, C75.8-C75.9

PDX Collection 325
C75.4-C75.9

PDX Collection 326
C74.00-C75.9

PDX Collection 327
C45.7-C45.9, C76.8, C78.00-C78.39, C79.89-C79.9, C7A.00, C7A.098-C7B.00, C7B.09-C7B.8, C80.0-C80.2, D49.81-D49.9

PDX Collection 328
C45.7-C45.9, C76.8, C78.1, C78.30-C78.39, C79.89-C79.9, C7A.00, C7A.098-C7B.00, C7B.09-C7B.8, C80.0-C80.2, D49.81-D49.9

PDX Collection 329
C45.7-C45.9, C76.8, C78.2-C78.39, C79.89-C79.9, C7A.00, C7A.098-C7B.00, C7B.09-C7B.8, C80.0-C80.2, D49.81-D49.9, J91.0

PDX Collection 330
C45.7-C45.9, C76.8, C78.00-C78.39, C79.89-C79.9, C7A.00, C7A.098-C7B.00, C7B.09-C7B.8, C80.0-C80.2, D49.81-D49.9

PDX Collection 331
C45.7-C45.9, C76.8, C78.4, C78.80-C78.89, C79.89-C79.9, C7A.00, C7A.098-C7B.00, C7B.09-C7B.8, C80.0-C80.2, D49.81-D49.9

PDX Collection 332
C45.7-C45.9, C76.8, C78.5, C78.80-C78.89, C79.89-C79.9, C7A.00, C7A.098-C7B.00, C7B.09-C7B.8, C80.0-C80.2, D49.81-D49.9

PDX Collection 333
C45.7-C45.9, C76.8, C78.6, C78.80-C78.89, C79.89-C79.9, C7A.00, C7A.098-C7B.00, C7B.04-C7B.8, C80.0-C80.2, D49.81-D49.9

PDX Collection 334
C45.7-C45.9, C76.8, C78.7-C78.89, C79.89-C79.9, C7A.00, C7A.098-C7A.8, C7B.00, C7B.02, C7B.09-C7B.8, C80.0-C80.2, D49.81-D4.99

PDX Collection 335
C45.7-C45.9, C76.8, C78.4-C78.89, C79.89-C79.9, C7A.00, C7A.098-C7B.00, C7B.02, C7B.04-C7B.8, C80.0-C80.2, D49.81-D49.9

PDX Collection 336
C45.7-C45.9, C76.8, C79.00-C79.19, C79.89-C79.9, C7A.00, C7A.098-C7B.00, C7B.09-C7B.8, C80.0-C80.2, D49.81-D49.9

PDX Collection 337
C45.7-C45.9, C76.8, C79.2, C79.89-C79.9, C7A.00, C7A.098-C7B.00, C7B.09-C7B.8, C80.0-C80.2, D49.81-D49.9

PDX Collection 338
C45.7-C45.9, C76.8, C79.31, C79.89-C79.9, C7A.00, C7A.098-C7B.00, C7B.09-C7B.8, C80.0-C80.2, D49.81-D49.9

PDX Collection 339
C45.7-C45.9, C76.8, C79.32-C79.49, C79.89-C79.9, C7A.00, C7A.098-C7B.00, C7B.09-C7B.8, C80.0-C80.2, D49.81-D49.9

PDX Collection 340
C45.7-C45.9, C76.8, C79.51-C79.52, C79.89-C79.9, C7A.00, C7A.098-C7B.00, C7B.03, C7B.09-C7B.8, C80.0-C80.2, D49.81-D49.9

PDX Collection 341
C45.7-C45.9, C76.8, C79.60-C79.62, C79.89-C79.9, C7A.00, C7A.098-C7B.00, C7B.09-C7B.8, C80.0-C80.2, D49.81-D49.9

PDX Collection 342
C45.7-C45.9, C76.8, C79.70-C79.72, C79.89-C79.9, C7A.00, C7A.098-C7B.00, C7B.09-C7B.8, C80.0-C80.2, D49.81-D49.9

PDX Collection 343
C45.7-C45.9, C76.8, C79.81, C79.89-C79.9, C7A.00, C7A.098-C7B.00, C7B.09-C7B.8, C80.0-C80.2, D49.81-D49.9

PDX Collection 344
C45.7-C45.9, C76.8, C79.82-C79.9, C7A.00, C7A.098-C7B.00, C7B.09-C7B.8, C80.0-C80.2, D49.81-D49.9

PDX Collection 345
C45.7-C45.9, C76.8, C79.89-C79.9, C7A.00, C7A.098-C7B.00, C7B.09, C7B.1-C7B.8, C80.0-C80.2, D49.81-D49.9

PDX Collection 346
C45.7-C45.9, C76.8, C79.89-C79.9, C7A.00-C7B.00, C7B.09-C7B.8, C80.0-C80.2, D49.81-D49.9

PDX Collection 347
C17.0, C17.8-C17.9, C26.0, C26.9, C45.7-C45.9, C46.4, C76.8, C7A.00-C7B.00, C7B.1, C80.0-C80.2, D49.0, D49.81-D49.9

PDX Collection 348
C17.1, C17.8-C17.9, C26.0, C26.9, C45.7-C45.9, C46.4, C76.8, C7A.00-C7B.00, C7B.1, C80.0-C80.2, D49.0, D49.81-D49.9

PDX Collection 349
C17.2, C17.8-C17.9, C26.0, C26.9, C45.7-C45.9, C46.4, C76.8, C7A.00-C7B.00, C7B.1, C80.0-C80.2, D49.0, D49.81-D49.9

PDX Collection 350
C17.8-C17.9, C26.0, C26.9, C45.7-C45.9, C46.4, C76.8, C7A.00-C7B.00, C7B.1, C80.0-C80.2, D49.0, D49.81-D49.9

PDX Collection 351
C18.1, C18.8-C18.9, C26.0, C26.9, C45.7-C45.9, C46.4, C76.8, C7A.00-C7B.00, C7B.1, C80.0-C80.2, D49.0, D49.81-D49.9

PDX Collection 352
C18.0, C18.8-C18.9, C26.0, C26.9, C45.7-C45.9, C46.4, C76.8, C7A.00-C7B.00, C7B.1, C80.0-C80.2, D49.0, D49.81-D49.9

PDX Collection 353
C18.2, C18.8-C18.9, C26.0, C26.9, C45.7-C45.9, C46.4, C76.8, C7A.00-C7B.00, C7B.1, C80.0-C80.2, D49.0, D49.81-D49.9

PDX Collection 354
C18.4, C18.8-C18.9, C26.0, C26.9, C45.7-C45.9, C46.4, C76.8, C7A.00-C7B.00, C7B.1, C80.0-C80.2, D49.0, D49.81-D49.9

PDX Collection 355
C18.6, C18.8-C18.9, C26.0, C26.9, C45.7-C45.9, C46.4, C76.8, C7A.00-C7B.00, C7B.1, C80.0-C80.2, D49.0, D49.81-D49.9

PDX Collection 356
C18.7-C18.9, C26.0, C26.9, C45.7-C45.9, C46.4, C76.8, C7A.00-C7B.00, C7B.1, C80.0-C80.2, D49.0, D49.81-D49.9

PDX Collection 357
C20, C21.2-C21.8, C26.0, C26.9, C45.7-C45.9, C46.4, C76.8, C7A.00-C7B.00, C7B.1, C80.0-C80.2, D49.0, D49.81-D49.9

PDX Collection 358
C18.8-C18.9, C26.0, C26.9, C45.7-C45.9, C46.4, C76.8, C7A.00-C7B.00, C7B.1, C80.0-C80.2, D49.0, D49.81-D49.9

PDX Collection 359
C34.80-C34.92, C39.9, C45.7-C45.9, C46.50-C46.52, C76.8, C7A.00-C7B.00, C7B.1, C80.0-C80.2, D49.1, D49.81-D49.9

PDX Collection 360
C37, C7A.00-C7A.8

PDX Collection 361
C16.0-C16.9, C26.0, C26.9, C45.7-C45.9, C46.4, C49.A2, C76.8, C7A.00-C7B.00, C7B.1, C80.0-C80.2, D49.0, D49.81-D49.9

PDX Collection 362
C45.7-C45.9, C64.1-C65.9, C68.8-C68.9, C76.8, C7A.00-C7B.00, C7B.1, C80.0-C80.2, D49.511-D49.59, D49.81-D49.9

PDX Collection 363
C45.7-C45.9, C46.3, C76.8-C77.9, C7A.00, C7A.098-C7B.8, C80.0-C80.2, D49.81-D49.9

PDX Collection 364
C45.7-C45.9, C76.8, C78.7-C78.89, C79.89-C79.9, C7A.00, C7A.098-C7B.8, C80.0-C80.2, D49.81-D49.9

PDX Collection 365
C45.7-C45.9, C76.8, C79.51-C79.52, C79.89-C79.9, C7A.00, C7A.098-C7B.8, C80.0-C80.2, D49.81-D49.9

PDX Collection 366
C45.7-C45.9, C76.8, C78.6, C78.80-C78.89, C79.89-C79.9, C7A.00, C7A.098-C7B.8, C80.0-C80.2, D49.81-D49.9

PDX Collection 367
C45.7-C45.9, C76.8, C79.89-C79.9, C7A.00, C7A.098-C7B.8, C80.0-C80.2, D49.81-D49.9

PDX Collection 368
C81.00-C81.09, C81.40-C81.49, C81.90, C81.98, D49.81-D49.9

PDX Collection 369
C81.00-C81.01, C81.08-C81.09, C81.40-C81.41, C81.48-C81.49, C81.90-C81.91, C81.98, D49.81-D49.9

PDX Collection 370
C81.00-C81.02, C81.08-C81.09, C81.40-C81.42, C81.48-C81.49, C81.90-C81.92, C81.98, D49.81-D49.9

PDX Collection 371
C81.00, C81.03, C81.08-C81.09, C81.40, C81.43, C81.48-C81.49, C81.90, C81.93, C81.98, D49.81-D49.9

PDX Collection 372
C81.00, C81.04, C81.08-C81.09, C81.40, C81.44, C81.48-C81.49, C81.90, C81.94, C81.98, D49.81-D49.9

PDX Collection 373
C81.00, C81.05, C81.08-C81.09, C81.40, C81.45, C81.48-C81.49, C81.90, C81.95, C81.98, D49.81-D49.9

PDX Collection 374
C81.00, C81.06, C81.08-C81.09, C81.40, C81.46, C81.48-C81.49, C81.90, C81.96, C81.98, D49.81-D49.9

PDX Collection 375
C81.00, C81.07-C81.09, C81.40, C81.47-C81.49, C81.90, C81.97-C81.98, D49.81-D49.9

PDX Collection 376
C81.10-C81.19, C81.90, C81.98, D49.81-D49.9

PDX Collection 377
C81.10-C81.11, C81.18-C81.19, C81.90-C81.91, C81.98, D49.81-D49.9

PDX Collection 378
C81.10, C81.12, C81.18-C81.19, C81.90, C81.92, C81.98, D49.81-D49.9

PDX Collection 379
C81.10, C81.13, C81.18-C81.19, C81.90, C81.93, C81.98, D49.81-D49.9

PDX Collection 380
C81.10, C81.14, C81.18-C81.19, C81.90, C81.94, C81.98, D49.81-D49.9

PDX Collection 381
C81.10, C81.15, C81.18-C81.19, C81.90, C81.95, C81.98, D49.81-D49.9

PDX Collection 382
C81.10, C81.16, C81.18-C81.19, C81.90, C81.96, C81.98, D49.81-D49.9

PDX Collection 383
C81.10, C81.17-C81.19, C81.90, C81.97-C81.98, D49.81-D49.9

PDX Collection 384
C81.20-C81.29, C81.90, C81.98, D49.81-D49.9

PDX Collection 385
C81.20-C81.21, C81.28-C81.29, C81.90-C81.91, C81.98, D49.81-D49.9

PDX Collection 386
C81.20, C81.22, C81.28-C81.29, C81.90, C81.92, C81.98, D49.81-D49.9

PDX Collection 387
C81.20, C81.23, C81.28-C81.29, C81.90, C81.93, C81.98, D49.81-D49.9

PDX Collection 388
C81.20, C81.24, C81.28-C81.29, C81.90, C81.94, C81.98, D49.81-D49.9

PDX Collection 389
C81.20, C81.25, C81.28-C81.29, C81.90, C81.95, C81.98, D49.81-D49.9

PDX Collection 390
C81.20, C81.26, C81.28-C81.29, C81.90, C81.96, C81.98, D49.81-D49.9

PDX Collection 391
C81.20, C81.27, C81.28-C81.29, C81.90, C81.97, C81.98, D49.81-D49.9

PDX Collection 392
C81.30-C81.39, C81.90, C81.98, D49.81-D49.9

PDX Collection 393
C81.30-C81.31, C81.38-C81.39, C81.90-C81.91, C81.98, D49.81-D49.

PDX Collection 394
C81.30, C81.32, C81.38-C81.39, C81.90, C81.92, C81.98, D49.81-D49.9

PDX Collection 395
C81.30, C81.33, C81.38-C81.39, C81.90, C81.93, C81.98, D49.81-D49.9

PDX Collection 396
C81.30, C81.34, C81.38-C81.39, C81.90, C81.94, C81.98, D49.81-D49.9

PDX Collection 397
C81.30, C81.35, C81.38-C81.39, C81.90, C81.95, C81.98, D49.81-D49.9

PDX Collection 398
C81.30, C81.36, C81.38-C81.39, C81.90, C81.96, C81.98, D49.81-D49.9

PDX Collection 399
C81.30, C81.37, C81.38-C81.39, C81.90, C81.97, C81.98, D49.81-D49.9

PDX Collection 400
C81.30-C81.39, C81.98, D49.81-D49.9

PDX Collection 401
C81.70-C81.79, C81.90, C81.98, D49.81-D49.9

PDX Collection 402
C81.70-C81.71, C81.78-C81.79, C81.90-C81.91, C81.98, D49.81-D49.9

PDX Collection 403
C81.70, C81.72, C81.78-C81.79, C81.90, C81.92, C81.98, D49.81-D49.9

PDX Collection 404
C81.70, C81.73, C81.78-C81.79, C81.90, C81.93, C81.98, D49.81-D49.9

PDX Collection 405
C81.70, C81.74, C81.78-C81.79, C81.90, C81.94, C81.98, D49.81-D49.9

PDX Collection 406
C81.70, C81.75, C81.78-C81.79, C81.90, C81.95, C81.98, D49.81-D49.9

PDX Collection 407
C81.70, C81.76, C81.78-C81.79, C81.90, C81.96, C81.98, D49.81-D49.9

PDX Collection 408
C81.70, C81.77, C81.78-C81.79, C81.90, C81.97, C81.98, D49.81-D49.9

PDX Collection 409
C81.90-C81.98, D49.81-D49.9

PDX Collection 410
C81.90-C81.91, C81.98, D49.81-D49.9

PDX Collection 411
C81.90, C81.92, C81.98, D49.81-D49.9

PDX Collection 412
C81.90, C81.93, C81.98, D49.81-D49.9

PDX Collection 413
C81.90, C81.94, C81.98, D49.81-D49.9

PDX Collection 414
C81.90, C81.95, C81.98, D49.81-D49.9

PDX Collection 415
C81.90, C81.96, C81.98, D49.81-D49.9

PDX Collection 416
C81.90, C81.97-C81.98, D49.81-D49.9

PDX Collection 417
C82.00-C82.50, C82.59-C82.99, C83.10, C83.19, C84.40, C84.49, C84.60, C84.69-C84.70, C84.79, C84.A0, C84.A9, C84.Z0, C84.Z9, C84.90, C84.99-C85.10, C85.19-C85.20, C85.29-C85.80, C85.89-C85.90, C85.99, C86.4, C88.4, C96.4, C96.9, C96.Z, D49.81-D49.9

PDX Collection 418
C82.00-C82.01, C82.08-C82.11, C82.18-C82.21, C82.28-C82.31, C82.38-C82.41, C82.48-C82.49, C82.51, C82.60-C82.61, C82.68-C82.81, C82.88-C82.91, C82.98-C82.99, C83.11, C84.41, C84.61, C84.71, C84.A1, C84.Z1, C84.91, C85.11, C85.21, C85.81, C85.91, C86.0, D49.81-D49.9

PDX Collection 419
C82.00, C82.02, C82.08-C82.10, C82.12, C82.18-C82.20, C82.22, C82.28-C82.30, C82.32, C82.38-C82.40, C82.42, C82.48-C82.49, C82.52, C82.60, C82.62, C82.68-C82.80, C82.82, C82.88-C82.90, C82.92, C82.98-C82.99, C83.12, C84.42, C84.62, C84.72, C84.92, C84.A2, C84.Z2, C85.12, C85.22, C85.82, C85.92, D49.81-D49.9

PDX Collection 420
C82.00, C82.03, C82.08-C82.10, C82.13, C82.18-C82.20, C12.23, C82.28-C82.30, C82.33, C82.38-C82.40, C82.43, C82.48-C82.49, C82.53, C82.60, C82.63, C82.68-C82.80, C82.83, C82.88-C82.90, C82.93, C82.98-C82.99, C83.13, C84.43, C84.63, C84.73, C84.93, C84.A3, C84.Z3, C85.13, C85.23, C85.83, C85.93, C86.2, C86.3, D49.81-D49.9

PDX Collection 421
C82.00, C82.04, C82.08-C82.10, C82.14, C82.18-C82.20, C82.24, C82.28-C82.30, C82.34, C82.38-C82.40, C82.44, C82.48-C82.49, C82.54, C82.60, C82.64, C82.68-C82.80, C82.84, C82.88-C82.90, C82.94, C82.98-C82.99, C83.14, C84.44, C84.64, C84.74, C84.94, C84.A4, C84.Z4, C85.14, C85.24, C85.84, C85.94, D49.81-D49.9

PDX Collection 422
C82.00, C82.05, C82.08-C82.10, C82.15, C82.18-C82.20, C82.25, C82.28-C82.30, C82.35, C82.38-C82.40, C82.45, C82.48-C82.49, C82.55, C82.60, C82.65, C82.68-C82.80, C82.85, C82.88-C82.90, C82.95, C82.98-C82.99, C83.15,

C84.45, C84.65, C84.75, C84.95, C84.A5, C84.Z5, C85.15, C85.25, C85.85, C85.95, D49.81-D49.9

PDX Collection 423
C82.00, C82.06, C82.08-C82.10, C82.16, C82.18-C82.20, C82.26, C82.28-C82.30, C82.36, C82.38-C82.40, C82.46, C82.48-C82.49, C82.56, C82.60, C82.66, C82.68-C82.80, C82.86, C82.88-C82.90, C82.96, C82.98-C82.99, C83.16, C84.46, C84.66, C84.76, C84.96, C84.A6, C84.Z6, C85.16, C85.26, C85.86, C85.96, D49.81-D49.9

PDX Collection 424
C82.00, C82.07, C82.08-C82.10, C82.17-C82.20, C82.27-C82.30, C82.37-C82.40, C82.47-C82.49, C82.57, C82.60, C82.67-C82.80, C82.87-C82.90, C82.97-C82.99, C83.17, C84.47, C84.67, C84.77, C84.97, C84.A7, C84.Z7, C85.17, C85.27, C85.87, C85.97, C86.1, D49.81-D49.9

PDX Collection 425
C82.00-C82.49, C82.58, C82.60-C82.99, C83.18, C84.48, C84.68, C84.78, C84.98, C84.A8, C84.Z8, C85.18, C85.28, C85.88, C85.98, D49.81-D49.9

PDX Collection 426
C82.50-C82.59, C83.10-C83.19, C84.40-C84.49, C84.60-C84.79, C84.90-C84.99, C84.A0-C84.Z9, C85.10-C86.4, C88.4, C96.4, C96.9, C96.Z, D49.81-D49.9

PDX Collection 427
C82.50-C82.51, C82.58-C82.59, C83.10-C83.11, C83.18-C83.19, C84.40-C84.41, C84.48-C84.61, C84.68-C84.71, C84.78-C84.79, C84.90-C84.91, C84.98-C84.99, C84.A0-C84.A1, C84.A8-C84.A9, C84.Z0-C84.Z1, C84.Z8-C84.Z9, C85.10-C85.11, C85.18-C85.21, C85.28-C85.81, C85.88-C85.91, C85.98-C85.99, C86.0, C86.4, C88.4, D49.81-D49.9

PDX Collection 428
C82.50, C82.52, C82.58-C82.59, C83.10, C83.12, C83.18-C83.19, C84.40, C84.42, C84.48-C84.60, C84.62, C84.68-C84.70, C84.72, C84.78-C84.79, C84.90, C84.92, C84.98-C84.99, C84.A0, C84.A2, C84.A8-C84.A9, C84.Z0, C84.Z2, C84.Z8-C84.Z9, C85.10, C85.12, C85.18-C85.20, C85.22, C85.28-C85.80, C85.82, C85.88-C85.90, C85.92, C85.98-C85.99, C86.4, C88.4, D49.81-D49.

PDX Collection 429
C82.50, C82.53, C82.58-C82.59, C83.10, C83.13, C83.18-C83.19, C84.40, C84.43, C84.48-C84.60, C84.63, C84.68-C84.70, C84.73, C84.78-C84.79, C84.90, C84.93, C84.98-C84.99, C84.A0, C84.A3, C84.A8-C84.A9, C84.Z0, C84.Z3, C84.Z8-C84.Z9, C85.10, C85.13, C85.18-C85.20, C85.22, C85.28-C85.80, C85.83, C85.88-C85.90, C85.93, C85.98-C85.99, C86.2-C86.4, C88.4, D49.81-D49.9

PDX Collection 430
C82.50, C82.54, C82.58-C82.59, C83.10, C83.14, C83.18-C83.19, C84.40, C84.44, C84.48-C84.60, C84.64, C84.68-C84.70, C84.74, C84.78-C84.79, C84.90, C84.94, C84.98-C84.99, C84.A0, C84.A4, C84.A8-C84.A9, C84.Z0, C84.Z4, C84.Z8-C84.Z9, C85.10, C85.14, C85.18-C85.20, C85.24, C85.28-C85.80, C85.84, C85.88-C85.90, C85.94, C85.98-C85.99, C86.4, C88.4, D49.81-D49.9

PDX Collection 431
C82.50, C82.55, C82.58-C82.59, C83.10, C83.15, C83.18-C83.19, C84.40, C84.45, C84.48-C84.60, C84.65, C84.68-C84.70, C84.75, C84.78-C84.79, C84.90, C84.95, C84.98-C84.99, C84.A0, C84.A5, C84.A8-C84.A9, C84.Z0, C84.Z5, C84.Z8-C84.Z9, C85.10, C85.15, C85.18-C85.20, C85.25, C85.28-C85.80, C85.85, C85.88-C85.90, C85.95, C85.98-C85.99, C86.4, C88.4, D49.81-D49.9

PDX Collection 432
C82.50, C82.56, C82.58-C82.59, C83.10, C83.16, C83.18-C83.19, C84.40, C84.46, C84.48-C84.60, C84.66,

C84.68-C84.70, C84.76, C84.78-C84.79, C84.90, C84.96, C84.98-C84.99, C84.A0, C84.A6, C84.A8-C84.A9, C84.Z0, C84.Z6, C84.Z8-C84.Z9, C85.10, C85.16, C85.18-C85.20, C85.26, C85.28-C85.80, C85.86, C85.88-C85.90, C85.96, C85.98-C85.99, C86.4, C88.4, D49.81-D49.9

PDX Collection 433
C82.50, C82.57, C82.58-C82.59, C83.10, C83.17, C83.18-C83.19, C84.40, C84.47-C84.49, C84.60, C84.67, C84.68-C84.69, C84.70, C84.77, C84.78-C84.79, C84.90, C84.97-C84.99, C84.A0, C84.A7-C84.A9, C84.Z0, C84.Z7, C84.Z8-C84.Z9, C85.10, C85.17-C85.20, C85.27-C85.29, C85.80, C85.87-C85.90, C85.97-C85.99, C86.1, C86.4, C88.4, D49.81-D49.9

PDX Collection 434
C82.50-C82.59, C83.10-C83.19, C84.40-C84.49, C84.60-C84.79, C84.90-C84.99, C84.A0-C84.Z9, C85.10-C86.4, C88.4, D49.81-D49.9

PDX Collection 435
C83.00-C83.09, C83.80-C83.99, C86.5-C86.6, D49.81-D49.9

PDX Collection 436
C83.00-C83.01, C83.08-C83.09, C83.80-C83.81, C83.88-C83.91, C83.98-C83.99, C86.5-C86.6, D49.81-D49.9

PDX Collection 437
C83.00, C83.02, C83.08-C83.09, C83.80, C83.82, C83.88-C83.89, C83.90, C83.92, C83.98-C83.99, C86.5-C86.6, D49.81-D49.9

PDX Collection 438
C83.00, C83.03, C83.08-C83.09, C83.80, C83.83, C83.88-C83.89, C83.90, C83.93, C83.98-C83.99, C86.5-C86.6, D49.81-D49.9

PDX Collection 439
C83.00, C83.04, C83.08-C83.09, C83.80, C83.84, C83.88-C83.89, C83.90, C83.94, C83.98-C83.99, C86.5-C86.6, D49.81-D49.9

PDX Collection 440
C83.00, C83.05, C83.08-C83.09, C83.80, C83.85, C83.88-C83.89, C83.90, C83.95, C83.98-C83.99, C86.5-C86.6, D49.81-D49.9

PDX Collection 441
C83.00, C83.06, C83.08-C83.09, C83.80, C83.86, C83.88-C83.89, C83.90, C83.96, C83.98-C83.99, C86.5-C86.6, D49.81-D49.9

PDX Collection 442
C83.00, C83.07-C83.09, C83.80, C83.87-C83.89, C83.90, C83.97-C83.99, C86.5-C86.6, D49.81-D49.9

PDX Collection 443
C83.30-C83.39, D49.81-D49.9

PDX Collection 444
C83.30-C83.31, C83.38-C83.39, D49.81-D49.9

PDX Collection 445
C83.30, C83.32, C83.38-C83.39, D49.81-D49.9

PDX Collection 446
C83.30, C83.33, C83.38-C83.39, D49.81-D49.9

PDX Collection 447
C83.30, C83.34, C83.38-C83.39, D49.81-D49.9

PDX Collection 448
C83.30, C83.35, C83.38-C83.39, D49.81-D49.9

PDX Collection 449
C83.30, C83.36, C83.38-C83.39, D49.81-D49.9

PDX Collection 450
C83.30, C83.37-C83.39, D49.81-D49.9

PDX Collection 451
C83.50-C83.59, D49.81-D49.9

PDX Collection 452
C83.50-C83.51, C83.58-C83.59, D49.81-D49.9

PDX Collection 453
C83.50, C83.52, C83.58-C83.59, D49.81-D49.9

PDX Collection 454
C83.50, C83.53, C83.58-C83.59, D49.81-D49.9

PDX Collection 455
C83.50, C83.54, C83.58-C83.59, D49.81-D49.9

PDX Collection 456
C83.50, C83.55, C83.58-C83.59, D49.81-D49.9

PDX Collection 457
C83.50, C83.56, C83.58-C83.59, D49.81-D49.9

PDX Collection 458
C83.50, C83.57-C83.59, D49.81-D49.9

PDX Collection 459
C83.70-C83.79, D49.81-D49.9

PDX Collection 460
C83.70-C83.71, C83.78-C83.79, D49.81-D49.9

PDX Collection 461
C83.70, C83.72, C83.78-C83.79, D49.81-D49.9

PDX Collection 462
C83.70, C83.73, C83.78-C83.79, D49.81-D49.9

PDX Collection 463
C83.70, C83.74, C83.78-C83.79, D49.81-D49.9

PDX Collection 464
C83.70, C83.75, C83.78-C83.79, D49.81-D49.9

PDX Collection 465
C83.70, C83.76, C83.78-C83.79, D49.81-D49.9

PDX Collection 466
C83.70, C83.77-C83.79, D49.81-D49.9

PDX Collection 467
C82.50, C82.59, C83.10, C83.19, C84.00-C84.09, C84.40,
C84.49, C84.60, C84.69-C84.70, C84.79, C84.90, C84.99,
C84.A0, C84.A9-C84.Z0, C84.Z9, C85.10, C85.19-C85.20,
C85.29-C85.80, C85.89-C85.90, C85.99, C86.4, C88.4, C96.4,
C96.9, C96.Z, D49.81-D49.9

PDX Collection 468
C82.51, C83.11, C84.00-C84.01, C84.08-C84.09, C84.41,
C84.61, C84.71, C84.91, C84.A1, C84.Z1, C85.11, C85.21,
C85.81, C85.91, C86.0, D49.81-D49.9

PDX Collection 469
C82.52, C83.12, C84.00, C84.02, C84.08-C84.09, C84.42,
C84.62, C84.72, C84.92, C84.A2, C84.Z2, C85.12, C85.22,
C85.82, C85.92, D49.81-D49.9

PDX Collection 470
C82.53, C83.13, C84.00, C84.03, C84.08-C84.09, C84.43,
C84.63, C84.73, C84.93, C84.A3, C84.Z3, C85.13, C85.23,
C85.83, C85.93, C86.2-C86.3, D49.81-D49.9

PDX Collection 471
C82.54, C83.14, C84.00, C84.04, C84.08-C84.09, C84.44,
C84.64, C84.74, C84.94, C84.A4, C84.Z4, C85.14, C85.24,
C85.84, C85.94, D49.81-D49.9

PDX Collection 472
C82.55, C83.15, C84.00, C84.05, C84.08-C84.09, C84.45,
C84.65, C84.75, C84.95, C84.A5, C84.Z5, C85.15, C85.25,
C85.85, C85.95, D49.81-D49.9

PDX Collection 473
C82.56, C83.16, C84.00, C84.06, C84.08-C84.09, C84.46,
C84.66, C84.76, C84.96, C84.A6, C84.Z6, C85.16, C85.26,
C85.86, C85.96, D49.81-D49.9

PDX Collection 474
C82.57, C83.17, C84.00, C84.07, C84.08-C84.09, C84.47,
C84.67, C84.77, C84.97, C84.A7, C84.Z7, C85.17, C85.27,
C85.87, C85.97, D49.81-D49.9

PDX Collection 475
C82.58, C83.18, C84.00-C84.09, C84.48, C84.68, C84.78,
C84.98, C84.A8, C84.Z8, C85.18, C85.28, C85.88, C85.98,
D49.81-D49.9

PDX Collection 476
C82.50, C82.59, C83.10, C83.19, C84.10-C84.19, C84.40,
C84.49-C84.60, C84.69-C84.70, C84.79, C84.90, C84.99,
C84.A0, C84.A9-C84.Z0, C84.Z9, C85.10, C85.19-C85.20,
C85.29-C85.80, C85.89-C85.90, C85.99, C86.4, C88.4, C96.4,
C96.9, C96.Z, D49.81-D49.9

PDX Collection 477
C82.51, C83.11, C84.10-C84.11, C84.18-C84.19, C84.41,
C84.61, C84.71, C84.91, C84.A1, C84.Z1, C85.11, C85.21,
C85.81, C85.91, C86.0, D49.81-D49.9

PDX Collection 478
C82.52, C83.12, C84.10, C84.12, C84.18-C84.19, C84.42,
C84.62, C84.72, C84.92, C84.A2, C84.Z2, C85.12, C85.22,
C85.82, C85.92, D49.81-D49.9

PDX Collection 479
C82.53, C83.13, C84.10, C84.13, C84.18-C84.19, C84.43,
C84.63, C84.73, C84.93, C84.A3, C84.Z3, C85.13, C85.23,
C85.83, C85.93, C86.2-C86.3, D49.81-D49.9

PDX Collection 480
C82.54, C83.14, C84.10, C84.14, C84.18-C84.19, C84.44,
C84.64, C84.74, C84.94, C84.A4, C84.Z4, C85.14, C85.24,
C85.84, C85.94, D49.81-D49.9

PDX Collection 481
C82.55, C83.15, C84.10, C84.15, C84.18-C84.19, C84.45,
C84.65, C84.75, C84.95, C84.A5, C84.Z5, C85.15, C85.25,
C85.85, C85.95, D49.81-D49.9

PDX Collection 482
C82.56, C83.16, C84.10, C84.16, C84.18-C84.19, C84.46,
C84.66, C84.76, C84.96, C84.A6, C84.Z6, C85.16, C85.26,
C85.86, C85.96, D49.81-D49.9

PDX Collection 483
C82.57, C83.17, C84.10, C84.17-C84.19, C84.47, C84.67,
C84.77, C84.97, C84.A7, C84.Z7, C85.17, C85.27, C85.87,
C85.97, C86.1, D49.81-D49.9

PDX Collection 484
C82.58, C83.18, C84.10-C84.19, C84.48, C84.68, C84.78,
C84.98, C84.A8, C84.Z8, C85.18, C85.28, C85.88, C85.98,
D49.81-D49.9

PDX Collection 485
C88.2-C88.3, C88.8-C90.02, C90.10-C90.12,
C90.20-C90.22, C90.30-C90.32, C91.00-C91.02,
C91.10-C91.12, C91.30-C91.32, C91.50-C91.52,
C91.60-C91.62, C91.90-C91.92, C91.A0-C91.A2,
C91.Z0-C91.Z2, C92.00-C92.02, C92.10-C92.12,
C92.20-C92.22, C92.30-C92.32, C92.40-C92.42,
C92.50-C92.52, C92.60-C92.62, C92.90-C92.92,
C92.A0-C92.A2, C92.Z0-C92.Z2, C93.00-C93.02,
C93.10-C93.12, C93.30-C93.32, C93.90-C93.92,
C93.Z0-C93.Z2, C94.00-C94.02, C94.20-C94.22,
C94.30-C94.32, C94.80-C94.82, C95.00-C95.02,
C95.10-C95.12, C95.90-C95.92, D49.81-D49.9

PDX Collection 486
C88.2-C88.3, C88.8-C90.02, C90.10-C90.12,
C90.20-C90.22, C90.30-C90.32, C91.00-C91.02,
C91.10-C91.12, C91.30-C91.32, C91.40-C91.42,
C91.50-C91.52, C91.60-C91.62, C91.90-C91.92,

C91.A0-C91.A2, C91.Z0-C91.Z2, C92.00-C92.02,
C92.10-C92.12, C92.20-C92.22, C92.30-C92.32,
C92.40-C92.42, C92.50-C92.52,
C92.60-C92.62, C92.90-C92.92,
C92.A0-C92.A2, C92.Z0-C92.Z2, C93.00-C93.02,
C93.10-C93.12, C93.30-C93.32, C93.90-C93.92,
C93.Z0-C93.Z2, C94.00-C94.02, C94.20-C94.22,
C94.30-C94.32, C94.40-C94.42, C94.6, C94.80-C94.82,
C95.00-C95.02, C95.10-C95.12, C95.90-C95.92, D45-D46.22,
D46.4, D46.9, D46.A-D46.Z, D47.01-D47.09, D47.3, D47.9,
D47.Z2, D47.Z9, D48.7-D48.9, D49.81-D49.9

PDX Collection 487
C82.50, C82.59, C83.10, C83.19, C84.40,
C84.49-C84.60, C84.69-C84.70, C84.79, C84.90, C84.99,
C84.A0, C84.A9-C84.Z0, C84.Z9, C85.10, C85.19-C85.20,
C85.29-C85.80, C85.89-C85.90, C85.99, C86.4, C88.4,
C91.40-C91.42, C96.4, C96.9, C96.Z, D49.81-D49.9

PDX Collection 488
C88.2-C88.3, C88.8-C88.9, C90.10-C90.11,
C90.20-C90.21, C90.30-C90.31, C91.00-C91.02,
C91.10-C91.12, C91.30-C91.32, C91.40-C91.42,
C91.50-C91.52, C91.60-C91.62, C91.90-C91.92,
C91.A0-C91.A2, C91.Z0-C91.Z2, C92.00-C92.02,
C92.10-C92.12, C92.20-C92.22, C92.30-C92.32,
C92.40-C92.42, C92.50-C92.52,
C92.60-C92.62, C92.90-C92.92,
C92.A0-C92.A2, C92.Z0-C92.Z2, C93.00-C93.02,
C93.10-C93.12, C93.30-C93.32, C93.90-C93.92,
C93.Z0-C93.Z2, C94.00-C94.02, C94.20-C94.22,
C94.30-C94.32, C94.40-C94.42, C94.6, C94.80-C94.82,
C95.00-C95.02, C95.10-C95.12, C95.90-C95.92, D45-D46.22,
D46.4, D46.9, D46.A-D46.Z, D47.01-D47.1, D47.3, D47.9,
D47.Z2, D47.Z9, D48.7-D48.9

PDX Collection 489
C82.50, C82.59, C83.10, C83.19, C84.40,
C84.49-C84.60, C84.69-C84.70, C84.79, C84.90, C84.99,
C84.A0, C84.A9-C84.Z0, C84.Z9, C85.10, C85.19-C85.20,
C85.29-C85.80, C85.89-C85.90, C85.99, C86.4, C88.4, C96.0,
C96.4, C96.9, C96.Z, D49.81-D49.9

PDX Collection 490
C82.50, C82.59, C83.10, C83.19, C84.40,
C84.49-C84.60, C84.69-C84.70, C84.79, C84.90, C84.99,
C84.A0, C84.A9-C84.Z0, C84.Z9, C85.10, C85.19-C85.20,
C85.29-C85.80, C85.89-C85.90, C85.99, C86.4, C88.4,
C96.20-C96.29, C96.4, C96.9, C96.Z, D49.81-D49.9

PDX Collection 491
C96.4, C96.9, C96.Z, D49.81-D49.9

PDX Collection 492
E71.310-E71.32, E71.40-E71.548, E80.4-E80.7, E88.40-E88.49,
H49.811-H49.819

PDX Collection 493
C82.50, C82.59, C83.10, C83.19, C84.40,
C84.49-C84.60, C84.69-C84.70, C84.79, C84.90, C84.99,
C84.A0, C84.A9-C84.Z0, C84.Z9, C85.10, C85.19-C85.20,
C85.29-C85.80, C85.89-C85.90, C85.99, C86.4, C88.4, C96.4,
C96.9, C96.A, C96.Z, D49.81-D49.9

PDX Collection 494
C88.8, C94.40-C94.42, C94.6, D45-D46.22, D46.4, D46.9,
D46.A-D46.C, D46.Z, D47.01-D47.1, D47.3, D47.9, D47.Z2,
D47.Z9, D75.81, Z51.0

PDX Collection 495
D47.Z1, D78.81-D78.89, E89.810-E89.89, H59.011-H59.019,
H59.031-H59.099, H59.811-H59.89, H95.811-H95.89, I97.3,
M96.89, N98.1-N98.9, T86.850-T86.99

PDX Collection 496
D47.4, D50.0-D64.9, D68.312, D68.51-D68.69, D75.81, D75.89-D75.9, D77, D89.2

PDX Collection 497
D50.0-D64.9, D75.9, P61.2-P61.4

PDX Collection 498
D50.0-D64.9, D75.9, P61.2-P61.4

PDX Collection 499
D50.0-D64.9, D69.3-D69.49, D75.9, P61.2-P61.4

PDX Collection 500
D60.0-D60.9, D61.1-D64.9, D70.0-D70.9, D72.810-D72.820, D72.823, D72.825-D72.829, D75.9-D76.3, P61.2

PDX Collection 501
D47.4, D50.0-D64.9, D68.312, D68.51-D68.69, D75.81, D75.89-D75.9, D77, D89.2, T79.2XX[A]

PDX Collection 502
D47.4, D65-D69.9, D75.81-D75.9, D77, D89.2

PDX Collection 503
D47.4, D65-D69.9, D75.82-D75.9, D77, D89.2

PDX Collection 504
D47.4, D68.311-D68.318, D68.51-D68.69, D70.0-D72.9, D73.81, D75.81, D75.89-D77, D89.2

PDX Collection 505
D47.4, D68.312, D68.51-D68.69, D70.0-D72.9, D73.81, D75.81, D75.89-D77, D89.2

PDX Collection 506
D56.4, D58.2-D59.2, D59.4-D59.9, D64.4-D64.9, D74.0-D74.9, D75.9

PDX Collection 507
D60.0-D60.9, D61.1-D61.9, D65, D69.3-D70.9, D72.818-D72.819, D75.82, D75.9

PDX Collection 508
D78.01-D78.02, D78.21-D78.89, H95.811-H95.89, I85.01, I85.11, I97.3, K21.9, K22.8, K23-K25.0, K25.2, K25.4, K25.6, K26.0, K26.2, K26.4, K26.6, K27.0, K27.2, K27.4, K27.6, K28.0, K28.2, K28.4, K28.6, K29.01, K29.21, K29.31, K29.41, K29.51, K29.61, K29.71, K29.81, K29.91, K31.811, K55.21, K57.01, K57.11, K57.13, K57.21, K57.31, K57.33, K57.41, K57.51, K57.53, K57.81, K57.91, K57.93, K62.5, K92.0-K92.2, M96.89, N98.1-N98.9, P54.1-P54.3, T81.10X-T81.19X[A], T81.82X[A], T81.89X-T81.9XX[A]

PDX Collection 509
D78.11-D78.12, D78.81-D78.89, E36.11-E36.8, E89.810-E89.89, G96.11, G97.41-G97.49, H59.011-H59.019, H59.031-H59.099, H59.211-H59.229, H59.811-H59.89, H95.31-H95.32, H95.811-H95.89, I97.3, I97.51-I97.52, J95.71-J95.72, K91.71-K91.72, L76.11-L76.12, L76.81-L76.82, M96.820-M96.821, M96.89, N98.1-N98.9, N99.71-N99.72, T81.82X[A], T81.89X-T81.9XX[A]

PDX Collection 510
D78.81-D78.89, H95.811-H95.89, I97.3, M96.89, N98.1-N98.9, T81.82X[A], T81.89X-T81.9XX[A]

PDX Collection 511
D80.0, D80.3-D81.4, D81.6-D81.7, D81.89-D84.0, D84.8-D84.9, D89.3-D89.9

PDX Collection 512
D80.0-D81.2, D81.4, D81.6-D81.7, D81.89-D84.0, D84.8-D84.9, D89.3-D89.9

PDX Collection 513
D81.3, D81.5, D81.810, D84.1, E76.01-E76.9, E79.1-E80.29, E80.4-E80.7, E88.81

PDX Collection 514
D78.81-D78.89, D89.810-D89.813, E89.810-E89.89, H59.011-H59.019, H59.031-H59.099, H59.811-H59.89, H95.811-H95.89, I97.3, M96.89, N98.1-N98.9, T86.00-T86.09

PDX Collection 515
B15.0-B19.9, E03.5, E08.00-E08.59, E08.618-E09.59, E09.618-E10.59, E10.618-E10.649, E10.69-E11.59, E11.618-E11.649, E11.69-E13.59, E13.618-E16.2, E89.1, G32.89, G89.0-G89.4, G93.81-G93.9, G96.8-G96.9, G98.0-G98.8, G99.8, I60.00-I62.9, K72.91, R29.700-R29.742, R40.0-R40.2124, R40.2210-R40.2224, R40.2310-R40.2324, R40.2340-R40.2344, R40.3-R41.3, R41.82, R41.9-R42, R44.8-R44.9, R45.83-R45.84, R46.0-R46.89, R52, R55, R68.0-R68.83, R68.89-R69, S02.0XX-S02.19X[A,B], S02.91X, S06.0X1[A], S06.0X9-S06.9X9[A]

PDX Collection 516
A17.9, A18.81-A18.82, A18.84, A18.89, E00.0-E03.4, E03.8-E07.1, E07.89-E07.9, E30.9, E34.1, E34.50-E35, E89.0

PDX Collection 517
E06.0-E06.9

PDX Collection 518
E08.00-E08.59, E08.618-E09.59, E09.618-E10.52, E10.59, E10.618-E10.649, E10.69-E11.59, E11.618-E11.649, E11.69-E13.59, E13.618-E16.2, E30.9, E34.1, E34.8-E35, E89.1

PDX Collection 519
G89.0-G89.4, I70.261-I70.269, I96, R41.0-R41.3, R41.82, R41.9, R44.8-R44.9, R45.83-R45.84, R46.0-R46.89, R52, R68.0-R68.19, R68.81-R68.83, R68.89-R69

PDX Collection 520
E08.00-E08.59, E08.618-E09.59, E09.618-E10.59, E10.618-E10.649, E10.69-E11.59, E11.618-E11.649, E11.69-E13.59, E13.618-E16.2, E30.9, E34.1, E34.50-E35, E89.1

PDX Collection 521
E22.1-E22.9

PDX Collection 522
E22.0-E23.7, E24.1, E30.9, E34.1, E34.4, E34.8-E35, E89.3

PDX Collection 523
E22.0-E23.7, E24.1, E30.9, E34.1, E34.4-E35, E89.3

PDX Collection 524
E22.1-E23.7, E24.1, E30.9, E34.1, E34.50-E35, E89.3

PDX Collection 525
E24.0, E24.2-E26.9, E30.9, E34.1, E34.50-E35

PDX Collection 526
A17.9, A18.7, A18.82, A18.84, A18.89, E27.0-E27.9, E30.9, E34.1, E34.50-E35, E89.6

PDX Collection 527
E30.9, E32.0-E32.9, E34.1, E34.50-E35

PDX Collection 528
E30.9, E34.0-E34.2, E34.50-E35

PDX Collection 529
E36.01-E36.02, E36.8, E89.810-E89.89, H95.811-H95.89, I85.01, I85.11, I97.3, K21.9, K22.8, K23-K25.0, K25.2, K25.4, K25.6, K26.0, K26.2, K26.4, K26.6, K27.0, K27.2, K27.4, K27.6, K28.0, K28.2, K28.4, K28.6, K29.01, K29.21, K29.31, K29.41, K29.51, K29.61, K29.71, K29.81, K29.91, K31.811, K55.21, K57.01, K57.11, K57.13, K57.21, K57.31, K57.33, K57.41, K57.51, K57.53, K57.81, K57.91, K57.93, K62.5, K92.0-K92.2, M96.89, N98.1-N98.9, P54.1-P54.3, T81.10X-T81.19X[A], T81.82XA, T81.89X-T81.9XX[A]

PDX Collection 530
E40-E46, E64.0

PDX Collection 531
D81.818-D81.819, E51.11-E53.9, E56.0, E56.8-E63.9, E64.8-E64.9

PDX Collection 532
E55.0-E63.9, E64.3-E64.9, M83.0-M83.9

PDX Collection 533
E66.2, I27.0-I27.81, I27.83, I27.89-I27.9

PDX Collection 534
C88.0, D47.2, D89.0-D89.1, E70.0-E71.30, E72.00-E72.02, E72.04-E74.9, E75.21-E75.249, E75.3, E75.5-E75.6, E77.0-E78.70, E78.79-E78.9, E88.09-E88.2, E88.89

PDX Collection 535
C96.5-C96.6, E71.39-E71.548, E80.3, E88.40-E88.49, E88.89, H49.811-H49.819

PDX Collection 536
C96.5-C96.6, E71.310-E71.448, E80.3-E80.7, E88.40-E88.49, E88.89, H49.811-H49.819

PDX Collection 537
E75.00-E75.19, E75.4, F84.2, G13.2-G13.8, G30.0-G31.82, G31.84-G31.9, G91.4, G94

PDX Collection 538
E75.00-E75.19, E75.23, E75.25-E75.29, E75.4, F84.2, G13.2-G13.8, G31.2-G31.82, G32.89, G91.4, G93.81, G93.89-G94, G96.8-G96.9, G98.0-G98.8, G99.8

PDX Collection 539
D81.3, D81.5, D81.810, D84.1, E76.01-E76.9, E79.1-E80.29, E80.4-E80.7, E85.0, E85.9, E88.81

PDX Collection 540
E78.71-E78.72, Q87.1-Q87.89, Q89.8, Q99.2

PDX Collection 541
E84.0-E84.9

PDX Collection 542
E85.0-E85.9, E88.81

PDX Collection 543
E86.0-E87.8

PDX Collection 544
E08.21-E08.29, E09.21-E09.29, E88.3, N00.0-N01.9, N02.8-N02.9, N04.7-N05.1, N05.6-N06.1, N06.6-N07.1, N07.6-N08, N14.0-N15.0, N15.8-N17.9

PDX Collection 545
C96.5-C96.6, E71.310-E71.548, E80.3-E80.7, E88.89

PDX Collection 546
E36.8, E89.810-E89.89, H95.811-H95.89, I97.3, M96.89, N98.1-N98.9, T81.82XA, T81.89X-T81.9XX[A]

PDX Collection 547
F01.51

PDX Collection 548
F02.81, F03.91

PDX Collection 549
F05, R45.851

PDX Collection 550
F02.80-F02.81, F04-F06.8, F10.10-F11.19, F11.21-F13.19, F13.21-F14.19, F14.21-F15.19, F15.21-F16.19, F16.21-F17.209, F17.213-F17.219, F17.223-F17.229, F17.293-F18.19, F18.21-F19.19, F19.21-F19.99, F53-F55.8, R78.0

PDX Collection 551
F07.0-F07.81, F07.9-F09, F20.0-F51.03, F51.12, F51.19, F51.3-F51.9, F52.5, F54, F59-F63.2, F63.81-F63.9, F68.10-F80.4, F80.82-F84.0, F84.3-F99, G44.201-G44.229, H93.25, R45.1-R45.2, R45.5-R45.82, R45.86-R45.87

PDX Collection 552
F30.13, F30.2, F31.13-F31.2, F31.4-F31.5, F31.63-F31.64

PDX Collection 553
F31.13-F31.2, F31.63-F31.64

PDX Collection 554
F31.13-F31.2, F31.4-F31.5, F31.63-F31.64

PDX Collection 555
F32.0-F32.3, F33.0-F33.40, F33.9

PDX Collection 556
F45.9, F50.00-F50.9, F59, F98.21-F98.3

PDX Collection 557
F50.00-F50.9, F98.21-F98.29

PDX Collection 558
F72-F73

PDX Collection 559
A02.21, A17.0-A17.1, A27.81, A39.0, A50.41, A51.41, A52.13, A54.82, A54.84, A54.89-A54.9, A87.0-A87.9, B00.3, B02.1, B26.1, B37.5, B38.4, B45.1, B58.2, G00.0-G03.9, G04.2, G32.89, G61.0, G96.8-G96.9, G98.0-G98.8, G99.8

PDX Collection 560
A02.21, A17.0-A17.1, A17.82, A27.81, A39.0, A50.41-A50.42, A51.41, A52.13-A52.14, A54.82, A54.84, A54.89-A54.9, A81.1, A81.82-A81.89, A83.0-A85.8, A87.0-A88.0, A88.8, A92.1-A92.8, A93.0, A96.2, A98.3-A98.4, B00.3-B00.4, B00.89-B01.11, B01.81-B02.23, B02.29, B02.7-B02.9, B04, B06.01, B08.04-B08.09, B08.20-B08.22, B08.60-B08.79, B09-B10.89, B26.1-B26.2, B27.00-B27.99, B33.1, B33.24, B33.4-B33.8, B34.1-B34.2, B34.4, B34.8, B37.5, B38.4, B45.1-B58.2, B92, B94.2, B94.8-B94.9, B97.10, B97.19-B97.29, B97.5-B97.6, B97.81-B97.89, G00.0-G04.01, G04.2, G04.31, G04.81-G05.4, G32.89, G37.0, G37.4-G37.5, G61.0, G96.8-G96.9, G98.0-G98.8, G99.8, J09.X3-J09.X9, J10.2-J10.89, J11.2-J11.89, L44.4, P35.2-P35.9, P37.0-P37.4, P37.8-P37.9

PDX Collection 561
G04.1, G11.0-G12.9, G32.0-G37.3, G37.5-G37.9, G80.0-G80.2, G80.4-G80.9, G81.00-G83.9, G90.01-G90.09, G90.2, G90.4, G90.50-G90.9, G92, G93.40-G93.49, G93.81, G93.89-G95.9, G96.8-G96.9, G98.0-G99.8, I67.83, R53.2

PDX Collection 562
A17.82, A28.1, A50.42, A52.14, A75.9, A79.9, A81.1, A81.82-A81.89, A83.0-A85.8, A87.2, A88.0, A88.8, A92.1-A92.8, A93.0, B00.4, B00.82, B01.11-B01.12, B04, B06.01, B08.09, B08.20-B08.22, B08.60-B08.79, B09, B10.01-B10.09, B26.2, B27.00-B27.99, B33.1, B45.0, B45.2-B45.9, B54, B58.2, B75, B97.10, B97.21, G04.00-G04.01, G04.31, G04.81-G05.4, G37.0, G37.4-G37.5, H66.40-H66.43, J09.X3-J09.X9, J10.2-J10.89, J11.2-J11.89, L44.4, M1A.10X0-M1A.19X1, M32.0-M32.9, P35.2-P35.9, P37.0-P37.9, T56.0X1-T56.0X4[A]

PDX Collection 563
A06.6, A17.81, E08.40-E08.49, E08.618-E08.638, E08.649-E08.8, E09.40-E09.49, E09.618-E09.638, E09.649-E09.8, E10.40-E10.49, E10.618-E10.638, E10.649, E10.69-E10.8, E11.40-E11.49, E11.618-E11.638, E11.649, E11.69-E11.8, E13.40-E13.49, E13.618-E13.638, E13.649-E13.8, G06.0-G08, G93.81, G93.89-G93.9

PDX Collection 564
A06.6, A17.81, E08.40-A08.49, E08.618-E08.638, E08.649-E08.8, E09.40-E09.49, E09.618-E09.638, E09.649-E09.8, E10.40-E10.49, E10.618-E10.638, E10.649, E10.69-E10.8, E11.40-E11.49, E11.618-E11.638, E11.649, E11.69-E11.8, E13.40-E13.49, E13.618-E13.638, E13.649-E13.8, G06.1

PDX Collection 565
A06.6, A17.81, E08.40-E08.49, E08.618-E08.638, E08.649-E08.8, E09.40-E09.49, E09.618-E09.638, E09.649-E09.8, E10.40-E10.49, E10.618-E10.638, E10.649, E10.69-E10.8, E11.40-E11.49, E11.618-E11.638, E11.649, E11.69-E11.8, E13.40-E13.49, E13.618-E13.638, E13.649-E13.8, G06.0-G06.2, G07-G08

PDX Collection 566
G04.1, G20, G21.11-G21.9, G32.89-G37.9, G80.0-G80.2, G80.4-G80.9, G82.20-G83.0, G92, G93.1, G93.40-G93.6, G93.81, G93.89-G93.9, G96.8-G96.9, G98.0-G98.8, G99.8, I67.83, R53.2

PDX Collection 567
G04.1, G10-G12.9, G21.0, G23.0-G25.79, G25.82-G26, G32.0-G37.9, G80.0-G83.9, G90.01-G90.09, G90.2-G90.9, G92-G93.1, G93.40-G93.49, G93.81, G93.89-G95.9, G96.8-G96.9, G98.0-G99.8, I67.83, R53.2

PDX Collection 568
G04.1, G10-G12.9, G21.0, G23.0-G25.79, G25.82-G26, G32.0-G37.3, G37.5-G37.9, G80.0-G83.9, G90.01-G90.09, G90.2-G90.9, G92, G93.1, G93.40-G93.49, G93.81, G93.89-G93.9, G95.0-G95.9, G96.12-G96.9, G97.1, G98.0-G99.8, I67.83, R53.2

PDX Collection 569
G11.0-G11.9, G32.81

PDX Collection 570
E08.40-E08.49, E08.618-E08.638, E08.649-E08.8, E09.40-E09.49, E09.618-E09.638, E09.649-E09.8, E10.40-E10.49, E10.618-E10.638, E10.649, E10.69-E10.8, E11.40-E11.49, E11.618-E11.638, E11.649, E11.69-E11.8, E13.40-E13.49, E13.618-E13.638, E13.649-E13.8, G11.3, G11.8-G12.9, G32.0, G32.89, G90.01-G90.09, G90.2, G90.4, G90.50-G90.9, G95.0-G95.9, G96.8-G96.9, G98.0-G99.8

PDX Collection 571
G10, G21.0, G23.0-G25.79, G25.82-G26, G80.3, G81.00-G81.94, G90.3, G93.2, G93.40-G93.49, I67.83

PDX Collection 572
G20, G21.11-G21.9

PDX Collection 573
G20, G21.11-G21.9, G90.01-G90.09, G93.40-G93.49, I67.83

PDX Collection 574
G20, G21.11-G21.9, G25.70-G25.79, G25.89-G26, G80.3, G93.40, G93.41-G93.49, I67.83

PDX Collection 575
G04.1, G10, G12.22, G20-G21.9, G24.01-G25.79, G25.82-G26, G32.89-G37.2, G37.5-G37.9, G80.0-G80.9, G82.20-G83.0, G92, G93.1, G93.40-G93.6, G93.81, G93.89-G93.9, G96.8-G96.9, G98.0-G98.8, G99.8, I67.83, R53.2

PDX Collection 576
G04.1, G11.3, G11.8-G12.9, G32.0, G32.89-G37.3, G37.5-G37.9, G80.0-G83.9, G90.01-G90.09, G90.2, G90.4-G90.9, G93.1, G93.40-G93.49, G95.0-G96.9, G97.1, G98.0-G99.8, I67.83, R53.2

PDX Collection 577
G36.0, G93.40-G93.49, I67.83

PDX Collection 578
G04.1, G10-G12.9, G21.0, G24.01-G25.79, G25.82-G26, G32.0-G37.3, G37.5, G37.8-G37.9, G80.0-G83.9, G90.01-G90.09, G90.2, G90.4-G90.9, G92, G93.40-G93.49, G93.81, G93.89-G95.9, G96.8-G96.9, G98.0-G99.8, I67.83, R53.2

PDX Collection 579
A92.30-A92.39, B97.21, G93.40-G93.49, I67.83

PDX Collection 580
A02.21, A17.0-A27.81, A39.0, A50.41, A51.41, A52.13, A54.82, A54.84, A54.89-A54.9, A87.0-A87.9, A96.2, A98.3-A98.4, B00.3, B00.89-B00.9, B02.0-B02.29, B02.7-B02.9, B10.81-B10.89, B26.1, B33.24-B33.8, B34.1-B34.2, B34.4-B34.8, B37.5, B38.4, B45.1, B58.2, B92, B94.2-B94.9, B97.10, B97.19, B97.29, B97.5-B97.6, B97.81-B97.89, E08.40-E08.49, E09.40-E09.49, E10.40-E10.49, E11.40-E11.49, E13.40-E13.49, G00.0-G03.9, G04.1-G04.2, G11.3, G11.8-G12.9, G32.0, G32.89-G37.2, G37.5-G37.9, G61.0, G80.0-G80.2, G80.4-G83.9, G90.01-G90.09, G90.2, G90.4-G90.9, G93.1, G93.40-G93.49, G95.0-G95.9, G96.12-G96.9, G97.1, G98.0-G99.8, I67.83, R53.2

PDX Collection 581
G32.89, G40.001-G40.319, G40.401-G40.919, G40.A01-G40.B19, G93.40-G93.49, G93.9, G96.8-G96.9, G98.0-G98.8, G99.8. I67.83, R56.1

PDX Collection 582
E08.40-E08.49, E09.40-E09.49, E10.40-E10.49, E11.40-E11.49, E13.40-E13.49, G32.89, G40.001-G40.319, G40.401-G40.919, G40.A01-G40.A19, G40.B01-G40.B19, G93.81, G93.89-G93.9, G96.8-G96.9, G98.0-G98.8, G99.8, R56.1

PDX Collection 583
E08.40-E08.49, E08.618-E08.638, E08.649-E08.8, E09.40-E09.49, E09.618-E09.638, E09.649-E09.8, E10.40-E10.49, E10.618-E10.638, E10.649, E10.69-E10.8, E11.40-E11.49, E11.618-E11.638, E11.649, E11.69-E11.8, E13.40-E13.49, E13.618-E13.638, E13.649-E13.8, G32.89, G40.001-G40.319, G40.401-G40.419, G40.501-G40.919, G40.A01-G40.B19, G93.81, G93.89-G93.9, G96.8-G96.9, G98.0-G98.8, G99.8, R56.1

PDX Collection 584
G43.601-G43.619, I63.00-I66.9

PDX Collection 585
G43.601-G43.619, I63.00-I66.9

PDX Collection 586
E08.51-E08.59, E08.618-E08.638, E08.649-E08.8, E09.51-E09.59, E09.618-E09.638, E09.649-E09.8, E10.51-E10.59, E10.618-E10.638, E10.649, E10.69-E10.8, E11.51-E11.59, E11.618-E11.638, E11.649, E11.69, E11.8, E13.51-E13.59, E13.618-E13.638, E13.649-E13.8, G45.0-G45.2, G45.8-G46.2, I63.00-I63.039, I63.09, I63.139, I63.19-I63.239, I63.29, I65.01-I65.9, I67.841-I67.848, I87.8-I87.9, I99.8-I99.9

PDX Collection 587
G45.3, H34.00-H34.9

PDX Collection 588
E11.42, G13.0, G13.1, G50.0-G65.2, M34.83

PDX Collection 589
G51.0-G54.5, G54.8-G60.9, G61.81-G61.89, G62.81-G62.89, G64

PDX Collection 590
G51.0-G54.5, G54.8-G60.9, G61.81-G61.9, G62.81, G62.89-G62.9, G64

PDX Collection 591
E08.40-E08.49, E08.618-E08.638, E08.649-E08.8, E09.40-E09.49, E09.618-E09.638, E09.649-E09.8, E10.40-E10.49, E10.618-E10.638, E10.649, E10.69-E10.8, E11.40-E11.49, E11.618-E11.638, E11.649, E11.69-E11.8, E13.40-E13.49, E13.618-E13.638, E13.649-E13.8, G32.89, G70.00-G70.01, G70.80-G70.81, G73.1-G73.3, G96.8-G96.9, G98.0-G98.8, G99.8

PDX Collection 592
E08.40-E08.49, E08.618-E08.638, E08.649-E08.8, E09.40-E09.49, E09.618-E09.638, E09.649-E09.8,

E10.40-E10.49, E10.618-E10.638, E10.649, E10.69-E10.8,
E11.40-E11.49, E11.618-E11.638, E11.649, E11.69-E11.8,
E13.40-E13.49, E13.618-E13.638, E13.649-E13.8, G32.89,
G71.0, G71.2, G96.8-G96.9, G98.0-G98.8, G99.8

PDX Collection 593
G32.89, G70.00-G71.0, G71.11-G72.3, G72.81-G73.7,
G96.8-G96.9, G98.0-G98.8, G99.8

PDX Collection 594
G70.1-G72.3, G72.81-G73.7

PDX Collection 595
E08.40-E08.49, E08.618-E08.638, E08.649-E08.8,
E09.40-E09.49, E09.618-E09.638, E09.649-E09.8,
E10.40-E10.49, E10.618-E10.638, E10.649, E10.69-E10.8,
E11.40-E11.49, E11.618-E11.638, E11.649, E11.69-E11.8,
E13.40-E13.49, E13.618-E13.638, E13.649-E13.8, G04.1,
G32.89, G80.0-G80.2, G80.4-G83.9, G90.1, G93.81,
G93.89-G93.9, G96.8-G96.9, G98.0-G98.8, G99.8,
Q06.0-Q06.1, Q06.3, Q06.8-Q06.9, Q07.8-Q07.9, R53.2

PDX Collection 596
G80.1, G93.40-G93.49, I67.83

PDX Collection 597
G80.2, G93.40-G93.49, I67.83

PDX Collection 598
G20, G21.11-G21.9, G25.70-G25.79, G25.89-G26,
G80.0-G80.9, G93.40-G93.49, I67.83

PDX Collection 599
G32.89, G82.50-G83.0, G83.5-G83.9, G96.8-G96.9,
G98.0-G98.8, G99.8, R53.2

PDX Collection 600
G04.1, G32.89, G82.20-G82.54, G83.10-G83.14, G83.4-G83.9,
G96.8-G96.9, G98.0-G98.8, G99.8, R53.2

PDX Collection 601
G04.1, G32.89, G80.0-G83.9, G92, G93.40-G93.49, G93.81,
G93.89-G93.9, G96.8-G96.9, G98.0-G98.8, G99.8, I67.83,
R53.2

PDX Collection 602
G90.50-G90.59

PDX Collection 603
E08.40-E08.49, E09.40-E09.49, E10.40-E10.49, E11.40-E11.49,
E13.40-E13.49, G04.1, G11.3, G11.8-G12.9, G32.0,
G32.89-G37.3, G37.5-G37.9, G80.0-G80.2, G80.4-G83.9,
G90.01-G90.09, G90.2, G90.4-G90.9, G93.1, G93.40-G93.49,
G95.0-G95.9, G96.12-G96.9, G97.1, G98.0-G99.8, I67.83,
R53.2

PDX Collection 604
G91.0-G91.3, G91.8-G91.9

PDX Collection 605
E08.40-E08.49, E08.618-E08.638, E08.649-E08.8,
E09.40-E09.49, E09.618-E09.638, E09.649-E09.8,
E10.40-E10.49, E10.618-E10.638, E10.649, E10.69-E10.8,
E11.40-E11.49, E11.618-E11.638, E11.649, E11.69-E11.8,
E13.40-E13.49, E13.618-E13.638, E13.649-E13.8,
G13.2-G13.8, G31.2, G31.83-G31.9, G90.1, G91.0-G91.9,
G93.81, G93.89-G94, Q03.0-Q03.9, Q04.4-Q04.8,
Q05.0-Q05.4, Q05.9-Q06.1, Q06.3, Q06.8-Q06.9,
Q07.02-Q07.9

PDX Collection 606
A17.82, A17.9, A18.82, A18.84, A18.89, A39.81, A50.42,
A52.14, A83.0-A85.1, A85.8-A86, A88.8-A89, B00.4,
B01.11, B10.01-B10.09, B26.2, B58.2, E08.40-E08.49,
E08.618-E08.638, E08.649-E08.8, E09.40-E09.49,
E09.618-E09.638, E09.649-E09.8, E10.40-E10.49,
E10.618-E10.638, E10.649, E10.69-E10.8, E11.40-E11.49,
E11.618-E11.638, E11.649, E11.69-E11.8, E13.40-E13.49,
E13.618-E13.638, E13.649-E13.8, G04.00-G04.01, G04.31,

G04.81-G05.4, G32.89, G37.3-G37.4, G92, G93.40-G93.49,
G93.81, G93.89-G93.9, G96.8-G96.9, G98.0-G98.8, G99.8,
I67.83

PDX Collection 607
E08.40-E08.49, E08.618-E08.638, E08.649-E08.8,
E09.40-E09.49, E09.618-E09.638, E09.649-E09.8,
E10.40-E10.49, E10.618-E10.638, E10.649, E10.69-E10.8,
E11.40-E11.49, E11.618-E11.638, E11.649, E11.69-E11.8,
E13.40-E13.49, E13.618-E13.638, E13.649-E13.8, G32.89,
G93.1-G93.2, G96.8-G96.9, G98.0-G98.8, G99.8

PDX Collection 608
G21.0, G83.5, G93.41-G93.49, I67.83

PDX Collection 609
G21.0, G83.5, G93.40-G93.49, I67.83

PDX Collection 610
G21.0, G83.5, G93.40, G93.41

PDX Collection 611
G81.90, G93.82

PDX Collection 612
G93.6, G93.82

PDX Collection 613
G93.7

PDX Collection 614
G04.1, G11.3, G11.8-G12.9, G32.0, G32.89-G37.3,
G37.5-G37.9, G80.0-G80.2, G80.4-G83.9, G90.01-G90.09,
G90.2, G90.4-G90.9, G93.40-G93.49, G93.81, G93.89-G93.9,
G95.0-G95.9, G96.12-G96.9, G97.1, G98.0-G99.8, I67.83,
R53.2

PDX Collection 615
E08.40-E08.49, E09.40-E09.49, E10.40-E10.49, E13.40-E13.49,
G04.1, G11.3-G12.9, G32.0, G32.89, G35-G37.9, G80.0-G83.9,
G90.01, G90.09, G90.2, G90.4-G90.9, G93.1, G93.40-G93.49,
G95.11-G95.9, G96.12-G96.9, G97.1, G98.0-G99.8, I67.83,
R53.2

PDX Collection 616
E08.40-E08.49, E08.618-E08.638, E08.649-E08.8,
E09.40-E09.49, E09.618-E09.638, E09.649-E09.8,
E10.40-E10.49, E10.618-E10.638, E10.649, E10.69-E10.8,
E11.40-E11.49, E11.618-E11.638, E11.649, E11.69-E11.8,
E13.40-E13.49, E13.618-E13.638, E13.649-E13.8, G32.89,
G96.0, G96.8-G96.9, G98.0-G98.8, G99.8

PDX Collection 617
D78.81-D78.89, E36.8, E89.810-E89.89, G97.0, G97.2-G97.32,
G97.81-G97.82, H59.011-H59.019, H59.031-H59.099,
H59.811-H59.89, H95.811-H95.89, I97.3, I97.810-I97.821,
L76.81-L76.82, M96.89, N98.1-N98.9, T81.82XA,
T81.89X-T81.9XX[A]

PDX Collection 618
G97.0, G97.2-G97.32, G97.81-G97.82, H95.811-H95.89,
I97.3, I97.810-I97.821, M96.89, N98.1-N98.9, T81.82XA,
T81.89X-T81.9XX[A]

PDX Collection 619
97.51-G97.52, G97.61-G97.64, H95.811-H95.89, I85.01,
I85.11, I97.3, K21.9, K22.8, K23-K25.0, K25.2, K25.4, K25.6,
K26.0, K26.2, K26.4, K26.6, K27.0, K27.2, K27.4, K27.6,
K28.0, K28.2, K28.4, K28.6, K29.01, K29.21, K29.31, K29.41,
K29.51, K29.61, K29.71, K29.81, K29.91, K31.811, K55.21,
K57.01, K57.11, K57.13, K57.21, K57.31, K57.33, K57.41,
K57.51, K57.53, K57.81, K57.91, K57.93, K62.5, K92.0-K92.2,
M96.89, N98.1-N98.9, P54.1-P54.3, T81.10X-T81.19X[A],
T81.82X-T81.9XX[A]

PDX Collection 620
G90.01, G90.09, G90.2, G90.50-G90.9, G93.40-G93.49,
G99.0, I67.83

PDX Collection 621
H05.00-H05.049

PDX Collection 622
A02.24, A17.9, A18.03-A18.09, A18.82, A18.84, A18.89,
H05.021-H05.029, M46.20-M46.39, M86.00-M86.9

PDX Collection 623
A02.24, A17.9, A18.03-A18.09, A18.82, A18.84, A18.89,
H05.031-H05.039, M46.20-M46.39, M86.00-M86.9

PDX Collection 624
A18.54, H20.00-H20.9

PDX Collection 625
H20.051-H20.059, H21.331-H21.339, H33.121-H33.129,
H44.001-H44.029, H44.121-H44.129, H44.19

PDX Collection 626
H30.001-H30.93

PDX Collection 627
H31.301-H32

PDX Collection 628
H33.001-H33.119, H33.191-H33.8, H35.70-H35.739

PDX Collection 629
H35.60-H35.63, H35.81-H35.89

PDX Collection 630
H40.211-H40.219

PDX Collection 631
H16.241-H16.249, H21.331-H21.339, H33.121-H33.129,
H44.001-H44.19

PDX Collection 632
H44.111-H44.119, H44.131-H44.139

PDX Collection 633
H46.00-H46.9

PDX Collection 634
A17.9, A18.50-A18.59, A18.82, A18.84, A18.89, A39.82,
E08.311-E08.39, E08.618-E08.638, E08.649-E08.8,
E09.311-E09.39, E09.618-E09.638, E09.649-E09.8,
E10.311-E10.39, E10.618-E10.638, E10.649, E10.69-E10.8,
E11.311-E11.39, E11.618-E11.638, E11.649, E11.69-E11.8,
E13.311-E13.39, E13.618-E13.638, E13.649-E13.8,
H47.10-H47.13, H47.231-H47.239, H47.331-H47.339,
H57.8-H57.9, H59.40-H59.43, Q11.3, Q15.8-Q15.9

PDX Collection 635
H47.41-H47.539

PDX Collection 636
H47.611-H47.9

PDX Collection 637
H53.10-H53.139, H53.16, R44.1, R48.3

PDX Collection 638
H59.011-H59.019, H59.031-H59.099, H59.811-H59.89,
H95.811-H95.89, I97.3, M96.89, N98.1-N98.9, T81.82XA,
T81.89X-T81.9XX[A]

PDX Collection 639
H59.011-H59.019, H59.031-H59.129, H59.311-H59.329,
H59.331-H59.369, H59.811-H59.89, H95.811-H95.89, I85.01,
I85.11, I97.3, K21.9, K22.8, K23-K25.0, K25.2, K25.4, K25.6,
K26.0, K26.2, K26.4, K26.6, K27.0, K27.2, K27.4, K27.6,
K28.0, K28.2, K28.4, K28.6, K29.01, K29.21, K29.31, K29.41,
K29.51, K29.61, K29.71, K29.81, K29.91, K31.811, K55.21,
K57.01, K57.11, K57.13, K57.21, K57.31, K57.33, K57.41,
K57.51, K57.53, K57.81, K57.91, K57.93, K62.5, K92.0-K92.2,
M96.89, N98.1-N98.9, P54.1-P54.3, T81.10X-T81.19X[A],
T81.82X[A], T81.89X-T81.9XX[A]

PDX Collection 640
H60.20-H60.23, H70.001-H70.13

PDX Collection 641

A17.9, A18.6, A18.82, A18.84, A18.89, H70.001-H70.213, H70.219-H70.93, H75.00-H75.83, H93.8X1-H93.93, H94.80-H95.199, Q16.1, Q16.9, Q17.3-Q17.9

PDX Collection 642

H95.21-H95.22, H95.41-H95.89, I85.01, I85.11, I97.3, K21.9, K22.8, K23-K25.2, K25.4, K25.6, K26.0, K26.2, K26.4, K26.6, K27.0, K27.2, K27.4, K27.6, K28.0, K28.2, K28.4, K28.6, K29.01, K29.21, K29.31, K29.41, K29.51, K29.61, K29.71, K29.81, K29.91, K31.811, K55.21, K57.01, K57.11, K57.13, K57.21, K57.31, K57.33, K57.41, K57.51, K57.53, K57.81, K57.91, K57.93, K62.5, K92.0-K92.2, M96.89, N98.1-N98.9, P54.1-P54.3, T81.10X-T81.19X[A], T81.82XA, T81.89X-T81.9XX[A]

PDX Collection 643

D78.81-D78.89, E36.8, E89.810-E89.89, H59.011-H59.019, H59.031-H59.099, H59.811-H59.89, H95.811-H95.89, I97.3, L76.81-L76.82, M96.89, N98.1-N98.9, T81.82XA, T81.89X-T81.9XX[A]

PDX Collection 644

A01.00-A01.09, A39.51, A52.03, A78, B33.21, B37.6, I00, I01.1, I01.8-I02.0, I05.0-I07.9, I08.1-I08.3, I08.9, I09.1, I09.89-I09.9, I33.0-I39, I42.4, I87.8-I87.9, I99.8-I99.9, Q22.2, Q23.8-Q23.9, Q24.8, T82.6XXA

PDX Collection 645

I01.0-I09.9, I50.20-I50.43

PDX Collection 646

I01.0-I09.9

PDX Collection 647

I00, I01.2-I01.9, I09.0, I09.9, I23.0-I23.3, I23.6-I23.8, I40.0-I41, I51.0, I51.4, I87.8-I87.9, I99.8-I99.9

PDX Collection 648

I09.81, I09.9, I11.0, I50.1-I50.9, I87.8-I87.9, I99.8-I99.9

PDX Collection 649

I10-I16.9, I87.8-I87.9, I99.8-I99.9, N18.6, N26.2

PDX Collection 650

I10-I16.9, I87.8-I87.9, I99.8-I99.9, N26.2

PDX Collection 651

I09.81, I11.0, I13.0, I13.2, I20.0-I22.9, I24.0, I24.8-I24.9, I25.5-I25.6, I25.82-I25.83, I25.89-I25.9, I50.1, I50.810-I50.9, I87.8-I87.9, I99.8-I99.9, R57.0, R57.9

PDX Collection 652

I20.0-I22.9, I24.0, I24.8-I24.9, I25.5-I25.6, I25.89-I25.9, I87.8-I87.9, I99.8-I99.9

PDX Collection 653

I21.01-I22.9, I87.8-I87.9, I99.8-I99.9

PDX Collection 654

E78.71-E78.72, I23.0-I23.8, I40.0-I41, I51.0-I51.2, I51.4, I87.8-I87.9, I97.0-I97.191, I99.8-I99.9, P29.30-P29.38, Q20.0-Q21.9, Q23.8-Q23.9, Q24.8-Q24.9, Q27.30, Q27.4, Q28.0-Q28.1, Q28.8-Q28.9, Q87.1-Q87.89, Q89.7-Q89.8, Q99.2

PDX Collection 655

I23.0-I23.4, I23.6-I23.8, I51.0-I51.1, I87.8-I87.9, I99.8-I99.9

PDX Collection 656

I23.0-I23.3, I23.5-I23.8, I51.0, I51.2, I87.8-I87.9, I99.8-I99.9

PDX Collection 657

I20.0-I22.9, I24.0-I24.9, I25.5-I25.6, I25.89-I25.9, I87.8-I87.9, I99.8-I99.9

PDX Collection 658

I24.0-I24.9, I87.8-I87.9, I99.8-I99.9

PDX Collection 659

I25.3-I25.41

PDX Collection 660

I25.42, I67.0, I77.2-I77.3, I77.5-I77.6, I77.70, I77.75-I77.79, I77.89-I77.9, M31.8-M31.9

PDX Collection 661

I09.381, I11.0, I13.2, I20.0-I22.9, I24.0, I24.8-I25.119, I25.5-I25.739, I25.760-I25.799, I25.812-I25.9, I50.1, I50.810-I50.9, I87.8-I87.9, I99.8-I99.9, R57.0, R57.9

PDX Collection 662

I25.10-I25.119, I25.700-I25.739, I25.760-I25.799, I25.812-I25.84

PDX Collection 663

I09.81, I11.0, I13.0, I13.2, I20.0-I22.9, I24.0, I24.8-I25.119, I25.5-I25.799, I25.811-I25.9, I50.1, I50.810-I50.9, I87.8-I87.9, I99.8-I99.9, R57.0, R57.9

PDX Collection 664

I25.10-I25.119, I25.700-I25.799, I25.811-I25.84

PDX Collection 665

I09.81, I11.0, I13.0, I13.2, I20.0-I22.9, I24.0, I24.8-I25.119, I25.5-I25.759, I25.790-I25.799, I25.811, I25.82-I25.9, I50.1, I50.810-I50.9, I87.8-I87.9, I99.8-I99.9, R57.0, R57.9

PDX Collection 666

I25.10-I25.119, I25.700-I25.759, I25.790-I25.799, I25.811, I25.82-I25.84

PDX Collection 667

I26.01-I26.99, I27.20-I27.9, I74.01-I74.10, I74.19, I87.8-I87.9, I99.8-I99.9

PDX Collection 668

I26.01-I26.99, I27.82, I74.01-I74.10, I74.19, I87.8-I87.9, I99.8-I99.9, T80.0XX[A], T81.718A, T81.72XA, T82.817-T82.818[A]

PDX Collection 669

I26.01-I26.99, I27.82, I74.01-I74.10, I74.19, I87.8-I87.9, I99.8-I99.9

PDX Collection 670

I26.01-I26.99, I27.82, I74.01-I74.10, I74.19, I87.8-I87.9, I99.8-I99.9, T80.0XXA, T81.718A, T81.72XA, T82.817-T82.818[A]

PDX Collection 671

E66.2, I27.0, I27.20-I27.9, I28.8-I28.9, I87.8-I87.9, I99.8-I99.9

PDX Collection 672

I28.0-I28.9

PDX Collection 673

I01.0, I09.2, I30.0-I30.9, I31.3-I32, I87.8-I87.9, I99.8-I99.9

PDX Collection 674

I31.0-I31.9, I87.8, I99.8-I99.9

PDX Collection 675

I01.1, I08.1-I08.3, I09.1, I33.0-I33.9, I38-I39, I87.8-I87.9, I99.8-I99.9

PDX Collection 676

I38-I39, I87.8-I87.9, I99.8-I99.9

PDX Collection 677

I01.2, I09.0, I23.0-I23.3, I23.6-I23.8, I40.0-I41, I51.0, I51.4, I87.8-I87.9, I99.8-I99.9

PDX Collection 678

I09.81, I11.0, I13.0, I13.2, I25.10-I25.119, I25.5-I25.799, I25.811-I25.9, I42.0-I44.1, I44.30-I44.39, I45.2-I45.4, I45.81-I45.89, I48.0-I49.1, I49.3-I49.8, I50.1, I50.810-I50.9, I87.8-I87.9, I99.8-I99.9, Q24.6, R00.0-R00.2, R57.0, R57.9

PDX Collection 679

I44.0-I49.02, I49.2, I49.8, I87.8-I87.9, I99.8-I99.9, R00.1

PDX Collection 680

I46.2-I49.02, I49.2, I87.8-I87.9, I99.8-I99.9

PDX Collection 681

I09.81, I11.0, I50.1-I50.9, I87.8-I87.9, I99.8-I99.9

PDX Collection 682

I09.81, I11.0, I50.1-I50.9, I87.8-I87.9, I99.8-I99.9, J81.0

PDX Collection 683

I09.81, I11.0, I50.1-I50.9, I51.81, I51.9-I52, I87.8-I87.9, I99.8-I99.9

PDX Collection 684

E03.5, G93.82, I60.0-I62.9, I87.8-I87.9, I99.8-I99.9, R40.0-R40.2224, R40.2310-R40.2324, R40.2340-R40.2344, R40.3-R40.4, S02.0XX[A,B], S02.101-S02.102[A,B], S02.109[A,B], S02.110-S02.19X[A,B], S02.91X[A,B], S06.0X0-S06.0X1[A], S06.0X9-S06.9X9[A]

PDX Collection 685

E08.51-E08.59, E08.618-E08.638, E08.649-E08.8, E09.51-E09.59, E09.618-E09.638, E09.649-E09.8, E10.51-E10.59, E10.618-E10.638, E10.649, E10.69-E10.8, E11.51-E11.59, E11.618-E11.638, E11.649, E11.69-E11.8, E13.51-E13.59, E13.618-E13.638, E13.649-E13.8, G43.601-G43.619, I63.00-I63.29, I65.01-I65.9, I87.8-I87.9, I99.8, I99.9

PDX Collection 686

E08.51-E08.59, E08.618-E08.638, E08.649-E08.8, E09.51-E09.59, E09.618-E09.638, E09.649-E09.8, E10.51-E10.59, E10.618-E10.638, E10.649, E10.69-E10.8, E11.51-E11.59, E11.618-E11.638, E11.649, E11.69-E11.8, E13.51-E13.59, E13.618-E13.638, E13.649-E13.8, G43.601-G43.619, I63.00-I63.29, I65.01-I65.9, I87.8-I87.9, I99.8-I99.9

PDX Collection 687

E08.51-E08.59, E08.618-E08.638, E08.649-E08.8, E09.51-E09.59, E09.618-E09.638, E09.649-E09.8, E10.51-E10.59, E10.618-E10.638, E10.649, E10.69-E10.8, E11.51-E11.59, E11.618-E11.638, E11.649, E11.69-E11.8, E13.51-E13.59, E13.618-E13.638, E13.649-E13.8, G43.601-G43.619, I63.00-I63.29, I65.01-I65.9, I87.8-I87.9, I99.8-I99.9

PDX Collection 688

E08.51-E08.59, E08.618-E08.638, E08.649-E08.8, E09.51-E09.59, E09.618-E09.638, E09.649-E09.8, E10.51-E10.59, E10.618-E10.638, E10.649, E10.69-E10.8, E11.51-E11.59, E11.618-E11.638, E11.649, E11.69-E11.8, E13.51-E13.59, E13.618-E13.638, E13.649-E13.8, G43.601-G43.619, I63.30-I63.9, I66.01-I66.9, I87.8-I87.9, I99.8-I99.9

PDX Collection 689

I77.2-I77.3, I77.5-I77.6, I77.89-I77.9, M31.8-M31.9

PDX Collection 690

E08.51-E08.59, E08.618-E08.638, E08.649-E08.8, E09.51-E09.59, E09.618-E09.638, E09.649-E09.8, E10.51-E10.59, E10.618-E10.638, E10.649, E10.69-E10.8, E11.51-E11.59, E11.618-E11.638, E11.649, E11.69-E11.8, E13.51-E13.59, E13.618-E13.638, E13.649-E13.8, I67.4, I87.8-I87.9, I99.8-I99.9

PDX Collection 691

E08.51-E08.59, E08.618-E08.638, E08.649-E08.8, E09.51-E09.59, E09.618-E09.638, E09.649-E09.8, E10.51-E10.59, E10.618-E10.638, E10.649, E10.69-E10.8, E11.51-E11.59, E11.618-E11.638, E11.649, E11.69-E11.8, E13.51-E13.59, E13.618-E13.638, E13.649-E13.8, I67.5, I87.8-I87.9, I99.8-I99.9

PDX Collection 692

E08.51-E08.59, E08.618-E08.638, E08.649-E08.8, E09.51-E09.59, E09.618-E09.638, E09.649-E09.8, E10.51-E10.59, E10.618-E10.638, E10.649, E10.69-E10.8, E11.51-E11.59, E11.618-E11.638, E11.649, E11.69-E11.8,

E13.51-E13.59, E13.618-E13.638, E13.649-E13.8, I67.6,
I87.8-I87.9, I99.8-I99.9

PDX Collection 693
E08.51-E08.59, E08.618-E08.638, E08.649-E08.8,
E09.51-E09.59, E09.618-E09.638, E09.649-E09.8,
E10.51-E10.59, E10.618-E10.638, E10.649, E10.69-E10.8,
E11.51-E11.59, E11.618-E11.638, E11.649, E11.69-E11.8,
E13.51-E13.59, E13.618-E13.638, E13.649-E13.8, I67.7, I68.2,
I87.8-I87.9, I99.8-I99.9

PDX Collection 694
E08.51-E08.59, E08.618-E08.638, E08.649-E08.8,
E09.51-E09.59, E09.618-E09.638, E09.649-E09.8,
E10.51-E10.59, E10.618-E10.638, E10.649, E10.69-E10.8,
E11.51-E11.59, E11.618-E11.638, E11.649, E11.69-E11.8,
E13.51-E13.59, E13.618-E13.638, E13.649-E13.8,
G45.0-G45.2, G45.8-G46.2, I60.00-I62.9, I63.30-I63.9,
I66.01-I66.9, I67.81-I67.82, I67.841-I67.89, I87.8-I87.9,
I99.8-I99.9

PDX Collection 695
I69.051-I69.052, I69.151-I69.152, I69.251-I69.252,
I69.351-I69.352, I69.851-I69.852, I69.951-I69.952

PDX Collection 696
I69.053-I69.054, I69.153-I69.154, I69.253-I69.254,
I69.353-I69.354, I69.853-I69.854, I69.953-I69.954

PDX Collection 697
I69.059, I69.159, I69.259, I69.359, I69.859, I69.959

PDX Collection 698
I70.231-I70.25, L44.8-L45, L94.2, L94.4, L97.101-L97.929,
L98.411-L98.499, L98.7, L98.7-L99

PDX Collection 699
I70.92, I73.81-I74.19, .I74.2-I77.2, I77.5-I77.6,
I77.810-I77.819, I79.1-I79.8, M31.8-M31.9

PDX Collection 700
E08.51-E08.59, E08.618-E08.638, E08.649-E08.8,
E09.51-E09.59, E09.618-E09.638, E09.649, E09.65-E09.8,
E10.51-E10.59, E10.618-E10.638, E10.649, E10.69-E10.8,
E11.51-E11.59, E11.618-E11.638, E11.649, E11.69-E11.8,
E13.51-E13.59, E13.618-E13.638, E13.649-E13.8,
I71.00-I71.9, I77.810-I77.819, I79.0, I87.8-I87.9, I99.8-I99.9

PDX Collection 701
E08.51-E08.59, E08.618-E08.638, E08.649-E08.8,
E09.51-E09.59, E09.618-E09.638, E09.649, E09.65-E09.8,
E10.51-E10.59, E10.618-E10.638, E10.649, E10.69-E10.8,
E11.51-E11.59, E11.618-E11.638, E11.649, E11.69-E11.8,
E13.51-E13.59, E13.618-E13.638, E13.649-E13.8, I74.11,
I74.8-I74.9, I76, I87.8-I87.9, I99.8-I99.9

PDX Collection 702
E08.51-E08.59, E08.618-E08.638, E08.649-E08.8,
E09.51-E09.59, E09.618-E09.638, E09.649, E09.65-E09.8,
E10.51-E10.59, E10.618-E10.638, E10.649, E10.69-E10.8,
E11.51-E11.59, E11.618-E11.638, E11.649, E11.69-E11.8,
E13.51-E13.59, E13.618-E13.638, E13.649-E13.8, I74.2,
I74.8-I74.9, I76, I87.8-I87.9, I99.8-I99.9

PDX Collection 703
E08.51-E08.59, E08.618-E08.638, E08.649-E08.8,
E09.51-E09.59, E09.618-E09.638, E09.649, E09.65-E09.8,
E10.51-E10.59, E10.618-E10.638, E10.649, E10.69-E10.8,
E11.51-E11.59, E11.618-E11.638, E11.649, E11.69-E11.8,
E13.51-E13.59, E13.618-E13.638, E13.649-E13.8, I74.3-I74.4,
I74.8-I74.9, I76, I87.8-I87.9, I99.8-I99.9

PDX Collection 704
E08.51-E08.59, E08.618-E08.638, E08.649-E08.8,
E09.51-E09.59, E09.618-E09.638, E09.649, E09.65-E09.8,
E10.51-E10.59, E10.618-E10.638, E10.649, E10.69-E10.8,
E11.51-E11.59, E11.618-E11.638, E11.649, E11.69-E11.8,

E13.51-E13.59, E13.618-E13.638, E13.649-E13.8, I74.5-I74.9,
I76, I87.8-I87.9, I99.8-I99.9

PDX Collection 705
E08.51-E08.59, E08.618-E08.638, E08.649-E08.8,
E09.51-E09.59, E09.618-E09.638, E09.649, E09.65-E09.8,
E10.51-E10.59, E10.618-E10.638, E10.649, E10.69-E10.8,
E11.51-E11.59, E11.618-E11.638, E11.649, E11.69-E11.8,
E13.51-E13.59, E13.618-E13.638, E13.649-E13.8, I74.8-I74.9,
I76, I87.8-I87.9, I99.8-I99.9

PDX Collection 706
E08.51-E08.59, E08.618-E08.638, E08.649-E08.8,
E09.51-E09.59, E09.618-E09.638, E09.649, E09.65-E09.8,
E10.51-E10.59, E10.618-E10.638, E10.649, E10.69-E10.8,
E11.51-E11.59, E11.618-E11.638, E11.649, E11.69-E11.8,
E13.51-E13.59, E13.618-E13.638, E13.649-E13.8,
I74.8-I75.019, I76, I87.8-I87.9, I99.8-I99.9

PDX Collection 707
E08.51-E08.59, E08.618-E08.638, E08.649-E08.8,
E09.51-E09.59, E09.618-E09.638, E09.649, E09.65-E09.8,
E10.51-E10.59, E10.618-E10.638, E10.649, E10.69-E10.8,
E11.51-E11.59, E11.618-E11.638, E11.649, E11.69-E11.8,
E13.51-E13.59, E13.618-E13.638, E13.649-E13.8, I74.8-I74.9,
I75.021-I75.029, I76, I87.8-I87.9, I99.8-I99.9

PDX Collection 708
E08.51-E08.59, E08.618-E08.638, E08.649-E08.8,
E09.51-E09.59, E09.618-E09.638, E09.649, E09.65-E09.8,
E10.51-E10.59, E10.618-E10.638, E10.649, E10.69-E10.8,
E11.51-E11.59, E11.618-E11.638, E11.649, E11.69-E11.8,
E13.51-E13.59, E13.618-E13.638, E13.649-E13.8, I74.8-I74.9,
I75.81, I76, I87.8-I87.9, I99.8-I99.9

PDX Collection 709
E08.51-E08.59, E08.618-E08.638, E08.649-E08.8,
E09.51-E09.59, E09.618-E09.638, E09.649, E09.65-E09.8,
E10.51-E10.59, E10.618-E10.638, E10.649, E10.69-E10.8,
E11.51-E11.59, E11.618-E11.638, E11.649, E11.69-E11.8,
E13.51-E13.59, E13.618-E13.638, E13.649-E13.8, I74.8-I74.9,
I75.89, I76, I87.8-I87.9, I99.8-I99.9

PDX Collection 710
I25.42, I67.0, I77.2, I77.70, I77.72-I77.79

PDX Collection 711
I77.4

PDX Collection 712
I77.5, M31.8-M31.9

PDX Collection 713
E08.51-E08.59, E08.618-E08.638, E08.649-E08.8,
E09.51-E09.59, E09.618-E09.638, E09.649, E09.65-E09.8,
E10.51-E10.59, E10.618-E10.638, E10.649, E10.69-E10.8,
E11.51-E11.59, E11.618-E11.638, E11.649, E11.69-E11.8,
E13.51-E13.59, E13.618-E13.638, E13.649-E13.8,
I80.00-I80.9, I87.8-I87.9, I99.8-I99.9

PDX Collection 714
E08.51-E08.59, E08.618-E08.638, E08.649-E08.8,
E09.51-E09.59, E09.618-E09.638, E09.649, E09.65-E09.8,
E10.51-E10.59, E10.618-E10.638, E10.649, E10.69-E10.8,
E11.51-E11.59, E11.618-E11.638, E11.649, E11.69-E11.8,
E13.51-E13.59, E13.618-E13.638, E13.649-E13.8, I81,
I82.210-I82.291, I82.401-I82.729, I82.811-I82.91,
I82.A11-I82.C29, I87.8-I87.9, I99.8-I99.9

PDX Collection 715
E08.51-E08.59, E08.618-E08.638, E08.649-E08.8,
E09.51-E09.59, E09.618-E09.638, E09.649, E09.65-E09.8,
E10.51-E10.59, E10.618-E10.638, E10.649, E10.69-E10.8,
E11.51-E11.59, E11.618-E11.638, E11.649, E11.69-E11.8,
E13.51-E13.59, E13.618-E13.638, E13.649-E13.8, I82.0,
I82.210-I82.291, I82.401-I82.729, I82.811-I82.91,
I82.A11-I82.C29, I87.8-I87.9, I99.8-I99.9

PDX Collection 716
E08.51-E08.59, E08.618-E08.638, E08.649-E08.8,
E09.51-E09.59, E09.618-E09.638, E09.649, E09.65-E09.8,
E10.51-E10.59, E10.618-E10.638, E10.649, E10.69-E10.8,
E11.51-E11.59, E11.618-E11.638, E11.649, E11.69-E11.8,
E13.51-E13.59, E13.618-E13.638, E13.649-E13.8, I82.1,
I82.210-I82.291, I82.401-I82.729, I82.811-I82.91,
I82.A11-I82.C29, I87.8-I87.9, I99.8-I99.9

PDX Collection 717
E08.51-E08.59, E08.618-E08.638, E08.649-E08.8,
E09.51-E09.59, E09.618-E09.638, E09.649, E09.65-E09.8,
E10.51-E10.59, E10.618-E10.638, E10.649, E10.69-E10.8,
E11.51-E11.59, E11.618-E11.638, E11.649, E11.69-E11.8,
E13.51-E13.59, E13.618-E13.638, E13.649-E13.8,
I82.210-I82.291, I82.401-I82.729, I82.811-I82.91,
I82.A11-I82.C29, I87.8-I87.9, I99.8-I99.9

PDX Collection 718
E08.51-E08.59, E08.618-E08.638, E08.649-E08.8,
E09.51-E09.59, E09.618-E09.638, E09.649, E09.65-E09.8,
E10.51-E10.59, E10.618-E10.638, E10.649, E10.69-E10.8,
E11.51-E11.59, E11.618-E11.638, E11.649, E11.69-E11.8,
E13.51-E13.59, E13.618-E13.638, E13.649-E13.8,
I82.210-I82.291, I82.401-I82.729, I82.811-I82.91,
I82.A11-I82.C29, I87.8-I87.9, I99.8-I99.9

PDX Collection 719
E08.51-E08.59, E08.618-E08.638, E08.649-E08.8,
E09.51-E09.59, E09.618-E09.638, E09.649, E09.65-E09.8,
E10.51-E10.59, E10.618-E10.638, E10.649, E10.69-E10.8,
E11.51-E11.59, E11.618-E11.638, E11.649, E11.69-E11.8,
E13.51-E13.59, E13.618-E13.638, E13.649-E13.8,
I82.210-I82.291, I82.3, I82.401-I82.729, I82.811-I82.91,
I82.A11-I82.C29, I87.8-I87.9, I99.8-I99.9

PDX Collection 720
I83.001-I83.229, I83.90-I83.93

PDX Collection 721
I16.4, I85.00-I85.01, I85.11, I87.8-I87.9, I99.8-I99.9, K22.6,
K25.0-K28.9, K29.01, K29.21, K29.31, K29.41, K29.51,
K29.61, K29.71, K29.81, K29.91, K31.811, K92.0-K92.2

PDX Collection 722
I16.4, I85.01, I85.11, I87.8-I87.9, I99.8-I99.9,
K22.10-K22.11, K22.6-K22.70, K22.710-K22.719,
K25.0-K28.9, K29.01, K29.21, K29.31, K29.41, K29.51,
K29.61, K29.71, K29.81, K29.91, K31.811, K55.21, K57.01,
K57.11, K57.13, K57.21, K57.31, K57.33, K57.41, K57.51,
K57.53, K57.81, K57.91, K57.93, K62.5, K92.0-K92.2

PDX Collection 723
I16.4, I85.01, I85.10-I85.11, I87.8-I87.9, I99.8-I99.9, K22.6,
K25.0-K28.9, K29.01, K29.21, K29.31, K29.41, K29.51,
K29.61, K29.71, K29.81, K29.91, K31.811, K92.0-K92.2

PDX Collection 724
I85.01, I85.11, I87.8-I87.9, I99.8-I99.9

PDX Collection 725
I80.00-I80.9

PDX Collection 726
I87.1

PDX Collection 727
I83.001-I83.229, I83.90-I83.93, I87.2, I87.8-I87.9, I99.8-I99.9

PDX Collection 728
D78.81-D78.89, E36.8, E89.810-E89.89, H59.011-H59.019,
H59.031-H59.099, H59.811-H59.89, H95.811-H95.89,
I97.110-I97.191, I97.3, I97.710-I97.791, I97.88-I97.89,
L76.81-L76.82, M96.89, N98.1-N98.9, T81.82XA,
T81.89X-T81.9XX[A]

PDX Collection 729
H95.811-H95.89, I85.01, I85.11, I97.3-I97.42,
I97.610-I97.648, K21.9, K22.8, K23-K25.0, K25.2, K25.4,
K25.6, K26.0, K26.2, K26.4, K26.6, K27.0, K27.2, K27.4,
K27.6, K28.0, K28.2, K28.4, K28.6, K29.01, K29.21,
K29.31, K29.41, K29.51, K29.61, K29.71, K29.81, K29.91,
K31.811, K55.21, K57.01, K57.11, K57.13, K57.21, K57.31,
K57.33, K57.41, K57.51, K57.53, K57.81, K57.91, K57.93,
K62.5, K92.0-K92.2, M96.89, N98.1-N98.9, P54.1-P54.3,
T81.10X-T81.19X[A], T81.82XA, T81.89X-T81.9XX[A]

PDX Collection 730
A15.8-A15.9, A17.9, A18.82, A18.84, A18.89, J04.10-J04.2,
J05.10-J05.11, J22, J98.8-J98.9

PDX Collection 731
A15.8-A15.9, A17.9, A18.82, A18.84, A18.89, J04.0-J04.2,
J05.10-J05.11, J22, J98.8-J98.9

PDX Collection 732
J04.31, J05.10-J05.11

PDX Collection 733
A15.0-A15.6, A15.8-A15.9, A17.9, A18.82, A18.84, A18.89,
A21.2, A22.1, A31.0, A37.01, A37.11, A37.81, A37.91, A42.0,
A43.0, A48.1, B25.0, B39.0-B39.2, B44.0, B58.3, B59, B67.1,
J09.X1-J09.X2, J10.00-J10.1, J11.00-J11.1, J12.0-J12.3,
J12.89-J18.1, J18.8-J18.9, J22, J44.0-J44.9, J45.21-J45.22,
J45.31-J45.32, J45.41-J45.42, J45.51-J45.902, J47.0-J70.4,
J70.8-J70.9, J98.4, J98.8-J99, Q33.4, R91.1

PDX Collection 734
A15.0-A15.6, A15.8-A15.9, A17.9, A18.82, A18.84, A18.89,
A20.2, A21.1, A22.1, A31.0, A37.01, A37.11, A37.81, A37.91,
A42.0, A43.0, A48.1, B25.0, B39.0-B39.2, B44.0, B58.3,
B59, B67.1, J09.X1-J09.X2, J10.00-J10.1, J11.00-J11.1,
J12.0-J12.3, J12.81-J18.1, J18.8-J18.9, J22, J60-J70.4,
J70.8-J70.9, J98.4, J98.8-J99, R91.1

PDX Collection 735
A15.0-A15.6, A15.8-A15.9, A17.9, A18.82, A18.84, A18.89,
A21.2, A22.1, A31.0, A37.01, A37.11, A37.81, A37.91, A42.0,
A43.0, A48.1, B25.0, B39.0-B39.2, B44.0, B58.3, B59, B67.1,
J09.X1-J09.X2, J10.00-J10.1, J11.00-J11.1, J12.0-J12.3,
J12.81-J18.1, J18.8-J18.9, J22, J44.9, J47.0-J70.4,
J70.8-J70.9, J98.4, J98.8-J99, Q33.4, R91.1

PDX Collection 736
J18.2, J22, J81.1, J98.4, J98.8-J99, R91.1

PDX Collection 737
J21.0

PDX Collection 738
J20.0-J21.9

PDX Collection 739
J22, J36, J98.8-J98.9

PDX Collection 740
J22, J39.0-J39.1, J98.8-J98.9

PDX Collection 741
J10.08, J41.1-J42, J44.0-J44.1

PDX Collection 742
J10.08, J22, J45.20-J45.998, J98.4, J98.8-J99, R91.1

PDX Collection 743
A17.9, A18.82, A18.84, A18.89, J09.X2, J10.08, J11.1, J44.9,
J47.0-J47.1, J68.1, J68.4-J68.9, Q33.4

PDX Collection 744
J22, J80, J96.00-J96.92, J98.8-J98.9, R09.2

PDX Collection 745
I09.81, I50.1-I50.9, J22, J81.0, J98.8-J98.9

PDX Collection 746
A15.0-A15.6, A15.8-A15.9, A17.9, A18.82, A18.84, A18.89,
A20.2, A21.1, A22.1, A31.0, A37.01, A37.11, A37.81, A37.91,

A42.0, A43.0, A48.1, B25.0, B39.0-B39.2, B44.0, B58.3,
B59, B67.1, J09.X1-J09.X2, J10.00-J10.1, J11.00-J11.1,
J12.0-J12.3, J12.89-J18.1, J18.8-J18.9, J22, J47.0-J70.4,
J70.8-J70.9, J82, J98.4, J98.8-J99, Q33.4, R91.1

PDX Collection 747
A15.0-A15.6, A15.8-A15.9, A17.9, A18.82, A18.84, A18.89,
J22, J44.9, J47.0-J70.4, J70.8-J70.9, J84.01-J84.82,
J84.89-J84.9, J98.4, J98.8-J99, Q33.4, R91.1

PDX Collection 748
J84.83-J84.848, P22.0-P28.5, P28.89-P29.2, P29.4,
P29.89-P29.9, P84, P94.1-P96.0, P96.3-P96.5, P96.82-P96.89

PDX Collection 749
A06.5, A15.0-A15.6, A15.8-A15.9, A17.9, A18.82, A18.84,
A18.89, J22, J85.0-J85.2, J98.8-J98.9

PDX Collection 750
J22, J85.3, J98.8-J98.9

PDX Collection 751
J22, J86.0-J86.9, J98.4, J98.8-J99, R91.1

PDX Collection 752
A15.0-A15.6, A15.8-A15.9, A17.9, A18.82, A18.84, A18.89,
J22, J90-J92.9, J94.0-J94.9, J98.4, J98.8-J99, R09.1, R91.1

PDX Collection 753
C45.7-C45.9, C76.8, C78.2-C78.39, C79.89-C79.9, C7A.00,
C7A.098, C7A.1-C7B.00, C7B.09-C7B.8, C80.0-C80.2,
D49.81-D49.9, J90-J91.0, J94.0, J94.2

PDX Collection 754
J22, J93.0-J93.9, J95.811-J95.812, J98.4, J98.8-J99, R91.1

PDX Collection 755
J22, J93.8, J95.00-J95.09, J98.01-J98.09, J98.8-J98.9

PDX Collection 756
J22, J95.1-J95.3, J95.821-J95.822, J98.8-J98.9

PDX Collection 757
D78.81-D78.89, E36.8, E89.810-E89.89, H59.011-H59.019,
H59.031-H59.099, H59.811-H59.89, H95.811-H95.89, I97.3,
J95.4-J95.5, J95.84, J95.851-J95.89, L76.81-L76.82, M96.89,
N98.1-N98.9, T81.82XA, T81.89X-T81.9XX[A]

PDX Collection 758
H95.811-H95.89, I85.01, I85.11, I97.3, J95.61-J95.62,
J95.830-J95.831, J95.860-J95.863, K21.9, K22.8,
K23-K25.0, K25.2, K25.4, K25.6, K26.0, K26.2, K26.4,
K26.6, K27.0, K27.2, K27.4, K27.6, K28.0, K28.2, K28.4,
K28.6, K29.01, K29.21, K29.31, K29.41, K29.51, K29.61,
K29.71, K29.81, K29.91, K31.811, K55.21, K57.01, K57.11,
K57.13, K57.21, K57.31, K57.33, K57.41, K57.51, K57.53,
K57.81, K57.91, K57.93, K62.5, K92.0-K92.2, M96.89,
N98.1-N98.9, P54.1-P54.3, T81.10X-T81.19X[A], T81.82XA,
T81.89X-T81.9XX[A]

PDX Collection 759
J95.850, Z99.0-Z99.12, Z99.81-Z99.89

PDX Collection 760
J22, J98.11-J98.19, J98.8-J98.9

PDX Collection 761
K00.0-K08.9, M26.00-M26.9, M27.61-M27.69

PDX Collection 762
K11.0-K11.9, K31.89-K31.9, K92.81, R68.2

PDX Collection 763
K12.1-K12.39, K14.0, K14.2

PDX Collection 764
K22.11, K22.8-K23, K31.82

PDX Collection 765
E16.4, I85.01, K22.10-K22.11, K22.6-K22.719, K25.0-K28.9,
K29.01, K29.21, K29.31, K29.41, K29.51, K29.61, K29.71,
K29.81, K29.91, K31.811, K31.89-K31.9, K55.21, K57.01,

K57.11, K57.13, K57.21, K57.31, K57.33, K57.41, K57.51,
K57.53, K57.81, K57.91, K57.93, K62.5, K92.0-K92.81

PDX Collection 766
K21.9, K22.3, K22.6, K22.8-K23

PDX Collection 767
E16.4, I85.01, K21.9, K22.10-K22.11, K22.3, K22.6-K28.9,
K29.01, K29.21, K29.31, K29.41, K29.51, K29.61, K29.71,
K29.81, K29.91, K31.811, K55.21, K57.01, K57.11, K57.13,
K57.21, K57.31, K57.33, K57.41, K57.51, K57.53, K57.81,
K57.91, K57.93, K62.5, K92.0-K92.2

PDX Collection 768
E16.4, I85.01, K22.10-K22.11, K22.6-K22.719, K25.0-K28.9,
K29.01, K29.21, K29.31, K29.41, K29.51, K29.61, K29.71,
K29.81, K29.91, K31.5, K31.811, K31.89-K31.9, K55.21,
K57.01, K57.11, K57.13, K57.21, K57.31, K57.33,
K57.41, K57.51, K57.53, K57.81, K57.91, K57.93, K62.5,
K92.0-K92.81

PDX Collection 769
E16.4, I85.01, K22.6, K25.0-K28.9, K29.01, K29.21, K29.31,
K29.41, K29.51, K29.61, K29.71, K29.81, K29.91, K31.5,
K31.811, K31.82, K31.89-K31.9, K55.21, K57.01, K57.11,
K57.13, K57.21, K57.31, K57.33, K57.41, K57.51, K57.53,
K57.81, K57.91, K57.93, K62.5, K92.0-K92.81

PDX Collection 770
E16.4, I85.01, K22.10-K22.11, K22.6-K22.719, K25.0-K28.9,
K29.01, K29.21, K29.31, K29.41, K29.51, K29.61, K29.71,
K29.81, K29.91, K31.811, K55.21, K57.01, K57.11, K57.13,
K57.21, K57.31, K57.33, K57.41, K57.51, K57.53, K57.81,
K57.91, K57.93, K62.5, K92.0-K92.2

PDX Collection 771
K31.0

PDX Collection 772
K30-K31.1, K31.5, K31.84, Q38.5, Q40.0, Q40.8-Q41.9,
Q43.4-Q43.9

PDX Collection 773
K31.5, Q38.5, Q40.8-Q41.9, Q43.4-Q43.9

PDX Collection 774
K31.6, Q38.5, Q40.8-Q40.9, Q43.4-Q43.9

PDX Collection 775
E16.4, I85.01, K22.10-K22.11, K22.6-K22.719, K25.0-K28.9,
K29.01, K29.21, K29.31, K29.41, K29.51, K29.61, K29.71,
K29.81, K29.91, K31.811, K31.82, K55.21, K57.01, K57.11,
K57.13, K57.21, K57.31, K57.33, K57.41, K57.51, K57.53,
K57.81, K57.91, K57.93, K62.5, K92.0-K92.2

PDX Collection 776
K31.89-K38.9, K92.81

PDX Collection 777
K31.89-K31.9, K40.00-K40.91, K45.0, K45.8-K46.0, K92.81

PDX Collection 778
K31.89-K31.9, K41.00-K41.91, K45.0, K45.8-K46.0, K92.81

PDX Collection 779
K31.89-K31.9, K41.10-K41.21, K41.40-K41.91, K45.0,
K45.8-K46.0, K92.81

PDX Collection 780
K42.0-K42.1, K43.0-K43.1, K43.3-K43.4, K43.6-K43.7, K45.0,
K45.8-K46.0

PDX Collection 781
K31.89-K31.9, K42.0-K43.9, K45.0, K45.8-K46.0, K46.9,
K92.81

PDX Collection 782
K44.0-K46.0

PDX Collection 783
K40.00-K46.9

PDX Collection 784
K31.89-K31.9, K40.00-K46.9, K92.81

PDX Collection 785
K50.00-K51.919

PDX Collection 786
K50.00-K50.919

PDX Collection 787
K51.00-K51.919

PDX Collection 788
K52.0

PDX Collection 789
K52.1

PDX Collection 790
K55.011-K55.1, K55.30-K55.33

PDX Collection 791
K55.011-K55.069, K55.1, K55.30-K55.33, K55.8-K55.9

PDX Collection 792
K56.0-K56.3, K56.49-K56.7, K63.4, K63.89-K63.9,
K91.30-K91.32, K92.89-K92.9, R11.13

PDX Collection 793
K57.00-K57.13

PDX Collection 794
K57.20-K57.93

PDX Collection 795
K58.0-K58.9, K59.1-K59.9, K91.0-K91.1

PDX Collection 796
K61.0-K61.4

PDX Collection 797
K62.6

PDX Collection 798
K63.0

PDX Collection 799
K63.1

PDX Collection 800
K63.2

PDX Collection 801
K63.3

PDX Collection 802
E16.4, I85.01, K22.10-K22.11, K22.6-K22.719, K25.0-K28.9,
K29.01, K29.21, K29.31, K29.41, K29.51, K29.61, K29.71,
K29.81, K29.91, K31.811, K55.21, K57.01, K57.11, K57.13,
K57.21, K57.31, K57.33, K57.41, K57.51, K57.53, K57.81,
K57.91, K57.93, K62.5, K63.81, K92.0-K92.2

PDX Collection 803
K63.4, K63.89-K63.9, K65.0-K65.9, K67, K68.19-K68.9,
K92.89-K92.9, R11.13

PDX Collection 804
K66.1

PDX Collection 805
D78.81-D78.89, E36.8, E89.810-E89.89, H59.011-H59.019,
H59.031-H59.099, H59.811-H59.89, H95.811-H95.89, I97.3,
K68.11, L76.81-L76.82, M96.89, N98.1-N98.9, T81.4XXA,
T81.82XA, T81.89X-T81.9XX[A]

PDX Collection 806
K68.12, M60.00-M60.19, M61.00-M61.19, M61.30-M61.59,
M62.3, M62.50-M62.59, M62.84, M62.89, M72.6

PDX Collection 807
K72.91, K76.5, K76.89-K76.9 K72.00-K72.01, K76.2-K76.3,
K76.5, K76.89-K76.9

PDX Collection 808
K72.00-K72.01, K76.2-K76.3, K76.5, K76.89-K76.9

PDX Collection 809
A06.4, K75.0-K75.1, K76.5, K76.89-K76.9

PDX Collection 810
K72.91, K76.5-K76.6, K76.89-K76.9

PDX Collection 811
K76.5, K76.7, K76.89-K76.9

PDX Collection 812
K80.00-K80.21, K80.40, K80.44, K80.62-K80.63,
K80.66-K80.67, K80.80, K81.0-K81.9, K82.9, K83.5-K83.9,
K87

PDX Collection 813
K80.00-K80.21, K80.62-K80.63, K80.66-K80.67, K80.80,
K81.0-K81.9, K82.9, K83.5-K83.9, K87

PDX Collection 814
K83.0, K83.5-K83.9, K87

PDX Collection 815
K80.30-K80.71, K80.81-K81.9, K83.5-K83.9, K87

PDX Collection 816
K80.62-K80.63, K81.0-K81.9, K82.9, K83.5-K83.9, K87

PDX Collection 817
K80.66-K80.67, K81.0-K81.9, K82.9, K83.5-K83.9, K87

PDX Collection 818
K80.00, K80.12, K80.62-K80.63, K80.66-K80.67, K81.0-K81.9,
K82.9, K83.5-K83.9, K87

PDX Collection 819
K81.0-K81.9, K82.9, K83.5-K83.9, K87

PDX Collection 820
K82.0-K82.9, K83.5-K83.9, K87

PDX Collection 821
K80.31, K80.33, K80.35, K80.37, K80.41, K80.43, K80.45,
K80.47, K80.51, K80.81, K83.1, K83.5-K83.9, K87,
Q44.2-Q44.3

PDX Collection 822
K83.2-K83.3, K83.5-K83.9, K87

PDX Collection 823
B25.2, E16.8, K85.00-K86.9

PDX Collection 824
K86.2-K86.9

PDX Collection 825
E84.19, K90.0-K90.49, K90.89-K90.9, K91.2

PDX Collection 826
K90.81

PDX Collection 827
K90.3-K90.49, K90.89-K90.9, K91.2

PDX Collection 828
D78.81-D78.89, E36.8, E89.810-E89.89, H59.011-H59.019,
H59.031-H59.099, H59.811-H59.89, H95.811-H95.89,
I97.3, K91.81-K91.83, K91.850-K91.89, K94.20-K95.89,
L76.81-L76.82, M96.89, N98.1-N98.9, T81.710A, T81.82XA,
T81.89X-T81.9XX[A]

PDX Collection 829
H95.811-H95.89, I85.01, I85.11, I97.3, K21.9, K22.8,
K23-K25.0, K25.2, K25.4, K25.6, K26.0, K26.2, K26.4,
K26.6, K27.0, K27.2, K27.4, K27.6, K28.0, K28.2, K28.4,
K28.6, K29.01, K29.21, K29.31, K29.41, K29.51, K29.61,
K29.71, K29.81, K29.91, K31.811, K55.21, K57.01,
K57.11, K57.13, K57.21, K57.31, K57.33, K57.41, K57.51,
K57.53, K57.81, K57.91, K57.93, K62.5, K91.61-K91.62,
K91.840-K91.841, K91.870-K91.873, K92.0-K92.2, M96.89,
N98.1-N98.9, P54.1-P54.3, T81.10X-T81.19X[A], T81.82XA,
T81.89X-T81.9XX[A]

PDX Collection 830
K94.00-K94.19

PDX Collection 831
D78.81-D78.89, E36.8, E89.810-E89.89, H59.011-H59.019,
H59.031-H59.099, H59.811-H59.89, H95.811-H95.89,
I97.3, K91.81-K91.83, K91.850-K91.89, K94.00-K95.89,
L76.81-L76.82, M96.89, N98.1-N98.9, T81.710A, T81.82XA,
T81.89X-T81.9XX[A]

PDX Collection 832
A17.9, A18.4, A18.82, A18.84, A18.89, A48.2-A48.4,
A48.8-A49.9, B78.1, B95.0-B96.89, E83.2, L02.11,
L02.811-L02.818, L02.91, L03.221-L03.222, L03.811-L03.91,
L08.0-L08.9, L44.8-L45, L73.2, L88, L92.8, L94.2, L94.4,
L98.0, L98.3, L98.7, L98.8, L99, Z16.10-Z16.39

PDX Collection 833
A17.9, A18.4, A18.82, A18.84, A18.89, A48.2-A48.4,
A48.8-A49.9, B78.1, B95.0-B96.89, E83.2, L02.211-L02.219,
L02.811-L02.818, L02.91, L03.311-L03.316, L03.319-L03.326,
L03.329-L03.91, L08.0, L08.81-L08.9, L44.8-L45, L73.2,
L88, L92.8, L94.2, L94.4, L98.0, L98.3, L98.7, L98.8, L99,
Z16.10-Z16.39

PDX Collection 834
A17.9, A18.4, A18.82, A18.84, A18.89, A48.2-A48.4,
A48.8-A49.9, B78.1, B95.0-B96.89, E83.2, L02.31,
L02.811-L02.818, L02.91, L03.317, L03.327, L03.811-L03.91,
L08.0, L08.81-L08.9, L44.8-L45, L73.2, L88, L92.8, L94.2,
L94.4, L98.0, L98.3, L98.7, L98.8, L99, Z16.10-Z16.39

PDX Collection 835
A17.9, A18.4, A18.82, A18.84, A18.89, A48.2-A48.4,
A48.8-A49.9, B78.1, B95.0-B96.89, E83.2, L02.411-L02.414,
L02.811-L02.818, L02.91, L03.111-L03.114, L03.121-L03.124,
L03.811-L03.91, L08.0, L08.81-L08.9, L44.8-L45, L73.2,
L88, L92.8, L94.2, L94.4, L98.0, L98.3, L98.7, L98.8, L99,
Z16.10-Z16.39

PDX Collection 836
A17.9, A18.4, A18.82, A18.84, A18.89, A48.2-A48.4,
A48.8-A49.9, B78.1, B95.0-B96.89, E83.2, L02.415-L02.419,
L02.811-L02.818, L02.91, L03.115-L03.119, L03.125-L03.129,
L03.811-L03.91, L08.0, L08.81-L08.9, L44.8-L45, L73.2,
L88, L92.8, L94.2, L94.4, L98.0, L98.3, L98.7, L98.8, L99,
Z16.10-Z16.39

PDX Collection 837
A17.9, A18.4, A18.82, A18.84, A18.89, A48.2-A48.4,
A48.8-A49.9, B78.1, B95.0-B96.89, E83.2, L02.511-L02.519,
L02.811-L02.818, L02.91, L03.811-L03.91, L08.0,
L08.81-L08.9, L44.8-L45, L73.2, L88, L92.8, L94.2, L94.4,
L98.0, L98.3, L98.7, L98.8, L99, Z16.10-Z16.39

PDX Collection 838
A17.9, A18.4, A18.82, A18.84, A18.89, A48.2-A48.4,
A48.8-A49.9, B78.1, B95.0-B96.89, E83.2, L02.611-L02.619,
L02.811-L02.818, L02.91, L03.811-L03.91, L08.0,
L08.81-L08.9, L44.8-L45, L73.2, L88, L92.8, L94.2, L94.4,
L98.0, L98.3, L98.7, L98.8, L99, Z16.10-Z16.39

PDX Collection 839
A17.9, A18.4, A18.82, A18.84, A18.89, A48.2-A48.4,
A48.8-A49.9, B78.1, B95.0-B96.89, E83.2, L02.811-L02.818,
L02.91, L03.811-L03.91, L08.0, L08.81-L08.9, L44.8-L45,
L73.2, L88, L92.8, L94.2, L94.4, L98.0, L98.3, L98.7, L98.8,
L99, Z16.10-Z16.39

PDX Collection 840
A17.9, A18.4, A18.82, A18.84, A18.89, A48.2-A48.4,
A48.8-A49.9, B78.1, B95.0-B96.89, E83.2, L02.811-L02.818,
L02.91, L03.211, L03.213, L03.811-L03.91, L08.0,
L08.81-L08.9, L44.8-L45, L73.2, L88, L92.8, L94.2, L94.4,
L98.0, L98.3, L98.7, L98.8, L99, Z16.10-Z16.39

PDX Collection 841
L05.01-L05.92, L44.8-L45, L94.2, L94.4, L98.7, L98.8, L99

PDX Collection 842
L10.0-L10.9, L12.0-L12.1, L12.8-L12.9, L13.8-L14, L44.8-L45, L94.2, L94.4, L98.7, L98.8, L99

PDX Collection 843
L00, L12.30-L12.35, L26, L30.4, L44.8-L45, L51.0-L54, L71.0-L71.9, L92.0, L93.0-L93.2, L94.2, L94.4, L95.1, L98.2, L98.7, L98.8, L99

PDX Collection 844
L49.3

PDX Collection 845
L49.4

PDX Collection 846
L49.5

PDX Collection 847
L49.6

PDX Collection 848
L49.7

PDX Collection 849
L49.8

PDX Collection 850
L49.9

PDX Collection 851
L12.30-L12.35, L44.8-L45, L51.0-L53.3, L71.0-L71.9, L93.0-L93.2, L94.2, L94.4, L98.7, L98.8, L99

PDX Collection 852
H95.811-H95.89, I85.01, I85.11, I97.3, K21.9, K22.8, K23, K25.0, K25.2, K25.4, K25.6, K26.0, K26.2, K26.4, K26.6, K27.0, K27.2, K27.4, K27.6, K28.0, K28.2, K28.4, K28.6, K29.01, K29.21, K29.31, K29.41, K29.51, K29.61, K29.71, K29.81, K29.91, K31.811, K55.21, K57.01, K57.11, K57.13, K57.21, K57.31, K57.33, K57.41, K57.51, K57.53, K57.81, K57.91, K57.93, K62.5, K92.0-K92.2, L76.01-L76.02, L76.21-L76.82, M96.89, N98.1-N98.9, P54.1-P54.3, T81.10X-T81.19X[A], T81.82XA, T81.89X-T81.9XX[A]

PDX Collection 853
L08.0, L08.81, L88

PDX Collection 854
L89.000-L89.95, L97.101-L97.929, L98.411-L98.499

PDX Collection 855
A17.9, A18.02, A18.09, A18.82, A18.84, A18.89, A39.83-A39.84, A54.40, A54.42-A54.43, A54.82, A54.84, A54.89-A54.9, B06.82, M00.00-M02.30, M02.319, M02.329, M02.339, M02.349, M02.359, M02.369, M02.379-M02.9, M05.40-M05.59, M05.70-M06.09, M06.20-M07.69, M11.00-M11.9, M12.10-M15.0, M15.3-M15.9, M16.2-M16.9, M17.2-M17.9, M18.2-M19.93, M24.10-M24.176, M25.00, M25.08-M25.18, M25.40-M25.676, M25.80-M25.9, M35.2, M36.1-M36.4, R26.2, R29.4

PDX Collection 856
A17.9, A18.02, A18.09, A18.82, A18.84, A18.89, A39.83-A39.84, A54.40, A54.42-A54.43, A54.82, A54.84, A54.89-A54.9, B06.82, M00.00-M02.30, M02.319, M02.38-M02.819, M02.88-M02.9, M05.40-M05.59, M05.70-M06.09, M06.20-M07.69, M11.00-M11.9, M11.20-M11.219, M11.28-M11.819, M11.88-M11.9, M12.10-M15.0, M15.3-M15.9, M19.011-M19.019, M19.111-M19.119, M19.211-M19.219, M19.90-M19.93, M24.10-M24.119, M25.00, M25.011-M25.019, M25.08-M25.119, M25.18, M25.40-M25.419, M25.48-M25.519, M25.541-M25.549, M25.60-M25.619, M25.80-M25.819, M25.9, M35.2, M36.1-M36.4, R26.2

PDX Collection 857
A17.9, A18.02, A18.09, A18.82, A18.84, A18.89, A39.83-A39.84, A54.40, A54.42-A54.43, A54.82, A54.84, A54.89-A54.9, B06.82, M00.00-M02.30, M02.329,

M02.38-M02.80, M02.821-M02.829, M02.88-M02.9, M05.40-M05.59, M05.70-M07.60, M07.621-M07.629, M07.68-M07.69, M11.00, M11.021-M11.029, M11.08-M11.10, M11.121-M11.129, M11.18-M11.20, M11.221-M11.229, M11.28-M11.80, M11.821-M11.829, M11.88-M11.9, M12.10, M12.121-M12.129, M12.18-M12.20, M12.221-M12.229, M12.28-M12.30, M12.321-M12.329, M12.38-M12.40, M12.421-M12.429, M12.48-M12.50, M12.521-M12.529, M12.58-M12.80, M12.821-M12.829, M12.88-M12.9, M13.0-M13.10, M13.121-M13.129, M13.80, M13.821-M13.829, M13.88-M13.89, M14.60-M15.9, M19.021-M19.029, M19.121-M19.129, M19.221-M19.229, M19.90-M19.93, M24.10, M24.121-M24.129, M25.00, M25.021-M25.029, M25.08-M25.10, M25.121-M25.129, M25.18, M25.40, M25.421-M25.429, M25.48-M25.50, M25.521-M25.529, M25.541-M25.549, M25.60, M25.621-M25.629, M25.80, M25.821-M25.829, M25.9, M35.2, M36.1-M36.4, R26.2

PDX Collection 858
A17.9, A18.02, A18.09, A18.82, A18.84, A18.89, A39.83-A39.84, A54.40, A54.42-A54.43, A54.82, A54.84, A54.89-A54.9, B06.82, M00.00-M02.30, M02.339, M02.38-M02.80, M02.831-M02.839, M02.88-M02.9, M05.40-M05.59, M05.70-M07.60, M07.631-M07.639, M07.68-M07.69, M11.00, M11.031-M11.039, M11.08-M11.10, M11.131-M11.139, M11.18-M11.20, M11.231-M11.239, M11.28-M11.80, M11.831-M11.839, M11.88-M11.9, M12.10, M12.131-M12.139, M12.18-M12.20, M12.231-M12.239, M12.28-M12.30, M12.331-M12.339, M12.38-M12.40, M12.431-M12.439, M12.48-M12.50, M12.531-M12.539, M12.58-M12.80, M12.831-M12.839, M12.88-M12.9, M13.0-M13.10, M13.131-M13.139, M13.80, M13.831-M13.839, M13.88-M15.9, M19.031-M19.039, M19.131-M19.139, M19.231-M19.239, M19.90-M19.93, M24.10, M24.131-M24.139, M25.00, M25.031-M25.039, M25.08-M25.10, M25.131-M25.139, M25.18, M25.40, M25.431-M25.439, M25.48-M25.50, M25.531-M25.539, M25.541-M25.549, M25.60, M25.631-M25.639, M25.80, M25.831-M25.839, M25.9, M35.2, M36.1-M36.4, R26.2

PDX Collection 859
A17.9, A18.02, A18.09, A18.82, A18.84, A18.89, A39.83-A39.84, A54.40, A54.42-A54.43, A54.82, A54.84, A54.89-A54.9, B06.82, M00.00, M00.041-M00.049, M00.08-M00.10, M00.141-M00.149, M00.18-M00.20, M00.241-M00.249, M00.28-M00.80, M00.841-M00.849, M00.88-M01.X0, M01, X41-M01.X49, M01.X8-M02.10, M02.141-M02.149, M02.18-M02.30, M02.349, M02.38-M02.80, M02.841-M02.849, M02.88-M02.9, M05.40-M05.59, M05.70-M06.09, M06.20-M07.60, M07.641-M07.649, M07.68-M07.69, M11.00, M11.041-M11.049, M11.08-M11.10, M11.141-M11.149, M11.18-M11.20, M11.241-M11.249, M11.28-M11.80, M11.841-M11.849, M11.88-M11.9, M12.10, M12.141-M12.149, M12.18-M12.20, M12.241-M12.249, M12.28-M12.30, M12.341-M12.349, M12.38-M12.40, M12.441-M12.449, M12.48-M12.50, M12.541-M12.549, M12.58-M12.80, M12.841-M12.849, M12.88-M13.10, M13.141-M13.149, M13.80, M13.841-M13.849, M13.88-M15.9, M18.0-M18.9, M19.041-M19.049, M19.141-M19.149, M19.241-M19.249, M19.90-M19.93, M24.10, M24.141-M24.149, M25.00, M25.08-M25.10, M25.141-M25.149, M25.18, M25.40, M25.441-M25.449, M25.48-M25.50, M25.541-M25.549, M25.60, M25.641-M25.649, M25.80, M25.841-M25.849, M25.9, M35.2, M36.1-M36.4, R26.2

PDX Collection 860
A17.9, A18.02, A18.09, A18.82, A18.84, A18.89, A39.83-A39.84, A54.40, A54.42-A54.43, A54.82, A54.84,

A54.89-A54.9, B06.82, M00.00, M00.051-M00.059, M00.08-M00.10, M00.151-M00.159, M00.18-M00.20, M00.251-M00.259, M00.28-M00.29, M00.80, M00.851-M00.859, M00.88-M00.9, M01.X0, M01.X51-M01.X59, M01.X8-M02.10, M02.151-M02.159, M02.18-M02.30, M02.359, M02.38-M02.80, M02.851-M02.9, M05.40-M05.59, M05.70-M06.09, M06.20-M06.39, M06.80-M07.60, M07.651-M07.659, M07.68-M07.69, M11.00, M11.051-M11.059, M11.08-M11.10, M11.151-M11.159, M11.18-M11.20, M11.251-M11.259, M11.28-M11.80, M11.851-M11.859, M11.88-M12.10, M12.151-M12.159, M12.18-M12.20, M12.251-M12.259, M12.28-M12.30, M12.351-M12.359, M12.38-M12.40, M12.451-M12.459, M12.48-M12.50, M12.551-M12.559, M12.58-M12.80, M12.851-M12.859, M12.88-M13.10, M13.151-M13.159, M13.80, M13.851-M13.859, M13.88-M15.0, M15.3-M16.9, M19.90-M19.93, M24.10, M24.151-M24.159, M25.00, M25.051-M25.059, M25.08-M25.10, M25.151-M25.159, M25.18, M25.40, M25.451-M25.459, M25.48-M25.559, M25.60, M25.651-M25.659, M25.80, M25.851-M25.859, M25.9, M35.2, M36.1-M36.4, R26.2, R29.4

PDX Collection 861
A17.9, A18.02, A18.09, A18.82, A18.84, A18.89, A39.83-A39.84, A54.40, A54.42-A54.43, A54.82, A54.84, A54.89-A54.9, B06.82, M00.00, M00.061-M00.069, M00.08-M00.10, M00.161-M00.169, M00.18-M00.20, M00.261-M00.269, M00.28-M00.29, M00.80, M00.861-M00.869, M00.88-M00.9, M01.X0, M01.X61-M01.X69, M01.X8-M02.10, M02.161-M02.169, M02.18-M02.30, M02.369, M02.38-M02.80, M02.861-M02.869, M02.88-M02.9, M05.40-M05.59, M05.70-M06.09, M06.20-M06.39, M06.80-M07.60, M07.661-M07.669, M07.68-M07.69, M11.00, M11.061-M11.069, M11.08-M11.10, M11.161-M11.169, M11.18-M11.20, M11.261-M11.269, M11.28-M11.80, M11.861-M11.869, M11.88-M12.10, M12.161-M12.169, M12.18-M12.20, M12.261-M12.269, M12.28-M12.30, M12.361-M12.369, M12.38-M12.40, M12.461-M12.469, M12.48-M12.50, M12.561-M12.569, M12.58-M12.80, M12.861-M12.869, M12.88-M13.10, M13.161-M13.169, M13.80, M13.861-M13.869, M13.88-M15.0, M15.3-M15.9, M17.0-M17.9, M19.90-M19.93, M24.10, M25.00, M25.061-M25.069, M25.08-M25.10, M25.161-M25.169, M25.18, M25.40, M25.461-M25.469, M25.48-M25.50, M25.541-M25.549, M25.561-M25.569, M25.60, M25.661-M25.669, M25.80, M25.861-M25.869, M25.9, M35.2, M36.1-M36.4, R26.2

PDX Collection 862
A17.9, A18.02, A18.09, A18.82, A18.84, A18.89, A39.83-A39.84, A54.40, A54.42-A54.43, A54.82, A54.84, A54.89-A54.9, B06.82, M00.00, M00.071-M00.079, M00.08-M00.10, M00.171-M00.179, M00.18-M00.20, M00.271-M00.279, M00.28-M00.29, M00.80, M00.871-M00.879, M00.88-M00.9, M01.X0, M01.X71-M01.X79, M01.X8-M02.10, M02.171-M02.179, M02.18-M02.9, M05.40-M05.59, M05.70-M06.09, M06.20-M06.39, M06.80-M07.60, M07.671-M07.679, M07.68-M07.69, M11.00, M11.071-M11.079, M11.08-M11.10, M11.171-M11.179, M11.18-M11.20, M11.271-M11.279, M11.28-M11.80, M11.871-M11.879, M11.88-M11.9, M12.10, M12.171-M12.179, M12.18-M12.20, M12.271-M12.279, M12.28-M12.30, M12.371-M12.379, M12.38-M12.40, M12.471-M12.479, M12.48-M12.50, M12.571-M12.579, M12.58-M12.80, M12.871-M12.879, M12.88-M13.10, M13.171-M13.179, M13.80, M13.871-M13.879, M13.88-M15.0, M15.3-M15.9, M19.071-M19.079, M19.171-M19.179, M19.271-M19.279, M19.90-M19.93, M24.10, M24.171-M24.176, M25.00, M25.071-M25.10,

M25.171-M25.18, M25.40, M25.471-M25.50,
M25.541-M25.549, M25.571-M25.60, M25.671-M25.676,
M25.80, M25.871-M25.9, M35.2, M36.1-M36.4, R26.2

PDX Collection 863

A02.23, A17.9, A18.02, A18.09, A18.82, A18.84, A18.89,
A39.83-A39.84, A54.40, A54.42-A54.43, A54.82, A54.84,
A54.89-A54.9, B06.82, M00.00, M00.011-M02.30,
M02.319, M02.329, M02.339, M02.349, M02.359, M02.369,
M02.379, M02.38-M02.9, M05.40-M05.59, M05.70-M07.69,
M11.00-M15.0, M15.3-M15.9, M16.2-M16.9, M17.2-M17.9,
M18.2-M18.9, M19.111-M19.93, M24.10-M24.176, M25.00,
M25.08-M25.18, M25.40-M25.676, M25.80-M25.9, M35.2,
M36.1-M36.4, R29.4

PDX Collection 864

A02.23, A17.9, A18.02, A18.09, A18.82, A18.84, A18.89,
A39.83-A39.84, A54.40, A54.42-A54.43, A54.82, A54.84,
A54.89-A54.9, B06.82, M00.00, M00.011-M02.30,
M02.319, M02.329, M02.339, M02.349, M02.359, M02.369,
M02.379, M02.38-M02.9, M05.40-M05.59, M05.70-M07.69,
M11.00-M15.0, M15.3-M15.9, M16.2-M16.9, M17.2-M17.9,
M18.2-M18.9, M19.111-M19.93, M24.10-M24.176, M25.00,
M25.08-M25.18, M25.40-M25.676, M25.80-M25.9, M35.2,
M36.1-M36.4, R29.4

PDX Collection 865

A02.23, A17.9, A18.02, A18.09, A18.82, A18.84, A18.89,
A39.83-A39.84, A54.40, A54.42-A54.43, A54.82, A54.84,
A54.89-A54.9, B06.82, M00.00, M00.011-M02.30,
M02.319, M02.329, M02.339, M02.349, M02.359, M02.369,
M02.379, M02.38-M02.9, M05.40-M05.59, M05.70-M07.69,
M11.00-M15.0, M15.3-M15.9, M16.2-M16.9, M17.2-M17.9,
M18.2-M18.9, M19.111-M19.93, M24.10-M24.176, M25.00,
M25.08-M25.18, M25.40-M25.676, M25.80-M25.9, M35.2,
M36.1-M36.4, R29.4

PDX Collection 866

A02.23, A17.9, A18.02, A18.09, A18.82, A18.84, A18.89,
A39.83-A39.84, A54.40, A54.42-A54.43, A54.82, A54.84,
A54.89-A54.9, B06.82, M00.00, M00.011-M02.30,
M02.319, M02.329, M02.339, M02.349, M02.359, M02.369,
M02.379, M02.38-M02.9, M05.40-M05.59, M05.70-M07.69,
M11.00-M15.0, M15.3-M15.9, M16.2-M16.9, M17.2-M17.9,
M18.2-M18.9, M19.111-M19.93, M24.10-M24.176, M25.00,
M25.08-M25.18, M25.40-M25.676, M25.80-M25.9, M35.2,
M36.1-M36.4, R29.4

PDX Collection 867

E08.40-E08.49, E08.618-E08.638, E08.649-E08.8,
E09.40-E09.49, E09.618-E09.638, E09.649-E09.8,
E10.40-E10.49, E10.618-E10.638, E10.649, E10.69-E10.8,
E11.40-E11.49, E11.618-E11.638, E11.649, E11.69-E11.8,
E13.40-E13.49, E13.618-E13.638, E13.649-E13.8, G32.89,
G70.00-G72.3, G72.81-G73.7, G96.8-G96.9, G98.0-G98.8,
G99.8

PDX Collection 868

M25.00-M25.08, T79.A11A-T79.A29A

PDX Collection 869

M25.00-M25.039, M25.08, T79.A11-T79.A19[A]

PDX Collection 870

M25.00-M25.029, M25.08, T79.A11-T79.A19[A]

PDX Collection 871

M25.00-M25.049, M25.08, T79.A11-T79.A19[A]

PDX Collection 872

M25.00, M25.031-M25.049, M25.08, T79.A11-T79.A19[A]

PDX Collection 873

M25.00, M25.061-M25.08, T79.A21-T79.A29[A]

PDX Collection 874

E08.51-E08.59, E08.618-E08.638, E08.649-E08.8,
E09.51-E09.59, E09.618-E09.638, E09.649-E09.8,

E10.51-E10.59, E10.618-E10.638, E10.649, E10.69-E10.8,
E11.51-E11.59, E11.618-E11.638, E11.649, E11.69-E11.8,
E13.51-E13.59, E13.618-E13.638, E13.649-E13.8, I87.8-I87.9,
I99.8-I99.9, M30.0-M31.7

PDX Collection 875

I87.8-I87.9, I99.8-I99.9, M30.0-M31.7

PDX Collection 876

M33.00-M33.19, M33.90-M33.99, M36.0

PDX Collection 877

E08.40-E08.49, E08.618-E08.638, E08.649-E08.8,
E09.40-E09.49, E09.618-E09.638, E09.649-E09.8,
E10.40-E10.49, E10.618-E10.638, E10.649, E10.69-E10.8,
E11.40-E11.49, E11.618-E11.638, E11.649, E11.69-E11.8,
E13.40-E13.49, E13.618-E13.638, E13.649-E13.8, G32.89,
G70.00-G72.3, G72.81-G73.7, G96.8-G96.9, G98.0-G98.8,
G99.8, M33.00-M33.19, M33.90-M33.99, M36.0

PDX Collection 878

M33.20-M33.29

PDX Collection 879

E08.40-E08.49, E08.618-E08.638, E08.649-E08.8,
E09.40-E09.49, E09.618-E09.638, E09.649-E09.8,
E10.40-E10.49, E10.618-E10.638, E10.649, E10.69-E10.8,
E11.40-E11.49, E11.618-E11.638, E11.649, E11.69-E11.8,
E13.40-E13.49, E13.618-E13.638, E13.649-E13.8, G32.89,
G70.00-G72.3, G72.81-G73.7, G96.8-G96.9, G98.0-G98.8,
G99.8, M33.20-M33.29

PDX Collection 880

G72.41-G72.49, M35.1, M35.5, M35.8

PDX Collection 881

A02.24, A17.9, A18.03, A18.09, A18.82, A18.84, A18.89,
M46.20-M46.39, M86.00-M86.9

PDX Collection 882

A17.9, A18.01, A18.03, A18.09, A18.82, A18.84, A18.89,
M46.20-M46.39, M86.00-M86.9

PDX Collection 883

M47.011-M47.029, M47.11-M47.13, M47.21-M47.23,
M47.811-M47.813, M47.891-M47.893

PDX Collection 884

M25.78, M47.011-M47.16, M47.20-M47.9, M48.10-M48.38,
M48.9

PDX Collection 885

M47.14-M47.15

PDX Collection 886

M46.40, M46.46-M46.49, M47.16, M47.26-M47.28,
M47.816-M47.818, M47.896-M47.898, M51.06, M51.26-M51.27,
M51.36-M51.37, M51.46-M51.47, M51.86-M51.9

PDX Collection 887

M48.30-M48.38

PDX Collection 888

M48.40X-M48.58X[A], M80.00X-M80.88X[A],
M84.30X-M84.68X[A], M84.750-M84.759[A]

PDX Collection 889

M50.00-M50.03, M50.20-M50.23

PDX Collection 890

M51.04-M51.05, M51.24-M51.25

PDX Collection 891

M51.06, M51.24-M51.25

PDX Collection 892

K68.12, M60.000-M60.19, M61.00-M61.19, M61.30-M61.59,
M62.3, M62.50-M62.59, M62.82, M62.84, M62.89, M72.6

PDX Collection 893

M70.80-M70.99, M79.81-M79.9, R29.898,
S45.301-S45.899[A], S55.201-S55.899[A],
S65.801-S65.899[A]

PDX Collection 894

M70.80-M70.99, M79.81-M79.9, R29.898,
S75.801-S75.899[A], S85.201-S85.899[A],
S95.001-S95.099[A], S95.201-S95.899[A]

PDX Collection 895

S31.001A, S31.011A, S31.021A, S31.031A, S31.041A,
S31.051-S31.159[A], S31.600-S31.659[A],
S31.831-S31.839[A], S36.00X-S37.599[A],
S37.812-S37.99X[A], S38.3XX[A], S39.021-S39.023[A],
T07.XXX-T14.91X[A], T79.8XX-T79.9XX[A]

PDX Collection 896

S31.001A, S31.011A, S31.021A, S31.031A, S31.041A,
S31.051A, S31.600-S31.659[A], S36.81X-S36.899[A]

PDX Collection 897

M80.00X-M80.88X[K,P], M84.30X-M84.68X[K,P],
M84.750-M84.759[K,P], S02.0XX-S02.92X[K],
S12.000-S12.691[K], S22.000-S22.9XX[K],
S32.000-S32.9XX[K], S42.001-S42.92X[K,P],
S49.001-S49.199[K,P], S52.001-S52.92X[K,M,N,P,Q,R],
S59.001-S59.299[K,P], S62.001-S62.92X[K,P],
S72.001-S72.92X[K,M,N,P,Q,R], S79.001-S79.199[K,P],
S82.001-S82.92X[K,M,N,P,Q,R], S89.001-S89.399[K,P],
S92.001-S92.919[K,P]

PDX Collection 898

A17.9, A18.03-A18.09, A18.82, A18.84, A18.89,
M46.20-M46.39, M86.00-M86.9

PDX Collection 899

A17.9, A18.03-A18.09, A18.82, A18.84, A18.89,
M46.20-M46.39, M86.00, M86.08-M86.10, M86.18-M86.20,
M86.28-M86.319, M86.38-M86.419, M86.48-M86.519,
M86.58-M86.619, M86.68-M86.8X1, M86.8X8-M86.9

PDX Collection 900

A17.9, A18.03-A18.09, A18.82, A18.84, A18.89,
M46.20-M46.39, M86.00, M86.08-M86.10, M86.18-M86.20,
M86.28-M86.30, M86.321-M86.329, M86.38-M86.40,
M86.421-M86.429, M86.48-M86.50, M86.521-M86.529,
M86.58-M86.60, M86.621-M86.629, M86.68-M86.69,
M86.8X0, M86.8X2, M86.8X8-M86.9

PDX Collection 901

A17.9, A18.03-A18.09, A18.82, A18.84, A18.89,
M46.20-M46.39, M86.00, M86.08-M86.10, M86.18-M86.20,
M86.28-M86.30, M86.331-M86.339, M86.38-M86.40,
M86.431-M86.439, M86.48-M86.50, M86.531-M86.539,
M86.58-M86.60, M86.631-M86.639, M86.68-M86.8X0,
M86.8X3, M86.8X8-M86.9

PDX Collection 902

A17.9, A18.03-A18.09, A18.82, A18.84, A18.89,
M46.20-M46.39, M86.00, M86.08-M86.10, M86.18-M86.20,
M86.28-M86.30, M86.341-M86.349, M86.38-M86.40,
M86.441-M86.449, M86.48-M86.50, M86.541-M86.549,
M86.58-M86.60, M86.41-M86.649, M86.68-M86.69, M86.8X0,
M86.8X4, M86.8X8-M86.9

PDX Collection 903

A17.9, A18.03-A18.09, A18.82, A18.84, A18.89,
M46.20-M46.39, M86.00, M86.08-M86.10, M86.18-M86.20,
M86.28-M86.30, M86.351-M86.359, M86.38-M86.40,
M86.451-M86.459, M86.48-M86.50, M86.551-M86.559,
M86.58-M86.60, M86.651-M86.659, M86.68-M86.8X0,
M86.8X5, M86.8X8-M86.9

PDX Collection 904

A17.9, A18.03-A18.09, A18.82, A18.84, A18.89,
M46.20-M46.39, M86.00, M86.08-M86.10, M86.18-M86.20,
M86.28-M86.30, M86.361-M86.369, M86.38-M86.40,
M86.461-M86.469, M86.48-M86.50, M86.561-M86.569,
M86.58-M86.60, M86.661-M86.669, M86.68-M86.8X0,
M86.8X6, M86.8X8-M86.9

PDX Collection 905

A17.9, A18.03-A18.09, A18.82, A18.84, A18.89,
M46.20-M46.39, M86.00, M86.08-M86.10, M86.18-M86.20,
M86.28-M86.30, M86.371-M86.379, M86.38-M86.40,
M86.471-M86.479, M86.48-M86.50, M86.571-M86.579,
M86.58-M86.60, M86.671-M86.679, M86.68-M86.8X0,
M86.8X7-M86.9

PDX Collection 906

M46.20-M46.39, M86.30-M86.9, M88.0-M88.9,
M90.60-M90.69

PDX Collection 907

M87.00-M87.9, M90.50-M90.59

PDX Collection 908

M87.00-M87.9, M90.50-M90.59

PDX Collection 909

M87.00-M87.9, M90.50-M90.59

PDX Collection 910

M87.00, M87.031-M87.819, M87.831-M87.849,
M87.861-M87.9, M90.50, M90.521-M90.549,
M90.561-M90.59

PDX Collection 911

D78.81, D78.89, E36.8, E89.810-E89.89, H59.011-H59.019,
H59.031-H59.819, H59.88-H59.89, H95.811-H95.89,
I97.3, L76.81-L76.82, M96.621-M96.69, M96.89,
M97.01X-M97.9XX[A], N98.1-N98.9, T81.82XA,
T81.89X-T81.9XX[A], T84.010-T84.039[A],
T84.050-T84.9XX[A]

PDX Collection 912

H95.811-H95.89, I85.01, I85.11, I97.3, K21.9, K22.8,
K23-K25.2, K25.4, K25.6, K26.0, K26.2, K26.4, K26.6,
K27.0, K27.2, K27.4, K27.6, K28.0, K28.2, K28.4, K28.6,
K29.01, K29.21, K29.31, K29.41, K29.51, K29.61, K29.71,
K29.81, K29.91, K31.811, K55.21, K57.01, K57.11, K57.13,
K57.21, K57.31, K57.33, K57.41, K57.51, K57.53, K57.81,
K57.91, K57.93, K62.5, K92.0-K92.2, M96.810-M96.811,
M96.830-M96.89, N98.1-N98.9, P54.1-P54.3,
T81.10X-T81.19X[A], T81.82XA, T81.89X-T81.9XX[A]

PDX Collection 913

M99.10-M99.11, S03.8XX-S03.9XX[A], S12.000-S12.691[A,B],
S12.9XX-S13.4XX[A], S13.8XX[A], S14.0XX-S14.108[A],
S14.111-S14.118[A], S14.121-S14.128[A],
S14.131-S14.138[A], S14.141-S14.148[A],
S14.151-S14.158[A], S16.1XX[A], S29.011-S29.019[A],
S38.3XX[A], S39.011-S39.013[A], T07.XXX-T14.91X[A],
T79.A0X-T79.9XX[A]

PDX Collection 914

M99.18, S43.201-S43.226[A]

PDX Collection 915

A17.9, A18.10-A18.11, A18.13, A18.82, A18.84,
A18.89, A54.21, A54.29, A54.82, A54.84, A54.89-A54.9,
A59.00, A59.8-A59.9, B37.41-B37.49, E08.21-E08.29,
E08.618-E08.638, E08.649, E08.65-E08.8, E09.21-E09.29,
E09.618-E09.638, E09.649-E09.8, E10.21-E10.29,
E10.618-E10.638, E10.649, E10.69-E10.8, E11.21-E11.29,
E11.618-E11.638, E11.649, E11.69-E11.8, E13.21-E13.29,
E13.618-E13.638, E13.649-E13.69, E13.8, E88.3,
M10.30-M10.39, N10, N11.10, N11.8, N11.9, N13.0-N13.39,
N13.6, N14.0-N19, N25.0-N27.9, N28.1-N29, N36.41-N36.43,
N36.8-N36.9, N39.8-N39.9, R31.0-R31.9

PDX Collection 916

A17.9, A18.10-A18.11, A18.13, A18.82, A18.84, A18.89,
A54.21, A54.29, A54.82, A54.84, A54.89-A54.9, A59.00,
A59.8-A59.9, B37.41-B37.49, E09.21-E09.29,
E88.3, M10.30-M10.39, N00.0-N13.39, N13.6, N14.0-N19,
N25.0-N27.9, N28.1-N29, N36.41-N36.43, N36.8-N36.9,
N39.8-N39.9, R31.0-R31.9

PDX Collection 917

A17.9, A18.10-A18.11, A18.13, A18.82, A18.84,
A18.89, A54.21, A54.29, A54.82, A54.84, A54.89-A54.9,
A59.00, A59.8-A59.9, B37.41-B37.49, E08.21-E08.29,
E08.618-E08.638, E08.649, E08.65-E08.8, E09.21-E09.29,
E09.618-E09.638, E09.649-E09.8, E10.21-E10.29,
E10.618-E10.638, E10.649, E10.69-E10.8, E11.21-E11.29,
E11.618-E11.638, E11.649, E11.69-E11.8, E13.21-E13.29,
E13.618-E13.638, E13.649-E13.69, E13.8, M10.30-M10.39,
N00.0-N13.39, N13.6, N14.0-N19, N25.0-N27.9, N28.1-N29,
N36.41-N36.43, N36.8-N36.9, N39.8-N39.9, R31.0-R31.9

PDX Collection 918

A17.9, A18.10-A18.11, A18.13, A18.82, A18.84, A18.89,
A54.21, A54.29, A54.82, A54.84, A54.89-A54.9, A59.00,
A59.8-A59.9, A98.5, B37.41-B37.49, E08.21-E08.29,
E08.618-E08.638, E08.649, E08.65-E08.8, E09.21-E09.29,
E09.618-E09.638, E09.649-E09.8, E10.21-E10.29,
E10.618-E10.638, E10.649, E10.69-E10.8, E11.21-E11.29,
E11.618-E11.638, E11.649, E11.69-E11.8, E13.21-E13.29,
E13.618-E13.638, E13.649-E13.69, E13.8, M10.30-M10.39,
N00.0-N13.39, N13.6, N14.0-N19, N25.0-N27.9, N28.1-N29,
N36.41-N36.43, N36.8-N36.9, N39.8-N39.9, R31.0-R31.9

PDX Collection 919

A17.9, A18.10-A18.11, A18.13, A18.82, A18.84,
A18.89, A54.21, A54.29, A54.82, A54.84, A54.89-A54.9,
A59.00, A59.8-A59.9, B37.41-B37.49, E08.21-E08.29,
E08.618-E08.638, E08.649, E08.65-E08.8, E09.21-E09.29,
E09.618-E09.638, E09.649-E09.8, E10.21-E10.29,
E10.618-E10.638, E10.649, E10.69-E10.8, E11.21-E11.29,
E11.618-E11.638, E11.649, E11.69-E11.8, E13.21-E13.29,
E13.618-E13.638, E13.649-E13.69, E13.8, M10.30-M10.39,
N00.0-N13.39, N13.6, N14.0-N19, N25.0-N27.9, N28.1-N29,
N36.41-N36.43, N36.8-N36.9, N39.0, N39.8-N39.9,
R31.0-R31.9, R82.71

PDX Collection 920

N11.1, N13.4-N13.5, N13.8-N13.9, N28.82, N28.89-N30.91,
N32.89-N33, N36.41-N36.43, N36.8-N36.9, N39.0,
N39.8-N39.9, Q62.4-Q62.8, Q64.10-Q64.19, Q64.8-Q64.9,
R31.0-R31.9, R82.71, Z90.6

PDX Collection 921

A17.9, A18.10-A18.11, A18.13, A18.82, A18.84, A18.89,
A54.21, A54.29, A54.82, A54.84, A54.89-A54.9, A59.00,
A59.8-A59.9, A98.5, B37.41-B37.49, E08.21-E08.29,
E08.618-E08.638, E08.649, E08.65-E08.8, E09.21-E09.29,
E09.618-E09.638, E09.649-E09.8, E10.21-E10.29,
E10.618-E10.638, E10.649, E10.69-E10.8, E11.21-E11.29,
E11.618-E11.638, E11.649, E11.69-E11.8, E13.21-E13.29,
E13.618-E13.638, E13.649-E13.69, E13.8, M10.30-M10.39,
N00.0-N13.39, N13.6, N14.0-N19, N25.0-N27.9, N28.1-N29,
N36.41-N36.43, N36.8-N36.9, N39.8-N39.9, O23.01-O23.03,
O23.11-O23.13, O23.21-O23.23, O23.31-O23.33,
O23.41-O23.43, O23.511-O23.513, O23.521-O23.523,
O23.591-O23.593, O23.91-O23.93, O86.11, O86.13-O86.29,
R31.0-R31.9

PDX Collection 922

A17.9, A18.10-A18.11, A18.13, A18.82, A18.84, A18.89,
A54.21, A54.29, A54.82, A54.84, A54.89-A54.9, A59.00,
A59.8-A59.9, B37.41-B37.49, E08.21-E08.29, E09.21-E09.29,
M10.30-M10.39, N00.0-N13.39, N13.6, N14.0-N19,
N25.0-N27.9, N28.1-N29, N36.41-N36.43, N36.8-N36.9,
N39.0, N39.8-N39.9, R31.0-R31.9, R82.71

PDX Collection 923

N11.1, N13.4-N13.5, N13.8-N13.9, N28.82, N28.89-N30.91,
N32.89-N33, N36.41-N36.43, N36.8-N36.9, N39.0,
N39.8-N39.9, Q62.4-Q62.8, Q64.10-Q64.19, Q64.8-Q64.9,
R31.0-R31.9, R82.71

PDX Collection 924

E08.21-E08.29, E08.618-E08.638, E08.649-E08.8,
E09.21-E09.29, E09.618-E09.638, E09.649-E09.8,
E10.21-E10.29, E10.618-E10.638, E10.649, E10.69-E10.8,
E11.21-E11.29, E11.618-E11.638, E11.649, E11.69-E11.8,
E13.21-E13.29, E13.618-E13.638, E13.649-E13.8, E88.3,
M10.30-M10.39, N00.0-N13.39, N13.6, N14.0-N19,
N25.0-N27.9, N28.1-N29, N36.41-N36.43, N36.8-N36.9,
N39.8-N39.9, Q60.0-Q62.39, Q63.0-Q63.9, Q64.8-Q64.9,
R31.0-R31.9

PDX Collection 925

E08.21-E08.29, E08.618-E08.638, E08.649-E08.8,
E09.21-E09.29, E09.618-E09.638, E09.649-E09.8,
E10.21-E10.29, E10.618-E10.638, E10.649, E10.69-E10.8,
E11.21-E11.29, E11.618-E11.638, E11.649, E11.69-E11.8,
E13.21-E13.29, E13.618-E13.638, E13.649-E13.8, E88.3,
M10.30-M10.39, N00.0-N13.39, N13.6, N14.0-N19,
N25.0-N27.9, N28.1-N29, N36.41-N36.43, N36.8-N36.9,
N39.8-N39.9, R31.0-R31.9

PDX Collection 926

E08.21-E08.29, E08.618-E08.638, E08.649-E08.8,
E09.21-E09.29, E09.618-E09.638, E09.649-E09.8,
E10.21-E10.29, E10.618-E10.638, E10.649, E10.69-E10.8,
E11.21-E11.29, E11.618-E11.638, E11.649, E11.69-E11.8,
E13.21-E13.29, E13.618-E13.638, E13.649-E13.8,
M10.30-M10.39, N00.0-N13.39, N13.6, N14.0-N19,
N25.0-N27.9, N28.1-N29, N36.41-N36.43, N36.8-N36.9,
N39.8-N39.9, Q60.0-Q62.39, Q63.0-Q63.9, Q64.8-Q64.9,
R31.0-R31.9

PDX Collection 927

E08.21-E08.29, E08.618-E08.638, E08.649-E08.8,
E09.21-E09.29, E09.618-E09.638, E09.649-E09.8,
E10.21-E10.29, E10.618-E10.638, E10.649, E10.69-E10.8,
E11.21-E11.29, E11.618-E11.638, E11.649, E11.69-E11.8,
E13.21-E13.29, E13.618-E13.638, E13.649-E13.8, I12.9,
M10.30-M10.39, N00.0-N13.39, N13.6, N14.0-N19,
N25.0-N27.9, N28.1-N29, N36.41-N36.43, N36.8-N36.9,
N39.8-N39.9, Q60.0-Q62.39, Q63.0-Q63.9, Q64.8-Q64.9,
R31.0-R31.9

PDX Collection 928

N11.1, N13.4-N13.5, N13.8-N13.9, N20.0-N22, N28.82,
N28.89-N29, N36.41-N36.43, N36.8-N36.9, N39.8-N39.9,
R31.0-R31.9

PDX Collection 929

A17.9, A18.10-A18.11, A18.13, A18.82, A18.84, A18.89,
A54.21, A54.29, A54.82, A54.84, A54.89-A54.9, A59.00,
A59.8-A59.9, A98.5, B37.41-B37.49, E08.21-E08.29,
E08.618-E08.638, E08.649, E08.65-E08.8, E09.21-E09.29,
E09.618-E09.638, E09.649-E09.8, E10.21-E10.29,
E10.618-E10.638, E10.649, E10.69-E10.8, E11.21-E11.29,
E11.618-E11.638, E11.649, E11.69-E11.8, E13.21-E13.29,
E13.618-E13.638, E13.649-E13.69, E13.8, M10.30-M10.39,
N00.0-N13.6, N14.0-N19, N25.0-N27.9, N28.1-N29,
N36.41-N36.43, N36.8-N36.9, N39.8-N39.9, R31.0-R31.9

PDX Collection 930

A17.9, A18.10-A18.11, A18.13, A18.82, A18.84, A18.89,
A54.21, A54.29, A54.82, A54.84, A54.89-A54.9, A59.00,
A59.8-A59.9, A98.5, B37.41-B37.49, E08.21-E08.29,
E08.618-E08.638, E08.649, E08.65-E08.8, E09.21-E09.29,
E09.618-E09.638, E09.649-E09.8, E10.21-E10.29,
E10.618-E10.638, E10.649, E10.69-E10.8, E11.21-E11.29,
E11.618-E11.638, E11.649, E11.69-E11.8, E13.21-E13.29,
E13.618-E13.638, E13.649-E13.69, E13.8, M10.30-M10.39,
N00.0-N13.39, N13.6, N14.0-N19, N25.0-N27.9, N28.1-N29,
N36.41-N36.43, N36.8-N36.9, N39.8-N39.9, R31.0-R31.9

PDX Collection 931

N13.70-N13.739, N28.0, N28.9-N29

PDX Collection 932
A17.9, A18.10, A18.12-A18.13, A18.82, A18.84, A18.89,
A54.00-A54.02, A54.09-A54.1, A54.82, A54.84, A54.89-A54.9,
A59.00, A59.8-A59.9, B37.41-B37.49, N11.1, N13.4-N13.5,
N13.8-N13.9, N28.82, N28.89-N30.91, N32.89-N33,
N36.41-N36.43, N36.8-N36.9, N39.0, N39.8-N39.9,
R31.0-R31.9, R82.71

PDX Collection 933
A54.00-A54.02, A54.09-A54.1, A54.82, A54.84, A54.89-A54.9,
N32.1-N32.2, N32.89-N33, N36.41-N36.43, N36.8-N36.9,
N39.8-N39.9, R30.0, R30.9, R31.0-R31.9

PDX Collection 934
A54.00-A54.02, A54.09-A54.1, A54.82, A54.84, A54.89-A54.9,
A59.00, A59.03, A59.8-A59.9, B37.41-B37.49, N13.9,
N34.0-N34.3, N35.111-N35.9, N36.41-N36.43, N36.8-N39.0,
N39.8-N39.9, N44.1-N44.8, N47.6, N48.1-N48.9, N49.1-N49.9,
N50.3-N50.89, N51, N53.11-N53.9, Q54.0-Q55.9, Q64.0,
Q64.2-Q64.9, R30.0, R30.9-R31.9, R82.71

PDX Collection 935
N13.9, N34.0, N34.2-N36.43, N36.5-N37, N39.8-N39.9,
N44.1-N44.8, N47.6, N48.1-N48.9, N49.1-N49.9, N50.3-N50.89,
N51, N53.11-N53.9, N99.110-N99.115, Q54.0-Q55.21,
Q55.23-Q55.9, Q64.0, Q64.8-Q64.9, R30.0, R30.9-R31.9

PDX Collection 936
A54.82, A54.84, A54.89-A54.9, A59.00, A59.8-A59.9,
B37.41-B37.49, N10, N11.9-N13.39, N13.6, N13.9, N15.1,
N28.82, N28.84-N30.91, N34.1, N36.41-N36.43, N36.8-N36.9,
N39.0, N39.8-N39.9, N99.511, R30.0, R30.9-R31.9, T83.511A

PDX Collection 937
A18.14, A54.22, A54.82, A54.84, A54.89-A54.9, A59.00,
A59.02, A59.8-A59.9, B37.41-B37.49, N40.0-N42.9

PDX Collection 938
A59.00, A59.8-A59.9, B37.41-B37.49, N43.0-N43.3

PDX Collection 939
N44.00-N44.04

PDX Collection 940
A54.23, A54.82, A54.84, A54.89-A54.9, A59.00, A59.8-A59.9,
B26.0, B37.41-B37.49, N45.1-N45.4

PDX Collection 941
N47.6, N48.0-N48.9, N52.01-N52.9

PDX Collection 942
A17.9, A18.10, A18.16-A18.18, A18.82, A18.84, A18.89,
A54.03, A54.24, A54.82, A54.84, A54.89-A54.9, A59.00,
A59.8-A59.9, B37.41-B37.49, N70.01-N71.9, N73.0-N74,
N75.9, N76.5, N76.81-N76.89, N90.810-N90.818,
N94.818-N94.9, N96, Q55.0-Q55.4, Q55.7-Q55.9

PDX Collection 943
A17.9, A18.10, A18.16-A18.18, A18.82, A18.84, A18.89,
A54.03, A54.24, A54.82, A54.84, A54.89-A54.9, A59.00,
A59.8-A59.9, B37.41-B37.49, N70.01-N71.9, N72, N73.0-N74,
N75.9, N76.5, N76.81-N76.89, N85.8-N85.9, N90.810-N90.818,
N94.818-N94.9, N96, Q55.0-Q55.4, Q55.7-Q55.9

PDX Collection 944
A17.9, A18.10, A18.16-A18.18, A18.82, A18.84, A18.89,
A59.00-A59.01, A59.8-A59.9, B37.3-B37.49, N75.0-N77.1,
N84.3, N90.3, N90.60-N90.9, N94.810-N94.9, N96,
Q55.0-Q55.4, Q55.7-Q55.9

PDX Collection 945
N72, N75.9, N76.5, N76.81-N76.89

PDX Collection 946
N82.0-N82.9

PDX Collection 947
N83.00-N83.53, N83.6-N83.9, N99.83

PDX Collection 948
N98.0, T80.211-T80.29X[A], T82.7XXA, T88.0XXA

PDX Collection 949
D78.81-D78.89, E36.8, E89.810-E89.89, H59.011-H59.019,
H59.031-H59.099, H59.811-H59.89, H95.811-H95.89,
I97.3, L76.81-L76.82, M96.89, N32.89, N33, N98.1-N98.9,
N99.510-N99.518, T81.82XA, T81.89X-T81.9XX[A], T83.010A,
T83.020A, T83.030A, T83.090A, T83.110-T83.29X[A],
T83.410-T83.69X[A], T83.712-T83.714[A], T83.718A,
T83.719A, T83.722-T83.724[A], T83.728-T83.9XX[A],
T85.310-T85.311[A], T85.320-T85.321[A],
T85.390-T85.391[A], T85.510-T85.9XX[A], T85.810D,
T85.820D, T85.830D, T85.840D, T85.850D, T85.860D,
T85.890D, T86.820-T86.829, T86.842-T86.849

PDX Collection 950
D78.81-D78.89, E36.8, E89.810-E89.89,
H59.011-H59.019, H59.031-H59.099, H59.811-H59.89,
H95.811-H95.89, I97.3, L76.81-L76.82, M96.89,
N32.89, N33, N39.0, N98.1-N98.9, N99.510-N99.518,
R82.71, T81.82XA, T81.89X-T81.9XX[A], T83.010A,
T83.020A, T83.030A, T83.090A, T83.110-T83.29X[A],
T83.410-T83.69X[A], T83.712-T83.714[A], T83.718A,
T83.719A, T83.722-T83.724[A], T83.728-T83.9XX[A],
T85.310-T85.311[A], T85.320-T85.321[A],
T85.390-T85.391[A], T85.510-T85.9XX[A], T85.810D,
T85.820D, T85.830D, T85.840D, T85.850D, T85.860D,
T85.890D, T86.842-T86.849

PDX Collection 951
D78.81-D78.89, E36.8, E89.810-E89.89, H59.011-H59.019,
H59.031-H59.099, H59.811-H59.89, H95.811-H95.89,
I97.3, L76.81-L76.82, M96.89, N32.89, N33, N98.1-N98.9,
N99.510-N99.518, T81.82XA, T81.89X-T81.9XX[A], T83.010A,
T83.020A, T83.030A, T83.090A, T83.110-T83.29X[A],
T83.410-T83.69X[A], T83.712-T83.714[A], T83.718A,
T83.719A, T83.722A-T83.724A, T83.728-T83.9XX[A]

PDX Collection 952
H95.811-H95.89, I85.01, I85.11, I97.3, K21.9, K22.8,
K23-K25.0, K25.2, K25.4, K25.6, K26.0, K26.2, K26.4, K26.6,
K27.0, K27.2, K27.4, K27.6, K28.0, K28.2, K28.4, K28.6,
K29.01, K29.21, K29.31, K29.41, K29.51, K29.61, K29.71,
K29.81, K29.91, K31.811, K55.21, K57.01, K57.11, K57.13,
K57.21, K57.31, K57.33, K57.41, K57.51, K57.53, K57.81,
K57.91, K57.93, K62.5, K92.0-K92.2, M96.89, N98.1-N98.9,
N99.61-N99.62, N99.820-N99.821, N99.840-N99.843,
P54.1-P54.3, T81.10X-T81.19X[A], T81.82XA,
T81.89X-T81.9XX[A]

PDX Collection 953
O00.00-O00.91

PDX Collection 954
003.0-007.4, 011.4-011.5, 012.04-012.05, 012.14-012.15,
012.24-012.25, 013.4-013.5, 014.04-014.05,
014.14-014.15, 014.24-014.25, 014.94-014.95,
016.4-016.5, 020.0-020.9, 025.10-025.3, 026.10-026.13,
026.30-026.43, 026.63, 026.711-026.819, 026.841-026.86,
026.891-026.93, 029.011-029.93, 035.7XX-, 044.00-044.63,
045.8X1-045.93, 075.4, 075.81, 075.89-075.9, 080, 090.89,
099.111-099.285, 099.330-099.335, 099.350-099.355,
099.511-099.73, 099.820-099.825, 099.840-09A.53, Z33.2

PDX Collection 955
003.0-007.4, 011.4, 011.5, 012.04, 012.05, 012.14,
012.15, 012.24, 012.25, 013.4, 013.5, 014.04, 014.05,
014.14, 014.15, 014.24, 014.25, 014.94, 014.95, 016.4,
016.5, 020.0-020.9, 025.10-025.3, 026.10-026.13,
026.30-026.43, 026.63-026.819, 026.841-026.86,
026.891-026.93, 029.011-029.93, 035.7XX0-035.7XX9,
044.00-044.13, 044.20-044.53, 045.8X1-045.93, 075.4,
075.81, 075.89-075.9, 080, 090.89, 099.111-099.285,
099.330-099.335, 099.350-099.355, 099.511-099.73,
099.820-099.825, 099.840-09A.53, Z33.2

PDX Collection 956
003.0-007.4, 011.4, 011.5, 012.04, 012.05, 012.14,
012.15, 012.24, 012.25, 013.4, 013.5, 014.04, 014.05,
014.14, 014.15, 014.24, 014.25, 014.94, 014.95, 016.4,
016.5, 020.0-020.9, 025.10-025.3, 026.10-026.13,
026.30-026.43, 026.63-026.819, 026.841-026.86,
026.891-026.93, 029.011-029.285, 035.7XX9-035.7XX9,
044.00-044.13, 044.20-044.53, 045.8X1-045.93, 075.4,
075.81, 075.89-075.9, 080, 090.89, 099.111-099.285,
099.330-099.335, 099.350-099.355, 099.511-099.73,
099.820-099.825, 099.840-09A.53, Z33.2

PDX Collection 957
003.0-007.4, 011.4, 011.5, 012.04, 012.05, 012.14,
012.15, 012.24, 012.25, 013.4, 013.5, 014.04, 014.05,
014.14, 014.15, 014.24, 014.25, 014.94, 014.95, 016.4,
016.5, 020.0-020.9, 025.10-025.3, 026.10-026.13,
026.30-026.43, 026.63-026.819, 026.841-026.86,
026.891-026.93, 029.011-029.93, 035.7XX0-035.7XX9,
044.00-044.13, 044.20-044.53, 045.8X1-045.93, 075.4,
075.81, 075.89-075.9, 080, 090.89, 099.111-099.285,
099.330-099.335, 099.350-099.355, 099.511-099.73,
099.820-099.825, 099.840-09A.53, Z33.2

PDX Collection 958
003.0-007.4, 011.4, 011.5, 012.04, 012.05, 012.14,
012.15, 012.24, 012.25, 013.4, 013.5, 014.04, 014.05,
014.14, 014.15, 014.24, 014.25, 014.94, 014.95, 016.4,
016.5, 020.0-020.9, 025.10-025.3, 026.10-026.13,
026.30-026.43, 026.63-026.819, 026.841-026.86,
026.891-026.93, 029.011-029.93, 035.7XX0-035.7XX9,
044.00-044.13, 044.20-044.53, 045.8X1-045.93, 075.4,
075.81, 075.89-075.9, 080, 090.89, 099.111-099.285,
099.330-099.335, 099.350-099.355, 099.511-099.73,
099.820-099.825, 099.840-09A.53, Z33.2

PDX Collection 959
003.0-007.4, 011.4, 011.5, 012.04, 012.05, 012.14,
012.15, 012.24, 012.25, 013.4, 013.5, 014.04, 014.05,
014.14, 014.15, 014.24, 014.25, 014.94, 014.95, 016.4,
016.5, 020.0-020.9, 025.10-025.3, 026.10-026.13,
026.30-026.43, 026.63-026.819, 026.841-026.86,
026.891-026.93, 029.011-029.93, 035.7XX0-035.7XX9,
044.00-044.13, 044.20-044.53, 045.8X1-045.93, 075.4,
075.81, 075.89-075.9, 080, 090.89, 099.111-099.285,
099.330-099.335, 099.350-099.355, 099.511-099.73,
099.820-099.825, 099.840-09A.53, Z33.2

PDX Collection 960
003.0-007.4, 011.4, 011.5, 012.04, 012.05, 012.14,
012.15, 012.24, 012.25, 013.4, 013.5, 014.04, 014.05,
014.14, 014.15, 014.24, 014.25, 014.94, 014.95, 016.4,
016.5, 020.0-020.9, 025.10-025.3, 026.10-026.13,
026.30-026.43, 026.63-026.819, 026.841-026.86,
026.891-026.93, 029.011-029.93, 035.7XX0-035.7XX9,
044.00-044.13, 044.20-044.53, 045.8X1-045.93, 075.4,
075.81, 075.89-075.9, 080, 090.89, 099.111-099.285,
099.330-099.335, 099.350-099.355, 099.511-099.73,
099.820-099.825, 099.840-09A.53, Z33.2

PDX Collection 961
003.0-007.4, 011.4, 011.5, 012.04, 012.05, 012.14,
012.15, 012.24, 012.25, 013.4, 013.5, 014.04, 014.05,
014.14, 014.15, 014.24, 014.25, 014.94, 014.95, 016.4,
016.5, 020.0-020.9, 025.10-025.3, 026.10-026.13,
026.30-026.43, 026.63-026.819, 026.841-026.86,
026.891-026.93, 029.011-029.93, 035.7XX0-035.7XX9,
044.00-044.13, 044.20-044.53, 045.8X1-045.93, 075.4,
075.81, 075.89-075.9, 080, 090.89, 099.111-099.285,
099.330-099.335, 099.350-099.355, 099.511-099.73,
099.820-099.825, 099.840-09A.53, Z33.2

PDX Collection 962

008.1-008.81, 008.83-008.9, 011.4, 011.5, 012.04, 012.05, 012.14, 012.15, 012.24, 012.25, 013.4, 013.5, 014.04, 014.05, 014.14, 014.15, 014.24, 014.25, 014.94, 014.95, 016.4, 016.5, 020.0-020.9, 025.10-025.3, 026.10-026.13, 026.30-026.43, 026.63-026.819, 026.841-026.86, 026.891-026.93, 029.011-029.93, 035.7XX0-035.7XX9, 044.00-044.13, 044.20-044.53, 045.8X1-045.93, 075.4, 075.81, 075.89-075.9, 080, 090.89, 099.111-099.285, 099.330-099.335, 099.350-099.355, 099.511-099.73, 099.820-099.825, 099.840-09A.53

PDX Collection 963

008.2-008.81, 008.83-008.9, 011.4, 011.5, 012.04, 012.05, 012.14, 012.15, 012.24, 012.25, 013.4, 013.5, 014.04, 014.05, 014.14, 014.15, 014.24, 014.25, 014.94, 014.95, 016.4, 016.5, 020.0-020.9, 025.10-025.3, 026.10-026.13, 026.30-026.43, 026.63-026.819, 026.841-026.86, 026.891-026.93, 029.011-029.93, 035.7XX0-035.7XX9, 044.00-044.13, 044.20-044.53, 045.8X1-045.93, 075.4, 075.81, 075.89-075.9, 080, 090.89, 099.111-099.285, 099.330-099.335, 099.350-099.355, 099.511-099.73, 099.820-099.825, 099.840-09A.53

PDX Collection 964

010.011-012.03, 012.04, 012.05, 012.14, 012.15, 012.20-016.9, 025.10-026.13, 026.30-026.43, 026.63-026.819, 026.841-026.86, 026.891-026.93, 029.011-029.93, 035.7XX0-035.7XX9, 075.4, 075.81, 075.89-075.9, 080, 090.89, 099.111-099.285, 099.330-099.335, 099.350-099.355, 099.511-099.73, 099.820-099.825, 099.840-09A.53

PDX Collection 965

011.5, 012.05, 012.11-012.13, 012.15, 012.21-012.23, 012.25, 013.5, 014.05, 014.15, 014.25, 014.95, 016.5, 026.831-026.833, 090.89

PDX Collection 966

011.4, 011.5, 012.04, 012.05, 012.14, 012.15, 012.24, 012.25, 013.4, 013.5, 014.04, 014.05, 014.14, 014.15, 014.24, 014.25, 014.94, 014.95, 016.4, 016.5, 020.0-020.9, 025.10-025.3, 026.10-026.13, 026.30-026.43, 026.63-026.819, 026.841-026.86, 026.891-026.93, 029.011-029.93, 035.7XX0-035.7XX9, 044.00-044.13, 044.20-044.53, 075.4, 075.81, 075.89-075.9, 080, 090.89, 099.111-099.119, 099.12-099.285, 099.330-099.335, 099.350-099.355, 099.511-099.73, 099.820-099.825, 099.840-09A.53

PDX Collection 967

011.4, 011.5, 012.04, 012.05, 012.14, 012.15, 012.24, 012.25, 013.4, 013.5, 014.04, 014.05, 014.14, 014.15, 014.24, 014.25, 014.94, 014.95, 016.4, 016.5, 022.20-022.93, 025.10-025.3, 026.10-026.13, 026.30-026.43, 026.63-026.819, 026.841-026.86, 026.891-026.93, 029.011-029.93, 035.7XX0-035.7XX9, 075.4, 075.81, 075.89-075.9, 080, 087.0-087.9, 090.89, 099.111-099.119, 099.12-099.285, 099.330-099.335, 099.350-099.355, 099.511-099.73, 099.820-099.825, 099.840-09A.53

PDX Collection 968

011.4, 011.5, 012.04, 012.05, 012.14, 012.15, 012.24, 012.25, 013.4, 013.5, 014.04, 014.05, 014.14, 014.15, 014.24, 014.25, 014.94, 014.95, 016.4, 016.5, 023.00-023.93, 025.10-025.3, 026.10-026.13, 026.30-026.43, 026.63-026.819, 026.841-026.86, 026.891-026.93, 029.011-029.93, 035.7XX0-035.7XX9, 075.4, 075.81, 075.89-075.9, 080, 086.11, 086.13-086.29, 090.89, 099.111-099.285, 099.330-099.335, 099.350-099.355, 099.511-099.73, 099.820-099.825, 099.840-09A.53

PDX Collection 969

011.4, 011.5, 012.04, 012.05, 012.14, 012.15, 012.24, 012.25, 013.4, 013.5, 014.04, 014.05, 014.14, 014.15, 014.24, 014.25, 014.94, 014.95, 016.4, 016.5, 024.011-024.33, 024.811-025.3, 026.10-026.13, 026.30-026.43, 026.63-026.819, 026.841-026.86, 026.891-026.93, 029.011-029.93, 035.7XX0-035.7XX9, 075.4, 075.81, 075.89-075.9, 080, 090.89, 099.111-099.285, 099.330-099.335, 099.350-099.355, 099.511-099.73, 099.820-099.825, 099.840-09A.53

PDX Collection 972

011.4, 011.5, 012.04, 012.05, 012.14, 012.15, 012.24, 012.25, 013.4, 013.5, 014.04, 014.05, 014.14, 014.15, 014.24, 014.25, 014.94, 014.95, 016.4, 016.5, 025.10-025.3, 026.10-026.13, 026.30-026.43, 026.611-026.819, 026.841-026.86, 026.891-026.93, 029.011-029.93, 035.7XX0-035.7XX9, 075.4, 075.81, 075.89-075.9, 080, 090.89, 099.111-099.285, 099.330-099.335, 099.350-099.355, 099.511-099.73, 099.820-099.825, 099.840-09A.53

PDX Collection 973

026.872-026.879, 034.31-034.33

PDX Collection 976

030.001-030.019, 030.031-031.23X9, 031.31X0-032.9XX9, 080

PDX Collection 977

033.0

PDX Collection 978

036.0110-036.0139, 036.0910-036.0939

PDX Collection 979

036.4XX0-036.4XX9

PDX Collection 982

041.01X0-041.03X9

PDX Collection 983

041.1010-041.1039, 041.1210-041.1239, 041.1410-041.1439

PDX Collection 985

011.4, 011.5, 012.04, 012.05, 012.14, 012.15, 012.24, 012.25, 013.4, 013.5, 014.04, 014.05, 014.14, 014.15, 014.24, 014.25, 014.94, 014.95, 016.4, 016.5, 025.10-025.3, 026.10-026.13, 026.30-026.43, 026.63-026.819, 026.841-026.86, 026.891-026.93, 029.011-029.93, 035.7XX0-035.7XX9, 045.001-045.099, 046.001-046.93, 067.0-067.9, 075.4, 075.81, 075.89-075.9, 080, 090.89, 099.111-099.285, 099.330-099.335, 099.350-099.355, 099.511-099.73, 099.820-099.825, 099.840-09A.53

PDX Collection 986

011.4, 011.5, 012.04, 012.05, 012.14, 012.15, 012.24, 012.25, 013.4, 013.5, 014.04, 014.05, 014.14, 014.15, 014.24, 014.25, 014.94, 014.95, 016.4, 016.5, 020.0-020.9, 025.10-025.3, 026.10-026.13, 026.30-026.43, 026.63-026.819, 026.841-026.86, 026.891-026.93, 029.011-029.93, 035.7XX0-035.7XX9, 044.00-044.13, 044.20-044.53, 045.8X1-045.8X3, 045.91-045.93, 075.4, 075.81, 075.89-075.9, 080, 090.89, 099.111-099.285, 099.330-099.335, 099.350-099.355, 099.511-099.73, 099.820-099.825, 099.840-09A.53

PDX Collection 987

011.4, 011.5, 012.04, 012.05, 012.14, 012.15, 012.24, 012.25, 013.4, 013.5, 014.04, 014.05, 014.14, 014.15, 014.24, 014.25, 014.94, 014.95, 016.4, 016.5, 025.10-025.3, 026.10-026.13, 026.30-026.43, 026.63-026.819, 026.841-026.86, 026.891-026.93, 029.011-029.93, 035.7XX0-035.7XX9, 047.00-047.9, 060.00-060.23X9, 075.4, 075.81, 075.89-075.9,

080, 090.89, 099.111-099.285, 099.330-099.335, 099.350-099.355, 099.511-099.73, 099.820-099.825, 099.840-09A.53

PDX Collection 988

011.4, 011.5, 012.04, 012.05, 012.14, 012.15, 012.24, 012.25, 013.4, 013.5, 014.04, 014.05, 014.14, 014.15, 014.24, 014.25, 014.94, 014.95, 016.4, 016.5, 025.10-025.3, 026.10-026.13, 026.30-026.43, 026.63-026.819, 026.841-026.86, 026.891-026.93, 029.011-029.93, 035.7XX0-035.7XX9, 036.8120-036.8199, 063.9, 071.00-071.1, 071.5, 071.81, 071.89-071.9, 075.4, 075.81, 075.89-075.9, 080, 090.89, 099.111-099.285, 099.330-099.335, 099.350-099.355, 099.511-099.73, 099.820-099.825, 099.840-09A.53

PDX Collection 989

068, 076, P03.811

PDX Collection 990

011.4, 011.5, 012.04, 012.05, 012.14, 012.15, 012.24, 012.25, 013.4, 013.5, 014.04, 014.05, 014.14, 014.15, 014.24, 014.25, 014.94, 014.95, 016.4, 016.5, 025.10-025.3, 026.10-026.13, 026.30-026.43, 026.63-026.819, 026.841-026.86, 026.891-026.93, 029.011-029.93, 035.7XX0-035.7XX9, 036.8120-036.8199, 070.4, 071.00-071.1, 071.5, 071.81, 071.89-071.9, 075.4, 075.81, 075.89-075.9, 080, 090.89, 099.111-099.285, 099.330-099.335, 099.350-099.355, 099.511-099.73, 099.820-099.825, 099.840-09A.53

PDX Collection 991

011.4, 011.5, 012.04, 012.05, 012.14, 012.15, 012.24, 012.25, 013.4, 013.5, 014.04, 014.05, 014.14, 014.15, 014.24, 014.25, 014.94, 014.95, 016.4, 016.5, 025.10-025.3, 026.10-026.13, 026.30-026.43, 026.63-026.819, 026.841-026.86, 026.891-026.93, 029.011-029.93, 035.7XX0-035.7XX9, 036.8120-036.8199, 070.3, 071.00-071.1, 071.5, 071.81, 071.89-071.9, 075.4, 075.81, 075.89-075.9, 080, 090.89, 099.111-099.285, 099.330-099.335, 099.350-099.355, 099.511-099.73, 099.820-099.825, 099.840-09A.53

PDX Collection 992

011.4, 011.5, 012.04, 012.05, 012.14, 012.15, 012.24, 012.25, 013.4, 013.5, 014.04, 014.05, 014.14, 014.15, 014.24, 014.25, 014.94, 014.95, 016.4, 016.5, 025.10-025.3, 026.10-026.13, 026.30-026.43, 026.63-026.819, 026.841-026.86, 026.891-026.93, 029.011-029.93, 035.7XX0-035.7XX9, 036.8120-036.8199, 070.20-070.23, 070.4, 071.00-071.1, 071.5, 071.81, 071.89-071.9, 075.4, 075.81, 075.89-075.9, 080, 090.89, 099.111-099.285, 099.330-099.335, 099.350-099.355, 099.511-099.73, 099.820-099.825, 099.840-09A.53

PDX Collection 993

011.4, 011.5, 012.04, 012.05, 012.14, 012.15, 012.24, 012.25, 013.4, 013.5, 014.04, 014.05, 014.14, 014.15, 014.24, 014.25, 014.94, 014.95, 016.4, 016.5, 025.10-025.3, 026.10-026.13, 026.30-026.43, 026.63-026.819, 026.841-026.86, 026.891-026.93, 029.011-029.93, 035.7XX0-035.7XX9, 036.8120-036.8199, 071.00-071.1, 071.5, 071.81, 071.89-071.9, 075.4, 075.81, 075.89-075.9, 080, 090.89, 099.111-099.285, 099.330-099.335, 099.350-099.355, 099.511-099.73, 099.820-099.825, 099.840-09A.53

PDX Collection 994

011.4, 011.5, 012.04, 012.05, 012.14, 012.15, 012.24, 012.25, 013.4, 013.5, 014.04, 014.05, 014.14, 014.15, 014.24, 014.25, 014.94, 014.95, 016.4, 016.5, 025.10-025.3, 026.10-026.13, 026.30-026.43, 026.63-026.819, 026.841-026.86, 026.891-026.93, 029.011-029.93, 035.7XX0-035.7XX9, 036.8120-036.8199,

O71.ØØ-O71.2, O71.5, O71.81, O71.89-O71.9, O75.4,
O75.81, O75.89-O75.9, O8Ø, O9Ø.89, O99.111-O99.285,
O99.33Ø-O99.335, O99.35Ø-O99.355, O99.511-O99.73,
O99.82Ø-O99.825, O99.84Ø-O9A.53

PDX Collection 995
O11.4, O11.5, O12.Ø4, O12.Ø5, O12.14, O12.15, O12.24,
O12.25, O13.4, O13.5, O14.Ø4, O14.Ø5, O14.14,
O14.15, O14.24, O14.25, O14.94, O14.95, O16.4,
O16.5, O25.1Ø-O25.3, O26.1Ø-O26.13, O26.3Ø-O26.43,
O26.63-O26.819, O26.841-O26.86, O26.891-O26.93,
O29.Ø11-O29.93, O35.7XXØ-O35.7XX9, O36.812Ø-O36.8199,
O71.ØØ-O71.1, O71.3, O71.5, O71.81, O71.89-O71.9, O75.4,
O75.81, O75.89-O75.9, O8Ø, O9Ø.89, O99.111-O99.285,
O99.33Ø-O99.335, O99.35Ø-O99.355, O99.511-O99.73,
O99.82Ø-O99.825, O99.84Ø-O9A.53

PDX Collection 996
O11.4, O11.5, O12.Ø4, O12.Ø5, O12.14, O12.15, O12.24,
O12.25, O13.4, O13.5, O14.Ø4, O14.Ø5, O14.14,
O14.15, O14.24, O14.25, O14.94, O14.95, O16.4,
O16.5, O25.1Ø-O25.3, O26.1Ø-O26.13, O26.3Ø-O26.43,
O26.63-O26.819, O26.841-O26.86, O26.891-O26.93,
O29.Ø11-O29.93, O35.7XXØ-O35.7XX9, O36.812Ø-O36.8199,
O71.ØØ-O71.1, O71.4, O71.5, O71.81, O71.89-O71.9, O75.4,
O75.81, O75.89-O75.9, O8Ø, O9Ø.89, O99.111-O99.285,
O99.33Ø-O99.335, O99.35Ø-O99.355, O99.511-O99.73,
O99.82Ø-O99.825, O99.84Ø-O9A.53

PDX Collection 997
O11.4, O11.5, O12.Ø4, O12.Ø5, O12.14, O12.15, O12.24,
O12.25, O13.4, O13.5, O14.Ø4, O14.Ø5, O14.14,
O14.15, O14.24, O14.25, O14.94, O14.95, O16.4,
O16.5, O25.1Ø-O25.3, O26.1Ø-O26.13, O26.3Ø-O26.43,
O26.63-O26.819, O26.841-O26.86, O26.891-O26.93,
O29.Ø11-O29.93, O35.7XXØ-O35.7XX9, O36.812Ø-O36.8199,
O71.ØØ-O71.1, O71.5-O71.6, O71.81, O71.89-O71.9, O75.4,
O75.81, O75.89-O75.9, O8Ø, O9Ø.89, O99.111-O99.285,
O99.33Ø-O99.335, O99.35Ø-O99.355, O99.511-O99.73,
O99.82Ø-O99.825, O99.84Ø-O9A.53

PDX Collection 998
O11.4, O11.5, O12.Ø4, O12.Ø5, O12.14, O12.15, O12.24,
O12.25, O13.4, O13.5, O14.Ø4, O14.Ø5, O14.14,
O14.15, O14.24, O14.25, O14.94, O14.95, O16.4,
O16.5, O25.1Ø-O25.3, O26.1Ø-O26.13, O26.3Ø-O26.43,
O26.63-O26.819, O26.841-O26.86, O26.891-O26.93,
O29.Ø11-O29.93, O35.7XXØ-O35.7XX9, O36.812Ø-O36.8199,
O71.ØØ-O71.1, O71.5, O71.7, O71.81, O71.89-O71.9, O75.4,
O75.81, O75.89-O75.9, O8Ø, O9Ø.89, O99.111-O99.285,
O99.33Ø-O99.335, O99.35Ø-O99.355, O99.511-O99.73,
O99.82Ø-O99.825, O99.84Ø-O9A.53

PDX Collection 999
O11.4, O11.5, O12.Ø4, O12.Ø5, O12.14, O12.15, O12.24,
O12.25, O13.4, O13.5, O14.Ø4, O14.Ø5, O14.14,
O14.15, O14.24, O14.25, O14.94, O14.95, O16.4,
O16.5, O25.1Ø-O25.3, O26.1Ø-O26.13, O26.3Ø-O26.43,
O26.63-O26.819, O26.841-O26.86, O26.891-O26.93,
O29.Ø11-O29.93, O35.7XXØ-O35.7XX9, O36.812Ø-O36.8199,
O71.ØØ-O71.1, O71.5, O71.81, O71.89-O71.9, O72.Ø, O75.4,
O75.81, O75.89-O75.9, O8Ø, O9Ø.89, O99.111-O99.285,
O99.33Ø-O99.335, O99.35Ø-O99.355, O99.511-O99.73,
O99.82Ø-O99.825, O99.84Ø-O9A.53

PDX Collection 1ØØØ
O11.4, O11.5, O12.Ø4, O12.Ø5, O12.14, O12.15, O12.24,
O12.25, O13.4, O13.5, O14.Ø4, O14.Ø5, O14.14,
O14.15, O14.24, O14.25, O14.94, O14.95, O16.4,
O16.5, O25.1Ø-O25.3, O26.1Ø-O26.13, O26.3Ø-O26.43,
O26.63-O26.819, O26.841-O26.86, O26.891-O26.93,
O29.Ø11-O29.93, O35.7XXØ-O35.7XX9, O36.812Ø-O36.8199,

O71.ØØ-O71.1, O71.5, O71.81, O71.89-O71.9, O72.1, O75.4,
O75.81, O75.89-O75.9, O8Ø, O9Ø.89, O99.111-O99.285,
O99.33Ø-O99.335, O99.35Ø-O99.355, O99.511-O99.73,
O99.82Ø-O99.825, O99.84Ø-O9A.53

PDX Collection 1ØØ1
O11.4, O11.5, O12.Ø4, O12.Ø5, O12.14, O12.15, O12.24,
O12.25, O13.4, O13.5, O14.Ø4, O14.Ø5, O14.14,
O14.15, O14.24, O14.25, O14.94, O14.95, O16.4,
O16.5, O25.1Ø-O25.3, O26.1Ø-O26.13, O26.3Ø-O26.43,
O26.63-O26.819, O26.841-O26.86, O26.891-O26.93,
O29.Ø11-O29.93, O35.7XXØ-O35.7XX9, O36.812Ø-O36.8199,
O71.ØØ-O71.1, O71.5, O71.81, O71.89-O71.9, O72.2, O75.4,
O75.81, O75.89-O75.9, O8Ø, O9Ø.89, O99.111-O99.285,
O99.33Ø-O99.335, O99.35Ø-O99.355, O99.511-O99.73,
O99.82Ø-O99.825, O99.84Ø-O9A.53

PDX Collection 1ØØ2
O11.4, O11.5, O12.Ø4, O12.Ø5, O12.14, O12.15, O12.24,
O12.25, O13.4, O13.5, O14.Ø4, O14.Ø5, O14.14,
O14.15, O14.24, O14.25, O14.94, O14.95, O16.4,
O16.5, O25.1Ø-O25.3, O26.1Ø-O26.13, O26.3Ø-O26.43,
O26.63-O26.819, O26.841-O26.86, O26.891-O26.93,
O29.Ø11-O29.93, O35.7XXØ-O35.7XX9, O75.1, O75.4,
O75.81, O75.89-O75.9, O8Ø, O9Ø.89, O99.111-O99.285,
O99.33Ø-O99.335, O99.35Ø-O99.355, O99.511-O99.73,
O99.82Ø-O99.825, O99.84Ø-O9A.53

PDX Collection 1ØØ3
O75.2

PDX Collection 1ØØ4
O11.4, O11.5, O12.Ø4, O12.Ø5, O12.14, O12.15, O12.24,
O12.25, O13.4, O13.5, O14.Ø4, O14.Ø5, O14.14,
O14.15, O14.24, O14.25, O14.94, O14.95, O16.4,
O16.5, O25.1Ø-O25.3, O26.1Ø-O26.13, O26.3Ø-O26.43,
O26.63-O26.819, O26.841-O26.86, O26.891-O26.93,
O29.Ø11-O29.93, O35.7XXØ-O35.7XX9, O75.3-O75.4,
O75.81, O75.89-O75.9, O8Ø, O9Ø.89, O99.111-O99.285,
O99.33Ø-O99.335, O99.35Ø-O99.355, O99.511-O99.73,
O99.82Ø-O99.825, O99.84Ø-O9A.53

PDX Collection 1ØØ5
O11.4, O11.5, O12.Ø4, O12.Ø5, O12.14, O12.15,
O12.24, O12.25, O13.4, O13.5, O14.Ø4, O14.Ø5,
O14.14, O14.15, O14.24, O14.25, O14.94, O14.95,
O16.4, O16.5, O25.1Ø-O25.3, O26.1Ø-O26.13,
O26.3Ø-O26.43, O26.63-O26.819, O26.841-O26.86,
O26.891-O26.93, O26.899-O26.93, O29.Ø11-O29.93,
O35.7XXØ-O35.7XX9, O75.4, O75.81, O75.89, O75.9, O8Ø,
O85, O86.12, O86.81-O86.89, O9Ø.89, O99.111-O99.285,
O99.33Ø-O99.335, O99.35Ø-O99.355, O99.511-O99.73,
O99.82Ø-O99.825, O99.84Ø-O9A.53

PDX Collection 1ØØ6
O11.4, O11.5, O12.Ø4, O12.Ø5, O12.14, O12.15, O12.24,
O12.25, O13.4, O13.5, O14.Ø4, O14.Ø5, O14.14,
O14.15, O14.24, O14.25, O14.94, O14.95, O16.4,
O16.5, O22.2Ø-O22.93, O25.1Ø-O25.3, O26.1Ø-O26.13,
O26.3Ø-O26.43, O26.63-O26.819, O26.841-O26.86,
O26.891-O26.93, O29.Ø11-O29.93, O35.7XXØ-O35.7XX9,
O75.4, O75.81, O75.89-O75.9, O8Ø, O86.4-O87.9, O9Ø.89,
O99.111-O99.285, O99.33Ø-O99.335, O99.35Ø-O99.355,
O99.511-O99.73, O99.82Ø-O99.825, O99.84Ø-O9A.53

PDX Collection 1ØØ7
O11.4, O11.5, O12.Ø4, O12.Ø5, O12.14, O12.15, O12.24,
O12.25, O13.4, O13.5, O14.Ø4, O14.Ø5, O14.14,
O14.15, O14.24, O14.25, O14.94, O14.95, O16.4,
O16.5, O25.1Ø-O25.3, O26.1Ø-O26.93, O29.Ø11-O29.93,
O35.7XXØ-O35.7XX9, O75.4, O75.81-O8Ø, O88.Ø11-O88.83,
O9Ø.89, O99.111-O9A.53

PDX Collection 1ØØ8
O11.4, O11.5, O12.Ø4, O12.Ø5, O12.14, O12.15, O12.24,
O12.25, O13.4, O13.5, O14.Ø4, O14.Ø5, O14.14,
O14.15, O14.24, O14.25, O14.94, O14.95, O16.4,
O16.5, O25.1Ø-O25.3, O26.1Ø-O26.13, O26.3Ø-O26.43,
O26.63-O26.819, O26.841-O26.86, O26.891-O26.93,
O29.Ø11-O29.93, O35.7XXØ-O35.7XX9, O75.4, O75.81,
O75.89-O75.9, O8Ø, O9Ø.3, O9Ø.89, O99.111-O99.285,
O99.33Ø-O99.335, O99.35Ø-O99.73, O99.82Ø-O99.825,
O99.84Ø-O9A.53

PDX Collection 1ØØ9
O11.4, O11.5, O12.Ø4, O12.Ø5, O12.14, O12.15, O12.24,
O12.25, O13.4, O13.5, O14.Ø4, O14.Ø5, O14.14,
O14.15, O14.24, O14.25, O14.94, O14.95, O16.4,
O16.5, O25.1Ø-O25.3, O26.1Ø-O26.13, O26.3Ø-O26.43,
O26.63-O26.819, O26.841-O26.86, O26.891-O26.93,
O29.Ø11-O29.93, O35.7XXØ-O35.7XX9, O75.4, O75.81,
O75.89-O75.9, O8Ø, O9Ø.4, O9Ø.89, O99.111-O99.285,
O99.33Ø-O99.335, O99.35Ø-O99.355, O99.511-O99.73,
O99.82Ø-O99.825, O99.84Ø-O9A.53

PDX Collection 1Ø11
O11.4, O11.5, O12.Ø4, O12.Ø5, O12.14, O12.15, O12.24,
O12.25, O13.4, O13.5, O14.Ø4, O14.Ø5, O14.14,
O14.15, O14.24, O14.25, O14.94, O14.95, O16.4,
O16.5, O25.1Ø-O25.3, O26.1Ø-O26.13, O26.3Ø-O26.43,
O26.63-O26.819, O26.841-O26.86, O26.891-O26.93,
O29.Ø11-O29.93, O35.7XXØ-O35.7XX9, O75.4, O75.81,
O75.89-O75.9, O8Ø, O9Ø.89, O98.Ø11-O98.Ø3,
O99.111-O99.285, O99.33Ø-O99.335, O99.35Ø-O99.355,
O99.511-O99.73, O99.82Ø-O99.825, O99.84Ø-O9A.53

PDX Collection 1Ø12
O26.11-O26.13, O26.31-O26.33, O26.41-O26.43,
O26.63-O26.713, O26.72-O26.813, O26.86,
O26.891-O26.893, O26.9Ø-O26.93, O29.Ø11-O29.Ø13,
O29.Ø21-O29.Ø23, O29.Ø91-O29.Ø93, O29.111-O29.113,
O29.121-O29.123, O29.191-O29.193, O29.211-O29.213,
O29.291-O29.293, O29.3X1-O29.3X3, O29.41-O29.5X3,
O29.61-O29.8X3, O29.91-O29.93, O35.7XXØ-O35.7XX9,
O98.111-O98.33, O99.351-O99.353, O99.355, O99.89

PDX Collection 1Ø13
O98.411-O98.613, O98.711-O98.93, O99.83Ø-O99.835

PDX Collection 1Ø14
O11.4, O11.5, O12.Ø4, O12.Ø5, O12.14, O12.15, O12.24,
O12.25, O13.4, O13.5, O14.Ø4, O14.Ø5, O14.14,
O14.15, O14.24, O14.25, O14.94, O14.95, O16.4,
O16.5, O25.1Ø-O25.3, O26.1Ø-O26.13, O26.3Ø-O26.43,
O26.63-O26.819, O26.841-O26.86, O26.891-O26.93,
O29.Ø11-O29.93, O35.7XXØ-O35.7XX9, O75.4, O75.81,
O75.89-O75.9, O8Ø, O9Ø.89, O98.411-O98.93,
O99.111-O99.285, O99.33Ø-O99.335, O99.35Ø-O99.355,
O99.511-O99.73, O99.82Ø-O9A.53

PDX Collection 1Ø15
O11.4, O11.5, O12.Ø4, O12.Ø5, O12.14, O12.15, O12.24,
O12.25, O13.4, O13.5, O14.Ø4, O14.Ø5, O14.14,
O14.15, O14.24, O14.25, O14.94, O14.95, O16.4,
O16.5, O25.1Ø-O25.3, O26.1Ø-O26.13, O26.3Ø-O26.43,
O26.63-O26.819, O26.841-O26.86, O26.891-O26.93,
O29.Ø11-O29.93, O35.7XXØ-O35.7XX9, O75.4, O75.81,
O75.89-O75.9, O8Ø, O9Ø.89, O98.611-O98.63,
O99.111-O99.285, O99.33Ø-O99.335, O99.35Ø-O99.355,
O99.511-O99.73, O99.82Ø-O9A.53

PDX Collection 1Ø16
O25.11-O25.3, O99.281-O99.285, O99.511-O99.513,
O99.52-O99.613, O99.62-O99.713, O99.72-O99.73,
O99.82Ø-O99.825, O9A.111-O9A.113, O9A.12-O9A.213,
O9A.22-O9A.313, O9A.32-O9A.413, O9A.42-O9A.513,
O9A.52-O9A.53

PDX Collection 1017
O25.10, O99.280, O99.519, O99.619, O99.719, O9A.119,
O9A.219, O9A.319, O9A.419, O9A.519

PDX Collection 1018
O11.4, O11.5, O12.04, O12.05, O12.14, O12.15, O12.24,
O12.25, O13.4, O13.5, O14.04, O14.05, O14.14,
O14.15, O14.24, O14.25, O14.94, O14.95, O16.4,
O16.5, O25.10-O25.3, O26.10-O26.13, O26.30-O26.43,
O26.63-O26.819, O26.841-O26.86, O26.891-O26.93,
O29.011-O29.93, O35.7XX0-O35.7XX9, O75.4, O75.81,
O75.89-O75.9, O80, O90.89, O99.111-O99.285,
O99.320-O99.335, O99.350-O99.355, O99.511-O99.73,
O99.820-O99.825, O99.840-O9A.53

PDX Collection 1019
O11.4, O11.5, O12.04, O12.05, O12.14, O12.15, O12.24,
O12.25, O13.4, O13.5, O14.04, O14.05, O14.14,
O14.15, O14.24, O14.25, O14.94, O14.95, O16.4,
O16.5, O25.10-O25.3, O26.10-O26.13, O26.30-O26.43,
O26.63-O26.819, O26.841-O26.86, O26.891-O26.93,
O29.011-O29.93, O35.7XX0-O35.7XX9, O75.4, O75.81,
O75.89-O75.9, O80, O90.3, O90.89, O99.111-O99.285,
O99.330-O99.335, O99.350-O99.73, O99.820-O99.825,
O99.840-O9A.53

PDX Collection 1020
P10.0-P10.1, P10.4-P11.2, P11.9, P15.0-P15.9, P29.0-P29.2,
P29.4, P29.89-P29.9, P52.4, P52.6-P52.9, P94.1-P94.9, P96.0,
P96.3-P96.5, P96.82-P96.89

PDX Collection 1021
P10.2-P10.3, P29.0-P29.2, P29.4, P29.89-P29.9, P50.0-P50.9,
P52.0-P52.3, P52.5, P53-P54.0, P54.6-P54.9, P60-P61.9,
P94.1-P94.9, P96.0, P96.3-P96.5, P96.82-P96.89

PDX Collection 1022
P10.2-P10.3, P29.0-P29.2, P29.4, P29.89-P29.9, P50.0-P50.9,
P52.0-P52.3, P52.5, P53-P54.0, P54.6-P54.9, P60-P61.9,
P91.2, P94.1-P94.9, P96.0, P96.3-P96.5, P96.82-P96.89

PDX Collection 1023
P10.0-P10.1, P10.4-P11.2, P11.9-P12.2, P15.0-P15.9,
P29.0-P29.2, P29.4, P29.89-P29.9, P52.4, P52.6-P52.9,
P94.1-P94.9, P96.0, P96.3-P96.5, P96.82-P96.89

PDX Collection 1024
P22.8-P22.9, P28.2-P28.4, P28.81-P28.9, R06.81, R23.0

PDX Collection 1025
P22.8-P22.9, P28.2, P28.4, P28.81-P28.9, R06.81

PDX Collection 1026
P22.8-P22.9, P28.2-P28.4, P28.81-P28.9, R06.81

PDX Collection 1027
P22.1-P22.9, P24.00, P24.10, P24.20, P24.30, P24.80,
P28.2-P28.5, P28.89-P28.9, P29.81, R06.81, R09.2

PDX Collection 1028
I27.0, I27.20-I27.81, I27.83-I27.9

PDX Collection 1029
P29.81

PDX Collection 1030
P29.0-P29.2, P29.4, P29.89-P35.9, P37.0-P37.4, P37.8-P37.9,
P94.1-P94.9, P96.0, P96.3-P96.5, P96.82-P96.89

PDX Collection 1031
P29.0-P29.2, P29.4, P29.89-P29.9, P36.0-P36.9, P37.5,
P38.1-P39.9, P53, P60-P61.9, P94.1-P94.9, P96.0,
P96.3-P96.5, P96.82-P96.89

PDX Collection 1032
P39.2, P39.4-P39.9

PDX Collection 1033
A02.1, A20.7, A22.7, A39.2-A39.4, A40.9-A41.59,
A41.81-A41.9, A42.7, A48.2, A48.4, A48.8-A49.9, B00.7, B92,
B94.2-B96.89, P39.2-P39.9, P95, P96.9, R78.81

PDX Collection 1034
A49.9, N10-N11.0, N11.8-N12, N13.6, N15.1, N28.82,
N28.84-N30.31, N30.80-N30.91, N36.9-N39.0, N39.9,
N99.511, P39.2, P39.4-P39.9, R30.0, R30.9, T83.511A

PDX Collection 1035
P29.0-P29.2, P29.4, P29.89-P29.9, P53, P60-P61.9,
P94.1-P96.0, P96.3-P96.5, P96.82-P96.89

PDX Collection 1036
P29.0-P29.2, P29.4, P29.89-P29.9, P50.0-P50.9, P53-P54.9,
P60-P61.9, P94.1-P96.0, P96.3-P96.5, P96.82-P96.89

PDX Collection 1037
P29.0-P29.2, P29.4, P29.89-P29.9, P55.0-P57.0, P94.1-P96.0,
P96.3-P96.5, P96.82-P96.89

PDX Collection 1038
P29.0-P29.2, P29.4, P29.89-P29.9, P57.8-P59.9, P94.1-P96.0,
P96.3-P96.5, P96.82-P96.89

PDX Collection 1039
D50.0-D55.9, D56.4, D57.00-D57.3, D57.80-D64.9, D75.9,
P61.2-P61.4

PDX Collection 1040
D50.1-D53.9, D56.4, D57.00-D57.20, D57.3,
D57.811-D57.819, D58.2, D59.0-D59.1, D59.3, D60.0-D61.9,
D63.0-D64.9, D75.9, P61.5, P61.8-P61.9

PDX Collection 1041
P29.0-P29.2, P29.4, P29.89-P29.9, P70.0-P71.9, P72.1,
P72.9-P74.4, P74.9, P94.0-P94.9, P96.0, P96.3-P96.5,
P96.82-P96.89

PDX Collection 1042
P70.0-P70.4, P70.9-P71.9, P72.1, P72.9-P74.4, P74.9, P94.0

PDX Collection 1043
P76.0-P78.9

PDX Collection 1044
P29.0-P29.2, P29.4-P29.9, P76.0-P78.9, P94.1-P96.0,
P96.3-P96.5, P96.82-P96.89

PDX Collection 1045
P83.0, P83.30-P83.39

PDX Collection 1046
P29.0-P29.2, P29.4, P29.89-P29.9, P83.2, P94.1-P96.0,
P96.3-P96.5, P96.82-P96.89

PDX Collection 1047
P80.0-P83.0, P83.30-P83.39

PDX Collection 1048
P29.0-P29.2, P29.4, P29.89-P29.9, P90, P91.811-P91.9,
P94.1-P96.0, P96.3-P96.5, P96.82-P96.89

PDX Collection 1049
P90-P91.1, P91.3-P91.5, P91.811-P91.9

PDX Collection 1050
P84, P91.60-P91.63

PDX Collection 1051
P92.01-P92.09

PDX Collection 1052
P93.0-P93.8, P96.1-P96.2

PDX Collection 1053
Q00.0-Q00.2

PDX Collection 1054
Q01.0-Q02, Q04.0-Q04.8

PDX Collection 1055
Q04.4-Q04.8

PDX Collection 1056
E78.71-E78.72, G90.1, Q05.0-Q06.1, Q06.3, Q06.8-Q07.9,
Q87.1-Q87.89, Q89.7-Q89.8, Q99.2

PDX Collection 1057
E78.71-E78.72, I23.0-I23.3, I23.6-I23.8, I51.0, P29.30-P29.38,
Q20.0-Q21.9, Q23.8-Q23.9, Q24.8-Q24.9, Q27.30, Q27.4,
Q28.0-Q28.1, Q28.8-Q28.9, Q87.1-Q87.89, Q89.7-Q89.8,
Q99.2

PDX Collection 1058
E78.71-E78.72, I23.0-I23.3, I23.6-I23.8, I51.0, Q20.0-Q20.9,
Q21.1-Q21.9, Q23.8-Q23.9, Q24.8-Q24.9, Q27.30, Q27.4,
Q28.0-Q28.1, Q28.8-Q28.9, Q87.2-Q87.3, Q87.5-Q87.89,
Q89.7-Q89.8

PDX Collection 1059
E78.71-E78.72, P29.30-P29.38, Q20.9, Q22.0-Q22.3,
Q23.8-Q23.9, Q24.8-Q24.9, Q27.30, Q27.4, Q28.0-Q28.1,
Q28.8-Q28.9, Q87.1-Q87.89, Q89.7-Q89.8, Q99.2

PDX Collection 1060
E78.71-E78.72, Q20.9, Q22.0-Q22.3, Q23.8-Q23.9,
Q24.8-Q24.9, Q27.30, Q27.4, Q28.0-Q28.1, Q28.8-Q28.9,
Q87.2-Q87.3, Q87.5-Q87.89, Q89.7-Q89.8

PDX Collection 1061
E78.71-E78.72, P29.30-P29.38, Q20.9, Q22.4-Q23.9,
Q24.8-Q24.9, Q27.30, Q27.4, Q28.0-Q28.1, Q28.8-Q28.9,
Q87.1-Q87.89, Q89.7-Q89.8, Q99.2

PDX Collection 1062
E78.71-E78.72, Q20.9, Q23.8-Q24.4, Q24.8-Q24.9,
Q27.30, Q27.4, Q28.0-Q28.1, Q28.8-Q28.9, Q87.2-Q87.3,
Q87.5-Q87.89, Q89.7-Q89.8

PDX Collection 1063
E78.71-E78.72, P29.30-P29.38, Q20.9, Q23.8-Q23.9,
Q24.2-Q24.4, Q24.8-Q24.9, Q27.30, Q27.4, Q28.0-Q28.1,
Q28.8-Q28.9, Q87.1-Q87.89, Q89.7-Q89.8, Q99.2

PDX Collection 1064
Q20.9, Q23.8-Q23.9, Q24.5, Q24.8-Q24.9

PDX Collection 1065
E78.71-E78.72, P29.30-P29.38, Q20.9, Q23.8-Q23.9,
Q24.6-Q24.9, Q27.30, Q27.4, Q28.0-Q28.1, Q28.8-Q28.9,
Q87.1-Q87.89, Q89.7-Q89.8, Q99.2

PDX Collection 1066
Q25.0, Q27.30, Q27.4, Q28.0-Q28.1, Q28.8

PDX Collection 1067
E78.71-E78.72, Q25.1-Q25.3, Q27.30, Q27.4, Q28.0-Q28.1,
Q28.8-Q28.9, Q87.2-Q87.3, Q87.5-Q87.89, Q89.7-Q89.8

PDX Collection 1068
E78.71-E78.72, P29.30-P29.38, Q25.1-Q25.3, Q27.30, Q27.4,
Q28.0-Q28.1, Q28.8-Q28.9, Q87.1-Q87.89, Q89.7-Q89.8,
Q99.2

PDX Collection 1069
E78.71-E78.72, Q25.1-Q25.49, Q25.8-Q25.9, Q27.30, Q27.4,
Q28.0-Q28.1, Q28.8-Q28.9, Q87.2-Q87.3, Q87.5-Q87.89,
Q89.7-Q89.8

PDX Collection 1070
Q25.5-Q25.79, Q27.30, Q27.4, Q28.0-Q28.1, Q28.8-Q28.9

PDX Collection 1071
Q26.0-Q26.1, Q26.8, Q27.30, Q27.4, Q28.0-Q28.1,
Q28.8-Q28.9

PDX Collection 1072
Q26.2, Q27.30, Q27.4, Q28.0-Q28.1, Q28.8-Q28.9

PDX Collection 1073
Q26.3-Q26.4, Q27.30, Q27.4, Q28.0-Q28.1, Q28.8-Q28.9

PDX Collection 1074
Q26.9, Q27.30, Q27.4, Q28.0-Q28.1, Q28.8-Q28.9

PDX Collection 1075
Q20.0-Q20.8, Q21.0-Q21.9, Q27.30, Q27.4, Q28.0-Q28.1,
Q28.8

PDX Collection 1076
Q27.30, Q27.4, Q28.0-Q28.9

PDX Collection 1077
Q20.0-Q28.9

PDX Collection 1078
J39.8, J45.990, J98.09, Q31.1-Q32.4, Q34.0-Q34.9

PDX Collection 1079
Q33.0-Q34.9

PDX Collection 1080
J44.9, J47.0-J47.9, J68.1, J68.4-J68.9, Q33.4

PDX Collection 1081
Q39.0-Q39.9, Q45.8-Q45.9

PDX Collection 1082
Q39.5-Q39.9, Q45.8-Q45.9

PDX Collection 1083
Q41.0-Q41.9, Q45.8-Q45.9

PDX Collection 1084
Q42.0-Q42.9, Q45.8-Q45.9

PDX Collection 1085
Q43.1-Q43.2, Q45.8-Q45.9

PDX Collection 1086
Q43.3-Q43.9

PDX Collection 1087
Q41.0-Q43.9

PDX Collection 1088
Q44.0-Q44.7

PDX Collection 1089
Q44.2-Q44.3, Q45.8-Q45.9

PDX Collection 1090
Q44.0-Q44.1, Q44.4-Q44.7

PDX Collection 1091
Q45.0-Q45.9

PDX Collection 1092
N13.9, Q60.0-Q60.6

PDX Collection 1093
N13.9, Q61.00, Q61.9

PDX Collection 1094
N13.9, Q61.01

PDX Collection 1095
N13.9, Q61.02, Q61.5-Q61.8

PDX Collection 1096
N13.9, Q61.11-Q61.3

PDX Collection 1097
N13.9, Q61.4

PDX Collection 1098
N13.9, Q62.0-Q62.2, Q62.39

PDX Collection 1099
N13.9, Q64.10-Q64.19, Q64.8-Q64.9

PDX Collection 1100
N13.9, Q64.2-Q64.39, Q64.8-Q64.9

PDX Collection 1101
Q67.5, Q76.3, Q76.425-Q76.429

PDX Collection 1102
Q67.6-Q67.8, Q68.1, Q74.3

PDX Collection 1103
Q76.5-Q76.9, Q77.2

PDX Collection 1104
Q77.3, Q77.6, Q78.0-Q78.3, Q78.5-Q78.9

PDX Collection 1105
Q40.1, Q79.0-Q79.1

PDX Collection 1106
Q79.2-Q79.59

PDX Collection 1107
Q79.6

PDX Collection 1108
Q85.1-Q85.9, Q89.7, Q89.9

PDX Collection 1109
Q85.8-Q85.9, Q89.9

PDX Collection 1110
E78.71-E78.72, Q85.8-Q85.9, Q87.1-Q87.89, Q89.7-Q89.9, Q99.2

PDX Collection 1111
Q89.01-Q89.09, Q89.9

PDX Collection 1112
Q89.3, Q89.7, Q89.9

PDX Collection 1113
Q89.4-Q89.7, Q89.9

PDX Collection 1114
Q90.0-Q99.1, Q99.8-Q99.9

PDX Collection 1115
Q90.0-Q99.1, Q99.8-Q99.9

PDX Collection 1116
Q90.0-Q99.1, Q99.8-Q99.9

PDX Collection 1117
Q90.0-Q99.1, Q99.8-Q99.9

PDX Collection 1118
Q90.0-Q99.1, Q99.8-Q99.9

PDX Collection 1119
R04.2-R04.9, R09.3, R68.13

PDX Collection 1120
J22, J80, J96.00-J96.92, J98.8-J98.9, R06.3, R06.81, R09.2

PDX Collection 1121
G89.0-G89.4, J80, J96.00-J96.92, R09.01-R09.02, R09.2, R29.700-R29.742, R41.0-R41.3, R41.82, R41.9, R44.8-R44.9, R45.83-R45.84, R46.0-R46.89, R52, R68.0-R68.19, R68.81-R68.83, R68.89-R69

PDX Collection 1122
P57.8-P59.9, R17, R23.8-R23.9

PDX Collection 1123
G89.0-G89.4, R18.0-R19.09, R19.30-R19.37, R29.700-R29.742, R41.0-R41.3, R41.82, R41.9, R44.8-R44.9, R45.83-R45.84, R46.0-R46.89, R52, R68.0-R68.19, R68.81-R68.83, R68.89-R69

PDX Collection 1124
A33, A35, G10-G11.2, G11.4, G20-G25.79, G25.82-G26, G32.81, G80.3, G81.10-G81.14, G89.0-G89.4, G90.3, R29.0, R29.700-R29.742, R41.0-R41.3, R41.82, R41.9, R44.8-R44.9, R45.83-R45.84, R46.0-R46.89, R52, R68.0-R68.19, R68.81-R68.83, R68.89-R69

PDX Collection 1125
R29.1, R29.810

PDX Collection 1126
R29.5, R29.810

PDX Collection 1127
R30.1, R39.0, R39.2-R39.9

PDX Collection 1128
R29.3, R29.6-R29.890, R29.90-R29.91, R41.4

PDX Collection 1129
G89.0-G89.4, R29.700-R29.742, R41.0-R41.3, R41.82, R41.9-R42, R44.0, R44.2-R44.9, R45.83-R45.84, R46.0-R46.89, R52, R68.0-R68.19, R68.81-R68.83, R68.89-R69

PDX Collection 1130
F05

PDX Collection 1131
F80.1, F80.81, I62.00-I66.9, R47.01-R47.9, R49.0-R49.9

PDX Collection 1132
G32.89, G40.001-G40.319, G40.401-G40.919, G40.A01-G40.B19, G89.0-G89.4, G93.81, G93.89-G93.9, G96.8-G96.9, G98.0-G98.8, P90, P91.811-P91.9, R29.700-R29.742, R41.0-R41.3, R41.82, R41.9, R44.8-R44.9, R45.83-R45.84, R46.0-R46.89, R52, R56.00-R56.9, R68.0-R68.19, R68.81-R68.83, R68.89-R69

PDX Collection 1133
G89.0-G89.4, R09.89, R29.700-R29.742, R41.0-R41.3, R41.82, R41.9, R44.8-R44.9, R45.83-R45.84, R46.0-R46.89, R52, R57.0-R57.9, R65.21, R68.0-R68.19, R68.81-R68.83, R68.89-R69

PDX Collection 1134
G89.0-G89.4, R29.700-R29.742, R41.0-R41.3, R41.82, R41.9, R44.8-R44.9, R45.83-R45.84, R46.0-R46.89, R52, R64, R68.0-R68.19, R68.81-R68.83, R68.89-R69

PDX Collection 1135
D62, D64.4-D64.9

PDX Collection 1136
B34.9, E07.81, G89.0-G89.4, R29.700-R29.742, R41.0-R41.3, R41.82, R41.9, R44.8-R44.9, R45.83-R45.84, R46.0-R46.89, R52, R68.0-R68.19, R68.81-R68.83, R68.89-R69, R70.1, R77.0-R77.9, R78.1-R78.6, R78.81, R78.9, R79.1-R79.89, R97.20, R97.21

PDX Collection 1137
G89.0-G89.4, R29.700-R29.742, R41.0-R41.3, R41.82, R41.9, R44.8-R44.9, R45.83-R45.84, R46.0-R46.89, R52, R68.0-R68.19, R68.81-R68.83, R68.89-R69, R82.0, R82.5-R82.99

PDX Collection 1138
G89.0-G89.4, R29.700-R29.742, R41.0-R41.3, R41.82, R41.9, R44.8-R44.9, R45.83-R45.84, R46.0-R46.89, R52, R68.0-R68.19, R68.81-R68.83, R68.89-R69, R82.1, R82.3, R82.5-R82.99

PDX Collection 1139
S01.101-S01.159[A], S05.20X-S05.8X9[A], S05.91X-S05.92X[A], S38.3XXA, T07.XXX-T14.91X[A], T79.A0X-T79.9XX[A]

PDX Collection 1140
S01.90X-S01.95X[A], S02.0XX-S02.19X[A,B,S], S02.2XX-S02.82X[S], S02.91X[A,B,S], S02.92XS, S06.0X0-S07.9XX[A], S08.89XA, S09.10X-S09.19X[A], S09.8XX-S09.90X[A], S09.92X-S09.93X[A], S16.8XX-S19.9XX[A], S38.3XX[A], T07.XXX-T14.91X[A], T79.A0XA-T79.9XX[A]

PDX Collection 1141
S01.90X-S01.95X[A], S02.0XX-S02.2XX[A,B,S], S02.30X-S02.413[S], S02.42X-S02.82X[S], S02.91X[A,B,S], S02.92XS, S06.0X0-S07.9XX[A], S08.89XA, S09.10X-S09.19X[A], S09.8XX-S09.90X[A], S09.92X-S09.93X[A], S16.8XX-S19.9XX[A], S38.3XXA, S92.811-S92.819[A,B], T07.XXX-T14.91X[A], T79.A0X-T79.8XX[A]

PDX Collection 1142
S01.90X-S01.95X[A], S02.0XX[A,B,S], S02.101-S02.2XX[A,B,S], S02.30X-S02.32X[A,B,S], S02.400-S02.413[S], S02.42X[A,B,S], S02.5XX-S02.69X[S], S02.80X-S02.92X[A,B,S], S06.0X0-S07.9XX[A], S08.89XA, S09.10X-S09.19X[A], S09.8XX-S09.919X[A], S09.8XX-S09.90X-S09.3X[A], S16.8XX-S19.9XX[A], S38.3XX[A], T07.XXX-T14.91X[A], T79.8XX-T79.9XX[A], T79.A0X-T79.A9X[A]

PDX Collection 1143
S01.90X- S01.95X[A], S02.0XX[A,B,S],
S02.101-S02.413[A,B,S], S02.42XS, S02.5XXS,
S02.600[A,B,S]-S02.69X[A,B,S], S02.91[A,B,S], S02.92XS,
S06.0X0-S07.9XX[A], S08.89X[A], S09.10X-S09.19X[A],
S09.8XX-S09.90X[A], S09.92X-S09.93X[A],
S16.8XX-S19.9XX[A], S38.3XXA, T07.XXX-T14.91X[A],
T79.8XX-T79.9XX[A], T79.A0X-T79.A9X[A]

PDX Collection 1144
S04.011-S04.049[A], S04.811-S04.9XX[A]

PDX Collection 1145
S04.10X-S04.12X[A], S04.811-S04.9XX[A]

PDX Collection 1146
S04.20X-S04.22X[A], S04.811-S04.9XX[A]

PDX Collection 1147
S04.30X-S04.32X[A], S04.811-S04.9XX[A]

PDX Collection 1148
S04.40X-S04.42X[A], S04.811-S04.9XX[A]

PDX Collection 1149
S04.50X-S04.52X[A], S04.811-S04.9XX[A]

PDX Collection 1150
S04.60X-S04.62X[A], S04.811-S04.9XX[A]

PDX Collection 1151
S04.70X-S04.9XX[A]

PDX Collection 1152
S04.811-S04.9XX[A]

PDX Collection 1153
S01.101-S01.159[A], S05.20X-S05.8X9[A],
S05.91X-S05.92X[A], S38.3XXA, T07.XXX-T14.91X[A],
T79.8XX-T79.9XX[A]

PDX Collection 1154
S01.90X-S01.95X[A], S02.0XX-S02.19X[A,B,S],
S02.2XX-S02.82X[S], S02.91X[A,B,S], S02.92XS,
S06.0X0-S07.9XX[A], S08.89X-S09.19X[A],
S09.8X-S09.90X[A]. S09.92X-S09.93X[A],
S16.8XX-S19.9XX[A], S38.3XXA. T07.XXX-T14.91X[A],
T79.A0X-T79.9XX[A]

PDX Collection 1155
G93.6, G93.82, S01.90X-S01.95X[A], S02.0XX-S02.19X[A,B,S],
S02.2XXS-S02.82X[S], S02.91X[A,B,S], S02.92X[S],
S06.0X0-S07.9XX[A], S08.89X-S09.19X[A],
S09.8XX-S09.90X[A], S09.92X-S09.93X[A],
S16.8XX-S19.9XX[A], S38.3XX[A], T07.XXX-T14.91X[A],
T79.8XX-T79.9XX[A], T79.A0X-T79.A9X[A]

PDX Collection 1156
S01.90X-S01.95X[A], S02.0XX-S02.92X[S],
S07.0XX-S07.9XX[A], S08.89X-S09.19X[A],
S09.8XX-S09.90X[A], S09.92X-S09.93X[A],
S16.8XX-S19.9XX[A], T07.XXX-T14.91X[A],
T79.8XX-T79.9XX[A], T79.A0X-T79.A9X[A]

PDX Collection 1157
S09.0XXA, S15.101-S15.199[A], S15.8XX-S15.9XX[A],
T07.XXX-T14.91X[A], T79.8XX-T79.9XX[A],
T79.A0X-T79.A9X[A]

PDX Collection 1158
S01.301-S01.359[A], S08.111-S08.129[A],
S09.20X-S09.399[A], S09.91X[A], S38.3XX[A],
T07.XXX-T14.91X[A], T79.8XX-T79.9XX[A]

PDX Collection 1159
S11.011-S11.039[A], S11.80X-S11.95X[A], S13.4XXA,
S13.8XX[A], S16.1XX-S16.2XX[A], S38.3XX[A],
T07.XXX-T14.91X[A], T79.8XX-T79.9XX[A],
T79.A0X-T79.A9X[A]

PDX Collection 1160
S11.10X-S11.15X[A], S11.80X-S11.95X[A], S13.4XX[A],
S13.8XXA, S16.1XX-S16.2XX[A], S38.3XXA,
T07.XXX-T14.91X[A], T79.8XX-T79.9XX[A]

PDX Collection 1161
S11.10X-S11.15X[A], S11.80X-S11.95X[A],
S13.4XX[A], S13.8XXA, S16.1XX-S16.2XX[A],
S38.3XXA, T07.XXX-T14.91X[A], T79.8XX-T79.9XX[A],
T79.A0X-T79.A9X[A]

PDX Collection 1162
S11.20X-S11.95X[A], S13.4XXA, S13.8XXA,
S16.1XX-S16.2XX[A], S38.3XXA, T07.XXX-T14.91X[A],
T79.8XX-T79.9XX[A]

PDX Collection 1163
S11.20X-S11.95X[A], S13.4XX[A], S13.8XXA,
S16.1XX-S16.2XX[A], S38.3XXA, T07.XXX-T14.91X[A],
T79.8XX-T79.9XX[A], T79.A0X-T79.A9X[A]

PDX Collection 1164
M48.40X-M48.58X[S], M80.08X[S], M80.88X[S], M84.350[S],
M84.454[S], M84.550[S], M84.58X[S], M84.650[S],
M99.10-M99.11, M99.15-M99.17, M99.19, S03.1XX[A],
S03.8XX-S03.9XX[A], S12.000-S12.691[A,B,S], S12.8XXS,
S12.9XX[A,S], S13.0XX-S13.4XX[A], S13.8XX-S14.159[A],
S16.1XXA, S22.000-S22.9XX[S], S23.20X-S23.29X[A],
S23.9XX[A], S24.109A, S24.119A, S24.139A, S24.149A,
S24.159A, S29.001-S29.019[A], S29.091-S29.9XX[A],
S32.000-S32.9XX[S], S33.30X-S33.39X[A], S33.9XXA,
S38.1XXA, S38.3XX-S39.013[A], S39.091-S39.94X[A],
T07.XXX-T14.91X[A], T79.8XX-T79.9XX[A],
T79.A0X-T79.A9X[A]

PDX Collection 1165
S03.8XX-S03.9XX[A], S12.8XXA, S29.011-S29.019[A],
S38.3XXA, S39.011-S39.013[A], T07.XXX-T14.91X[A],
T79.8XX-T79.9XX[A], T79.A0X-T79.A9X[A]

PDX Collection 1166
M48.40X-M48.58X[S], M80.08XS, M80.88XS,
M84.350S, M84.454S, M84.550S, M84.58XS, M84.650S,
M99.10-M99.11, M99.15-M99.17, M99.19, S03.1XXA,
S12.000-S12.691[A,B,S], S12.8X[S, S12.9XX[A,
S], S13.0XX-S13.29X[A], S13.9XX-S14.159[A],
S22.000-S22.9XX[S], S23.20X-S23.29X[A], S23.9XXA,
S24.109A, S24.119A, S24.139A, S24.149A, S24.159A,
S29.001-S29.009[A], S29.091-S29.9XX[A],
S32.000-S32.9XX[S], S33.30X-S33.39X[A], S33.9XXA,
S38.1XXA, S39.001-S39.003[A], S39.091-S39.94X[A],
T07.XXX-T14.91X[A], T79.8XX-T79.9XX[A],
T79.A0X-T79.A9X[A]

PDX Collection 1167
S09.0XXA, S15.009A, S15.02[A, S15.099-S15.199[A],
S15.8XX-S15.9XX[A], T07.XXX-T14.91X[A],
T79.8XX-T79.9XX[A], T79.A0X-T79.A9X[A]

PDX Collection 1168
S21.101-S21.159[A], S21.301-S21.95X[A], S23.3XX[A],
S23.8XX[A], S27.50X-S27.69X[A], S27.892A-S28.1XX[A],
S29.021A, S29.029A, S38.3XXA, T07.XXX-T14.91X[A],
T79.7XXA, T79.8XX-T79.9XX[A], T79.A0X-T79.A9X[A]

PDX Collection 1169
S21.101-S21.159[A], S21.301A-S21.95X[A],
S27.50X-S27.69X[A], S27.892-S27.9XX[A], S28.1XXA,
S29.021A, S29.029A, S38.3XXA, T07.XXX-T14.91X[A],
T79.7XXA, T79.8XX-T79.9XX[A], T79.A0X-T79.A9X[A]

PDX Collection 1170
S21.101A-S21.159[A], S21.301-S21.95X[A],
S27.0XX-S27.2XX[A], S27.309A, S27.329A,
S27.339A, S27.409A, S27.50X-S27.69X[A], S27.803A,
S27.892-S28.1XX[A], S29.021A, S29.029A, S38.3XXA,
T07.XXX-T14.91X[A], T79.7XXA, T79.8XX-T79.9XX[A],
T79.A0X-T79.A9X[A]

PDX Collection 1171
M48.40X-M48.58X[S], M80.08XS, M80.88XS,
M83.50S, M84.454S, M84.550S, M84.58XS, M84.650S,
M99.12, M99.15-M99.17, M99.19, S03.1XXA,
S03.8XX-S03.9XX[A], S12.000-S12.9XX[S], S13.9XXA,
S14.109A, S14.119A, S14.129A, S14.139A, S14.149A,
S14.159A, S22.000-S22.089[A,B,S], S22.20XS-S23.3XX[A],
S23.8XX-S24.159[A], S29.001-S29.019[A],
S29.091-S29.9XX[A], S32.000-S32.9XX[S], S32.9XXS,
S33.30X-S33.39X[A], S33.9XXA, S38.1XXA,
S38.3XXA, S39.001-S39.013[A], S39.091-S39.94X[A],
T07.XXX-T14.91X[A], T79.8XX-T79.9XX[A],
T79.A0X-T79.A9X[A]

PDX Collection 1172
S03.8XX-S03.9XX[A], S22.20X-S22.24X[A,B], S22.5XX[A,B],
S29.011-S29.019[A], S38.3XXA, S39.011-S39.013[A],
T07.XXX-T14.91X[A], T79.8XX-T79.9XX[A],
T79.A0X-T79.A9X[A]

PDX Collection 1173
S03.8XX-S03.9XX[A], S22.20X-S22.5XX[A,B],
S29.011-S29.019[A], S38.3XXA, S39.011-S39.013[A],
T07.XXX-T14.91X[A], T79.8XX-T79.9XX[A],
T79.A0X-T79.A9X[A]

PDX Collection 1174
S03.8XX-S03.9XX[A], S22.31X-S22.5XX[A,B],
S29.011-S29.019[A], S38.3XX[A], S39.011-S39.013[A],
T07.XXX-T14.91X[A], T79.8XX-T79.9XX[A],
T79.A0X-T79.A9X[A]

PDX Collection 1175
S03.8XX-S03.9XX[A], S22.20X-S22.5XX[A,B],
S29.011-S29.019[A], S38.3XXA, S39.011-S39.013[A],
T07.XXX-T14.91X[A], T79.8XX-T79.9XX[A],
T79.A0X-T79.A9X[A]

PDX Collection 1176
M80.00X-M80.019[A], M80.041A-M80.049[A],
M80.80X-M80.819[A], M80.841-M80.849[A],
M84.40X-M84.419[A], M84.441-M84.446[A],
M84.454A, M84.474-M84.519[A], M84.541-M84.550[A],
M84.574-M84.576[A], M84.60X-M84.619[A],
M84.641-M84.650[A], M84.674-M84.68[A],
S03.8XX-S03.9XX[A], S22.9XX-S22.9XX[A,B],
S29.011-S29.019[A], S32.301-S32.9XX[A,B], S33.4XX[A],
S33.6XX-S33.8XX[A], S38.3XXA, S39.011-S39.013[A],
S73.001-S73.199[A], S76.001-S76.019[A],
S76.091-S76.119[A], S76.191-S76.219[A],
S76.291-S76.319[A], S76.391-S76.819[A],
S76.891-S76.919[A], S76.991-S76.999[A],
S79.811-S79.929[A], T07.XXX-T14.91X[A],
T79.8XX-T79.9XX[A], T79.A9X[A]

PDX Collection 1177
M48.40X-M48.58X[S], M80.08X[S], M80.88XS,
M84.350S, M84.454S, M84.550S, M84.58S, M84.650S,
M99.15-M99.17, M99.19, S03.1XXA, S12.000-S12.9XX[S],
S13.9XXA, S14.109A, S14.119A, S14.129A,
S14.139A, S14.149A, S14.159A, S22.000-S22.9XX[S],
S23.20X-S23.29X[A], S23.9XX-S24.159[A],
S29.001-S29.009[A], S29.091-S29.9XX[A],
S32.000-S32.9XX[S], S33.30X-S33.39X[A], S33.9XXA,
S38.1XXA, S39.001-S39.003[A], S39.091-S39.94X[A],
T07.XXX-T14.91X[A], T79.8XX-T79.9XX[A],
T79.A0X-T79.A9X[A]

PDX Collection 1178
S25.00XA-S25.09X[A], T07.XXX-T14.91X[A],
T79.8XX-T79.9XX[A], T79.A0X-T79.A9X[A]

PDX Collection 1179
S25.101-S25.199[A], T07.XXX-T14.91X[A],
T79.8XX-T79.9XX[A], T79.A0X-T79.A9X[A]

PDX Collection 1180
S25.20X-S25.29X[A], T07.XXX-T14.91X[A],
T79.8XX-T79.9XX[A], T79.A0X-T79.A9X[A]

PDX Collection 1181
S25.301-S25.399[A], T07.XXX-T14.91X[A],
T79.8XX-T79.9XX[A], T79.A0X-T79.A9X[A]

PDX Collection 1182
S25.401-S25.499[A], T07.XXX-T14.91X[A],
T79.8XX-T79.9XX[A], T79.A0X-T79.A9X[A]

PDX Collection 1183
S25.401[A]-S25.499[A], T07.XXX-T14.91X[A],
T79.A0X[A]-T79.9XX[A]

PDX Collection 1184
S25.501-S25.899[A]

PDX Collection 1185
S25.00X-S25.99X[A]

PDX Collection 1186
S21.301-S21.459[A], S26.00X-S26.99X[A],
S27.50X-S27.69X[A], S27.892-S27.9XX[A],
T07.XXX-T14.91X[A]

PDX Collection 1187
S21.101-S21.159[A], S21.301-S21.95X[A],
S26.00X-S26.99X[A], S27.50X-S27.69X[A],
S27.892-S27.9XX[A], S28.1XX[A], S29.021A, S29.029A,
S38.3XXA, T07.XXX-T14.91X[A], T79.7XX-T79.9XX[A],
T79.A0X-T79.A9X[A]

PDX Collection 1188
S21.101-S21.159[A], S21.301-S21.95X[A],
S27.0XX-S27.399[A], S27.50X-S27.69X[A],
S27.892-S27.9XX[A], S28.1XXA, S29.021A, S29.029A[A],
S38.3XX[A], T07.XXX-T14.91X[A], T79.7XX-T79.9XX[A],
T79.A0X-T79.A9X[A]

PDX Collection 1189
S21.101-S21.159[A], S21.301-S21.95X[A],
S27.301-S27.399[A], S27.50X-S27.69X[A],
S27.892-S27.9XX[A], S28.1XXA, S29.021A, S29.029A,
S38.3XXA, T07.XXX-T14.91X[A], T79.7XX-T79.9XX[A],
T79.A9XA

PDX Collection 1190
S21.101-S21.159[A], S21.301-S21.95X[A],
S27.301-S27.399[A], S27.50X-S27.69X[A],
S27.892-S27.9XX[A], S28.1XXA, S29.021A, S29.029A,
S38.3XXA, T07.XXX-T14.91X[A], T79.7XX-T79.9XX[A],
T79.A0X-T79.A9X[A]

PDX Collection 1191
S21.101-S21.159[A], S21.301-S21.95X[A],
S27.401-S27.69X[A], S27.892-S27.9XX[A], S28.1XXA,
S29.021A, S29.029A, S38.3XXA, T07.XXX-T14.91X[A],
T79.7XX-T79.9XX[A], T79.A0X-T79.A9X[A]

PDX Collection 1192
S21.101-S21.159[A], S21.301-S21.95X[A],
S27.50X-S27.809[A], S27.892-S27.9XX[A], S28.1XX[A],
S29.021A, S29.029A, S38.3XXA, T07.XXX-T14.91X[A],
T79.7XX-T79.9XX[A], T79.A9XA

PDX Collection 1193
S21.101-S21.159[A], S21.301-S21.95X[A],
S27.50X-S27.69X[A], S27.812-S27.9XX[A], S28.1XXA,
S29.021A, S29.029A, S38.3XXA, T07.XXX-T14.91X[A],
T79.7XX-T79.9XX[A], T79.A0X-T79.A9X[A]

PDX Collection 1194
S21.101-S21.159[A], S21.301-S21.95X[A],
S27.50X-S27.69X[A], S27.892-S27.9XX[A], S28.1XXA,
S29.021A, S29.029A, S38.3XXA, T07.XXX-T14.91X[A],
T79.7XX-T79.9XX[A], T79.A3X-T79.A9X[A]

PDX Collection 1195
S31.001[A], S31.011[A], S31.021[A], S31.031[A], S31.041[A],
S31.051[A], S31.100-S31.159[A], S31.600-S31.659[A],
S31.831-S31.839[A], S36.81X-S36.99X[A],
S38.3XXA, S39.021-S39.023[A], T07.XXX-T14.91X[A],
T79.8XX-T79.9XX[A], T79.A0X-T79.A9X[A]

PDX Collection 1196
M48.40X-M48.58X[S], M80.08XS, M80.88XS,
M84.350S, M84.454S, M84.550S, M84.58XS, M84.650S,
M99.13, M99.15-M99.17, M99.19, S03.1XXA,
S03.8XX-S03.9XX[A], S12.000-S12.9XX[S], S13.9XXA,
S14.109A, S14.119A, S14.129A, S14.139A, S14.149A,
S14.159A, S22.000-S22.9XX[S], S23.20X-S23.29X[A],
S23.9XXA, S24.109A, S24.119A, S24.139A, S24.149A,
S24.159A, S29.001-S29.019[A], S29.091-S29.9XX[A],
S32.000-S32.059[A,B,S], S32.10X-S32.9XX[S],
S33.0XX-S33.141[A], S33.30X-S33.39X[A],
S33.5XXA, S33.9X[A, S34.01XA, S34.101-S34.129[A],
S38.1XXA, S38.3XX-S39.013[A], S39.091-S39.94X[A],
T07.XXX-T14.91X[A], T79.8XX-T79.9XX[A],
T79.A0X-T79.A9X[A]

PDX Collection 1197
M48.40X-M48.58X[S], M80.08XS, M80.88XS, M84.350S,
M84.454S, M84.550S, M84.58XS, M84.650S, M99.14-M99.17,
M99.19, S03.1XXA, S03.8XX-S03.9XX[A], S12.000-S12.9XX[S],
S13.9XXA, S14.109A, S14.119A, S14.129A, S14.139A,
S14.149A, S14.159A, S22.000-S22.9XX[S], S23.20XA,
S23.29XA, S23.9XXA, S24.109A, S24.119A,
S24.139A, S24.149A, S24.159A, S29.001-S29.019[A],
S29.091-S29.9XX[A], S32.000-S32.059[S],
S32.10X-S32.2XX[A,B,S], S32.301-S32.9XX[S],
S33.2XX-S33.4XX[A], S33.6XX-S33.9XX[A],
S34.02X[A], S34.131-S34.3XX[A], S38.1XXA,
S38.3XXA, S39.001-S39.013[A], S39.091-39.94X[A],
T07.XXX-T14.91X[A], T79.8XX-T79.9XX[A],
T79.A0X-T79.A9X[A]

PDX Collection 1198
M48.40X-M48.58X[A], M80.00X-M80.88X[A],
M84.30X-M84.68X[A], M84.750-M84.759[A],
S03.8XX-S03.9XX[A], S22.9XX[A,B], S29.011-S29.019[A],
S32.301-S32.399[A,B], S32.810-S32.9XX[A,B], S33.4XXA,
S33.6XX-S33.8XX[A], S38.3XXA, S39.011-S39.013[A],
S73.001-S73.199[A], S76.001-S76.019[A],
S76.091-S76.119[A], S76.191-S76.219[A],
S76.291-S76.319[A], S76.391-S76.819[A],
S76.891-S76.919[A], S76.991-S76.999[A],
S79.811-S79.929[A], T07.XXX-T14.91X[A],
T79.8XX-T79.9XX[A], T79.A0X-T79.A9X[A]

PDX Collection 1199
M48.40X-M48.58X[A], M80.00X-M80.88X[A],
M84.30X-M84.68X[A], M84.750-M84.759[A],
S03.8XX-S03.9XX[A], S22.9XX[A,B], S29.011-S29.019[A],
S32.401-S32.499[A,B], S32.810-S32.811[A,B],

S32.89X-S32.9XX[A,B], S33.4XXA, S33.6XX-S33.8XX[A],
S38.3XXA, S39.011-S39.013[A], S73.001-S73.199[A],
S76.001-S76.019[A], S76.091-S76.119[A],
S76.191-S76.219[A], S76.291-S76.319[A],
S76.391-S76.819[A], S76.891-S76.919[A],
S76.991-S76.999[A], S79.811-S79.829[A],
S79.911-S79.929[A], T07.XXX-T14.91X[A],
T79.8XX-T79.9XX[A], T79.A0X-T79.A9X[A]

PDX Collection 1200
S03.8XX-S03.9XX[A], S22.9XX[A,B], S29.011-S29.019[A],
S32.401-S32.499[A,B], S32.810-S32.811[A,B],
S32.89X-S32.9XX[A,B], S33.4XXA, S33.6XX-S33.8XX[A],
S38.3XXA, S39.011-S39.013[A], S73.001-S73.199[A],
S76.001-S76.019[A], S76.091-S76.119[A], S76.191-S76.219[A],
S76.291-S76.319[A], S76.391-S76.819[A], S76.891-S76.919[A],
S76.991-S76.999[A], S79.811-S79.929[A], T07.XXX-T14.91X[A],
T79.A0X-T79.A9X[A], T79.8XX-T79.9XX[A]

PDX Collection 1201
M48.40X-M48.58X[A], M80.00X-M80.88X[A],
M84.30X-M84.68X[A], M84.750-M84.759[A],
S03.8XX-S03.9XX[A], S22.9XX[A,B], S29.011-S29.019[A],
S32.501-S32.599[A,B], S32.810-S32.811[A,B],
S32.89X-S32.9XX[A,B], S33.4XXA, S33.6XX-S33.8XX[A],
S38.3XX-S39.013[A], S73.001-S73.199[A], S76.001-S76.019[A],
S76.091-S76.119[A], S76.191-S76.219[A], S76.291-S76.319[A],
S76.391-S76.819[A], S76.891-S76.919[A], S76.991-S76.999[A],
S79.811-S79.929[A], T07.XXX-T14.91X[A],T79.A0X-T79.A9X[A],
T79.8XX-T79.9XX[A]

PDX Collection 1202
S32.601-S32.699[A]

PDX Collection 1203
M48.40X-M48.58X[A], M80.00X-M80.88X[A],
M84.30X-M84.68X[A], M84.750-M84.759[A],
S03.8XX-S03.9XX[A], S22.9XX[A,B], S29.011-S29.019[A],
S32.601-S32.811[A,B], S32.89X-S32.9XX[A,B], S33.4XX[A],
S33.6XX-S33.8XX[A], S38.3XXA, S39.011-S39.013[A],
S73.001-S73.199[A], S76.001-S76.019[A], S76.091-S76.119[A],
S76.191-S76.219[A], S76.291-S76.319[A], S76.391-S76.819[A],
S76.891-S76.919[A], S76.991-S76.999[A], S79.811-S79.929[A],
T07.XXX-T14.91X[A], T79.A0X-T79.A9X[A], T79.8XX-T79.9XX[A]

PDX Collection 1204
M48.40X-M48.58X[A], M80.00X-M80.88X[A],
M84.30X-M84.68X[A], M84.750-M84.759[A],
S03.8XX-S03.9XX[A], S22.9XX[A,B], S29.011-S29.019[A],
S32.301-S32.811[A,B], S32.89X-S32.9XX[A,B], S33.4XXA,
S33.6XX-S33.8XX[A], S38.3XXA, S39.011-S39.013[A],
S73.001-S73.199[A], S76.001-S76.019[A], S76.091-S76.119[A],
S76.191-S76.219[A], S76.291-S76.319[A], S76.391-S76.819[A],
S76.891-S76.919[A], S76.991-S76.999[A], S79.811-S79.929[A],
T07.XXX-T14.91X[A], T79.A0X-T79.A9X[A], T79.8XX-T79.9XX[A]

PDX Collection 1205
S32.89XA

PDX Collection 1206
M48.40X-M48.58X[A], M80.00X-M80.88X[A],
M84.30X-M84.68X[A], M84.750-M84.759[A],
S03.8XX-S03.9XX[A], S22.9XX[A,B], S29.011-S29.019[A],
S32.301-S32.9XX[A,B], S33.4XXA, S33.6XX-S33.8XX[A],
S38.3XXA, S39.011-S39.013[A], S73.001-S73.199[A],
S76.001-S76.019[A], S76.091-S76.119[A], S76.191-S76.219[A],
76.291-S76.319[A], S76.391-S76.819[A], S76.891-S76.919[A],
S76.991-S76.999[A], S79.811-S79.929[A], T07.XXX-T14.91X[A],
T79.A0X-T79.A9X[A], T79.8XX-T79.9XX[A]

PDX Collection 1207
M48.40X-M48.58X[S], M80.08XS, M80.88XS, M84.350S,
M84.454S, M84.550S, M84.58XS, M84.650S, M99.15-M99.17,
M99.19, S03.1XXA, S12.000-S12.9XX[S], S13.9XXA,
S14.109A, S14.119A, S14.129A, S14.139A, S14.149A,
S14.159A, S22.000-S22.9XX[S], S23.20XA, S23.29XA,
S23.9XXA, S24.109A, S24.119A, S24.139A, S24.149A,
S24.159A, S29.001-S29.009[A], S29.091-S29.9XX[A],
S32.000-S32.9XX[S], S33.30X-S33.39X[A],
S33.9XX-S34.01X[A], S34.101-S34.129[A],
S38.1XX[A], S39.001-S39.003[A], S39.091-S39.94X[A],
T07.XXX-T14.91X[A], T79.A0X-T79.A9X[A],
T79.8XX-T79.9XX[A]

PDX Collection 1208
M48.40X-M48.58X[S], M80.08XS, M80.88XS, M84.350S,
M84.454S, M84.550S, M84.58XS, M84.650S, M99.15-M99.17,
M99.19, S03.1XXA, S12.000-S12.9XX[S], S13.9XXA,
S14.109A, S14.119A, S14.129A, S14.139A, S14.149A,
S14.159A, S22.000-S22.9XX[S], S23.20X-S23.29X[A],
S23.9XXA, S24.109A, S24.119A, S24.139A, S24.149A,
S24.159A, S29.001-S29.009[A], S29.091-S29.9XX[A],
S32.000-S32.9XX[S], S33.30X-S33.39X[A], S33.9XXA,
S34.02XA, S34.131-S34.139[A], S34.3XXA, S38.1XXA,
S39.001-S39.003[A], S39.091-S39.94X[A],
T07.XXX-T14.91X[A], T79.A0X-T79.A9X[A],
T79.8XX-T79.9XX[A]

PDX Collection 1209
S35.00X-S35.09X[A], S35.8X1-S35.99X[A],
T07.XXX-T14.91X[A], T79.A0X-T79.A9X[A],
T79.8XX-T79.9XX[A]

PDX Collection 1210
S35.10X-S35.19X[A], S35.8X1-S35.99X[A],
T07.XXX-T14.91X[A], T79.A0X-T79.A9X[A],
T79.8XX-T79.9XX[A]

PDX Collection 1211
S35.211-S35.219[A], S35.8X1-S35.99X[A],
T07.XXX-T14.91X[A], T79.A0X-T79.A9X[A],
T79.8XX-T79.9XX[A]

PDX Collection 1212
S35.221-S35.229[A], S35.8X1-S35.99X[A],
T07.XXX-T14.91X[A], T79.A0X-T79.A9X[A],
T79.8XX-T79.9XX[A]

PDX Collection 1213
S35.231-S35.239[A], S35.8X1-S35.99X[A],
T07.XXX-T14.91X[A], T79.A0X-T79.A9X[A],
T79.8XX-T79.9XX[A]

PDX Collection 1214
S35.291[A], S35.8X1-S35.99X[A], T07.XXX-T14.91X[A],
T79.8XX-T79.9XX[A], T79.A0XA, T79.A3X-T79.A9X[A]

PDX Collection 1215
S35.292-S35.298[A], S35.8X1-S35.99X[A],
T07.XXX-T14.91X[A], T79.A0X-T79.A9X[A],
T79.8XX-T79.9XX[A]

PDX Collection 1216
S35.299A, S35.8X1-S35.99X[A], T07.XXX-T14.91X[A],
T79.A0X-T79.A9X[A], T79.8XX-T79.9XX[A]

PDX Collection 1217
S35.311-S35.319[A], S35.8X1-S35.99X[A],
T07.XXX-T14.91X[A], T79.A0X-T79.A9X[A],
T79.8XX-T79.9XX[A]

PDX Collection 1218
S35.321-S35.329[A], S35.8X1-S35.99X[A],
T07.XXX-T14.91X[A], T79.A0X-T79.A9X[A],
T79.8XX-T79.9XX[A]

PDX Collection 1219
S35.331-S35.339[A], S35.8X1-S35.99X[A],
T07.XXX-T14.91X[A], T79.A0X-T79.A9X[A],
T79.8XX-T79.9XX[A]

PDX Collection 1220
S35.341-S35.349[A], S35.8X1-S35.99X[A],
T07.XXX-T14.91X[A], T79.A0X-T79.A9X[A],
T79.8XX-T79.9XX[A]

PDX Collection 1221
S35.401-S35.403[A], S35.411-S35.413[A], S35.491-S35.493[A],
S35.8X1-S35.99X[A], T07.XXX-T14.91X[A], T79.A0X-T79.A9X[A],
T79.8XX-T79.9XX[A]

PDX Collection 1222
S35.404-S35.406[A], S35.414-S35.416[A], S35.494-S35.496[A],
S35.8X1-S35.99X[A], T07.XXX-T14.91X[A], T79.A0X-T79.A9X[A],
T79.8XX-T79.9XX[A]

PDX Collection 1223
S35.50X-S35.516[A], S35.59X-S35.99X[A],
T07.XXX-T14.91X[A], T79.A0X-T79.A9X[A],
T79.8XX-T79.9XX[A]

PDX Collection 1224
S35.50X-S35.513[A], S35.59X-S35.99X[A],
T07.XXX-T14.91X[A], T79.A0X-T79.A9X[A],
T79.8XX-T79.9XX[A]

PDX Collection 1225
S35.50XA, S35.514-S35.516[A], S35.59X-S35.99X[A],
T07.XXX-T14.91X[A], T79.A0X-T79.A9X[A],
T79.8XX-T79.9XX[A]

PDX Collection 1226
S35.50XA, S35.531-S35.533[A], S35.59X-S35.99X[A],
T07.XXX-T14.91X[A], T79.8XX-T79.9XX[A], T79.A0X[A],
T79.A3X-T79.A9X[A]

PDX Collection 1227
S35.50X[A], S35.534-S35.536[A], S35.59X-S35.99X[A],
T07.XXX-T14.91X[A], T79.8XX-T79.9XX[A], T79.A0XA,
T79.A3X-T79.A9X[A]

PDX Collection 1228
S35.8X1-S35.99X[A], T07.XXX-T14.91X[A],
T79.8XX-T79.9XX[A], T79.A0XA, T79.A3X-T79.A9X[A]

PDX Collection 1229
S35.00X-S35.99X[A], T07.XXX-T14.91X[A],
T79.8XX-T79.9XX[A], T79.A0XA, T79.A3X-T79.A9X[A]

PDX Collection 1230
S31.001A, S31.011A, S31.021A, S31.031A, S31.041A,
S31.051A, S31.100-S31.159[A], S31.600-S31.659[A],
S31.831-S31.839[A], S36.00X-S36.09[A],
S36.81X-S36.99[A], S38.3XXA, S39.021-S39.023[A],
T07.XXX-T14.91X[A], T79.8XX-T79.9XX[A],
T79.A0X-T79.A9X[A]

PDX Collection 1231
S31.001A, S31.011A, S31.021A, S31.031A, S31.041A,
S31.051A, S31.100-S31.159[A], S31.600-S31.659[A],
S31.831-S31.839[A], S36.112-S36.119[A],
S36.81X-S36.99[A], S38.3XXA, S39.021-S39.023[A],
T07.XXX-T14.91X[A], T79.8XX-T79.9XX[A],
T79.A0X-T79.A9X[A]

PDX Collection 1232
S31.001A, S31.011A, S31.021A, S31.031A, S31.041A,
S31.051A, S31.100-S31.159[A], S31.600-S31.659[A],
S31.831-S31.839[A], S36.122-S36.13[A],
S36.81X-S36.99[A], S38.3XXA, S39.021-S39.023[A],
T07.XXX-T14.91X[A], T79.8XX-T79.9XX[A],
T79.A0X-T79.A9X[A]

PDX Collection 1233
M79.A3, S31.001A, S31.011A, S31.021A, S31.031A, S31.041A,
S31.051A, S31.100-S31.159[A], S31.600-S31.659[A],
S31.831-S31.839[A], S36.200-S36.299[A],
S36.81X-S36.99[A], S38.3XX[A], S39.021-S39.023[A],
T07.XXX-T14.91X[A], T79.8XX-T79.9XX[A],
T79.A3X-T79.A9X[A]

PDX Collection 1234
M79.A3, S31.001A, S31.011A, S31.021A, S31.031A, S31.041A,
S31.051A, S31.100-S31.159[A], S31.600-S31.659[A],
S31.831-S31.839[A], S36.30X-S36.39[A],
S36.81X-S36.99[A], S38.3XXA, S39.021-S39.023[A],
T07.XXX-T14.91X[A], T79.8XX-T799.XX[A],
T79.A3X-T79.A9X[A]

PDX Collection 1235
M79.A3, S31.001A, S31.011A, S31.021A, S31.031A, S31.041A,
S31.051A, S31.100-S31.159[A], S31.600-S31.659[A],
S31.831-S31.839[A], S36.400-S36.499[A],
S36.81X-S36.99[A], S38.3XX[A], S39.021-S39.023[A],
T07.XXX-T14.91X[A], T79.8XX-T79.9XX[A],
T79.A3X-T79.A9X[A]

PDX Collection 1236
M79.A3, S31.001A, S31.011A, S31.021A, S31.031A, S31.041A,
S31.051A, S31.100-S31.159[A], S31.600-S31.659[A],
S31.831-S31.839[A], S36.500-S36.99[A],
S38.3XXA, S39.021-S39.023[A], T07.XXX-T14.91X[A],
T79.8XX-T79.9XX[A], T79.A3X-T79.A9X[A]

PDX Collection 1237
S31.001A, S31.011A, S31.021A, S31.031A, S31.041A,
S31.051A, S31.100-S31.159[A], S31.600-S31.659[A],
S31.831-S31.839[A], S36.81X-S37.099[A],
S38.3XXA, S39.021-S39.023[A], T07.XXX-T14.91X[A],
T79.8XX-T79.9XX[A], T79.A0X-T79.A9X[A]

PDX Collection 1238
S31.001A, S31.011A, S31.021A, S31.031A, S31.041A,
S31.051A, S31.100-S31.159[A], S31.600-S31.659[A],
S31.831-S31.839[A], S36.81X-S36.99[A],
S37.10X-S37.19[A], S37.401-S37.599[A],
S37.822-S37.99[A], S38.3XXA, S39.021-S39.023[A],
T07.XXX-T14.91X[A], T79.8XX-T79.9XX[A],
T79.A0X-T79.A9X[A]

PDX Collection 1239
S31.001A, S31.011A, S31.021A, S31.031A, S31.041A,
S31.051A, S31.100-S31.159[A], S31.600-S31.659[A],
S31.831-S31.839[A], S36.81X-S36.99[A],
S37.20X-S37.599[A], S37.822-S37.99[A],
S38.3XXA, S39.021-S39.023[A], T07.XXX-T14.91X[A],
T79.8XX-T79.9XX[A], T79.A0X-T79.A9X[A]

PDX Collection 1240
S31.001A, S31.011A, S31.021A, S31.031A, S31.041A,
S31.051A, S31.100-S31.159[A], S31.600-S31.659[A],
S31.831-S31.839[A], S36.81X-S36.99[A],
S37.401-S37.69[A], S37.822-S37.99[A],
S38.3XXA, S39.021-S39.023[A], T07.XXX-T14.91X[A],
T79.8XX-T79.9XX[A], T79.A0X-T79.A9X[A]

PDX Collection 1241
S31.001A, S31.011A, S31.021A, S31.031A, S31.041A,
S31.051A, S31.100-S31.159[A], S31.600-S31.659[A],
S31.831-S31.839[A], S36.81X-S36.99[A],
S37.812-S37.819[A], S38.3XXA, S39.021-S39.023[A],
T07.XXX-T14.91X[A], T79.8XX-T799.XX[A],
T79.A0X-T79.A9X[A]

PDX Collection 1242
S31.001A, S31.011A, S31.021A, S31.031A, S31.041A,
S31.051A, S31.100-S31.159[A], S31.600-S31.659[A],
S31.831-S31.839[A], S36.81X-S36.99[A],

S37.401-S37.599[A], S37.822-S37.99X[A],
S38.3XXA, S39.021-S39.023[A], T07.XXX-T14.91X[A],
T79.8XX-T79.9XX[A], T79.A0X-T79.A9X[A]

PDX Collection 1243

S42.001-S42.036[A,B], S62.90XB

PDX Collection 1244

S42.101-S42.199[A,B], S62.90XB

PDX Collection 1245

S42.201[A,B], S42.202B, S42.209-S42.211[A,B], S42.212[B],
S42.213-S42.214[A,B], S42.215[B], S42.216-S42.221[A,B],
S42.222[B], S42.223-S42.224[A,B], S42.225[B],
S42.226-S42.231[A,B], S42.232[B], S42.239-S42.241[A,B],
S42.242[B], S42.249-S42.251[A,B], S42.252[B],
S42.253-S42.254[A,B], S42.255[B], S42.256-S42.261[A,B],
S42.262[B], S42.263-S42.264[A,B], S42.265[B],
S42.266[A,B], S42.271A, S42.279A, S42.291[A,B], S42.292B,
S42.293-S42.294[A,B], S42.295B, S42.296-S42.301[A,B],
S42.302B, S42.309[A,B], S42.311A, S42.319A,
S42.321[A,B], S42.322B, S42.323-S42.324[A,B], S42.325B,
S42.326-S42.331[A,B], S42.332B, S42.333-S42.334[A,B],
S42.335B, S42.336-S42.341[A,B], S42.342B,
S42.343-S42.344[A,B], S42.345B, S42.346-S42.351[A,B],
S42.352B, S42.353-S42.354[A,B], S42.355B,
S42.356-S42.361[A,B], S42.362B, S42.363-S42.364[A,B],
S42.365B, S42.366-S42.391[A,B], S42.392B,
S42.399-S42.401[A,B], S42.402B, S42.409-S42.411[A,B],
S42.412B, S42.413-S42.414[A,B], S42.415B,
S42.416-S42.421[A,B], S42.422B, S42.423-S42.424[A,B],
S42.425B, S42.426-S42.431[A,B], S42.432B,
S42.433-S42.434[A,B], S42.435B, S42.436-S42.441[A,B],
S42.442B, S42.443-S42.444[A,B], S42.445B,
S42.446-S42.447[A,B], S42.448B, S42.449-S42.451[A,B],
S42.452B, S42.453-S42.454[A,B], S42.455B,
S42.456-S42.461[A,B], S42.462B, S42.463-S42.464[A,B],
S42.465B, S42.466-S42.471[A,B], S42.472B,
S42.473-S42.474[A,B], S42.475B, S42.476[A,B], S42.481A,
S42.489A, S42.491[A,B], S42.492B, S42.493-S42.494[A,B],
S42.495B, S42.496-S42.92X[A,B], S49.001A,
S49.009-S49.011[A], S49.019-S49.021[A], S49.029-S49.031[A],
S49.039-S49.041[A], S49.049-S49.091[A], S49.099-S49.101[A],
S49.109-S49.111[A], S49.119-S49.121[A], S49.129-S49.131[A],
S49.139-S49.141[A], S49.149-S49.191[A], S49.199A

PDX Collection 1246

S42.201-S42.266[B], S42.291-S42.296[B],
S42.301-S42.309[A,B], S42.311-S42.319[A],
S42.321-S42.476[A,B], S42.481-S42.489[A],
S42.491-S42.92X[A,B], S49.101-S49.199[A], S62.90X[B]

PDX Collection 1247

S42.201B, S42.202-S42.209[A,B], S42.211B,
S42.212-S42.213[A,B], S42.214B, S42.215-S42.216[A,B],
S42.221B, S42.222-S42.223[A,B], S42.224B,
S42.225-S42.226[A,B], S42.231B, S42.232-S42.239[A,B],
S42.241B, S42.242-S42.249[A,B], S42.251B,
S42.252-S42.253[A,B], S42.254B, S42.255-S42.256[A,B],
S42.261B, S42.262-S42.263[A,B], S42.264B,
S42.265-S42.266[A,B], S42.272-S42.279[A], S42.291B,
S42.292-S42.293[A,B], S42.294B, S42.295-S42.296[A,B],
S42.301B, S42.302-S42.309[A,B], S42.312-S42.319[A],
S42.321B, S42.322-S42.323[A,B], S42.324B,
S42.325-S42.326[A,B], S42.331B, S42.332-S42.333[A,B],
S42.334B, S42.335-S42.336[A,B], S42.341B,
S42.342-S42.343[A,B], S42.344B, S42.345-S42.346[A,B],
S42.351B, S42.352-S42.353[A,B], S42.354B,
S42.355-S42.356[A,B], S42.361B, S42.362-S42.363[A,B],
S42.364B, S42.365-S42.366[A,B], S42.391B,
S42.392-S42.399[A,B], S42.401B, S42.402-S42.409[A,B],
S42.411B, S42.412-S42.413[A,B], S42.414B,

S42.415-S42.416[A,B], S42.421B, S42.422-S42.423[A,B],
S42.424B, S42.425-S42.426[A,B], S42.431B,
S42.432-S42.433[A,B], S42.434B, S42.435-S42.436[A,B],
S42.441B, S42.442-S42.443[A,B], S42.444B,
S42.445-S42.446[A,B], S42.447B, S42.448-S42.449[A,B],
S42.451B, S42.452-S42.453[A,B], S42.454B,
S42.455-S42.456[A,B], S42.461B, S42.462-S42.463[A,B],
S42.464B, S42.465-S42.466[A,B], S42.471B,
S42.472-S42.473[A,B], S42.474B, S42.475-S42.476[A,B],
S42.482-S42.489[A], S42.491B, S42.492-S42.493[A,B],
S42.494B, S42.495-S42.92X[A,B], S49.002-S49.009[A],
S49.012-S49.019[A], S49.022-S49.029[A], S49.032-S49.039[A],
S49.042-S49.049[A], S49.092-S49.099[A], S49.102-S49.109[A],
S49.112-S49.119[A], S49.122-S49.129[A], S49.132-S49.139[A],
S49.142-S49.149[A], S49.192-S49.199[A]

PDX Collection 1248

S42.201-S42.266[A,B], S42.271-S42.279[A],
S42.291-S42.309[A,B], S42.311-S42.319[A],
S42.321-S42.476[A,B], S42.481-S42.489[A],
S42.491-S42.92X[A,B], S49.001-S49.199[A]

PDX Collection 1249

S42.311A, S42.319-S42.321[A], S42.323-S42.324[A],
S42.326-S42.331[A], S42.333-S42.334[A],
S42.336-S42.341[A], S42.343-S42.344[A],
S42.346-S42.351[A], S42.353-S42.354[A],
S42.356-S42.361[A], S42.363-S42.364[A],
S42.366-S42.391[A], S42.399A

PDX Collection 1250

S42.312-S42.319[A], S42.322-S42.323[A],
S42.325-S42.326[A], S42.332-S42.333[A],
S42.335-S42.336[A], S42.342-S42.343[A],
S42.345-S42.346[A], S42.352-S42.353[A],
S42.355-S42.356[A], S42.362-S42.363[A],
S42.365-S42.366[A], S42.392-S42.399[A]

PDX Collection 1251

S42.311-S42.399[A]

PDX Collection 1252

M99.18, S43.201A, S43.203-S43.204[A], S43.206A,
S43.211A, S43.213-S43.214[A], S43.216A, S43.221A,
S43.223-S43.224[A], S43.226A

PDX Collection 1253

M99.18, S43.202-S43.203[A], S43.205-S43.206[A],
S43.212-S43.213[A], S43.215-S43.216[A],
S43.222-S43.223[A], S43.225-S43.226[A]

PDX Collection 1254

S45.001A, S45.009-S45.011[A], S45.019-S45.091[A],
S45.099A, S45.301A, S45.309-S45.311[A],
S45.319-S45.391[A], S45.399-S45.801[A],
S45.809-S45.811[A], S45.819-S45.891[A],
S45.899-S45.901[A], S45.909-S45.911[A],
S45.919-S45.991[A], S45.999[A], S55.201A,
S55.209-S55.211[A], S55.219-S55.291[A],
S55.299-S55.801[A], S55.809-S55.811[A],
S55.819-S55.891[A], S55.899-S55.901[A],
S55.909-S55.911[A], S55.919-S55.991[A], S55.999A,
S65.801A, S65.809-S65.811[A], S65.819-S65.891[A],
S65.899-S65.901[A], S65.909-S65.911[A],
S65.919-S65.991[A], S65.999A

PDX Collection 1255

S45.002-S45.009[A], S45.012-S45.019[A],
S45.092-S45.099[A], S45.302-S45.309[A],
S45.312-S45.319[A], S45.392-S45.399[A],
S45.802-S45.809[A], S45.812-S45.819[A],
S45.892-S45.899[A], S45.902-S45.909[A],
S45.912-S45.919[A], S45.992-S45.999[A],
S55.202-S55.209[A], S55.212-S55.219[A],

S55.292-S55.299[A], S55.802-S55.809[A],
S55.812-S55.819[A], S55.892-S55.899[A],
S55.902-S55.909[A], S55.912-S55.919[A],
S55.992-S55.999[A], S65.802-S65.809[A],
S65.812-S65.819[A], S65.892-S65.899[A],
S65.902-S65.909[A], S65.912-S65.919[A],
S65.992-S65.999[A]

PDX Collection 1256

S45.001-S45.099[A], S45.301-S45.399[A],
S45.801-S45.999[A], S55.201-S55.999[A],
S65.801-S65.999[A]

PDX Collection 1257

S45.101A, S45.109-S45.111[A], S45.119-S45.191[A],
S45.199-S45.201[A], S45.209A-S45.211[A],
S45.219-S45.291[A], S45.299-S45.301[A],
S45.309-S45.311[A], S45.319-S45.391[A],
S45.399-S45.801[A], S45.809-S45.811[A],
S45.819-S45.891[A], S45.899-S45.901[A],
S45.909-S45.911[A], S45.919-S45.991[A], S45.999A,
S55.201[A], S55.209-S55.211[A], S55.219-S55.291[A],
S55.299-S55.801[A], S55.809-S55.811[A],
S55.819-S55.891[A], S55.899-S55.901[A],
S55.909-S55.911[A], S55.919-S55.991[A], S55.999A,
S65.801A, S65.809-S65.811[A], S65.819-S65.891[A],
S65.899-S65.901[A], S65.909-S65.911[A],
S65.919-S65.991[A], S65.999A

PDX Collection 1258

S45.102-S45.109[A], S45.112-S45.119[A],
S45.192-S45.199[A], S45.202-S45.209[A],
S45.212-S45.219[A], S45.292-S45.299[A],
S45.302-S45.309[A], S45.312-S45.319[A],
S45.392-S45.399[A], S45.802-S45.809[A],
S45.812-S45.819[A], S45.892-S45.899[A],
S45.902-S45.909[A], S45.912-S45.919[A],
S45.992-S45.999[A], S55.202-S55.209[A],
S55.212-S55.219[A], S55.292-S55.299[A],
S55.802-S55.809[A], S55.812-S55.819[A],
S55.892-S55.899[A], S55.902-S55.909[A],
S55.912-S55.919[A], S55.992-S55.999[A],
S65.802-S65.809[A], S65.812-S65.819[A],
S65.892-S65.899[A], S65.902-S65.909[A],
S65.912-S65.919[A], S65.992-S65.999[A]

PDX Collection 1259

S45.101-S45.999[A], S55.201-S55.999[A],
S65.801-S65.999[A]

PDX Collection 1260

S45.301A, S45.309-S45.311[A], S45.319-S45.391[A],
S45.399-S45.801[A], S45.809-S45.811[A],
S45.819-S45.891[A], S45.899-S45.901[A],
S45.909-S45.911[A], S45.919-S45.991[A], S45.999A,
S55.001A, S55.009-S55.011[A], S55.019-S55.091[A],
S55.099A, S55.201A, S55.209-S55.211[A],
S55.219-S55.291[A], S55.299-S55.801[A],
S55.809-S55.811[A], S55.819-S55.891[A],
S55.899-S55.901[A], S55.909-S55.911[A],
S55.919-S55.991[A], S55.999A, S65.001A,
S65.009-S65.011[A], S65.019-S65.091[A], S65.099A,
S65.201A, S65.209-S65.211[A], S65.219-S65.291[A],
S65.299-S65.301[A], S65.309-S65.311[A],
S65.319-S65.391[A], S65.399-S65.401[A],
S65.409-S65.411[A], S65.419-S65.491[A],
S65.499-S65.500[A], S65.502A, S65.504A, S65.506A,
S65.508-S65.510[A], S65.512A, S65.514A, S65.516A,
S65.518-S65.590[A], S65.592A, S65.594A, S65.596A,
S65.598-S65.801[A], S65.809-S65.811[A],
S65.819-S65.891[A], S65.899-S65.901[A],
S65.909-S65.911[A], S65.919-S65.991[A], S65.999A

PDX Collection 1261
S45.302-S45.309[A], S45.312-S45.319[A],
S45.392-S45.399[A], S45.802-S45.809[A],
S45.812-S45.819[A], S45.892-S45.899[A],
S45.902-S45.909[A], S45.912-S45.919[A],
S45.992-S45.999[A], S55.002-S55.009[A],
S55.012-S55.019[A], S55.092-S55.099[A],
S55.202-S55.209[A], S55.212-S55.219[A],
S55.292-S55.299[A], S55.802-S55.809[A],
S55.812-S55.819[A], S55.892-S55.899[A],
S55.902-S55.909[A], S55.912-S55.919[A],
S55.992-S55.999[A], S65.002-S65.009[A],
S65.012-S65.019[A], S65.092-S65.099[A],
S65.202-S65.209[A], S65.212-S65.219[A],
S65.292-S65.299[A], S65.302-S65.309[A],
S65.312-S65.319[A], S65.392-S65.399[A],
S65.402-S65.409[A], S65.412-S65.419[A],
S65.492-S65.499[A], S65.501A, S65.503A, S65.505A,
S65.507-S65.509[A], S65.511A, S65.513A, S65.515A,
S65.517-S65.519[A], S65.591A, S65.593A, S65.595A,
S65.597-S65.599[A], S65.802-S65.809[A],
S65.812-S65.819[A], S65.892-S65.899[A],
S65.902-S65.909[A], S65.912-S65.919[A],
S65.992-S65.999[A]

PDX Collection 1262
S45.301-S45.999[A], S55.001-S55.099[A],
S55.201-S55.999[A], S65.001-S65.099[A],
S65.201-S65.999[A]

PDX Collection 1263
S41.001A, S41.009-S41.011[A], S41.019-S41.021[A],
S41.029-S41.031[A], S41.039-S41.041[A],
S41.049-S41.051[A], S41.059-S41.101[A],
S41.109-S41.111[A], S41.119-S41.121[A],
S41.129-S41.131[A], S41.139-S41.141[A],
S41.149-S41.151[A], S41.159A, S46.021A, S46.029A,
S46.121A, S46.129A, S46.221A, S46.229A, S46.321A,
S46.329A, S46.821A, S46.829A, S46.921A, S46.929A

PDX Collection 1264
S41.002-S41.009[A], S41.012-S41.019[A],
S41.022-S41.029[A], S41.032-S41.039[A],
S41.042-S41.049[A], S41.052-S41.059[A],
S41.102-S41.109[A], S41.112-S41.119[A],
S41.122-S41.129[A], S41.132-S41.139[A],
S41.142-S41.149[A], S41.152-S41.159[A],
S46.022-S46.029[A], S46.122-S46.129[A],
S46.222-S46.229[A], S46.322-S46.329[A],
S46.822-S46.829[A], S46.922-S46.929[A]

PDX Collection 1265
S41.001-S41.159[A], S46.021-S46.029[A],
S46.121-S46.129[A], S46.221-S46.229[A],
S46.321-S46.329[A], S46.821-S46.829[A],
S46.921-S46.929[A]

PDX Collection 1266
S41.001A, S41.009-S41.011[A], S41.019-S41.021[A],
S41.029-S41.031[A], S41.039-S41.041[A], S41.049-S41.051[A],
S41.059-S41.101[A], S41.109-S41.111[A], S41.119-S41.121[A],
S41.129-S41.131[A], S41.139-S41.141[A], S41.149-S41.151[A],
S41.159A, S46.021A, S46.029A, S46.121A, S46.129A, S46.221A,
S46.229A, S46.321A, S46.329A, S46.821A, S46.829A, S46.921A,
S46.929A, S48.011A, S48.019-S48.021[A], S48.029-S48.111[A],
S48.119-S48.121[A], S48.129-S48.911[A], S48.919-S48.921[A],
S48.929A, S51.001A, S51.009-S51.011[A], S51.019-S51.021[A],
S51.029-S51.031[A], S51.039-S51.041[A], S51.049-S51.051[A],
S51.059-S51.801[A], S51.809-S51.811[A], S51.819-S51.821[A],
S51.829-S51.831[A], S51.839-S51.841[A], S51.849-S51.851[A],
S51.859A, S56.021A, S56.029A, S56.121A, S56.123A, S56.125A,
S56.127A, S56.129A, S56.221A, S56.229A, S56.321A, S56.329A,

S56.421A, S56.423A, S56.425A, S56.427A, S56.429A, S56.521A,
S56.529A, S56.821A, S56.829A, S56.921A, S56.929A, S58.011A,
S58.019-S58.021[A], S58.029-S58.111[A], S58.119-S58.121[A],
S58.129-S58.911[A], S58.919-S58.921[A], S58.929A, S61.001A,
S61.009-S61.011[A], S61.019-S61.021[A], S61.029-S61.031[A],
S61.039-S61.041[A], S61.049-S61.051[A], S61.059-S61.101[A],
S61.109-S61.111[A], S61.119-S61.121[A], S61.129-S61.131[A],
S61.139-S61.141[A], S61.149-S61.151[A], S61.159-S61.200[A],
S61.202A, S61.204A, S61.206A, S61.208-S61.210[A],
S61.212A, S61.214A, S61.216A, S61.218-S61.220[A], S61.222A,
S61.224A, S61.226A, S61.228-S61.230[A], S61.232A,
S61.234A, S61.236A, S61.238-S61.240[A], S61.242A,
S61.244A, S61.246A, S61.248-S61.250[A], S61.252A, S61.254A,
S61.256A, S61.258-S61.300[A], S61.302A, S61.304A,
S61.306A, S61.308-S61.310[A], S61.312A, S61.314A,
S61.316A, S61.318-S61.320[A], S61.322A, S61.324A,
S61.326A, S61.328-S61.330[A], S61.332A, S61.334A,
S61.336A, S61.338-S61.340[A], S61.342A, S61.344A,
S61.346A, S61.348-S61.350[A], S61.352A, S61.354A, S61.356A,
S61.358-S61.401[A], S61.409-S61.411[A], S61.419-S61.421[A],
S61.429-S61.431[A], S61.439-S61.441[A], S61.449-S61.451[A],
S61.459-S61.501[A], S61.509-S61.511[A], S61.519-S61.521[A],
S61.529-S61.531[A], S61.539-S61.541[A], S61.549-S61.551[A],
S61.559A, S66.021A, S66.029A, S66.120A, S66.122A, S66.124A,
S66.126A, S66.128-S66.129[A], S66.221A, S66.229A, S66.320A,
S66.322A, S66.324A, S66.326A, S66.328-S66.329[A],
S66.421A, S66.429A, S66.520A, S66.522A, S66.524A, S66.526A,
S66.528-S66.529[A], S66.821A, S66.829A, S66.921A, S66.929A,
S68.011A, S68.019-S68.021[A], S68.029-S68.110[A],
S68.112A, S68.114A, S68.116A, S68.118-S68.120[A], S68.122A,
S68.124A, S68.126A, S68.128-S68.411[A], S68.419-S68.421[A],
S68.429-S68.511[A], S68.519-S68.521[A], S68.529-S68.610[A],
S68.612A, S68.614A, S68.616A, S68.618-S68.620[A], S68.622A,
S68.624A, S68.626A, S68.628-S68.711[A], S68.719-S68.721[A],
S68.729[A], T07.XXX-T14.91X[A], T79.A0X-T79.9XX[A]

PDX Collection 1267
S41.002-S41.009[A], S41.012-S41.019[A], S41.022-S41.029[A],
S41.032-S41.039[A], S41.042-S41.049[A], S41.052-S41.059[A],
S41.102-S41.109[A], S41.112-S41.119[A], S41.122-S41.129[A],
S41.132-S41.139[A], S41.142-S41.149[A], S41.152-S41.159[A],
S46.022-S46.029[A], S46.122-S46.129[A], S46.222-S46.229[A],
S46.322-S46.329[A], S46.822-S46.829[A], S46.922-S46.929[A],
S48.012-S48.019[A], S48.022-S48.029[A], S48.112-S48.119[A],
S48.122-S48.129[A], S48.912-S48.919[A], S48.922-S48.929[A],
S51.002-S51.009[A], S51.012-S51.019[A], S51.022-S51.029[A],
S51.032-S51.039[A], S51.042-S51.049[A], S51.052-S51.059[A],
S51.802-S51.809[A], S51.812-S51.819[A], S51.822-S51.829[A],
S51.832-S51.839[A], S51.842-S51.849[A], S51.852-S51.859[A],
S56.022-S56.029[A], S56.122A, S56.124A, S56.126A,
S56.128-S56.129[A], S56.222-S56.229[A], S56.322-S56.329[A],
S56.422A, S56.424A, S56.426A, S56.428-S56.429[A],
S56.522-S56.529[A], S56.822-S56.829[A], S56.922-S56.929[A],
S58.012-S58.019[A], S58.022-S58.029[A], S58.112-S58.119[A],
S58.122-S58.129[A], S58.912-S58.919[A], S58.922-S58.929[A],
S61.002-S61.009[A], S61.012-S61.019[A], S61.022-S61.029[A],
S61.032-S61.039[A], S61.042-S61.049[A], S61.052-S61.059[A],
S61.102-S61.109[A], S61.112-S61.119[A], S61.122-S61.129[A],
S61.132-S61.139[A], S61.142-S61.149[A], S61.152-S61.159[A],
S61.201A, S61.203A, S61.205A, S61.207-S61.209[A],
S61.211A, S61.213A, S61.215A, S61.217-S61.219[A], S61.221A,
S61.223A, S61.225A, S61.227-S61.229[A], S61.231A,
S61.233A, S61.235A, S61.237-S61.239[A], S61.241A, S61.243A,
S61.245A, S61.247-S61.249[A], S61.251A, S61.253A,
S61.255A, S61.257-S61.259[A], S61.301A, S61.303A,
S61.305A, S61.307-S61.309[A], S61.311A, S61.313A,
S61.315A, S61.317-S61.319[A], S61.321A, S61.323A,
S61.325A, S61.327-S61.329[A], S61.331A, S61.333A,

S61.335A, S61.337-S61.339[A], S61.341A, S61.343A, S61.345A,
S61.347-S61.349[A], S61.351A, S61.353A, S61.355A,
S61.357-S61.359[A], S61.402-S61.409[A], S61.412-S61.419[A],
S61.422-S61.429[A], S61.432-S61.439[A], S61.442-S61.449[A],
S61.452-S61.459[A], S61.502-S61.509[A], S61.512-S61.519[A],
S61.522-S61.529[A], S61.532-S61.539[A], S61.542-S61.549[A],
S61.552-S61.559[A], S66.022-S66.029[A], S66.121[A],
S66.123A, S66.125A, S66.127-S66.129[A], S66.222-S66.229[A],
S66.321A, S66.323A, S66.325A, S66.327-S66.329[A],
S66.422-S66.429[A], S66.521A, S66.523A, S66.525A,
S66.527-S66.529[A], S66.822-S66.829[A], S66.922-S66.929[A],
S68.012-S68.019[A], S68.022-S68.029[A], S68.111A, S68.113A,
S68.115A, S68.117-S68.119[A], S68.121A, S68.123A, S68.125A,
S68.127-S68.129[A], S68.412-S68.419[A], S68.422-S68.429[A],
S68.512-S68.519[A], S68.522-S68.529[A], S68.611A, S68.613A,
S68.615A, S68.617-S68.619[A], S68.621A, S68.623A, S68.625A,
S68.627-S68.629[A], S68.712-S68.719[A], S68.722-S68.729[A],
T07.XXX-T14.91X[A], T79.A0X-T79.9XX[A]

PDX Collection 1268
S41.001-S41.159[A], S46.021-S46.029[A],
S46.121-S46.129[A], S46.221-S46.229[A],
S46.321-S46.329[A], S46.821-S46.829[A],
S46.921-S46.929[A], S48.011-S48.929[A],
S51.001-S51.859[A], S56.021-S56.029[A],
S56.121-S56.129[A], S56.221-S56.229[A],
S56.321-S56.329[A], S56.421-S56.429[A],
S56.521-S56.529[A], S56.821-S56.829[A],
S56.921-S56.929[A], S58.011-S58.929[A],
S61.001-S61.559[A], S66.021-S66.029[A],
S66.120-S66.129[A], S66.221-S66.229[A],
S66.320-S66.329[A], S66.421-S66.429[A],
S66.520-S66.529[A], S66.821-S66.829[A],
S66.921-S66.929[A], S68.011-S68.729[A],
T07.XXX-T14.91X[A], T79.A0X-T79.9XX[A]

PDX Collection 1269
S52.001-S52.009[B,C], S52.021-S52.109[B,C],
S52.121-S52.189[B,C], S52.201-S52.209[A,B,C],
S52.211-S52.219[A], S52.221-S52.266[A,B,C],
S52.271-S52.279[B,C], S52.281-S52.309[A,B,C],
S52.311-S52.319[A], S52.321-S52.516[A,B,C],
S52.531-S52.616[A,B,C], S52.691-S52.92X[A,B,C],
S59.001-S59.099[A], S59.201-S59.299[A], S62.90XB

PDX Collection 1270
S52.001 [A,B,C], S52.002[B,C], S52.009 [A,B,C],
S52.011[A], S52.019[A], S52.021[A,B,C], S52.022[B,C],
S52.023-S52.024[A,B,C], S52.025[B,C], S52.026-S52.031[A,B,C],
S52.032[B,C], S52.033-S52.034[A,B,C], S52.035[B,C],
S52.036-S52.041[A,B,C], S52.042[B,C], S52.043-S52.044[A,B,C],
S52.045[B,C], S52.046-S52.091[A,B,C], S52.092[B,C],
S52.099-S52.101[A,B,C], S52.102[B,C], S52.109[A,B,C],
S52.111A, S52.119A, S52.121[A,B,C], S52.122[B,C],
S52.123-S52.124[A,B,C], S52.125[B,C], S52.126-S52.131[A,B,C],
S52.132[B,C], S52.133-S52.134[A,B,C], S52.135[B, C],
S52.136-S52.181[A,B,C], S52.182[B,C], S52.189-S52.201[A,B,C],
S52.202[B,C], S52.209[A,B,C], S52.211A, S52.219A,
S52.221[A,B,C], S52.222[B,C], S52.223-S52.224[A,B,C],
S52.225[B,C], S52.226-S52.231[C], S52.232[B,C],
S52.233-S52.234[A,B,C], S52.235[B,C], S52.236-S52.241[C],
S52.242[B,C], S52.243-S52.244[A,B,C], S52.245[B,C],
S52.246-S52.251[A,B,C], S52.252[B,C], S52.253-S52.254[A,B,C],
S52.255[B,C], S52.256-S52.261[A,B,C], S52.262[BC],
S52.263-S52.264[A,B,C], S52.265[B,C], S52.266-S52.271[A,B,C],
S52.272[B,C], S52.279-S52.281[A,B,C], S52.282[B,C],
S52.283-S52.291[A,B,C], S52.292[B,C], S52.299-S52.301[A,B,C],
S52.302[B,C], S52.309[A,B,C], S52.311A, S52.319A,
S52.321[A,B,C], S52.322[B,C], S52.323-S52.324[A,B,C],

S52.325[B,C], S52.326-S52.331[A,B,C], S52.332[B,C],
S52.333-S52.334[A,B,C], S52.335[B,C], S52.336-S52.341[A,B,C],
S52.342[B,C], S52.343-S52.344[A,B,C], S52.345[B,C],
S52.346-S52.351[A,B,C], S52.352[B,C], S52.353-S52.354[A,B,C],
S52.355[B,C], S52.356-S52.361[A,B,C], S52.362[B,C],
S52.363-S52.364[A,B,C], S52.365[B,C], S52.366-S52.371[A,B,C],
S52.372[B,C], S52.379-S52.381[A,B,C], S52.382[B,C],
S52.389-S52.391[A,B,C], S52.392[B,C], S52.399-S52.501[A,B,C],
S52.502[B,C], S52.509-S52.511[A,B,C], S52.512[B,C],
S52.513-S52.514[A,B,C], S52.515[B,C], S52.16[A,B,C],
S52.521[A], S52.529[A], S52.531[A,B,C], S52.532[B,C],
S52.539-S52.541[A,B,C], S52.542[B,C], S52.549-S52.551[A,B,C],
S52.552[B,C], S52.559-S52.561[A,B,C], S52.562[B,C],
S52.569-S52.571[A,B,C], S52.572[B,C], S52.579-S52.591[A,B,C],
S52.592[B,C], S52.599-S52.601[A,B,C], S52.602[B,C],
S52.609-S52.611[A,B,C], S52.612[B,C], S52.613-S52.614[A,B,C],
S52.615[B,C], S52.616[A,B,C], S52.621[A], S52.629A,
S52.691[A,B,C], S52.692[B,C], S52.699-S52.92X[A,B,C],
S59.001A, S59.009-S59.011[A], S59.019-S59.021[A],
S59.029-S59.031[A], S59.039-S59.041[A], S59.049-S59.091[A],
S59.099-S59.101[A], S59.109-S59.111[A], S59.119-S59.121[A],
S59.129-S59.131[A], S59.139-S59.141[A], S59.149-S59.191[A],
S59.199-S59.201[A], S59.209-S59.211[A], S59.219-S59.221[A],
S59.229-S59.231[A], S59.239-S59.241[A], S59.249-S59.291[A],
S59.299A

PDX Collection 1271
S52.001[B,C], S52.002-S52.009[A,B,C], S52.012-S52.019[A],
S52.021[B,C], S52.022-S52.023[A,B,C], S52.024[B,C],
S52.025-S52.026[A,B,C], S52.031[B,C], S52.032-S52.033[A,B,C],
S52.034[B,C], S52.035-S52.036[A,B,C], S52.041[B,C],
S52.042-S52.043[A,B,C], S52.044[B,C], S52.045-S52.046[A,B,C],
S52.091[B,C], S52.092-S52.099[A,B,C], S52.101[B,C],
S52.102-S52.109[A,B,C], S52.112-S52.119[A], S52.121[B,C],
S52.122-S52.123[A,B,C], S52.124[B,C], S52.125-S52.126[A,B,C],
S52.131[B,C], S52.132-S52.133[A,B,C], S52.134[B,C],
S52.135-S52.136[A,B,C], S52.181[B,C], S52.182-S52.189[A,B,C],
S52.201[B,C], S52.202-S52.209[A,B,C], S52.212-S52.219[A],
S52.221[B,C], S52.222-S52.223[A,B,C], S52.224[B,C],
S52.225-S52.226[A,B,C], S52.231[B,C], S52.232-S52.233[A,B,C],
S52.234[B,C], S52.235-S52.236[A,B,C], S52.241[B,C],
S52.242-S52.243[A,B,C], S52.244[B,C], S52.245-S52.246[A,B,C],
S52.251[B,C], S52.252-S52.253[A,B,C], S52.254[B,C],
S52.255-S52.256[A,B,C], S52.261[B,C], S52.262-S52.263[A,B,C],
S52.264[B,C], S52.265-S52.266[A,B,C], S52.271[B,C],
S52.272-S52.279[A,B,C], S52.281[B,C], S52.282-S52.283[A,B,C],
S52.291[B,C], S52.292-S52.299[A,B,C], S52.301[B,C],
S52.302-S52.309[A,B,C], S52.312-S52.319[A], S52.321[B,C],
S52.322-S52.323[A,B,C], S52.324[B,C], S52.325-S52.326[A,B,C],
S52.331[B,C], S52.332-S52.333[A,B,C], S52.334[B,C],
S52.335-S52.336[A,B,C], S52.341[B,C], S52.342-S52.343[A,B,C],
S52.344[B,C], S52.345-S52.346[A,B,C], S52.351[B,C],
S52.352-S52.353[A,B,C], S52.354[B,C], S52.355-S52.356[A,B,C],
S52.361[B,C], S52.362-S52.363[A,B,C], S52.364[B,C],
S52.365-S52.366[A,B,C], S52.371[B,C], S52.372-S52.379[A,B,C],
S52.381[B,C], S52.382-S52.389[A,B,C], S52.391[B,C],
S52.392-S52.399[A,B,C], S52.501[B,C], S52.502-S52.509[A,B,C],
S52.511[B,C], S52.512-S52.513[A,B,C], S52.514[B,C],
S52.515-S52.516[A,B,C], S52.522-S52.529[A], S52.531[B,C],
S52.532-S52.539[A,B,C], S52.541[B,C], S52.542-S52.549[A,B,C],
S52.551[B,C], S52.552-S52.559[A,B,C], S52.561[B,C],
S52.562-S52.569[A,B,C], S52.571[B,C], S52.572-S52.579[A,B,C],
S52.591[B,C], S52.592-S52.599[A,B,C], S52.601[B,C],
S52.602-S52.609[A,B,C], S52.611[B,C], S52.612-S52.613[A,B,C],
S52.614[B,C], S52.615-S52.616[A,B,C], S52.622-S52.629[A],
S52.691[B,C], S52.692-S52.92X[A,B,C], S59.002-S59.009[A],
S59.012-S59.019[A], S59.022-S59.029[A], S59.032-S59.039[A],
S59.042-S59.049[A], S59.092-S59.099[A], S59.102-S59.109[A],

S59.112-S59.119[A], S59.122-S59.129[A], S59.132-S59.139[A],
S59.142-S59.149[A], S59.192-S59.199[A], S59.202-S59.209[A],
S59.212-S59.219[A], S59.222-S59.229[A], S59.232-S59.239[A],
S59.242-S59.249[A], S59.292-S59.299[A]

PDX Collection 1272
S52.001-S52.009[A,B,C], S52.011-S52.019[A],
S52.021-S52.109[A,B,C], S52.111-S52.119[A],
S52.121-S52.209[A,B,C], S52.211-S52.219[A],
S52.221-S52.309[A,B,C], S52.311-S52.319[A],
S52.321-S52.516[A,B,C], S52.521-S52.529[A],
S52.531-S52.616[A,B,C], S52.621-S52.629[A],
S52.691-S52.92X[A,B,C], S59.001-S59.299[A]

PDX Collection 1273
S52.001-S52.009[BC], S52.021-S52.109[BC],
S52.121-S52.189[BC], S52.201-S52.209[ABC],
S52.211-S52.219[A], S52.221-S52.266[ABC],
S52.271-S52.279[BC], S52.281-S52.309[ABC],
S52.311-S52.319[A], S52.321-S52.516[ABC],
S52.531-S52.549[BC], S52.551-S52.616[ABC],
S52.691-S52.92X[ABC], S59.001-S59.099[A],
S59.201-S59.299[A], S62.90XB

PDX Collection 1274
S45.301A, S45.309-S45.311[A], S45.319-S45.391[A],
S45.399-S45.801[A], S45.809-S45.811[A],
S45.819-S45.891[A], S45.899-S45.901[A],
S45.909-S45.911[A], S45.919-S45.991[A], S45.999A,
S55.001A, S55.009-S55.011[A], S55.019-S55.091[A],
S55.099A, S55.201A, S55.209-S55.211[A],
S55.219-S55.291[A], S55.299-S55.801[A],
S55.809-S55.811[A], S55.819-S55.891[A],
S55.899-S55.901[A], S55.909-S55.911[A],
S55.919-S55.991[A], S55.999A, S65.001A,
S65.009-S65.011[A], S65.019-S65.091[A], S65.099A,
S65.801A, S65.809-S65.811[A], S65.819-S65.891[A],
S65.899-S65.901[A], S65.909-S65.911[A],
S65.919-S65.991[A], S65.999A

PDX Collection 1275
S45.302-S45.309[A], S45.312-S45.319[A],
S45.392-S45.399[A], S45.802-S45.809[A],
S45.812-S45.819[A], S45.892-S45.899[A],
S45.902-S45.909[A], S45.912-S45.919[A],
S45.992-S45.999[A], S55.002-S55.009[A],
S55.012-S55.019[A], S55.092-S55.099[A],
S55.202-S55.209[A], S55.212-S55.219[A],
S55.292-S55.299[A], S55.802-S55.809[A],
S55.812-S55.819[A], S55.892-S55.899[A],
S55.902-S55.909[A], S55.912-S55.919[A],
S55.992-S55.999[A], S65.002-S65.009[A],
S65.012-S65.019[A], S65.092-S65.099[A],
S65.802-S65.809[A] S65.812-S65.819[A],
S65.892-S65.899[A], S65.902-S65.909[A],
S65.912-S65.919[A], S65.992-S65.999[A]

PDX Collection 1276
S45.301-S45.999[A], S55.001-S55.099[A],
S55.201-S55.999[A], S65.001-S65.099[A],
S65.801-S65.999[A]

PDX Collection 1277
S45.301A, S45.309-S45.311[A], S45.319-S45.391[A],
S45.399-S45.801[A], S45.809-S45.811[A],
S45.819-S45.891[A], S45.899-S45.901[A],
S45.909-S45.911[A], S45.919-S45.991[A], S45.999A,
S55.101A, S55.109-S55.111[A], S55.119-S55.191[A],
S55.199-S55.201[A], S55.209-S55.211[A],
S55.219-S55.291[A], S55.299-S55.801[A],
S55.809-S55.811[A], S55.819-S55.891[A],
S55.899-S55.901[A], S55.909-S55.911[A],

S55.919-S55.991[A], S55.999A, S65.101A,
S65.109-S65.111[A], S65.119-S65.191[A], S65.199A,
S65.801A, S65.809-S65.811[A], S65.819-S65.891[A],
S65.899-S65.901[A], S65.909-S65.911[A],
S65.919-S65.991[A], S65.999A

PDX Collection 1278
S45.302-S45.309[A], S45.312-S45.319[A],
S45.392-S45.399[A], S45.802-S45.809[A],
S45.812-S45.819[A], S45.892-S45.899[A],
S45.902-S45.909[A], S45.912-S45.919[A],
S45.992-S45.999[A], S55.102-S55.109[A],
S55.112-S55.119[A], S55.192-S55.199[A],
S55.202-S55.209[A], S55.212-S55.219[A],
S55.292-S55.299[A], S55.802A-S55.809[A],
S55.812-S55.819[A], S55.892-S55.899[A],
S55.902-S55.909[A], S55.912-S55.919[A],
S55.992-S55.999[A], S65.102-S65.109[A],
S65.112-S65.119[A], S65.192-S65.199[A],
S65.802-S65.809[A], S65.812-S65.819[A],
S65.892-S65.899[A], S65.902-S65.909[A],
S65.912-S65.919[A], S65.992-S65.999[A]

PDX Collection 1279
S45.301-S45.999[A], S55.101-S55.999[A],
S65.101-S65.199[A], S65.801-S65.999[A]

PDX Collection 1280
S51.001[A], S51.009-S51.011[A], S51.019-S51.021[A],
S51.029-S51.031[A], S51.039-S51.041[A],
S51.049-S51.051[A], S51.059-S51.801[A],
S51.809-S51.811[A], S51.819-S51.821[A].
S51.829-S51.831[A], S51.839-S51.841[A],
S51.849-S51.851[A], S51.859A, S56.021A, S56.029A,
S56.121A, S56.123A, S56.125A, S56.127A, S56.129A,
S56.221A, S56.229A, S56.321A, S56.329A, S56.421A,
S56.423A, S56.425A, S56.427A, S56.429A, S56.521A,
S56.529A, S56.821A, S56.829A, S56.921A, S56.929A,
S61.501A, S61.509-S61.511[A], S61.519-S61.521[A],
S61.529-S61.531[A], S61.539-S61.541[A],
S61.549-S61.551[A], S61.559A

PDX Collection 1281
S51.002-S51.009[A], S51.012-S51.019[A],
S51.022-S51.029[A], S51.032-S51.039[A],
S51.042-S51.049[A], S51.052-S51.059[A],
S51.802-S51.809[A], S51.812-S51.819[A],
S51.822-S51.829[A], S51.832-S51.839[A],
S51.842-S51.849[A], S51.852-S51.859[A],
S56.022-S56.029[A], S56.122A, S56.124A, S56.126A,
S56.128-S56.129[A], S56.222-S56.229[A],
S56.322-S56.329[A], S56.422A, S56.424A, S56.426A,
S56.428-S56.429[A], S56.522-S56.529[A],
S56.822-S56.829[A], S56.922-S56.929[A],
S61.502-S61.509[A], S61.512-S61.519[A],
S61.522-S61.529[A], S61.532-S61.539[A],
S61.542-S61.549[A], S61.552-S61.559[A]

PDX Collection 1282
S51.001-S51.859[A], S56.021-S56.029[A],
S56.121-S56.129[A], S56.221-S56.229[A],
S56.321-S56.329[A], S56.421-S56.429[A],
S56.521-S56.529[A], S56.821-S56.829[A],
S56.921-S56.929[A], S61.501-S61.559[A]

PDX Collection 1283
S62.001-S62.186[A,B]

PDX Collection 1284
S62.201-S62.399[B], S62.90X[A]

PDX Collection 1285
S62.501-S62.669[A,B], S62.90XA, S62.91X-S62.92X[A,B]

PDX Collection 1286
S42.201-S42.266[A,B], S42.271-S42.279[A],
S42.291-S42.309[A,B], S42.311-S42.319[A],
S42.321-S42.476[A,B], S42.481-S42.489[A],
S42.491-S42.92X[A,B], S49.001-S49.199[A],
S52.001-S52.009[A,B,C], S52.021-S52.109[A,B,C],
S52.121-S52.209[A,B,C], S52.211-S52.219[A],
S52.221-S52.309[A,B,C], S52.311-S52.319[A],
S52.321-S52.616[A,B,C], S52.691-S52.92X[A,B,C],
S59.001-S59.299[A], S62.001-S62.92X[A,B]

PDX Collection 1287
S62.501-S62.669[A,B], S62.90X[B], S62.91X-S62.92X[A,B]

PDX Collection 1288
S45.301[A], S45.309-S45.311[A], S45.319-S45.391[A],
S45.399-S45.801[A], S45.809-S45.811[A],
S45.819-S45.891[A], S45.899-S45.901[A],
S45.909-S45.911[A], S45.919-S45.991[A], S45.999A,
S55.201A, S55.209-S55.211[A], S55.219-S55.291[A],
S55.299-S55.801[A], S55.809-S55.811[A],
S55.819-S55.891[A], S55.899-S55.901[A],
S55.909-S55.911[A], S55.919-S55.991[A], S55.999[A],
S65.201A, S65.209-S65.211[A], S65.219-S65.291[A],
S65.299-S65.301[A], S65.309-S65.311[A], S65.319-
S65.391[A], S65.399A, S65.801A, S65.809-S65.811[A],
S65.819-S65.891[A], S65.899-S65.901[A],
S65.909-S65.911[A], S65.919-S65.991[A], S65.999A

PDX Collection 1289
S45.302-S45.309[A], S45.312-S45.319[A],
S45.392-S45.399[A], S45.802-S45.809[A],
S45.812-S45.819[A], S45.892-S45.899[A],
S45.902-S45.909[A], S45.912-S45.919[A],
S45.992-S45.999[A], S55.202-S55.209[A],
S55.212-S55.219[A], S55.292-S55.299[A],
S55.802-S55.809[A], S55.812-S55.819[A],
S55.892-S55.899[A], S55.902-S55.909[A],
S55.912-S55.919[A], S55.992-S55.999[A],
S65.202-S65.209[A], S65.212-S65.219[A],
S65.292-S65.299[A], S65.302-S65.309[A],
S65.312-S65.319[A], S65.392-S65.399[A],
S65.802-S65.809[A], S65.812-S65.819[A],
S65.892-S65.899[A], S65.902-S65.909[A],
S65.912-S65.919[A], S65.992-S65.999[A]

PDX Collection 1290
S45.301-S45.999[A], S55.201-S55.999[A],
S65.201-S65.399[A], S65.801-S65.999

PDX Collection 1291
S45.301A, S45.309-S45.311[A], S45.319-S45.391[A],
S45.399-S45.801[A], S45.809-S45.811[A],
S45.819-S45.891[A], S45.899-S45.901[A],
S45.909-S45.911[A], S45.919-S45.991[A], S45.999A,
S55.201A, S55.209-S55.211[A], S55.219-S55.291[A],
S55.299-S55.801[A], S55.809-S55.811[A],
S55.819-S55.891[A], S55.899-S55.901[A],
S55.909-S55.911[A], S55.919-S55.991[A], S55.999A,
S65.401A, S65.409-S65.411[A], S65.419-S65.491[A],
S65.499-S65.500[A], S65.502A, S65.504A, S65.506A,
S65.508-S65.510[A], S65.512A, S65.514A, S65.516A,
S65.518-S65.590[A], S65.592A, S65.594A, S65.596A,
S65.598-S65.801[A], S65.809-S65.811[A],
S65.819-S65.891[A], S65.899-S65.901[A],
S65.909-S65.911[A], S65.919-S65.991[A], S65.999A

PDX Collection 1292
S45.302-S45.309[A], S45.312-S45.319[A],
S45.392-S45.399[A], S45.802-S45.809[A],
S45.812-S45.819[A], S45.892-S45.899[A],
S45.902-S45.909[A], S45.912-S45.919[A],
S45.992-S45.999[A], S55.202-S55.209[A],

S55.212-S55.219[A], S55.292-S55.299[A],
S55.802-S55.809[A], S55.812-S55.819[A],
S55.892-S55.899[A], S55.902-S55.909[A],
S55.912-S55.919[A], S55.992-S55.999[A],
S65.402-S65.409[A], S65.412-S65.419[A],
S65.492-S65.499[A], S65.501A, S65.503A, S65.505A,
S65.507-S65.509[A], S65.511A, S65.513A, S65.515A,
S65.517-S65.519[A], S65.591A, S65.593A, S65.595A,
S65.597-S65.599[A], S65.802-S65.809[A],
S65.812-S65.819[A], S65.892-S65.899[A],
S65.902-S65.909[A], S65.912A, S65.919A, S65.992A,
S65.999A

PDX Collection 1293
S45.301-S45.999[A], S55.201-S55.999[A],
S65.401-S65.999[A]

PDX Collection 1294
S61.401A, S61.409-S61.411[A], S61.419-S61.421[A],
S61.429-S61.431[A], S61.439-S61.441[A],
S61.449-S61.451[A], S61.459A, S66.021A,
S66.029A, S66.120A, S66.122A, S66.124A, S66.126A,
S66.128-S66.129[A], S66.221A, S66.229A, S66.320A,
S66.322A, S66.324A, S66.326A, S66.328-S66.329[A],
S66.421A, S66.429A, S66.520A, S66.522A, S66.524A,
S66.526A, S66.528-S66.529[A], S66.821A, S66.829A,
S66.921A, S66.929A

PDX Collection 1295
S61.402-S61.409[A], S61.412-S61.419[A],
S61.422-S61.429[A], S61.432-S61.439[A],
S61.442-S61.449[A], S61.452-S61.459[A],
S66.022-S66.029[A], S66.121A, S66.123A, S66.125A,
S66.127-S66.129[A], S66.222-S66.229[A],
S66.321A, S66.323A, S66.325[A], S66.327-S66.329A,
S66.422-S66.429[A], S66.521A, S66.523A, S66.525A,
S66.527-S66.529[A], S66.822-S66.829[A],
S66.922-S66.929[A]

PDX Collection 1296
S61.401-S61.459[A], S66.021-S66.029[A],
S66.120-S66.129[A], S66.221-S66.229[A],
S66.320-S66.329[A], S66.421-S66.429[A],
S66.520-S66.529[A], S66.821-S66.829[A],
S66.921-S66.929[A]

PDX Collection 1297
M48.40X-M48.58X[A], M80.00X-M80.88X[A],
M84.30X-M84.68X[A], M84.750-M84.759[A],
S03.8XX-S03.9XX[A], S29.011-S29.019[A],
S38.3XXA, S39.011-S39.013[A], S72.001[A,B,C],
S72.002[B,C], S72.009-S72.011[A,B,C],
S72.012[B,C], S72.019-S72.021[A,B,C],
S72.022[B,C], S72.023-S72.024[A,B,C],
S72.025[B,C], S72.026-S72.031[A,B,C],
S72.032[B,C], S72.033-S72.034[A,B,C],
S72.035[B,C], S72.036-S72.041[A,B,C],
S72.042[B,C], S72.043-S72.044[A,B,C],
S72.045[B,C], S72.046-S72.051[A,B,C],
S72.052[B,C], S72.059-S72.061[A,B,C],
S72.062[B,C], S72.063-S72.064[A,B,C],
S72.065[B,C], S72.066-S72.091[A,B,C],
S72.092[B,C], S72.099-S72.101[A,B,C],
S72.102[B,C], S72.109-S72.111[A,B,C],
S72.112[B,C], S72.113-S72.114[A,B,C],
S72.115[B,C], S72.116-S72.121[A,B,C],
S72.122[B,C], S72.123-S72.124[A,B,C],
S72.125[B,C], S72.126-S72.131[A,B,C],
S72.132[B,C], S72.133-S72.134[A,B,C],
S72.135[B,C], S72.136-S72.141[A,B,C],
S72.142[B,C], S72.143-S72.144[A,B,C],
S72.145[B,C], S72.146-S72.301[A,B,C],

S72.302[B,C], S72.309-S72.321[A,B,C],
S72.322[B,C], S72.323-S72.324[A,B,C], S72.325[B,C],
S72.326-S72.331[A,B,C], S72.332[B,C],
S72.333-S72.334[A,B,C], S72.335[B,C],
S72.336-S72.341[A,B,C], S72.342[B,C],
S72.343-S72.344[A,B,C], S72.345[B,C],
S72.346-S72.351[A,B,C], S72.352[B,C],
S72.353-S72.354[A,B,C], S72.355[B,C],
S72.356-S72.361[A,B,C], S72.362[B,C],
S72.363-S72.364[A,B,C], S72.365[B,C],
S72.366-S72.391[A,B,C], S72.392[B,C],
S72.399-S72.401[A,B,C], S72.402[B,C],
S72.409-S72.411[A,B,C], S72.412[B,C],
S72.413-S72.414[A,B,C], S72.415[B,C],
S72.416-S72.421[A,B,C], S72.422[B,C],
S72.423-S72.424[A,B,C], S72.425[B,C],
S72.426-S72.431[A,B,C], S72.432[B,C],
S72.433-S72.434[A,B,C], S72.435[B,C],
S72.436-S72.441[A,B,C], S72.442[B,C],
S72.443-S72.444[A,B,C], S72.445[B,C],
S72.446-S72.451[A,B,C], S72.452[B,C],
S72.453-S72.454[A,B,C], S72.455[B,C],
S72.456-S72.461[A,B,C], S72.462[B,C],
S72.463-S72.464[A,B,C], S72.465[B,C], S72.466[A,B,C],
S72.471A, S72.479A, S72.491[A,B,C], S72.492[B,C],
S72.499-S72.92X[A,B,C], S73.101A, S73.109-S73.111[A],
S73.119-S73.121[A], S73.129-S73.191[A], S73.199A,
S76.001A, S76.009-S76.011[A], S76.019A, S76.091A,
S76.099-S76.101[A], S76.109-S76.111[A],
S76.119A, S76.191A, S76.199-S76.201[A],
S76.209-S76.211[A], S76.219A, S76.291A,
S76.299-S76.301[A], S76.309-S76.311[A], S76.319A,
S76.391A, S76.399-S76.801[A], S76.809-S76.811[A],
S76.819A, S76.891A, S76.899-S76.901[A],
S76.909-S76.911[A], S76.919A, S76.991A, S76.999A,
S79.001A, S79.009-S79.011[A], S79.019-S79.091[A],
S79.099-S79.101[A], S79.109-S79.111[A],
S79.119-S79.121[A], S79.129-S79.131[A],
S79.139-S79.141[A], S79.149-S79.191[A],
S79.199-S79.811[A], S79.819-S79.821[A],
S79.829-S79.911[A], S79.919-S79.921[A], S79.929A,
S82.90X-S82.92X[A,B,C], T07.XXX-T14.91X[A],
T79.A0X-T79.9XX[A]

PDX Collection 1298
M48.40X-M48.58X[A], M80.00X-M80.88X[A],
M84.30X-M84.68X[A], M84.750-M84.759[A],
S03.8XX-S03.9XX[A], S29.011-S29.019[A], S38.3XX[A],
S39.011-S39.013[A], S72.001-S72.466[A,B,C],
S72.471-S72.479[A], S72.491-S72.92X[A.B.C],
S73.101-S73.199[A], S76.001-S76.019[A],
S76.091-S76.119[A], S76.191-S76.219[A],
S76.291-S76.319[A], S76.391-S76.819[A],
S76.891-S76.919[A], S76.991-S76.999[A],
S79.001-S79.929[A], S82.90X-S82.92X[A,B,C],
T07.XXX-T14.91X[A], T79.A0X-T79.9XX[A]

PDX Collection 1299
M48.40X-M48.58X[A], M80.00X-M80.88X[A],
M84.30X-M84.68X[A], M84.750-M84.759[A],
S03.8XX-S03.9XX[A], S29.011-S29.019[A], S38.3XXA,
S39.011-S39.013[A], S72.001[B,C], S72.002-S72.009[A,B,C],
S72.011[B,C], S72.012-S72.019[A,B,C],
S72.021[B,C], S72.022-S72.023[A,B,C],
S72.024[B,C], S72.025-S72.026[A,B,C],
S72.031[B,C], S72.032-S72.033[A,B,C],
S72.034[B,C], S72.035-S72.036[A,B,C],
S72.041[B,C], S72.042-S72.043[A,B,C],
S72.044[B,C], S72.045-S72.046[A,B,C],
S72.051[B,C], S72.052-S72.059[A,B,C],

S72.061[B,C], S72.062-S72.063[A,B,C],
S72.064[B,C], S72.065-S72.066[A,B,C],
S72.091[B,C], S72.092-S72.099[A,B,C],
S72.101[B,C], S72.102-S72.109[A,B,C],
S72.111[B,C], S72.112-S72.113[A,B,C],
S72.114[B,C], S72.115-S72.116[A,B,C],
S72.121[B,C], S72.122-S72.123[A,B,C],
S72.124[B,C], S72.125-S72.126[A,B,C],
S72.131[B,C], S72.132-S72.133[A,B,C],
S72.134[B,C], S72.135-S72.136[A,B,C],
S72.141[B,C], S72.142-S72.143[C], S72.144[B,C],
S72.145-S72.146[A,B,C], S72.21X-S72.26X[A,B,C],
S72.301[B,C], S72.302-S72.309[A,B,C],
S72.321[B,C], S72.322-S72.323[A,B,C], S72.324[B,C],
S72.325-S72.326[A,B,C], S72.331[B,C],
S72.332-S72.333[A,B,C], S72.334[B,C],
S72.335-S72.336[A,B,C], S72.341[B,C],
S72.342-S72.343[A,B,C], S72.344[B,C],
S72.345-S72.346[A,B,C], S72.351[B,C],
S72.352-S72.353[A,B,C], S72.354[B,C],
S72.355-S72.356[A,B,C], S72.361[B,C],
S72.362-S72.363[A,B,C], S72.364[B,C],
S72.365-S72.366[A,B,C], S72.391[B,C],
S72.392-S72.399[A,B,C], S72.401[B,C],
S72.402-S72.409[A,B,C], S72.411[B,C],
S72.412-S72.413[A,B,C], S72.414[B,C],
S72.415-S72.416[A,B,C], S72.421[B,C],
S72.422-S72.423[A,B,C], S72.424[B,C],
S72.425-S72.426[A,B,C], S72.431[B,C],
S72.432-S72.433[A,B,C], S72.434[B,C],
S72.435-S72.436[A,B,C], S72.441[B,C],
S72.442-S72.443[A,B,C], S72.444[B,C],
S72.445-S72.446[A,B,C], S72.451[B,C],
S72.452-S72.453[A,B,C], S72.454[B,C],
S72.455-S72.456[A,B,C], S72.461[B,C],
S72.462-S72.463[A,B,C], S72.464[B,C],
S72.465-S72.466[A,B,C], S72.472-S72.479[A], S72.491[B,C],
S72.492-S72.92X[A,B,C], S73.102-S73.109[A],
S73.112-S73.119[A], S73.122-S73.129[A],
S73.192-S73.199[A], S76.002-S76.009[A],
S76.012-S76.019[A], S76.092-S76.099[A],
S76.102-S76.109[A], S76.112-S76.119[A],
S76.192-S76.199[A], S76.202-S76.209[A],
S76.212-S76.219[A], S76.292-S76.299[A],
S76.302-S76.309[A], S76.312-S76.319[A],
S76.392-S76.399[A], S76.802-S76.809[A],
S76.812-S76.819[A], S76.892-S76.899[A],
S76.902-S76.909[A], S76.912-S76.919[A],
S76.992-S76.999[A], S79.002-S79.009[A],
S79.012-S79.019[A], S79.092-S79.099[A],
S79.102-S79.109[A], S79.112-S79.119[A],
S79.122-S79.129[A], S79.132-S79.139[A],
S79.142-S79.149[A], S79.192-S79.199[A],
S79.812-S79.819[A], S79.822-S79.829[A],
S79.912-S79.919[A], S79.922-S79.929[A],
S82.90X-S82.92X[A,B,C], T07.XXX-T14.91X[A], T79.8XXA
T79.A0X-T79.9XX[A]

PDX Collection 1300
M80.00X-M80.019[A], M80.041-M80.059[A],
M80.80X-M80.819[A], M80.841-M80.859[A],
M84.40X-M84.419[A], M84.441-M84.459[A],
M84.474-M84.519[A], M84.541-M84.559[A],
M84.574-M84.576[A], M84.60X-M84.619[A],
M84.641-M84.659[A], M84.674-M84.68X[A],
M84.750-M84.759[A], S03.8XX-S03.9XX[A],
S29.011-S29.019[A], S38.3XX[A], S39.011-S39.013[A],
S72.001[A,B,C], S72.002[B,C], S72.009-S72.011[A,B,C],
S72.012[B,C], S72.019-S72.021[A,B,C],

S72.022[B,C], S72.023-S72.024[A,B,C],
S72.025[B,C], S72.026-S72.031[A,B,C],
S72.032[B,C], S72.033-S72.034[A,B,C],
S72.035[B,C], S72.036-S72.041[A,B,C],
S72.042[B,C], S72.043-S72.044[A,B,C],
S72.045[B,C], S72.046-S72.051[A,B,C],
S72.052[B,C], S72.059-S72.061[A,B,C], S72.062[B,C],
S72.063-S72.064[A,B,C], S72.065[B,C],
S72.066-S72.091[A,B,C], S72.092[B,C],
S72.099-S72.101[C], S72.102[B,C], S72.109-S72.111[A,B,C],
S72.112[B,C], S72.113-S72.114[A,B,C],
S72.115[B,C], S72.116-S72.121[A,B,C],
S72.122[B,C], S72.123-S72.124[A,B,C],
S72.125[B,C], S72.126-S72.131[A,B,C],
S72.132[B,C], S72.133-S72.134[A,B,C],
S72.135[B,C], S72.136-S72.141[A,B,C],
S72.142[B,C], S72.143-S72.144[A,B,C],
S72.145[B,C], S72.146-S72.301[A,B,C],
S72.302[B,C], S72.309-S72.321[A,B,C],
S72.322[B,C], S72.323-S72.324[A,B,C],
S72.325[B,C], S72.326-S72.331[A,B,C],
S72.332[B,C], S72.333-S72.334[A,B,C],
S72.335[B,C], S72.336-S72.341[A,B,C],
S72.342[B,C], S72.343-S72.344[A,B,C],
S72.345[B,C], S72.346-S72.351[A,B,C],
S72.352[B,C], S72.353-S72.354[A,B,C],
S72.355[B,C], S72.356-S72.361[A,B,C],
S72.362[B,C], S72.363-S72.364[A,B,C],
S72.365[B,C], S72.366-S72.391[A,B,C],
S72.392[B,C], S72.399-S72.401[A,B,C],
S72.402[B,C], S72.409-S72.411[A,B,C],
S72.412[B,C], S72.413-S72.414[A,B,C], S72.415[B,C],
S72.416-S72.421[A,B,C], S72.422[B,C],
S72.423-S72.424[A,B,C], S72.425[B,C],
S72.426-S72.431[A,B,C], S72.432[B,C],
S72.433-S72.434[A,B,C], S72.435[B,C],
S72.436-S72.441[A,B,C], S72.442[B,C],
S72.443-S72.444[A,B,C], S72.445[B,C],
S72.446-S72.451[A,B,C], S72.452[B,C],
S72.453-S72.454[A,B,C], S72.455[B,C],
S72.456-S72.461[A,B,C], S72.462[B,C],
S72.463-S72.464[A,B,C], S72.465[B,C], S72.466[A,B,C],
S72.471A, S72.479A, S72.491[A,B,C], S72.492[B,C],
S72.499-S72.92X[A,B,C], S73.101A, S73.109-S73.111[A],
S73.119-S73.121[A], S73.129-S73.191[A], S73.199A,
S76.001A, S76.009-S76.011[A], S76.019A, S76.091A,
S76.099-S76.101[A], S76.109-S76.111[A],
S76.119A, S76.191A, S76.199-S76.201[A],
S76.209-S76.211[A], S76.219A, S76.291A,
S76.299-S76.301[A], S76.309-S76.311[A], S76.319A,
S76.391A, S76.399-S76.801[A], S76.809-S76.811[A],
S76.819A, S76.891A, S76.899-S76.901[A],
S76.909-S76.911[A], S76.919A, S76.991A, S76.999A,
S79.001A, S79.009-S79.011[A], S79.019-S79.091[A],
S79.099-S79.101[A], S79.109-S79.111[A],
S79.119-S79.121[A], S79.129-S79.131[A],
S79.139-S79.141[A], S79.149-S79.191[A],
S79.199-S79.811[A], S79.819-S79.821[A],
S79.829-S79.911[A], S79.919-S79.921[A], S79.929A,
S82.90X-S82.92X[A,B,C], T07.XXX-T14.91X[A],
T79.A9X-T79.9XX[A]

PDX Collection 1301
M80.00X-M80.019[A], M80.041-M80.059[A],
M80.80X-M80.819[A], M80.841-M80.859[A],
M84.40X-M84.419[A], M84.441-M84.459[A],
M84.474-M84.519[A], M84.541-M84.559[A],
M84.574-M84.576[A], M84.60X-M84.619[A],
M84.641-M84.659[A], M84.674-M84.68X[A],

M84.750-M84.759[A], S03.8XX-S03.9XX[A],
S29.011-S29.019[A], S38.3XXA, S39.011-S39.013[A],
S72.001-S72.466[A,B,C], S72.471-S72.479[A],
S72.491-S72.92X[A,B,C], S73.101-S73.199[A],
S76.001-S76.019[A], S76.091-S76.119[A],
S76.191-S76.219[A], S76.291-S76.319[A],
S76.391-S76.819[A], S76.891-S76.919[A],
S76.991-S76.999[A], S79.001-S79.929[A],
S82.90X-S82.92X[A,B,C], T07.XXX-T14.91X[A],
T79.A9X-T79.9XX[A]

PDX Collection 1302
M80.00X-M80.019[A], M80.041-M80.059[A],
M80.80X-M80.819[A], M80.841-M80.859[A],
M84.40X-M84.419[A], M84.441-M84.459[A],
M84.474-M84.519[A], M84.541-M84.559[A],
M84.574-M84.576[A], M84.60X-M84.619[A],
M84.641-M84.659[A], M84.674-M84.68X[A],
M84.750-M84.759[A], S03.8XX-S03.9XX[A],
S29.011-S29.019[A], S38.3XX[A], S39.011-S39.013[A],
S72.001[B,C], S72.002-S72.009[A,B,C],
S72.011[B,C], S72.012-S72.019[A,B,C],
S72.021[B,C], S72.022-S72.023[A,B,C],
S72.024[B,C], S72.025-S72.026[A,B,C],
S72.031[B,C], S72.032-S72.033[A,B,C],
S72.034[B,C], S72.035-S72.036[A,B,C],
S72.041[B,C], S72.042-S72.043[A,B,C],
S72.044[B,C], S72.045-S72.046[A,B,C],
S72.051[B,C], S72.052-S72.059[A,B,C],
S72.061[B,C], S72.062-S72.063[A,B,C],
S72.064[B,C], S72.065-S72.066[A,B,C],
S72.091[B,C], S72.092-S72.099[A,B,C],
S72.101[B,C], S72.102-S72.109[A,B,C],
S72.111[B,C], S72.112-S72.113[A,B,C], S72.114[B,C],
S72.115-S72.116[A,B,C], S72.121[B,C],
S72.122-S72.123[A,B,C], S72.124[B,C],
S72.125-S72.126[A,B,C], S72.131[B,C],
S72.132-S72.133[A,B,C], S72.134[B,C],
S72.135-S72.136[A,B,C], S72.141[B,C],
S72.142-S72.143[A,B,C], S72.144[B,C],
S72.145-S72.146[A,B,C], S72.21X-S72.26X[A,B,C],
S72.301[B,C], S72.302-S72.309[A,B,C],
S72.321[B,C], S72.322-S72.323[A,B,C], S72.324[B,C],
S72.325-S72.326[A,B,C], S72.331[B,C],
S72.332-S72.333[A,B,C], S72.334[B,C],
S72.335-S72.336[A,B,C], S72.341[B,C],
S72.342-S72.343[A,B,C], S72.344[B,C],
S72.345-S72.346[A,B,C], S72.351[B,C],
S72.352-S72.353[A,B,C], S72.354[B,C],
S72.355-S72.356[A,B,C], S72.361[B,C],
S72.362-S72.363[A,B,C], S72.364[B,C],
S72.365-S72.366[A,B,C], S72.391[B,C],
S72.392-S72.399[A,B,C], S72.401[B,C],
S72.402-S72.409[A,B,C], S72.411[B,C],
S72.412-S72.413[A,B,C], S72.414[B,C],
S72.415-S72.416[A,B,C], S72.421[B,C],
S72.422-S72.423[A,B,C], S72.424[B,C],
S72.425-S72.426[A,B,C], S72.431[B,C],
S72.432-S72.433[A,B,C], S72.434[B,C],
S72.435-S72.436[A,B,C], S72.441[B,C],
S72.442-S72.443[A,B,C], S72.444[B,C],
S72.445-S72.446[A,B,C], S72.451[B,C],
S72.452-S72.453[A,B,C], S72.454[B,C],
S72.455-S72.456[A,B,C], S72.461[B,C],
S72.462-S72.463[A,B,C], S72.464[B,C],
S72.465-S72.466[A,B,C], S72.472-S72.479[A], S72.491[B,C],
S72.492-S72.92X[A,B,C], S73.102-S73.109[A],
S73.112-S73.119[A], S73.122-S73.129[A],
S73.192-S73.199[A], S76.002-S76.009[A],

S76.012-S76.019[A], S76.092-S76.099[A],
S76.102-S76.109[A], S76.112-S76.119[A],
S76.192-S76.199[A], S76.202-S76.209[A],
S76.212-S76.219[A], S76.292-S76.299[A],
S76.302-S76.309[A], S76.312-S76.319[A],
S76.392-S76.399[A], S76.802-S76.809[A],
S76.812-S76.819[A], S76.892-S76.899[A],
S76.902-S76.909[A], S76.912-S76.919[A],
S76.992-S76.999[A], S79.002-S79.009[A],
S79.012-S79.019[A], S79.092-S79.099[A],
S79.102-S79.109[A], S79.112-S79.119[A],
S79.122-S79.129[A], S79.132-S79.139[A],
S79.142-S79.149[A], S79.192-S79.199[A],
S79.812-S79.819[A], S79.822-S79.829[A],
S79.912-S79.919[A], S79.922-S79.929[A],
S82.90X-S82.92X[A,B,C], T07.XXX-T14.91X[A],
T79.A9X-T79.9XX[A]

PDX Collection 1303
M80.00X-M80.019[A], M80.041-M80.059[A],
M80.80X-M80.819[A], M80.841-M80.859[A],
M84.40X-M84.419[A], M84.441-M84.459[A],
M84.474-M84.519[A], M84.541-M84.559[A],
M84.574-M84.619[A], M84.641-M84.659[A],
M84.674-M84.68X[A], M84.750-M84.759[A],
S03.8XX-S03.9XX[A], S29.011-S29.019[A], S38.3XXA,
S39.011-S39.013[A], S72.491-S72.499[B,C],
S73.101-S73.199[A], S76.001-S76.019[A],
S76.091-S76.119[A], S76.191-S76.219[A],
S76.291-S76.319[A], S76.391-S76.819[A],
S76.891-S76.919[A], S76.991-S76.999[A],
S79.811-S79.929[A], S82.001-S82.099[A,B,C],
S82.90X-S82.92X[A,B,C], T07.XXX-T14.91X[A],
T79.A9X-T79.9XX[A]

PDX Collection 1304
M99.16-M99.17, M99.19, S03.1XXA, S33.30X-S33.39X[A],
S73.001A, S73.003-S73.004[A], S73.006A, S73.041A,
S73.043-S73.044[A], S73.046A

PDX Collection 1305
M99.16-M99.17, M99.19, S03.1XXA, S33.30X-S33.39X[A],
S73.002-S73.003[A], S73.005-S73.006[A],
S73.042-S73.043[A], S73.045-S73.046[A]

PDX Collection 1306
M99.16-M99.17, M99.19, S03.1XXA, S33.30X-S33.39X[A],
S73.001-S73.006[A], S73.041-S73.046[A]

PDX Collection 1307
M99.16-M99.17, M99.19, S03.1XXA, S33.30X-S33.39X[A],
S73.011A, S73.013-S73.014[A], S73.016A

PDX Collection 1308
M99.16-M99.17, M99.19, S03.1XXA, S33.30X-S33.39X[A],
S73.012-S73.013[A], S73.015-S73.016[A]

PDX Collection 1309
M99.16-M99.17, M99.19, S03.1XXA, S33.30X-S33.39X[A],
S73.011-S73.016[A]

PDX Collection 1310
M99.16-M99.17, M99.19, S03.1XXA, S33.30X-S33.39X[A],
S73.021A, S73.023-S73.024[A], S73.026A

PDX Collection 1311
M99.16-M99.17, M99.19, S03.1XXA, S33.30X-S33.39X[A],
S73.022-S73.023[A], S73.025-S73.026[A]

PDX Collection 1312
M99.16-M99.17, M99.19, S03.1XXA, S33.30X-S33.39X[A],
S73.021-S73.026[A]

PDX Collection 1313
M99.16-M99.17, M99.19, S03.1XXA, S33.30X-S33.39X[A],
S73.031A, S73.033-S73.034[A], S73.036A

PDX Collection 1314
M99.16-M99.17, M99.19, S03.1XXA, S33.30X-S33.39X[A],
S73.032-S73.033[A], S73.035-S73.036[A]

PDX Collection 1315
M99.16-M99.17, M99.19, S03.1XXA, S33.30X-S33.39X[A],
S73.031-S73.036[A]

PDX Collection 1316
S75.001A, S75.009-S75.021[A], S75.029-S75.091[A],
S75.099A, S75.801A, S75.809-S75.811[A],
S75.819-S75.891[A], S75.899-S75.901[A],
S75.909-S75.911[A], S75.919-S75.991[A], S75.999A,
S85.201A, S85.209-S85.211[A], S85.219-S85.291[A],
S85.299A, S85.801A, S85.809-S85.811[A],
S85.819-S85.891[A], S85.899-S85.901[A],
S85.909-S85.911[A], S85.919-S85.991[A], S85.999A,
S95.001A, S95.009-S95.011[A], S95.019-S95.091[A],
S95.099A, S95.201A, S95.209-S95.211[A],
S95.219-S95.291[A], S95.299-S95.801[A],
S95.809-S95.811[A], S95.819-S95.891[A],
S95.899-S95.901[A], S95.909-S95.911[A],
S95.919-S95.991[A], S95.99[A]

PDX Collection 1317
S75.002-S75.009[A], S75.012-S75.019[A],
S75.022-S75.029[A], S75.092A, S75.099A,
S75.802-S75.809[A], S75.812-S75.819[A],
S75.892-S75.899[A], S75.902-S75.909[A],
S75.912-S75.919[A], S75.992-S75.999[A],
S85.202-S85.209[A], S85.212-S85.219[A],
S85.292-S85.299[A], S85.802-S85.809[A],
S85.812-S85.819[A], S85.892-S85.899[A],
S85.902-S85.909[A], S85.912-S85.919[A],
S85.992-S85.999[A], S95.002-S95.009[A],
S95.012-S95.019[A], S95.092-S95.099[A],
S95.202-S95.209[A], S95.212-S95.219[A],
S95.292-S95.299[A], S95.802-S95.809[A],
S95.812-S95.819[A], S95.892-S95.899[A],
S95.902-S95.909[A], S95.912-S95.919[A],
S95.992-S95.999[A]

PDX Collection 1318
S75.001-S75.099[A], S75.801-S75.999[A],
S85.201-S85.299[A], S85.801-S85.999[A],
S95.001-S95.099[A], S95.201-S95.999[A]

PDX Collection 1319
S75.101A, S75.109-S75.111[A], S75.119-S75.121[A],
S75.129-S75.191[A], S75.199[A], S75.801A,
S75.809-S75.811[A], S75.819-S75.891[A],
S75.899-S75.901[A], S75.909-S75.911[A],
S75.919-S75.991[A], S75.999[A], S85.201A,
S85.209-S85.211[A], S85.219-S85.291[A], S85.299A,
S85.801A, S85.809-S85.811[A], S85.819-S85.891[A],
S85.899-S85.901[A], S85.909-S85.911[A],
S85.919-S85.991[A], S85.999A, S95.001A,
S95.009-S95.011[A], S95.019-S95.091[A], S95.099A,
S95.201A, S95.209-S95.211[A], S95.219-S95.291[A],
S95.299-S95.801[A], S95.809-S95.811[A],
S95.819-S95.891[A], S95.899-S95.901[A],
S95.909-S95.911[A], S95.919-S95.991[A], S95.999A

PDX Collection 1320
S75.102-S75.109[A], S75.112-S75.119[A],
S75.122-S75.129[A], S75.192-S75.199[A],
S75.802-S75.809[A], S75.812-S75.819[A],
S75.892-S75.899[A], S75.902-S75.909[A],
S75.912-S75.919[A], S75.992-S75.999[A],
S85.202-S85.209[A], S85.212-S85.219[A],
S85.292-S85.299[A], S85.802-S85.809[A],
S85.812-S85.819[A], S85.892-S85.899[A],
S85.902-S85.909[A], S85.912-S85.919[A],

S85.992-S85.999[A], S95.002-S95.009[A],
S95.012-S95.019[A], S95.092-S95.099[A],
S95.202-S95.209[A], S95.212-S95.219[A],
S95.292-S95.299[A], S95.802-S95.809[A],
S95.812-S95.819[A], S95.892-S95.899[A],
S95.902-S95.909[A], S95.912-S95.919[A],
S95.992-S95.999[A]

PDX Collection 1321
S75.101-S75.199[A], S75.801-S75.999[A],
S85.201-S85.299[A], S85.801-S85.999[A],
S95.001-S95.099[A], S95.201-S95.999[A]

PDX Collection 1322
S75.201A, S75.209-S75.211[A], S75.219-S75.221[A],
S75.229-S75.291[A], S75.299-S75.801[A],
S75.809-S75.811[A], S75.819-S75.891[A],
S75.899-S75.901[A], S75.909-S75.911[A],
S75.919-S75.991[A], S75.999A, S85.201A, S85.209A,
S85.211A, S85.219-S85.291[A], S85.299-S85.301[A],
S85.309-S85.311[A], S85.319-S85.391[A],
S85.399-S85.401[A], S85.409-S85.411[A],
S85.419-S85.491[A], S85.499A, S85.801A, S85.809A,
S85.811A, S85.819-S85.891[A], S85.899-S85.901[A],
S85.909-S85.911[A], S85.919-S85.991[A], S85.999A,
S95.001A, S95.009-S95.011[A], S95.019-S95.091[A],
S95.099A, S95.201A, S95.209-S95.211[A],
S95.219-S95.291[A], S95.299-S95.801[A],
S95.809-S95.811[A], S95.819-S95.891[A],
S95.899-S95.901[A], S95.909-S95.911[A],
S95.919-S95.991[A], S95.999A

PDX Collection 1323
S75.202-S75.209[A], S75.212-S75.219[A],
S75.222-S75.229[A], S75.292-S75.299[A],
S75.802-S75.809[A], S75.812-S75.819[A],
S75.892-S75.899[A], S75.902-S75.909[A],
S75.912-S75.919[A], S75.992-S75.999[A],
S85.202-S85.209[A],S85.212-S85.219[A],
S85.292-S85.299[A], S85.302-S85.309[A],
S85.312-S85.319[A], S85.392-S85.399[A],
S85.402-S85.409[A], S85.412-S85.419[A],
S85.492-S85.499[A], S85.802-S85.809[A],
S85.812-S85.819[A], S85.892-S85.899[A],
S85.902-S85.909[A], S85.912-S85.919[A],
S85.992-S85.999[A], S95.002-S95.009[A],
S95.012-S95.019[A], S95.092-S95.099[A],
S95.202-S95.209[A], S95.212-S95.219[A],
S95.292-S95.299[A], S95.802-S95.809[A],
S95.812-S95.819[A], S95.892-S95.899[A],
S95.902-S95.909[A], S95.912-S95.919[A],
S95.992-S95.999[A]

PDX Collection 1324
S75.201-S75.999[A], S85.201-S85.499[A],
S85.801-S85.999[A], S95.001-S95.099[A],
S95.201-S95.999[A]

PDX Collection 1325
M79.A21-M79.A29, S75.001A, S75.009-S75.011[A],
S75.019-S75.021[A], S75.029-S75.091[A],
S75.099-S75.101[A], S75.109-S75.111[A],
S75.119-S75.121[A], S75.129-S75.191[A],
S75.199-S75.201[A], S75.209-S75.211[A],
S75.219-S75.221[A], S75.229-S75.291[A],
S75.299-S75.801[A], S75.809-S75.811[A],
S75.899-S75.901[A], S75.909-S75.911[A],
S75.919-S75.991[A], S75.999A, S85.001A,
S85.009-S85.011[A], S85.019-S85.091[A],
S85.099-S85.101[A], S85.109-S85.111[A],
S85.119-S85.121[A], S85.129-S85.131[A],
S85.139-S85.141[A], S85.149-S85.151[A],

S85.159-S85.161[A], S85.169-S85.171[A],
S85.179-S85.181[A], S85.189-S85.201[A],
S85.209-S85.211[A], S85.219-S85.291[A],
S85.299-S85.301[A], S85.309-S85.311[A],
S85.319-S85.391[A], S85.399-S85.401[A],
S85.409-S85.411[A], S85.419-S85.491[A],
S85.499-S85.501[A], S85.509-S85.511[A],
S85.519-S85.591[A], S85.599-S85.801[A],
S85.809-S85.811[A], S85.819-S85.891[A],
S85.899-S85.901[A], S85.909-S85.911[A],
S85.919-S85.991[A], S85.999A, S95.001A,
S95.009-S95.011[A], S95.019A, S95.091A,
S95.099-S95.101[A], S95.109-S95.111[A], S95
119-S95.191[A], S95.199-S95.201[A], S95.209-S95.211[A],
S95.219-S95.291[A], S95.299-S95.801[A],
S95.809-S95.811[A]. S95.819-S95.891[A],
S95.899-S95.901[A], S95.909-S95.911[A],
S95.919-S95.991[A], S95.999A

PDX Collection 1326
M79.A21-M79.A29, S75.002-S75.009[A], S75.012-S75.019[A],
S75.022-S75.029[A], S75.092-S75.099[A],
S75.102-S75.109[A], S75.112-S75.119[A],
S75.122-S75.129[A], S75.192-S75.199[A],
S75.202-S75.209[A], S75.212-S75.219[A],
S75.222-S75.229[A], S75.292-S75.299[A],
S75.802-S75.809[A], S75.812-S75.819[A],
S75.892-S75.899[A], S75.902-S75.909[A],
S75.912-S75.919[A], S75.992-S75.999[A],
S85.002-S85.009[A], S85.012-S85.019[A],
S85.092-S85.099[A], S85.102-S85.109[A],
S85.112-S85.119[A], S85.122-S85.129[A],
S85.132-S85.139[A], S85.142-S85.149[A],
S85.152-S85.159[A], S85.162-S85.169[A],
S85.172-S85.179[A], S85.182-S85.189[A],
S85.202-S85.209[A], S85.212-S85.219[A],
S85.292-S85.299[A], S85.302-S85.309[A],
S85.312-S85.319[A], S85.392-S85.399[A],
S85.402-S85.409[A], S85.412-S85.419[A],
S85.492-S85.499[A], S85.502-S85.509[A],
S85.512-S85.519[A], S85.592-S85.599[A],
S85.802-S85.809[A], S85.812-S85.819[A],
S85.892-S85.899[A], S85.902-S85.909[A],
S85.912-S85.919[A], S85.992-S85.999[A],
S95.002-S95.009[A], S95.012-S95.019[A],
S95.092-S95.099[A], S95.102-S95.109[A],
S95.112-S95.119[A], S95.192-S95.199[A],
S95.202-S95.209[A], S95.212-S95.219[A],
S95.292-S95.299[A], S95.802-S95.809[A],
S95.812-S95.819[A], S95.892-S95.899[A],
S95.902-S95.909[A], S95.912-S95.919[A],
S95.992-S95.999[A]

PDX Collection 1327
M79.A21-M79.A29, S75.001-S75.999[A], S85.001-S85.999[A],
S95.001-S95.999[A]

PDX Collection 1328
S71.001A, S71.009-S71.011[A], S71.019-S71.021[A],
S71.029-S71.031[A], S71.039-S71.041[A],
S71.049-S71.051[A], S71.059-S71.101[A],
S71.109-S71.111[A], S71.119-S71.121[A],
S71.129-S71.131[A], S71.139-S71.141[A],
S71.149-S71.151[A], S71.159A, S76.021A, S76.029A,
S76.121A, S76.129A, S76.221A, S76.229A, S76.321A,
S76.329A, S76.821A, S76.829A, S76.921A, S76.929A

PDX Collection 1329
S71.002-S71.009[A], S71.012-S71.019[A],
S71.022-S71.029[A], S71.032-S71.039[A],

S71.042-S71.049[A], S71.052-S71.059[A],
S71.102-S71.109[A], S71.112-S71.119[A],
S71.122-S71.129[A], S71.132-S71.139[A],
S71.142-S71.149[A], S71.152-S71.159[A],
S76.022-S76.029[A], S76.122-S76.129[A],
S76.222-S76.229[A],S76.322-S76.329[A],
S76.822-S76.829[A], S76.922-S76.929[A]

PDX Collection 1330
S71.001-S71.159[A], S76.021-S76.029[A],
S76.121-S76.129[A], S76.221-S76.229[A],
S76.321-S76.329[A], S76.821-S76.829[A],
S76.921-S76.929[A]

PDX Collection 1331
S77.00X-S77.02X[A], S77.20X-S77.22X[A]

PDX Collection 1332
S77.10X-S77.22X[A]

PDX Collection 1333
S71.001A, S71.009-S71.011[A], S71.019-S71.021[A],
S71.029-S71.031[A], S71.039-S71.041[A],
S71.049-S71.051[A], S71.059-S71.101[A],
S71.109-S71.111[A], S71.119-S71.121[A],
S71.129-S71.131[A], S71.139-S71.141[A],
S71.149-S71.151[A], S71.159A, S76.021A, S76.029A,
S76.121A, S76.129A, S76.221A, S76.229A, S76.321A,
S76.329A, S76.821A, S76.829A, S76.921A, S76.929A,
S78.011A, S78.019-S78.021[A], S78.029-S78.111[A],
S78.119-S78.121[A], S78.129-S78.911[A],
S78.919-S78.921[A], S78.929A, S81.001A,
S81.009-S81.011[A], S81.019-S81.021[A],
S81.029-S81.031[A], S81.039-S81.041[A],
S81.049-S81.051[A], S81.059-S81.801[A],
S81.809-S81.811[A], S81.819-S81.821[A],
S81.829-S81.831[A], S81.839-S81.841[A],
S81.849-S81.851[A], S81.859A, S86.021A, S86.029A,
S86.121A, S86.129A, S86.221A, S86.229A, S86.321A,
S86.329A, S86.821A, S86.829A, S86.921A, S86.929A,
S88.011A, S88.019-S88.021[A], S88.029-S88.111[A],
S88.119-S88.121[A], S88.129-S88.911[A],
S88.919-S88.921[A], S88.929A, S91.001A,
S91.009-S91.011[A], S91.019-S91.021[A],
S91.029-S91.031[A], S91.039-S91.041[A],
S91.049-S91.051[A], S91.059-S91.101[A],
S91.103-S91.104[A], S91.106-S91.111[A],
S91.113-S91.114[A], S91.116-S91.121[A],
S91.123-S91.124[A], S91.126-S91.131[A],
S91.133-S91.134[A], S91.136-S91.141[A],
S91.143-S91.144[A], S91.146-S91.151[A],
S91.153-S91.154[A], S91.156-S91.201[A],
S91.203-S91.204[A], S91.206-S91.211[A],
S91.213-S91.214[A], S91.216-S91.221[A],
S91.223-S91.224[A], S91.226-S91.231[A],
S91.233-S91.234[A], S91.236-S91.241[A],
S91.243-S91.244[A], S91.246-S91.251[A],
S91.253-S91.254[A], S91.256-S91.301[A],
S91.309-S91.311[A], S91.319-S91.321[A],
S91.329-S91.331[A], S91.339-S91.341[A],
S91.349-S91.351[A], S91.359A, S96.021A,
S96.029A, S96.121A, S96.129A, S96.221A, S96.229A,
S96.821A, S96.829A, S96.921A, S96.929A, S98.011A,
S98.019-S98.021[A], S98.029-S98.111[A],
S98.119-S98.121[A], S98.129-S98.131[A],
S98.139-S98.141[A], S98.149-S98.211[A],
S98.219-S98.221[A], S98.229-S98.311[A],
S98.319-S98.321[A], S98.329-S98.911[A],
S98.919-S98.921[A], S98.929[A], T07.XXX-T14.91X[A],
T79.8XX-T79.9XX[A], T79.A0X-T79.A9X[A]

PDX Collection 1334
S71.002-S71.009[A],
S71.012-S71.019[A], S71.022-S71.029[A],
S71.032-S71.039[A], S71.042-S71.049[A],
S71.052-S71.059[A],S71.102-S71.109[A],
S71.112-S71.119[A], S71.122-S71.129[A],
S71.132-S71.139[A], S71.142-S71.149[A],
S71.152-S71.159[A], S76.022-S76.029[A],
S76.122-S76.129[A], S76.222-S76.229[A],
S76.322-S76.329[A], S76.822-S76.829[A],
S76.922-S76.929[A], S78.012-S78.019[A],
S78.022-S78.029[A], S78.112-S78.119[A],
S78.122-S78.129[A], S78.912-S78.919[A],
S78.922-S78.929[A], S81.002-S81.009[A],
S81.012-S81.019[A], S81.022-S81.029[A],
S81.032-S81.039[A], S81.042-S81.049[A],
S81.052-S81.059[A], S81.802-S81.809[A],
S81.812-S81.819[A], S81.822-S81.829[A],
S81.832-S81.839[A], S81.842-S81.849[A],
S81.852-S81.859[A], S86.022-S86.029[A],
S86.122-S86.129[A], S86.222-S86.229[A],
S86.322-S86.329[A], S86.822-S86.829[A],
S86.922-S86.929[A], S88.012-S88.019[A],
S88.022-S88.029[A], S88.112-S88.119[A],
S88.122-S88.129[A], S88.912-S88.919[A],
S88.922-S88.929[A], S91.002-S91.009[A],
S91.012-S91.019[A], S91.022-S91.029[A],
S91.032-S91.039[A], S91.042-S91.049[A],
S91.052-S91.059[A], S91.102-S91.103[A],
S91.105-S91.109[A], S91.112-S91.113[A],
S91.115-S91.119[A], S91.122-S91.123[A],
S91.125-S91.129[A], S91.132-S91.133[A],
S91.135-S91.139[A], S91.142-S91.143[A],
S91.145-S91.149[A], S91.152-S91.153[A],
S91.155-S91.159[A], S91.202-S91.203[A],
S91.205-S91.209[A], S91.212-S91.213[A],
S91.215-S91.219[A], S91.222-S91.223[A],
S91.225-S91.229[A], S91.232-S91.233[A],
S91.235-S91.239[A], S91.242-S91.243[A],
S91.245-S91.249[A], S91.252-S91.253[A],
S91.255-S91.259[A], S91.302-S91.309[A],
S91.312-S91.319[A], S91.322-S91.329[A],
S91.332-S91.339[A], S91.342-S91.349[A],
S91.352-S91.359[A], S96.022-S96.029[A],
S96.122-S96.129[A], S96.222-S96.229[A],
S96.822-S96.829[A], S96.922-S96.929[A],
S98.012-S98.019[A], S98.022-S98.029[A],
S98.112-S98.119[A], S98.122-S98.129[A],
S98.132-S98.139[A], S98.142-S98.149[A],
S98.212-S98.219[A], S98.222-S98.229[A],
S98.312-S98.319[A], S98.322-S98.329[A],
S98.912-S98.919[A], S98.922-S98.929[A],
T07.XXX-T14.91X[A], T79.8XX-T79.9XX[A],
T79.A0X-T79.A9X[A]

PDX Collection 1335
S71.001-S71.159[A], S76.021-S76.029[A],
S76.121-S76.129[A], S76.221-S76.229[A],
S76.321-S76.329[A], S76.821-S76.829[A],
S76.921-S76.929[A], S78.011-S78.929[A],
S81.001-S81.859[A], S86.021-S86.029[A],
S86.121-S86.129[A], S86.221-S86.229[A],
S86.321-S86.329[A], S86.821-S86.829[A],
S86.921-S86.929[A], S88.011-S88.929[A],
S91.001-S91.359[A], S96.021-S96.029[A],
S96.121-S96.129[A], S96.221-S96.229[A],
S96.821-S96.829[A], S96.921-S96.929[A],
S98.011-S98.929[A], T07.XXX-T14.91X[A],
T79.8XX-T79.9XX[A], T79.A0X-T79.A9X[A]

PDX Collection 1336
S82.001-S82.099[A,B,C]

PDX Collection 1337
M80.00X-M80.019[A], M80.041-M80.049[A],
M80.80X-M80.819[A], M80.841-M80.849[A],
M84.40X-M84.419[A], M84.441-M84.446[A],
M84.454A, M84.474-M84.519[A], M84.541-M84.550[A],
M84.574-M84.576[A], M84.60X-M84.619[A],
M84.641-M84.650[A], M84.674-M84.68X[A],
S03.8XX-S03.9XX[A], S29.011-S29.019[A],
S38.3XXA, S39.011-S39.013[A], S73.101-S73.199[A],
S76.001-S76.019[A], S76.091-S76.119[A],
S76.191-S76.219[A], S76.291-S76.319[A],
S76.391-S76.819[A], S76.891-S76.919[A],
S76.991-S76.999[A], S79.811-S79.929[A],
S82.001-S82.099[B,C], S82.101-S82.156[A,B,C],
S82.191-S82.299[A,B,C], S82.401-S82.499[A,B,C],
S82.831-S82.839[A,B,C], S82.861-S82.866[A,B,C],
S82.90X-S82.92X[A,B,C], S89.001-S89.099[A],
S89.201-S89.299[A], T07.XXX-T14.91X[A],
T79.8XX-T79.9XX[A], T79.A9XA

PDX Collection 1338
S82.001[B,C], S82.002-S82.009[A,B,C], S82.011[B,C],
S82.012-S82.013[A,B,C], S82.014-S82.021[B,C],
S82.022-S82.023[A,B,C], S82.024[B,C],
S82.025-S82.026[A,B,C], S82.031-S82.033[A,B,C],
S82.034[B,C], S82.035-S82.036[A,B,C],
S82.041[B,C], S82.042-S82.043[A,B,C], S82.044[B,C],
S82.045-S82.046[A,B,C], S82.091[B,C],
S82.092-S82.099[A,B,C]

PDX Collection 1339
S82.001-S82.099[A,B,C]

PDX Collection 1340
M80.00X-M80.019[A], M80.041-M80.049[A],
M80.061-M80.819[A], M80.841-M80.849[A],
M80.861-M80.879[A], M84.40X-M84.419[A],
M84.441-M84.446[A], M84.454A, M84.461-M84.519[A],
M84.541-M84.550[A], M84.561-M84.619[A],
M84.641-M84.650[A], M84.661-M84.68X[A],
S03.8XX-S03.9XX[A], S29.011-S29.019[A], S38.3XXA,
S39.011-S39.013[A], S73.101A, S73.109-S73.111[A],
S73.119-S73.121[A], S73.129-S73.191[A],
S73.199[A], S76.001[A], S76.009-S76.011[A],
S76.019A, S76.091A, S76.099-S76.101[A],
S76.109-S76.111[A], S76.119A, S76.191A,
S76.199-S76.201[A], S76.209-S76.211[A], S76.219A,
S76.291A, S76.299-S76.301[A], S76.309-S76.311[A],
S76.319A, S76.391A, S76.399-S76.801[A],
S76.809-S76.811[A], S76.819A, S76.891A,
S76.899-S76.901[A], S76.909-S76.911[A], S76.919A,
S76.991A, S76.999A, S79.811A, S79.819-S79.821[A],
S79.829A, S79.911A, S79.919-S79.921[A], S79.929A,
S82.101[A,B,C], S82.102[B,C], S82.109-S82.111[A,B,C],
S82.112[B,C], S82.113-S82.114[A,B,C], S82.115[B,C],
S82.116-S82.121[A,B,C], S82.122[B,C],
S82.123-S82.124[A,B,C], S82.125[B,C],
S82.126-S82.131[A,B,C], S82.132[B,C],
S82.133-S82.134[A,B,C], S82.135[B,C],
S82.136-S82.141[A,B,C], S82.142[B,C],
S82.143-S82.144[A,B,C], S82.145[B,C],
S82.146-S82.151[A,B,C], S82.152[B,C],
S82.153-S82.154[A,B,C], S82.155[B,C], S82.156[A,B,C],
S82.191[A,B,C], S82.192[B,C], S82.199-S82.201[A,B,C],
S82.202[B,C], S82.209-S82.221[A,B,C],
S82.222[B,C], S82.223-S82.224[A,B,C], S82.225[B,C],
S82.226-S82.231[A,B,C], S82.232[B,C],
S82.233-S82.234[A,B,C], S82.235[B,C],

S82.236-S82.241[A,B,C], S82.242[B,C],
S82.243-S82.244[A,B,C], S82.245[B,C],
S82.246-S82.251[A,B,C], S82.252[B,C],
S82.253-S82.254[A,B,C], S82.255[B,C],
S82.256-S82.261[A,B,C], S82.262[B,C],
S82.263-S82.264[A,B,C], S82.265[B,C],
S82.266-S82.291[A,B,C], S82.292[B,C], S82.299[A,B,C],
S82.401[A,B,C], S82.402[B,C], S82.409-S82.421[A,B,C],
S82.422[B,C], S82.423-S82.424[A,B,C], S82.425[B,C],
S82.426-S82.431[A,B,C], S82.432[B,C],
S82.433-S82.434[A,B,C], S82.435[B,C],
S82.436-S82.441[A,B,C], S82.442[B,C],
S82.443-S82.444[A,B,C], S82.445[B,C],
S82.446-S82.451[A,B,C], S82.452[B,C],
S82.453-S82.454[A,B,C], S82.455[B,C],
S82.456-S82.461[A,B,C], S82.462[B,C],
S82.463-S82.464[A,B,C], S82.465[B,C],
S82.466-S82.491[A,B,C], S82.492[B,C], S82.499[A,B,C],
S82.831[A,B,C], S82.831-S82.832[B,C], S82.839[A,B,C],
S82.861[A,B,C], S82.862[B,C], S82.863-S82.864[A,B,C],
S82.865[B,C], S82.866[A,B,C], S82.90X-S82.92X[A,B,C],
S89.001A, S89.009-S89.011[A], S89.019-S89.021[A],
S89.029-S89.031[A], S89.039-S89.041[A],
S89.049-S89.091[A], S89.099A, S89.201A,
S89.209-S89.211[A], S89.219-S89.221[A],
S89.229-S89.291[A], S89.299A, T07.XXX-T14.91X[A],
T79.8XX-T79.9XX[A], T79.A9XA

PDX Collection 1341
M80.00X-M80.019[A], M80.041-M80.049[A],
M80.061-M80.819[A], M80.841-M80.849[A],
M80.861-M80.879[A], M84.40X-M84.419[A],
M84.441-M84.446[A], M84.454A, M84.461-M84.519[A],
M84.541-M84.550[A], M84.561-M84.619[A],
M84.641-M84.650[A], M84.661-M84.68X[A],
S03.8XX-S03.9XX[A], S29.011-S29.019[A],
S38.3XXA, S39.011-S39.013[A], S73.101-S73.199[A],
S76.001-S76.019[A], S76.091-S76.119[A],
S76.191-S76.219[A], S76.291-S76.319[A],
S76.391-S76.819[A], S76.891-S76.919[A],
S76.991-S76.999[A], S79.811-S79.929[A],
S82.101-S82.156[A,B,C], S82.191-S82.299[A,B,C],
S82.401-S82.499[A,B,C], S82.831-S82.839[A,B,C],
S82.861-S82.866[A,B,C], S82.90X-S82.92X[A,B,C],
S89.001-S89.099[A], S89.201-S89.299[A],
T07.XXX-T14.91X[A], T79.8XX-T79.9XX[A], T79.A9XA

PDX Collection 1342
M80.00X-M80.019[A], M80.041-M80.049[A],
M80.061-M80.819[A], M80.841-M80.849[A],
M80.861-M80.879[A], M84.40X-M84.419[A],
M84.441-M84.446[A], M84.454[A], M84.461-M84.519[A],
M84.541-M84.550[A], M84.561-M84.619[A],
M84.641-M84.650[A], M84.661-M84.68X[A],
S03.8XX-S03.9XX[A], S29.011-S29.019[A],
S38.3XXA, S39.011-S39.013[A], S73.102-S73.109[A],
S73.112-S73.119[A], S73.122-S73.129[A],
S73.192-S73.199[A], S76.002-S76.009[A],
S76.012-S76.019[A], S76.092-S76.099[A],
S76.102-S76.109[A], S76.112-S76.119[A],
S76.192-S76.199[A], S76.202-S76.209[A],
S76.212-S76.219[A], S76.292-S76.299[A],
S76.302-S76.309[A], S76.312-S76.319[A],
S76.392-S76.399[A], S76.802-S76.809[A],
S76.812-S76.819[A], S76.892-S76.899[A],
S76.902-S76.909[A], S76.912-S76.919[A],
S76.992-S76.999[A], S79.812-S79.819[A],
S79.822-S79.829[A], S79.912-S79.919[A],
S79.922-S79.929[A], S82.101[B,C], S82.102-S82.109[A,B,C],

S82.111[B,C], S82.112-S82.113[A,B,C], S82.114[B,C],
S82.115-S82.116[A,B,C], S82.121[B,C],
S82.122-S82.123[A,B,C], S82.124[B,C],
S82.125-S82.126[A,B,C], S82.131[B,C],
S82.132-S82.133[A,B,C], S82.134[B,C],
S82.135-S82.136[A,B,C], S82.141[B,C],
S82.142-S82.143[A,B,C], S82.144[B,C],
S82.145-S82.146[A,B,C], S82.151[B,C],
S82.152-S82.153[A,B,C], S82.154[B,C],
S82.155-S82.156[A,B,C], S82.191[B,C],
S82.192-S82.199[A,B,C], S82.201[B,C],
S82.202-S82.209[A,B,C], S82.221[B,C],
S82.222-S82.223[A,B,C], S82.224[B,C],
S82.225-S82.226[A,B,C], S82.231[B,C],
S82.232-S82.233[A,B,C], S82.234[B,C],
S82.235-S82.236[A,B,C], S82.241[B,C],
S82.242-S82.243[A,B,C], S82.244[B,C],
S82.245-S82.246[A,B,C], S82.251[B,C],
S82.252-S82.253[A,B,C], S82.254[B,C],
S82.255-S82.256[A,B,C], S82.261[B,C],
S82.262-S82.263[A,B,C], S82.264[B,C],
S82.265-S82.266[A,B,C], S82.291[B,C],
S82.292-S82.299[A,B,C], S82.401[B,C],
S82.402-S82.409[A,B,C], S82.421[B,C],
S82.422-S82.423[A,B,C], S82.424[B,C],
S82.425-S82.426[A,B,C], S82.431[B,C],
S82.432-S82.433[A,B,C], S82.434[B,C],
S82.435-S82.436[A,B,C], S82.441[B,C],
S82.442-S82.443[A,B,C], S82.444[B,C],
S82.445-S82.446[A,B,C], S82.451[B,C],
S82.452-S82.453[A,B,C], S82.454[B,C],
S82.455-S82.456[A,B,C], S82.461[B,C],
S82.462-S82.463[A,B,C], S82.464[B,C],
S82.465-S82.466[A,B,C], S82.491[B,C],
S82.492-S82.499[A,B,C], S82.831[B,C],
S82.832-S82.839[A,B,C], S82.861[B,C],
S82.862-S82.863[A,B,C], S82.864[B,C],
S82.865-S82.866[A,B,C], S82.90X-S82.92X[A,B,C],
S89.002-S89.009[A], S89.012-S89.019[A],
S89.022-S89.029[A], S89.032-S89.039[A],
S89.042-S89.049[A], S89.092-S89.099[A],
S89.202-S89.209[A], S89.212-S89.219[A],
S89.222-S89.229[A], S89.292-S89.299[A],
T07.XXX-T14.91X[A], T79.8XX-T79.9XX[A], T79.A9XA

PDX Collection 1343
S82.101[A,B,C], S82.102[B,C], S82.109-S82.111[A,B,C],
S82.112[A,B], S82.113-S82.114[A,B,C],
S82.115[B,C], S82.116-S82.121[A,B,C], S82.122[B,C],
S82.123-S82.124[A,B,C], S82.125[B,C],
S82.126-S82.131[A,B,C], S82.132[B,C],
S82.133-S82.134[A,B,C], S82.135[B,C],
S82.136-S82.141[A,B,C], S82.142[B,C],
S82.143-S82.144[A,B,C], S82.145[B,C],
S82.146-S82.151[A,B,C], S82.152[B,C],
S82.153-S82.154[A,B,C], S82.155[B,C],
S82.156[A,B,C], S82.161A, S82.169A, S82.191[A,B,C],
S82.192[B,C], S82.199-S82.201[A,B,C],
S82.202[B,C], S82.209-S82.221[A,B,C],
S82.222[B,C], S82.223-S82.224[A,B,C], S82.225[B,C],
S82.226-S82.231[A,B,C], S82.232[B,C],
S82.233-S82.234[A,B,C], S82.235[B,C],
S82.236-S82.241[A,B,C], S82.242[B,C],
S82.243-S82.244[A,B,C], S82.245[B,C],
S82.246-S82.251[A,B,C], S82.252[B,C],
S82.253-S82.254[A,B,C], S82.255[B,C],
S82.256-S82.261[A,B,C], S82.262[B,C],
S82.263-S82.264[A,B,C], S82.265[B,C],

S82.266-S82.291[A,B,C], S82.292[B,C],
S82.299[A,B,C], S82.311A, S82.319A, S82.401[A,B,C],
S82.402[B,C], S82.409-S82.421[A,B,C],
S82.422[B,C], S82.423-S82.424[A,B,C], S82.425[B,C],
S82.426-S82.431[A,B,C], S82.432[B,C],
S82.433-S82.434[A,B,C], S82.435[B,C],
S82.436-S82.441[A,B,C], S82.442[B,C],
S82.443-S82.444[A,B,C], S82.445[B,C],
S82.446-S82.451[A,B,C], S82.452[B,C],
S82.453-S82.454[A,B,C], S82.455[B,C],
S82.456-S82.461[A,B,C], S82.462[B,C],
S82.463-S82.464[A,B,C], S82.465[B,C],
S82.466-S82.491[A,B,C], S82.492[B,C], S82.499[A,B,C],
S82.811A, S82.819-S82.821[A], S82.829[A], S82.831[A,B,C],
S82.832[B,C], S82.839[A,B,C], S82.861[A,B,C],
S82.862[B,C], S82.863-S82.864[A,B,C], S82.865[B,C],
S82.866[A,B,C], S89.001A, S89.009-S89.011[A],
S89.019-S89.021[A], S89.029-S89.031[A],
S89.039-S89.041[A], S89.049-S89.091[A], S89.099A,
S89.201A, S89.209-S89.211[A], S89.219-S89.221[A],
S89.229-S89.291[A], S89.299A

PDX Collection 1344
S82.101[B,C], S82.102-S82.109[A,B,C],
S82.111[B,C], S82.112-S82.113[A,B,C], S82.121[B,C],
S82.122-S82.123[A,B,C], S82.124[B,C],
S82.125-S82.126[A,B,C], S82.131[B,C],
S82.132-S82.133[A,B,C], S82.134[B,C],
S82.135-S82.136[A,B,C], S82.141[B,C],
S82.142-S82.143[A,B,C], S82.144[B,C],
S82.145-S82.146[A,B,C], S82.151[B,C],
S82.152-S82.153[A,B,C], S82.154[B,C],
S82.155-S82.156[A,B,C], S82.162-S82.169[A],
S82.191[B,C], S82.192-S82.199[A,B,C],
S82.201[B,C], S82.202-S82.209[A,B,C],
S82.221[B,C], S82.222-S82.223[A,B,C], S82.224[B,C],
S82.225-S82.226[A,B,C], S82.231[B,C],
S82.232-S82.233[A,B,C], S82.234[B,C],
S82.235-S82.236[A,B,C], S82.241[B,C],
S82.242-S82.243[A,B,C], S82.244[B,C],
S82.245-S82.246[A,B,C], S82.251[B,C],
S82.252-S82.253[A,B,C], S82.254[B,C],
S82.255-S82.256[A,B,C], S82.261[B,C],
S82.262-S82.263[A,B,C], S82.264[B,C],
S82.265-S82.266[A,B,C], S82.291[B,C],
S82.292-S82.299[A,B,C], S82.312-S82.319[A],
S82.401[B,C], S82.402-S82.409[A,B,C],
S82.421[B,C], S82.422-S82.423[A,B,C], S82.424[B,C],
S82.425-S82.426[A,B,C], S82.431[B,C],
S82.432-S82.433[A,B,C], S82.434[B,C],
S82.435-S82.436[A,B,C], S82.441[B,C],
S82.442-S82.443[A,B,C], S82.444[B,C],
S82.445-S82.446[A,B,C], S82.451[B,C],
S82.452-S82.453[A,B,C], S82.454[B,C],
S82.455-S82.456[A,B,C], S82.461[B,C],
S82.462-S82.463[A,B,C], S82.464[B,C],
S82.465-S82.466[A,B,C], S82.491[B,C],
S82.492-S82.499[A,B,C], S82.812-S82.819[A],
S82.822-S82.829[A], S82.831[B,C], S82.832-S82.839[A,B,C],
S82.861[B,C], S82.862-S82.863[A,B,C], S82.864[B,C],
S82.865-S82.866[A,B,C], S89.002-S89.009[A],
S89.012-S89.019[A], S89.022-S89.029[A],
S89.032-S89.039[A], S89.042-S89.049[A],
S89.092-S89.099[A], S89.202-S89.209[A],
S89.212-S89.219[A], S89.222-S89.229[A],
S89.292-S89.299[A]

PDX Collection 1345
S82.101-S82.156[A,B,C], S82.161-S82.169[A],
S82.191-S82.299[A,B,C], S82.311-S82.319[A],
S82.401-S82.499[A,B,C], S82.811-S82.829[A],
S82.831-S82.839[A,B,C], S82.861-S82.866[A,B,C],
S89.001-S89.099[A], S89.201-S89.299[A]

PDX Collection 1346
M80.00X-M80.019[A], M80.041-M80.049[A],
M80.061-M80.819[A], M80.841-M80.849[A],
M80.861-M80.879[A], M84.40X-M84.419[A],
M84.441-M84.446[A], M84.454[A], M84.461-M84.519[A],
M84.541-M84.550[A], M84.561-M84.576[A],
M84.60X-M84.619[A], M84.641-M84.650[A],
M84.661-M84.68X[A], S03.8XX-S03.9XX[A],
S29.011-S29.019[A], S38.3XXA, S39.011-S39.013[A],
S73.101A, S73.109-S73.111[A], S73.119-S73.121[A],
S73.129-S73.191[A], S73.199A, S76.001A,
S76.009-S76.011[A], S76.019A, S76.091A,
S76.099-S76.101[A], S76.109-S76.111[A],
S76.119A, S76.191A, S76.199-S76.201[A],
S76.209-S76.211[A], S76.219A, S76.291A,
S76.299-S76.301[A], S76.309-S76.311[A], S76.319A,
S76.391A, S76.399-S76.801[A], S76.809-S76.811[A],
S76.819A, S76.891A, S76.899-S76.901[A],
S76.909-S76.911[A], S76.919A, S76.991A, S76.999A,
S79.811A, S79.819-S79.821[A], S79.829-S79.911[A],
S79.919-S79.921[A], S79.929A, S82.101[A,B,C],
S82.102[B,C], S82.109-S82.111[A,B,C],
S82.112[B,C], S82.113-S82.114[A,B,C], S82.115[B,C],
S82.116-S82.121[A,B,C], S82.122[B,C],
S82.123-S82.124[A,B,C], S82.125[B,C],
S82.126-S82.131[A,B,C], S82.132[B,C],
S82.133-S82.134[A,B,C], S82.135[B,C],
S82.136-S82.141[A,B,C], S82.142[B,C],
S82.143-S82.144[A,B,C], S82.145[B,C],
S82.146-S82.151[A,B,C], S82.152[B,C],
S82.153-S82.154[A,B,C], S82.155[B,C],
S82.156[A,B,C], S82.161A, S82.169A, S82.191[A,B,C],
S82.192[B,C], S82.199-S82.201[A,B,C],
S82.202[B,C], S82.209-S82.221[A,B,C],
S82.222[B,C], S82.223-S82.224[A,B,C], S82.225[B,C],
S82.226-S82.231[A,B,C], S82.232[B,C],
S82.233-S82.234[A,B,C], S82.235[B,C],
S82.236-S82.241[A,B,C], S82.242[B,C],
S82.243-S82.244[A,B,C], S82.245[B,C],
S82.246-S82.251[A,B,C], S82.252[B,C],
S82.253-S82.254[A,B,C], S82.255[B,C],
S82.256-S82.261[A,B,C], S82.262[B,C],
S82.263-S82.264[A,B,C], S82.265[B,C],
S82.266-S82.291[A,B,C], S82.292[B,C],
S82.299[A,B,C], S82.311A, S82.319A, S82.401[A,B,C],
S82.402[B,C], S82.409-S82.421[A,B,C],
S82.422[B,C], S82.423-S82.424[A,B,C], S82.425[B,C],
S82.426-S82.431[A,B,C], S82.432[B,C],
S82.433-S82.434[A,B,C], S82.435[B,C],
S82.436-S82.441[A,B,C], S82.442[B,C],
S82.443-S82.444[A,B,C], S82.445[B,C],
S82.446-S82.451[A,B,C], S82.452[B,C,],
S82.453-S82.454[A,B,C], S82.455[B,C],
S82.456-S82.461[A,B,C], S82.462[B,C],
S82.463-S82.464[A,B,C], S82.465[B,C],
S82.466-S82.491[A,B,C], S82.492[B,C], S82.499[A,B,C],
S82.811A, S82.819-S82.821[A], S82.829A, S82.831[A,B,C],
S82.832[B,C], S82.839[A,B,C], S82.861[A,B,C], S82.862[B,C],
S82.863-S82.864[A,B,C], S82.865[B,C], S82.866[A,B,C],
S82.90X-S82.92X[A,B,C], S89.001A, S89.009-S89.011[A],

S89.019-S89.021[A], S89.029-S89.031[A],
S89.039-S89.041[A], S89.049-S89.091[A],
S89.099A, S89.201A, S89.209A, S89.211-S89.219[A],
S89.221-S89.229[A], S89.291-S89.299[A],
T07.XXX-T14.91X[A], T79.A9X-T79.9XX[A]

PDX Collection 1347
M80.00X-M80.019[A], M80.041-M80.049[A],
M80.061-M80.819[A], M80.841-M80.849[A],
M80.861-M80.879[A], M84.40X-M84.419[A],
M84.441-M84.446[A], M84.454A, M84.461-M84.519[A],
M84.541-M84.550[A], M84.561-M84.576[A],
M84.60X-M84.619[A], M84.641-M84.650[A],
M84.661-M84.68X[A], S03.8XX-S03.9XX[A],
S29.011-S29.019[A], S38.3XXA, S39.011-S39.013[A],
S73.101-S73.199[A], S76.001-S76.019[A],
S76.091-S76.119[A], S76.191-S76.219[A],
S76.291-S76.319[A], S76.391-S76.819[A],
S76.891-S76.919[A], S76.991-S76.999[A],
S79.811-S79.929[A], S82.301-S82.309[A,B,C],
S82.391-S82.399[A,B,C], S82.51X-S82.56X[B,C],
S82.61X-S82.66X[A,B,C], S82.841-S82.856[A,B,C],
S82.871-S82.876[B,C], S82.891-S82.92X[A,B,C],
S89.101-S89.199[A], S89.301-S89.399[A],
T07.XXX-T14.91X[A], T79.A9X-T79.9XX[A]

PDX Collection 1348
S72.001-S72.92X[A,B,C], S79.001-S79.199[A],
S82.001-S82.156[A,B,C], S82.191-S82.309[A,B,C],
S82.391-S82.66X[A,B,C], S82.831-S82.92X[A,B,C],
S89.001-S89.399[A], S92.001-S92.599[A,B],
S92.811-S92.919[A,B]

PDX Collection 1349
S75.801A, S75.809-S75.811[A], S75.819-S75.891[A],
S75.899-S75.901[A], S75.909-S75.911[A],
S75.919-S75.991[A], S75.999A, S85.001A,
S85.009-S85.011[A], S85.019-S85.091[A], S85.099A,
S85.201A, S85.209-S85.211[A], S85.219-S85.291[A],
S85.299A, S85.801A, S85.809-S85.811[A],
S85.819-S85.891[A], S85.899-S85.901[A],
S85.909-S85.911[A], S85.919-S85.991[A], S85.999A,
S95.001A, S95.009-S95.011[A], S95.019-S95.091[A],
S95.099-S95.201[A], S95.209-S95.211[A],
S95.219-S95.291[A], S95.299-S95.801[A],
S95.809-S95.811[A], S95.819-S95.891[A],
S95.899-S95.901[A], S95.909-S95.911[A],
S95.919-S95.991[A], S95.999A

PDX Collection 1350
S75.802-S75.809[A], S75.812-S75.819[A],
S75.892-S75.899[A], S75.902-S75.909[A],
S75.912-S75.919[A], S75.992-S75.999[A],
S85.002-S85.009[A], S85.012-S85.019[A],
S85.092-S85.099[A], S85.202-S85.209[A],
S85.212-S85.219[A], S85.292-S85.299[A],
S85.802-S85.809[A], S85.812-S85.819[A],
S85.892-S85.899[A], S85.902-S85.909[A],
S85.912-S85.919[A], S85.992-S85.999[A],
S95.002-S95.009[A], S95.012-S95.019[A],
S95.092-S95.099[A], S95.202-S95.209[A],
S95.212-S95.219[A], S95.292-S95.299[A],
S95.802-S95.809[A], S95.812-S95.819[A],
S95.892-S95.899[A], S95.902-S95.909[A],
S95.912-S95.919[A], S95.992-S95.999[A]

PDX Collection 1351
S75.801A-S75.999[A], S85.001-S85.099[A],
S85.201-S85.299[A], S85.801-S85.999[A],
S95.001-S95.009[A], S95.201-S95.999[A]

PDX Collection 1352
S75.801A, S75.809-S75.811[A], S75.819-S75.891[A],
S75.899-S75.901[A], S75.909-S75.911[A],
S75.919-S75.991[A], S75.999A, S85.101A,
S85.109-S85.111[A], S85.119-S85.121[A], S85.129A,
S85.201A, S85.209-S85.211[A], S85.219-S85.291[A],
S85.299A, S85.801A, S85.809-S85.811[A],
S85.819-S85.891[A], S85.899-S85.901[A],
S85.909-S85.911[A], S85.919-S85.991[A], S85.999A,
S95.001A, S95.009-S95.011[A], S95.019-S95.091[A],
S95.099-S95.201[A], S95.209-S95.211[A],
S95.219-S95.291[A], S95.299-S95.801[A],
S95.809-S95.811[A], S95.819-S95.891[A],
S95.899-S95.901[A], S95.909-S95.911[A],
S95.919-S95.991[A], S95.999A

PDX Collection 1353
S75.802-S75.809[A], S75.812-S75.819[A],
S75.892-S75.899[A], S75.902-S75.909[A],
S75.912-S75.919[A], S75.992-S75.999[A],
S85.102-S85.109[A], S85.112-S85.119[A],
S85.122-S85.129[A], S85.202-S85.209[A],
S85.212-S85.219[A], S85.292-S85.299[A],
S85.802-S85.809[A], S85.812-S85.819[A],
S85.892-S85.899[A], S85.902-S85.909[A],
S85.912-S85.919[A], S85.992-S85.999[A],
S95.002-S95.009[A], S95.012-S95.019[A],
S95.092-S95.099[A], S95.202-S95.209[A],
S95.212-S95.219[A], S95.292-S95.299[A],
S95.802-S95.809[A], S95.812-S95.819[A],
S95.892-S95.899[A], S95.902-S95.909[A],
S95.912-S95.919[A], S95.992-S95.999[A]

PDX Collection 1354
S75.801-S75.999[A], S85.101-S85.129[A],
S85.201-S85.299[A], S85.801-S85.999[A],
S95.001-S95.099[A], S95.201-S95.999[A]

PDX Collection 1355
S75.801A, S75.809-S75.811[A], S75.819-S75.891[A],
S75.899-S75.901[A], S75.909-S75.911[A],
S75.919-S75.991[A], S75.999A, S85.131A,
S85.139-S85.141[A], S85.149-S85.151[A], S85.159A,
S85.201A, S85.209-S85.211[A], S85.219-S85.291[A],
S85.299A, S85.801A, S85.809-S85.811[A],
S85.819-S85.891[A], S85.899-S85.901[A],
S85.909-S85.911[A], S85.919-S85.991[A], S85.999A,
S95.001A, S95.009-S95.011[A], S95.019-S95.091[A],
S95.099-S95.201[A], S95.209-S95.211[A],
S95.219-S95.291[A], S95.299-S95.801[A],
S95.809-S95.811[A], S95.819-S95.891[A],
S95.899-S95.901[A], S95.909-S95.911[A],
S95.919-S95.991[A], S95.999A

PDX Collection 1356
S75.802-S75.809[A], S75.812-S75.819[A],
S75.892-S75.899[A], S75.902-S75.909[A],
S75.912-S75.919[A], S75.992-S75.999[A],
S85.132-S85.139[A], S85.142-S85.149[A],
S85.152-S85.159[A], S85.202-S85.209[A],
S85.212-S85.219[A], S85.292-S85.299[A],
S85.802-S85.809[A], S85.812-S85.819[A],
S85.892-S85.899[A], S85.902-S85.909[A],
S85.912-S85.919[A], S85.992-S85.999[A],
S95.002-S95.009[A], S95.012-S95.019[A],
S95.092-S95.099[A], S95.202-S95.209[A],
S95.212-S95.219[A], S95.292-S95.299[A],
S95.802-S95.809[A], S95.812-S95.819[A],
S95.892-S95.899[A], S95.902-S95.909[A],
S95.912-S95.919[A], S95.992-S95.999[A]

PDX Collection 1357
S75.801-S75.999[A], S85.131-S85.159[A],
S85.201-S85.299[A], S85.801-S85.999[A],
S95.001-S95.099[A], S95.201-S95.999[A]

PDX Collection 1358
S75.801A, S75.809-S75.811[A], S75.819-S75.891[A],
S75.899-S75.901[A], S75.909-S75.911[A],
S75.919-S75.991[A], S75.999A, S85.161A,
S85.169-S85.171[A], S85.179-S85.181[A], S85.189A,
S85.201A, S85.209-S85.211[A], S85.219-S85.291[A],
S85.299A, S85.801A, S85.809-S85.811[A],
S85.819-S85.891[A], S85.899-S85.901[A],
S85.909-S85.911[A], S85.919-S85.991[A], S85.999A,
S95.001A, S95.009-S95.011[A], S95.019-S95.091[A],
S95.099-S95.201[A], S95.209-S95.211[A],
S95.219-S95.291[A], S95.299-S95.801[A],
S95.809-S95.811[A], S95.819-S95.891[A],
S95.899-S95.901[A], S95.909-S95.911[A],
S95.919-S95.991[A], S95.999A

PDX Collection 1359
S75.802-S75.809[A], S75.812-S75.819[A],
S75.892-S75.899[A], S75.902-S75.909[A],
S75.912-S75.919[A], S75.992-S75.999[A],
S85.162-S85.169[A], S85.172-S85.179[A],
S85.182-S85.189[A], S85.202-S85.209[A],
S85.212-S85.219[A], S85.292-S85.299[A],
S85.802-S85.809[A], S85.812-S85.819[A],
S85.892-S85.899[A], S85.902-S85.909[A],
S85.912-S85.919[A], S85.992-S85.999[A],
S95.002-S95.009[A], S95.012-S95.019[A],
S95.092-S95.099[A], S95.202-S95.209[A],
S95.212-S95.219[A], S95.292-S95.299[A],
S95.802-S95.809[A], S95.812-S95.819[A],
S95.892-S95.899[A], S95.902-S95.909[A],
S95.912-S95.919[A], S95.992-S95.999[A]

PDX Collection 1360
S75.801-S75.999[A], S85.161-S85.189[A],
S85.201-S85.299[A], S85.801-S85.999[A],
S95.001-S95.099[A], S95.201-S95.999[A]

PDX Collection 1361
S75.801[A], S75.809-S75.811[A], S75.819-S75.891[A],
S75.899-S75.901[A], S75.909-S75.911[A],
S75.919-S75.991[A], S75.999A, S85.201A,
S85.209-S85.211[A], S85.219-S85.291[A], S85.299A,
S85.501A, S85.509-S85.511[A], S85.519-S85.591[A],
S85.599A, S85.801A, S85.809-S85.811[A],
S85.819-S85.891[A], S85.899-S85.901[A],
S85.909-S85.911[A], S85.919-S85.991[A], S85.999A,
S95.001A, S95.009-S95.011[A], S95.019-S95.091[A],
S95.099-S95.201[A], S95.209-S95.211[A],
S95.219-S95.291[A], S95.299-S95.801[A],
S95.809-S95.811[A], S95.819-S95.891[A],
S95.899-S95.901[A], S95.909-S95.911[A],
S95.919-S95.991[A], S95.999A

PDX Collection 1362
S75.802-S75.809[A], S75.812-S75.819[A],
S75.892-S75.899[A], S75.902-S75.909[A],
S75.912-S75.919[A], S75.992-S75.999[A],
S85.202-S85.209[A], S85.212-S85.219[A],
S85.292-S85.299[A], S85.502-S85.509[A],
S85.512-S85.519[A], S85.592-S85.599[A],
S85.802-S85.809[A], S85.812-S85.819[A],
S85.892-S85.899[A], S85.902-S85.909[A],
S85.912-S85.919[A], S85.992-S85.999[A],
S95.002-S95.009[A], S95.012-S95.019[A],
S95.092-S95.099[A], S95.202-S95.209[A],
S95.212-S95.219[A], S95.292-S95.299[A],

S95.802-S95.809[A], S95.812-S95.819[A],
S95.892-S95.899[A], S95.902-S95.909[A],
S95.912-S95.919[A], S95.992-S95.999[A]

PDX Collection 1363
S75.801-S75.999[A], S85.201-S85.299[A],
S85.501-S85.599[A], S85.801-S85.999[A],
S95.001-S95.099[A], S95.201-S95.999[A]

PDX Collection 1364
S81.001A, S81.009-S81.011[A], S81.019-S81.021[A],
S81.029-S81.031[A], S81.039-S81.041[A],
S81.049-S81.051[A], S81.059-S81.801[A],
S81.809-S81.811[A], S81.819-S81.821[A],
S81.829-S81.831[A], S81.839-S81.841[A],
S81.849-S81.851[A], S81.859A, S86.021A, S86.029A,
S86.121A, S86.129A, S86.221A, S86.229A, S86.321A,
S86.329A, S86.821A, S86.829-S86.921[A], S86.929A,
S91.001A, S91.009A, S91.011A, S91.019-S91.021[A],
S91.029-S91.031[A], S91.039-S91.041[A],
S91.049-S91.051[A], S91.059A, S96.021A, S96.029A,
S96.121A, S96.129A, S96.221A, S96.229A, S96.821A,
S96.829A, S96.921A, S96.929A

PDX Collection 1365
S81.002-S81.009[A], S81.012-S81.019[A],
S81.022-S81.029[A], S81.032-S81.039[A],
S81.042-S81.049[A], S81.052-S81.059[A],
S81.802-S81.809[A], S81.812-S81.819[A],
S81.822-S81.829[A], S81.832-S81.839[A],
S81.842-S81.849[A], S81.852-S81.859[A],
S86.022-S86.029[A], S86.122-S86.129[A],
S86.222-S86.229[A], S86.322-S86.329[A],
S86.822-S86.829[A], S86.922-S86.929[A],
S91.002-S91.009[A], S91.012-S91.019[A],
S91.022-S91.029[A], S91.032-S91.039[A],
S91.042-S91.049[A], S91.052-S91.059[A],
S96.022-S96.029[A], S96.122-S96.129[A],
S96.222-S96.229[A], S96.822-S96.829[A],
S96.922-S96.929[A]

PDX Collection 1366
S81.001-S81.859[A], S86.021-S86.029[A],
S86.121-S86.129[A], S86.221-S86.229[A],
S86.321-S86.329[A], S86.821-S86.829[A],
S86.921-S86.929[A], S91.001-S91.059[A],
S96.021-S96.029[A], S96.121-S96.129[A],
S96.221-S96.229[A], S96.821-S96.829[A],
S96.921-S96.929[A]

PDX Collection 1367
M80.00X-M80.019[A], M80.041-M80.049[A],
M80.061-M80.819[A], M80.841-M80.849[A],
M80.861-M80.879[A], M84.40X-M84.419[A],
M84.441-M84.446[A], M84.454A, M84.461-M84.519[A],
M84.541-M84.550[A], M84.561-M84.576[A],
M84.60X-M84.619[A], M84.641-M84.650[A],
M84.661-M84.68X[A], S03.8XX-S03.9XX[A],
S29.011-S29.019[A], S38.3XXA, S39.011-S39.013[A],
S73.101-S73.199[A], S76.001-S76.019[A],
S76.091-S76.219[A], S76.291-S76.319[A],
S76.391-S76.819[A], S76.891-S76.919[A],
S76.991-S76.999[A], S79.811-S79.929[A],
S82.90X-S82.92X[A,B,C], S92.001-S92.066[B],
S92.101-S92.356[A,B], S92.811-S92.819[A,B],
S92.901-S92.909[A,B], T07.XXX-T14.91X[A],
T79.A9X-T79.9XX[A]

PDX Collection 1368
M80.00X-M80.019[A], M80.041-M80.049[A],
M80.80X-M80.819[A], M80.841-M80.849[A],
M84.40X-M84.419[A], M84.441-M84.446[A],
M84.454A, M84.474-M84.519[A], M84.541-M84.550[A],

M84.574-M84.576[A], M84.60X-M84.619[A],
M84.641-M84.650[A], M84.674-M84.68X[A],
S03.8XX-S03.9XX[A], S29.011-S29.019[A],
S38.3XXA, S39.011-S39.013[A], S73.101-S73.199[A],
S76.001-S76.019[A], S76.091-S76.219[A],
S76.291-S76.319[A], S76.391-S76.819[A],
S76.891-S76.919[A], S76.991-S76.999[A],
S79.821-S79.929[A], S82.90X-S82.92X[A,B,C],
S92.001-S92.066[B], S92.101-S92.356[A,B],
S92.811-S92.819[A,B], S92.901-S92.909[A,B],
T07.XXX-T14.91X[A], T79.A9X-T79.9XX[A]

PDX Collection 1369
S92.001-S92.919[A,B]

PDX Collection 1370
S75.801A, S75.809-S75.811[A], S75.819-S75.891[A],
S75.899-S75.901[A], S75.909-S75.911[A],
S75.919-S75.991[A], S75.999A, S85.201A,
S85.209-S85.211[A], S85.219-S85.291[A], S85.299A,
S85.801A, S85.809-S85.811[A], S85.819-S85.891[A],
S85.899-S85.901[A], S85.909-S85.911[A],
S85.919-S85.991[A], S85.999A, S95.001A,
S95.009-S95.011[A], S95.019-S95.091[A],
S95.099-S95.201[A], S95.209-S95.211[A],
S95.219-S95.291[A], S95.299-S95.801[A],
S95.809-S95.811[A], S95.819-S95.891[A],
S95.899-S95.901[A], S95.909-S95.911[A],
S95.919-S95.991[A], S95.999A

PDX Collection 1371
S75.802-S75.809[A], S75.812-S75.819[A],
S75.892-S75.899[A], S75.902-S75.909[A],
S75.912-S75.919[A], S75.992-S75.999[A],
S85.202-S85.209[A], S85.212-S85.219[A],
S85.292-S85.299[A], S85.802-S85.809[A],
S85.812-S85.819[A], S85.892-S85.899[A],
S85.902-S85.909[A], S85.912-S85.919[A],
S85.992-S85.999[A], S95.002-S95.009[A],
S95.012-S95.019[A], S95.092-S95.099[A],
S95.102-S95.109[A], S95.112-S95.119[A],
S95.192-S95.199[A], S95.202-S95.209[A],
S95.212-S95.219[A], S95.292-S95.299[A],
S95.802-S95.809[A], S95.812-S95.819[A],
S95.892-S95.899[A], S95.902-S95.909[A],
S95.912-S95.919[A], S95.992-S95.999[A]

PDX Collection 1372
S75.801-S75.999[A], S85.201-S85.299[A],
S85.801-S85.999[A], S95.001-S95.099[A],
S95.101-S95.999[A]

PDX Collection 1373
T17.400-T17.498[A]

PDX Collection 1374
T17.400-T17.998[A]

PDX Collection 1375
T20.30XA, T20.39XA, T20.70XA, T20.79XA

PDX Collection 1376
T20.311-T20.319[A], T20.39XA, T20.711-T20.719[A],
T20.79XA

PDX Collection 1377
T20.32XA, T20.39XA, T20.72XA, T20.79XA

PDX Collection 1378
T20.33XA, T20.39XA, T20.73XA, T20.79XA

PDX Collection 1379
T20.34XA, T20.39XA, T20.74XA, T20.79XA

PDX Collection 1380
T20.35XA, T20.39XA, T20.75XA, T20.79XA

PDX Collection 1381
T20.36XA, T20.39XA, T20.76XA, T20.79XA

PDX Collection 1382
T20.37X-T20.39X[A], T20.77X-T20.79X[A]

PDX Collection 1383
T20.30X-T20.39X[A], T20.70X-T20.79X[A]

PDX Collection 1384
T21.30XA, T21.39XA, T21.70XA, T21.79XA

PDX Collection 1385
T21.30X-T21.31X[A], T21.39XA, T21.70X-T21.71X[A],
T21.79XA

PDX Collection 1386
T21.30XA, T21.32XA, T21.39XA, T21.70XA, T21.72XA,
T21.79XA

PDX Collection 1387
T21.30XA, T21.33X-T21.35X[A], T21.39XA, T21.70XA,
T21.73X-T21.75X[A], T21.79XA

PDX Collection 1388
T21.30XA, T21.36X-T21.39X[A], T21.70XA,
T21.76X-T21.79X[A]

PDX Collection 1389
T22.30XA, T22.391-T22.399[A], T22.70XA,
T22.791-T22.799[A]

PDX Collection 1390
T22.30X-T22.319[A], T22.391-T22.399[A],
T22.70X-T22.719[A], T22.791-T22.799[A]

PDX Collection 1391
T22.30XA, T22.321-T22.329[A], T22.391-T22.399[A],
T22.70XA, T22.721-T22.729[A], T22.791-T22.799[A]

PDX Collection 1392
T22.30XA, T22.331-T22.339[A], T22.391-T22.399[A],
T22.70XA, T22.731-T22.739[A], T22.791-T22.799[A]

PDX Collection 1393
T22.30XA, T22.341-T22.349[A], .T22.391-T22.399[A],
T22.70XA, T22.741-T22.749[A], T22.791-T22.799[A]

PDX Collection 1394
T22.30XA, T22.351-T22.359[A], T22.391-T22.399[A],
T22.70XA, T22.751-T22.759[A], T22.791-T22.799[A]

PDX Collection 1395
T22.30XA, T22.361-T22.369[A], T22.391-T22.399[A],
T22.70XA, T22.761-T22.769[A], T22.791-T22.799[A]

PDX Collection 1396
T23.301-T23.309[A], T23.391-T23.399[A],
T23.701-T23.709[A], T23.791-T23.799[A]

PDX Collection 1397
T23.301-T23.319[A], T23.391-T23.399[A],
T23.701-T23.719[A], T23.791-T23.799[A]

PDX Collection 1398
T23.301-T23.309[A], T23.321-T23.329[A],
T23.391-T23.399[A], T23.701-T23.709[A],
T23.721-T23.729[A], T23.791-T23.799[A]

PDX Collection 1399
T23.301-T23.309[A], T23.331-T23.339[A],
T23.391-T23.399[A], T23.701-709[A], T23.731-T23.739[A],
T23.791-T23.799[A]

PDX Collection 1400
T23.301-T23.309[A], T23.341-T23.349[A],
T23.391-T23.399[A], T23.701-T23.709[A],
T23.741-T23.749[A], T23.791-T23.799[A]

PDX Collection 1401
T23.301-T23.309[A], T23.351-T23.359[A],
T23.391-T23.399[A], T23.701-T23.709[A],
T23.751-T23.759[A], T23.791-T23.799[A]

PDX Collection 1402
T23.301-T23.309[A], T23.361-T23.369[A],
T23.391-T23.399[A], T23.701-T23.709[A],
T23.761-T23.769[A], T23.791-T23.799[A]

PDX Collection 1403
T23.301-T23.309[A], T23.371-T23.379[A],
T23.391-T23.399[A], T23.701-T23.709[A],
T23.771-T23.779[A], T23.791-T23.799[A]

PDX Collection 1404
T24.301-T24.309[A], T24.391-T24.399[A],
T24.701-T24.709[A], T24.791-T24.799[A],
T25.391-T25.399[A], T25.791-T25.799[A]

PDX Collection 1405
T24.301-T24.309[A], T24.311-T24.319[A],
T24.391-T24.399[A], T24.701-T24.709-T24.719[A],
T24.791-T24.799[A], T25.391-T25.399[A],
T25.791-T25.799[A]

PDX Collection 1406
T24.301-T24.309[A], T24.321-T24.329[A],
T24.391-T24.399[A], T24.701-T24.709[A],
T24.721-T24.729[A], T24.791-T24.799[A],
T25.391-T25.399[A], T25.791-T25.799[A]

PDX Collection 1407
T24.301-T24.309[A], T24.331-T24.339[A],
T24.391-T24.399[A], T24.701-T24.709[A],
T24.731-T24.739[A], T24.791-T24.799[A],
T25.391-T25.399[A], T25.791-T25.799[A]

PDX Collection 1408
T24.301-T24.309[A], T24.391-T24.399[A],
T24.701-T24.709[A], T24.791-T24.799[A],
T25.311-T25.319[A], T25.391-T25.399[A],
T25.711-T25.719[A], T25.791-T25.799[A]

PDX Collection 1409
T24.301-T24.309[A], T24.391-T24.399[A],
T24.701-T24.709[A], T24.791-T24.799[A],
T25.321-T25.329[A], T25.391-T25.399[A],
T25.721-T25.729[A], T25.791-T25.799[A]

PDX Collection 1410
T24.301-T24.309[A], T24.391-T24.399[A],
T24.701-T24.709[A], T24.791-T24.799[A],
T25.331-T25.339[A], T25.391-T25.399[A],
T25.731-T25.739[A], T25.791-T25.799[A]

PDX Collection 1411
T27.0XX-T27.7XX[A], T28.3XX-T28.49X[A],
T28.8XX-T28.99X[A]

PDX Collection 1412
T28.1XXA, T28.3XX-T28.49X[A], T28.6XXA,
T28.8XX-T28.99X[A]

PDX Collection 1413
T28.2XX-T28.49X[A], T28.7XX-T28.99X[A]

PDX Collection 1414
T31.0-T32.99

PDX Collection 1415
T33.011-T33.42X[A], T33.60X-T33.72X[A],
T33.90X-T34.42X[A], T34.60X-T34.72X[A],
T34.90X-T34.99X[A]

PDX Collection 1416
T33.011-T34.99X[A], T69.021-T69.029[A]

PDX Collection 1417
T33.2XX-T33.72X[A], T33.90X-T33.99X[A],
T34.2XX-T34.72X[A], T34.90X-T34.99X[A]

PDX Collection 1418
T33.2XX-T33.42X[A], T33.60X-T33.99X[A],
T34.2XX-T34.42X[A], T34.60X-T34.99X[A]

PDX Collection 1419
T67.0XX-T67.9XX[A]

PDX Collection 1420
T33.2XX-T33.42X[A], T33.60X-T33.72X[A],
T33.90X-T33.99X[A], T34.2XX-T34.42X[A],
T34.60X-T34.72X[A], T34.90X-T34.99X[A],
T69.021-T69.029[A]

PDX Collection 1421
T70.3XX-T70.9XX[A]

PDX Collection 1422
T71.111-T71.9XX[A]

PDX Collection 1423
T74.01X-T74.92X[A], T76.01X-T76.92X[A]

PDX Collection 1424
T74.91XA, T76.91XA

PDX Collection 1425
T75.1XXA

PDX Collection 1426
T78.00X-T78.09X[A]

PDX Collection 1427
D78.81-D78.89, E36.8, E89.810-E89.89, H59.011-H59.019,
H59.031-H59.039, H59.091-H59.099, H59.811-H59.89,
H95.811-H95.89, I97.3, L76.81-L76.82, M96.89, N98.1-N98.9,
T07.XXX-T14.91X[A], T79.0XXA, T79.A0X-T79.9XX[A],
T80.0XXA, T81.82XA, T81.89X-T81.9XX[A]

PDX Collection 1428
D78.81-D78.89, E36.8, E89.810-E89.89, H59.011-H59.019,
H59.031-H59.039, H59.091-H59.099, H59.811-H59.89,
H95.811-H95.89, I97.3, L76.81-L76.82, M96.89, N98.1-N98.9,
T07.XXX-T14.91X[A], T79.0XXA, T79.A0X-T79.9XX[A],
T81.82XA, T81.89X-T81.9XX[A]

PDX Collection 1429
D78.81-D78.89, E36.8, E89.810-E89.89, H59.011-H59.019,
H59.031-H59.039, H59.091-H59.099, H59.811-H59.89,
H95.811-H95.89, I97.3, L76.81-L76.82, M96.89, N98.1-N98.9,
T07.XXX-T14.91X[A], T79.2XXA, T79.A0X-T79.9XX[A],
T81.82X-T81.9XX[A]

PDX Collection 1430
D78.81-D78.89, E36.8, E89.810-E89.89, H59.011-H59.019,
H59.031-H59.039, H59.091-H59.099, H59.811-H59.89,
H95.811-H95.89, I97.3, L76.81-L76.82, M96.89, N98.1-N98.9,
T07.XXX-T14.91X[A], T79.4XXA, T79.A0X-T79.9XX[A],
T81.82X-T81.9XX[A]

PDX Collection 1431
D78.01-D78.02, D78.21-D78.22, D78.31-D78.34,
D78.81-D78.89, E36.01-E36.02, E36.8, E89.810-E89.89,
G97.51-G97.52, G97.61-G97.64, H59.011-H59.019,
H59.031-H59.039, H59.091-H59.099, H59.111-H59.129,
H59.311-H59.329, H59.331-H59.369, H59.811-H59.819,
H59.88-H59.89, H95.21-H95.22, H95.41-H95.42,
H95.51-H92.52, H95.551-H95.554, H95.811-H95.819,
H95.88-H95.89, I97.3-I97.42, I97.610-I97.648,
J95.61-J95.62, J95.830-J95.831, J95.860-J95.863,
K91.61-K91.62, K91.840-K91.841, K91.870-K91.873,
L76.01-L76.02, L76.21-L76.22, L76.31-L76.34, L76.81-L76.82,
M96.810-M96.811, M96.830-M96.89, N98.1-N98.9,
N99.61-N99.62, N99.820-N99.821, N99.840-N99.843,
T07.XXX-T14.91X[A], T79.5XXA, T79.A0X-T79.9XX[A],
T81.10X-T81.19X[A], T81.82X-T81.9XX[A], T88.2XXA

PDX Collection 1432
D78.81-D78.89, E36.8, E89.810-E89.89, H59.011-H59.019,
H59.031-H59.039, H59.091-H59.099, H59.811-H59.89,
H95.811-H95.89, I97.3, L76.81-L76.82, M96.89,
N98.1-N98.9, S21.101-S21.159[A], S21.301-S21.459[A],

S21.90X-S21.95X[A], S27.0XX-S27.399[A],
S27.50X-S27.809[A], S27.892-S27.9XX[A],
S28.1XX[A], S29.021-S29.029[A], T07.XXX-T14.91X[A],
T79.7XX-T79.9XX[A], T81.82X-T81.9XX[A]

PDX Collection 1433
M70.80-M70.99, M79.81-M79.9, R29.898

PDX Collection 1434
S31.001A, S31.011A, S31.021A, S31.031A, S31.041A,
S31.051A, S31.100-S31.159[A], S31.600-S31.659[A],
S31.831-S31.839[A], S36.00X-S37.599[A],
S37.812-S37.99X[A], S38.3XXA, S39.021-S39.023[A],
T07.XXX-T14.91X[A], T79.8XX-T79.9XX[A]

PDX Collection 1435
T79.0XXA, T80.0XXA

PDX Collection 1436
T80.1XXA, T80.810-T80.818[A], T80.90XA

PDX Collection 1437
T80.30X-T80.A9X[A], T80.910-T80.92X[A]

PDX Collection 1438
T80.30X-T80.419[A], T80.910-T80.92X[A], T80.A9XA

PDX Collection 1439
T80.51X-T80.69X[A]

PDX Collection 1440
T80.61X-T80.69X[A]

PDX Collection 1441
D78.01-D78.02, D78.21-D78.22, D78.31-D78.34,
D78.81-D78.89, E36.01-E36.02, E36.8, E89.810-E89.89,
G97.51-G97.52, G97.61-G97.64, H59.011-H59.019,
H59.031-H59.039, H59.091-H59.099, H59.111-H59.129,
H59.311-H59.369, H59.331-H59.349, H59.811-H59.819,
H59.88-H59.89, H95.21-H95.22, H95.41-H95.42,
H59.51-H59.54, H95.811-H95.819, H95.88-H95.89,
I97.3-I97.42, I97.610-I97.648, J95.61-J95.62,
J95.830-J95.831, J95.860-J95.863, K91.61-K91.62,
K91.840-K91.841, K91.870-K91.873, L76.01-L76.02,
L76.21-L76.22, L76.31-L76.34, L76.81-L76.82,
M96.810-M96.811, M96.830-M96.89, N98.1-N98.9,
N99.61-N99.62, N99.820-N99.821, N99.840-N99.843,
T79.4XXA, T81.10X-T81.19X[A], T81.82X-T81.9XX[A],
T88.2XXA

PDX Collection 1442
D78.81-D78.89, E36.8, E89.810-E89.89, H59.011-H59.019,
H59.031-H59.039, H59.091-H59.099, H59.811-H59.89,
H95.811-H95.89, I97.3, L76.81-L76.82, M96.89, N98.1-N98.9,
T81.30X-T81.33X[A], T81.82X-T81.9XX[A]

PDX Collection 1443
D78.81-D78.89, E36.8, E89.810-E89.89, H59.011-H59.019,
H59.031-H59.039, H59.091-H59.099, H59.811-H59.89,
H95.811-H95.89, I97.3, L76.81-L76.82, M96.89, N98.1-N98.9,
T81.500-T81.599[A], T81.82X-T81.9XX[A]

PDX Collection 1444
D78.81-D78.89, E36.8, E89.810-E89.89, H59.011-H59.019,
H59.031-H59.039, H59.091-H59.099, H59.811-H59.89,
H95.811-H95.89, I97.3, L76.81-L76.82, M96.89, N98.1-N98.9,
T81.60X-T81.69X[A], T81.82X-T81.9XX[A]

PDX Collection 1445
D78.81-D78.89, E36.8, E89.810-E89.89, H59.011-H59.019,
H59.031-H59.039, H59.091-H59.099, H59.811-H59.89,
H95.811-H95.89, I97.3, L76.81-L76.82, M96.89, N98.1-N98.9,
T81.710-T81.72X[A], T81.82X-T81.9XX[A]

PDX Collection 1446
D78.81-D78.89, E36.8, E89.810-E89.89, H59.011-H59.019,
H59.031-H59.039, H59.091-H59.099, H59.811-H59.89,

H95.811-H95.89, I97.3, L76.81-L76.82, M96.89, N98.1-N98.9,
T81.718-T81.72X[A], T81.82X-T81.9XX[A]

PDX Collection 1447
D78.81-D78.89, E36.8, E89.810-E89.89, H59.011-H59.019,
H59.031-H59.039, H59.091-H59.099, H59.811-H59.89,
H95.811-H95.89, I97.3, L76.81-L76.82, M96.89, N98.1-N98.9,
T81.82X-T81.9XX[A]

PDX Collection 1448
D78.81-D78.89, E36.8, E89.810-E89.89, H59.011-H59.019,
H59.031-H59.039, H59.091-H59.099, H59.811-H59.89,
H95.811-H95.89, I97.3, L76.81-L76.82, M96.89, N98.1-N98.9,
T81.82X-T81.9XX[A], T82.01X-T82.09X[A]

PDX Collection 1449
D78.81-D78.89, E36.8, E89.810-E89.89, H59.011-H59.019,
H59.031-H59.039, H59.091-H59.099, H59.811-H59.89,
H95.811-H95.89, I97.3, L76.81-L76.82, M96.89,
N98.1-N98.9, T81.82X-T81.9XX[A], T82.110-T82.111[A],
T82.120-T82.121[A], T82.190-T82.191[A]

PDX Collection 1450
D78.81-D78.89, E36.8, E89.810-E89.89, H59.011-H59.019,
H59.031-H59.039, H59.091-H59.099, H59.811-H59.89,
H95.811-H95.89, I97.3, L76.81-L76.82, M96.89, N98.1-N98.9,
T81.82X-T81.9XX[A], T82.118A, T82.128A, T82.198A,
T82.221-T82.228[A], T82.512A, T82.522A, T82.532A,
T82.592A, T82.594A, T82.598A

PDX Collection 1451
D78.81-D78.89, E36.8, E89.810-E89.89, H59.011-H59.019,
H59.031-H59.039, H59.091-H59.099, H59.811-H59.89,
H95.811-H95.89, I97.3, L76.81-L76.82, M96.89, N98.1-N98.9,
T81.82X-T81.9XX[A], T82.211-T82.218[A]

PDX Collection 1452
D78.81-D78.89, E36.8, E89.810-E89.89, H59.011-H59.019,
H59.031-H59.039, H59.091-H59.099, H59.811-H59.89,
H95.811-H95.89, I97.3, L76.81-L76.82, M96.89,
N98.1-N98.9, T81.82X-T81.9XX[A], T82.310-T82.538[A],
T82.590-T82.595[A]

PDX Collection 1453
D78.81-D78.89, E36.8, E89.810-E89.89, H59.011-H59.019,
H59.031-H59.039, H59.091-H59.099, H59.811-H59.89,
H95.811-H95.89, I97.3, L76.81-L76.82, M96.89,
N98.1-N98.9, T81.82X-T81.9XX[A], T82.519A, T82.539A,
T82.599-T82.9XX[A], T85.9XXA

PDX Collection 1454
D78.81-D78.89, E36.8, E89.810-E89.89, H59.011-H59.019,
H59.031-H59.039, H59.091-H59.099, H59.811-H59.89,
H95.811-H95.89, I97.3, L76.81-L76.82, M96.89,
N98.1-N98.9, T81.82X-T81.9XX[A], T82.01X-T82.118[A],
T82.120-T82.128[A], T82.190-T82.198[A],
T82.211-T82.9XX[A], T85.310-T85.311[A],
T85.320-T85.321[A], T85.390-T85.391[A],
T85.510-T85.738[A], T85.7XXA, T85.810[A,D], T85.820[A,D],
T85.830[A,D], T85.840[A,D], T85.850[A,D], T85.860[A,D],
T85.890[A,D], T86.820-T86.829, T86.842-T86.849

PDX Collection 1455
D78.81-D78.89, E36.8, E89.810-E89.89, H59.011-H59.019,
H59.031-H59.039, H59.091-H59.099, H59.811-H59.89,
H95.811-H95.89, I97.3, L76.81-L76.82, M96.89,
N98.1-N98.9, T81.82X-T81.9XX[A], T82.01X-T82.118[A],
T82.120-T82.128[A], T82.190-T82.198[A],
T82.221-T82.9XX[A], T85.310-T85.311[A],
T85.320-T85.321[A], T85.390-T85.391[A],
T85.510-T85.738[A], T85.79XA, 85.810[A,D], T85.820[A,D],
T85.830[A,D], T85.840[A,D], T85.850[A,D], T85.860[A,D],
T85.890[A,D], T85.9XXA, T86.820-T86.829, T86.842-T86.849

PDX Collection 1456
D78.81-D78.89, E36.8, E89.810-E89.89, H59.011-H59.019,
H59.031-H59.039, H59.091-H59.099, H59.811-H59.89,
H95.811-H95.89, I97.3, L76.81-L76.82, M96.89, N98.1-N98.9,
N99.510-N99.518, T81.82A, T81.89-T81.9[A], T83.010A,
T83.020A, T83.030A, T83.090A, T83.110-T83.29X[A],
T83.410-T83.69[A], T83.712-T83.714[A], T83.718A, T83.719A,
T83.722-T83.724[A], T83.728-T83.9XX[A]

PDX Collection 1457
D78.81-D78.89, E36.8, E89.810-E89.89, H59.011-H59.019,
H59.031-H59.039, H59.091-H59.099, H59.811-H59.89,
H95.811-H95.89, I97.3, L76.81-L76.82, M96.89, N98.1-N98.9,
N99.510-N99.518, R82.71, T81.82X-T81.9XX[A], T83.010A,
T83.020A, T83.030A, T83.090A, T83.110-T83.29X[A],
T83.410-T83.498[A], T83.510-T83.518[A],
T83.590-T83.598[A], T83.61X-T83.69X[A],
T83.712-T83.719[A], T83.722-T83.729[A], T83.79XA,
T83.81X-T83.9XX[A], T85.310-T85.311[A],
T85.320-T85.321[A], T85.390-T85.391[A],
T85.510-T85.79X[A], T85.810[A,D], T85.820[A,D],
T85.830[A,D], T85.840[A,D], T85.850[A,D], T85.860[A,D],
T850.890[A,D], T85.9XXA, T86.842-T86.849

PDX Collection 1458
D78.81-D78.89, E36.8, E89.810-E89.89,
H59.011-H59.019, H59.031-H59.039, H59.091-H59.099,
H59.811-H59.89, H95.811-H95.89, I97.3, L76.81-L76.82,
M96.89, N39.0, N98.1-N98.9, N99.510-N99.518,
T81.82X-T81.9XX[A], T83.010A, T83.020A, T83.030A,
T83.090A, T83.110-T83.29X[A], T83.410-T83.498[A],
T83.510-T83.518[A], T83.590-T83.598[A],
T83.61X-T83.69X[A], T83.712-T83.719[A],
T83.722-T83.729[A], T83.79XA, T83.81X-T83.9XX[A],
T85.310-T85.738[A], T85.79XA, T85.810[A,D], T85.820[A,D],
T85.830[A,D], T85.840[A,D], T85.850[A,D], T85.860[A,D],
T850.890[A,D], T85.9XXA, T86.820-T86.849

PDX Collection 1459
D78.81-D78.89, E36.8, E89.810-E89.89, H59.011-H59.019,
H59.031-H59.039, H59.091-H59.099, H59.811-H59.89,
H95.811-H95.89, I97.3, L76.81-L76.82, M96.621-M96.69,
M96.89, M97.01X-M97.02X[A], M97.11X-M97.12X[A],
M97.21X-M97.22X[A], M97.31X-M97.32X[A],
M97.41X-M97.42X[A], M97.8XXA, M97.9XXA,
N98.1-N98.9, T81.82X-T81.9XX[A], T84.010-T84.039[A],
T84.050-T84.9XX[A], T85.310-T85.311[A],
T85.320-T85.321[A], T85.390-T85.391[A],
T85.510-T85.738[A], T85.79XA, T85.810[A,D], T85.820[A,D],
T85.830[A,D], T85.840[A,D], T85.850[A,D], T85.860[A,D],
T85.890[A,D],T85.9XXA, T86.820-T86.829, T86.842-T86.849

PDX Collection 1460
D78.81-D78.89, E36.8, E89.810-E89.89, H59.011-H59.019,
H59.031-H59.039, H59.091-H59.099, H59.811-H59.89,
H95.811-H95.89, I97.3, L76.81-L76.82, M96.89, N98.1-N98.9,
T81.82X-T81.9XX[A], T85.01X-T85.199[A]

PDX Collection 1461
D78.81-D78.89, E89.810-E89.89, H59.011-H59.019,
H59.031-H59.039, H59.091-H59.099, H59.811-H59.89,
H95.811-H95.89, I97.3, M96.89, N98.1-N98.9,
T85.21X-T85.29X[A]

PDX Collection 1462
H59.011-H59.019, H59.031-H59.819, H59.88-H59.89,
H95.811-H95.89, I97.3, M96.89, N98.1-N98.9,
T85.310-T85.311[A], T85.320-T85.321[A],
T85.390-T85.391[A], T85.612A, T85.615A, T85.618A,
T85.622A, T85.625A, T85.628A, T85.635A, T85.638A,
T85.692A, T85.695A, T85.698-T85.738[A], T85.79XA,
T85.810[A,D], T85.820[A,D], T85.830[A,D], T85.840[A,D],

T85.850[A,D], T85.860[A,D], T85.890[A,D], T85.9XX[A],
T86.842-T86.849

PDX Collection 1463
D78.81-D78.89, E89.810-E89.89, H59.011-H59.019,
H59.031-H59.039, H59.091-H59.099, H59.811-H59.89,
H95.811-H95.89, I97.3, M96.89, N98.1-N98.9,
T85.41X-T85.49X[A]

PDX Collection 1464
H95.811-H95.89, I97.3, M96.89, N98.1-N98.9,
T85.510-T85.598[A], T85.612A, T85.615A, T85.618A,
T85.622A, T85.625A,T85.628A, T85.635A, T85.638A, T85.692A,
T85.695A, T85.698-T85.738[A], T85.79XA, T85.810[A,D],
T85.820[A,D], T85.830[A,D], T85.840[A,D], T85.850[A,D],
T85.860[A,D], T85.890[A,D], T85.9XXA

PDX Collection 1465
H95.811-H95.89, I97.3, M96.89, N98.1-N98.9, T85.610A,
T85.612A, T85.615A, T85.618-T85.620A, T85.622A, T85.625A,
T85.628-T85.630A, T85.635A, T85.638-T85.690[A], T85.692A,
T85.695A, T85.698-T85.738[A], T85.79XA, T85.810[A,D],
T85.820[A,D], T85.830[A,D], T85.840[A,D], T85.850[A,D],
T85.860[A,D], T85.890[A,D], T85.9XXA

PDX Collection 1466
H95.811-H95.89, I97.3, M96.89, N98.1-N98.9,
T85.611-T85.612[A], T85.614-T85.618[A],
T85.621-T85.622[A], T85.624-T85.628[A],
T85.631-T85.638[A], T85.691-T85.692[A],
T85.694-T85.738[A], T85.79XA, T85.810[A,D], T85.820[A,D],
T85.830[A,D], T85.840[A,D], T85.850[A,D], T85.860[A,D],
T85.890[A,D], T85.9XXA

PDX Collection 1467
D78.81-D78.89, E89.810-E89.89, H59.011-H59.019,
H59.031-H59.039, H59.091-H59.099, H59.811-H59.89,
H95.811-H95.89, I97.3, M96.89, N98.1-N98.9,
T85.310-T85.311[A], T85.320-T85.321[A],
T85.390-T85.391[A], T85.510-T85.738A, T85.79XA,
T85.810[A,D], T85.820[A,D], T85.830[A,D], T85.840[A,D],
T85.850[A,D], T85.860[A,D], T85.890[A,D], T85.9XXA,
T86.842-T86.849

PDX Collection 1468
H95.811-H95.89, I97.3, M96.89, N98.1-N98.9,
T85.612-T85.613[A], T85.615A, T85.618[A],
T85.622-T85.623[A], T85.625A, T85.628[A], T85.635A,
T85.638[A], T85.692-T85.693[A], T85.695A,
T85.698-T85.738[A], T85.79XA, T85.810[A,D], T85.820[A,D],
T85.830[A,D], T85.840[A,D], T85.850[A,D], T85.860[A,D],
T85.890[A,D], T85.9XXA, T86.820-T86.829

PDX Collection 1469
H95.811-H95.89, I97.3, M96.621-M96.89,
M97.01X-M97.9XX[A], N98.1-N98.9, N99.510-N99.518,
T81.82X-T81.9XX[A], T82.01X-T82.118[A],
T82.120-T82.128[A], T82.192-T82.198[A],
T82.211-T83.010[A], T83.020[A], T83.030[A],
T83.090A, T83.110-T83.29X[A], T83.410-T83.69X[A],
T83.712-T83.714[A], T83.718A, T83.719A,
T83.722-T83.724[A], T83.728-T83.9XX[A],
T84.010-T84.039[A], T84.050-T85.29X[A],
T85.41X-T85.49X[A], T85.611-T85.618[A],
T85.621-T85.622[A], T85.624-T85.628[A],
T85.631-T85.638[A], T85.691-T85.692[A],
T85.694-T85.738[A], T85.79XA, T85.810[A,D], T85.820[A,D],
T85.830[A,D], T85.840[A,D], T85.850[A,D], T85.860[A,D],
T85.890[A,D], T85.9XXA, T86.820-T86.829

PDX Collection 1470
D78.81-D78.89, E36.8, E89.810-E89.89,
H59.011-H59.019, H59.031-H59.039, H59.091-H59.099,
H59.811-H59.89, H95.811-H95.89, I97.3,

L76.81-L76.82, M96.621-M96.89, M97.01X-M97.9XX[A],
N98.1-N98.9, N99.510-N99.518, T81.82X-T81.9XX[A],
T82.01X-T82.118[A], T82.120-T82.128[A],
T82.192-T82.198[A], T82.211-T83.29X[A],
T83.410-T83.69X[A], T83.712-T83.714[A], T83.718A,
T83.719A, T83.722-T83.724[A], T83.728-T83.9XX[A],
T84.010-T84.039[A], T84.050-T85.738[A], T85.79XA,
T85.810[A,D], T85.820[A,D], T85.830[A,D], T85.840[A,D],
T85.850[A,D], T85.860[A,D], T85.890[A,D], T85.9XXA,
T86.820-T86.849

PDX Collection 1471
D78.81-D78.89, E89.810-E89.89, H59.011-H59.019,
H59.031-H59.039, H59.091-H59.099, H59.811-H59.89,
H95.811-H95.89, I97.3, M96.89, N98.1-N98.9, T86.10-T86.19

PDX Collection 1472
D78.81-D78.89, E89.810-E89.89, H59.011-H59.019,
H59.031-H59.039, H59.091-H59.099, H59.811-H59.89,
H95.811-H95.89, I97.3, M96.89, N98.1-N98.9, T86.20-T86.39

PDX Collection 1473
D78.81-D78.89, E89.810-E89.89, H59.011-H59.019,
H59.031-H59.039, H59.091-H59.099, H59.811-H59.89,
H95.811-H95.89, I97.3, M96.89, N98.1-N98.9, T86.40-T86.49

PDX Collection 1474
D78.81-D78.89, E89.810-E89.89, H59.011-H59.019,
H59.031-H59.039, H59.091-H59.099, H59.811-H59.89,
H95.811-H95.89, I97.3, M96.89, N98.1-N98.9, T86.5,
T86.830-T86.839

PDX Collection 1475
D78.81-D78.89, E89.810-E89.89, H59.011-H59.019,
H59.031-H59.039, H59.091-H59.099, H59.811-H59.89,
H95.811-H95.89, I97.3, M96.89, N98.1-N98.9,
T86.810-T86.819

PDX Collection 1476
D78.81-D78.89, E89.810-E89.89, H59.011-H59.019,
H59.031-H59.039, H59.091-H59.099, H59.811-H59.89,
H95.811-H95.89, I97.3, M96.89, N98.1-N98.9, T85.613A,
T85.623A, T85.693A, T86.820-T86.829

PDX Collection 1477
H95.811-H95.89, I97.3, M96.89, N98.1-N98.9, T86.5,
T86.830-T86.839

PDX Collection 1478
H59.011-H59.019, H59.031-H59.099, H59.811-H59.89,
H95.811-H95.89, I97.3, M96.89, N98.1-N98.9, T85.318A,
T85.328A, T85.398A, T85.810[A,D], T85.820[A,D],
T85.830[A,D], T86.840-T86.841

PDX Collection 1479
H59.011-H59.019, H59.031-H59.039, H59.091-H59.099,
H59.811-H59.89, H95.811-H95.89, I97.3, M96.621-M96.89,
M97.01X-M97.9XX[A], N98.1-N98.9, N99.510-N99.518,
T81.82XA, T81.89X-T81.9XX[A], T82.01X-T82.118[A],
T82.120-T82.128[A], T82.192-T82.198[A],
T82.211-T83.010[A], T83.020A, T83.030A, T83.090A,
T83.110-T83.29X[A], T83.410-T83.69X[A],
T83.712A-T83.714A, T83.718A, T83.719A, T83.722-T83.724[A],
T83.728-T84.039[A], T84.050-T85.49X[A], T85.612A,
T85.615A, T85.618A, T85.622A, T85.625A, T85.628A,
T85.635A, T85.638A, T85.692A, T85.695A, T85.698, T85.738A,
T85.79XA, T85.810[A,D], T85.820[A,D], T85.830[A,D],
T85.840[A,D], T85.850[A,D], T85.860[A,D], T85.890[A,D],
T85.9XXA, T86.820-T86.829, T86.840-T86.849

PDX Collection 1480
D78.81-D78.89, E89.810-E89.89, H59.011-H59.019,
H59.031-H59.039, H59.091-H59.099, H59.811-H59.89,
H95.811-H95.89, I97.3, M96.89, N98.1-N98.9,
T86.890-T86.899

PDX Collection 1481
D78.81-D78.89, E36.8, E89.810-E89.89, H59.011-H59.019,
H59.031-H59.039, H59.091-H59.099, H59.811-H59.89,
H95.811-H95.89, I97.3, L76.81-L76.82, M96.89, N98.1-N98.9,
T81.82X-T81.9XX[A], T87.0X1-T87.0X9

PDX Collection 1482
D78.81-D78.89, E36.8, E89.810-E89.89, H59.011-H59.019,
H59.031-H59.039, H59.091-H59.099, H59.811-H59.89,
H95.811-H95.89, I97.3, L76.81-L76.82, M96.89, N98.1-N98.9,
T81.82X-T81.9XX[A], T87.1X1-T87.1X9

PDX Collection 1483
D78.81-D78.89, E36.8, E89.810-E89.89, H59.011-H59.019,
H59.031-H59.039, H59.091-H59.099, H59.811-H59.89,
H95.811-H95.89, I97.3, L76.81-L76.82, M96.89, N98.1-N98.9,
T81.82X-T81.9XX[A], T87.2

PDX Collection 1484
D78.81-D78.89, E36.8, E89.810-E89.89, H59.011-H59.019,
H59.031-H59.039, H59.091-H59.099, H59.811-H59.89,
H95.811-H95.89, I97.3, L76.81-L76.82, M96.89, N98.1-N98.9,
T81.82X-T81.9XX[A], T87.40-T87.9

PDX Collection 1485
T88.1XXA

PDX Collection 1486
D78.01-D78.02, D78.21-D78.89, E36.01-E36.02, E36.8,
E89.810-E89.89, G97.51-G97.52, G97.61-G97.64,
H59.011-H59.019, H59.031-H59.039, H59.091-H59.099,
H59.111-H59.129, H59.311-H59.329, H59.331-H59.369,
H59.811-H59.89, H95.21-H95.22, H95.41-H95.42,
H95.51-H95.54, H95.811-H95.89, I97.3-I97.42,
I97.610-I97.648, J95.61-J95.62, J95.830-J95.831,
J95.860-J95.863, K91.61-K91.62, K91.840-K91.841,
K91.870-K91.873, L76.01-L76.02, L76.21-L76.22,
L76.31-L76.34, L76.81-L76.82, M96.810-M96.811,
M96.830-M96.89, N98.1-N98.9, N99.61-N99.62,
N99.820-N99.821, T79.4XXA, T81.10X-T81.19X[A], T81.82XA,
T81.89X-T81.9XX[A], T88.2XX-T88.3XX[A]

PDX Collection 1487
Z43.1

PDX Collection 1488
D47.Z1, T86.20-T86.39, T86.850-T86.859, T86.90-T86.99,
Z94.1, Z94.3, Z94.89-Z94.9

PDX Collection 1489
D47.Z1, T86.10-T86.19, T86.850-T86.859, T86.90-T86.99,
Z94.0, Z94.89-Z94.9

PDX Collection 1490
D47.Z1, T86.40-T86.49, T86.850-T86.859, T86.90-T86.99,
Z94.4, Z94.89, Z94.9

PDX Collection 1491
D47.Z1, T86.810-T86.819, T86.850-T86.859, T86.90-T86.99,
Z94.2, Z94.89-Z94.9

PDX Collection 1492
D47.Z1, D89.810-D89.813, T86.00-T86.09, T86.850-T86.859,
T86.90-T86.99, Z94.9

PDX Collection 1493
E66.01-E66.1, E66.8-E66.9, Z68.1-Z68.54

PDX Collection 1494
E65-E66.1, E66.8-E66.9, Z68.1-Z68.54

PDX Collection 1495
D47.Z1, T86.830-T86.839, T86.90-T86.99, Z94.82,
Z94.89-Z94.9

PDX Collection 1496
D47.Z1, T86.850-T86.859, T86.890-T86.99, Z94.83, Z94.9

PDX Collection 1497
D47.Z1, T86.850-T86.859, T86.90-T86.99, Z94.9

PDX Collection 1498
D47.Z1, T86.20-T86.39, T86.850-T86.99, Z94.1, Z94.3,
Z95.811-Z95.812

MAKE THE MOST *of your* PHYSICIAN CODING EXAM Review!

ELSEVIER

1. Assess! Take the Pre-Exam

Use the Pre-Exam located on the companion Evolve site to gauge your strengths and weaknesses, develop a plan for focused study, and gain a better understanding of the testing process.

2018 PHYSICIAN CODING EXAM REVIEW
The Certification Step

Carol J. Buck
MS, CPC, CCS-P

ELSEVIER

2. Study!

Use the quizzes in this book to sharpen your skills and build competency.

4. Test! Take the Final Exam

Gauge your readiness for the actual physician coding exam with the Final Exam. Boost your test-taking confidence and ensure certification success.

3. Apply! Take the Post-Exam

After studying, apply your knowledge to the Post-Exam located on the companion Evolve site. When finished, you'll receive scores for both the Pre- and Post-Exams and a breakdown of incorrect answers to help you identify areas where you need more detailed study and review.

ISBN: 978-0-323-43078-4

Perfect *your* understanding *and* prepare for certification
— START YOUR REVIEW NOW!

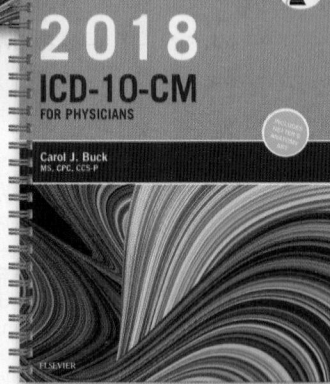

STEP 4: PROFESSIONAL

"Nothing is particularly hard if you divide it into small jobs."
— HENRY FORD

WE WANT TO APPLAUD YOU FOR TAKING THIS STEP IN YOUR CAREER.
Medical coding is a fine profession that has the ability to intrigue and captivate
you for a lifetime. Practice your craft carefully, with due diligence, patience for
the process, and always the highest ethical standards.

TRACK YOUR PROGRESS!

*See the checklist in the front of this
book to learn more about your next
step toward coding success!*

Author and Educator
Carol J. Buck, MS, CPC, CCS-P

Lead Technical Collaborator
Jackie Grass Koesterman, CPC

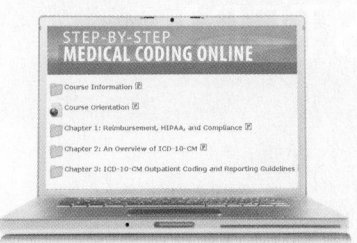

Trust Carol J. Buck and Elsevier to take you through the **levels** *of* CODING SUCCESS

STEP4:
PROFESSIONAL

STEP3: CERTIFY

STEP2: PRACTICE

STEP1: LEARN

With the resources you need for every level of coding success, Carol J. Buck and Elsevier are with you every step of your coding career. From beginning to advanced, from the classroom to the workplace, from application to certification, the Step Series products are your guides to greater opportunities and successful career advancement.

Keep climbing with the most trusted names in medical coding.

Author and Educator
Carol J. Buck, MS, CPC, CCS-P

Lead Technical Collaborator
Jackie Grass Koesterman, CPC